W9-AHG-821

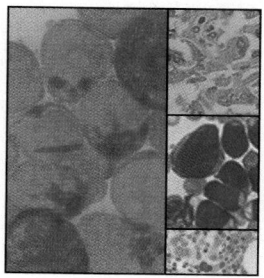

CLINICAL ONCOLOGY

Third Edition

MARTIN D. ABELOFF, MD
Eli Kennerly Marshall, Jr. Professor of Oncology
Professor of Medicine, Johns Hopkins University School of Medicine
Director, The Sidney Kimmel Comprehensive Cancer Center
at Johns Hopkins, Baltimore, MD

JAMES O. ARMITAGE, MD
Joe Shapiro Professor of Medicine, Department of Internal Medicine,
University of Nebraska Medical Center, Omaha, NE

JOHN E. NIEDERHUBER, MD
Professor, Departments of Surgery and Oncology, Wattawa Professor-
Bascom, University of Wisconsin-Madison, Madison, WI

MICHAEL B. KASTAN, MD, PHD
Chair, Department of Hematology/Oncology, St. Jude Children's
Research Hospital; Professor, Department of Pediatrics, University of
Tennessee School of Medicine, Memphis, TN

W. GILLIES MCKENNA, MD, PHD
Henry K. Pancoast Professor and Chair, Department of Radiation
Oncology, University of Pennsylvania School of Medicine, Philadelphia, PA

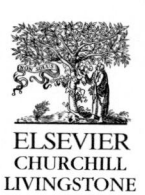

ELSEVIER
CHURCHILL
LIVINGSTONE

ELSEVIER
CHURCHILL
LIVINGSTONE

The Curtis Center
170 S Independence Mall W 300E
Philadelphia, Pennsylvania 19106

CLINICAL ONCOLOGY

ISBN 0-443-06629-9

Copyright © 2004, Elsevier Inc. All rights reserved.

No part of this publication may be reproduced or transmitted in any form or by any means, electronic or mechanical, including photocopying, recording, or any information storage and retrieval system, without permission in writing from the publisher. Permissions may be sought directly from Elsevier's Health Sciences Rights Department in Philadelphia, PA, USA: phone: (+1) 215 238 7869, fax: (+1) 215 238 2239, e-mail: healthpermissions@elsevier.com. You may also complete your request on-line via the Elsevier homepage (http://www.elsevier.com), by selecting 'Customer Support' and then 'Obtaining Permissions'.

Distributed in the United Kingdom by Churchill Livingstone, Robert Stevenson House, 1-3 Baxter's Place, Leith Walk, Edinburgh EH1 3AF, Scotland, and by associated companies, branches, and representatives throughout the world.

NOTICE

Medicine is an ever-changing field. Standard safety precautions must be followed, but as new research and clinical experience broaden our knowledge, changes in treatment and drug therapy may become necessary or appropriate. Readers are advised to check the most current product information provided by the manufacturer of each drug to be administered to verify the recommended dose, the method and duration of administration, and contraindications. It is the responsibility of the licensed prescriber, relying on experience and knowledge of the patient, to determine dosages and the best treatment for each individual patient. Neither the publisher nor the authors assume any liability for any injury and/or damage to persons or property arising from this publication.

Previous editions copyright 2000, 1995

International Standard Book Number 0-443-06629-9

Acquisitions Editor: Dolores Meloni
Developmental Editor: Donna Morrissey
Designer: Karen O'Keefe Owens
Executive Publisher: Susan F. Pioli

Printed in the United States of America.
Last digit is the print number: 9   8   7   6   5   4   3   2   1

To my wife Diane and my family, who have provided encouragement and enormous support during this project and throughout my career. To my colleagues and patients, who have taught me a great deal about science, medicine, and life.
MARTIN D. ABELOFF, MD

To my wife and my family.
JAMES O. ARMITAGE, MD

To my wife Tracey who recently lost her battle with cancer and whose memory inspires all who knew her to work a little harder each day toward the elimination of the pain and suffering from this disease. To my son, Matthew, who is teaching me so much about the living of one's life. To my many friends, colleagues, students, and patients who provide constant inspiration for projects such as this.
JOHN E. NIEDERHUBER, MD

To the cornerstones of my life: my wife Kathy and my sons, Benjamin, Nathaniel, and Jonathan. Kathy, I am so proud of the way that you have taken a negative turn in life and made it into such a positive and productive force at the national level. Boys, I am very proud of the young men that you are becoming and watching your futures develop is my greatest joy. Thank you all for being so supportive of my career. A special note of gratitude is extended to my teachers, colleagues, and patients, from whom I have learned so much.
MICHAEL B. KASTAN, MD, PhD

To my wife and collaborator Ruth Muschel and my friend and mentor Eli Glatstein.
W. GILLIES MCKENNA, MD, PhD

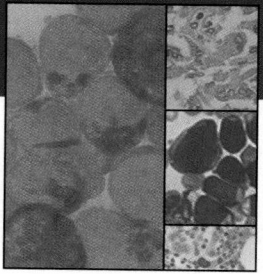

Contributors

JAMES L. ABBRUZZESE, MD
M. G. and Lillie A. Johnson Chair for Cancer Treatment and Research, Chair, Department of Gastrointestinal Medical Oncology, Professor of Medicine, University of Texas M.D. Anderson Cancer Center, Houston, TX.

MARTIN D. ABELOFF, MD
Eli Kennerly Marshall, Jr. Professor of Oncology, Professor of Medicine, Johns Hopkins University School of Medicine; Director, Sidney Kimmel Comprehensive Cancer Center, Johns Hopkins Hospital, Baltimore, MD.

GHASSAN K. ABOU-ALFA, MD
Clinical Assistant Attending, Memorial Sloan-Kettering Cancer Center; Weill Medical College, Cornell University, New York, NY.

JANET L. ABRAHM, MD
Associate Professor of Medicine and Anesthesia, Harvard Medical School; Director, Pain and Palliative Care Program, Dana-Farber Cancer Institute and Brigham and Women's Hospital, Boston, MA.

JEFFREY S. ABRAMS, MD
Associate Chief, Clinical Investigations Branch, National Cancer Institute, Bethesda, MD.

GEZA ACS, PhD
Assistant Professor, Pathology and Laboratory Medicine, Hospital of the University of Pennsylvania, Philadelphia, PA.

JOSEPH AISNER, MD
Professor of Medicine, Professor of Environmental and Community Medicine, Professor and Chief, Medical Oncology, Robert Wood Johnson Medical School, University of Medicine and Dentistry of New Jersey; Associate Director for Clinical Sciences, The Cancer Institute of New Jersey, New Brunswick, NJ.

SEENA C. AISNER, MD
Professor and Vice Chair Pathology, Chief, Anatomical Pathology, Department of Pathology, New Jersey Medical School, University of Medicine and Dentistry of New Jersey, New Brunswick, NJ.

RHODA M. ALANI, MD
Assistant Professor of Oncology, Dermatology, Molecular Biology, and Genetics, The Sidney Kimmel Comprehensive Cancer Center, Johns Hopkins University School of Medicine, Baltimore, MD.

STEVEN R. ALBERTS, MD
Associate Professor of Oncology, Mayo Clinic College of Medicine; Consultant in Medical Oncology, Mayo Clinic, Rochester, MN.

RICCARDO ALESSANDRO, PhD
Assistant Professor, Department of Biopathology and Biomedical Methods, Faculty of Medicine, University of Palermo, Palermo, Italy.

RICHARD F. AMBINDER, MD, PhD
Professor, Departments of Oncology, Pharmacology, and Pathology, Johns Hopkins School of Medicine; Director of Hematologic Malignancies, The Sidney Kimmel Comprehensive Cancer Center, Johns Hopkins Hospital, Baltimore, MD.

CLAY M. ANDERSON, MD
Associate Professor of Clinical Medicine, Department of Medicine, Division of Hematology/Oncology, University of Missouri–Columbia School of Medicine; University of Missouri–Columbia Hospital Ellis Fischel Cancer Center, Columbia, MO.

KENNETH C. ANDERSON, MD
Kraft Family Professor of Medicine, Harvard Medical School; Chief, Division of Hematologic Neoplasia, Director, Jerome Lipper Multiple Myeloma Center, Dana-Farber Cancer Institute, Boston, MA.

FREDERICK R. APPELBAUM, MD
Professor and Head, Division of Medical Oncology, University of Washington School of Medicine; Member and Director, Clinical Research Division, Fred Hutchinson Cancer Research Center, Seattle, WA.

JAMES O. ARMITAGE, MD
Joe Shapiro Professor of Medicine, Department of Internal Medicine, University of Nebraska Medical Center, Omaha, NE.

MOHAMMED BAGHERI, MD
Fellow, Mohs Micrographic Surgery, Department of
Plastic Surgery, University of Wisconsin, Madison, WI;
private practice, Hemet, CA.

GOPAL BAJAJ, MD
Resident in Radiation Oncology, Department of Radiation
Oncology and Molecular Radiation Science, The Sidney
Kimmel Cancer Center at Johns Hopkins, Baltimore, MD.

CHARLES M. BALCH, MD
Professor of Surgery and Oncology, Johns Hopkins School
of Medicine, Baltimore, MD; Executive Vice President and
Chief Executive Officer, American Society of Clinical
Oncology, Alexandria, VA.

LODOVICO BALDUCCI, MD
Professor of Oncology and Medicine, University of South
Florida College of Medicine; Program Leader, Senior Adult
Oncology Program, H. Lee Moffitt Cancer Center and
Research Institute, Tampa, FL.

DAVID S. BARDENSTEIN, MD
Assistant Professor of Ophthalmology and Pathology,
Case Western Reserve University School of Medicine,
Cleveland, OH.

CLAUDIA BEGHÉ, MD
Associate Professor, University of South Florida College of
Medicine; Chief, Nursing Home, James A. Haley Veterans
Hospital, Tampa, FL.

FREDERICK G. BEHM, MD
University of Tennessee College of Medicine; St. Jude
Children's Research Hospital, Memphis, TN.

CHANDRA P. BELANI, MD
Professor of Medicine, University of Pittsburgh; Director,
Lung and Esophageal Cancer Program, University of
Pittsburgh Cancer Institute, Pittsburgh, PA.

CHARLES L. BENNETT, MD, PhD, MPP
Professor of Medicine, Feinberg School of Medicine at
Northwestern University; Associate Director, Midwest
Center for Health Services Research and Policy Studies,
VA Chicago Healthcare System, Chicago IL.

JOHN M. BENNETT, MD
Professor of Medicine, Emeritus, University of Rochester;
Clinical In-Patient Director, Strong Memorial Hospital,
Rochester, NY.

GEROLD BEPLER, MD, PhD
Professor of Medicine and Oncology, Program Leader,
Thoracic Oncology, H. Lee Moffitt Cancer Center and
Research Institute, Tampa, FL.

ROSS STUART BERKOWITZ, MD
William H. Baker Professor of Gynecology, Harvard
Medical School; Director of Gynecologic Oncology,
Co-Director, New England Trophoblastic Disease Center,
Brigham and Women's Hospital Dana-Farber Cancer
Institute, Boston, MA.

MICHAEL R. BISHOP, MD
Experimental Transplantation and Immunology Branch,
National Cancer Institute, National Institutes of Health,
Bethesda, MD.

LESLIE BLUMGART, MD, FACS, FRCS
Professor of Surgery, Weill Medical College of Cornell
University; Enid A. Haupt Chair in Hepatobiliary Surgery,
Chief, Hepatobiliary Service, Memorial Sloan-Kettering
Cancer Center, New York, NY.

MICHAEL BOROWITZ, MD, PhD
Professor of Pathology and Oncology, Johns Hopkins
University School of Medicine; Director, Hematologic
Pathology, Johns Hopkins Hospital, Baltimore, MD.

JULIENNE E. BOWER, PhD
Assistant Professor, Department of Psychiatry and
Biobehavioral Sciences, David Geffen School of Medicine,
University of California–Los Angeles; Cousins Center for
Psychoneuroimmunology, UCLA Neuropsychiatric
Institute, Los Angeles, CA.

JULIE R. BRAHMER, MD
Assistant Professor of Oncology, The Sidney Kimmel
Comprehensive Cancer Center at Johns Hopkins,
Baltimore, MD.

VIVIEN H. C. BRAMWELL, PhD, MBBS, MRCP, FRCP, FRCPC
Professor, Division of Medical Oncology, Department of
Oncology, University of Calgary; Director, Department of
Medicine, Tom Baker Cancer Centre; Head, Division of
Medical and Radiation Oncology, Department of
Medicine, Calgary Health Region/University of Calgary,
Foothills Medical Centre, Calgary Health Region, Calgary,
Alberta, Canada.

EDUARDO BRUERA, MD
Professor, University of Texas–Houston; Chair,
Department of Palliative Care and Rehabilitation, M.D.
Anderson Cancer Center, Houston, TX.

THERESA M. BUSCH, PhD
Assistant Professor, Department of Radiation Oncology,
University of Pennsylvania, Philadelphia, PA.

MITCHELL S. CAIRO, MD
Professor of Pediatrics, Medicine, and Pathology, Chief,
Division of Pediatric Hematology and Blood and Marrow
Transplantation, Columbia University; Director, Blood and
Marrow Transplantation, Morgan Stanley Children's
Hospital of New York–Presbyterian, New York, NY.

DARIO CAMPANA, MD, PhD
Professor, Department of Pediatrics, University of
Tennessee Health Science Center, College of Medicine;
Member, Departments of Hematology, Oncology, and
Pathology, St. Jude Children's Research Hospital,
Memphis, TN.

H. BALLENTINE CARTER, MD
Professor of Urology and Oncology, Johns Hopkins School of Medicine, Baltimore, MD.

DANIEL W. CHAN, PhD
Professor of Pathology, Oncology, Radiology, and Urology, Johns Hopkins University School of Medicine; Director, Clinical Chemistry Division, Johns Hopkins Hospital, Baltimore, MD.

ALFRED E. CHANG, MD
Professor of Surgery, Chief, Division of Surgical Oncology, University of Michigan, Ann Arbor, MI.

BRUCE D. CHESON, MD
Professor of Medicine, Georgetown University; Head of Hematology, Lombardi Comprehensive Cancer Center, Washington, DC.

NAI-KONG V. CHEUNG, MD, PhD
Professor of Pediatrics, Weil Medical College of Cornell University; Enid A. Haupt Chair in Pediatric Oncology, Memorial Sloan-Kettering Cancer Center; Attending Pediatrician, Memorial Hospital, New York, NY.

MICHAELE C. CHRISTIAN, MD
Associate Director, Division of Cancer Treatment and Diagnosis, Cancer Therapy Evaluation Program, National Cancer Institute, Bethesda, MD.

CHRISTINA CHU, MD
Assistant Professor, Department of Obstetrics and Gynecology, Gynecologic Oncology, Clinical Practices of the University of Pennsylvania, Philadelphia, PA.

TIMOTHY CLAIR, MS
Chemist, Laboratory of Pathology, National Cancer Institute, National Institutes of Health, Bethesda, MD.

MICHAEL F. CLARKE, MD
Professor of Internal Medicine and Cell and Developmental Biology, University of Michigan Cancer Center, Ann Arbor, MI.

ANTHONY J. CMELAK, MD
Associate Professor, Department of Radiation Oncology, Vanderbilt University School of Medicine, Nashville, TN.

PETER F. COCCIA, MD
Ittner Professor of Pediatrics, Vice Chairman, Department of Pediatrics, Chief, Section of Pediatric Hematology/ Oncology and Stem Cell Transplantation, University of Nebraska Medical Center, Omaha, NE.

ALFRED M. COHEN, MD
Professor of Surgery, University of Kentucky College of Medicine; Director and CEO, Markey Cancer Center, Lexington, KY.

BERTRAND COIFFIER, MD, PhD
Professor of Hematology, Université Claude Bernard; Head, Department of Hematology, Hospices Civils de Lyon, Lyon, France.

CAROLYN E. COLE, MSN, MM
Associate Director, Colon Cancer Prevention Program, University of Wisconsin Comprehensive Cancer Center, Madison, WI.

ROBERT E. COLEMAN, MD, FRCP
Professor of Medical Oncology, University of Sheffield; Professor of Medical Oncology/Honorary Consultant, Cancer Research Centre, Weston Park Hospital, Sheffield, UK.

JOSEPH M. CONNORS, MD
Clinical Professor of Medicine, University of British Columbia; Medical Oncologist, British Columbia Cancer Agency, Vancouver, British Columbia, Canada.

LINDA D. COOLEY, RN, MD
Associate Professor, University of Missouri Kansas City Medical School; Director, Cytogenetic Laboratory, Children's Mercy Hospital, Kansas City, MO.

LYNN COPPAGE, MD
Assistant Professor, H. Lee Moffitt Cancer Center and Research Institute at the University of South Florida, Tampa, FL.

KENNETH H. COWAN, MD, PhD
Director, Eppley Institute for Cancer Research; Director, UNMC Eppley Cancer Center, University of Nebraska Medical Center, Omaha, NE.

DANIEL J. CULKIN, MD
Professor and Chair, Department of Urology, Oklahoma University College of Medicine; Chief, Urology Services, Oklahoma University Medical Center; Chief, Urology Section, VA Medical Center, Oklahoma City, OK.

JOSEP DALMAU, MD, PhD
Associate Professor, Department of Neurology, Hospital of the University of Pennsylvania, Philadelphia, PA.

GIULIO J. D'ANGIO, MD
Professor (Emeritus), University of Pennsylvania School of Medicine; Hospital of the University of Pennsylvania; Children's Hospital of Philadelphia, PA.

STEVEN R. DEITCHER, MD
Head, Section of Hematology and Coagulation Medicine, Department of Hematology and Medical Oncology, The Cleveland Clinic Foundation, Cleveland, OH.

GEORGE D. DEMETRI, MD
Associate Professor of Medicine, Harvard Medical School; Director, Center for Sarcoma and Bone Oncology, Dana-Farber Cancer Institute, Boston, MA.

PHILIP DeSIMONE, MD
Professor of Medicine, University of Kentucky College of Medicine; Markey Cancer Center, Lexington, KY.

THEODORE L. DeWEESE, MD
Professor of Radiation Oncology, Oncology, and Urology; Chair Department of Radiation Oncology and Molecular Radiation Sciences, The Johns Hopkins University School of Medicine, Baltimore, MD.

KATHLEEN M. DIEHL, MD
Assistant Professor of Surgery, University of Michigan Medical Center, Ann Arbor, MI.

SUBBA R. DIGUMARTHY, MD
Fellow, Department of Radiology, Massachusetts General Hospital, Boston, MA.

DONALD C. DOLL, MD
Professor of Medicine, Division of Hematology and Medical Oncology, Ellis Fischel Cancer Center, University of Missouri–Columbia, Columbia, MO.

JEFFREY S. DOME, MD
Assistant Professor, Department of Pediatrics, University of Tennessee Memphis College of Medicine; Assistant Member, Department of Hematology/Oncology, St. Jude Children's Research Hospital, Memphis, TN.

ROSS C. DONEHOWER, MD
Professor of Oncology and Medicine, Director, Division of Medical Oncology, Johns Hopkins University School of Medicine; Virginia and D. K. Ludwig Professor of Clinical Investigation of Cancer, Sidney Kimmel Comprehensive Cancer Center at Johns Hopkins, Baltimore, MD.

JOHN H. DONOHUE, MD
Professor of Surgery, Mayo Clinic College of Medicine; Consultant in Surgery, Mayo Clinic, Rochester, MN.

JEFFREY A. DREBIN, MD, PhD
Professor of Surgery and Molecular Biology and Pharmacology, Washington University School of Medicine; Attending Surgeon, Barnes-Jewish Hospital and Siteman Cancer Center, St Louis, MO.

BRIAN J. DRUKER, MD
JELD-WEN Chair of Leukemia Research, Oregon Health and Science University Cancer Institute; Investigator, Howard Hughes Medical Institute, Portland, OR.

LINDA R. DUSKA, MD
Assistant Professor of Gynecology, Obstetrics, and Reproductive Biology, Harvard Medical School; Assistant in Gynecology and Obstetrics, Massachusetts General Hospital, Gillette Center for Women's Cancers, Boston, MA.

MARIO A. EISENBERGER, MD
R. Dale Hughes Professor of Oncology and Urology, Division of Medical Oncology, The Sidney Kimmel Comprehensive Cancer Center at Johns Hopkins, Baltimore, MD.

VICTOR M. ELNER, MD PhD
Associate Professor of Ophthalmology, Department of Ophthalmology, W. D. Kellogg Eye Center, University of Michigan; Assistant Professor of Pathology, Department of Pathology, University of Michigan Hospital, Ann Arbor, MI.

REBECCA L. ELSTROM, MD
Instructor, University of Pennsylvania School of Medicine; Abramson Family Cancer Research Institute, University of Pennsylvania, Philadelphia, PA.

MICHAEL S. EWER, MD, PhD, JD
Professor of Medicine, University of Texas M.D. Anderson Cancer Center, Houston, TX.

STEFAN FADERL, MD
Assistant Professor, University of Texas M.D. Anderson Cancer Center, Houston, TX.

MARWAN FAKIH, MD
Assistant Professor of Medicine, State University of New York–Buffalo; Assistant Professor of Medicine and Gastrointestinal Oncology, Roswell Park Cancer Institute, Buffalo, NY.

ERIC R. FEARON, MD, PhD
Department of Internal Medicine, Human Genetics, and Pathology, University of Michigan Medical School, Ann Arbor, MI.

MICHAEL FELDMAN, MD, PhD
Assistant Professor of Pathology, University of Pennsylvania Health System, Philadelphia, PA.

ALESSANDRO FICHERA, MD
Assistant Professor of Surgery, The University of Chicago Pritzker School of Medicine, Chicago, IL.

ISAIAH J. FIDLER, DVM, PhD
Professor and Chair, Department of Cancer Biology, M.D. Anderson Cancer Center, University of Texas, Houston, TX.

ALEXANDRA H. FILIPOVICH, MD
Professor of Pediatrics, University of Cincinnati; Ralph J. Stolle Chair in Clinical Immunology, Professor of Pediatrics, Director, Immunodeficiency and Histocytosis Program, Medical Director, Hematology/Oncology Diagnostic Laboratory, Cincinnati Children's Hospital Medical Center, Cincinnati, OH.

ROBERT L. FOOTE, MD
Professor of Oncology, Mayo Medical School; Consultant, Department of Oncology, Division of Radiation Oncology, Mayo Clinic, Rochester, MN.

ARLENE A. FORASTIERE, MD
Professor of Oncology, Johns Hopkins University, Sidney Kimmel Comprehensive Cancer Center at Johns Hopkins, Baltimore, MD.

JAMES M. FORD, MD
Assistant Professor of Medicine, Genetics, and Pediatrics, Divisions of Oncology and Medical Genetics, Stanford University School of Medicine, Stanford, CA.

ROBIN S. FREEDBERG, MD
Associate Professor of Medicine, New York University Medical Center, New York, NY.

ALISON G. FREIFELD, MD
Associate Professor of Internal Medicine, University of Nebraska Medical Center, Omaha, NE.

DANIELLE M. FRIEDRICHSEN, PhD
Postdoctoral Fellow, Divisions of Clinical Research and Human Biology, Fred Hutchinson Cancer Research Center, Seattle, WA.

ARLAN F. FULLER, Jr., MD
Assistant Professor of Gynecology, Obstetrics, and Reproductive Biology, Harvard Medical School; Chief, Division of Gynecologic Oncology, Massachusetts General Hospital, Gillette Center for Women's Cancers, Boston, MA.

SHIRISH M. GADGEEL, MD
Assistant Professor, Wayne State University/Thoracic Program, Karamanos Cancer Institute, Detroit, MI.

PATRICIA A. GANZ, MD
Professor, UCLA School of Public Health, Department of Health Services, Professor, David Geffen School of Medicine at UCLA, Department of Medicine, University of California–Los Angeles; Director, Division of Cancer Prevention and Control Research, Jonsson Comprehensive Cancer Center at UCLA, Los Angeles, CA.

JORGE A. GARCIA, MD
Urologic Oncology Fellow, University of California Comprehensive Cancer Center, San Francisco, CA.

DENNIS A. GASTINEAU, MD
Associate Professor of Medicine, Mayo Medical School; Director, Human Cell Therapy Laboratory, Mayo Clinic, Rochester, MN.

MANISH GHARIA, MD
Clinical Assistant Professor, University of Wisconsin, Madison, WI; Clinical Assistant Professor, Medical College of Wisconsin, Milwaukee, WI.

MARK R. GILBERT, MD
Associate Professor, M.D. Anderson Cancer Center, University of Texas, Houston, TX.

KATRINA Y. GLOVER, MD
Medical Oncology Fellow, University of Texas M.D. Anderson Cancer Center, Houston, TX.

JOHN M. GOLDMAN, DM, FRCP, FRCPath
Professor of Leukaemia Biology, Imperial College; Consultant Haematologist, Hammersmith Hospital, London, UK.

DONALD PETER GOLDSTEIN, MD
Professor of Obstetrics, Gynecology, and Reproductive Biology, Harvard Medical School; Co-Director, New England Trophoblastic Disease Center, Brigham and Women's Hospital; Dana Farber Cancer Institute, Boston, MA.

MARCELO P. V. GOMES, MD
Research Associate, Section of Hematology and Coagulation Medicine, Department of Hematology and Medical Oncology, The Cleveland Clinic, Cleveland, OH.

ANNE KATHRYN GOODMAN, MD
Associate Professor of Gynecology, Obstetrics, and Reproductive Biology, Harvard Medical School; Associate Director, Division of Gynecologic Oncology, Massachusetts General Hospital, Gillette Center for Women's Cancers, Boston, MA.

ELLEN GORDON, MD
Dermatologic Surgeon, Department of Dermatology, Marshfield Clinic, Marshfield, WI.

DANIEL M. GREEN, MD
Professor of Pediatrics, School of Medicine and Biomedical Sciences, University at Buffalo, State University of New York; Attending Physician, Roswell Park Cancer Institute, Pediatrics, Buffalo, NY.

LOUISE GROCHOW, MD
Investigation Drug Branch, National Cancer Institute, National Institutes of Health, Bethesda, MD.

THOMAS G. GROSS, MD, PhD
Associate Professor of Pediatrics, Director, Division of Hematology/Oncology/BMT, Children's Hospital, Ohio State University, Columbus, OH.

STUART A. GROSSMAN, MD
Professor of Oncology, Medicine, and Neurosurgery, Johns Hopkins University and Sidney Kimmel Comprehensive Cancer Center at Johns Hopkins, Baltimore, MD.

LEONARD L. GUNDERSON, MD
Getz Family Professor and Chair Department of Radiation Mayo Clinic College of Medicine and Mayo Clinic, Deputy Director for Clinical Affairs, Scottsdale, AZ.

THOMAS R. HABERMANN, MD
Professor of Medicine, Mayo Clinic College of Medicine; Consultant, Division of Hematology, Department of Medicine, Mayo Clinic, Rochester, MN.

STEPHEN M. HAHN, MD
Associate Professor, Department of Radiation Oncology, University of Pennsylvania, Philadelphia, PA.

JOHN D. HAINSWORTH, MD
Director of Clinical Research, Sarah Cannon Cancer Center, Nashville, TN.

WILLIAM D. HAIRE, MD
Professor, Department of Internal Medicine, Section of Oncology and Hematology, University of Nebraska Medical Center, Omaha, NE.

DANIEL HALLER, MD
Professor and Associate Chief for Clinical Affairs, Division of Hematology–Oncology, Department of Medicine, University of Pennsylvania School of Medicine, Philadelphia, PA.

NADER HANNA, MD
Assistant Professor of Surgery, University of Kentucky College of Medicine, Lexington, KY.

ELEANOR E. R. HARRIS, MD
Assistant Professor, Department of Radiation Oncology, Gynecologic Oncology, Clinical Practices of the University of Pennsylvania, Philadelphia, PA.

WAYNE B. HARRIS, MD
Winship Cancer Institute, Emory University School of Medicine, Atlanta, GA.

NANCY H. HEIDEMAN, PharmD
Assistant Professor, College of Pharmacy, University of New Mexico, Albuquerque, NM.

RICHARD L. HEIDEMAN, MD
Professor of Pediatrics, University of New Mexico, Albuquerque, NM.

RICHARD F. HEITMILLER, MD
Associate Professor of Surgery, Johns Hopkins Medical Institutions; Chief of Surgery, Union Memorial Hospital, Baltimore, MD.

KATHY J. HELZLSOUER, MD, MHS
Professor, Department of Epidemiology, Johns Hopkins University Bloomberg School of Public Health; The Sidney Kimmel Comprehensive Cancer Center, Baltimore, MD.

DIANE HERSHOCK, MD, PhD
Assistant Professor of Medicine, Hematology/Oncology Division, Hospital of the University of Pennsylvania, Philadelphia Veterans Hospital, Philadelphia, PA.

TERU HIDESHIMA, MD, PhD
Principal Associate, Dana-Farber Cancer Institute, Boston, MA.

LESLIE R. HOLMES, MD
Assistant Professor, Department of Radiation Oncology, Emory University School of Medicine; Assistant Professor, Department of Radiation Oncology, Loughlin Radiation Oncology Center, Atlanta, GA.

KIM HUANG, MD
Resident, University of California, San Francisco, CA.

JAMES N. IHLE, PhD
Investigator, Howard Hughes Medical Institute; Chair, Department of Biochemistry, St. Jude Children's Research Institute, Memphis, TN.

RUSSELL F. JACOBY, MD
Associate Professor of Medicine, University of Wisconsin; Director, Colon Cancer Prevention Program, University of Wisconsin Comprehensive Cancer Center, Madison, WI.

ELAINE S. JAFFE, MD
Clinical Professor of Pathology, George Washington University School of Medicine, Washington, DC; Chief, Hematopathology Section, Deputy Chief, Laboratory of Pathology, National Cancer Institute, Bethesda, MD.

RAKESH K. JAIN, PhD
Andrew Werk Cook Professor, Department of Radiation Oncology, Harvard Medical School, Cambridge, MA; Director, Edwin L. Steele Laboratory of Tumor Biology, Department of Radiation Oncology and MGH Cancer Center, Massachusetts General Hospital, Boston, MA.

DAVID H. JOHNSON, MD
Professor of Medicine, Director, Division of Hematology–Oncology, Deputy Director, Vanderbilt-Ingram Cancer Center, Vanderbilt University School of Medicine, Nashville, TN.

HEATHER JONES, MD
Clinical Instructor, University of Pennsylvania School of Medicine, Philadelphia, PA; Clinical Instructor, Netherlands Cancer Institute, Amsterdam, The Netherlands.

KEVIN D. JUDY, MD
Associate Professor, Department of Neurosurgery, University of Pennsylvania School of Medicine; Staff Physician, Hospital of the University of Pennsylvania, Philadelphia, PA.

CARL H. JUNE, MD
Professor, Department of Pathology and Laboratory Medicine, University of Pennsylvania School of Medicine, Philadelphia, PA.

ANDRE KALIL, MD
Assistant Professor, University of Nebraska Medical Center; Associate Director, Immunocompromised Host Infectious Diseases Program, Nebraska Medical Center, Omaha, NE.

JEFFREY A. KANT, MD PhD
Professor, Pathology and Human Genetics, University of Pittsburgh; Director, Division of Molecular Diagnostics, University of Pittsburgh Medical Center Health System, Pittsburgh, PA.

HAGOP M. KANTARJIAN, MD
Professor of Medicine, Chair, Department of Leukemia, University of Texas M. D. Anderson Cancer Center, Houston, TX.

MICHAEL B. KASTAN, MD, PhD
Professor of Pediatrics, Chief, Division of Pediatric Hematology/Oncology, University of Tennessee; Chair, Hematology/Oncology, Co-Director, Molecular Oncology Program, St. Jude Children's Research Hospital, Memphis, TN.

MARGARET KEMENY, MD, FACS
Professor of Surgery, Mt. Sinai School of Medicine, New York, NY; Director, Queens Cancer Center, Queens Hospital, Jamaica, NY.

NANCY E. KEMENY, MD
Professor of Medicine, Weill Medical College of Cornell University; Attending Physician, Memorial Sloan-Kettering Cancer Center, New York, NY.

THOMAS W. KENSLER, PhD
Professor, Johns Hopkins Bloomberg School of Public Health, Baltimore, MD.

LAWRENCE R. KLEINBERG, MD
Assistant Professor, Department of Radiation Oncology and Molecular Sciences, Johns Hopkins University, Baltimore, MD.

ELISE C. KOHN, MD
Head, Molecular Signaling Section, Laboratory of Pathology, Chair, Gynecologic Malignancies Faculty, Center for Cancer Research, National Cancer Institute, National Institutes of Health, Bethesda, MD.

RAMI KOMROKJI, MD
Senior Instructor of Medicine, University of Rochester, Rochester, NY.

PETER A. KOUIDES, MD
Attending Hematologist, Rochester General Hospital/ The Lipson Blood and Cancer Center; Associate Professor of Medicine, University of Rochester School of Medicine; Research Director, Mary M. Gooley Hemophilia Center, Rochester, NY.

OMER KUCUK, MD
Professor of Medicine, Wayne State University; Population Studies and Prevention Program, Karamanos Cancer Institute, Detroit, MI.

PAUL F. LAMBERT, PhD
Professor, Department of Oncology, McArdle Laboratory for Cancer Research, University of Wisconsin, Madison, WI.

JULIE R. LANGE, MD, ScM
Assistant Professor of Surgery, Johns Hopkins Medical Institutions, Baltimore, MD.

PAUL O. LARSON, MD
Associate Professor, Department of Surgery, Division of Plastic Surgery, Mohs Surgery Clinic, University of Wisconsin Medical School, Madison, WI.

JANESSA LASKIN, MD
Assistant Professor of Medicine, University of British Columbia; Medical Oncologist, B. C. Cancer Agency, Vancouver, British Columbia, Canada.

THEODORE S. LAWRENCE, MD, PhD
Professor and Chair of Radiation Oncology, University of Michigan, Ann Arbor, MI.

FRED T. LEE, JR., MD
Associate Professor of Radiology, University of Wisconsin, Madison, WI.

SUSANNA I. LEE, MD, PhD
Instructor in Radiology, Harvard Medical School; Staff Radiologist, Department of Radiology, Massachusetts General Hospital, Boston, MA.

TODD LEE, PharmD, PhD
Research Assistant Professor, Department of General Internal Medicine, Division of Medicine, Northwestern University, Feinberg School of Medicine; Adjunct Assistant Professor, Center for Pharmacoeconomic Research, Department of Pharmacy Practice, College of Pharmacy, University of Illinois at Chicago, Chicago, IL; Senior Investigator, Midwest Center for Health Services and Policy Research, Hines VA Hospital, Hines, IL.

RENATO LENZI, MD
Associate Professor of Medicine, University of Texas M.D. Anderson Cancer Center, Houston, TX.

CARYN LERMAN, PhD
Professor, Annenberg Public Policy Center and Department of Psychiatry, University of Pennsylvania; Director, Tobacco Use Research Center, Associate Director, Population Science and Cancer Control, University of Pennsylvania Health System, Philadelphia, PA.

ALLEN S. LICHTER, MD
Professor of Radiation Oncology, Dean, College of Medicine, University of Michigan Medical Center, Ann Arbor, MI.

LANCE A. LIOTTA, MD, PhD
Chief, Laboratory of Pathology, Center for Cancer Research, National Cancer Institute, National Institutes of Health, Bethesda, MD.

ALLAN LIPTON, MD
Professor of Medicine and Oncology, Milton S. Hershey Medical Center, Hershey, PA.

T. ANDREW LISTER, MD, FRCP, FRCPath, FRCR
Professor of Medical Oncology, Queen Mary's School of Medicine; Professor of Medical Oncology, Director of

Cancer Services, Honorary Consultant, St. Bartholomew's Hospital, London, UK.

FULVIO LONARDO, MD
Assistant Professor of Pathology, Wayne State University School of Medicine; Department of Pathology, Harper University Hospital; Karmanos Cancer Institute, Detroit, MI.

CHARLES L. LOPRINZI, MD
Professor, Mayo Medical School, Rochester, MN.

JOHN S. MACDONALD, MD
Professor of Medicine, New York Medical College; Medical Director, St. Vincent's Comprehensive Cancer Center, New York, NY.

MITCHELL MACHTAY, MD
Associate Professor of Radiation Oncology, Bodine Cancer Center, Thomas Jefferson University Hospital, Philadelphia, PA.

AMIT MAITY, MD, PhD
Assistant Professor, Department of Radiation Oncology, University of Pennsylvania School of Medicine; Staff Physician, Hospital of the University of Pennsylvania, Philadelphia, PA.

UZMA MALIK, MD
Assistant Professor, University of Kentucky College of Medicine, Lexington, KY.

JOHN C. MANSOUR, MD
Surgical Resident, Department of Surgery, University of Wisconsin Hospitals and Clinics, Madison, WI.

BERYL McCORMICK, MD
Associate Professor of Radiation Oncology in Medicine, Weill Medical College of Cornell University; Attending Physician, Memorial Sloan-Kettering Cancer Center, New York, NY.

CHARLES J. McDONALD, MD
Professor and Chair, Department of Dermatology, Brown University Medical School; Chair, Department of Dermatology, Rhode Island Hospital, Providence RI.

I. ROSS McDOUGALL, MD, PhD
Professor of Radiology, Department of Nuclear Medicine, Stanford University, Stanford, CA.

W. GILLIES McKENNA, MD, PhD
Henry K. Pancoast Professor and Chair, Department of Radiation Oncology, University of Pennsylvania School of Medicine, Philadelphia, PA.

STEVEN G. MERANZE, MD
Associate Professor of Radiology and Radiological Sciences, Associate Professor of Surgery, Director, Interventional Radiology, Vanderbilt University Medical Center, Nashville, TN.

ADAM R. METWALLI, MD
Resident, Department of Urology, Oklahoma University Health Sciences Center, Oklahoma City, OK.

JAMES M. METZ, MD
Assistant Professor, Department of Radiation Oncology, University of Pennsylvania, Philadelphia, PA.

FRANK L. MEYSKENS, Jr., MD
Professor of Medicine and Biological Chemistry, Director, Chao Family Comprehensive Cancer Center, University of California, Irvine, CA.

FABRIZIO MICHELASSI, MD
Professor of Surgery, The University of Chicago Pritzker School of Medicine, Chicago, IL.

MICHAEL C. MILONE, MD, PhD
Postdoctoral Fellow, University of Pennsylvania School of Medicine, Philadelphia, PA.

VICTORIA MOCK, DNSc
Director, Center for Nursing Research, Johns Hopkins University; Associate Professor, Johns Hopkins University School of Nursing; Joint Position in Oncology, Johns Hopkins School of Medicine; Director of Nursing Research, The Sidney Kimmel Comprehensive Cancer Center, The Johns Hopkins Hospital, Baltimore, MD.

MOHAMMED MOHIUDDIN, MD
Professor, University of Kentucky College of Medicine, Lexington, KY.

JAMES E. MONTIE, MD
Professor and Chairman, Department of Urology, Valassis Professor of Urologic Oncology, University of Michigan, Ann Arbor, MI.

MARGARET MOONEY, MD
Senior Investigator, Clinical Investigations Branch, Cancer Therapy Evaluation Program, Division of Cancer Treatment and Diagnosis, National Cancer Institute, Bethesda, MD.

A. ROSS MORTON, MD, FRCP, FRCPC
Professor of Medicine, Queen's University; Consultant Nephrologist, Kingston General Hospital, Kingston, Ontario, Canada.

JOHN E. MUNZENRIDER, MD
Associate Professor, Harvard University School of Medicine, Cambridge, MA; Associate Radiation Oncologist, Department of Radiation Oncology, Massachusetts General Hospital, Boston, MA.

JAMES R. NEFF, MD
Professor of Orthopaedic Surgery and Pathology, University of Nebraska College of Medicine; Professor of Orthopaedic Surgery and Pathology, University of Nebraska Medical Center, Omaha, NE.

WILLIAM G. NELSON, MD, PhD
Professor of Oncology, Urology, Pharmacology and Molecular Sciences, Medicine, Pathology, and Radiation Oncology and Molecular Radiation Sciences, Sidney Kimmel Comprehensive Cancer Center, Brady Institute of Urology, Johns Hopkins University School of Medicine, Baltimore, MD.

SUZANNE NESBIT, PharmD, BCPS
Clinical Coordinator, Cancer Pain Service, Sidney Kimmel Comprehensive Cancer Center at Johns Hopkins; Clinical Pharmacy Specialist, Pain Management, Department of Pharmacy, Johns Hopkins Hospital, Baltimore, MD.

JOHN E. NIEDERHUBER, MD
Professor, Departments of Surgery and Oncology, Wattawa Professor–Bascom, University of Wisconsin–Madison, Madison, WI.

TRACEY O'CONNOR, MD
Assistant Professor of Clinical Medicine, State University of New York at Buffalo; Assistant Professor of Clinical Medicine, Roswell Park Cancer Institute, Buffalo, NY.

KENNETH OFFIT, MD, MPH
Associate Professor of Medicine and Public Health, Cornell University Medical College; Chief, Clinical Genetics Service, Department of Medicine, Associate Attending Physician, Department of Medicine, Memorial Sloan-Kettering Cancer Center, New York, NY.

EILEEN M. O'REILLY, MD
Assistant Professor of Medicine, Weill Medical College of Cornell University, New York Presbyterian Hospital; Assistant Attending Physician, GI Medical Oncology, Memorial Sloan-Kettering Cancer Center, New York, NY.

ELAINE A. OSTRANDER, PhD
Affiliate Professor, Departments of Biology and Genome Science, University of Washington; Member, Divisions of Clinical Research and Human Biology, Fred Hutchinson Cancer Research Center, Seattle, WA.

BRIAN O'SULLIVAN, MD
Professor, Princess Margaret Hospital, Ontario Cancer Institute, Toronto, Ontario, Canada.

TEDDY D. PAN, MD
Clinical Assistant Professor, Department of Dermatology, Brown Medical School; Physician, Rhode Island Hospital, Miriam Hospital, Providence, RI; Physician, Newton-Wellesley Hospital, Newton, MA.

HARPREET PANNU, MD
Assistant Professor, Department of Radiology, Johns Hopkins University, Baltimore, MD.

DREW M. PARDOLL, MD, PhD
Professor of Oncology, Sidney Kimmel Comprehensive Cancer Center, Johns Hopkins University School of Medicine, Baltimore, MD.

DAVID ROSS PARKINSON, MD
Vice President, Research, Head, Oncology Therapeutic Area, Amgen, Inc., Thousand Oaks, CA.

HARVEY I. PASS, MD
Professor of Surgery and Oncology, Wayne State University, Karmanos Cancer Institute; Chief of Thoracic Oncology, Karmanos Cancer Institute; Chief of Thoracic Surgery, John D. Dingell Veterans Hospital of Detroit, Detroit, MI.

FREDA PATTERSON, MS
Project Manager, Tobacco Use Research Center, University of Pennsylvania Health System, Philadelphia, PA.

MICHAEL C. PERRY, MD, FRCP
Professor and Director, Divisions of Hematology and Medical Oncology, Department of Internal Medicine; Nellie B. Smith Chair of Oncology, Ellis Fischel Cancer Center, University of Missouri–Columbia, Columbia, MO.

LoANN C. PETERSON, MD
Professor, Feinberg School of Medicine, Northwestern University; Director of Hematopathology, Northwestern Memorial Hospital, Chicago, IL.

MARK R. PETTELKOW, MD
Professor, Departments of Dermatology and Biochemistry and Molecular Biology, Mayo Clinic College of Medicine, Rochester, MN.

PETER C. PHILLIPS, MD
Professor, Department of Neurology, University of Pennsylvania School of Medicine; Schoemaker Professor and Director of Neuro-Oncology, Children's Hospital of Philadelphia, Philadelphia, PA.

STEVEN PIANTADOSI, MD, PhD
Professor of Oncology Biostatistics, Sidney Kimmel Comprehensive Cancer Center at Johns Hopkins; Joint Appointments, Biostatistics and Epidemiology, Bloomberg School of Public Health, Johns Hopkins University, Baltimore, MD.

JENNIFER A. PIETENPOL, PhD
Professor, Department of Biochemistry, Associate Director for Basic Research Programs, Vanderbilt-Ingram Cancer Center, Vanderbilt University School of Medicine, Nashville, TN.

PETER W. T. PISTERS, MD, FACS
Professor of Surgery, University of Texas M. D. Anderson Cancer Center, Houston, TX.

JULIAN JOSEPH PRIBAZ, MD
Professor of Surgery, Harvard Medical School; Brigham and Women's Hospital; Children's Hospital, Boston, MA.

AMY A. PRUITT, MD
Associate Professor, Department of Neurology, University of Pennsylvania School of Medicine; Staff Physician, Hospital of the University of Pennsylvania, Philadelphia, PA.

CHING-HON PUI, MD
Professor, Department of Pediatrics, University of Tennessee Health Science Center College of Medicine; Director, Leukemia/Lymphoma Division, Department of Hematology-Oncology, Fahad Nassar Al-Rashid Chair of Leukemia Research, American Cancer Society FM Kirby Clinical Research Professor, St. Jude Children's Research Hospital, Memphis, TN.

HARRY QUON, MD
Assistant Professor, University of Pennsylvania School of Medicine; Director, Head and Neck Radiation Oncology, Associate Director, Center for Head and Neck Cancer, Hospital of the University of Pennsylvania, Philadelphia, PA.

MARTIN N. RABER, MD
Clinical Professor of Medicine, University of Texas M. D. Anderson Cancer Center, Houston, TX.

WILLIAM F. REGINE, MD
Professor and Chair, Department of Radiation Oncology, University of Maryland School of Medicine, Baltimore, MD.

PAUL RICHARDSON, MD
Assistant Professor in Medicine, Harvard Medical School; Clinical Director, Jerome Lipper Multiple Myeloma Center, Dana-Farber Cancer Institute, Boston, MA.

MARK RITTER, MD, PhD
Associate Professor, Department of Human Oncology, University of Wisconsin–Madison, Madison, MI.

JOHN ROBERTS, MD
Assistant Professor of Surgery, Department of Cardiac and Thoracic Surgery, Section of Surgical Sciences, Vanderbilt University School of Medicine, Nashville, TN.

LESLIE ROBINSON-BOSTOM, MD
Department of Dermatology, Brown University Medical School; Director of Dermatopathology, Rhode Island Hospital, Providence, RI.

CARLOS RODRIGUEZ-GALINDO, MD
Assistant Professor, University of Tennessee Health Sciences Center; Assistant Member, St. Jude Children's Research Hospital, Memphis, TN.

MYRNA R. ROSENFELD, MD, PhD
Professor, University of Pennsylvania; Associate Professor, Hospital of the University of Pennsylvania, Philadelphia, PA.

NADIA ROSENTHAL, PhD
Head, Mouse Biology Programme, European Molecular Biology Laboratory, Monterotondo (Rome), Italy.

ROBERT D. RUBENS, MD, FRCP
Professor of Clinical Oncology, University of London; Guy's Hospital, London, UK.

EDWARD B. RUBENSTEIN, MD
Senior Vice President of Medical and Commercial Development, MGI Pharma, Inc., Bloomington, MN.

JAMES L. RUBENSTEIN, MD, PhD
Assistant Adjunct Professor, Hematology/Oncology, Department of Medicine, Attending Physician, University of California, San Francisco, CA.

BRIAN P. RUBIN, MD, PhD
Assistant Professor of Pathology, University of Washington, Seattle, WA.

JOHN C. RUCKDESCHEL, MD
Professor of Medicine, Wayne State University School of Medicine; President and CEO, Karmanos Cancer Institute, Detroit, MI.

VALERIE W. RUSCH, MD
Professor of Surgery, Cornell University Medical College; Chief, Thoracic Division, Department of Surgery, William G. Cahan Chair of Surgery, Memorial Sloan-Kettering Cancer Center, New York, NY.

ANTHONY H. RUSSELL, MD
Associate Professor of Radiation Oncology, Harvard Medical School; Director of Gynecologic Radiotherapy, Department of Radiation Oncology, Massachusetts General Hospital, Boston, MA.

HOWARD M. SANDLER, MD
Professor, Departments of Radiation Oncology and Urology, University of Michigan Medical School, Ann Arbor, MI.

JOHN T. SANDLUND, MD
University of Tennessee College of Medicine; St. Jude Children's Research Hospital, Memphis, TN.

FRED SANFILIPPO, MD, PhD
Professor of Pathology, Dean, College of Medicine and Public Health, Senior Vice President for Health Science, Ohio State University; Chief Executive Officer, Ohio State University Medical Center, Columbus, OH.

VICTOR SANTANA, MD
University of Tennessee Health Sciences Center College of Medicine; Director, Solid Tumor Division, Member, Department Hematology–Oncology, St. Jude Children's Research Hospital, Memphis, TN.

ANN G. SCHWARTZ, MD, MPH
Associate Center Director for Population Sciences, Karamanos Cancer Institute, Detroit, MI.

MICHAEL V. SEIDEN, MD, PhD
Assistant Professor in Medicine, Harvard Medical School; Associate Physician in Medicine, Massachusetts General Hospital, Boston, MA.

DUANE SEWELL, MD
Assistant Professor, Department of Otolaryngology, University of Pennsylvania, Philadelphia, PA.

WILLIAM H. SHARFMAN, MD
Assistant Professor of Oncology, Johns Hopkins School of Medicine; Director of Cutaneous Oncology, The Sidney Kimmel Comprehensive Cancer Center at Johns Hopkins, Baltimore, MD.

RINA SIDDIQUI, MD
Weill Medical College of Cornell University; Fellow, Clinical Genetics Service, Department of Medicine, Memorial Sloan-Kettering Cancer Center, New York, NY.

JONATHAN W. SIMONS, MD
Director, Winship Cancer Institute; Professor and Chair Department of Hematology and Oncology, The Robert W. Woodruff Health Sciences Center, Emory University School of Medicine, Atlanta, GA.

ERIC J. SMALL, MD
Professor of Medicine and Urology, University of California Comprehensive Cancer Center, San Francisco, CA.

DAVID C. SMITH, MD
Associate Professor of Medicine and Urology, University of Michigan, Ann Arbor, MI.

RYAN P. SMITH, MD
Instructor, University of Pennsylvania Medical Center; Attending Physician, Department of Radiation Oncology, Hospital of the University of Pennsylvania, Philadelphia, PA.

PENNY K. SNEED, MD
Professor in Residence, University of California, San Francisco, CA.

STEPHEN N. SNOW, MD, MBA
Professor, Department of Surgery, Division of Plastic Surgery, Mohs Surgery Clinic, University of Wisconsin Medical School; Professor, Mohs Surgery Clinic, University of Wisconsin Hospital and Clinics, Madison, WI.

LORI J. SOKOLL, PhD
Assistant Professor of Pathology, Oncology, and Urology, Johns Hopkins University; Associate Director, Clinical Chemistry Division, Johns Hopkins Hospital, Baltimore, MD.

JAMES L. SPEYER, MD
Professor of Clinical Medicine, New York University; Associate Director of Clinical and Hospital Operations, New York University School of Medicine, New York, NY.

ALEXANDER I. SPIRA, MD, PhD
Staff, Hematology/Oncology, Inova Fairfax Hospital, Farifax, VA.

SHERI L. SPUNT, MD
Assistant Professor, University of Tennessee College of Medicine; Assistant Member, Department of Hematology–Oncology, St. Jude Children's Research Hospital, Memphis, TN.

PAUL T. STRICKLAND, PhD
Professor, Johns Hopkins Bloomberg School of Public Health, Baltimore, MD.

BILL SUGDEN, PhD
Professor, Department of Oncology, McArdle Laboratory for Cancer Research, University of Wisconsin–Madison, Madison, WI.

ANNETTE SUNGA, MD
Clinical Instructor, State University of New York at Buffalo; Clinical Instructor, Roswell Park Cancer Institute, Buffalo, NY.

MARTIN S. TALLMAN, MD
Professor of Medicine, Division of Hematology/Oncology, Northwestern University Feinberg School of Medicine; Attending Physician, Northwestern Memorial Hospital, Co-Director, Hematologic Malignancy Program, Robert H. Lurie Comprehensive Cancer Center, Chicago, IL.

JAMES E. TALMADGE, PhD
Professor, Department of Pathology and Microbiology, Director, Laboratory of Transplantation, University of Nebraska Medical Center, Omaha, NE.

RUDRANATH TALUKDAR, MBBS
Instructor, M. D. Anderson Cancer Center, University of Texas, Houston, TX.

AYALEW TEFFERI, MD
Professor of Hematology and Medicine, Mayo College of Medicine, Rochester, MN.

JAMES TATE THIGPEN, MD
Director, of Oncology, Professor, Department of Medicine, Division of Oncology, University of Mississippi Medical Center, Jackson, MS.

CRAIG B. THOMPSON, MD
Scientific Director, Abramson Family Cancer Research Institute, University of Pennsylvania, Philadelphia, PA.

TRAVIS L. THOMPSON, MD
Chief Resident, Department of Radiation Oncology and Molecular Radiation Sciences, Johns Hopkins Hospital, Baltimore, MD.

KENSEI TOBINAI, MD, PhD
Chief, Hematology Division, National Cancer Center Hospital, Tokyo, Japan.

FRANK TORTI, MD
Professor and Director, Comprehensive Cancer Center at Wake Forest University, Winston-Salem, NC.

DONALD L. TRUMP, MD
Professor of Medicine, State University of New York at Buffalo; Chair, Department of Medicine, Senior Vice President, Clinical Research, Roswell Park Cancer Institute, Buffalo, NY.

JO-ANNE VAN BURIK, MD, FACP
Assistant Professor, Department of Medicine, Division of Infectious Disease and International Medicine, Head, Infections of Immunocompromised Host, Non-HIV, University of Minnesota, Minneapolis, MN.

GAURI R. VARADHACHARY, MD
Assistant Professor of Medicine, Department of Gastrointestinal Medical Oncology, University of Texas M. D. Anderson Cancer Center, Houston, TX.

KALA VISVANATHAN, MBBS, FRACP, MHS
Assistant Professor of Epidemiology and Oncology, Johns Hopkins University Bloomberg School of Public Health, Baltimore, MD.

JULIE M. VOSE, MD
Neumann M. and Mildred E. Harris Professor, Chief, Section of Hematology/Oncology, University of Nebraska Medical Center, Omaha, NE.

HENRY WAGNER, MD
Division Director, Radiation Oncology, Penn State Milton S. Hershey Center, Hershey, PA.

RICHARD L. WAHL, MD
Professor of Radiology and Oncology, Henry N. Wagner, Jr. Professor of Nuclear Medicine, Director of Nuclear Medicine, Vice Chairman for Technology and New Business Development, Russell H. Morgan Department of Radiology and Radiological Sciences, Johns Hopkins University School of Medicine, Baltimore, MD.

TOSHIKI WATANABE, MD, PhD
Associate Professor, Institute of Medical Sciences, University of Tokyo, Tokyo, Japan.

BARBARA L. WEBER, MD
Professor and Director, Cancer Genomics Program at Abramson Family Cancer Research Institute, University of Pennsylvania, Philadelphia, PA.

RANDAL S. WEBER, MD
Hubert and Olive Stringer Professor and Chair, Department of Head and Neck Surgery, University of Texas M.D. Anderson Cancer Center, Houston.

SHARON WEBER, MD
Assistant Professor, University of Wisconsin Hospital, Madison, WI.

S. JACK WEI, MD
Chief Resident, Department of Radiation Oncology, Hospital of the University of Pennsylvania, Philadelphia, PA.

RONALD J. WEIGEL, MD, PhD
Professor of Surgery, Vice Chair, Department of Surgery, Thomas Jefferson University, Philadelphia, PA.

IRVING L. WEISSMAN, MD
Professor of Pathology and Developmental Biology, Director, Cancer and Stem Cell Biology Institute, Stanford University School of Medicine, Stanford, CA.

WILLIAM WESTRA, MD
Associate Professor of Pathology, Johns Hopkins University School of Medicine; Associate Professor of Pathology, Otolaryngology-Head and Neck Surgery, and Dermatology, Associate Director, Division of Surgical Pathology, The Johns Hopkins Hospital, Baltimore, MD.

MICHAEL J. WEYANT, MD
Fellow in Thoracic Surgery, Memorial Sloan-Kettering Cancer Center and New York Presbyterian Hospital, New York, NY.

ANTONIO C. WOLFF, MD
Assistant Professor of Oncology, Johns Hopkins University School of Medicine; The Sidney Kimmel Comprehensive Cancer Center at Johns Hopkins, Baltimore, MD.

GARY S. WOOD, MD
Johnson Professor and Chairman, Department of Dermatology, University of Wisconsin; Chief of Dermatology, Middleton VA Medical Center, Madison, WI.

WILLIAM C. WOOD, MD
Professor, Emory University School of Medicine; Chair, Department of Surgery, Emory University School of Medicine, Atlanta, GA.

JAMES E. WOOLDRIDGE, MD
Assistant Professor, Department of Internal Medicine, University of Iowa; Assistant Professor, University of Iowa College of Medicine, Iowa City, IA.

ANTOINETTE J. WOZNIAK, MD
Professor of Medicine and Oncology, Wayne State University; Head, Multidisciplinary Lung Cancer Clinic, Karmanos Cancer Institute, Detroit, MI.

LANCE EVERETT WYATT, MD
Chief Resident in Plastic and Reconstructive Surgery, Harvard Plastic Surgery Residency Training Program, Department of Surgery, Brigham and Women's Hospital, Boston, MA.

ANAADRIANA ZAKARIJA, MD
Fellow, Northwestern University Feinberg School of Medicine, Chicago, IL.

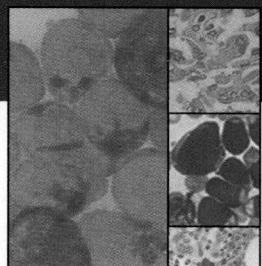

REVIEWERS

The publisher wishes to acknowledge the following individuals, who previewed advance materials for *Clinical Oncology*, 3rd Edition.

Po-Min Chen, MD, DMS, Taipei-Veterans General Hospital, and National Yang-Ming University, Taipei, Taiwan

Professor G. Giaccone, Head, Division of Medical Oncology, Vrije Universiteit Medical Center, Amsterdam, The Netherlands

Robert Hawkins, Cancer Research UK, Professor and Director of Medical Oncology, Christie CRC Research Centre, Manchester, UK

Professor S. B. Kaye, MD FRCP, Professor of Medical Oncology, Royal Marsden Hospital, London, UK

Professor (Dr.) Purvish M. Parikh, MD, DNB, FICP, PhD, Head of Medical Oncology, Tata Memorial Hospital, Parel, Mumbai, India

Dr. T. Rajkumar, MD (General Medicine), DM (Medical Oncology), PhD (London), Scientific Director, Cancer Institute (WIA), Adyar, Chennai, India

Professor John F. Smyth, Cancer Research UK, University of Edinburgh, Cancer Research Centre, Edinburgh, UK; Editor-in-Chief, European Journal of Cancer

Professor Penella J. Woll, FRCP, PhD, University of Sheffield, Sheffield, UK

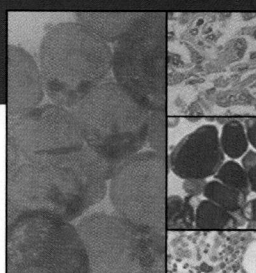

PREFACE

The field of clinical oncology is experiencing rapid advancement, which is the result of impressive accomplishments in both laboratory and clinical science. The genetic mechanisms underlying cancer and their downstream effects are quickly becoming understood. The development of therapies, such as antibodies and small molecules aimed at specific molecular targets key in the neoplastic process, provide the promise of less toxic and more effective therapeutic options. Cancer prevention as a clinical science is making advances both in eliminating known carcinogens (e.g., tobacco) and in the development of drugs that inhibit carcinogenesis. The cumulative effect of these advances is, for the first time, a sustained reduction in the age-adjusted death rate from cancer in the United States.

This third edition of *Clinical Oncology* reflects these exciting changes. In addition to simply providing new knowledge, this information is now presented in a more attractive and useful way. Each chapter begins with summaries that highlight the key points that would, for example, allow one to pass a board exam. In each chapter, in addition to a critical analysis of the literature, the authors present their own opinions in specially identified boxes and algorithms. The use of color throughout the text makes the material more easily understood.

As the editors gathered to begin the planning for the third edition of *Clinical Oncology*, we were faced with the challenge of replacing a dear and respected colleague whose new responsibilities as Dean precluded his continued participation in this project. Alan Lichter was a driving force for all of us during the inaugural first edition and the significantly enhanced second edition. Many of the design concepts of *Clinical Oncology* stem from Alan's vision of creating something new and unique that emphasizes a user friendly approach.

For the third edition, with Alan's assistance, we have recruited an outstanding new partner to continue the multidisciplinary approach. W. Gillies McKenna is one of the country's leaders in the field of radiation oncology and has brought new energy and ideas to the development of this edition. We have added Michael Kastan, a nationally and internationally recognized physician-scientist as our "basic science editor" to provide more rigorous guidance in preparing the critically important section on the biology of cancer. Having a comprehensive background in the molecular basis of cancer is becoming increasingly critical for all that encompasses the prevention, diagnosis, and treatment of this complex disease.

The multidisciplinary nature of cancer care is reflected in our editors, whose expertise includes pediatric oncology, surgical oncology, radiation oncology, medical oncology, and hematologic malignancies. The editors are deeply indebted to our outstanding authors who, in a most diligent and thoughtful way, have brought a wide range of interests and disciplines to this volume on clinical oncology.

Our goal is to provide a textbook that is *the* most useful, understandable, attractive, and thorough in presenting the principles of clinical oncology. It is meant to be equally useful to students and trainees, experts in the various disciplines of oncology, and as a reference text for physicians in other disciplines who also see patients with cancer. It is our hope that our readers will find this a scholarly textbook properly balanced among the disciplines of science, clinical medicine, and humanism that will serve them in their important efforts to prevent, diagnose, and treat more effectively the many diseases that are known as cancer.

ACKNOWLEDGMENTS

The third edition of this book represents a highly collaborative and dynamic effort between the editors and Elsevier. We are greatly indebted to Dolores Meloni for her creative input and guidance and for sharing the editors' commitment and determination to make this third edition even better than its predecessors. Donna Morrissey and Nancy Lombardi are acknowledged for their truly exceptional support of this project. The expert support provided by Michele Pass, Elaine Ryan, Margaret Hall, Nancy Bernard, and April Meiller is also greatly appreciated. Finally, we want to express our gratitude to the many authors for their superb contributions and for their generosity and friendship.

Martin D. Abeloff, MD
James O. Armitage, MD
John E. Niederhuber, MD
Michael B. Kastan, MD, PhD
W. Gillies McKenna, MD, PhD

CONTENTS

PART II • PROBLEMS COMMON TO CANCER AND ITS THERAPY   713

PART III • SPECIFIC MALIGNANCIES 1345

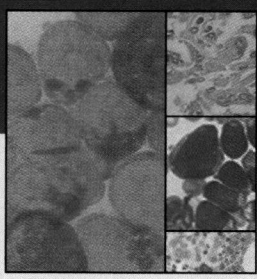

PART I

SCIENCE OF CLINICAL ONCOLOGY

BIOLOGY AND CANCER
Molecular Tools in Cancer Research
Intracellular Signaling
The Cellular Microenvironment
Biology of Cancer Metastases
Control of the Cell Cycle
Cell Life and Cell Death
Immunology and Cancer
Stem Cells, Cell Differentiation, and
 Cancer
Vascular and Interstitial Biology of
 Tumors

THE GENESIS OF CANCER
Environmental Factors
DNA Damage Response Pathways and
 Cancer
Viruses and Human Cancer
Genetic Factors: Hereditary Cancer
 Predisposition Syndromes

Genetic Factors: Finding Cancer
 Susceptibility Genes
Progressing from Gene Mutations to
 Cancer
Immunodeficiency and Cancer

DIAGNOSING CANCER
Pathology and Laboratory Medicine
  A. Surgical Pathology
  B. Flow Cytometry in Oncologic
    Diagnosis
  C. Cytogenetics
  D. Molecular Diagnostics
  E. Clinical Chemistry: Tumor Markers
Imaging

PREVENTING AND TREATING CANCER
Biostatistics for Clinical Trials
Structures Supporting Cancer Clinical
 Trials
Economic Analysis of Cancer Treatment

Epidemiology and Population Sciences
Cancer Prevention, Screening, and Early
 Detection
Smoking Cessation: Current Treatments
 and Future Directions
Chemotherapy
The Basics of Radiation Therapy
Surgical Interventions in Cancer
Bone Marrow Transplantation
Gene Therapy in Oncology
The Present and Future of Molecularly
 Targeted Therapy
Photodynamic Therapy
Therapeutic Antibodies and Immunologic
 Conjugates
Cancer Vaccines
Complementary and Alternative Medicine

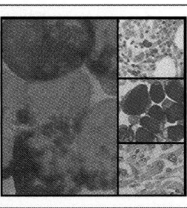

MOLECULAR TOOLS IN CANCER RESEARCH

Nadia Rosenthal

SUMMARY OF KEY POINTS

- This chapter covers basic principles of molecular biology, explains the most frequently used laboratory techniques in cancer research, describes recent developments in animal models of human cancer, and discusses current and prospective clinical applications.

- It provides the necessary conceptual and technical background to grasp the central principles and methods of modern molecular genetics underpinning current cancer research. The scale of the problem is reflected in the massive volume of molecular information now available

through genome databases and tumor profiling. A basic understanding by generalist and specialist alike will be critical to realize the full potential of this information and to revolutionize cancer treatment through molecular diagnostics and pharmaceuticals.

INTRODUCTION

The last decade has seen an unprecedented decline in rates of cancer-related death. Although new epidemiologic insights and the incremental improvements in survival through increasingly complex and lengthy treatments have contributed largely to this achievement, equally important advances are being made in basic research on prevention and early detection. Although the diagnosis of cancer previously depended on morphologic and other phenotypic criteria, now highly sensitive molecular techniques allow pathologists to follow specific genetic changes in particular tumors and detect occult malignant cells in normal tissues.

New avenues for treatment tailoring and patient surveillance are promised by gene-based diagnostics. Genome-wide profiling of gene expression with the use of DNA microarrays represents one of the latest breakthroughs in cancer research and provides an unprecedented opportunity to dissect the biologic processes underlying tumor progression by monitoring the changes in a tumor cell's transcriptional landscape. When applied on a larger scale, these assays can optimize pharmaceutical intervention by targeting therapeutic approaches to specific patient populations.

Molecular biology also provides the basic tools with which to study genes involved in cancer growth patterns and tumor suppression. An advanced understanding of the processes governing cell growth and differentiation has revolutionized the diagnosis and prognosis of malignant disorders. Discovery of the mechanisms responsible for genetic instability may lead to more reliable tests for hereditary susceptibility to cancer, and ultimately, to more effective therapies.

LOOKING AT DNA

The discovery of the double helical structure of DNA 50 years ago marked the beginning of a revolution in our understanding of heredity and evolution, and of the mutations that underlie cell dysfunction and disease. Tumors arise from the clonal progeny of a single cell carrying multiple sites of acquired and, sometimes, inherited DNA damage that all its progeny share. During the early steps of tumor formation, mutations that lead to an intrinsic genetic instability allow additional deleterious DNA alterations to accumulate. These genetic changes confer selective advantages on the clone of tumor cells by disrupting the control of cell proliferation, favoring the growth of the tumor and its subclones. The identification of specific mutations characterizing a tumor provides a tool for analyzing the neoplastic progression and remission of the disease.

DNA consists of two long strands of polynucleotides that twist around each other clockwise in a double helix (Fig. 1-1). Nucleic acid bases attached to the sugar groups of each strand face each other within the helix, perpendicular to its axis. These comprise only four bases: the purines, adenine and guanine (A and G), and the pyrimidines, cytosine and thymine (C and T). During assembly of the double helix, stable pairings of nucleotides from either strand are made between A and T or between G and C. Each base pair forms one of the billions of rungs in the long, unbroken ladder of DNA forming a chromosome. Exploitation of the exquisite sequence specificity of certain bacterial DNA endonucleases, called *restriction enzymes*, allows the systematic cleavage of very large DNA molecules into predictable, manageable subfragments. These can be identified by hybridization

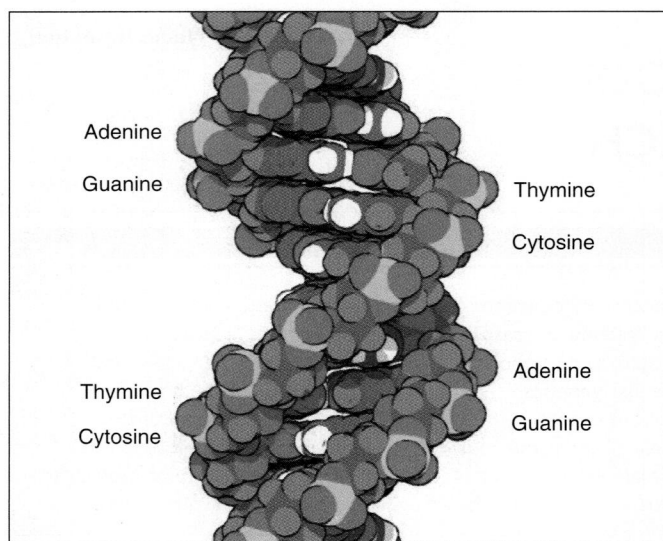

Figure 1-1. The DNA double helix. The sequence of four bases (guanine, adenine, thymine, and cytosine) in the DNA helix determines the specificity of genetic information. The bases face inward from the sugar-phosphate backbone and form pairs with complementary bases on the opposing strand for specific recognition. The arrangement of chemical groups is unique for each base pair, allowing base pairs to be specifically targeted by transcription factors, polymerases, restriction enzymes, and other DNA-binding proteins. (Modified from Goodsell DS: The molecular perspective: DNA. Oncologist 2000;5:81–82.)

of a short, specific DNA or RNA oligonucleotide probe to its complementary base sequence, or target, in the fractionated genomic material. In most applications, the enzyme-digested sample of DNA is size-fractionated by gel electrophoresis and transferred onto a nylon membrane (Southern blotting; Fig. 1-2) to which the labeled probe is then applied. DNA fragments containing sequences that hybridize with a radioactively labeled probe can be detected by autoradiography, or alternatively, by nonisotopic colorimetric or chemiluminescent systems.

THE VARIABLE GENOME

The functional unit of inherited information in DNA, the gene, is most often represented by a discrete section of sequence necessary to encode a particular protein structure. Because protein synthesis occurs in the cytoplasm, genetic information is transported out of the nucleus by a copy of the gene, messenger RNA (mRNA), constructed base by base from the DNA template by a polymerase enzyme. In the cytoplasm, proteins are then synthesized, or translated, in macromolecular complexes called *ribosomes* that read the mRNA sequence and convert the nucleic acid code, based on three-base segments, or codons, into a 20–amino-acid code to form the corresponding protein.

In the human nucleus, each of the 23 tightly compacted chromosomes has a characteristic size and structure and a distinctive base sequence that carries unique protein coding information. Other noncoding DNA sequences are

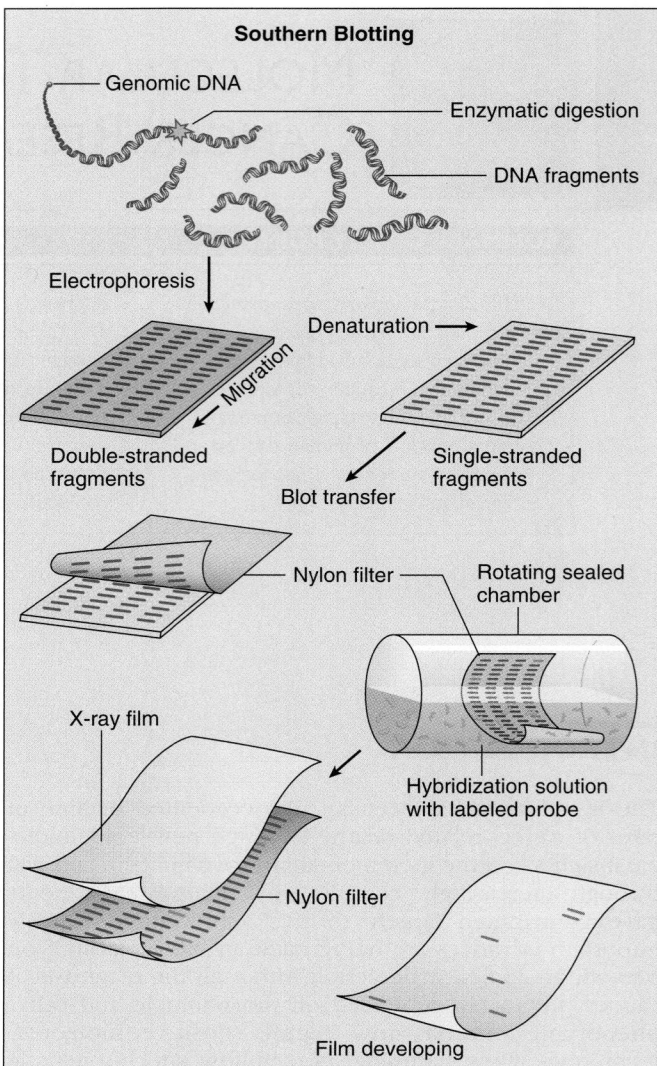

Figure 1-2. Analysis of DNA by gel electrophoresis and Southern blotting. Genomic DNA is cut with restriction enzymes into fragments before being separated according to size by gel electrophoresis. The four lanes on the gel represent the digestion of the DNA with four different restriction enzymes. In Northern blotting, total cellular RNA, including messenger RNA, can also be separated according to size. After electrophoresis, the nucleic acids in the gel are transferred directly onto a charged nylon filter to which they are tightly bound. Thus the filter contains a precise replica of the nucleic acid distribution in the gel. The filter is then hybridized in a rotating sealed chamber with a DNA or RNA probe specific for the target of interest (in this case, sequences in a microbial pathogen). Probes have traditionally been radioactively labeled with nucleotides containing phosphorus 32; however, the use of nonradiolabeled probes is becoming more common. After the probe has hybridized to its target sequence, the nonhybridized probe is washed away, and the filter is exposed to x-ray film. A DNA sequence complementary to the probe is seen as a dark band on the developed film. The position of the hybridized target sequence in each lane is unique to the restriction enzyme used to digest the DNA. This procedure is termed *Southern blotting* when DNA is analyzed and *Northern blotting* when RNA is analyzed. (Modified from Naber SP: Molecular pathology—diagnosis of infectious disease. N Engl J Med 1994;331:1212–1215.)

used for directing the transcription of neighboring genes through complex regulatory circuits involving protein binding and modification of the DNA itself or through shifting of its chromosomal packaging. Loss, gain, or re-arrangement of chromosomal segments through deletion or translocation is a common form of neoplastic mutation, as protein-coding segments from different genes are combined or regulatory sequences are brought into new proximity to genes they do not normally control. Gross changes in DNA arrangement can be detected by cyto-genetic analysis of chromosomal features on metaphase spreads. Fluorescent in situ hybridization provides greater resolution by localizing specific chromosomal DNA sequences corresponding to fluorescently labeled probes (Fig. 1-3), and it can be used to track specific alterations in chromosomal structure in which known genes are involved.

Although cytogenetic techniques are useful in detect-ing consistent, nonrandom structural abnormalities of clonal tumor cells, they require cell culture, which can limit their usefulness, particularly in analysis of solid tumors. Application of the polymerase chain reaction (PCR) allows the detection of specific changes in small tumor samples. Two chemically synthesized single-stranded DNA fragments, or primers, match chromosomal DNA sequences flanking the segment in which a mutation is suspected. With the addition of nucleotide building blocks and a heat-stable DNA polymerase, the primers initiate synthesis of new DNA strands by using the chromosomal material as a template. Each successive copying cycle, initiated by "melting" the resulting double-stranded products with heat, doubles the number of DNA segments in the reaction (Fig. 1-4). The technique is exceptionally sensitive: Millions of identical DNA copies can be generated in a matter of hours with PCR by using a single DNA molecule as the starting material. Changes in the size of the resulting fragment caused by addition or loss of DNA bases can be detected by gel electrophoresis, and subtler single-base mutations can be identified by automated DNA sequencing techniques.

The complete set of DNA sequences carried on all the chromosomes is known as the *genome*, which varies little among individuals. The strict base-pairing rule that dictates DNA structure is critical for the storage, retrieval, and transfer of genetic information. The duplicated genetic information in the two strands of DNA not only permits the repair of a damaged coding sequence but also forms the basis for the replication of DNA. During cell division, polymerase enzymes unwind the DNA strands and copy them, using the base sequences as a template for constructing a new helix so that the dividing cell passes its entire genetic content on to its progeny. Errors in this process are rare, and person-to-person differences comprise only about 0.1% of the human genome. These genetic variations, or polymorphisms, are inherited if they occur in the germline. Most genetic variation is of no phenotypic consequence, occurring in regions that do not encode protein or do not alter the regulation of nearby genes. Given the disruptive effects that even subtle mutations may have on the expression of a protein product, it is important to distinguish these changes from benign polymorphisms.

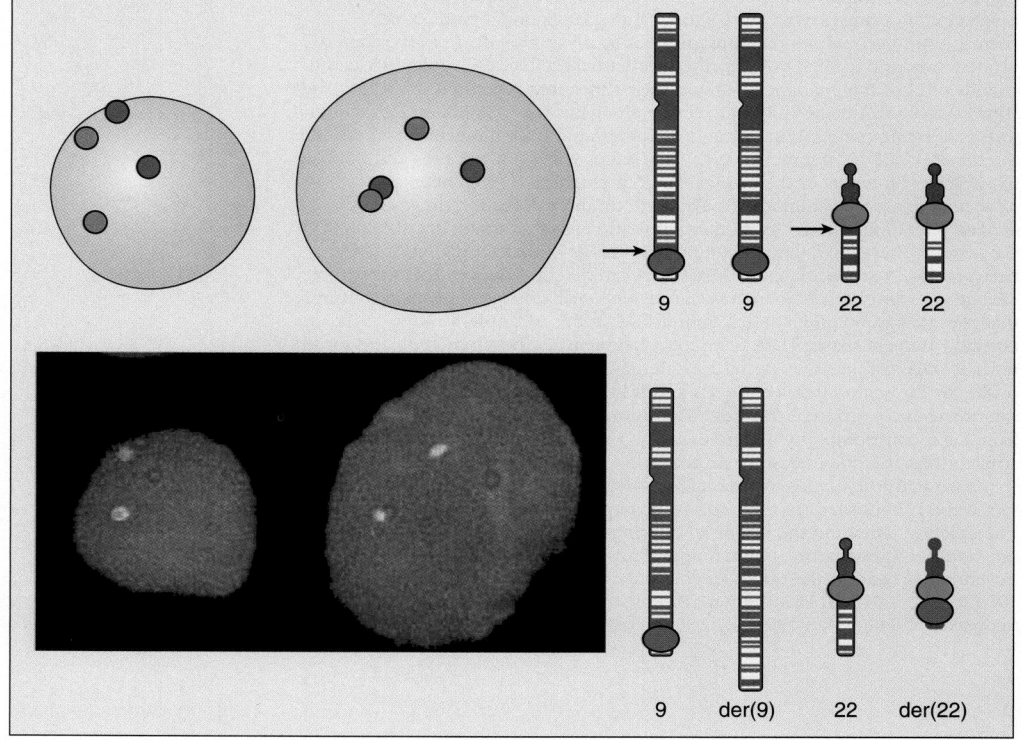

Figure 1-3. Detection of chromosomal translocations in interphase cells by fluorescent in situ hybridization (FISH). FISH technology uses a labeled DNA segment as a probe to search homologous sequences in interphase chromosomes for the t(9;22)(q34;q11) translocation, associated with chronic myeloid leukemia. On the left, patient nuclei were hybridized with probes for chromosome 9 (labeled with SpectrumRed fluorophore) and chromosome 22 (labeled with SpectrumGreen). (Modified from Varella-Garcia M: Molecular cytogenetics in solid tumors: Laboratory tool for diagnosis, prognosis, and therapy. Oncologist 2003;8:45–58.)

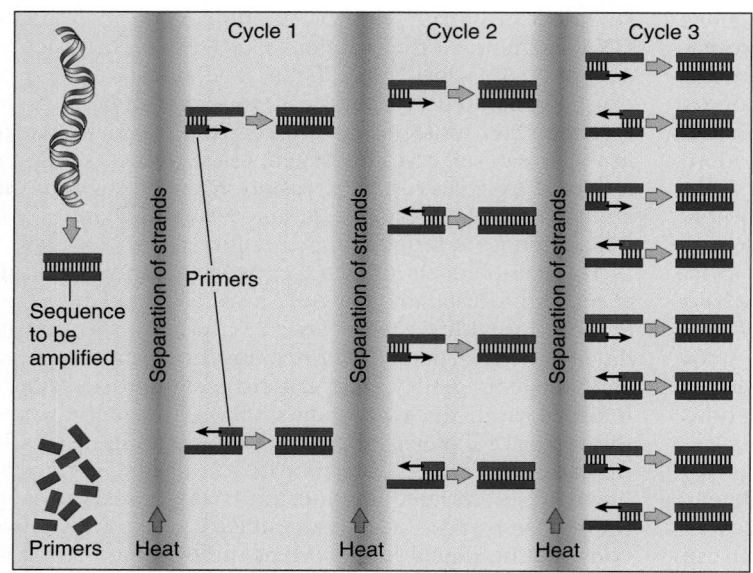

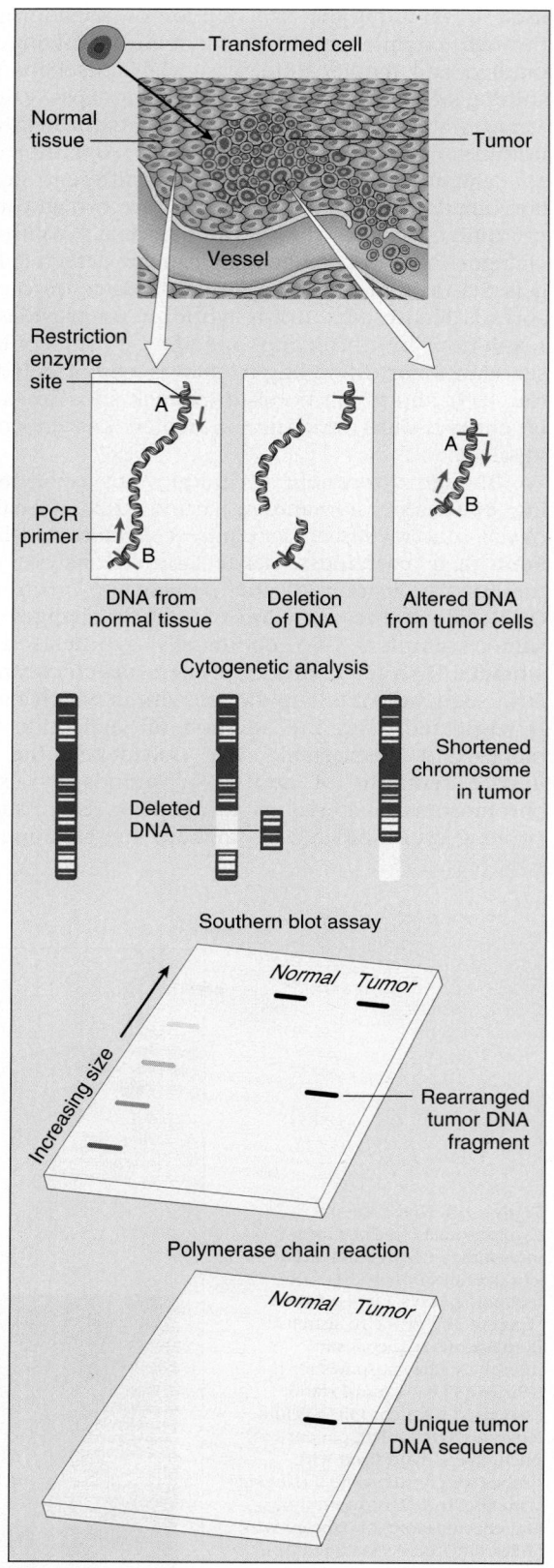

Figure 1-4. A, Amplification of DNA by PCR. The DNA sequence to be amplified is selected by primers, which are short, synthetic oligonucleotides that correspond to sequences flanking the DNA to be amplified. After an excess of primers is added to the DNA, together with a heat-stable DNA polymerase, the strands of both the genomic DNA and the primers are separated by heating and allowed to cool. A heat-stable polymerase elongates the primers on either strand, thus generating two new, identical double-stranded DNA molecules and doubling the number of DNA fragments. Each cycle takes just a few minutes and doubles the number of copies of the original DNA fragment. **B,** Cytogenetic and molecular analyses of tumor cells. Three methods of detecting the specific genetic alterations shared by all the neoplastic cells in a tumor are shown. (1) If the genetic alteration is large enough, as in the deletion of a region of DNA between loci A and B, cytogenetic analysis can detect grossly visible karyotypic changes. (2) Southern blot analysis can detect small changes in gene structure that routine karyotyping studies cannot find. In this example, a probe to locus A normally detects a large DNA restriction fragment, as shown by the band for the normal DNA sample. Because of the deleted DNA segment in the tumor cells, the probe for the region between loci A and B hybridizes to a smaller, rearranged, tumor-specific restriction fragment. The normal, larger band shown on the blot is from DNA contributed by non-neoplastic stromal and reactive cells. (3) In many applications, the polymerase chain reaction (PCR) can detect alterations in DNA structure with the highest degree of sensitivity. Here, the primers that anneal to loci A and B in normal DNA are too far apart to yield an amplified PCR product. The deletion shown in the tumor DNA brings the two annealing sites close to one another, allowing the generation of a novel, amplified PCR product. (**A,** From Rosenthal N: Tools of the trade—recombinant DNA. N Engl J Med 1994:331:315–317. **B,** From Naber SP: Molecular pathology—detection of neoplasia. N Engl J Med 1994;331:1508–1510.)

Our ability to detect those polymorphisms that exist in human populations is one of the most important concepts in modern medical genetics. Even when DNA polymorphisms are not directly involved in a disease, they provide markers for clonality and for the loss or rearrangement of specific chromosomal segments in growing tumors, particularly when the alterations are too small to be detected by cytogenetic analysis. When a polymorphism occurs in the recognition site of a restriction enzyme, lost or rearranged DNA produces a change in the enzyme cleavage pattern, and these restriction fragment length polymorphisms can be detected by Southern blot analysis.

More than 90% of human genetic variation can be traced to single-nucleotide polymorphisms (SNPs). These are highly abundant, stable, and distributed throughout the genome and are associated with racial diversity, individual traits, and susceptibility to diseases. Tracking thousands of SNPs has identified medically relevant genes predisposing families to common forms of cancer. Although PCR with specific primer pairs, or amplicons, has been extensively used to characterize SNPs in selected genomic regions, novel methods for large-scale SNP detection include single-nucleotide primer extension, allele-specific hybridization, oligonucleotide ligation assay, and invasive signal amplification, all of which detect polymorphisms directly from genomic DNA without the requirement of PCR amplification.

MANIPULATING GENES

The engineering of genes by recombinant DNA technology evolved from methods initially devised to provide sequences in amounts sufficient for biochemical analysis. In the original protocol, the desired segment is clipped from the surrounding DNA and inserted into a bacterial or viral vector, which is then amplified millions of times in a host bacterium (Fig. 1-5). With the use of recombinant DNA, genetic engineering can routinely produce industrial quantities of pure, therapeutically important products in a cost-effective way. For diagnostic purposes, it is easier and faster to amplify a known genomic DNA sequence directly from a patient sample with PCR, but the classic approach is still applied to the construction of recombinant DNA libraries.

To be useful, a DNA library must be as complete as possible, with recombinant members, or clones, sufficiently numerous to include all the sequences in an individual genome. For certain kinds of gene-linkage analysis that require long, uninterrupted stretches of DNA, special vectors, such as yeast artificial chromosomes, can carry foreign DNA fragments of enormous lengths. Chromosomal segments represented in genomic DNA libraries can contain the structure of an entire gene, including the information that regulates its expression, and form the starting material for sequencing the human genome.

Figure 1-5. Recombinant DNA. The DNA segment to be amplified is separated from surrounding genomic DNA by cleavage with a restriction enzyme. The enzymatic cuts often produce staggered or "sticky" ends. In the example shown here, the restriction enzyme *Eco*RI recognizes the sequence GAATTC and cuts each strand between *G* (guanine) and *A* (adenine); the two strands of the genomic DNA are shown as blue and purple (*C* denotes cytosine, and *T*, thymine). The same restriction enzyme cuts the circular plasmid DNA (tan) at a single site, generating sticky ends that are complementary to the sticky ends of the genomic DNA fragment. The cut genomic DNA and the remainder of the plasmid, when mixed together in the presence of a ligase enzyme, form smooth joints on each side of the plasmid–genomic DNA junction. This new molecule—recombinant DNA—is carried into bacteria, which replicate the plasmid as they grow in culture. (From Rosenthal N: Tools of the trade—recombinant DNA. N Engl J Med 1994;331:315–317.)

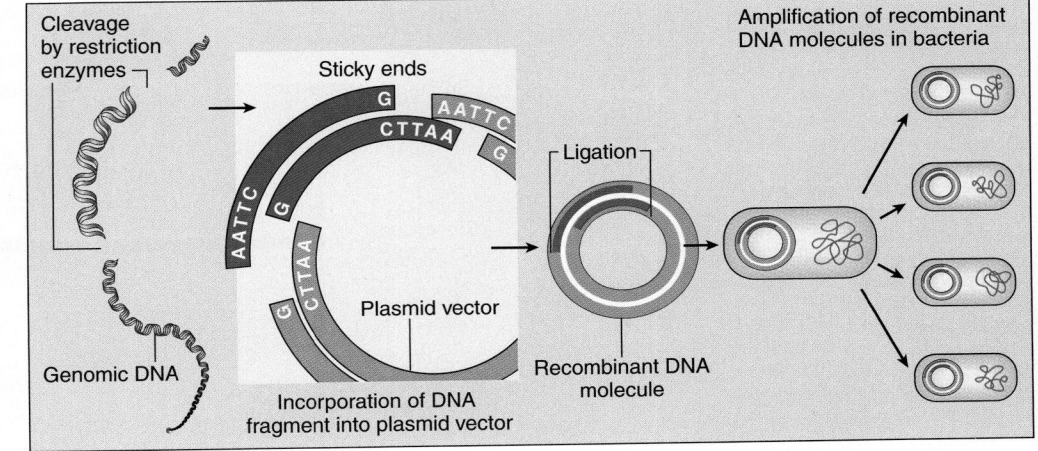

Science of Clinical Oncology

For some applications, construction of partial libraries, which contain only the DNA sequences transcribed by a particular tissue or type of cell, is sufficient. The starting material in this case is mRNA. For cloning purposes, the enzyme reverse transcriptase can convert mRNA into complementary DNA (cDNA). Advanced techniques for acquiring full-length copies of RNA transcripts include rapid amplification of cDNA ends (RACE). The cDNA ends are then incorporated into vectors, much the same way as genomic DNA fragments are. The number of clones in a cDNA library is much smaller than that in a genomic library, because a cDNA library represents only the genes expressed by the tissue of interest. Furthermore, cDNA libraries contain only the coding portion of genes. Screening of DNA libraries for a specific gene usually involves mass growth of bacterial hosts on agar, transfer of replicates to nylon filter, and exposure to a specific DNA probe. The probe's unique sequence of nucleotides ensures that it hybridizes only to a nucleic acid molecule with the complementary sequence, which marks the position of the target clone. Cloning vectors can also be modified to drive the expression of their payload,

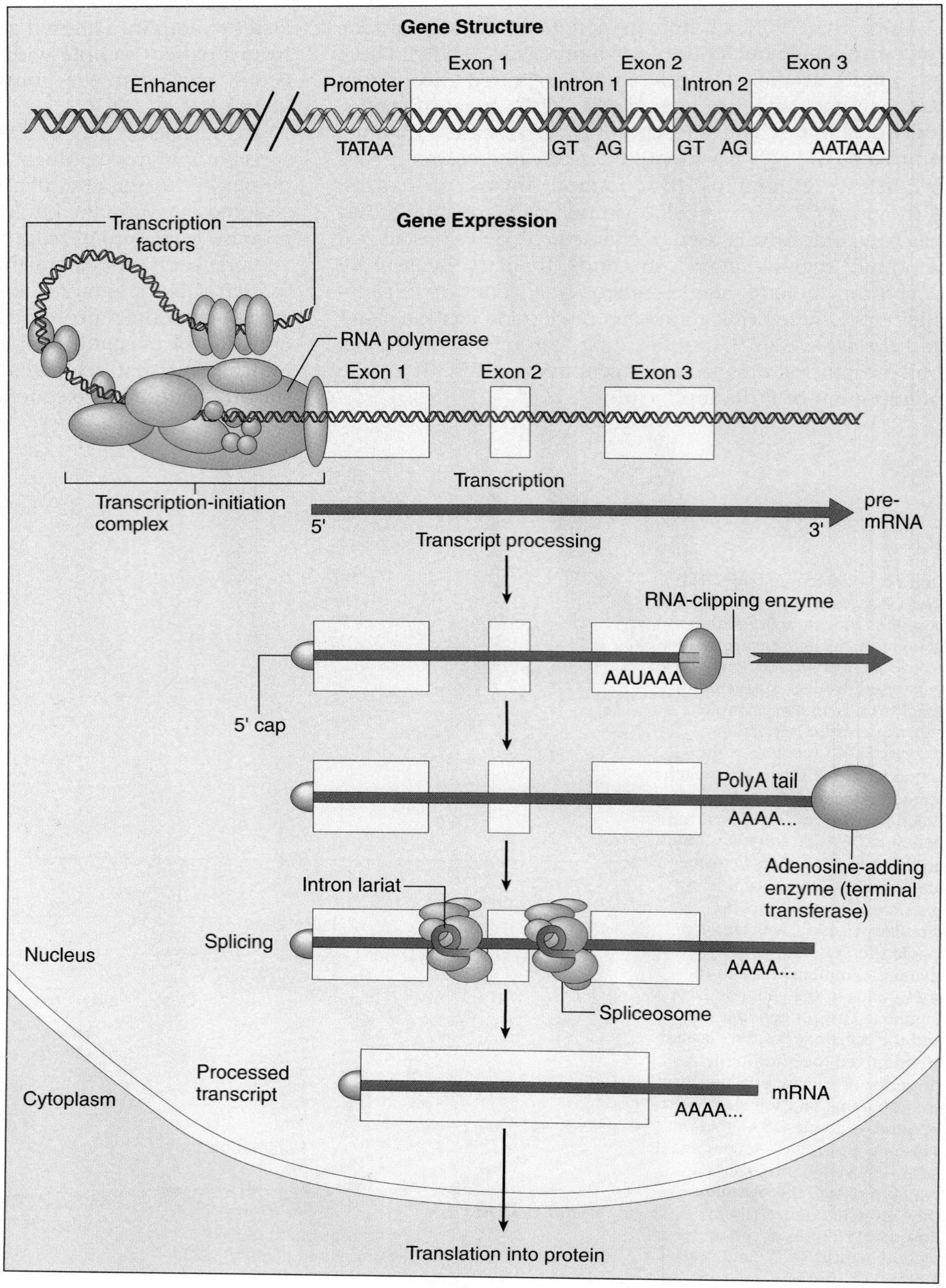

Figure 1-6. Mammalian gene structure and expression. The DNA sequences that are transcribed as RNA are collectively called the *gene* and include exons (expressed sequences) and introns (intervening sequences). Introns invariably begin with the nucleotide sequence GT and end with AG. An AT-rich sequence in the last exon forms a signal for processing the end of the RNA transcript. Regulatory sequences that make up the promoter and include the TATA box occur close to the site where transcription starts. Enhancer sequences are located at variable distances from the gene. Gene expression begins with the binding of multiple protein factors to enhancer sequences and promoter sequences. These factors help form the transcription-initiation complex, which includes the enzyme RNA polymerase and multiple polymerase-associated proteins. The primary transcript (pre-mRNA) includes both exon and intron sequences. Post-transcriptional processing begins with changes at both ends of the RNA transcript. At the 5' end, enzymes add a special nucleotide cap; at the 3' end, an enzyme clips the pre-mRNA about 30 base pairs (bp) after the AAUAAA sequence in the last exon. Another enzyme adds a polyA tail, which consists of up to 200 adenine nucleotides. Next, spliceosomes remove the introns by cutting the RNA at the boundaries between exons and introns. The process of excision forms lariats of the intron sequences. The spliced mRNA is now mature and can leave the nucleus for protein translation in the cytoplasm. (From Rosenthal N: Regulation of gene expression. N Engl J Med 1994;331:931–932.)

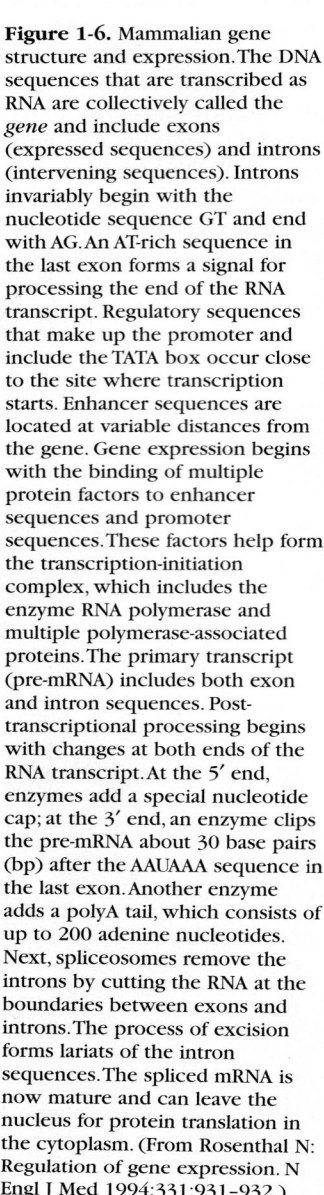

producing "expression" libraries in bacteria that can be screened for protein production by using specific antibodies.

CONTROLLING GENE EXPRESSION

Genes encode information that specifies functional products, either RNA molecules or proteins used for various cellular functions. By contrast, regulatory sequences do not encode a product. Yet without them, a cell could not coordinate the expression of the hundreds of thousands of genes in its nucleus, could not select only certain genes for expression, and could not activate or repress them in response to precise internal or external signals. Our understanding of gene expression and its perturbation in cancer has increased greatly over the past two decades. The primary level of gene control is the transcription of DNA into RNA. Nucleotide sequences that influence transcription are common to many genes and lie in regions of DNA upstream of the transcription start site (Fig. 1-6). Collectively called the *promoter* of a gene, these proximal sequences comprise binding sites for the RNA polymerase and its numerous cofactors. Although the position of the promoter with regard to the transcription start site is relatively inflexible, other DNA regulatory elements, known as *enhancers*, occur in unpredictable locations, often at a considerable distance from the gene they control.

DNA regulatory elements contain binding sites for multiple proteins, called *transcription factors*, which interact to form regulatory networks controlling gene transcription. Their function can be altered by signals that induce modifications such as phosphorylation or by interactions with other regulators such as steroid hormones. Many of the cell's responses to a wide variety of external stimuli, such as neurotransmitters, antigens, cytokines, and growth factors are mediated through transcription factors.

Some transcription factors bind to particular regions of enhancers and drive their associated genes in many types of cells, whereas others, active in only a limited variety of cells, maintain a tissue-specific pattern of gene expression. Enhancers are often responsible for the aberrant expression of genes after chromosomal translocation associated with specific forms of cancer. A normally quiescent gene, promoting cell growth that is dislocated to a position near a strong enhancer, may be activated inappropriately.

Enhancers and promoters have been assigned specific roles by means of cell culture assays, in which putative regulatory DNA sequences are introduced into cell cultures on special vectors carrying test or *reporter* genes and are examined for their ability to activate expression of the reporter gene. By assessing the effects of deleting, adding, or changing DNA sequences within the regulatory element, a researcher is often able to pinpoint the precise nucleotides that are critical for recognition by transcription factors.

The interaction between protein and DNA is also used to identify transcription factor binding sites in a regulatory region. The electrophoretic mobility shift assay (EMSA), also referred to as a *gel-shift assay*, depends on gel electrophoresis to determine whether a labeled DNA fragment binds nuclear proteins and the extent to which this binding is sequence-specific (Fig. 1-7). Another method,

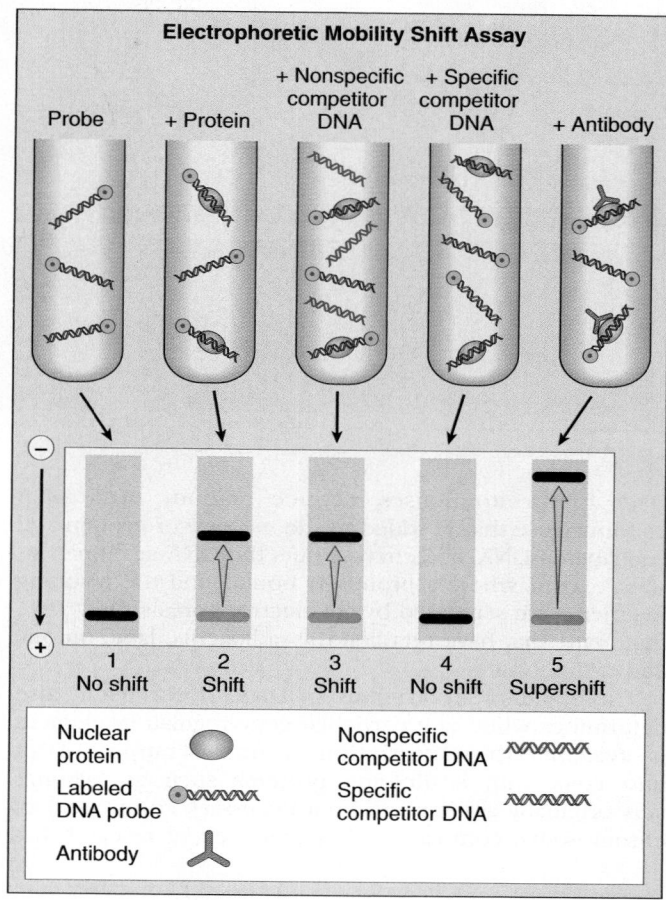

Figure 1-7. Electrophoretic mobility shift assay. This assay uses nuclear protein and a radioactive DNA probe to detect interactions between protein and DNA, which appear as a shifted band in a gel. A labeled genomic DNA fragment carrying the suspected protein-binding sites is combined with a crude preparation of nuclear proteins from the cell type of interest. After a brief incubation to allow the protein and the DNA to interact, the mixture is loaded onto a gel for electrophoresis to separate molecular complexes of different sizes. A control sample contains only the radioactive DNA. The gel is electrophoresed under nondenaturing conditions, so that noncovalently bound complexes of protein and DNA remain intact. Autoradiography of the gel reveals the radiolabeled DNA, either by itself (*lane 1*) or in protein-DNA complex (*lane 2*). The addition of competitor DNAs defines the specificity of the interaction between the protein and the DNA probe (*lanes 3* and *4*). These competitor DNAs bear no radioactive tag. They are incubated individually (in amounts that are larger than that of the radiolabeled DNA fragment) with the mixtures of radioactive DNA probe and nuclear protein. If the original interaction between labeled DNA and protein was specific, an unrelated nonspecific competitor should not interfere with the appearance of the shifted band on the gel (*lane 3*). Another variation of the method uses an antibody against a nuclear protein. The antibody binds to the protein, adding its size to that of the radiolabeled DNA–nuclear protein complex. After electrophoresis, the mobility of the supershifted complex and the complex formed in the absence of antibody can be compared (*lane 2* vs. *lane 5*). (From Rosenthal N: Recognizing DNA. N Engl J Med 1995;333:925–927.)

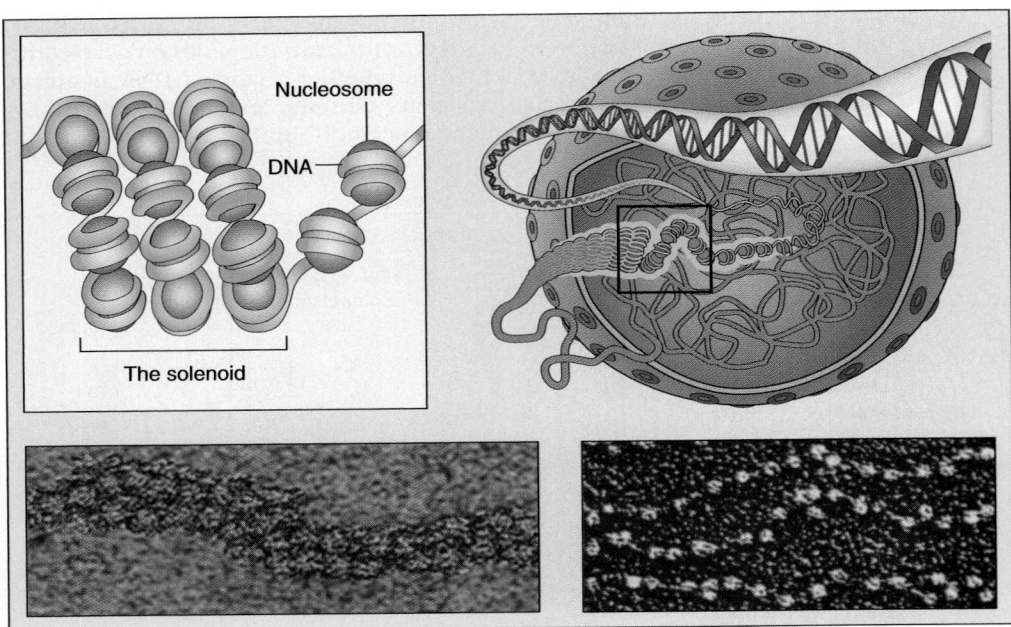

Figure 1-8. Chromatin packaging of DNA. The 4 meters of DNA in every human cell must be compressed in the nucleus, reaching compaction ratios of 1:400,000. This is achieved by wrapping the DNA (blue) around histone protein complexes (green), forming nucleosomes connected by a thread of free linker DNA. Each nucleosome, together with its linker, packages about 200 bp (66 nm) of DNA. The nucleosomes are then coiled into chromatin, a rope of nucleoprotein about 30 nm thick (bottom left EM). To allow DNA to be accessed by transcription and replication apparatus, chromatin is relaxed (bottom right electron micrograph). (Courtesy of Jakob Waterborg www.umkc.edu/sbs/waterborg/chromat/chromatn.html © 1998 Jakob Waterborg.)

DNA footprinting, uses a trace amount of a DNA endonuclease that is added to the mixture of protein and end-labeled DNA. The enzyme cuts the DNA at numerous sites, except where a protein is bound, and the resulting fragments are separated by gel electrophoresis. Only DNA fragments that have retained the radioactive label on one end will be visible.

The higher-order structure of DNA, or chromatin, also determines whether a particular gene regulatory element is available to transcription factors. Wrapping DNA into coils with scaffolding proteins such as histones was originally assumed to be a necessary component of chromosomal compaction, but more recent research has linked rearrangement of chromatin and associated DNA methylation with the inactivation of tumor suppressor genes and neoplastic transformation (Fig. 1-8). Epigenetic modifications of the nuclear environment that determine the accessibility of a gene can persist during cell division, because inherited patterns of methylation provide permanent marks for altered chromatin configuration in daughter cells. These multiple levels of control are necessary to ensure the correct gene expression so central to the normal function of the cell.

Once transcribed, the RNA transcript is modified at both ends and then undergoes a highly regulated process called *splicing*. In higher organisms, most protein-

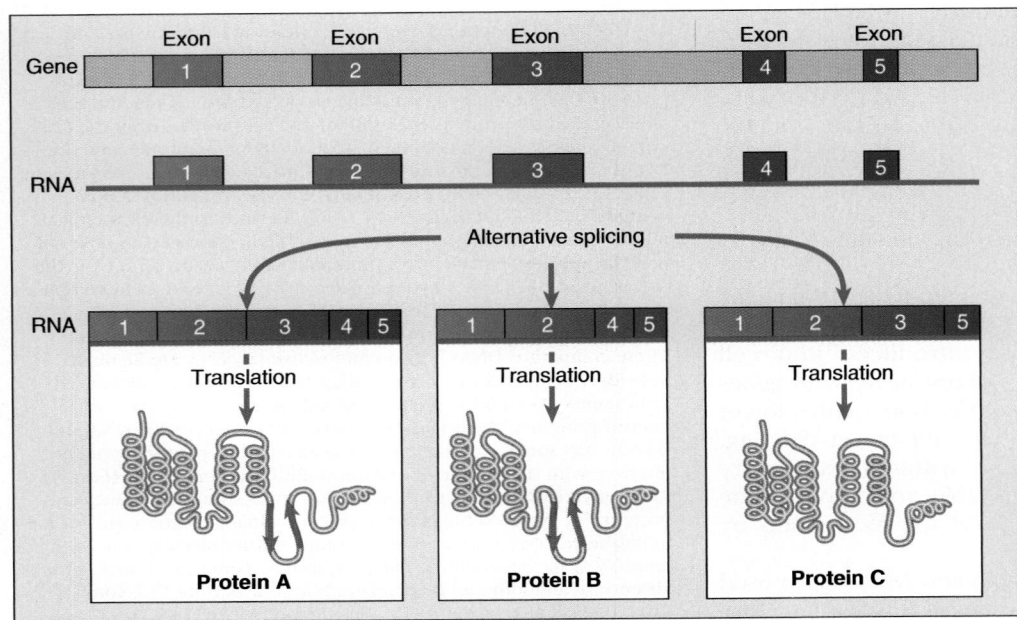

Figure 1-9. Alternate splicing produces multiple related proteins, or isoforms, from a single gene. (From Guttmacher AE, Collins F: Genomic medicine—A primer. N Engl J Med 2002;347:1512–1520.)

coding gene sequences are unexpectedly interrupted by stretches of noncoding sequences, called *introns*. The genetic machinery must remove these introns to form a continuous chain of coding sequences, or *exons*, which subsequently undergo translation into protein. The splicing process requires absolute precision, because the deletion or addition of a single nucleotide at the splice junction would throw the three-base coding sequence out of frame. The biologic importance of RNA splicing is not entirely understood, but the fact that many medically relevant genes have alternate splice patterns—in which different combinations of exons are chosen for the final mRNA transcript—means that one gene can encode many different proteins (Fig. 1-9). Splicing also has important implications for the manipulation of genetic information. For example, cDNA libraries from a particular tissue can provide important information about the products of alternate splicing in a way that a genomic DNA library cannot.

Monitoring of global gene expression patterns of cells with DNA microarrays allows the simultaneous evaluation of thousands of gene transcripts and their relative expression during the progression of malignancy. Microarrays allow high-throughput differential screens of mRNA expression from two sources (such as tumor and normal cells), by using cDNA or oligonucleotide libraries that are arranged in extremely high density on microchips. These are probed with a mixture of fluorescently tagged cDNA fragments generated from the tumor and from normal samples, resulting in a differential staining of each gene spot. The relative intensity of the two different colors reflects the RNA expression level of each gene, and is analyzed with a laser confocal scanner. With microarrays, single genes that constitute diagnostic, prognostic, or therapeutically relevant markers can be systematically monitored. Alternatively, the entire set of expressed genes can be collectively analyzed by using powerful statistical methods to classify tumors by their transcriptional profiles (Fig. 1-10). Microarray analysis has already dramatically improved our ability to explore the genetic changes associated with cancer etiology and development and is providing new tools for disease diagnosis, prognosis prediction, and, ultimately, individualized therapy.

Serial analysis of gene expression (SAGE) provides a simultaneous, comprehensive evaluation of mRNA species. SAGE does not require prior knowledge of the genes of interest and provides quantitative and qualitative data for potentially every transcribed sequence in a particular tissue or cell type. Furthermore, SAGE can quantify low-abundance transcripts and reliably detect relatively small differences in transcript concentrations between cell populations. The SAGE method generates a short-sequence tag that comprises a unique identifier of a transcript, derived from a defined location within that transcript. Many transcript tags are concatenated into a single molecule and then sequenced, revealing the identity of multiple tags simultaneously. The relative presentation of each member of a SAGE tag library is proportional to the corresponding mRNA abundance in the original transcript population. Comparative expression profiles can then be deduced by comparing

the abundance of individual tags within each sample set. This allows changes in global expression profiles of normal or malignant tissues under different therapeutic conditions to be rapidly evaluated.

PROTEINS TO THE FORE

Recent advances in protein analytic techniques over the last decade have made it possible to identify and examine the expression of most proteins and to envision large-scale protein analysis on the level of gene-based screens. Various systematic methods have contributed to the current explosion of information on the proteome, the protein complement of the genome, and are currently being compared for their ability to provide suitable platforms for generating databases on protein structural features, interaction maps, activity profiles, and regulatory modifications. The yeast two-hybrid system is a popular genetics-based approach for detecting protein-protein interactions inside a cell (Fig. 1-11). One protein fused to the DNA-binding domain (bait) and a different protein fused to the activation domain of a transcriptional activator (prey) are expressed together in yeast cells. If the bait and prey interact, transcription of a reported gene is induced and typically detected by a color reaction that reflects the transactivation of the reporter gene, and by proxy, the interaction of the two test proteins. The method can also be used for large-scale protein interactions, determination of RNA-protein interactions, and protein-ligand binding.

As a complementary proteomics tool, mass spectrometry provides an accurate mass measurement of charged peptides isolated by two-dimensional gel electrophoresis, producing a mass-to-charge ratio of charged samples under vacuum that can be used to determine the sequence identity of peptides. Combined with a specific proteolytic cleavage step, mass spectroscopy can be used for peptide mass mapping. Automation of this process has made mass spectroscopy the analytic tool of choice for many proteomics projects.

After a decade of development proteomics is still primarily a basic research activity, yet in the near future, this technology is likely to have a profound impact on medicine. A precise diagnosis of cancer with the use of proteomics could be envisioned, based on highly discriminating patterns of proteins in easily accessible patient samples (e.g., blood or saliva). Proteomics information also promises to provide sophisticated mathematical models of the molecular events underlying a process as complex as neoplastic transformation, which will capture the dynamics of the disease with unprecedented power.

ANIMAL MODELS OF CANCER

Once the genetic basis of a particular cancer has been identified, creating animal models becomes critical to

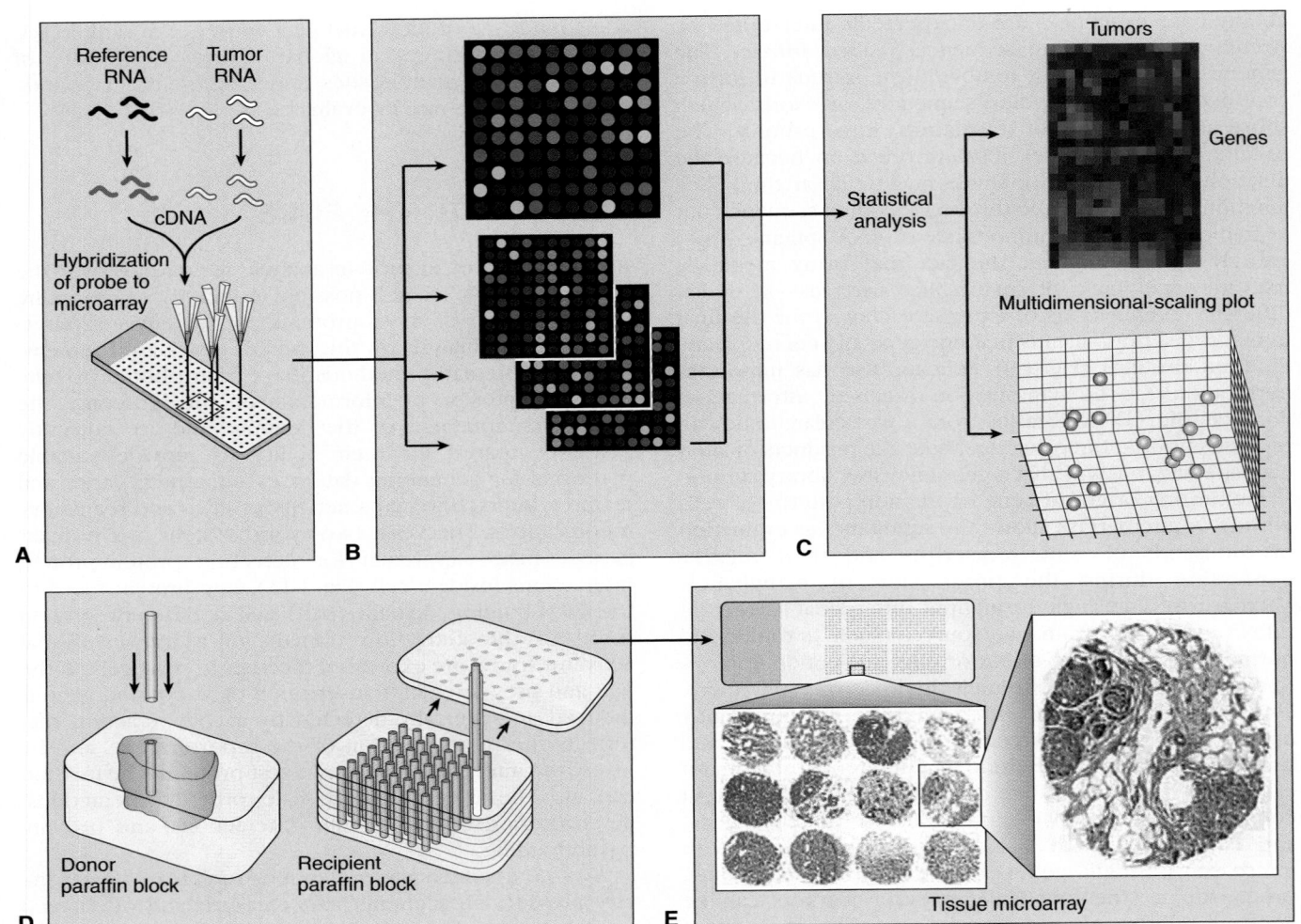

Figure 1-10. Microarrays of complementary DNA (cDNA) and breast tumor tissue. **A,** Reference RNA and tumor RNA are labeled by reverse transcription with different fluorescent dyes (green for the reference cells and red for the tumor cells) and hybridized to a cDNA microarray containing robotically printed cDNA clones. **B,** The slides are scanned with a confocal laser scanning microscope, and color images are generated with RNA from the tumor and reference cells for each hybridization. Genes up-regulated in the tumors appear red, whereas those with decreased expression appear green. Genes with similar levels of expression in the two samples appear yellow. Genes of interest are selected on the basis of the differences in the level of expression by known tumor classes (e.g., *BRCA1*-mutation–positive and *BRCA2*-mutation–positive). Statistical analysis determines whether these differences in the gene expression profiles are greater than would be expected by chance. **C,** The differences in the patterns of gene expression between tumor classes can be portrayed in the form of a color-coded plot, and the relations between tumors can be portrayed in the form of a multidimensional-scaling plot. Tumors with similar gene-expression profiles cluster close to one another in the multidimensional-scaling plot. **D,** Particular genes of interest can be further studied through the use of a large number of arrayed, paraffin-embedded tumor specimens, referred to as *tissue microarrays*. **E,** Immunohistochemical analyses of hundreds or thousands of these arrayed biopsy specimens can be performed in order to extend the microarray findings. (From Hedenfalk I, Duggan D, Chen Y, et al: Gene expression profiles in hereditary breast cancer. N Engl J Med 2001;344:539–548.)

further study its pathophysiology and to design therapeutic strategies. Integrating an oncogene that causes malignancy into the genome of a mouse without altering the mouse's own genes generates a transgenic, cancer-prone mouse that transmits this trait to its offspring with a dominant pattern of inheritance. Although species differences in tumor susceptibility and disease remission exist between mice and humans, the tools for genetic manipulation in the mouse are superior to those in other mammals, and useful information about the function of oncogenes can be gained by targeted expression of mutant protein products in mouse tissues.

The technology for producing transgenic mice joins recombinant DNA methods with standard techniques that are used today by in vitro fertilization clinics, relying on our understanding of mammalian reproduction and the development of protocols to harvest, manipulate, and re-implant eggs and early embryos (Fig. 1-12). The transgene is constructed so that the gene product will be expressed under appropriate spatial and temporal control. In addition to all the standard signals necessary for efficient transcription and translation of the gene, transgenes contain a promoter, or regulatory region, that drives transcription in either a ubiquitous or tissue-restricted

Figure 1-11. Exploring protein-protein interactions with the yeast two-hybrid system. Two-hybrid technology exploits the fact that transcriptional activators are modular in nature. Two physically distinct functional domains are necessary to get transcription: a DNA-binding domain that binds to the DNA of the promoter and an activation domain that binds to the basal transcription apparatus and activates transcription. **A,** The known gene encoding *protein A* is cloned into the "bait" vector, fused to the gene encoding a DNA-binding domain from some transcription factor. When placed into a yeast system with a reporter gene, this fusion protein can bind to the reporter gene promoter, but it cannot activate transcription. **B,** Separately, a second gene (or a library of cDNA fragments encoding potential interactors), *protein B*, is cloned into the "prey" vector, fused to an activation domain of a different transcription factor. When placed into a yeast strain containing the reporter gene, it cannot activate transcription because it has no DNA-binding domain. **C,** When the two vectors are placed into the same yeast, a transcription factor is formed that can activate the reporter gene if protein B, made by the second plasmid, binds to protein A. **D,** Screening a yeast two-hybrid library. The plate on the left holds 96 different yeast strains in patches (or colonies), each of which expresses a different bait protein (*top*). The plate on the right holds 96 patches, each of the same yeast strain (prey strain) that expresses a protein fused to an activation domain (prey). The plate of bait strains and the plate of prey strains are each pressed to the same replica velvet, and the impression is lifted with a plate containing YPD medium. After one day of growth on the YPD plate, during which time the two strains mate to form diploids, the YPD plate is pressed to a new replica velvet, and the impression is lifted with a plate containing diploid selection medium and an indicator such as X-Gal. Blue patches (dark spots) on the X-Gal plate indicate that the lacZ reporter is transcribed, suggesting that the prey interacts with the bait at that location. (**C,** Text after http://www.invitrogen.com/catalog_project/cat_hybrid.html [July, 2000]; figure retrieved from http://www.nature.com/.../journal/v403/n6770/full/403601a0_r.html. **D,** From Bartel PL, Fields S (eds): The Yeast Two-Hybrid System. New York, Oxford University Press, 1997; Finley RL Jr, Brent R: Two-hybrid analysis of genetic regulatory networks. Retrieved from http://www.genetics.wayne.edu/finlab/YTHnetworks.html.)

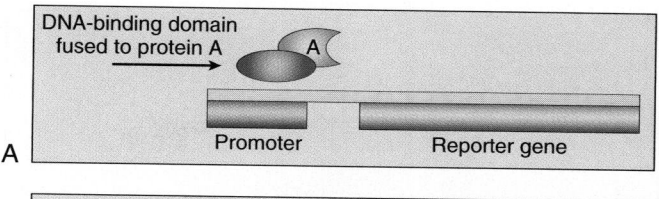

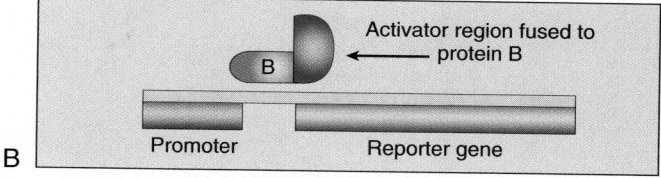

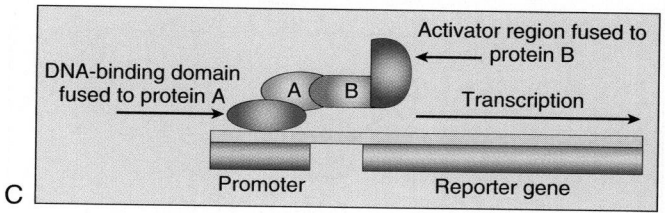

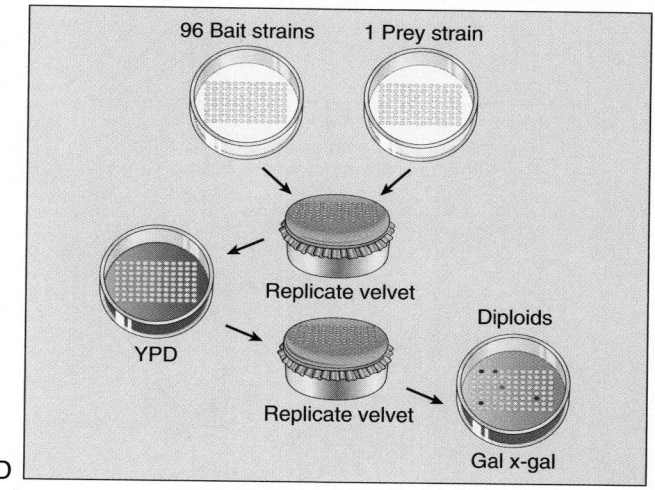

pattern. This requires an extensive knowledge of genetic regulation in the target cells.

The transgene is then injected into the male pronucleus of a fertilized mouse egg, obtained from a female mouse in which hyperovulation has been hormonally induced. The injected eggs are cultured to the two-cell stage and then implanted in the oviduct of another recipient female mouse. Transgenic pups are identified by the presence of the transgene in their genomic DNA (obtained from the tip of the tail and analyzed by PCR). Typically, several copies of the transgene are incorporated in a head-to-tail orientation into a single random site in the mouse genome. About 30% of the resulting pups will have integrated the transgene into their germline DNA, and they constitute the founders of the transgenic lines. RNA analysis of their progeny determines the level of transgene expression and whether the transgene is being expressed in the desired location or at the appropriate time. Given

the variability in transgene number and chromosomal location, transgene expression patterns and levels can diverge considerably among different founder lines carrying the same transgene.

In general, transgenesis is optimal for modeling oncogenic mutations that cause a gain of function, producing disease even when they occur in only one of a gene's two alleles. For example, an activating mutation in a growth factor that causes abnormal cell proliferation can be mimicked by introducing a transgenic version of the mutated growth factor gene under the control of an appropriate regulatory sequence for expression in the tissue of interest. The relative susceptibility of such a transgenic mouse to tumorigenesis can help distinguish between a primary and secondary role of the mutant factor, and established lines of these animals can be used for testing new therapeutic protocols.

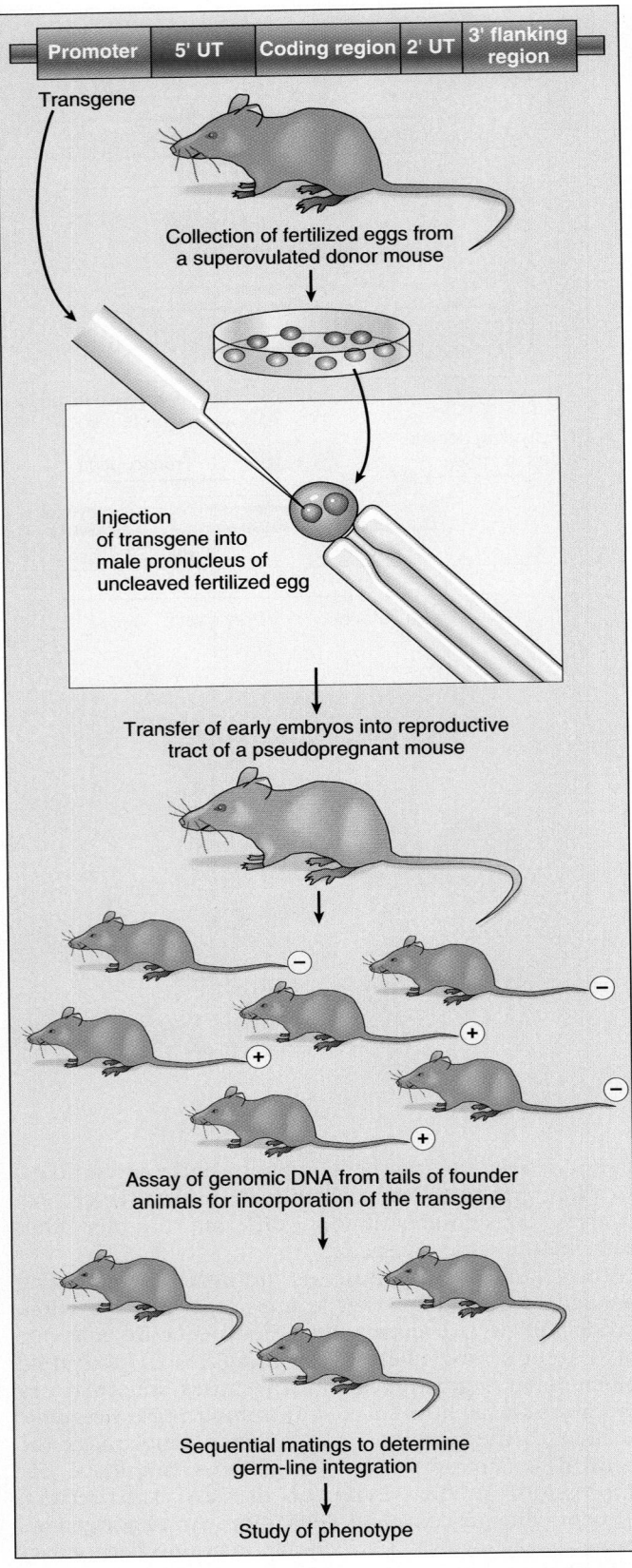

Figure 1-12. Generation of transgenic mice. The transgene containing the DNA sequences necessary for the expression of a functional protein is injected into the male (larger) pronucleus of uncleaved fertilized eggs through a micropipette. The early embryos are then transferred into the reproductive tract of a mouse rendered "pseudopregnant" by hormonal therapy. The resulting pups (founders) are tested for incorporation of the transgene by assaying genomic DNA from their tails. Founder animals that have incorporated the transgene (+) are mated with nontransgenic mice, and their offspring are mated with each other to confirm germ-line integration and to establish a line of homozygous transgenic mice. Several transgenic lines that have incorporated different numbers of transgenes at different integration sites (and thus express various amounts of the protein of interest) are usually studied. UT, untranslated. (From Schuldiner AR: Transgenic animals. N Engl J Med 1996;334:653–655.)

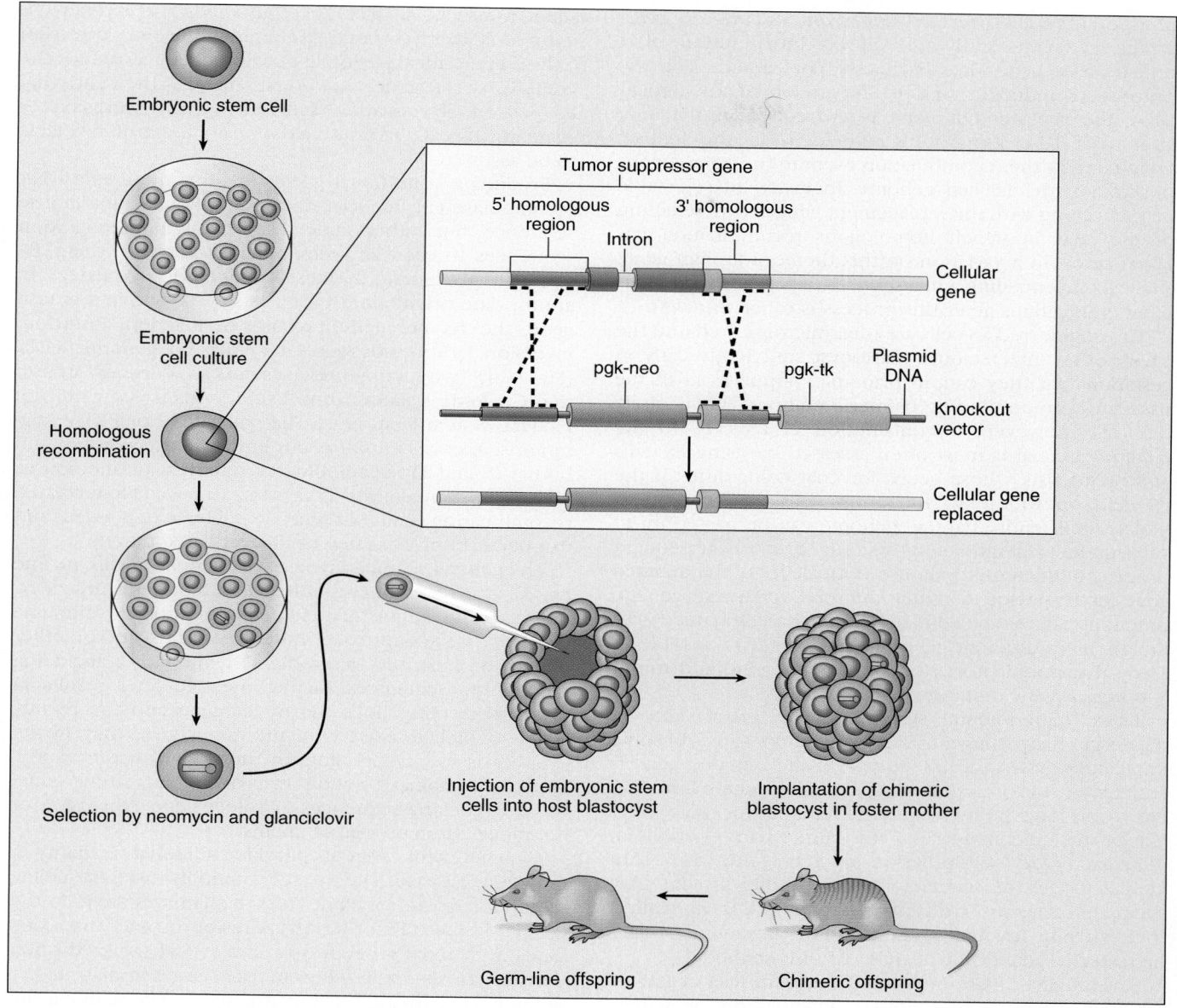

Figure 1-13. Homologous recombination between a cellular gene and a knockout vector to create mice lacking a tumor suppressor gene. Embryonic stem cells (*upper left panel*) contain the tumor suppressor cellular gene (*upper right panel*), which consists of exon 1 (olive green, a 5′ noncoding region), an intron, and exon 2 (red, a protein-coding region, and yellow, a 3′ noncoding region). A knockout vector—consisting of a collinear assembly of a DNA flanking segment 5′ to the cellular gene (blue), the phosphoglycerate kinase–bacterial neomycin gene (pgk-neo, violet), a 3′ segment of the cellular gene (yellow), a DNA flanking segment 3′ to the cellular gene (green), and the phosphoglycerate kinase–viral thymidine kinase gene (pgk-tk, orange)—is created and introduced into the embryonic–stem cell culture. Double recombination occurs between the cellular gene and the knockout vector in the 5′ homologous regions and the 3′ homologous regions (*dashed lines*), resulting in the incorporation of the inactive knockout vector, including pgk-neo but not pgk-tk, into the cellular genomic locus of the embryonic stem cell. The presence of pgk-neo and the absence of pgk-tk in these replaced genes will allow survival of these embryonic stem cells after positive–negative selection with neomycin and ganciclovir. The clone of mutant embryonic stem cells is injected into a host blastocyst, which is implanted into a pseudopregnant foster mother, and subsequently develops into a chimeric offspring (*bottom panel*). The contribution of the embryonic stem cells to the germ cells of the chimeric mouse results in germline transmission of the embryonic stem cell genome to offspring that are heterozygous for the mutated tumor suppressor allele. The heterozygotes are mated to produce mutant, cancer-prone mice homozygous for tumor suppressor deficiency. (Modified from Mazjoub JA, Muglia LJ: Knockout mice. N Engl J Med 1996;334:904–906.)

In contrast to disorders caused by dominantly acting oncogenes, recessive genetic disorders, such as loss-of-function mutations in the tumor suppressor gene, require both copies (alleles) of a gene to be inactivated. The methods needed to produce animal models of recessive genetic disease differ from those used to study dominant traits. Gene knockout technology has been developed to generate mice in which one allele of an endogenous gene is removed or altered in a heritable pattern (Fig. 1-13). Gene disruption or replacement is first engineered in

Science of Clinical Oncology

pluripotential cells, termed *embryonic stem (ES) cells*, which are genetically altered by introduction of a replacement gene that is inactive or mutant. For the purpose of reducing random integration of the foreign DNA, the replacement gene is embedded into a long stretch of DNA from its native locus in the mouse, which targets the recombination event to the homologous position in the ES cell genome. Inclusion of selectable markers along with the replacement gene allows selection of the cells in which homologous recombination has taken place. In a variation on this theme, a foreign gene, such as one encoding a marker, can be placed in the locus of an endogenous gene; this process is called *knock-in*.

The engineered ES cells are then microinjected into the cavity of an intact mouse blastocyst sufficiently early in gestation that they can, in principle, populate all of the tissues of the developing chimeric embryo. This is rarely the case, however, so contribution of ES cells to the resulting animal is most often assessed by using ES cells and blastocysts whose genes for coat color differ. If the ES cells contribute to the germ cells of the founder mouse, their entire haploid genome can be passed on to subsequent generations. By mating together subsequent progeny of the founder mouse, both alleles of the mutated gene can be passed to a single animal. Overlapping genetic functions can also be defined by cross-breeding mice with mutations in different genes. In this way it is possible to study the combinatorial effects of oncogene and tumor suppressor gene mutations.

These experimental systems are of great value in dissecting the pathogenesis of many tumor types. In some knockout studies, the phenotype of the mutated gene is anticipated by prior knowledge of the gene's function. However, unexpected mutant phenotypes may help clarify the mechanism of the underlying neoplasia. Pharmacologic manipulation of transgenic knockout animal models of cancer will prove useful in screening therapeutic agents with potential for study in clinical trials. Therapy involving gene or cell replacement can also be tested in genetically engineered disease models.

Several caveats are important when the use of knockout technology is considered. Inactivation of widely expressed genes with multiple functions may have complex phenotypes. Conversely, if the functions of two genes overlap, a mutation in one of the genes may not produce an abnormal phenotype because of compensation by the unaltered partner. Perhaps the greatest drawback lies in the disruption of development by mutation of a gene essential for embryogenesis, preventing further study of its action in the adult.

CONTROLLING THE GENOME

Recent advances in manipulating the mouse genome have resulted in more sophisticated models of human cancer. Site-specific recombinase systems combined with gene targeting techniques in ES cells afford an added level of control over the mouse genome, inducing single-point mutations or site-specific chromosomal rearrangements in a tissue- and time-restricted pattern, or activating a silent transgene at will. These methods can circumvent embryonic death by targeted alteration of gene expression only after a critical period in development and reduce the complexity of gene functional analysis by restricting its pattern of activation. Inducible gene expression or silencing also allows acute, as opposed to chronic, effects to be assessed.

Producing conditional alleles in mice requires a DNA recombinase enzyme that does not recognize any mouse sequence, but rather targets short, foreign recognition sequences to catalyze recombination between them. By strategic placement of these recognition sequences in appropriate orientations either beside or within a mouse gene, the recombination results in deletion, insertion, inversion, or translocation of associated genomic DNA (Fig. 1-14). Two recombinase systems are currently in use: the Cre-loxP system from bacteriophage P1 and the Flp-FRT system from yeast. The 34-bp loxP or FRT recognition sequences do not occur in the mouse genome, and both Cre and Flp recombinases function autonomously, without the need for cofactors. Cre- or Flp-mediated recombination is not distance- or cell-type–dependent and can occur in proliferating or differentiated tissues.

The general scheme involves two mouse lines. One line carries the recombinase either as a transgene driven by tissue-specific regulatory elements or knocked into one allele of a gene expressed in the desired tissue. The other mouse line harbors a modified gene target including recognition sequences. Mating the two lines results in progeny carrying both the target gene and the recombinase, which interact with the target gene only in the desired tissues. Depending on the design of the experiment, recombinase action can delete an entire gene, remove blocking sequences to induce gene expression, or rearrange chromosomal segments.

Gene-inducible systems provide additional flexibility in modeling disease. The most commonly used inducible method is the tetracycline (tet) regulatory system. In the classic design (tTA or tet-off), a fusion protein that combines a bacterial tet repressor and a viral transactivation domain drives expression of the target transgene by binding to upstream tet operator sequences flanking the transgene transcription start site. In the presence of the antibiotic inducer, the fusion protein is dissociated from the operator sequences, inactivating the transgene. In a complementary design, called *reverse'tTA* (rtTA or tet-on), structural modification of the tet repressor makes the antibiotic an active requirement for binding of the fusion protein to the operator sequences, such that its administration activates transgene expression at any time during the life span of the mouse, whereas withdrawal results in down-regulation of the gene. It is important that the transgene integrates into a genomic locus that permits proper tTA or rtTA regulation, so that the system exhibits minimal "intrinsic leakiness" and good antibiotic responsiveness.

Another recently developed conditional method is based on the activation of nuclear hormone receptors to control gene expression. Two current systems involve activation of a mammalian estrogen receptor; an estrogen analog, 4-hydroxy-tamoxifen; or an insect hormone

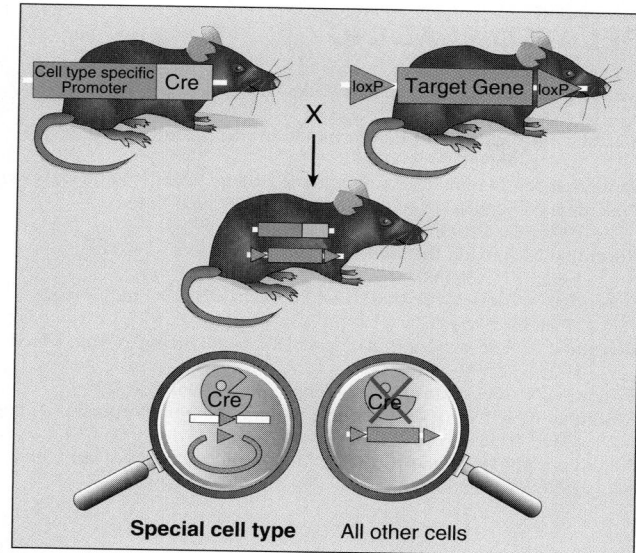

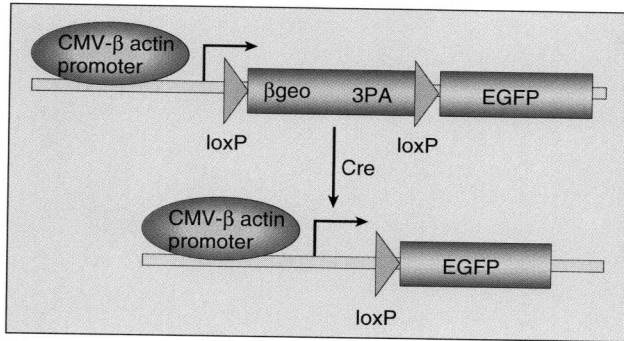

Figure 1-14. Conditional mutagenesis schemes demonstrated with the Cre-loxP system. **A,** Two mouse lines are required for conditional gene deletion. First, a conventional transgenic mouse line with Cre targeted to a specific tissue or cell type, and second, a mouse strain that embodies a target gene (endogenous gene or transgene) flanked by two loxP sites in a direct orientation ("floxed gene"). Recombination (excision and consequently inactivation of the target gene) occurs only in those cells expressing Cre recombinase. Hence, the target gene remains active in all cells and tissues that do not express the Cre recombinase. **B,** The Z/EG double reporter system. These transgenic mice constitutively express lacZ under the control of the cytomegalovirus enhancer/chicken actin promoter. Expression is widespread, with notable exceptions being liver and lung tissue. Expression is observed throughout all embryonic and adult stages. When crossed with a Cre recombinase-expressing strain, lacZ expression is replaced with enhanced green fluorescent protein expression in tissues expressing Cre. This double reporter system makes it possible to distinguish a lack of reporter expression from a lack of Cre recombinase expression while providing a means to assess Cre excision activity in live animals and cells. (**A,** Courtesy of Kay-Uwe Wagner, National Institutes of Health. **B,** From Novak A, Guo C, Yang W, Nagy A, Lobe CG: Z/EG, a double reporter mouse line that expresses enhanced green fluorescent protein upon Cre-mediated excision. Genesis 2000;28:147–155.)

receptor with the corresponding ligand, ecdysone. Although several variations on these hormone-receptor systems are currently under study, the underlying principle is the same. A regulatory protein, such as a transcription factor, is fused with the ligand-binding domain from a nuclear hormone receptor protein. The resulting chimeric transgene is placed under the control of a promoter that directs expression to the tissue of interest, and transgenic animals are generated. In the absence of the hormone or an analog, the fusion protein accumulates in the desired tissue but is rendered inactive through its association with resident heat shock proteins. Hormone, administered either systemically or topically, binds to the ligand-binding domain moiety of the fusion protein, dissociates it from the heat shock protein, and allows the transcriptional regulatory component to find its natural DNA targets and activate expression of the corresponding genes. Removal of hormone leads to inactivation of the fusion protein and gene down-regulation. If the ligand-binding domain is fused to a recombinase, administration of hormone leads to the rearrangement of target sequences. This reaction is not reversible but provides additional temporal control over the recombinase-based mutation.

The genetic construction of cancer-prone mice with the capacity to control transgene expression in vivo provides new avenues to determine the role of oncogenes in tumor generation and maintenance. Conditional expression systems have already been developed to generate hematopoietic, leukemogenic, and lympho-magenic mutations, as well as solid tumors, in the mouse. These inducible cancer models can be exploited to identify oncogenic signals that influence host-tumor interactions, to establish the role of a given oncogenic lesion in advanced tumors, and to evaluate therapies targeted to cancer-causing mutations. Potential clinical applications of inducible systems include targeting virally delivered transgene expression to malignant tissues by the use of specific inducible regulatory elements, restricting the expression of transgenes exclusively to affected tissues, and increasing the therapeutic index of the vectors, particularly in the context of solid tumors. In all cases, a basic knowledge of the specific mutations involved in the molecular genetics of malignancies is required, because it is often unclear whether the causal mutation underlying the genesis of neoplasia continues to play a central role in the progression to the fully transformed state. This is particularly important in modeling cancers characterized by genetic plasticity, in which drug resistance can arise after primary tumor formation.

These evolving techniques of gene manipulation in vivo constitute major advances in cancer research. They have enabled the integration of underlying molecular biologic principles of malignancy with pathophysiologic consequences, generating an invaluable resource for understanding the complex genetics of tumor formation, which holds great promise for improved treatment of human cancer.

RECOMMENDED TEXTS

Alberts B, Johnson A, Lewis J, Raff M, Roberts K, Weller P: Molecular biology of the cell, 4th ed. London, UK, Taylor and Francis Group, 2002.

Mendelsohn J, Israel MA, Liotta LA, Howley PM. Molecular basis of cancer, 2nd ed. Philadelphia, PA, Elsevier Science, 2001.

RECOMMENDED READING

Albanese C, Hulit J, Sakamaki T, Pestell RG: Recent advances in inducible expression in transgenic mice. Semin Cell Dev Biol 2002;13:129–141.

Guttmacher AE, Collins FS: Genomic medicine: A primer. N Engl J Med 2002;347:1512–1520.

Hahn WC, Weinberg RA: Mechanisms of disease: Rules for making human tumor cells. N Engl J Med 2002;347:1593–1603.

Jonkers J, Berns A: Conditional mouse models of sporadic cancer. Nat Rev Cancer 2002;2:251–265.

RELATED READING

Krontiris TG: Molecular medicine: Oncogenes. N Engl J Med 1995;333:303–306.

Majzoub JA, Muglia LJ: Molecular medicine: Knockout mice. N Engl J Med 1996;334:904–907.

Rosenthal N: DNA and the genetic code. N Engl J Med 1994;331:39–41.

Rosenthal N: Regulation of gene expression. N Engl J Med 1994;331:931–933.

Rosenthal N: Stalking the gene: DNA libraries. N Engl J Med 1994;331:599–600.

Rosenthal N: Tools of the trade: Recombinant DNA. N Engl J Med 1994;331:315–317.

Rosenthal N: Fine structure of a gene: DNA sequencing. N Engl J Med 1995;332:589–591.

Rosenthal N: Recognizing DNA. N Engl J Med 1995;333:925–927.

Rosenthal N, Schwartz RS: In search of perverse polymorphisms. N Engl J Med 1998;333:122–124.

Schuldiner AR: Molecular medicine: Transgenic animals. N Engl J Med 1996;334:653–655.

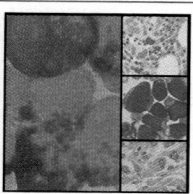

James N. Ihle

INTRACELLULAR SIGNALING

SUMMARY OF KEY POINTS

- Transition of normal cells to malignant cells almost always includes alteration of intracellular signaling pathways.
- The steps of cellular signaling usually include ligand binding to cell surface receptors; activation of the receptors; recruitment of adapter proteins; activation of one or more signaling pathways, usually involving alterations in phosphorylation status of one or more target proteins; and frequently activation of transcription factors.
- Signaling pathways are the mechanisms by which changes in the extracellular environment affect intracellular function. Examples of changes in the extracellular environment that entail this approach include alterations in integrins and extracellular matrix; alterations in levels of hormones, circulating growth factors, and cytokines; and alterations in antigen binding.
- Alteration of signaling pathways can result in both enhanced proliferation and inappropriate survival of tumor cells. Thus altered signaling pathways can contribute to tumor development, tumor metastasis, and resistance of tumor cells to therapeutic intervention.

CELL SIGNALING AND CANCER

Many studies of intracellular signaling have their origins in studies of cancer. One of the first identified human cancer genes, mutated *ras,* has been a focus of pathways of intracellular signaling for decades. The first identified cellular gene acquired by a retrovirus and capable of directly inducing transformation was the c-*myc* gene—a gene that is transcriptionally activated in response to a variety of intracellular signaling pathways. Since discovery of these initial examples, most oncogenes have been shown to be involved in intracellular signaling ranging from activation of members of almost all receptor families to participation in almost all intracellular signaling pathways.

The close relation between cellular transformation and intracellular signaling emphasizes the critical role of intracellular signaling in cell behavior. From the earliest organisms, it has been critical to sense the environment and to change patterns of gene expression accordingly. This requirement became more important with development of multicellular organisms and the need for spatial orientation of cells during development and for control of their extent of growth. Added to the complexity of cellular communication associated with development came the requirement for sensing a wide spectrum of physiologic states, including hormonal clues, immunologic commands, and defense responses associated with innate immunity. Consideration of the number of intracellular signaling pathways should make it clear that any mammalian cell is being instructed about how to behave in a constant, dynamic manner. It should be equally apparent that alterations in this regulation are some of the central

characteristics of a transformed cell. In addition, dynamic regulation of cell behavior has potential therapeutic implications.

GENERAL PRINCIPLES OF INTRACELLULAR SIGNALING

The specifics of intracellular signaling can appear overwhelming because of the number of pathways and the complex and unique properties of individual pathways. Identification of overriding principles shared among pathways facilitates understanding and places in perspective individual signaling pathways and events in the pathways. As illustrated by description of various receptor systems, many receptor systems have relatively dedicated intracellular signaling pathways, and families of receptors have strikingly similar requirements.

In almost all receptor systems, engagement of ligand induces aggregation or altered physical structure of the receptor and initiates the sequence of events leading to intracellular signaling. One characteristic response involves recruitment of one or more proteins to the receptor complex through recognition of the altered receptor structure or through modification of receptor or membrane residues. These recruitments are mediated through a spectrum of docking domains that enable recognition and specificity. Formation of the receptor complex ultimately results in activation of intracellular signaling events. In some cases the pathways are relatively simple, as in the transcription factors Stat (signal transducer and activator of transcription) and Smad (Sma plus Mad, see later), both of which are activated at the receptor complex, translocate to the nucleus, and activate gene transcription. Other cases are more complex, including activation of transcription factors such as the ets proteins, NFAT (nuclear factor of activated T cells) transcription factors, or nuclear factor κB (NF-κB), all of which require a receptor-initiated signal to be propagated through a sequence of cellular events (Fig. 2-1).

In study of the mammalian families of genes that participate in intracellular signaling, a useful concept is that the mammalian genome evolved from two duplications of the genome that characterizes *Drosophila*. Thus for a large number of gene families, a single gene in *Drosophila* is represented by four genes in the mammalian genome. However, three loci frequently are present, a finding consistent with loss of the genomic region containing the fourth gene. In many cases, however, the basic two duplications have undergone further modification by extensive duplication within a genomic region. The result often is a locus containing a number of highly related genes. Interesting examples of both events are the loci associated with the Stat family of transcription factors. The single gene of *Drosophila* is represented by three loci in the mammalian genome. At each locus, two Stat genes exist in tandem (Stat1/Stat4, Stat2/Stat6, Stat3/Stat5), representing duplication of the initial locus before the genomic duplications. Moreover, at one locus, duplication of the Stat5 gene occurred after genomic duplication, giving rise to the tandem linked Stat5a and Stat5b genes. As might be imagined, existence of four copies of a gene has allowed a variety of evolutionary opportunities, all of which are observed. All loci may retain redundant functions, or one locus may retain the primary function while the other three loci evolve. Evolution of loci may give rise to nonfunctional loci, loci

that acquire lineage-specific functions, or loci that may be needed for functions that have been lost during evolution. Therefore the concept of conservation of the gene does not ensure a function at the present point in evolution.

An emerging concept in intracellular signaling is that there is considerable "noise" in signaling. In particular, receptor engagement may result in a variety of biochemical changes and activation of intracellular signaling pathways. Although it might seem intuitive that if a pathway is activated or a protein is modified it must have a functional consequence, experimental evidence strongly indicates that this is not the case. Although numerous examples exist to support this concept, one particularly striking example involves the intracellular signaling associated with the four structurally related receptors for growth hormone (GH), prolactin, erythropoietin (Epo), and thrombopoietin (Tpo). Each receptor has an essential nonredundant function in its specific physiologic role, and, as discussed later, all require the same receptor-associated tyrosine kinase Jak2 (Janus family of protein tyrosine kinases 2). Activation of the receptors results in receptor tyrosine phosphorylation, recruitment of a number of adapter proteins, and activation of numerous signaling pathways, including activation of the highly related transcription factors Stat5a and Stat5b. It is not possible to differentiate receptors biochemically by the changes occurring after receptor activation. The receptors are functionally redundant. Thus the prolactin receptor, which is physiologically critical for mammary gland development and ovarian function, can mediate all the functions normally provided by the Epo receptor in erythropoiesis. Given these observations, it is striking that deletion of one pathway, activation of Stat5a/b, completely

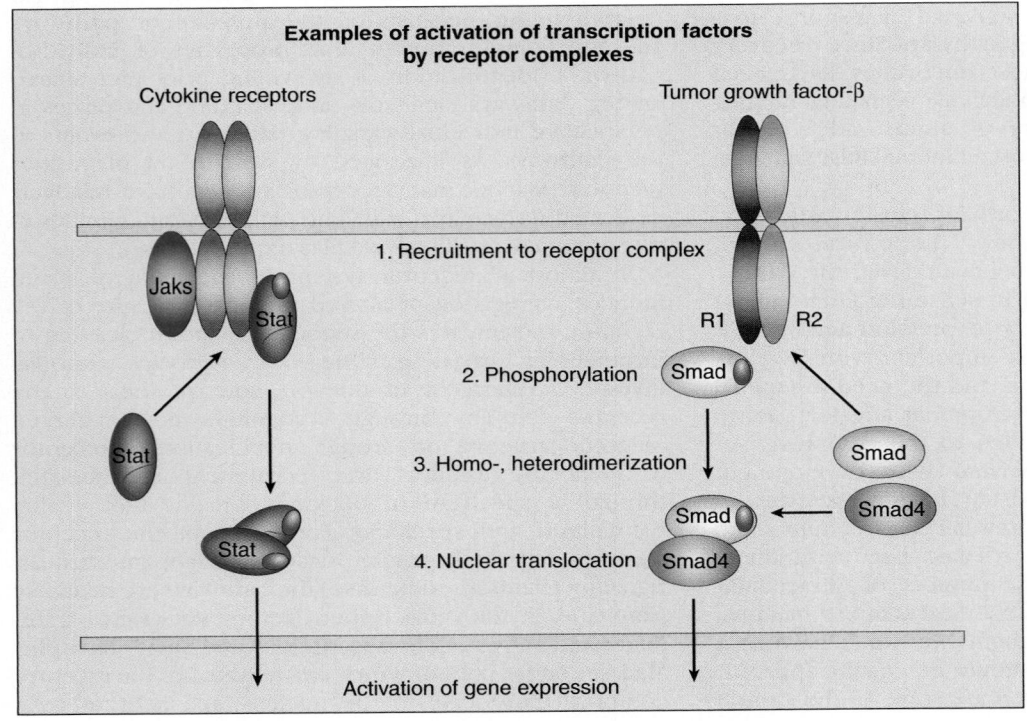

Examples of activation of transcription factors by receptor complexes

Cytokine receptors   Tumor growth factor-β

Jaks
Stat
Stat   R1   R2

1. Recruitment to receptor complex
2. Phosphorylation   Smad

3. Homo-, heterodimerization   Smad
                            Smad4
Stat   Smad
4. Nuclear translocation   Smad4

Activation of gene expression

Figure 2-1. Direct activation of transcription factors by receptor complexes. Several intracellular signaling pathways entail relatively direct mechanisms of activation of gene expression after receptor engagement. Two examples are the Stat family of transcription factors and the Smad family of transcription factors. In both cases, resident, cytoplasmic proteins are recruited to the activated receptor complex through interactions facilitated by receptor modifications by phosphorylation. Once recruited to the complex, the latent transcription factors are phosphorylated at the critical residues required for activation. As a consequence of modification, the proteins either homodimerize (Stat) or heterodimerize (Stat, Smad) and are translocated to the nucleus. In the nucleus, the homodimerized, heterodimerized proteins have the ability to bind DNA in a sequence-specific manner to activate gene expression.

eliminates the physiologic mechanisms associated with prolactin and GH while having only subtle effects on the physiologic mechanisms associated with Epo or Tpo. This example illustrates the importance of knowing the consequences of gene deletions in assessment of the role of a particular signaling pathway in a specific physiologic setting. Throughout this chapter, emphasis is placed on providing this information when available.

In study of genes associated with cancer, the ability to transform cells is frequently equated with the concept that the gene must play a central role in cell growth or differentiation. In reality, mutation of a gene may bestow on that gene properties not characteristic of the cellular gene; amplification of a gene may change affinity considerations to reveal new substrates; dominant negatives may associate with proteins of unrelated pathways; or activating mutations may affect pathways not normally affected. Examples are indicated throughout the chapter, although one example has particular relevance—the *ras* gene. H-*ras* was one of the first mutated genes found to be associated with cancer and, as a consequence, for decades has been a focal point for studies of intracellular signaling. Therefore it is notable that deletion of H-*ras* in mice causes no phenotypic changes. Moreover, deletion of H-*ras* and N-*ras* together causes no phenotypic changes. Among the *ras* family members, only deletion of K-*ras* causes phenotypic changes that are lineage specific.[1,2] Although there has been considerable emphasis on the *ras* pathway in intracellular signaling, it is not clear that the critical pathways involve either H-*ras* or N-*ras*.

Current research in cancer biology often has taken the course of gene profiling to provide information about tumors. The goal has been identification of properties that provide diagnostic information or are predictors of response to therapy. Almost all the intracellular signaling pathways discussed affect gene expression. For example, hundreds of genes have been identified whose expression is affected by the Stat transcription factors activated in interferon (IFN) signaling. This pathway is only one of many under dynamic regulation and potentially altered by a number of factors. It might be proposed that the environment of the cell may be as predicted by the gene pattern as are the genetic changes associated with transformation. Therefore any consideration of gene profiling should take into consideration the contributions of intracellular signaling.

The following sections are an overview of the many intracellular signaling pathways. Throughout the chapter references are provided that contain additional details of a particular pathway. For example, a more detailed review of the Jak/Stat pathway is contained in a review in *Current Opinion in Cell Biology*.[3]

RECEPTOR SYSTEMS UTILIZING INDUCTION OF TYROSINE PHOSPHORYLATION

A variety of ligand recognition systems share activation of protein tyrosine kinases. In all cases, ligand binding changes the physical state of a receptor complex and often recruits and activates receptor-associated protein tyrosine kinases. Tyrosine kinase activation invariably involves phosphorylation of sites with the kinase domain in what is termed the *activation loop*, which is essential for activation of kinase activity. Once activated, the kinase phosphorylates additional sites on the receptor and receptor-associated proteins. These sites recruit additional substrates into the receptor complex through interaction of sites of tyrosine phosphorylation. Protein domains specific for such sites include the SH2 domain (Src homology 2 domain) and the PTB (phosphotyrosine-binding) domain. The chemical structures of many of these domains interacting with their specific phosphorylated tyrosines have been determined. Among the various receptor systems activating tyrosine phosphorylation, common substrates often are recruited, although some substrates are more specific for specific families.

Tyrosine Kinase Receptor Signaling

One of the largest families of proteins involved in signal transduction, the receptor tyrosine kinases, share an extracellular ligand-binding domain, a transmembrane, and a cytoplasmic domain containing a protein tyrosine kinase catalytic domain. The family consists of approximately 60 genes divided into 20 subfamilies defined by similarity in structure of ligands and the receptors.[4] The receptors control survival, differentiation, and proliferation of cells of almost all lineages. For example, the four highly related fibroblast growth factor receptors (FGFR1, FGFR2, FGFR3, and FGFR4) and the approximately 20 ligands all play essential, unique roles in early embryonic development, as established by production of strains of mice lacking the individual receptors. Similarly, the four highly related EGR (early growth response) receptors have numerous ligands that play essential roles in development. The largest subfamily consists of the Eph receptors and their ligands, the ephrins, most of which are involved in neuronal development.

In cancer, there exist numerous examples in which chromosomal translocations have resulted in altered expression or expression of structurally altered and activated kinases of all subfamilies. One of the first molecularly identified virally transduced oncogenes (*fms*) was shown to be a derivative of protein tyrosine kinase receptor genes (colony-stimulating factor 1 [CSF-1] receptor). In a number of cases, translocations fuse the kinase domain with a dimerization domain. The result is constitutive activation of the kinase catalytic domain by transphosphorylation or constitutive activation of the kinase domain due to overexpression. Irrespective of the mechanisms, the consequences are activation of intracellular signaling pathways. Although the pathways activated often are those normally associated with ligand-regulated signaling, activated receptors also can phosphorylate substrates that are normally not substrates and thereby inappropriately activate intracellular signaling pathways.

Activation of signaling by tyrosine kinase receptors involves several well-characterized steps. Ligand induces oligomerization of the receptor, a process that results in juxtaposition of the cytoplasmic, catalytic domains in a manner that allows transphosphorylation and activation of kinase activity.[5-9] The mechanisms by which ligand induces oligomerization can be one of several. The ligand may exist normally as a dimer and therefore bind two receptor chains in a symmetrical manner, as is the case for CSF-1 and stem cell factor (SCF). An alternative is that a ligand has two binding sites for the receptor. Last, many ligands are cell associated and thereby can induce receptor oligomerization. Irrespective of the mechanism, the key function of the ligand is to drive receptor oligomerization.

The mechanism of activation of receptor tyrosine kinases almost invariably involves transphosphorylation of a critical tyrosine in the kinase domain in a region referred to as the *activation loop*. Determination of the molecular structure of receptor tyrosine kinase catalytic domains has provided insights into the basis for activation. In the case of the insulin receptor,[10] the critical, regulatory tyrosine resides in a loop that is very near the substrate binding site and thereby can interfere with the ability of the adenosine triphosphate (ATP) binding loop to gain access to the catalytic site. Phosphorylation of the tyrosine is speculated to lead to a change of conformation that results in swinging out of this inhibitory loop from the catalytic site. This process allows binding and phosphorylation of substrates. The structure of the FGFR has been solved.[10,11] Although orientation of the tyrosine relative to the substrate binding site and the ATP binding loop is somewhat different, the unphosphorylated form can be hypothesized to primarily interfere with access of the ATP binding loop to the catalytic site. The structure of the kinase domain and the critical role of tyrosine phosphorylation in receptor activation provide important target sites for small-molecule inhibitors. This theme also appears to apply to kinases that associate with receptors of the cytokine receptor superfamily.

Activation of kinase activity is followed by phosphorylation of a variety of sites within the cytoplasmic domain of the receptor. These sites serve as "docking" sites for a variety of proteins that are either substrates for the kinases or are activated through recruitment into the receptor complex.[12] Most of the proteins recruited to the receptor complex are recruited through interaction between SH2 domains and specific sites of tyrosine phosphorylation. SH2 domains consist of 100-amino-acid domains that contain a binding pocket that recognizes phosphotyrosine and generally three to six carboxyl-located amino acid residues that allow specificity of interaction. The structures of several SH2 domains have been solved and provide important insights into the interactions involved in phosphotyrosine binding and specificity.[13,14] A second domain, termed the *phospho-tyrosine-binding domain* (PTB) domain, has been identified.[15,16] The binding properties of PTB domains are quite different from those of SH2 domains, and PTB domains are much less frequently encountered than are SH2 domains.

The concept of receptor recruitment of substrates has two important consequences. First, the requirement to recruit substrates to a site of active tyrosine phospho-rylation leads to an essential mechanism of providing specificity for signaling. Only those pathways are activated for which the components can be recruited to the receptor complex. Second, the requirement for receptor tyrosine phosphorylation ensures that phosphorylation of signaling components occurs only within the context of ligand-driven receptor activation. Thus the critical requirements are met for both ligand-dependent and ligand/receptor-specific activation. The importance of this mechanism is readily evident in comparisons of the properties of the wild-type receptors with those of altered receptors that are mutated or fused with aggregation-inducing partners, as occurs in a variety of transformed cells. In these cases activation of kinase activity is independent of ligand and frequently results in phosphorylation and activation of substrates that are not seen in responses to normal ligand.

Beyond activation there is a requirement for deactivation of ligand-activated receptor complexes. One mechanism of inactivation is internalization of the ligand-receptor complex. This mechanism often involves internalization through clathrin-coated pits and internalization to the endosomes. In the endosomes, receptor-ligand complexes dissociate, and either the complexes are degraded or the receptor is cycled back to the membrane.[17] In some cases ligand-induced receptor activation results in ubiquitination of the receptor that targets it for degradation by the proteosomes. Last, dephosphorylation of the receptor, particularly dephosphorylation of the critical tyrosines in the activation loop, may be responsible for downregulation of the receptor. Of particular interest in this regard are the tyrosine phosphatases that contain SH2 domains and therefore can be specifically recruited to the receptor complex. Although some evidence supports such a mechanism for the tyrosine protein receptor kinases,[18] a critical role for such phosphatases is evident in the function of the cytokine receptor superfamily.

The Cytokine Receptor Superfamily

A wide variety of cytokines affecting a broad spectrum of cell lineages can be functionally grouped through their use of structurally and functionally related receptors of the cytokine receptor superfamily.[19] This evolving group of ligands and receptors is relatively new, as evidenced by the existence of only one cytokine and one receptor of the cytokine receptor superfamily in *Drosophila*. Members of the family have acquired physiologic roles as diverse as regulation of expansion of erythroid lineage cells (Epo) and megakaryocytes (Tpo) and regulation of physiologic mechanisms affecting growth (GH), mammary gland development, and ovarian function during pregnancy (prolactin). The receptors for Epo, Tpo, GH, and prolactin are very related in protein sequence and likely evolved from a common progenitor. In addition to cytokines, the receptors for the IFNs are members of this family and are frequently referred to as type II cytokine receptors.

The cytokine receptors consist of related receptor chains of variable numbers that frequently have common chains. The structural homology includes four positionally conserved cysteine residues in the extracellular domain and a WSXWS motif located, normally, near the transmembrane domain. The simplest receptors consist of a single receptor chain that includes the Tpo, Epo, GH, and prolactin receptors. A number of cytokine receptors associated with regulation of the lymphoid lineages consist of unique receptor chains that associate with a common receptor γ chain. These cytokine receptors include the interleukin 2 (IL-2) receptor, which consists of an essential unique β chain, the common γ chain, and an α chain, which, curiously, does not have the conserved motifs associated with the other cytokine receptor chains but which can increase affinity of the receptor β/γ receptor complex for IL-2.

The crystal structures for several cytokine receptors complexed with ligands have been ascertained. The GH receptor structure was the first determined.[20] The structure was somewhat surprising in revealing that GH ligates the receptor through interaction with two different sites. The extracellular domains of the receptors consist of a tandem repeat of fibronectin type III–like modules, each containing the characteristic cysteines. The role of the WSXWS motif cannot be deduced from the structure. The structure of GH complexed to the prolactin receptor also has been determined.[21] This structure has remarkable similarity to that of the GH receptor, although the two receptors contain only 28% identical amino acids in the extracellular domain. The structure of the Epo receptor has been determined. This receptor is ligated with a peptide capable of activating receptor function.[22] Again, the structure emphasizes the remarkable similarity of the overall structure of the extracellular domain to the other cytokine receptors and shows that relatively few contacts are involved in binding of the peptide mimic. This finding led to the suggestion that activation of cytokine receptors may be accomplished by relatively small-molecule hormone mimics.

Despite the similarity of the extracellular domains, the cytokine receptors have cytoplasmic domains that vary considerably in both structure and size. The most disappointing observation has been that none of the receptors contain any obvious catalytic domains in the cytoplasmic domain; thus it is not apparent how these receptors might function. The only structural similarity has been limited to the membrane proximal domain and consists of what often is referred to as the *box 1* and *box 2 motifs.*[23] These motifs are very loosely defined. The box 1 "conserved" motif is limited to a pro, any amino acid, pro (PxP) motif. Irrespective of the limited conservation of the sequence, mutational analysis of this region of all the receptors examined has indicated that this region is essential for all receptor functions.

For all the cytokine receptor superfamily members, the consequence of ligand binding is induction of tyrosine phosphorylation of a variety of substrates. In all cases this tyrosine phosphorylation depends on the presence of one or more members of the four members of the Janus family of protein tyrosine kinases (Jaks) in the receptor complex.[24] Single-chain receptors, including Epo/Tpo/GH/prolactin associate specifically with Jak2. In the case of the IL-2 receptor family, the unique receptor chain associates with Jak1, whereas the common γ chain associates with Jak3. The IL-6 receptor family associates with Jak1, and the fourth Jak family member (Tyk2) participates only in the IFN-α/β and IL-12 receptor complexes. In all cases, ligation of the receptor complex results in transphosphorylation of receptor-associated kinases on sites within the activation loop of the kinase domain, the result being activation of kinase activity. The essential role of the Jak kinases in cytokine receptor signaling has been most dramatically illustrated by derivation of mouse strains lacking individual or multiple members. The absence of specific Jaks results in loss of function of specific subsets of cytokine receptors with which Jaks associate. For example, in the absence of Jak2, Epo receptor function is completely lost, and absence of either Jak1 or Jak3 results in loss of function of the IL-2 receptor family members. Naturally occurring deficiencies of Jak3 exist in humans and result in varying degrees of severe combined immunodeficiency resulting from loss of function of receptors for IL-7 and IL-2, among others. In contrast to the essential role of these kinases in cytokine receptor signaling, activation in the context of other receptor systems is not critical.

Activation of Jaks after ligation of the receptors results in tyrosine phosphorylation of a number of sites on the receptor. As with all receptor systems that entail tyrosine phosphorylation, additional substrates are recruited to the complex through interaction between PTB domains (SH2 and protein tyrosine kinase domains) and specific sites. Through recruitment of proteins to the receptor complex, a variety of shared intracellular pathways are activated (see later). For example, both phospholipase C γ1 (PLC-γ1) and PLC-γ2 are recruited to most cytokine receptor complexes. In addition, the adapter protein Shc is recruited and initiates a series of protein interactions and phosphorylations that ultimately result in activation of mitogen-activated protein kinases (MAPKs). Most receptors also recruit the regulatory subunit of the phosphatidylinositol 3-kinase (PI3K) complex p85 and thereby recruit active PI3K activity to receptor-associated membrane sites (see later). All cytokine receptors recruit and activate one or more members of the Stat family of transcriptional factors. The specificity for recruitment and activation of Stats by individual cytokines depends on sites of tyrosine phosphorylation on the receptor. Although the concept is well established that receptor tyrosine phosphorylation is essential for initiation of much intracellular signaling, it is less clear that activation of the pathways, in some settings, is physiologically necessary. For example, mutant mouse strains have been developed that have truncated Epo receptors that contain only half of the cytoplasmic domain and no tyrosines.[25] It was certainly unexpected that substantial loss of cytoplasmic domain and absence of tyrosines would have no consequences for receptor function.

A major family of proteins regulating cytokine signaling is the suppressor of cytokine signaling (SOCS) proteins.[26] The family consists of structurally related proteins that contain a central SH2 domain and a carboxyl-terminal shared domain referred to as the *SOCS box.* The SH2 domains target the various family members to sites of tyrosine phosphorylation on the receptor or to sites of tyrosine phosphorylation of the receptor-associated Jak kinases. The SOCS box interacts with the elongin B/C complex and thereby is hypothesized to mediate ubiquitination and degradation of the targeted protein.[27] From results of the first studies of the proteins it was speculated that binding and potential targeting for degradation were important in downregulating signaling. This concept has been supported by the phenotypic consequences of deletion of one or more of the family members. For example, within 3 weeks after birth, mice lacking SOCS1 die of a complex pathologic condition that results from inability to suppress IFN-γ signaling. The perinatal lethality can be spared by placing the SOCS1 deficiency on an IFN-γ deficiency.[28,29] Similarly, deletion of SOCS3 produces embryonic lethality due to loss of negative regulation of leukemia inhibitory factor (LIF) signaling in trophoblasts of the placenta.[30,31] In contrast, deletions of other family members have caused no phenotypic changes (CIS) or have more subtle consequences (SOCS2, SOCS6).[32,33] The remarkably different phenotypes and extent of physiologic relevance of the SOCS family members emphasize the need to establish early in studies of gene function the consequences of deleting the gene.

Fc Receptor Signaling

A large group of structurally and functionally related receptors include the antigen-specific receptors on T and B cells that are referred to as the *Fc receptor family.*[34–38] In addition to antigen-specific receptors, this family includes such diverse receptors as the collagen receptor on platelets, receptors for Fc domains of immunoglobulins on a variety of cells, and the receptors used by natural killer (NK) cells. As with all tyrosine kinase–based receptor systems, the function of ligand is to drive aggregation of the receptor complex and allow activation of receptor-associated kinases. In the case of the Fc receptor family, the ligand-induced receptor complex contains a number of components and often is referred to as a *signalsome.* The inherent nature of the complex is almost identical among the various receptor complexes, the diversity largely due to use of different family members of the proteins composing the complex. One of the most important functional consequences of receptor complex activation is induction of a calcium flux that activates a variety of cellular responses.

Initiation of tyrosine phosphorylation in Fc receptor complexes depends on ligand-mediated aggregation of the receptor complex and initial activation of an Src family member protein kinase.[39] In T-cell receptors, Lck associates with the receptor complex, and Lyn is involved in B-cell receptor signaling. Activation also depends on the presence of members of the Tec family of protein tyrosine kinases, including Btk in B-cell receptor complexes and the family members Rlk and Itk redundantly in the case of the T-cell receptor.[40,41] As a consequence of kinase activation, sites are phosphorylated on the receptor chains or receptor-associated chains. Many receptor complexes contain related sites of phosphorylation that are referred to as *immunoreceptor tyrosine-based activation domains*

(ITAMs) or *immunoreceptor tyrosine-based inhibitory domains* (ITIMs).[42,43] Phosphorylation of ITIM sequences is associated with recruitment of SH2 domain–containing tyrosine phosphatases and downregulation of the receptor complex. ITAMs recruit SH2 domain–containing adapter proteins that further coordinate assembly of an activated receptor complex.

Essential additional kinases recruited to the complex are structurally related kinases ZAP-70 in the case of the T-cell receptor complex and Syk in the case of the B-cell receptor complex, as well as other Fc receptor complexes[44,45] (Fig. 2-2). The essential role of each of these kinases in receptor function has been established through derivation of mouse strains deficient in each of the kinases. In addition, a form of hypogammaglobulinemia in humans is associated with mutations in Btk. One of the key consequences of activation of tyrosine phosphorylation is recruitment and tyrosine phosphorylation of an adapter protein. In the case of the B-cell receptor complex, the adapter protein is Slp56 (also called *BLNK*),[46,47] and in the case of the T-cell receptor complex, the adapter protein is Slp76.[48] Recruitment and phosphorylation of these adapter proteins is essential for subsequent recruitment and activation of PLC-γ1 in T-cell receptors and PLC-γ2 in B-cell receptors and other Fc receptor complexes (see Fig. 2-2). Recruitment depends on interaction between the SH2 domains of the enzymes and sites of phosphorylation on the adapter proteins. It is

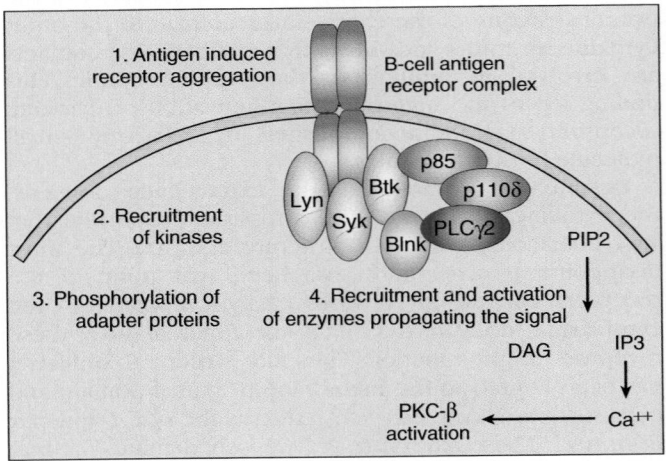

Figure 2-2. Intracellular signaling from the B-cell receptor complex. Engagement of the B-cell receptor by ligands initiates formation of a receptor complex critical to propagation of a cellular response. The first events after ligand binding are recruitment and activation of tyrosine kinases of at least three distinct families (Lyn, Syk, Btk). The activated kinases phosphorylate adapter proteins, such as BLNK and p85, that recruit enzymes that including phosphatidylinositol 3-kinase p110δ and phospholipase C γ2 (PLCγ2). The complex is assembled through protein interactions mediated by interaction between SH2 domains and sites of tyrosine phosphorylation and interaction between pleckstrin homology (PH) domains and sites of membrane lipid phosphorylation. The ultimate function of the complex is generation of diacylglycerol (DG) and inositol 1,4,5-triphosphate (IP3), which activate protein kinase Cβ (PKC-β). The result is activation of a variety of downstream signaling pathways. PIP2, phosphatidylinositol 4,5-bisphosphate.

hypothesized that tyrosine phosphorylation of the enzymes also may be required for functional activation.

Formation of a stable, activated receptor complex depends on membrane modifications, including phosphorylation of the 3′ hydroxyl on phosphatidylinositol (PI). In the case of the B-cell receptor complex, the kinase responsible for PI phosphorylation is p110δ, which is recruited to the complex by the adapter-regulatory subunit p85 through interaction between its SH2 domain and sites of phosphorylation in the receptor complex. Genetic deletion of either p85 or p110δ dramatically reduces receptor-induced signaling.[49] Phosphorylation of the 3′ site of inositol creates a binding site for pleckstrin homology (PH) domains. In the context of the Fc receptor family members, this process produces membrane docking sites for both Btk and p110δ, both of which contain PH domains essential for function in the context of the receptor complex. Conversely, the lipid phosphatase and tensin homologue (PTEN) specifically dephosphorylates the 3′ inositol site and is essential to ultimate disassembly of the receptor complex.

After recruitment and activation, PLC-γ1 or PLC-γ2 hydrolyzes membrane lipids, and this process releases inositol 1,4,5-triphosphate (IP$_3$) and diacylglycerol (DAG). The IP$_3$ generated interacts with its intracellular receptor to promote calcium release from endogenous stores. DAG and calcium then activate members of the protein kinase C (PKC) family of serine/threonine kinases. The essential PKC in the case of the B-cell receptor is the classic PKC-β1, whereas in T cells the critical family member is nontypical PKC-θ. The consequences of activation of PKCs in intracellular signaling are likely to be many, although one consequence is activation of a kinase complex involved with regulation of the transcription factors of the NF-κB family (see later). In T cells, activation of calcium flux is critical for activation of a sequence of events that regulates members of the NFAT family of transcription factors.

Integrin Signaling

Sensing the environment has been an essential capability of cells throughout evolution. The possibility that cell adhesion might be important in regulating cell behavior first came from studies of tumor cells. Subsequently, regulation of a number of cellular responses has been shown to be mediated through recognition of the extracellular environment and specifically through receptor-mediated recognition of extracellular matrix proteins. This recognition is provided through a family of integrin receptors that consist of a core recognition unit containing one of 8 β subunits associated with one of 18 α subunits, giving rise to at least 24 distinct integrin receptors.[50] The integrins are unique in their linkage to the actin-based microfilament system and thereby their ability to control cellular properties, such as membrane motion, cellular movement, and cell adherence. The integrin receptors are unique in their bidirectional regulation. Intracellular signaling events can modify integrin receptor structure to allow the receptor to recognize ligand. Conversely, ligand binding initiates cellular signaling events that control a variety of cellular responses. Integrin-regulated events have been shown or proposed to contribute to many of the altered properties of tumors cells.[51]

As with many receptor systems, the initial consequences of ligand binding are a change in receptor structure and, in the case of the integrins, induction of clustering. The clustered integrins rapidly recruit the tyrosine kinase focal adhesion kinase (FAK) that becomes activated by transphosphorylation of an activation-loop tyrosine and goes on to phosphorylate a number of additionally recruited substrates. FAK is a widely expressed kinase that is evolutionarily conserved and is related to the FAK-related kinase proline-rich tyrosine kinase 2 (PYK2). Recruitment of FAK requires a unique carboxyl-terminal domain termed the *focal adhesion targeting domain* (FAT domain), which interacts with the focal adhesion complex component paxillin, which binds directly to the cytoplasmic domains of integrin receptors. Once recruited to the complex and tyrosine phosphorylated, c-*src* is recruited to the sites of FAK tyrosine phosphorylation through SH2 domain interactions. Deletion of either FAK[52] or paxillin[53] results in an embryonic lethal phenotype associated with defects in cell migration consistent with their proposed roles. Interestingly, PYK2 has a much more restricted role in vivo and functions primarily in macrophage and B-cell migration.[54]

As with almost all receptor complexes containing or recruiting tyrosine protein kinases, the integrin receptor complexes recruit a number of adapter/linker proteins that couple to activation of shared pathways. For example, PI3K, PLCγ, Shc, Grb2, and Grb7 are recruited through SH2 interactions. The result is activation of pathways that affect cell survival and promote cell growth. Of particular importance to integrin receptor systems is the ability to regulate activity of the Rho family of small guanosine triphosphatases (GTPases), including Rho, Cdc42, and Rac, all of which play critical roles in formation and organization of cortical actin networks in cells. Although the precise details of activation are still being investigated, some participants are emerging. For example, activation of Rac, a critical event promoting cell migration, depends on FAK/Src recruitment and tyrosine phosphorylation of an adapter protein, Cas, that recruits Crk, which is required for recruitment of Dock180. Experimental evidence suggests that Dock180 directly increases guanosine triphosphate (GTP)-bound Rac. Paxillin, in addition to recruiting FAK, recruits p21-activated kinase (PAK), adapter protein Nck, and members of the Cdc42/Rac GTP exchange factors (PIX/Cool), which further contribute to membrane changes.

SIGNALING PATHWAYS ACTIVATED BY TYROSINE KINASE–BASED RECEPTOR SYSTEMS

All receptor-signaling systems that activate tyrosine phosphorylation function in signal transduction with similar mechanisms and frequently use similar signaling pathways. The central concept is recruitment of appropriate substrates to the receptor complex through interaction of phosphotyrosine recognition domains with sites of tyrosine phosphorylation on the activated kinase receptor chains or adapter proteins recruited to the complex and tyrosine phosphorylated. This interaction may occur through SH2 domains, which bind phosphotyrosine with a specificity defined by the amino acid sequence 1 to 6 residues carboxyl to the phosphotyrosine or through PTB domains, which bind phosphotyrosine, the specificity being defined by the amino acid sequence 3 to 5 residues amino-terminal of phosphotyrosine. In addition, many proteins recruited to receptor complexes contain additional domains that help recruit or stabilize the proteins within the complex or play a role in activation. In particular, proteins may be myristylated to facilitate membrane localization or may contain a transmembrane domain that targets them to the membrane. Many proteins recruited to receptor complexes contain PH domains that specifically recognize the 3′ phosphate site of membrane-localized phosphatidylinositol (3,4,5) triphosphate [PI(3,4,5)P$_3$]. This presence of a 3′ binding site is highly regulated through recruitment of the kinases responsible for phosphorylation as well as the phosphatase (PTEN) that dephosphorylates the site (see later).

Signal Transducers and Activators of Transcription

Members of the signal transducers and activators of transcription (Stat) family of proteins are primarily involved in mediating the biologic affects of the cytokine receptors but also are frequently found to be activated in the context of other receptor systems that rely on tyrosine phosphorylation. The family consists of seven members localized at three chromosomal loci: Stat1, Stat4 (chromosome 1), Stat2, Stat6, and Stat3 and two highly related genes encoding Stat5a and Stat5b. The Stats contain an essential carboxyl-region SH2 domain that defines the specificity with which a particular cytokine receptor complex recruits the protein into the complex. In the case of cytokine receptor systems, recruitment is invariably directed by sites of tyrosine phosphorylation on the receptor chains, whereas receptor tyrosine kinases recruit Stats through sites of tyrosine phosphorylation outside the kinase domain. Once recruited to the complex, Stats are tyrosine phosphorylated at a critical site carboxyl to the SH2 domain. In a remarkable and unique manner, these sites of tyrosine phosphorylation are recognized by the Stat SH2 domain to allow stable formation of a homodimer or heterodimer, the structure of which has been determined.[55,56] Dimerization depends on sequences in the amino-terminal domain. Once dimerized, the Stat is translocated to the nucleus by an unknown mechanism and, as a dimer, can bind a unique DNA sequence specific for each Stat to activate gene transcription. In some cases, activity of the activated Stats can be further enhanced by serine phosphorylation in the carboxyl-terminal, transactivation domain.

The biologic functions of the Stats have been defined through derivation of mouse strains lacking individual as well as multiple family members (reviewed in 3). Results of these studies have indicated that individual Stats play remarkably specific roles in mediating the function of cytokines. For example, Stat1-deficient mice are viable and overtly normal. However, their ability to respond to IFNs is almost completely eliminated. The result is extreme sensitivity to viral infections and exhibition of an increased rate of tumor induction, presumably due to loss of the tumor surveillance associated with IFNs. Deletion of either Stat4 or Stat6 similarly does not cause any loss of viability, but the functions of IL-4 and IL-6 in modifying immune responses are completely lost. Stat5a and Stat5b play essential roles in the physiologic mechanisms of GH and prolactin. In this regard, absence of Stat5a and Stat5b phenocopies deletions of the GH and prolactin receptors. In addition, Stat5a and Stat5b are essential for peripheral T-cell function and for more subtle functions of stem cells.

A number of studies have described constitutive activation of one or more Stat family members in tumors. On the basis of these observations, it has been proposed that activation of Stats can contribute to transformation or malignant progression.[57] However, constitutive activation in a fraction of tumors does not ensure that activation has relevance to transformation. For example, Stat5a and Stat5b are constitutively activated in chronic myeloid leukemia (CML) or tumors induced with the Bcr-Abl fusion kinase associated with CML.[58] However, studies with Stat5a/b-deficient mice have shown that the ability of Bcr-Abl to cause transformation of B-cell lineage cells is independent of Stat5a/b.[59] This finding does not imply, however, that Stat5a/b might not be critical in some forms of tumors. Induction of a myeloproliferative disease by another fusion kinase, Tel-Jak2, does require Stat5a/b, and this requirement is the result of induced expression of the cytokine oncostatin M by activated Stat5a/b.[60] These examples demonstrate the unique ability of gene deletions in mice to establish, or negate, the role of suspected genes in tumorigenesis.

Adapter Proteins in Tyrosine Phosphorylation–Based Signaling

One of the common features in signal transduction from receptor complexes that use protein tyrosine phosphorylation is the participation of adapter proteins. Adapter proteins can be present in the receptor complex or recruited to the receptor complex through interactions with receptor chains. As a consequence of receptor activation, adapter proteins are frequently highly phosphorylated and play an essential role in recruiting or activating the next step in the signaling pathways. Although frequently identified in the context of a specific receptor system, most adapter proteins also are found to be present in a variety of receptor systems. Essential to understanding the roles of individual adapters has been the derivation of mutant strains of mice lacking the genes. Such studies have frequently shown that physiologically significant participation may occur in only a subset of receptor systems in which the genes are present. The following examples illustrate the common properties as well as the unique functional specificity that exists.

The Adapter Protein Shc and Coupling to Ras Activation

One of the first adapter proteins identified was Shc. This protein was isolated in a search for novel SH2 domain–containing proteins.[61] There are three mammalian Shc family members, ShcA, ShcB, and ShcC. All have a carboxyl SH2 domain and an amino-terminal PTB domain. Importantly, the PTB domain of the Shc proteins is structurally similar to that of PH domains and, like PH domains, binds phosphoinositols. The central region contains a domain that is tyrosine phosphorylated and becomes a docking site for the Grb2:Sos complex. The model that has emerged from a variety of studies is that various receptors recruit Shc to the complex, where it becomes tyrosine phosphorylated and recruits the Grb2:Sos complex by recognition of phosphotyrosines on Shc by the SH2 domain of Grb2. Formation of the complex and possibly recruitment of the complex to the membrane result in activation of guanine nucleotide exchange factor activity of Sos and thereby an increase in the amount of GTP-Ras. The physiologic requirements for the Shc proteins have been addressed in derivation of mutant strains of mice lacking one or more proteins. Strikingly, deletion of ShcB or ShcC, either alone or combined, has a subtle phenotype that consists of a loss of survival of specific subsets of neurons unique for each family member.[62] In contrast, deletion of ShcA results in an embryonic lethal phenotype that includes defects in cardiovascular development and may have roles in other lineages.[63]

Insulin Response Substrates: Adapters Critical for Insulin Signaling

The insulin response substrates (IRS-1, IRS-2, IRS-3, and IRS-4) were initially identified as substrates of tyrosine phosphorylation mediated by the insulin receptor and are typical receptor adapter proteins.[64,65] Although these substrates were identified in the context of insulin signaling, studies have shown they are substrates of tyrosine phosphorylation in the context of many tyrosine kinase–based receptor systems. All the IRS proteins contain an amino-terminal PH domain and an adjacent PTB domain and function as classic adapter proteins in recruiting a variety of signaling proteins to receptor complexes through multiple sites of tyrosine phosphorylation. The critical role of IRS-1 and IRS-2 in insulin responses and growth in general has been well established through derivation of mice lacking one or both of the genes. In particular, deletion of *IRS-2* results in subtle growth reduction and impaired peripheral insulin signaling and pancreatic β-cell function.[66] Deletion of *IRS-1* results in severe growth reduction.[67,68] Mice containing haploinsufficiency of each gene on an insufficiency of the second gene give partial responses consistent with the existence of both unique and overlapping functions. Although the gene deletions have nicely substantiated the roles of IRS-1 and IRS-2 in insulin and insulin-like growth factor signaling, a potential essential role in the context of other receptor systems in which IRS proteins are phosphorylated has not been evident.

The Gab Family of Adapter Proteins

The Gab family of adapter proteins similarly contains an amino-terminal PH domain and is found to be inducibly tyrosine phosphorylated in the context of many tyrosine phosphorylation-based receptor systems.[69,70] To date, three family members have been identified—Gab1, Gab2, and Gab3—all of which uniquely also contain proline-rich domains that can serve as a binding domain for SH3 domain–containing proteins. Each family member has a distinct pattern of unique and overlapping sites of expression. As with most adapters, sites of tyrosine phosphorylation on the Gab proteins are associated with activation of PI3K activity by recruitment of p85, recruitment of SHP2 (Src homology protein tyrosine phosphatase 2), and recruitment of other adapter proteins, including Crk. Deletion of Gab1 results in an embryonic lethal phenotype, and cells lacking Gab1 have reduced MAPK activation in response to epidermal growth factor (EGF) or platelet-derived growth factor (PDGF). In contrast, deletion of Gab2 results in a much more subtle change in phenotype, consisting of impaired allergic reactions as a consequence of defects in immunoglobulin E receptor signaling.

Dok Adapter Proteins

The Dok family consists of three closely related mammalian genes—Dok-1, Dok-2, and Dok-3—and two more distantly related proteins Dok-4 and Dok-5.[71-74] The initial family member was identified as a highly tyrosine-phosphorylated protein in CML cells that associated with the negative regulator of Ras signaling, RasGAP. It later was found that Dok proteins are inducibly tyrosine phosphorylated in the context of a variety of receptor systems. The proteins have a PH domain at the amino terminus that is followed by a PTB domain. Tyrosine phosphorylation occurs at numerous sites at the carboxyl terminus. Several studies have shown that the Dok family members negatively regulate signaling through a variety of receptors, including several members of the Fc receptor superfamily.

FRS2 Proteins as Adapter Proteins

The adapter protein FRS2α was identified in the context of signaling through the fibroblast growth factor (FGF) and is somewhat different among the adapter proteins in using myristylation at the amino terminus and a PTB domain to recruit the protein to membrane-localized receptor complexes.[75] The family currently consists of two members, FRS2α and FRS2β. However, as with all adapter proteins, tyrosine phosphorylation occurs at multiple sites on the protein that serve as docking sites for downstream activators of signaling pathways. Deletion of the *Frs2α* gene in mice results in early embryonic lethality consistent with the hypothesis that this gene plays a critical role in FGF signaling. Cells lacking FRS2α are defective in a specific subset of signaling events associated with FGF, including MAPK activation and PI3K activation, which contribute to cellular defects in chemotactic responses and cell proliferation. Interesting functions, such as recruitment of Shc or PLC-γ1, are not affected. Chemotaxis and proliferation in response to EGF or PDGF also are not affected. These findings demonstrate the often remarkable specificity of adapter proteins in individual receptor complexes in activation of specific pathways.

Vav Adapters as Critical Regulators of T- and B-Cell Signaling

Vav-1 was initially identified by the ability of a fusion protein containing Vav-1 to induce transformation of fibroblasts in cell culture. Soon thereafter it was shown that Vav-1 becomes highly tryosine phosphorylated in the context of a wide variety of receptors.[76–78] Recruitment of Vav to receptor complexes is mediated by an SH2 domain essential to Vav function. However, like most adapter proteins, Vav proteins also contain a PH domain and SH3 domains. The three highly related mammalian family members, Vav-1, Vav-2, and Vav-3, belong to a larger family of approximately 40 Dbl proteins characterized functionally as guanine-nucleotide exchange factors for the Rho family of small GTPases. Although Vav adapters are activated in the context of a variety of receptor systems, mice lacking individual or combinations of Vav family members have shown that these substances have an essential role in signaling from T- or B-cell receptors. Deletion of Vav-1 results in severe impairment of T-cell development and function, whereas deletion of Vav-2 results in slight impairment of T-cell function. However, both B-cell function and T-cell function are severely affected in mice lacking both Vav-1 and Vav-2. Although the precise functions of Vav in the context of T-cell and B-cell receptors is not known, absence of either affects the extent to which receptor engagement induces calcium flux, a known critical event in receptor signaling. Because of similarities between Vav deficiency and deficiency of other components of the T/B-cell receptor signalosomes, it has been proposed that Vav functions to stabilize the complexes.

Fc Receptor Superfamily Adapter Proteins

Members of the Fc receptor superfamily use a number of very specific adapter proteins. In the context of the T-cell receptor, the adapter proteins SLP-76 (SH2 domain containing leukocyte phosphoprotein of 76 kd) and LAT (linker for activation of T cells) are essential for efficient receptor signaling. Deletion of either gene in mice results in profound loss of T-cell receptor signaling.[79,80] SLP-76 is recruited to the receptor complex through SH2 domains. LAT is localized in the receptor complex by membrane targeting the protein with a transmembrane domain. In many Fc receptors, including the B-cell immunoglobulin receptor, the adapter protein BLNK, also called *SLP-56* to denote its similarity to SLP-76, plays an essential, non-redundant role. Importantly, BLNK is one of the few adapter proteins that has been shown to be mutated in humans and associated with pathologic processes.[47] In all cases, these adapter proteins are required for formation of a functional signalosome that can couple receptor

engagement to the induction of calcium flux and are specifically proposed to be required for recruitment of PLC-γ1 and PLC-γ2 to the receptor complex.

Formation of a functional receptor complex often requires participation of adapter proteins, which function in various ways. In some cases, adapter proteins play an essential role in forming or stabilizing the receptor complex, in essence providing glue to hold the complex together. In many cases, however, adapter proteins are needed to provide binding sites for recruitment of additional receptor components, allowing activation of specific pathways. Perhaps because of the natural membrane localization of adapter proteins, potential to be recruited to the membrane, and proximity to multiple receptors, recruitment and tyrosine phosphorylation of adapter proteins is promiscuous. Consequently, the ability to be recruited or phosphorylated in the context of a specific receptor cannot be used to imply an essential role. Fortunately, most of the genes for adapter proteins have been deleted in mice, and deletion mutants can frequently be used to critically address physiologic significance.

Tyrosine Phosphatases in Receptor Signaling

As might be predicted from the critical role of tyrosine phosphorylation in initiating and propagating intracellular signaling, tyrosine phosphatases play an equally important role in controlling the activity of tyrosine phosphorylation–based receptor systems. Tyrosine phosphatases share a structurally conserved protein tyrosine phosphatase catalytic domain. These phosphatases typically have been subdivided into three groups, including the classic phosphatases, the dual-specificity phosphatases, and the low-molecular-weight phosphatases. Among the classic protein tyrosine phosphatases, 37 distinct mammalian genes have been identified that can be further divided into 17 subtypes on the basis of catalytic domain structure. Approximately half of these enzymes are cytoplasmic; the others are membrane-associated phosphatases. Curiously, a number of the membrane-associated phosphatases contain two catalytic domains. As illustrated by the following examples, tyrosine phosphatases have been found to play critical roles in both negative and positive regulation of intracellular signaling.

The two phosphatases that have been consistently implicated in signal transduction through tyrosine kinase–based receptor systems are SHP-1 and SHP-2. Both enzymes contain a carboxyl-terminal catalytic domain and two amino-terminal SH2 domains. Both are recruited to a variety of receptor systems through recognition provided by the SH2 domain, most frequently involving the more amino-terminal SH2 domain. Binding in the receptor complex results in activation of the phosphatase activity of SHP-1. Through dephosphorylation of sites within the receptor complex, it has been speculated that down-regulation of the complex would occur. In the case of SHP-1, this model has been largely confirmed by characterization of a naturally occurring mutation of the gene in mice. Termed *motheaten*, this mutation is a protein null mutation. The phenotype is perinatal lethal, in which there is excessive proliferation of a variety of hematopoietic lineages, including macrophages, which can contribute to the lethal phenotype.[81,82] The phenotype is consistent with the concept that recruitment of SHP-1 to a variety of receptor complexes is critical in downregulation.

The role of SHP-2 in intracellular signaling is hypothesized to be a positive mediator of signaling rather than a negative mediator. Detailed structural studies are available for SHP-2 that provide insights into its regulation.[83] The structure has revealed that the amino-terminal SH2 domain binds intramolecularly to the catalytic domain and blocks the phosphatase active site. Binding to a site of tyrosine phosphorylation by the amino-terminal SH2 domain releases this inhibition and stimulates phosphatase catalytic activity approximately 10-fold. Further binding to the second SH2 domain increases catalytic activity 100-fold. Although studies have shown an essential role for enzymatic activity in signaling, precisely what substrates are involved, particularly the role of SHP-2 in activation of the MAPK pathway, has not been determined. An essential role in signaling is evident from the embryonic lethality associated with deletion of the gene. Developmental defects are numerous, but midgestation lethality is associated with defects in mesodermal patterning and body organization.[84]

One of the first transmembrane protein tyrosine phosphatases identified was CD45, a phosphatase highly expressed on all hematopoietic cells.[85] Studies of the precise functions and targets of CD45 illustrate some of the difficulties in studying enzymes that might function quite differently in different cells and in the context of different receptor systems. Deletion of CD45 has its major effect on T cells. The consequences include defects in early thymic development, substantial reduction in positive selection, and lesser consequences in negative selection. Downstream signaling from the T-cell receptor complex is compromised. Although there are subtle effects of CD45 deletion on B-cell function, signaling downstream of the B-cell complex is less affected. In T cells, the altered phenotypes can be directly related to loss of dephosphorylation of the negative regulatory site of the Src kinase Lck. In particular, the defects can be corrected by transgenic expression of an Lck mutated at the Y^{505} regulatory site. In addition, CD45 can dephosphorylate the activation loop site of Lck to reduce kinase activity. Studies have indicated that CD45 also may function as a Jak tyrosine kinase phosphatase and thereby negatively regulate cytokine receptor signaling.

The Phospholipid Cycle

A variety of receptor systems couple into membrane modifications that are key to intracellular signaling. An interest in these modifications arose with the demonstration that PIK activity existed in a transforming complex containing polyoma middle T and c-*src*. The critical modifications involve phosphorylation-dephosphorylation of inositol-containing lipids. Phosphatidylinositol 3-phosphate (PI3P) is constitutively present in cell membranes. However, the 3,4 and 3,4,5 phosphorylated forms are normally at very low levels but can be rapidly produced in response to a variety of growth factors and can play essential roles in intracellular signaling. Modification of PI is mediated by a series of enzymes that have specificity for the site and substrate and are grouped into three classes.[86,87] A single enzyme (Vps34p) constitutes the class III PI3Ks and is primarily involved in generation of PI3P, which plays an essential role in membrane trafficking to the lysosome. The activity or membrane localization of Vps34p is regulated by an associated serine threonine kinase, p150. The class II enzymes consist of three family members, PI3KCα, PI3KCβ, and PI3KCγ, and contain a conserved carboxyl terminal C2 domain that characterizes the family. Activity of these enzymes is largely restricted to phosphorylation of PI and PI4P.

Unlike class II and III enzymes, members of the class I family of enzymes have been consistently implicated in intracellular signaling. The family consists of four genes, *p110α*, *p110β*, *p110γ*, and *p110δ*. The gene *p110γ* functions in the context of heterotrimeric G-protein–coupled receptors. Through derivation of mice deficient in the enzyme, the function of *p110γ* has been shown to be critical for leukocyte function. The other three enzymes share an association with a regulatory subunit of 85 kd or 55 kd. In mammals three genes—*p85α* (which encodes proteins of 55 and 50 kd as well as the 85-kd isoform), *p85β*, and *p55γ*—encode regulatory subunits.[88] The regulatory subunits are proposed to regulate enzyme activity, but equally important, they contain two SH2 domains that target the enzymatic complex to the receptor complexes. In addition, *p85α* and *p85β* contain an N-terminal SH3 domain. The critical role of each component in signal transduction is illustrated by the striking, but often distinct, consequences of deleting the genes. For example, deletion of either *p110α* or *p110β* results in very early embryonic lethality due to severe proliferative defects in many tissues. The gene *p110γ*, in contrast to *p110α* and *p110β*, which are broadly expressed, is expressed primarily in hematopoietic cells. Deletion of *p110γ* in mice has demonstrated the essential, nonredundant role of this gene in signaling through the B-cell receptor complex. Disruption of the p85α gene results in a comparable defect in B-cell receptor signaling, indicating that the p85α/p110δ complex is uniquely critical for signaling through the B-cell receptor complex. This phenomenon is particularly striking when one considers that two of the critical components of the complex, Btk and PLC-γ2, contain PH domains known to be critical in signaling.

Another example of pathways activated after generation of PI(3,4)P$_2$ or PI(3,4,5)P$_3$ is cascades involving serine/threonine kinases. One central enzyme in this regard is phosphoinositide-dependent protein kinase 1 (PDK1).[89] PDK1 has both an N-terminal and a C-terminal PH domain that bind PI(3,4,5)P$_3$ with high affinity. Binding does not appear to alter the kinase activity of PDK1. Recruitment to the membrane brings PDK1 in contact with critical substrates activated by PDK1-dependent phosphorylation within the activation loop of their kinase domains. The substrates of PDK1 include many members of the AGC group of kinases. The critical role of PDK1 in activating several of these kinases, including Akt, S6-kinase, and ribosomal S6 kinase (RSK), has been demonstrated by use of embryonic stem cells deficient in PDK1. The embryonic stem cells grow normally, indicating that in this cell lineage, these pathways are not critical for cellular proliferation or survival. However, deletion of PDK1 results in an early embryonic lethal phenotype in which many cell lineages are dramatically affected.

One of the critical substrates of PDK1 is the kinase Akt (also called *PKB*). In mammals, the Akt family of kinases includes Akt1, Akt2, and Akt3, all of which are approximately 85% identical.[90,91] Akt1, as are other Akts, is recruited to the membrane through a PH domain and is activated by PDK1-dependent phosphorylation of Thr^{308} in the activation loop. Further phosphorylation occurs independently of PDK1 at Ser^{374} and results in full activation of kinase activity. Once activated, Akt1 phosphorylates a variety of proteins, including GSK3, BAD, mTOR, IRS-1, BRCA1, and members of the Forkhead family of transcription factors. A physiologic consequence of Akt activation is stimulation of protein synthesis, cell growth, and cell cycle progression. Although Akt has been implicated in a variety of fundamental cellular responses, derivation of mice lacking Akt1 or Akt2 has suggested very limited functions. Akt1-deficient mice are viable although smaller than wild-type animals. In contrast, Akt2-deficient mice are diabetic, establishing a critical role for this enzyme in insulin-dependent control of carbohydrate metabolism.

The critical role of PI3Ks in generating PH domain interacting sites and thereby allowing recruitment or stabilization of signaling complexes suggests that downregulation of the complexes might require dephosphorylation of the sites. Numerous studies have shown that the lipid phosphatase PTEN is a critical negative regulator of signaling.[92-94] PTEN specifically dephosphorylates the 3′ position of $PI(3,4,5)P_3$ and $PI(3,4)P_2$. Because PTEN is relatively constantly expressed and its activity is not regulated, formation of receptor complexes and recruitment of PH domain–containing proteins depend on the ability to overcome the constitutive activity of PTEN. The proposed role of PTEN is consistent with the phenotype of mice lacking PTEN or having reduced levels of PTEN activity. Loss of PTEN correlates with an increase in PI(3) derivatives in all cells that have been examined. More generally, complete loss of PTEN results in an embryonic lethal phenotype associated with gross developmental defects. Haploinsufficiency of PTEN results in a variety of phenotypes, including hyperproliferation of a variety of cell types, such as B cells, and leads to emergence of a variety of tumor types consistent with a role as a tumor suppressor gene.

In addition to PTEN, the PI phosphatases SHIP1 and SHIP2 have been implicated in intracellular signaling. *SHIP* is an acronym for SH2 domain–containing inositol-5-phosphatase.[95] These proteins contain an amino-terminal SH2 domain and two PTB domains and hydrolyze the 5′ position of $PI(3,4,5)P_3$. SHIP1 is primarily expressed in the hematopoietic lineages, whereas SHIP2 is more generally expressed. SHIP1 and SHIP2 are recruited to a variety of receptor complexes. Binding into the complex results in

activation of phosphatase activity. Although precisely how these enzymes link to signaling events is unknown, the consequences of their deletion in mice have remarkably distinct and specific affects. Deletion of SHIP1 leads to rapid perinatal death with massive myeloid cell infiltration in various tissues, including the lungs. In addition, the response of hematopoietic cells to cytokines is enhanced, consistent with a role of SHIP1 in negative regulation of signaling. In contrast, loss of SHIP2 leads to increased sensitivity to insulin and perinatal death consistent with a specific role of SHIP2 in negative regulation of signaling through the insulin receptor. Haploinsufficiency of SHIP2 is sufficient to cause increased sensitivity to insulin.

RECEPTOR SYSTEMS INDUCING SERINE/THREONINE PHOSPHORYLATION

Although used less than tyrosine phosphorylation as an initial biochemical response to initiate intracellular signaling, two notable receptor systems initiate signaling through activation of serine and threonine phosphorylation. The central properties are remarkably similar to the tyrosine phosphorylation–based receptor systems in that receptor aggregation results in recruitment or activation of kinases, and this activation is essential for propagation of all the downstream signaling events. The two families of receptors, however, function quite differently. The Toll/IL-1 receptors recruit a kinase to the complex and activate pathways used by a number of receptor systems. In contrast, the transforming growth factor β (TGF-β) receptor family consists of transmembrane proteins containing a kinase catalytic domain that functions primarily to activate members of the Smad family of transcriptional regulators.

Toll/Interleukin-1 Receptor Family Signaling

The receptor for IL-1 was the first receptor characterized as a member of what is now called the *Toll/IL-1 receptor family*.[96,97] The family currently consists of the receptors for IL-1 and IL-18 as well as six receptors termed *Toll-like receptors* (TLR1-6). Whereas the IL-1 and IL-18 receptors bind the cytokine ligands, the specificity of the Toll-related receptors is unknown, or the receptors bind distinct bacterial cell-wall components speculated to be important in innate immunity. *Drosophila* has a single receptor, Toll, related to the mammalian family from which the family name was derived. The *Drosophila* gene is critical for establishment of dorsoventral polarity during development and is involved in recognition of microorganisms. Irrespective of the binding specificity, activation of the receptors results in almost identical intracellular signaling events, which result in activation of the NF-κB and the c-Jun N-terminal kinases (JNKs). Activity of the receptor family depends on a domain of approximately 200 amino acids in the cytoplasmic domain containing three conserved boxes and termed the *TIR domain*.

The intracellular signaling mediated by the *Drosophila* Toll receptor has been extensively characterized and forms the paradigm for signaling by mammalian receptors. Critical to Toll signaling is recruitment of a receptor adapter protein called *Tube* and a serine/threonine kinase called *Pelle*. A consequence of receptor activation is activation of Dorsal, the fly homologue of the mammalian NF-κB family of transcription factors. The mammalian receptors similarly require an adapter protein, MyD88, which, on the basis of the phenotype of mice in which the gene was disrupted, is essential for receptor function. Another potentially important adapter protein associated with the complex is Tollip. The mammalian homologues of Pelle are the four members of the IRAK (IL-1 receptor–associated kinases) family of serine/threonine kinases (IRAK-1, IRAK-2, IRAK-M, IRAK-4). These kinases are characterized by an amino-terminal death domain (DD) and a centrally located kinase domain. The DD is critical for interaction with Myd88 and thereby targeting the kinase to the receptor complex.

The four Jak kinases play critical roles in specific subsets of cytokine receptors. Evolution of the mammalian IRAKs has taken a completely different course. Two of the kinases (IRAK-2 and IRAK-M) are catalytically inactive owing to mutation of a critical lysine in the ATP binding pocket. Moreover, deletion of IRAK-1 only reduces receptor function, and this reduction can be restored by a catalytically inactive IRAK-1 protein. However, deletion of IRAK-4 inactivates the activity of all the receptors.[98] The model that is emerging is one in which IRAK-4 is recruited to the complex and one of its functions is to phosphorylate IRAK-1. IRAK-1 serves as an adapter protein critical for recruitment of TRAF6 (tumor necrosis factor receptor–associated factor 6) into the complex. The essential role of TRAF6 in receptor signaling is evident from the phenotype of mice in which the gene has been deleted. The next series of events in signal propagation has not been ascertained. The primary consequences of signal transduction are activation of NF-κB and activation of the JNK and p38 family of kinases.

The Transforming Growth Factor-β Receptor Family and Smads in Intracellular Signaling

TGF-β was identified a number of years ago as a factor that could promote tumor cell growth. Since that time, it has become clear that the TGF-β factors (TGF-β1, 2, and 3) have both growth-promoting and growth-inhibiting functions, depending on cell lineage. Moreover, the TGF-β factors are members of a large family of approximately 30 related ligands that also includes the activins, inhibins, and bone morphogenetic proteins (BMPs). The members of the family play essential roles in regulating developmental events and contribute to systemic homeostasis.

The TGF-β family of receptors consists of membrane-spanning proteins containing a cytoplasmic serine/threonine kinase catalytic domain. The receptors mediate physiologic responses to a number of important ligands involved in development and to environmental changes associated with production of TGF-β. Curiously, although

TGF-β was initially identified as a tumor growth factor, the responses to TGF-β are highly cell line– and lineage-specific. Developmentally, the TGF-β receptor family members mediate responses to activins, inhibins, and BMPs. The TGF-β–related factors bind to receptors that consist of two distinct serine/threonine kinase domain–containing transmembrane proteins. Type I receptors are characterized by containing a glycine/serine-rich domain (GS domain) in the juxtamembranous region. Type II receptors do not contain this domain. Ligand initially binds to the type II receptor chain, and ligation allows recruitment of the type I receptor into the complex. The type II receptor phosphorylates the type I receptor in the GS domain and activates its catalytic activity. Mammals contain seven type I receptors, which can variably associate with one of the five type II receptors.[99]

The TGF-β receptor family has been reported to activate a number of pathways common to many receptor systems, including the MAPK/JNK/p38 pathways. However, most intracellular signaling mediated by the TGF-β receptor family can be accounted for by activation of members of the Smad family of transcription factors. Conversely, the Smad family members exclusively mediate the physiologic mechanisms associated with the TGF-β receptor family. Much like the Stat proteins, Smads mediate a membrane signal directly to the nucleus and mediate gene transcription. The term *Smad* is a fusion the names for related transcription factors identified in *Drosophila* (Mad, for "mothers against decapentaplegic") and *Caenorhabditis elegans* (Sma). The family consists of eight mammalian proteins of 40 to 60 kd that share a carboxyl-terminal homology domain referred to as the *MH2 domain*. The molecular structure of the MH2 domain of Smad4 has been determined.[100] In addition, several Smads contain a related amino-terminal domain that has DNA-binding activity and is referred to as the *MH1 domain*. The MH1 and MH2 domains are connected by a region called the *linker*.

The Smads have been divided into three functional groups. The R-Smads (Smad-1, -2, -3, -5, and -8) are receptor regulated through phosphorylation, confer receptor specificity, and contain an MH1 domain. The C-Smad (Smad-4) is a common Smad required for function of the R-Smads, as described later. The human Smad4 was initially identified as a tumor suppressor gene (DPC4) on chromosome 18q21.1 and is associated with pancreatic and possibly other human cancers.[101] Last, inhibitory Smads (Smad-6 and -7) suppress receptor signaling and are characterized by the absence of the MH1 domain. The MH1 domain has been shown to bind DNA, whereas the MH2 domain is required for transcriptional activation. The linker region contains sites of phosphorylation by MAPKs that are hypothesized to inhibit translocation to the nucleus and thus suppress TGF-β signaling.

Although not all the details of activation have been elucidated, a remarkably simple picture of intracellular signaling is emerging. The R-Smads are initially recruited to the receptor complex through interaction between a small domain in the carboxyl domain of the Smads and the receptor complex. Receptor recognition is defined by as little as a two-amino-acid difference in the domain.[102]

Once recruited to the receptor complex, Smads are directly phosphorylated by the type II receptor kinase and translocate to the nucleus and activate or, in some cases, suppress gene transcription.[99,103] Phosphorylation of the R-Smads occurs in the carboxyl terminal at a characteristic Ser-Ser-X-Ser motif. Translocation and transcriptional activation require association of the common Smad, Smad4, with the activated Smads. Smad4, unlike the other Smads, does not contain the Ser-Ser-X-Ser motif and has not been shown to be recruited into the receptor complex. Thus the model that is emerging is that pathway receptor–regulated Smads (1, 2, 3, 5, 9) are recruited to the receptor complex through their ability to recognize specific receptor complexes, are phosphorylated, and associate with the common mediator, Smad4, to translocate and regulate gene expression.

Inhibitory Smads have been identified and are characterized by the absence of the MH2 domain. These Smads often are induced by TGF-β signaling and are hypothesized to control the extent and duration of signaling. The mechanism of repression by Smad6 and Smad7 appears to involve binding to type I receptors and thereby interference with phosphorylation of receptor-specific Smads.[104,105] The inability of these Smads to dissociate from the receptor complex is speculated to be due to absence of the canonical phosphorylation site in the carboxyl terminus.

INTRACELLULAR SIGNALING BY THE FRIZZLED FAMILY OF RECEPTORS

The initial mammalian introduction to the Frizzled family of receptors started with identification of a transforming gene, *int-1*, associated with retrovirus-transduced mammary tumors.[106,107] The *int-1* gene was the mammalian homologue of a ligand termed *wingless* (Wnt) initially identified in *Drosophila*, and the receptor in Flys for Wnt was termed *Frizzled*. Since its initial description, a growing class of receptors related to Frizzled has been identified that mediate the physiologic responses for ligands of the Wnt family. The Frizzled receptors share an amino-terminal signal sequence followed by a domain of approximately 120 amino acids with an invariant pattern of 10 conserved cysteine residues. Following a seven membrane-spanning domain, all the receptors share conserved carboxyl-terminal cytoplasmic domains.

The participants in signal transduction through the Frizzled receptors have been identified both genetically and by biochemical studies.[108–110] The critical components include proteins related to the *Drosophila* gene *armadillo*. These components includes β-catenin in vertebrates, proteins related to the *Drosophila* gene product Disheveled, glycogen synthase kinase 3β (GSK-3β), and the tumor suppressor gene *adenomatous polyposis coli* (*APC*). β-Catenin normally exists in a complex with the tumor suppressor protein, APC, the protein Axin, and the kinase GSK-3β. The APC gene was initially identified as a gene that when mutated was associated with a familial adenomatous polyposis syndrome in which patients have large numbers of benign polyps of the colorectal epithelium

that progress to invasive tumors and metastasize. It was subsequently demonstrated that a number of colorectal tumors have both alleles deleted.[111] In the complex, the interaction between Axin, APC, and GSK-3β facilitates efficient phosphorylation of β-catenin. Phosphorylation of β-catenin marks the protein for degradation by ubiquitination and subsequent degradation by the proteosome. Engagement of the Frizzled receptors modifies the function of the complex through another protein termed *Disheveled* to inhibit GSK-3β function and thereby to allow accumulation and nuclear translocation of β-catenin.

The target proteins for β-catenin are the family of four mammalian high-mobility group (HMG) domains containing DNA-binding proteins: Lef-1 (lymphoid enhancer factor), Tcf-1 (T-cell factor), Tcf-3, and Tcf-4. These proteins are the mammalian homologues of the single *Drosophila* Tcf gene.[112] Binding of β-catenin to an amino-terminal domain enables these DNA-binding proteins to activate gene transcription. In the absence of β-catenin, the proteins can suppress gene expression. The essential role of TCFs in gene regulation is evident from the phenotypes of mice in which individual and multiple family members have been deleted. Lef-1–deficient mice have multiple developmental defects, including hair follicle, tooth, and mammary gland defects. Loss of Tcf-1 affects T-cell development, whereas absence of Tcf-4 causes defects in proliferation of the epithelial cells of the colon. The latter is of particular importance, because loss of APC and thus increasing levels of β-catenin and Tcf-4 activity are associated with increased proliferation of these cells.

The foregoing process represents what is commonly referred to as the *canonical Wnt intracellular signaling pathway*. However, GSK-3β activity and β-catenin stability may be regulated by other pathways in less-defined ways. In addition, Wnt signaling involves β-catenin/Tcf-independent signaling pathways. In particular, the Frizzled receptors may function very similarly to G-coupled receptors. For example, studies have shown that some members of the receptor superfamily can stimulate PI signaling through a conventional heterotrimeric G-protein complex.[113] The ability to activate Gβγ and Gα subunits suggests that these receptors could couple Wnt binding to activation of a number of additional pathways, including activation of PKCs through a calcium-dependent pathway. Consistent with this hypothesis, Wnt signaling has been implicated in activation of the NFAT transcription factors through a calcineurin-dependent pathway. Details of this pathway are described later. Wnt signaling also has been implicated in activation of Rho GTPases and JNKs.[114]

NOTCH RECEPTOR SIGNALING

Introduction to the mammalian Notch receptor family started with demonstration that the chromosomal translocation t(7;9)(q34;q34.3) in T-cell lymphoblastic leukemia involves fusion of the T-cell receptor β locus with the cytoplasmic domain of a mammalian Notch homologue, now referred to as the *mammalian Notch1 gene.*[115] Before identification in mammals, the family was identified in *Drosophila,* in which it is involved in cell-fate decisions during differentiation.[116] Three additional mammalian family members have been identified— Notch2, Notch3, and Notch4. Notch1 also is activated in thymic lymphoma by retroviral insertions.[117] Notch2 has been implicated in feline leukemia virus–induced lymphoma, and Notch4 was identified as the gene associated with a common mammary tumor virus integration site in tumors (Int3). Notch3 has been implicated in a hereditary, adult-onset condition causing stroke and dementia.[118]

The Notch receptors are large transmembrane proteins of approximately 300 kd that contain 36 tandem EGF-like repeats and three repeats of a motif called the *Lin-12 repeat* in the extracellular domain. The cytoplasmic domain characteristically consists of a number of ankyrin-like repeats, a glutamine-rich domain, and a region rich in glutamine, serine, and threonines, the *PEST domain.* Transformation of various cell types by Notch family members is associated with overexpression of the cytoplasmic domain. The ligands for the mammalian Notch receptors include Delta; Delta-like1, 3, and 4; and Jagged1 and 2. The ligands contain several unique motifs and properties. The amino terminal contains a signal peptide followed by a novel motif shared with the *Drosophila* serrate (DSL) and 16 EGF-like repeats comparable with those in the receptors. The extracellular portion contains a cysteine-rich domain followed by the transmembrane domain. The cytoplasmic domain consists of approximately 130 amino acids without distinguishing motifs. Both Jagged1 and Jagged2 are expressed in a variety of tissues. The cell membrane association of the ligands and the existence of a relatively large cytoplasmic domain suggest the interesting possibility that the ligand may also initiate intracellular signaling events.

The Notch receptors are speculated to signal by a unique mechanism. Ligand binding is proposed to induce intracellular cleavage, releasing the cytoplasmic domain. This domain translocates the nucleus and regulates gene transcription through its interaction with a DNA-binding protein variably termed *RBP-Jκ* (recombination signal sequence binding protein for Jκ genes), CBF1 (C-promoter binding factor 1), or KBF2 (κ binding factor 2). RBP-Jκ binds the promoters of several viral and cellular genes and suppresses their transcription. RBP-Jκ is the mammalian homologue of a DNA-binding protein Suppressor of Hairless [Su(H)], which has been implicated in signaling by the *Drosophila* Notch receptor. The current model[119] suggests that the intracellular cleavage product of Notch interacts with a repression domain of RBP-Jκ through the membrane proximal region. Association with RBP-Jκ both suppresses Notch activity as a repressor of transcription and may provide transcriptional activator activity. Gene disruption studies have demonstrated that RBP-Jκ is critical for early embryonic development.[120] Numerous studies, however, have failed to provide convincing evidence of nuclear localization of the cytoplasmic domain of the Notch receptors.[121]

The functions of the mammalian Notch receptors are many and are consistent with controlling cell fate in a number of cell lineages. For example, studies have shown that Notch1 signaling is essential for commitment of cells to the T-cell lineage at the stage of the common lymphoid precursor.[122] The proposed target of Notch signaling, CSL/RBP-J [CSL indicates CBF-1, Su(H), Lag-1], when deleted at this stage of lymphoid lineage development similarly interferes with T-lineage commitment. In addition, however, the targeted mutation of Notch1 in mice results in embryonic lethality on day 9 due to defects in somite segmentation. The mutation also plays a critical role in neurogenesis.[123,124]

G PROTEIN–COUPLED RECEPTOR SYSTEMS

Much intracellular signaling relies on G protein–coupled receptors. The G protein–coupled signaling system was one of the first pathways discovered. Research on this system solved the central question about the mechanisms by which a variety of hormones were able to induce increases in the intracellular second messenger, cyclic adenosine monophosphate (cAMP). G protein–coupled receptors, of which there are more than 1000, are known to transduce the response to a variety of agents, including those involved in light perception, taste, smooth-muscle status, a variety of hormones, and neural transmitters, to name some of the agents. One particularly large subgroup of receptors is those that mediate the diverse biologic effects of chemokines.[125-128] All the receptors involved in G protein–coupled signaling share the structural property of containing seven membrane-spanning α helical domains. The extracellular loops are involved in ligand binding, and the intracellular loops are involved in G-protein recognition. Binding of ligand to the extracellular domain alters the cytoplasmic domain in such a manner as to facilitate interaction of the G-protein complex with the receptor and promote its activation.

The diversity of cellular responses mediated by G protein–coupled receptors is controlled in part by the combinatorial nature of the G-protein complex that associates with specific receptors. G-protein complexes consist of three subunits and are frequently referred to as *heterotrimeric G-protein complexes.* The subunits consist of an α effector subunit, which is the guanine nucleotide binding subunit, and the β and γ subunits, which, as a complex, also mediate signaling events. There are 16 α subunits, 4 β subunits, and 7 γ subunits. In the absence of ligand, the α subunit binds guanosine diphosphate (GDP) and forms a stable complex with the β/γ subunit. On ligand binding, the trimeric complex is recruited to the cytoplasmic domains of the receptor. The result is exchange of GDP with GTP on the α subunit. The "activated" G-protein complex then dissociates from the receptor and the GTP-α subunit, and the β/γ complexes are available to activate their target proteins. Activity of the GTP-α subunit is terminated by hydrolysis of GTP. This process allows the GDP-α subunit to reassociate with the β/γ subunit, and the signaling ground state is reestablished.

The G-protein effectors are differentiated from a variety of monomeric G proteins, such as Ras, by their regulation by β/γ complexes. It has been suggested that evolutionarily this acquisition provided important features for signal transduction.[129] In the absence of ligand, the β/γ association with the GDP-containing α subunit stabilizes the ground state. Second, ligand engagement results in release of the β/γ complex, providing a potential second regulator of downstream events. Third, once activated, dissociation of the GTP–α subunit complex from the β/γ complex further ensures dissociation of the GTP-activated α subunit from the receptor. Last, the higher affinity of the α subunit for GTP relative to GDP ensures that signal termination occurs only by hydrolysis of bound GTP.

The diversity of responses observed with G protein–coupled receptors is largely determined by which α and β/γ subunits associate with the receptor. Early studies to define the biochemical pathways in G protein–coupled receptor signaling focused on specific biochemical responses, such as cellular increases in cAMP. During these studies, it was found that cholera toxin and pertussis toxin were potent inhibitors of these responses. It is now established that this inhibition is due to toxin modification of specific α subunits. One of the first substrates for G-protein activation identified was adenylyl cyclase, which when activated by binding of GTP-bound α subunits is activated to produce cAMP. As discussed later, cAMP, one of the first second messengers identified, has the potential to interact with and change the activity of a variety of cellular proteins.

A number of G protein–coupled receptors couple ligand binding to activation of one subfamily of the phospholipase C family members, PLC-β. Tyrosine kinase–based signaling systems often couple to activation of PLC-γ1 or PLC-γ2, which, among the PLC family members, uniquely contain SH2 and SH3 domains. The PLC-β subfamily consists of four family members that contain the typical catalytic domain, an EF domain, and the PH domain that characterize all PLC family members. In addition, these family members have a unique carboxyl domain that contains the site for α-subunit interaction or for interaction with the β/γ complex. Activation of the PLC-β family members results in hydrolysis of membrane-associated PI(4,5) and generation of inositol (1,4,5)-trisphosphate (IP$_3$) and DAG. The released IP$_3$ interacts with its specific receptors to induce a transient increase in calcium that can mediate a variety of responses, including activation of protein kinases.

G protein–coupled receptors also couple to activation of cyclic guanosine monophosphate (cGMP) phosphodiesterase. For example, the G protein–coupled receptor rhodopsin is activated by light-induced isomerization of retinal protein. Activation results in release of GTP-bound α subunit from the transducin–G protein complex, which activates phosphodiesterase. This process leads to a decrease in cGMP level. The result is changes in ion channel activity and nerve impulses. In addition to this sequence, a number of ion channels are directly regulated by G proteins. Other cellular responses regulated by G-protein complexes include exocytosis, vesicular traffic, and tyrosine phosphatase activity.

TUMOR NECROSIS FACTOR RECEPTOR INTRACELLULAR SIGNALING

The TNF receptor (TNFR) family was first identified as the receptors for the tumor necrosis factors (TNFs) and the Fas ligand. The conserved motif defining the family resides in the extracellular domain and consists of a six-cysteine-containing domain.[19] The family includes approximately 25 receptors for approximately 18 ligands, including CD40, CD30, CD27, OX-40, the TNFs, and Fas ligand.[130] Among the receptors, a subfamily that includes TNFR1, Fas, and nerve growth factor receptor (NGFR) p75 contain a conserved cytoplasmic domain referred to as the *death domain* (DD). This domain is essential to the ability of these receptors to couple ligand binding to induction of apoptosis. The receptors for TRAMP (transgenic adenocarcinoma mouse prostate; DR3), TRAIL (tumor necrosis factor–related apoptosis-inducing ligand; DR4), and a related receptor, DR5, also have been shown to contain cytoplasmic DDs. The DDs can be moved among various receptors and retain their ability to induce apoptosis. As with all receptor systems, ligand drives aggregation of the receptors. The result is an altered receptor confirmation, which allows recruitment of various proteins to the receptor complex (Fig. 2-3). The chief consequences of activation of TNFRs are two contrasting responses. In the case of DD-containing receptors, the primary physiologic response is induction of apoptosis. With all the TNFR family members, receptor engagement induces activation of NF-κB transcription factor, which is associated with protection from apoptosis. Many of the molecular details of activation of these pathways have been elucidated in the last few years, largely through derivation of strains of mice lacking individual components of the intracellular signaling pathways.

The ability to induce apoptosis depends on the presence of the DD, a domain of approximately 60 amino acids that contains 6 conserved α helical regions. The DD in the receptor tails recruits adapter proteins that also contain DD, including the TNFR-associated death domain (TRADD) and the Fas-associated death domain (FADD) proteins. The roles of both proteins have been investigated by derivation of mutant strains of mice lacking the genes. FADD deficiency results in an embryonic lethal phenotype, although the precise basis is not known.[131] In addition, apoptosis induced by several receptors (TNFR1, Fas, DR3) is dramatically reduced, demonstrating the essential role of this adapter in signaling. FADD contains a death effector domain (DED), which interacts with a homologous domain on caspase 8. Ligand-induced recruitment and aggregation of caspase 8 result in processing of the proenzyme to the active enzyme by autoproteolytic cleavage. Mutant mice lacking caspase 8 phenotypically copy the FADD-deficient mice and similarly are resistant to apoptosis by several death-inducing ligands.[132] Activated caspase 8 activates other caspases and substrates of the caspases. One intriguing substrate is the inhibitor of caspase-activated DNAase.[133,134] Cleavage of the inhibitor liberates active DNAase, which cleaves DNA. The result is the nucleosomal degradation that has long characterized cells undergoing induced apoptosis.

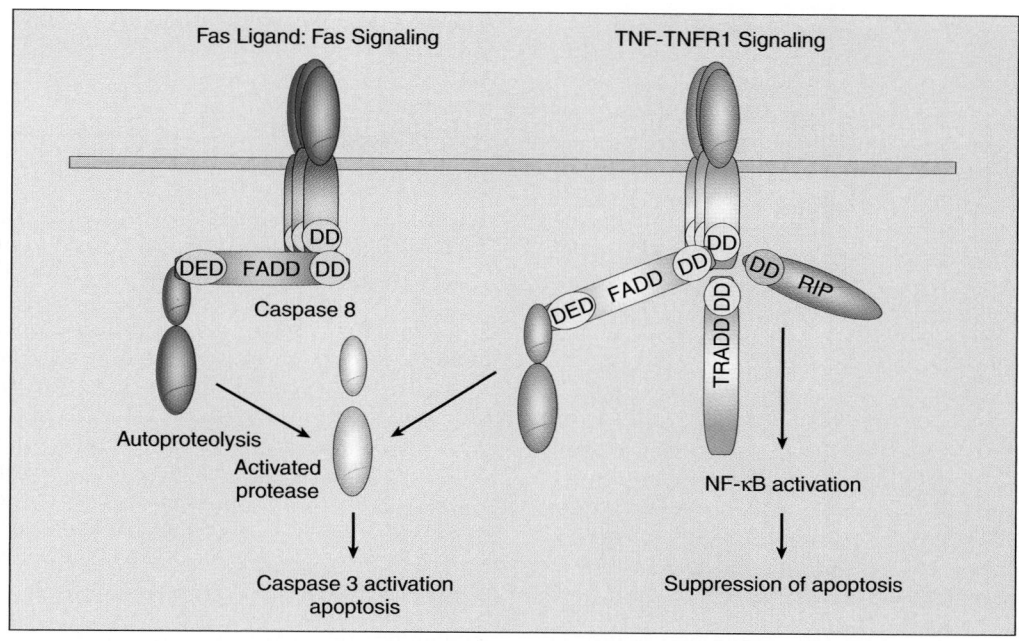

Figure 2-3. Intracellular signaling by tumor necrosis factor (TNF)/Fas ligands. Members of the tumor necrosis factor receptor (TNFR) family mediate activation of proteases responsible for apoptotic cell death. The receptor for Fas ligand, Fas, contains death domains (DD) in the cytoplasmic domain that, when in an aggregated state as a consequence of ligand binding, recruit another DD-containing adapter protein termed *FADD* (Fas-associated death domain). FADD contains a death effector domain (DED) that recruits the protease caspase 8. Caspase 8 is activated by autoproteolytic cleavage and proteolytically activates other members of the caspase family, including caspase 3, which is a key mediator of cell death by apoptosis. TNFR1 mediates activation of the apoptotic pathway through initial recruitment of the adapter protein TRADD (TNF receptor–associated death domain) and subsequent recruitment of FADD. The activated receptor complex also recruits kinase receptor–interacting protein (RIP), which activates an intracellular signaling pathway that results in activation of nuclear factor κB (NF-κB), a step that regulates expression of genes capable of suppressing apoptosis. Unlike intracellular signaling mediated by Fas, the outcome of signaling through the TNFR1 receptor may or may not result in cell death.

The caspase family is centrally linked to apoptotic programs of intracellular signaling. The family consists of 10 family members, caspases 1 through 10, many of which, when overexpressed, mediate cell death. The caspases share a conserved catalytic site motif that includes a critical cysteine residue that contributes to the active site. The caspases are synthesized as proenzymes that require proteolytic cleavage for activation. Activation and amplification of the caspases result in degradation of a number of target proteins that together mediate the characteristic pattern of apoptotic cell death. The first member identified was IL-1β–converting enzyme (ICE).[135] After cloning of ICE, a gene (*ced3*) involved in apoptosis during differentiation in nematodes was cloned and was found related structurally to ICE.[136] The unique role of ICE in regulating IL-1 release is nicely illustrated by the phenotype of mutant mice lacking ICE.[137] The mice develop normally but have a major defect in production of IL-1β in response to stimulation. This inability is speculated to be the basis of resistance of the mice to lipopolysaccharide (LPS)-induced endotoxic shock. The phenotype also illustrates the lack of a nonredundant role for this member of the family in other cellular systems. Studies of mutant mice lacking caspase 3[138] have similarly demonstrated the central role of caspase 3 in apoptosis is that of a target for a variety of intracellular pathways associated with apoptosis. These pathways include the FADD/caspase 8 pathway and the Apaf-1/caspase 9 pathway, which is activated under conditions of release of cytochrome C from mitochondria.[139]

TRADD was isolated by its ability to bind to TNFR1. TNFR1 intracellular signaling differs from Fas signaling in that receptor engagement may or may not induce apoptosis. The distinction is related to the proteins recruited to the receptor complex. Induction of apoptosis results from TRADD-dependent recruitment of FADD to the complex and its subsequent recruitment of caspase 8. In competition with these events, however, are recruitment of TRAFs and receptor-interacting protein (RIP) and activation of NF-κB with its induction of antiapoptotic genes. RIP was initially identified as a protein that interacted with the receptor Fas.[140] RIP consists of an amino-terminal kinase domain, an α-helical center domain, and a carboxyl DD. Again, derivation of mice lacking RIP has led to a view somewhat different from that initially derived from biochemical studies.[141] RIP-deficient mice are normal at birth but fail to thrive and die at 1 to 3 days. Unexpectedly, extensive apoptosis occurs in both lymphoid and adipose tissues, and the cells are highly sensitive to TNF-induced cell death. TNF is not capable of inducing NF-κB activation in the cells. Thus RIP is presumably in the receptor complex and is essential for the signaling pathway that results in activation of NF-κB.

The TRAF family is characterized by a conserved carboxyl-terminal (TRAF-C) domain and an α-helical domain, the TRAF-N domain. In addition, all but TRAF1 contain an amino-terminal RING finger domain, a domain found in a variety of proteins. The TRAF family currently consists of six members, and one family member has been shown to be involved in IL-1 signaling.[142] Overexpression of many of the members of the family can induce NF-κB activation. The precise role of the TRAF family members is being examined by derivation of mutant mice. Mice that lack TRAF3 die soon after birth.[143] The mice are runts and peripheral white blood cell counts decrease dramatically within a few days after birth. Fetal liver cells can completely reconstitute the hematopoietic system, but the T cells are defective in such mice. The phenotype of the T cells is consistent with the hypothesis that TRAF3 is critical for a T-cell proliferative response. The phenotype of the T-cell defects suggests that CD30 may be the receptor with which TRAF3 interacts. TRAF2 deletion also results in early lethality, and TRAF2-deficient cells show increased apoptosis with TNF stimulation.[144] However, this increased sensitivity occurs without loss of ability to activate NF-κB and may involve JNK-dependent pathways. Thus TRAF2 and RIP function through independent, essential pathways to negate the apoptotic response. The properties of TRAF6-deficient mice suggest a function for this family member in CD40 signaling, although deletion of TRAF6 also suggests a much broader range of functions in intracellular signaling, including a role in responses to IL-1 and LPS.[145]

Several additional gene products control the apoptotic responses initiated by TNFR family members. For example, FLIP (cellular FADD-like IL-1β–converting enzyme [c-FLICE] inhibitory protein, also called Casper) is structurally similar to caspase 8 in containing a DD and a caspase-like domain. However, the protein lacks enzymatic activity and thus can function as a dominant negative to block recruitment of functional caspase 8 to the receptor complex. Consistent with this mechanism, FLIP-deficient cells are highly sensitive to DD-containing receptors.[146] Both FLIP and FADD have embryonic lethal phenotypes not associated with apoptosis, a feature that demonstrates they have functions that are independent of their roles in TNF intracellular signaling. Another example is A20, a zinc finger gene whose deletion results in greatly increased sensitivity to TNF-induced apoptosis.[147] Although the mechanisms are not fully detailed, absence of A20 is associated with lack of recruitment of RIP and TRAF2 to the complex.

The foregoing examples demonstrate the complex protein interactions that initiate the intracellular signaling involving in obtaining a physiologic response. They also illustrate the dynamic interactions that can lead to competition for pathway activation and the dramatic consequences that can occur in subtle shifts in complex formation. The unique position of TNFR intracellular signaling pathways in initiation of cell death clearly identifies these pathways as targets for drugs that may be useful in managing cancer. Similarly, the critical role of NF-κB in controlling proapoptotic responses has prompted studies to determine whether inhibition NF-κB may make cells more susceptible to manipulation of the apoptotic pathways.

INTRACELLULAR RECEPTORS: EXTERNAL AND INTERNAL SENSORS

One of the larger families of proteins involved in intracellular signaling is the nuclear receptors, which has approximately 50 family members.[148] This family of receptors was identified initially as the mediators for signaling cellular responses to the steroid hormones, including testosterone, estradiol, progesterone, thyroid hormone, and retinoic acid. Receptors related to the receptors for these hormones later were identified and called *orphan receptors* because the ligands initially were unknown. However, the ligands for many of the receptors have since been identified and support the concept that this family of receptors has evolved to sense and allow specific responses to a variety of conditions. For example, a number of the receptors have fatty acids as ligands and play essential roles in, for example, adipogenesis. Other subfamilies of receptors recognize bile acids, oxysterols, and xenobiotic compounds. Involvement of this family of receptors in cancer is best illustrated by the role of fusion of the *PML* gene with the retinoic acid receptor alpha (RARα) in promyelocytic leukemia with t(15;17)(q22;q21). The remarkable response of these patients to treatment with all-*trans*-retinoic acid represents the first model of targeted therapy.

The receptors consist of an amino-terminal ligand-independent transcriptional activation domain (AF-1). The central region of the protein contains a DNA-binding domain consisting of two zinc-finger domains. The carboxyl region contains the ligand-binding domain and a ligand-dependent transcriptional activation domain. The steroid receptors function as homodimers, whereas most of the orphan receptors function as heterodimers with the retinoic acid receptors RARα, β, and γ. With many of the steroid receptors, ligand binding promotes DNA-binding activity. In many cases, however, the nonligated receptors bind DNA and repress gene expression by recruiting repressors to the promoter. Binding of ligand disrupts binding to the repressors and promotes binding to coactivators to induce gene expression.

COMMON TARGETS OF INTRACELLULAR SIGNALING

Intracellular Signaling Involving the Nuclear Factor κB Family

One of the most common events during intracellular signaling in a variety of receptor systems is activation of members of the NF-κB transcription factor family. The relevance of activating the pathway has been most dramatically illustrated by the diverse consequences observed when members of the family are deleted in mice. These consequences include embryonic lethality due to defects in liver development, development of multiorgan inflammation and myeloid hyperplasia due to altered T-cell function, and defects in B-cell development.[149-155] Consistent with these roles, the family members regulate expression of a variety of genes, including cytokine and chemokine genes, genes involved in controlling cell cycle progression, genes contributing to protecting cells from apoptosis, and genes affecting cell adhesion and migration. In addition, the founding member of the family was initially identified as the oncogene (v-*rel*) transduced by a retrovirus and capable of inducing hematopoietic tumors. Consistent with a role in cancer, members of the family are frequently amplified in tumors, and transformed cells frequently have activated NF-κB transcriptional complexes.[156]

The NF-κB family of proteins consists of the initial complex consisting of a 50-kd component (NF-κB1) and a 65-kd component (RelA). In addition, mammalian species contain RelB, c-*rel,* and NF-κB2. The family members are characterized by an amino-terminal *rel*-homology domain of approximately 300 amino acids. This domain is required for dimerization of family members, their nuclear translocation, DNA-binding activity, and the ability to activate gene expression. NF-κB1 and B2 are synthesized as precursors of 105 kd and 100 kd processed to the transcriptionally active forms of p50 and p52. All intracellular signaling events regulating the function of NF-κB family members involve initiation of events that result in nuclear translocation of the transcription complexes (Fig. 2-4).

The essential regulators of NF-κB function are the inhibitors of κB (IκB) proteins that bind the dimers and retain them as inactive complexes in the cytoplasm. The inhibitors are characterized by multiple ankyrin repeats that mediate protein-protein interactions. The inhibitors include IκBα, IκBβ, and IκBε, and the c-terminal domains of p100 and p105. Translocation of the active NF-κB dimers to the nucleus depends on phosphorylation of the IκB proteins at two amino-terminal serine residues that targets them for ubiquitination and subsequent degradation. Phosphorylation is mediated by an IκB kinase complex consisting of the two related kinases IκB kinase α (IKKα) and IKKβ and the regulatory protein IKKγ (also called Nemo). Production of mice deficient in each component has demonstrated the essential role of IKKβ and IKKγ in the complex for activation of all NF-κB family members.[157,158] Curiously, however, deletion of IKKα has shown that this component is essential for functions associated with epidermal development that is independent of NF-κB functions.[159] In addition, IKKα is required for efficient processing, in a yet to be defined manner, of NF-κ precursors in response to some ligands.

Although the role of the IKK complex in initiating the events required for activation of NF-κB transcription factors is well established, the upstream activators are less well defined. The difficulty is likely due in part to the fact that there may be many ways of activating the complex and that different initiating signals use distinct but different activators. For example, on the basis of the phenotype of PKC-θ–deficient mice, activation of the IKK complex in response to signaling through the T-cell receptor depends on PKC-θ.[160] In B cells, activation of the IKK complex depends on PKC-β,[161] and activation of PKC-β depends on signaling from the B-cell receptor complex involving generation of a calcium flux that releases DAG. Although these two cases entail members of the PKC superfamily of kinases, it is not established that all pathways leading to activation of the IKK complex and activation of NF-κB transcription factors involve kinases of this family.

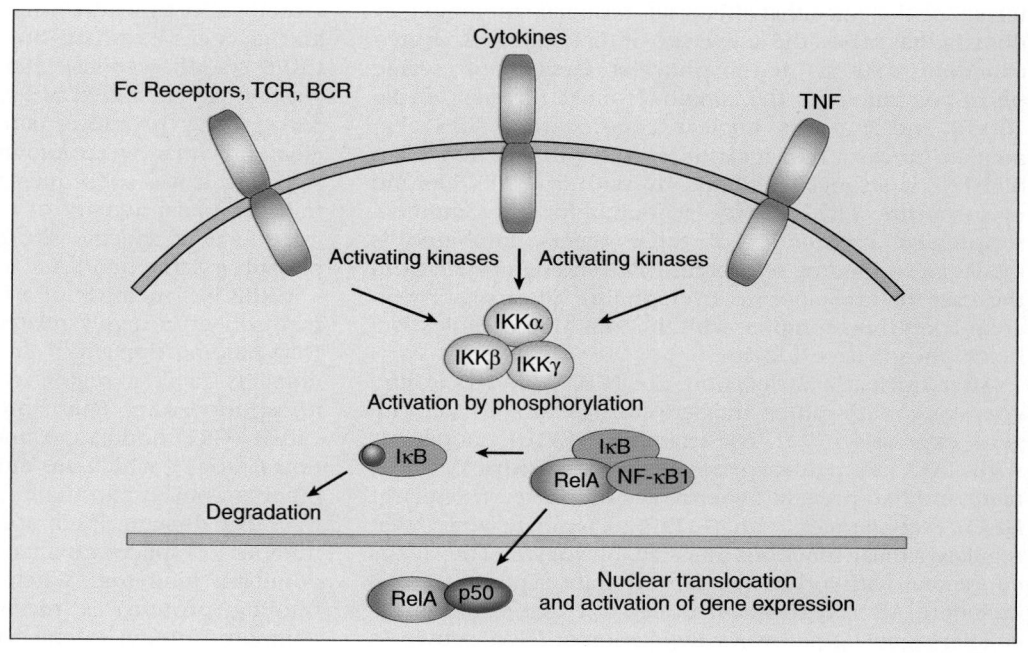

Figure 2-4. Intracellular signaling events in activation of nuclear factor κB (NF-κB). A variety of receptors are capable of activating members of the NF-κB family of transcription factors. The central event in activation involves phosphorylation and activation of the inhibitors of NF-κB kinase complex. The complex consists of two kinases, α and β, and an adapter protein γ. Activation can be mediated by a variety of kinases that are activated during receptor engagement. The function of the complex is to phosphorylate inhibitor of κB (IκB) and target it for destruction by the proteosome. In the absence of IκB, the dimeric complex is released from the cytoplasm, translocates to the nucleus, and activates expression of a variety of genes affecting cell function. BCR, B-cell receptor; IKK, IκB kinase; TCR, T-cell receptor; TNF, tumor necrosis factor.

NFAT Transcription Factors: Targets of Multiple Signaling Pathways

Although NFAT (nuclear factor of activated T cells) was initially identified in the context of regulation of cytokine gene expression after T-cell activation, studies of NFAT-deficient mice have shown the family members are essential for the intracellular signaling that controls a spectrum of developmental events. The family consists of four members, NFATc1 through NFATcc4, characterized by highly related DNA-binding domains related to the *rel* DNA-binding domain of NF-κB transcription factors. In addition, an amino-terminal region contains serine-rich or serine/proline-rich domains and domains required for binding of calcineurin. Activation of NFAT transcriptional activity depends on upstream signaling events that induce a Ca^{2+} flux. In the case of the T-cell receptor, one of the functions of the receptor signalsome is to recruit PLC-γ1, which hydrolyzes membrane lipids to yield IP_3 and DAG. IP_3 interacts with specific intracellular receptors (IP_3R) to induce release of Ca^{2+} from intracellular stores. The release from intracellular stores also triggers influx of extracellular Ca^{2+}. The combination gives rise to the sustained increase in intracellular Ca^{2+} that is required for NFAT activation.

Increases in intracellular Ca^{2+} result in activation of a number of enzymes that contribute to the spectrum of intracellular signaling events associated with the increases.[162] One particularly interesting gene is *Dream* a Ca^{2+}-regulated transcriptional repressor. Deletion of *Dream* in mice produces a phenotype in which there is marked attenuation of the mice to sense pain from a variety of stimuli.[163] Regulation of NFAT activity is mediated by Ca^{2+} binding to calmodulin (CaM) and to a regulatory subunit of calcineurin (CnB) in a complex containing the phosphatase catalytic subunit of calcineurin (CnA). The family of calcineurin genes includes *CnAα,β,γ* and *CnBα,β*. Binding of Ca^{2+} results in a conformational change that affects a C-terminal autoinhibitory domain that masks the active site of the enzyme. Activated calcineurin then dephosphorylates sites of serine phosphorylation in the amino-terminal domain of the NFATs and exposes nuclear translocation sites that mediate nuclear translocation of the protein. Activation of NFAT is strongly inhibited by two drugs, FK506 and cyclosporine. This activity accounts for the immunosuppressive capabilities of these agents. Inhibition is mediated by binding to proteins (FK-binding protein or, in the case of cyclosporine, cyclophilin). The drug-protein complexes then complex with the CnA/CnB complex and block phosphatase activity.

After nuclear translocation, the NFATs bind DNA and cooperate with other transcription factors to activate gene expression.[164,165] For example, NFATc4 cooperates with GATA4 to regulate genes involved in cardiac development and that prevent hypertrophy of the heart. Similarly, NFATc1 cooperates with GATA2 to regulate genes that regulate similar functions in skeletal myocytes. The NFATs cooperate with other families of transcription factors, including AP-1, regulated through the Ras-MAPK intracellular signaling pathways. Regulation of NFAT activity is

highly dynamic, and nuclear phosphorylation is constantly causing the proteins to return to the cytoplasm through highly efficient nuclear export signals. Although a number of kinases have been suggested as regulating this aspect, genetic evidence provides convincing data supporting a critical role for GSK-3β.[166,167] This kinase is also a critical mediator in the Wnt signaling pathway.

The physiologic roles of signaling involving the NFATs have been established through derivation of mutant strains of mice lacking individual NFATs as well as multiple family members.[165,168] These studies have demonstrated a spectrum of both redundant and nonredundant roles in a spectrum of physiologic processes. NFATc1 is essential for cardiac morphogenesis, NFATc2 has roles in the immune system and in chondrogenesis, and NFATc3 deficiency is associated with defects in thymic development and results in T-cell hyperproliferation. Deficiency of NFATc4 alone produces no defects, although in combination with a deficiency in NFATc3, it reveals a redundant role in controlling vascular patterning. Deficiencies of both NFATc1 and NFATc2 result in profound T-cell proliferation defects and cytokine production.

CREB/CREM/ATF-1: Targets of Multiple Signaling Pathways

The concept that extracellular triggering would initiate a series of biochemical events that propagate the cellular response was developed in elegant studies that defined the role of cAMP as a second messenger in signaling. One of the major signaling pathways initiated by G protein–coupled receptors is activation of adenylyl cyclase, which catalyzes formation of cAMP from ATP. Many of the signaling consequences of production of cAMP result from binding of cAMP to the regulatory subunit of protein kinase A (PKA) and release of the catalytic subunit, which phosphorylates a series of target proteins. Targets of PKA include a number of enzymes that directly affect metabolism, such as phosphorylase kinase and glycogen synthase but also the transcription factor CREB (cAMP response element binding protein). CREB was initially identified as a transcription factor capable of recognizing promoter sites (CRE [cAMP responsive element]) that were known to be regulated by cAMP signaling. It was subsequently found that activation of the transcriptional activity of CREB depended on phosphorylation at a specific site (S^{133}) and that this site was phosphorylated by PKA.

CREB is a member of a family of transcription factors that contain a highly related basic-leucine zipper (bZip) DNA-binding domain.[169] In addition, two glutamine-rich domains flank a region containing the critical site of phosphorylation. The family members include CREB, CREM (CRE modulator), and ATF-1 (activating transcription factor-1), which are most highly similar in the DNA-binding domain and share far less sequence homology in the other domains. Each of the family members exhibits a number of splice variants, some of which function as dominant inhibitors. When phosphorylated, CBP (CREB binding protein) is recruited to the transcriptional complex through interaction between the KID (kinase-inducible domain) of CREB and the KIX domain of CBP. CBP and a highly related protein, p300, are large proteins that contain a number of domains that target interaction with a wide spectrum of transcription factors. Their function as critical coactivators has been particularly emphasized by the observation that deletion of either results in an early embryonic lethal phenotype. Moreover, the observations that deficiency of both is more severe and that haploinsufficiency for both is lethal indicate a redundancy for many critical functions.[170]

CREB family members can be activated by a variety of intracellular signaling pathways besides the cAMP/PKA pathway. For example, Ca^{2+} can activate CREB-responsive genes and is most likely activated by one or more of the CaM-dependent kinases CaMKI (CaM kinase I), CaMKII, or CaMKIV. CREB function also is activated in responses to a number of growth factors. A number of different kinases have been proposed as proximal activators, including Akt, the RSK kinases, and mitogen- and stress-activated protein kinase 1 and 2 (MSK1/2). On the basis of the spectrum of intracellular signaling pathways capable of activating CREB family members, it might have been anticipated that deletion of individual genes might have catastrophic consequences. However, CREB null embryos are born but die soon after birth, and the deficiencies primarily affect the nervous system.[171] Further studies have established a critical role in the nervous system.[172] CREM-deficient mice are viable but have defects in spermatogenesis associated with germ-cell aplasia.[173]

The Mitogen-Activated Protein Kinase Cascade

One of the most frequently observed events in intracellular signaling through a variety of pathways is activation of kinases of the MAPK family (Fig. 2-5). The complexity associated with the events upstream of activation, unfortunately, is matched only by the incredibly ill-developed nomenclature associated with the system. The cascade consists of several related and overlapping pathways of kinase activation that are highly conserved in evolution and that are activated in the context of a variety of cytokines and growth factors as well as conditions of cellular stress. The initiating event for activation of MAPKs can be derived from a variety of types of growth factor receptor signaling (see later), from cellular stress, or from receptors that mediate proinflammatory responses. Irrespective of the nature of the initial input, the primary function is activation of a kinase that has the ability to activate another kinase of the family of related kinases, the MKKs (MAPK kinases), which activate the structurally and functionally related Erk, Jnk, and p38 kinases. The latter, when activated, can translocate to the nucleus and phosphorylate transcription factors and thereby regulate gene expression.

The principle function of the kinase cascades is to induce tyrosine and threonine phosphorylation of a group of structurally and functionally related kinases that include the extracellular signal-regulated kinases (Erk1, Erk2, Erk5), the c-*jun* kinases (Jnk1, Jnk2, Jnk3), and the p38 group of kinases (p38α, p38β, p38γ, p38δ). Collectively, these kinases are referred to as the *mitogen-activated protein kinases* (MAPKs). The kinases are structurally similar, relatively small kinases ranging from 38 kd to approximately 45 kd with specificity for threonine/serine phosphorylation. All share the property that their activity is dramatically affected by phosphorylation of a threonine and tyrosine within the activation loop of the kinase catalytic domain. The essential sequence for Erks is a TEY; in Jnks the sequence is TPY; and in p38 kinases, the sequence is TGY. Phosphorylation of these sites can increase catalytic activity 1000 fold. The mechanism is hypothesized to be very similar to phosphorylation within the activation loop of the kinase domain of tyrosine kinases. In particular, in Erk2, binding of its activating kinase, Mek, alters the confirmation of the subdomain VIII loop and exposes Y^{185} for phosphorylation. Phosphorylation would then release the block for substrate binding with subsequent T^{183} phosphorylation, further activating the enzyme by facilitating correct alignment of the catalytic residues. Once they are phosphorylated, MAPKs translocate to the nucleus through a mechanism that involves dimer formation[174] and phosphorylate a number of substrates.

Figure 2-5. Mitogen-activated protein kinase (MAPK) cascades. Intracellular signaling from various receptors involves activation of members of the mitogen-activated kinases. The MAPKs consist of three families of related kinases (Erks, p38s, Jnks). Activation of MAPKs is mediated by phosphorylation by a series of related kinases, MKKs (MAPK kinases), which are activated by a broad spectrum of kinases through phosphorylation. Activated MAPKs translocate to the nucleus and phosphorylate a variety of structurally unrelated transcription factors. The transcription factors and gene expression thus are activated.

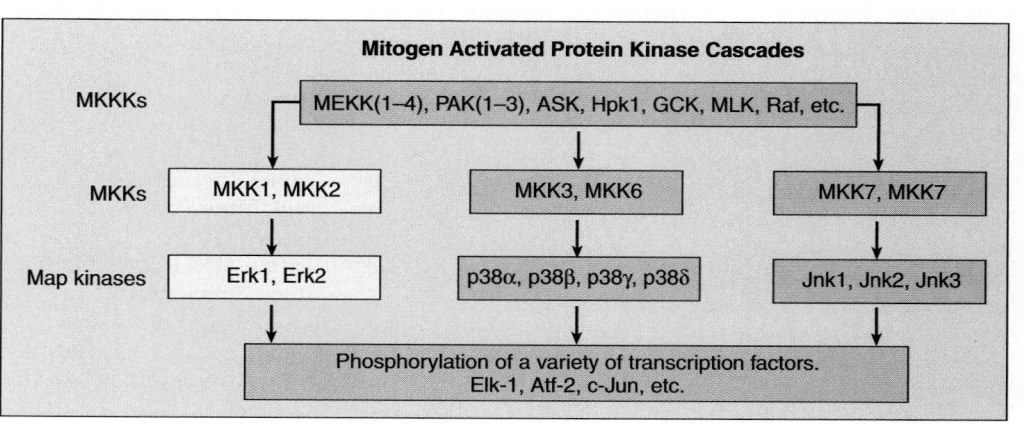

The activated Erks, Jnks, and p38 kinases phosphorylate a variety of substrates, many of which are transcriptional factors. Some of the substrates are unique for a particular family member, whereas other substrates can be phosphorylated by more than one family member. A few examples illustrate the function and importance of the pathways. The classic example is regulation of the immediate early gene, c-fos, a gene highly and transiently induced in response to a variety of cellular stimulants. Serum-induced expression of c-fos depends on a serum response element (SRE), an element that binds a serum response factor (SRF). Induction of c-fos expression requires recruitment to SRF of a factor to form a ternary complex. The recruited factor is an ets family member, Sap-1, or the highly related family member, Elk-1.[175] The ability of Elk-1 or Sap-1 to be recruited into the complex depends on phosphorylation of a cluster of serine and threonine in the carboxyl-terminal region. These phosphorylations can be mediated by both Erk family members[176,177] and Jnk members.[178] Thus within the context of serum stimulation, growth factors, or cytokines, c-fos activation is mediated by the Erks, whereas induction of c-fos by ultraviolet light, stress, TNF-α, IL-1, or osmotic shock is mediated by the Jnks. Another transcription factor activated after serine phosphorylation at two sites in the amino terminal is c-jun. The Jnks were initially identified from cloning of novel Erk-related kinases that could mediate this phosphorylation.[179,180] Other transcription factors regulated by phosphorylation include ATF2 by the Jnks,[181] CHOP by p38,[182] and MEF2C by p38[183] as well as by Erk5.[184] Last, two intracellular receptors, the estrogen receptor[185] and the PPARg receptor,[186] are functionally modified by phosphorylation by the MAPKs.

The activities of MAPKs are regulated through phosphorylation and dephosphorylation. Dephosphorylation is mediated by a group of dual-specificity phosphatases capable of dephosphorylating both tyrosine and threonine at the activation domain of the MAPKs. The first MAPK phosphatases (MKPs) were identified as immediate early genes in response to growth factors or serum.[187-189] Thus it is curious that serum induces activation of the MAPKs and that this pathway, or others, induces transcription of genes that encode the phosphatases that will inactivate the pathway. Many of the phosphatases have remarkable specificity for particular MAPKs. This phenomenon appears to be due to the requirement for interaction between a noncatalytic domain of the phosphatase and MAPK. This interaction is required for activation of phosphatase activity.[190] There are as many as nine mammalian dual-specificity phosphatases, including MKP-1, MKP-2, MKP-3, MKP-4, and PAC-1 (phosphatase of activated cells 1), all of which are specific for MAPKs.

Activation of MAPKs is mediated by a family of dual-specificity kinases capable of phosphorylating the critical threonine and tyrosine residues in the activation domain. The kinases of this family are generally referred to as *MAPK kinases* (MKK), although a variety of terms exist, such as MEK and MAPKK. The MKKs exhibit varying specificities for the various MAPKs. MKK1 and MKK2 specifically phosphorylate the Erk MAPKs. MKK3 and MKK6 phosphorylate the p38 MAPKs. MKK4 and MKK7 phosphorylate the Jnk MAPKs. Mice deficient in MKK4 (also called SEK1, JNKK) have been generated. The absence of MKK4 results in embryonic lethality relatively late in development, day 14.[191] The ability of heat shock or the protein synthesis inhibitor anisomycin to induce JNK activation is lost, demonstrating the essential, nonredundant role of MKK4 in these signaling pathways. However, ability to activate JNK in response to a number of additional inducers has not been affected. The role of MKK4 in lymphoid cells was examined in chimeric rag$^{-/-}$ mice.[192,193] Relatively minor phenotypes were observed that suggested CKK4 might be involved in aspects of CD28-mediated IL-2 production or provide a slight degree of protection from Fas- and CD3-mediated apoptosis.

The MKKs are activated by a variety of kinases, at least 14, that are activated in response to growth factors and stress. At this level, the terminology becomes even more complex, and a consistent nomenclature has not emerged. A number of examples illustrate the classic pathways and the newly emerging kinases capable of activating one or more of the MAPK pathways. The classic pathway is growth factor–associated *ras/raf* activation of the Erks. Activation of the pathway begins with recruitment of an "adapter" protein to an activated receptor complex. In the case of tyrosine kinase receptors, the adapter protein is most frequently Grb2, whereas in the case of most cytokine receptors, the adapter protein Shc is recruited to the receptor complex. In either case, recruitment involves recognition of specific sites of tyrosine phosphorylation on the receptor by the SH2 domains of the adapter protein. In recruitment of Shc, the adapter is phosphorylated, and Grb2 is recruited to the complex through its interaction with tyrosine phosphorylated Shc. Grb2 subsequently recruits the GTP exchange factor SOS (son of sevenless) to the complex, a process that results in exchange of GDP for GTP on *ras*. In an unspecified manner, GTP-*ras* recruits Raf-1 to the membrane and mediates its activation.[194,195] Simply targeting Raf-1 to the membrane results in its activation and subsequent activation of the pathway.[196]

A series of protein kinases—MEKK1, MEKK2, MEKK3, and MEKK4—have been identified on the basis of homology with yeast kinases involved in MAPK signaling pathways. MEKK1 specifically activates the Erk MAPK pathway through phosphorylation of MKK1,[197] and the Jnk MAPK pathway through MKK4.[198,199] Activation of MEKK1 binds Ras in a GTP-dependent manner and binds Cdc42 and Rac. Evidence exists to indicate that activation of MEKK1 by EGF requires *ras*. In distinct contrast from this mechanism, MEKK1 has been shown to be activated by cleavage by caspases.[200] In this case, activation of MEKK1 is associated with induction of apoptosis. Last, Nck-interacting kinase (NIK) has been identified as binding to adapter protein Nck and is capable of activating MEKK1.[201] It can be anticipated that derivation of mice deficient in MEKKs will help to resolve the biologic roles of these kinases and provide insights into their role in activation of the various MAPK pathways.

Another group of kinases involved in activation of MAPK pathways, possibly through phosphorylation of

CLINICAL RELEVANCE

Alterations in signaling pathways contribute to

TUMOR DEVELOPMENT

Examples include overexpression of growth factor receptors (e.g., Her2neu), constitutive activation of secondary signaling molecules (e.g., *ras*), and chromosomal translocations (e.g., *bcr/abl*)

TUMOR RESISTANCE TO THERAPY

Can be caused by increased cellular survival signals (e.g., EGF receptor amplification), inhibition of cell death signals (e.g., *bcl-2* overexpression), blockade of negative growth signals (e.g., TGF-β pathway), and potentially increased repair of DNA damage.

MKKs, are the PAKs (p21-activated kinases) (PAK1, PAK2, PAK3). PAKs regulate morphologic and cytoskeletal changes in a variety of cell types. Their activity is regulated by Rac and Cdc42. PAK2 has been shown to be activated by caspase cleavage.[202] Activated forms of PAKs have been shown to activate the Jnk and p38, but not the Erk, MAPK pathways.[201] This mechanism may be independent of Rac and Cdc42 activation.[203]

Other kinases implicated in activation of the MAPK pathways include apoptosis signal–regulating kinase (Ask1),[204] the proto-oncogene Tpl-2,[205] hematopoietic progenitor kinase 1 (Hpk1),[186,206] members of the mixed lineage kinases (MLK),[207] and germinal center kinase (GCK).[208] In addition, Tab1 and Tak1 are implicated in TGF-β–induced activation of MAPK pathways. These examples illustrate the complexity of defining the kinase cascades involved in intracellular signaling.

SUMMARY AND CONCLUSIONS

The examples described illustrate the incredibly dynamic events that occur in intracellular signaling. It is clear that the behavior of a particular cell is defined by its environment. During development, environmental clues provide signals to guide cell movement and to control whether a cell will proliferate or undergo apoptosis. Evolution has used a variety of receptor systems to recognize the clues and has integrated them into intracellular signaling pathways that often converge to mediate comparable outcomes. Following development, environmental clues are necessary to maintain homeostasis, and many lineages or tissues require tightly regulated stem cell reproduction and functional differentiation to maintain organisms. Beyond these fundamental functions, intracellular signaling is involved in sensing the metabolic state of an organism. Central to cancer is the concept that cells lose the ability to sense and respond appropriately to these environmental clues. The complexity of changes associated with cancer can be anticipated to be as complex as the intracellular signaling pathways involved in normal regulation of cells. As our understanding of intracellular signaling grows, our ability to precisely define the changes that occur in cancer improves. Perhaps more important is that as our understanding of intracellular signaling pathways and their precise physiologic roles increases, we may be able to use these pathways in therapeutic approaches to the control of cancer cells.

REFERENCES

1. Johnson L, Greenbaum D, Cichowski K, et al: K-ras is an essential gene in the mouse with partial functional overlap with N-ras [published erratum appears in Genes Dev 1997;11:3277]. Genes Dev 1997;11:2468–2481.
2. Esteban LM, Vicario-Abejon C, Fernandez-Salguero P, et al: Targeted genomic disruption of H-ras and N-ras, individually or in combination, reveals the dispensability of both loci for mouse growth and development. Mol Cell Biol 2001;21:1444–1452.
3. Ihle JN: The Stat family in cytokine signaling. Curr Opin Cell Biol 2001;13:211–217.
4. Heldin CH: Protein tyrosine kinase receptors. Cancer Surv 1996;27:7–24.
5. Heldin CH, Ostman A: Ligand-induced dimerization of growth factor receptors: Variations on the theme. Cytokine Growth Factor Rev 1996;7:3–10.
6. Weiss FU, Daub H, Ullrich A: Novel mechanisms of RTK signal generation. Curr Opin Genet Dev 1997;7:80–86.
7. Lemmon MA, Schlessinger J: Regulation of signal transduction and signal diversity by receptor oligomerization. Trends Biochem Sci 1994;19:459–463.
8. Ullrich A, Schlessinger J: Signal transduction by receptors with tyrosine kinase activity. Cell 1990;61:203–212.
9. Heldin CH: Dimerization of cell surface receptors in signal transduction. Cell 1995;80:213–223.
10. Hubbard SR, Wei L, Ellis L, et al: Crystal structure of the tyrosine kinase domain of the human insulin receptor. Nature 1994;372:746–754.
11. Mohammadi M, Schlessinger J, Hubbard SR: Structure of the FGF receptor tyrosine kinase domain reveals a novel autoinhibitory mechanism. Cell 1996;86:577–587.
12. Pawson T: Protein modules and signalling networks. Nature 1995;373:573–580.
13. Booker GW, Breeze AL, Downing AK, et al: Structure of an SH2 domain of the p85 alpha subunit of phosphatidylinositol-3-OH kinase. Nature 1992;358:684–687.
14. Waksman G, Kominos D, Robertson DR, et al: Crystal structure of the phosphotyrosine recognition domain SH2 of v-src complexed with tyrosine-phosphorylated peptides. Nature 1992;358:646–653.
15. Kavanaugh WM, Williams LT: An alternative to SH2 domains for binding tyrosine-phosphorylated proteins. Science 1995;266:1862–1865.
16. van der Geer P, Pawson T: The PTB domain: A new protein module implicated in signal transduction. Trends Biochem Sci 1995;20:277–280.
17. Sherr CJ: Colony-stimulating factor-1 receptor. Blood 1990;75:1–12.
18. Kozlowski M, Larose L, Lee F, et al: SHP-1 binds and negatively modulates the c-Kit receptor by interaction with tyrosine 569 in the c-Kit juxtamembrane domain. Mol Cell Biol 1998;18:2089–2099.
19. Bazan JF: Emerging families of cytokines and receptors. Curr Biol 3:603–606, 1997.
20. De Vos AM, Ultsch M, Kossiakoff AA: Human growth hormone and extracellular domain of its receptor: Crystal structure of the complex. Science 1992;255:306–312.
21. Somers W, Ultsch M, De Vos AM, et al: The x-ray structure of a growth hormone-prolactin receptor complex. Nature 1994;372:478–481.
22. Livnah O, Stura EA, Johnson DL, et al: Functional mimicry of a protein hormone by a peptide agonist: The EPO receptor complex at 2.8 Å. Science 1996;273:464–471.

23. Murakami M, Narazaki M, Hibi M, et al: Critical cytoplasmic region of the interleukin 6 signal transducer gp130 is conserved in the cytokine receptor family. Proc Natl Acad Sci USA 1991;88:11349–11353.

24. Ihle JN: Janus kinases in cytokine signalling. Philos Trans R Soc Lond B Biol Sci 1996;351:159–166.

25. Zang H, Sato K, Nakajima H, et al: The distal region and receptor tyrosines of the Epo receptor are non-essential for in vivo erythropoiesis. EMBO J 2001;20:3156–3166.

26. Starr R, Hilton DJ: SOCS: Suppressors of cytokine signalling. Int J Biochem Cell Biol 1998;30:1081–1085.

27. Zhang JG, Farley A, Nicholson SE, et al: The conserved SOCS box motif in suppressors of cytokine signaling binds to elongins B and C and may couple bound proteins to proteasomal degradation. Proc Natl Acad Sci USA 1999;96:2071–2076.

28. Marine JC, Topham DJ, McKay C, et al: SOCS1 deficiency causes a lymphocyte-dependent perinatal lethality. Cell 1999;98:609–616.

29. Alexander WS, Starr R, Fenner JE, et al: SOCS1 is a critical inhibitor of interferon gamma signaling and prevents the potentially fatal neonatal actions of this cytokine. Cell 1999;98:597–608.

30. Roberts AW, Robb L, Rakar S, et al: Placental defects and embryonic lethality in mice lacking suppressor of cytokine signaling 3. Proc Natl Acad Sci USA 2001;98:9324–9329.

31. Takahashi Y, Carpino N, Cross JC, et al: SOCS3: An essential regulator of LIF receptor signaling in trophoblast giant cell differentiation. EMBO J 2003;22:372–384.

32. Metcalf D, Greenhalgh CJ, Viney E, et al: Gigantism in mice lacking suppressor of cytokine signalling-2. Nature 2000;405:1069–1073.

33. Krebs DL, Uren RT, Metcalf D, et al: SOCS-6 binds to insulin receptor substrate 4, and mice lacking the SOCS-6 gene exhibit mild growth retardation. Mol Cell Biol 2002;22:4567–4578.

34. Daeron M: Fc receptor biology. Annu Rev Immunol 1997;15:203–234.

35. Davis RS, Dennis G Jr, Odom MR, et al: Fc receptor homologs: Newest members of a remarkably diverse Fc receptor gene family. Immunol Rev 2002;190:123–136.

36. Nadler MJ, Matthews SA, Turner H, et al: Signal transduction by the high-affinity immunoglobulin E receptor Fc epsilon RI: Coupling form to function. Adv Immunol 2000;76:325–355.

37. Ravetch JV, Bolland S: IgG Fc receptors. Annu Rev Immunol 2001;19:275–290.

38. Monteiro RC, van de Winkel JG: IgA Fc receptors. Annu Rev Immunol 2003;21:177–204.

39. Zamoyska R, Basson A, Filby A, et al: The influence of the src-family kinases, Lck and Fyn, on T cell differentiation, survival and activation. Immunol Rev 2003;191:107–118.

40. Miller AT, Berg LJ: New insights into the regulation and functions of Tec family tyrosine kinases in the immune system. Curr Opin Immunol 2002;14:331–340.

41. Schaeffer EM, Debnath J, Yap G, et al: Requirement for Tec kinases Rlk and Itk in T cell receptor signaling and immunity. Science 1999;284:638–641.

42. Isakov N: ITIMs and ITAMs: The yin and yang of antigen and Fc receptor-linked signaling machinery. Immunol Res 1997;16:85–100.

43. Watson SP, Gibbins J: Collagen receptor signalling in platelets: Extending the role of the ITAM. Immunol Today 1998;19:260–264.

44. Elder ME: ZAP-70 and defects of T-cell receptor signaling. Semin Hematol 1998;35:310–320.

45. Chu DH, Morita CT, Weiss A: The Syk family of protein tyrosine kinases in T-cell activation and development. Immunol Rev 1998;165:167–180.

46. Pappu R, Cheng AM, Li B, et al: Requirement for B cell linker protein (BLNK) in B cell development. Science 1999;286:1949–1954.

47. Minegishi Y, Rohrer J, Coustan-Smith E, et al: An essential role for BLNK in human B cell development. Science 1999;286:1954–1957.

48. Clements JL, Yang B, Ross-Barta SE, et al: Requirement for the leukocyte-specific adapter protein SLP-76 for normal T cell development. Science 1998;281:416–419.

49. Fruman DA, Cantley LC: Phosphoinositide 3-kinase in immunological systems. Semin Immunol 2002;14:7–18.

50. Hynes RO: Integrins: bidirectional, allosteric signaling machines. Cell 2002;110:673–687.

51. Ruoslahti E: Fibronectin and its integrin receptors in cancer. Adv Cancer Res 1999;76:1–20.

52. Ilic D, Furuta Y, Kanazawa S, et al: Reduced cell motility and enhanced focal adhesion contact formation in cells from FAK-deficient mice. Nature 1995;377:539–544.

53. Hagel M, George EL, Kim A, et al: The adaptor protein paxillin is essential for normal development in the mouse and is a critical transducer of fibronectin signaling. Mol Cell Biol 2002;22:901–915.

54. Guinamard R, Okigaki M, Schlessinger J, et al: Absence of marginal zone B cells in Pyk-2-deficient mice defines their role in the humoral response. Nat Immunol 2000;1:31–36.

55. Becker S, Groner B, Müller CW: Three-dimensional structure of the Stat3β homodimer bound to DNA. Nature 1998;394:145–151.

56. Chen X, Vinkemeier U, Zhao Y, et al: Crystal structure of a tyrosine phosphorylated STAT-1 dimer bound to DNA. Cell 1998;93:827–839.

57. Darnell JE Jr: Transcription factors as targets for cancer therapy. Nat Rev Cancer 2002;2:740–749.

58. Chai SK, Nichols GL, Rothman P: Constitutive activation of JAKs and STATs in BCR-Abl-expressing cell lines and peripheral blood cells derived from leukemic patients. J Immunol 1997;159:4720–4728.

59. Sexl V, Piekorz R, Moriggl R, et al: Stat5a/b contribute to interleukin 7-induced B-cell precursor expansion, but abl- and bcr/abl-induced transformation are independent of stat5 [abstract]. Blood 2000;96:2277–2283.

60. Schwaller J, Parganas E, Wang D, et al: Stat5 is essential for the myelo- and lymphoproliferative disease induced by TEL/JAK2. Mol Cell 2000;6:693–704.

61. Ravichandran KS: Signaling via Shc family adapter proteins. Oncogene 2001;20:6322–6330.

62. Sakai R, Henderson JT, O'Bryan JP, et al: The mammalian ShcB and ShcC phosphotyrosine docking proteins function in the maturation of sensory and sympathetic neurons. Neuron 2000;28:819–833.

63. Zhang L, Camerini V, Bender TP, et al: A nonredundant role for the adapter protein Shc in thymic T cell development. Nat Immunol 2002;3:749–755.

64. Myers MG Jr, Xiao JS, White MF: The IRS-1 signaling system. Trends Biochem Sci 1994;19:289–293.

65. Yenush L, White MF: The IRS-signalling system during insulin and cytokine action. Bioessays 1997;19:491–500.

66. Withers DJ, Gutierrez JS, Towery H, et al: Disruption of IRS-2 causes type 2 diabetes in mice. Nature 1998;391:900–904.

67. Araki E, Lipes MA, Patti ME, et al: Alternative pathway of insulin signalling in mice with targeted disruption of the IRS-1 gene. Nature 1994;372:186–190.

68. Tamemoto H, Kadowaki T, Tobe K, et al: Insulin resistance and growth retardation in mice lacking insulin receptor substrate-1. Nature 1994;372:182–186.

69. Gu H, Neel BG: The "Gab" in signal transduction. Trends Cell Biol 2003;13:122–130.

70. Liu Y, Rohrschneider LR: The gift of Gab. FEBS Lett 2002;515:1–7.

71. Lemay S, Davidson D, Latour S, et al: Dok-3, a novel adapter molecule involved in the negative regulation of immunoreceptor signaling. Mol Cell Biol 2000;20:2743–2754.

72. Di Cristofano A, Carpino N, Dunant N, et al: Molecular cloning and characterization of p56dok-2 defines a new family of RasGAP-binding proteins. J Biol Chem 1998;273:4827–4830.

73. Carpino N, Wisniewski D, Strife A, et al: p62(dok): A constitutively tyrosine-phosphorylated, GAP-associated protein in chronic myelogenous leukemia progenitor cells. Cell 1997;197–204.

74. Grimm J, Sachs M, Britsch S, et al: Novel p62dok family members, dok-4 and dok-5, are substrates of the c-Ret receptor tyrosine kinase and mediate neuronal differentiation. J Cell Biol 2001;154:345–354.

75. Lax I, Wong A, Lamothe B, et al: The docking protein FRS2alpha controls a MAP kinase–mediated negative feedback mechanism for signaling by FGF receptors. Mol Cell 2002;10:709–719.

76. Bustelo XR: Regulation of Vav proteins by intramolecular events. Front Biosci 2002;7:d24–d30.

77. Turner M, Billadeau DD: VAV proteins as signal integrators for multi-subunit immune-recognition receptors. Nat Rev Immunol 2002;2:476–486.

78. Turner M: The role of Vav proteins in B cell responses. Adv Exp Med Biol 2002;512:29–34.

79. Jordan MS, Singer AL, Koretzky GA: Adaptors as central mediators of signal transduction in immune cells. Nat Immunol 2003;4:110–116.

80. Yablonski D, Weiss A: Mechanisms of signaling by the hematopoietic-specific adaptor proteins, SLP-76 and LAT and their B cell counterpart, BLNK/SLP-65. Adv Immunol 2001;79:93–128.

81. Shultz LD, Schweitzer PA, Rajan TV, et al: Mutations at the murine motheaten locus are within the hematopoietic cell protein tyrosine phosphatase (Hcph) gene. Cell 1993;73:1445–1454.

82. Tsui HW, Siminovitch KA, de Souza L, et al: Motheaten and viable motheaten mice have mutations in the haematopoietic cell phosphatase gene. Nat Gen 1993;4:124–129.

83. Hof P, Pluskey S, Dhe-Paganon S, et al: Crystal structure of the tyrosine phosphatase SHP-2. Cell 1998;92:441–450.

84. Saxton TM, Henkemeyer M, Gasca S, et al: Abnormal mesoderm patterning in mouse embryos mutant for the SH2 tyrosine phosphatase Shp-2. EMBO J 1997;16:2352–2364.

85. Alexander DR: The CD45 tyrosine phosphatase: A positive and negative regulator of immune cell function. Semin Immunol 2000;12:349–359.

86. Vanhaesebroeck B, Leevers SJ, Panayotou G, et al: Phosphoinositide 3-kinases: A conserved family of signal transducers. Trends Biochem Sci 1997;22:267–272.

87. Vanhaesebroeck B, Stein RC, Waterfield MD: The study of phosphoinositide 3-kinase function. Cancer Surv 1996;27:249–270.

88. Cantley LC: The phosphoinositide 3-kinase pathway. Science 2002;296:1655–1657.

89. Vanhaesebroeck B, Alessi DR: The PI3K-PDK1 connection: More than just a road to PKB. Biochem J 2000;346:561–576.

90. Brazil DP, Park J, Hemmings BA: PKB binding proteins. Getting in on the Akt. Cell 2002;111:293–303.

91. Nicholson KM, Anderson NG: The protein kinase B/Akt signalling pathway in human malignancy. Cell Signal 2002;14:381–395.

92. Comer FI, Parent CA: PI 3-kinases and PTEN: How opposites chemoattract. Cell 2002;109:541–544.

93. Leslie NR, Downes CP: PTEN: The down side of PI 3-kinase signalling. Cell Signal 2002;14:285–295.

94. Parsons R, Simpson L: PTEN and cancer. Methods Mol Biol 2003;222:147–166.

95. Backers K, Blero D, Paternotte N, et al: The termination of PI3K signaling by SHIP1 and SHIP2 inositol 5-phosphatases. Adv Enyzme Regul 2003;43:15–28.

96. Janssens S, Beyaert R: Functional diversity and regulation of different interleukin-1 receptor- associated kinase (IRAK) family members. Mol Cell 2003;11:293–302.

97. Medzhitov R: Toll-like receptors and innate immunity. Nat Rev Immunol 2001;1:135–145.

98. Suzuki N, Suzuki S, Duncan GS, et al: Severe impairment of interleukin-1 and Toll-like receptor signalling in mice lacking IRAK-4. Nature 2002;416:750–756.

99. Massague J: TGFbeta signaling: Receptors, transducers, and Mad proteins. Cell 1996;85:947–950.

100. Shi Y, Hata A, Lo RS, et al: A structural basis for mutational inactivation of the tumour suppressor Smad4. Nature 1997;388:87–93.

101. Hahn SA, Schutte M, Hoque AT, et al: DPC4, a candidate tumor suppressor gene at human chromosome 18q21.1. Science 1996;271:350–353.

102. Lo RS, Chen YG, Shi Y, et al: The L3 loop: A structural motif determining specific interactions between SMAD proteins and TGF-beta receptors. EMBO J 1998;17:996–1005.

103. Heldin CH, Miyazono K, Dijke P: TGF-beta signalling from cell membrane to nucleus through SMAD proteins. Nature 1997;390:465–471.

104. Nakao A, Afrakhte M, Moren A, et al: Identification of Smad7, a TGF-beta-inducible antagonist of TGF-beta signalling. Nature 1997;389:631–635.

105. Imamura T, Takase M, Nishihara A, et al: Smad6 inhibits signalling by the TGF-beta superfamily. Nature 1997;389:622–626.

106. Nusse R, van Ooyen A, Cox D, et al: Mode of proviral activation of a putative mammary oncogene (int-1) on mouse chromosome 15. Nature 1984;307:131–136.

107. Rijsewijk F, Schuermann M, Wagenaar E, et al: The Drosophila homolog of the mouse mammary oncogene int-1 is identical to the segment polarity gene wingless. Cell 1987;50:649–657.

108. Nusse R: A versatile transcriptional effector of Wingless signaling. Cell 1997;89:321–323.

109. Siegfried E, Wilder EL, Perrimon N: Components of wingless signaling in Drosophila. Nature 1994;367:76–80.

110. Cadigan KM, Nusse R: wingless signaling in the Drosophila eye and embryonic epidermis. Development 1996;122:2801–2812.

111. Bienz M, Clevers H: Linking colorectal cancer to Wnt signaling. Cell 2000;103:311–320.

112. Eastman Q, Grosschedl R: Regulation of LEF-1/TCF transcription factors by Wnt and other signals. Curr Opin Cell Biol 1999;11:233–240.

113. Slusarski DC, Corces VG, Moon RT: Interaction of Wnt and a Frizzled homologue triggers G-protein-linked phosphatidylinositol signalling. Nature 1997;390:410–413.

114. Pandur P, Maurus D, Kuhl M: Increasingly complex: New players enter the Wnt signaling network. Bioessays 2002;24:881–884.

115. Ellisen LW, Bird J, West DC, et al: TAN-1, the human homolog of the Drosophila notch gene, is broken by chromosomal translocations in T lymphoblastic neoplasms. Cell 1991;66:649–661.

116. Artavanis-Tsakonas S, Matsuno K, Fortini ME: Notch signaling. Science 1995;268:225–232.

117. Girard L, Hanna Z, Beaulieu N, et al: Frequent provirus insertional mutagenesis of Notch1 in thymomas of MMTVD/myc transgenic mice suggests a collaboration of c-myc and Notch1 for oncogenesis. Genes Dev 1996;10:1930–1944.

118. Joutel A, Corpechot C, Ducros A, et al: Notch3 mutations in CADASIL, a hereditary adult-onset condition causing stroke and dementia. Nature 1996;383:707–710.

119. Jarriault S, Brou C, Logeat F, et al: Signalling downstream of activated mammalian Notch. Nature 1995;377:355–358.

120. Oka C, Nakano T, Wakeham A, et al: Disruption of the mouse RBP-J kappa gene results in early embryonic death. Development 1995;121:3291–3301.

121. Artavanis-Tsakonas S, Rand MD, Lake RJ: Notch signaling: Cell fate control and signal integration in development. Science 1999;284:770–776.

122. Pear WS, Radtke F: Notch signaling in lymphopoiesis. Semin Immunol 2003;15:69–79.

123. Conlon RA, Reaume AG, Rossant J: Notch1 is required for the coordinate segmentation of somites. Development 1995;121:1533–1545.

124. Pompa JL, Wakeham A, Correia KM, et al: Conservation of the Notch signalling pathway in mammalian neurogenesis. Development 1997;124:1139–1148.

125. Offermanns S, Simon MI: Organization of transmembrane signalling by heterotrimeric G proteins. Cancer Surv 1996;27:177–198.

126. Baggiolini M, Dewald B, Moser B: Human chemokines: An update. Annu Rev Immunol 1997;15:675–705.

127. Simon MI, Strathmann MP, Gautam N: Diversity of G proteins in signal transduction. Science 1991;252:802–808.

128. Offermanns S, Simon MI: Genetic analysis of mammalian G-protein signalling. Oncogene 1998;17:1375–1381.

129. Conklin BR, Bourne HR: Structural elements of G alpha subunits that interact with G beta gamma, receptors, and effectors. Cell 1993;73:631–641.

130. Locksley RM, Killeen N, Lenardo MJ: The TNF and TNF receptor superfamilies: Integrating mammalian biology. Cell 2001;104:487–501.

131. Yeh WC, de la Pompa JL, McCurrach ME, et al: FADD: Essential for embryo development and signaling from some, but not all, inducers of apoptosis. Science 1998;279:1954–1958.

132. Varfolomeev EE, Schuchmann M, Luria V, et al: Targeted disruption of the mouse Caspase 8 gene ablates cell death induction by the TNF receptors, Fas/Apo1, and DR3 and is lethal prenatally. Immunity 1998;9:267–276.

133. Sakahira H, Enari M, Nagata S: Cleavage of CAD inhibitor in CAD activation and DNA degradation during apoptosis. Nature 1998;391:96–99.

134. Enari M, Sakahira H, Yokoyama H, et al: A caspase-activated DNase that degrades DNA during apoptosis, and its inhibitor ICAD. Nature 1998;391:43–50.

135. Cerretti DP, Kozlosky CJ, Mosley B, et al: Molecular cloning of the interleukin-1 beta converting enzyme. Science 1992;256:97–100.

136. Yuan J, Shaham S, Ledoux S, et al: The C. elegans cell death gene ced-3 encodes a protein similar to mammalian interleukin-1β-converting enzyme. Cell 1993;75:641–652.

137. Li P, Allen H, Banerjee S, et al: Mice deficient in IL-1β-converting enzyme are defective in production of mature IL-1β and resistant to endotoxic shock. Cell 1995;80:401–411.

138. Woo M, Hakem R, Soengas MS, et al: Essential contribution of caspase 3/CPP32 to apoptosis and its associated nuclear changes. Genes Dev 1998;12:806–819.

139. Yoshida H, Kong YY, Yoshida R, et al: Apaf1 is required for mitochondrial pathways of apoptosis and brain development. Cell 1998;94:739–750.

140. Stanger BZ, Leder P, Lee T-H, et al: RIP: A novel "death domain"-containing protein kinase that interacts with Fas/APO-1 (CD95) and causes cell death. Cell 1995;81:513–523.

141. Kelliher MA, Grimm S, Ishida Y, et al: The death domain kinase RIP mediates the TNF-induced NF-κB signal. Immunity 1998;8:297–303.

142. Cao Z, Xiong J, Takeuchi M, et al: TRAF6 is a signal transducer for interleukin-1. Nature 1996;383:443–446.

143. Xu Y, Cheng G, Baltimore D: Targeted disruption of TRAF3 leads to postnatal lethality and defective T-dependent immune responses. Immunity 1996;5:407–415.

144. Yeh WC, Shahinian A, Speiser D, et al: Early lethality, functional NF-kappa-B activation, and increased sensitivity to TNF-induced cell death in TRAF2-deficient mice. Immunity 1997;7:715–725.

145. Lomaga MA, Henderson JT, Elia AJ, et al: Tumor necrosis factor receptor-associated factor 6 (TRAF6) deficiency results in exencephaly and is required for apoptosis within the developing CNS. J Neurosci 2000;20:7384–7393.

146. Yeh WC, Itie A, Elia AJ, et al: Requirement for Casper (c-FLIP) in regulation of death receptor-induced apoptosis and embryonic development. Immunity 2000;12:633–642.

147. Lee EG, Boone DL, Chai S, et al: Failure to regulate TNF-induced NF-kappa-B and cell death responses in A20-deficient mice. Science 2000;289:2350–2354.

148. Chawla A, Repa JJ, Evans RM, et al: Nuclear receptors and lipid physiology: Opening the X-files. Science 2001;1866–1870.

149. Weih F, Carrasco D, Durham SK, et al: Multiorgan inflammation and hematopoietic abnormalities in mice with a targeted disruption of RelB, a member of the NF-kappa-B/Rel family. Cell 1995;80:331–340.

150. Weih F, Durham SK, Barton DS, et al: Both multiorgan inflammation and myeloid hyperplasia in RelB-deficient mice are T cell dependent. J Immunol 1996;157:3974–3979.

151. Sha WC, Liou H-C, Tuomanen EI, et al: Targeted disruption of the p50 subunit of NF-kappa-B leads to multifocal defects in immune responses. Cell 1995;80:321–330.

152. Beg AA, Sha WC, Bronson RT, et al: Embryonic lethality and liver degeneration in mice lacking the RelA component of NF-kappa B. Nature 1995;376:167–170.

153. Gerondakis S, Strasser A, Metcalf D, et al: Rel-deficient T cells exhibit defects in production of interleukin 3 and granulocyte-macrophage colony-stimulating factor. Proc Natl Acad Sci USA 1996;93:3405–3409.

154. Kontgen F, Grumont RJ, Strasser A, et al: Mice lacking the c-rel proto-oncogene exhibit defects in lymphocyte proliferation, humoral immunity, and interleukin-2 expression. Genes Dev 1995;9:1965–1977.

155. Beg AA, Sha WC, Bronson RT, et al: Constitutive NF-kappa B activation, enhanced granulopoiesis, and neonatal lethality in I kappa B alpha-deficient mice. Genes Dev 1995;9:2736–2746.

156. Karin M, Cao Y, Greten FR, et al: NF-kappa-B in cancer: from innocent bystander to major culprit. Nat Rev Cancer 2002;2:301–310.

157. Li Q, Van Antwerp D, Mercurio F, et al: Severe liver degeneration in mice lacking the I-kappa-B kinase 2 gene. Science 1999;284:321–325.

158. Rudolph D, Yeh WC, Wakeham A, et al: Severe liver degeneration and lack of NF-kappa-B activation in NEMO/IKK-gamma-deficient mice. Genes Dev 2000;14:854–862.

159. Hu Y, Baud V, Delhase M, et al: Abnormal morphogenesis but intact IKK activation in mice lacking the IKK-alpha subunit of I-kappa-B kinase. Nature 2001;410:710–714.

160. Sun Z, Arendt CW, Ellmeier W, et al: PKC-theta is required for TCR-induced NF-kappa-B activation in mature but not immature T lymphocytes. Nature 2000;404:402–407.

161. Saijo K, Mecklenbrauker I, Santana A, et al: Protein kinase C beta controls nuclear factor kappa-B activation in B cells through selective regulation of the I-kappa-B kinase alpha. J Exp Med 2002;195:1647–1652.

162. Ikura M, Osawa M, Ames JB: The role of calcium-binding proteins in the control of transcription: structure to function. Bioessays 2002;24:625–636.

163. Cheng HY, Pitcher GM, Laviolette SR, et al: DREAM is a critical transcriptional repressor for pain modulation. Cell 2002;108:31–43.

164. Crabtree GR: Calcium, calcineurin, and the control of transcription. J Biol Chem 2001;276:2313–2316.

165. Crabtree GR, Olson EN: NFAT signaling: Choreographing the social lives of cells. Cell 2002;109(suppl):S67–S79.

166. Hoeflich KP, Luo J, Rubie EA, et al: Requirement for glycogen synthase kinase-3-beta in cell survival and NF-kappa-B activation. Nature 2000;406:86–90.

167. Beals CR, Sheridan CM, Turck CW, et al: Nuclear export of NF-ATc enhanced by glycogen synthase kinase-3. Science 1997;275:1930–1933.

168. Horsley V, Pavlath GK: NFAT: Ubiquitous regulator of cell differentiation and adaptation. J Cell Biol 2002;156:771–774.

169. Servillo G, Della Fazia MA, Sassone-Corsi P: Coupling cAMP signaling to transcription in the liver: Pivotal role of CREB and CREM. Exp Cell Res 2002;275:143–154.

170. Kung AL, Rebel VI, Bronson RT, et al: Gene dose-dependent control of hematopoiesis and hematologic tumor suppression by CBP. Genes Dev 2000;14:272–277.

171. Rudolph D, Tafuri A, Gass P, et al: Impaired fetal T cell development and perinatal lethality in mice lacking the cAMP response element binding protein. Proc Natl Acad Sci USA 1998;95:4481–4486.

172. Lonze BE, Ginty DD: Function and regulation of CREB family transcription factors in the nervous system. Neuron 2002;35:605–623.

173. Nantel F, Monaco L, Foulkes NS, et al: Spermiogenesis deficiency and germ-cell apoptosis in CREM-mutant mice. Nature 1996;380:159–162.

174. Khokhlatchev AV, Canagarajah B, Wilsbacher J, et al: Phosphorylation of the MAP kinase ERK2 promotes its homodimerization and nuclear translocation. Cell 1998;93:605–615.

175. Hill CS, Treisman R: Transcriptional regulation by extracellular signals: mechanisms and specificity. Cell 1995;80:199–211.

176. Gille H, Sharrocks AD, Shaw PE: Phosphorylation of transcription factor p62^{TCF} by MAP kinase stimulates ternary complex formation at c-fos promoter. Nature 1992;358:414–417.

177. Gille H, Kortenjann M, Thomae O, et al: ERK phosphorylation potentiates Elk-1-mediated ternary complex formation and transactivation. EMBO J 1995;14:951–962.

178. Cavigelli M, Dolfi F, Claret FX, et al: Induction of c-fos expression through JNK-mediated TCF/Elk-1 phosphorylation. EMBO J 1995;14:5957–5964.

179. Derijard B, Hibi M, Wu IH, et al: JNK1: A protein kinase stimulated by UV light and Ha-Ras that binds and phosphorylates the c-Jun activation domain. Cell 1994;76:1025–1037.

180. Hibi M, Lin A, Smeal T, et al: Identification of an oncoprotein- and UV-responsive protein kinase that binds and potentiates the c-Jun activation domain. Genes Dev 1993;7:2135–2148.

181. Gupta S, Campbell D, Derijard B, et al: Transcription factor ATF2 regulation by the JNK signal transduction pathway. Science 1995;267:389–393.

182. Wang XZ, Ron D: Stress-induced phosphorylation and activation of the transcription factor CHOP (GADD153) by p38 MAP Kinase. Science 1996;272:1347-1349.

183. Han J, Jiang Y, Li Z, et al: Activation of the transcription factor MEF2C by the MAP kinase p38 in inflammation. Nature 1997;386:296-299.

184. Kato Y, Kravchenko VV, Tapping RI, et al: BMK1/ERK5 regulates serum-induced early gene expression through transcription factor MEF2C. EMBO J 1997;16:7054-7066.

185. Kato S, Endoh H, Masuhiro Y, et al: Activation of the estrogen receptor through phosphorylation by mitogen-activated protein kinase. Science 1995;270:1491-1494.

186. Hu MC, Qiu WR, Wang X, et al: Human HPK1, a novel human hematopoietic progenitor kinase that activates the JNK/SAPK kinase cascade. Genes Dev 1996;10:2251-2264.

187. Charles CH, Sun H, Lau LF, et al: The growth factor-inducible immediate-early gene 3CH134 encodes a protein-tyrosine-phosphatase. Proc Natl Acad Sci USA 1993;90:5292-5296.

188. Sun H, Charles CH, Lau LF, et al: MKP-1 (3CH134), an immediate early gene product, is a dual specificity phosphatase that dephosphorylates MAP kinase in vivo. Cell 1993;75:487-493.

189. Yoon JK, Lau LF: Involvement of JunD in transcriptional activation of the orphan receptor gene *nur*77 by nerve growth factor and membrane depolarization in PC12 cells. Mol Cell Biol 1994;14:7731-7743.

190. Camps M, Nichols A, Gillieron C, et al: Catalytic activation of the phosphatase MKP-3 by ERK2 mitogen-activated protein kinase. Science 1998;280:1262-1265.

191. Yang D, Tournier C, Wysk M, et al: Targeted disruption of the MKK4 gene causes embryonic death, inhibition of c-Jun NH2-terminal kinase activation, and defects in AP-1 transcriptional activity. Proc Natl Acad Sci USA 1997;94:3004-3009.

192. Nishina H, Bachmann M, Oliveira DSA, et al: Impaired CD28-mediated interleukin 2 production and proliferation in stress kinase SAPK/ERK1 kinase (SEK1)/mitogen-activated protein kinase kinase 4 (MKK4)-deficient T lymphocytes. J Exp Med 1997;186:941-953.

193. Nishina H, Fischer KD, Radvanyi L, et al: Stress-signalling kinase Sek1 protects thymocytes from apoptosis mediated by CD95 and CD3. Nature 1997;385:350-353.

194. Vojtek AB, Hollenberg SM, Cooper JA: Mammalian ras interacts directly with the serine/threonine kinase raf. Cell 1993;74:205-214.

195. Zhang XF, Settleman J, Kyriakis JM, et al: Normal and oncogenic p21ras proteins bind to the amino-terminal regulatory domain of c-Raf-1. Nature 1993;364:308-313.

196. Stokoe D, Macdonald SG, Cadwallader K, et al: Activation of raf as a result of recruitment to the plasma membrane. Science 1994;264:1463-1467.

197. Lange-Carter CA, Pleiman CM, Gardner AM, et al: A divergence in the MAP kinase regulatory network defined by MEK kinase and Raf. Science 1993;260:315-319.

198. Yan M, Dai T, Deak JC, et al: Activation of stress-activated protein kinase by MEKK1 phosphorylation of its activator SEK1. Nature 1994;372:798-800.

199. Minden A, Lin A, Claret FX, et al: Selective activation of the JNK signaling cascade and c-Jun transcriptional activity by the small GTPases Rac and Cdc42Hs. Cell 1995;81:1147-1157.

200. Pharr PN, Hofbauer A: Loss of flk-2/flt3 expression during commitment of multipotent mouse hematopoietic progenitor cells to the mast cell lineage. Exp Hematol 1997;25:620-628.

201. Su YC, Han J, Xu S, et al: NIK is a new Ste20-related kinase that binds NCK and MEKK1 and activates the SAPK/JNK cascade via a conserved regulatory domain. EMBO J 1997;16:1279-1290.

202. Rudel T, Bokoch GM: Membrane and morphological changes in apoptotic cells regulated by caspase-mediated activation of pak2. Science 1997;276:1571-1574.

203. Lamarche N, Tapon N, Stowers L, et al: Rac and Cdc42 induce actin polymerization and G1 cell cycle progression independently of p65PAK and the JNK/SAPK MAP kinase cascade. Cell 1996;87:519-529.

204. Ichijo H, Nishida E, Irie K, et al: Induction of apoptosis by ASK1, a mammalian MAPKKK that activates SAPK/JNK and p38 signaling pathways. Science 1997;275:90-94.

205. Salmeron A, Ahmad TB, Carlile GW, et al: Activation of MEK-1 and SEK-1 by Tpl-2 proto-oncoprotein, a novel MAP kinase kinase. EMBO J 1996;15:817-826.

206. Kiefer F, Tibbles LA, Anafi M, et al: HPK1, a hematopoietic protein kinase activating the SAPK/JNK pathway. EMBO J 1996;15:7013-7025.

207. Rana A, Gallo K, Godowski P, et al: The mixed lineage kinase SPRK phosphorylates and activates the stress-activated protein kinase activator, SEK-1. J Biol Chem 1996;271:19025-19028.

208. Pombo CM, Kehrl JH, Sanchez I, et al: Activation of the SAPK pathway by the human STE20 homologue germinal centre kinase. Nature 1995;377:750-754.

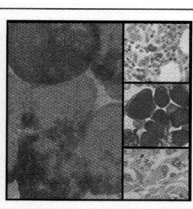

3

THE CELLULAR MICROENVIRONMENT

Riccardo Alessandro

Timothy Clair

Lance A. Liotta

Elise C. Kohn

SUMMARY OF KEY POINTS

- The success of cancer development and dissemination is caused and regulated by interactions with the microenvironment. Paget described the role of the "seed," the cancer cell, and the "soil," the local microenvironment.[1]
- Advances in cell and molecular biology have resulted from the study of communication between the cancer cell (seed) and the microenviroment (soil) that drives

production of autocrine and paracrine factors, drives vascular outgrowth, stimulates production of invasion factors by the stroma and the host, causes immune modulation, and results in a favorable environment for the malignancy to the detriment of normal cells.
- Local stromal and inflammatory cells are altered in function and cell-cell interactions in response to the

presence of the tumor.
- Tumor cell interactions with the cellular and noncellular locale can augment signals for survival, proliferation, and migration within the tumor.
- Understanding the components of the microenvironment and their interplay will assist in the development of more logical, targeted therapies for cancer.

INTRODUCTION

The structures of tissues in an organism are the result of combinations of cell births, cell migration, and cell deaths that occur during the process of development. A cell, within the society of cells comprising mature tissue, displays a phenotype that depends on its developmental history and its response to its environment. This includes the capacity to interact constructively with other cell populations in the process of tissue formation. Cancer is the evolution of a population of cells that has become independent of the processes that regulate normal development. To progress toward full malignancy, a cancer cell acquires changes[2] that make it relatively independent of normal intrinsic self-regulation and interaction with its environment. This environment is a rich source of the surrounding extracellular matrix (ECM), autocrine secretions of the tumor, and the paracrine secretions of other cellular components of the particular tissue. However, cancer cells are not isolated and autonomous but interact dynamically with their environment through-out the disease process.[3] This heterotypic perspective drives much of current cancer research and is supported by a great deal of recent evidence regarding the interaction of cancer and surrounding stromal tissue, which contains fibroblasts, myofibroblasts, inflammatory cells, blood vessels, and ECM components.

Interactions between tumor cells and the host connective tissue represent a violation of the normal tissue boundaries that physiologically prevent intermixing of cells from different tissues. As a consequence of this interaction, a highly modified local host microenviron-ment is produced in which a multitude of cytokines and bioactive molecules provide structural and functional

cues for several steps of the tumorigenic and metastatic cascade (Fig. 3-1). This activated stroma deeply influences tumor development, leading to deranged cell proliferation and survival, as well as increased ability to migrate beyond the original location into other sites to form metastases. What are the molecular mechanisms by which this altered microenvironment can modulate the malignant phenotype? The answer to this question requires review of the processes that underlie the physiologic functioning of tissue-cell societies.[3]

Maintenance of normal cell and tissue homeostasis requires signal integration and regulation between growth factors and their receptors, cell-cell adhesion molecules, cell-matrix receptors, and intracellular signaling proteins (Fig. 3-2). Each cell type presents an array of surface receptors appropriate for its local environment. Activation of signaling pathways through growth factors, cell contact, and/or interaction with molecules of the ECM results in modifications of cell shape, behavior, and response to soluble molecules. These signals may be switched on and off in normal cells, depending on the presence or absence of appropriate stimuli. As a consequence, complex processes requiring a dynamic modification of cellular phenotype are finely tuned and self-limiting; the invasive phenotypes expressed by normal cells during development, wound healing, and immune function are instructive examples. These phenotypes occur in response to a variety of molecules and stimuli that activate defined signaling pathways, leading to the expression of genes involved in cell proliferation, adhesion, motility, and proteolysis.[4,5] When a wound is repaired or inflammation is arrested, the molecular relay is switched off and the invasive behavior stops.

Disruption of this fine balance can therefore enhance aberrant cell proliferation, survival, migration, and

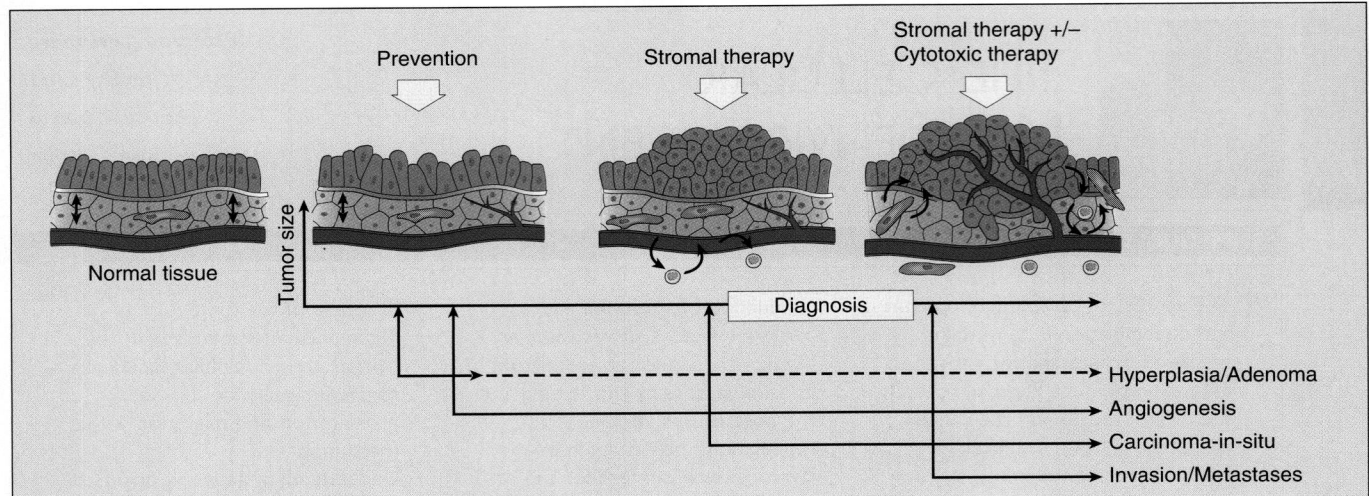

Figure 3-1. Tumor-host microenvironment cross-talk is involved at all stages during tumor progression and can be a molecular target for intervention. Interaction between the stroma and epithelium is part of the process that maintains normality. Stresses including genetic disturbances, metabolic disturbances, and illness alter this interaction and can promote development of malignancy. Changes in the interaction between the stroma and the transforming and invading epithelium can be targeted therapeutically and may be useful for prevention, as well as treatment.

function that might promote tumor development. This disruption occurs coupled with and in part as a consequence of mutations in genes that, according to the functional classification proposed by Kinzler and Vogelstein,[6] monitor growth (gatekeeper genes) or regulate genomic stability (caretaker genes) of the cells. The molecular background that characterizes the growing tumor mass can also be modulated by the signals coming from the surrounding stroma where normal cells, such as myofibroblasts, endothelial cells, and immune cells, cannot be considered mere bystanders but are active components that alter the properties of tumors. In addition to gatekeeper and caretaker gene products, another category of genes affecting carcinogenesis has been described: the

landscaper genes[6] (Table 3-1). The products of these genes are implicated in the regulation of signaling pathways activated after binding of autocrine or paracrine mediators on the tumor cell surface. Defects in these genes have been involved in hereditary syndromes predisposing cancer development.

Juvenile polyposis syndrome is an example in which an autosomal dominant mutation in a critical gene has a proliferative phenotype at one point, but the lesions can progress to carcinoma over time. Juvenile polyposis syndrome is characterized by the presence of numerous

Figure 3-2. Normal cell function is the result of appropriate cues and responses from genome and environment. Genomic and genetic changes and different environmental events alter the balance of signaling, and thus the behavior of the stromal and tumor cells. Genetic aberrations shift production of growth factors and cytokines in the tumor cell and thus drive the responses in the tumor and stromal cells. This further dysregulates the local microenvironmental milieu to drive migration, reorganization, and survival signals for the tumor and the local stromal components.

TABLE 3-1

Classification of Cancer Genes

Gatekeeper Genes

Rb	Cell proliferation, cell cycle
P53	Angiogenesis, apoptosis
NF1	Angiogenesis
VHL	Angiogenesis
MEN II	Cell migration
PTEN	Motility, cell-cell adhesion, survival
BRCA1, 2	DNA repair, angiogenesis
APC	Cell-cell adhesion
CDKN2A	Cell cycle, apoptosis

Caretaker Genes

HMSH2	Target genes of mismatch repair system are:
HMLH1	TGFβ receptor II, IGFII receptor, Bax, Caspase 5,
PMS1	MMP2. Deregulation of these genes can affect cell
PMS2	growth, ECM production, cell adhesion, angiogenesis, and apoptosis

Landscaper Genes

Gene	Cell functions affected at tumor-host interface
SMAD4	Cell proliferation, ECM production, angiogenesis
BMPR1A	

gastrointestinal hamartomatous polyps in the colon at a young age. These polyps are composed of stromal cells—mainly smooth muscle cells, myofibroblasts, and immune cells—wherein epithelial cells are enmeshed forming cystically dilated glands. It has also been suggested that mutations in the stromal cells of the hamartomatous formation may modulate epithelial cell proliferation through altered cross-talk between stromal cells and epithelial cells.[7] Germline mutations in different members of the transforming growth factor-β (TGF-β) superfamily have been observed in 5% to 35% of cases of juvenile polyposis syndrome.[8,9] Most mutations produce truncated proteins that have lost their function as intracellular signaling mediators in the TGF-β pathway.[10] Inactivation of different components of TGF-β signaling pathway has been found in sporadic cases of gastric and colorectal cancers as well.[11] TGF-β is a multifunctional cytokine; it mediates its effects on cells through a heteromeric receptor complex that consists of type I (RI) and type II (RII) components. RI and RII are serine-threonine kinases that phosphorylate downstream signaling proteins of the *mothers against dpp* (SMAD) *Drosophila* protein family.[12] SMAD2 and SMAD3 then translocate to the nucleus and transcriptionally regulate the expression of genes involved in cell proliferation, survival, and ECM production.[13] These functions are not only an integral part of tissue homeostasis, they are also logical targets for dysregulation in nonhereditary carcinogenesis.

Both epithelial and stromal cells can be modulated by TGF-β, and frequently, this interaction between carcinoma and stroma is reciprocal. In general, epithelial cells are growth-inhibited and mesenchymal cells are growth-stimulated by this cytokine.[14,15] TGF-β, is overexpressed in many human cancers, including prostate cancer, and can stimulate phenotypic switching of fibroblasts to myofibroblasts; this desmoplastic stromal reaction has been observed in precancerous prostatic intraepithelial neoplasia lesions.[16] Conversely, stroma derived from carcinoma can induce carcinogenic changes in prostate epithelial cells, demonstrating a stromal contribution to epithelial-mesenchymal transition.[17] In fact, independent genetic alterations have been detected in both stromal and epithelial cells from breast tumor tissue, suggesting that some genetic alterations in stromal cells may precede genotypic changes in the epithelial cells.[18] Increased production of TGF-β was observed to increase the ability of certain tumors to metastasize.[19,20] This excess of TGF-β can act in a paracrine fashion on the peritumoral stroma by recruiting inflammatory cells and/or tumor vasculature, thus promoting tumor progression.

Therefore tumoral host stroma represents a very particular microenvironment in which complex dynamic relations between cancer cells and normal cells occur. Tumor development must be considered not just as the transformation of normal cells into malignant cells but also, more appropriately, as the conversion of a complex tissue-like structure into a neoplasm. The specific events underlying this revolution in our thinking about cancer are now beginning to be understood in terms of altered signaling affecting proliferation, cell-cell contacts, motility, cell survival, and angiogenesis.

THE MALIGNANT INVASIVE PHENOTYPE

Acquisition of migratory and invasive properties is a turning point in malignant tumor development. Invasion through glandular and vascular basement membrane occurs during transition from benign neoplasm and in situ cancer to invasive and potentially metastatic carcinomas. As a primary tumor grows, it recruits new blood vessels that can support the metabolic needs, as well as provide access to the body's circulatory blood system. Tumor-driven angiogenesis represents an early event in cancer progression[21,22]; the local tumor microenvironment is saturated with soluble mitogens and motility factors that attract endothelial cells, as well as fibroblasts and inflammatory cells that contribute to the modification of stroma[23,24] (Fig. 3-3). Degradative and synthetic processes concomitantly occur at the tumor-host interface. Digestion of ECM components by tumor-secreted proteases produces bioactive fragments that facilitate the malignant invasive process.[3,25] Besides tumor cell-induced degradative processes, an intense and enhanced deposition of ECM, the desmoplastic response, characterizes the area around primary or metastatic tumor epithelium.[26] This process, which has been always considered as a defense mechanism to restrain tumor growth, could conversely provide a fertile ground that would support the proliferation and invasion of cancer cells. Quantitative and qualitative alteration of ECM molecules at the tumor-stroma interface has been described in different cancers including breast, colon, and pancreas carcinomas.[27-30] Tumor-specific isoforms of fibronectin, collagen, and other ECM components found in desmoplasia have been shown to induce cancer cell proliferation and migration and collagenase production[31-33]

Moreover, stroma derived from carcinoma can induce carcinogenic changes in epithelial cells, demonstrating a stromal contribution to epithelial-mesenchymal transition that is observed during tumorigenesis.[17] Olumi and colleagues[34] have demonstrated that primary, phenotypically normal fibroblasts associated with neoplasia stimulate tumor progression of initiated nontumorigenic epithelial cells both in an in vivo tissue recombination system and in an in vitro co-culture system. These carcinoma-associated fibroblasts did not form tumors when grafted or inoculated alone and did not have the same effect on normal primary prostate epithelium. The molecular mechanisms responsible for the effect exerted by the stroma on epithelial carcinogenesis have not been fully elucidated, but the production and secretion of soluble molecules, as well as ECM components, from mesenchymal cells have been proposed.

The cellular composition at the tumor-host interface is profoundly modified by the normal stroma-epithelium interface.[3] Endothelial cells from microvessels in the surrounding stroma are induced to migrate into the tumor where they proliferate and form new blood vessels in response to numerous tumor-secreted angiogenic factors such as basic fibroblast growth factor (bFGF), TGF-β, vascular endothelial growth factor (VEGF), and platelet-

Science of Clinical Oncology

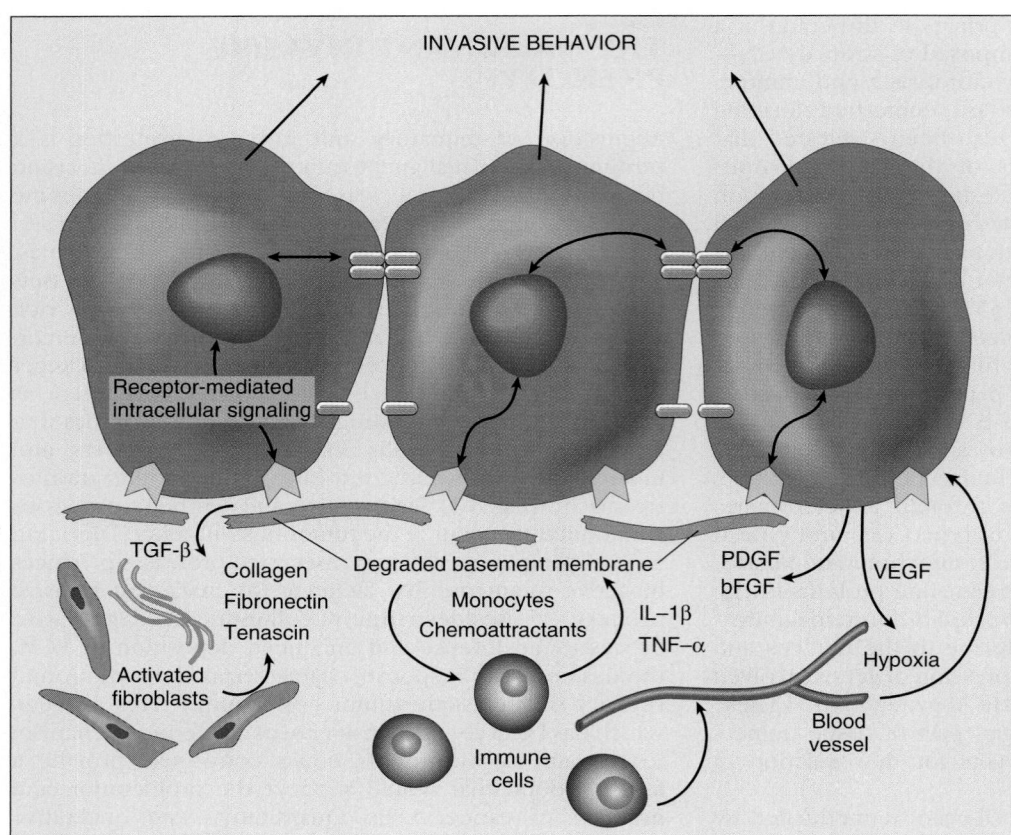

INVASIVE BEHAVIOR

Receptor-mediated
intracellular signaling

TGF-β

Collagen
Fibronectin
Tenascin

Degraded basement membrane

PDGF
bFGF

VEGF

Monocytes
Chemoattractants

IL–1β
TNF–α

Hypoxia

Activated
fibroblasts

Immune
cells

Blood
vessel

Figure 3-3. Interaction with the microenvironment plays a critical role in the development of the malignant phenotype. Host fibroblasts, immune cells, and endothelial cells are recruited at the invasive front by factors secreted from premalignant and malignant tumor cells. This heterogeneous cell population participates in the modification of the extracellular matrix (ECM) by producing cytokines and proteases. Hypoxia in the local environment stimulates the production and secretion of vascular endothelial growth factor (VEGF) and interleukin (IL)-8, recruiting endothelial and inflammatory cells and leading to capillary formation and further production of activating growth factors and cytokines. Growth factors, ECM molecules, and bioactive fragments derived by degradation of ECM components stimulate the expression of the invasive and motile phenotypes of both the malignant cell and the activated stromal components. bFGF, Basic fibroblast growth factor; PGDF, platelet-derived growth factor; TGF-β, transforming growth factor-β; TNF-α, tumor neccrosis factor-α.

derived growth factor (PDGF).[35] Evidence indicates that these factors may be produced by activated stromal cells, as well as carcinoma cells, again demonstrating an interactive relationship between host stroma and growing tumor mass.[36,37] These molecules also attract other cell types such as myofibroblasts, activated fibroblasts, and inflammatory cells that are commonly found adjacent to the tumor mass.[3,24] This varied cell population and the changed composition of local connective tissue represent a source of signals that affect tumor development.

Lastly, the tumor-host interface is the site of action of the invasive, motile tumor cell. Histologic observations indicate the presence of invasive clusters of cells in epithelial tumors, as well as in blood and lymph vessels. The leading edge of such clusters in vitro in three-dimensional collagen matrices is composed of highly motile "pathfinder" cells, and the cells in the trailing edge are passive, suggesting that tumor cell clusters may be organized as coherent tissue that contains cells with specialized (e.g., invasive) functions.[38-40]

SIGNALING CROSS-TALK AT THE TUMOR-STROMA INTERFACE

A complex environment is found at the leading edge of invasive tumors (see Fig. 3-3). A plethora of signaling molecules, produced both by tumor and local stromal cells, interacts with cell surface receptors and stimulates

intracellular signaling events that lead to changes in cell function and gene expression. Furthermore, amplification of these signaling events can occur through signal network cross-talk that becomes dysregulated in the malignant background or that is induced by the new microenvironment generated in the tumor-stroma interface. Illustrative examples are provided by the analysis of the cross-talk between the biochemical pathways mediated by integrins and growth factor receptors, and cell-cell adhesion receptors with growth factor receptors.

Cross-Talk Between Cell Adhesion and Growth Factor Receptors

Invading cancer cells are faced with a modified and activated host stroma. Cell-matrix adhesion receptors, notably integrins, are distributed normally on the basal cell surface of normal epithelium, where they have access to and bind basement membrane components such as laminin, fibronectin, and collagen type IV.[41] During invasion, these receptors delocalize across the tumor cell surface and bind different ECM components such as interstitial collagens, tenascin, and elastin. This alteration of topographic distribution of integrins and the inappropriate or noncontextual outside-in signaling stimulated by ECM components activate intracellular pathways, allowing cancer cells to survive in a foreign soil (Fig. 3-4).

Several groups have shown the involvement of integrins in tumor progression, invasive growth, and metastasis formation.[41-46] It has often been difficult to demonstrate a positive or negative correlation between tumor progression and integrin expression.[47] For the purpose of explaining these results, it is appropriate to consider the complex microenvironment at the tumor stroma interface where the integrin can communicate and synergize with activated growth factor receptors and cytokine signal transduction pathways. For example, human pancreatic carcinoma cells adhere to vitronectin through integrin $\alpha_v\beta_5$ yet are unable to migrate to this ligand. In these cells, epidermal growth factor (EGF) receptor activation leads to de novo $\alpha_v\beta_5$-dependent tumor cell migration to vitronectin.[48] Brooks and colleagues[49] have shown, in support of these findings, that stimulation of $\alpha_v\beta_5$-expressing CS-1 melanoma cells with either insulin or insulin-like growth factor (IGF)-1 promotes vitronectin-dependent motility. The same group showed that tumor cells readily metastasize to the lungs of either chick embryos or severe combined immunodeficient (SCID) mice after stimulation with either insulin or IGF-1.[49] Moro and colleagues[50] have recently demonstrated that integrins, c-src, a cytoplasmic kinase, and EGF receptor kinases form a multimolecular complex and that this association is required for EGF receptor phosphorylation. Moreover, they showed that the integrin-induced pattern of EGF receptor phosphorylation is distinct from that induced by EGF.[50] These data demonstrate that integrin-stimulated pathways and growth factor–activated signaling intersect and modulate cell activities critical for tumor cell invasion.

EGF receptor (EGF-R), a prototypic receptor tyrosine kinase (RTK), illustrates the ramification and intersection of receptor cross-talk with downstream signaling driving cell motility, survival, and proliferation (growth factor signaling cross-talk; see Fig. 3-4). The first signaling cascade to be defined downstream of EGF-R activation was the *ras*-mitogen-activated protein kinase (MAPK) pathway.[51] MAPK activation has been shown in response to integrin binding in a variety of tumor cell lines,[52,53] and a synergistic effect from EGF-R and β_1-integrin stimulation has been demonstrated for the activation of MAPK signaling pathway in A431 human carcinoma cell line.[54] EGF-R-mediated MAPK signaling is also activated in tumor cells after stimulation with lysophosphatidic acid (LPA).[55,56] LPA binds the edg family of G protein–coupled receptors and induces various cellular responses including cytoskeletal rearrangements, cell proliferation, suppression of apoptosis, and cell motility.[55,57] Cross-talk between G protein–coupled receptors and EGF-Rs further illustrates the complexity of signaling events at the plasma membrane level in invading tumor cells.

Integrin–growth factor receptor interactions are not restricted to the EGF receptor. It has been shown that cell-matrix interaction stimulates phosphorylation of the scatter factor/hepatocyte growth factor receptor, c-met,[58] PDGF receptors,[59] recepteur d'origine nantais kinase

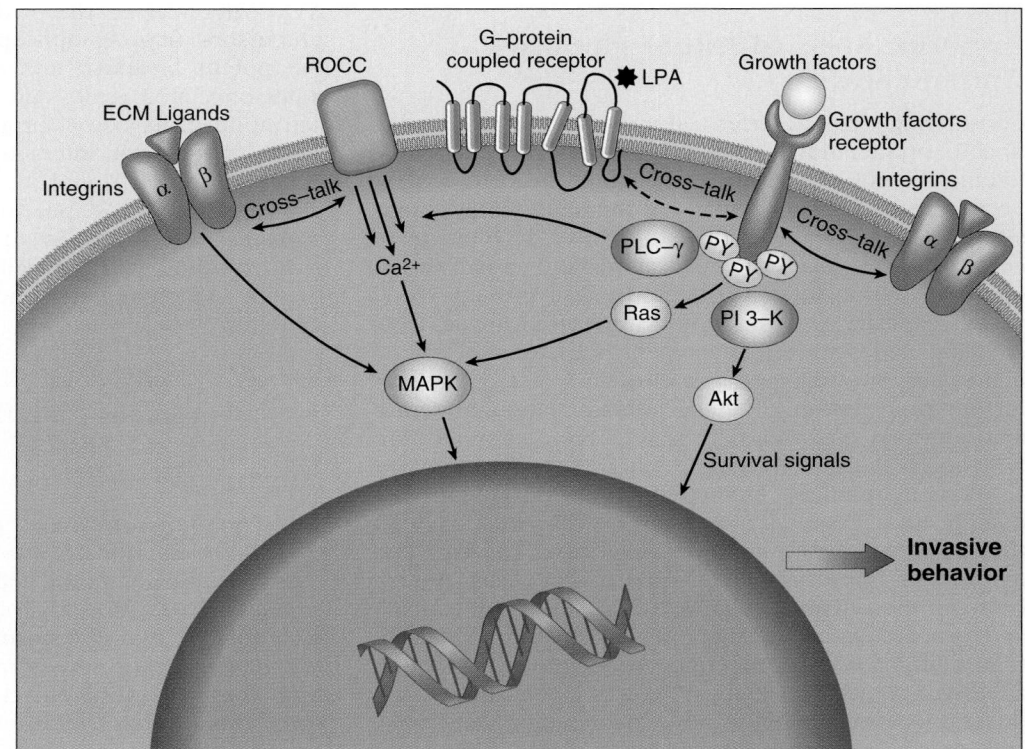

Figure 3-4. Focal signaling networks involve integrin and growth factor receptor cooperation. A simplified version of the key elements of the signaling network activated by integrin and growth factor cooperation is shown. Integrins bind extracellular matrix (ECM) molecules and cluster at focal contacts where signaling molecules and ion channels participate in a multimolecular signalosome. Activation of growth factor receptors (GFRs) by ligand causes a transient association of the complex with the multimolecular signaling structures. GFR activation may also be modulated by regulatory inputs from G protein–coupled receptors. The different signal transduction pathways overlap, and their integration thus affects migration, invasion, and cell survival. A central role in this signaling pathway appears to be played by mitogen-activated protein kinase (MAPK) for invasion and motility and by Akt for invasion and survival. LPA, lysophosphatidic acid; PI 3-K, phosphatidylinositol 3-kinase PLC-γ, phospholipase C-γ; ROCCs, receptor-operated calcium channels.

(RON),[60] and VEGF receptor.[61] This suggests that activation of growth factor receptors in the absence of their specific ligands can be a broadly used mechanism in different types of tumors, enabling cancer cells to rapidly adapt to rapidly changing environmental conditions.

Most of the RTKs also recruit phospholipase C-γ (PLC-γ) and activate it by phosphorylation. PLC-γ is involved in RTK-induced motility in several cell types, including stromal and endothelial cells.[62] Activation of PLC-γ is required for motility stimulated by EGF, PDGF, and IGF-1.[63] Chen and colleagues[64] showed that PLC-γ activation mobilizes the actin-regulatory protein, gelsolin, thus facilitating cytoskeletal reorganization for cell migration. Moreover, PLC-γ–mediated production of inositol trisphosphate and diacylglycerol activates protein kinase C and increases cytosolic calcium concentration.[65] Transient increases in intracellular calcium, through PLC-γ or other sources, have been demonstrated to affect tumor and endothelial cell adhesion, spreading, and motility.[66-68]

Ca^{2+} influx is one of the first signaling events affected after stimulation of integrin receptors in most cells of the tumor microenvironment.[32] β_1-Integrin ligation by collagen type IV in A2058 melanoma cells was shown to modulate tumor cell motility by finely regulating the intracellular Ca^{2+} concentration.[69,70] Modulation of intracellular calcium has been shown to affect proliferation, adhesion, protease secretion, and metastatic abilities of A2058 melanoma cells.[71,72] This has also been shown to regulate the invasive response of activated endothelial cells during angiogenesis.[66-68,73,74] Derangement of complex networks occurring between parallel pathways may then produce mechanisms for signal augmentation, thus leading to increased metastatic potentials of progressive tumors.

Paracrine Stromal-Tumor Motility Communication

Considering what a cancer cell must accomplish in addition to proliferation to become a successful metastatic lesion, it is not surprising that it would need to acquire properties of self-sufficiency and locomotion. The metastatic sequence is understood to involve detachment of cells within a primary tumor, local migration and invasion of stromal tissue, intravasation and transit through blood vessels, capillary bed arrest and extravasation, further local crawling and invasion, attachment, formation of micrometastases, survival, perhaps dormancy, and eventually further proliferation.[75,76] Successful migration of tumor and activated endothelial cells requires communication with and response to the local milieu.

Microenvironment interaction occurs throughout this complicated progression as cancer cells conspire with their stromal cell neighbors to grow, survive, and metastasize. These interactions are mediated by contact between the cell and the ECM, by direct cell-cell contact, and by secreted factors. Migration and invasion of cells in tumor stroma result from cooperation among protrusive, adhesive, contractile, and proteolytic mechanisms and occur under the combined influence of tumor and stromal cells on the content and architecture of the ECM and on the autocrine and paracrine production and activation of proteinases and chemotactic factors. This complex microenvironment contains migration-stimulating factors such as scatter factor/hepatocyte growth factor produced by fibroblasts, VEGF and bFGF produced by tumor cells, matrix metalloproteinases and urokinase plasminogen activator produced by fibroblasts and endothelial cells, TGF-β produced by tumor cells or released from the ECM by proteinase activity, EGF and PDGF produced by tumor cells, cytokines produced by inflammatory cells, and chemokines from inflammatory and stromal cells.[3]

The exoenzyme autotaxin (ATX) illustrates the complexity of signaling in this mixture of effectors. Originally identified as a melanoma cell autocrine motility factor, ATX stimulates the migration of a variety of cells in the local tumor microenvironment, including cancer cells, fibroblasts, and vascular smooth muscle cells. Expression of ATX in *ras*-transformed fibroblasts augments their in vitro invasive potential, as well as the size, number, and vascularity of tumors formed in mice.[77] Inclusion of ATX or ATX-secreting cells elicits an angiogenic response in Matrigel plugs inserted subcutaneously in mice,[78] including the formation of blood vessels that contain both endothelial cells and pericytes. ATX stimulates a tubulogenic response in endothelial cells but does not stimulate a strong migration response in chemotaxis assays. The angiogenic activity of ATX may affect nonendothelial cell targets, including pericytes, which can stabilize new vessels. Vascular smooth muscle cells, as well as endothelial cells stimulated with the angiogenic factor bFGF, secrete ATX, raising the possibility that three different cell types contribute to the angiogenic response by secreting ATX into a mutually attractive environment. The biologic effects of ATX depend on its enzymatic activity,[79] and ATX can catalyze the hydrolysis of lysophospholipid precursors (e.g., lysophosphatidylcholine) to produce the potent bioactive mediator, LPA.[80,81] LPA can elicit mitogenic, motogenic, and survival responses through activation of its edg G protein–coupled receptor family alone or through interaction with RTKs.[82] The local expression of ATX and its substrates may regulate the bioavailability of LPA, providing additional regulatory and signaling complexity in the tumor microenvironment. ATX may also be an extracellular target for pharmacologic therapy, which requires the design of specific enzyme inhibitors.

Signaling Cross-Talk Between Soluble Factors and Cell-Cell Adhesion Molecules Affects Invasive Phenotype in Cancer Cells

The acquisition of migratory properties and the weakening of cell-cell adhesion are crucial for tumor cell metastasis. Loss of expression of the cell-cell adhesion molecules and increased expression and/or activation of growth factor receptors are two molecular events observed in invading cancer cells. There are some indications that signaling from these two different classes of receptors can interconnect and cooperate to activate cell functions critical to metastasis formation (Fig. 3-5).

Figure 3-5. Cell-cell adhesion molecules and growth factor receptors cooperate to activate multiple signaling pathways and cell functions. An additional source of stimulation and regulation of normal and malignant microenvironmental events is cell-cell interaction and its cross-talk with intracellular signaling events. Ligand binding to growth factor receptors triggers both a permissive signaling to the mitogen-activated protein kinase (MAPK) cascade and destabilization of the β-catenin and α-catenin complex. An augmentation of β-catenin in the cytoplasm causes its translocation to the nucleus where it interacts with members of tcf transcription factor family and regulates the expression of genes related to the invasive phenotype. Increased receptor tyrosine kinase activity and loss of E-cadherin function lead to deranged intracellular signaling seen in tumor cells at the invasive front. MT-MMPS, Membrane-bound-metalloproteinase; PI-3K, phosphatidylinositol 3-kinase.

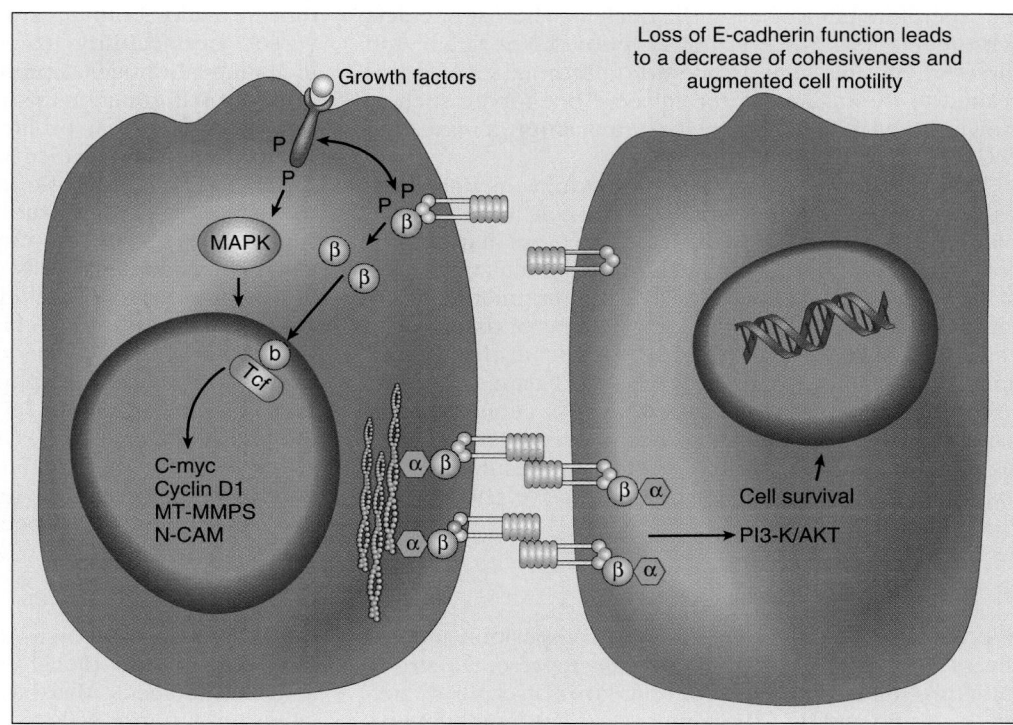

E-cadherin, a calcium-dependent cell-cell adhesion molecule that is critical to the functional integrity of the adherens junction, plays a role in the establishment and maintenance of epithelial morphology and differentiation.[83] The majority of epithelial tumors show reduced E-cadherin expression. A correlation between reduced E-cadherin expression, loss of tumor differentiation, and increased invasiveness has been found,[84] although E-cadherin mutations have been detected in only a minority of tumors.[85] Accumulating evidence suggests that E-cadherin plays an important role in outside-in signal transduction. For instance, E-cadherin can induce ligand-independent activation of EGF-Rs in an immortalized human keratinocyte cell line, which in turn leads to the stimulation of MAPKs.[86] N-cadherin, an E-cadherin–related adhesion molecule, and a receptor of fibroblast growth factor (FGFR) have been shown to cooperate to activate a signaling cascade that results in tumor invasion. N-cadherin associates with FGFR, protecting it from ligand-induced downregulation. The sustained expression of FGFR at the plasma membrane thus leads to continued MAPK activation, collagenase expression, and tumor cell invasion.[87]

Other studies have shown that E-cadherin–based cell-cell contacts trigger activation of another signaling pathway that is critical in tumor invasion: the phosphatidylinositol 3-kinase/Akt survival pathway.[88] Fuchs and colleagues[89] have demonstrated that transfection of MDA-MB-435s mammary carcinoma cells with tumor-associated mutations of E-cadherin enhance random cell movement compared with wild-type E-cadherin–expressing cells.

The motility-increasing activity of mutant E-cadherin was inhibited by treatment of the cells with EGF-R and phosphatidylinositol 3-kinase inhibitors, thus showing the interconnection of E-cadherin downstream signaling with growth factor–stimulated pathways.[89] Other transfection studies have demonstrated that changes in the expression levels of growth factor RTKs and E-cadherin may be coordinated. For instance, transfection with the Her2/neu oncogene downregulated E-cadherin expression in a mammary epithelial cell line.[90] It appears that increased RTK activity, such as that observed at the tumor-host interface, and loss of E-cadherin function may be related cellular events that are critical for tumor progression.

Activation of receptor tyrosine kinases has been shown to affect the adhesive function of E-cadherin by phosphorylation of regulatory catenin proteins. Three catenins, β-catenin, plakoglobin/γ-catenin, and p120cas bind to the cytoplasmic domain of cadherins.[91-93] They are involved in connecting the cadherins to the cell cytoskeleton, as well as in outside-in signaling activated by cell-cell contacts.[94] The catenins are heavily tyrosine-phosphorylated in Src-transformed cells and in response to growth factors such as EGF,[95] PDGF,[96] FGF,[97] and hepatocyte growth factor.[98] In vitro studies have demonstrated loss of cell polarity and reduced intercellular adhesion on stimulation of tumor cells with EGF through the activation of tyrosine kinase activity of EGF-R.[99] Phosphorylation of the EGF-R cytoplasmic domain and of β-catenin and γ-catenin appears to cause destabilization of the complex and its dissociation from the actin cytoskeleton, leading to a rise in the β-catenin concentration in the cell cytoplasm. β-Catenin may therefore translocate to the nucleus where it interacts with members of the Tcf transcription factor family and directly regulates gene expression of a number of genes related to the malignant and invasive phenotype such as c-myc, cyclin D1, membrane-type metalloproteinase, and N-CAM[56,100,101] (see Fig. 3-5).

These examples show how signal transduction pathways activated independently by cell-cell adhesion and binding of ligands to growth factor receptors may overlap and synergize inside the cells, thus modulating gene expression and cell function. The tumor microenvironment is characterized by the derangement of tissue social rules that regulate and correctly coordinate the cell-cell and ECM-cell interactions, as well as the balanced production of and response to growth factors. As a consequence, cancer cells have dysregulation of the receptor-mediated signaling cross-talk, which ultimately results in the expression of a more malignant and invasive phenotype.

Microenvironmental Cross-Talk in Tumor Angiogenesis

Microenvironmental changes in ECM composition and cell diversity at the tumor host interface represent a strong initiating milieu for the development of a capillary network around and into the tumor mass. This complex process is regulated by the balance of angiogenesis inducers and angiogenesis inhibitors in the local extracellular environment.[35] These factors may be secreted from cancer or stromal cells, may be mobilized from the ECM, or may be a structural component of ECM. Site-specific regulation of angiogenic factors, such as bFGF and VEGF in tumors,[102,103] has been demonstrated in xenografts of gastric cancer, brain tumor, and human melanoma cell lines among others, thus supporting the concept of influence of host stroma in tumor progression. Numerous cytokines and growth factors produced by cells in the local microenvironment can induce expression of angiogenic factors by tumor cells.[104] For instance, addition of interleukin (IL)-1β and IGF-1 to human colon cancer cells regulates VEGF expression by increasing its transcription.[105,106] Claffey and colleagues[107] showed that bFGF strongly induces the expression of VEGF in stromal cells in vivo, as well as in fibroblasts in vitro. In situ hybridization experiments to study the expression of the VEGF and VEGF receptors flt-1 and KDR, as well as the ECM components thrombospondin-1, collagen type I, and fibronectin and the proteoglycans versican and decorin on frozen sections of normal breast tissue, in situ carcinomas, invasive carcinomas, and metastatic carcinomas revealed that the formation of vascular stroma preceded tumor invasion. These data confirm the hypothesis that tumor cells do not invade normal stroma but rather a richly vascular stroma that they have induced.[36]

As the tumor mass grows, the local tumor tissue microenvironment tends to be hypoxic, hypoglycemic, and acidic, triggering stimuli for production of proangiogenic cytokines.[108,109] VEGF expression is induced by hypoxia through the action of the transcription factor, hypoxia-inducible factor-1.[110] Not only is VEGF a potent molecule that stimulates endothelial cell proliferation, motility, and tube formation both in vitro and in vivo,[111] it also increases vessel permeability to circulating macromolecules including fibrinogen, fibronectin, and clotting factors.[112] This fibrin-fibronectin matrix attracts macrophages and stimulates fibroblast proliferation, which in turn further induces angiogenesis (see Fig. 3-1).

VEGF plays a key role in maintaining the integrity of blood vessels through the activation of endothelial cell survival through antiapoptotic signaling. VEGF is a survival factor for endothelial cells, and it inhibits their apoptosis in part by activating the antiapoptotic kinase, Akt/PKB, via a phosphatidylinositol 3-kinase–dependent pathway.[113,114] Treatment of endothelial cells with VEGF induces the expression of the antiapoptotic proteins Bcl-2 and A1, which inhibit activation of upstream caspases.[115] Endothelial cell survival by VEGF signaling may be enhanced by a synergistic effect with $\alpha_v\beta_3$-mediated signaling. Cross-talk between the two systems is proven by the findings that VEGF receptor has been reported to associate selectively with $\alpha_v\beta_3$ and that VEGF mitogenicity and receptor activity were enhanced by endothelial adhesion to the $\alpha_v\beta_3$ ligand, vitronectin.[116]

VEGF is also known to induce the expression of E-selectin on endothelial cells.[117] E-selectin is a cell-cell adhesion molecule that has been shown to facilitate the adhesion of tumor cells to endothelial cells, thus allowing transendothelial migration during metastasis.[118,119] Recent studies have demonstrated that E-selectin may modulate the expression of properties related to malignant phenotype in colon cancer cells such as cytoskeleton rearrangement, motility, and protease secretion.[120] These effects were mediated by stimulation of calcium influx in the cancer cells though receptor-operated calcium channels.[121] These findings demonstrate how heterotypic cross-signaling, occurring at the tumor-host interface, can affect several steps of tumor progression.

IMPACT ON CANCER ETIOLOGY, PREVENTION, DIAGNOSIS, AND TREATMENT

Understanding the complex interactions of the local tumor microenvironment will alter the horizon of scientific directions and clinical decision making for cancer prevention, diagnosis, and treatment. The data presented argue that the local microenvironment is activated early, reflects paracrine events between the tumor and the stromal components, and may be localized to this specialized component of the tumor. Thus studies into the etiology of tumor development and progression have led to the recognition of this being a critically bioactive arena of the microenvironment.

The key area of greatest local activity within the tumor, against which preventive and therapeutic agents can be targeted, is this zone of local microenvironment interaction. Data are accumulating to indicate that the cellular and signaling cross-talk that is stimulated and dysregulated within this interaction zone provides a unique and productive milieu for therapeutic targeting.[3] Stromal therapy, directed at the complex events ongoing in this region

Our current approach to cancer therapy is to categorize cancers by organ (e.g., breast cancer or ovarian cancer), then by histology (e.g., papillary serous ovarian cancer), then by stage and grade. These are the descriptive terms that we use to make treatment decisions. However, when we look carefully, we find that all papillary serous ovarian cancers of defined stage and grade are not alike genetically, functionally, or clinically. This observation is not limited to ovarian cancer but occurs across the spectrum of solid tumors. It is no wonder that each patient with a solid tumor responds differently to interventions and that not all patients respond successfully to "standard" treatment approaches. As we begin to understand the complexities of the microenvironments of the primary organ and the secondary sites, we will learn how to selectively direct clinical interventions to those sites. For these reasons, we may find that different therapeutic regimens are required for primary disease and secondary disseminated disease. Treating cancer as a foreign seed in a foreign soil, rather than as a cell in which the proliferation machinery has gone awry, means focusing on the molecular, cellular, and local environmental changes that have occurred as part of the transformation and dissemination tumor package. This type of treatment will reduce the generic toxicity profiles occurring from DNA damaging agents, such as most chemotherapy, but may create new profiles as we alter cell signaling behaviors. Targeting molecular events that are selectively activated in the local cancer milieu should focus the intervention on the biochemical event that is altered and reduce collateral toxicity. Combination with cytotoxic treatments such as radiation therapy and chemotherapy may be required to extirpate tumor, but as individual modalities, may stabilize and limit the cancer. Focusing development of therapeutics to biologic behavior is the new paradigm of molecular medicine and stromal therapy intervention; targeting the local microenvironment of the host and tumor cells, will further narrow that spectrum.

where the stromal cells and tumor cells have created a rich paracrine and autocrine resource, could be considered a method for prevention therapy because of the early and substantial activation profile that occurs in premalignant and/or preinvasive disease. Furthermore, stromal therapy is logical in the treatment of disease but may need to be complemented by combination approaches with other signal or molecularly targeted agents or with chemotherapeutic agents. Emerging data (see also chapter 4 by Fidler) indicate that combinations of inhibitors of activated signaling proteins and chemotherapy may selectively attack the vasculature of the microenvironment with bystander effects against the tumor caused by loss of nutrient supply and metastasis conduits. If treatment is directed to the activated pathways, the therapeutic intervention could be targeted to the most biologically active area, and the potential for adverse events could be reduced. Further, treatment directed to the active pathways should provide a new and improved opportunity for development of biomarkers and surrogate markers of treatment benefit or failure that may allow us to determine early in the course of disease who might benefit. This triage would allow clinical researchers to optimize therapy for the patients and also more correctly fit patients to potential trials.

IMPLICATIONS FOR THE FUTURE

The more knowledge we accumulate on the molecular, biochemical, and local events underlying the development and progression of malignancy, the more logical and successful will be our preclinical and clinical development of biomarkers for diagnosis, prognostication, and of therapies for prevention and treatment. Understanding how cancer coordinates and processes its information should guide construction of molecularly targeted therapeutics and optimal treatment schedules and methods of administration. Most noninfectious or nontraumatic pathologic conditions of adulthood and childhood are chronic (e.g., rheumatic diseases, degenerative diseases, and biochemical diseases such as diabetes). The field of medicine considers the long-term medical intervention(s) that have turned these previously deadly and/or disabling diseases into survivable diseases with improved and prolonged life to be successful. Application of this concept to cancer, to make cancer a chronic disease rather than to focus strictly on curing it, could have the greatest cost-benefit implications for the future and the lives of many patients. The continued collaboration of clinician-scientists, scientist-clinicians, and basic clinicians and scientists is necessary to make this vision happen. Understanding the local tumor microenvironment and targeting its unique attributes are key steps in that direction.

ACKNOWLEDGEMENT

The authors acknowledge support for travel and international scientific exchange from the Italian Association for Cancer Research (AIRC) and University of Palermo (International Cooperation).

REFERENCES

1. Paget S: The distribution of secondary growths in cancer. Lancet 1889;1:571–573.
2. Hanahan D, Weinberg, RA: The hallmarks of cancer. Cell 2000;100:57–70.
3. Liotta LA, Kohn EC: The microenvironment of the tumour-host interface. Nature 2001;411:375–379.
4. Boyer B, Valles AM, Edme N: Induction and regulation of epithelial-mesenchymal transitions. Biochem Pharmacol 2000;60:1091–1099.
5. Stupack DG, Cho SY, Klemke RL: Molecular signaling mechanisms of cell migration and invasion. Immunol Res 2000;21:83–88.
6. Kinzler KW, Vogelstein B: Landscaping the cancer terrain. Science 1998;280:1036–1037.
7. Wirtzfeld DA, Petrelli NJ, Rodriguez-Bigas MA: Hamartomatous

polyposis syndromes: Molecular genetics, neoplastic risk, and surveillance recommendations. Ann Surg Oncol 2001;8:319-327.

8. Wu TT, Rezai B, Rashid A, et al: Genetic alterations and epithelial dysplasia in juvenile polyposis syndrome and sporadic juvenile polyps. Am J Pathol 1997;150:939-947.

9. Houlston R, Bevan S, Williams A, et al: Mutations in DPC4 (SMAD4) cause juvenile polyposis syndrome, but only account for a minority of cases. Hum Mol Genet 1998;7:1907-1912.

10. Roth S, Sistonen P, Salovaara R, et al: SMAD genes in juvenile polyposis. Genes Chromosomes Cancer 1999;26:54-61.

11. Gold LI: The role for transforming growth factor-beta (TGF-beta) in human cancer. Crit Rev Oncog 1999;10:303-360.

12. Attisano L, Wrana JL: Signal transduction by the TGF-beta superfamily. Science 2002;296:1646-1647.

13. Moustakas A, Souchelnytskyi S, Heldin CH: Smad regulation in TGF-beta signal transduction. J Cell Sci 2001;114:4359-4369.

14. Reynisdottir I, Polyak K, Iavarone A, et al: Kip/Cip and Ink4 Cdk inhibitors cooperate to induce cell cycle arrest in response to TGF-beta. Genes Dev 1995;9:1831-1845.

15. Moustakas A, Pardali K, Gaal A, et al: Mechanisms of TGF-beta signaling in regulation of cell growth and differentiation. Immunol Lett 2002;82:85-91.

16. Tuxhorn JA, Ayala GE, Smith MJ, et al: Reactive stroma in human prostate cancer: Induction of myofibroblast phenotype and extracellular matrix remodeling. Clin Cancer Res 2002;8:2912-2923.

17. Cunha GR, Hayward SW, Wang YZ: Role of stroma in carcinogenesis of the prostate. Differentiation 2002;70:473-485.

18. Moinfar F, Man YG, Arnould L, et al: Concurrent and independent genetic alterations in the stromal and epithelial cells of mammary carcinoma: Implications for tumorigenesis. Cancer Res 2000;60:2562-2566.

19. Weeks BH, He W, Olson KL, et al: Inducible expression of transforming growth factor beta1 in papillomas causes rapid metastasis. Cancer Res 2001;61:7435-7443.

20. Ananth S, Knebelmann B, Gruning W, et al: Transforming growth factor beta1 is a target for the von Hippel-Lindau tumor suppressor and a critical growth factor for clear cell renal carcinoma. Cancer Res 1999;59:2210-2216.

21. Brandvold KA, Neiman P, Ruddell A: Angiogenesis is an early event in the generation of myc-induced lymphomas. Oncogene 2000;19:2780-2785.

22. Theurillat JP, Hainfellner J, Maddalena A, et al: Early induction of angiogenetic signals in gliomas of GFAP-v-src transgenic mice. Am J Pathol 1999;154:581-590.

23. Tuxhorn JA, Ayala GE, Rowley DR: Reactive stroma in prostate cancer progression. J Urol 2001;166:2472-2483.

24. Elenbaas B, Weinberg RA: Heterotypic signaling between epithelial tumor cells and fibroblasts in carcinoma formation. Exp Cell Res 2001;264:169-184.

25. Xu J, Rodriguez D, Petitclerc E, et al: Proteolytic exposure of a cryptic site within collagen type IV is required for angiogenesis and tumor growth in vivo. J Cell Biol 2001;154:1069-1079.

26. Walker RA: The complexities of breast cancer desmoplasia. Breast Cancer Res 2001;3:143-145.

27. Pucci Minafra I, Minafra S, Tomasino RM, et al: Collagen changes in the ductal infiltrating (scirrhous) carcinoma of the human breast. A possible role played by type I trimer collagen on the invasive growth. J Submicrosc Cytol Pathol 1986;18:795-805.

28. Iacobuzio-Donahue CA, Argani P, Hempen PM, et al: The desmoplastic response to infiltrating breast carcinoma: Gene expression at the site of primary invasion and implications for comparisons between tumor types. Cancer Res 2002;62:5351-5357.

29. Iacobuzio-Donahue CA, Ryu B, Hruban RH, et al: Exploring the host desmoplastic response to pancreatic carcinoma: Gene expression of stromal and neoplastic cells at the site of primary invasion. Am J Pathol 2002;160:91-99.

30. Halvorsen TB, Seim E: Association between invasiveness, inflammatory reaction, desmoplasia and survival in colorectal cancer. J Clin Pathol 1989;42:162-166.

31. Ioachim E, Charchanti A, Briasoulis E, et al: Immunohistochemical expression of extracellular matrix components tenascin, fibronectin, collagen type IV and laminin in breast cancer: Their prognostic value and role in tumour invasion and progression. Eur J Cancer 2002;38:2362-2370.

32. Scarpino S, Stoppacciaro A, Pellegrini C, et al: Expression of EDA/EDB isoforms of fibronectin in papillary carcinoma of the thyroid. J Pathol 1999;188:163-167.

33. Schillaci R, Luparello C, Minafra S: Type I and I-trimer collagens as substrates for breast carcinoma cells in culture. Effect on growth rate, morphological appearance and actin organization. Eur J Cell Biol 1989;48:135-141.

34. Olumi AF, Grossfeld GD, Hayward SW, et al: Carcinoma-associated fibroblasts direct tumor progression of initiated human prostatic epithelium. Cancer Res 1999;59:5002-5011.

35. Folkman J: Role of angiogenesis in tumor growth and metastasis. Semin Oncol 2002;29:15-18.

36. Brown LF, Guidi AJ, Schnitt SJ, et al: Vascular stroma formation in carcinoma in situ, invasive carcinoma, and metastatic carcinoma of the breast. Clin Cancer Res 1999;5:1041-1056.

37. Valkovic T, Dobrila F, Melato M, et al: Correlation between vascular endothelial growth factor, angiogenesis, and tumor-associated macrophages in invasive ductal breast carcinoma. Virchows Arch 2002;440:583-588.

38. Liotta LA, Saidel MG, Kleinerman J: The significance of hematogenous tumor cell clumps in the metastatic process. Cancer Res 1976;36:889-894.

39. Friedl P, Noble PB, Walton PA, et al: Migration of coordinated cell clusters in mesenchymal and epithelial cancer explants in vitro. Cancer Res 1995;55:4557-4560.

40. Ruiter DJ, van Krieken JH, van Muijen GN, et al: Tumour metastasis: Is tissue an issue? Lancet Oncol 2001;2:109-112.

41. Mays RW, Nelson WJ, Marrs JA: Generation of epithelial cell polarity: Roles for protein trafficking, membrane-cytoskeleton, and E-cadherin-mediated cell adhesion. Cold Spring Harb Symp Quant Biol 1995;60:763-773.

42. Natali PG, Nicotra MR, Bartolazzi A, et al: Integrin expression in cutaneous malignant melanoma: Association of the alpha 3/beta 1 heterodimer with tumor progression. Int J Cancer 1993;54:68-72.

43. Oshita F, Kameda Y, Ikehara M, et al: Increased expression of integrin beta1 is a poor prognostic factor in small-cell lung cancer. Anticancer Res 2002;22:1065-1070.

44. Grossman HB, Lee C, Bromberg J, et al: Expression of the alpha6beta4 integrin provides prognostic information in bladder cancer. Oncol Rep 2000;7:13-16.

45. Demeure MJ, Doffek KM, Rezaee M, et al: Diminished expression of the alpha 5 beta 1 integrin (fibronectin receptor) by invasive clones of a human follicular thyroid cancer cell line. World J Surg 1994;18:569-575; discussion 575-566.

46. Barr LF, Campbell SE, Bochner BS, et al: Association of the decreased expression of alpha3beta1 integrin with the altered cell: Environmental interactions and enhanced soft agar cloning ability of c-myc-overexpressing small cell lung cancer cells. Cancer Res 1998;58:5537-5545.

47. Mizejewski GJ: Role of integrins in cancer: Survey of expression patterns. Proc Soc Exp Biol Med 1999;222:124-138.

48. Klemke RL, Yebra M, Bayna EM, et al: Receptor tyrosine kinase signaling required for integrin alpha v beta 5-directed cell motility but not adhesion on vitronectin. J Cell Biol 1994;127:859-866.

49. Brooks PC, Klemke RL, Schon S, et al: Insulin-like growth factor receptor cooperates with integrin alpha v beta 5 to promote tumor cell dissemination in vivo. J Clin Invest 1997;99:1390-1398.

50. Moro L, Dolce L, Cabodi S, et al: Integrin-induced epidermal growth factor (EGF) receptor activation requires c-Src and p130Cas and leads to phosphorylation of specific EGF receptor tyrosines. J Biol Chem 2002;277:9405-9414.

51. Maruta H, Burgess AW: Regulation of the Ras signalling network. Bioessays 1994;16:489-496.

52. Miyamoto S, Teramoto H, Gutkind JS, et al: Integrins can collaborate with growth factors for phosphorylation of receptor tyrosine kinases and MAP kinase activation: Roles of integrin aggregation and occupancy of receptors. J Cell Biol 1996;135:1633-1642.

53. Moro L, Venturino M, Bozzo C, et al: Integrins induce activation of EGF receptor: Role in MAP kinase induction and adhesion-dependent cell survival. EMBO J 1998;17:6622-6632.

54. Kawahara E, Nakada N, Hikichi T, et al: EGF and beta1 integrin

convergently regulate migration of A431 carcinoma cell through MAP kinase activation. Exp Cell Res 2002;272:84–91.

55. Kranenburg O, Moolenaar WH: Ras-MAP kinase signaling by lysophosphatidic acid and other G protein-coupled receptor agonists. Oncogene 2001;20:1540–1546.

56. Shtutman M, Zhurinsky J, Simcha I, et al: The cyclin D1 gene is a target of the beta-catenin/LEF-1 pathway. Proc Natl Acad Sci USA 1999;96:5522–5527.

57. Fishman DA, Liu Y, Ellerbroek SM, et al: Lysophosphatidic acid promotes matrix metalloproteinase (MMP) activation and MMP-dependent invasion in ovarian cancer cells. Cancer Res 2001;61:3194–3199.

58. Rusciano D, Lorenzoni P, Burger MM: Constitutive activation of c-Met in liver metastatic B16 melanoma cells depends on both substrate adhesion and cell density and is regulated by a cytosolic tyrosine phosphatase activity. J Biol Chem 1996;271:20763–20769.

59. Sundberg C, Rubin K: Stimulation of beta1 integrins on fibroblasts induces PDGF independent tyrosine phosphorylation of PDGF beta-receptors. J Cell Biol 1996;132:741–752.

60. Danilkovitch-Miagkova A, Angeloni D, Skeel A, et al: Integrin-mediated RON growth factor receptor phosphorylation requires tyrosine kinase activity of both the receptor and c-Src. J Biol Chem 2000;275:14783–14786.

61. Wang JF, Zhang XF, Groopman JE: Stimulation of beta 1 integrin induces tyrosine phosphorylation of vascular endothelial growth factor receptor-3 and modulates cell migration. J Biol Chem 2001;276:41950–41957.

62. Gschwind A, Zwick E, Prenzel N, et al: Cell communication networks: Epidermal growth factor receptor transactivation as the paradigm for interreceptor signal transmission. Oncogene 2001;20:1594–1600.

63. Bornfeldt KE, Raines EW, Nakano T, et al: Insulin-like growth factor-I and platelet-derived growth factor-BB induce directed migration of human arterial smooth muscle cells via signaling pathways that are distinct from those of proliferation. J Clin Invest 1994;93:1266–1274.

64. Chen P, Xie H, Sekar MC, et al: Epidermal growth factor receptor-mediated cell motility: Phospholipase C activity is required, but mitogen-activated protein kinase activity is not sufficient for induced cell movement. J Cell Biol 1994;127:847–857.

65. Janmey PA: Phosphoinositides and calcium as regulators of cellular actin assembly and disassembly. Annu Rev Physiol 1994;56:169–191.

66. Alessandro R, Masiero L, Lapidos K, et al: Endothelial cell spreading on type IV collagen and spreading-induced FAK phosphorylation is regulated by Ca2+ influx. Biochem Biophys Res Commun 1998;248:635–640.

67. Kohn EC, Alessandro R, Spoonster J, et al: Angiogenesis: Role of calcium-mediated signal transduction. Proc Natl Acad Sci USA 1995;92:1307–1311.

68. Masiero L, Lapidos KA, Ambudkar I, et al: Regulation of the RhoA pathway in human endothelial cell spreading on type IV collagen: Role of calcium influx. J Cell Sci 1999;112(Pt 19):3205–3213.

69. Hodgson L, Dong C: Ca2+]i as a potential downregulator of alpha2beta1-integrin-mediated A2058 tumor cell migration to type IV collagen. Am J Physiol Cell Physiol 2001;281:C106–C113.

70. Hodgson L, Kohn EC, Dong C: Extracellular lipid-mediated signaling in tumor-cell activation and pseudopod protrusion. Int J Cancer 2000;88:593–600.

71. Kohn EC, Jacobs W, Kim YS, et al: Calcium influx modulates expression of matrix metalloproteinase-2 (72-kDa type IV collagenase, gelatinase A). J Biol Chem 1994;269:21505–21511.

72. Kohn EC, Sandeen MA, Liotta LA: In vivo efficacy of a novel inhibitor of selected signal transduction pathways including calcium, arachidonate, and inositol phosphates. Cancer Res 1992;52:3208–3212.

73. Alessandro R, Masiero L, Liotta LA, et al: The role of calcium in the regulation of invasion and angiogenesis. In Vivo 1996;10:153–160.

74. Sjaastad MD, Nelson WJ: Integrin-mediated calcium signaling and regulation of cell adhesion by intracellular calcium. Bioessays 1997;19:47–55.

75. Chambers AF, Groom AC, MacDonald IC: Dissemination and growth of cancer cells in metastatic sites. Nat Rev Cancer 2002;2:563–572.

76. Woodhouse EC, Chuaqui RF, Liotta LA: General mechanisms of metastasis. Cancer 1997;80:1529–1537.

77. Nam SW, Clair T, Campo CK, et al: Autotaxin (ATX), a potent tumor motogen, augments invasive and metastatic potential of ras-transformed cells. Oncogene 2000;19:241–247.

78. Nam SW, Clair T, Kim YS, et al: Autotaxin (NPP-2), a metastasis-enhancing motogen, is an angiogenic factor. Cancer Res 2001;61:6938–6944.

79. Lee HY, Clair T, Mulvaney PT, et al: Stimulation of tumor cell motility linked to phosphodiesterase catalytic site of autotaxin. J Biol Chem 1996;271:24408–24412.

80. Moolenaar WH: Lysophospholipids in the limelight: Autotaxin takes center stage. J Cell Biol 2002;158:197–199.

81. Umezu-Goto M, Kishi Y, Taira A, et al: Autotaxin has lysophospholipase D activity leading to tumor cell growth and motility by lysophosphatidic acid production. J Cell Biol 2002;158:227–233.

82. Moolenaar WH: Bioactive lysophospholipids and their G protein-coupled receptors. Exp Cell Res 1999;253:230–238.

83. Steinberg MS, McNutt PM: Cadherins and their connections: Adhesion junctions have broader functions. Curr Opin Cell Biol 1999;11:554–560.

84. Takeichi M: Cadherins in cancer: Implications for invasion and metastasis. Curr Opin Cell Biol 1993;5:806–811.

85. Becker KF, Atkinson MJ, Reich U, et al: E-cadherin gene mutations provide clues to diffuse type gastric carcinomas. Cancer Res 1994;54:3845–3852.

86. Pece S, Gutkind JS: Signaling from E-cadherins to the MAPK pathway by the recruitment and activation of epidermal growth factor receptors upon cell-cell contact formation. J Biol Chem 2000;275:41227–41233.

87. Suyama K, Shapiro I, Guttman M, et al: A signaling pathway leading to metastasis is controlled by N-cadherin and the FGF receptor. Cancer Cell 2002;2:301–314.

88. Pece S, Chiariello M, Murga C, et al: Activation of the protein kinase Akt/PKB by the formation of E-cadherin-mediated cell-cell junctions. Evidence for the association of phosphatidylinositol 3-kinase with the E-cadherin adhesion complex. J Biol Chem 1999;274:19347–19351.

89. Fuchs M, Hutzler P, Brunner I, et al: Motility enhancement by tumor-derived mutant E-cadherin is sensitive to treatment with epidermal growth factor receptor and phosphatidylinositol 3-kinase inhibitors. Exp Cell Res 2002;276:129–141.

90. D'Souza B, Taylor-Papadimitriou J: Overexpression of ERBB2 in human mammary epithelial cells signals inhibition of transcription of the E-cadherin gene. Proc Natl Acad Sci USA 1994;91:7202–7206.

91. Gumbiner BM: Signal transduction of beta-catenin. Curr Opin Cell Biol 1995;7:634–640.

92. Gottardi CJ, Gumbiner BM: Adhesion signaling: How beta-catenin interacts with its partners. Curr Biol 2001;11:R792–R794.

93. Reynolds AB, Daniel J, McCrea PD, et al: Identification of a new catenin: The tyrosine kinase substrate p120cas associates with E-cadherin complexes. Mol Cell Biol 1994;14:8333–8342.

94. Conacci-Sorrell M, Zhurinsky J, Ben-Ze'ev A: The cadherin-catenin adhesion system in signaling and cancer. J Clin Invest 2002;109:987–991.

95. Hazan RB, Norton L: The epidermal growth factor receptor modulates the interaction of E-cadherin with the actin cytoskeleton. J Biol Chem 1998;273:9078–9084.

96. Downing JR, Reynolds AB: PDGF, CSF-1, and EGF induce tyrosine phosphorylation of p120, a pp60src transformation-associated substrate. Oncogene 1991;6:607–613.

97. El-Hariry I, Pignatelli M, Lemoine NR: FGF-1 and FGF-2 regulate the expression of E-cadherin and catenins in pancreatic adenocarcinoma. Int J Cancer 2001;94:652–661.

98. Shibamoto S, Hayakawa M, Takeuchi K, et al: Tyrosine phosphorylation of beta-catenin and plakoglobin enhanced by hepatocyte growth factor and epidermal growth factor in human carcinoma cells. Cell Adhes Commun 1994;1:295–305.

99. Shiozaki H, Kadowaki T, Doki Y, et al: Effect of epidermal growth factor on cadherin-mediated adhesion in a human oesophageal cancer cell line. Br J Cancer 1995;71:250–258.

100. Takahashi M, Tsunoda T, Seiki M, et al: Identification of membrane-type matrix metalloproteinase-1 as a target of the beta-catenin/Tcf4 complex in human colorectal cancers. Oncogene 2002;21:5861–5867.

101. Conacci-Sorrell ME, Ben-Yedidia T, Shtutman M, et al: Nr-CAM is a target gene of the beta-catenin/LEF-1 pathway in melanoma and colon cancer and its expression enhances motility and confers tumorigenesis. Genes Dev 2002;16:2058–2072.

102. Singh RK, Bucana CD, Gutman M, et al: Organ site-dependent expression of basic fibroblast growth factor in human renal cell carcinoma cells. Am J Pathol 1994;145:365–374.

103. Tsuzuki Y, Mouta Carreira C, Bockhorn M, et al: Pancreas microenvironment promotes VEGF expression and tumor growth: Novel window models for pancreatic tumor angiogenesis and microcirculation. Lab Invest 2001;81:1439–1451.

104. Fidler IJ: The organ microenvironment and cancer metastasis. Differentiation 2002;70:498–505.

105. Akagi Y, Liu W, Xie K, et al: Regulation of vascular endothelial growth factor expression in human colon cancer by interleukin-1beta. Br J Cancer 1999;80:1506–1151.

106. Akagi Y, Liu W, Zebrowski B, et al: Regulation of vascular endothelial growth factor expression in human colon cancer by insulin-like growth factor-I. Cancer Res 1998;58:4008–4014.

107. Claffey KP, Abrams K, Shih SC, et al: Fibroblast growth factor 2 activation of stromal cell vascular endothelial growth factor expression and angiogenesis. Lab Invest 2001;81:61–75.

108. Leonard EJ, Yoshimura T: Neutrophil attractant/activation protein-1 (NAP-1[Interleukin-8]). Am J Respir Cell Mol Biol 1990;2:479–486.

109. Xu L, Fidler IJ: Acidic pH-induced elevation in interleukin 8 expression by human ovarian carcinoma cells. Cancer Res 2000;60:4610–4616.

110. Harris AL: Hypoxia—a key regulatory factor in tumour growth. Nat Rev Cancer 2002;2:38–47.

111. Ferrara N: Role of vascular endothelial growth factor in physiologic and pathologic angiogenesis: therapeutic implications. Semin Oncol 2002;29:10–14.

112. Senger DR, Brown LF, Claffey KP, et al: Vascular permeability factor, tumor angiogenesis and stroma generation. Invasion Metastasis 1994;14:385–394.

113. Thakker GD, Hajjar DP, Muller WA, et al: The role of phosphatidylinositol 3-kinase in vascular endothelial growth factor signaling. J Biol Chem 1999;274:10002–10007.

114. Gerber HP, McMurtrey A, Kowalski J, et al: Vascular endothelial growth factor regulates endothelial cell survival through the phosphatidylinositol 3'-kinase/Akt signal transduction pathway. Requirement for Flk-1/KDR activation. J Biol Chem 1998;273:30336–30343.

115. Gerber HP, Dixit V, Ferrara N: Vascular endothelial growth factor induces expression of the antiapoptotic proteins Bcl-2 and A1 in vascular endothelial cells. J Biol Chem 1998;273:13313–13316.

116. Soldi R, Mitola S, Strasly M, et al: Role of alphavbeta3 integrin in the activation of vascular endothelial growth factor receptor-2. EMBO J 1999;18:882–892.

117. Aoki M, Kanamori M, Yudoh K, et al: Effects of vascular endothelial growth factor and E-selectin on angiogenesis in the murine metastatic RCT sarcoma. Tumour Biol 2001;22:239–246.

118. Kitayama J, Tsuno N, Sunami E, et al: E-selectin can mediate the arrest type of adhesion of colon cancer cells under physiological shear flow. Eur J Cancer 2000;36:121–127.

119. Zhang GJ, Adachi I: Serum levels of soluble intercellular adhesion molecule-1 and E-selectin in metastatic breast carcinoma: Correlations with clinicopathological features and prognosis. Int J Oncol 1999;14:71–77.

120. Flugy AM, D'Amato M, Russo D, et al: E-selectin modulates the malignant properties of T84 colon carcinoma cells. Biochem Biophys Res Commun 2002;293:1099–1106.

121. D'Amato M, Flugy AM, Alaimo G, et al: Role of calcium in E-selectin induced phenotype of T84 colon carcinoma cells. Biochemical Biophysical Research Communications 2003;301:907–914.

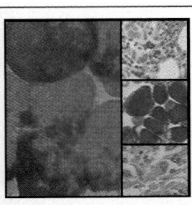

4

Isaiah J. Fidler

BIOLOGY OF CANCER METASTASIS

SUMMARY OF KEY POINTS

- The major cause of death from cancer is metastases that are resistant to conventional therapy.
- By the time of initial diagnosis, malignant neoplasms are far advanced in their natural history.
- Neoplastic cells are genetically unstable, and hence, primary human neoplasms are heterogeneous for a large number of biologic properties that include invasion and metastasis.
- The process of metastasis consists of sequential and selective steps that are highly selective. To produce a metastasis, tumor cells must

complete all steps, including proliferation, induction of angiogenesis, motility, invasion, entrance into the circulation, arrest in distant organ vascular bed, extravasation into the organ parenchyma, proliferation, and induction of neovasculature. At all steps, the tumor cells must evade destruction by host-specific and nonspecific defense mechanisms.
- Metastases are clonal in origin and can originate from one surviving metastatic cell.

- Metastatic cells usurp homeostatic mechanisms for their survival and growth in specific organ microenvironments.
- The "cross-talk" between tumor cells ("seeds") and host factors ("soil") provides new approaches for therapy of metastases, that is, targeting homeostatic factors that are favorable to the survival and growth of metastatic cells.

INTRODUCTION

Once a diagnosis of cancer is established, the urgent and fearful question is whether it is localized or has already spread to regional lymph nodes and visceral organs. This fear is well justified. Despite improvements in early diagnosis, surgical techniques, general patient care, and local and systemic adjuvant therapies, most deaths of patients with cancer result from the relentless growth of metastases that are resistant to conventional therapies. Surgical excision of primary neoplasms is not curative in many patients because by that time, metastasis may well have occurred.[1] Metastases can be located in different organs and in different regions of the same organ. The organ microenvironment can alter the efficiency of delivering anticancer agents and also directly modify the metastatic tumor cells' response to therapy. The major challenge for treatment of metastases is the biologic heterogeneity of cancer cells in primary lesions and especially in metastases. This heterogeneity is exhibited in a wide range of genetic, biochemical, immunologic, and biologic characteristics, such as cell-surface receptors, enzymes, karyotypes, cell morphologies, growth properties, sensitivities to various therapeutic agents, and ability to invade and produce metastasis.[1-5]

Improvements in the treatment of metastasis depend on a better understanding of the mechanisms responsible for the development of biologic heterogeneity in cancer and metastases and the pathogenesis of the metastatic process. This chapter reviews some basic concepts of the mechanisms of tumor progression, generation of biologic heterogeneity, and pathogenesis of cancer metastasis.

THE PROCESS OF CANCER METASTASIS

The process of cancer metastasis consists of a series of sequential interrelated steps, each of which is rate-limiting, since a failure at any of the steps aborts the process.[2] The outcome of the process is dependent on both the intrinsic properties of the tumor cells and the responses of the host; the balance of these interactions can vary among different patients.[6-10] In principle, the steps or events in the pathogenesis of a metastasis are similar in all tumors (Fig. 4-1).

The major steps in the formation of a metastasis are as follows: (1) *Transformation of normal cells into tumor cells and their growth* after the initial transforming event. Growth of neoplastic cells must be progressive, with nutrients for the expanding tumor mass initially supplied by simple diffusion. (2) *Extensive vascularization*, that is, angiogenesis, must occur if a tumor mass is to exceed 1 mm in diameter.[11] The production and secretion of proangiogenic factors by tumor cells and host cells play a major role in establishing a capillary network from the surrounding host tissue. (3) *Local invasion* of the host stroma by some tumor cells occurs by several parallel mechanisms. Thin-walled venules, like lymphatic channels, offer very little resistance to penetration by tumor cells and provide the most common pathways for tumor cell entry into the circulation. (4) *Detachment and embolization* of single tumor cells or aggregates occurs next, with the vast majority of circulating tumor cells being rapidly destroyed. (5) Once the tumor cells have *survived* the circulation, they must (6) *arrest* in the capillary beds of

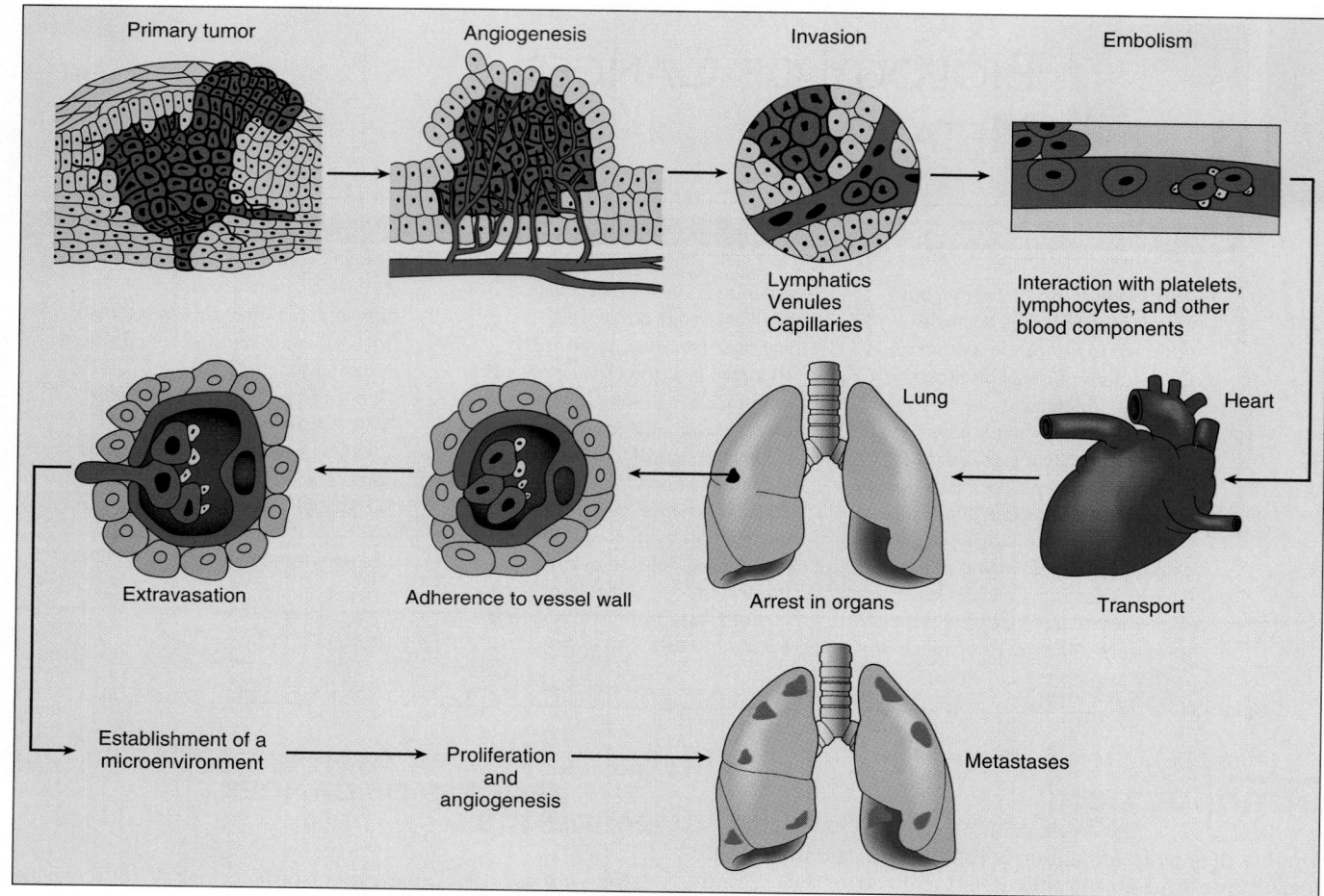

Figure 4-1. The process of metastasis consists of sequential linked steps. Metastatic cells must complete all of these steps if a clinically relevant lesion is to develop. If a disseminating tumor cell fails to survive any of these steps, it will not produce a metastasis.

distant organs, by *adhering* either to capillary endothelial cells or to subendothelial basement membrane, which may be exposed. (7) *Extravasation* occurs next, probably by mechanisms similar to those operative during invasion. (8) *Proliferation* within the organ parenchyma completes the metastatic process. To continue growing beyond the size of 0.2 mm in diameter, the micrometastasis must develop a vascular network and evade destruction by host defenses. The cells can then invade blood vessels, enter the circulation, and produce additional metastases.

Growth at a Primary Site

The growth and survival of cells is dependent on an adequate supply of oxygen and nutrients and the removal of toxic products. Oxygen can diffuse radially from capillaries for only 150 to 200 µm. When distances exceed this, cell death follows.[11-13] Thus the expansion of tumor masses beyond 1 mm in diameter depends on the development of a new blood supply, or angiogenesis.[14-16]

The induction of angiogenesis is mediated by multiple molecules that are released by both tumor cells and host cells. Among these molecules are members of the fibroblast growth factor (FGF) family, vascular endothelial cell growth factor (VEGF) also called *vascular permeability factor* (*VPF*), interleukin-8, angiogenin, angiotropin, epidermal growth factor (EGF), fibrin, platelet-derived growth factor, transforming growth factor-α (TGF-α), TGF-β, and tumor necrosis factor-α.[14-16] The formation of new vasculature consists of sequential steps: endothelial cells must proliferate, migrate, and penetrate host stroma and extracellular matrix (ECM). The endothelial cells must also undergo morphogenesis. The vasculature of many solid tumors is not identical to that in normal tissues. There are differences in cellular composition, permeability, vessel stability, and regulation of growth.[17] The extent of angiogenesis is determined by the balance between factors that stimulate and those that inhibit new blood vessel growth and survival. Although in normal tissues the inhibitory influence predominates,[18] in tumors many neoplastic cells switch from an angiogenesis-inhibiting to an angiogenesis-stimulating phenotype, which coincides with the loss of the wild-type allele of the p53 tumor suppressor gene and is the result of reduced production of the antiangiogenic factor thrombospondin.[19]

Angiogenesis can occur by either sprouting or non-sprouting processes.[20] Sprouting angiogenesis occurs by branching (true sprouting) of new capillaries from preexisting vessels. Nonsprouting angiogenesis results from the enlargement, splitting, and fusion of preexisting vessels produced by the proliferation of endothelial cells within the wall of a vessel. Transcapillary pillars (or transluminal bridges) are sometimes observed in enlarged vessels produced by nonsprouting angiogenesis.[20] This type of angiogenesis can occur concurrently with sprouting angiogenesis in the vascularization of organs or tissues such as the lungs and heart.[20] The mechanism of nonsprouting angiogenesis in metastasis is not yet known, but VEGF, which plays a pivotal role in developmental, physiologic, and pathologic neovascularization,[21] is a candidate effector molecule. VEGF stimulates the proliferation and migration of endothelial cells and induces the expression of metalloproteinases and plasminogen activity by these cells.[22,23] Moreover, overexpression of VEGF in tumor cells enhances tumor growth and metastasis in several animal models by stimulating vascularization (increased microvessel density).[24]

Benign neoplasms are sparsely vascularized, whereas malignant neoplasms are highly vascular.[1] The increase in vasculature also increases the probability that tumor cells will enter the circulation and produce metastasis.[25] Many[26,27] but not all[28,29] recent studies indicated that increased microvessel density in the areas of most intense neovascularization is a significant and independent prognostic indicator in early-stage breast cancer. Studies with other neoplasms such as prostate cancer,[30,31] melanoma,[32] ovarian carcinoma,[33] gastric carcinoma,[34] and colon carcinoma[35] also support the conclusion that the vascular density, that is, the angiogenesis index, is a useful prognostic factor (see Chapter 9).[36]

TUMOR CELL INVASION

To reach blood vessels or lymphatics, tumor cells must penetrate host stroma that includes basement membrane. The interaction with the basement membrane consists of attachment, matrix dissolution, motility, and penetration.[9] At least three nonmutually exclusive mechanisms can be involved in tumor cell invasion of tissues. First, mechanical pressure produced by rapidly proliferating neoplasms may force cords of tumor cells along tissue planes of least resistance.[37-39] Second, increased cell motility can contribute to tumor cell invasion. Most tumor cells possess the necessary cytoplasmic machinery for active locomotion[40,41] and increased tumor cell motility is preceded by a loss of cell-to-cell cohesive forces. In epithelial cells, the loss of cell-to-cell contact is associated with down-regulation of the expression of E-cadherin, a cell surface glycoprotein involved in calcium-dependent homotypic cell-to-cell cohesion.[42,43] E-cadherin is localized at the epithelial junction complex and is responsible for the organization, maintenance, and morphogenesis of epithelial tissues.[43,44] Reduced levels of E-cadherin are associated with a decrease in cellular/tissue differentiation and increased grade in carcinomas.[43-48] Many differen-

tiated carcinomas express higher levels of E-cadherin messenger RNA, as do adjacent normal epithelial cells, whereas poorly differentiated carcinomas do not.[48,49] Mutations in the E-cadherin gene[50] and abnormalities of α-catenin, which is an E-cadherin–associated protein, have been associated with the transition of cells from the noninvasive to the invasive phenotype.[51,52] Moreover, the transfection of E-cadherin–encoding complementary DNA into invasive cancer cells has been shown to inhibit their motility,[53,54] which is associated with the alteration of cytoskeletal elements and the response to the cytokine automotility factor,[55-59] scatter factor,[60,61] thromboplastin,[62] ECM,[63] and monocyte-derived monokines.[64]

Third, invasive tumor cells secrete enzymes capable of degrading basement membranes, which constitute a barrier between epithelial cells and the stroma. Epithelial cells and stromal cells produce a complex mixture of collagens, proteoglycans, and other molecules, which contains ligands for adhesion receptors and is permeable to molecules but not to cells.[65-71] Colon cancer cells also produce and secrete basement membrane components such as laminin.[72] Well-differentiated human colon carcinomas produce a large amount of laminin, whereas poorly differentiated colon carcinomas produce discontinuous basement membranes that are low in laminin.[73] A decrease in laminin content has also been demonstrated in basement membranes of dysplastic adenomatous polyps, but discontinuity of basement membranes was noted only in colon carcinomas.[72-75] Proteoglycans—including chondroitin sulfate, heparin sulfate, hyaluronate, and heparin—are other major constituents of the ECM whose major function may be serving as a reservoir for growth factors,[76] which can be released in an active form by degradation of the ECM.[77]

To invade the basement membrane, a tumor cell must first attach to ECM components by a receptor-ligand interaction. One group of such cell surface receptors is the integrins, which specifically bind cells to laminin, collagen, or fibronectin.[78,79] Many integrins that bind to different components of the ECM are expressed on the surface of human carcinoma cells.[79-81] Tumor progression has been associated with a gradual decrease of integrin expression, suggesting that the loss of integrins, coupled with the loss of E-cadherin, may facilitate detachment from a primary neoplasm.[80]

Other proteins that bind to ECM components are the lectins. Normal intestinal epithelial cells contain two highly conserved galactins with molecular weights of 31.0 and 14.5 kd.[82,83] The expression of the 31-kd lectin is increased in carcinomas, absent in adenomas, and weak in normal epithelium. Its intramural content is significantly associated with carcinoembryonic antigen (CEA).[84] CD44, a receptor responsible for lymphocyte homing,[85,86] binds to ECM components and to CEA.[86,87] It is expressed as a 90-kd protein in lymphocytes and as a 150- to 180-kd protein in epithelial cells.[87] The production of CD44 gene transcript is markedly increased in some human cancer cells.[88] CD44 may regulate migration through the ECM, and an abnormal pattern of activity of the CD44 gene has been reported in metastatic human colon carcinomas.[89]

Science of Clinical Oncology

Subsequent to binding, tumor cells can degrade connective-tissue ECM and basement membrane components.[90] The production of enzymes such as type IV collagenase (gelatinase, matrix metalloproteinase) and heparinase in metastatic tumor cells correlates with invasive capacity of human carcinoma cells. Type IV collagenolytic metalloproteinases with apparent molecular masses of 98, 92, 80, 68, and 64 kd have been detected in highly metastatic cells. Poorly metastatic cells, on the other hand, appear to secrete very low amounts of only the 92-kd metalloproteinase.[91]

Under experimental conditions, collagenase activity can be stimulated by purified mucin products, which are associated with poor prognosis.[92] Human cancer cells can also secrete a plasminogen activator, urokinase, which activates the serine protease plasmin from plasminogen. Plasmin induces degradation of laminin and, hence, tumor cell invasion. Plasmin also activates collagenase type IV, which in turn will deplete the membrane of both laminin and collagen type IV.[93] Furthermore, plasmin acts as chemoattractant for tumor cells.[94]

LYMPHATIC METASTASIS

Early clinical observations led to the impression that carcinomas spread mainly by the lymphatic route and tumors of mesenchymal origin spread mainly through the bloodstream. The reality, however, invalidates this belief.[95] The lymphatic and vascular systems have numerous connections,[96] and disseminating tumor cells may pass from one system to the other.[96-99] For these reasons, the division of metastatic routes into lymphatic spread and hematogenous spread is arbitrary. During invasion, tumor cells can easily penetrate small lymphatic vessels and can be passively transported in the lymph. Tumor emboli may be trapped in the first lymph node encountered on their route, or they may bypass regional draining lymph nodes to form distant nodal metastases ("skip metastasis"). Although this phenomenon was recognized by Stephen Paget in 1889,[100] its implications for treatment were frequently ignored in the development of surgical approaches to treatment of cancers.[101]

Regional lymph nodes (RLNs) in the area of a primary neoplasm may become enlarged as a result of reactive hyperplasia or growth of tumor cells. Although the use of morphologic criteria for assessing prognosis on the basis of lymph node appearance is debatable, lymphocyte-depleted lymph nodes are believed to indicate a less favorable prognosis than those demonstrating reactive inflammatory characteristics.[101] Whether the RLNs can retain tumor cells and serve as a temporary barrier for cell dissemination has been controversial.[102-104] In most experimental animal systems used to investigate this question, normal lymph nodes were subjected to a single challenge with a large number of tumor cells, a situation that may not be analogous to RLNs at the early stages of cancer spread in humans, when small numbers of cancer cells continuously enter the lymphatics.[102] This issue is important because of practical considerations for surgical management of such neoplasms as cutaneous melanoma.[101]

It calls into question whether elective prophylactic lymph node dissection can prevent metastasis to visceral organs. For example, the biologic justification for elective lymph node dissection in patients with melanoma presumes that metastasis of some cutaneous melanomas occurs first in the RLNs and that only later do tumor cells gain access to the circulation to reach distant organs. If this is the case, and RLNs can act as a temporary barrier to the spread of cancer, removing the RLNs with micrometastases could clearly increase the cure rate in subgroups of patients with melanoma. Some evidence exists that patients with melanomas of intermediate thickness (1 to 4 mm) have an improved survival rate subsequent to elective lymph node dissection.[105,106] In colorectal cancers, more radical operations that include removal of RLNs have been associated with improved survival rates.[107] In contrast, in breast cancer, removal of the axillary lymph nodes in a randomized prospective study was not associated with improved survival rates.[108]

Recent advances in mapping of the lymphatics draining cutaneous melanoma (by the use of dyes or radioactive tracers) have allowed surgeons to identify the lymph node draining the tumor site (i.e., the sentinel lymph node).[109] The presence of melanoma micrometastases in sentinel lymph nodes is correlated with poor prognosis and hence indicates a need for wide field of dissection. In a series of more than 500 melanoma cases with longer than 4 years' median clinical follow-up, investigators concluded that absence of disease in sentinel lymph node correlates with increased disease-free status (in other nodes) and few or no skip metastases.[110-112] These data suggest that elective lymph node dissection when metastatic cells are present in sentinel lymph nodes produces beneficial results in patients with melanoma.

HEMATOGENOUS METASTASIS

To produce a metastasis via the bloodstream, tumor cells must survive transport in the circulation, adhere to small blood vessels or capillaries, either grow locally or invade the vessel wall, and grow in the organ parenchyma. Most tumor cells released into the bloodstream are eliminated rapidly, and therefore the mere presence of tumor cells in the circulation does not predict that metastasis will occur.[10,113,114] Using radiolabeled tumor cells, Fidler[113] found that by 24 hours after entry into the circulation, less than 0.1% of the cells were viable, and less than 0.01% of tumor cells placed into the circulation eventually survived to grow into lung metastases.

Although most tumor cells are destroyed in the bloodstream, it seems that the greater the number of cells released by a primary tumor, the greater is the probability that some cells will survive to form metastases. The number of tumor emboli in the circulation appears to correlate well with the size and clinical duration of the primary tumor,[21,22,115] and the development of necrotic and hemorrhagic areas in large tumors facilitates this process by providing access to the circulation.[15] To a large degree, the rapid death of most circulating tumor cells is probably due to blood turbulence. The survival of tumor cells in the circulation can be increased by aggregation with each other[116] or with host cells, such as platelets[117] and lymphocytes.[118]

Once metastatic cells reach the microcirculation, they interact with cells of the vascular endothelium. These interactions include nonspecific mechanical lodgment of tumor cell emboli,[119] as well as interactions between proteins expressed on the cell surface of circulating tumor cells and receptors expressed on the surface of endothelial cells.[120,121] The organ distribution of metastatic foci is believed to depend, in part, on the ability of blood-borne malignant cells to adhere to specific endothelium and produce endothelial cell retraction.[119-121]

Tumor emboli must attach firmly (in contrast to passive lodgment) to endothelial cells and the internal layer of the intima of a vessel, and after attachment, the successful tumor cells must penetrate the vessel wall to reach and grow in the extravascular tissues.[122] The shedding of endothelial cells from the capillary wall is a normal and continuous physiologic event. Thus the wear and tear of endothelium may lead to temporary gaps that expose the basement membrane. Tumor cells can attach firmly to a vessel wall if the endothelium is damaged or contains gaps.[123,124] Because tumor cells can interact with platelets during transport in the circulation,[117,125,126] any damage to endothelium may lead to adherence of platelets, which is enhanced by the early deposition of fibrinogen on the endothelial cell surface.[125,126] The initial arrest there of a tumor-platelet-lymphocyte clump could be the crucial first step in lodgment and could occur by means of the adherence of platelets associated with tumor cells to platelets adhering to the damaged endothelium.[124-126] The formation of fibrin clots at sites of tumor cell arrest in the microcirculation can damage blood vessels.[127] The increased coagulability often observed in the blood of patients with cancer may be related to the high levels of thromboplastin found in certain tumors, to the production of high levels of procoagulant-A activity,[128] or to the presence of phosphatidylserine in the outer leaflet of tumor cell membranes.[129] Other factors such as mechanical trapping of large tumor cell aggregates in small-diameter vessels must also be considered. If the resulting emboli are large, a greater proportion of implanted cells survive to produce metastases.[21,22,115] Tumor cells with high metastatic potential tend to aggregate with each other (homotypic clumps) or with lymphocytes and platelets (heterotypic clumps).[117,118] Clumps of tumor cells can be arrested in the vasculature simply by a wedging process.[123] Tumor cell attachment in the microvasculature can also be enhanced by localized trauma. Tissue damaged physically, chemically, or even by reduction of oxygen tension provides a better site for attachment.[119]

The adhesion of tumor cells to the vascular endothelium is regulated by mechanisms similar to those used by leukocytes. The initial attachment of leukocytes to vascular endothelial cells is regulated by the selectin family of adhesion molecules, which consists of three closely related cell-surface molecules.[130] E-selectin, which is expressed by endothelial cells, mediates initial attachment of lymphocytes (and tumor cells) by interaction with specific carbohydrate ligands that contain sialylated fucosylated lactosamines.[131] The expression of mucin-type carbohydrates on the surface of human colon carcinoma has been correlated with their metastatic potential,[132] perhaps through differential interaction with E-selectins expressed on specific endothelial cells.[125,133] The development of firm adhesion requires the interaction of other adhesion molecules, another selective process in metastasis. Several classes of cell-to-cell adhesion molecules regulate this adhesion. These include the hyaluronate receptor CD44 and its splice variants,[134-136] the integrins $\alpha5\beta1, \alpha6\beta1,$ and $\alpha6\beta4$,[137,138] and the galactoside-binding galectin-3.[139] The arrest of tumor cells in capillary beds leads to the retraction of endothelial cells[121] and the exposure of the tumor cells to the ECM. The adhesion of metastatic cells to components of the ECM, such as fibronectin, laminin, and thrombospondin, facilitates metastasis to specific tissues[140,141]; and peptides containing sequences of these components of the ECM can reduce formation of hematogenous metastases.[129,141]

After they arrest or adhere, tumor cells may traverse the vessel wall to reach the extravascular tissues. Tumor cells can grow and destroy the surrounding vessel, invade by penetrating the endothelial basement membrane, or follow migrating white blood cells.[142] Malignant cells frequently penetrate thin-walled capillaries but rarely invade arteries or arteriole walls, which are rich in elastin fibers.[98,142,143] The extravasation of malignant cells at particular secondary sites also involves their responses to tissue or organ factors. Tumor cells can recognize tissue-specific motility factors that direct their movement and invasion.[144]

Tumor Cell Proliferation

The final steps in metastasis are tumor cell proliferation at secondary sites coupled with induction of angiogenesis. During the interaction of metastatic cells with host tissues, autocrine, paracrine, or endocrine signals influence tumor cell proliferation, and growth is dependent on the net balance of positive and negative signals,[1] which can explain site-specific metastasis.[145] Several organ-derived growth factors have been isolated and purified to homogeneity. A potent growth-stimulating factor was isolated from lung-conditioned medium,[146] and stromal cells in the bone have been shown to produce a factor that stimulates the growth of human prostatic carcinoma cells.[147] Conversely, a number of tissue-specific inhibitors have been isolated and purified, including TGF-β,[148] mammastatin,[149] and amphiregulin.[150]

Different concentrations of hormones in individual organs, differentially expressed local factors, or paracrine growth factors may all influence the growth of malignant cells.[145,151] For example, insulin-like growth factor-I (IGF-I) is synthesized in most mammalian tissue with the highest concentration in the liver.[152] IGF-I stimulates cell growth by controlling cell cycle progression.[153] The growth of carcinoma cells metastatic to the liver is stimulated by hepatocyte-derived IGF-I, correlating with IGF-I–receptor density on the cells.[154] Another example is TGF-β. Many transformed cells produce increased levels of TGF-β and become refractory to its growth inhibitory effects.[155]

Clonal stimulation or inhibition of human colon and renal carcinoma cells by TGF-β_1 has been reported in correlation with differential expression of its receptors.[156]

Autocrine or paracrine host growth factors that control organ repair and regeneration may also affect the proliferation of malignant tumor cells. Human colon cancer and human renal cancer cells were transplanted into nude mice that had been subjected to hepatectomy, nephrectomy, or abdominal surgery (used as a trauma control).[157] After partial hepatectomy, the liver undergoes regeneration associated with an increased expression of TGF-α that regulates division of hepatocytes[158] and normal colonic epithelial cells.[159] TGF-α exerts its effect through interaction with the epidermal growth factor receptor (EGF-R), a plasma membrane glycoprotein that has within its cytoplasmic domain a tyrosine-specific protein tyrosine kinase (PTK) activity. The binding of TGF-α to the EGF-R stimulates a series of rapid responses, including phosphorylation of tyrosine residues within the EGF-R itself and within many other cellular proteins, hydrolysis of phosphatidyl inositol, release of Ca^{2+} from intracellular stores, elevation of cytoplasmic pH, and morphologic changes.[160] After 10 to 12 hours in the continuous presence of EGF or TGF-α, cells are committed to synthesize DNA and to divide.[160,161] Colon cancer cells demonstrated accelerated growth in partially hepatectomized mice but not in nephrectomized mice. Renal cancer cells underwent a significant growth acceleration subsequent to unilateral nephrectomy but not hepatectomy.[157] Similar data have been reported for rat colon carcinoma cells injected intraportally. The incidence and size of liver metastases were significantly increased in hepatectomized rats as compared with sham-operated controls.[158] TGF-α mRNA was shown to increase approximately twofold in rat hepatocytes during the first 8 to 24 hours after partial hepatectomy, coinciding with an increase in EGF-R mRNA and a downregulation of these receptor proteins, as well as a loss of EGF-R protein kinase activity.[162] These results suggest that TGF-α is a physiologic regulator of liver regeneration by means of an autocrine mechanism.[159] Moreover, TGF-α production by hepatocytes might also have a paracrine role, stimulating proliferation of adjacent nonparenchymal cells or tumor cells.[163] These results indicate that metastatic cells can respond to physiologic signals produced when homeostasis is disturbed and that tumor cells that either originate from or have an affinity for growth in a particular organ can usurp these physiologic signals.

Hepatocyte growth factor (HGF), another liver mitogen, is synthesized and secreted from nonparenchymal liver cells (endothelial and Kupffer cells). Subsequent to liver damage, a rapid increase is observed in HGF mRNA in Kupffer cells, paralleling the downregulation of its receptor, the *c-met* protooncogene, in hepatocytes.[164] Like EGF-R, *c-met* belongs to the tyrosine kinase family of receptors.[165] HGF is a potent mitogen for hepatocytes, melanocytes, and prostate cells; and it enhances the invasive capacity of carcinomas.[166] Levels of TGF-β mRNA increase in normal nonparenchymal liver cells, coinciding with hepatocyte DNA replication and mitosis, and TGF-β inhibits EGF-stimulated DNA synthesis, implying that it

may be a component of a paracrine regulatory loop that controls hepatocyte replication in the late stages of liver regeneration.[158]

EGF-Rs are present on many normal and tumor cells.[160] Increased levels and/or amplification of EGF-R have been found in many human tumors and cell lines, including breast cancer,[167] gliomas,[168] lung cancer,[169] bladder cancer,[170] epidermoid carcinoma,[171] and colon carcinoma,[172] suggesting that the high expression level of the EGF-R tyrosine kinase may contribute to abnormal cell growth. Analyses of human colon cancer (HCC) cells isolated from surgical specimens that differed in malignant potential showed no amplification or rearrangements in the genes encoding EGF-R.[173] In contrast, highly metastatic human colon cancer variant cells (either Dukes' stage D or cells selected for metastatic potential in nude mice from a Dukes' stage B2 tumor) expressed significantly more EGF-R mRNA transcripts when compared with low-metastatic human colon cancer cell types.[174] The in vitro growth stimulation of cells with high or low metastatic potential by TGF-α demonstrated the functional significance of increased EGF-R numbers on metastatic cells.

The EGF-Rs expressed on metastatic HCC cells were functional as determined by in vitro growth stimulation assays with picogram concentrations of TGF-α and to be specific as shown by neutralization with anti–EGF-R or anti–TGF-α antibodies. Moreover, EGF-R–associated PTK activity also paralleled the observed EGF-R levels. Immunohistochemical analysis of the low metastatic parental HCC cells demonstrated heterogeneity in the EGF-R–specific staining pattern, with only a few of the cells staining intensely for EGF-R; whereas cells selected for high metastatic potential exhibited uniform, intense staining. Western blotting confirmed the presence of higher EGF-R protein levels in the metastatic cell lines than in the low metastatic cell line. Finally, isolation of low and high EGF-R–expressing cells by fluorescence-activated cell sorting directly correlated with production of hepatic metastases.[174]

The analyses described show a direct correlation between expression of EGF-R and ability to produce liver metastases in nude mice. These findings were confirmed by analysis of formalin-fixed, paraffin-embedded colon carcinoma surgical specimens for EGF-R transcripts with a rapid colorimetric mRNA in situ hybridization (ISH) technique.[174] Cell-surface hybridization with EGF-R–antisense hyperbiotinylated oligonucleotide probes in primary and metastatic colon carcinoma specimens directly correlated with immunohistochemistry and Northern blot analyses.

In human tissues, the highest levels of *c-met* mRNA expression are found in the liver, kidneys, stomach, and thyroid. Studies with anti-*c-met* antibodies have revealed that receptor protein levels are high in hepatocytes and in gastric and intestinal epithelium (including the colon and rectum), indicating a role for HGF and *c-met* in the growth and turnover of epithelial tissues.[175] High levels of *c-met* are expressed by HCC cells and cell lines that have been adapted to grow in culture from Dukes' stage B2 or stage D or from liver metastases. Analyses of mRNA isolated directly from HCC specimens and normal colon mucosa also suggest the presence of more *c-met* transcripts in the tumor tissues.[174]

METASTASIS OF METASTASES

The tumor cells proliferating within metastases can invade host stroma, penetrate blood vessels, and enter the circulation to produce secondary metastases, the so-called metastasis of metastases.[176-178] Hart and Fidler[179] used the preferential growth of B16 melanoma metastases in specific organs. After the intravenous injection of B16 melanoma cells into syngeneic mice, tumor growths developed in the lungs and in fragments of lung or ovarian tissue implanted intramuscularly into the quadriceps femoris but not in renal tissue implanted as a control. Tumor growth in the specific transplanted organ could have been caused by the arrest and growth of tumor cells immediately after intravenous injection, that is, "initial metastases." Alternatively, tumor cells injected intravenously could have been arrested in the lungs, where they developed; once metastases had been established, tumor cells could enter the circulation to be arrested at other organs and produce "secondary metastases."[176,178,180] To distinguish between these possibilities, Fidler and Nicolson[178] performed several experiments: Two weeks after normal, tumor-free mice were joined parabiotically to metastasis-bearing mice, there was no evidence of any tumor growth in the "guest" animals. However, when the parabiont animals were allowed to survive for 4 weeks after separation from the metastasis-bearing animals, 40% developed lung metastases. Because the host mice did not have primary tumors at the time of parabiosis, the metastases in the guest mice could have only arisen as metastasis from metastases (Fig. 4-2).

THE BIOLOGIC HETEROGENEITY OF NEOPLASMS

Only a few cells in a primary tumor can give rise to a metastasis.[1] This is due in part to the elimination of any disseminating tumor cell that fails to complete any step in the metastatic process. The data raise the question of whether the development of metastases represents the fortuitous survival and growth of a very few neoplastic cells or the selective growth of unique subpopulations of malignant cells endowed with special properties. In other words, can all cells growing in a primary neoplasm produce secondary lesions, or do only specific and unique cells possess the appropriate properties that would enable them to survive the potentially destructive journey from the primary tumor to the sites of future metastases? Most data show that neoplasms are biologically heterogeneous and that the process of metastasis is selective.

Clinical observations of human neoplasms have suggested that the lesions tend to undergo a series of changes during the course of the disease; for example, a growth that initially appeared to be a benign tumor can change into a malignant, lethal tumor. Foulds[181] describes this phenomenon of tumor evolution as "neoplastic progression" and defines it as "acquisition of permanent, irreversible qualitative changes in one or more characteristics of a neoplasm." This evolution of tumors is gradual, and tumor cells proceed toward increased autonomy from their host by a temporal change in various properties. The acquisition and loss of various characteristics are likely to be independent of each other.[182] Moreover, because tumor progression can occur over periods of months or even years, the behavior of a neoplasm in any given individual may vary at different stages of the disease. Finally, because neoplasms are not independent of their host, tumor pro-

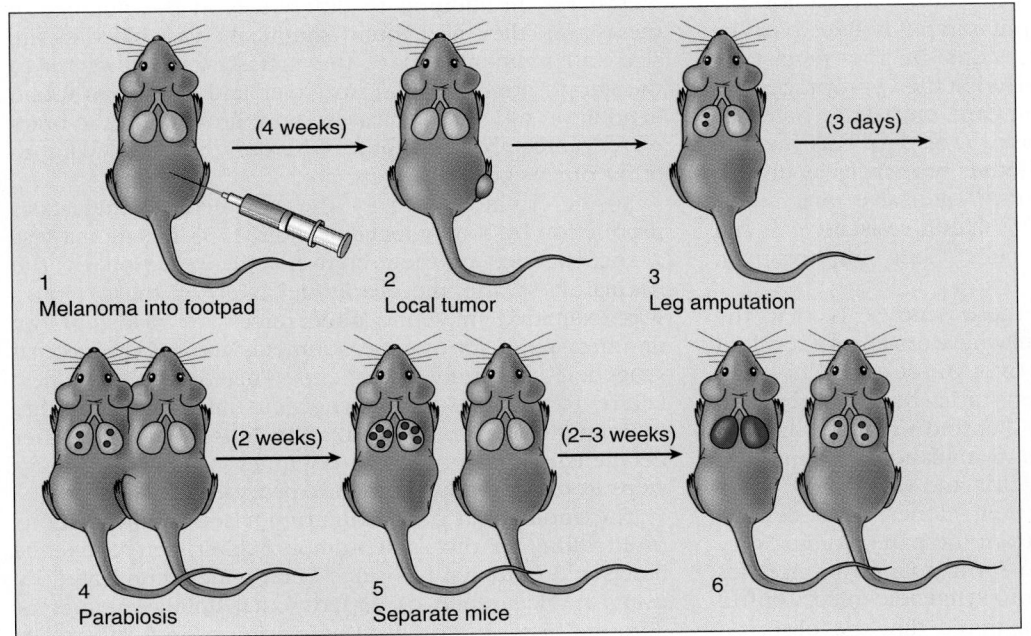

1 Melanoma into footpad   (4 weeks)   2 Local tumor   3 Leg amputation   (3 days)

4 Parabiosis   (2 weeks)   5 Separate mice   (2–3 weeks)   6

Figure 4-2. Metastasis of a metastasis. Design of the experiment that demonstrated that metastases metastasize. Melanoma cells were implanted into the footpads of syngeneic mice. The leg with tumor was amputated and the mice were parabiosed to normal syngeneic animals. Two weeks later, the mice were separated. The fact that the "guest" mouse had lung metastases proves that lung metastases can give rise to additional metastases.

gression is influenced by host homeostatic mechanisms, that is, selection pressures.[183-190]

Many techniques, ranging from karyotype analysis to molecular probes, have been used to study the origin of human neoplasms. The majority of human cancers result from the proliferation of a single transformed cell,[188-198] and the generation of biologic diversity in such tumors must therefore reflect a complex pattern of clonal diversification during tumor progression.[183-185]

HETEROGENEITY OF THE METASTATIC PHENOTYPE

Cells with different metastatic properties have been isolated from the same parent tumor, thus supporting the hypothesis that not all the cells in a primary tumor can successfully disseminate. Two general approaches have been used to isolate populations of cells that differ from the parent neoplasm in metastatic capacity. In the first approach, metastatic cells are selected in vivo: Tumor cells are implanted subcutaneously, intramuscularly, or into other organs, and metastasis is allowed to occur. The metastatic lesions are harvested, and the cells that are recovered can first be expanded in culture or used immediately to repeat the process. The cycle is repeated several times. The behavior of the cycled cells is compared with that of the cells of the parent tumor to determine whether the selection process enhanced metastatic capacity,[199] and in two studies the increase in metastatic capacity of the recovered cells was not found to result from the adaptation of tumor cells to preferential growth in a particular organ.[200,201] This procedure was originally used to isolate the B16-F10 line from the wild-type B16 melanoma[199] (Fig. 4-3). It has also been successfully used to produce tumor cell lines with increased metastatic capacity from many of the experimental tumors tested.[202,203]

In the second approach, cells are selected for the enhanced expression of a phenotype believed to be important in one or more steps of the metastatic sequence, and then they are tested in the appropriate host to determine whether concomitant metastatic potential has been increased or decreased (Fig. 4-4). This method has been used to examine whether properties as diverse as resistance to T lymphocytes,[118] adhesive characteristics,[204] invasive capacity,[203,205,206] lectin resistance,[207] and resistance to natural killer cells[208] are important in metastasis.

An obvious criticism of these studies is that the surviving isolated tumor line may have arisen as a result of adaptive rather than selective processes. The first experimental proof for metastatic heterogeneity in neoplasms was provided by Fidler and Kripke[209] in 1977 in work with the mouse B16 melanoma. Using the modified fluctuation assay of Luria and Delbruck,[210] they showed that different tumor cell clones, each derived from individual cells isolated from the parent tumor, vary dramatically in their ability to form pulmonary nodules after intravenous inoculation into syngeneic mice. Control subcloning procedures demonstrated that the observed

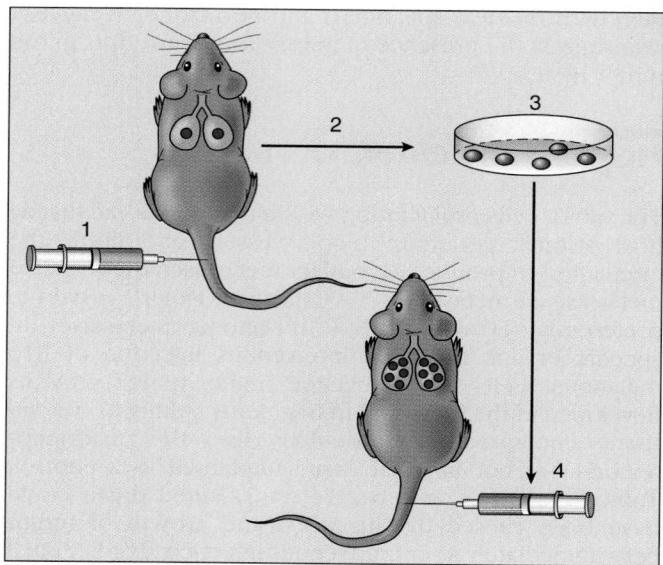

Figure 4-3. In vivo enrichment for metastatic cells. Heterogeneous parental neoplasms are injected intravenously or subcutaneously (1). Metastases are harvested (2) and cells are grown in culture (3). The metastatic potential of the cells isolated from metastasis is determined subsequent to injection into mice (4).

diversity was not a consequence of the cloning procedure[209] (Fig. 4-5, p. 68).

To exclude the possibility that the metastatic heterogeneity found in the B16 melanoma might have been introduced as a result of the lengthy in vivo and in vitro cultivation, Fidler and colleagues[211] studied the biologic and metastatic heterogeneity in a mouse melanoma induced in mice by long-term exposure to UVB radiation and painting with croton oil.[212] Fidler and colleagues[211] found that clones differed greatly from each other and from the parent tumor in their ability to produce metastases. In addition to differences in the number of metastases, they also found significant variability in the size and pigmentation of the metastases. Metastases to the lymph nodes, brain, heart, liver, and skin were found in addition to lung metastases; those growing in the brain were uniformly melanotic, whereas those growing in other organs generally were not.

To determine whether the absence of metastasis production by some clones of the K-1735 melanoma was a consequence of their immunologic rejection by the normal host, the metastatic behavior of these clones was examined in young nude mice.[213-216] Most of the nonmetastatic clones were nonmetastatic in both normal syngeneic and nude recipients. Therefore, the clones' failure to metastasize in syngeneic mice was not due to immunologic rejection by the host,[214] but to other deficiencies that prevented completion of one or more steps in the complex metastatic process.

The finding that preexisting tumor cell subpopulations proliferating in the same tumor exhibit heterogeneous metastatic potential has since been widely confirmed by using a wide range of experimental animal tumors of different histories and histologic origins. Similarly, studies

Figure 4-4. In vitro selection for metastatic cells. Heterogeneous parental neoplasm cells (1) are placed on a membrane (2). Subsequent to invasion, the invading cells are expended in culture (3) and cloned (4). The invasive and metastatic potential of the clones are tested in mice (5) and compared with that of original unselected parental cells.

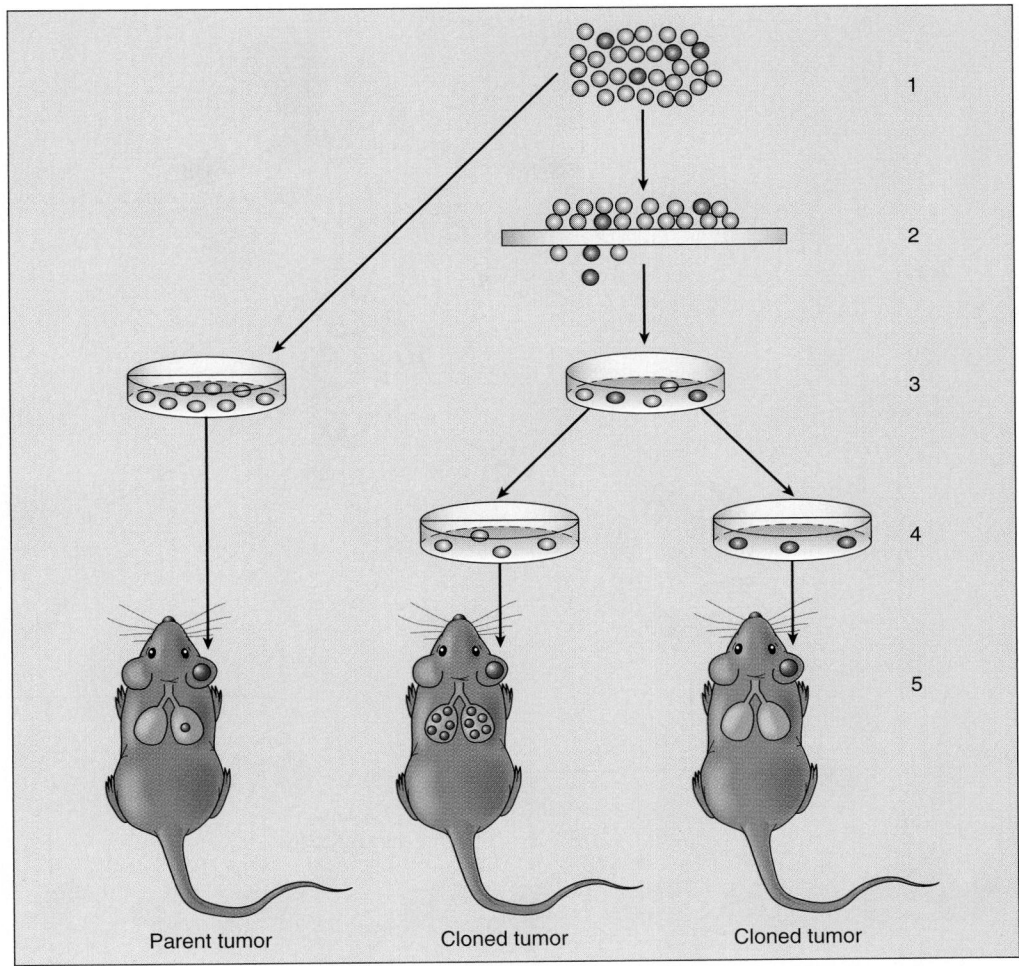

Parent tumor   Cloned tumor   Cloned tumor

in which young nude mice were used have indicated that human tumors, such as colon carcinoma, renal carcinoma, prostate carcinoma, gastric cancer, lung cancer, and melanoma also contain subpopulations of cells with widely differing metastatic properties.[91,217-226]

Fidler and colleagues[215,216] also determined whether the cells that survive to form metastases possess a greater metastatic capacity than most cells in an unselected neoplasm. Most lines derived from metastatic deposits produced significantly more metastases than cells of the parent line (Fig. 4-6, p. 69). Studies with heterogeneous, unselected neoplasms have therefore led Fidler and associates[216-222] to conclude that metastasis is a selective process regulated by a number of different mechanisms.

CLONAL ORIGIN AND DEVELOPMENT OF BIOLOGIC HETEROGENEITY IN CANCER METASTASES

Like primary neoplasms, metastases may have a unicellular or a multicellular origin. Pathologists know that neoplasms frequently exhibit different morphologic appearances in different areas. For this reason, the malignant or benign nature of a tumor cannot be determined with confidence unless multiple sections from all parts of the tumor are examined. The zonal differences in tumors are not restricted to structure alone but include biologic characteristics such as growth rates, sensitivity to cytotoxic drugs, antigenicity, and pigmentation.[227] Because primary tumors are not uniform, it is possible that tumor cell aggregates entering the circulation from one zone of the tumor may be different from those entering from another zone. If an embolic aggregate originates from a primary tumor's homogeneous zone, regardless of whether only one cell or several cells has survived to proliferate in distant organs, the resulting metastasis will be like that of a primary tumor of unicellular origin. If a mixed embolus derived from an area of zonal junctions enters the circulation, the unicellular or multicellular origin of the metastasis would depend on whether a single cell or multiple cells survived to proliferate. To determine whether individual metastases are clonal and whether different metastases can be produced by different progenitor cells, Talmadge and colleagues[228] performed a series of experiments based on the fact that x-irradiation of tumor cells induces random chromosome breaks and rearrangements. Analyzing the karyotype composition

Science of Clinical Oncology

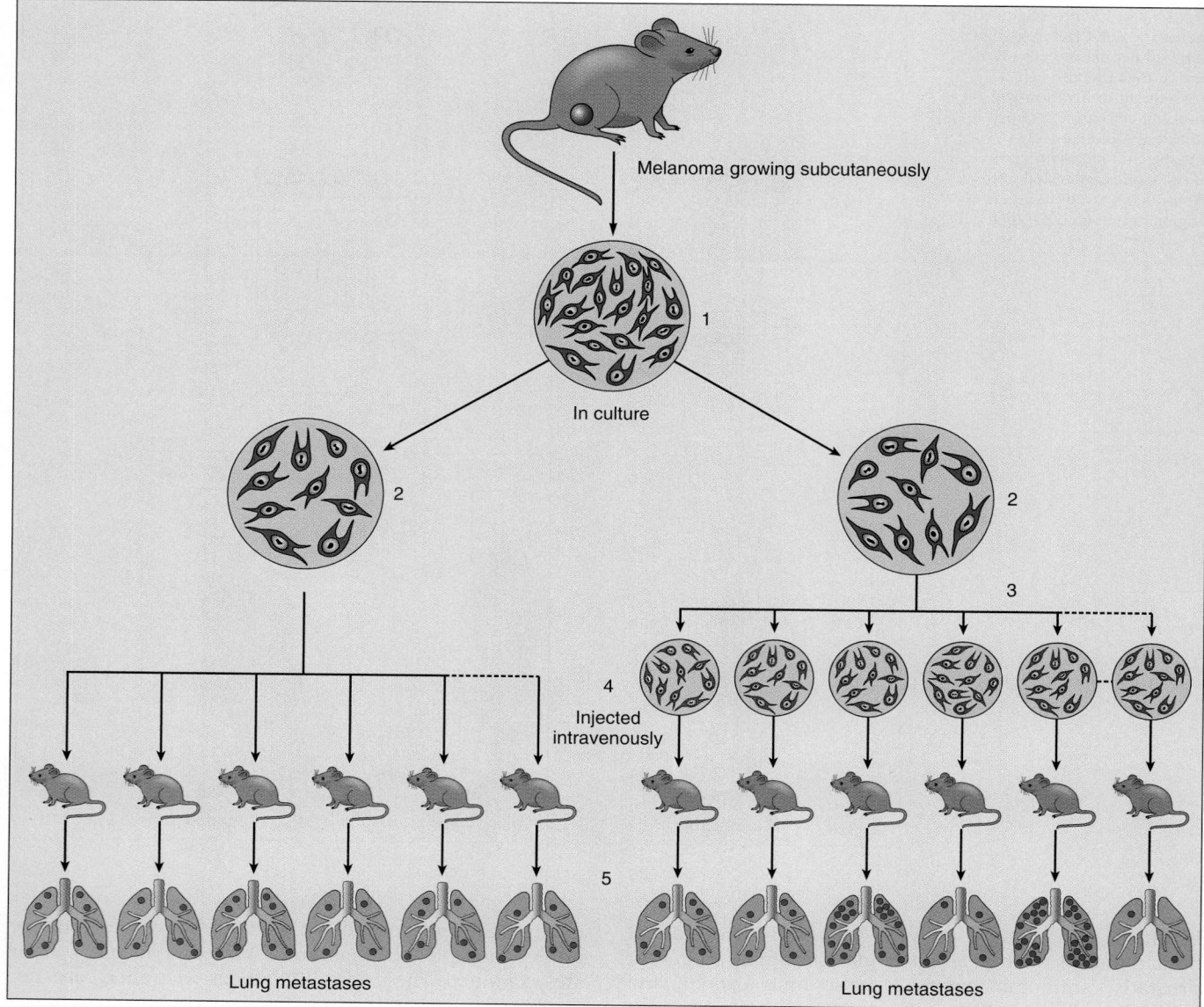

Figure 4-5. Design of the experiment demonstrating that neoplasms are heterogeneous for metastatic properties and that metastatic cells preexist within the primary neoplasm. A heterogeneous parental neoplasm is grown in culture (1) and divided into 2 aliquots (2). One culture is cloned (3). Cells from unselected parental tumor *(left panel)* and cells from individual clones *(right panel)* are injected into syngeneic mice (4). Metastatic potential is determined several weeks later.

of 21 individual melanoma lung metastases after cultivating cells from individual lesions, this research group found unique karyotypic patterns of abnormal, marker chromosomes in most of the lines established from metastases, which suggested that each metastasis originated from a single progenitor cell. Similar results have been obtained in other rodent tumor systems.[229-232] These studies revealed that the majority of metastases are of clonal origin. Moreover, variant clones with diverse phenotypes are formed, rapidly resulting in the generation of significant cellular diversity within individual metastases.[233,234]

Cancer metastases of a clonal origin can be produced by two different mechanisms, proliferation of a single cell or proliferation of many cells. In the case of the second possibility, the cell aggregate at the metastatic site must have a homogeneous composition. Subsequent experiments demonstrated that even when heterogeneous clumps of two different melanoma cells reached the lung vasculature, the resultant metastases were all of single-cell origin.[235] Thus, regardless of whether an embolus is initially homogeneous or heterogeneous, metastases can be unicellular in origin. Collectively, these observations indicate that different metastases arise from different progenitor cells. Nevertheless, heterogeneity develops rapidly to create significant intralesional heterogeneity.

The cellular composition of different metastases in the same host is heterogeneous, both within a single meta-

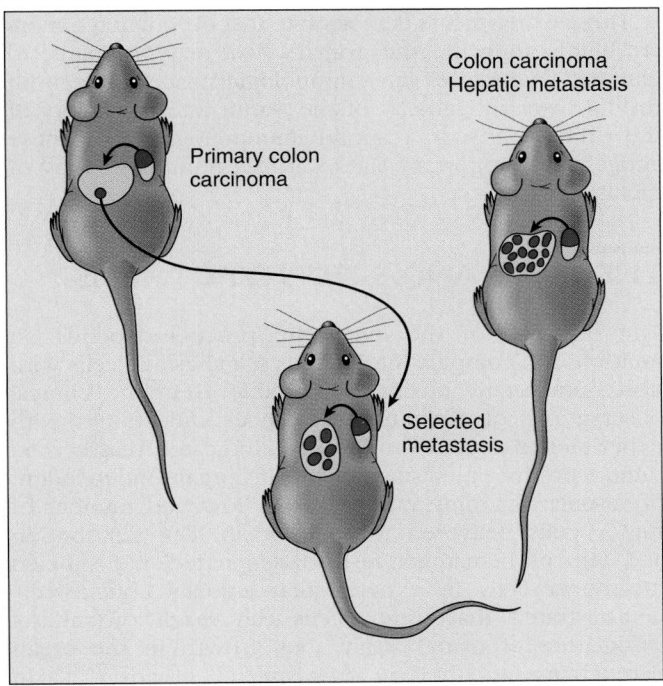

Figure 4-6. Selection for metastatic colon carcinoma cells. An experiment demonstrating that hepatic metastases produced by colon carcinoma cells consist of cells with increased metastatic potential. Cells from a primary human carcinoma are injected into the spleens of nude mice. The cells from liver metastases produced as many lesions (on reinjection) as did cells from hepatic metastasis recovered from a patient.

stasis (intralesional heterogeneity) and among different metastases (interlesional heterogeneity). This heterogeneity reflects two major processes: the selective nature of the metastatic process and the rapid evolution and phenotypic diversification of clonal tumor cell populations during progressive tumor growth (which itself results from the inherent genetic and phenotypic instability of many clonal populations of tumor cells).

Karyotypic analysis of primary tumors, and especially of metastases, reveals gross structural alterations (deletions, rearrangements, aneuploidy) and increased ploidy in comparison with normal cells.[236] Cells that populate metastases frequently exhibit altered karyotype and ploidy as compared with cells in primary tumors.[237,238] Similarly, cellular heterogeneity with respect to gene amplification, gene rearrangement, and point mutations in cellular gene and proto-oncogene sequences of tumor cells has been reported.[239-242]

To explain the process of tumor evolution and progression as originally defined by Foulds in 1954, Nowell[183-185] suggest that acquired genetic variability within developing clones of tumors, coupled with host selection pressures, can result in the emergence of new tumor cell variants that exhibit increasing growth autonomy or malignancy. Nowell's hypothesis predicted that accelerating tumor progression toward malignancy can be accompanied by increasing genetic instability of the evolving cells. To test this hypothesis, Cifone and

Fidler[243] have examined the rates of mutation of paired metastatic and nonmetastatic cloned lines isolated from four different mouse neoplasms. They found that highly metastatic cells were phenotypically less stable than their nonmetastatic counterparts. Moreover, in highly metastatic clones, the rate of spontaneous mutation was found to be severalfold higher than that in low metastatic clones.[243] Similar data have been reported for other neoplasms.[244-246]

Collectively, these studies suggest that the more metastatic a tumor cell population is, the greater the likelihood that the cells will undergo rapid phenotypic diversification and thus escape various therapeutic modalities. This process may well be further exaggerated by the mutagenic action of many of the chemotherapeutic drugs used in current treatment regimens.[247]

CLONAL INTERACTIONS WITHIN METASTASES

Subpopulations of tumor cells within a neoplasm are not autonomous units but are influenced by other neoplastic and normal host cells in close proximity. Subpopulations of mammary tumor cells have been shown to affect the growth patterns, immunogenicity, and chemosensitivity of each other.[248-252] Similar regulatory control may exist for the metastatic phenotype of different cells within mixed tumors of different etiologic and histologic origins. The demonstration of interclonal stabilization for expression of immunogenicity[253] also supports the concept that individual subpopulations of cells regulate each other's phenotype.

Thus different subpopulations of tumor cells stabilize and impose an equilibrium on each other.[252] Selection pressures such as host immunity, depletion of an essential nutrient, or chemotherapy can lead to the emergence of a clonal population with a growth advantage, that is, clonal dominance.[254,255] Clonality, however, is not synonymous with homogeneity. In fact, strong selection pressures also lead to removal of the polyclonal stabilization effects and, hence, to rapid biologic diversification of primary and metastatic lesions.[256,257]

HOST IMMUNITY AND CANCER METASTASIS

Any discussion of the role of the immune system in metastasis must address three issues: the antigenic heterogeneity of neoplasms, the intrinsic immunogenicity of metastatic cells, and the ability of the host to recognize and destroy autochthonous tumor cells.

The heterogeneous nature of neoplasms with regard to antigenicity, immunogenicity, and susceptibility to antibody-dependent cellular cytotoxicity and to natural killer (NK) cells, T cells, lymphokine-activated killer (LAK) cells, tumor-infiltrating leukocyte (TIL), or cytotoxic T-lymphocyte (CTL) therapy is now well recognized.[213,214,258-265] Moreover, antigenicity differs between primary tumors and their metastases and among different metastatic lesions.[266-270] Similarly, tumors recurring at the site of excision of an original tumor can be antigenically distinct.[271] In fact, vaccination against polyclonal tumors failed because only the dominant subpopulation's growth was restricted. The minor subpopulations, which did not constitute a sufficient mass in the vaccine to stimulate the immune response, proceeded to proliferate after the vaccination and eventually became the dominant population.[271]

Another issue that should be considered is whether the relative antigenicity of malignant cells influences their metastatic potential. Experimental studies on the role of the immune response in cancer metastasis have yielded contradictory results. In some tumor systems, depression of immunologic reactivity has been shown to increase the incidence of both spontaneous and experimental metastasis, whereas in other systems, depression of host immunity has been shown to decrease or prevent formation of metastases.[214] In yet another series of tumors, alterations of immunologic reactivity did not seem to influence the growth of local or disseminated tumors.[272] These conflicting reports cannot be readily reconciled. Obviously, the role of the immune system in experimental metastasis varies for different tumors, and no predictive generalizations regarding the role of host immunity can be made from a single tumor system.

Syngeneic sensitized lymphocytes may interact with antigenic tumor cells at several different steps of the metastatic process.[1] How efficiently the cells of a particular tumor traverse these steps will influence the extent to which they will be affected by immunologic processes. Moreover, the immune system itself has both inhibiting and stimulating effects on tumor growth, and these effects can be exerted simultaneously. These stimulating effects may result, as Prehn[272] has suggested, from a direct effect of lymphoid cells or their products on tumor growth. The factors that determine whether a stimulating or inhibiting immune response will predominate are still not known for certain, but they are likely to involve such variables as the characteristics of the tumor antigen, the mode of antigen presentation, and the initial site of interaction with host immune cells.

Metastatic cells can successfully evade host immune surveillance mechanisms when host immunity is suppressed. UV light–induced skin tumors are highly immunogenic and are rejected on transplantation into normal syngeneic hosts.[211,213,273] How, then, do these tumors grow in the original host? A series of experiments by Donawho and Kripke[274] has shown that exposure of mice to UV light leads to generation of suppressor T lymphocytes, which can then prevent the immunologic destruction of these highly immunogenic tumor cells. Pretreatment of normal syngeneic hosts with UV light before inoculation of these highly immunogenic UV light–induced tumor cells allows the progressive growth of tumors as though they were inoculated into immuno-deficient hosts. UV radiation also influences the susceptibility of mice to systemic tumor challenge as shown by the fact that UV light–induced tumors form more pulmonary metastases in UV-irradiated mice than in normal syngeneic recipients.[275]

These experiments demonstrate that even when tumors are highly antigenic, the primary host may be unable to eliminate metastases by immunologic means. Thus, both the intrinsic antigenicity of the tumor and the ability of the primary host to respond immunologically to these antigens are important factors in the immunotherapy of metastases.

THE "SEED AND SOIL" HYPOTHESIS

The outcome of the metastatic process depends on multiple and complex interactions of metastatic cells with host homeostatic mechanisms (Table 4-1).[276,277] Clinical observations of patients with cancer and studies with experimental rodent tumors have indicated that certain tumors produce metastasis to specific organs independent of vascular anatomy, rate of blood flow, and number of tumor cells delivered to each organ. The distribution and fate of hematogenously disseminated, radiolabeled melanoma cells in experimental animals conclusively demonstrated that tumor cells can reach the micro-vasculature of many organs, but growth in the organ parenchyma occurred in only specific organs.[278-280] In 1889, Stephen Paget[100] researched the mechanisms that regulate organ-specific metastasis (i.e., pattern of metastasis by different cancers). Paget questioned whether the organ distribution of metastases produced by different human neoplasms was due to chance and analyzed more than 700 autopsy records of women with breast cancer. His research documented a nonrandom pattern of visceral (and bone) metastasis. This finding suggested to Paget that the process was not a result of chance but, rather, certain tumor cells (the "seed") had a specific affinity for the

TABLE 4-1

Tumor Cell Properties and Host Factors That Regulate

I. Tumor Cell Properties

  A. *Facilitation of Metastasis*
   1. Production of growth factors and their receptors
   2. Production of angiogenic factors
   3. Motility, invasiveness
   4. Aggregation, deformability
   5. Specific cell surface receptors and adhesion molecules
  B. *Inhibition of Metastasis*
   1. Antigenicity
   2. Production of angiogenic inhibitors
   3. Tissue inhibitors of degradative enzymes
   4. Cohesion (E-cadherin)

II. Host Factors

  A. *Facilitation of Metastasis*
   1. Neovascularization
   2. Paracrine and endocrine growth factors
   3. Platelets and their products
   4. Immune cells and their products
  B. *Inhibition of Metastasis*
   1. Tissue barriers
   2. Blood turbulence, endothelial cells
   3. Tissue inhibitors of degradative enzymes
   4. Tissue antiproliferative factors
   5. Immune cells and their products

milieu of certain organs (the "soil"). Metastases resulted only when the seed and soil were compatible.[100]

In 1929, J. Ewing[281] challenged Paget's seed and soil theory and hypothesized that metastatic dissemination occurs by purely mechanical factors that are a result of the anatomic structure of the vascular system. These explanations have been evoked separately and together to explain the metastatic site preference of certain types of neoplasms. In a review of clinical studies on site preferences of metastases produced by different human neoplasms, Sugarbaker[282] concluded that common *regional* metastatic involvements could be attributed to anatomic or mechanical considerations, such as efferent venous circulation or lymphatic drainage to regional lymph nodes, but that metastasis in *distant* organs from numerous types of cancers were site specific.

Experimental data supporting the "seed and soil" hypothesis of Paget were derived from studies on the preferential invasion and growth of B16 melanoma metastases in specific organs.[179] In vitro experiments demonstrating organ-selective adhesion, invasion, and growth and experiments with organ tissue–derived soluble growth factors indicate that "soil" factors can have profound effects on certain tumor cell subpopulations also support Paget's hypothesis.[277]

There is no question that the circulatory anatomy influences the dissemination of many malignant cells[6,7,10]; however, it cannot, as Ewing[281] proposed, fully explain the patterns of distribution of numerous tumors. Ethical considerations prevent the experimental analysis of cancer metastasis in patients as studied in laboratory animals, by which either Paget or Ewing might be proved correct. The introduction of peritoneovenous shunts for palliation of malignant ascites has, however, provided an opportunity to study some of the factors affecting metastatic spread in humans. Tarin and colleagues[283,284] have described the outcome in patients with malignant ascites draining into the venous circulation, with the resulting entry of viable tumor cells into the jugular veins. Good palliation with minimal complications was reported for 29 patients with different neoplasms. The autopsy findings in 15 patients substantiated the clinical observations that the shunts do not significantly increase the risk of metastasis. In fact, despite continuous entry of millions of tumor cells into the circulation, metastases in the lungs (the first capillary bed encountered) were rare. These results provide compelling verification of the venerable "seed and soil" hypothesis.[100]

An interesting demonstration of organ-specific metastasis comes from studies of experimental brain metastasis. Schackert and Fidler[285,286] and Fujimaki and colleagues[287] have described the development of a mouse model with which to study cerebral metastasis after injection of syngeneic tumor cells into the internal carotid artery. A direct, intracranial injection of tumor cells was used to determine tumorigenicity. The injection of cells into the internal carotid artery of mice simulates the hematogenous spread of tumor emboli to the brain. Thus this technique can be used to examine the last steps of the metastatic process: release of tumor cells into the circulation, arrest of tumor cells in capillaries, penetration and extravasation of the tumor cells into the brain through the blood-brain barrier, and continuous growth of the cells in the tissue.

The two melanomas differed in patterns of brain metastasis: The K-1735 melanoma produced lesions only in the brain parenchyma, whereas the B16 melanoma produced only meningeal growths.[286,287] Similarly, different human melanomas[288,289] and carcinomas[290] injected into the internal carotid artery of nude mice produce unique patterns of brain metastasis. These results demonstrate specificity for metastatic growth in different regions within a single organ. The results from site distribution analysis of radiolabeled murine melanoma cells injected into the internal carotid artery ruled out that the patterns of initial cell arrest in the microvasculature of the brain predicted the eventual sites of growth. Thus an alternative explanation for the different sites of tumor growth involves interactions between the metastatic cells and the organ environment, possibly in terms of specific binding to endothelial cells and responses to local growth factors. In other words, organ-specific metastases are produced by tumor cells that are receptive to their new environment.

THE "SEED AND SOIL" HYPOTHESIS: 2003

A current definition of the "seed and soil" hypothesis consists of three principles. First, neoplasms are biologically heterogeneous and contain subpopulations of cells with different angiogenic, invasive, and metastatic properties. Second, the process of metastasis is selective for cells that succeed in invasion, embolization, survival in the circulation, arrest in a distant capillary bed, and extravasation into and multiplication within the organ parenchyma. Although some of the steps in this process contain stochastic elements, as a whole, metastasis favors the survival and growth of a few subpopulations of cells that preexist within the parent neoplasm (Fig. 4-7). Third, and perhaps most important for the design of new cancer therapies, is that the outcome of metastasis depends on multiple interactions ("cross-talk") of metastatic cells with homeostatic mechanisms, which the tumor cells can usurp.[277] The successful metastatic cell, referred to years ago as the *decathlon champion*,[1,291] must today also be viewed as a cell receptive to its environment. Therefore in the treatment of metastasis, not only tumor cells but also the homeostatic factors that promote tumor cell growth, survival, angiogenesis, invasion, and metastasis can be targeted (see Chapter 3).

Modulation of Cancer Cell Response to Chemotherapy

Clinical observations have suggested that the organ environment can influence the response of tumors to chemotherapy. For example, in women with breast cancer, lymph node and skin metastases respond to chemotherapy better than lung or bone metastases. Experimental systems suggested a basis for this observation.[292,293] Studies by Staroselsky and colleagues[294] have shown that a

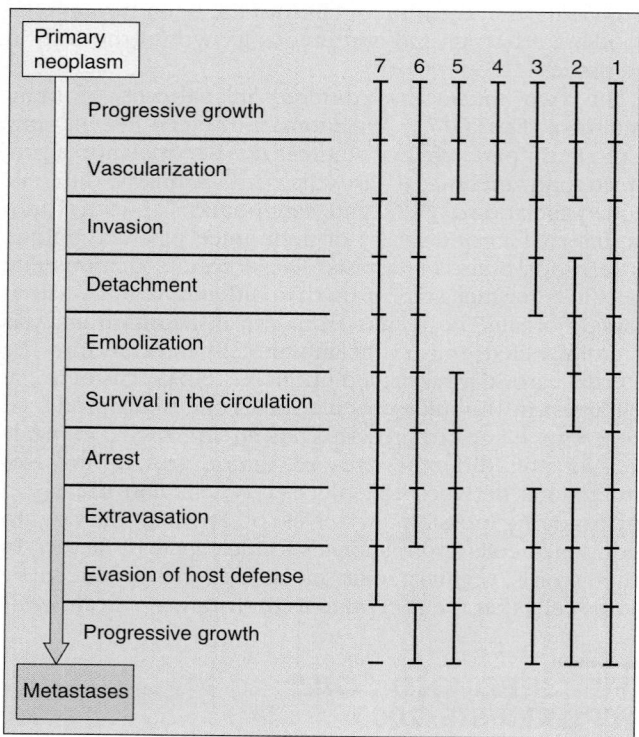

Figure 4-7. Sequential steps in the pathogenesis of cancer metastasis. Each discrete step of metastasis is likely to be regulated by transient or permanent changes in DNA, RNA, or proteins of multiple genes. Since nonmetastatic cells fail to produce metastasis because of one or more deficiencies, induction of metastatic competence in different nonmetastatic cells may involve inactivation or deactivation of different genes. Examples are (1) metastasis-competent cells; (2) deficiency in invasion or extravasation step; (3) deficiency in aggregation, survival in circulation, and arrest; (4 and 5) multiple deficiencies; (6) high immunogenicity and antigenicity; and (7) deficiency in ability to grow at metastatic sites.

mouse fibrosarcoma growing subcutaneously in syngeneic mice was sensitive to systemic administration of doxorubicin (DXR), whereas lung metastases were not. Wilmanns and colleagues[295] and Yoon and colleagues[296] obtained similar results with the CT-26 murine colon cancer and the B16 melanoma, respectively: Subcutaneous tumors were sensitive to DXR, whereas metastases growing in the liver or lung were not.

Several intrinsic properties of tumor cells can render them resistant to chemotherapeutic drugs, including increased expression of the *mdr* genes, leading to overproduction of the transmembrane transport protein P-gp.[297] Increased levels of P-gp can be induced by selecting tumor cells for resistance to natural product amphiphilic anticancer drugs. Elevated expression of P-gp accompanied by development of the MDR phenotype has also been found in many solid tumors of the colon, kidney, and liver that had not been exposed to chemotherapy.[298]

Dong and associates[299] investigated whether specific organ microenvironments can influence the response of tumor cells and regulate the expression level of P-gp in the tumor cells and, hence, their response to chemotherapy. In this study, murine CT-26 colon cancer cells growing in

the lungs of syngeneic mice were refractory to systemic administration of DXR, whereas the same cells growing subcutaneously were sensitive to the drug. CT-26 cells harvested from lung metastases expressed high levels of *mdr*-1 mRNA and exhibited increased resistance to DXR (but not to 5-fluorouracil) as compared with cells harvested from subcutaneous tumors or parental cells maintained in culture, which expressed low levels of *mdr*-1 mRNA. The drug resistance and accompanying elevated expression of *mdr*-1 found for cells growing in the lungs were dependent on interaction with the specific organ environment. Once removed from the lung, the cells reverted to a sensitive phenotype.[299]

The findings of organ-specific response to DXR are not restricted to CT-26 cells. UV-2237 mouse fibrosarcoma cells,[294] human KM12 colon carcinoma cells,[295] and murine B16 melanoma cells[296] also showed significant differences in resistance to DXR (but not 5-fluorouracil) between subcutaneous tumors (sensitive) and lung or liver metastases (resistant). In patients with colon carcinoma, high-level P-gp expression is found on the invasive edge of the primary tumor (growing in the colon) in lymph node, lung, and liver metastases.[300]

Collectively, the data demonstrate that the organ environment can induce the P-gp–associated MDR phenotype in tumor cells. The expression of P-gp is transient: Once removed from the environment (lung), the cells' resistance reverts to that of the sensitive parent cells. This environmental regulation of the MDR phenotype may explain, in part, the polarized expression of *mdr*-1 in colon carcinomas[301] and the discrepancy between in vitro and in vivo expression levels of the MDR phenotype.

Predicting the Malignant Potential of Human Carcinomas

To produce a clinically relevant metastasis, metastatic cells must complete all the steps outlined in Figure 1. The failure of most tumor cells to produce a metastasis can be due to different single or multiple deficiencies, such as inability to invade host stroma, inability to arrest in the capillary bed, and failure to grow in a distant organ's parenchyma. Searching for a uniform factor that prevents tumor cells from producing metastasis is therefore unproductive. Each discrete step of metastasis (e.g., invasion or extravasation) can be regulated by transient or permanent changes at the DNA or RNA level in different genes or by the activation/deactivation of many specific genes. The identification of tumor cells capable of producing metastasis therefore requires a multiparametric analysis.

Bucana and co-workers[302] developed a rapid technique for detecting the activity of genes involved in the formation of metastasis: vascularization, invasion, adhesion, and proliferation. This technique, colorimetric ISH, can detect specific mRNA transcripts in cultured cells, frozen tissues, and formalin-fixed, paraffin-embedded specimens.[174,300,302–304] The expression level of several genes that regulate different steps of the metastatic process correlated with the metastatic potential of human colon carcinoma cells. The mRNA expression level for EGF-R (growth), basic FGF (bFGF) and interleukin-8 (angiogenesis), type IV collagenase (invasion), E-cadherin (cohesion) and CEA (adhesion) and multidrug resistance (*mdr*)-1 (drug resistance) in the human colon carcinoma cell lines and clones with different metastatic potential was measured by Northern blot analysis and by ISH. Highly metastatic cells growing in culture uniformly expressed high levels of EGFR, bFGF, and CEA mRNA; whereas cultures of low metastatic cells displayed heterogeneous patterns.[303,304]

Kitadai and colleagues[300,304] examined the expression of metastasis-related genes in surgical specimens of human colon carcinomas. Dukes' stage C and D tumors exhibited a higher level of expression for EGFR, bFGF, type IV collagenase, and *mdr*-1 mRNA than Dukes' stage B tumors. The expression level of E-cadherin did not correlate with the stage of disease. The ISH technique revealed intertumoral heterogeneity for expression of several genes among Dukes' stage B neoplasms. Moreover, Kitadai and associates[304] found intratumoral heterogeneous staining for bFGF and type IV collagenase in some Dukes' stage B tumors, with the highest expression level at their invasive edge. In Dukes' stage C and D tumors, the expression of these genes was more uniform.[300,304]

In the final set of experiments, Kitadai and co-workers[300] examined the expression level of EGF-R, bFGF, type IV collagenase, E-cadherin, and *mdr*-1 in formalin-fixed, paraffin-embedded archival specimens of primary human colon carcinomas from patients with at least 5 years of follow-up. The ISH technique revealed inter-tumoral and intratumoral heterogeneity for expression of the metastasis-related genes. The expression of bFGF, collagenase type IV, EGF-R, and *mdr*-1 mRNA was higher in Dukes' stage D tumors than in Dukes' stage B tumors. Among the 22 Dukes' stage B neoplasms, five specimens exhibited a high expression level of EGF-R, bFGF, and collagenase type IV. Clinical outcome data (5-year follow-up) revealed that all five patients with Dukes' stage B tumors had distant metastasis (recurrent disease), whereas the other 17 patients with Dukes' stage B tumors expressing low levels of the metastasis-related genes were disease-free. Multivariate analysis identified high levels of expression of collagenase type IV and low levels of expression of E-cadherin as independent factors significantly associated with metastasis or recurrent disease. More specifically, metastatic or recurrent disease was associated with a high ratio of expression of collagenase type IV to E-cadherin. Collectively, these data show that multiparametric ISH analysis for metastasis-related genes may predict the metastatic potential, and hence, the clinical outcome, of individual lymph node–negative human colon cancers.[300]

Research published by different investigators affiliated with Fidler's laboratory also found an inverse correlation between expression of collagenase type IV and E-cadherin in formalin-fixed, paraffin-embedded specimens of human gastric carcinoma,[303] human prostate carcinoma,[305,306] human pancreatic carcinoma,[307] and human lung adeno-carcinoma[308] by using an mRNA ISH technique. The ISH technique revealed intertumoral heterogeneity for expression of E-cadherin and collagenase in early gastric cancer and advanced gastric cancer. In the majority of the tumors, the investigators reported an inverse relationship between the reactivities of E-cadherin and collagenase type IV. Specifically, E-cadherin was expressed at higher levels in the center of a neoplasm than in its periphery, whereas collagenase type IV was expressed at a higher level on the periphery (invasive edge) than in the center. Advanced cancers with high levels of expression for collagenase type IV on the periphery had a higher incidence of distant metastasis than those with low expression.

CONCLUSIONS

Before diagnosis, tumors in internal organs may grow to 1 cm^3 (1 g) and consist of approximately 10^9 cells. Assuming that a neoplasm has developed from the proliferation of a single transformed cell, it must have doubled about 30 times to attain this size. When a neoplasm weighs 2 kg (believed to be the maximum tumor burden compatible with life), it contains 10^{12} cells. Although impressive, the increase from 1 g to 1 kg takes only 10 doublings. Therefore at diagnosis, malignant cancers are relatively far advanced in their natural history. The period over which this growth occurs depends on the doubling time of the cancer, but on average, human neoplasms are thought to double every 2 months. Rapidly growing lesions such as testicular cancer may double every month, whereas slow-growing tumors such as prostate cancer may double every year.[5]

Primary human neoplasms are heterogeneous for a large number of properties that include invasion and metastasis. The process of metastasis is sequential and selective, with every step of the process containing stochastic elements, and the growth of metastases represents the end point of many lethal events that only few tumor cells can survive. In fact, the successful metastatic cell, that many years ago Fidler[1,291] called the *decathlon champion*, must be viewed as a cell able to manipulate its new environment (see Fig. 4-7). For many years, all of the efforts to treat cancer have concentrated on the inhibition or destruction of tumor cells. Strategies to both treat the tumor cell (e.g., chemotherapy and immunotherapy) and modulate the host microenvironment (e.g., tumor vasculature) could provide an additional approach for cancer treatment. The recent advancements in understanding of the biologic basis of cancer metastasis present unprecedented possibilities for translating basic research to the clinical reality of cancer treatment.

The outcome of cancer metastasis depends on multiple interactions (cross-talk) between selected metastatic cells and homeostatic mechanisms unique to some organ microenvironments. The organ microenvironment can influence the biology of cancer growth, angiogenesis, and metastasis in several different ways. Treatment of metastasis therefore should be targeted not only against metastatic tumor cells, but also the homeostatic factors that are favorable to metastasis, growth, and survival of the metastatic cells. The recent advances in understanding of the biologic basis of cancer metastasis present unprecedented possibilities for translating basic research into the clinical reality of cancer treatment.

REFERENCES

1. Fidler IJ: Critical factors in the biology of human cancer metastasis: Twenty-eighth GHA Clowes Memorial Award Lecture. Cancer Res 1990;50:6130.
2. Poste G, Fidler IJ: The pathogenesis of cancer metastasis. Nature 1979;283:139.
3. Fidler IJ, Poste G: The cellular heterogeneity of malignant neoplasms: Implications for adjuvant chemotherapy. Semin Oncol 1985;12:207.
4. Fidler IJ: Modulation of the organ microenvironment for the treatment of cancer metastasis (editorial). J Natl Cancer Inst 1995;84:1588.
5. Radinsky R, Aukerman SL, Fidler IJ: The heterogeneous nature of metastatic neoplasms: Relevance to biotherapy. In Oldham RK (ed): Principles of cancer biotherapy, 3rd ed. Boston, Kluwer Academic, 1998, p 16.
6. Willis RA: The spread of tumors in the human body. London, Butterworth, 1972.
7. Sugarbaker EV: Cancer metastasis: A product of tumor-host interactions. Curr Probl Cancer 1979;3:1.
8. Hart IR, Goode NT, Wilson RE: Molecular aspects of the metastatic cascade. Biochim Biophys Acta 1989;989:65.
9. Liotta LA, Stetler-Stevenson WG: Tumor invasion and metastasis: An imbalance of positive and negative regulation. Cancer Res 1991;51:5054s.
10. Weiss L: Principles of metastasis. Orlando, Fla, Academic Press, 1985.
11. Folkman J: How is blood vessel growth regulated in normal and neoplastic tissue? GHA Clowes Memorial Award Lecture. Cancer Res 1986;46:467.
12. Jain RK: Barriers to drug delivery in solid tumors. Sci Am 1994;271:58.
13. Auerbach W, Auerbach R: Angiogenesis inhibition: A review. Pharmac Ther 1994;63:265.
14. Fidler IJ, Ellis LM: The implications of angiogenesis for the biology and therapy of cancer metastasis. Cell 1994;79:185,
15. Folkman J, Klagsbrun M: Angiogenic factors. Science 1987;235:444.
16. Nagy JA, Brown LF, Senger DR, et al: Pathogenesis of tumor stroma generation: A critical role for leaky blood vessels and fibrin deposition. Biochim Biophys Acta 1989;948:305.
17. Folkman J, Cotran R: Relation of vascular proliferation to tumor growth. Int Rev Exp Pathol 1976;16:207.
18. Folkman J: Angiogenesis in cancer, vascular, rheumatoid and other disease. Nature Med 1995;27.
19. Dameron KM, Volpert OV, Tainsky MA, Bouk N: Control of angiogenesis in fibroblasts by p53 regulation of thrombospondin-1. Science 1994;265:1502.
20. Risau W: Mechanisms of angiogenesis. Nature 1997;386:671.
21. Carmeliet P, Ferreira V, Breier G, et al: Abnormal blood vessel development and lethality in embryos lacking a single VEGF allele. Nature 1996;380:435.
22. Ferrera N, Carver-Moore K, Chen H, et al: Heterozygous embryonic lethality induced by targeted inactivation of the VEGF gene. Nature 1996;380:439.
23. Senger DR, Galli SJ, Dvorak AM, et al: Tumor cells secrete a vascular permeability factor that promotes accumulation of ascites fluid. Science 1983;219:983.
24. Kumar R, Yoneda J, Bucana CD, Fidler IJ: Regulation of distinct steps of angiogenesis by different angiogenic molecules. Int J Oncol 1998;12:749.
25. Liotta LA, Steeg PS, Stetler-Stevenson WG: Cancer metastasis and angiogenesis: An imbalance of positive and negative regulation. Cell 1991;64:327.
26. Weidner N, Folkman J, Pozza F, et al: Tumor angiogenesis: A new significant and independent prognostic indicator in early stage breast carcinoma. J Natl Cancer Inst 1992;84:1875.
27. Gasparini G, Harris AL: Clinical importance of the determination of tumor angiogenesis in breast carcinoma: Much more than a new prognostic tool. J Clin Oncol 1995;13:765.
28. Hall N, Fish D, Hunt N, et al: Is the relationship between angiogenesis and metastasis in breast cancer real? Surg Oncol 1992;1:223.
29. Van Hoef ME, Knox WF, Dhesi SS, et al: Assessment of tumour vascularity as a prognostic factor in lymph node negative invasive breast cancer. Eur J Cancer 1993;29A:1141.
30. Weidner N, Carroll PR, Flax J, Flumenfeld W, Folkman J: Tumor angiogenesis correlates with metastasis in invasive prostate carcinoma. Am J Pathol 1993;143:401.
31. Fregene TA, Khanuja PS, Noto AC, et al: Tumor-associated angiogenesis in prostate cancer. Anticancer Res 1993;13:2377.
32. Graham CH, Rivers J, Kerbel RS, et al: Extent of vascularization as a prognostic indicator in thin (<0.76 mm) malignant melanomas. Am J Pathol 1994;145:510.
33. Hollingsworth HC, Kohn EC, Steinberg SM, et al: Tumor angiogenesis in advanced stage ovarian carcinoma. Am J Pathol 1995;147:33.
34. Maeda K, Chung Y-S, Takatsuka S, et al: Tumour angiogenesis and tumour cell proliferation as prognostic indicators in gastric carcinoma. Br J Cancer 1995;72:319.
35. Takahashi Y, Kitadai Y, Bucana CD, et al: Expression of vascular endothelial growth factor and its receptor, KDR, correlates with vascularity, metastasis, and proliferation of human colon cancer. Cancer Res 1995;55:3964.
36. Fidler IJ: Angiogenic heterogeneity: Regulation of neoplastic angiogenesis by the organ microenvironment (editorial). J Natl Cancer Inst 2001;93:1040.
37. Gabbert H: Mechanisms of tumor invasion: Evidence from in vivo observations. Cancer Metastasis Rev 1985;4:283.
38. Mareel MM, Van Roy FM, Bracke ME: How and when do tumor cells metastasize? Crit Rev Oncog 1993;4:559.
39. Portella G, Liddell J, Crombie R, et al: Molecular mechanisms of invasion and metastasis during mouse skin tumour progression. Invasion Metastasis 1994–1995;14:7.
40. Volk T, Geiger B, Raz A: Motility and adhesive properties of high and low-metastatic murine neoplastic cells. Cancer Res 1984;44:811.
41. Doyle GM, Sharief Y, Mohler JL: Prediction of metastatic potential by cancer cell motility in the Dunning R-3327 prostatic adenocarcinoma in vivo model. J Urol 1992;147:514.
42. Takeichi M: Cadherin cell adhesion receptors as a morphogenetic regulator. Science 1990;251:1451.
43. Shimoyama Y, Hirohashi S, Hirano S, et al: Cadherin cell adhesion molecules in human epithelial tissues and carcinomas. Cancer Res 1989;49:2128.
44. Dorudi S, Sheffield JP, Poulsom R, et al: E-cadherin expression in colorectal cancer: An immunocytochemical and in situ hybridization study. Am J Pathol 1993;142:981.
45. Umbas R, Schalken JA, Alders TW, et al: Expression of the cellular adhesion molecule E-cadherin is reduced or absent in high-grade prostate cancer. Cancer Res 1992;52:5100.
46. Mayer B, Johnson JP, Leitl F, et al: E-cadherin expression in primary and metastatic gastric cancer: Downregulation correlates with cellular dedifferentiation and glandular disintegration. Cancer Res 1993;53:1690.
47. Oka H, Shiozaki H, Kobayashi H, et al: Expression of E-cadherin cell adhesion molecule in human breast cancer tissues and its relationship to metastasis. Cancer Res 1993;53:1696.
48. Kadowaki T, Shiozaki H, Inoue M, et al: E-cadherin and α-catenin expression in human esophageal cancer. Cancer Res 1994;54:291.
49. Schipper JH, Frixen UH, Behrens J, et al: E-cadherin expression in squamous carcinomas of the head and neck: Inverse correlation with tumor differentiation and lymph node metastasis. Cancer Res 1991;51:6328.
50. Oda T, Kanai Y, Oyama T, et al: E-cadherin gene mutations in human gastric carcinoma cell lines. Proc Natl Acad Sci USA 1994;91:1858.
51. Shiozaki H, Iihara K, Oka H, et al: Immunohistochemical detection of α-catenin expression in human cancers. Am J Pathol 1994;144:667.
52. Vermeulen SJ, Bruyneel EA, Bracke ME, et al: Transition from the noninvasive to the invasive phenotype and loss of α-catenin in human colon cancer cells. Cancer Res 1995;55:4722.
53. Frixen UH, Behrens J, Sachs M, et al: E-cadherin-mediated cell-cell adhesion prevents invasiveness of human carcinoma cells. J Cell Biol 1991;113:173.
54. Vleminckx K, Vakaet L Jr, Mareel M, et al: Genetic manipulation of E-cadherin expression by epithelial tumor cells reveals an invasion suppressor role. Cell 1991;66:107.

55. Liotta LA, Stracke ML, Aznavoorian SA, et al: Tumor cell motility. Semin Cancer Biol 1991;2:111.
56. Silletti S, Paku S, Raz A: Tumor autocrine motility factor responses are mediated through cell contact and focal adhesion rearrangement in the absence of new tyrosine phosphorylation in metastatic cells. Am J Pathol 1996;148:1649.
57. Lotan R, Amos B, Watanabe H, Raz A: Suppression of motility factor receptor expression by retinoic acid. Cancer Res 1992;52:4878.
58. Watanabe H, Shinozaki T, Raz A, Chigira M: Expression of autocrine motility factor receptor in serum- and protein-independent fibrosarcoma cells: Implications for autonomy in tumor-cell motility and metastasis. Int J Cancer 1993;53:689.
59. Silletti S, Yao JP, Pienta KJ, Raz A: Loss of cell-contact regulation and altered responses to autocrine motility factor correlate with increased malignancy in prostate cancer cells. Int J Cancer 1995;63:100.
60. Kenworthy P, Dowrick P, Baillie-Johnson H, et al: The presence of scatter factor in patients with metastatic spread to the pleura. Br J Cancer 1992;66:243.
61. Giordano S, Zhen Z, Medico E, et al: Transfer of mitogenic and invasive response to scatter factor/hepatocyte growth factor by transfection of human *MET* protooncogene. Proc Natl Acad Sci USA 1993;90:649.
62. Yabkowitz R, Mansfield PJ, Dixit VM, Suchard SJ: Motility of human carcinoma cells in response to thrombospondin: Relationship to metastatic potential and thrombospondin structural domains. Cancer Res 1993;53:378.
63. Ruoslahti E: Control of cell motility and tumour invasion by extracellular matrix interactions—The Walter Herbert Lecture. Br J Cancer 1992;66:239.
64. Jiang WG, Puntis MCA, Hallett MB: Monocyte-conditioned media possess a novel factor which increases motility of cancer cells. Int J Cancer 1993;53:426.
65. Behrens J: Cell contacts, differentiation, and invasiveness of epithelial cells. Invasion Metastasis 1994–1995;14:61.
66. Liotta LA: Tumor invasion and metastasis—role of the extracellular matrix: Rhoads Memorial Award Lecture. Cancer Res 1986;46:1.
67. Nakajima M, Chop AM: Tumor invasion and extracellular matrix degradative enzymes: Regulation of activity by organ factors. Semin Cancer Biol 1991;2:115.
68. Crawford HC, Matrisian LM: Tumor and stromal expression of matrix metalloproteinases and their role in tumor progression. Invasion Metastasis 1994–1995;14:234.
69. Moscatelli D, Rifkin DB: Membrane and matrix localization of proteinases: A common theme in tumor cell invasion and angiogenesis. Biochim Biophys Acta 1988;948:67.
70. Nicolson GL: Metastatic tumor cell interactions with endothelium, basement membrane, and tissue. Curr Opin Cell Biol 1989;1:1009.
71. Sloane BF: Cathepsin B and cystatins: Evidence for a role in cancer progression. Semin Cancer Biol 1990;1:137.
72. Forster SJ, Talbot IC, Critchley DR: Laminin and fibronectin in rectal adenocarcinoma: Relationship to tumor grade, stage, and metastasis. Br J Cancer 1984;50:51.
73. Daneker GW Jr, Mercurio AM, Guerra L, et al: Laminin expression in colorectal carcinomas varying in degree of differentiation. Arch Surg 1987;122:1470.
74. Remy L, Lissitsky JC, Daemi N, et al: Laminin expression by two clones isolated from the colon carcinoma cell line LoVo that differs in metastatic potential and basement membrane organization. Int J Cancer 1992;51:204.
75. Mafune K, Ravikumar TS: Anti-sense RNA of 32-kDa laminin-binding protein inhibits attachment and invasion of a human colon carcinoma cell line. J Surg Res 1992;52:340.
76. Andres JL, Ronnstrand L, Cheifetz J, Massague J: Purification of the transforming growth factor-beta (TGF-β) binding proteoglycan betaglycan. J Biol Chem 1991;266:23282.
77. Chakrabarty S, Fan D, Varani J: Modulation of differentiation and proliferation in human colon carcinoma cells by transforming growth factor β1 and β2. Int J Cancer 1990;46:493.
78. Ruoslahti E: Integrins. J Clin Invest 1991;87:1.
79. Koretz K, Schlag P, Boumsell L, Moller P: Expression of VLA-alpha 2, VLA-alpha 6, and VLA-beta 1 chains in normal mucosa and adenomas of the colon, and in colon carcinomas and their liver metastases. Am J Pathol 1991;138:741.
80. Pignatelli M, Smith MEF, Bodmer WF: Low expression of collagen receptors in moderate and poorly differentiated colorectal adenocarcinomas. Br J Cancer 1990;61:636.
81. Hemler ME, Crouse C, Sonnenberg A: Association of the VLA alpha 6 subunit with a novel protein. A possible alternative to the common VLA beta 1 subunit on certain cell lines. J Biol Chem 1989;264:6529.
82. Leffler H, Masiarz FR, Barondes SH: Soluble lactose-binding vertebrate lectins: A growing family. Biochemistry 1989;28:9222.
83. Gabius HJ, Engelhardt R, Hellmann T: Characterization of membrane lectins in human colon carcinoma cells by flow cytofluorometry, drug targeting and affinity chromatography. Anticancer Res 1987;2:109.
84. Byrn R, Medrek P, Thomas P: Effect of heterogeneity of CEA on liver cell membrane binding and its kinetics of removal from circulation. Cancer Res 1985;45:3137.
85. Culty M, Miyake K, Kincade PW, et al: The hyaluronate receptor is a member of the CD44 (H0CAM) family of cell surface glycoproteins. J Cell Biol 1990;111:2765.
86. Jalkanen S, Jalkanen M: Lymphocyte CD44 binds the COOH-terminal heparin-binding domain of fibronectin. J Cell Biol 1992;116:817.
87. Faassen AE, Schrager JA, Klein DJ, et al: A cell surface chondroitin sulfate proteoglycan, immunologically related to CD44, is involved in type I collagen-mediated melanoma cell motility and invasion. J Cell Biol 1992;116:521.
88. Stamenkovic I, Aruffo A, Amiot M, Seed B: The hematopoietic and epithelial forms of DC44 are distinct polypeptides with different adhesion potentials for hyaluronate bearing cells. EMBO J 1991;10:343.
89. Matsumura Y, Tarin D: Significance of CD44 gene products for cancer diagnosis and disease evaluation. Lancet 1992;340:1053.
90. Nakajima M, Irimura T, Nicolson GL: Heparanases and tumor metastasis. J Cell Biochem 1988;36:157.
91. Morikawa K, Walker SM, Nakajima M, et al: Influence of organ environment on the growth, selection, and metastasis of human colon carcinoma cells in nude mice. Cancer Res 1988;48:6863.
92. Schwartz B, Bresalier RS, Kim YS: The role of mucin in colon-cancer metastasis. Int J Cancer 1992;52:60.
93. Boyd D, Ziober B, Chakrabarty S, Brattain MG: Examination of urokinase protein/transcript levels and their relationship with laminin degradation in cultured colon carcinoma. Cancer Res 1989;49:816.
94. Terranova P, Maslow D, Markus G: Directed migration of murine and human tumor cells to collagenase and other proteases. Cancer Res 1989;49:4835.
95. Fisher ER, Fisher B: Recent observations on concepts of metastasis. Arch Pathol 1967;83:321.
96. Fisher B, Fisher ER: The interrelationship of hematogenous and lymphatic tumor cell dissemination. Surg Gynecol Obstet 1966;122:791.
97. del Regato JA: Pathways of metastatic spread of malignant tumors. Semin Oncol 1977;4:33.
98. Fisher B, Fisher ER: The organ distribution of disseminated ^{51}Cr-labeled tumor cells. Cancer Res 1967;27:412.
99. Carr I: Lymphatic metastasis. Cancer Metastasis Rev 1983;22:307.
100. Paget S: The distribution of secondary growths in cancer of the breast. Lancet 1889;1:571.
101. Fidler IJ, Balch CM: The biology of cancer metastasis and implications for therapy. Curr Probl Surg 1987;24:137.
102. Fisher B, Fisher ER: Studies concerning the regional lymph node in cancer. Cancer 1971;27:1001.
103. Fisher B, Fisher ER: Barrier function of lymph node to tumor cells and erythrocytes. I. Normal nodes. Cancer 1967;20:1907.
104. Zeidman I, Buss JM: Experimental studies on the spread of cancer in the lymphatic system. I. Effectiveness of the lymph node as a barrier to the passage of embolic tumor cells. Cancer Res 1954;14:403.
105. Balch CM: The role of elective lymph node dissection in melanoma: Rationale, results, and controversies. J Clin Oncol 1988;6:163.
106. Hein DW, Moy RL: Elective lymph node dissection in stage I malignant melanoma: A meta-analysis. Melanoma Res 1992;2:273.

Science of Clinical Oncology

107. Enker E, Laffer UT, Block GE: Enhanced survival of patients with colon and rectal cancer is based upon wide anatomic resection. Ann Surg 1979;190:350.

108. Fisher B, Redmond C, Fisher E, et al: Ten-year results of a randomized clinical trial comparing radical mastectomy and total mastectomy with or without radiation. N Engl J Med 1985;312:11:674.

109. Cox CE, Pendas S, Cox JM, et al: Guidelines for sentinel node biopsy and lymphatic mapping of patients with breast cancer. Ann Surg 1998;227:645.

110. Morton DL, Wen D-R, Wong JH, et al: Technical details of intraoperative lymphatic mapping for early stage melanoma. Arch Surg 1992;127:392.

111. Glass EC, Essner R, Morton DL: Kinetics of three lymphoscintigraphic agents in patients with cutaneous melanoma. J Nucl Med 1998;39:1185.

112. Joseph E, Brobeil A, Glass F, et al: Results of complete lymph node dissection in 83 melanoma patients with positive sentinel nodes. Ann Surg Oncol 1998;5:119.

113. Fidler IJ: Metastasis: Quantitative analysis of distribution and fate of tumor emboli labeled with ^{125}I-5-iodo-2′-deoxyuridine. J Natl Cancer Inst 1970;45:773.

114. Weiss L: Metastatic inefficiency: Causes and consequences. Cancer Rev 1986;3:1.

115. Fidler IJ: The relationship of embolic homogeneity, number, size and viability to the incidence of experimental metastasis. Eur J Cancer 1973;9:223.

116. Updyke TV, Nicolson GL: Malignant melanoma lines selective *in vitro* for increased homotypic adhesion properties have increased experimental metastatic potential. Clin Exp Metastasis 1986;:231.

117. Gasic GJ: Role of plasma, platelets and endothelial cells in tumor metastasis. Cancer Metastasis Rev 1984;3:99.

118. Fidler IJ, Bucana C: Mechanism of tumor cell resistance to lysis by syngeneic lymphocytes. Cancer Res 1977;37:3945.

119. Nicolson G: Cancer metastasis: Tumor cell and host organ properties important in metastasis to specify secondary sites. Biochim Biophys Acta 1988;948:175.

120. Arap W, Pasqualini R, Ruoslahti E: Cancer treatment by targeted drug delivery to tumor vasculature in a mouse model. Science 1998;279:377.

121. Pasqualini R, Koivunen E, Kain R, et al: Aminopeptidase N is a receptor for tumor-homing peptides and a target for inhibiting angiogenesis. Cancer Res 2000;60:722.

122. Weiss L, Orr FW, Honn KV: Interactions of cancer cells with the microvasculature during metastasis. FASEB J 1988;2:12.

123. Weiss L: Cell adhesion molecules: A critical examination of their role in metastasis. Invasion Metastasis 1994–1995;14:192.

124. El-Sabban ME, Pauli BU: Adhesion-mediated gap junctional communication between lung-metastatic cancer cells and endothelium. Invasion Metastasis 1994–1995;14:164.

125. Karpatkin S, Pearlstein E, Ambrogio C, Coller BS: Role of adhesive proteins in platelet tumor interaction in vitro and metastasis formation in vivo. J Clin Invest 1988;81:1012.

126. Karpatkin S, Pearlstein E: Role of platelets in tumor cell metastasis. Ann Intern Med 1981;95:636.

127. Dvorak HF, Seneger DR, Dvorak AM: Fibrin as a component of the tumor stroma: Origins and biological significance. Cancer Metastasis Rev 1983;2:41.

128. Cliffton EE, Grossi CE: The rationale of anticoagulants in the treatment of cancer. J Med 1974;5:107.

129. Fidler IJ: Macrophages and metastasis: a biological approach to cancer therapy: Presidential address. Cancer Res 1985;45:4714.

130. Hofmann M, Rudy W, Zoller M, et al: CD44 splice variants confer metastatic behavior in rats: Homologous sequences are expressed in human tumor cell lines. Cancer Res 1992;51:5292.

131. McCarthy JB, Skubitz APN, Lidy J, et al: Tumor cell adhesive mechanisms and their relationship to metastasis. Semin Cancer Biol 1991;2:155.

132. Mareel M, Vleminckx K, Vermeulen S, et al: Homotypic cell-cell adhesion molecules and tumor invasion. In Graumann W, Drukker J (eds): Progress in histo- and cytochemistry: Histochemistry of receptors, Vol 26. Stuttgart, Fischer Verlag, 1992, p 95.

133. Yamamura K, Kibbey MC, Kleinman HK: Melanoma cells selected for adhesion to laminin peptides have different malignant properties. Cancer Res 1993;53:423.

134. Birch M, Mitchell S, Hart IR: Isolation and characterization of human melanoma cell variants expressing high and low levels of CD44. Cancer Res 1991;51:6660.

135. Friedrichs K, Franke F, Lisboa B-W: CD44 isoforms correlate with cellular differentiation but not with prognosis in human breast cancer. Cancer Res 1995;55:5424.

136. Ponta H, Sleeman J, Dall P, et al: CD44 isoforms in metastatic cancer. Invasion Metastasis 1994–1995;14:82.

137. Nesbit M, Herlyn M: Adhesion receptors in human melanoma progression. Invasion Metastasis 1994–1995;14:131.

138. Ruoslahti E: Fibronectin and its α5β1 integrin receptor in malignancy. Invasion Metastasis 1994–1995;14:87.

139. Xu X-C, El-Naggar AK, Lotan R: Differential expression of galectin-1 and galectin-3 in thyroid tumors. Am J Pathol 1995;147:815.

140. Kim WH, Jun SH, Kibbey MC, et al: Expression of β1 integrin in laminin-adhesion-selected human colon cancer cell lines of varying tumorigenicity. Invasion Metastasis 1994–1995;14:147.

141. Terranova VP, Williams JE, Liotta LA, Martin GR: Modulation of the metastatic activity of melanoma cells by laminin and fibronectin. Science 1984;226:982..

142. Zeidman I: Metastasis: A review of recent advances. Cancer Res 1957;17:157.

143. Coman DR: Mechanisms responsible for the origin and distribution of blood-borne tumor metastasis: A review. Cancer Res 1953;13:397.

144. Hujanen ES, Terranova VP: Migration of tumor cells to organ-derived chemoattractants. Cancer Res 1985;45:3517.

145. Fidler IJ: "Seed and soil" revisited: Contribution of the organ microenvironment to cancer metastasis. In Brodt P (ed): Surgical oncology clinics of North America: Cancer metastasis: Biological and clinical aspects. Philadelphia, WB Saunders, 2001, p 257.

146. Cavanaugh PG, Nicolson GL: Purification and some properties of a lung-derived growth factor that differentially stimulates the growth of tumor cells metastatic to the lung. Cancer Res 1989;49:3928.

147. Chung LWK: Fibroblasts are critical determinants in prostatic cancer growth and dissemination. Cancer Metastasis Rev 1991;10:263.

148. Roberts AB, Thompson NL, Heine U, Flanders C, Sporn MB: Transforming growth factor β: Possible roles in carcinogenesis. Br J Cancer 1988;57:594–600.

149. Ervin PR, Kaminski MS, Cody RL, Wicha MS: Production of mammastatin, a tissue-specific growth inhibitor, by normal human mammary cells. Science 1989;244:1585.

150. Plowman GD, Green JM, McDonald VL, Neubauer MG, Disteche CM, Todaro GJ, et al: The amphiregulin gene encodes a novel epidermal growth factor-related protein with tumor-inhibitory activity. Mol Cell Biol 1981;10:1969.

151. Radinsky R: Growth factors and their receptors in metastasis. Semin Cancer Biol 1991;2:169.

152. Zarrilli R, Bruni CB, Riccio A: Multiple levels of control of insulin-like growth factor gene expression. Mol Cell Endocrinol 1994;101:R1.

153. Stiles CD, Capone GT, Scher CD, Antoniades HN, Van Wyk JJ, Pledger WJ: Dual control of cell growth by somatomedins and platelet-derived growth factor. Proc Natl Acad Sci USA 1979;76:1279.

154. Long L, Nip J, Brodt P: Paracrine growth stimulation by hepatocyte-derived insulin-like growth factor-1: A regulatory mechanism for carcinoma cells metastatic to the liver. Cancer Res 1994;54:3732.

155. Roberts AB, Sporn MB, Assoian RK, Smith JM, Roche NS, Wakefield LM, et al: Transforming growth factor type B: Rapid induction of fibrosis and angiogenesis in vivo and stimulation of collagen formation in vitro. Proc Natl Acad Sci USA 1986;83:4167.

156. Fan D, Chakrabarty S, Seid C, Bell CW, Schackert H, Morikawa K, et al: Clonal stimulation or inhibition of human colon carcinomas and human renal carcinoma mediated by transforming growth factor-β1. Cancer Commun 1989;1:117.

157. Gutman M, Singh RK, Price JE, Fan D, Fidler IJ: Accelerated growth

of human colon cancer cells in nude mice undergoing liver regeneration. Invasion Metastasis 1995;14:362.

158. Mead JE, Fausto N: Transforming growth factor α may be a physiological regulator of liver regeneration by means of an autocrine mechanism. Proc Natl Acad Sci USA 1989;86:1558.

159. Markowitz SD, Molkentin K, Gerbic C, et al: Growth stimulation by coexpression of transforming growth factor-α and epidermal growth factor receptor in normal an adenomatous human colon epithelium. J Clin Invest 1990;86:356.

160. van der Geer P, Hunter T, Lindberg RA: Receptor protein-tyrosine kinases and their signal transduction pathways. Annu Rev Cell Biol 1994;10:251.

161. Schlessinger J: Allosteric regulation of the epidermal growth factor receptor kinase. J Cell Biol 1986;103:2067.

162. van Dale P, Galand P: Effect of partial hepatectomy on experimental liver invasion by intraportally injected colon carcinoma cells in rats. Invasion Metastasis 1988;8:217.

163. Michalopoulos GK: Liver regeneration: Molecular mechanisms of growth control. FASEB J 1990;4:176.

164. Gherardi E, Stoker M: Hepatocyte growth factor-scatter factor: Mitogen, motogen, and *met*. Cancer Cells 1991;3:227.

165. Ullrich A, Schlessinger J: Signal transduction by receptors with tyrosine kinase activity. Cell 1990;61:203.

166. Furlong RA: The biology of hepatocyte growth factor/scatter factor. Bioessays 1992;14:613.

167. Sainsbury JR, Farndon JR, Harris AL, Sherbert GV: Epidermal growth factor receptors on human breast cancers. Br J Surg 1985;72:186–188.

168. Libermann TA, Nusbaum HR, Razon N, et al: Amplification, enhanced expression and possible rearrangement of EGF receptor gene in primary brain tumours of glial origin. Nature (Lond) 1985;313:144.

169. Harris AL, Neal DE: Epidermal growth factor and its receptor in human cancer. In Sluyser M (ed): Growth factors and oncogenes in breast cancer. Chichester, United Kingdom, Ellis Horwoo, Ltd, 1987, p. 60.

170. Berger MS, Greenfield C, Gullick WJ, et al: Evaluation of epidermal growth factor receptors in bladder tumours. Br J Cancer 1987;56:533.

171. Ullrich AL, Coussens L, Hayflick JS, et al: Human epidermal growth factor receptor cDNA sequence and aberrant expression of the amplified gene in A431 epidermoid carcinoma cells. Nature (Lond) 1984;309:418.

172. Gross ME, Zorbas MA, Daniels YJ, et al: Cellular growth response to epidermal growth factor in colon carcinoma cells with an amplified epidermal growth factor receptor derived from a familial adenomatous polyposis patient. Cancer Res 1991;51:1452.

173. Radinsky R, Risin S, Fan D, et al: Level and function of epidermal growth factor receptor predict the metastatic potential of human colon carcinoma cells. Clin Cancer Res 1995;1:19.

174. Radinsky R, Bucana CD, Ellis LE, et al: A rapid colorimetric in situ messenger RNA hybridization technique for analysis of epidermal growth factor receptor in paraffin-embedded surgical specimens of human colon carcinomas. Cancer Res 1993;53:937.

175. Bottaro DP, Rubin JS, Faletto DL, et al: Identification of the hepatocyte growth factor receptor as the *c-met* proto-oncogene product. Science 1991;215:802.

176. Sugarbaker EV, Cohen AM, Ketcham AS: Do metastases metastasize? Am Surg 1971;174:161.

177. Hoover HC, Ketcham AS: Metastasis of metastases. Am J Surg 1975;130:405.

178. Fidler IJ, Nicolson G: Organ selectivity for implantation survival and growth of B16 melanoma variant tumor lines. J Natl Cancer Inst 1976;57:1199.

179. Hart IR, Fidler IJ: Role of organ selectivity in the determination of metastatic patterns of B16 melanoma. Cancer Res 1981;41:1281.

180. Kinsey DL: An experimental study of preferential metastasis. Cancer 1960;13:874.

181. Foulds L: The experimental study of tumor progression. A review. Cancer Res 1954;14:327.

182. Klein G, Klein E: Immune surveillance against virus-induced tumors and nonrejectability of spontaneous tumors: Contrasting consequences of host-versus-tumor evolution. Proc Natl Acad Sci USA 1977;74:2121.

183. Nowell PC: The clonal evolution of tumor cell populations: Acquired genetic liability permits stepwise selection of variant sublines and underlies tumor progression. Science 1976;194:23.

184. Nowell PC: Chromosomal and molecular clues to tumor progression. Semin Oncol 1989;16:116.

185. Nowell PC: Mechanisms of tumor progression. Cancer Res 1986;46:2203.

186. Prehn RT: Tumor progression and homeostasis. Adv Cancer Res 1976;23:203.

187. Hart IR, Easty D: Tumor cell progression and differentiation in metastasis. Semin Cancer Biol 1991;2:87.

188. Failkow PJ: Clonal origin of human tumors. Annu Rev Med 1979;30:135.

189. Fearon ER, Hamilton SR, Vogelstein B: Clonal analysis of human colorectal tumors. Science 1987;238:193.

190. Muleris M, Salmon RJ, Dutrillaux B: Chromosomal study demonstrating the clonal evolution and metastatic origin of a metachronous colorectal carcinoma. Int J Cancer 1986;38:167.

191. Vogelstein B, Fearon ER, Hamilton SR, et al: Genetic alterations during colorectal tumorigenesis. Proc Am Assoc Cancer Res 1989;30:634.

192. Waghorne C, Thomas M, Lagarde A, et al: Genetic evidence for progressive selection and overgrowth of primary tumors by metastatic cell subpopulations. Cancer Res 1988;48:6109.

193. Noguchi S, Motomura K, Inaji H, et al: Clonal analysis of human breast cancer by means of the polymerase chain reaction. Cancer Res 1992;52:6594.

194. Jacobs IJ, Kohler MF, Wiseman RW, et al: Clonal origin of epithelial ovarian carcinoma: Analysis by loss of heterozygosity, p53 mutation, and x-chromosome inactivation. J Natl Cancer Inst 1992;84:1793.

195. Nakamine H, Masih AS, Okano M, et al: Characterization of clonality of Epstein-Barr virus-induced human B lymphoproliferative disease in mice and severe combined immunodeficiency. Am J Pathol 1993;142:139.

196. Sidransky D, Frost P, von Eschenbach A, et al: Clonal origin of bladder cancer. N Engl J Med 1992;326:737.

197. Vogelstein B, Fearon ER, Kern SE, et al: Allelotype of colorectal carcinomas. Science (Washington DC) 1989;244:207.

198. Staroselsky AN, Radinsky R, Fidler IJ, et al: The use of molecular genetic markers to demonstrate the effect of organ environment on clonal dominance in a human renal cell carcinoma grown in nude mice. Int J Cancer 1992;51:130.

199. Fidler IJ: Selection of successive tumor lines for metastasis. Nature 1973;242:148.

200. Raz A, Hanna N, Fidler IJ: In vivo isolation of a metastatic tumor cell variant involving selective and nonadaptive processes. J Natl Cancer Inst 1981;66:183.

201. Talmadge JE, Fidler IJ: Cancer metastasis is selective or random depending on the parent tumor population. Nature 1978;27:593.

202. Poste G: Experimental systems for analysis of the malignant phenotype. Cancer Metastasis Rev 1982;1:141.

203. Hart IR: The selection and characterization of an invasive variant of the B16 melanoma. Am J Pathol 1979;97:587.

204. Reading CL, Hutchins JT: Carbohydrate structure in tumor immunity. Cancer Metastasis Rev 1985;4:221.

205. Poste G, Doll J, Hart IR, Fidler IJ: In vitro selection of murine B16 melanoma variants with enhanced tissue invasive properties. Cancer Res 40:1636.

206. Sloane BF, Honn KV: Cysteine proteinase and metastasis. Cancer Metastasis Rev 1984;3:249.

207. Kerbel RS, Dennis JW, Lagarde AE, Frost P: Tumor progression in metastasis: An experimental approach using lectin-resistant tumor variants. Cancer Metastasis Rev 1982;1:99.

208. Hanna N: Role of natural killer cell in control of cancer metastasis. Cancer Metastasis Rev 1982;1:45.

209. Fidler IJ, Kripke ML: Metastasis results from pre-existing variant cells within a malignant tumor. Science 1977;197:893.

210. Luria SE, Delbruck M: Mutations of bacteria from virus sensitive to virus resistance. Genetics 1943;28:491.

211. Fidler IJ, Gruys E, Cifone MA, et al: Demonstration of multiple phenotype diversity in a murine melanoma of recent origin. J Natl Cancer Inst 1981;67:947.

212. Kripke ML: Speculation on the role of ultraviolet radiation in the development of malignant melanoma. J Natl Cancer Inst 1979;63:541.

213. Kripke ML: Immunoregulation and carcinogenesis: Past, present, and future. J Natl Cancer Inst 1988;80:722.

214. Fidler IJ, Kripke ML: Tumor cell antigenicity, host immunity, and cancer metastasis. Cancer Immunol Immunother 1980;7:201.

215. Aukerman SL, Price JE, Fidler IJ: Different deficiencies in the prevention of tumorigenic-low-metastatic murine K-1735 melanoma cells from producing metastases. J Natl Cancer Inst 1986;77:915.

216. Fidler IJ: Rationale and methods for the use of nude mice to study the biology and therapy of human cancer metastasis. Cancer Metastasis Rev 1986;5:29.

217. Giavazzi R, Jessup JM, Campbell DE, et al: Experimental nude mouse model of human colorectal cancer liver metastasis. J Natl Cancer Inst 1986;77:1303.

218. Kozlowski JM, Fidler IJ, Campbell D, et al: Metastatic behavior of human tumor cell lines grown in the nude mouse. Cancer Res 1984;44:3522.

219. Naito S, von Eschenbach AC, Giavazzi R, Fidler IJ: Growth and metastasis of tumor cells isolated from a human renal cell carcinoma implanted into different organs of nude mice. Cancer Res 1986;46:4109.

220. Morikawa K, Walker SM, Jessup JM, Fidler IJ: In vivo selection of highly metastatic cells from surgical specimens of different human colon carcinomas implanted into nude mice. Cancer Res 1988;48:1943.

221. Fidler IJ, Naito S, Pathak S: Orthotopic implantation is essential for the selection, growth and metastasis of human renal cell cancer in nude mice. Cancer Metastasis Rev 1990;9:149.

222. Fidler IJ: Orthotopic implantation of human colon carcinomas into nude mice provides a valuable model for the biology and therapy of cancer metastasis. Cancer Metastasis Rev 1991;10:229.

223. Pettaway CA, Pathak S, Greene G, et al: Selection of highly metastatic variants of different human prostatic carcinomas utilizing orthotopic implantation in nude mice. Clin Cancer Res 1996;2:1627.

224. Dinney CPN, Fishbeck R, Singh RK, et al: Isolation and characterization of metastatic variants from human transitional cell carcinoma passaged by orthotopic implantation in athymic nude mice. J Urol 1995;154:1532.

225. Gohji K, Nakajima M, Dinney CPN, et al: The importance of orthotopic implantation to the isolation and biological characterization of a metastatic human clear cell renal carcinoma in nude mice. Int J Oncol 1993;2:23.

226. Stephenson RA, Dinney CPN, Gohji K, et al: Metastatic model for human prostate cancer using orthotopic implantation in nude mice. J Natl Cancer Inst 1992;84:951.

227. Fidler IJ, Hart IR: Biological and experimental consequences of the zonal composition of solid tumors. Cancer Res 1981;41:3266.

228. Talmadge JE, Wolman SR, Fidler IJ: Evidence for the clonal origin of spontaneous metastasis. Science 1982;217:361.

229. Poste G, Tzeng J, Doll J, Greig R: Evolution of tumor cell heterogeneity during progressive growth of individual lung metastases. Proc Natl Acad Sci USA 1982;79:6574.

230. Hu F, Wang RY, Hsu TC: Clonal origin of metastasis in B16 murine melanoma: A cytogenetic study. J Natl Cancer Inst 1987;78:155.

231. Talmadge JE, Zbar B: Clonality of pulmonary metastases from the bladder 6 subline of the B16 melanoma studied by southern hybridization. J Natl Cancer Inst 1987;78:315.

232. Ootsuyama A, Tanaka K, Tanooka H: Evidence by cellular mosaicism for monoclonal metastasis of spontaneous mouse mammary tumors. J Natl Cancer Inst 1987;78:1223.

233. Kerbel RS, Waghorne C, Man MS, et al: Alteration of the tumorigenic and metastatic properties of neoplastic cells is associated with the process of calcium phosphate-mediated DNA transfection. Proc Natl Acad Sci USA 1987;84:1263.

234. Talmadge JE, Benedict K, Madsen J, Fidler IJ: The development of biological diversity and susceptibility to chemotherapy in cancer metastases. Cancer Res 1984;44:3801.

235. Fidler IJ, Talmadge JE: Evidence that intravenously derived murine pulmonary melanoma metastases can originate from the expansion of a single tumor cell. Cancer Res 1986;46:5167.

236. Sandberg AA, Turc-Carel C, Gemmill RM: Chromosomes in solid tumors and beyond. Cancer Res 1988;48:1049.

237. Balaban GB, Herlyn M, Clark WH, Nowell PC: Karyotypic evolution in human malignant melanoma. Cancer Genet Cytogent 1986;19:113.

238. Shapiro JR, Shapiro WR: The subpopulations and isolated cell types of freshly resected high grade human gliomas: Their influence on the tumor's evolution in vivo and behavior and therapy in vitro. Cancer Metastasis Rev 1985;4:107.

239. Wolman SR, McMorrow LE, Fidler IJ, Talmadge JE: Development and progression of karyotypic variability in melanoma K1735 following X-irradiation. Cancer Res 1985;45:1839.

240. Bos JL, Fearon ER, Hamilton SR, et al: Prevalence of *ras* gene mutations in human colorectal cancers. Nature 1987;327:293.

241. Vogelstein B, Fearon ER, Hamilton SR, et al: Genetic alterations during colorectal tumorigenesis. Proc Am Assoc Cancer Res 1989;30:634.

242. Fearon ER, Vogelstein B: A genetic model for colorectal tumorigenesis. Cell 1990;61:759.

243. Cifone MA, Fidler IJ: Increasing metastatic potential is associated with increasing genetic instability of clones isolated from murine neoplasms. Proc Natl Acad Sci USA 1982;78:6949.

244. Cillo C, Dick JE, Ling V, Hill RP: Generation of drug-resistant variants in metastatic B16 mouse melanoma cell lines. Cancer Res 1987;47:2604.

245. Hill RP, Chambers AF, Ling V, Harris JF: Dynamic heterogeneity: Rapid generation of metastatic variants in mouse B16 melanoma cells. Science 1984;224:998.

246. Bailly M, Bertrand S, Dore J-F: Increased spontaneous mutation rates and prevalence of karyotype abnormalities in highly metastatic human melanoma cell lines. Melanoma Res 1993;3:51.

247. Poste G, Greig R: On the genesis and regulation of cellular heterogeneity in malignant tumors. Invasion Metastasis 1982;2:137.

248. Heppner GH, Miller BE: Therapeutic implications of tumor heterogeneity. Semin Oncol 1989;16:91.

249. Miller BE, Miller FR, Wilburn DJ, Heppner GH: Analysis of tumour cell composition in tumours composed of paired mixtures of mammary tumour cell lines. Br J Cancer 1987;56:561.

250. Miller BE, Miller FR, Wilburn DJ, Heppner GH: Dominance of a tumor subpopulation line in mixed heterogeneous mouse mammary tumors. Cancer Res 1988;48:5747.

251. Hamada J, Takeichi N, Kobayashi H: Metastatic capacity and intercellular communication between normal cells and metastatic cell clones derived from a rat mammary carcinoma. Cancer Res 1988;48:5129.

252. Heppner GH: Cell-to-cell interaction in regulating diversity of neoplasms. Semin Cancer Biol 1991;2:97.

253. Itaya T, Judde JG, Hunt B, Frost P: Genotypic and phenotypic evidence of clonal interactions in murine tumor cells. J Natl Cancer Inst 1989;81:664.

254. Kerbel RS, Waghorne C, Korczak B, Breitman ML: Clonal changes in tumours during growth and progression evaluated by Southern gel analysis of random integrations of foreign DNA. Ciba Foundation Symposium 1988;141:123.

255. Newcomb EW, Silverstein SC, Silagi S: Malignant mouse melanoma cells do not form tumors when mixed with cells of a non-malignant subclone: Relationships between plasminogen activator expression by the tumor cells and the host's immune response. J Cell Physiol 1978;95:169.

256. Chambers AF, Harris JF, Ling V, Hill RP: Rapid phenotype variation in cells derived from lung metastases of KHT fibrosarcoma. Invasion Metastasis 1984;4:225.

257. Raz A: Regional emergence of metastatic heterogeneity in a growing tumor. Cancer Lett 1982;17:153.

258. Prehn RT: Immunostimulation of the lympho-dependent phase of neoplastic growth. J Natl Cancer Inst 1977;59:1043.

259. Fidler IJ, Gersten DM, Kripke ML: Influence of immune status on the metastasis of three murine fibrosarcomas of different immunogenicities. Cancer Res 1979;39:3816.

260. Gambacorti-Passerini C, Rivoltini L, Radvissani M, et al: Susceptibility of human and murine drug-resistant tumor cells to the lytic activity of rIL2-activated lymphocytes (LAK). Cancer Metastasis Rev 1988;7:335.

261. Gronberg A, Ferm M, Tsai L, Kjessling R: Interferon is able to reduce tumor cell susceptibility to human lymphokine-activated killer (LAK) cells. Cell Immunol 1989;118:10.

262. Loeffler D, Heppner G: Influence of tumor microenvironmental factors on NK and LAK cells. Proc Am Assoc Cancer Res 1989;30:365.

263. McCready DR, Balch CM, Fidler IJ, Murray JL: Lack of comparability between binding of monoclonal antibodies to melanoma cells in vitro and localization in vivo. J Natl Cancer Inst 1989;81:682.

264. Topalian SL, Rosenberg SA: Mechanism of melanoma resistance to lysis by tumor infiltrating lymphocytes (TIL). Proc Am Assoc Cancer Res 1989;30:377.

265. Wikstrand CJ, Grahmann FC, McComb RD, Bigner DD: Antigenic heterogeneity of human anaplastic gliomas and glioma-derived cell lines by monoclonal antibodies. J Neuropathol Exp Neurol 1981;44:229.

266. Albino AP, Lloyd KO, Houghton AN, et al: Heterogeneity in surface antigen and glycoprotein expression of cell lines derived from different melanoma metastases of the same patient. J Exp Med 1981;154:1764.

267. Bystryn JC, Bernstein P, Lui P, Valentine F: Immunophenotype of human melanoma cells in different metastases. Cancer Res 1985;45:5603.

268. Fogel M, Gorelik E, Segal S, Feldman M: Differences in cell surface antigens of tumor metastases and those of the local tumor. J Natl Cancer Inst 1979;62:585.

269. Kiger N: Heterogeneity in surface antigen of cell lines and clones from a murine carcinoma. Int J Cancer 1985;35:129.

270. Roth JA, Restrepo C, Scuderi P, et al: Analysis of antigenic expression by primary and autologous metastatic human sarcomas using murine monoclonal antibodies. Cancer Res 1984;44:5320.

271. Pimm MV, Baldwin RW: Antigenic differences between methylcholanthrene-induced rat sarcoma and post-surgical recurrences. Int J Cancer 1977;20:37.

272. Prehn RT: The immune reaction as a stimulator of tumor growth. Science 1972;176:170.

273. Kripke ML: Effects of UV radiation on tumor immunity. J Natl Cancer Inst 1990;82:1392.

274. Donawho CK, Kripke ML: Immunologic factors in melanoma. Clin Dermatol 1992;10:69.

275. Kripke ML, Fidler IJ: Enhanced experimental metastasis of ultraviolet light-induced fibrosarcomas in ultraviolet light-irradiated syngeneic mice. Cancer Res 1980;40:625.

276. Fidler IJ: Metastasis: Quantitative analysis of distribution and fate of tumor emboli labeled with 125I-5-iodo-2'-deoxyuridine. J Natl Cancer Inst 1970;45:773.

277. Fidler IJ: Modulation of the organ microenvironment for the treatment of cancer metastasis (editorial). J Natl Cancer Inst 1995;84:1588.

278. Price JE, Natio S, Fidler IJ: Growth in an organ microenvironment as a selective process in metastasis. Clin Expl Metastasis 1988;6:91.

279. Price JE, Aukerman SL, Fidler IJ: Evidence that the process of murine melanoma metastasis is sequential and selective and contains stochastic elements. Cancer Res 1986;46:5172.

280. Hart IR, Talmadge JE, Fidler IJ: Metastatic behavior of a murine reticulum cell sarcoma exhibiting organ-specific growth. Cancer Res 1981;41:1281.

281. Ewing J: Neoplastic diseases, 6th ed, Philadelphia, WB Saunders, 1928.

282. Sugarbaker EV: Cancer metastasis: A product of tumor-host interactions. Curr Probl Cancer 1979;3:1.

283. Tarin D, Price JE, Kettlewell MGW, et al: Mechanisms of human tumor metastasis studied in patients with peritoneovenous shunts. Cancer Res 1984;44:3584.

284. Tarin D, Price JE, Kettlewell MGW, et al: Clinicopathological observations on metastasis in man studied in patients treated with peritoneovenous shunts. Br Med J 1984;288:749.

285. Schackert G, Fidler IJ: Development of in vivo models for studies of brain metastasis. Int J Cancer 1988;41:589.

286. Schackert G, Fidler IJ: Site-specific metastasis of mouse melanomas and a fibrosarcoma in the brain or the meninges of syngeneic animals. Cancer Res 1988;48:3478.

287. Fujimaki T, Price JE, Fan D, et al: Selective growth of human melanoma cells in the brain parenchyma of nude mice. Melanoma Res 1996;6:363.

288. Zhang R, Price JE, Fujimaki T, Bucana CD, Fidler IJ: Differential permeability of the blood-brain barrier in experimental brain metastases produced by human neoplasms implanted into nude mice. Am J Pathol 1992;141:1115.

289. Schackert G, Price JE, Bucana CD, Fidler IJ: Unique patterns of brain metastasis produced by different human carcinomas in athymic nude mice. Int J Cancer 1989;44:892.

290. Schackert G, Price JE, Zhang RD, et al: Regional growth of different human melanoma as metastases in the brain of nude mice. Am J Pathol 1990;136:95.

291. Fidler IJ: Tumor heterogeneity and the biology of cancer invasion and metastasis. Cancer Res 1978;38:2651.

292. Smith KA, Begg AC, Denekamp J: Differences in chemosensitivity between subcutaneous and pulmonary tumors. Eur J Cancer Clin Oncol 1985;21:249.

293. Price JE, Naito S, Fidler IJ: Growth in an organ microenvironment as a selective process in metastasis. Clin Exp Metastasis 1988;6:91.

294. Staroselsky A, Fan D, O'Brian CA, et al: Site-dependent differences in response of the UV-2237 murine fibrosarcoma to systemic therapy with Adriamycin. Cancer Res 1990;40:7775.

295. Wilmanns C, Fan D, O'Brian CA, et al: Modulation of doxorubicin sensitivity and level of P-glycoprotein expression in human colon carcinoma cells by ectopic and orthotopic environments in nude mice. Int J Oncol 1993;3:412.

296. Yoon SS, Zhang RD, Bucana CD, et al: Epigenetic regulation of multidrug resistance and metastasis-related genes in human lung adenocarcinoma cells growing in ectopic and orthotopic organs of nude mice. Int J Oncol 1995;7:1261.

297. Tsuruo T: Mechanisms of multidrug resistance and implications for therapy. Gann 1988;79:285.

298. Weinstein RS, Kuszak IR, Kluskens LF, et al: P-glycoprotein in pathology: The multidrug resistance gene family in humans. Hum Pathol 1990;21:34.

299. Dong Z, Radinsky R, Fan D, et al: Organ-specific modulation of steady-state mdr gene expression and drug resistance in murine colon cancer cells. J Natl Cancer Inst 1994;86:913.

300. Kitadai Y, Ellis LM, Takahashi Y, et al: Multiparametric in situ mRNA hybridization analysis to detect metastasis-related genes in surgical specimens of human colon carcinoma. Clin Cancer Res 1995;1:1095.

301. Mizoguchi T, Yamada K, Furukawa T, et al: Expression of the mdr1 gene in human gastric and colorectal carcinomas. J Natl Cancer Inst 1990;82:1679.

302. Bucana CD, Radinsky R, Dong Z, et al: A rapid colorimetric in situ mRNA hybridization technique using hyperbiotinylated oligonucleotide probes for analysis of mdr-1 in mouse colon carcinoma cells. J Histochem Cytochem 1993;41:499.

303. Anzai H, Kitadai Y, Bucana CD, et al: Intratumoral heterogeneity and inverse correlation between expression of E-cadherin and collagenase type IV in human gastric carcinomas. Differentiation 1996;60:119.

304. Kitadai Y, Bucana CD, Ellis LM, et al: In situ mRNA hybridization technique for analysis of metastasis-related genes in human colon carcinoma cells. Am J Pathol 1995;147:1238.

305. Greene G, Kitadai Y, Pettaway CA, et al: Correlation of metastasis-related gene expression with metastatic potential in prostate carcinoma cells implanted in nude mice using an in situ mRNA hybridization technique. Am J Pathol 1997; 150:1571.

306. Kuniyasu H, Troncoso P, Johnston D, et al: Relative expression of type IV collagenase, E-cadherin, and VEGF/VPF in prostatectomy specimens distinguishes organ-confined from pathologically advanced prostate cancers. Clin Cancer Res 2000;6:2295.

307. Kuniyasu H, Ellis LM, Evans DB, et al: Relative expression of E-cadherin and type IV collagenase genes predicts disease outcome in patients with resectable pancreatic carcinoma. Clin Cancer Res 1999;5:25.

308. Herbst RS, Yano S, Kuniyasu H, et al: Differential expression of E-cadherin and type IV collagenase genes predicts outcome in patients with stage I non-small cell lung carcinoma. Clin Cancer Res 2000;6:790.

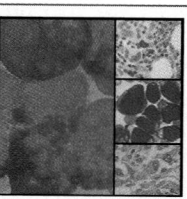

CONTROL OF THE CELL CYCLE

Jennifer A. Pietenpol

Michael B. Kastan

SUMMARY OF KEY POINTS

- Cells in most postnatal tissues are quiescent. Exceptions include cells of the hematopoietic system, skin, and gastrointestinal mucosa.
- Two major challenges for proliferating cells are to make an accurate copy of the three billion bases of DNA (S-phase) and to segregate the duplicated chromosomes equally into daughter cells (mitosis).
- Progression through the cell cycle is dependent on both extrinsic and intrinsic factors.
  - Extrinsic factors include cell-to-cell contact, basement membrane attachments, and growth factor or cytokine exposure.
  - The internal cell cycle machinery is controlled largely by oscillating levels of cyclin proteins and by modulation of cyclin-dependent kinase activity.
- One way in which growth factors regulate cell cycle progression is by affecting the levels of cyclin D in the G1 phase of the cell cycle. The "restriction point" of the cell cycle

occurs in late G1 and is the point beyond which the cell is committed to progress through the rest of the cell cycle.
- Cell cycle checkpoints are surveillance mechanisms that link the rate of cell cycle transitions to the timely and accurate completion of prior, dependent events.
- Cells can arrest at cell cycle checkpoints temporarily to allow for (a) the repair of cellular damage; (b) the dissipation of an exogenous cellular stress signal; or (c) availability of essential growth factors, hormones, or nutrients.
- Among the major functions of the p53 tumor suppressor protein are to modulate cellular responses to stress and to induce cell cycle arrest, senescence, or death as appropriate.
- A major objective of cell cycle arrests in the G_1 and S phases of the cell cycle after DNA damage is presumably to minimize replication of damaged DNA templates.

- Arrests in G_2 and M phases after DNA damage or mitotic spindle damage are presumably to prevent propagation of damaged chromosomes and to ensure appropriate segregation of chromosomes to daughter cells.
- Disruption of cell cycle controls is a pathognomonic feature of all malignant cells. Disruption can manifest as alterations of growth factor signaling pathways, dysregulation of cyclin protein expression, enhanced activity of cyclin-dependent kinases, altered expression or function of cyclin-dependent kinase inhibitors, and mutation of cell cycle checkpoint controls.
- Because cell cycle control is disrupted in virtually all tumor types, the cell cycle-related gene products that are mutated in tumors provide therapeutic targets that might preferentially affect tumor cells more than normal tissues.

INTRODUCTION

Although most cells in an adult human are quiescent or in a nonproliferative state, specialized cells, such as those of the hematopoietic system or those that line the gastrointestinal tract, maintain proliferation. On average, about two trillion cell divisions occur in an adult human every 24 hours (about 25 million per second). It is critically important that various cell types divide at a rate sufficient to produce the needed cells for growth and replacement. If, however, any given cell type divides more rapidly than is necessary, the normal organization and functions of the organism will be disrupted, as the rapidly dividing cells invade and interfere with specialized tissues. Such is the course of events in cancer.

Over the past two decades, unraveling the basic molecular events that control eukaryotic cell cycle transitions has been an area of intense research pursuit. Studies in a variety of organisms have identified an evolutionarily

conserved signal transduction system for controlling cell cycle transitions through regulation of the activity of key enzymes called cyclin-dependent kinases. Further, many investigations have focused on understanding how the signaling pathways that mediate the cell cycle transitions are regulated and modified after cellular stresses. Human cells are continuously exposed to external agents (e.g., reactive chemicals and UV light) and to internal agents (e.g., byproducts of normal intracellular metabolism, such as reactive oxygen intermediates) that can induce cell stress. Eukaryotic cells have evolved cell cycle machinery with a series of surveillance pathways—termed *cell cycle checkpoints*—to ensure that cells copy and divide their genomes with high fidelity during each replication cycle. Cell cycle arrest after DNA damage is critical for maintenance of genomic integrity, and loss of normal cell cycle checkpoint signaling is a hallmark of tumor cells. The ability to manipulate cell cycle checkpoint signaling also has important clinical implications, as modulation of the checkpoints in human tumor cells could enhance cellular sensitivity to chemotherapeutic regimens that induce DNA damage. This chapter focuses on the mechanics of the cell cycle and checkpoint signaling pathways and on how this knowledge might lead to more efficient use of current anticancer therapies and to the development of novel agents.

THE CELL CYCLE MACHINERY

Overview of Cell Cycle Phases

The cell cycle is the sequence of events by which a growing cell duplicates all its components and divides into two daughter cells, each with sufficient machinery to repeat the process. The most important components are the cell's chromosomes, which contain DNA in complex with proteins. Eukaryotic cell division is a highly regulated process. One round of cell division requires high-fidelity duplication of the three billion bases of DNA in each cell during S phase of the cell cycle and proper segregation of duplicated chromosomes during mitosis or M phase. Before and after S phase and M phase the cell transits through "gap" phases, termed G_1 and G_2 (Fig. 5-1). G_1 phase is a period after mitosis when cells prepare for successful DNA synthesis, and G_2 is a period after DNA synthesis when the cell prepares for successful mitosis. The cycle of DNA synthesis and sister chromatid separation runs in parallel with a growth cycle in which the

cell's macromolecules and organelles are also duplicated and partitioned, more or less evenly, between daughter cells. During normal cell proliferation, these two cycles occur at the same rate, so that each round of DNA synthesis and mitosis is balanced by doubling of all other macromolecules in the cell. In this way, the DNA/protein ratio of a cell is maintained within advantageous limits. Orderly progression through the cell cycle is ensured by intrinsic mechanisms that regulate the dependence of one cell cycle event on another. For example, replication of DNA cannot take place until cells have passed through mitosis. In addition, regulatory controls, called *checkpoints,* can modulate cell cycle progression in response to adverse conditions (such as those in the presence of damaged DNA) and will be discussed in a subsequent section. When cells encounter specific growth inhibitory signals or there is an absence of appropriate mitogenic signaling, cells can cease proliferation and enter a nondividing, quiescent state known as G_0, or they can undergo apoptosis.

Mechanics of the Cell Cycle Engine

Cell cycle progression is mediated by the activation of a highly conserved family of protein kinases, the cyclin-dependent kinases (cdks).[1,2] Activation of a cdk requires binding to a specific regulatory subunit, termed a *cyclin.* Cyclins were so named because of their fluctuating levels through the cell cycle. The presence of a 100-amino acid sequence, the "cyclin box," defines a protein as a cyclin family member.[1] The cyclin/cdk complexes are the central cell cycle regulators, with each complex controlling a specific cell cycle transition (see Fig. 5-1). To date, at least nine cdks and 15 cyclins have been described.[3] Extracellular stimuli, such as growth factors and hormones, elevate D-type cyclins (cyclins D1, D2, and D3), which bind to and activate cdk4 and cdk6 and stimulate quiescent cells to enter the cell cycle or proliferating cells to continue proliferation.[4-7] After elevation of D-type cyclins and activation of cdk4 or cdk6 in G_1, cyclin E levels increase and bind cdk2 in cell. The cyclin E/cdk complexes regulate the transition from G_1 into S phase.[8-10] Cyclin A is induced shortly after cyclin E and binds to cdk2 in S phase and to cdc2 (cdk1) in G_2 and mitosis.[11] Cyclin A is thought to be involved in the regulation of S phase entry, and it is also important in G_2 and M phases.[12] The entry into mitosis from G_2 is under the control of B-type cyclins, which also associate with cdc2.[13-15]

In normal cells, the cdks are expressed throughout the cycle; however, each cyclin protein has a restricted period of expression. The limited expression of each cyclin protein is due to cell cycle-dependent regulation of both cyclin gene transcription and protein degradation.[16,17] For cdks to become active, they must bind a cyclin and undergo site-specific phosphorylation. The cyclin/cdk complex is regulated by a number of phosphorylation and dephosphorylation events, resulting either in activation or inhibition of kinase activity.[1] Phosphorylation is carried out by cyclin-activating kinase, and dephosphorylation is mediated by members of the Cdc25 family of dual-specificity protein phosphatases.

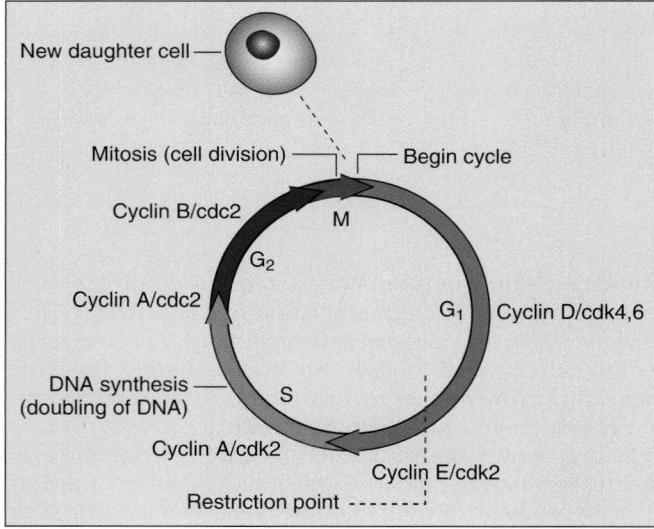

Figure 5-1. One round of cell division requires high-fidelity duplication of DNA during S phase of the cell cycle and proper segregation of duplicated chromosomes during mitosis or M phase. Before and after S phase and M phase, the cell transits through "gap" phases, termed G_1 and G_2. Extracellular stimuli, such as growth factors and hormones, elevate D-type cyclins that bind to and activate cdk4 and cdk6 and stimulate cells to transit through G_1 to the restriction point. At the restriction point, cyclin E levels increase and bind cdk2 in the cell. The cyclin E/cdk complexes regulate the G_1/S transition. Cyclin A is induced after cyclin E and binds cdk2 in S phase and cdc2 in G_2 and mitosis. The entry into mitosis is under the control of B-type cyclins, which also associate with cdc2.

The mammalian Cdc25 family consists of three members: Cdc25A, Cdc25B, and Cdc25C, which appear to have specificity for different cyclin/cdk complexes.[18-20] Cdc25A promotes entry into S phase by acting on cyclin A/cdk2 and cyclin E/cdk2 and is required for DNA replication.[21-24] Further, Cdc25A is a transcriptional target of c-Myc and E2F, and its RNA and protein levels increase as cells are stimulated to enter the cycle from quiescence.[24-26] Another important regulator of S phase progression is the Cdc25B phosphatase.[27] Cdc25B activation occurs during S phase and peaks during the G_2 phase, and Cdc25B activity is necessary for S phase completion in vivo.[28,29] Both Cdc25B and Cdc25B play roles in the G_2/M transition. Cdc25C dephosphorylates cyclin B1/cdc2 and is essential for progression through the G_2/M phase of the cell cycle.[18,30] Cdc25B appears to play a similar role, but with a different timing with respect to Cdc25C.[31]

G_1 Phase

G_1 is a phase in which cells make critical decisions about their fates, including the commitment to replicate DNA and complete the cell division cycle. If mitogens are available and the cellular milieu is favorable for proliferation, a decision to enter S phase is made at a time in mid-to-late G_1, called the *restriction point* (see Fig. 5-1). In unstressed cells, this commitment to replicate DNA and divide is irreversible until the next G_1 phase. The restriction point switch, from the growth factor-dependent early G_1 to the subsequent mitogen-independent phases, reflects the induction of broad transcription programs that regulate genes critical for G_1/S transition and coordination of S-G_2-M phase progress.

Integral to the molecular switch that controls transition from G_1 to S phase and key downstream targets of the G_1 phase cyclin/cdk complexes are the members of the retinoblastoma protein (RB) family: RB, p107, and p130.[32] During G_1 progression, RB is sequentially phosphorylated by cyclin D1/cdk4,6 and cyclin E/cdk2 complexes (Fig. 5-2).[33-35] Phosphorylated RB can function as either a transcriptional repressor or a transcriptional activator depending on its phosphorylation state and the proteins with which it binds.[36] Best understood is the role of RB as a transcriptional repressor in its hypophosphorylated state when bound to the E2F family of transcription factors.[36] The E2F family mediates transcription of genes required for DNA synthesis, including cyclin E, cyclin A, cyclin B, dihydrofolate reductase, and thymidine kinase (see Fig. 5-2).[37] The binding of hypophosphorylated RB to E2F inhibits E2F-dependent transcription of S phase genes and arrests cells at the G_1/S transition.[38] The ability of RB to function as a transcriptional repressor involves other protein families, including histone deacetylase and chromatin remodeling SWI/SNF complexes.[39] RB can also be regulated by acetylation, which is mediated by histone acetylases such as p300/CBP. The acetylases are under cell cycle control and prevent efficient RB phosphorylation by cyclin E/ckd2.[40] Sequential phosphorylation of RB by cyclin D/cdk4/6 and cyclinE/cdk2 complexes inhibits the repressor activity of RB, as it results in the dissociation of E2F and RB, and S phase entry (see Fig. 5-2). As cells progress into S phase, maintenance of RB hyperphosphor-

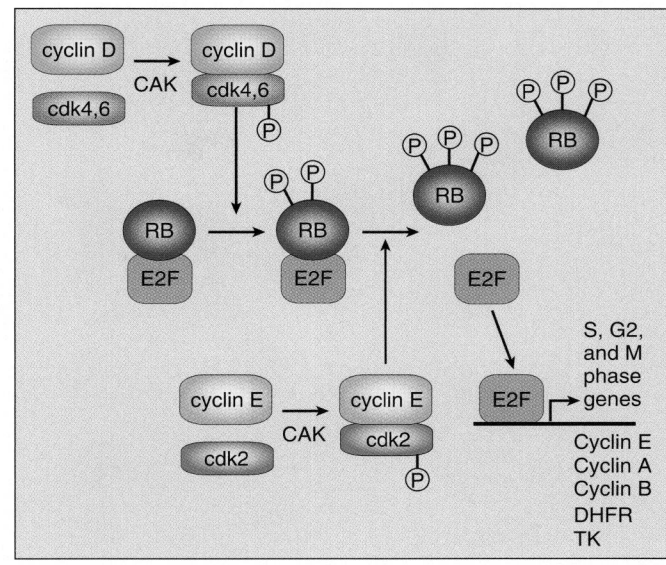

Figure 5-2. The G_1/S transition. During G_1 phase progression, activation of cyclin D/cdk4 and cyclin E/cdk2 complexes by cyclin activating kinase (CAK) leads to sequential phosphorylation of the transcription factor RB. Hypophosphorylated RB binds to the E2F transcription factor family to inhibit S phase entry. Once hyperphosphorylated, RB dissociates from E2F, resulting in activation of genes required for S phase entry.

ylation is necessary for the successful completion of DNA replication.[41] Cell cycle regulation by RB plays an important role in preventing tumorigenesis, as mutations that affect the RB signaling pathway have been identified in the majority of human cancers.[42]

In addition to regulation by phosphorylation and dephosphorylation events as described previously, cdks are regulated by a group of functionally related proteins called cdk inhibitors.[1] The cdk inhibitors fall into two families: the INK4 inhibitors and the Cip/Kip inhibitors. There are four known INK4 family members: p16^{INK4A}, p15^{INK4B}, p19^{INK4D}, and p18^{INK4C}, and three known Cip/Kip family members: p21$^{Waf1/Cip1}$, p27^{Kip1}, and p57^{Kip2}. The INK4 family specifically inhibits cdk4 and cdk6 activity during the G_1 phase of the cell cycle, while the Cip/Kip family can inhibit cdk activity during all phases of the cell cycle (Fig. 5-3). Both families of cdk inhibitors can arrest cells in the G1 phase of the cell cycle by inhibiting the activities of cdks and preventing their ability to phosphorylate and inactive RB and other RB-family proteins.[1] The levels, subcellular localization, and activity of these inhibitors can be regulated by various forms of cell stress and growth inhibitory signaling pathways.

S Phase

Biochemical and genetic approaches have brought major advances to our understanding of how DNA replication is controlled in the cell. The quest for the molecular mechanisms that ensure genome integrity by controlling once-per-cell cycle replication has resulted in the emergence of a fundamental model describing the control of DNA synthesis. Eukaryotic DNA replication is a complex

Science of Clinical Oncology

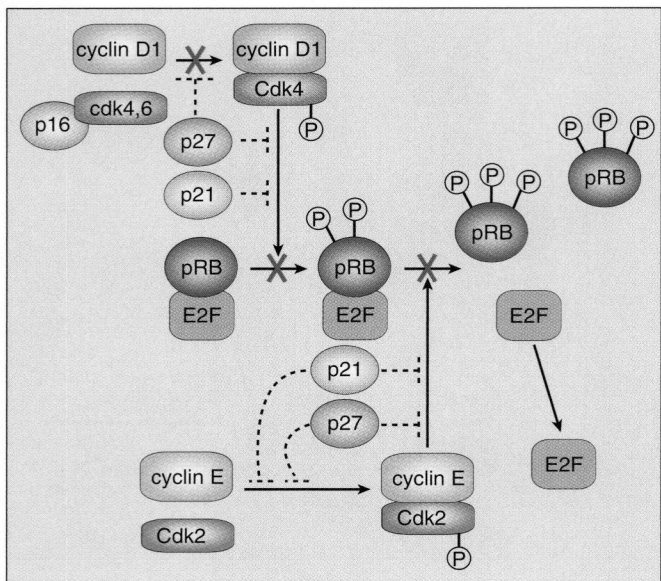

Figure 5-3. Role of cdk inhibitors in the G_1/S transition. Members of the INK4 and Cip/Kip cdk inhibitor families (represented by p16 and p21/27, respectively) can inhibit the cyclin/cdk kinase complexes to mediate a G_1/S cell cycle arrest. INK4 family members bind directly to cdk4 or cdk6 and inhibit binding to the cyclin, whereas p21 and p27 can bind to both the cyclin and cdk components with higher affinity for the cyclin.

process including the recognition of initiation sites on DNA, multistep preparation of DNA for duplication, and assembly of multiprotein complexes capable of beginning DNA synthesis at initiation sites. The process starts late in M phase as the cell completes its previous cycle and lasts until the appropriate time of DNA replication at each origin-of-replication initiation site. An interplay of multisubunit protein complexes occurs during S phase, involving proteins that bind to the origins of replication initiation, proteins with helicase activity, replication protein A, and DNA polymerase α.

The initiation of DNA replication during the S phase of the cell cycle takes place at multiple sites on the chromosomes, called the *origins of replication*. The state of eukaryotic replication origins changes during the cell cycle (Fig. 5-4).[43,44] It is proposed that replication origins are in two different states during the cell cycle. One state exists during G_1 phase, before DNA replication begins, when a multiprotein complex called the prereplicative complex (pre-RC) assembles on the origin. The second state exists from the initiation of S phase to the end of M phase, when a postreplicative complex (post-RC) is present at the replication origins. Cdk activity is thought to control each round of DNA replication. At the end of M phase, low cdk activity allows for the assembly of the pre-RC, a state competent for replication. When chromatin becomes replication-competent, it is referred to as *licensed*. Initiator proteins required for pre-RC formation include the Origin Recognition Complex (ORC), Cdc6, Cdt1, and MCM proteins (MCM2 to MCM7).[45-48] The six MCM proteins interact with each other to form a hexameric complex thought to function as a replicative helicase.[49] Cdc6 and

Cdt1 are required to load MCM proteins on chromatin.[50,51] Human Cdt1 is coassociated with geminin, which is a negative regulator of pre-RC formation that prevents the loading of MCM onto chromatin.[50] This sequential association of initiator proteins with origin DNA licenses chromatin for replication.

A model has been proposed to explain the coordination of chromatin licensing and the cell cycle (see Fig. 5-4). The ORC associates with replication origins, and this association persists throughout the cell cycle.[52] As cells complete mitosis, Cdc6 and Cdt1 are loaded on chromatin, and they in turn load the MCM complex on chromatin, at which point licensing is considered complete.[50] The multiprotein complex is considered to be the pre-RC.[43] This complex is activated at the G1/S transition, and DNA replication is initiated. Two protein kinases, cdk2 and HsDbf4-dependent kinase (hcdc7), are required to activate the licensed origins for initiation. The activity of the protein kinases is believed to result in changes in the pre-RC that promotes Cdc45 binding to the MCM complex, followed by the unwinding of replication origins. Subsequently, DNA replicating proteins such as RPA, DNA polymerase α and ε are recruited to initiation sites.[53-55] After activation of the replication origins, both the MCM complex and Cdc45 move together with replication enzymes assembled at replication forks to complete DNA replication.[56,57] Thus, an increase in cdk2 and hcdc7 activity at the G_1/S transition triggers initiation and converts the origin to the post-RC state. The reformation of pre-RC does not occur again until the end of mitosis.

To maintain genomic integrity, it is essential that origins do not fire a second time until mitosis has been completed. The cdk cycle controls the two states at replication origins, couples the initiation of S phase to the completion of M phase, and prevents re-replication events from occurring during a single round of the cell cycle.[58-60] The MCM complex is a key component of DNA replication; the cycle of cdk activity within the cell regulates the precise timing of loading and activation of the MCM complex and prevents its reloading before the completion of a cell cycle.

G_2/M Phase Transition

After duplication of the genome in S phase, cells transit through G_2 and prepare for mitosis. As cells enter into G_2 phase, cyclin B/cdc2 complexes form and are kept inactive by phosphorylation (Fig. 5-5). At the end of G_2 phase, cyclin B/cdc2 complexes are activated by dephosphorylation, and cells enter into mitosis.[61,62] Phosphorylation is carried out by the Wee1/Mik1 family of protein kinases.[63,64] The enzyme that dephosphorylates and activates cdc2 at the end of G_2 and initiates mitosis is Cdc25C.[65,66] Cdc25C is localized in the cytoplasm during interphase and enters the nucleus just before mitosis.[19] Although less well understood, Cdc25B also plays a role at the mitotic transition. The cyclin A/Cdc2 complex is likely regulated in a similar manner; however, further studies are necessary to define the role of cyclin A kinase activity in mitosis.

Another mechanism by which cyclin B1/cdc2 complexes are regulated is through a shift in their subcellular

Figure 5-4. S phase transition. The origin replication complex (ORC) associates with replication origins, and this association persists throughout the cell cycle. As the cells complete mitosis, Cdc6 and Cdt1 are loaded on chromatin, and they in turn load the MCM complex on chromatin, at which point licensing is considered complete and the multiprotein complex is considered to be the pre-RC. This complex is activated at the G1/S transition, and DNA replication is initiated. Two protein kinases—cdk and HsDbf4-dependent kinase—are required to activate the licensed origins for initiation. The activity of the protein kinases is believed to result in changes in the pre-RC, which promotes Cdc45 binding to the MCM complex, followed by the unwinding of replication origins. Subsequently, DNA replicating proteins such as RPA, DNA polymerase α, and DNA polymerase ε are recruited to initiation sites. An increase in cdk and hsDbf4 activity at the G$_1$/S transition triggers initiation and converts the origin to the post-RC state. The reformation of pre-RC does not occur again until the end of mitosis.

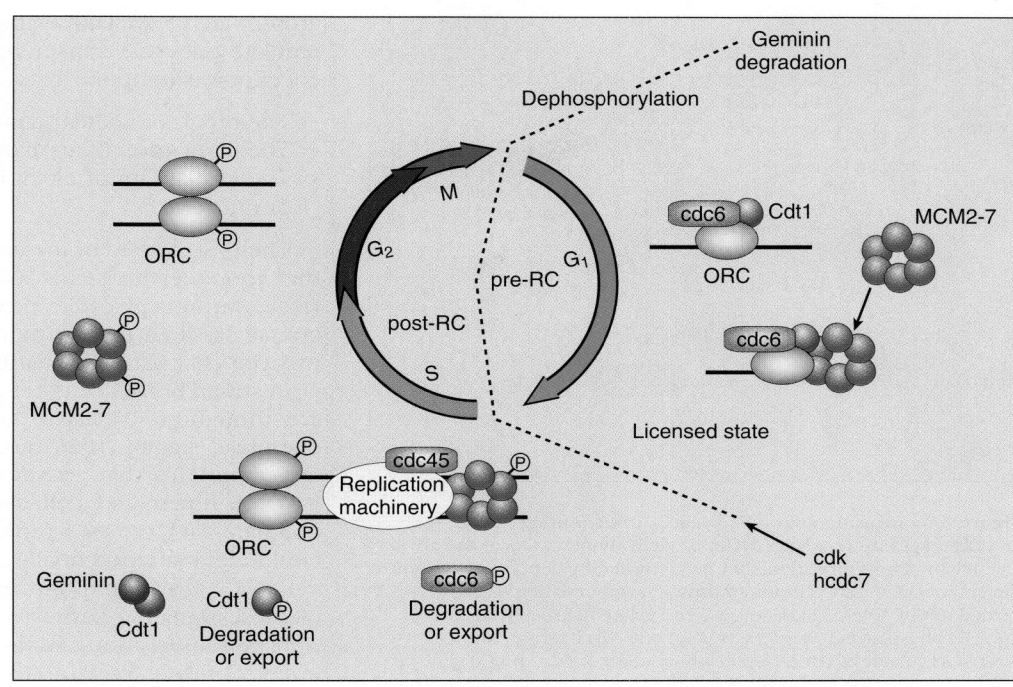

localization. For most cyclins, the scenario after biosynthesis is nuclear localization until cell cycle-mediated degradation occurs. In contrast, cyclin B1 is in the cytoplasm during S phase and G$_2$ phase and is translocated to the nucleus at the beginning of mitosis.[67] It is thought that the precise regulation of cyclin B1 localization prevents premature mitosis during interphase, while allowing regulated access of cyclin B1/cdc2 complexes to their nuclear substrates at the onset of mitosis.

M Phase

Mitosis is the process by which a cell ensures that each daughter cell will have a complete set of chromosomes. There are five key stages of mitosis (Fig. 5-6):

1. During prophase, the chromosomes become condensed, and proteins begin to bind the kinetochores, preparing for spindle attachment.
2. Upon breakdown of the nuclear envelope, the cell enters prometaphase, during which the mitotic spindle is formed and the chromosomes attach to microtubules in the spindle through their kinetochores. Once attached, the chromosomes align along the metaphase plate in the center of the spindle.
3. During metaphase, all of the chromosomes are attached to microtubules through their kinetochores and are aligned at the metaphase plate.
4. At anaphase onset, the sister chromatids separate and move toward the poles of the spindle.

5. During telophase, the parent cell is divided into two daughter cells by cytokinesis.

As cells enter mitosis, phosphorylation of key components causes significant changes in the architecture of the cell. This phosphorylation is due mainly to cyclin B/cdc2 activity.[68] Cyclin B/cdc2-mediated phosphorylation induces changes in the microtubule network, the actin microfilaments, and the nuclear lamina.[69-71] Other cyclin B/cdc2 substrates include histone H1 and microtubule-associated proteins such as MAP4, MAP2, and stathmin.[16,72] In addition to the central function of cdc2, the family of polo-like protein kinases (Plks) also plays a critical role in several mitotic events.[73,74] Several Plk homologs have been identified in mammalian cells.[75] In human cancer cells, injection of anti-Plk1 antibodies leads to a mitotic arrest with a monopolar spindle formed around a smaller than usual centrosome.[76] These findings suggest that Plks are critical for the formation of a bipolar spindle. It is proposed that Plks initiate the onset of mitosis by activating Cdc25C, although little is known about the exact trigger for Plk activation.[77] Plks are also important regulators of mitotic exit.

Mitotic exit requires sister chromatid separation, spindle disassembly, and cytokinesis. The initiation and coordination of these processes are controlled by degradation of key regulatory proteins. The mediator of this protein destruction is a multisubunit protein called the anaphase-promoting complex (APC) or cyclosome.[78,79]

Science of Clinical Oncology

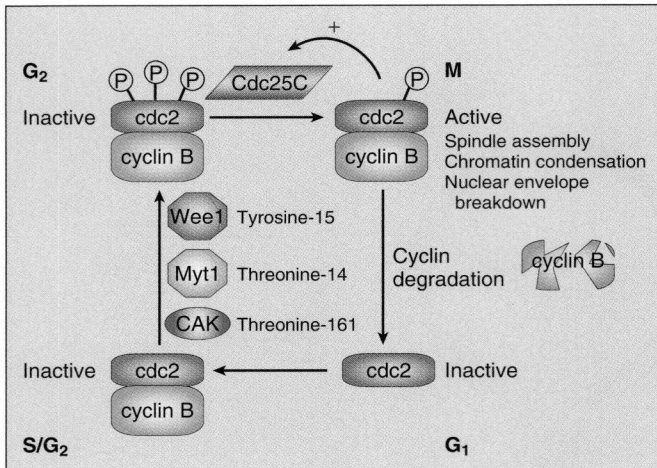

Figure 5-5. Regulation of cyclin B/cdc2 activity during the cell cycle. As cells enter into G_2 phase, cyclin B/cdc2 complexes form and are kept inactive by phosphorylation; they are activated by dephosphorylation at the end of G_2 to lead cells into mitosis. Phosphorylation of cdc2 is carried out by Wee-1 kinase and a Wee-1 related kinase, Myt1. The Cdc25C phosphatase counteracts Wee1 and Myt1 activity and is a positive regulator of cdc2. Dephosphorylation of cdc2 by Cdc25C in late G_2 activates the cyclin B/cdc2 complex and initiates mitosis. The cyclin B/cdc2 complex is thought to phosphorylate Cdc25C, which further activates Cdc25C, inducing the full activation of cyclin B/cdc2 by forming an autocatalytic feedback loop. At the end of mitosis, cyclin B is degraded by the APC, and cdc2 remains inactive until cyclin B levels increase again during late S and early G_2.

Key APC substrates are the mitotic A- and B-type cyclins. Cyclin A is degraded in metaphase, whereas B-type cyclins are degraded when cells enter anaphase.[80,81] Cyclin B1 destruction starts as soon as the last chromosomes are aligned on the metaphase plate and is complete by the end of metaphase.[82] Another group of APC substrates are proteins that function as anaphase inhibitors. During G_2, sister chromatids are held together by proteins called cohesins, which require inactivation by APC for anaphase initiation.[83,84] Overall, the APC regulates two different steps in mitosis. First, sister chromatid separation is triggered by destruction of the anaphase inhibitors, after which spindle disassembly and mitotic exit are initiated by the degradation of mitotic cyclins. These two steps allow the cell to couple the exit from mitosis to the prior completion of anaphase.

CELL CYCLE CHECKPOINTS

At key transitions during eukaryotic cell cycle progression, signaling pathways monitor the successful completion of events in one phase of the cell cycle before proceeding to the next phase. These regulatory pathways are commonly referred to as *cell cycle checkpoints*.[85] In a broader context, cell cycle checkpoints are signal transduction pathways that link the rate of cell cycle phase transitions to the timely and accurate completion of prior, dependent events. Checkpoint surveillance functions are not confined solely to nuclear events, as parameters such as

growth factor availability and cell mass accumulation also regulate cell cycle transition.[86] Cells can arrest at cell cycle checkpoints temporarily to allow for any of the following:

- The repair of cellular damage
- The dissipation of an exogenous cellular stress signal
- The availability of essential growth factors, hormones, or nutrients

The best studied of the cell cycle checkpoints are those that monitor the status and structure of chromosomal DNA during cell-cycle progression. These checkpoints contain, as their most proximal signaling elements, sensor proteins that scan chromatin for partially replicated DNA, DNA strand breaks, or other abnormalities. Sensor proteins are thought to translate DNA-derived stimuli into biochemical signals that modulate specific downstream target proteins that activate signaling pathways involved in DNA repair and cell cycle arrest.[87,88] Further, when cellular damage is irreparable, checkpoint signaling could eliminate potentially hazardous cells by permanent cell cycle arrest or apoptosis. The physiological relevance of these signaling pathways is supported by their evolutionary conservation and the finding that the major consequence of their alteration in humans is tumorigenesis.[87,88]

G_1/S Checkpoint

G_1 is a phase in which cells make critical decisions about their fates, including the commitment to replicate DNA and complete the cell division cycle. As discussed previously, if the cellular milieu is favorable for proliferation, a decision to enter S phase is made at a restriction point. In unstressed cells, this commitment to replicate DNA and divide is irreversible until the next G_1 phase. If DNA is damaged, however, the G_1/S checkpoint is integral for preventing transition of cells into S phase and replication of the damaged DNA template. In fact, if checkpoint signaling is activated in G_1, it can delay cell cycle progression even if cells have already passed the restriction point. Due to its essential and rate-limiting role in G_1/S transition, cyclin E/cdk2 is a key target for the DNA damage checkpoint.[35] Progression through G_1 can be halted at either the restriction point, by inhibition of RB phosphorylation, or closer to the S phase transition by inhibition of cyclin E/cdk2 activity. The activation of the G_1 and subsequent checkpoints during the cell cycle relies on a distinct network of signaling pathways that ultimately regulate the activity of the key enzymes of the cell cycle, the cdks.

Central to activation of the G_1/S cell cycle checkpoint and all those that follow is the ability of the cell to "sense" stress and activate the requisite signaling pathways. The stress that is best studied in human cells is that induced by DNA damage. For the G_1 checkpoint to be effective in blocking cell entry into S phase within minutes of exposure of cells to DNA damaging agents, machinery must be in place within cells that is poised to act without the time requirement of transcription and translation. Pathways that satisfy this requirement involve proteins that can "sense" DNA lesions and transduce this signal through phosphorylation to effectors that can signal rapidly to downstream targets.[87,88] How DNA lesions or

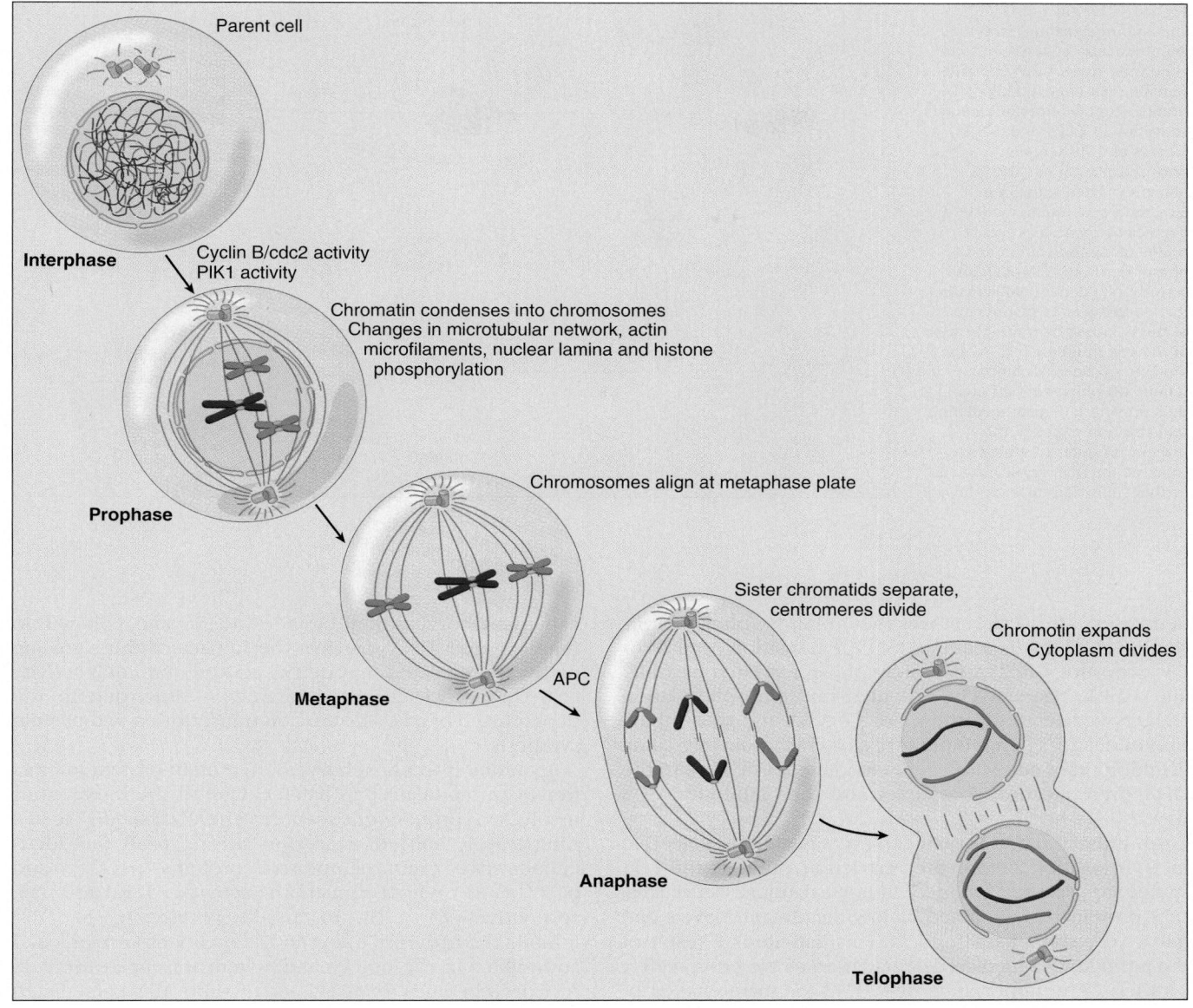

Interphase

Cyclin B/cdc2 activity
PIK1 activity

Chromatin condenses into chromosomes
Changes in microtubular network, actin
microfilaments, nuclear lamina and histone
phosphorylation

Prophase

Chromosomes align at metaphase plate

Metaphase

APC

Sister chromatids separate,
centromeres divide

Chromotin expands
Cytoplasm divides

Anaphase

Telophase

Figure 5-6. Key stages of mitosis. As the parent cell enters prophase, the chromosomes condense and proteins bind the kinetochores, preparing for spindle attachment. Upon nuclear envelope breakdown, the cell enters prometaphase, during which the mitotic spindle is formed and the chromosomes attach to microtubules in the spindle via their kinetochores. Once attached, the chromosomes align along the metaphase plate in the center of the spindle. During metaphase, all of the chromosomes are attached to microtubules via their kinetochores and are aligned at the metaphase plate. At anaphase onset, the sister chromatids separate and move toward the poles of the spindle. During telophase, the parent cell is divided into two daughter cells by cytokinesis.

blocks to DNA synthesis are "sensed" is not well understood; however, the key transducer proteins are members of the DNA-dependent protein kinase-like family that includes human ataxia telangiectasia mutated (ATM) and ATM-related (ATR).[89-91] These proteins are required for all checkpoints that are engaged by altered DNA structure and/or DNA lesions and activate effector kinases by phosphorylation. ATM was originally cloned as the gene mutation in ataxia telangiectasia (AT), an inherited disease that is characterized by predisposition to cancer.[92,93] ATM, ATR, and DNA-PK are thought to act at very early stages after the initiation of DNA damage. In human cells,

two effectors, kinases Chk2 and Chk1, are activated by phosphorylation in response to DNA damage and replication disturbances.[87,89-91] After exposure of cells to ionizing radiation, ATM phosphorylates Chk2 regardless of cell cycle position.[94,95] In response, however, to ultraviolet radiation or exposure of cells to agents that inhibit DNA replication (e.g., hydroxyurea), ATR activates Chk1 by phosphorylation.[96]

For cells in G_1 that are past the restriction point and near the G_1/S transition, a key target for checkpoint signaling is the cyclin E/cdk2 complex (Fig. 5-7). After exposure of cells to UV or IR, the level of Cdc25A phosphatase rapidly

Science of Clinical Oncology

I

Figure 5-7. Model of G_1/S checkpoint signaling after genotoxic stress. In response to genotoxic stress, the ATM/ATR signaling pathway is activated, leading to phosphorylation and activation of Chk1 and Chk2 kinases and subsequent phosphorylation of Cdc25A. Phosphorylated Cdc25A is targeted for ubiquitin-mediated degradation, which prevents cyclin E/cdk2 activation and S phase transition. ATM/ATR also activate p53-dependent signaling that contributes to maintenance of the G_1 arrest by transactivation of the cdk inhibitor p21, which binds to cyclin/cdk complexes to reduce RB phosphorylation and thus prevent E2F from mediating transcription of genes, the protein products of which are required for DNA replication and further transition through the cell cycle.

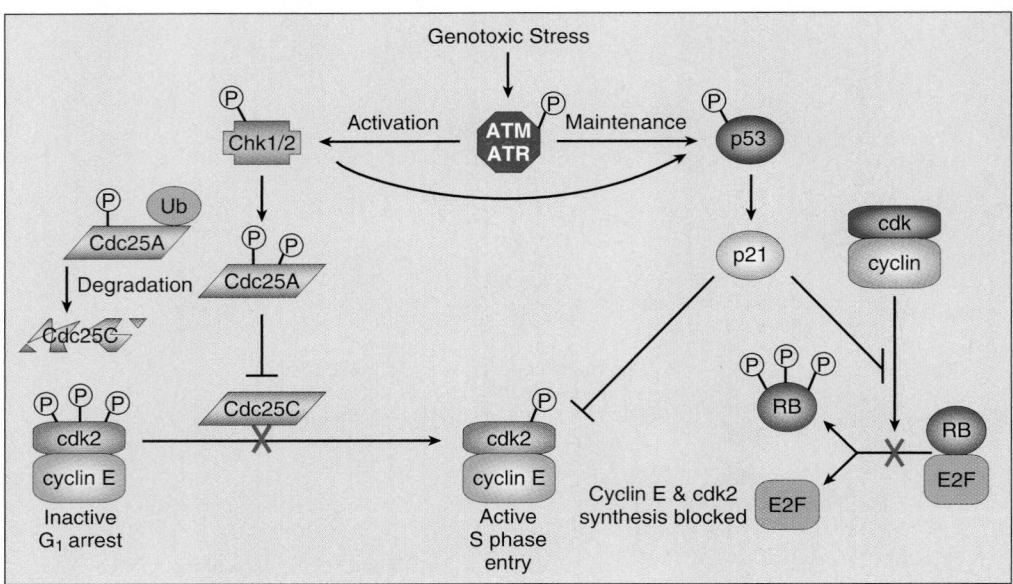

decreases.[35] Cdc25A removes the inhibitory phosphorylation on cdk2 that is required for G_1/S transition. After IR or UV exposure, Cdc25A is rapidly phosphorylated by Chk2 and Chk1, respectively. Chk-mediated phosphorylation triggers accelerated turnover of Cdc25A and thus inhibition of cdk2.[97,98] An endpoint of this checkpoint signaling is inhibition of cdk2-dependent loading of Cdc45 onto the DNA prereplication complexes and thus inhibition of S phase.[99]

An integral target for checkpoint signaling in cells that in G_1 transition before the restriction point is the p53 tumor suppressor protein.[100] In normal, nonstressed cells, p53 protein is maintained at low steady-state levels and has a very short half-life.[101-104] This half-life is a result of the rapid MDM2-mediated degradation of the protein after synthesis. The importance of MDM2 for maintenance of appropriate p53 levels in vivo is highlighted by the fact that absence of MDM2 in knock-out mice results in early embryonic lethality that is rescued by a dual knock-out of MDM2 and p53.[105,106]

After exposure of cells to stress (including DNA damage or oxidative stress), p53 phosphorylation changes, and protein levels increase significantly (see Fig. 5-7).[100] Identification of the kinases that phosphorylate p53 after genotoxic stress provided key links between the transducers and effector kinases of checkpoint signaling and the downstream target proteins such as p53. Upstream transducers that are required for p53-mediated maintenance of G_1 checkpoint arrest are the same as those required for activation of the checkpoint, namely the ATM/ATR and Chk2/Chk1 kinases. Phosphorylation leads to increased levels and activity of p53 as a transcriptional activator. Among the genes regulated by p53, the cdk inhibitor p21[WAF1/Cip1] plays a central role in G_1 checkpoint by inhibiting cdks that are essential for entry into S phase.[107-110] Thus, although ATM/ATR-mediated signaling

can phosphorylate key targets Cdc25A and p53 within minutes after DNA damage, the impact of the signaling pathways regulated by Cdc25A and p53 on cdk2 activity and G_1/S blockage are separated in time, due to the dependence of p53 signaling on transcription and protein synthesis.

In addition to phosphorylation, protein-protein interactions can modulate p53 half-life. One of the interactions involves a protein encoded by the INK4a/ARF locus. Alternatively spliced transcripts arising from this locus encode two tumor suppressor proteins, p16[INK4A] and p19[ARF] (ARF), which regulate the activities of RB and p53, respectively.[111,112] As discussed previously, p16[INK4A] inhibits the activities of cyclin D-dependent kinases, cdk4 and cdk6. On the other hand, when present in the cell, ARF protein binds to MDM2 and disrupts MDM2-mediated degradation of p53, leading to p53 stabilization and a p53-dependent transcriptional response.[113-116] ARF gene expression is induced by oncogenic stimuli such as viral oncoprotein expression or elevated levels of c-myc or ras.[117-119] The biological importance of ARF in the activation of p53 signaling pathways is exemplified by the finding that ARF-deficient mice develop spontaneous tumors and have accelerated tumor progression after carcinogen exposure, similar to p53-null mice.[120] These findings provide the molecular basis for the stabilization of p53 observed in cells after oncogenic stimulation and demonstrate that this signaling pathway is distinct from that activated by genotoxic stress.[121] Although the p53-mediated induction of the cdk inhibitor p21[WAF1/Cip1] contributes to ARF-induced growth arrest, ARF can prevent proliferation of p21[WAF1/Cip1]-null primary mouse embryo fibroblasts (MEFs), indicating that other ARF-inducible genes can compensate.[122,123] ARF also can inhibit proliferation of MEFs lacking both MDM2 and p53, implying that ARF can interact with targets other than

MDM2.[124] Consistent with these findings, mice lacking ARF, p53, and MDM2 develop multiple and more aggressive tumors than mice lacking either gene alone.[124] Thus, ARF is a major component of a regulatory pathway stimulated by oncogenic signals culminating in both p53-dependent and -independent signaling. Although the importance of this pathway has been established overtly in experimental animal oncology, it still must be documented further in human oncology to understand the full biological significance of ARF as a tumor suppressor in human cells.

Human cells also have evolved additional mechanisms to prolong a G_1 cell cycle checkpoint arrest. For example, after exposure of keratinocytes and melanocytes to physiological doses of UV radiation, there is an increase of the cdk inhibitor p16[INK4a].[125] Such secondary maintenance pathways act in a cell-type and stimulus-specific manner. Given the direct role that cdk inhibitors play in regulation of the G_1/S transition, it is not surprising that cdk inhibitor function is often compromised in human tumors. The p16[INK4A] gene is the frequent target of mutations that ablate its function, including point mutations, promoter methylation, or homozygous deletions.[126] Likewise, many human breast cancers have reduced p27[Kip1] protein expression or aberrant subcellular localization of the protein that has been correlated with more aggressive tumors.[127-130]

S Phase Checkpoint

If one of the major goals of cell cycle checkpoints is to prevent the deleterious consequences of replicating damaged DNA, the responses of cells that are already in S phase at the time of the DNA damage will be critical for optimal outcome of the cell. Because DNA replication is ongoing in S-phase cells, these cells must respond virtually instantaneously to halt initiation of new replication forks throughout S phase. In response to the introduction of DNA double-strand breaks, such as those introduced by ionizing irradiation, this instantaneous response is initiated by activation of the ATM protein kinase.[89] It has recently been demonstrated that just a few breaks in the cell's genome results in instantaneous activation of ATM protein throughout the cell, thus providing a mechanism by which the cell can respond quickly and completely to the presence of broken DNA.[131] This activation appears to occur through some aspect of chromatin structure that is altered by the presence of broken DNA and through autophosphorylation of the ATM protein. For responses to other types of DNA damage, such as base damage caused by exposure to ultraviolet (UV) light or alkylating agents, the ATR kinase, rather than the ATM kinase, appears to be important for initiating the relevant signal transduction pathways.[132]

Once ATM or ATR has been activated by the introduction of DNA damage, these protein kinases begin to phosphorylate substrates to help the cell arrest cell cycle progression or repair DNA (Fig. 5-8). As discussed previously, the phosphorylation of p53, mdm2, and Chk2 by ATM following DNA damage contributes to the arrest of cells in G1 before the restriction point. Among the proteins phosphorylated by ATM that contribute to arrest of cells in S phase are Nbs1, Brca1, SMC1, and FAncD2.[133-139] Once these proteins are phosphorylated, there is an immediate cessation of initiation of new replication forks for approximately 90 minutes, after which time replication begins to resume. It is not yet known how phosphorylation of these proteins prevents initiation of new replication forks, and mechanistic linkage of these signaling molecules to the DNA replication machinery remains a major gap in our knowledge. Nevertheless, the importance of this process in cancer formation in humans is suggested by the fact that many of these genes are mutated in familial cancer syndromes. For example, the cancer susceptibility syndromes Ataxia-telangiectasia, Nijmegen breakage syndrome, Fanconi's anemia, and familial breast/ovarian carcinoma syndrome are caused by inherited mutations in ATM, Nbs1, FAncD2, and Brca1, respectively.

G2 Checkpoint

In addition to activation of the G_1/S and S phase checkpoints, DNA damage also activates checkpoint arrest in G_2 to prevent the passage of DNA lesions to two daughter cells during mitosis. These DNA damage checkpoint pathways all share common upstream signaling pathways made up of the ATM/ATR transducer and Chk2/Chk1 effector kinases. The biochemical pathways involved in the DNA damage-induced G_2 arrest involve signaling cascades that converge to inhibit the activation of cdc2 through maintenance of tyrosine-15 phosphorylation.[140] By preventing dephosphorylation of this inhibitory site, cyclinB/cdc2 is not activated, and cells remain arrested in the G_2 phase of the cell cycle. Evidence for this is provided by the experimental use of cdc2 mutants that cannot be phosphorylated at tyrosine-15. When these mutants are expressed in human cells, the G_2 delay induced by DNA damage is abrogated.[141]

Activation of the G_2 checkpoint after genotoxic stress involves ATM-mediated phosphorylation and activation of the Chk1 and Chk2 kinases (Fig. 5-9).[142-144] Both Chk1 and Plk1 are proposed to play a key role in the G_2 arrest through targeting the cdc2-specific phosphatase, Cdc25C, for phosphorylation after DNA damage.[143,145,146] One working model is that Chk1-mediated phosphorylation of Cdc25C on serine-216, after DNA damage, creates a binding site for 14-3-3 proteins.[145] Because the 14-3-3 proteins are found in the cytoplasm in human cells, it is proposed that 14-3-3 proteins prevent cell transition into mitosis by sequestering Cdc25C in the cytoplasm.[147] Such nuclear export would separate the phosphatase from its substrate, cyclin B/cdc2. Recent studies in yeast, however, suggest that other levels of regulation of Cdc25C besides nuclear export might participate in the G_2 arrest induced by DNA damage.[88] It is proposed that direct inhibition of Cdc25 activity by Chk1 is sufficient for proficient checkpoint regulation of Cdc25 and that Cdc25C might be inhibited by another upstream kinase, Plk1.[146] The activity of Plk1 is inhibited in the G_2 phase of human tumor cells exposed to ionizing radiation, camptothecin, and doxorubicin. Further, expression of a mutant Plk1 in

Science of Clinical Oncology

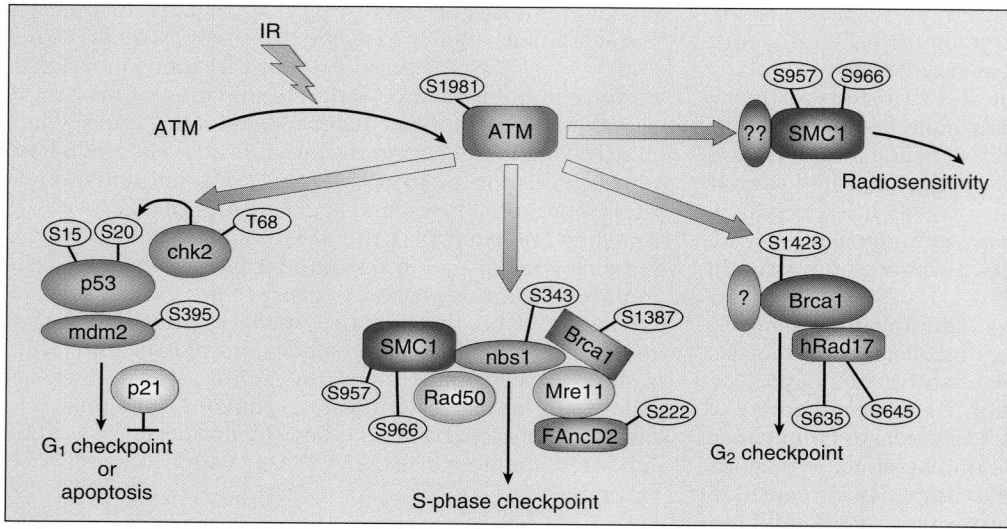

Figure 5-8. Schematic representation of the signal transduction pathways initiated by ATM after ionizing irradiation (IR) and the functional roles of the ATM targets. After IR, the specific activity of the ATM kinase increases, and it subsequently phosphorylates Chk2, p53, and mdm2 to initiate the G1 arrest; Nbs1, FancD2, Brca1, and SMC1 to initiate the S-phase arrest; and Brca1 and hRad17 to cause a G2 arrest. SMC1 is the only target of ATM where mutation of the ATM phosphorylation sites affects radiosensitivity.

which residues necessary for Plk1 activation are altered, prevents Plk1 inactivation and leads to G_2 override in cells treated with doxorubicin.[148] Studies have shown that normal epithelial cells and fibroblasts undergo G_2 arrest in response to Plk inactivation in the absence of DNA damage. Clearly, more investigation is required for a complete understanding of the role of Chk1 and Plk activity in G_2 checkpoint function. Further, there is not sufficient evidence at this time to rule out the role of other Cdc25 family members in the G_2 checkpoint.

In addition to a role in G_1/S checkpoint function, p53-mediated signaling plays an integral role in maintenance of the G_2 checkpoint delay after activation of the checkpoint. Both p53 and several of its downstream targets are necessary to maintain a G_2 arrest after DNA damage, and tumor cells lacking these proteins enter into mitosis with accelerated kinetics.[149] p53 is believed to exert G_2 checkpoint responses through transcriptional upregulation of the downstream target genes p21, 14-3-3σ, and GADD45 (see Fig. 5-9). Similar to its regulation of the cyclin D1/

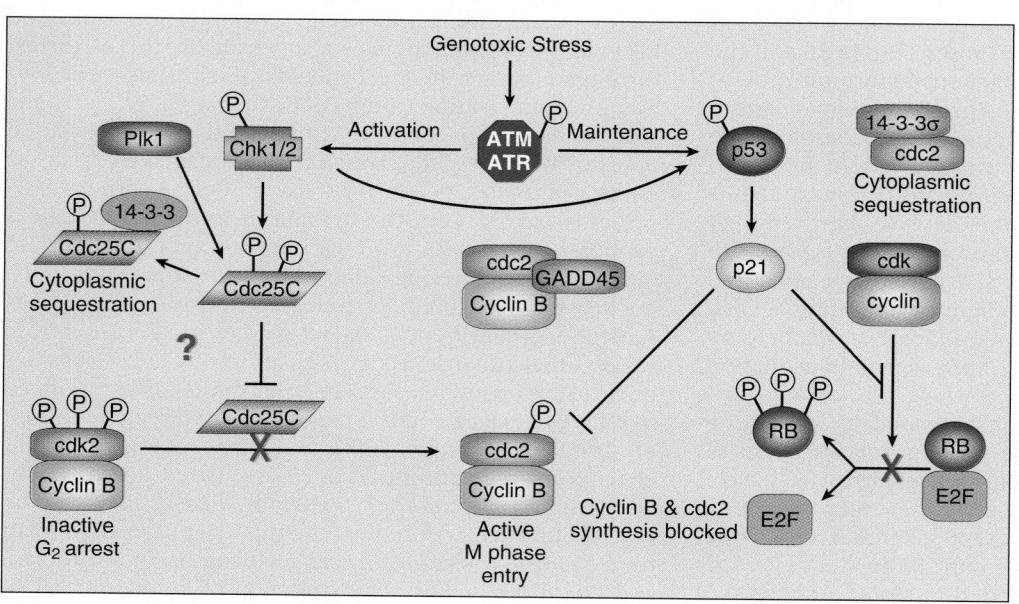

Figure 5-9. Model of G_2/M checkpoint signaling after genotoxic stress. In response to genotoxic stress, the ATM/ATR signaling pathway is activated, leading to phosphorylation and activation of Chk1 and Chk2 kinases and subsequent phosphorylation of Cdc25C. Plk1 can also phosphorylate Cdc25C. Phosphorylated Cdc25C can be sequestered in the cytoplasm by 14-3-3 proteins, preventing cyclin B/cdc2 activation and mitotic entry. ATM/ATR also activate p53-dependent signaling that contributes to maintenance of the G_2 arrest by upregulating the 14-3-3σ protein that sequesters cdk1 in the cytoplasm. The p53 gene also transactivates the cdk inhibitor p21, which binds to cyclin/cdk complexes to reduce RB phosphorylation and eventually prevents E2F from mediating synthesis of cyclin B and cdc2. The p21 gene also directly binds and inhibits cyclin B/cdk1 complexes to block mitotic entry. Upregulation of GADD45, mediated by p53, also can inhibit cyclin B/cdc2 activity through direct binding of the GADD45 to the complex.

cdk4,6 or cyclin E/cdk2 complexes at the G_1/S checkpoint, p21 can bind to and inhibit the cyclin B1/cdc2 complex and inhibit cyclin-activated kinase-mediated cdc2 activation.[150] The p53-dependent increase in 14-3-3σ modulates the subcellular localization of the cyclin B1/Cdc2 complex, as the binding of 14-3-3σ to cdc2 results in retention of the kinase in the cytoplasm.[151] Loss of 14-3-3σ also results in abrogation of the DNA damage G_2 checkpoint and premature mitotic entry.[151] The p53-mediated GADD45-dependent G_2 arrest is induced only after specific types of DNA damage, as lymphocytes from GADD45 knockout mice failed to arrest after exposure to UV radiation but retained the G_2 checkpoint initiated by ionizing radiation.[152] GADD45 can directly inhibit the cyclin B1/cdc2 complex.[153] In addition to direct inhibition of the cyclin B1/cdc2 complex by p21, p53 signaling can also mediate a reduction of cyclin B1 and cdc2 levels.[154-156] The reduced expression of cyclin B1/Cdc2 is mediated in part by p53-dependent transcriptional repression of the cyclin B1 and cdc2 promoters and is RB dependent.[155] The importance of p53-dependent regulation of cdc2 activity is exemplified by the findings that constitutive activation of cyclin B1/cdc2 activity overrides p53-mediated G_2 arrest.[157] Thus, human cells have evolved multiple signaling pathways to establish and maintain a G_2 arrest.

Spindle Checkpoint

The existence of the mitotic checkpoint could be of key importance to trap damaged cells that have escaped the prior checkpoints due to absence of functional upstream sensor or transducer proteins that regulate multiple checkpoint pathways throughout the cell cycle, such as ATM or p53. The mitotic spindle checkpoint monitors spindle microtubule structure, chromosome alignment on the spindle, and chromosome attachment to kinetochores during mitosis (Fig. 5-10).[158] The spindle checkpoint delays the onset of chromosome segregation during anaphase until any defects in the mitotic spindle are corrected. Unattached kinetochores are thought to be the source of the checkpoint signal, and mechanical tension at the kinetochore dictates whether the checkpoint is initiated or not.[159] Activation of the spindle checkpoint prevents mitotic progression through inhibition of the anaphase-promoting complex activator, Cdc20.[160]

Mediators of the spindle checkpoint pathway include the Mad2, Bub1, and Bub3 proteins.[158] Mad2 localizes to the kinetochores during prometaphase until alignment of the chromosomes occurs in metaphase and regulates mitotic exit by interaction with components of the APC machinery (such as Cdc20) that mediate anaphase entry.[72,161] Bub1 and Bub3 also localize to kinetochores and regulate chromosome/kinetochore interactions, and both are required for cell cycle arrest after disruption of microtubule dynamics during mitosis.[72] Expression of a dominant-negative Bub1 in cells abrogated spindle checkpoint function, as cells failed to undergo apoptosis and continued through the cell cycle despite mitotic spindle disruption.[162] Inactivating mutations in Bub1 have been identified in human colon carcinoma cell lines,

suggesting that disruption of the spindle checkpoint could occur during tumor progression.[163] Because aneuploidy is a shared feature of a majority of cancer cells, future studies could reveal that additional components of the spindle checkpoint pathway frequently are altered in tumors.

Integral to cell cycle regulation is the proper coordination of mitotic exit and subsequent S phase entry. After DNA synthesis, cells have a tetraploid (4N) DNA content that is reduced to a diploid (2N) DNA content in each daughter cell after successful completion of mitosis. Intact checkpoint pathways are needed to prevent the S phase entry of cells that have failed to properly segregate their chromosomes during mitosis. Cells with defective spindle checkpoint function can exit from mitosis with a 4N DNA content.[72] These cells can inappropriately continue to the next cell cycle division and, in the absence of a functional G_1/S checkpoint, enter S phase with a 4N DNA content; this process is known as endoreduplication. Endoreduplication results in the generation of polyploid cells—that is, cells with a 4N or greater DNA content after mitotic exit. Cells that are RB-, p53-, p21-, or p16-deficient can endoreduplicate after microtubule inhibitor treatment.[164-168] The G_1 cell cycle regulators, however, do not directly regulate the mitotic arrest induced by microtubule inhibitors; rather, absence of these proteins allows deregulated cdk2 activity, the precise control of which is required for normal cells to maintain proper coupling of mitotic exit and S-phase entry.[167,169] Thus, in addition to playing a role in checkpoint function after DNA damage, proteins that mediate the G_1/S checkpoint through regulation of cdk2 activity also prevent inappropriate S-phase entry after an abnormal mitotic exit and are critical to proper coordination of S phase and mitosis.

CELL CYCLE DYSREGULATION IN HUMAN CANCERS

Molecular analysis of human tumors demonstrates that alterations in components of the cell cycle machinery and checkpoint signaling pathways occur in the majority of human tumors (Table 5-1). This finding underscores how important maintenance of cell cycle control is in the prevention of human cancer. Alterations in the cell cycle machinery that occur most frequently include loss or mutation of the RB tumor suppressor, overexpression of cyclins, cdks, and Cdc25 phosphatases, and loss of expression cdk inhibitors. The most frequently altered cell cycle checkpoint signaling molecule is the p53 tumor suppressor. Proteins that reside upstream of p53 (including ATM and Chk2) are also targeted for mutation in human tumors, and their discovery and analysis have greatly deepened our insight on DNA damage response signaling pathways.

Mutations that affect the RB signaling pathway have been identified in the majority of human cancers.[42] RB function is defective in many human cancers, including retinoblastoma, breast, osteosarcoma, and lung.[170] The RB gene was the first tumor suppressor gene identified, and shortly after validation of the RB gene as the locus that

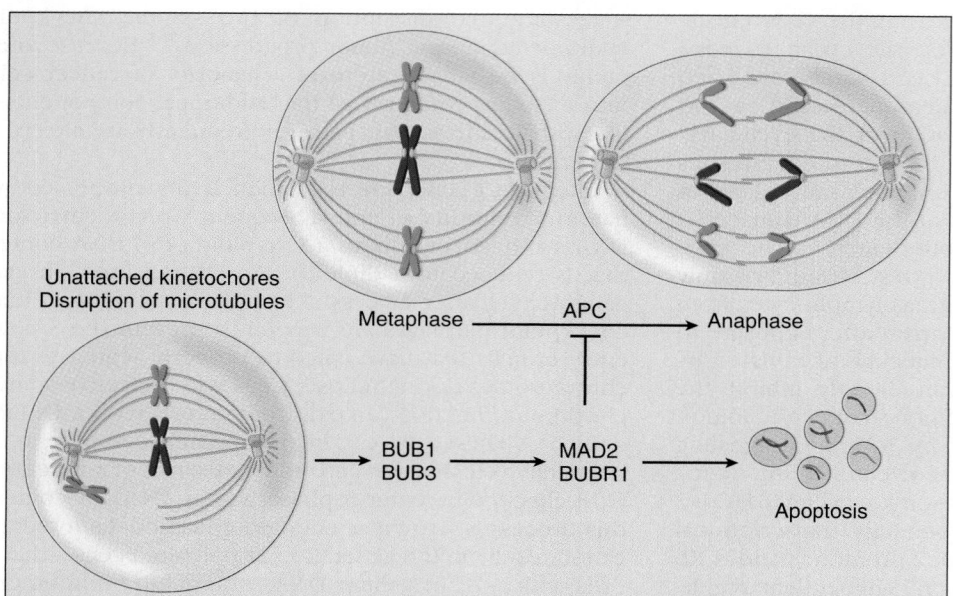

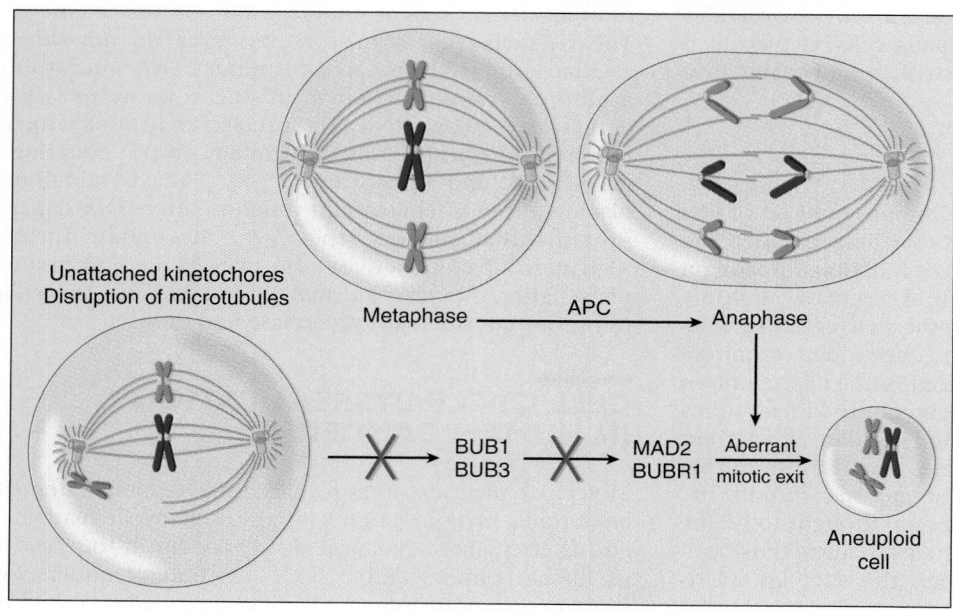

Figure 5-10. The spindle checkpoint. Improper chromosome alignment on the mitotic spindle, disruption of microtubule dynamics, or unattached kinetochores can activate the spindle checkpoint. Spindle checkpoint signaling is mediated by the Bub1, Bub3, BubR1, and Mad2 proteins, all of which localize to kinetochores. **A,** Intact spindle checkpoint signaling induces either metaphase arrest through inhibition of APC or induction of apoptosis. **B,** Defective spindle checkpoint function from either loss of Bub1- and Bub3-dependent signaling or abrogation of Mad2/BubR1-mediated APC inhibition can lead to aberrant mitotic exit and, in the absence of a functional G$_1$/S checkpoint, to the generation of aneuploid cells.

underlies the development of both familial and sporadic retinoblastoma, mutational inactivation of the RB gene was implicated in the etiology of lung cancer, with greater than 90% of small-cell lung cancers having defective RB.[171-173] The evidence linking alterations of RB activity with human lung tumorigenesis is unequivocal. The frequency of RB pathway inactivation in lung cancer is so high that it is reasonable to propose that disruption of this pathway (through the genetic or epigenetic targeting of one RB or upstream signaling components) is a requirement for the genesis of lung cancer.[174] It is important to note that inactivation of the parallel and interconnecting p14^{ARF}/p53 axis is also essential in functionally RB-deficient lung cells to bypass efficient apoptosis.[116]

In breast cancer, loss of normal RB function due to mutation is associated with 20% of tumors.[175] In the 80% of breast carcinomas in which RB gene mutation is not observed, alterations in components of the signaling pathways that regulate RB are frequently found, including cyclin D1 and cyclin E overexpression and cdk4 and cdk6 gene amplification.[170,176,177] Nearly 50% of invasive breast cancers have elevated cyclin D expression compared with surrounding normal breast epithelium, while transgenic mice with overexpression of human cyclin D1 or cyclin E in mammary cells develop mammary adenocarcinomas.[178-180] Similarly, cdk4 and cdk6 gene amplification occur in breast cancers, sarcomas, gliomas, and melanomas.[181]

CHECKPOINTS AND TUMORIGENESIS

To ensure high-fidelity DNA replication and division, mammalian cells have evolved checkpoint signaling pathways that execute several tasks: rapid induction of cell cycle delay, activation of DNA repair, maintenance of cell cycle arrest until repair is complete, reinitiation of cell cycle progression if repair occurred, or initiation of apoptosis if the damage was irreparable. The many checkpoints during the cell cycle provide a fail-safe mechanism by which cells are repaired or eliminated through apoptosis before the damaged DNA is transferred to daughter cells. Although a given individual cell in the human body would not benefit from undergoing apoptosis, this outcome would be highly beneficial to the outcome of the individual in the prevention of tumorigenesis.

Modifications of cdk inhibitors that are upstream regulators of RB activity are also commonly found in human tumors. The cdk inhibitor $p27^{KIP1}$ is often aberrantly expressed in human breast cancer, and reduced $p27^{KIP1}$ protein levels are correlated with more aggressive breast tumors.[127,128] Likewise, decreased expression of the cdk inhibitor $p57^{KIP2}$ is found in human bladder cancers.[182] Germline mutations in $p16^{INK4A}$ predispose individuals to melanoma, while deletion of the $p15^{INK4B}$ and $p16^{INK4A}$ genes is linked to the pathogenesis of lymphomas, mesotheliomas, and pancreatic cancers.[181,183] In tumor types in which $p16^{INK4A}$ and $p15^{INK4B}$ are not deleted, methylation of the gene locus leads to transcriptional repression and loss of gene expression. In some tumors, the hypermethylation-associated inactivation affects both $p16^{INK4a}$ and $p14^{ARF}$, which is encoded by an alternative reading frame of $p16^{INK4a}$.[184]

Both Cdc25A and Cdc25B phosphatases are overexpressed in more than 30% of primary breast tumors, 40% to 60% of non–small-cell lung cancers, 50% of head and neck tumors, and a significant fraction of non-Hodgkin's lymphomas.[185-187] Elevation of these oncogenic phosphatases can result in increased activation of cdk and override of checkpoint arrest. Cdc25B overexpression in a transgenic mouse model system results in increased susceptibility to carcinogen-induced mammary tumors.[188]

p53 gene mutation is the most frequently observed mutation in the majority of human tumors. The importance of p53-dependent signaling in tumor suppression is underscored by the frequency of mutation in sporadic tumors and the finding that germline mutations of the p53 gene result in Li-Fraumeni syndrome, a highly penetrant familial cancer syndrome associated with significantly increased rates of brain tumors, breast cancers, and sarcomas.[189,190] In human tumors that lack p53 gene mutation, p53 function may be disrupted by alterations in cellular proteins that modulate the levels, localization, and biochemical activity of p53. For example, in some tumors with wild-type p53 alleles, MDM2 gene amplification occurs, resulting in MDM2 protein overexpression and

TABLE 5-1

Mutations of Cell Cycle Checkpoint Regulators in Human Tumors*

GENE/PROTEIN	TUMORS ASSOCIATED WITH MUTATIONS OR ALTERED EXPRESSION	HEREDITARY SYNDROMES ASSOCIATED WITH GERMLINE MUTATIONS
ATM	Breast carcinomas, lymphomas, leukemias	Ataxia-telangiectasia
Bub1	Colorectal carcinomas	NR
BRCA1	Breast and ovarian carcinoma	Familial breast and ovarian cancer
Cdc25A	Carcinomas of breast, lung, head and neck, and lymphoma	NR
Cdc25B	Carcinomas of breast, lung, head and neck, and lymphoma	NR
Cdk4	Wide array of cancers	NR
Cdk6	Wide array of cancers	
Chk1	Colorectal and endometrial carcinomas	NR
Chk2	Carcinomas of breast, lung, colon, urogenital tract, and testis	Li-Fraumeni syndrome
Cyclin D1	Wide array of cancers	NR
Cyclin D2	Lymphoma and carcinomas of the colon, testis and ovary	NR
Cyclin D3	Lymphoma, pancreatic carcinoma	NR
Cyclin E	Wide array of cancers	NR
MDM2	Soft tissue tumors, osteosarcomas, esophageal carcinomas	NR
MRE11	Lymphoma	Ataxia-telangiectasia-like disorder
NBS	Lymphomas, leukemias	Nijmegen breakage syndrome
$p15^{INK4B}$	Wide array of cancers	NR
$p16^{INK4A}$	Wide array of cancers	Familial melanoma
$p27^{KIP1}$	Wide array of cancers	NR
p53	Wide array of cancers	Li-Fraumeni syndrome
$p57^{KIP2}$	Bladder carcinomas	NR
p130	Wide array of cancers	NR
RB	Wide array of cancers	Familial retinoblastoma

NR, not reported.
*Only alterations that are present in >10% of primary tumors are represented.

subsequent p53 inactivation.[191] In human papillomavirus-induced cervical carcinoma, the p53 gene is typically not mutated; however, the human papillomavirus E6 protein binds p53 and targets it for degradation, abrogating p53-dependent signaling.[192]

Mutation in components of the DNA damage response pathway also leads to enhanced tumorigenesis as discussed previously. For example, ATM mutations occur in ataxia telangiectasia, a disorder in which patients have increased sensitivity to radiation and an elevated incidence of leukemias, lymphomas, and breast cancer.[92,193] ATM-null mice exhibit growth retardation, neurologic dysfunction, infertility, defective T lymphocyte maturation, and sensitivity to ionizing radiation.[194,195] The majority of ATM-deficient animals develop malignant lymphomas by four months of age, while ATM-/- fibroblasts have abnormal radiation checkpoint function after exposure to ionizing radiation.[194,195] The DNA double-strand break repair gene MRE11 is mutated in individuals with an ataxia-telangiectasia-like disorder.[196] Mutations of Chk2 and Chk1 also arise in human cancers. Chk2 mutations have been reported in several cancers, including lung, while Chk1 mutations have been observed in human colon and endometrial cancers.[197,198] In addition, heterozygous alteration of Chk2 occurs in a subset of individuals with Li-Fraumeni syndrome that lack p53 gene mutations.[199] These findings support the theory that in human tumors where the p53 gene is intact, the function of the tumor suppressor might be disrupted by alterations in cellular proteins that modulate the levels or activity of p53.

Spindle checkpoint disruption has also been linked to the pathogenesis of several human tumors. Bub1 mutations have been identified in human colon carcinoma cells, and Bub1 mutation facilitates the transformation of cells lacking the breast cancer susceptibility gene, BRCA2.[163,200] Recent studies by Michel et al. demonstrate that Mad2 haplo-insufficiency results in significantly elevated rates of lung tumor development in Mad2+/– mice compared with age-matched wild-type mice.[201]

THERAPEUTIC MANIPULATION OF CELL CYCLE CONTROLS

Research over the past two decades has shown that alterations in cell cycle machinery and checkpoint signaling lead to tumorigenesis. These findings have important implications for the optimization of current therapeutic regimens and for the selection of novel cell cycle targets for the future development of anticancer agents. A leading goal of cancer-based research is to identify compounds that will target key cell cycle controls in a highly selective manner.

Targeting DNA Damage Response Proteins

Since many of the anticancer agents currently used clinically target the DNA of the tumor cell, it seems reasonable to build upon the insights gained in recent years of the molecular controls of cellular responses to DNA damage to design novel approaches that would either make tumor cells more sensitive or normal cells less sensitive to these agents. The former result should facilitate tumor cell kill, and the latter result should reduce normal tissue toxicity. For example, building upon the signal transduction pathways initiated by ionizing radiation (see Fig. 5-8), numerous different proteins could theoretically be targeted to enhance the radiation sensitivity of a tumor cell. Because it is easier to conceive of ways to inhibit enzymes like kinases than to restore function to proteins with structural defects, the ATM and Chk2 kinases provide tantalizing targets to alter radiosensitivity. Screens for small molecule inhibitors of these kinases are underway to develop such sensitizing agents. It is recognized that if such inhibitors are given systemically, sensitization of normal tissues could be a problem. But because therapeutic radiation can be delivered locally either with external beam radiation or with brachytherapy (delivered either through seeds or through antibody conjugates), it is easy to conceive of scenarios in which these irradiation treatments would become more effective tumoricidal approaches when used in combination with small molecule inhibitors of these kinases. Similar concepts would apply to almost any molecular target involved in controlling cellular responses to DNA damage. Alternatively, it is conceivable that augmenting cellular responses to DNA damage in normal tissues could reduce the toxicities normally associated with chemotherapy and radiation therapy.

Targeting cdk Activity

Because cdk activity—in particular cdk2 activity—is frequently elevated in human tumors, inhibition of cdk activity is a rational strategy for anticancer therapies. Conceptual and practical problems impact the development and introduction of such drugs for clinical use, however. Cdk2 is active throughout the cell cycle and plays multiple roles in progression through the cell cycle, as described previously. Also, it is likely that these effects differ among different tumor and normal tissues. As a result, inhibition of cdk2 is likely to have highly complex effects. Nonetheless, numerous pharmacological inhibitors of cdks have been developed, and several are in clinical testing.[202] Problems in development of inhibitors have been related to specificity of the agents and unpredictable toxicity profiles. One of the first compounds to be tested, flavopiridol, arrests cancer cells at the G_1/S and G_2/M transitions through inhibition of cdk2, cdk4, and cdc2 kinase activity.[203] Flavopiridol has potent antiproliferative activity against a variety of human cancer cell lines and has produced favorable clinical responses in Phase I and Phase II studies of patients with renal, colorectal, gastric, lung, and esophageal carcinomas.[204-206] Ongoing clinical trials are evaluating flavopiridol in non-Hodgkin's lymphoma and in breast and prostate cancers.[207] The clinical tests of flavopiridol and related chemical cdk inhibitors has spawned further research efforts to design mechanism-based cdk inhibitors through manipulation of the phosphorylation and cyclin-binding sites of cdk proteins. The specificity of cdk inhibitors, however, remains a limiting factor, as severe side effects were experienced by patients in Phase I and Phase II studies. Several studies demonstrate that flavopiridol binds and inactivates cytosolic aldehyde dehydrogenase and glycogen phosphorylase and inhibits global transcription, bringing into question flavopiridol's mechanism of action.[208-210]

Staurosporine is a nonspecific protein kinase inhibitor that can override DNA damage-induced G_2 delay in response to ionizing radiation.[211] The cytotoxicity of staurosporine has limited its potential clinical efficacy, however, leading to the development of staurosporine analogs with improved specificity and reduced cytotoxicity.[212] One such staurosporine derivative, UCN-01, is a cdk2 inhibitor but also a potent abrogator of the G_2 cell cycle checkpoint, and it increases the cytotoxic effect of DNA-damaging agents in human tumor cells.[213,214] UCN-01 significantly inhibits the growth of a variety of human tumors in mice xenograft tumor models and is currently in Phase I clinical trials showing promising results.[215-217] Preclinical studies have provided many mechanistic insights to UCN-01 activity. Treatment of tumor cells with UCN-01 results in Cdc25C activation, although these are indirect effects of UCN-01 inhibition of upstream kinases, including cdk2.[218] UCN-01 inhibits Chk1; however, the related Chk2 kinase and the upstream ATM kinase are refractory to inhibition by UCN-01.[219] As is the case for other cdk inhibitors, a major limitation of UCN-01 is lack of specificity.

New approaches are beginning to address the issue of chemical cdk inhibitor specificity through modification of screening procedures.[220,221] Also, several selective cdk2 inhibitors are currently under development.[202] This avenue of research will continue to reveal novel compounds that will be more potent and selective than those currently available, and it will identify other potential targets of cdk inhibitors that might be beneficial or antagonistic to therapeutic strategies.

Targeting Chromatin-Modifying Enzymes

Although many existing anticancer drugs target kinases involved in cell cycle or checkpoint signaling pathways, other agents are under development that can regulate tumor cell cycle transit through modulation of enzymes that modify the acetylation state of the histones that are an important component of cellular chromatin. Recent studies have identified molecular interaction between the cell-cycle regulatory apparatus and proteins that regulate histone acetylation and deacetylation. For example, RB binds both E2F proteins and histone deacetylase (HDAC) complexes.[222,223] HDACs play an important role in RB transcriptional repression. Acetylation of histones by a number of histone acetyl transfereases (HATs) also plays an integral role in coordinating gene expression required for cell cycle progression. For example, expression of cyclin D requires HAT activity.[224] Several components of the cell cycle and checkpoint machinery described previously are both regulated by HATs and bind directly to HATs (e.g., p53).[225] Cell cycle regulatory kinases can phosphorylate and inactive HDACs, coordinate gene expression, and bind to HATs.

Preclinical studies have shown that inhibiting HDAC activity can induce cell cycle arrest or differentiation in a significant fraction of tumor cell types.[226] Thus, the design of drugs to inhibit histone deacetylase activity has been pursued. These compounds increase the acetylation state of the chromatin, alter chromatin structure, and modulate gene expression required for cell cycle arrest. Histone deacetylase inhibitors can trigger a G_2 arrest in normal human cells; however, this G_2 arrest fails to occur in a diverse range of human tumor cells and they undergo apoptosis.[227] The histone deacetylase inhibitors FR901228 and MS-27-275 have potent in vitro and in vivo anticancer activity, and FR901228 has demonstrated efficacy against T-cell lymphoma in clinical trials.[228-230] Because subsets of HDACs bind and regulate specific sets of genes, it is likely that the identification of select HDAC inhibitors will provide anticancer effects that are selective for given genetic lesions in a tumor cell.

SUMMARY

Over the past several decades, investigators have uncovered a wealth of information about the proteins controlling cell growth and division in human cells. A key finding is that loss of cell cycle checkpoints is a universal alteration identified in human cancer.[231] Although numerous genetic alterations can result in loss of normal checkpoints, the hope is that common strategies will be developed against a wide variety of cancers. Even though several of the currently used anticancer therapies target nonselective and non–mechanism-based targets, their effectiveness, albeit limited in many cases, is likely due to the fact that they ultimately target cell cycle regulatory or DNA damage response signaling pathways, the status of which is different in normal cells vs. tumor cells. Identifying all the components of the cellular machinery that control the cell cycle both positively and negatively is vital to the continued development of anticancer agents that can preferentially eliminate cancer cells and minimize the toxicity to normal tissues. The information generated by the genomic and proteomic approaches using eukaryotic model systems will continue to reveal new cell cycle regulatory molecules. As our understanding of cell cycle regulation and checkpoint signaling increases, the goal is to use this knowledge in the design of mechanism-based therapeutics that will bring anticancer therapy to a new level. There can be little doubt of the value of targeting cell cycle in drug discovery.

REFERENCES

1. Sherr CJ, Roberts JM: CDK inhibitors: Positive and negative regulators of G_1-phase progression. Genes Dev 1999;13:1501–1512.
2. Miller ME, Cross FR: Cyclin specificity: How many wheels do you need on a unicycle? J Cell Sci 2001;114:1811–1820.
3. Morgan DO: Cyclin-dependent kinases: Engines, clocks, and microprocessors. Annu Rev Cell Dev Biol 1997;13:261–291.
4. Matsushime H, Ewen ME, Strom DK, et al: Identification and properties of an atypical catalytic subunit (p34^{PSK-J3}/cdk4) for mammalian D type G1 cyclins. Cell 1992;71:323–334.

5. Xiong Y, Zhang H, Beach D: D type cyclins associate with multiple protein kinases and the DNA replication and repair factor PCNA. Cell 1992;71:505-514.

6. Meyerson M, Harlow E: Identification of G₁ kinase activity for cdk6, a novel cyclin D partner. Mol Cell Biol. 1994;14:2077-2086.

7. Bates S, Bonetta L, MacAllan D, et al: CDK6 (PLSTIRE) and CDK4 (PSK-J3) are a distinct subset of the cyclin-dependent kinases that associate with cyclin D1. Oncogene 1994;9:71-79.

8. Koff A, Cross F, Fisher A, et al: Human cyclin E, a new cyclin that interacts with two members of the CDC2 gene family. Cell 1991;66:1217-1228.

9. Elledge SJ, Spottswood MR: A new human p34 protein kinase, CDK2, identified by complementation of a cdc28 mutation in Saccharomyces cerevisiae, is a homolog of Xenopus Eg1. Embo J 1991;10:2653-2659.

10. Ninomiya-Tsuji J, Nomoto S, Yasuda H, Reed SI, Matsumoto K: Cloning of a human cDNA encoding a CDC2-related kinase by complementation of a budding yeast cdc28 mutation. Proc Natl Acad Sci USA 1991;88:9006-9010.

11. Tsai LH, Harlow E, Meyerson M: Isolation of the human cdk2 gene that encodes the cyclin A- and adenovirus E1A-associated p33 kinase. Nature 1991;353:174-177.

12. Draetta G, Luca F, Westendorf J, Brizuela L, Ruderman J, Beach D: Cdc2 protein kinase is complexed with both cyclin A and B: Evidence for proteolytic inactivation of MPF. Cell 1989;56:829-838.

13. Draetta G, Brizuela L, Potashkin J, Beach D: Identification of p34 and p13, human homologs of the cell cycle regulators of fission yeast encoded by cdc2+ and suc1+. Cell 1987;50:319-325.

14. Draetta G, Beach D: Activation of cdc2 protein kinase during mitosis in human cells: Cell cycle-dependent phosphorylation and subunit rearrangement. Cell 1988;54:17-26.

15. Lee MG, Norbury CJ, Spurr NK, Nurse P: Regulated expression and phosphorylation of a possible mammalian cell-cycle control protein. Nature 1988;333:676-679.

16. Murray A, Hunt T: The Cell Cycle. Oxford, Oxford University Press, 1993.

17. Rolfe M, Chiu MI, Pagano M: The ubiquitin-mediated proteolytic pathway as a therapeutic area. J Mol Med 1997;75:5-17.

18. Sadhu K, Reed SI, Richardson H, Russell P: Human homolog of fission yeast cdc25 mitotic inducer is predominantly expressed in G2. Proc Natl Acad Sci USA 1990;87:5139-5143.

19. Heald R, McLoughlin M, McKeon F: Human wee1 maintains mitotic timing by protecting the nucleus from cytoplasmically activated Cdc2 kinase. Cell 1993;74:463-474.

20. Galaktionov K, Beach D: Specific activation of cdc25 tyrosine phosphatases by B-type cyclins: Evidence for multiple roles of mitotic cyclins. Cell 1991;67:1181-1194.

21. Jinno S, Suto K, Nagata A, et al: Cdc25A is a novel phosphatase functioning early in the cell cycle. Embo J 1994;13:1549-1556.

22. Saha P, Eichbaum Q, Silberman ED, Mayer BJ, Dutta A: p21CIP1 and Cdc25A: Competition between an inhibitor and an activator of cyclin-dependent kinases. Mol Cell Biol 1997;14:4338-4345.

23. Hoffmann I, Draetta G, Karsenti E: Activation of the phosphatase activity of human cdc25A by a cdk2-cyclin E dependent phosphorylation at the G1/S transition. Embo J 1994;13:4302-4310.

24. Blomberg I, Hoffmann I: Ectopic expression of Cdc25A accelerates the G₁/S transition and leads to premature activation of cyclin E- and cyclin A-dependent kinases. Mol Cell Biol 1999;19:6183-6194.

25. Galaktionov K, Chen XC, Beach D: Cdc25 cell-cycle phosphatase as a target of c-*myc*. Nature 1996;382:511-517.

26. Vigo E, Muller H, Prosperini E, et al: CDC25A phosphatase is a target of E2F and is required for efficient E2F-induced S phase. Mol Cell Biol 1999;19:6379-6395.

27. Nilsson I, Hoffmann I: Cell cycle regulation by the Cdc25 phosphatase family. Prog Cell Cycle Res 2000;4:107-114.

28. Lammer C, Wagerer S, Saffrich R, Mertens D, Ansorge W, Hoffmann I: The cdc25B phosphatase is essential for the G2/M phase transition in human cells. J Cell Sci 1998;111:2445-2453.

29. Garner-Hamrick PA, Fisher C: Antisense phosphorothioate oligonucleotides specifically down-regulate cdc25B causing S-phase delay and persistent antiproliferative effects. Int J Cancer 1998;76:720-728.

30. Strausfeld U, Fernandez A, Capony JP, et al: Activation of p34cdc2 protein kinase by microinjection of human cdc25C into mammalian cells. Requirement for prior phosphorylation of cdc25C by p34cdc2 on sites phosphorylated at mitosis. J Biol Chem 1994;269:5989-6000.

31. Karlsson C, Katich S, Hagting A, Hoffmann I, Pines J: Cdc25B and Cdc25C differ markedly in their properties as initiators of mitosis. J Cell Biol 1999;146:573-584.

32. Adams PD: Regulation of the retinoblastoma tumor suppressor protein by cyclin/cdks. Biochim Biophys Acta 2001;1471:M123-M133.

33. Lundberg AS, Weinberg RA: Functional inactivation of the retinoblastoma protein requires sequential modification by at least two distinct cyclin-cdk complexes. Mol Cell Biol 1998;8:753-761.

34. Morris EJ, Dyson NJ: Retinoblastoma protein partners. Adv Cancer Res 2001;82:1-54.

35. Bartek J, Lukas J: Pathways governing G1/S transition and their response to DNA damage. FEBS Lett 2001;490:117-122.

36. Sellers WR, Kaelin WG: pRB as a modulator of transcription. Biochim Biophys Acta 1996;1288:M1-M5.

37. Sladek TL: E2F transcription factor action, regulation, and possible role in human cancer. Cell Prolif 1997;30:97-105.

38. Wang JY: Retinoblastoma protein in growth suppression and death protection. Curr Opin Genet Dev 1997;7:39-45.

39. Harbour JW, Dean DC: The Rb/E2F pathway: Expanding roles and emerging paradigms. Genes Dev 2000;14:2393-2409.

40. Chan HM, Krstic-Demonacos M, Smith L, Demonacos C, La Thangue NB: Acetylation control of the retinoblastoma tumour-suppressor protein. Nat Cell Biol 2001;3:667-674.

41. Knudsen ES, Buckmaster C, Chen TT, Feramisco JR, Wang JYJ: Inhibition of DNA synthesis by RB: Effects on G₁/S transition and S-phase progression. Genes Dev 1998;12:2278-2292.

42. Sellers WR, Kaelin WGJ: Role of the retinoblastoma protein in the pathogenesis of human cancer. J Clin Oncol 1997;15:3301-3312.

43. Diffley JF: Eukaryotic DNA replication. Curr Opin Cell Biol 1994;6:368-372.

44. Rowley A, Dowell SJ, Diffley JF: Recent developments in the initiation of chromosomal DNA replication: a complex picture emerges. Biochim Biophys Acta 1994;1217:239-256.

45. Bell SP, Stillman B: ATP-dependent recognition of eukaryotic origins of DNA replication by a multiprotein complex. Nature 1992;357:128-134.

46. Stillman B, Bell SP, Dutta A, Marahrens Y: DNA replication and the cell cycle. Ciba Found Symp 1992;170:147-156; discussion 156-160.

47. Dutta A, Bell SP: Initiation of DNA replication in eukaryotic cells. Annu Rev Cell Dev Biol 1997;13:293-332.

48. Maine GT, Sinha P, Tye BK: Mutants of S. cerevisiae defective in the maintenance of minichromosomes. Genetics 1984;106:365-385.

49. Tye BK: MCM proteins in DNA replication. Annu Rev Biochem 1999;68:649-686.

50. Nishitani H, Lygerou Z: Control of DNA replication licensing in a cell cycle. Genes Cells 2002;7:523-534.

51. Bell SP, Dutta A: DNA replication in eukaryotic cells. Annu Rev Biochem 2002;71:333-374.

52. Liang C, Stillman B: Persistent initiation of DNA replication and chromatin-bound MCM proteins during the cell cycle in cdc6 mutants. Genes Dev 1997;11:3375-3386.

53. Walter J, Newport J: Initiation of eukaryotic DNA replication: origin unwinding and sequential chromatin association of Cdc45, RPA, and DNA polymerase alpha. Mol Cell 2000;5:617-627.

54. Zou L, Stillman B: Assembly of a complex containing Cdc45p, replication protein A, and Mcm2p at replication origins controlled by S-phase cyclin-dependent kinases and Cdc7p-Dbf4p kinase. Mol Cell Biol 2000;20:3086-3096.

55. Takisawa H, Mimura S, Kubota Y: Eukaryotic DNA replication: from pre-replication complex to initiation complex. Curr Opin Cell Biol 2000;12:690-696.

56. Labib K, Tercero JA, Diffley JF: Uninterrupted MCM2-7 function required for DNA replication fork progression. Science 2000;288:1643-1647.

57. Tercero JA, Labib K, Diffley JF: DNA synthesis at individual replication forks requires the essential initiation factor Cdc45p. Embo J 2000;19:2082-2093.

58. Wuarin J, Nurse P: Regulating S phase: CDKs, licensing and proteolysis. Cell 1996;85:785-787.

59. Diffley JF: Once and only once upon a time: Specifying and regulating origins of DNA replication in eukaryotic cells. Genes Dev 1996;10:2819-2830.

60. Stillman B: Cell cycle control of DNA replication. Science 1996;274:1659-1664.

61. Krek W, Nigg EA: Differential phosphorylation of vertebrate p34cdc2 kinase at the G1/S and G2/M transitions of the cell cycle: Identification of major phosphorylation sites. Embo J 1991;10:305-316.

62. Norbury C, Blow J, Nurse P: Regulatory phosphorylation of the p34cdc2 protein kinase in vertebrates. Embo J 1991;10:3321-3329.

63. Lundgren K, Walworth N, Booher R, Dembski M, Kirschner M, Beach D: Mik1 and wee1 cooperate in the inhibitory tyrosine phosphorylation of cdc2. Science 1991;270:86-90.

64. Parker LL, Piwnica-Worms H: Inactivation of p34^{cdc2}-cyclin B complex by the human WEE1 tyrosine kinase. Science 1992;257:1955-1957.

65. Coleman TR, Dunphy WG: Cdc2 regulatory factors. Curr Opin Cell Biol 1994;6:877-882.

66. Sebastian B, Kakizuka A, Hunter T: Cdc25M2 activation of cyclin-dependent kinases by dephosphorylation of threonine-14 and tyrosine-15. PNAS 1993;90:3521-3524.

67. Hagting A, Karlsson C, Clute P, Jackman M, Pines J: MPF localization is controlled by nuclear export. Embo J 1998;17:4127-4138.

68. Nigg EA: Targets of cyclin-dependent protein kinases. Curr Opin Cell Biol 1993;5:187-193.

69. Peter M, Nakagawa J, Doree M, Labbe JC, Nigg EA: In vitro disassembly of the nuclear lamina and M phase-specific phosphorylation of lamins by cdc2 kinase. Cell 1990;61:591-602.

70. Blangy A, Lane HA, d'Herin P, Harper M, Kress M, Nigg EA: Phosphorylation by p34cdc2 regulates spindle association of human Eg5, a kinesin-related motor essential for bipolar spindle formation in vivo. Cell 1995;83:1159-1169.

71. Yamashiro S, Yamakita Y, Ishikawa R, Matsumura F: Mitosis-specific phosphorylation causes 83K non-muscle caldesmon to dissociate from microfilaments. Nature 1990;344:675-678.

72. Sorger PK, Dobles M, Tournebize R, Hyman AA: Coupling cell division and cell death to microtubule dynamics. Curr Opin Cell Biol 1997;9:807-814.

73. Sunkel CE, Glover DM: Polo, a mitotic mutant of Drosophila displaying abnormal spindle poles. J Cell Sci 1988;89:25-38.

74. Llamazares S, Moreira A, Tavares A, et al: Polo encodes a protein kinase homolog required for mitosis in Drosophila. Genes Dev 1991;5:2153-2165.

75. Glover DM, Hagan IM, Tavares AAM: Polo-like kinases: A team that plays throughout mitosis. Genes Dev 1998;12:3777-3787.

76. Lane HA, Nigg EA: Antibody microinjection reveals an essential role for human Polo-like kinase 1 (Plk1) in the functional maturation of mitotic centrosomes. Nature Med 1996;2:630-631.

77. Kumagai A, Dunphy WG: Purification and molecular cloning of Plx1, a Cdc25-regulatory kinase from Xenopus egg extracts. Science 1996;273:1377-1380.

78. Cohen-Fix O, Koshland D: The metaphase-to-ananphase transition: Avoiding a mid-life crisis. Curr Opin Cell Biol 1997;9:800-806.

79. Morgan DO: Regulation of the APC and the exit from mitosis. Nat Cell Biol 1999;1:E47-E53.

80. Pines J, Hunter T: Human cyclins A and B1 are differentially located in the cell and undergo cell cycle-dependent nuclear transport. J Cell Biol 1991;115:1-17.

81. Gallant P, Nigg EA: Cyclin B2 undergoes cell cycle-dependent nuclear translocation and, when expressed as a non-destructible mutant, causes mitotic arrest in HeLa cells. J Cell Biol 1992;117:213-224.

82. Clute P, Pines J: Temporal and spatial control of cyclin B1 destruction in metaphase. Nat Cell Biol 1999;1:82-87.

83. Funabiki H, Yamano H, Kumada K, Nagao K, Hunt T, Yanagida M: Cut2 proteolysis required for sister-chromatid seperation in fission yeast. Nature 1996;381:438-441.

84. Ciosk R, Zachariae W, Michaelis C, Shevchenko A, Mann M, Nasmyth K: An ESP1/PDS1 complex regulates loss of sister chromatid cohesion at the metaphase to anaphase transition in yeast. Cell 1998;93:1067-1076.

85. Hartwell LH, Weinert TA: Checkpoints: Controls that ensure the order of cell cycle events. Science 1989;246:629-634.

86. Stocker H, Hafen E: Genetic control of cell size. Curr Opin Genet Dev 2000;10:529-535.

87. Zhou BBS, Elledge SJ: The DNA damage response: Putting checkpoints in perspective. Nature 2000;408:433-439.

88. Boddy MN, Russell P: DNA replication checkpoint. Curr Biol 2001;11:R953-R956.

89. Kastan MB, Lim DS: The many substrates and functions of ATM. Nat Rev Mol Cell Biol 2000;1:179-186.

90. Shiloh Y: ATM and ATR: Networking cellular responses to DNA damage. Curr Opin Genet Dev 2001;11:71-77.

91. Abraham RT: Cell cycle checkpoint signaling through the ATM and ATR kinases. Genes Dev 2001;15:2177-2196.

92. Taylor AM, Harnden DG, Arlett CF, et al: Ataxia telangiectasia: a human mutation with abnormal radiation sensitivity. Nature 1975;258:427-429.

93. Painter RB, Young BR: Radiosensitivity in ataxia-telangiectasia: a new explanation. Proc Natl Acad Sci USA 1980;77:7315-7317.

94. Matsuoka S, Rotman G, Ogawa A, Shiloh Y, Tamai K, Elledge SJ: Ataxia telangiectasia-mutated phosphorylates Chk2 in vivo and in vitro. Proc Natl Acad Sci USA 2000;97:10389-10394.

95. Matsuoka S, Huang M, Elledge SJ: Linkage of ATM to cell cycle regulation by the Chk2 protein kinase. Science 1998;282:1893-1897.

96. Liu Q, Guntuku S, Cui XS, et al: Chk1 is an essential kinase that is regulated by Atr and required for the G(2)/M DNA damage checkpoint. Genes Dev 2000;14:1448-1459.

97. Mailand N, Falck J, Lukas C, et al: Rapid destruction of human Cdc25A in response to DNA damage. Science 2000;288:1425-1429.

98. Falck J, Mailand N, Syljuåsen RG, Bartek J, Lukas J: The ATM-Chk2-Cdc25A checkpoint pathway guards against radioresistant DNA synthesis. Nature 2001;410:842-847.

99. Costanzo V, Robertson K, Ying CY, et al: Reconstitution of an ATM-dependent checkpoint that inhibits chromosomal DNA replication following DNA damage. Mol Cell 2000;6:649-659.

100. Kastan MB, Onyekwere O, Sidransky D, Vogelstein B, Craig RW: Participation of p53 protein in the cellular response to DNA damage. Cancer Res 1991;51:6304-6311.

101. Maltzman W, Czyzyk L: UV irradiation stimulates levels of p53 cellular tumor antigen in nontransformed mouse cells. Mol Cell Biol 1984;4:1689-1694.

102. Reich NC, Oren M, Levine AJ: Two distinct mechanisms regulate the levels of a cellular tumor antigen, p53. Mol Cell Biol 1983;3:2143-2150.

103. Reich NC, Levine AJ: Growth regulation of a cellular tumour antigen, p53, in nontransformed cells. Nature 1984;308:199-201.

104. Reihsaus E, Kohler M, Kraiss S, Oren M, Montenarh M: Regulation of the level of the oncoprotein p53 in non-transformed and transformed cells. Oncogene 1990;5:137-145.

105. Jones SN, Roe AE, Donehower LA, Bradley A: Rescue of embryonic lethality in Mdm2-deficient mice by absence of p53. Nature 1995;378:206-208.

106. Luna RMD, Wagner DS, Lozano G: Rescue of early embryonic lethality in mdm2-deficient mice by deletion of p53. Nature 1995;378:203-206.

107. Harper JW, Adami GR, Wei N, Keyomarsi K, Elledge SJ: The p21 Cdk-interacting protein Cip1 is a potent inhibitor of G1 cyclin-dependent kinases. Cell 1993;75:805-816.

108. Deng CX, Zhang PM, Harper JW, Elledge SJ, Leder P: Mice lacking p21$^{CIP1/WAF1}$ undergo normal development, but are defective in G1 checkpoint control. Cell 1995;82:675-684.

109. El-Deiry WS, Tokino T, Velculescu VE, et al: WAF1, a potential mediator of p53 tumor suppression. Cell 1993;75:817-825.

110. Waldman T, Kinzler KW, Vogelstein B: p21 is necessary for the p53-mediated G$_1$ arrest in human cancer cells. Cancer Res 1995;55:5187-5190.

111. Serrano M, Hannon GJ, Beach D: A new regulatory motif in cell-cycle control causing specific inhibition of cyclin D/CDK4. Nature 1993;366:704-707.

112. Quelle DE, Zindy F, Ashmun RA, Sherr CJ: Alternative reading frames of the INK4a tumor suppressor gene encode two unrelated proteins capable of inducing cell cycle arrest. Cell 1995;83:993–1000.

113. Zhang YP, Xiong Y, Yarbrough WG: ARF promotes MDM2 degradation and stabilizes p53: ARF-INK4a locus deletion impairs both the Rb and p53 tumor suppression pathways. Cell 1998;92:725–734.

114. Pomerantz J, Schreiber-Agus N, Liegeois NJ, et al: The Ink4a tumor suppressor gene product, p19^Arf, interacts with MDM2 and neutralizes MDM2's inhibition of p53. Cell 1998;92:713–723.

115. Kamijo T, Weber JD, Zambetti G, Zindy F, Roussel MF, Sherr CJ: Functional and physical interactions of the ARF tumor suppressor with p53 and Mdm2. Proc Natl Acad Sci USA 1998;95:8292–8297.

116. Sherr CJ: The INK4a/ARF network in tumour suppression. Nat Rev Mol Cell Biol 2001;2:731–737.

117. De Stanchina E, McCurrach ME, Zindy F, et al: E1A signaling to p53 involves the p19^ARF tumor suppressor. Genes Dev 1998;12:2434–2442.

118. Zindy F, Eischen CM, Randle DH, et al: Myc signaling via the ARF tumor suppressor regulates p53-dependent apoptosis and immortalization. Genes Dev 1998;12:2424–2433.

119. Palmero I, Pantoja C, Serrano M: p19^ARF links the tumour suppressor p53 to Ras. Nature 1998;395:125–126.

120. Kamijo T, Zindy F, Roussel MF, et al: Tumor suppression at the mouse INK4a locus mediated by the alternative reading frame product p19^ARF. Cell 1997;91:649–659.

121. Sherr CJ: Tumor surveillance via the ARF-p53 pathway. Genes and Development 1998;12:2984–2991.

122. Pantoja C, Serrano M: Murine fibroblasts lacking p21 undergo senescence and are resistant to transformation by oncogenic Ras. Oncogene 1999;18:4974–4982.

123. Modestou M, Puig-Antich V, Korgaonkar C, Eapen A, Quelle DE: The alternative reading frame tumor suppressor inhibits growth through p21-dependent and p21-independent pathways. Cancer Res 2001;61:3145–3150.

124. Weber JD, Jeffers JR, Rehg JE, et al: p53-independent functions of the p19^ARF tumor suppressor. Genes Dev 2000;14:2358–2365.

125. Pavey S, Conroy S, Russell T, Gabrielli B: Ultraviolet radiation induces p16CDKN2A expression in human skin. Cancer Res 1999;59:4185–4189.

126. Sharpless NE, DePinho RA: The INK4A/ARF locus and its two gene products. Curr Opin Gen 1999;9:22–30.

127. Porter PL, Malone KE, Heagerty PJ, et al: Expression of cell-cycle regulators p27Kip1 and cyclin E, alone and in combination, correlate with survival in young breast cancer patients. Nature Med 1997;3:222–225.

128. Catzavelos C, Bhattacharya N, Ung YC, et al: Decreased levels of the cell-cycle inhibitor p27^kip1 protein: Prognostic implications in primary breast cancer. Nat Med 1997;3:227–230.

129. Liang J, Zubovitz J, Petrocelli T, et al: PKB/Akt phosphorylates p27, impairs nuclear import of p27 and opposes p27-mediated G1 arrest. Nat Med 2002;8:1153–1160.

130. Viglietto G, Motti ML, Bruni P, et al: Cytoplasmic relocalization and inhibition of the cyclin-dependent kinase inhibitor p27^Kip1 by PKB/Akt-mediated phosphorylation in breast cancer. Nat Med 2002;8:1136–1144.

131. Bakkenist CJ, Kastan MB: DNA damage activates ATM through intermolecular autophosphorylation and dimer dissociation. Nature 2003;421:499–506.

132. Shiloh Y, Kastan MB: ATM: genome stability, neuronal development, and cancer cross paths. Adv Cancer Res 2001;83:209–254.

133. Lim DS, Kim ST, Xu B, et al: ATM phosphorylates p95/nbs1 in an S-phase checkpoint pathway. Nature 2000;404:613–614.

134. Wu X, Ranganathan V, Weisman DS, et al: ATM phosphorylation of Nijmegen breakage syndrome protein is required in a DNA damage response. Nature 2000;405:477–482.

135. Zhou BB, Chaturvedi P, Spring K, et al: Caffeine abolishes the mammalian G2/M DNA damage checkpoint by inhibiting ataxia-telangiectasia-mutated kinase activity. J Biol Chem 2000;275:10342–10348.

136. Taniguchi T, Garcia-Higuera I, Xu B, et al: Convergence of the fanconi anemia and ataxia telangiectasia signaling pathways. Cell 2002;109:459–472.

137. Kim ST, Xu B, Kastan MB: Involvement of the cohesin protein, Smc1, in Atm-dependent and independent responses to DNA damage. Genes Dev 2002;16:560–570.

138. Yazdi PT, Wang Y, Zhao S, Patel N, Lee EY, Qin J: SMC1 is a downstream effector in the ATM/NBS1 branch of the human S-phase checkpoint. Genes Dev 2002;16:571–582.

139. Xu B, O'Donnell AH, Kim ST, Kastan MB: Phosphorylation of serine 1387 in Brca1 is specifically required for the Atm-mediated S-phase checkpoint after ionizing irradiation. Cancer Res 2002;62:4588–4591.

140. Hwang A, Muschell RJ: Radiation and the G2 phase of the cell cycle. Radiat Res 1998;150:S52–S59.

141. Jin P, Gu Y, Morgan DO: Role of inhibitory CDC2 phosphorylation in radiation-induced G2 arrest in human cells. J Cell Biol 1996;134:963–970.

142. Matsuoka S, Huang M, Elledge SJ: Linkage of ATM to cell cycle regulation by the Chk2 protein kinase. Science 1998;282:1893–1897.

143. Sanchez Y, Wong S, Thoma RS, et al: Conservation of the Chk1 checkpoint pathway in mammals: Linkage of DNA damage to Cdk regulation through Cdc25C. Science 1997;277:1497–1501.

144. Furnari B, Rhind N, Russell P: Cdc25C mitotic inducer targeted by Chk1 DNA damage checkpoint kinase. Science 1997;277:1495–1497.

145. Peng CY, Graves PR, Thoma RS, Wu ZQ, Shaw AS, Piwnica-Worms H: Mitotic and G2 checkpoint control: Regulation of 14-3-3 protein binding by phosphorylation of Cdc25C on serine-216. Science 1997;277:1501–1505.

146. Smits VAJ, Medema RH: Checking out the G2/M transition. Biochim Biophys Acta Gene Struct Expr 2001;1519:1–12.

147. Lopez-Girona A, Furnari B, Mondesert O, Russell P: Nuclear localization of Cdc25C is regulated by DNA damage and a 14-3-3 protein. Nature 1999;397:172–175.

148. Smits VAJ, Klompmaker R, Arnaud L, Rijksen G, Nigg EA, Medema RH: Polo-like kinase-1 is a target of the DNA damage checkpoint. Nat Cell Biol 2000;2:672–676.

149. Bunz F, Dutriaux A, Lengauer C, et al: Requirement for p53 and p21 to sustain G2 arrest after DNA damage. Science 1998;282:1497–1501.

150. Innocente SA, Abrahamson JLA, Cogswell JP, Lee JM: p53 regulates a G2 checkpoint through cyclin B1. Proc Natl Acad Sci USA 1999;96:2147–2152.

151. Chan TA, Hermeking H, Lengauer C, Kinzler KW, Vogelstein B: 14-3-3Sigma is required to prevent mitotic catastrophe after DNA damage. Nature 1999;401:616–620.

152. Wang XW, Zhan QM, Coursen JD, et al: GADD45 induction of a G2/M cell cycle checkpoint. Proc Natl Acad Sci USA 1999;96:3706–3711.

153. Zhan QM, Antinore MJ, Wang XW, et al: Association with Cdc2 and inhibition of Cdc2/cyclin B1 kinase activity by the p53-regulated protein Gadd45. Oncogene 1999;18:2892–2900.

154. Innocente SA, Abrahamson JL, Cogswell JP, Lee JM: p53 regulates a G2 checkpoint through cyclin B1. Proc Natl Acad Sci USA 1999;96:2147–2152.

155. Flatt PM, Tang LJ, Scatena CD, Szak ST, Pietenpol JA: p53 regulation of G2 checkpoint is retinoblastoma protein dependent. Mol Cell Biol 2000;20:4210–4223.

156. Badie C, Bourhis J, Sobczak-Thépot J, et al: p53-dependent G2 arrest associated with a decrease in cyclins A2 and B1 levels in a human carcinoma cell line. Br J Cancer 2000;82:642–650.

157. Park M, Chae HD, Yun J, et al: Constitutive activation of cyclin B1-associated cdc2 kinase overrides p53-mediated G2-M arrest. Cancer Res 2000;60:542–545.

158. Burke DJ: Complexity in the spindle checkpoint. Curr Opin Genet Dev 2000;10:26–31.

159. Gorbsky GJ: The mitotic spindle checkpoint. Curr Biol 2001;11:R1001–R1004.

160. Kim SH, Lin DP, Matsumoto S, Kitazono A, Matsumoto T: Fission yeast Slp1: An effector of the Mad2-dependent spindle checkpoint. Science 1998;279:1045–1047.

161. Fang GW, Yu HT, Kirschner MW: The checkpoint protein MAD2 and the mitotic regulator CDC20 form a ternary complex with the anaphase-promoting complex to control anaphase initiation. Genes Dev 1998;12:1871–1883.

162. Taylor SS, McKeon F: Kinetochore localization of murine Bub1 is required for normal mitotic timing and checkpoint response to spindle damage. Cell 1997;89:727–735.

163. Cahill DP, Lengauer C, Yu J, et al: Mutations of mitotic checkpoint genes in human cancers. Nature 1998;392:300–303.

164. Cross SM, Sanchez CA, Morgan CA, et al: A p53-dependent mouse spindle checkpoint. Science 1995;267:1353–1356.

165. Khan SH, Wahl GM: p53 and pRb prevent rereplication in response to microtubule inhibitors by mediating a reversible G_1 arrest. Cancer Res 1998;58:396–401.

166. Pellegata NS, Antoniono RJ, Redpath JL, Stanbridge EJ: DNA damage and p53-mediated cell cycle arrest: A re-evaluation. Proc Natl Acad Sci USA 1996;93:15209–15214.

167. Stewart ZA, Leach SD, Pietenpol JA: p21[Waf1/Cip1] inhibition of cyclin E/Cdk2 activity prevents endoreduplication after mitotic spindle disruption. Mol Cell Biol 1999;19:205–215.

168. Di Leonardo A, Khan SH, Linke SP, Greco V, Seidita G, Wahl GM: DNA rereplication in the presence of mitotic spindle inhibitors in human and mouse fibroblasts lacking either p53 or pRb function. Cancer Res 1997;57:1013–1019.

169. Lanni JS, Jacks TS: Characterization of the p53-dependent postmitotic checkpoint following spindle disruption. Mol Cell Biol 1998;18:1055–1064.

170. Zheng L, Lee WH: The retinoblastoma gene: A prototypic and multifunctional tumor suppressor. Exp Cell Res 2001;264:2–18.

171. Friend SH, Bernards R, Rogelj S, et al: A human DNA segment with properties of the gene that predisposes to retinoblastoma and osteosarcoma. Nature 1986;323:643–646.

172. Lee W-H, Bookstein R, Hong F, Young L-J, Shew J-Y, Lee EV-HP: Human retinoblastoma susceptibility gene: Cloning, identification, and sequence. Science 1987;235:1394–1399.

173. Harbour JW, Lai S-L, Whang-Peng J, Gazdar AF, Minna JD, Kaye FJ: Abnormalities in structure and expression of the human retinoblastoma gene in SCLC. Science 1988;241:353–357.

174. Kaye FJ: RB and cyclin dependent kinase pathways: Defining a distinction between RB and p16 loss in lung cancer. Oncogene 2002;21:6908–6914.

175. Varley JM, Armour J, Swallow JE, et al: The retinoblastoma gene is frequently altered leading to loss of expression in primary breast tumours. Oncogene 1989;4:725–729.

176. Nobori T, Miura K, Wu DJ, Lois A, Takabayashi K, Carson DA: Deletions of the cyclin-dependent kinase-4 inhibitor gene in multiple human cancers. Nature 1994;368:753–756.

177. Ravaioli A, Bagli L, Zucchini A, Monti F: Prognosis and prediction of response in breast cancer: The current role of the main biological markers. Cell Prolif 1998;31:113–126.

178. Weinstat-Saslow DW, Merino MJ, Manrow RE, et al: Overexpression of cyclin D mRNA distinguishes invasive and in situ breast carcinomas from non-malignant lesions. Nature Med 1995;1:1257–1260.

179. Wang TC, Cardiff RD, Zukerberg L, Lees E, Arnold A, Schmidt EV: Mammary hyperplasia and carcinoma in MMTV-cyclin D1 transgenic mice. Nature 1994;369:669–671.

180. Bortner DM, Rosenberg MP: Induction of mammary gland hyperplasia and carcinomas in transgenic mice expressing human cyclin E. Mol Cell Biol 1997;17:453–459.

181. Elsayed YA, Sausville EA: Selected novel anticancer treatments targeting cell signaling proteins. The Oncologist 2001;6:517–537.

182. Oya M, Schulz WA: Decreased expression of p57(KIP2)mRNA in human bladder cancer. Br J Cancer 2000;83:626–631.

183. Cannon-Albright LA, Goldgar DE, Meyer LJ, et al: Assignment of a locus for familial melanoma, MLM, to chromosome 9p13-p22. Science 1992;258:1148–1152.

184. Esteller M, Herman JG: Cancer as an epigenetic disease: DNA methylation and chromatin alterations in human tumours. J Pathol 2002;196:1–7.

185. Galaktionov K, Lee AK, Eckstein J, et al: CDC25 phosphatases as potential human oncogenes. Science 1995;269:1575–1577.

186. Wu W, Fan YH, Kemp BL, Walsh G, Mao L: Overexpression of cdc25A and cdc25B is frequent in primary non-small cell lung cancer but is not associated with overexpression of c-myc. Cancer Res 1998;58:4082–4085.

187. Gasparotto D, Maestro R, Piccinin S, et al: Overexpression of CDC25A and CDC25B in head and neck cancers. Cancer Res 1997;57:2366–2368.

188. Yao Y, Slosberg ED, Wang L, et al: Increased susceptibility to carcinogen-induced mammary tumors in MMTV-Cdc25B transgenic mice. Oncogene 1999;18:5196–5166.

189. Nigro JM, Baker SJ, Preisinger AC, et al: Mutations in the p53 gene occur in diverse human tumour types. Nature 1989;342:705–708.

190. Ozbun MA, Butel JS: Tumor suppressor p53 mutations and breast cancer: A critical analysis. Adv Cancer Res 1995;66:71–142.

191. Momand J, Jung D, Wilczynski S, Niland J: The MDM2 gene amplification database. Nucl Acids Res 1998;26:3453–3459.

192. Scheffner M, Werness BA, Hulbregtse JM, Levine AJ, Howley PM: The E6 oncoprotein encoded by human papillomavirus types 16 and 18 promotes the degradation of p53. Cell 1990;63:1129–1136.

193. Khanna KK: Cancer risk and the ATM gene: A continuing debate. J Natl Cancer Inst 2000;92:795–802.

194. Barlow C, Hirotsune S, Paylor R, et al: ATM-deficient mice: A paradigm of ataxia telangiectasia. Cell 1996;86:159–171.

195. Xu Y, Ashley T, Brainerd EE, Bronson RT, Meyn MS, Baltimore D: Targeted disruption of ATM leads to growth retardation, chromosomal fragmentation during meiosis, immune defects, and thymic lymphoma. Genes Dev 1996;10:2411–2422.

196. Baker FL, Sanger LJ, Rodgers RW, Jabboury K, Mangini OR: Cell proliferation kinetics of normal and tumour tissue in vitro: Quiescent reproductive cells and the cycling reproductive fraction. Cell Prolif 1995;28:1–15.

197. Matsuoka S, Nakagawa T, Masuda A, Haruki N, Elledge SJ, Takahashi T: Reduced expression and impaired kinase activity of a Chk2 mutant identified in human lung cancer. Cancer Res 2001;61:5362–5365.

198. Bertoni F, Codegoni AM, Furlan D, Tibiletti MG, Capella C, Broggini M: CHK1 frameshift mutations in genetically unstable colorectal and endometrial cancers. Genes Chrom Cancer 1999;26:176–180.

199. Bell DW, Varley JM, Szydlo TE, et al: Heterozygous germ line hCHK2 mutations in Li-Fraumeni syndrome. Science 1999;286:2528–2531.

200. Lee H, Trainer AH, Friedman LS, et al: Mitotic checkpoint inactivation fosters transformation in cells lacking the breast cancer susceptibility gene, Brca2. Mol Cell 1999;4:1–10.

201. Michel LS, Liberal V, Chatterjee A, et al: MAD2 haplo-insufficiency causes premature anaphase and chromosome instability in mammalian cells. Nature 2001;409:355–359.

202. Wadler S: Perspectives for cancer therapies with cdk2 inhibitors. Drug Resist Updat 2001;4:347–367.

203. Buolamwini JK: Cell cycle molecular targets in novel anticancer drug discovery. Curr Pharm Des 2000;6:379–392.

204. Senderowicz AM: Flavopiridol: The first cyclin-dependent kinase inhibitor in human clinical trials. Invest New Drugs 1999;17:313–320.

205. Stadler WM, Vogelzang NJ, Amato R, et al: Flavopiridol, a novel cyclin-dependent kinase inhibitor, in metastatic renal cancer: A University of Chicago Phase II Consortium study. J Clin Oncol 2000;18:371–375.

206. Schwartz GK, Ilson D, Saltz L, et al: Phase II study of the cyclin-dependent kinase inhibitor flavopiridol administered to patients with advanced gastric carcinoma. J Clin Oncol 2001;19:1985–1992.

207. Sausville EA, Johnson J, Alley M, Zaharevitz D, Senderowicz AM: Inhibition of CDKs as a therapeutic modality. Ann NY Acad Sci 2000;910:207–222.

208. Schnier JB, Kaur G, Kaiser A, et al: Identification of cytosolic aldehyde dehydrogenase 1 from non-small cell lung carcinoma as a flavopiridol-binding protein. FEBS Letters 1999;454:100–104.

209. Oikonomakos NG, Schnier JB, Zographos SE, Skamnaki VT, Tsitsanou KE, Johnson LN: Flavopiridol inhibits glycogen phosphorylase by binding at the inhibitor site. J Biol Chem 2000;275:34566–34573.

210. Lam LT, Pickeral OK, Peng AC, et al: Genomic-scale measurement of mRNA turnover and the mechanisms of action of the anti-cancer drug flavopiridol. Genome Biology 2001;2:Research–41.

211. Tam SW, Schlegel R: Staurosporine overrides checkpoints for mitotic onset in BHK cells. Cell Growth Diff 1992;3:811–817.

212. Courage C, Snowden R, Gescher A: Differential effects of staurosporine analogues on cell cycle, growth, and viability in A549 cells. Br J Cancer 1996;74:1199–1205.

213. Wang Q, Fan S, Eastman A, Worland PJ, Sausville EA, O'Connor PM: UCN-01: A potent abrogator of G2 checkpoint function in cancer cells with disrupted p53. J Natl Cancer Inst 1996;88:956–965.

214. Bunch RT, Eastman A: Enhancement of cisplatin-induced cytotoxicity by 7-hydroxystaurosporine (UCN-01), a new G2-checkpoint inhibitor. Clin Cancer Res 1996;2:791–797.

215. Akinga S, Gomi K, Morimoto M, Tamaoki T, Okabe M: Antitumor activity of UCN-01, a selective inhibitor of protein kinase C, in murine and human tumor models. Cancer Res 1991;51:4888–4892.

216. Akinga S, Nomura K, Gomi K, Okabe M: Enhancement of antitumor activity of mitomycin C in vitro and in vivo by UCN-01, a selective inhibitor of protein kinase C. Cancer Chemother Pharmacol 1993;32:183–189.

217. Senderowicz AM, Sausville EA: Preclinical and clinical development of cyclin-dependent kinase modulators. J Natl Cancer Inst 2000;92:376–387.

218. Yu L, Orlandi L, Wang P, et al: UCN-01 abrogates G2 arrrest through a cdc2-dependent pathway that is associated with inactivation of the Wee1Hu kinase and activation of the cdc25c phosphatase. J Biol Chem 1998;273:33455–33464.

219. Graves PR, Yu LJ, Schwarz JK, et al: The Chk1 protein kinase and the Cdc25C regulatory pathways are targets of the anticancer agent UCN-01. J Biol Chem 2000;275:5600–5605.

220. Knockaert M, Greengard P, Meijer L: Pharmacological inhibitors of cyclin-dependent kinases. Trends Pharmacol Sci 2002;23:417–425.

221. Knockaert M, Meijer L: Identifying in vivo targets of cyclin-dependent kinase inhibitors by affinity chromatography. Biochem Pharmacol 2002;64:819–825.

222. Magnaghi-Jaulin L, Groisman R, Naguibneva I, et al: Retinoblastoma protein represses transcription by recruiting a histone deacetylase. Nature 1998;391:601–605.

223. Brehm A, Miska EA, McCance DJ, Reid JL, Bannister AJ, Kouzarides T: Retinoblastoma protein recruits histone deacetylase to repress transcription. Nature 1998;391:597–601.

224. Albanese C, D'Amico M, Reutens AT, et al: Activation of the cyclin D1 gene by the E1A-associated protein p300 through AP-1 inhibits cellular apoptosis. J Biol Chem 1999;274:34186–34195.

225. Gu W, Roeder RG: Activation of p53 sequence-specific DNA binding by acetylation of the p53 C-terminal domain. Cell 1997;90:595–606.

226. Wang C, Fu M, Mani S, Wadler S, Senderowicz AM, Pestell RG: Histone acetylation and the cell-cycle in cancer. Front Biosci 2001;6:D610–D629.

227. Ling Q, Burgess A, Fairlie DP, Leonard H, Parsons PG, Gabrielli BG: Histone deacetylase inhibitors trigger a G2 checkpoint in normal cells that is defective in tumor cells. Mol Biol Cell 2000;11:2069–2083.

228. Nakajima H, Kim YB, Terano H, Yoshida M, Horinouchi S: FR901228, a potent antitumor antibiotic, is a novel histone deacetylase inhibitor. Exp Cell Res 1998;241:126–133.

229. Saito A, Yamashita T, Mariko Y, et al: A synthetic inhibitor of histone deacetylase, MS-27-275, with marked in vivo antitumor activity against human tumors. Proc Natl Acad Sci USA 1999;96:4592–4597.

230. Piekarz RL, Robey R, Sandor V, et al: Inhibitor of histone deacetylation, depsipeptide (FR901228), in the treatment of peripheral and cutaneous T-cell lymphoma: A case report. Blood 2001;98:2865–2868.

231. Hartwell LH, Kastan MB: Cell cycle control and cancer. Science 1994;266:1821–1828.

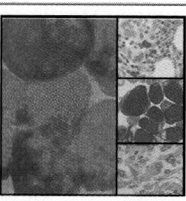

6

CELL LIFE AND CELL DEATH

Rebecca L. Elstrom

Craig B. Thompson

SUMMARY OF KEY POINTS

- Apoptosis control mechanisms appear to be impaired in virtually all tumors, suggesting that a required step in carcinogenesis is to disengage the apoptotic machinery.
- Two basic pathways of apoptosis have been described: the extrinsic or death receptor-mediated pathway

and the intrinsic or mitochondrial pathway.
- The fate of a cell is determined by the balance of proapoptotic and antiapoptotic factors within the cell.
- Oncogenic transformation promotes proapoptotic pathways. Cancer cells must disable tumor suppressor

molecules and/or activate survival signals to evade programmed cell death.
- Therapeutic strategies aimed at restoring tumor suppressors and interfering with survival factors are playing increasingly important roles in antineoplastic treatments.

INTRODUCTION

The evolution of a normal cell into cancer involves disruption and deregulation of a number of basic cellular processes. Multicellular organisms, in their evolution from simple, single cells, have developed redundant controls through which the homeostasis between different cell types is maintained. One of the safeguards that prevents excess cell accumulation is a cell-intrinsic program that can induce cell death through apoptosis. The growing understanding that transforming mutations can activate this intrinsic apoptotic response has emphasized the importance of this process in preventing cancer cell development. Apoptosis control mechanisms appear to be impaired in virtually all tumors, suggesting that a required step in carcinogenesis is to disengage the apoptotic machinery.

The concept that genes regulating cell death could play a role in tumorigenesis arose in the mid-1980s, when investigators first discovered that a translocation commonly found in follicular lymphoma, between chromosomes 14 and 18, brings a region on chromosome 18 called breakpoint cluster region 2 (Bcl-2) into close proximity with the immunoglobulin heavy chain enhancer on chromosome 14, resulting in overexpression of the Bcl-2 gene.[1] Later work showed that the Bcl-2 gene product promotes oncogenesis by a novel mechanism.[2,3] Instead of inducing cell proliferation or invasion, the Bcl-2 protein inhibits the normal programmed cell death of B cells, resulting in the failure to eliminate the clonal B cells as they accumulate in excess. These findings demonstrated for the first time that disarming death pathways within a cell could predispose to development of malignancy.

Since the description of Bcl-2, extensive progress has been made in understanding both the mechanisms of apoptosis and the ways in which this process contributes to tumorigenesis. The identification of a family of genes related to Bcl-2 that contribute to the balance between life

and death, together with the discovery of the critical role of mitochondria in cellular homeostasis and apoptosis, have broadened our understanding of the dynamic interplay of forces determining the fate of cells. Harnessing these forces will improve our capability not only to understand the mechanisms by which normal cells become malignant but also to prevent and treat cancer in humans.

FUNDAMENTAL SCIENCE

The process of apoptosis involves a cell-intrinsic suicide program that not only kills the cell but also stimulates the clearance and complete degradation of the corpse without inducing an inflammatory reaction. Apoptosis differs from other forms of cell death, such as necrosis, in that clearance of the cell is controlled through the activity of caspases—cysteine proteases with aspartate specificity that normally exist in an inactive, zymogen form. The initiator caspases 8 and 9 are activated by cellular signals (to be discussed shortly) and subsequently cleave downstream effector caspases, such as caspases 3, 6, and 7. These effector caspases set into motion the degradation of cellular components such as structural proteins, cell cycle machinery, and DNA. These processes result in the characteristic morphology of apoptotic cells, membrane blebbing, cell shrinkage, and DNA fragmentation. The end result is the disposal of the cell in a controlled manner, allowing turnover and phagocytosis without the inflammatory reaction to intracellular substances that accompanies death by necrosis.

As noted in the preceding discussion, the caspase cascade is initiated through specific cellular signals. These signals come through one of two major pathways: the extrinsic, receptor-mediated pathway, or the intrinsic, mitochondrial pathway. Although these pathways often are considered separately, extensive cross-talk exists between them.

Cell Death by Murder

In some cases, apoptosis is initiated through ligation of specific cell-surface receptors, the death receptors (Fig. 6-1). These molecules are members of the tumor necrosis factor receptor (TNFR) family. The best studied of these include Fas and TNFR1.[4,5] These receptors exist as trimers at the cell surface, which are activated on binding of ligand, Fas ligand (FasL) and TNF, respectively. The intracellular domains of these receptors contain death domains which, on activation of the receptor, can recruit a Death-Inducing Signaling Complex (DISC), which leads to activation of a caspase cascade. The Fas death domain binds the Fas-associated death domain (FADD) adapter protein, which directly recruits caspase 8 and allows its cleavage and activation.

Activation of TNFR1, on the other hand, has multiple potential downstream effects.[6] TNFR1 binds the TNF receptor-associated death domain (TRADD) adapter protein, which in turn might recruit FADD, resulting in caspase 8 activation and apoptosis, as with Fas. TRADD also, however, can bind TNF-Receptor Associated Factor-2 (TRAF-2), which may recruit inhibitor of apoptosis proteins (IAPs), which bind the DISC and inhibit activation of caspase 8. Alternatively, TRAF-2 may recruit components of the mitogen-activated protein kinase (MAPK) cascade, leading to activation of Jun-N-terminal kinase (JNK) and c-jun. Although in some systems JNK appears to promote TNFR1-induced apoptosis, these findings are inconsistent, and the role of JNK in receptor-mediated apoptosis is controversial. Finally, TRADD can bind receptor-interacting protein (RIP), resulting in activation of NF-kB, which antagonizes the apoptotic program. NF-kB is a transcription factor that activates expression of survival molecules such as inhibitor of apoptosis proteins (IAPs) and c-FLIP, a direct inhibitor of caspase 8 activation.[7] IAPs were first described in baculoviruses, where they were shown to inhibit apoptosis of host cells following viral infection.[8] Homologues such as XIAP and c-IAP-1 and -2 have since been identified in mammals; they appear to function by binding and inhibiting caspase activation in both the death receptor and mitochondrial pathways.[9-11]

Another ligand/receptor pair that is increasingly understood to play a role in both immune regulation and control of cancer is the TNF-related apoptosis inducing ligand, TRAIL, and its receptors, TRAIL-R1/DR4 and TRAIL-R2/DR5.[12,13] TRAIL induces apoptosis in a variety of transformed cells but is much less toxic to normal cells than to abnormal ones. The intracellular signaling pathways induced by TRAIL are similar to those of the TNFR1. TRAIL is expressed as a cell surface molecule on NK cells, and it has been shown in some models to inhibit tumor growth.[14] TRAIL might also bind to decoy receptors TRAIL-R3/DcR1 and TRAIL-R4/DcR2. These decoy receptors sequester TRAIL from the signaling receptors, blocking TRAIL-induced apoptosis.[15,16] Expression of these decoy receptors might provide the mechanism by which normal cells escape TRAIL-induced death, as many tumor cells show lower expression of the decoy receptors.

Cell Death by Suicide

The importance of mitochondria in apoptosis was demonstrated in 1996, when Liu and colleagues[17] demonstrated that cytochrome c, a component of the electron transport chain normally contained in the mitochondrial intermembrane space, could initiate programmed cell death when present in the cytosol. This finding led to the demonstration that the intrinsic, or mitochondria-dependent, cell death program resulted from loss of mitochondrial integrity with release of intermembrane space contents (Fig. 6-2). Cytochrome c, on release into the cytosol, forms a complex with Apaf-1 and ATP. This complex, known as the apoptosome, binds and activates procaspase 9.[18] Other mitochondrial contents also participate in apoptosis. For example, Smac/DIABLO,[19,20] Htra2,[21] apoptosis inducing factor (AIF), and endonuclease (endo) G also contribute to the cell death program.[22-24] Inhibitory proteins such as XIAP and cIAPs-1 and -2 bind to the apoptosome and inhibit activation of caspases. Smac/DIABLO and Htra2 function by inhibiting the inhibitors, which allows apoptosis to proceed. The progression of the cell death program appears to depend on the relative ratios of apoptosis promoters and inhibitors. Evidence suggests that AIF, on the other hand, might function independently of caspase activity. On release from

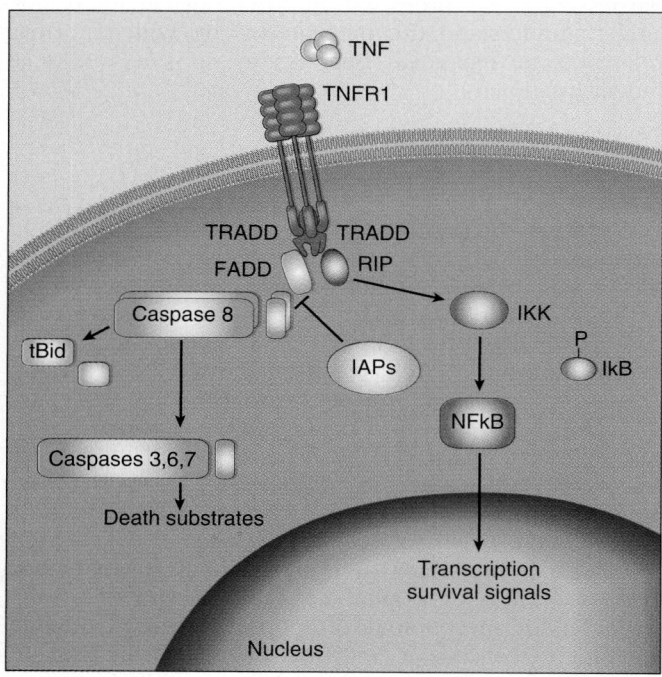

Figure 6-1. Death receptors can initiate apoptosis or promote cell survival. On ligation of the death receptor, adaptors are recruited. For TNFR1, the outcome of ligand binding depends on the state of the cell. TRADD might bind the FADD molecule, which recruits caspase 8, resulting in its oligomerization and activation. Active caspase 8 in turn cleaves and activates effector caspases and the BH3 only molecule Bid, initiating an apoptotic cascade. This process is inhibited by IAPs. Alternatively, binding of TNFR1 might induce recruitment of RIP and IkB kinase (IKK), resulting in release of the NFkB transcription factor from its inhibitor, IkB. NFkB then enters the nucleus, activating transcription of survival genes such as IAPs, therefore antagonizing the proapoptotic factors.

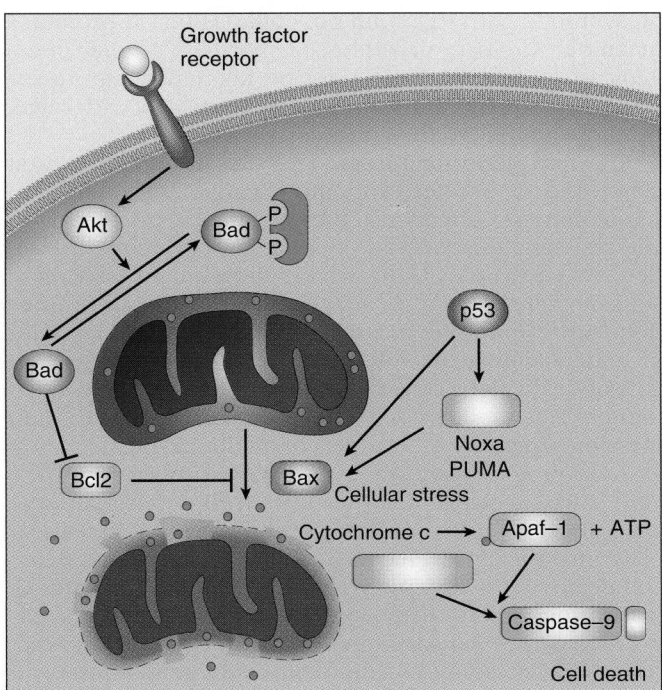

Figure 6-2. Mitochondria-dependent apoptosis. Under conditions of cellular stress, the proapoptotic molecules Bax and/or Bak oligimerize at the mitochondria and induce release of mitochondrial contents, including cytochrome c. Cytochrome c then binds Apaf-1, and in combination with ATP forms the apoptosome. The apoptosome induces cleavage and activation of caspase 9, which activates a caspase cascade culminating in cell death. This process might be stimulated by DNA damage, which results in activation of p53, which, among several functions, promotes transcription of the BH3-only molecules Noxa and PUMA. The apoptotic pathway is antagonized by Bcl-2, which can block cytochrome c release and mitochondrial dysfunction. Growth factor stimulation might also antagonize apoptosis, in part through activation of such survival factors as Akt, which can phosphorylate and inactivate proapoptotic molecules such as the BH3 protein, Bad.

mitochondria, AIF translocates to the nucleus, where, in cooperation with endo G, it can initiate large-scale fragmentation of DNA.

Controversy exists over the mechanism by which mitochondria lose integrity, resulting in release of their contents and initiation of the caspase cascade. General mechanisms proposed include mitochondrial dysfunction leading to matrix swelling and outer membrane rupture. Alternatively, loss of mitochondrial integrity could involve formation of specific pores large enough to release the intermembrane components.[25] Another controversy exists over the importance of caspases in the actual death of cells following mitochondrial compromise as opposed to their role of simply orchestrating cellular disposal. Some investigators have shown that once mitochondria lose integrity, cells will die even in the absence of caspase activation.[26] This finding is consistent with the idea that release of mitochondrial contents proceeds from large-scale catastrophe to the mitochondria, with cellular viability impossible in the absence of mitochondrial function. Others have suggested that, under some circumstances, cells can recover even following cytochrome c release if

caspases are held in check.[27] The function of IAPs in preventing apoptosome activity suggests that in some cases death can be prevented, but the role of caspases likely varies with different apoptotic stimuli.

The Bcl-2 Family

Bcl-2 family proteins play a key role in regulation of mitochondrial integrity and programmed cell death. The Bcl-2 family includes proteins with both antiapoptotic and proapoptotic function. Bcl-2, the first identified member of this family, acts to prevent apoptosis, as do Bcl-X_L and Mcl-1. Bax and Bak antagonize the function of the antiapoptotic family members and are critical in promoting apoptosis through the mitochondrial pathway. All these family members have multiple domains, termed Bcl-2 Homology (BH) domains. A third type of Bcl-2 family member, exemplified by Bad, Bim, and others, consist of a single BH domain and are termed BH3-only molecules. The BH3-only family members also play a key role in promoting apoptosis.

Extensive progress has been made in understanding the mechanisms by which these Bcl-2 family members regulate mitochondrial integrity and apoptosis, though many questions remain. The antiapoptotic molecules Bcl-2 and Bcl-X_L localize to the mitochondria and maintain mitochondrial integrity. This could occur through promotion of exchange of metabolic substrates across the mitochondrial membrane, allowing maintenance of respiration.[28] Alternatively, antiapoptotic Bcl-2 family members might bind and inhibit the function of proapoptotic family members.[29] The multidomain proapoptotic molecules, Bax and Bak, are required for mitochondrial apoptosis initiated through most stimuli.[30] Mice with targeted knockouts of either of these molecules show largely normal apoptotic function, but loss of both Bax and Bak results in a severe defect in apoptosis.[31] This finding suggests that although these two molecules might have largely redundant functions, presence of one or the other is critical to allowing apoptosis to proceed. The BH3-only molecules, in contrast, appear to have a signaling function. Various apoptotic stimuli induce expression and/or activation of specific BH3-only family members, which translocate to the mitochondria and initiate Bax/Bak-dependent apoptosis (Fig. 6-3). They could operate either by activating Bax and Bak or by inhibiting the antiapoptotic function of Bcl-2 and Bcl-Xl. It has been suggested that different members of this group could have distinct functions: some directly binding and activating Bax/Bak, and others indirectly activating these proapoptotic molecules by binding and antagonizing Bcl-2/Bcl-X_L.[32]

The BH3-only protein Bid provides an example of cross-talk between the receptor-mediated and mitochondrial pathways of apoptosis. Bid is a target of active caspase 8.[33,34] Once cleaved, this truncated form of the protein, tBid, can translocate to mitochondria, inducing cytochrome c release and amplification of the apoptotic signal. Although in some cell types death receptor engagement can kill cells independently of mitochondrial participation, in other cell types, this amplification step is critical to effect cell death.

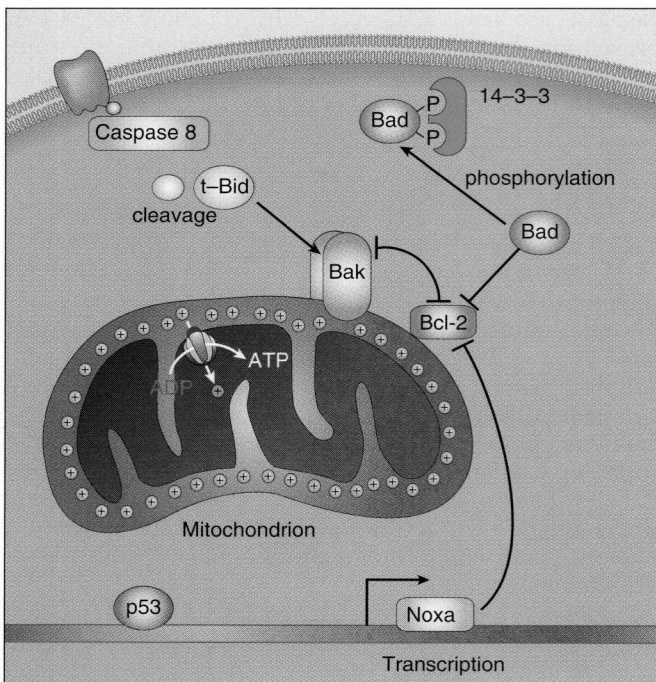

Figure 6-3. BH3-only proteins initiate apoptosis. Several BH3-only proteins exist and could function in various ways to promote apoptosis. Bid is cleaved by caspase 8 on death receptor stimulation and subsequently translocates to mitochondria, where it can activate oligomerization of Bax and Bak. Other proteins, such as Bad and Noxa, function by inhibiting antiapoptotic Bcl-2 molecules. Noxa is transcriptionally regulated by p53, and Bad is regulated by inhibitory phosphorylation, which is growth factor dependent.

APOPTOSIS IN CANCER

The events that can lead to mitochondrial apoptosis are varied. These include loss of normal survival-promoting extrinsic signals, DNA damage, metabolic stress such as hypoxia and nutrient limitation, oncogenic stresses, and toxins. Under normal circumstances, cells require extrinsic signals to promote cellular homeostasis and survival. These signals include growth factors and cell-cell or cell-matrix contact. Survival signals demonstrate to the cell that it is in an appropriate location and that cells like it are present in an appropriate number. Loss of these signals can occur if the cell finds itself in an ectopic position (loss of cell-cell or cell-matrix contact) or when specific cell types are in excess numbers (causing competition for growth factors), resulting in apoptosis.

Oncogenes as Triggers of Apoptosis

Oncogenic stresses, such as activation of Myc or loss of Rb with subsequent uncontrolled activation of the cell cycle machinery, can induce mitochondrially mediated apoptosis. The mechanisms by which this occurs are not clear, but it is well demonstrated that oncogenesis through these pathways requires the additional step of inhibition of programmed cell death. As Myc promotes activity of

biosynthetic pathways, one possibility is that it promotes metabolic stress, to be discussed shortly.[35,36] Other oncogenic stresses, such as loss of the Rb tumor suppressor with subsequent activation of E2F, or DNA damage, promote activity of the tumor suppressor p53.[37]

Research performed in recent years has demonstrated clearly the importance of apoptotic pathways in control of tumorigenesis. Cancer cells, through inappropriate growth and proliferation, outstripping of resources, and translocation to environments to which they are not adapted, subject themselves to death triggers and therefore must disable the apoptotic response to survive. A critical point in understanding the role of apoptosis in cancer is that lack of death alone does not suffice to make a cancer cell. Rather, tumors must activate proliferative, growth, and invasion programs—the targets of traditional oncogenes. It is these programs and their tendency to overwhelm the cell's survival signals that place the cell under apoptotic stress. Disabling of apoptotic pathways makes the cancer cells intrinsically defective in initiation of programmed cell death; such disabling promotes resistance to antineoplastic therapy but also suggests that many cancer cells live constantly "on the edge" of death. It is possible that restoration of apoptotic function could suffice for, or at least contribute to, the elimination of a tumor.

Tumor Suppressors Promote Apoptosis

p53

p53 is one of the best studied tumor suppressors, and its function is lost in at least half of human solid tumors. p53 activity is induced through stabilization of the protein in response to various oncogenic signals (including DNA damage), resulting in inhibition of cell growth through either cell cycle arrest or induction of apoptosis.[38] The specific mechanisms by which one or the other response occurs are not completely clear but could include duration of activity or the prevailing state of the cell. The activity of p53 appears to be mediated largely through its ability to act as a transcription factor, and p53 might play the roles of both transcriptional activator and repressor for different targets.

p53 activity and levels are controlled by its upstream regulator, MDM2. MDM2 protein binds p53 and exports it from the nucleus, blocking its ability to act as a transcriptional regulator. MDM2 also targets p53 for proteasome-dependent degradation through its activity as a ubiquitin ligase. MDM2, in turn, is inhibited in its inhibition by p14ARF. In the absence of loss of p53 itself, overexpression of MDM2 can act as an oncogene, functionally suppressing p53 activity. MDM2 is overexpressed in multiple human tumor types, including lung cancer, brain cancers, and breast cancers.[39,40] p14ARF, conversely, has been shown to be lost in various tumors, including colon cancers.[41] Abnormalities of these upstream regulators tend to occur in tumors that retain wild-type p53, demonstrating that dismantling of the p53/MDM2/p14ARF pathway might play a key role in tumorigenesis.

The antitumor activity of p53 is mediated largely through its transcriptional effects. p53-dependent genes play multiple roles in apoptosis. For example, several proapoptotic Bcl-2 family members are transcriptionally activated by p53, including Bax and the BH3-only proteins Noxa and PUMA.[42,43] Whereas Bax activity is also post-translationally regulated through control of subcellular localization, the activity of Noxa and PUMA might be constitutive upon expression. Expression of Apaf-1, another important element in the mitochondrial pathway, is induced through p53 activity. p53 promotes death receptor pathways through activation of Fas transcription, and it inhibits survival signaling through induction of PTEN.[38] Although this list of antitumor effects of p53 is far from exhaustive, the foregoing examples provide insight into the importance of this pathway in blocking tumorigenesis. Nontranscriptional roles for p53 in apoptotic regulation have also been proposed.[44,45]

Proapoptotic Bcl-2 Family Members

In contrast to the oncogenic effects of the antiapoptotic Bcl-2 family members, proapoptotic family members, particularly Bax, have been implicated as tumor suppressors. Bax and its functional homolog, Bak, are critical in mediating apoptosis through the mitochondrial pathway induced by many cellular stresses.[30,46] Experimental models have suggested that Bax and Bak might have p53-independent function in suppression of tumorigenesis and might act as bona fide tumor suppressors.[47] In one study, murine cells expressing adenoviral E1A, a proliferative factor, and dominant negative p53 were unable to form tumors in mice. Additional loss of Bax and Bak, however, resulted in the formation of highly invasive tumors, emphasizing the capability of these molecules to inhibit carcinogenesis. Furthermore, mutations in Bax and Bak have been identified in many colon cancers, especially those with microsatellite instability, and gastric cancers.[48,49]

BH3-only proteins could also be important in preventing tumorigenesis. Although evidence implicating them as bona fide tumor suppressors is scant, BH3-only proteins play a role in the response to apoptotic stimuli of various death pathways, including p53 and death receptors.

PTEN

The activity of the survival pathway mediated through PI3K and Akt, discussed subsequently, is antagonized by phosphatase and tensin homolgous on chromosome 10 (PTEN), a dual-specificity (protein and lipid) phosphatase that degrades phosphatidylinositol-3,4,5-triphosphate [Ptd(3,4,5)P3] back to the bisphosphate form, terminating the signal of PI3K. PTEN was first discovered in the search for a tumor suppressor on chromosome 10 that is frequently lost in glioblastoma and prostate cancer. Since its discovery, researchers have shown that PTEN acts as a negative regulator of Akt.[50] Tumorigenesis in response to loss of PTEN appears to depend in part on deregulation of Akt activity.[51]

The frequency of PTEN loss in human tumors is exceeded only by that of p53. PTEN function is abnormal in the majority of glioblastomas and prostate cancers and has been described in many other human cancers, including breast cancer and endometrial cancer. Further-more, mice bearing an inactive allele of PTEN develop tumors in multiple organ systems.[52,53] The loss of a single allele of PTEN appears to be sufficient to promote tumorigenesis, as haploinsufficient mice frequently do not lose the second allele upon development of tumors, and loss of the second allele is a late event in many tumors.

Survival Factors Prevent Apoptosis in Cancer Cells

Antiapoptotic Bcl-2 Family Members

The central role of Bcl-2 family members in control of apoptosis suggests that these proteins may be appropriate targets of dysregulation in tumorigenesis, and, as predicted, many tumors show alterations in these proteins. The earliest description of antiapoptotic activity in cancer was that of overexpression of Bcl-2 in follicular lymphoma. This overexpression is brought about by the t(14;18) translocation, which brings the Bcl-2 gene locus into juxtaposition with the immunoglobulin heavy chain enhancer, an abnormality found in at least 85% of follicular lymphomas. Since this discovery, Bcl-2 overexpression has been found in a multitude of different cancers, including other types of lymphoma and solid tumors such as breast cancer.[54]

The importance of Bcl-2 in the pathogenesis of cancer has also been demonstrated in experimental models. For example, mice expressing transgenic c-Myc in B cells develop lymphoma with a long latency period, suggesting the need for other transforming mutations for tumorigenesis. Co-expression of Bcl-2 markedly shortens the latency period, demonstrating synergy of these two molecules in lymphomagenesis.[2] Myc activation in cell lines induces apoptosis, in part through activation of p53. These experiments imply that a critical step in Myc-induced transformation is inhibition of apoptosis, and that Bcl-2 can provide this function. Bcl-Xl, another antiapoptotic family member with function similar to Bcl-2, also appears to play a role in both experimental and naturally-occurring human tumors.[55-57]

Mice expressing transgenic Bcl-2 and Bcl-X$_L$ illustrate the important concept that inhibition of apoptosis alone does not induce tumorigenesis. Enforced expression of these molecules in B lymphocytes of mice leads to accumulation of lymphocytes, but lymphoma develops only rarely.[58] Instead, Bcl-2 and Bcl-X$_L$ facilitate lymphomagenesis by inhibiting the death that normally accompanies oncogenic activation. Likewise, lymphocytes bearing the t(14;18) can be detected in some healthy people with no evidence of lymphoma.[58] Taken together, these points of evidence emphasize the fact that although suppression of apoptosis is an important step in transformation, it is not sufficient to drive carcinogenesis.

NFkB

Another pathway through which tumor cells might suppress apoptosis is the NFkB pathway. As discussed previously, activation of NFkB during death receptor stimulation sets into motion a transcriptional program that inhibits apoptosis and promotes survival. NFkB, under normal circumstances, is held in check by binding of the inhibitor of NFkB, IkB. NFkB is released on phosphorylation of IkB through activity of two IkB kinases, IKKalpha and IKKbeta.[59] Phosphorylation targets IkB for ubiqitination and degradation by the 26S proteasome, releasing NFkB to translocate to the nucleus and activate its target genes (Fig. 6-4). Oncogenic stimuli, as well as survival signals, might promote NFkB activation. For example, Ras-mediated transformation could stimulate transcriptional activity of NFkB through an unknown mechanism.[60] Furthermore, the Bcr-Abl fusion protein, a causative mutation in chronic myeloid leukemia, activates NFkB by promoting nuclear translocation.[61] Virally induced transformation by HTLV-1 is dependent in part on Tax-mediated activation of the IKKs.[62]

The proto-oncogene Bcl-3 was identified on one arm of a translocation found in some lymphoid malignencies, t(14;19). This translocation brings the Bcl-3 gene in proximity to the immunoglobulin heavy chain enhancer, resulting in its overexpression. The Bcl-3 gene encodes a member of the IkB family, but this gene product appears to function differently from other IkBs.[63] Specifically, Bcl-3 localizes to the nucleus and modifies the function of NFkB subunits.[64] When overexpressed in normal T cells, Bcl-3 promotes survival following cellular activation, and expression appears to be induced on treatment with

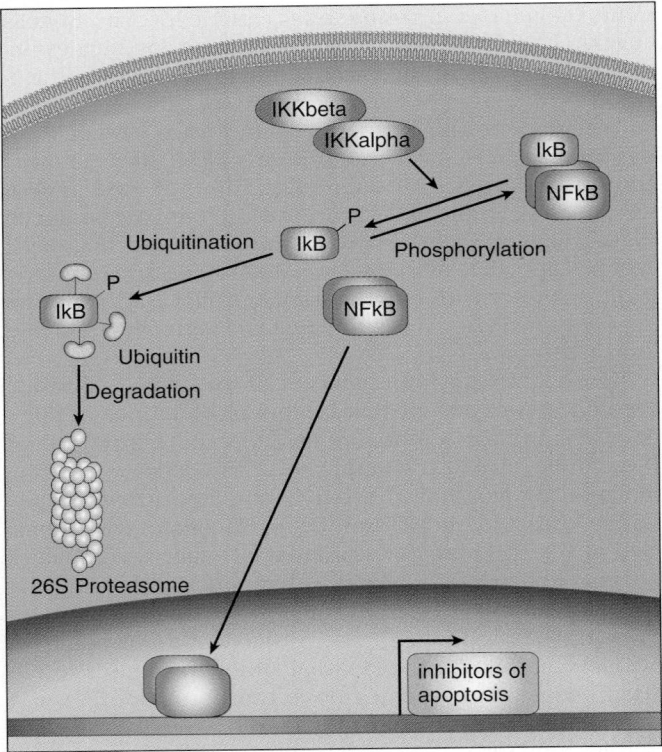

Figure 6-4. NFkB is a transcriptional activator of multiple antiapoptotic genes. Under resting conditions, NFkB is bound by its inhibitor, IkB, which prevents its transcriptional activity by maintaining it in the cytoplasm. Activation signals stimulate activity of IkB kinases (IKK), which phosphorylate IkB. Phosphorylated IkB can then be ubiquitinated and targeted to the proteasome for degradation. This process releases NFkB to enter the nucleus, where it activates transcription from its target promoters.

immunologic adjuvants, suggesting a physiological survival role for it in the immune system.[65] Mice expressing a Bcl-2 transgene in B lymphocytes do not develop lymphoma, but they do show accumulation of B cells and hyper-responsiveness of the immune system, similar to the findings in Bcl-2 transgenic mice.

PI3K/Akt

Many tumors lose extracellularly-derived survival signals during pathogenesis, either by outstripping limited growth factors or by translocating to inappropriate environments. One signaling pathway that has been implicated in provision of survival signals is the phosphotidylinositol-3-kinase (PI3K) pathway.[66,67] Many growth factors, including interleukin-2, interleukin-3, platelet-derived growth factor (PDGF), and insulin-like growth factor (IGF), signal in part through PI3K. PI3K phosphorylates phosphotidylinositide-4,5-bisphosphate (Ptd(4,5)P2) to Ptd(3,4,5)P3, which acts as a second messenger, activating downstream effectors such as the serine/threonine kinase Akt, also known as protein kinase B (PKB) (Fig. 6-5). Akt appears to be a critical survival factor in many cell types, and its activity might promote survival through multiple functions, such as phosphorylation and inactivation of the BH3-only protein Bad, and through the Forkhead family transcription factor FKHRL1.[50,68] In addition, Akt acts in the insulin signaling pathway to promote glucose uptake, and it appears to play a similar role in non-insulin responsive cells, promoting glucose uptake and glycolysis upon growth factor stimulation. It has been proposed that this metabolism-promoting effect of Akt might protect mitochondrial integrity through maintenance of substrate availability, thereby preventing apoptosis.[69,70]

Multiple studies have demonstrated the importance of Akt activity in tumorigenesis, either through amplification of one of the three AKT genes, or through loss of PTEN function. Amplification of Akt results in a similar phenotype to PTEN loss and has been found in gastric cancers, breast cancers, and other tumor types.[71-73] Furthermore, animal models also have demonstrated the role of Akt in tumorigenesis. Mice expressing constitutively active Akt in T cells develop thymic lymphoma at a high rate.[74]

Epigenetic Gene Silencing

Inhibition of expression of tumor suppressor genes through epigenetic mechanisms is emerging as an important mechanism by which tumor cells might disable proapoptotic pathways. Promoter methylation at CpG islands could repress transcription of genes in the absence of mutation (Fig. 6-6). In addition, histone deacetylation might also turn off gene expression, possibly by inhibiting access of transcription factors. For example, Soengas and colleagues[75] have shown that many melanoma cells (both primary tumors and cell lines) suppress Apaf-1 expression. This results in inhibition of p53-dependent apoptosis in these cells and renders them resistant to chemotherapy. Apaf-1 suppression is mediated not by mutation of Apaf-1, but rather through methylation, as treatment with the methylation inhibitor 5-azacytidine restores both Apaf-1

Figure 6-5. The PI3K-Akt pathway is activated by multiple growth factor receptors and oncogenes and plays a critical role in promoting cell survival. PI3K is activated by growth factor stimulation or intracellular signals such as activated ras or the oncogene BCR-Abl. Active PI3K phosphorylates phosphotidylinositols to PIP3 at the plasma membrane. PIP3 recruits Akt and its activating kinases, PDK1 and an uncharacterized PDK2, to the membrane, where Akt is phosphorylated and activated. Akt then promotes survival functions such as Bad and Forkhead inactivation, activation of NFkB and MDM2, and glucose metabolism. PI3K activity is antagonized by the phosphatase PTEN, which degrades PIP3.

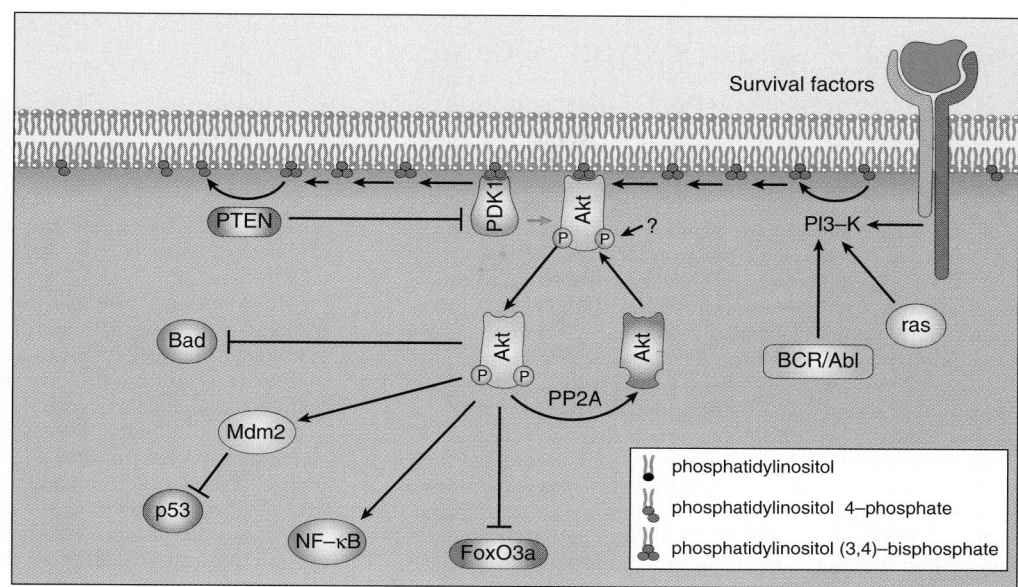

expression and chemosensitivity. Methylation appears to play an important role in suppression of tumor suppressors in other tumors as well. For example, childhood neuroblastomas show loss of expression of caspase 8 through methylation of its promoter at high frequency.[76] Finally, promoter methylation of the p14ARF locus might suppress its expression in multiple tumor types.[77]

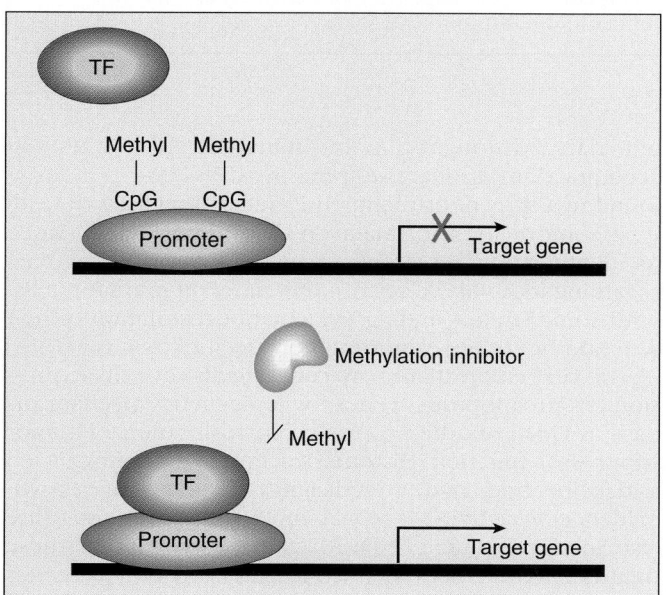

Figure 6-6. Epigenetic gene silencing is a mechanism by which cancer cells turn off tumor suppressor gene expression. In the process of development or oncogenesis, genes might be silenced through promoter methylation. In tumors, promoters of tumor suppressor genes such as Apaf-1 and caspase 8 are frequent targets of methylation. Methylation inhibitors, such as 5-azacytidine, reactivate expression of these tumor suppressor genes, potentially contributing to anticancer therapy.

MANIPULATING APOPTOSIS IN CANCER TREATMENT

As discussed previously, cancer cells must dismantle or inhibit apoptotic pathways in order to maintain their transformed phenotype. Many transformation-inducing mutations also have the effect of promoting programmed cell death, and cells are unable to pass through these initial changes to become cancer unless apoptosis is inhibited. This fact has two correlates. First, most traditional cancer chemotherapies act through induction of apoptosis, and the intrinsic apoptotic defects of these cells could make them inherently resistant to chemotherapy. On the other hand, cancer cells are constantly living "on the edge," pushed beyond the normal limits of cell viability. This fact might make tumor cells profoundly susceptible to apoptosis if either the defect can be corrected or another death pathway can be activated. This reasoning is the basis of the many attempts currently in progress to design therapies that will attain one of these objectives.

Restoration of Apoptotic Capability

Restoration of lost apoptotic pathways can be accomplished by several methods. First, if a proapoptotic gene, such as p53, is mutated, gene therapy provides a direct way in which to restore expression of the missing protein. This approach has been tried in several settings. The most common approach has been to attempt to deliver the gene in question via an adenoviral vector. This approach has been used with p53 in tumors of the head and neck, and in lung tumors using the INGN201 construct from Introgen Therapeutics;[78] some success has been seen with intratumoral injections. Another such construct is Schering-Plough's SCH58500, which has shown evidence of activity in advanced ovarian cancer.[79] Systemic therapy

Science of Clinical Oncology

METABOLIC DEREGULATION IN CANCER

Cells that lose survival signals fail to maintain themselves and undergo progressive atrophy. Loss of survival-inducing signal transduction leads to downregulation of cell surface nutrient transporters (e.g., glucose transporters) and to a decreased rate of glucose metabolism, as evidenced by decreased levels of hexokinase and phosphofructokinase, two key regulatory enzymes in the glycolytic pathway.[69,100-102] The loss of glycolytic products reduces delivery of substrate to the mitochondria, resulting in mitochondrial damage. Nutrient limitation might have similar metabolic effects when cells accumulate in excess of the existing vascular supply.

In the 1920s, Warburg observed that cancer cells metabolize glucose at a higher rate than their normal counterparts. Furthermore, he found that the malignant cells relied on glycolysis for a disproportionate amount of their ATP production, with comparatively little energy produced by oxidative phosphorylation. Warburg hypothesized that this shift to aerobic glycolysis resulted from defects in mitochondrial function in the cancer cells.

Other researchers have subsequently confirmed Warburg's findings of increased aerobic glycolysis in cancer cells. The high rate of glucose uptake in tumors has formed the basis of a novel imaging modality, positron emission tomography (PET), using an 18-fluorine-labeled glucose analog. A study evaluating PET scanning in lymphoma showed that more than 90% of lymphomas—including very indolent tumors—metabolize glucose at an abnormally high rate.[103] Although several research groups have found mutations in genes that encode mitochondrial enzymes in cancer cells, the fact that normal lymphocytes are unable to maintain glucose uptake and glycolysis in the face of dropping ATP levels suggests an alternative hypothesis. In this scenario, normal cells lack the ability to take up sufficient glucose to maintain themselves and instead are dependent on extrinsic signal transduction to maintain the expression and function of nutrient transporters. As a corollary, mutations that activate such signaling pathways could enable the cell to take up glucose in excess of that needed for bioenergetic or synthetic activities. Under such conditions, cells would secrete the excess glucose as lactate and have sufficient bioenergetic reserves to support entry into and progression through the cell cycle.

These findings raise the possibility that cancer cells, in the process of transformation, turn on signaling pathways that allow autonomous access to nutrients and metabolic pathways, rendering the cells independent of the extracellular signals normally required to maintain nutrient uptake. This facilitated access to nutrients would provide substrate to mitochondria, allowing maintenance of mitochondrial function and suppression of apoptosis even in the absence of growth factor signaling. If this hypothesis is true, autonomous access to nutrients is likely accomplished in multiple ways by different tumors. One potential contributor to this goal is Akt. Akt is critical in the insulin signaling pathway to activate glucose uptake in insulin-responsive tissues, and it appears to play a similar role in non–insulin-responsive cells on growth factor stimulation. Although the role of Akt as an oncogene might include several functions, it clearly has the potential to promote glucose transporter expression and activity of glycolytic enzymes.

The role of metabolic control in tumorigenesis is poorly understood. Elucidation of this fundamental process in cancer might offer greater appreciation for the mechanisms of carcinogenesis. Furthermore, the recognition of the importance of metabolic control in cancer could offer new therapeutic targets, improving our chances of defeating cancer in the future.

---

poses an additional challenge, however, in terms of both feasibility and safety. The effect of gene therapy with p53 would be expected to be seen only in cells in which the transgene is expressed, requiring that every cell be infected by the vector. Furthermore, the safety of adenovirus vectors remains at issue.

Another, similar approach has been to target cancer cells lacking p53 by taking advantage of the fact that adenovirus must inactivate p53 in order to replicate in cells. Usually this is accomplished through the activity of the virus's E1Bp55 protein, which binds and inactivates p53. A virus that lacks E1Bp55 is unable to replicate in normal cells. Cancer cells that lack p53 present a viable target, however, allowing the virus to accomplish its lytic life cycle and killing the cell. This approach is being used clinically with the drug ONYX-015, which, similar to p53 gene therapy, has shown success with intratumoral injection in combination with chemotherapy in head and neck cancers.[80] Once again, systemic delivery appears more problematic.

In addition to genetic approaches, the p53 pathway has been targeted using small molecules designed to restore p53 function. This approach takes advantage of the fact that, in most cancers, p53 is inactivated not by deletion but rather through a point mutation that results in accumulation of inactive protein. CP-31398 is a drug found in a screen for therapeutic agents that restore wild-type conformation to mutant p53 in tumor cells.[81] Since its identification, researchers have found conflicting data regarding its ability to restore p53 function in tumor cells, with some studies finding evidence of restoration of p53 function but others reporting nonspecific toxicity.[82,83]

The realization that many cancer cells turn off expression of proapoptotic genes by epigenetic mechanisms has provided another approach to restoration of tumor suppressor function. Histone deacetylase inhibitors, such as depsipeptide, have entered clinical trials and have shown evidence of activity.[84,85] DNA methylation inhibitors are also in development.[86] The lack of specificity of these treatments raise theoretical concerns, however, that genes which have been silenced in differentiation (e.g., hTERT, the human telomerase gene that might play a role in tumor promotion) or other tumor promoting genes could be turned on through demethylation or deacetylation. Silencing of TRAIL decoy receptors through methylation has been demonstrated in cancer cells.[87] The end result of these therapies could depend on the balance of genes silenced through epigenetic mechanisms in each cancer.

Inhibition of Survival Factors

Small molecule inhibitors might also show activity in the inhibition of survival factors expressed in cancer cells. PI3K inhibitors, for example, have shown synergy with chemotherapy agents in vitro, and translation to a clinical setting could offer promising therapy.[88] Farnesyltransferase inhibitors, which inhibit activation of Ras and therefore of PI3K, are currently in clinical trials. Although early results have been disappointing, their use in appropriate combinations with other therapies might lead to better results. The 26S proteasome is important in myriad cellular pathways, but its importance in activation of NFkB, through degradation of IkB, has raised the possibility that inhibition of proteasomal degradation could have specifically proapoptotic effects in cancer cells. Akt has also been reported to phosphorylate the tumor suppressor genes TSC-1 and TSC-2 and target them for proteasomal degradation.[89] PS-341, a proteasomal inhibitor, is also in clinical trials at the time of this writing and could have clinical activity in some hematologic malignancies, notably multiple myeloma.[90]

Antisense strategies are in development to target various antiapoptotic molecules. Antisense oligonucleotides act by binding to specific mRNAs, forming dsRNA complexes. These complexes might inhibit expression of the target mRNAs, either by blocking translation or through targeting them for destruction by the cell through recognition of abnormal dsRNA. The most developed of these antisense oligonucleotides is the one targeted against Bcl-2.[91-93] The antisense Bcl-2 currently in use is oblimersen, also known as Genasense. Trials in hematologic malignancies and in several solid tumors are ongoing at the time of this writing. Activity has been seen, particularly in the context of combination therapy with traditional chemotherapeutic agents.

Other survival factors have also been targeted for downregulation through the use of antisense oligonucleotides. Ha-ras, which promotes survival in part through activation of PI3K and Akt, provides the target for ISIS 2503.[94] Other antisense targets include MDM2, which targets p53 for nuclear export and degradation, and XIAP.[95,96] All of these constructs have shown antitumor activity in either preclinical or clinical trials. One concern, which is also a concern with gene therapy, regards the ability to deliver drug in vivo to a meaningful number of the cancer cells. The early success seen with Bcl-2 antisense provides some encouragement that the antisense therapy approach could, in fact, prove to be feasible.

Death Receptor Activation

As discussed in previous sections, death receptor signaling appears to play an important role in some tumors. Initial studies examined the use of Fas and TNF as death-inducing ligands. Yet, although these molecules demonstrated antitumor activity, their utility as therapeutic agents has been compromised by toxicity, with both normal cells and malignant cells targeted for death.

Investigations of TRAIL have raised the possibility that this ligand might be more selective for tumor cells. Most normal cells express decoy receptors that sequester TRAIL, preventing it from sending an intracellular death signal. Tumor cells appear to be uniquely sensitive to the apoptotic stimulus of TRAIL; one reason might be downregulation of decoy receptor expression, possibly by promoter methylation.[87] Studies in mice and nonhuman primates have demonstrated minimal toxicity to normal cells with administration of TRAIL.[97,98] When researchers examined the effects of TRAIL on human hepatocytes in vitro, however, it was found to cause significant cell death, raising the question of whether TRAIL, like its counterparts Fas and TNF, might be too toxic for use in humans.[99] The use of TRAIL as a therapeutic agent remains under investigation.

SUMMARY

Understanding of apoptosis and its importance in tumorigenesis is evolving rapidly. Much of the research discussed in this chapter is new at the time of this writing, and our understanding and interpretation of these findings will almost certainly undergo revision as more information constantly becomes available. The current appreciation for these processes, however, already has provided opportunities for advancement of patient care.

In the future, research further clarifying the basic mechanisms of apoptosis—including events mediating mitochondrial demise along with a better understanding of the nature of death signals—will continue to improve our arsenal of potential weapons against cancer. As has been found with traditional antineoplastic therapies, success will most likely be found with a combination of therapeutic approaches. These might include the addition of apoptosis-based therapies to traditional agents, combining proapoptotic with antisurvival approaches, along with strategies to manipulate apoptosis that await development as knowledge of the complex process evolves.

REFERENCES

1. Tsujimoto Y, Finger LR, Yunis J, Nowell PC, Croce CM: Cloning of the chromosome breakpoint of neoplastic B cells with the t(14;18) chromosome translocation. Science 1984;226:1097–1099.
2. Vaux DL, Cory S, Adams JM: Bcl-2 gene promotes haemopoietic cell survival and cooperates with c-myc to immortalize pre-B cells. Nature 1988;335:440–4422.
3. McDonnell TJ, Deane N, Platt FM, et al: bcl-2-immunoglobulin transgenic mice demonstrate extended B cell survival and follicular lymphoproliferation. Cell 1989;57:79–88.
4. Chen G, Goeddel DV: TNF-R1 signaling: A beautiful pathway. Science 2002;296:1634–1635.
5. Wajant H: The Fas signaling pathway: More than a paradigm. Science 2002;296:1635–1636.
6. Hsu H, Xiong J, Goeddel DV: The TNF receptor 1-associated protein TRADD signals cell death and NF-kappa B activation. Cell 1995;81:495–504.
7. Wang CY, Mayo MW, Korneluk RG, Goeddel DV, Baldwin AS Jr: NF-kappaB antiapoptosis: Induction of TRAF1 and TRAF2 and c-IAP1 and c-IAP2 to suppress caspase-8 activation. Science 1998;281:1680–1683.

8. Clem RJ, Miller LK: Control of programmed cell death by the baculovirus genes p35 and iap. Mol Cell Biol 1994;14:5212-5222.

9. Liston P, Roy N, Tamai K, et al: Suppression of apoptosis in mammalian cells by NAIP and a related family of IAP genes. Nature 1996;379:349-353.

10. Rothe M, Pan MG, Henzel WJ, Ayres TM, Goeddel DV: The TNFR2-TRAF signaling complex contains two novel proteins related to baculoviral inhibitor of apoptosis proteins. Cell 1995;83:1243-1252.

11. Uren AG, Pakusch M, Hawkins CJ, Puls KL, Vaux DL: Cloning and expression of apoptosis inhibitory protein homologs that function to inhibit apoptosis and/or bind tumor necrosis factor receptor-associated factors. Proc Natl Acad Sci USA 1996;93:4974-4978.

12. Wiley SR, Schooley K, Smolak PJ, et al: Identification and characterization of a new member of the TNF family that induces apoptosis. Immunity 1995;3:673-682.

13. Pitti RM, Marsters SA, Ruppert S, Donahue CJ, Moore A, Ashkenazi A: Induction of apoptosis by Apo-2 ligand, a new member of the tumor necrosis factor cytokine family. J Biol Chem 1996;271:12687-12690.

14. Takeda K, Hayakawa Y, Smyth MJ, et al: Involvement of tumor necrosis factor-related apoptosis-inducing ligand in surveillance of tumor metastasis by liver natural killer cells. Nat Med 2001;7:94-100.

15. Pan G, Ni J, Wei YF, Yu G, Gentz R, Dixit VM: An antagonist decoy receptor and a death domain-containing receptor for TRAIL. Science 1997;277:815-818.

16. Sheridan JP, Marsters SA, Pitti RM, et al: Control of TRAIL-induced apoptosis by a family of signaling and decoy receptors. Science 1997;277:818-821.

17. Liu X, Kim CN, Yang J, Jemmerson R, Wang X: Induction of apoptotic program in cell-free extracts: requirement for dATP and cytochrome c. Cell 1996;86:147-157.

18. Li P, Nijhawan D, Budihardjo I, et al: Cytochrome c and dATP-dependent formation of Apaf-1/caspase-9 complex initiates an apoptotic protease cascade. Cell 1997;91:479-489.

19. Verhagen AM, Ekert PG, Pakusch M, et al: Identification of DIABLO, a mammalian protein that promotes apoptosis by binding to and antagonizing IAP proteins. Cell 2000;102:43-53.

20. Du C, Fang M, Li Y, Li L, Wang X: Smac, a mitochondrial protein that promotes cytochrome c-dependent caspase activation by eliminating IAP inhibition. Cell 2000;102:33-42.

21. Suzuki Y, Imai Y, Nakayama H, Takahashi K, Takio K, Takahashi R: A serine protease, HtrA2, is released from the mitochondria and interacts with XIAP, inducing cell death. Mol Cell 2001;8:613-621.

22. Joza N, Susin SA, Daugas E, et al: Essential role of the mitochondrial apoptosis-inducing factor in programmed cell death. Nature 2001;410:549-554.

23. Parrish J, Li L, Klotz K, Ledwich D, Wang X, Xue D: Mitochondrial endonuclease G is important for apoptosis in C. elegans. Nature 2001;412:90-94.

24. Li LY, Luo X, Wang X: Endonuclease G is an apoptotic DNase when released from mitochondria. Nature 2001;412:95-99.

25. Hewick RM, Waterfield MD, Miller LK, Fried M: Correlation between genetic loci and structural differences in the capsid proteins of polyoma virus plaque morphology mutants. Cell 1977;11:331-338.

26. Wang X: The expanding role of mitochondria in apoptosis. Genes Dev 2001;15:2922-2933.

27. Waterhouse NJ, Goldstein JC, von Ahsen O, Schuler M, Newmeyer DD, Green DR: Cytochrome c maintains mitochondrial transmembrane potential and ATP generation after outer mitochondrial membrane permeabilization during the apoptotic process. J Cell Biol 2001;153:319-328.

28. Vander Heiden MG, Chandel NS, Schumacker PT, Thompson CB: Bcl-xL prevents cell death following growth factor withdrawal by facilitating mitochondrial ATP/ADP exchange. Mol Cell 1999;3:159-167.

29. Hengartner MO: The biochemistry of apoptosis. Nature 2000;407:770-776.

30. Wei MC, Zong WX, Cheng EH, et al: Proapoptotic BAX and BAK: A requisite gateway to mitochondrial dysfunction and death. Science 2001;292:727-730.

31. Lindsten T, Ross AJ, King A, et al: The combined functions of proapoptotic Bcl-2 family members bak and bax are essential for normal development of multiple tissues. Mol Cell 2000;6:1389-1399.

32. Letai A, Bassik MC, Walensky LD, Sorcinelli MD, Weiler S, Korsmeyer SJ: Distinct BH3 domains either sensitize or activate mitochondrial apoptosis, serving as prototype cancer therapeutics. Cancer Cell 2002;2:183-192.

33. Luo X, Budihardjo I, Zou H, Slaughter C, Wang X: Bid, a Bcl2 interacting protein, mediates cytochrome c release from mitochondria in response to activation of cell surface death receptors. Cell 1998;94:481-490.

34. Li H, Zhu H, Xu CJ, Yuan J: Cleavage of BID by caspase 8 mediates the mitochondrial damage in the Fas pathway of apoptosis. Cell 1998;94:491-501.

35. Johnston LA, Prober DA, Edgar BA, Eisenman RN, Gallant P: Drosophila myc regulates cellular growth during development. Cell 1999;98:779-790.

36. Iritani BM, Eisenman RN: c-Myc enhances protein synthesis and cell size during B lymphocyte development. Proc Natl Acad Sci USA 1999;96:13180-13185.

37. Nahle Z, Polakoff J, Davuluri RV, et al: Direct coupling of the cell cycle and cell death machinery by E2F. Nat Cell Biol 2002;4:859-864.

38. Vousden KH, Lu X: Live or let die: the cell's response to p53. Nat Rev Cancer 2002;2:594-604.

39. Bueso-Ramos CE, Manshouri T, Haidar MA, et al: Abnormal expression of MDM-2 in breast carcinomas. Breast Cancer Res Treat 1996;37:179-188.

40. Eymin B, Gazzeri S, Brambilla C, Brambilla E: Mdm2 overexpression and p14(ARF) inactivation are two mutually exclusive events in primary human lung tumors. Oncogene 2002;21:2750-2761.

41. Burri N, Shaw P, Bouzourene H, et al: Methylation silencing and mutations of the p14ARF and p16INK4a genes in colon cancer. Lab Invest 2001;81:217-229.

42. Yu J, Zhang L, Hwang PM, Kinzler KW, Vogelstein B: PUMA induces the rapid apoptosis of colorectal cancer cells. Mol Cell 2001;7:673-682.

43. Nakano K, Vousden KH: PUMA, a novel proapoptotic gene, is induced by p53. Mol Cell 2001;7:683-694.

44. Caelles C, Helmberg A, Karin M: p53-dependent apoptosis in the absence of transcriptional activation of p53-target genes. Nature 1994;370:220-223.

45. Mihara M, Erster S, Zaika A, et al: p53 has a direct apoptogenic role at the mitochondria. Mol Cell 2003;11:577-590.

46. Zong WX, Lindsten T, Ross AJ, MacGregor GR, Thompson CB: BH3-only proteins that bind pro-survival Bcl-2 family members fail to induce apoptosis in the absence of Bax and Bak. Genes Dev 2001;15:1481-1486.

47. Degenhardt K, Chen G, Lindsten T, White E: BAX and BAK mediate p53-independent suppression of tumorigenesis. Cancer Cell 2002;2:193-203.

48. Rampino N, Yamamoto H, Ionov Y, et al: Somatic frameshift mutations in the BAX gene in colon cancers of the microsatellite mutator phenotype. Science 1997;275:967-969.

49. Kondo S, Shinomura Y, Miyazaki Y, et al: Mutations of the bak gene in human gastric and colorectal cancers. Cancer Res 2000;60:4328-4330.

50. Stambolic V, Suzuki A, de la Pompa JL, et al: Negative regulation of PKB/Akt-dependent cell survival by the tumor suppressor PTEN. Cell 1998;95:29-39.

51. Stiles B, Gilman V, Khanzenzon N, et al: Essential role of AKT-1/protein kinase B alpha in PTEN-controlled tumorigenesis. Mol Cell Biol 2002;22:3842-3851.

52. Podsypanina K, Ellenson LH, Nemes A, et al: Mutation of Pten/Mmac1 in mice causes neoplasia in multiple organ systems. Proc Natl Acad Sci USA 1999;96:1563-1568.

53. Di Cristofano A, Pesce B, Cordon-Cardo C, Pandolfi PP: Pten is essential for embryonic development and tumour suppression. Nat Genet 1998;19:348-355.

54. Olopade OI, Adeyanju MO, Safa AR, et al: Overexpression of BCL-x protein in primary breast cancer is associated with high tumor grade and nodal metastases. Cancer J Sci Am 1997;3:230-237.

55. Chao DT, Linette GP, Boise LH, White LS, Thompson CB, Korsmeyer SJ: Bcl-XL and Bcl-2 repress a common pathway of cell death. J Exp Med 1995;182:821–828.

56. Pena JC, Thompson CB, Recant W, Vokes EE, Rudin CM: Bcl-xL and Bcl-2 expression in squamous cell carcinoma of the head and neck. Cancer 1999;85:164–170.

57. Packham G, White EL, Eischen CM, et al: elective regulation of Bcl-XL by a Jak kinase-dependent pathway is bypassed in murine hematopoietic malignancies. Genes Dev 1998;12:2475–2487.

58. Strasser A, Harris AW, Cory S: E mu-bcl-2 transgene facilitates spontaneous transformation of early pre-B and immunoglobulin-secreting cells but not T cells. Oncogene 1993;8:1–9.

59. Richmond A: Nf-kappa B, chemokine gene transcription and tumour growth. Nat Rev Immunol 2002;2:664–674.

60. Finco TS, Westwick JK, Norris JL, Beg AA, Der CJ, Baldwin AS Jr: Oncogenic Ha-Ras-induced signaling activates NF-kappaB transcriptional activity, which is required for cellular transformation. J Biol Chem 1997;272:24113–24116.

61. Reuther JY, Reuther GW, Cortez D, Pendergast AM, Baldwin AS Jr: A requirement for NF-kappaB activation in Bcr-Abl-mediated transformation. Genes Dev 1998;12:968–981.

62. Chu ZL, DiDonato JA, Hawiger J, Ballard DW: The tax oncoprotein of human T-cell leukemia virus type 1 associates with and persistently activates IkappaB kinases containing IKKalpha and IKKbeta. J Biol Chem 1998;273:15891–15894.

63. Kerr LD, Duckett CS, Wamsley P, et al: The proto-oncogene bcl-3 encodes an I kappa B protein. Genes Dev 1992;6:2352–2363.

64. Zhang Q, Didonato JA, Karin M, McKeithan TW: BCL3 encodes a nuclear protein which can alter the subcellular location of NF-kappa B proteins. Mol Cell Biol 1994;14:3915–3926.

65. Mitchell TC, Hildeman D, Kedl RM, et al: Immunological adjuvants promote activated T cell survival via induction of Bcl-3. Nat Immunol 2001;2:397–402.

66. Kauffmann-Zeh A, Rodriguez-Viciana P, Ulrich E, et al: Suppression of c-Myc-induced apoptosis by Ras signalling through PI(3)K and PKB. Nature 1997;385:544–548.

67. Kennedy SG, Wagner AJ, Conzen SD, et al: The PI 3-kinase/Akt signaling pathway delivers an anti-apoptotic signal. Genes Dev 1997;11:701–713.

68. Dudek H, Datta SR, Franke TF, et al: Regulation of neuronal survival by the serine-threonine protein kinase Akt. Science 1997;275:661–665.

69. Vander Heiden MG, Plas DR, Rathmell JC, Fox CJ, Harris MH, Thompson CB: Growth factors can influence cell growth and survival through effects on glucose metabolism. Mol Cell Biol 2001;21:5899–5912.

70. Plas DR, Talapatra S, Edinger AL, Rathmell JC, Thompson CB: Akt and Bcl-xL promote growth factor-independent survival through distinct effects on mitochondrial physiology. J Biol Chem 2001;276:12041–12048.

71. Cheng JQ, Godwin AK, Bellacosa A, et al: AKT2, a putative oncogene encoding a member of a subfamily of protein-serine/threonine kinases, is amplified in human ovarian carcinomas. Proc Natl Acad Sci USA 1992;89:9267–9271.

72. Cheng JQ, Ruggeri B, Klein WM, et al: Amplification of AKT2 in human pancreatic cells and inhibition of AKT2 expression and tumorigenicity by antisense RNA. Proc Natl Acad Sci USA 1996;93:3636–3641.

73. Staal SP: Molecular cloning of the akt oncogene and its human homologues AKT1 and AKT2: Amplification of AKT1 in a primary human gastric adenocarcinoma. Proc Natl Acad Sci USA 1987;84:5034–5037.

74. Malstrom S, Tili E, Kappes D, Ceci JD, Tsichlis PN: Tumor induction by an Lck-MyrAkt transgene is delayed by mechanisms controlling the size of the thymus. Proc Natl Acad Sci USA 2001;98:14967–4972.

75. Soengas MS, Capodieci P, Polsky D, et al: Inactivation of the apoptosis effector Apaf-1 in malignant melanoma. Nature 2001;409:207–211.

76. Teitz T, Wei T, Valentine MB, et al: Caspase 8 is deleted or silenced preferentially in childhood neuroblastomas with amplification of MYCN. Nat Med 2000;6:529–535.

77. Esteller M, Cordon-Cardo C, Corn PG, et al: p14ARF silencing by promoter hypermethylation mediates abnormal intracellular localization of MDM2. Cancer Res 2001;61:2816–2821.

78. Merritt JA, Roth JA, Logothetis CJ: Clinical evaluation of adenoviral-mediated p53 gene transfer: review of INGN 201 studies. Semin Oncol 2001;28:105–114.

79. Zhang JY: Apoptosis-based anticancer drugs. Nat Rev Drug Discov 2002;1:101–102.

80. Khuri FR, Nemunaitis J, Ganly I, et al: a controlled trial of intratumoral ONYX-015, a selectively-replicating adenovirus, in combination with cisplatin and 5-fluorouracil in patients with recurrent head and neck cancer. Nat Med 2000;6:879–885.

81. Foster BA, Coffey HA, Morin MJ, Rastinejad F: Pharmacological rescue of mutant p53 conformation and function. Science 1999;286:2507–2510.

82. Rippin TM, Bykov VJ, Freund SM, Selivanova G, Wiman KG, Fersht AR: Characterization of the p53-rescue drug CP-31398 in vitro and in living cells. Oncogene 2002;21:2119–2129.

83. Takimoto R, Wang W, Dicker DT, Rastinejad F, Lyssikatos J, el-Deiry WS: The mutant p53-conformation modifying drug, CP-31398, can induce apoptosis of human cancer cells and can stabilize wild-type p53 protein. Cancer Biol Ther 2002;1:47–55.

84. Richon VM, O'Brien JP: Histone deacetylase inhibitors: A new class of potential therapeutic agents for cancer treatment. Clin Cancer Res 2002;8:662–664.

85. Piekarz RL, Robey R, Sandor V, et al: Inhibitor of histone deacetylation, depsipeptide (FR901228), in the treatment of peripheral and cutaneous T-cell lymphoma: A case report. Blood 2001;98:2865–2868.

86. Flynn J, FAng JY, Mikovits JA, Reich NO: A potent cell-active allosteric inhibitor of murine DNA cytosine C5 methyltransferase. J Biol Chem 2003;278:8238–8243.

87. van Noesel MM, van Bezouw S, Salomons GS, et al: Tumor-specific down-regulation of the tumor necrosis factor-related apoptosis-inducing ligand decoy receptors DcR1 and DcR2 is associated with dense promoter hypermethylation. Cancer Res 2002;62:2157–2161.

88. Ng SSW, Tsao MS, Chow S, Hedley DW: Inhibition of phosphatidylinositide 3-kinase enhances gemcitabine- induced apoptosis in human pancreatic cancer cells. Cancer Res 2002;60:5451–5455.

89. Plas DR, Thompson CB: Akt activation promotes degradation of tuberin and FOXO3a via the proteasome. J Biol Chem 2003;278:12361–12366.

90. Orlowski RZ, Stinchcombe TE, Mitchell BS, et al: Phase I trial of the proteasome inhibitor PS-341 in patients with refractory hematologic malignancies. J Clin Oncol 2002;20:4420–4427.

91. Webb A, Cunningham D, Cotter F, et al: BCL-2 antisense therapy in patients with non-Hodgkin lymphoma. Lancet 1997;349:1137–1141.

92. Jansen B, Wacheck V, Heere-Ress E, et al: Chemosensitisation of malignant melanoma by BCL2 antisense therapy. Lancet 2000;356:1728–1733.,

93. Marcucci G, Byrd JC, Dai G, et al: Phase 1 and pharmacodynamic studies of G3139, a Bcl-2 antisense oligonucleotide, in combination with chemotherapy in refractory or relapsed acute leukemia. Blood 2003;101:425–432.

94. Cunningham CC, Holmlund JT, Geary RS, et al: A Phase I trial of H-ras antisense oligonucleotide ISIS 2503 administered as a continuous intravenous infusion in patients with advanced carcinoma. Cancer 2001;92:1265–1271.

95. Capoulade C, Mir LM, Carlier K, et al: Apoptosis of tumoral and nontumoral lymphoid cells is induced by both mdm2 and p53 antisense oligodeoxynucleotides. Blood 2001;97:1043–1049.

96. Sasaki H, Sheng Y, Kotsuji F, Tsang BK: Down-regulation of X-linked inhibitor of apoptosis protein induces apoptosis in chemoresistant human ovarian cancer cells. Cancer Res 2000;60:5659–5666.

97. Ashkenazi A, Pai RC, Fong S, et al: Safety and antitumor activity of recombinant soluble Apo2 ligand. J Clin Invest 1999;104:155–162.

98. Walczak H, Miller RE, Ariail K, et al: Tumoricidal activity of tumor necrosis factor-related apoptosis-inducing ligand in vivo. Nat Med 1999;5:157–163.

99. Jo M, Kim TH, Seol DW, et al: Apoptosis induced in normal human hepatocytes by tumor necrosis factor- related apoptosis-inducing ligand. Nat Med 2000;6:564–567.

100. Rathmell JC, Vander Heiden MG, Harris MH, Frauwirth KA, Thompson CB: In the absence of extrinsic signals, nutrient utilization by lymphocytes is insufficient to maintain either cell size or viability. Mol Cell 2000;6:683–692.

101. Deckwerth TL, Johnson EM, Jr.: Temporal analysis of events associated with programmed cell death (apoptosis) of sympathetic neurons deprived of nerve growth factor. J Cell Biol 1993;123:1207–1222.

102. Gottlob K, Majewski N, Kennedy S, Kandel E, Robey RB, Hay N: Inhibition of early apoptotic events by Akt/PKB is dependent on the first committed step of glycolysis and mitochondrial hexokinase. Genes Dev 2001;15:1406–1418.

103. Elstrom R, Guan L, Nakhoda K, et al: Utility of FDG-PET scanning in lymphoma by WHO classification. Blood 2003;101:3875–3876.

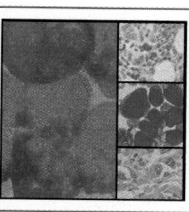

Drew M. Pardoll

IMMUNOLOGY AND CANCER

SUMMARY OF KEY POINTS

- Although the classic immune surveillance hypothesis has not been experimentally validated, evidence is accumulating that some newly developing tumors induce natural immune responses that eliminate them before they become clinically detectable.
- To survive in the host, tumors must develop active mechanisms that enable them to invade tissues without activating immune responses that would destroy them. Successful tumors, therefore, have developed mechanisms to shift the immunologic balance from activation to tolerance induction. Breaking immune tolerance is a central goal

of active immunotherapy. The first successful immunotherapeutic approaches used monoclonal antibodies targeted at tumors.
- There is clear evidence that despite the capacity of tumors to induce immunologic tolerance to their antigens, adoptive transfer protocols demonstrate that tumor-specific T cells do indeed exist in humans. Advances in the understanding of T-cell regulation offer a stunning variety of new opportunities to enhance T cell–based antitumor immunity.
- Emerging appreciation for the central role of dendritic cells (DC)

in initiating immune responses has led to development of DC-based vaccines and new strategies to load DC more effectively with tumor antigens.
- Elucidation of both costimulatory pathways for T-cell activation and immunologic checkpoints that negatively regulate immune responses provides a number of opportunities to amplify normally weak immune responses. Ultimately, successful immunotherapy of cancer will require rationally designed combined approaches that target key regulatory points in the immune response in a coordinated fashion.

INTRODUCTION

The interaction between developing tumors and their immunologic environment is active, not passive. As tumors develop, they acquire genetic alterations and alter gene expression patterns, providing a large number of potential tumor antigens capable of being recognized by the immune system. A fundamental question in cancer immunology is how the immune system recognizes these antigens—specifically, whether it responds to them by becoming activated or becoming tolerant of them as it does to self-tissue antigens.

For well over a century, investigators have appreciated the potential of the immune system to combat cancer. In the 1880s Paul Ehrlich coined the term "magic bullet" in reference to the capacity of antibodies to recognize and target both infectious organisms and cancer cells.[1] In the 1890s, William Coley, a New York surgeon, recognized that some of his cancer patients who developed systemic infections then experienced regression of their tumors. Coley postulated that the systemic infections nonspecifically activated immune responses, which, in turn, attacked the patients' tumors. Coley began to treat cancers with extracts from specific bacteria that had been associated with tumor regressions.[2] These bacterial extracts, called Coley's toxins, raised tremendous excitement at the time based on their occasional ability to induce dramatic regressions of large tumors; however, the

nonspecific toxicities induced by these toxins caused tremendous morbidity. Ultimately, Coley's toxins were abandoned because of their high toxicity and because the absence of understanding of their mechanism of action precluded rational modifications that would mitigate toxicity while maintaining antitumor efficacy. (Of historical note, the term "Coley's toxins" actually was coined by Coley's nemesis and antagonist, James Ewing— the Ewing of Ewing sarcoma—who believed that Coley overdramatized the antitumor responses and minimized the toxicities associated with his bacterial extracts.) Although promise and skepticism continue to characterize the field of cancer immunotherapy, certain features of the immune system do make it extremely attractive as a potential anticancer weapon.

THE IMMUNE SYSTEM'S POTENTIAL FOR ANTITUMOR ACTIVITY

The wide diversity of the components of the adaptive immune response provides the potential for exquisite specificity. Both antibodies and T-cell receptors can distinguish between biochemical structures that differ by as little as a single methyl group. Therefore, the combination of antibodies and T cells offers the capacity to recognize even subtle biochemical differences that are either specific or selective to tumor cells relative to their normal counterparts (Fig. 7-1).

Diversity
T cells - 10^{18}
Antibodies - 10^{22}

Specificity
Can distinguish a
single methyl group

Weaponry
NO, superoxides,
HOCl, H202,
FasL, TRAIL,
Perforin,
Granzyme B,
Myeloperoxidase
complement
phagocytes

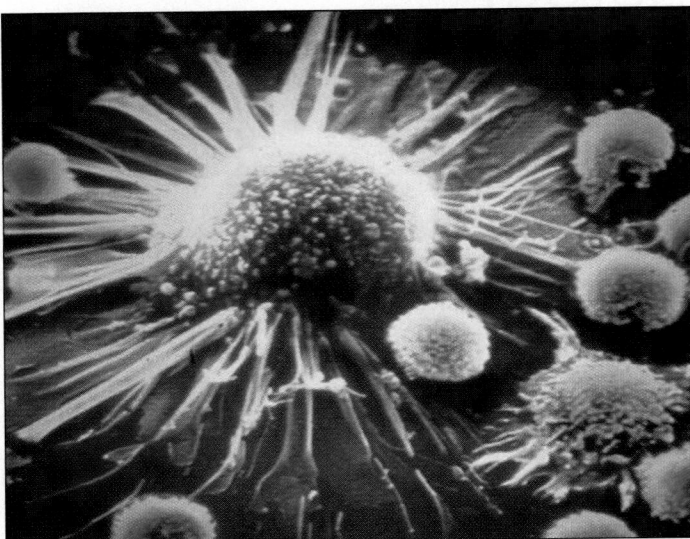

Figure 7-1. Many features of the immune system make it a potentially effective anticancer agent. This electron micrograph shows a tumor cell being recognized by a tumor-specific cytotoxic T lymphocyte (*lower right*). Other lymphocytes in the vicinity are not specific for any of the antigens expressed by the tumor and, therefore, do not engage the tumor cell. The tumor-specific lymphocyte has recognized cognate peptide–MHC complexes on the tumor cell and engaged these complexes through upregulation and activation of various adhesion molecules. The cytotoxic lymphocyte is creating pores in the tumor cell membrane by elaboration of perforin. These perforin pores allow the entry of various proteases, such as granzyme-B, into the tumor cell. Granzyme-B and other cytotoxic granule enzymes cleave effector caspaces and initiate a death program in the target cell. In general, the immune system possesses both tremendous diversity and tremendous weaponry. T cells, via their T-cell receptors, can generate 10^{18} different potential specificities. B cells, using a similar mechanism of diversity generation, can produce roughly 10^{23} potential different antibody specificities. Both T-cell receptors and immunoglobulins can recognize molecular differences as small as a single methyl group. The various components of the immune system—both innate and adaptive—utilize many different cytocidal molecules. These include superoxides and nitric oxide as well as other reactive oxygen species. Additional effectors include Fas ligand and TRAIL, which induce target cell death through specific receptors of the extrinsic apoptosis pathway. Other systems, such as the complement system and cellular cytotoxicity mechanisms mediated by activated natural killer (NK) cells and macrophages, round out a diverse and potent cytotoxic repertoire.

T cells also offer the capacity to recognize intracellular antigens in essentially any cellular compartment because T cells, via their T-cell receptors, recognize peptide-major histocompatibility complex (MHC) complexes on the cell surface. Most of the peptides presented by MHC molecules on the cell surface are derived from processing of proteins in intracellular compartments. These intracellular processing pathways, which have been worked out at the molecular level, result in loading of nascent MHC class I molecules in the endoplasmic reticulum and nascent MHC class II molecules in endosome-like compartments. Following loading, the peptide MHC complexes are transported to the cell surface for recognition by T cells. Therefore, the MHC system acts like a conveyer belt bringing pieces of intracellular antigens to the surface for recognition by T cells.

The cytotoxic mechanisms of the immune system are diverse and extremely potent. Once bound to their targets, antibodies can efficiently fix complement as well as mediate antibody-dependent cellular cytotoxicity mechanisms mediated by activated natural killer cells and macrophages. Cytotoxic T cells that recognize target cells expressing cognate peptide-MHC complexes efficiently form pores in target cell membranes through secretion of perforin. It is now estimated that three or even fewer cognate peptide MHC complexes on a cell can render it

targetable by an activated cytotoxic T lymphocyte (CTL). Perforin-dependent pores allow for the injection of granzyme-B, which induces caspase activation cascades, which lead to target cell apoptosis. Additional cytocidal effector pathways utilized by the immune system include the elaboration of nitric oxide, superoxides, hydrogen peroxide, hypochlorate, and inducers of extrinsic apoptosis pathways such as Fas ligand and tumor necrosis factor-related apoptosis-inducing ligand. In fact, a number of studies have demonstrated that tumor cells that develop multidrug resistance to all standard chemotherapeutic agents continue to be susceptible to killing by various immunologic effector mechanisms.

The major form of immunotherapy that has reached fruition in the modern era uses monoclonal antibodies targeted at cell membrane proteins selectively expressed by tumor cells. The application of antibodies and immunologic conjugates for cancer therapy is covered in detail in Chapter 32. Immunotherapeutic approaches such as adoptive immunotherapy and active immunotherapy (i.e., cancer vaccines, see Chapter 33) have yet to become "standard" therapy for cancer patients, despite a large amount of both animal modeling and clinical trials activity. However, analysis of clinical trials performed during the past two decades clearly demonstrates that these trials have failed to incorporate some of the most promising approaches based on the relatively recent molecular and cellular definition of immune regulation. Nonetheless, the success of allogeneic bone marrow transplantation in many hematologic tumors is now recognized to be based on the anticancer effect of T cells transferred into conditioned recipients along with the bone marrow graft—the "graft vs. tumor" effect. Essentially all curative responses in allogeneic bone marrow transplantation can be attributed in large part to the T cell–mediated graft vs. tumor effect rather than the chemoradiation therapy incorporated into the conditioning regimen for the recipient.

RELATION BETWEEN CANCER CELLS AND THE IMMUNE SYSTEM

Ultimately, successful immunotherapy of cancer will require an understanding of the relation between the immune system and tumors as they transform, invade, and metastasize. There is evidence that immune responses against tumor antigens are similar in some ways (but not in all) to immune responses against "self" tissue antigens. Because tumors are transformations of normal cells, it is not surprising that immune responses to tumors would in many ways resemble those to normal tissues. Indeed, immune tolerance to tumors has been demonstrated to mimic the natural mechanisms of immune tolerance to normal tissues in a number of systems. However, dissection of the molecular and cellular events of tumor transformation, combined with increased understanding of the pathophysiology of tumor progression, illustrates that there are important features that distinguish cancer cells from their normal counterparts. Some of these differences significantly affect the nature of the interaction between developing cancers and the immune system, and these features may well provide the immunologic window to be exploited therapeutically.

Tumors differ fundamentally from their normal cell counterparts in antigenic composition and biologic behavior. The molecular hallmark of carcinogenesis is genetic instability. Genetic instability in cancers is a consequence of deletion or mutational inactivation of genome guardians, such as p53 (see Chapters 5 and 15). In fact, many of the genetically defined familial cancer syndromes, such as hereditary nonpolyposis colon cancer and familial breast cancer, are due to mutations in genes that mediate responses to DNA damage (see Chapters 11 and 13). The genetic instability of cancer cells means that new antigens are constantly being generated in tumors as they develop and progress. The accumulation of karyotypic abnormalities in advanced undifferentiated cancers emphasizes the level of genetic instability in tumors. This genetic instability does not occur in normal nontransformed tissues, which maintain their genome guardians and therefore a stable biochemical and antigenic profile. In addition to the thousands of mutational events that occur during tumorigenesis, hundreds of genes that are either inactive or expressed at relatively low levels in the normal tissue counterparts, are upregulated significantly in cancers. Although these epigenetic changes do not formally create tumor-specific neoantigens, they raise the concentration on encoded proteins dramatically, and thereby affect the antigenic profile of the tumor cell.

Another biologic feature of tumors that distinguishes them from normal cells is their capacity to invade across normal tissue barriers and metastasize. Both of these processes are associated with massive disruption of tissue architecture. At the cellular level, normal cell–cell adhesions and cell–tissue matrix interactions are disrupted. One of the important consequences of tissue disruption, whether caused by infectious or mechanical mechanisms, is the elaboration of proinflammatory signals. These signals, in the form of cytokines and chemokines, are critical initiators of both innate and adaptive immune responses. Unlike normal tissues, therefore, cancers are constantly confronted with inflammatory responses as they invade tissues and metastasize through the body. How they handle and modulate these responses dictates their interplay with the host's immune system. Recent insights in both basic immunology and cancer immunology are leading to the realization that while immune tolerance represents a major barrier to successful anticancer therapy, cancer patients themselves contain significant repertoires of both T cells and B cells specific for tumor antigens. Insights into the molecules and signaling pathways that regulate decisions between immunologic activation and tolerance provide exciting new opportunities to reverse tumor-specific tolerance and harness these components of the immune system for successful therapy.

THE NATURAL IMMUNE RESPONSE TO TUMORS: SURVEILLANCE VERSUS TOLERANCE

The past half-century has witnessed a vigorous and ongoing debate between tumor immune surveillance and immune tolerance hypotheses (Fig. 7-2). At the heart of this debate is the question of whether the immune system naturally responds to tumors arising spontaneously within the body. In 1959, Lewis Thomas initially proposed the immune surveillance hypothesis, suggesting that a natural role of the immune system was to recognize newly arising tumors via their expression of tumor-specific neoantigens and eliminate them.[3] Burnet subsequently refined this hypothesis to suggest that tumors arise about as often as infection with pathogens and that the immune system constantly recognizes and eliminates these tumors based on their expression of tumor-associated antigens (TAAs).[4] Originally, the existence of TAAs was hypothesized based on the finding that experimental tumors induced in animals often were rejected when transplanted to syngeneic hosts, whereas transplants of normal tissue between syngeneic hosts were accepted. Modern molecular oncology provides a basis for TAAs as consequences of the genetic and epigenetic alterations fundamental to cancer cells. Not surprisingly, both spontaneously arising and chemically induced tumors in animal systems display diverse immunologic properties on transplantation, with some being rejected effectively (regressor tumors)

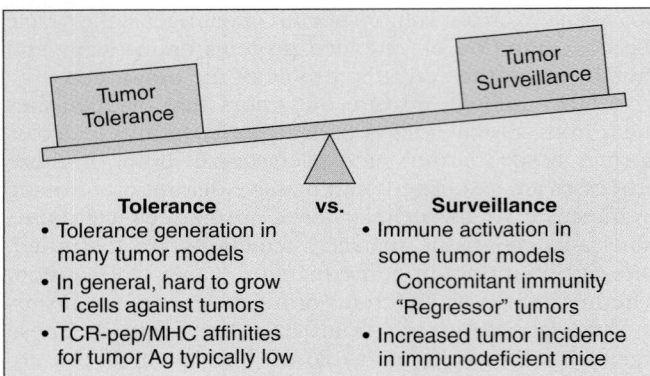

Figure 7-2. The natural relationship between tumors and the immune system represents a balance between immune surveillance and immune tolerance. Evidence for the capacity of tumors to induce immune tolerance comes from multiple animal models in which antigen-specific tolerance can be demonstrated directly on introduction or natural formation of a tumor. Immune tolerance induction by tumors is evidenced further by the extreme difficulty in propagating tumor-specific T cells from most cancer patients. Under circumstances in which tumor-specific T cells can be propagated, the affinity of their T-cell receptor for cognate tumor peptide/MHC ligands typically is much lower than that of T cells specific for viral antigens. This suggests that the high-affinity T cells specific for tumor antigens have been tolerized in vivo. On the other hand, some evidence favors an immune surveillance component of the immune system. Many tumors that are generated by carcinogen induction or other means are rejected by the immune system when transplanted into syngeneic recipients. This contrasts with the acceptance of syngeneic grafts of normal tissues and organs. In addition, recent studies in mice rendered immunodeficient by gene knockout demonstrate an increased incidence of both spontaneous and carcinogen-induced cancers.

and others growing progressively (progressor tumors) after transplantation to syngeneic hosts.[5-9] A corollary to the immune surveillance hypotheses is that clinically progressive cancers are not eliminated because they develop active mechanisms of either immune escape or resistance.

The primary challenges to the immune surveillance hypothesis came from both experimental and epidemiologic data addressing a fundamental prediction of this hypothesis, namely that immunodeficient individuals should display a dramatic increase in tumor incidence. This prediction was first evaluated by analyzing the incidence of tumors in nude mice, which have defective thymic epithelial development and, therefore, significantly reduced numbers of T cells and T cell–dependent immune responses.[10-14] These studies revealed no increased incidence of tumors in nude mice relative to their immunocompetent syngeneic counterparts. A caveat to the interpretation of these experiments is that nude mice still produce diminished numbers of T cells and are therefore capable of some T cell–dependent immunity. In addition, nude mice often display a compensatory increase in innate immunity, including natural killer cell function.

In the 1970s and 1980s, epidemiologic studies of patients with heritable immune deficiencies revealed a more complex pattern of cancer incidence.[15,16] A significantly increased frequency of uncommon cancers such as

B-cell lymphoblastic lymphomas and Kaposi sarcoma was observed. However, there was no increased incidence of the common epithelial cancers seen in adulthood, with the exception of stomach cancer. As more was learned about the viral etiology of some malignancies, it became clear that the cancers most commonly found in immunodeficient individuals were virus-associated (see Chapters 12 and 16 for a more detailed analysis of the viral etiology of cancer and cancers in immunodeficient patients, respectively). Essentially all of the B-cell lymphomas observed in immunodeficient patients are caused by Epstein-Barr virus, resulting from a failure of T cells to control Epstein-Barr virus–transformed B cells.[17] Kaposi sarcoma is the result of failure to respond to human herpes virus-8–infected cells.[18] Other virus-associated cancers (such as cervical cancer caused by human papillomavirus) also are observed at increased frequency in immunodeficient persons.[19,20] It is likely that the increased incidence of stomach cancer in immunodeficient patients relates to aberrant or ineffective immune responses to *Helicobacter pylori* infection.[21]

From these studies, the notion emerged that immune surveillance indeed protects against certain pathogen (mostly virus)–associated cancers, either by preventing infection or by limiting chronic infection by viruses that eventually can lead to cancer. However, failure to observe an altered incidence of cancers with no viral or bacterial association was taken as a strong argument against the classic immune surveillance hypothesis.

A number of recent studies re-evaluating tumor incidence in genetically manipulated mouse models has revealed new evidence that various components of the immune system can at least modify both carcinogen-induced and spontaneous carcinogenesis. In a series of studies by Schreiber and colleagues, cancer incidence was examined in mice rendered immunodeficient via genetic knockout of either the RAG-1 gene, the gamma interferon (γ-IFN) receptor gene, or the STAT-1 gene (Fig. 7-3).[22,23] RAG-1 is a critical molecule for recombination of both T-cell receptor and immunoglobulin genes during development; RAG-1–deficient mice, therefore, produce absolutely no T cells or B cells. The γ-IFN receptor knockout mice are incapable of transducing signals by γ-IFN, which is one of the most important T cell–dependent immunologic effector molecules, mediating many T cell–dependent responses. Signal transducer for activation of transcription-1 (STAT-1) is a critical intracellular signal transducer for both type 1 and type 2 interferon receptors as well as other proinflammatory stimuli. As a result, γ-IFN-receptor knockout mice and STAT-1 knockout mice have impaired innate and adaptive immunity. When tumor incidence was monitored in either RAG-1-/- or γ-IFN-receptor-/- mice either treated with carcinogens or crossed onto a cancer-prone p53-/- background, the incidence of observable cancers was increased slightly but significantly relative to nonimmunodeficient counterparts when observed over an extended period (greater than 1 year). Furthermore, γ-IFN-/- × p53-/- mice also developed a broader spectrum of tumors in mice lacking p53 alone. Transplantation studies suggested that direct γ-IFN sensitivity by the tumor played a significant role

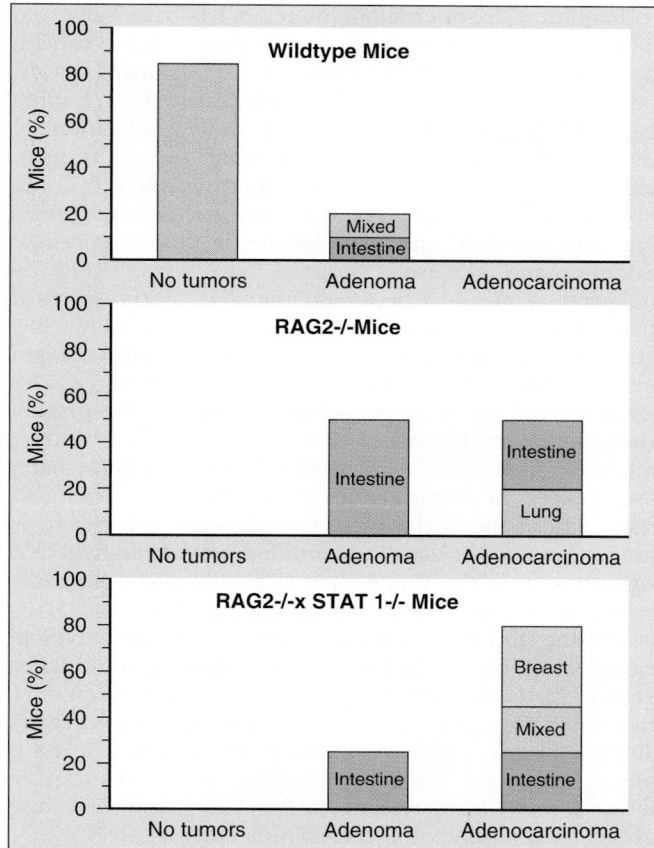

Figure 7-3. Increased incidence of spontaneous tumors in mice lacking T and B cells and interferon signaling pathways. Shankaran and colleagues[23] followed wild-type, Rag-1 KO (incapable of rearranging T-cell receptor or immunoglobulin genes) or Rag-1 KO/Stat-1 KO (incapable of transmitting interferon signals) mice over their 2-year life span. Although wild-type mice eventually were found to develop adenomas, none of them developed malignant adenocarcinomas. However, a large proportion of Rag-1 knockout mice followed beyond 1 year of age did develop adenocarcinomas, usually involving the gut and the lungs. When Rag-1 knockout were crossed to Stat-1 knockout mice, these double-deficient animals developed tumors in virtually all cases. They demonstrated tumor development in additional tissue sites, including the breast. In addition, a significant proportion of animals displayed multiple sites of adenocarcinoma development (mixed). These studies demonstrate that the immune system can play a role in modifying the incidence and type of tumors that develop spontaneously.

in the defect in immune surveillance. These results prompted an analysis of γ-IFN sensitivity of human tumors. Although loss of γ-IFN sensitivity has been documented in a number of cases, the overall incidence in human cancer appears to be quite low. A follow-up study further evaluated the –/–/–/–. Tumor incidence was not increased in young RAG-1– or STAT-1–deficient mice; however, when animals were followed over their normal 2-year life span, an increased tumor incidence was indeed observed, particularly in the RAG-1–/– and RAG-1–/– × STAT-1 –/– mice. Of note, whereas RAG-deficient mice predominantly developed intestinal epithelial tumors, double RAG/STAT-1 knockout mice had a high incidence of breast cancers frequency as well. All tumors from these

animals displayed a regressor phenotype in that they were rejected after transplant into immune competent mice, further suggesting that their development in the original host was related to defects in immune surveillance.

Smyth and colleagues recently have reported similar results, noting an increase in both lymphomas and epithelial tumors in mice deficient in γ-IFN or perforin. Taken together, these recent studies in immunodeficient mice have led to a modified version of the immune surveillance hypothesis, termed "immune editing." The immune editing hypothesis posits that the immune system has a more subtle role in modifying tumorigenesis than originally envisioned by Thomas and Burnett. A recent study by Dranoff and colleagues raises an important caveat to be borne in mind when interpreting tumor incidence in genetically manipulated immunodeficient mice. This group documented an increased incidence of carcinogenesis (in particular, lung and gastrointestinal cancer) in GM-CSF –/– × γ-IFN –/– mice. However, they also noted an increase in the incidence of infection with a bacterium not commonly found in immunocompetent mice. Follow-up studies demonstrated that when GM-CSF–/– × γ-IFN–/– mice were maintained on antibiotics, the increased incidence of tumorigenesis was no longer observed.[24] These studies raised the possibility that the increased tumor incidence in all of the analyses of immunodeficient mice are the consequence of pathogen-associated carcinogenesis due to a lack of immune surveillance against the pathogen rather than newly developing tumors. Ultimately, observations of tumor incidence in genetically immunodeficient mice raised under notobiotic conditions will be necessary to resolve this issue.

Intraepithelial Lymphocytes in Tumor Immune Surveillance

Because epithelial linings in many organs represent a major site of carcinogenesis and are indeed the origin for most of the common adult cancers, a potentially important immunologic component in surveying for transformed cells may be the system of intraepithelial lymphocytes (IELs). These IELs represent a unique subset of lymphocytes found interspersed in diverse epithelial tissues.[25-27] Classic IELs display features of both adaptive and innate immune systems. The IELs of the gut are 50% γδ-TCR–expressing and 50% αβ-TCR–expressing. In the mouse, essentially all skin IELs express the γδ-T cell receptor (TCR) and an extremely limited TCR repertoire.[28,29] The IELs are less evident in human skin, although there have been recent reports that such a population enriched with γδ-TCR–expressing cells does indeed exist.[30] Although the ligands for the TCRs of IELs have not been well defined, there is evidence that they are self-antigens whose expression may be enhanced under stress or inflammatory conditions.[31]

The best evidence that epidermal IELs can serve a role in tumor immune surveillance comes from recent studies demonstrating that both γδ- and αβ-knockout mice were much more susceptible than their wild-type counterparts to development of skin cancer on skin painted with

Science of Clinical Oncology

carcinogen-promoter regimens.[32] At the molecular level, a confluence of findings points to the NKG2D receptor as a central player in the immunologic sensing of carcinogenic events in the skin, gut, and possibly other sites as well. NKG2D originally was defined as an activating natural killer (NK) cell (NK receptor).[33-35] Intraepithelial lymphocytes express particularly high levels of NKG2D.[36-39]

The first evidence that NKG2D might play a role in tumor immune surveillance came from the finding that both normal colonic epithelium as well as a significant proportion of tumors could express the two defined human ligands for NKG2D—MICA and MICB.[40-42] Mouse NKG2D does bind to products of the retinoic acid inducible gene family, RAE-1α-ε as well as to the product of the H60 gene.[38,39] Although the RAE-1 and H60 genes are not induced obviously by heat shock, they are indeed upregulated in mouse skin after application of carcinogens.[32]

Several groups have provided evidence in mice and humans that RAE-1 and H60 are indeed involved in immune recognition and tumor surveillance in mice. Recognition and killing of murine skin keratinocytes or intestinal epithelial cells by γδ IEL requires expression of NKG2D ligands and is blocked by anti-NKG2D antibodies.[32] In related studies on systemic cancers, transfection of mouse tumors that do not naturally express RAE-1α and H60 with these genes leads to NK-dependent immune rejection of the transfectants in vivo and also, in some cases, to activation of antigen specific CD8+ αβ T cells.[43-45]

The emerging data on NKG2D function in IELs together with the potentially stress-inducible nature of its ligands suggests an intraepithelial system of immune surveillance that may indeed be relevant to carcinogenesis as well as infectious challenges. The major initiating event of carcinogenesis in the skin—ultraviolet light—is a potent source of DNA damage or genotoxic stress. The major guardians of genomic damage are endogenous cell autonomous pathways such as the ATM-p53 pathway, but it certainly is reasonable to hypothesize that such stress could activate an extrinsic immunologic suppressor pathway via expression of NKG2D ligands that would, in turn, rapidly activate adjacent IELs.

Immune Escape and Resistance Mechanisms Employed by Tumors

As indicated in the preceding section, a primary corollary to the immune surveillance hypothesis is that successful development of tumors requires that they develop mechanisms of escape from detection or resistance to killing by the immune system. Although much work has been done on tumor resistance mechanisms, virtually all of the evidence is circumstantial and does not prove that the observed alterations in antigen processing machinery or expression of immune inhibitory molecules is a response on the part of the tumor to activate antitumor immunity. Downregulation of the antigen processing machinery—particularly the MHC class I pathway—has been documented extensively in a large variety of tumors. In humans, downregulation of the MHC class I molecules

or deletion of β2-microglobulin genes has been observed in a range of tumor types, particularly breast cancer, prostate cancer, and lung cancer.[46-69] In many cases, individual HLA alleles are lost selectively. This finding has been suggested to represent downmodulation of the presentation of immunodominant tumor antigen; however, this theory has never been proved directly at the level of specific antigen recognition. Loading of peptides onto nascent MHC class I molecules in the endoplasmic reticulum requires processing of cytosolic antigens by the proteosome into peptides, followed by transport of these peptides across the endoplasmic reticulum (ER) membrane by the transporter associated with antigen presentation (TAP) complex. Downregulation of TAP genes as well as those encoding subunits of the proteosome necessary for generation of MHC class I binding peptides (such as LMP-2 and LMP-7) likewise have been documented in a number of tumor types.[70-75] In most cases where the MHC class I processing machinery is downmodulated, it usually is rapidly upregulated by γ-IFN, suggesting that the diminished expression is epigenetic in origin and reversible. Downmodulation of the MHC processing and presentation machinery is not a typical feature of all cancer. In fact, tumors often express higher levels of MHC class I molecules and processing machinery than their normal tissue of origin. For example, virtually all renal cancers express quite high levels of MHC class I, whereas normal renal epithelium expresses barely detectable levels of surface MHC class I and very low levels of TAP until exposed to stimuli such as γ-IFN.

Attempts to correlate levels of MHC expression with clinical prognosis in humans or tumor growth rates in the mouse have generated inconsistent outcomes, depending on the tumor type or system.[63] Some human studies suggest that expression of MHC molecules by the tumor is a poor prognostic indicator; other studies, however, have suggested the opposite. An example of a human cancer in which MHC class I level is consistently downmodulated by multiple mechanisms in the progression from premalignant lesions to malignancy is cervical cancer.[76-78]

Because NK cells demonstrate enhanced recognition and killing of cells with low MHC class I levels,[79,80] downmodulation of the MHC class I processing machinery would not necessarily represent an effective strategy by the tumor to cloak itself from recognition by the immune system. Indeed, although some reports have suggested that increasing the level of MHC expression resulted in diminished in vivo tumor growth of some murine tumors,[81-83] other tumors demonstrate exactly the opposite outcome—that is, diminished growth with lower levels of MHC expression consequent to enhanced NK cell recognition.[84,85] In conclusion, although the modulation of MHC levels and antigen processing machinery often is observed during the progression of cancer, it is still unclear whether this is a true consequence of development of immune resistance in response to a robust immune surveillance system.

Arguments about loss of TAAs as an escape mechanism from immune surveillance are equally inconclusive. Heterogeneity of TAA expression and attempts to correlate TAA loss are well documented in murine tumor models with transplantation of immunogenic tumors or after vaccination.[86-92] Likewise, Yee and coworkers[92] demonstrated specific loss of cognate melanoma antigens in relapsing tumors from patients treated with adoptive transfer of melanoma antigen–specific CD8+ T cells. Similarly, there are anecdotal reports of specific antigen loss after treatment of melanoma patients with peptide vaccines.[93-95] Taken together, these reports support the concept of TAA loss as a mechanism to escape immunotherapeutically induced antitumor responses. However, despite attempts to document TAA loss with natural tumor progression in humans (particularly in melanoma),[50,52,96-100] there is no clear evidence that TAA loss is a tumor escape response to immune surveillance in the unmanipulated host.

The other major mechanism for putative immune resistance by tumors is the expression of secreted or cell surface molecules that either kill or inhibit cellular components of the effector immune response. Examples include TGF-β[101-103] and FasL.[104-109] FasL also has been shown to display proinflammatory effects, so its role in tumor immune protection is questionable.[110-112]

Induction of Antigen-specific Immune Tolerance by Tumors

Since the early 1990s, murine models of cancer immunity have demonstrated that, in striking contrast to immune surveillance, tumors possess a potent capacity to induce immune tolerance to their antigens. Tolerance appears to be operative predominantly at the level of T cells; B-cell tolerance to tumors is less certain because there is ample evidence for the induction of antibody responses in animals bearing tumors as well as human patients with tumors. With the exception of antibodies against membrane receptors directly involved in tumor growth (e.g., members of the epidermal growth factor receptor family), there is little evidence that the bulk of the humoral response to tumors provides significant or relevant antitumor immunity. In contrast, numerous adoptive transfer studies have demonstrated the potent capacity of T cells to kill growing tumors, either directly through CTL activity or indirectly through multiple CD4-dependent effector mechanisms. It is thus likely that from the standpoint of the tumor, induction of antigen-specific tolerance among T cells is of paramount importance for survival.

The most clearcut evidence for induction of T cell tolerance by tumors has come from the analysis of responses to tumor antigens using TCR transgenic T cells.[113-116] Tolerance induction has been demonstrated in both the CD4 and the CD8 compartment. In general, initial activation of tumor antigen–specific T cells is observed commonly; however, the activated state of T cells typically is not sustained, with failure of tumor elimination as a common consequence.[117-123] In most cases, tolerance induction among tumor antigen specific T cells is an active process involving antigen recognition. Virtually all investigators who have explored the mechanisms of tumor antigen recognition by T cells have found that the predominant pathway of recognition is instead through cross-presentation by host bone marrow–derived antigen-presenting cells.[116,124-126] A recent analysis of mesothelin-specific CD8 responses induced by an allogeneic cell-based pancreatic cancer vaccine demonstrates robust cross-priming in a human tumor model.[127]

The goal of defining the outcome of T-cell recognition of tumor antigens has been emphasized. As stated earlier, the most common consequence of antigen recognition appears to be tolerance induction, although activation of tumor-specific T cells sometimes is observed. Although the initial experiments were done using transplantable tumors, the most relevant analyses are in tumor-prone transgenic mouse systems in which immunity to tumor antigens can be followed during the endogenous transformation from normal cells to tumors. In these systems, tumor development sometimes has been associated with immune activation and, in other cases, induction of tolerance.[126,128] Analysis of the consequences of transformation in additional tumor transgenic mouse systems will be critical to understanding the varied consequences of tumorigenesis in different tissues with regard to immune activation vs. tolerance. A common theme among all these experiments is that the nature of immune responses to tumors is either tolerance (via ignorance, anergy, or deletion) or a level of activation that is insufficient to eliminate progressing tumors.

Clearcut documentation of antigen-specific immune tolerance induction in human cancer is much more difficult owing to the small number of well-defined human tumor antigens (other than melanoma) and the unavailability of clean transgenic approaches to quantify antigen-specific immune responses. Nonetheless, the fact that it is so much more difficult to culture tumor-specific T-cell lines from cancer patients than virus-specific T cells suggests that high-avidity tumor-specific T cells have been tolerized.

Induction of Regulatory T Cells by Tumors

One of the most important new dimensions to be added the T-cell tolerance question has come from the rebirth of the suppressor cell field.[129-131] T cells that were able to suppress immune responses were first described in the 1970s.[132] Back then, suppressor T cells were thought to be a specialized population of CD8 cells, the effects of which were mediated by secreted antigen-specific factors. Robert North described CD4+ suppressor cells as inhibitors of antitumor immunity in the 1970s and early 1980s, although little attention was paid to this particular aspect of the early chapter of suppressor T cells.[133] Failure to clone antigen-specific suppressor factors or purify them biochemically led to the demise of this entire field by the mid-1980s. Sakaguchi and colleagues created a renaissance in T cell–mediated suppression through their work in the mid-1990s. They demonstrated that a small population of thymically derived CD4 cells that coexpress the interleukin-2 receptor (IL-2R) alpha chain (CD25) is crucial for control of autoreactive T cells in vivo.

There is relatively little specific information on the role of Treg cells in inducing or maintaining tumor tolerance under normal circumstances. However, evidence is beginning to emerge that strongly supports the notion that they are induced by tumors as part of tolerance induction and that they significantly limit the efficacy of cancer immunotherapies. In one study by van Elsas and associates, a combination of a GM-CSF transduced tumor vaccine plus anti-CTLA4 was much more effective at eliminating established tumors when animals were treated with anti-CD25 antibodies before vaccination and anti-CTLA4 treatment.[134,135] In a second set of studies, Jaffee and colleagues demonstrated that treatment of mice with low-dose Cytoxan prior to vaccination enhanced the ability of HER-2/neu/GM-CSF vaccines to protect HER-2/neu transgenic mice from challenge with HER-2/neu–expressing tumors.[136] Because the Cytoxan and vaccine treatments were performed before the tumor challenge, the enhanced effect of Cytoxan could not be explained by a direct antitumor effect. Indeed, low-dose Cytoxan treatment has long been touted to inhibit or kill suppressor cells, although this effect more recently had been attributed to creation of lymphoid "space." However, adoptive transfer experiments with CD4+/CD25+ cells from non-Cytoxan–treated HER-2/neu transgenic mice proved that the effect of Cytoxan was indeed due to inhibition of Treg cells. Many additional demonstrations for an important role of Treg cells in blunting or blocking antitumor immunity probably will be seen, most likely because they are a natural consequence of tolerance induction. They represent a very tempting target for inhibition as part of combination immunotherapy strategies.

Can the Evidence for Tumor Immune Surveillance and Tolerance Be Reconciled?

The apparently disparate concept of a natural immune surveillance system for tumors together with the remarkable capacity of tumors to induce tolerance to their antigens is a fundamental paradox in cancer immunology. Any unifying hypothesis must take into account the diverse nature of the genetic and epigenetic changes occurring during the progressive stages of the tumor transformation growth and metastasis.

The hallmark of cancer is tissue invasion and metastasis. Both processes are highly disruptive of tissue architecture. In fact, the tumor itself represents a tissue with highly disrupted architecture. Whenever tissue architecture is disturbed, strong proinflammatory signals in the form of cytokines such as TNF and type 1 interferons and chemokines such as RANTES are elaborated. In addition, disruption of epithelial linings of the gut, skin, and bronchi allows bacterial products such as lipopolysaccharide to infiltrate tissues. These cytokines and chemokines, as well as bacterial products, not only activate components of innate immunity (e.g., neutrophils, NK cells, and macrophages) but also activate dendritic cells. Dendritic cells are the critical antigen-presenting cell that initiates immune responses by naïve T cells. To activate T cells, DCs must themselves be activated to "mature" from an immature precursor state. Dendritic cell maturation, which is induced by the same endogenous stimuli (cytokines and chemokines) and exogenous

stimuli (bacterial and fungal products such as LPS—collectively known as pathogen-associated molecular patterns [PAMPs]) that activate innate immunity, results in enhanced antigen presentation and elaboration of costimulatory signals necessary for activating T cells (Fig. 7-4).

If, in the course of tissue invasion, a developing tumor generates a neoantigen consequent to genetic instability, it is possible that the neoantigen would be presented to the immune system in the context of the proinflammatory, immunologically activating environment associated with tissue disruption. According to the "danger" model of immune activation versus tolerance, such a neoantigen would be viewed as foreign, inducing a strong T-cell response that, together with innate responses, could

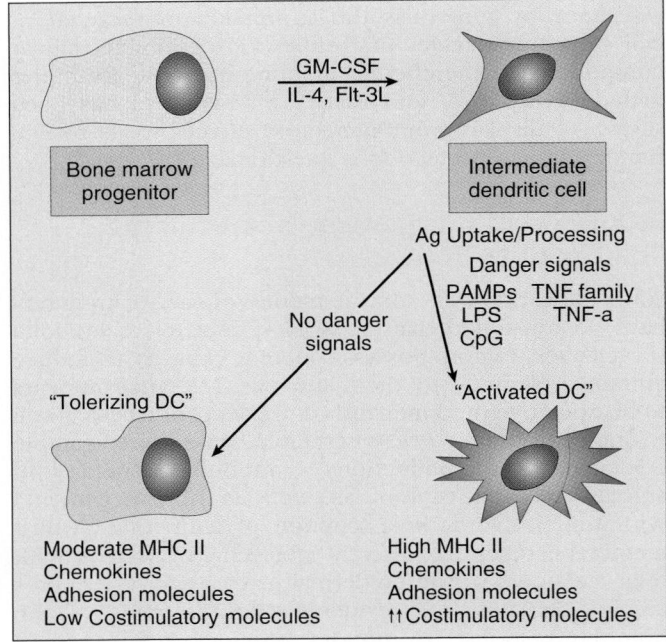

Figure 7-4. Two different pathways of dendritic cell differentiation. Dendritic cells are the critical immunologic sensors that ultimately determine whether the immune system will become activated or tolerized. Initially, intermediate dendritic cells differentiate from bone marrow progenitors under control of cytokines such as GM-CSF, FLT-3 ligand, and interleukin-4. Intermediate dendritic cells are specialized for antigen uptake and processing in the periphery. In the presence of various proinflammatory cytokines or pathogen-derived molecular species (pathogen-associated molecular patterns [PAMPs]), the intermediate dendritic cells mature as they traffic from the periphery to the secondary lymphoid tissues (lymph nodes and periarteriolar lymphatic sheaths of the spleen). Dendritic cell maturation involves the traffic of peptide/MHC complexes to the cell surface, production of chemokines that attract naïve T cells, upregulation of adhesion molecules, and upregulation of multiple costimulatory molecules in the B7 family as well as the TNF family. A highly activated dendritic cell is the critical antigen-presenting cell to initiate the activation of T-cell responses. In the absence of infection or proinflammatory signals, a steady-state process is operative in which dendritic cells from the periphery traffic to secondary lymphoid tissues and are capable of presenting antigens to T cells in a tolerogenic fashion. Because these dendritic cells do not express significant levels of costimulatory molecules, the result of antigen presentation is induction of anergy or deletion among T cells that results in tolerance. This pathway represents a natural pathway for induction and maintenance of tolerance to peripheral self-antigens.

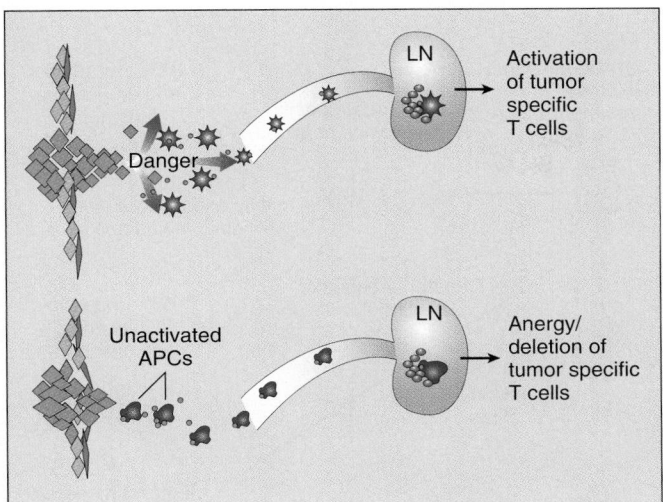

Figure 7-5. Two potential immunologic outcomes of tumor development are immune activation or tolerance generation. When tumors first develop, they disrupt natural tissue barriers as part of the early stages of invasion and metastasis. This tissue invasion and disruption can result in the generation of proinflammatory and immunologic danger signals. These proinflammatory signals, including the release of PAMPs (e.g., from gut bacteria in the case of colon cancer) and local induction of proinflammatory cytokines such as TNF and type 1 interferons, can result in activation of dendritic cells as well as components on innate immunity. Activated dendritic cells can carry neoantigens released by the tumor to the draining lymph node, where they can activate tumor specific T cells (*top*). For a tumor to progress, including tissue invasion and metastases, it must invade tissues in a manner that does not incite an immunologically productive immune response. If it succeeds in doing so, a default pathway becomes operative in which tumor-specific neoantigens are taken up by tolerizing dendritic cells (i.e., those that fail to be appropriately activated). These tolerizing dendritic cells traffic into draining lymph nodes and present tumor antigens to T cells in a tolerogenic fashion (see Fig. 7-4). It is postulated that the initiation of this tolerogenic process by tumor cells may involve the active participation of oncogenic pathways that inhibit both the release and sensing of immunologic danger signals in the environment of the invading tumor (*bottom*).

eliminate the tumor (Fig. 7-5). Such an early transformation event would thus be terminated prior to becoming clinically evident in an immunocompetent individual. These abortive events, which are relatively uncommon, are observed as increased tumor incidence when components of the immune system are inactivated, such as in the RAG knockout and STAT-1 or γ-IFN receptor knockout mice evaluated by Schreiber and colleagues.[23] It is notable that the major site of tumorigenesis in the RAG- and STAT-1–deficient mice was in the gut, the major source of proinflammatory PAMPs such as LPS. This model does not invoke the existence of a specific tumor immune surveillance system, but, rather, suggests that the occasional naturally activated antitumor responses are a consequence of the proinflammatory effects of tumor invasion together with neoantigen expression. In contrast, the NKG2D-based system for IELs may represent a more specific mechanism to detect early consequences of genotoxic stress in epithelial cells. Such a system putatively would synergize with the endogenous cellular systems that induce apoptosis of cells whose DNA has been damaged beyond repair.

It is now well established that for tumors to progress and take advantage of genetic instability with its consequent mutations and alterations in gene expression. Intrinsic suppressors must be inactivated, by either mutation, deletion, or—in some cases—promoter methylation. By analogy, it is reasonable to imagine that in the same way tumors may develop specific mechanisms to inhibit induction of immune responsiveness so as to avoid activating innate and adaptive components of immunity specific for their antigens (see Fig. 7-5). Indeed, recent work by Yu and colleagues suggests that natural oncogenic pathways may indeed have these very specific immunologic consequences. They evaluated the immunologic role of activation of STAT-3 in tumor cells. STAT-3 is activated constitutively in a large proportion of tumors of diverse histologic types and appears to represent a true oncogenic pathway, inducing cell cycle regulatory genes such as cyclin D1 and anti-apoptotic genes such as BCL-Xl.[137] Wang and colleagues have demonstrated that blockade of STAT-3 signaling in tumor cells with a constitutively activated STAT-3 pathway results in upregulation of multiple proinflammatory cytokines and chemokines. Therefore, one of the apparent roles of STAT-3 activation in tumor cells is to suppress the release of proinflammatory danger signals, thereby enhancing the potential ability of a tumor to invade and metastasize without alarming the immune system.[138] In addition, STAT-3 activation in tumor cells induces the elaboration of multiple factors that inhibit dendritic cell differentiation, one of which is VEGF.[139,140] Thus, activated STAT-3, an oncogenic event in tumor cells, also inhibits the sensing of proinflammatory danger signals by antigen-presenting cells. It is likely that other oncogenic pathways will be found to have immunologic consequences as well.

Thus, one can picture tumor progression as a process that has a dichotomous outcome with regard to interactions with the immune system, analogous to the cellular responses to DNA damage, the ultimate initiator of carcinogenesis. To invade tissues successfully and metastasize without activating immune responses that would be lethal to the tumor, the tumor probably needs to activate systems that diminish proinflammatory danger signal production and sensing. In addition to the pleotropic effects of STAT-3 activation, the TGF-β commonly produced by tumors additionally down-modulates diverse inflammatory processes.[141-143] The consequence would then be a transition in the immune response from activation to tolerance induction, because, in the absence of proinflammatory danger signals (or failure to sense them) DCs present antigens to T cells in a fashion that induces tolerance, putatively because they do not express adequate costimulatory molecules[144-147] (see Fig. 7-4). Therefore, although immune surveillance probably works to eliminate some early-stage transformed cells, the tumors that reach clinical attention because of their advanced progression and metastases are likely to have developed mechanisms that enable them to spread without inducing a level of immunity that would be lethal to them. In other words, clinically advanced tumors probably have developed active mechanisms to shift the balance of immunity from surveillance to tolerance.

Science of Clinical Oncology

RATIONALE FOR ACTIVE IMMUNOTHERAPY OF CANCER

In the face of the mounting evidence presented earlier that successfully developing tumors induce tolerance to their antigens, a fundamental question that arises in considering immunotherapy of cancer is whether this tolerance can be broken. In the case of antibody-based therapy, tolerance can be bypassed easily by producing monoclonal antibodies in mice against candidate cell membrane tumor antigens for human tumors (such as HER-2/neu) and then "humanizing" them genetically (see Chapter 32). The critical challenge in immunotherapy strategies involving T cells is to break tolerance in the existing repertoire of tumor-reactive T cells within the cancer patient's body. Understanding the state of tumor-specific T cell repertoire once tolerance has been imposed is critical to the design of strategies to break tumor tolerance. For example, if all high affinity T cells have been deleted, tolerance is not reversible. Fortunately, the murine studies described earlier suggest that tolerance induction by tumors usually involves a component of T cell anergy in which T cells remain but are in a somewhat paralyzed state. In humans, the most informative analyses regarding the state of tumor-specific T cells involve adoptive transfer of T cells removed from patients and activated and expanded in vitro before reinfusion. Although these adoptive transfer studies are difficult to apply reproducibly in large numbers of patients, they are informative regarding the potential of the endogenous antitumor T-cell repertoire.

Two recent adoptive transfer studies in patients with melanoma bear consideration. In one study, Yee and coworkers treated patients with melanoma with CD8 T-cell clones from patients with melanoma specific for two melanocyte/melanoma antigens—MART-1/melan A or gp100 (Fig. 7-6).[92] In parallel studies, Rosenberg and colleagues also have evaluated the efficacy of adoptively transferred melanoma-specific T cells from populations of tumor-infiltrating lymphocytes (TIL).[148] A number of important conclusions can drawn at least be tentatively from these two adoptive T-cell transfer studies. First, they both indicate that tumor-reactive T cells do exist in cancer patients and that when appropriately activated, they are indeed capable of trafficking into even large metastatic tumor deposits and eliminating tumor cells expressing the target antigen. Secondly, unless the T cells are specific for a target critical to tumor growth and persistence, a monovalent specificity to the immunotherapy probably will be insufficient in patients with a large tumor burden. This conclusion is strongly supported by the frequent development of antigen loss variants subsequent to adoptive therapy with individual T-cell clones. It is highly likely that at least some of the enhanced clinical success of the TIL study relates to the mixed specificities of the infused TIL cultures. Consequently, future immunotherapy strategies need to focus on the generation of combined CD4 and CD8 T-cell activation.

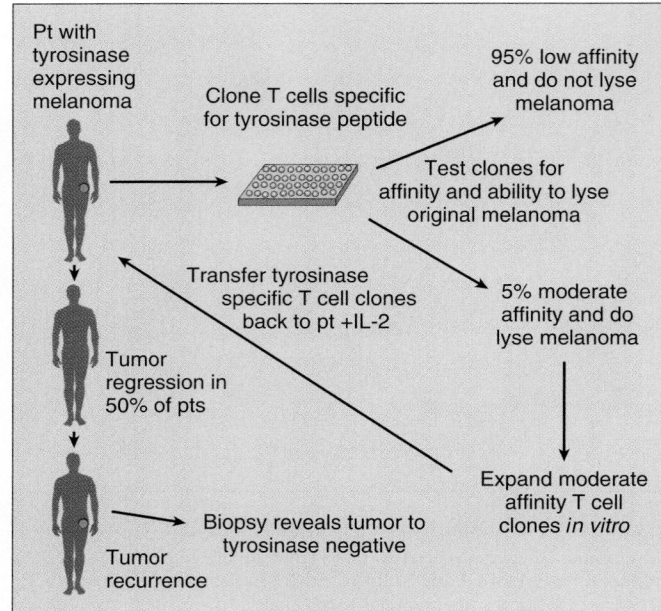

Figure 7-6. There is evidence that cancer patients possess tumor-specific T cells. In a set of adoptive transfer experiments, Yee and colleagues generated T-cell clones from melanoma patients specific for the melanocyte/melanoma antigen tyrosinase.[92] CD8 T-cell clones specific for HLA-A2–restricted tyrosinase peptides were grown in culture. By analyzing binding of tyrosinase peptide/HLA-A2 tetramers, Yee and colleagues were able to derive a set of relative TCR affinity values for individual clones. They found that the majority of tyrosinase-specific CD8 T-cell clones bound tetramer very weakly, indicating that their T-cell receptor had a low affinity for cognate tyrosinase peptide/HLA-A2. These T-cell clones efficiently lysed peptide-loaded target cells; however, they failed to lyse tyrosinase-positive melanoma cells. A small fraction of the tyrosinase-specific T-cell clones bound tyrosinase/HLA-A2 tetramers to a higher degree, indicating that they possessed intermediate affinities for the tyrosinase/HLA-A2 complex. These T-cell clones successfully lysed melanoma cells in addition to peptide-loaded target cells. When these intermediate-affinity T-cell clones were reinfused into patients, together with low doses of interleukin-2, a significant proportion of the patients generated temporary regressions in some of their tumors. However, all of the patients eventually demonstrated tumor recurrence. Biopsy analysis of tumors before adoptive T-cell therapy and also after recurrence revealed the specific loss of tyrosinase in response to adoptive T-cell therapy. When similar treatments were done with T cells specific for a different melanoma antigen, gp100, the recurrences were associated with loss of gp100 rather than tyrosinase. These clinical studies demonstrate definitively that melanoma patients possess T cells capable of being activated to kill their melanoma cells. However, targeting a single antigen whose expression is not necessary for the tumor growth or survival will result in the selection of antigen loss variants by the tumor.

The Dendritic Cell as a Target for Therapeutic Vaccines

Studies in mouse models, as well as T-cell adoptive transfer studies in humans such as those described earlier in this chapter, clearly demonstrate that cancer patients maintain a latent population of tumor-reactive T cells. In part because of the technical difficulties of ex vivo T-cell culture and adoptive transfer, the major initiatives in immunotherapy have involved attempts to activate these latent T-cell populations in vivo through active immunotherapy strategies. The most common theme among active immunotherapy strategies is enhancement or modulation of antigen-presenting cell (APC) function. Presentation of antigen by APCs is the critical initial step in initiation of adaptive immunity. The quantitative and qualitative characteristics of T-cell responses to antigen depend on the signals they receive from the APC. Elucidation of the molecular events of APC proliferation, differentiation, and activation, together with the molecular definition of signals communicated between APCs and T cells, is transforming the design of therapeutic vaccines. Among the major bone marrow–derived APC subtypes (B cells, macrophages and dendritic cells), the DC has emerged as the most potent APC type responsible for initiating immune responses. Because virtually all phases of DC differentiation and function can be modulated by engineered vaccines, it is important to understand the molecular signals that regulate their role in activation of T cell–dependent immunity.[149-151]

At sites of infection and inflammation, bone marrow–derived progenitor cells (either circulating or resident in the tissue) respond to both proliferative and differentiative signals to develop into mature DCs.[152-156] Initially, immature DCs pass through a stage of differentiation that is specialized for antigen uptake and processing but not for presentation to T cells. Antigen uptake occurs through both micropinocytosis ("drinking of fluid-phase antigens") and receptor-mediated endocytosis, dependent on lectin-like membrane molecules such as CD36 and DEC-205.[157,158] Once in endosomal compartments, antigens are digested into peptide, peptidoglycan, and glycolipid fragments, which are shunted to lysosome-like compartments where they associate with MHC class II as well as class Ib molecules. In addition to processing within vesicular compartments, antigens also are transferred out of endosomes and into the cytosol where they can undergo proteosome-dependent processing and TAP-dependent transport into the ER for association with MHC class I molecules.[149,159]

Once they have ingested antigens at inflammatory sites in the tissue, immature DCs differentiate in response to a number of distinct maturation signals (see Fig. 7-4). Many diverse molecules induce DC maturation, but most appear to signal DCs via binding to two classes of receptor—the toll-like receptors (TLR) and the TNF receptor (TNFR) family. The TLRs are pattern recognition receptors (PRR), which bind common chemical moieties expressed by pathogens, termed pathogen-associated molecular patterns (PAMPs).[160] The TNFR family members deliver maturation signals in response to endogenously produced ligands. The two best-characterized endogenous DC maturation factors are TNF-α itself and CD40L.[161-163]

One of the first consequences of DC maturation is the expression of chemokine receptors such as CCR7, which cause migration from the peripheral tissues to the draining lymph nodes via afferent lymphatics.[164] Once the DC is in the draining lymph node, full maturation transforms DC function from antigen uptake and processing into antigen presentation to T cells. This maturation phase involves the traffic of MHC class II molecules from MHC loading compartments onto the cell surface, where they present peptides derived from antigens ingested during the immature tissue phase.[165,166] Presentation of MHC class II-restricted antigens to CD4 cells in the paracortical regions of the lymph node sets up a cross-talk in which CD4 cells further activate DCs through CD40 as well as CD40-independent pathways.[167-170] These activated DCs are particularly potent in presenting antigens to and activating CD8 cells. Mature DCs also produce chemokines, thereby selectively attracting immature T cells to their surface. This function, together with expression of high levels of adhesion molecules such as ICAM-1, can be observed through clustering of as many as 100 T cells onto the surface of a single dendritic cell.[171]

In addition to provision of high densities of peptide–MHC complexes for T-cell stimulation (termed *signal 1*), DCs regulate T-cell activation and differentiation through provision of costimulatory signals in the form of soluble and membrane-bound ligands (collectively termed *signal 2*). The best-characterized soluble signal delivered to T cells by DCs is the cytokine IL-12, which induces γ-IFN production and promotes Th1 differentiation via a STAT-4–dependent pathway. The best-characterized membrane-bound costimulatory ligands are represented by the B7 family (Fig. 7-7).[172-181]

In addition to the B7 family members, other TNF family members expressed by DCs costimulate T cells. Two examples of this category of costimulatory signals are 4-1BBL and OX40-L.[182-184] The ever-expanding panoply of costimulatory signals used by DCs to instruct T cells as to their pathway of differentiation and effector function adds a high degree of complexity to the communication between APC and T cells (see Fig. 7-7). Evidence is accumulating that, in the absence of maturation signals that activate DCs, a steady-state process occurs in which DCs carry antigens from the periphery to the secondary lymphoid tissues, presenting them to T cells in a fashion that induces tolerance. Although the absolute characteristics of the "tolerizing" DC are not absolutely determined, it appears that they express low levels of critical costimulatory molecules, including B7.2 (see Fig. 7-4). Each of the molecular events involved in proliferation, antigen presentation, and costimulation represents a potential target that is being exploited in the design of immunotherapy approaches. Dendritic cell–based vaccines, an active area of immunotherapy research, will have to be carefully examined to characterize the nature of antigen presentation and costimulatory molecule expression by the relevant DC subtypes.

The Potential of Dendritic Cell Vaccines

The ability to culture DCs ex vivo led to a burst of studies of ex vivo antigen-loaded DCs as tumor vaccines. Initially, it was demonstrated that loading of ex vivo cultured DCs with either MHC class I–restricted peptides or whole proteins followed by administration back into the animal led to the generation of immune responses against

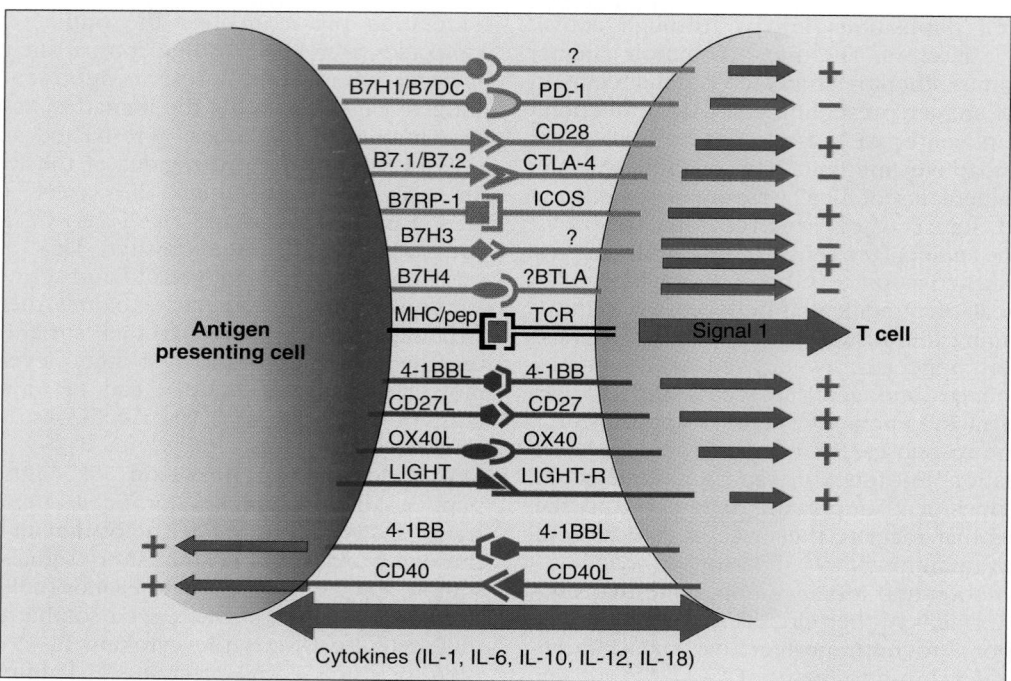

Figure 7-7. The immunologic synapse involves multiple signals between antigen-presenting cell and T cell. At its simplest level, T-cell activation requires two signals. Signal 1 is delivered through the T-cell receptor after engagement by a peptide–MHC complex displayed on the antigen-presenting cell. Signal 2—the costimulatory signal—is now appreciated to represent multiple ligand receptor interactions that transmit both positive and negative signals to the T cell. In general, costimulatory signals fall into three categories—the B7 family, the TNF family, and cytokines. There are now seven known members of the B7 family, some of which have two receptors with opposing signaling pathways. The best examples are B7.1 and B7.2, which transmit positive costimulatory signals to T cells via the CD28 receptor and counterregulatory negative signals via CTLA-4. Multiple TNF family members transmit signals via specific cognate TNF receptor family members. The B7 family appears to predominantly transmit signals unidirectionally from antigen presenting cell to T cell, but various interactions between the TNF family and the TNF-R family transmit signals from T cell to antigen-presenting cell. Cytokines also transmit signals bidirectionally between antigen-presenting cell and T cell. This complex crosstalk, which occurs in a highly organized fashion at the interaction surface between antigen-presenting cell and T cell, is called the *immunologic synapse*. This analogy to neural transmission is apt, because cell differentiation and activation decisions are made based on integration of the multiple signals transmitted by these ligand–receptor interactions.

the loaded antigen.[185] Significant antitumor responses subsequently were demonstrated after injection of DCs loaded with either tumor-derived peptides or tumor lysates.[186-188] More recently, the advent of more efficient gene transfer vectors has led to approaches in which ex vivo cultured DCs are transduced with genes encoding relevant viral or tumor antigens.[189-191] A number of recombinant replication–defective viruses have been used to transduce DCs. In addition, Gilboa and colleagues have demonstrated that purified RNA can be used effectively to transduce DCs, with resultant presentation of encoded antigens.[192] This strategy offers the interesting possibility that DCs could be transduced with the entire amplified transcriptome of a tumor cell, even when only a tiny amount of tumor tissue is available. Another approach aimed at providing DCs with a full complement of tumor antigens has been DC tumor fusion vaccines.[193] The concept behind this approach is to fuse autologous tumor cells with dendritic cells, thereby allowing for the coexpression of all relevant tumor antigens together with all relevant DC molecules within the same cell. In another approach, DCs loaded with antigen were transduced with genes encoding GM-CSF and CD40L to create an autocrine DC stimulation loop. These genetically

modified DCs resulted in much more potent stimulation of antitumor immunity than immunization with only DCs loaded with antigen.[194] A major issue with regard to ex vivo loaded DC vaccines is the degree of maturation that is induced in vitro and its relevance to homing and function of loaded DCs after reinjection. Steinman, Bardwaj, and colleagues have demonstrated that immunization of patients with antigen-loaded immature DCs actually can result in tolerance or suppression of antigen-specific responses as compared with activation induced by immunization with antigen-loaded DCs matured in vitro prior to injection.[195] Ex vivo loaded DC vaccines currently are under active clinical development, so the therapeutic value of various DC manipulations soon may be sorted out. Currently the lack of direct comparative studies leaves open the question of which method of loading DCs ex vivo will be the most effective.

The elucidation of specific molecules that induce DC proliferation and maturation has provided an important base for the engineering of vaccines with enhanced therapeutic potency based on in vivo DC activation. The prototypical example has been the incorporation of GM-CSF into cell-based tumor vaccines (see Fig. 7-2). Before the discovery of GM-CSF transduced tumors as potent vaccines, a large number of genetically modified tumor vaccines had been evaluated. Genes introduced into tumor cells included MHC genes, genes encoding foreign antigens (i.e., xenogenization),[196-198] costimulatory genes,[199-201] and cytokine genes.[202-211] GM-CSF–transduced vaccines were shown further to cure animals of established micrometastatic tumors.[212,213] Because GM-CSF is strictly a DC differentiation and proliferation factor, it is unclear what stimuli induce DC maturation in this vaccine approach. The most likely maturation stimulus in GM-CSF–transduced vaccines comes from endogenous factors released by dying cells, such as heat shock proteins. Indeed, recent reports have demonstrated that transduction of tumor cells with the hsp-70 gene, significantly increasing the concentration of intracellular hsp-70, enhanced tumor cell immunogenicity.[214,215] Another example of vaccine engineering using a combination of DC proliferative and maturation stimuli was provided by Colombo and colleagues. They found that vaccination with tumor cells cotransduced with GM-CSF and CD40L genes generated a dramatic increase in activated DCs at the vaccine site as well as enhanced vaccine potency.[216]

A number of early stage clinical trials using both autologous[217,218] and allogeneic[219] GM-CSF gene-transduced cell-based vaccines have demonstrated both immunization and occasional clinical responses in diverse cancer types, including renal, prostate, melanoma, and pancreatic cancer. These results are promising, but they must be viewed with caution, particularly since earlier generations of BCG-based cancer vaccines that showed promise in initial reports failed to demonstrate significant clinical benefit in larger multicenter randomized clinical trials.[220-222] Two principles form the basis for application of allogeneic genetically modified vaccines. First, tumor antigen discovery studies in human cancer—particularly melanoma—have demonstrated that a significant proportion of recognized antigens are shared.[223,224] Second, as mentioned earlier in this chapter, a number of murine studies have demonstrated that the critical pathway for processing of tumor antigens is cross-presentation by bone marrow–derived APCs.[116,124-126] It is not necessary, therefore, to match HLA alleles between patient and allogeneic vaccine lines. In fact, a recent analysis of immune responses generated after vaccination with an allogeneic GM-CSF–transduced pancreatic vaccine definitively demonstrated the cross-priming pathway.[127]

Tumor-specific and Tumor-selective Antigens in Antigen-specific Immunotherapy of Cancer

A major advantage of cell-based vaccines is the diversity of expressed tumor antigens and the fact that it is not

---

ANTIGEN-SPECIFIC VERSUS TUMOR CELL–BASED IMMUNOTHERAPY STRATEGIES

Cancer immunotherapy strategies can be subdivided into those that use the tumor cell itself as a source of antigen versus antigen-specific approaches that target specific tumor antigens for immunity. Relatively little information was available on candidate tumor antigens recognizable by T cells before the 1990s; therefore, essentially all immunotherapy strategies used either irradiated tumor cells or tumor cell extracts mixed with adjuvants such as BCG (Bacillus Calmette-Guérin). When Boon and colleagues developed and applied expression cloning approaches to identify the first T cell–recognized human tumor antigen—Mage-1—a wave of human tumor antigen identification efforts was begun and, with that, the prospects for antigen-specific immunotherapy improved. By the mid-1990s, it was expected that antigen-specific immunotherapy approaches would rapidly make obsolete any whole tumor cell–based immunotherapy approaches, owing to the capacity of antigen-specific strategies to target tumor cells more selectively. In particular, the finding that many of the identified tumor antigens were expressed selectively in the tumor and the testes (sometimes referred to as cancer-testes antigens) suggested that targeting these antigens could provide a high degree of tumor selectivity. Although antigen-specific immunotherapy approaches using either adoptive T-cell therapy or recombinant vaccines remain an exciting area of investigation, clinical results to date with antigen-specific immunotherapy approaches have been largely disappointing. The current failures of antigen-specific immunotherapy approaches can be attributed to three factors:

1. Existing T-cell responses against some of the tumor antigens used in clinical trials may be relatively weak and of low affinity.

2. Limitations in delivery systems for the immunizing antigen may not target antigen to appropriately activated dendritic cells sufficiently, thereby limiting the induction of T-cell responses to that antigen.

3. Most of the antigens used in clinical trials are not necessary for the tumor's survival. Therefore, they allow for the development of antigen-loss variants that permit the tumor to escape even an effective immune response.

Whole cell–based immunotherapy strategies provide an advantage over antigen-specific immunotherapy strategies at the level of antigen diversity. By definition, immunotherapies based on whole tumor or tumor extracts provide a high degree of polyvalency that includes every antigen expressed by the tumor. For approaches that rely on autologous tumor cells, unique antigens that are the consequence of tumor-specific mutations and other genetic alterations likewise are available to induce immune responses. Obviously, an associated disadvantage of immunotherapy approaches that use whole tumor cells is that a myriad of normal tissue antigens are included as well, raising the prospect that a highly active vaccination approach could produce significant autoimmune sequelae. Currently, the single "best" immunotherapy approach—whether antigen-specific or tumor-based—has yet to be defined. Likewise, there is still much work to do to elucidate which specific tumor antigens represent the best targets and are capable of generating the most effective immune responses.

necessary to know the immunorelevant tumor antigens for a given patient's cancer. However, the continuing elucidation of specific immunodominant antigens at the molecular level allows for new generations of antigen-specific vaccines that previously were possible only in vaccines for infectious diseases. Antigen-based immunotherapy of cancer is critically dependent on the identification of relevant tumor antigens. As has become clear from cancer biology, genetic and epigenetic events in the tumor cell provide a virtually limitless number of potential tumor antigens. Immunologically relevant tumor antigens can be divided according to which are identified with antibodies and which are recognized by T cells. Ongoing efforts beginning more than 20 years ago to generate tumor-specific monoclonal antibodies have yielded a few tumor-specific antibodies and defined many cell surface determinants that are not tumor-specific but are expressed at higher levels on the tumor than on nontransformed cells. Monoclonal antibodies against important growth factor receptors such as HER-2/Neu and EGFR as well as lineage-specific molecules such as CD20 (expressed on normal B cells and B-cell lymphomas) have generated significant clinical responses and have invigorated this immunotherapeutic approach. The largest number of immunologically defined tumor antigens has been identified from serologic screening of phage display libraries from tumors using cancer patients' serum.[225]

The primary approach to identifying tumor antigens recognizable by T cells, screening of tumor libraries using tumor-reactive T cells from cancer patients, generally is considered a superior approach to identification of tumor rejection antigens but requires established T-cell lines and clones.[223,224] Although most of the information on human tumor antigens recognized by T cells has been acquired in the context of melanoma, the growing experience with other human cancers suggests a general paradigm in which tumor antigens fall into one of four categories:

1. Unique tumor-specific antigens that are the products of mutation. Many of these mutations are physiologically relevant to the cancer (e.g., inactivating mutations in cdk-4 or activating mutations in ras).[226-228] Mutated tumor antigens may generate the most potent antitumor immunity of all but have the distinct disadvantage that immunotherapies that incorporate them must be individualized to the specific patient. Nonetheless, clinical trials using individually constructed idiotypic vaccines for B-cell lymphoma have demonstrated significant antitumor responses in a significant number of patients.[229]
2. Viral antigens in virus-associated cancers. Viral antigens such as HPV-16 E6 and E7 are highly promising antigens that are shared among a large proportion of the tumors that express these viruses.[230,231] Other important viruses such as hepatitis B and C probably are better targets for treatment of premalignant disease.[232,233]
3. Tissue-specific differentiation antigens. The most commonly identified melanoma antigens are not tumor-specific but, rather, melanocyte-specific. Examples include tyrosinase, tyrosinase-related protein (TRP)-1,

TRP-2, gp100, and MART-1/Melan-A.[223,224] All are melanosomal proteins and most are involved in melanin biosynthesis. The observed correlation between induction of vitiligo, which is depigmentation of the skin from immune attack on melanocytes, and antimelanoma responses in both murine and human immunotherapy trials suggests that, under some circumstances, tolerance to tissue-specific differentiation antigens can be broken, with therapeutically beneficial outcomes.[234,235]

4. Tumor-selective antigens. Many normal genes expressed at very low (or undetectable) levels in normal tissues are upregulated in tumors due to epigenetic effects that alter DNA methylation and histone acetylation. Differential expression of antigens in tumors provides potential therapeutic windows, even when expression is not completely tumor-specific. A large number of tumor antigens in this category (including the MAGE family, BAGE, GAGE and NY-eso-1) have been identified as targets of T-cell responses from patients with melanoma and other tumor types.[236]

Manipulation of Tumor Antigens for Antigen-specific Immunotherapy of Cancer

The elucidation of specific receptors on DCs that are responsible for receptor-mediated endocytosis provides a strategy to modify antigens so that they can be bound to these DC uptake receptors more efficiently. Levy and colleagues demonstrated that fusion proteins of idiotype with GM-CSF enhanced vaccine potency to the greatest extent relative to fusion of idiotype proteins to other cytokines such as IL-2.[237] In these fusion vaccines, GM-CSF serves a dual role in enhancing DC proliferation and also targeting of antigen to endosomal antigen-processing compartments after binding to its receptor on DC progenitors.

More direct antigen-targeting approaches have used fusion genes between antigen and immunoglobulin Fc regions to enhance Fc receptor-mediated antigen uptake by APCs.[238,239] Approaches that modify antigens so that they can be targeted selectively to DC receptors such as CD36 and DEC-205 ultimately may provide more effective priming.[240] A recent study demonstrated that conjugation of antigens to anti–DEC-205 antibodies dramatically enhanced the targeting of antigen to DEC-205+ DCs. Importantly, this maneuver alone failed to produce sustained antigen-specific immunity because of the failure to activate DCs in vivo. Addition of an activating anti-CD40 antibody to the DEC-205-antigen conjugate did produce sustained immunity, demonstrating the importance of combining MHC targeting and APC activation strategies.

The heat shock proteins represent another interesting category of proteins that may target antigen effectively to DCs and, furthermore, into MHC processing pathways. It is now well established that complexing of peptide antigens to certain heat shock proteins such as gp96, hsp-70, calreticulin and hsp-110 enhances their immunogenicity significantly.[241] Heat shock proteins were first used as tumor vaccines by extracting them from tumor cells followed by immunization with the purified heat

HOW TO DEFINE A GOOD TUMOR ANTIGEN

Antigen-based immunotherapy of cancer is critically dependent on the identification of tumor rejection antigens. The criteria and strategies for identification of tumor antigens vary significantly and are a subject of persistent debate. Although a large number of candidate tumor antigens have been serologically defined by screening of phage-display libraries from tumors using cancer patients' serum, this approach does not provide insights into which of these antigens would generate effective antitumor immunity. Screening of tumor libraries using tumor-reactive T cells from cancer patients generally is considered a superior approach to identification of tumor rejection antigens but requires established T-cell lines and clones. A good tumor rejection antigen must display sufficiently high levels of expression on tumor cells to be recognized by T cells (or antibodies, in the case of membrane antigens). An adequate repertoires of lymphocytes bearing receptors with sufficiently high affinities for the antigen that have not been rendered completely anergic so as to be incapable of activation also must be available. Thus, mechanisms of tolerance to candidate tumor antigens profoundly affect the ability of vaccines to generate effective immunity against them. With the exception of human melanoma, most vaccines deveoped thus far have used antigens whose immunologic status is not well understood.

Selective expression by the tumor relative to normal tissues often is considered an important feature; however, tissue-specific differentiation antigens also are potential targets in tumors of dispensable tissues, such as melanoma and prostate cancer. One might imagine that there would be strong tolerance to tissue-specific antigens; however, some tissues represent sites of relative "immune privilege" in that normally they are ignored by the immune system. These antigens may be more "exposed" when expressed by tumors.

One of the most important parameters of a T-cell response is the affinity between the T-cell receptor and its cognate peptide-MHC ligand. Low-affinity T cells do not function efficiently in either killing target cells (in the case of CD8 CTL) or producing high levels of cytokine (in the case of CD4 helper T cells). T-cell receptor affinity rarely is measured with tumor-reactive T cells. In cases where affinities have been measured, the affinities of most T cells were significantly lower than those of typical virus-specific T cells. However, epitope engineering can generate enhanced immunity at the level of TCR affinity for peptide MHC. In summary, it will be critical to define the potential repertoire of T cells against specific tumor-associated antigens as well as their state of activation or tolerance before choosing the "best" antigens for antigen-specific immunotherapy.

---

shock protein. Heat shock proteins isolated from tumors are naturally complexed with a whole array of tumor-associated peptides. Other approaches to link antigen to heat shock protein have included the production of recombinant fusion proteins in which antigenic peptides are linked to the heat shock protein as well as nucleic acid-based vaccines in which fusion genes between antigen and heat shock protein gene are incorporated.[242,243] Immunogenic heat shock proteins complexed with antigenic peptides have been shown to load the MHC class I processing pathway efficiently.[244] Although the intracellular pathway by which heat shock proteins effectively load MHC class I molecules with their associated peptides has not yet been elucidated, Srivastava and colleagues have identified CD91, the α2 macro-globulin receptor, as an important receptor for multiple types of heat shock protein (gp96, hsp-70, hsp-90).[245] One report has suggested that hsp-70 can activate macrophages via CD14/TLR-4 (LPS receptor)–dependent and –independent pathways.[246] Heat shock proteins also have been reported to activate DCs, but the receptors that mediate these putative activation functions not yet been elucidated.[247]

Another approach to enhancing peptide-MHC ligand density on DCs is to enhance the targeting of antigens into the MHC processing pathways. For example, grafting of the endosomal/lysosomal targeting signal in the cytoplasmic tail of the LAMP-1 protein onto the E7 gene resulted in enhanced CD4 responses and ultimate antitumor potency of both recombinant vaccinia and recombinant nucleic acid vaccines.[248-250] A number of MHC class I targeting approaches also have resulted in enhanced immunization potency.[243,251,252] Another strategy for enhanced MHC class I processing has been

the construction of "epitopes on a string." This approach separates out individual epitopes from a given antigen and strings them together, separated by linkers that encode basic amino acids that are good substrates for proteosome cleavage.[253] A number of these strategies probably function via distinct mechanisms, so it is likely that maximal loading of MHC on APCs will be achieved through combining different targeting signals (see Fig. 7-3).

Manipulation of Costimulatory Pathways

Qualitative and quantitative elements of T-cell activation and differentiation are determined in large part by signals delivered by costimulatory molecules (see Fig. 7-7). Three primary approaches have been used to build costimulatory molecules into immunotherapeutic approaches. One involves the transduction of tumor cells with B7 genes to enhance their immunogenicity as vaccines.[199-201] The original concept behind introducing B7 genes into tumors came from the idea that tumors fail to stimulate immune responses against them under normal circumstances because they did not express costimulatory molecules. Therefore, presentation of signal 1 (peptide/MHC) in the absence of costimulatory signals would result in either failure to effectively activate tumor-specific T cells or tolerance induction. Transduction of tumor cells with the genes encoding either B7.1 or B7.2 would reconstitute costimulation and, therefore, might activate antitumor immune responses through direct presentation. Indeed, multiple studies have confirmed that B7-transduced tumor cells are effectively rejected when B7 levels that are high enough are achieved. However, more detailed analysis of the mechanisms of both rejection and immune priming by B7-transduced tumors supports the emerging view that direct presentation by tumor cells to the immune system is a relatively minor pathway compared with the indirect presentation pathway via bone marrow–derived APCs (cross-priming).[254] A more promising application of B7 molecules to vaccine design has been the inclusion of B7 genes in recombinant nucleic acid and viral vaccine vectors for antigen-specific vaccination.[255,256] The basis for the inclusion of B7 genes in recombinant nucleic acid or viral vaccines comes from the idea that one of the methods by which these vaccines immunize is through direct transduction or infection of APCs. Theoretically, even though professional APCs (i.e., dendritic cells) naturally express B7 molecules, the increased expression provided by B7 genes engineered into recombinant vaccines as well as altered patterns or ratios of expression of the different B7 family members could significantly modify the ultimate outcome of T-cell priming in vivo. A number of studies have demonstrated that incorporation of either B7.1 or B7.2 into DNA vaccines as well as recombinant vaccinia vaccines enhances the generation of CTL responses and, in some cases, antibody responses against the specific antigen expressed by the recombinant vaccine. Another approach that has been used to enhance immunization with the B7 costimulatory molecules has been the infusion of B7-Ig dimers, either systemically or mixed with vaccine formulations.[257] Chimeric immunoglobulin-B7 fusion molecules, which display B7 as a dimer, are extremely potent costimulators for T cells in vitro and have been shown to enhance the potency of tumor vaccines in vivo. The list of potential TNF receptor family molecules expressed by T cells that may participate in modifying T-cell responses (either upward or downward) continues to grow. Two very interesting candidate costimulatory receptors of the TNFR family are 4-1BB and OX40. Administration of putatively agonist anti-4-1BB and anti-OX40 antibodies has been shown to induce antitumor immunity when administered either alone or in the context of a vaccine.[182-184] CD27 and CD30 are two additional TNF receptor family members on T cells that may represent interesting targets for either activation or inhibition of antigen-specific responses.[258,259]

Cytokines in Immune Regulation and Cancer Immunotherapy

Cytokines are by far the largest category of immuno-regulatory molecules. They have been used as systemic agents, as local agents, and as components of both genetically modified cell-based and recombinant antigen-specific vaccines. Rather than discussing the detailed application of cytokines to immunotherapy, a topic covered in numerous reviews, some general principles and a few selected examples of cytokine application to immunotherapy are covered here. The major clinical application of cytokines has been in the form of systemic administration of the recombinant cytokine protein. In general, systemic administration of cytokines as single agents in cancer immunotherapy has been quite disappointing. Of the many cytokines tested, interleukin-2 (IL-2) has an established track record in patients with metastatic renal cancer and melanoma and has been

demonstrated to induce durable, complete responses in these two cancers in between 3% and 10% of patients.[260] Unfortunately, the toxicity of systemically administered cytokines (including IL-2) is quite high and significantly limits their widespread application. The therapeutic effects of IL-2 in murine tumor systems as well as in human melanoma and renal cancer are immunologically mediated, because IL-2 has no direct effect on the tumor cells themselves. However, it is unclear whether systemically administered IL-2, particularly at higher doses, enhances antigen-specific antitumor immunity when administered as a single systemic agent. Indeed, the serum concentrations achieved with high dose IL-2 are high enough to bind to the intermediate-affinity IL-2 receptor expressed on NK cells (IL-2Rβ). Likewise, the antitumor effects of high-dose IL-12 in mice are mediated at least partially by NK and NKT cells without clear evidence that antigen-specific T-cell immunity is enhanced. Application of systemic IL-2 in conjunction with vaccination may be found to be a more effective way to utilize IL-2 to enhance systemic antigen-specific T-cell immunity. When T cells initially are activated by their cognate antigen, they express a high-affinity IL-2 receptor consisting of the IL-2Rα and IL-2Rβ subunits (together with the non–IL-2 binding IL-2Rγ signaling subunit). Thus, antigen-specific T cells activated in response to a vaccine should respond transiently to lower doses of IL-2 based on their expression of the high affinity IL-2 receptor. Indeed, preliminary studies combining vaccination with lower doses of IL-2 have demonstrated evidence of synergy between these two agents.

One of the disappointing surprises in systemic cytokine administration has been the large differences in tolerability of systemic cytokines between mice and humans. Cytokines such as IL-2, TNF-α, and IL-12, which induce regressions of established tumors in mice at high systemic doses, are lethal to humans at doses that achieve therapeutic serum concentrations in mice. For example, the LD50 for systemic IL-2 in mice is estimated to be roughly 50-fold higher than that in humans whereas the LD50 for TNF-α is roughly 300-fold higher in mice than in humans. Toxicity determinations for IL-12 are more complicated because lower doses of IL-12 can "tolerize" individuals to higher doses of IL-12. Nonetheless, the maximal tolerable doses of IL-12 in humans are significantly below the doses that achieve significant antitumor responses in mice.

Virtually all cytokines behave physiologically as auto-crine or paracrine factors, so it is not surprising that applying them as systemic agents results in unacceptable toxicities and side effects owing to the loss of geographical specificity that is so critical to normal cytokine physiology. The primary motivation for building cytokines into tumor cell vaccines as well as recombinant nucleic acid or viral vectors is to maximize the expression of the cytokine at the site of antigen delivery. In the case of cytokine gene-transduced tumor vaccines, introduction of genes encoding cytokines targeted at the T cell have been less successful in priming immune responses than transduction of cytokines aimed at APCs, particularly dendritic cells.

The paracrine physiology of cytokines is just as critical for the function of effector cells at sites of metastatic tumor in the periphery as it is for the initiation of immune responses. Proof of the principle behind the efficacy of targeting cytokines to tumor metastases has come from studies by Reisfeld and colleagues, who have linked cytokines such as IL-2 to the Fc regions of antitumor antibodies.[261] Although the antitumor antibodies themselves demonstrate limited efficacy, owing to limited penetration into solid tumors by most monoclonal antibodies infused systemically, there is enough concentration in the tumors to increase the local concentration of IL-2, thereby enhancing antitumor immune responses in a T cell–dependent fashion. It will be of great interest in the future to evaluate combination vaccination approaches that would generate an increased population of tumor-specific T cells expressing high-affinity IL-2 receptors together with IL-2–linked antitumor antibodies. Engineering approaches to maximize the efficacy of cytokine signaling during the effector phase of antitumor immunity also have been applied to adoptive T-cell transfer approaches.[262-264]

Possibly the most promising application of T-cell costimulatory or proliferative cytokines is their incorporation as genes into recombinant nucleic acid and viral vaccines (see Fig. 7-3). Multiple studies have demonstrated that incorporation of cytokine genes to recombinant vaccines of this sort not only can enhance T-cell responses quantitatively but also can alter the differentiation pattern of antigen-specific T cells. Again, this approach is based on the notion that both nucleic acid and viral vaccines act in part through direct infection of antigen presenting cells, thereby maximizing the paracrine effect of the cytokine on T cells to which the infected or transduced APC is presenting antigen. For example, Bersofsky and colleagues performed a detailed analysis of the type of immune responses generated by nucleic acid vaccines in which multiple different cytokine genes were incorporated. They found that GM-CSF, which acts on APCs, generated the greatest level of T-cell immunity, though the characteristics of the responses were mixed TH1 and TH2. When interleukin-12 was incorporated into the nucleic acid vaccine, antigen-specific responses were predominantly TH1 in character, whereas when IL-4 or IL-10 was incorporated into the vaccine, TH1 responses were quenched, and the predominant response was TH2 in character.[265]

Microbial Vectors in Antigen-specific Immunotherapy of Cancer

For all of the added value that recombinant DNA technology provides in engineering elements into vaccine constructs that enhance their potency, nature itself provides a virtually limitless array of delivery systems in the form of diverse microbes with potent intrinsic immunologic properties (Fig. 7-8). Many specific examples of recombinant microbial based cancer vaccines are covered in Chapter 33 on cancer vaccines; here we cover some general principles of viral and bacterial vaccine design. Viruses are the most diverse and efficient gene transfer agents, and their natural cell tropism and biologic

Vaccine type	Advantages	Disadvantages
Ex vivo loaded dendritic cells	Potential to load large #s of DCs with specific Ags	Hard to generate DCs in a consistent fashion
Peptide	Easy to produce Safe	Low potency HLA specific
Protein + adjuvant	Mod. easy to produce Many poss. adjuvants	Generally good for Ab but weak CTL
Recombinant DNA	Easy to produce, stable **Construct versatility Safe**	Weaker vaccines
Recombinant virus or bacteria	**Construct versatility Multiple species-> opportunities to increase potency**	Safety an issue

Figure 7-8. Different approaches to antigen-specific vaccine design. Some of the more common approaches to construction of antigen-specific vaccines—ex vivo loaded dendritic cells, peptide, protein, recombinant DNA, and recombinant virus and bacteria—are presented. Each has specific advantages and disadvantages. Currently, there is no single gold standard for vaccine vector or composition.

features can significantly enhance the immunogenicity of antigens carried within them.[266-270,272,273] Elements of viruses that can diminish their potency as vaccine vectors include the presence of virally encoded inhibitors of immunity.[271] These include molecules that block processing and presentation in the MHC class I pathway (e.g., TAP inhibitors and inhibitors of MHC class I traffic out of the endoplasmic reticulum) and cytokine decoys, among others. Thus, deleting immunologic inhibitory genes from recombinant viruses may enhance their vaccine potency while attenuating their virulence.

The diverse set of bacteria whose immunopathogenesis is becoming understood has led to the development of a number of interesting and promising recombinant bacterial vaccines. Genetic engineering of intracellular bacteria has produced enhanced immune responses in the case of BCG, *Salmonella* spp, *Shigella* spp, and *Listeria* spp.[274-279] More recently, recombinant bacteria have been appreciated as an interesting new vector for delivery of nucleic acid vaccines.[280-282] Thus, engineering plasmids with eukaryotic promoter and enhancer elements driving the antigen gene results in more potent immunity induction then when the plasmids utilize prokaryotic promoters. These results indicate that the bacteria can transfer plasmids directly into eukaryotic transcriptional compartments within infected APCs.

Amplification of Immunity Through Blockade of Inhibitory Pathways and Regulatory T Cells

As engineered immunotherapeutic agents continue to become more sophisticated, a potency ceiling will be reached because of the presence of hardwired inhibitory pathways that negatively regulate lymphocyte responses—the so-called immunologic checkpoints. It is now clear that the quantitative response to antigen is balanced by both positive (costimulatory) and negative (checkpoint) signaling pathways (Fig. 7-9). In the case of T-cell responses, a number of these pathways appear to have components that are either exclusively or at least selectively expressed by T cells. As they are elucidated, the signaling molecules of immunologic checkpoints will represent a major target for antibody-based as well as pharmacologic intervention. Among the best studied of these counter regulatory pathways is the one initiated by engagement of CTLA-4. Naive T cells express the costimulatory B7 receptor CD28, whose engagement amplifies TCR-dependent responses in a number of ways including increased cytokine gene transcription rates, increased cytokine mRNA stability and inhibition of activation-induced cell death. Subsequent to T-cell activation, a second B7 receptor, CTLA-4 becomes expressed. CTLA-4 has a much higher affinity for B7.1 and B7.2 then does CD28. CTLA-4 delivers inhibitory signals to T cells that oppose the costimulatory signals delivered by CD28.[283] Allison and colleagues have demonstrated that transient in vivo blockade of CTLA-4 with a blocking antibody administered at the time of tumor vaccination can enhance vaccine potency and subsequent antitumor immunity.[284-286]

Dissection of signaling pathways in T cells has revealed a number of additional potential targets for inhibitors of immunologic checkpoints. PD-1, a membrane molecule induced subsequent to T-cell activation, is a CTLA-4–like inhibitory molecule that decreases cytokine responses in T cells and may enhance activation-induced cell death of T cells. PD-1 is now appreciated to be a receptor for two of the newer B7 family members, B7-H1/PDL-1 and B7-DC/PDL-2.[177-180] Given that both B7-H1 and B7-DC can costimulate enhanced cytokine production by naive T cells, it is likely that PD-1 represents a counter regulatory inhibitory receptor matched against an as yet unidentified costimulatory receptor on naive T cells. PD-1 knockout mice do not develop the broad hyperimmune organ infiltrates that CTLA-4 knockout mice develop but, rather, display a more focal autoimmunity.[287-289] Recently, another inhibitory ligand for T-cell stimulation, termed B7-H4, has been discovered, which may signal through an ITIM-containing inhibitory receptor on T cells termed BTLA.[290-292]

A number of intracellular inhibitory signaling pathways in T cells represent promising targets for pharmacologic intervention. Some of the best candidates include Cbl-b, Cabin, and certain protein tyrosine phosphatases (PTPs), as well as the tyrosine kinase Csk. Among the phosphatases, SHiP-1, SHP-1, and SHP-2 have all been implicated in downmodulating signaling pathways activated by TCR engagement.[293] More recently, the CD45 PTP has been demonstrated to regulate immune responses negatively by inhibiting JAK-1 and 2 activation, thereby downmodulating responses to certain cytokines.[294] Downstream of the JAK kinases, activation of the STAT transcription factors is inhibited by the CIS/SOCS family.[295] Csk has been well demonstrated to inhibit or downmodulate TCR signaling through phosphorylation of regulatory tyrosines on the src family tyrosine kinases, which are critical for T-cell activation.[296] Cbl-b is an adaptor protein that appears to regulate T-cell activation negatively by antagonizing CD28-mediated costimulatory pathways. Thus, T cells from Cbl-b knockout mice are hypersensitive to low doses of T-cell stimulatory ligands and, furthermore, are relatively CD28-independent in their activation.[297,298] Cabin is a molecule that appears to have multiple functions, including acting as a scaffold for coordinating transcription factors. Cabin originally was identified as a molecule that binds to and inhibits calcineurin, a critical serine phosphatase that mediates TCR-dependent cytokine activation through dephosphorylation of NFAT-c, a critical step in nuclear translocation.[299] The calcineurin-inhibiting portion of Cabin has been localized and represents an interesting target for pharmacologic intervention.

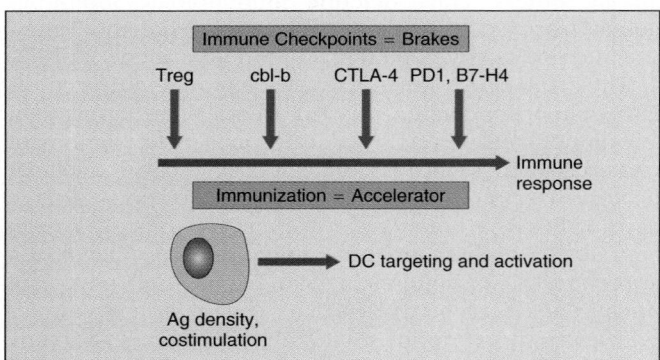

Figure 7-9. The amplitude and character of immune responses is determined by positive forces to initiate and amplify T-cell responses balanced by immunologic checkpoints. Initiation of T-cell activation by dendritic cells is determined largely by antigen density and expression of appropriate costimulatory signals. The optimal combination of high antigen density and high expression of costimulatory signals positively drives T-cell responses. The amplitude of these T-cell responses is muted by the activity of multiple inhibitory pathways, called *immunologic checkpoints*. These checkpoints, including regulatory T cells, intracellular inhibitors of TCR signaling such as cbl-b, and inhibitory pathways initiated by engagement of cell membrane molecules such as CTLA-4 and PD-1, downmodulate immune responses. The purpose of immunologic checkpoints is twofold. One is to help maintain peripheral self-tolerance; the second is to turn off immune response once the offending antigen has been cleared. Failure to engage immunologic checkpoints typically results in both pathologic hyperimmunity and autoimmunity. However, temporary blockade of immunologic checkpoints potentially could enhance the activation and potency of typically weak responses such as antitumor responses.

REALISTIC PROSPECTS FOR SUCCESSFUL IMMUNOTHERAPY OF CANCER

The weight of evidence that established cancers induce immune tolerance to their antigens defines the major challenge to successful immunotherapy. Although the mechanisms by which chronic viral infections avoid immune elimination are still largely unknown, it is likely that common mechanisms as well as distinct mechanisms relative to non–virus associated cancers will be operative. The barriers of immunologic tolerance, together with the failure of cancer vaccines as single agents to achieve sufficient success in randomized Phase III trials in patients

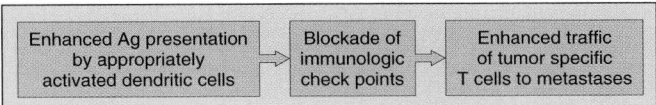

Figure 7-10. Successful immunotherapy will require combination approaches—there is no single "magic bullet." This figure depicts three important points of attack in the generation of combination immunotherapy approaches. The first involves efficient loading of appropriately activated dendritic cells. This is accomplished through new generations of vaccines that selectively target antigens more efficiently to dendritic cells. The second component involves temporary blockade of immunologic checkpoints that blunt the amplitude of T-cell activation. Finally, approaches that enhance the traffic and function of tumor-specific T cells to sites of tumor involvement may be critical for successful therapy, particularly under circumstances where specific organs are affected by metastatic disease.

with advanced cancer, has raised a significant degree of skepticism about immunotherapy of cancer in general. However, the most promising vaccination strategies—indeed, most of those described in this chapter—have only just begun to enter early stage clinical trials. It is therefore premature to conclude that the cryptic repertoire of tumor-specific (and virus-specific) T cells known to exist in patients with cancer and chronic viral disease cannot be mobilized with therapeutic success.

A major theme that has emerged from the growing preclinical animal model immunotherapy investigations is the importance of combination approaches that target different regulatory points in the immune response from priming to amplification to effector function (Fig. 7-10). The most clearcut benefits of combination approaches are those demonstrated by the synergy observed with vaccination and CTLA-4 blockade as well as vaccination after elimination or inhibition of T regulatory cells. In addition, vaccination in the context of bone marrow transplantation shows great promise due to the effects of BMT on multiple elements of T cell–dependent immune responses. Innovative combinatorial immunotherapies are becoming a major focus of translational efforts in many different cancer types.

REFERENCES

1. Ehrlich P, Sulek K: Prize in 1908 awarded to P. Ehrlich and E. Metchnikoff for their work in immunology. Wiad Lek 1967;20:1117–1118.
2. Coley WB: The treatment of malignant tumors by repeated inoculations of erysipelas. With a report of ten original cases. 1893. Clin Orthop 1991;262:3–11.
3. Thomas L: In Lawrence HS (ed): Discussion of Cellular and Humoral Aspects of the Hypersensitive States. New York, Hoeber-Harper, 1959, pp 529–532.
4. Burnet FM: The concept of immunological surveillance. Prog Exp Tumor Res 1970;13:1–27.
5. Gross L: Intradermal immunization of C3H mice against a sarcoma that originated in an animal of the same line. Cancer Res 1943;3: 326–333.
6. Foley EJ: Antigenic properties of methylcholanthrene-induced tumors in mice of the strain of origin. Cancer Res 1953;13:835–837.
7. Baldwin RW: Immunity to methylcholanthrene-induced tumors in inbred rats following atrophy and regression of implanted tumors. Br J Cancer 1955;9:652–665.
8. Prehn RT: Immunity to methylcholanthrene-induced sarcomas. J Natl Cancer Inst 1957;18:769–778.
9. Old LJ, et al: Antigenic properties of chemically-induced tumors. Ann NY Acad Sci 1962;101:80–106.
10. Stutman O: Tumor development after 3-methylcholanthrene in immunologically deficient athymic nude mice. Science 1979;183:534–536.
11. Outzen HC, Custer RP, Eaton JP, Johnson FN: Spontaneous and induced tumor incidence in germfree "nude" mice. J Reticuloendothel Soc 1975;17:1–9.
12. Rygaard J, Povlsen CO: The nude mouse vs. the hypothesis of immunological surveillance. Transplant Rev 1976;28:43–61.
13. Moller G: Experiments and the concept of immunological surveillance. Transplant Rev 1976;28:1–97.
14. Holland JM, et al: Survival and cause of death in aging germfree athymic nude and normal inbred C3Hf/He mice. J Natl Cancer Inst 1978;61:1357–1361.
15. Penn I: Tumors of the immunocompromised patient. Ann Rev Med 1988;39:63–73.
16. List AF, Greco FA, Vogler LB: Lymphoproliferative diseases in immunocompromised hosts: the role of Epstein-Barr virus. J Clin Oncol 1987;5:1673–1689.
17. Gaidano G,. Dalla FR: Biologic aspects of human immunodeficiency virus-related lymphoma. Curr Opin Oncol 1992;4: 900–906.
18. Mesri EA, Mesri M, Liversidge J, Forrester JV: Human herpesvirus-8/Kaposi's sarcoma-associated herpesvirus is a new transmissible virus that infects B cells. J Exp Med 1996;183:2385–2390.
19. Boshart M, Gissman L, Ikenberg H, Kleinheinz A, Scheurlen W, zur Hausen H: A new type of papillomavirus DNA, its presence in genital cancer biopsies and in cell lines derived from cervical cancer. EMBO J 1984;3:1151–1157.
20. Beaudenon S, et al: Plurality of genital human papillomaviruses: characterization of two new types with distinct biological properties. Virology 1987;161:374–384.
21. McFarlane GA, Munro A: Helicobacter pylori and gastric cancer. Br J Surg 1997;84:1190–1199.
22. Kaplan DH, Shankaran V, Dighe AS, et al: Demonstration of an interferon gamma-dependent tumor surveillance system in immunocompetent mice. Proc Natl Acad Sci USA 1998;95: 7556–7561.
23. Shankaran VIH, Bruce AT, White JM, Swanson PE, Old LJ, Schreiber RD: IFN-gamma and lymphocytes prevent primary tumour development and shape tumour immunogenicity. Nature 2001;410:1107–1111.
24. Enzler T, Gillesson S, Manis JP, et al: Deficiencies of GM-CSF and interferon gamma link inflammation and cancer. J Exp Med 2003;197:1213–1219.
25. Lefrancois L, Fuller B, Huleatt JW, Olson S, Puddington L: On the front lines: intraepithelial lymphocytes as primary effectors of intestinal immunity. Springer Semin Immunopathol 1997;18: 463–475.
26. Allison JP, Asarnow DM, Bonyhadi M, et al: Gamma delta T cells in murine epithelia: origin, repertoire, and function. Adv Exp Med Biol 1991;292:63–69.
27. Nandi D, Allison JP: Phenotypic analysis and gamma delta-T cell receptor repertoire of murine T cells associated with the vaginal epithelium. J Immunol 1991;147:1773–1778.
28. Asarnow DM, Kuziel WA, Bonyhadi M, Tigelaar RE, Tucker PW, Allison JP: Limited diversity of gamma delta antigen receptor genes of Thy-1+ dendritic epidermal cells. Cell 1988;55:837–847.
29. Asarnow DM, Goodman T, Le Francois L, Allison JP: Distinct antigen receptor repertoires of two classes of murine epithelium-associated T cells. Nature 1989;341:60–62.
30. Holtmeier W, Pfander M, Hennemann A, Zollner TM, Kaufmann R, Caspary WF: The TCR-delta repertoire in normal human skin is restricted and distinct from the TCR-delta repertoire in the peripheral blood. J Invest Dermatol 2001;116:275–280.
31. Havran WL, Chien YH, Allison JP: Recognition of self antigens by skin-derived T cells with invariant gamma delta antigen receptors. Science 1991;252:1430–1432.
32. Girardi M, Steele CR, Lewis JM, et al: Regulation of cutaneous malignancy by (gamma) (delta) T cells. Science 2001;294: 605–609.

33. Lanier LL: NK cell receptors. Annu Rev Immunol 1998;16: 359-393.

34. Bakker AB, Wu J, Phillips JH, Lanier LL: NK cell activation: distinct stimulatory pathways counterbalancing inhibitory signals. Hum Immunol 2000;61:18-27.

35. Moretta A, Bottino C, Vitale M, et al: Activating receptors and coreceptors involved in human natural killer cell-mediated cytolysis. Annu Rev Immunol 2001;19:197-223.

36. Bauer S, Groh V, Wu J, et al: Activation of NK cells and T cells by NKG2D, a receptor for stress-inducible MICA. Science 1999;285:727-729.

37. Wu J, Song Y, Bakker AB, Bauer S, Spies T, Lanier LL Phillips JH: An activating immunoreceptor complex formed by NKG2D and DAP10. Science 1999;285:730-732.

38. Cerwenka A, Bakker AB, McClanahan T: Retinoic acid early inducible genes define a ligand family for the activating NKG2D receptor in mice. Immunity 2000;12:721-727.

39. Diefenbach A, Jamieson AM, Liu SD, Shastri N, Raulet DH: Ligands for the murine NKG2D receptor: expression by tumor cells and activation of NK cells and macrophages. Nat Immunol 2000;1: 119-126.

40. Groh V, Bahram S, Bauer S, Herman A, Beauchamp M, Spies T: Cell stress-regulated human major histocompatibility complex class I gene expressed in gastrointestinal epithelium. Proc Natl Acad Sci USA 1996;93:12445-12450.

41. Groh V, Steinle A, Bauer S, Spies T: Recognition of stress-induced MHC molecules by intestinal epithelial gamma delta T cells. Science 1998;279:1737-1740.

42. Groh V, Rhinehart R, Secrist H, Bauer S, Grabstein KH, Spies T: Broad tumor-associated expression and recognition by tumor-derived gamma delta T cells of MICA and MICB. Proc Natl Acad Sci USA 1999;96:6879-6884.

43. Diefenbach A, Jensen ER, Jamieson AM, Raulet DH: Rae1 and H60 ligands of the NKG2D receptor stimulate tumour immunity. Nature 2001;413:165-171.

44. Cerwenka A, Baron JL, Lanier LL: Ectopic expression of retinoic acid early inducible-1 gene (RAE-1) permits natural killer cell-mediated rejection of a MHC class I-bearing tumor in vivo. Proc Natl Acad Sci USA 2001;98:11521-11526.

45. Jamieson AM, Diefenbach A, McMahon CW, Xiong N, Carlye JR, Raulet DH: The role of the NKG2D immunoreceptor in immune cell activation and natural killing. Immunity 2002;17:19-29.

46. Esteban F, Concha A, Delgado M, Perez-Ayala M, Ruiz-Cabello F, Garrido F: Lack of MHC class I antigens and tumour aggressiveness of the squamous cell carcinoma of the larynx. Br J Cancer 1990;62:1047-1051.

47. Esteban F, Concha A, Huelin C, et al: Histocompatibility antigens in primary and metastatic squamous cell carcinoma of the larynx. Int J Cancer 1989;43:436-442.

48. Esteban F, Redondo M, Delgado M, Garrido F, Ruiz-Cabello F: MHC class I antigens and tumour-infiltrating leucocytes in laryngeal cancer: long-term follow-up. Br J Cancer 1996;74:1801-1804.

49. Ferrone S, Marincola FM: Loss of HLA class I antigens by melanoma cells: molecular mechanisms, functional significance and clinical relevance. Immunol Today 1995;16:487-494.

50. Natali PG, Bigotti A, Nicotra MR, Viora M, Manfredi D, Ferrone S: Distribution of human Class I (HLA-A,B,C) histocompatibility antigens in normal and malignant tissues of nonlymphoid origin. Cancer Res 1984;44:4679-4687.

51. Natali P, Bigotti A, Cavaliere R, et al: Heterogeneous expression of melanoma-associated antigens and HLA antigens by primary and multiple metastatic lesions removed from patients with melanoma. Cancer Res 1985;45:2883-2889.

52. Natali PG, Cavaliere R, Bigotti A, et al: Antigenic heterogeneity of surgically removed primary and autologous metastatic human melanoma lesions. J Immunol 1983;130:1462-1466.

53. Natali PG, Nicotra MR, Bigotti A, et al: Selective changes in expression of HLA class I polymorphic determinants in human solid tumors. Proc Natl Acad Sci USA 1989;86:6719-6723.

54. Perez M, Cabrera T, Lopez MA, et al: Heterogeneity of the expression of class I and II HLA antigens in human breast carcinoma. J Immunogenet 1986;13:247-253.

55. Whitwell HL, Hughes HP, Moore M, Ahmed A: Expression of major histocompatibility antigens and leucocyte infiltration in benign and malignant human breast disease. Br J Cancer 1984;49: 161-172.

56. Zuk JA, Walker RA: Immunohistochemical analysis of HLA antigens and mononuclear infiltrates of benign and malignant breast. J Pathol 1987;152:275-285.

57. Ruiz-Cabello F, Lopez Nevot MA, Gatierrez J, et al: Phenotypic expression of histocompatibility antigens in human primary tumours and metastases. Clin Exp Metastasis 1989;7:213-226.

58. Ruiz-Cabello F, Perez-Ayala M, Gomez O, et al: Molecular analysis of MHC-class-I alterations in human tumor cell lines. Int J Cancer 1991;6(Suppl):123-130.

59. Cabrera T, Angustas Fernandez M, Sierra A, et al: High frequency of altered HLA class I phenotypes in invasive breast carcinomas. Hum Immunol 1996;50:127-134.

60. Cabrera T, Collado A, Fernandez MA, et al: High frequency of altered HLA class I phenotypes in invasive colorectal carcinomas. Tissue Antigens 1998;52:114-123.

61. van den Ingh HF, Ruiter DJ, Griffioen G, van Murjen GN, Ferrone S: HLA antigens in colorectal tumours—low expression of HLA class I antigens in mucinous colorectal carcinomas. Br J Cancer 1987;55:125-130.

62. van Driel WJ, Tjiong MY, Hilders CG, Trimbs BJ, Fleuren GJ: Association of allele-specific HLA expression and histopathologic progression of cervical carcinoma. Gynecol Oncol 1996;62:33-41.

63. Marincola F, Jaffe EM, Hicklin BJ, Ferrone S: Escape of human solid tumors from T-cell recognition: molecular mechanisms and functional significance. Adv Immunol 2000;74:181-273.

64. D'Urso CM, Wang ZG, Cao Y, Tatake R, Zeff RA, Ferrone S: Lack of HLA class I antigen expression by cultured melanoma cells FO-1 due to a defect in B2m gene expression. J Clin Invest 1991;87:284-292.

65. Wang Z, Cao Y, Albino AP, Zeff RA, Houghton A, Ferrone S: Lack of HLA class I antigen expression by melanoma cells SK-MEL-33 caused by a reading frameshift in beta 2-microglobulin messenger RNA. J Clin Invest 1993;91:684-692.

66. Bicknell DC, Rowan A, Bodmer WF: Beta 2-microglobulin gene mutations: a study of established colorectal cell lines and fresh tumors. Proc Natl Acad Sci USA 1994;91:4751-4756.

67. Benitez R, Godelaine D, Lopez-Nevot MA, et al: Mutations of the beta2-microglobulin gene result in a lack of HLA class I molecules on melanoma cells of two patients immunized with MAGE peptides. Tissue Antigens 1998;52:520-529.

68. Blanchet O, Bourge JF, Zinszer H, et al: Altered binding of regulatory factors to HLA class I enhancer sequence in human tumor cell lines lacking class I antigen expression. Proc Natl Acad Sci USA 1992;89:3488-3492.

69. Doyle A, Martin WJ, Funa K, et al: Markedly decreased expression of class I histocompatibility antigens, protein, and mRNA in human small-cell lung cancer. J Exp Med 1985;161:1135-1151.

70. Restifo NP, Marincola FM, Kawakami Y, Taubenberger J, Yanelli JR, Rosenberg SA: Loss of functional beta 2-microglobulin in metastatic melanomas from five patients receiving immunotherapy. J Natl Cancer Inst 1996;88:100-108.

71. Rowe M, Khanna R, Jacob CA, et al: Restoration of endogenous antigen processing in Burkitt's lymphoma cells by Epstein-Barr virus latent membrane protein-1: Coordinate up-regulation of peptide transporters and HLA-class I antigen expression. Eur J Immunol 1995;25:1374-1384.

72. Sanda MG, Restifo NP, Walsh JC, et al: Molecular characterization of defective antigen processing in human prostate cancer. J Natl Cancer Inst 1995;87:280-285.

73. Alpan RS, Zhang M, Pardee AB: Cell cycle-dependent expression of TAP1, TAP2, and HLA-B27 messenger RNAs in a human breast cancer cell line. Cancer Res 1996;56:4358-4361.

74. Seliger B, Hohne A, Knuth A, et al: Reduced membrane major histocompatibility complex class I density and stability in a subset of human renal cell carcinomas with low TAP and LMP expression. Clin Cancer Res 1996;2:1427-1433.

75. Hilders CG, Houbiers JG, Krul EJ, Fleuren GJ: The expression of histocompatibility-related leukocyte antigens in the pathway to cervical carcinoma. Am J Clin Pathol 1994;101:5-12.

76. Koopman L, Koopman LA, Corver WE, van der Slik AR, Giphart MJ, Fleuren GJ: Multiple genetic alterations cause frequent and

heterogeneous human histocompatibility leukocyte antigen class I loss in cervical cancer. J Exp Med 2000;191:961–976.

77. Clarke B, Chetty R: Postmodern cancer: the role of human immunodeficiency virus in uterine cervical cancer. Mol Pathol 2002;55:19–24.

78. Moretta A, Biassoni R, Bottino C: Major histocompatibility complex class I-specific receptors on human natural killer and T lymphocytes. Immunol Rev 1997;155:105–117.

79. Lanier LL, Phillips JH: Inhibitory MHC class I receptors on NK cells and T cells. Immunol Today 1996;17:86–91.

80. Hui K, Grosveld F, Festenstein H: Rejection of transplantable AKR leukaemia cells following MHC DNA-mediated cell transformation. Nature 1984;311:750–752.

81. Wallich R, Bulbuc N, Hammerling GJ, Katzav S, Segal S, Feldman M: Abrogation of metastatic properties of tumour cells by de novo expression of H-2K antigens following H-2 gene transfection. Nature 1985;315:301–305.

82. Haywood GR, McKhann CF: Antigenic specificities on murine sarcoma cells. Reciprocal relationship between normal transplantation antigens (H-2) and tumor- specific immunogenicity. J Exp Med 1971;133:1171–1187.

83. Ljunggren HG, Karre K: Host resistance directed selectively against H-2-deficient lymphoma variants. Analysis of the mechanism. J Exp Med 1985;162:1745–1759.

84. Karre K, Ljunggren HG, Piontek G, Kiessling R: Selective rejection of H-2-deficient lymphoma variants suggests alternative immune defense strategy. Nature 1986;319:675–678.

85. Urban JL, Burton RC, Holland JM, Kripke ML, Schreiber H: Mechanisms of syngeneic tumor rejection. Susceptibility of host-selected progressor variants to various immunological effector cells. J Exp Med 1982;155:557–573.

86. Uyttenhove C, Maryanski J, Boon T: Escape of mouse mastocytoma P815 after nearly complete rejection is due to antigen-loss variants rather than immunosuppression. J Exp Med 1983;157: 1040–1052.

87. Wortzel RD, Philipps C, Schreiber H: Multiple tumour-specific antigens expressed on a single tumour cell. Nature 1983;304: 165–167.

88. Urban JL, Kripke ML, Schreiber H: Stepwise immunologic selection of antigenic variants during tumor growth. J Immunol 1986;137:3036–3041.

89. Ward PL, Koeppen H, Hurteau T, Schreiber H: Tumor antigens defined by cloned immunological probes are highly polymorphic and are not detected on autologous normal cells. J Exp Med 1989;170:217–232.

90. Ward PL, Koeppen HK, Hurteau T, Rowley DA, Schreiber H: Major histocompatibility complex class I and unique antigen expression by murine tumors that escaped from CD8+ T-cell-dependent surveillance. Cancer Res 1990;50:3851–3858.

91. Lethe B, van den Eynde B, van Pel A, Corradin C, Boon T: Mouse tumor rejection antigens P815A and P815B: two epitopes carried by a single peptide. Eur J Immunol 1992;22:2283–2288.

92. Yee C, Thompson JA, Byrd D, et al: Adoptive T cell therapy using antigen-specific CD8+ T cell clones for the treatment of patients with metastatic melanoma: In vivo persistence, migration, and anti-tumor effect of transferred T cells. Proc Natl Acad Sci USA 2002;99:15840–15842.

93. Jager E, Ringhoffer M, Altmannsberger M, et al: Immunoselection in vivo: Independent loss of MHC class I and melanocyte differentiation antigen expression in metastatic melanoma. Int J Cancer 1997;71:142–147.

94. Ohnmacht GA, Wang E, Mocellin S, et al: Short-term kinetics of tumor antigen expression in response to vaccination. J Immunol 2001;167:1809–1820.

95. de Vries T, Fourkour A, Wobbes T, Verkroost G, Ruiter DJ, van Murijen GN: Heterogeneous expression of immunotherapy candidate proteins gp100, MART-1, and tyrosinase in human melanoma cell lines and in human melanocytic lesions. Cancer Research 1997;57:3223–3229.

96. Cormier JN, Abati A, Fetsch P, et al: Comparative analysis of the in vivo expression of tyrosinase, MART-1/Melan-A, and gp100 in metastatic melanoma lesions: Implications for immunotherapy. J Immunother 1998;21:27–31.

97. Cormier J, Panelli MC, Hackett JA, et al: Natural variation of the expression of HLA and endogenous antigen modulates CTL recognition in an in vitro melanoma model. Int J Cancer 1999;80:781–790.

98. Riker A, Cormier J, Panelli M, et al: Immune selection after antigen-specific immunotherapy of melanoma. Surgery 1999;126:112–120.

99. Scheibenbogen C, Weyers I, Ruiter D, Wilhauck M, Bittinger A, Keilholz U: Expression of gp100 in melanoma metastases resected before or after treatment with IFN alpha and IL-2. J Immunother Emphasis Tumor Immunol 1996;19:375–380.

100. Schmid P, Itin P, Rufli T: In situ analysis of transforming growth factor-beta s (TGF-beta 1, TGF-beta 2, TGF-beta 3), and TGF-beta type II receptor expression in malignant melanoma. Carcinogenesis 1995;16:1499–1503.

101. Moretti S, Pinzi C, Berti E, et al: In situ expression of transforming growth factor beta is associated with melanoma progression and correlates with Ki67, HLA-DR and beta 3 integrin expression. Melanoma Res 1997;7:313–321.

102. Van Belle P, Rodeck U, Naumah I, Halpern AC, Elder DE: Melanoma-associated expression of transforming growth factor-beta isoforms. Am J Pathol 1996;148:1887–1894.

103. Wojtowicz-Praga S, Verma UN, Wakefield L, et al: Modulation of b16 melanoma growth and metastasis by anti-transforming growth factor beta antibody and interleukin-2. Immunotherapy 1996;19:169–175.

104. Hahne M, Rimoldi D, Schroter M, et al: Melanoma cell expression of Fas (Apo-1/CD95) ligand: Implications for tumor immune escape. Science 1996;274:1363–1366.

105. Gratas C, Tohma Y, van Meir EG, et al: Fas ligand expression in glioblastoma cell lines and primary astrocytic brain tumors. Brain Pathol 1997;7:863–869.

106. Bennett MW, O'Connell J, O'Sullivan GC, et al: The Fas counterattack in vivo: Apoptotic depletion of tumor-infiltrating lymphocytes associated with Fas ligand expression by human esophageal carcinoma. J Immunol 1998;160:5669–5675.

107. Niehans GA, Brunner T, Frizelle SP, et al: Human lung carcinomas express Fas ligand. Cancer Res 1997;57:1007–1012.

108. O'Connell J, O'Sullivan GC, Collins JK, Shanahan F: The Fas counterattack: Fas-mediated T cell killing by colon cancer cells expressing Fas ligand. J Exp Med 1996;184:1075–1082.

109. Shiraki K, Tsuji N, Shioda T, Isselbacher KJ, Takahashi H: Expression of Fas ligand in liver metastases of human colonic adenocarcinomas. Proc Natl Acad Sci USA 1997;94:6420–6425.

110. Chappell DB, Zaks TZ, Rosenberg SA, Restifo NP: Human melanoma cells do not express Fas (Apo-1/CD95) ligand. Cancer Res 1999;59:59–62.

111. Seino K, Kayagaki N, Okumura K, Yagita H: Antitumor effect of locally produced CD95 ligand. Nat Med 1997;3:165–170.

112. Arai H, Gordon D, Nabel EG, Nabel GJ: Gene transfer of Fas ligand induces tumor regression in vivo. Proc Natl Acad Sci USA 1997;94:13862–13867.

113. Bogen B, Munthe L, Sollien A, et al: Naive CD4+ T cells confer idiotype-specific tumor resistance in the absence of antibodies. Eur J Immunol 1995;25:3079–3086.

114. Bogen B: Peripheral T cell tolerance as a tumor escape mechanism: deletion of CD4+ T cells specific for a monoclonal immunoglobulin idiotype secreted by a plasmacytoma. Eur J Immunol 1996;26:2671–2679.

115. Staveley-O'Carroll K, Sotomayor E, Montgomery J, et al: Induction of antigen-specific T cell anergy: An early event in the course of tumor progression. Proc Natl Acad Sci USA 1998;95:1178–1183.

116. Sotomayor EM, Borrello I, Rattis FM, et al: Cross-presentation of tumor antigens by bone marrow-derived antigen-presenting cells is the dominant mechanism in the induction of T-cell tolerance during B-cell lymphoma progression. Blood 2001;98:1070–1077.

117. Wick M, Dubey P, Koeppen H, et al: Antigenic cancer cells grow progressively in immune hosts without evidence for T cell exhaustion or systemic anergy. J Exp Med 1997;186:229–238.

118. Speiser DE, Miranda R, Zakarian A, et al: Self antigens expressed by solid tumors do not efficiently stimulate naive or activated T cells: Implications for immunotherapy. J Exp Med 1997;186:645–653.

119. Doan T, Herd KA, Lambert PF, Fernando GJ, Street MD, Tindle RW: Peripheral tolerance to human papillomavirus E7 oncoprotein

occurs by cross-tolerization, is largely Th-2-independent, and is broken by dendritic cell immunization. Cancer Res 2000;60: 2810-2815.

120. den Boer AT, Diehl L, van Mierlo CJ, et al: Longevity of antigen presentation and activation status of APC are decisive factors in the balance between CTL immunity versus tolerance. J Immunol 2001;167:2522-2528.

121. Shrikant P, Khoruts A, Mescher MF: CTLA-4 blockade reverses CD8+ T cell tolerance to tumor by a CD4+ T cell- and IL-2-dependent mechanism. Immunity 1999;11:483-493.

122. Schell TD, Knowles BB, Tevethia SS: Sequential loss of cytotoxic T lymphocyte responses to simian virus 40 large T antigen epitopes in T antigen transgenic mice developing osteosarcomas. Cancer Res 2000;60:3002-3012.

123. Ochsenbein AF, Sierro S, Odermatt B, et al: Roles of tumour localization, second signals and cross priming in cytotoxic T-cell induction. Nature 2001;411:1058-1064.

124. Huang AY, Golumbek P, Ahmadzadeh M, Jaffee E, Pardoll D, Levitsky H: Role of bone marrow-derived cells in presenting MHC class I-restricted tumor antigens. Science 1994;264:961-965.

125. Robinson B, Scott BM, Lake RA, et al: Lack of ignorance to tumor antigens: Evaluation using nominal antigen transfection and T-cell receptor transgenic lymphocytes in Lyons-Parish analysis—implications for tumor tolerance. Clin Cancer Res 2001;7(Suppl 3): 811S-817S.

126. Nguyen LT, Elford AR, Marakami K, et al: Tumor growth enhances cross-presentation leading to limited T cell activation without tolerance. J Exp Med 2002;195:423-435.

127. Morck A, et al: Functional genomics identifies mesothelin as an immunodominant pancreatic cancer antigen. Submitted 2002.

128. Drake C, et al: Prostate tumorigenesis induces tolerance in prostate specific T cells. Submitted 2002.

129. Sakaguchi S, Sakaguchi N, Shimizu J, et al: Immunologic tolerance maintained by CD35+CD4+ regulatory cells: their common role in controlling autoimmunity, tumor immunity, and transplantation tolerance. Immunol Rev 2001;182:18-32.

130. Shevach E: CD4+ CD25+ suppressor T cells: more questions than answers. Nat Rev Immunol 2002;2:389-400.

131. Maloy K, Powrie F: Regulatory T cells in the control of immune pathology. Nat Immunol 2001;2:816-822.

132. Gershon R, Kondo K: Infectious immunological tolerance. Immunology 1971;21:903-914.

133. North R, Bursuker I: Generation and decay of the immune response to a progressive fibrosacrcoma. I. Ly-1+2 -suppressor T cells down-regulate the generation of Ly-1-2+ effector T cells. J Exp Med 1984;159:1295-1311.

134. Sutmuller R, van Duivenvoorde LM, van Elsas A, et al: Synergism of cytotoxic T lymphocyte-associated antigen 4 blockade and depletion of CD25+ regulatory cells in antitumor therapy reveals alternative pathways for suppression of autoreactive cytotoxic T lymphocyte responses. J Exp Med 2001;194:823-832.

135. van Elsas A, Sutmuller RP, Hurwitz AA, et al: Elucidating the autoimmune and antitumor effector mechanisms of a treatment based on cytotoxic T lymphocyte antigen-4 blockade in combination with a B16 melanoma vaccine: comparison of prophylaxis and therapy. J Exp Med 2001;194:481-489.

136. Ercolini AM, Machiels JP, Chen YC, et al: Inhibition of T regulatory cells by Cytoxan releases high avidity T cells specific for immunodominant epitopes of HER-2/neu. J Immunol 2003;170: 4273-4280.

137. Catlett-Galcone R, et al: Constitutive activation of Stat3 signaling confers resistance to apoptosis in human U266 myeloma cells. Immunity 1999;10:105-115.

138. Wang T, et al: Regulation of the innate and adaptive immune responses by Stat3 signaling in tumors. Submitted 2002.

139. Gabrilovich DI, Chen HL, Girgis KR, et al: Production of vascular endothelial growth factor by human tumors inhibits the functional maturation of dendritic cells. Nat Med 1996;2:1096-1103.

140. Niu G, Wright KL, Huang M, et al: Constitutive Stat3 activity up-regulates VEGF expression and tumor angiogenesis. Oncogene 2002;21:2000-2008.

141. Kulkarni A, Karlsson S: Transforming growth factor-beta 1 knockout mice. A mutation in one cytokine gene causes a dramatic inflammatory disease. Am J Pathol 1993;143:3-9.

142. Leveen P, Larsson J, Ehinger M, et al: Induced disruption of the transforming growth factor beta type II receptor gene in mice causes a lethal inflammatory disorder that is transplantable. Blood 2002;100:560-568.

143. Chen W, Wahl S: TGF-beta: receptors, signaling pathways and autoimmunity. Curr Dir Autoimmun 2002;5:62-91.

144. Adler AJ, Marsh DW, Yochum GS, et al: CD4+ T cell tolerance to parenchymal self-antigens requires presentation by bone marrow-derived antigen-presenting cells. J Exp Med 1998;187:1555-1564.

145. Steinman R, Turley S, Mellman I, Inaba K: The induction of tolerance by dendritic cells that have captured apoptotic cells. J Exp Med 2000;191:411-416.

146. Legge K, Gregg RK, Maldonado-Lopez R, et al: On the role of dendritic cells in peripheral T cell tolerance and modulation of autoimmunity. J Exp Med 2002;196:217-227.

147. Steinman R, Nussenzweig M: Avoiding horror autotoxicus: the importance of dendritic cells in peripheral T cell tolerance. Proc Natl Acad Sci USA 2002;99:351-358.

148. Dudley M, Wunderlich JR, Robbins PF, et al: Cancer regression and autoimmunity in patients after clonal repopulation with antitumor lymphocytes. Science 2002;298:850-854.

149. Mellman I, Steinman R: Dendritic cells: specialized and regulated antigen processing machines. Cell 2001;106:255-258.

150. Steinman RM: The dendritic cell system and its role in immunogenicity. Annu Rev Immunol 1991;9:271-296.

151. Bancherau J, Steinman RM: Dendritic cells and the control of immunity. Nature 1998;392:245-252.

152. Inaba K, Steinman RM, Pack MW, et al: Identification of proliferating dendritic cell precursors in mouse blood. J Exp Med 1992;175:1157-1167.

153. Caux C, Dezutter-Dambuyant C, Schmitt D, Bancherau J: GM-CSF and TNF-alpha cooperate in the generation of dendritic Langerhans cells. Nature 1992;360:258-261.

154. Kiertscher SM, Roth MD: Human CD14+ leukocytes acquire the phenotype and function of antigen-presenting dendritic cells when cultured in GM-CSF and IL-4. J Leukoc Biol 1996;59:208-218.

155. Romani N, Reider D, Heuer M, et al: Generation of mature dendritic cells from human blood. An improved method with special regard to clinical applicability. J Immunol Methods 1996;196:137-151.

156. Maraskovsky E, Brasel K, Teepe M, et al: Dramatic increase in the numbers of functionally mature dendritic cells in Flt3 ligand-treated mice: multiple dendritic cell subpopulations identified. J Exp Med 1996;184:1953-1962.

157. Ren Y, Silverstein RL, Allen J, Savill J: CD36 gene transfer confers capacity for phagocytosis of cells undergoing apoptosis. J Exp Med 1995;181:1857-1862.

158. Nussenzweig MC, Steinman RM, Witmer MD, Gutchinov B: A monoclonal antibody specific for mouse dendritic cells. Proc Natl Acad Sci USA 1982;79:161-165.

159. Yewdell J, Norbury C, Bennink J: Mechanisms of exogenous antigen presentation by MHC class I molecules in vitro and in vivo: implications for generating CD8+ T cell responses to infectious agents, tumors, transplants and vaccines. Adv Immunol 1999;73:1-77.

160. Akira S, Takeda K, Kaisho T: Toll-like receptors: critical proteins linking innate and acquired immunity. Nat Immunol 2001;2:675-680.

161. Sallusto F, Lanzavecchia A: Efficient presentation of soluble antigen by cultured human dendritic cells is maintained by granulocyte/macrophage colony-stimulating factor plus interleukin 4 and downregulated by tumor necrosis factor alpha. J Exp Med 1994; 179:1109-1118.

162. Caux C, Massacrier C, Vanbervliet B, et al: Activation of human dendritic cells through CD40 cross-linking. J Exp Med 1994;180:1263-1272.

163. Cella M, Scheidegger D, Palmer-Lehmann K, Lane P, Lanzavecchia A, Alber G: Ligation of CD40 on dendritic cells triggers production of high levels of interleukin-12 and enhances T cell stimulatory capacity: T-T help via APC activation. J Exp Med 1996;184: 747-752.

164. Saeki H, Moore AM, Brown MJ, Hwang ST: Cutting edge: secondary lymphoid-tissue chemokine (SLC) and CC chemokine receptor 7

(CCR7) participate in the emigration pathway of mature dendritic cells from the skin to regional lymph nodes. J Immunol 1999;162: 2472-2475.

165. Cella M, Engering A, Pinet V, Pieters J, Lanzavecchia A: Inflammatory stimuli induce accumulation of MHC class II complexes on dendritic cells. Nature 1997;388:782-787.

166. Pierre P, Turley SJ, Gatti E, et al: Developmental regulation of MHC class II transport in mouse dendritic cells. Nature 1997;388: 787-792.

167. Schoenberger SP, Toes RE, van der Voort EI, Offringa R, Melief CJ: T help for CTL is mediated by CD40-CD40L interactions. Nature 1998;393:480-483.

168. Bennett SR, Carbone FR, Karamalis R, Flavell RA, Miller JFAP, Heath WR: Help for cytotoxic-T-cell responses is mediated by CD40 signalling. Nature 1998;393:478-480.

169. Ridge JP, DiRosa F, Matzinger P: A conditioned dendritic cell can be a temporal bridge between a CD4+ T-helper and a T-killer cell. Nature 1998;393:474.

170. Lu Z, Yuan L, Zhou X, Sotomayor E, Levitsky HI, Pardoll DM: CD40-independent pathways of T cell help for priming of CD8(+) cytotoxic T lymphocytes. J Exp Med 2000;191:541-550.

171. Chang C, Furue M, Tamaki K: Selective regulation of ICAM-1 and major histocompatibility complex class I and II molecular expression on epidermal Langerhans cells by some of the cytokines released by keratinocytes and T cells. Eur J Immunol 1994;24:2889-2895.

172. Linsley PS, Brady W, Urnes M, et al: Binding of the B cell activation antigen B7 to CD28 costimulates T cell proliferation and interleukin 2 mRNA accumulation. J Exp Med 1991;173: 721-730.

173. Schwartz RH: Costimulation of T lymphocytes: the role of CD28, CTLA-4, and B7/BB1 in interleukin-2 production and immuno-therapy. Cell 1992;71:1065-1068.

174. Shahinian A, Pfeffer K, Lee KP, et al: Differential T cell costimu-latory requirements in DC28-deficient mice. Science 1993;261: 609-612.

175. Borriello F, Setha MP, Boyd SD, et al: B7-1 and B7-2 have overlapping, critical roles in immunoglobulin class switching and germinal center formation. Immunity 1997;6:303-313.

176. Caux C, Vanbervliet B, Massacrier C, et al: B70/B7-2 is identical to CD86 and is the major functional ligand for CD28 expressed on human dendritic cells. J Exp Med 1994;180:1841-1847.

177. Dong H, Zhu G, Tamada K, Chen L: B7-H1, a third member of the B7 family, co-stimulates T-cell proliferation and interleukin-10 secretion [see comments]. Nat Med 1999;5:1365-1369.

178. Freeman GJ, Long AJ, Iwai Y, et al: Engagement of the PD-1 immunoinhibitory receptor by a novel B7 family member leads to negative regulation of lymphocyte activation. J Exp Med 2000;192:1027-34.

179. Tseng SY, Otsuji M, Gorski K, et al: B7-DC, a new dendritic cell molecule with unique costimulatory properties for T cells. J Exp Med 2001;193:839-846.

180. Latchman Y, Wood CR, Chernova T, et al: PD-L2 is a second ligand for PD-I and inhibits T cell activation. Nat Immunol 2001;2:261-268.

181. Chapoval AI, Ni J, Lau JS, et al: B7-H3: a costimulatory molecule for T cell activation and IFN-gamma production. Nat Immunol 2001;2:269-274.

182. Melero I, Shufford WW, Newby SA, et al: Monoclonal antibodies against the 4-1BB T-cell activation molecule eradicate established tumors. Nat Med 1997;3:682-685.

183. Weinberg AD, Rivera MM, Prell R, et al: Engagement of the OX-40 receptor in vivo enhances antitumor immunity. J Immunol 2000;164:2160-2169.

184. Bansal-Pakala P, Jember AG, Croft M: Signaling through OX40 (CD134) breaks peripheral T-cell tolerance. Nat Med 2001;7:907-912.

185. Porgador A, Gilboa E,: Bone marrow-generated dendritic cells pulsed with a class I-restricted peptide are potent inducers of cytotoxic T lymphocytes. J Exp Med 1995;182:255-260.

186. Mayordomo JI, Zorina T, Storkus WJ, et al: Bone marrow-derived dendritic cells pulsed with synthetic tumour peptides elicit protective and therapeutic antitumour immunity. Nat Med 1995;1:1297-1302.

187. Lambert LA, Gibson GR, Maloney M, Barth RJ Jr: Equipotent generation of protective antitumor immunity by various methods of dendritic cell loading with whole cell tumor antigens. J Immunother 2001;24:232-236.

188. Shimizu K, Thomas EK, Griedlin M, Mule JJ: Enhancement of tumor lysate- and peptide-pulsed dendritic cell-based vaccines by the addition of foreign helper protein. Cancer Res 2001;61: 2618-2624.

189. Song W, Kong HL Carpenter H, et al: Dendritic cells genetically modified with an adenovirus vector encoding the cDNA for a model tumor antigen induce protective and therapeutic antitumor immunity. J Exp Med 1997;186:1247-1256.

190. Specht JM, Wang G, Do MT, et al: Dendritic cells retrovirally transduced with a model tumor antigen gene are therapeutically effective against established pulmonary metastases. J Exp Med 1997;186:1213-1221.

191. Dyall J, Latouche JB, Schnell S, Sadelain M: Lentivirus-transduced human monocyte-derived dendritic cells efficiently stimulate antigen-specific cytotoxic T lymphocytes. Blood 2001;97:114-121.

192. Boczkowski D, Nair SK, Snyder D, Gilboa E: Dendritic cells pulsed with RNA are potent antigen-presenting cells in vitro and in vivo. J Exp Med 1996;184:465-472.

193. Gong J, Chen D, Kashiwaba M, Kufe D: Induction of antitumor activity immunization with fusion of dendritic and carcinoma cells. Nat Med 1997;3:558-561.

194. Klein C, Bueler H, Mulligan RC: Comparative analysis of genetically modified dendritic cells and tumor cells as therapeutic cancer vaccines. J Exp Med 2000;191:1699-1708.

195. Dhodapkar MV, Steinman RM, Krasovosky J, Munz C, Bhardwaj N: Antigen-specific inhibition of effector T cell function in humans after injection of immature dendritic cells. J Exp Med 2001;193: 233-238.

196. Fearon ER, Itaya T, Hunt B, Vogelstein B, Frost P: Induction in a murine tumor of immunogenic tumor variants by transfection with a foreign gene. Cancer Res 1988;48:2975-2980.

197. Itaya T, Yamagiwa S, Okada F, et al: Xenogenization of a mouse lung carcinoma (3LL) by transfection with an allogeneic class I major histocompatibility complex gene (H-2Ld). Cancer Res 1987;47: 3136-3140.

198. Plautz GE, Yang ZY, Wu BY, Gao X, Huang L, Nabel GJ: Immunotherapy of malignancy by in vivo gene transfer into tumors [see comments]. Proc Natl Acad Sci USA 1993;90: 4645-4649.

199. Townsend SE, Allison JP: Tumor rejection after direct costimu-lation of CD8+ T cells by B7-transfected melanoma cells. Science 1993;259:368-370.

200. Chen L, Ashe S, Brady WA, et al: Costimulation of antitumor immunity by the B7 counterreceptor for the T lymphocyte molecules CD28 and CTLA-4. Cell 1992;71:1093-1102.

201. Baskar S, Ostrand-Rosenberg S, Nabavi N, Nadler LM, Freeman GJ, Glimcher CH: Constitutive expression of B7 restores immunogenicity of tumor cells expressing truncated major histocompatibility complex class II molecules. Proc Natl Acad Sci USA 1993;90:5687-5690.

202. Golumbek PT, Lazenby AJ, Levitski HI, et al: Treatment of established renal cancer by tumor cells engineered to secrete interleukin-4. Science 1991;254:713-716.

203. Restifo NP, Spiess PJ, Karp SE, Mule JJ, Rosenberg SA: A nonimmunogenic sarcoma transduced with the cDNA for interferon gamma elicits CD8+ T cells against the wild-type tumor: correlation with antigen presentation capability. J Exp Med 1992;175:1423-1431.

204. Asher M, Mule J, Kasid A: Murine tumor cells transduced with the gene for tumor necrosis factor-α. J. Immunol 1991;146:3227-3229.

205. Bannerji R, Arroyo CD, Cordon-Cardo C, Gilboa E: The role of IL-2 secreted from genetically modified tumor cells in the establish-ment of antitumor immunity. J Immunol 1994;152: 2324-2332.

206. Gansbacher B, Bannerji R, Daniels B: Retroviral vector-mediated gamma-interferon gene transfer into tumor cells generates potent and long lasting antitumor immunity. Cancer Res 1990;50:7820-7826.

207. Li WQ, Diamantstein T, Blankenstein T: Lack of tumorigenicity of interleukin 4 autocrine growing cells seems related to the

anti-tumor function of interleukin 4. Mol Immunol 1990;27:1331-1337.

208. Hock H, Diamantstein T, Blankstein T: Interleukin 7 induces CD4+ T cell-dependent tumor rejection. J Exp Med 1991;174:1291-1298.

209. Colombo MP, Ferrari G, Stoppacciaro A, et al: Granulocyte colony-stimulating factor gene transfer suppresses tumorigenicity of a murine adenocarcinoma in vivo. J Exp Med 1991;173:889-897.

210. Porgador A, Tzehoval E, Katz A, et al: Interleukin 6 gene transfection into Lewis lung carcinoma tumor cells suppresses the malignant phenotype and confers immunotherapeutic competence against parental metastatic cells. Cancer Res 1992;52:3679-3686.

211. Blankenstein T, Qin Z, Uberla K: Tumor suppression after tumor cell-targeted tumor necrosis factor via gene transfer. J Exp Med 1991;173:1047-1052.

212. Dranoff G, Jaffee E, Lazenby A, et al: Vaccination with irradiated tumor cells engineered to secrete murine granulocyte-macrophage colony-stimulating factor stimulates potent, specific, and long-lasting anti-tumor immunity. Proc Natl Acad Sci USA 1993;90:3539-3543.

213. Pardoll D, Jaffee E: Genetically modified tumor vaccines. In Rosenberg SA (ed): Principles and Practice of Biologic Therapy of Cancer. Charlottesville, VA: Silverchair, 1999, pp 647-662.

214. Okamoto M, Tazawa K, Kawagoshi, T, et al: The combined effect against colon-26 cells of heat treatment and immunization with heat treated colon-26 tumour cell extract. Int J Hyperthermia 2000;16:263-273.

215. Wang X, Li Y, Manjili MH, Repasky EA, Pardoll DM, Subjeck JR: Hsp110 overexpression increases the immunogenicity of the murine CT26 colon tumor. Cancer Immunol Immunother 2002;51:311-319.

216. Chiodoni C, Paglia P, Stoppacciaro A, Rodolfo, M, Parenza M, Colmbo MP: Dendritic cells infiltrating tumors cotransduced with granulocyte/macrophage colony-stimulating factor (GM-CSF) and CD40 ligand genes take up and present endogenous tumor-associated antigens, and prime naive mice for a cytotoxic T lymphocyte response. JExp Med 1999;190:125-133.

217. Simons JW, Jaffee EM, Weber CE, et al: Bioactivity of autologous irradiated renal cell carcinoma vaccines generated by ex vivo granulocyte-macrophage colony-stimulating factor gene transfer. Cancer Res 1997;57:1537-1546.

218. Soiffer R, Lynch T, Mih M, et al: Vaccination with irradiated autologous melanoma cells engineered to secrete human granulocyte-macrophage colony-stimulating factor generates potent antitumor immunity in patients with metastatic melanoma. Proc Natl Acad Sci USA 1998;95:13141-13146.

219. Jaffee EM, Hruban RH, Riedrzycki B, et al: Novel allogeneic granulocyte-macrophage colony-stimulating factor-secreting tumor vaccine for pancreatic cancer: a phase i trial of safety and immune activation. J Clin Oncol 2001;19:145-156.

220. Wittes R: Bacille Calmette-Guerin vaccine. Clin Infect Dis 2000;31(Suppl 3):S115-S121.

221. Foon K: Immunotherapy for colorectal cancer. Curr Oncol Rep 2001;3:116-126.

222. Zeh H, Stavely-O'Carroll K, and Choti M: Vaccines for colorectal cancer. Trends Mol Med 2001;7:307-313.

223. Boon T, Old LJ: Cancer tumor antigens. Curr Opin Immunol 1997;9:681-683.

224. Robbins PF, Kawakami Y: Human tumor antigens recognized by T cells. Curr Opin Immunol 1996;8:628-636.

225. Sahin U, Tureci O, Schmitt H, et al: Human neoplasms elicit multiple specific immune responses in the autologous host. Proc Natl Acad Sci USA 1995;92:11810-11813.

226. Wolfel T, Hauer M, Schneider J, et al: A p16INK4a-insensitive CDK4 mutant targeted by cytolytic T lymphocytes in a human melanoma. Science 1995;269:1281-1284.

227. Fossum B, Breivik J, Meling GI, et al: A K-ras 13Gly→Asp mutation is recognized by HLA-DQ7 restricted T cells in a patient with colorectal cancer. Modifying effect of DQ7 on established cancers harbouring this mutation? Int J Cancer 1994;58:506-511.

228. Fossum B, Gedde-Dahl T 3rd, Breivik J, et al: p21-ras-peptide-specific T-cell responses in a patient with colorectal cancer. CD4+

and CD8+ T cells recognize a peptide corresponding to a common mutation (13Gly→Asp). Int J Cancer 1994;56:40-45.

229. Kwak LW, Young HA, Pennington RW, Weeks SD: Vaccination with syngeneic, lymphoma-derived immunoglobulin idiotype combined with granulocyte/macrophage colony-stimulating factor primes mice for a protective T-cell response. Proc Natl Acad Sci 1996;93:10972-10977.

230. Galloway DA, Jenison SA: Characterization of the humoral immune response to genital papillomaviruses. Mol Biol Med 1990;7:59-72.

231. Howley PM: Papillomavirinae and their replication. In fields BN, Knipe DM (eds): Fundamental Virology. New York: Raven Press, 1991:743-763.

232. Beasley RP, Hwang LY, Lin CC, Chien CS: Hepatocellular carcinoma and hepatitis B virus. A prospective study of 22,707 men in Taiwan. Lancet 1981;2:1129-1133.

233. Brechot C: What is the role of hepatitis B virus in the appearance of hepatocellular carcinomas in patients with alcoholic cirrhosis? Gastroenterol Clin Biol 1982;6:727-730.

234. Overwijk WW, Lee DS, Surman DR, et al: Vaccination with a recombinant vaccinia virus encoding a "self" antigen induces autoimmune vitiligo and tumor cell destruction in mice: requirement for CD4+ T lymphocytes. Proc Natl Acad Sci USA 1999;96:2982-2987.

235. Rosenberg SA, White DE: Vitiligo in patients with melanoma: normal tissue antigens can be targets for cancer immunotherapy. J Immunother Emphasis Tumor Immunol 1996;19:81-84.

236. van der Bruggen P, Traversari C, Chomez P, et al: A gene encoding an antigen recognized by cytolytic T lymphocytes on a human melanoma. Science 1991;254:1643-1647.

237. Tao MH, Levy R: Idiotype/granulocyte-macrophage colony-stimulating factor fusion protein as a vaccine for B-cell lymphoma. Nature 1993;362:755-758.

238. Boyle JS, Brady JL, Lew AM: Enhanced responses to a DNA vaccine encoding a fusion antigen that is directed to sites of immune induction. Nature 1998;392:408-411.

239. You Z, Huang X, Hester J, Toh HC, Chen SY: Targeting dendritic cells to enhance DNA vaccine potency. Cancer Res 2001;61:3704-3711.

240. Mahnke K, Cuo M, Lee S, et al: The dendritic cell receptor for endocytosis, DEC-205, can recycle and enhance antigen presentation via major histocompatibility complex class II-positive lysosomal compartments. J Cell Biol 2000;151:673-684.

241. Srivastava PK: Roles of heat shock proteins in innate and adaptive immunity. Nat Rev Immunol 2002;2:185-194.

242. Castellino F, Boucher PE, Eichelberg K, et al: Receptor-mediated uptake of antigen/heat shock protein complexes results in major histocompatibility complex class I antigen presentation via two distinct processing pathways. J Exp Med 2000;191:1957-1964.

243. Chen CH, Wang TL, Huang CF, et al: Enhancement of DNA vaccine potency by linkage of antigen gene to an HSP70 gene. Cancer Res 2000;60:1035-1042.

244. Suto R, Srivastava PK: A mechanism for the specific immuno-genicity of heat shock protein-chaperoned peptides. Science 1995;269:1585-1588.

245. Basu S, Binder RJ, Ramalingam T, Srivastava PK: CD91 is a common receptor for heat shock proteins gp96, hsp90, hsp70, and calreticulin. Immunity 2001;14:303313.

246. Asea A, Kraeft SK, Kurt-Jones EA, et al: SK, HSP70 stimulates cytokine production through a CD14-dependent pathway, demonstrating its dual role as a chaperone and cytokine. Nat Med 2000;6:435-442.

247. Kuppner MC, Gastpar R, Gelwer S, et al: The role of heat shock protein (hsp70) in dendritic cell maturation: hsp70 induces the maturation of immature dendritic cells but reduces DC differentiation from monocyte precursors. Eur J Immunol 2001;31:1602-1609.

248. Wu TC, Guarnieri FG, Stavely-O'Carroll KF, et al: Engineering an intracellular pathway for major histocompatibility complex class II presentation of antigens. Proc Natl Acad Sci USA 1995;92:11671-11675.

249. Lin KY, Guarnieri FG, Stavely-O'Carroll KF, et al: Treatment of established tumors with a novel vaccine that enhances major histocompatibility class II presentation of tumor antigen. Cancer Res 1996;56:21-26.

250. Ji H, Wang TL, Chen CH, et al: Targeting human papillomavirus type 16 E7 to the endosomal/lysosomal compartment enhances the antitumor immunity of DNA vaccines against murine human papillomavirus type 16 E7-expressing tumors. Hum Gene Ther 1999;10:2727–2740.

251. Hung CF, Cheng WF, Chai CY, et al: Improving vaccine potency through intercellular spreading and enhanced MHC class I presentation of antigen. J Immunol 2001;166:5733–5740.

252. Hung CF, Cheng WF, Hsu KF, et al: Cancer immunotherapy using a DNA vaccine encoding the translocation domain of a bacterial toxin linked to a tumor antigen. Cancer Res 2001; 61:3698–3703.

253. Livingston BD, Newman M, Crimi C, McKenney D, Chestnut R, Sette A: Optimization of epitope processing enhances immunogenicity of multiepitope DNA vaccines. Vaccine 2001;19:4652–4660.

254. Huang AY, Bruce AT, Pardoll DM, Levitsky HI: Does B7-1 expression confer antigen-presenting cell capacity to tumors in vivo? J Exp Med 1996;183:769–776.

255. Kim JJ, Bagarazzi ML, Trivedi N, et al: Engineering of in vivo immune responses to DNA immunization via codelivery of costimulatory molecule genes. Nat Biotechnol 1997;15:641–646.

256. Agadjanyan MG, Kim JJ, Trivedi N, et al: CD86 (B7-2) can function to drive MHC-restricted antigen-specific CTL responses in vivo. J Immunol 1999;162:3417–3427.

257. Sturmhoefel K, Lee K, Gray GS, et al: Potent activity of soluble B7-IgG fusion proteins in therapy of established tumors and as vaccine adjuvant. Can Res 1999;58:4964–4972.

258. Schmitter D, Bolliger U, Hallek M, Pichert G: Involvement of the CD27-CD70 co-stimulatory pathway in allogeneic T-cell response to follicular lymphoma cells. Br J Haematol 1999;106:64–70.

259. Watts T, DeBenedette M: T cell co-stimulatory molecules other than CD28. Curr Opin Immunol 1999;11:286–293.

260. Atkins MB, Lotze MT, Dutcher JP, et al: High-dose recombinant interleukin 2 therapy for patients with metastatic melanoma: analysis of 270 patients treated between 1985 and 1993. J Clin Oncol 1999;17:2105–2116.

261. Lode HN, Xiang R, Gillies SD, Becker JC, Reisfeld RA: Immunocytokines: A promising approach to cancer immunotherapy. Pharmacol Ther 1998;80:277–292.

262. Cheever M, Thompson JA, Kern DE, Greenberg PD: Interleukin 2(IL-2) administered in vivo: influence of IL-2 route and timing on T cell growth. J Immunol 1985;134:3895–3900.

263. Kern D, Klarnet JP, Cheever MA, Greenberg PD: Requirements for the generation of a Lyt-2+ T cell proliferative response to a syngeneic tumor in the absence of L3T4 + T cells. Cancer Res 1990;50:6256–6263.

264. Evans L, Witte PR, Feldhaus AL, et al: Expression of chimeric granulocyte-macrophage colony-stimulating factor/interleukin 2 receptors in human cytotoxic T lymphocyte clones results in GMCSF-dependent growth. Human Gene Ther 1999;10: 1941–1951.

265. Ahlers JD, Dunlop N, Alling DW, Nara PL, Berzofsky JA: Cytokine-in-adjuvant steering of the immune response phenotype to HIV-1 vaccine constructs: granulocyte-macrophage colony-stimulating factor and TNF-alpha synergize with IL-12 to enhance induction of cytotoxic T lymphocytes. J Immunol 1997;158: 3947–3958.

266. Smith GL, Murphy BR, Moss B: Construction and characterization of an infectious vaccinia virus recombinant that expresses the influenza hemagglutinin gene and induces resistance to influenza virus infection in hamsters. Proc Natl Acad Sci USA 1983;80: 7155–7159.

267. Panicali D, Paoletti E: Construction of poxviruses as cloning vectors: insertion of the thymidine kinase gene from herpes simplex virus into the DNA of infectious vaccinia virus. Proc Natl Acad Sci USA 1982;79:4927–4931.

268. Moss B: Genetically engineered poxviruses for recombinant gene expression, vaccination, and safety. Proc Natl Acad Sci USA 1996;93:11341–11348.

269. Carroll MW, Overwijk WW, Chamberlin RS, Moss B, Rosenberg SA, Restifo NP: Highly attenuated modified vaccinia virus Ankara (MVA) as an effective recombinant vector: A murine tumor model. Vaccine 1997;15:387–394.

270. Paoletti E, Taylor J, Meignier B, Meric C, Tarlaglia J: Highly attenuated poxvirus vectors: NYVAC, ALVAC and TROVAC. Dev Biol Stand 1995;84:159–163.

271. Velders MP, McElhiney S, Cassetti MC, et al: Eradication of established tumors by vaccination with Venezuelan equine encephalitis virus replicon particles delivering human papillomavirus 16 e7 RNA. Cancer Res 2001;61:7861–7867.

272. Elzey BD, Siemens DR, Ratliff TL, Lubaroff DM: Immunization with type 5 adenovirus recombinant for a tumor antigen in combination with recombinant canarypox virus (alvac) cytokine gene delivery induces destruction of established prostate tumors. Int J Cancer 2001;94:842–849.

273. Gewurz BE, Gaudet R, Tortorella D, Wang EW, Ploegh H: Virus subversion of immunity: A structural perspective. Curr Opin Immunol 2001;13:442–450.

274. Irvine KR, Chamberlin RS, Shulman EP, Surman DK, Rosenberg SA, Restifo NP: Enhancing efficacy of recombinant anticancer vaccines with prime/boost regimens that use two different vectors. J Natl Cancer Inst 1997;89:1595–1601.

275. Ramshaw IA, Ramsay AJ: The prime-boost strategy: exciting prospects for improved vaccination. Immunol Today 2000;21:163–165.

276. Pan ZK, Ikonomidis G, Lazenby A, Pardoll D, Paterson Y: A recombinant Listeria monocytogenes vaccine expressing a model tumour antigen protects mice against lethal tumour cell challenge and causes regression of established tumours. Nat Med 1995;1: 471–477.

277. Thole JE, van Dalen PJ, Havenith CE, et al: Live bacterial delivery systems for development of mucosal vaccines. Curr Opin Mol Ther 2000;2: 94–99.

278. Killeen K, Spriggs D, Mekalanos J: Bacterial mucosal vaccines: Vibrio cholerae as a live attenuated vaccine/vector paradigm. Curr Top Microbiol Immunol 1999;236:237–254.

279. Ohara N, Yamada T: Recombinant BCG vaccines. Vaccine 2001;19:4089–4098.

280. Shata MT, Stevceva L, Agwales S, Lewis GK, Hone DM: Recent advances with recombinant bacterial vaccine vectors. Mol Med Today 2000;6:66–71.

281. Sizemore DR, Branstrom AA, Sadoff JC: Attenuated Shigella as a DNA delivery vehicle for DNA-mediated immunization. Science 1995;270:299–302.

282. Darji A, Gazman CA, Gerstel B, et al: Oral somatic transgene vaccination using attenuated S. typhimurium. Cell 1997;91:765–775.

283. Chambers CA, Kuhn MS, Egen JC, Allison JP: CTLA-4-mediated inhibition in regulation of T cell responses: Mechanisms and manipulation in tumor immunotherapy. Annu Rev Immunol 2001;19:565–594.

284. van Elsas A, Hurwitz AA, Allison JP: Combination immunotherapy of B16 melanoma using anti-cytotoxic T lymphocyte-associated antigen 4 (CTLA-4) and granulocyte/macrophage colony-stimulating factor (GM-CSF)-producing vaccines induces rejection of subcutaneous and metastatic tumors accompanied by autoimmune depigmentation. J Exp Med 1999;190:355–366.

285. Hurwitz AA, Yu TF, Leach DR, Allison JP: CTLA-4 blockade synergizes with tumor-derived granulocyte-macrophage colony-stimulating factor for treatment of an experimental mammary carcinoma. Proc Natl Acad Sci USA 1998;95:10067–10071.

286. Hurwitz AA, Foster BA, Kwon ED, et al: Combination immunotherapy of primary prostate cancer in a transgenic mouse model using CTLA-4 blockade. Cancer Res 2000;60:2444–2448.

287. Nishimura H, Okazaki T, Tanaka Y, et al: Autoimmune dilated cardiomyopathy in PD-1 receptor-deficient mice. Science 2001;291:319–322.

288. Dong H, Strome SE, Salomao DR, et al: Tumor-associated B7-H1 promotes T-cell apoptosis: a potential mechanism of immune evasion. Nat Med 2002;8:793–800.

289. Shin T, Kennedy G, Gorski K, et al: Cooperative B7-1/2 (DC80/CD86) and B7-DC costimulation of CD4 + T cells independent of the PD-1 receptor. J Exp Med 2003;198:31–38.

290. Sica GL, Choi IH, Zhu G, et al: B7-H4, a molecule of the B7 family, negatively regulates T cell immunity. Immunity 2003;18:849–861.

291. Prasad D, Richards S, Mai XM, Dong C: B7S1, a novel B7 family member that negatively regulates T cell activation. Immunity 2003;18:863–873.

Science of Clinical Oncology

I

292. Watanabe N, Gavrieli M, Sedy JR, et al: BTLA is a lymphocyte inhibitory receptor with similarities to CTLA-4 and PD-1. Nat Immunol 2003;4:670–679.

293. Ibarra-Sanchez MJ, Simoncic PD, Nestel FR, Duplay P, Lapp WS, Tremblay ML: The T-cell protein tyrosine phosphatase. Semin Immunol 2000;12:379–386.

294. Irie-Sasaki J, Sasaki T, Matsumoto W, et al: CD45 is a JAK phosphatase and negatively regulates cytokine receptor signalling. Nature 2001;409:349–354.

295. Greenhalgh CJ, Hilton DJ: Negative regulation of cytokine signaling. J Leukoc Biol 2001;70:348–356.

296. Vang T, Torgersen KM, Sundvold V, et al: Activation of the COOH-terminal Src kinase (Csk) by cAMP-dependent protein kinase inhibits signaling through the T cell receptor. J Exp Med 2001;193:497–507.

297. Chiang YJ, Kole HK, Brown K, et al: Cbl-b regulates the CD28 dependence of T-cell activation. Nature 2000;403:216–220.

298. Bachmaier K, Krawczyk C, Kozieradzki I, et al: Negative regulation of lymphocyte activation and autoimmunity by the molecular adaptor Cbl-b. Nature 2000;403:211–216.

299. Sun L, Youn HD, Loh C, Stolow M, He W, Liu JO: Cabin 1, a negative regulator for calcineurin signaling in T lymphocytes. Immunity 1998;8:703–711.

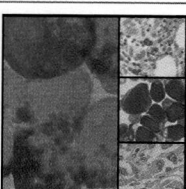

STEM CELLS, CELL DIFFERENTIATION, AND CANCER

Michael F. Clarke

Irving L. Weissman

SUMMARY OF KEY POINTS

- Most cancers arise in tissues (such as the gut, breast, prostate, lungs, and bone marrow) that contain a stem cell population.
- Stem cells have three fundamental properties: the ability to divide and give rise to a new stem cell in a process called *self-renewal*, the ability to give rise to the differentiated cells of an organ, and genetic constraints on expansion.
- The fact that stem cells are the only long-lived cells in most tissues in which cancers arise suggests that early mutations that lead to cancer accumulate in stem cells.
- Because oncogenic mutations accumulate in stem cells and because stem cells, like cancer cells,

- are the only cells in the tissue that have the intrinsic ability to self-renew, stem cells can be target cells for neoplastic transformation.
- In addition to classes of oncogenes that affect cell survival and proliferation, there is a class of oncogenes that permits cells to self-renew. Thus in some cancers, the target cells for neoplastic transformation may be progenitor cells that have acquired the ability to self-renew as a result of one or more mutations.
- New data suggest that in both leukemia and breast cancer, a small, phenotypically distinct subset of cancer cells has the exclusive ability to form tumors.

- At present, therapeutic targets are selected based on the proposition that all of the cancer cells within a particular tumor are capable of driving tumor formation and metastasis. However, because the bulk of the cancer cells in the tumor are unable to form tumors, these cells are the targets of many therapies.
- To be effective, therapies must target the critical tumorigenic cancer cell population.
- The ability to prospectively identify tumorigenic cancer cells should allow the identification of new diagnostic markers and therapeutic targets.

INTRODUCTION

Common cancers arise in tissues that contain a large subpopulation of proliferating cells that are responsible for replenishing the short-lived mature cells. In such organs, cell maturation is arranged in a hierarchy in which a rare population of stem cells gives rise to the mature cells, which perpetuate themselves through a process called *self-renewal*.[1-11] Because of their rarity, stem cells must be isolated prospectively to study their biologic, molecular, and biochemical properties. Although it is likely that they give rise to most tissues, stem cells have been rigorously identified and purified in only a few. The stem cells that give rise to the lymphohematopoietic system, called *hematopoietic stem cells* (HSCs), have been isolated from mice and humans and are the best characterized stem cells. The utility of tissue containing HSCs has been demonstrated in cancer therapy with its extensive use for bone marrow transplantation to regenerate the hematolymphoid system after myeloablative protocols.[12] The prospective isolation of HSCs from patients can result in a population of cancer-free cells for autologous transplantation.[13-17]

Understanding the cellular biology of the tissues in which cancers arise, and specifically of the stem cells residing in those tissues, could provide new insights into cancer biology. Several aspects of stem cell biology are relevant to cancer. First, both normal stem cells and cancer stem cells undergo self-renewal, and emerging evidence suggests that similar molecular mechanisms regulate self-renewal in normal stem cells and their malignant counterparts. Next, it is quite likely that mutations that lead to cancer accumulate in normal stem cells. Finally, as stated previously, it is likely that tumors contain a rare "cancer stem cell" population with indefinite proliferative potential that drives the growth and metastasis of tumors.[18-27]

PROPERTIES OF NORMAL STEM CELLS

HSCs are the most studied and best understood somatic stem cell population and serve as a model for stem cells from other tissues.[1,9,26,28,29] Hematopoiesis is a tightly regulated process in which a pool of HSCs eventually gives rise to the lymphohematopoietic system consisting of the formed blood elements (e.g., red blood cells, platelets, granulocytes, macrophages, and B and T lymphocytes). These cells are important for oxygenation, prevention of bleeding, immunity, and fighting infections, respectively. In the adult, HSCs have three fundamental properties. First, HSCs need to self-renew to maintain the stem cell pool. Self-renewal is not synonymous with proliferation. Self-renewal is a cell division in which one or both of the daughter cells remain undifferentiated and have the ability to give rise to another stem cell, as well as the spectrum of differentiated mature progeny. Second, they must undergo differentiation to maintain a constant pool of mature cells in normal conditions and to produce increased numbers of a particular lineage in response to stresses such as bleeding or infection. Third, the total number of HSCs is under strict genetic regulation.[30]

In the mouse hematopoietic system, multipotent cells constitute 0.05% of bone marrow cells and are heterogeneous with respect to their ability to self-renew. There are three different populations of multipotent cells: long-term self-renewing HSCs, short-term self-renewing HSCs, and multipotent progenitors without detectable self-renewal potential.[7,31] These populations form a hierarchy in which the long-term HSCs give rise to short-term HSCs, which in turn give rise to multipotent progenitors[7] (Fig. 8-1). As HSCs mature from the long-term self-renewing pool to multipotent progenitors, they become more mitotically active but lose the ability to self-renew. Only long-term HSCs can give rise to mature hematopoietic cells for the lifetime of the animal, whereas short-term HSCs and multipotent progenitors reconstitute lethally irradiated mice for less than 8 weeks.[7]

Despite the fact that the phenotypic and functional properties of mouse and human HSCs have been extensively characterized,[2] understanding of the fundamental stem cell property, self-renewal, is minimal.[26,28,32] In most cases, HSCs differentiate when exposed to combinations of growth factors that can induce extensive proliferation in long-term cultures.[33] Although recent progress has been made in identifying culture conditions that maintain HSC activity in culture for a limited period,[34] it has proven to be exceedingly difficult to identify tissue culture conditions that promote a significant and prolonged expansion of progenitors with transplantable HSC activity.

Genetic Regulation of Self-Renewal in Normal Stem Cells and Cancer Cells

Maintenance of a tissue or a tumor is determined by a balance of cell proliferation and cell death.[35] As would be expected, many of the mutations that drive tumor expansion regulate either cell proliferation or survival. For example, the prevention of apoptosis by enforced expression of the oncogene Bcl-2 promotes the development of lymphoma and also results in increased numbers of HSCs in vivo, suggesting that cell death plays a role in regulating the homeostasis of HSCs.[36,37] In fact, the progression to experimental acute myelogenous leukemia (AML) in mice requires at least three, and likely four, independent events to block the several intrinsically triggered and extrinsically induced programmed cell death pathways of meloid cells.[38] Proto-oncogenes such as c-*myb* and c-*myc* that drive proliferation of tumor cells are also essential for HSC development.[39-42]

Self-renewal is critical for both normal stem cells and cancer stem cells. In a normal tissue, stem cell numbers are under tight genetic regulation, resulting in the maintenance a constant number of stem cells in the organ.[30,43,44] In contrast, cancer stem cells have escaped this homeostatic regulation, and the number of cells within a tumor with the ability to self-renew is constantly expanding, resulting in the inevitable growth of the tumor. Because cancer cells and normal stem cells share the ability to self-renew, it is not surprising that a number of genes classically associated with cancer may also regulate normal stem cell development.[26,45] In combination with other growth factors, sonic hedgehog (Shh) signaling has also been implicated in the regulation of self-renewal by the finding that cells highly enriched for human HSCs (CD34$^+$Lin$^-$CD38$^-$) exhibit increased

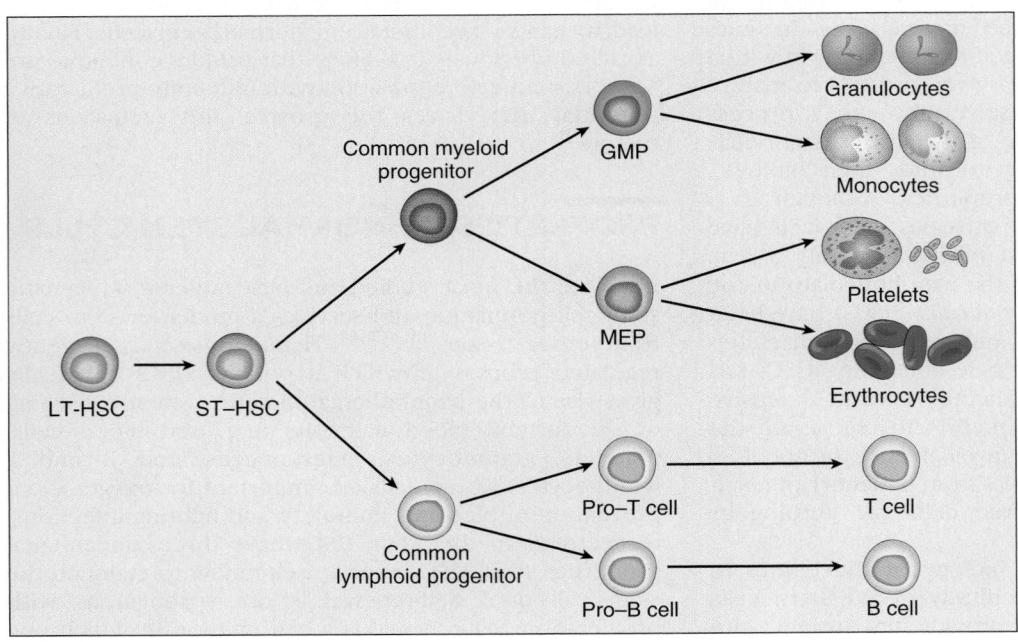

Figure 8-1. Blood development hierarchy. All of the diverse mature blood cells arise from the hematopoeitic stem cells (HSCs). The cells capable of multilineage reconstitution of a lethally irradiated mouse are contained within two identifiable and separate populations of cells: the long-term hematopoietic stem cells HSCs (LT-HSCs) and the short-term hematopoietic stem cells HSCs (ST-HSCs). Only the LT-HSCs are capable of self-renewal for the lifetime of the animal. In contrast, other cells, even the ST-HSCs that can give rise to large numbers of mature blood cells, have very limited life spans (measured in hours to 1 or 2 months). GMP, granulocyte-macrophage progenitors; MEP, myeloid-erythroid progenitors.

self-renewal in response to Shh stimulation in vitro.[46] Several other genes related to oncogenesis have been shown to be important for stem cell function. For example, mice deficient for *tal-1/SCL*, which is involved in some cases of human acute myeloid leukemia, lack embryonic hematopoiesis,[47] suggesting that *tal-1/SCL* is required for intrinsic or extrinsic events necessary to initiate hematopoiesis, for maintenance of the earliest definitive blood cells, or for the formation of blood cells downstream of embryonic HSCs.[47,48] Members of the Hox family have also been implicated in human leukemia, and enforced expression of *HoxB4* can affect stem cell functions.[49,50] One of the major targets of the p53 tumor suppressor gene is p21^{cip1}. Bone marrow from p21^{cip1}-deficient mice has a reduced ability to serially reconstitute lethally irradiated recipients. Failure at serial transfer could result from exhaustion of the stem cell pool, loss of telomeres, or loss of transplantability.[51] Thus many genes involved in stem cell fate decisions are also involved in malignant transformation.

The notion that the function of certain oncogenes is to regulate self-renewal is perhaps best illustrated by studies of the oncogene *bmi-1*. In mice, *bmi-1* cooperates with *c-myc* to induce lymphoma.[52,53] The number of HSCs is markedly reduced in postnatal *bmi-1$^{-/-}$* mice, and transplanted *bmi-1$^{-/-}$* fetal liver and bone marrow cells are able to contribute only transiently to hematopoiesis, indicating a cell autonomous defect of HSC self-renewal in *bmi-1$^{-/-}$* mice.[54] The expression of stem cell–associated genes,[3] cell survival genes, transcription factors, and genes modulating proliferation including *p16^{Ink4a}* and *p19^{Arf}* is altered in bone marrow cells of *bmi-1$^{-/-}$* mice. This suggests that the function of *bmi-1* is to regulate a cascade of genes that modulate stem cell self-renewal. In a mouse model of leukemia, leukemic cells lacking expression of *bmi-1* eventually undergo proliferation arrest associated with signs of differentiation and apoptosis when transplanted in syngenic hosts. Infection of the cells with a *bmi-1* retrovirus completely rescues the proliferative defect of the *bmi-1$^{-/-}$* leukemic stem cells.[55] These studies conclusively demonstrate that malignant transformation requires not only activation of proliferation pathways, as well as inactivation of cell death and cell cycle arrest pathways, but also activation of self-renewal pathways.

Two other signaling pathways implicated in oncogenesis in both mice and humans, the Wnt/β-catenin and Notch pathways, may play central roles in the self-renewal of both normal and cancer stem cells. The Notch family of receptors was first identified in *Drosophila* species and has been implicated in development and differentiation.[56] In *Caenorhabditis elegans*, Notch plays a role in germ cell self-renewal.[57] In neural development, transient Notch activation initiates an irreversible switch from neurogenesis to gliogenesis by embryonic neural crest stem cells.[10] Notch activation of HSCs in culture with either of the Notch ligands Jagged-1 or Delta transiently increases the primitive progenitor activity both in vitro and in vivo, suggesting that Notch activation promotes either the maintenance of progenitor cell multipotentiality or HSC self-renewal.[58,59] Although the Notch pathway plays a

central role in development and the mouse oncogene *int-3* is a truncated Notch4,[60] the role of Notch in de novo human cancer is complex and less well understood. Various members of the Notch signaling pathway are expressed in cancers of epithelial origin, and activation of the Notch pathway by chromosomal translocation is involved in some cases of leukemia.[61-65] Microarray analysis has shown that members of the Notch pathway are often overexpressed by tumor cells.[62,63] A truncated Notch4 messenger RNA is expressed by some breast cancer cell lines.[66] Overexpression of Notch1 leads to growth arrest of a small cell lung cancer cell line, whereas inhibition of Notch1 signals can induce leukemia cell lines to undergo apoptosis.[56,58,67] Elegant work by Miele and colleagues[68] showed that activation of Notch1 signaling maintains the neoplastic phenotype in Ras-transformed human cells. They also found that in de novo cancers, cells with an activating Ras mutation also demonstrate increased expression of Notch1 and Notch4.

Wnt/β-catenin signaling also plays a pivotal role in the self-renewal of normal stem cells and malignant transformation.[69-71] The Wnt pathway was first implicated in mouse mammary tumor virus (MMTV)–induced breast cancer in which deregulated expression of Wnt-1 caused by proviral insertion resulted in mammary tumors.[72,73] Subsequently, it has been shown that Wnt proteins play a central role in pattern formation. Wnt-1 belongs to a large family of highly hydrophobic secreted proteins that function by binding to their cognate receptors, members of the Frizzled and low-density lipoprotein receptor-related protein families, resulting in activation of β-catenin.[45,62,69,74,75] In the absence of receptor activation, β-catenin is marked for degradation by a complex consisting of the adenomatous polyposis coli (APC), Axin, and glycogen synthase kinase-3β proteins.[62,70,71,76-79] Wnt proteins are expressed in the bone marrow, and activation of Wnt/β-catenin signaling by Wnt proteins in vitro or by expression of a constitutively active β-catenin expands the pool of early progenitor cells and enriched normal transplantable HSCs in tissue culture and in vivo.[26,71,76] Inhibition of Wnt/β-catenin by ectopic expression of Axin, an inhibitor of β-catenin signaling, leads to inhibition of stem cell proliferation both in vitro and in vivo. Other studies suggest that the Wnt/β-catenin pathway mediates stem or progenitor cell self-renewal in other tissues.[77,78,80,81] The level of β-catenin in a particular keratinocyte directly correlates with its proliferative capacity.[77,78,81] As in their normal HSC counterparts, enforced expression of an activated β-catenin in epidermal stem cells increases their ability to self-renew and decreases their ability to differentiate. Mice that fail to express TCF-4, one of the transcription factors that is activated when bound to β-catenin, soon exhaust their undifferentiated crypt epithelial progenitor cells, further suggesting that Wnt signaling is involved in the self-renewal of epithelial stem cells.[45,80]

Activation of β-catenin in colon cancer by inactivation of the protein degradation pathway, most frequently by mutation of APC, is common.[45,62,70,79] Expression of certain Wnt genes is increased in some other epithelial cancers, suggesting that activation of β-catenin might be secondary to ligand activation in such cancers.[69,82-87] There is evidence that constitutive activation of the Wnt/β-catenin pathway may confer a stem/progenitor cell phenotype to cancer cells. Inhibition of β-catenin/TCF-4 in a colon cancer cell line induced the expression of the cell cycle inhibitor $p21^{cip-1}$ and induced the cells to stop proliferating and acquire a more differentiated phenotype.[87] Enforced expression of the proto-oncogene c-myc, which is transcriptionally activated by β-catenin/TCF-4, inhibited the expression of $p21^{cip-1}$ and allowed the colon cancer cells to proliferate when β-catenin/TCF-4 signaling was blocked, linking Wnt signaling to c-myc in the regulation of cell proliferation and differentiation.[87]

The implication of roles for genes such as Notch, Wnt, c-myc, and Shh in the regulation of self-renewal of HSCs, and perhaps of stem cells, from multiple tissues suggests that there may be common self-renewal pathways in many types of normal somatic stem cells and cancer stem cells. It will be important to identify the molecular mechanisms by which these pathways work and to determine whether the pathways interact to regulate the self-renewal of normal stem cells and cancer stem cells.

Target Cells for Malignant Transformation

If oncogenic mutations often target signaling pathways that regulate proliferation and self-renewal, then are stem cells, highly proliferative progenitor cells, or both the target of neoplastic transformation? Several lines of evidence suggest that stem cells may be involved in the evolution of a cancer. First, the fact that multiple mutations are necessary for a cell to become cancerous[88,89] suggests that in many cases mutations accumulate in a stem cell. Progenitor cells have a very limited life span, making it less likely that all of the mutations occur during the life of these relatively short-lived cells.[1,7,8,26,28,90,91] Second, the regulation of stem cell expansion and self-renewal is under strict genetic regulation by multiple genes, and unregulated expansion of stem cells would, in essence, result in a cancer.[30,43,44] Third, most cancers arise in tissues that contain stem cells that have the intrinsic ability to self-renew. Because cancer cells must undergo self-renewal, this suggests that stem cells may more easily undergo malignant transformation than progenitor cells that lack this fundamental property and must therefore activate these self-renewal pathways to become malignant. In the hematopoietic system, the only cells with the ability to self-renew are HSCs and mature lymphocytes. The common blood cancers, acute leukemias and lymphomas, may arise from the HSCs or lymphocytes, respectively, via constitutive activation of mitogenic pathways associated with the proliferation of normal cells.[26,35,92,93] Although it may be easier for stem cells to undergo malignant transformation, it is possible, if not likely, that in many cases progenitor cells give rise to cancer. For example, the initial mutations that occur in the stem cell could permit a single mutation to transform a progenitor cell. It is also possible that certain oncogenic mutations such as bmi-1 could confer the property of self-renewal to a progenitor cell.

The target cells for transformation are best understood in hematopoietic malignancies because the developmental hierarchy of the blood is well established. One of the most frequent mutations in AML is the t(8;21) mutation, which results in the expression of a chimeric AML-ETO transcript in the leukemic cells.[94-96] $CD34^+Thy1^+CD38^-$ Lin^- HSCs can be isolated from patients in clinical remission and up to 90% of the time are found to express the chimeric AML-1-ETO transcript.[96] When these HSCs were analyzed by means of in vitro differentiation assays, the HSCs gave rise to normal progeny, demonstrating that the mutation was present in the otherwise normal stem cells. In these patients, the $Thy1^-$ subset of $CD34^+CD38^-$ Lin^- cells gave rise to leukemic colonies in vitro; this could represent HSCs that lost Thy1 expression or downstream multipotent progenitors that have gained self-renewal capacity.[74] Taken together, these observations support the notion that mutations accumulate in stem cells, and subsequent mutations in either the stem cells or their progeny result in overt leukemia.

Although stem cells are frequently the target of mutations that lead to malignant transformation, it is likely that progenitor cells may be transformed by subsequent genetic events that confer immortality, self-renewal potential, or both to these normally non–self-renewing cells (Fig. 8-2). In patients with chronic myelogenous leukemia (CML), the BCR-ABL mutation is present in both normal and leukemic stem cells. In otherwise normal hematopoietic cells, the BCR-ABL mRNA is expressed solely by the progenitor cells.[2,97,98] In a mouse model of CML, BCR-ABL expression targeted to myeloid progenitor cells by the hMRP-8 promoter resulted in CML-like disease in a subset of the mice. Furthermore, when $hMRP8p210^{BCR/ABL}$ mice were crossed with hMRP8bcl-2 mice, a proportion of the mutant mice developed a disease resembling AML.[99] Although the expression of transforming genes was targeted to early progenitor cells, the appearance of the leukemia cells and clinical course resembled human CML and AML in the $hMRP8p210^{BCR/ABL}$ mice and the $hMRP8p210^{BCR/ABL}$/hMRP8bcl-2 mice, respectively. In a mouse model of high-grade glioblastoma, enforced expression of the epidermal growth factor receptor (EGF-R)–enriched populations in either Ink4a/Arf null neuronal stem cells or Ink4a/Arf null astrocytes led to malignant glioblastomas when the cells were injected orthotopically into mice.[100] Notably, in the majority of the cases, the transformed astrocytes appeared to acquire an immature phenotype in the brains of the mice, suggesting that there was "dedifferentiation."[100] There are two other possible explanations for these results. First, the astrocyte tissue culture cells could have contained a rare population of neuronal stem cells that were transformed, and these stem cells were responsible for generating the tumors. Second, it is possible that the tissue culture conditions could have caused the dedifferentiation of the astrocytes and that unless the astrocytes are grown in tissue culture, they cannot give rise to glioblastomas in an animal. The observations in humans and mice support the notion that oncogenic mutations accumulate in the stem cells, but expression of the mutated gene by progenitors downstream of the stem cells can lead to their neoplastic

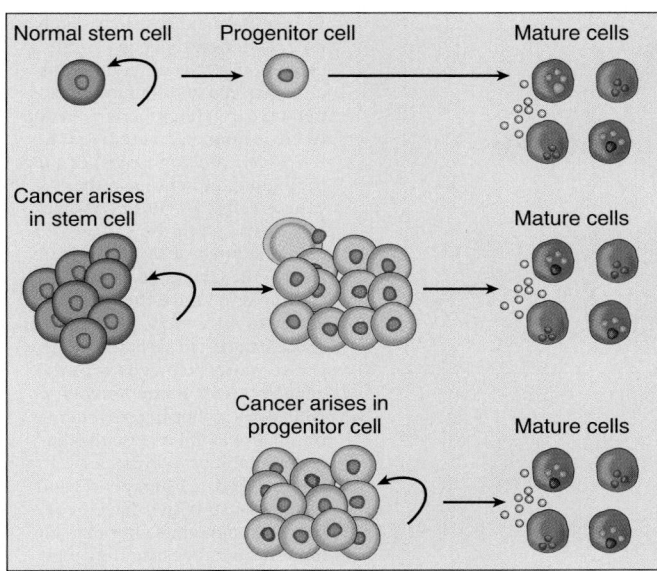

Figure 8-2. Target cells for neoplastic transformation. In many tissues in which cancers arise, the stem cells are the only long-lived cells and are the only cells capable of self-renewal. Because they are already capable of extensive self-renewal, they are good targets for neoplastic transformation. Dysregulation of the self-renewal process may be simpler in these cells than in progenitor cells that lack this ability. In order for progenitor cells to undergo malignant transformation, they must acquire the ability to undergo extensive self-renewal as a result of oncogenic mutations.

transformation of progenitor cells. These observations have implications for targeted therapies.

It is possible that only a minority of the mice whose progenitors express BCR-ABL develop leukemia because the progenitors must acquire an additional mutation that causes deregulated self-renewal. There are two lines of evidence that support this notion. First, expression of *bmi-1* is necessary for the self-renewal of adult HSCs, and the blast cells of patients with AML express large amounts of this protein.[92] Although expression of HoxA9 and Meis1 induces transplantable AML in normal mice, expression of these genes in the absence of *bmi-1* does not.[54,55] This suggests that both normal HSCs and leukemic stem cells require *bmi-1* to self-renew. Second, deregulated β-catenin signaling occurs in many de novo human cancers and causes cancer in transgenic mouse models. Because expression of a constitutively active β-catenin can promote the self-renewal of normal HSCs, as well as stem cells from other tissues, it is quite plausible that activation of this pathway promotes self-renewal of the cancer cells.* From these results, it is evident that future studies focusing on the molecular regulation of the self-renewal of normal stem cells and cancer cells will likely lead to more effective therapies for cancer.

Evidence for Cancer Stem Cells

It has long been known that cancers consist of phenotypically heterogeneous populations of cancer cells.[22-25,103-106]

*See references 2, 26, 80, 81, 87, 93, 97, 99, 101, 102.

These phenotypically distinct cell populations could arise in part from sequential mutations caused by genetic instability, environmental factors, or both (Fig. 8-3A). Alternatively, a tumor can be viewed as an aberrant organ containing a tumorigenic (stem cell) population that drives tumor growth. These tumorigenic cells would have acquired oncogenic mutations that result in unregulated self-renewal and would also give rise to phenotypically diverse populations of tumor cells that lack the ability to self-renew (Fig. 8-3B). Several lines of evidence suggest that this latter model accounts for some of the cellular heterogeneity seen in tumors, although genetic instability and environmental factors could also contribute to the variability in phenotypes.[107,108] It is well documented that many types of cancer contain heterogeneous populations of cells that variably express differentiation markers that reflect the tissues from which the tumors originate, as well as cancer cells that have an immature appearance.[104,109,110] Examples of this include the variable expression of milk proteins by some breast cancers and the variable expression of myeloid markers, lymphoid markers, or both in CML and AML. Perhaps the most striking example of abnormal differentiation in cancer is the variable expression of diverse tissues in some germ cell tumors. Mature tissues such as teeth, skin, and hair are present in some cases of teratocarcinomas (Fig. 8-4). In contrast, in some tumors only a minority of the cancer cells express immature cell markers such as α-fetoprotein (see Fig. 8-4). Because the terminally differentiated cells that form the teeth and hair in the tumors are unlikely to be able to proliferate and form new tumors, these data suggest that the minority population of α-fetoprotein–expressing cancer cells has the exclusive ability to form new tumors consisting of more tumorigenic cells, as well as the phenotypically diverse populations of non–self-renewing abnormally differentiated cells. If this is true, these cells can thus be considered cancer stem cells.

If a tumor is viewed as an abnormal organ, then the principles of stem cell biology can be applied to better understand the biology of these diseases.[1,8,9] It was first shown in hematopoietic malignancies and subsequently in solid cancers that only a subset of cancer cells were clonogenic when placed in tissue culture or injected into immunodeficient mice.[20,22-24,104,106,111,112] For example, only 1 in 100 to 1 in 10,000 mouse myeloma cells obtained from ascites fluid formed in vitro colony-forming assays. Similarly, only 1% to 4% of leukemic cells formed spleen colonies when transplanted into mice. In solid cancers, only 1 in 1000 to 1 in 5000 ovarian cancer or lung cancer cells formed colonies in soft agar. Because only a minority of normal bone marrow cells was also clonogenic, the clonogenic cancer cells were described as *cancer stem cells*, implying that only a distinct population of cancer cells was able to proliferate extensively in these assays. However, an alternative explanation is that all the cancer cells had an intrinsic ability to proliferate extensively, but only a minority of cells did so in a particular assay.[106]

To prove that a phenotypically distinct population of cancer cells is solely responsible for perpetuating the disease, it is necessary to isolate different populations of

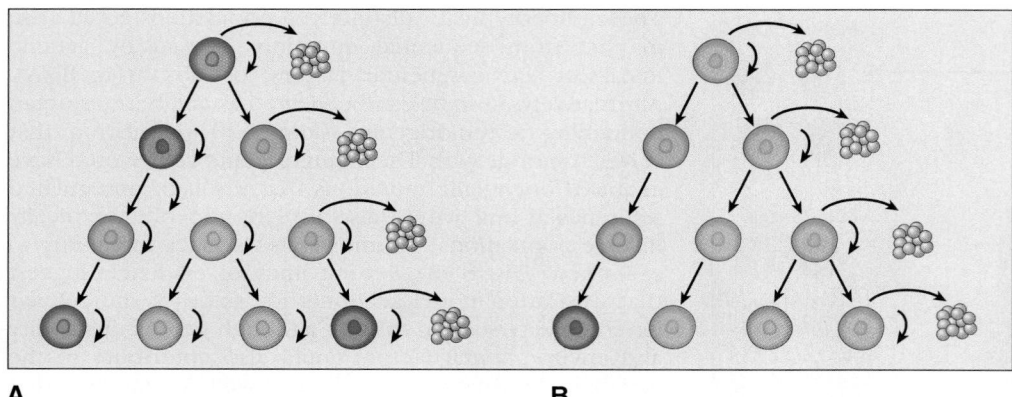

Figure 8-3. The two most likely models of heterogeneity of the cancer cells, shown as different colored cells within a tumor, are depicted. **A,** Heterogeneity is due to environmental factors (*gold, red, green,* and *blue cells*) or due to ongoing mutations in the cancer cells (*magenta cells*). In this model, all of the cancer cells have the intrinsic ability to form tumors. **B,** Cancer stem cells (*yellow cells*) have the exclusive ability to self-renew. As in normal tissues, the stem cells would give rise to more stem cells with the capacity to form new tumors, as well as the other heterogeneous populations of cancer cells that lack the ability to form new tumors. To date, therapeutic and diagnostic strategies have been based on model (**A**) but may be limited since because they may not target the rare population of cancer stem cells depicted in model (**B**).

cancer cells and demonstrate that one or more groups are enriched for the ability to initiate disease and other populations lack this ability. This was done in the case of AML, when it was shown that in most cases of human AML, a leukemic tumor initiating subpopulations of cells could be identified prospectively and purified from the bone marrow of multiple patients. In most cases of AML, the minority population of $CD34^+CD38^-$ cells was the only group of cells capable of establishing human AML in the bone marrow of nonobese diabetic/severe combined immunodeficient (NOD/SCID) mice.[113,114] Remarkably, within the $CD34^+CD38^-$ population are $Thy1^+$ $CD34^+CD38^-$ normal HSCs.[2,90,96,113-116] Because normal HSCs, but not their leukemic initiating cell counterparts, express Thy 1, it is likely that the early mutations occurred in the HSCs and the final transforming mutations occurred either in early downstream progenitors or in HSCs, if, as a consequence of neoplastic transformation, Thy 1 expression was lost.[96]

Recently, tumorigenic and nontumorigenic subsets of cancer cells have been isolated from human breast cancer tumors. When a similar model for human breast cancer in which isolated cells were grown in immunocompromised mice was used, a minority population of breast cancer cells that possessed the ability to form new tumors was identified.[18] Tumorigenic cells could be distinguished from nontumorigenic cancer cells on the basis of surface marker expression. In eight of nine patients, tumorigenic cells could be prospectively identified and isolated as $CD44^+CD24^{-/low}Lineage^-$ cells.[18] As few as 100 $CD44^+CD24^{-/low}Lineage^-$ cells were able to form tumors, whereas tens of thousands of cells from other populations of cells within the tumor failed to form tumors in NOD/SCID mice. These tumorigenic cells could be serially passaged in mice, and each time cells within this population generated new tumors containing additional

$CD44^+CD24^{-/low}Lineage^-$ tumorigenic cells, as well as phenotypically mixed populations of other nontumorigenic cancer cells. These data demonstrate the presence of a hierarchy of cells within a breast cancer tumor in which only a fraction of the cells have the ability to proliferate extensively and other cells have only a limited proliferative potential, suggesting that the tumorigenic cells can both self-renew and differentiate. The phenotype of the tumorigenic breast cancer cells may be similar to normal breast epithelial stem or progenitor cells, because early multipotent epithelial progenitor cells have been reported to express epithelial cell antigen (ESA) and CD44.[117-119]

The $CD44^+CD24^{-/low}Lineage^-$ tumorigenic breast cancer cell and the $CD34^+CD38^-$ leukemia-initiating cells share with normal stem cells the abilities to proliferate extensively and to give rise to diverse cell types with reduced developmental or proliferative potential.[5,18] The extensive proliferative potential of the tumorigenic breast cancer cell population was demonstrated by the ability of as few as 200 tumorigenic breast cancer cells or several thousand leukemia-initiating cells to give rise to tumors that could be serially transplanted in NOD/SCID mice. This extensive proliferative potential contrasts with the bulk of the breast cancer cells that lack the ability to form detectable tumors. Not only was the $CD44^+CD24^{-/low}Lineage^-$ population of cells able to give rise to additional tumorigenic $CD44^+CD24^{-/low}Lineage^-$ cells, it was also able to give rise to phenotypically diverse nontumorigenic cells that comprised the bulk of the tumors. Thus both tumorigenic breast cancer cells and leukemia-initiating cells from most tumors appear to exhibit properties of cancer stem cells. However, before these cells can definitively be called *cancer stem cells*, new assays are needed to demonstrate that a single transplanted cell gives rise to all of the diverse populations of cancer cells within a tumor.

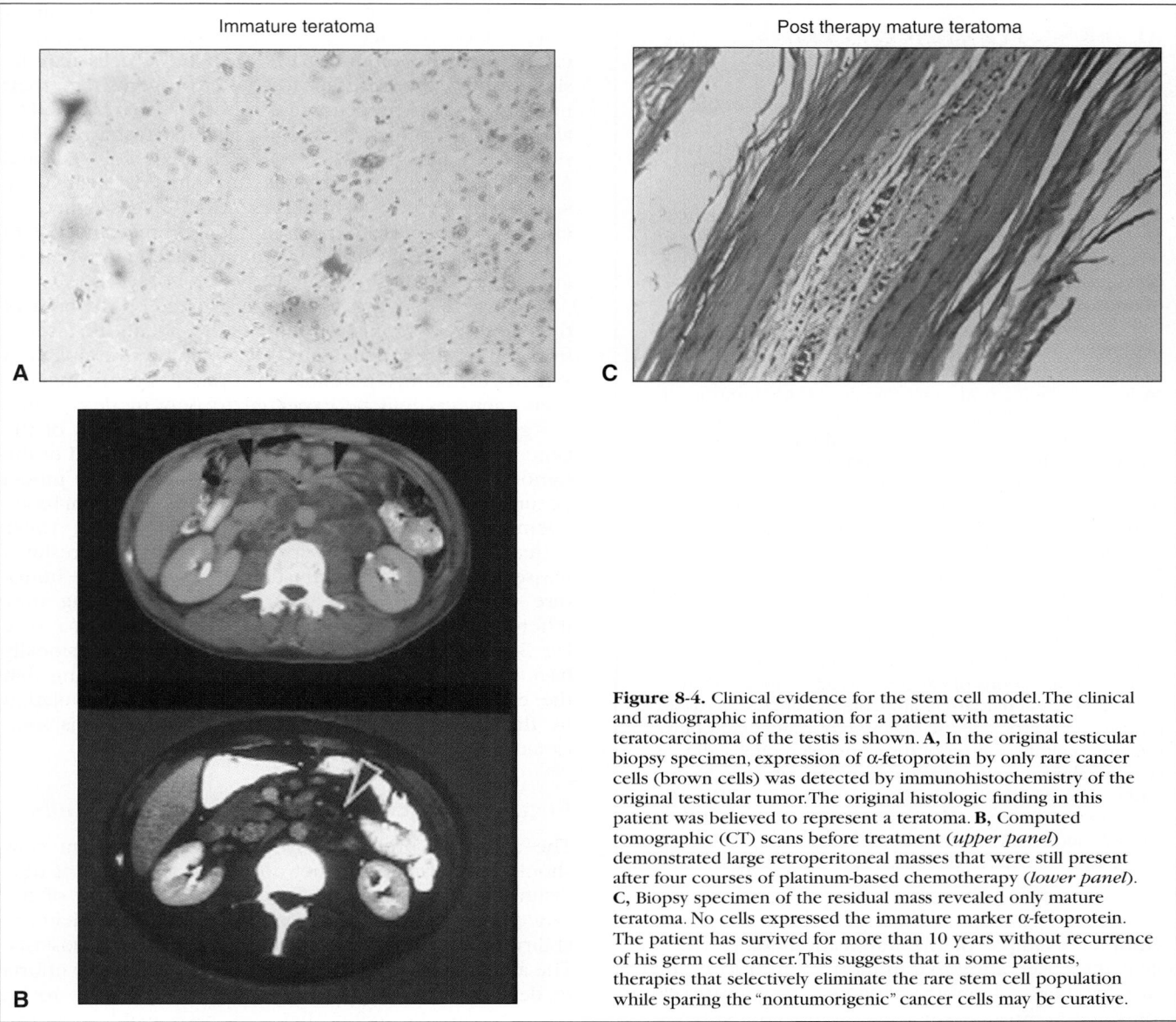

Figure 8-4. Clinical evidence for the stem cell model. The clinical and radiographic information for a patient with metastatic teratocarcinoma of the testis is shown. **A,** In the original testicular biopsy specimen, expression of α-fetoprotein by only rare cancer cells (brown cells) was detected by immunohistochemistry of the original testicular tumor. The original histologic finding in this patient was believed to represent a teratoma. **B,** Computed tomographic (CT) scans before treatment (*upper panel*) demonstrated large retroperitoneal masses that were still present after four courses of platinum-based chemotherapy (*lower panel*). **C,** Biopsy specimen of the residual mass revealed only mature teratoma. No cells expressed the immature marker α-fetoprotein. The patient has survived for more than 10 years without recurrence of his germ cell cancer. This suggests that in some patients, therapies that selectively eliminate the rare stem cell population while sparing the "nontumorigenic" cancer cells may be curative.

Implications of Cancer Stem Cells for the Diagnosis and Treatment of Cancer

Although the immunocompromised mouse model provides compelling evidence in support of the stem cell model of cancer, the ultimate confirmation of the hypothesis requires proof in humans. If the growth of solid cancers is driven by cancer stem cells, this would have profound implications for the diagnosis and treatment of cancer. At present, all of the phenotypically diverse cancer cells are treated as if they possess the ability to form tumors and the ability to metastasize. However, if in most tumors only a small population of cancer cells has the ability to self-renew and other populations of cancer cells have only limited ability to proliferate, then this would explain several conundrums of cancer biology. For example, for many years it has been recognized that disseminated cytokeratin-positive breast cancer cells can be detected in the bone marrow of patients who never experience relapse, even without adjuvant therapy.[120-127] One possibility is that the cancer cells lie dormant until some unknown event triggers them to proliferate. Another explanation is that the cancer cells in the bone marrow in this group of patients arose from the spread of nontumorigenic cancer cells, and only when the cancer stem cells metastasize and subsequently self-renew will frank tumors form. Thus the development of diagnostic reagents that allow cancer stem cells to be identified may have prognostic significance for patients with breast cancer.

ALTERNATIVE CANCER CELL HETEROGENITY MODELS

An alternative explanation for the engraftment of the ability of single, phenotypically unique population of AML cells or breast cancer cells to engraft in NOD/SCID mice is that all cancer cells are tumorigenic in humans but that only the CD34+CD38−Thy1−Lin− AML cells or the CD44+CD24−/lowLineage− breast cancer cells are able to proliferate in mice. However, there are several reasons that this appears unlikely. First, NOD/SCID mice have previously been validated as in vivo models for the growth of normal human HSCs and human neural stem cells.[2,9,115,139-141] Second, tumors passaged in mice contain heterogeneous cancer cells that are phenotypically similar to the cancer cells present in the original tumors from patients, including both tumorigenic and nontumorigenic fractions.[18,19,114,115] This demonstrates that the mouse environment is not incompatible with the survival of the nontumorigenic cell fractions. Third, in the case of breast cancers, both the tumorigenic and nontumorigenic fractions of cancer cells exhibit a similar cell-cycle distribution in mouse tumors, demonstrating that the nontumorigenic cells are able to divide in mice.[18] Thus based on these data and the data obtained for other types of normal and malignant human stem cells, the NOD/SCID mouse model reliably supports the engraftment of clonogenic human progenitors. However, human data are required to completely exclude the possibility that different populations of cancer cells are clonogenic in mice than those that are clonogenic in humans. Because ethical issues preclude the injection of cancer cells into humans, unequivocal proof the stem cell model, will require clinical studies that confirm that therapeutic agents that effectively target cancer stem cells in the immunodeficient mice also eliminate cancer stem cells in patients and result in clinical cures.

Another example of the implications of cancer stem cells is the observation that in most solid cancers such as breast cancers, chemotherapy can frequently shrink tumors, but in most patients, the tumors rapidly recur and there is only a small impact on patient survival.[13,128,129] Most of the cancer therapeutic agents in current use have been developed largely for their ability to shrink a tumor. If only a minority of the cancer cells are tumorigenic and are responsible for driving tumor growth and metastasis, then tumor shrinkage must reflect primarily the elimination of the bulk population of nontumorigenic cells. If a substantial number of tumor stem cells were spared, then the tumors would regenerate from these cells. In support of this model, many patients treated with chemotherapy realize an initial shrinkage of their tumors, but tumors recur in sites of prior disease.

The similarities of the AML tumor-initiating cells and normal HSCs suggest that the AML tumor-initiating cells may be more resistant to chemotherapy than the bulk population of leukemic blasts. Compared with their differentiated progeny, normal HSCs express high levels of genes that make them more resistant to cytotoxic agents including antiapoptotic members of the bcl-2 family, as well as members of the ABC transporters that pump many drugs out of the cell.[29,37,130-133] If the same is true for their cancer stem cell counterparts, then these cells may be significantly more resistant to cytotoxic agents than their nontumorigenic progeny. In support of this possibility, although the chemotherapeutic agent cytosine arabinoside very efficiently killed leukemic blast cells isolated from many patients, the leukemia-initiating cells were selectively spared.[134] This observation suggests that the effect of a particular therapeutic agent on the cancer stem cell population must be taken into account when its curative potential is evaluated.[135]

Because therapeutic agents are selected on the basis of their ability to rapidly shrink tumors, agents that selectively target the cancer stem cells could be overlooked in screens to identify potential therapeutic agents. Initially, such agents would be expected to only modestly slow the growth of a tumor. However, the elimination of the cancer stem cells would eventually halt the spread of the tumor. Perhaps the best clinical evidence of this model occurs in patients with teratocarcinoma. Platinum-based chemotherapy is curative in the majority of these patients[136]; however, many patients are left with residual masses (see Fig. 8-4). After surgical resection, the immature cancer cells have been eliminated, leaving only differentiated cancer cells in a mature teratoma (see Fig. 8-4). Patients with mature teratomas only occasionally have metastases and most are cured, demonstrating that the elimination of the presumed stem cell population by the chemotherapy is sufficient for curing this solid cancer.

Future Implications of Cancer Stem Cells

The ability to prospectively identify cancer stem cells should have a major impact on the development of new diagnostic and therapeutic agents. At present, all of the cancer cells within a tumor are treated as if they had the ability to drive tumor growth, invasion, and metastasis. The ability to identify these crucial cells will allow efforts to develop new diagnostic marker and therapies to be focused on the cells that are responsible for the maintenance of the malignancy—the cancer stem cells. For example, in efforts to identify the genes and proteins expressed by cancer cells, either whole tumors or all of the phenotypically diverse cancer cells within a tumor are presently used. Because the cancer stem cells represent only a minority of the cancer cells in most tumors, it is nearly impossible to identify diagnostic markers or therapies that target these cells. However, directing expression analyses to enriched populations of cancer stem cells should allow the identification of novel diagnostic markers and novel therapeutic targets that can be exploited to more effectively diagnose and treat cancer. This principle is illustrated by the observation that BCR/ABL oncogene mRNA is not expressed by HSCs that carry the mutation in their DNA[97-99]; such an approach may have implications even when oncogenic mutations are targeted.

As illustrated for AML leukemia-initiating cells, the ability to prospectively identify the cancer stem cells

THERAPEUTIC IMPLICATIONS OF THE STEM CELL MODEL

The stem cell model of cancer has major implications for new cancer therapeutics that are directed against new targets, even mutations that contribute to the malignant phenotype. The expression of many genes by normal stem cells and their more differentiated progeny can differ. This includes genes that have been implicated in neoplastic transformation such as BCR/ABL and Flt3-ITD (an internal duplication of the signaling domain of Flt3 [Flk-2] that is found in the AML blasts in some patients), which have been implicated in CML and AML, respectively. Evidence suggests that neither of these genes is expressed by HSCs, but normal, early hematopoietic progenitors express both genes.[31,97-99] The cellular mechanism by which mutations of these genes drive tumor formation would therefore determine the efficacy of therapeutic agents against these targets. As illustrated in Figure 8-5, in the context of a multiple mutation model of cancer, there are four possible ways in which these mutations could be expressed by the leukemogenic (tumorigenic) and nontumorigenic cancer cells. In model A, all of the mutations occur in stem cells, but as a consequence of the other mutations, mRNA and protein are expressed by the leukemic stem cells. Because the leukemic stem cells in model A maintain the sole ability to self-renew, agents that target this pathway would have curative potential. In model B, mutations accumulate in the HSC, but an Flt3-ITD mutation

in a progenitor cell allows the cell to gain the ability to self-renew. Again, because the self-renewing cancer cells would express the Flt3-ITD mRNA and protein, agents that target this pathway would have curative potential. In model C, the mutations accumulate in the stem cells, but as in their normal counterparts, Flt3 mRNA and protein are expressed by progeny, resulting in increased proliferation of the leukemic progenitor cells and consequent tumor formation (i.e., leukemia). However, because the self-renewing leukemic stem cells, which contain but do not express the mutated gene, would be spared, therapies against these targets would result in tumor shrinkage but would not be curative. In model D, the mutations accumulate in the stem cells, and the initial mutation results in the expansion of the stem cell pool. However, the final Flt3 mutation is expressed only by the progenitor cells and confers the ability to self-renew to an early progenitor cell. In this scenario, because there are now two phenotypically distinct populations of cancer cells that can self-renew (the original stem cell and an early progenitor cell), some of the self-renewing cells (the self-renewing progenitor cells) would express the target but others would not (the original stem cells). As in model C, in this scenario, agents that target Flt3 would fail to be curative because they would spare a large number of the cancer stem cells.

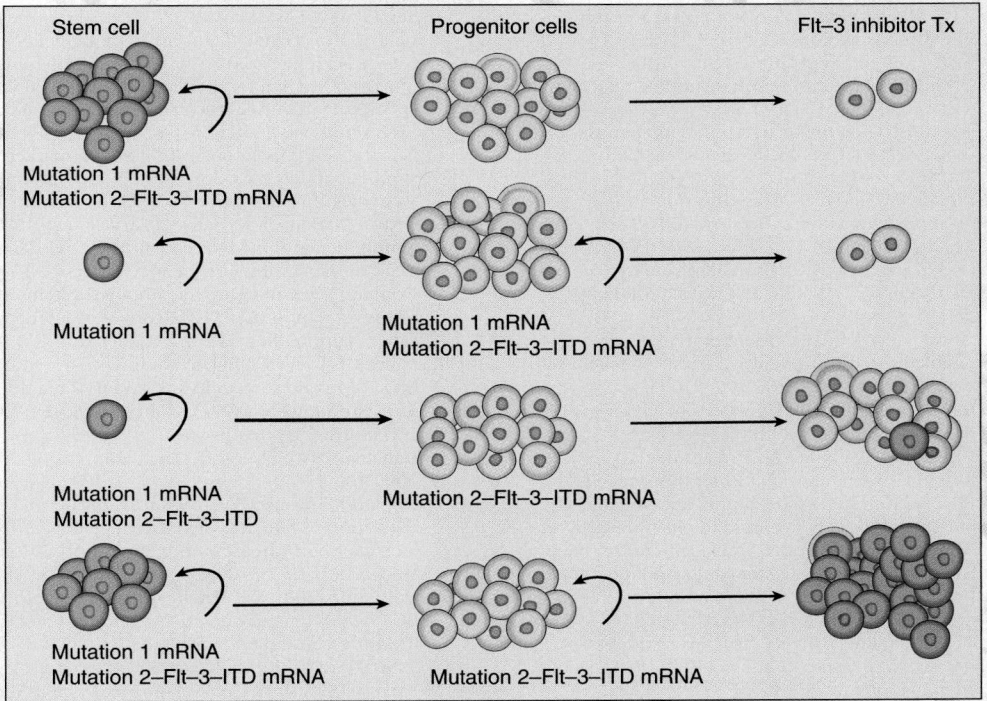

Figure 8-5. Models of expression of oncogenes in cancer cells. In the figure, cancer cells that correspond to developmentally normal stem cells or normal progenitor cells are depicted as red and pink cells, respectively. The presence of a mutation in each cell type is shown for each model. Expression of the mutant gene by each population of cells in the different models is shown. The curved arrows indicate the ability of a population of cells to self-renew.

should also improve the ability to evaluate the curative potential of new therapeutic agents. Although cancer cell lines are useful for the evaluation of particular biologic pathways, they have proven to be somewhat unreliable when used in attempts to predict the clinical efficacy of a particular therapeutic agent in patients.[137,138] Because the tumors that arise in immunodeficient mouse models of human cancer appear to more closely recapitulate the phenotypic diversity of patients' original tumors, including the generation of tumorigenic and nontumorigenic cells, these models might more effectively predict the potential usefulness of a particular drug. New agents could be tested for their ability to eliminate the tumorigenic (cancer stem cell) component of tumors from multiple patients, allowing the agents with the greatest curative potential to proceed to human clinical trials.

REFERENCES

1. Akashi K, Weissman, IL: Developmental biology of hematopoiesis. In Zon LI (ed). New York, Oxford University Press, 2001.
2. Baum CM, Weissman IL, Tsukamoto AS, Buckle AM, Peault B: Isolation of a candidate human hematopoietic stem-cell population. Proc Natl Acad Sci USA 1992;89:2804-2808.
3. Morrison S, Hemmati H, Wandycz A, Weissman I: The purification and characterization of fetal liver hematopoietic stem cells. Proc Natl Acad Sci USA 1995;92:10302-10306.
4. Morrison S, Prowse K, Ho P, Weissman I: Telomerase activity in hematopoietic cells is associated with self-renewal potential. Immunity 1996;5:207-216.
5. Morrison SJ, Uchida N, Weissman IL: The biology of hematopoietic stem cells. Annu Rev Cell Dev Biol 1995;11:35-71.
6. Morrison SJ, Wandycz AM, Hemmati HD, Wright DE, Weissman IL: Identification of a lineage of multipotent hematopoietic progenitors. Development 1997;124:1929-1939.
7. Morrison SJ, Weissman IL: The long-term repopulating subset of hematopoietic stem cells is deterministic and isolatable by phenotype. Immunity 1994;1: 661-673.
8. Spangrude GJ, Heimfeld S, Weissman IL: Purification and characterization of mouse hematopoietic stem cells. Science 1988;241:58-62.
9. Uchida N, Buck DW, He D, et al: Direct isolation of human central nervous system stem cells. Proc Natl Acad Sci USA 2000;97: 14720-14725.
10. Morrison S, Perez SE, Qiao Z, et al: Transient Notch activation initiates an irreversible switch from neurogenesis to gliogenesis by neural crest stem cells. Cell 2000;101:499-510.
11. Morrison SJ, Shah NM, Anderson DJ: Regulatory mechanisms in stem cell biology. Cell 1997;88:287-298.
12. Baum C, Uchida N, Peault B, Weissman IL: Isolation and characterization of hematopoietic progenitor and stem cells. In Forman SJ, Blume KG, Thomas E D (eds): Bone Marrow Transplantation. Boston, Blackwell Scientific Publications, 1994.
13. Negrin RS, Atkinson K, Leemhuis T, et al: Transplantation of highly purified CD34+Thy-1+ hematopoietic stem cells in patients with metastatic breast cancer. Biol Blood Marrow Transplant 2000;6: 262-271.
14. Voena C, Locatelli G, Castellino C, et al: Qualitative and quantitative polymerase chain reaction detection of the residual myeloma cell contamination after positive selection of CD34+ cells with small- and large-scale Miltenyi cell sorting system. Br J Haematol 2002;117:642-645.
15. Michallet M, Philip T, Philip I, et al: Transplantation with selected autologous peripheral blood CD34+Thy1+ hematopoietic stem cells (HSCs) in multiple myeloma: Impact of HSC dose on engraftment, safety, and immune reconstitution. Exp Hematol 2000;28:858-870.
16. Tricot G, Gazitt Y, Leemhuis T, et al: Collection, tumor contamination, and engraftment kinetics of highly purified hematopoietic progenitor cells to support high dose therapy in multiple myeloma. Blood 1998;91:4489-4495.
17. Barbui A, Galli M, Dotti G, et al: Negative selection of peripheral blood stem cells to support a tandem autologous transplantation programme in multiple myeloma. Br J Haematol 2002;116: 202-210.
18. Al-Hajj M, Wicha M, Morrison SJ, Clarke MF: Prospective identification of breast cancer cells. Proc Natl Acad Sci USA 2003;100:3983-3988.
19. Al-Hajj M, Wicha M, Morrison SJ, Clarke MF: Prospective identification of breast cancer cells. Proc Natl Acad Sci USA 2002.
20. Park CH, Bergsagel DE, McCulloch EA: Mouse myeloma tumor stem cells: A primary cell culture assay. J Natl Cancer Inst 1971;46:411-422.
21. Bruce WR, Gaag H: A quantitative assay for the number of murine lymphoma cells capable of proliferation in vivo. Nature 1963;199:79-80.
22. Wodinsky I, Swiniarski J, Kensler CJ: Spleen colony studies of leukemia L1210.I. Growth kinetics of lymphocytic L1210 cells in vivo as determined by spleen colony assay. Cancer Chemother Rep 1967;51:415-421.
23. Bergsagel DE, Valeriote FA: Growth characteristics of a mouse plasma cell tumor. Cancer Res 1968;28:2187-2196.
24. Southam C, Brunschwig A: Quantitative studies of autotransplantation of human cancer. Cancer 1961;14:971-978.
25. Hamburger AW, Salmon SE: Primary bioassay of human tumor stem cells. Science 1977;197:461-463.
26. Reya T, Morrison SJ, Clarke MF, Weissman IL: Stem cells, cancer, and cancer stem cells. Nature 2001;414:105-111.
27. Lagasse E, Weissman IL: bcl-2 inhibits apoptosis of neutrophils but not their engulfment by macrophages. J Exp Med 1994;179: 1047-1052.
28. Weissman IL: Translating stem and progenitor cell biology to the clinic: Barriers and opportunities. Science 2000;287:1442-1446.
29. Terskikh AV, Easterday MC, Li L, et al: From hematopoiesis to neuropoiesis: Evidence of overlapping genetic programs. Proc Natl Acad Sci USA 2001;98:7934-7939.
30. Morrison SJ, Qian D, Jerebek L, et al: A genetic determinant that specifically regulates the frequency of hematopoietic stem cells. J Immunol 2002;168:635-642.
31. Christensen JL, Weissman IL: Flk-2 is a marker in hematopoietic stem cell differentiation: A simple method to isolate long-term stem cells. Proc Natl Acad Sci USA 2001;98:14541-14546.
32. Osawa M, Hanada K, Hamada H, Nakauchi H. Long-term lymphohematopoietic reconstitution by a single CD34-low/negative hematopoietic stem cell. Science 1996;273:242-245.
33. Domen J, Weissman IL: Hematopoietic stem cells need two signals to prevent apoptosis; BCL-2 can provide one of these, Kitl/c-Kit signaling the other. J Exp Med 2000;192:1707-1718.
34. Miller CL, Eaves CJ: Expansion in vitro of adult murine hematopoietic stem cells with transplantable lympho-myeloid reconstituting ability. Proc Natl Acad Sci USA 1997;94: 13648-13653.
35. Hanahan D, Weinberg RA: The hallmarks of cancer. Cell 2000;100:57-70.
36. Domen J, Cheshier SH, Weissman IL: The role of apoptosis in the regulation of hematopoietic stem cells: Overexpression of BCL-2 increases both their number and repopulation potential. J Exp Med 2000;191:253-264.
37. Domen J, Gandy KL, Weissman IL: Systemic overexpression of BCL-2 in the hematopoietic system protects transgenic mice from the consequences of lethal irradiation. Blood 1998;91:2272-2282.
38. Traver D, Akashi K, Weissman IL, Lagasse E: Mice defective in two apoptosis pathways in the myeloid lineage develop acute myeloblastic leukemia. Immunity 1998;9:47-57.
39. Mucenski ML, McLain K, Kier AB, et al: A functional c-myb gene is required for normal murine fetal hepatic hematopoiesis. Cell 1991;65:677-689.
40. Clarke MF, Kukowska-Latallo JF, Westin E, Smith M, Prochownik EV: Constitutive expression of a c-myb cDNA blocks Friend murine

erythroleukemia cell differentiation. Mol Cell Biol 1988;8: 884–892.

41. Danish R, el-Awar O, Weber BL, et al: c-myb effects on kinetic events during MEL cell differentiation. Oncogene 1992;7: 901–907.

42. Prochowinik E, Kukowska J: Deregulated expression of c-myc by murine erythroleukaemia cells prevents differentiation. Nature 1986;322:848–850.

43. Phillips RL, Reinhart AJ, Van Zant G: Genetic control of murine hematopoietic stem cell pool sizes and cycling kinetics. Proc Natl Acad Sci USA 1992;89:11607–11611.

44. Muller-Sieburg CE, Cho RH, Sieburg HB, Kupriyanov S, Riblet R: Genetic control of hematopoietic stem cell frequency in mice is mostly cell autonomous. Blood 2000;95:2446–2448.

45. Taipale J, Beachy PA: The Hedgehog and Wnt signalling pathways in cancer. Nature 2001;411:349–354.

46. Bhardwaj G, Murdoch B, Wu D, et al: Sonic hedgehog induces the proliferation of primitive human hematopoietic cells via BMP regulation. Nat Immunol 2001;2:172–180.

47. Shivdasani R, Mayer E, Orkin S: Absence of blood formation in mice lacking the T-cell leukaemia oncoprotein tal-1/SCL. Nature 1995;373:432–434.

48. Porcher C, Swat W, Rockwell K, Fujiwara Y, Alt F, Orkin SH: The T cell leukemia oncoprotein SCL/tal-1 is essential for development of all hematopoietic lineages. Cell 1996;86:47–57.

49. Buske C, Feuring-Buske M, Abramovich C, et al: Deregulated expression of HOXB4 enhances the primitive growth activity of human hematopoietic cells. Blood 2002;100:862–868.

50. Antonchuk JSG, Humphries RK: HOXB4-induced expansion of adult hematopoietic stem cells ex vivo. Cell 2002;109:39–45.

51. Cheng T, Rodrigues N, Shen H, et al: Hematopoietic stem cell quiescence maintained by p21cip1/waf1. Science 2000;287: 1804–1808.

52. van Lohuizen M, Frasch M, Wientjens E, Berns A: Sequence similarity between the mammalian bmi-1 proto-oncogene and the *Drosophila* regulatory genes Psc and Su(z)2. Nature 1991;353: 353–355.

53. van der Lugt NM, Domen J, Linders K, et al: Posterior transformation, neurological abnormalities, and severe hematopoietic defects in mice with a targeted deletion of the bmi-1 proto-oncogene. Genes Dev 1994;8:757–769.

54. Park IK, Qian D, Kiel M, et al: Bmi-1 is required for the maintenance of self-renewing adult hematopoietic stem cells. Nature 2003;423:302–305.

55. Lessard J, Sauvageau G: Bmi-1 determines the proliferative capacity of normal and leukaemic stem cells. Nature 2003;423:255–260.

56. Artavanis-Tsakonas S, Rand MD, Lake RJ: Notch signaling: cell fate control and signal integration in development. Science 1999;284: 770–776.

57. Berry L, Westlund B, Schedl T: Germ-line tumor formation caused by activation of glp-1, a *Caenorhabditis elegans* member of the Notch family of receptors. Development 1997;124:925–936.

58. Shelly LL, Fuchs C, Miele L: Notch-1 inhibits apoptosis in murine erythroleukemia cells and is necessary for differentiation induced by hybrid polar compounds. J Cell Biochem 1999;73:164–175.

59. Varnum-Finney B, Xu L, Brashem-Stein C, et al: Pluripotent, cytokine-dependent, hematopoietic stem cells are immortalized by constitutive Notch1 signaling. Nat Med 2000;6: 1278–1281.

60. Gallahan D, Callahan R: The mouse mammary tumor associated gene INT3 is a unique member of the NOTCH gene family (NOTCH4). Oncogene 1997;14:1883–1890.

61. Zagouras P, Stifani S, Blaumueller C, Carcangiu M, Artavanis-Tsakonas S: Alterations in Notch signaling in neoplastic lesions of the human cervix. Proc Natl Acad Sci USA 1995;92: 6414–6418.

62. Leethanakul C, Patel V, Gillespie J, et al: Distinct pattern of expression of differentiation and growth-related genes in squamous cell carcinomas of the head and neck revealed by the use of laser capture microdissection and cDNA arrays. Oncogene 2000;19:3220–3224.

63. Liu Y, Dehni G, Purcell KJ, et al: Epithelial expression and chromosomal location of human TLE genes: Implications for notch signaling and neoplasia. Genomics 1996;31:58–64.

64. Capobianco AJ, Zagouras P, Blaumueller CM, Artavanis-Tsakonas S, Bishop JM: Neoplastic transformation by truncated alleles of human NOTCH1/TAN1 and NOTCH2. Mol Cell Biol 1997;17: 6265–6273.

65. Ellisen LW, Bird J, West DC, et al: TAN-1, the human homolog of the *Drosophila* notch gene, is broken by chromosomal translocations in T lymphoblastic neoplasms. Cell 1991;66: 649–661.

66. Imatani A, Callahan R: Identification of a novel NOTCH-4/INT-3 RNA species encoding an activated gene product in certain human tumor cell lines. Oncogene 2000;19:223–231.

67. Jehn BM, Bielke W, Pear WS, Osborne BA: Cutting edge: Protective effects of notch-1 on TCR-induced apoptosis. J Immunol 1999; 162:635–638.

68. Weizen S, Rizzo P, Braid M, et al: Activation of Notch-1 signaling maintains the neoplastic phenotype in human Ras-transformed cells. Nat Med 2002;8:979–986.

69. Cadigan KM, Nusse R: Wnt signaling: A common theme in animal development. Genes Dev 1997;11:3286–3305.

70. Spink KE, Polakis P, Weis WI: Structural basis of the Axin-adenomatous polyposis coli interaction. EMBO J 2000;19: 2270–2279.

71. Austin TW, Solar GP, Ziegler FC, Liem L, Matthews W: A role for the Wnt gene family in hematopoiesis: Expansion of multilineage progenitor cells. Blood 1997;89:3624–3635.

72. Tsukamoto AS, Grosschedl R, Guzman RC, Parslow T, Varmus HE: Expression of the int-1 gene in transgenic mice is associated with mammary gland hyperplasia and adenocarcinomas in male and female mice. Cell 1988;55:619–625.

73. Nusse R, Brown A, Papkoff J, et al: A new nomenclature for int-1 and related genes: The Wnt gene family. Cell 1991;64:231.

74. Reya T, O'Riordan M, Okamura R, et al: Wnt signaling regulates B lymphocyte proliferation through a LEF-1 dependent mechanism. Immunity 2000;13:15–24.

75. Wu C, Zeng Q, Blumer KJ, Muslin AJ: RGS proteins inhibit Xwnt-8 signaling in Xenopus embryonic development. Development 2000;127:2773–2784.

76. Van Den Berg DJ, Sharma AK, Bruno E, Hoffman R: Role of members of the Wnt gene family in human hematopoiesis. Blood 1998;92:3189–3202.

77. Gat U, DasGupta R, Degenstein L, Fuchs E: De novo hair follicle morphogenesis and hair tumors in mice expressing a truncated beta-catenin in skin. Cell 1998;95:605–614.

78. Chan EF, Gat U, McNiff JM, Fuchs E: A common human skin tumour is caused by activating mutations in beta-catenin. Nat Genet 1999;21:410–413.

79. Hedgepeth CM, Deardorff MA, Rankin K, Klein PS: Regulation of glycogen synthase kinase 3beta and downstream Wnt signaling by Axin. Mol Cell Biol 1999;19:7147–7157.

80. Korinek V, Barker N, Moerer P, et al: Depletion of epithelial stem-cell compartments in the small intestine of mice lacking Tcf-4. Nat Genet 1998;19:379–383.

81. Zhu AJ, Watt FM: Beta-catenin signalling modulates proliferative potential of human epidermal keratinocytes independently of intercellular adhesion. Development 1999;126:2285–2298.

82. Nusse R: The Wnt gene family in tumorigenesis and in normal development. J Steroid Biochem Mol Biol 1992;43:9–12.

83. Weeraratna AT, Jiang Y, Hostetter G, et al: Wnt5 signaling directly affects cell motility and invasion of metastatic melanoma. Cancer Cell 2002;1:279–288.

84. Saitoh T, Mine T, Katoh M: Up-regulation of WNT8B mRNA in human gastric cancer. Int J Oncol 2002;20:343–348.

85. Saitoh T, Mine T, Katoh M: Frequent up-regulation of WNT5A mRNA in primary gastric cancer. Int J Mol Med 2002;9:515–519.

86. Kirikoshi H, Inoue S, Sekihara H, Katoh M: Expression of WNT10A in human cancer. Int J Oncol 2001;19:997–1001.

87. van de Wetering M, Sancho E, Verweij C, et al: The beta-catenin/TCF-4 complex imposes a crypt progenitor phenotype on colorectal cancer cells. Cell 2002;111:241–250.

88. Knudson AG Jr, Strong LC, Anderson DE: Heredity and cancer in man. Prog Med Genet 1973;9:113–158.

89. Fearon ER, Vogelstein B: A genetic model for colorectal tumorigenesis. Cell 1990;61:759-767.

90. Uchida N, Weissman IL: Searching for hematopoietic stem cells: Evidence that Thy-1.1lo Lin- Sca-1+ cells are the only stem cells in C57bL/Ka-Thy1.1 bone marrow. J Exp Med 1992;175:175-184.

91. Kondo M, Weissman I, Akashi K: Identification of clonogenic common lymphoid progenitors in mouse bone marrow. Cell 1997;91:661-672.

92. Park IK, Qian D, Kiel M, et al: Bmi-1 is required for the maintenance of self-renewing adult hematopoietic stem cells. Nature 2002;423:302-305.

93. Wechsler-Reya R, Scott MP: The developmental biology of brain tumors. Annu Rev Neurosci 2001;24:385-428.

94. Kowenz-Leutz E, Twamley G, Ansieau S, Leutz A: Novel mechanism of C/EBP beta (NF-M) transcriptional control: Activation through derepression. Genes Dev 1994;8:2781-2791.

95. Rhoades KL, Hetherington CJ, Harakawa M, et al: Analysis of the role of AML1-ETO in leukemogenesis, using an inducible transgene mouse model. Blood 2000;96:2108-2115.

96. Miyamoto T, Weissman IL, Akashi K: AML1/ETO-expressing nonleukemic stem cells in acute myelogenous leukemia with 8;21 chromosomal translocation. Proc Natl Acad Sci USA 2000;97:7521-7526.

97. Negrin RS, Weissman IL: Hematopoietic stem cells in normal and malignant states. Bone Marrow Transplantation 1992;2:23-26.

98. Bedi A, Zehnbauer BA, Collector MI, et al: BCR-ABL gene rearrangement and expression of primitive hematopoietic progenitors in chronic myeloid leukemia. Blood 1993;81:2898-2902.

99. Jaiswal S, Traver D, Miyamoto T, Akashi K, Lagasse E, Weissman IL: Expression of BCR/ABL and BCL-2 in myeloid progenitors leads to myeloid leukemias. Proc Natl Acad Sci USA 2003;100:1000-10007.

100. Bachoo RM, Maher EA, Ligon KL, et al: Epidermal growth factor receptor and Ink4a/Arf: Convergent mechanisms governing terminal differentiation and transformation along the neural stem cell to astrocyte axis. Cancer Cell 2002;1:269-277.

101. Platt FM, Cebra-Thomas JA, Baum CM, Davie JM, McKearn JP: Monoclonal antibodies specific for novel murine cell surface markers define subpopulations of germinal center cells. Cell Immunol 1992;143:449-466.

102. Kyoizumi S, Baum CM, Kaneshima H, et al: Implantation and maintenance of functional human bone marrow in SCID-hu mice. Blood 1992;79:1704-1711.

103. Ozols RF, et al: Inhibition of human ovarian cancer colony formation by Adriamycin and its major metabolites. Cancer Res 1980;40:4109-4112.

104. Heppner GH: Tumor heterogeneity. Cancer Res 1984;44:2259-2265.

105. Nowell PC: Mechanisms of tumor progression. Cancer Res 1986;46:2203-2207.

106. Weisenthal L, Lippman ME: Clonogenic and nonclonogenic in vitro chemosensitivity assays. Cancer Treatment Reports 1985;69:615-632.

107. Aubele M, Werner M: Heterogeneity in breast cancer and the problem of relevance of findings. Anal Cell Pathol 1999;19:53-58.

108. Golub TR: Genome-wide views of cancer. N Engl J Med 2001;344:601-602.

109. Fidler IJ, Kripke ML: Metastasis results from preexisting variant cells within a malignant tumor. Science 1977;197:893-895.

110. Fidler IJ, Hart IR: Biological diversity in metastatic neoplasms: Origins and implications. Science 1982;217:998-1003.

111. Salsbury AJ: The significance of the circulating cancer cell. Cancer Treat Rev 1975;2:55-72.

112. Henrique D, Hirsinger E, Adam J, et al: Maintenance of neuroepithelial progenitor cells by Delta-Notch signalling in the embryonic chick retina. Curr Biol 1997;7:661-670.

113. Bonnet D, Dick J: Human acute myeloid leukemia is organized as a hierarchy that originates from a primitive hematopoietic cell. Nat Med 1997;3:730-737.

114. Lapidot T, Sirard C, Vormoor J, et al: A cell initiating human acute myeloid leukaemia after transplantation into SCID mice. Nature 1994;17:645-648.

115. Bhatia M, Wang JC, Kapp U, Bonnet D, Dick JE: Purification of primitive human hematopoietic cells capable of repopulating immune-deficient mice. Proc Natl Acad Sci USA 1997;94:5320-5325.

116. George AA, Franklin J, Kerkof K, et al: Detection of leukemic cells in the CD34(+)CD38(-) bone marrow progenitor population in children with acute lymphoblastic leukemia. Blood 2001;97:3925-3930.

117. Liu A, True LD, Tracy L, et al: Cell-cell interaction in prostate gene regulation and cytodifferentiation. Proc Natl Acad Sci USA 1997;94:10705-10710.

118. Stingl J, Eaves C, Kuusk U, Emerman J: Phenotypic and functional characterization in vitro of a multipotent epithelial cell present in the normal adult human breast. Differentiation 1998;63:201-213.

119. Gudjonsson T, Villadsen R, Bissell M, et al: Isolation, immortalization, and characterization of a human breast epithelial cell line with stem cell properties. Genes Dev 2002;16:693-706.

120. Manegold C, Krempien B, Kaufmann M, Schwechheimer K, Schettler G: The value of bone marrow examination for tumor staging in breast cancer. J Cancer Res Clin Oncol 1988;114:425-428.

121. Stadtmauer EA, Tsai DE, Sickles CJ, et al: Stem cell transplantation for metastatic breast cancer: Analysis of tumor contamination. Med Oncol 1999;16:279-288.

122. Datta YH, Adams PT, Drobyski WR, et al: Sensitive detection of occult breast cancer by the reverse-transcriptase polymerase chain reaction. J Clin Oncol 1994;12:475-482.

123. Braun S, Pantel K: Prognostic significance of micrometastatic bone marrow involvement. Breast Cancer Res Treat 1998;52:201-216.

124. Janni W, Gastroph S, Hepp F, et al: Prognostic significance of an increased number of micrometastatic tumor cells in the bone marrow of patients with first recurrence of breast carcinoma. Cancer 2000;88:2252-2259.

125. Braun S, Pantel K: Micrometastatic bone marrow involvement: Detection and prognostic significance. Med Oncol 1999;16:154-165.

126. DiStefano A, Tashima CK, Yap HY, Hortobagyi GN: Bone marrow metastases without cortical bone involvement in breast cancer patients. Cancer 1979;44:196-198.

127. Ingle JN, Tormey DC, Bull JM, Simon RM: Bone marrow involvement in breast cancer: Effect on response and tolerance to combination chemotherapy. Cancer 1977;39:104-111.

128. Schultz LB, Weber BL: Recent advances in breast cancer biology. Curr Opin Oncol 1999;11:429-434.

129. Lippman ME: High-dose chemotherapy plus autologous bone marrow transplantation for metastatic breast cancer. N Engl J Med 2000;342:1119-1120.

130. Harrison DE, Lerner CP: Most primitive hematopoietic stem cells are stimulated to cycle rapidly after treatment with 5-fluorouracil. Blood 1991;78:1237-1240.

131. Peters R, Leyvraz S, Perey L: Apoptotic regulation in primitive hematopoietic precursors. Blood 1998;92:2041-2052.

132. Feuerhake F, Sigg W, Hofter EA, Dimpfl T, Welsch U: Immunohistochemical analysis of Bcl-2 and Bax expression in relation to cell turnover and epithelial differentiation markers in the non-lactating human mammary gland epithelium. Cell Tissue Res 2000;299:47-58.

133. Zhou S, Schuetz JD, Bunting KD, et al: The ABC transporter Bcrp1/ABCG2 is expressed in a wide variety of stem cells and is a molecular determinant of the side-population phenotype. Nat Med 2001;7:1028-1034.

134. Guzman ML, Neering S, Upchurch D, et al: Nuclear factor-kappaB is constitutively activated in primitive human acute myelogenous leukemia cells. Blood 2001;98:2301-2307.

135. Guzman ML, Swiderski CF, Howard DS, et al: Preferential induction of apoptosis for primary human leukemic stem cells. Proc Natl Acad Sci USA 2002;99:16220-16225.

136. Williams SD, Birch R, Einhorn LH, Irwin L, Greco FA, Loeher PJ: Treatment of disseminated germ-cell tumors with cisplatin, bleomycin, and either vinblastine or etoposide. N Engl J Med 1987;316:1435-1440.

137. Hoffman RM: Orthotopic metastatic mouse models for anticancer

drug discovery and evaluation: A bridge to the clinic. Invest New Drugs 1999;17:343–359.

138. Brown JM: NCI's anticancer drug screening program may not be selecting for clinically active compounds. Oncol Res 1997;9:213–215.

139. Bhatia M, Bonnet D, Murdoch B, Gan OI, Dick JE: A newly discovered class of human hematopoietic cells with SCID-repopulating activity. Nat Med 1998;4:1038–1045.

140. Larochelle A, Vormoor J, Hanenberg H, et al: Identification of primitive human hematopoietic cells capable of repopulating NOD/SCID mouse bone marrow: Implications for gene therapy. Nat Med 1996;2:1329–1337.

141. Rosu-Myles M, Gallacher L, Murdoch B, et al: The human hematopoietic stem cell compartment is heterogeneous for CXCR4 expression. Proc Natl Acad Sci USA 2000;97:14626–14631.

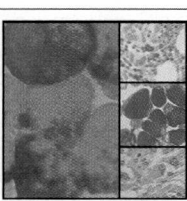

VASCULAR AND INTERSTITIAL BIOLOGY OF TUMORS

Rakesh K. Jain

SUMMARY OF KEY POINTS

- A solid tumor is an organ composed of neoplastic cells and host stromal cells nourished by the vasculature made of endothelial cells—all embedded in an extracellular matrix. The interactions among these cells and between these cells, their surrounding matrix, and their local microenvironment, control the expression of various genes. The products encoded by these genes, in turn, control the pathophysiologic characteristics of the tumor. The tumor pathophysiology governs not only tumor growth, invasion, and metastasis but also the response to various therapies.
- Tumor vasculature is made of host vessels co-opted by tumor cells and by new vessels formed by the

- processes of vasculogenesis and angiogenesis. A constellation of positive and negative regulators of angiogenesis governs the process of neovascularization.
- Tumor vessels are abnormal in terms of their organization, structure, and function. These abnormalities contribute to heterogeneous vascular permeability, blood flow, and microenvironment.
- Tumor interstitial matrix is formed by proteins secreted by host and tumor cells and by those leaked from the nascent blood vessels.
- Tumor interstitium is heterogeneous, with some regions fairly permeable and others difficult to penetrate.
- Interstitial hypertension is a hallmark of solid tumors and results

- from vessel leakiness, lack of functional lymphatics, and compression of vessels by proliferating cancer cells.
- Cancer therapy is plagued by two major problems: physiological resistance to drug delivery and oxygen and drug resistance driven by genetic and epigenetic mechanisms. Anti-angiogenic therapy has the potential to overcome these problems. Furthermore, judicious application of this therapy can normalize the tumor vessels and make them more efficient for delivery of oxygen and drugs. Combined anti-angiogenic and conventional therapies appear promising in the clinic.

INTRODUCTION

A solid tumor is an organ comprised of neoplastic cells and host stromal cells nourished by the vasculature made of endothelial cells—all embedded in an extracellular matrix (Fig. 9-1). The interactions among these cells and between these cells, their surrounding matrix, and their local microenvironment, control the expression of various genes. The products encoded by these genes, in turn, control the pathophysiologic characteristics of the tumor. The tumor pathophysiology governs not only the tumor growth, invasion, and metastasis but also the response to various therapies. In this chapter, we will discuss various pathophysiological parameters that characterize the vascular and extravascular compartments of a tumor and the mechanisms governing the formation and function of these compartments.

VASCULAR COMPARTMENT

Neoplastic cells, like normal cells, need oxygen and other nutrients for their survival and growth. Every normal cell in our body is located within 100–200 μm from a blood capillary so that it can receive oxygen and other nutrients by the process of diffusion. Likewise, cells undergoing

neoplastic transformation depend on nearby capillaries for growth. These preneoplastic (i.e., hyperplastic or dysplastic) cells can grow as a spherical or ellipsoidal cellular aggregate. Once the size of the cellular aggregate reaches the diffusion limit for critical nutrients and oxygen, however, the aggregate as a whole can become dormant. Indeed, human tumors can remain dormant for a number of years due to a balance between proliferation and apoptosis. Once they have access to new blood vessels formed by angiogenesis, however, they may grow and metastasize. What triggers the growth of new vessels? What molecular and cellular mechanisms are involved? How do these vessels compare with normal vessels with respect to structure and function?

Angiogenesis

The fact that the vascular system is associated with tumor growth in animals and humans has been known for nearly a century.[1] Powerful insights into the neovascularization of transplanted tumors using the transparent window techniques were developed in the 1940s.[2-6] The possibility that tumors produce an "angiogenic" substance was suggested in 1968.[7,8] The hypothesis that blocking angiogenesis should block tumor growth and metastasis was proposed shortly thereafter in 1971.[9] The concept that a tissue acquires angiogenic capacity during

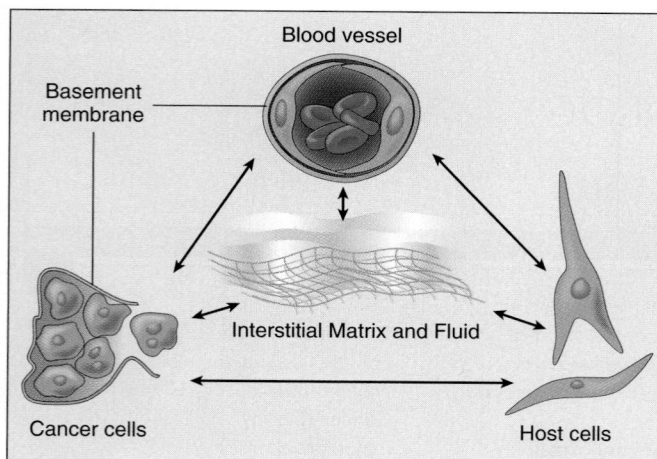

Figure 9-1. Schematic representation of a solid tumor. The key components include cancer cells, host cells, and vasculature made of endothelial cells—all embedded in a matrix bathed in interstitial fluid. Arrows indicate interactions between the components. (Adapted from Jain RK: Angiogenesis and lymphangiogenesis in tumor: Insights from intravital microscopy. In Stillman B [ed]: Cold Spring Harbor Symposium on Quantitative Biology [The Cardiovascular System], 2002, pp 239–248.)

neoplastic transformation—and, by extension, that anti-angiogenesis could be used to prevent cancer—was put forward in 1976.[10] At present, various anti- and pro-angiogenesis strategies are being evaluated clinically to prevent or treat a large number of diseases, including cancer.[11,12]

Both normal and pathological angiogenic processes are governed by the net balance between pro- and anti-angiogenic factors.[13,14] This balance is spatially and temporally regulated under physiological conditions, so that the "angiogenic switch" is "on" when needed (e.g., during embryonic development, wound healing, forma-

tion of the corpus luteum) and "off" otherwise. During neoplastic transformation and tumor progression, this regulation is deranged, and blood vessels form ectopically to support a growing tumor mass.

Cellular Mechanisms

At least four cellular mechanisms are involved in the vascularization of tumors: co-option, intussusception, sprouting (angiogenesis), and vasculogenesis (Fig. 9-2). Tumor cells can co-opt and grow around existing vessels to form "perivascular" cuffs. However, as stated earlier, these cuffs can not grow beyond the diffusion limit of critical nutrients, and may actually cause the collapse of the vessels due to the growth pressure (referred to as "solid stress"). Alternatively, an existing vessel may enlarge in response to the growth factors released by tumors, and an interstitial tissue column may grow in the enlarged lumen and partition the lumen to form an expanded vascular network. This mode of intussusceptive microvascular growth has been observed during tumor growth, wound healing and gene therapy.[15-18]

"Sprouting" angiogenesis is perhaps the most widely studied mechanism of vessel formation. During sprouting angiogenesis, the existing vessels become leaky in response to growth factors released by normal cells or cancer cells; the basement membrane and the interstitial matrix dissolve; pericytes dissociate from the vessel; endothelial cells (EC) migrate and proliferate to form an array/sprout; a lumen is formed in the sprout (a process referred to as *canalization*); branches and loops are formed by confluence and anastomoses of sprouts to permit blood flow; and finally, these immature vessels are invested in basement membrane and pericytes. During physiological angiogenesis, these vessels differentiate into mature arterioles, capillaries, and venules, whereas in tumors they might remain immature.[4,12,19,20]

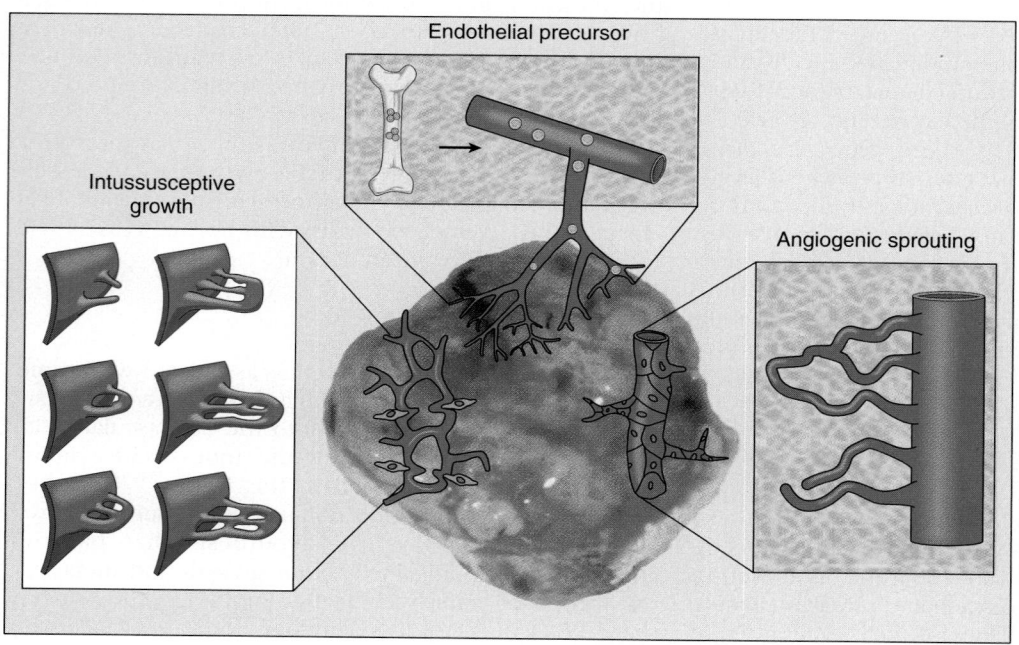

Figure 9-2. Cellular mechanisms of vascularization in tumors. At least four mechanisms are involved: (1) intussusception—tumor vessels enlarge and an interstitial tissue column grows in the enlarged lumen, expanding the network; (2) vasculogenesis—endothelial precursor cells mobilized from the bone marrow or peripheral blood contribute to the endothelial lining of tumor vessels; (3) "sprouting" angiogenesis—the existing vascular network expands by forming sprouts or bridges; and (4) co-option (not shown)—tumor cells grow around existing vessels to form "perivascular" cuffs. (Adapted from Jain RK, Carmeliet PF: Angiogenesis in cancer and other diseases. Nature 2000;407:249–257.)

During embryonic development, a primitive vascular plexus is formed from endothelial precursor cells (EPC, also known as hemangioblasts) by a process referred to as vasculogenesis. Circulating EPCs mobilized from the bone marrow or peripheral blood also can contribute to postnatal vasculogenesis in tumors and other tissues.[21,22] The current challenge is to discern the relative contribution of each of the four mechanisms of neo-angiogenesis to the formation of tumors to optimize anti-angiogenic treatment of cancer.[23]

Molecular Mechanisms

Various pro- and anti-angiogenic molecules that orchestrate different steps in vessel formation, along with their functions, are listed in Table 9-1. Vascular endothelial growth factor (VEGF) is perhaps the most critical pro-angiogenic molecule. Originally discovered in 1983 as the vascular permeability factor (VPF) and cloned in 1989, VEGF increases vascular permeability, promotes migration and proliferation of ECs, serves as an EC survival factor, and is known to upregulate leukocyte adhesion molecules on ECs.[18,24-26] During tumor progression, the number of distinct angiogenic molecules produced by a tumor can increase.[27,28] Thus, after VEGF signaling is blocked, a tumor might rely on other, alternative angiogenic molecules (e.g., basic fibroblast growth factor [bFGF], interleukin-8 [IL-8]). Other positive regulators of angiogenesis include the angiopoietins that are involved in stabilizing vessels and controlling vascular permeability; various proteases involved in dissolving/remodeling matrix and releasing growth factors; and recently discovered organ-specific angiogenic stimulators (e.g., endocrine gland VEGF).[20,29,30]

Angiogenesis inhibitors include soluble receptors of various pro-angiogenic ligands and molecules that downregulate the expression of stimulators (e.g., interferons) or that interfere with the release of the stimulators or binding with their receptors (e.g., platelet factor 4). Thrombospondins are among the first and most well characterized endogenous inhibitors that interfere with the growth, adhesion, migration, and survival of ECs.[13] Other endogenous inhibitors include fragments of various plasma or matrix proteins (e.g., angiostatin, a fragment of plasminogen; endostatin, a fragment of collagen XVIII; tumstatin, a fragment of collagen IV).[31-33] Neither the mechanisms of action of the matrix-derived inhibitors nor their physiological role are well understood.[34]

TABLE 9-1

Angiogenesis Activators and Inhibitors*

ACTIVATORS	FUNCTION	INHIBITORS	FUNCTION
VEGF family members[†‡]	Stimulate angio/vasculogenesis, permeability, leukocyte adhesion	VEGFR-1; soluble VEGFR-1; soluble neuropilin-1 (NRP-1)	Sink for VEGF, VEGF-B, PlGF
VEGFR[‡], NRP-1, NRP-2	Integrate angiogenic and survival signals	Ang 2[†‡]	Antagonist of Ang 1
EG-VEGF	Stimulate growth of endothelial cells derived from endocrine glands	TSP-1,2	Inhibit endothelial migration, growth, adhesion, and survival
Ang 1 and Tie 2[†‡]	Stabilize vessels	Angiostatin and related plasminogen kringles	Inhibit endothelial migration and survival
PDGF-BB and receptors	Recruit smooth muscle cells	Endostatin (collagen XVIII fragment)	Inhibit endothelial survival and migration
TGF-β1[§], endoglin, TGF-β receptors	Stimulate extracellular matrix production	Tumstatin (collagen IV fragment)	Inhibit endothelial protein synthesis
FGF, HGF, MCP-1	Stimulate angio/arteriogenesis	Vasostatin; calreticulin	Inhibit endothelial growth
Integrins $\alpha_v\beta_3, \alpha_v\beta_5, \alpha_5\beta_1$	Receptors for matrix macromolecules and proteinases	Platelet factor-4	Inhibit binding of bFGF and VEGF
VE-cadherin; PECAM (CD31)	Endothelial junctional molecules	Tissue-inhibitors of MMP (TIMPs); MMP-inhibitors; PEX	Suppress pathologic angiogenesis
Ephrins[‡]	Regulate arterial/venous specification	Meth-1; Meth-2	Inhibitors containing MMP-, TSP-, and disintegrin-domains
Plasminogen activators, MMPs	Remodel matrix, release growth factor	IFN-α, -β, -γ; IP-10, IL-4, IL-12, IL-18	Inhibit endothelial migration; downregulate bFGF
PAI-1	Stabilize nascent vessels	Prothrombin kringle-2; anti-thrombin III fragment	Suppress endothelial growth
NOS; COX-2	Stimulate angiogenesis and vasodilation	16 kD-prolactin	Inhibit bFGF/VEGF
AC133	Regulate angioblast differentiation	VEGI	Modulate cell growth
Chemokines[§]	Pleiotropic role in angiogenesis	Fragment of SPARC	Inhibit endothelial binding and activity of VEGF
Id1/Id3	Inhibit differentiation	Osteopontin fragment	Interfere with integrin signaling
		Maspin	Protease inhibitor
		Canstatin, proliferin-related protein, restin	Mechanisms unknown

*Selected list updated from ref. 11; for complete function and references, see supplementary information (http://steele.mgh.harvard.edu).
[†]Also present in or affecting nonendothelial cells.
[‡]See ref. 20.
[§]Opposite effect in some contexts.
Note: See text for explanation of abbreviations.

The generation of pro- and anti-angiogenic molecules can be triggered by metabolic stress (e.g., low pO_2, low pH, or hypoglycemia), mechanical stress (e.g., shear stress, solid stress), immune/inflammatory cells that have infiltrated the tissue, and genetic mutations (e.g., activation of oncogenes or deletion of suppressor genes that control the production of angiogenesis regulators).[13,14,35-37] These molecules can emanate from cancer cells, endothelial cells, stromal cells, blood, and extracellular matrix (Fig. 9-3).[38-41] Because the normal host cells differ among organs, the detailed mechanisms of angiogenesis might depend on the specific host-tumor interactions operating within a given tissue.[42-48] Furthermore, because the tumor micro-environment is likely to change during tumor growth, regression, and relapse, profiles of pro- and anti-angiogenic molecules are likely to change with time and space.[49,50] The challenge currently is to develop a unified conceptual framework to describe the temporal and spatial profiles of this increasingly diverse array of angiogenesis regulators with the aim of developing effective therapeutic strategies.[51]

Vascular Architecture

In a normal tissue, blood flows from an artery to arterioles to capillaries to venules to a vein. Although the tumor vasculature originates from these host vessels and the mechanisms of angiogenesis are similar, its organization may differ dramatically, depending on the tumor type, its location, and whether it is growing, regressing, or relapsing.[52-54] In general, tumor vessels are dilated, saccular, tortuous, and chaotic in their patterns of interconnection.[55] For example, whereas normal vasculature is characterized by dichotomous branching, tumor vasculature has many trifurcations and branches with uneven diameters.[56,57] The fractal dimensions and minimum path lengths of tumor vasculature are different from those of normal host vasculature.[52-54,58]

The molecular mechanisms of this abnormal vascular architecture are not understood, but it seems reasonable to hypothesize that the imbalance of VEGF and angiopoietins is a key contributor.[20,59] "Normalization" of the tumor vasculature observed during therapies that reduce VEGF (e.g., hormone withdrawal from a hormone-dependent tumor), interfere with VEGF signaling (e.g., treatment with anti-VEGF receptor-2 antibody) (Fig. 9-4), or mimic an anti-angiogenic cocktail (e.g., Herceptin treatment of a HER2 overexpressing tumor) is in concert with this molecular hypothesis.[12,49,50,60] Mechanical stress generated by proliferating tumor cells also can lead to the partially compressed or totally collapsed vessels often found in tumors.[61,62] The decompression of blood vessels observed after induction of apoptosis in perivascular cells supports this mechanical hypothesis.[63] Perhaps the combination of both molecular and mechanical factors renders the tumor vasculature abnormal, and, thus, both types of factors must be taken into account when designing novel strategies for cancer treatment.

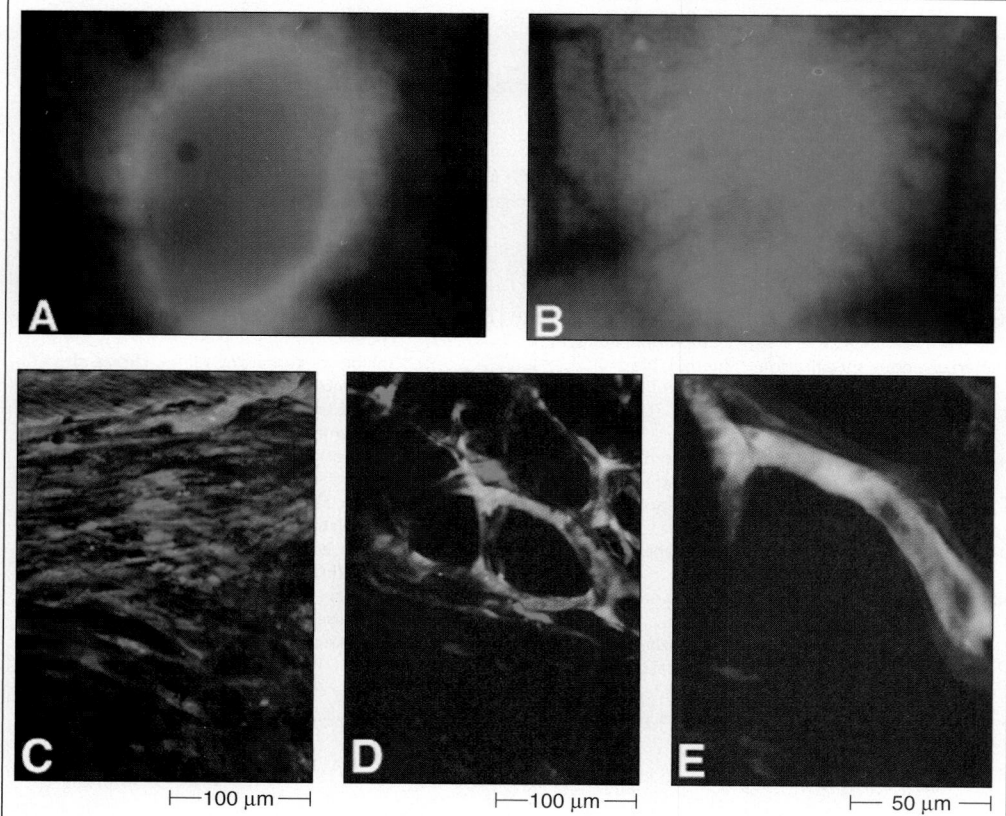

├─100 μm─┤   ├─100 μm─┤   ├─ 50 μm ─┤

Figure 9-3. Tumor induction of host promoter activity in stromal cells. The expression of VEGF in host cells can be examined using transgenic mice expressing a green fluorescent protein (GFP) under the control of the VEGF promoter. **A,** A murine mammary carcinoma xenograft shows host cell VEGF expression mainly at the periphery of the tumor after one week. **B,** After two weeks, the VEGF-expressing host cells have infiltrated the tumor. **C,** A GFP-expressing layer of host cells can be seen at the tumor-host interface. **D** and **E,** The VEGF-expressing host cells colocalize with the angiogenic tumor vessels. (**A** and **B,** From Fukumura D, Xavier R, Sugiura T, et al: Tumor induction of VEGF promoter activity in stromal cells. Cell 1998;94:715–725. **C–E,** From Brown EB, Campbell RB, Tsuzuki Y, et al: In vivo measurement of gene expression, angiogenesis and physiological function in tumors using multiphoton laser scanning microscopy. Nature Med 2001;7:1069.)

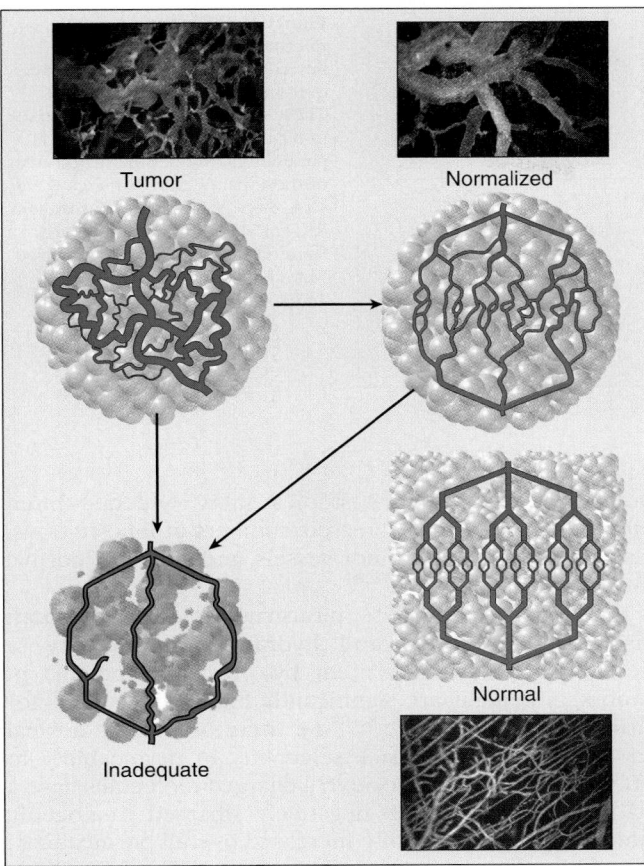

Figure 9-4. Normalization of tumor vasculature. Normal vessels are well organized with even diameters. In contrast, tumor vessels are tortuous, with increased vessel diameter, length, density, and permeability. Anti-angiogenic therapies "normalize" the tumor vascular network and could ultimately reduce the vasculature to the point at which it provides inadequate support for tumor growth. (Adapted from Jain RK: Normalizing tumor vasculature with anti-angiogenic therapy: A new paradigm for combination therapy. Nature Med 2001;7:987–989; Jain RK: Angiogenesis and lymphangiogenesis in tumor: Insights from intravital microscopy. In Stillman B [ed]: Cold Spring Harbor Symposium on Quantitative Biology [The Cardiovascular System], 2002, pp 239–248; Jain RK, Cameliet PF: Vessels of death or life. Sci Am 2001;285:38.)

Blood Flow and Microcirculation

Blood flow in a vascular network, whether normal or abnormal, is governed by the arterio-venous pressure difference and flow resistance. Flow resistance is a function of the vascular architecture (referred to as *geometric resistance*) and of the blood viscosity(rheology, referred to as *viscous resistance*).[55] Abnormalities in both vasculature and viscosity increase the resistance to blood flow in tumors.[56,64-66] As a result, overall perfusion rates (blood flow rate per unit volume) in tumors are lower than in many normal tissues.[67-69]

Both macroscopically and microscopically, tumor blood flow is temporally and spatially chaotic. Macroscopically, four spatial regions can be recognized in a tumor:

1. An avascular necrotic region
2. A semi-necrotic region
3. A stabilized microcirculation region
4. An advancing front (Fig. 9-5)[70,71]

At the microscopic level, in normal tissues, RBC velocity is dependent on vessel diameter, but there is no such dependence in most tumors.[42,44,72] Furthermore, the average RBC velocity can be an order of magnitude lower in some tumors compared to that of normal host tissue (Fig. 9-6).[42] In a given vessel within a tumor, blood flow fluctuates with time and can reverse its direction.[70,72,73]

In addition to the elevated geometric and viscous (rheologic) resistance, other molecular and mechanical factors contribute to this spatial and temporal heterogeneity. These include imbalance between pro- and anti-angiogenic molecules; "solid stress" generated by proliferating cancer cells; vascular remodeling by intussusception; and coupling between luminal and interstitial fluid pressure via hyperpermeability of tumor vessels.[15,51,54,61-63,74-76] As we will learn later, this heterogeneity contributes to both acute and chronic hypoxia in tumors—a major cause of resistance to radiation and other therapies.

Considerable effort has gone into increasing tumor blood flow for improving radiation therapy, or decreasing tumor perfusion in the case of hyperthermia. This has been difficult to achieve reproducibly because tumor vasculature consists of both vessels co-opted from the pre-existing host vasculature and vessels resulting from the angiogenic response of host vessels to cancer cells. The former are invested in normal contractile perivascular cells, whereas the latter lack these perivascular cells or these cells are abnormal.[41,55,77] Presumably as a result, efforts to increase the tumor blood flow by pharmacological or physical agents have not always been reproducible or successful.[55,68] On the other hand, the strategy of decreasing or shutting down the tumor blood flow—by "stealing" blood away from the "passive component" of the tumor vasculature by vasodilators, by vascular targeting, or by intravascular coagulation—has shown promise in experimental systems.[68,69,78-80] It also appears that judiciously applied anti-angiogenic therapy could "normalize" the abnormal tumor microcirculation by pruning the immature vessels (see Fig. 9-4), thus rendering the remaining vasculature more responsive to vasoactive agents.[81]

Vascular Permeability

Once a blood-borne molecule has reached an exchange vessel, its extravasation occurs by diffusion, convection, and, to some extent, presumably by transcytosis.[24,82] The diffusive permeability, P, of a molecule depends on the size, shape, charge, and flexibility of the molecule, and on the size, shape, charge, and dynamics of the transvascular transport pathway. In normal vessels, these pathways include diffusion along the EC membrane (for lipophilic solutes), trans-EC diffusion, inter-endothelial junctions (< 7 nm), open or closed fenestrations (< 10 nm), and transendothelial channels (including vesicles or vesico-vacuolar channels, VVOs).[24,82] Some of these anatomical pathways may be lined with glycocalyx on EC, thus effectively reducing the size of the pathway. A basement membrane (BM) may further retard the movement of

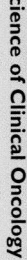

Science of Clinical Oncology

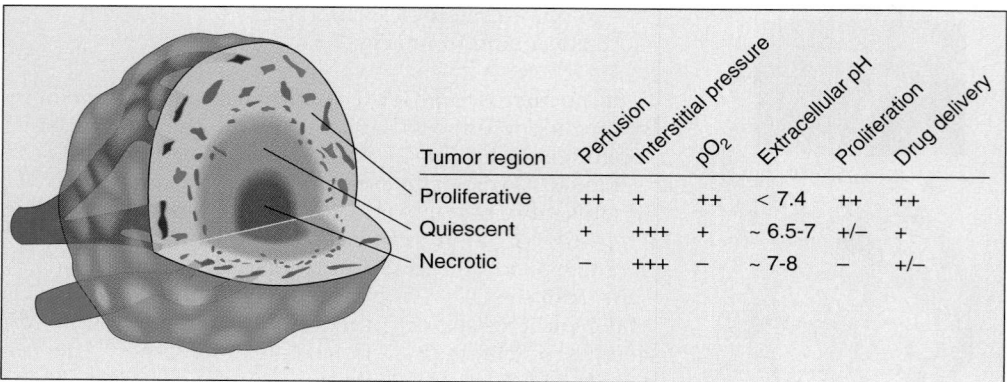

Figure 9-5. The tumor microenvironment is heterogeneous with proliferative, quiescent, and necrotic regions. These regions can be characterized in terms of various physiological parameters. Decreasing magnitude of these parameters is indicated as +++, ++, +, +/–, and –/–. (From Jain RK, Forbes NS: Can engineered bacteria help control cancer? Proc Nat Acad Sci USA 2001;98: 14748–14750.)

Tumor region	Perfusion	Interstitial pressure	pO2	Extracellular pH	Proliferation	Drug delivery
Proliferative	++	+	++	< 7.4	++	++
Quiescent	+	+++	+	~ 6.5-7	+/–	+
Necrotic	–	+++	–	~ 7-8	–	+/–

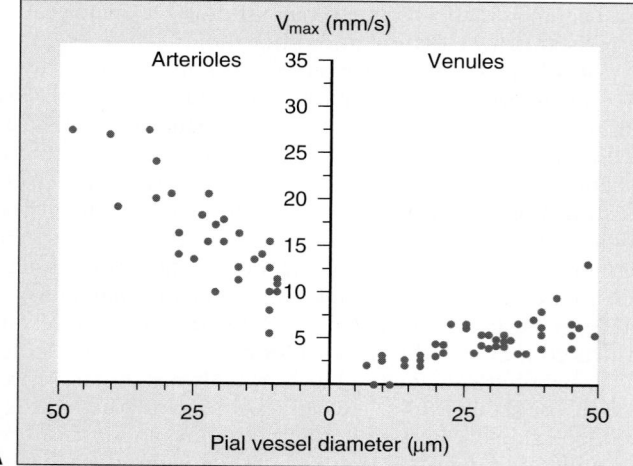

A

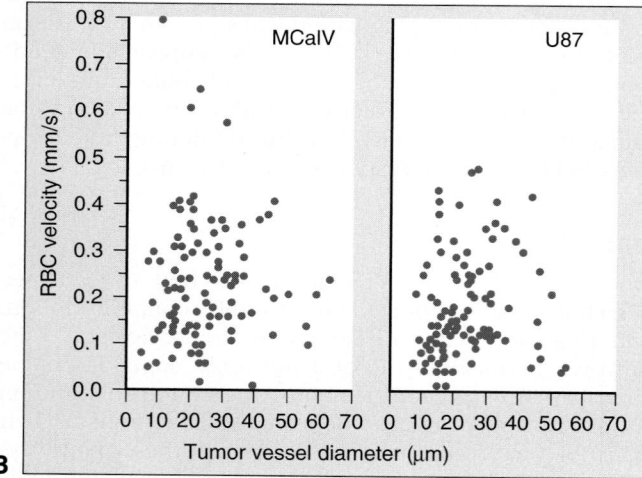

B

Figure 9-6. Blood velocity as a function of vessel diameter. **A,** Normal pial vessels. **B,** MCaIV (mammary carcinoma) and U87 (glioma) tumors xenografted on the pial surface. The measured tumor blood velocities are an order of magnitude lower than the velocities in the normal host tissue and are not related to the vessel density. (From Yuan F, Salehi HA, Boucher Y, Vasthare US, Tuma RF, Jain RK: Vascular permeability and microcirculation of gliomas and mammary carcinomas transplanted in rat and mouse cranial windows. Cancer Res 1994;54:4564–4568.)

molecules. Ultrastructure studies show widened interendothelial junctions, increased numbers of fenestrations, vesicles, and VVOs in tumor vessels, and a lack of normal BM and pericytes.[24,45,77,82,83]

In concert with these ultrastructural findings, both vascular permeability and hydraulic conductivity (a measure of water movement by pressure gradient) of tumors, in general, are significantly higher than those for various normal tissues.[42,84-88] Furthermore, unlike normal vessels, tumor vessels lack selectivity in permeability to different molecules.[89] Positively charged molecules have a higher affinity for the negatively charged angiogenic tumor vessels.[90-92] Despite increased overall permeability, not all blood vessels of a tumor are leaky (Fig. 9-7A). Even the leaky vessels have a finite pore size that is tumor-dependent (Fig. 9-7B), and ultrastructural studies show that the larger pore size in tumors represent wide interendothelial junctions.[45,83] Not only do the vascular permeability and pore size vary from one tumor to the next (see Figs. 9-7A–C), but within the same tumor they vary spatially and temporally, as they do during tumor growth, regression, and relapse.[45,49,50]

The local microenvironment plays an important role in controlling vascular permeability (Fig. 9-7D). For example, a human glioma (HGL21) has fairly leaky vessels when grown subcutaneously in immunodeficient mice, but it exhibits blood-brain barrier properties in the cranial window.[42,59] Such site-dependent differences for other tumors have been observed in other orthotopic sites.[44,47,48] One possible explanation is that the host-tumor interactions control the production and secretion of cytokines associated with permeability increase (e.g., VEGF) and decrease (e.g., angiopoietin 1).[20,29,59,93,94] A better understanding of the molecular mechanisms of permeability regulation in tumors is likely to yield strategies for improved delivery of molecular medicine to tumors.

Movement of Cells Across Vessel Walls

Both cancer cells and immune cells frequently move across the walls of blood vessels—the former in the process of metastasis and the latter during immune response or cell-based immunotherapy. Both transendothelial (through ECs) and periendothelial (between ECs)

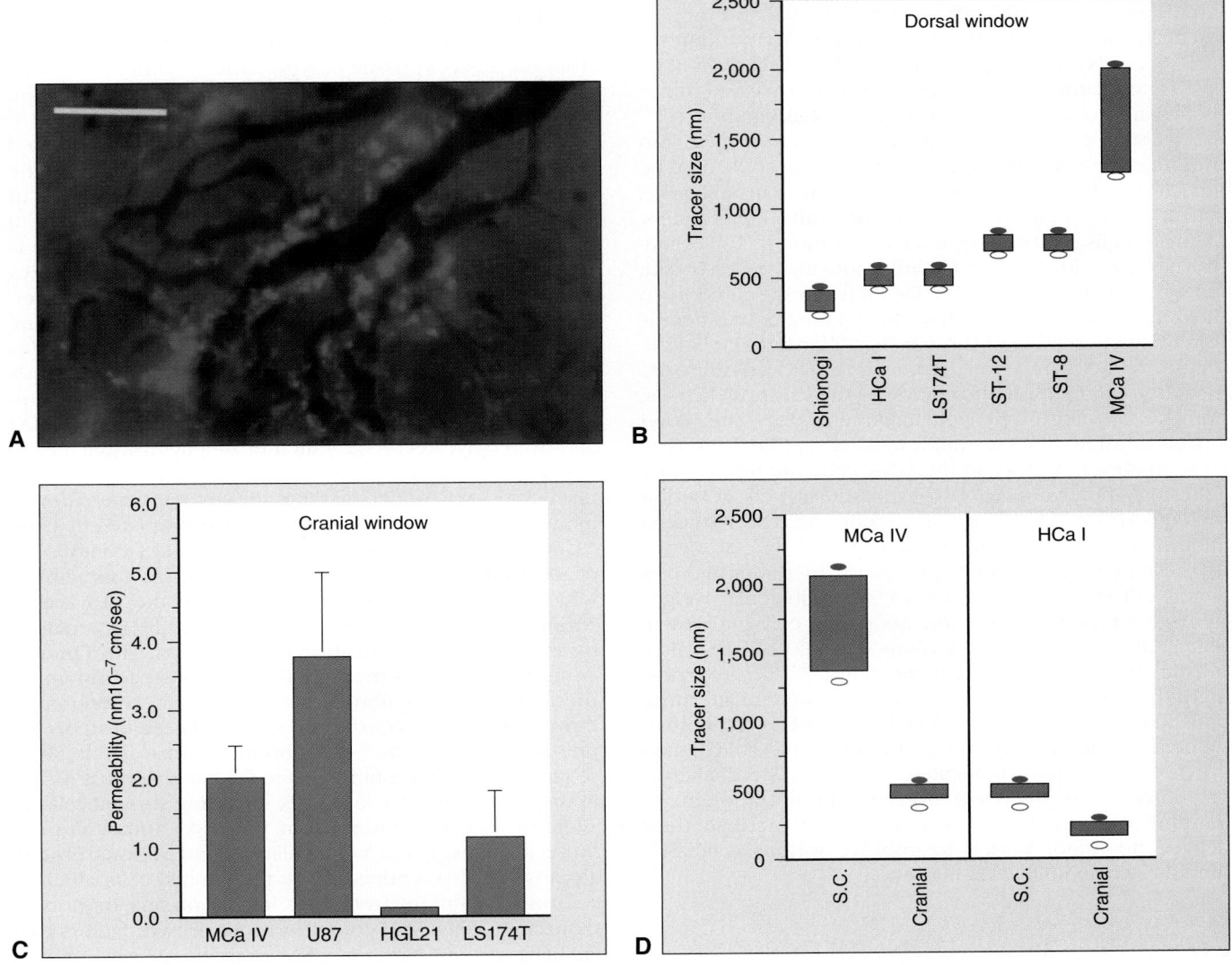

Figure 9-7. Heterogeneous permeability of tumor vessels. Vessel permeability varies spatially within a given tumor; between tumors of identical type implanted in different host organ environments; and between different tumor types in the same organ environment. **A,** Vessels within a given tumor are leaky in some areas and relatively impermeable in others. **B** and **C,** Tumors of different types grown in the same environment show variations in both vessel pore size and permeability. Pore sizes are measured by the largest tracer particle able to permeate the vessel wall. **D,** MCaIV and HCaI tumors implanted in two different sites (subcutaneous and cranial) have vessels with different pore sizes. For both tumor types, larger pore sizes are observed in the subcutaneous (sc) tumors compared with the cranial tumors. (**A** and **C,** From Yuan F, Leunig M, Huang SK, Berk DA, Papahadjopoulos D, Jain RK: Microvascular permeability and interstitial penetration of sterically stabilized [stealth] liposomes in a human tumor xenograft. Cancer Res 1994;54:3352–3356. **B** and **D,** From Hobbs SK, Monsky WL, Yuan F, et al: Regulation of transport pathways in tumor vessels: Role of tumor type and microenvironment. Proc Nat Acad Sci USA 1998;95:4607–4612.)

pathways have been proposed as a route for intravasation and extravasation of cells. Very little is known about intravasation except that tumors might shed more than a million cells per gram per day and most of these are not clonogenic.[95-97] More is known about the molecular and cellular mechanisms of extravasation.[98] When a cell enters a blood vessel, it can continue to move with the flowing blood, collide with the vessel wall, adhere transiently or stably, and finally extravasate. These interactions are governed both by local hydrodynamic forces and adhesive forces. The former are determined by the vessel diameter and fluid velocity and the latter by the expression, strength,

and kinetics of bond formation between adhesion molecules and by the surface area of contact.[99-103] Deformability of cells affects both types of forces.[104]

Rolling of endogenous leukocytes is generally low in tumor vessels, whereas stable adhesion (≥ 30 sec) is comparable between normal vessels and tumor vessels.[105] On the other hand, both rolling and stable adhesion are nearly zero in angiogenic vessels induced in collagen gels by bFGF or VEGF, two of the most potent angiogenic factors.[43] Whether this observation is due to a low flux of leukocytes into angiogenic vessels and/or to downregulation of adhesion molecules in these immature vessels is currently not known. The age of the animal also plays an important role in leukocyte-endothelial interactions.[106]

Further insight into the types of cells that adhere to tumor vessels comes from studies on the localization of IL-2 activated natural killer (A-NK) cells in normal and tumor tissues in mice using positron emission tomography.[107,108] After systemic injection, these cells localized primarily in the lungs immediately after injection and could not be detected in the tumor.[107] Increased rigidity caused by IL-2 activation might contribute to the mechanical entrapment of these cells in the lung microcirculation.[109,110] Constitutive expression of certain adhesion molecules in the lung vasculature might also facilitate their retention in the lungs.[98] One approach to reducing lung entrapment is to reduce the rigidity of these cells.[104,111] Alternatively, the lung can be circumvented by injecting A-NK cells directly into the blood supply of tumors. In this case, A-NK cells, both xenogenic and syngeneic, adhered to some blood vessels in three different tumor models via CD18 and very large antigen-4 (VLA-4) on the A-NK cells and intercellular adhesion molecule-1 (ICAM-1), vascular cell adhesion molecule-1 (VCAM-1), and E-selectin on the activated endothelium of angiogenic vessels.[26,108,112-115]

These molecules can be upregulated by tumor necrosis factor-α (TNF-α) and a protein of 90kD molecular weight (p90) that is secreted by some neoplastic cells and downregulated by transforming growth factor-β (TGF-β)—also, presumably, secreted by cancer cells.[46,99,116-120] Surprisingly, the pro-angiogenic VEGF also can upregulate these molecules, presumably via VEGFR1 (a VEGF receptor), whereas another pro-angiogenic molecule, bFGF, can downregulate these molecules.[26,40,49,60,121] The challenge currently is to decrease nonspecific entrapment of immune cells in normal vessels and to increase their delivery to tumor vessels to improve various cell-based therapies, including gene therapy.

EXTRAVASCULAR COMPARTMENT

Composition and Origin

The extravascular compartment of a solid tumor consists of neoplastic cells (parenchyma) and host cells (e.g., inflammatory cells, fibroblasts) residing in an interstitial matrix bathed by the interstitial fluid (see Fig. 9-1). Depending on the tumor type and its stage of differentiation, neoplastic cells might be dispersed in the matrix as individual cells (e.g., lymphomas, melanomas) or as clumps, sheets, or nests (e.g., carcinomas). More than 80% of tumors are carcinomas arising from epithelial cells. The remaining include sarcomas arising from mesenchymal cells (e.g., bone or muscle cells); lymphomas arising from lymphoid tissue; leukemias arising from hematopoietic cells; and hemangiomas arising from endothelial cells. In a poorly differentiated carcinoma, the cancer cells might be packed loosely in clumps, whereas in a well differentiated carcinoma, the cells might be connected with intercellular junctions and tightly packed in a nest enveloped by a basement membrane. With tumor progression, cancer cells can invade the basement membrane and spread to other regions.[24]

These various types of normal host cells must migrate into the tumor from normal tissue. Inflammatory cells might enter the tumor via blood vessels or might infiltrate from the adjacent tissue or lymphatics.[98] Other host cells, such as fibroblasts, might proliferate and migrate from the adjacent connective tissue.[20,38,41]

The interstitial subcompartment of a tumor is bounded by the walls of the blood vessels on one side and by the membranes of cancer and stromal cells on the other. In normal tissues, the blood vessels are surrounded by a basement membrane, which, as discussed previously, is defective in tumors.[20] In addition, functional lymphatics might be confined to the tumor margin.[122,123] The interstitial space of tumors, like that of normal tissues, is composed of a collagen and elastin fiber network that provides structural support to the tissue. Interdispersed in this cross-linked structure are the interstitial fluid (IF) and macromolecular constituents (polysaccharides hyaluronan [HA] and proteoglycans [PG]), which form a hydrophilic gel.

Compared with our understanding of blood vessel formation, our understanding of stroma generation is minimal. Dvorak and coworkers[24] have proposed that the extravasated plasma protein fibrinogen, a key component of the tumor interstitial fluid (TIF), clots to form fibrin, which serves as a major component of the provisional stroma. This provisional stroma eventually is replaced by more mature connective tissue stroma. The TIF also contains several other RGD (arg-gly-asp)-containing proteins, including fibronectin, vitronectin, osteopontin, thrombospondin, decorin, and tenacin. These proteins are present in both free and bound forms. Their RGD sequence provides a binding site for adhesion that assists in the migration of various cells, including stromal cells. In addition to extravasating from the leaky tumor vessels, these proteins, along with collagen and various proteoglycans, are also synthesized by the stromal cells, albeit in a form that differs from that in the plasma or normal tissues.[24] TIF also can contain various growth factors that facilitate stroma formation. For example, in vitro studies suggest that platelet-derived growth factor-β (PDGF-β) is involved in the recruitment of fibroblasts to tumors, and TGF-β induces the production of collagen and other matrix molecules in tumors.[20,124] With the increasing interest in using the fragments of matrix constituents for controlling angiogenesis, our understanding of the molecular and cellular mechanisms of stroma generation in tumors will increase.[34]

Interstitial Transport

Once a molecule has extravasated, its movement through the interstitial space occurs by diffusion and convection.[125] Diffusion is proportional to the concentration gradient in the interstitium, and convection is proportional to the interstitial fluid velocity, which, in turn, is proportional to the pressure gradient in the interstitium. Just as the interstitial diffusion coefficient, D (cm^2/s), relates the diffusive flux to the concentration gradient, the interstitial hydraulic conductivity, K (cm^2/mm Hg · s), relates the interstitial velocity to the pressure gradient.[125] Values of these transport coefficients are governed by the

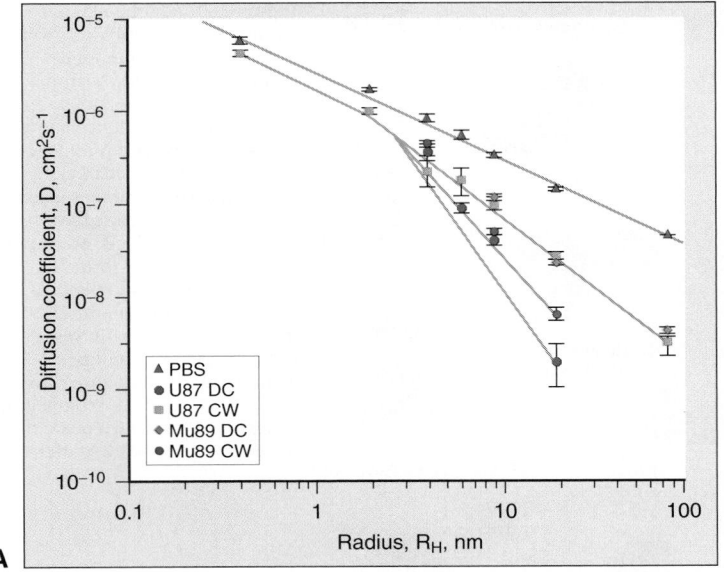

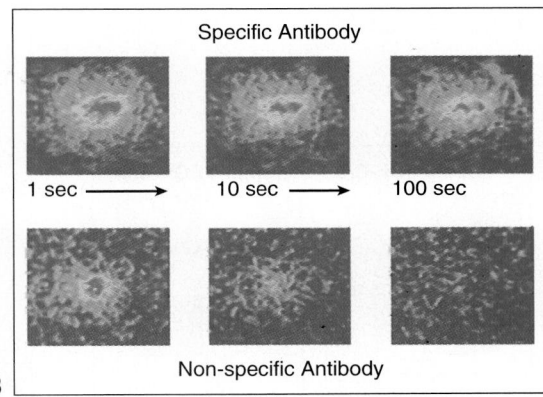

Figure 9-8. Interstitial transport in tumors. Transport of molecules through a tumor is affected by several factors. **A,** Diffusivity of a molecule in a tumor decreases with increasing molecular weight and is dependent on the host-tumor interaction. The diffusivity of macromolecules is lower in subcutaneous (sc) tumors (-) than in cranial (cw) tumors (—), and both are less than in water (PBS). **B,** Interstitial transport is also reduced by binding. The fluorescence of a photo-bleached spot recovers much more slowly with a specific antibody than with a nonspecific antibody. The binding of the specific antibody hinders the transport of the molecule into the photo-bleached spot, slowing the fluorescence recovery. (**A,** From Pluen A, Boucher Y, Ramanujan S, et al: Role of tumor-host interactions in interstitial diffusion of macromolecules: Cranial vs. subcutaneous tumors. Proc Nat Acad Sci USA 2001;98:4628–4633. **B,** Adapted from Berk DA, Yuan F, Leunig M, Jain RK: Direct in vivo measurement of targeted binding in a human tumor xenograft. Proc Nat Acad Sci USA 1997;94:1785–1790.)

structure and composition of the interstitial compartment and by the physicochemical properties of the solute molecule.[126-136]

The value of K for a human colon carcinoma xenograft (LS174T), measured using two different methods, was found to be higher than that of a hepatoma, which, in turn, was higher than that of the normal liver.[132,137,138] Using fluorescence recovery after photobleaching (FRAP), D of various molecules in tumors was found to be about 1/3 that in water and higher than the values in the host tissue (Fig. 9-8A).[127,139] Collagen content and structure have a significant effect on D in tumors.[134-136,140,141] This is surprising because hyaluronan and proteoglycans, not collagen, account for most of the resistance to transport in normal tissues. Because collagen is produced by host cells (e.g., fibroblasts), the penetrability into a tumor depends on the host-tumor interaction (see Fig. 9-8A). Thus, agents that interfere with collagen synthesis and/or organization (e.g., Relaxin) might increase interstitial transport in tumors.[136]

The time constant for a molecule with diffusion coefficient D to diffuse across a distance L is approximately $L^2/4D$. For diffusion of IgG in tumors, this time constant is on the order of one hour for a 100-μm distance, days for a 1-mm distance, and months for a 1-cm distance. So for a 1-mm distance in tumor, diffusional transport would take days, and for a 1-cm distance in tumor, it would take months. If the central vessels have collapsed completely due to cellular proliferation and interstitial matrix rearrangement, the reduced delivery of macromolecules by blood flow would make diffusion the primary mechanism

of delivery to this necrotic center.[61,63] Binding of a low- or high-molecular-weight drug to plasma proteins and various tissue components could further retard their transport in tumors.[139,142-148] The role of binding is clearly illustrated in Figure 9-8B, which compares the rate of fluorescence recovery of a photobleached spot in tumor tissue injected with a nonspecific vs. a specific IgG. In addition to the heterogeneity of D in tumors, the most unexpected result of these photobleaching studies was the large extent (30%–40%) of nonspecific binding.[139] These results collectively suggest that the interstitial compartment of a tumor can be a formidable barrier to the uniform delivery of therapeutic macromolecules (e.g., antibodies, genes) in tumors, and strategies are needed to modify this barrier.

Lymphangiogenesis and Lymphatic Transport

In most normal tissues, extravasated plasma and macromolecules are taken up by the lymphatics and brought back to the central circulation. It is widely accepted that lymphatic vessels are present in the tumor margin and the peritumoral tissue (Fig. 9-9A). Indeed, invasion of peritumoral lymphatics is considered to be a poor prognostic factor for a number of tumors (e.g., breast, colorectal, and endometrial cancers), and lymphatic metastasis is a major cause of morbidity and mortality for others (e.g., melanoma, head and neck cancer, lung cancer, and cervical cancer) (www.uptodate.com). The hotly debated issue for nearly a century has been whether

Science of Clinical Oncology

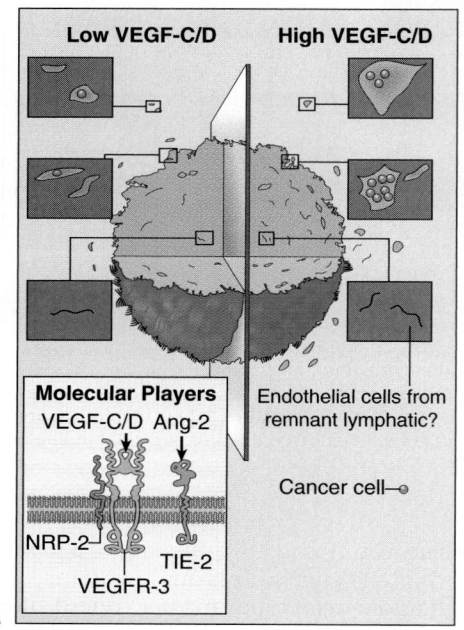

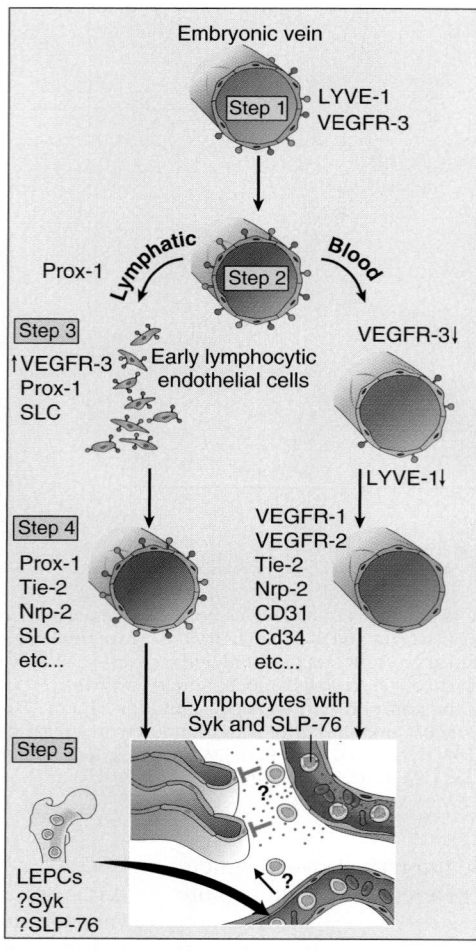

Figure 9-9. A, Schematic of lymphatics in tumors. It is widely accepted that peritumoral lymphatics exist and that metastasis can occur via these lymphatic vessels. Recent evidence shows that structures within tumors that stain for lymphatic markers are not functional. The lower-left insert shows the molecular players in lymphangiogenesis. **B,** Mechanisms of lymphatic vessel formation and separation from blood vessels. (**A,** From Jain RK, Fenton BT: Intratumoral lymphatic vessels: A case of mistaken identity or malfunction? J Nat Cancer Inst 2002;94:417–421. **B,** From Jain RK, Padera TP: Lymphatics make the break. Science 2003;299:209–210.)

anatomically defined lymphatic vessels are present within solid tumors and, if so, whether they function (see Fig. 9-9A).[67,149] Currently available immunohistochemical markers stain for structures in some tumors that resemble lymphatic vessels. Because many of these markers lack specificity, however, it is not clear whether they stain functional lymphatic vessels, endothelial cells from remnant lymphatic vessels, or some other structures (e.g., preferential fluid channels).[122,123,137,150] It is likely that the "mechanical" stress induced by proliferating cancer cells compress and impair lymphatic vessels that are co-opted or formed within a tumor.[61] The impaired lymphatic vessels, in turn, contribute to the interstitial hypertension characteristic of animal and human tumors (to be discussed shortly).

Embryonic lymphatic vessels originate primarily from blood vessels according to the following process (Fig. 9-9B).[151-153]

1. In the early embryo, endothelial cells of the cardinal vein express lymphatic vascular endothelial receptor-1 (LYVE-1) and VEGFR3, molecules observed primarily (but not exclusively) on lymphatic vessels in normal adult tissues.
2. A yet unknown signal triggers the expression of the homeobox gene *Prox* 1 so that the protein is displayed in a polarized fashion in the endothelial cells of the cardinal vein. This marks the first stage of commitment to the lymphatic lineage.
3. These LYVE-1-VEGFR3-Prox 1 positive cells then start to bud, again in a polarized fashion.
4. At this stage, these early lymphatic endothelial cells start expressing secondary lymphoid chemokine (SLC) and increased levels of VEGFR3, markers of mature lymphatic endothelial cells.
5. They then begin to form the lymphatic system.

Members of the angiopoietin family (Ang 2) and its receptor (Tie 2) are presumably involved in the maturation and patterning of these nascent lymphatic vessels.[154] The hematopoietic signaling pathway, Syk/SLP-76, contributes to the separation of lymphatics from blood vessels.[153]

The molecules involved in angiogenesis are also involved in lymphangiogenesis. For example, vascular endothelial growth factor (VEGF) -C and -D can induce both angiogenesis and lymphangiogenesis and are associated with lymphogenic metastasis in a variety of tumors.[122] Their receptor VEGFR3 is present in both lymphatic and vascular endothelium. As is the case with vascular angiogenesis, other positive and negative regulators (e.g., angiopoietins) and other receptors (e.g.,

TABLE 9-2

Interstitial Fluid Pressure (mmHg) in Normal and Neoplastic Tissues in Patients

TISSUE TYPE	N	MEAN	RANGE	REFERENCES
Normal skin	5	0.4	−1.0 – 3.0	(166)
Normal breast	8	0.0	−0.5 – 3.0	(166)
Head and neck carcinomas	27	19.0	1.5 – 79.0	(165)
Cervical carcinomas	12	15.7	10.0 – 26.0	(163)
Cervical carcinomas	102	19.0[†]	−3.0 – 48.0	(172)
Lung carcinomas	26	10.0	1.0 – 27.0	(123)
Metastatic melanomas	14	21.0	0.0 – 60.0	(167)
Metastatic melanomas	12	14.5	2.0 – 41.0	(162)
Breast carcinomas	13	29.0	5.0 – 53.0	(169)
Breast carcinomas	8	15.0	4.0 – 33.0	(166)
Brain tumors*	17	7.0	2.0 – 15.0	(168)
Brain tumors*	11	1.0	−0.5 – 8.0	(171)
Colorectal liver metastasis	8	21.0	6.0 – 45.0	(166)
Lymphomas	7	4.5	1.0 – 12.5	(167)
Renal cell carcinoma	1	38.0	—	(166)

*Patients were treated with anti-edema therapy.
[†]IFP given is a median value.

chemokine receptors and neuropilins) could be involved in lymphangiogenesis, and as discussed previously, mechanisms analogous to co-option, intussusception, sprouting, and vasculogenesis might operate in lymphatic growth.[11,154] Similar to the recently discovered organ-specific angiogenic molecule (EG-VEGF) and endothelial precursor cells, there could be organ-specific lymphangiogenic molecules and lymphatic endothelial precursor cells that contribute to tumor-associated lymphangiogenesis.[22,30,153] Moreover, the proteolytic processing of lymphangiogenic molecules and the phenotype and function of the resulting lymphatics might depend not only on the tumor type but also on the host organ in which the tumor is growing.[60,151,153,155]

The mechanical and/or molecular signals that could trigger the lymphangiogenic switch are unknown. Because lymphatic vessels help maintain the balance of fluid in tissues, hydrostatic pressure is a likely trigger. Whether the hyperplasia and the increased density of lymphatic vessels seen in the tumor margins are a response to elevated hydrostatic pressure in tumors and whether the newly formed lymphatics are able to remain open and carry cancer cells are open questions. Techniques such as microlymphangiography, reagents that block signaling of VEGF-C and -D, and yet-to-be-discovered lymphangiogenic factors will allow us to answer these important questions.[6,153,155-160]

Interstitial Hypertension

Unlike normal tissues, in which the interstitial fluid pressure (IFP) is around zero mmHg, both animal and human tumors exhibit interstitial hypertension (Table 9-2).[123,125,138,161-173] The tumor IFP begins to increase as soon as the host vessels become leaky in response to angiogenic molecules such as VEGF, and, thus, IFP can be lowered by antibodies against VEGF or VEGFR2 (unpublished data).[174,175] The IFP increases with tumor size in some tumors and remains independent of tumor size in others.[161,162,165,166]

Three mechanisms contribute to interstitial hypertension in tumors. In normal tissues, the lymphatics maintain the fluid homeostasis; thus, the lack of functional lymphatics in tumors is a key contributor. Indeed, DiResta and colleagues[176] have been able to lower the IFP by placing "artificial lymphatics" in tumors. The second contributor is the high permeability of tumor vessels. As a result, the hydrostatic and oncotic (colloid osmotic) pressures become almost equal between the intravascular and extravascular spaces.[164,177] At least two pieces of evidence support this hypothesis. First, reducing permeability by blocking VEGF signaling lowers IFP.[175] Second, IFP goes up and down with the microvascular pressure within seconds.[178-180] The two mechanisms described thus far can only explain interstitial hypertension up to 20–30 mmHg, the microvascular pressure of most exchange vessels (the hydrostatic pressure within the lumina of capillaries) in our bodies, but IFPs as high as 94 mmHg have been measured in human tumors.[163] Because microvascular pressure (MVP) is the driving force for IFP in tumors, these tumors must have a high MVP. Indeed, this is the case.[164] There are two possible explanations for elevated MVP in tumors: the tumor vessels have reduced arterial resistance so that the MVP becomes closer to arterial pressure, and/or the tumor vessels have increased venous resistance due to compression and tortuousity so that the whole intratumor vascular network is under hypertension. Indirect evidence for the latter comes from the decrease in IFP after decompression of tumor vessels by taxol-induced apoptosis of perivascular cells.[63]

The elevated pressure can compromise the tumor microcirculation and delivery of therapeutics in three ways:

1. Reduced transmural pressure gradients due to equilibrium between MVP and IFP reduce convection across

tumor vessel walls and thus compromise the transport of macromolecules.[164,180,181]

2. Because IFP is nearly uniform throughout a tumor and drops precipitously in the tumor margin, the interstitial fluid oozes out of the tumor into the surrounding normal tissue, carrying macromolecules with it (Fig. 9-10A).[161,181,182]

3. Finally, transmural coupling between IFP and MVP due to high permeability of tumor vessels can lead to blood flow stasis in tumors without physically occluding the vessels.[74-76]

Thus, decreasing vascular permeability might restore the transmural pressure gradients and potentially resume/reestablish blood flow in the nonperfused regions of tumors. Some direct and indirect anti-angiogenic therapies might "normalize" the tumor vasculature through this mechanism (see Fig. 9-4).[81]

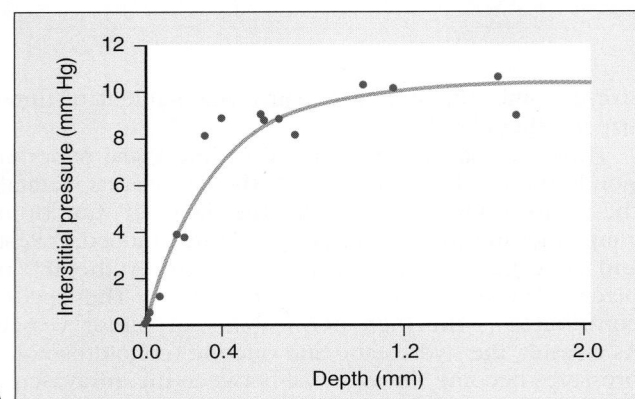

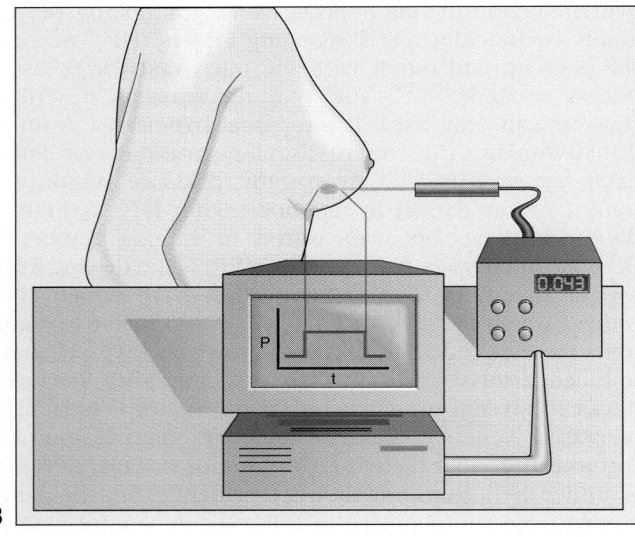

Figure 9-10. Interstitial fluid pressure (IFP) profile in a tumor and its potential application. **A,** IFP is elevated and nearly uniform in the bulk of the tumor and drops precipitously in the tumor margin. **B,** This elevated pressure can be exploited to determine the location of a tumor precisely. (**A,** Adapted from Boucher Y, Baxter LT, Jain RK: Interstitial pressure gradients in tissue-isolated and subcutaneous tumors: Implications for therapy. Cancer Res 1990;50:4478-4484. **B,** From Jain RK, Boucher Y, Stacey-Clear A, Moore D, Kopans D: Method for locating tumors prior to needle biopsy. Patent #5,396,897. USA, 1995.)

Metabolic Environment

Hypoxia

A key function of the vasculature is to provide adequate levels of nutrients and oxygen to the parenchymal cells and to remove waste products. Based on the anatomy of the capillary bed and a mathematical model of oxygen diffusion and consumption, the Nobel laureate August Krogh introduced the concept of a diffusion limit for oxygen of 100–200 μm nearly a century ago.[183] This unit of tissue—a single capillary surrounded by a 100–200 μm radius cylinder—is referred to as a "Krogh cylinder" in physiology. Nearly 50 years later, Thomlinson and Gray[184] identified similar "cords" in human lung cancer and found necrotic cells beyond 180 μm away from blood vessels, presumably due to lack of oxygen. This is referred to as "chronic hypoxia" or "diffusion-limited" hypoxia. Although various hypoxia markers and microelectrodes have suggested these gradients, the first direct measurements of these perivascular gradients, along with pO_2 and blood flow rate of the same vessels, became possible only recently with the development of phosphorescence quenching microscopy (Fig. 9-11A).[185,186]

As discussed previously, blood flow in tumor vessels is intermittent, and, thus, some regions of a tumor are starved for oxygen periodically. The resulting hypoxia is referred to as "acute hypoxia" or "perfusion-limited hypoxia."[187,188] A necessary consequence of intermittent blood flow is the resumption of blood flow after shutdown, and the resulting production of free radicals can lead to "reperfusion injury" or "reoxygenation injury", applying additional selection pressure on cancer cells.

Low pH

Another consequence of the abnormal microcirculation of the tumor is low extracellular pH. There are at least two sources of H^+ ions in tumors—lactic acid and carbonic acid.[189] The former results from glycolysis and the latter from conversion of CO_2 and H_2O via carbonic anhydrase. The intracellular pH of cancer cells remains neutral or alkaline (pH 7.4), however, in spite of the acidic extracellular pH. Because carbonic anhydrase-9, various glucose transporters (GLUT1, 3), and enzymes in the glycolytic pathway are upregulated by hypoxia, one would expect low extracellular pH and hypoxia to track each other and to colocalize with regions of low blood flow.[190] Surprisingly, there is a lack of spatial correlation among these parameters (Fig. 9-11B), a discovery made possible by recent developments in optical techniques that permit the simultaneous high-resolution mapping of multiple physiological parameters.[186] A potential explanation for this lack of concordance is that some perfused tumor vessels carry hypoxic blood.[186] Thus, although they might not be able to deliver adequate oxygen to the surrounding cells, they may be able to carry away the waste products (e.g., lactic acid).

Molecular, Cellular, and Therapeutic Consequences

The presence of oxygen during irradiation makes the damage to DNA produced by radiation-induced free radicals permanent, whereas such damage can be repaired under hypoxic conditions.[191] Therefore, hypoxia in solid

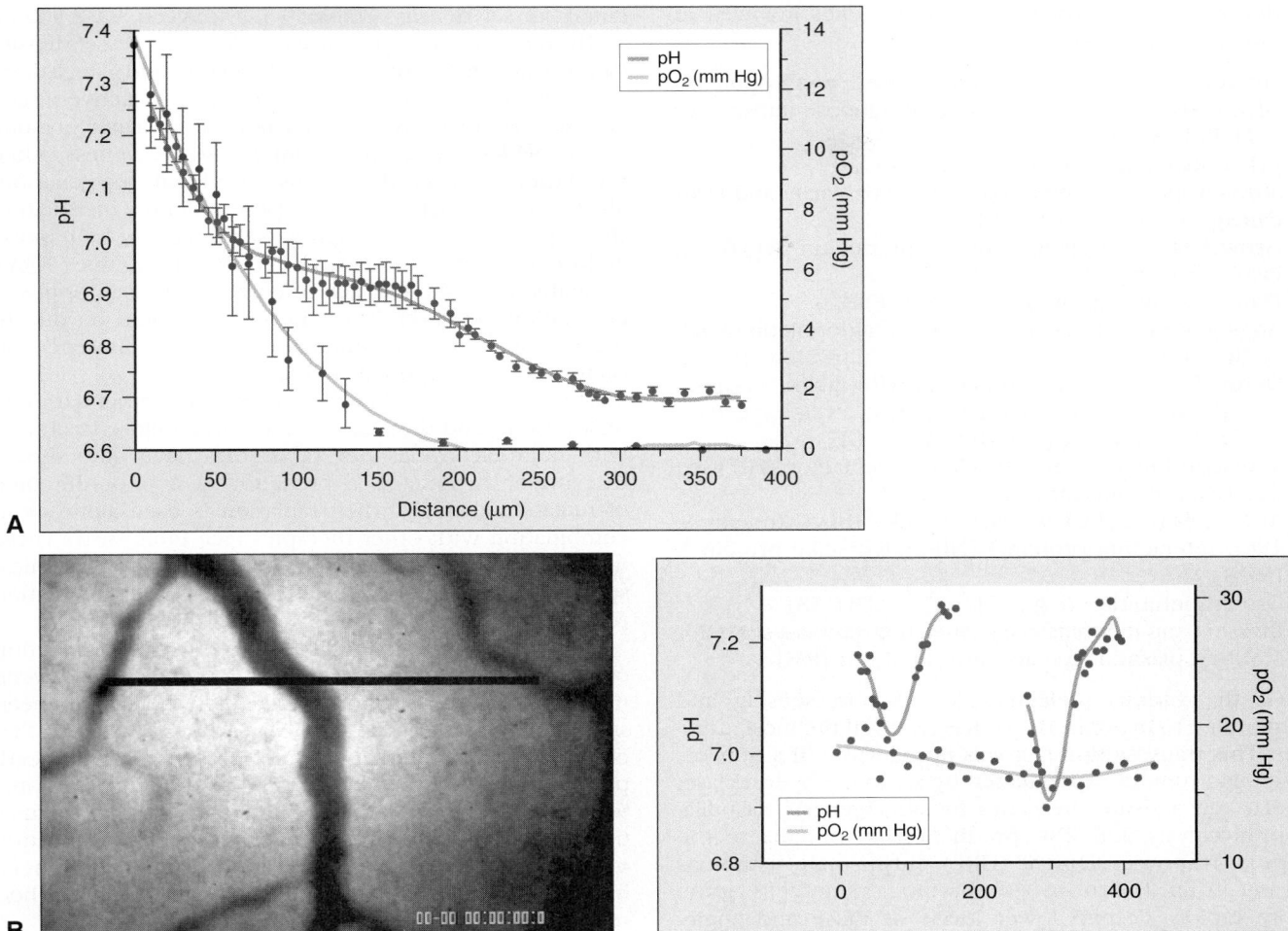

Figure 9-11. A, pH and pO_2 as a function of distance from a blood vessel in a tumor. The tumor environment becomes progressively more hypoxic and acidic further away from a blood vessel. **B,** Lack of correlation between pH and pO_2 in tumors. (From Helmlinger G, Yuan F, Dellian M, et al: Interstitial pH and pO_2 gradients in solid tumors in vivo: High-resolution measurements reveal a lack of correlation. Nature Med 1997;3:177.)

tumors significantly reduces their radiation sensitivity. Tumor hypoxia is also associated with resistance to some chemotherapeutics.[191] Similarly, low extracellular pH can affect the cellular uptake and cytotoxicity of some therapeutics adversely or favorably.[192-194] As a result, for nearly half a century, considerable preclinical and clinical efforts have been focused on alleviating hypoxia by improving tumor perfusion with various therapies, including:

- Mild hyperthermia or drugs
- Increasing oxygen content of the blood (via hyperbaric oxygenation, for example)
- Increasing hemoglobin/hematocrit (via erythropoeitin, for example)
- Developing radiation sensitizers

Unfortunately, the clinical outcome has not met expectations for multiple reasons. These include the inability to increase pO_2 in all regions of tumors to optimal levels and/or to deliver radiation sensitizers or chemotherapeutic drugs to all regions of a tumor at therapeutically effective levels.

As a result, two broad strategies are emerging:

1. Use hypoxia and/or low pH to activate drugs or to attract anaerobic bacteria.
2. Dissect hypoxia-induced pathways to identify novel targets for drug development.

The first strategy has led to the development of drugs such as Tirapazamine and to the rejuvenation of interest in bacteriolytic therapy; both approaches are in clinical trials.[71,191] The second strategy has revealed several molecular determinants of the physiological and pathophysiological responses to hypoxia.[190] The balance between hypoxia-induced apoptosis/necrosis on one hand, and the increased resistance to cell death mediated by various hypoxia-induced pathways on the other, determines whether a tumor can survive and even grow under hypoxic conditions. Ultimately, hypoxia might select for tumor cells that are more malignant, more invasive and genetically unstable, and less susceptible to apoptosis, thus rendering them resistant to various therapies. Therefore, several molecules in the hypoxia-induced pathways are now being targeted in the development of diagnostic and therapeutic agents.

Science of Clinical Oncology

Hypoxia-induced pathways include genes involved in the following processes:

- Oxygen delivery (e.g., heme oxygenase 1, erythropoietin)
- Glycolysis and glucose uptake (e.g., glucose transporter (GLUT)-1, -3, hexokinas-1, -2)
- pH control (e.g., carbonic anhydrase-9, -12)
- Stress-response pathways (e.g., growth arrest- and DNA damage-induced gene GADD 153)
- Growth-factor signaling (e.g., interleukin (IL)-6, -8, insulin-like growth factor (IGF)-2
- Platelet-derived growth factor (PDGF)-B)
- Angiogenesis (e.g., VEGF-A, VEGFR1, angiopoietin [Ang]-2, Tie-2 (an angiopoietin receptor), fibroblast growth factor [FGF]-3, transforming growth factor [TGF]-β, -β1, -β3, nitric oxide synthase [NOS], cyclooxygenase [COX]-2, hepatocyte growth factor [HGF])
- Transcription (e.g., hypoxia-inducible factor (HIF)-1α, 2α, JUN, FOS, nuclear factor (NF)-κB)
- Apoptosis (e.g., BCL-interacting killer [BIK], Annexin V, 19kD interacting protein-3 [NIP3], NIP3-like protein X [NIX])
- Growth inhibition (e.g., p21, p27, GADD153)
- Invasion and metastasis (e.g., metalloproteinases [MMP], MMP-13, plasminogen activator inhibitor [PAI]-1)[190]

Of the various molecules involved in sensing and responding to hypoxia, HIF1α has received the most attention. This transcription factor is upregulated in a number of human tumors.[190] Regulated by a proline hydroxylase, HIF1α can activate the genes for angiogenesis, vasodilation, glycolysis, and RBC production by binding to the hypoxia-response element (HRE). Surprisingly, teratomas arising from HIF1α(-/-) embryonic stem cells grow more rapidly despite lower levels of VEGF and angiogenesis.[40,195] This counter-intuitive finding could be a result of the ability of HIF1α(-/-) cells to survive under hypoxic conditions instead of undergoing apoptosis.[41] Interestingly, other HIF1α(-/-) cancer cells lead to slowly growing tumors. As a result, molecular therapies that target HIF1α or HRE are under intensive investigation for cancer detection and treatment.[190]

CLINICAL IMPLICATIONS

Two major problems currently plague the nonsurgical treatment of malignant solid tumors. First, physiological barriers within tumors impede the delivery of therapeutics and oxygen (a key sensitizer to ionizing radiation) at effective concentrations to all cancer cells.[196,197] Second, inherent or acquired resistance resulting from genetic and epigenetic mechanisms reduces the effectiveness of both conventional and novel therapies.[198] Can we take advantage of the unique pathophysiology of tumors to overcome these problems for better management of cancer? As discussed next, recent clinical data offer some hope.

Prognostic Implications

In the setting of radiation therapy, three indices of the pathophysiology of tumors have been evaluated as potential predictors of the treatment outcome in the clinic: vessel density (Table 9-3A), oxygen level (Table 9-3B), and interstitial pressure (Table 9-3C). Vessel density can be evaluated in pretreatment biopsies and is measured either in "hot spots" (i.e., regions of most active angiogenesis) or in the tissue as a whole. The former presumably provides a measure of tumor's aggressiveness, while the latter reflects the status of global oxygenation. Most studies to date show that poor outcome of radiation therapy correlates with high vessel density in "hot spots" and/or low overall microvessel density (Table 9-3A). Several studies show a lack of correlation or an opposite correlation, however. This discrepancy could be due to the morphometric techniques used or to differences in tumor types or treatment schedules.

The oxygen levels in a tumor also have potential prognostic value, and they can be measured before treatment with microelectrodes. Several studies have now shown that tumor hypoxia is a predictor of a poor outcome of radiation therapy when radiation is used alone or in combination with other therapies (see Table 9-3B). These findings are consistent with in vitro and in vivo preclinical studies showing the adverse effect of hypoxia on radiation responses.

Finally, because interstitial fluid pressure is a reflection of the global physiology of tumors, a correlation between tumor IFP and the response to radiation therapy has been suggested. One study of cervical cancer has shown that elevated tumor interstitial fluid pressure can, indeed, predict a poor outcome of radiation therapy (see Table 9-3C). Further studies are needed to evaluate the prognostic significance of IFP in tumors. One potential application of the steep rise of pressure at the tumor periphery, however, is improved localization of tumors before their removal (see Fig. 9-10B).[199]

The aforementioned parameters also seem to be important in predicting the outcome of surgery and chemotherapy. Data on the adverse predictive value of increased microvascular density in "hotspots" has recently been summarized for a range of tumor types.[200] Tumor hypoxia correlated with poor outcome even when surgery was the only treatment and is now considered as a prognostic factor for overall tumor aggressiveness and resistance to therapy.[201,202]

Although each of these prognostic approaches has its advantages, a key disadvantage is that they are all invasive. With the rapid developments taking place in the field of noninvasive imaging, it is likely that the measurement of various physiological parameters in tumors will become more convenient and more comfortable for patients, and then it will become possible to tailor therapies for individual patients based on the physiological and molecular profiles of their tumors. Such noninvasive techniques will also allow us to monitor tumor response in the course of therapy and to modify the therapy if necessary.

Therapeutic Implications

Given the physiological barriers to the delivery and effectiveness of various conventional and novel therapeutics, one strategy that is gaining increasing interest is to target the tumor vasculature. This strategy has the advantage of targeting tumor endothelial cells that are easily accessible

TABLE 9-3

A. Correlation of Tumor Microvessel Density with Poor Outcome of Radiotherapy

TUMOR SITE/TYPE	NO. OF PATIENTS	TREATMENT ENDPOINT	LEVEL OF TUMOR VASCULARITY		REFERENCES
			IN "HOT SPOTS"	MEAN	
Carcinoma of the	105	LC		L	Kolstad et al[a]
uterine cervix	47	LC		L	Awwad et al[b]
	95	5-year survival		L	Siracka et al[c]
	111	LC, overall survival	H	NS	Cooper et al[d]
	40	LC, disease-free/overall survival	NS	NS	Sundfor et al[e]
	146	LC	H	L	West et al[f]
Oral squamous cell	26	LC		H	Lauk et al[g]
carcinoma	34	LC, overall survival	H		
		Histopathological response to radiation	NS		Brun et al[h]
	100	LC, disease-free/overall survival	H		Aebersold et al[i]
Carcinoma of the head	23	LC, overall survival	L		Zatterstrom et al[j]
and neck	71	Complete remission	H		Gasparini et al[k]
	15	LC, disease-free survival		L	Kaanders et al[l]

H, correlation with high vascularity; L, correlation with low vascularity; LC, local/locoregional control; NS, no statistically significant dependence of vascularity.

[a]Kolstad P: Intercapillary distance oxygen tension and local recurrent in cervic cancer. Scand J Clin Invest 1968;S22:145–157.
[b]Awwad HK, el Naggar M, Mocktar N, Barsoum M: Intercapillary distance measurement as an indicator of hypoxia in carcinoma of the cervix uteri. Int J Radiat Oncol Biol Phys 1986;12:1329–1333.
[c]Siracka E, Revesz L, Kovac R, Siracky J: Vascular density in carcinoma of the uterine cervix and its predictive value for radiotherapy. Int J Cancer 1988;41:819–822.
[d]Cooper RA, Wilks DP, Logue JP, et al: High tumor angiogenesis is associated with poorer survival in carcinoma of the cervix treated with radiotherapy. Clin Cancer Res 1998;4:2795–2800.
[e]Sundfor K, Lyng H, Trope CG, Rofstad EK: Treatment outcome in advanced squamous cell carcinoma of the uterine cervix: Relationships to pretreatment tumor oxygenation and vascularization. Radiother Oncol 2000;54:101–107.
[f]West CM, Copper RA, Loncaster JA, Wilks DB, Bromley M: Tumor vascularity: A histological measure of angiogenesis and hypoxia. Cancer Res 2001;61:2907–2910.
[g]Lauk S, Skates S, Goodman M, Suit D: A morphometric study of the vascularity of oral squamous-cell carcinomas and its relation to outcome of radiation therapy. Eur J Cancer Clin Oncol 1989;25:1431–1440.
[h]Brun E, Zatterstrom U, Kjellen E, et al: Prognostic value of histopathological response to radiotherapy and microvessel density in oral squamous cell carcinomas. Acta Oncol 201;40:491–496.
[i]Aebersold DM, Beer KT, Laissue J, et al: Intratumoral microvessel density predicts local treatment failure of radically irradiated squamous cell cancer of the oropharyns. Int J Radiat Oncol Biol Phys 2000;48:17–25.
[j]Zatterstrom UK, Brun E, Willen R, Kjellen E, Wennerberg J: Tumor angiogenesis and prognosis in squamous cell carcinoma, of the head and neck. Head Neck 1995;17:312–318.
[k]Gasparini G, Bevilacqua P, Bonoldi E, et al: Predictive and prognostic markers in a series of patients with head and neck squamous cell invasive carcinoma treated with concurrent chemoradiation therapy. Clin Cancer Res 1995;1:1375–1383.
[l]Kaanders JH, Wijffels KI, Marres HA, et al: Pimonidazole binding and tumor vascularity predict for treatment outcome in head and neck cancer. Cancer Res 2002;62:7066–7074.

B. Significance of Tumor Hypoxia as a Predictor of Poor Outcome of Radiotherapy*

TUMOR SITE/TYPE	NO. OF PATIENTS	THERAPEUTIC ENDPOINT (YRS OF FOLLOW-UP)	CRITERION OF A LOW-OXYGENATED TUMOR	REFERENCES
Cancers of the uterine cervix	42	Disease-free/overall survival (6)	Median pO_2 < 10 mmHg	Hockel et al[m] Hockel et al[n]
	74	Disease-free/overall survival (3)	HF5 > 50%	Fyles et al[o]
	106	Disease-free survival (5)	HFS > 50%	Fyles et al[p]
	51	Disease-free/overall survival (3)	Median pO_2 < 10 mmHg, HF5 > 20%	Knocke et al[q]
	40	Disease-free/overall survival (5)	HF5 below the overall median	Sundfor et al[e]
Carcinoma of the head and neck	66	Locoregional control (2)	HF2.5 below the overall median, HF2.5 > 15%	Nordsmark et al[r] Nordsmark et al[s]
	28	Disease-free/overall survival (2)	Median pO_2 < 10 mmHg	Brizel et al[t]
	41	Overall survival (3)	HF2.5 below the overall median	Rudat et al[u]
Soft tissue sarcoma	22	Disease-free survival (1.5)	Median pO_2 < 10 mmHg	Brizel et al[v]
	28[†]	Disease-free/overall survival (5)	Median pO_2 below the overall median	Nordsmark et al[w]

pO_2, oxygen partial pressure; mmHg, millimeters of mercury; HF2.5 and HF5, the fractions of pO_2 readings below 2.5 and 5 mmHg, respectively.
* All measurements were performed before or at the beginning of radiotherapy using Eppendorf histography system (Eppendorf, Hamburg, Germany).
[†] Radiation was combined with hyperthermia.
[m]Hockel M, Schalenger K, Aral B, Mitze M, Schaffer U, Vaupel P: Association between tumor hypoxia and malignant progression in advanced cancer of the uterine cervix. Cancer Res 1996;56:4509–4515.
[n]Hockel M, Knoop C, Schlenger K, et al: Intratumoral pO_2 predicts survival in advanced cancer of the uterine cervix. Radiother Oncol 1993;26:45–50.
[o]Fyles AW, Milosevic M, Wong R, et al: Oxygenation predicts radiation response and survival in patients with cervix cancer. Radiother Oncol 1998;48:149–156.
[p]Fyles A, Milosevic M, Hedley D, et al: Tumor hypoxia has independent predictor impact only in patients with node-negative cervix cancer. J Clin Oncol 2002;20:860–687.
[q]Knocke TH, Weitmann HD, Feldmann HJ, Selzer E, Potter R: Intratumoral pO2-measurements as predictive assay in the treatment of carcinoma of the uterine cervix. Radiother Oncol 1999;53:99–104.
[r]Nordsmark M, Overgaard M, Overgaard J: Pretreatment oxygenation predicts radiation response in advanced squamous cell carcinoma of the head and neck. Radiother Oncol 1996;41:31–39.
[s]Nordsmark M, Overgaard J: A confirmatory prognostic study on oxygenation status and loco-regional control in advanced head and neck squamous cell carcinoma treated by radiation therapy. Radiother Oncol 2000;57:39–43.

TABLE 9-3, *cont'd*

[t]Brizel DM, Sibley GS, Prosnitz LR, Scher RL, Dewhirst MW: Tumor hypoxia adversely affects the prognostic of carcinoma of the head and neck. Int J Radiat Oncol Biol Phys 1997;38:285–289.

[u]Rudat V, Vanselow B, Wollensack P, et al: Repeatability and prognostic impact of the pretreatment pO_2 histography in patients with advanced head and neck cancer. Radiother Oncol 2000;57:31–37.

[v]Brizel DM, Scully SP, Harrelson JM et al: Tumor oxygenation predicts for the likelihood of distant metastases in human soft tissue sarcoma. Cancer Res 1996;56:941–943.

[w]Nordsmark M, Alsner J, Keller J, et al: Hypoxia in human soft tissue sarcomas: Adverse impact on survival and no association with p53 mutations. Br J Cancer 2001;84:1070–1075

C. Interstitial Fluid Pressure in Cervical Carcinoma for Prediction of Poor Radiation Response[‡]

NO. OF PATIENTS	TREATMENT ENDPOINT	INITIAL IFP	ΔIFP	REFERENCES
7	Tumor regression		≥ 0	(163)
102	Disease-free survival (3 years)	High (> 19 mmHg)		(172), §
40	Local control	Low (< 10 mmHg)	≥ 0	(173)

IFP, interstitial fluid pressure.

[‡] The measurements were performed by "wick-in-needle" technique. The initial IFP was measured in a tumor before or at the beginning of radiotherapy; a "post-treatment" evaluation of IFP was performed in the same tumor at the end of or after radiotherapy; ΔIFP, the difference between posttreatment and initial IFP.

§ Milosevic MF, Fyles AW, Wong R, et al: Interstitial fluid pressure in cervical carcinoma: Within tumor heterogeneity, and relation to oxygen tension. Cancer 1998;82:2418–2426.

to a blood-borne drug and are presumably genetically stable. In addition, each EC supports multiple cancer cells, thus providing "therapeutic amplification." The inability to target all ECs in a tumor, however, can reduce the effectiveness of antivascular therapy. Similarly, the responsiveness of ECs to multiple alternative angiogenic molecules can limit the effectiveness of various anti-angiogenic therapies when used alone; however, combining these therapies with conventional cytotoxic therapies has led to long-term tumor cure in mice.[11,12,200,203–205] For example, using two human tumor xenografts in nude mice, a VEGFR2-blocking antibody decreased the dose of fractionated radiation that controlled 50% of the tumors locally by 24% and 41%, respectively, without changing skin reaction in the field of tumor irradiation.[203]

Because the anti-angiogenic agents in current use are unable to destroy the tumor vasculature completely, they must be used in combination with radiation and chemotherapy. The challenge at present is to combine anti-angiogenic and conventional therapies optimally. Delivery of drugs and oxygen can be compromised if the therapies completely destroy the tumor vasculature. On the other hand, judiciously applied anti-angiogenic therapy can prune the inefficient vessels of a tumor and render the remaining vasculature more efficient (see Fig. 9-4).[81] This "normalization" of the tumor vasculature has been demonstrated in various preclinical models.[49,50,60,93] Whether this can be accomplished in human tumors with various anti-angiogenic agents and monitored with noninvasive imaging awaits the results of ongoing clinical trials. The recent encouraging results on a VEGF-neutralizing antibody combined with chemotherapy in patients with metastatic colorectal cancer show promise for this combined treatment approach.[206,207]

ACKNOWLEDGMENTS

I would like to thank Sergey Kozin, Stephany Lin, Timothy Padera, Brian Stoll, and Patrick Au for their invaluable assistance and critical input in the preparation of this chapter; and Bruce Chabner and Robert Weinberg for critically reviewing this chapter.

This chapter is an updated and expanded version of a chapter entitled: Molecular pathophysiology of tumors. In: Perez CA, Brady LW, Halperin EC, Schmidt-Ullrich R (eds), Principles and Practice of Radiation Therapy. New York, Lippincott, Williams & Wilkins, 2003.

The work summarized here has been supported by continuous support from the National Cancer Institute since 1980.

REFERENCES

1. Goldman E: The growth of malignant disease in man and the lower animals with special reference to the vascular system. Lancet 1907;2:1236–1240.
2. Ide AG, Baker NH, Warren SL: Vascularization of the Brown-Pearce rabbit epithelioma transplant as seen in the transplant ear chamber. Am J Radiol 1939;42:891–899.
3. Algire GH, Chalkley HW: Vascular reactions of normal and malignant tissues in vivo. I. Vascular reactions of mice to wounds and to normal and neoplastic transplants. J Natl Cancer Inst 1945;6:73–85.
4. Jain RK, Schlenger K, Hockel M, Yuan F: Quantitative angiogenesis assays: Progress and problems. Nature Med 1997;3:1203–1208.
5. Jain RK, Munn LL, Fukumura D: Transparent window models and intravital microscopy: Imaging gene expression, physiological function and drug delivery in tumors. In Teicher BA (ed): Tumor Models in Cancer Research. Totowa, NJ, Humana Press, 2001, pp 647–672.
6. Jain RK, Munn LL, Fukumura D: Dissecting tumour pathophysiology using intravital microscopy. Nature Rev Cancer 2002;2:266–276.
7. Greenblatt M, Shubi P: Tumor angiogenesis: Transfilter diffusion studies in the hamster by the transparent chamber technique. J Natl Cancer Inst 1968;41:111–124.
8. Ehrmann RL, Knoth M: Choriocarcinoma—Transfilter stimulation of vasoproliferation in hamster cheek pouch studied by light and electron microscopy. J Natl Cancer Inst 1968;41:1329–1341.
9. Folkman J: Tumor angiogenesis. In Holland JF, Frei E, III, Bast RC Jr, et al (eds): Cancer Medicine, 5th ed. Ontario, Canada, BC Decker, 2000, pp 132–152.
10. Gullino PM: Angiogenesis and oncogenesis. J Natl Cancer Inst 1978;61:639–643.
11. Carmeliet P, Jain RK: Angiogenesis in cancer and other diseases. Nature 2000;407:249–257.
12. Jain RK, Carmeliet PF: Vessels of death or life. Sci Am 2001;285:38–45.

13. Bouck N, Stellmach V, Hsu SC: How tumors become angiogenic. In Vande Woude G, Klein G (eds): Advances in Cancer Reasearch, vol. 69. San Diego, CA, Academic Press, 1996, pp 135-174.

14. Hanahan D, Weinberg RA: The hallmarks of cancer. Cell 2000;100:57-70.

15. Patan S, Munn LL, Jain RK: Intussusceptive microvascular growth in a human colon adenocarcinoma xenograft: A novel mechanism of tumor angiogenesis. Microvasc Res 1996;51:260-272.

16. Patan S, Munn LL, Tanda S, Roberge S, Jain RK, Jones RC: Vascular morphogenesis and remodeling in a model of tissue repair—Blood vessel formation and growth in the ovarian pedicle after ovariectomy. Circ Res 2001;89:723-731.

17. Patan S, Tanda S, Roberge S, Jones RC, Jain RK, Munn LL: Vascular morphogenesis and remodeling in a human tumor xenograft—Blood vessel formation and growth after ovariectomy and tumor implantation. Circ Res 2001;89:732-739.

18. Dvorak HF: Vascular permeability factor/vascular endothelial growth factor: A critical cytokine in tumor angiogenesis and a potential target for diagnosis and therapy. J Clin Oncol 2002;20:4368-4380.

19. Carmeliet P: Mechanisms of angiogenesis and arteriogenesis. Nature Med 2000;6:389-395.

20. Jain RK: Molecular regulation of vessel maturation. Nature Med 2003;9:685-693.

21. Isner JM: Myocardial gene therapy. Nature 2002;415:234-239.

22. Rafii S, Lyden D, Benezra R, Hattori K, Heissig B: Vascular and haematopoietic stem cells: Novel targets for anti-angiogenesis therapy? Nature Rev Cancer 2002;2:826-835.

23. Stoll BR, Migliorini C, Kadambi A, Munn LL, Jain RK: A mathematical model of the contribution of endothelial progenitor cells to angiogenesis in solid tumors: Implications for anti-angiogenic therapy. Blood 2003. (Published on line May 29, 2003; DOI 10.1182/blood-2003-D2-0365.)

24. Dvorak HF, Nagy JA, Feng D, Dvorak AM: Tumor architecture and targeted delivery. In Abrams PG, Fritzberg AR (eds): Radioimmunotherapy of Cancer, New York, Marcel Dekker, 2002, pp 107-135.

25. Ferrara N: VEGF and the quest for tumour angiogenesis factors. Nature Rev Cancer 2002;2:795-803.

26. Melder RJ, Koenig GC, Witwer BP, Safabakhsh N, Munn LL, Jain RK: During angiogenesis, vascular endothelial growth factor and basic fibroblast growth factor regulate natural killer cell adhesion to tumor endothelium. Nature Med 1996;2:992-997.

27. Yoshiji H, Harris SR, Thorgeirsson UP: Vascular endothelial growth factor is essential for initial but not continued in vivo growth of human breast carcinoma cells. Cancer Res 1997;57:3924-3928.

28. Fidler IJ: Angiogenic heterogeneity: Regulation of neoplastic angiogenesis by the organ microenvironment. J Natl Cancer Inst 2001;93:1040-1041.

29. Yancopoulos GD, Davis S, Gale NW, Rudge JS, Wiegand SJ, Holash J: Vascular-specific growth factors and blood vessel formation. Nature 2000;407:242-248.

30. LeCouter J, Kowalski J, Foster J, et al: Identification of an angiogenic mitogen selective for endocrine gland endothelium. Nature 2001;412:877-884.

31. O'Reilly MS, Holmgren L, Shing Y, et al: Angiostatin: A novel angiogenesis inhibitor that mediates the suppression of metastases by a Lewis lung carcinoma. Cell 1994;79:315-328.

32. O'Reilly MS, Boehm T, Shing Y, et al: Endostatin: An endogenous inhibitor of angiogenesis and tumor growth. Cell 1997;88:277-285.

33. Maeshima Y, Sudhakar A, Lively JC, et al: Tumstatin, an endothelial cell-specific inhibitor of protein synthesis. Science 2002;295:140-143.

34. Kalluri R: Basement membranes: Structure, assembly and role in tumour angiogenesis. Nature Rev Cancer 2003;6:422-433.

35. Kerbel RS: Tumor angiogenesis: Past, present and the near future. Carcinogenesis 2000;21:505-515.

36. Fukumura D, Xu L, Chen Y, Gohongi T, Seed B, Jain RK: Hypoxia and acidosis independently up-regulate vascular endothelial growth factor transcription in brain tumors in vivo. Cancer Res 2001;61:6020-6024.

37. Xu L, Fukumura D, Jain RK: Acidic extracellular pH induces vascular endothelial growth factor (VEGF) in human glioblastoma cells via ERK1/2 MAPK signaling pathway—Mechanism of low pH-induced VEGF. J Biol Chem 2002;277:11368-11374.

38. Fukumura D, Xavier R, Sugiura T, et al: Tumor induction of VEGF promoter activity in stromal cells. Cell 1998;94:715-725.

39. Helmlinger G, Endo M, Ferrara N, Hlatky L, Jain RK: Formation of endothelial cell networks. Nature 2000;405:139-141.

40. Tsuzuki Y, Fukumura D, Oosthuyse B, Koike C, Carmeliet P, Jain RK: Vascular endothelial growth factor (VEGF) modulation by targeting hypoxia-inducible factor-1 alpha -> hypoxia response element -> VEGF cascade differentially regulates vascular response and growth rate in tumors. Cancer Res 2000;60:6248-6252.

41. Brown EB, Campbell RB, Tsuzuki Y, et al: In vivo measurement of gene expression, angiogenesis and physiological function in tumors using multiphoton laser scanning microscopy. Nature Med 2001;7:1069.

42. Yuan F, Salehi HA, Boucher Y, Vasthare US, Tuma RF, Jain RK: Vascular permeability and microcirculation of gliomas and mammary carcinomas transplanted in rat and mouse cranial windows. Cancer Res 1994;54:4564-4568.

43. Dellian M, Witwer BP, Salehi HA, Yuan F, Jain RK: Quantitation and physiological characterization of angiogenic vessels in mice—Effect of basic fibroblast growth factor vascular endothelial growth factor vascular permeability factor, and host microenvironment. Am J Pathol 1996;149:59-71.

44. Fukumura D, Yuan F, Monsky WL, Chen Y, Jain RK: Effect of host microenvironment on the microcirculation of human colon adenocarcinoma. Am J Pathol 1997;151:679-688.

45. Hobbs SK, Monsky WL, Yuan F, et al: Regulation of transport pathways in tumor vessels: Role of tumor type and microenvironment. Proc Nat Acad Sci USA 1998;95:4607-4612.

46. Gohongi T, Fukumura D, Boucher Y, et al: Tumor-host interactions in the gallbladder suppress distal angiogenesis and tumor growth: Involvement of transforming growth factor beta 1. Nature Med 1999;5:1203-1208.

47. Tsuzuki Y, Mouta Carreira C, Bockhorn M, Xu L, Jain RK, Fukumura D: Pancreas microenvironment promotes VEGF expression and tumor growth: Novel window models for pancreatic tumor angiogenesis and microcirculation. Lab Invest 2001;81:1439-1451.

48. Monsky WL, Mouta Carreira C, Tsuzuki Y, Gohongi T, Fukumura D, Jain RK: Role of host microenvironment in angiogenesis and microvascular functions in human breast cancer xenografts: Mammary fat pad versus cranial tumors. Clin Cancer Res 2002;8:1008-1013.

49. Jain RK, Safabakhsh N, Sckell A, et al: Endothelial cell death, angiogenesis, and microvascular function after castration in an androgen-dependent tumor: Role of vascular endothelial growth factor. Proc Nat Acad Sci USA 1998;95:10820-10825.

50. Izumi Y, Xu L, di Tomaso E, Fukumura D, Jain RK: Herceptin acts as an anti-angiogenic cocktail. Nature 2002;416:279-280.

51. Ramanujan S, Koenig GC, Padera TP, Stoll BR, Jain RK: Local imbalance of proangiogenic and antiangiogenic factors: A potential mechanism of focal necrosis and dormancy in tumors. Cancer Res 2000;60:1442-1448.

52. Gazit Y, Berk DA, Leunig M, Baxter LT, Jain RK: Scale-invariant behavior and vascular network formation in normal and tumor-tissue. Phys Rev Let 1995;75:2428-2431.

53. Gazit Y, Baish JW, Safabakhsh N, Leunig M, Baxter LT, Jain RK: Fractal characteristics of tumor vascular architecture during tumor growth and regression. Microcirculation 1997;4:395-402.

54. Baish JW, Jain RK: Fractals and cancer. Cancer Res 2000;60:3683-3688.

55. Jain RK: Determinants of tumor blood flow: A review. Cancer Res 1988;48:2641-2658.

56. Less JR, Skalak TC, Sevick EM, Jain RK: Microvascular architecture in a mammary carcinoma: Branching patterns and vessel dimensions. Cancer Res 1991;51:265-273.

57. Less JR, Posner MC, Skalak TC, Wolmark N, Jain RK: Geometric resistance and microvascular network architecture of human colorectal carcinoma. Microcirculation 1997;4:25-33.

58. Baish JW, Jain RK: Cancer, angiogenesis and fractals. Nature Med 1998;4:984.

59. Jain RK, Munn LL: Leaky vessels? Call Ang1! Nature Med 2000;6:131-132.

60. Kadambi A, Mouta Carreira C, Yun C, et al: Vascular endothelial growth factor (VEGF)-C differentially affects tumor vascular function and leukocyte recruitment: Role of VEGF-receptor 2 and host VEGF-A. Cancer Res 2001;61:2404-2408.

Science of Clinical Oncology

61. Helmlinger G, Netti PA, Lichtenbeld HC, Melder RJ, Jain RK: Solid stress inhibits the growth of multicellular tumor spheroids. Nature Biotechnol 1997;15:778-783.

62. Koike C, McKee TD, Pluen A, et al: Solid stress facilitates spheroid formation: Potential involvement of hyaluronan. Br J Cancer 2002;86:947-953.

63. Griffon-Etienne G, Boucher Y, Brekken C, Suit HD, Jain RK: Taxane-induced apoptosis decompresses blood vessels and lowers interstitial fluid pressure in solid tumors: Clinical implications. Cancer Res 1999;59:3776-3782.

64. Sevick EM, Jain RK: Geometric resistance to blood flow in solid tumors perfused ex vivo: Effects of tumor size and perfusion pressure. Cancer Res 1989;49:3506-3512.

65. Sevick EM, Jain RK: Viscous resistance to blood flow in solid tumors: Effect of hematocrit on intratumor blood viscosity. Cancer Res 1989;49:3513-3519.

66. Sevick EM, Jain RK: Effect of red blood cell rigidity on tumor blood flow: Increase in viscous resistance during hyperglycemia. Cancer Res 1991;51:2727-2730.

67. Gullino PM: Extracellular compartments of solid tumors. In Becker FF (ed): Cancer. New York, Plenum, 1975, pp 327-354.

68. Jain RK, Ward-Hartley K: Tumor blood flow: Characterization, modifications, and role in hyperthermia. IEEE Trans Sonics Ultrason 1984;31:504-526.

69. Vaupel P, Kallinowski F, Okunieff P: Blood-flow, oxygen and nutrient supply, and metabolic microenvironment of human-tumors—A review. Cancer Res 1989;49:6449-6465.

70. Endrich B, Reinhold HS, Gross JF, Intaglietta M: Tissue perfusion inhomogeneity during early tumor-growth in rats. J Natl Cancer Inst 1979;62:387-395.

71. Jain RK, Forbes NS: Can engineered bacteria help control cancer? Proc Nat Acad Sci USA 2001;98:14748-14750.

72. Leunig M, Yuan F, Menger MD, et al: Angiogenesis, microvascular architecture, microhemodynamics, and interstitial fluid pressure during early growth of human adenocarcinoma LS174T in SCID mice. Cancer Res 1992;52:6553-6560.

73. Brizel DM, Klitzman B, Cook JM, Edwards J, Rosner G, Dewhirst MW: A comparison of tumor and normal tissue microvascular hematocrits and red cell fluxes in a rat window chamber model. Int J Radiat Oncol Biol Phys 1993;25:269-276.

74. Netti PA, Roberge S, Boucher Y, Baxter LT, Jain RK: Effect of transvascular fluid exchange on pressure-flow relationship in tumors: A proposed mechanism for tumor blood flow heterogeneity. Microvasc Res 1996;52:27-46.

75. Baish JW, Netti PA, Jain RK: Transmural coupling of fluid flow in microcirculatory network and interstitium in tumors. Microvasc Res 1997;53:128-141.

76. Mollica F, Jain RK, Netti PA: A model for temporal heterogeneities of tumor blood flow. Microvasc Res 2003;65:56-60.

77. Morikawa S, Baluk P, Kaidoh T, Haskell A, Jain RK, McDonald DM: Abnormalities in pericytes on blood vessels and endothelial sprouts in tumors. Am J Pathol 2002;160:985-1000.

78. Dolmans D, Kadambi A, Hill JS, et al: Vascular accumulation of a novel photosensitizer, MV6401, causes selective thrombosis in tumor vessels after photodynamic therapy. Cancer Res 2002;62:2151-2156.

79. Huang X, Molema G, King S, Watkins L, Edington TS, Thorpe PE: Tumor infarction in mice by antibody-directed targeting of tissue factor to tumor vasculature. Science 1997;275:547-550.

80. Ruoslahti E: Specialization of tumor vasculature. Nature Rev Cancer 2002;2:83-90.

81. Jain RK: Normalizing tumor vasculature with anti-angiogenic therapy: A new paradigm for combination therapy. Nature Med 2001;7:987-989.

82. Jain RK: Transport of molecules across tumor vasculature. Cancer Metastasis Rev 1987;6:559-593.

83. Hashizume H, Baluk P, Morikawa S, et al: Openings between defective endothelial cells explain tumor vessel leakiness. Am J Pathol 2000;156:1363-1380.

84. Gerlowski LE, Jain RK: Microvascular permeability of normal and neoplastic tissues. Microvasc Res 1986;31:288-305.

85. Sevick EM, Jain RK: Measurement of capillary filtration coefficient in a solid tumor. Cancer Res 1991;51:1352-1355.

86. Yuan F, Leunig M, Berk DA, Jain RK: Microvascular permeability of albumin, vascular surface area, and vascular volume measured in human adenocarcinoma LS174T using dorsal chamber in SCID mice. Microvasc Res 1993;45:269-289.

87. Lichtenbeld HC, Yuan F, Michel CC, Jain RK: Perfusion of single tumor microvessels: Application to vascular permeability measurement. Microcirculation 1996;3:349-357.

88. Endo M, Jain RK, Witwer B, Brown D: Water channel (aquaporin 1) expression and distribution in mammary carcinomas and glioblastomas. Microvasc Res 1999;58:89-98.

89. Yuan F, Dellian M, Fukumura D, et al: Vascular permeability in a human tumor xenograft: molecular size-dependence and cut-off size. Cancer Res 1995;55:3752-3756.

90. Thurston G, McLean JW, Rizen M, et al: Cationic liposomes target angiogenic endothelial cells in tumors and chronic inflammation in mice. J Clin Invest 1998;101:1401-1413.

91. Dellian M, Yuan F, Trubetskoy VS, Torchilin VP, Jain RK: Vascular permeability in a human tumour xenograft: molecular charge dependence. Br J Cancer 2000;82:1513-1518.

92. Campbell RB, Fukumura D, Brown EB, et al: Cationic charge determines the distribution of liposomes between the vascular and extravascular compartments of tumors. Cancer Res 2002;62:6831-6836.

93. Yuan F, Chen Y, Dellian M, Safabakhsh N, Ferrara N, Jain RK: Time-dependent vascular regression and permeability changes in established human tumor xenografts induced by an anti-vascular endothelial growth factor vascular permeability factor antibody. Proc Nat Acad Sci USA 1996;93:14765-14770.

94. Monsky WL, Fukumura D, Gohongi T, et al: Augmentation of transvascular transport of macromolecules and nanoparticles in tumors using vascular endothelial growth factor. Cancer Res 1999;59:4129-4135.

95. Gullino PM: Techniques in tumor pathophysiology. In Busch H (ed): Methods in Cancer Research. New York, Academic Press, 1970, pp 45-92.

96. Swartz MA, Kristensen CA, Melder RJ, et al: Cells shed from tumours show reduced clonogenicity, resistance to apoptosis, and in vivo tumorigenicity. Br J Cancer 1999;81:756-759.

97. Chang YS, di Tomaso E, McDonald DM, Jones R, Jain RK, Munn LL: Mosaic blood vessels in tumors: Frequency of cancer cells in contact with flowing blood. Proc Nat Acad Sci USA 2000;97:14608-14613.

98. Jain RK, Koenig GC, Dellian M, Fukumura D, Munn LL, Melder RJ: Leukocyte-endothelial adhesion and angiogenesis in tumors. Cancer Metastasis Rev 1996;15:195-204.

99. Melder RJ, Munn LL, Yamada S, Ohkubo C, Jain RK: Selectin- and integrin-mediated T-lymphocyte rolling and arrest on TNF-α-activated endothelium: Augmentation by erythrocytes. Biophys J 1995;69:2131-2138.

100. Munn LL, Melder RJ, Jain RK: Role of erythrocytes in leukocyte-endothelial interactions: Mathematical model and experimental validation. Biophys J 1996;71:466-478.

101. Melder RJ, Yuan J, Munn LL, Jain RK: Erythrocytes enhance lympho-cyte rolling and arrest in vivo. Microvasc Res 2000;59:316-322.

102. Yuan J, Melder RJ, Jain RK, Munn LL: Lateral view flow system for studies of cell adhesion and deformation under flow conditions. Biotechniques 2001;30:388-394.

103. Migliorini C, Qian Y, Chen H, Brown EB, Jain RK, Munn LL: Red blood cells augment leukocyte rolling in a virtual blood vessel. Biophys J 2002;83:1834-1841.

104. Melder RJ, Kristensen CA, Munn LL, Jain RK: Modulation of A-NK cell rigidity: In vitro characterization and in vivo implications for cell delivery. Biorheology 2001;38:151-159.

105. Fukumura D, Salehi HA, Witwer B, Tuma RF, Melder RJ, Jain RK: Tumor-necrosis-factor-α-induced leukocyte adhesion in normal and tumor vessels: effect of tumor type, transplantation site, and host strain. Cancer Res 1995;55:4824-4829.

106. Yamada S, Melder RJ, Leunig M, Ohkubo C, Jain RK: Leukocyte rolling increases with age. Blood 1995;86:4707-4708.

107. Melder RJ, Brownell AL, Shoup TM, Brownell GL, Jain RK: Imaging of activated natural-killer-cells in mice by positron emission tomography: preferential uptake in tumors. Cancer Res 1993;53:5867-5871.

108. Melder RJ, Elmaleh D, Brownell AL, Brownell GL, Jain RK: A method for labeling cells for positron emission tomography (PET) studies. J Immunol Meth 1994;175:79-87.

109. Sasaki A, Jain RK, Maghazachi AA, Goldfarb RH, Herberman RB: Low

deformability of lymphokine-activated killer cells as a possible determinant of in vivo distribution. Cancer Res 1989;49:3742–3746.

110. Melder RJ, Jain RK: Kinetics of interleukin-2 induced changes in rigidity of human natural killer cells. Cell Biophys 1992;20:161–176.

111. Melder RJ, Jain RK: Reduction of rigidity in human activated natural-killer-cells by thioglycolate treatment. J Immunol Meth 1994;175:69–77.

112. Melder RJ, Salehi HA, Jain RK: Interaction of activated natural-killer-cells with normal and tumor vessels in cranial windows in mice. Microvasc Res 1995;50:35–44.

113. Sasaki A, Melder RJ, Whiteside TL, Herberman RB, Jain RK: Preferential localization of human adherent lymphokine-activated killer cells in tumor microcirculation. J Natl Cancer Inst 1991;83:433–437.

114. Munn LL, Koenig GC, Jain RK, Melder RJ: Kinetics of adhesion molecule expression and spatial organization using targeted sampling fluorometry. Biotechniques 1995;19:622–626, 628–631.

115. Munn LL, Melder RJ, Jain RK: Analysis of cell flux in the parallel-plate flow chamber: Implications for cell capture studies. Biophys J 1994;67:889–895.

116. Jallal B, Powell J, Zachwieja J, et al: Suppression of tumor growth in vivo by local and systemic 90K level increase. Cancer Res 1995;55:3223–3227.

117. Melder RJ, Koenig GC, Munn LL, Jain RK: Adhesion of activated natural killer cells to tumor necrosis factor-α-treated endothelium under physiological flow conditions. Nat Immun 1996;15:154–163.

118. Gamble JR, Vadas MA: Endothelial adhesiveness for blood neutrophils is inhibited by transforming growth factor-β. Science 1988;242:97–99.

119. Gamble JR, Vadas MA: Endothelial-cell adhesiveness for human T-lymphocytes is inhibited by transforming growth-factor-β. J Immunol 1991;146:1149–1154.

120. Gamble JR, Khew-Goodall Y, Vadas MA: Transforming growth-factor-β inhibits e-selectin expression on human endothelial-cells. J Immunol 1993;150:4494–4503.

121. Detmar M, Brown LF, Schon MP, et al: Increased microvascular density and enhanced leukocyte rolling and adhesion in the skin of VEGF transgenic mice. J Invest Dermatol 1998;111:1–6.

122. Jain RK, Fenton BT: Intratumoral lymphatic vessels: A case of mistaken identity or malfunction? J Nat Cancer Inst 2002;94: 417–421.

123. Padera TP, Kadambi A, di Tomaso E, et al: Lymphatic metastasis in the absence of functional intratumor lymphatics. Sci 2002;296:1883–1886.

124. Elenbaas B, Weinberg RA: Heterotypic signaling between epithelial tumor cells and fibroblasts in carcinoma formation. Exper Cell Res 2001;264:169–184.

125. Jain RK: Transport of molecules in the tumor interstitium: A review. Cancer Res 1987;47:3039–3051.

126. Berk DA, Yuan F, Leunig M, Jain RK: Fluorescence photobleaching with spatial fourier-analysis: Measurement of diffusion in light-scattering media. Biophys J 1993;65:2428–2436.

127. Chary SR, Jain RK: Direct measurement of interstitial convection and diffusion of albumin in normal and neoplastic tissues by fluorescence photobleaching. Proc Natl Acad Sci USA 1989;86:5385–5389.

128. Johnson EM, Berk DA, Jain RK, Deen WM: Diffusion and partitioning of proteins in charged agarose gels. Biophys J 1995;68:1561–1568.

129. Johnson EM, Berk DA, Jain RK, Deen WM: Hindered diffusion in agarose gels: Test of effective medium model. Biophys J 1996;70:1017–1023.

130. Johnson ME, Berk DA, Blankschtein D, Golan DE, Jain RK, Langer RS: Lateral diffusion of small compounds in human stratum corneum and model lipid bilayer systems. Biophys J 1996;71:2656–2668.

131. Nugent LJ, Jain RK: Extravascular diffusion in normal and neoplastic tissues. Cancer Res 1984;44:238–244.

132. Swabb EA, Wei J, Gullino PM: Diffusion and convection in normal and neoplastic tissues. Cancer Res 1974;34:2814–2822.

133. Pluen A, Netti PA, Jain RK, Berk DA: Diffusion of macromolecules in agarose gels: Comparison of linear and globular configurations. Biophys J 1999;77:542–552.

134. Pluen A, Boucher Y, Ramanujan S, et al: Role of tumor-host interactions in interstitial diffusion of macromolecules: Cranial vs. subcutaneous tumors. Proc Nat Acad Sci USA 2001;98:4628–4633.

135. Davies Cde L, Berk DA, Pluen A, Jain RK: Comparison of IgG diffusion and extracellular matrix composition in rhabdomyo-

136. Brown EB, McKee TD, di Tomaso E, Seed B, Boucher Y, Jain RK: Dynamic imaging of collagen and its modulation in tumors in vivo using second harmonic generation. Nature Med, 2003;9:796–800.

137. Boucher Y, Brekken C, Netti PA, Baxter LT, Jain RK: Intratumoral infusion of fluid: Estimation of hydraulic conductivity and implications for the delivery of therapeutic agents. Br J Cancer 1998;78:1442–1448.

138. Znati CA, Rosenstein M, McKee TD, et al: Irradiation reduces interstitial fluid transport and increases the collagen content in tumors. Clin Cancer Res (in press).

139. Berk DA, Yuan F, Leunig M, Jain RK: Direct in vivo measurement of targeted binding in a human tumor xenograft. Proc Nat Acad Sci USA 1997;94:1785–1790.

140. Netti PA, Berk DA, Swartz MA, Grodinsky AJ, Jain RK: Role of extracellular matrix assembly in interstitial transport in solid tumors. Cancer Res 2000;60:2497–2503.

141. Ramanujan S, Pluen A, McKee TD, Brown EB, Boucher Y, Jain RK: Diffusion and convection in collagen gels: Implications for transport in the tumor interstitium. Biophys J 2002;83:1650–1660.

142. Baxter LT, Jain RK: Transport of fluid and macromolecules in tumors. III. Role of binding and metabolism. Microvasc Res 1991;41:5–23.

143. Baxter LT, Jain RK: Transport of fluid and macromolecules in tumors. IV. A microscopic model of the perivascular distribution. Microvasc Res 1991;41:252–272.

144. Juweid M, Neumann R, Paik C, et al: Micropharmacology of monoclonal-antibodies in solid tumors: Direct experimental-evidence for a binding-site barrier. Cancer Res 1992;52:5144–5153.

145. Kaufman EN, Jain RK: Quantification of transport and binding parameters using fluorescence recovery after photobleaching. Potential for in vivo applications. Biophys J 1990;58:873–885.

146. Kaufman EN, Jain RK: Measurement of mass transport and reaction parameters in bulk solution using photobleaching: Reaction limited binding regime. Biophys J 1991;60:596–610.

147. Kaufman EN, Jain RK: Effect of bivalent interaction upon apparent antibody affinity: Experimental confirmation of theory using fluorescence photobleaching and implications for antibody binding assays. Cancer Res 1992;52:4157–4167.

148. Kaufman EN, Jain RK: In vitro measurement and screening of monoclonal antibody affinity using fluorescence photobleaching. J Immunol Meth 1992;155:1–17.

149. Leu AJ, Berk DA, Lymboussaki A, Alitalo K, Jain RK: Absence of functional lymphatics within a murine sarcoma: A molecular and functional evaluation. Cancer Res 2000;60:4324–4327.

150. Mouta Carreira C, Nasser SM, di Tomaso E, et al: LYVE-1 is not restricted to the lymph vessels: Expression in normal liver blood sinusoids and down-regulation in human liver cancer and cirrhosis. Cancer Res 2001;61:8079–8084.

151. Alitalo K, Carmeliet P: Molecular mechanisms of lymphangiogenesis in health and disease. Cancer Cell 2002;1:219–227.

152. Oliver G, Detmar M: The rediscovery of the lymphatic system: Old and new insights into the development and biological function of the lymphatic vasculature. Genes Dev 2002;16:773–783.

153. Jain RK, Padera TP: Lymphatics make the break. Science 2003;299:209–210.

154. Gale NW, Thurston G, Hackett SF, et al: Angiopoietin-2 is required for postnatal angiogenesis and lymphatic patterning, and only the latter role is rescued by angiopoietin-1. Dev Cell 2002;3:411–423.

155. Jain RK, Padera TP: Prevention and treatment of lymphatic metastasis by antilymphangiogenic therapy. J Nat Cancer Inst 2002;94:785–787.

156. Leu AJ, Berk DA, Yuan F, Jain RK: Flow velocity in the superficial lymphatic network of the mouse tail. Am J Physiol Heart Circ Physiol 1994;36:H1507–H1513.

157. Swartz MA, Berk DA, Jain RK: Transport in lymphatic capillaries. I. Macroscopic measurements using residence time distribution theory. Am J Physiol Heart Circ Physiol 1996;39:H324–H329.

158. Berk DA, Swartz MA, Leu AJ, Jain RK: Transport in lymphatic capillaries. II. Microscopic velocity measurement with fluorescence photobleaching. Am J Phys Heart Circ Physiol 1996;39:H330–H337.

159. Jeltsch M, Kaipainen A, Joukov V, et al: Hyperplasia of lymphatic vessels in VEGF-C transgenic mice. Science 1997;276:1423–1425.

160. Padera TP, Stoll BS, So PTC, Jain RK: High-speed intravital multi-photon scanning laser microscopy of microvasculature, lymphatics, and leukocyte-endothelial interactions. Molec Imag 2002;1:9-15.

161. Boucher Y, Baxter LT, Jain RK: Interstitial pressure gradients in tissue-isolated and subcutaneous tumors: Implications for therapy. Cancer Res 1990;50:4478-4484.

162. Boucher Y, Kirkwood JM, Opacic D, Desantis M, Jain RK: Interstitial hypertension in superficial metastatic melanomas in humans. Cancer Res 1991;51:6691-6694.

163. Roh HD, Boucher Y, Kalnicki S, Buchsbaum R, Bloomer WD, Jain RK: Interstitial hypertension in carcinoma of uterine cervix in patients: Possible correlation with tumor oxygenation and radiation response. Cancer Res 1991;51:6695-6698.

164. Boucher Y, Jain RK: Microvascular pressure is the principal driving force for interstitial hypertension in solid tumors: Implications for vascular collapse. Cancer Res 1992;52:5110-5114.

165. Gutmann R, Leunig M, Feyh J, et al: Interstitial hypertension in head and neck tumors in patients: Correlation with tumor size. Cancer Res 1992;52:1993-1995.

166. Less JR, Posner MC, Boucher Y, Borochovitz D, Wolmark N, Jain RK: Interstitial hypertension in human breast and colorectal tumors. Cancer Res 1992;52:6371-6374.

167. Curti BD, Urba WJ, Alvord WG, et al: Interstitial pressure of subcutaneous nodules in melanoma and lymphoma patients: Changes during treatment. Cancer Res 1993;53:2204-2207.

168. Arbit E, Lee J, DiResta GR: Interstitial hypertension in human brain tumors: Possible role in peritumoral edema formulation. In Nagai H, Kamiya K, Ishi S (eds): Intracranial Pressure, vol IX: Tokyo, Springer-Verlag, 1994, pp 604-614.

169. Nathanson SD, Nelson L: Interstitial fluid pressure in breast-cancer, benign breast conditions, and breast parenchyma. Ann Surg Oncol 1994;1:333-338.

170. Boucher Y, Lee I, Jain RK: Lack of general correlation between interstitial fluid pressure and oxygen partial-pressure in solid tumors. Microvas Res 1995;50:175-182.

171. Boucher Y, Salehi H, Witwer B, Harsh GR 4th, Jain RK: Interstitial fluid pressure in intracranial tumours in patients and in rodents. Br J Cancer 1997;75:829-836.

172. Milosevic M, Fyles A, Hedley D, et al: Interstitial fluid pressure predicts survival in patients with cervix cancer independent of clinical prognostic factors and tumor: Oxygen measurements. Cancer Res 2001;61:6400-6405.

173. Znati CA, Gerszten K, Faul C, et al: Changes in interstitial fluid pressure in patients undergoing radiation therapy for carcinoma of the uterine cervix. (In preparation.)

174. Boucher Y, Leunig M, Jain RK: Tumor angiogenesis and interstitial hypertension. Cancer Res 1996;56:4264-4266.

175. Lee CG, Heijn M, di Tomaso E, et al: Anti-vascular endothelial growth factor treatment augments tumor radiation response under normoxic or hypoxic conditions. Cancer Res 2000;60:5565-5570.

176. DiResta GR, Lee J, Healey JH, Levchenko A, Larson SM, Arbit E: "Artificial lymphatic system": A new approach to reduce interstitial hypertension and increase blood flow, pH and pO(2) in solid tumors. Ann Biomed Eng 2000;28:543-555.

177. Stohrer M, Boucher Y, Stangassinger M, Jain RK: Oncotic pressure in solid tumors is elevated. Cancer Res 2000;60:4251-4255.

178. Zlotecki RA, Boucher Y, Lee I, Baxter LT, Jain RK: Effect of angiotensin II induced hypertension on tumor blood flow and interstitial fluid pressure. Cancer Res 1993;53:2466-2468.

179. Netti PA, Baxter LT, Boucher Y, Skalak R, Jain RK: Time-dependent behavior of interstitial fluid pressure in solid tumors: Implications for drug-delivery. Cancer Res 1995;55:5451-5458.

180. Netti PA, Hamberg LM, Babich JW, et al: Enhancement of fluid filtration across tumor vessels: Implication for delivery of macromolecules. Proc Nat Acad Sci USA 1999;96:3137-3142.

181. Jain RK, Baxter LT: Mechanisms of heterogeneous distribution of monoclonal antibodies and other macromolecules in tumors: Significance of elevated interstitial pressure. Cancer Res 1988;48:7022-7032.

182. Butler TP, Grantham FH, Gullino PM: Bulk transfer of fluid in interstitial compartment of mammary tumors. Cancer Res 1975;35:3084-3088.

183. Krogh A: The Anantomy and Physiology of Capillaries. New York, Yale University Press, 1922.

184. Thomlinson RH, Gray LH: The histological structure of some human lung cancers and the possible implications for radiotherapy. Br J Cancer 1955;9:539-549.

185. Torres Filho IP, Leunig M, Yuan F, Intaglietta M, Jain RK: Noninvasive measurement of microvascular and interstitial oxygen profiles in a human tumor in scid mice. Proc Nat Acad Sci USA 1994;91:2081-2085.

186. Helmlinger G, Yuan F, Dellian M, Jain RK: Interstitial pH and pO_2 gradients in solid tumors in vivo: High-resolution measurements reveal a lack of correlation. Nature Med 1997;3:177-182.

187. Brown JM, Giaccia AJ: The unique physiology of solid tumors: Opportunities (and problems) for cancer therapy. Cancer Res 1998;58:1408-1416.

188. Dewhirst MW: Concepts of oxygen transport at the microcirculatory level. Sem Radiat Oncol 1998;8:143-150.

189. Helmlinger G, Sckell A, Dellian M, Forbes NS, Jain RK: Acid production in glycolysis-impaired tumors provides new insights into tumor metabolism. Clin Cancer Res 2002;8:1284-1291.

190. Harris AL: Hypoxia: A key regulatory factor in tumour growth. Nature Rev Cancer 2002;2:38-47.

191. Brown JM: The hypoxic cell: A target for selective cancer therapy—Eighteenth Bruce F. Cain Memorial Award lecture. Cancer Res 1999;59:5863-5870.

192. Vukovic V, Tannock IF: Influence of low pH on cytotoxicity of paclitaxel, mitoxantrone and topotecan. Br J Cancer 1997;75:1167-1172.

193. Cowan DS, Tannock IF: Factors that influence the penetration of methotrexate through solid tissue. Int J Cancer 2001;91:120-125.

194. Kozin SV, Shkarin P, Gerweck LE: The cell transmembrane pH gradient in tumors enhances cytotoxicity of specific weak acid chemotherapeutics. Cancer Res 2001;61:4740-4743.

195. Carmeliet P, Dor Y, Herbert JM, et al: Role of HIF-1alpha in hypoxia-mediated apoptosis, cell proliferation and tumour angiogenesis. Nature 1998;394:485-490.

196. Jain RK: Barriers to drug delivery in solid tumors. Sci Am 1994;271:58-65.

197. Jain RK: The next frontier of molecular medicine: Delivery of therapeutics. Nature Med 1998;4:655-657.

198. McCormick F: New-age drug meets resistance. Nature 2001;412:281-282.

199. Jain RK, Boucher Y, Stacey-Clear A, Moore R, Kopans D: Method for locating tumors prior to needle biopsy. Patent #5,396,897. USA, March 14, 1995.

200. Kerbel R, Folkman J: Clinical translation of angiogenesis inhibitors. Nature Rev Cancer 2002;2:727-739.

201. Hockel M, Schlenger K, Aral B, Mitze M, Schaffer U, Vaupel P: Association between tumor hypoxia and malignant progression in advanced cancer of the uterine cervix. Cancer Res 1996;56:4509-4515.

202. Hockel M, Vaupel P: Tumor hypoxia: Definitions and current clinical, biologic, and molecular aspects. J Nat Cancer Inst 2001;93:266-276.

203. Kozin SV, Boucher Y, Hicklin DJ, Bahlen P, Jain RK, Suit HD: Vascular endothelial growth factor receptor-2-blocking antibody potentiates radiation-induced long-term control of human tumor xenografts. Cancer Res 2001;61:39-44.

204. Klement G, Baruchel S, Rak J, et al: Continuous low-dose therapy with vinblastine and VEGF receptor-2 antibody induces sustained tumor regression without overt toxicity. J Clin Invest 2000;105:R15-R24.

205. Browder T, Butterfield CE, Kraling BM, et al: Antiangiogenic scheduling of chemotherapy improves efficacy against experimental drug-resistant cancer. Cancer Res 2000;60:1878-1886.

206. Hurwitz H, Fehrenbacher L, Cartwright T, et al: Bevacizumab (Avastin, a monoclonal antibody to vascular endothelial growth factor) prolongs survival in first-line colorectal cancer (CRC): Results of a Phase III trial of Bevacizumab in combination with bolus IFL (Irinotecan, 5-Fluorouracil, Leucovorin) as first-line therapy in subjects with metastatic CRC. Proc Am Soc Clin Oncol 2003;22:1207.

207. Willett CG, Boucher Y, di Tomaso E, et al: Direct evidence that the VEGF-specific antibody Bevacizumab has antivascular effects in human rectal cancer. Nat Med 2004;10:145-147.

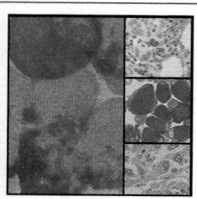

ENVIRONMENTAL FACTORS

Paul T. Strickland

Thomas W. Kensler

SUMMARY OF KEY POINTS

HISTORY OF IDENTIFICATION OF HUMAN CARCINOGENS

- The carcinogenic effects of many environmental and occupational agents were first described in humans.
- Beginning in the twentieth century with the advent of animal bioassay programs, evidence of carcinogenicity in experimental animals has preceded evidence from epidemiologic or case studies in humans.
- The majority of human cancers likely result from the interaction of several or more carcinogenic influences (none of which singly is readily detectable) along with intrinsic factors (inherited genes, hormones, immune status).

ROLE OF ENVIRONMENTAL AGENTS IN THE ETIOLOGY OF HUMAN CANCER

- Although the causes of most human cancers remain unidentified, data

supports the opinion that environmental agents are the principal causes of human cancers.
- Cigarette smoking could be responsible for 25% of all cancers in the United States.
- Chemical carcinogens include aromatic amines, benzene, aflatoxins, tobacco chemicals, and chemotherapeutic agents.
- Radiation carcinogens include ultraviolet radiation, ionizing radiation, and radon.
- A number of metal carcinogens have been identified, including arsenic, nickel, cadmium, and chromates. These have been associated largely with occupational exposures.
- Fibers (asbestos, silica) and dusts are well established as etiologic agents in lung cancers.
- Many components in the diet can influence the development of cancer through carcinogenic or anticarcinogenic mechanisms.

EXPOSURE BIOMARKERS AND SUSCEPTIBILITY FACTORS/ CHEMOPREVENTION

- The identification of molecular biologic markers of exposure, effect, and susceptibility (reflecting events prior to clinical disease) will help to further our understanding of human carcinogenesis.
- The characterization of the human genome has enabled study of the roles of common polymorphisms in carcinogen metabolism or of DNA repair genes in susceptibility to cancer.
- Primary and secondary approaches to the prevention of cancer will be greatly facilitated by the development of noninvasive biomarkers that identify high-risk individuals.
- Tertiary prevention might also be enhanced by characterizing cancers with respect to etiology, genetic profile, or metabolic capacity.

INTRODUCTION

The carcinogenic effects of a sizable number of environmental or industrial chemicals have first been described in humans. The influences of occupation and lifestyle in cancer occurrence were observed at least as early as the sixteenth century. Ramazzini in 1700 noted that nuns exhibited a higher frequency of breast cancer than was observed among other women. Also in that century, Paracelsus and Agricola described *Bergkrankheiten* in miners in the Schneeberg and Joachimstal regions of Europe. *Bergkrankheiten* was later recognized as lung cancer, probably caused by uranium and its decay product radon.[1] Subsequently, in 1761 Hill associated the use of tobacco snuff with cancer in the nasal passage, and in 1775 Pott noted the occurrence of soot-related scrotal cancer among chimney sweeps. In 1895 Rehn published evidence that occupational exposure to aromatic amines was associated with bladder cancer, while Unna in 1894 associated sunlight exposure with skin cancer. It was not until the early 20th century that animal models for chemical carcinogenesis were developed. For example,

Yamagiwa and Ichikawa reported in 1915 on the production of skin tumors following topical application of crude coal tar to the ears of rabbits, and Sasaki and Yoshida reported in 1935 that feeding of azo dyes to rats led to the development of liver tumors. In the intervening decades, there has been substantial growth in our understanding of the roles of chemicals (both manufactured and naturally occurring), radiation, and viruses in the cancer process. Of particular importance has been the recognition that these extrinsic factors interact with intrinsic factors (e.g., inherited genes, hormones, immune status) to determine overall susceptibility and risk. A central role of diet in these interactions is featured by observations that dietary factors can both enhance and inhibit tumor formation.

Contrary to experiences in earlier centuries, with the advent of animal bioassay programs, evidence of carcinogenicity in experimental animals has preceded evidence obtained from epidemiologic studies or case reports in many instances. Although the term *carcinogen* means "giving rise to carcinomas" (e.g., epithelial malignancies) in general, broader operational definitions are used for carcinogens in animal bioassays. A carcinogen may be defined as an agent whose administration to previously untreated animals leads to a statistically significant increased incidence of malignant neoplasms, compared with the incidence in appropriate untreated control animals, whether the control animals have a low or high spontaneous incidence of the neoplasms in question. Chemicals, radiation, and viruses are the primary agents identified. Synthetic and naturally occurring chemicals comprise the largest group of known human carcinogens. More than 60 chemicals, chemical mixtures, and industrial processes have been classified as human carcinogens (Table 10-1) and more than 300 chemicals have been identified as animal carcinogens to date. These figures evolve from an environmental milieu of perhaps 10^7 chemicals, although the vast majority of these agents have not been evaluated for carcinogenicity.

Chemical carcinogens comprise a diverse array of chemical structures, including both organic and inorganic compounds. Relatively few carcinogens are direct acting, as the innate reactivity of such compounds also tends to make them unstable. Rather, most carcinogens require metabolic activation to reactive species. These activated *procarcinogens* are more stable in the environment and are of greater concern for exposures to the general population. Once formed, the reactive intermediates can interact with DNA to produce genetic lesions that can result in mutation of critical cellular genes, including oncogenes and tumor suppressor genes. Metabolic pathways can be influenced strongly by a variety of extrinsic and intrinsic factors and are important determinants of both interindividual and target organ susceptibilities to carcinogens. Carcinogenesis is a dynamic, multistage

TABLE 10-1

Agents and Processes Considered Carcinogenic in Humans by the International Agency for Cancer Research

AGENT OR PROCESS	COMMON ORGAN OR TISSUE SITES OF CANCER
Ambient and Dietary Exposure	
Aflatoxins	Liver
Arsenic and arsenic compounds	Lung, skin
Erionite	Pleura, peritoneum
Cultural Habits	
Alcoholic beverages	Oral cavity, pharynx, larynx, esophagus, liver
Betel quid with tobacco	Oral cavity
Tobacco products, smokeless	Oral cavity
Tobacco smoke	Respiratory tract, urinary bladder, renal pelvis, pancreas
Salted fish, Chinese style	Nasopharynx
Solar radiation	Skin
Occupational	
Aluminum production	Lung, urinary bladder
4-Aminobiphenyl	Urinary bladder
Asbestos	Lung, pleura, peritoneum, larynx, gastrointestinal tract
Auramine, manufacture of	Urinary bladder
Benzene	Leukemia
Benzidine	Urinary bladder
Beryllium	Lung
Bis(chloromethyl)ether and chloromethyl methyl ether	Lung
Boot and shoe manufacture and repair	Nasal sinus
Cadmium	Lung
Chromium[VI] compounds	Lung
Coal gasification	Lung, urinary bladder, scrotum
Coal-tar pitches	Skin, scrotum, lung
Coal tars	Skin, lung
Coke production	Skin, scrotum, lung, urinary bladder
Dioxin	All cancers combined
Ethylene oxide	Lymphatic, hematopoietic
Furniture and cabinet making	Nasal sinus
Iron and steel founding	Lung
Isopropyl alcohol manufacture (strong acid process)	Nasal sinus
Magenta, manufacture of	Urinary bladder
Mineral oils (untreated and mildly treated)	Skin, scrotum
Mustard gas	Lung, larynx/pharynx
2-Naphthylamine	Urinary bladder
Nickel and nickel compounds	Lung, nasal sinus
Painting	Lung
Rubber industry	Urinary bladder, leukemia
Shale oils	Skin, scrotum
Silica, crystalline	Lung
Soots	Skin, scrotum, lung

TABLE 10-1

Agents and Processes Considered Carcinogenic in Humans by the International Agency for Cancer Research—cont'd	
AGENT OR PROCESS	**COMMON ORGAN OR TISSUE SITES OF CANCER**
Strong inorganic acid mists containing sulfuric acid	Larynx
Talc containing asbestiform fibers	Lung
Underground mining with exposure to radon	Lung
Vinyl chloride	Liver, lung, gastrointestinal tract, brain
Wood dust	Nasal cavities, paranasal sinuses
Therapeutic Use	
Analgesics mixtures containing phenacetin	Renal, urinary bladder
Azathioprine	Leukemia
N,N-Bis(2-chloroethyl)-2-naphthylamine	Urinary bladder
1,4-Butanediol dimethanesulfonate	Leukemia
Chlorambucil	Leukemia
Cyclosporine	Lymphoma
Cyclophosphamide	Urinary bladder, leukemia
Estrogen replacement therapy	Endometrium, breast
Estrogen, nonsteroidal	Cervix/vagina, breast, endometrium, testes
Estrogens, steroidal	Endometrium, breast
Melphalan	Leukemia
8-Methoxypsoralen plus UV radiation	Skin
Methyl-CCNU	Leukemia
MOPP	Leukemia
Oral contraceptives (combined)	Liver
Oral contraceptives (sequential)	Endometrium
Tamoxifen	Endometrium
Thiotepa	Leukemia
Treosulfan	Leukemia
Infectious Agents	
Epstein-Barr virus	Lymphoma
Helicobacter pylori	Stomach
Hepatitis B virus	Liver
Hepatitis C virus	Liver
Human immunodeficiency virus type 1	Kaposi's sarcoma
Human papilloma viruses types 16, 18	Cervical
Human T-cell lymphotropic virus type 1	Adult T-cell leukemia/lymphoma
Opisthorchis viverrini	Cholangiocarcinoma
Schistosoma haematobium	Urinary bladder

Data from International Agency for Research on Cancer: IARC monographs on the evaluation of carcinogenic risk to humans, vol 1–82, Lyon, IARC, 1970-2002. An updated listing of the overall evaluation of carcinogenicity to humans can be accessed on the Internet at http://193.51.164.11/monoeval/grlist.html or through www.iarc.fr. (Note: For examples of carcinogenic ionizing radiations, see Table 10-3).

process through which a normal cell is converted into a malignant neoplasm. Although our understanding of the neoplastic process is incomplete, current knowledge provides considerable insight into the critical actions of carcinogens. The goal of this chapter is to highlight the roles of discrete chemical and physical agents in the etiology of human cancers. In turn, fuller understanding of the mechanistic basis for the actions of these carcinogenic agents will allow for more effective means to identify other carcinogens in our environment and to develop preventive strategies to interrupt, block, or reverse the neoplastic process.

ROLE OF ENVIRONMENTAL AGENTS IN THE ETIOLOGY OF HUMAN CANCERS

The causes of most human cancers remain unidentified; however, considerable evidence suggests that "extraconstitutional" or environmental and lifestyle factors are important contributors. For example, cigarette smoking could be responsible for 25% of all cancers in the United States. The opinion that environmental agents are the principal causes of human cancers is derived largely from the following series of epidemiologic observations:

1. Although the overall incidence of cancer is reasonably constant between countries, incidences of specific tumor types can vary up to several hundredfold.
2. There are large differences in tumor incidence within populations of a single country.
3. Migrant populations assume the cancer incidence of their new environment within one to two generations.
4. Cancer rates within a population can change rapidly.

Although the extent to which environmental agents contribute to human carcinogenesis remains to be defined precisely, a considerable number of epidemiologic studies indicate important roles for the various naturally occurring and manufactured chemicals, radiations, metals, and fibers found in our individual environments.

Chemicals

Polycyclic Aromatic Hydrocarbons

The English surgeon Percival Pott[2] was among the first to document the association of an environmental agent with cancer. During the late 18th century, he determined that the unusually high incidence of scrotal cancer among chimney sweeps was due to their occupational exposure to soot and tar. As a consequence, recommendations for bathing and use of protective clothing were promulgated by chimney sweepers' guilds in parts of Europe, but not in England. Subsequent decreases in the incidence of scrotal cancer were observed in continental Europe, demonstrating the efficacy of simple prevention efforts. It was not until the present century that the active carcinogens in soot and coal tar were shown to be polycyclic aromatic hydrocarbons (PAHs).[3] This was accomplished through the application of coal tar and fractions thereof to the skins of test animals that subsequently developed malignant skin tumors. Although many PAHs were identified in coal tar, most of the carcinogenic activity was attributed to the PAH benzo[a]pyrene.

Humans are exposed to PAHs from a variety of sources that include occupation, smoking, diet, and air.[4] PAHs are readily absorbed into the body through the skin, lungs, and gastrointestinal tract. Occupational and medicinal exposures constitute the highest levels of human PAH exposure (albeit in small groups within the population), whereas diet and smoking are the major sources of exposure to PAHs in the general population. Air concentrations of greater than 10 μg benzo[a]pyrene/m^3 are characteristic of topside gas and coke works. Broiled, barbecued, or smoked meats and fish contain relatively high concentrations of benzo[a]pyrene (1 to 20 μg/kg).

Cutaneous occupational exposure to PAHs has been associated with increased risk of skin and scrotal cancers in chimney sweeps and in individuals exposed to unrefined lubricating oils in the textile and machining industries.[1] Scrotal cancer among mule spinners in the Manchester cotton industry was attributed to the saturation of the workers' trousers with lubricating oil. A review of all admissions for scrotal cancer to the Royal Manchester Infirmary from 1902 to 1922 indicated that 49% had worked as mule spinners, while 16% had worked with tar or paraffin. As the textile industry declined in the middle 20th century, an increasing proportion of scrotal cancer was associated with cutting oils used in metal machining.

An excess of lung cancer has been demonstrated among individuals with substantial inhalation exposure to PAHs, including roofers and pavers, coke oven workers, certain steel and iron manufacturing workers, and aluminum production workers.[5] In addition, several studies suggest that workers highly exposed through inhalation might also be at increased risk of cancer at sites other than skin and lung. The strongest evidence for such an association is for bladder cancer, where a dose-response relationship has been demonstrated between PAH exposure and bladder cancer risk in aluminum workers after adjustment for smoking. Other sites with suggestive increases in risk include the pancreas and upper gastrointestinal tract.

Several biochemical pathways are involved in the metabolism of PAHs and of benzo[a]pyrene in particular (Fig. 10-1).[3] The initial step in benzo[a]pyrene metabolism involves the epoxidation of an aromatic double bond by one of the cytochrome P-450 mono-oxygenases (P450 1A1). The epoxide-benzo[a]pyrene intermediates might form phenols or glutathione conjugates or be further oxidized by epoxide hydrolase to form dihydrodiol-benzo[a]pyrene. This latter metabolite can undergo a second oxidation step, resulting in the highly reactive 7,8-dihydrodiol-9,10-epoxidebenzo[a]pyrene. Many studies have indicated a role for aryl hydrocarbon hydroxylase (P450 1A1) in the oxygenation of PAHs in animal models, and recent studies using human liver tissue suggest that nifedipine oxidase (P450 3A3/4) activates 7,8-dihydro-7,8-dihydroxybenzo[a]pyrene to a genotoxic species.

Experimental studies demonstrate that cultured human lung or colon tissue metabolizes benzo[a]pyrene to the proximate carcinogen 7,8-dihydro-7,8-dihydroxybenzo[a]-pyrene and that benzo[a]pyrene metabolites bind to DNA in cultured tissue. Oral administration of benzo[a]pyrene to rodents produces benzo[a]pyrene-DNA adducts in liver, stomach, colon, and intestine and cancers of the esophagus, forestomach, intestine, lungs, and mammary gland.

Aromatic Amines

The occurrence of bladder cancer among dye industry workers was reported in 1895 by the German physician Ludwig Rehn, who suggested a causal relationship. With the rapid expansion of the chemical industry during and after World War I, increased risk of bladder cancer was observed among workers employed in chemical manufacturing and textile dyeing.[6] An industrywide study of workers exposed to dyes in England and Wales demonstrated increased risks of bladder cancer among men exposed to 1-naphthylamine (observed [O]/expected [E] = 8.6), benzidine (O/E = 13.9), 2-naphthylamine (O/E = 86.7), or mixed dyes (O/E = 54.7). The International Agency for Research on Cancer (IARC) subsequently considered that the cancer hazard associated with exposure to 1-naphthylamine was due to the likely contamination of commercial grade 1-naphthylamine with 4%–10% 2-naphthylamine.[7] Additional studies in the dye industry identified auramine and magenta as human bladder carcinogens. Increased risk of bladder cancer among rubber workers and in the electric cable industry has been attributed to the naphthylamine added to rubber as an antioxidant.

Excess risk of bladder cancer has been observed in the silk-dyeing industry, in which benzidine-based dyes are used extensively. Elevated incidence of bladder cancer associated with benzidine manufacturing and production in the United States and Japan is complicated by probable co-exposure to 2-naphthylamine and o-toluidine. The production of these aromatic amines has declined in recent years; the result has been a considerable reduction in bladder cancer among workers in these industries.

Aromatic amines are metabolized and excreted through a process involving acetylation by N-acetyltransferase.[8]

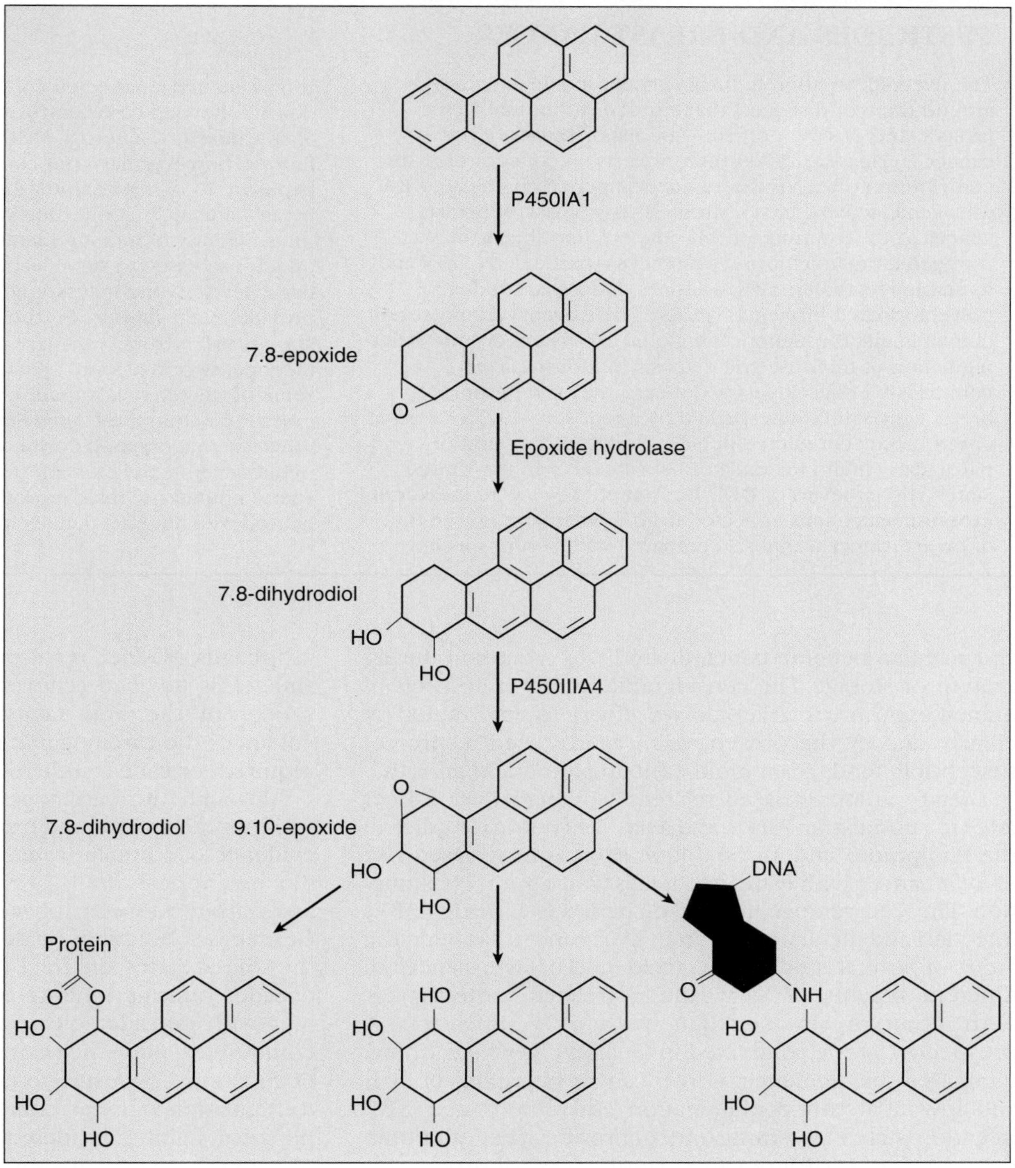

Figure 10-1. Metabolic activation of benzo[a]pyrene and formation of DNA and protein adducts.

Genetic variation in one of the genes, *NAT2,* coding for this enzyme produces either rapid or slow metabolic phenotypes in humans. Analysis of the *NAT2* phenotypes of patients with bladder cancer from the dye industry indicates that individuals exhibiting the slow phenotype could be more susceptible to bladder cancer caused by aromatic amines.

Benzene

Exposure to benzene was suspected to be the cause of leukemia in a number of individual cases and case series reported worldwide between 1928 and 1976.[1] Case-control studies indicated increased risks of non-lymphocytic leukemia among workers in Sweden exposed to benzene-containing petroleum products and for lymphomas among workers in New York State exposed to benzene. Prospective studies conducted in the rubber

industry provide the most convincing evidence for an association between benzene exposure and leukemia. Most of the excess leukemia in this industry is found among rubber workers exposed to solvents, including benzene. Excess mortality from leukemia has been observed among former employees of a rubber film production plant (O/E = 4.7) and a rubber coating plant (O/E = 3.7).

Aflatoxins

The hepatotoxic effect of aflatoxins was first recognized when aflatoxin-contaminated feed was inadvertently fed to poultry. Subsequent animal studies demonstrated the carcinogenic potential of the aflatoxins, particularly aflatoxin B_1. The aflatoxins are produced by the fungal strains *Aspergillus flavus* and *A. paraciticus*. Grains and foodstuffs for human consumption such as corn, peanuts,

PESTICIDES AND BREAST CANCER

The five-fold variation in breast cancer incidence rates around the world suggest that extraconstitutional factors—lifestyle and/or environment—are major causes of breast cancer. During the 1990s, there was rising concern over the contribution of exposures to environmental chemicals with estrogenic activity (xenoestrogens) to the risk of breast cancer. At the forefront of this concern have been the weakly estrogenic organochlorine pesticides—particularly DDT and its stable metabolite, DDE—and the industrial products, polychlorinated biphenyls (PCBs). These agents are persistent contaminants throughout the global ecosystem despite strict regulation of their use and disposal in industrialized countries for over 20 years. Concern over the pesticide-breast cancer link was sparked by a report in 1993 of a case-control study conducted in New York State, a region of particularly high incidence of breast cancer in the United States. Higher levels of DDE, but not of PCBs, were measured in serum specimens collected from women around the time of breast cancer diagnosis compared with serum specimens from matched, unaffected control subjects.[29] Nearly a half dozen follow-up case-control studies conducted in Massachusetts, California, Mexico, and several regions of Europe, however, have not confirmed the hypothesis that exposure to either DDT and/or PCBs increases the risk of breast cancer.[30,31] A question with all these studies, though, is the suitability of measurements of organochlorines in blood or adipose tissue to serve as proper surrogates for target tissue levels. Nonetheless, epidemiological studies also fail to provide much support for the hypothesis. Differences in known risk factors (e.g., parity, age at menarche and menopause, and alcohol consumption) appear to account for some of the regional variation in breast cancer incidence and mortality within the United States. It should be kept in mind, however, that organochlorine xenoestrogens do remain a public health concern with regard to worldwide decreases in sperm counts and male reproductive capacity, and increased neurodevelopmental deficits in children.

and rice can become contaminated with aflatoxin during growth or storage. The considerable variation in levels of human exposure to aflatoxin worldwide is determined by climate and by the preventive measures used to protect susceptible foods from mold contamination and growth.[9]

Dietary aflatoxin is correlated with high liver cancer rates in sub-Saharan Africa and Asia. Case-control studies in the Philippines and Mozambique show an increased risk of liver cancer with estimated levels of aflatoxin consumption. The cocarcinogenic role of hepatitis B virus (HBV) infection and dietary aflatoxin in liver cancer has been the focus of several studies. The incidence of liver cancer in different regions of Swaziland correlated more closely with aflatoxin intake than with HBV infection. A prospective study conducted in Guangxi Province, China, compared the incidence of liver cancer in regions of high and low aflatoxin contamination and determined HBV infection status.[9] A strong interaction between aflatoxin exposure and HBV-positive status was observed for relative risk of liver cancer. Among HBV-positive individuals, the incidence of liver cancer was 649 per 100,000 in the high aflatoxin region and 66 per 100,000 in the low aflatoxin region, whereas among HBV-negative individuals, the incidence of liver cancer was 99 per 100,000 and 0 per 100,000 in high or low aflatoxin regions, respectively.

The new techniques of molecular dosimetry for human carcinogen exposure have been applied in populations exposed to aflatoxin. With individual exposures often in excess of 10–100 µg/d, the presence of aflatoxin metabolites and DNA adducts can be quantified in the urine after exposure. The association of urinary aflatoxin-DNA adducts with risk of liver cancer has also been demonstrated in a prospective epidemiologic study.[10]

Tobacco Chemicals

Tobacco use causes more cancer deaths worldwide than any other human activity. Cigarette smoking is associated with cancers of the lung, oral cavity, pharynx, larynx, esophagus, bladder, renal pelvis, and pancreas. The use of smokeless tobacco (chewing tobacco or snuff) leads to cancer of the oral cavity. Thus, although combustion enhances the carcinogenic properties of tobacco, it is not required for cancer induction.

Although the carcinogenic properties of tobacco tar were first demonstrated experimentally during the 1920s, evidence of a human cancer risk from the use of tobacco did not appear until 1939, when Muller[11] reported an association between tobacco use and lung carcinoma in Germany. Subsequent epidemiologic studies conducted in the United States and the United Kingdom during the next decade confirmed this causal relationship. These findings met with considerable resistance in both the scientific community and the general public, however. Unlike occupational exposure to carcinogens, which was subject to regulation in many countries, tobacco exposure was a personal habit considered by many users to be more pleasurable than dangerous. Unfortunately, the addictive characteristics of nicotine, a major constituent of tobacco, made it more difficult for tobacco users to reduce their consumption. Societal acceptance of a causal association with lung cancer was advanced by the first reports from the Royal College of Physicians in the United Kingdom (1962) and from the Surgeon General in the United States (1964) regarding the risks of tobacco use. By contrast, the tobacco industry has steadfastly resisted attempts to educate the public to the health hazards of tobacco use and has continued to market cigarettes aggressively, particularly in developing countries. Explosive increases in the incidence of lung cancer, probably even outracing those already occurring in the United States, can be anticipated in these countries over the next few decades. Based on tobacco usage trends, it is estimated that more than one million new cases per year of lung cancer will occur in China in the 21st century.[11]

More than 3000 chemicals have been identified in cigarette smoke, of which at least 30 are known to be carcinogenic in animals (Table 10-2). The gas phase of tobacco smoke contains several carcinogenic or tumor-promoting compounds, including dimethylnitrosamine, dialkylnitrosamines, vinyl chloride, acrolein, and benzene. Most of the carcinogenic activity of cigarette smoke is

TABLE 10-2

Tumorigenic Agents in Tobacco Smoke

COMPOUNDS	MAINSTREAM SMOKE (PER CIGARETTE)
PAHs	
Benzo[a]anthracene	20–70 ng
Benzo[b]fluoranthene	4–22 ng
Benzo[f]fluoranthene	6–21 ng
Benzo[k]fluoranthene	6–12 ng
Benzo[a]pyrene	20–40 ng
Chrysene	40–60 ng
Dibenz[a,h]anthracene	4 ng
Dibenzo[a,i]pyrene	1.7–3.2 ng
Dibenzo[a],[l]pyrene	Detectable
Indenol[1,2,3][c,d]pyrene	4–20 ng
5-Methylchrysene	0.6 ng
Aza-arenes	
Quinoline	1–2 μg
Dibenz[a,h]acridine	0.1 ng
Dibenz[a,j]acridine	3–10 ng
7H-Dibenzo[c,g]carbazole	0.7 ng
N-Nitrosamines	
N-Nitrosodimethylamine	0.1–180 ng
N-Nitrosethylmethylamine	3–13 ng
N-Nitrosodiethylamine	0–25 ng
N-Nitrosopyrrolidine	1.5–110 ng
N-Nitrosodiethanolamine	0–36 ng
N(-Nitrosonornicotine	0.12–2.7 μg
4-(Methylnitrosamine)-1-(3-pyridyl)-1-butanone	0.08–0.77 μg
N(-Nitrosoanabasine	0.14–4.6 μg
Aromatic Amines	
2-Toluidine	30–200 ng
2-Naphthylamine	1–22 ng
4-Aminobiphenyl	2–5 ng
Aldehydes	
Formaldehyde	70–100 μg
Acetaldehyde	18–1400 ng
Crotonaldehyde	10–20 μg
Miscellaneous Organic Compounds	
Benzene	12–48 μg
Acrylonitrile	3.2–15 μg
2-Nitropropane	0.73–1.21 μg
Ethylcarbamate	20–38 ng
Vinyl chloride	1–16 ng
Inorganic Compounds	
Hydrazine	24–43 ng
Arsenic	40–120 ng
Nickel	0–600 ng
Chromium	4–70 ng
Cadmium	41–62 ng
Polonium-210	0.03–1.0 pCi

From Reducing the Health Consequences of Smoking: 25 Years of Progress. Washington, DC, U.S. Department of Health and Human Services, 1989.

found in the particulate phase. This phase includes carcinogenic and co-carcinogenic PAHs, methylated PAHs, heterocyclic hydrocarbons, chlorinated hydrocarbons, phenols, catechols, and metals. Organ-specific carcinogens in the particulate phase include N-nitrosamines (and precursors), which have been associated with esophageal and pancreatic cancers, and aromatic amines, which are associated with kidney and bladder cancers. An important finding from experimental studies is the strong interactive effect observed when certain mixtures of these compounds are assayed for carcinogenic potential.

Chemotherapeutic Agents

The systemic toxicity of sulfur mustard gas among soldiers exposed during World War I led to investigations of the mechanism of action of nitrogen mustard compounds. The cytotoxic effect observed in lymphatic tissues was subsequently replicated and studied in experimental animal models. This property of nitrogen mustards and other alkylating compounds prompted their use as antineoplastic drugs during the 1940s. Several other types of drugs were developed at that time for use in the treatment of cancer, including the antibiotic actinomycin A and the antimetabolite methotrexate. Later decades saw the introduction of a variety of alkylating agents (e.g., chlorambucil, cyclophosphamide, bis-chloroethylnitrosourea, busulfan, cisplatin), anti-metabolites (5-fluorouracil, 6-meracptopurine), antibiotics (adriamycin, bleomycin, daunomycin), and mitotic inhibitors (vincristine, vinblastine) as antineoplastics.

As early as 1948, the carcinogenic properties of the anticancer drug 4-aminostilbene and its metabolites were reported by Haddow and colleagues.[12] This and subsequent findings by Elizabeth and John Weisbuger led to the institution of carcinogenesis bioassays for new anticancer drugs under development by the National Cancer Institute (NCI).

Preneoplastic dysplasias were frequently observed in the epithelial tissues of patients with cancer undergoing chemotherapy. The appearance of frank second malignancies among patients treated by chemotherapy was reported during the 1970s.[13] In addition, renal transplant patients receiving anticancer drugs for immunosuppression exhibited excess risks of mesenchymal and epithelial cancers.

The successful treatment of Hodgkin's disease with multiagent chemotherapy is associated with the long-term complication of acute myeloid leukemia (AML) and non-Hodgkin's lymphoma. Increased risk of AML among patients treated for non-Hodgkin's lymphoma, ovarian cancer, multiple myeloma, or small cell carcinoma of the lung has also been attributed to antineoplastic therapy. The risk of AML is most strongly associated with the alkylating antineoplastics—particularly cyclophosphamide, melphalan, busulfan, treosulfan, and semustine (methyl-CCNU)—or with combination chemotherapies that include alkylating agents.

A large case-control study conducted in collaboration with 11 population-based cancer registries and two large oncology hospitals in Europe and Canada identified

Science of Clinical Oncology

114 cases of leukemia among 99,113 ovarian cancer survivors.[14] Patients receiving chemotherapy alone had a relative risk for leukemia of 12 compared with patients treated by surgery alone. By contrast, patients receiving radiation therapy alone (compared with surgery alone) had no significant increase in the risk of leukemia. In order of decreasing leukemogenic potency, the drugs melphalan, thiotepa, chlorambucil, cyclophosphamide, and treosulfan were independently associated with significantly increased risk of leukemia. Combination treatment with Adriamycin and cisplatinum also increased the risk of leukemia, indicating that one or both of these drugs is leukemogenic in humans.

Radiation

Ultraviolet

Solar ultraviolet (UV) radiation is the major physical carcinogen in our environment and the primary cause of skin cancer in humans. More than 600,000 individuals will develop new basal cell carcinoma or squamous cell carcinoma of the skin each year in the United States, making nonmelanoma skin cancer the most common cancer.[7] The incidence of both nonmelanoma and melanoma skin cancer among light-skinned individuals is increasing at 3%–5% per year in the United States. This increase has been attributed to changing life-style and leisure habits over the past four decades, resulting in an increase in the number of people receiving greater exposure to sunlight. Although basal cell carcinoma occurs more frequently than squamous cell carcinoma (the ratio of basal cell to squamous cell carcinoma is approximately 4:1), the incidence of squamous cell carcinoma appears to be increasing more rapidly than that of basal cell carcinoma. In addition, squamous cell carcinoma metastasizes more frequently and is responsible for more deaths than are caused by basal cell carcinoma.

The relationship between solar UV exposure and skin cancer in humans has been demonstrated from incidence data in human populations residing at different latitudes. The incidence of nonmelanoma skin cancer (basal and squamous cell carcinomas) exhibits a generally increasing trend with decreasing latitude among individuals with similar skin types.[7] Nonmelanoma skin cancers and the premalignant skin neoplasm, actinic keratosis, are also associated with cumulative lifetime UV exposure estimated from outdoor activities. This is particularly apparent among those with outdoor occupations such as farmers and sailors. The anatomic distribution of these skin neoplasms, primarily on sun-exposed areas, including the face, ears, neck, and hands, is consistent with a solar etiology. The phenotypic characteristics of light skin complexion, ease of sunburning (skin type), and light hair color are known to enhance the risk of nonmelanoma skin cancer. Pigmentation of the skin, either constitutive or induced (as in tanning), clearly plays an important role in protecting skin from the carcinogenic effects of UV radiation. Individuals with moderately to heavily pigmented skin (Latin, Hispanic, Negroid) exhibit much lower rates of skin cancer than do those with poorly or nonpigmented skin (Celtic, albino). The importance of pigmentation is

also demonstrated by the finding that susceptibility to sunburn is a strong indicator of risk of both basal and squamous cell carcinoma.

Molecular evidence also supports an etiologic role of solar UV in human skin cancer. Increased levels of DNA photodamage are detected in the normal epidermis of individuals following exposure to solar UV radiation. In addition, analysis of mutational spectra in human non-melanoma skin cancer DNA shows that mutations specific for UV radiation (dipyrimidine mutations) are frequently present.

Animal studies confirm the carcinogenic effects of UV radiation and indicate that the UV-B portion (280–320 nm) of the solar spectrum is primarily responsible for the carcinogenic properties of sunlight. This wave band encompasses the long-wavelength end of the absorbance spectrum of DNA (Fig. 10-2) and has been shown to cause mutations in mammalian cells. Stratospheric ozone efficiently absorbs UV-B wavelengths below 300 nm, thereby determining the short-wavelength end of the solar spectrum reaching the earth's surface. Concern over the destruction of stratospheric ozone due to environmental pollution with chlorofluorocarbons, resulting in increased intensity of UV-B radiation at the earth's surface, has encouraged the refinement of risk estimates for human skin cancer under conditions of reduced atmospheric ozone.

Ionizing

The discovery and manipulation of ionizing radiation in the early 20th century led to detrimental health effects among many researchers. Toxicity, radiation burns, and cancer were observed among handlers of radioactive materials. The deaths of Marie Curie and Thomas Edison's assistant from cancer have been attributed to severe radiation exposure. The use of radium in luminous paint during the 1930s led to a high incidence of osteosarcoma

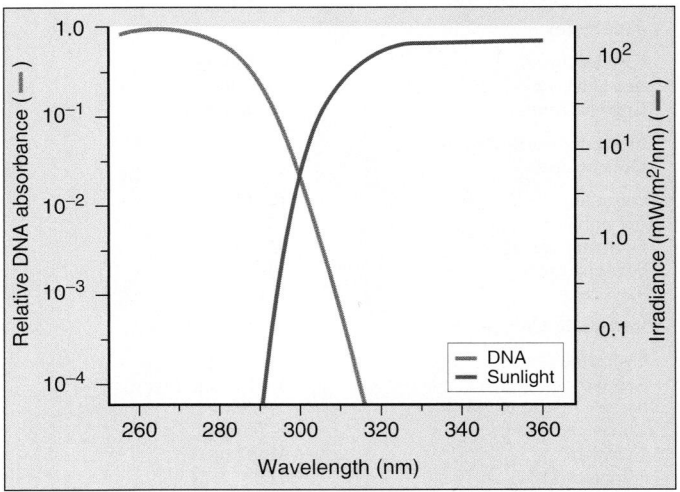

Figure 10-2. Overlap between the wavelengths of solar ultraviolet radiation reaching the earth's surface and the absorbance spectrum of DNA.

among dial painters who inadvertently ingested radium when shaping their brush tips with the tongue.[1] By the 1940s, an elevated incidence of leukemia was observed among radiologists. After World War II, excess leukemia was observed among atomic bomb survivors and among patients treated with x-rays.

Epidemiologic studies of populations exposed to high doses of radiation indicate increased risks for a variety of cancers, depending on the type of radiation and route of exposure (Table 10-3). Among atomic bomb blast survivors, excess leukemias appeared within several years of exposure, whereas excess cancers of the breast, lung, esophagus, thyroid, colon, bladder, ovary, and multiple myeloma appeared only 20–25 years later. In contrast, populations exposed to nuclear weapons fallout exhibit only excess risk of thyroid cancer due to radioactive iodine. Heavy exposure to x-rays for diagnostic or therapeutic procedures has been associated with increased risk of the following types of cancers:

- Leukemia after in utero exposure
- Breast cancer after repeated chest exposure
- Leukemia, lung, stomach, and esophagus after spinal exposure
- Thyroid, skin, and neck after scalp or thymus exposure[5]

The use of cobalt 60 x-ray treatment for cervical cancer is associated with leukemia and cancers of the stomach, rectum, bladder, vagina, buccal cavity, nasopharynx, and lung. Because most radiation exposure in ambient or occupational environments occurs as protracted low-dose exposure, an important public health concern is the cancer risk from low-level exposure. Most of these risk estimates are extrapolated from high to low doses and from acute to chronic exposures and are therefore subject to a number of assumptions that profoundly influence the resulting low-level risk estimates. Populations with potential (or known) low-level radiation exposures include employees in the nuclear industry, individuals living near nuclear production or storage facilities, military personnel participating in atmospheric nuclear weapons tests or living near test sites, patients receiving diagnostic radiation, and residents of buildings with radon contamination. In addition, nuclear accidents such as the Chernobyl incident in the former Soviet Union produce both acute and chronic exposure to local and distant populations.

Radon

Radon gas is encountered in hard rock mining for iron, tin, fluorspar, and uranium.[7] The radioactive decay of radon and its products produces alpha particles. The earliest reports defining an association between lung cancer and mining described the high rate of lung cancers among uranium miners in the Schneeberg region of Czechoslovakia in the late nineteenth century. A variety of potential causes were proposed, including radon inhalation. Studies of lung cancer mortality among Colorado uranium miners demonstrated dose-related increases in lung cancer risk in miners with protracted

TABLE 10-3

Examples of Radiation-Induced Cancers		
SOURCES OF EXPOSURE	**EXPOSURE CIRCUMSTANCES**	**CANCER TYPES**
Explosions of Nuclear Weapons		
Blast	Atomic bombing survivors in Hiroshima and Nagasaki	Leukemia, breast, lung, thyroid, stomach, colon, multiple myeloma, esophagus, ovary
Fallout	Populations exposed through atmospheric testing, including Marshall Islanders, veterans in the Pacific, general population in Nevada, Utah	Thyroid
Diagnostic Procedures		
X-rays	Children exposed in utero	Leukemia
Thorotrast	Cerebral and limb angiography; of biliary passages	Liver
Fluoroscopic x-ray	Monitoring of lung infections in patients with tuberculosis	Breast
Therapeutic Procedures		
X-ray	Postpartum mastitis	Breast
X-ray	Ankylosing spondylitis	Leukemia, lung, stomach, esophagus
Cobalt-60	Treatment for cancer of the cervix	Leukemia, stomach, rectum, bladder, vagina, female genital, lung, buccal cavity, nasopharynx, esophagus
X-ray	Treatment of benign head and neck conditions	Thyroid, skin, central nervous system
Radium-224	Ankylosing spondylitis, bone tuberculosis	Bone sarcoma
Professional Exposures		
X-ray	Early radiologists	Skin, leukemia
Radon	Uranium, hard-rock miners	Lung cancer
X-ray, γ-rays, neutrons	Nuclear industry	Multiple myeloma
Radium isotopes	Radium dial painters	Bone, head sarcoma

Adapted from Higginson J, Muir CS, Munoz N: Human cancer: Epidemiology and environmental causes. Cambridge monographs on cancer reseach. Cambridge, Cambridge University Press, 1992.

exposure to radon.[1] In addition, small cell undifferentiated carcinomas predominated in highly exposed miners, in contrast to the typical distribution of pulmonary cancer pathology in the general United States population. Elevated risk of lung cancer has also been reported for iron ore miners in England, France, and Sweden; however, the proportion of risk attributable to radon in these populations is difficult to assess.

Analysis of lung cancer mortality and smoking in Colorado uranium miners suggests a greater than additive mortality rate for cumulative radon exposure and cumulative cigarette smoking.[7] In other words, the increased risk of lung cancer among miners compared with nonminers is larger when comparing smokers than when comparing nonsmokers. Interestingly, among atomic bomb survivors, cigarette smoking and radiation exposure have only an additive effect of lung cancer risk. This anomaly has been attributed to the different exposure patterns experienced by atomic bomb survivors (acute) and uranium miners (protracted).

Metals

Arsenic

Medicinal use of inorganic arsenic was associated with skin cancers in the early 20th century. More recently, excess skin cancer has been observed in populations exposed to arsenic-contaminated drinking water, whereas excess lung cancer has been found in populations with occupational exposure to inorganic arsenic compounds.[1] An increased risk of lung cancer of six- to 14-fold was reported for gold miners in Rhodesia, where the ore contains arsenic. Chronic arsenism was also prevalent among these miners. Several studies in Japan, Sweden, and the United States have documented excess lung cancers among workers involved in copper smelting. Inorganic arsenic is a byproduct of the smelting process and is also used as a hardener. Two large retrospective studies of copper smelters have shown that lung cancer mortality is related to estimated arsenic exposure.

Another source of occupational exposure is the manufacture and use of arsenical pesticides.[1] An early study of mortality among workers at a factory manufacturing arsenical sheep dip in Wales found an excess of skin and lung cancers, particularly among those directly involved in the chemical processes. Case control studies in two United States plants manufacturing arsenical pesticides found arsenic dose-related increases in risk of lung cancer. Reports of skin and lung cancers among vineyard workers with exposure to arsenic fungicides and pesticides appeared during the late 1950s. An autopsy series of 82 vineyard workers exposed in Germany found 61 deaths from cancer, including 44 respiratory tract cancers; multiple skin cancers and Bowen's disease were also reported.

Nickel

The nickel refining industry was established in South Wales around 1900. During the subsequent 40 years, evidence accumulated for increased rates of nasal cancer, and later, lung cancer among workers in nickel refineries.[7]

Several prospective studies in England and Wales found elevated risks of nasal cancer (O/E = 12) and lung cancer (O/E = 16), particularly among process workers in the refinery. The highest cancer risk was associated with the calcination of impure nickel copper sulfate. Further studies indicated that the cancer risk began to decline when environmental controls were introduced in the industry during the 1930s. Evidence of excess cancer risk associated with nickel exposure as late as the 1950s was reported in a refinery in Norway, however. Excess nasal, laryngeal, and lung cancers were observed; smoking and nickel exposure appeared to contribute to lung cancer risk in an additive manner.

Cadmium

Elevated risk of prostate and lung cancer among workers exposed to cadmium has been reported. Cadmium exposure has a stronger association with lung cancer than with prostate cancer.[7] Several small historical prospective studies of cadmium smelters and battery workers show increased risks of prostate cancer (O/E = 1.2 to 3.5) and lung cancer (O/E = 1.35); however, a larger study of 7000 workers exposed to cadmium for at least one year showed no increased risk of prostate cancer. A major nonoccupational source of cadmium exposure is from cigarette smoke, which contains 1–2 μg cadmium per pack of cigarettes.

Chromates

Several reports of lung cancer in chromate industry workers appeared in Germany during the 1930s. Subsequent epidemiologic investigations examined this association in workers involved in chromate production, chromate pigment manufacture, and chrome plating.[7] Excess lung cancer was found among workers in three chromate production plants in England (threefold excess) and in a production plant in Baltimore (twofold excess). Exposure to lead and zinc chromate pigments, but not to lead pigment alone, was related to excess lung cancer in a British study. Confirmatory results have been reported for workers exposed to lead and zinc chromates in the Netherlands, West Germany, and Norway. Experimental investigations indicate that the hexavalent salts of chromium are highly carcinogenic, whereas trivalent chromium is not carcinogenic.

Fibers and Dusts

Asbestos

The appearance of lung cancer in asbestosis patients was first reported in the 1930s. Over the next 50 years, a variety of study complications were recognized and overcome in the process of determining the lung cancer risk associated with the naturally occurring silicate fiber, asbestos.[5] A major problem was exposure assessment, as many workers were mobile, having variable levels of exposure in a variety of industries or worksites. Furthermore, measurement techniques for asbestos fibers were also variable, making the use of historical measurements suspect. Some studies did not report asbestos type; that is, chrysotile, amosite, anthophyllite, or crocidolite. The long latency period between first exposure and lung cancer reported by Selikoff[15] complicates risk estimates. Misdiagnosis of the cancer pathologies specific to asbestos (mesothelioma) is a potential problem, especially in studies that depend on death certificates.

More than 30 epidemiologic studies have been mounted to examine lung cancer risk in workers with potential exposure to asbestos during mining, milling, manufacturing, insulating, and shipbuilding.[1] In general, these studies demonstrate enhanced risk of lung cancer, and possibly enhanced risk of laryngeal cancer. The association between asbestos exposure and mesothelioma of the lung, a relatively rare cancer, was reported in the early 1960s. This finding was confirmed among insulation workers, asbestos manufacturing workers, and other occupationally exposed populations.

Cases of pleural malignancies in Denmark and Germany in the 1930s were reported to be concentrated in seaport towns rather than in other urban areas. Later studies of the geographic distribution of mesothelioma deaths in England and Wales demonstrated a correlation between mesothelioma and areas of high asbestos use related to shipbuilding, gas mask manufacture, or asbestos manufacturing. Further studies led to the conclusion that risk of mesothelioma was not limited to the workers but extended to members of their household and to residents living in the vicinity of asbestos-related industries.

Evidence of a synergistic effect of asbestos and smoking for lung cancer risk was found among insulation workers in New York.[7] The age-standardized mortality ratio for lung cancer was 5.2 for nonsmoking asbestos-exposed workers (compared with nonexposed nonsmokers), 10.8 for nonexposed smokers, and 53.2 for asbestos-exposed smokers. Thus, the risk of lung cancer from both smoking and exposure to asbestos is much greater than the sum of the risks associated with either exposure. A similar result was reported for female workers at a British asbestos factory, but the results for male workers at the same factory could not distinguish between additive or multiplicative effects.

Silica

Exposure to silica dusts occurs in several occupational groups, including foundry workers, pottery workers, miners, and quarrymen. Examination of occupational mortality statistics and high-exposure segments of these industries consistently show an increased risk for lung cancer among silica-exposed workers.[1] Two studies using silicosis registries have shown an association between silicosis and lung cancer. Excess mortality from lung cancer (O/E = 2.8) was found among 3,600 men recorded in the Swedish silicosis registry from 1931 to 1969. An excess of lung cancer deaths (O/E = 2.0) was also found among 1,910 miners registered with silicosis in Ontario from 1940 to 1975. Pottery workers in the United States exhibited a significant excess of lung cancer among men whose work entailed making ceramic plumbing fixtures.

Wood Dusts

The cancer risk associated with wood dust has been investigated in furniture workers, carpenters, wood-workers, lumberjacks, sawmill workers, and paper or pulp mill workers.[7] Excess nasal adenocarcinoma is found consistently among furniture workers in several countries, primarily with exposure in the 1920s and 1930s. The highest risk is seen among those with exposure to hardwood dusts, and after a latent period of 30 years. Small increases in risk of larynx cancer, lung cancer, and Hodgkin's disease have also been reported among persons with these occupations.

DIETARY MODIFIERS OF CARCINOGENESIS: NATURALLY OCCURRING CARCINOGENS AND ANTICARCINOGENS

Most of the known human carcinogens discussed in the foregoing sections have been identified from occupational and iatrogenic exposures; however, such agents are rather minor contributors to the current overall cancer burden. Exposures to many of these agents have been typically at high doses in small, well-defined cohorts. Most human cancers likely result from interactions of several or more carcinogenic influences, none of which singly is readily detectable. The carcinogenic process is subject to influence by many modifying factors, which in the aggregate probably represent the largest determinant of human cancer. These factors can be constitutive, including age, gender, immunologic status, and genetic composition. Extraconstitutional factors are also very important, particularly diet and lifestyle habits such as smoking and alcohol consumption. Many epidemiologic studies indicate that general increases in consumption of fiber-rich cereals, fruits, and vegetables and decreased consumption of fat-rich foods and excessive alcohol will serve as prudent approaches to reducing overall cancer risk.

Many components in the diet can contribute to carcinogenesis. Two major influences are fat and calorie consumption. Fat consumption is most strongly associated with the hormone-dependent cancers (breast, ovary, and endometrium in females and prostate in males) and the gastrointestinal cancers (gallbladder, colon, and rectum in both sexes). It is not known whether these relationships are causal and, if so, whether they relate to the type of fat (saturated, unsaturated, polyunsaturated) or to the overall caloric content of the diet. Dietary fat intervention studies such as the Women's Health Trial might provide direct information on the effects of reducing dietary fat consumption on the incidences of cancer and other diseases. Decreased fat consumption could exert protective effects through both direct and indirect means. Fats can promote tumor development directly and are also a major source of calories. Animals fed high-fat diets consistently demonstrated enhanced tumorigenic outcomes. Conversely, it has been recognized for decades that caloric restriction has a very powerful, general inhibitory effect on carcinogenesis in many induced and spontaneous laboratory animal tumor models. The behavioral changes required to affect comparable population-wide reductions in fat and/or calorie consumption, however, pose formidable challenges.

Many minor dietary components act as carcinogens or anticarcinogens.[16] Dozens of natural mutagens and carcinogens derived from plant, fungal, and bacterial sources have been described, which present a significant carcinogenic challenge to humans. These natural carcinogens, however, are opposed by an equally expansive array of food-derived anticarcinogens. These anticarcinogens consist of both nutrient (e.g., vitamins, minerals) and non-nutrient components, many of which function as antioxidants. In addition to scavenging oxidants, many of the non-nutrient anticarcinogens in plants alter the balance between the metabolic activation and inactivation of chemical carcinogens. Inverse epidemiologic associations between risk of cancer at several sites and ingestion of fruits and vegetables have been observed.[17] These associations might be linked to β-carotene, other carotenoids, folate, fiber, vitamin C, and other antioxidants, and to other components of the fruits and vegetables. Although a protective role of specific nutrients has been difficult to establish in many instances, inverse relationships between intake of vitamin C-rich foods and oral, esophageal, and gastric cancer incidence and between β-carotene intake and lung cancer incidence have been described. A fuller understanding of the role of dietary factors in human carcinogenesis is destined to have a significant impact on disease incidence.

EXPOSURE BIOMARKERS AND SUSCEPTIBILITY FACTORS

Assessing Human Exposure: Role for Intermediate Biomarkers

Increased understanding of the mechanistic basis of carcinogenesis provides opportunities for the identification of molecular biologic markers reflecting events occurring between exposure and clinical disease. These molecular biologic markers can be classified into three major categories:

1. Markers of exposure reflecting either an internal or a biologically effective dose of carcinogen
2. Markers of effect indicating a biologic response to an exposure
3. Markers of susceptibility that characterize the inherent susceptibility of an individual to a carcinogenic agent[18]

It is anticipated that the use of biologic markers will help define the roles of environmental agents (particularly in complex mixtures) in the etiology of human cancer.

The interaction of a carcinogen with macromolecules was demonstrated by Miller and Miller in 1947, when they showed that azo dye bound to the liver protein of treated

---

DO CARCINOGENS IN FRIED AND BROILED MEATS CONTRIBUTE TO RISK OF COLON CANCER?

The risk of colon cancer is strongly associated with consumption of red meat and animal fat. This association has been observed in a number of international correlative studies and case-control studies. A prospective study of colon cancer risk among women demonstrated an association with consumption of red meat and animal fat (but not with vegetable fat), independent of total energy intake.[36] The increased risk associated with animal fat was due primarily to meat intake as opposed to dairy product intake. The relative risk of colon cancer in women who consumed beef, pork, or lamb daily was 2.5 (95% confidence interval, 1.2–5.0) compared with those who consumed these meats less than once a month. In another study that addressed cooking practices, consumption of fried foods and barbecued, broiled, or smoked meats was associated with increased risk of cancer at specific colorectal subsites in men.[37]

Despite these observations, and despite rapid advances in the molecular genetics of susceptibility and predisposition, the specific chemical etiologies of colon and other diet-associated cancers remain unclear. Several hypotheses have been proposed to explain the strong association of colon cancer risk with red meat and animal fat. Diets high in fat increase the incidence of chemically induced colon cancers in rats and also increase the excretion of primary bile acids, which are converted to secondary bile acids by bacterial metabolism. Some secondary bile acids (e.g., deoxycholic and lithocholic acid) are colon tumor promoters in animal models. Thus, it has been hypothesized that increased animal fat in the human diet leads to promotion of colon tumors by secondary bile acids. An alternative (or complementary) hypothesis is that carcinogens in cooked meats contribute to

colon carcinogenesis. The cooking of meat produces at least two major classes of carcinogens—polycyclic aromatic hydrocarbons (PAHs) and heterocyclic aromatic amines—which induce genotoxic damage or cancer in the gastrointestinal tracts of animals receiving these compounds orally.[38] Cooked meats are a major source of animal fat in Western diets; it has been suggested that cooking-induced carcinogens in meat, rather than animal fat, play a causative role in colon cancer. Estimates of average daily ingestion of PAHs and heterocyclic amines from diet are comparable (0.1–10 mg/d).

In addition to PAHs, highly mutagenic heterocyclic amine compounds are formed during the broiling or frying of meat and fish due to pyrolysis of amino acids and proteins. More than a dozen heterocyclic amines have been identified; the most common forms are quinolines, quinoxalines, pyridines, and carbolines.[38] Examples include 2-amino-3-methylimidazo(4,5-f)quinoline (IQ), 2-amino-3,8-dimethylimidazo(4,5-f)quinoxaline (8-MeIQx), 2-amino-1-methyl-6-phenylimidazo(4,5-b)pyridine (PhIP), and 3-amino-1,4-dimethyl-5H-pyrido(4,3-b)indole (Trp-P-1). These compounds are highly mutagenic in bacteria and carcinogenic in animals, causing colon cancer, mammary cancer, liver cancer, prostate cancer, and lymphoma. PhIP is one of the most common heterocyclic amines formed in broiled and fried meats, occurring at levels comparable to or greater than those of benzo[a]pyrene. Male rats fed PhIP develop colon adenocarcinomas, whereas female rats develop mammary adenocarcinomas. The role of heterocyclic amine compounds and PAHs in the etiology of human colon cancer, however, is still under investigation and remains to be determined.

rats. Later studies indicated the importance of carcinogen modification of DNA (either directly or after metabolic activation) in the cancer process. The measurement of carcinogen metabolites, carcinogen-DNA adducts, or carcinogen-protein adducts in human tissues or fluids provide the basis for molecular dosimetry research and the rapidly expanding field of "molecular" cancer epidemiology. The potential advantage of this approach is that more accurate assessments of individual or group dose may be achieved than through estimates of carcinogen exposure in the environment or workplace.

Carcinogen-DNA and carcinogen-protein adducts have been detected in tissues from a variety of human populations with known or suspected carcinogen exposure.[9,19] PAH-DNA adducts are elevated in white blood cells from individuals occupationally exposed to airborne PAHs, including coke oven workers, foundry workers, and aluminum plant workers. Increased levels of PAH-DNA adducts have also been reported in lung tissue from heavy smokers. DNA isolated from exfoliated bladder epithelial cells of cigarette smokers has been shown to contain 4-aminobiphenyl adducts. Alkylation damage has been detected in DNA from esophageal tissue of persons living in regions with documented dietary exposure to nitrosamines. Aflatoxin adducts are found in hepatic DNA following dietary exposure to this mycotoxin. Cisplatin-DNA intrastrand adducts have been measured in white blood cells of patients undergoing cancer chemotherapy.

Carcinogen-DNA adducts excreted in urine provide a noninvasive means for quantifying DNA damage. Urinary concentration of aflatoxin-guanine adducts is strongly correlated with dietary aflatoxin intake. In addition to their use as indicators of previous carcinogen exposure, DNA adducts have the potential for use as direct indicators of future cancer risk. The first prospective test of this application appeared in 1992, when detectable levels of aflatoxin-guanine adducts, as well as several other aflatoxin metabolites, in urine were shown to be predictive of liver cancer development.[10] Furthermore, an interactive effect for liver cancer risk was seen between urinary aflatoxin biomarkers and HBV infection history.

Carcinogen-protein adducts have also proved useful as biomarkers of human exposure. Alkylation damage in hemoglobin has been used as an exposure index in risk assessment analyses of individuals occupationally exposed to ethylene oxide. 4-aminobiphenyl adducts in hemoglobin are highly specific (and sensitive) markers of exposure to cigarette smoke.[9] The level of 4-aminobiphenyl hemoglobin adducts is related to the number of cigarettes smoked, the type of tobacco, and the metabolic phenotype of the smoker. The levels of these adducts drop markedly after smoking cessation.

Unreacted carcinogen metabolites excreted in urine are also used to monitor human exposure to and uptake of carcinogens and related compounds. Concentrations of hydroxylated PAHs (e.g., 1-hydroxypyrene) in urine are elevated in smokers, in patients after topical treatment with coal-tar, in road pavers, in coke-oven workers, in aluminum plant workers, and in individuals ingesting PAHs from food.[20] In occupational settings, the concentration of urinary 1-hydroxypyrene is highly correlated with estimated or measured concentrations of airborne PAHs. This noninvasive approach to exposure assessment has potential application as a routine biomonitoring tool. In all these studies, significant differences in adduct or metabolite levels are observed between individuals with similar carcinogen exposure. These differences have been attributed to several factors, including individual biologic variability, exposure misclassification, and confounding variables such as diet, physical activity, smoking, or personal environment. An understanding of the true basis for these differences will be useful in elucidating the determinants of individual susceptibility to cancer. By identifying specific modulators that enhance or inhibit carcinogen metabolism and the formation of adducts, it will be possible to examine their effects on human cancer risk.

Metabolic Polymorphisms and Human Susceptibility

Another major area of research in molecular cancer epidemiology is the study of individual metabolic phenotypes and their roles in determining biomarker levels and human susceptibility to environmental carcinogens.[21] Certain cytochrome P-450 metabolic enzymes are known to be involved in the activation of specific human carcinogens, and some have been linked to increased cancer risk. For example, inducible P450 1A1 activity is higher in cultured lymphocytes from lung cancer cases than in controls. Two genetic polymorphisms in the P450 1A1 structural gene have also been tentatively associated with lung cancer risk in Japan.

Hepatic arylamine N-acetyltransferase correlates with individual differences in susceptibility to both bladder and colorectal cancers in humans.[21] A series of genetic polymorphisms of this enzyme exist in humans, resulting in slow- and rapid-acetylator phenotypes. Interestingly, the rapid-acetylator phenotype appears to protect aromatic amine-exposed individuals from bladder cancer; however, the same rapid phenotype might enhance risk of colorectal cancer. These results are attributed to the fact that N-acetylation of arylamines competes against the formation of reactive arylamine metabolites that reach the bladder, whereas acetyltransferase in the colonic mucosa can O-acetylate N-hydroxyarylamine metabolites to highly reactive derivatives.

A recent meta-analysis of 22 case-control studies in the general population examined the effect of slow acetylation on risk of bladder cancer.[22] Overall, the slow acetylation phenotype/genotype was found to increase risk of bladder cancer by about 40% compared with rapid acetylators (odds ratio of 1.4, with 95% confidence interval of 1.2–1.6). This is the clearest example of a common metabolically modified cancer risk in the general population. The carcinogenic exposure in this case is, presumably, due to aryl amine compounds from various sources, including cigarette smoke.

DNA Repair and Human Susceptibility

An important mechanism that protects the genome from mutagenic effects of carcinogens is the repair of cellular

DNA. The importance of this protection is perhaps best illustrated by the unusually severe effects of sunlight on individuals who are deficient in DNA repair.[23] The rare inherited disorder xeroderma pigmentosum (XP) is characterized by various levels of DNA-repair deficiencies. Individuals with XP exhibit an unusually high incidence of multiple skin cancers and might not live beyond early adulthood in the absence of protective measures against sunlight. The median age of onset for nonmelanoma skin cancers among XP patients is approximately eight years of age, compared with about 60 years of age in the general population. In addition, the prevalence of melanoma of the skin is unusually high among XP patients.

Several other inherited diseases exhibit altered cellular response to DNA damage.[24] Ataxia telangiectasia (AT), Bloom syndrome, and Fanconi's anemia are autosomal recessive genetic disorders characterized by chromosomal instability, with patients developing malignancies more frequently and at younger age than occurs in the general population. Approximately 10% of AT patients develop malignancies, primarily of the lymphoreticular system, before the age of 20. Heterozygous relatives of AT patients and Fanconi's anemia patients are also at moderately increased risk of cancer compared with unrelated persons.

Although these diseases clearly represent unusual cases, some forms of these diseases (e.g., complementation group XP-E) exhibit only moderate deficiencies in DNA repair—approximately 60%–90% of normal–yet remain unusually susceptible to cancer. This finding suggests that small reductions in DNA repair efficiency could lead to considerable increases in cancer susceptibility. Interestingly, significant variability in DNA repair proficiency has been demonstrated among disease-free "normal" individuals. This variability in the general population could contribute to differences in susceptibility not only to skin cancer but also to cancers of other organs.

PUBLIC HEALTH APPROACHES TO CANCER PREVENTION

An aging population and a decline in mortality from cardiovascular disease could herald the emergence of cancer as the major cause of death in the United States. Moreover, the curative treatment of many established (and especially disseminated) malignancies remains an enigmatic problem for which progress is measured in small steps. Clearly, the optimal way for dealing with virtually all diseases, including cancer, is prevention. As a consequence, the challenge to public health professionals is to devise and implement preventive measures against cancer.

As presented in Figure 10-3, the prevention of cancer can take several forms. Primary prevention targets healthy individuals and can be achieved by avoiding exposure to risk factors. Another approach is to stimulate the defense mechanisms of the host to interfere with the carcinogenic

HEALTH EFFECTS AND CONTROL OF SMOKING

A series of reports from the U.S. Surgeon General since 1964 have argued that cigarette smoking is the most significant source of preventable morbidity and premature mortality in developed countries. An estimated annual excess mortality of 350,000 is attributed to cigarette smoking in the United States. These deaths are the result of coronary heart disease, cancer, and various respiratory diseases.[32] Cancers associated with smoking or smokeless tobacco use include those of the lung, oral cavity, esophagus, larnyx, and bladder. Weaker associations have been reported for cancers of the pancreas, kidney, and cervix. The overall increase in risk of disease among smokers compared with nonsmokers is about tenfold for lung cancer, sixfold for chronic obstructive pulmonary disease, and twofold for myocardial infarction. The combined effect of smoking-related diseases on the average life expectancy of smokers is a reduction of five to eight years.

On a worldwide basis, the data is equally disturbing. An estimated three million deaths in 1995 were attributed to tobacco use; roughly two million of these were in developed countries and one million in developing countries. If current usage trends continue unabated, estimates as high as 10 million deaths due to tobacco use annually could be expected by the year 2025.[33] The majority of these deaths (seven million) are expected to occur in developing countries, where tobacco use is increasing rapidly. Whereas percentage of world tobacco consumption in developing countries was 49% in 1974–1976, this figure increased to 61% in 1984–1986 and was projected to rise to 71% by the year 2000.[34] Per capita consumption of cigarettes is increasing most rapidly in developing Asian countries.

Although the majority of tobacco is produced in developing countries, the declining market in developed countries has refocused the efforts of producers in these countries toward developing countries for continued growth.

The addictive properties of tobacco smoking, due primarily to nicotine, cause both physiological and psychological dependence. Withdrawal symptoms can be severe and include irritability, aggressiveness, hostility, depression, difficulty concentrating and a craving for tobacco. These pharmacological factors are reinforced by social factors such as peer pressure, emulation of family role models, and cultural influences. Because most smokers begin smoking, and often form lifelong smoking habits, in their teenage years, much of the advertising effort of tobacco companies is aimed at this age group.

Smoking control measures use various strategies: cessation programs, clinical or community interventions, governmental or private-sector regulations, taxation of tobacco products, and smoking prevention programs.[35] Although the majority of ex-smokers have achieved abstinence without extensive personal assistance from organized cessation programs, other control measures (national health education programs, physician counseling, indoor smoking regulations) and family pressure are important influences contributing to smoking cessation. Smoking prevention programs, particularly in schools, and government taxation have been somewhat effective in reducing the initiation of smoking among children and adolescents in developing countries. These approaches will need to be applied in developing countries to stem the expansion of smoking worldwide.

Figure 10-3. Strategies for prevention of multistage carcinogenesis.

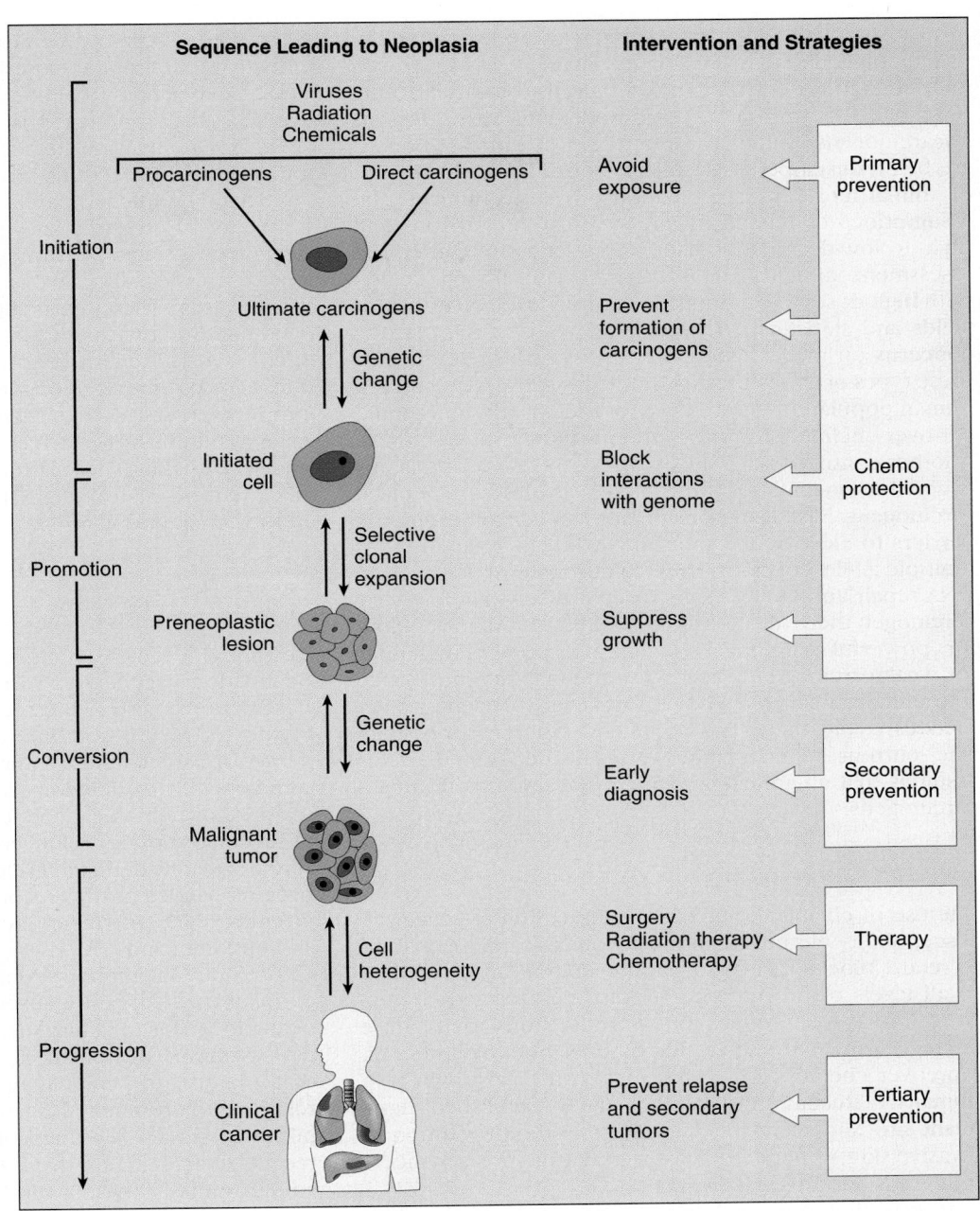

process. Secondary prevention measures use early detection and intervention before pathologic conditions are clinically apparent. The success of these strategies will be greatly facilitated by the development of noninvasive biomarkers that identify high-risk individuals. Finally, tertiary prevention is aimed at minimizing the effect of existing disease and consequent disability by avoiding development of new cancers and complications or relapses after therapy for initial malignancies.

Identifying Human Carcinogens

The major current strategy for cancer prevention is the avoidance of exposure to environmental, industrial, and social hazards. Identification of human carcinogens takes

two forms. In several instances (e.g., soot and coal tars, aromatic amines, vinyl chloride, and benzene), carcinogenic compounds were discovered after they were suspected of being involved in the development of cancers in humans. Most carcinogenic substances, however, are identified in the course of long-term toxicologic studies in animals. The value of this approach is buttressed by the fact that for those chemicals identified as being causally associated with human cancer, and for which there has been adequate experimental evaluation, all have been shown to cause cancer in laboratory animals.[25] However, animal bioassays for carcinogenicity are very costly (several million dollars per compound) and time consuming (five years). Therefore, much attention is being directed toward the development and validation of short-

Science of Clinical Oncology

1

term tests for carcinogens. Many assays for genotoxicity using mutagenesis, chromosome damage, or DNA repair as endpoints are used to screen chemicals for carcinogenic potential. Short-term assays for modifying factors such as cocarcinogens, tumor promoters, and anticarcinogens are being developed as well. A major difficulty in the use of animal bioassays is estimation of risk to humans. The assumptions contained in interspecies comparisons and high- to low-dose extrapolations render a straightforward assessment difficult. Bioassays are typically conducted with high doses of carcinogens to provide adequate tumor yields and statistical strength; however, there are strong concerns on mechanistic grounds as to the relevance of these types of exposures to chronic low-dose exposures in human populations. Protective host-defense systems could be overwhelmed in these aberrant exposure settings. Another controversial issue in dose-response relationships is whether no-effect or threshold levels exist for chemical carcinogens. Based on considerations of metabolism, the barriers to electrophiles reaching critical targets in DNA, multiple alleles for transforming and/or suppressor genes, DNA repair, and other factors, it seems likely that for every carcinogen there must be a threshold. It could be very low for powerful carcinogens and correspondingly higher for weak carcinogens. Faced with the inability in practice to define human thresholds, however, prudent policy dictates avoidance of carcinogens wherever possible. The current regulatory posture in the United States assumes that all animal carcinogens are potential human carcinogens.

Cancer Chemoprevention

The use of chemical or dietary interventions to alter the susceptibility of humans to the actions of carcinogens and to retard, block, or reverse carcinogenesis can be applied to all levels of prevention and has been termed chemoprevention.[26] There are many indications that these strategies are extremely effective in laboratory animals. Moreover, chemoprevention against cancer also works in humans.[27] Recent investigations have established significant site- and agent-specific effects in the prevention of invasive skin, upper aerodigestive tract, and breast cancers in high-risk groups.

It was first observed in the early part of the 20th century that carcinogenesis could be modified by discrete chemical agents. These initial experiments demonstrated that the formation of skin tumors in rodents could be blocked by local application of chemopreventive agents. The protective agents used in these early studies, however, were typically carcinogens or toxins themselves. Consequently, their application to humans did not appear to be practical. Thus, the field of cancer chemoprevention did not receive significant attention until the early 1970s, when Wattenberg demonstrated that dietary antioxidants could protect against tumor formation. The experimental observations that seemingly innocuous preservatives found in the Western diet could dramatically protect against diverse carcinogens at distal sites sparked the development of chemoprevention as a viable strategy for the reduction of human cancers. To date, more than 20

classes of discrete chemicals have been shown to be effective inhibitors of experimental carcinogenesis.[28]

The expectation that effective chemoprotection against cancer can be achieved is supported by the view that cancer is unlikely to be the exception to the history of other major (infectious and noninfectious) diseases of humans, in which the mortality began to decline as a result of protective and preventive measures far in advance of specific treatments. Cancer chemoprevention could be especially valuable in populations at high risk of certain neoplasms, particularly as improved molecular techniques allow for the identification of these high-risk individuals. Preventive strategies can employ both prescriptive interventions with specific nutrients, non-nutrients, and drugs in selected populations at high risk of cancer, and lifestyle changes that include altered nutrition and social habits. These latter approaches might ultimately play an even greater role in the overall reduction of cancer in the general population.

SUMMARY

The carcinogenic effects of many environmental and occupational agents were first described in humans. These observations were replicated in animal models beginning in the early 20th century. Carcinogenic agents come in many forms, including naturally occurring and manufactured chemicals, radiations, metals, fibers, and viruses. The majority of human cancers likely result from interactions of several or more carcinogenic influences, none of which singly is readily detectable. Elucidation of the carcinogenic process has led to the recognition that extrinsic factors interact with intrinsic factors to determine overall susceptibility and risk.

The identification of molecular biologic markers of exposure, effect, and susceptibility, reflecting events occurring prior to clinical disease, will help to further our understanding of human carcinogenesis. It is anticipated that the use of biologic markers will help define the roles of environmental agents (particularly in complex mixtures) in the etiology of human cancers. With the recent characterization of the human genome, much attention has focused on the role of common polymorphisms in carcinogen metabolism or of DNA repair genes and susceptibility to cancer. By identifying specific factors that enhance or inhibit carcinogen metabolism and biomarker formation, it will be possible to examine their effects on human cancer risk.

Primary and secondary approaches to the prevention of cancer will be greatly facilitated by the development of noninvasive biomarkers that identify high-risk individuals. Tertiary prevention might also be enhanced by characterizing cancers with respect to etiology, genetic profile, or metabolic capacity. The use of chemical or dietary interventions to alter the susceptibility of humans to the actions of carcinogens and to retard, block, or reverse carcinogenesis can be applied to all levels of prevention and has been termed chemoprevention. Preventive strategies can employ both prescriptive interventions with specific nutrients, non-nutrients and drugs in selected populations at high risk of cancer, and lifestyle changes that include altered nutrition and social habits.

The major current strategy for cancer prevention is the avoidance of exposure to environmental, industrial, and social hazards that increase the risk of cancer. Currently, most carcinogenic substances are identified in the course of long-term toxicologic studies in animals. Much attention is also directed toward the development and validation of short-term tests for carcinogens, such as mutagenicity, chromosome damage, or DNA repair.

REFERENCES

1. Alderson M: Occupational Cancer. London, Butterworth, 1986.
2. Waldron HA: A brief history of scrotal cancer. Br J Ind Med 1983;40:390–401.
3. Dipple A, Moschel RC, Bigger CAH: Polynuclear aromatic carcinogens. In Searle CE (ed): Chemical Carcinogens, vol 2 (ACS Monograph 182). Washington, DC, American Chemical Society, 1984, p 41.
4. Sontag JM: Carcinogens in Industry and the Environment. New York, Marcel Dekker, 1981.
5. Higginson J, Muir CS, Munoz N: Human Cancer: Epidemiology and Environmental Causes. Cambridge Monographs on Cancer Research. Cambridge, Cambridge University Press, 1992.
6. Case RAM, Hosker ME, McDonald DB, Pearson JT: Tumours of the urinary bladder in workers engaged in the manufacture and use of certain dyestuff intermediates in the British chemical industry. Br J Prev Social Med 1954;11:75.
7. International Agency for Research on Cancer: IARC Monographs on the Evaluation of Carcinogenic Risk to Humans. Vol. 1–83. Lyon, IARC, 1970–2003.
8. Hein DW: Molecular genetics and function of NAT1 and NAT2: Role in aromatic amine metabolism and carcinogenesis. Mut Res 2002;506/507:65–77.
9. Kensler T, Qian GS, Chen JG, Groopman JD: Translational strategies for cancer prevention in liver. Nature Rev Cancer 2003;3:321–329.
10. Ross RK, Yuan JM, Yu MC, et al: Urinary aflatoxin biomarkers and risk of hepatocellular carcinoma. Lancet 1992;339:943–946.
11. Zaridze DG, Peto R (eds): Tobacco: A Major International Health Hazard. (IARC Scientific Publ No. 74). Lyon, International Agency for Cancer Research, 1986.
12. Haddow A, Harris R, Kon G, Roe E: The growth inhibitory and carcinogenic properties of 4-aminostilbene and derivatives. Philos Trans R Soc Lond Biol 1948;1948A:241.
13. Reimer RR, Hoover R, Fraumeni JF: Acute leukemia after alkylating agent therapy of ovarian cancer. N Engl J Med 1977;297:177–181.
14. Kaldor JM, Day NE, Pettersson F, et al: Leukemia following chemotherapy for ovarian cancer: A study of 114 cases and their matched controls. N Engl J Med 1990;322:1–6.
15. Selikoff FJ, Hammond EC, Churg J: Asbestos exposure, smoking, and neoplasia. JAMA 1968;204:106.
16. Ames BN: Dietary carcinogens and anticarcinogens. Science 1983;221:1256–1264.
17. World Cancer Research Fund/American Institute for Cancer Research: In: Food, Nutrition and the Prevention of Cancer: A Global Perspective. Washington, DC, AICR, 1997.
18. Schulte PA, Perera F (eds): Molecular Epidemiology: Principles and Practices. San Diego, Calif., Academic Press, 1993.
19. Groopman JD, Kensler TW: The light at the end of the tunnel for chemical-specific biomarkers: Daylight or headlight? Carcinogenesis 1999;20:1–11.
20. Strickland P, Kang D, Sithisarankul P: Polycyclic aromatic hydrocarbon metabolites in urine as biomarkers of exposure and effect. Environ Health Perspec 1996;104(Suppl 5):927–932.
21. d'Errico A, Taioli E, Chen X, Vineis P: Genetic metabolic polymorphisms and the risk of cancer: A review of the literature. Biomarkers 1996;1:149.
22. Marcus PM, Vineis P, Rothman N: NAT2 slow acetylation and bladder cancer risk: A meta-analysis of 22 case-control studies conducted in the general population. Pharmacogenetics 2000;10:115–122.
23. Moriwaki S, Kraemer KH: Xeroderma pigmentosum—Bridging a gap between clinic and laboratory. Photodermatol Photoimmunol Photomed 2001;17:47–54.
24. Friedberg EC, Walker GC, Siede W: DNA Repair and Mutagenesis. Washington DC, ASM Press, 1995.
25. Huff J: Chemicals causally associated with cancers in humans and in laboratory animals. In Waalkes MP, Ward JM (eds): Carcinogenesis. New York, Raven Press, 1994.
26. Kelloff GJ, Sigman CC, Greenwald P: Cancer chemoprevention: Progress and promise. Eur J Cancer 1999;35:2031–2038.
27. Lippman SM, Hong WK: Cancer prevention by delay: Commentary re: JA O'Shaughnessy et al, Treatment and prevention of intraepithelial neoplasia: An important target for accelerated new agent development. Clin Cancer Res 2002;8:314–346.
28. Prevention of cancer in the next millennium: Report of the Chemoprevention Working Group to the American Association for Cancer Research. Cancer Res 1999;59:4743.
29. Wolff MS, Toniolo PG, Lee EW, Rivera M, Dubin N: Blood levels of organochlorine residues and risk of breast cancer. J Nat Cancer Inst 1993;85:648–652.
30. Hunter DJ, Hankinson SE, Laden F, et al: Plasma organochlorine levels and the risk of breast cancer. N Eng J Med 1997;337:1253–1258.
31. Safe SH: Xenoestrogens and breast cancer. N Eng J Med 1997;337:1303–1304.
32. Smoking and Health: A Report of the Surgeon General. Washington, DC, U.S. Department of Health, Education and Welfare, 1979.
33. Peto R. Smoking and death: The past 40 years and the next 40. BMJ 1994;309:937–939.
34. The Food and Agriculture Organization of the United Nations. Tobacco Supply, Demand and Trade Projections 1995 and 2000. Rome, Food and Agriculture Organization, 1990.
35. Fielding JE: Smoking: health effects and control. In Last JM (ed): Public Health and Preventive Medicine. Norwalk, CT, Appleton Century Crofts, 1986, p 999.
36. Willett WC, Stampfer MJ, Colditz GA, Rosner BA, Speizer FE: Relation of meat, fat, and fiber intake to risk of colon cancer in a prospective study of women. N Engl J Med 1990;323:1664–1672.
37. Peters RK, Garabrant DH, Yu MC, Mack TM: A case-control study of occupational and dietary factors in colorectal cancer in young men by subsite. Cancer Res 1989;49:5459–5468.
38. Knize MG, Kulp KS, Salmon CP, Keating GA, Felton JS: Factors affecting human heterocyclic amine intake and the metabolism of PhIP. Mutat Res 2002;506/507:153–162.

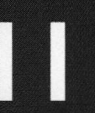
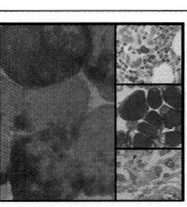

DNA DAMAGE RESPONSE PATHWAYS AND CANCER

James M. Ford

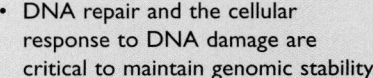

SUMMARY OF KEY POINTS

- DNA repair and the cellular response to DNA damage are critical to maintain genomic stability.
- Defects in the repair or response to DNA damage encountered from endogenous or external sources results in an increased rate of genetic mutations, often leading to the development of cancer.
- Inherited mutations in DNA damage response pathway genes often result in cancer susceptibility.
- The major active pathways for DNA repair in humans are nucleotide excision repair, base excision repair, mismatch DNA repair, and

- homologous recombination or non-homologous end-joining processes for double-strand break repair.
- Defects in nucleotide excision repair lead to the skin cancer–prone syndrome xeroderma pigmentosum, as well as Cockayne syndrome and trichothiodystrophy.
- Defects in base excision repair can result in enhanced colon adenomas and cancers.
- Defects in mismatch repair result in hereditary nonpolyposis colorectal cancer syndrome.
- Defects in DNA double-strand break repair and response pathways

- underlie a number of cancer prone disorders, including ataxia-telangiectasia, Nijmegen breakage syndrome, Bloom syndrome, Werner syndrome, Rothmund-Thompson syndrome, and Fanconi anemia.
- The highly cancer prone Li-Fraumeni syndrome, due to inherited p53 mutations, and breast-ovarian cancer syndrome, due to inherited mutations of the BRCA1 and BRCA2 genes, exhibit defects in multiple DNA repair and DNA damage response pathways.

INTRODUCTION

Cancer is a genetic disease, caused by the accumulation over time of changes to our DNA resulting in altered function of genes important for normal cellular functions and growth properties, including many proto-oncogenes and tumor suppressor genes. Nearly all cancers are clonal in origin; that is, they originate from a single progenitor cell rather than a group of cells. Although this observation provides evidence favoring a genetic rather than an infectious or environmental etiology, it also is now clear that development of cancer in a particular cell type or tissue is caused by a series of specific mutations, each of which could be caused by DNA replication errors, endogenous or exogenous DNA damage, or the result of inherited mutations. For most common cancers, during the process of carcinogenesis multiple genetic events occur in many different genes, suggesting that an early and perhaps necessary event in the cancer process is an underlying defect in mechanisms that should maintain genomic stability. In fact, alterations in the specific genes required for recognizing, processing, and responding to DNA damage may result in an enhanced rate of accumulation of additional mutations, recombinational events, chromosomal abnormalities, and gene amplification.[1] Therefore, DNA repair is essential not only for the basic processes of transcription and replication necessary for cellular survival, but also for maintaining genomic stability and avoiding the development of malignancies. Numerous links have been identified between oncogenesis and acquired or inherited defects in genomic stability that cause a "mutator" phenotype, highlighting the key role of DNA protection systems in tumor prevention. This chapter reviews the major DNA repair mechanisms active in mammalian cells, and our emerging understanding of DNA damage-signaling pathways that integrate with other cellular processes regulating transcription, replication, cell division, and apoptosis in response to DNA damage. The relevance of these mechanisms to cancer is explored by focusing on several human cancer predisposition syndromes caused by underlying defects in DNA damage processing.

Advances in molecular biology and cancer genetics have defined three general groups of genes involved in the development of human cancers: oncogenes, tumor suppressor genes, and DNA damage repair and response genes. The latter set of genes, in particular, are important for inherited cancer susceptibility, due to their direct involvement in genomic stability. Much of what we know regarding cancer genes in sporadic tumors comes from the study of relatively rare inherited familial cancer syndromes caused by mutations passed along in the germ-line DNA of families and predisposing to the development of cancers, often at a very young age and at a high incidence, in affected carriers. Individuals who inherit a germ-line mutation in genes involved in or required for DNA repair usually are at increased risk for the development of cancer due to the enhanced frequency of mutations and increased genomic instability. Susceptibility to cancer is also affected by environmental factors and low-penetrance modifier genes.

191

Many recently converging lines of experimental evidence reveal the complexity of the cellular responses to DNA damage and their role in malignant transformation.[2] A number of interrelated biochemical pathways exist that influence the following actions:

1. The metabolism of potentially mutagenic or carcinogenic agents
2. The efficiency and manner by which damaged DNA is recognized and repaired
3. Cell cycle progression and the coordination of DNA replication and cell division relative to the repair of lesions
4. The decision point determining survival or the active induction of programmed death of cells carrying different types and amounts of DNA damage

Many cellular pathways have evolved that require hundreds of gene products for the direct repair of DNA damage and involve excision of damaged DNA bases and joining of broken DNA strands (Table 11-1). The central role of DNA damage responses in neoplastic transformation has been highlighted by the discovery that mutations in several classes of genes required for DNA repair and the maintenance of genomic integrity result in a predisposition to the development of certain malignancies.[3] In fact, a number of rare, inherited disorders have been described that appear to be caused by defects in the repair of DNA lesions (Table 11-2), and many of these are associated with an increased risk of developing certain cancers.[4]

TYPES OF DNA DAMAGE

DNA undergoes several types of spontaneous modifications, and it also can react with many physical and chemical agents, some of which are endogenous products of normal cellular metabolism (e.g., reactive oxygen species) whereas others, including ionizing radiation and ultraviolet light, are threats from the external environment (Fig. 11-1). One pronounced example is exposure to genotoxic compounds in cigarette smoke, which currently are responsible for the most common cancers in Western countries. Most active chemotherapeutic agents function by damaging DNA through alkylation, cross-linking, and other means, and mechanisms to repair these lesions also may determine the sensitivity of a tumor to such

treatments. Damage to DNA can cause genetic alterations (termed *mutations* when they are deleterious), and these mutations can lead to the development of cancer. DNA damage also may result in cell death, which can have serious consequences for the organism of which the cell is a part—for example, loss of irreplaceable neurons in the brain. Accumulation of damaged DNA also has been thought to contribute to some of the features of aging. Therefore, it is not surprising that a complex set of cellular surveillance and repair mechanisms has evolved to reverse or limit potentially deleterious DNA damage. Some of these DNA repair systems are so important that life cannot be sustained without them. An increasing number of human hereditary diseases that are characterized by severe developmental problems or a predisposition to cancer have been found to be linked to deficiencies in DNA repair (see Table 11-2).

CONSEQUENCES OF DNA DAMAGE

The results of DNA damage are diverse and usually adverse. Acute effects arise from disturbed DNA metabolism, triggering cell-cycle arrest or cell death. Long-term effects result from irreversible mutations that contribute to oncogenesis and inherited genetic disorders. Many lesions block transcription: this has elicited the development of a dedicated repair system, transcription-coupled repair (TCR), which displaces or removes the stalled RNA polymerase and ensures preferential repair of lesions within the transcribed strand of expressed genes.[5-7] Transcriptional stress due to DNA lesions that block the RNA polymerase, and DNA strand breaks caused by DNA damage or stalled replication forks, may constitute two major signals for DNA damage–inducible responses, including apoptosis,[8-10] which may be a significant anticancer mechanism. Lesions also may interfere with DNA replication. Recently, a growing class of at least nine specialized DNA polymerases, termed ζ (zeta) to σ (sigma), that seems devoted specifically to overcoming damage-induced replicational stress was discovered.[11,12] These special polymerases take over temporarily from the blocked replicative DNA polymerases (δ [delta], ε [epsilon]). They have more flexible base-pairing properties permitting translesion synthesis, with each polymerase probably designed for a specific category of injury.

TABLE 11-1

Human DNA Repair Pathways

DNA REPAIR PATHWAY	TYPE OF DNA DAMAGE	APPROXIMATE NO. OF GENES
Nucleotide excision repair	Bulky or helix-distorting DNA adducts, e.g., ultraviolet photoproducts, carcinogen adducts	37
Base excision repair	Oxidative DNA damage Spontaneous depurination	40
Mismatch repair	Mispaired nucleotides 1–15 nucleotide insertion-deletion loops	26
Homologous recombination	Double-strand DNA breaks, DNA crosslinks	20
Nonhomologous end joining	Double-strand DNA breaks	10

TABLE 11-2

Human Genetic Diseases Involving Defects in DNA Damage Response Pathways

SYNDROME	GENE(S)	BIOLOGIC FUNCTIONS	CLINICAL FEATURES	HYPERSENSITIVITIES
Xeroderma pigmentosum	XPA–XPG XPV	Nucleotide excision repair Translesional DNA synthesis	Sunlight hypersensitivity Neurologic defects Skin cancers	UV, chemical carcinogens
Cockayne syndrome	CSA, CSB XPB, XPD, XPG	Transcription-coupled repair	Growth retardation Mental retardation Premature aging Sunlight hypersensitivity	UV, chemical carcinogens Reactive oxygen species
Trichothiodystrophy	XPB, XPD, TTDA	Nucleotide excision repair Transcription	Sulfur-deficient brittle hair Dry, scaly skin Mental and physical retardation Sunlight sensitivity	UV
Hereditary nonpolyposis Colorectal cancer (lynch syndrome)	MLH1, MSH2, MSH6, PMS1, PMS2	Mismatch repair	Colorectal, endometrial, gastric, bile duct cancers	6-Thioguanine and cisplatin resistance
Ataxia telangiectasia	ATM	DNA damage-responsive kinase	Cerebellar ataxia Telangiectasia Immunodeficiency Lymphomas	Ionizing radiation
Ataxia telangiectasia-like disease	MRE11	Double-strand break repair	Similar to AT	
Nijmegen breakage syndrome	NBS1	Double-strand break repair	Microcephaly Immunodeficiency Lymphomas, neuroblastoma Rhabdomyosarcoma	Ionizing radiation
Bloom syndrome	BLM	DNA helicase Homologous recombination at stalled replication forks?	Sunlight hypersensitivity Growth retardation Leukemias, lymphomas Breast and intestinal cancers	UV, hydroxyurea
Werner syndrome	WRN	DNA helicase Homologous recombination? Translesional synthesis?	Premature aging Atherosclerosis Soft tissue sarcomas Melanoma, thyroid cancer	4-NQO, camptothetin Hydroxyurea
Rothmund-Thompson syndrome	RECQL4	DNA helicase	Growth deficiency Sunlight sensitivity Osteogenic sarcomas Squamous cell carcinomas	UV
Fanconi anemia	FANCA – G BRCA2	Interstrand crosslink repair Homologous recombination	Growth retardation Anatomic defects Bone marrow failure Myeloid leukemia Squamous cell cancers	Bifunctional alkylating agents Ionizing radiation
Li-Fraumeni syndrome	p53	Apoptosis Cell cycle checkpoints Nucleotide excision repair	Breast cancer Brain cancers Adrenocortical carcinoma Leukemia Bone and soft tissue sarcomas	?
Li-Fraumeni–like syndrome	Chk2	DNA damage responsive kinase	Similar to Li-Fraumeni syndrome	
Breast–ovarian cancer syndrome	BRCA1 BRCA2	Double-strand break repair Nucleotide excision repair	Breast cancer Ovarian cancer	Ionizing radiation? UV, cisplatin?

UV, ultraviolet.

However, this solution to replication blocks comes at the expense of a higher error rate. Nevertheless, translesion polymerases still protect the genome. For instance, inherited defects in pol η (eta), encoded for by the XPV/POLH/RAD30 gene, which specializes in relatively error-free bypassing of UV-induced cyclobutane pyrimidine dimers, causes a variant form of the skin cancer–prone disorder xeroderma pigmentosum.[13,14] Therefore, detection of DNA lesions may occur by blocked transcription, replication, or specialized sensors. Although the precise molecular mechanisms by which the cell senses altered DNA remain obscure, such signals result in a complex cellular response including cell cycle checkpoints, DNA repair, and apoptosis.

DNA DAMAGE RESPONSE PATHWAYS

DNA damage checkpoints initially were defined as regulatory pathways that control the ability of cells to arrest the cell cycle in response to DNA damage, allowing time for repair.[15] However, in addition to controlling cell cycle

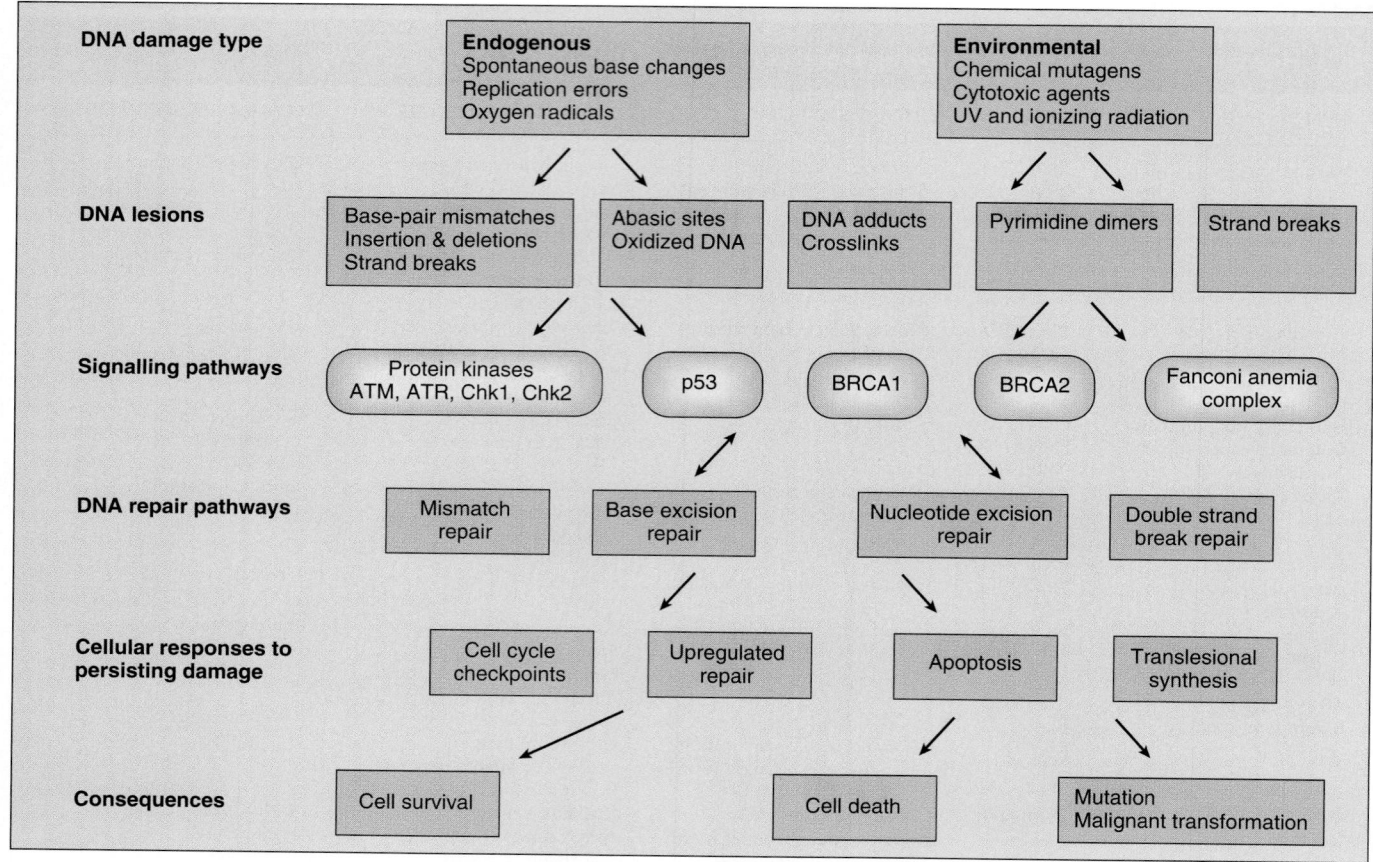

Figure 11-1. Cellular responses to DNA damage. Different types of DNA damage cause a variety of different types of lesions, and these, in turn, are dealt with by a variety of DNA repair mechanisms and signal various cellular response pathways. The outcome of DNA damage may be survival of a normal cell, cell death, or mutagenesis, possibly leading toward malignant transformation.

arrest, proteins involved in these pathways have been shown to control the activation of DNA repair pathways,[2,16-20] the movement of DNA repair proteins to sites of DNA damage,[21-25] and activation of transcriptional responses.[26-28] When damage is too significant, a cell may opt for the ultimate mode of rescue by initiating apoptosis at the expense of a whole cell.[29-31] As the DNA damage response pathway has been better defined at a molecular level, it has been discovered to be a complex network of interacting pathways that together execute the response. Initial recognition of DNA damage occurs by detection of a variety of damage-specific DNA binding proteins that either by themselves or together with complexes of associated proteins not directly involved in DNA repair may signal the DNA damage response.[32] Transduction and amplification of the DNA damage signal often is carried out by an overlapping set of conserved protein kinases, including the phosphoinositide-3-kinase-related proteins, which include ataxia-telangiectasia mutated (ATM) and ATM-Rad3-related (ATR) proteins, the checkpoint kinases Chk1 and Chk2, and others.[2,33-38] Many of these protein kinases are themselves targets for phosphorylation and activation; they then further target downstream genes critical to oncogenesis, such as p53 and BRCA1.[33,39-41] The ultimate targets of this highly regulated DNA damage response include mechanisms for DNA repair, and

although much of DNA repair is constitutive, a number of regulatory connections between the DNA damage response pathway and DNA repair have emerged.[2] In mammals, a large number of genes involved in DNA repair are transcriptionally induced in response to DNA damage, suggesting that many facets of repair are inducible, similar to the RecA-dependent SOS response that enhances DNA repair and mutagenesis following DNA damage in bacteria.[2,20,42] In fact, the p53 tumor suppressor gene is a central mediator of the DNA damage-inducible transcriptional response in humans, and p53-deficient fibroblasts are deficient in several aspects of DNA repair.[16,17] Therefore, the mammalian DNA damage-inducible response pathway is highly regulated, and is fine-tuned to determine if a particular cell type proceeds to a cell cycle checkpoint and DNA repair, or cell death, following a significant damage insult. Defects at any level of these pathways can alter repair and result in carcinogenesis (see Fig. 11-1).

TYPES OF DNA REPAIR AND THEIR CONTRIBUTION TO CANCER

DNA repair may be defined as those cellular responses associated with the restoration of the normal nucleotide sequence following events which damage or alter the genome.[43] Given the wide variety of DNA damage a cell encounters, it is not surprising that there are an equally large number of repair systems available to handle these insults. Indeed, many of the repair systems are broadly overlapping and interacting, with several sharing certain strategies and even specific gene products. Much of what is known regarding the basic mechanisms of many types of DNA repair comes from the study of lower organisms, such as bacteria and yeast, since these pathways have been highly conserved through evolution. Inherited defects in any of the major DNA repair pathways in humans, in general, predisposes to malignancy, and several of these syndromes will be discussed, in detail. In humans, a great deal has been learned regarding DNA repair from the often rare, autosomal recessive hereditary syndromes associated with defects in DNA repair genes.[4]

Nucleotide Excision Repair

The most versatile and ubiquitous mechanisms for DNA repair are those in which the damaged or incorrect part of a DNA strand is excised and then the resulting gap is filled by repair replication using the complementary strand as template. The redundancy of genetic information provided by the duplex DNA structure is essential to the maintenance of the genome by this "cut and patch" mode known as *excision repair*. Each DNA strand can serve as a template for repairing the other strand, as well as for replicating it. Excision repair was discovered in the early 1960s through basic studies on the effects of ultraviolet (UV) irradiation on DNA synthesis and repair replication in bacteria.[44-46] Nucleotide excision repair (NER) functions to remove many types of lesions, including bulky base adducts of chemical carcinogens, intrastrand cross-links, and UV-induced cyclobutane pyrimidine dimers and 6-4 photoproducts. Such lesions may serve as structural blocks to transcription and replication due to distortion of the helical conformation of DNA, and they also may result in mutations if translesional replication occurs or if they are not repaired correctly. The sequential steps for NER include (1) recognition of the damaged site, (2) incision of the damaged DNA strand near the site of the defect, (3) removal of a stretch of the affected strand containing the lesion, (4) repair replication to replace the excised region with a corresponding stretch of normal nucleotides using the complementary strand as a template, and (5) ligation to join the repair patch at its 3' end to the contiguous parental DNA strand (Fig. 11-2).[47,48] This excision repair pathway, which can remove DNA damage from sites throughout the genome, is termed *global genomic repair (GGR)*. The majority of human NER genes have been identified and cloned, and many have been shown to be mutated in hereditary NER-deficient, cancer-prone diseases.[49]

A unique problem arises if a bulky lesion is encountered by a translocating RNA polymerase making messenger RNA before repair enzymes have removed the damage and restored intact DNA. The polymerase may be arrested at the site of the lesion, and that also prevents access to the damage by repair enzymes. Furthermore, the arrest of transcription in human cells can trigger apoptosis. In this situation, a dedicated excision repair

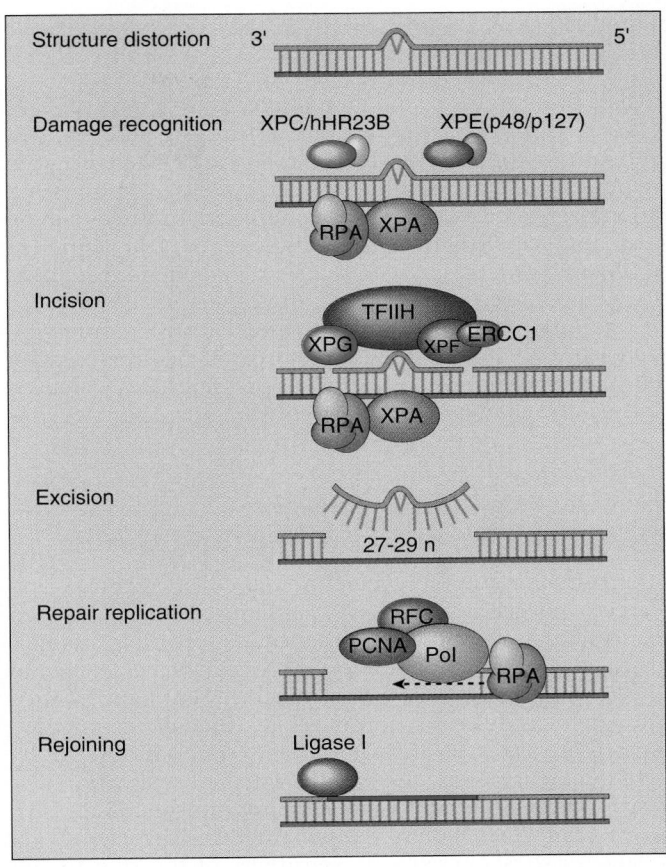

Figure 11-2. Mechanism for human nucleotide excision repair. Ultraviolet irradiation–induced adducts in genomic DNA are recognized by the XPE and XPC/hHR23B protein heteroduplexes that recruit the XPA/RPA complex and the larger TFIIH protein complex. Dimers that occur in the transcribed strand of an expressed gene result in a blocked RNA polymerase II molecule, which together with the CSA and CSB gene products serves to recruit the downstream repair machinery. The TFIIH complex contains helicases, including XPB and XPD, that unwind the DNA and allow the other repair proteins access for incision and excision of the damaged DNA oligonucleotide. After excision, repair replication occurs based on the normal DNA template and ligation of the newly synthesized DNA sequence. In total, more than 25 proteins participate in NER.

pathway known as transcription-coupled repair (TCR) comes to the rescue and displaces the RNA polymerase, and then efficiently repairs the blocking lesion so that transcription may resume—and so that the cell may survive.[42] The existence of a mechanism to facilitate the preferential repair of the transcribed strand of active genes in both eukaryotes and prokaryotes raises a number of questions as to its evolutionary role. Certainly, one could presume that strand-specific repair of active genes would be important for maintaining genomic stability in multicellular organisms by helping to avoid transforming mutations in expressed proto-oncogenes and tumor suppressor genes in humans. However, the lack of an increased incidence of malignancy in individuals with Cockayne syndrome (CS), a disease in which TCR has been selectively lost but GGR retained, argues against the idea that this NER pathway is critical in the process of transformation. The existence of TCR in unicellular and prokaryotic organisms suggests that its function may be more important to the basic processes of transcription and replication required for cellular survival than for avoidance of transforming mutations.

Recently, it has been understood that the GGR subpathway of NER is inducible following DNA damage, in concert with damage-inducible cell cycle checkpoints and apoptosis.[2,42] In fact, the p53 gene, central to maintaining genomic stability in human cells, is required for efficient GGR of UV light–induced and carcinogen-induced DNA damage, and functions as a DNA damage–activated transcription factor that directly regulates the expression of several NER genes.[18-20] Therefore, the GGR pathway of NER may be more relevant to suppressing DNA damage–induced malignancy, and highly regulated by genes involved in tumor suppression.

Human Nucleotide Excision Repair–Deficient Syndromes and Cancer

A direct correlation between unrepaired DNA damage and carcinogenesis in humans was first established when James Cleaver found that the cancer-prone hereditary disease xeroderma pigmentosum (XP) involved a defect in the repair of DNA lesions produced by UV light.[50] Since then, at least three syndromes have been attributed to inborn errors in NER: XP, CS, and trichothiodystrophy (TTD), all characterized by exquisite sun sensitivity.

Xeroderma pigmentosum is a rare, autosomal recessive disease in which homozygous individuals display several characteristics: (1) extreme sensitivity of the skin to sun exposure evident by 1 year of age; (2) pigmentation abnormalities and premalignant lesions in sun-exposed skin; (3) increases up to 4000-fold in incidence of skin cancers (predominantly squamous and basal cell carcinomas, but also melanomas) and ocular neoplasms, occurring 3 to 5 decades earlier than in the general population; and (4) a 10- to 20-fold increased incidence of internal cancers in non–sun-exposed sites.[4,51,52] Overall, the lifespan is reduced by approximately 30 years among patients with XP, and many die due to malignancies.[53] Approximately 20% of patients with XP also display progressive neurologic degeneration, characterized by peripheral neuropathy, sensorineural deafness, progressive mental retardation, and cerebellar and pyramidal tract involvement.[54] Xeroderma pigmentosum occurs worldwide, in all ethnic groups and with a frequency varying from one to ten patients per million.

The biochemical defect in cells from most XP individuals is in NER,[50] although in a small number of cases (known as XP-variants), excision repair appears normal and a defect exists in bypass replication at unrepaired lesions due to a mutation in the pol η (eta) translesional synthesis gene (XPV).[55] Complementation analysis via fusion of cells from different patients has demonstrated genetic heterogeneity within XP and provided evidence for the existence of at least seven excision-deficient complementation groups, termed XP-A to XP-G, in addition to XP-variant.[4]

Cockayne syndrome is another autosomal recessive disease that is associated with defective TCR of UV-damaged and oxidative-damaged DNA.[56-58] It is characterized by cutaneous photosensitivity, cachectic dwarfism, skeletal abnormalities, retinal degeneration, cataracts, severe mental retardation, and neurologic degeneration characterized by primary demyelination.[54,59] In contrast to patients with XP, those with CS are not at increased risk for developing skin cancers. The average lifespan of individuals with CS is only 12 years, with most patients succumbing to infectious or renal complications rather than cancer.[60] Cockayne syndrome is characterized by the existence of at least three complementation groups. Several patients have been described in XP groups B, D and G who share the DNA repair defects and clinical features of CS together with the cutaneous manifestations of XP.[61,62]

Trichothiodystrophy is an autosomal recessive condition sharing many of the signs and symptoms of CS, with the additional hallmark of brittle hair and nails due to reduced sulfur content in the component proteins. As with CS, several of the responsible genes implicated are XPB and XPD, but there is a third complementation group, TTD-A, for which no gene has been identified. The favored model for TTD is that of a transcription deficiency with respect to the genes relevant to the phenotype, including sulfur-containing proteins.[63] It also is conceivable that TTD and CS could be diseases of "premature cell death" in which the transcription deficiency and deficiency in TCR could cause the apoptosis of certain classes of metabolically active cells that sustain significant endogenous oxidative damage (e.g., neurons).

Analysis of the specific abnormalities in NER displayed by the various genetic complementation groups of XP, CS, and TTD allow correlations to be drawn with their heterogeneous clinical features. Specifically, only those subgroups of patients who display a defect in GGR are at significantly increased risk for developing UV-induced malignancies. In contrast, the neurologic symptoms and developmental abnormalities associated with other complementation groups of XP and CS are found only in those groups that are defective in TCR. The fact that the TFIIH complex, containing the XPB and XPD proteins, is common to both core NER and transcriptional initiation, supports the suggestion that the clinical phenotype of patients with defects in TCR may actually be due to abnormalities in transcription rather than in repair itself.[63]

Although these observations may explain the molecular basis for many of the clinical characteristics of XP and CS, they present an apparent paradox with regard to these patients' cancer risk. Many currently recognized oncogenes and tumor suppressor genes are known to possess important cellular functions, and to be actively expressed in normal cells. Because CS cells are defective in the repair of actively expressed genes, it would be reasonable to expect be that these patients would acquire mutations in genes, leading to transformation more readily than normal patients. However, this is not supported be the clinical picture. It has been demonstrated that defects in TCR specifically activate DNA damage–induced apoptosis,[8,9] which may eliminate potentially mutagenic, premalignant cells.

Another puzzling aspect of the clinical phenotype of XP is why these patients do not appear to be at a greater risk for developing neoplasms other than skin cancers. Although a disproportionate number of relatively rare tumors such as brain sarcomas and extraglossal carcinomas of the oral cavity have been described in patients with XP who are under 40 years of age,[51] individuals with XP do not appear to be at significantly increased risk for more common solid or hematologic malignancies. It may be that the early mortality experienced by XP patients, or a decreased exposure to non-UV environmental carcinogens during their early life, may partially explain these observations. However, modest alterations in NER activity caused by functional polymorphisms in XP genes may contribute to solid tumor cancer risk.[64,65]

Base Excision Repair

A major source of DNA damage to cellular genomes arises from normal metabolism in the cytoplasmic environment through hydrolysis and exposure to reactive metabolites that cause oxidation and alkylation of DNA. The repair system primarily involved in identifying and removing such lesions, as well as dealing with the spontaneous loss of purines from DNA, is the base excision repair (BER) pathway.[66,67] The essential nature of BER for viability is highlighted by the fact that although a number of BER proteins have been discovered, only recently has a single human hereditary disease been identified that appears to result from an apparent mutation in a gene unique to this pathway.[68-70] The enormous task required for BER is exemplified by the fact that in 1 hour a human being spontaneously loses on the order of a trillion guanines from his or her DNA, and each of these must be replaced. Similarly, a large number of cytosines become deaminated spontaneously and the resulting product, uracil, must be removed and replaced with cytosine to restore the correct nucleotide sequence. In most cases BER is initiated by one of a set of lesion-specific glycosylases that recognize the altered or inappropriate base and cleave it from its sugar moiety in the DNA (Fig. 11-3). Different DNA glycosylases remove different kinds of damage, conferring specificity to the process. Once the base is removed, the apurinic/apyrimidinic (AP) site is removed by an AP-endonuclease or an AP-lyase, which cleaves the DNA strand 5′ or 3′ to the AP site, respectively. The remaining deoxyribose phosphate residue is excised by a phosphodiesterase, with the resulting gap filled by a DNA polymerase and the strand sealed by DNA ligase. The major oxidized purine lesion is 8-oxo-7,8-dihydroguanine (8-oxoG), which is abundant and has strong mutagenic properties. Oxidized pyrimidines include thymine glycol, 5-hydroxycytosine, and formamidopyrimidines. Oxidized bases, including both 8-oxoG and thymine glycol, share the property of blocking DNA replication and transcription, and must be repaired efficiently to maintain genomic stability.[71,72]

In mammalian cells, the gene functions responsible for the strand incision steps of BER include the glycosylases hNTH1 (homologous to bacterial endonuclease III), which removes oxidized pyrimidines; hOGG1, which targets oxidized purines; and MYH (Mut Y homolog), which removes adenines mispaired with an 8-oxoG, together with AP endonuclease 1 (APE1).[73] Recent evidence

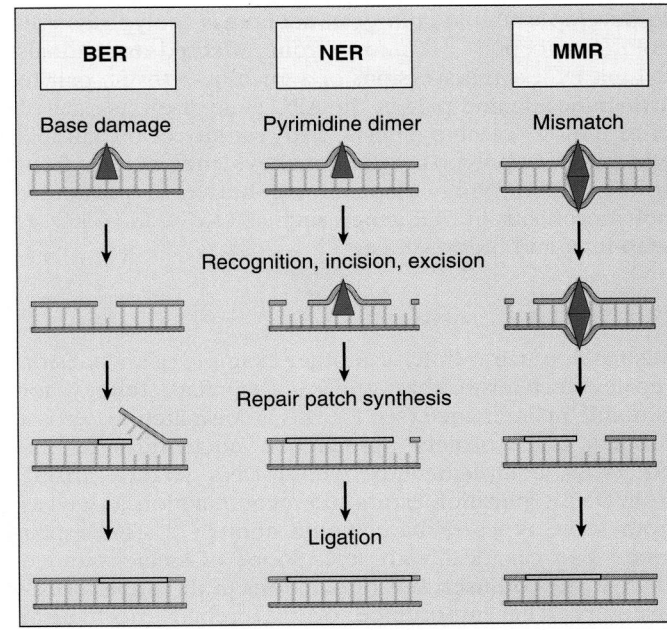

Figure 11-3. Excision repair pathways for DNA damage. The three main excision repair pathways in human cells—base excision repair (BER), nucleotide excision repair (NER), and mismatch repair (MMR)—proceed through similar steps to restore the normal DNA sequence. Following recognition of altered DNA bases, employing lesion-specific glycosylases for BER, XP proteins for NER, and MutS homologs for MMR, incision of DNA is achieved by endonucleases and displacement or degradation of single-stranded sections of DNA that contain the damage by enzymes with helicase and exonuclease activity. Repair replication of the resulting DNA gap and strand ligation results in the repaired double-stranded DNA molecule. The many repair enzymes involved in each specific step are tightly coupled, and may be regulated or inducible by DNA damage response pathways.

suggests that a transcription-coupled BER of oxidized bases may occur, analogous to TCR of UV-photoproducts, particularly for thymine glycol and 8-oxoG lesions, and that requires several NER enzymes as well, including XPG, TFIIH and CSB.[71] In addition, it recently has been noted that, similar to NER, p53 may participate in the regulation of BER, potentially by directly interacting with the BER complex.[74,75]

Attempts to engineer mice deficient in the core enzymes required for BER typically have resulted in early embryonic death, whereas knockout of individual glycosylases produces mice with no overt phenotype at all.[76] This attests to the importance of the repair of DNA lesions from endogenous causes during embryonic development, as well as the likely redundancy between individual glycosylases and overlap with TCR. It also is consistent with the near-absence of known human hereditary diseases characterized by defects in BER genes.

However, given the mutagenic and cytotoxic potential of the classes of DNA damage that are BER substrates, it seems likely that altered activity in these pathways would result in enhanced cancer risk. The most direct evidence for a role for BER in cancer comes from the recent discovery that germline mutations in the MYH gene, which is involved in processing 8-oxoG lesions, is associated with recessive inheritance of a predisposition to develop multiple colorectal adenomas (polyposis) and colon cancers.[68-70] Tumors from affected individuals exhibit excess transversions of a guanine-cytosine pair to a thymine-adenine pair in the APC gene, itself associated with colon carcinogenesis and causative of familial adenomatous polyposis. Additional evidence derives from studies identifying associations between particular polymorphisms in BER genes, such as OGG1 and XRCC1, with lung and breast cancers.[65,77,78]

Mismatch Repair

Mismatch repair (MMR) is another example of an excision repair mechanism that utilizes a similar strategy for genomic maintenance (see Fig. 11-3). Mismatch repair is a process that corrects mismatched nucleotides in the otherwise complementary paired DNA strands arising from DNA replication errors and recombination, as well as from some types of base modifications.[79-81] This repair mode also can deal with small loops of single-stranded DNA at sites of insertions or deletions in the duplex DNA structure. The importance of this repair mechanism in maintaining genetic stability is illustrated by the observation that its absence results in a large increase in the frequency of spontaneously occurring mutations, particularly in microsatellite sequences of highly repetitive DNA.[82] Some of these spontaneous mutations arise from mistakes introduced during DNA replication, in spite of the operation of a "proofreading" system that also helps to ensure the high fidelity of replication. In humans, genetic defects in several mismatch repair genes have been linked to hereditary nonpolyposis colon cancer (HNPCC), as well as to sporadic cancers that exhibit instability in regions of DNA containing short repetitive sequences of nucleotides, a feature known as microsatellite instability (MSI).

As with other modes of excision repair, four principal steps are required for MMR: (1) mismatch recognition; (2) recruitment of additional MMR factors; (3) identification of the newly synthesized DNA strand containing the mismatched nucleotides, followed by their excision; and (4) resynthesis of the excised tract and ligation. The biochemical workings of this pathway are best understood in bacteria, but a similar set of events occurs in human cells. Based on functional homologies to their bacterial counterparts and sequence homology to corresponding yeast genes, a number of human genes have been cloned that participate in MMR, including those homologous to

---

THE CENTRAL ROLE OF DNA DAMAGE IN CANCER DEVELOPMENT: IMPLICATIONS FOR CANCER PREVENTION

Despite many decades of investigation, the exact cause of most cancers remains unknown, with a few important exceptions (e.g., certain cancers of the lung, skin, cervix). Rather, cancer is associated with a broad and heterogeneous group of genetic and environmental influences, making the development of schemes for targeted prevention difficult.

However, 30 years ago, prior to much of our current understanding of the specific molecular and genetic changes associated with cancer, Dr. Larry Loeb proposed that a common early event in the development of many cancers is the expression of a "mutator phenotype" resulting from mutations in genes that normally function to maintain genetic stability. Based on calculations of the estimated fidelity of DNA replication and repair in normal human cells, and the rarity of spontaneous mutations that occur in normal cells, Loeb noted the statistical unlikelihood that the large number of chromosomal aberrations and genetic mutations observed in human malignancies would occur by chance in a single cell. He speculated that if a cell exhibited unusual levels of genetic instability due to inherited or acquired mutations in the genes that regulate the processes of DNA replication and repair, the rate of additional mutations occurring in other genes important for carcinogenesis will be dramatically elevated. As is obvious from the many specific examples discussed in this chapter, Loeb's prediction has been born out by many subsequent studies of multistep carcinogenesis and the identification of cancer susceptibility syndromes caused by inherited mutations in DNA repair genes. More recently, this hypothesis has also derived support from studies demonstrating that variability in normal DNA repair capacity between individuals may correlate with cancer risk, suggesting that subtle functional alterations due to genetic polymorphisms in DNA repair genes may be predictive of cancer susceptibility.

The mutator phenotype theory also has major implications for the prevention of cancers. Although it may be impossible to avoid initial genetic alterations in genes controlling genetic stability, reducing the amount of DNA damage to which these premalignant cells are particularly vulnerable could slow the accumulation of additional mutations. Certainly, reducing exposure to known environmental carcinogens is important in this goal, but the majority of DNA damage likely occurs due to endogenous reactants of normal cellular metabolism, such as oxygen reactive species, activated lipids, metal cations, and so forth. In fact, it has been estimated that oxidative radicals generate up to 10,000 DNA damage events per cell per day. Therefore, means to reduce the amount of oxidative DNA damage, or enhance its repair, may slow the carcinogenic process sufficiently to prevent the clinical occurrence of some cancers. Indeed, evidence from several fields suggests that anti-oxidants may have chemopreventative properties. For example, epidemiological evidence suggests that diets rich in the common trace element selenium may be associated with reduced cancer risk. Recent experimental studies suggest that selenium possesses several properties that make it attractive for cancer prevention targeted at the mutator phenotype. Selenium can function as a scavenger of oxygen free radicals and may also enhance some DNA repair activities regulated by the p53 gene product. Although the identification of specific pharmacologic agents for cancer prevention in humans remains investigational, our rapidly increasing understanding of processes for the prevention and repair of DNA damage provides many new targets for rational drug development.

the bacterial MutS mismatch recognition protein (hMSH2, hMSH3 and hMSH6) and to the bacterial MutL gene (hMLH1 and hPMS2).[83-85] In humans, heterodimers of the MSH2/6 proteins recognize single base-pair mismatches and short insertion-deletion loops, whereas MSH2/3 dimers recognize longer loops. Heterodimeric complexes of MLH1/PMS2 and MLH1/PMS1 interact with the MSH complexes and replication factors, for strand discrimination and DNA excision. Similar to NER and BER, additional proteins are then recruited for repair replication based on the original DNA template.

The MMR system also may interact with DNA damage due to certain alkylators and intercalating agents that assume similar structural alterations in DNA as mismatches, and actually result in erroneous or futile MMR cycles, resulting ultimately in apoptosis. Thus, intact MMR may confer chemosensitivity to these chemotherapeutic agents, and MMR-defective tumors may exhibit resistance to certain drugs.[86]

Human Mismatch Repair Deficiency and Cancer

Hereditary nonpolyposis colon cancer, also known as Lynch syndrome types I and II, is the most common form of colon cancer with an inherited predisposition.[87] It is an autosomal dominant inherited condition with an incidence of 1:1000 in the general population. HNPCC accounts for about 5% of all colorectal cancers, patients with HNPCC also are at elevated risk for cancers of the endometrium, ovary, stomach, small bowel, and other sites. Patients with HNPCC have an 80% lifetime risk for colorectal cancer and a 50% lifetime risk for endometrial cancer. The discovery of MSI, that is, the frequent alteration in the tract lengths of certain short repetitive nucleotide sequences, in some hereditary colorectal cancers provided the first indication that the etiology of these cancers might involve a problem in the MMR system.[88] The finding of germline MMR gene defects in patients with HNPCC established that these defects are the cause of the enhanced incidence of cancer.[83-85] Germline mutations in MLH1and MSH2 together account for more than half of all cases of HNPCC. Defects in MSH6 cause a late-onset HNPCC phenotype. No hMSH3 mutations have been reported in families with a predilection to colon cancer, but PMS1 mutations have been implicated in a very few families. This finding is consistent with the notion that loss of hMLH1 and hMSH2 is associated with complete inactivation of MMR, whereas defects in the other proteins cause only a partial MMR deficiency. No strong genotype-phenotype correlations have been observed to date, but mutations in the MSH2 gene do appear to be associated with more extracolonic manifestations than are mutations in the MLH1 gene.

Microsatellite instability has been identified as a source of the genomic instability driving tumorigenesis in a number of sporadic tumor types, in addition to those that arise in the context of inherited germline mutations of MMR genes.[88,89] For example, up to 20% of sporadic colon cancers exhibit MSI, particularly those that present in the ascending colon and in individuals less than 50 years old,

the majority of which are due to epigenetic silencing of MLH1 gene expression by promoter hypermethylation.[90,91] Whether through genetic or epigenetic inactivation, loss of MMR results in an elevated rate of mutations, particularly at microsatellite sequences, several of which occur in the coding sequences of other genes often found mutated in cancers, including TGF beta type II receptor, BAX and the mismatch repair genes MSH3 and MSH6, themselves. Therefore, clear genetic evidence demonstrates that the phenotype of genetic instability associated with defects in MMR results in the genotype of tumors that arise due to these defects. Intriguingly, the survival of patients with MSI-associated colorectal cancer is better than that of those with more typical tumors exhibiting chromosomal instability.[92-94] These tumors also demonstrate different biologic and pathological characteristics. Whether their more favorable outcome reflects differences in clinical behavior, responsiveness to therapy, or both, remains to be fully determined.

Double-Strand Break Repair

Double-strand breaks (DSBs) in DNA induced by x-rays or chemicals or during replication of single-strand breaks, and presumably during repair of interstrand DNA crosslinks, usually are dealt with through the recombination machinery (Fig. 11-4). An unrepaired DSB is a highly lethal event, and even a single occurrence in the entire genome is thought to be sufficient to signal cell cycle checkpoints that prevent attempted DNA synthesis or cell division until repair has been completed in certain cells, or apoptosis in other cell types. Double-strand breaks also pose problems during mitosis, because intact chromosomes are a prerequisite for proper chromosome segregation during cell division. Thus, these lesions often induce various sorts of chromosomal aberrations, including aneuploidy, deletions (loss of heterozygosity), and chromosomal translocations—all of which are intimately associated with carcinogenesis. Genetic recombination is the principal mechanism for dealing with DSBs that involve homologous stretches of nucleotide at the ends to be joined. If no such homology is present, however, there is another system for nonhomologous end joining, which is more error-prone. Recent studies have identified a cascade of protein kinases involved in signaling cellular processes in response to DSBs. Many of these have been found defective in cancer-prone disorders exhibiting genomic instability, such as the ATM protein[38] and the Chk2 protein kinase associated with a Li-Fraumeni–like cancer susceptibility syndrome.[95-97] A major target for these kinase activities is the p53 tumor suppressor gene. This gene, when phosphorylated, is activated and involved in G1 arrest and apoptosis following ionizing radiation[33,34,98-101]; when found mutated in the germline, it results in the Li-Fraumeni cancer susceptibility syndrome. Many enzymes that may be involved in the actual DNA transactions necessary for DSB repair have been found in cancer-prone disorders, including MRE11 (AT-like disorder), NBS1 (Nijmegen breakage syndrome), BRCA1 and BRCA2 (breast-ovarian cancer syndrome), and the RecQ-like helicases (Werner, Bloom, and Rothmund Thomson syndromes).

Science of Clinical Oncology

1

Figure 11-4. Mechanisms for DNA double-strand break (DSB) repair. The repair of DNA DSBs is carried out by two mechanisms. *Left,* The rapid, but error-prone, nonhomologous end-joining that directly seals breaks but may result in the gain or loss of several nucleotides due to short areas of microhomologies used for annealing prior to ligation. Exposed DNA ends are recognized by the Ku70/80 heterodimer that recruits the DNA-dependent protein kinase catalytic subunit and other proteins assisting in strand alignment. The XRCC4-ligase IV heteroduplex joins the breaks. *Right,* The high-fidelity, homologous recombination of sister chromatids at sites of DSBs is the less prominent mode in mammalian cells. This DNA repair pathway is mediated by RAD51-associated proteins, including RAD52, which recognizes single-strand DNA ends and together with other proteins results in short nuclease-mediated resection. RAD51 then forms a nucleoprotein filament on the exposed strand, and, probably with BRCA2 and other proteins, promotes strand invasion and displacement at homologous sequences. Thus, the undamaged sister molecule acts as a template for the resynthesis of the missing nucleotides.

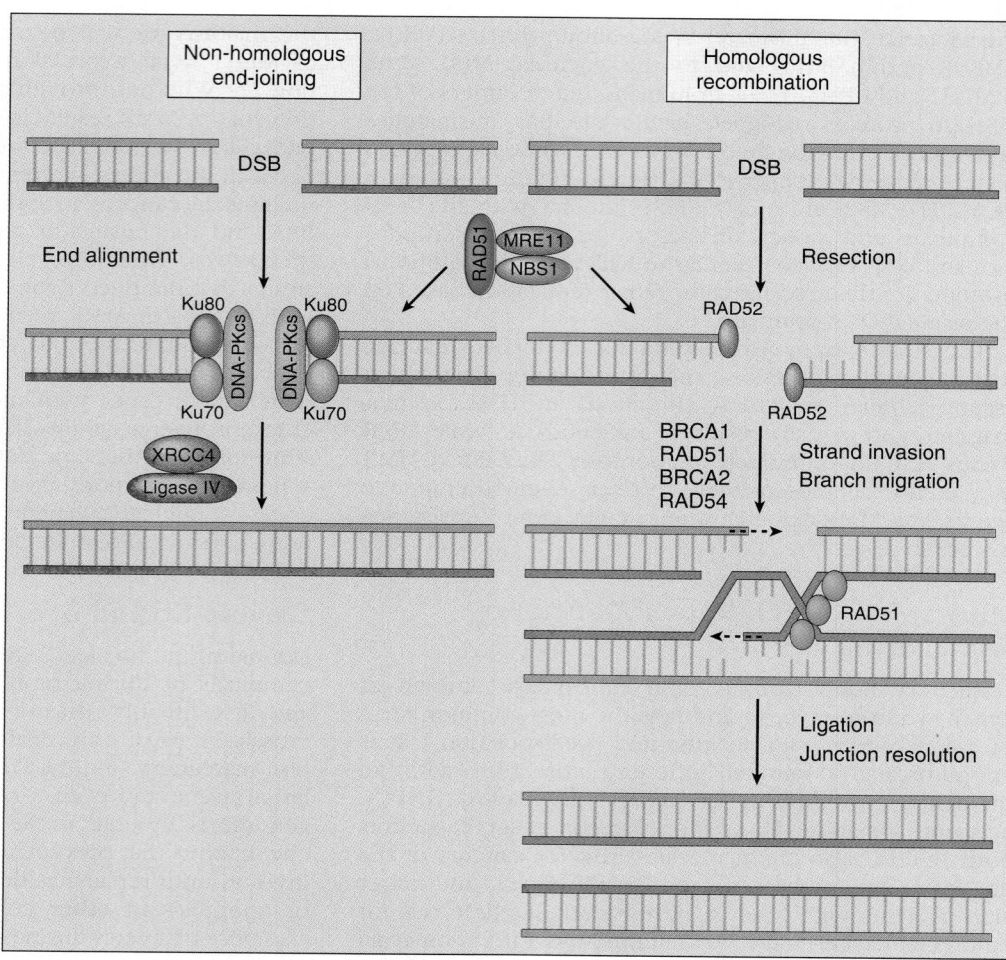

Ataxia Telangiectasia

Ataxia telangiectasia (AT) originally was identified in humans with a severe sensitivity to ionizing radiation. Later it was learned that AT also affects the immune system and the cerebellum. The neurologic defect causes progressive loss of motor control, leading to lack of coordination and balance. Respiratory infections develop in children with this disease as a consequence of the deficiency in the immune system. A single gene, ATM, is responsible for the multiple and surprisingly diverse symptoms of this disease, including a predisposition to lymphoma and leukemia. Over 10% of AT patients develop cancer at an early age. Ataxia telangiectasia is an autosomal recessive disease with an incidence of nearly one in 100,000 live births. Persons who are heterozygous for AT, about 1% of the general population, may have an increased predisposition to cancer, in particular breast cancers, especially those individuals expressing an ATM with missense mutations resulting in a dominant-negative effect on their wild-type ATM gene.[102-104] ATM is a central signaling protein in the DNA damage response, and cells lacking ATM fail to execute many critical cellular responses to DNA damage. For example, one hallmark of AT is what has been termed x-ray–resistant DNA synthesis. It is now know that the ATM gene product is a key element in delaying the initiation of DNA replication following DNA damage resulting in strand breaks. In addition, ATM directly phosphorylates the NBS1 protein, resulting in its association with the MRE11 and RAD50 gene products, which together are required for both nonhomologous end-joining and homologous recombination of DSBs.[105] Inherited germline mutations of the NBS1 and MRE11 genes themselves result in clinical variants of AT, termed *Nijmegen breakage syndrome* and *AT-like disorder,* respectively.[106] Therefore, ATM is central to a DNA damage response pathway critical for regulating recombination and repair following DSBs. Defects in many of the component proteins in the pathway result in genomic instability and a predisposition to cancer.

OTHER CANCER-PRONE DISORDERS ASSOCIATED WITH GENOMIC INSTABILITY

Diseases Involving Homologues of *recQ*

There are at least three cancer-prone diseases in humans in which the defect is in a homologue of the gene *recQ*, originally discovered in bacteria.[107] The product of *recQ* is a helicase, which in *Escherichia coli* is involved in processing the nascent DNA at arrested replication forks. Helicases are enzymes that separate the complementary strands of nucleic acid duplexes using energy derived from ATP hydrolysis. In humans, recQ helicases are thought to function at the interface between DNA replication and recombination in dealing with damaged replication forks, and interact with many other nuclear proteins that are required for DNA metabolism.[108] The biologic and clinical effects of the homozygous deficiency of these genes can be quite dramatic and profound. Thus, Bloom syndrome is characterized by an extremely high frequency of genetic exchanges (so-called sister chromatid exchanges) that cause genomic instability and lymphoma, leukemias, and solid tumors of the GI tract and breast.[109,110] Of interest, recent studies have identified an increased risk that individuals who are heterozygous for a BLM mutation will develop colorectal cancer, potentially due to haploinsufficiency.[111,112] In Werner syndrome the deficiency in another recQ homologue results in remarkable features of premature aging as well as a predisposition to sarcomas, melanoma, and cancers of the thyroid.[113–115] Yet another recQ homologue defect is Rothmund-Thompson syndrome, which is characterized by growth deficiency and predisposition to cancer, in particular to osteogenic sarcomas.[116,117]

p53 gene and Li-Fraumeni Syndrome

The discovery of the p53 tumor suppressor gene more than 20 years ago inspired widespread investigations with the aim of understanding the basic biology behind its role in maintaining genomic stability and the cellular response to DNA damage. p53 is one of the most commonly mutated genes in human cancers,[118] and its product is a multifunctional protein that regulates several physiologic processes including cell cycle checkpoints, apoptosis, and DNA repair.[20,98,99,119] The primary role of p53 in tumor suppression has been attributed to its function as a transcription factor, regulating expression of over 100 different cellular genes.[28] In response to a variety of genotoxic stimuli, p53 protein is stabilized through a series of post-translational modifications,[120] is activated for sequence-specific DNA binding, and transcriptionally regulates downstream target genes that contain a consensus p53 response element in their promoter or intronic segments. These p53 target genes include those important for cell cycle checkpoints, such as p21[121]; apoptosis, such as BAX and PERP[122]; and DNA repair, such as the DDB2 and XPC genes required for NER.[18–20]

Patients with the rare autosomal dominant Li-Fraumeni syndrome (LFS) are at increased risk for developing a number of common tumors at an early age due to an inherited germline defect in one allele of the p53 gene, including soft tissue and osteosarcomas, breast cancer, brain tumors, lymphomas, leukemia, and adrenocortical carcinomas. Mutations in the p53 tumor suppressor gene account for 70% to 85% of classic LFS cases.[123–125] Recently, mutations in the Chk2 gene have been shown to occur in the germline of LFS-like families that do not contain p53 mutations.[95–97] Although the heterozygote carriers of a defective p53 allele do not appear to have

clinical problems or DNA repair defects, when the second allele has been mutated or lost, the absence of functional p53 results in severe problems for the cell. First of all, the p53-controlled pathway of apoptosis is disengaged, so severely damaged cells will survive and be at risk for carcinogenic transformation because of their genomic instability. That genomic instability derives from the fact that p53 also is an important regulator of cell cycle checkpoints. Thus, as with the situation in AT, the cells continue to progress through their growth cycle, rather than pausing to allow time for DNA lesions to be repaired. Finally, p53 serves an important regulatory function in NER, and in its absence some important mutagenic lesions simply are not repaired. That, of course, is a major contributor to the genomic instability and the consequent development of tumors.

BRCA1, BRCA2, and Breast-Ovarian Cancer Susceptibility

Hereditary breast cancer includes a broad group of hereditary predisposition conditions in which breast cancer is a component tumor, and account for approximately 5% to 10% of all breast cancer cases. Hereditary syndromes of breast and ovarian cancer susceptibility have been particularly associated with germline mutations of two genes, BRCA1 and BRCA2, as well as rare cases due to mutations in the p53 gene in LFS and the PTEN gene in Cowden disease. Recent experimental data suggest that both of the BRCA genes may be involved in multiple DNA repair activities.[126–130]

The BRCA1 and 2 genes are large and complex. Many hundreds of different germline mutations have been detected in each, but only rare sporadic breast or ovarian cancers have been found to harbor BRCA1 mutations. The exact biochemical functions of these proteins remain unknown, but increasing evidence suggests they may be involved in various aspects of DNA repair and DNA damage-response pathways. For example, BRCA1 is phosphorylated after exposure to DNA-damaging agents by ATM, ATR and Chk2; associates with a number of DNA repair proteins including MSH2, MSH6, ATM, RAD51, and the RAD50-MRE11-NBS1 protein complex following DNA damage; and localizes to nuclear foci with these proteins after treatment with ionizing radiation and UV radiation.[23,131,132] The association of BRCA1 with RAD51, an enzyme involved in the coordination of recombination, suggests its involvement in DSB repair, and strong data exist implicating BRCA1 in homologous recombination.[133] Other studies suggest that BRCA1 may regulate cellular processes through transcriptional coactivation. Recently, BRCA1 has been shown to transcriptionally regulate the NER genes XPC, DDB2 and GADD45 and affect GGR of UV- and cisplatin-induced DNA damage.[129,134,135] Chromosomal instability also is characteristic of breast tumors that harbor BRCA2 mutations, probably due to defective recombination-mediated DSB repair. BRCA2 has been shown to bind to the RAD51 protein, an enzyme involved in the coordination of recombination, and together they colocalize to nuclear sites containing DNA strand breaks

DNA REPAIR AND CANCER TREATMENT

As discussed in this chapter, many genes implicated in the development of cancer play roles in DNA repair. The mechanism of action for most cancer chemotherapeutic drugs, as well as radiation therapy, is thought to be through DNA damage. Therefore, it seems logical that cancers that acquired defects in DNA repair during the tumorigenic process would also be particularly susceptible to the cytotoxic effects of DNA damaging therapeutic agents. However, for most common cancers, the clinical experience suggests otherwise. It is likely that the frequently concurrent inactivation of cell cycle checkpoints and apoptotic processes during tumorigenesis obscures the effect of DNA repair defects, and thus the response of clinical tumors to various treatments remains very difficult to predict, even with genetic information. Nevertheless, several examples have emerged in which a detailed understanding of the DNA repair defects present in a particular tumor type may allow for the rational selection of certain treatment approaches likely to be more effective.

One example relates to the function of the BRCA1 gene that is involved in several types of DNA repair, including double-strand break repair, nucleotide excision repair, and DNA crosslink repair. Germline mutations in the BRCA1 gene predispose individuals to a very high risk for developing breast and ovarian cancers, and somatic inactivation of BRCA1 activity has also been observed in sporadic breast and ovarian cancers due to promoter methylation of the BRCA1 or FANCF genes. Clinical and experimental data are now emerging that indicate that tumors deficient in BRCA1 function may be particularly sensitive to the chemotherapeutic drug cisplatin, which causes DNA damage repaired through the nucleotide excision and crosslink repair pathways and ionizing radiation, which causes double-strand DNA breaks.

A quite different example relates to the 15%–20% of colorectal cancers that have inactivated the mismatch repair pathway and exhibit microsatellite instability (MSI). It has been appreciated for some time that individuals with colorectal cancer expressing high levels of MSI have longer survival than stage matched patients with colorectal cancer without MSI. However, whether these prognostic differences related to differences in tumor biology or to sensitivity to chemotherapy was unclear. Recently, though, clinical studies suggest that patients with surgically resected stage II or III MSI–positive colorectal cancer do not benefit from 5-Fluorouracil-based adjuvant chemotherapy, as do patients with mismatch repair intact colorectal cancers, but, nevertheless, have better outcomes even without additional therapy. Experiments with mismatch repair defective colon cancer cell lines suggest that they are also resistant to the cytotoxic effects of oxaliplatin (in fact, an intact mismatch repair pathway may be necessary to confer the apoptotic effects of platinum induced DNA damage), but are susceptible to the topoisomerase I inhibitor, CPT-11. Since both these drugs are now being used for the treatment of colorectal cancer, concurrent diagnostic testing of tumors for MSI and mismatch repair activity may help guide their selection and use in individual patients.

These examples and others suggest that our rapidly improving knowledge of the role of specific cancer genes in DNA repair pathways may have significant impact on the treatment of human cancers. Efforts to obtain genotypic and phenotypic information from individual tumors should allow for tailored, rational selection of therapies for cancer treatment, an approach that is central to the emerging field of pharmacogenomics.

---

caused by ionizing radiation. Structural studies of BRCA2 DNA-binding domains suggest that BRCA2 may facilitate interactions of RAD51 with single-stranded DNA during recombination.[136,137] The genomic instability associated with mutations of BRCA1 and BRCA2, therefore, may be due in part to the intact but error-prone nonhomologous end-joining repair pathway.[127]

Fanconi Anemia, Cancer, and Interstrand Cross-link Repair

The centrality and interwoven nature of DNA repair pathways for genomic stability have been highlighted by recent findings regarding Fanconi anemia, a rare, autosomal recessive disease that confers an increased risk of acute myeloid leukemia; squamous cell carcinomas of the head, neck, and esophagus; gynecologic carcinomas; and liver tumors at a young age.[138,139] At least eight subtypes of Fanconi anemia have been determined by complementation analyses, and germline mutations in seven different genes have been identified. Surprisingly, it recently was reported that germline homozygous inactivating mutations of the BRCA2 gene may be the cause of this disease in the D1 and possibly also the B complementation groups.[140] In addition, the FANCD2 gene product links Fanconi anemia proteins to BRCA1 in the response to DNA damage. Following ionizing radiation, FANCD2 becomes monoubiquitinated by a complex of five other Fanconi anemia proteins and binds to and colocalizes with BRCA1 to nuclear sites occupied by RAD51 and BRCA2.[141] This process also is regulated by the ATM protein kinase, which phosphorylates FANCD2 in response to DNA damage.[142] It has long been appreciated that cells from patients with Fanconi anemia are hypersensitive to DNA crosslinking agents, such as mitomycin C and cisplatin, in addition to being modestly sensitive to ionizing radiation. Although DNA crosslink repair in mammalian cells is poorly understood, it has been proposed that it utilizes components of both the excision repair and DSB repair systems to sequentially incise DNA near the site of a crosslink followed by homologous recombination or nonhomologous end-joining.[139] Therefore, the Fanconi anemia proteins appear to function at an interface between several DNA repair and DNA damage response pathways.

CONCLUSIONS AND FUTURE DIRECTIONS

Recent molecular biology and genetic research has provided ample evidence to support the longstanding prediction that genomic instability is a major factor driving the onset and progression of carcinogenesis.[143]

Overlapping and interacting mechanisms for DNA repair and the cellular response to DNA damage are critical components for the maintenance of genomic stability. Alterations in these pathways often are early events in the multistep acquisition of genetic mutations leading to cancer development. Continued exploration of the DNA damage response will prove important for our improved understanding of cancer etiology, prevention, genetic susceptibility, diagnosis, and treatment.

REFERENCES

1. Loeb LA, Loeb KR, Anderson JP: Multiple mutations and cancer. Proc Natl Acad Sci USA 2003;100:776-781.
2. Zhou BB, Elledge SJ: The DNA damage response: putting checkpoints in perspective. Nature 2000;408:433-439.
3. Hoeijmakers JH: Genome maintenance mechanisms for preventing cancer. Nature 2001;411:366-374.
4. Ford JM, Hanawalt PC: Role of DNA excision repair gene defects in the etiology of cancer. Curr Top Microbiol Immunol 1997;221:47-70.
5. Bohr VA, Smith CA, Okumoto DS, Hanawalt PC: DNA repair in an active gene: removal of pyrimidine dimers from the DHFR gene of CHO cells is much more efficient than in the genome overall. Cell 1985;40:359-369.
6. Mellon I, Bohr VA, Smith CA, Hanawalt PC: Preferential DNA repair of an active gene in human cells. Proc Natl Acad Sci USA 1986;83:8878-8882.
7. Mellon I, Spivak G, Hanawalt PC: Selective removal of transcription-blocking DNA damage from the transcribed strand of the mammalian DHFR gene. Cell 1987;51:241-249.
8. Yamaizumi M, Sugano T: U.V.-induced nuclear accumulation of p53 is evoked through DNA damage of actively transcribed genes independent of the cell cycle. Oncogene 1994;9:2775-2784.
9. Ljungman M, Zhang F: Blockage of RNA polymerase as a possible trigger for UV light-induced apoptosis. Oncogene 1996;13:823-831.
10. Nelson WG, Kastan MB: DNA strand breaks: the DNA template alterations that trigger p53-dependent DNA damage response pathways. Mol Cell Biol 1994;14:1815-1823.
11. Friedberg EC, Wagner R, Radman M: Specialized DNA polymerases, cellular survival, and the genesis of mutations. Science 2002;296:1627-1630.
12. Kunkel TA: Considering the cancer consequences of altered DNA polymerase function. Cancer Cell 2003;3:105-110.
13. Masutani C, Kusumoto R, Yamada A, et al: The XPV (xeroderma pigmentosum variant) gene encodes human DNA polymerase eta. Nature 1999;399:700-704.
14. Johnson RE, Kondratick CM, Prakash S, Prakash L: hRAD30 mutations in the variant form of xeroderma pigmentosum. Science 1999;285:263-265.
15. Weinert TA, Hartwell LH: The RAD9 gene controls the cell cycle response to DNA damage in Saccharomyces cerevisiae. Science 1988;241:317-322.
16. Ford JM, Hanawalt PC: Li-Fraumeni syndrome fibroblasts homozygous for p53 mutations are deficient in global DNA repair but exhibit normal transcription-coupled repair and enhanced UV resistance. Proc Natl Acad Sci USA 1995;92:8876-8880.
17. Ford JM, Hanawalt PC: Expression of wild-type p53 is required for efficient global genomic nucleotide excision repair in UV-irradiated human fibroblasts. J Biol Chem 1997;272:28073-28080.
18. Hwang BJ, Ford JM, Hanawalt PC, Chu G: Expression of the p48 xeroderma pigmentosum gene is p53-dependent and is involved in global genomic repair. Proc Natl Acad Sci USA 1999;96:424-428.
19. Adimoolam S, Ford JM: p53 and DNA damage-inducible expression of the xeroderma pigmentosum group C gene. Proc Natl Acad Sci USA 2002;19:12985-12990.
20. Adimoolam S, Ford JM: p53 and regulation of DNA damage recognition during nucleotide excision repair. DNA Repair 2003;2(9):947-954.
21. Scully R, Chen J, Ochs RL, et al: Dynamic changes of BRCA1 subnuclear location and phosphorylation state are initiated by DNA damage. Cell 1997;90:425-435.
22. Scully R, Chen J, Plug A, et al: Association of BRCA1 with Rad51 in mitotic and meiotic cells. Cell 1997;88:265-275.
23. Cortez D, Wang Y, Qin J, Elledge SJ: Requirement of ATM-dependent phosphorylation of brca1 in the DNA damage response to double-strand breaks. Science 1999;286:1162-1166.
24. Wu X, Ranganathan V, Weisman DS, et al: ATM phosphorylation of Nijmegen breakage syndrome protein is required in a DNA damage response. Nature 2000;405:477-482.
25. Fitch ME, Cross IV, Ford JM: p53 responsive nucleotide excision repair gene products p48 and XPC, but not p53, localize to sites of UV-irradiation-induced DNA damage, in vivo. Carcinogenesis 2003;24:843-850.
26. Smith ML, Fornace AJ Jr: Mammalian DNA damage-inducible genes associated with growth arrest and apoptosis. Mutat Res 1996;340:109-124.
27. Fornace AJ Jr, Amundson SA, Bittner M, et al: The complexity of radiation stress responses: analysis by informatics and functional genomics approaches. Gene Expr 1999;7:387-400.
28. Zhao R, Gish K, Murphy M, et al: Analysis of p53-regulated gene expression patterns using oligonucleotide arrays. Genes Dev 2000;14:981-993.
29. Lowe SW, Schmitt EM, Smith SW, Osborne BA, Jacks T: p53 is required for radiation-induced apoptosis in mouse thymocytes. Nature 1993;362:847-849.
30. Lowe SW, Ruley HE, Jacks T, Housman DE: p53-dependent apoptosis modulates the cytotoxicity of anticancer agents. Cell 1993;74:957-967.
31. Clarke AR, Purdie CA, Harrison DJ, et al: Thymocyte apoptosis induced by p53-dependent and independent pathways. Nature 1993;362:849-852.
32. Cline SD, Hanawalt PC: Who's on first in the cellular response to DNA damage? Nat Rev Mol Cell Biol 2003;4:361-73.
33. Canman CE, Lim DS, Cimprich KA, et al: Activation of the ATM kinase by ionizing radiation and phosphorylation of p53. Science 1998;281:1677-1679.
34. Kastan MB, Lim DS: The many substrates and functions of ATM. Nat Rev Mol Cell Biol 2000;1:179-186.
35. Shieh SY, Ahn J, Tamai K, Taya Y, Prives C: The human homologs of checkpoint kinases Chk1 and Cds1 (Chk2) phosphorylate p53 at multiple DNA damage-inducible sites. Genes Dev 2000;14:289-300.
36. Matsuoka S, Huang M, Elledge SJ: Linkage of ATM to cell cycle regulation by the Chk2 protein kinase. Science 1998;282:1893-1897.
37. Liu Q, Guntuku S, Cui XS, et al: Chk1 is an essential kinase that is regulated by Atr and required for the G(2)/M DNA damage checkpoint. Genes Dev 2000;14:1448-1459.
38. Shiloh Y: ATM and related protein kinases: safeguarding genome integrity. Nat Rev Cancer 2003;3:155-168.
39. Tibbetts RS, Brumbaugh KM, Williams JM, et al: A role for ATR in the DNA damage-induced phosphorylation of p53. Genes Dev 1999;13:152-157.
40. Xu B, O'Donnell AH, Kim ST, Kastan MB: Phosphorylation of serine 1387 in Brca1 is specifically required for the ATM-mediated S-phase checkpoint after ionizing irradiation. Cancer Res 2002;62:4588-4591.
41. Bakkenist CJ, Kastan MB: DNA damage activates ATM through intermolecular autophosphorylation and dimer dissociation. Nature 2003;421:499-506.
42. Hanawalt PC: Subpathways of nucleotide excision repair and their regulation. Oncogene 2002;21:8949-8956.

43. Friedberg EC: DNA Repair. New York, WH Freeman, 1985.

44. Setlow RB, Carrier W: The disappearance of thymidine dimers from DNA: an error correcting mechanism. Proc Natl Acad Sci USA 1964;51:226–231.

45. Boyce R, Howard-Flanders P: Release of UV light-induced thymidine dimers from DNA in E. coli. Proc Natl Acad Sci USA 1964;51:293–300.

46. Pettijohn D, Hanawalt PC: Evidence for repair-replication of UV damage in bacteria. J Mol Biol 1964;9:395–402.

47. Wood RD: Nucleotide excision repair in mammalian cells. J Biol Chem 1997;272:23465–23468.

48. de Laat WL, Jaspers NG, Hoeijmakers JH: Molecular mechanism of nucleotide excision repair. Genes Dev 1999;13:768–785.

49. Wood RD, Mitchell M, Sgouros J, Lindahl T: Human DNA repair genes. Science 2001;291:1284–1289.

50. Cleaver JE: Defective repair replication of DNA in xeroderma pigmentosum. Nature 1968;218:652–656.

51. Kraemer KH, Lee MM, Scotto J: DNA repair protects against cutaneous and internal neoplasia: evidence from xeroderma pigmentosum. Carcinogenesis 1984;5:511–514.

52. Cleaver JE, Kraemer KH: Xeroderma pigmentosum. In Scriver CR, Beudet AL, Sly WS, Valle D (eds): Metabolic Basis of Inherited Disease. New York, McGraw-Hill, 1989, pp 2949–2971.

53. Kraemer KH, Slor H: Xeroderma pigmentosum. Clin Dermatol 1985;3:33–69.

54. Robbins JH: Xeroderma pigmentosum: defective DNA repair causes skin cancer and neurodegeneration. JAMA 1988;260:384–388.

55. Wang YC, Maher VM, Mitchell DL, McCormick JJ: Evidence from mutation spectra that the UV hypermutability of xeroderma pigmentosum variant cells reflects abnormal, error-prone replication on a template containing photoproducts. Mol Cell Biol 1993;13:4276–4283.

56. Schmickel RD, Chu EHY, Trosko JE: Cockayne syndrome: a cellular sensitivity to ultraviolet light. Pediatrics 1977;60:135–139.

57. Venema J, Mullenders LHF, Natarajan AT, Van Zeeland AA, Mayne LV: The genetic defect in Cockayne syndrome is associated with a defect in repair of UV-induced DNA damage in transcriptionally active DNA. Proc Natl Acad Sci USA 1990;87:4707–4711.

58. Cooper PK, Nouspikel T, Clarkson SG, Leadon SA: Defective transcription-coupled repair of oxidative base damage in Cockayne syndrome patients from XP group G. Science 1997;275:990–993.

59. Timme TL, Moses RE: Review: diseases with DNA damage-processing defects. Am J Med Sci 1988;295:40–48.

60. Nance MA, Berry SA: Cockayne syndrome: review of 140 cases. Am J Med Gen 1992;42:68–84.

61. Robbins JH, Kraemer KH, Lutzner MA, Festoff BW, Coon HG: Xeroderma pigmentosum: an inherited disease with sun sensitivity, multiple cutaneous neoplasms and abnormal repair. Ann Intern Med 1974;80:221–228.

62. Vermeulen W, Scott RJ, Rodgers S, et al: Clinical heterogeneity within xeroderma pigmentosum associated with mutations in the DNA repair and transcription gene ERCC3. Am J Hum Genet 1994;54:191–200.

63. Lehmann AR: The xeroderma pigmentosum group D (XPD) gene: one gene, two functions, three diseases. Genes Dev 2001;15:15–23.

64. Benhamou S, Sarasin A: ERCC2/XPD gene polymorphisms and cancer risk. Mutagenesis 2002;17:463–469.

65. Mohrenweiser HW, Wilson DM, Jones IM: Challenges and complexities in estimating both the functional impact and the disease risk associated with the extensive genetic variation in human DNA repair genes. Mutat Res 2003;526:93–125.

66. Demple B, Harrison L: Repair of oxidative damage to DNA: enzymology and biology. Annu Rev Biochem 1994;63:915–948.

67. Seeberg E, Eide L, Bjoras M: The base excision repair pathway. Trends Biochem Sci 1995;20:391–397.

68. Al-Tassan N, Chmiel NH, Maynard J, et al: Inherited variants of MYH associated with somatic G:C→T:A mutations in colorectal tumors. Nat Genet 2002;30:227–232.

69. Jones S, Emmerson P, Maynard J, et al: Biallelic germline mutations in MYH predispose to multiple colorectal adenoma and somatic G:C→T:A mutations. Hum Mol Genet 2002;11:2961–2967.

70. Halford SE, Rowan AJ, Lipton L, et al: Germline mutations but not somatic changes at the myh locus contribute to the pathogenesis of unselected colorectal cancers. Am J Pathol 2003;162:1545–1548.

71. Le Page F, Kwoh EE, Avrutskaya A, et al: Transcription-coupled repair of 8-oxoguanine: requirement for XPG, TFIIH, and CSB and implications for Cockayne syndrome. Cell 2000;101:159–171.

72. Bohr VA: Repair of oxidative DNA damage in nuclear and mitochondrial DNA, and some changes with aging in mammalian cells. Free Radic Biol Med 2002;32:804–812.

73. Morland I, Rolseth V, Luna L, Rognes T, Bjoras M, Seeberg E: Human DNA glycosylases of the bacterial Fpg/MutM superfamily: an alternative pathway for the repair of 8-oxoguanine and other oxidation products in DNA. Nucleic Acids Res 2002;30:4926–4936.

74. Seo YR, Fishel ML, Amundson S, Kelley MR, Smith ML: Implication of p53 in base excision DNA repair: in vivo evidence. Oncogene 2002;21:731–737.

75. Smith ML, Seo YR: p53 regulation of DNA excision repair pathways. Mutagenesis 2002;17:149–156.

76. Friedberg EC, Meira LB: Database of mouse strains carrying targeted mutations in genes affecting biological responses to DNA damage. Version 5. DNA Repair (Amst) 2003;2:501–530.

77. Divine KK, Gilliland FD, Crowell RE, et al: The XRCC1 399 glutamine allele is a risk factor for adenocarcinoma of the lung. Mutat Res 2001;461:273–278.

78. Goode EL, Ulrich CM, Potter JD: Polymorphisms in DNA repair genes and associations with cancer risk. Cancer Epidemiol Biomarkers Prev 2002;11:1513–1530.

79. Kolodner R: Biochemistry and genetics of eukaryotic mismatch repair. Genes Dev 1996;10:1433–1442.

80. Kolodner RD, Marsischky GT: Eukaryotic DNA mismatch repair. Curr Opin Genet Dev 1999;9:89–96.

81. Jiricny J, Nystrom-Lahti M: Mismatch repair defects in cancer. Curr Opin Genet Dev 2000;15:157–161.

82. Peltomaki P: Role of DNA mismatch repair defects in the pathogenesis of human cancer. J Clin Oncol 2003;21:1174–1179.

83. Fishel R, Lescoe MK, Rao MRS, et al: The human mutator gene homolog MSH2 and its association with hereditary nonpolyposis colon cancer. Cell 1993;75:1027–1038.

84. Hemminki A, Peltomaki P, Mecklin JP, et al: Loss of the wild type MLH1 gene is a feature of hereditary nonpolyposis colorectal cancer. Nat Genet 1994;8:405–410.

85. Papadopoulos N, Nicolaides NC, Wei YF, et al: Mutation of a mutL homolog in hereditary colon cancer. Science 1994;263:1625–1629.

86. Karran P, Bignami M: DNA damage tolerance, mismatch repair and genome instability. Bioessays 1994;16:833–839.

87. Lynch HT, Smyrk T: Hereditary nonpolyposis colorectal cancer (Lynch syndrome). An updated review. Cancer 1996;78:1149–1167.

88. Parsons R, Li GM, Longley MJ, et al: Hypermutability and mismatch repair deficiency in RER+ tumor cells. Cell 1993;75:1227–1236.

89. Thibodeau SN, Bren G, Schaid D: Microsatellite instability in cancer of the proximal colon. Science 1993;260:816–819.

90. Kuismanen SA, Holmberg MT, Salovaara R, et al: Epigenetic phenotypes distinguish microsatellite-stable and -unstable colorectal cancers. Proc Natl Acad Sci USA 1999;96:12661–12666.

91. Nakagawa H, Nuovo GJ, Zervos EE, et al: Age-related hypermethylation of the 5′ region of MLH1 in normal colonic mucosa is associated with microsatellite-unstable colorectal cancer development. Cancer Res 2001;61:6991–6995.

92. Gryfe R, Kim H, Hsieh ET, et al: Tumor microsatellite instability and clinical outcome in young patients with colorectal cancer. N Engl J Med 2000;342:69–77.

93. Hemminki A, Mecklin JP, Jarvinen H, Aaltonen LA, Jooensuu H: Microsatellite instability is a favorable prognostic indicator in patients with colorectal cancer receiving chemotherapy. Gastroenterology 2000;119:921–928.

94. Samowitz WS, Curtin K, Ma KN, et al: Microsatellite instability in sporadic colon cancer is associated with an improved prognosis at the population level. Cancer Epidemiol Biomarkers Prev 2001;10:917–923.

95. Bell DW, Varley JM, Szydlo TE, et al: Heterozygous germ line hCHK2 mutations in Li-Fraumeni syndrome. Science 1999;286:2528–2531.

96. Meijers-Heijboer H, van den Ouweland A, Klijn J, et al: Low-penetrance susceptibility to breast cancer due to CHEK2(*)1100delC in noncarriers of BRCA1 or BRCA2 mutations. Nat Genet 2002;31:55–59.

97. Vahteristo P, Bartkova J, Eerola H, et al: A CHEK2 genetic variant contributing to a substantial fraction of familial breast cancer. Am J Hum Genet 2002;71:432–438.

98. Kastan MB, Onyekwere O, Sidransky D, Vogelstein B, Craig RW: Participation of p53 protein in the cellular response to DNA damage. Cancer Res 1991;51:6304–6311.

99. Kuerbitz SJ, Plunkett BS, Walsh WV, Kastan MB: Wild-type p53 is a cell cycle checkpoint determinant following irradiation. Proc Natl Acad Sci USA 1992;89:7491–7495.

100. Khanna KK, Keating KE, Kozlov S, et al: ATM associates with and phosphorylates p53: mapping the region of interaction. Nat Genet 1998;20:398–400.

101. Banin S, Moyal L, Shieh S, et al: Enhanced phosphorylation of p53 by ATM in response to DNA damage. Science 1998;281:1674–1677.

102. Gatti RA, Tward A, Concannon P: Cancer risk in ATM heterozygotes: a model of phenotypic and mechanistic differences between missense and truncating mutations. Mol Genet Metab 1999;68:419–423.

103. Dork T, Bendix R, Bremer M, et al: Spectrum of ATM gene mutations in a hospital-based series of unselected breast cancer patients. Cancer Res 2001;61:7608–7615.

104. Scott SP, Bendix R, Chen P, Clark R, Dork T, Lavin MF: Missense mutations but not allelic variants alter the function of ATM by dominant interference in patients with breast cancer. Proc Natl Acad Sci USA 2002;99:925–930.

105. Carney JP, Maser RS, Olivares H, et al: The hMre11/hRad50 protein complex and Nijmegen breakage syndrome: linkage of double-strand break repair to the cellular DNA damage response. Cell 1998;93:477–486.

106. Stewart GS, Maser RS, Stankovic T, et al: The DNA double-strand break repair gene hMRE11 is mutated in individuals with an ataxia-telangiectasia-like disorder. Cell 1999;99:577–587.

107. Nakayama H, Nakayama K, Nakayama R, Irino N, Nakayama Y, Hanawalt PC: Isolation and genetic characterization of a thymineless death-resistant mutant of Escherichia coli K12: identification of a new mutation (recQ1) that blocks the RecF recombination pathway. Mol Gen Genet 1984;195:474–480.

108. Hickson ID: RecQ helicases: Caretakers of the genome. Nat Rev Cancer 2003;3:169–178.

109. Ellis NA, Groden J, Ye TZ, et al: The Bloom's syndrome gene product is homologous to RecQ helicases. Cell 1995;83:655–666.

110. Ellis NA, German J: Molecular genetics of Bloom's syndrome. Hum Mol Genet 1996;5:1457–1463.

111. Gruber SB, Ellis NA, Scott KK, et al: BLM heterozygosity and the risk of colorectal cancer. Science 2002;297:2013.

112. Goss KH, Risinger MA, Kordich JJ, et al: Enhanced tumor formation in mice heterozygous for Blm mutation. Science 2002;297:2051–2053.

113. Yu CE, Oshima J, Fu YH, et al: Positional cloning of the Werner's syndrome gene. Science 1996;272:258–262.

114. Oshima J: The Werner syndrome protein: an update. Bioessays 2000;22:894–901.

115. Shen JC, Loeb LA: The Werner syndrome gene: the molecular basis of RecQ helicase-deficiency diseases. Trends Genet 2000;16:213–220.

116. Kitao S, Shimamoto A, Goto M, et al: Mutations in RECQL4 cause a subset of cases of Rothmund-Thomson syndrome. Nat Genet 1999;22:82–84.

117. Wang LL, Gannavarapu A, Kozinetz CA: Association between osteosarcoma and deleterious mutations in the RECQL4 gene in Rothmund-Thomson syndrome. J Natl Cancer Inst 2003;95:669–674.

118. Hollstein M, Sidranksky D, Vogelstein B, Harris CC: p53 mutations in human cancers. Science 1991;253:49–53.

119. Levine, AJ: p53, the cellular gatekeeper for growth and division. Cell 1997;88:323–331.

120. Oren M: Regulation of the p53 tumor suppressor protein. J Biol Chem 1999;274:36031–36034.

121. El-Deiry WS, Tokino T, Velculescu VE, et al: WAF1, a potential mediator of p53 tumor suppression. Cell 1993;75:817–825.

122. Vousden KH, Lu X: Live or let die: the cell's response to p53. Nat Rev Cancer 2002;2:594–604.

123. Malkin D, Li FP, Strong LC, et al: Germ line p53 mutations in a familial syndrome of breast cancer, sarcomas and other neoplasms. Science 1990;250:1233–1238.

124. Srivastava S, Zou ZQ, Pirollo K, Blattner W, Chang EH: Germ-line transmission of a mutated p53 gene in a cancer-prone family with Li-Fraumeni syndrome. Nature 1990;348:747–749.

125. Frebourg T, Barbier N, Yan YX, et al: Germ-line p53 mutations in 15 families with Li-Fraumeni syndrome. Am J Hum Genet 1995;56:608–615.

126. Jasin M: Homologous repair of DNA damage and tumorigenesis: the BRCA connection. Oncogene 2002;21:8981–8993.

127. Venkitaraman AR: Cancer susceptibility and the functions of BRCA1 and BRCA2. Cell 2002;108:171–182.

128. Venkitaraman AR: A growing network of cancer-susceptibility genes. N Engl J Med 2003;348:1917–1919.

129. Hartman AR, Ford JM: BRCA1 and p53: Compensatory roles in DNA repair. J Mol Med 2003;81:700–707.

130. Wooster R, Weber BL: Breast and ovarian cancer. N Engl J Med 2003;348:2339–2347.

131. Xu B, Kim S, Kastan MB: Involvement of Brca1 in S-phase and G(2)-phase checkpoints after ionizing irradiation. Mol Cell Biol 2001;21:3445–3450.

132. Wang Y, Cortez D, Yazdi P, Neff N, Elledge SJ, Qin J: BASC, a super complex of BRCA1-associated proteins involved in the recognition and repair of aberrant DNA structures. Genes Dev 2000;14:927–939.

133. Moynahan ME, Chiu JW, Koller BH, Jasin M: Brca1 controls homology-directed DNA repair. Mol Cell 1999;4:511–518.

134. Harkin DP, Bean JM, Miklos D, et al: Induction of GADD45 and JNK/SAPK-dependent apoptosis following inducible expression of BRCA1. Cell 1999;97:575–586.

135. Hartman AR, Ford JM: BRCA1 induces DNA damage recognition factors and enhances nucleotide excision repair. Nat Genet 2002;32:180–184.

136. Pellegrini L, Yu DS, Lo T, et al: Insights into DNA recombination from the structure of a RAD51-BRCA2 complex. Nature 2002;420:287–293.

137. Yang H, Jeffrey PD, Miller J, et al: BRCA2 function in DNA binding and recombination from a BRCA2-DSS1-ssDNA structure. Science 2002;297:1837–1848.

138. Alter BP: Cancer in Fanconi anemia, 1927–2001. Cancer 2003;97:425–440.

139. D'Andrea AD, Grompe M: The Fanconi anaemia/BRCA pathway. Nat Rev Cancer 2003;3:23–34.

140. Howlett NG, Taniguchi T, Olson S, et al: Biallelic inactivation of BRCA2 in Fanconi anemia. Science 2002;297:606–609.

141. Garcia-Higuera I, Taniguchi T, Ganesan S, et al: Interaction of the Fanconi anemia proteins and BRCA1 in a common pathway. Mol Cell 2001;7:249–262.

142. Taniguchi T, Garcia-Higuera I, Xu B, et al: Convergence of the Fanconi anemia and ataxia telangiectasia signaling pathways. Cell 2002;109:459–472.

143. Loeb LA: Mutator phenotype may be required for multistage carcinogenesis. Cancer Res 1991;51:3075–3079.

Science of Clinical Oncology

I

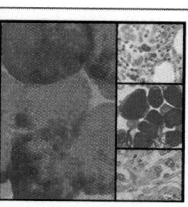

12

VIRUSES AND HUMAN CANCER

Paul F. Lambert

Bill Sugden

SUMMARY OF KEY POINTS

- The last 25 years have revealed the existence of human tumor viruses.
- Human tumor viruses contribute to at least 15% of all human cancers.
- The mechanisms by which viruses contribute to development of associated cancers have illuminated nonviral causes of human cancer.

- Specific viral targets for development of antiviral therapies can be identified through detailed understanding of these mechanisms.
- Understanding the modes of transmission of tumor viruses has led to public health measures to stop the spread of the viruses and

to development and use of effective vaccines.
- The study of human tumor viruses has become an underappreciated paradigm for the goal of cancer research: to understand the cause of a specific cancer so that the cancer can be prevented.

INTRODUCTION

Viruses cause cancer in people. Approximately 15% of all human cancers are thought to have a viral cause,[1] and this fraction is likely to grow as we investigate additional cancers for a potential viral cause and identify new human viruses. Identifying a human cancer as having a viral cause has substantive consequences both for treatment and for prevention. The known virally caused human cancers often express virally encoded products in the tumor cells. These viral products are potential targets for antiviral, tumor-specific therapies. Viral infections can be prevented by vaccines; therefore it may be possible to eliminate human cancers that require viral contributions for development.

The search for human tumor viruses has been propelled by a long appreciation that viruses can cause cancers in birds and rodents. Viruses were isolated as filterable extracts from avian tumors in the first decade of the last century and were shown to induce tumors in susceptible animals.[2,3] Parallel findings were made in mice in the 1940s.[4] These animal tumor viruses were in the retrovirus family and led researchers to look for retroviruses as human tumor viruses in the 1960s and 1970s. However, most of the human tumor viruses subsequently identified are in different virus families and do not conform to some of the expectations derived from study of highly oncogenic animal retroviruses. For example, highly oncogenic tumor viruses induce tumors in animals rapidly. Inoculation of Rous sarcoma virus into the wing web of newborn chicks can induce fatal sarcoma within 2 weeks in 100% of susceptible animals.[5] In addition, highly oncogenic tumor viruses are oncogenic because they have acquired and express potent derivatives of cellular proto-oncogenes. In fact, many of the known human proto-oncogenes were first identified as homologues of the oncogenes transduced by the highly

oncogenic animal retroviruses.[6] Known human tumor viruses, however, usually do not induce cancers rapidly; often 15 to 50 years elapse between the primary infection and tumor development. Nor do human tumor viruses express cellularly derived oncogenes; rather, some of them have evolved to inhibit cellular tumor suppressor genes. These differences between highly oncogenic animal viruses and human tumor viruses probably have contributed to reticence in our recognizing that viruses do cause cancers in people.

A second obstacle in our recognizing that viruses can be tumorigenic in their human hosts is that we lack convincing animal models in which to test these viruses directly. For all practical purposes, all known human tumor viruses infect only people. In addition, we now know that human viruses found not to be tumorigenic in people are tumorigenic when experimentally introduced into test animals. For example, human adenovirus 12, which causes only respiratory infections in people, is highly oncogenic when inoculated into newborn hamsters.[7] The lack of an experimentally tractable animal host for human tumor viruses has required multiple lines of evidence to affirm that a given virus can contribute to a given human cancer. In particular, epidemiologic findings have been combined with genetic and molecular analyses in cell culture to identify human tumor viruses. Experiments with mice transgenic for viral genes also have supported these identifications.

We introduce the six known human tumor viruses, the tumors with which they are associated, data that support these associations, and models to explain the viral contributions to these tumors. These viruses are discussed in the order of discovery; early findings often have provided insight for analysis of subsequently identified viruses. Finally, we outline the kinds of virus-specific therapies it is possible to develop and the likelihood of developing vaccines to human tumor viruses to limit or eliminate specific human cancers.

EPSTEIN-BARR VIRUS

Epstein-Barr Virus (EBV) was identified through the insight and advocacy of Dennis Burkitt, who as a young surgeon, having identified Burkitt's lymphoma as a new disease entity, analyzed the geographic and climatic distribution of this childhood lymphoma, determined that it overlapped with that of malaria, and posited it to have an infectious cause.[8] At Burkitt's urging and with his proffered biopsy samples, Michael Anthony Epstein, Yvonne Barr, and their colleagues identified EBV in Burkitt's lymphoma–derived cells.[9] To do so, these investigators developed the expertise to propagate these cells in culture.[10] Cell lines derived from EBV-positive Burkitt's lymphoma proved powerful tools for associating EBV with various human diseases. Different EBV-positive cell lines express different viral antigens and thereby have served as test samples for patients' expression of antibodies to EBV-encoded antigens.

Results of serologic analysis of these antibodies led the Henles in Philadelphia to propose EBV as the cause of infectious mononucleosis.[11,12] A colleague in their laboratory who had lacked antibodies to EBV-encoded antigens developed those antibodies on contracting infectious mononucleosis. The etiologic role of EBV in this "self-limiting lymphoproliferation" was subsequently established by careful, prospective epidemiologic studies in which serologic analysis was used to demonstrate that only immunologically naive people were at risk of development of infectious mononucleosis. When mononucleosis developed, these people would first express antibodies to EBV-encoded antigens of the immunoglobulin M (IgM) class, and only later to those of the IgG class.[13] Thus approximately 85% of infectious mononucleosis cases were shown to arise from a primary infection with EBV. Serologic studies also allowed the Henles to propose that nasopharyngeal carcinoma (NPC) might be caused by EBV, because NPC patients were characterized by having atypically high titers to EBV-associated antigens.[14] However, the data that linked EBV causally to Burkitt's lymphoma and NPC by the early 1970s was only "guilt by association." Although EBV caused most cases of infectious mononucleosis upon primary infection, serologic evidence had demonstrated that children in the parts of Africa in which Burkitt's lymphoma is endemic and adults in the parts of China in which NPC is prevalent all had been infected with EBV, that is, were EBV seropositive, long before these cancers developed.

Serologic analysis of EBV in the 1960s and 1970s illustrated a conundrum for viruses and human cancers: How can many people be infected with a given virus, and yet how can that virus contribute to tumor development in only a few infected subjects after long periods of time? This apparent paradox applies to most cancers associated with human tumor viruses and explains a major reluctance to consider viruses as etiologic agents for human cancer. The World Health Organization, without resolving this conundrum, sponsored a prospective epidemiologic survey in Uganda that entailed serologic testing of 42,000 youngsters for evidence for or against the etiologic contribution of EBV to Burkitt's lymphoma. The region studied had a high incidence of this cancer. Blood samples were collected from children, and the serum was stored. Blood samples were obtained from children later identified as having Burkitt's lymphoma, and titers to EBV antigens were determined. In this prospective survey, investigators found 14 youngsters in whom Burkitt's lymphoma developed over the 5 years their cases were followed. Before tumor development, children in whom lymphoma developed had, on average, a 3.4-fold higher titer of antibodies to one class of EBV antigens than did children who did not have lymphoma.[15] That is, for children in parts of the world in which EBV-associated Burkitt's lymphoma is endemic, a high titer of antibodies to a given set of EBV-encoded antigens represents a 30-fold risk factor for development of Burkitt's lymphoma.[15]

Do these findings prove that EBV causes Burkitt's lymphoma? No. Proof in such cases for which direct experiments are not feasible ultimately comes from accretion of supporting findings in the absence of confounding data. The results of the World Health Organization study do, however, suggest it is unlikely that EBV is a passenger virus that merely replicates well in tumor cells, because the antibody titers were elevated 7 to 54 months before tumor detection.[15] Similar prospective surveys were performed in China and identified as a risk factor for development of NPC the presence of antibodies of the IgA class to the same set of EBV antigens.[16]

The association of EBV with Burkitt's lymphoma and NPC and the demonstration that EBV causes most cases of infectious mononucleosis have led researchers to consider other diseases with which EBV might be associated. During the last 20 years, EBV has been linked to post-transplantation lymphoproliferative disease (PTLD),[17] oral hairy leukoplakia,[18] approximately one third to one half of cases of Hodgkin's disease,[19,20] and one tenth of cases of gastric carcinoma.[21] These linkages have been made not only through serologic analysis but also by molecular genetic analyses that render the linkages more robust. The latter analyses have been made possible by elucidation of the molecular virologic features of EBV in cell culture.[22]

EBV is a herpesvirus. It has a double-stranded DNA of 165,000 to 170,000 base pairs (bp)[23] and encodes approximately 80 genes[24] (Fig. 12-1). Like other herpesviruses, EBV has two distinct phases to its life cycle. It can infect cells, express a small subset of its genes (see Fig. 12-1), and cohabit with the cell, without killing it. This is the latent phase. EBV also can emerge from its latency, express all or most of its genes, amplify its DNA, assemble progeny virions, and kill its host cell by lysis. This is the lytic phase. Unlike neurotropic herpesviruses such as herpes simplex virus type 1 (HSV-1) and varicella-zoster virus, EBV in its latent phase need not be maintained in a nonproliferating host cell. Rather, it has the capacity to both initiate and maintain proliferation in at least the B lymphocytes it infects in cell culture and at early stages of primary infection in vivo.[25,26] It is its ability to affect proliferation and survival of the infected host cell that likely renders EBV oncogenic.

Figure 12-1. Map of the Epstein-Barr (EBV) genome. The genome of the B95-8 strain of EBV in its circular double-stranded DNA form of 165 kilobase pairs (kbp) is depicted as it is found in latently infected B cells. The genome is a linear DNA within the viral particle and is circularized on infection at its terminal repeat (TR) elements found at the 5′ and 3′ ends of the linear molecule. The EBV genome encodes approximately 80 genes. The exons (*yellow boxes*) for coding segments of the viral genes expressed in B cells infected in vitro, including *EBNA1*, *EBNA2*, *EBNA3a/b/c*, *EBNA-LP*, *LMP1*, and *LMPA/B*. The yellow boxes designated EBERs are the two small RNAs encoded by EBV. *Dashed lines* represent primary transcripts originating from viral promoters denoted *p*. Also shown are the positions of the origins of replication, OriP and OriLyt, which support the latent and lytic replication of the viral genome, respectively. (See Kieff and Rickinson[22] for details of the genome and life cycle of EBV.)

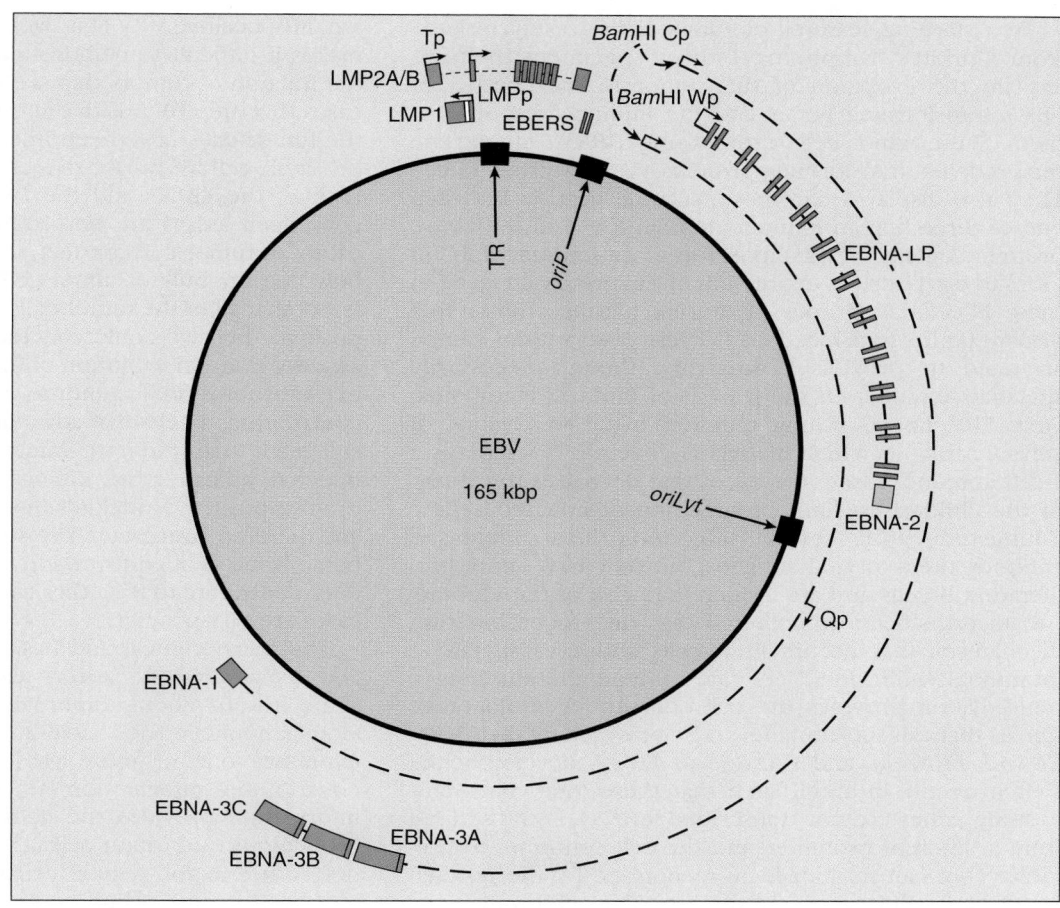

EBV induces and maintains infected B lymphocytes to proliferate by maintaining its DNA extrachromosomally and expressing at least five viral genes that regulate expression of both viral and cellular genes and control viral DNA replication.[27] EBV-infected cells that contain intact viral DNA and express two or more viral genes are hallmarks of all EBV-associated diseases. Identification of viral DNA and of viral gene products, our gradual appreciation of the functions of these viral gene products, and immune responses to them now constitute much of the persuasive evidence linking EBV causally to its associated cancers.

EBV clearly can induce and maintain proliferation of infected B cells. Genetic experiments in which two viral genes, *EBNA2* and *LMP1* (see Fig. 12-1), within the context of the virus are expressed conditionally demonstrate that each gene product assayed alone must function for infected B cells to continue to proliferate.[28,29] These observations are particularly telling because they help to explain the multistep evolution of Burkitt's lymphoma. Many other genetic analyses have shown that three additional viral genes—*EBNA1*, *EBNA3a*, and *EBNA3c* (see Fig. 12-1)—contribute to some facet of cell proliferation.[27] *EBNA1* has been found to be required for survival of infected cells and, at least indirectly, to be required to maintain cell proliferation as well.[30] *EBNA3a* acts at the stage of initiation of proliferation.[31] All of these viral

transforming genes except for *EBNA1* are recognized by the cytotoxic T-cell response of the host.[32] *EBNA1* encodes a stretch of gly, gly, ala residues that inhibits its proteolytic degradation and subsequent presentation by class I HLA molecules.[33] The cytotoxic response of the host is sufficiently robust that patients recovering from infectious mononucleosis lack B cells that express RNA encoding these transforming genes. The surviving EBV-infected B cells are in distinct, differentiated states in which they no longer proliferate and express only another detectable viral protein, *LMP2*, a viral gene product not required for cellular proliferation (see Fig. 12-1).[34,35]

Failure of this robust immune response to EBV's transforming proteins contributes to PTLD. The infected proliferating B cells in these immunosuppressed patients express all five of the transforming proteins.[36] Two kinds of successful therapy for PTLD demonstrate the critical role of the patient's immune response in failing to limit this "iatrogenic" tumor. First, if immunosuppression can be reduced for the patient such that a transplant is still tolerated, PTLD may regress. Second, several groups have amplified the donor's T cells cytotoxic for EBV's transforming proteins before bone marrow transplantation. Treatment of PTLD patients with these syngenic, specific killer T cells has been curative.[37] These encouraging findings underscore the important role of the immune response in limiting survival of EBV-infected cells.

Science of Clinical Oncology

Two startling features of tumor cells freshly isolated from Burkitt's lymphoma biopsy specimens help to explain the evolution of this tumor in the context of EBV's transforming genes and the immune response to them. These tumor cells express only *EBNA1* among the required viral transforming proteins, yet they proliferate.[38] They also display a chromosomal translocation between one of three human immunoglobulin loci and the c-*myc* proto-oncogene.[39,40] Juxtaposition of an immunoglobulin locus to c-*myc* drives expression of the proto-oncogene in these B cells as it does in murine plasmacytomas that display similar translocations.[41] These observations can be arranged to provide a satisfying, though necessarily speculative model for the genesis of Burkitt's lymphoma. First, EBV infects young children living in regions of central Africa in which malaria is endemic.[42] Malaria is a T-cell immunosuppressive agent that decreases the ability of the children to limit proliferation of infected cells.[43] Youngsters with severe infections have increased antibody titers to viral antigens, but they have more proliferating B cells and are at increased risk of the chromosomal translocation, fostered by the recombination mechanism, that occurs in B cells and uses signals at immunoglobulin loci.[44] A rare immunoglobulin/c-*myc* translocation provides the cell constitutive proliferative signals that can substitute for those provided by the *LMP1*, *EBNA2*, *EBNA3a*, and *EBNA3c* of EBV. A developmental switch occurs in a cell such that these four viral transforming genes are not transcribed. *EBNA1* is transcribed from a different promoter; and the cell continues to proliferate but can no longer be recognized by the residual cytotoxic T-cell response of the host. The cell proliferates, acquires additional mutations (often mutations inactivating p53), and evolves rapidly into Burkitt's lymphoma.[45] This model fits well with what we know today. Each of the cancers with which EBV is causally associated is sufficiently idiosyncratic, however, to make it impractical to extend this model beyond Burkitt's lymphoma.

All EBV-associated cancers contain EBV DNA and express *EBNA1* and EBERs (see Fig. 12-1), which are small viral RNAs. Some of the cancers also express *LMP1*.[36] We know less about the genesis of these other tumors, but findings on NPC provide evidence for an unexpected contribution of EBV to its causation. Huang and her colleagues have shown that EBV infects cells that already can be distinguished as being preneoplastic in the evolution of NPC.[46] This finding might lead one to believe that EBV is merely a passenger in this tumor. However, 100% of NPC tumors are infected with EBV, making it likely that the virus contributes some selective advantage to infected, preneoplastic cells such that they are the ones that evolve into tumors. It is not known what this selective advantage is, but it is reasonable to hypothesize that EBV could provide these cells proliferative or survival signals, as it does to Burkitt's lymphoma cells during their evolution.

Two additional cancers associated with EBV differ dramatically from Burkitt's lymphoma, NPC, and PTLD in viral association. Whereas effectively all cases of Burkitt's lymphoma in Africa, all of NPC, and all PTLD are EBV-positive, only approximately 30% to 50% of cases of Hodgkin's disease and 10% of cases of gastric carcinoma are EBV-positive.[21,47] This lack of a general association makes it difficult to demonstrate a causal role for EBV in the fraction of tumors that are virus-positive. However, in cases that are EBV-positive, it has been claimed that all of the tumor cells have been infected. This finding depends on single-cell assays for detection of viral gene products such as the EBERs and the *LMP1* protein in the tumor cells. Such assays are not 100% efficient, nor is identification of tumor cells perfect, so it is accurate to conclude only that the bulk of tumor cells are infected. Were we to know that all of the tumor cells in a given patient are EBV-positive, then we could conclude that viral infection was an early event in evolution of that tumor. Retention of this extrachromosomal genome would favor the virus's contributing a selective advantage to the evolving tumor cell such that the rare infected cell outgrew any uninfected, precancerous siblings. Any contributions of EBV to virus-positive Hodgkin's disease and gastric carcinoma are, therefore, uncertain. The strongest evidence for there being some viral contribution is the recognition that EBV does contribute to the other cancers for which most or all cases are EBV-positive.

The many clinical and basic scientific studies of EBV and its associated cancers can be extracted to yield some lessons about tumor viruses in general. First, the viral genomic nucleic acid remains in tumor cells and expresses one or more viral genes. Second, the virus contributes information to infected cells, and the information provides the cells a selective advantage in evolving toward tumor cells. This information is, however, not sufficient for tumor formation. Additional, multiple, rare events must occur in the infected cells for them to evolve into tumors. These additional essential events explain both why the associated tumors develop in only a fraction of people infected with a given tumor virus and why they usually develop only after long delays.

HEPATITIS B VIRUS

Hepatitis B virus (HBV) was identified because it was recognized as an antigen in serum of donors by antibodies in serum of other infected donors.[48] Thoughtful analyses by Blumberg and his colleagues correlated the presence of the antigen with hepatitis, a correlation strengthened by seroconversion of a laboratory worker who contracted hepatitis.[48] By the late 1960s blood donated to blood banks was screened for the antigen, positive samples were removed, and only negative samples were used for transfusions. This early insightful intervention led to a significant reduction in transfusion-associated hepatitis.[49] Blumberg and his colleagues also demonstrated a striking association between HBV, antibodies to its antigens, and hepatocellular carcinoma (HCC).[48] These early findings have been built upon to demonstrate that HBV does cause HCC, which is either the fifth or sixth most common cancer in people today. Of the approximately 500,000 new cases of HCC in the world each year, HBV is estimated to cause between 50% and 70%.[50,51] Most of the rest of these cases are attributable to hepatitis C virus (HCV), a member of the flavivirus family.

Two kinds of data have established the causal role of HBV in HCC. A prospective survey of 22,707 male civil servants in Taiwan was initiated at the end of 1975.[52] Of these subjects, 3454 were found to have positive results for HBV surface antigen (HBsAg), findings that indicated chronic infection with HBV. The entire group of 22,707 members was observed for an average of 8.9 years. By the end of 1986, 152 of the 3454 HBsAg-positive men had HCC, whereas only 9 of the 19,253 HBsAg-negative men had it. The relative risk in the HBsAg-positive cohort for development of HCC was therefore 100 times greater than that for the HBsAg-negative group.[53] This prospective epidemiologic study provided robust data that the presence of HBV is strongly associated with development of HCC.

The second kind of data demonstrating that HBV can cause HCC has been derived by removing HBV from a population and determining whether the incidence of HCC declines. Taiwan began vaccinating children in 1984, first with a plasma-derived antigen and eventually with a recombinant antigen. Between 1984 and 1994, the incidence of infection as monitored by the presence of HBsAg had decreased from 9.8% to 1.3% among children 12 years or younger.[54] Similar results were found in The Gambia, where among children vaccinated during the first year, the number of 9-year-olds with chronic infection was only 10% of that among unvaccinated children.[55] HCC is a cancer that peaks in persons between 50 and 60 years of age but does occur rarely in children 6 to 14 years of age. The incidence of HCC in the latter population in Taiwan decreased from 0.64 per 100,000 per year averaged from 1981 to 1990 to 0.36 per 100,000 per year averaged between 1990 and 1994 and is statistically significant ($P < .01$).[56] This decline presumably reflects the eightfold reduction in chronic HBV infection in children at risk of development of HCC. That removing a virus from a population decreases the incidence of an associated cancer in that population is compelling evidence that the virus contributes causally to the cancer. We can expect that a decline of HCC in the vaccinated adult population will be more striking in decades to come.

Although it is clear that HBV causes HCC in people, it is not clear how it does so. Researchers now invoke two distinct contributions, direct or indirect, to explain the oncogenesis of HBV. HBV encodes one gene, pX (Fig. 12-2), which can affect viral and cellular transcription and has been proposed to contribute directly to oncogenesis. HCC in general evolves in patients with marked liver cirrhosis. HBV can contribute to cirrhosis by providing targets for T-cell killing and thereby may contribute indirectly to oncogenesis.

Molecular virologic study of HBV has illuminated the viral life cycle but has yet to identify the mode of oncogenesis.[57] HBV is a small, enveloped virus with a double-stranded DNA genome, one strand of which is incomplete. The complete viral duplex DNA is 3.2 kbp long (see Fig. 12-2), serves as a template for transcription by RNA polymerase II, and is replicated by reverse transcription of a more than full-length RNA transcript of approximately 3.4 kb. All members of the hepadnavirus family preferentially infect hepatocytes. This tropism is apparently

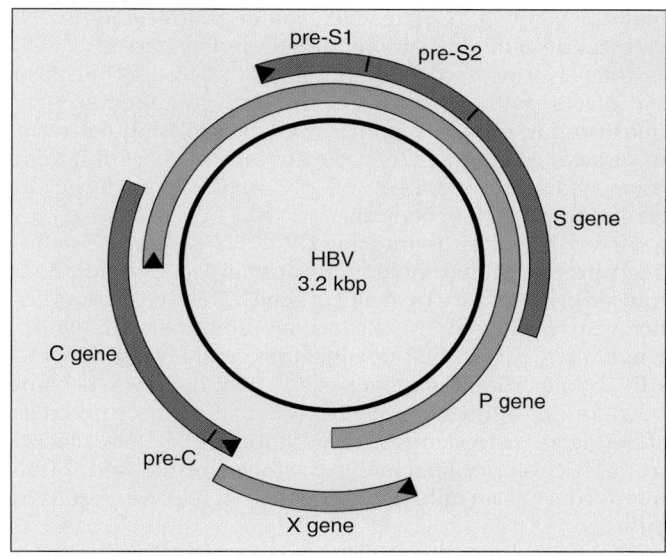

Figure 12-2. Map of the hepatitis B virus (HBV) genome. The 3200–base pair genome of HBV is a circular double-stranded DNA in infected cells (*black*). The genome in the viral particle is partially double-stranded DNA because of an incomplete extension of the plus strand by the viral DNA polymerase (P). *Colored boxes* indicate the coding segments for the structural (*blue*) and nonstructural (*yellow*) viral genes. *Arrowheads* represent the sites at which translation of the viral proteins begins. These viral proteins are translated from multiple messenger RNAs: one for Pre-S1, Pre-S2, and S; one for Pre-S2 and S; one for core and P; and one for x. (See Ganem D, Schneider R: Hepadnaviridae: The viruses and their replication. In Fields BN, Howley PM, Griffin DE, et al [eds]: Virology, vol 2, 4th ed. Philadelphia, Lippincott Williams & Wilkins, 2001, pp 2923–2969 for details of the genome and life cycle of HBV.)

mediated by a cellular receptor expressed in hepatocytes and by viral transcription, being controlled in part by cellular transcription factors principally expressed in hepatocytes. Unlike most DNA viruses, HBV undergoes its complete life cycle to yield progeny virions, which exit from hepatocytes by secretory pathways without killing the host cell. This anomalous behavior of hepadnaviruses means that, in the absence of an exogenous function of the host, an infected hepatocyte could survive, carry out its normal functions, and release large amounts of infectious HBV for long periods of time. Accordingly, some persons with chronic infection have large amounts of HBV in their serum.

Mammalian hepadnaviruses encode pX, which is not found in the avian species; only the mammalian members are known to cause HCC in their hosts. This correlation has focused interest on pX as being likely to contribute to the oncogenesis of mammalian hepadnaviruses. It is difficult to gauge the potential role of pX in the oncogenesis of HBV. Much information exists in the literature, but no ready synthesis of this information explains such a role. Most HCC tumor biopsy specimens retain viral sequences encoding pX,[58] but few express the protein detectably.[59] It has been proposed that pX associates with *p53* and inhibits its activation of apoptosis[60]; however, pX is not detected in HCC biopsies,[59] and between 30% and 90% of such biopsy specimens have

Science of Clinical Oncology

mutations in *p53*.[58,59] The viral protein pX in studies in cell culture can bind one subunit of RNA polymerase II as well as transcription factor IIB (TF-IIB).[61,62] This protein also associates with Smad4, an integral member of the transforming growth factor b (TGF-b) signaling pathway, to foster signaling in this pathway.[63] How these different transcriptional activities of pX might contribute to evolution of HCC is unclear.

HBV DNA often is integrated in HCC tumors.[64] It has been proposed that integration of viral DNA could affect transcription of nearby cellular genes. This suggestion has been strengthened by the recognition that the woodchuck member of the hepadnavirus family contributes to HCC by insertional mutagenesis.[65] HBV, however, has not been found to integrate at sites that can be interpreted as affecting its oncogenesis. In addition, HBV DNA cloned from HCC biopsy specimens has been tested and found not to score as an enhancer sequence in hepatoma cells in culture.[66]

The hypothesis that HBV indirectly contributes to the development of HCC by inducing rounds of cirrhosis and subsequent liver regeneration is appealing. HBV infection can be acute or chronic. It appears that acute infection correlates with a robust cytotoxic T-cell response to all viral antigens, whereas chronic infection correlates with a weak T-cell response.[67] These cytotoxic responses lead to death of hepatocytes; however, results of experiments with mice transgenic for HBV genes and with infected chimpanzees indicate there also is a potent noncytotoxic mechanism for limiting viral expression in infected hepatocytes.[68,69] In these experiments, immune cells release interferon γ, which by some means inhibits viral gene expression and promotes loss of viral DNA from infected cells.[68,69] Administration of interleukin 18 (IL-18) limits viral replication efficiently in a transgenic mouse model by inducing production of both type 1 and type 2 interferons.[70] Chronic, not acute, infection correlates with eventual development of HCC. How these two modes of eliminating infected cells would be balanced to yield long-term or chronic infection, the resulting cirrhosis, and the concomitant hepatocellular regeneration required for accumulation of mutations predisposing to HCC are not known.

A role for cytotoxic T cells in the evolution of HCC has been modeled in mice transgenic for HBV surface proteins (see Fig. 12-2). These mice are tolerant of these viral antigens, but when the mice are reconstituted with syngeneic, nontransgenic bone marrow and challenged with syngeneic, immune, nontransgenic splenocytes, they contract cirrhosis and maintain cytotoxic T cells specific for HbsAg.[71] These animals have long-term liver damage and by 18 to 20 months of age have HCC.

There are two consequences of the model in which HBV contributes indirectly to HCC. The first is that the oncogenesis of HBV should be limited to liver, because the process depends on the capacity of the liver to regenerate to enable the proliferation required to accumulate mutations predisposing to cancer. HBV causes only HCC. Second, no function of HBV would be required to maintain proliferation of tumor cells. The latter consequence would mean that therapies targeting functions, such as pX enhancement of transcription, would be ineffective.

HUMAN PAPILLOMAVIRUSES

Cervical cancer is caused by human papillomaviruses (HPVs). Approximately 200 genotypes of HPVs have been identified. Most HPV genotypes infect squamous epithelium lining the skin. A subset are mucosotropic and infect stratified, squamous epithelium lining the anogenital tract and oral cavity. A subset of these mucosotropic HPVs, the so-called high-risk HPVs, are associated with more than 99% of cases of human cervical cancer, other anogenital cancers, and a subset of squamous carcinomas of the head and neck, particularly those of the oropharynx. HPV-16 and HPV-18, the high-risk HPVs most common in cancer, are present in more than 85% of cases of human cervical carcinoma. The mucosotropic HPVs are thought to be transmitted sexually. The association between specific mucosotropic HPVs and human cancers was first recognized in the 1980s when Harald zur Hausen and associates at the German Cancer Research Institute in Heidelberg detected the presence of then novel HPV genotypes in human cervical cancers and in cell lines derived from such cancers.[72,73] In these cell lines, which include HeLa cells, HPV DNA often is integrated into the host genome, and only a subset of viral genes, *E6* and *E7*, are expressed.[74,75] This discovery led to the hypothesis that HPV *E6* and *E7* genes contribute to cervical cancer, a premise now well supported by experimental research.

An association between papillomaviruses and cancer was first demonstrated in the early 1930s with the recognition that a subcellular, transmittable (i.e., infectious) agent causes squamous carcinoma in cottontail rabbits.[76] The agent was later identified to be a virus, cottontail rabbit papillomavirus (CRPV), which induces warts in the rabbits. In a subset of these infected rabbits, cancer develops at the original site of CRPV infection. Other animal papillomaviruses induce frank cancer. Bovine papillomavirus (BPV), which represents a class of papillomaviruses that induce fibropapilloma, characterized by hyperplasia of both the dermal fibroblasts and epidermal epithelial cells, can induce epithelial tumors of the alimentary canal in cows.[77] Such tumors are thought to arise when animals ingest bracken fern, which contains the potent chemical carcinogen quercetin.[78-80] Thus papillomaviruses and chemical carcinogens act together to induce tumors in cattle.

Study of papillomaviruses in the laboratory began in earnest in the late 1970s, when Lowy, Howley, and their colleagues at the National Institutes of Health discovered that BPV-1 infects and transforms a mouse fibroblast cell line, C127, in cell culture.[81-83] The parental C127 cells, although immortalized, are contact inhibited. Infection by BPV-1 or transfection of C127 cells with a bacterial recombinant plasmid containing the entire BPV-1 genome yields foci of cells that are no longer contact inhibited. Transformed C127 cells harbor the viral genome as a nuclear plasmid and express viral early genes. The viral gene products *E5* (*E* referring to *early*, *5* referring to the fifth largest translational open reading frame), *E6*, and *E7*[84-89] contribute to this transformation (Fig. 12-3). By the time HPVs were recognized as potential etiologic agents

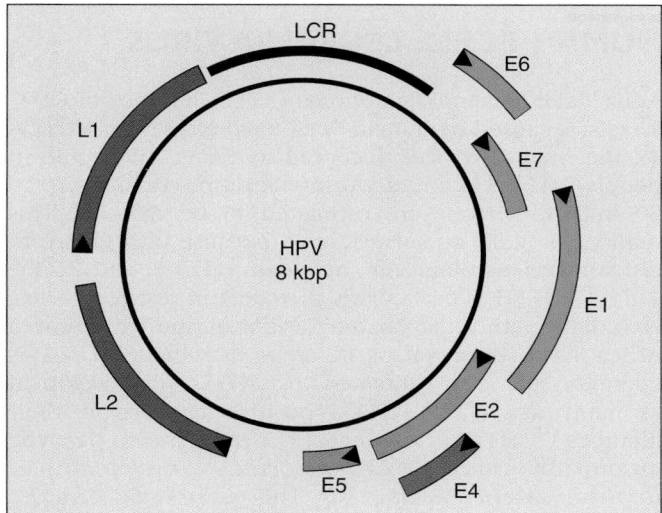

Figure 12-3. Map of the human papillomavirus (HPV) genome. The *circle* indicates the approximately 7900–base pair (bp) circular double-stranded DNA genome of HPV-16 as found in viral particles and infected cells. The *boxes outside the circle* indicate the various translational open reading frames (ORFs) that encode the viral proteins. These include the early (E) and late (L) ORFs. Most early ORFs (*yellow*) are expressed throughout the viral life cycle within stratified squamous epithelium, whereas late ORFs, which encode the capsid proteins (*blue*), and *E4* (*green*) are selectively expressed in the productively infected, terminally differentiated epithelial cells. Among the early ORFs are *E6* and *E7*, the two ORFs encoding like-named oncoproteins commonly found expressed in HPV-associated anogenital and oral cancers. RNA synthesis of papillomaviruses is complex, yielding many potential messenger RNAs, all of which terminate at polyadenylation sites located at the end of the *E5* and *L1* open reading frames. The long control region (LCR) encodes multiple *cis*-acting elements that regulate viral transcription and synthesis of viral DNA. (See Howley PM, Lowry DR: Paillomaviruses and their replication. In Fields BN, Howley PM, Griffin DE, et al [eds]: Virology, vol 2, 4th ed. Philadelphia, Lippincott Williams & Wilkins, 2001, pp 2197–2229 for details of the genome and life cycle of HPV.)

in human cervical cancer in the mid 1980s, a wealth of information pointing to the transforming potential of animal papillomaviruses in tissue culture had been established.

The seminal studies of zur Hausen and colleagues in the early to mid 1980s, in which the investigators identified HPV DNA in cell lines derived from cervical cancer, checkmated a long-argued role for HSV-2 in human cervical cancer. The posited role for HSV-2 in cervical cancer arose from findings that patients with cervical cancer often had antibodies to HSV-2, a sexually transmitted agent. However, their tumor cells lack HSV-2 DNA, and today it is accepted that HSV-2 does not contribute causally to cervical cancer. This early error provides an important lesson to researchers and epidemiologists trying to identify biologic agents that contribute to cancer. Proof by today's standards requires a smoking gun (in this case, the gun includes the viral genome and its expression of viral genes in cancer cells).

In 1985, both the zur Hausen and the Howley laboratories reported that HPV DNA (see Fig. 12-3) is integrated in chromosomal DNA in cell lines derived from cervical cancer.[74,75] This finding initially led to speculation that

HPVs contribute to cervical cancer by integrating in or nearby to disrupt the function of cellular genes that protect against cancer (i.e., tumor suppressor genes) or activate cellular genes that can promote cancers (i.e., proto-oncogenes), akin to the mechanism of oncogenesis by certain oncogenic avian and rodent retroviruses. However, a role of HPV as an insertional mutagen in cancer is not consistent with its different sites of integration in different cancers, which have not been found to be near known or suspected tumor suppressor genes or proto-oncogenes. Rather, it is likely that integration of the HPV genome leads to selective upregulation of expression of two viral genes, *E6* and *E7* (see Fig. 12-3), which encode gene products that directly contribute to cancer. The mechanism of this upregulation remains poorly understood but may reflect (1) derepression of *E6* and *E7* expression from the viral promoter resulting from disruption of a viral transcription factor, *E2*, which can repress their transcription,[90] (2) an increase in the stability of *E6* and *E7* messenger RNA (mRNA) resulting from disruption on integration of an mRNA instability element present in the 3′ end of the *E6* and *E7* mRNA,[91] or (3) increased transcriptional initiation from the viral promoter directing expression of *E6* and *E7* after integration of the viral DNA. Recognition of increased expression of *E6* and *E7* in cervical carcinoma, coupled with the knowledge that *E6* and *E7* contribute to the transforming potential of BPV-1 in mouse fibroblasts, provided the impetus for examination of the tumorigenic activities of these two viral genes.

Evidence of a critical role of increased expression of HPV *E6* and *E7* in the genesis of cervical cancer comes from numerous studies: (1) Cervical epithelial cells harboring integrated HPV-16 DNA have a selective growth advantage over cells harboring normal extrachromosomal viral genomes, and this growth advantage correlates with increased expression of *E6* and *E7*.[92] (2) *E6* and *E7* bind and inactivate the tumor suppressor gene products *p53* and *pRB*, respectively.[93,94] (3) *p53* and *pRB* are wild-type in cell lines derived from HPV-positive cervical cancers, whereas they are mutated in HPV-negative, cervical cancer–derived cell lines.[95] (4) Expression of the *E6* and *E7* viral genes is required for survival of cervical cancer–derived cell lines.[96-101] Together these observations strongly support the hypothesis that *E6* and *E7* contribute causally to human cervical cancer, at least by blocking the functions of cellular tumor suppressors.

The *E6* and *E7* genes from the high-risk HPVs are transforming in tissue culture. They act independently or synergistically to immortalize multiple cell types, including human foreskin keratinocytes, cervical epithelial cells, and mammary epithelial cells.[102-107] In addition, *E7* cooperates with an activated *ras* to transform baby rat kidney or human cervical epithelial cells.[108-110] The oncogenic properties of high-risk HPV *E6* and *E7* in vivo have been validated through characterization of HPV transgenic mice.[111-118]

E6 and *E7* are best known for their ability to associate with the cellular tumor suppressors *p53* and *pRB*, respectively.[93,94] Discovery of these interactions represents a major advance in our understanding of the mechanisms

Science of Clinical Oncology

of oncogenesis: inhibition of tumor suppressors predisposes cells to evolve into tumors. *E6* induces degradation of *p53* via recruitment of a ubiquitin ligase, *E6-AP*.[119,120] *E6* inhibits the transcriptional regulatory activities of *p53* protein in tissue culture cells.[121,122] Association of *E7* with *pRB* also promotes degradation of *pRB*[123,124] and disrupts the capacity of *pRB* to bind and functionally inactivate the cellular *E2F* transcription factors.[110,125] Whereas these abilities of *E6* and *E7* to inactivate *p53* and *pRB*, respectively, likely play an important role in their oncogenic potentials, it is important to recognize that *E6* and *E7* both can bind additional cellular factors, and these interactions may contribute to HPV-associated carcinogenesis. Which of these many interactions contribute to oncogenic potential remains to be determined.

There is growing appreciation of the role of HPVs not only in anogenital cancers such as cervical cancer but also in head and neck cancers of the oral cavity and in skin cancers.[126-129] The multiple interactions of *E6* and *E7* with cellular proteins that have regulatory functions is consistent with the contribution of *E6* and *E7* to cancers through multiple mechanisms. Studies in tissue culture strongly support the hypothesis that continued expression of *E6* and *E7* is required for continued growth of cervical cancer cells[96-100] and, perhaps, other cancers to which HPVs contribute causally.

Cervical cancer takes decades to arise in most patients after initial infection with high-risk HPV. During this time, the HPV must persist in the patient. Strategies that interfere with viral persistence may prove effective in preventing the development of cancer. *E6* and *E7* are important to the replicative phase of the HPV life cycle and, therefore, for viral persistence, indicating they also are appropriate targets for antiviral and antitumor drug development. Studies have been conducted in which organotypic tissue culturing has been used to recapitulate the life cycle of HPVs in fully differentiating, stratified squamous epithelial cells. Results of these studies have implicated *E7* in reprogramming cells within the terminally differentiating compartment of the epithelium to support amplification of the viral DNA genome, likely through its inactivation of *pRB*.[130] Inactivation of *p53* by *E6* may be necessary for viral replication through inhibition of cellular stress responses elicited by inactivation of *pRB* by *E7*.[131] At least two more HPV proteins, *E1* and *E2* (see Fig. 12-3), contribute to replication of the viral genome.[132] *E1* and *E2* bind to an origin-of-DNA replication on the viral genome.[133] *E1* is a DNA helicase that unwinds the viral double-stranded DNA genome at its origin and, together with *E2*, recruits cellular DNA replication proteins that then synthesize the viral DNA.[133-135] Thus *E1* and *E2* both represent potentially useful targets for intervening in the viral life cycle.

One desirable, long-term public health strategy for dealing with this and other human tumor viruses is generation of an effective, prophylactic vaccine for prevention of initial infection. Generation of such a vaccine is well along in the case of the mucosotropic HPVs implicated in cervical cancer, although several issues complicate the potential success of this strategy. This candidate vaccine is discussed later.

HUMAN T-CELL LEUKEMIA VIRUS I

Adult T-cell leukemia/lymphoma (ATLL), a tumor of CD4+ T cells, is caused by human T-cell leukemia virus 1 (HTLV-1), the only retrovirus accepted as being oncogenic in people. HTLV-1 is found worldwide; approximately 10 to 20 million persons are estimated to be infected. This number is likely an overestimate because of a failure to differentiate serologically between HTLV-1 and HTLV-2.[136,137] HTLV-1 is particularly prevalent in restricted sites, including southern Japan, the Caribbean, and West Central Africa. ATLL is prevalent in areas in which HTLV-1 is common, and it is estimated that ATLL will develop in as many as 5% of HTLV-1–positive carriers in their lifetimes.[138] HTLV-1 also causes a progressive, paralytic myelopathy called *HTLV-1–associated myelopathy* or *tropical, spastic paraparesis*. This neurologic disorder appears to arise preferentially in patients whose HLA haplotypes fail to limit viral load.[139]

The data that link HTLV-1 causally to ATLL are varied. ATLL can occur in familial clusters. It is characterized by an average age at onset of 56 years and proves rapidly fatal, 50% of patients dying within 6 months of diagnosis.[138] Patients generally have antibodies to HTLV-1–encoded proteins.[140] In 88 of 88 primary biopsy specimens of ATLL examined, all had single copies of integrated HTLV-1 proviruses.[141] The presence of the provirus of HTLV-1 in all of the tumors makes it likely that infection with the virus is an early, contributing event in evolution of the tumor. The presence of ATLL in familial clusters is consistent with the routes of transmission of HTLV-1. HTLV-1 is passed from male to female via semen and from mother to child by breast milk. The latter route has been demonstrated prospectively. Encouraging carrier mothers to refrain from breast-feeding has decreased transmission of HTLV-1 to their children by 80%.[142] It appears highly likely that this form of public health intervention will lead to a corresponding decrease in ATLL in Japan. Such a decrease would constitute formal proof of the oncogenic role of HTLV-1 in ATLL.

HTLV-1 clearly differs from the highly oncogenic animal retroviruses that encode oncogenes derived from cellular proto-oncogenes. HTLV-1 is a complex retrovirus that encodes multiple open reading frames in addition to the *gag*, *pol*, and *env* genes common to simple retroviruses (Fig. 12-4). However, none of these additional viral genes is obviously related to known proto-oncogenes, and all are thought to affect the viral life cycle either directly or indirectly by affecting the host cell.[143,144] It is accepted that one viral protein, Tax (see Fig. 12-4), which regulates both viral and cellular gene expression, is a major contribution of HTLV-1 to leukemogenesis. It also is evident that viral infection precedes onset of ATLL by 50 years or more, that many cells are infected, and that this clonal tumor develops in only a minority of infected persons. These combined observations indicate that multiple rare events in an HTLV-1–infected CD4+ T cell must occur for that cell to evolve into ATLL.

Several approaches demonstrate that Tax can transform cells in culture and be oncogenic in animal models.

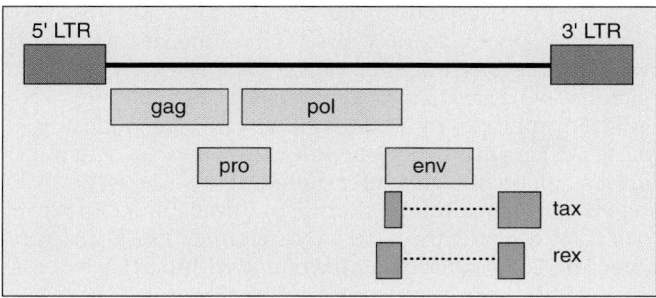

Figure 12-4. Map of the human T-cell leukemia virus 1 (HTLV-1) genome shows the approximately 9000–base pair DNA proviral form of the HTLV-1 genome as it is found integrated into the host genome. The genome as present in the viral particle consists of two copies of a single-stranded positive-strand RNA. Long terminal repeats (LTRs; *green*) flank the unique region that contains the translational open reading frames (*boxes*) for structural (*blue*) and nonstructural (*yellow*) viral proteins. The LTRs contain *cis*-acting elements required for transcription and replication of the viral genome. The structural genes are transcribed late in the viral life cycle from the 5′ LTR, whereas the nonstructural proteins are transcribed early from the 5′ LTR from different, spliced transcripts. (See Green PL, Chen ISY: Human T-cell leukemia viruses type 1 and 2. In Fields BN, Howley PM, Griffin DE, et al [eds]: Virology, vol 2, 4th ed. Philadelphia, Lippincott Williams & Wilkins, 2001, pp 1941–1969 for details of the genome and life cycle of HTLV-1.)

Introduction of a vector expressing Tax into established, adherent rodent cells can transform them to grow in an anchorage-independent manner.[145] Strains of rodent cells can be transformed with Tax in combination with the *ras* oncogene to yield cells tumorigenic in nude mice.[146] Tax also has been recombined into herpesvirus saimiri and introduced into resting human T cells. These infected cells can proliferate and yield infected, immortalized progeny, whereas the Tax-negative parental virus cannot do so.[147] In accord with these data, variants of HTLV-1 from which the Tax gene has been deleted no longer can immortalize human T cells in culture.[148] These results in culture are paralleled and bolstered by others in transgenic animal models. Expression of Tax from the HTLV-1 long terminal repeat (LTR, the viral promoter), in transgenic mice leads to mesenchymal tumors.[149] When expression of Tax is directed at lymphoid cells, leukemia develops in transgenic animals.[150] The exact means by which Tax transforms cells in culture or is oncogenic in animal models is not obvious.

Tax can be considered a paradigm for viral proteins that affect host cells in that it has multiple, distinct functions not found in any one cellular protein. During its evolution HTLV-1 apparently has assimilated multiple cellular activities in this one gene product. Tax can be viewed as having at least three kinds of activities: it activates transcription through nuclear factor κB (NF-κB) and CBP (CREB-binding protein, CREB indicating cyclic adenosine monophosphate response element–binding protein); it inhibits transcription, perhaps through binding histone deacetylase 1 (HDAC1); and it inhibits several tumor suppressor gene products.[143,151-155] Tax potently activates transcription from the HTLV-1 LTR[156] and activates the promoters for IL-2, IL-2 receptor α chain, and c-*fos*.[157-159]

This transcriptional activation may contribute to proliferation of an infected T cell. It also can activate the promoter for *bcl*-x and thereby help to inhibit apoptosis.[160] Tax can positively regulate transcription by binding CREB and CBP as well as some members of the NF-κB family.[161-163] Tax not only binds members of the NF-κB family directly but also can activate homing of NF-κB to the nucleus by binding to IκBα and promoting its degradation.[164,165] Some of the protein-protein associations of Tax have been functionally validated through chromatin immunoprecipitations that have documented binding of Tax, CREB, and CBP to the LTR of HTLV-1 in intact, HTLV-1–transformed T cells.[166]

Tax can inhibit transcription. It has been shown to inhibit both expression of the β-DNA polymerase gene[151] and some promoters regulated by CBP/p300.[167] It has been proposed that the latter inhibition occurs by binding of Tax to CBP and effective sequestering of CBP such that CBP is unavailable to bind other DNA-binding, transcription factors. It has been shown that Tax binds HDAC1 as measured by coimmunoprecipitation.[152] Were Tax to tether HDAC1 to a promoter, the resulting localized histone deacetylation would presumably inhibit transcription of that promotor.[168]

A third activity of Tax is inhibition of some cellular tumor suppressors. Tax has been shown to bind to and inhibit the function of p16^{INK4A}.[153] p16^{INK4A} binds cyclin-dependent kinase 4 (CDK4), a kinase that when activated can phosphorylate pRb, yielding release of *E2F* transcription factors and promotion of the G$_1$ to S transition of the cell cycle. Tax on binding p16^{INK4A} can increase the kinase activity of CDK4.[153] p16^{INK4A} often is found to be mutationally inactivated in tumors. Consistent with functional inactivation of p16^{INK4A} by Tax, p16^{INK4A} was shown to be wild-type in sequence in two HTLV-1–infected T-cell lines in which Tax is expressed but to be deleted in four uninfected T-cell lines.[153] Tax also appears to bind cyclin D3 and may thereby foster, by a second means, activity of CDK4 and CDK6.[154] Binding of Tax to p16^{INK4A} and cyclin D3 would inhibit control of the cell cycle and promote cell proliferation. Tax also can inhibit the transcriptional activity of *p53* by an NF-κB–dependent mechanism that culminates in phosphorylation of *p53* at certain residues.[155,169] Such inhibition of *p53* is likely to limit its induction of apoptosis and increase the rate of survival of HTLV-1–infected, proliferating T cells.

The multiple activities of Tax likely contribute to the associated leukemogenesis of HTLV-1 but must be insufficient for development of ATLL. Multiple T cells are initially infected by HTLV-1, but over the course of the 50 to 60 years of its development, only one infected cell and its progeny give rise to the tumor. The additional genetic and epigenetic events necessary for this evolution are not known. It is clear that expression of viral genes in infected cells is surprisingly low. Measurement of RNA encoding Tax indicates that between 0.1% and 10% of freshly harvested, infected T cells express a Tax message in vivo.[170] These findings indicate that regulation of HTLV-1 expression, be it at the level of T-cell development or immune response to viral antigens, is likely also to be critical to development of ATLL.

HUMAN HEPATITIS C VIRUS

Human hepatitis C virus (HCV) is accepted as an etiologic agent for HCC along with HBV. Approximately one half of cases of HCC in the United States are ascribed to HCV infection.[171] Infection with HCV constitutes a 20-fold risk of development of HCC among men in Taiwan.[172] HCV represents the most common chronic viral infection among blood-borne pathogens in the United States, where the rate of infection during the period from 1988 to 1994 was estimated to be 1.8%.[173] The World Health Organization estimates the worldwide infection rate at 3%, yielding more than 170 million infected persons.[174] The rates of infection vary widely, the rate being as low as 0.01% to 0.1% in Scandinavia and the United Kingdom and as high as 17% to 26% in Egypt.[173] Infection is thought to arise from contaminated blood, use of shared needles among users of intravenous drugs, organ transplantation, hemodialysis, sexual transmission, and vertical transmission. Establishment of sensitive tests for identifying contaminated blood and blood products has greatly reduced the rate of infection in the general population. As with people chronically infected with HBV, HCC in HCV-positive persons correlates with chronic hepatitis and cirrhosis. Di Bisceglie[175] estimated that in each decade cirrhosis develops in 20% of persons with chronic HCV infection and that over two decades HCC develops in 2% to 7% of persons with chronic infection. The hyperproliferative state induced by chronic hepatitis and cirrhosis is argued to lead to accumulation of genetic changes and to contribute to the onset of liver cancer. The specific contribution of HCV to this scheme is not known.

HCV is a flavivirus. This status indicates the virus is unique among human tumor viruses for having RNA as its only genetic material (Fig. 12-5). HCV was identified in 1989 during a search for the causal agent of non-A, non-B hepatitis.[176] This flavivirus contains a 9.6-kb, positive-stranded RNA as its genome, which encodes a single translation product of approximately 3000 amino acids (see Fig. 12-5). This polyprotein is cleaved by both cellularly and virally encoded proteases to yield at least 10 proteins.[177] Study of HCV has been daunting for at least two reasons. The sequence of the virus varies in infected persons such that there are six recognized genotypes with multiple subtypes among patients and a spectrum of quasispecies within any one infected person.[178] Members of these quasispecies within one patient vary 1% to 2% in sequence.[179] In addition, there is no available cell culture for HCV. Researchers have made heroic efforts to overcome the latter hurdle and have met with partial success.

In 1999 Bartenschlager and colleagues described replication of a subgenomic derivative of HCV in a cell line derived from human HCC.[180] These subgenomic replicons were difficult to establish but once established exhibited bona fide characteristics of flaviviral nucleic acid replication. One thousand to 5000 molecules of plus-strand RNA were present in each cell. Minus-strand RNA was present at 10% to 20% of the level of the plus-strand, and this viral RNA replication was insensitive to treatment of cells with actinomycin D. This mode of nucleic acid replication in cells will allow elucidation of the *cis* and *trans* elements it requires, but with an unexpected twist. Efficient replication of the subgenomic derivatives of HCV requires mutation of at least two viral genes that enhance replication in cells but abrogate infectivity of intact HCV RNA.[181] Chimpanzees are the only nonhuman host for HCV. The parental strain of HCV used to derive the subgenomic replicons is infectious in this primate host, although a derivative of it, containing the mutations required for efficient replication of the subgenomic replicons, is not. This finding must limit conclusions drawn from analysis of replication of these mutated subgenomic replicons in cells. The findings also indicate that generation of the many sequence variants that constitute the quasispecies within any one infected patient may contribute to successful replication of HCV.

Lack of a cell culture host for infection with HCV and of a practicable animal host has led researchers to seek chimeric animal models of infection. Researchers formerly developed a chimeric animal model for HBV that has been adapted to study of HCV. Mice transgenic for the plasminogen activator urokinase (uPA), which is expressed in the liver, have hepatocytes with a selective disadvantage such that transplanted, nontransgenic hepatocytes repopulate the liver.[182] When these animals are crossed with nu/nu mice, they not only tolerate rat hepatocytes but also support rat hepatocytes reconstituting their livers.[183] These findings paved the way for Rogler and his colleagues to cross mice transgenic for uPA with mice null for Rag-2, which eliminates their B- and T-cell responses, and to repopulate the livers with woodchuck hepatocytes.[184] These chimeric animals supported infection with woodchuck HBV and became chronically infected with 10^6 to 10^{11} virions per milliliter of serum. Human hepatocytes also can repopulate the livers of uPA-transgenic animals as long as the xenograft is not rejected. SKID mice homozygously transgenic for uPA accept human hepatocytes such that 50% or more of their hepatocytes are of human origin.[185] These animals can be infected with HCV such that 75% of them become persistently infected with 10^4 to 10^6 viral RNA molecules per milliliter of serum, and

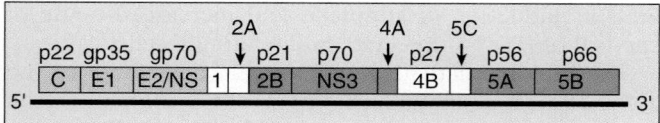

		2A		4A	5C	
p22	gp35 gp70	↓ p21	p70	↓ p27 ↓	p56	p66
C	E1	E2/NS	1	2B	NS3	4B	5A	5B

5′ ——————————————————————————————— 3′

Figure 12-5. Map of the hepatitis C virus (HCV) genome. The 9500-nucleotide-long positive-strand RNA of HCV is shown in *black*. It encodes a single 3000-amino-acid polyprotein that is proteolytically cleaved into mature proteins (*labeled boxes*, alternative names indicated above the boxes) by cellularly and virally encoded proteases (NS3/4A and possibly 2B). At the 5′ and 3′ ends are short noncoding regions (NCR) that contain signals for replication of the viral genome. The 5′ NCR also contains an internal ribosome entry site. *Blue* indicates structural proteins *Yellow* indicates nonstructural proteins, including proteases, helicases, and RNA polymerase. (See Major ME, Rehermann B, Feinstone SM: Hepatitis C viruses. In Fields BN, Howley PM, Griffin DE, et al [eds]: Virology, vol 1, 4th ed. Philadelphia, Lippincott Williams & Wilkins, 2001, pp 1127–1161 for details of the genome and life cycle of HCV.)

the infection can be passaged serially in them. These reconstituted animals are difficult to generate but should provide insight into the life cycle of HCV and may serve as models in which to test inhibitors of HCV infection.

Evidence of a direct role of HCV in HCC has come from studies of the HCV core protein. The HCV core protein can cooperate with an activated form of the *ras* oncogene to transform primary rodent cells in tissue culture.[186] HCC develops in mice transgenic for HCV core protein.[187] Several potential mechanisms have been invoked to explain the transforming potential of HCV core protein. It has been found to enhance cell proliferation through stimulation of mitogen-activated protein kinase.[188,189] In addition, HCV core protein can inactivate a transcription factor, IZIP, and this inactivation correlates with transformation in rodent cells.[190] The core protein has been found to activate Stat3 (signal transducer and activator of transcription 3), and this activation may contribute to its transforming potential.[191] Whether the HCV core protein contributes directly to human HCC is uncertain. Neither replication of subgenomic replicons in cell culture nor infection of chimeric mice populated with human hepatocytes allows ready testing of the possible role of the core protein in the oncogenesis of HCV.

Current therapies for HCV infection are unsatisfactory. The combination of interferon α plus ribavirin, a general antiviral nucleotide analog, has supported clearance of detectable HCV in 40% of a treated group over 1 year. Those who responded had higher titers of the virus.[192] These observations may indicate that treatments with multiple, independently acting drugs are the most likely route to successful therapy for HCV infection.[193] In the United States, approximately 10,000 deaths are attributed to HCV each year, and today infection with HCV is the leading indication for liver transplantation.[173] This mode of treatment is not practical for most persons with infection. Lack of satisfactory therapy for chronic HCV infection and associated HCC make it important to continue development of tractable means for studying the life cycle of HCV and for elucidating the mode of its oncogenesis.

KAPOSI'S SARCOMA HERPESVIRUS

Identification of Kaposi's sarcoma herpesvirus (KSHV) represents the culmination of much scientific detective work. Kaposi's sarcoma (KS) was known before the acquired immunodeficiency syndrome epidemic,[194,195] but the incidence increased markedly among human immunodeficiency virus (HIV)-positive persons. Researchers therefore looked for molecular evidence of an infectious agent present in KS lesions. In 1994, Chang and Moore and their colleagues used a newly developed enrichment procedure based on polymerase chain reaction to identify DNA sequences present in KS but absent in normal cells. The investigators identified a new herpesvirus, KSHV (also called *human herpesvirus 8*), which is related to EBV and herpesvirus saimiri.[196] Results of retrospective studies indicated that KSHV was prevalent in different parts of the world before the spread of HIV and that in Africa, for example, the prevalence of KSHV has not changed. What

has changed is the incidence of KS, so that in regions where this tumor was formerly infrequent, the incidence increased threefold between 1988 and 1996.[197] Similarly, the frequency of infection with KSHV among certain cohorts in the United States has not altered with the advent of HIV,[198] but the incidence of KS has.[199] KSHV has been detected in one class of lymphoma, called *body-cavity–based lymphoma* or *primary effusion lymphoma* (PEL)[200] and in an atypical lymphoproliferative disorder called *multicentric Castleman's disease*.[201]

KSHV is now accepted as contributing causally to KS and PEL. Each of these malignant lesions has intriguing features likely to reflect their viral causation. Single-cell assays of early KS lesions have detected KSHV in a minority of cells that surround their vascular spaces, whereas in the more advanced, nodular lesions, more than 90% of the spindle cells characteristic of these lesions are KSHV antigen–positive.[202] The viral antigen–positive cells also stain with antibodies against vascular endothelial growth factor (VEGF) receptor 3, indicating they are lymphatic or proliferating endothelial cells. That only a subset of the cells characteristic of early KS lesions appear to be infected with KSHV likely indicates that infected cells affect development of their neighbors. This possibility is supported by the existence of multiple cellular homologues of cytokines and receptors encoded by KSHV that may allow infected cells to interact with adjacent, uninfected cells.[203,204] PEL cells are B cells in origin. In six of seven cases studied, PEL cells have nongermline immunoglobulin mRNA, indicating they are likely derived from B cells that have encountered antigen.[205] These cells often, however, fail to express B-cell activation antigens.[206] PEL cells usually but not always are coinfected with EBV.[200,206] The etiologic role of EBV in this lymphoma is not yet determined. However, because it often is retained in these cells as they are propagated in vitro and is maintained in them in vivo, EBV is likely to provide the tumor cells some selective advantage.

KSHV encodes many genes with clear homology to cellular genes, some of which are candidates for contributing to viral oncogenesis (Fig. 12-6). Three categories of these cellular homologues are particularly likely to be important for tumor development: cyclins, inhibitors of apoptosis, and cytokines and receptors. KSHV encodes its own cyclin. Cellular cyclins bind specific, dependent kinases (CdK) the activities of which promote progression through the cell cycle and are controlled by cellular inhibitors, including p16^{INK4A}, p21^{CIP1}, and p27^{Kip1}. KSHV-encoded cyclin can promote cellular proliferation in part by overcoming these cellular inhibitors. It does so apparently by extending the substrates phosphorylated by Cdk6 to include p27^{Kip1}.[207,208] Phosphorylation of p27^{Kip1} at position 187 leads to its downregulation and promotes passage through the G$_1$ phase of the cell cycle. One measure of the activity of the KSHV cyclin Cdk6 complex is that it can foster progression of nuclei isolated from cells in G$_1$ to undergo DNA synthesis.[209] The KSHV cyclin can also induce cells to undergo apoptosis.[210] It is striking that in cells lacking *p53*, expression of KSHV cyclin promotes cells both to become aneuploid and to survive so that they continue to proliferate. In fact, mice that are

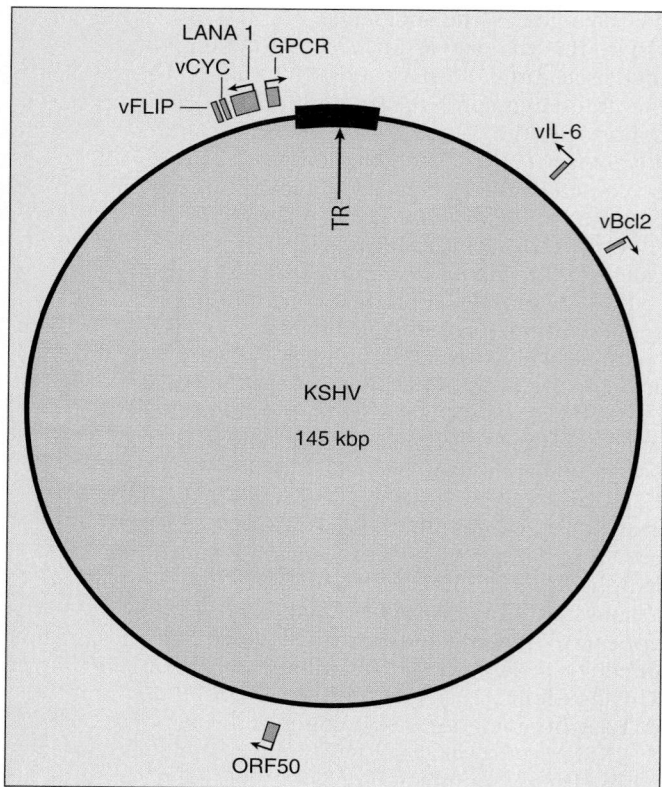

Figure 12-6. Map of the Kaposi's sarcoma herpesvirus (KSHV) genome. The genome of KSHV consists of approximately 145 kilobase pairs (kbp) of linear double-stranded DNA in the viral particle. The viral genome becomes circularized on infection through the terminal repeats found at the 5′ and 3′ ends of the linear genome. The terminal repeats also contain the origin of plasmid replication used during the latent phase of the viral life cycle. *Yellow boxes* indicate positions of viral genes expressed during latency or thought to contribute to oncogenesis by KSHV. *Arrows* indicate the positions from which the RNA encoding the labeled proteins is expressed. Several of these primary transcripts are polycistronic. (See Moore PS, Chang Y: Kaposi's sarcoma–associated herpesvirus. In Fields BN, Howley PM, Griffin DE, et al [eds]: Virology, vol 2, 4th ed. Philadelphia, Lippincott Williams & Wilkins, 2001, pp 2803–2833 for details of the genome and life-cycle of KSHV.)

transgenic for KSHV cyclin and are *p53*-null develop T- and B-cell lymphomas with a mean latency of 3 months, a latency shorter than that for *p53*-null mice alone.[211]

KSHV encodes its own inhibitors of apoptosis, viral Bcl-2 and viral FLIP (an inhibitor of cellular FLICE, a protein mediating Fas ligand–induced cell death) (see Fig. 12-6). Viral Bcl-2 shares its limited sequence homology with cellular Bcl-2 in regions critical for inhibiting apoptosis and fails to dimerize with cellular Bcl-2 and Bcl-X_L, thus avoiding regulation by potential cell-binding partners.[212] Viral Bcl-2 can inhibit apoptosis induced by efficient expression of KSHV cyclin.[213] Viral FLIP can inhibit apoptosis mediated by the Fas pathway and induced by cytotoxic T lymphocytes.[214]

Finally, KSHV encodes homologues of cytokines and cytokine receptors (see Fig. 12-6). Its viral IL-6 may promote proliferation of PEL cells, although these cells appear to be dependent on cellular IL-6 and not viral IL-6 for continued growth.[215] KSHV also encodes a G protein–coupled receptor (viral GPCR), which is likely to be pivotal for development of KS. Expression of viral GPCR in endothelial cells in mice leads to KS-like tumors, whereas individual expression of KSHV cyclin, KSHV Bcl-2, or KSHV FLIP does not.[216] What is particularly exciting is that cells inoculated into mice that express viral GPCR promote tumor formation by coinoculated cells that individually express viral cyclin or viral FLIP, or both.[216] These findings support a model in which viral GPCR contributes to the development of KS by affecting neighboring cells not infected by KSHV. The model also is supported by the findings that viral GPCR induces expression of cellular VEGF receptor 2 in endothelial cells that proliferate in the presence of VEGF and that viral GPCR induces expression of VEGF.[217,218] These observations define an autostimulatory loop in which KSHV GPCR alone can maintain proliferation of endothelial cells. These collected observations help to explain the viral contributions to KS and perhaps PEL. These explanations are not yet complete, however, because several of these putative viral oncogenes, including viral IL-6, viral Bcl-2, and viral GPCR, are expressed during the lytic phase of the life cycle of KSHV. The lytic phase of a herpesvirus is thought traditionally to lead to death of the host cell. How these putative viral oncogenes can affect oncogenesis and be expressed only in cells destined to die soon is an enigma yet to be resolved.

Studies of cell lines derived from PEL and human endothelial cells are providing the foundation for understanding infections by KSHV in vivo. PEL cells maintain KSHV DNA extrachromosomally and consistently express the viral protein LANA-1 (see Fig. 12-6), which is required for viral plasmid replication.[219,220] In general, these cells support the latent phase of the KSHV life cycle and express the viral cyclin and the viral inhibitor of cellular FLICE, FLIP, but few other viral proteins. Some PEL cell lines support inefficient spontaneous conversion to the lytic phase of the viral cycle, which can be further induced by treatment of cells with tetradecanoyl phorbol acetate or introduction of a plasmid including ORF50 (see Fig. 12-6), a viral inducer of the lytic cycle.[221] The released virus is infectious on human dermal microvascular endothelial cells (DMVEC).[222,223] These DMVEC cultures can be passaged to yield populations in which all cells are infected, express LANA-1, assume a spindle-cell morphology, and can proliferate indefinitely.[223] The spindle shape is characteristic of cells in KS lesions in vivo. Staining of these infected DMVEC-derived spindle cells indicates that 5% to 10% of them spontaneously support early stages of the lytic cycle of KSHV, and 1% to 2% express genes diagnostic of the late stages of the viral life cycle.[223] If endothelial cells infected in vivo by KSHV display a similar distribution of cells supporting the latent, early, and late lytic phases of the viral life cycle, then the enigma of the oncogenic contribution of viral genes expressed only during the lytic cycle may be resolved. Sustained, spontaneous conversion of 5% to 10% of KSHV-infected cells to support the viral lytic cycle may allow enough infected cells to express enough KSHV GPCR to promote the bystander-dependent tumor evolution proposed by Bais and colleagues.[218]

MANAGEMENT AND PREVENTION OF VIRAL TUMORS

Tumors associated causally with viruses are treated variously: surgical resection, when appropriate, is used in combination with chemotherapy and/or radiation therapy. These treatments are disappointing in that overall survival rates often are low and so far have not been able to capitalize on any specific antiviral therapies. Current survival rates after different therapies obviously vary with the malignant disease, its stage, and the setting in which the patient is treated. For example, youngsters with Burkitt's lymphoma have a 4-year overall survival rate of 65%.[224] After treatment approximately 45% of NPC patients remain disease-free for 10 years, but this value is highly dependent on the stage at which NPC is diagnosed.[225] In the United States, 26% of HBV-positive patients with surgically resected HCC have a 5-year, local disease-free survival rate; the rate for the analogous HCV-positive group is 38%.[226] In a retrospective study in Germany, investigators found a median survival time of 7 years among patients with a mix of HBV- and HCV-associated HCC.[227] The 5-year median survival rate for patients with cervical carcinoma ranges from 65%[228] to 75% to 90%[229] in different studies. The median survival time once the diagnosis of ATLL is made is only 10 months.[230] The overall survival rates among KS patients who are HIV-positive have changed with introduction of highly active antiretroviral therapies (HAART). Before this therapy was developed, the median overall survival time was 13 months. With HAART, the survival period surpasses 28 months.[231] The median survival for PEL patients has been described as "dismal," but there are case reports that indicate some combination therapies are helpful.[232] These actuarial findings indicate that development of antiviral therapies directed at viral gene products that maintain tumor phenotypes is a highly desirable goal. It is also desirable to develop vaccines to prevent infection by tumor viruses. Development of effective vaccines that can prevent initial infection or induce elimination of viral persistence is being pursued for all human tumor viruses. Success or the glimmer of success has been achieved for two of them.

Hepatitis B Virus Vaccine

Although there are four serotypes of HBV, highly effective vaccines for HBV have been developed that consist only of its surface antigen, HBsAg. Today this subunit vaccine usually is synthesized with recombinant DNA expressed in yeast. Vaccines for HBV began to be used in the early 1980s, and since 2001, 129 countries routinely vaccinate infants and/or adolescents against HBV.[233] These vaccinations are effective. The fraction of children infected with HBV has been reported to have declined between 7.5- and 10-fold in Taiwan and The Gambia, respectively.[54,55] This decline has been paralleled by a detectable decrease in the frequency of HCC in children in Taiwan, an age group for which this viral tumor is rare.[56]

The current HBV vaccines apparently are free of unwanted side effects but can select for variants of HBV resistant to the neutralizing antibodies they elicit.[233] One domain of HBsAg in particular elicits neutralizing antibodies efficiently, and mutations in it can allow viral escape. The frequency of these escape mutants in populations of vaccinated children has increased significantly.[234] One means of overcoming selection for such escape mutants would be to generate vaccines for HBV that include more than the HBsAg as an immunogen; such vaccines are being developed.

Human Papillomavirus Vaccine

The second family of human tumor viruses for which an effective prophylactic vaccine can be envisioned is HPVs associated with cervical cancer, other anogenital cancers, and certain head and neck cancers, in particular HPV-16 and HPV-18. These two viruses account for approximately 85% of cases of cervical cancer worldwide and, as found in one study, 16% of new infections.[235] Several HPV prophylactic vaccines designed to prevent or eliminate acute infection by HPV-16 and HPV-18 are in clinical trials.[236] These vaccines are based on production of virus-like particles (VLPs) composed of the major capsid protein of HPV-16 and HPV-18, L1, which self-assembles into icosahedrons (see Fig. 12-3). These L1-based VLPs induce neutralizing antibodies in vaccinated persons. Pre-clinical studies with CRPV and canine oral papillomavirus (COPV) demonstrated the effectiveness of VLP-based vaccines in protecting animals from CRPV and COPV infection.[237,238] Phase I and phase II clinical trials likewise demonstrated the effectiveness of HPV-16 VLP-based vaccines in inducing neutralizing antibodies specific for HVP-16 and in preventing HPV-16 infection.[239,240] One issue relevant to the effectiveness of these vaccines is the specificity of immune responses invoked by VLP-based vaccines for specific HPV genotypes. Approximately two dozen HPV genotypes are associated with anogenital cancers. VLP-based vaccines induce protective immunity that is highly specific for the genotype from which the VLP is generated. This specificity has led to development of polyvalent vaccines composed of a mixture of VLPs generated with L1 proteins from multiple mucosotropic HPV genotypes. These multivalent vaccines are composed of HPV-16, HPV-18, HPV-6, and HPV-11 VLPs. HPV-6 and HPV-11 are low-risk mucosotropic HPVs that induce genital warts but do not contribute to cervical cancer. It remains to be seen whether, once a population is protected from HPV-16– and HPV-18–induced cancers, other HPV genotypes arise to induce a greater incidence of cervical cancer than they currently cause. Studies in progress are designed to increase the cross-genotype neutralizing capacity of the VLP-based vaccines. Incorporation of the minor capsid protein, L2, may contribute to this property, because neutralizing antibodies induced against L2 tend to be more generally effective at neutralizing multiple genotypes.[241] There is a concern whether the HPVs, particularly HPV-16 and HPV-18, will evolve to

Science of Clinical Oncology

become resistant to VLP-based vaccines. Assuming the high effectiveness of the vaccines currently under development and their worldwide distribution, and given the long latency of cervical cancer, the World Health Organization estimates prophylactic HPV vaccines will lead to a reduction of deaths due to cervical cancer no earlier than 2040.

REFERENCES

1. Parkin D, Pisani P, Munoz N, Ferlay J: The global health burden of infection associated cancers. Cancer Surv 1999;33:5–33.
2. Ellerman V, Bang OB: Experimentelle Leukämie bei Hühnern. Zentralbl Bakteriol Parasitenkd Infectionskr Hyg Abt Orig 1908;46:595–609.
3. Rous P: A sarcoma of the fowl transmissible by an agent separable from the tumor cells. J Exp Med 1911;13:397–411.
4. Gross L: "Spontaneous" leukemia developing in CH3 mice following inoculation in infancy, with AK-leukemic extracts, or AK-embryos. Proc Soc Exp Biol Med 1951;76:27–32.
5. Payne LN, Purchase HP: Leukosis/sarcoma group. In Calnek BW (ed): Diseases of Poultry, 9th ed. Ames, Iowa, Iowa State University Press, 1991, pp 386–439.
6. Cooper GM: Oncogenes, 2nd ed. Boston, Jones & Bartlett, 1995.
7. Trentin JJ, Yabe Y, Taylor G: The quest for human cancer viruses. Science 1962;137:835–849.
8. Burkitt D: A children's cancer dependent upon climatic factors. Nature 1962;194:232–234.
9. Epstein M, Achong BG, Barr YM: Virus particles in cultured lymphoblasts from Burkitt's lymphoma. Lancet 1964;1:702–703.
10. Epstein M, Barr YM: Cultivation in vitro of human lymphoblasts from Burkitt's lymphoma. Lancet 1964;1:252–253.
11. Henle G, Henle W, Diehl V: Relation of Burkitt's tumor–associated herpes-type virus to infectious mononucleosis. Proc Natl Acad Sci USA 1968;59:94–101.
12. Niederman JC, McCollum RW, Henle G, Henle W: Infectious mononucleosis: Clinical manifestations in relation to EB virus antibodies. JAMA 1968;203:205–209.
13. Evans AS, Niederman JC: Epstein Barr virus. In Evans AS (ed): Viral Infections of Humans, 3rd ed. New York, Plenum Press, 1989, pp 265–292.
14. Henle W, Henle G, Ho HC, et al: Antibodies to Epstein-Barr virus in nasopharyngeal carcinoma, other head and neck neoplasms, and control groups. J Natl Cancer Inst 1970;44:225–231.
15. de-The G, Geser A, Day NE, et al: Epidemiological evidence for causal relationship between Epstein-Barr virus and Burkitt's lymphoma from Ugandan prospective study. Nature 1978;274:756–761.
16. Zeng Y, Zhang LG, Wu YC, et al: Prospective studies on nasopharyngeal carcinoma in Epstein-Barr virus IgA/VCA antibody-positive persons in Wuzhou City, China. Int J Cancer 1985;36:545–547.
17. Crawford DH, Thomas JA, Janossy G, et al: Epstein Barr virus nuclear antigen positive lymphoma after cyclosporin A treatment in patient with renal allograft. Lancet 1980;1:1355–1356.
18. Greenspan JS, Greenspan D, Lennette ET, et al: Replication of Epstein-Barr virus within the epithelial cells of oral "hairy" leukoplakia, an AIDS-associated lesion. N Engl J Med 1985;313:1564–1571.
19. Evans AS, Gutensohn NM: A population-based case-control study of EBV and other viral antibodies among persons with Hodgkin's disease and their siblings. Int J Cancer 1984;34:149–157.
20. Weiss LM, Strickler JG Warnke RA, Purtilo DT, Sklar J: Epstein-Barr viral DNA in tissues of Hodgkin's disease. Am J Pathol 1987;129:86–91.
21. Imai S, Koizumi S, Sugiura M, et al: Gastric carcinoma: Monoclonal epithelial malignant cells expressing Epstein-Barr virus latent infection protein. Proc Natl Acad Sci USA 1994;91:9131–9135.
22. Kieff E, Rickinson AB: Epstein Barr virus and its replication. In Fields BN, Howley PM, Griffin DE, et al (eds): Fields Virology, vol 2, 4th ed. Philadelphia, Lippincott Williams & Wilkins, 2001, pp 2511–2573.
23. Bloss TA, Sugden B: Optimal lengths for DNAs encapsidated by Epstein-Barr virus. J Virol 1994;68:8217–8222.
24. Baer R, Bankier AT, Biggin MD, et al: DNA sequence and expression of the B95-8 Epstein-Barr virus genome. Nature 1984;310:207–211.
25. Henle W, Diehl V, Kohn G, Zur Hausen H, Henle G: Herpes-type virus and chromosome marker in normal leukocytes after growth with irradiated Burkitt cells. Science 1967;157:1064–1065.
26. Robinson JE, Smith D, Niederman J: Plasmacytic differentiation of circulating Epstein-Barr virus-infected B lymphocytes during acute infectious mononucleosis. J Exp Med 1981;153:235–244.
27. Bornkamm GW, Hammerschmidt W: Molecular virology of Epstein-Barr virus. Philos Trans R Soc Lond B Biol Sci 2001;356:437–459.
28. Kempkes B, Spitkovsky D, Jansen-Durr P, et al: B-cell proliferation and induction of early G1-regulating proteins by Epstein-Barr virus mutants conditional for EBNA2. EMBO J 1995;14:88–96.
29. Kilger E, Kieser A, Baumann M, Hammerschmidt W: Epstein-Barr virus–mediated B-cell proliferation is dependent upon latent membrane protein 1, which simulates an activated CD40 receptor. EMBO J 1998;17:1700–1709.
30. Kennedy G, Komano J, Sugden B: Epstein-Barr virus provides a survival factor to Burkitt's lymphomas. Proc Natl Acad Sci USA (in press).
31. Kempkes B, Pich D, Zeidler R, Sugden B, Hammerschmidt W: Immortalization of human B lymphocytes by a plasmid containing 71 kilobase pairs of Epstein-Barr virus DNA. J Virol 1995;69:231–238.
32. Moss DJ, Burrows SR, Silins SL, Misko I, Khanna R: The immunology of Epstein-Barr virus infection. Philos Trans R Soc Lond B Biol Sci 2001;356:475–488.
33. Levitskaya J, Coram M, Levitsky V, et al: Inhibition of antigen processing by the internal repeat region of the Epstein-Barr virus nuclear antigen-1. Nature 1995;375:685–688.
34. Babcock GJ, Decker LL, Volk M, Thorley-Lawson DA: EBV persistence in memory B cells in vivo. Immunity 1998;9:395–404.
35. Qu L, Rowe DT: Epstein-Barr virus latent gene expression in uncultured peripheral blood lymphocytes. J Virol 1992;66:3715–3724.
36. Crawford DH: Biology and disease associations of Epstein-Barr virus. Phil Trans R Soc Lond B Biol Sci 2001;356:461–473.
37. Aguilar LK, Rooney CM, Heslop HE: Lymphoproliferative disorders involving Epstein-Barr virus after hemopoietic stem cell transplantation. Curr Opin Oncol 1999;11:96–101.
38. Rowe M, Rowe DT, Gregory CD, et al: Differences in B cell growth phenotype reflect novel patterns of Epstein-Barr virus latent gene expression in Burkitt's lymphoma cells. EMBO J 1987;6:2743–2751.
39. Zech L, Haglund U, Nilsson K, Klein G: Characteristic chromosomal abnormalities in biopsies and lymphoid-cell lines from patients with Burkitt and non-Burkitt lymphomas. Int J Cancer 1976;17:47–56.
40. Taub R, Kirsch I, Morton C, et al: Translocation of the c-myc gene into the immunoglobulin heavy chain locus in human Burkitt lymphoma and murine plasmacytoma cells. Proc Natl Acad Sci USA 1982;79:7837–7841.
41. Stanton LW, Watt R, Marcu KB: Translocation, breakage and truncated transcripts of c-myc oncogene in murine plasmacytomas. Nature 1983;303:401–406.
42. Morrow RH, Kisuule A, Pike MC, Smith PG: Burkitt's lymphoma in the Mengo districts of Uganda: Epidemiologic features and their relationship to malaria. J Natl Cancer Inst 1976;56:479–483.
43. Whittle HC, Brown J, Marsh K, et al: T-cell control of Epstein-Barr virus–infected B cells is lost during P. falciparum malaria. Nature 1984;312:449–450.
44. Lam KM., Syed N, Whittle H, Crawford DH: Circulating Epstein-Barr virus–carrying B cells in acute malaria. Lancet 1991;337:876–878.
45. Gaidano G, Ballerini P, Gong JZ, et al: p53 mutations in human lymphoid malignancies: Association with Burkitt lymphoma and chronic lymphocytic leukemia. Proc Natl Acad Sci USA 1991;88:5413–5417.
46. Chan AS, To KF, Lo KW, et al: High frequency of chromosome 3p deletion in histologically normal nasopharyngeal epithelia from southern Chinese. Cancer Res 2000;60:5365–5370.

47. Grasser FA, Murray PG, Kremmer E, et al: Monoclonal antibodies directed against the Epstein-Barr virus-encoded nuclear antigen 1 (EBNA1): Immunohistologic detection of EBNA1 in the malignant cells of Hodgkin's disease. Blood 1994;84:3792-3798.

48. Blumberg BS: Australia antigen and the biology of hepatitis B. Science 1977;197:17-25.

49. Senior JR, Sutnick AI, Goeser E, London WT, Dahlke MB, Blumberg BS: Reduction of post-transfusion hepatitis by exclusion of Australia antigen from donor blood in an urban public hospital. Am J Med Sci 1974;267:171-177.

50. Wild CP, Hall AJ: Primary prevention of hepatocellular carcinoma in developing countries. Mutat Res 2000;462:381-393.

51. Monto A, Wright TL: The epidemiology and prevention of hepatocellular carcinoma. Semin Oncol 2001;28:441-449.

52. Beasley RP, Hwang LY, Lin CC, Chien CS: Hepatocellular carcinoma and hepatitis B virus: A prospective study of 22,707 men in Taiwan. Lancet 1981;2:1129-1133.

53. Beasley RP: Hepatitis B virus: The major etiology of hepatocellular carcinoma. Cancer 1988;61:1942-1956.

54. Chen HL, Chang MH, Ni YH, et al: Seroepidemiology of hepatitis B virus infection in children: Ten years of mass vaccination in Taiwan. JAMA 1996;276:906-908.

55. Montesano R: Hepatitis B immunization and hepatocellular carcinoma: The Gambia Hepatitis Intervention Study. J Med Virol 2002;67:444-446.

56. Chang MH, Chen CJ, Lai MS, et al: Universal hepatitis B vaccination in Taiwan and the incidence of hepatocellular carcinoma in children. Taiwan Childhood Hepatoma Study Group. N Engl J Med 1997;336:1855-1859.

57. Seeger C, Mason WS: Hepatitis B virus biology. Microbiol Mol Biol Rev 2000;64:51-68.

58. Unsal H., Yakicier C, Marcais C, et al: Genetic heterogeneity of hepatocellular carcinoma. Proc Natl Acad Sci USA 1994;91:822-826.

59. Henkler F, Waseem N, Golding MH, Alison MR, Koshy R: Mutant p53 but not hepatitis B virus X protein is present in hepatitis B virus-related human hepatocellular carcinoma. Cancer Res 1995;55:6084-6091.

60. Wang XW, Gibson MK, Vermeulen W, et al: Abrogation of p53-induced apoptosis by the hepatitis B virus X gene. Cancer Res 1995;55:6012-6016.

61. Lin Y, Nomura T, Cheong J, Dorjsuren D, Iida K, Murakami S: Hepatitis B virus X protein is a transcriptional modulator that communicates with transcription factor IIB and the RNA polymerase II subunit 5. J Biol Chem 1997;272:7132-7139.

62. Haviv I, Shamay M, Doitsh G, Shaul Y: Hepatitis B virus pX targets TFIIB in transcription coactivation. Mol Cell Biol 1998;18:1562-1569.

63. Lee DK, Park SH, Yi Y, et al: The hepatitis B virus encoded oncoprotein pX amplifies TGF-beta family signaling through direct interaction with Smad4: Potential mechanism of hepatitis B virus-induced liver fibrosis. Genes Dev 2001;15:455-466.

64. Buendia MA: Hepatitis B viruses and hepatocellular carcinoma. Adv Cancer Res 1992;59:167-226.

65. Fourel G, Couturier J, Wei Y, Apiou F, Tiollais P, Buendia MA: Evidence for long-range oncogene activation by hepadnavirus insertion. EMBO J 1994;13:2526-2534.

66. Pineau P, Marchio A, Mattei MG, et al: Extensive analysis of duplicated-inverted hepatitis B virus integrations in human hepatocellular carcinoma. J Gen Virol 1998;79:591-600.

67. Chisari FV, Ferrari C: Hepatitis B virus immunopathogenesis. Annu Rev Immunol 1995;13:29-60.

68. Guidotti LG, Ando K, Hobbs MV, et al: Cytotoxic T lymphocytes inhibit hepatitis B virus gene expression by a noncytolytic mechanism in transgenic mice. Proc Natl Acad Sci USA 1994;91:3764-3768.

69. Guidotti LG, Rochford R, Chung J, Shapiro M, Purcell R, Chisari FV: Viral clearance without destruction of infected cells during acute HBV infection. Science 1999;284:825-829.

70. Kimura K, Kakimi K, Wieland S, Guidotti LG, Chisari FV: Interleukin-18 inhibits hepatitis B virus replication in the livers of transgenic mice. J Virol 2002;76:10702-10707.

71. Nakamoto Y, Guidotti LG, Kuhlen CV, Fowler P, Chisari FV: Immune pathogenesis of hepatocellular carcinoma. J Exp Med 1998;188:341-350.

72. Boshart M, Gissmann L, Ikenberg H, Kleinheinz A, Scheurlen W, zur Hausen H: A new type of papillomavirus DNA, its presence in genital cancer biopsies and in cell lines derived from cervical cancer. EMBO J 1984;3:1151-1157.

73. Durst M, Gissmann L, Ikenberg H, zur Hausen H: A papillomavirus DNA from a cervical carcinoma and its prevalence in cancer biopsy samples from different geographic regions. Proc Natl Acad Sci USA 1983;80:3812-3815.

74. Schwarz E, Freese UK, Gissmann L, et al: Structure and transcription of human papillomavirus sequences in cervical carcinoma cells. Nature 1985;314:111-114.

75. Yee C, Krishnan HI, Baker CC, Schlegel R, Howley PM: Presence and expression of human papillomavirus sequences in human cervical carcinoma cell lines. Am J Pathol 1985;119:361-366.

76. Shope RE: A transmissible tumor-like condition in rabbits. J Exp Med 1932;56:793-802.

77. Jarrett WF, Murphy J, O'Neil BW, Laird HM: Virus-induced papillomas of the alimentary tract of cattle. Intl J Cancer 1978;22:323-328.

78. Campo MS, Moar MH, Sartirana ML, Kennedy IM, Jarrett WF: The presence of bovine papillomavirus type 4 DNA is not required for the progression to, or the maintenance of, the malignant state in cancers of the alimentary canal in cattle. EMBO J 1985;4:1819-1825.

79. Jarrett WF, McNeil PE, Grimshaw WT, Selman IE, McIntyre WI: High incidence area of cattle cancer with a possible interaction between an environmental carcinogen and a papilloma virus. Nature 1978;274:215-217.

80. Pennie WD, Campo MS: Synergism between bovine papillomavirus type 4 and the flavonoid quercetin in cell transformation in vitro. Virology 1992;190:861-865.

81. Dvoretzky I, Shober R, Chattopadhyay SK, Lowy DR: A quantitative in vitro focus assay for bovine papilloma virus. Virology 1980;103:369-375.

82. Law MF, Lowy DR, Dvoretzky I, Howley PM: Mouse cells transformed by bovine papillomavirus contain only extrachromosomal viral DNA sequences. Proc Natl Acad Sci USA 1981;78:2727-2731.

83. Lowy DR, Dvoretzky I, Shober R, Law MF, Engel L, Howley PM: In vitro tumorigenic transformation by a defined sub-genomic fragment of bovine papilloma virus DNA. Nature 1980;287:72-74.

84. Androphy EJ, Schiller JT, Lowy DR: Identification of the protein encoded by the E6 transforming gene of bovine papillomavirus. Science 1985;230:442-445.

85. Nakabayashi Y, Chattopadhyay SK, Lowy DR: The transforming function of bovine papillomavirus DNA. Proc Natl Acad Sci USA 1983;80:5832-5836.

86. Sarver N, Rabson MS, Yang YC, Byrne JC, Howley PM: Localization and analysis of bovine papillomavirus type 1 transforming functions. J Virol 1984;52:377-388.

87. Schiller JT, Vass WC, Vousden KH, Lowy DR: E5 open reading frame of bovine papillomavirus type 1 encodes a transforming gene. J Virol 1986;57:1-6.

88. Schlegel R, Wade GM, Rabson MS, Yang YC: The E5 transforming gene of bovine papillomavirus encodes a small, hydrophobic polypeptide. Science 1986;233:464-467.

89. Yang YC, Okayama H, Howley PM: Bovine papillomavirus contains multiple transforming genes. Proc Natl Acad Sci USA 1985;82:1030-1034.

90. Thierry F, Yaniv M: The BPV1-E2 trans-acting protein can be either an activator or a repressor of the HPV18 regulatory region. EMBO J 1987;6:3391-3397.

91. Jeon S, Lambert PF: Integration of human papillomavirus type 16 DNA into the human genome leads to increased stability of E6 and E7 mRNAs: Implications for cervical carcinogenesis. Proc Natl Acad Sci USA 1995;92:1654-1658.

92. Jeon S, Allen-Hoffmann BL, Lambert PF: Integration of human papillomavirus type 16 into the human genome correlates with a selective growth advantage of cells. J Virol 1995;69:2989-2997.

93. Dyson N, Howley PM, Munger K, Harlow E: The human papilloma virus-16 E7 oncoprotein is able to bind to the retinoblastoma gene product. Science 1989;243:934-937.

94. Werness BA, Levine AJ, Howley PM: Association of human papillomavirus types 16 and 18 E6 proteins with p53. Science 1990;248:76–79.

95. Scheffner M, Munger K, Byrne JC, Howley PM: The state of the p53 and retinoblastoma genes in human cervical carcinoma cell lines. Proc Natl Acad Sci USA 1991;88:5523–5527.

96. Francis DA, Schmid SI, Howley PM: Repression of the integrated papillomavirus E6/E7 promoter is required for growth suppression of cervical cancer cells. J Virol 2000;74:2679–2686.

97. Goodwin EC, DiMaio D: Repression of human papillomavirus oncogenes in HeLa cervical carcinoma cells causes the orderly reactivation of dormant tumor suppressor pathways. Proc Natl Acad Sci USA 2000;97:12513–12518.

98. Goodwin EC, Yang E, Lee CJ, Lee HW, DiMaio D, Hwang ES: Rapid induction of senescence in human cervical carcinoma cells. Proc Natl Acad Sci USA 2000;97:10978–10983.

99. Hwang ES, Riese DJ 2nd, Settleman J, et al: Inhibition of cervical carcinoma cell line proliferation by the introduction of a bovine papillomavirus regulatory gene. J Virol 1993;67:3720–3729.

100. Nishimura A, Ono T, Ishimoto A, et al: Mechanisms of human papillomavirus E2-mediated repression of viral oncogene expression and cervical cancer cell growth inhibition. J Virol 2000;74:3752–3760.

101. Wells SI, Francis DA, Karpova AY, Dowhanick JJ, Benson JD, Howley PM: Papillomavirus E2 induces senescence in HPV-positive cells via pRB- and p21(CIP)-dependent pathways. EMBO J 2000;19:5762–5771.

102. Band V, Zajchowski D, Kulesa V, Sager R: Human papilloma virus DNAs immortalize normal human mammary epithelial cells and reduce their growth factor requirements. Proc Natl Acad Sci USA 1990;87:463–467.

103. Durst M, Dzarlieva PR, Boukamp P, Fusenig NE, Gissmann L: Molecular and cytogenetic analysis of immortalized human primary keratinocytes obtained after transfection with human papillomavirus type 16 DNA. Oncogene 1987;1:251–256.

104. Hawley-Nelson P, Vousden KH, Hubbert NL, Lowy DR, Schiller JT: HPV16 E6 and E7 proteins cooperate to immortalize human foreskin keratinocytes. EMBO J 1989;8:3905–3910.

105. Hudson JB, Bedell MA, McCance DJ, Laiminis LA: Immortalization and altered differentiation of human keratinocytes in vitro by the E6 and E7 open reading frames of human papillomavirus type 18. J Virol 1990;64:519–526.

106. Kaur P, McDougall JK, Cone R: Immortalization of primary human epithelial cells by cloned cervical carcinoma DNA containing human papillomavirus type 16 E6/E7 open reading frames. J Gen Virol 1989;70:1261–1266.

107. Pirisi L, Creek KE, Doniger J, DiPaolo JA: Continuous cell lines with altered growth and differentiation properties originate after transfection of human keratinocytes with human papillomavirus type 16 DNA. Carcinogenesis 1988;9:1573–1579.

108. Crook T, Storey A, Almond N, Osborn K, Crawford L: Human papillomavirus type 16 cooperates with activated ras and fos oncogenes in the hormone-dependent transformation of primary mouse cells. Proc Natl Acad Sci USA 1988;85:8820–8824.

109. Matlashewski G, Schneider J, Banks L, Jones N, Murray A, Crawford L: Human papillomavirus type 16 DNA cooperates with activated ras in transforming primary cells. EMBO J 1987;6:1741–1746.

110. Phelps WC, Bagchi S, Barnes JA, et al: Analysis of trans activation by human papillomavirus type 16 E7 and adenovirus 12S E1A suggests a common mechanism. J Virol 1991;65:6922–6930.

111. Arbeit JM, Howley PM, Hanahan D: Chronic estrogen-induced cervical and vaginal squamous carcinogenesis in human papillomavirus type 16 transgenic mice. Proc Natl Acad Sci USA 1996;93:2930–2935.

112. Elson DA, Riley RR, Lacey A, Thordarson G, Talamantes FJ, Arbeit JM: Sensitivity of the cervical transformation zone to estrogen-induced squamous carcinogenesis. Cancer Res 2000;60:1267–1275.

113. Greenhalgh DA, Rothnagel JA, Quintanilla MI, et al: Induction of epidermal hyperplasia, hyperkeratosis, and papillomas in transgenic mice by a targeted v-Ha-ras oncogene. Mol Carcinog 1993;7:99–110.

114. Herber R, Liem A, Pitot H, Lambert PF: Squamous epithelial hyperplasia and carcinoma in mice transgenic for the human papillomavirus type 16 E7 oncogene. J Virol 1996;70:1873–1881.

115. Lambert PF, Pan H, Pitot HC, Liem A, Jackson M, Griep AE: Epidermal cancer associated with expression of human papillomavirus type 16 E6 and E7 oncogenes in the skin of transgenic mice. Proc Natl Acad Sci USA 1993;90:5583–5587.

116. Pan H, Griep AE: Altered cell cycle regulation in the lens of HPV-16 E6 or E7 transgenic mice: Implications for tumor suppressor gene function in development. Genes Dev 1994;8:1285–1299.

117. Song S, Liem A, Miller JA, Lambert PF: Human papillomavirus types 16 E6 and E7 contribute differently to carcinogenesis. Virology 2000;267:141–150.

118. Song S, Pitot HC, Lambert PF: The human papillomavirus type 16 E6 gene alone is sufficient to induce carcinomas in transgenic animals. J Virol 1999;73:5887–5893.

119. Huibregtse JM., Scheffner M, Howley PM: A cellular protein mediates association of p53 with the E6 oncoprotein of human papillomavirus types 16 or 18. EMBO J 1991;10:4129–4135.

120. Scheffner M, Huibregtse JM, Vierstra RD, Howley PM: The HPV-16 E6 and E6-AP complex functions as a ubiquitin-protein ligase in the ubiquitination of p53. Cell 1993;75:495–505.

121. Lechner MS, Mack DH, Finicle AB, Crook T, Vousden KH, Laimins LA: Human papillomavirus E6 proteins bind p53 in vivo and abrogate p53-mediated repression of transcription. EMBO J 1992;11:3045–3052.

122. Mietz JA, Unger T, Huibregtse JM, Howley PM: The transcriptional transactivation function of wild-type p53 is inhibited by SV40 large T-antigen and by HPV-16 E6 oncoprotein. EMBO J 1992;11:5013–5020.

123. Boyer SN, Wazer DE, Band V: E7 protein of human papilloma virus-16 induces degradation of retinoblastoma protein through the ubiquitin-proteasome pathway. Cancer Res 1996;56:4620–4624.

124. Jones DL, Alani RM, Munger K: The human papillomavirus E7 oncoprotein can uncouple cellular differentiation and proliferation in human keratinocytes by abrogating p21Cip1-mediated inhibition of cdk2. Genes Dev 1997;11:2101–2111.

125. Chellappan S, Kraus VB, Kroger B, et al: Adenovirus E1A, simian virus 40 tumor antigen, and human papillomavirus E7 protein share the capacity to disrupt the interaction between transcription factor E2F and the retinoblastoma gene product. Proc Natl Acad Sci USA 1992;89:4549–4553.

126. Andl T, Kahn T, Pfuhl A, et al: Etiological involvement of oncogenic human papillomavirus in tonsillar squamous cell carcinomas lacking retinoblastoma cell cycle control. Cancer Res 1998;58:5–13.

127. Biliris KA, Koumantakis E, Dokianakis DN, Sourvinos G, Spandidos DA: Human papillomavirus infection of non-melanoma skin cancers in immunocompetent hosts. Cancer Lett 2000;161:83–88.

128. Gillison ML, Koch WM, Capone RB, et al: Evidence for a causal association between human papillomavirus and a subset of head and neck cancers. J Natl Cancer Inst 2000;92:709–720.

129. Kiviat NB: Papillomaviruses in non-melanoma skin cancer: Epidemiological aspects. Semin Cancer Biol 1999;9:397–403.

130. Flores ER, Allen-Hoffmann BL, Lee D, Lambert PF: The human papillomavirus type 16 E7 oncogene is required for the productive stage of the viral life cycle. J Virol 2000;74:6622–6631.

131. Park RB, Androphy EJ: Genetic analysis of high-risk E6 in episomal maintenance of human papillomavirus genomes in primary human keratinocytes. J Virol 2002;76:11359–11364.

132. Ustav M, Stenlund A: Transient replication of BPV-1 requires two viral polypeptides encoded by the E1 and E2 open reading frames. EMBO J 1991;10:449–457.

133. Mohr IJ, Clark R, Sun S, Androphy EJ, MacPherson P, Botchan MR: Targeting the E1 replication protein to the papillomavirus origin of replication by complex formation with the E2 transactivator. Science 1990;250:1694–1699.

134. Sedman J, Stenlund A: Co-operative interaction between the initiator E1 and the transcriptional activator E2 is required for replicator specific DNA replication of bovine papillomavirus in vivo and in vitro. EMBO J 1995;14:6218–6228.

135. Yang L, Mohr I, Fouts E, Lim DA, Nohaile M, Botchan M: The E1 protein of bovine papilloma virus 1 is an ATP-dependent DNA helicase. Proc Natl Acad Sci USA 1993;90:5086–5090.

136. de The G, Bomford R: An HTLV-I vaccine: Why, how, for whom? AIDS Res Hum Retrovir 1993;9:381–386.

137. Madeleine MM, Wiktor SZ, Goedert JJ, et al: HTLV-I and HTLV-II

world-wide distribution: Reanalysis of 4,832 immunoblot results. Int J Cancer 1993;54:255-260.

138. Tajima K: Malignant lymphomas in Japan: Epidemiological analysis of adult T-cell leukemia/lymphoma (ATL). Cancer Metastasis Rev 1988;7:223-241.

139. Jeffery KJ, Usuku K, Hall SE, et al: HLA alleles determine human T-lymphotropic virus-I (HTLV-I) proviral load and the risk of HTLV-I-associated myelopathy. Proc Natl Acad Sci USA 1999;96:3848-3853.

140. Hinuma Y, Nagata K, Hanaoka M, et al: Adult T-cell leukemia: Antigen in an ATL cell line and detection of antibodies to the antigen in human sera. Proc Natl Acad Sci USA 1981;78:6476-6480.

141. Yoshida M, Seiki M, Yamaguchi K, Takatsuki K: Monoclonal integration of human T-cell leukemia provirus in all primary tumors of adult T-cell leukemia suggests causative role of human T-cell leukemia virus in the disease. Proc Natl Acad Sci USA 1984;81:2534-2537.

142. Hino S, Katamine S, Miyata H, Tsuji Y, Yamabe T, Miyamoto T: Primary prevention of HTLV-1 in Japan. Leukemia 1997; 11(Suppl 3):57-59.

143. Yoshida M: Multiple viral strategies of HTLV-1 for dysregulation of cell growth control. Annu Rev Immunol 2001;19:475-496.

144. Albrecht B, Lairmore MD: Critical role of human T-lymphotropic virus type 1 accessory proteins in viral replication and pathogenesis. Microbiol Mol Biol Rev 2002;66:396-406.

145. Tanaka A, Takahashi C, Yamaoka S, Nosaka T, Maki M, Hatanaka M: Oncogenic transformation by the tax gene of human T-cell leukemia virus type I in vitro. Proc Natl Acad Sci USA 1990;87:1071-1075.

146. Pozzatti R, Vogel J, Jay G: The human T-lymphotropic virus type I tax gene can cooperate with the ras oncogene to induce neoplastic transformation of cells. Mol Cell Biol 1990;10:413-417.

147. Grassmann R, Berchtold S, Radant I, et al: Role of human T-cell leukemia virus type 1 X region proteins in immortalization of primary human lymphocytes in culture. J Virol 1992;66:4570-4575.

148. Ross TM, Pettiford SM, Green PL: The tax gene of human T-cell leukemia virus type 2 is essential for transformation of human T lymphocytes. J Virol 1996;70:5194-5202.

149. Nerenberg M, Hinrichs SH, Reynolds RK, Khoury G, Jay G: The tat gene of human T-lymphotropic virus type 1 induces mesenchymal tumors in transgenic mice. Science 1987;237:1324-1329.

150. Grossman WJ, Kimata J, Wong FH, Zutter M, Ley TJ, Ratner L: Development of leukemia in mice transgenic for the tax gene of human T-cell leukemia virus type I. Proc Natl Acad Sci USA 1995;92:1057-1061.

151. Jeang KT, Widen SG, Semmes OJ 4th, Wilson SH: HTLV-I trans-activator protein, tax, is a trans-repressor of the human beta-polymerase gene. Science 1990;247:1082-1084.

152. Ego T, Ariumi Y, Shimotohno K: The interaction of HTLV-1 Tax with HDAC1 negatively regulates the viral gene expression. Oncogene 2002;21:7241-7246.

153. Suzuki T, Kitao S, Matsushime H, Yoshida M: HTLV-1 Tax protein interacts with cyclin-dependent kinase inhibitor p16INK4A and counteracts its inhibitory activity towards CDK4. EMBO J 1996;15:1607-1614.

154. Neuveut C, Low KG, Maldarelli F, et al: Human T-cell leukemia virus type 1 Tax and cell cycle progression: Role of cyclin D-cdk and p110Rb. Mol Cell Biol 1998;18:3620-3632.

155. Pise-Masison CA, Radonovich M, Sakaguchi K, Appella E, Brady JN: Phosphorylation of p53: A novel pathway for p53 inactivation in human T-cell lymphotropic virus type 1-transformed cells. J Virol 1998;72:6348-6355.

156. Felber BK, Paskalis H, Kleinman-Ewing C, Wong-Staal F, Pavlakis GN: The pX protein of HTLV-I is a transcriptional activator of its long terminal repeats. Science 1985;229:675-679.

157. Cross SL, Feinberg MB, Wolf JB, Holbrook NJ, Wong-Staal F, Leonard WJ: Regulation of the human interleukin-2 receptor alpha chain promoter: Activation of a nonfunctional promoter by the transactivator gene of HTLV-I. Cell 1987;49:47-56.

158. Siekevitz M, Feinberg MB, Holbrook N, Wong-Staal F, Greene WC: Activation of interleukin 2 and interleukin 2 receptor (Tac) promoter expression by the trans-activator (tat) gene product of

human T-cell leukemia virus, type I. Proc Natl Acad Sci USA 1987;84:5389-5393.

159. Fujii M, Sassone-Corsi P, Verma IM: c-Fos promoter trans-activation by the tax1 protein of human T-cell leukemia virus type I. Proc Natl Acad Sci USA 1988;85:8526-8530.

160. Tsukahara T, Kannagi M, Ohashi T, et al: Induction of Bcl-x(L) expression by human T-cell leukemia virus type 1 Tax through NF-kappaB in apoptosis-resistant T-cell transfectants with Tax. J Virol 1999;73:7981-7987.

161. Kwok RP, Laurance ME, Lundblad JR, et al: Control of cAMP-regulated enhancers by the viral transactivator Tax through CREB and the co-activator CBP. Nature 1996;380:642-646.

162. Suzuki T, Hirai H, Fujisawa J, Fujita T, Yoshida M: A trans-activator Tax of human T-cell leukemia virus type 1 binds to NF-kappa B p50 and serum response factor (SRF) and associates with enhancer DNAs of the NF-kappa B site and CArG box. Oncogene 1993;8:2391-2397.

163. Suzuki T, Hirai H, Yoshida M: Tax protein of HTLV-1 interacts with the Rel homology domain of NF-kappa B p65 and c-Rel proteins bound to the NF-kappa B binding site and activates transcription. Oncogene 1994;9:3099-3105.

164. Suzuki T, Hirai H, Murakami T, Yoshida M: Tax protein of HTLV-1 destabilizes the complexes of NF-kappa B and I kappa B-alpha and induces nuclear translocation of NF-kappa B for transcriptional activation. Oncogene 1995;10:1199-1207.

165. Maggirwar SB, Harhaj E, Sun SC: Activation of NF-kappa B/Rel by Tax involves degradation of I kappa B alpha and is blocked by a proteasome inhibitor. Oncogene 1995;11:993-998.

166. Lemasson I, Polakowski NJ, Laybourn PJ, Nyborg JK: Transcription factor binding and histone modifications on the integrated proviral promoter in human T-cell leukemia virus-I–infected T-cells. J Biol Chem 2002;277:49459-49465.

167. Suzuki T, Uchida-Toita M, Yoshida M: Tax protein of HTLV-1 inhibits CBP/p300-mediated transcription by interfering with recruitment of CBP/p300 onto DNA element of E-box or p53 binding site. Oncogene 1999;18:4137-4143.

168. Knoepfler PS, Eisenman RN: Sin meets NuRD and other tails of repression. Cell 1999;99:447-450.

169. Pise-Masison CA, Mahieux R, Jiang H, et al: Inactivation of p53 by human T-cell lymphotropic virus type 1 Tax requires activation of the NF-kappaB pathway and is dependent on p53 phosphorylation. Mol Cell Biol 2000;20:3377-3386.

170. Kinoshita T, Shimoyama M, Tobinai K, et al: Detection of mRNA for the tax1/rex1 gene of human T-cell leukemia virus type I in fresh peripheral blood mononuclear cells of adult T-cell leukemia patients and viral carriers by using the polymerase chain reaction. Proc Natl Acad Sci USA 1989;86:5620-5624.

171. Yao F, Terrault N: Hepatitis C and hepatocellular carcinoma. Curr Treat Options Oncol 2001;2:473-483.

172. Sun CA, Wu DM, Lin CC, et al: Incidence and cofactors of hepatitis C virus–related hepatocellular carcinoma: A prospective study of 12,008 men in Taiwan. Am J Epidemiol 2003;157:674-682.

173. Yen T, Keefe EB, Ahmed A: The epidemiology of hepatitis C virus infection. J Clin Gastroenterol 2003;36:47-53.

174. WHO: WHO Global Surveillance and control of hepatitis C: Report of a WHO consultation organized in collaboration with the viral Hepatitis Prevention Board. J Viral Hepat 1999;6:35-47.

175. Di Bisceglie AM: Hepatitis C and hepatocellular carcinoma. Hepatology 1997;26:34S-38S.

176. Choo QL, Kuo G, Weiner AJ, Overby LR, Bradley DW, Houghton M: Isolation of a cDNA clone derived from a blood-borne non-A, non-B viral hepatitis genome. Science 1989;244:359-362.

177. Rosenberg S: Recent advances in the molecular biology of hepatitis C virus. J Mol Biol 2001;313:451-464.

178. Smith DB, Pathirana S, Davidson F, et al: The origin of hepatitis C virus genotypes. J Gen Virol 1997;78:321-328.

179. Bukh J, Miller RH, Purcell RH: Genetic heterogeneity of hepatitis C virus: Quasispecies and genotypes. Semin Liver Dis 1995;15:41-63.

180. Lohmann V, Körner F, Koch JO, Herian U, Theilmann L, Bartenschlager R: Replication of subgenomic hepatitis C virus RNAs in a hepatoma cell line. Science 1999;285:110-113.

181. Bukh J, Pietschmann T, Lohmann V, et al: Mutations that permit efficient replication of hepatitis C virus RNA in Huh-7 cells

prevent productive replication in chimpanzees. Proc Natl Acad Sci USA 2002;99:14416-14421.

182. Rhim JA, Sandgren EP, Degen JL, Palmiter RD, Brinster RL: Replacement of diseased mouse liver by hepatic cell transplantation. Science 1994;263:1149-1152.

183. Rhim JA, Sandgren EP, Palmiter RD, Brinster RL: Complete reconstitution of mouse liver with xenogenic hepatocytes. Proc Natl Acad Sci USA 1995;92:4942-4946.

184. Petersen J, Dandri M, Gupta S, Rogler CE: Liver repopulation with xenogenic hepatocytes in B and T cell-deficient mice leads to chronic hepadnavirus infection and clonal growth of hepatocellular carcinoma. Proc Natl Acad Sci USA 1998;95:310-315.

185. Mercer DF, Schiller DE, Elliott JF, et al: Hepatitis C virus replication in mice with chimeric human livers. Nat Med 2001;7:927-933.

186. Ray R, Lagging L, Meyer K, Ray R: Hepatitis C virus core protein cooperates with ras and transforms primary rat embryo fibroblasts to tumorigenic phenotype. J Virol 1996;70:4438-4443.

187. Moriya K, Fujie H, Shintani Y, et al: The core protein of hepatitis C virus induces hepatocellular carcinoma in transgenic mice. Nat Med 1998;4:1065-1067.

188. Aoki H, Hayashi J, Moriyama M, Arakawa Y, Hino O: Hepatitis C virus core protein interacts with the 14-3-3 protein and activates the kinase Raf-1. J Virol 2000;74:1736-1741.

189. Hayashi J, Aoki H, Kajino K, Moriyama M, Arakawa Y, Hino O: Hepatitis C virus core protein activates the MAPK/ERK cascade synergistically with tumor promoter TPA, but not with EGF or TGFalpha. Hepatology 2000;32:958-961.

190. Jin D, Wang H, Zhou Y, et al: Hepatitis C virus core protein-induced loss of LZIP function correlates with cellular transformation. EMBO J 2000;19:729-740.

191. Yoshida T, Hanada T, Tokuhisa T, et al: Activation of STAT3 by the hepatitis C virus core protein leads to cellular transformation. J Exp Med 2002;196:641-653.

192. Reichard O, Norkrans G, Frydén A, Braconier JH, Sönnerborg A, Weiland O: Randomised, double-blind, placebo-controlled trial of interferon a-2b with and without ribavirin for chronic hepatitis C. Lancet 1998;351:83-87.

193. Brown JL: Efficacy of combined interferon and ribavirin for treatment of hepatitis C. Lancet 1998;351:78-79.

194. Cook-Mozaffari P, Newton R, Beral V, Burkitt DP: The geographical distribution of Kaposi's sarcoma and of lymphomas in Africa before the AIDS epidemic. Br J Cancer 1998;78:1521-1528.

195. Geddes M, Franceschi S, Barchielli A, et al: Kaposi's sarcoma in Italy before and after the AIDS epidemic. Br J Cancer 1994;69: 333-336.

196. Chang Y, Cesarman E, Pessin MS, et al: Identification of herpesvirus-like DNA sequences in AIDS-associated Kaposi's sarcoma. Science 1994;266:1865-1869.

197. Dedicoat M, Newton R: Review of the distribution of Kaposi's sarcoma-associated herpesvirus (KSHV) in Africa in relation to the incidence of Kaposi's sarcoma. Br J Cancer 2003;88:1-3.

198. Osmond DH, Buchbinder S, Cheng A, et al: Prevalence of Kaposi sarcoma-associated herpesvirus infection in homosexual men at beginning of and during the HIV epidemic. JAMA 2002;287: 221-225.

199. Jacobson LP, Jenkins FJ, Springer G, et al: Interaction of human immunodeficiency virus type 1 and human herpesvirus type 8 infections on the incidence of Kaposi's sarcoma. J Infect Dis 2000;181:1940-1949.

200. Cesarman E, Chang Y, Moore PS, Said JW, Knowles DM: Kaposi's sarcoma-associated herpesvirus-like DNA sequences in AIDS-related body-cavity-based lymphomas. N Engl J Med 1995;332: 1186-1191.

201. Soulier J, Grollet L, Oksenhendler E, et al: Kaposi's sarcoma-associated herpesvirus-like DNA sequences in multicentric Castleman's disease. Blood 1995;86:1276-1280.

202. Dupin N, Fisher C, Kellam P, et al: Distribution of human herpesvirus-8 latently infected cells in Kaposi's sarcoma, multicentric Castleman's disease, and primary effusion lymphoma. Proc Natl Acad Sci USA 1999;96:4546-4551.

203. Moore PS, Chang Y: Kaposi's sarcoma-associated herpesvirus-encoded oncogenes and oncogenesis. J Natl Cancer Inst Monogr 1998;(23):65-71.

204. Jenner RG, Boshoff C: The molecular pathology of Kaposi's sarcoma-associated herpesvirus. Biochim Biophys Acta 2002;1602:1-22.

205. Matolcsy A, Nador RG, Cesarman E, Knowles DM: Immunoglobulin VH gene mutational analysis suggests that primary effusion lymphomas derive from different stages of B cell maturation. Am J Pathol 1998;153:1609-1614.

206. Nador RG, Cesarman E, Chadburn A, et al: Primary effusion lymphoma: A distinct clinicopathologic entity associated with the Kaposi's sarcoma-associated herpes virus. Blood 1996;88: 645-656.

207. Mann DJ, Child ES, Swanton C, Laman H, Jones N: Modulation of p27(Kip1) levels by the cyclin encoded by Kaposi's sarcoma-associated herpesvirus. EMBO J 1999;18:654-663.

208. Ellis M, Chew YP, Fallis L, et al: Degradation of p27(Kip) cdk inhibitor triggered by Kaposi's sarcoma virus cyclin-cdk6 complex. EMBO J 1999;18:644-653.

209. Laman H, Coverley D, Krude T, Laskey R, Jones N: Viral cyclin-cyclin-dependent kinase 6 complexes initiate nuclear DNA replication. Mol Cell Biol 2001;21:624-635.

210. Ojala PM, Tiainen M, Salven P, et al: Kaposi's sarcoma-associated herpesvirus-encoded v-cyclin triggers apoptosis in cells with high levels of cyclin-dependent kinase 6. Cancer Res 1999;59: 4984-4989.

211. Verschuren EW, Klefstrom J, Evan GI, Jones N: The oncogenic potential of Kaposi's sarcoma-associated herpesvirus cyclin is exposed by p53 loss in vitro and in vivo. Cancer Cell 2002;2:229-241.

212. Cheng EH, Nicholas J, Bellows DS, et al: A Bcl-2 homolog encoded by Kaposi sarcoma-associated virus, human herpesvirus 8, inhibits apoptosis but does not heterodimerize with Bax or Bak. Proc Natl Acad Sci USA 1997;94:690-694.

213. Ojala PM, Yamamoto K, Castanos-Velez E, Biberfeld P, Korsmeyer SJ, Makela TP: The apoptotic v-cyclin-CDK6 complex phosphorylates and inactivates Bcl-2. Nat Cell Biol 2000;2:819-825.

214. Djerbi M, Screpanti V, Catrina AI, Bogen B, Biberfeld P, Grandien A: The inhibitor of death receptor signaling, FLICE-inhibitory protein defines a new class of tumor progression factors. J Exp Med 1999;190:1025-1032.

215. Asou H, Said JW, Yang R, et al: Mechanisms of growth control of Kaposi's sarcoma-associated herpes virus-associated primary effusion lymphoma cells. Blood 1998;91:2475-2481.

216. Montaner S, Sodhi A, Molinolo A, et al: Endothelial infection with KSHV genes in vivo reveals that vGPCR initiates Kaposi's sarcomagenesis and can promote the tumorigenic potential of viral latent genes. Cancer Cell 2003;3:23-36.

217. Bais C, Santomasso B, Coso O, et al: G-protein-coupled receptor of Kaposi's sarcoma-associated herpesvirus is a viral oncogene and angiogenesis activator. Nature 1998;391:86-89.

218. Bais C, Van Geelen A, Eroles P, et al: Kaposi's sarcoma associated herpesvirus G protein-coupled receptor immortalizes human endothelial cells by activation of the VEGF receptor-2/KDR. Cancer Cell 2003;3:131-143.

219. Ballestas ME, Kaye KM: Kaposi's sarcoma-associated herpesvirus latency-associated nuclear antigen 1 mediates episome persistence through cis-acting terminal repeat (TR) sequence and specifically binds TR DNA. J Virol 2001;75:3250-3258.

220. Hu J, Garber AC, Renne R: The latency-associated nuclear antigen of Kaposi's sarcoma-associated herpesvirus supports latent DNA replication in dividing cells. J Virol 2002;76:11677-11687.

221. Gradoville L, Gerlach J, Grogan E, et al: Kaposi's sarcoma-associated herpesvirus open reading frame 50/Rta protein activates the entire viral lytic cycle in the HH-B2 primary effusion lymphoma cell line. J Virol 2000;74:6207-6212.

222. Moses AV, Fish KN, Ruhl R, et al: A: Long-term infection and transformation of dermal microvascular endothelial cells by human herpesvirus 8. J Virol 1999;73:6892-6902.

223. Ciufo DM, Cannon JS, Poole LJ, et al: Spindle cell conversion by Kaposi's sarcoma-associated herpesvirus: Formation of colonies and plaques with mixed lytic and latent gene expression in infected primary dermal microvascular endothelial cell cultures. J Virol 2001;75:5614-5626.

224. Cairo MS, Sposto R, Perkins SL, et al: Burkitt's and Burkitt-like

lymphoma in children and adolescents: A review of the Children's Cancer Group experience. Br J Haematol 2003;120:660–670.

225. Lee SS, Weiss RS, Javier RT: Binding of human virus oncoproteins to hDlg/SAP97, a mammalian homolog of the Drosophila discs large tumor suppressor protein. Proc Natl Acad Sci USA 1997;94:6670–6675.

226. Ahmad SA, Bilimoria MM, Wang X, et al: Hepatitis B or C virus serology as a prognostic factor in patients with hepatocellular carcinoma. J Gastrointest Surg 2001;5:468–476.

227. Rabe C, Pilz T, Klostermann C, et al: Clinical characteristics and outcome of a cohort of 101 patients with hepatocellular carcinoma. World J Gastroenterol 2001;7:208–215.

228. Wang H, Chia KS, Du WB, et al: Population-based survival for cervical cancer in Singapore, 1968–1992. Am J Obstet Gynecol 2003;188:324–329.

229. Donato DM: Surgical management of stage IB-IIA cervical carcinoma. Semin Surg Oncol 1999;16:232–235.

230. Yamaguchi K, Watanabe T: Human T lymphotropic virus type-I and adult T-cell leukemia in Japan. Int J Hematol 2002;76(Suppl 2):240–245.

231. Tam HK, Zhang ZF, Jacobson LP, et al: Effect of highly active antiretroviral therapy on survival among HIV-infected men with Kaposi sarcoma or non-Hodgkin lymphoma. Int J Cancer 2002;98:916–922.

232. Ghosh SK, Wood C, Boise LH, et al: Potentiation of TRAIL-induced apoptosis in primary effusion lymphoma through azidothymidine-mediated inhibition of NF-kappa B. Blood 2003;101:2321–2327.

233. Rizzetto M, Zanetti AR: Progress in the prevention and control of viral hepatitis type B: Closing remarks. J Med Virol 2002;67:463–466.

234. Zuckerman JN, Zuckerman AJ: Current topics in hepatitis B. J Infect Dis 2000;41:130–136.

235. Winer RL, Lee SK, Hughes JP, Adam DE, Kiviat NB, Koutsky LA: Genital human papillomavirus infection: Incidence and risk factors in a cohort of female university students. Am J Epidemiol 2003;157:218–226.

236. Frazer I: Vaccines for papillomavirus infection. Virus Res 2002;89:271–274.

237. Christensen ND, Reed CA, Cladel NM, Han R, Kreider JW: Immunization with viruslike particles induces long-term protection of rabbits against challenge with cottontail rabbit papillomavirus. J Virol 1996;70:960–965.

238. Suzich JA, Ghim SJ, Palmer-Hill FJ, et al: Systemic immunization with papillomavirus L1 protein completely prevents the development of viral mucosal papillomas. Proc Natl Acad Sci USA 1995;92:11553–11557.

239. Harro CD, Pang YY, Roden RB, et al: Safety and immunogenicity trial in adult volunteers of a human papillomavirus 16 L1 virus-like particle vaccine. J Natl Cancer Inst 2001;93:284–292.

240. Koutsky LA, Ault KA, Wheeler CM, et al: A controlled trial of a human papillomavirus type 16 vaccine. N Engl J Med 2002;347:1645–1651.

241. Roden RB, Yutzy WH 4th, Fallon R, Inglis S, Lowy DR, Schiller JT: Minor capsid protein of human genital papillomaviruses contains subdominant, cross-neutralizing epitopes. Virology 2000;270:254–257.

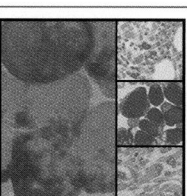

GENETIC FACTORS: HEREDITARY CANCER PREDISPOSITION SYNDROMES

Kenneth Offit

Rina Siddiqui

SUMMARY OF KEY POINTS

- The discovery of inherited mutations of oncogenes and tumor suppressor genes associated with increased risk for cancer has opened up a new field of cancer medicine. The impact of these recent breakthroughs in molecular genetics has been felt in three areas of clinical oncology: cancer diagnosis, cancer prognosis, and cancer prevention based on prediction of inherited cancer risk.

- These areas of oncology constitute the foundation for the study of clinical cancer genetics (Fig. 13-1).[1]

- Genetic tests to diagnose cancers are included in clinical evaluations by practicing oncologists with increasing frequency. Cancer genetic tests that predict outcome after treatment are being incorporated into the care of patients by a range of cancer specialists. The continued development of genetic tests that predict familial cancer risk accurately has given rise to the new discipline of cancer genetic counseling.

- Medical, surgical, and radiation oncologists and allied professionals have played a leading role in integration of genetics into clinical practice. This chapter reviews the major applications of genetic technologies in the presymptomatic management of patients with or at risk for cancer.

GENETICS IN CANCER PREDISPOSITION

One of the most challenging developments in clinical oncology is the availability of testing for inherited mutations of cancer predisposition genes. As these genes have been identified and characterized, guidelines for the responsible clinical translation of this information have been developed by medical and surgical subspecialty societies (e.g., the Statements of the American Society of Clinical Oncology).[2,3] These guidelines emphasize that in the process of offering a predictive genetic "test" to a patient or family affected by cancer, both the provider and the individual being tested must be prepared to deal with all of the medical, psychological, and social consequences of a positive, negative, or ambiguous result.

The need to understand and act effectively on genetic information cuts across the fields of medical genetics, primary care medicine, oncology, public health, behavioral science, and public policy.[1] Current concerns about the widespread commercial availability of cancer susceptibility tests relate both to the clinical validity of the tests and to the potential for misuse and misinterpretation of data.

The Content of Clinical Cancer Genetics Consultations

Cancer risk counseling is most frequently requested for families with the most common hereditary neoplasms: breast, ovarian, prostate, and colon cancers. In general, counseling should be offered to families with multiple cases of related cancers in several generations, multiple related cancers in the same individual, or cancers at an early age.

A selected set of syndromes of cancer predisposition, listed in Table 13-1, is reviewed in this chapter. More detailed discussion of breast and colon cancer susceptibilities are found in the chapters discussing these tumors (see Chapters 11, 14, 80, and 94). A more comprehensive list of syndromes and genetic features is provided in Table 13-2.

The need for physician education in cancer genetics has been emphasized. A study of physicians offering colon

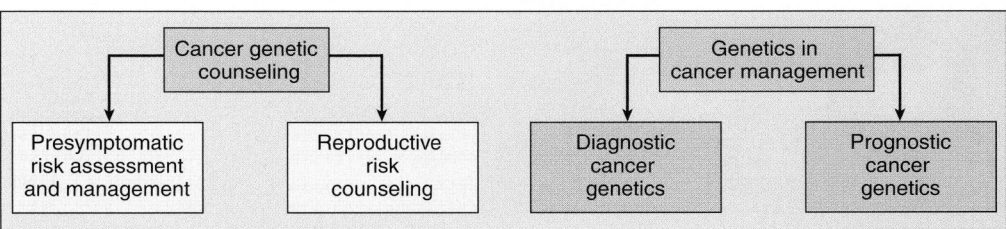

Figure 13-1. The components of clinical cancer genetics. (From Offit K: Clinical Cancer Genetics: Risk Counseling and Management. New York, John Wiley & Sons, 1998.)

227

TABLE 13-1

Selected Cancer Predisposition Syndromes

SYNDROME	GENE
I. The Major Cancer Predisposition Syndromes	
A. Hereditary breast and ovarian cancer syndromes	BRCA1, BRCA2
B. Familial adenomatous polyposis	APC
C. Hereditary nonpolyposis colon cancer syndrome	MSH2, MLH1, MSH6
D. Hereditary prostate cancer	Multiple loci
E. Multiple endocrine neoplasias (I, II)	MEN1, RET
F. Hereditary melanoma syndromes	CDKN2^{p16}, CDK4
G. Familial retinoblastoma	RB1
H. Neurofibromatosis I, II	NF1, NF2
I. von Hippel-Lindau syndrome	VHL
II. Recently Described Cancer Predisposition Syndromes	
A. Gorlin syndrome	PTCH
B. Carney complex	PRKAR1A
C. Cowden syndrome	PTEN
D. Birt-Hogg-Dubé syndrome	BHD
E. Rhabdoid predisposition syndrome	SNF5/INI1

TABLE 13-2

Syndromes of Inherited Cancer Predisposition in Clinical Oncology

SYNDROME (OMIM* ENTRY)	COMPONENT MALIGNANCIES	MODE OF INHERITANCE	GENES
1. Hereditary Breast Cancer Syndromes			
Hereditary breast and breast cancer Ovarian cancer syndrome 113705 600185	Ovarian cancer Colon cancer Prostate cancer Pancreatic cancer	Dominant	BRCA1 BRCA2
Li-Fraumeni syndrome soft tissue sarcoma 151623	Breast cancer Osteosarcoma Leukemia Brain tumors Adrenocortical carcinoma	Dominant	p53 CHK2
Cowden syndrome 158350	Breast cancer Thyroid cancer Other cancers	Dominant	PTEN
Bannayan-Riley-Ruvalcaba syndrome 153480	Breast cancer Meningioma Thyroid follicular cell tumors	Dominant	PTEN
Ataxia telangiectasia 208900	Leukemia Lymphoma Ovarian cancer Gastric cancer Brain tumors Colon cancer	Recessive	ATM
2. Hereditary Gastrointestinal Malignancies			
Hereditary nonpolyposis colon cancer, including "Lynch II" syndrome (HNPCC) 120435 120436 114500 114400	Colon cancer Endometrial cancer Ovarian cancer Pancreatic cancer Stomach and small bowel cancers	Dominant	MSH2 MLH1 MSH6
Familial polyposis (including attenuated phenotype and Ashkenazi low-penetrance phenotype) 175100	Colon cancer	Dominant	APC
Familial attenuated polyposis 175100	Colon cancer	Dominant	APC

TABLE 13-2

Syndromes of Inherited Cancer Predisposition in Clinical Oncology—cont'd

SYNDROME (OMIM* ENTRY)	COMPONENT MALIGNANCIES	MODE OF INHERITANCE	GENES
Hereditary gastric cancer 137215	Stomach cancers	Dominant	CDH1
Juvenile polyposis 174900	Gastrointestinal cancers Pancreatic cancer	Dominant	PTEN SMAD4/DPC4 BMPR1A
Peutz-Jeghers syndrome 175200	Colon cancer Small bowel cancer Breast cancer Ovarian cancer Pancreatic cancer	Dominant	STK11
Hereditary melanoma pancreatic cancer syndrome 606719	Pancreatic cancer Melanoma	Dominant	CDKN2A/p16
Hereditary pancreatitis 167800	Pancreatic cancer	Dominant	PRSS1
Turcot syndrome 276300	Colon cancer Basal cell carcinoma Ependymoma Medulloblastoma Glioblastoma Papillary thyroid carcinoma Leukemia	Dominant	MLH1 APC PMS2
Familial gastrointestinal stromal tumor 606764	Gastrointestinal stromal Tumors	Dominant	c-KIT
3. Genodermatoses with Cancer Predisposition			
Melanoma syndromes 155600 155601	Malignant melanoma	Dominant	CDKN2 (p16) CDK4 CMM
Basal cell cancers (Gorlin syndrome) 109400	Basal cell cancers Brain tumors	Dominant	PTCH
Cowden syndrome	See above	Dominant	PTEN
Neurofibromatosis 1 162200	Neurofibrosarcomas Pheochromocytomas Optic gliomas	Dominant	NF1
Neurofibromatosis 2 101000	Vestibular schwannomas	Dominant	NF2
Tuberous sclerosis 191100	Myocardial rhabdomyoma Multiple bilateral renal angiomyolipoma Ependymoma Renal cancer Giant cell astrocytoma	Dominant	TSC1 TSC2
Carney complex 160980	Myxoid subcutaneous tumors Primary adrenocortical nodular hyperplasia Testicular Sertoli cell tumor Pituitary adenoma Mammary ductal fibroadenoma Schwannoma Pheochromocytoma	Dominant	PRKAR1A
Muir-Torre syndrome 158320	Sebaceous carcinoma Sebaceous epitheliomas Sebaceous adenomas Basal cell carcinoma Colon cancer Duodenal carcinoma Laryngeal carcinoma Malignant gastrointestinal tract tumors Malignant genitourinary tract tumors Breast cancer	Dominant	MLH1 MSH2
Xeroderma pigmentosum 278730 278700 278720 278760	Skin cancer Melanoma Leukemia	Recessive	XPA XPC XPD(ERCC2) XPF

Science of Clinical Oncology

Continued

TABLE 13-2

Syndromes of Inherited Cancer Predisposition in Clinical Oncology—cont'd

SYNDROME (OMIM* ENTRY)	COMPONENT MALIGNANCIES	MODE OF INHERITANCE	GENES
Rothmund-Thomson syndrome 268400	Basal cell carcinoma Squamous cell carcinoma Osteogenic sarcoma	Recessive	RECQL4 RECQL5
4. Leukemia/Lymphoma Predisposition Syndromes			
Bloom syndrome 210900	Leukemia Carcinoma of the tongue Esophageal carcinoma Wilms tumor Colon cancer	Recessive	BLM
Fanconi's anemia 227650	Leukemia Esophageal cancer Skin carcinoma Hepatoma	Recessive	FACA FACC FACD1 FACD2 FACE FACF FACG
Schwachman-Diamond syndrome 260400	Myelodysplasia Acute myelogenous leukemia	Recessive	SBDS
Nijmegen breakage syndrome 251260	Lymphoma Glioma Medulloblastoma Rhabdomyosarcoma	Recessive	NBS1
Cannale-Smith syndrome 601859	Lymphoma	Dominant	FAS FASL
Immunodeficiency syndromes:			
Wiskott-Aldrich 301000	Hematopoietic malignancies	X-linked recessive	WASP
Common variable immune deficiency 240500	Lymphomas	Recessive Dominant	Unknown Unknown
Severe combined immune deficiency 102700 300400 202500	B-cell lymphoma	X-linked recessive Recessive	IL2RG ADA JAK3 RAG1 RAG2 IL7R CD45 Unknown
X-linked lymphoproliferative syndrome 308240	Lymphoma	X-linked recessive	SH2D1A
5. Genitourinary Cancer Predisposition Syndromes			
Hereditary prostate cancer 176807 601518	Prostate cancer	Dominant	HPC1 HPCX PCAP PCBC PRCA
Simpson-Golabi-Behmel syndrome 312870	Embryonal tumors Wilms' tumor	X-linked recessive	GPC3
von Hippel-Lindau syndrome 193300	Hemangioblastomas of retina and central nervous system Renal cell cancer Pheochromocytomas	Dominant	VHL
Beckwith-Wiedemann syndrome 130650	Wilms' tumor Hepatoblastoma Adrenal carcinoma Gonadoblastoma	Dominant	CDKN1C
Wilms' tumor syndrome 194070	Nephroblastoma	Dominant	WT1
WAGR (Wilms' tumor, aniridia, growth retardation) 194072	Wilms' tumor	Dominant	WT1
Birt-Hogg-Dubé syndrome 135150	Renal tumors	Dominant	FLCL
Papillary renal cancer syndrome 605074 164860	Renal cancer	Dominant	MET

TABLE 13-2

Syndromes of Inherited Cancer Predisposition in Clinical Oncology—cont'd

SYNDROME (OMIM* ENTRY)	COMPONENT MALIGNANCIES	MODE OF INHERITANCE	GENES
Constitutional t(3;8) t(3;8) translocation 603046	Renal cell cancer	Dominant	TRC8
Hereditary bladder cancer 109800	Bladder cancer	Sporadic	Unknown
Hereditary testicular cancer 273300	Testicular cancer Possibly recessive	Possibly X-linked	Unknown Unknown
Rhabdoid predisposition syndrome 601607	Rhabdoid tumors (see below)	Dominant	SNF5/INI1
6. Central Nervous System/Vascular Cancer Predisposition Syndromes			
Hereditary paraganglioma 185470 115310	Paraganglioma Pheochromocytoma	Dominant	SDHD SDHC SDHB
Retinoblastoma 180200	Retinoblastoma Osteosarcoma	Dominant	RB1
Rhabdoid predisposition syndrome 601607	Rhabdoid tumors Medulloblastoma Choroid plexus tumors Primitive neuroectodermal tumors	Dominant	SNF5/INI1
7. Sarcoma/Bone Cancer Predisposition Syndromes			
Multiple exostoses 133700 133701	Chondrosarcoma	Dominant	EXT1 EXT2
Leiomyoma/renal cancer syndrome 605839	Papillary renal cell carcinoma Uterine leiomyosarcomas	Dominant	FH
Carney's complex	See above	Dominant	PRKAR1A
Werner's syndrome 277700	Sarcoma/osteosarcoma Meningioma	Recessive	WRN RECQL2 RECQL3
8. Endocrine Cancer Predisposition Syndromes			
MEN1 131100	Pancreatic islet cell tumors Pituitary adenomas Parathyroid adenomas	Dominant	MEN1
MEN2 171400	Medullary thyroid cancers Pheochromocytoma Parathyroid hyperplasia	Dominant	RET
Hereditary papillary thyroid cancer 188500	Papillary thyroid cancer	Dominant	RET

*OMIM, On-Line Mendelian Inheritance in Man: http://www3.ncbi.nlm.nih.gov/Omim/

cancer genetic testing from one commercial laboratory revealed that almost a third of the providers misinterpreted the results. There were no differences in ability to interpret the test results among subspecialty groups, and only 19% offered genetic counseling before the test.[4]

Whether performed as part of a research study or in the course of routine clinical care, genetic testing for inherited cancer risk requires careful informed consent. The elements of informed consent for genetic testing are summarized in Table 13-3.

Elements of Cancer Genetic Counseling

Genetic counseling has been defined as "a communication process which deals with the human problems associated with the occurrence, or risk of occurrence, of a genetic disorder in a family."[5,6] For a number of reasons—

including the strong presumption of benefit of cancer screening and early detection options—the counselor's role is to educate and enumerate options, answer questions about what is known, and suggest appropriate referrals for cancer screening or preventive options.

Several elements are involved in a typical cancer genetic counseling session:

1. The first phase is called *contracting*, during which the goals and expectations of the session are reviewed between counselor and consultand ("*proband*"). During this discussion, it is often helpful to elicit the *baseline risk perception* of the individual.
2. *Pedigree construction* consists of assembly of pedigree information using standardized symbols. The full family structure, which includes all healthy and affected relatives, should be represented. The relative's name,

TABLE 13-3

The Elements of Informed Consent for Cancer Genetic Testing

1. *What the test is intended to do*—that is, determine whether a mutation can be detected in a specific cancer susceptibility gene.
2. *What can be learned from both a positive and negative test*, including information on the magnitude of health risks associated with a positive test, and the risks that could remain even after a negative test.
3. *The possibility that no additional risk information will be obtained* after testing, or that the test will result in a finding of unknown significance (e.g., a polymorphism) that would require further studies.
4. *The options for approximation of risk without genetic testing*, e.g., using empiric risk tables for breast cancer given differing family histories.
5. *The risk of passing a mutation on to children.*
6. *The importance of notification of family members that they might share a hereditary risk for cancer*, with every effort made to assist in contacting of family members and providing them access to counseling and testing.
7. *The medical options and limited proof of efficacy for surveillance and cancer prevention for individuals with a positive test*, and the accepted recommendations for cancer screening even if genetic testing is negative.
8. *The technical accuracy of the test*—the sensitivity and specificity of the analytic methodology.
9. *The risks of psychological distress and family disruption*, whether or not a mutation is found.
10. *The risk of employment and/or insurance discrimination* following disclosure of genetic test results; and the *level of confidentiality of results* compared with other medical tests and procedures.
11. *The risks that nonrelatedness of family members will be discovered*, and how this information will be disclosed (or not disclosed).
12. *The fees and costs of testing*, including the laboratory test and the associated consultation by the health professional providing pretest education, results disclosure, and follow-up, and the costs of preventive procedures, which might not be covered by third-party payers.

age when affected by cancer, current age or age at death, type of cancer(s), and other medical conditions should be noted. Information on type of treatment and the hospital where the diagnostic biopsy was performed should also be obtained. The process of documenting the pedigree by obtaining necessary records is often aided by the family.

3. *Medical history* focuses on reference to known preneoplastic lesions (e.g., polyps, dysplastic nevi, in situ breast lesions). Associated congenital abnormalities and related medical conditions are noted. The medical history should include an occupational history and an exposure history, either of which might be causally related to familial cancer clusters.

4. The *physical examination* should identify congenital abnormalities or other physical findings (e.g., facial trichilemmomas in Cowden syndrome or sebaceous adenomas in Muir-Torre syndrome) associated with cancer predisposition.

5. Interpreting the factors just discussed, *risk assessment* is based on the pedigree and on the availability of empiric risk data. A number of empiric databases are available to provide risk estimates to families with breast, ovarian, or colon cancers. Individuals' interest in and ability to receive quantitative risk estimates will vary greatly. The communication and explanation of genetic risks for cancer often requires a review of basic concepts of Mendelian genetics and a simplified presentation of the "two-hit" hypothesis (see Chapter 15).

6. The most challenging aspect of cancer risk counseling is the formulation and discussion of options for early detection and prevention. In most cases, these options include cancer screening by radiographic, endoscopic, or other means of physical examination or laboratory testing. Although most of these options have been proven to be effective in the average-risk population (e.g., mammography, colonoscopy), they are only presumed to be of benefit in the high-risk population. The most dramatic option for cancer prevention—the

removal of healthy organs—is now an established part of the management of syndromes such as familial polyposis, MEN2a, and, increasingly, inherited breast/ovarian and colon cancer syndromes. Referral to a variety of surgical or medical subspecialists is a component of the counseling session. (It should be noted that the foregoing discussion can be provided without recourse to genetic testing. In those instances in which genetic testing is appropriate, *pretest genetic counseling* is indicated. This discussion requires an educational effort to convey the potential impact of any test results, whether positive, negative, or ambiguous. The components of *informed consent* as part of pretest counseling were summarized in Table 13-3. The potential risks of genetic testing are primarily psychological and include nonmedical potential liabilities such as genetic discrimination.)

7. Finally, genetic counseling should provide a forum for *response to questions, support*, and *plans for follow-up*. Although it is a truism that counseling should be "supportive," such an outcome could require significant preparation and considerable counseling experience.

Syndromes of Cancer Predisposition

Genes whose alteration results in hereditary predisposition to human cancers can be divided into oncogenes and tumor suppressor genes. The molecular mechanisms of these two classes of genes are presented in previous chapters of this book (see Chapter 15). A small minority of human cancer predisposition syndromes result from inherited mutations of oncogenes. The majority of cancer predisposition syndromes are due to inherited defects in tumor suppressor genes. The tumor suppressor genes can be further subdivided into "gatekeepers" such as *APC, p53, Rb*, and *VHL*, which directly prevent runaway cell growth, and "caretakers" such as *ATM, MSH2, MLH1*, defects of which act indirectly to cause neoplasia by leading to increased mutation of other critical genes. Yet a third class of genes, which includes *PTEN* and *SMAD4*, act as "landscapers," as defects of these genes cause alterations in the terrain for epithelial cell growth, leading to eventual neoplastic changes. Complicating this model, however, is the observation that the same gene might act as a "landscaper" for one tumor system and as a "gatekeeper" for another, violating the principle of Occam's razor.[7] Thus, in practice, this etiologic nosology of genetic mechanisms is of less clinical relevance than the shared phenotypes of these cancer susceptibility syndromes. For this reason, Table 13-2 and the discussion that follows are grouped by the major component tumors by the organ system that is primarily affected. The syndromes included in this chapter are those most commonly encountered in oncologic practice, along with several recently defined entities that have been associated with mutations of novel cancer susceptibility genes. The most common of these syndromes, which result in predisposition to cancers of the breast, ovary, colon, and prostate, affect tens of thousands of Americans diagnosed with cancers of these sites each year in the United States and also result in increased risk for a second neoplasm for the millions of cancer survivors. Recently, a number of rarer syndromes have been characterized at the molecular level and could also be encountered in the practice of cancer medicine.

THE MAJOR SYNDROMES OF CANCER PREDISPOSITION

Breast and Ovarian Cancer Syndromes

Clinical Features

Although only about 18,000 cases of breast cancer each year are associated with an obvious hereditary predisposition, more than 200,000 breast cancer survivors in the United States developed their primary cancers as a result of a hereditary predisposition, and these individuals remain at risk for secondary cancers. When detected at an early stage, more than 90% of breast cancers are curable. These statistics underscore the rationale for the clinical interest in the use of genetics in clinical oncology.

From one in 150 to one in 800 individuals in the population carry a genetic susceptibility to breast cancer, and in certain ethnic groups the prevalence is much higher.[8-10] Syndromes of breast cancer susceptibility have been linked to mutations of *BRCA1* and *BRCA2*, and a smaller number of cases has been linked with germline mutations of *p53*, *PTEN*, *CHK2*, and rarer syndromes. In Cowden syndrome (described in detail in the discussion that follows), there is dominant inheritance of multiple hamartomatous lesions, including papillomas of the lips and mucous membranes, acral keratoses of the skin, and germline mutations of *PTEN*.[11] In Li-Fraumeni syndrome, early-onset breast cancer occurs along with soft-tissue sarcomas, osteosarcoma, leukemia, brain tumors, adrenocortical tumors, and other cancers. Rarely, a typical breast-ovarian kindred might be found to have a germline *p53* mutation.[12] In Northern European families, mutations of *CHK2* could be associated with familial breast cancer

mutations[13]; however, we did not find this allele to be of clinical relevance in a North American cohort.[14]

Both benign and malignant breast tumors occur in Muir-Torre syndrome, a variant of hereditary nonpolyposis colon cancer (HNPCC) that is associated with germline mutations of *MSH2* and *MLH1*. Women with Peutz-Jeghers syndrome carry germline mutations in the *STK11* gene and are at increased risk for breast cancer. Although they are the subject of much controversy, recent studies of selected kindreds have demonstrated that carriers of some *ATM* mutations have an elevated risk of breast cancer.[15]

All told, linkage studies suggest that about 50% of breast cancer kindreds are linked to *BRCA1*, 30% to *BRCA2*, and the remainder to *BRCA3* and other as yet unidentified genes.[16] Up to two thirds of families with both male and female breast cancer were due to *BRCA2* mutations, while more than 80% of families with both breast and ovarian cancer were due to inherited *BRCA1* mutations.[17]

Compared with the 10% risk for breast cancer among women in the general population, estimates of the breast cancer risk conferred by a common susceptibility gene ranged from 67% to 69% by age 70 based on epidemiologic analyses.[18,19] Genetic linkage studies of families selected because of the occurrence of early-onset breast or ovarian cancer gave risk estimates as high as 70%–90% in families segregating mutations of either of these two genes.[16,20-22] Ovarian cancer risks in these families varied from 10% to 80%, and risk for a second breast cancer ran as high as 64% by age 70. More recent estimates based on population studies of isolated populations led to slightly lower risk estimates, with lifetime risk of breast cancer estimated at 56% by age 70 (confidence interval 40%–73%), with ovarian cancer risk estimated as 16%.[23] Penetrance estimates derived from a clinic-based ascertainment of families revealed a 64% risk for breast or ovarian cancer by age 70.[24] The role of ascertainment bias in deriving these and similar estimates has been reviewed.[25]

Prior studies had also noted a fourfold increased relative risk of colorectal cancer in *BRCA* carriers, and a similar risk of developing prostate cancer in males. An increased risk of pancreatic cancer also emerged from studies of specific *BRCA* mutations in Ashkenazi Jewish individuals.[23,26,27] The risk for breast cancers in males is clearly elevated in *BRCA2* carriers, and there is the suggestion that the risk of ovarian cancer could be somewhat lower in this group and that the risk of breast cancer at a younger age might also be lower in some *BRCA2* heterozygotes.[28] We have shown recently that, in addition to Fanconi anemia, individuals who are compound heterozygotes for two *BRCA2* mutations develop medulloblastomas in early childhood.[29]

Genetics

BRCA1 is a large gene, spanning more than 100,000 bases of genomic DNA with 22 coding and two noncoding exons. *BRCA2* is also a large gene, consisting of 27 exons distributed over 70 kb of genomic DNA. Both genes, by coincidence, share a large exon 11. An update of mutations reported in these genes can be accessed through the Internet at http://www.nhgri.nih.gov/Intramural_research/Lab_transfer/Bic

Of the *BRCA1* mutations identified, the large majority cause premature truncation of the peptide by frameshift or nonsense sequence changes; however, 5%–10% of *BRCA* mutations are missense mutations, many of which are problematic for the clinician because they are of unknown clinical significance. The proportion of these variants of unknown significance was as high as 10%–23% in some series, and this poses counseling challenges.[30,31] The role of *BRCA1* and *BRCA2* in DNA damage response and homologous recombination is reviewed elsewhere in this text (see Chapter 11) and in recent reviews.[32]

"Founder" *BRCA* mutations have been documented in geographically isolated populations. In North American families, the most common founder mutations occur in individuals of Ashkenazi Jewish origin. These include a two-base pair deletion in codon 23 (termed *185delAG*), another *BRCA1* mutation 5382insC, and the 6174delT mutation of *BRCA2*.[26,28,33-35] About 1 in 40 Ashkenazi Jews harbors one of the common mutations of *BRCA1* or *BRCA2*, a relatively high carrier frequency for an inherited cancer predisposition syndrome.[23,26,35] Other mutations in *BRCA1* and *BRCA2* occur in the Ashkenazim; 16 out of 737 (2%) Ashkenazi Jews tested as part of a clinic-based ascertainment had a nonfounder mutation.[36] In another study of Ashkenazi individuals with a personal history of breast or ovarian cancer who had previously been shown not to have a founder mutation, 3 of 70 participants (4.3%) had a deleterious nonfounder mutation.[37] Founder mutations in populations other than the Ashkenazim have also been observed.[38-40]

BRCA1-linked cases have been associated with medullary subtype and higher mitotic indices.[41] *BRCA1*-linked tumors are of higher grade and are more frequently negative for estrogen and progesterone receptors.[42,43] They display features suggestive of a more "aggressive" phenotype, including a higher proportion of cells in S phase and other indices of higher histologic grade.[41,43-46]

Clinical Management

Three elements of breast surveillance recommended to *BRCA* heterozygotes include-self-examination, clinician examination, and mammography. These recommendations are of presumed but still unproven efficacy.[47] It has been estimated that for a woman in the general population who begins screening at age 35 and continues to age 75, the benefit is at least 25 times greater than the potential radiation risk.[48] Sensitivity to diagnostic radiation remains a possibility for heterozygotes for *BRCA* mutations. Investigational approaches to breast cancer screening of *BRCA* mutation carriers includes magnetic resonance imaging (MRI).[49-51] Based on our observation of "kinetic failures" (i.e., interval cancers) in *BRCA* mutation carriers, we recommend twice annual breast screening in *BRCA* carriers.[52]

For women at the highest hereditary risk for breast cancer, or for those whose breasts are difficult to examine or who have had biopsies showing atypia, it is appropriate to discuss the option of removing the healthy breasts as a preventative measure (prophylactic mastectomy). Retrospective studies support the risk-reducing role for surgery in "high-risk" patients.[53] A recent prospective study has also shown the efficacy of this approach.[54]

Because of their antiestrogen properties, tamoxifen, raloxifene, and a newer class of "synthetic" estrogen receptor modulators have emerged as candidate hormonal chemopreventive agents in *BRCA*-linked families. The safety of these drugs for premenopausal women remains to be established. In April of 1998, the NSABP Breast Cancer Prevention Trial was halted because of a reported 45% decrease in breast cancer across all age groups taking tamoxifen in a trial of women at increased risk for breast cancer. Two smaller European trials failed to confirm these results, however, and one of these studies was restricted to women with family histories of breast cancer.[55,56] Similarly, in carriers of *BRCA1* and *BRCA2* mutations, the two studies that have examined the impact of tamoxifen on subsequent breast cancer risk have shown conflicting conclusions, although only one of these studies was sufficiently powered to reach significant results.[57,58] Interestingly, smoking (possibly because of its antiestrogenic effects) has also been shown to decrease breast cancer risk in carriers of *BRCA* mutations.[59]

The indications for and limitations of ovarian screening remain controversial.[60,61] The standard recommendations for individuals at increased risk for ovarian cancer have included pelvic examination, ultrasound imaging, and serum tumor markers. Small trials have demonstrated the ability of ultrasound with Doppler and CA-125 to find early stage ovarian cancers.[52,62] The American College of Physicians has recommended a combination of ultrasound and CA-125 screening, preferably in a research setting, for women with a family history of ovarian cancer.[63] A common recommendation is to screen twice yearly using these modalities, starting at an early age.[64]

Prophylactic removal of the ovaries is generally presented as an option to women with two first-degree relatives with ovarian cancer or in families linked to *BRCA1* or *BRCA2*, or to women considering hysterectomy in the setting of a germline mutation associated with HNPCC. Recent studies have confirmed that such surgeries might not only decrease incidence of subsequent breast and ovarian cancer but also might find occult early-stage ovarian neoplasms.[65,66] These studies also have confirmed that serous surface carcinoma, also called papillary serous carcinoma, still can occur following "prophylactic" oophorectomy, leading some authors to use the term *risk-reducing salpingo-oophorectomy*.[67,68]

Combination oral contraceptives (COC) containing estrogen and high-dose progestin result in a time-dependent, protective effect against ovarian cancer in some, but not all studies of *BRCA* mutation carriers.[69-71] There remains concern about a small increased risk of breast cancer due to oral contraceptives in this group, particularly those with *BRCA1* mutations.[72]

Common Colon Cancer Predisposition Syndromes

Highly penetrant dominant susceptibility syndromes account for about 5% of colon cancers. The most common of these syndromes is hereditary nonpolyposis colon cancer (HNPCC), with familial adenomatous polyposis (FAP) as a rarer familial syndrome. For adults, genetic epidemiologic analyses have suggested the presence of a common susceptibility allele for both colon cancer and adenomatous polyps that account for at least 15% and possibly half of all colon cancer cases.[73,74]

Familial Adenomatous Polyposis

Clinical Features. Familial adenomatous polyposis (FAP) is also referred to as adenomatous polyposis coli (*APC*). Children present with hundreds to thousands of adenomatous polyps at a young age. Virtually all affected individuals exhibit polyposis by age 35 years, and all will go on to develop colon cancer. Colon cancer is thus inevitable if the colon is not removed and occurs at an average age of 39 years. Flexible sigmoidoscopy at early age establishes the diagnosis, and prophylactic colectomy is performed during the teen years. Patients remain at risk for primary adenomas and carcinomas of the duodenum and rectum and for desmoid tumors, osteomas, thyroid carcinoma, hepatoblastoma, and other hepatopancreatic tumors.[75]

Genetics. FAP arises from germline mutations in the *APC* gene.[76] Genotype-phenotype correlations have been described for this syndrome, particularly for congenital hypertrophy of the retinal epithelium and the number of polyps observed.[77] An attenuated form of FAP is associated with mutations at the extreme 5′ and 3′ ends of the gene.[78] Recently, it was reported that up to 30% of patients with multiple adenomas (15–100 adenomas) who have tested negative for *APC* mutations might carry a biallelic mutation in *MYH*.[79]

Clinical Management. FAP is the paradigm for preventive removal of the end-organ prior to tumor development in a cancer syndrome. In classic FAP, *APC* gene testing should be performed by ages 10 to 12 years, about the time that sigmoidoscopy would begin. Unaffected individuals who have wild-type *APC* but who have an affected family member with a known mutation are not subjected to intensive surveillance but instead follow the screening recommendations for the general population.[80] In the case of attenuated FAP, in which adenomas might not occur until the third or fourth decade, the age at which genetic testing and clinical surveillance should begin is not as clearly defined. Once an *APC* gene mutation has been identified and adenomas are found, prophylactic colectomy is performed, usually during the teen years.[81] Sulindac, a nonsteroidal anti-inflammatory drug, has been used to reduce adenoma development in individuals with FAP, and similar effects have been noted with celecoxib, a COX-2 inhibitor; however, the possibility of delaying colectomy while patients are treated pharmacologically has not yet been established.[82,83] Patients require lifelong surveillance for extracolonic tumors, including those of the upper GI tract as well as of the ileal pouch (if proctocolectomy has been performed).[84]

Hereditary Nonpolyposis Colon Cancer

Clinical Features. A constellation of colon and endometrial cancers has become known as "Lynch syndrome" or "hereditary nonpolyposis colon cancer" (HNPCC)[85] Five additional tumor sites have demonstrated increased observed/expected (O/E) ratios in HNPCC kindreds: cancers of the stomach (O/E = 4.1), ovary (O/E = 3.5), small intestine (O/E = 25), ureter (O/E = 22), and kidney (O/E = 3.2).[86] There is a 70% to 75% risk of colon cancer by age 65 in HNPCC families.[87,88] The penetrance was shown to be 92% by age 60 in one series, while a median age at diagnosis for colon cancer was only 44 to 46 years.[89] A 20% to 30% risk of endometrial cancer by age 70 was reported, with a median age of onset from the late forties to the early fifties.[90] In a study of 50 molecularly confirmed HNPCC families and 360 mutation carriers, the cumulative incidence of endometrial cancer (60%) exceeded that of colorectal cancer (54%) in the female mutation carriers.[91] This risk should be compared to the risk for endometrial cancer of 3% in the general population.

At a 1991 meeting in Amsterdam, the International Collaborative Group on HNPCC defined the syndrome as:

1. Histologically verified colorectal cancer in three or more relatives, one of whom is a first-degree relative of the other two
2. Colorectal cancer involving at least two generations
3. One or more colorectal cancer cases diagnosed before 50 years of age

In a subsequent meeting, the "Amsterdam II criteria" for HNPCC were defined to include extracolonic cancers associated with HNPCC.[92] In 1996, a set of guidelines known as the Bethesda criteria were defined to delineate individuals who might be at risk for HNPCC and for whom molecular genetic analysis could be appropriate.[93]

Although there do not appear to be defining histologic features of HNPCC tumors, mucinous types appear to be more common. Adenomas, like the cancers in HNPCC, appear more commonly on the right side. The adenomas appear as multiple lesions in about 20% of at-risk individuals. Fewer than 100 polyps are generally present in these patients.[94] Tumors of HNPCC patients show a diploid genotype, consistent with the improved survival of patients that is also noted.[94,95]

A variant of HNPCC with multiple (50–100) small adenomas was described in six members of an HNPCC kindred.[96] This syndrome, termed *flat adenoma syndrome* in an earlier report, is now felt to be an attenuated form of familial adenomatous polyposis.[97]

Genetics. Initial studies revealed that two genes on chromosomes 2p and 3p account for the majority of HNPCC kindreds.[98] About 45% to 70% of HNPCC families were associated with mutations in one of the three known genes: *MSH2*, *MLH1*, and *MSH6*.[99-102] Mutations in two other genes, *PMS1* and *PMS2*, have also been speculated to cause the HNPCCC syndrome; however, this association has not been fully confirmed.[103] Of these, mutations of *MSH2* and *MLH1* were far more frequent than the others, accounting for about 30% each of families meeting Amsterdam criteria for HNPCC. More than 75% of reported mutations of *MSH2* and *MLH1* have been inactivating insertions, deletions, alterations in premessenger RNA splicing signals, and nonsense mutations; however, 23% of 120 mutations surveyed were missense mutations.[104] The most common *MSH2* mutation observed was an in-frame deletion of most of exon 5 from nucleotides 793 to 942. The remainder of *MSH2* mutations have been scattered across the gene.[104]

Mutations of *MSH6* less frequently result in the replication error repair (RER) phenotype of the other HNPCC genes and could account for a small number of familial colon cancer families.[105] The RER phenotype is most commonly detected as microsatellite instability utilizing PCR screening of tumors with microsatellite markers. The RER phenotype is present in about 80% of HNPCC-associated colon cancers and in about 15% of sporadic colon tumors, as well as in other tumors associated with HNPCC (e.g. uterine, gastric cancers).[106,107]

In young patients (less than 35 years of age), the detection of the RER phenotype is quite common (seen in 58%) and could be associated with detectable HNPCC gene mutations in only half of the cases with the RER phenotype.[108] Testing for RER is recommended for all patients with colorectal cancer diagnosed before age 50 years, a family history of colon or endometrial cancer, or a personal history of metachronous colon or endometrial cancers.[98,109] A multivariate analysis of 184 families revealed that three factors predicted the probability of finding an *MSH2* or *MLH1* mutation: young age at diagnosis, presence of the Amsterdam criteria, and presence of endometrial cancer.[102]

A case report has documented a germline *MLH1* mutation and somatic loss of wild-type *MLH1* expression in the breast tumor of a woman in an HNPCC kindred with both colon and breast cancer, and an *MLH* compound heterozygote had breast cancer.[110,111] Breast cancers are not statistically over-represented in HNPCC kindreds, however.[86,111]

Lack of expression of either *MLH1* or *MSH2* in tumors is correlated with MSI in the tumor, allowing use of immunohistochemistry along with MSI analysis.[112] Lack of expression of the MLH1 protein can direct germline testing to begin with the *MLH1* gene. Similarly, if there is no expression of *MSH2*, the germline testing strategy should begin with the *MSH2* gene. Immunohistochemical analysis can also now be used to evaluate for *MSH6* and *PMS2* protein expression. In older patients affected with colorectal cancer, hypermethylation of the promoter of *MLH1* could account for lack of protein expression of *MLH1*.[113] Indeed, this epigenetic (nonhereditary) mechanism of *MLH1* promoter hypermethylation appears to be responsible for the majority of the remaining patients whose tumors are characterized by defective DNA mismatch repair.[114]

Clinical Management. The commonly recommended option for HNPCC family members has been screening colonoscopy at a frequent interval, ranging from 1 to 2 years, with annual screening being the most conservative recommendation, and the one we recommend. A 7.4% difference in colorectal cancer incidence was observed in 133 members of HNPCC kindreds undergoing 3-year colonoscopy or barium enema, compared with 118

HNPCC controls without screening.[115,116] Polypectomies are more likely to yield tumors in patients with HNPCC.[117] Despite the presumptive beneficial effect of polypectomy in the HNPCC group, four cancers emerged between the screening intervals, suggesting that more frequent surveillance is most prudent.[117] Indeed, polyp recurrences have anecdotally been noted within a year of colonoscopy, confirming the rationale for frequent surveillance.[118]

A suggested age to begin colonoscopy screening in the unaffected mutation-carrier is 20 to 25, based on data regarding the frequency of the mutation in early-onset cases. Because of the very high rate of synchronous and metachronous colon cancers in HNPCC kindreds, subtotal colectomy has been recommended at the first diagnosis of colon cancer in a member of an HNPCC family.[119] Prophylactic colectomy in HNPCC gene carriers remains a controversial recommendation.[120]

Women in HNPCC kindreds should be screened via pelvic exams as well as via transvaginal ultrasound. The ovaries and kidneys, also organs at risk, can be visualized during the ultrasound examination. Currently recommended measures include annual transvaginal ultrasound (to measure endometrial thickness) and/or endometrial aspirate.[121] If these measures are used, most experts recommend that they begin by age 25 to 35 years; however, the sensitivity and specificity of these measures have not been demonstrated, and their benefits remain unproven. In addition, urinalysis may be performed due to the increased risk of urinary tract cancers in HNPCC. Upper endoscopy is also appropriate in HNPCC families with a known history of gastric cancer. For women with mutations of one of the HNPCC-associated genes, prophylactic hysterectomy and bilateral salpingo-oophorectomy remains a viable option to consider after childbearing, or around age 35 to 40.[122] Recommendations for members of families with Muir-Torre syndrome are generally similar to those for HNPCC.

Due to the very subtle, flat nature of some adenomas that characterize HNPCC, a barium enema and roentgenologic examination is generally not considered a suitable alternative to colonoscopy. Flexible sigmoidoscopy is not recommended due to the high risk of right-sided tumors. For endometrial cancer, surveillance is less well established, largely because of the technical limitations of the available surveillance modalities.

Prostate Cancer

Clinical Features

Of the approximately one quarter of a million men diagnosed with prostate cancer in 2004, about 5% to 10% will be associated with a strong family history of the disease. One estimated frequency of a prostate cancer susceptibility allele was .003 to .006, meaning that about one in 170 to one in 85 individuals has an inherited a genetic mutation, which, in males, confers a susceptibility to prostate cancer. The penetrance for this dominant syndrome of prostate cancer susceptibility was quite high, estimated to be 88% by age 85. The syndrome was estimated to account for 43% of prostate cancers diagnosed before age 56 and 9% by age 85.[123,124] Although it was estimated that only 2% of prostate cancer in the general population was diagnosed before age 56, this proportion has been increasing with the introduction of newer screening modalities. The clinical features, stage, histology, and PSA at diagnosis are comparable in hereditary and nonhereditary cases.[125]

Genetics

A linkage analysis of 91 kindreds containing 600 individuals affected by prostate cancer revealed linkage to a locus on chromosome 1q24-25. Individuals linked to this gene, called *HPC1*, demonstrated an 88% lifetime probability of developing prostate cancer, with an average age at diagnosis of 66 years.[126] Subsequent studies by other groups have failed to reproduce these results, however, which suggests genetic heterogeneity and broadens the search for other prostate cancer susceptibility alleles.[127-129] A case-control study demonstrated an increased risk of prostate cancer among individuals carrying polymorphisms in the genes encoding the androgen receptor (AR) and vitamin D receptors (VDR).[130] An earlier study associated a Taq I polymorphism in the *VDR* gene with a threefold increase in prostate cancer risk.[131] A slightly increased risk of prostate cancer was associated with germline mutations of *BRCA*, and this observation has generally been confirmed.[132]

More recent segregation analyses of families with prostate cancer have revealed that familial aggregation of prostate cancer can best be explained by the autosomal dominant inheritance of a rare susceptibility gene, with a the risk of prostate cancer between 89% and 97% by the age of 85.[124] Other studies also have indicated that a subset of hereditary prostate cancers could be X-linked or recessive.[133]

Because the prevalence of prostate cancer is extremely high, it is difficult to recognize phenocopies in segregation studies. The late age of onset of prostate cancer results in a lack of available samples from multiple generations in a family. There is also a paucity of defining clinical features associated with hereditary prostate cancer.[134,135]

As shown in Table 13-4, several loci for prostate cancer susceptibility genes have been identified. The first of these, *HPC1*, was identified by Smith and colleagues[135] after a genome-wide scan of 66 high-risk prostate cancer families. Linkage to 1q24-25 was noted.[136] Germline mutations in the *RNASEL* gene on chromosome 1q25 were identified in high-risk prostate cancer families. In 2001, Tavtigian and coworkers[137] performed a study of high-risk prostate cancer families from the Utah Population Database that provided evidence for linkage to a locus on chromosome 17p, called *HPC2*. Mutations of *ELAC2* segregated with prostate cancer in two of the pedigrees. Other studies were unable to confirm linkage to *HPC2* or an association between prostate cancer risk and mutations in the *ELAC2* gene, and these studies suggest genetic heterogeneity. Other loci on chromosomes 1 and 20, as well as an X-liked locus, have been identified and have been reviewed elsewhere.[134]

Clinical Management

The normal concentration of prostate specific antigen (PSA) in the serum is 0 to 4 ng/mL. Values greater than 10 ng/mL are more likely to be associated with cancer. Transrectal ultrasound is commonly performed in the setting of an increased PSA, with transrectal needle biopsy of any suspicious area guided by ultrasound or digital rectal examination (DRE). Current recommendations by the American Cancer Society and a number of professional societies include DRE and PSA screening offered to men between the ages of 50 and 70.[138] Initial evidence for the efficacy of this approach in decreasing mortality was demonstrated in a trial of 45,000 men.[139]

A study of individuals at increased risk for prostate cancer by virtue of a family history demonstrated the value of "intensive" screening (PSA, DRE, transrectal ultrasound, and systematic and directed core biopsies).[140] Future options for those at hereditary risk for prostate cancer include hormonal chemoprevention.[141] A large-scale trial of finasteride, however, showed a modest delay in the appearance of prostate cancer but also sexual side effects and an increased risk of high-grade prostatic neoplasms.[142]

Multiple Endocrine Neoplasias

Multiple Endocrine Neoplasia Type 1

Clinical Features. The most common features of multiple endocrine neoplasias (MEN) type 1 (MEN1) cancers are parathyroid adenomas (seen in about 90% of cases) and pancreatic islet cell tumors (seen in about 50%–75% of cases). The latter might present as a gastrinoma, VIPoma, glucagonoma, or insulinoma, with about one quarter of the pancreatic tumors found to be nonfunctional. Pituitary adenomas are seen in 25% to 65% of cases and can be non-functional or functional, most often as prolactinomas.[143,144] Malignant neuroendocrine tumors of thymic origin are also observed as part of the spectrum of MEN1 tumors.

Genetics. The *MEN1* gene contains 10 exons. Analysis of 15 kindreds revealed 12 different mutations.[145] With the recent availability of direct mutation detection, more widespread genetic screening for this condition is now possible.

TABLE 13-4

Putative Prostate Cancer Susceptibility Genes

LOCUS	LOCATION	POSSIBLE GENE
PC1	1q24-q25	RNASEL
PC2	17p11	ELAC2
PCAP	1q42-q43	
CAPB	1p36	
PCX	Xq27-q28	
PC20	20q13	

From Nwosu V, Carpten J, Trent JM, Sheridan R: Heterogeneity of genetic alterations in prostate cancer: Evidence of the complex nature of the disease. Hum Mol Genet 2001;10:2313–2318.

Clinical Management. In the setting of a family with documented MEN1, screening of offspring commonly begins at an early age (between ages 5 and 10) and is continued at regular intervals thereafter. Screening should include, at a minimum, serum ionized calcium and prolactin determinations. Many specialists recommend full screening, with measurement of pituitary (GH, ACTH, FSH, TSH, prolactin), parathyroid (PTH), and pancreatic hormones (insulin, somatostatin, glucagon, pancreatic polypeptide, VIP, neurotensin), as well as radiographic imaging to assess pituitary size.[146] Guidelines for the management of these patients have been published.[147]

Multiple Endocrine Neoplasia Type 2

Clinical Features. Multiple endocrine neoplasia type 2 (MEN2a) is characterized by multiple cases of endocrine tumors, particularly medullary thyroid carcinoma and pheochromocytoma. There is also hyperplasia of the parathyroid in one quarter of the cases. Hypertension is the common presenting symptom, with diagnosis classically made by measurement of urinary VMA and metanephrine. Routine screening for MEN2a has been directed to the thyroid medullary lesions, with a pentagastrin challenge given to measure calcitonin response.[148] Measurement of serum ionized calcium has also been included in the diagnostic evaluation.

MEN2b is a variant of MEN2a characterized by an earlier age of onset, enlarged and nodular lips, a Marfanoid habitus, ganglioneuromatosis of the intestine, and a variety of other abnormalities.[149] This phenotype is also accompanied by medullary carcinoma of the thyroid (which could be more clinically aggressive) and pheochromocytoma. Parathyroid disease is less common in MEN2b than in MEN2a.

Medullary carcinoma of the thyroid runs in families about 25% of the time, either as a syndrome of site-specific familial medullary carcinoma of the thyroid (FMCT) or as MEN2.[150] The cases usually present in the third and fourth decades and are usually bilateral and multifocal. Familial papillary thyroid cancer is distinct from FMCT and has also been associated with an increased incidence of colorectal cancer.[151]

Genetics. In 1993, it was observed that mutations in the *RET* gene were associated with MEN2a, MEN2b, and FMCT.[152,153] Specific mutations of the *RET* gene have been associated with MEN2a, MEN2b, and FMCT.[152,154-156] *RET* testing of sporadic cases of medullary carcinoma of the thyroid will yield a relatively low (5%) rate of diagnosis of MEN2a in the absence of a family history of the disease, C-cell hyperplasia, or multifocality.[157,158] Nonetheless, *RET* testing is more sensitive than traditional biochemical screening. It was observed that asymptomatic children with *RET* mutations and normal plasma calcitonin levels already had small foci of medullary carcinoma of the thyroid at the time of "prophylactic" surgery.[159] These findings were confirmed in a large study in the United States.[160]

A study of 477 MEN2a families showed an association between codon 634 mutations and pheochromocytoma,

mutations at codons 768 and 804, and FMTC, whereas codon 918 mutation is MEN2b-specific. Rare families with both MEN 2 and Hirschsprung's disease were found to have MEN2-specific codon mutations.[161] A 611 codon mutation appears to be associated with a rather mild and slow-progression form of MTC. The classic M918T mutation in exon 16 is found in MEN2b, and a less common mutation in *RET* codon 883 has also been reported.[162,163]

Clinical Management. These results have established *RET* testing as the gold standard for MEN2a screening and prophylactic thyroidectomy as the primary preventative intervention. The age at which surgery is best performed is now thought to be 3 to 5 years in most centers. Genetic testing should thus be performed by this age and perhaps even earlier in families with MEN2b, as the thyroid cancers can occur at an earlier age.[164] Heterozygotes for *RET* mutations in the setting of MEN2a are generally screened with abdominal ultrasound and CT, as well as via 24-hour urine studies through the adult years, at least to age 35. Recently, plasma screening for the pheochromocytomas has been suggested (see the section of this chapter on von Hippel-Lindau syndrome). The treatment of choice for patients with MEN2a or MEN2b and a unilateral pheochromocytoma is unilateral resection, as substantial morbidity and significant mortality are associated with the Addisonian state after bilateral adrenalectomy.[165]

Melanoma Syndromes

Clinical Features

Approximately 10% to 15% of the 30,000 new cases of cutaneous malignant melanoma each year have a family history of the disease. Familial melanoma syndromes have been referred to variously as familial atypical mole malignant melanoma syndrome (FAMMM), B-K mole syndrome, or hereditary dysplastic nevus syndrome (DNS).[166-169] In many of these families, there is an association between melanoma and a precursor lesion (dysplastic nevus).[170]

Genetics

Melanoma kindreds, some with dysplastic nevi, demonstrated genetic linkage to chromosomes 1p and 9p12-22, suggesting genetic heterogeneity.[171-173] A 65% penetrance by age 80 was predicted for gene carriers.[174] Candidate gene investigations identified *CDKN2* as a likely candidate for the melanoma predisposing gene (also called *MLM*), with subsequent studies documenting germline mutations of the gene *CDKN2* encoding *p16* in most, but not all, 9p21-linked families.[175] *CDKN2* normally generates a protein product, $p16^{INK4}$, which is an inhibitor of the cyclin D1-dependent kinase 4 complex.

Germline mutations of *CDK4* have also been observed in melanoma-prone kindreds and also in association with breast cancers.[176] Thus, at least three genes—*CDKN2(p16)*, *CDK4*, a 1p-linked gene—and probably others contribute to the genetic heterogeneity of hereditary melanoma syndromes. A syndrome of melanoma and pancreatic cancer has been associated with germline mutations of *CDKN2*, and in addition to pancreatic cancer, breast cancers have also been seen in these kindreds.[177-179]

The lifetime risk of melanoma in *CDKN2A* carriers is estimated to be approximately 70%; however, the risk varies with population incidence. In Australia, the penetrance can be as high as 90%, and in Europe as low as 13%.[180] Within families in which a mutation has been identified, dysplastic nevi have been observed in relatives who have a wild-type familial mutation, complicating the clinical interpretation of testing in this setting.

Clinical Management

In the setting of a germline mutation of one of these genes, careful surveillance offers the promise of cure of early-stage lesions. Surveillance for those at familial risk for melanoma is generally accomplished by twice-yearly total-body skin examination and serial photography. Because the minority of melanoma-prone families carries mutations in the *CDKN2A* gene, however, a negative result for a mutation in this gene in an individual without a known familial *CDKN2A* mutation does not imply lack of genetic susceptibility. Furthermore, as many as one third of the families strongly linked to 9p have been found not to carry mutations in *CDKN2A*. This could be due to mutations in noncoding regions, epigenetic mechanisms of gene inactivation (e.g., methylation), or another undiscovered gene at or near this locus. Some individuals who carry the familial mutation in *CDKN2A* might never develop melanoma. Most significantly, families have been studied in which two siblings—one mutation positive and the other mutation negative—both developed dysplastic nevi and melanoma. Because of the genetic heterogeneity of the familial melanoma syndromes and environmental interactions, genetic testing is of limited predictive value and for this reason is less frequently offered on a clinical basis.[181,182]

Retinoblastoma

Clinical Features

Although it is the most common primary malignant tumor of the eye in children, retinoblastoma accounts for only 1% of pediatric malignancies. There are about 200 cases diagnosed each year, and, of these, fewer than 100 will be linked to hereditary factors.

The tumor is generally diagnosed before the age of 4 years, with the median age of $1^{1}/_{2}$ years at diagnosis. Unilateral tumors present around 2 years of age, while bilateral tumors present at a median age of 8 months. In hereditary cases in which there is a known risk of bilateral disease, it is usually possible to preserve both eyes. The critical importance of early diagnosis is a strong justification to offer genetic counseling to all affected patients.[183] Rarely, children might present with "trilateral retinoblastoma," the occurrence of bilateral retinoblastoma with pineoblastoma, occurring either at time of diagnosis of retinoblastoma or months to years after retinoblastoma diagnosis.[184]

Genetics

In 1971, based on the observation of an earlier age of onset in heritable retinoblastomas, Knudson[185] derived the "two-hit" model of tumorigenesis (see Chapter 15). The *RB1* gene, identified in 1986, spans 27 exons and 180 kb of genomic DNA. This large size and the lack of "hotspots" in the more than 100 known mutations, complicate routine analysis.[186] A survey of germline mutations in 119 patients with bilateral or hereditary retinoblastoma revealed germline mutations in 99 (83%).[187] In some cases, "lower-penetrance" mutations resulting in skipped generations have been observed.[188,189] The spectrum of somatic and germline mutations in *RB* is dominated by small mutations, with more than 368 documented and available for review in a locus-specific database available at http://www.d-lohmann.de/*Rb*/mutations.html.[190] Particular splice-site mutations might result in low-penetrance retinoblastoma. Missense mutations also might be associated with low penetrance and are clustered around exon 20.[191]

Clinical Management

The use of genetic diagnosis can serve as a critical resource in the counseling of these families, as has now been documented in clinical series.[192] In addition, genetic testing has now been used for preimplantation diagnosis.[193] In the event that a child of an affected parent does not inherit a mutation, an enormous savings of both cost and risk will result from cancellation of the routine examinations under general anesthesia that these children require.[194] In the setting of a positive test, early diagnosis can lead to treatments that preserve the eyes. Second primary tumors are observed in patients with germline RB mutations, with a risk approaching 26%. Second cancers may occur from one to 40 years after treatment.[195,196] The tumors include osteosarcoma and other types of sarcoma, malignant melanoma, brain tumors, and possibly other common tumors such as breast cancer or leukemia. In a follow-up of 1458 patients, the cumulative mortality from second neoplasms at 40 years after follow-up was greater than 30% in the radiotherapy group, compared with 6% in the group that did not receive radiotherapy.[197] In addition to soft-tissue sarcomas and osteosarcomas, adult-onset lipomas have also been observed at increased frequency in survivors of hereditary retinoblastoma. The detection of lipomas in these patients might predict the occurrence of other secondary tumors.[198]

Neurofibromatosis

NF1

Clinical Features. Although it is one of the most common of the single-gene disorders, with an incidence of approximately 1 in 3000, patients with neurofibromatosis 1 (NF1) have a small excess risk for malignancy. Results of proportionate mortality ratio (PMR) analyses showed that persons with NF1 were 34 times more likely (PMR = 34.3, 95% confidence interval [CI] 30.8–38.0) to have a malignant connective or other soft-tissue neoplasm listed on their death certificates than were persons without NF1.[199] Despite this, the syndrome is not frequently encountered by cancer geneticists. Diagnostic criteria for NF1 include two or more of the following features:

- Six or more cafe au lait macules greater than 15 mm in size in adults and greater than 5 mm in children
- Two or more neurofibromas or one plexiform neurofibroma
- Axillary or inguinal freckling
- Optic glioma
- Two or more hamartomas of the iris (Lisch nodules)
- Characteristic osseous lesion (e.g. sphenoid dysplasia long bone cortical thinning)
- A first-degree relative with NF1

The overall risk for malignancy in patients with NF1 is higher than for the general population, and the distribution of tumors is unusual, including astrocytomas, malignant peripheral nerve sheath tumors (MPNST), rhabdomyosarcoma, leiomyosarcoma, pheochromocytoma, leukemia, optic glioma, and carcinoma of the ampulla of Vater.[200,201]

Genetics. The very large size of the *NF1* gene—57 exons spanning 350 kb of genomic DNA—has posed diagnostic difficulties. Approximately 100 germline mutations have been observed, with most predicted to result in premature translational truncation.[202] Mutation detection using standard techniques might miss large gene deletions, which have been documented as de novo events and can be detected using intragenic markers or molecular cytogenetic techniques.[203] More recent surveys have reported a higher sensitivity of mutation detection.[204]

Clinical Management. Patients with NF1 are perhaps best managed in specialty clinics, although specific medical interventions are not necessary for many patients. In the absence of options for prevention of the CNS tumors, there is also a limited role for preventive oncologic counseling of patients. Brain tumors in NF1 kindreds tend to have a more indolent course than in the general population and hence are best managed conservatively. MPNST, in contrast, do not respond to standard chemotherapy or radiation therapy; the most effective treatment appears to be early diagnosis and surgery.[205]

NF2

Clinical Features. NF2 is a very rare disorder, with an incidence of approximately 1 in 35,000. The diagnostic criteria for NF2 include bilateral vestibular schwannomas (also called acoustic neuromas), or a first-degree relative with NF2, or unilateral vestibular schwannoma and addition features, including meningioma, glioma, neurofibroma, schwannoma, posterior subcapsular lenticular opacities, or cerebral calcification.[206] More recent diagnostic criteria have been proposed.[207] The growth of the tumor causes progressive compression of cranial nerve VIII, producing progressive hearing loss and tinnitus. Some manifestation of the disease is usually evident by the age of 40. As with NF1, the new mutation rate for NF2 is estimated to be about 50%.

Genetics. The *NF2* gene has 16 exons, and its protein product showed significant homology to moesin, ezrin, and radixin-like proteins, hence the name "merlin."[208] Of 50 mutations of *NF2* initially described, most were large deletions or other mutations leading to a truncated protein.[209,210] The truncating mutations are correlated with a more severe phenotype.[211]

Clinical Management. Management of the NF2 patient is surgical and is best performed in large centers by experienced neurosurgeons and otolaryngologists.[212,213] Unfortunately, there is substantial surgery-related morbidity after resection of intracranial meningiomas and/or spinal tumors.[214] Genetic testing can now be considered at an early age, with the absence of a familial mutation in an offspring precluding the need for special radiographic or other surveillance.[215] The elucidation of the molecular mechanisms of this syndrome offers promise for improved medical management.[214]

von Hippel-Lindau Disease

About 2% of the 30,000 patients with renal cell cancers occurring each year will have a family history of the disease. The most common hereditary form of renal cell carcinoma in adults is von Hippel-Lindau (VHL) syndrome.

Clinical Features

VHL syndrome is a rare hereditary syndrome associated with both cancer predisposition and a tendency to form cysts.[216] The most common manifestations of the syndrome are cerebellar, spinal, and medullary hemangioblastomas, retinal angiomas, renal cell carcinomas, and pheochromocytomas. Of these, the retinal and cerebellar lesions are the most common and are seen in the majority of cases.[217] They commonly present at an early age (25–30 years) with symptoms of visual abnormalities or occipital or frontal headaches.[218-220]

Renal cell carcinomas are observed in about one quarter of VHL cases.[221] The renal tumors present at around age 45, compared with 62 years of age in the general population.[222,223] The majority of VHL patients will probably develop renal cell carcinoma if they survive the other manifestations of the syndrome. The renal tumors are frequently multifocal, bilateral, and recurrent.[224,225] The pheochromocytomas are less common and are observed in about 10% to 26% of cases but also can be multifocal.[221,226] The observation of familial pheochromocytoma should lead to the consideration of the diagnosis of VHL.[227] Pancreatic tumors are also observed but are much less common. About 90% of individuals in VHL kindreds are affected by age 45, and 99% affected by age 65.[228,229] More rarely observed in VHL syndrome are meningiomas and lung cancers, reviewed by Decker and associates.[230] Papillary adenocarcinomas of the endolymphatic sac are more common than originally thought in this syndrome and are observed in up to 11% of patients with VHL, accounting for hearing loss at a median age of 22 in these patients.[231]

Zbar and others[232-234] have grouped VHL into four subtypes based on the likelihood of pheochromocytoma or renal cell carcinoma. These subtypes are:

1. VHL type 1: All VHL syndrome-related tumors except pheochromocytoma
2. VHL type 2A, with a reduced risk of renal cell carcinoma or pancreatic cysts and pheochromocytoma
3. VHL syndrome type 2B, with renal cell carcinoma and pancreatic cysts (and pheochromocytoma)
4. VHL syndrome type 2C, with pheochromocytoma only

Because of heterogeneity, these classifications should not be used as a rationale to alter the recommended clinical screening protocol for individuals at risk for VHL.

Genetics

The *VHL* gene mapped to 3p25-6 was identified in 1993.[235] About 40% of mutations resulted in a truncated protein, while the remainder were missense mutations.[236] Pheochromocytoma appeared to be more common among patients with missense mutations, compared with those with deletions, insertions, or nonsense mutations.[227,237] The *VHL* gene product, pVHL, is a component of an E3 ubiquitin ligase that targets the alpha subunits of the HIF (hypoxia-inducible factor) transcription factor for destruction in the presence of oxygen. Consequently, tumor cells lacking pVHL overproduce the products of HIF target genes such as vascular endothelial growth factor and transforming growth factor alpha.[238] Approximately 96% to 97% of patients with truncating or null mutations in the *VHL* gene (i.e., deletions or frameshift, nonsense, or splice site mutations) have VHL syndrome type 1 (i.e., VHL syndrome without pheochromocytoma). On the other hand, 69% to 98% of the patients with VHL syndrome and pheochromocytoma (VHL syndrome type 2) have missense mutations.[232,234,239] Mutations associated with subtypes of VHL are *VHL2A: Y98H, Y112H, V116F, L188V; VHL2B: R167Q, R167W; VHL2C: V155L, R238W*. Mutations observed in *VHL* have been compared in North America, Europe, and Japan.[234]

Risk Management Recommendations

VHL is a hereditary syndrome for which genetic testing and screening as described next is considered part of the standard management for at-risk family members.[240] Ophthalmological screening should begin by age 5 years, as should annual blood pressure monitoring and measurement of urinary catecholamine metabolites. Annual abdominal and pelvic imaging (e.g., ultrasound and/or CT examination) should begin during the teen years. CT scan or MRI can also be used to screen for CNS tumors, pheochromocytomas, and endolymphatic sac tumors. Recently, the sensitivity of plasma normetanephrine and metanephrine (especially normetanephrine) has been shown to be high enough to warrant consideration for substitution for urinary measurements when screening patients with VHL for pheochromocytomas.[241] Finally, prenatal diagnosis is now possible if a *VHL* mutation is identified in either of the parents, and preimplantation genetic diagnosis (PGD) has recently been offered for couples with an inherited predisposition for late-onset disorders.[242]

RECENTLY CHARACTERIZED CANCER PREDISPOSITION SYNDROMES

Gorlin Syndrome/Nevoid Basal Cell Carcinoma Syndrome

Basal cell carcinomas are the most common malignancy in humans, with three quarters of a million cases occurring each year. In a small subset of families, basal cell carcinomas occur at early age and in great numbers. The nevoid basal cell carcinoma syndrome (NBCCS) consists of multiple basal cell carcinomas, usually presenting after puberty, accompanied by odontogenic jaw cysts, congenital skeletal abnormalities, ectopic calcification of the falx cerebri, and characteristic "pits" in the skin of the palms and soles.[243,244]

A hallmark of the syndrome is the increased susceptibility of the skin to the damaging and tumor-inducing effects of ionizing radiation.[245] Multiple basal cell carcinomas have developed within 6 to 36 months after radiation therapy. Unlike Bloom syndrome or ataxia telangiectasia, there is no in vitro evidence of chromosome fragility.

One estimate of the prevalence of the syndrome (1 in 57,000) comes from a study of a U.K. population of 4 million in northwest England.[246] As described by Gorlin[247] in 1987, penetrance for the syndrome is virtually 100% over the course of a lifetime. NBCCS is diagnosed in individuals with two major and one minor criterion or one major and three minor criteria.[248] Major criteria include the following:

- Lamellar calcification of the falx before 20 years of age;
- Jaw keratocyst
- Palmar/plantar pits (two or more)
- Multiple (>5) basal cell carcinomas or a basal cell carcinoma before the age of 30 years
- A first-degree relative with NBCCS

Minor criteria include the following:

- Childhood medulloblastoma (also called primitive neuro-ectodermal tumor [PNET])
- Lympho-mesenteric or pleural cysts
- Macrocephaly
- Cleft lip or palate
- Vertebral anomalies observed on chest x-ray and/or spinal x-ray: bifid/splayed/extra ribs, bifid vertebrae, or polydactyly that is either preaxial or postaxial
- Ovarian/cardiac fibroma
- Ocular anomalies (cataract, developmental defects, and pigmentary changes of the retinal epithelium)

One study showed that approximately 5% of patients with Gorlin syndrome will develop medulloblastoma in the first few years of life, and that 10% of patients with medulloblastoma diagnosed at 2 years of age or less have Gorlin syndrome.[249]

Genetics

In 1996, Johnson and coworkers[250] found mutations in exon 15 of the human homolog of the Drosophila *patched* gene (called *PTH* or *PTCH*) in two of 60 typical NBCC kindreds. An analysis of 71 unrelated individuals with NBCCS revealed 26 with mutations scattered throughout the 23 exons of the gene. In 86% of the individuals, the mutations caused a truncated protein.[251] NBCCS is caused by germline mutations of the gene *PTCH* mapped to chromosomal locus 9q22.3. The *PTCH* gene consists of 23 exons and encodes an integral membrane protein with 12 transmembrane regions and two extracellular loops and a putative sterol-sensing domain. Mutations of *PTCH* are the only known genetic alterations known to be associated with NBCCS.[252] For kindreds with diagnostic clinical findings of NBCCS who test negative for a mutation by sequence analysis, Southern blot analysis may be performed to detect large deletions. About 70% to 80% of probands have inherited the condition from a parent, and about 20% to 30% of probands have a de novo mutation.

Risk Management Recommendations

Life expectancy in NBCCS is not significantly different from average. The major clinical issues revolve around the cosmetic effect of treatment of multiple skin tumors and jaw keratocysts, which can recur. The jaw cysts also can undergo malignant transformation.[253] Interactions with oral and plastic surgeons and dermatologists are important. Because of early-onset risk of disease (e.g., for medulloblastomas), genetic testing of children is appropriate for this condition. Evaluation of members of NBCC kindreds generally includes, in addition to skin examination and measurement of head circumference, radiographic examination of the skull, spine, ribs, and jaws.[254] In addition, ophthalmologic and dental examination and radiographic monitoring of the jaw cysts (oropantomography) may be performed on affected individuals. MRI scans of at-risk children offers a means to diagnose medulloblastomas, although it is unclear whether this will improve outcome. If no physical or radiographic stigmata are noted by 5 years of age in the child of an affected patient, the chances that the child is a heterozygote are small.[248] As mentioned, radiotherapy for large basal cell cancers should be avoided, as this can lead to the development of thousands of BCCs in the radiation field.[246,255] Prenatal testing for NBCCS is possible if the disease-causing mutation has been identified in an affected family member.

Carney Complex

Clinical Features

Carney complex (CNC) is a multiple-neoplasia syndrome that has been referenced in the medical genetics literature by acronyms such as "NAME" syndrome and "LAMB" syndrome.[256,257] As described by Carney and associates[258] in 1985, the complex is characterized by myxomas, skin pigment abnormalities, endocrine tumors, and schwannomas. The median age at diagnosis for CNC has been reported as 20 years, with spotty skin pigmentation and heart myxomas being the most common initial clinical manifestations.[259] The skin abnormalities involve the lips,

conjunctiva, inner or outer canthi, and the mucosa of the vagina or penis. Atrial myxomas are by far of greatest clinical concern, as they usually result in a decreased life span and account for the major causes of mortality in affected individuals; cardiac myxoma can cause stroke and death.[260] Ductal adenoma of the breast, myxoid fibroadenomas, and other breast findings on breast imaging have been described in the literature as a part of the Carney complex.[261] Large-cell calcifying Sertoli cell tumor (LCCSCT), a frequent component of CNC in men, has been associated with infertility due to hormonal imbalance. It has been detected as early as at 2 years of age.[262]

Primary pigmented nodular adrenocortical disease (PPNAD) occurs most frequently in association with the Carney complex. A study by Stratakis and colleagues[263] in 1999 showed that for 95% of the patients, PPNAD occurred as a component of the Carney complex, and 14% of these patients had Cushing's syndrome. Thus, the diagnosis of PPNAD should prompt screening for the Carney complex. Other organs involved in CNC are the thyroid gland and ovaries. Lesions associated with thyroid gland involvement include follicular hyperplasia, follicular adenoma, and follicular and papillary carcinomas. Ultrasonography is useful tool in screening and diagnosis of these lesions.[264] Ovarian involvement in CNC with serous cystadenomas has been described in the literature, suggesting that pelvic ultrasound could be indicated as a part of initial evaluation in women with CNC-related possible risk for malignancy.[265]

Diagnostic criteria for the syndrome require two or more of the manifestations or one major manifestation and one of the minor criteria. Major criteria include:

- Skin pigmentary abnormalities (multiple lentigines of the face, blue nevus, or epithelioid blue nevus)
- Myxoma (cutaneous myxoma or mucosal myxomatosis)
- Cardiac myxoma
- Endocrine tumors or endocrine overactivity (primary pigmented nodular adrenocortical disease as a micronodular form of adrenal hyperplasia, growth hormone-producing pituitary adenoma, large-cell calcifying Sertoli cell tumor, or thyroid adenoma or carcinoma)
- Psammomatous melanotic schwannoma
- Thyroid carcinoma or multiple nodules on thyroid ultrasound in a young patient
- Multiple ductal adenomas of the breast
- Osteochondromyxoma[266]

To make the diagnosis, an individual must have two of the components listed, one of the manifestations in addition to an affected first-degree relative, or an inactivating mutation of the *PRKAR1A* gene. A malignant neoplasm is a relatively uncommon finding in affected patients.

Genetics

Mutations in *PRKAR1A* (17q23-q24) are identified in about 40% of individuals with CNC.[267] *PRKAR1A* codes for the RI-alpha subunit of *PKA*, a critical cellular component of a number of cyclic nucleotide-dependent signaling pathways and maps to chromosome 17q24.[268] *PRKAR1-α* frameshift mutations can cause haploinsufficiency of R1-α and manifest as Carney complex. As predicted by the Knudson "two-hit" hypothesis, loss of heterozygosity of the normal allele supports the model that RI-α might have tumor suppression function in the target tissues in this syndrome.

Clinical Management

Recommendations for patients with CNC include the following measures:

- Annual echocardiography
- Annual measurement of urinary-free cortisol
- Testicular sonogram for male patients at their initial visit
- Thyroid ultrasound at initial visit and as needed thereafter
- Pelvic ultrasound for female patients at their initial visit
- Breast imaging

Children should have echocardiography during the first 6 months of life and annually thereafter to detect the potentially lethal myxomas. Children with LCCSCT could require monitoring of growth rate and puberal status bone age determination, and further laboratory evaluation could be necessary if gynecomastia is present.[266]

Cowden Syndrome

Clinical Features

Cowden syndrome (CS) is an autosomal dominant disorder characterized by multiple hamartomas with a high risk of benign and malignant tumors of the thyroid, breast, and endometrium. Consensus criteria for Cowden syndrome establish three diagnostic categories: pathognomic criteria, major criteria, and minor criteria.[269]

- *Pathognomonic criteria* include mucocutaneous lesions, facial trichilemmomas, acral keratoses, papillomatous lesions, and mucosal lesions.
- *Major criteria* include breast cancer, thyroid cancer (especially follicular histology), macrocephaly, Lhermitte-Duclos disease (LDD) (defined as presence of a cerebellar dysplastic gangliocytoma), and endometrial carcinoma.[270]
- *Minor criteria* include other thyroid lesions (e.g., goiter), mental retardation, hamartomatous intestinal polyps, fibrocystic disease of the breast, lipomas, fibromas, genitourinary tumors (e.g., uterine fibroids, renal cell carcinoma), or genitourinary malformation.

The diagnosis of CS is made if an individual meets any one of the following criteria:

- Pathognomonic mucocutaneous lesions alone if there are six or more facial papules, of which three or more must be trichilemmoma, or cutaneous facial papules and oral mucosal papillomatosis
- Oral mucosal papillomatosis and acral keratoses
- Six or more palmo-plantar keratoses

Alternatively, the individual may fulfill two major criteria, one of which must be either macrocephaly or LDD. Alternatively, the individual may fulfill one major and three minor criteria or four minor criteria.

The palmar and plantar hyperkeratotic pits usually become evident later in childhood. Subcutaneous lipomas and cutaneous hemangiomas can also be seen in CS but with low frequency.[271] An increased risk of early-onset male breast cancer has been noted in mutation carriers.[272]

Genetics

The gene for CS has been mapped to 10q22-23 and was identified as *PTEN*.[273] *PTEN* acts as a tumour suppressor gene by mediating cell cycle arrest or apoptosis or both.[274] Full sequencing and molecular testing by Southern blot analysis are available clinically and on a research basis, respectively.

Heterozygous germline mutations in *PTEN* are responsible for most cases of Cowden syndrome. Nonsense and missense mutations that disrupt the protein tyrosine/dual-specificity phosphatase domain of this gene are also identified in certain families.[275] A *PTEN* gene mutation can be detected in about 80% of the patients with CS.[276]

Risk Management Recommendations

Individuals with known germline *PTEN* mutations should undergo appropriate cancer screening.[269,277] Female patients with CS should be screened for breast cancer, starting clinical breast exam at age 25 and annual mammography at age 30 or 5 years younger than the earliest age of breast cancer diagnosis in the family. Men should perform monthly breast self-examination. Female patients should receive endometrial cancer screening beginning approximately at age 35 years or 5 years before the youngest endometrial cancer diagnosis in the family, and they should undergo comprehensive annual physical examinations starting at age 18 years with screening for skin and thyroid lesions (including a baseline thyroid ultrasound). Individuals with CS should undergo a baseline colonoscopy at age 50 years and annual urinalysis to detect renal carcinoma. Finally, prenatal testing for CS can be performed if a mutation has been described in a parent.

Birt-Hogg-Dubé Syndrome

Clinical Features

Birt-Hoge-Dubé syndrome is a recently molecularly characterized cancer predisposition syndrome that was first described in 1977.[278] This rare genodermatosis is comprised of a triad of findings:

- Fibrofolliculomas, which appear as white or skin-colored papules on the face and upper torso
- Spontaneous pneumothorax
- Kidney tumors[279]

Approximately 15% to 30% of patients with cutaneous BHD syndrome develop renal tumors. A recent review of 130 solid renal tumors resected from 30 patients with BHD in 19 different families revealed that renal tumors were multiple and bilateral and were noted at an early age (mean age, 50.7 years). The vast majority were hybrid oncocytic neoplasms that had areas reminiscent of chromophobe renal cell carcinoma and oncocytoma, while a significant number were chromophobe renal cell carcinomas, and a minority were conventional clear cell renal carcinomas.[280,281] The cutaneous lesions usually appear in the region of the head, neck, and upper part of the trunk in the third or fourth decade of life, and about 15% to 30% of patients with the skin lesions of BHD syndrome develop renal tumors. A review of 130 solid renal tumors resected from 30 patients with BHD in 19 different families revealed that renal tumors were multiple and bilateral and were noted at an early age (mean 50.7 years). Khoo and colleagues[282] described an association with colorectal neoplasia in some families with BHD; however, other reports did not confirm this finding.[283] Individuals with BHD syndrome are at markedly increased risk of spontaneous pneumothoraces, and the syndrome has also been associated with a progressive flecked chorioretinopathy with constricted visual fields.[284]

Genetics

BHD is inherited in an autosomal dominant manner. The BHD gene has been mapped to chromosome 17p11.2 and has recently been identified as expressing a novel protein, folliculin.[285,286] The exact function of this protein is not known. Affected individuals exhibit loss of protein function, usually due to a frameshift mutation in the coding sequence.

Risk Management

Patients with BHD syndrome and their relatives should undergo abdominal computed tomography and renal ultrasound screening for renal tumors. The lung cysts are best seen on CT scans. Dermatologic consultation is advised. Ophthalmologic examination should be performed on patients with DHB syndrome due to the high incidence of chorioretinopathy.

Rhabdoid Predisposition Syndrome

Clinical Features

Rhabdoid predisposition syndrome (RPS) was initially described in 1999 by Sevenet and coworkers.[287] The syndrome results in pediatric cancer predisposition, including renal and extrarenal malignant rhabdoid tumors, choroid plexus carcinomas, central primitive neuro-ectodermal tumors, and medulloblastomas.[288,289] In the families that have been described with RPS, the penetrance appears to be quite high at a very young age. In the initial study, all of the first cancers occurred before the age of 3 years in mutation carriers, and no mutation carriers were unaffected.[287] Pediatric brain tumors are emerging as an important component of this syndrome.[290] The spectrum of cancers observed in RPS overlaps somewhat with Li-Fraumeni syndrome; pediatric medulloblastomas also can occur in Gorlin syndrome and in compound BRCA2 heterozygotes, as noted in previous sections of this chapter.

Genetics

Rhabdoid predisposition syndrome is caused by mutation of hSNF5/INI1 at 2q11.2. Most mutations in the hSNF5/INI1 gene are truncating mutations.[291] The hSNF5/INI1 gene encodes a subunit of the SWI/SNF family of chromatin-remodeling complexes. The spectrum of tumors encompassed by the somatic mutations of hSNF5/INI1 is similar to the spectrum of tumors seen in the hereditary syndrome.[292]

Risk Management Recommendation

Because this syndrome has been described only recently, clinical management is still evolving. As with Li-Fraumeni syndrome, the value of screening for component tumors is unproven. The average survival of infants after diagnosis of malignant rhabdoid tumors with abnormalities of chromosome 22q11 is less than 6 weeks.[293] Less than 25% of infants and young children with rhabdoid tumor of the kidney survive.[290,294,295]

Other Familial Neoplasms

Familial aggregations of individuals affected by Wilms' tumors, leukemias, lymphomas, gastric cancer, testicular cancer, lung cancer, and other malignancies have been described. A group of autosomal recessive disorders, including Bloom syndrome, Fanconi anemia, ataxia telangiectasia, and xeroderma pigmentosum, are associated with increased susceptibility to a variety of neoplasms. An additional number of hereditary syndromes are characterized by both nonmalignant (congenital) features and by a predisposition to cancer (see Offit[1] for a review). With the identification of genes associated with many of these syndromes, presymptomatic testing and counseling will become available.

The highly penetrant susceptibility alleles associated with the syndromes reviewed in this chapter account for a minority of human cancers. Nonetheless, the number of molecularly characterized, highly penetrant cancer syndromes has continued to grow. A larger proportion of human cancers might be associated with genetic polymorphisms that confer a lesser cancer risk. It was predicted, based on the Utah genealogies, that inherited susceptibility to cancer was documented even in carcinogen-associated tumors (e.g., head and neck, lung, leukemia), and these observations would emerge as a major focus for the next era of research at the interphase of genetics and clinical oncology.[296] Recent reviews of genetic polymorphisms and cancer risk have begun to lay the foundation for genomic approaches to low-penetrance cancer predisposition and interactions between genetics and the environment.[297]

ACKNOWLEDGMENTS

The authors are indebted to Colleen-Anne Campbell, who assisted in the research and referencing of recently described cancer predisposition syndromes, and to Dr. Noah Kauff for his critical review of the manuscript.

REFERENCES

1. Offit K: Clinical cancer genetics: Risk counseling and management, 2nd ed. New York, Wiley Liss, 2004.

2. American Society of Clinical Oncology: Statement of the American Society of Clinical Oncology: Genetic testing for cancer susceptibility. J Clin Oncol 1996;14:1730–1736.

3. American Society of Clinical Oncology: American Society of Clinical Oncology policy statement update: Genetic testing for cancer susceptibility. J Clin Oncol 2003;21:2397–2406.

4. Giardiello FM, Brensinger JD, Petersen GM, et al: The use and interpretation of commercial APC gene testing for familial adenomatous polyposis. New Engl J Med 1997;336:823–827.

5. Epstein CJ: Forward. In Kessler S (ed): Genetic Counseling: Psychological Dimensions. New York, Academic Press, 1979, pp i–xiii.

6. Kessler S: The processes of communication, decision making, and coping in genetic counseling. In Kessler S (ed): Genetic Counseling: Psychological Dimensions. New York, Academic Press, 1979, pp 35–51.

7. Kinzler KW, Vogelstein B: Landscaping the cancer terrain. Science 1998;280:1036–1037.

8. Claus EB, Risch N, Thompson WD, et al: Genetic analysis of breast cancer in the cancer and steroid hormone study. Am J Hum Genet 1991;48:232–242.

9. Whittemore AS, Gong G, Itnyre J, et al: Prevalence and contribution of BRCA1/2 mutations in breast cancer and ovarian cancer: Results from three U.S. population based case-control studies of ovarian cancer. Am J Hum Genet 1997;60:496–504.

10. Ford D, Easton DF: The genetics of breast and ovarian cancer. Br J Cancer 1995;72:805–812.

11. Starink TM: Cowden's disease: Analysis of fourteen new cases. J Am Acad Dermatol 1984;11:1127–1141.

12. Sidransky D, Tokino T, Helzlsouer K, et al: Inherited p53 mutations in breast cancer. Cancer Res 1992;52:2984–2986.

13. Meijers-Heijboer H, van den Ouweland A, Klijn J, et al: Low-penetrance susceptibility to breast cancer due to CHEK2(*)1100delC in noncarriers of BRCA1 or BRCA2 mutations. Nat Genet 2002;31:55–59.

14. Offit K, Pierce H, Kirchhoff T, et al: Frequency of CHEK2*1100delC in New York breast cancer cases and controls. BMC Med Genet 2003;4:1.

15. Chenevix-Trench G, Spurdle AB, Gatei M, et al: Dominant negative ATM mutations in breast cancer families. J Natl Cancer Inst 2002;94:205–215.

16. Ford D, Easton DF, Stratton M, et al: Genetic heterogeneity and penetrance analysis of the BRCA1 and BRCA2 genes in breast cancer families. Am J Hum Genet 1998;62:676–689.

17. Frank TS, Deffenbaugh AM, Reid JE, et al: Clinical characteristics of individuals with germline mutations in BRCA1 and BRCA2: Analysis of 10,000 individuals. J Clin Oncol 2002;20:1480–1490.

18. Claus EB, Risch N, Thompson WD, et al: Genetic analysis of breast cancer in the cancer and steroid Hormone Study. Am J Hum Genet 1991;48:232–242.

19. Whittemore AS, Gong G, Itnyre J, et al: Prevalence and contribution of BRCA1/2 mutations in breast cancer and ovarian cancer: Results from three U.S. population based case-control studies of ovarian cancer. Am J Hum Genet 1997;60:496–504.

20. Wooster R, Mangion J, Eeles R, et al: A germline mutation in the androgen receptor gene in two brothers with breast cancer and Reifenstein syndrome. Nat Genet 1992;2:132–134.

21. Easton DF, Ford D, Bishop DT (Breast Cancer Linkage Consortium): Breast and ovarian cancer incidence in BRCA1-mutation carriers. Am J Hum Genet 1995;56:265–271.

22. Ford D, Easton DF, Bishop DT, Narod SA, Goldgar DE (Breast Cancer Linkage Consortium): Risks of cancer in BRCA1-mutation carriers. Lancet 1994;343:692–695.

23. Struewing JP, Abeliovich D, Peretz T, et al: The carrier frequency of the BRCA1 185delAG mutation is approximately 1% in Ashkenazi Jewish individuals. Nat Genet 1995;11:198–200.

24. Levy-Lahad E, Catane R, Eisenberg S, et al: Founder BRCA1 and BRCA2 mutations in Ashkenazi Jews in Israel: Frequency and differential penetrance in ovarian cancer and in-breast-ovarian cancer families. Am J Hum Genet 1997;60:1059–1067.

25. Begg CB: On the use of familial aggregation in population-based case probands for calculating penetrance. J Natl Cancer Inst 2002;94:1221–1226.

26. Tonin P, Weber B, Offit K, et al: Frequency of recurrent BRCA1 and BRCA2 mutations in Ashkenazi Jewish breast cancer families. Nat Med 1997;2:1179–1183.

27. Ozcelik H, Schmocker B, Di Nicola N, et al: Germline BRCA2 6174delT mutations in Ashkenazi Jewish pancreatic cancer patients. Nat Genet 1997;16:17–18.

28. Oddoux C, Struewing JP, Clayton CM, et al: The carrier frequency of the BRCA2 6174delT mutation among Ashkenazi Jewish individuals is approximately 1%. Nat Genet 1996;14:188–190.

29. Offit K, Levran O, Hanenberg H, et al: Shared genetic susceptibility to breast cancer, brain tumors, and Fanconi anemia. J Natl Cancer Inst 2003;95:1548–1551.

30. Peshkin BN, DeMarco TA, Brogan BM, Lerman C, Isaacs C: BRCA1/2 testing: Complex themes in result interpretation. J Clin Oncol 2001;19:2555–2565.

31. Stoppa-Lyonnet D, Laurent-Puig P, Essioux L, et al: BRCA1 sequence variations in 160 individuals referred to a breast/ovarian family cancer clinic. Am J Hum Genet 1997;60:1021–1030.

32. Venkitaraman AR: Cancer susceptibility and the functions of BRCA1 and BRCA2. Cell 2002;108:171–182.

33. Offit K, Gilewski T, Norton L, et al: Germline BRCA1 185delAG mutations in Jewish women with breast cancer. Lancet 1996;347:1643–1646.

34. Benjamin B, Roa AA, Boyed KV, Richard SC: Ashkenazi Jewish population frequencies for common mutations in BRCA1 and BRCA2. Nat Genet 1996;14:185–187.

35. Neuhausen S, Gilewski T, Norton L, et al: Recurrent BRCA2 6174delT mutations in Ashkenazi Jewish women affected by breast cancer. Nat Genet 1996;13:126–128.

36. Frank TS, Deffenbaugh AM, Reid JE, et al: Clinical characteristics of individuals with germline mutations in BRCA1 and BRCA2: Analysis of 10,000 individuals. J Clin Oncol 2002;20:1480–1490.

37. Kauff ND, Perez-Segura P, Robson ME, et al: Incidence of non-founder BRCA1 and BRCA2 mutations in high-risk Ashkenazi breast and ovarian cancer families. J Med Genet 2002;39:611–614.

38. Szabo CI, King MC: Population genetics of BRCA1 and BRCA2. Am J Hum Genet 1997;60:1013–1021.

39. Khoo US, Chan KY, Cheung AN, et al: Recurrent BRCA1 and BRCA2 germline mutations in ovarian cancer: A founder mutation of BRCA1 identified in the Chinese population. Hum Mutat 2002;19:307–308.

40. Thorlacius S, Sigurdsson S, Bjarnadottir H, et al: Study of a single BRCA2 mutation with high carrier frequency in a small population. Am J Hum Genet 1997;60:1079–1084.

41. Lakhani SR, Sloane JP, Gusterson BA, et al: The pathology of familial breast cancer: Evidence for differences between breast cancers developing in carriers of BRCA1 mutations, BRCA2 mutations and sporadic cases. Lancet 1997;349:1488–1510.

42. Johannsson OT, Idvall I, Anderson C, et al: Tumor biological features of BRCA1-induced breast and ovarian cancer. Eur J Cancer 1997;33:362–371.

43. Robson M, Rajan P, Rosen PP, et al: BRCA-associated Breast Cancer: Absence of a characteristic immunophenotype. Cancer Res 1998;58:1839–1842.

44. Bignon YJ, Fonck Y, Chassagne MC, et al: Histoprognostic grade in tumours from families with hereditary predisposition to breast cancer. Lancet 1995;346:258.

45. Jacquemier J, Eisinger F, Birnbaum D, Sobol H: Histoprognostic grade in BRCA1-associated breast cancer. Lancet 1995;345:1503.

46. Marcus JN, Watson P, Page DL, et al: Hereditary breast cancer: Pathobiology, prognosis, and BRCA1 and BRCA2 gene linkage. Cancer 1996;77:697–709.

47. Burke W, Daly M, Garber J, et al: Recommendations for follow-up care of individuals with an inherited predisposition to cancer: BRCA1 and BRCA2. JAMA 1997;277:997–1003.

48. Mettler FA, Upton A, Kelsey CA, et al: Benefits vs. risks from mammography. Cancer 1996;77:903–909.

49. Kuhl CK, Schrading S, Leutner CC, et al: Surveillance of high risk women with proven or suspected familial (hereditary) breast

cancer: First mid-term results of a multi-modality clinical screening trial [abstract]. Proc Amer Soc Clin Oncol 2003;22:4a.

50. Kriege M, Brekelmans CTM, Boetes C, et al: MRI screening for breast cancer in women with high familial and genetic risk: First results of the Dutch MRI screening study (MRISC) [abstract]. Proc Amer Soc Clin Oncol 2003;22:5a.

51. Robson ME, Morris E, Kauff N, et al: Breast cancer screening utilizing magnetic resonance imaging (MRI) in carriers of *BRCA* mutations [abstract]. Proc Amer Soc Clin Oncol 2003;22:362a.

52. Scheur L, Kauff N, Robson M, et al: Outcome of preventive surgery and screening for breast and ovarian cancer in *BRCA* mutation carriers. J Clin Oncology 2002;20:1260-1268.

53. Hartmann LC, Sellers TA, Schaid DJ, et al: Efficacy of bilateral prophylactic mastectomy in *BRCA1* and *BRCA2* gene mutation carriers. J Natl Cancer Inst 2001;93:1633-1637.

54. Meijers-Heijboer H, Van Geel B, Van Putten WL, et al: Breast cancer after prophylactic bilateral mastectomy in women with a *BRCA1* or *BRCA2* mutation. N Engl J Med 2001;345:159-164.

55. Veronesi V, Maisonneuve P, Costa A, et al: Prevention of breast cancer with tamoxifen;preliminary findings of the Italian randomised trial among hysterectomised women. Lancet 1998;352:93-97.

56. Powles T, Eeles R, Ashley S, et al: Interim analysis of the incidence of breast cancer in the Royal Marsden tamoxifen randomised hemoprevention trial. Lancet 1998;358:98-101.

57. Narod SA, Brunet JS, Ghadirian P, et al: Tamoxifen and risk of contralateral breast cancer in *BRCA1* and *BRCA2* mutation carriers: A case-control study. Hereditary breast cancer clinical study group. Lancet 2000;356:1876-1881.

58. King MC, Wieand S, Hale K, et al: Tamoxifen and breast cancer incidence among women with inherited mutations in *BRCA1* and *BRCA2*. National surgical adjuvant breast and bowel project (NSABP-P1) breast cancer prevention trial. JAMA 2001;286:2251-2256.

59. Brunet JS, Ghadirian P, Rebbeck T, et al: Effect of smoking on breast cancer in carriers of mutant *BRCA1* or *BRCA2* genes. J Natl Cancer Inst 1998;90:761-765.

60. Kramer BS, Gohagan J, Prorok PC, Smart C: A National Cancer Institute sponsored screening trial for prostatic, lung, colorectal and ovarian cancers. Cancer 1993;71:589-593.

61. NIH consensus conference. Ovarian cancer: Screening, treatment, and follow-up. JAMA 1995;273:491-497.

62. Bourne TH, Campbell S, Reynolds KM, et al: Screening for early familial ovarian cancer with transvaginal ultrasonography and color blood flow imaging. BMJ 1993;306:1025-1029.

63. American College of Physicians: Screening for ovarian cancer: Recommendations and rationale. Ann Intern Med 1994;121:141-142.

64. Lynch HT, Albano WA, Lynch JF, Lynch PM, Campbell A: Surveillance and management of patients at high genetic risk for ovarian carcinoma. Obstet Gynecol 1982;59:589-596.

65. Kauff ND, Satagopan JM, Robson ME, et al: Risk-reducing salpingo-oophorectomy in women with a *BRCA1* or *BRCA2* mutation. N Engl J Med 2002;346:1609-1615.

66. Rebbeck TR, Lynch HT, Neuhausen SL, et al: Prophylactic oophorectomy in carriers of *BRCA1* or *BRCA2* mutations. N Engl J Med 2002;346:1616-1622.

67. Struewing JP, Watson P, Easton DF, Ponder BAJ, Lynch HT, Tucker MA: Prophylactic oophorectomy in inherited breast/ovarian cancer families. J Natl Cancer Inst Monogr 1995;17:33-35.

68. Chen KT, Schooley JL, Flam MM: Peritoneal carcinomatosis after prophylactic oophorectomy in familial ovarian cancer syndrome. Obstet Gynecol 1985;66:93S-94S.

69. Modan B, Hartge P, Hirsh-Yechezkel G, et al: Parity, oral contraceptives, and the risk of ovarian cancer among carriers and noncarriers of a *BRCA1* or *BRCA2* mutation. N Engl J Med 2001;345:235-240.

70. Narod SA, Risch HA, Moslehi R, et al: Oral contraceptives and the risk of hereditary ovarian cancer. N Engl J Med 1998;339:424-428.

71. Narod SA, Sun P, Risch HA, et al: Ovarian cancer, oral contra-ceptives, and *BRCA* mutations. N Engl J Med 2001;345:1706-1707.

72. Narod SA, Dube M, Klijn J, et al: Oral contraceptives and the risk of breast cancer in *BRCA1* and *BRCA2* Carriers. J Natl Cancer Inst 2002;94:1773-1779.

73. Cannon-Albright LA, Skolnick MH, Bishop DT, Lee RG, Burt RW: Common inheritance of susceptibility to colonic adenomatous polyps and associated colorectal cancers. New Engl J Med 1988;319:533-537.

74. Houlston RS, Collins A, Slack J, Morton ME: Dominant genes for colorectal cancer are not rare. Ann Hum Genet 1992;56:99-103.

75. Campbell WJ, Spence RA, Parks TG: Familial adenomatous polyposis. Br J Surg 1994;81:1722-1733.

76. Kinzler KW, Nilbert MC, Su LK, et al: Identification of *FAP* locus genes from chromosome 5q21. Science 1991;253:661-665.

77. Bertario L, Russo A, Sala P, et al: Hereditary colorectal tumor registry multiple approach to the exploration of genotype-phenotype correlations in familial adenomatous polyposis. J Clin Oncol 2003;21:1698-1707.

78. Spirio L, Olschwang S, Groden J, et al: Alleles of the *APC* gene: an attenuated form of familial polyposis. Cell 1993;75:951-957.

79. Sieber OM, Lipton L, Crabtree M, et al: Multiple colorectal adenomas, classic adenomatous polyposis, and germ-line mutations in *MYH*. N Engl J Med 2003;348:791-799.

80. King JE, Dozois RR, Lindor NM, Ahlquist DA: Care of patients and their families with familial adenomatous polyposis. Mayo Clin Proc 2000;75:57-67.

81. Jagelman DG: Clinical management of familial adenomatous polyposis. Cancer Surv 1989;8:159-167.

82. Giardiello FM, Yang VW, Hylind LM, et al: Primary chemoprevention of familial adenomatous polyposis with sulindac. N Engl J Med 2002;346:1054-1059.

83. Steinbach G, Lynch PM, Phillips RK, et al: The effect of celecoxib, a cyclooxygenase-2 inhibitor, in familial adenomatous polyposis. N Engl J Med 2000;342:1946-1952.

84. Parc YR, Olschwang S, Desaint B, Schmitt G, Parc RG, Tiret E: Familial adenomatous polyposis: Prevalence of adenomas in the ileal pouch after restorative proctocolectomy. Ann Surg 2001;233:360-364.

85. Marra G, Boland CR: Hereditary nonpolyposis colorectal cancer: The syndrome, the genes, and historical perspectives. J Natl Cancer Inst 1995;87:1114-1125.

86. Watson P, Lynch HT: Extracolonic cancer in hereditary nonpolyposis colorectal cancer. Cancer 1993;71:677-685.

87. Bailey-Wilson JE, Elston RC, Schuelke GS, et al: Segregation analysis of hereditary nonpolyposis colorectal cancer. Genet Epidemiol 1986;3:27-38.

88. Scapoli C, Ponz de Leon M, Sassatelli R, et al: Genetic epidemiology of hereditary non-polyposis colorectal cancer syndromes in Modena, Italy: Results of a complex segregation analysis. Ann Hum Genet 1994;58:275-295.

89. Vasen HF, Taal BG, Griffioen G, et al: Clinical heterogeneity of familial colorectal cancer and its influence on screening protocols. Gut 1994;35:1262-1266.

90. Watson P, Vasen HF, Mecklin JP, Jarvinen H, Lynch HT: The risk of endometrial cancer in hereditary nonpolyposis colorectal cancer. Am J Med 1994;96:516-520.

91. Aarnio M, Sankila R, Pukkala E, et al: Cancer risk in mutation carriers of DNA-mismatch-repair genes. Int J Cancer 1999;81:214-218.

92. Vasen HF, Watson P, Mecklin JP, Lynch HT: New clinical criteria for hereditary nonpolyposis colorectal cancer (HNPCC, Lynch syndrome) proposed by the international collaborative group on HNPCC: Gastroenterology 1999;116:1453-1456.

93. Rodriguez-Bigas M, Boland CR, Hamilton S, et al: A National Cancer Institute workshop on hereditary non-polyposis colorectal cancer: Meeting highlights and Bethesda guidelines. J Natl Cancer Inst 1997;23:6-10.

94. Kouri M, Laasonen A, Mecklin JP, Jarvinen H, Franssila K, Pyrhonen S: Diploid predominance in hereditary non-polyposis colorectal carcinoma evaluated by flow cytometry. Cancer 1990;65:1825-1829.

95. Sanikila R, Aaltonen LA, Jarvinen H, Mecklin JP: Better survival rates in patients with *MLH1*-complex associated hereditary colorectal cancer. Gastroenterology 1996;110:682-687.

96. Lynch HT, Smyrk T, Lanspa SJ, et al: Flat adenomas in a colon cancer-prone kindred. J Natl Cancer Inst 1988;80:278-282.

97. Muto T, Kamiya J, Sawada T, et al: Small flat adenoma of the large bowel with special reference to its clinical pathologic features. Dis Colon Rectum 1985;28:847-851.

98. Nyström-Lahti M, Parsons R, Sistonen P, et al: Mismatch repair genes on chromosomes 2p and 3p account for a major share of hereditary nonpolyposis colorectal cancer families evaluable by linkage. Am J Hum Genet 1994;55:659-665.

99. Leach FS, Nicholaides NC, Papadappoulos N, et al: Mutations of the *MutS* homolog in hereditary non-polyposis colorectal cancer. Cell 1993;75:1215-1225.

100. Bronner CE, Baker SM, Morrison PT, et al: Mutation in the DNA mismatch repair gene homologue *HMLH1* is associated with hereditary non-polyposis colon cancer. Nature 1994;368:258-261.

101. Liu B, Parsons R, Papadopoulos N, et al: Analysis of mismatch repair genes in hereditary non-polyposis colorectal cancer patients. Nat Med 1996;2:169-174.

102. Wijnen J, Vasen H, Khan PM, et al: Clinical findings with implications for genetic testing in families with clustering of colorectal cancer. N Engl J Med 1998;339:511-518.

103. Liu T, Yan H, Kuismanen S, et al: The role of *hPMS1* and *hPMS2* in predisposing to colorectal cancer. Cancer Res 2001;61:7798-7802.

104. Papadopoulous N, Lindblom A: Molecular basis of HNPCC: Mutations of *MMR* genes. Hum Mutat 1997;10:89-99.

105. Edelman W, Yang K, Umar A, et al: Mutation in the mismatch repair gene *MSH6* causes cancer susceptibility. Cell 1997;91:467-477.

106. Aaltonen LA, Peltomaki P, Leach FS, et al: Clues to the pathogenesis of colon cancer. Science 1993;260:812-816.

107. Thibodeau SN, Bren G, Schald D, et al: Microsatellite instability in cancer of the proximal colon. Science 1993;260:816-819.

108. Liu B, Farrington SM, Petersen GM, et al: Genetic instability occurs in the majority of young patients with colorectal cancer. Nat Med 1995;1:348-352.

109. Aaltonen LA, Salovaara R, Kristo P, et al: Incidence of hereditary non-polyposis colorectal cancer and the feasibility of molecular screening for the disease. N Engl J Med 1998;338:1481-1487.

110. Hackman P, Tannergard P, Osei-Mensa S, et al: A human compound heterozygote for two *MLH1* missense mutations. Nat Genet 1997;17:135-136.

111. Risinger JI, Barrett JC, Watson P, Lynch HT, Boyd J: Molecular genetic evidence of the occurrence of breast cancer as an integral tumor in patients with the hereditary nonpolyposis colorectal carcinoma syndrome. Cancer 1996;77:1836-1843.

112. Lindor NM, Burgart LJ, Leontovich O, et al: Immunohistochemistry versus microsatellite instability testing in phenotyping colorectal tumors. J Clin Oncol 2002;20:1043-1048.

113. Cunningham JM, Christensen ER, Tester DJ, et al: Hypermethylation of the *hMLH1* promoter in colon cancer with microsatellite instability. Cancer Res 1998;58:3455-3460.

114. Cunningham JM, Kim CY, Christensen ER, et al: The frequency of hereditary defective mismatch repair in a prospective series of unselected colorectal carcinomas. Am J Hum Genet 2001;69:780-790.

115. Winawer SJ, Zauber AG, O'Brien MJ, et al: Randomized comparison of surveillance intervals after colonoscopic removal of newly diagnosed adenomatous polyps. N Engl J Med 1993;328:901-906.

116. Winawer SJ, Zauber AG, Ho MN, et al: Prevention of colorectal cancer by colonoscopic polypectomy. New Eng J Med 1993;329:1977-1981.

117. Jarvinen HJ, Mecklin JP, Sistonen P, et al: Screening reduces colorectal cancer rate in families with hereditary nonpolyposis colorectal cancer. Gastroenterology 1995;108:1405-1411.

118. Vasen HF, Nagengast FM, Khan PM, et al: Interval cancers in hereditary non-polyposis colorectal cancer (Lynch syndrome). Lancet 1995;345:1183-1184.

119. Lynch HT, Smyrk T, Lynch J: An update of HNPCC (Lynch syndrome). Cancer Genet Cytogenet 1997;93:84-99.

120. Rodriguez-Bigas MA: Prophylactic colectomy for gene carriers in hereditary non-polyposis colorectal cancer. Cancer 1996;78:199-201.

121. Giardiello FM, Brensinger JD, Petersen GM: AGA technical review on hereditary colorectal cancer and genetic testing. Gastroenterology 2001;121:198-213.

122. Burke W, Petersen G, Lynch P, et al: Recommendations for follow-up care of individuals with an inherited predisposition to cancer. I: Hereditary nonpolyposis colon cancer. JAMA 1997;277:915-919.

123. Carter BS, Beaty TH, Steinberg GD, Childs B, Walsh PC: Mendelian inheritance of familial prostate cancer. Proc Natl Acad Sci USA 1992;89:3367-3371.

124. Schaid DJ, McDonnell SK, Blute ML, Thibodeau SN: Evidence for autosomal dominant inheritance of prostate cancer. Am J Hum Genet 1998;62:1425-1438.

125. Carter BS, Bova GS, Beaty TH, et al: Hereditary prostate cancer: Epidemiologic and clinical features. J Urol 1993;150:797-802.

126. Smith JR, Freije D, Carpten JD, et al: Major susceptibility locus for prostate cancer on chromosome 1 suggested by a genome-wide search. Science 1996;274:1371-1374.

127. Gibbs M, McIdoe RA, Stanford JL, et al: Linkage analysis of the *HPC* region in high risk prostate cancer families [abstract]. Am J Hum Genet 1997;61:71a.

128. Eeles RA, Durocher F, Edwards S, et al: Linkage analysis of chromosome 1q markers in 136 prostate cancer families. Am J Hum Genet 1998;62:653-658.

129. Berthon P, Valeri A, Cohen-Akenine A, et al: Predisposing gene for early-onset prostate cancer, localized on chromosome 1q42.2-43. Am J Hum Genet 1998;62:1416-1424.

130. Ingles SA, Ross RK, Yu MC, et al: Association of prostate cancer risk with genetic polymorphisms in vitamin D receptor and androgen receptor. J Natl Cancer Inst 1997;89:166-170.

131. Taylor JA, Hirvonen A, Watson M, Pittman G, Mohler JL, Bell DA: Association of prostate cancer with vitamin D receptor gene polymorphism. Cancer Res 1996;56:4108-4110.

132. Langston AA, Stanford JL, Wicklund KG, Thompson JD, Blazej RG, Ostrander EA: Germ-line *BRCA1* mutations in selected men with prostate cancer. Am J Hum Genet 1996;58:881-884.

133. Monroe KR, Yu MC, Kolonel LN, et al: Evidence of an X-linked or recessive genetic component to prostate cancer risk. Nat Med 1995;1:827-829.

134. Nwosu V, Carpten J, Trent JM, Sheridan R: Heterogeneity of genetic alterations in prostate cancer: Evidence of the complex nature of the disease. Hum Mol Genet 2001;10:2313-2318.

135. Smith JR, Freije D, Carpten JD, et al: Major susceptibility locus for prostate cancer on chromosome 1 suggested by a genome-wide search. Science 1996;274:1371-1374.

136. Carpten J, Nupponen N, Isaacs S, et al: Germline mutations in the *ribonuclease L* gene in families showing linkage with *HPC1*. Nat Genet 2002;30:181-184.

137. Tavtigian SV, Simard J, Teng DH, et al: A candidate prostate cancer susceptibility gene at chromosome 17p. Nat Genet 2001;27:172-180.

138. Littrup PJ, Goodman AC, Mettlin CJ: The benefit and cost of prostate cancer early detection. CA Cancer J Clin 1993;43:134-149.

139. Labrie F, Dupont A, Candas B, et al:, Decrease of prostate cancer death by screening: First data from the Quebec prospective and randomized study [abstract]. Proc Amer Soc Clin Oncol 1998;17:4a.

140. McWhorter WP, Hernandez AD, Meikle AW, et al: A screening study of prostate cancer in high risk families. J Urol 1992;148:826-828.

141. Donodeo F: Prevention trial for prostate cancer piques public interest. J Natl Cancer Inst 1993;85:1801-1802.

142. Thompson IM, Goodman PJ, Tangen CM, et al: The influence of finasteride on the development of prostate cancer. N Engl J Med 2003;349:215-224.

143. Pang JT, Thakker RV: Multiple endocrine neoplasia Type 1 (MEN 1). Eur J Cancer 1994;30:1961-1968.

144. Thakker RV: The molecular genetics of the multiple endocrine neoplasia syndromes. Clin Endocrinol 1993;38:1-14.

145. Chandrasekharappa SC, Guru S, Manickam P, et al: Positional cloning of the gene for multiple endocrine neoplasia type 1. Science 1997;276:404-407.

146. Vasen HF, Lamers CB, Lips CJ, et al: Screening for multiple endocrine neoplasia syndrome type 1. A study of 11 kindreds in The Netherlands. Arch Intern Med 1989;149:2717-2722.

147. Brandi ML, Gagel RF, Angeli A, et al: Guidelines for diagnosis and therapy of MEN type 1 and type 2. J Clin Endocrinol Metab 2001;86:5658-5671.

148. Telenius-Berg M, Berg B, Hamberger B, et al: Impact of screening on prognosis in the multiple endocrine neoplasia type 2 syndromes: Natural history and treatment results in 105 patients. Henry Ford Hosp Med J 1984;32:225-231.

Science of Clinical Oncology

149. Vasen HF, Van Der Feltz M, Raue F, et al: The natural course of multiple endocrine neoplasia type IIb: A study of 18 cases. Arch Intern Med 1992;152:1250-1252.

150. Farndon JR, Dilley WG, Baylin SB, et al: Familial medullary thyroid carcinoma without associated endocrinopathies: A distinct clinical entity. Br J Surg 1986;73:278-281.

151. Stoffer SS, Van Dyke DL, Bach JV, Szpunar W, Weiss L: Familial papillary carcinoma of the thyroid. Am J Hum Genet 1986;25:775-782.

152. Mulligan LM, Eng C, Healey CS, et al: Specific mutations of the *RET* proto-oncogene are related to disease phenotype in MEN2A and FMTC. Nat Genet 1994;6:70-74.

153. Eng C: The *RET* proto-oncogene in multiple endocrine neoplasia type 2 and Hirschsprung's disease. N Engl J Med 1996;335:943-951.

154. Mulligan LM, Kwok JB, Healey CS, et al: Germ-line mutations of the *RET* proto-oncogene in multiple endocrine neoplasia type 2A. Nature 1993;363:458-460.

155. Donis-Keller H, Dou S, Chi D, et al: Mutations in the *RET* protooncogene are associated with MEN2a and FMTC. Hum Mol Genet 1993;2:851-856.

156. Schuffenecker I, Ginet N, Goldgar D, et al: Prevalence and parental origin of de novo *RET* mutations in multiple endocrine neoplasia type 2a and familial medullary cancer of the thyroid. Am J Hum Genet 1997;60:233-237.

157. Eng C, Mulligan LM, Smith DP, et al: Low frequency of germline mutations in the *RET* proto-oncogene in patients with apparently sporadic medullary carcinoma of the thyroid. Clin Endocrinol 1995;43:123-127.

158. Decker RA, Peacock ML, Borst MJ, Sweet JD, Thomson NW: Progress in genetic screening of multiple endocrine neoplasia type 2a: Is calcitonin testing obsolete? Surgery 1995; 118:257-264.

159. Lips CJ, Landsvater RM, Höppener JW, et al: Clinical screening as compared with DNA analysis in families with multiple endocrine neoplasia type 2A. N Engl J Med 1994;331:828-835.

160. Wells SA Jr., Chi DD, Toshima K, et al: Predictive DNA testing and prophylactic thyroidectomy in patients at risk for multiple endocrine neoplasia type 2A. Ann Surg 1994;220:237-247.

161. Eng C, Clayton D, Schuffenecker I, et al: The relationship between specific *RET* proto-oncogene mutations and disease phenotype in multiple endocrine neoplasia type 2. International *RET* mutation consortium analysis. JAMA 1996;276:1575-1579.

162. Leboulleux S, Travagli JP, Caillou B, et al: Medullary thyroid carcinoma as part of a multiple endocrine neoplasia type 2B syndrome: Influence of the stage on the clinical course. Cancer 2002;94:44-50.

163. Smith DP, Houghton C, Ponder BA: Germline mutation of *RET* codon 883 in two cases of de novo MEN 2B. Oncogene 1997;15:1213-1217.

164. Skinner MA, DeBenedetti MK, Moley JF, Norton JA, Wells SA: Medullary thyroid cancer in children with multiple endocrine neoplasia type 2a and 2b. J Pediatr Surg 1996;31:177-181.

165. Lairmore TC, Ball DW, Baylin SB, Wells SA: Management of pheochromocytomas in patients with multiple endocrine neoplasia type 2 syndromes. Ann Surg 1993;217:595-601.

166. Reimer RR, Clark WH, Greene MH, et al: Precursor lesions in familial melanoma: A new genetic preneoplastic syndrome. JAMA 1978;239:744-746.

167. Lynch HT, Fusaro RM, Danes BS, et al: A review of hereditary malignant melanoma including biomarkers in familial atypical multiple mole melanoma syndrome. Cancer Genet Cytogenet 1983;8:325-358.

168. Greene MH, Clark WH Jr, Tucker MA, et al: Acquired precursors of cutaneous malignant melanoma: The familial dysplastic nevus syndrome. N Engl J Med 1985;312:91-97.

169. Tucker MA: Individuals at high risk of melanoma. Pigment Cell 1988;9:95-109.

170. Clurman BE, Groudine M: The *CDKN2A* tumor-suppressor locus—a tale of two proteins. N Engl J Med 1998;338:910-912.

171. Bale SJ, Dracopoli NC, Tucker MA, et al: Mapping the gene for hereditary cutaneous malignant melanoma-dysplastic nevus syndrome to chromosome 1p. N Eng J Med 1989;320:1367-1372.

172. Goldstein AM, Dracopoli NC, Ho EC, et al: Further evidence for a locus for cutaneous malignant melanoma-dysplastic nevus (CMM/DN) on chromosome 1p and evidence for genetic heterogeneity. Am J Hum Genet 1993;52:537-550.

173. Cannon-Albright LA, Goldgar DE, Meyer LJ, et al: Assignment of a locus for familial melanoma, *MLM,* to chromosome 9p13-22. Science 1992;258:1148-1152.

174. Cannon-Albright LA, Meyer LJ, Goldgar DE, et al: Penetrance and expressivity of the chromosome 9p melanoma susceptibility locus (*MLM*). Cancer Res 1994;54:6041-6044.

175. Kamb A, Shattuck-Eidens D, Eeles R, et al: Analysis of the *p16* gene (*CDKN2*) as a candidate for the chromosome 9p melanoma susceptibility locus. Nat Genet 1994;8:23-26.

176. Zuo L, Weger J, Yang Q, et al: Germline mutations in the *p16INK4a* binding domain of *CDK4* in familial melanoma. Nat Genet 1996;12:97-99.

177. Goldstein AM, Fraser MC, Struewing JP, et al: Increased risk of pancreatic cancer in melanoma-prone kindreds with *p16INK4* mutations. N Engl J Med 1995;333:970-974.

178. Whelan AJ, Bartsch D, Goodfellow P, et al: Brief report: A familial syndrome of pancreatic cancer and melanoma with a mutation in the *CDKN2* tumor suppressor gene. N Engl J Med 1995;333:975-977.

179. Borg A, Sandberg T, Nilsson K, et al: High frequency of multiple melanomas and breast and pancreas carcinomas in *CDKN2A* mutation-positive melanoma families. J Natl Cancer Inst 2000;92:1260-1266.

180. Bishop DT, Demenais F, Goldstein AM, et al: Geographical variation in the penetrance of *CDKN2A* mutations for melanoma. J Natl Cancer Inst 2002;94:894-903.

181. Goldstein AM, Tucker MA: Screening for *CDKN2A* mutations in hereditary melanoma. J Natl Cancer Inst 1997;19:676-678.

182. Kefford RF, Newton Bishop JA, Bergman W, Tucker MA: Counseling and DNA testing for individuals perceived to be genetically predisposed to melanoma: A consensus statement of the melanoma genetics consortium. J Clin Oncol 1999;17:3245-3251.

183. Gallie B, Dunn J, Chan H, Hamel P, Phillips R: The genetics of retinoblastoma: Relevance to the patient. Pediatr Clin North Am 1991;38:299-315.

184. Marcus DM, Brooks SE, Leff G, et al: Trilateral retinoblastoma: Insights into histogenesis and management. Surv Ophthalmol 1998;43:59-70.

185. Knudson AG: Mutation and cancer: Statistical study of retinoblastoma. Proc Natl Acad Sci USA 1971;68:820-823.

186. Friend SH, Bernards R, Rogelj S, et al: A human DNA segment with properties of the gene that predisposes to retinoblastoma and osteosarcoma. Nature 1986;323:643-646.

187. Lohmann DR, Brandt B, Hopping W, Passarge E, Horsthemke B: The spectrum of *RB1* germ-line mutations in hereditary retinoblastoma. Am J Hum Genet 1996;58:940-949.

188. Yandell DW, Herrera GE, Dayton SH, Dryja TP, Ludeke BI: Penetrance of *RB* mutations: Two families with a low-penetrance form of hereditary retinoblastoma carry the same missense mutation. Am J Hum Genet 1991;49:45.

189. Onadim Z, Hungerford J, Cowell JK, et al: Follow-up of retinoblastoma patients having prenatal and perinatal predictions for mutant gene carrier status using intragenic polymorphic probes from the *RB1* gene. Br J Cancer 1992;65:711-716.

190. Lohmann DR: *RB1* gene mutations in retinoblastoma. Hum Mutat 1999;14:283-288.

191. Harbour JW: Molecular basis of low-penetrance retinoblastoma. Arch Ophthalmol 2001;119:1699-1704.

192. Cohen JG, Dryja TP, Davis KB, et al: *RB1* genetic testing as a clinical service: A follow-up study. Med Pediatr Oncol 2001;37:372-378.

193. Girardet A, Hamamah S, Anahory T, et al: First preimplantation genetic diagnosis of hereditary retinoblastoma using informative microsatellite markers. Mol Hum Reprod 2003;9:111-116.

194. Noorani HZ, Khan HN, Gallie BL, Detsky AS: Cost comparison of molecular versus conventional screening of relatives at risk for retinoblastoma. Am J Hum Genet 1996;59:301-307.

195. Sanders BM, Jay M, Draper CJ, Roberts EM: Non-ocular cancer in relatives of retinoblastoma patients. Br J Cancer 1989;60:358-365.

196. Eng C, Li FP, Abramson DH, et al: Mortality from second tumors among long-term survivors of retinoblastoma. J Natl Cancer Inst 1993;85:1121-1128.

197. Li FP, Abramson DH, Tarone RE, Kleinerman RA, Fraumeni JF, Boice JD: Hereditary retinoblastoma, lipoma, and second primary cancers. J Natl Cancer Inst 1997;89:83–84.

198. Zbar B, Tory K, Merino M, et al: Hereditary papillary renal cell carcinoma. J Urol 1994;151:561–566.

199. Rasmussen SA, Yang Q, Friedman JM, et al: Mortality in neurofibromatosis 1: An analysis using U.S. death certificates. Am J Hum Genet 2001;68:1110–1118.

200. Sorensen SA, Mulvihill JJ, Nielsen A, et al: Long-term follow-up of Von Recklinghausen neurofibromatosis: Survival and malignant neoplasms. N Engl J Med 1986;314:1010–1015.

201. Huson SM, Harper PS, Compston DA, et al: Von Recklinghausen neurofibromatosis: A clinical and population study in South East Wales. Brain 1988;111:1355–1381.

202. Colman SD, Wallace MR: Neurofibromatosis Type 1. Eur J Cancer 1994;30:1974–1981.

203. Rasmussen SA, Colman SD, Abernathy CR, Schwartz CE, Arn PH, Wallace MR: Prevalence of large *NF1* gene deletions in neurofibromatosis type 1 (*NF1*) [abstract]. Am J Hum Genet 1996;59:37a.

204. Messiaen LM, Callens T, Mortier G, et al: Exhaustive mutation analysis of the *NF1* gene allows identification of 95% of mutations and reveals a high frequency of unusual splicing defects. Hum Mutat 2000;15:541–555.

205. Korf, BR: Malignancy in neurofibromatosis type 1. Oncologist 2000;5:477–485.

206. Evans DG, Huson SM, Donnai D, et al: A genetic study of type 2 neurofibromatosis in the United Kingdom. II: Guidelines for genetic counseling. J Med Genet 1992;29:847–852.

207. Baser ME, Friedman JM, Wallace AJ, et al: Evaluation of clinical diagnostic criteria for neurofibromatosis 2. Neurology 2002;59:1759–1765.

208. Trofatter JA, MacCollin MM, Rutter JL, et al: A novel moesin-, ezrin-, radixin-like gene is a candidate for the neurofibromatosis 2 tumor suppressor. Cell 1993;72:791–800.

209. Thomas G, Merel P, Sanson M, et al: Neurofibromatosis type 2. Eur J Cancer 1994;30:1981–1987.

210. Parry D, MacCollin MM, Kaiser-Kupfer MI, et al: Germ-line mutations in the neurofibromatosis 2 gene: Correlations with disease severity and retinal abnormalities. Am J Hum Genet 1996;59:529–539.

211. Evans DG, Trueman L, Wallace A, Collins S, Strachan T: Genotype/phenotype correlations in type 2 neurofibromatosis (NF2): Evidence for more severe disease associated with truncating mutations. J Med Genet 1998;35:450–455.

212. Evans DG, Ramsden R, Huson SM, et al: Type 2 neurofibromatosis: The need for supraregional care? J Laryngol Otol 1993;107:401–406.

213. Baser ME, Friedman JM, Aeschliman D, et al: Predictors of the risk of mortality in neurofibromatosis 2. Am J Hum Genet 2002;71:715–723.

214. Evans DG, Sainio M, Baser ME: Neurofibromatosis type 2. J Med Genet 2000;37:897–904.

215. Guttman DG, Aylsworth A, Carey JC, et al: The diagnostic evaluation and multidisciplinary management of neurofibromatosis 1 and neurofibromatosis 2. JAMA 1997;276:51–65.

216. Clifford SC, Maher ER: Von Hippel-Lindau disease: Clinical and molecular perspectives. Adv Cancer Res 2001;82:85–105.

217. Maher ER, Yates JR, Harries R, et al: Clinical features and natural history of Von Hippel-Lindau disease. Q J Med 1990;77:1151–1163.

218. Webster AR, Maher ER, Moore AT: Clinical characteristics of ocular angiomatosis in Von Hippel-Lindau disease and correlation with germline mutation. Arch Ophthalmol 1999;117:371–378.

219. Wanebo JE, Lonser RR, Glenn GM, Oldfield EH: The natural history of central nervous system hemangioblastomas in patients with Von Hippel-Lindau disease. J Neurosurg 2003;98:82–94.

220. Dollfus H, Massin P, Taupin P, et al: Retinal hemangioblastoma in Von Hippel-Lindau disease: A clinical and molecular study. Invest Ophthalmol Vis Sci 2002;43:3067–3074.

221. Lonser RR, Glenn GM, Walther M, et al: Von Hippel-Lindau disease. Lancet 2003;361:2059–2067.

222. Maher ER, Yates JR, Ferguson-Smith MA: Statistical analysis of the two stage mutation model in Von Hippel-Lindau disease. J Med Gene 1990;27:311–314.

223. Maher ER, Kaelin WG: Von Hippel-Lindau disease. Medicine (Baltimore) 1997;76:381–391.

224. Walther MM, Lubensky IA, Venzon D, Zbar B, Linehan WM: Prevalence of microscopic lesions in grossly normal renal parenchyma from patients with Von Hippel-Lindau disease, sporadic renal cell carcinoma and no renal disease: Clinical implications. J Urol 1995;154:2010–2014.

225. Choyke PL, Glenn GM, Walther MM, et al: The natural history of renal lesions in Von Hippel-Lindau disease: A serial CT study in 28 patients. AJR Am J Roentgenol 1992;159:1229–1234.

226. Walther MM, Reiter R, Keiser HR, et al: Clinical and genetic characterization of pheochromocytoma in Von Hippel-Lindau families: Comparison with sporadic pheochromocytoma gives insight into natural history of pheochromocytoma. J Urol 1999;162:659–664.

227. Crossey PA, Richards FM, Foster K, et al: Identification of intragenic mutations in the Von Hippel Lindau disease tumor suppressor gene and correlation with disease phenotype. Hum Mol Genet 1994;3:1303–1308.

228. Maher ER, Iselius L, Yates JR, et al: Von-Hippel Lindau disease: A genetic study. J Med Genet 1991;28:443–447.

229. Maher ER, Webster AR, Woodward ER, Richards FM, Moore AT: Allelic heterogeneity and modifier effects determine expression in Von Hippel-Lindau disease [abstract]. Am J Hum Genet 1996;59:394a.

230. Decker HJ, Weidt EJ, Brieger J: The Von Hippel-Lindau tumor suppressor gene. Cancer Genet Cytogenet 1997;93:74–83.

231. Manski TJ, Heffner DK, Glenn GM, et al: Endolymphatic sac tumours: A source of morbid hearing loss in Von Hippel-Lindau disease. JAMA 1997;277:1461–1466.

232. Chen F, Kishida T, Yao M, et al: Germline mutations in the Von Hippel-Lindau disease tumor suppressor gene: Correlations with phenotype. Hum Mutat 1995;5:66–75.

233. Zbar B: Von Hippel-Lindau disease and sporadic renal cell carcinoma. Cancer Surv 1995;25:219–232.

234. Zbar B, Kishida T, Chen F, et al: Germline mutations in the Von Hippel-Lindau (*VHL*) gene in families from North America, Europe and Japan. Hum Mutat 1996;8:348–357.

235. Latif F, Tory K, Gnarra J, et al: Identification of the Von Hippel-Lindau disease tumor suppressor gene. Science 1993;260:1317–1320.

236. Maher ER: Von Hippel-Lindau disease. Eur J Cancer 1994;30:1987–1990.

237. Beroud C, Joly D, Gallou C, Staroz F, Orfanelli MT, Junien C: Software and database for the analysis of mutations in the *VHL* gene. Nucleic Acids Res 1998;26:256–258.

238. Kondo K, Kaelin WG Jr: The Von Hippel-Lindau tumor suppressor gene. Exp Cell Res 2001;264:117–125.

239. Stolle C, Glenn G, Zbar B, et al: Improved detection of germline mutations in the Von Hippel-Lindau disease tumor suppressor gene. Hum Mutat 1998;12:417–423.

240. Lonser RR, Glenn GM, Walther M, et al: Von Hippel-Lindau disease. Lancet 2003;361:2059–2067.

241. Eisenhofer G, Lenders JW, Linehan WM, et al: Plasma normetanephrine and metanephrine for detecting pheochromocytoma in Von Hippel-Lindau disease and multiple endocrine neoplasia type 2. N Engl J Med 1999;340:1872–1879.

242. Rechitsky S, Verlinsky O, Chistokhina A, et al: Preimplantation genetic diagnosis for cancer predisposition. Reprod Biomed Online 2002;5:148–155.

243. Gorlin RJ, Goltz RW: Multiple nevoid basal-cell epithelioma, jaw cysts and bifid rib: A syndrome. New Engl J Med 1960;262:908–912.

244. Gorlin RJ: Nevoid basal-cell carcinoma syndrome. Medicine 1987;66:98–113.

245. Strong LC: Genetic and environmental interactions. Cancer 1977;40:1861–1866.

246. Evans DG, Farndon PA, Burnell LD, Gattamaneni HR, Birch JM: The incidence of Gorlin syndrome in 173 consecutive cases of medulloblastoma. Br J Cancer 1991;64:959–961.

247. Gorlin RJ: Nevoid basal-cell carcinoma syndrome. Medicine (Baltimore) 1987;66:98–113.

248. Evans DG, Ladusans EJ, Rimmer S, Burnell LD, Thakker N, Farndon PA: Complications of the naevoid basal cell carcinoma syndrome: Results of a population based study. J Med Genet 1993;30: 460-464.

249. Cowan R, Hoban P, Kelsey A, Birch JM, Gattamaneni R, Evans DG: The gene for the naevoid basal cell carcinoma syndrome acts as tumour-suppressor gene in medulloblastoma. Br J Cancer 1997;76:141-145.

250. Johnson RL, Rothman AL, Xie J, et al: Human homolog of PATCHED, a candidate gene for the Basal cell nevus syndrome. Science 1996;272:1666-1671.

251. Wicking C, Shanley S, Smyth I, et al: Most germ-line mutations in the nevoid basal cell carcinoma syndrome lead to a premature termination of the PATCHED protein, and no genotype-phenotype correlations are evident. Am J Hum Genet 1997;60:21-26.

252. Tate G, Li M, Suzuki T, Mitsuya T, et al: A new germline mutation of the PTCH gene in a Japanese patient with nevoid basal cell carcinoma syndrome associated with meningioma. Jpn J Clin Oncol 2003;33:47-50.

253. Anand VK, Arrowood JP Jr, Krolls SO, et al: Malignant potential of the odontogenic keratocyst. Otolaryngol Head Neck Surg 1994;111:124-129.

254. Bitar GJ: Basal cell nevus syndrome: guidelines for early detection. Am Fam Physician 2002;65:2501-2504.

255. Strong LC: Genetic and environmental interactions. Cancer 1977;40:1861-1866.

256. Atherton DJ, Pitcher DW, Wells RS, MacDonald DM: A syndrome of various cutaneous pigmented lesions, myxoid neurofibromata and atrial myxoma: the NAME syndrome. Br J Dermatol 1980;103: 421-429.

257. Rhodes AR, Silverman RA, Harrist TJ, Perez-Atayde AR: Mucocutaneous lentigines, cardiomucocutaneous myxomas, and multiple blue nevi: The LAMB syndrome. J Am Acad Dermatol 1984;10:72-82.

258. Carney JA, Gordon H, Carpenter PC, Shenoy BV, Go VL: The complex of myxomas, spotty pigmentation, and endocrine overactivity. Medicine (Baltimore) 1985;64:270-283.

259. Stratakis CA, Carney JA, Lin JP, et al: Carney complex, a familial multiple neoplasia and lentiginosis syndrome: Analysis of 11 kindreds and linkage to the short arm of chromosome 2. J Clin Invest 1996;97:699-705.

260. Carney JA, Young WF: Primary pigmented nodular adrenocortical disease and its associated conditions. Endocrinologist 1992;2: 6-21.

261. Courcoutsakis NA, Chow CK, Shawker TH, Carney JA, Stratakis CA: Syndrome of spotty skin pigmentation, myxomas, endocrine overactivity, and schwannomas (Carney complex): Breast imaging findings. Radiology 1997;205:221-227.

262. Premkumar A, Stratakis CA, Shawker TH, Papanicolaou DA, Chrousos GP: Testicular ultrasound in Carney complex. J Clin Ultrasound 1997;25:211-214.

263. Stratakis CA, Sarlis NJ, Kirschner LS, et al: Paradoxical response to dexamethasone assists with the diagnosis of primary pigmented nodular adrenocortical disease (PPNAD). Ann Intern Med 1999;131:585-591.

264. Stratakis CA, Courcoutsakis NA, Abati A, et al: Thyroid gland abnormalities in patients with the syndrome of spotty skin pigmentation, myxomas, endocrine overactivity, and schwannomas (Carney complex). J Clin Endocrinol Metab 1997;82:2037-2043.

265. Stratakis CA, Papageorgiou T, Premkumar A, et al: Ovarian lesions in Carney complex: Clinical genetics and possible pre-disposition to malignancy. J Clin Endocrinol Metab 2000;85: 4359-4366.

266. Stratakis CA, Kirschner LS, Carney JA: Clinical and molecular features of the Carney complex: Diagnostic criteria and recommendations for patient evaluation. J Clin Endocrinol Metab 2001;86:4041-4046.

267. Kirschner LS, Sandrini F, Monbo J, Lin JP, Carney JA, Stratakis CA: Genetic heterogeneity and spectrum of mutations of the PRKAR1A gene in patients with Carney complex. Hum Mol Genet 2000;9:3037-3046.

268. Casey M, Vaughan CJ, He J, et al: Mutations in the protein kinase A R1—a regulatory subunit cause familial cardiac myxomas and Carney complex. J Clin Invest 2000;106:R31-R38.

269. Eng C: Will the real Cowden syndrome please stand up: Revised diagnostic criteria. J Med Genet 2000;37:828-830.

270. Eng C, Murday V, Seal S, et al: Cowden syndrome and Lhermitte-Duclos disease in a family: A single genetic syndrome with pleiotropy? J Med Genet 1994;31:458-461.

271. Hanssen AM, Fryns JP: Cowden syndrome. J Med Genet 1995;32:117-119.

272. Fackenthal JD, Marsh DJ, Richardson AL, et al: Male breast cancer in Cowden syndrome patients with germline PTEN mutations. J Med Genet 2001;38:159-164.

273. Li J, Yen C, Liaw D, et al: PTEN, a putative protein tyrosine phosphatase gene mutated in human brain, breast and prostate cancer. Science 1997;275:1943-1947.

274. Eng, C: Role of PTEN, a lipid phosphatase upstream effector of protein kinase B, in epithelial thyroid carcinogenesis. Ann N Y Acad Sci 2002;968:213-221.

275. Liaw D, Marsh DJ, Li J, et al: Germline mutations of the PTEN gene in Cowden syndrome, an inherited breast and thyroid cancer syndrome. Nat Genet 1997;16:64-67.

276. Marsh DJ, Kum JB, Lunetta KL, et al: PTEN mutation spectrum and genotype-phenotype correlations in Bannayan-Riley-Ruvalcaba syndrome suggest a single entity with Cowden syndrome. Hum Mol Genet 1999;8:1461-1472.

277. NCCN practice guidelines: Genetics/familial high risk cancer. Oncology 1999;13:161-186.

278. Birt AR, Hogg GR, Dube WJ: Hereditary multiple fibrofolliculomas with trichodiscomas and acrochordons. Arch Dermatol 1977;113:1674-1677.

279. Toro JR, Glenn G, Duray P, et al: Birt-Hogg-Dube syndrome: A novel marker of kidney neoplasia. Arch Dermatol 1999;135: 1195-1202.

280. Pavlovich CP, Walther MM, Eyler RA, et al: Renal tumors in the Birt-Hogg-Dube syndrome. Am J Surg Pathol 2002;26:1542-1552.

281. Durrani OH, Ng L, Bihrle W, et al: Chromophobe renal cell carcinoma in a patient with the Birt-Hogg-Dube syndrome. J Urol 2002;168:1484-1485.

282. Khoo SK, Giraud S, Kahnoski K, et al: Clinical and genetic studies of Birt-Hogg-Dube syndrome. J Med Genet 2002;39:906-912.

283. Zbar B, Alvord WG, Glenn G, et al: Risk of renal and colonic neoplasms and spontaneous pneumothorax in the Birt-Hogg-Dube syndrome. Cancer Epidemiol Biomarkers Prev 2002;11: 393-400.

284. Walter P, Kirchhof B, Korge B, Heimann K: Flecked chorio-retinopathy associated with Birt-Hogg-Dube syndrome. Graefes Arch Clin Exp Ophthalmol 1997;235:359-361.

285. Khoo SK, Bradley M, Wong FK, Hedblad MA, Nordenskjold M, Teh BT: Birt-Hogg-Dube syndrome: Mapping of a novel hereditary neoplasia gene to chromosome 17p12-q11.2. Oncogene 2001;20:5239-5242.

286. Nickerson ML, Warren MB, Toro JR, et al: Mutations in a novel gene lead to kidney tumors, lung wall defects, and benign tumors of the hair follicle in patients with the Birt-Hogg-Dube syndrome. Cancer Cell 2002;2:157-164.

287. Sevenet N, Sheridan E, Amram D, Schneider P, Handgretinger R, Delattre O: Constitutional mutations of the hSNF5/INI1 gene predispose to a variety of cancers. Am J Hum Genet 1999; 65:1342-1348.

288. Lee HY, Yoon CS, Sevenet N, Rajalingam V, Delattre O, Walford NQ: Rhabdoid tumor of the kidney is a component of the rhabdoid predisposition syndrome. Pediatr Dev Pathol 2002;5:395-399.

289. Taylor MD, Gokgoz N, Andrulis IL, Mainprize TG, Drake JM, Rutka JT: Familial posterior fossa brain tumors of infancy secondary to germline mutation of the hSNF5 gene. Am J Hum Genet 2000;66:1403-1406.

290. Savla J, Chen TT, Schneider NR, Timmons CF, Delattre O, Tomlinson GE: Mutations of the hSNF5/INI1 gene in renal rhabdoid tumors with second primary brain tumors. J Natl Cancer Inst 2000;92: 648-650.

291. Sevenet N, Lellouch-Tubiana A, Schofield D, et al: Spectrum of hSNF5/INI1 somatic mutations in human cancer and genotype-phenotype correlations. Hum Mol Genet 1999;8:2359-2368.

292. Sévenet N, Lellouch-Tubiana A, Amram D, Schneider P, Jouvet A, Delattre O: HSNF5/INI1, a component of the SWI/SNF complex,

demonstrates loss of function mutations in various cancers. Cancer Detect Prev 2000;24(S).

293. White FV, Dehner LP, Belchis DA, et al: Congenital disseminated malignant rhabdoid tumor: A distinct clinicopathologic entity demonstrating abnormalities of chromosome 22q11. Am J Surg Pathol 1999;23:249-256.

294. Palmer NF, Sutow W: Clinical aspects of the rhabdoid tumor of the kidney: A report of the national Wilms' tumor study group. Med Pediatr Oncol 1983;11:242-245.

295. Tomlinson G, Breslow N, Moksness J, Beckwith B, D'Angio G, Green DM: Prognostic factors in rhabdoid tumors of the kidney: Results of the national Wilms' tumor study group. Proc ASCO 1996;15:460.

296. Cannon-Albright LA, Thomas A, Goldgar DE, et al: Familiality of cancer in Utah. Cancer Res 1994;54:2378-2385.

297. Goode EL, Ulrich CM, Potter JD: Polymorphisms in DNA repair genes and associations with cancer risk. Cancer Epidemiol Biomarkers Prev 2002;11:1513-1530.

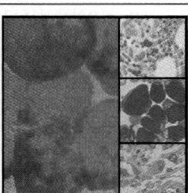

14

GENETIC FACTORS: FINDING CANCER SUSCEPTIBILITY GENES

Elaine A. Ostrander

Danielle M. Friedrichsen

SUMMARY OF KEY POINTS

- The identification of cancer susceptibility genes by either linkage studies within families or association studies in populations is a useful way to understand defining events in tumor development and to identify cellular pathways that are likely to be important in cancer.
- Cancer susceptibility genes can be either strongly penetrant, where individuals born with a mutant allele have a high probability of developing cancer, or weakly penetrant, for which the probability of developing cancer is lower.

- Ideal families for linkage studies are large, include many affected individuals who can be readily examined and interviewed and include individuals with similar clinical features of disease from multiple generations. This allows large data sets associated with genetic heterogeneous forms of cancer to be stratified into homogenous subsets, thus increasing the power to detect genes.
- Linkage between polymorphic markers and a disease state is assessed using a number of statistical tools, including the

parametric lod score and nonparametric NPL score.
- Association studies that include populations of affected cases and controls are useful for testing hypotheses about candidate genes and alleles that may be disease associated. A well-defined set of cases and matched controls is important.
- Association studies and linkage-based studies both require collection of accurate clinical and family history data by clinicians, and both offer the future hope for genetic testing.

INTRODUCTION

Cancer susceptibility genes are those that, when mutated, increase an individual's risk of having cancer. If an individual is born with one mutant copy of a cancer susceptibility gene, subsequent mutations in the wild-type allele within the relevant tissues can result in a lack of functional gene product, leading to tumor formation.[1] Genetic mapping of cancer susceptibility genes allows identification of both genes and pathways that play a role in cancer susceptibility. Although the direct public health impact associated with cloning any specific cancer gene may be minimal, the contributions to understanding of tumor development and metastasis that such advances make are potentially enormous.

Population-based studies reveal excess familial cancer aggregation for most organ sites.[2] However, cancer susceptibility genes have been mapped for only a few cancer sites to date, and cloned for even fewer. Several studies suggest that the overall percentage of cancers in the general population that are caused by inherited mutations is low, likely less than a few percent, even when all organ sites are considered.[3] For breast and prostate cancer, the numbers are probably among the most well supported; 5% to 10% of cases of each are thought to be due to mutations in inherited susceptibility loci.[4-7] The remaining cancer cases, making up the majority, are considered sporadic in nature. They are probably caused by a mixture of specific genetic and environmental

factors, with genetic background playing a poorly understood role.

Cancer susceptibly alleles associated with a given gene may be either strongly penetrant, leading to a high probability that individuals born with a mutant allele will have the disease in question, or weakly penetrant, with carriers having a proportionately lower probability of having the disease. Allele penetrance associated with susceptibility alleles is often age-dependent, with the probability of having the disease increasing with each decade of life. Genetic mapping of cancer susceptibility genes is extremely difficult, in part because genetic background and environmental exposures are likely to affect penetrance. In addition, both highly and weakly penetrant alleles can be associated with the same gene. The same allele can be associated with widely varying age-dependent penetrance within a single family.

Highly penetrant disease alleles are best identified by family-based linkage analysis studies. The segregation of a defined chromosomal segment with affected individuals in multiple families suggests the presence of a cancer susceptibility gene within the genomic region tested. Statistical analysis that is performed after genotyping of appropriate numbers of families with markers defining regions of interest allows researchers to calculate the probability that any given chromosomal region carries a susceptibility gene. Weakly penetrant alleles are more easily identified by association tests after analysis of DNA from two distinct populations, for example, patients with cancer together with an appropriately matched set of control subjects. Weak alleles are hypothesized to be more common in the general human population and are therefore likely to account for a higher percentage of cancer in the population overall. In this chapter, we investigate the ways that both highly and weakly penetrant disease alleles are identified and studied.

FUNDAMENTAL SCIENCE

Hereditary Cancer Families

Strong and Amos[8] have defined a general paradigm for population studies that can be applied to identifying genes important in predisposition to cancer. The hypothesis that a particular cancer has an identifiable genetic component usually occurs through family history analysis of sequential cancer cases, general clinical observations, and finally, epidemiologic studies. Epidemiologic studies assess whether there is significant evidence for an increased cancer risk at a particular organ site that can be associated with a family history of the disease. If so, a segregation analysis may be undertaken to identify features of the putative susceptibility loci. Typical analyses address mode of inheritance (dominant, recessive, or X-linked) and estimate frequency and penetrance of the disease allele in the general population, age-dependent penetrance, and potential number of genes contributing to the disease. In the event that genetic linkage studies are eventually undertaken, data from the segregation analysis are key in developing statistical models for analyzing subsequent linkage data.

Familial aggregation is a general term that describes the occurrence of multiple cases of cancer within a family (Fig. 14-1). Such clustering may be due to shared environment, shared alleles of particular genes, or simply chance if the tumor is very common in the population. The successful mapping of cancer susceptibility genes for breast, colon, and prostate cancer has led to the development of a strictly defined term, *hereditary cancer*,

which describes families with three or more first-degree relatives with a given cancer, three successive generations with cancer, or at least two siblings with the same cancer detected at a relatively young age.[4] *First degree relatives* are defined as parents and offspring or sets of siblings.

Many epidemiologic studies indicate that a family history of a specific cancer within first-degree relatives is associated with a doubling or more of risk among relatives.[9] In the case of prostate cancer, for instance, studies of selected hospital-based patient populations,[10,11] population-based case-control studies,[12-14] and cohort studies[2,15] all demonstrate that a family history of disease increases an individual's risk. If the affected family members are first-degree relatives (e.g., brothers or fathers and sons), the risk increases from 1.7-fold to 3.7-fold. Younger ages at diagnosis and multiple affected relatives with the disease tend to be associated with even higher relative risk (RR). For example, men with three or more first-degree relatives with prostate cancer have almost an 11-fold increased risk of the disease compared with men who have no family history of the disease.[10] For this reason, families ascertained for linkage analysis studies tend to be large, have multiple affected individuals, and feature people who were given a diagnosis of the disease at a comparatively young age.

Linkage Mapping and Finding Cancer Susceptibility Genes

Several requirements must be met to successfully identify cancer susceptibility genes. First, a large number of so-called high risk families must be ascertained by using appropriate guidelines for human subjects. Clinical features and family history data must be recorded, and DNA samples must be obtained. Second, DNA samples from appropriate family members need to be screened by using a set of *polymorphic markers* that span the genome at a high density. Historically, genome scans have used markers distributed approximately every 10 million base pairs. Recent studies suggest that a denser scan with markers every 5 million base pairs may be preferable. Finally, the data must be interpreted or analyzed in the context of the disease in question. Creating stratified data sets, which allow analysis of families with a common disease or family history features, is important and may increase the chance of finding a susceptibility-associated locus. These issues are each discussed in turn in the following sections.

Family Collection

Cancer is a heterogeneous disease involving multiple susceptibility genes. In a statistically ideal situation, a given set of affected individuals within a family would all have cancer for the same reason; that is each member would have inherited a mutated copy of the same gene. But in truth, for common cancers such as those of the breast, prostate, and colon, any given family may have individuals whose disease is due to mutations in multiple different genes, some highly and some weakly penetrant, as well as family members whose disease is sporadic.[16] Often disease presentation is similar in genetic and sporadic

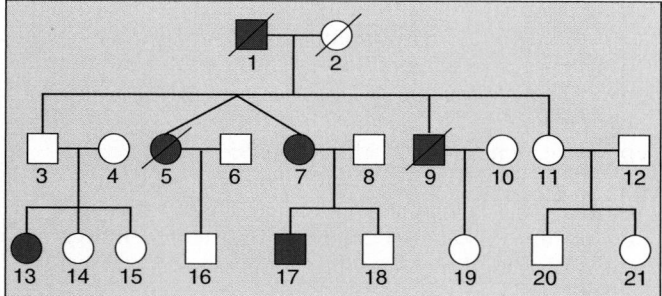

Figure 14-1. Theoretical pedigree of a family segregating an autosomal dominant disorder. Individuals are numbered 1 to 21. Males are indicated by squares and females are indicated by circles. Symbols for affected individuals are filled (numbers 1, 5, 7, etc.). A diagonal line through the symbol indicates that individual is deceased (1, 2, 5, and 9). A horizontal line between symbols indicates a mating (1+2; 3+4; etc.). Perpendicular lines drawn from mating lines indicate children (e.g., 13, 14, and 15 are all daughters of 3 and 4). Siblings are designated as shown for individuals 3, 5, 7, and 9; and individuals 5 and 7 are twins.

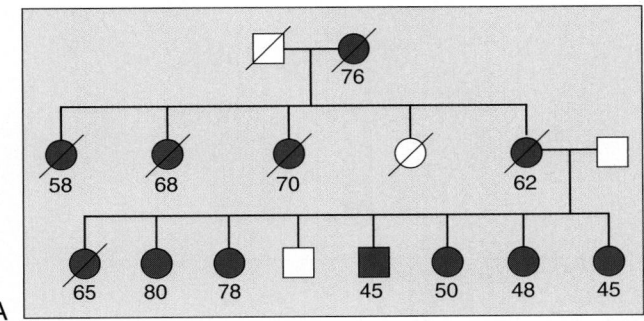

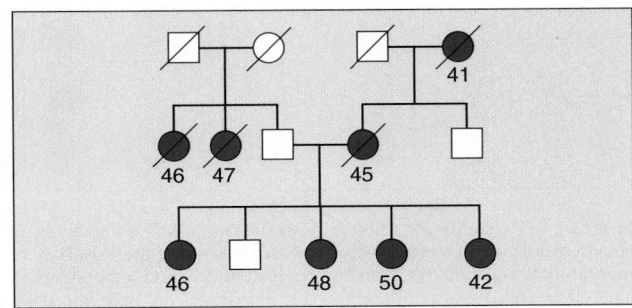

Figure 14-2. Two theoretical breast cancer families. Age at diagnosis is indicated below the symbol; males are indicated by squares, and females, by circles. **A,** The family has many members affected with breast cancer, but some were given diagnoses relatively early in life (<50 years), whereas others were much older at diagnosis (>70 years). The utility of this family for genetic mapping studies is thus limiting, because it likely contains individuals with both sporadic and hereditary breast cancer. **B,** All individuals were affected at an early age, but breast cancer, caused by mutations in either the same or different genes, is present on both sides of the family. Because there is no way to distinguish the number of mutant genes, a priori, the utility of this family for a genome-wide scan is also somewhat limited.

cases, and examination of clinical features is uninformative for determining whether a specific patient represents a genetic or sporadic case.

Figure 14-2 demonstrates two types of seemingly useful families for linkage mapping studies. Both include a significant number of affected members. The first family, in particular, has a large number of affected individuals (Fig. 14-2A). However, some individuals were affected very early in life, whereas others were given diagnoses at later ages. It is likely that some individuals have the disease because they inherited mutated copies of a particular gene, whereas others have the disease for sporadic reasons unrelated to the disease allele segregating in the family. Ideally, age at onset provides some guidance as to which individuals are more likely to have hereditary versus sporadic forms of the disease; but this is not absolute, and in the case of a disease with age-dependent penetrance, some people will be affected late in life, even though they carry a mutant allele, and others will be affected early in life for sporadic reasons. The family shown in Figure 14-2B also appears to be informative for and conducive to linkage mapping studies. There are several affected individuals in the family and all were affected at a relatively early age. However, the presence of disease segregating on both sides of the family should be

noted. The affected individuals in the youngest generation could have cancer because they inherited mutant alleles from one or both sides of their family. Therefore, the family is of limited utility for mapping studies.

Obtaining good clinical information for all individuals in a family mapping study gives geneticists the power to stratify the data into more homogenous subsets. This increases statistical power for finding the genes associated with any one particular aspect of a phenotype. If a subset of individuals in the family in Figure 14-2B all had tumors of similar stage and grade, this homogenous subset of data could be considered in isolation from the rest of the affected cases, reducing heterogeneity and increasing power. In addition to clinical features of disease, family history, age at onset, and presence or absence of other cancers are all ways to stratify data into homogenous subsets and improve the likelihood of finding causative genes.

Identification of cancer families and collection of critical medical information including family history, medical record data, and DNA samples are generally regulated by institutional review boards (IRBs). Families must be identified in a way that is neither intrusive nor coercive. For these reasons, genetic epidemiologists are increasingly turning to advertisement in periodicals such as supplements to popular newspapers or widely read periodicals[17] to recruit families eligible for a particular study. A particularly innovative approach used by investigators trying to find hereditary prostate cancer families was to establish a toll-free phone number, which was then advertised on a popular syndicated television talk show.[18] Listeners whose family history matched that described were encouraged to call for a preliminary phone screening and to obtain more information about the study.

For linkage-based approaches to finding genes to be useful, rigorous quantitative data regarding strength of phenotype must be available for multiple generations of the family. Medical record data must be carefully and systematically extracted into well-protected databases. Family history data must also be obtained redundantly from multiple members of the family, and care must be taken to resolve discrepancies. Consent to contact other family members regarding the study is needed, as is permission to obtain medical records. Individual privacy must also be protected, and personal identifiers such as names and addresses must remain confidential.

Locus Heterogeneity

If a particular trait is controlled by a large number of genes, each of which contributes only minimally to the final complex phenotype, it will be difficult to dissect the contributions of any one gene by studying a small number of families. If, however, the phenotype is controlled largely by a small number of genes, the underlying genetics will be much easier to resolve. The breast cancer susceptibility genes *BRCA1* and *BRCA2* were likely among the first to be mapped for several reasons related to this point.[19,20] First, only two genes appear to control the majority of the hereditary breast cancer in the general population.[21] Had the number been larger, the task would have been proportionately greater. Second, large and well-characterized families had been meticulously ascertained. This ensured that there was sufficient statistical power to undertake the genome scan. Third, the power of any given data set can be increased dramatically by identifying families in which several members share minor disease features, thus making it likely that their disease is due to mutations in the same gene. The presence of ovarian cancer in some families and not others and the presence of breast cancer in some male carriers allowed for creation of data sets enriched for the *BRCA1* and *BRCA2* genes, respectively.[19,20] Finally, it is always useful to remove from a data set families whose disease is known to be caused by any given gene. The identification of the *BRCA1* gene and subsequent removal of *BRCA1*-linked families from remaining data sets provided further useful enrichment for *BRCA2*-linked families.[20,22]

Initially, in the case of breast cancer, investigators did not know the number of genes likely to be involved in genetic susceptibility. Detailed *segregation analysis* had suggested that the gene or genes responsible for breast cancer were likely to be highly penetrant and autosomal and to produce patterns of age-dependent penetrance. A segregation analysis typically involves interviewing a large number of sequential case patients who share common features of the disease. Once a segregation analysis is complete, the resulting data can be factored into the resulting genome-wide scan. This allows data from some individuals to be weighed more significantly. Segregation analyses have now been done for nearly all types of cancer,[4,7,23-26] providing investigators with an array of clues with which to begin their search for genes of interest.

After families are designated for a genome-wide scan, a power analysis is performed to determine whether there is sufficient statistical power in a specific group of families to identify a marker or set of markers linked to the trait, given a certain set of assumptions. The assumptions include how many markers are being tested, how informative each marker is likely to be, and the composition of the families in question. The scenario in which a given set of families offers sufficient power to find a gene only if one of the markers is extremely close to the locus occurs frequently and is particularly associated with diseases such as cancer, for which locus heterogeneity is common. The power to find genes decreases dramatically as the number of genes that contribute to a phenotype increases.[27]

Principles of Genetic Linkage Analysis

The principles of meiotic recombination are key to understanding linkage analysis. In meiosis, the cell division leading to gamete formation, homologous chromosomes are paired. Each chromosome consists of two identical strands (chromatids), with each chromosome pairing composed of four strands. Homologous chromosomes separate from each other during the process of meiosis except at one or two zones of contact in a process that leads to *genetic recombination* (Fig. 14-3). Mendel's second law, independent assortment, states that alleles of genes at different loci segregate or assort independently of one another. Deviations from independent assortment occur when genes are located close to one another, and

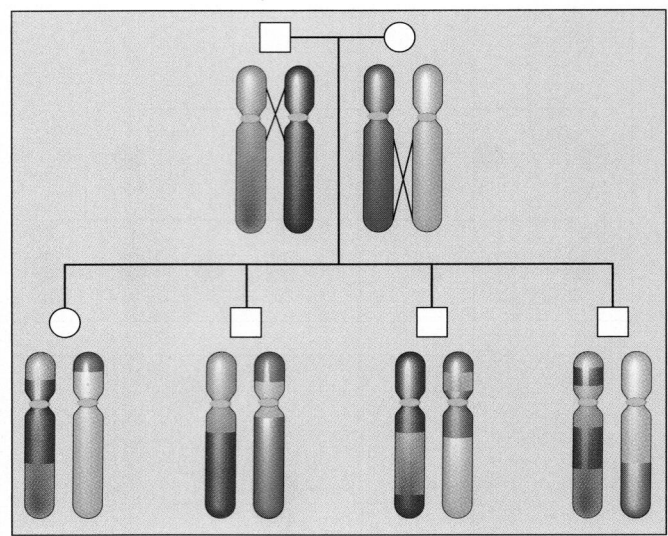

Figure 14-3. Genetic recombination is the process of exchanging genetic information between two chromatids during meiosis. The recombination events for a single chromosome within a family are illustrated. The father's homologous chromosomes are light and dark purple, and the mother's are light and dark green. Recombination events occurring during meiosis create unique parental chromosomes.

alleles assort together more than 50% of the time. In this case, the associated loci are said to be *linked*. However, if two loci are located on different chromosomes or far apart on the same chromosome, their alleles will assort randomly, with a given set of alleles being transmitted to the same gamete 50% of the time. Such loci are *unlinked*.

For any given chromosomal segment, the probability of a genetic recombination event occurring between a pair of markers or a marker and a gene is proportional to the distance between them. This probability is expressed as a recombination frequency (q) where:

$$\theta = \text{Number of recombinant offspring/Number of total offspring}$$

Recombination frequency ranges from 0 for genes that are so closely linked that crossover events essentially never occur to 0.5 for genes that assort randomly. Within small intervals, when the probability of multiple crossovers is negligible and the relationship between the recombination fraction (θ) and the distance between two genes (x), is simply $x = \theta$.[28] After a minor mathematical adjustment for the possibility of double recombinants is made, recombination fractions are expressed in units called *centimorgans* (*cM*), named after the geneticist Thomas Hunt Morgan.[29] One percent recombination ($\theta = 0.01$) is equal to 1 cM, which corresponds to about one million base pairs. The entire human genome is estimated to be about 3300 cM.

Genetic linkage mapping queries whether any given portion of the genome is consistently inherited with the disease status. The ordered set of alleles associated with a particular part of the genome received by an offspring from one parent is called a *haplotype* (Fig. 14-4). Recombinant haplotypes are generated when a crossover occurs between two linked markers (see Fig. 14-3). In

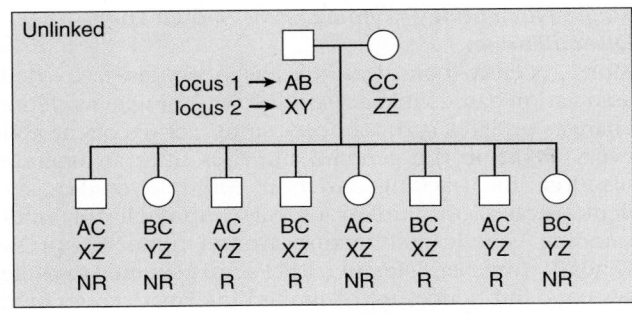

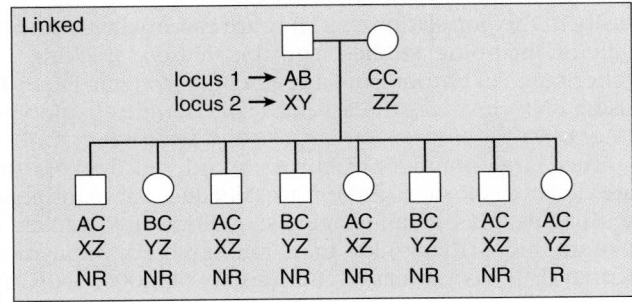

Figure 14-4. Linked and unlinked markers segregating in two families. Below the symbols, the genotypes for both markers are listed. Offspring have either recombinant (R) or nonrecombinant (NR) haplotypes. The father is heterozygous for marker 1, AB, and marker 2, XY; and the mother is homozygous for both markers, CC and ZZ. **A,** If the markers were unlinked, there would be equal numbers of R and NR haplotypes from the father (AX, BY, AY, and BX). **B,** There is an excess of NR haplotypes (AX and BY), and only one R haplotype appears. Therefore these loci are linked.

Figure 14-4, the father is a heterozygote for two loci (AB for locus 1 and XY for locus 2). The mother is homozygous at both of the same loci, but with different alleles (CC and ZZ), and as a result, all offspring will inherit the C, Z haplotype. If these two markers are unlinked, as they would be if they were on different chromosomes or far apart on the same chromosome, four types of gametes would be expected from the father (*A,X; B,Y; A,Y; and B,X*) in approximately equal proportions (Fig. 14-4*A*). However, if the markers are linked (Fig. 14-4*B*), the father would be expected to produce an excess of the two "parental" haplotypes (*A,X* and *B,Y*), over a smaller number of the "nonparental" or "recombinant" haplotypes (*A,Y* and *B,X*).

Undertaking Genome-Wide Scans

Marker Informativeness

Key to the success of any genome scan is the development of a well-defined set of markers that completely spans the genome at defined intervals. The number of markers used sets the resolution of the resulting scan. A 10-cM genome scan, for instance, will only allow localization of a disease locus to within 5 million base pairs, whereas a 1-cM density scan, composed of approximately 3000 markers, will localize a gene to within half a million base pairs.

A genetic marker, by definition, has two or more alleles. If the frequency of the most common allele is less than

95%, the marker is said to be *polymorphic*. One measure of polymorphism is called *polymorphism information content (PIC)*.[30] PIC defines the probability that the genotype of a specific offspring will be sufficiently informative to determine which of two parental alleles has been inherited. Markers are assigned PIC values between 0 (minimally informative) and 1.0 (perfectly informative). A second measure of polymorphism is called *heterozygosity*. Heterozygosity (H) is calculated as: $H = 1 - \Sigma (Pi)^2$. Pi is a measure of the allele frequencies for a given marker in the population under consideration.[31]

There are currently several thousand well-characterized markers with assigned PIC values whose chromosomal locations in the human genome are well known.[32] Sets of markers known to be very polymorphic and to have 5-cM or 10-cM spacing, and thus optimized for genome-wide scans, are commercially available for the human, mouse, rat, and dog genomes. The advantage of using commercially prepared marker sets is that the markers have often been multiplexed; therefore, it is usually possible to analyze several markers simultaneously (Fig. 14-5).

Several different types of markers for genetic linkage mapping are currently in use. In the late 1980s, the most frequently used markers for genetic mapping were based on restriction fragment length polymorphisms (RFLPs),[33] which could be assayed by a technique called *Southern blotting*.[34] RFLP mapping is based on the idea that a single base change in DNA sequence will create or destroy a bacterial restriction enzyme site. After digestion with an appropriate purified enzyme and electrophoretic separation through a gel matrix, digested DNA is transferred to a membrane and probed for the presence or absence of sequence-defining enzyme sites by using radioactively labeled DNA fragments or probes. After its introduction in

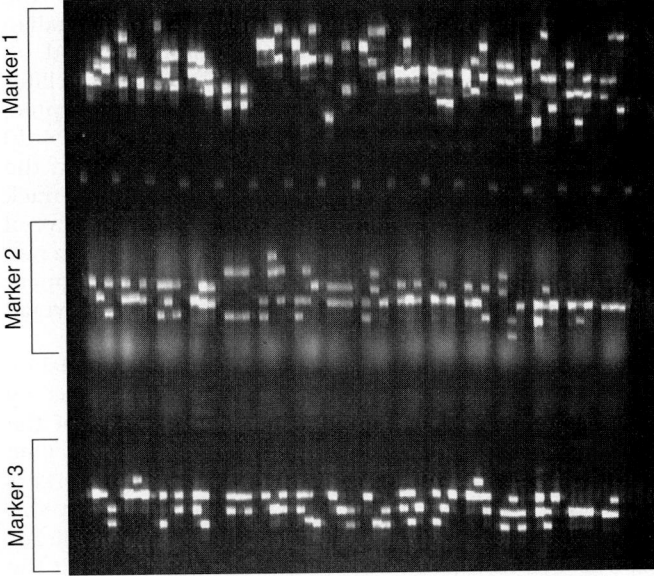

Figure 14-5. Image of data from a denaturing acrylamide gel run on a LICOR automated sequencer. Each sample lane contains results from a single individual. From top to bottom the three groupings of horizontal bands indicate microsatellite markers 1, 2, and 3. Every fourth lane (left to right) contains size standards used to automatically size each allele.

Science of Clinical Oncology

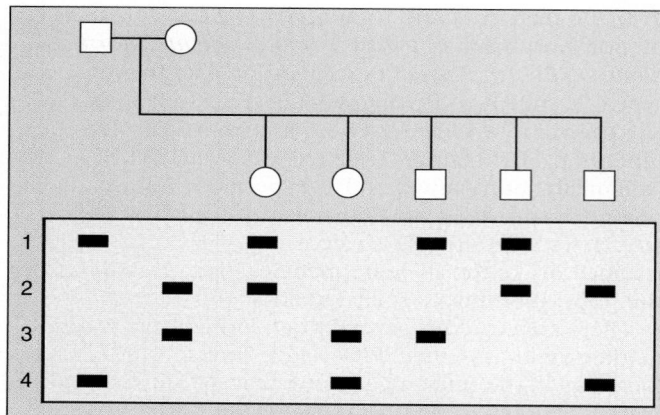

Figure 14-6. Schematic agarose gel electrophoresis of a microsatellite marker analyzed on a single family. Males are indicated by squares and females by circles. Four alleles are segregating; the father has alleles 1 and 4 and the mother carries alleles 2 and 3. Each child has inherited one allele from each parent, together with the surrounding genomic information.

the early 1980s, RFLP mapping rapidly gained popularity because it allowed researchers to scan nearly any region of the genome of interest within 2 to 3 days.[35] The approach fell from popularity in the late 1980s with the discovery of polymerase chain reaction–based methods,[36] which offered investigators comparatively quicker and more precise ways to detect DNA sequence variation.[37,38]

For the last several years, most genome-wide scans have exclusively used microsatellite-based markers. Microsatellites are small stretches of repetitive DNA, composed of repeated motifs of mono-, di-, tri-, or tetranucleotides, such as (CA)n or (GAG)n, located randomly in the genome.[39-41] They occur frequently in mammalian populations, with a dinucleotide (CA)n repeat found, on average, every 30 to 60 kilobases (kb).[41,42] Microsatellites occurring in human DNA are extremely polymorphic, with a given marker occasionally having in excess of 20 alleles. Microsatellite alleles are sufficiently stable in the population and therefore can be reliably used to track inheritance of chromosomal segments through several generations in a family. Yet with an estimated mutation rate of 5×10^{-4} to 10^{-5} per allele per meiosis, new alleles appear frequently in the population, contributing to their overall utility as genetic markers.[43]

Individual microsatellite markers are distinguished from one another after amplification of the locus by polymerase chain reaction (PCR) and separation of the resulting alleles by electrophoresis[37,38] (Fig. 14-6). One disadvantage of (CA)n repeat-based microsatellite markers is that the resulting variant alleles are so similar in size that they can sometimes be hard to separate on a gel. For this reason, most genome scans today are done with the use of commercially prepared sets of markers based largely on tri- and tetra-nucleotide repeats. Although less frequent than (CA)n repeats, they are easier to automate, and the resulting data are assessed with generally lower error rates.

Single Nucleotide Polymorphisms and Linkage Disequilibrium

More recently, consideration has been given to doing association-based linkage studies with single nucleotide changes or SNPs (pronounced "snips"). SNPs occur about every 11 kb in the genome and thus offer an unending resource for tracking variation. Multiple studies have demonstrated the utility of this approach for understanding genetic architecture around tumor suppressor genes.[44] However, SNPs, like RFLPs, are generally two-allele systems, and hence, are of limited informativeness in any genome scan. In addition, many changes occur with such rarity in the population that they are essentially useless for genetic mapping studies. For this reason, tracking the inheritance of chromosomal segments through a family by using SNPs involves the assembly of data into haplotypes (Fig. 14-7).

Very large numbers of correctly ordered markers that are spaced close together are needed to map genes with SNPs.[45] Because linkage disequilibrium is unlikely to extend more than 3 kb in a random-bred population, Kruglyak[45] has estimated that some 500,000 SNPs are required for whole-genome studies of families collected from an outbreed population. To reduce the workload, researchers are focusing increasingly on studying families from inbred populations. The advantages of examining inbred populations are two-fold. First, fewer disease alleles are predicted to segregate with a particular phenotype in a restricted population. Second, nonrandom mapping and restriction of the gene pool make it likely that only a few alleles, and occasionally even only one highly penetrant allele, will be responsible for a particular disease in the population.

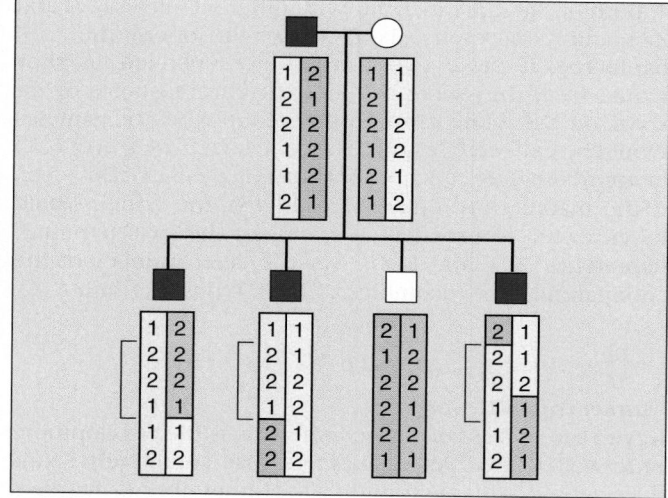

Figure 14-7. SNP haplotypes in a prostate cancer family. Males are indicated by squares and females by circles. Each individual's haplotype for a chromosomal region of interest is drawn below the symbols. The father's two haplotypes are blue or green and the mother's are red or yellow. The three affected brothers and father all share the haplotype shaded blue, whereas the unaffected brother has inherited the haplotype shaded green. There are recombination events in brothers 2 and 4, restricting the region of interest to that defined by SNPs 2, 3, and 4 (indicated by the brackets).

Studies of colon cancer in Finland and studies of breast cancer in Iceland and in Ashkenazi Jewish populations illustrate the advantages of studying restricted populations very well. In Finland, two mutations in the DNA mismatch repair gene, *MLH1*, termed *mutations 1* and *2*, account for 51% of all Finnish families with verified or putative cases of hereditary nonpolyposis colorectal cancer.[46] Nineteen *mutation 1* and six *mutation 2* families were further investigated by haplotype analysis, by using 15 microsatellite markers surrounding the *MLH1* locus. The presence of a large conserved disease haplotype in both *mutation 1* and *mutation 2* families indicated that these families are likely to descend from two common ancestors (one with *mutation 1* and one with *mutation 2*) born in the sixteenth century and eighteenth century, respectively.[46]

For the breast cancer susceptibility genes, *BRCA1* and *BRCA2*, several founder mutations have been identified in different populations.[47] For instance, a single *BRCA2* mutation, 999del5, was found in 16 of 21 Icelandic breast cancer families.[48] All 16 of these families share a *BRCA2* haplotype, suggesting a common population origin. Studies of breast cancer in Jewish families have also demonstrated this point, contributing enormously to our knowledge of founding mutations in both the *BRCA1* and *BRCA2* genes.[49,50] The three common founder mutations in this population, *BRCA1*-185delAG, 5382insC, and *BRCA2*-6174delT, have a combined prevalence of 2% to 2.5%. This is 10 to 50 times higher than the general population frequency of these alleles.[47,49,51,52] With these observations in mind, investigators have frequently sought families for genetic mapping studies from regions of the world where marriage between related individuals is not taboo and where geographic barriers have restricted gene flow. Even more desirable are populations, like that of Finland, in which the number of founders is small.[53] This is especially true for prostate cancer, which is a heterogeneous disease, and the relative genetic homogeneity of Finland may help confirm the role of two hereditary prostate cancer loci, HPC1 and HPCX. Support for the HPCX locus, but not the HPC1 locus, was found in a subset of Finnish families, suggesting that the HPCX locus may contain a founder mutation in Finland.[54]

Genotyping

Once a set of markers has been selected and DNA samples from the families in the study have been isolated, several automated methods are available for genotyping DNA samples. Among the most popular is the Applied Biosystems (ABI) Capillary system. The GeneScan software displays the peaks for all four fluorescent dyes: red, yellow, green, and blue (Fig. 14-8A). In Figure 14-8A, there are 10 microsatellite markers multiplexed in a single run. Genotyper software will display results from the four dyes individually (Fig. 14-8B), as well as assign the marker names, allele sizes, and band intensities for each peak.

Measures of Linkage

Calculating Lod Scores

On completion of a genome-wide scan, extensive checking is done by using programs such as PEDCHECK,

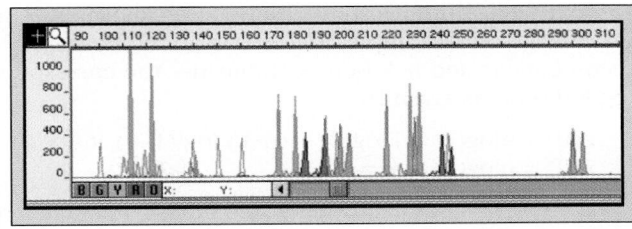

A

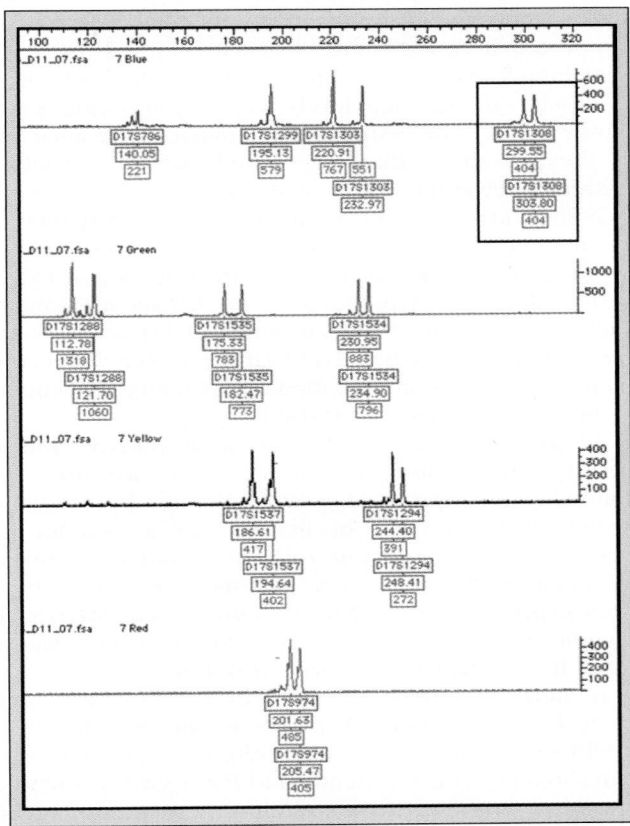

B

Figure 14-8. Genotyping data from the Applied Biosystems (ABI) Capillary sequencer. **A,** The output from GeneScan analysis. Output shows the signal peaks from one individual for the 10 microsatellite markers multiplexed in this specific run. The peaks are displayed according to color and size from 90 base pairs (bp) on the left to 310 bp on the right. **B,** The Genotyper program output shown assigns genotypes for each of the microsatellite markers. Information about the peaks is listed below the graph. The yellow boxes list marker names, green boxes indicate allele sizes, and the red box shows peak intensity. The box indicates one microsatellite marker, D17S1308. This individual is a heterozygote with 300 bp and 304 bp alleles.

PREST, and RELPAIR to detect potential genotyping errors by checking, for instance, Mendelian inheritance.[55-57] Data are then analyzed to determine which, if any, markers are closely linked to a putative disease locus. The likelihood for linkage ($\theta < 0.5$) versus the likelihood for recombination ($\theta = 0.5$) is calculated based on the number of observed recombinant and nonrecombinant offspring produced by a given mating. Conventionally, the logarithm of the likelihood ratio, or lod score, is

$$Z(\theta) = \log_{10} [L(\theta) / L(0.5)]$$

and is used as the measure of support for linkage versus nonlinkage. For example, if n observations consist of k recombinants and n–k nonrecombinants, the corresponding lod score is given by

$$Z(\theta) = n\log(2) + k\log(\theta) + (n-k) \log (1-\theta), \text{ if } \theta > 0.$$
$$Z(\theta) = n\log(2), \text{ if } \theta = 0.$$

It is often stated that linkage is "found;" that is, a marker under consideration is said to be linked to a putative disease locus when a recombination fraction of $\theta < 0.5$ is supported by a lod score of at least 3.0.[58] However, in searching for genes, it is important to distinguish between pointwise significance levels and genome-wide significance levels.[59] The pointwise or nominal significance level is the probability that one would encounter such an extreme deviation at a specific locus by chance. The genome-wide significance level is the probability that one would encounter such a deviation somewhere in the whole genome scan. The former is an evaluation of a single test of the null hypothesis of no linkage (testing for linkage of a favorite candidate gene to a disease locus); the latter involves screening over a large number of tests (i.e., running a large number of markers spanning the genome) to find the most significant result.

In assessing the significance of a putative linkage result, Lander and Kruglyak[59] have assigned the following descriptors. *Suggestive linkage* is that which would be expected to occur one time at random in a genome scan. *Significant linkage* would be expected to occur 0.05 times in a genome-wide scan. *Highly significant linkage* that is considered statistically significant is expected to occur 0.001 times in a genome scan. It is generally the norm to report all regions with a nominal *P* value of $P = .05$ in a complete genome scan. These may indicate places in the genome where additional families, markers, or both are needed. A lod threshold of 3.3, corresponding to $P = 5 \times 10^5$, is the value that is now accepted as indicating a genome-wide significance level of 5%. Thus in the context of a genome-wide scan, a marker is said to be linked to a disease locus if a lod score of 3.3 is achieved.[59]

Limitations and Sources of Error

Linkage analysis is an inherently error-prone approach. It is fairly easy to arrive at an incorrect conclusion because of the large number of assumptions that must be made in the calculation. For instance, calculation of lod scores is dependent on accuracy of the linkage model.[60] In addition, studies have shown that lod score analysis of a small number of families is very sensitive to changes in a few key data points. Small errors in genotyping or misclassification of affected status have the potential to artificially inflate or deflate a particular lod score. Consider, for example, age at onset. The linkage calculation will weigh the value of information provided by any given family member compared with that of every other person in the study. So if early onset of disease is a defining part of the phenotype associated with a proposed breast cancer locus, the genotyping data from a woman who had breast cancer at the age of 30 years will be considered more readily than that from a woman who had the disease at age 80. The latter represents an age at which approximately one in ten women will have breast cancer for reasons not associated with highly penetrant alleles. Therefore it is vitally important that the clinician participating in the study obtain the most current and accurate information available from any patient who is likely to be a study participant, including the age at which various family members had cancer.

One additional problem with this type of calculation is the loss of power associated with missing data. In principle, an individual who is a heterozygote at two loci A and B (*AaBa*) could have received his or her *A* allele in coupling with either the *B* or the *b* allele from one parent. To distinguish recombinants from nonrecombinants, the parental and nonparental haplotypes must be known. If the A and B alleles were inherited together on the same chromosome, they are said to be in *phase*. Unfortunately, when mapping diseases such as cancer with older ages of onset, two generation families are typically all that are available for sampling, thus limiting the ability to determine phase. However, collection and analysis of data from spouses or offspring of deceased affected individuals is often a way to reassemble the genotype of the deceased individual. Similarly, collection of DNA samples from unaffected siblings can be very useful for establishing parental phase.

Nonparametric Analysis

Because calculation of lod scores is dependent on models of linkage that are notoriously difficult to derive,[61] researchers are turning toward nonparametric linkage (NPL), or nonmodel-based approaches for mapping genes.[62] Such approaches use only the data from affected individuals; thus no assumptions are made as to whether an unaffected person is more or less likely to have cancer, and if so at what age. In an NPL analysis, haplotypes are built across the relevant regions of the genome by using

---

It is noteworthy that there is frequent confusion in the literature about lod scores versus probability measures. Again, according to the example provided by Lander and Kruglyak, a lod score of 3.0 means the observed data are 1000 times more likely to arise under a specific hypothesis of linkage than under the null hypothesis of independent assortment. A *P* value of 10^{-3} means that the probability of encountering as large a lod score as is observed is 10^{-3} under the null hypothesis.

Clinicians often choose to participate in studies that are aimed at confirmation of previously published linkage reports. For confirmation of published findings of linkage in an independent data set, a nominal *P* value of .01 is required. Because linkage from any previously published reports may hinge on precise features of the clinical diagnosis or stratification of the data set based on features of family history, it is vital that participating physicians record their clinical observations as accurately as possible.

computer programs such as GENEHUNTER.[62] The data are compared, and *P* values are calculated to assess the degree of significance observed between inheritance of a disease state and a specific haplotype.

Nonparametric approaches have the disadvantage of being less powerful than lod score–based approaches, because data from unaffected individuals, which could have contributed to the lod score, do not contribute to the NPL score. For diseases that are genetically heterogeneous, such as common cancers, this is more than made up for by the lack of reliance on incomplete or inaccurate linkage models.

One final consideration is that of age at diagnosis versus age at onset, which, depending on the disease and available diagnostics, can differ by several years. Diagnosis of prostate cancer by prostate specific antigen (PSA) testing provides an interesting example. The widespread use of screening for prostate cancer by serum PSA measurements, as well as digital rectal examination, has dramatically changed the patterns of disease incidence in the United States.[63] Rates increased rapidly between 1986 and 1993, in part because of the detection of latent prostate tumors in the general population as a result of PSA screening.[64] It is generally believed that PSA can detect tumors from 2 to 5 years earlier than previous methods.[65-67] Therefore, data from a man given a diagnosis of prostate cancer at age 65 in 1995 should contribute differentially to a genome scan than data from a man given the diagnosis at the same age in 1975. The man given the diagnosis in 1975, assuming he participated in screening, would probably have been given the diagnosis in his early sixties if he were alive today.

It is also important to note the difference between untested and unaffected individuals. Patients are more likely know that they are truly unaffected with a disease such as prostate cancer (as defined by PSA status) than they are likely to know they are truly unaffected with other cancers, such as pancreatic or ovarian cancer, for which vigilant screening is not the norm. For this reason, in some genome-wide scans for cancer susceptibly genes, clinical status of putatively unaffected individuals may be coded as "unknown" rather then "unaffected." It is important that the interviewing physician make the distinction when recording any patient's family and medical history.

Positional Cloning Resources

Meiotic linkage studies may define a region of interest as small as a few thousand bases or as big as several million bases. The latter may span more than a hundred genes[68,69] and must be further reduced before mutation scanning can realistically begin. Several strategies exist for narrowing the search. Among the most common is the search for genomic rearrangements in tumors, which may indicate chromosomal regions where cancer susceptibility genes are likely to be located. Genomic rearrangements in tumors can be assayed in a variety of ways, with an overall goal of defining minimal regions of genomic loss and then selecting candidate genes for further study. These are discussed in the following sections.

Loss of Heterozygosity in Tumors

One assay commonly used for this purpose is loss of heterozygosity (LOH). LOH detects chromosomal deletions within tumor cell populations by comparing allele patterns from a single individual's normal cells and tumor cells at a set of ordered genetic markers. Most LOH studies to date have focused on a limited number of chromosomes. For best use of the technique, high-density, genome-wide scans of 300 to 400 markers are needed. The point at which a pattern changes from two haplotypes, representing the heterozygous state of the normal cell, to a single haplotype, representing the loss of all or part of one chromosomal arm containing a putative cancer gene, is used to define the boundaries of LOH for a single tumor. To date, multiple regions of LOH have been defined for essentially all tumor types, in some situations facilitating understanding of the function of the underlying genes. In some cases, the delineation of LOH boundaries has been a useful way to narrow a region of interest initially defined by genetic linkage analysis.

Comparative Genome Hybridization

If more information is desired, comparative genome hybridization (CGH) can be used to look at gains and losses of chromosomal regions in tumors.[70,71] CGH allows investigators to perform genome-wide analysis of DNA sequence copy number in a single tissue. In this procedure, differentially labeled genomic DNA from a "test" and a "reference" cell population are cohybridized to normal metaphase chromosome spreads. Blocking DNA is added to the experimental mix to suppress repetitive sequences. Regions of gain or loss of DNA sequences, such as deletions, duplications, or amplifications, are seen as changes in the ratio of the intensities of the two fluorochromes. The procedure works because the ratio of fluorescence intensities along the length of the chromosome is proportional to the ratio of the copy numbers of the corresponding DNA sequences in the test and reference genomes at each point in the chromosome. More recent innovations with this technique allow investigators to circumvent the low resolution associated with metaphase spreads and very precisely determine DNA copy number by combining traditional CGH with arrays.[72]

Tissue Banks and Expression Arrays

One problem not infrequently associated with LOH and CGH studies is lack of reproducibility across studies. This is due to both the limited number of tumors typically available for studies and the heterogeneity in the tumors themselves, reflecting in all likelihood genetic heterogeneity of the disease. One way to circumvent both problems is to develop tumor banks in which investigators can deposit well-characterized tissues for a variety of research purposes.[73] One potential complication is the rigor with which such banks must be maintained. It is important that complete pathologic records accompany each tissue and that the tissue deposited be as free as possible of adjacent noncancerous tissue. Toward this end, researchers have turned increasingly to the use of laser capture microdissection as a way to isolate virtually pure populations of tumor for LOH and CGH studies.[74]

One other method for refining linkage data before proceeding with candidate genome analysis is the use of expression arrays. Expression arrays analyze differences in gene expression on a large scale by assaying thousands of genes in one experiment. For one type, DNA microarrays, DNA sequences from the coding regions of known or putative genes are assayed with probes made from messenger RNA, which determines an expression profile of genes for a certain cell type or experimental condition. In terms of cancer genomics, normal cells may express different portions of the genome or different genes at different levels when compared with their neoplastic counterparts, which may indicate biologic networks or pathways involved in disease pathogenesis.[75] Microarray experiments have led to molecular classification of many cancer types according to differences in gene expression, including breast cancer,[76] lymphomas,[77] and soft-tissue tumors.[78] Integration of DNA microarray data with genetic mapping results will help to prioritize candidate genes in regions of known linkage.

Finally, it is worth noting that even in these days of human genome sequence availability and vast amounts of expression data, refinement of any specific region of interest before candidate gene assessment may require classic positional cloning techniques.[79] BAC or YAC physical contigs may need to be made across a region of interest, and then techniques such as exon trapping or direct hybridization may be used to find the coding sequences of interest.[80] As single gene traits are defined and researchers' interest turns increasingly to multigene traits, a combination of traditional and twenty-first century approaches will most likely define the genes of interest.[81]

Assessment of Candidate Genes

Once a candidate gene is proposed, it is important to determine whether sequence level changes in the gene are associated with the disease of interest. Association studies are distinct from linkage analysis in that a specific alteration in a candidate gene is assessed in both affected and unaffected individuals to determine whether the variant is found more often in individuals with the disease and whether the observation is statistically significant.

Candidate genes are identified in a variety of ways. For instance, the biologic function of a known gene may suggest a role in cancer susceptibility. Alternatively, the sequence of the gene may suggest it is a member of a protein family known to play a role in cancer biology. Genes that are important in DNA repair, apoptosis, and cell cycle regulation are all likely candidates. Finally, the gene in question may be located at a locus identified by linkage analysis of high-risk families. Thus it may be one of a large number of genes under consideration.

The breast cancer susceptibility loci *BRCA1* and *BRCA2* again provide an interesting example. Both were identified after a large number of other candidate genes within the linked regions of chromosomes 17 and 13, respectively, were analyzed.[20,22] In both cases, protein-truncating mutations were found to segregate with affected women in multiple high-risk families,[82-84] and protein-truncating mutations in both genes were

determined to be rare in women drawn from the general population.[85-87] Still to be determined is the relative importance of a large number of missense changes in both genes that have been reported in individual women with breast cancer.[88,89] However, in each case, the analysis of high-risk families allowed investigators to easily conclude that the disease-causing genes had been identified.

Association Studies

Unfortunately, the certain identification of a cancer susceptibility gene is seldom as straightforward as that described previously. For these reasons, association studies are frequently performed to determine whether alleles of a particular gene are disease-associated. Two primary types of study design are typically used: cohort and case-control studies. In a cohort study, subjects are selected on the basis of an exposure of interest and monitored over time to determine whether and when they will develop cancer and the degree to which the exposure is associated with disease. In genetic epidemiology, the "exposure" is the gene variant under consideration. This type of cohort study is prospective in nature; both the exposure and the health outcomes (presence or absence of cancer over time) occur after the enrollment of study subjects. The advantages of cohort studies include minimized bias and the ability to calculate RR directly. RR is the risk of developing a disease given a particular exposure and is calculated as the likelihood of developing cancer among a set of individuals with a particular genotype, divided by the likelihood of developing cancer among a set of individuals who do not carry that genotype. Disadvantages include the fact that prospective cohort studies are time-consuming and large numbers of study subjects are typically required to obtain sufficient power to determine associations. Loss of subjects to long-term follow-up over time is also an issue because it may affect ability to draw conclusions and is an issue over which investigators have little control.

Cohort studies may also be retrospective in nature, when the exposure and subsequent development of the disease occur before the study begins. For the purpose of finding associations between disease status and genotype, retrospective cohorts depend on existing medical records to identify individuals with cancer and therefore are subject to recall bias,[90-93] which can introduce error into the study.[94] Fortunately, the exposure in genetic epidemiology is a particular genotype, which does not change over time and therefore is not subject to recall bias.

Case-control studies differ from cohort studies in that the selection of subjects is based on their disease status. Case-control studies can use smaller sample sizes than an equivalent cohort study and have the potential to examine multiple risk factors simultaneously. Two very popular case-control designs are population-based and hospital-based. For each, it is important to select case patients and control subjects who are similar in all variables including age, race, socioeconomic status, and ethnic background.[95-100]

Population-based, case-control studies draw on a well-defined source population such as a particular geographic region defined by state, county, or city for ascertainment of both case patients and unaffected control subjects. Popular mechanisms include use of cancer registries, such as Surveillance Epidemiology and End Results (SEER), or health care provider databases. Control subjects should be selected from the same source population or geographic region by a method designed to randomly sample individuals, such as random digit telephone dialing.[101] Selection bias, in which selection of case patients, control subjects, or both is influenced by prior exposures, is a particular concern in case-control studies.[98-100,102,103] Proper design of the selection process can help reduce this problem. Multiple studies have shown, for instance, that nonparticipants in such studies are more likely to smoke than individuals who agree to participate.[103]

In comparison, hospital-based, case-control studies enlist a sequential series of patients who are admitted to the hospital or clinic during a specific period. Case patients are enrolled because they have the cancer of interest, whereas control subjects are determined to be cancer-free, although they may be patients at the same clinic or hospital for unrelated reasons. Significantly more potential for bias exists in hospital-based case-control studies. Depending on the clinic or hospital from which patients are drawn, disease presentation, severity, and treatment outcome may be nonrandom among study subjects. Often cases are drawn from so called "high risk" clinics. In such situations, both case patients and control subjects may be more likely to carry a specific genotype. They may have been referred to a high-risk clinic because of their family history status. Thus, it may be difficult to generalize results from a hospital-based case-control study to the general population.

Confounders and Sources of Bias

Confounders are any factors that are associated with the exposure, as well as the disease, and are outside of the causal pathway of the exposure. In the study of genetic risk factors and disease, an important confounder is ethnic background. For example, in a study of the association between human leukocyte antigen (HLA) genotypes and cervical cancer, ethnic background must be addressed as a potential confounder because HLA genotypes can vary by ethnic background, and lifestyle factors that contribute to disease can be associated with ethnic differences.[104] When the association between HLA genotype and cancer was calculated, ethnic background was adjusted to minimize the potential for bias caused by this confounder.[104]

Another source of bias specific to case-control studies and retrospective cohorts is recall bias.[94] Study subjects may find it difficult to correctly remember information related to subjective factors that are potentially important in disease susceptibility such as those related to diet, exercise, and stress.[105] Recall bias can lead to incorrect or incomplete measurement of a potential confounder. This introduces error into the calculation of the association between the exposure and the disease because of the inability to fully adjust for the effects of confounders.

SNP Genotyping and Association Studies

In an ideal situation, collection of blood samples from all study subjects is undertaken as part of any genetic

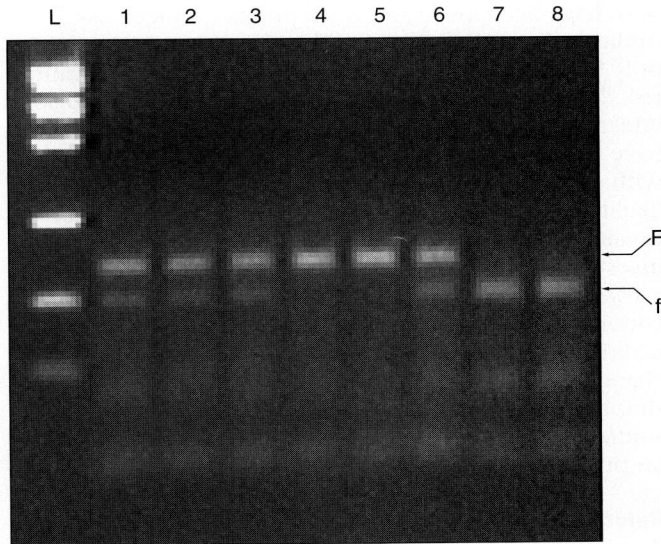

Figure 14-9. Restriction fragment SNP gel for the *FokI* vitamin D receptor polymorphism. The L lane is a size standard ladder, and lanes 1 to 8 are individual samples. There are two bands indicated by arrows. The smaller fragment (f) is cleaved by the *FokI* enzyme, whereas the larger band (F) is uncut by *FokI*. Lanes 4 and 5 have homozygous FF individuals. Alternatively, lanes 7 and 8 are ff homozygous, and the remaining individuals are heterozygous, Ff.

epidemiology study. The resulting DNA samples can then be used to assay for association of candidate genes and features of disease. In the literature to date, two types of assays have been frequently used. The presence of a particular SNP will frequently create or destroy a restriction enzyme site. To assay, DNA samples can be amplified by PCR, the resulting amplicon digested with an appropriate restriction enzyme, and the products separated by electrophoresis on agarose gels (Fig. 14-9). In situations in which a restriction enzyme assay is not possible and in cases involving small insertions or deletions, PCR primers are used to amplify the region of interest, and the resulting product is examined by direct sequencing.

SNPs that introduce nonsense changes, causing premature termination of the protein, and SNPs that alter a key amino acid sequence in the encoded protein are the focus of much of the current literature on nearly all cancers.[106] Other SNPs of interest change single amino acids in key protein motifs or occur in splice regions. Much less well understood are SNPs found to be in association with the disease state but located in noncoding regions of the gene.[107-109] Association studies are observational in nature and define genotypes or exposures that are simply "associated" with a particular disease, but they may not actually cause the disease of interest. In such situations, the SNP is thought to be in linkage disequilibrium with an as yet unidentified disease-causing mutation.

SNPs within the vitamin D receptor (VDR) gene provide a set of interesting examples. Single base changes in intron 8 and within exon 9 affect recognition sites for the restriction enzymes *BsmI* and *TaqI*. Neither variant apparently affects the resulting protein sequence, but both have been associated with prostate cancer risk.[107,109] Additionally, variation in the 3′ untranslated region of the poly A tail is similarly associated with prostate cancer risk,[108] but the alteration appears to have no obvious effect on mRNA stability.[110] All three polymorphisms have been reported to be in at least partial association with one another in a subset of studies, and in all likelihood, serve as markers for an undiscovered disease-causing variant.[110,111] In addition to these variants, some investigators report a variant in exon 2, which creates a *FokI* restriction enzyme site and results in a new start codon for the protein, generating a transcript with three additional amino acids.[112] It is unknown whether this change itself is disease-associated or whether it, too, is simply a marker for an unknown variant. Functional studies are needed to test the role of all of these variants on protein function.

Relative Risks

Results of an association study are evaluated by calculation of a RR or odds ratio (OR). Values greater than 1.0 indicate that the exposure (in this case a particular genotype) is associated with an increased risk of the cancer under consideration. In comparison, values between 0 and 1 indicate a decreased risk for the disease associated with that genotype. In cohort studies, RR can be calculated directly as the likelihood of developing cancer among a set of individuals with a particular genotype, divided by the likelihood of developing cancer among a set of individuals who do not carry that genotype. Thus the RR is the risk of developing cancer in the general source population, given a particular genotype.

A different statistical method is used for assessing risk in case-control studies, because subjects are selected according to disease status and not exposure, as they would be in a cohort study. The OR can be an estimation of the RR and is calculated as the odds of exposure for cases divided by the odds of exposure for controls. For both RR and OR, 95% confidence intervals are typically calculated. Statistically significant associations are those in which the 95% confidence interval excludes the null hypothesis or 1.0.

Logistic regression is used to calculate ORs when multiple factors are expected to affect the risk of the disease. Such calculations are done after adjustments are made to account for the contribution of other disease-associated factors. If high-quality information about other characteristics of subjects is collected, data sets can be stratified by age, family history, or clinical features of the disease before calculating the association between genotype and disease, as a way of identifying important modifiers of risk in relation to genotype.

Genetic Testing

Patients will frequently approach clinicians with questions about genetic testing opportunities for specific cancers. If appropriate tests are available, identifying a person with increased risk for a particular cancer is useful for at least three reasons. First, it can suggest a particular clinical course that will reduce the chance of having cancer, such as treatment with tamoxifen or prophylactic surgery for women at risk for hereditary breast cancer.[113-115] Second, it can induce patients at risk to undergo more vigilant screening, such as frequent colonoscopy examinations for patients at risk for colon cancer. Finally, an individual's quality of life can sometimes be improved by having specific knowledge about the true risk for disease or recurrence. Such information is frequently sought by unaffected individuals who perceive themselves to be at increased risk as a consideration in family planning. In addition, patients with cancer often seek information about mutations they may carry to better understand the risks faced by their offspring.

The American Society of Human Genetics defines genetic counseling as a "communication process which deals with the human problems associated with the occurrence or risk of occurrence of a genetic disorder in a family." Therefore it should only be offered in consultation with certified genetic counselors who serve to (1) help patients comprehend the medical facts and risks associated with their disease; (2) help patients understand their alternatives for dealing with both risk of disease and recurrence; (3) help patients choose a clinical course that best meets their needs; and (4) provide support and guidance for patients experiencing difficulty in dealing with unexpected results. Patients often approach genetic testing with strong preconceived notions about the likelihood that they have an inherited mutation. Thus, "unexpected" is likely to apply to both carriers and noncarriers.

In advising patients whether it is appropriate to consider genetic testing, it is important to remember that many currently available tests have limitations. *Clinical validity* is the term used to describe the predictive value of a test for clinical outcomes.[116] It is affected by both the sensitivity and the specificity of the test, as well as a host of factors that are beyond laboratory control such as penetrance of the mutant allele. The latter may itself be a function of genetic background, environmental exposures, or both. Most mutations associated with cancer susceptibility genes are not fully penetrant. So, even a person living into his or her eighties is unlikely to experience a 100% probability of having cancer, even if he or she carries protein-truncating mutations in a particular gene. Helping patients understand these concepts may be difficult.

One additional concern is what to tell patients who do not have obvious protein-truncating mutations but who do carry missense changes in the coding region of a cancer susceptibility gene. Again, particularly interesting examples are provided by the *BRCA1* gene. More than 300 independent missense changes have been reported for *BRCA1* to date.[88] Disease association status is known for only a fraction of these, such as those occurring in the RING finger domain[117] and the C-terminal region of the protein.[118,119] In the case of RING finger mutations, these conclusions are supported by the existence of dozens of families in which RING finger mutations are shown to closely segregate with disease state.[120,121] Other single amino acid changes are known to be inconsequential polymorphisms that clearly do not affect protein function.

For instance, some 40% of the population is heterozygous for the substitution of leucine for proline at position 871, as reported in the canonical sequence. Both residues are hydrophobic, and the location is not one that is well conserved evolutionarily; and this is likely to be an inconsequential polymorphism in the gene. Of particular concern, rather, are the large number of missense changes reported in patients with breast cancer, whose disease association status is unknown. Phylogenetic analysis provides some insight as to which are likely to be important,[122] and functional assays are useful for testing mutations in some regions of the gene.[119,123] However, at this time little guidance is available for most patients carrying such changes.

Implications for the Future

The sequence of the human genome has been referred to as an "instruction book for human biology."[124] Locked within the sequence of each individual's DNA is the genetic code necessary to develop a complete and healthy individual, but encoded as well is the sequence level variation that will determine each person's susceptibility to a host of diseases. Variation is important in defining the field of genomic medicine. A more complete understanding of the molecular pathways involved in cancer susceptibility will suggest avenues for the development of both methods of diagnosis and treatment. Identification of specific genes offers the promise of genetic testing to individuals at risk, as well as the hope for targeted therapeutics. Finally, understanding the specific variation offers the promise of twenty-first century "personalized medicine" in which lifestyle, diet, and preventative therapies come together to offer patients a full spectrum of choices for maintaining their personal health.

It is clear that the Human Genome Project has had and will continue to have an effect on human health and biology.[124] What remains to be seen is the rate at which the successes of the Human Genome Project will move from bench to bedside. In a sense, that rate will be determined by practicing physicians. Knowledge of the underlying principles of genetic analysis is fundamental to today's practicing clinician. The ability to accurately record family history and medical record data affects the integrity of all subsequent studies for which those data are used. An understanding by physicians of the findings generated through both association studies and family-based linkage studies is key to both moving research forward and prioritizing new hypotheses for researchers to consider. Finally, as twentieth century–born patients struggle to make personal health care choices in the twenty-first century, communicating what genomic medicine has to offer is a vital task at which every physician must now excel.

REFERENCES

1. Knudson AG: Chasing the cancer demon. Annu Rev Genet 2000;34:1–19.
2. Goldgar DE, Easton DF, Cannon-Albright LA, Skolnick MH: Systematic population-based assessment of cancer risk in first-degree relatives of cancer probands. J Natl Cancer Inst 1994;86:1600–1608.
3. Easton D, Peto J: The contribution of inherited predisposition to cancer incidence. Cancer Surv 1990;9:395–416.
4. Carter BS, Beaty TH, Steinberg GD, Childs B, Walsh PC: Mendelian inheritance of familial prostate cancer. Proc Natl Acad Sci USA 1992;89:3367–3371.
5. Schaid DJ, McDonnell SK, Blute ML, Thibodeau SN: Evidence for autosomal dominant inheritance of prostate cancer. Am J Hum Genet 1998;62:1425–1438.
6. Grönberg H, Damber L, Damber J-E, Iselius L: Segregation analysis of prostate cancer in Sweden: Support for dominant inheritance. Am J Epidemiol 1997;146:552–557.
7. Claus EB, Risch N, Thompson WD: Genetic analysis of breast cancer in the cancer and steroid hormone study. Am J Hum Genet 1991;48:232–242.
8. Strong LC, Amos C: Inherited susceptibility. In Schottenfeld D, Fraumeni JF (eds): Cancer epidemiology and prevention, 2nd ed. New York, Oxford University Press, 1996, pp 559–583.
9. Ross R, Schottenfeld D: Prostate cancer. In Schottenfeld D, Fraumeni JF (eds): Cancer epidemiology and prevention, 2nd ed. New York, Oxford University Press, 1996, pp 1180–1126.
10. Steinberg GD, Carter BS, Beaty TH, Childs B, Walsh PC: Family history and the risk of prostate cancer. Prostate 1990;17:337–347.
11. Spitz MR, Currier RD, Fueger JJ, Babaian RJ, Newell GR: Familial patterns of prostate cancer: A case control analysis. J Urol 1991;146:1305–1307.
12. Whittemore A, Wu A, Kolonel L, et al: Family history and prostate cancer risk in black, white, and Asian men in the United States and Canada. Am J Epidemiol 1995;141:732–740.
13. Hayes RB, Liff JM, Pottern LM, et al: Prostate cancer risk in US blacks and whites with a family history of cancer. Int J Cancer 1995;60:361–364.
14. Ghadirian P, Howe GR, Hislop TG, Maisonneuve P: Family history of prostate cancer: A multi-center case-control study in Canada. Int J Cancer 1997;70:679–681.
15. Cerhan JR, Parker AS, Putnam SD, et al: Family history and prostate cancer risk in a population-based cohort of Iowa men. Cancer Epidemiol Biomarkers Prev 1999;8:53–60.
16. Ostrander EA, Stanford JL: Genetics of prostate cancer: Too many loci, too few genes. Am J Hum Genet 2000;67:1367–1375.
17. Smith JR, Freije D, Carpten JD, et al: Major susceptibility locus for prostate cancer on chromosome 1 suggested by a genome-wide search. Science 1996;274:1371–1374.
18. Gibbs M, Stanford JL, McIndoe RA, et al: Evidence for a rare prostate cancer-susceptibility locus at chromosome 1p36. Am J Hum Genet 1999;64:776–787.
19. Hall JM, Lee MK, Newman B, et al: Linkage of early onset familial breast cancer to chromosome 17q21. Science 1990;250:1684–1689.
20. Wooster R, Neuhausen SL, Mangion J, et al: Localization of a breast cancer susceptibility gene, BRCA2, to chromosome 13q12-13. Science 1994;265:2088–2090.
21. Peto J, Collins N, Barfoot R, et al: Prevalence of BRCA1 and BRCA2 gene mutations in patients with early-onset breast cancer. J Natl Cancer Inst 1999;91:943–949.
22. Miki Y, Swensen J, Shattuck-Eidens D, et al: A strong candidate for the breast and ovarian cancer susceptibility gene BRCA1. Science 1994;266:66–71.
23. Presciuttini S, Strigini P: Genetic epidemiology of colorectal cancer. Tumori 1996;82:107–113.
24. Sellers TA, Chen PL, Potter JD, Bailey-Wilson JE, Rothschild H, Elston RC: Segregation analysis of smoking-associated malignancies: Evidence for Mendelian inheritance. Am J Med Genet 1994;52:308–314.
25. Malmer B, Iselius L, Holmberg E, Collins A, Henriksson R, Grönberg H: Genetic epidemiology of glioma. Br J Cancer 2001;84:429–434.
26. Banke MG, Mulvihill JJ, Aston CE: Inheritance of pancreatic cancer in pancreatic cancer-prone families. Med Clin North Am 2000;84:677–690, x–xi.
27. Jarvik GP, Stanford JL, Goode EL, et al: Confirmation of prostate cancer susceptibility genes using high risk families. Monogr Natl Cancer Inst 1999;26:81–88.

28. Morgan TH: The theory of genes. New Haven, Conn., Yale University Press, 1928.

29. Morgan TH: Random segregation versus coupling in Mendelian inheritance. Science 1911;34:384.

30. Botstein D, White RL, Skolnick M, Davis RW: Construction of a genetic linkage map in man using restriction fragment length polymorphisms. Am J Hum Genet 1980;32:314-331.

31. Ott J: Genetic loci and genetic polymorphisms. In: Analysis of Human Genetic Linkage, 3rd ed. Baltimore, John Hopkins University, 1999, pp 24-36.

32. Broman KW, Murray JC, Sheffield VC, White RL, Weber JL: Comprehensive human genetic maps: Individual and sex-specific variation in recombination. Am J Hum Genet 1998;63:861-869.

33. White R, Lalouel JM: Chromosome mapping with DNA markers. Sci Am 1988;258:40-48.

34. Southern EM: Detection of specific sequences among DNA fragments separated by gel electrophoresis. J Mol Biol 1975;98:503-517.

35. Wyman AR, White R: A highly polymorphic locus in human DNA. Proc Natl Acad Sci USA 1980;77:6754-6758.

36. Saiki RK, Gelfand DH, Stoffel S, et al: Primer-directed enzymatic amplification of DNA with a thermostable DNA polymerase. Science 1988;239:487-491.

37. Weber JL, May PE: Abundant class of human DNA polymorphisms which can be typed using the polymerase chain reaction. Am J Hum Genet 1989;44:388-396.

38. Litt M, Luty JA: A hypervariable microsatellite revealed by in vitro amplification of a dinucleotide repeat within the cardiac muscle actin gene. Am J Hum Genet 1989;44:397-401.

39. Hamada H, Kakunaga T: Potential Z-DNA forming sequences are highly dispersed in the human genome. Nature 1982;298:396-398.

40. Miesfeld R, Krystal M, Arnheim N: A member of a new repeated sequence family which is conserved throughout eucaryotic evolution is found between the human delta and beta globin genes. Nucleic Acids Res 1981;9:5931-5947.

41. Stallings RL, Ford AF, Nelson D, Torney DC, Hildebrand CE, Moyzis RK: Evolution and distribution of (GT)n repetitive sequences in mammalian genomes. Genomics 1991;10:807-815.

42. Ostrander EA, Sprague GF Jr, Rine J: Identification and characterization of dinucleotide repeat (CA)n markers for genetic mapping in dog. Genomics 1993;16:207-213.

43. Kwiatkowski DJ, Henske EP, Weimer K, Ozelius L, Gusella JF, Haines J: Construction of a GT polymorphism map of human 9q. Genomics 1992;12:229-240.

44. Bonnen PE, Wang PJ, Kimmel M, Chakraborty R, Nelson DL: Haplotype and linkage disequilibrium architecture for human cancer-associated genes. Genome Res 2002;12:1846-1853.

45. Kruglyak L: Prospects for whole-genome linkage disequilibrium mapping of common disease genes. Nat Genet 1999;22:139-144.

46. Moisio AL, Sistonen P, Weissenbach J, de la Chapelle A, Peltomaki P: Age and origin of two common MLH1 mutations predisposing to hereditary colon cancer. Am J Hum Genet 1996;59:1243-1251.

47. Neuhausen SL: Ethnic differences in cancer risk resulting from genetic variation. Cancer 1999;86(suppl 8):1755-1762.

48. Thorlacius S, Olafsdottir G, Tryggvadottir L, et al: A single BRCA2 mutation in male and female breast cancer families from Iceland with varied cancer phenotypes [see comments]. Nat Genet 1996;13:117-119.

49. Struewing JP, Abeliovich D, Peretz T, et al: The carrier frequency of the *BRCA1* 185delAG mutation is approximately 1 percent in Ashkenazi Jewish individuals. Nat Genet 1995;11:198-200.

50. Neuhausen S, Gilewski T, Norton L, et al: Recurrent BRCA2 6174delT mutations in Ashkenazi Jewish women affected by breast cancer. Nat Genet 1996;13:126-128.

51. Oddoux C, Struewing JP, Clayton CM, et al: The carrier frequency of the BRCA2 6174delT mutation among Ashkenazi Jewish individuals is approximately 1%. Nat Genet 1996;14:188-190.

52. Roa BB, Boyd AA, Volcik K, Richards CS: Ashkenazi Jewish population frequencies for common mutations in BRCA1 and BRCA2. Nat Genet 1996;14:185-187.

53. de la Chapelle A, Wright FA: Linkage disequilibrium mapping in isolated populations: The example of Finland revisited. Proc Natl Acad Sci USA 1998;95:12416-12423.

54. Schleutker J, Matikainen M, Smith J, et al: A genetic epidemiological study of hereditary prostate cancer (HPC) in Finland: Frequent HPCX linkage in families with late-onset disease. Clin Cancer Res 2000;6:4810-4815.

55. O'Connell JR, Weeks DE: PedCheck: A program for identification of genotype incompatibilities in linkage analysis. Am J Hum Genet 1998;63:259-266.

56. Sun L, Wilder K, McPeek MS: Enhanced pedigree error detection. Hum Hered 2002;54:99-110.

57. Epstein MP, Duren WL, Boehnke M: Improved inference of relationship for pairs of individuals. Am J Hum Genet 2000;67:1219-1231.

58. Morton N: Sequential tests for the detection of linkage. Am J Hum Genet 1955;7:277-318.

59. Lander E, Kruglyak L: Genetic dissection of complex traits: Guidelines for interpreting and reporting linkage results. Nat Genet 1995;11:241-247.

60. Risch N, Giuffra L: Model misspecification and multipoint linkage analysis. Hum Hered 1992;42:7-92.

61. Clerget-Darpoux F, Bonaiti-Pellie C, Hochez J: Effects of misspecifying genetic parameters in lod score analysis. Biometrics 1986;42:393-399.

62. Kruglyak L, Daly MJ, Reeve-Daly MP, Lander ES: Parametric and nonparametric linkage analysis: A unified multipoint approach. Am J Hum Genet 1996;58:1347-1363.

63. Potosky AL, Miller BA, Albertsen PC, Kramer BS: The role of increasing detection in the rising incidence of prostate cancer. JAMA 1995;273:548-552.

64. Stanford J, Stephenson R, Coyle L, et al: Prostate cancer trends 1973-1995, SEER Program, National Cancer Institute. Vol. 99. Bethesda, Md., National Institutes of Health, 1999, p 4543.

65. Gann PH, Hennekens CH, Stampfer MJ: A prospective evaluation of plasma prostate-specific antigen for detection of prostatic cancer [see comments]. JAMA 1995;273:289-294.

66. Pearson J, Luderer A, Metter E, et al: Longitudinal analysis of serial measurement of free and total PSA among men with and without prostatic cancer. Urology 1996;48(suppl 6A):4-9.

67. Whittemore AS, Lele C, Friedman GD, Stamey T, Vogelman JH, Orentreich N: Prostate-specific antigen as predictor of prostate cancer in black men and white men. J Natl Cancer Inst 1995;87:354-360.

68. Venter JC, Adams MD, Myers EW, et al: The sequence of the human genome. Science 2001;291:1304-1351.

69. Lander ES, Linton LM, Birren B, et al: Initial sequencing and analysis of the human genome. Nature 2001;409:860-921.

70. Kallioniemi A, Kallioniemi OP, Sudar D, et al: Comparative genomic hybridization for molecular cytogenetic analysis of solid tumours. Science 1992;258:818-821.

71. Kallioniemi OP, Kallioniemi A, Piper J, et al: Optimizing comparative genomic hybridization for analysis of DNA sequence copy number changes in solid tumors. Genes Chromosomes Cancer 1994;10:231-243.

72. Pinkel D, Segraves R, Sudar D, et al: High resolution analysis of DNA copy number variation using comparative genomic hybridization to microarrays. Nat Genet 1998;20:207-211.

73. Grizzle WE, Aamodt R, Clausen K, LiVolsi V, Pretlow TG, Qualman S: Providing human tissues for research: How to establish a program. Arch Pathol Lab Med 1998;122:1065-1076.

74. Craven RA, Banks RE: Laser capture microdissection and proteomics: Possibilities and limitation. Proteomics 2001;1:1200-1204.

75. Nelson PS, Stanford JL, Ostrander EA: Prostate cancer research in the post-genome era. Epidemiol Rev 2001;23:187-190.

76. Perou CM, Jeffrey SS, van de Rijn M, et al: Distinctive gene expression patterns in human mammary epithelial cells and breast cancers. Proc Natl Acad Sci USA 1999;96:9212-9217.

77. Alizadeh AA, Ross DT, Perou CM, van de Rijn M: Towards a novel classification of human malignancies based on gene expression patterns. J Pathol 2001;195:41-52.

78. Nielsen TO, West RB, Linn SC, et al: Molecular characterisation of soft tissue tumours: A gene expression study. Lancet 2002;359:1301-1307.

79. Collins FS: Positional cloning: Let's not call it reverse anymore. Nat Genet 1992;1:3-6.

80. Duyk GM, Kim SW, Myers RM, Cox DR: Exon trapping: A genetic screen to identify candidate transcribed sequences in cloned mammalian genomic DNA. Proc Natl Acad Sci USA 1990;87: 8995–8999.

81. Collins FS: Positional cloning moves from perditional to traditional. Nat Genet 1995;9:347–350.

82. Castilla LH, Couch FJ, Erdos MR, et al: Mutations in the BRCA1 gene in families with early-onset breast and ovarian cancer. Nat Genet 1994;8:387–391.

83. Friedman LS, Ostermeyer EA, Szabo CI, et al: Confirmation of BRCA1 by analysis of germline mutations linked to breast and ovarian cancer in ten families. Nat Genet 1994;8:399–404.

84. Couch FJ, Farid LM, DeShano ML, et al: BRCA2 germline mutations in male breast cancer cases and breast cancer families. Nat Genet 1996;13:123–125.

85. Malone KE, Daling JR, Neal C, et al: Frequency of BRCA1/BRCA2 mutations in a population-based sample of young breast cancer cases. Cancer 2000;88:1393–1402.

86. Newman B, Mu H, Butler LM, Millikan RC, Moorman PG, King MC: Frequency of breast cancer attributable to BRCA1 in a population-based series of American women [see comments]. JAMA 1998;279:915–921.

87. Whittemore AS, Gong G, Itnyre J: Prevalence and contribution of BRCA1 mutations in breast cancer and ovarian cancer: Results from three U.S. population-based case-control studies of ovarian cancer. Am J Hum Genet 1997;60:496–504.

88. Szabo C, Masiello A, Ryan JF, Brody LC: The breast cancer information core: Database design, structure, and scope. Hum Mutat 2000;16:123–131.

89. Shen D, Vadgama JV: BRCA1 and BRCA2 gene mutation analysis: Visit to the Breast Cancer Information Core (BIC). Oncol Res 1999;11:63–69.

90. Aitken J, Bain C, Ward M, Siskind V, MacLennan R: How accurate is self-reported family history of colorectal cancer? Am J Epidemiol 1995;141:863–871.

91. Berwick M, Chen YT: Reliability of reported sunburn history in a case-control study of cutaneous malignant melanoma. Am J Epidemiol 1995;141:1033–1037.

92. Parent ME, Ghadirian P, Lacroix A, Perret C: Accuracy of reports of familial breast cancer in a case-control series. Epidemiology 1995;6:184–186.

93. Kaye WE, Hall HI, Lybarger JA: Recall bias in disease status associated with perceived exposure to hazardous substances. Ann Epidemiol 1994;4:393–397.

94. Barry D: Differential recall bias and spurious associations in case/control studies. Stat Med 1996;15:2603–2616.

95. Greenland S: Response and follow-up bias in cohort studies. Am J Epidemiol 1977;106:184–187.

96. Criqui MH: Response bias and risk ratios in epidemiologic studies. Am J Epidemiol 1979;109:394–399.

97. Criqui MH, Austin M, Barrett-Connor E: The effect of non-response on risk ratios in a cardiovascular disease study. J Chronic Dis 1979;32:633–638.

98. Heilbrun LK, Nomura A, Stemmermann GN: The effects of nonresponse in a prospective study of cancer. Am J Epidemiol 1982;116:353–363.

99. Bergstrand R, Vedin A, Wilhelmsson C, Wilhelmsen L: Bias due to non-participation and heterogenous sub-groups in population surveys. J Chronic Dis 1983;36:725–728.

100. Benfante R, Reed D, MacLean C, Kagan A: Response bias in the Honolulu Heart Program. Am J Epidemiol 1989;130:1088–1100.

101. Waksberg J: Sample methods for random digit dialing. J Am Stat Soc 1978;73:40–46.

102. Wilhelmsen L, Ljungberg S, Wedel H, Werko L: A comparison between participants and non-participants in a primary preventive trial. J Chronic Dis 1976;29:331–339.

103. Carter WB, Elward K, Malmgren J, Martin ML, Larson E: Participation of older adults in health programs and research: A critical review of the literature. Gerontologist 1991;31:584–592.

104. Maciag PC, Schlecht NF, Souza PS, Franco EL, Villa LL, Petzl-Erler

ML: Major histocompatibility complex class II polymorphisms and risk of cervical cancer and human papillomavirus infection in Brazilian women. Cancer Epidemiol Biomarkers Prev 2000;9:1183–1191.

105. Smith-Warner SA, Spiegelman D, Yaun SS, et al: Intake of fruits and vegetables and risk of breast cancer: A pooled analysis of cohort studies. JAMA 2001;285:769–776.

106. Webb T: SNPs: Can genetic variants control cancer susceptibility? J Natl Cancer Inst 2002;94:476–478.

107. Ingles SA, Coetzee GA, Ross RK, et al: Association of prostate cancer with vitamin D receptor haplotypes in African-Americans. Cancer Res 1998;58:1620–1623.

108. Ingles SA, Ross RK, Yu MC, et al: Association of prostate cancer risk with genetic polymorphisms in vitamin D receptor and androgen receptor. J Natl Cancer Inst 1997;89:166–170.

109. Taylor JA, Hirvonen A, Watson M, Pittman G, Mohler JL, Bell DA: Association of prostate cancer with vitamin D receptor gene polymorphism. Cancer Res 1996;56:4108–4110.

110. Durrin LK, Haile RW, Ingles SA, Coetzee GA: Vitamin D receptor 3'-untranslated region polymorphisms: Lack of effect on mRNA stability. Biochim Biophys Acta 1999;1453:311–320.

111. Ingles SA, Haile RW, Henderson BE, et al: Strength of linkage disequilibrium between two vitamin D receptor markers in five ethnic groups: Implications for association studies. Cancer Epidemiol Biomarkers Prev 1997;6:93–98.

112. Gross C, Eccleshall TR, Malloy PJ, Villa ML, Marcus R, Feldman D: The presence of a polymorphism at the translation initiation site of the vitamin D receptor gene is associated with low bone mineral density in postmenopausal Mexican-American women. J Bone Miner Res 1996;11:1850–1855.

113. King MC, Wieand S, Hale K, et al: Tamoxifen and breast cancer incidence among women with inherited mutations in BRCA1 and BRCA2: National Surgical Adjuvant Breast and Bowel Project (NSABP-P1) Breast Cancer Prevention Trial. JAMA 2001;286:2251–2256.

114. Haffty BG, Harrold E, Khan AJ, et al: Outcome of conservatively managed early-onset breast cancer by BRCA1/2 status. Lancet 2002;359:1471–1477.

115. van Roosmalen MS, Verhoef LC, Stalmeier PF, Hoogerbrugge N, van Daal WA: Decision analysis of prophylactic surgery or screening for BRCA1 mutation carriers: A more prominent role for oophorectomy. J Clin Oncol 2002;20:2092–2100.

116. Grann VR, Jacobson JS: Population screening for cancer-related germline gene mutations. Lancet Oncol 2002;3:341–348.

117. Brzovic PS, Meza JE, King MC, Klevit RE: BRCA1 RING domain cancer-predisposing mutations. Structural consequences and effects on protein-protein interactions. J Biol Chem 2001;276: 41399–41406.

118. Monteiro AN, August A, Hanafusa H: Evidence for a transcriptional activation function of BRCA1 C-terminal region. Proc Natl Acad Sci USA 1996;93:13595–13599.

119. Vallon-Christersson J, Cayanan C, Haraldsson K, et al: Functional analysis of BRCA1 C-terminal missense mutations identified in breast and ovarian cancer families. Hum Mol Genet 2001;10:353–360.

120. Serova O, Montagna M, Torchard D, et al: A high incidence of BRCA1 mutations in 20 breast-ovarian cancer families. Am J Hum Genet 1996;58:42–51.

121. Szabo CI, King MC: Inherited breast and ovarian cancer. Hum Mol Genet 1995;4:1811–1817.

122. Fleming MA, Potter JD, Ramirez CJ, Ostrander GK, Ostrander EA: Understanding missense mutations in the BRCA1 gene: An evolutionary approach. Proc Natl Acad Sci USA 2003;100: 1151–1156.

123. Hayes F, Cayanan C, Barilla D, Monteiro AN: Functional assay for BRCA1: Mutagenesis of the COOH-terminal region reveals critical residues for transcription activation. Cancer Res 2000;60: 2411–2418.

124. Collins FS, McKusick VA: Implications of the Human Genome Project for medical science. JAMA 2001;285:540–544.

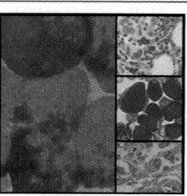

Eric R. Fearon

PROGRESSING FROM GENE MUTATIONS TO CANCER

SUMMARY OF KEY POINTS

- A root cause of cancer is the accumulation of defects in genes that play critical roles in regulating cell proliferation, differentiation, and cell death (apoptosis). The mutations in cancer cells are of two types—gain-of-function mutations in oncogenes and loss-of-function mutations in tumor suppressor genes.

- Not infrequently in cancer cells, epigenetic mechanisms can alter expression of proto-oncogenes and tumor suppressor genes substantially, leading to essentially the same consequences as if the structure and/or sequence of the genes were affected by mutation.

- Clinical and pathologic studies have long indicated that cancers arise from preexisting benign lesions. Based on epidemiologic studies of the age-incidence patterns of benign and malignant lesions, it was estimated that roughly six to seven rate-limiting events were needed for development of a clinically recognizable cancer, and the rate-limiting events were proposed to represent the stepwise accumulation of mutations in precancerous cells. The molecular descriptive work carried out on cancers supports the view that multiple mutations and gene expression changes accumulate in a cancer cell during its development, and benign lesions generally have fewer alterations than their malignant counterparts.

- A process termed clonal selection plays a critical role in determining the particular constellation of genetic and epigenetic defects present in a cancer cell. In brief, clonal selection is essentially a punctuated evolutionary process that promotes the outgrowth of precancerous and cancerous cells carrying those mutations and gene expression changes that confer the most potent proliferative and survival properties upon the cancer cells, in a given context.

- Though a diverse array of mutations and gene expression changes has been implicated in cancer pathogenesis, the defects appear to affect a relatively limited number of conserved signaling pathways or networks. Certain genes are targeted recurrently by mutations in one or a few tumor types, while other genes in the signaling pathway might be much more frequently mutated in other cancer types. The basis for the differences in mutation frequency in genes that function in a signaling pathway and that should have essentially similar effects when mutated presumably reflects the fact that the signaling pathways are considerably more branched and complex than is currently recognized. Nevertheless, the proto-oncogenes and tumor suppressor genes targeted by recurrent somatic gene defects in cancer more than likely represent particularly critical nodes in the cell's regulatory circuitry.

- Although cancer represents a very heterogeneous collection of diseases, the development of all cancers, regardless of type, appears to be critically dependent on the acquisition of certain traits that allow the cancer cells to acquire the ability not only to grow in an unchecked fashion in their tissue of origin but also to grow as metastatic lesions in distant sites in the body. Nine distinct signature traits are likely to be inherent to the majority if not all cancer cells Some gene defects in cancer cells could contribute predominantly to a few or perhaps even only one of the signature traits of cancer cells. Many of the gene defects and expression changes, however, might have been selected for in large part because they exert pleiotropic effects on the cancer cell phenotype.

- Despite the fact that some gene defects arise early in the development of certain cancer types, there is evidence that advanced cancer cells might remain critically dependent on the "early gene defects" for continued growth and survival. Such findings imply that agents that specifically target key signaling pathways and proteins could have utility in advanced cancers, even if the signaling pathway defect arose very early in cancer development.

- Future studies will further clarify the role of gene defects in cancer phenotype, allowing more definitive and specific strategies for inhibiting cancer cells.

INTRODUCTION

A genetic basis for human cancer has been recognized for perhaps more than a century and has been supported by data from familial and epidemiologic studies and animal studies. Only in the past 25 years, however, has molecular evidence been obtained to support the view that cancer is a genetic disease. Studies from many different fields—including tumor virology, chemical carcinogenesis, molecular biology, somatic cell genetics, and genetic epidemiology—have provided fundamental insights into mechanisms underlying cancer development. Although environmental and dietary factors and other genes undoubtedly play substantial roles in cancer development, it is now well established that the accumulation of multiple mutations in a single cell is fundamental to the pathogenesis of cancer. The mutations occur in two distinct classes of cellular genes: oncogenes and tumor suppressor genes. As noted in Chapters 13 and 14, some mutations could be present in the germline of individuals and could predispose to particular cancers. Such mutations can also be passed on to future generations. The nature and role of germline mutations in cancer development are of great interest to cancer biologists, because the mutations provide powerful clues about the identity of genes and pathways that play particularly critical roles in the conversion of normal cells to malignancy. Nevertheless, germline mutations in oncogenes or tumor suppressor genes are likely have a major contributing role in only a small fraction of cancers, and the vast majority of mutations in cancer are somatic (i.e., present only in the tumor cells).

A subset of the cellular genes affected by inherited and somatic mutations in human cancer will be discussed in greater detail in this chapter. Brief mention will be made here of some general properties of the genes. Oncogenes, when mutated, act in a positive fashion to promote tumorigenesis. Their normally functioning cellular counterparts, termed proto-oncogenes, have been found to be important regulators of many aspects of cell growth. The proteins encoded by various proto-oncogenes can be found in virtually all subcellular compartments, including the nucleus, the cytoplasm, and at the cell surface. The term *proto-oncogene* does not imply that genes of this class lie dormant in the cell with the purpose of promoting tumorigenesis. Rather, the terminology reflects the fact that mutations in cancer cells alter the normal structure and/or expression pattern of the proto-oncogene, generating oncogenic variant forms with altered function. In genetic terms, oncogenic alleles have "gain-of-function" mutations conferring enhanced or novel functions.

In contrast to the activating mutations in oncogenes, loss-of-function defects in tumor suppressor genes are found in cancer cells. The term "anti-oncogenes" has sometimes been used with respect to the tumor suppressor class of genes. The term suggests the primary function of the genes might be to act in direct opposition to activated oncogenes. Although some of the proteins encoded by tumor suppressor genes do in fact bind to and regulate the

function proto-oncogenes or function in pathways that directly regulate proto-oncogene activity, such action is not a general principle for these genes. Hence, genes that contribute to cancer by virtue of inactivating or loss-of-function mutations in human cancers will be referred to here as tumor suppressor genes. The normal functions of tumor suppressor genes, like those of the proto-oncogenes, are diverse, and the proteins encoded by these genes are found in essentially all compartments of the cell. Compared with the vast array of oncogenic alleles seen in human cancer, a more limited number of tumor suppressor genes has been identified at the molecular level thus far. This finding might not be an accurate representation of the prevalence of oncogene vs. tumor suppressor gene mutations in cancer. Rather, it could reflect the practical difficulties associated with experimental strategies to identify genes that negatively regulate the growth of cells.

Much evidence indicates that mutations in genes that regulate the recognition and repair of DNA damage play critical roles in tumorigenesis. The DNA damage recognition and repair genes could be considered to constitute a distinct class of cancer genes. But because DNA repair genes appear uniformly to be affected by loss-of-function mutations in cancer, they will be classified here as tumor suppressor genes. Nevertheless, on the basis of certain features, DNA damage recognition and repair genes might constitute a potentially unique subset of tumor suppressor genes. Specifically, compared with the presumed direct role of many tumor suppressor genes in the regulation of cell growth and programmed cell death, at least some of the DNA repair proteins could have more passive roles in growth, differentiation, and cell survival. Their inactivation in tumor cells might lead predominantly to the acquisition of a "mutator phenotype," with a resultant increased rate of mutations in other cellular genes having rate-determining roles in the cancer process (i.e., oncogenes and tumor suppressor genes).

In addition to the well established role of oncogene and tumor suppressor gene mutations in cancer, there is large and growing body of data indicating that epigenetic mechanisms could play critical roles in altering the patterns and levels of expression of certain proto-oncogenes and tumor suppressor genes in cancer. For instance, in some cancers, defects in transcriptional regulatory mechanisms can lead to markedly increased levels of proto-oncogene expression akin to that seen in cancer cells, with mutational defects altering the structure or copy number of the proto-oncogene. Conversely, gene silencing mechanisms can exert dramatic effects on the expression of certain tumor suppressor genes in cancer cells, essentially rendering the genes functionally inactive in the absence of any mutations.

Given the enormous advances over the past two decades in defining oncogene and tumor suppressor gene mutations and gene expression defects in cancer, it will not be possible in this chapter to review in a comprehensive fashion the vast array of gene defects identified in human cancers. Neither will it be possible to discuss in great detail the possible contributions of the many different gene defects to alterations in cell signaling and cell physiology. Rather, the primary aim of this chapter will be to offer a framework for understanding the relationship between gene defects in cancer cells and the impact of the accumulated defects on the cancer cell phenotype. Though some details on the identity and nature of gene defects in cancer will be offered here, the emphasis will be on concepts likely to have biologic and clinical significance.

CANCERS ARISE FROM THE ACCUMULATION OF MULTIPLE GENE DEFECTS

Based on a simple consideration of the large number of mutations likely to be encountered by normal cells during the many years of life, it would seem improbable that cancers arise as the result of any single gene defect. Even in individuals strongly predisposed to cancer as a result of a germline mutation in a specific oncogene or tumor suppressor gene, the vast majority of cells in the individual never develop into cancer or even display definitive morphologic changes akin to those seen in benign tumors. In fact, depending on the inherited cancer syndrome, a significant fraction of those individuals carrying germline mutations never develop cancer. Therefore, any model for cancer must incorporate these data suggesting that cancers likely arise as the result of the accumulation of multiple gene defects in an affected cell. Another issue to consider prior to formulating genetic models for cancer development is that clinical and histopathologic data suggest that the development of nearly all cancers, regardless of the organ site, is often if not invariably preceded by precancerous phases or stages in which the neoplastic cells manifest increasingly disordered patterns of differentiation and morphology.

Given this background, it would appear that there is compelling if not unequivocal evidence that cancers arise from accumulated defects in several genes and that precancerous (benign) precursor lesions contain, by necessity, fewer of the key gene defects. The question then becomes: How many rate-limiting defects or "hits" are required for cancer development? Although no definitive answer to this question can be given at this point, some estimates can be offered. Most common cancers show dramatically increased incidence with increasing age. Based on analysis of the age-specific incidence of a number of common cancers and some straightforward assumptions about the rate of mutations and the size of the target cell population, it was argued as early as the mid-1950s that most common epithelial cancers arise as the result of four to seven rate-limiting events.[1-4] It was inferred that these rate-limiting events represented mutational events. Moreover, benign lesions were inferred to arise as the result of fewer gene defects, consistent with the fact that recognizable benign lesions often demonstrate an age-incidence distribution shifted roughly one to two decades earlier in life than cancers arising in the corresponding organ/tissue sites. Nevertheless, questions about certain key biologic assumptions underlying the multi-hit models confounded the use of age-incidence

data to model the number of rate-limiting mutations. Given the attendant uncertainties about estimates of rate-limiting mutation numbers based solely on age-incidence data and the practical difficulties in defining the nature and significance of all inherited and somatic gene defects in cancer, a definitive answer to the number of rate-determining mutations for a particular cancer type has not yet been obtained. At the very least, however, it is encouraging to note that molecular analyses of a number of common cancers, such as those of the colon, lung, and pancreas, indicate that five or more gene defects are not infrequently seen in cancers, and that fewer of the gene defects are seen in precancerous precursor lesions.[5-9]

CLONAL SELECTION AND EVOLUTION IN CANCER

As discussed previously, most, if not all, cancers are thought to arise from preexisting precancerous populations of cells, and multiple rate-limiting mutations (events) are likely needed for conversion of a normal cell to a cancerous cell. Molecular studies of cancers of various types and their corresponding associated precancerous lesions have yielded some fundamental insights into the processes likely to be critical in emergence of the cancer:

1. First, whereas normal tissues and tissues from non-cancerous disease states display polyclonal (balanced) cell populations, the neoplastic component present in benign lesions and cancers invariably displays a clonally related cell population, consistent with the notion that neoplastic transformation of one or at most a few cells within a tissue give rise to all daughter cells present in the tumor.
2. Second, in those tumors in which it has been possible to analyze both cancer cells and associated precancerous cell populations, a subset of the somatic gene defects present in the cancer are represented clonally in the precancerous cell population. Other somatic gene defects appear to be acquired during progression from the precancer subclones to the dominant subclone in the cancer.

These molecular findings in benign and malignant tumors are essentially consistent with a model proposed initially by Foulds[10] and subsequently advanced by Nowell[11] (Fig. 15-1). In brief, the clonal evolution model predicts that cancers arise as the result of successive expansions of clonally related cell populations. The successive expansions are driven by the punctuated acquisition of mutations and gene expression changes that endow a particular cell and its progeny with selective growth and survival advantages over cells that do not harbor the gene defects. Clonal selection is thus essentially an evolutionary process that allows the outgrowth of precancerous and cancerous cells carrying mutations and gene expression changes that confer the most potent proliferative and survival properties upon the cancer cells. It is important to recognize that the specific constellation of genetic and epigenetic changes present in

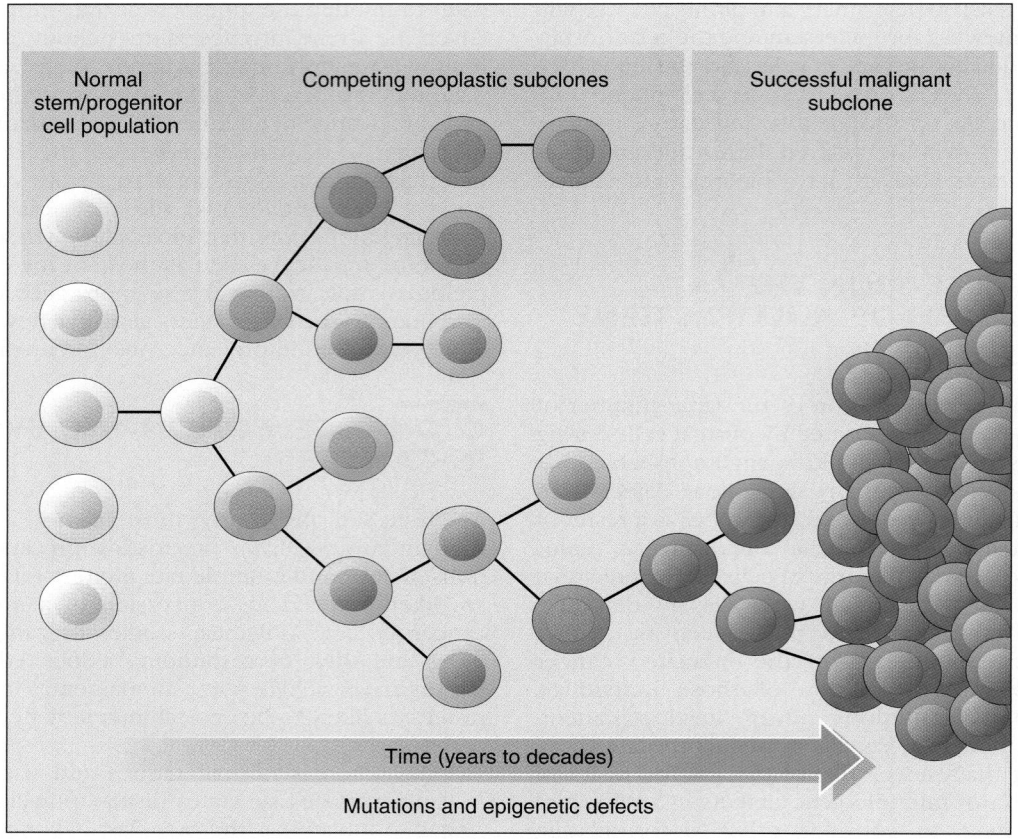

Figure 15-1. Role of clonal selection in cancer development and progression. Clonal selection is essentially a punctuated evolutionary process promoting outgrowth of precancerous and cancerous cells carrying those mutations and gene expression changes that confer the most potent proliferative and survival properties on the cancer cells in a given context. The schematic diagram indicates that the stepwise emergence of benign and malignant cells over time is critically influenced by mutations and epigenetic defects. Neoplasms most likely arise from a stem cell or progenitor cell population that is capable of additional cell divisions and acquisition of certain differentiated characteristics. Following the accumulation of a particular constellation of mutations and epigenetic defects in oncogenes and tumor suppressor genes, a successful malignant subclone will outgrow the various competing neoplastic subclones. Further genetic heterogeneity within the malignant subclone (not depicted) is possible, and the genetic heterogeneity in the malignant subclone might give rise to new subclones that display increased invasive and metastatic potential. (Modified from Kern SE: Progressive genetic abnormalities in human neoplasia. In Mendelsohn J, Howley PM, Israel MA, Liotta LA [eds]: The Molecular Basis of Cancer, 2nd ed. Philadelphia, WB Saunders, 2001, pp 41–69.)

precancerous and cancerous cells is context dependent. This constellation likely varies considerably from one cancer type to another and perhaps even to a significant degree among cancers that display similar clinical and histopathologic features. The basis for the context-dependent relationship of the changes that confer a selective growth advantage in a particular cancer might reflect any or all of the following:

- Physiologic differences in organ site and even micro-environment within the organ site;
- The identities of the preceding somatic gene defects in the precancerous or cancerous clone; and even
- The constitutional sequence variations and gene expression patterns present in non-neoplastic tissues of the patient.

This issue of context-dependent effects of gene defects that promote clonal selection will be addressed further in the sections that follow.

The clonal evolution model has some important biologic and clinical ramifications, just a few of which will be mentioned here:

1. The clonal gene defects present in a cancer can be traced in precancerous lesions from the same organ site with a goal of attempting to clarify the preferred order in which gene defects arise in the natural history of a particular cancer type. The particular order in which defects accumulate during the initiation and subsequent progression of one cancer type often differs from the progression in another cancer type. As a result, a genetic or epigenetic change critical in tumor initiation in one cancer type might contribute to tumor progression in another tumor type and vice versa.
2. Defects arising at "early" stages of tumorigenesis could play a vital role not only in tumor initiation but also in the aggressive behavior of advanced-stage cancers.
3. The model predicts that further genetic heterogeneity will be a common and important factor in primary

cancer lesions and metastases. Genetic heterogeneity likely plays a significant role in resistance to chemotherapy and the emergence of aggressive cell populations in patients with advanced cancer.

4. Finally, it is important to note that clonal somatic mutations are often presumed to have a causal role in promoting further tumor outgrowth and/or progression, because somatic mutations can become clonal (i.e., present in all neoplastic cells) by only a limited number of mechanisms. For instance, the genetic alteration itself could have been selected for because it provided the neoplastic cell with a growth advantage, allowing it to become the predominant cell type in the tumor (clonal expansion). Alternatively, a somatic mutation, when detected, might have arisen essentially coincident with another, perhaps undetected, alteration that was the crucial change underlying clonal outgrowth.

Nevertheless, given this perspective on the potential uncertainties associated with linking somatic mutations to cancer development, it is perhaps apparent why it is even more problematic to assign causal significance to gene expression changes in precancerous and cancerous cells. Specifically, the ambiguities in assigning a causal role to gene expression changes in the absence of mutations are in large part due to difficulties in determining whether the gene expression changes merely reflect or are causally involved in the cancer process. Nonetheless, if a specific gene defect can be shown to promote tumorigenesis or neoplastic transformation in in vitro models or animal model experiments, or if the same gene or chromosomal region is altered recurrently in tumors, then it could be reasonable to infer that the particular defect might indeed have a causal role in tumorigenesis.

ONCOGENE AND TUMOR SUPPRESSOR GENE DEFECTS IN CANCER TARGET CONSERVED SIGNALING PATHWAYS

Recurrent Mutational Targets in Cancer

As discussed previously, oncogenic alleles have "gain-of-function" mutations in genetic terms. Oncogenic variant alleles present in cancer are generated from the normal counterpart proto-oncogenes by various mutational mechanisms, including point or localized mutations, gross chromosomal rearrangements, or gene amplification. Some representative oncogene mutations in human cancer are summarized in Table 15-1. From a brief review of the data in Table 15-1, several generalizations are apparent:

1. The mutations affect proteins functioning in various compartments of the cell, including growth factor receptors, cytoplasmic signal tranducers, and nuclear proteins, such as transcription factors.

2. Although some oncogene mutations—such as the specific chromosomal translocations and resultant fusion proteins seen in cancers of hematopoietic origin (e.g., BCR-ABL translocation seen in chronic myelogenous leukemia and a subset of acute lymphoid leuke-

mias, and the PML-RARα translocation seen in acute promyelocytic leukemia)—might be unique to cancers of a particular type, other mutations, such as those in K-RAS, β-catenin, and c-MYC genes, are found in a broad spectrum of different cancer types.

3. Oncogene mutations in cancer are nearly always somatic, as only a very few germline mutations in proto-oncogenes have been linked to cancer predisposition thus far.

4. Some proto-oncogenes, such as K-RAS or BCL2, have been found to be altered only by mutations of essentially a single type in cancer—namely, by point mutations in the K-RAS gene and chromosomal translocations affecting the BCL2 gene. In contrast, other proto-oncogenes, such as c-MYC, could be affected by more than one activating mechanism in cancer, including both chromosomal translocation and gene amplification. Both mutational mechanisms lead to increased levels of c-MYC transcripts and protein.

In contrast to the activating mutations that generate oncogenic alleles from proto-oncogenes, inactivation of the normal function of tumor suppressor genes is critical in tumorigenesis. Akin to the proto-oncogenes, the functions of tumor suppressor genes are diverse, and proteins encoded by these genes reside in practically all subcellular compartments (Table 15-2). Many tumor suppressor genes were identified by virtue of the fact that they are mutated in the germline of individuals affected by a known Mendelian cancer syndrome or who at the very least display a markedly elevated risk of cancer. The link between germline inactivating mutation in a purported tumor suppressor gene and cancer predisposition provides highly persuasive evidence of the functional significance of the gene in the cancer process. Nevertheless, for the vast majority of tumor suppressor genes, in terms of their magnitude, somatic inactivating mutations play a far more significant role in cancer development than do germline mutations.

Another important point to consider is that much of the attention to tumor suppressor genes has been focused on demonstrating that cancer cells carry bi-allelic inactivating mutations. Clearly, a diverse array of mechanisms can inactivate gene function, including nonsense, frameshift, and nonconservative missense mutations, as well as gross deletions of the gene or even the chromosome region containing the gene. In a number of cases, studies of the chromosomal mechanisms associated with tumor suppressor gene inactivation in cancer tissues—such as loss of the parental heterozygosity (i.e., LOH) that is present in normal tissues—have even been used to infer the existence of tumor suppressor genes in particular chromosomal regions, prior to the actual identification of the tumor suppressor gene of interest. The emphasis on defining bi-allelic inactivating mutations in tumor suppressor genes has been stimulated in large part by the Knudson hypothesis,[4,12,13] which predicted that recessive genetic determinants played a critical role in retinoblastoma and many other cancers and that inactivation of both alleles of a tumor suppressor gene was needed to abrogate tumor suppressor gene activity. Nevertheless, as

TABLE 15-1

Representative Oncogene Mutations in Cancer

GENE	ACTIVATION MECHANISM	PROTEIN PROPERTIES	TUMOR TYPES
K-RAS	Point mutation	Signal transducer (p21 GTPase)	Pancreatic, colorectal, lung (adeno), endometrial, other carcinomas
N-RAS	Point mutation	Signal transducer (p21 GTPase)	Myeloid leukemia, colorectal cancer
H-RAS	Point mutation	Signal transducer (p21 GTPase)	Bladder carcinoma
EGFR (ERBB)	Amplification	Growth factor (EGF) receptor	Gliomas
NEU (HER2/ERBB2)	Amplification	Growth factor receptor	Breast, ovarian, gastric, other carcinomas
c-MYC	Chromosome translocation amplification	Transcription factor	Burkitt's lymphomas
			Small cell lung carcinoma (SCLC); other carcinomas; glioblastoma
N-MYC	Amplification	Transcription factor	Neuroblastoma, SCLC; glioblastoma
L-MYC	Amplification	Transcription factor	SCLC, ovarian carcinoma
BCL-2	Chromosome translocation	Anti-apotosis protein	B-cell lymphoma (follicular type)
CYCD1	Amplification, chromosome translocation	Cyclin D, cell cycle control	Breast and other carcinomas
			B-cell lymphoma, parathyroid adenoma
BCR-ABL	Chromosome translocation tyrosine kinase	Chimeric nonreceptor	CML, ALL (T cell)
RET	Chromosome translocation point mutation	GDNF receptor tyrosine kinase	Thyroid cancer (papillary type)
			Thyroid cancer (medullary type—germline mutations)
CDK4	Amplification point mutation	Cyclin-dependent kinase	Sarcoma, glioblastoma
			Melanoma (germline mutations)
MET	Point mutation	Hepatocyte growth factor (HGF) receptor	Renal carcinoma (papillary type—germline mutations)
SMO	Point mutations	Transmembrane signaling molecule in sonic hedgehog pathway	Basal cell skin cancer
β-CAT (CTNNB1)	Point mutation, in-frame deletion	Transcriptional co-activator, links E-cadherin to cytoskeleton	Melanoma; colorectal, endometrial, ovarian, hepatocellular, and other carcinomas; hepatoblastoma; Wilms' tumor
HST	Amplification	Growth factor (FGF-like)	Gastric carcinoma
PML-RARα	Chromosome translocation	Chimeric transcription factor	APL
E2A-PBX1	Chromosome translocation	Chimeric transcription factor	Pre-B ALL
MDM-2	Amplification	p53 binding protein	Sarcoma
GLI	Amplification	Transcription factor	Sarcoma, glioma
TTG	Chromosome translocation	Transcription factor	T-cell ALL
AKT2	Amplification	Signal transducer (Serine/threonine kinase; downstream effector of PI3K)	Pancreatic and ovarian carcinoma
PIK3CA	Amplification	Catalytic subunit of PI3K	Ovarian carcinoma
STK15	Amplification	Centrosome-associated kinase	Breast, colon, ovarian, and prostate carcinomas; gliomas

ALL, acute lymphocytic leukemia; APL, acute promyelocytic leukemia; CML, chronic myelogenous leukemia; EGF, epidermal growth factor; FGF, fibroblast growth factor; GDNF, glial-derived neurotrophic factor; GTPase, guanine trinucleotide phosphatase; HGF, hepatocyte growth factor; PI3K, phosphatidylinositol 3-kinase; SCLC, small cell carcinoma of the lung.

will be discussed in more detail following, a variety of observations suggest that epigenetic (nonmutational) mechanisms could play a prominent role in inactivating tumor suppressor gene function in sporadic tumors. Furthermore, for certain tumor suppressor genes, inactivation of only one of the two alleles of a tumor suppressor gene could significantly impair cell growth regulation or programmed cell death. For example, p53 proteins carrying missense mutations in the central (DNA-binding region) of the protein can often potently interfere via dominant negative mechanisms with the wild-type p53 protein in the cell, because p53 functions as a homo-tetrameric protein and all subunits must be wild type for intact p53 function in transcriptional regulation.[14,15] For other proteins, such as the cyclin-dependent kinase inhibitory protein p27, reduction of protein levels to 50% of the levels present in normal cells could result in

significant detrimental effects on the ability of the cell to regulate growth appropriately.[16,17]

Epigenetic Mechanisms of Proto-oncogene Activation and Tumor Suppressor Inactivation

The foregoing discussion has largely emphasized the role and significance of somatic and germline mutations in proto-oncogenes and tumor suppressor genes in cancer. The rationale for focusing on the role of genetic alterations in cancer initiation and progression is based chiefly on the view that it is arguably more straightforward to ascribe a causal role in cancer to specific alterations in the tumor cell genome than it is to attribute a causal role in cancer to apparent changes in the levels and/or patterns of gene expression in cancer cells.

TABLE 15-2

Representative Tumor Suppressor Gene Mutations in Cancer

GENE	ASSOCIATED INHERITED CANCER SYNDROME	CANCERS WITH SOMATIC MUTATIONS	PRESUMED FUNCTION OF PROTEIN
RB1	Familial retinoblastoma	Retinoblastoma, osteosarcoma, SCLC, breast, prostate, bladder, pancreas, esophageal, others	Transcriptional regulator; E2F binding
TP53	Li-Fraumeni syndrome	Approx. 50% of all cancers (rare in some types, such as prostate carcinoma and neuroblastoma)	Transcription factor; regulates cell cycle and apoptosis
p16/INK4A	Familial melanoma, familial pancreatic carcinoma	Approx. 25%–30% of many different cancer types (e.g., breast, lung, pancreatic, bladder)	Cyclin-dependent kinase inhibitor (i.e., Cdk4 and Cdk6)
p14^{Arf} (p19^{Arf})	Familial melanoma	Approx. 15% of many different cancer types	Regulates Mdm-2 protein stability and hence p53 stability; alternative reading frame of p16/INK4A gene
APC	Familial adenomatous polyposis coli (FAP), Gardner syndrome, Turcot's syndrome	Colorectal carcinomas, desmoid tumors, hepatocellular carcinoma, breast (rare)	Regulates levels of β-catenin protein in the cytsol; binding to EB1 and microtubules
WT-1	WAGR, Denys-Drash Syndrome	Wilms' tumor	Transcription factor
NF-1	Neurofibromatosis type 1	Melanoma, neuroblastoma	p21ras-GTPase
NF-2	Neurofibromatosis type 2	Schwannoma, meningioma, ependymoma	Juxtamembrane link to cytoskeleton at adherens junction
VHL	von Hippel-Lindau syndrome	Renal (clear cell type), hemangioblastoma	Regulator of protein stability
BRCA1	Inherited breast and ovarian cancer	Ovarian (~10%), rare in breast cancer	DNA repair; complexes with Rad 51 and BRCA2; transcriptional regulation
BRCA2	Inherited breast (both female and male), pancreatic cancer, others	Rare mutations in pancreatic, others	DNA repair; complexes with Rad 51 and BRCA1
MEN-1	Multiple endocrine neoplasia type 1	Parathyroid adenoma, pituitary adenoma, endocrine tumors of the pancreas	Nuclear protein; unknown function
PTCH	Gorlin syndrome, hereditary basal cell carcinoma syndrome	Basal cell skin carcinoma, medulloblastoma	Transmembrane receptor for sonic hedgehog factor; negative regulator of smoothened protein
PTEN/MMAC1	Cowden's syndrome; sporadic cases of juvenile polyposis syndrome	Glioma, breast, prostate, follicular thyroid carcinoma, head and neck squamous carcinoma	Phosphoinositide 3-phosphatase; protein tyrosine phosphatase
SMAD4	Familial juvenile polyposis syndrome	Pancreatic (~50%), approx. 10%–15% of colorectal cancers, rare in others	Transcriptional factor in TGF-β signaling pathway
BMPR1A	Familial juvenile polyposis syndrome	Not known	Receptor for bone morphogenetic protein
MSH2, MLH1, PMS1, PMS2, MSH6	Hereditary nonpolyposis colorectal cancer	Colorectal, gastric, endometrial, ovarian	DNA mismatch repair
CDH1	Familial diffuse-type gastric cancer	Gastric (diffuse type), lobular breast carcinoma, rare in other types (e.g., ovarian)	E-cadherin cell-cell adhesion molecule
LKB1/STK11	Peutz-Jeghers syndrome	Lung adenocarcinoma (~30%); rare pancreas cancers; absent in most other cancers	Serine/threonine protein kinase
EXT1	Hereditary multiple exostoses	Not known	Glycosyltransferase; heparan sulfate chain elongation
EXT2	Hereditary multiple exostoses	Not known	Glycosyltransferase; heparan sulfate chain elongation
TSC1	Tuberous sclerosis	Not known	Hamartin; binds tuberin (TSC2); regulates cell size by inhibiting target of rapamycin (TOR) function and protein synthesis
TSC2	Tuberous sclerosis	Not known	Tuberin—see above regarding TSC1

Potential difficulties in assigning a causal role in cancer to changes in the expression of various proto-oncogenes or tumor suppressor genes include uncertainties about whether the apparent differences in gene expression reflect true changes in gene expression or simply reflect the possibility that the cancer could have arisen from neoplastic transformation of a cell type that had strikingly different gene expression than the majority of normal cells in the tissue from which the cancer originated. In spite of the fact that changes solely in the expression (but not in the structure or sequence) of proto-oncogenes and tumor suppressor genes have been more difficult to implicate definitively in the cancer process, genuine progress in the area of cancer epigenetics has been made. Arguably, the most compelling data for assigning a critical (and likely causal) role to changes in gene expression in the cancer process are for those genes that have already been well established in prior studies to function as tumor suppressor genes. For instance, as noted previously, persuasive evidence of tumor suppressor gene function in a particular type of cancer might be provided by virtue of the fact that definitive germline and/or somatic inactivating mutations in the genes can be identified in a subset of tumors. Hence, the emphasis here will be placed on illustrating how epigenetic mechanisms have been assigned a causal role in silencing tumor suppressor genes in cancer. This emphasis is due largely to space limitations and not simply because of the absence of data implicating epigenetic mechanisms in proto-oncogene activation in cancer. Indeed, a priori, there is no reason why epigenetic mechanisms cannot lead to substantial increases in the expression of proto-onconcogenes, with expression changes perhaps on the order of those seen in cancers with high-copy amplification of the respective proto-oncogene. In some cases, epigenetic mechanisms likely do lead to overexpression of certain proto-oncogenes in a variety of cancer types, such as for c-MYC, the epidermal growth factor receptor (EGFR), and the aurora-2 kinase and very closely related kinases.[18-20]

As summarized in Table 15-2, somatic inactivation of tumor suppressor genes resulting from well established genetic mechanisms has been seen in many cancers. There is also a robust and growing body of data, however, to support the view that epigenetic mechanisms somatically inactivate selected tumor suppressor genes in certain cancer types (Fig. 15-2).[21,22] Although data are only now emerging on the specific transcriptional and chromatin remodeling mechanisms responsible for epigenetic silencing of tumor suppressor genes, it has been demonstrated in many studies that increases in the methylation of CpG-rich sequences ("CpG islands") in the

regulatory regions (i.e., promoter/enhancer regions) of tumor suppressor genes are often linked to loss of tumor suppressor gene expression. For instance, although the *VHL* gene is inactivated by mutational mechanisms in roughly 80% of renal carcinomas of clear cell type, in the majority of the cell clear renal carcinomas where specific *VHL* mutations cannot be detected, loss of *VHL* gene expression appears to be tightly linked to hypermethylation of the *VHL* promoter.[22,23] For some other tumor suppressor genes—including the $p16^{INK4a}$, *BRCA1*, and *MLH1* genes—promoter hypermethylation has also been implicated as key mechanism of inactivation.[22] In fact, based on studies of genes displaying extensive CpG island methylation and decreased or absent gene expression in cancer cells of one type or another, it has been suggested that aberrant CpG methylation could play a broad and important role in the cancer process.[22] Some of the established and candidate tumor suppressor genes suggested to be commonly inactivated in cancer as a result of CpG island methylation in cancer are listed in Table 15-3.

Nevertheless, at this point, it might be reasonable to offer a few cautionary comments regarding the linkages between CpG island methylation, gene silencing, and tumor suppressor genes. One issue to reflect on is the high degree of uncertainty about what fraction of the genes whose promoters show increased methylation in

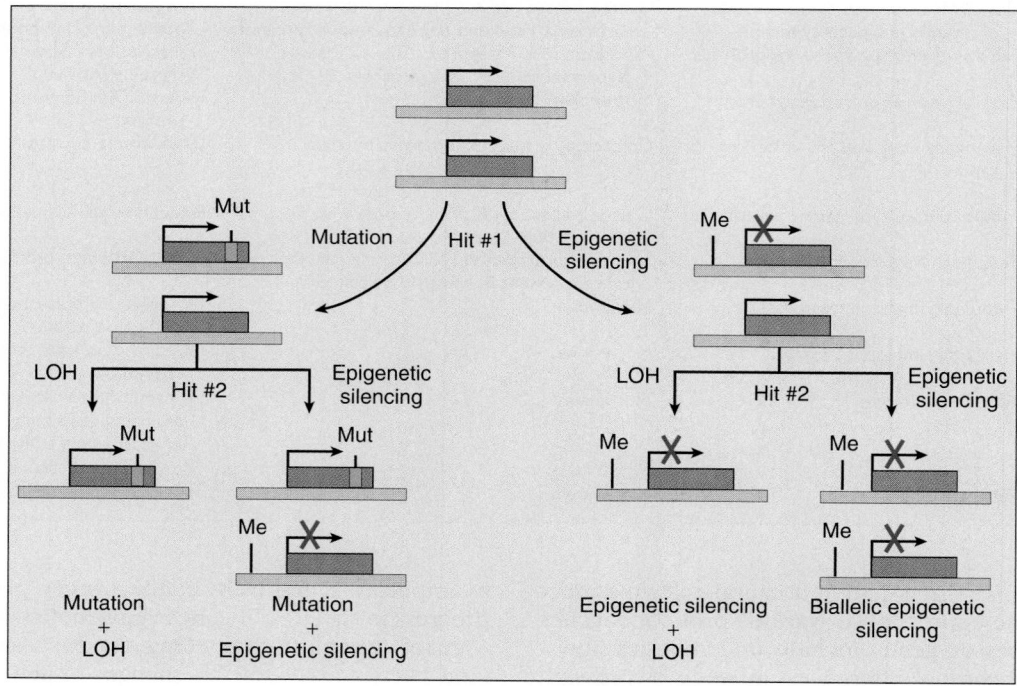

Figure 15-2. Knudson's two-hit hypothesis revised. In brief, Knudson's hypothesis predicted that both alleles of a tumor suppressor gene would need to be inactivated by germline and/or somatic mutations to elicit critical phenotypic alterations associated with cancer development. The revised version of Knudson's two-hypothesis considers the possibility that tumor suppressor gene inactivation can result from either genetic (mutation) or epigenetic silencing events. The two functional alleles of a given tumor suppressor gene are indicated by the two purple boxes (*top*). The first inactivating event affecting one of the two tumor suppressor gene alleles could either be a mutation, such as the localized defect indicated by the yellow box (*left*), or transcriptional silencing associated with or caused by hypermethylation of CpG-rich sequences in the promoter/regulatory region (*right*). The inactivating event for the second tumor suppressor gene allele (i.e., "Hit #2") could be a nondisjunction event resulting in loss of the chromosome containing the wild-type tumor suppressor gene allele (loss of heterozygosity, LOH) or epigenetic silencing. (Modified from Jones PA, Laird PW: Cancer epigenetics comes of age. Nat Genet 1999;21:163–167.)

TABLE 15-3

Representative Genes Affected by Promoter Hypermethylation and Silencing in Cancer

GENE	IDENTITY/FUNCTION	GERMLINE MUTATIONS IN CANCER?	SOMATIC MUTATIONS IN CANCER?	HYPERMETHYLATED IN CANCER ONLY?
TP73	p53-related transcription factor	No	No	Yes
VHL	VHL protein; regulator of HIF-1	Yes	Yes	No
MLH1	Mismatch repair	Yes	Yes	No
RASSF1A	Ras effector homologue	No	No	Yes
O6MGMT	DNA damage repair	No	No	Yes
DAPK	Death associated protein kinase	No	No	Yes
Caspase 8	Programmed cell death	No	No	Yes
Apaf-1	Programmed cell death	No	No	Yes
FHIT	Diadenosine polyphosphate hydrolase	Yes	Yes	No
SMARCA3	SWI/SNF-related chromatin factor	No	No	Yes
RIZ1	Retinoblastoma-binding histone methylase	No	Yes	No
p16^{INK4a}	Cyclin-dependent kinase inhibitor	Yes	Yes	No
GSTP1	DNA damage repair	No	No	Yes
RB	E2F inhibitor; cell cycle control	Yes	Yes	No
CDH1	E-cadherin cell-cell adhesion molecule	Yes	Yes	No
HIC1	Zinc finger transcription factor	No	No	Yes
BRCA1	Breast cancer predisposition; DNA repair	Yes	Yes	No
LKB1 (STK11)	Serine/threonine kinase	Yes	Yes	No
TIMP3	Tissue inhibitor of metalloproteinase	No	No	Yes

Data from Rountree MR, et al: DNA methylation, chromatin inheritance, and cancer. Oncogene 2001;20:3156–3165, table 1 and Jones PA, Baylin SB: The fundamental role of epigenetic events in cancer. Nature Rev Genet 2002;3:415–428, figure 2.

cancers actually function in vivo as tumor suppressor genes. Promoter hypermethylation and loss of gene expression might perhaps be best considered as potentially useful but insufficient criteria for establishing tumor suppressor gene function in the absence of other supporting data. For instance, additional, supportive evidence of tumor suppressor gene function might include data indicating that the methylation status of a promoter is tightly linked to its expression in a large panel of primary cancer specimens, and data showing that gene expression can be readily and fully restored by treatment of cancer cells with demethylating and/or chromatin remodeling agents, such as histone deacetylase inhibitors. In addition, data showing that bi-allelic inactivation of the methylated gene occurs by mutational mechanisms (e.g., localized mutation and LOH) or a combination of mutational and epigenetic mechanisms in at least some cancers might also represent a potentially critical set of observations. Yet another caveat to be aware of is that because several transcription factors that specifically repress tumor suppressor gene expression have been identified (e.g., the Snail and Slug proteins and their ability to repress E-cadherin in breast cancer and the bmi-1 oncoprotein and its repression of p16^{INK4a} and p19^{ARF}), in some cases promoter hypermethylation might be principally a reflection rather than a proximal cause of tumor suppressor gene inactivation in cancer.[24-26]

Alterations In Cancer Target Conserved Signaling Pathways and Networks

As described previously and summarized in Tables 15-1 and 15-2, the protein products of proto-oncogenes and tumor suppressor genes have been implicated in diverse cellular processes. In light of the potentially vast complexity suggested by the diverse array of gene defects in cancer, it is somewhat reassuring to note that some general concepts have emerged with respect to the means by which genetic and epigenetic alterations contribute to cancer initiation and progression. Perhaps the principal overarching theme is that the protein products of oncogenes and tumor suppressor genes function in highly conserved signaling pathways and regulatory networks.

One of the best studied of these regulatory networks is the one in which the pRb protein functions.[27] The pRb protein appears to play an important role in regulating cell cycle progression, in large part via its ability to bind to E2F transcription factor proteins. The binding of pRb to E2F proteins allows pRb to silence expression of E2F-regulated or "target" genes, such as those needed for the DNA synthetic (S) phase of the cell cycle. The ability of the pRb protein to bind to E2F proteins and to function in transcriptional repression appears to be tightly linked to its phosphorylation status, with the hyperphosphorylated forms of pRb incapable of binding to and regulating E2F proteins. Strong evidence indicates that the cyclin D1 protein and its associated protein kinase, cyclin dependent kinase 4 (Cdk4), negatively regulate pRb by phosphorylating it, and that the p16 tumor suppressor protein is a critical inhibitor of the Cdk4/cyclin D1 complex (Fig. 15-3). As noted in Table 15-2, a subset of sporadic cancers of various types has inactivating mutation in the RB1 gene.[28] In other cancers, pRb function appears to be critically compromised as a result of mutations in other components of the network/pathway.[28] For example, in many cancers lacking RB1

Science of Clinical Oncology

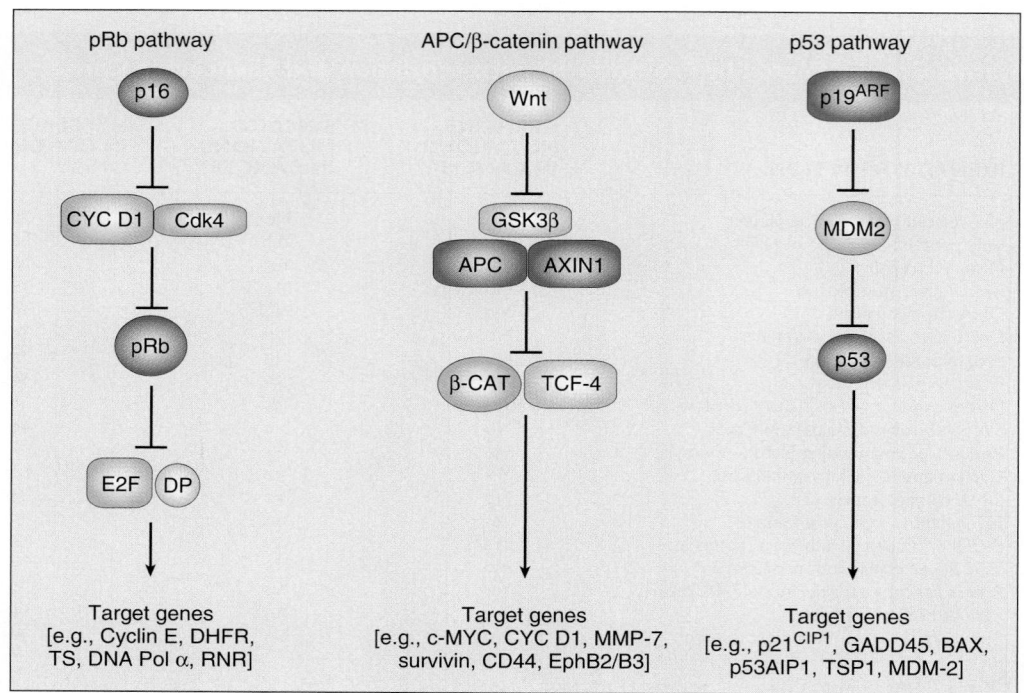

Figure 15-3. Recurrent gene defects in conserved signaling pathways in cancer. Three signaling pathways commonly affected by mutations in various cancers are shown. Selected interactions between components of the pRb pathway (*left*), APC/β-catenin (*middle*), and p53 pathways (*right*) are shown. Tumor suppressor proteins are indicated with red symbols, oncogene products are indicated by green, and those proteins not known to be affected by mutational or epigenetic defects in human cancer are indicated in yellow. Inhibitory interactions between proteins are indicated by perpendicular lines, and activating effects are indicated by arrows. Presumptive downstream genes whose expression is affected by the pathways are noted. APC, adenomatous polyposis coli; β-CAT, β-catenin; Cdk4, cyclin-dependent kinase 4; CYC D1, cyclin D1; DHFR, dihydrofolate reductase; DNA Polα, DNA polymerase α; GADD45, growth arrest and DNA damage inducible gene 45; GSK3β, glycogen synthase 3β; MMP-7, matrix metalloproteinase7, p21^{CIP1}, p21 cdk-interacting protein 1; p53AIP1, p53-regulated apoptosis-inducing protein 1; RNR, ribonucleotide reductase; TCF-4, T cell factor-4; TS, thymidylatesynthase; TSP1, thrombospondin 1.

mutations, inactivating mutations in the *p16^INK4a* gene have been noted. In other cancers lacking *RB1* mutations (including some breast cancers), gene amplification and overexpression of cyclin D1 is found. In yet other cancers lacking *RB1* mutations, such as some glioblastomas and sarcomas, amplification and overexpression of the *CDK4* gene has been seen frequently. The net effect of mutations in the pRb pathway—whether in *RB1* itself or in other genes, such as *p16^INK4a*, *cyclin D1*, or *CDK4*—is to inactivate pRb function and its ability to regulate expression of critical E2F target genes (Fig. 15-3).

Studies of other proto-oncogenes and tumor suppressor genes have also supported the existence of conserved regulatory networks in which multiple different tumor suppressor gene and proto-oncogene protein products function. A key function of the APC (adenomatous polyposis coli) tumor suppressor protein is to participate in a multiprotein complex that regulates the levels of the β-catenin protein in the cytoplasm and nucleus (see Fig. 15-3).[29] Components of the multiprotein complex regulating β-catenin include not only the APC protein but also another tumor suppressor protein known as AXIN1, and a kinase known as glycogen synthase kinase 3β (GSK3β). Inactivation of APC or AXIN1 function in cancer cells appears to lead to an inability to phosphorylate β-catenin and hence target it for recognition and subsequent ubiquitination by the βTrCP1 ubiquitin ligase, and

ultimately to its destruction by the proteasome. As a result, cancer cells with APC or AXIN1 inactivation display increased levels of β-catenin in the cytoplasm and nucleus, and essentially constitutive complexing of β-catenin with transcription factors of the T cell factor (TCF) family, such as TCF-4. When bound to TCF-4, β-catenin can function as a transcriptional co-activator, and in cancers with APC inactivation (e.g., colorectal carcinomas) or cancers with AXIN1 inactivation (e.g., hepatocellular carcinomas), TCF transcriptional activity clearly is deregulated. In a subset of the colorectal carcinomas lacking APC inactivation and in a variety of other cancer types (see Table 15-1), activating (oncogenic) mutations in the β-catenin protein have been found.[30] These missense and in-frame deletion mutations affect key phosphorylation sites in the N-terminus of β-catenin, essentially rendering β-catenin resistant to regulation by the APC/AXIN1/GSK3β complex; the mutant β-catenin protein accumulates in the cell and deregulates TCF transcription. It is worthy of interest that transcription of several proto-oncogenes, including the *c-MYC* and cyclin D1 genes, appears to be activated directly by the β-catenin/TCF complex.[29,31,32] Other tumor suppressor gene regulatory networks have been defined, including the p53/MDM2/p19^Arf pathway (see Fig. 15-3), the PTCH/SMO/GLI pathway, and the MSH2/MLH1/PMS2 DNA mismatch recognition and repair pathway. Similar to the situation for the pRb, APC/β-catenin, and p53 pathways, mutations in cancer cells not infrequently target the PTCH/SMO/GLI and MSH2/MLH1/PMS2 pathways, either activating an oncogene within the pathway (e.g., SMO or GLI for the PTCH/SMO/GLI pathway) or inactivating one of the key tumor suppressors (e.g., either MLH1 or MSH2 in the mismatch repair pathway).

Although a large collection of genetic and biochemic data support the proposed protein functions and interactions depicted in Figure 15-3, it seems likely that the situation in vivo is far more complex. For example, based on the regulatory scheme outlined for the pRb pathway in Figure 15-3, it might appear that the phenotypic consequences of pRb or p16^{INK4a} inactivation are functionally equivalent. Patients with germline mutations inactivating pRb are predisposed to retinoblastomas and osteosarcomas, however, whereas those with germline defects in p16^{INK4a} are predisposed predominantly to melanoma and pancreatic cancer.[33] Moreover, while those with germline mutations affecting pRb or p16^{Ink4a} are predisposed to a rather limited spectrum of cancers, somatic defects in the pRb pathway (e.g., including mutations in pRb, p16Ink4a, cyclin D1, and Cdk4) are seen in the majority of a broad array of cancer types.[28] Unfortunately, there is no compelling mechanistic explanation for these observations at present, but a general explanation can perhaps be offered. Specifically, the genetic pathways in which certain oncogenes and tumor suppressor genes function are probably not simply linear pathways as indicated schematically in Figure 15-3, but more likely represent much more complex networks. The branches of the network might even vary considerably, depending on cell type and developmental context, though it seems reasonable to predict that the genes and the protein products affected recurrently by mutation in human cancer represent particularly critical nodes in the pathways and networks.

CONTRIBUTION OF GENE DEFECTS TO THE SIGNATURE TRAITS OF CANCER CELLS

Defining Signature Traits of Cancer Cells

Cancer represents a highly heterogeneous collection of diseases. In total, in excess of 100 diseases are termed cancer. Each cancer type has distinct biologic and clinical features and a variable prognosis. Even cancers arising in a single organ site, such as the ovary, kidney, or the lung, represent a hodgepodge of different diseases. Morphologic features often allow the particular cancer types to be distinguished to some degree from one another. Yet, even for patients whose cancers have essentially identical gross and microscopic appearances and similar clinical manifestations, there can be vast differences in outcome. In spite of this complexity, the development of all cancers, regardless of type, is likely to be critically dependent on the acquisition of certain phenotypic features that allow the cancer cells not only to grow in an unchecked fashion in their tissue of origin but also to gain the ability

to disseminate into surrounding tissues and organs, lymphatics, and the bloodstream and ultimately to grow as metastatic lesions in distant sites in the body. As indicated in Figure 15-4, among the signature traits likely to be inherent to the majority if not all cancer cells are the following:

- An increased tendency to manifest a stem cell or progenitor-like phenotype
- An enhanced response to growth-promoting signals
- A relative resistance to growth-inhibitory cues
- An increased mutation rate to allow for the rapid generation of new variant daughter cells
- The ability to attract and support a new blood supply (angiogenesis)
- The capacity to minimize an immune response and/or evade destruction by immune effector cells
- The capacity for essentially limitless cell division
- A failure to respect tissue boundaries, allowing for invasion into adjacent tissues, organs, blood vessels, and lymphatics
- The ability to grow in organ sites with microenvironments markedly different from the one in which the cancer cells arose

The development of some of these traits is likely to be associated with specific stages of the tumorigenesis (see Fig. 15-4), although acquisition of the signature traits in cancers of one type or another is far more likely to show a preferred order than an invariant order.[34] Furthermore, many of the signature traits of cancer cells elaborated in the foregoing list represent highly complex biologic capabilities (e.g., angiogenic activity, immune evasion/resistance, metastatic competence). Therefore, it is likely that substantial changes in a number of cell-signaling pathways might be needed for the cancer cell to develop many of the signature traits.

An exhaustive cataloguing of the observations linking specific gene defects to the altered phenotype of cancer cells will not be offered here, in part because of space limitations and in part because of uncertainties about the significance of some of the linkages between single gene defects and cancer phenotype that have been suggested in the literature to date. Nonetheless, some general concepts regarding the relationships between gene defects and cancer cell phenotype have emerged, and two of these concepts will offered here:

1. First, although some of the specific mutations and major gene expression defects seen in cancer cells could contribute predominantly to a few or perhaps even only one of the signature traits of cancer cells listed previously, it seems likely that many of the gene defects and expression changes could have been selected for in large part because they exert pleiotropic effects on the cancer cell phenotype.
2. Second, for some tumor types, it has been possible to gain insights into the apparent order in which genetic and epigenetic changes might arise and contribute to cancer pathogenesis. The data suggest that defects in certain genes and signaling pathways could strongly be selected for at certain point in cancer development

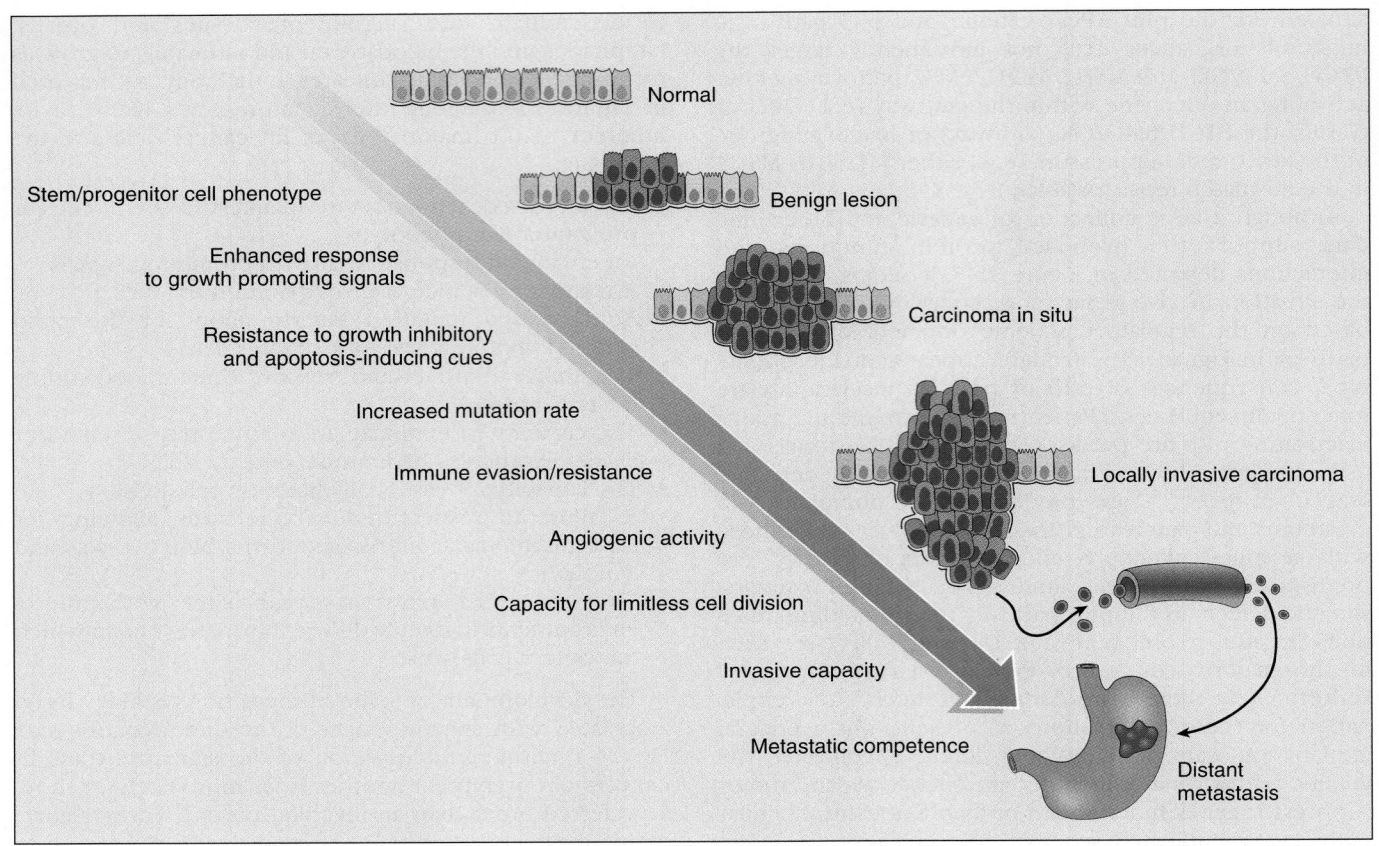

Figure 15-4. Acquisition of signature traits in neoplastic cells during cancer progression. Depicted in the figure are representative stages in the development of a cancer, perhaps a typical epithelial cancer, such as those typically arising in the lung, colon, breast, or prostate. The schema suggests that most advanced cancers arise via clonal selection from subclones present in earlier stage benign and localized lesions (e.g., carcinoma in situ and locally invasive carcinoma). Some of the properties of advanced cancer cells are depicted by the ability of the cells to enter the bloodstream and to seed and grow in distant organ sites, such as the liver (*bottom*). Nine signature traits of cancer cells are listed. The relative time at which neoplastic cells acquire some of the traits is uncertain, though it seems likely that some traits, such as the expression of a stem/progenitor cell phenotype or enhanced response to growth-promoting signals, may be acquired earlier in cancer development. Other traits, such as invasive capacity and/or metastatic competence, may be acquired later. Many signature traits of cancer cells are in fact complicated biological capabilities (e.g., angiogenic activity, immune evasion/resistance, metastatic competence) and likely depend on defects in a number of different factors and signaling pathways.

and progression, perhaps in large part because the alterations allow the precancerous or cancerous cells to acquire certain critical phenotypic features.

It is of some interest that gene defects that could be nearly uniformly present in early stage lesions of one tumor type might arise preferentially in later-stage tumors in another organ site. These data suggest that cellular and tissue context have critical, albeit poorly understood, modifying effects on the specific genetic defects that give rise to neoplastic transformation and clonal outgrowth. These two concepts—the often pleiotropic effects of the gene defects present in cancer cells and the context-dependent effects of the gene defects—will be expanded on shortly, with presentation of some concrete examples.

Contribution of APC Inactivation and β-catenin Deregulation to Cancer Phenotype

As discussed earlier, mutational defects leading to deregulation of the signaling activity of the β-catenin

protein are present in broad array of cancer types, including colorectal tumors, where upwards of 90% of colorectal adenomas and carcinomas harbor inactivating mutations in APC or the AXIN1 homologue AXIN2, or gain-of-function mutations in β-catenin itself.[29] Based on the observation that germline inactivating mutations in APC markedly increase the rate at which adenomatous lesions arise in the colon and rectum and on extensive descriptive molecular studies showing that somatic mutations in APC or β-catenin are present in even microscopic adenomatous lesions in the colon, it appears that dysregulation of β-catenin likely plays a central role in the earliest stages of colon cancer development.[29,30] In other cancer types in which β-catenin is often deregulated by mutational mechanisms, such as hepatocellular and endometrial cancers, the timing of β-catenin mutations in the natural history of disease is less certain.[30]

Given this background, what might be the contribution of β-catenin defects to the development and biologic behavior of colon and perhaps other cancers? As highlighted previously, β-catenin, upon its association with TCF

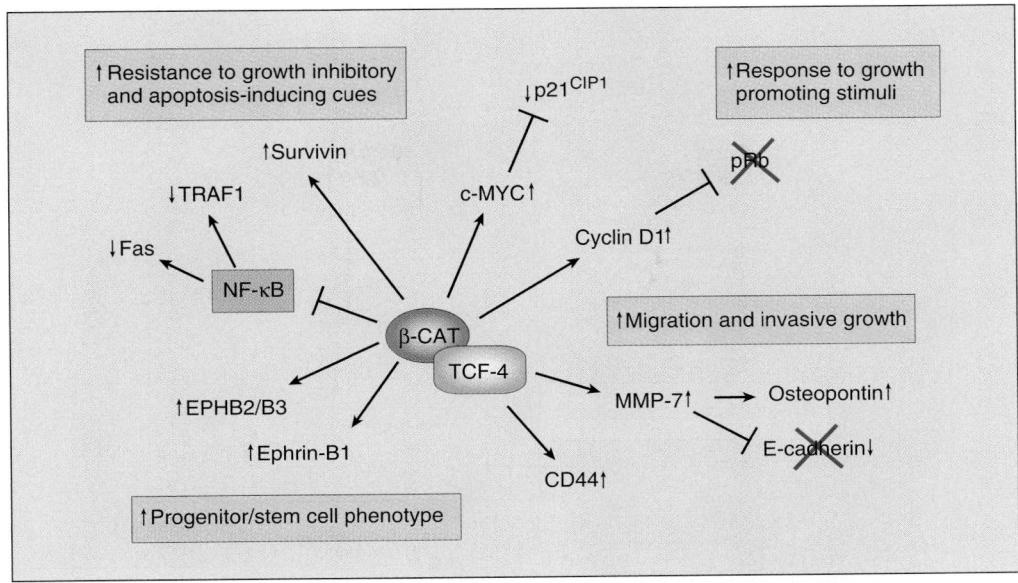

Figure 15-5. Potential contributions of β-catenin deregulation to cancer cell signature traits. Inactivation of the APC tumor suppressor protein or activating (oncogenic) mutations in β-catenin can lead to marked increases in the levels of free β-catenin protein in the cytoplasm and nucleus, enhanced binding of β-catenin to the TCF-4 (T cell factor-4) transcription factor, and activation of β-catenin/TCF-4 regulated genes. Some of the genes that may be directly regulated by the β-catenin–TCF-4 transcription process include the genes for c-MYC, cyclin D1, MMP-7, survivin, CD44, the EPHB2 and EPHB3 receptors, and their ligand Ephrin-B1. Some of the potential effects resulting from activation of these target genes are indicated. In addition to β-catenin's role in activating expression of TCF-4–related genes, β-catenin appears to inhibit the activity of NF-κB and NF-κB's ability to activate genes with potential roles in apoptosis, such as Fas and TRAF1. The potential contributions of β-catenin to cancer cell traits is discussed in more detail in the text.

transcription factors, has been implicated in activating expression of genes (including cyclin D1 and c-MYC) that likely play critical roles in stimulating progression through the G1-S transition. Effects of cyclin D1 activation on the pRb pathway and progression through the G1-S phase of the cell cycle have been mentioned earlier. As indicated in Figure 15-5, one of the apparent consequences of c-MYC activation of colon cancer cells is repression of the expression of the p21^{CIP1} cyclin-dependent kinase inhibitor, and inhibition of p21^{CIP1} might contribute to defective cell cycle control.[15,35-37] In addition to effects on cyclin D1 and c-MYC, deregulation of β-catenin/TCF transcription has been implicated in activation of a number of genes that might play a role in maintaining or inducing a progenitor cell or stem cell-like phenotype in colon cells that should otherwise be destined for differentiation or apoptosis (see Fig. 15-5).[35] Genes that could play a role in conferring a progenitor cell phenotype include the cell surface protein CD44 and the EphB2 and EphB3 receptors and their ligand ephrin-B1.[35,38] Either individually or collectively along with other molecules, the cell surface proteins might exert potent effects on colonic epithelial cell fate, perhaps in part by inhibiting appropriate migration of cells in the crypt and hence favoring response to proliferation-inducing signals over differentiation-inducing cues.[35]

Another presumptive β-catenin/TCF target gene with a potential role in acquisition of several critical cancer phenotypic traits is the matrix metalloproteinase-7 (MMP-7, also known as matrilysin) (see Fig. 15-5).[39] MMP-7 itself has a number of potential roles in cancer pro-

gression, including the ability to cleave and down-regulate the activity of the E-cadherin tumor suppressor protein and the ability to cleave osteopontin and apparently activate osteopontin's cell migration-stimulating activity.[40-42] Besides the role of dysregulated βb-catenin in activating transcription of TCF target genes, there is evidence that elevated levels of nuclear β-catenin in cancer cells can interfere with NF-kB function and NF-kB's ability to activate key downstream effectors of apoptosis, such as Fas and TRAF1 (see Fig. 15-5).[43] Finally, the carboxyl-terminal region of the APC tumor suppressor protein confers binding to the EB1 protein (a microtubule-binding protein) and to microtubules.[44] Given the apparent role of EB1 in regulating microtubule dynamics, cell polarity, and chromosome stability and the evidence that APC inactivation in certain cellular contexts could confer a chromosome instability phenotype, it is possible that APC inactivation also contributes to a chromosomal instability phenotype in colorectal cancer cells.[44,45]

Contribution of RAS Signaling Pathway Defects to Cancer Phenotype

RAS gene mutations were the first somatic gene defects to be characterized at the molecular level in cancer cells, and we now know that mutations in the three RAS genes—H-RAS, K-RAS, and N-RAS—are among the most common oncogene defects in cancer, with an estimated 20% of all cancers carrying a point-mutated, activated RAS allele.[46,47] RAS proteins appear to play key roles in several important signaling pathways (Fig. 15-6), and proteins that

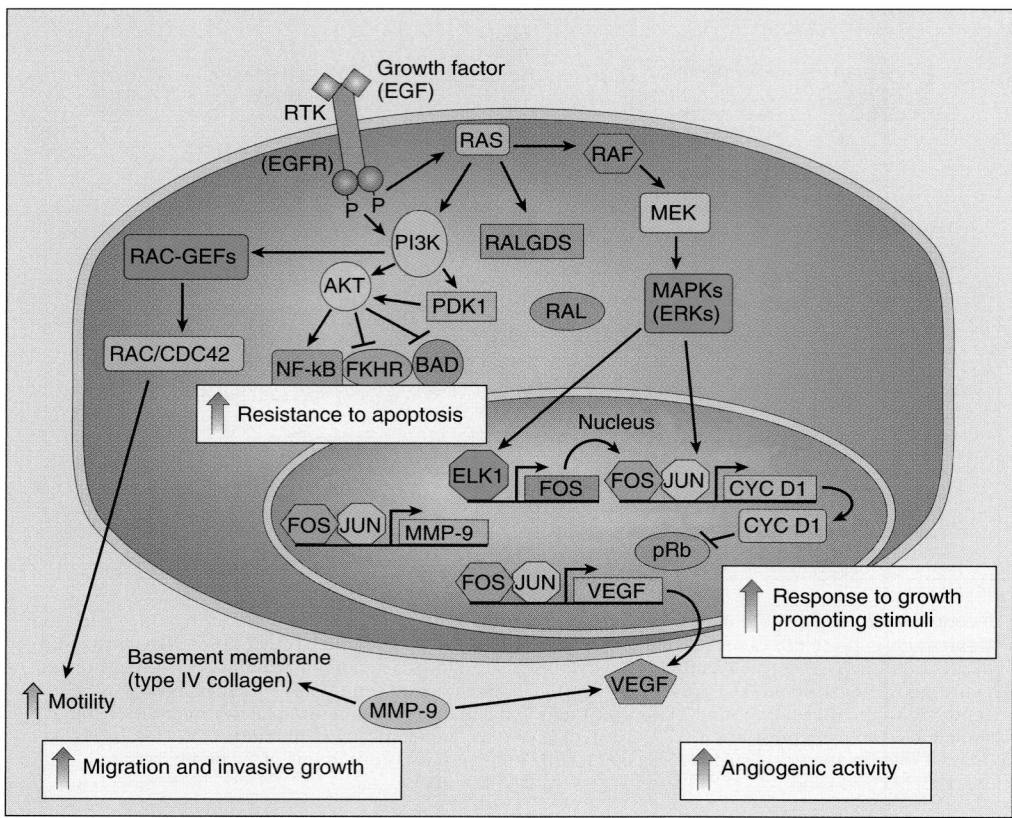

Figure 15-6. Potential contribution of RAS pathway defects to the cancer cell phenotype. The RAS protein is indicated near the top of the figure, and selected upstream and downstream factors are also indicated relative to their likely location in the cell. RAS pathway signaling interactions are complex and only selected functional interactions upstream and downstream of RAS are indicated. As indicated in the figure and discussed in more detail in the text, RAS pathway activation can likely enhance the response to growth-promoting stimuli via effects on cyclin D1 (CYC D1) expression and pRb phosphorylation and activity. These effects on cyclin D1 expression are likely to be mediated by the RAF/MAPK (mitogen activated protein kinase) signaling cascade and its effects on downstream conscription factors, including JUN and the ETS-related protein ELK1, which activates expression of JUN's dimeric partner, FOS. RAS pathway activation also likely acts to increase resistance to apoptosis in some settings, through effects on AKT and its ability to inhibit factors with pro-apoptotic roles (e.g., Forkhead in human rhabdomyosarcoma [FKHR] or BAD) or AKT's ability to activate NF-κB's survival function. Besides these effects, RAS pathway activation may act to stimulate vascular endothelial growth factor (VEGF) production and angiogenesis. RAS can enhance cell migration and invasion via RAC/CDC42-mediated effects on the cytoskeleton and possibly FOS/JUN-mediated increases in the expression of some matrix metalloproteases, such as MMP-9. Finally, MMP-9 can also promote release of VEGF from extracellular reservoirs, perhaps further enhancing VEGF effects on angiogenesis.

function upstream or downstream of the RAS proteins are affected by mutations in certain cancers. For instance, mutational activation and/or overexpression of growth factors upstream of RAS, such as EGFR and/or ERBB2 (also known as HER2/Neu), can commonly be seen in a number of epithelial cancers, including breast and ovarian carcinomas and others (see Table 15-1). Mutations downstream of RAS can also be seen in cancers, including defects in the mitogen-activated protein kinase (MAPK) pathway as a result of BRAF gene mutations, or defects in phosphatidylinositol 3-kinase (PI3K) signaling, as result of amplification and overexpression of AKT2 or inactivating mutations in the PTEN (phosphatase and tensin homologue) tumor suppressor gene.[46,48,49]

The consequences of RAS mutations specifically and RAS signaling pathway defects more generally are varied and undoubtedly dependent on cell context, because constitutive activation of RAS signaling in certain contexts can promote apoptosis rather than cell proliferation or neoplastic transformation.[50,51] In brief, activated mutant RAS alleles have been implicated in enhanced response to proliferative cures, perhaps to a certain extent due to the ability of RAS-MAPK activation to enhance expression of cyclin D1, and to cyclin D1's ability to inactivate pRb function via phosphorylation (see Fig. 15-6).[46,51] RAS pathway activation also can interfere with the induction of apoptosis, perhaps in part via activation of the PI3K pathway and its ability to antagonize the pro-apoptotic factor BAD and perhaps other molecules important in promoting programmed cell death (see Fig. 15-6).[46,49] In addition to the potential ability of RAS pathway activation to enhance cell proliferation and inhibit programmed cell death, RAS activation has been implicated in transcriptional activation in cancer cells of vascular endothelial growth factor (VEGF), a potent stimulator of angiogenesis.[52] Moreover, RAS activation has been linked to increased invasive potential in cancer cells.[46] The role of RAS in promoting invasiveness might be mediated through RAC-dependent effects on the cytoskeleton and through MAPK pathway-dependent activation of matrix metalloproteinases (e.g., MMP-9), which can function in degradation of the basement membrane component type IV collagen (see Fig. 15-6).[40,46] Interestingly, MMP-9 has also been implicated in promoting angiogenesis in some settings, via its ability to stimulate release of VEGF from poorly defined extracellular reservoirs.[53]

Role of Tissue and Context Differences in the Contributions of Gene Defects to Cancer Cell Phenotype

The published literature on the potential contributions of gene defects to the altered phenotype of cancer cells has offered some suggestions about how to consider the role of the gene defects in cancer pathogenesis. For instance, terms like *gatekeeper* and *caretaker* have been used to classify the contributions of genes to cancer development.[54] "Gatekeeper" genes have been suggested to be those genes that play particularly critical roles in regulating cell proliferation and inhibiting cancer development in certain tissues (e.g., the APC gene in colorectal cancer), and the tumor suppressive function of the genes must be overcome for cancers to arise in a given tissue or organ site.[54] "Caretakers" have been generally defined as those genes that do not play direct roles in growth control but rather likely play important roles in a number of tissues in maintaining the fidelity of the genome, via their role in DNA damage recognition and repair processes. The MLH1 and MSH2 mismatch repair genes have been proposed to be representative caretaker genes, and some researchers have suggested that perhaps the BRCA1 and BRCA2 genes might also represent caretaker genes.[54,55] The use of terms like *gatekeeper* and *caretaker* might have some merit. As will be illustrated shortly, however, given the apparently important role of "gatekeeper" gene defects in cancers arising in various organ sites, but the quite variable timing of "gatekeeper" gene defects in the natural history of one cancer type vs. another, the term *gatekeeper* might be more confusing than illuminating. In the case of some presumed "caretaker" genes, the genes might not be playing the passive role in the cancer process that has been assigned to them. This view is based on three lines of argument:

1. The apparent tissue specificity of the tumors that arise in individuals harboring germline mutations in the "caretaker" genes, such as in those individuals affected by HNPCC and germline MLH1 or MSH2 mutations;
2. The likely variable time in cancer development at which "caretaker" mutations could arise from one tumor to the next, with sporadic colon tumors not usually manifesting mismatch repair gene inactivation and microsatellite instability until the carcinoma stage, despite the fact that adenomas in those with HNCC often show high-frequency microsatellite instability; and
3. The evidence that "caretaker" genes might actually play key roles in regulating cell proliferation and promoting apoptosis in certain contexts.[56-59]

In general, those individuals who harbor a germline mutation in specific tumor suppressor genes or proto-oncogenes are predisposed to a limited spectrum of cancer types. This observation is puzzling for a couple of reasons. The majority of genes affected by germline mutations in specific inherited cancer syndromes are essentially ubiquitously expressed in adult tissues. Furthermore, for a number of the tumor suppressor genes, mutations are often found to inactivate the gene in a much broader collection of sporadic cancer types than the types commonly arising in germline mutation carriers. Children who carry a germline mutation in the *RB1* gene have a highly elevated risk of developing retinoblastoma and a more modest risk of developing osteosarcoma, but no dramatic increase in the risk of most common adult cancers. Yet, somatic defects in pRb have been found and are believed critical in the development of many different cancers, such as small cell lung carcinomas (SCLCs), where the vast majority of SCLCs have pRb defects.[28,59]

There are potential explanations for these puzzling observations. For instance, although pRb could have an essential role in regulating retinoblast cell proliferation and/or differentiation, in other tissues (e.g., lung or breast epithelial cells), pRb might have a redundant role in growth control, perhaps because of the contribution of pRb-related proteins such as p107 and p130.[27] Under this scenario, pRb inactivation in most cell types might not promote neoplastic growth unless other defects, such as those in pRb-related proteins, are also present. An alternative and perhaps more likely possibility is that somatic inactivation of pRb could trigger programmed cell death or apoptosis in many cell types, unless other somatic gene defects have arisen previously and these other defects interfere with the cell's ability to undergo apoptosis after disruption of *RB1* function (Fig. 15-7). Evidence that pRb inactivation can act in a context-dependent fashion to promote apoptosis vs. neoplastic transformation has been offered.[60,61] The tissue specificity of cancers seen in individuals carrying germline mutations in inherited cancer genes is not restricted to the case of pRb. Germline *p53* mutations predispose primarily to osteosarcoma, soft-tissue sarcoma, leukemia, brain tumors, and breast cancer in women, and *p16INK4a* germline mutations predispose primarily to melanoma and pancreatic cancer. In spite of the relatively limited spectrum of cancer types seen in those carrying germline p53 or *p16INK4a* mutations, the *p53* and *p16INK4a* genes represent perhaps the two most commonly altered genes in human cancer described thus far, with each of the genes inactivated in upwards of 35%–50% of many different sporadic cancer types.

Finally, some genes with prominent roles in the development of a variety of different cancer types are sometimes presumed to have essentially singular functions in the cancer process, in spite of data that suggest otherwise. As an example, the E-cadherin protein plays an important role in cell-to-cell adhesion via the ability of its extracellular domain to form adhesive interactions with E-cadherin molecules on opposing cell surfaces and via the ability of the E-cadherin cytoplasmic domain to link to the actin cortical cytoskeleton through interactions with catenin proteins at the plasma membrane.[62] Early functional studies have suggested that

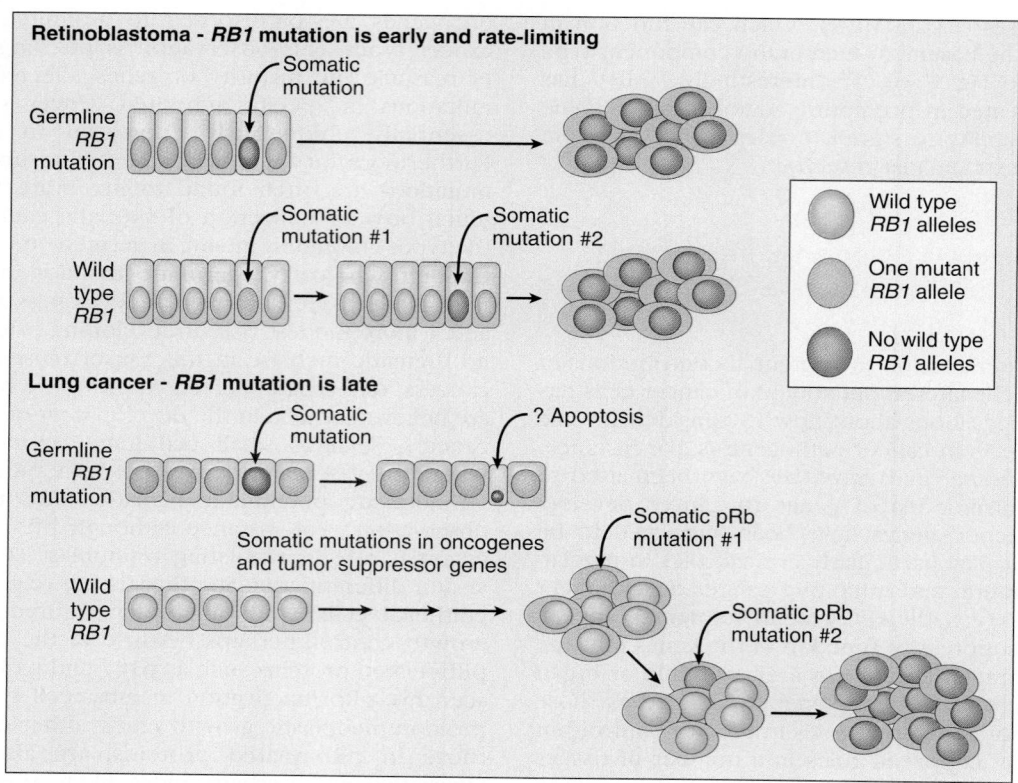

Figure 15-7. Mutations in the retinoblastoma tumor suppressor gene (*RB1*) contribute to inherited and sporadic cancers. The figure indicates that cell context affects the contribution of *RB1* mutations to cancer development. In individuals carrying a germline mutation in one *RB1* allele, somatic inactivation of the remaining *RB1* allele is an early and rate-limiting event in retinoblastoma formation. Sporadic forms of retinoblastoma are dependent on inactivation of both *RB1* alleles. Because somatic inactivation of both *RB1* alleles must occur in a single developing retinoblast before tumor formation can ensue, retinoblastoma is a rare disease in those who do not carry a germline *RB1* mutation (i.e., the general population). Those who carry a germline *RB1* mutation do not manifest a markedly increased risk to many common cancers, such as lung cancer, despite the fact that *RB1* mutations are frequently observed in sporadic forms of lung cancer (e.g., small cell lung carcinoma). These observations imply that *RB1* mutations might contribute to tumor progression rather than tumor initiation in most cancer types other than retinoblastoma and perhaps osteosarcoma. Possible explanations for this phenomenon include the possibility that inactivation of both *RB1* alleles prior to the acquisition of defects in other oncogenes or tumor suppressor genes is not associated with any growth advantage and *RB1* activation in some contexts may even induce apoptosis. (Modified from Haber DA, Fearon ER: The promise of cancer genetics. Lancet, 1998;351[suppl 2]:1–8.)

restoration of E-cadherin in cancer cells that had endogenous E-cadherin defects interfered with the invasive properties of cancer cells in selected in vitro assays.[63] Perhaps in large part because of these observations, the loss of E-cadherin expression in cancer has nearly invariably been assigned a role in promoting invasive behavior in advanced cancer cells. Although loss of E-cadherin function might indeed contribute to invasive behavior in cancers arising in vivo, it is worth bearing in mind that defects in E-cadherin could in fact play a distinct role in altering cell growth very early in the neoplastic transformation process in some tumor types, such as in the gastric carcinomas arising in patients carrying germline E-cadherin mutations.[64]

CLINICAL IMPLICATIONS

Based on review of the data on the apparent contributions of gene defects to cancer phenotype, some clinical implications are apparent. The genes and the protein products recurrently altered by mutations and/or epigenetic defects

in human cancer more than likely represent particularly critical nodes in the pathways and networks regulating cell growth, differentiation, and programmed cell death. Hence, efforts to target the proteins and pathways with apparently central roles in the pathogenesis of a number of different cancer types would appear potentially to offer the broadest impact. Additionally, because the gene defects that promote clonal selection during cancer development might have particularly pleiotropic effects on the cancer cell phenotype, targeting of the central pathways in cancer might also be expected to have some of the most dramatic effects on cancer cells. For example, in light of the important role of RAS pathway defects in a broad array of cancer types and the view that RAS pathway deregulation exerts pleiotropic effects on the cancer cell phenotype, drugs that inhibit the activity of Raf, MEK, or MAPK could have potent anticancer activity in a subset of the many cancers with RAS pathway defects.[65] Moreover, even though RAS pathway defects can arise at early-to-intermediate stages of tumor development in some cancer types (e.g., colorectal cancer), it is encouraging to learn that dramatic effects on the growth of advanced cancer cells can be seen when the activity of the mutant RAS protein is antagonized.[66-68]

In spite of the generally optimistic view that is offered as a result of our rapidly expanding understanding of the nature and contribution of gene defects in cancer pathogenesis, some significant challenges remain if novel and specific new anticancer therapies are to be achieved in the near term. In particular, for a fair number of the specific signaling pathways commonly disrupted in cancer, it might prove difficult to define readily tractable targets for therapeutic intervention. For instance, in the case of the p53 pathway, it is unclear how one might effectively restore p53 function in proteins carrying missense substitutions or p53 functional activity in tumors in which the p53 protein is intact and simply antagonized by upstream defects (e.g., p19[ARF] or MDM2 defects). In the case of cancers with mutations leading to β-catenin deregulation, a potential goal might be to define agents that specifically interfere with the nuclear function of β-catenin in transcriptional activation of β-catenin/ TCF-regulated target genes. Although this is not an unreasonable notion, it could be extremely challenging— given the rather limited successes to date in defining small molecules that specifically affect transcription factor complexes—to target β-catenin via conventional pharmacologic approaches. Similar concerns could perhaps be raised regarding the merits of attempting to target other specific nuclear proteins and transcription factors that are deregulated in cancer cells.

Given these concerns regarding the likelihood of success in defining small molecules that effectively target some of the pathways most commonly deregulated in cancer, emphasis for therapeutic targeting in the near term might be placed on potentially more promising molecular targets in cancer, such as Cdk4 (e.g., for cancers with an intact pRb protein, but defects in p16[INK4a], cyclin D1, or Cdk4) or various effector molecules in the PI3K-AKT pathway, such as the AKT or mTOR proteins (e.g., for cancers with PTEN defects).[49] Although the success of approaches to target cancer cells more selectively remains to be broadly established, it is obvious that the efforts to understand the relationship between gene defects, altered cell signaling and physiology, and cancer phenotype have already and will continue to shape our views of how best to proceed with novel therapeutic interventions.

REFERENCES

1. Nordling CE: A new theory on the cancer-inducing mechanism. Br J Cancer 1953;6:68-72.
2. Armitage P, Doll R: The age distribution of cancer and a multi-stage theory of carcinogenesis. Br J Cancer 1954;8:1-12.
3. Renan MJ: How many mutations are required for tumorigenesis? Implications from human data. Mol Carcinogenesis 1993;7:139-146.
4. Knudson AG: Two genetic hits (more or less) to cancer. Nature Rev Cancer 2001;1:157-162.
5. Fearon ER, Vogelstein B: A genetic model for colorectal tumorigenesis. Cell 1990;61:759-767.
6. Kinzler KW, Vogelstein B: Lessons from hereditary colorectal cancer. Cell 1996;87:159-170.
7. Yokota J, Wada M, Shimosato Y, Terada M, Sugimura T: Loss of heterozygosity on chromosomes 3, 13, and 17 in small-cell carcinoma and on chromosome 3 in adenocarcinoma of the lung. Proc Natl Acad Sci USA;1987, 84:9252-9256.
8. Mitsuuchi Y, Testa JR: Cytogenetics and molecular genetics of lung cancer. Am J Med Genet 2002;115:183-188.
9. Jaffee EM, Hruban RH, Canto M, Kern SE: Focus on pancreas cancer. Cancer Cell 2002;2:25-28.
10. Foulds L: The natural history of cancer. J Chronic Dis 1958;8:2-37.
11. Nowell P: The clonal evolution of tumor cell populations. Science 1976;194:23-28.
12. Knudson AG: Mutations and cancer: statistical study of retinoblastoma. Proc Natl Acad Sci USA 1971;68:820-823.
13. Knudson AG: Mutation and human cancer. Adv Cancer Res 1973;17:317-352.
14. Ko LJ, Prives C: p53: Puzzle and paradigm. Genes Dev 1996;10:1054-1072.
15. Vousden KH, Lu X: Live or let die: The cell's response to p53. Nature Rev Cancer 2002;2:594-604.
16. Fero ML, Randel E, Gurley KE, Roberts JM, Kemp CJ: The murine gene p27Kip1 is haplo-insufficient for tumour suppression. Nature 1998;396:177-180.
17. Philipp-Staheli J, Payne SR, Kemp CJ: p27(Kip1): Regulation and function of a haploinsufficient tumor suppressor and its misregulation in cancer. Exp Cell Res 2001;264:148-168.
18. Pelengaris S, Khan M, Evan G: c-MYC: More than just a matter of life and death. Nat Rev Cancer 2002;2:764-776.
19. Ritter CA, Arteaga CL: The epidermal growth factor receptor-tyrosine kinase: A promising therapeutic target in solid tumors. Semin Oncol 2003;30:3-11.
20. Katayama H, Brinkley WR, Sen S: The Aurora kinases: Role in cell transformation and tumorigenesis. Cancer Metast Rev 2003;22:451-464.
21. Jones PA, Laird PW: Cancer epigenetics comes of age. Nat Genet 1999;21:163-167.
22. Jones PA, Baylin SB: The fundamental role of epigenetic events in cancer. Nature Rev Genet 2002;3:415-428.
23. Herman JG, Latif F, Weng Y, et al: Silencing of the VHL tumor-suppressor gene by DNA methylation in renal carcinoma. Proc Natl Acad Sci USA 1994;91:9700-9704.
24. Hajra KM, Chen DY, Fearon ER: The SLUG zinc-finger protein represses E-cadherin in breast cancer. Cancer Res 2002;62:1613-1618.
25. Jacobs JJ, Kieboom K, Marino S, DePinho RA, van Lohuizen M: The oncogene and Polycomb-group gene bmi-1 regulates cell proliferation and senescence through the ink4a locus. Nature 1999;397:164-168.
26. Vonlanthen S, Heighway J, Altermatt HJ, et al: The bmi-1 oncoprotein is differentially expressed in non-small cell lung cancer and correlates with INK4A-ARF locus expression. Br J Cancer 2001;84:1372-1376.
27. Classon M, Harlow E: The retinoblastoma tumour suppressor in development and cancer. Nature Rev Cancer 2002;2:910-917.
28. Sellers WR, Kaelin WG Jr: Role of the retinoblastoma protein in the pathogenesis of human cancer. J Clin Oncol 1997;15:3301-3312.
29. Bienz M, Clevers H: Linking colorectal cancer to Wnt signaling. Cell 2000;103:311-320.
30. Polakis P: Wnt signaling and cancer. Genes Dev 2000;14:1837-1851.
31. He TC, Sparks AB, Rago C, et al: Identification of c-MYC as a target of the APC pathway. Science 1998;281:1509-1512.
32. Tetsu O, McCormick F: Beta-catenin regulates expression of cyclin D1 in colon carcinoma cells. Nature 1999;398:422-426.
33. Fearon ER: Human cancer syndromes: Clues to the origin and nature of cancer. Science 1997;278:1043-1050.
34. Hanahan D, Weinberg RA: The hallmarks of cancer. Cell 2000;100:57-70.
35. van de Wetering M, Sancho E, Verweij C, et al: The beta-catenin/ TCF-4 complex imposes a crypt progenitor phenotype on colorectal cancer cells. Cell 2002;111:241-250.
36. Seoane J, Le HV, Massague J: Myc suppression of the p21(Cip1) Cdk inhibitor influences the outcome of the p53 response to DNA damage. Nature 2002;419:729-734.
37. Vousden KH. Switching from life to death: The Miz-ing link between Myc and p53. Cancer Cell 2002;2:351-352.

38. Batlle E, Henderson JT, Beghtel H, et al: Beta-catenin and TCF mediate cell positioning in the intestinal epithelium by controlling the expression of EphB/ephrinB. Cell 2002;111:251–263.

39. Crawford HC, Fingleton BM, Rudolph-Owen LA, et al: The metalloproteinase matrilysin is a target of beta-catenin transactivation in intestinal tumors. Oncogene 1999;18:2883–2891.

40. Lynch CC, Matrisian LM: Matrix metalloproteinases in tumor-host cell communication. Differentiation 2002;70:561–573.

41. Noe V, Fingleton B, Jacobs K, et al: Release of an invasion promoter E-cadherin fragment by matrilysin and stromelysin-1. J Cell Sci 2001;114:111–118.

42. Agnihotri R, Crawford HC, Haro H, Matrisian LM, Havrda MC, Liaw L: Osteopontin, a novel substrate for matrix metalloproteinase-3 (stromelysin-1) and matrix metalloproteinase-7 (matrilysin). J Biol Chem 2001;276:28261–28267.

43. Deng J, Miller SA, Wang HY, et al: Beta-catenin interacts with and inhibits NF-kappa B in human colon and breast cancer. Cancer Cell 2002;2:323–334.

44. Fodde R, Smits R, Clevers H: APC, signal transduction and genetic instability in colorectal cancer. Nat Rev Cancer 2001;1:55–67.

45. Fodde R, Kuipers J, Rosenberg C, et al: Mutations in the APC tumour suppressor gene cause chromosomal instability. Nat Cell Biol 2001;3:433–438.

46. Downward J: Targeting ras signaling pathways in cancer therapy. Nature Rev Cancer 2003;3:11–22.

47. Malumbres M, Barbacid M: RAS oncogenes: The first 30 years. Nature Rev Cancer 2003;3:459–465.

48. Davies H, Bignell GR, Cox C, et al: Mutations of the BRAF gene in human cancer. Nature 2002;417:949–954.

49. Vivanco I, Sawyers CL: The phosphatidylinositol 3-kinase-AKT pathway in human cancer. Nat Rev Cancer 2002;2:489–501.

50. Mayo MW, Wang CY, Cogswell PC, et al: Requirement of NF-kappaB activation to suppress p53-independent apoptosis induced by oncogenic Ras. Science 1997;278:1812–1815.

51. Pruitt K, Der CJ: Ras and Rho regulation of the cell cycle and oncogenesis. Cancer Lett 2001;171:1–10.

52. Rak J, Kerbel RS: Ras regulation of vascular endothelial growth factor and angiogenesis. Methods Enzymol 2001;333:267–283.

53. Bergers G, Brekken R, McMahon G, et al: Matrix metalloproteinase-9 triggers the angiogenic switch during carcinogenesis. Nat Cell Biol 2000;2:737–744.

54. Kinzler KW, Vogelstein B: Cancer susceptibility genes. Gatekeepers and caretakers. Nature 1997;386:761–763.

55. Levitt NC, Hickson ID: Caretaker tumour suppressor genes that defend genome integrity. Trends Mol Med 2002;8:179–186.

56. Lynch HT, de la Chapelle A: Genetic susceptibility to non-polyposis colorectal cancer. J Med Genet 1999;36:801–818.

57. Young J, Leggett B, Gustafson C, et al: Genomic instability occurs in colorectal carcinomas but not in adenomas. Hum Mutat 1993;2:351–354.

58. Aaltonen LA, Peltomäki P, Mecklin J-P, et al: Replication errors in benign and malignant tumors from hereditary nonpolyposis colorectal cancer patients. Cancer Res 1994;54:1645–1648.

59. Kaye FJ: RB and cyclin dependent kinase pathways: Defining a distinction between RB and p16 loss in lung cancer. Oncogene 2002;21:6908–6914.

60. Morgenbesser SD, Williams BO, Jacks T, DePinho RA: p53-dependent apoptosis produced by Rb-deficiency in the developing mouse lens. Nature 1994;371:72–74.

61. Lipinski MM, Jacks T: The retinoblastoma gene family in differentiation and development. Oncogene 1999;18:7873–7882.

62. Takeichi M: Morphogenetic roles of classic cadherins. Curr Opin Cell Biol 1995;7:619–627.

63. Vleminckx K, Vakaet L Jr, Mareel M, Fiers W, van Roy F: Genetic manipulation of E-cadherin expression by epithelial tumor cells reveals an invasion suppressor role. Cell 1991;66:107–119.

64. Guilford P, Hopkins J, Harraway J, et al: E-cadherin germline mutations in familial gastric cancer. Nature 1998;392:402–405.

65. Sebolt-Leopold JS: Development of anticancer drugs targeting the MAP kinase pathway. Oncogene 2000;19:6594–6599.

66. Shirasawa S, Furuse M, Yokoyama N, Sasazuki T: Altered growth of human colon cancer cell lines disrupted at activated Ki-ras. Science 1993;260:85–88.

67. Mukhopadhyay T, Tainsky M, Cavendaer AC, Roth JA: Specific inhibition of K-ras expression and tumorigenicity of lung cancer cells by antisense RNA. Cancer Res 1991;51:1744–1748.

68. Brummelkamp TR, Bernards R, Agami R: Stable suppression of tumorigenicity by virus-mediated RNA interference. Cancer Cell 2002;2:243–247.

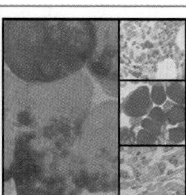

16 | IMMUNODEFICIENCY AND CANCER

Alexandra H. Filipovich

Thomas G. Gross

SUMMARY OF KEY POINTS

- Neoplasms are the second most common cause of mortality (after infections) among patients with primary and acquired immunodeficiencies.
- Infections, whether de novo, reactivated, or chronic, play a pivotal role in promoting development of both lymphomas and carcinomas. Examples include:
  - Epstein-Barr virus associated with lymphoproliferative disorders
  - *H. Pylori* associated with gastric carcinomas and maltomas
  - Human papilloma virus associated with skin and cervical carcinomas
- Categories of genetic

immunodeficiencies with increased risk of developing tumors include:
- Combined defects with T-cell dysfunction (e.g., Wiskott-Aldrich syndrome)
- Defects that inhibit lymphoid apoptosis (e.g., autoimmune lymphoproliferative syndrome [ALPS])
- Defects of genomic instability (e.g., ataxia telangiectasia)
- Categories of acquired immunodeficiencies with increased risk of developing tumors include:
  - Recipients of solid organ allografts, especially children receiving liver or bowel transplants
  - Recipients of T-cell–depleted

mismatched allogeneic hematopoietic stem cells
- Transplant recipients
- HIV/AIDS patients
- The risk of lymphoproliferative disorders in immunodeficient hosts can be reduced by:
  - Correction of primary immunodeficiencies with bone marrow transplant (BMT)
  - Reduction of immune suppression in allograft recipients
  - Close monitoring of transplant recipients with sensitive polymerase chain reaction (PCR) techniques for Epstein-Barr virus and preemptive treatment with anti-CD20 antibodies.

INTRODUCTION

Retrospective surveys of patients with primary and acquired immune deficiencies have revealed several patterns of increased risk for specific cancer types. In the majority of immunodeficiency conditions—whether de novo, reactivated, or chronic—localized infections play a pivotal role in promoting the development of both lymphomas and carcinomas. Specifically, patients with primary (genetically determined) or acquired immune deficiencies that affect T-cell function are at increased risk of developing lymphomas after exposure to Epstein-Barr virus (EBV). This risk group includes patients who are immune suppressed after solid organ allografting, after hematopoietic stem cell transplantation, or secondary to HIV infection. Chronic immune suppression also increases the risk for carcinomas that are linked to infection with viruses, such as herpes family viruses associated with Kaposi's sarcoma (increased risk for HIV-infected subjects and solid organ allograft recipients) or human papilloma virus (HPV) associated with squamous cell carcinoma of the skin and cervical cancer (increased risk for solid organ allograft recipients). Patients with congenital humoral immune defects (especially IgA deficiency) who are persistently colonized with *Helicobacter pylori* experience a higher rate of gastric carcinomas and gastric maltomas. A minor, but biologically instructive, category of

patients at increased risk of tumors of both hematopoietic and epithelial origin are individuals with inherited defects of genomic instability, which lead to both immunodeficiency and propensity to tumor development. Examples of such disorders include ataxia telangiectasia and Bloom's syndrome.

Although tumors in immune-deficient persons remain a major cause of morbid and fatal complications, progress has been made in reducing the risk of malignant transformation in many patients through better understanding of the etiopathogenesis. The risk of life-threatening "lymphomas" can be reduced substantially by correcting the underlying primary immune defect via hematopoietic stem cell transplantation and by reducing immune suppression in recipients of solid organ transplants. More recently, the availability of sensitive methods for monitoring reactivation of EBV in immune-compromised populations using quantitative polymerase chain reaction (PCR) techniques, combined with the preemptive or therapeutic use of anti-CD20 antibodies to thwart EBV infection, have led to successful control of post-transplant "lymphomas." Newer antiretroviral therapies and other approaches that maintain and strengthen cell-mediated immunity in HIV-infected individuals have reduced their risk of "opportunistic" lymphomas. Rapid and reliable diagnosis of *H. pylori* infection and appropriate antibiotic treatment for susceptible hosts diminishes the risks of both carcinomas and lymphomas of the stomach.

History

In 1959, Lewis Thomas[1] proposed the concept that immune surveillance was an active process controlling the emergence of malignant clones from somatic cells that undergo precancerous mutations during the lifetime of a normal, immune-competent individual. This hypothesis predicted that immune-deficient subjects should experience much higher rates of all types of cancers compared with the general population. Surveys of patients with primary and acquired immune deficiencies, however, have not substantiated an increased risk of all cancer types.[2] Retrospective clinical investigations have revealed several patterns of association between increased risk of certain malignancies and underlying disease types. In many cases, de novo, reactivated, or chronic localized infections play a substantial role in driving tumor development. Specifically, patients with primary (genetically determined) or acquired immune deficiencies that affect T-cell function are at increased risk of developing lymphomas after exposure to Epstein-Barr virus.[3,4] This risk group includes patients who are immune suppressed after solid organ allografting or hematopoietic stem cell transplantation or secondary to HIV infection. Chronic immune suppression also increases patients' risk of developing carcinomas that are linked to infection with viruses. For example, HIV-infected subjects and solid organ allograft recipients run an increased risk of Kaposi's sarcoma, which is associated with herpes family viruses; solid organ allograft recipients are also at greater risk of developing squamous cell carcinoma of the skin and cervical cancer because of the association of these with human papilloma virus (HPV). Persons with congenital humoral immune defects (especially IgA deficiency) who are persistently colonized with *H. pylori* experience higher rates of gastric carcinomas and gastric maltomas. The third category of patients at increased risk of tumors of hematopoietic and epithelial origin is individuals with inherited defects of genomic instability, which lead to both immune deficiency and propensity to tumor development.[5]

Even among classic primary immunodeficiencies, the array of tumors observed varies among the different immunodeficiency diagnoses. The recent delineation of precise genetic causes for the majority of primary immune deficiencies has made possible initial molecular dissection of affected pathways of lymphocyte proliferation and programmed cell death in distinct disorders and has helped to reconcile the differences in tumors seen among patients with those disorders.

Although tumors in immune-deficient persons remain a major cause of morbid and fatal complications, progress has been made in reducing the risk of malignant transformation in many patients through better understanding of the etiopathogenesis. The risk of life-threatening "lymphomas" can be reduced substantially by correcting the underlying primary immune defect via hematopoietic stem cell transplantation and by reducing immune suppression in recipients of solid organ transplants.[6,7] More recently, the availability of sensitive methods for monitoring reactivation of EBV in immune-compromised populations using quantitative PCR techniques, combined with the preemptive or therapeutic use of anti-CD20 antibodies to thwart EBV infection, have led to successful control of post-transplant "lymphomas."[8-10] Newer anti-retroviral therapies and other approaches that maintain and strengthen cell-mediated immunity in HIV-infected individuals have reduced their risk of "opportunistic" lymphomas. Rapid and reliable diagnosis of *H. pylori* infection and appropriate antibiotic treatment for susceptible hosts diminishes the risks of both carcinomas and lymphomas of the stomach.[11,12]

At the same time, new medical advances could create new populations of patients at risk for lymphoid tumors in particular. Use of ever more intensive therapies to eradicate cancer in adults, highly immune-suppressive "minitransplants" in elderly individuals, and use of immune-ablative chemotherapy in the setting of autologous transplants for underlying autoimmune diseases place subjects at risk for reactivation of EBV for many months or years after these procedures.[13,14] In all of these settings, there is a significant probability of prolonged erasure of the immune repertoire "memory," with a limited capacity to restore thymopoiesis. Finally, genetic manipulation of the immune system that bypasses normal regulatory mechanisms has the potential to create rather than reduce lymphoproliferative consequences, as is seen in murine and human trials of gene therapy for primary immunodeficiencies.[15,16]

LYMPHOMAS AND IMMUNODEFICIENCY

Factors That Contribute to the Increased Risk of Lymphoproliferative Disorders in Primary and Secondary Immunodeficiencies

Three general biologic circumstances, often occurring in concert, predispose individuals with primary or acquired immunodeficiencies to the development of lymphoproliferative disorders. These are:

1. The endemic incidence of EBV infection
2. The predominance of type 2 cytokine production in susceptible hosts, and, in the case of primary immune defects
3. Disruption of normal pathways that regulate lymphocyte cell cycling and survival by genetic mutations

EBV is a major cofactor in many lymphomas (lymphoproliferative tumors) in the setting of immune compromise, due to the unique properties of EBV as a transforming agent of B cells and its expression of genes that inhibit human cell–mediated immunity. Because of the ubiquitous presence of EBV, most people become infected with it during their lifetime. During evolution, EBV has established its (normally) commensal relationship with humans, wherein primary infection is not fatal but rather leads to a state of lifelong viral latency. The latent state of EBV is maintained by host-specific, cell-mediated immune responses (conferred by T and NK cells) to viral antigens that are expressed whenever the virus becomes activated or re-enters the replicative phase. In cases in which cell-mediated control of EBV latency is inadequate (due to genetic immunodeficiency) or fails (after immune suppression or destruction), EBV-immortalized B cells resume and continue proliferation.[17] Repeated cell divisions increase the probability of sequential loss of heterozygosity mutations and frank cytogenetic re-arrangements. These acquired genetic changes in the B cells render them less responsive to normal regulatory stimuli and favor malignant transformation. The emergence and persistence of EBV-transformed B cells and resultant lymphoproliferative disorders is further favored by a type 2 skewed cytokine milieu, which occurs in a number of immunodeficient settings.[18] Increased relative concentrations of IL-4 and IL-10 support B-cell activation and proliferation while inhibiting the type 1 cellular immunity that is essential for the control of EBV-bearing B cells. Type 2 cytokine skewing has been observed in patients with a number of primary immune defects characterized by compromised quantity, maturity, diversity, and/or responsiveness of T cells. Disorders such as Omenn's syndrome (a form of severe combined immunodeficiency [SCID]) and Wiskott-Aldrich syndrome are examples of such primary immunodeficiencies. Patients recovering from hematopoietic stem cell transplantation and solid organ allograft recipients immunosuppressed with tacrolimus (FK506) or cyclosporine also develop type 2 skewing, as do HIV-infected patients, who demonstrate progressive loss of CD4 cells.

Identification of many of the specific molecular defects responsible for primary immunodeficiencies reveal additional mechanisms that could contribute to lymphomagenesis in some of the diseases. Some of these defects are discussed in detail later in this chapter.

Clinical Characteristics of Lymphomas in Primary Immune Deficiencies

Advances in prevention and treatment of opportunistic infections now allow patients with primary immuno-deficiencies to enjoy longer median survival rates than ever before; however, neoplastic disorders—particularly lymphoproliferative complications—remain the second most common cause of premature mortality (still preceded by infections).[19] The incidence of tumors in patients with certain immunodeficiency diseases, such as Wiskott-Aldrich syndrome (WAS), ataxia telangiectasia (AT), and common variable immunodeficiency (CVID), is estimated at between 15% and 25%, with a substantially increased risk of developing lymphoma that increases with advancing age.[20,21]

An important early contribution to the relationship between primary immunodeficiency and cancer was provide by the international Immunodeficiency Cancer Registry (ICR), which evolved in the 1970s as an outgrowth of the observations of Drs. Good and Gatti[22] regarding cancers diagnosed in immunodeficient children. This voluntary registry was pivotal in the description of the distribution of tumor types in patients with primary immunodeficiencies, pointing to the remarkable predominance of lymphomas across virtually all diagnoses. Table 16-1 is a reproduction of earlier publications of the ICR data listing tumor types reported for various immuno-deficiency diseases. In recent times, with the advantage of retrospective review of clinical and pathologic materials from the early cases, we recognize imperfections in the original cataloging. For example, it is likely that a significant proportion of the boys listed as having hypogammaglobulinemia who developed lymphomas were actually affected with X-linked severe combined

Science of Clinical Oncology

TABLE 16-1

Immunodeficiency Cancer Registry Cases: Distribution of Tumors and Immunodeficiencies

IMMUNODEFICIENCY	ADENO-CARCINOMA	LYMPHOMA	HODGKIN'S DISEASE	LEUKEMIA	OTHER TUMORS	TOTAL
Severe combined immunodeficiency	1 (2.4%)	31 (73.8%)	4 (9.5%)	5 (11.9%)	1 (2.4%)	42 (8.4%)
X-linked agammaglobulinemia	3 (14.3%)	7 (33.3%)	3 (14.3%)	7 (33.3%)	1 (4.8%)	21 (4.2%)
Common variable immunodeficiency	20 (16.7%)	55 (45.8%)	8 (6.7%)	8 (6.7)	29 (24.2%)	120 (24.0%)
IgA deficiency	8 (21.1%)	6 (15.8%)	3 (7.9%)	0 (0%)	21 (55.3%)	38 (7.6%)
Hyper-IgM syndrome	0 (0%)	9 (56.3%)	4 (25.0%)	0 (0%)	3 (18.8%)	16 (3.2%)
Wiskott-Aldrich syndrome	0 (0%)	59 (75.6%)	3 (3.8%)	7 (9.0%)	9 (11.5%)	78 (15.6%)
Ataxia telangiectasia	13 (8.7%)	69 (46.0%)	16 (10.7%)	32 (21.3%)	20 (13.3%)	150 (30.0%)
Other immunodeficiencies	1 (4.0%)	12 (48.0%)	1 (4.0%)	4 (16.0%)	7 (28.0%)	25 (5.0%)
Total immunodeficiency categories	46 (9.2%)	252 (50.4%)	43 (8.6%)	63 (12.6%)	96 (19.2%)	500 (100%)

immunodeficiency (XSCID). Similarly, review of slides from cases of "leukemia" in patients with SCID, hypo-gammaglobulinemia, and WAS suggest that these were actually disseminated lymphoproliferative disorders of mature B cells. Nonetheless, the general outline of tumor types and their proportional distribution among patients with various immunodeficiencies that was provided by the ICR has withstood the test of time.

The descriptive information provided by the ICR has made possible a comparison of clinical characteristics and response to chemotherapy for non–Hodgkin's lymphomas (NHL) and Hodgkin's disease (HD) between patients with primary immunodeficiencies and the general population, guiding clinicians with these unique cases. Table 16-2, also a reproduction of previously published ICR data, summarizes clinical characteristics of reported cases of NHL. The data highlight several features, including:

- Male predominance, even in patients with n autosomal recessive disorders such as AT
- Young median age at diagnosis
- High frequency of extranodal presentation involving predominantly gastrointestinal, central nervous system (CNS), or disseminated sites

EBV has been identified as a common cofactor in the predominant B-cell phenotypes but also in cases of T-cell NHL and HD. In contrast to tumors in patients with other types of immunodeficiency, lymphomas in patients with AT are usually EBV negative. This finding is consistent with the hypothesis that genetic predisposition to tumorigenesis in patients with AT occurs due to mutations arising from the chromosomal repair defect.

Lymphoproliferative disorders or "lymphomas" in both primary and secondary immunodeficient states span the spectrum from reactive hyperplasias through frank malignancy. Not all lymphomas in immunodeficient hosts, despite clonal origin or malignant histologic appearance,

require intensive chemotherapy to regress. Resolution has occurred with antibiotic therapy in maltomas and with steroids, interferon α, low-dose chemotherapy, or rituximab in EBV-positive tumors.[9,23-25]

Historically, treatment of NHL with conventional doses of chemotherapy and radiation met with limited success in immunodeficient patients.[26] Tumor responses were reported as inferior to those observed in the general population for reasons that remain quite obscure, although the major reported causes of early mortality in the 1950s to 1980s were opportunistic infections. In the current era, improved antiviral and antifungal therapies allow most patients with immunodeficiencies who have cancer to be treated aggressively. Ideally, achievement of remission should be followed by reconstituting hematopoietic stem cell transplantation if a suitable donor is available.

Based on ICR reporting, Hodgkin's disease accounts for approximately 10% of tumors arising in patients with immunodeficiencies and occurs at an early median age—less than 10 years of age.[27] A case-control study performed by the ICR in the late 1980s compared the immunodeficiency cases with other pediatric cases from a multi-institutional international cooperative study group. Immunodeficient patients with HD presented earlier in life (mean age, 7.8 years vs. 11.5 years in the general population) and were significantly less likely to achieve initial remission. HD in immunodeficient patients far more commonly presented with histologies of mixed cellularity and lymphocyte depletion (now recognized as representing feeble immune response to the true malignant population) when compared with presumed nonimmunodeficient subjects.[27] For immunodeficient patients who achieved remission of HD, the 5-year probability of survival was 53% (vs. 86% for patients in the general population). Immunodeficient patients who achieve remission of HD should be considered for allogeneic bone marrow transplantation.

TABLE 16-2

Characteristics of non-Hodgkin's Lymphomas in the Immunodeficiency Cancer Registry*

| IMMUNODEFICIENCY | N | SEX[†] (M:F) | MEDIAN AGE AT DIAGNOSIS (YRS) | PRIMARY TUMOR SITES (%)[‡] | | | |
				CNS	GASTROINTESTINAL TRACT	LYMPH NODE	MULTIPLE
Severe combined immunodeficiency	31	23:7	1.6	6.5	3.2	9.7	48.4
X-linked agammaglobulinemia	7	7:0	1.2	0	14.3	14.3	14.3
Common variable immunodeficiency	55	30:23	23.0	1.8	12.7	12.7	25.5
IgA deficiency	6	4:1	9.4	16.7	0	0	0
Hyper-IgM syndrome	9	7:2	7.8	11.1	22.2	22.2	0
Wiskott-Aldrich syndrome	59	59:0	6.2	23.7	6.8	8.5	20.3
Ataxia telangiectasia	69	40:24	8.5	0	8.7	10.1	14.5
Other immunodeficiencies	4	4:0	4.0	0	0	0	0
Total immunodeficiency categories	240	174:57	7.1	7.9	8.8	10.4	21.7

ICR, Immunodeficiency Cancer Registry.
*This table excludes cases of non-Hodgkin's lymphoma in immunodeficiency categories with fewer than two cases reported.
[†]Sex reported where known.
[‡]For 51.3% of ICR cases, primary tumor site is other or unknown.

TABLE 16-3

Primary Immunodeficiencies: Predominant Reported Tumors

DISORDERS	INHERITANCE	GENE DEFECT	INCREASED SUSCEPTIBILITY TO EBV	TYPE 2 CYTOKINE SKEWING	DISRUPTION OF NORMAL APOPTOSIS	TUMORS
Severe combined immunodeficiency						
X-SCID	X	Common Gamma chain[†]	+			Lymphoma
Omenn's	AR	RAG 1/2[‡]	+	+		Lymphoma
PNP deficiency	AR	PNP[§]	+	+		Lymphoma
Wiskott-Aldrich syndrome	X	WASP	+	+	+	Lymphoma*
CD40-L deficiency	X	CD40 L	+		+	HD, biliary tract tumors
X-linked lymphoproliferative syndrome	X	SH2D1	+			Lymphoma*
Chédiak-Highashi syndrome	AR	LYST[16]	+			Lymphoma*
ALPS	AD, AR	FAS[21]			+	Lymphoma
Hyper IgE syndrome	AD	?		+		Lymphoma
IgA deficiency/CVID	AD, S	?				Lymphoma* GI carcinoma

AD, autosomal dominant; ALPS, autoimmune lymphoproliferative syndrome; AR, autosomal recessive; CVID, common variable immunodeficiency; EBV, Epstein-Barr virus; GI, gastrointestinal; HD, Hodgkin's disease; PNP, purine nucleoside phosphorylase; S, sporadic; SCID, severe combined immunodeficiency; X, X-linked.
*Frequently associated with EBV
[†]From Noguchi M, Yi H, Rosenblatt HM, et al: Interleukin-2 receptor gamma chain mutation results in X-linked severe combined immunodeficiency in humans. Cell 1993;73:147–157.
[‡]From Villa A, Sobacchi C, Notarangelo LD, et al: V(D)J recombination defects in lymphocytes due to RAG mutations: Severe immunodeficiency with a spectrum of clinical presentations. Blood 2001;97:81–88.
[§]From Markert ML: Purine nucleoside phosphorylase deficiency. Immunodefic Rev 1991;3:45–81.

Primary Immunodeficiencies Associated with Lymphomas

Table 16-3 lists some of the primary immunodeficiencies associated with lymphomas and epithelial cancers, identifying the underlying molecular defects and other biologic characteristics associated with predisposition to lymphoma development.

Severe Combined Immunodeficiencies

SCID is a collection of more than a dozen genetically distinct disorders with severe impairment of both cellular and humoral immune function, leading to early mortality from opportunistic infections during infancy in the absence of aggressive medical intervention.[28] SCID patients who have developed lymphomas share the characteristics of presence of B cells (targets for EBV transformation) and severe quantitative or qualitative defects in T cells. Examples of such conditions include the following:

- XSCID, in which loss of function mutations in the X-linked common gamma chain gene of multiple interleukin receptors block T-cell development, but B-cell numbers are generally plentiful.
- Purine nucleoside phosphorylase (PNP) deficiency, in which T-cell expansion and function are impaired by accumulation of toxic intracellular metabolites, with lesser effects on B cells.

- Omenn's syndrome, caused by mutations in *RAG1* genes predominantly, which severely restricts both B- and T-cell repertoire development and results in marked skewing toward a type 2 cytokine production.

Wiskott-Aldrich Syndrome

Wiskott-Aldrich syndrome (WAS), an X-linked disorder of broad-ranging and variable immunodeficiency and micro-thrombocytopenia, results from mutations in the WASP gene.[29] The WASP gene encodes a large intracellular protein with several functional domains involved with cytoskeletal integrity and signal transduction. Several molecules reported to be associated with WASP are involved in normal progression through the cell cycle. WASP is expressed in cells of hematopoietic origin and in the thymus. Experimental evidence suggests that WAS B cells are relatively resistant to apoptosis, and rare reports of EBV-negative B-cell lymphomas have surfaced, especially among adult males with clinically milder forms of WAS that are sometimes termed *X-linked thrombo-cytopenia* (XLT).

X-Linked Lymphoproliferative Syndrome

X-linked lymphoproliferative syndrome (XLP), long recognized as a condition with exquisite sensitivity to fatal complications of EBV infection and a high risk of lymphoma, results from mutations in the SH2D1A or SAP (slam associated protein) gene on the X chromosome.[30] Clinical features of XLP include an excessively intense

Science of Clinical Oncology

immune reaction to EBV associated with hemophago-cytosis and liver failure, lymphomas, aplastic anemia, and/or acquired hypogammaglobulinemia. SAP, an adaptor protein linked to at least four known regulatory molecules, can alter T and NK cell functions in both activating and downregulating directions and is thought to be involved in T-to-B-cell interactions through cytokine regulation.[31] Analyses from the XLP (Purtilo) registry indicate that many of the lymphomas occurring in patients with XLP are EBV negative, contrary to early predictions. This suggests an independent lymphomagenic diathesis in XLP.[32] More recently, cases of boys who have developed separate, clonally distinct tumors years apart have been found to be due to XLP.

Chédiak-Higashi Syndrome

Chédiak-Higashi syndrome (CHS) is an autosomal recessive disorder characterized by recurrent bacterial infections, oculocutaneous albinism, abnormal platelets, varied neurologic dysfunction, and a 90% probability of developing a lethal hemophagocytic complication asso-ciated with EBV infection (referred to as the accelerated phase) before age 20.[33] As part of the "accelerated phase," some patients develop disseminated lymphoproliferative disorder. CHS is caused by mutations in the LYST gene (lysosomal trafficking regulator), and giant lysosomes are characteristic findings in leucocytes on blood smear. Because lysosomes are the key storage compartments for cytolytic proteins (including perforin and Granzyme B), the cytotoxic effector function of NK and T cells is typically impaired in CHS, presenting a vulnerability to control of EBV infection.[34] A transport defect inhibiting peptide loading and antigen presentation by HLA class II molecules on EBV-transformed CHS B lymphocytes has also been proposed as an additional mechanism contrib-uting to escape of transformed B cells from immunologic control.

X-Linked Hyper IgM Syndrome (XHIM, X-Linked CD40 Ligand Deficiency)

XHIM results in failure of immunoglobulin switching by B cells (which requires signaling through CD40) and in decreased development and maintenance of type 1 cell-mediated responses (including NK cell function) due to impaired responsiveness of CD40 expressing monocyte-derived antigen presenting cells (APCs).[35] Patients with XHIM appear to have an increased risk of lymphomas, but especially of HD associated with EBV infection. Presumably, depressed cell-mediated function required for control of EBV is responsible for this occurrence. Patients with XHIM are also at increased risk for biliary carcinomas, as there is a high rate of sclerosing cholangitis in patients with a history of chronic cryptosporidiosis.[36] In parts of the world where cryptosporidial infection is less prevalent, this complication of XHIM is rarely observed.

Autoimmune Lymphoproliferative Syndrome

Autoimmune lymphoproliferative syndrome (ALPS) represents a constellation of genetic apoptosis defects associated with mutations in FAS, Fas ligand, and Caspase 8 genes.[37] Most of the cases described have had hetero-zygous, dominant negative mutations involving FAS. Characteristic clinical features of the syndrome present in early childhood or even at birth. These include chronic multifocal lymphadenopathy, splenomegaly, autoimmune hemolytic anemia (and often other immune cytopenias), with increased proportions of circulating senescent T cells (CD3+, αβ T-cell receptor [TCR]–, CD4–CD8–), so-called double-negative T cells. The majority of patients expe-rience symptomatic improvement with steroid therapy, and generally, autoimmune complications lessen in severity with advancing age. The estimated risk of lymphoma in such patients ranges around 30%, however, and some patients have developed more than one lymphoid tumor over time. Patients who have the most severe forms of ALPS should be considered for correction with hematopietic stem cell transplantation. Recently, use of rituximab and fansidar, agents that induce apoptosis in the senescent lymphocytes bypassing the FAS/FAS ligand signal, have been shown to reduce lymphadenopathy and autoimmune symptoms in patients with ALPS.[38] Whether such strategies will ultimately reduce the risk of lymphomas remains to be determined.

Clinical Characteristics of Lymphoproliferative Disorders in Acquired Immunodeficiencies

Patients recovering from hematopoietic stem cell trans-plantation (HSCT) or solid organ allografting and patients with HIV infection all demonstrate rates of lymphoproli-ferative complications substantially exceeding those seen in the general population.

EBV Post-transplant Lymphoma After Hematopoietic Stem Cell Transplantation

After HSCT, the incidence of post-transplant lymphoma (PTLD) ranges from approximately 1% or less after un-manipulated matched sibling donor transplants or auto-logous transplants to greater than 30% after T-depleted haploidentical (mismatched) transplants in patients with certain underlying immunodeficiencies (e.g., WAS).[39] Virtually all cases of PTLD are associated with EBV and generally present during the first 6 months after trans-plantation—the period when T-cell immune reconstitu-tion is still very poor. The majority of cases of PTLD occur in donor-derived EBV-transformed B cells, although occa-sionally, EBV reactivation in host cells is demonstrated. Several risk factors for development of PTLD—both host-and transplant-related—have been identified in multivariate analyses. These include the following:

- T-cell depletion of the stem cell product (a procedure aimed at decreasing the risk of graft-vs.-host disease [GVHD] after allogeneic transplantation)
- HLA mismatching
- Older age of the transplant recipient

In univariate analyses, chronic GVHD (which is asso-ciated with prolonged immunodeficiency after transplant) and use of anti–T-cell antibody treatments also emerge as predisposing variables.[40] The incidence of PTLD after unrelated umbilical cord blood transplantation (an immunologically naive graft) also appears to be increased compared with T-replete transplants from adult donors.

Methods of T-cell depletion that also remove or inactivate donor B cells are associated with reduced risk of PTLD.[41] PTLD after HSCT has several symptomatic presentations. The most common is a syndrome reminiscent of acute infectious mononucleosis with fever, relative lymphocytosis, lymphadenopathy, and lymphoid swelling in the oral cavity, with detectable EBV in the blood by PCR techniques. Average time to symptomatic presentation of this form of PTLD is approximately day 70 after transplant.[42] Rapid diagnosis and treatment with rituxan can be life-saving in such situations. Adjunctive use of ganciclovir could also be helpful in this setting. Failure to treat patients early and effectively can lead to dissemination with B-cell infiltration of the marrow, lungs, reticuloendothelial system, and CNS. In other cases, the symptomatic onset can be more indolent, with limited extranodal accumulations of transformed B cells. Of note, lymphadenopathy in the first few months after allogeneic transplantation is a very rare occurrence and should lead one to strongly consider the diagnosis of PTLD. Lymphoid aggregates are not easily visualized on plain chest radiographs, so computed tomography scans of the head, neck, chest, and abdomen are recommended in suspected cases.

Sustained remission of PTLD has been shown to coincide with the development of donor-type EBV-specific cytotoxic T lymphocytes (CTLs). Although rituxan is considered the treatment of choice for PTLD currently, high-dose steroids, low-dose cyclophosphamide, α-interferon, and donor lymphocyte infusions have been applied with success in anecdotal cases.[43] It is likely that many cases of PTLD still go unrecognized premortem, and given the low rate of autopsy in post-transplant deaths, the actual incidence has probably been underestimated.

PTLD After Solid Organ Grafting

The use of immunosuppression after allografting heightens the risk of PTLD in previously immunocompetent subjects. Rates of PTLD range from 1% to 5% after kidney transplantation (increased 30–50-fold over age- and sex-matched general population) to as high as 25% after visceral organ transplants (liver and small bowel), especially in EBV-seronegative pediatric recipients of EBV-positive organs, who showed a threefold higher rate of PTLD than adult liver transplant recipients.[44,45] In adult transplant recipients, the risk of PTLD increases with older age at transplant (>50 years), presence of hepatitis C, and underlying alcoholic cirrhosis.[46] Use of more intensive and prolonged immunosuppression—especially use of OKT3 monoclonal antibody for treatment of graft rejection—was reported to further increase PTLD risk in patients with all types of organ transplants.[47] In more recent series with close monitoring of tacrolimus immune suppression and preemptive screening for EBV reactivation, the incidence of PTLD has declined substantially in all patient groups but remains the second major cause of post-transplant mortality, following sepsis. As with HSCT, PTLD after solid organ transplantation is virtually 100% EBV positive. Pediatric recipients who were EBV seronegative often develop symptoms of a systemic mono-

nucleosis-like infection, whereas adult recipients might present with solid lymphoid lesions (often in extranodal sites that include the CNS) or even with disseminated, stage III to IV lymphoma. Histologies range from B-cell hyperplasia to oligoclonal and (most often) monotypic and monoclonal tumors with various gene rearrangements, oncogene mutations, and/or loss of heterozygosity mutations.

Although the incidence of PTLD as a complication of immune suppression after organ transplantation has declined, the mortality rate from this cause remains at approximately 50% in affected patients.[48] The critical role of intact cell-mediated immunity in control of EBV-associated PTLD is demonstrated in cases in which regression occurs after reduction in immune suppression, at the risk of organ rejection. Surgical excision and/or radiation of limited disease is associated with a high rate of durable remissions. In more aggressive or persistent tumors, rituxan and other anti–B-cell therapies, low-dose cyclophosphamide, and α-interferon therapy have been applied successfully, although as many as half of the patients relapse and likely eventually die of PTLD complications.[9,49]

Lymphomas Associated with HIV Infection

The incidence of lymphomas among HIV-infected adults during the early years of the worldwide epidemic was reported to exceed 20%.[50] More recent estimates have been revised to between 4% to 10% and could drop even lower for individuals receiving multidrug antiviral regimens and protease inhibitors. A recent review of causes of death in a U.S.-based population that had received HAART (highly active antiretroviral therapy) shows increasing proportions of death from non–AIDS-defining malignancies and chronic disorders of adulthood.[51] Although the reported association of lymphomas with EBV in HIV-infected persons ranges between 30% and 60%, extranodal and CNS sites are more frequent in HIV-infected patients than in age- and gender-matched controls in the general population.[52] Response to conventional chemotherapy protocols is less successful in this patient group than in nonimmunodeficient hosts.

CARCINOMAS ASSOCIATED WITH IMMUNE DEFICIENCIES

Gastric Carcinomas and Maltomas

A relationship between gastric atrophy, long-standing dyspepsia and gastric ulcer disease, and the development of gastric carcinomas in adults with common variable immunodeficiency was observed decades before the discovery of a causal link to chronic *H. pylori* infestation.[53] A retrospective study of banked sera from a group of presumed nonimmunodeficient adult patients diagnosed with gastric carcinoma revealed an increased incidence of IgA deficiency in cancer-bearing subjects (1 in 20) compared with the general blood donor pool (1 in 400), further implicating defective humoral immunity as a contributing factor to this unusual type of tumor.[54]

It is now recognized that *H. pylori* infection is the most common cofactor for gastric carcinoma and is associated with maltomas in nonimmunodeficient whites.[55] Chronic inflammation from *H. pylori* incites local cytokine production, which alters adhesive properties of local epithelial surfaces and promotes ectopic lymphoid proliferation. Mucosa-associated lymphoid tissue is not present in healthy gastric mucosa, but it can develop in sites of long-persisting inflammation.[56] Maltomas are generally monoclonal and can take on the appearance of aggressive, large B-cell lymphomas. These tumors are reported not only in adults with primary immunodeficiency but also in immunosuppressed organ transplant recipients. Organ transplant recipients also carry an increased risk of gastric carcinoma, to the extent that diagnostic endoscopy is now recommended as part of the post-transplant follow-up for symptomatic individuals.[57] Fortunately, effective eradication of *H. pylori* with antibiotics, antacid therapy, and (occasionally) surgical excision is highly curative for both gastric carcinomas and maltomas.[58] Presumably, surveillance for *H. pylori* infection and antibiotic suppression can prevent these tumors in immune-deficient populations in the future.

Carcinomas After Allografting

The risk of post-transplant carcinomas after bone marrow transplantation is impacted by several factors—the strongest of which is likely the patient's inherent susceptibility to carcinogenesis. For example, patients who have an underlying systemic defect in DNA repair (e.g., Fanconi anemia) might be "cured" of their marrow failure or acute leukemia by replacement of genetically normal hematopoietic stem cells but remain at high risk for epithelial cancers, especially in areas of transplant-related radiation such as the head and neck.[59] Even among patients without obvious susceptibility to DNA damage, differences in response to the radiation commonly used in transplant treatment of patients with hematologic malignancies could account for future risk of skin, bone, and CNS tumors.

The cumulative risk of cancer in solid organ transplant recipients rises to more than 50% at 20 years after transplant.[60] Many of these cancers involve the skin and are enhanced by increased sun exposure (i.e., time to development of skin cancer decreases with increasing latitude). Compared with the general population, the risk of developing cancer after organ transplantation is increased three- to fivefold. Table 16-4 tallies the relative increased risks of certain carcinomas in organ transplant recipients as collected through the Israel Penn Tumor Transplant Registry in Cincinnati, Ohio.

Skin and lip cancers account for nearly 40% of all post-transplant cancers, showing a male predominance of 2:1. With close surveillance, deaths are infrequent. An unusual "skin" cancer diagnosed in transplant recipients is Merkel Cell Cancer (MCC), a highly aggressive neuroendocrine tumor arising principally in the head and neck region. No clear association with an inciting pathogen is known for this unusual tumor, which is usually seen in elderly whites; organ transplant recipients account for nearly 8% of the less than 1000 cases of MCC reported worldwide.[61]

Kaposi's sarcoma (KS) has long been identified as one of the "opportunistic tumors" in organ transplant recipients, with a nearly 1000-fold increase over the general population, although it is not reported after hematopoietic stem cell transplantation or in primary immunodeficiencies. KS is more commonly reported after renal transplantation and in patients of "Mediterranean" descent, such as Greeks, Italians, Turks, and Arabs. In this setting, it is usually not associated with HIV infection. Other de novo sarcomas also account for some of the post-transplant risk of malignancy and appear to have a particularly aggressive biologic activity.[62]

Cervical cancer accounts for about 10% of post-transplant cancers in women. Fortunately, 75% of the lesions are in situ. It is hoped that future vaccine interventions against HPV can lower the rate of this complication for women in general. The number of breast cancer cases after allografting is comparable to that expected among women of like age; however, a higher mortality has been observed among stage III and IV patients when

TABLE 16-4

Incidence of Carcinomas Following Solid Organ Transplantation		
TUMOR TYPE	**INCIDENCE VS. GENERAL POPULATION**	**FACTOR INCREASING RISK**
Skin cancer		
Squamous cell carcinoma	40–50-fold	Sun exposure, latitude
Basal cell carcinoma	tenfold	
Melanoma	fivefold	
Cervical cancer*	14-fold	Human papilloma virus infection
Endometrial cancer	twofold	
Bladder cancer	fourfold	
Kidney cancer	eightfold	Usually developing in native kidney
Ureteral cancer	1000-fold	
Kaposi's sarcoma	1000-fold	Kidney transplant, Mediterranean descent

*Majority in situ
Data provided by the Israel Penn Transplant Tumor Registry, Cincinnati, Ohio.

FOSTERING AWARENESS ABOUT CARCINOMAS IN ORGAN TRANSPLANT RECIPIENTS

The cumulative risk of cancer in solid organ transplant recipients exceeds 50% 20 years after grafting. Compared with the general adult population, the risk of developing cancer after organ transplantation increases three- to fivefold. Patient education about specific cancer risks and preventive lifestyle, coupled with regular medical exams screening for early malignancy, might reduce cancer mortality in organ recipients. The skin and lips are the most common sites of cancer in allograft recipients; development of squamous cell carcinomas is markedly accelerated by sun exposure in this population. In addition to squamous cell carcinoma, unusual skin cancers such as Merkel cell cancer and Kaposi's sarcoma occur with markedly increased incidence after organ transplantation. Cervical cancer accounts for 10% of cases of post-transplant cancers in women; although the rate of breast cancer does not appear to increase, mortality from more advanced stage disease is increased. De novo lung cancer in immune-suppressed individuals carries a particularly poor prognosis regardless of histologic type. Thus, recommendations regarding avoidance to sun exposure, regular dermatologic and gynecologic screening, and intervention to achieve sustained smoking cessation should be included as part of routine long-term transplant follow-up.

compared with nonimmunesuppressed women.[63] Thus, more frequent screening, if it identifies earlier, lower-grade malignancies, could be indicated for female organ transplant recipients.

De novo lung cancer in immune-suppressed renal transplant recipients is an aggressive, invasive lesion with poor prognosis irrespective of histologic type or treatment modality.[64] Prospective organ recipients should receive strong encouragement and intervention to achieve sustained cigarette smoking cessation.

Immunodeficiency and Cancer in Genetic Disorders of DNA Repair

Table 16-5 lists several rare genetic disorders of DNA repair in which resultant immune deficiency and intrinsic susceptibility to carcinomas have been identified. DNA is constantly exposed to potentially damaging insults, both external (e.g., environmental radiation) and intrinsic (e.g., byproducts of cellular metabolism). A number of molecular strategies have evolved to maintain genomic stability. Mechanisms utilized in eukaryotes include those involved in the following processes:

- Recognition and direct repair of DNA damage
- Cell cycle checkpoints that pause cell cycle progression in the presence of damage, allowing the time needed for repair
- Mechanisms for removal of irreversibly damaged cells, such as the triggering of apoptosis (discussed previously in the section on ALPS)

DNA double-strand breaks represent the most potentially serious damage to the genome. Two major pathways exist to repair such damage: homologous recombination repair and nonhomologous end joining (NHEJ). Defects in either of these pathways can result in chromosomal rearrangements, loss of heterozygosity, and gene mutations leading to cancers.

On the other hand, generation of immunologic diversity among both B and T cells requires a well-orchestrated "creation" of DNA breaks followed by rearrangement of immunoglobulin and T-cell receptor gene sequences and repair to stabilize the final genetic product. In this process of gene rearrangement, sequence changes such as mutations and additions, which contribute to the desired diversity of new coding regions, occur frequently. Mechanisms creating this immunologic diversity likely include helicases, polymerases, and DNA ligases. Several of the known genetic defects associated with immunodeficiency and predisposition to cancers are described in the following sections. Many other rare cases with immunodeficiency and cancers have been identified, but the specific molecular defects are still unknown.

Ataxia Telangiectasia

Ataxia telangiectasia (AT) is an autosomal recessive disorder with cancer predisposition that has variable and profound immunologic and other systemic manifestations, principally cerebellar degeneration.[65] For some time, it has been recognized that AT cells fail to activate cell-cycle checkpoints normally after exposure to γ irradiation or radiomimetic agents. The mutant gene in AT (ATM) is a member of the phosphotidyl inositol kinase (PIK) family of molecules involved in signal transduction

TABLE 16-5

Genetic Disorders Associated with Chromosomal Instability That Result in Immunodeficiency and Predisposition to Cancer			
DISORDER	**GENE DEFECT**	**IMMUNE DEFECTS**	**CANCERS REPORTED**
Ataxia telangiectasia	ATM[66]	IgA deficiency, ↓T cells	Lymphoma, leukemia, hepatocarcinoma, Genitourinary carcinoma, skin cancer
Nijmegen breakage syndrome	NBS1[70]	Hypogammaglobulinemia Lymphopenia	Myeloid leukemia, lymphoma
Bloom's syndrome	BLM[71]	Hypogammaglobulinemia NK cell deficiency	Lymphoma, epithelial cancer
Werner's syndrome	WRN[72]	Antibody deficiency?	Lymphoma

and has also been implicated in meiotic recombination.[66] ATM appears to act as a sensor of double-stranded DNA breakage (e.g., in response to oxidative stress), activating numerous damage repair pathways, including cell cycle checkpoint control, p53 activation, and DNA repair. Mutations in ATM lead to accelerated telomere loss and premature aging.[67] In the context of normal lymphopoiesis, ATM is clearly involved in control of productive gene rearrangements of the B- and T-cell immune receptor molecules, as AT lymphocytes demonstrate a 25-fold increase in nonrandom rearrangements of immunoglobulin and TCR genes compared with lymphocytes from normal individuals.[68] Thymic output in AT is very reduced. The consequent restricted T-cell repertoire emerges from oligoclonal post-thymic expansion.[69] Some of the nonrandom rearrangements involve translocation of Ig chains with c-myc, reflecting, in magnified proportion, commonly seen cytogenetic rearrangements in general lymphomagenesis. In addition to the predominant lymphoid tumors (both lymphomas and leukemias), patients with AT experience high rates of epithelial cancers involving the skin, gastrointestinal tract, genitourinary tract, and central nervous systems. Multiple tumors can be present simultaneously or can develop sequentially. Early reports from the ICR discussed concordance of histologies in tumors affecting AT siblings from the same family—an intriguing but still mysterious observation. The extent of response of tumors in AT patients to conventional chemotherapy remains controversial; however, the frequent development of chronic lung disease in AT and the tendency by treating physicians to reduce chemotherapy intensity could contribute to poorer outcomes.

Nijmegen Breakage Syndrome

Nijmegen breakage syndrome (NBS) is another rare autosomal recessive syndrome, which, like AT, is associated with both humoral and T-cell defects, clinical radiosensitivity, chromosomal instability, and predisposition to lymphoid and epithelial cancers.[70] Other characteristics of patients with NBS are growth retardation, microcephaly, and "birdlike" facies. The protein defective in NBS—NBS1, nibrin, or p95—appears to function together with ATM to "sense" DNA double-strand breaks and activate a diversity of corrective actions. As in AT, lymphocytes of patients with NBS display frequent chromosomal aberrations at the sites of TCR and IgH rearrangement.

Bloom's Syndrome

Bloom's syndrome (BS) has autosomal recessive inheritance involving mutations in the BLM gene.[71] In addition to immunodeficiency—especially humoral defects and predisposition to cancer—patients with BS experience growth retardation, progeria, impaired fertility, sunsensitive erythema of the face, and chronic lung disease (similar to patients with AT). The protein defective in Bloom's syndrome is a member of the RecQ helicase family and appears to function during DNA replication or in the postreplication process to resolve aberrancies incurred during replication. The BLM protein colocalizes with a gene, *hMLH1*, which is linked to mismatch repair. A propensity to colonic adenomas, epidermal carcinomas,

and acute myeloid leukemia has been reported in patients with BS.

Werner's Syndrome

Werner's syndrome (WS), an autosomal recessive disorder with features of progeria and multiple endocrine neoplasias, results from loss of function mutations in the WRN gene, which encodes a helicase/exonuclease.[72] Reports of immunodeficiency are not well substantiated, but predilection to sinopulmonary infections is noted. Genomic instability in WS is typified by elevated illegitimate recombination events and accelerated loss of telomerase sequences.

REFERENCES

1. Thomas L: Cellular and Humoral Aspects of Hypersensitivity States. New York, Hoeber, 1959.
2. Filipovich A, Spector BD, Frizzera G, Kersey JH: Malignancies in the immunocompromised human. In Giraldo G, Beth E (eds): The Role of Viruses in Human Cancer. New York, Elsevier North Holland, 1980, pp 237–253.
3. Filipovich AH, Mather A, Kamat D, Kersey JH, Shapiro RS: Lymphoproliferative disorders and other tumors complicating immunodeficiencies. Immunodeficiency 1994;5:91–112.
4. Filipovich AH, Mather A, Kamat D, Shapiro RS: Primary immunodeficiencies: Genetic risk factors for lymphoma. Cancer Res 1992;52:5465S–5467S.
5. Gennery AR, Cant AJ, Jeggo PA: Immunodeficiency associated with DNA repair defects. Clin Exp Immunol 2000;121:1–7.
6. Neudorf S, Filipovich A, Kersey JH: Immunoreconstitution by Bone Marrow Transplantation Decreases Lymphoreticular Malignancies in Wiskott-Aldrich and Severe Combined Immune Deficiency Syndromes. New York, Plenum Press, 1984.
7. Penn I: The price of immunotherapy. Curr Probl Surg 1981;18:681–751.
8. Holmes RD, Orban-Eller K, Karrer FR, Rowe DT, Narkewicz MR, Sokol R: Response of elevated Epstein-Barr virus DNA levels to therapeutic changes in pediatric liver transplant patients: 56-month follow up and outcome. Transplantation 2002;74:367–372.
9. Berney T, Delis S, Kato T, et al: Successful treatment of post-transplant lymphoproliferative disease with prolonged rituximab treatment in intestinal transplant recipients. Transplantation 2002;74:1000–1006.
10. Kuehnle I, Huls MH, Liu Z, et al: CD20 monoclonal antibody (rituximab) for therapy of Epstein-Barr virus lymphoma after hemopoietic stem-cell transplantation. Blood 2000;95:1502–1505.
11. Laheij RJ, van Rossum LG, Verbeek AL, Jansen JB: Helicobacter pylori infection treatment of nonulcer dyspepsia: An analysis of meta-analyses. J Clin Gastroenterol 2003;36:315–320.
12. Alsolaiman MM, Bakis G, Nazeer T, MacDermott RP, Balint JA: Five years of complete remission of gastric diffuse large B cell lymphoma after eradication of Helicobacter pylori infection. Gut 2003;52:507–509.
13. Hakim FT, Cepeda R, Kalemi S, et al: Constraints on CD4 recovery postchemotherapy in adults: Thymic insufficiency and apoptotic decline of expanded peripheral CD4 cells. Blood 1997;90:3789–3798.
14. Wulffraat M, de Kleer I, Brinkman D, et al: Autologous stem cell transplantation for refractory juvenile idiopathic arthritis: Current results and perspectives. Transplant Proc 2002;34:2925–2926.
15. Hacein-Bey-Abina S, von Kalle C, Schmidt M, et al: A serious adverse event after successful gene therapy for X-linked severe combined immunodeficiency. N Engl J Med 2003;348:255–256.
16. Brown MP, Topham DJ, Sangster MY, et al: Thymic lymphoproliferative disease after successful correction of CD40 ligand deficiency by gene transfer in mice. Nat Med 1998;4:1253–1260.
17. Okano M, Gross TG: From Burkitt's lymphoma to chronic active Epstein-Barr virus (EBV) infection: An expanding spectrum of EBV-associated diseases. Pediatr Hematol Oncol 2001;18:427–442.

18. Mathur A, Kamut DM, Filipovich AH, Steinbuch M, Shapiro RS: Immunoregulatory abnormalities in patients with Epstein-Barr virus- associated B cell lymphoproliferative disorders. Transplantation 1994;57:1042–1045.

19. Filipovich AH, Heinitz KJ, Robison LL, Frizzera G: The immunodeficiency cancer registry. A research resource. Am J Pediatr Hematol Oncol 1987;9:183–184.

20. Morrell DE, Cromartie, E, Swift M: Mortality and cancer incidence in 263 patients with ataxia-telangiectasia. J Natl Cancer Inst 1986;77:89–92.

21. Perry GS 3rd, Spector BD, Schuman LM, et al: The Wiskott-Aldrich syndrome in the United States and Canada (1892–1979). J Pediatr 1980;97:72–78.

22. Gatti RA, Good RA: Occurrence of malignancy in immuno-deficiency diseases. A literature review. Cancer 1971;28:89–98.

23. Urakami Y, Sano T: Long-term follow-up of gastric metaplasia after eradication of Helicobacter pylori. J Med Invest 2003;50:48–54.

24. Shapiro RFA: Successful therapy for EBV associated B cell lymphoproliferative disorder in immunodeficiency using alpha interferon and intravenous immunoglobulin. In Ablashi D, Faggioni A, Krugeret G, et al (eds): Epstein-Barr Virus and Human Disease II. Clifton, NJ, Humana, 1989, p 355.

25. Gross TG: Low-dose chemotherapy for children with post-transplant lymphoproliferative disease. Recent Results Cancer Res 2002;159:96–103.

26. Mueller BPP: Medical progress: Cancer in children with primary or secondary immunodeficiencies. J Pediatr 1995;126:1.

27. Robison LL, Stoker V, Frizzera G, Heinitz K, Meadows AT, Filipovich AH: Hodgkin's disease in pediatric patients with naturally occurring immunodeficiency. Am J Pediatr Hematol Oncol 1987;9:189–192.

28. Fischer A: Primary immunodeficiency diseases: An experimental model for molecular medicine. Lancet 2001;357:1863–1869.

29. Derry JM, Ochs HD, Francke U: Isolation of a novel gene mutated in Wiskott-Aldrich syndrome. Cell 1994;78:635–644.

30. Coffey AJ, Brooksbank RA, Brandan O, et al: Host response to EBV infection in X-linked lymphoproliferative disease results from mutations in an SH2-domain encoding gene. Nat Genet 1998;20:129–135.

31. Sayos J, Wu C, Morra M, et al: The X-linked lymphoproliferative-disease gene product SAP regulates signals induced through the co-receptor SLAM. Nature 1998;395:462–469.

32. Sumegi J, Huang D, Lanyi D, et al: Correlation of mutations of the SH2D1A gene and Epstein-Barr virus infection with clinical phenotype and outcome in X-linked lymphoproliferative disease. Blood 2000;96:3118–3125.

33. Barbosa MD, Nguyen QA, Tchernev VT, et al: Identification of the homologous beige and Chediak-Higashi syndrome genes. Nature 1996;382:262–265.

34. Ward DM, Shiflett SL, Kaplan J: Chediak-Higashi syndrome: A clinical and molecular view of a rare lysosomal storage disorder. Curr Mol Med 2002;2:469–477.

35. Notarangelo LD, Duse M, Ugazio AG: Immunodeficiency with hyper-IgM (HIM). Immunodefic Rev 1992;3:101–121.

36. Hayward AR, Levy J, Facchetti F, et al: Cholangiopathy and tumors of the pancreas, liver, and biliary tree in boys with X-linked immunodeficiency with hyper-IgM. J Immunol 1997;158:977–983.

37. Rieux-Laucat F, Le Diest F, Hivroz C, et al: Mutations in Fas associated with human lymphoproliferative syndrome and autoimmunity. Science 1995;268:1347–1349.

38. van der Werff Ten Bosch J, Schotte P, Ferster A, et al: Reversion of autoimmune lymphoproliferative syndrome with an antimalarial drug: Preliminary results of a clinical cohort study and molecular observations. Br J Haematol 2002;117:176–188.

39. Filipovich AJH: Immune Mediated Hematologic and Oncologic Disorders, Including Epstein-Barr Virus Infection. Philadelphia, WB Saunders, 1996.

40. Gross TG, Steinbuch M, DeFor T, et al: B cell lymphoproliferative disorders following hematopoietic stem cell transplantation: Risk factors, treatment and outcome. Bone Marrow Transplant 1999;23:251–258.

41. Gross TG, Loechelt BJ: Epstein-Barr virus associated disease following blood or marrow transplant. Pediatr Transplant 2003;7(Suppl 3):44–50.

42. Shapiro RS, McClain K, Frizzera G, et al: Epstein-Barr virus associated B cell lymphoproliferative disorders following bone marrow transplantation. Blood 1988;71:1234–1243.

43. Papadopoulos EB, Ladanyi M, Emmanuel D, et al: Infusions of donor leukocytes to treat Epstein-Barr virus-associated lymphoproliferative disorders after allogeneic bone marrow transplantation. N Engl J Med 1994;330:1185–1191.

44. Dotti G, Fiocchi R, Motta T, et al: Lymphomas occurring late after solid-organ transplantation: Influence of treatment on the clinical outcome. Transplantation 2002;74:1095–1102.

45. Jain D, Hui P, McNamara J, Schwartz D, German J, Reyes-Mugica M: Bloom syndrome in sibs: First reports of hepatocellular carcinoma and Wilms tumor with documented anaplasia and nephrogenic rests. Pediatr Dev Pathol 2001;4:585–589.

46. Duvoux C, Pageaux GP, Vanlemmens C, et al: Risk factors for lymphoproliferative disorders after liver transplantation in adults: An analysis of 480 patients. Transplantation 2002;74:1103–1109.

47. McCaughan GW, Strasser S, Dolan P, Sheil AG: Liver allograft rejection: Analysis of OKT3 rescue therapy. Transplant Proc 1992;24:2250–2251.

48. Ramalingam P, et al: Post-transplant lymphoproliferative disorders in lung transplant recipients: The Cleveland Clinic experience. Mod Pathol 2002;15:647–656.

49. Gross TG: Treatment of Epstein-Barr virus-associated post-transplant lymphoproliferative disorders. J Pediatr Hematol Oncol 2001;23:7–9.

50. Knowles DM: Pathology and Pathogenesis of Non-Hodgkin's Lymphomas Associated with HIV Infection, 2nd ed. New York, Arnold, 1997, p 471.

51. Louie JK, Hsu LC, Osmond DH, Katz MH, Schwarcz SK: Trends in causes of death among persons with acquired immunodeficiency syndrome in the era of highly active antiretroviral therapy, San Francisco, 1994–1998. J Infect Dis 2002;18:1023–1027.

52. Goedert JJ, Cote TR, Virgo P, et al: Spectrum of AIDS-associated malignant disorders. Lancet 1998;351:1833–1839.

53. Filipovich AH, Shapiro RS: Tumor in patients with common variable immunodeficiency. Estratto dalla rivista EOS 1991;11:43–46.

54. den Hartog G, van der Meer JW, Jansen JB, van Furth R, Lamers CB: Decreased gastrin secretion in patients with late-onset hypogammaglobulinemia. N Engl J Med 1988;318:1563–1567.

55. Correa P: Helicobacter pylori infection and gastric cancer. Cancer Epidemiol Biomarkers Prev 2003;12:238S–241S.

56. Kusic B, Gasparov S, Katicic M, Dominis M, Antica M: Monoclonality in Helicobacter pylori-positive gastric biopsies: An early detection of mucosa-associated lymphoid tissue lymphoma. Exp Mol Pathol 2003;74:61–67.

57. Buell JF, Husted T, Hanaway MJ, et al: Gastric cancer in transplant recipients: Detection of malignancy [correction of malignacy] by aggressive endoscopy. Transplant Proc 2002;34:1784–1785.

58. Aull MJ, Buell JF, Peddi VR, et al: Maltoma: a Helicobacter pylori-associated malignancy in transplant patients: A report from the Israel Penn International Transplant Tumor Registry with a review of published literature. Transplantation 2003;75:225–228.

59. Socie G, Devergie A, Grinski T, et al: Transplantation for Fanconi's anaemia: Long-term follow-up of fifty patients transplanted from a sibling donor after low-dose cyclophosphamide and thoraco-abdominal irradiation for conditioning. Br J Haematol 1998;103:249–255.

60. Sheil AG, Disney AP, Mathew TH, Amiss N: De novo malignancy emerges as a major cause of morbidity and late failure in renal transplantation. Transplant Proc 1993;25:1383–1384.

61. Buell JF, Trofe J, Hanaway MJ, et al: Immunosuppression and Merkel cell cancer. Transplant Proc 2002;34:1780–1781.

62. Husted TL, Buell JF, Hanaway MJ, et al: De novo sarcomas in solid organ transplant recipients. Transplant Proc 2002;34:1786–1787.

63. Buell JF, Hanaway MJ, Trofe J, et al: De novo breast cancer in renal transplant recipients. Transplant Proc 2002;34:1778–1779.

64. Kelly BS, Buell JF, Merchent TB, et al: De novo lung cancer in renal transplant recipients. Israel Penn International Transplant Tumor Registry. ASTS, 2003.

65. Shiloh Y, Rotman G: Ataxia-telangiectasia and the ATM gene: Linking neurodegeneration, immunodeficiency, and cancer to cell cycle checkpoints. J Clin Immunol 1996;16:254–260.

66. Shiloh Y: ATM and related protein kinases: Safeguarding genome integrity. Nat Rev Cancer 2003;3:155–168.

67. Wong KK, Maser RS, Bachoo RM, et al: Telomere dysfunction and Atm deficiency compromises organ homeostasis and accelerates ageing. Nature 2003;421:643–648.

68. Hecht F, Hecht BK: Chromosome changes connect immuno-deficiency and cancer in ataxia-telangiectasia. Am J Pediatr Hematol Oncol 1987;9:185–188.

69. Giovannetti A, Mazetta F, Caprini E, et al: Skewed T-cell receptor repertoire, decreased thymic output, and predominance of terminally differentiated T cells in ataxia telangiectasia. Blood 2002;100:4082–4089.

70. Tauchi H, Matsura S, Kobayashi J, Sakamoto S, Komatsu K: Nijmegen breakage syndrome gene, NBS1, and molecular links to factors for genome stability. Oncogene 2002;21:8967–8980.

71. Langland G, Elliott J, Li Y, Creaney J, Dixon K, Groden J: The BLM helicase is necessary for normal DNA double-strand break repair. Cancer Res 2002;62:2766–2770.

72. Orren DK, Theodore S, Machwe A: The Werner syndrome helicase/exonuclease (WRN) disrupts and degrades D-loops in vitro. Biochemistry 2002;41:13483–13488.

7

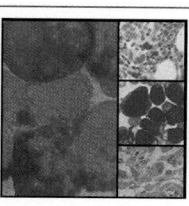

PATHOLOGY AND LABORATORY MEDICINE

Michael Borowitz

William Westra

Linda D. Cooley

Jeffrey A. Kant

Lori J. Sokoll

Daniel W. Chan

Fred Sanfilippo

SUMMARY OF KEY POINTS

- The range of diagnostic modalities useful in the characterization of cancer has expanded significantly in recent decades.
- The challenge is to utilize the appropriate technique or the right indication; this invariably requires

the expertise and oversight of the experienced pathologist–laboratorian.
- This chapter reviews cancer diagnostics grouped into five categories.

1. Surgical pathology
2. Flow cytometry
3. Cytogenetics
4. Molecular diagnostics
5. Clinical chemistry

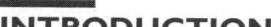

INTRODUCTION

The number and types of diagnostic modalities available to characterize cancer have increased dramatically over the past few decades. From histologic evaluation that began more than a century ago, to flow cytometry and cytogenetics in the 1970s and 1980s, and to molecular pathology more recently, the armamentarium of tests now available presents both opportunity and challenge. The opportunity is to provide better and more accurate methods for detecting and defining the presence of cancer. The challenge is to use the right techniques for the right indications to improve sensitivity for screening and specificity for diagnosis.

The availability of a wide range of test methods, applications, and costs has brought other factors into consideration for the clinician. The overuse of highly sensitive tests results in increased false-positive diagnoses, whereas using highly specific tests inappropriately increases false-negative diagnoses. The cost implications of inappropriate intervention due to inappropriate testing go far beyond the simple expense of the test. Thus the right algorithm of test use is critical to getting the right diagnosis in the most cost-effective and timely manner to optimize patient outcome.

The expertise of the diagnostic pathologist–laboratorian is critical in both the selection and the interpretation of

modern tests for cancer diagnosis. For more subjective tests such as routine histology, flow cytometry, or cytogenetics, experience and skill are well recognized as key determinants for accurate interpretation. More analytically precise tests such as serum tumor marker assays or molecular diagnostics also require a high degree of sophistication by the laboratory director to ensure that the data obtained are accurate and not the result of artifact or sampling error. Experience and skill in both test use and interpretation are critically important in dealing with analytic as well as biologic predictive value.

This chapter provides the clinical oncologist with an understanding of the use and interpretation of the current diagnostic modalities available for the evaluation of cancer patients. The goal is not to provide an exhaustive review of tests and details that would be more appropriate for pathologists. We have somewhat arbitrarily grouped the many cancer diagnostics that are now available into five categories: surgical pathology, flow cytometry, cytogenetics, molecular diagnostics, and clinical chemistry. Each section outlines the methods, applications, and interpretation of the tests in that area. We hope this chapter will provide insight into the best use of tests in different settings and the pitfalls in interpretation, so as to be of value to the clinical oncologist in interacting with patients as well as colleagues in pathology and laboratory medicine.

Surgical Pathology

SUMMARY OF KEY POINTS

KEY METHOD
- Routine histopathologic examination is the cornerstone of cancer diagnosis.
- Immunohistochemistry is an important adjunct that allows more precision in diagnosis and classification.

- Fine-needle aspiration, when used properly, is very valuable to guide treatment decisions.

SPECIFIC ROLES OF PATHOLOGIC EXAMINATION OF TISSUES
- Histologic diagnosis and classification of cancer.

- Assignment of pathologic grade and stage.
- Frozen-section examination to direct a surgical procedure and ensure that appropriate diagnostic tissue is obtained.
- Triage of tissue for specialized testing, and banking for research purposes.

"… in addition to applied microscopy, there is scientific microscopy. What will in the end be of importance in the development of medicine is whether the microscope proves to be an agent merely of diagnosis or truly of reform."[1]

Rudolph Virchow, 1855

The inception of pathology as a medical discipline can be traced back to Renaissance Italy, when the autopsy was valued for correlating clinical history with pathologic findings.[2] Pathology would develop as a hybrid specialty, a scientific foundation for understanding disease mechanisms and a backbone for clinical practice. During the nineteenth century, pathologists were primarily academicians who studied and taught the causes, mechanisms, and consequences of disease. Direct diagnostic application was, at best, a peripheral concern bestowed on a small group of full-time autopsy pathologists whose primary role was to confirm a diagnosis in the dead rather than to formulate a diagnosis in the living.[3] At the turn of the twentieth century, pathology became a more clinically relevant discipline for several reasons.[4] Technical innovations permitted detailed microscopic descriptions of tissue patterns and cell structures that, in turn, dramatically improved diagnostic capabilities. The introduction of anesthesia and aseptic technique allowed surgeons to perform longer and more complicated procedures that required improved diagnostic skills. Finally, an enlightened medical community and the public at large came to recognize that small and subtle tumors were easier to eradicate than were large and conspicuous ones.[5]

Given this new emphasis on early cancer detection and treatment, oncologic surgeons could no longer rely on their own clinical skills and gross observations to evaluate the presence and full extent of tumor growth. Instead, a new breed of physician/pathologist evolved with specialized training in the histologic characteristics of tumors. In 1926, the American College of Surgeons insisted on properly staffed hospital laboratories under the direction of physicians trained in clinical pathology and called for the mandatory systematic examination of all surgical specimens to culminate in a report detailing the pathologic findings.

METHODS AND APPLICATIONS

The surgical pathology evaluation of a presumptive tumor specimen strives to specify clearly and comprehensively the presence, nature, and extent of a tumor in a way that guides further therapy, measures results, and predicts future outcome. The report integrates the macroscopic findings, the microscopic findings, and increasingly, the results of immunohistochemistry and even molecular genetic analysis. The scope and complexity of the surgical pathology report have increased dramatically over recent years, and groups such as the Association of Directors of Anatomic and Surgical Pathologists and the Cancer Committee of American Pathologists recently issued a number of standardized protocols that are organ/tumor specific.[6-10]

Whatever the style and format, the contents of the surgical pathology report should invariably include information regarding the presence or absence of tumor, histologic classification, pathologic staging, adequacy of tumor removal (i.e., status of the surgical margins), and tumor grade.[11] Increasingly, these anatomic measurements are supplemented by relevant immunohistochemical, cytogenetic, and molecular biologic information to refine tumor classification and to guide the selection of therapeutic options.

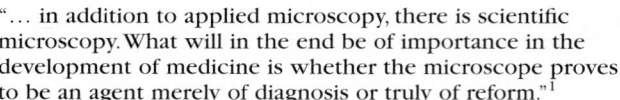

Tumor Classification

As strategies for the treatment of oncology patients become increasingly sophisticated and tumor specific, current classification schemes aim to categorize tumors in ways that are precise, reproducible, and clinically relevant. The classification of tumors is hierarchical; progressing from fundamental distinctions in biologic potential (e.g., benign vs. premalignant vs. malignant) to broad separation in cellular differentiation (e.g., epithelial vs. mesenchymal vs. lymphoid vs. melanocyctic) to much finer dissection of phenotypic expression (e.g., squamous vs. glandular, chondroid vs. osteoid, B cell vs. T cell).

Standardized international nomenclature for tumor classification has been successfully promoted by a variety of professional organizations. Most notably, the Armed Forces Institute of Pathology (AFIP) continues to update its highly influential series on tumor pathology, the *Atlas of Tumor Pathology*, in an effort to "promote a consistent, unified, and biologically sound nomenclature; guide the surgical pathologist in the diagnosis of the various tumors and tumor-like lesions; and provide relevant histogenetic, pathogenetic, and clinicopathologic information on these entities."[12] The World Health Organization also implemented a program with similar aims. Its recent collection of books on the classification of tumors has taken a more deliberate approach to incorporate relevant genetic data as a component in naming and characterizing tumors.[13]

Pathologic Staging

Stage and grade have traditionally been used as parameters to characterize the clinical severity of a tumor. Stage usually outweighs grade in importance as an indicator of patient outcome for most cancers, with the notable exception of many soft tissue sarcomas. Stage is a measure of tumor growth. It takes into account the size of a tumor and the extent to which it has anatomically spread. Tumor staging permits valid comparison between groups of patients, facilitates exchange of information among treatment centers, guides selection of therapy, and makes possible the empirical estimation of patient outcome.[14] The widely used TNM system uses three components to express anatomic extent of disease: "T" is a measure of the local extent of tumor spread; "N" indicates the presence or absence of metastatic spread to regional lymph nodes; and "M" specifies the presence or absence of metastatic spread to distant sites. T, N, and M classifications are combined to provide a stage grouping.

Clinical staging (designated as cTNM) defines the anatomic extent of a tumor based on clinical evidence before the initiation of treatment. It incorporates the findings obtained from the physical examination, imaging studies, surgical exploration, and tissue biopsy. Clinical stage is used as a guide for the selection of primary therapy. In contrast, pathologic staging (designated pTNM) is based on examination of the surgically resected specimen. Assessment of pathologic stage is contingent on the recognition and removal of tumor to allow meaningful anatomic assessment of tumor origin and local extension. Thus the pathologist's ability to render an accurate pathologic stage is sometimes compromised by the surgical approach, especially when a tumor is fragmented or removed through the laparoscope. Pathologic staging is used mainly to direct adjuvant therapy, estimate prognosis, and report results, but does not invalidate the clinical stage (and vice versa).

Tumor Grading

Tumor grade is a semiquantitative measurement of histologic differentiation from the normal tissue from which the tumor arises. Well-differentiated tumors (grade 1) closely resemble their non-neoplastic counterpart; poorly differentiated tumors (grade 3 or 4) do not. As a rule of thumb, the more poorly differentiated a tumor, the more aggressive its behavior; but the impact of tumor grade on tumor behavior is highly tumor specific. For example, the expected behavior and treatment of soft tissue sarcomas is profoundly influenced by tumor grade. In contrast, most lung carcinomas are uniformly aggressive, irrespective of histologic grade. For other tumor types, the utility of histologic grading falls somewhere between these two extremes.

No single uniform scheme exists for the histologic grading of malignant neoplasms; grading schemes are tumor specific. For some tumors, histologic classification defines tumor grade. Small cell carcinoma of the lung, anaplastic carcinoma of the thyroid, and Ewing's sarcoma are, by definition, high-grade (i.e., poorly differentiated) tumors; whereas carcinoid tumor of the lung, polymorphous low-grade carcinoma of the salivary glands, and small lymphocytic lymphoma are, by definition, low-grade (i.e., well-differentiated) tumors. Some tumor types are graded based on the severity of cytologic atypia (e.g., leiomyosarcoma, renal cell carcinoma); others, on the basis of architectural growth patterns (e.g., adenocarcinoma of the prostate); and still others, by the combination of cellular atypia and architectural disarray (e.g., ductal carcinoma of the breast). Effective grading strategies strive to minimize inconsistency in application and maximize the prognostic significance of tumor stratification.

Intraoperative Frozen-Section Consultation

The "frozen section" is a method whereby fresh tissue is frozen, thinly sectioned, stained, and examined under the microscope. To benefit fully from the diagnostic value of the frozen section, the surgeon and the pathologist must have a balanced appreciation for its strengths and limitations.[15]

In four common situations, requests for frozen section are appropriate:[16]

1. To establish a diagnosis or determine pathologic stage to guide the type and/or extent of the operation. Frozen-section detection of metastatic carcinoma in sentinel lymph nodes, for example, now makes possible the selection of patients who would benefit from one-step lymph node dissections.
2. To determine the adequacy of tumor removal. Frozen-section analysis of surgical margins provides assurance of complete tumor removal at the time of surgery and thus minimizes the need for additional operations for revisions of positive margins.
3. To confirm the nature of the lesion. This is important to guide fresh tissue distribution for appropriate laboratory studies such as to the microbiology laboratory for culture studies, to the flow-cytometry laboratory for immunophenotypic analysis, and to the genetics laboratory for cytogenetic or molecular analysis.
4. To assess the presence and quality of lesional tissue before the operation is completed. In this instance, the frozen section serves not to establish an intraoperative diagnosis but to ensure that adequate tissue has been secured such that a definite diagnosis can be rendered on permanent histologic examination.

Science of Clinical Oncology

APPROPRIATE USE OF FROZEN SECTIONS IN SURGICAL PATHOLOGY

Frozen section, used appropriately, is an important tool in the management of a cancer patient. Several important indications can lead to a specific action on the part of the surgeon, but inappropriate uses run the risk of compromising care.

Frozen sections *should* be used

- To establish a diagnosis or pathologic stage, and thereby determine the type and extent of the operation needed.
- To establish the status of the surgical margin to determine if a wider local excision is necesssary.
- To establish the presence and nature of appropriate lesional tissue to distribute fresh tissue for additional laboratory studies, such as microbiology culture, flow cytometry, or molecular assays.
- To establish the adequacy of a biopsy, thereby ensuring that a definitive diagnosis will be rendered on permanent histology.

Frozen sections *should not* be used

- For curiosity with no clear-cut plan to use results, as this is unnecessarily costly and may also tie up pathology resources needed for other more appropriate frozen sections occurring at the same time.
- To establish a diagnosis when there is a threat of irreparable damage to tissue architecture that would preclude a definite diagnosis on permanent histology.
- To document a focal microscopic finding in a large specimen, as sampling error may lead to an erroneous conclusion and inappropriate surgical approach.

Accurate frozen-section diagnosis is compromised by inherent limitations of the technique,[17,18] especially suboptimal preservation of cytologic and histologic detail. Tissue fragmentation due to the presence of fat, bone, or foreign material and tissue distortion secondary to ice-crystal formation cause distortions that may obscure the true identity of the pathologic process. Some specimens, particularly delicate tissue fragments in which important diagnostic distinctions are made on the basis of subtle architectural and cytologic alterations, are particularly susceptible to frozen section–induced morphologic alterations. In these cases, frozen-section analysis may be counterproductive and may compromise an accurate tissue diagnosis. For example, frozen-section evaluation of nonpalpable breast lesions, once a routine practice, is no longer encouraged because of a high error rate and a propensity to obscure irrevocably the subtle morphologic distinction between benign hyperplasia and intraductal carcinoma.

Accuracy of the frozen section also is limited by time constraints so that a cursory microscopic evaluation of large specimens is highly vulnerable to sampling error. Thus invasion within a large villous adenoma of the colorectum, transcapsular extension of an encapsulated follicular neoplasm of the thyroid, or malignant trans-formation within a benign mixed tumor of the parotid may easily elude detection when microscopic examination is limited to one or two frozen sections.

When the frozen section is used properly, its diagnostic accuracy now routinely exceeds 97% in both academic centers and general practice settings.[19,20] Diagnostic accuracy is especially high when the frozen section is used to make broad and fundamental distinction between pathologic processes (e.g., presence of tumor vs. absence of tumor, inflammatory process vs. neoplastic process, benign tumor vs. malignant tumor). Conversely, accuracy diminishes with increasing demands for precise tumor subclassification. Regardless of the situation, accuracy is improved when the pathologist is provided with appropriate clinical information and the indication for the consult.

Immunohistochemistry

Immunohistochemistry (IHC) is a method for localizing specific constituents in tissues based on antibody recognition of tissue antigens. Initially developed by Coons in 1940 as an investigative immunofluorescence technique to detect antigens in frozen tissue sections,[21] technical advances over the past two decades have thrust the technique into the forefront of diagnostic pathology.[22] The development of nonfluorescent chromogens has allowed visualization of antigen-antibody binding by using the conventional light microscope. The introduction of various amplification steps (e.g., peroxidase-antiperoxidase method, avidin-biotin conjugate method, polymerase-based labeling system) has significantly improved sensitivity. The discovery of means to "unmask" antigens (e.g., enzyme digestion, heat-induced epitope retrieval) has permitted consistency in staining despite variations in tissue fixation and processing. Finally, the development of techniques to manufacture highly specific monoclonal antibodies has greatly expanded the arsenal of probes that can target virtually any immunogenic marker.[23] By adapting the technique to formalin-fixed and paraffin-embedded tissues, IHC is now compatible with standard tissue-processing procedures and can even be performed in a retrospective fashion on tissue blocks that have been archived for many years. IHC is now used routinely to address a range of key diagnostic questions.[24]

Is It a Tumor?

In some specific instances, markers identified by IHC can help make the fundamental distinction between a malignant tumor and some benign process. For example, the demonstration of κ or λ light-chain restriction by IHC is a good indicator of monoclonality in B-cell processes, and can help distinguish malignant lymphoma from an inflammatory process. In the prostate, the absence of high-molecular-weight cytokeratin and p63 by IHC labeling points to the absence of a basal cell layer, helping to distinguish an adenocarcinoma from benign adenosis.[25] As the molecular genetic basis of human tumors becomes increasingly understood, antibodies to products of oncogenes and tumor-suppressor genes hold much promise in recognizing neoplastic processes.

What Type of Tumor Is It?

The most basic application of IHC is tumor classification. For tumors that show no specific differentiation at the light-microscopic level, IHC is fundamental in making critical distinctions among epithelial, mesenchymal, lymphoid, melanocyctic, and germ cell neoplasms. Even for differentiated tumors, IHC provides a detailed phenotypic description that goes well beyond the resolution capabilities of the standard light microscope. In studies emphasizing the importance of second-opinion surgical pathology, the application of IHC has been identified as a key factor resulting in major therapeutic and prognostic modifications for patients sent to large referral hospitals for oncologic surgery (Fig. 17-1).[26,27] Hematopathology is one example of a field that has become increasingly reliant on IHC, where the availability of antibodies to lineage-restricted antigens has made possible high-resolution and clinically relevant classification of hematolymphoid neoplasms.[28] IHC is having a similar impact on soft tissue sarcomas, primitive round blue cell tumors, and other areas of diagnostic pathology in which precise tumor classification is beyond the reach of conventional hematoxylin and eosin (H&E) histology.[29,30]

Where Did the Tumor Arise?

The expression of some markers is so highly tissue specific that a single IHC stain can sometimes establish the most likely primary site for a neoplasm of unknown origin. Unfortunately, there are few situations in which the site of origin be established by a single marker. However, most tumors display a distinctive pattern of IHC staining against a selected array of antibody probes, a pattern sometimes referred to as an "immunohistochemical profile." For example, the difficult distinction between malignant mesothelioma and peripheral lung adenocarcinoma is aided by unique IHC fingerprints for a panel of antibody probes.[31] With the regular introduction of new antibodies into the diagnostic armamentarium, these profiles are becoming increasingly elaborate. Internet-accessible databases have become very useful in disseminating updated information regarding IHC profiles of various tumor types based on published data.[32]

Has the Tumor Metastasized?

IHC can optimize detection of micrometastases when traditional microscopic examination is too crude to detect scattered individual tumor cells. Staining of sentinel lymph nodes with cytokeratin to detect metastatic breast carcinoma and HMB-45 to detect metastatic melanoma is now routinely used for the accurate pathologic staging of regional lymph nodes.[33,34]

How Will the Tumor Behave?

IHC can help to measure determinants of disease outcome. For various tumor types, a high proliferation rate portends aggressive tumor behavior and poor outcome. The traditional practice of counting mitotic figures as a crude measure of tumor proliferation is now being replaced by more quantitative assessment of proliferation activity as measured by IHC detection of certain nuclear antigens that are expressed during stages of active cell division (e.g., Ki-67).[35] Perhaps more important, IHC can help predict tumor response to certain therapies. Detection of estrogen receptor, progesterone receptor, and HER-2/*neu* has direct and immediate therapeutic implications, and these findings are now routinely incorporated into surgical pathology reports of invasive breast carcinomas.[36,37] A wave of new antibody probes against oncogene products, tumor-suppressor gene products, and various cellcycle signaling proteins (e.g., activated kinases) may help individualize treatment regimens based on specific expression profiles.[38] However, the application of these markers to prognosis will require standardized technical protocols, defined cutoff values for positive results, and clinical validation studies with uniform treatment arms and adequate follow-up.[39]

Fine Needle Aspiration

In contrast to tissue histopathology with its strong reliance on architectural patterns of tumor growth, cytopathology extracts diagnostic information from the appearance of individual cells and cell clusters. Although its use has surged over the last two decades, cytopathology is far from novel. Indeed, attempts to define distinctions between benign and malignant cells scraped from the surfaces of tumors constitute the origin, not the pinnacle, of contemporary diagnostic pathology.[3] George Papanicolaou (1883–1962) is generally credited with the rediscovery of cytopathologic examination. Not only did he demonstrate its value regarding diagnostic accuracy, but he launched its routine use as a highly effective means of reducing cancer-related morbidity and mortality.

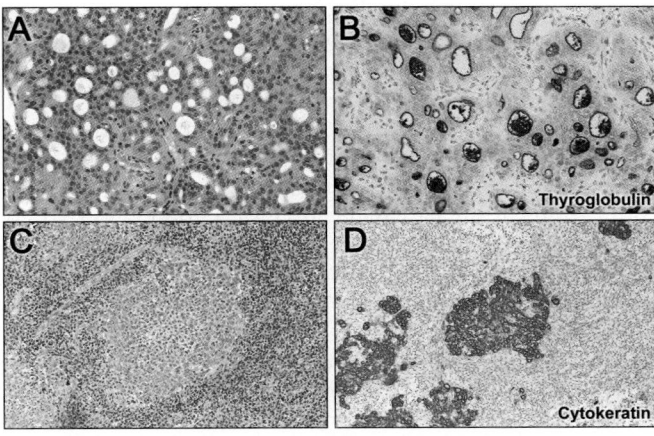

Figure 17-1. Impact of immunohistochemistry on tumor classification. **A,** The submitting pathologist diagnosed this neck mass as metastatic adenocarcinoma of salivary gland origin (H&E stain). **B,** A second-opinion diagnosis of metastatic thyroid carcinoma was confirmed by immunohistochemistry (thyroglobulin stain). **C,** The submitting pathologist diagnosed this tonsillar mass as a malignant lymphoma (H&E stain). **D,** A second-opinion diagnosis of undifferentiated carcinoma was confirmed by immunohistochemistry (cytokeratin stain). (From Westra WH, Kronz JD, Eisele DW: The impact of second opinion surgical pathology on the practice of head and neck surgery: A decade experience at a large referral hospital. Head Neck 2002;24:684–693, with permission).

Fine needle aspiration (FNA) is a procedure that uses a fine gauge needle to remove cells from a suggestive mass for microscopic examination. Its primary role is to guide treatment decisions, and in this role, FNA offers several significant advantages over the frozen section:

1. It provides a preoperative rather than intraoperative diagnosis. Some estimate that up to 80% of all thyroid surgery can be avoided by routinely aspirating thyroid nodules.[40]
2. It is cost-effective. FNA is a simple technique that is inherently economical and often circumvents the need for a much more costly surgical intervention.
3. It is safe. FNA eliminates the need for general anesthesia and minimizes the risk of complications associated with more invasive procedures for tumor acquisition.

With notable exceptions (e.g., testicular masses, ovarian masses, primary malignant melanomas), FNA is no longer believed to facilitate tumor spread or induce severe hemorrhage, an occasional complication of larger bore needles.[41]

Although reported accuracy rates range from 90% to 99%, divergent opinions persist about the reliability of the FNA and its role in clinical management. Most authorities, however, would concede the following generalities:[42]

1. Accuracy is related to the site and nature of the neoplasm. FNA is not very useful in those situations in which tumor classification depends less on cytologic features and more on architectural patterns, such as locally invasive tumor growth. When dealing with encapsulated neoplasms of the thyroid, for example, FNA is notoriously inaccurate in separating follicular adenomas from follicular carcinomas because a diagnosis of malignancy is contingent on the histologic demonstration of tumor invasion.
2. Accuracy is related to the scope of the clinical question. FNA is highly reliable when grappling with broad distinctions (e.g., presence of tumor vs. absence of tumor, inflammatory process vs. neoplastic process, benign tumor vs. malignant tumor), but accuracy diminishes for precise tumor subclassification. Moreover, largely due to the impact of limited tumor sampling by FNA, a malignant tumor is more likely to be misdiagnosed as benign (i.e., false-negative result) than a benign tumor is to be misdiagnosed as malignant (i.e., false-positive result).
3. Accuracy is related to the experience of the cytopathologist and the quality of the slide preparations.

Because of the combined impact of these three factors, FNA is best used as an adjunctive diagnostic tool. It should serve to complement, not supplant, the clinical, radiographic, and laboratory findings.

FUTURE DIRECTIONS

Breakneck developments in molecular biology, biotechnology, and bioinformatics are driving a molecular revolution in pathology. Contemporary research resulting in the identification of tens of thousands of new genes and providing insight into the function and complex interaction of these genes will present the pathologist with new opportunities for solving old diagnostic problems. The technologic armamentarium of the surgical pathologist, once reliant solely on the light microscope to detect phenotypic alterations, is now equipped with sophisticated tools to isolate and compare single cell populations in a tumor and to detect submicroscopic alterations in gene integrity, gene expression, and gene translation.[43,44]

The direct application of molecular techniques to diagnostic oncologic pathology has only just begun, but, as discussed in subsequent sections, a growing number of examples bolster the bold claims that molecular analysis will profoundly aid the diagnoses, prognosis, and treatment of tumors. For hematologic neoplasms, delineation of various chromosomal translocations has allowed more clinically relevant classification of leukemias and lymphomas.[45,46] Genetic analysis is having a similar impact on soft tissue tumors.[47] Increased access to detailed genetic information also will provide a clearer picture of patient outcome and help individualize treatment plans. For hematopoietic neoplasms, detection of specific translocations already provides prognostic information independent of morphologic and immunophenotypic characterization. Moreover, the products of these transforming genes provide attractive targets for promising new therapeutic agents.

For sporadic epithelial neoplasms, the molecular genetic makeup of a tumor is not currently integrated into the inventory of more classic prognostic and predictive determinants. Efforts to do so have been stalled by the number and complexity of genetic alterations, the absence of standardized methods to measure and interpret test results, the high cost and limited availability of the technology, and the absence of well-designed clinical studies to assess clinical utility.[48] The application of such techniques is well appreciated in breast cancer, for which quantitative measures of hormone-receptor expression and HER-2/*neu* gene amplification are now routinely incorporated to assess outcome and guide therapy. These applications in breast cancer forecast a coming era when pharmacologic and radiation sensitivity profiles based on molecular genetic alterations will permit customized treatment of individual patients.

The molecular revolution will certainly enhance the role of the surgical pathologist in the multidisciplinary approach to the patient with cancer, not replace it. Advances in basic tumor research clearly are dependent on the involvement of well-trained pathologists not just to characterize tumors accurately with respect to site of origin and pathologic grade but also to distinguish normal and neoplastic tissue, and identify subtle degrees of morphologic changes in an individual section. With all the developments of new technology and approaches, classic light microscopy remains the cornerstone of tumor diagnostics and the starting point for the application of any new prognostic or therapeutic marker.

Flow Cytometry in Oncologic Diagnosis

SUMMARY OF KEY POINTS

KEY METHODS
- Fluorescently conjugated antibodies, bound to cell-surface or intracellular proteins, allow enumeration and detailed characterization of subsets of cells in heterogeneous mixtures.
- Fluorescent DNA-binding dyes allow determination of tumor ploidy and can assess cell-cycle characteristics of tumors.

APPLICATIONS
Acute Leukemia
- Used for lineage assignment and classification of leukemia.

- Certain phenotypes correlate with molecular abnormalities.
- Minimal residual disease detection is prognostic in both acute lymphoblastic leukemia (ALL) and acute myelogenous leukemia (AML).

Lymphoma and Chronic Lymphoproliferative Disorders
- Suitable for use on cell suspensions of tissue, fine-needle aspirates, fluids, as well as blood and marrow.
- Clonality of B-cell processes readily

detected by light-chain restriction assay.
- Many lymphoid disorders are defined by phenotypic profiles.

Solid Tumors
- DNA ploidy and S-phase fraction can be detected.
- Prognostic significance is controversial, but measurement has value in certain tumors.
- Methodologic difficulties have contributed to lack of acceptance.

Flow cytometry is a technology used to study attributes of individual cells in a suspension. Over the past two decades, flow cytometry has become increasingly sophisticated; high-speed sorters and analyzers capable of detecting more than a dozen colors simultaneously have kept flow cytometry in the forefront as a tool for the fundamental investigation into cancer. At the same time, flow cytometry has matured from a research technology to one that is part of the routine clinical laboratory. This chapter focuses on diagnostic aspects of flow cytometry.

METHODS

A flow cytometer analyzes large numbers of cells one at a time. As such, it is an ideal tool for examination of properties of populations of cells. It is best thought of as a technique that is complementary to imaging: it does not provide as much detail about individual cells, but provides much better statistical measurements, and has the great strength of being able to characterize different groups of cells in heterogeneous mixtures. It also can physically sort specific subpopulations of cells. Although a detailed discussion of the workings of a flow cytometer is outside the scope of this chapter, discussion of a few general principles is in order.

Functional Components

A flow cytometer has three separate components: a fluidics system, an optical platform, and signal-processing electronics. The fluidic system aspirates the sample, mixes it with a sheath fluid to produce laminar flow, and conducts the cell suspension past the sensing zone where individual cells are examined. The optical platform consists of the laser light source(s), lenses to focus the light on the passing cell stream, band-pass filters to capture light of restricted wavelengths, and photo-multiplier tubes (PMTs) that capture the emitted signals. The electronics convert photons to electrical signals in proportion to the total light contacting the PMTs, and amplify and scale the signals so that data can be readily analyzed. The value of each collected parameter is "quantitized" and assigned to a particular *channel*. Higher channels reflect brighter signals. Current software packages reprocess collected data electronically in a variety of formats; this flexibility of data analysis is critical to the utility of this technology.

Electronically reprocessed data are displayed by software programs in the form of *dot plots* or *histograms*. The most useful displays generally correlate one parameter with another, where each dot represents a single event (cell) with the x- and y-channel values for the two chosen parameters. In addition to fluorescence, *forward scatter*, and *right angle*, or *side scatter* can be displayed. The former parameter is roughly proportional to the size of the cells, whereas the latter is a measure of internal cellular complexity, which for hematopoietic cells generally means granularity. Typically, dot plots of either forward versus side scatter, or scatter versus fluorescence, are used to identify populations of interest in a process called gating, and additional displays show additional fluorescence or scatter characteristics of these populations. Because scatter measurements are made in parallel to, and independent of, the fluorescence measurements, four-color flow cytometry, for example, is equivalent to six-parameter cytometry. The term *multiparameter flow cytometry* is typically used to define simultaneous analysis of five or more parameters on individual cells.

Fluorochromes and Fluorescence

Fluorochromes are compounds that have spectral characteristics that allow them to absorb light of certain wavelengths and then to emit light at longer wavelengths. Emission is a specific characteristic of the compound, is not limited to a fixed wavelength, but rather constitutes a spectrum, with variable numbers of photons emitted at different wavelengths. Different fluorochromes, including fluorescein isothiocyanate (FITC) and phycoerythrin (PE) as well as others, all have the capacity of absorbing light at 488 nm but emit at different wavelengths, thereby making it possible to perform multicolor flow cytometry with a single laser emitting at 488 nm. So-called tandem conjugates, which covalently couple two fluorochrome molecules, allow emitted light to be transferred from one to the other and can greatly increase the number of colors that can be detected with a single laser. Additional dyes such as allophycocyanin, which emit longer wavelengths, cannot be excited by a 488-nm laser but require a second light source, most frequently one emitting light at 635 nm.

APPLICATIONS OF FLOW CYTOMETRY TO CLINICAL ONCOLOGY

Currently flow cytometry plays a significant role in the diagnosis, classification, and management of patients with acute leukemia, chronic lymphoproliferative disorders, and non-Hodgkin's lymphoma. The early promise of this technology in the management of patients with solid tumors has not been completely realized, but it still plays a role in certain areas. Each of these areas is discussed in detail separately.

Acute Leukemia

Flow-cytometric immunophenotyping has become a standard practice in the evaluation of new patients with acute leukemia. The most obvious role of flow cytometry is in the distinction of lymphoid from myeloid leukemia, but many ways exist in which flow cytometry can help in the diagnosis and management of these patients (Table 17-1).

Lineage Assignment in Acute Leukemia

Phenotypic analysis of a bone marrow that is completely replaced by blasts is an almost trivial problem. Multiparameter flow cytometry, however, can dissect and categorize all populations in bone marrow, and, most important, can distinguish leukemic cells from normal, even when these are not the majority population. The antibody panel used to study patients with acute leukemia typically contains representative markers of all lineages, with some redundancy to allow recognition and classification because many antigens may be aberrantly lost or acquired in leukemic cells.[49,50] No standard combinations of antibodies are used by all laboratories. However, certain combinations have proved particularly useful not only for the most economic classification of leukemia, but also for their ability to demonstrate characteristic aberrant

TABLE 17-1

Applications of Flow Cytometry in Hematologic Neoplasia

Acute Leukemia

Distinction of myeloid and lymphoid leukemia
Distinction of T-ALL from precursor B-ALL
Subclassification of lymphoid and myeloid leukemia
Identification of phenotypes associated with characteristic molecular and cytogenetic abnormalities
Identification and enumeration of blasts in heterogeneous samples
Identification of abnormal phenotypes for purposes of monitoring patients after therapy (minimal residual disease)
Identification of hyperdiploidy in pediatric ALL
Identification of abnormal patterns of myeloid maturation in myelodysplastic syndromes

Lymphoma and Lymphoproliferative Disorders

Identification of clonal B-cell proliferations
Subclassification of B-cell lymphomas and leukemias
    Diagnosis of chronic lymphocytic leukemia
    Diagnosis of hairy cell leukemia
    Identification of characteristic phenotypes in other lymphomas
Prognosis of CLL (CD38 expression)
Identification of phenotypically abnormal T cells
Subclassification of T-cell lymphoproliferative disorders
Diagnosis of plasma cell dyscrasias
Identification of abnormal phenotypes for purposes of monitoring patients after therapy (minimal residual disease)

ALL, acute lymphoblastic leukemia; CLL, chronic lymphocytic leukemia.

patterns that may be extremely useful for the detection of residual disease in follow-up samples (see later).

Difficulties encountered in the interpretation of flow-cytometry data derive largely from two problems. First, in cases in which leukemic cells are not an obviously dominant population, it is important to ensure that the cells of interest are analyzed. The most useful general approach for this takes advantage of the fact that the common leukocyte antigen CD45 is differentially expressed on different types of hematopoietic cells, and, when combined with side scatter, produces a display in which blasts occupy a unique position not occupied by normal cells (Fig. 17-2).[51] Thus combining CD45 in one color with multiple combinations of antibodies in additional colors allows the detailed characterization of blast populations in marrow even when they are present only in low numbers.

Failure to select the leukemic population for analysis, or including a mixture of leukemic and normal cells in a gate, may give rise to confusion in the reporting of flow-cytometry results. It is best to identify the leukemic population visually and to provide a detailed description of the antigens expressed on the leukemic population. This is particularly true in myeloid leukemias, in which the dynamic patterns of maturation associated with morphologic variation in AML are reflected in changes in both light scatter and antigen expression as leukemic cells mature. Tabular arrays of "percentage positive" are not recommended as part of a flow-cytometry report, as they cannot reflect this complexity and may cause confusion.[52]

The second problem in interpreting flow-cytometry results in leukemia derives from the fact that most of the

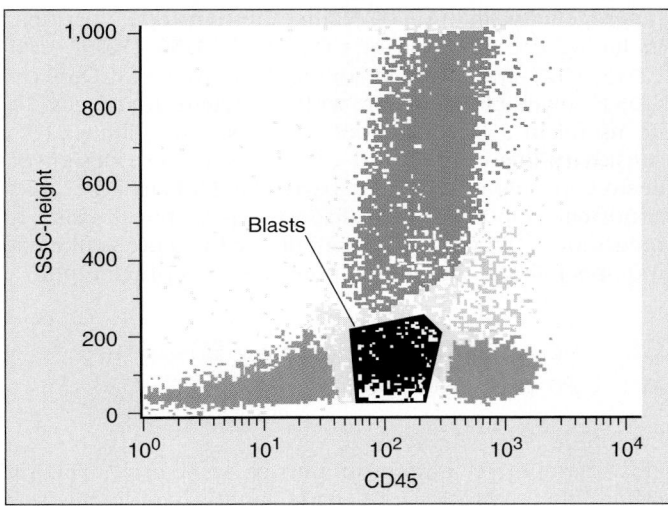

Figure 17-2. CD45 gating in acute leukemia. Dual-parameter display of CD45 and side scatter of bone marrow containing increased blasts. These two parameters can readily separate lymphocytes (*yellow*), granulocytes (*blue*), monocytes (*light blue*), and nucleated red cells (*pink*). In normal marrow, a "hole" is found with few events in the low side scatter (SSC)/intermediate CD45 region, but in this case, a distinct population can be identified. This allows gating and analysis of antigen expression on just the blast population.

reagents used in classifying leukemia are only relatively rather than absolutely specific. Thus correct classification requires not only a panel with some redundancy, but also an understanding of patterns of reactivity of the antibodies. Markers like CD13 and CD33, which are considered "myeloid antigens" because they were originally produced against myeloid leukemia cells, are found on up to half of cases of lymphoid leukemia,[53] and interpretation of leukemias positive for these markers continues to be a cause of confusion today.[54] Generally speaking, the most specific markers of a given lineage are not highly sensitive, and the most sensitive ones are not specific. This is more true of myeloid markers than of lymphoid ones, such that lymphoid leukemias can usually be recognized precisely, whereas poorly differentiated myeloid leukemias are usually defined by the presence of myeloid markers in the absence of specific lymphoid antigens.

Acute Leukemias of Indeterminate or Ambiguous Lineage

Although the great majority of cases of acute leukemia can be easily categorized as to lineage, the lack of absolute specificity of most markers, and the promiscuity of their expression, implies that some cases cannot easily be resolved. Unfortunately, considerable controversy exists about the use of the term *mixed lineage* or *biphenotypic* leukemia. Clearly, leukemias that express myeloid- and lymphoid-associated markers in combination represent a heterogeneous group of diseases. A scoring system has been proposed[55] that assigns various point values to different antigens, with a diagnosis of "biphenotypic leukemia" rendered if the score is high for more than one

lineage. Although this is an objective method of defining lineage, it has the misfortune of mixing different kinds of cases with different molecular abnormalities. The scoring system, as originally conceived, also does not distinguish between cases in which blasts coexpress antigens of different lineages and those in which there are distinct leukemic blast populations. The latter situation is much less common, but properly can be thought of as true mixed-lineage leukemia. Certain of these, such as the combination of B-precursor ALL and AML in patients with the Philadelphia chromosome, represent distinct entities.

Association of Immunophenotype and Molecular Abnormalities

Many phenotypes in both ALL and AML are highly associated with characteristic cytogenetic abnormalities.[56–62] The most specific phenotypic association in ALL is probably one that predicts a mixed leukemia lineage (MLL) rearrangement,[57,58] whereas other translocations such as E2A-PBX1 or TEL-AML1 show strong but not specific associations.[59,60] In AML, the most important link is in promyelocytic leukemia with the t(15;17). Whereas lack of HLA-DR is the best-known abnormality, only about half of cases of DR-negative AMLs turn out to be acute promyleocytic leukemia (APL), and other combinations of marker expression are much more sensitive and specific for APL.[61] Other common translocations also show phenotypic associations. AML with the t(8;21), with dim CD19, bright CD34, and frequent TdT expression[62] is probably the most predictive. AML associated with myelodysplastic syndrome is almost always CD34 positive, and generally shows significant aberrant abnormalities in blast antigen expression.[63] However, none of these findings, by itself, is specific for MDS-related AML. MDS, however, also is associated with characteristic abnormalities in granulocyte maturation.[64] Finding these in conjunction with a minor phenotypically abnormal myeloid blast population makes MDS likely; however, large-scale studies on the sensitivity and specificity of diagnoses of MDS by flow cytometry have yet to be performed.

Minimal Residual Disease Detection in Acute Leukemia

In recent years, several studies have demonstrated that finding residual leukemic cells in the marrows of patients in clinical and morphologic remission is a very strong adverse prognostic factor.[65–72] Although the most extensive data exist in childhood ALL,[65–68] the principle has also been shown to apply to adult ALL[69,70] and to AML.[71,72]

Both molecular and flow-based methods have been used to detect MRD. For leukemias associated with specific translocations, it is clear that molecular methods that detect unique fusion transcripts are significantly more sensitive than flow-based methods. However, molecular methods based on detecting clone-specific rearrangements of immunoglobulin or T-cell receptor genes in ALL are only slightly, if at all, more sensitive than flow assays; these have sensitivities on the order of 10^{-4} to 10^{-5}[65,66] whereas flow-based technologies can also achieve 10^{-4} sensitivities in the majority of cases.[68,73–75] Both methods are about equally capable of predicting outcome, at least in ALL.

Science of Clinical Oncology

Flow-based assays of MRD are based on the principle that nearly all leukemias show a pattern of expression of antigens that is aberrant when compared with the pattern seen in normal differentiation.[73-75] This aberrancy can take several forms. Some leukemic cells can abnormally express antigens of a different lineage or show loss of expression of a normal lineage marker. What is seen more commonly, however, is expression of normal differentiation antigens, but at an intensity that is different from that expected for a particular stage of differentiation. This latter attribute makes flow MRD analysis applicable to the great majority of cases of leukemia. Nonetheless, recognizing these deviations requires a clear understanding of patterns of maturation in normal differentiation, including marrow regeneration, as viewed in multiparameter space.

The pattern of antigen acquisition and loss during B-cell maturation in the bone marrow has been very well characterized, and certain markers are particularly useful for distinguishing normal and leukemic maturation. Consideration of markers including intensity of CD45, CD34, CD10, and TdT or aberrant coexpression of myeloid or other unexpected antigens can allow detection of as few as 1×10^4 leukemic cells even when normal B-cell precursors are present in significant numbers (Fig. 17-3).[73,74] Marrow T–ALL is even more easily distinguished from normal T cells, most readily by coexpression of cytoplasmic CD3 and TdT, which is never seen on any normal cell.[75] Detection of myeloid MRD is generally a more elaborate process because of the greater phenotypic

heterogeneity in AML. Certain aberrant combinations, including coexpression of CD34 and CD56, CD117 and CD15, CD7 and myeloid antigens, or loss of CD38 on CD34$^+$ myeloblasts occur with sufficient frequency to be useful in a large number of cases.[72] To achieve 10^{-4} sensitivity in essentially all cases may require design of custom panels unique to a particular leukemia. Because abnormal populations at diagnosis may not persist at recurrence,[76] monitoring patients with acute leukemia requires following more than one aberrant phenotype.

Chronic Lymphoproliferative Disorders and Lymphoma

Lymphoid Tissue Analysis

Flow-cytometric immunophenotyping plays a major role in the evaluation of a patient with lymphoma (see Table 17-1).[77-80] The techniques used to approach such patients are generally similar to those with acute leukemia, although some differences are found in the most useful panels of antibodies. Lymphoid tissue must first be disaggregated to produce a cell suspension suitable for flow-cytometric analysis. Although this is readily accomplished in most low-grade lymphomas, high-grade lymphomas may give a nonrepresentative sample because of the greater fragility of the neoplastic cells compared with residual normal ones. Fibrosis also may make disaggregation difficult or result in disruption of neoplastic cells. Consequently, flow-cytometric analysis of lymphoma requires careful gating to ensure that the cells of interest are analyzed.

In contrast to the situation with acute leukemias, no single antibody serves as a useful surrogate for the neoplastic population. However, in B-cell malignancies, neoplastic B cells generally greatly outnumber normal ones (although there may be normal T cells), so that use of a pan–B-cell antibody such as CD19 or CD20 can help to isolate the neoplastic cells for analysis. In addition, forward scatter, as a marker of cell size, may be a very useful parameter to help distinguish frequently larger neoplastic cells from smaller normal counterparts.

Because lymphoma phenotyping by flow cytometry may be difficult, some laboratories consider tissue immunohistochemistry the preferred method for phenotyping. However, the two techniques are complementary. The principle advantages of flow cytometry relate to its speed and its ability to identify and phenotype precisely the neoplastic elements in a heterogeneous sample. A complete phenotypic characterization, and in many cases, a diagnosis can be achieved within a few hours from the time of biopsy, rather than the days needed for histopathologic examination and immunostaining. Flow cytometry is also far better than immunohistochemistry for demonstrating light-chain restriction, and therefore clonality, in B-cell neoplasms.[79,80]

The disadvantages of flow cytometry come from the architectural disruption created by making a cell suspension and the aforementioned possible loss of cells of interest. Hodgkin's lymphoma in particular can

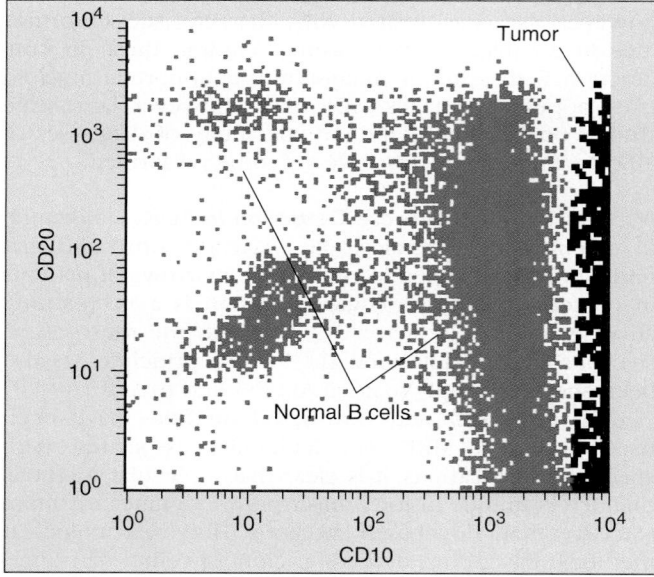

Figure 17-3. Minimal residual disease detection in acute lymphoblastic leukemia. Normal B cells have a fixed pattern of expression of different antigens as they mature. Leukemic cells depart from this normal pattern. In this case, the residual leukemic cells, which constituted less than 0.05% of the total sample, are easily recognized because they have much brighter CD10 expression than do normal B-cell precursors.

essentially never be diagnosed with flow cytometry. Even in non-Hodgkin's lymphoma, grading may be difficult from flow-cytometric immunophenotyping alone, and precise classification can only rarely be accomplished; lymphoma classification still relies heavily on morphology, and this must be correlated with flow-cytometric information.

Classification of lymphoma, and grading in particular, can be improved by assessment of DNA content by flow cytometry (see later), because S-phase fraction is closely correlated with grade.[79-81] Burkitt's lymphoma, which has the highest S fraction of any neoplasm, can generally be reliably identified by flow cytometry. However, in lesions like follicular lymphoma, grading systems still are based on morphologic criteria, and although there might be reason to expect that flow-based methods might be more objective, these have not been validated in large series to the point at which they are generally accepted.

One of the most fruitful applications of flow cytometry in the diagnosis of lymphoma is in the analysis of specimens from fine-needle aspirates (FNA).[82,83] Cells obtained by FNA are already in suspension, and flow-cytometric analysis contributes significantly to the cytopathologic diagnosis of lymphoma, which is notoriously difficult. Although FNA has been used for years in the evaluation of recurrent adenopathy in patients with known lymphoma, when combined with flow cytometry, it can serve as a primary diagnostic modality in lymphoma. The majority of non-Hodgkin's lymphomas can be recognized and graded, and, importantly, lymphomas also can usually be excluded. Optimal application of this technology, however, requires close collaboration between the cytopathologist and flow cytometrist, a clear understanding of the strengths and limitations of the two techniques, and a willingness to revert to open biopsy in ambiguous cases.

Blood and Marrow Analysis

Limitations attendant on generating cell suspensions do not apply to patients with blood or marrow involvement by chronic lymphoproliferative disorders.[77,80,84-86] Subclassification of these lesions relies heavily on flow cytometry. Chronic lymphocytic leukemia (CLL) is now essentially defined by its immunophenotypic characteristics. Expression of CD38, as assessed by flow cytometry, has recently been recognized as a powerful prognostic marker in CLL; patients with positive leukemic cells fare much worse than do those who are negative.[87-89] Other B-cell lymphoproliferative disorders have characteristic, if not always absolutely specific, phenotypes.[77,80,84,85,90,91] Mantle cell lymphoma can often be recognized in leukemic phase, although the most specific marker, cyclin D1, is very difficult to detect by flow with current techniques. Hairy cell leukemia, conversely, has not only a characteristic but also a highly specific phenotype[80,92]; occasionally patients with unexplained pancytopenia can be determined to have hairy cell leukemia when only a tiny number of blood cells with the classic phenotype are identified[92] (Fig. 17-4).

One of the most important attributes of flow cytometry is its ability to demonstrate clonality in B-cell populations, based on restricted expression of one type of immuno-

globulin light chain.[77,79,80] This is particularly valuable in the evaluation of patients with unexplained lymphocytosis.[93,94] This feature also is useful for staging patients with B-cell non-Hodgkin's lymphoma,[95,96] as the presence of as little as 0.5% to 1% of a clonal B-cell population, or even less, can be demonstrated in the marrow or blood of some patients. The high sensitivity of flow cytometry for detecting clonal populations has, however, demonstrated small clonal B-cell populations in some patients without obvious lymphoma or leukemia.[93,94] Thus finding a small marrow clone, in the absence of other evidence of lymphoma, should be interpreted with caution, in analogy to finding a monoclonal gammopathy in a patient without evidence of myeloma.

Some controversy exists about the applicability of flow cytometry to patients with myeloma. Whereas plasma cells have a characteristic phenotype, including very bright expression of CD38 and expression of CD138,[97,98] plasma cells are under-represented on marrow aspirates studied by flow compared with the prevalence of cells on films or in biopsies. Nevertheless, the unique phenotype of plasma cells makes them easy to recognize, and by using membrane-permeabilization techniques, it is easy to demonstrate cytoplasmic immunoglobulin (Ig) light-chain restriction.[98] Of more significance is that neoplastic plasma cells usually have abnormal phenotypes.[99-102] Although no single specific phenotypic abnormality permits distinction between benign monoclonal gammopathy and myeloma, the relative proportion of abnormal versus normal plasma cells has been suggested to be a predictor of behavior.[100,101] Moreover, persistence of an abnormal phenotype after therapy is predictive of outcome in patients with myeloma.[101,102]

In contrast to B-cell lymphoproliferative disorders, no widely accepted and straightforward method is used to demonstrate that a T-cell population is clonal, although recent work on the flow-cytometric demonstration of restriction of V-beta gene use in T-cell leukemias has shown promise.[103,104] However, T-cell malignancies often show abnormal T-cell phenotypes, most often characterized by loss of a normal pan-T antigen, or expression of a T-cell antigen at abnormal intensity.[113;159-161] Because certain small unusual T-cell populations may be seen in small numbers in non-neoplastic conditions, this technique has more limited sensitivity than demonstration of a clonal B-cell population. However, when abnormal T cells account for more than a few percent of cells, multiparameter flow cytometry can easily demonstrate these and plays a significant role in categorizing these uncommon tumors.

Residual Disease Detection in Chronic Lymphoproliferative Disorders

MRD has not been studied in chronic lymphoproliferative disorders to the extent that it has in acute leukemia. In part this reflects the overall more indolent nature of these diseases, and also the fact that molecular markers, such as immunoglobulin gene rearrangement, are used in many cases. However, the same principles applied to acute leukemia can be used in CLL. Although detection of light-

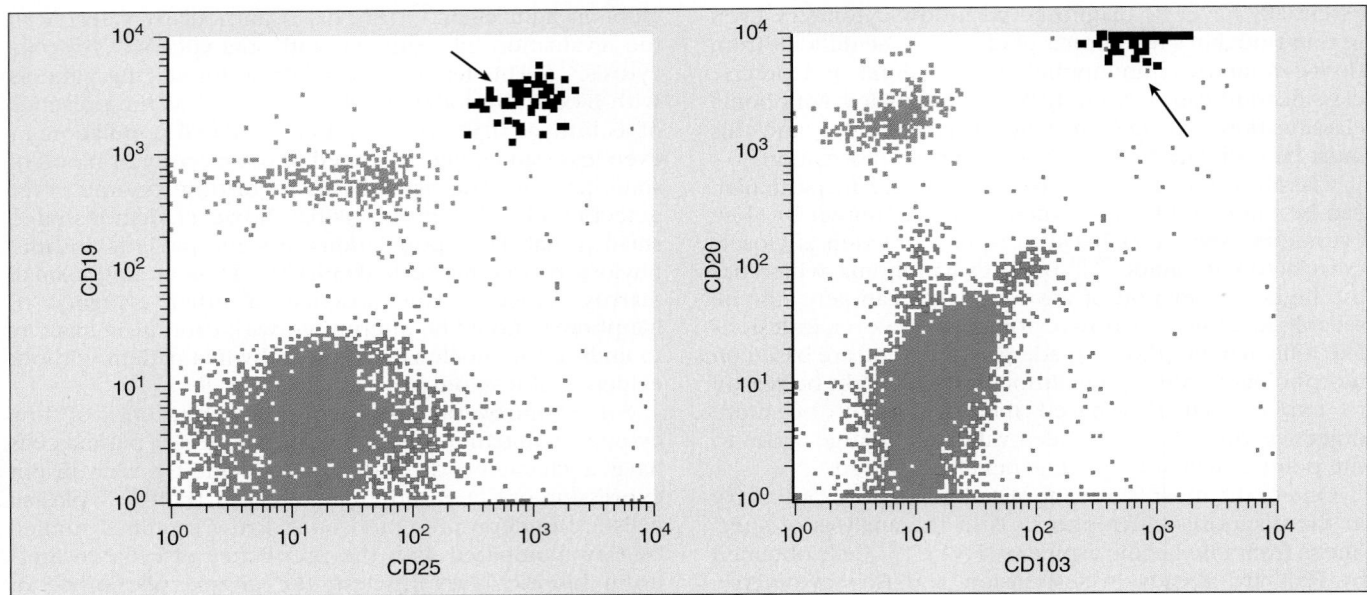

Figure 17-4. Flow-cytometric detection of hairy cell leukemia. A small population (*arrows*) accounts for less than 1% of this peripheral blood sample and can readily be recognized. Expression of CD19 and CD20 is brighter than the background normal B cells (*blue*), and the abnormal cells also express CD103 and CD25.

chain-restricted clones is difficult much below the level of 0.1%, aberrant phenotypes that allow detection with a sensitivity of at least 1×10^{-4} can be detected in most cases of CLL.[106,107] Just as in acute leukemia, presence of MRD in patients considered to be in remission by standard criteria is associated with an adverse prognosis.[107]

Solid Tumors: Analysis for DNA Content

Numerous fluorescent dyes bind stoichiometrically to cellular DNA and can thus provide an accurate assessment of DNA content of cells. In a single-parameter fluorescence histogram, tumors with abnormal numbers of chromosomes will show a distinct peak separate from the normal G_0/G_1 peak of diploid cells. Such tumors are referred to as *aneuploid*. Moreover, cells progressing through the cell cycle will show incrementally increased levels of DNA while they are in S phase, and those in G_2 or in mitosis will show exactly twice the amount of DNA as that represented by the G_0/G_1 population. Thus integration of the area under the curve between the G_0/G_1 and G_2/M peaks gives the proportion of cells in S phase, commonly referred to as S-phase fraction. A variety of software packages are available to calculate S-phase fraction from these histograms.

DNA content analysis in tumors was one of the earliest applications of flow cytometry in tumors. Huge numbers of studies have attempted to define the prognostic significance of either ploidy or S-phase fraction in a large number of different solid tumors. This proliferation of studies was made possible by the finding that fixed, paraffin-embedded tissue sections could be used for DNA analysis by flow, which resulted in many retrospective studies on archival material for which outcome was already known.[108] However, the literature is confusing and contradictory, and the early promise of this measurement as an important diagnostic and prognostic marker in cancer has not been realized.

A DNA Cytometry Consensus Conference held in 1992 attempted both to indicate the problems with the technology and to describe the most promising areas for its application.[109-112] Several studies performed with these recommendations in mind confirmed the prognostic significance of either ploidy or S-phase fraction with bladder, prostate, and breast cancer, most often highlighted as the most promising tumor systems.[113-115] However, many conflicting studies exist, and in general, the technology has not been widely embraced in clinical oncology. In some practices, it is occasionally used to help manage certain subgroups of patients with some cancers. For example, some might use S-phase fraction to help manage patients with early-stage, node-negative breast cancer, whereas others use ploidy of superficial bladder cancers to help identify patients whose tumors might progress. It is worth noting, however, that one reason for the lack of acceptance of this measurement is the difficulties that have been encountered in standardization. S-phase fraction in particular has shown very poor interlaboratory reproducibility.[116] The ultimate effect of these technical problems is that it is very difficult for an individual laboratory to offer clinicians a test result that helps them decide how to manage a particular patient. The inability of this technology to make significant inroads in the clinic is unfortunate because recent studies, by using highly sophisticated analytic methods, suggest that in breast cancer at least, both ploidy and S-phase fraction are powerful independent prognostic markers.[117] A detailed summary of all the controversies is outside the scope of this chapter, but several reviews are available.[118,119]

FUTURE OF FLOW CYTOMETRY IN CLINICAL ONCOLOGY

Flow cytometry in the clinical laboratory is at something of a crossroads. On the one hand, improvements in standardization and the technology itself have made it possible to develop easy-to-operate instruments that fit well with the model of the clinical laboratory. At the same time, with the possible exception of MRD assessment, no significant growth has occurred in the applicability of this technology to cancer. Empirical classification of leukemia and lymphoma with new markers has, with few exceptions such as CD38 in CLL, not been fruitful. At the same time, technologic advances in cancer diagnosis seem currently to focus on methods of assessing genetic lesions in cancer. However, although genetic abnormalities clearly produce cancer, they do so through production of abnormal proteins, and detection of a number of different proteins in specific cell populations is what flow cytometry does best.

Thus it would appear that flow cytometry is well suited to validate, and to translate into clinical practice, many of the exciting findings that derive from genomics. This proof of principle has already been applied to ALL, in which, in a comparison of DNA microarray profiles of normal and leukemic B-cell precursors, CD58 emerged as an important discriminating marker, and flow cytometry validated this observation.[120] As new markers are discovered, the ease of flow-cytometric analysis and the general acceptability of this technology in clinical practice will make this an ideal platform on which to develop new tests to help diagnose and manage patients with cancer.

Linda D. Cooley

Cytogenetics

SUMMARY OF KEY POINTS

KEY METHODS
- Karyotyping using chromosome banding methods provides comprehensive analysis of structural and numeric chromosomal abnormalities; this requires dividing cells.
- Molecular cytogenetics or fluorescence in situ hybridization (FISH) can assess for specific genetic abnormalities and does not require viable tumor.
- Additional methods include multicolor (M)-FISH, spectral karyotyping (SKY), or comparative genomic hybridization (CGH).

APPLICATIONS
Myeloid Disorders
- Chronic myeloid leukemia is defined by a specific translocation.
- FISH is important for monitoring response to therapy in CML.
- Karyotyping provides critical prognostic information in acute myeloid leukemia and myelodysplasia.

Lymphoid Disorders
- Subsets of acute lymphoid leukemia are defined by structural or numeric abnormalities of chromosomes.

- Translocations seen in many lymphomas help to define the diseases.

Solid Tumors
- Certain soft tissue sarcomas are defined by specific translocations.
- Gene amplification of HER-2/*neu*, detected by FISH, is of importance in breast cancer.
- Cytogenetic abnormalities aid in the diagnosis of many brain tumors.
- Some epithelial tumors have prognostically significant cytogenetic abnormalities.

Cytogenetic analysis is a laboratory method that uses tissue culture and specialized techniques to provide genetic information about cells and tissues of interest. Cancer cytogenetic analysis focuses on defining the genetic aberrations of neoplastic tissues. As early as 1890, David von Hansemann speculated that the abnormal mitotic figures in cancer biopsies were important to the origin and development of malignancy, and in 1914, Theodor Boveri[121] published a systematic somatic muta- tion theory of cancer suggesting that chromosome abnormalities were responsible for cellular changes that caused normal cells to become malignant. However, it was not until the 1960s that the first nonrandom chromosome abnormality was associated with a particular neoplastic disorder.

In 1960, Nowell and Hungerford[122] noted a very small "deleted" chromosome in cases of chronic myelocytic leukemia. Methods for banding and identifying individual chromosomes developed in the early 1970s made it possible to identify this chromosome, termed the *Philadelphia chromosome*, as a deleted chromosome 22. Rowley[123] showed in 1973 that the del(22) was part of a reciprocal translocation with chromosome 9 [i.e., t(9;22)]. Since that discovery just 30 years ago, the field of cancer genetics and the understanding of tumorigenesis have evolved dramatically. Today, the entire genome is mapped,[124] and numerous methods are available to look at the sequence of DNA base pairs, mutations in genes, and so on, to determine normal versus abnormal states and their significance.

Cytogenetic analysis is a powerful tool for the diagnosis and classification of tumors. The detection of an acquired clonal chromosome abnormality in tumor tissue confirms that the process is neoplastic, thereby ruling out a reactive or non-neoplastic disorder. Chromosomal anomalies that are disease or disease-subtype specific can be diagnostic when histopathologic parameters are inconclusive. Many anomalies are prognostic and are useful in making therapeutic decisions.

This section on cytogenetics includes a brief overview of cytogenetics, clinical indications for conventional and molecular cytogenetic testing, and a synopsis of what the clinician can expect from a cytogenetic laboratory. A summary of the known diagnostic and prognostic values of certain chromosome abnormalities in clinical practice is provided in tabular form.

METHODS AND APPLICATIONS

Data from cytogenetic studies of neoplasias have demonstrated that rearrangement, loss, duplication, and imbalance of genetic material are consistent findings and that the genetic anomalies are nonrandom.[125] Cytogenetic information obtained from studying hematologic disorders has facilitated discovery of genes located at sites of recurrent chromosomal rearrangements.[126] Molecular investigations of these genes have led to the discovery that alteration of genes as a result of chromosomal rearrangement contributes to the pathogenesis of malignancies. Characterization of the affected genes has led to understanding of gene function, mechanisms of mutation, and more recently to designing tumor-specific therapy.[127] Solid tumors, although less extensively studied than hematologic disorders, now consistently show nonrandom chromosome aberrations with diagnostic and therapeutic specificities.[125,128]

Specimens

Successful cytogenetic studies of neoplastic tissues and cells require an adequate specimen of viable tumor cells, pertinent patient information, and prompt delivery to the processing laboratory. Tumor cell viability is crucial, as metaphase chromosomes for cytogenetic analysis can be obtained only from dividing cells. Although tumor cells may be long lived in the human body, once removed, they quickly lose their viability, making quick delivery to the laboratory a necessity. Appropriate specimen processing is dependent on the information that accompanies the sample. Critical information includes patient demographics, differential diagnosis, symptoms, and other laboratory findings. The cytogenetics laboratory uses the information to choose the best methods for the suspected disease process. In the absence of adequate information, the specimen may not be processed optimally to yield the malignant clone.

For hematologic tumors, 2 to 3 mL of bone marrow aspirate (BMA) collected in sodium heparin is the ideal specimen. In situations in which a BMA cannot be obtained because of marrow fibrosis, a packed marrow, or other reasons, a bone marrow biopsy or a peripheral blood (PB) specimen may be successful. However, for a specimen to yield information about clonal chromosome abnormalities, the PB white cell differential must be abnormal (i.e., abnormal or immature cells must be present). The laboratory will need the white blood cell count and differential to inoculate the cell cultures correctly with appropriate numbers of cells. For routine studies of neoplastic hematologic disorders, no cell mitogens are used in culture. The malignant cell population will spontaneously divide to yield metaphase cells. Only when the disease process is known to be a T-cell or a B-cell disorder will T- or B-cell mitogens, respectively, be used in one of several initiated cultures.

Depending on the disease process, other specimen types may be appropriate for cytogenetic analysis. Virtually all body fluids and tissues are candidates for tissue culture and capture of metaphase cells. Examples of useful sources are ascitic and pleural fluids, effusions, and occasionally cerebrospinal fluid. Tissues with solid aggregates of tumor cells (e.g., spleen, lymph node, chloroma) also can be used. Such specimens and solid-tumor samples should be acquired in a sterile fashion and placed in medium supplied by the cytogenetic laboratory for transport. The sample of tissue should be selected to contain viable tumor, avoiding normal and necrotic tissues. Adequate sample size is variable, but if available, a sample volume of 500 mg or a sample measuring in aggregate $0.5 \times 0.5 \times 0.5$ cm is recommended.

Assays

Conventional cytogenetic analysis uses *chromosome-banding* methods to bring out the A-T and G-C rich bands that are inherent in chromosomes. The banding pattern of each chromosome is unique. The distinct banding pattern permits cytogeneticists to distinguish chromosomes and to identify normal and abnormal chromosomes (Fig. 17-5). Each chromosome is divided into numbered regions and bands. The numbered bands allow identification of where specific breaks occur in the chromosome, thus making possible recognition of recurrent rearrangements. In addition to band numbering, a nomenclature[129] was instituted in 1971 (and updated in 1995) to facilitate description and communication of chromosome abnormalities (Table 17-2).

Flow-cytometry studies of tumor cells, as discussed earlier, can be performed to determine DNA content or "ploidy" of the tumor cells. Normal diploid cells with 46

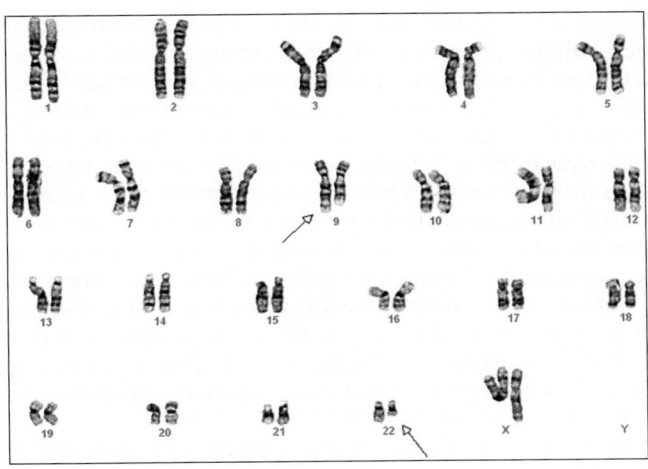

Figure 17-5. Karotype to illustrate standard arrangement and Giemsa-trypsin banding of chromosomes in a female patient with chronic myelocytic leukemia. The karyotype nomenclature is written as 46,XX,t(9;22)(q34;q11.2) (*arrows* to derivative chromosomes 9 and 22).

chromosomes have a DNA index or DI of 1.0 (see Table 17-2). The DI of aneuploid tumor cells can be used to approximate the number of chromosomes per cell [e.g., a tumor with a DI of 1.15 will have ~53 chromosomes (1.15 × 46 = 52.9)].

The clinician can expect final cytogenetic results in the majority of cases within a reasonable time: 5 to 7 days for hematologic disorders; 2 weeks for solid tumors; 1 to 2 days for STATs or molecular cytogenetic studies. The final report will describe all clonal chromosome abnormalities

TABLE 17-2

Cytogenetic Nomenclature

Nomenclature Abbreviations

t(9;22)(q34;q11.2) example
t, translocation
(9;22), chromosomes involved
(q34;q11.2), breakpoints of chromosomes involved
q34, breakpoint of chromosome 9
q11.2, breakpoint of chromosome 22
q, long arm
p, short arm
del, deletion
dup, duplication
inv, inversion
add, added unidentified material
mar, marker; unidentified chromosome
+ or –, gain or loss of chromosome noted
XX, female
XY, male

Tumor Cell DNA Content: "Ploidy"

Diploid, 2n or 46 chromosomes
Haploid, 1n or 23 chromosomes
DNA Index (DI), DNA content of cell
46 chromosomes, DNA Index of 1.0
Pseudodiploid, 46 chromosome with abnormalities
Aneuploid, chr number not exact multiple of haploid set
Tetraploid, 4n or 92 chromosomes

by using current cytogenetic nomenclature (ISCN, 1995), a narrative interpretation of the abnormalities, and a commentary that correlates the cytogenetic findings with pertinent histopathologic findings, clinical diagnosis, and/or known prognostic or therapeutic significance.

Molecular cytogenetic analysis or *fluorescence in situ hybridization* (FISH) can be performed when viable tumor material is unavailable, conventional cytogenetic analysis is unsuccessful, or specific genetic events must be assessed at the molecular level. FISH[130] uses known fluorochrome-labeled DNA sequences or *probes* to hybridize to cells under investigation. The natural tendency for a DNA strand to hybridize with its complementary DNA sequence is the basis for the test. The specificity of the hybridization provides explicit information about the region probed. FISH is commonly used in laboratories to detect gene rearrangements, chromosome deletions or duplications, gene amplification, chromosome aneuploidy, or to clarify unbalanced chromosome rearrangements. FISH is frequently performed by using cytogenetically prepared metaphase cells and/or interphase cells. However, FISH analysis also can be performed by using paraffin-embedded tissue samples, touch preparations, cytospin preparations, and blood and bone marrow smears.

Other molecular cytogenetic methods such as *comparative genomic hybridization*[131] (CGH), *multicolor FISH*[132] (M-FISH), and *spectral karyotyping*[133] (SKY) are found primarily in research laboratories because of their high cost. The CGH method uses labeled tumor DNA and labeled normal reference DNA hybridized to normal metaphase chromosomes to detect regional genomic DNA gains and losses. This computer-based method gives a picture of the DNA of all chromosomes and allows analysis of tumor DNA when chromosomes cannot be obtained. Both SKY and M-FISH methods use multiple fluorochrome labels and computer software to "paint" each chromosome a different color. When the chromosomes are hybridized to the abnormal tumor metaphase-cell chromosomes, computer analysis of the painted chromosomes can detect rearrangements and provide information about unidentified marker chromosomes and chromosome rearrangements not recognized by conventional G-band cytogenetic analysis.

FISH studies are now commonly part of the routine laboratory test menu. Often FISH studies are used to complement conventional cytogenetic analysis to provide the most detailed and relevant information about the tumor under investigation. Tables 17-3 and 17-4 list the indications, benefits, and disadvantages of using conventional cytogenetic and FISH studies.

Cytogenetic Aberrations

Chromosomal aberrations in neoplasia can be grouped according to type. In the first type, no loss of genetic material occurs. Rearrangements of this type include reciprocal translocations and inversions that are known to relocate genes with resultant expression of altered gene products.[134] The second type results in loss or gain of genetic material, and the pathogenic effect depends on which genes are gained or lost. Included in this type are nonreciprocal translocations, deletions, and duplications, as well as loss or gain of whole chromosomes. A third type of aberration results in amplification of genetic material from a specific gene or gene region. This is seen at the chromosome level as double minute chromosomes (small paired dot-like acentric chromosomes) or as homogeneously stained regions within a chromosome.[135] Gene amplification, an infrequent aberration, is associated with specific neoplasias and most often correlated with aggressive disease.[135]

The karyotype of a tumor may show single or multiple aberrations. Some tumors demonstrate a single anomaly such as a reciprocal translocation or a gain of an extra chromosome. Other tumors show many anomalies that may include reciprocal or nonreciprocal translocations, deletions, loss, or gain of chromosomes, and so forth. For some types of tumors, a complex karyotype indicates advanced or aggressive disease. However, the prognostic significance of a karyotype depends on the specific aberrations present. Whereas some tumors have characteristic single anomalies, some tumors have characteristic patterns of chromosome aberrations. An example of the former would be the reciprocal t(9;22) in poor-prognosis childhood acute lymphoblastic leukemia (ALL), and the latter example could be the favorable-prognosis hyperdiploid karyotype of childhood ALL that consistently shows 54 chromosomes and extra copies of chromosomes X, 4, 6, 10, 14, 17, 18, and 21.[136]

The utility of a cytogenetic analysis of tumor tissue depends on finding the abnormal population of cells that represents the neoplastic process. Cytogenetically, a clone is present when two or more cells with the same chromosomal anomaly are found. A subclone is a second population of cells that contains the original chromosome anomaly and one or more additional anomalies in two or more cells. A subclone indicates clonal evolution and may portend a change to a more aggressive disease state. For instance, chronic-phase CML with the t(9;22) often shows clonal evolution when the disease transforms to the accelerated phase by the gain of an extra der(22) or "Ph" chromosome, trisomy 8, or an isochromosome 17q[137] (Fig. 17-6).

Cytogenetic analysis is a valuable tool in the workup of a patient with a neoplastic process. In addition to defining the clonal chromosome abnormality of a tumor at diagnosis, conventional and molecular cytogenetic studies are indispensable tools for assessing disease status after therapy or transplantation and at disease relapse.

A description of chromosome aberrations that have been documented by repeated investigations to be useful in neoplasia is given in Tables 17-5, 17-6, and 17-7. In some

---

TABLE 17-3

 Cytogenetic Analysis

Indications

- Provide diagnostic and prognostic information
- Evaluate and subtype myeloid disorders
- Subclassify lymphoproliferative disorders
- Distinguish prognostic groups in childhood ALL
- Differentiate small round cell tumors
- Differentiate sarcomas
- Subtype solid tumors
- Obtain information for follow-up testing
- Detect clone after therapy or after transplantation
- Determine donor cell engraftment status
- Reassess clone at relapse for new anomalies

Benefits

- Visualize entire karyotype
- Detect disease progression

Disadvantages

- Turn-around time is days to weeks (solid tumors)

ALL, acute lymphoblastic leukemia.

TABLE 17-4

FISH Analysis

Indications

- Identify specific diagnostic and/or prognostic anomalies
- Detect reciprocal translocations, rearrangements
- Detect deletions, duplications
- Detect chromosome or gene copy number
- Identify unrecognized chromosomes material
- Identify clonal abnormality for follow-up testing
- Assess donor cell engraftment (opposite-sex donor)
- Assess remission status
- Detect recurrent disease
- Detect minimal residual disease

Benefits

- Analyze dividing and nondividing cells
- Easy to examine large numbers of cells
- Rapid turnaround

Disadvantages

- Provides information only for locus of probe tested
- Requires knowledge of chromosome anomaly or diagnosis

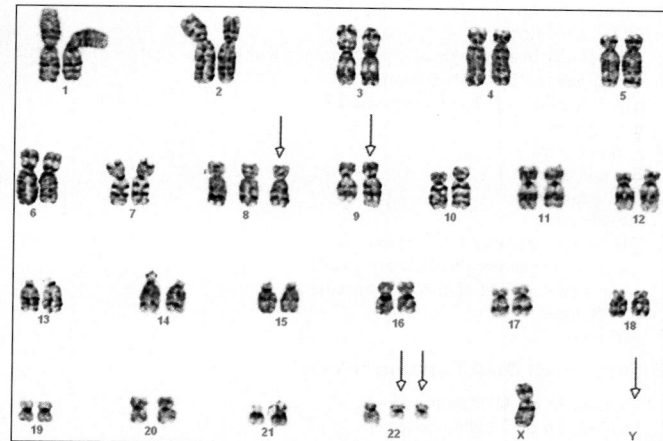

Figure 17-6. Karotype to illustrate clonal evolution in a male patient with chronic myelocytic leukemia in blast crisis. The karyotype is written as 47,X,-Y,+8,t(9;22)(q34;q11.2), +der(22)t(9;22)(q34;q11.2) (*arrows* to derivative chromosomes 9 and 22, extra copy of chromosome 8, and missing sex chromosome).

TABLE 17-5

Myeloid Disorders: Chromosome Abnormalities That Are Diagnostic or Prognostic

DISEASE ENTITY	CHROMOSOME ABNORMALITY	GENES INVOLVED	FISH	PROGNOSIS	COMMENT	REFERENCES
AML	t(8;21)(q22;q22)	ETO/AML1	++	Good		Jaffe et al;[a] Slovak et al;[b] Grimwade et al;[c] Woods et al;[d] Raimondi et al[e]
	inv(16)/t(16;16)	CBFB/MYH11	++	Good	Increased risk of CNS disease	Jaffe et al;[a] Slovak et al;[b] Grimwade et al;[c] Woods et al;[d] Raimondi et al[e]
	t(15;17)(q22;q21)	PML/RARA	++	Good	Good; responsive to ATRA	Raimondi et al;[e] Melnick and Licht[f]
	t(11;17)(q23.1;q21)	PLZF/RARA	+		Variant translocation, poor response to ATRA	Jaffe et al;[a] Slovak et al;[b] Grimwade et al;[c] Melnick and Licht[f]
	t(11q23;v)	MLL	++	Poor	Increased risk of CNS disease	Slovak et al;[b] Grimwade et al[c]
	t(1;22)(p13;q13)	OTT/MAL	+		Defines infant AML-M7 subgroup	Dastugue et al[g]
MDS and AML	5q- sole abnormality		++	Good	5q- Syndrome in elderly with macrocytic anemia	Boultwood et al;[h] Greenberg et al[i]
	-7		++	Poor		Greenberg et al;[i] Pedersen B[j]
	-5/5q-;-7/7q- together		++	Poor	Often in complex karyotype	Jaffe et al;[a] Slovak et al;[b] Grimwade et al;[c] Greenberg et al[i]
	+8		++	Intermed	Intermediate <60 yr; Poor >60 yr	Jaffe et al;[a] Slovak et al;[b] Grimwade et al;[c] Greenberg et al[i]
	t/del(11q)	MLL	++	Inter poor	Intermediate to poor	Jaffe et al;[a] Slovak et al;[b] Grimwade et al;[c] Greenberg et al[i]
	3q26, inv(3)(q21q26),t(3;21)	EVI1 or EAP	+	Poor		Jaffe et al;[a] Slovak et al;[b] Grimwade et al;[c] Greenberg et al[i]
	complex k'type (≥3 abn)			Poor		Jaffe et al;[a] Slovak et al;[b] Grimwade et al;[c] Greenberg et al[i]
	20q-,-Y		++	Good		Greenberg et al[i]
Therapy-related AML/MDS						
More topoisomerase II inhibitors	Inv(16), t(15/17)	CBFB, RARA	++	Good	t(8;21) longer survival than other 21q22 abnormalities	Rowley and Olney[k]
	21q22	AML1	++	Intermed		Rowley and Olney[k]
	11q23	MLL	+	Poor		Rowley and Olney[k]
More radiation exposure and alkylating agents	3q26 abnormalities	EVI1	++	Poor		Rowley and Olney[k]
	5/7 abnormalities		++	Poor		Rowley and Olney[k]
CML	t(9;22)(q34;q11.2)	BCR/ABL	++	Poor	Reduced survival with del ABL/BCR/ASS	Huntly et al;[l] Sinclair et al[m]
	t(9;22) + del(9q)	ASS deletion	++	Poor		Johansson et al[n]
	t(9;22) + Ph,+8,+19,i(17q)		++		Indicates transition to blast phase	Jaffe et al[a]
MPD other than CML	13q-, 20q-,+9, +8,+1q		++		Distinguish CML from other MPDs	
MM/MF	20q-,13q-		++	Good	Favorable in myelofibrosis	Tefferi et al[o]

BOLD, Chromosome abnormalities that diagnose or characterize the disease process; ++, FISH probes commercially available, +, FISH performed for abnormality by research lab or with home-brew probes; AML, acute myeloidleukemia; ATRA, all-trans retinoic acid; MDS, myelodysplastic syndrome; AA, aplastic anemia; CML, chronic myeloid leukemia; MPD, myeloproliferative disorders; CIMF, chronic idiopathic myelofibrosis; CNS, central nervous system.

[a]Jaffe ES, Harris NL, Stein H,Vardiman JW (eds):World Health Organization Classification of Tumors. Pathology and Genetics of Haematopoietic and Lymphoid Tissues. Lyon, France, IARC Press, 2001.
[b]Slovak ML, Kopecky KJ, Cassileth PA, et al: Karyotypic analysis predicts outcome of preremission and postremission therapy in adult acute myeloid leukemia:A Southwest Oncology Group/Eastern Cooperative Oncology Group study. Blood 2000;96:4075.
[c]Grimwade D,Walker H, Harrison G, et al:The predictive value of hierarchical cytogenetic classification in older adults with acute myeloid leukemia (AML):Analysis of 1065 patients entered into the United Kingdom Medical Research Council AML11 trial. Blood 2001;98:1312.
[d]Woods WG, Neudorf S, Gold S, et al:A comparison of allogeneic bone marrow transplantation, autologous bone marrow transplantation, and aggressive chemotherapy in children with acute myeloid leukemia in remission:A report from the Children's Cancer Group. Blood 2001;97:56.
[e]Raimondi SC, Chang MN, Ravindranath Y, et al:Chromosomal abnormalities in 478 children with acute myeloid leukemia: Clinical characteristics and treatment outcome in a cooperative Pediatric Oncology Group study–POG 8821. Blood 1999;94:3707.
[f]Melnick A, Licht JD: Deconstructing a disease: RARalpha, its fusion partners, and their roles in the pathogenesis of acute promyelocytic leukemia. Blood 1999;93:3167.
[g]Dastugue N, Lafage-Pochitaloff M, Pages M-P, et al: Cytogenetic profile of childhood and adult megakaryoblastic leukemia (M7):A study of the Groupe Francais de Cytogenetique Hematologique (GFCH). Blood 2002;100:618.
[h]Boultwood J, Fidler C, Strickson AJ, et al: Narrowing and genomic annotation of the commonly deleted region of the 5q- syndrome. Blood 2002;99:4638.
[i]Greenberg P, Cox C, LeBeau MM, et al: International Scoring System for evaluating prognosis in myelodysplastic syndromes. Blood 1997;89:2079.
[j]Pedersen B, Koch J, Bendix Hansen K, et al:The monosomy 7 clone in interphase and metaphase cell population:A combined chromosome and primed in situ labeling study.Acta Haematol 1997;97:216.
[k]Rowley JD, Olney HJ: International Workshop on the relationship of prior therapy to balanced chromosome aberrations in therapy-related myelodysplastic syndromes and acute leukemia: Overview report. Genes Chrom Cancer 2002;33:331.
[l]Huntly BJP, Reid AG, Bench AJ, et al: Deletions of the derivative chromosome 9 occur at the time of the Philadelphia translocation and provide a powerful and independent prognostic indicator in chronic myeloid leukemia. Blood 2001;98:1732.
[m]Sinclair PB, Nacheva EP, Leversha M, et al: Large deletions at the t(9;22) breakpoint are common and may identify a poor-prognosis subgroup of patients with chronic myeloid leukemia.Acta Haematol 2002;107:76.
[n]Johansson B, Fioretos T, Mitelman F: Cytogenetic and molecular genetic evolution of chronic myeloid leukemia. Acta Haematol 2002;107:76.
[o]Tefferi A, Mesa RA, Schroeder G, et al: Cytogenetic findings and their clinical relevance in myelofibrosis with myeloid metaplasia. Br J Haematol 2001;113:763.

Science of Clinical Oncology

1

TABLE 17-6

Lymphoid Disorders: Chromosome Abnormalities That Are Diagnostic or Prognostic

DISEASE ENTITY	CHROMOSOME ABNORMALITY	GENES INVOLVED	FISH	PROGNOSIS	COMMENT	REFERENCES
ALL B-precursor	t(9;22)(q34;q11.2)	BCR/ABL	++	Poor	Very poor with high WBC	Harrison;[a] Pui;[b] Secker-Walker et al[c]
	-7, t(9;22)(q34;q11.2)	BCR/ABL	++	Poor	Often infants	Harrison;[a] Pui;[b] Secker-Walker et al[c]
	t(4;11)(q21;q23)/t(11q;v)	AF4/MLL	+	Poor		Harrison;[a] Pui;[b] Secker-Walker et al[c]
	t(12;21)(p13;q22)	TEL/AML1L	++	Good	Improved therapy has improved outcome	Jamil et al[d]
	t(1;19)(q23)p13.3)	E2A/PBX1	+	Intermed		Harrison;[a] Pui;[b] Secker-Walker et al[c]
	t(8;14)(q24;q32) or variants	c-MYC/IgH	++		Burkitt lymphoma therapy	Harrison;[a] Pui;[b] Secker-Walker et al[c]
	54-65 chr with +4,+10,+17,+18		++	Good		Harrison;[a] Pui;[b] Secker-Walker et al;[c] Trueworthy et al[e]
	<44 chr		++	Poor		Harrison;[a] Pui;[b] Secker-Walker et al[c]
CLL	+12		++		Atypical lymphoplasmacytic morphology; CLL/PL	Hjalmar et al;[f] Dohner et al[g]
	del(13q14) or -13	RB1	++	Good	When present as the sole anomaly	Dohner et al[g]
	del(11q21)	ATM	++	Poor		Dohner et al[g]
	del(17p13)	TP53	++	Poor		Dohner et al[g]
	t(14;19)(q32;q13)	BCL3	+		Often young adults	Michaux et al[h]
MM/PCL	Hyperdiploid +3,5,7,9,11,15,19		++	Better	Longer OS and EFS	Smadja et al;[i] Sawyer et al[j]
	Hypodiploid/Pseudodiploid		++	Poor	<46, 46, and >81 chromosomes	Smadja et al[i]
	-13 or del(13q14)	DBM/RB1	++		Most common translocation in MM	Sawyer et al;[j] Facon et al;[k] Avet-Loiseau et al[l]
	t(11;14)(q13;q32)	CCND1/IgH	++		Present in ~15% of MM	Avet-Loiseau et al[l]
	t(8;14) & variants	c-MYC/IgH	+		Most common in PCL	Avet-Loiseau et al[l]
	t(4;14)(p16;q32)	IgH	+	Poor	Most common in PCL	Smadja et al[m]
	t(14;16)(q32;q24)	IgH	+	Poor		Smadja et al[m]
Mature B-cell lymphomas						
Follicular	**t(14;18)(q32;q21)**	IgH/BCL2	++			Tilly et al[n]
MALT	**t(11;18)(q21;q21)**	API2/MLT	+		Resistant to *Helicobacter pylori* therapy	Remstein et al;[o] Liu et al[p]
Mantle cell	**t(11;14)(q13;q32)**	CCND1/IgH	++		Distinguish MCL from CLL	Li et al[q]
Burkitt	**t(8;14)(q24;q32)**	c-MYC/IgH	++			Magrath[r]
	t(8;22)(q24;q11.2)	c-MYC/IgL	+			Magrath[r]
	t(2;8)(p11.2;q24)	c-MYC/IgK	+			Magrath[r]
T-cell LPDs	t(14q11), t(7q35)	TCR sites				Jaffe et al[s]
Anaplastic large cell	**t(2;5)(p23;q35) and variants**	ALK/NPM	++	Good	ALK+ tumors show better survival	Cataldo et al;[t] Gascoyne et al[u]

BOLD, Chromosome abnormalities that diagnose or characterize the disease process; +, FISH performed for abnormality by research lab or with home-brew probes; ++, FISH probes commercially available; +, FISH performed for abnormality by research lab or with home-brew probes; ALL, acute lymphoblastic leukemia; CLL, chronic lymphocytic leukemia; PL, prolymphocytic leukemia; MM, multiple myeloma; PCL, plasma cell leukemia; OS, overall survival; EFS, event-free survival; MALT, mucosa-associated lymphoid tissue; LPD, lymphoproliferative disorder; FISH, fluorescence in situ hybridization.

[a] Harrison C: The detection and significance of chromosomal abnormalities in childhood acute lymphoblastic leukemia. Blood Rev 2001;15:49.
[b] Pui CH: Acute lymphoblastic leukemia in children. Curr Opin Oncol 2000;12:3.
[c] Secker-Walker LM, Prentice HG, Richards S, et al: Cytogenetics adds independent prognostic information in adults with acute lymphoblastic leukaemia on MRC trial UKALL XA:MRC Adult Leukaemia Working Parry. Br J Haematol 1997;96:601.
[d] Jamil A, Theil KS, Kahwash S, et al: TEL/AML1 fusion gene: Its frequency and prognostic significance in childhood acute lymphoblastic leukemia. Cancer Genet Cytogenet 2000;122:73.
[e] Trueworthy R, Shuster J, Look T, et al: Ploidy of lymphoblasts is the strongest predictor of treatment outcome in B progenitor cell ALL of childhood:A Pediatric Oncology Group study. J Clin Oncol 1992;10:606-613.
[f] Hjalmar V, Kimby E, Matutes E, et al: Trisomy 12 and lymphoplasmacytoid lymphocytes in chronic leukemia B-cell disorders. Haematologica 1998;83:602.
[g] Dohner H, Stilgenbauer S, Benner A, et al: Genomic aberrations and survival in chronic lymphocytic leukemia. N Engl J Med 2000;343:1910.
[h] Michaux L, Dierlamm J, Wlodarska I, et al: t(14;19)/BCL3 Rearrangements in lymphoproliferative disorders:A review of 23 cases. Cancer Genet Cytogenet 1997;94:36.
[i] Smadja NV, Bastard C, Brigaudeau C, et al: Hypodiploidy is a major prognostic factor in multiple myeloma. Blood 2001;98:2229.
[j] Sawyer JR, Waldron JA, Jagannath S, Barlogie B: Cytogenetic findings in 200 patients with multiple myeloma. Cancer Genet Cytogenet 1995;82:41.
[k] Facon T, Aver-Loiseau H, Guillerm G, et al: Chromosome 13 abnormalities identified by FISH analysis and serum beta2-microglobulin produce a powerful myeloma staging system for patients receiving high-dose therapy. Blood 2001;97:1566.
[l] Avet-Loiseau H, Facon T, Grosbois B, et al: Oncogenesis of multiple myeloma: 14q3 and 13q chromosomal abnormalities are not randomly distributed, but correlated with natural history, immunological features, and clinical presentation. Blood 2002;99:2191.
[m] Smadja NV, Bastard C, Brigaudeau C: Primary plasma cell leukemia and multiple myeloma: One or two diseases according to the methodology. Blood 1999;94:3607.
[n] Tilly H, Rossi A, Stamatoullas A, et al: Prognostic value of chromosomal abnormalities in follicular lymphoma. Blood 1994;84:1043.
[o] Remstein ED, James CD, Kurtin PJ: Incidence and subtype specificity of API2-MALT1 fusion translocations in extranodal, nodal, and splenic marginal zone lymphomas. Am J Pathol 2000;156:1183.
[p] Liu H, Ye H, Ruskone-Fourmestraux A, et al: t(11;18) is a marker for all stage gastric MALT lymphoma that will not respond to H. pylori eradication. Gastroenterology 2002;286.
[q] Li JY, Gaillard F, Moreau A, et al: Detection of translocation t(11;14)(q13;q32) in mantle cell lymphoma by fluorescence in situ hybridization. Am J Pathol 1999;154:1449.
[r] Magrath I: The pathogenesis of Burkitt's lymphoma. Adv Cancer Res 1990;55:133.
[s] Jaffe ES, Harris NL, Stein H, Vardiman JW (eds): World Health Organization classification of Tumors. Pathology and Genetics of Tumors of Haematopoietic and Lymphoid Tissues. Lyon, France, IARC Press, 2001.
[t] Cataldo KA, Jalal SM, Law ME, et al: Comparison of immunohistochemical studies, FISH, and RT-PCR in paraffin-embedded tissue. Am J Surg Pathol 1999;23:1386.
[u] Gascoyne RD, Aoun P, Wu D, et al: Prognostic significance of anaplastic lymphoma kinase (ALK) protein expression in adults with anaplastic large cell lymphoma. Blood 1999;93:3913.

TABLE 17-7

Solid Tumors: Chromosome Abnormalities That Are Diagnostic or Prognostic

DISEASE ENTITY	CHROMOSOME ABNORMALITY	GENES INVOLVED	FISH	PROGNOSIS	COMMENT	REFERENCES
Kidney/Bladder						
RCC, papillary	+7, +17, t(X;1)(p11.2;q21)	VHL, other	++		Characterize papillary RCC	Kovacs et al;[a] Kattar et al[b]
RCC, clear cell	-3 or del(3p)		+		Characterize nonpapillary RCC	Martinez et al;[c] Gnarra et al[d]
Bladder	+7, loss of 9p21, +17		++		Detect recurrent disease	Jung et al;[e] Sarosdy et al;[f] Watters et al[g]
WT	16q-, +1q, 1p-, -22, 17p-	TP53, other	++	Poor		Klamt et al;[h] Dome et al;[i] Brown et al[j]
Prostate	8p22 loss, 8q24 gain	LPL, c-MYC	++		Increased recurrence risk	Sato et al;[k] Tsuchiya et al;[l] Matsuyama et al[m]
Breast	d-min, hsr	HER2/neu	++		+ Tumors; therapeutic implications	Xu et al;[n] Diaz;[o] Seidman et al;[p] Perez et al[q]
Brain						
Glioblastoma	10q-, +7, 9p-, EGFR amplific	PTEN (10q23)	+	Poor	PTEN loss or mutation poor prognostic factor	Bigner et al;[r] Tada et al;[s] Smith et al;[t]
Oligodendroglioma	del(1p36), del((19q13.3)		+	Good	Favorable response to therapy	Bigner et al;[u] Cairncross;[v] Ueki et al[w]
MB/PNET	i(17q)		++		i(17q) characteristic of MB/PNET	Gilbertson et al;[x] Aldosari[y]
	c-MYC amplification	c-MYC	++	Poor	10% have c-MYC amplification	Biegel et al[z]
AT/RT	-22 or del(22q)	INI1	+	Poor	Distinguish AT/RT from MB/PNET	Bruch et al[aa]
Meningioma	-22 or del(22q11.2)	NF2	++	Benign	1p/14q deletions in anaplastic tumors	Cai et al[bb] Ketter et al[cc]
Small Round Cell Tumors						
Alveolar RMS	t(2;13)(q37;q14)	PAX3/FKHR	+		Older youth, truncal location, poorer outcome	Sorensen et al;[dd] Anderson et al[ee]
Alveolar RMS	t(1;13)(p36;q14)	PAX7/FKHR	+		Younger child, extremity location	Sorensen et al;[dd] Anderson et al[ee]
Embryonal RMS	hyperdiploid	None	++		Distinguish from alveolar subtype	Shapiro et al;[ff] Pappo et al[gg]
NB	del(1p), +17q, dmin, hsr	n-MYC	++	Poor		Fong et al;[hh] Maris J[ii]
EWS/pPNET	t(11;22)(q24;q12) & variants	FLI1/EWS	+			Ginsberg et al;[jj] Peter et al;[kk] Hattinger et al[ll]
DSRCT	t(11;22)(p13;q12)	WT1/EWS	+			Gerald et al;[mm] Gerald et al[mn]
CCS	t(12;22)(q13;q12)	ATF1/EWS	+		Distinguish cutaneous melanoma from CCS	Antonescu et al;[oo] Panagopoulos et al[pp]
Soft Tissue Tumors						
CFS/CMN	t(12;15)(p12;q25),+11,+17,+20	ETV6/NTRK3	+			Knezevich et al;[qq] Rubin et al[rr]
SS	t(X;18)(p11;q11)	SSX/SYT	+		SSX1, biphasic; SSX2, monophasic	Ladanyi et al;[ss] Kawai et al[tt]
Liposarcoma	t(12;16)(q13;p11)	FUS/CHOP	+			Dei Tos[uu]
Myxoid chondrosarcoma	t(9;22)(q22;q12)	CHN/EWS	+			Clark et al[vv]

BOLD, Chromosome abnormalities that diagnose or characterize the disease process; ++, FISH probes commercially available; +, FISH performed for abnormality by research lab or with home-brew probes; RCC, renal cell carcinoma; WT, Wilms tumor; MB, medulloblastoma; PNET, primitive neuroectodermal tumor; AT/RT, atypical teratoid/rhabdoid tumor; RMS, rhabdomyosarcoma; NB, neuroblastoma; EWS, Ewing's sarcoma; DSRCT, desmoplastic small round cell tumor; CCS, clear cell sarcoma; CFS, congenital fibrosarcoma; CMN, congenital mesoblastic nephroma; SS, synovial sarcoma; FISH, fluorescence in situ hybridization.

[a]Kovacs G, Fuzesi L, Emanual A, Kung HF: Cytogenetics of papillary renal cell tumors. Genes Chromosomes Cancer 1991;3:249.
[b]Kattar MM, Grignon DJ, Wallis T, et al: Clinicopathologic and interphase cytogenetic analysis of papillary (chromophilic) renal cell carcinoma. Mod Pathol 1997;10:1143.
[c]Martinez A, Fullwood P, Kondo K, et al: Role of chromosome 3p12-p21 tumor suppressor genes in clear renal cell carcinoma: analysis of VHL dependent and VHL independent pathways to tumorigenesis. Mod Pathol 2000;53:137.
[d]Gnarra JR, Tory K, Weng Y, et al: Mutation of the VHL tumour suppressor gene in renal carcinoma. Nat Genet 1994;7:85.
[e]Jung I, Reeder JE, Cox C, et al: Chromosome 9 monosomy by fluorescence in situ hybridization of bladder irrigation specimens is predictive of tumor recurrence. J Urol 1999;162:1900.
[f]Sarosdy MF, Schellhammer P, Bokinsky G, et al: Clinical evaluation of a multi-target fluorescence in situ hybridization assay for detection of bladder cancer. J Urol 2002;168:1950.
[g]Watters AD, Ballantyne SA, Going JJ, et al: Aneusomy of chromosomes 7 and 17 predicts the recurrence of transitional cell carcinoma of the urinary bladder. BJU Int 2000;85:42.
[h]Klamt B, Schulze M, Thate C, et al: Allele loss in Wilms tumors of chromosome arms 11q, 16, and 22q correlate with clinicopathological parameters. Genes chromosomes Cancer 1998;22:287.
[i]Dome JS, Coppes MJ: Recent advances in Wilms tumor genetics: Curr Opin Pediatr 2002;14:5.
[j]Bown N, Cotterill SJ, Roberts P, et al: Cytogenetic abnormalities and clinical outcome in Wilms tumor: A study by the U.K. Cancer Cytogenetics Group and the U.K. Children's Cancer Study Group. Med Pediatr Oncol 2002;38:11.

Continued

Science of Clinical Oncology

1

TABLE 17-7

Solid Tumors: Chromosome Abnormalities That Are Diagnostic or Prognostic—cont'd

[k]Sato K, Qian J, Slezak JM, et al: Clinical significance of alterations of chromosome 8 in high-grade, advanced, nonmetastatic prostate carcinoma. J Natl Cancer Inst 1999;91:1574.

[l]Tsuchiya N, Slezak JM, Lieber MM, et al: Clinical significance of alterations of chromosome 8 detected by fluorescence in situ hybridization analysis in pathologic organ-confined prostate cancer. Genes Chromosomes Cancer 2002;34:363.

[m]Matsuyama H, Pan Y, Oba K, et al: Deletions on chromosome 8p22 may predict disease progression as well as pathological staging in prostate cancer. Clin Cancer Res 2001;7:3139.

[n]Xu R, Perle MA, Inghirami G, et al: Amplification of Her-2/neu gene in Her-2/neu-overexpressing and -nonexpressing breast carcinomas and their synchronous benign, premalignant, and metastatic lesions detected by FISH in archival material. Mod Pathol 2002;15:116.

[o]Diaz NM: Laboratory testing for HER2/neu in breast carcinoma: an evolving strategy to predict response to targeted therapy. Cancer Control 8:415.

[p]Seidman AD, Fornier MN, Esteva FJ, et al: Weekly trastuzamab and paclitaxel therapy for metastatic breast cancer with analysis of efficacy by HER2 immunophenotype and gene amplification. J Clin Oncol 2001;19:2587.

[q]Perez EA, Roche PC, Jenkins RB, et al: HER2 testing in patients with breast cancer: poor correlation between weak positivity by immunohistochemistry and gene amplification by fluorescence in situ hybridization. Mayo Clin Proc 2002;77:148.

[r]Bigner SH, Mark H, Burger PC, et al: Specific chromosomal abnormalities in malignant human gliomas. Cancer Res 1988;48:405.

[s]Tada K, Shiraishi S, Kamiryo T, et al: Analysis of loss of heterozygosity chromosome 10 in patients with malignant astrocytic tumors: Correlation with patient age and survival. J Neurosurg 2001;95:651.

[t]Smith JS, Tachibana I, Passe SM, et al: PTEN mutation, EGFR amplification, and outcome in patients with anaplastic astrocytoma and glioblastoma multiforme. J Natl Cancer Inst 2001;93:1246.

[u]Bigner SH, Matthews MR, Rasheed BKA, et al: Molecular genetic aspects of oligodendrogliomas including analysis by comparative genomic hybridization. Am J Pathol 1999;155:375.

[v]Cairncross JG, Ueki K, Zlatescu MC, et al: Specific genetic predictors of chemotherapeutic response and survival in patients with anaplastic oligodendrogliomas. J Natl Cancer Inst 1998;90:1473.

[w]Ueki K, Nishikawa R, Nakazato Y, et al: Correlation of histology and molecular genetic analysis of 1p, 19, 10q, TP53, EGFR, CDK4, and CDKN2A in 91 astrocytic and oligodendroglial tumors. Clin Cancer Res 2002;8:196.

[x]Gilbertson R, Wickramasinghe C, Hernan R, et al: Clinical and molecular stratification of disease risk in medulloblastoma. Br J Cancer 2001;85:705.

[y]Aldosari N, Bigner SH, Burger PC, et al: MYCC and MYCN oncogene amplification in medulloblastoma: A fluorescence in situ hybridization study on paraffin sections from the Children's Oncology Group. Arch Pathol Lab Med 2002;126:540.

[z]Biegel JA, Fogelgren B, Zhou JY, et al: Mutations of the INI1 rhabdoid tumor suppressor gene in medulloblastomas and primitive neuroectodermal tumors of the central nervous system. Clin Cancer Res 2000;6:2759.

[aa]Bruch LA, Hill DA, Cai DX, et al: A role for fluorescence in situ hybridization detection of chromosome 22q dosage in distinguishing atypical teratoid/rhabdoid tumors from medulloblastoma/central primitive neuroectodermal tumors. Hum Pathol 2001;32:156.

[bb]Cai DX, Banerjee R, Scheithauer BW, et al: Chromosome 1p and 14q FISH analysis in clinicopathologic subsets of meningioma: Diagnosis and prognostic implications. J Neuropathol Exp Neurol 2001;60:628.

[cc]Ketter R, Henn W, Niedermayer I, et al: Predictive value of progression-associated chromosomal aberrations for the prognosis of meningiomas: A retrospective study of 198 cases. J Neurosurg 2001;95:601.

[dd]Sorensen PH, Lynch JC, Qualman SJ, et al: PAX3-FKHR and PAX7-FKHR gene fusions are prognostic indicators in alveolar rhabdomyosarcoma: A report from the Children's Oncology Group. J Clin Oncol 2002;20:2672.

[ee]Anderson J, Gordon T, McManus A, et al: Detection of the PAX3-FKHR fusion gene in paediatric rhabdomyosarcoma: A reproducible predictor of outcome? Br J Cancer 2001;85:831.

[ff]Shapiro DN, Parham DM, Douglass EC, et al: Relationship of tumor-cell ploidy to histologic subtype and treatment outcome in children and adolescents with unresectable rhabdomyosarcoma. J Clin Oncol 1991;9:159.

[gg]Pappo AS, Crist WM, Kuttesch J, et al: Tumor-cell DNA content predicts outcome in children and adolescents with clinical group III embryonal rhabdomyosarcoma: The Intergroup Rhabdomyosarcoma Study Committee of the Children's Cancer Group and the Pediatric Oncology Group. J Clin Oncol 1993;11:1901.

[hh]Fong CT, Dracopoli NC, White PS, et al: Loss of heterozygosity for chromosome 1p in human neuroblastomas: Correlation with N-myc amplification. Proc Natl Acad Sci USA 1989;86:3753.

[ii]Maris JM, Weiss MJ, Guo C, et al: Loss of heterozygosity at 1p36 independently predicts for disease progression but not decreased overall survival probability in neuroblastoma patients: a Children's Oncology Group Study. J Clin Oncol 2000;18:1888.

[jj]Ginsberg JP, de Alava E, Ladanyi M, et al: EWS-FLI1 and EWS-ERG gene fusions are associated with similar clinical phenotypes in Ewing's sarcoma. J Clin Oncol 1999;17:1809.

[kk]Peter M, Couturier J, Pacquement H, et al: A new member of the ETS family fused to EWS in Ewing tumors. Oncogene 1997;14:1159.

[ll]Hattinger CM, Potschger U, Tarkkanen M, et al: Prognostic impact of chromosomal aberrations in Ewing tumours. Br J Cancer 86:2002;1763.

[mm]Gerald WL, Ladanyi M, de Alava E, et al: Clinical, pathologic, and molecular spectrum of tumors associated with t(11;22)(p13;q12): Desmoplastic small round-cell tumor and its variants. J Clin Oncol 1998;16:3028.

[nn]Gerald WL, Rosai J, Ladanyi M: Characterization of the genomic breakpoint and chimeric transcripts in the EWS-WT1 gene fusion of desmoplastic small round cell tumor. Proc Natl Acad Sci USA 1995;92:1028.

[oo]Antonescu CR, Tschernyavsky SJ, Woodruff JM, et al: Molecular diagnosis of clear cell sarcoma: Detection of EWS-ATF1 and MITF-M transcripts and histopathological and ultrastructural analysis of 12 cases. J Mol Diagn 2002;4:44.

[pp]Panagopoulos I, Mertens F, Debiec-Rychter M, et al: Molecular genetic characterization of the EWS/ATF1 fusion gene in clear cell sarcoma of tendons and aponeuroses. Int J Cancer 2002;99:560.

[qq]Knezevich SR, McFadden DE, Tao W, et al: A novel ETV6-NTRK3 gene fusion in congenital fibrosarcoma. Nat Genet 1998;18:184.

[rr]Rubin BP, Chen CJ, Morgan TW, et al: Congenital mesoblastic nephroma t(12;15) is associated with ETV6-NTRK3 gene fusion: Cytogenetic and molecular relationship to congenital (infantile) fibrosarcoma. Am J Pathol 1998;153:1451.

[ss]Ladanyi M, Antonescu CR, Leung DH, et al: Impact of SYT-SSX fusion type on the clinical behavior of synovial sarcoma: A multi-institutional restrospective study of 243 patients. Cancer Res 2002;62:135.

[tt]Kawai A, Woodruff J, Healey JH, et al: SYT-SSX gene fusion as a determinant of morphology and prognosis in synovial sarcoma. N Engl J Med 1998;338:153.

[uu]Dei Tos AP: Liposarcoma: New entities and evolving concepts. Ann Diagn Pathol 2000;4:252.

[vv]Clark J, Benjamin H, Gill S, et al: Fusion of the EWS gene to CHN, a member of the steroid/thyroid receptor gene superfamily, in a human myxoid chondrosarcoma. Oncogene 1996;12:229.

circumstances, as in CML, the associations are so clearly established that the abnormalities define the disease process. In others, such as AML with recurring translocations, they define distinct subsets of a heterogeneous disease. Some other abnormalities provide important prognostic information within a disease category. No attempt is made to include all known chromosomal aberrations or their associations, and the reader is referred to other excellent references for comprehensive reviews[138,139] and to the OMIM (Online Mendelian Inheritance in Man) website for continually updated information on human genes and disorders.[140] Many of these abnormalities are discussed in more detail in the discussion of specific tumors elsewhere in this book.

SUMMARY

Cytogenetic analysis of tumor cells provides an opportunity to visualize all genetic material in a cell as chromosomes. The vast majority of all neoplasias have shown cytogenetic abnormalities, and many of these chromosomal aberrations are disease-type and subtype specific. In addition to providing diagnostic information, clonal chromosomal abnormalities provide information important to prognosis and therapeutic management.

Cytogenetic abnormalities in tumor cells are acquired, nonrandom, and clonal. The chromosomal abnormalities are present only in the tumor tissues. One or more chromosomal abnormalities present in two or more cells define a clone. Subclonal populations contain the abnormality or abnormalities of the stemline clone plus additional abnormalities, thus indicating clonal evolution.

Clonal evolution correlates with increasingly aggressive tumor biology.

Cytogenetic analysis of any tissue type may be accomplished with viable, fresh tissue. For best results, the processing laboratory must receive the sample with appropriate patient information as soon as possible after sample acquisition. When fresh tissue is not available, paraffin-embedded tissue, touch preparations, cytospin preparations, and blood or bone marrow smears may often be used for specific molecular cytogenetic studies.

Molecular cytogenetic analysis or FISH uses DNA probes to hybridize to specific regions in the genome, thereby providing information about the region that is probed. Limited but specific genetic information may be obtained by using available probes. CGH provides information about regional genomic DNA gains and losses. Technologies using multiple-color FISH methods (SKY, M-FISH) may provide information about unidentified marker chromosomes and chromosome rearrangements not recognized by conventional G-band cytogenetic analysis. With the newer methods, the most detailed information about the tumor under investigation is often obtained by using a combination of conventional and molecular cytogenetic methods.

Cytogenetic information about tumor tissues has been accumulating since the 1960s. Today, cytogenetic studies are used to provide information about a patient's particular disease process, how it can best be managed, and what outcomes can be expected. Not all disease processes yield specific diagnostic or prognostic information, but sufficient information is obtained to warrant some type of cytogenetic study at the time of diagnosis for all childhood hematopoietic disorders and solid tumors, all adult hematopoietic disorders, sarcomas, central nervous system tumors, and selected epithelial tumors.

Molecular Diagnostics

SUMMARY OF KEY POINTS

KEY METHODS
- Polymerase chain reaction (PCR) is a cornerstone method for most applications.
- Automated and quantitative methods now exist that improve reproducibility and clinical application.
- Southern blot is valuable for detection of gene rearrangements and chromosomal translocations.
- Direct sequencing methods and screening for genetic mutations play an increasing role.

APPLICATIONS
Hematologic Malignancies
- Demonstrate clonality, with immunoglobulin or T-cell–receptor gene rearrangements.

- Can be used to assess specific molecular translocations that define many leukemias or lymphomas.
- Sensitive and quantitative assessment of minimal residual disease.
- Used in transplantation, both for human leukocyte antigen matching and for assessment of engraftment and chimerism.

Solid Tumors
- Numerous hereditary cancer syndromes can be identified by presence of specific mutations.
- Many soft tissue tumors can be diagnosed and classified based on specific translocations.

- Prognostically significant subsets of many tumors can be identified based on specific genetic markers.

ASSAYS IN DEVELOPMENT
- Gene profiling by using DNA microarrays shows tremendous promise in improving classification and identifying therapeutic targets.
- DNA methylation assays may help diagnose and classify tumors.
- New molecular approaches to early detection or detection of residual disease show promise.
- Proteomic profiling also may allow improved diagnosis and classification.

Characteristic markers involved in the molecular pathogenesis of various cancers have been described with increasing regularity over the last three decades. The term *molecular diagnostics* applied to cancer is generally regarded as the analysis of nucleic acids from patient samples to detect characteristic findings to assist in the diagnosis of neoplasia and in some cases to provide prognostic information. For hereditary cancers due to germline mutations, molecular testing may yield predictive information presymptomatically, which has great significance for management and counseling of not only the individual at risk but also potentially other as-yet-unaffected family members.

Molecular markers also provide sensitive ways to track residual cancer or bone marrow engraftment and thus assist with tailoring therapy to detect agents of etiologic interest in the assessment of cancer [e.g., human T-cell leukemia virus (HTLV), Epstein-Barr virus (EBV), human herpesvirus (HHV8)], as well as in the selection of specific cellular therapeutic products as with high-resolution tissue typing for bone marrow transplantation. Because the functional manifestation of most nucleic acid changes is through normal or altered proteins produced (or not) from affected genes, the definition of molecular diagnostics has recently begun to expand to include applications that involve the analysis of proteins (proteomics).

METHODS

Specimens

Assays start with a process that extracts the target nucleic acid from a sample by disrupting cells. Because nucleated cells are the primary source of DNA, paucicellular samples of bone marrow and blood or even tumors after therapy may not reflect the state of a diagnostic sample. After taking necessary tissue for histopathologic examination or other studies, it is crucial to set aside if possible a portion of the "diagnostic" specimen for nucleic acid preparation or storage, on which assays can be performed subsequently if desired. Blood, bone marrow, and certain body-fluid samples must be adequately anticoagulated because appreciable numbers of nucleated cells are lost in clots. Ethylenediaminetetraacetic acid (EDTA) or citrate generally is preferable to heparin as an anticoagulant because heparin may bind to extracted nucleic acids and interfere with subsequent steps in various molecular assays. However, heparin is the anticoagulant of choice for cytogenetic analysis, so it may be necessary to obtain two samples or split the sample into separate tubes. Tissue (≥ 100 to 200 mg) can be frozen at $-80°C$ or in liquid nitrogen and processed subsequently for nucleic acid or protein. DNA (and RNA) can be obtained from archival paraffin-embedded specimens, but appreciable fragmentation and/or degradation of nucleic acid occurs in such specimens, and without question, the preferred sample for molecular diagnostic analysis is a fresh sample.

Samples should be submitted to the laboratory in a timely fashion, particularly if RNA is the nucleic acid targeted. Late Friday and weekend blood or bone marrow samples from which DNA (and often RNA) will be extracted subsequently often perform satisfactorily when stored for several days at refrigerator (not freezer) temperatures. Generally 4 to 6 mg of DNA is obtained per 1,000,000 nucleated cells, so obtaining sufficient nucleic acid is generally not a problem unless samples are quite hypocellcular. Hypocellular samples (e.g., cerebrospinal fluid or bone marrow after aggressive treatment) may yield insufficient DNA to perform certain assays (e.g., Southern blotting; see later).

Polymerase Chain Reaction

Polymerase chain reaction (PCR)[141] underlies the vast majority of molecular assays performed for clinical purposes, in many cases as a "front-end" to generate sufficient nucleic acid to analyze by additional techniques like DNA sequencing. Amplification of DNA enables both the analysis of samples with small numbers of cells and the generation of abundant "clean" material to analyze from normal samples. The amount of input nucleic acid for PCR varies with the assay, but one to several assays can be performed generally for each microgram of DNA obtained.

For highly sensitive qualitative detection of unique DNA constructs such as chromosomal translocations, *nested PCR* can be performed, in which an aliquot of an initial amplification reaction undergoes a second round of PCR by using a new set of primers located internal to those for the first reaction. Increasingly, PCR reactions are being done on real-time platforms, which offer broad linear ranges and provide either qualitative or quantitative measures for a target in a specimen.[142] PCR assays generally have no problem amplifying DNA regions up to several kilobases in size.

For PCR assays in which RNA is the starting material (RT-PCR), RNA is first incubated with the enzyme reverse transcriptase (RT) in the presence of either general or specific oligonucleotide primers. RT is capable of making a DNA copy strand (cDNA) off the RNA template. The cDNA products are then subjected to standard PCR amplification. If nucleotide sequence is the desired assay information, as, for example, when looking for deleterious changes (mutations), direct *DNA sequencing* is performed from primary PCR products.[143]

Southern Blotting

Southern blotting is a long-standing technique useful for clonality assessment in hematolymphoid neoplasms, as well as for identification of chromosomal translocations in both hematologic and solid tumors (Fig. 17-7).[144] Physical restructuring of a chromosomal region by translocation, or the physiologic elimination during lymphocyte development of DNA segments from immunoglobulin and T-cell receptor (TcR) genes, leads to restriction endonuclease–generated DNA fragments of new lengths, which characterize the clonal cells that have expanded to form the cancer. Fragments with sequences of interest are detected by probes that are capable of exposing X-ray film.

Southern blot assays have a number of disadvantages clinically. They require substantial amounts of nucleic acid, generally several micrograms per lane evaluated. Thus a full (three) restriction enzyme evaluation for immunoglobulin heavy chain or TcR β-chain gene rearrangement generally requires 6 to 15 μg of DNA. Southern blots also are labor intensive, technically demanding, and typically

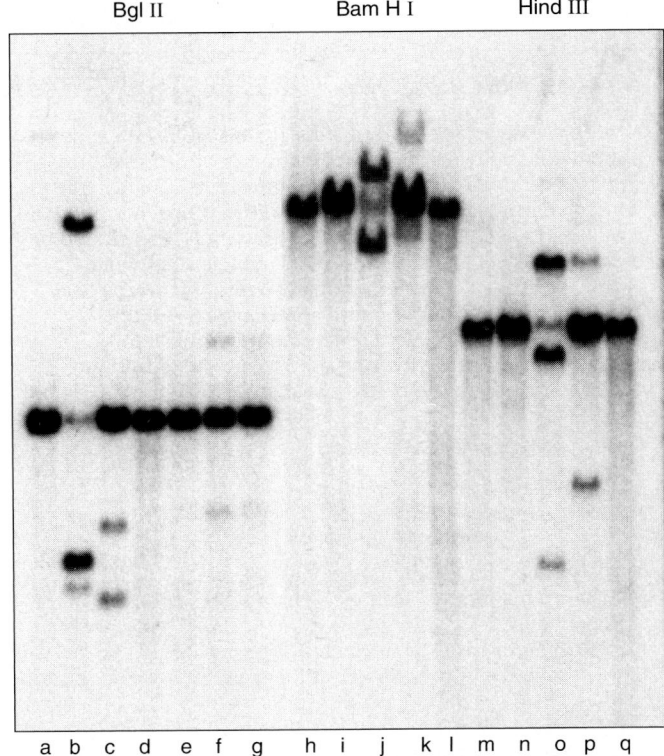

Figure 17-7. Immunoglobulin heavy-chain gene assessment by Southern blot. Typical three restriction enzyme analysis (enzymes indicated at the top) of five patient specimens (1, lanes a, h, m; 2, lanes b, j, o; 3, lanes c, k, p; 4, lanes d, i, n; 5, lanes e, l, q). Note the different order of patients for *Bgl*II versus the other enzymes. A single germline band is seen in all enzyme digests for the normal control (patient 1). Lanes f and g are mixtures of 10% and 4% B-cell lymphoma DNA in normal DNA (note faint rearranged alleles above and below the germline band on the *Bgl*II digest); these serve as positive and sensitivity controls. Two rearranged alleles for both immunoglobulin heavy-chain genes are seen in patient samples 2 and 3. Patient 2 demonstrates an additional faint band, with enzymes *Bgl*II and *Hin*dIII supporting clonal evolution. Note also reduced intensity of the germline allele for patient 2, indicating that this sample contains a high fraction of neoplastic cells. Patients 4 and 5 are normal for all enzyme digests.

take 5 to 7 days to deliver an answer. Because of time constraints and limited sample volumes, many laboratories run Southern blot assays once or twice a week.

Other DNA Assays

Numerous di-, tri-, and tetranucleotide sequences spread throughout the human genome provide a variety of length polymorphisms known as *simple tandem repeats (STRs)*—also called *microsatellite* markers—which generally are of different lengths on maternally and paternally inherited alleles. Such markers are occasionally useful in linkage analysis to follow "at-risk" chromosomes passed in the germline from one parent or the other, in the assessment of bone marrow engraftment, and in the comparison of the relative abundance of STRs in tumor and normal tissues to determine allelic loss (loss of heterozygosity, LOH).

ANCILLARY LABORATORY TESTS IN HEMATOLOGIC MALIGNANCIES

A wide variety of specialized tests are available for the study of hematologic malignancies. Selection of appropriate tests depends on the disease and sometimes on the manner in which a particular disease may be followed up. The following grouping indicates a rough priority in which tests should be ordered in particular diseases. This listing is somewhat artificial, because obviously in many cases, the diagnosis is not known, or not known until some specialized test is performed. Thus more than one path might have to be followed for diagnosis, or some tests performed in stages once the results of the first are available.

CHRONIC MYELOID LEUKEMIA

At Diagnosis
Karyotyping and either FISH or PCR

Monitoring
FISH with quantitative PCR used once FISH becomes negative
Karyotyping in cases of suspected progression
Flow cytometry in progression or blast crisis, not in chronic phase

ACUTE MYELOID LEUKEMIA

At Diagnosis
Karyotyping and flow cytometry
PCR or FISH for PML-RARa in cases that are morphologically or phenotypically suggestive of APL

Monitoring
Flow cytometry
Karyotyping
PCR in APL but not for other translocations

ACUTE LYMPHOID LEUKEMIA

At Diagnosis
Flow cytometry
FISH or PCR for BCR-ABL
FISH or PCR for TEL-AML1 (pediatric)
Ploidy or FISH for trisomies (pediatric)
Karyotyping
PCR for TcR or immunoglobulin (Ig) only if minimal residual disease (MRD) studies planned or if a diagnostic dilemma

Monitoring
Flow cytometry
PCR for BCR-ABL if positive
PCR for Ig/TcR for MRD studies
PCR for other translocations less well established

CHRONIC LYMPHOCYTIC LEUKEMIA

At Diagnosis
Flow cytometry
FISH
Routine karyotyping less frequently used

Monitoring
Flow cytometry
FISH
IgH/TCR PCR rarely used for MRD studies

MYELODYSPLASTIC SYNDROME

At Diagnosis
Karyotyping
Flow cytometry controversial, probably more in high-grade than in low-grade MDS

Monitoring
Karyotyping
Flow cytometry in disease progression

NON-HODGKIN'S LYMPHOMA

At Diagnosis
Immunophenotyping, either by flow cytometry or immunohistochemistry
FISH for specific translocations in morphologically and phenotypically suggestive lesions, especially CCND1-IgH or MYC-IgH
PCR for IgH/TcR in difficult cases or if MRD studies planned
PCR for bcl2-IgH if MRD studies planned in follicular lymphoma
Routine karyotyping rarely performed

Monitoring
Flow cytometry in staging, especially of marrow
PCR or flow cytometry in MRD studies

HODGKIN'S LYMPHOMA

At Diagnosis
Immunohistochemistry
Flow cytometry only to exclude other things

Monitoring
Usually none, or limited immunohistochemistry

MULTIPLE MYELOMA

At Diagnosis
Serum protein electrophoresis and immunofixation
FISH
Flow cytometry

Monitoring
Serum protein electrophoresis
Flow cytometry for MRD studies

New gene chip technologies that use high-density arrays of oligonucleotides or cDNA probes spotted on glass surfaces allow *expression profiling* of tumors by providing a relative assessment of the levels of expressions of thousands of different genes by tumor cells and the sorting of these dense and complex patterns by software-clustering programs into groups that preliminary studies indicate may identify the origin or behavioral profile of a tumor, or even its genetic origin.[145-147]

APPLICATIONS

Applications currently exist for two large classes of cancers, hematolymphoid neoplasms, for which a large variety of molecular tests have evolved over the last 20 years, and solid tumors, for which clinically useful assays are more recent and limited. Currently the vast majority of molecular oncology assays are "home-brew" methods, developed by individual laboratories such that little standardization exists. The lack of standarization reflects the reality of relatively low test volumes, and thus little incentive for commercial entities to develop and seek Food and Drug Administration–approved assays. This is not a major barrier to the use of these tests, but it has had an impact on the availability of tests and places an additional onus on the clinician to understand what information can be obtained from assays.

Hematolymphoid Neoplasms

Molecular assays for hematolymphoid neoplasms are not necessary in all cases if information from histology, immunophenotype, and cytogenetic assessment is sufficient for diagnosis.[148] Moreover, the relative value of molecular assays differs in different diseases and clinical situations. Molecular assay results should not be used by themselves, but rather evaluated in conjunction with clinical, histologic, immunophenotypic, and other information to arrive at the best picture of a patient's disease. This is generally best done by a hematopathologist. Properly chosen assays can help in both the diagnosis and classification of neoplasms.

Clonality assays are first-line tests for suspected hematolymphoid neoplasms; these are directed at populations that demonstrate immunoglobulin heavy chain (IgH) or TcR gene rearrangement or a specific chromosomal translocation.[149,150]

Gene-Rearrangement Assays

Gene-rearrangement assays look for the presence of a significant clonal B- or T-lymphoid population by detecting a predominant gene rearrangement. Each tumor cell generally contains the same rearranged IgH or TcR gene, and Southern or PCR-based assays can detect down to 1% to 5% tumor cells. IgH gene rearrangement is assessed for B cells, because this gene undergoes rearrangement first during B-lymphoid development. The TcR β- or γ-chain genes are commonly examined for T-lymphoid cells, the β more commonly in Southern blot analysis. Assays for

rearrangement of Ig light chain, TcR α or TcR δ-chains genes are less common.

The gold-standard assay for IgH and TcR-β gene clonal assessment is Southern blot analysis, in which a labeled probe that recognizes the IgH or TcR gene is hybridized to restriction-endonuclease–digested sample DNA. New hybridizing bands of different size indicate clones with rearranged IgH or TcR alleles (see Fig. 17-7). Rearrangement must be seen with two (or more) restriction enzymes for the sample to be scored as positive.[151] Clonal evolution within a neoplasm may sometimes be observed as new hybridizing bands in the presence of previously demonstrated ones.

PCR assays (Fig. 17-8) for hematolymphoid neoplasms can be performed quickly to look for clonal rearrangements of the IgH and TcR genes. Relatively conserved framework regions of variable (V) region gene segments serve as targets for upstream PCR primers, whereas similarly conserved regions in joining (J) or adjacent sequences are targeted by downstream primers. The IgH gene is generally evaluated for B lymphocytes, and the TcR γ-chain gene for T lymphocytes. The sensitivity of PCR assays is similar to and perhaps a bit better than Southern assays.[152]

PCR assays offer advantages and disadvantages. A major plus is the ability to analyze a sample within 24 hours, or even the same day. A second advantage of PCR is that smaller input of DNA is required, thus expanding the range of evaluable samples. A limitation of both IgH and TcR PCR assays is decreased sensitivity, because only a subset of Southern-blot rearranged samples will be clonal by the PCR assay. This arises because the PCR primers do not bind equally well with all V- or J-region gene segments that may participate in clonal rearrangement. Typically IgH PCR assays directed at a single region of V region genes will detect 75% to 85% of IgH gene rearrangements.[153,154]

Low-level expansions of normal B or T cells may occur in response to antigen or other factors yielding low-predominance clonal results on both Southern and PCR assays. The polyclonal ladder pattern seen in IgH PCR assays (Fig. 17-8A) is an example of this phenomenon. Such clones are presumably under host control, and it is important to interpret low-level clonal bands in the broader context of a case. Conditions that enhance immune "reactivity," such as autoimmune disease, may provide particular challenges. Important interpretive elements of clonality assays, and especially PCR assays, are given in Table 17-8.

Chromosomal Translocations

Detection of a translocation helps anchor a diagnosis and also potentially provides a sensitive marker for monitoring disease burden (Fig. 17-8C). As discussed in the previous section, molecular cytogenetic tools, such as FISH, may comfortably substitute for DNA- or RNA-based assays to look quickly for chromosomal translocations in diagnostic samples. However, PCR can detect a much smaller percentage of tumor cells in a population of normal cells, allowing a search for *minimal residual disease* (MRD). Because translocations generally are present only in tumor

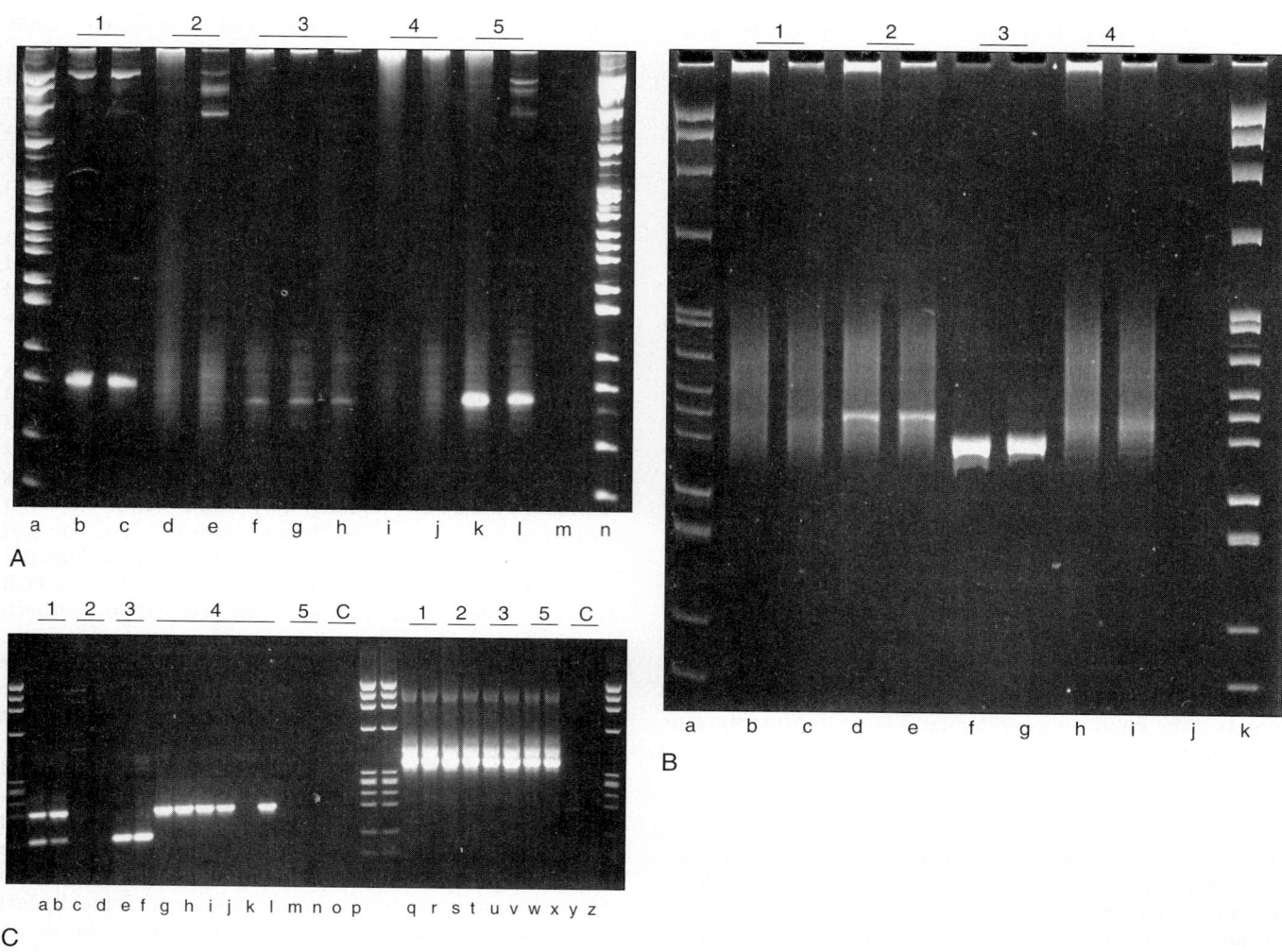

Figure 17-8. Polymerase chain reaction (PCR) and reverse transcriptase–PCR (RT-PCR) analysis in hematolymphoid neoplasia. **A,** Immunoglobulin heavy-chain gene PCR analysis. Testing is done at two or more different DNA concentrations for each of five patients. Lanes a and n are molecular size standards; lane m, a minus-DNA control to rule out potential PCR contamination. Patients 4 and 5 are known reactive (polyclonal) and lymphoma (monoclonal) samples, respectively. Patient 1 has a monoclonal process involving most cells in the specimen; patient 2 has a polyclonal process; and patient 3 has a subtle monoclonal process in a polyclonal background. **B,** T-cell receptor γ-chain gene PCR analysis. Patients 3 and 4 are known lymphoma and reactive samples. Patient 1 is polyclonal; patient 2 has a monoclonal process in a polyclonal background. **C,** Bcr-abl RT-PCR analysis for major breakpoint region (mbr) of bcr gene. Patient 4 has RNA from the K562 cell line; patient 5 is known negative for the Philadelphia chromosome. Six dilutions from 10^{-3} to 10^{-8} parts of K562 RNA in normal RNA are assayed as sensitivity/positive controls; "dropout" as seen at the 10^{-7} dilution in this sample can happen. Patient 1 is positive (b3a2 fusion product); patient 2, negative; and patient 3, positive (b2a2 fusion product) for bcr-abl translocation. The presence of both b3a2 and b2a2 fusion products in patient 1 reflects alternative RNA splicing. Lanes r–z represent RT-PCR amplification for porphobilinogen deaminase, a housekeeping gene, to ensure specimen RNA integrity. Lanes o, p, y, and z are minus RNA controls to rule out contamination.

cells (see caveat later), and no background products exist as for IgH or TcR genes, MRD studies can be conducted down to one tumor cell in 10,000 to 1,000,000 normal cells (Table 17-9). Most MRD assays currently use real-time quantitative PCR or RT-PCR and follow the increase or decrease of the ratio of a specific tumor marker to a reference gene, which presumably is expressed uniformly in both tumor and normal cells. Quantitative PCR and RT-PCR methods that use internal controls to indicate sample integrity are the preferred method to assess residual disease. Real-time (RQ) methods are becoming the widespread method of choice, as they are less cumbersome than competitive methods, although the latter may offer

slightly greater detection sensitivity. Several clinical studies have shown that PCR-negative status after chemotherapy is correlated with a lower rate of relapse, and that apparently cured patients in long-term clinical remission may still remain PCR positive with sensitive assays. Change from PCR-negative to PCR-positive status often heralds relapse several months later.[155-160]

High-sensitivity PCR studies are not suitable for screening for presence of disease. What appear to be false-positive molecular results for the bcl2-IgH and bcr-abl genes have been described at a low level in normal individuals and raise at least theoretical cautions for the interpretation of MRD.[161-165] Such results presumably

Science of Clinical Oncology

TABLE 17-8

Interpretative Cautions for Clinicians Ordering Hematolymphoid Clonality Assays

- Negative PCR results for IgH and TcR gene rearrangement or chromosomal translocation assays do not fully exclude the possibility of neoplasia because not all rearrangements or translocations may be detected by the assay.
- Make sure if results are negative and the case is suggestive of neoplasia that laboratory reports indicate controls have been performed to exclude inhibitors of PCR amplification.
- Results described as "oligoclonal" for IgH or TcR gene rearrangement PCR assays should be interpreted conservatively. These may reflect self-limited reactive expansions of lymphocytes.
- "Nested" PCR or RT-PCR qualitative assays for certain chromosomal translocations (e.g., bcl2-IgH, bcr-abl) may be positive in normal individuals.

IgH, immunoglobulin heavy chain; PCR, polymerase chain reaction; RT, reverse transcriptase; TcR, T-cell receptor.

indicate small populations of cells that have undergone translocations that precede cancer, but have not progressed through subsequent mutational or transformation steps necessary for the development of neoplasia.

Assays in Marrow Transplantation

The human leukocyte antigen (HLA) histocompatibility locus on human chromosome 6 is an extraordinarily diverse region with more than 1300 known alleles identified to date.[166,167] HLA matching of donors and recipients for bone marrow transplantation at class I and class II loci is a complex but important application of molecular diagnostics in clinical oncology, and millions of potential donors have been pretyped through programs such as the National Marrow Donor Program in the United States or similar ones in other countries. Families of molecularly discrete alleles that share the same serologic (or antigenic) activity have been identified, and it is clear that molecular typing to match donors and recipients closely offers benefits over serologic typing for graft survival as well as graft-versus-host disease.[168] Matching for class II alleles is particularly important, although a single molecularly mismatched class I allele appears to be well tolerated.[169]

STRs or variable number of tandem repeat (VNTR) markers are routinely used to assess engraftment and

TABLE 17-9

Comparison of Methods for Minimal Residual Disease Assessment

METHOD	SENSITIVITY
Cytogenetics, conventional	1%–10%
Cytogenetics, FISH	0.2%–10%
Southern blot	1%–10%
Flow cytometry	$1/10^3$–$1/10^4$
PCR/RT-PCR, quantitative	$1/10^3$–10^5
PCR/RT-PCR, nested	$1/10^5$–10^6

FISH, fluorescence in site hybridization; PCR, polymerase chain reaction; RT, reverse transcriptase.

potential mixed chimerism after bone marrow transplantation.[170] These types of identity markers, also used in forensic, paternity, and linkage applications, permit unambiguous determination of donor and recipient alleles and low levels of mixed chimerism down to several percentage points. This information is useful in making decisions for pancytopenic patients regarding levels of immunosuppressive therapy as well as treatment for infection or recurrent disease.

Other Applications in Hematolymphoid Neoplasms

PCR can easily be performed to look for specific viral agents in association with bone marrow failure or neoplasia. PCR applications are straightforward for detection of parvovirus B19, type 6 and type 8 human herpes viruses, types 1 and 2 human T-cell leukemia viruses (HTLV), as well as Epstein-Barr virus (EBV). Although titers may fluctuate and cases may occur in the absence of significant levels of EBV, some reports suggest that quantitative PCR assessment of EBV viral DNA levels may be a useful indicator to follow for possible emergence of post-transplant lymphoproliferative disease (PTLD) after solid organ transplantation.[171] Southern-blot assessment of clonal or polyclonal integration of EBV viral DNA may also be useful in assessing potential PTLD cases for neoplastic risk.[172]

Microarray-based assays are currently investigational tools for hematolymphoid neoplasms, but expression profiling studies have demonstrated impressive power in the assessment of a variety of leukemias and lymphomas.[173-177]

SOLID TUMORS

The definition of molecular markers useful in the diagnosis and management of patients with solid tumors has lagged behind that for hematolymphoid neoplasms, although some areas have a rich literature, particularly pediatric sarcomas and mutational detection in hereditary cancers. The range of abnormalities that can be detected in solid tumors include translocations, point mutations, allelic loss, gene amplification, microsatellite instability, and abnormalities in DNA methylation of genes. Some of these, such as chromosomal translocations in sarcomas, or amplification of HER-2/*neu* in breast cancer, can be detected by FISH as well as by PCR or Southern-based methods (see Table 17-7 for a list of tumors associated with genetic lesions that can be detected with either method). However, additional molecular abnormalities can be detected in a greater range of solid tumors.

Mutations and Hereditary Cancer Syndromes

A variety of hereditary cancer syndromes that demonstrate autosomal dominant inheritance lend themselves to molecular genetic testing in patients whose family history and/or clinical phenotype suggest that testing may be useful. It is important that patients receive appropriate pre- and post-test counseling and written informed consent be obtained; consider using a medical geneticist or genetic counselor if appropriate.

Hereditary cancers with mendelian inheritance are a small subset (<5%) of solid tumors, but the detection of a disease-causing mutation can be of enormous benefit to patients and physicians, as well as to immediate and extended family. Major disease groups include hereditary breast and ovarian cancer due to mutations of the BRCA1, BRCA2, Tp53, and CHEK2 genes, hereditary colorectal cancer associated with hereditary polyposis due to mutations of the APC gene, and hereditary nonpolyposis colorectal carcinoma associated primarily with mutations of the h-MSH2 and h-MLH1 genes. It is likely that other genes contribute to familial cases of breast cancer that test negative for mutations in these genes, presumably through different penetrances and interactions with hormonal and environmental factors.

Hereditary cancers are particularly challenging disorders for molecular diagnostics laboratories because many mutations spread over large areas or the entirety of the causative genes have been described for most. This necessitates whole gene sequencing (or at least screening) of many exons as well as intron/exon junctions. Abnormalities usually include a range of missense mutations with single amino acid changes, and many prematurely truncated proteins resulting from nonsense, frameshift, and split-site mutations that lead to STOP codons.

Because of the large size of many genes responsible for hereditary cancer syndromes, screening assays are often done first. These assays examine PCR-amplified regions of the entire gene by using techniques like *single-strand conformation polymorphism* (SSCP) analysis or *denaturing high-pressure liquid chromatography* (DHPLC). Screening assays are quite effective, detecting more than 95% of point mutations in many genes. Screening and sequencing methods generally do not detect major structural changes such as partial gene deletions or duplications, because no unique DNA nucleotide changes are present. Major structural changes are believed to constitute up to 15% to 20% of cases in certain disorders such as hereditary breast cancer due to BRCA1.[178] A number of novel methods recently have been identified that permit straightforward and comprehensive screening for duplications and deletions, generally focused on changes in copy number of exons in the BRCA1 gene,[179,180] where structural rearrangements are more common than for the BRCA2 gene. Because of high complexity, and in some cases exclusive intellectual property positions (see later), molecular testing for most hereditary disorders is generally concentrated in relatively few commercial and academic reference centers, sometimes in single laboratories.

Many other hereditary cancer syndromes can be assessed clinically or on a research basis. A selected group with genes that can be analyzed focusing on fewer than 10 exons includes MEN-2, type 2 multiple endocrine neoplasia (c-ret)[181]; hereditary paraganglioma (SDHD, SDHB)[182]; Li-Fraumeni syndrome (p53)[183]; Von-Hippel Lindau syndrome (VHL)[184]; type 1 multiple endocrine neoplasia (MEN1)[185]; and Cowden syndrome (PTEN).

Allele Loss (Loss of Heterozygosity) as a Tumor Signature

The development of neoplasia is commonly accompanied by genetic instability leading to the deletion of small or larger regions of DNA from various chromosomes.[186] By using PCR assays directed at highly polymorphic length markers (usually STRs) throughout the genome, it is possible to "scan" in a general fashion for regional losses by comparing the ratio of different-sized alleles in a sample of interest with the ratio obtained from normal (frequently adjacent) tissue of the same individual. These ratios should be approximately 1.0 normally. Theoretically in a pure tumor population, a marker may be lost entirely. However, normal connective, vascular, and inflammatory cells within a tumor would be expected to contribute normal cells, and conservative allele ratios of around less than 2/3 or greater than 1.5 are typically used to determine whether there is LOH. LOH studies can be conducted on fresh or archival (paraffin-embedded) tissue, and their specificity may be augmented by enrichment of tumor cells by using a dissection microscope or laser-capture microdissection.[187]

A particularly useful clinical application of LOH analysis has been in the evaluation of oligodendrogliomas, in which LOH for markers on the short arm of chromosome 1 and the long arm of chromosome 19 are both diagnostic and prognostic.[188,189] Other possible applications of LOH analysis are being piloted to include comparison of "signature" patterns of LOH to identify de novo second primary tumors from intraparenchymal metastatic spread of a single primary tumor.[190] Straightforward genotyping of small tissue fragments by using STR alleles also may be useful to resolve the vexing question of whether a tissue "floater" from another specimen has somehow become included in the paraffin block of another tissue specimen.[191]

Colorectal Cancer

Several applications related to colorectal carcinoma are in regular or investigational use. The potential to look for mutations from desquamated adenoma or carcinoma cells in stool as a screening approach for colonic cancer has been entertained for some time,[192] and DNA seems to be stable for reasonable amounts of time as it traverses the colon and in collected stool. Mutations have been shown to be detectable at modest sensitivity and high specificity by using digital protein truncation.[193] A kit targeting 15 mutations has been developed and tested on a selected series of carcinoma, adenoma, and normal patients.[194] Results demonstrated reasonably good sensitivity and specificity, and larger trials of this screening approach are in progress.

Microsatellite alleles are present in two copies in most individuals. Some tumors demonstrate *microsatellite instability* (MSI), in which additional, often minor, bands of different size are noted in addition to germline alleles seen in normal cells (Fig. 17-9). MSI bands reflect insertions or deletions of nucleotides within the microsatellite repeat sequence; these additional atypical

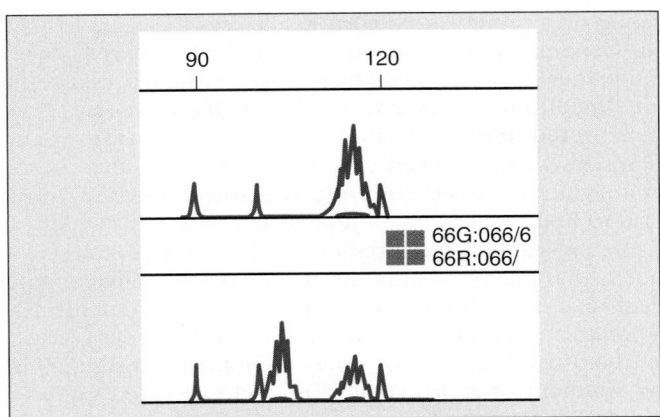

Figure 17-9. Microsatellite instability (MSI) assessment of ascending colon carcinoma specimen. Capillary electrophoresis tracing shows normal (*upper*) and tumor (*lower*) analysis by single tandem repeat (BAT26) analysis. The "jagged" peak in the upper tracing represents apparent homozygosity for a single allele. The jagged appearance arises from "stutter" during polymerase chain reaction amplification. Note the novel smaller (left-shifted) allele in the tumor. This sample showed additional MSI with other markers; immunohistochemistry demonstrated MSH2 protein expression in normal colonic epithelium but not in tumor cells. (Courtesy of Antonia Sepulveda, MD)

alleles are believed to result from defects in mismatch repair (MMR) systems under control of such genes as MSH2, MLH1, or others. The study of MSI has been particularly intense in the area of colon carcinoma,[195] where it appears to provide a powerful prognostic factor for improved survival, although some controversy exists.[196,197] MSI is the starting point for analysis of colon tumors if hereditary nonpolyposis colon cancer (HNPCC) is a consideration. A positive result is suggestive of HNPCC and often triggers further DNA-sequencing studies to search for causative mutations (see hereditary cancer syndromes earlier). A small percentage (~15%) of sporadic colon tumors also demonstrate MSI.

NEWER DIAGNOSTIC TECHNIQUES AND POTENTIAL APPLICATIONS

DNA Methylation

The ability of the nucleotide cytosine to undergo methylation to 5-methylcytosine has been correlated with important consequences for normal and altered cell function to include X-chromosome inactivation, gene expression, development, genetic imprinting, and cancer.[198] Alterations of methylation are acquired (or epigenetic) changes associated with virtually all types of cancer. Gene silencing associated with methylation of promoter regions of tumor-suppressor[199] or DNA-repair genes[200] may be either causal for or linked to mutational changes that play important roles in the development of cancer[201] and are potentially important in a wide range of sporadic cancers. Specific methylation markers or panels have not been validated yet for clinical use, but they show

promise. Methylation markers may be useful for tumor diagnosis or subclassification.[202] More exciting are possibilities that early epigenetic changes associated with cancer could be screened from organs at risk through analysis of exfoliated and excreted cells or even by using circulating peripheral blood cells to look for the same epigenetic abnormality.[203]

Expression Profiling/Microarrays

As with hematopoietic neoplasms, microarray-based expression profiling studies hold enormous potential in the management of patients with solid tumors. It is particularly encouraging that profiling studies of solid tumors have provided exciting results despite the seemingly greater challenge of analyzing samples in which variable amounts of non-neoplastic vascular, stromal, and inflammatory cells are present. Studies have shown the ability to distinguish normal from different types of prostate disease, to distinguish different grades of prostate cancer, and to define prognostic subgroups of breast cancer.[204-208] As microarray-based assays are validated, standardized, and become more prevalent, pathologists and surgeons accustomed to placing specimens routinely in formalin or other fixatives for morphologic and immunohistochemical analysis will need to adapt, because RNA from fresh tissues is likely to provide the highest quality results. Further developments that permit the performance of microarray-based methods on small tissue biopsies or sample obtained by FNA also will be important.

Cancer-specific Detection at Low Levels in Tissue, Blood, and Bone Marrow

For some time, investigators have probed the utility of "tumor-specific" molecular markers to identify metastatic carcinoma in sentinel or other lymph nodes or circulating in the blood with the hope of using such assays to determine patient prognosis and, in some cases, management decisions.[209,210] Some groups are attempting to develop rapid PCR methods that would allow such markers to be used intraoperatively.[211] Although progress has been made, these types of applications do not appear to be ready for clinical application. Difficulties have included false-positive results due to a lack of specific expression or expression from pseudogenes. False-positive results also have been noted in normal control samples.

Proteomics

The ability to analyze complex mixtures of proteins, the final effector molecules for most cellular processes, would seem to offer an essential tool for diagnosis, treatment, and early detection of cancer. Samples for analysis can be established tumors, secretions/excretions from organs at risk for neoplasia like breast[212] or bowel, or blood itself. Methods used include 2D gels, with spots analyzed by mass spectrometry, and increasingly sophisticated computer software,[213] or analysis of ionized peptides released by laser excitation of mixtures of proteins bound to chips [surface-enhanced laser desorption ionization (SELDI)[214] or matrix-assisted laser desorption ionization (MALDI)],[215] coupled to time-of-flight (TOF) mass spectrometry. Several studies show promise in the ability of these techniques to identify protein profiles associated with specific cancers,[216-218] but further validation studies are needed before these algorithms can be used clinically.

BUSINESS, REGULATORY, AND ETHICAL ISSUES AND MOLECULAR DIAGNOSTICS

Several business and regulatory trends are likely to have a significant impact on molecular diagnostic testing in oncology for at least the next decade. The first is intellectual property positions on discoveries relating to molecular pathogenesis, tumor markers, and their use in patient care.[218,219] Despite increasing concern throughout medicine, patents filed and granted on nucleic acid sequences, genes, molecular techniques, and clinical applications have grown dramatically over the last decade.[220] The best-known example in oncology is the BRCA1 and BRCA2 genes. Patents to both genes are held by a single entity, and full gene analysis is restricted to a single laboratory run by the patent holder. Many laboratorians are concerned that if useful focused panels of molecular markers emerge from current research using microarrays or other technologies, it will be difficult or impossible to offer these clinically because of multiple and perhaps conflicting patent positions.

The second is an increasing interest by government and the lay community in stricter regulation of molecular testing, including better understanding by patients of tests performed on them. Under guidelines currently being considered for implementation in revisions to CLIA-88 (the Clinical Laboratory Improvement Act of 1988) in the United States, it is quite possible that most molecular oncology assays could be regarded as "genetic" tests, whether assays are for hereditary (germline) or acquired (somatic) markers of cancer. The primary importance of these guidelines is the expected requirement for more rigorous standards to establish clinical validity and clinical utility of assays, particularly as regards an impact of the assay result on a decision for patient management. It also is likely that signed informed consent for the specific test(s) performed will be required of the patient (and the

requesting physician) before results can be released by the laboratory. To date, federal and third-party payor guidelines in the United States have presumed that tests are "medically necessary," but it is likely this will be interpreted more strictly in the future. Appropriate reimbursement for even clearly indicated molecular tests is a significant issue currently, and this could very well lead to limited offering of molecular assays.

A long-standing requirement in the United States has been that assay results used in patient-management decisions or to counsel patients must be generated in a laboratory licensed under CLIA, and for molecular assays, a laboratory licensed for "high complexity" testing. This requirement was previously underappreciated by the research laboratories that developed many of these assays, but is likely to lead to closer collaborations between research and clinical laboratories in the future. It also is possible that standardized FDA-approved assays will become commercially attractive to develop, particularly for cancers that are more common, especially if a test result is linked to a specific decision on therapy.

SUMMARY

Over the next two decades, molecular diagnostic assays will be increasingly important tools for the determination of tumor diagnosis, prognosis, and residual presence, as well as initial and follow-up therapy. Targeted molecular markers will likely remain useful and be the predominant tests for the near future. However, validated panels of markers or expression profiling of tumors by using microarrays or proteomic methods show potential to supplement or replace single markers dramatically in determining diagnosis, prognosis, and whether available therapies will be beneficial. New understandings of molecular pathogenesis in cancer will continue to grow, with valuable contributions from microarray and proteomics studies, we hope leading to targeted therapies and opportunities to monitor therapy with molecular assays. Intellectual property positions may limit the rate at which useful clinical applications can be developed because of licensing and cost considerations. Increasing demands will be placed on physicians to ensure that patients understand the impact molecular tests on decisions for their management.

i J. Sokoll and Daniel W. Chan

Clinical Chemistry: Tumor Markers

SERUM TUMOR MARKERS SUMMARY

KEY METHODS
- Radioimmunoassay and more recently enzyme-linked immunosorbent assay (ELISA) are cornerstones of methods.
- Monoclonal antibodies have been produced against a wide variety of secreted antigens.

APPLICATIONS
Screening and Early Detection
- In most tumor systems, low prevalence of disease means that routine population screening is not possible, although screening can be combined with other approaches to improve specificity.
- In some high-prevalence situations tumor marker screening is appropriate, for example, PSA for prostate cancer.

Diagnosis
- Levels of particular markers are useful adjuncts to diagnosis in many tumor systems including ovarian cancer, germ cell tumors, or neuroendocrine tumors.

- In some tumor systems, serum markers contribute to staging information and help direct therapy.

Monitoring
- Most serum tumor markers are useful to monitor treatement or progression of cancer.
- Decrease of tumor marker levels can be used as a means to assess successful surgery or chemotherapy.
- Increase in a tumor marker can be a harbinger of relapse or disease progression.

Tumor markers, also called cancer markers, biomarkers, and, in some instances, cancer-associated antigens, are substances present in or produced by a tumor itself or produced by the host in response to a tumor that can be used to differentiate a tumor from normal tissue or to determine the presence of a tumor based on measurement in the blood or secretions. Such substances can be found in cells, tissues, or body fluids. They can be measured qualitatively or quantitatively by chemical, immunologic, or molecular biologic methods to identify the presence of a cancer. A wide spectrum of molecules is classified as tumor markers including enzymes, hormones, oncofetal antigens, carbohydrate markers, blood group antigens, proteins, receptors, and genes or gene products.[221] Although strictly speaking, tumor markers can be recovered from any tissue or fluid and identified by use of proteomic testing (see previous section), this chapter is devoted largely to those that are secreted and detectable in serum.

The first recognized tumor marker was the Bence-Jones protein, discovered in 1847 by precipitation of a protein in acidified boiled urine. This protein, the monoclonal light chain of immunoglobulins secreted by tumor plasma cells, is still in use in the diagnosis of multiple myeloma. The first half of the twentieth century included the discovery of hormones, such as human chorionic gonadotropin (hCG), and enzymes, such as acid phophatase (for prostate cancer), and isoenzymes and proteins that have altered concentrations in biologic fluids in malignancy. The discoveries of α-fetoprotein (AFP) and carcinoembryonic antigen (CEA) in the 1960s led to the use of tumor markers for monitoring and to the use of the term *onco-developmental markers* because of the production of these markers in fetal development and in tumors.

An ideal tumor marker should be specific for a given type of cancer and undetectable in healthy people or in those with benign disease, as well as sensitive enough to detect small tumors for early diagnosis or during screening. Unfortunately, most known tumor markers are neither specific nor sensitive enough for these purposes. Other desirable characteristics include concentrations proportional to tumor volume, short half-lives to allow early assessment of response to therapy, predictable increases and decreases in concentration responding to cancer progression and regression, and ability to be measured in a standardized and reproducible fashion in easily accessible specimens. Tumor markers are most useful in evaluating the progression of disease status after the initial therapy, and monitoring the effectiveness of subsequent treatment.[221-223]

Despite the numerous tumor markers that have been reported, relatively few are in routine clinical use. Practice guidelines and recommendations for the use of tumor markers in a range of cancers have been developed by groups of scientists and clinicians from the National Academy of Clinical Biochemistry[224] and the European Group on Tumor Markers,[225] although scientist and clinician viewpoints on the use of tumor markers do not always agree. The use of tumor markers is also included in Practice Guidelines in Oncology from the National Comprehensive Cancer Network[226] and the American Society for Clinical Oncology has published recommendations for selected cancers.[227] Practice guidelines from these and other national and international organizations are summarized by Fleisher and colleagues[224] and Sturgeon.[228]

Tumor marker use in the United States is limited in comparison to that in other countries as a result of required approval by regulatory agencies such as the Food and Drug Administration (FDA), which influences reimbursement. In addition, the FDA, which uses the term *tumor-associated antigens immunologic tests*, typically

TABLE 17-10

FDA-Approved Tumor Markers

ANALYTE	ASSOCIATED CANCER	DESIGNATED INDICATION
Serum, Plasma		
CA15-3, CA27.29	Breast	Monitoring; recurrence
HER-2/neu	Breast	Monitoring
CA125	Ovarian	Monitoring; second-look evaluation
CA19-9	Pancreatic	Monitoring
Total PSA, complexed PSA (cPSA)	Prostate	Detection in men aged 50 years or older in conjunction with digital rectal examination (DRE); monitoring; prognosis
Free PSA	Prostate	Aid in distinguishing prostate cancer from benign prostate conditions in men 50 yaers or older with a total PSA of 4–10 ng/mL and nonsuggestive DRE in conjunction with total PSA (% free PSA)
Prostatic acid phosphatase	Prostate	Monitoring
Carcinoembryonic antigen (CEA)	Colorectal, breast, lung	Monitoring; prognosis
α-Fetoprotein (AFP)	Nonseminomatous testicular	Monitoring
Thyroglobulin	Thyroid	Monitoring (in patients without thyroglobulin autoantibodies)
β-Human chorionic gonadotropin (β-hCG)	None	Detection of pregnancy (not approved as a tumor marker)
Urine		
BTA *stat,* BTA TRAK, FDP	Bladder	Management in conjunction with cystoscopy
NMP-22	Bladder	Diagnosis in symptomatic patients or those with risk factors; recurrence
Tissue		
Estrogen and progesterone receptors	Breast	Assessing the likelihood of response to therapy; prognosis and management
HER-2/neu	Breast	Assessment of patients for whom herceptin (transtuzumab) treatment is being considered

BTA bladder tumor antigen; FDA, Food and Drug Administration; FDP, Fibrin Degradation Products; NMP, nucleus matrix protein; PSA, prostate specific antigen.

approves assays for specific clinical applications that may limit their use in other clinical settings. Currently approved markers and associated cancers and applications are listed in Table 17-10.

METHODS

The introduction of *radioimmunoassay* in the 1960s and of *enzyme-linked immunosorbant assays* (ELISAs) and monoclonal antibodies in the 1970s was instrumental in the tumor-marker field with respect to marker measurement and discovery. New cell-surface antigens identified with the use of monoclonal antibodies, including the carbohydrate antigens CA125, CA15-3, and CA19-9, have improved clinical sensitivity and specificity compared with the oncofetal antigens. Recently, studies of oncogenes and tumor-suppressor genes, as well as development of molecular techniques such as recombinant DNA technology, polymerase chain reaction (PCR), and automated sequencing, have resulted in the understanding and use of tumor markers at the molecular level.[221,222] New methods, such as those using the proteomic technique SELDI (surface-enhanced laser desorption/ionization), which combines ProteinChip arrays with time-of-flight mass spectrometry,[216,229] will have a significant impact not only on the discovery of new tumor markers, but also on the way they are measured.

CLINICAL APPLICATIONS OF TUMOR MARKERS

Screening and Early Detection

When screening for a disease, several factors must be taken into account. The disease must be important, common, and cause substantial morbidity and mortality. An understanding of the natural history of the disease must assure that early detection can play a role in reversal of the clinical course, and effective treatment must be available. The testing method also should be economical and noninvasive. When deciding to apply screening techniques, particularly if biochemical or immuno-chemical markers are used, an understanding of the analytic sensitivity (lowest detectable limit) and analytic specificity (extraneous interference) is essential. The precision of the assay (ability to reproduce the results) also must be known and acceptable for use in large population studies. In addition to high analytic sensitivity and specificity, and acceptable clinical sensitivity and specificity, it is important that there be a high prevalence of the disease in the population, as this affects the positive predictive value.[230]

Screening programs can be successful in regions or populations where specific cancers are highly prevalent. AFP concentrations have been used as a screening test for germ cell tumors in high-incidence areas including China, Japan, Taiwan, Africa, and Alaska. With a cutoff in the range of 10 to 20 μg/L, AFP has been shown to have a sensitivity of between 60% and 90% and a corresponding specificity of 70% to 80%, although hepatitis and cirrhosis also may be considered possible causes of elevated values.[221,223] The American Cancer Society (ACS) has published specific recommendations for the early detection of breast, colorectal, prostate, and cervical cancers,[231] although among these cancers, the only serum tumor marker that is part of any screening algorithm is PSA (see later).

Because individual tumor markers cannot be used for screening in a population in which the prevalence of the disease is low, an approach to improve their utility is to combine analysis of the marker with other procedures. In ovarian cancer, for example, strategies have included combining CA125 with ultrasound or using a two-stage strategy in which ultrasonography is performed only if CA125 concentrations are elevated. In a study of 4000 women, specificity of CA125 plus ultrasound was 99.9% compared with 98.3% for CA125 alone. Other strategies that have been proposed to improve the specificity of CA125 include the use of multiple markers, including OVX1 and M-CSF. However, requiring elevation of all markers, while increasing specificity, sacrifices sensitivity; similarly, if elevation of only one marker is used as an indicator of disease, then specificity is lost.[232,233]

As noted earlier, probably the best tumor marker for screening is PSA. Although it is for all intents and purposes organ specific, it is not cancer specific. PSA may be elevated (>4 ng/mL) in men with benign prostatic disease such as benign prostatic hyperplasia (BPH). PSA elevations also may occur with aging and with conditions such as prostatitis. Thus a number of methods have been proposed to increase the clinical utility of PSA for the early detection and diagnosis of prostate cancer, particularly in the diagnostic gray zone of 4 to 10 ng/mL, where there is significant overlap in PSA concentrations between prostate cancer and BPH. These approaches include age-specific reference ranges, PSA density, PSA velocity, and PSA molecular forms.[234,235] The premise behind age-specific references (0 to 2.5, 3.5, 4.5, and 6.5 for age ranges 40 to 49, 50 to 59, 60 to 69, and 70 to 79 years, respectively) is that lowering the upper end of the reference range in younger men would potentially increase sensitivity and aid in detecting organ-confined tumors earlier when surgery may be curative, whereas extending the range in older men would increase specificity, taking into account small increases in prostate volume, and PSA production and secretion with aging. However, because extending the range in older men may miss significant cancers, the use of age-adjusted ranges is controversial.

Assessment of *PSA density*, the ratio of PSA to prostate volume determined by transrectal ultrasound, is another method to increase PSA specificity; this assessment attempts to adjust for the increased volume often found in BPH. Limitations to PSA density include inaccuracies in measurement of prostate size and reduced sensitivity of prostate cancer detection. *PSA velocity*, similar to an approach used with CA125 for ovarian cancer, is defined as the change in PSA concentrations over time. A velocity

of 0.75 ng/mL per year or more is suggestive of cancer. At least three PSA measurements 12 to 18 months apart are needed to calculate velocity. The effectiveness of this approach may be diminished by interassay and inter-laboratory variation.

The most successful approach to increase the clinical utility of PSA in the 4- to 10-ng/mL range is assessment of the free and complexed forms of the PSA molecule. In the early 1990s, it was discovered that the majority of PSA measured in serum is complexed to protease inhibitors (~80% to 90%), with only a small portion in the free or unbound form. It also was discovered that men with prostate cancer, benign prostate disease, and no disease may differ in the proportions of free PSA and PSA bound to α_1-antichymotrypsin. Although the mechanism is at present unknown, patients with prostate cancer have a lower percentage of free PSA (free PSA/total PSA) compared with men with benign disease. By using a cutoff of 25% in men with a negative digital rectal examination (DRE), 95% of cancers can be detected while sparing 20% of unnecessary biopsies.[234]

Tumor Markers in Diagnosis

Lack of sensitivity and specificity limits the use of tumor markers for cancer diagnosis, although in contrast to screening, prevalence of disease is likely to be higher in diagnostic situations. In most cases, histologic confirmation in tissue remains the gold standard for primary diagnosis, although tumor markers can still play a useful role in conjunction with other measures or procedures. For instance, tumor markers may aid in differentiating benign and malignant disease, or in identifying histologic tumor type.[223]

Despite the controversy over the use of CA125 in the early detection of ovarian cancer, CA125 is more accepted as an adjunct in distinguishing benign from malignant disease in women, particularly in postmenopausal women with ovarian masses,[236] where elevated concentrations of CA125 greater than 95 U/mL in postmenopausal women can discriminate malignant from benign pelvic masses with a positive predictive value of 95%.[233] In premenopausal women, benign conditions resulting in elevated CA125 levels may be a confounding factor. The multiple-markers approach has been applied to the preoperative discrimination of malignant and benign pelvic masses by using a number of analytic techniques.[237,238]

AFP can play a useful role in the classification of germ cell tumors. AFP is the major serum protein of the early fetus synthesized by the fetal gut, liver cells, and yolk sac, and hCG, which is a glycoprotein consisting of two distinct subunits and synthesized and secreted by the placental syncytiotrophoblast, of tumor type. In seminomas, AFP is not elevated, whereas hCG is present in 10% to 30% of cases. Either hCG or AFP or both are produced by 60% to 90% of nonseminomatous germ cell testicular tumors at the time of diagnosis. Both markers are elevated in embryonal carcinoma (hCG, >65%; AFP, >70%), whereas these markers are not useful in teratomas. AFP is elevated in yolk sac tumors, whereas hCG is elevated in choriocarcinomas, and therefore useful in gestational trophoblastic disease as well. Typical reference values for AFP are 10 to 15 µg/L, whereas 5 IU/L is often used as a cutoff for hCG in testicular cancer. Total β-hCG assays, measuring both intact hCG and the free β-subunit, may be preferable because of the production of free β-subunits in cancer.[221]

Other tumor markers play a role in testicular cancers. Placental alkaline phosphatase, another oncodevelopmental marker, can be elevated in seminomas in addition to a number of other cancers. Sensitivity is increased when it is combined with the nonspecific enzyme marker lactate dehydrogenase (LDH). LDH concentrations further correlate with tumor burden and therefore prognosis.[221,239]

Tumor markers also may play a role in the diagnosis of neuroendocrine tumors.[221,223,240] For example, the diagnosis of pheochromocytoma is usually established with an increase in the urinary excretion of catecholamines or catecholamine metabolites. Similarly, catecholamine metabolites vanillylmandelic acid (VMA) and homovanillic acid (HVA) are beneficial in neuroblastoma. Calcitonin is used in medullary thyroid cancer, with increased diagnostic sensitivity resulting from stimulation of calcitonin release with pentagastrin, whereas urinary 5-hydroxyindoleacetic acid (5-HIAA) is the primary test for overproduction of serotonin in carcinoid tumors, and specific circulating serum tumor markers may aid in the diagnosis of pancreatic endocrine tumors. It also has been suggested that neuron-specific enolase (NSE), an isoenzyme of the glycolytic enzyme enolase found predominantly in neurons and neuroendocrine cells and elevated in neuroendocrine tumors, may be helpful in the diagnosis of small cell lung cancer in the small percentage of cases in which it is not possible to establish a final diagnosis by biopsy.

Prognosis/Prediction of Therapeutic Response

The clinical staging of cancer can be aided by tumor markers, because the serum level of the marker reflects tumor burden. The marker value at the time of diagnosis may be used as a prognostic indicator for disease progression and patient survival. This is possible for an individual patient, but different levels of markers produced by different tumors do not usually allow the clinician to determine the prognosis of a tumor from the initial level or to assign specific therapies.[221] However, tumor markers may be included as staging criteria for some cancers, as, for example, with CEA and colorectal cancer,[241] LDH in lymphoma,[242] or LDH, hCG, and AFP in testicular germ cell tumors.[243]

Monitoring Disease

Most serum tumor markers are used to monitor treatment and progression of cancer. Markers may be used to determine the success of the initial treatment (e.g., surgery or radiation), detect the recurrence of cancer, and monitor the effectiveness of treatment.[241] To determine the success of surgery, an elevated marker level before surgery should decrease after a successful operation. The rate of decrease is predicted by using the half-life of the marker. If the half-life after treatment is longer than the expected half-life, it can be assumed that the treatment has not been successful in removing the tumor. The magnitude of marker reduction may, however, reflect the degree of success of the treatment or the extent of disease involvement. PSA is particularly useful for determining the success of initial surgical or radiation treatment of prostate cancer. After radical prostatectomy, PSA concentrations should decrease to undetectable levels if the tumor was organ confined and all prostatic tissue was removed. After allowing for sufficient clearance of pretreatment PSA (total PSA half-life of 2 to 3 days), finding detectable post-treatment PSA suggests remaining prostate tissue or the presence of metastases.[234]

With the recurrence of cancer after a successful initial treatment, marker values may not appear within the normal half-life. They may decrease to a steady level that is higher than normal, or remain within the reference interval for healthy individuals. A subsequent increase in the marker values suggests recurrence of the cancer.[221] Serum tumor markers may detect recurrence of disease before clinical evidence, so-called biochemical recurrence. Ultrasensitive PSA assays allow earlier detection of prostate cancer after radical prostatectomy. In breast cancer patients receiving adjuvant chemotherapy, the breast cancer marker CA27.29 has been shown to detect recurrent disease before any clinical evidence appears. Early detection of cancer recurrence may be helpful to initiate early treatment or change therapy, although it is useful only if effect treatment is available.[230]

Levels of most tumor marker correlate with the effectiveness of treatment and response to therapy. In breast cancer, the concentration of markers such as CA27.29 changes with the treatment and the clinical outcome of the patient, as does CEA in colorectal cancer and CA125 in ovarian cancer. Marker values usually increase with progressive disease, decrease with remission, and do not change significantly with stable disease. Tumor-marker kinetics are generally more important than individual values, although interpretation of kinetic changes may be complicated. For example, marker values in response to treatment may show an initial delay before demonstrating the expected pattern of change.[244]

The Working Group on Tumor Marker Criteria of the International Society for Oncodevelopmental Biology and Medicine has published the following criteria for the interpretation of changes in tumor marker values.[245] "If no therapy is given, at least a linear increase in three consecutive samples (i.e., two time intervals) on a log scale should be registered to establish a recurrence. Usual intervals could be 3 months but are clinically determined. After a first increase, next samples should be taken after 2 to 4 weeks, irrespective of the absolute level." If therapy is given, the changes in marker values should reflect the clinical progression of the disease. "Progressive disease is defined by an increase in the marker level of at least 25%. Sampling should be repeated within 2 to 4 weeks for additional evidence. The sampling interval during therapy may depend on the type of tumor and should be related to clinical follow-up." A decrease in marker value of at least 50% is indicative of partial remission "with the concept that tumor load is related to the changes in serum tumor marker levels." The Working Group also provided a general opinion that "a complete remission cannot be determined by tumor marker levels, but if tumor marker levels are elevated, the clinical decision of complete remission based on conventional methods should be considered incorrect unless an explanation for the presence of an elevated level is given."

ANALYTIC CONSIDERATIONS

A number of clinical and analytic limitations should be considered in the interpretation and use of tumor markers.[244,246] Physiological influences to be considered include biologic variability, effects of aging and menopause, and half-life and route of elimination. Tumor markers can be elevated as result of renal failure, liver failure, and cholestasis, depending on whether the marker is eliminated through glomerular filtration or metabolized by the liver. For example, serum CEA concentrations may elevated in patients with liver disease. False-positive marker results may reflect, for example, prostatitis with PSA, or inflammation of serous membranes or biliary ducts with CA125 and CA19-9, respectively.[246] Smokers have higher concentrations of CEA in comparison to non-smokers, and reference ranges for CEA in lung cancer typically are stratified by smoking status. This underscores the importance of selection of cutoff values with respect to selection of reference groups. Knowledge of the reference group as healthy individuals or patients with benign diseases will influence interpretation.[244]

Knowledge of the tumor-marker level before surgery is important for subsequent use in monitoring because markers are not 100% sensitive, even in advanced disease, and tumors can be nonsecreting. For example, CA19-9, a sialylated derivative of the Lewis[a] blood group antigen, is not expressed in the estimated 3% to 5% of population with the Lewis[a-b-] genotype.[221] Treatment also may influence marker concentrations, with increased release with chemotherapy or surgery, such as the spike observed in CA125 concentrations after abdominal surgery.[223] Tumor manipulation also can influence concentrations, as evidenced by the increased PSA concentrations observed after prostate biopsy, transurethral resection, prostate massage, or other procedures. Although influence of DRE is thought to be minimal, it is recommended that blood for PSA measurements be drawn before the procedure or a minimum of 1 week after the DRE.[247]

One of the most critical analytic considerations affecting tumor-marker result interpretation is the fact that different assays, specifically immunoassays, may give different values for the same marker. Therefore values cannot be used interchangeably, and it is recommended that patients be followed up by using the same laboratory method. Clinicians also should be informed when laboratories change tumor-marker assay methods and be offered a crossover period and an explanation of the

association between the old and new assays. Differing results among assays can be attributed to calibration differences resulting from different materials, value assignments, antibody types and specificities, assay designs and kinetics, variations in reference ranges or cutoffs, and assay robustness.[246,248,249]

Factors affecting assay robustness include assay measuring range, encompassing the detection limit and upper limit where sample dilution is not required, accuracy and precision of dilutional linearity, high dose-hook effect, and interferences from endogenous antibodies. Endogenous antibodies include anti-analyte antibodies such as thyroglobulin autoantibodies and anti-reagent antibodies such as heterophile and human anti-mouse antibodies (HAMAs). HAMAs, which may occur as a result of treatment with monoclonal antibodies or immunoscintigraphy with antibodies similar to assay antibodies, can bind to reagent antibodies with resulting falsely high or low values, depending on assay design. HAMA can be minimized by using chimeric antibodies in vivo and at the assay level by choice of assay antibodies and inclusion of nonimmune animal serum as a blocking technique.[221,249]

FUTURE DIRECTIONS

With current advances in proteomic and genomic technology, the diagnosis of disease in the future will be based on the combination of methods, with classification based on molecular as opposed to morphologic features. Unique gene or protein profiles of multiple biomarkers, accounting for cancer heterogeneity, will be measured in tissue, cells, and body fluids. The analysis of panels of protein biomarkers may be performed by traditional ELISA, antibody-based protein chips, or microarrays. Furthermore, many more diagnostic tests will be generated as the result of genomic and proteomic discoveries. For example, serum biomarkers for a number of cancers recently have been identified by using SELDI-TOF.[216,217,229,250] Integrated diagnostic tools that combine these methods with molecular imaging techniques will be used, and bioinformatics will play a key role. The rapid translation of tests from the laboratory to the bedside will elevate the importance of laboratory testing in cancer diagnosis and care of the cancer patient.

REFERENCES

1. Virchow RL: Disease, Life and Man; Selected Essays. Stanford, CA, Stanford University Press, 1958.
2. Rosai J: Some considerations on the origin, evolution, and outlook of American surgical pathology. In Rosai J (ed): Guiding the Surgeon's Hand: The History of American Surgical Pathology. Washington, DC, American Registry of Pathology, Armed Forces Institute of Pathology, 1997, pp 1-5.
3. Fechner RE: The birth and evolution of American surgical pathology. In Rosai J (ed): Guiding the Surgeon's Hand: The History of American Surgical Pathology. Washington, DC, American Registry of Pathology, Armed Forces Institute of Pathology, 1997, pp 7-21.
4. Wright JR Jr: The development of the frozen section technique:

The evolution of surgical biopsy, and the origins of surgical pathology. Bull Hist Med 1985;59:295–326.

5. Bloodgood JC: Prevention, diagnosis and treatment of cancer in its earliest stages. South Med J 1926;19:287–292.

6. Rosai J: Standardized reporting of surgical pathology diagnoses for the major tumor types: A proposal. The Department of Pathology, Memorial Sloan-Kettering Cancer Center. Am J Clin Pathol 1993;100:240–255.

7. Association of Directors of Anatomic and Surgical Pathology: Recommendations for reporting soft tissue sarcomas. Am J Clin Pathol 1999;111:594–598.

8. Association of Directors of Anatomic and Surgical Pathology: Recommendations for the reporting of specimens containing oral cavity and oropharynx neoplasms. Am J Clin Pathol 2000;114:336–338.

9. Association of Directors of Anatomic and Surgical Pathology Agency: Recommendations for the reporting of resected prostate carcinomas. Hum Pathol 1996;27:321–323.

10. Association of Directors of Anatomic and Surgical Pathology: Recommendations for the reporting of breast carcinoma. Hum Pathol 1996;27:220–223.

11. Westra WH: General approach to surgical pathology specimens. In Hruban RH, Westra WH, Phelps TH, Isacson C (eds): Surgical Pathology Dissection: An Illustrated Guide. New York, Springer-Verlag, 1996, pp 1–13.

12. Rosai J, Sobin LH (eds): Atlas of Tumor Pathology, 3rd series. Washington, DC: Armed Forces Institute of Pathology, 1991.

13. Kleihues P, Sobin LH (eds): World Health Organization Classification of Tumors. Lyon, France, IARC Press, 2000.

14. Greene FL, Page DL, Fleming ID, et al. (eds): AJCC Cancer Staging Manual, 6th ed. Philadelphia, Lippincott Williams & Wilkins, 2002.

15. Ackerman LV, Ramirez GA: The indications for and limitations of frozen section diagnosis: A review of 1,269 consecutive frozen section diagnoses. Br J Surg 1959;46:336–350.

16. Zarbo RJ, Schmidt WA, Bachner P, et al: Indications and immediate patient outcomes of pathology intraoperative consultations: College of American Pathologists/Centers for Disease Control and Prevention Outcomes Working Group Study. Arch Pathol Lab Med 1996;120:19–25.

17. Westra WH, Pritchett DD, Udelsman R: Intraoperative confirmation of parathyroid tissue during parathyroid exploration: A retrospective evaluation of the frozen section. Am J Surg Pathol 1998;22:538–544.

18. Wick MR: Intraoperative consultations in pathology: A current perspective. Am J Clin Pathol 1995;104:239–242.

19. Ferreiro JA, Myers JL, Bostwick DG: Accuracy of frozen section diagnosis in surgical pathology: Review of a 1-year experience with 24,880 cases at Mayo Clinic Rochester. Mayo Clin Proc 1995;70:1137–1141.

20. Zarbo RJ, Hoffman GG, Howanitz PJ: Interinstitutional comparison of frozen-section consultation: A College of American Pathologists Q-Probe study of 79,647 consultations in 297 North American institutions. Arch Pathol Lab Med 1991;115:1187–1194.

21. Coons AH, Creech HJ, Jones RN: Immunological properties of an antibody containing a fluorescent group. Exp Biol Med 1941;47:200.

22. Chan JK: Advances in immunohistochemistry: impact on surgical pathology practice. Semin Diagn Pathol 2000;17:170–177.

23. Taylor CR, Shi S-R, Barr NJ, Wu N: Techniques of Immunohistochemistry: Principles, Pitfalls, and Standardization. In Dabbs DJ (ed): Diagnostic Immunohistochemistry. New York, Churchill Livingstone, 2002, pp 3–43.

24. Wick MR, Ritter JH, Swanson PE: The impact of diagnostic immunohistochemistry on patient outcomes. Clin Lab Med 1999;19:797–814, vi.

25. Shah RB, Zhou M, LeBlanc M, Snyder M, Rubin MA: Comparison of the basal cell-specific markers, 34betaE12 and p63, in the diagnosis of prostate cancer. Am J Surg Pathol 2002;26:1161–1168.

26. Kronz JD, Westra WH, Epstein JI: Mandatory second opinion surgical pathology at a large referral hospital. Cancer 1999;86:2426–2435.

27. Westra WH, Kronz JD, Eisele DW: The impact of second opinion surgical pathology on the practice of head and neck surgery: A

decade experience at a large referral hospital. Head Neck 2002;24:684–693.

28. Chu PG, Chang KL, Arber DA, Weiss LM: Immunophenotyping of hematopoietic neoplasms. Semin Diagn Pathol 2000;17:236–256.

29. Devoe K, Weidner N: Immunohistochemistry of small round-cell tumors. Semin Diagn Pathol 2000;17:216–224.

30. Suster S: Recent advances in the application of immuno-histochemical markers for the diagnosis of soft tissue tumors. Semin Diagn Pathol 2000;17:225–235.

31. Moran CA, Wick MR, Suster S: The role of immunohistochemistry in the diagnosis of malignant mesothelioma. Semin Diagn Pathol 2000;17:178–183.

32. *Immunoquery* [Dennis M. Frisman] [Online] 10/27/02—last updated. Available: http://www.immunoquery.com [Accessed 1/2003]

33. Yared MA, Middleton LP, Smith TL, et al: Recommendations for sentinel lymph node processing in breast cancer. Am J Surg Pathol 2002;26:377–382.

34. Baisden BL, Askin FB, Lange JR, Westra WH: HMB-45 immuno-histochemical staining of sentinel lymph nodes: A specific method for enhancing detection of micrometastases in patients with melanoma. Am J Surg Pathol 2000;24:1140–1146.

35. Brown DC, Gatter KC: Ki67 protein: the immaculate deception? Histopathology 2002;40:2–11.

36. Nunes RA, Harris LN: The HER2 extracellular domain as a prognostic and predictive factor in breast cancer. Clin Breast Cancer 2002;3:125–135.

37. Hayes DF, Thor AD: c-ErbB-2 in breast cancer: Development of a clinically useful marker. Semin Oncol 2002;29:231–245.

38. Griffin J: The biology of signal transduction inhibition: Basic science to novel therapies. Semin Oncol 2001;28:3–8.

39. Seidal T, Balaton AJ, Battifora H: Interpretation and quantification of immunostains. Am J Surg Pathol 2001;25:1204–1207.

40. Gharib H: Fine-needle aspiration biopsy of thyroid nodules: Advantages, limitations, and effect. Mayo Clin Proc 1994;69:44–49.

41. Amedee RG, Dhurandhar NR: Fine-needle aspiration biopsy. Laryngoscope 2001;111:1551–1557.

42. Ellis GL, Auclair PL: Fine-needle aspiration biopsy of salivary glands. In Ellis GL, Auclair PL (eds): Tumors of the Salivary Glands. Washington, DC, Armed Forces Institute of Pathology, 1995, p 441.

43. El-Naggar AK: Methods in molecular surgical pathology. Semin Diagn Pathol 2002;19:56–71.

44. Gabrielson E, Berg K, Anbazhagan R: Functional genomics, gene arrays, and the future of pathology. Mod Pathol 2001;14:1294–1299.

45. Chan JK: The new World Health Organization classification of lymphomas: The past, the present and the future. Hematol Oncol 2001;19:129–150.

46. Sen F, Vega F, Medeiros LJ: Molecular genetic methods in the diagnosis of hematologic neoplasms. Semin Diagn Pathol 2002;19:72–93.

47. Singer S: New diagnostic modalities in soft tissue sarcoma. Semin Surg Oncol 1999;17:11–22.

48. Jones D, Fletcher CD: How shall we apply the new biology to diagnostics in surgical pathology? J Pathol 1999;187:147–153.

49. Braylan RC, Orfao A, Borowitz MJ, et al: Optimal number of reagents required to evaluate hematolymphoid neoplasias: Results of an international consensus meeting. Cytometry 2001;46:23–27.

50. Stewart CC, Behm FG, Carey JL, et al: U.S.–Canadian Consensus recommendations on the immunophenotypic analysis of hematologic neoplasia by flow cytometry: Selection of antibody combinations. Cytometry 1997;30:231–235.

51. Borowitz MJ, Guenther KL, Shults KE, Stelzer GT: Immunophenotyping of acute leukemia by flow cytometric analysis: use of CD45 and right angle light scatter to gate on leukemic blasts Am J Clin Pathol 1993;100:534–540.

52. Braylan RC, Atwater SK, Diamond L, et al: U.S.–Canadian Consensus recommendations on the immunophenotypic analysis of hematologic neoplasia by flow cytometry: Data reporting. Cytometry 1997;30:245–248.

53. Khalidi HS, Chang KL, Medeiros LJ, et al: Acute lymphoblastic leukemia: Survey of immunophenotype, French-American-British classification, frequency of myeloid antigen expression, and

karyotypic abnormalities in 210 pediatric and adult cases. Am J Clin Pathol 1999;111:467-476.

54. Boldt DH, Kopecky KJ, Head D, et al: Expression of myeloid antigens by blast cells in acute lymphoblastic leukemia of adults: The Southwest Oncology Group experience. Leukemia 1994;8:2118-2126.

55. Bene MC, Castoldi G, Knapp W, et al: Proposals for the immunological classification of acute leukemias: European Group for the Immunological Characterization of Leukemias (EGIL). Leukemia 1995;9:1783-1786.

56. Hrusak O, Porwit-MacDonald A: Antigen expression patterns reflecting genotype of acute leukemias. Leukemia 2002;16:1233-1258.

57. Ludwig WD, Bartram CR, Harbott J, et al: Phenotypic and genotypic heterogeneity in infant acute leukemia, I: Acute lymphoblastic leukemia. Leukemia 1989;3:431-439.

58. Wuchter C, Harbott J, Schoch C, et al: Detection of acute leukemia cells with mixed lineage leukemia (MLL) gene rearrangements by flow cytometry using monoclonal antibody 7.1. Leukemia 2000;14:1232-1238.

59. Borowitz MJ, Rubnitz J, Nash M, et al: Surface antigen phenotype can predict TEL-AML1 rearrangement in childhood B-precursor ALL: A Pediatric Oncology Group study. Leukemia 1998;12:1764-1770.

60. Borowitz MJ, Hunger SP, Carroll AJ, et al: Predictability of the t(1;19)(q23;p13) from surface antigen phenotype: Implications for screening cases of childhood acute lymphoblastic leukemia for molecular analysis: A Pediatric Oncology Group study. Blood 1993;82:1086-1091.

61. Orfao A, Chillon MC, Bortoluci AM, et al: The flow cytometric pattern of CD34, CD15 and CD13 expression in acute myeloblastic leukemia is highly characteristic of the presence of PML-RARalpha gene rearrangements. Haematologica 1999;84:405-412.

62. Porwit-MacDonald A, Janossy G, Ivory K, et al: Leukemia-associated changes identified by quantitative flow cytometry. IV. CD34 overexpression in acute myelogenous leukemia M2 with t(8;21). Blood 1996;87:1162-1169.

63. Ogata K, Nakamura K, Yokose N, et al: Clinical significance of phenotypic features of blasts in patients with myelodysplastic syndrome. Blood 2002;100:3887-3896.

64. Stetler-Stevenson M, Arthur DC, Jabbour N, et al: Diagnostic utility of flow cytometric immunophenotyping in myelodysplastic syndrome. Blood 2001;98:979-987.

65. van Dongen JJ, Seriu T, Panzer-Grumayer ER, et al: Prognostic value of minimal residual disease in acute lymphoblastic leukaemia in childhood. Lancet 1998;352:1731-1738.

66. Cave H, van der Werff ten Bosch J, Suciu S, et al: Clinical significance of minimal residual disease in childhood acute lymphoblastic leukemia: European Organization for Research and Treatment of Cancer—Childhood Leukemia Cooperative Group. N Engl J Med 1998;339:591-598.

67. Dworzak MN, Froschl G, Printz D, et al: Prognostic significance and modalities of flow cytometric minimal residual disease detection in childhood acute lymphoblastic leukemia. Blood 2002;99:1952-1958.

68. Campana D, Neale GA, Coustan-Smith E, Pui CH: Detection of minimal residual disease in acute lymphoblastic leukemia: the St Jude experience. Leukemia 2001;15:278-279.

69. Sanchez J, Serrano J, Gomez P, et al: Clinical value of immunological monitoring of minimal residual disease in acute lymphoblastic leukaemia after allogeneic transplantation. Br J Haematol 2002;116:686-694.

70. Krampera M, Vitale A, Vincenzi C, et al: Outcome prediction by immunophenotypic minimal residual disease detection in adult T-cell acute lymphoblastic leukaemia. Br J Haematol 2003;120:74-79.

71. San Miguel JF, Vidriales MB, Lopez-Berges C, et al: Early immunophenotypical evaluation of minimal residual disease in acute myeloid leukemia identifies different patient risk groups and may contribute to postinduction treatment stratification. Blood 2001;98:1746-1751.

72. San Miguel JF, Martinez A, Macedo A, et al: Immunophenotyping investigation of minimal residual disease is a useful approach for predicting relapse in acute myeloid leukemia patients. Blood 1997;90:2465-2470.

73. Weir EG, Cowan K, LeBeau P, Borowitz MJ: A limited antibody panel can distinguish B-precursor acute lymphoblastic leukemia from normal B precursors with four color flow cytometry: Implications for residual disease detection. Leukemia 1999;13:558-567.

74. Lucio P, Gaipa G, van Lochem EG, et al: BIOMED-I concerted action report: flow cytometric immunophenotyping of precursor B-ALL with standardized triple-stainings: BIOMED-1 Concerted Action Investigation of Minimal Residual Disease in Acute Leukemia: International Standardization and Clinical Evaluation. Leukemia 2001;15:1185-1192.

75. Campana D, Coustan-Smith E, Janossy G: The immunologic detection of minimal residual disease in acute leukemia. Blood 1990;76:163-171.

76. Tomova A, Babusikova O: Shifts in expression of immunological cell markers in relapsed acute leukemia. Neoplasma 2001;48:164-168.

77. Stetler-Stevenson M, Braylan RC: Flow cytometric analysis of lymphomas and lymphoproliferative disorders. Semin Hematol 2001;38:111-123.

78. Echeverri C, Fisher S, King D, Craig D: Immunophenotypic variability of B-cell non-Hodgkin lymphoma: a retrospective study of cases analyzed by flow cytometry. Am J Clin Pathol 2002;117:615-620.

79. Tbakhi A, Edinger M, Myles J, Pohlmann B, Tubbs RR: Flow cytometric immunophenotyping of non-Hodgkin's lymphomas and related disorders. Cytometry 1996;25:113-124.

80. DiGiuseppe JA, Borowitz MJ: Clinical utility of flow cytometry in the chronic lymphoid leukemias. Semin Oncol 1998;25:6-10.

81. Duque RE, Andreeff M, Braylan RC, Diamond LW, Peiper SC: Consensus review of the clinical utility of DNA flow cytometry in neoplastic hematopathology. Cytometry 1993;14:492-496.

82. Dong HY, Harris NL, Preffer FI, Pitman MB: Fine-needle aspiration biopsy in the diagnosis and classification of primary and recurrent lymphoma: a retrospective analysis of the utility of cytomorphology and flow cytometry. Mod Pathol 2001;14:472-481.

83. Nicol TL, Silberman M, Rosenthal DL, Borowitz MJ: The accuracy of combined cytopathologic and flow cytometric analysis of fine-needle aspirates of lymph nodes. Am J Clin Pathol 2000;114:18-28.

84. Garcia DP, Rooney MT, Ahmad E, Davis BH: Diagnostic usefulness of CD23 and FMC-7 antigen expression patterns in B-cell lymphoma classification. Am J Clin Pathol 115:258-265.

85. Xu Y, McKenna RW, Kroft SH: Assessment of CD10 in the diagnosis of small B-cell lymphomas: A multiparameter flow cytometric study. Am J Clin Pathol 2002;117:291-300.

86. Sanchez ML, Almeida J, Vidriales B, et al: Incidence of phenotypic aberrations in a series of 467 patients with B chronic lymphoproliferative disorders: basis for the design of specific four-color stainings to be used for minimal residual disease investigation. Leukemia 2002;16:1460-1469.

87. Durig J, Naschar M, Schmucker U, et al: CD38 expression is an important prognostic marker in chronic lymphocytic leukaemia. Leukemia 2002;16:30-35.

88. Del Poeta G, Maurillo L, Venditti A, et al: Clinical significance of CD38 expression in chronic lymphocytic leukemia. Blood 2001;98:2633-2639.

89. Ibrahim S, Keating M, Do KA, et al: CD38 expression as an important prognostic factor in B-cell chronic lymphocytic leukemia. Blood 2001;98:181-186.

90. Criel A, Verhoef G, Vlietinck R, et al: Further characterization of morphologically defined typical and atypical CLL: Clinical, immunophenotypic, cytogenetic and prognostic study on 390 cases. Br J Haematol 1997;97:383-391.

91. Frater JL, McCarron KF, Hammel JP, et al: Typical and atypical chronic lymphocytic leukemia differ clinically and immunophenotypically. Am J Clin Pathol 2001;116:655-664.

92. Cornfield DB, Mitchell Nelson DM, Rimsza LM, Molker Pah D, Braylan RC: The diagnosis of hairy cell leukemia can be established by flow cytometric analysis of peripheral blood, even in patients with low levels of circulating malignant cells. Am J Hematol 2001;67:223-226.

Science of Clinical Oncology

93. Rawstron AC, Green MJ, Kuzmicki A, et al: Monoclonal B lymphocytes with the characteristics of "indolent" chronic lymphocytic leukemia are present in 3.5% of adults with normal blood counts. Blood 2002;100:635–639.

94. Wang C, Amato D, Rabah R, Zheng J, Fernandez B: Differentiation of monoclonal B lymphocytosis of undetermined significance (MLUS) and chronic lymphocytic leukemia (CLL) with weak CD5 expression from CD5(-) CLL. Leuk Res 2002;26:1125–1129.

95. Sah SP, Matutes E, Wotherspoon AC, Morill R, Catovsky D: A comparison of flow cytometry, bone marrow biopsy, and bone marrow aspirates in the detection of lymphoid infiltration in B cell disorders. J Clin Pathol 2003;56:129–132.

96. Duggan PR, Easton D, Luider J, Aver IA: Bone marrow staging of patients with non-Hodgkin lymphoma by flow cytometry: correlation with morphology. Cancer 2000;88:894–899.

97. Chilosi M, Adami F, Lestani M, et al: CD138/syndecan-1: a useful immunohistochemical marker of normal and neoplastic plasma cells on routine trephine bone marrow biopsies. Mod Pathol 1999;12:1101–1106.

98. Chang CC, Schur BC, Kampalath B, LIndholm P, Becker CG, Vesole DH: A novel multiparametric approach for analysis of cytoplasmic immunoglobulin light chains by flow cytometry. Mod Pathol 2001;14:1015–1021.

99. Sezer O, Heider U, Zavrski I, Possinger K: Differentiation of monoclonal gammopathy of undetermined significance and multiple myeloma using flow cytometric characteristics of plasma cells. Haematologica 2001;86:837–843.

100. Ocqueteau M, Orfao A, Almeida J, et al: Immunophenotypic characterization of plasma cells from monoclonal gammopathy of undetermined significance patients: Implications for the differential diagnosis between MGUS and multiple myeloma. Am J Pathol 1998;152:1655–1665.

101. San Miguel JF, Almeida J, Mateo G, et al: Immunophenotypic evaluation of the plasma cell compartment in multiple myeloma: A tool for comparing the efficacy of different treatment strategies and predicting outcome. Blood 2002;99:1853–1856.

102. Rawstron AC, Davies FE, DasGupta R, et al: Flow cytometric disease monitoring in multiple myeloma: The relationship between normal and neoplastic plasma cells predicts outcome after transplantation. Blood 2002;100:3095–3100.

103. Schwab C, Willers J, Niederer E, et al: The use of anti-T-cell receptor-Vbeta antibodies for the estimation of treatment success and phenotypic characterization of clonal T-cell populations in cutaneous T-cell lymphomas. Br J Haematol 2002;118:1019–1026.

104. Langerak AW, van Den BR, Wolvers-Tettero IL, et al: Molecular and flow cytometric analysis of the Vbeta repertoire for clonality assessment in mature TCRalphabeta T-cell proliferations. Blood 2001;98:165–173.

105. Gorczyca W, Weisberger J, Liu Z, et al: An approach to diagnosis of T-cell lymphoproliferative disorders by flow cytometry. Cytometry 2002;50:177–190.

106. Garcia VJ, Delgado I, Benito L, et al: CD79b expression in B cell chronic lymphocytic leukemia: Its implication for minimal residual disease detection. Leukemia 1999;13:1501–1505.

107. Rawstron AC, Kennedy B, Evans PA, et al: Quantitation of minimal disease levels in chronic lymphocytic leukemia using a sensitive flow cytometric assay improves the prediction of outcome and can be used to optimize therapy. Blood 2001;98:29–35.

108. Hedley DW, Friedlander ML, Taylor IW, Rugg CA, Musgrove EA: Method for analysis of cellular DNA content of paraffin-embedded pathological material using flow cytometry. J Histochem Cytochem 1983;31:1333–1335.

109. Wheeless LL, Badalament RA, der ver White RW, Fradet Y, Tribukait B: Consensus review of the clinical utility of DNA cytometry in bladder cancer: Report of the DNA Cytometry Consensus Conference. Cytometry 1993;14:478–481.

110. Hedley DW, Clark GM, Cornelisse CJ, Killander D, Kute T, Merkel D: Consensus review of the clinical utility of DNA cytometry in carcinoma of the breast: Report of the DNA Cytometry Consensus Conference. Cytometry 1993;14:482–485.

111. Bauer KD, Bagwell CB, Giaretti W, et al: Consensus review of the clinical utility of DNA flow cytometry in colorectal cancer. Cytometry 1993;14:486–491.

112. Shankey TV, Kallioniemi OP, Koslowski JM, et al: Consensus review of the clinical utility of DNA content cytometry in prostate cancer. Cytometry 1993;14:497–500.

113. Bergers E, Baak JP, van Diest PJ, et al: Prognostic value of DNA ploidy using flow cytometry in 1301 breast cancer patients: Results of the prospective Multicenter Morphometric Mammary Carcinoma Project. Mod Pathol 1997;10:762–768.

114. Ross JS, Sheehan CE, Ambros RA, et al: Needle biopsy DNA ploidy status predicts grade shifting in prostate cancer. Am J Surg Pathol 1999;23:296–301.

115. Alderisio M, Cenci M, Valli C, et al: Nm23-H1 protein, DNA-ploidy and S-phase fraction in relation to overall survival and disease free survival in transitional cell carcinoma of the bladder. Anticancer Res 1998;18:4225–4230.

116. Coon JS, Paxton H, Lucy L, Homburger H: Interlaboratory variation in DNA flow cytometry: Results of the College of American Pathologists' Survey. Arch Pathol Lab Med 1994;118:681–685.

117. Bagwell CB, Clark GM, Spyratos F, et al: DNA and cell cycle analysis as prognostic indicators in breast tumors revisited. Clin Lab Med 2001;21:875–895.

118. Wenger CR, Clark GM: S-phase fraction and breast cancer: A decade of experience. Breast Cancer Res Treat 1998;51:255–265.

119. Ross JS: DNA ploidy and cell cycle analysis in cancer diagnosis and prognosis. Oncology 1996;10:867–882, 887.

120. Chen JS, Coustan-Smith E, Suzuki T et al: Identification of novel markers for monitoring minimal residual disease in acute lymphoblastic leukemia. Blood 1997;97:2115.

121. Boveri T: Zur Frage der Entwicklung maligner Tumoren. Jena, Gustav Fischer-Verlag, 1914.

122. Nowell PC, Hungerford DA: A minute chromosome in human chronic granulocytic leukemia. Science 1960;132:1497.

123. Rowley JD: A new consistent chromosomal abnormality in chronic myelogenous leukemia identified by quinicrine fluorescence and Giemsa staining. Nature 1973;243:290–293.

124. Cheung VG, Nowak N, Jang W, et al: Integration of cytogenetic landmarks into the draft sequence of the human genome. Nature 2001;409:953.

125. Heim S, Mitelman F: Cancer Cytogenetics: Chromosomal and Molecular Genetic Aberrations of Tumor Cells, 2nd ed. New York, Wiley-Liss, 1995.

126. Bernard OA, Berger R: Location and function of critical genes in leukemogenesis inferred from cytogenetic abnormalities in hematologic malignancies. Semin Hematol 2000;37:412–419.

127. Druker BJ, Tamura S, Buchdunger E, et al: Effects of a selective inhibitor of the Abl tyrosine kinase on the growth of Bcr-Abl positive cells. Nat Med 1996;2:561–566.

128. Mitelman F, Johansson B, Mertens F (eds): Mitelman Database of Chromosome Aberrations in Cancer (2003) http://cgap.nci.nih.gov/Chromosomes/Mitelman.

129. Mitelman F (ed): An International System for Human Cytogenetic Nomenclature. Basel, Karger, 1995.

130. Cremer T, Lichter P, Borden J, Ward DK, Manvelidis L: Detection of chromosome aberrations in metaphase and interphase tumor cells by in situ hybridization using chromosome-specific library probes. Hum Genet 1988;80:235–246.

131. Kallioniemi A, Kallioniemi OP, Sudar D, et al: Comparative genomic hybridization for molecular cytogenetic analysis of solid tumors. Science 1992;258:818–821.

132. Speicher MR, Gwyn-Ballard ST, Ward DC: Karyotyping human chromosomes by combinatorial multicolor FISH. Nat Genet 1996;2:368–375.

133. Schrock E, duManoir S, Veldman T, et al: Multicolor spectral karyotyping of human chromosomes. Science 1996;273:494–497.

134. Mitelman F, Mertens F, Johansson B: A breakpoint map of recurrent chromosomal rearrangements in human neoplasia. Nat Genet 1997;15:417–474.

135. Seeger RC, Brodeur GM, Sather H, et al: Association of multiple copies of the N-myc oncogene with rapid progression of neuroblastomas. N Engl J Med 1985;313:1111–1116.

136. Harrison C: The detection and significance of chromosomal abnormalities in childhood acute lymphoblastic leukemia. Blood Rev 2001;15:49–59.

137. Johansson B, Fioretos T, Mitelman F: Cytogenetic and molecular genetic evolution of chronic myeloid leukemia. Acta Haematol 2002;107:76–94.

138. Look AT: Genes altered by chromosomal translocations in leukemias and lymphomas. In Vogelstein B, Kinzler KW (eds): The Genetic Basis of Human Cancer, 2nd ed. New York, McGraw-Hill, 2002, pp 57–92.

139. Olopade OI, Sobulo OM, Rowley JD: Recurring chromosome rearrangements in human cancer. In Bast RC, Kufe DW, Pollock RE, et al (eds): Cancer Medicine, 5th ed. New York, Decker, 2000, pp 88–107.

140. Inheritance in Man. http://www3.ncbi.nlm.nih.gov/Omim/.

141. Mullis K, Faloona F, Scharf S, Saiki R, Horn G, Erlich H: Specific enzymatic amplification of DNA in vitro: the polymerase chain reaction. Cold Spring Harb Symp Quant Biol 1986;51 Pt 1:263–273.

142. Bernard PS, Wittwer CT: Real-time PCR technology for cancer diagnostics. Clin Chem 2002;48:1178–1185.

143. Franca LT, Carrilho E, Kist TB: A review of DNA sequencing techniques. Q Rev Biophys 2002;35:169–200.

144. Southern EM: Detection of specific sequences among DNA fragments separated by gel electrophoresis. J Mol Biol 1975;98:503–517.

145. Schena M, Shalon D, Davis RW, Brown PO: Quantitative monitoring of gene expression patterns with a complementary DNA microarray. Science 1995;270:467–470.

146. Golub TR, Slonim DK, Tamayo P, et al: Molecular classification of cancer: Class discovery and class prediction by gene expression monitoring. Science 1999;286:531–537.

147. Liotta LA, Espina V, Mehta AI, et al: Protein microarrays: Meeting analytical challenges for clinical applications. Cancer Cell 2003;3:317–325.

148. Langerak AW, van Krieken JH, Wolvers-Tettero IL, et al: The role of molecular analysis of immunoglobulin and T cell receptor gene rearrangements in the diagnosis of lymphoproliferative disorders. J Clin Pathol 2001;54:565–567.

149. Coad JE, Olson DJ, Lander TA, McGlennan RC: Molecular assessment of clonality in lymphoproliferative disorders, I: Immunoglobulin gene rearrangements. Mol Diagn 1996;1:335–355.

150. Coad JE, Olson DJ, Lander TA, McGlennan RC: Molecular assessment of clonality in lymphoproliferative disorders, II: T-cell receptor gene rearrangements. Mol Diagn 1996;2:69–81.

151. NCCLS: Immunoglobulin and T-Cell Receptor Gene Rearrangement Assays; Approved Guideline, 2nd ed., 2002.

152. Greiner TC, Rubocki RJ: Effectiveness of capillary electrophoresis using fluorescent-labeled primers in detecting T-cell receptor gamma gene rearrangements. J Mol Diagn 2002;4:137–143.

153. Theriault C, Galoin S, Valmary S, et al: PCR analysis of immunoglobulin heavy chain (IgH) and TcR-gamma chain gene rearrangements in the diagnosis of lymphoproliferative disorders: Results of a study of 525 cases. Mod Pathol 2000;13:1269–1279.

154. Fodinger M, Winkler K, Mannhalter C, Cho HA: Combined polymerase chain reaction approach for clonality detection in lymphoid neoplasms. Diagn Mol Pathol 1999;8:80–91.

155. Uckun FM, Herman-Hatten K, Crotty ML, et al: Clinical significance of MLL-AF4 fusion transcript expression in the absence of a cytogenetically detectable t(4;11)(q21;q23) chromosomal translocation. Blood 1998;92:810–821.

156. Olavarria E, Kanfer E, Szydlo R, et al: Early detection of BCR-ABL transcripts by quantitative reverse transcriptase-polymerase chain reaction predicts outcome after allogeneic stem cell transplantation for chronic myeloid leukemia. Blood 2001;97:1560–1565.

157. Hochhaus A: Minimal residual disease in chronic myeloid leukaemia patients. Best Pract Res Clin Haematol 2002;15:159–178.

158. Grimwade D: The significance of minimal residual disease in patients with t(15;17). Best Pract Res Clin Haematol 2002;15:137–158.

159. Radich JP: Molecular measurement of minimal residual disease in Philadelphia-positive acute lymphoblastic leukaemia. Best Pract Res Clin Haematol 2002;15:91–103.

160. Liu Yin JA: Minimal residual disease in acute myeloid leukemia. Best Pract Res Clin Haematol 2002;15:119–135.

161. Limpens J, de Jong D, van Krieken JH, et al: Bcl-2/JH rearrangements in benign lymphoid tissues with follicular hyperplasia. Oncogene 1991;6:2271–2276.

162. Limpens J, Stad R, Vos C, et al: Lymphoma-associated translocation t(14;18) in blood B cells of normal individuals. Blood 1995;85:2528–2536.

163. Ji W, Qu GZ, Ye P, Zhang XY, Halabi S, Erlich M: Frequent detection of bcl-2/JH translocations in human blood and organ samples by a quantitative polymerase chain reaction assay. Cancer Res 1995;55:2876–2882.

164. Bose S, Deininger M, Gora-Tybor J, Goldman JM, Melo JV: The presence of typical and atypical BCR-ABL fusion genes in leukocytes of normal individuals: Biologic significance and implications for the assessment of minimal residual disease. Blood 1998;92:3362–3367.

165. Summers KE, Goff LK, Wilson AG, Gupta RK, Lister TA, Fitzgibbon J: Frequency of the Bcl-2/IgH rearrangement in normal individuals: Implications for the monitoring of disease in patients with follicular lymphoma. J Clin Oncol 2001;19:420–424.

166. Williams TM: Human leukocyte antigen gene polymorphism and the histocompatibility laboratory. J Mol Diagn 2001;3:98–104.

167. Rubinstein P: HLA matching for bone marrow transplantation—how much is enough? N Engl J Med 2001;345:1842–1844.

168. Petersdorf EW, Gooley TA, Anasetti C, et al: Optimizing outcome after unrelated marrow transplantation by comprehensive matching of HLA class I and II alleles in the donor and recipient. Blood 1998;92:3515–3520.

169. Petersdorf EW, Hansen JA, Martin PJ, et al: Major-histocompatibility-complex class I alleles and antigens in hematopoietic-cell transplantation. N Engl J Med 2001;345:1794–1800.

170. Van Deerlin VM, Leonard DG: Bone marrow engraftment analysis after allogeneic bone marrow transplantation. Clin Lab Med 2000;20:197–225.

171. Campe H, Jaeger G, Abou-Ajram C, et al: Serial detection of Epstein-Barr virus DNA in sera and peripheral blood leukocyte samples of pediatric renal allograft recipients with persistent mononucleosis-like symptoms defines patients at risk to develop post-transplant lymphoproliferative disease. Pediatr Transplant 2003;7:46–52.

172. Brown NA, Liu CR, Wang YF, et al: B-cell lymphoproliferation and lymphomagenesis are associated with clonotypic intracellular terminal regions of the Epstein-Barr virus. J Virol 1988;62:962–969.

173. Alizadeh AA, Eisen MB, Davis RE, et al: Distinct types of diffuse large B-cell lymphoma identified by gene expression profiling. Nature 2000;403:503–511.

174. Staudt LM: Molecular diagnosis of the hematologic cancers. N Engl J Med 2003;348:1777–1785.

175. Shipp MA, Ross KN, Tamayo P, et al: Diffuse large B-cell lymphoma outcome prediction by gene-expression profiling and supervised machine learning. Nat Med 2002;8:68–74.

176. Ferrando AA, Neuberg DS, Staunton J, et al: Gene expression signatures define novel oncogenic pathways in T cell acute lymphoblastic leukemia. Cancer Cell 2002;1:75–87.

177. Yeoh EJ, Ross ME, Shurtleff SA, et al: Classification, subtype discovery, and prediction of outcome in pediatric acute lymphoblastic leukemia by gene expression profiling. Cancer Cell 2002;1:133–143.

178. Unger MA, Nathanson KL, Calzone K, et al: Screening for genomic rearrangements in families with breast and ovarian cancer identifies BRCA1 mutations previously missed by conformation-sensitive gel electrophoresis or sequencing. Am J Hum Genet 2000;67:841–850.

179. Hogervorst FB, Nederlof PM, Gille JJ, et al: Large genomic deletions and duplications in the BRCA1 gene identified by a novel quantitative method. Cancer Res 2003;63:1449–1453.

180. Casilli F, Di Rocco ZC, Gad S, et al: Rapid detection of novel BRCA1 rearrangements in high-risk breast-ovarian cancer families using multiplex PCR of short fluorescent fragments. Hum Mutat 2002;20:218–226.

181. Eng C, Clayton D, Schuffenecker I, et al: The relationship between specific RET proto-oncogene mutations and disease phenotype in multiple endocrine neoplasia type 2. International RET mutation consortium analysis. JAMA 1996;276:1575–1579.

182. Baysal BE: Hereditary paraganglioma targets diverse paraganglia. J Med Genet 2002;39:617–622.

Science of Clinical Oncology

183. Varley JM: Germline TP53 mutations and Li-Fraumeni syndrome. Hum Mutat 2003;21:313–320.

184. Hes FJ, Lips CJ, van der Luijt RB: Molecular genetic aspects of Von Hippel-Lindau (VHL) disease and criteria for DNA analysis in subjects at risk. Neth J Med 2001;59:235–243.

185. Tsukada T, Yamaguchi K, Kameya T: The MEN1 gene and associated diseases: An update. Endocr Pathol 2001;12:259–273.

186. Vogelstein B, Fearon ER, Kern SE, et al: Allelotype of colorectal carcinomas. Science 1989;244:207–211.

187. Emmert-Buck MR, Bonner RF, Smith PD, et al: Laser capture microdissection. Science 1996;274:998–1001.

188. Feeley KM, Fullard JF, Heneghan MA, et al: Microsatellite instability in sporadic colorectal carcinoma is not an indicator of prognosis. J Pathol 1999;188:14–17.

189. Smith JS, Perry A, Borell TJ, et al: Alterations of chromosome arms 1p and 19q as predictors of survival in oligodendrogliomas, astrocytomas, and mixed oligoastrocytomas. J Clin Oncol 2000;18:636–645.

190. Finkelstein SD, Marsh W, Demetris AJ, et al: Microdissection-based allelotyping discriminates de novo tumor from intrahepatic spread in hepatocellular carcinoma. Hepatology 2003;37:871–879.

191. Hunt JL, Swalsky P, Sasatomi E, Niehouse L, Bakker A, Finkelstein SD: A microdissection and molecular genotyping assay to confirm the identity of tissue floaters in paraffin-embedded tissue blocks. Arch Pathol Lab Med 2003;127:213–217.

192. Sidransky D, Tokino T, Hamilton SR, et al: Identification of ras oncogene mutations in the stool of patients with curable colorectal tumors. Science 1992;256:102–105.

193. Traverso G, Shuber A, Levin B, et al: Detection of APC mutations in fecal DNA from patients with colorectal tumors. N Engl J Med 2002;346:311–320.

194. Ahlquist DA, Skoletsky JE, Boynton KA, et al: Colorectal cancer screening by detection of altered human DNA in stool: feasibility of a multitarget assay panel. Gastroenterology 2000;119:1219–1227.

195. Boland CR, Thibodeau SN, Hamilton SR, et al: A National Cancer Institute Workshop on Microsatellite Instability for cancer detection and familial predisposition: Development of international criteria for the determination of microsatellite instability in colorectal cancer. Cancer Res 1998;58:5248–5257.

196. Gryfe R, Kim H, Hsieh ET, et al: Tumor microsatellite instability and clinical outcome in young patients with colorectal cancer. N Engl J Med 2000;342:69–77.

197. Feeley KM, Fullard JF, Heneghan MA, et al: Microsatellite instability in sporadic colorectal carcinoma is not an indicator of prognosis. J Pathol 1999;188:14–17.

198. Laird PW: The power and the promise of DNA methylation markers. Nat Rev Cancer 2003;3:253–266.

199. Jones PA, Baylin SB: The fundamental role of epigenetic events in cancer. Nat Rev Genet 2002;3:415–428.

200. Mukai T, Sekiguchi M: Gene silencing in phenomena related to DNA repair. Oncogene 2002;21:9033–9042.

201. Nephew KP, Huang TH: Epigenetic gene silencing in cancer initiation and progression. Cancer Lett 2003;190:125–133.

202. Ahluwalia A, Yan P, Hurteau JA, et al: DNA methylation and ovarian cancer, I: Analysis of CpG island hypermethylation in human ovarian cancer using differential methylation hybridization. Gynecol Oncol 2001;82:261–268.

203. Cui H, Cruz-Correa M, Giardiello FM, et al: Loss of IGF2 imprinting: a potential marker of colorectal cancer risk. Science 2003;299:1753–1755.

204. Best CJ, Leiva IM, Chuaqui RF, et al: Molecular differentiation of high- and moderate-grade human prostate cancer by cDNA microarray analysis. Diagn Mol Pathol 2003;12:63–70.

205. Dhanasekaran SM, Barrette TR, Ghosh D, et al: Delineation of prognostic biomarkers in prostate cancer. Nature 2001;412:822–826.

206. van't Veer LJ, Dai H, van de Vijver MJ, et al: Gene expression profiling predicts clinical outcome of breast cancer. Nature 2002;415:530–536.

207. van de Vijver MJ, He YD, van't Veer LJ, et al: A gene-expression signature as a predictor of survival in breast cancer. N Engl J Med 2002;347:1999–2009.

208. Kallioniemi A: Molecular signatures of breast cancer: Predicting the future. N Engl J Med 2002;347:2067–2068.

209. Klein A, Fishman A, Zemer R, Zimlichman S, Altaras MM: Detection of tumor circulating cells by cytokeratin 20 in the blood of patients with endometrial carcinoma. Gynecol Oncol 2000;78:352–355.

210. Hara N, Kasahara T, Kawasaki T, et al: Reverse transcription-polymerase chain reaction detection of prostate-specific antigen, prostate-specific membrane antigen, and prostate stem cell antigen in one milliliter of peripheral blood: value for the staging of prostate cancer. Clin Cancer Res 2002;8:1794–1799.

211. Raja S, Luketich JD, Kelly LA, Gooding WE, Finkelstein SD, Godfrey TE: Rapid, quantitative reverse transcriptase-polymerase chain reaction: Application to intraoperative molecular detection of occult metastases in esophageal cancer. J Thorac Cardiovasc Surg 2002;123:475–482; discussion pp 482–483.

212. Sauter ER, Zhu W, Fan XJ, Wassel RP, Chervoneva I, Du Bois GC: Proteomic analysis of nipple aspirate fluid to detect biologic markers of breast cancer. Br J Cancer 2002;86:1440–1443.

213. Righetti PG, Castagna A, Antonucci F, et al: The proteome: Anno Domini 2002. Clin Chem Lab Med 2002;41:425–438.

214. Issaq HJ, Veenstra TD, Conrads TP, et al: The SELDI-TOF MS approach to proteomics: protein profiling and biomarker identification. Biochem Biophys Res Commun 2002;292:587–592.

215. Aebersold R, Mann M: Mass spectrometry-based proteomics. Nature 2003;422:198–207.

216. Petricoin EF, Ardekani AM, Hitt BA, et al: Use of proteomic patterns in serum to identify ovarian cancer. Lancet 2002;359:572–577.

217. Petricoin EF, 3rd, Ornstein DK, Paweletz CP, et al: Serum proteomic patterns for detection of prostate cancer. J Natl Cancer Inst 2002;94:1576–1578.

218. ACOG. Committee opinion: number 277, November 2002. Patients, medicine and the interests of patients: Applying general principles to gene patenting. Obstet Gynecol 2002;100:1051–1056.

219. Cho MK, Illangasekare S, Weaver MA, Leonard DG, Merz JF: Effects of patents and licenses on the provision of clinical genetic testing services. J Mol Diagn 2003;5:3–8.

220. Malakoff D, Service RF: Genomania meets the bottom line. Science 2001;291:1193–1203.

221. Chan DW, Sell S: Tumor markers. In Burtis CA, Ashwood ER (eds): Tietz Texbook of Clinical Chemistry, 3rd ed. Philadelphia, WB Saunders, 1999, pp 722–749.

222. Diamandis EP: Tumor Markers: Past, Present, and Future. In Diamandis EP, Fritsche HA, Lilja H, et al. (eds): Tumor Markers. Physiology, Pathobiology, Technology, and Clinical Applications. Washington, DC, AACC Press, 2002, pp 3–8.

223. Duffy MJ: Clinical uses of tumor markers: a critical review. Crit Rev Clin Lab Sci 2001;38:225–262.

224. Fleisher M, Dnistrian AM, Sturgeon CM, Lamerz R, Witliff JL: Practice guidelines for the use of tumor markers in the clinic. In Diamandis EP, Fritsche HA, Lilja H, et al.(eds): Tumor Markers. Physiology, Pathobiology, Technology, and Clinical Applications. Washington, DC, AACC Press, 2002, pp 33–63.

225. European Group for Tumor Markers (EGTM): Consensus recommendations. Anticancer Res 1999;19:2785–2820.

226. National Comprehensive Cancer Network. http://www.nccn.org/

227. Bast RC Jr, Ravdin P, Hayes DF, et al: 2000 update of recommendations for the use of tumor markers in breast and colorectal cancer: Clinical practice guidelines of the American Society of Clinical Oncology. J Clin Oncol 2001;19:1865–1878.

228. Sturgeon C: Practice guidelines for tumor marker use in the clinic. Clin Chem 2002;48:1151–1159.

229. Li J, Zhang Z, Rosenzweig J, Wang YY, Chan DW: Proteomic and bioinformatics approaches for identification of serum biomarkers. Clin Chem 2002;48:1296–1304.

230. Chan DW, Schwartz MK: Tumor Markers: Introduction and General Principles. In Diamandis EP, Fritsche HA, Lilja H, et al. (eds): Tumor Markers: Physiology, Pathobiology, Technology, and Clinical Applications. Washington, DC, AACC Press, 2002, pp 9–17.

231. Smith RA, Cokkinides V, Eyre HJ: American Cancer Society guidelines for the early detection of cancer, 2003. CA Cancer J Clin 2003;53:27–43.

232. Bast RC Jr, Urban N, Shridhar V, et al. Early detection of ovarian cancer: Promise and reality. Cancer Treat Res 2002;107:61–97.

233. Bast RC Jr, Xu F-J, Yu Y-H, Barnhill S, Zhang Z, Mills GB: CA 125: The past and the future. Int J Biol Markers 1998;13:179–187.
234. Polascik TJ, Oesterling JE, Partin AW: Prostate specific antigen: a decade of discovery: What we have learned and where we are going. J Urol 1999;162:293–306.
235. Sokoll LJ, Chan DW: Total, free, and complexed PSA: Analysis and clinical utility. J Clin Ligand Assay 1998;21:171–179.
236. NIH Consensus Conference Development Panel of Ovarian Cancer: Ovarian cancer. Screening, treatment, and follow-up. JAMA 1995;273:491–497.
237. Woolas RP, Conway MR, Xu F, et al: Combinations of multiple serum markers are superior to individual assays for discriminating malignant from benign pelvic masses. Gynecol Oncol 1995;59: 111–116.
238. Zhang Z, Barnhill SD, Zhang H, Xu F, et al: Combination of multiple serum markers using an artificial neural network to improve specificity in discriminating malignant from benign pelvic masses. Gynecol Oncol 1999;73:56–61.
239. Einhorn LH, Lowitz BB. Testicular Cancer. In Casciato DA, Lowitz BB (eds): Manual of Clinical Oncology, 3rd ed. Boston: Little, Brown, 1995, pp 228–236.
240. Oberg K, Stridsberg M: Neuroendocrine tumors. In Diamandis EP, Fritsche HA, Lilja H, et al (eds): Tumor Markers. Physiology, Pathobiology, Technology, and Clinical Applications. Washington, DC, AACC Press, 2002, pp 339–349.
241. Compton CC, Fenoglio-Presier CM, Pettigrew N, Fielding LP: American Joint Committee on Cancer prognostic factors consensus conference: colorectal working group. Cancer 2000;124:1739–1757.
242. The International Non-Hodgkin's Lymphoma Prognostic Factors Project: A predictive model for aggressive non-Hodgkin's lymphoma. N Engl J Med 1993;329:987–994.
243. Sobin LH, Wittekind C (eds): Testis: TNM Classification of Malignant Tumors, 5th ed. New York, Wiley-Liss, 1997, pp 174–179.
244. Fateh-Moghadam A, Stieber P: Sensible use of tumour markers, 2nd ed. Marloffstein-Rathsberg, Hartmann Verlag, 1993, pp 11–31.
245. Bonfrer JMG: Working group on tumor marker criteria (WGTMC). Tumor Biol 1990;11:287–288.
246. Basuyau J-P. Leroy M, Brunelle P: Determination of tumor markers in serum: Pitfalls and good practice. Clin Chem Lab Med 2001; 39:1227–1233.
247. Price CP, Allard J, Davies G, et al: Pre- and post-analytical factors that may influence use of serum prostate specific antigen and its isoforms in a screening programme for prostate cancer. Ann Clin Biochem 2001;38:188–216.
248. Sturgeon CM, Seth J: Why do immunoassays for tumor markers giver differing results? A view from the UK national External Quality Assessment Schemes. Eur J Clin Chem Clin Biochem 1996;34:755–759.
249. Sturgeon CM: Limitations of Assay Techniques for Tumor Markers. In Diamandis EP, Fritsche HA, Lilja H, et al(eds): Tumor Markers: Physiology, Pathobiology, Technology, and Clinical Applications. Washington, DC, AACC Press, 2002, pp 65–81.
250. Rai AJ, Zhang Z, Rosenzweig J, et al: Proteomic approaches to tumor marker discovery: Identification of biomarkers for ovarian cancer. Arch Pathol Lab Med 2002;126:1518–1526.

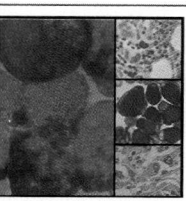

18 IMAGING

Richard L. Wahl

Harpreet Pannu

SUMMARY OF KEY POINTS

- Noninvasive medical imaging is increasingly essential to cancer management at multiple time points in the course of the illness.
- Examples of current usage of imaging include screening to detect cancer, characterizing lesions, performing locoregional and systemic staging, providing prognostic information, assessing response during and after therapy, restaging after treatment, performing follow-up of patients for recurrence, and precisely guiding therapies such as external beam radiation, brachytherapy, or thermal ablation.
- More invasive interventional radiologic procedures can also guide and monitor vascular or intraluminal delivery of treatments such as radioactive microspheres, embolic materials, thermal ablation, and therapeutic drugs.
- Imaging methods range from the traditional anatomic methods, such as x-ray, computed tomography (CT), and ultrasound, to the more functional methods of magnetic resonance imaging (MRI) and nuclear medicine methods, including positron emission tomography (PET) and single-photon-emission computed tomography (SPECT), and planar nuclear imaging. Optical imaging is promising, but limited by penetration of tissues to superficial structures in most cases.
- Plain films and mammography remain useful techniques, with mammography the only imaging method clearly proven effective when applied in the screening setting.
- CT remains the cornerstone technology for most oncologic imaging, and CT technology allowing for rapid-sequence angiography is growing in application as well as

- three-dimensional reconstruction of CT data sets.
- MRI is the imaging tool of choice for central nervous system, spinal, and musculoskeletal neoplasms, and is very useful in some head and neck cancers as well as in assessing vascular and hepatobiliary and pelvic lesions.
- Bone scans using single-photon methods (^{99m}Tc methylene diphosphonate) remain the dominant procedure for detecting suspected bone metastases; however, this technology is probably less sensitive than MRI and PET techniques in detecting bone metastases of many tumors.
- PET and PET/CT technology using ^{18}fluorodeoxyglucose (FDG) is growing rapidly in application and is increasingly routine in the management of patients with cancer at varying states of the disease process. PET is used with increasing frequency in the staging and follow-up of lung, colorectal, and head and neck cancers, as well as lymphomas and other types of tumors. PET with non-FDG tracers is a promising research area with growing clinical applications.
- The fusion of anatomic and functional images to create hybrid "anatomolecular images" with software or dedicated instruments such as PET/CT or SPECT/CT devices is also seeing rapid growth in applications in cancer imaging.
- Imaging management for staging lung cancer and characterizing solitary pulmonary nodules often includes PET in addition to CT when the technology is available because PET has high accuracy in lung cancer assessments vs. CT.
- Imaging management of suspected recurrences of colorectal, head and neck, lymphoma, and several other

- cancers often now includes the use of PET in addition to CT. Use of PET at earlier stages in the workup is increasingly applied.
- In prostate cancer, available imaging methods remain suboptimal for detection of primary tumor and early determination of whether tumor has spread from the prostate locally and systemically.
- Visceral angiography for diagnostic purposes is being supplanted by CT and MRI methods; however, it remains important as a tool for delivering therapies intravascularly such as chemotherapy, coils, or radioactive microspheres.
- CT, ultrasound, fluoroscopy, and innovative MRI systems can guide interventional procedures such as thermal and cryotherapeutic lesion ablations.
- Highly specific probe systems are being developed to allow for optical and radionuclide imaging of transfected gene biodistribution and function.
- Combined anatomic and functional information is being applied to allow for more precise planning of external beam radiation therapy including IMRT and conformal therapy, methods that potentially allow for increasing dose escalation and minimization of toxicity to normal tissues.
- Emerging imaging methods are increasingly providing information on the physiology and molecular characteristics of lesions, so that a multiparametric biologic imaging phenotype for tumors is provided that can more precisely guide tumor treatment on an individualized basis in specific patients to yield a higher probability of success without excessive toxicity for treatment of a selected neoplastic process.

INTRODUCTION

Noninvasive and invasive imaging is of fundamental and increasing importance in the daily management of the patient with cancer. Although physical examination and laboratory tests remain key for planning treatment, for solid tumor management, imaging tests represent a key objective metric of disease activity and are generally used at multiple times during the course of the disease to monitor the efficacy (or lack of efficacy) of treatment. Imaging tumor size is an objective endpoint in disease management and in comparing results of cancer treatments across institutions and types of treatment. Imaging is also increasingly applied in the drug development process and to aid in developing new cancer therapies.

Specific clinical questions addressed by imaging include screening for the presence of cancer, characterizing anatomic lesions as malignant or benign, determining the size and local extent of a primary lesion, and determining whether a tumor is localized or locoregionally or systemically metastatic (staging). Such studies are key to determining whether the patient is a candidate for surgical resection, identifying the extent of the field for radiation therapy, and determining whether systemic chemotherapy is appropriate. Initial staging of tumor size and extent can also provide important prognostic data. During the course of treatment, imaging is used to determine whether the cancer has responded to treatment. Imaging is also used to follow patients for recurrence or second malignancies. Imaging is increasingly being used as a method to allow for minimally invasive therapeutic procedures to be delivered to ablate cancers and more precisely guide the dosing of therapeutic drugs, including radiopharmaceuticals.[1]

Imaging is often the best means of noninvasively identifying and assessing tumors. By answering these questions, treatment decisions can be made with greater certainty and the prognosis of patients can be made more precisely. Before discussing the varying imaging methods available for cancer, it is important to consider some general principles applicable to all imaging tests.

Tasks for Imaging

The major roles of imaging in the current practice of cancer management are shown in Table 18-1.

GENERAL CONSIDERATIONS

Performance of Imaging Tests

Noninvasive imaging is used to perform a wide variety of important tasks. Although the best way to determine the medical utility of a diagnostic test can be argued, a few key concepts are required to understand and compare diagnostic tests for one of the most basic tasks (i.e., determining whether tumor is present). However, these same concepts can be applied in terms of the ability of imaging to predict resectability or response to treatment.

TABLE 18-1

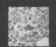
Imaging in Cancer: Key Current Clinical Uses in Cancer Management

Screening

Lesion characterization: Malignant or benign, size, local invasion
Tumor staging: Locoregional, systemic, at initial presentation or on retreatment
Size and extent of tumor: To plan radiation or other local therapy
Prognostic information

Defining sites for biopsy and subsequent analysis by pathology
Guidance of interventional therapy

Assessment of response to treatment
Restaging tumor after treatment

Assessment of normal organ function or status before, during, and after treatment
Assessment for toxicity or complications of treatment

Sensitivity

Sensitivity describes how often the imaging test would give a "positive result" in a patient with cancer (i.e., true-positive [TP] finding). Ideally, the test precisely detects and locates one or multiple cancers in a given patient. Thus, % Sensitivity = 100 × (Test positive/Disease present). Sensitivity can be calculated on a per-patient basis or a per-malignant lesion basis. The per-patient basis is most commonly used in screening studies for early diagnosis, whereas the per-lesion basis may be used in patients expected to have multiple sites of tumor. Per-lesion detection analyses can be misleading because they can be heavily biased by a single patient's results if that patient has multiple tumor foci.

It can sometimes be difficult to understand how good a test is by reading the literature. Sensitivity is supposed to be substantially independent of study composition, but as discussed in the next section, certain imaging tests may be insensitive for some very early-stage disease, but very, very sensitive for more advanced disease. Thus, the patient population and, very often, the tumor burden and average tumor size can make a difference in the sensitivity of a test. Virtually all noninvasive imaging tests are less sensitive for small-volume disease than for large-volume disease. For example, if an imaging test is used in a patient population in which patients have advanced disease before seeking medical attention (e.g., they are symptomatic at presentation), the imaging test may have far greater sensitivity than if it were used in patients with earlier-stage, smaller tumors. For example, positron emission tomography (PET) with [18]fluorodeoxyglucose (FDG) has been reported to be more than 90% sensitive for detecting metastatic melanoma, but is less than 20% sensitive in detecting early nodal metastases of melanoma at initial surgical resection. A test with high sensitivity has a low number of false-negative (FN) results. The false-negative fraction is commonly expressed as 1 – Sensitivity.[2]

Specificity

Specificity is the frequency with which a test result is negative if no disease is present or the true-negative (TN) ratio. As a percentage, specificity is 100 × (Test negative/Disease negative). Again, specificity can be calculated on a per-patient basis or a per-lesion or per-region basis. The per-patient calculations are commonly performed in the screening setting. They can also be done per region of the body (i.e., Is the liver free of tumor? Are the draining lymph nodes free of tumor?) This parameter is supposed to be independent of the prevalence of disease in the population, but can be affected substantially if there is a population characteristic that can result in false-positive (FP) results for the imaging test. For example, inflammatory and infectious lung disease, such as active tuberculosis (TB) or sarcoidosis, if present in a population, can result in false-positive findings on PET or computed tomography (CT) scans. In this situation, the specificity of PET with FDG, and likely of CT, for staging the mediastinum for cancer would vary. Thus, the specificity of PET for assessing mediastinal lymph nodes may be much lower in areas of the world with endogenous TB than in developed areas without TB or sarcoidosis. Therefore, an imaging test that is very useful in one part of the world may be far less useful in another part of the world. A highly specific test has a low frequency of false-positive results (i.e., a low frequency of a positive test result in the patient population that does not have the disease).[2]

Accuracy of Imaging

For detection of disease, a binary, yes-or-no answer as to whether disease is present is desirable. When such binary answers can be provided, it is simple to mathematically provide an accuracy value for a diagnostic imaging test. Thus, accuracy is 100(TP + TN/TP + FP + TN + FN). A highly accurate test with a low prevalence of false-positive and false-negative results has an accuracy approaching 100%.

Positive and Negative Predictive Values

Sensitivity and specificity define a test well, but its performance in a specific patient is affected by the population characteristics from which the patient is drawn. Thus, the referring physician often really wants to know whether an individual patient has cancer and, if so, where the tumor is located. Another important question is whether the tumor is localized or metastatic. The correct answer is a binary one in most cases, either yes or no, but imaging does not always indicate the true status of an individual patient. Thus, the statistical likelihood of the accuracy of the result might be conveyed in the report. This statistical likelihood will be related to the accuracy of the test as well as to the patient population characteristics. Thus, the positive predictive value is often of considerable clinical relevance. For example, the positive predictive value of a test with 90% sensitivity and 90% specificity will vary markedly depending on the frequency of disease in the population. With these test performance characteristics, two different conclusions could be reached by the clinician regarding the same imaging test.

90% SENSITIVE AND SPECIFIC TEST

50% Prevalence of cancer in the population imaged:
  1000 Independent scans
  50 False-positive findings in healthy patients (10% of 500)
  450 True-positive findings in patients with disease (90% of 500)
Positive predictive value (Disease positive/Test positive): 450/500 (90%)
Possible conclusion: ***An excellent test!***

90% SENSITIVE AND SPECIFIC TEST

10% Prevalence of cancer in the population imaged:
  1000 Independent scans
  90 False-positive findings in healthy patients (10% of 900)
  90 True-positive findings in patients with disease (10% of 1000)
Positive predictive value (Disease positive/Test positive): 50/100 (50%)
Possible conclusion: ***A rather lousy test!***

But these are the same test!

Thus, a test that is effective in a patient population with a high prevalence of a disease may be far less valuable in a patient population with a lower prevalence of the same disease. The most effective use of imaging technology is in groups of patients in whom the imaging characteristics are expected to be robust enough to allow for predictions in individual patients. These challenges are particularly apparent when a test that was developed in a patient population with disease is used to evaluate individuals with a low prevalence of tumor (e.g., screening). In this situation, the number of false-positive findings may rise dramatically, negating the value of the test.[3]

Receiver Operator Characteristic Curves

Imaging tests are interpreted by imaging specialists, often radiologists. Like all of medicine, there is considerable science involved in image interpretation, but there is also the human element, or "art," as it is referred to in some settings. In developed countries, medical specialty boards have been established to assure that practitioners have a basal level of training and knowledge, thereby providing a level of uniformity to image interpretations. However, even with board certification and extensive training, not all imaging specialists interpret a given imaging study in the same manner. Thus, although the goal of an imaging test is often a simple binary "yes, there is tumor" or "no, there is not tumor" answer, there are varying degrees of certainty in the interpretation of an image in most instances. Some readers read with high sensitivity, whereas others read with high specificity. Unless a test is very robust, it is hard to achieve both high sensitivity and high specificity.[4]

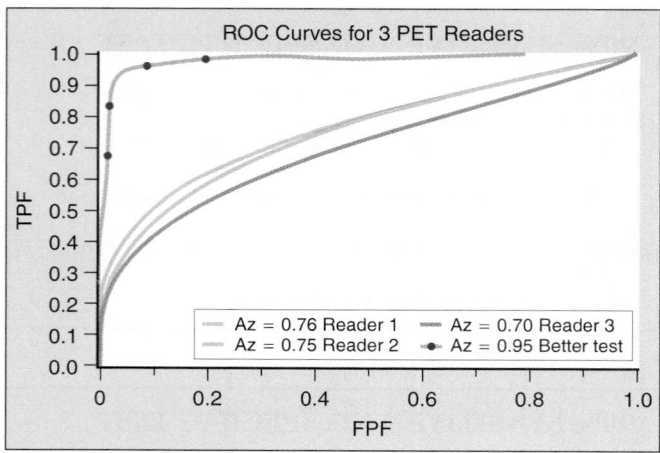

Figure 18-1. Receiver operator characteristic (ROC) curves plotting the true-positive fraction (TPF) [sensitivity] vs. the false-positive fraction (FPF) [1 – Specificity] for the three independent readers of the entire analysis data set. A hypothetical curve for the test if it had 95% accuracy is also shown. Az, estimated area under the ROC curve.

An example of a receiver operator characteristic (ROC) curve is shown in Figure 18-1. This set of curves reflects the performance of PET imaging in detecting axillary metastases in patients with newly diagnosed breast cancer. The axes of the curves are the true-positive fraction (Sensitivity/100) [y-axis] and the false-positive fraction (1 – Specificity/100) [x-axis], on a scale of 0 to 1. Thus, a perfect diagnostic test would have no false-positive or false-negative results. The results from three readers who graded PET scans using a five-point certainty scale are shown. The three readers had similar ROC curves, indicating that they were of generally comparable accuracy. The greater the area under an ROC curve, the greater the accuracy of the test. For the same test, however, two readers may be reading at different points on the ROC curve, meaning that one is more sensitive and one is more specific, but both are of equal accuracy. An excellent reader may have a greater area under the ROC curve than a less skilled reader, meaning that the more experienced reader is both more sensitive and more specific than a less experienced reader. Nonetheless, virtually none of our imaging tests is perfect, and varying "cut points" between disease and normalcy are often made, affecting the overall performance of the test. The area under the curve (AUC) of 0.7 to 0.76 was not viewed as sufficiently good for the task of nodal detection of metastatic cancer spread to the axilla. A higher, hypothetical curve, with an AUC of 0.9, is shown for a more robust test, such as a higher-resolution PET system devoted to imaging the axilla. In practice, sentinel node sampling, often guided by imaging or a radionuclide-sensitive probe system, is assuming a very important role in this area of tumor staging.[5]

Other Approaches to Assessing the Value of Imaging

Although sensitivity, specificity, and accuracy are commonly used to characterize the tumor detection process, other metrics may be of greater importance. For example, some studies have focused on how often imaging changes management substantially. This kind of study is of great practical interest, but the optimal methods to assess such changes in treatment decisions are evolving. Ideally, one would like to show that the use of imaging, especially a new imaging technology, when applied randomly to half of the study population, provided a reduction in the number of adverse events in the imaged population. As an example, a reduction in the number of "futile thoracotomies" has been proposed as a metric of success for PET vs. CT in planning the treatment of newly diagnosed lung cancer.[6] Ideally, randomization of patients to imaged vs. not imaged groups can be shown to improve survival. However, performance of randomized trials in which half of the patients undergo imaging and the other patients do not (or they obtain different kinds of imaging), with an endpoint of survival, will be of great interest. Unfortunately, such studies are complex because management of patients after imaging may be altered markedly. Thus, it can be difficult to separate the imaging study effect from the treatment effect. However, ultimately, for some imaging studies to be adopted, such evaluations of survival will be needed. This point is particularly relevant to screening, as discussed later.

Screening Concepts and Challenges

Screening programs for cancer have often taken the form of laboratory tests such as the Pap smear, or more recently, blood tests for tumor markers. The success of the Pap smear in reducing societal mortality rates from cervical cancer is incontrovertible. The use of imaging in screening for cancer is an example of success and considerable interest, but also a source of considerable controversy. As discussed in detail in the breast cancer section of this text (see Chapter 94), screening mammography programs have been shown capable of saving lives in women older than 50 years of age. These programs may also save lives in women 40 to 50 years of age, but the data are less compelling.[7] Studies have been initiated in which CT scanning is used to detect small pulmonary nodules. These studies clearly can find early lung cancers, but whether they improve survival remains to be determined by prospective study.[8]

Other areas in which screening by noninvasive imaging has been performed include colorectal cancer, where virtual colonoscopy can be used to look for early colon cancers, and in the pelvis in women who are at risk for ovarian cancer. More recently, screening CT centers offering a virtual evaluation of the entire body have become available, and even more recently, MRI and PET screening have been offered in some locales. The drivers of this growth are emotional and economic, but these tests are not yet well-founded scientifically in this screening setting.

Screening carries with it challenges, risks, and costs beyond the scope of this overview chapter. However, several key points apply to screening approaches, including those with noninvasive imaging. These points include whether a screening program is reasonable to consider, lead time bias, length bias, and the overall cost implications of screening, especially the costs of investigating false-positive results.

The requirements that must be met for a screening program to be considered "reasonable" may differ substantially based on the specific society's values and a specific individual's perception of risk. However, in general, the following characteristics are important for cancer screening: The cancer must have a considerable public health effect, the disease must have an asymptomatic period in which detection by imaging is possible, and a therapeutic intervention that can lead to better survival or quality of life must be available. Further, the prevalence of the disease must be sufficient in the population being screened to justify screening (especially the cost), medical treatment must be available for the early-stage cancer identified by screening, and there must be a high likelihood that the patients in whom early cancer is identified by image-based screening will go on to have a suitable therapeutic intervention. Further, the imaging test itself must be acceptable to patients (in terms of level of discomfort and cost), and it must be sufficiently sensitive to identify cancer often and sufficiently specific to minimize false-positive results. Finally, the costs of the screening process must be compatible with the society's or the individual's economic evaluation system, and the screening procedure must pose little or no risk to the patient.[3]

Another important consideration in screening programs is lead time bias. This concept, simply stated, indicates that if the natural history of a disease is unchanged, but the diagnosis is made earlier in the course of the illness, the apparent survival will be improved. For example, let us assume that tumor X has a 6-year natural history from its beginning until the death of the patient, and that treatment was ineffective. The disease might become clinically detectable after 4 years and lead to death in 6 years, a 2-year survival after diagnosis. With screening, if the tumor is detected 3 years after the onset of disease and no improvement in treatment occurs, then the survival in the screened population would appear to increase from 2 to 3 years after diagnosis. This illusion of improved survival in the screened population is a considerable concern and can lead to inappropriate enthusiasm for screening programs.[3]

Another important consideration in screening is the possibility of length bias. This is a more complex concept, but it may be related to the types of cancer that can be detected by screening programs. A possibility is that very rapidly growing and presumably highly lethal cancers are less likely to be detected by annual screening programs, whereas more slowly growing cancers, which have an intrinsically better prognosis, may be detected more frequently by screening. If so, the patients with cancers identified in the screened population could appear to have a better survival than the patients with cancers identified in the unscreened population.

Collectively, these two factors, lead time bias and length bias, generally make screening programs appear to improve the survival of patients with cancer. Because of these major biases intrinsic in screening, large studies are required to show that overall cancer-specific mortality (and ideally mortality from all causes) declines as a result of screening programs. Large, randomized trials are required to prove that this effect occurs, and few have been performed with imaging. Although many anecdotes exist regarding screening, the efficacy of these approaches is largely undocumented.

Costs of Screening

Determining whether a screening program is valuable depends on its cost and benefit. The concept of quality-adjusted life-years (QALYs) is often applied. This concept is the economic cost to society to result in 1 additional year of quality life for a member of the society. In many western countries, a figure of $50,000 has been considered a useful guide, with QALYs lower than this amount considered cost-effective. Such a guideline, however, does not necessarily apply when individuals make their own determinations as to whether to pay for a screening test. For example, it is reasonable to expect that those with greater disposable income would be willing to pay more per QALY than those with less disposable income. Thus, it can be difficult to generalize about the cost efficacy of screening procedures.[9]

Even when people choose to undergo a screening test at their own expense, there can be considerable costs transferred to society as a result of the screening program. For example, if a screening test has a high frequency of false-positive results, a substantial number of follow-up biopsies or procedures will occur and can cost a great deal of money. Such costs can dramatically raise the total cost per QALY. Particularly invasive procedures can also increase the likelihood of morbidity or death as a result of additional investigations. Such costs and risks must be considered, in addition to the cost of the imaging procedure, to determine the true cost per QALY associated with screening. Thus, screening remains an area of great promise, but also of considerable controversy.

Size of Detectable Lesions

Noninvasive imaging methods in humans cannot detect a single malignant cell. Imaging methods are improving, however, and detection of a much smaller number of cells is possible in small animal models. However, it has been estimated that by the time a tumor reaches 3 to 5 mm in diameter, which is the lower limit in size for detection by the best current noninvasive methods in humans, the tumor has undergone more than 25 doublings and contains 0.1 to 1 billion cells, depending on their size.[1] In contrast, a cytologist, on a very good day, may be able to identify a single cell as malignant using a microscope.

Realistically, even for histologic assessment of malignancy, typically a group of tumor cells must be present before cancer is diagnosed. However, light microscopy and more sensitive techniques such as immunohistochemistry and polymerase chain reactions mean that pathologic techniques potentially will be more sensitive than imaging methods. However, a very important proviso is that for pathologic methods to be effective, actual examination of the malignant cells is required; the sample containing the tumor must be cut appropriately and viewed under a microscope. This task may be impossible because 8-μm sections that are used for pathologic examination typically are taken only from a small portion of a tumor or lymph node, whereas most of the tumor or node will be unexamined (e.g., to assess a 1-cm node using 8-μm-thick sections, approximately 125 sections would be required). This large number of sections is not typically obtained. Despite the markedly superior sensitivity of histologic methods over noninvasive imaging, there is a major sampling error issue, and paradoxically, imaging in some diseases is more sensitive for cancer than is histologic examination. When tumors are imaged by noninvasive methods, the entire tumor is visualized, not just a small portion. So, paradoxically, imaging, despite limited resolution, can be more sensitive than pathology. However, if exhaustive and thorough sampling is performed, with microscopic examination of tissue, there is usually greater sensitivity for tumor than there is with current noninvasive imaging techniques.

Stage Migration

One of the major goals of noninvasive imaging is to precisely stage the tumor to allow the clinician to best choose treatment and determine the prognosis. The evolving concepts of tumor staging are discussed elsewhere in this text, but improvements in detection technology can change the understanding of the natural history of a given stage of disease. Patients with small or microscopic metastases to the mediastinum are likely to do better than patients with bulky metastases, but both may have the same stage of disease. As the sensitivity for detecting small lesions improves, it becomes possible to identify more patients with small primary tumors and small metastases to the lymph nodes or systemic disease. Thus, when primary tumors are detected at ever earlier and less advanced stages as imaging methods improve, patients are assigned to a higher stage than was used historically. Their presence in the advanced-stage group appears to improve survival and outcome in that group. Unfortunately, fewer and fewer patients are assigned to the lowest-stage groups, and overall survival may not be changed because of the higher proportion of patients in the higher-stage groups.[3]

MAJOR IMAGING MODALITIES

Broadly stated, cancer imaging can be performed using anatomic or functional imaging methods.[1] The traditional imaging of the patient with cancer, and the most established method, is based on anatomic imaging. However, there is an increasing move toward cancer imaging to be performed with more functional methods. Hybrid images, derived from and displaying both functional and anatomic data, are also becoming more widely available, often coming from the same hybrid imaging machine.[10,11] Imaging data are increasingly digital or digitized and suitable for postprocessing and image exchange. The major imaging modalities are discussed next.

Plain Film X-Rays

The traditional x-ray remains an important part of cancer imaging. It is commonly used to detect bone tumors and can be used to detect lung cancers in the thorax. The method displays mainly water and calcium density and is affected by overlapping tissue in front of or behind the lesion. X-rays have become increasingly digitized in the last few years, with the introduction of film digitization and phosphor screen capture devices. X-rays offer exceptional resolution, but relatively little image contrast. The radiation dose from a plain film x-ray is dependent on the portion of the body being examined.[12]

Mammography

Mammography is a specialized form of plain x-rays. Very high-resolution images of the breast are obtained using specialized devices optimized for breast cancer detection. Digital mammography is now available, and offers greater flexibility of image display because of the digital image format. A limitation of the digital format is the field of view of the imaging phosphor, which may be too small to fully include some breast tissue.[13]

Computed Tomography

CT is now established as the dominant imaging technique for cancer detection and follow-up. CT scanners acquire images using an x-ray source and digital detector elements. The x-ray source rotates rapidly around the patient. Faster and faster rotation speeds of the scanners, along with detectors capable of imaging multiple slice thicknesses in a rapid spiral motion, are being used. These faster scanners can potentially evaluate the entire body in a few seconds. Although such evaluations provide key information about lesion size, some lesions may elude detection unless contrast is given intravenously, orally, or both. With such devices, it is also possible to capture contrast in arteries or veins to provide superior visualization of these structures, which can then be displayed three-dimensionally or in a volume-rendered fashion. A disadvantage of CT is its cost, both technically and in terms of the radiation dose. Although CT is an exceptional technique, it remains a predominantly anatomic imaging method. All CT images are digital. A major challenge with CT is the large amount of image data generated for analysis, data that can take a long time to interpret fully.[14]

Angiography

Historically, angiography has been performed after intravascular insertion of catheters into arteries, followed by rapid injection of iodinated contrast media, along with rapid-sequence filming of the images. The improving ability of rapid-sequence CT scanning to show the vascular anatomy (CT angiography) is rapidly replacing the use of angiography for diagnostic purposes. Angiography can still be used to produce the most precise maps of vascular anatomy before organ transplantation or radical cancer surgery. Most angiography is now performed using digital image-capture devices known as digital angiography. Angiographic delivery of therapy is, however, an important area, because this form of imaging can allow for therapeutic delivery of embolization materials such as coils, delivery of chemotherapeutic agents regionally, or delivery of radioactive microspheres, for example. Angiography has high resolution, but typically delivers a high dose of radiation energy to the patient.[15]

Ultrasound

Ultrasound is an imaging method that does not involve the use of ionizing radiation, but uses reflected beams of high-frequency sound to generate images. Ultrasound provides high resolution and some functional information, specifically about the presence and direction of blood flow in tissues. Ultrasound provides some tissue characterization properties, and is very effective in determining whether a tissue is cystic or solid. Ultrasound can guide biopsies effectively and provides real-time imaging capability to guide biopsies and procedures. Ultrasound is less effective in the evaluation of deeper structures, and requires access to a sonographic window. Thus, it has only a modest role in evaluating deep abdominal structures. Ultrasound is commonly used in evaluations of the pelvis, neck (including the thyroid), and gallbladder and liver areas. Agents that can enhance the visualization of vessels, or can be specifically retained in clots, are under evaluation, suggesting that ultrasound can offer some functional information beyond the purely anatomic.[16]

Magnetic Resonance Imaging and Magnetic Resonance Spectroscopy

Magnetic resonance imaging (MRI), as applied in imaging most cancers, is a predominantly anatomic imaging method that does not use ionizing radiation. MRI offers superb contrast resolution between tissues and excellent spatial resolution. However, MRI does not offer the level of temporal resolution, in general, as seen with ultrasound, fluoroscopy, or recent-generation, multiple-slice CT scanners. However, MRI technology has inexorably moved forward, and rapid-pulse sequences allowing gating of images are now available for several types of scanners. MRI images can be of a variety of pulse sequences, allowing visualization of several parameters. However, visualization of hydrogen nuclei is the major approach with conventional 1.5 T and 3 T (Tesla) machines. Visualization of blood, especially with contrast materials such as gadolinium chelates, and of altered vascular permeability is routinely applied.[17]

MRI is used as the procedure of choice in evaluating neoplasms of the brain and spinal cord regions as well as musculoskeletal tumors. MRI is also used with increasing frequency in the evaluation of tumors of the extremities such as sarcomas. With gadolinium contrast enhancement, MRI can also be useful in locating tumors of the breast, which appear as areas of contrast enhancement. MRI can also provide valuable information about tumors in close proximity to vascular structures as well as in the liver and upper abdomen. Tumors in the upper abdomen and liver can be degraded in their appearance on MRI because of respiratory motion artifacts. Therefore, this approach is less commonly applied than in other situations, such as in the lower pelvis, where there often is less respiratory motion artifact. Research is ongoing to develop agents that can facilitate specific MRI contrast enhancement. More rapid whole-body MRI acquisition methods are also under evaluation, which may broaden the use of MRI.

Magnetic resonance spectroscopy (MRS) is an exciting method by which tissue characterization can be achieved by sampling its magnetic spectrum at 1.5 T. Some devices now provide a 3 T or higher field strength signal for evaluation, offering the possibility of more refined tissue characterization. Opportunities to detect increased content of choline (often increased in tumor foci) vs. other substituents can be helpful in separating tumor from nonmalignant tissues in the brain and elsewhere. Spectroscopy can also provide information on lactate concentration and pH, among other parameters. A limitation of spectroscopy is resolution, which is typically not nearly as fine as that of MRI itself. Thus, spectroscopy has only limited application in most oncologic practice.[18]

Nuclear Medicine and Positron Emission Tomography

Radionuclide methods can provide a great deal of functional information, but often with limited anatomic resolution. Broadly, there are single-photon and positron-emitting isotopes. Single-photon emitters typically have longer half-lives than positron emitters, and decay in a different fashion. Depending on the ligand attached to the radioactive isotope, a wide variety of processes can be imaged. For single-photon imaging, the most common isotope is ^{99m}Tc, which can be used to image bone (bone scan with ^{99m}Tc methylene diphosphonate) or thyroid (technetium pertechnetate), for example. With positron emitters, the most commonly used tracer is F18, which is used as the radiolabel for FDG, an agent that images glycolysis in vivo. Because tumors have increased glycolytic metabolism in general, this agent is seeing very rapid growth in its application to tumor imaging, especially in lung and colorectal tumors and lymphomas.[19]

Both PET and SPECT have very high sensitivity for a small number of radioactive molecules in vivo as well as the ability to quantitate the radioactivity concentration precisely. Thus, these methods have importance as both clinical and research tools. The intrinsic lack of anatomic resolution for PET and SPECT can be partly addressed by fusing the PET or SPECT images to CT using computer software. More recently, dedicated hybrid imaging devices, including both PET and CT or SPECT and CT in a single device, have been applied to the imaging practice of cancer.

Higher doses of radioactive isotopes can also be therapeutic. For example, ^{131}I is used for the treatment of thyroid cancer as sodium iodide. The same isotope, conjugated to an anti-CD20 monoclonal antibody, has recently been approved by the U.S. Food and Drug

Administration to treat low-grade and transformed B-cell non-Hodgkin's lymphoma that is considered refractory to standard treatments. The tracer doses are used to guide the treatment doses in such instances.[20]

Optical Imaging Methods

Optical imaging methods are applied in a variety of ways. For example, the external physical examination of a patient involves visual interrogation of reflected light. Infrared and transmitted light are also used to a limited extent in evaluating small parts of the body. Optical imaging has the limited penetration depth of a variety of forms of light in the body. Thus, this type of approach may prove of greatest utility in evaluating small animals as part of experimental studies, or for superficial organs, such as the breast. The possibility of constructing light-emitting contrast media is a real one, and optical imaging has the potential to provide remarkable sensitivity and resolution in superficial structures. However, it is not routinely applied, with the exception of visualization of the interior of the eye, visualization of the cervix, and endoscopy from above and below.[21] The strengths and weaknesses of the major imaging methods are contrasted in Table 18-2.

ANATOMIC VERSUS FUNCTIONAL IMAGING

Limitations of Anatomic Imaging of Cancer

Anatomic imaging has been the fundamental approach to cancer imaging for more than 100 years. The robustness of anatomic methods is supported by their daily use in managing individual patients with cancer. However, anatomic imaging detects a phenotypic alteration that is sometimes, but not invariably, associated with cancer—a mass. However, with anatomic imaging, we often do not know whether masses are the result of malignant or benign etiologies such as in solitary pulmonary nodules or borderline-size lymph nodes. Similarly, small cancers are undetectable with traditional anatomic methods, because they have not yet formed a mass. After surgery, it is even more difficult to assess for the presence of recurrent

tumor with anatomic methods. Post-treatment scans are complicated by the need for comparisons with normal anatomy to detect altered morphologic findings as a result of cancer. Anatomic methods do not predict the response to treatment and do not quickly document tumors responding to therapy.[22] Despite these challenges, anatomic images remain routine in cancer management. PET, a functional imaging method, helps to address many of the limitations of anatomic imaging, and when combined with anatomic images in fusion images, is emerging as a particularly valuable tool, providing both anatomic precision and functional information in a single image set.[3]

Molecular and Functional Alterations in Cancer

The molecular bases of neoplasia are increasingly well defined. Mutations in genomic DNA precede the development of overt neoplasia.[23] With sufficient alterations in genotype, phenotypic changes occur. These genotypic and phenotypic changes in cancer antedate the development of a discrete mass lesion, and represent potential targets for innovative imaging agents. The concepts of altered "genome" and "proteome" resulting in alterations in metabolism, consistent with an altered "metabolosome," are increasingly recognized as present in cancers. PET, because of its superb sensitivity to low signal levels, can detect signals from tracers, targeting such alterations that are preferentially present in cancer.

PET has led the growing field of molecular imaging to the clinic, in part because of the quantitative capabilities of PET and the sensitivity of electronic collimation, but also because of the choice of a proper radiotracer for cancer imaging. Although a wide variety of molecular, proteomic, and metabolic alterations occur in cancers, and many of these can or may ultimately be imaged with PET, the most useful target in the clinical practice of PET is the increased glucose metabolism present in most cancers. Other PET tracers, such as those targeting hypoxia, proliferation, amino acid transport, blood-brain barrier permeability, and protein synthesis, are discussed in the following sections. The challenge with all imaging modalities is how to best integrate them into clinical practice. The next section addresses these issues.

TABLE 18-2

Imaging Methods

MODALITY	RESOLUTION	SENSITIVITY	SPECIFICITY	FUNCTIONAL IMAGING ABILITY
Magnetic resonance imaging	3 mm	Moderate	Moderate	Moderate with spectroscopy
Computed tomography	2 mm	Moderate	Moderate	Low, except angiography
Radiographs	2 mm	Low	Moderate	Very little
Single-photon-emission computed tomography	1 cm	High	Moderate	Excelllent
Positron emission tomography	5 mm	High	Relatively high	Excellent
Ultrasound	5 mm	Low	Low	Some, especially with contrast
Mammography	2 mm	Moderate	Relatively low	None
Angiography	2 mm	Moderate	Moderate	Low

Bragg DG, Rubin P, Hricak H: Imaging strategies for oncologic diagnosis and multidisciplinary treatment. In Bragg D, Rubin P, Hricak H (eds): Oncologic Imaging, 2nd ed. Philadelphia, WB Saunders, 2002, pp 3–20.

DISEASE-SPECIFIC IMAGING RECOMMENDATIONS

Brief discussions of the role and possible role of imaging in managing several common cancers follow. There is great variation in the imaging workup of specific types of tumors, depending on the type of therapy planned. In general, the more aggressive and radical the planned treatment the more critical the need for accurate determination of the location of all foci of tumor through imaging. Similarly, the intensity and frequency of follow-up imaging examinations must be guided by the potential importance of the information gained. For example, if no effective salvage therapy is available, intensive surveillance for recurrent tumor makes little sense, except to provide reassurance to patients when test results are negative. This may seem self-evident, but it is surprising how practice patterns vary.

Lung Cancer

The initial diagnosis of lung cancer is often based on incidental detection of an abnormality on an imaging study, although more advanced lung cancer can cause hemoptysis, cough, weight loss, hoarseness, infection, or shortness of breath. If a solitary pulmonary nodule 1 to 3 cm in diameter is identified on a chest x-ray or on screening CT, the workup to determine whether it represents lung cancer can take a variety of forms. Comparison with old anatomic images is essential, but if none are available, a decision must be made whether to perform a biopsy or remove the tumor or follow the abnormality. A variety of factors can be considered, including patient age, smoking history, lesion size, and history of exposure to potential infectious agents.

The morphology of the nodule is examined to determine whether it has characteristics that suggest malignancy or benignity. The margin and internal density of the lesion are examined. Smooth, well-defined margins suggest a benign nodule, but can also be seen in 21% of malignant nodules.[24] A lobulated margin suggests cells of different lines with uneven growth, but can be seen in 25% of benign nodules. A spiculated margin is highly suggestive of malignancy. Both benign and malignant nodules can be homogeneous and can cavitate. A cavity with a wall thickness of 4 mm or less is likely benign in 95% of cases, a wall thickness of 5 to 15 mm is indeterminate, and a wall thickness of more than 15 mm is likely malignant in 95% of cases.[24] If the lesion contains fat, it is specific for a hamartoma, and 50% of hamartomas have fat on CT.

Benign calcifications are central in the lesion, diffuse and solid, laminated, or popcorn-like. Calcification is seen in 6% of lung cancers on CT, and tends to be eccentric or amorphous.[24] Thus, calcification alone does not indicate benignity in a lung nodule. If contrast is administered and the lesion is monitored over 5 minutes, enhancement of less than 15 HU (Hounsfield Units) suggests a benign lesion and enhancement of greater than 20 HU suggests a malignant lesion, with reported sensitivity of as high as 98%, specificity of 73%, and accuracy of 85%.[25] However, these CT criteria rely on very small changes in CT attenuation levels. These subtle changes may be insufficient to allow for reliable stratification of nodules as malignant or benign, because timing of the CT bolus is also an important consideration. The growth rate of the lesion can also be evaluated, but this is difficult for subcentimeter lesions. Computer programs for nodule detection are being developed that also provide lesion volume, and this may prove useful in follow-up.

However, for a significant number of patients, the risk of cancer remains intermediate. For such patients, PET imaging with FDG may be useful. PET has been reported to have sensitivity of approximately 96% for detecting cancer in solitary pulmonary nodules (predominantly ≥1 cm in diameter) in a retrospective meta-analysis,[26] with specificity of approximately 80%. However, some lesion histologies are less well detected, such as bronchiolo-alveolar carcinomas. Nonetheless, the PET scan can help to determine which patients require immediate biopsy or excision of a nodule (i.e., a nodule with intense FDG uptake) vs. those who can be observed (some of those with low or no tracer uptake). The use of PET varies widely, but it can be a valuable tool for helping to determine which patients need invasive procedures for pulmonary nodules. Because false-negative findings occur, however, patients who do not have surgery should be followed up regularly for up to 2 years to ensure that there has been no lesion growth. An example of a patient with both "hot" and "cold" nodules is shown in Figure 18-2A.

Once lung cancer is diagnosed, an appropriate staging workup should be undertaken. The workup for non–small cell lung cancer is often done to determine whether the patient is a candidate for surgery. Because PET imaging with FDG is at least 20% more accurate than CT imaging, PET is commonly recommended as a staging procedure for the mediastinum and for systemic evaluation for metastases.[27] In a prospective randomized trial, PET reduced the number of futile thoracotomies by half, from 41% to 21%, vs. algorithms in which PET was not performed.[28] This occurred in part by identifying remote foci of metastatic disease that were not identified by standard staging methods. There is not yet complete consensus on how PET should be used in staging non–small cell lung cancer, but performing PET before surgery is increasingly recommended. It is generally considered wise to perform a biopsy on FDG-avid lymph nodes to prove that they represent cancer. In contrast, many would argue that mediastinoscopy is no longer essential for patients who have negative mediastinal PET and CT scans, although in some patients, cancer in nodes is detected only surgically. An example of a positive PET scan with ipsilateral and contralateral mediastinal tumor involvement is shown in Figure 18-2B.

For mediastinal nodes, a short-axis diameter of greater than 1 cm is considered abnormal on CT. Larger nodes can be reactive and subcentimeter nodes can contain tumor, leading to sensitivity of 40% to 67% and specificity of 79% to 86% for metastatic disease.[29]

Early studies have shown the hybrid PET/CT technology to be superior to PET alone for the staging

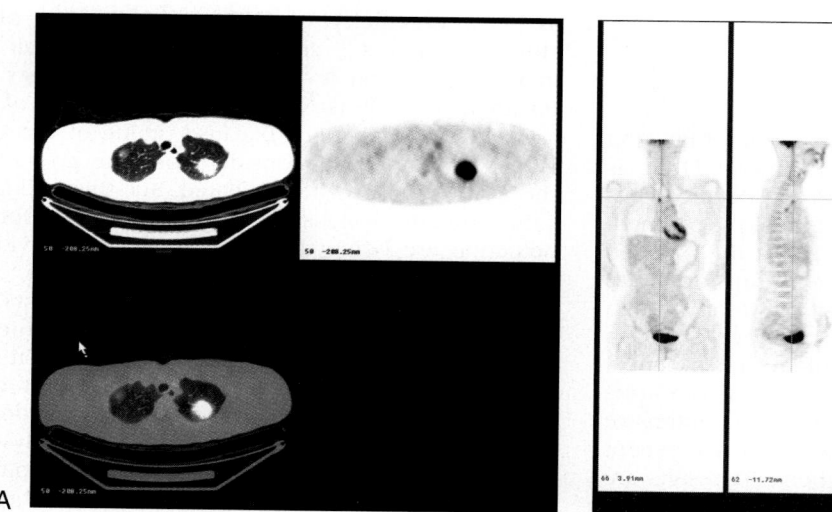

Figure 18-2. A, Positron emission tomography (PET) and computed tomography (CT) images. The upper left image is CT, the upper right image is PET, and the lower left image is PET and CT data fused. The CT scan shows a smaller right apical nodule and a large left upper lung nodule. PET shows increased uptake of [18]fluorodeoxyglucose (FDG) in the left apical nodule, consistent with cancer, whereas only minimal uptake is seen in the right apical lesion, consistent with benign disease. Fused PET and CT images confirm the location of increased apical FDG uptake, as in the left lung nodule. **B,** Whole-body images from PET scans of the patient shown in **(A).** The images include coronal, sagittal, transverse, and "projection" whole-body views, from left to right. They show cancer in the left upper lung, mediastinal involvement, and a right paratracheal tumor focus. Normal uptake is seen in the heart, brain, and excretory system (bladder).

of lung cancer.[30] The best algorithm for staging the mediastinum is evolving, but PET and PET/CT are the most accurate noninvasive methods. Some argue that mediastinoscopy is necessary in each case, however, because PET may produce false-negative results in patients with a low tumor burden, although the negative predictive value of a negative PET scan and a negative CT scan is approximately 95%. However, others would argue that patients with a low tumor burden, below the level of detectability with PET and CT, may be suitable candidates for surgery without the need for mediastinoscopy. Positive PET scans for metastases generally require tissue confirmation of the most advanced site of tumor to avoid false-positive imaging findings that a tumor is not resectable. Examples of detection of lung cancer on CT and the use of reformatted virtual images are shown in Figure 18-3.

For imaging the brain, MRI with contrast is recommended. In general, this is performed if patients have larger primary tumors or any symptoms that suggest

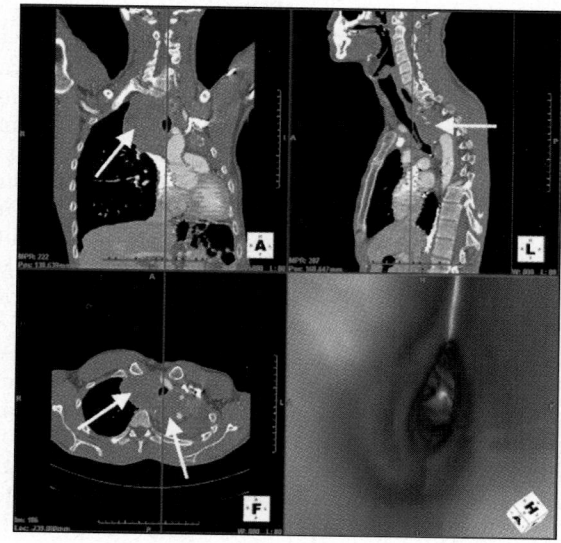

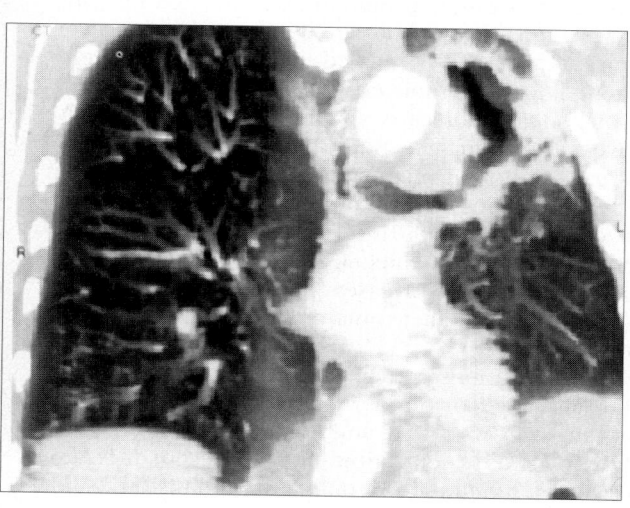

Figure 18-3. Lung cancer. **A,** Axial computed tomography (CT) image (*lower left*) shows a mediastinal mass (*arrows*) narrowing the airway. Coronal (*top left*) and sagittal (*top right*) reconstructed images show narrowing of the airway by mass (*arrows*). Virtual bronchoscopy image (*lower right*) shows an endoluminal view of the narrowed airway. **B,** Coronal reconstruction of CT data in a different patient shows a cavitating mass in the left upper lobe. (Courtesy of Dr. Leo Lawler, Johns Hopkins University.)

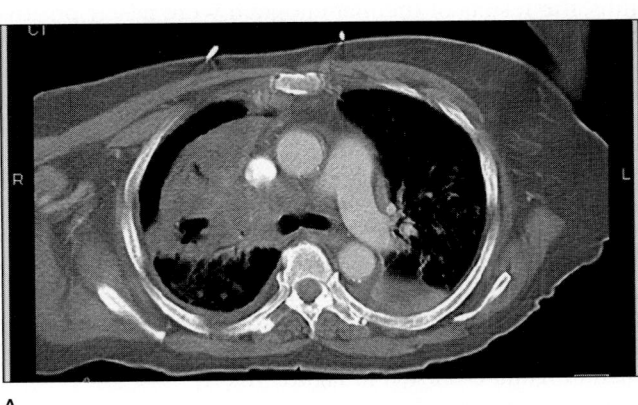
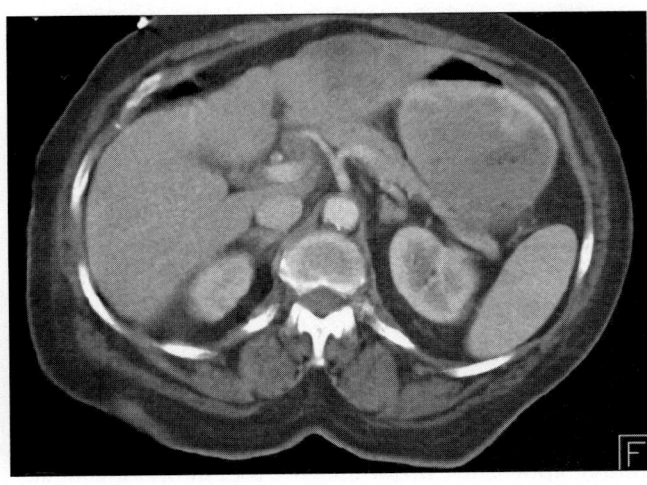

A   B

Figure 18-4. Lung cancer. **A,** Axial computed tomography (CT) scan of the chest with IV contrast shows a mass obstructing the right upper lobe bronchus. **B,** CT scan of the abdomen shows a metastatic hypodense lesion in the left lobe of the liver.

central nervous system involvement, although in some centers, MRI with contrast is performed in each patient in whom resection for cure is planned for lung cancer. Evaluation for bone metastases is currently performed by bone scan. Any patient with bone pain or an elevated alkaline phosphatase level should undergo this study. In practice, where PET is available, bone scans are gradually being replaced by PET scans. This area is evolving, and the bone scan remains the routine procedure in most centers when bone metastases are suspected.

In institutions that do not have PET available, bone scan, MRI of the brain, and CT of the chest and abdomen, to include the adrenals, are recommended. The abdominal CT should be performed with contrast to best evaluate the liver. An example of a patient with extensive mediastinal disease and liver metastases is shown in Figure 18-4.

For small cell lung cancer, a determination of whether the disease is extensive or localized must be made to determine the form of therapy. CT is essential for the chest and upper abdomen. MRI is typically performed of the brain, and a bone scan is done to search for bone metastases. PET scans show promise in small cell lung cancer, but are not yet routinely used for this type of staging in many centers. In addition, the literature is much less extensive than for non–small cell lung cancer.

Evaluation of the Adrenal

Adrenal masses occur in approximately 9% of the population. These masses can be benign adenomas, metastatic disease from primary tumors such as lung cancer, or primary adrenal cortical carcinoma. CT and MRI are used to distinguish adenomas from malignant lesions in the adrenals. Adrenal adenomas have low attenuation on noncontrast CT as a result of elevated lipid content. If a threshold value of 0 HU is used, sensitivity is 47% and specificity is 100% for the diagnosis of adenoma.[31] If a threshold value of 10 HU is used, sensitivity is 71% and specificity is 98% for the diagnosis of adenoma.

Adenomas take up contrast material, but the washout of contrast material from an adenoma is faster than from a metastatic lesion. On 10-minute delayed images obtained after contrast injection, greater than 50% decrease in the density of the lesion is specific for an adenoma.[31] If the lesion is atypical on CT, chemical shift imaging on MRI is used to determine whether it is an adenoma. An adenoma has both lipid and water content, and decreases in signal are seen on out-of-phase T1-weighted images. PET has a growing role in evaluating the adrenals, with accuracy of 90% and greater reported in some series. An example of detection of adrenal and systemic metastases is shown in Figure 18-5.

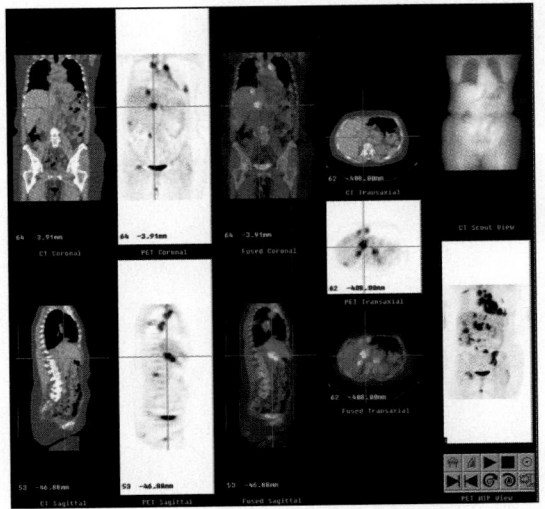

Figure 18-5. Positron emission tomography (PET) and computed tomography (CT) image panel shows a variety of PET, CT, and fused images that show diffusely metastatic lung carcinoma. Notable are adrenal metastases that are best seen on the transverse images, although many metastases are visible in a variety of locations. This image also shows the multiple types of images available from a PET and CT system.

Science of Clinical Oncology

PET is also useful in the evaluation of small cell lung cancers and mesotheliomas, although the data are evolving, and CT is the established method for this type of evaluation. For follow-up of lung cancer, the guidelines are more challenging because the available therapeutic options are often more limited. PET has a growing role because it can better separate residual scarring from viable tumor than can CT.

Thus, in lung cancer, both anatomic and functional imaging techniques are very important. PET is growing rapidly in use, and where available, is a routine part of the workup of many patients with solitary pulmonary nodules and primary lung cancers.

Breast Cancer

Mammography is the major imaging tool in breast cancer, allowing for early detection of tumors. When properly used, mammographic screening programs have been shown to save lives vs. unscreened populations, and these programs are routinely implemented in many countries.[32]

Although mammography is a reasonably sensitive and specific procedure, the relatively low prevalence of cancer means that many image-directed biopsies show no tumor; thus, the results of the mammogram were falsely positive. Stereotactic biopsy devices have greatly facilitated nonsurgical breast biopsies. Although other techniques can detect breast cancer, only ultrasound is used fairly commonly in the breast in most imaging centers to help to separate cystic from solid lesions or to help to locate and evaluate palpable but mammographically negative lesions. MRI with gadolinium contrast is used because it is a very sensitive technique and can help to determine whether disease is unifocal or multicentric. PET methods are occasionally applied in the breast, but these are infrequently used for diagnosis and are generally used in disseminated disease. An example of a positive mammogram is shown in Figure 18-6A.

Breast cancer often metastasizes first to locoregional lymph nodes. The evaluation of the axillary nodes is not done effectively with current noninvasive imaging methods. However, imaging can help to define which

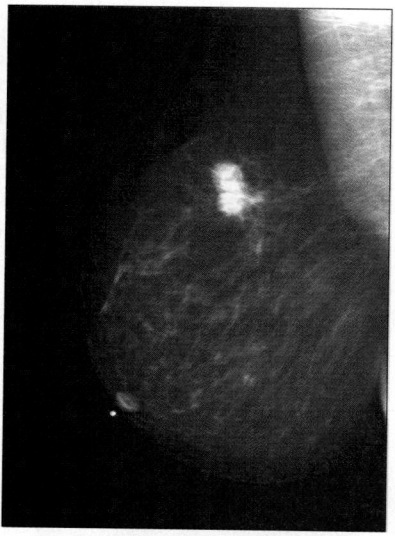

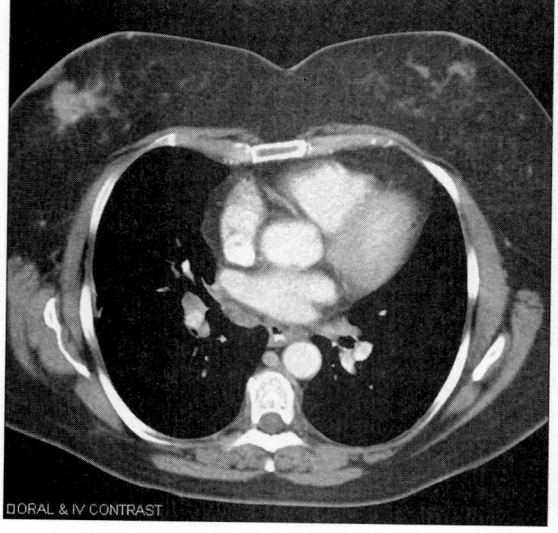

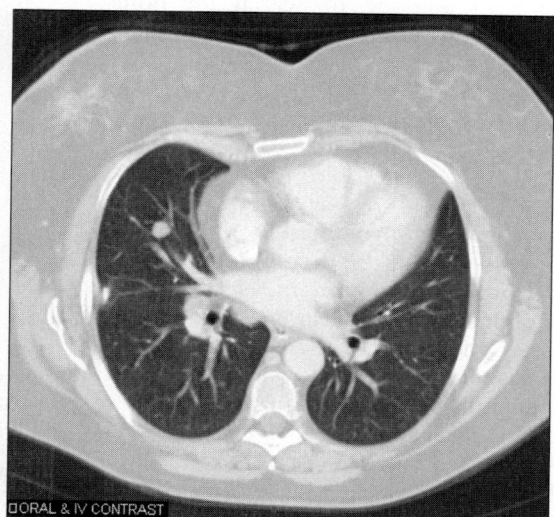

Figure 18-6. Breast cancer. **A,** Mammogram of the right breast shows cancer. **B,** Axial computed tomography (CT) image shows an irregular soft tissue primary mass in the right breast in a different patient. **C,** Axial CT image with a lung window shows a metastatic nodule in the right lung. (**A,** Courtesy of Dr. Nagi Khouri, Johns Hopkins University.)

lymph nodes should be resected for histologic sampling. Sentinel node imaging or detection using a probe system is playing an ever-increasing role in axillary assessment of patients with breast cancer. This procedure is discussed in more detail elsewhere in the text, but imaging is used, especially in European centers, to help better localize the axillary nodes for intraoperative assessment and determine atypical routes of lymphatic drainage. Studies have shown sentinel node sampling procedures to be at least 90% sensitive relative to axillary dissection, which is considered useful sensitivity, and is 100% specific.[33]

The extent of systemic imaging required in the initial workup of a patient with breast cancer depends on the size of the primary tumor and the status of the axillary nodes at biopsy. For patients with positive nodes, it can be argued that the likelihood of systemic metastatic disease is higher; thus, more intensive evaluation may be more appropriate. Some would suggest a baseline bone scan and CT of the chest and abdomen at this time. The frequency of follow-up is debated, given the improbability of curing recurrent systemic disease, and some have advocated only limited biochemical follow-up. However, this is a controversial area. Examples of the use of CT in imaging primary and metastatic breast cancers are shown in Figure 18-6B and C. PET imaging can detect, using FDG, disseminated cancers; however, the optimal role of PET in imaging is evolving. PET is a highly effective tool for evaluating soft tissue involvement and quickly assessing treatment response.[34]

Prostate Cancer

The role of imaging in newly diagnosed prostate cancer is evolving.

Evaluation of the Prostate

Unfortunately, intraprostate carcinoma is not particularly well detected by imaging with ultrasound or other methods. Although transrectal ultrasound has been used to guide biopsies, up to 40% of prostate cancers are isoechoic (and thus undetectable) by this method. Similarly, the positive predictive value of hypoechoic lesions of the prostate is typically well less than 50%. Ultrasound can be used to detect abnormalities and guide biopsy of the entire prostate because it does an excellent job of defining the overall shape, size, and location of the prostate for purposes of systematic biopsy. A sextant approach is often used to sample the base, middle, and apex of the prostate bilaterally, in addition to biopsy of any suspicious areas. Although this technique is less than perfect in accuracy for detecting prostate cancers, on ultrasound, tumors in the peripheral zone are more readily visible than tumors in the inner gland. The peripheral zone is echogenic, and tumors that are hypoechoic to it (approximately 60%) can be detected.[35] However, hypoechoic lesions can also be caused by inflammatory processes, and the positive predictive value of ultrasound is approximately 18% to 52%.[35] Similarly, on MRI, cancers that are hypointense on T2-weighted images are seen, but the findings are not specific for tumor. Extension of cancer beyond the prostate capsule is suggested on

ultrasound when the capsule margin is irregular or the seminal vesicles are abnormal in morphology; however, sensitivity of as low as 20% has been reported. The sensitivity of MRI for extracapsular invasion is approximately 50%, and specificity is 95%.[35] Patients at intermediate risk for invasion, with a prostate-specific antigen (PSA) level of 10 to 20 ng/mL and a Gleason score of 5 to 7, may benefit from MRI staging of local extension.[35] MRI methods are considered to be improving, especially with the use of spectroscopy.[35,36]

CT has no established role in evaluating the prostate itself or local invasion (25% sensitivity for capsular invasion), although tumors can sometimes be seen on CT (Fig. 18-7A). CT is used to detect bladder and rectal invasion, adenopathy, and distant metastases, and MRI is used to assess local extent. Similarly, the sensitivity for detecting nodal metastases has been reported to be as low as 30% with CT. Higher sensitivity can be achieved, but with lower specificity. Generally, pathologic proof is desirable before it is concluded that a patient has metastatic disease to the lymph nodes, and if it is demonstrated, radical prostatectomy is considered inappropriate. Large nodal metastases are easily detected on CT imaging, however (Fig. 18-7B). It is not clear that MRI is better than CT; however, recent data with a node-specific paramagnetic contrast agent has shown very high sensitivity and accuracy in the detection of nodal metastases.[36] Given the low sensitivity of CT and MRI (traditionally) to nodal metastases, it has been recommended that the serum PSA level be at least 20 ng/mL before CT is performed. If the CT findings are positive, then biopsy can be performed of the enlarged node or nodal sampling can be performed before radical prostatectomy. CT is also the test of choice for visceral metastases.

For bone metastases, a bone scan is a sensitive technique relative to x-rays. The results of a bone scan can be positive when radiographs of bone are essentially normal. It is currently recommended that a radionuclide bone scan be performed only if the serum PSA level at presentation is greater than 10 ng/mL. It is very rare for a bone scan to be positive for tumor at lower levels at the time of diagnosis. Some argue that for large primary tumors or very high Gleason scores a bone scan may still be appropriate at staging.

Thus, imaging is used selectively in patients with newly diagnosed prostate cancer. For recurrent prostate cancer, a bone scan is commonly used whenever the PSA level begins to rise. New PET methods are promising in prostate cancer, but are not in widespread use. Similarly, MRS has shown promise in evaluating the prostate gland and determining whether the tumor has spread beyond the prostate.

Much monitoring of prostate cancer now involves sequential blood tests to measure the PSA level. When the PSA level rises persistently, recurrence of tumor has occurred, but determining the site of recurrence is often problematic. Bone scans and CT are often used, with radioantibody imaging for anti-PMSA (prostate membrane specific antigen) antibodies used only infrequently because of limited diagnostic accuracy, although some

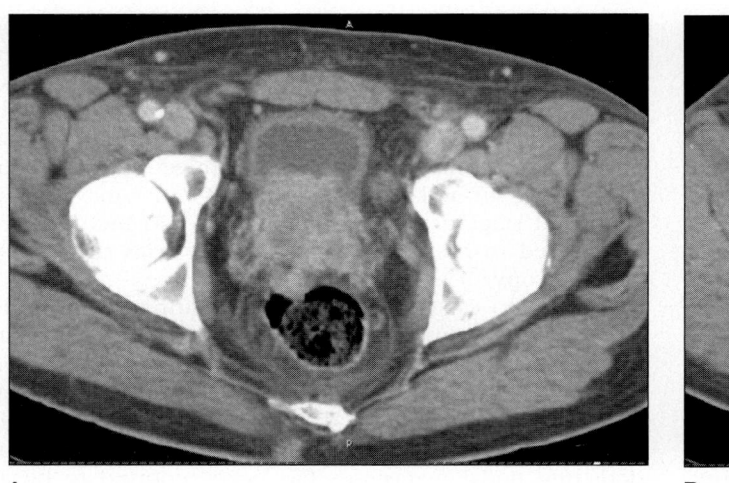

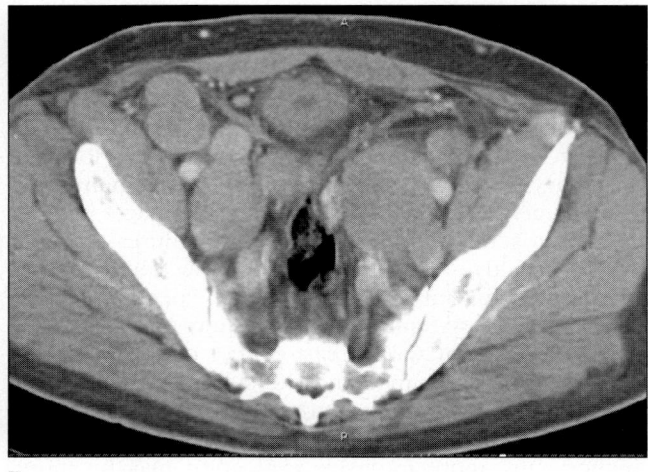

A   B

Figure 18-7. Prostate cancer. **A,** Axial computed tomography (CT) image shows an enlarged prostate with an enhancing mass and irregular margins. **B,** More superior image shows enlarged bilateral pelvic nodes from metastatic disease.

promising results have been obtained by experienced groups.

Colon Cancer

The role of noninvasive imaging in the diagnosis of the primary lesion has changed over the last several decades. Barium enema studies were at one time used extensively to search for colorectal cancer. They have been replaced, in large measure, by fiberoptic colonoscopy. However, there is a growing level of interest in virtual colonoscopy, which is performed using CT scanning and per-rectum insufflation after thorough bowel preparation. This procedure is used to a limited extent for screening. The technique faces challenges because it requires bowel preparation and is quite time-consuming to interpret. This is an area of considerable opportunity for noninvasive imaging. Infrequently, these cancers can be detected by other methods such as ultrasound.

The extent of preoperative imaging performed before resection of primary colon cancer is variable, based on the institution. In general, the larger the primary tumor the more aggressive the staging procedure. In most instances, however, the primary tumor must be surgically resected for palliation (or cure), even if metastatic tumor is present. For staging, the most common studies include CT scan with contrast of the abdomen and pelvis, CT scan of the thorax (or chest radiograph), and bowel imaging to exclude the presence of a second primary colon cancer. In institutions in which PET imaging is available, PET is used somewhat more frequently at presentation; however, it is much more commonly applied in the setting of suspected recurrence.

For colorectal cancer, many advocate regular imaging studies after surgery for "cure," because isolated metastases or oligometastases of colorectal cancer can be resected from the liver or lungs; in some instances, the patient is disease-free for a long period. Thus, before such removal of a limited number of metastases is contemplated, a thorough imaging procedure is undertaken. Generally, this includes CT of the abdomen and pelvis with contrast and CT of the thorax without contrast. CT of the thorax may be replaced by a chest x-ray, but chest x-rays are less sensitive for pulmonary metastases.

PET is very often applied in this setting and in the setting of a rising carcinoembryonic antigen level after surgery. The precise timing of follow-up studies can be variable, but the frequency is often every 6 to 12 months in the early years after surgery. There is considerable evidence that PET can detect more metastatic foci than CT in the setting of a rising carcinoembryonic antigen level.[37] An example of a patient initially believed to have only a limited number of liver metastases is shown in Figure 18-8; however, more extensive disease was identified (Fig. 18-8B).

Although immunoscintigraphy has been used, it is used relatively infrequently because of the availability of PET. PET with FDG often does not detect small (<5 mm) tumors, and is known to be less sensitive for tumors of mucinous histology.

Ultrasound can detect many liver lesions, and is a very useful technique for guiding biopsies of the liver. Many patients with liver metastases have intraoperative ultrasound to assess the extent and location of hepatic metastases. For liver metastases, CT is still the most commonly used procedure, but in a recent meta-analysis, PET was a more robust test to identify the presence and location of hepatic metastases of colorectal cancer, compared with CT, MRI, or ultrasound methods.[38]

Gynecologic Neoplasms

Screening for gynecologic neoplasms is generally not performed by imaging, except for very limited programs that have evaluated the use of either transabdominal or, more commonly, transvaginal ultrasound of the pelvis to detect masses that may be appropriate for removal

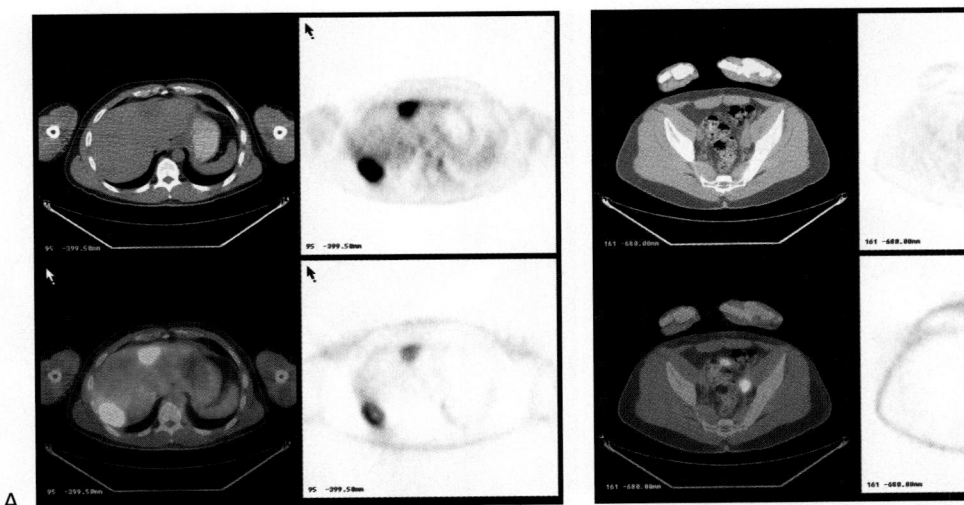

Figure 18-8. Colon cancer. **A,** Positron emission tomography (PET) and computed tomography (CT) image display of a patient with two [18]fluorodeoxyglucose (FDG)-avid lesions in the liver. These are seen on the CT (*upper left*) scan, attenuation-corrected PET (*upper right*) scan, non-attenuation-corrected PET (*lower right*) scan, and fused images (*lower left*). **B,** PET and CT images of the pelvis, oriented as in **(A),** show increased FDG uptake in a left external iliac lymph node metastasis.

because they could represent ovarian cancer. However, such programs have not been proven cost-effective and are not widely applied, but they warrant further study, because this is a very important health problem.

Cervical carcinoma is one of the diseases in which screening using the Pap smear has a large effect in terms of lowering mortality rates by detecting premalignant changes and early-stage disease. Although much of the staging of cervical carcinoma is performed by physical examination, for larger primary tumors, imaging has an important role. CT and MRI are both used in the pelvis; however, there is growing use of PET for tumor staging.

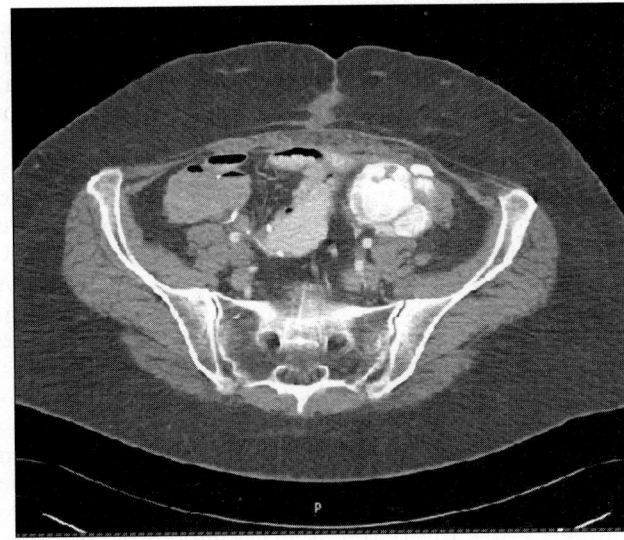

Figure 18-9. Ovarian cancer. Axial computed tomography image shows a dense, calcified mass in the left pelvis, compatible with a metastatic implant from ovarian cancer.

As in other tumors, PET appears to be more sensitive than anatomic imaging methods. Emerging data show PET to provide better prognostic value than anatomic imaging in cervical cancer.[39]

In ovarian cancer, no technique is able to detect microscopic metastatic disease. Ultrasound is the main method by which these tumors are identified at their earliest stages; however, the unfortunate fact is that these tumors are usually diagnosed at an advanced stage. Imaging can be used in an attempt to determine how extensive the surgical procedure should be. CT and MRI are both used to assess the extent of ovarian cancer, with CT the preferred method (Fig. 18-9). PET is not sensitive to tumor foci smaller than 8 mm to 1 cm, but is reliable in detecting larger tumor foci. For this reason, some advocate the use of PET to determine whether tumor debulking should be performed. PET has a role in the setting of a rising CA125 level in patients with normal CT findings.[40]

For surveillance after ovarian carcinoma surgery, the use of serum markers and imaging is recommended. The aggressivity of imaging follow-up is dependent on the treatments available. PET has an emerging role in this setting, although practice patterns vary widely.

Lymphoma

For both Hodgkin's and non-Hodgkin's lymphomas, accurate staging is important. For both types of lymphoma, accurate definition of the tumor burden is needed for effective treatment planning, especially treatment with external beam radiation. CT is the accepted method for noninvasive staging of lymphoma, with PET seeing increasing use because it is capable of locating more tumor foci than CT in many studies.[41] An example of CT imaging of abdomino-pelvic lymphoma is shown in Figure 18-10.

Science of Clinical Oncology

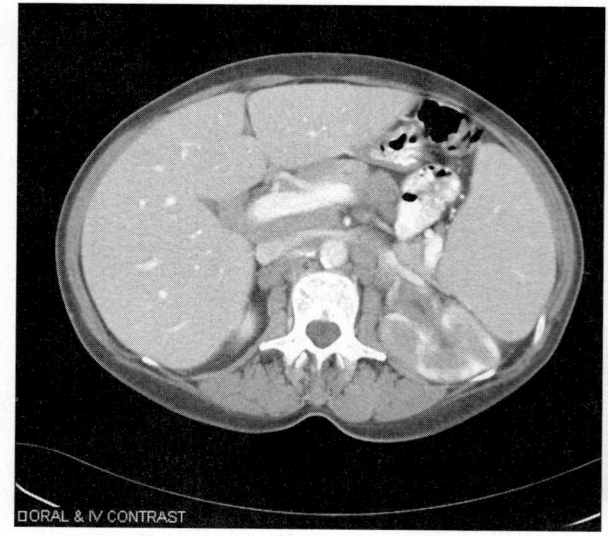

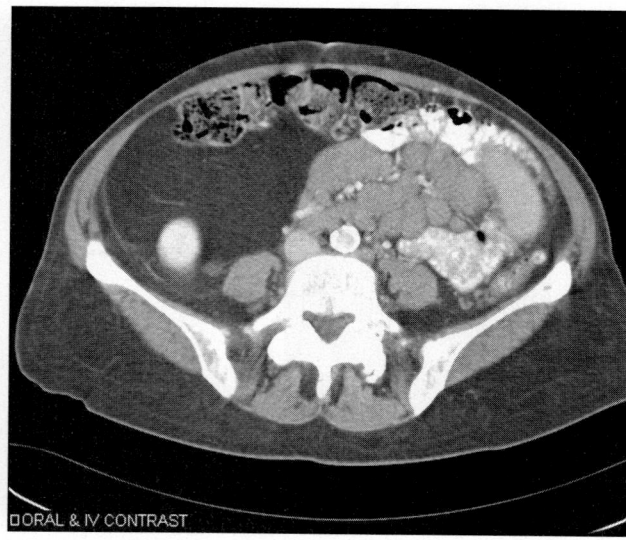

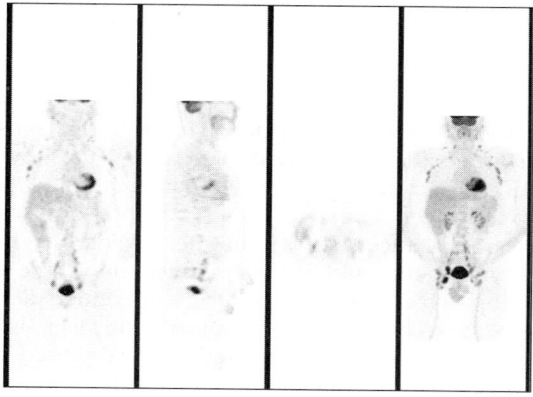

Figure 18-10. Lymphoma. **A,** Axial computed tomography image with oral and IV contrast shows para-aortic adenopathy and infiltration of the left kidney by lymphoma. **B,** Image of the lower abdomen in the same patient shows enlarged mesenteric nodes. **C,** Positron emission tomography–only images (left to right, coronal, sagittal, transverse, and anterior projections) show focal areas of increased [18]fluorodeoxyglucose uptake in multiple lymph node groups, including the axillary, inguinal, and iliac regions, consistent with disseminated lymphoma.

For follow-up of lymphoma, CT is traditionally applied, and there are clear response criteria in place to follow lymphoma therapy. One of the challenges in lymphoma is that large masses often do not normalize in size after treatment, leading to questions in interpretation of a residual mass lesion. Determining whether these lesions contain a viable tumor is an important issue because it defines whether more treatment is needed. Data indicate that ^{67}Ga scintigraphy can be an effective method for assessing the viability of residual Hodgkin's lymphoma and intermediate- and high-grade non-Hodgkin's lymphoma. However, even though data are limited, PET with FDG is rapidly supplanting the role of ^{67}Ga scintigraphy in assessing the viability of residual masses of lymphoma. If a residual mass of lymphoma shows increased FDG uptake, it is virtually always indicative of residual viable tumor; however, scans can also be falsely negative because some tumor foci may be smaller than the resolution of PET imaging.[42]

Positive midtreatment ^{67}Ga and PET scans predict a poor outcome from therapy, and positive PET scans at the conclusion of a therapeutic regimen also indicate a poor prognosis. PET can detect disease in the bone marrow and spleen in some instances.[43]

Challenges associated with PET include reactive lymph nodes and nodes involved with inflammatory processes such as sarcoidosis, which can be very FDG-avid. Similarly, uptake of FDG in brown fat in the neck and thymus can be confusing in some instances.

Thus, anatomic imaging has been the key for lymphoma assessments and remains so in most centers. However, PET imaging and PET/CT imaging, providing additional functional information, is of growing utility. A limitation of PET-only methods is the lack of a standardized set of response criteria. It is generally true that tracer activity in PET images decreases more rapidly than tumor shrinkage occurs (i.e., anatomic changes of treatment lag behind metabolic changes detectable by PET). For these reasons, PET scans may appear normal before CT scans do. A concern is that there is not strong evidence showing that a negative PET scan should be used to truncate the duration of lymphoma therapy. As an example, if a PET scan became negative after two cycles of treatment, this would not justify, based on current data, discontinuing treatment. However, if a treatment involved a standard of four possible courses of treatment and PET became negative after these courses were completed, available data suggest that this portends a very good prognosis vs. a positive PET scan.

It can be argued that PET is not essential in all patients with lymphoma. However, the use of PET and PET/CT is becoming increasingly the norm in centers with this technology available. Because PET can find some lymphomatous tumors that are undetectable by CT, this method is increasingly finding routine application in the care of patients with lymphoma. Examples of PET images of lymphoma are shown in Figure 18-10C.

Melanoma

The imaging management of melanoma varies based on the stage of disease. The use of lymphoscintigraphy to locate lymphatic drainage routes, and thus lymph nodes with the potential for metastatic involvement, is commonly performed for primary melanomas of intermediate thickness. Although practice patterns vary, it is typical to use this method for melanomas that are more than 1 mm thick without other evidence of metastases. If the sentinel node identified by surgery (often using radionuclide guidance) is involved with tumor, then additional staging procedures are often done. These procedures most commonly include CT of the chest and abdomen, and of the pelvis as well if the melanoma affected the lower extremities. If there are systemic metastases, brain imaging is performed, using MRI with and without gadolinium contrast enhancement.

PET with FDG is also a potent method for detecting metastatic melanoma, often detecting more tumor foci than CT. PET is particularly good for soft tissue metastases, but cannot detect microscopic disease. Thus, sentinel lymph node biopsy is used in preference to PET for detecting early metastases. There is some evidence that ultrasound can detect small nodal metastases of melanoma, but it is not widely applied. However, PET can detect most tumor foci larger than 6 mm and sometimes can detect smaller tumor foci. CT is a more robust technique for small pulmonary nodules than is PET.[44]

When melanoma metastases occur, especially if they are localized, they can be resected surgically. However, identifying whether only one or two, vs. many, metastases are present is a major challenge. Certainly, aggressive surgical procedures are not appropriate if there are disseminated metastases. For these reasons, staging imaging procedures are performed aggressively before major surgery is undertaken to resect melanoma metastases. PET is commonly part of such a staging evaluation. For systemically metastatic melanoma, PET has been reported to be approximately 90% sensitive. Thus, although anatomic imaging dominates, PET has a growing role in melanoma assessment.[45] For bone metastases, radionuclide bone scanning is an important diagnostic procedure as well.

Bladder Carcinoma

Bladder carcinoma often presents at an early stage, and no imaging evaluation is performed to determine whether there are locoregional or systemic metastases. However, ultrasound has been used to determine the depth of penetration of primary bladder carcinomas. An important consideration in bladder carcinomas is that uroepithelial tumors are often multicentric. Thus, intravenous pyelogram examinations to evaluate the entire genitourinary system are quite commonly performed early in the diagnostic algorithm. Although ultrasound can detect many bladder cancers 5 mm and larger, transurethral sonography is more sensitive, but obviously is invasive. MRI is more commonly used than CT for assessing primary bladder lesions because of its superior soft tissue contrast characterization abilities.[46]

For larger primary tumors that are invasive, imaging evaluation is important to help to determine whether surgery is appropriate. Metastatic disease to locoregional nodes or systemic metastases indicate disease with a poorer prognosis, and tumor invading local structures or metastatic to nodes or systemically is often considered unresectable. CT is most commonly used for local nodal staging, but MRI can also be used. Small nodal metastases are commonly not detected using CT, because they have not enlarged the lymph nodes sufficiently to allow the tumor-involved nodes to be detectable. CT has a reported sensitivity of 60% to 70%. Biopsy is commonly used to determine whether an enlarged node seen on CT truly contains tumor. MRI is probably more sensitive than CT in detecting nodal metastases, and new contrast agents that accumulate in normal nodes are potentially important for enhancing the diagnostic accuracy of MRI in detecting nodal metastases.[47]

PET with FDG has been used and is promising in this disease; however, images of the pelvis can be degraded by intense F18 activity in the bladder. For bone metastases, radionuclide bone scan remains the procedure of choice, and MRI can also be sensitive.

Follow-up of bladder carcinoma usually involves the use of CT scans. Follow-up for new or recurrent bladder carcinoma within the bladder usually requires direct visualization of the bladder by cystoscopy.

Head and Neck Cancer

Head and neck tumors are often associated with cigarette smoking and alcohol use or abuse. Most are of squamous cell etiology. A key issue in these lesions is determining whether the disease is localized to the head and neck or whether metastatic disease or a second primary lesion is present. Thus, imaging the lungs is usually done to exclude a primary or metastatic lung tumor. To assess a primary lesion in the head and neck, physical examination is very important. However, CT and MRI are both very potent methods. MRI typically is performed before and after gadolinium contrast is administered. CT is usually performed after contrast enhancement. MRI is subject to respiratory and motion artifacts. Thus, CT is somewhat more commonly used in the initial staging of these tumors.[48] An example of a positive CT scan in the head and neck is shown in Figure 18-11A.

CT and MRI can characterize the extent of primary tumors; however, CT is clearly more effective than MRI in assessing the extent of involvement of cartilage or bone. For nodal metastases, current diagnostic schemes are mainly based on nodal size. Nodal size is an imperfect indicator of tumor involvement, however.

Science of Clinical Oncology

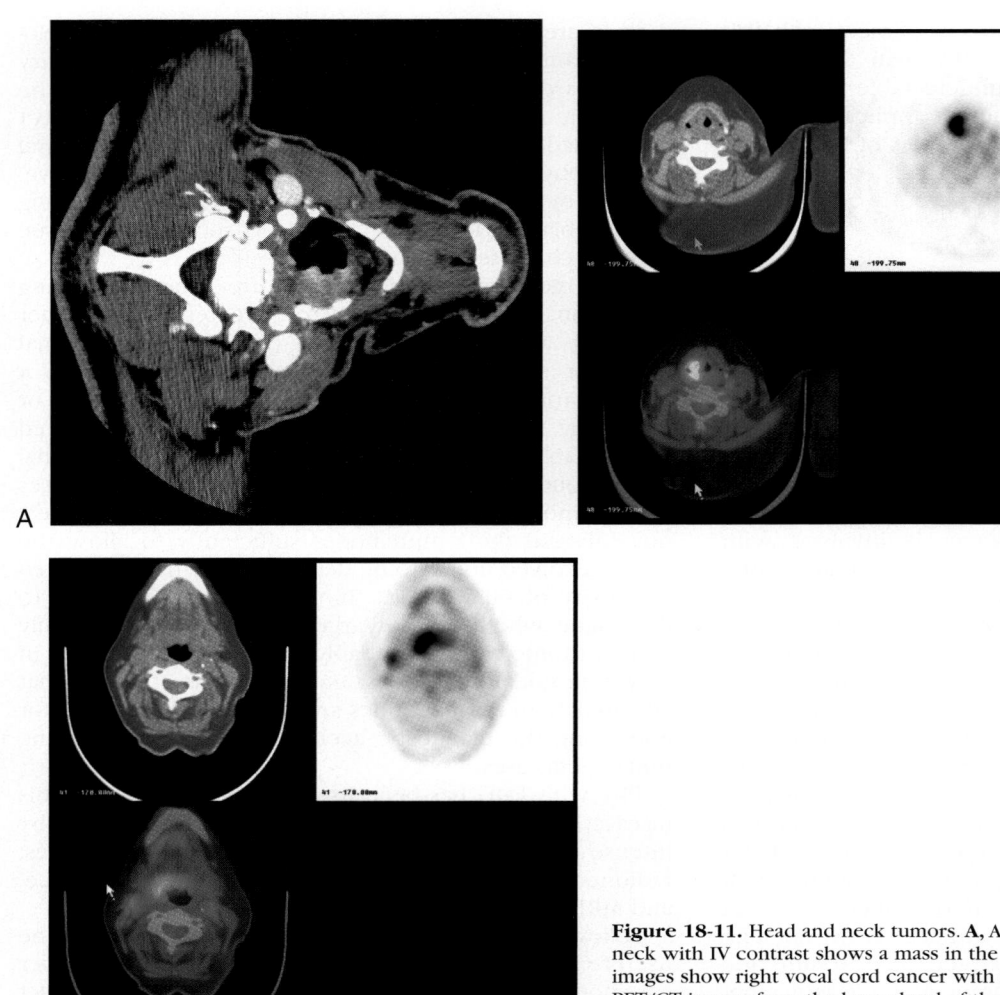

Figure 18-11. Head and neck tumors. **A,** Axial computed tomography image of the neck with IV contrast shows a mass in the left piriform sinus. **B,** PET and PET/CT images show right vocal cord cancer with intense tracer uptake. **C,** PET and PET/CT images from the lower level of the neck show nodal tracer uptake consistent with metastases. (Courtesy of Dr. David Yousem, Johns Hopkins University.)

Increasingly, PET with FDG is being applied to the assessment of head and neck cancers. Although several studies have suggested that PET, MRI, and CT have similar sensitivity, more recent studies suggested that PET is more accurate in staging (Fig. 18-11B and C). However, PET can detect increased glucose uptake in nonmalignantly involved inflamed nodes (false-positive findings). These can occur in patients with head and neck or gingival infection or the common cold. Defining the precise extent of tumor is important to determine whether surgery or radiation therapy should be performed. More extensive tumors are less amenable to surgical resection.

Occasionally, head and neck cancers present as isolated nodal metastases without the location of the primary tumor being evident. Imaging has a role in such cases. Often MRI is performed as well as extensive inspection and biopsies; however, PET with FDG has also been applied. This method can detect perhaps 15% to 30% of primary tumors.

For recurrent tumors, PET appears to be a more robust test than MRI or CT, especially when timed properly, probably because contrast enhancement can be seen in both postoperative changes (and postradiation tissue) and tumors. In general, FDG uptake is a more reliable predictor of tumor than the anatomic methods. PET is useful in surveillance for the recurrence of these tumors, but it is not yet considered the standard of care.

Thus, for head and neck cancers, MRI offers excellent contrast resolution for soft tissues, but can be degraded substantially by motion. For this reason, CT with contrast is much more commonly performed. PET with FDG is assuming a growing role in cancer management, especially for recurrence and for assessment of response to treatment. PET with CT is increasingly used to stage and monitor these tumors during and after treatment, and may increasingly become the standard of care.[49]

Pancreatic Carcinoma

The standard of care for the imaging diagnosis of pancreatic cancers is CT scanning. Although MRI can be useful, CT, including CT angiography, is the main method used for staging and assessing tumor invasion of vessels (Fig. 18-12). Some studies have shown PET with FDG to

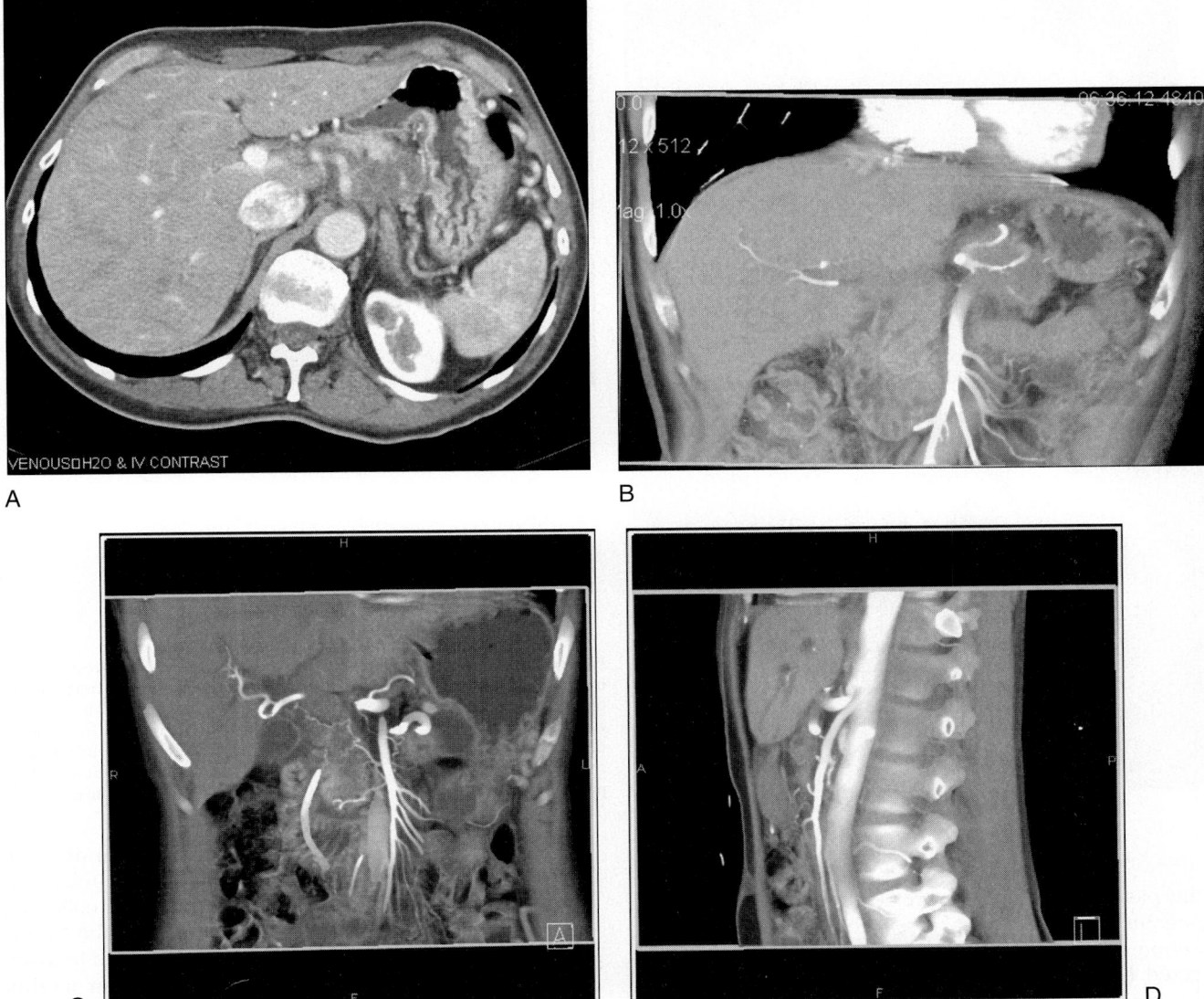

Figure 18-12. Pancreatic cancer. **A,** Axial computed tomography (CT) image showing a mass in the pancreatic body, encasing the splenic artery. **B,** Coronal volume-rendered three-dimensional CT image showing tumor encasing the splenic and left gastric arteries. **C,** Coronal volume-rendered coronal maximum-intensity projection. **D,** Sagittal volume-rendered three-dimensional CT images showing a mass in the pancreatic head without invasion of the superior mesenteric artery or vein. A common bile duct stent is also seen.

be somewhat more sensitive for detecting tumors and to have moderately high accuracy, approximately 85%, in characterizing pancreatic lesions as malignant or benign.[50,51] Ultrasound is used to assess cystic lesions. After treatment, salvage therapy is ineffective and the aggressivity of monitoring of these patients is often less than in other, more treatable cancers. Neuroendocrine tumors of the pancreas can often be detected using ^{111}In pentetreotide (Octreoscan), a SPECT procedure.

Liver Cancer

Hepatic malignancies, especially hepatomas, are common worldwide. Both CT and MRI can be very effective in detecting these lesions. They are sometimes challenging to assess, because they can overlap in appearance between cirrhosis with regenerating nodules and tumors. Multiphase CT imaging, CT angiography, and MRI with and without gadolinium contrast are commonly used in hepatomas. PET is less reliable, because approximately half—and sometimes more—of hepatomas are not FDG-avid. Ultrasound can also be used to assess the liver and guide biopsies.

Metastatic lesions to the liver are also common, especially in the United States. For most tumors, CT is the initial method used for assessing whether tumor is present. However, PET with FDG is more sensitive than CT in detecting liver metastases in common cancers such as colorectal.[37,38] Thus, PET is seeing greater application in assessing suspected liver metastases, although ultrasound, CT, and MRI are also important methods and are more commonly applied in many centers (Fig. 18-13).

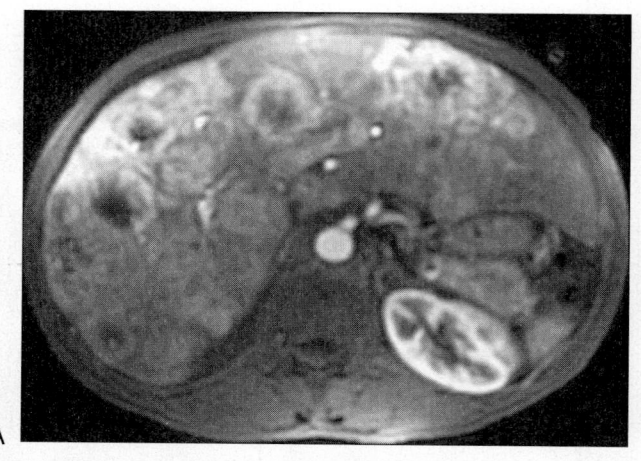

A

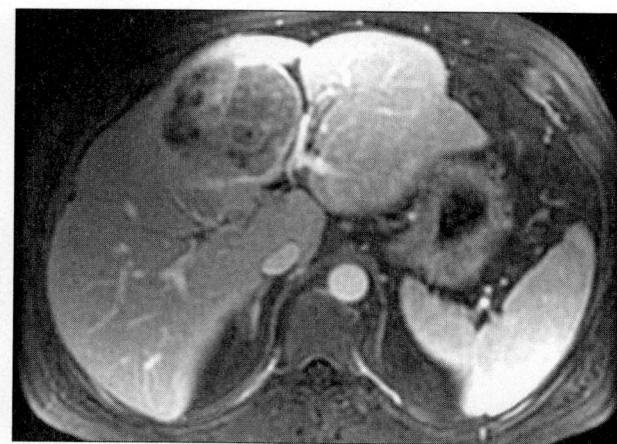

B

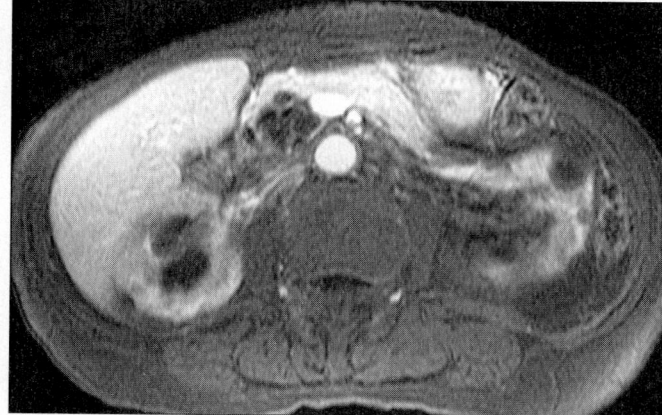

C

Figure 18-13. Liver. **A,** Carcinoid metastases. Axial magnetic resonance image with gadolinium shows multiple enhancing masses in both lobes of the liver. **B,** Hepatoma. Axial magnetic resonance image with gadolinium shows a solid mass in the left lobe of the liver. **C,** Intraductal papillary mucinous tumor of the pancreas. Axial T1-weighted image of the abdomen shows a low-signal-intensity cystic mass in the head of the pancreas. (Courtesy of Dr. Ihab Kamel, Johns Hopkins University.)

Kidney Cancer

In the past, renal cancers were detected by intravenous pyelograms; however, the most common method for detection now is CT. Renal cell cancer is commonly detected incidentally because of the widespread use of cross-sectional imaging. Between 25% and 50% of surgically treated renal cell cancers are discovered incidentally.[52] Renal lesions are classified as cysts or solid masses, depending on their characteristics as shown by imaging. Renal cysts are fluid-filled and appear anechoic with increased through transmission on ultrasound. They show water density without enhancement on CT, and appear hyperintense on T2-weighted images also without enhancement on MRI. Renal masses are typically evaluated by CT as a result of short examination times and ease of evaluation, even in patients with a large body habitus, which can make ultrasound difficult. MRI is typically used for problem-solving. Multiphasic scanning is performed on CT to evaluate the density of lesions before contrast and as contrast filters from the cortex into the medulla and collecting system. An increase in density by greater than 20 HU corresponds to lesion enhancement and confirms the presence of a solid mass. CT is used to stage the tumor by determining the presence of renal vein invasion, adenopathy, local extension, and distant metastases. The accuracy of CT for staging is 91%.[52] For resectable lesions, CT can provide information on whether the lesion is amenable to nephron-sparing surgery or partial nephrectomy. Lesions that are smaller than 4 cm, polar, and cortical, and do not involve the renal hilum or collecting system may be candidates for partial nephrectomy. Although CT, MRI, and ultrasound can all be used to assess renal lesions, CT with contrast is the dominant method (Fig. 18-14). PET is useful only when the tumor is FDG-avid. However, the normal excretion of FDG by the kidneys makes evaluation of the kidneys more challenging than other tissues, and some renal masses are not very FDG-avid. Thus, PET with FDG is not currently recommended for renal cancers.

Endocrine Tumors

Imaging is used to study several types of endocrine tumors in a variety of locations. For adrenal tumors, CT is the procedure of choice, with meta-iodobenzyl guanidine [123]I (MIBG) scanning and MRI scanning also proving useful for lesion characterization.[53] MIBG accumulates selectively in pheochromocytomas. Adrenal masses with low Hounsfield Units (<10 HU) are typically adenomas, which are lipid-rich. For the thyroid gland, radioiodine imaging is commonly used. For non–radioiodine-avid thyroid cancers, PET with FDG is very useful for lesion detection and is recommended in the setting of a rising serum thyroglobulin level with a normal ^{131}I or [23]I scan (Fig. 18-15). For neuroendocrine tumors such as carcinoid

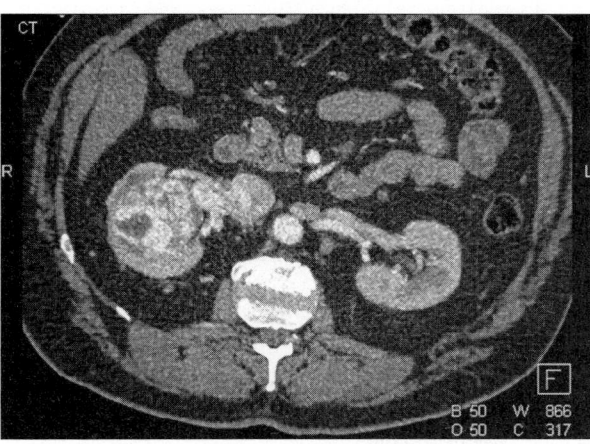

Figure 18-14. Renal cancer. Axial computed tomography images of the abdomen with IV contrast, showing enhancing renal cell carcinoma in the right kidney. Enhancing tumor invades the right renal vein.

tumors, CT and radiolabeled octreotide analogs are very useful.

Brain Tumors

The dominant method for the assessment of brain tumors is the MRI scan. This is the preferred method for initial detection, assessment of extent of disease, and assessment of efficacy of therapy. The superior soft tissue contrast provided by MRI places it ahead of CT for lesion characterization (Fig. 18-16).

Unfortunately, even sophisticated MRI techniques, often relying on tumor enhancement using gadolinium, cannot detect microscopic disease. MRI findings, although fairly specific for tumor, are not completely specific. Thus, occasionally infarcts, infections, and foci of

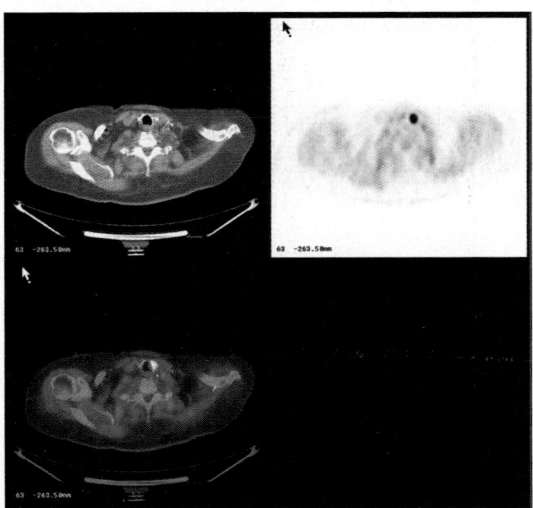

Figure 18-15. Thyroid cancer. Positron emission tomography and computed tomography image panel showing an intense [18]fluorodeoxyglucose uptake focus near clips in the left thyroid bed, consistent with recurrent thyroid cancer.

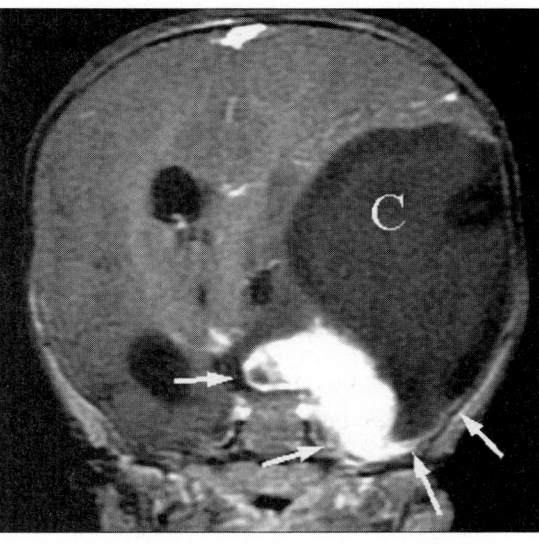

Figure 18-16. Coronal magnetic resonance image with gadolinium of the brain shows a mass with peripheral enhancement *(arrows)*, compatible with tumor, and a more hypointense necrotic area.

demyelination can mimic tumor foci on MRI. PET has a very limited role but can be useful in assessing residual tumor after radiation therapy and determining whether residual masses are caused by tumor or tumor necrosis.

MRS can also be useful in evaluating this issue because tumors typically have high levels of choline and low levels of NAA (N-acetyl-aspartate). Angiography, although a historically useful method, is less frequently performed for diagnostic purposes in brain tumors. MRI, CT, and PET can guide biopsies. Further, MRI can be used intraoperatively to guide therapy.[54]

Pediatric Tumors

CT is generally the method of choice for evaluation. For tumors of the central nervous system and for sarcomas, MRI is preferred. FDG has a growing role, especially for lymphomas and sarcomas. MIBG scanning is often used in neuroblastomas. CT scanning should be performed with a reduced tube current and energy to minimize the radiation dose while preserving the quality of the diagnostic image. Multiphase CT should be avoided in children unless it is clearly indicated to minimize the radiation dose to the child.[55]

Esophageal and Gastric Cancer

CT scanning is the method of choice for initial staging. Endoscopic ultrasound is the most sensitive and accurate method for determining whether tumor has invaded the wall of the esophagus or involved the periesophageal nodes. PET scanning is very sensitive in determining whether there is stage IV disease, and is typically performed as part of the initial staging evaluation, at least for esophageal cancer, to identify patients who are clearly not candidates for surgery.[56]

Science of Clinical Oncology

Sarcomas

MRI is the method of choice for detection and assessment of soft tissue sarcomas. Gadolinium contrast enhancement is commonly used as well. PET imaging with FDG has been useful in assessing primary sarcomas for their aggressivity and defining possible sites for biopsy as well as for defining prognosis and grade.[57,58]

DEFINING NORMAL ORGAN FUNCTION FOR CANCER THERAPY

Several tests are used to determine whether a patient is a suitable candidate for aggressive therapy. These tests include myocardial perfusion imaging at stress to determine whether ischemia is present. If present it could increase the risk for a major surgical procedure. Echocardiography is also used for this purpose. Determinations of myocardial function are also often performed before chemotherapy is given. This may take the form of a myocardial blood pool study or, less commonly, an echocardiogram to determine chamber size and ejection fraction.

Pulmonary function is usually determined by pulmonary ventilatory function tests; however, split lung function and regional function may be determined by pulmonary perfusion imaging with ^{99m}Tc MAA (macro-aggregated albumin; i.e., a quantitative lung scan). Regional ventilation can also be assessed quantitatively. Such determinations help to predict the level of pulmonary function expected after surgery. Split assessment of renal function is sometimes performed before removal of a renal cancer to ensure that the remaining kidney will be functional.

The location of eloquent brain activity can be identified, and motor cortex function can be evaluated by functional imaging as well. Functional imaging can also help to guide brain tumor surgery by avoiding key areas of the brain.

GUIDANCE OF RADIATION THERAPY

Radiation therapy can be palliative, or may be performed with curative intent. In general, the goal is to deliver maximum radiation to the tumor while minimizing radiation delivery to normal tissues. This is a delicate balance, and is achieved through increasingly sophisticated dose delivery systems. The anatomic location of a tumor is most commonly defined by treatment-planning CT. The CT data are used to define tumor and normal tissues with a therapy-planning system. The planning potentially can be enhanced by better definition of the gross tumor volume (or biologic tumor volume) vs. anatomic tumor volume. These are sometimes not identical. PET with FDG is beginning to be used to better define the biologic tumor volume, often with data from PET/CT. Although this is hardly the norm, it is clear that imaging is key to the optimal planning of radiation therapy ports. The potential to target areas of tumor that are not iden-

tified on CT (expand port size) or reduce ports to areas that are not involved with tumor is substantial, because the goal is to irradiate tumor, but not normal tissues.[59]

INTERVENTIONAL PROCEDURES

Increasingly, imaging is being combined with a therapeutic procedure to provide minimally invasive therapeutics. Examples include the use of CT to guide thermal ablation of the liver or lung and the use of MRI to guide ablation of brain and prostate tumors (through heat and cold). The ability to locate tumors and follow, in near real time, the response to treatment is of tremendous potential.

Catheter-based delivery systems are also important. For example, angiographic catheters can be used to deliver regional chemotherapy, emboli, or radioactive or chemical microspheres to treat tumors. This is an area of growing application.

EMERGING OPPORTUNITIES IN IMAGING

Functional imaging methods such as PET are being used increasingly to assess treatment response early after treatment is begun. Beyond this, a variety of imaging methods are being developed to image key aspects of tumor biology (Table 18-3). For example, the interest in gene therapeutic approaches has led to attempts to determine, through imaging, whether genes, when delivered, actually reach tumors and, more importantly, whether they express in vivo the desired levels of gene product expected to be required to achieve a therapeutic effect. For example, dopamine receptors have been transfected into cells and imaged with radioligands capable of binding to the D2 dopamine receptor. Similarly, genes have been transfected that express viral thymidine kinase. This agent is suitable for gene therapy

TABLE 18-3

 Emerging Uses of Imaging

Individual Patient Management Decisions

Phenotyping of the Tumor and Host

Tumor
Viability, proliferation, extent of necrosis or apoptosis, hypoxia, prognosis, type of treatment most likely to be effective based on receptors or presence of imageable pathways

Host
Individualized assessment of pharmacokinetics of the drug and of organ function and pharmacodynamics

Drug Development
Does the tumor have a relevant target?
Does the drug reach the target?
Is the target pathway affected by treatment?
Is the proper dose of drug being given?
Does alteration of the target pathway alter the tumor biology?

and can be imaged with radiolabeled substrates such as filauradine.[60]

Similarly, a great deal of interest has been expressed in stem cell biology and the potential for stem cells to allow for regeneration of tissues. Tracking these stem cells in vivo and determining their biodistribution and ultimate proliferation are exceptional opportunities for imaging. These goals have been achieved with both nuclear medicine and MRI methods.

Small animal imaging devices of a variety of types are now being used to help in drug development. Small animal PET, SPECT, MRI, and CT scanners have been used to assess treatment response and aspects of tumor biology. Such methods are of critical importance for assessing the response of cancers to treatment with newer agents and understanding therapeutic effects. Even combined human PET/CT devices have been used for imaging and can provide useful information for drug development in cancer.

Some methods are of tremendous importance in preclinical studies, but will be more difficult to extend to human studies. An example is optical imaging. Such methods are capable of tremendous sensitivity and excellent resolution in vivo in small animals. A variety of approaches can be used, with emitted light, transmitted light, and reflected light. With bioluminescence approaches, a very small number of cancer cells can be identified in vivo in small animals. Similarly, very small tumor foci can be resolved with GFP (green fluorescent protein) expression. However, such approaches, although very potent in vivo in small animals and capable of being combined with radionuclide and other methods, are not likely to be effectively translated into humans because of the limited penetration in tissue of light photons. Thus, small animal imaging is a key element of progress in this area.

SUMMARY

Anatomic imaging of cancer using x-rays has proven very useful for more than 100 years and still is by far the dominant approach to imaging the patient with cancer. Anatomic methods, although very potent, have clear limitations. These methods reliably show whether a large mass is present, but not the composition of the mass. In addition, they can be insensitive to small tumor foci, are slow to change in response to therapy, are not predictive of response, and may not be useful in evaluating the postoperative patient. Imaging additional phenotypic alterations of the altered genotype of cancers with functional imaging methods such as PET adds what is often clinically valuable information for patient management in several common cancers. Although many molecular alterations are present in cancer, the one that is by far most exploited in clinical practice and research is the accelerated glucose metabolism present in most cancers. This process is well imaged with the radiotracer FDG. The ability to localize spatially the molecular alterations of cancer, through qualitative cognitive methods performed by the imaging specialist, computer fusion of image sets, or fused "anatomolecular" image sets using dedicated PET/CT, is key to optimal use of the imaging methods. Functional, "molecular" imaging methods such as PET, SPECT, and varying methods of MRI, in addition to optical and ultrasound imaging and technical improvements in CT and interventional techniques, are expected to enhance the care of the patient with cancer.

REFERENCES

1. Bragg DG, Rubin P, Hricak H: Imaging strategies for oncologic diagnosis and multidisciplinary treatment. In Bragg D, Rubin P, Hricak H: Oncologic Imaging, 2nd ed. Philadelphia, WB Saunders, 2002, pp 3-20.
2. Bossuyt PM, Reitsma JB, Bruns DE, et al: Toward complete and accurate reporting of studies of diagnostic accuracy: The STARD initiative. Acad Radiol 2003;10:664-669.
3. Gates TJ: Screening for cancer: Evaluating the evidence. Am Fam Physician 2001;63:513-522.
4. Hanley JA: Receiver operating characteristic (ROC) methodology: The state of the art. Crit Rev Diagn Imaging 1989;29:307-335.
5. Wahl RL, Siegel BA, Coleman RE, Gatsonis CG: Prospective multicenter study of axillary nodal staging by positron emission tomography in breast cancer. J Clin Oncol 2004;22:277-285.
6. Verboom P, Van Tinteren H, Hoekstra OS, et al: Cost-effectiveness of FDG-PET in staging non-small cell lung cancer: The PLUS study. Eur J Nucl Med Mol Imaging 2003;30(11):1444-1449.
7. de Koning HJ: Mammographic screening: Evidence from randomised controlled trials. Ann Oncol 2003;14:1185-1189.
8. Henschke CI, Yankelevitz DF, McCauley DI, et al: Guidelines for the use of spiral computed tomography in screening for lung cancer. Eur Respir J 2003;39:45s-51s.
9. Ubel PA, Hirth RA, Chernew ME, Fendrick AM: What is the price of life and why doesn't it increase at the rate of inflation? Arch Intern Med 2003;163:1637-1641.
10. Wahl RL, Quint LE, Cieslak RD, et al: "Anatometabolic" tumor imaging: Fusion of FDG PET with CT or MRI to localize foci of increased activity. J Nucl Med 1993;34:1190-1197.
11. Cohade C, Wahl RL: Applications of positron emission tomography/computed tomography image fusion in clinical positron emission tomography: Clinical use, interpretation methods, diagnostic improvements. Semin Nucl Med 2003;33:228-237.
12. Gourtsoyiannis N, Grammatikakis J, Prassopoulos P: Role of conventional radiology in the diagnosis and staging of gastro-intestinal tract neoplasms. Semin Surg Oncol 2001;20:91-108.
13. Shah AJ, Wang J, Yamada T, Fajardo LL: Digital mammography: A review of technical development and clinical applications. Clin Breast Cancer 2003;4:63-70.
14. Miles KA: Functional computed tomography in oncology. Eur J Cancer 2002;38:2079-2084.
15. Singh K: Interventional radiology in the gynaecological oncology patient. Best Pract Res Clin Obstet Gynaecol 2001;15:279-290.
16. DePriest PD, DeSimone CP: Ultrasound screening for the early detection of ovarian cancer. J Clin Oncol 2003;21(Suppl 10):194-199.
17. Laking GR, Price PM, Sculpher MJ: Assessment of the technology for functional imaging in cancer. Eur J Cancer 2002;38:2194-2199.
18. Kwock L, Smith JK, Castillo M, et al: Clinical applications of proton MR spectroscopy in oncology. Technol Cancer Res Treat 2002;1:17-28.
19. Jerusalem G, Hustinx R, Beguin Y, Fillet G: PET scan imaging in oncology. Eur J Cancer 2003;39:1525-1534.
20. Kaminski MS, Zelenetz AD, Press OW, et al: Pivotal study of iodine I 131 tositumomab for chemotherapy-refractory low-grade or transformed low-grade B-cell non-Hodgkin's lymphomas. J Clin Oncol 2001;19:3918-3928.
21. Bremer C, Ntziachristos V, Weissleder R: Optical-based molecular imaging: Contrast agents and potential medical applications. Eur Radiol 2003;13:231-243.
22. Wahl RL: Anatomolecular imaging of cancer. Mol Imag Biol 2003; 5(2):49-56.

23. Zhang W, Laborde PM, Coombes KR, et al: Cancer genomics: Promises and complexities. Clin Cancer Res 2001;7:2159–2167.

24. Erasmus JJ, Connolly JE, McAdams HP, Roggli VL: Solitary pulmonary nodules: Part I. Morphologic evaluation for differentiation of benign and malignant lesions. Radiographics 2000;20:43–58.

25. Erasmus JJ, McAdams HP, Connolly JE: Solitary pulmonary nodules: Part II. Evaluation of the indeterminate nodule. Radiographics 2000;20:59–66.

26. Gould MK, Maclean CC, Kuschner WG, et al: Accuracy of positron emission tomography for diagnosis of pulmonary nodules and mass lesions: A meta-analysis. JAMA 2001;285:914–924.

27. Dwamena BA, Sonnad SS, Angobaldo JO, Wahl RL: Metastases from non-small cell lung cancer: Mediastinal staging in the 1990s. Meta-analytic comparison of PET and CT. Radiology 1999;213:530–536.

28. van Tinteren H, Hoekstra OS, Smit EF, et al: Effectiveness of positron emission tomography in the preoperative assessment of patients with suspected non-small-cell lung cancer: The PLUS multicentre randomised trial. Lancet 2002;359(9315):1388–1393.

29. Beadsmoore CJ, Screaton NJ: Classification, staging and prognosis of lung cancer. Eur J Radiol 2003;45:8–17.

30. Lardinois D, Weder W, Hany TF, et al: Staging of non-small-cell lung cancer with integrated positron-emission tomography and computed tomography. N Engl J Med 2003;348:2500–2507.

31. Mayo-Smith WW, Boland GW, Noto RB, Lee MJ: State-of-the-art adrenal imaging. Radiographics 2001;21:995–1012.

32. Smith RA, Saslow D, Sawyer KA, et al: American Cancer Society guidelines for breast cancer screening: Update 2003. CA Cancer J Clin 2003;53:141–169.

33. Veronesi U, Paganelli G, Viale G, et al: A randomized comparison of sentinel-node biopsy with routine axillary dissection in breast cancer. N Engl J Med 2003;349:546–553.

34. Wu D, Gambhir SS: Positron emission tomography in diagnosis and management of invasive breast cancer: Current status and future perspectives. Clin Breast Cancer 2003;4(Suppl 1):55–63.

35. Yu KK, Hricak H: Imaging prostate cancer. Radiol Clin North Am 2000;38:59–85.

36. Harisinghani MG, Barentsz J, Hahn PF, et al: Noninvasive detection of clinically occult lymph-node metastases in prostate cancer. N Engl J Med 2003;348:2491–2499.

37. Chin BB, Wahl RL: 18F-Fluoro-2-deoxyglucose positron emission tomography in the evaluation of gastrointestinal malignancies. Gut 2003;52(Suppl 4):23–29.

38. Kinkel K, Lu Y, Both M, Warren RS, Thoeni RF: Detection of hepatic metastases from cancers of the gastrointestinal tract by using noninvasive imaging methods (US, CT, MR imaging, PET): A meta-analysis. Radiology 2002;224:748–756.

39. Singh AK, Grigsby PW, Dehdashti F, et al: FDG-PET lymph node staging and survival of patients with FIGO stage IIIb cervical carcinoma. Int J Radiat Oncol Biol Phys 2003;56:489–493.

40. Zimny M, Siggelkow W, Schroder W, et al: 2-[Fluorine-18]-fluoro-2-deoxy-d-glucose positron emission tomography in the diagnosis of recurrent ovarian cancer. Gynecol Oncol 2001;83:310–315.

41. O'Doherty MJ, Macdonald EA, Barrington SF, et al: Positron emission tomography in the management of lymphomas. Clin Oncol (R Coll Radiol) 2002;14:415–426.

42. Spaepen K, Stroobants S, Dupont P, et al: Prognostic value of positron emission tomography (PET) with fluorine-18 fluorodeoxyglucose ([18F]FDG) after first-line chemotherapy in non-Hodgkin's lymphoma: Is [18F]FDG-PET a valid alternative to conventional diagnostic methods? J Clin Oncol 2001;19:414–419.

43. Front D, Bar-Shalom R, Mor M, et al: Hodgkin disease: Prediction of outcome with 67Ga scintigraphy after one cycle of chemotherapy. Radiology 1999;210:487–491.

44. Cobben DC, Koopal S, Tiebosch AT, et al: New diagnostic techniques in staging in the surgical treatment of cutaneous malignant melanoma. Eur J Surg Oncol 2002;28:692–700.

45. Swetter SM, Carroll LA, Johnson DL, Segall GM: Positron emission tomography is superior to computed tomography for metastatic detection in melanoma patients. Ann Surg Oncol 2002;9:646–653.

46. Barentsz JO, Witjes JA, Ruijs JH: What is new in bladder cancer imaging? Urol Clin North Am 1997;24:583–602.

47. Lawler LP: MR imaging of the bladder. Radiol Clin North Am 2003;41:161–177.

48. Zinreich J: Imaging in laryngeal cancer: Computed tomography, magnetic resonance imaging, positron emission tomography. Otolaryngol Clin North Am 2002;35:971–991.

49. Wong RJ, Lin DT, Schoder H, et al: Diagnostic and prognostic value of [(18)F]fluorodeoxyglucose positron emission tomography for recurrent head and neck squamous cell carcinoma. J Clin Oncol 2002;20:4199–4208.

50. Kalra MK, Maher MM, Boland GW, et al: Correlation of positron emission tomography and CT in evaluating pancreatic tumors: Technical and clinical implications. Am J Roentgenol 2003;181:387–393.

51. Hanbidge AE: Cancer of the pancreas: The best image for early detection. CT, MRI, PET or US? Can J Gastroenterol 2002;16:101–105.

52. Sheth S, Scatarige JC, Horton KM, et al: Current concepts in the diagnosis and management of renal cell carcinoma: Role of multidetector C and three-dimensional CT. Radiographics 2001;21:237–254.

53. Pocaro AB, Cavalleri S, Ballista C, et al: Modern imaging methods and preoperative management of pheochromocytoma: Review of the literature and case report. Arch Esp Urol 2000;53:749–753.

54. Jacobs AH, Winkler A, Dittmar C, et al: Molecular and functional imaging technology for the development of efficient treatment strategies for gliomas. Technol Cancer Res Treat 2002;1:187–204.

55. Frush DP: Pediatric CT: Practical approach to diminish the radiation dose. Pediatr Radiol 2002;32:714–717.

56. Reed CE, Eloubeidi MA: New techniques for staging esophageal cancer. Surg Clin North Am 2002;82:697–710.

57. Hoffer FA: Primary skeletal neoplasms: Osteosarcoma and Ewing sarcoma. Top Magn Reson Imaging 2002;13:231–239.

58. Brenner W, Bohuslavizki KH, Eary JF: PET imaging of osteosarcoma. J Nucl Med 2003;44:930–942.

59. Ling CC, Humm J, Larson S, et al: Towards multidimensional radiotherapy (MD-CRT): Biological imaging and biological conformality. Int J Radiat Oncol Biol Phys 2000;47:551–560.

60. Tjuvajev JG, Avril N, Oku T, et al: Imaging herpes virus thymidine kinase gene transfer and expression by positron emission tomography. Cancer Res 1998;58:4333–4341.

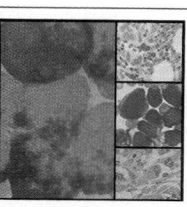

19

BIOSTATISTICS FOR CLINICAL TRIALS

Steven Piantadosi

SUMMARY OF KEY POINTS

SOURCE OF UNCERTAINTY IN CLINICAL TRIALS

- Uncertainty in trials can be classified as systematic error (bias) or random error.
- These types of errors can be controlled principally through the design of the medical study but not reliably through analysis alone.
- The strength of the evidence produced by a clinical trial depends on its design, primarily the amount and nature of the bias and random error that it controls.

DEVELOPMENTAL CLINICAL TRIALS

- Clinical trials are designed primarily to meet specific developmental questions.
- An early developmental question is the relationship between dose and safety (phase I).
- These studies also address mechanistic questions such as pharmacokinetics and pharmacodynamics.
- The second major developmental question is providing evidence of

safety and activity, usually in a disease specific cohort (phase II).
- These middle developmental trials provide evidence to support or discourage definitive, long-term, and expensive comparative trials.

COMPARATIVE STUDIES

- Comparative trials (phase III) often use randomization to remove treatment selection bias.
- Clinically definitive endpoints, such as disease progression and survival, are employed.
- Other systematic effects can be minimized by using masking.
- Random errors are minimized by employing sufficiently large sample sizes. These studies also require sophisticated infrastructures for data management, study monitoring, and multisite coordination.

ANALYSIS

- The most appropriate methods to apply for analysis of a clinical trial depend strongly on the purpose and the design used for the study.

- All analyses begin with quality control data and sophisticated descriptive views of the data.
- Comparative studies require estimates of clinically relevant quantities such as risks or relative risks of the defined outcomes.
- Design flaws cannot be reliably corrected by sophisticated analyses.
- As a general principle analyses unconditionally include all patients who meet the eligibility criteria and are based on treatment assignment.

REPRESENTATION OF EVIDENCE

- The most clinically relevant summary of evidence from a trial is the estimate of the magnitude of treatment effect.
- In addition to magnitude, the precision with which an effect is estimated is often useful (e.g., 95% confidence interval).
- P-values are deficient as measures of strength of evidence and should not be the primary currency of clinical trial results.

INTRODUCTION

The purpose of this chapter is to review biostatistical concepts that are helpful to clinicians in planning, conducting, and assessing clinical trials in oncology. I describe areas in which a statistical perspective can improve the design, execution, analysis, and interpretation of clinical studies. Several good texts and expository articles provide additional details regarding these concepts. These include history and policy,[1,2] general discussions,[3-14] cancer trials,[15-21] ethics,[22-25] prognostic factor analyses,[26,27] and reporting.[28-33]

Much of this chapter pertains to study design, implementation, and quality control. I emphasize these, because a well-designed and well-executed trial addressing an important therapeutic or management question will

usually provide cogent evidence without an elaborate analysis. Statistical analysis can do little to make the results of a poorly designed or executed trial compelling. This is not to trivialize analysis; an improper one can distort the findings of a well-designed and well-executed trial.

My first topic is outlining some of the sources of uncertainty in inferences from clinical trials including dose finding (phase I) studies, safety and activity (phase II) studies, and comparative (phase III) studies. After this, I discuss five areas of statistical activity that are important to the success of a program of studies in the management of oncologic disease: (1) formulation and refinement of an important therapeutic question through the use of developmental trials, (2) design of comparative trials, (3) implementation of a trial and quality control, (4) data analysis, and (5) description of results and preparation of publications.

SOURCES OF UNCERTAINTY IN CLINICAL TRIALS

The most convincing clinical trials use methods to control and minimize relevant sources of uncertainty. Two types of uncertainty or errors can result when making inferences about treatment effects in medical studies: bias (systematic error) and random error. Both types of error can be controlled by using proper design. However, neither type of error can be reliably controlled by analysis alone.

Bias

Numerous sources and types of bias exist in clinical trials, for example, see Sackett[34] or Chalmers.[35] All biases produce systematically high or low misestimates of the true treatment effect. The relative magnitude of bias and random error is important. Because, in human studies, we are often interested in treatment effects that are about the same magnitude as potential biases, control of systematic errors is important. Unfortunately, investigators seldom know the relative magnitude or direction of bias. Consequently, we routinely attempt to eliminate it through the appropriate use of eligibility criteria, randomization, and treatment masking.

Patients who agree to participate in a clinical trial are usually not perfectly representative of the population with the disease (selection bias). Although this can affect the external validity of the study, it is unlikely to affect the estimates of treatment *differences*. When the comparison group is subject to the same selection effect, as in randomized studies, relative treatment effects are estimated without bias and are likely to generalize to patients who do not meet the eligibility criteria. More clinically significant biases arise from exclusion of patients after study entry, loss of data for reasons associated with outcome or prognosis, differential assessment of outcomes in treatment groups, and retrospective definitions or analyses. For example, it often seems clinically appropriate to exclude patients because of "non-evaluability" or "noncompliance" with the study. However, these definitions are applied after registration or randomization and are therefore both outcomes and predictors. One cannot reliably make exclusions based on such outcomes without the potential for bias.

Some data can be missing for reasons associated with outcome, for example, when a recurrence or death event is not observed because the patient has not returned to clinic for follow-up visits. Commonly used life-table methods assume that such study subjects are censored at the time of last follow-up. This "informative censoring" results in an underreporting of events and can be corrected only by actively ascertaining the status of all patients.

Random Errors

In later sections of this chapter, I emphasize estimation of effects and confidence intervals as being the most

TABLE 19-1

Random Errors from Hypothesis Tests

RESULT OF HYPOTHESIS TEST	TRUE STATE OF NATURE	
	H_0 TRUE	H_0 FALSE
Reject H_0	Type I error	No error
Do not reject H_0	No error	Type II error

clinically useful summary of data. However, because statistical hypothesis tests have had a prominent role in the design and analysis of trials and still provide a useful perspective on errors of inference, I discuss errors attributable to chance in these traditional terms. The two types of random error that can result from a formal hypothesis test are shown in Table 19-1. The type I error is a "false positive" result and occurs if no treatment effect or difference exists, but the investigators wrongly conclude that there is. The chance of making a type I error is frequently under the control of the investigator, even into the analysis stage of a clinical trial. This is true because the type I error can usually be controlled through the level of significance chosen for statistical tests.

In one general circumstance, the type I error must be carefully considered when designing a clinical trial. This occurs when multiple statistical tests are to be performed, a process that inflates the overall type I error. This happens when investigators intend to examine accumulating data and repeatedly perform statistical tests, as is done in sequential or group sequential interim monitoring of clinical trials. Failing to account properly for the effect of such repeated hypothesis tests can greatly increase the type I error rate. This point is expanded later in a discussion of sequential methods.

The type II error is a false negative and occurs when we fail to detect a treatment effect or difference that is actually present. The power of a clinical trial is the chance of declaring a treatment effect of a specified size to be statistically significant (i.e., not making a type II error). The type II error can only be controlled by proper design, specifically a sufficiently large sample size, and not by any procedures used in the analysis of the study. This point is frequently missed.

A small study may yield a high power to detect a large treatment difference. However, clinicians may be genuinely interested in modest sized or small treatment effects. A small study will usually have low power to detect such differences reliably. It makes little sense to undertake a trial when the chance of missing a clinically important effect is larger than the chance of finding it.

After a comparative clinical trial is completed, it is not helpful to consider the power that the study had against the observed difference, so-called post hoc power, although this commonly is done. If the observed treatment difference is smaller than anticipated and not statistically significant, the power of the trial against that difference will be low. Post hoc power is not helpful, because a power calculation is a probability statement that conditions on a hypothetical treatment effect. After the study, the treatment effect from the trial is no longer hypothetical. A power calculation regarding a *new* clinical trial will be useful to the extent that anyone intends to perform a new study in the same circumstance. We should rely on the estimated treatment effect and confidence interval to summarize the data, rather than the properties of a hypothesis test that is no longer relevant.

Strength of Evidence

Many medical advances have been, and continue to be, made without conducting formal clinical trials. For example, when treatment effects are large, they usually become evident despite the variability and bias present in less formal methods of evaluation. However, many important treatment effects are characterized by natural variability of about the same magnitude as the treatment effect itself. In these circumstances, only careful design and conduct of clinical trials will separate treatment effect from bias and error reliably. Well-designed studies will estimate the magnitude of important clinical effects, quantify errors resulting from chance, reduce or eliminate bias, provide a high degree of credibility and reproducibility in results, and influence future clinical practice.

To meet these goals, investigators often conduct a variety of types of clinical studies. It is helpful to distinguish clinical trials from other types of medical investigations on the basis of who controls three essential components of design: treatment or exposure of the subjects, end-point ascertainment (i.e., collection of outcome data), and analysis. True experiments place all three components under the control of the investigator. For example, a case report is relatively weak evidence because it is a demonstration only that some event of clinical interest is possible. A case series is a demonstration of possibly related clinical events but is subject to large selection biases. In a database analysis, treatment is determined not by design but by patient or physician preference, permitting large biases. In an "observational" study, the investigator takes advantage of natural exposures or treatment selection and chooses an appropriate comparison group by design. However, confounders may not be controlled adequately. In a clinical trial, treatment assignment is by design, and end-point ascertainment is actively performed on all subjects.

With this type of hierarchy, one can see that the strength of evidence in medical studies is directly related to the amount of prospective design in the investigation. The more control exerted by the investigators over the essential components, the stronger will be the design and the more credible will be the results. See Byar[36] for a general discussion of this topic.

DEVELOPMENTAL TRIALS

The use of clinical trials in oncology is similar to that in medical disciplines studying prevention, drugs, and devices. During the developmental stages of new therapies, physicians evaluate evidence concerning related treatments and perform noncomparative clinical trials. Statistical thinking can be of great benefit in areas such as critical review of relevant literature, overviews of previous trial results, design of dose-finding and toxicity studies, and design of studies to estimate treatment effects and feasibility.

Literature Review

A critical review of relevant literature is usually needed before carrying out preliminary studies to determine whether a particular therapeutic approach is feasible and promising. For example, before launching a major comparative clinical trial to determine whether a patient with apparently nonresectable cancer can be helped by preoperative radiation and/or chemotherapy, we need preliminary studies to adjust dose schedules, to see if the treatments are well tolerated and that subsequent surgery is relatively free of complications, and to obtain preliminary data on the likelihood of a successful resection. Once a potentially useful treatment has gone through this pilot phase of development, a comparative trial can be designed to determine if the new procedure performs as well as, or better than, standard therapy.

Overviews of Previous Trial Results

Overviews of comparative clinical trials are often used to summarize results and to increase statistical power when individual trials are too small to detect small effects or seem to yield inconsistent results. However, similar analyses are useful when developing new treatments, especially while planning studies. Even an informal overview can show if, or where, a new study is likely to contribute knowledge.

Recently overviews of results, or "meta-analyses" as they are sometimes called, have become common tools for assessing treatment effects when individual trials do not yield convincing evidence.[36] However, to facilitate design, such formal methods are seldom required.

Dose Finding

Clinical trials that focus primarily on the relation between dose and safety of new drugs or biologicals are often termed "phase I" trials. Their purpose is to study drug distribution, metabolism, excretion, and toxicity and, in the case of cytotoxic drugs, to determine the dose associated with tolerable and reversible side effects. Until recently, statistical thinking has contributed relatively little to the design of these studies.

In oncology, these studies are often done in patients who have been previously treated with standard therapies. The concepts in classic phase I designs include (1) selection, in advance, of a small set of drug doses to be tried; (2) treatment of a small number (e.g., three) patients at each dose with toxicity monitoring; (3) decision rules for stopping the trial based on clinical outcomes; and (4) decision rules for escalating or de-escalating the dose in a subsequent cohort. Often, a few additional patients are studied at the final dose, with the total number of patients treated being usually fewer than 25 to 30.

This type of design alleviates certain practical and ethical problems in administering agents with unknown properties to humans. For example, it tends to minimize the number of patients treated at high (toxic) doses of the drug. It also tends to treat relatively larger numbers of patients at lower (ineffective) doses. Such designs are inefficient. These properties tend to select conservative doses for later developmental testing.

Recently, improved phase I designs have been suggested that correct such problems.[37-39] In some of these designs, doses are not prespecified but are determined from the current results and a mathematical model of the dose-to-toxicity curve. The final sample size of the trial is not fixed in advance but depends on the toxicities observed.

Safety and Activity

After determining the pharmacologic properties of a new drug and a clinically useful dose, trials focus on obtaining evidence of treatment safety and activity. These are conventionally termed "phase II" trials or "safety and activity" trials. The principal question to be addressed in this step of development is whether the new treatment has enough promise to warrant testing against standard therapy in a large comparative trial (i.e., a rigorous study with an internal control group). In this middle developmental step, the study design usually chosen to answer this question is a single-cohort trial with an external control group. The control-group comparison is usually based on the literature, prior investigator experience, or consensus opinion as to what constitutes a worthwhile level of activity in a given disease.

Such studies also usually use surrogate clinical outcomes rather than definitive outcomes such as survival. Surrogate outcomes are chosen because ideally they are known soon after treatment, are easily and accurately measured, and are thought to be informative with respect to later definitive outcomes. Tumor shrinkage (response rate) is a classic surrogate outcome for activity in this setting, based on the cytotoxic model, in which it would imply tumor cell killing.

Unfortunately, tumor shrinkage is a poor surrogate for survival. Furthermore, some therapies would not be expected to produce tumor shrinkage in the usual cytotoxic model. An example might be cytostatic agents. Some caution must be exercised when making developmental decisions on the basis of surrogate outcomes. For certain agents, safety and activity trials should use definitive outcomes such as survival (overall failure rate), making them somewhat larger and lengthier than conventional designs.

Two types of designs are commonly used in middle development: fixed sample size and staged. In fixed sample size trials, the number of study subjects is chosen in advance (e.g., to yield a specified precision in the estimated response rate). Staged designs use a treatment evaluation after groups of subjects have been entered, permitting early termination of accrual if high or low response rates are observed. Excellent working designs can be obtained from only two stages.[40]

Numerous other statistical issues arise in the design and evaluation of phase II trials. Questions include patient selection, how to evaluate response quantitatively, patient exclusions, and the role of randomization. Space does not permit discussing these issues here. Reviews can be found in Buyse and colleagues.[7]

Sample Size for Middle Developmental Trials

Consider a phase II trial in which patients with esophageal cancer are treated with chemotherapy before surgical resection. A complete response is defined as the absence of macroscopic and microscopic tumor at the time of surgery. We suspect that this might occur 35% of the time and would like the 95% confidence interval of our estimate to be ±15%. Approximate 95% confidence intervals for a proportion, P, are

$$P\text{-}p \pm 1.96 \times \sqrt{[P(1 - P)/n]},$$

where n is the number of patients tested and 1.96 is the quantile from the normal distribution corresponding to a two-sided probability of 5%. Substituting into this formula yields

$$0.15 = 1.96 \times \sqrt{[0.35(1 - 0.35)/n\}]}$$

or $n = 39$ patients required to meet the requirements for precision. Because 35% is just an estimate of the proportion and some patients may not complete the study, the actual sample size might be increased slightly. Expected accrual rates may be used to estimate the required duration of this study in a straightforward fashion.

A useful, but rough, rule of thumb for estimating sample sizes needed for proportions may be derived in the same way. Because $P(1 - P)$ is maximal for $P = 0.5$, an approximate and conservative relation between n, the sample size, and w, the width of the 95% confidence interval is $n = 1/w^2$. Thus to achieve a precision of ±10% (.10) requires 100 patients, and a precision of ±20% (.20) requires 25 patients. This inverse-square relation demands large sample sizes for high precision. This rule of thumb is not valid for proportions that deviate greatly from .5. For example, for proportions less than about .2 or greater than about .8, exact binomial methods should be used to estimate precision and sample size.

Similarly, consider a middle developmental trial in which a definitive outcome such as reduction in the overall failure rate is required. On a log scale, the confidence interval for the hazard ratio is $\log\Delta$ plus or minus Z_α/Δ, where Δ is the hazard ratio, d is the total number of failures, and $Z_\alpha = 1.96$ for a two-sided 95% interval. Like that for a response rate, this confidence interval can be made as small (precise) as necessary by observing more events.

Compared with a reference failure rate on standard therapy, a reduction of 33% on a new treatment (hazard = 0.2; ratio = 0.67) might be considered a useful improvement. If the reference failure rate is 0.3 per person-year (corresponding to median failure time of 2.3 years) and accrual proceeds at 75 subjects per year for 2 years with 1 additional year of follow-up, then we would expect to observe about 48 failures. This number of events would yield a precision of about ±0.06 (95% confidence interval) in the observed failure rate. Thus such a study has to be larger and longer than a conventional safety and activity trial with a surrogate outcome.

COMPARATIVE STUDIES

Helping to design a comparative trial is a major responsibility for the biostatistician. The process involves detailed discussions with other investigators to resolve issues such as (1) what population should be studied; (2) are the treatment methods unambiguously defined; (3) how will patients be assigned to treatment groups; (4) how will outcomes be measured, and what can be done to assure that measurements will be obtained uniformly on all patients regardless of treatment assignment; and (5) what can be done to minimize loss to follow-up and to promote compliance with the treatment protocol.

In the sections that follow, I outline some points of good design (Table 19-2), which are not intended to be taken chronologically. Many of them must proceed simultaneously. However, attention to each of these items will likely result in a stronger trial.

Dual Roles of the Physician

Physicians who develop new treatments have two roles that are sometimes dissonant with each other. The first is as an advocate for the care and interests of the individual patient. The second is as a scientist representing the needs of others. The conduct of clinical trials is one of many areas in which these roles can, but do not necessarily, conflict. From a clinical trials perspective, physician advocacy for the individual patient is an ideal and not an exclusive standard of conduct. This ideal is not met in circumstances of triage, allocation of scarce and expensive technologies such as organ transplantation, training of new physicians, and vaccination. All of these

circumstances knowingly place some patients at risk for the benefit of others.

Even if we accept the individual advocacy ideal, some patients will always receive an inferior treatment because of physician error. Failure to learn from such mistakes can hardly be considered ethical. It is incumbent on physicians to learn quickly and convincingly from the inevitable use of less-effective treatments so that their scope of application is minimized. Controlled experiments in the proper clinical setting are the most reliable way to accomplish this. Conversely, we must learn about efficacious new therapies as quickly as possible so that they can be used broadly.

Although clinical trials are conducted worldwide, concerns are voiced frequently about the ethics of randomization.[41] Although any medical technology can be used inappropriately in specific instances, nothing is inherently unethical in randomization when it is used because physicians lack knowledge about the superiority of treatments and to eliminate bias so that the best possible evidence can be gathered. Circumstances of collective uncertainty will always exist in which randomized treatment comparisons are the most ethical course of action.

In some circumstances, evidence becomes available during the conduct of the trial that one treatment is superior. This can happen, for example, if one treatment is unexpectedly better or worse or has unacceptable side effects.

Investigators are ethically bound to learn of such circumstances as early as possible by monitoring the accumulating data and closing the inferior treatment arm if necessary. The administrative and statistical plans to meet this contingency require planning during the design phase of the trial.

Quantify Objectives

An important task in designing a clinical trial and drafting the study protocol is to convert clinical objectives into quantitative measurements of outcome variables. For example, we might be interested to know if a certain therapy "results in lower morbidity." However, the measurement of morbidity is not automatically well defined, particularly if the study involves more than one investigator. At least three aspects of morbidity must be defined. The first is a window of time during which adverse events can plausibly be attributed to the therapy. The second is a list of specific diagnoses or complications to be included. The third is a list of procedures required to establish each diagnosis definitively.

Define the Study Population by Using Eligibility and Exclusion Criteria

Differences in eligibility criteria probably explain many of the discrepant results in the clinical literature from seemingly identical clinical trials. Even when several institutions use the same protocol, differences in interpretation of eligibility criteria and types of patients referred contribute to differences in outcomes. As a

TABLE 19-2

STEP	CONCEPT
Ten Concepts in Comparative Trial Design	
1	Review ethical issue and consent
2	Quantify objectives
3	Define the study population by using eligibility and exclusion criteria
4	Assess accrual resources
5	Specify treatments
6	Define end points and methods of assessment
7	Calculate quantitative properties of the design
8	Establish procedures for managing data
9	Establish procedures for monitoring
10	Control treatment allocation and bias

Science of Clinical Oncology

consequence, trials from different institutions and or times may not be comparable even if the eligibility criteria are the same. This is one argument in favor of randomized concurrent controls.

To some extent, study results can be shaped by the eligibility and exclusion criteria. Consider how drug toxicity or operative morbidity can be reduced by the careful selection of patients. Age restrictions can reduce the number and severity of many chemotherapy toxicities, although such restrictions are seldom made explicit. Eligibility criteria can be used to define a more homogeneous study population, reducing the interpatient variability in outcomes. However, this will not necessarily reduce the size of a trial. For example, patients with poor prognosis may respond to treatment in the same way as those with good prognosis. If so, a trial excluding poor–prognosis patients would be needlessly prolonged.

In many instances, end points may be evaluated more easily if certain complicating factors are prevented by patient exclusion. For example, if patients with recent nonpulmonary malignancies are excluded from a lung cancer trial, evaluation of tumor recurrences and second primaries might be made simpler.

Ethical considerations also suggest that patients who are unlikely to benefit from the treatment (e.g., because of organ system dysfunction) not be allowed to participate in the trial. Whenever possible, quantitative parameters such as laboratory values should be used to make these definitions rather than qualitative clinical assessments. Some studies in patients with advanced cancer call for a "life expectancy of at least 6 months." A more useful and reproducible criterion might be Karnofsky performance status greater than, say, 8.

Assess Accrual Resources

One unfortunate and preventable mistake made in clinical trials is to plan and initiate a study, only to have it terminate early because of low accrual. This situation can be avoided with some advance planning. First, investigators should be aware of the accrual rate required to complete a study in a certain fixed period. This is a best-case projection. Most researchers would like to see comparative treatment trials completed within 5 years and pilot or feasibility studies finished within 1 to 2 years. Disease-prevention trials may take longer. In any case, the accrual rate required to complete a study within the time targeted can be estimated easily from the total sample size required.

Second, investigators must obtain realistic estimates of accrual rates. The raw number of patients with a specific diagnosis can often be determined easily from hospital or clinic records but is a large overestimate of potential study accrual. It must be reduced by the proportion of subjects likely to meet the eligibility criteria, and again by the proportion of those willing to participate in the trial (e.g., consenting to randomization). This latter proportion is usually less than half. Study duration can then be projected based on this potential accrual rate, which might be one fourth to half of the patient population.

Third, investigators can project trial duration based on a worst-case accrual. The study may still be feasible under such plans. If not, plans for terminating the trial because of low accrual must be made so as not to waste resources. In particular, accrual estimates from participating institutions other than the investigators' own are suspect. How long will the study take as a single-institution trial?

To estimate accrual more accurately, a formal survey of participants can be done before accrual starts. As patients are seen over a certain period, a record can be kept to see whether they match the eligibility criteria. To estimate the proportion willing to give consent, one could briefly explain the proposed study and ask if they would hypothetically be willing to participate.

Treatment Specification

Control of treatments and their allocation is a defining characteristic of true experimental designs. In practical situations, explicit plans are needed for modifications in the treatment of individual patients. To satisfy scientific objectives, essential components of the therapy should be guided by the protocol, but modifications that are unlikely to affect the outcome should be left to the treating physician.

Physicians participating in trials are always obligated to replace protocol treatments with others when they believe that it is in the best interests of the patient. However, sufficient flexibility in the treatment specification, especially concerning complications, toxicity, or side effects, may permit most patients to continue following the protocol. This could contribute more information to the trial results and enhance the credibility of the study report.

Defining End Points and Methods of Assessment

Selection of end points and the use of prospective methods of assessment greatly affect the strength of a trial. Important characteristics of the end point are that it correspond to the scientific objectives of the trial. The method of assessing end points should be accurate and free of bias. This is helpful for both subjective end points and for objective ones such as survival and recurrence time. Even when using well-defined event times, incomplete follow-up can create bias.

From a biostatistical perspective, three types of end points are likely to be used widely in oncology trials. These are (1) continuously varying measurements, (2) dichotomous outcomes, and (3) event times. I will briefly discuss each of these.

Continuously Varying Measurements

Measurements that can theoretically vary continuously over some range are common and useful types of assessments. Examples include many laboratory values, blood or tissue levels, functional disability measures, or physical dimensions. In a study population, these measurements have a distribution, often characterized by a mean or other location parameter, and variance or other dispersion parameter. Consequently, these outcomes will be most useful when the primary effect of a treatment is to raise or lower the average measure in a population. Typical statistical tests that can detect differences such as these include the *t* test or a nonparametric analog and analyses of variance (for more than two groups). To control the effect of confounders or prognostic factors on these outcomes, linear regression models might be used.

Dichotomous Measures

Some assessments have only two possible values (i.e., present or absent). Examples include some imprecise measurements such as tumor size, which might be described only as responding or not, and outcomes like infection, which is either present or not. Inaccuracy in measurement can make a continuous value ordinal or dichotomous. In the study population, these outcomes will be frequently summarized as a proportion. Comparing proportions might lead to tests such as the χ^2 or exact conditional tests. Another useful population summary is the odds or log-odds. The effect of prognostic factors or confounders on this outcome can often be modeled by using logistic regression.

Event Times

Event times are common and useful outcome measurements in clinical trials. Survival time and disease-free or recurrence time are well-known examples. However, many other intervals might be of clinical importance, such as time to hospital discharge or time spent on a ventilator. The distinguishing feature of event-time outcomes is the possibility of censoring. This means that some subjects under observation may not experience the event by the end of the study. Using the information in the censored observation time requires some special statistical procedures. In the study population, event-time or "survival" distributions (e.g., life tables) might be used to summarize the data. Clinicians are also accustomed to seeing medians or fixed time proportions used to summarize these outcomes. Perhaps the most useful summary is the hazard, which can be thought of as a proportion adjusted for follow-up time. The effect of prognostic factors or confounders on hazard rates can often be modeled by using survival regression models.

Other End Points

Several other types of end points are important for some medical studies but are not used frequently in oncology. These include counts, multiple category outcomes, ordered categories, disease–intensity measures, and repeated measurements. For example, units of blood used might be described as a count, and chemotherapy toxicities are often described in ordered categories. Much discussion among clinical trialists recently has concerned the use of "intermediate end points," which become known early after treatment but are very reliably associated with definitive outcomes. Examples include premalignant lesions in cancer-prevention studies and CD4 lymphocyte counts in acquired immunodeficiency syndrome (AIDS). Intermediate end points are probably not so relevant to oncologic studies as to these others

areas of study. One notable exception is the use of prostate specific antigen (PSA) to monitor prostate cancer recurrence.

Control Treatment Allocation and Bias

Randomization

Randomization is one of the most effective means for reducing bias because it guarantees that treatment assignment will not be based on patients' prognostic factors. The benefits derived from randomized treatment assignment are well known.[35,36] After randomization, treatment differences can be attributed to the true treatment effect plus random variability.

One argument against randomization is that it is unnecessary because confounders can be controlled in the analysis by using statistical adjustment procedures. The extent to which this can be done relies on two additional assumptions: (1) the investigators have measured the confounders in the experimental subjects, and (2) the assumptions of the statistical models or other adjustment procedures are known to be correct. Randomization is a more reliable method than adjustment because it controls bias without these assumptions. Moreover, it controls the effects of confounders whether they are known to the investigator or not. Critics of randomization often overlook this last point, which provides randomized studies with their high degree of credibility.

Blinding or Masking

Masking (blinding) is another bias-reducing technique in which the patient (single blind), physician (double blind), and perhaps the monitors (triple blind) in a clinical trial are unaware of the individual patient–treatment assignments. As a result of blinding, treatment assessments can be made without prejudice, increasing the utility of both objective and subjective outcomes. Masking of drugs is often simple to implement, particularly with the assistance of a hospital pharmacy or pharmaceutical company. In oncology, treatment masking is frequently possible, although sometimes logisitically impractical.

Calculate Quantitative Properties of the Design (Precision, Power, Duration)

Questions regarding the quantitative properties of clinical trial designs are among those most frequently asked by clinicians. It is not possible to specify a universally valid approach to answering such questions. Instead, I provide some basic ideas and examples. For a more statistically oriented review, see Donner.[42] Although computer software is available to perform many power and sample-size calculations, most programs are written for a statistical user.

Two basic considerations in estimating precision and power are the purpose of the trial and its primary end point. For noncomparative designs, the goals of the study are often to estimate some useful clinical quantity with a specified precision. Examples of end points with clinical interest are average blood or tissue levels of a drug, the proportion of patients responding or meeting other predefined criteria, or population failure rates. A useful measure of precision is the confidence interval of the estimate. For example, narrow 95% confidence intervals indicate a higher degree of certainty about the location of a true effect than do wide 95% confidence intervals. Because confidence intervals depend on the number of subjects studied, targets for precision can often be translated into requirements for sample size.

Comparative clinical trials require more complicated methods to estimate sample size and power. Often comparative studies are designed to yield statistical hypothesis tests with desirable properties, such as a high power to detect important clinical differences reliably. In trials with survival time as the primary end point, the power of the study depends on the number of events (e.g., recurrences or deaths). Confusion can arise over the number of patients placed on study versus the number of events required for the trial to have the intended statistical properties. As a test of equality between treatment groups, it is common to compare the ratio of hazard (or failure) rates (defined later) versus 1.0. Under fairly flexible assumptions, the size of such a study should satisfy

$$d = [(Z_\alpha + Z_\beta)^2(\Delta + 1)^2]/(\Delta - 1)^2$$

where d is the total number of events need on the study, Δ is the ratio of hazards in the two treatment groups, and Z_α and Z_β are the normal quantiles for the type I and II error rates.[43]

For example, with this formula, to detect a hazard rate of 1.75 as being statistically significantly different from 1.0 by using a two-sided .05 α-level test with 90% power requires

$$[(1.96 + 1.282)^2(1.75 + 1)^2]/(1.75 - 1)2 = 141 \text{ events.}$$

This is not the final sample size, as suggested by the safety and activity trial example discussed earlier. A sufficient number of patients must be placed in the study to yield 141 events in an interval of time appropriate for the trial. For example, if 50% of patients remain event free (censored) at the end of the trial, 282 subjects are required. In general, the sample size, n, is

$$n = d/(1 - p),$$

where p is the proportion censored.

TRIAL IMPLEMENTATION

Establish Procedures for Managing Data

All trials require certain minimal standards for collecting, quality controlling, and reporting data. Although many investigators use their own staff to perform such duties, sufficient skill is required to suggest that these activities be housed in groups dedicated to the purpose. Resources for this might exist on a departmental or institutional level. In other circumstances, an external or privately run coordinating center might be used. In no case should this reduce access to the data or substitute for skilled

translation of data elements from clinical and laboratory sources to study database.

At least five conceptual components to processing information from patients are found in a clinical trial: (1) eligibility check and registration/randomization; (2) data acquisition from the clinical record; (3) editing, error checking, building a database, and quality control; (4) interim reporting; and (5) analysis. Each of these, when properly performed, will reduce the frequency and severity of certain types of errors. Although one could write extensively about this subject, I summarize only a few important points about each component.

The eligibility check and registration is a simple but important quality-control point. Even the knowledge that eligibility will be impartially checked causes many investigators to take entry criteria more seriously. Usually a phone call requiring only a few moments is all that is needed. By using this opportunity, an identifying number can be assigned, a database record can be started, the pharmacy can be notified (if necessary), and other study bookkeeping can be initiated.

Data acquisition from the clinical record must be performed by an individual with sufficient clinical, protocol, and medical record knowledge. In some cases, this requires the investigator's expertise, whereas in other circumstances, a research nurse or data specialist can succeed. Unless studies are subject to external auditing, it is uncommon to catch errors made at this stage. Thus the principle investigator can have a major beneficial impact on the quality of data by being active here.

A simple and straightforward system for building and managing a database might begin with paper records or data forms that contain the information of clinical importance to the study. It is not necessary to record all the information needed for the care of the patient but rather only those items that correspond to the outcomes and objectives of the study. Ideally, one would not collect any items that do not need analysis. Information from these forms can be transcribed onto an appropriate computer database. Numerous quality-control checks and edits are necessary to be certain that the database produced from paper records accurately represents the clinical record. For example, audits may compare the database with the chart. Within a single patient's record, computerized checks of bounds and internal consistency can be performed. When reviewed by a knowledgeable person, lists and summaries of the data can trap many errors.

In recent years, personal computer–based software has made some of these tasks more simple and reliable. Many investigators use spreadsheets to assist with these tasks in small studies, although database software is more powerful. When existing databases and human resources are available, investigators should attempt to use them rather than building a system for each study independently. In any case, the investigator should understand the flow of data from the clinical record through the final analysis.

Interim reporting serves several purposes. It provides an opportunity for the investigators to review accumulating data related to administrative aspects of the study, such as accrual rates and delinquent observations. Complication and toxicity rates can be reviewed to be certain that the type, frequency, and severity of such events is reasonable. Efficacy end points can be reviewed, following appropriate statistical guidelines, to satisfy ethical concerns. Much has been written about these subjects, and I discuss more details later.

Establish Procedures for Monitoring

Plans for monitoring and early stopping of accrual are another element of good trial design that can greatly alleviate problems in conducting studies. Researchers have an ethical obligation to learn about treatment differences as quickly as possible and to minimize the number of patients who are placed on a convincingly inferior treatment. By planning for early termination of accrual when unexpectedly large differences are observed, investigators can make a clinical trial more acceptable to other researchers and patients. A full discussion of sequential and group sequential methods for use in this context is beyond the scope of this chapter. These methods are now commonly practiced by using well-described techniques.[44-48] Investigators can ensure that monitoring methods are effectively implemented by having the accumulating data reviewed formally at intervals by a monitoring committee.

Repeatedly performing statistical significance tests on accumulating data increases the overall type I error. If 10 interim analyses were conducted with the conventional significance level of .05, the resulting overall type I error might be as high as 15%. This inflation of the type I error can be even higher if many interim looks at the data are performed. To compensate for this and control the type I error, investigators must prospectively plan the analysis points and the significance level for each analysis.

To control the overall type I error at 5%, each interim look should use a significance level smaller than .05. For example, in a clinical trial comparing response rates and two-sided testing for significance 5 times, a frequently used group sequential method[57] indicates that the analyses should be conducted with significance levels of approximately .0000075, .0013, .0085, .023, and .041, to control the overall type I error at the conventional 5%. With this method, note that the final analysis is conducted by using a significance level near, but less than, the usual 5%. Early in the trial, achieving statistical significance is more difficult.

Unplanned interim analyses may have undesirable properties and can pose serious problems in interpretation for researchers and regulators. Attempts have been made to alleviate this problem by retrospectively applying group sequential methods, although this has difficulties of its own. Another alternative for monitoring is the use of bayesian statistical methods, which have much appeal to clinicians but have not gained as widespread use as other methods.[49] For a general discussion of monitoring alternatives, see Gail,[50] and for a practical discussion, see O'Fallon[51] or DeMets.[52] In any case, the time to plan properly for trial monitoring is during the design phase of the study.

A second reason for terminating a trial early is that interim analyses demonstrate the near equivalence of the treatments, and continuing the trial would be unlikely to demonstrate clinically significant differences. In this circumstance, early stopping has been based on "conditional power" calculations.[53] Using this technique reduces the size and length of trials that show no effect or treatment difference but still yields clinically useful information.

ANALYSIS

The exact procedures necessary for analyzing a clinical trial depend on the design and purposes of the study. For example, pharmacologic studies might require modeling and estimation of physiological parameters in each patient to meet their objectives, whereas comparative trials usually require summaries of relative treatment effects and confidence intervals. Analyses for these differing types of studies seem to have very little in common. However, when we consider that all trials should inform us about the population being studied, the need for unbiased statistical estimation of clinical effects, and the need to summarize data in the most clinically useful form, much common ground is evident.

The approach I recommend to analysis and reporting emphasizes estimation rather than hypothesis testing.[54-60] Measuring and reporting clinical effects and associated estimates of variability (or confidence intervals) is more informative and useful than focusing attention on formal tests of statistical hypotheses and P values.

A simple example should make the difference clear. Suppose a clinical trial is performed comparing two treatments, A and B, and the major outcome is survival. Investigators might perform a statistical hypothesis test comparing treatments A and B and report "survival on treatment A is significantly longer than on B ($P < .05$)." Alternatively, when emphasizing estimation, investigators might report "the estimated hazard ratio (A vs B) for death was 2.0 (95% confidence limits, 1.5–2.3)." In the first case, the reader is left only with a P value to summarize the data, whereas in the second case, the treatment difference is described more completely.

Some journals have adopted guidelines for reporting.[28-33] Our recommendations are similar in spirit to those. Although I have suggested some specific statistical methods and summaries for certain kinds of data, additional or alternative analytic procedures must be adopted in special cases, and I do not seek to limit analyses or reports. However, the basic concepts and approaches outlined here should prove to be helpful both clinically and statistically for correctness, lack of bias, completeness, and consistency.

In this spirit, I offer 10 basic steps in the accompanying box in the analysis of clinical trials. I emphasize that these steps are conceptual and do not necessarily occur in the order listed. Some steps are relevant only to randomized or comparative trials.

TEN CONCEPTS IN TRIAL ANALYSIS

1. Approach the trial as a test of treatment policy, not a test of treatment received. This is the "intent-to-treat" principle.
2. Include all patients who meet the eligibility criteria.
3. Examine the data and correct errors.
4. Describe the population on the study.
5. Verify the comparability of treatment groups.
6. Estimate the effect of treatment and other prognostic factors on the major outcome (univariate analyses), as well as confidence intervals.
7. Use standard statistical methods or models (e.g., linear, logistic, or proportional hazards regression), to re-estimate the treatment effect while adjusting for (a) statistically significantly imbalanced prognostic factors; (b) strong or influential prognostic factors, whether imbalanced or not; and (c) any prognostic factor for which it is important to demonstrate convincing control.
8. Consult the biostatistician concerning special methods to address secondary clinical questions. Any analyses not protected by the randomization should correspond to clinical hypotheses stated as study objectives. Control prognostic factors.
9. Consider repeating steps 1 through 6 after excluding ineligible patients (i.e., patients who are ineligible based on entry criteria).
10. Cautiously conduct exploratory or hypothesis-generating analyses: (a) any analysis suggested by the data and not by hypothesis, (b) any analysis that excludes patients based on postentry criteria, and (c) subset analyses. These should never be the "primary" analysis.

Intention to Treat

It is unfortunate that investigators conducting clinical trials cannot guarantee that the patients who participate will definitely complete (or even receive) the treatment assigned. Thus a clinical trial can be viewed as a test of treatment policy, not a test of treatment received. Many factors contribute to patients' failing to complete the intended therapy, including severe side effects, disease progression, strong preference for a different treatment, and a change of mind. Many such factors are strongly correlated with outcome, which can render a strong bias if such patients are removed from the analysis.

From a clinical perspective, postentry exclusion of eligible patients is essentially an attempt to use information from the future. When selecting a therapy for a new patient, the physician is primarily interested in the unconditional probability that the treatment will benefit the patient. Because the physician has no knowledge of whether the patient will complete the treatment intended, inferences that depend on events in the patient's future (i.e., adherence to therapy) are not helpful to that goal. In other words, adherence is both an outcome of the trial as well as a potential predictor. These two roles of adherence cannot be disentangled by removing patients from consideration. Consequently, the physician will be most interested in clinical trial results that include all patients who were assigned to the therapy.

To be certain that the trial results closely reflect the effect of the treatment, the eligibility criteria should exclude patients with characteristics that might prevent them from completing the therapy. For example, if the therapy is lengthy, perhaps only good-performance-status patients should be eligible. If the treatment is highly toxic, only patients with normal function in major organ systems will be likely to complete the therapy.

After these considerations, the most important analysis includes all patients registered or randomized on the trial regardless of postentry events. This analysis is the intention-to-treat analysis. It is possible to exclude patients who were retrospectively found not to meet the eligibility criteria (i.e., those who were mistakenly placed in the study) without creating bias. Ideally, such patients would not have entered the study because they would have been found to be ineligible. However, only eligibility or pre-entry criteria should be used to make such exclusions. If patients are excluded based on "evaluability" or other postentry criteria, the possibility of bias increases. Evaluability criteria are outcomes, no matter how well-defined clinically. If we exclude subjects based on outcomes, the potential for bias is great.

Examine the Data

The first practical step in any analysis is to look at the data. This includes examining lists and other simple tabulations that might highlight incorrect data values. Many problems in analyzing clinical trials can be prevented by correcting errors that become apparent in this way. This is also a step that knowledgeable investigators can perform quickly but very efficiently. With the widespread use of computers and automated analysis procedures to manage clinical information, it is possible to produce results from clinical studies without carefully examining the data. This is unfortunate because even a cursory examination of raw data by a technically knowledgeable person can detect many errors of importance to the analysis.

Some of the errors that are amenable to detection by inspection include (1) incorrectly missing data (patient had level measured but not recorded in the database); (2) incorrect decimal points (80 recorded instead of 8.0); (3) failure to convert numeric codes for special values (calcium becomes 99 instead of "missing"); (4) out-of-range or impermissible values (0.0 recorded instead of 8.0); (5) mislabeled variables (age is mistaken for calcium and vice versa); and (6) coding and recoding errors (0 should mean normal, and 1 should mean abnormal, but values are reversed).

Inspection of the data is particularly important for small- or single-investigator studies in which the data-management techniques are not subject to regular quality-control procedures, as might be the case in multi-institutional cooperative group studies. Errors in small studies can be particularly influential. Many times, small studies are recorded entirely on paper, with transcription to a computer at a later time, creating another opportunity for errors. Other times, data are stored on computers by using convenient but unsophisticated software such as spreadsheets rather than database management programs that permit validation and checking. Fortunately, the quantity of data from such small studies is often very amenable to checking by inspection. It is embarrassing, frustrating, and bad for morale to have to ask that analyses be repeated because data errors were discovered late.

Describe the Study Population

Clinical trials are studies of particularly well defined and often relatively small cohorts. Although the eligibility criteria define a target population of particular interest, the patients actually accrued on a trial may differ because of chance or subtle institutional characteristics. Investigators will want to describe the observed cohort, particularly with regard to important prognostic factors. Simple population measures and summary statistics usually suffice for this purpose. This process is also both a by-product of and valuable in error checking.

Verify the Comparability of Treatment Groups

In reports of many randomized studies, the first table presented is often intended to show the comparability of treatment groups. Actually, a lack of statistically significant differences between the treatment groups does not guarantee the absence of influential imbalances but only demonstrates the effectiveness of randomization. Even so, this is important because readers will have increased confidence in the validity of the findings if imbalances are either absent or detected and controlled in the analyses. Although we will take note of any statistically significant differences between groups, nonsignificant imbalances in strong prognostic factors can influence treatment comparisons. This is discussed more completely in deciding when to adjust (later section). Second, and conversely, statistically significant imbalances are not necessarily influential: the imbalance may occur in an inconsequential factor. For the clinician comparing groups, the magnitude of the difference is more important than the *P* value.

Estimate Treatment and Prognostic Effects

As mentioned earlier, some outcomes that are likely to be useful in oncology trials are group averages (or differences between group averages), probability of response (or odds ratios), and hazards (or hazard ratios). I omit discussion of methods for group averages because they are well known and focus on dichotomous outcomes and event times. These outcomes have similarities with respect to their summary statistics and presentation. Odds ratios are useful

TABLE 19-3

Responses on Treatments for Solid Tumors		
	OUTCOME	
TREATMENT	**RESPONSE**	**NO RESPONSE**
Group A	38	63
Group B	18	81

summaries of data to describe the effects of dichotomous variables. For example, differences in the probability of response might be described by an odds ratio. Similarly, hazard ratios are useful for describing differences in risk of failure over time. For example, differences in recurrence or survival curves might be described by a hazard ratio.

To illustrate these and other aspects of the estimation of clinical effects, I consider simulated data from a hypothetical randomized trial comparing two treatments (A and B) for treatment of solid tumors (Table 19-3). Simple randomization was used in this study with 101 patients on treatment A and 99 patients on treatment B. Data on response to treatment were collected as an example of a dichotomous outcome, and patients were followed up for survival as an example of an event-time endpoint. Differences in response and survival attributable to sex also are thought to be important. Nonparametric estimates of survival for subgroups defined by treatment/sex combinations are shown in Figure 19-1.

The advantage to using simulated data, aside from convenience, is that the "true" treatment and covariate effects are known. In this case, the true treatment effects were a fourfold odds of response and a twofold risk of death in favor of treatment A. For sex, the odds of response was twofold, and the risk of death was 1.5-fold, both in favor of female subjects. Response and survival were independent of one another. In what follows, the estimated effects will differ from these values because of random variation.

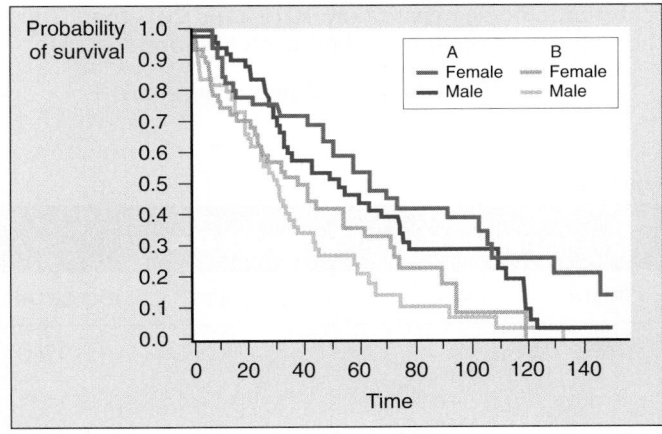

Figure 19-1. Survival by treatment group and sex on a hypothetical clinical trial.

TABLE 19-4

Example of Odds Summary Data

GROUP	SEX	PATIENTS	RESPONSES	RESPONSE ODDS
A	Males	53	15	.395
	Females	48	23	.920
	Overall	101	38	.603
B	Males	51	8	.186
	Females	48	10	.263
	Overall	99	18	.222

Odds and Hazard Ratios

The simulated response data for the two treatment groups are shown in Table 19-4. The estimated response rate (probability) on treatment A was 0.376 compared with 0.182 on treatment B. The odds of response for treatment A is

$$odds_A = P/(1 - P) = 0.376/0.624 = 0.063.$$

A more useful quantity for judging the relative effect of treatment on response is the odds ratio. The estimate of the overall odds ratio for group A versus group B, $\widehat{OR}_{AB}$ is

$$\widehat{OR}_{AB} = (38 \times 81)/(18 \times 63) = 2.71.$$

Because the odds of response on treatment A is almost threefold higher than on treatment B, this might be a clinically important difference. The decision to use the odds ratio of A versus B or (vice versa) is purely a matter of convenience. The data relating sex and response are shown in Table 19-4.

In treatment group A, the odds ratio for males versus females is 0.395/0.920 = 0.429. In group B, the corresponding ratio is 0.707. Thus it appears that male subjects are less likely to respond than female subjects, and I explore this further later in the analysis.

For event-time end points, the quantities of interest are the number of events in the groups and the total follow-up or exposure time (in years; Table 19-5).

The total exposure time is obtained by summing all follow-up times without regard to censoring. This represents the aggregate time at risk for the group. Thus the estimated overall hazard of death in group A, λ_A, is

$$\lambda_A = 70/5,614 = 0.012 \text{ per person-year,}$$

and for group B, is

$$\lambda_\beta = 77/3,434 = 0.022 \text{ per person-year.}$$

From these data, I would conclude that the risk of death after treatment B is higher and that this difference might be of clinical importance. Here also, sex appears to influence the risk of death. The estimated hazard ratios for male versus female subjects are 1.27 and 1.37 on treatments A and B. The effect of sex is explored later in more detail.

This example has shown the utility of odds and hazard ratios in summarizing clinical effects. The next section illustrates additional utility for confidence intervals.

Confidence Intervals

Informally, a confidence interval is a region in which we are confident that a true parameter or effect lies. Although this notion is not too misleading, confidence intervals are really probability statements about an estimate and not about the true parameter value. A 95% confidence interval indicates the region that would contain the true parameter value 95% of the time if we repeated the experiment. In other words, given the estimates resulting from a series of experiments, the true value will fall within the 95% confidence regions 95% of the time.

The value of confidence intervals is that they convey both the magnitude of the estimated clinical effect and a sense of its precision. In many cases, simple hypothesis tests are analogous to the confidence interval. In summaries of results from several studies, estimates and confidence intervals are more useful than P values.

Continuing with the example of the randomized clinical trial introduced in the section on treatment and prognostic effects, I first consider confidence intervals for the probability of response. An approximate 95% confidence interval for the probability of response on treatment A is

$$0.376 \pm 1.96 \times \sqrt{[0.376(1 - 0.376)/101]}$$
$$= 0.376 \pm 0.094 = [0.282\text{--}0.470].$$

Similarly, an approximate 95% confidence interval for response on treatment B is $0.182 \pm 0.076 = [0.106\text{--}0.258]$. Because of the large sample size and the intermediate size of the probabilities, these intervals are close to those that would be obtained by using exact binomial methods, which are [0.282–0.478] and [0.111–0.272] for groups A and B, respectively.

TABLE 19-5

Example of Hazard Summary Data

GROUP	SEX	PATIENTS	EXPOSURE TIME	DEATHS	HAZARD
A	Males	53	2,768	40	.014
	Females	48	2,846	30	.011
	Overall	101	5,614	70	.012
B	Males	51	1,632	42	.026
	Females	48	1,802	35	.019
	Overall	99	3,434	77	.022

For odds and hazard ratios, calculating confidence intervals on a log scale is relatively simple. An approximate confidence interval for the *log* odds ratio for A versus B is

$$\log\{2.71\} \pm Z_\alpha \times \sqrt{[1/63 + 1/38 + 1/81 + 1/18]}$$

where Z_α is the point on normal distribution exceeded with probability $\alpha/2$ (e.g., for $\alpha = 0.05$, $Z_\alpha = 1.96$). This yields a confidence interval of [0.35–1.65] for the log odds ratio or [1.41–5.21] for the odds ratio. Because the 95% confidence interval for $\hat{o}R_{AB}$ excludes 1.0, the difference is "statistically significant." The statistical test of the null $H_O : \hat{o}R_{AB} = 1.0$ is rejected with significance level $P = .003$.

A similar method can be used for the hazard ratio. An approximate confidence interval for the log hazard ratio is

$$\log\{1.83\} \pm Z_\alpha \times \sqrt{[1/77 + 1/70]}.$$

This yields a confidence interval of [0.264–0.911] for the log hazard ratio or [1.30–2.49] for the hazard ratio. Again, the confidence interval excludes 1.0, indicating a statistically significant difference in the death rates between the groups ($P < .001$).

Problems with P Values

In many circumstances, *P* values are useful, particularly in well-designed hypothesis tests. However, *P* values have properties that make them poor summaries of clinical effects.[61–67] In particular, *P* values do not convey the magnitude of a clinical effect. The size of the *P* value is a consequence of two things: the magnitude of the estimated treatment difference and its estimated variability (which is itself a consequence of sample size). Thus the *P* value partially reflects the size of the experiment, which has no biologic importance. The *P* value also hides the size of the treatment difference, which does have major biologic importance.

Some investigators conclude things like "the effect might be statistically significant in a larger sample." This, of course, misses the point, because any effect other than zero will be statistically significant in a large enough sample. The investigators really should be talking about the size and clinical significance of an estimated treatment effect rather than its *P* value. In summary, *P* values only quantify the type I error and incompletely characterize the biologically important effects in the data.

To illustrate the advantage of estimation and confidence intervals over *P* values, consider the recent discussion over the prognostic effect of perioperative blood transfusion in lung cancer.[54–60] Several studies (not clinical trials) of this phenomenon have been performed because of firm evidence in other malignancies and diseases that blood transfusion has a clinically important immuno-suppressive effect. Disagreement over the study results has stemmed, in part, from too strong an emphasis on hypothesis tests instead of accepting the estimated risk ratios and confidence limits. Some study results are shown in Table 19-6. Although the authors of the various reports came to different conclusions about the risk of blood transfusion because of differing *P* values, the estimated risk ratios adjusted for extent of disease appear to be consistent across studies. Based on these results, one might be justified in concluding that perioperative blood

TABLE 19-6

Summary of Studies Examining the Perioperative Effect of Blood Transfusion in Lung Cancer

STUDY	ENDPOINT	HAZARD RATIO	95% CONFIDENCE LIMITS
Tartter et al.[55]	Survival	1.99	1.09–3.64
Hyman et al.[56]	Survival	1.25	1.04–1.49
Pena et al.[57]	Survival	1.30	0.80–2.20
Keller et al.[58]	Recurrence		
	Stage I	1.24	0.67–1.81
	Stage II	1.92	0.28–3.57
Moores et al.[59]	Survival	1.57	1.14–2.16
	Recurrence	1.40	1.01–1.94

All hazard ratios are transfused versus untransfused patients and are adjusted for extent of disease.

transfusion has a modest adverse effect on lung cancer patients.

Adjustments

Not all clinical trial statisticians agree on the need for adjusted analyses in clinical trials. However, many investigators believe that the difference in estimated treatment effects before and after adjustment often conveys useful knowledge. Furthermore, nonrandomized studies, such as cohort studies, are invariably analyzed with adjustment for confounders or prognostic factors. The same kinds of systematic errors that can arise in observational studies can arise in clinical trials by chance. This seems to provide a firm rationale for examining the results of adjusted analyses.

One of the principal advantages of using statistical models to help analyze trial results is the straightforward generalization to multiple regressions suitable for adjusted analyses. With these methods, investigators can estimate the treatment effect while adjusting for prognostic factors. One should consider adjusting for variables that meet any of three criteria:

1. Prognostic factors that are statistically significantly imbalanced between the treatment groups
2. Strong or influential prognostic factors, whether imbalanced or not
3. To prove that a particular prognostic factor does not artificially create the treatment effect

The philosophy underlying adjusting in these circumstances is to be certain that the observed treatment effect is not due to confounding. The effects of clinical interest with adjustment are changes in relative-risk parameters rather than changes in *P* values.

Regression Methods

Regression is an unfortunate historically anomalous name for a very important statistical method. A more descriptive name might be *statistical modeling of multiple effects*. In any case, the essential idea is to relate an outcome of interest to one or more predictor variables by using a statistical model. The theoretical components of the

TABLE 19-7

MODEL	VARIABLE	ODDS RATIO	95% CONFIDENCE LIMITS	P VALUE
Logistic Regression Models Illustrating Adjusted Treatment Effects				
1	B vs. A	0.368	0.19–0.71	.003
2	Male vs. female	0.542	0.29–1.01	.055
3	B vs. A	0.358	0.19–0.69	.002
	Male vs. female	0.520	0.27–0.99	.046

model are its deterministic form (structural equation), probabilistic form (how it models errors), and parameters (biologic constants), whereas the empirical components are the observed data. If the model is approximately correct, it should predict the observed data "well" provided we choose appropriate parameter values. Conversely, we can choose those parameter values that make the predictions and observations (data) "close" in some well-defined way. This latter sense is the way in which most statistical models are used. Trustworthy fitting methods exist, such as maximum likelihood, to estimate the best parameter values.

If the model has been constructed so that the parameters also correspond to clinically interesting effects, it yields a way of estimating simultaneously the influence of several factors on the outcome. In practice, models also provide a means for obtaining confidence intervals, testing hypotheses, and even revising the model itself.

Statistical models such as logistic regression for dichotomous outcomes and survival regression for event times are likely to be useful both for estimating odds and hazard ratios and performing multiple regression adjustments. Provided the assumptions of these models are met, they can provide estimates of the appropriate relative risk parameter(s), confidence limits, and P values.

I return to the hypothetical randomized clinical trial introduced in the section on estimating treatment and prognostic effects, in which sex appeared to influence response rate and survival. For response, an appropriate statistical model is the logistic regression model, the results of which are shown in Table 19-7.

Models 1 and 2 show the overall odds ratios, confidence limits, and P values for Treatment and Sex considered individually. Model 3 shows the joint effects of Sex and Treatment group on response. When the effect of Treatment is taken into account, female subjects are seen to have a higher response odds. Because the estimated odds ratios do not change very much after adjustment, this suggests that Sex and Treatment have nearly independent effects on response.

For the survival end point, the results of proportional hazards regression models are shown in Table 19-8. The estimated hazard ratios are quantitatively similar to those determined earlier and show a higher risk for male subjects. Differences are due to different methods of calculation. The effect of treatment controlling for sex is significant. The adjusted hazard ratios (model 3) also suggest independent effects for Sex and Treatment on survival time.

Special Methods

Frequently, special analyses are needed to address specific clinical questions or secondary goals of the trial. In some prognostic factor studies, special regression models may be needed, such as time–dependent covariate models, to account correctly for the effects of predictors that change over time. Other examples of situations that may require sophisticated analytic methods are repeated longitudinal measurements, bayesian methods, nonindependent observations, and accounting for restricted randomization schemes. Aside from the lack of software for many needs, extra care is required to be certain that the assumptions of the analytic methods are met.

Repeated Analyses

Although I have tried to be firm about the value of the intention-to–treat analysis, in some circumstances, one would like to know if the exclusion of some patients on the basis of clinical criteria affects the results. One such situation is the exclusion of ineligible patients in a randomized trial. Actually, exclusions based on eligibility criteria do not violate the intention-to-treat principle. However, investigators may sometimes feel the need to exclude eligible patients. One can consider repeating steps one through six after doing so. Provided the fraction of patients excluded is small, say 5%, and affects both treatment groups (if the trial is comparative), it is likely that the results will agree with the intention-to-treat analysis. This is as much an argument not to exclude patients as it is to allow exclusions.

Data Exploration

Clinicians generally need very little encouragement to conduct exploratory analyses of their data. By exploratory

TABLE 19-8

MODEL	VARIABLE	HAZARD RATIO	95% CONFIDENCE LIMITS	P VALUE
Proportional Hazards Regression Models Illustrating Adjusted Treatment Effects				
1	B vs. A	1.91	1.36–2.66	<.001
2	Male vs. female	1.32	0.95–1.82	.100
3	B vs. A	1.92	1.37–2.68	<.001
	Male vs. female	1.34	0.96–1.85	.083

analyses, I mean those that do not follow directly from the design of the experiment. Such analyses are neither automatically inappropriate nor wrong. However, the conclusions derived from these analyses can be unreliable. Therefore they should serve only to generate hypotheses to be tested more rigorously in the future. Exploratory analyses may be unreliable for the following reasons.

1. A comparison suggested by the data and not by prior hypothesis is likely to have a type I error larger than the nominal P value. This occurs because investigators have a tendency to test only those differences that are large, most of which are probably due to chance.
2. An analysis that excludes patients based on postentry criteria (responses) will likely produce biased results.
3. Subset analyses are likely to be influenced by uncontrolled prognostic factors.
4. Investigating large numbers of subsets can lead to "significant" differences purely by chance (i.e., inflated type I error).

By relying on estimation of clinical effects rather than unplanned tests of statistical hypotheses, the utility of these exploratory analyses might be increased. Investigators might be less likely to misinterpret the results or to exaggerate their clinical utility. In any case, these types of exploratory analyses should never be the primary analysis of a clinical trial.

PUBLICATION AND INTERPRETATION

As with analysis, the most informative summaries and amount of detail to report from a clinical trial will depend largely on the nature of the clinical hypotheses being studied. This section outlines basic reporting guidelines that follow an estimation and confidence-interval approach and that should be helpful for reporting many types of clinical trials. These guidelines should also be useful for reviewing and interpreting published reports of trials and prognostic factor analyses.

Reports of clinical trial results may be subject to constraints that analyses are not. For example, reports often require a consensus among investigators and must undergo an imperfect editorial process before publication. I can offer little help here in navigating these difficulties, except to suggest a certain minimal content and structure.

Describe the Study Population

Clinically relevant descriptions of both the study and target populations should be reported. It also may be important to describe patients who met the eligibility criteria but chose not to participate in the trial, when this information is available. The need for this might arise when patients from a large group are asked to participate, but many refuse. As pointed out earlier, it may be difficult to generalize from these situations. For nonrandomized designs, even detailed descriptions of the study group may not provide a convincing basis on which to make comparisons with other studies. Thus comparison is not the motivation, but thoroughness is.

Treatment and Eligibility Failures

As mentioned earlier, it is acceptable to perform statistical analyses on only the subset of eligible patients, even when eligibility is corrected in retrospect. This does not create bias in the estimate of relative effects within the trial. Investigators should report those patients who were retrospectively found to have failed the eligibility criteria as well as those patients who failed to complete the assigned treatment.

In some situations, a large fraction of patients complete the assigned therapy but may receive additional therapy not specified by the protocol or design of the trial. For example, patients with esophageal cancer may undergo resection and chemotherapy and have a variety of second-line treatments if signs of disease progression or recurrence are observed. If some of these latter treatments are active, the results of an initial treatment comparison based on recurrence or survival may be skewed. In general, it is difficult or impossible to use the statistical information in studies that permit "crossovers" either to new treatments or to the other treatment arm.

TEN CONCEPTS IN REPORTING

1. Report all clinically relevant descriptions of the trial population including patients who met the eligibility criteria but chose not to participate.
2. Describe those patients who were retrospectively found to have failed the eligibility criteria and those patients who failed to complete the assigned treatment.
3. Report all statistical methods and assumptions made.
4. For univariate analyses, report estimated treatment effects (log-odds ratios or hazard ratios), confidence intervals, and significance levels of tests of no treatment effect (P values).
5. Report adjusted estimates of treatment effects, confidence intervals, and P values.
6. When no treatment effect is found, do not report the power of the study. Instead use point estimates and confidence limits.
7. Report any differences between "intention-to-treat" analyses and "eligible patient" analyses.
8. Results with strong biologic or clinical justification and P values near .05 could be called "statistically significant."
9. Results without biologic or clinical backup or those that seem contradictory should be reported but interpreted with caution.
10. Represent exploratory or hypothesis-generating analyses accurately.

One cannot exclude these patients but can use only the information up to the time of stopping the assigned treatment.

Statistical Methods and Assumptions

Readers should be made aware of any assumptions made in both the design and analysis of a clinical trial. For a discussion of some practical issues, see DerSimonian and associates.[33] The assumptions and limitations of many common statistical procedures are well understood by clinicians. However, the readers of clinical trial reports should be convinced that the data analyst has verified all important assumptions and reported the methods in detail for less well known statistical procedures. Examples of assumptions that are often made in analysis, often violated by the data, and also likely to be consequential are distributional assumptions underlying the t test or other statistical hypothesis tests, error distributions in linear regression analyses, and proportionality of hazards in life-table regressions.

For example, the t test assumes that the distributions being compared are normal with equal variances. It can yield incorrect results when either of these assumptions is false, particularly if distributions are not symmetric. Proportional hazards regression models most often assume that the effects of predictors is to multiply a baseline risk and that the multiplicative factor is constant over time. Although the model is robust to departures from this assumption (i.e., it will often yield the correct estimates of relative risk and significance levels anyway), it is helpful to validate the assumptions.

Univariate Analyses

It is likely that the data analyst will test the effect of all potentially important prognostic variables on the major outcomes. For these univariate analyses, investigators should report estimated treatment effects (odds ratios or hazard ratios), confidence intervals, and significance levels of tests of no treatment effect (P values). This does not preclude presenting other displays of univariate analyses (e.g., survival curves or 2×2 tables) if these analyses are especially relevant. However, the investigators should keep in mind that univariate analyses, particularly in uncontrolled studies, are subject to confounding. Consequently, these analyses should probably not be emphasized or presented in excessive detail.

Adjusted Analyses

In a randomized trial, the univariate comparison of treatment groups is a simple and valid summary. However, many investigators attempt to show that the treatment effect is not due to any measured confounders by using adjusted analyses. The best style of reporting multivariate analyses is the same as or similar to that for univariate effects. However, the adjusted analyses reported are usually selected from a larger set of less informative or preliminary results. As an example, consider a life-table regression model attempting to predict time to cancer recurrence. The "best" (most predictive but parsimonious) model might be built by using a step-down procedure from a large set of potential prognostic factors. Each step in the analysis need not be reported, but the final model is a major objective of the analysis.

For multiple regression analyses, investigators usually report adjusted estimates of treatment effects, confidence intervals, and P values. Not all prognostic factors retained in multiple regression models must be "statistically significant." It is often useful to keep nonsignificant effects in a multiple regression model to demonstrate convincingly that the treatment effect persists in their presence.

Negative Findings

When no statistically significant treatment effect or difference is found, the power of the study is sometimes called into question. However, the absence of a significant difference is not the same as evidence of no effect. Because clinical effects are measured by risk ratios rather than P values, guidelines given earlier emphasizing estimated treatment differences rather than hypothesis tests are important. Helpful advice regarding negative clinical trials is provided by Detsky and Sackett.[68] Power calculations performed after the study is completed are rarely, if ever, helpful.

The Effect of Patient Exclusions

Although I have emphasized the value of the intent-to-treat principle and related analyses, in practice, many exploratory analyses will be done. Investigators should report any differences between "intention-to-treat" analyses and "eligible patient" analyses. If subset analyses are performed, discrepancies between these and the major analyses of the clinical trial should be reported.

What Is Significant?

The P value should not be the only criterion for "significance." Results with strong biologic or clinical justification and P values near .05 are "statistically significant." When biologic justification is strong, effect estimates are large, and confidence intervals or P values indicate significance near conventional levels, it seems appropriate to label these results "statistically significant." Conversely, results with no biologic or clinical justification or those that seem paradoxical should be reported and interpreted with caution, even when P values are smaller than .05. No way exists to separate type I errors from truly significant results, except to rely on additional evidence and biologic rationale. It is wise to report cautiously results that seem not to make sense.

Exploratory Analyses

Exploratory or hypothesis-generating analyses should be only informally reported. They should not be emphasized as the primary findings of a clinical trial unless supported by the design and a priori hypothesis.

SUMMARY AND CONCLUSIONS

In developing new cancer treatments, investigators are often interested in treatment effects and differences that are about the same size as the variability or the bias that is a part of all clinical studies. The only solution for making valid inferences in the face of these potential errors is to design, conduct, and analyze clinical trials properly. A small number of important design considerations help control bias and random errors, including the use of randomization, blinding, stratification, minimizing postentry exclusions, adequate sample size, and planned interim monitoring.

Clinical trials have limitations, partly because of the rigor required to implement them. Investigators contemplating the use of these important scientific tools should focus most efforts on the design aspects of the study and concern themselves little with analysis. This is because most of the serious errors that can be made when performing clinical trials can be prevented or minimized by correct design. In this regard, consultation with an experienced clinical trial methodologist early in the design stage of an investigation will be of enormous benefit.

When analyzing and reporting the results of clinical trials, investigators should follow a simple approach. The purpose of a trial is to estimate an effect or treatment difference that if present would have clinical utility when treating new patients. Procedures or methods that do not facilitate estimating and reporting the treatment effect with precision and without bias are likely to mislead investigators. Often in clinical trials, investigators are interested in estimates of odds or hazard ratios between treatment groups.

These ideas suggest that the most useful results from clinical trials will be estimated risk ratios and their confidence limits. Especially in oncology studies, in which disease progression, recurrence, and death are of interest, estimates of risk difference are very relevant. Hypothesis tests and associated P values, although often (or exclusively) reported, are of lesser utility because they do not fully summarize the data. These recommendations are similar to those in many journals.

Despite some technical disagreement among statisticians regarding the need for adjusted analyses for imbalanced prognostic factors, I believe that it is wise to see if treatment effects change after accounting for imbalances. When this occurs, it seems likely that it will be of clinical interest. Although I discourage analyses that exclude any patients who meet the eligibility criteria, some circumstances will require that this be done (e.g., when a patient refuses to participate after randomization). Investigators should report, and emphasize as primary, those analyses that include all eligible patients.

REFERENCES

1. Bull JP: The historical development of clinical therapeutic trials. J Chronic Dis 1959;10:218-248.
2. Office of Technology Assessment, US Congress. The Impact of Randomized Clinical Trials on Health Policy and Medical Practice: Background Paper. Washington, DC, U.S. Government Printing Office, OTA-BP-H-22, 1983.
3. Meinert CL: Clinical Trials. Oxford, Oxford University Press, 1986.
4. Silverman WA: Human Experimentation: A Guided Step into the Unknown. Oxford, University Press, 1985.
5. Shapiro SH, Louis TA: Clinical Trials: Issues and Approaches. New York, Marcel Dekker, 1983.
6. Pocock SJ: Clinical Trials: A Practical Approach. New York, John Wiley, 1996.
7. Buyse ME, Staquet MJ, Sylvester RJ (eds): Cancer Clinical Trials. Methods and Practice. Oxford, Oxford University Press, 1984.
8. Leventhal BG, Wittes RE: Research Methods in Clinical Oncology. New York, Raven Press, 1988.
9. Freidman LM, Furberg CD, DeMets DL: Fundamentals of Clinical Trials. Boston, John Wright, 1981.
10. Armitage P: The design of clinical trials. Aust J Stat 1979;21:266-281.
11. Louis TA, Mosteller F, McPeek B: Timely topics in statistical methods for clinical trials. Annu Rev Biophys Bioeng 1982;11:81-104.
12. Lewis JA: Clinical trials: Statistical developments of practical benefit to the pharmaceutical industry (with discussion). J R Stat Soc A 1983;146:362-393.
13. Piantadosi S: Clinical Trials: A Methodologic Perspective. New York, John Wiley and Sons, 1997.
14. Piantadosi S: Principles of clinical trial design. Semin Oncol 1988;15:423-433.
15. Peto R, Pike MC, Armitage P, et al: Design and analysis of randomized clinical trials requiring prolonged observation of each patient, I: Introduction and design. Br J Cancer 1976;34:585-612.
16. Peto R, Pike MC, Armitage P, et al: Design and analysis of randomized clinical trials requiring prolonged observations of each patient, II: Analysis and examples. Br J Cancer 1977;35:1-39.
17. Byar DP, Simon RM, Friedewald WT, et al: Randomized clinical trials: Perspectives on some recent ideas. N Engl J Med 1976;295:74-80.
18. Piantadosi S, Saijo N, Tamura T: Basic design considerations for clinical trials in oncology. Jpn J Cancer Res 1992;83:547-558.
19. Armitage P, Berry G: The Design of Experiments. In: Statistical Methods in Medical Research, 3rd ed., Oxford, Blackwell, 1987, pp 172-175.
20. Simon RM: Design and Conduct of Clinical Trials. In DeVita VT Jr, Hellman S, Rosenberg SA, (eds): Cancer, 6th ed. Baltimore, Md., Lippincott Williams & Wilkins, 2001, pp 521-538.
21. Green SB: Randomized clinical trials: design and analysis. Semin Oncol 1981;8:417-423.
22. Taves DR: A new method of assigning patients to treatment and control groups. Clin Pharmacol Ther 1974;15:443-453.
23. Schafer A: The ethics of the randomized clinical trial. N Engl J Med 1977;307:719-724.
24. Burkhardt R, Kienle G: Basic problems in controlled trials. J Med Ethics 1983;9:80-84.
25. Vere DW: Problems in controlled trials: A critical response. J Med Ethics 1983;9:85-89.
26. Byar DP: Identification of prognostic factors. In Buyse ME, Staquet MJ, Sylvester RJ (eds): Cancer Clinical Trials: Methods and Practice. Oxford, Oxford University Press, 1984, pp 210-222.
27. George SL: Identification and assessment of prognostic factors. Semin Oncol 1988;15:462-471.
28. International Committee of Medical Journal Editors. Uniform requirements for manuscripts submitted to biomedical journals. Ann Intern Med 1988;108:258-265.
29. Bailar J, Mosteller F: Guidelines for statistical reporting for medical journals: Amplifications and explanations. Ann Intern Med 1988;108:266-273.
30. Altman D, Gore S, Gardner M, Pocock S: Statistical guidelines for contributors to medical journals. Br Med J 1983;286:1489-1493.
31. Mosteller F, Gilbert J, McPeek B: Reporting standards and research strategies for controlled clinical trials; Agenda for the editor. Cont Clin Trials 1980;1:37-58.
32. Berry G: Statistical guide-lines and statistical guidance. Med J Aust 1987;146:408-409.
33. DerSimonian R, Charette IJ, McPeek B, Mosteller F: Reporting on methods in clinical trials. N Engl J Med 1982;306:1332-1337.
34. Sackett DL: Bias in analytic research. J Chronic Dis 1979;32:51-63.

35. Chalmers TC: The control of bias in clinical trials. In Shapiro SH, Louis TA (eds): Clinical Trials: Issues and Approaches. New York, Marcel Dekker, 1983, pp 115-127.

36. Byar DP: Why data bases should not replace randomized clinical trials. Biometrics 1980;36:337-342.

37. Petitti D: Meta-Analysis, Decision Analysis, and Cost-Effectiveness Analysis. Oxford, Oxford University Press, 1994.

38. O'Quigley J, Chevret S: Methods for dose finding studies in cancer clinical trials: A review and results of a Monte Carlo study. Stat Med 1991;10:1647-1664.

39. Goodman S, Zahurak M, Piantadosi S: Some practical improvements in the continual reassessment method for phase I studies. Stat Med 1995;14:1149-1161.

40. Simon R: Optimal two-stage designs for phase II clinical trials. Control Clin Trials 1989;10:1-10.

41. Royall R: Ethics and statistics in randomized clinical trials. Stat Sci 1991;6:52-88.

42. Donner A: Approaches to sample size estimation in the design of clinical trials: A review. Stat Med 1984;3:199-214.

43. Freedman L: Tables of the number of patients required in clinical trials using the log-rank test. Stat Med 1982;1:121-129.

44. Anscombe FJ: Sequential medical trials. J Am Stat Assoc 1963;58:365-383.

45. Armitage P, McPherson CK, Rowe BC: Repeated significance tests on accumulating data. J R Stat Soc A 1969;132:235-244.

46. Pocock SJ: Group sequential methods in the design and analysis of clinical trials. Biometrika 1977;64:191-199.

47. O'Brien PC, Fleming TR: A multiple testing procedure for clinical trials. Biometrics 1979;35:549-556.

48. Hughes MD, Pocock SJ: Stopping rules and estimation problems in clinical trials. Stat Med 1988;7:1231-1242.

49. Berry DA: Interim analyses in clinical trials: Classical versus Bayesian approaches. Stat Med 1985;4:521-526.

50. Gail MH: Monitoring and stopping clinical trials. In Mike V, Stanley KE (eds): Statistics in Medical Research. New York, Wiley, 1982.

51. O'Fallon JR: Policies for interim analysis and interim reporting of results. Cancer Treat Rep 1985;69:1101-1106.

52. DeMets DL: Practical aspects in data monitoring: A brief review. Stat Med 1987;6:753-760.

53. Lan KKG, Simon R, Halperin M: Stochastically curtailed tests in long-term clinical trials. Comm Stat Cl 1982;1:207-219.

54. Piantadosi S: The adverse effect of blood transfusion in lung cancer [editorial]. Chest 1992;102:6-8.

55. Tartter PI, Burrows L, Kirschner P: Perioperative blood transfusion adversely affects prognosis after resection of stage I (subset N0) non-oat cell lung cancer. J Thorac Cardvasc Surg, 1984;88:659-662.

56. Hyman NH, Foster RS, DeMeules JE, Costanza MC: Blood transfusions and survival after lung cancer resection. Am J Surg 1985;149:502-507.

57. Pena CM, Rice TW, Ahmad M, Medendorp SV: The significance of perioperative blood transfusions in patients undergoing resection of stage I and II non-small cell lung cancers. Chest 1992;102:84-88.

58. Keller SM, Groshen S, Martini N, Kaiser LR: Blood transfusion and lung cancer recurrence. Cancer 1988;62:606-610.

59. Moores DWO, Piantadosi S, McKneally MF: Effect of perioperative blood transfusion on outcome in patients with surgically resected lung cancer. Ann Thorac Surg 1989;47:346-351.

60. Piantadosi S: The adverse effect of blood transfusion in lung cancer (editorial). Chest 1992;102:6-8.

61. Berry G, Statistical significance and confidence intervals. Med J Aust 1986;144:618-619.

62. Simon R: Confidence intervals for reporting results of clinical trials. Ann Intern Med 1986;105:429-435.

63. Gardner MJ, Altman DG: Confidence intervals rather than P values: Estimation rather than hypothesis testing. Br Med J 1986;292:746-750.

64. Braitman L: Confidence intervals extract clinically useful information from data. Ann Intern Med 1988;108:296-298.

65. Berger J: Are p-values reasonable measures of accuracy? In Francis BI, Manly Lam FC (eds): Pacific Stat. Congress. North Holland, Elsevier, 1986.

66. Berger J, Sellke T: Testing a point null hypothesis: The irreconcilability of p-values and evidence. J Am Stat Assoc 1987;82:112-139.

67. Rothman K: Significance questing. Ann Intern Med 1986;105:445-447.

68. Detsky AS, Sackett DL: When was a "negative" clinical trial big enough? Arch Intern Med 1986;145:709.

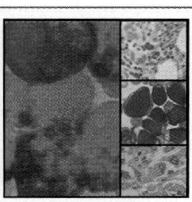

20

STRUCTURES SUPPORTING CANCER CLINICAL TRIALS

Michaele C. Christian

Jeffrey S. Abrams

David Ross Parkinson

SUMMARY OF KEY POINTS

- Cancer clinical trials provide the evidence on which sound oncology practice is based.
- Fewer than 5% of adult cancer patients participate in cancer clinical trials.
- Providing greater access to clinical trials has been a major goal of the National Cancer Institute, cancer centers, and patient advocacy groups.
- There are now many opportunities for physicians in private practice to participate in clinical trials sponsored by the National Cancer Institute and/or the biopharmaceutical industry.
- Critical components for successful participation in clinical trials include:

- The attitude and commitment of the physician.
- Sufficient preparation and infrastructure.
- Trained staff, including at least some of the following:
  - Clinical research nurse
  - Clinical research associate
  - Pharmacist
- Affiliation with an institution or network that provides the protocol and scientific and administrative support, such as:
  - Cooperative Group
  - Cancer Trials Support Unit
  - Cancer center network
  - Biopharmaceutical industry network
  - Research institution

- Access to an authorized Institutional Review Board.
- Access to adequate laboratory facilities to process protocol-required specimens.
- Adherence to good clinical practices.
- Accurate and timely data reporting:
  - Proper maintenance of primary source documentation.
  - Adequate preparation for on-site audits.
- There are now many organizations that provide access to clinical trials and/or provide the necessary training and certification; relevant Web sites are included in this chapter.

INTRODUCTION

Sound modern oncology practice is founded on the results from thousands of clinical trials conducted over the last four decades; thousands more clinical trials are ongoing at any given time and provide the evidence base for the rapidly changing therapeutic practices of this specialty. Motivations for the decision by an oncologist to participate actively in this extensive system of medical and scientific inquiry range from the ability to offer patients state-of-the-art treatments available through well-designed clinical trials, to the personal satisfaction and benefits achieved from participation in this process. The commitment of time and resources necessary to participate effectively in such clinical research, however— and, sometimes, unfamiliarity with the requirements and procedures—prevents many oncologists from taking part. It has been estimated that only 3%–5% of adult cancer patients in the United States are treated in clinical trials, with even lower rates of participation in many other countries. The lack of patient participation has been due in part to inadequate understanding of the clinical trials process. Fortunately—due to intense publicity and educational programs by both patient advocacy groups and clinical trials organizations and widespread access to clinical trials information on the Internet—a growing number of patients now expect that available clinical trials

will be included in the discussion of options for the treatment of their cancers. The purpose of this chapter is to describe some of the requirements, resources, and structures that are available to enable practicing oncologists to participate in clinical trials, and to discuss the responsibilities that come with such participation. Numerous opportunities now exist for practicing physicians and their patients to participate in cancer clinical trials, including treatment, prevention, and cancer control trials, whether conducted by the National Cancer Institute (NCI), cancer treatment institutions, or the biopharmaceutical industry. Widespread access to the Internet has revolutionized communication and made it possible to provide regulatory information, educational and training materials, data forms, and documents online. A wide array of structures and resources are now available to assist physicians and their staffs in placing their patients in clinical trials.

NATIONAL CANCER INSTITUTE-SPONSORED CLINICAL TRIALS ACTIVITIES

The National Cancer Institute (NCI) supports the development of nearly 150 agents (many in collaboration with pharmaceutical and biotechnology companies) and has an extensive clinical trials system that encompasses

USEFUL WEB SITES FOR CLINICAL TRIALS RESOURCES AND INFORMATION

Cancer.gov	http://cancer.gov/
Cancer Trials Support Unit (including links to cooperative groups)	http://www.ctsu.org
Cancer Therapy Evaluation Program (CTEP)	http://ctep.info.nih.gov/
Community Clinical Oncology Program (CCOP)	http://www3.cancer.gov/prevention/ccop/
Cancer Centers Program	http://www3.cancer.gov/cancercenters
Central IRB	http://www.ncicirb.org/
Physician's Data Query (PDQ)	http://cancer.gov/cancerinfo/pdq/

treatment, prevention, and control studies. More than 800 trials are active at a given time, and several hundred new trials open each year. In the treatment area, the NCI has programs for early therapeutics development (primarily phase I and II trials), including many sites with grants and contracts to complete these early trials. The NCI also supports a large program of clinical trials Cooperative Groups that conduct later trials, predominantly pilot studies and phase III trials. Phase III trials are conducted nationally, and participation in them is now possible even for oncology physicians who are not Cooperative Group members. Clinical Trials Cooperative Groups funded by the NCI (Table 20-1) provide a standing mechanism for performing large-scale multicenter treatment and prevention trials. Over the years, this system has supported an experienced cadre of clinical researchers, biostatisticians, and research support staff who can respond to new clinical discoveries by organizing definitive phase III clinical trials. Because of their size and complexity, these trials require extensive infrastructure support to manage the necessary regulatory and data reporting tasks. Although these Cooperative Group trials have provided a significant proportion of the evidence on which oncology practice is based, public advocacy for more rapid progress, increasing fiscal pressures on medical practice, and the accelerated pace of drug discovery caused the NCI to review and restructure aspects of its clinical trials program in 1998. One of the major goals of the restructuring was to increase access to NCI trials for patients and their physicians and to eliminate barriers to participation in clinical trials.

From the mid-1980s to the mid-1990s, accrual to Cooperative Group treatment trials reached a plateau at about 20,000 patients annually. Whereas the pediatric Groups consistently enrolled about 70% of all cancer patients, the adult Groups were only able to accrue fewer than 2% of all cases. Phase III trials in the adult Groups took an average of 4.5 years to enroll patients and an additional three to four years of follow-up before a result was known. This approximately eight-year cycle before potential treatment advances could be confirmed was clearly too long. It became imperative, therefore, to enable more rapid accrual to clinical trials.

Surveys among physicians and the public found that the obstacles to accrual in adult oncology were multifactorial (Table 20-2).[1-5] With these barriers in mind, the NCI undertook an extensive review of the clinical trials system, involving a wide range of stakeholders that included Cooperative Group and cancer center leaders, patient advocates, and government staff. The detailed reports of these reviews are available online (http://ctep.cancer.gov/forms/ArmitageReport.pdf). Several pilot projects aimed at modernizing the clinical trials regulatory and data collection systems, opening access to trials to more patients and investigators, and simplifying the role of local institutional review boards in multi-institutional clinical trials, are ongoing. New opportunities have been created for community physicians to participate in a broad array of clinical trials, and new tools have been created to enable this. Two major initiatives—the Cancer Trials Support Unit and the Central Institutional Review Board— are now becoming integral parts of NCI's clinical trials system and are described next.[6]

Cancer Trials Support Unit

The Cancer Trials Support Unit (CTSU) is designed to facilitate one-stop online access to a broad menu of predominantly phase III trials by a national network of NCI investigators. The network investigators include not only members of Cooperative Groups but also physicians in practice with no prior Group affiliation. They can access the CTSU menu of treatment trials from the public website (www.ctsu.org). The menu consists primarily of Cooperative Group phase III trials, although selected internationally-led phase III trials, Cooperative Group phase II trials, and some trials led by U.S. cancer centers are also available. The scientific leadership for each study remains within the organization that developed the trial

TABLE 20-1

Barriers to Clinical Trial Participation

PHYSICIAN RELATED	PATIENT RELATED
• Inadequate funding for data management personnel	• Doctor never discussed or offered
• Burdensome regulatory requirements	• Unaware of trials as option
Institutional Review Board	• Concerns about insurance coverage
Informed consent	• Fear of receiving placebo
Conflict of interest	
• Inadequate reimbursement	
• Lack of time	
• Resistance by third-party payers	

TABLE 20-2

NCI Funded Cooperative Groups and Web Site URLS

American College of Radiology Imaging Network (ACRIN)	http://www.acrin.org/
American College of Surgeons Oncology Group (ACOSOG)	http://www.acosog.org/
Cancer and Leukemia Group B (CALGB)	http://www.calgb.org/
Children's Oncology Group (COG)	http://www.childrensoncologygroup.org
Eastern Cooperative Oncology Group (ECOG)	http://www.ecog.org/
European Organization for Research and Treatment of Cancer (EORTC)	http://www.eortc.be/default.htm
Gynecologic Oncology Group (GOG)	http://www.gog.org/
National Cancer Institute of Canada Clinical Trials Group (NCIC-CTG)	http://www.ctg.queensu.ca/
North Central Cancer Treatment Group (NCCTG)	http://ncctg.mayo.edu/
National Surgical Adjuvant Breast and Bowel Project (NSABP)	http://www.nsabp.pitt.edu/
Radiation Therapy Oncology Group (RTOG)	http://www.rtog.org/
Southwest Oncology Group (SWOG)	http://www.swog.org/

(as will be described shortly), but patient enrollments can come from any network physician across the country. By providing more physicians and their patients the opportunity to choose from a broader menu of trials, the CTSU promotes faster accrual to individual trials, allows increased access and broader treatment options to more patients nationwide, and renders trials in uncommon cancers more feasible.

Although the clinical trials menu is the most visible aspect of the CTSU, another major function of the CTSU is its centralized regulatory database. For all Cooperative Group members and nonmember physicians in the network, the CTSU maintains important demographic information about their sites or practices, including Cooperative Group(s) and academic/practice affiliation(s), Office for Human Research Protection (OHRP) assurance numbers for their sites, Institutional Review Board approvals for specific protocols, and Conflict of Interest forms for investigators. This enables physicians, nurses, and clinical research associates to register once annually, instead of having to do this for each Group or trial in which they participate. Initiated in 2002, the Regulatory Support System requires that investigators complete a 1572 investigational drug form once yearly, along with a supplemental information form and a conflict of interest form.[7] Nurses and clinical research associates (CRAs) who participate in Group trials also register once annually online (registration available at https://iapps-ctep.nci.nih.gov/ctepar/main.html?Reset). Information from this registration database is accessible to all Cooperative Groups, as the CTSU Web-based system is shared and maintained in a coordinated manner with all the Cooperative Group operations offices. Centralizing regulatory data has reduced the workload for investigators in the field, consolidated duplicative work, and allowed Cooperative Group staff to partially offload this activity to the CTSU and focus instead on protocol development and analysis.

CTSU Trial Services

The CTSU maintains a public Web site that provides patients with information about all the clinical trials on the menu. The site links trials to participating physicians in a patient's local area and also provides links to medical insurance plans so that patients can verify whether the physician belongs to their insurance plan.

The widespread availability of Internet access in physician offices has made it possible for the CTSU to make the necessary documents, forms, and tools readily available. For physicians and their staffs, a password-protected members site contains the information needed to enroll a patient in one of the trials on the menu. Online access is provided to the protocol, case report forms, adverse event reporting forms, NCI pharmacy forms, site registration documents, patient enrollment documents, and education and training materials. Informed consent documents with Spanish and French translations are also available. In addition, detailed Institutional Review Board (IRB) application packets can be downloaded to make the process of obtaining local IRB approval much less time consuming.

Regardless of which organization is leading a protocol on the CTSU menu, the CTSU will manage site registration, protocol eligibility checks, and treatment randomization, obviating the need to interact with multiple different Cooperative Groups to treat patients on a variety of different protocols. Local site registrars can verify online that their site has successfully completed all the registration requirements for a specific protocol. In addition to the documents needed to conduct the study, the CTSU provides abstracted Time and Events Calendars and Protocol Schemas to assist medical staff with protocol adherence, a PowerPoint slide presentation to help physicians promote the trial, and patient education materials that provide information about both clinical trials in general and the specific trial under consideration. Physicians can also obtain quarterly accrual reports by study and by site and can order copies of investigator brochures when trials involve experimental drugs.

Data collection has been standardized on CTSU trials across all different Cooperative Groups and across diseases, to the extent possible, to facilitate ease of reporting, data sharing, and exchange. This has been possible because of the development of Common Data Elements (CDEs) through a project that NCI began several years ago in collaboration with the Cooperative Groups. For each disease, there now exists a set of commonly defined terms and values that are used to report information in a uniform manner. CDEs have now been developed for all the diseases treated in phase III studies by the adult Groups and are currently being developed for pediatric and phase I and II trials. Currently, data collection is done using paper case report forms. A pilot program is underway at selected sites, however, to utilize an electronic remote data capture system. The common CDE vocabulary system has made rapid development of electronic case report forms more feasible. If this pilot proves successful, electronic data reporting will be made available to all Groups and to the CTSU network in the future. Electronic data reporting should improve speed and data accuracy by providing real-time data queries when data are initially submitted, thereby reducing time-consuming follow-up queries weeks to months later when patient information might be less readily retrievable.

The CTSU handles all questions from the sites at the CTSU Help Desk (1-888-823-5923) and contacts the study principal investigator and reports back to the site when questions require medical expertise. Once again, this one-stop approach is designed to save time for the sites. The CTSU attempts to add value to the process by tracking questions and providing a Frequently Asked Questions (FAQs) section on the Web site.

Two additional tasks, auditing and research reimbursement, are also managed by the CTSU. Trials performed via the CTSU are audited in a fashion similar to other Cooperative Group trials (see the audit section) to verify data accuracy and quality by comparing the primary record with the research forms submitted by the site. Given that sites may now participate in trials led by multiple Groups, the CTSU patient charts are simply added to a scheduled audit when a Group is visiting a member site, to avoid burdening sites with multiple Cooperative Group audits. Depending on the number of CTSU accruals at a site, the audit team is sometimes supplemented with members from other Groups or CTSU staff to ensure sufficient expertise. Similarly, existing contractual relationships between Groups and their members have been used by the CTSU to forward payments to Group members who have participated in trials via the CTSU. Physicians who are not Group members are supported via direct contracts and are paid by the CTSU directly.

CTSU and Cooperative Group Interactions

The introduction of the CTSU is the first major structural change to NCI's multicenter trials system since its inception more than 50 years ago. Despite early growing pains, the CTSU is assuming a major role as a support structure that complements the work of the Cooperative Groups. The CTSU is not a scientific structure and does not develop or analyze the studies it supports. Rather, all the data it receives are passed on to the Group leading the trial for analysis. By reducing the duplicative administrative work that was done traditionally at each Group Operations Office, and by offering more clinical trials to each Group member, the CTSU allows the Groups to focus on their prime missions—developing important clinical trial questions and analyzing these trials rigorously.

CENTRAL INSTITUTIONAL REVIEW BOARD

Background

In NCI multicenter trials, the identical protocol is carried out at many sites, averaging about 100 (range 4–809), with each site requiring its own local institutional review board (LIRB) to conduct an initial full-board review and subsequent annual reviews, adverse event reviews, and amendment reviews. These multiple IRB reviews create a largely redundant, time-consuming workload at these sites, compounding the ever-mounting pressures on the nation's IRB system, which have been well documented.[8] To provide an idea of the scope of the duplicative effort that occurs, NCI has more than 10,000 registered investigators at more than 3000 sites. On average, there are 160 ongoing phase III trials and 30 new trials entering the NCI system annually, resulting in approximately 16,000 IRB reviews (3000 initial reviews) conducted each year.[9] In addition, investigators often mention that the amount of time, paperwork, and (more recently) funding required of them to obtain IRB approval is a serious barrier to opening trials. These factors provided the impetus for the NCI to develop a new, centralized approach to human subjects protection for its large, phase III trials program.

Customarily, central institutional review boards (CIRB) models were instituted when LIRBs were lacking. In these cases, for-profit central IRBs contract their services to institutions without IRBs and maintain close contact with the sites by sending staff for frequent visits, thereby fulfilling the OHRP requirement that the IRB of record have knowledge of the local context. By contrast, LIRBs exist throughout the NCI system, and this fact led NCI to use a model in which responsibility is shared between the CIRB and LIRB. The CIRB provides the initial full-board review and then transmits its decision and detailed minutes of the meeting to the LIRB participants via a confidential Web site. These sites have the option to perform a facilitated review, whereby a LIRB Chair (or a designated subcommittee) can review the CIRB documents rapidly, determine whether or not there are local issues that should be addressed, and then expeditiously approve the protocol, without the need for a full board review at the local level. If facilitated review is accepted by the local site, then the CIRB becomes the IRB of record for that protocol. This means that the CIRB will perform the continuing annual reviews, adverse event reviews from all sites participating in the trial, and the amendment reviews. This process relieves the LIRB of the burden of review for these multicenter trials, but the LIRB still has the responsibility to review adverse events that occur at the local site (but can now view them in the context of the overall adverse event review provided by the CIRB). The LIRB also retains responsibility for the medical and ethical conduct of the investigators and their staffs at their institution. To formalize this division of responsibility, a written agreement is signed by the LIRB when they join the CIRB Initiative (available at http://www.ncicirb.org).

NCI's CIRB is composed of a distinguished panel of oncology physicians, nurses, and patient representatives and includes a pharmacist, an ethicist, and a lawyer. The CIRB reviews all phase III studies from the Adult Cooperative Groups, as well as any phase III trials opened in the CTSU. Unlike most LIRBs, the CIRB is focused exclusively on cancer trials and has sufficient time and expertise to review each protocol in detail. In addition, compared with LIRBs, the CIRB by design has more leverage to request changes in the protocol and informed consent, as NCI requires that studies obtain CIRB approval before they can open.

More experience is needed to gauge the effectiveness of this new model for human subjects protection in multicenter trials. A major goal will be a significant reduction in review workload for LIRBs while still preserving their role as the primary overseers of the actual conduct of the research at the local site. Patients and investigators should benefit from the ability to open trials rapidly using this mechanism and from the likely greater availability of trials that results.

OTHER NCI-SPONSORED STRUCTURES SUPPORTING CLINICAL TRIALS

Although the CTSU and the CIRB represent new mechanisms to reduce barriers and facilitate broader clinical trials participation by practicing oncologists, there are a number of other important mechanisms that provide additional options for support and participation (Fig. 20-1).

Clinical Trials Cooperative Groups

For physicians who wish to be more actively involved in the intellectual and scientific aspects of clinical trials, and who can commit to accruing at least 5–10 patients per year to Group studies, actually joining a Cooperative Group should be a strong consideration. Most Groups have an affiliate program that allows community sites to partner or affiliate with a main member who assumes a number of the management and monitoring responsibilities for the affiliate. Procedures for joining can be found on the Groups' Web sites (see Table 20-2). Affiliate members attend the semi-annual meetings of the Groups and are actively involved in the scientific agenda, protocol development, and publications of the Group. In addition to intellectual satisfaction, career development, and networking opportunities, members have access to a broader array of clinical trials for their patients, including phase I, II, and pilot trials that are not available on the CTSU menu and which, therefore, are not accessible to nonmembers. Cooperative Groups also provide training and networking opportunities for research staff, including research nurses and CRAs, at Group meetings and in other venues.

Community Clinical Oncology Program

For practices or groups or networks of practices that already have research experience, and that can commit to enrolling significant numbers of patients in clinical trials, NCI grant funding through the Community Clinical Oncology Program (CCOP) mechanism offers many opportunities. CCOPs must document the ability to enroll 50 patients in cancer treatment studies plus 50–75 patients in prevention studies and/or trials focused on symptom management and cancer control. The grants provide important up-front funding to enable sites to hire critical staff from the start to support the substantial patient accrual that is required. In addition, special Minority-based CCOPs (MB-CCOPs) are funded and

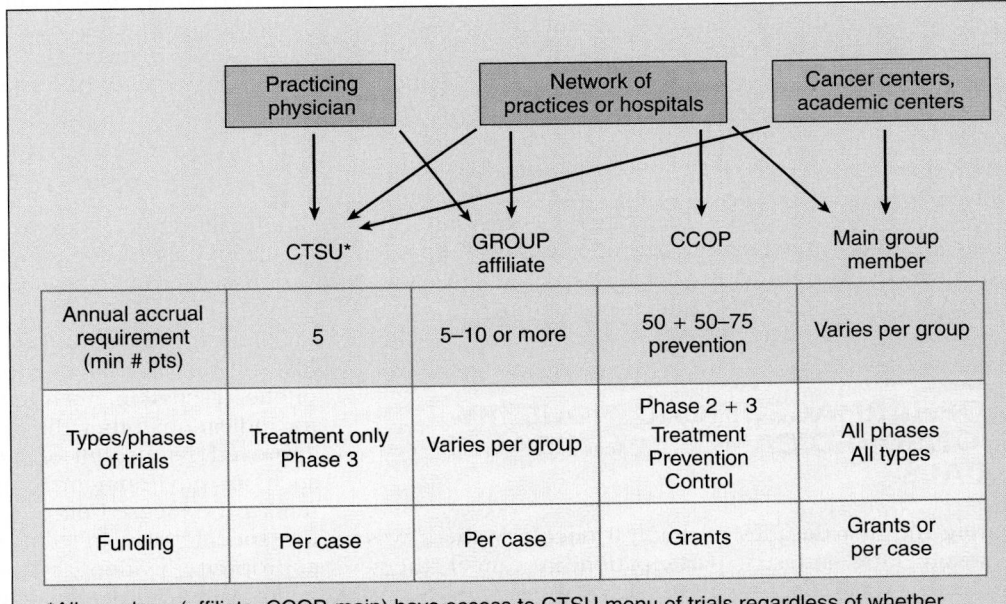

Figure 20-1. Mechanisms for participating in NCI-sponsored clinical trials.

	CTSU*	GROUP affiliate	CCOP	Main group member
Annual accrual requirement (min # pts)	5	5–10 or more	50 + 50–75 prevention	Varies per group
Types/phases of trials	Treatment only Phase 3	Varies per group	Phase 2 + 3 Treatment Prevention Control	All phases All types
Funding	Per case	Per case	Grants	Grants or per case

*All members (affiliate, CCOP, main) have access to CTSU menu of trials regardless of whether they are members of the group leading the trial.

Science of Clinical Oncology

provide additional support for groups or networks that serve predominantly minority populations. MB-CCOPs strive to increase cancer prevention and control activities in minority and under-served communities in addition to increasing access to clinical trials for minority patients. The CCOP program, funded by the NCI's Division of Cancer Prevention (DCP), has been in existence since 1983 and now funds 61 research sites in 34 states. Details regarding these programs can be found on the DCP Web site (http://www3.cancer.gov/prevention/ccop/).

Children's Oncology Group

Tremendous strides have been made over the past 50 years in the treatment of childhood cancers, transforming a once-fatal disease of children into a highly curable one. This success has been due in large part to the participation of large numbers of children with cancer in clinical trials. It is estimated that some 70% of children diagnosed are entered into clinical trials, and this has been a key factor in the rapid progress that has been made. In March 2000, four NCI-sponsored pediatric groups—the Children's Cancer Group (CCG), the Pediatric Oncology Group (POG), the Intergroup Rhabdomyosarcoma Study Group (IRSG), and the National Wilms' Study Group (NWTSG) B agreed to consolidate their efforts and formed the Children's Oncology Group (COG). COG has more than 230 member institutions, which include all major U.S. universities and teaching hospitals, as well as sites in Europe and Australia. Individual practices seeking affiliate membership can receive information at http://www.childrensoncologygroup.org.

NCI Cancer Centers Program

NCI-designated Cancer Centers exist in nearly every state and are funded by NCI to support a broad research infrastructure, including the personnel and physical resources to conduct a variety of clinical trials. While serving as tertiary referral centers, the Cancer Centers increasingly have recognized the desirability of forging links with community practitioners. The resultant research networks enable Cancer Centers to complete trials more quickly while providing practitioners and their patients with access to new drugs and techniques at an early stage of their development. These partnerships are flourishing in some areas of the country, and the model is likely to be replicated widely. For more information about Cancer Centers in your area, consult http://www3.cancer.gov/cancercenters.

BIOPHARMACEUTICAL INDUSTRY-SPONSORED CANCER CLINICAL TRIALS

During the first decades of medical oncology, there was relatively little industry participation in cancer thera-peutics development. In part, this was a reflection of the complexity of therapeutics development in the field, during a period when the lack of a sufficiently detailed understanding of cancer biology prevented a fully rational basis for new drug development. This relative lack of industry involvement, coupled with the significant public health problem presented by cancer, was responsible for the development of the large NCI-sponsored clinical trials apparatus described in detail in this chapter. The past decade, however, has seen a significant increase in biopharmaceutical investment in cancer discovery research and a parallel increase in both the extent and sophistication of industry sponsorship of clinical trials for the development of new cancer therapeutics. Hundreds of new agents are currently in different stages of clinical evaluation by the industry, either alone or in cooperation with the National Cancer Institute or similar organizations in other parts of the world.

Purpose and Nature of Industry-Sponsored Clinical Trials

The primary goal of therapeutic agent investigation by the biopharmaceutical industry is the evaluation of promising agents for eventual registration and commercialization. Because registration of a new cancer drug requires the demonstration of safety and efficacy for the new agent in the context of currently available therapy for the cancer being treated, the spectrum of clinical trials sponsored by industry often overlaps with the range of trials conducted by the Cooperative Groups. Furthermore, there is a long tradition of industry providing investigational agents for the conduct of clinical investigations through NCI-sponsored mechanisms, and there are many examples of new agents or indications that have received FDA approval on the basis of NCI-sponsored clinical trials. Ethical considerations regarding human investigation, and expectations regarding adherence to standards for the conduct of clinical trials, do not differ between NCI-sponsored and industry-sponsored clinical trials; therefore, the fundamental processes of conducting clinical trials are similar in both cases. Despite these similarities, however, there are some differences between industry trials and those sponsored by NCI.

Particular Characteristics of Industry-Sponsored Trials

Biopharmaceutical development proceeds in a heavily regulated environment, with detailed regulations from various government agencies covering the spectrum of activities ranging from those related to preparing an agent for first entry into humans, through the years of clinical investigation in patients, to post-approval restrictions on public discussion regarding possible uses of the agent for indications other than those for which the drug was approved. As a result of the requirements of working in such an environment, corporate clinical investigations tend to be focused on the "clinical development plan"—the specific plan of clinical trials that will produce an appropriate evidentiary base to allow for regulatory review of the safety and efficacy profile of the agent. During the investigational phase of an agent's life cycle, therefore, companies might restrict the general availability of the agent to individual investigators for clinical study. This perceived need for containment and control can lead to tension between the investigative community and the industrial sponsor. Other potential sources of tension in the interaction between companies and investigators relate to the investigators' perceptions of the need for independence and objectivity in the conduct of multicenter trials. Historically, for example, many companies have generated phase III protocols internally, although usually with considerable input from both external advisors and regulatory bodies. The trial would be conducted by company personnel, and authorship would be conferred on the principal investigator of the largest accruing site. Increasingly, a new model is emerging in which a recognized expert is appointed as the principal investigator; this individual has a much greater role in the design, monitoring, and eventual analysis and publication of the trial than might have been the case historically. Similarly, recent years have seen the almost universal adoption of independent Data and Safety Monitoring Committees for late-stage clinical trials to oversee safety-related information as it emerges from the ongoing trial, and to make recommendations to company staff about appropriate actions.

The Impact of Globalization on Pharmaceutical Development

Pharmaceutical products increasingly are marketed globally, and large multinational pharmaceutical companies, therefore, need to conduct clinical development from a global perspective. In 1999, clinical trials with investigational agents with which the FDA was involved were being conducted in 79 countries. This tendency toward global development has been greatly accelerated by the International Committee on Harmonization (ICH) process, which facilitated standardization of many of the activities involved in preparing agents for clinical investigation, conducting those investigations, and then preparing the information for registration. Now, a single set of standards exists for the conduct of industry-sponsored trials worldwide. Attempts are made, therefore, to harmonize the development process to produce a globally accepted drug registration package to the greatest extent possible.

Models for the Conduct of Industry Clinical Trials

Biopharmaceutical industry sponsors usually produce the investigational agent in their own facilities, as they anticipate eventually being responsible for the commercial production and distribution of the agent. They also can conduct the series of required clinical trials directly using their own clinical trials personnel, which may include internal company physicians, statisticians, monitors, data managers, quality assurance auditors, and the rest of the required infrastructure, such as company standard operating procedures (SOPs), company information system support, and drug distribution apparatus. Alternatively, drug sponsors may utilize a contract research organization (CRO) to perform the actual clinical trials. In fact, for large development programs, it is not unusual for large companies to coordinate clinical trials programs using a mixture of both internal and externally acquired resources. CROs are companies in the business of conducting clinical trials. Over the last decade, following the explosion in growth of biopharmaceutical clinical investigation, a large number of such companies have been created, some capable of conducting global trials. The actual arrangement, either direct or indirect, utilized by a drug sponsor for a particular clinical trial, is important to the investigator and staff at the clinical trial site because it determines the predominant source of interactions and contact during the actual conduct of the trial.

Different models exist, as well, for investigator participation in clinical trials with industry. Traditionally, pharmaceutical sponsors have dealt either with individual investigators or with individual institutions, as in the case of academic centers. Clinical trial contract budgets have included direct-trial related costs such as performing additional laboratory studies that are not being done as part of usual medical care, plus direct site-related costs associated with the time spent on the trial by the various participating staff, and indirect costs for institutional overhead. Recent years have seen the emergence of consortia of investigators (sometimes under the rubric of a "Site Management Organization") or consortia of institutions presenting themselves to companies as clinical trial entities, often linked by a single central IRB, and often offering the advantage of working under a single negotiated contract. In addition, individual academic centers sometimes have formed networks of oncologists within their referral area for the purpose of presenting themselves as more efficient entities for interaction. New models continue to evolve. These new models make it easier for companies to engage the several hundred sites required to conduct major phase III registration-directed trials in a much more efficient manner.

Good Clinical Practice and Other Issues

One area of drug development that has been the focus of ICH activities is the development of Good Clinical Practice (GCP) Guidelines for the conduct of clinical trials. Good Clinical Practice describes international ethical and scientific quality standards for designing, conducting, recording, and reporting trials that involve the participation of human subjects. The very useful and informative document "ICH E6 Consolidated Guidance for Good Clinical Practice for Industry" (available at http://www.fda.gov/cder/guidance/index.htm) represents a summary of GCP guidance for the generation of clinical trial data intended for submission to regulatory authorities. This document comprehensively summarizes the responsibilities of IRBs, investigators, and sponsors, as well as issues regarding the clinical protocol, investigator's brochure, and the documents essential in the conduct of a trial. Although investigators participating in an industry-sponsored clinical trial can expect help in the preparation of the required documents, it is important that they

Science of Clinical Oncology

I

understand their responsibilities both to their patients and to the drug sponsor within the context of a global registration program.

Recent concerns regarding investigator conflict of interest in new drug development have led many institutions to develop policies regarding the extent of financial involvement by investigators in companies sponsoring trials in which the investigators are participating. Industry sponsors have also developed conflict-of-interest policies. In addition, as part of drug approval submissions in the United States, companies must now provide financial disclosure statements from individual investigators participating in the registration-directed trials.

The Changing Nature of Oncology Trials: Impact on Infrastructure

The same explosion in understanding cancer biology that has led to the increase in the number of new agents under development brings with it a realization that the most appropriate tests of those biologically-targeted agents are clinical trials in which the patients entered have tumors that are biologically appropriate for the agent. For example, Gleevec administered to all newly diagnosed patients with any form of leukemia would have a response rate much less than in the biologically appropriate group of newly diagnosed patients with chronic myelogenous leukemia; selection of CML patients allows for a focused development program leading to rapid initial registration. The same considerations can logically be extended to matching any biologically directed agent with any cancer patient population and argues strongly for more complete biological characterization and continued monitoring of patients entering cancer clinical trials. Regardless of whether such characterization is prospective or retrospective in clinical trial design and analysis, it can be expected that the increased need for collection of peripheral blood for germline DNA studies, plasma for proteomics studies, fresh tumor tissue for DNA, RNA, and/or protein studies, tumor tissue blocks for DNA or immunohistochemical studies, or for specialized imaging studies, will all place new demands on the infrastructure required to conduct trials. These requirements will also introduce new challenges for quality control on sample collection and storage and will increase the resource requirements for trials. It is also likely, however, that such clinical trials will become much more informative. The potential exists in the future for smaller, more definitive trials in more biologically homogeneous groups of patients than is possible with the classic histopathology used currently to characterize patients; this potential should lead to more effective and well-tailored treatments.

Challenges to the Conduct of Industry Oncology Clinical Trials

Numerous challenges exist both to the oncologist looking to participate in the clinical trials process and to the corporate sponsor wishing to conduct such registration-directed trials. From the individual oncologist's perspective, the bureaucratic hurdles associated with the clinical trials administration process can appear daunting, particularly when added to the responsibilities of using investigational agents in patients. Acquiring sufficient trained personnel to conduct such trials is a challenge. Unless participation in a particular trial is part of a broader commitment to the clinical trials process with supportive infrastructure in place and experience in the conduct of several simultaneous ongoing trials, successful participation is unlikely. For these reasons, oncologists who are already participating in Cooperative Group trials through one or another mechanism already have in place some of the required infrastructure for the local conduct of industry-sponsored clinical trials.

The corporate sponsors of oncology drugs undergoing development face their own challenges and uncertainties. Cancer drug development traditionally has been a high-risk field. Many agents fail in late-stage development, a time when significant time and resources have already been expended. Although it is hoped that the kind of increased linkage of biological study with therapeutics development will eventually make this whole process more predictable, the development of new cancer drugs remains an expensive and a high-risk activity. Development is carried out through a clinical trials process that remains highly inefficient and lacking in standardized information collection, systems, and processes, and without many biological markers to aid in decision-making early enough in the clinical trials process to decrease risks in development. Continued improvements in efficiency and productivity of the clinical trials system remain a high priority in order to accelerate the delivery of effective new agents to patients.

EXPECTATIONS OF CLINICAL RESEARCH SITES

A number of components are critical for an effective research practice. These include:

- The presence of committed physicians willing to devote the time and energy necessary to conduct clinical research and to accept conscientiously the significant responsibility inherent in the conduct of human research.
- The availability of suitably trained staff (preferably an experienced research nurse) with enough time to assist in screening patients for protocol eligibility and for following patients on protocol treatment.
- The availability of suitable staff to administer the required treatments in the protocol-prescribed manner; increasingly, this might include administration of a wide range of potential therapeutics including, but not limited to, more conventional intravenous chemotherapy and, in some cases, radiation.
- Adequate and committed pharmacy capabilities to handle and account for investigational agents if these are part of the protocol treatment.
- Adequate data management staff to handle the data reporting requirements for patients treated on protocols.

- Access to an Institutional Review Board (IRB) with OHRP (Office for Human Research Protections) assurances to approve the protocol and monitor the progress of the research.
- Access to suitable laboratory facilities to complete the studies required by the protocol.
- Willingness to comply with certain federal regulatory requirements, including adequate privacy procedures and training in human subjects protection (available as an online course through NIH at http://cme.cancer.gov/c01/).

The number and precise composition of the necessary staff depends on the number of patients enrolled on clinical trials and the nature of the practice. In some settings, in which the number of patients on studies is small, one good research nurse can perform many of the required functions. At more active sites, research nurses, CRAs, and research pharmacists perform separate functions. For budgeting purposes, for example, it is often estimated that one full-time CRA can handle 25 new patients and up to 50 patients in follow-up in a year. Some of the structures supporting clinical trials participation, such as the CCOP program, provide substantial up-front funding to support salaries for the necessary staff in return for a commitment to substantial accrual. Many others, including the CTSU and the Cooperative Groups, provide a small amount of funding when each patient is accrued. The latter approach allows sites to introduce clinical research into their practices at a more gradual pace.

Quality Assurance and Audits

Because the accuracy of the data collected on clinical trials is critical to the validity of the conclusions from the trials, all clinical trials organizations include quality assurance and audit programs. Although these are structured somewhat differently depending on the mechanism of participation (with industry conducting the most frequent and extensive audits), all such programs have certain features in common. All send queries to the site when discrepancies or suspected errors are noted in submitted information, and all compare data submitted from the sites to the primary medical or research record for verification at on-site audits. NCI audits are typically conducted every three years and review a sample of patients enrolled on a variety of protocols. In addition to verifying data accuracy and protocol adherence, informed consents are reviewed, as are adverse event reporting compliance, pharmacy practices, and timeliness of required IRB submissions and approvals. Preparation for audits is time consuming for the sites, as all relevant records—including laboratory studies and films (CT, MRI, etc.) required to document tumor measurements and response verification—must be gathered for the audit team. Some consider this work onerous; however, audits fulfill an important educational role in addition to ensuring the quality of the data and clinical trial procedures at participating sites. Data quality initially became a concern when clinical trial participation moved beyond academic sites to community practices. A

number of evaluations in the 1980s, however, documented the ability of community sites to perform at a level comparable to academic institutions in terms of data quality, protocol adherence, and patient outcome.[10,11] Indeed, over 30% of the accrual to adult Cooperative Group trials now comes from community practices in the Community Clinical Oncology Program (CCOP), and additional accrual comes from Cooperative Group affiliates, predominantly community sites.

As noted previously, although regulatory standards regarding the conduct of clinical trials impose similar overall expectations, for its own reasons industry monitoring is both more extensive and frequent than the usual cooperative group monitoring. The basic tenet of monitoring for both industry- and NCI-sponsored clinical trials is similar—the need to verify data accuracy by comparing case report forms, whether submitted by paper or electronically, with source data in the patient's medical record. The sponsor-assigned clinical trial monitor will visit the site regularly, educate the involved staff about the goals and particular details of the protocol, and then track the progress of protocol-related activities throughout the conduct of the trial. Monitoring responsibilities include confirmation of appropriate local IRB review, investigator registration via completion of the FDA 1572 form, the existence of timely informed consent documents for each patient, inspection of drug accountability records, confirmation of timely and complete submission of serious adverse events reports, and ensuring appropriate and timely handling of amendments. These activities all fall within the responsibility of the clinical trial monitor, whether the monitor is provided directly from the company sponsor or through a contract research organization. Furthermore, regardless of whether the clinical trial is conducted directly by its own organization or by a CRO, biopharmaceutical companies often conduct their own quality assurance audits and monitoring associated with the trial, to further assure the integrity of the submitted data. The intensity of clinical trial monitoring tends to increase as clinical trials mature, and the data management group prepares to officially "lock" the database before the conduct of prespecified analysis and reporting activities. The intensity of quality assurance auditing also increases for a particular clinical trial when it has been identified as part of a New Drug Application (NDA) or Biologic Licensing Application (BLA) for drug registration with the FDA. Monitoring and data management activities are evolving with the widespread introduction of electronic data collection and submission systems that are replacing traditional paper-based case report form approaches.

Educational and Training Tools

As has been described previously, participation in clinical trials adds many complexities to care of cancer patients and can require that physicians, nurses, and other office staff acquire new and different skills. Fortunately, because of the widespread interest in clinical trials in the cancer community, there are many resources for gaining information about clinical trials and for acquiring the necessary skills. Professional societies are a good source for educational programs and materials, and some, like the Oncology Nursing Society (http://www.oncc.org/), the Society of Clinical Research Associates (SOCRA) (http://www.socra.org/), and the American Society of Health-System Pharmacists (http://www.ashp.org/) actually offer certification programs that can serve as important career development incentives to office staff. The American Society of Clinical Oncology (ASCO) (http://www.asco.org) also has a very useful Web site with links to a variety of sites that provide information about available clinical trials and detailed information about chemotherapy agents for physicians and nurses. NCI-sponsored Cooperative Groups provide regular educational activities for physicians, statisticians, nurses, and data managers participating in their trials. Furthermore, the biopharmaceutical industry sponsors a wide range of educational activities conducted by both academic institutions and professional societies (e.g., ASCO and the American Association of Cancer Research [AACR]) about the clinical trials process in general and about the responsibilities of the individual clinical investigator.

The Web site (http://cancer.gov/) provides a gateway to the many Web sites at the NCI and provides links to many other useful sites. It contains extensive information about cancer in general and cancer statistics, as well as detailed information about clinical trials with direct links to the Physician Data Query (PDQ). PDQ (http://cancer.gov/cancerinfo/pdq/) is a database maintained by the NCI that provides a comprehensive listing of NCI-sponsored clinical trials, along with extensive and detailed listings of trials (including international trials) that are submitted voluntarily by cancer centers, private hospitals, and the pharmaceutical and biotechnology industries. The PDQ search engine allows searches by geographic location and site or investigators, as well as tumor type, stage, and other relevant categories, and it provides contact information to facilitate patient referral when appropriate. In addition, PDQ provides detailed information about the treatment of many cancers, as well as information on screening, prevention, genetics, and supportive care. Useful information on insurance coverage for patients on clinical trials, including the coverage offered by specific insurance carriers, can also be obtained from cancer.gov.

The cancer.gov site also provides a link to the Cancer Therapy Evaluation Program (CTEP), which coordinates NCI-funded clinical trials in treatment across the country. The CTEP Web site contains detailed information related to the conduct of clinical trials, including the following:

- Human research protections and the required online course for all research teams conducting NIH funded research.
- The Investigators' Handbook and other tools for protocol development.
- Information on data reporting requirements and about the monitoring and auditing of clinical trials.

The Web site of the Division of Cancer Prevention (http://www3.cancer.gov/prevention/) provides similar information on the conduct of cancer prevention and control studies.

Other NCI resources include the Cancer Information Service (1-800-4-CANCER), a telephone service that provides information in both English and Spanish, answers many patient questions, and refers callers to other resources when appropriate.

CONCLUDING REMARKS

Although the involvement of oncologists in clinical trials introduces additional complexities to their practice of oncology, it also provides substantial benefits to all participants and ultimately contributes to the goals of improving cancer treatment and prevention. A growing number of clinical practices have been able to integrate active clinical research into their activities successfully. To help facilitate this participation, the NCI in 1998 began a small pilot project called the Expanded Participation Project (EPP) to engage previously uninvolved physicians in clinical trials.[12] A number of sites became involved successfully, and NCI developed a number of tools now available through the CTSU based on this EPP experience. These tools include IRB submission packets, protocol calendars, and summaries, among others. The sites in the EPP reported all study data electronically and rated the electronic system highly. It is envisioned that the availability of a central IRB nationally and an electronic data reporting system in the near future will eliminate critical barriers and will make it easier for community physicians to participate. Similarly, the biopharmaceutical industry continually seeks interested, conscientious physicians to participate in its trials. The shortage of such physicians creates a potentially serious limitation on the rate of development of new treatments for cancer. Surveys done under the auspices of the Coalition of National Cooperative Groups suggest that the attitude of the treating physician is, perhaps, the most critical factor in patient enrollment in clinical trials.[2,5] With the right attitude, an increasing number of resources and tools are now available to make access to clinical trials a reality for many more patients, with the potential to benefit both themselves and future patients with cancer.

REFERENCES

1. Taylor K, Feldstein M, Skeel R, Pandya KJ, Ng P, Carbone PP: Fundamental dilemmas of the randomized clinical trials process: Results of a survey of the 1,737 Eastern Cooperative Oncology Group Investigators. J Clin Oncol 1994;12:1796–1805.
2. Fleming ID: Barriers to clinical trials: Part I B Reimbursement problems. Cancer 1994;74:2662–2665.
3. Schain WS: Barriers to clinical trials: Part II—Knowledge and attitudes of potential participants. Cancer 1994;74:2666–2671.
4. Mansour EG: Barriers to clinical trials: Part III B Knowledge and attitudes of health care providers. Cancer 1994;74:2672–2675.
5. Comis RL, Aldige CR, Stovall EL, Krebs LU, Risher PJ, Taylor HJ: A quantitative survey of public attitudes towards cancer clinical trials. Available at http://www.cancertrialshelp.org/static_binary/308.pdf (accessed on 7/10/03).
6. Clinical Trials: A Blueprint for the Future. Bethesda, MD, National Institutes of Health Publication No. 99-4524, 1999.

7. Abrams JS, Cummings C: Implementing clinical trials in your practice: Getting started and what's new. In Perry MC (ed): Am Soc Clin Onc 2002 Educational Booklet. Alexandria, VA, 2002, pp 273-282.

8. Sung NS, Crowley WF Jr, Genel M, et al: Central challenges facing the national research enterprise. JAMA 2003;289:1278-1287.

9. Christian MC, Goldberg JL, Killen J, et al: Sounding board: A central institutional review board for multi-institutional trials. N Engl J Med 2002;346: 1405-1408.

10. Koretz MM, Jackson PM, Torti FM, Carter SK: A comparison of the quality of community affiliates and that of universities in the Northern California Oncology Group. J Clin Oncol 1983;1:640-644.

11. Begg CB, Carbone PP, Elson PJ, Zelen M: Participation of community hospitals in clinical trials: Analysis of five years of experience in the Eastern Cooperative Oncology Group. New Engl J Med 1982;306:1076-1080.

12. Saxman S, Vena D, Nasim G, et al: A National Cancer Institute pilot study to enhance enrollment in clinical trials: The Expanded Participant Project (EPP). Proc Am Soc Clin Oncol 2003;22:2108a.

Science of Clinical Oncology

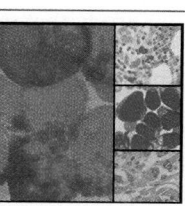

ECONOMIC ANALYSIS OF CANCER TREATMENT

Charles L. Bennett

Todd Lee

21

SUMMARY OF KEY POINTS

- Cancer care accounts for the largest number of dollars spent on any medical condition in the United States.
- Cancer accounts for 10% of all Medicare expenditures.
- Medicare does not reimburse for most outpatient pharmaceuticals, although exceptions exist for some cancer drugs.
- Patient care costs on clinical trials are only 10% greater than those in the nonclinical trial setting.

- Fewer than half of the states have passed legislation mandating coverage of clinical trials.
- Cost-benefit, cost-effectiveness, cost-utility, and cost-identification are the main methods for evaluating the economics of clinical interventions.
- Empirical studies have found that results of cost-effectiveness studies are associated with pharmaceutical versus not-for-profit funding, although quality is not.

- Economic studies rarely are incorporated into clinical trials sponsored by the National Cancer Institute (NCI).
- To date, only seven NCI-sponsored clinical trials have included economic assessments.

CANCER CARE IS EXPENSIVE

Health care expenditures continue to rise in the United States and now account for almost 15% of the total gross domestic product, representing $1.6 trillion in annual expenditures. The costs of treating patients with cancer contribute substantially to overall health care expenditures. In fact, the economic burden of cancer is the largest imposed by any medical illness in the United States.[1] The high expense associated with cancer is related to a number of factors, including an increase in the prevalence of cancer as people live longer, the high rate of comorbid medical illness in cancer patients, and high costs associated with diagnosis, treatment, and end-of-life and palliative care as new, more expensive treatments become available. The direct costs of cancer care made up 4.8% of medical care costs in 1985 and 4.9% in 1995, accounting for $18.1 billion and $41.2 billion, respectively.[1,2] In 2002, cancer care accounted for $61 billion in direct medical costs.

Cost is a major determinant of the type and intensity of cancer care, particularly related to reimbursement of high-tech and high-cost procedures and pharmaceutical products for cancer patients.[3] The physician has a large role in determining the medical costs incurred by individual patients. Medical costs are categorized into four areas: (1) direct medical costs, i.e., amounts spent for direct medical care in the prevention, screening, diagnosis, treatment, and palliation related to cancer care; (2) direct nonmedical costs, i.e., amounts spent for caregivers, travel, and other aspects of supportive care; (3) indirect costs, i.e., the economic value of lost productivity due to illness, disability, and death (mortality); and (4) intangible costs, i.e., those costs associated with pain,

suffering, and grief. Although several studies have evaluated the direct costs of various types of cancers, few include estimates of direct nonmedical, indirect, and intangible costs. Pilot studies indicate that these costs may be as high as 75% of the total cost of cancer care.[4,5]

In addition to considering total costs, it is important to consider the value provided by the intervention in exchange for the amount expended (Table 21-1). The number of articles addressing cost-effectiveness of cancer treatments has increased dramatically in the past few years, with a large number of these studies addressing supportive care agents.[6,7] Oncologists, insurers, and policymakers increasingly are addressing questions of costs, cost-effectiveness, and quality of life. Many changes have been made in this area since the late 1990s. Previously, the national mandate to evaluate the effectiveness of health care, including cancer care, was designed to incorporate cost-effectiveness assessments. The Agency for Health Research and Quality (formerly the Agency for Health Care Policy and Research) was given a mandate

TABLE 21-1

Types of Economic Analyses Used in Oncology

Type of economic analysis	Units used to measure costs and clinical outcomes
Cost-benefit	Costs and benefits are measured in the same terms (usually monetary)
Cost-effectiveness	Costs measured in monetary terms, effectiveness in clinical terms
Cost-identification	Costs measured in monetary terms, no effectiveness measurement
Cost-utility	Costs measured in monetary terms, utility measured in terms of utility

by Congress to evaluate medical care by preparing evidence-based practice guidelines. These guidelines also addressed cost considerations. Cancer-related topics included prostate and breast cancer. This mandate later was modified to focus on evidence-based technology assessments, which could then be incorporated by relevant persons in the medical community into guidelines produced by physicians or medical societies. Cost considerations were no longer addressed explicitly in this revised mandate. Nonetheless, economic assessments of cancer care have been developed by other sources.

Clinical Trials and Costs

The costs of cancer clinical trials have become an important issue related to cancer treatment and costs over the past decade. Six pilot studies have provided information about 1309 patients who received care on phase II/III clinical trials (Tables 21-2 and 21-3).[6-12] Costs of care for these patients have been matched with costs for controls who received standard oncology care. Cost estimates ranged from 10% lower to 23% higher for clinical trials in comparison to standard medical care. In response to these reports, Medicare, 16 states, and several private insurers now cover the costs of patient care in "qualifying" clinical trials.[11] The Association of American Cancer Institutes/Northwestern University Clinical Trials

Costs and Charges Project proposed a study that evaluates the costs of 100 patients enrolled on phase I clinical trials conducted at tertiary cancer centers with an equal number of matched controls.[11]

Primarily because of economic considerations, federal policies were not supportive of clinical trial reimbursement during the 1990s.[11] The previous administrator for Medicare, the Health Care Financing Agency (HCFA), excluded coverage of routine care costs associated with clinical trial participation, on the basis that such treatment was experimental or investigational.[13] However, the General Accounting Office found that fewer than 4% of claims for clinical trial costs incurred by Medicare beneficiaries were denied and that oncologists often submitted bills for components of complex treatments without specifying the procedure itself. It was estimated that Medicare had paid 50% to 90% of routine patient care costs in clinical trials.[14] In 1993, the Office of the Inspector General of the Department of Health and Human Services found that Medicare was being billed millions of dollars for patients who received care in clinical trials. However, quickly passed legislation prevented HCFA from collecting from the hospitals.[11]

A 1993 bill, the Cancer Treatment Improvement Act, never made it past committee. In 1996, 1997, 1998, and 1999, unsuccessful proposals were made for the Medicare Cancer Clinical Trial Coverage Act, introduced in the

TABLE 21-2

Estimates of Costs of Clinical Trials*

STUDY LOCATION OR SPONSOR	MEMORIAL SLOAN-KETTERING CANCER CENTER	AACI/ NORTHWESTERN UNIVERSITY	KAISER PERMANENTE	CBO/MAYO CLINIC	GROUP HEALTH COOPERATIVE	RAND/ NCI
First author	Quirk et al[10]	Bennett et al[9]	Fireman et al[7]	Wagner et al[6]	Barlow et al[8]	Goldman et al[12]
No. patients on clinical trials	77	35	135	61	49 breast/20 colorectal	932
Years	1995	1996–1998	1994–1996	1988–1994	1990–1996	1998–1999
Phase	II/III	II	III	II/III	II/III	I/II/III
Cost data						
Units used to measure costs	Costs	Charges	Costs	Costs	Costs	Costs
6 months						
Control group	$30.8	$63.7	$9.9	$10.1		
Clinical trial group	$37.1	$57.5	$12.2	$12.2	–	
% difference	17%	(–10%)	23%	21%		
12 months						
Control group			$15.5	$14.8		
Clinical trial group	–	–	$17.0	$16.8	–	
% difference			10%	14%		
24 months						
Control group				$25.0†		$33.2 (30
Clinical trial group	–	–	–	$30.0		$35.4 months)
% difference					20%	6.5%
60 months						
Control group				$26.8		
Clinical trial group	–	–	–	$27.1	–	
% difference				1%		

AACI, American Association of Cancer Institutes; CBO, Congressional Budget Office.
*Costs measured in units of $1,000.
†26 closely matched breast cancer patients only; other diseases did not show a remarkable cost difference.

TABLE 21-3

Methodologies of the Five Economic Assessments of Clinical Trials

STUDY	NO. CANCER CENTERS	PAYMENT SYSTEM	NO. CANCER TYPES	CASE SELECTION	BMT CASES	CONTROL SELECTION-MATCHING	EXCLUDED RESOURCES	COSTS	ANALYSIS
CBO and Mayo Clinic	1	Fee-for-service	9	All possible cases	No	Performance status	Outpatient prescription drugs	Costs: 5 years	Paired t test
Kaiser Permanente	17	Managed care	9	All possible cases	Yes	Eligibility for trial	None	Costs: 1 year	Univariate regression
Memorial Sloan-Kettering Cancer Center	1	Medicare	7	Patients treated primarily at the cancer center	No	Survival	Resources used outside of MSKCC	Costs: 6 months	Unpaired t test
AACI/ Northwestern University	5	Fee-for-service	5	Patients treated primarily at the cancer center	Yes	Eligibility for trial	Resources used outside of the AACI center	Charges: 6 months	Paired t test
Group Health Cooperative	NA	Managed care	2	GH members on SWOG studies	Not stated	Comorbidity, eligibility for trial (26 patients with breast cancer)	Not stated	Costs: 2 years	Not stated
RAND/NCI	83	Fee-for-service/ Medicare/ Medicaid	8	All possible cases	Yes	Eligibility for trial	None	Cost: 2.5	Multivariate regression

AACI, American Association of Cancer Institutes; BMT, bone marrow transplantation; CBO, Congressional Budget Office; MSKCC, Memorial Sloan-Kettering Cancer Center; SWOG, Southwest Oncology Group.

Senate, and the Medicare Cancer Clinical Trial Demonstration Act in the House. These proposals would have allocated $750 million to cover cancer clinical trials sponsored by the National Institutes of Health, the Department of Defense, and the Department of Veterans Affairs. The proposals required development of federal regulations that would define "routine patient care costs" and would have authorized a study of the impact of clinical trials reimbursement on group health insurance plans. In 2000, following years of lobbying by individuals, patient groups, health care workers, and organizations who were concerned about reimbursement denials of clinical trial costs and the low rates of accrual to clinical trials, then President Clinton issued an executive order stating that the Medicare administrator was authorized to cover the costs of cancer clinical trials. This benefit included a broad definition of "qualified" clinical trials. The Final National Coverage Determination extended the definition of qualified clinical trials beyond those funded or conducted by government bodies to trials that satisfied qualifying criteria.

Efforts to pass broad clinical trial legislation moved forward in 2001. A bill dealing specifically with coverage of patient care costs of cancer clinical trials was introduced in the House by Rep. Deborah Pryce (R-Ohio) as the Access to Cancer Clinical Trials Act of 2001 (H.R. 967). This bill is in line with the Medicare National Coverage Decision and mandates coverage of all phases of federally funded cancer prevention, diagnostic, and treatment trials; trials approved and funded by "qualified nongovernmental research entity identified in the guidelines issued by the National Institutes of Health for center support grants"; and investigational new drug (IND)–exempt investigator-initiated trials. During debate over the McCain-Kennedy-Edwards legislation, the Senate approved a nonbinding "sense of the Senate" amendment on clinical trials by an 89 to 1 vote. The amendment states that individuals with life-threatening diseases should have the opportunity to participate in federally approved or funded clinical trials. All versions of the proposed legislations state that qualified individuals are those who have life-threatening or serious illnesses "for which no standard treatment is effective," and that participation in the trial offers "meaningful potential for significant clinical benefit." This language raises concern that patients might be excluded from clinical trials if the standard therapies seem to be a reasonable option. President Bush has voiced support for coverage of patient care costs for treatment in "qualified" clinical trials. Thus, the prospects for passage of comprehensive federal legislation supporting clinical trial reimbursement during the Bush administration are good.

As of December 2002, 16 states had passed laws mandating coverage of patient care costs associated with treatment provided in specified categories of cancer clinical trials.[11] The question put before state legislatures has been whether insurance barriers to clinical research are best removed through voluntary action of health insurers or formal legislation. In 1995, Rhode Island became the first state to legislate insurance coverage for clinical trials. The original bill supported coverage of phase III and IV cancer treatment trials. An amended bill, in 1997, covered phase II, prevention, and screening clinical trials. Georgia mandated insurance for selected pediatric cancer trials in 1998. In 1999, Maryland and Virginia mandated insurance for cancer trials conducted in in-state academic institutions, Maine passed a law requiring coverage of NIH-sponsored trials in cooperative groups or NCI-designated cancer centers, and Louisiana passed a law including these trials as well as trials sponsored by the Food and Drug Administration (FDA), the Department of Defense, the Veterans Administration, and the Coalition of National Cancer Cooperative Groups. Several other states followed suit in 2000 and 2001. Illinois extended its guarantee of coverage to all "seriously ill patients for which no standard therapy is available," but required only that insurers had to offer this as an option, not that employers had to buy the benefit as part of their employee health coverage package. Many of the coverage initiatives excluded phase I trials, partly because no data existed on costs, little data existed on the investigative treatments, and the treatments had little chance of being therapeutic. Most initiatives limit coverage to cancer clinical trials, in part because the national infrastructure surrounding cancer trials is the most established and comprehensive of any disease and cancer clinical trials are subject to high levels of controls, monitoring, and oversight. State legislative efforts do not pertain to employees of self-insured corporations as defined under The Employee Retirement Security Act (ERISA) of 1974. Concern over variable scientific quality has led many state legislatures to limit reimbursement to trials funded by federal agencies. Institutional review boards ensure that a trial is designed and conducted ethically, but they do not assess scientific validity. This policy excludes a great many high-quality clinical trials that are funded by sources other than the federal government.

Private insurers have addressed policies related to reimbursement for clinical trials. In the early 1990s, private insurers who refused reimbursement for bone marrow transplants for breast cancer paid large jury awards and settlements to families of the affected individuals. Subsequently, many states and private insurers adopted policies to reimburse for the procedure. In 1999, a study reported no clinical benefit with bone marrow transplantation for breast cancer, and most insurers denied reimbursement for this treatment. The reports had been delayed by several years because poor clinical trial accrual had led to the extension of the study period.

As of 2002, several large private health insurers were reimbursing for medical care costs that occur with clinical trials. These insurers included the New Jersey Association of Health Plans, OhioMed, United Healthcare, and the Mayo Health Plan.[11] The New Jersey Association of Health Plans agreement is unique in that it is the first instance for which all private insurers in a single state voluntarily agreed to provide cancer clinical trial coverage. The agreement was the result of a collaborative effort of a working group consisting of insurers, consumers, and physicians. Michigan and Minnesota followed New Jersey's example and encouraged establishment of collaborative task forces to work with private insurers voluntarily to pursue clinical trial coverage.

Economic Assessments in Cancer Care

Economic issues in cancer care are paramount in planning for optimal use of scarce resources and in responding to the increased economic pressures faced by the health care system. Economic factors are a major determinant of the type and intensity of cancer care, because payers are concerned that expensive treatments may not be cost-effective. Physicians and health policymakers should make judgments on the effectiveness and cost-effectiveness of cancer care based on explicit assessments of the costs and benefits of alternative management strategies. To understand the financial impact of alternative cancer management strategies more clearly, it is essential to understand the basic terminology of economic studies in health care: costs, benefits, cost-effectiveness, cost-utility, and cost-minimization. It also is important to explain the methods used by policymakers and oncology researchers when they evaluate the costs of cancer care.

When Are Economic Assessments Likely to Be Helpful (Or Unhelpful)?

Assessments of the costs of cancer care can be considered when significant resources are being used; when resource considerations have a direct impact on patient care; and when resource allocation decisions are likely to be made.[15] Examples of situations in which a large amount of resources are used include supportive care agents such as antiemetics, erythropoietin, granulocyte colony-stimulating factor (GCSF), and genetic predictors. Resource considerations played a prominent role in the decision to support high-dose chemotherapy with stem cell transplantation for breast cancer before reports of unfavorable results were received from several randomized clinical trials. Economic analyses are unlikely to be helpful in cases in which a treatment works well but only a small number of individuals are affected. For example, advanced testicular cancer routinely is treated with chemotherapy. The cure rate is high, but the number of cases is less than 10,000 per year. Similarly, data have been collected on the economic implications of high-dose chemotherapy with stem cell transplantation for breast cancer, but will not be useful to policymakers because this procedure has not been found to be clinically effective.

Types of Economic Analyses

Economic evaluations provide information on the value of an intervention or therapy in relation to its costs when compared to a competing alternative. Economic evaluations provide information on the incremental benefit of a new intervention or therapy compared to an alternative, where, ideally, the alternative is the current standard of care. Economic evaluations of cancer interventions can range from decision analytic models to retrospective database comparisons to analyses conducted alongside clinical trials. However, all of the economic analyses of clinical interventions can be grouped into four categories based on the measure of effectiveness used in the analysis: cost-benefit; cost-effectiveness; cost-utility; and cost-identification (see Table 21-1).[16]

Cost-benefit analysis compares the incremental cost of a medical intervention with its incremental benefit, with both terms measured in monetary units. Therefore, interventions with positive net benefits, in which the value of the incremental benefits is greater than the incremental costs, are cost-beneficial compared to the alternative. In theory, cost-benefit analysis allows for the comparison of health interventions with other programs or interventions from nonhealth care sectors that may be competing for the same dollars. That is, with a cost-benefit analysis, a government could compare whether to spend monies on a new after-school program for children or use the same monies to fund a breast cancer screening program. However, difficulties in valuing all the relevant factors (e.g., years of life lost and quality of life) in monetary terms limits the use of cost-benefit analysis.

More commonly, economic evaluations in cancer care involve cost-effectiveness analysis. Cost-effectiveness provides information on the value of an intervention or therapy in relation to its costs when compared to a competing alternative when effectiveness is measured in clinical terms. The analysis compares two or more interventions to each other and provides information on the differences in costs and effects between comparators. The results are summarized into a ratio that provides the results in terms of the costs per unit of effect. This ratio is referred to as the incremental cost-effectiveness ratio, because it is assessing incremental differences between alternative treatments. Because it is a cost-effectiveness analysis, the denominator of the ratio is valued in natural units, such as years of life, and is calculated by finding the difference in the effectiveness measure between the alternatives. For example, many cost-effectiveness analyses in cancer treatments report the incremental cost per year of life saved.

Cost-utility analysis is a subset of cost-effectiveness analysis in which the measure of effectiveness is a utility, or value. Utilities provide a measure of overall quality of life and are applicable across different types of cancer. The measure is intended to incorporate both positive and negative aspects of treatment. The utility is combined with information on survival to estimate quality-adjusted life years, which are used as the measure of effectiveness in cost-utility analyses. Thus, cost-utility analyses provide an estimate of the cost per quality-adjusted life year gained. In principle, this method can be used to compare the value of screening programs to new chemotherapeutic agents to gauge the relative value of an alternative.

The final type of clinical economic analysis used in cancer studies is cost identification. This technique reports the total types and amounts of resources used in providing medical care, without formal assessments of the clinical benefits of the treatment. This technique is an integral part of the other economic evaluations in that it provides the cost estimate used in the numerator. However, with this method the benefits are not compared formally among alternatives.

It is important to emphasize that in all types of economic analyses the way monetary units are assigned to treatments can make important differences. Specifically, costs differ markedly from charges.[17] Costs represent the true opportunity cost of a resource, whereas charges represent the amount that is billed for that resource. There may be little connection between costs and charges, with charges typically being much greater than the actual costs. Therefore, it is important to be aware of whether costs or charges are being used to derive the economic estimates.

CANCER COSTS: ESTIMATES FROM MEDICARE POPULATIONS

Total medical care expenditures for oncology account for 10% of all Medicare expenditures.[1,2] Recent studies have incorporated economic analyses for various cancers experienced by the Medicare population.[1,2,18] These analyses are based on data that is disaggregated to include information on cancer site, stage of diagnosis, and type of treatment and are evaluated over long periods of time. The Surveillance Epidemiology and End Results (SEER) database includes detailed clinical data elements for cancer patients who received care in 11 geographic regions of the country (see http://seer.cancer.gov). Medicare databases include detailed information for inpatient services (part A) and payments for outpatient services (part B). Part A covers inpatient hospital care, skilled nursing facilities, home health services following a hospitalization, and hospice care. Almost all Medicare beneficiaries are entitled to part A benefits. Part B of the Medicare program covers physician services, outpatient services, diagnostic tests, emergency room visits, durable medical equipment, laboratory services, home health care that does not follow a hospital stay, and other medical services and supplies. Cancer screening services are covered for cervical, breast, colorectal, and prostate cancer. Approximately 95% of Medicare beneficiaries are eligible for part B benefits.

Medicare does not cover most prescription drugs, although it does provide coverage under part B for many types of chemotherapy and related treatments. Medicare Health Maintenance Organizations (HMOs) provide comprehensive care, including pharmaceuticals. Medicare does not cover routine nursing home care, which usually is covered by Medicaid or private insurance plans. The skilled nursing facility benefit applies to skilled nursing and rehabilitation services, but only if preceded by a hospitalization of 3 days or more. The Medicare-SEER cost files were generated by reviewing monthly cost files for each cancer patient identified in the SEER database. Cost data are entered based on costs in current year dollars. Prices are adjusted using the Medicare per capita index and Medicare-based price indices that account for differences in health care purchasing power over time and location. Costs are evaluated for the initial phase, the primary course of therapy, and any adjuvant therapy; continuing care, including surveillance activities for detecting recurrences and new cancers; and the terminal care phase.

These data were used to provide estimates of national expenditures for 1996 according to type of cancer and gender.[1] The most costly cancers for men were prostate, followed by lung and colorectal cancer. For women, the most costly cancers were breast, followed by colorectal and lung cancer.

Quality Assessment of Economic Analyses

Controversy exists over the quality of economic analyses of medical treatments and has led to the development of grading systems for economic evaluations.[19,20] The data and the models used in these analyses are the major determinants of the results. Additional items that are considered in the quality of economic evaluations include the objective and perspective of the analysis, data sources, type of comparison, handling of uncertainty, the time horizon of the analysis, and the discount rate.[20] Other important considerations are the outcome measure used in the analysis, measurement of costs, measurement of effectiveness, and the overall transparency of the analysis (i.e., were the assumptions explicitly stated?).[20]

Another item that is included in the grading system and that recently has been receiving more attention is the sponsor of the analysis. Concern has been raised over the potential for conflict of interest to affect the design and interpretation of economic analyses of medical therapies.[21-23] The newness of pharmacoeconomics research and its potential effects on pharmaceutical company revenue make it particularly vulnerable to financial conflicts of interest. Two papers have examined the effects of conflict of interest on pharmacoeconomic research in oncology.[21,22] The studies were based on reviews of economic analyses pertaining to three breakthrough areas in oncology—hematopoietic colony-stimulating factors, antiemetics, and taxanes. Articles were classified according to qualitative conclusion, quantitative result, timing of study initiation, and funding source. Correlations were evaluated between funding source and qualitative cost assessment; timing of study initiation; and discrepancies between qualitative conclusions and quantitative results. Favorable conclusions were reached by 81% of the pharmaceutical company–sponsored studies and 48% of the nonprofit-sponsored studies ($p < 0.009$). All of the studies that reached unfavorable conclusions had been sponsored by nonprofit organizations. Although nearly one fourth of the studies gave qualitative conclusions that overstated their quantitative results, this was not significantly greater for pharmaceutical company–sponsored studies than for nonprofit-sponsored studies.[21] More than 80% of economic studies funded by all sources were conducted after favorable clinical trial results were known. The findings of the study demonstrated a strong association between pharmaceutical company sponsorship and favorable economic assessments. Although there is no evidence of bias in individual articles, the results raised concerns about potential bias in pharmacoeconomic studies. Unfavorable cost profiles probably are underreported, and qualitative overstatements about the cost-effectiveness of new agents are not uncommon.

The second study addressed variations in study quality when the 44 pharmaceutical and not-for profit funded cost-effectiveness studies of the six breakthrough drugs in oncology were compared.[22] Two blinded investigators rated specific aspects of study reporting based on criteria from the U.S. Public Health Service Panel on Cost-effectiveness in Health and Medicine. Dissemination strategies were evaluated using impact factor scores from the Science Citation Index. The study found that the operational aspects of pharmaceutical manufacturer–sponsored study reporting were better overall than those associated with nonprofit-sponsored studies, with respect to the following criteria: the results were more likely to be reported based on data obtained from randomized clinical trials or detailed cost-models (90% vs 70%); to include descriptions of the source of cost differences (90% vs 79%); to state whether the study was carried out from a societal, governmental, or insurer perspective (70% vs 42%); and to indicate clearly the time period over which costs were evaluated (65% vs 50%). However, nonprofit-sponsored studies were more likely than pharmaceutical-sponsored studies to report the generalizability of the findings, including being more likely: to include information about how the data could be extrapolated to other clinical settings (58% vs 35%), to include statements on the statistical significance of the findings (38% vs 20%), and to clearly outline the cost per unit and data sources for the cost analyses (67% vs 45%). A similar percentage of pharmaceutical- and nonprofit-sponsored studies reported background and conclusions, as follows: about 89% provided literature comparisons of the results and discussed the limitations of the findings (75% for pharmaceutical manufacturer–sponsored and 67% for nonprofit-sponsored studies). Most studies were published in low impact factor, peer-reviewed journals, and journal impact factor scores were similar between pharmaceutical- and nonprofit-sponsored studies. Overall, the study found differences in study reporting, but not in types of journals where studies were published. These results, particularly with respect to differences in generalizability, may account in part for the finding that pharmaceutical manufacturer–sponsored studies were less likely to report unfavorable conclusions.

Strategies for Conducting Economic Analyses in Oncology

Economic assessments are potentially useful as secondary endpoints in clinical trials of new cancer therapies or technologies.[15] These analyses require additional time, effort, and funds. Cost analyses have been proposed alongside pivotal trials or new technologies, when investigational therapies are resource-intensive, or when new technologies or treatments are likely to be used by large numbers of cancer patients. In most cases, these analyses are associated with phase III clinical trials, although inclusion into phase II trials can facilitate collection of pilot data that can assist with study design for phase III trials. Phase IV studies also are possible sources of data for clinical and economic analyses. Estimates of the potential difference in costs between treatment arms should be included in the original study design.

The perspective of the economic analysis varies in many of the reported cost-effectiveness analyses. Most commonly, the perspective is that of the third-party payer. However, many analysts suggest that the societal perspective should be preferred. Many clinical trials report economic data that is based on a "modified" societal perspective—i.e., direct medical costs are quantified as societal costs, while direct nonmedical and productivity costs are not evaluated. Data collection can be prospective or retrospective. Prospective studies allow for timely assessment of clinical and economic outcomes at the end of the study. Detailed information on direct medical, direct nonmedical, productivity, and intangible costs can be obtained if careful planning is done before the study begins. Retrospective economic assessments are far less costly to conduct, but they include information on only a limited perspective (generally the third-party payer perspective). The time horizon in cost-effectiveness analyses alongside clinical trials represents the time interval from randomization to follow-up. The time horizon can influence the findings of the economic analysis, if follow-up is short. Ideally, the time horizon should be the same for the clinical and the economic analysis. The cost analysis is based on a review of final outcomes, which usually is set as survival. These outcomes should be identified prospectively. Despite increasing discussion about methodologies and practical approaches to conducting economic analyses alongside randomized clinical trials, remarkably few of these assessments have been reported in the literature (Tables 21-4 and 21-5). The National Cancer Institute–sponsored Cooperative Trials Groups have reported only one prospective economic analysis alongside clinical trials and six retrospective economic analyses.[24-30]

Conducting economic studies alongside clinical trials requires targeted funding, a large staff, and cooperation between clinical and economic analysts. Cost data should be considered as important as clinical data, and should be subjected to quality control assessments. The pharmaceutical industry has supported most of the economic analyses conducted to date. U.S. Healthcare funded the economic assessment of the autologous stem cell transplant studies for breast cancer, but the economic findings were not reported after the clinical trial results were reported as negative. A third option is the use of cancer control credits, similar to strategies used for quality-of-life studies. This option has not been implemented successfully in the cooperative group setting. Overall, most of the literature related to cost analyses in cancer has been based on retrospective assessments of clinical trials, and these retrospective reviews generally have been funded by the pharmaceutical industry.

Economic Analyses Conducted by Cancer Clinical Trials Groups

During the 1990s the NCI supported efforts to integrate economic analyses into cancer clinical trials.[15,16] In 1994, the NCI sponsored a conference with representatives of cancer centers and cooperative groups that addressed the importance, appropriateness, and complexity of these evaluations. In 1995, the American Society of Clinical

TABLE 21-4

Proposed Economic Analyses to Be Conducted by NCI-sponsored Clinical Trials Groups

STUDY	TREATMENT ARMS	EFFECTIVENESS TIMEFRAME	COSTS	RECOMMENDATION	OUTCOME
Gynecologic Oncology Group	Whole abdominal radiation therapy vs doxorubicin–cisplatin	Years (survival)	Years	Probably should not complete	Not done
National Wilms' Tumor Study	Intensive vs standard chemotherapy regimen with dactinomycin + doxorubicin	Years (2-year relapse-free survival and overall survival)	Years	Model treatment costs; toxicity costs not evaluated, because hospital days were similar for each arm	Buxton* (modeling effort)
Southwest Oncology Group	GCSF vs placebo for older patients with acute myeloid leukemia	Months (survival, complete remission)	Months	Cost-effectiveness or cost-utility study	Bennett et al[27] (cost-minimization)
Cancer and Leukemia Group B	High-dose chemotherapy with autologous bone marrow vs lower-dose chemotherapy for advanced breast cancer	Years	Years	Measure long-term costs	Clinical trial was negative
Cancer and Leukemia Group B proposed study	Laparoscopic vs open colectomy for colon cancer	Weeks	Weeks	Measure quality of life, operative and perioperative costs	In progress
Eastern Cooperative Oncology Group	Cisplatin + etoposide vs cisplatin + paclitaxel for advanced non–small cell lung cancer	Months	Months	Measure costs	Not done
VA Prostate Intervention vs Observation Trial (PIVOT)	Radical prostatectomy vs observation for localized prostate cancer	Years	Years	Study will be too difficult to conduct	Not done

*Buxton MJ: National Wilms' Tumor Study: Economic perspective. J Natl Cancer Inst Monogr 1995;19:27–29.

TABLE 21-5

Completed Economic Analyses Conducted by NCI-sponsored Clinical Trials Groups

STUDY	TREATMENT ARMS	EFFECTIVENESS TIMEFRAME	ECONOMIC TIMEFRAME	METHOD	OUTCOME
Southwest Oncology Group 9509	Vinorelbine + cisplatin vs paclitaxel + carboplatin for non–small cell lung cancer	Months	24 months	Cost-minimization	Cisplatin + vinorelbine is less costly (Ramsey et al, 2002[24])
Southwest Oncology Group 9031	GCSF vs placebo for adults with AML	Weeks	Weeks	Cost-minimization	GCSF did not add additional costs, and decreased hospital stay (Bennett et al, 2001[27])
Eastern Cooperative Oncology Group 1490	GM-CSF vs placebo for older adults with AML	Weeks	Weeks	Cost-minimization	GM-CSF was cost saving, and decreased infections (Bennett[29])
Pediatrics Oncology Group	GCSF vs control for children with leukemia	Weeks	Weeks	Cost-miminization	G-CSF did not add additional costs, and was associated with shortened duration of neutropenia (Bennett et al, 2000[30])
Children's Cancer Study Group	GCSF vs placebo for children with leukemia	Weeks	Weeks	Cost-minimization	G-CSF did not add additional costs, and was associated with shortened duration of neutropenia (Pui et al, 1997[26])
Radiation Therapy Oncology Group 90-03 and 91-04	Brain metastases; head and neck cancer	Not measured	Months	Cost estimation	90-03 costs estimated well; 91-04 costs not estimated very well (Owen et al, 2001[31])
Children's Cancer Study Group 1881, 1882, 1891, 1901, 1922, 1941	Acute leukemia–various treatments	Years	Months	Cost-effectiveness	Delayed intensification, augmented therapy, and dexamethasone therapy cost-effective vs treatment of first relapse (Gaynon et al, 2001[25])

AML, acute myelogenous leukemia; GCSF, granulocyte colony-stimulating factor; GM-CSF, granulocyte macrophage colony-stimulating factor.

Oncology (ASCO) established a Health Outcomes Working Group, which was charged with developing specific guidelines for implementing economic evaluations in cancer clinical trials.[16] In 1996, the NCI and ASCO convened a second meeting to consider the practical implementation of economic evaluation in cancer clinical trials. This meeting was attended by experts from the NCI-sponsored cooperative groups, NCI staff, and experts in the field of health economics. In 1998, a workbook that served as a developing guide designed to be used as practical reference for subsequent economic analyses of cancer clinical trials was published.[15] Subsequent to the publication of the workbook, the first articles describing economic analyses alongside clinical trials conducted by the NCI sponsored cooperative groups were published.

The first cost-effectiveness study of an NCI-sponsored cooperative group trial was reported in 1997 by investigators who were affiliated with the Children's Cancer Study Group.[26] The clinical trial evaluated the clinical and cost-effectiveness of granulocyte colony-stimulating factor as an adjunctive therapy for children with acute lymphoblastic leukemia. The study randomized 164 children and found a reduction in the duration of neutropenia (5.3 versus 12.7 days) and duration of hospitalization (6 versus 10 days). Cost-minimization

analyses indicated that GCSF did not add additional costs. Clinical and economic data were obtained directly from the clinical trial participants.

The second cost-effectiveness study of an NCI-sponsored cooperative group trial was reported in 1999 by investigators who were affiliated with the Eastern Cooperative Oncology Group.[29] The clinical trial, the ECOG 1490 study, was an FDA licensing study that evaluated the clinical effectiveness of the hematopoietic cytokine, granulocyte macrophage colony-stimulating factor (GM-CSF), as an adjunctive therapy for persons 55 years of age or older who were receiving induction chemotherapy for acute myeloid leukemia. The study randomized 119 patients to receive GM-CSF or placebo and found a 72% reduction in severe infections, four fewer days with an absolute neutrophil count lower than 500 cells/mL, but no significant difference in the duration of hospitalization. Decision analytic modeling was used to analyze the costs of GM-CSF use during induction therapy. Clinical probabilities of acquiring an infection were obtained from the clinical trial data. Economic data on hospital costs per day for infected and uninfected patients were obtained from billing data from seven sites that participated in the clinical trial. The significant improvements in rates of severe infections were associated with an estimated $2310 in cost savings per patient. The reduction in costs was particularly evident among individuals who received two cycles of induction chemotherapy. The study design and operations were efficient. Because the clinical data were submitted to the FDA in support of a licensing application, the clinical data base was obtained directly from the pharmaceutical manufacturer of GM-CSF. Most of the costs for the economic analyses were accounted for by obtaining resource and cost data. The study was conducted over a 6-month period, with funding for the study provided by the pharmaceutical manufacturer.

In 2000, an economic analysis of a clinical trial conducted by the former Pediatrics Oncology Group was published.[30] A retrospective analysis compared the costs of inpatient supportive care for pediatric patients with T-cell leukemia and advanced lymphoblastic lymphoma. Patients ranging from 1 to 22 years of age were randomized to receive either GCSF (n = 45) or no GCSF (n = 43) following induction and two cycles of maintenance therapy. There were no significant differences in neutropenia-related outcomes during the induction phase. During maintenance therapy, the patients receiving GCSF had significantly fewer days to an absolute neutrophil count above 500 cells/μL and a trend toward fewer days of hospitalization. The study found that the total median costs of supportive care were similar for patients receiving GCSF versus those who did not. This study also was conducted in an efficient manner. Data on resource utilization were tabulated from case report forms. Costs were derived from national data on hospitalization costs, average wholesale prices of pharmaceuticals, and patient billing information from a single institution. The study was conducted over a 4-month period, with support from the Cooperative Clinical Trial Group and the pharmaceutical supplier of the study drug.

Another cost-effectiveness study from an NCI cooperative trial group, reported in 2001, evaluated GCSF as part of a clinical trial of older patients with acute myelogenous leukemia who received induction chemotherapy.[27] The clinical trial, conducted by the Southwest Oncology Group (SWOG), randomized 207 patients 56 years of age or older to receive GCSF or placebo. Clinical findings indicated no significant difference in infections and in days of hospitalization between treatment arms, but three fewer days with an absolute neutrophil count below 500 cells/mL (see Table 21-2). A decision analytic model was used to estimate the costs of GCSF use. Estimates of costs per day for patients hospitalized with or without an active infection requiring parenteral antibiotics were derived from patient billing records. Clinical probabilities of infections were obtained from the clinical trial database. The improvement in the duration of absolute neutropenia, infection, and antibiotic use was accompanied by only an increase of only $120 per patient in total costs in the GCSF arm. This study, conducted by the same economic analysts who reported the ECOG study, also was efficient. The study design and methods were modeled after those used in the ECOG study. Clinical data were obtained directly from the final study report.

The cost data were taken from previously derived estimates that had been reported in the ECOG study. The entire study was conducted over a 3-month period, without funding from the pharmaceutical supplier, the NCI, or SWOG.

In 2001, the Radiation Therapy Oncology Group (RTOG) addressed the issue of economic analyses alongside cooperative group clinical trials.[31] An initial pilot study addressed four aims: (1) measurement of radiation therapy treatment costs for patients treated in different arms of two randomized controlled clinical trials; (2) comparison of measured costs to those predicted by an economic model; (3) examination of the distribution of costs among patients treated on the same arm; and (4) assessment of the feasibility of retrospective data collection effort. The RTOG selected two phase III clinical trials to evaluate in this pilot effort. The first study, RTOG 91-04, compared standard treatment to a total dose of 30 Gy with a second arm of accelerated hyperfractionation to a total dose of 54.4 Gy for cancer patients with brain metastases. The second study, RTOG 90-03, was a phase III study of patients with squamous cell carcinomas of the head and neck who received either standard fractionation to a dose of 70 Gy, hyperfractionation to a dose of 81.6 Gy, accelerated fractionation with a split to a total dose of 67.2 Gy, and accelerated fractionation with a concomitant boost to a total dose of 72 Gy. Expected quantities of procedure codes and relative value units (RVUs) associated with Medicare billing efforts were modeled. The median and mean RVUs were within the range predicted by an economic model for all arms of the head and neck cancer study, but were above the predicted range for the brain cancer study. Some of the study institutions had significant difficulties collecting the retrospective economic data, suggesting that prospective data collection may be the better strategy for economic analysis of RTOG studies. Clinical trials with complex treatment protocols, such as the head and neck cancer study, appeared particularly difficult to include in retrospective economic analytic efforts.

In 2001, researchers affiliated with the former Children's Cancer Study Group reported on the feasibility of using duration of hospitalization as a surrogate for cost and event-free survival as a measure of effectiveness to estimate cost-effectiveness ratios of various treatment regimens evaluated in clinical trials of children with acute lymphoblastic leukemia.[25] Marginal cost-effectiveness estimates of 133 days per patient for delayed intensification, 117 days for double delayed intensification, and 41 days for augmented therapy were derived. Relapse-adjusted marginal costs were 68 days per patient for delayed intensification, 52 days for double-dose intensification, and a savings of 16 days with augmented therapy and 82 days with dexamethasone-based therapy. The clinical analyses included 4986 children between 2 and 21 years old who had participated in clinical trials between 1988 and 1995, which provided the data on durations of hospitalization and clinical outcomes. The cost-effectiveness models were based on cohorts with 100 patients. The study was supported by grants to the office of the cooperative group's chairman and indicated that

Science of Clinical Oncology

retrospective economic analyses were feasible, providing that the economic analyses focused on duration of hospitalization.

In 2002, researchers affiliated with the Southwest Oncology Group reported the results of the first prospective economic analysis of a randomized clinical trial conducted by an NCI-sponsored cooperative clinical trial group.[24] The clinical trial included patients who were randomized to receive cisplatin plus vinorelbine versus carboplatin plus paclitaxel. The cost analysis included detailed information on both protocol and nonprotocol lung cancer–related health care expenditures for 24 months after the initiation of therapy.[24] Nationally standardized costs were applied to each resource use. Multivariate regression was used to evaluate lifetime expenditures and 95% confidence intervals. The analyses found similar survival and quality of life outcomes for the two study arms, while mean costs were $40,292 for the cisplatin/vinorelbine arm versus $48,940 for the carboplatin/paclitaxel arm. The cost differences were attributed primarily to higher costs of both chemotherapy and medical procedures for the cisplatin/vinorelbine treatment arm. The study was supported by unrestricted grants from pharmaceutical companies whose products were being compared in the clinical trial. The study indicated that prospective economic analyses could be conducted alongside randomized clinical trials, although these efforts did require external funding and committed resources from the statistical operations center of the cooperative clinical trial group.

As a group, the first set of economic analyses of cooperative group clinical trials were published between 1997 and 2002. The studies were based primarily on retrospective economic analyses, with the exception of one study by the Southwest Oncology Group. Funding sources were diverse, with most of the analytic efforts being supported by pharmaceutical suppliers. In one case, the office of the chairman of the cooperative group funded the study. The reports are real-life examples of the methods and operational considerations addressed in two conferences conducted by ASCO and the NCI in the 1990s.

CONCLUSIONS

Costs of cancer care can be evaluated in a variety of clinical settings. Economic considerations have important practical implications for oncologists, and should be addressed for most new cancer treatments and procedures. Continuing economic pressures facing the health care system in the United States serve as an important reminder of the importance of unbiased cost analyses, particularly for cancer treatments. Despite nearly universal support for economic information, the paucity of cost-effectiveness analyses, especially studies that are not funded by the pharmaceutical industry, is particularly worrisome. Policymakers and physicians strive to make informed decisions about rational allocations of cancer resources. Economic data, if properly obtained, can assist with these decisions.

REFERENCES

1. Brown ML, Lipscomb J, Snyder C: The burden of illness of cancer: economic cost and quality of life. Annu Rev Pub Health 2001;22: 91–113.
2. Brown ML, Riley GF, Schusser N, Etzoni R: Estimating health care costs related to cancer treatment from SEER-Medicare data. Medical Care 2002;40S:IV-104–IV-117.
3. Schulman KA, Glick HA, Yabroff R, Eisenberg JM: Introduction to clinical economics: assessment of cancer therapies. J Natl Cancer Inst Monogr 1995;19:1–9.
4. Calhoun EA, Chang C-H, Welshman E, Fishman DA, Lurain JR, Bennett CL: Evaluating the total costs of chemotherapy-induced neutropenia: results from a pilot study with ovarian cancer patients. Oncologist 2001;6:441–445.
5. Calhoun EA, Bennett CL: Evaluating the total costs of cancer: the Northwestern University Costs of Cancer Program. Oncology 2003;17:109–114.
6. Wagner JL, Alberts SR, Sloan JA, et al: Incremental costs of enrolling patients in clinical trials: A population based study. J Natl Cancer Inst 1999; 91:847–853 (erratum: J Natl Cancer Inst 2000;92: 164–165).
7. Fireman BH, Fehrenbacher L, Gruskin EP, Ray GT: Cost of care for patients in cancer clinical trials. J Natl Cancer Inst 2000;92: 136–142.
8. Barlow WS, Taplin D, Seger J, et al: Medical care costs of cancer patients on protocol. Presented at the NCI Meeting, Bethesda, MD: July 7, 1998. Summarized in Institute of Medicine: Extending Medicare Reimbursement in Clinical Trials. Washington, DC: National Academy Press, 2000).
9. Bennett CL, Stinson TJ, Vogel V, et al: Evaluating the financial impact of clinical trials in oncology: results from a pilot study from the Association of American Cancer Institutes/Northwestern University Clinical Trials Costs and Charges Project. J Clin Oncol 2000;18: 2805–2810.
10. Quirk J, Schrag D, Radzyner M, et al: Clinical trial costs are similar to and may be less than standard care and inpatient charges at an academic medical center are similar to major, minor, and non-teaching hospitals. Proc Am Soc Clin Oncol 2000;19:433a.
11. Bennett CL, Adams JR, Knox KS, Kelahan AM, Silver SM, Bailes JS: Clinical trials: Are they a good buy? J Clin Oncol 2001;19: 4330–4339.
12. Goldman DP, Berry SH, McCabe MH, et al: Incremental costs in National Cancer Institute sponsored clinical trials. JAMA 2003;289:2970–2977.
13. Aaron HJ, Gelband H (eds): Institute of Medicine Institute Report: Extending Medicare Reimbursement in Clinical Trials. Washington, DC: National Academy Press, 2000.
14. US General Accounting Office: NIH Clinical Trials: Various Factors Affect Patient Participation. Washington, DC: US General Accounting Office, 1999. Publication No. GAO/HEHS-99-1821.
15. Brown M, McCabe M, Schulman KA: Integrating economic analysis into cancer clinical trials: the National Cancer Institute–American Society of Clinical Oncology Economics Workbook. J Natl Cancer Inst Monogr 1998;24:1–84.
16. Schulman KA, Glick HA, Yabroff R, Eisenberg JM: Introduction to clinical economics: assessment of cancer therapies. J Natl Cancer Inst Monogr 1995;19:1–9.
17. Finkler SA: The distinction between cost and charges. Ann Intern Med 1982;96:102–109.
18. Warren JL, Brown ML, Fay MP, et al: Costs of treatment for elderly women with early stage breast cancer in fee-for-service settings. J Clin Oncol 2001;20:307–316.
19. Gold MR, Siegal JE, Russel LB, Weinstein MC (eds): Cost-effectiveness in health and medicine. New York: Oxford University Press, 1996.
20. Chiou CF, Hay JW, Wallace JF, et al: Development and validation of a grading system for the quality of cost-effectiveness studies. Med Care 2003;41:32–44.
21. Friedberg M, Saffran B, Stinson TJ, Nelson W, Bennett CL: Evaluation of conflict of interest in economic analyses of new drugs used in oncology. JAMA 1999;282:1453–1457.
22. Knox KS, Adams JR, Djulbegovic B, Stinson TJ, Bennett CL: Quality

and dissemination of industry sponsored economic analyses of six novel drugs used in oncology. Ann Oncol 2000;11:1591-1595.

23. Azimi NA, Welch G: The effectiveness of cost-effectiveness analysis in containing costs. J Gen Intern Med 1998;13:664-669.

24. Ramsey SD, Moinpour CM, Lovato LC, et al: Economic analysis of vinorelbine plus cisplatin versus paclitaxel plus carboplatin for advanced non-small cell lung cancer. J Natl Cancer Inst 2002;94:291-297.

25. Gaynon PS, Bostrom BC, Hutchinson RJ, et al : Duration of hospitalization as a measure of cost on Children's Cancer Group acute lymphoblastic leukemia studies. J Clin Oncol 2001;19: 1916-1925.

26. Pui CH, Boyett JM, Hughes WT, et al: Human granulocyte colony stimulating factor after induction chemotherapy in children with acute lymphoblastic leukemia. N Engl J Med 1997;336:1781-1787.

27. Bennett CL, Hynes D, Godwin J, Stinson TJ, Golub RM, Appelbaum FR, Southwest Oncology Group: Economic analysis of granulocyte colony stimulating as adjunct therapy for older patients with acute myelogenous leukemia (AML): estimates from a Southwest Oncology Group clinical trial. Cancer Investigation 2001; 9:603-610.

28. Bennett CL, Golub R, Waters TM, Tallman MS, Rowe JM: Economic analyses of phase III cooperative cancer group clinical trials: are they feasible? Cancer Investigation 1997;15:227-236.

29. Bennett CL, Stinson TJ, Tallman MS, et al: Economic analysis of a randomized placebo-controlled phase III study of granulocyte macrophage colony stimulating factor in adult patients (>55 to 70 years of age) with acute myelogenous leukemia. Eastern Cooperative Oncology Group (E1490). Ann Oncol 1999;10:177-182.

30. Bennett CL, Stinson TJ, Lane D, Amylon M, Land VJ, Laver JH: A cost-analysis of filgrastim for the prevention of neutropenia in pediatric T-cell leukemia and advanced lymphoma: a case for prospective economic analysis in cooperative group trials. Med Pediatr Oncol 2000;34:92-96.

31. Owen JB, Grigsby PW, Caldwell TM, et al: Can costs be measured and predicted by modeling within a cooperative clinical trials group: economic methodologic pilot studies of the Radiation Therapy Oncology Group studies 90-03 and 91-04. Int J Radiat Oncol Biol Phys 2001;49:633-639.

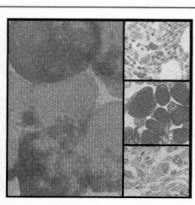

EPIDEMIOLOGY AND POPULATION SCIENCES

Kathy J. Helzlsouer

Kala Visvanathan

SUMMARY OF KEY POINTS

MEASURES OF RATES AND RISKS

- Cancer incidence is the number of new cases occurring in a population at risk for the disease over a specified period of time, usually 1 year. The cancer incidence rate is the measure of absolute risk of the disease.
- The annual cancer mortality rate is the number of deaths from cancer in 1 year per the population at risk during that period.
- Odds ratios and relative risks are measures of associations used to determine whether or not a characteristic is associated with a disease. The odds ratio is the odds that those with the disease were exposed compared to the odds that those without the disease were exposed. Odds ratios are the measure of association calculated in case-control studies. Relative risk is the ratio of the incidence (or mortality) rate in the exposed group to the incidence (or mortality) in the unexposed group. Relative risks and odds ratios can be calculated in prospective studies.

- The relative survival rate is the observed survival in people with the disease compared to the expected survival in the absence of the disease.

STUDY DESIGNS USED IN CLINICAL RESEARCH

- Case-control studies (retrospective) identify individuals with the disease (cases) and individuals without the disease (controls) and then compare the two groups on the proportion exposed and unexposed to the factors of interest. Controls should come from the same source population from which the cases arose. Population-based studies identify cases and controls from a well-defined region.
- Cohort studies (prospective studies) define groups according to an exposure and follow them for the development of disease. Cohort studies have the advantage of obtaining information on the exposure of interest prior to disease onset. Thus the presence of the disease does not influence the assessment of the exposure.

- Randomized controlled clinical trials compare the intervention to either a placebo or standard treatment using a process called randomization to make the treatment assignments.
- All of these study designs are subject to bias in their design and conduct. The highest-quality studies minimize potential biases in their design. All of these study designs are considered in evidence-based approaches to establishing clinical intervention guidelines.

TRANSLATING KNOWLEDGE TO CLINICAL PRACTICE: THE EVIDENCE-BASED APPROACH

- The U.S. Preventive Services Task Force and the Canadian Task Force on Preventive Health Care apply an evidence-based approach in making guidelines and recommendations regarding prevention and screening interventions.
- Evidence-based approaches consider the quality and strength of the evidence for both benefit and harms associated with an intervention.

INTRODUCTION

A question often asked by patients who have been diagnosed with cancer is "Why? What could have caused this?" Sometimes the question may be more specific: "Do you think the chemical I was exposed to contributed to this?" To answer these questions, the clinician should have an understanding of the etiology of cancer. Knowing the etiology also is the first step toward preventing cancer. Searching for the clues for cancer prevention, evaluating the success of interventions, and implementing the effective interventions in practice are accomplished using the tools of epidemiologic research. These tools range from ecological studies using available data on groups or populations to generate hypotheses to analytical studies such as case-control, cohort (prospective) studies, and clinical trials to test hypotheses. The knowledge gained

from these types of studies is used to determine the causes of cancer, select potential prevention intervention strategies, and then test them for efficacy and effectiveness. Epidemiology is the science underpinning clinical research and practice.

The logarithmic expansion of information on prevention, early detection, treatment, and prognosis of cancer requires a working knowledge of the principles of clinical research in order to evaluate new management approaches effectively and efficiently and determine which should be applied in the clinical setting. This chapter reviews the methods currently used for studying the etiology and prevention of cancer, reviews guidelines for determining what is a cause of cancer, and explains how the evidence is weighed to evaluate the effectiveness of specific interventions and their application in the clinical setting.

One of the first steps in answering the patient's question "Why did I get cancer?" is to examine the rates of cancer incidence and mortality. Is a specific cancer becoming more common? What changes may explain the change in rates? The approach of correlating disease rates with other factor trends, called *ecological studies*, serves to generate hypotheses to be tested in more rigorous study designs. For example, the increase in endometrial cancer rates in the 1970s was observed to coincide with an increasing rate of prescription of estrogen replacement therapy.[1] Further investigations confirmed that unopposed estrogen therapy caused an increased risk of endometrial cancer. Additional clinical studies have shown that adding progestin therapy eliminated the risk.[2] A change in rates of a specific cancer lead to the question of "Why?," and in this case the answer resulted in a strategy for prevention. Sometimes astute clinical observations provide clues to the etiology of cancer. It was a clinician's observation of occurrences of clear cell adenocarcinoma of the cervix, an unusual type of cervical cancer, that led to the discovery of the effect of in utero exposure to diethylstilbestrol (DES) on cancer and other health outcomes.[3]

Proving the link between an exposure and disease relies on information from well-designed and well-conducted observational studies. Further proof for a preventive factor comes from randomized clinical trials evaluating the efficacy of the intervention in lowering the risk of the disease. The evidence-based approach to clinical practice and formulating policies relies on weighing the evidence from multiple sources, with the greatest weight placed on clinical trials and population-based studies. This chapter discusses these study designs in the context of the evidence-based approach for clinical decision making that serves as the foundation for the art of medicine.

RATES AND RISK

Clues to the etiology of cancer often come from observing changes in rates of the disease over time. Examining trends in the incidence and mortality of cancer also can indicate whether prevention or treatment interventions are having an impact in the population. The incidence rates also provide an absolute risk or probability of cancer for the general population. To identify specific risk factors associated with cancer, other measures of risk, such as the relative risk, are needed. The measures or rates and risk are summarized in Table 22-1 and are described in the following paragraphs.

Cancer incidence is the number of new cases occurring in a population at risk for the disease over a specified period of time, usually 1 year. It usually is expressed as the number of cases per 100,000 population. For childhood cancers that are very rare compared to adult cancers, the number of cases usually is expressed per 1,000,000 population. Incidence rates can be calculated by sex, specific age groups, or race. For these specific rates, both the numerator and the denominator must be derived from the same restricted group.[4]

The annual cancer mortality rate is the number of deaths from cancer in 1 year per the population at risk during that period. Like cancer incidence rates, it usually is reported as the number per 100,000 population. Also like incidence rates, specific mortality rates, such as age- or sex-specific rates, can be calculated. In the United States, cause-specific mortality rates have been available for the entire population since 1930. Because these data are available and because it is thought that mortality rates are less subject to errors in classifying, these rates are

TABLE 22-1

Summary of Rates and Risk Measures

MEASUREMENT	DERIVATION
Annual cancer incidence rate	No. of new cases of a disease occurring in the population during 1 year divided by no. of persons at risk of developing the disease during that period of time per 100,000 population
Annual cancer mortality rate	No. of deaths due to cancer in the population during 1 year divided by no. of persons in the population at the midyear per 100,000
Lifetime risk of being diagnosed with cancer or dying from cancer	Calculated by applying cross-sectional age-specific cancer incidence rates (or mortality rates) to a hypothetical birth cohort of 10,000,000 individuals, taking into account deaths from other causes
Relative risk	Incidence in the exposed group divided by incidence in the nonexposed group
Relative odds (odds ratio)	Odds that those with the disease (cases) were exposed divided by odds that those without the disease (controls) were exposed
Observed survival	Proportion of cancer patients surviving (for a specified time)
Relative survival rate	Observed survival in people with cancer divided by expected survival if cancer were absent (for a specified time)
Prevalence—point prevalence	Number of cases of cancer present in the population at a specified time divided by number of persons in the population at that time
Period (partial prevalence)	Number of individuals in a population with the disease during a certain period.

Data from Gordis L: Epidemiology. Philadelphia, WB Saunders, 1996; and Ries LAG, Eisner MP, Kosary CL, et al (eds): SEER Cancer Statistics Review, 1975–2000. Bethesda, MD, National Cancer Institute; http://seer.cancer.gov/csr/1975_2000, 2003.

TABLE 22-2

Percent Diagnosed with All Cancers and Cancers of Selected Sites in 10-, 20-, and 30-Year Intervals and in Remaining Lifetime

	FOR 30-YEAR-OLDS				FOR 60-YEAR-OLDS			
	+10 YRS	+20 YRS	+30 YRS	EVENTUALLY	+10 YRS	+20 YRS	+30 YRS	EVENTUALLY
All Sites								
Men	0.72	2.57	8.57	46.34	15.91	33.92	43.70	45.63
Women	1.20	4.19	10.05	38.99	10.59	22.61	31.30	33.70
Lung and Bronchus								
Men	0.03	0.21	1.03	8.02	2.50	5.80	7.63	7.93
Women	0.03	0.18	0.81	5.90	1.71	3.93	5.25	5.49
Breast cancer (women)	0.40	1.83	4.49	13.72	3.81	7.53	9.81	10.36
Prostate cancer (men)	0.01	0.22	2.25	17.89	6.71	14.20	17.53	18.11

Data from Ries LAG, Eisner MP, Kosary CL, et al (eds): SEER Cancer Statistics Review, 1975–2000. Bethesda, MD, National Cancer Institute; http://seer.cancer.gov/csr/1975_2000, 2003

considered to be the best measure to use for gauging progress in the "war against cancer."[5-7]

Incidence and mortality rates are equivalent to the absolute risk of the disease. The absolute risks of developing cancer in the United States, by sex, race, and age groups, are published annually by the Surveillance Epidemiology and End Results (SEER) Program.[8] Examples of the probability of being diagnosed with cancer for two age groups, persons aged 30 and those aged 60, are shown in Table 22-2. The table shows the probability of being diagnosed with cancer over 10, 20, or 30 years, or eventually (i.e., at some point during the person's life), by age group and sex. For example, a 30-year-old man has a 0.72% risk of being diagnosed with cancer of any type in the next 10 years; the 10-year risk for a 60-year-old man is 15.91%. This demonstrates that the risk of getting cancer increases dramatically with age; the median age of diagnosis for all cancers in the United States is 68 years for men and 65 years for women.[8] For an average 30-year-old woman, the risk of developing breast cancer by the age of 60 is 4.49%; an average 60-year-old woman has a 10-year risk of 3.81% and an eventual risk of 10.36%. The probability of dying from cancer eventually is much lower than the probability of getting cancer: the lifetime risk of being diagnosed with any cancer is 45% for men and 39% for women, whereas the probability of dying from any cancer is 24% for men and 20% for women.[8] The age-specific and lifetime risks for developing cancer are based on the population risks and thus reflect an average absolute risk.

More refined estimates can be made by taking into account specific factors that influence an individual's risk of developing cancer. These models allow more refined risks to be given to an individual based on his or her specific risk factor profile and may be useful in clinical decision making. For example, the Gail model is a statistical model for predicting the risk of developing breast cancer taking into account age as well as other risk factors for breast cancer.[9] Using the Gail model, a 50-year-old woman whose mother had breast cancer and who had menarche at age 10, first birth at age 24, and a breast biopsy showing atypical hyperplasia falls into a group with a 5-year risk of 5.4% and a lifetime risk of 40%.[9] Compared to women without any risk factors, whose lifetime risk is 6.9%, or the general population risk of 11.9%, she falls into a high-risk group and the use of chemopreventive agents such as the selective estrogen receptor modulators could be considered.[10]

The absolute risk associated with a specific factor or exposure indicates the magnitude of the risk of developing cancer but does not indicate whether or not that factor is associated with the development of the disease. Determining whether or not the characteristic is a risk factor requires comparison of risks of disease in both the presence and absence of the characteristics being examined.

To determine whether or not a characteristic is associated with a disease, some measure of that association is needed. One such measure is relative risk (see Table 22-1). The relative risk compares the absolute risk of the disease in the exposed group to the absolute risk in the unexposed group. If this ratio is greater than 1—that is, the disease occurs more frequently in the exposed group—it is a risk factor. The greater the relative risk, the stronger the association with the exposure. If the relative risk is less than 1, the exposure is associated with a lower risk of developing the disease. Relative risks are calculated directly from cohort studies, which are prospective study designs that follow individuals, both exposed and unexposed to the factor or factors of interest, for disease occurrence. Odds ratios are estimates of the relative risk and are the measure of association used in case-control studies.

The survival rate is the number of individuals surviving for a specified time after diagnosis. Observed survival time measures the number of individuals surviving for a specified time after diagnosis regardless of the cause of death.[8] Relative survival rates are more often used in reporting cancer survival times. Relative survival rates compare the observed survival to that expected in the

Science of Clinical Oncology

1

ESTIMATION OF RISK/BENEFIT FROM CHEMOPREVENTION OF BREAST CANCER

A 42-year-old woman presents for evaluation of her risk of breast cancer and discussion of management options. She is Caucasian and premenopausal. Menarche occurred at the age of 12, and her first child was born when she was 28. Her mother had breast cancer, but there is no other family history of breast or other cancers on the maternal or paternal side of the family. She has had two breast biopsies, and neither has shown signs of atypical hyperplasia.

Because her family history is not suggestive of an inherited predisposition to cancer, it is appropriate to use the Gail model[1] to estimate her risk of breast cancer.[2] Use of this model leads to the findings that her risk of developing breast cancer over the next 5 years is 3.5%, and her risk to age 90 is 28.3%. The average 5-year and lifetime risks for her age group in the general population are 0.7% and 12.2%.

In discussing her risk she is told that out of 100 women with characteristics similar to hers, 28 eventually will go on to get breast cancer compared to 12 among women in the average risk group. Looking at it another way, 72 out of 100 women with characteristics similar to hers would not develop breast cancer. Because her 5-year risk is greater than the 1.7% risk used as the eligibility criteria in the Breast Cancer Prevention Trial, she is considered to be at high risk. The recommendations are to counsel women about

chemoprevention against breast cancer with selective estrogen receptor modifiers.[3] The Breast Cancer Prevention trial showed a 49% reduction in the risk of getting invasive breast cancer for women on tamoxifen versus those on placebo. Tamoxifen is approved for reducing the risk of breast cancer and can be used in premenopausal women.

Following the discussion of the potential risks and benefits of tamoxifen,[1] she raises concerns about the known side effects, including menopausal symptoms, risk of blood clots, and especially the risk of endometrial cancer. She decides against taking tamoxifen now but may change her mind if she must undergo another breast biopsy. She will continue screening with mammography and will revisit her decision about the use of chemoprevention in the future.

1. Gail MH, Constantino JP, Bryant J, et al: Weighing the risks and benefits of tamoxifen treatment for preventing breast cancer. J Natl Cancer Inst 1999;91:1829–1846. [Erratum in J Natl Cancer Inst 2000;92:275.]
2. National Cancer Institute Breast Cancer Risk Assessment Tool. Available at http://bcra.nci.nih.gov/brc/.
3. Breast Cancer—Chemoprevention. U.S. Preventive Services Task Force Update, 2002. Available at http://www.ahrq.gov/clinic/uspstf/uspsbrpv.htm.

---

absence of cancer. Thus it takes into account deaths from other causes.[8] This is especially important in older age groups, who have high mortality from other causes such as cardiovascular disease. Relative survival rates always are higher than observed survival rates. Interpretation of survival rates can be difficult, because they may be strongly influenced by methods of detection even if earlier detection does not lead to improved outcomes. For example, an individual may be diagnosed with screening and survive 6 years, but another who presented with clinical symptoms may only survive 4 years. Thus screening appears to extend survival by 2 years. However, it may be that screening only increased the lead time for diagnosis with no change in actual outcome. Thus, had the screened person waited for clinical symptoms to occur, for example, in 2 years, he or she would still have died at the same time and would have been a 4-year survivor from cancer. If not taken into consideration, this difference in lead time may lead to bias in assessment of the efficacy of methods of early detection in some observational study designs. Clinical trials using mortality as the measure of efficacy for a screening test eliminate the potential of lead time to bias the results.[4]

Prevalence of cancer is the number of people with cancer in a population at a specified time divided by the number of people in the population at that time. It is a function of both the incidence of the disease and the survival rate. *Partial* or *period prevalence* defines the number of individuals who have had the disease during a specified time period, for example, the number of individuals with or developing cancer in the past 5 years.[4,11] Prevalence indicates the overall burden of

disease in a population and may be most useful for planning for the availability and distribution of health care resources.

In the United States, cancer incidence, mortality, and survival rates are published annually basis by the SEER program.[8] The SEER program in the United States collects incidence and survival data from five states—Connecticut, Hawaii, Iowa, New Mexico, and Utah; four metropolitan regions—Detroit, Atlanta, San Francisco-Oakland, and Seattle-Puget Sound; Los Angeles County; the San Jose-Monterey area; and the Alaska Native Registry. The program was established in 1973 and is an outgrowth from earlier National Cancer Surveys. The regions in the SEER program are not a representative sampling of the U.S. population, but the registries cover approximately 14% of the U.S. population, include significant representation of minority groups, and provide high-quality data from an active surveillance system. Each year the SEER program publishes the Cancer Statistics Review,[8] which provides an excellent resource for data on cancer incidence and trends in the United States.

Another source for cancer incidence rates in the United States that eventually may cover the entire population is the National Program for Cancer Registries. The Centers for Disease Control and Prevention (CDC) oversees the National Program for Cancer Registries.[12,13] The goals of this program are to improve data collection and quality of data of state cancer registries and to help registries meet national standards established by the CDC regarding completeness, timeliness, and quality of the data. An increasing number of state and territory registries meet the standards necessary to be certified by the North

American Association of Central Cancer Registries,[12,13] and the National Program of Cancer Registries is rapidly approaching full coverage of the U.S. population. A joint report published by the CDC's National Program of Cancer Registries and the SEER program, *U.S Cancer Statistics: 2000 incidence,* covers 84% of the U.S. population (http://www.cdc.gov/cancer/npor/uscs2000/index.htm).

The International Agency for Research on Cancer (IARC) is part of the World Health Organization. Its mission is "to coordinate and conduct research on the causes of human cancer, the mechanisms of carcinogenesis, and to develop scientific strategies for cancer control" (http://www.iarc.fr/). The IARC publishes "Cancer Incidence in Five Continents,"[14] which provides high-quality information on cancer incidence from as many registries as possible worldwide.[11] This is an excellent resource for obtaining worldwide incidence rates. The World Health Organization also publishes a worldwide mortality base.[15]

Cancer Trends

Cancers of the lung, breast, and stomach are the three most commonly occurring cancers worldwide.[11] Because of their high survival rates, breast, colorectal, and prostate cancer are the three most prevalent cancers worldwide (Table 22-3).[11] The distribution of cancer types varies from country to country, and differences are most marked between developed and developing countries. For example, among men in developed countries prostate cancer is the second most common cancer and colorectal cancer the third most common cancer. Among men in developing countries, however, gastric cancer and liver cancer are the second and third most common cancers, after lung cancer. Among women, breast cancer is the most common cancer in developed and developing countries, but cervical cancer is the second most common cancer in developing countries, whereas colorectal, lung, stomach, and endometrial cancers exceed cervical cancer cases in developed countries.[11]

Trends in cancer mortality rates for men and women in the United States are shown in Figure 22-1. Death rates for lung and bronchus cancer in men have been declining for the last decade, after a peak around 1990, suggesting that preventive interventions such as smoking cessation have been effective. For women, the peak in rates came later than for men, with only a recent suggestion of a downturn in lung and bronchus cancer deaths rates. Death rates for cancers of the colon and rectum have declined for both men and women. Breast cancer death rates have declined for women in the last decade. Prostate cancer death rates increased, coinciding with the peak of incidence rates, and recently have declined, also coinciding with a decrease in incidence rates.[8] The acute rise in cancer death rates, preceded by the marked increased in incidence associated with uptake of screening and subsequent dramatic fall in cancer deaths, raises some questions on classification of death due to prostate cancer during this interval in addition to the possible impact of treatment and early detection.[16] Data from the SEER Program and the National Program of Cancer Registries were combined to examine trends in cancer incidence and deaths in the United States and to project future cancer burden. Total cancer incidence was stable from 1995 through 1999, and overall cancer deaths decreased for men and women from 1993 through 1999.[17] Trends in the incidence of specific cancers varied. For example, the incidence of breast cancer continued to increase during this period for women ages 50 to 64, as did prostate cancer for men. Assuming stable incidence rates, the total number of cancer cases in the United States is expected to double by 2050 due to the aging and increasing size of the population.[17]

The most common cancers also have good prospects for lowered risk through primary prevention or secondary prevention efforts with effective screening practices. Lung cancer remains the leading global cancer problem and reflects long-term trends in smoking rates. The most common trend is for rising rates in incidence and mortality, particularly among women in developed countries.[11] However, countries that have instituted strong antitobacco measures have noted marked declines in smoking-associated cancers, particularly lung cancer. Lung cancer deaths in the United Kingdom and Ireland have declined, and the trend is projected to continue.

Breast cancer is the second most common cancer in the world, with incidence rates increasing in developing as well as developed countries. Mortality rates from breast cancer are declining for some countries in North America and Europe, despite continued increases in incidence. This suggests an impact of screening, treatment, or both on improving breast cancer outcomes.

Cervical cancer remains a leading cause of cancer death among women worldwide, with declines in rates in developing countries lagging behind those seen in developed nations.[11] It has been shown that nationwide institution of cervical cancer screening practices is associated with subsequent declines in death from cervical cancer as well as the incidence of invasive forms of cervical cancer.[18] Following trends in invasive cervical cancer incidence and mortality can measure the impact of policies for screening, and, in the near future, the effectiveness of prevention through vaccines against the major cause of cervical cancer, human papillomavirus infection.

Most deaths from stomach cancer occur in developing countries. Rates vary greatly worldwide, but the overall trend is for declining mortality rates. Changes in incidence and mortality from colorectal cancer vary by country.

TABLE 22-3

Leading Causes of Cancer Incidence, Mortality, and Prevalence Worldwide		
INCIDENCE	**MORTALITY**	**PREVALENCE**
Lung	Lung	Breast
Breast	Stomach	Colorectal
Stomach	Liver	Prostate

Data from Parkin DM, Bray FI, Devesa SS: Cancer burden in the year 2000. The global picture. Eur J Cancer 2001; 8:S4–S66.

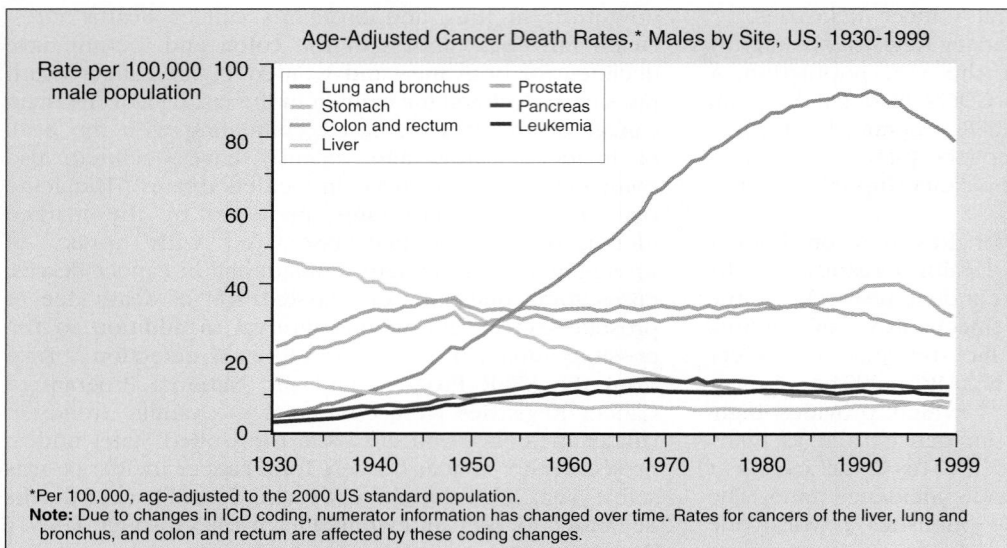

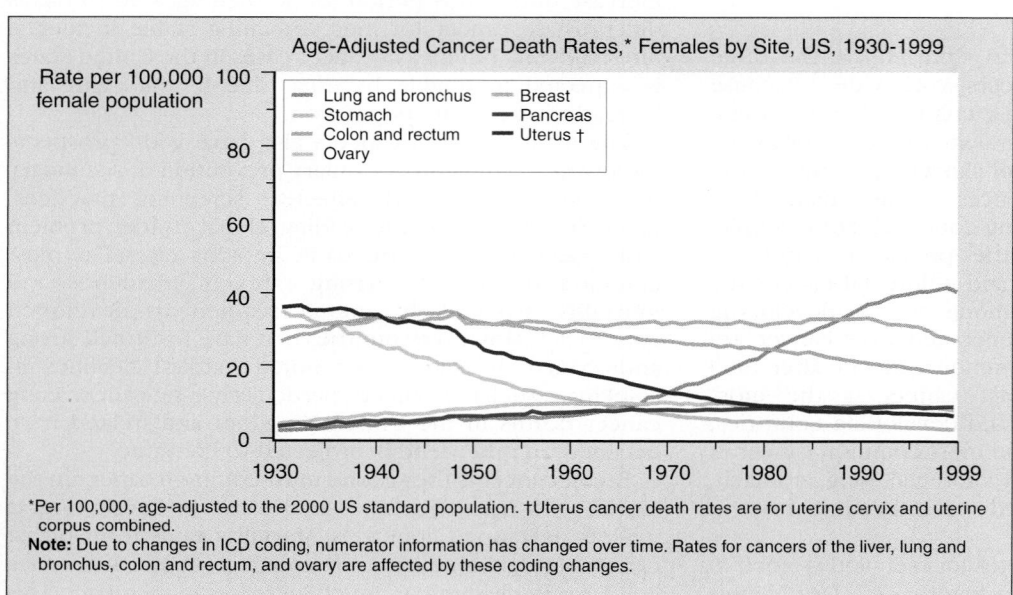

Figure 22-1. A, Age-adjusted cancer death rates in U.S. males per 100,000 population by site of cancer, 1930–1999. **B,** Age-adjusted cancer death rates in U.S. females per 100,000 population by site of cancer, 1930–1999. (From U.S. Mortality Public Use Data Tapes 1960–1999 and U.S. Mortality Volumes 1930–1959, National Center for Health Statistics, Centers for Disease Control and Prevention, 2002. http://www.cancer.org/docroot/STT/SH_O.asp)

Rates in traditionally low-risk countries, such as Japan, have increased markedly, and have been attributed to "westernization" of the diet, whereas rates in the United States have declined. Liver cancer rates may be on the rise, particularly in countries with increasing rates of hepatitis C virus infection.[11]

The rise in prostate cancer rates in a relatively short period indicates the rapid and widespread adoption of measurement of prostate-specific antigen (PSA) concentrations as a screening method (Fig. 22-2). As would be expected with the introduction and then persistence of a screening method, the rapid rise in the incidence of a cancer is followed by a decline to prescreening incidence rates. However, prostate cancer, like breast cancer, has been steadily increasing in incidence in the United States since the 1940s, suggesting changes in other underlying risk factors contributing to a real increase in disease rates. How much PSA screening is contributing to decreases in prostate cancer mortality is controversial. Results of trials to assess the efficacy of PSA testing on prostate cancer mortality are not yet available.[19]

Determining the Risk Factors for Cancer

Understanding the risk factors associated with a specific cancer is the first step in preventing the disease, because it enables us to learn more about the etiology of the disease and to identify high-risk groups who may benefit from interventions to prevent or detect the disease. Risk factors can be broadly divided into those that are

Figure 22-2. A, Age-adjusted incidence rate of prostate cancer reported by the SEER program, 1973–2000. **B,** Age-adjusted mortality rates for prostate cancer in the United States, 1969–2000. (**B,** From http://seer.cancer.gov/faststats/html/mor_prost.html)

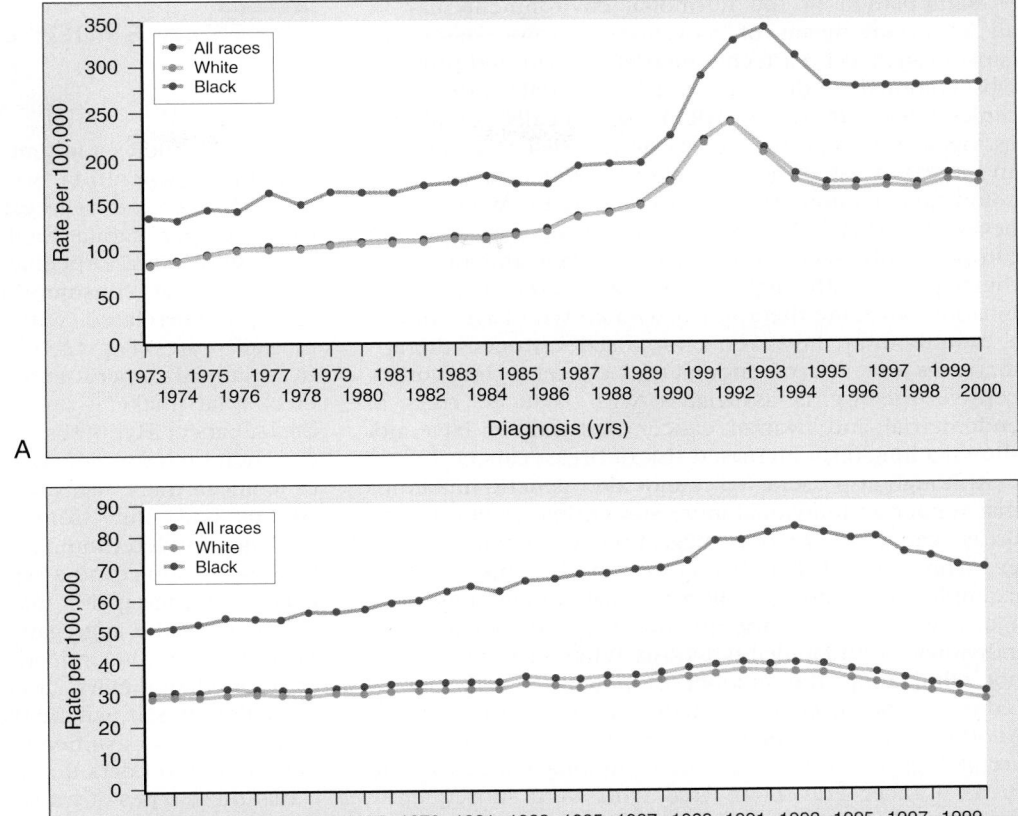

modifiable, including infectious agents, diet, and lifestyle habits, and those that are beyond our control, such as inherited genetic mutations. Focusing on those factors that are modifiable holds the most promise for having an impact on prevention. The following paragraphs present examples of the most common modifiable risk factors associated with cancer.

Tobacco use has been estimated to cause up to 30% of all cancers.[20] In countries where successful tobacco control steps have been undertaken, such as the United Kingdom and Ireland, rates of lung cancer have been decreasing.[11] On the other hand, in developing countries where tobacco use is on the rise, rates are increasing.

Diet is another factor that is associated with many cancer sites, although its contribution to overall cancer burden is less certain than that for tobacco.[20,21] Observational studies have suggested an association between dietary factors such as low dietary fiber intake and high red meat consumption and cancers such as colon cancer.[21] These associations have yet to be confirmed in clinical prevention trials.[22,23] It may be that factors associated with dietary intake, such as exercise, or other lifestyle factors underlie the protective association seen in observational studies and are not evaluated in the trial designs.

Infectious agents also contribute to the cancer burden. Human papillomavirus infection with oncogenic strains is the principle cause of cervical cancer.[24] Hepatitis B and hepatitis C infections are associated with liver cancer.[25,26] Infection with *Helicobacter pylori* is associated with gastric cancer. Although still a small contributor to the overall cancer burden, infections remain an important target for prevention through vaccines or antibiotic therapy, as in the case of *H. pylori*.[11] This information has particular relevance in developing countries, where infection-related cancers such as cervical and liver cancer remain leading preventable causes of cancer mortality.[11]

Sun exposure is a leading contributor to skin cancer and a major contributor to the observed worldwide increases in rates of melanoma. Preventive strategies such as encouraging young children and adults to wear a hat and use SPF 30 sunscreen may be working. A randomized trial in Canada comparing SPF 30 sunscreen to no intervention in schoolchildren if sun exposure was expected to last 30 minutes or longer demonstrated significantly fewer nevi (a precursor to melanoma) in the treated group than the controls.[27]

Although occupational exposures to carcinogens are a small contributor to the overall cancer burden, they are important for specific at-risk populations.[20] These, like the other factors mentioned previously, can be controlled, and exposures closely regulated.

Science of Clinical Oncology

Manipulation of the hormonal environment may be an important means of preventing hormone-associated cancers such as breast, endometrial, ovarian, and prostate. Observational studies and a clinical trial of hormone replacement therapy (HRT), specifically combined estrogen and progestin therapy, are consistent in showing an increased risk of breast cancer but a decreased risk of colon cancer among HRT users compared to women who never used HRT.[28] The risks of breast cancer may vary for estrogen only versus combined estrogen and progestin therapy,[29-31] with higher risks associated with combination hormone therapy. For women who have not had a hysterectomy, however, unopposed estrogen therapy increases the risk of endometrial cancer.[2] Oral contraceptive therapy is associated with reduced risks of endometrial and ovarian cancer, and studies have not shown a long-term increased risk of breast cancer.[32-35]

Although at present we cannot alter genetic mutations that render an individual more susceptible to developing breast cancer, there is a suggestion that environmental exposures and lifestyle habits may modify this risk. One example is Sulindac, a nonsteroidal anti-inflammatory agent, which reduces the number of polyps occurring in individuals with familial polyposis. Whether reducing, but not eliminating, the number of polyps is sufficient to reduce the occurrence of cancer is not known, however.[36] Another example is the use of tamoxifen by women who are at high risk for breast cancer. Among women in the Breast Cancer Prevention Trial who were subsequently determined to carry a mutation in BRCA1, tamoxifen use did not seem to alter the risk of breast cancer, but the numbers were small.[37] Additional inherited factors, such as polymorphisms resulting in functional changes in enzymes responsible for carcinogen metabolism or DNA repair, also may contribute to susceptibility to cancer.[38-40] These factors are likely to identify those in the population who can receive the most benefit from interventions that modify risk factors, such as smoking cessation or prevention programs.

TYPES OF STUDY DESIGNS

Time Trend Analysis and Ecological Studies

Ecological studies and time trend analyses are considered hypothesis-generating studies. Ecological studies use available data on aggregate measures of exposure, for example, per capita food consumption, and correlate these with disease-specific incidence data. For example, per capita fat consumption has been observed to be strongly correlated with international breast cancer mortality rates (Fig. 22-3).[41] This finding, along with results from animal experiments, supports the hypothesis that dietary fat intake is associated with risk of developing breast cancer. Hypotheses generated in ecological studies can then be tested in case-control studies, cohort studies, or clinical trials, using individual level data. Ecological studies and time trend analyses provide only weak evidence for determining causality, because these types of studies are subject to a type of bias called the ecological fallacy or aggregation bias. The ecological fallacy may occur when the aggregate group data do not reflect the association at the individual level. In the example just mentioned, of dietary fat consumption and breast cancer mortality rates, it may be that all the women who died of breast cancer consumed low levels of dietary fat and the per capita level data do not reflect this. Another concern is that these types of studies often fail to take into account other factors that differ among countries that may influence cancer rates. Prospective cohort studies have failed to confirm the hypothesis that dietary fat intake is associated with breast cancer risk.[42,43] Because of concerns that the range of fat intake in these cohort studies was not low enough to rule out an important effect of very low fat intake, the Women's Health Initiative, a randomized controlled clinical trial, is evaluating the impact of a low-fat diet on cancer and other disease as one of its aims.[28]

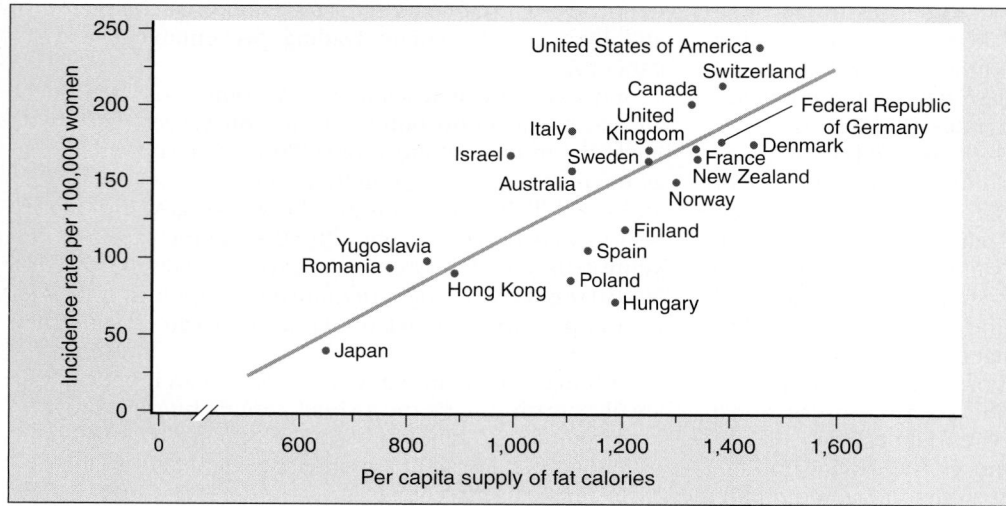

Figure 22-3. Correlation between dietary fat intake and breast cancer, by country. (From Prentice RL, Kakar F, Hursting S, et al: Aspects of the rationale for the Women's Health Trial. J Natl Cancer Inst 1988;80:802–814.)

TABLE 22-4

Comparison of Characteristics of Analytical Observation Studies

	CASE-CONTROL	COHORT STUDIES
Study groups	Defined by presence/absence of disease	Defined by presence/absence of exposure
Outcomes	Proportion of cases and controls exposed	Cancer incidence or mortality in the exposed and unexposed
Measures of association	Odds ratio	Absolute and relative risk
		Odds ratio can be calculated
		Attributable risk assessed directly
Multiple association	Can study multiple exposure—one study	Can study multiple disease outcomes with exposure
Duration of study	Short	Prospective cohorts for cancer outcomes—long duration
Sample size	Relatively small	Large for studies of cancer outcomes
Challenges	Control selection	Changes in factors over time
	Exposure assessment—especially recall bias	Surveillance bias

Data from Gordis L: Epidemiology. Philadelphia, WB Saunders, 1996.

Time trends analysis and ecological studies, although providing weak evidence to conclude that an association is causal, can identify important risk factors. The association between estrogen replacement therapy and endometrial cancer was first suggested by studies that showed a correlation between prescriptions for estrogen therapy and a rise in endometrial cancer incidence.[1] The association went on to be confirmed in case-control studies.

Analytical Observational Studies

Case-Control Studies

Case-control and cohort studies provide a higher level of evidence to support causal association than ecological studies. The characteristics of these study designs are outlined in Table 22-4. Case-control and cohort studies, as opposed to ecological studies, collect information on exposure and outcomes on the individual and then measure the degree of association (Fig. 22-4).

Case-control studies identify individuals with the disease (cases) and individual who are not affected with the disease (controls) and then compare the two groups by the proportion exposed and unexposed to factors of interest. Case-control studies also are called retrospective studies because one starts with the health outcomes and then looks back in time to assess the exposure. It is an efficient design, especially for rare diseases such as type-specific cancer, but a major challenge in case-control studies is to choose the most appropriate comparison

(control) group. The general rule is that controls should come from the same underlying population source from which the cases arose so that if the control subject becomes a case he or she would be in the study as a case. Multiple exposures can be studied in relation to one disease. However, a disadvantage of case-control studies is that it may be difficult to determine with certainty that the exposure preceded the onset of the disease. Another disadvantage relates to recall of the exposure. It may be difficult for cases and controls to recall specific exposures, timing, and duration. However, if cases and controls differ in their ability to recall, the result is a bias in the measure of an association.

The measure of association between the risk factor and disease calculated in a case-control study is the odds ratio (see Tables 22-1 and 22-4). The odds ratio is interpreted in the same way as a relative risk. If the odds ratio is greater than 1, the factor is associated with an increased risk of disease—or, put another way, cases are more likely to have been exposed to the factor than the controls. If the odds ratio is less than 1, then cases were less likely to be exposed than controls and the factor is, therefore, a protective factor. The odds ratio is a good estimate of the relative risk, which is calculated from cohort studies, when the disease is rare and when the history of exposure for the cases and controls is representative of that for all members of the source population.[4]

Case-case studies are a special type of study design in which cases with a specific characteristic, e.g., a specific gene mutation, are compared to cases of the same disease

Science of Clinical Oncology

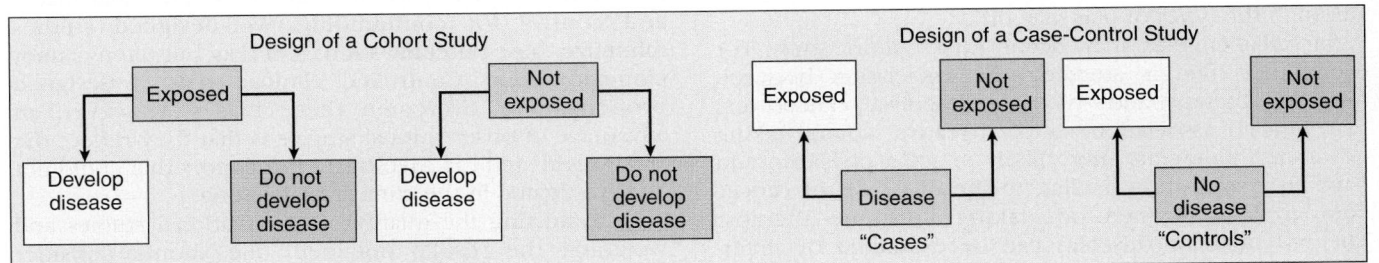

Figure 22-4. Comparison of cohort and case-control study designs. (From Gordis L: Epidemiology. Philadelphia, WB Saunders, 1996, p 163.)

without the characteristic. These types of studies are used to evaluate factors related to subtypes of a disease.[44] For example, a case-case study design of p53-positive and p53-negative ovarian cancer was used to examine the association between the number of ovulatory cycles and p53 overexpression.[45] Gene–environment interaction can be determined through this study design but the "main effect" association between the exposure and the development of cancer cannot be determined due to the lack of a nondisease control group.

Cohort Studies

Cohort studies define groups based on an exposure and follow the groups for the development of disease (see Fig. 22-4). Cohort studies are also referred to as prospective studies. A confusing term sometimes seen is *retrospective or nonconcurrent cohort studies*. This refers to cohort designs in which the cohort is formed and then available data on the exposure of interest are assembled and analyzed for the association with an outcome. This type of study design often is used in occupational cohort studies. The cohort of workers in an industry is identified and then work records of past exposure are obtained. A concurrent cohort design would identify the populations, assess exposure, and then follow the cohort forward in time for disease outcomes. In both types of cohort studies, the groups first are defined by exposures and then the incidence of disease is obtained.

A major advantage of cohort studies vis à vis other study designs such as case-control studies is the ability to quantify the absolute risk of disease and death associated with an exposure, in addition to determining the relative risk of disease (see Table 22-4). The prospective cohort design, unlike the case-control study design, allows these susceptibility factors to be characterized with respect to multiple disease outcomes. Another advantage to the cohort design is that exposure information (e.g., smoking, diet, alcohol intake) has been collected before the onset of disease. This eliminates the chance that the presence of disease alters the factor or biases ascertainment of exposure information, so recall bias is not a problem in cohort studies.

Potential Biases in Observational Studies

The highest-quality studies are designed to eliminate or minimize biases and to gather the necessary information needed to control for potential confounding. Biases are "systematic errors" that occur in the conduct of the study.[46] Observational studies and clinical trials are all subject to bias in the design and conduct of the study, although the types of bias may differ.

Surveillance bias may occur in a cohort study. For example, if one is studying the association between hormone therapy and risk of endometrial cancer, one may find an association, simply because women taking hormone therapy are more likely to see a physician and have an examination leading to the diagnosis of cancer compared to women not taking hormone therapy. The potential for this bias can be examined by determining the frequency of medical visits and routine medical care for all women.

Recall bias may occur in case-control studies if cases and controls recall the exposure differently. For example, because cases have a serious disease such as cancer, they may have given more thought to recalling past exposures and are more likely to remember that exposure than controls who are healthy, even if the proportions exposed are the same. In this situation a measured association between exposures and case status is biased by the differences in recall of that exposure of interest. Using similar probes to help stimulate memory for all participants and having well-trained interviewers asking the questions helps to eliminate or minimize this bias. Recall bias, a concern in case-control studies, is not an issue in cohort studies in which the exposure assessment precedes the onset of disease.

Selection bias may occur in all types of clinical studies, observational studies, and clinical trials. For example, hospital-based case-control studies may include only those individuals with a certain type of disease or an advanced stage of disease, or may be selected in some manner that is related to the exposure of interest. For example, if all cases from a certain manufacturing plant always refer to hospital X, a case-control study that includes only cases from this hospital may have an unrepresentative group of cases with a specific exposure history. Case-control and cohort studies that are population-based, recruiting all cases in a region, are less subject to selection bias.

Confounding can occur when a factor is associated with both the exposure of interest and the disease. Failure to take into account potential confounders of an association may lead to misleading interpretation of results. For example, a study of coffee consumption and cancer that fails to take into account smoking history may report an association between coffee and cancer, but the association may, in fact, be due to the fact that coffee drinkers may be more likely to smoke than non–coffee drinkers. Smoking is the true underlying cause of the cancer, and coffee is implicated only because it is associated with smoking: "guilt by association." A concern often cited in observational studies is the influence of potential confounding from unknown factors that then cannot be adjusted for either in the design or analysis. The influence of this potential bias is difficult to quantify. Stronger associations and those showing a dose response are less likely to be due to uncontrolled confounding, because for most studies, controlling for known confounders usually causes only minimal changes in the estimated relative risks.

Many challenges must be overcome in designing observational studies to eliminate these potential biases and control for confounding. Well-designed studies minimize these potential sources of bias, but often cannot eliminate them. Controlled clinical trials, if designed properly, may overcome these biases. However, an advantage of observational studies is that they reflect the "real world" and can investigate risk factors that could not be investigated in the clinical trial setting.

In evaluating the quality of observational studies and weighing the results obtained, one should consider whether studies are population-based and have taken steps to minimize potential confounding and biases such as selection bias, recall bias, information bias, and surveillance bias. Randomized controlled trials also are subject to some, but not all, of these biases. Through the experimental design in both observational studies and clinical trials, these biases can be markedly reduced, if not eliminated.

Randomized Controlled Clinical Trials

Randomized controlled clinical trials are the gold standard to evaluate the efficacy of an intervention or treatment on health outcomes and provide the highest level of evidence for judging effectiveness of an intervention.[16,47] The design of clinical trials should minimize the possibility of errors in selection, delivery of the intervention, adherence to the intervention, and assessment of outcomes. Figure 22-5 illustrates the major types of biases that may occur in clinical trials.[48] As in observational studies, selection bias and detection or surveillance bias may occur. High-quality trials are designed and conducted in ways to minimize these potential biases.

Selection bias occurs when there is a systematic difference in assignment to one of the treatment groups. The purpose of randomization is to prevent selection bias by allowing chance, rather than the investigator, to determine the treatment assignment. To be effective, the method of treatment allocation should not be transparent. For example, using odd days versus even days to allocate patients to an intervention allows treatment assignment to be easily predicted. Patients with more advanced disease may then be intentionally enrolled on a specific day, if, for example, the physician believes the new treatment to be more beneficial than the standard one.

A common misperception is that the randomization process is done to ensure comparability between the intervention groups in a trial. Comparability on characteristics of the subjects in the intervention group usually is achieved with randomization, but it is not guaranteed.

Imbalances in key characteristics, both known and unknown, may occur by chance, but the larger the number of subjects enrolled, the more likely it is that the group will be comparable. Thus, although uncontrolled confounding is less likely in a randomized clinical trial than in observational study design, it still may occur. If a factor such as age, gender, or stage of disease is likely to be associated with both the health outcome and the response to treatment, these factors should be taken into consideration in the randomization process to ensure that the groups are comparable with respect to the factor in question, particularly in trials with small sample sizes. For example, in the Breast Cancer Prevention Trial to evaluate the efficacy of tamoxifen for the prevention of breast cancer, age and estimated risk of developing breast cancer was taken into account during the randomization process.[49] Women were classified into age and risk groups, then randomized to tamoxifen or placebo, thus ensuring that the subjects in the intervention groups were comparable by age and risk of developing breast cancer.

Performance, attrition, and detection (or surveillance) biases can be minimized by masking of treatment assignment, standardizing protocols to ensure uniform administration of treatment and evaluation of outcomes, and monitoring trials to ensure adherence to the protocols. Masking treatment, as in placebo-controlled trials, helps to prevent systematic differences in measuring or determining outcomes in the two groups (see Fig. 22-5). Trials in which neither the participant nor the investigator knows the treatment assignment are known as "double-masked" trials. Masking of treatment assignment is particularly important when outcomes are subjective, such as quality of life or degree of pain. However, masking of treatment is not always possible, especially when evaluating treatments such as chemotherapy or radiation therapy or a screening intervention. In those situations, trial procedures should standardize measurement of outcomes and have outcomes assessed by individuals

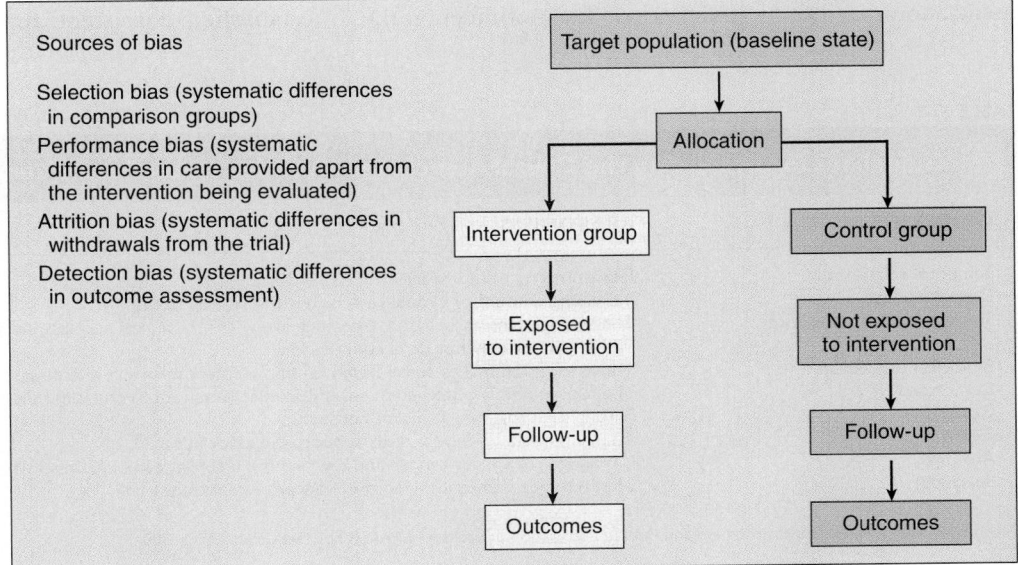

Figure 22-5. Possible sources of bias in randomized clinical trials. (From Clarke M, Oxman AD (eds): Cochrane Reviewers' Handbook 4.2.0 [updated March 2003]. Available at http://www.cochrane. dk/cochrane/handbook/handbook. htm.)

independent of the investigators to minimize error and bias. Data and Safety Monitoring Boards should be in place to oversee the conduct of the trial to ensure adherence to protocols as well as the safety of trial participants.

If the subjects in the study or the investigators are aware of the treatment assignment, this knowledge may influence drop-in or dropouts from the trial, independent of actual treatment-related side effects. A patient's belief that he or she is on a specific treatment may influence how symptoms that may or may not be related to the therapy are interpreted and then managed. Masking the treatment assignment helps to prevent this bias. In a masked study, differences in withdrawal from the study are more likely to be due to real differences in treatment effects.[48]

WEIGHING THE EVIDENCE

Etiology

Determining the causes of cancer and effectiveness of interventions to prevent or treat the disease requires judging and interpreting the available data, including animal experiments, human observational studies, and clinical trials. Guidelines for judging causality of the association between a risk factor and a chronic disease outcome such as cancer have emanated from Koch's postulates, which were established to help interpret causality for infectious agents.[50,51] Guidelines for interpreting causation (Table 22-5) include temporality, consistency, strength and dose response of the association, biological plausibility, experiment, analogy, coherence, and, perhaps least applicable to chronic diseases, specificity of the association.[50,51] These guidelines, along with assessment of the quality of study designs, are critical pieces used in the evidence-based approach to clinical decision making. It is not necessary for all of the guidelines to be met to make causal inferences. These are not strict criteria, but aids to the thought process.[51] For example, the biological mechanism underpinning an association may not be understood, thus not meeting the guideline of biological plausibility, yet it may be concluded that the factor is a cause of cancer. For example, John Snow's[4] conclusion that water was the source of the cholera epidemic in 18th-century London led to removal of the handle of the Broad Street pump and subsequently to a decline in the outbreak. This was done before the causal agent had been identified or the mechanism by which it worked (i.e., bacterial contamination) was understood. Similarly, the correct conclusion that tobacco use caused cancer was determined, based on human studies of exposure to tobacco and development of cancer, before the exact carcinogens and their method of action were identified.[52] It had been shown that smoking preceded the development of cancer in humans; multiple well-designed studies consistently observed a strong increased risk of developing cancer with an associated dose-response relationship, and animal models also were consistent with the human data. Smoking prevention and cessation were encouraged as a result, and they remain the most important means of lowering cancer rates.

For many factors associated with an increased risk of cancer, human experimental studies would not be ethical, so inferences concerning causality must rely on observational studies. However, for preventive and treatment interventions, the controlled clinical trial remains the gold standard for determining efficacy of the intervention. The efficient conduct of trials and observational studies will be a growing future challenge given limited health care resources. This is particularly true in the area of screening prevention trials, which require a large sample size and enormous resources.

Interventions: Translating to Clinical Practice

Translating knowledge into practice requires weighing the available evidence in a systematic fashion to help guide health care policies as well as individual clinical decisions. Several organizations, such as the Canadian Task Force on the Periodic Health Examination[53] and the U.S. Preventive Services Task Force (USPSTF),[54] have established consistent approaches to the evaluation of

TABLE 22-5

Guidelines for Evaluating the Causal Association Between a Risk Factor and Disease

GUIDELINE	REASONING
Temporal relationship	Exposure precedes disease
Dose response	Increasing amount of exposure = higher the risk of disease
Strength of the association	The stronger the association, the more likely it is to be real and less likely to be due to confounding factors that may or may not be accounted for.
Biological plausibility	The association makes sense based on known mechanisms of the disease.
Consistency	The association is observed in several studies (replication) and different populations.
Coherence	Putting it all together, it makes sense.
Experiment	Animal models or clinical trials support the association.
Analogy	Carcinogen X causes cancer and Y, which has a similar structure, also will cause cancer.
Specificity	The factor causes cancer and only cancer—the weakest link.

Adapted from Hill AB: The environment and disease: Association or causation? Proc R Soc Med 1965;58:295–300.

health care interventions.[53-55] This approach to weighing the evidence often is referred to as *evidence-based medicine*.[56] The evidence-based approach applies to preventive interventions, treatment, palliation, and counseling. Key principles in the evaluation process include assessing the quality of the studies, potential benefits of the intervention, and potential harms. Traditionally, a hierarchical ranking of study designs has been used in weighing the evidence, with the greatest weight given to well-designed, randomized clinical trials and the least given to expert opinion. However, this hierarchical ranking fails to account for the validity of the study design in a rigorous way. The third edition of the *Report of the U.S. Preventive Services Task Force*[54] has altered their methodology for reviewing and weighing the evidence to incorporate the quality of the study more formally, as well as the type of the study design. The emphasis is placed on internal validity of the studies, i.e., whether the studies are designed and conducted in such a way as to minimize potential biases. For example, the quality of a case-control study is judged by the following criteria:

- Accurate ascertainment of cases
- Nonbiased selection of cases/controls with exclusion criteria applied equally to both
- Response rate
- Diagnostic testing procedures applied equally to each group
- Appropriate attention to potential confounding variables[54]

The individual study is judged according to its internal validity based on the preceding criteria as well as the ability to generalize the results to other populations. Then coherence and consistency with other studies is examined in association with evidence for a direct effect on health. Studies of primary health outcomes, rather than surrogate or intermediate endpoints of health outcomes, are given more weight. The quality of the study design rather than the specific study design also receives more weight. Thus in this method of weighing the evidence, a well-designed and well-conducted prospective cohort study carries more weight than a poorly conducted randomized clinical trial. In addition to evaluating the benefits of the intervention for the primary health outcomes, its balance with potential harms also is considered.[54] The USPSTF methodology emphasizes that the quality of the study should not be confounded by magnitude of the observed effect. A large association or effect noted in a study may be meaningless if the study is poorly designed and conducted. Magnitude of the effect, quality of the evidence, and population burden of the condition are taken into consideration in making final recommendations. For example, recommendations for implementing the intervention into clinical practice could be made for low degrees of effect if the condition is common with a large population burden and for those interventions making a large impact on a rare condition that is associated with significant burden for the individual patient.[54] These elements are then used in grading the final recommendation. The final grading of the recommendations is listed in Table 22-6. A similar approach has

TABLE 22-6

Standard Recommendation Language: USPSTF 2003

Recommendation: A

Language: The USPSTF strongly recommends that clinicians routinely provide [the service] to eligible patients. (The USPSTF found good evidence that [the service] improves important health outcomes and concludes that benefits substantially outweigh harms.)

Recommendation: B

Language: The USPSTF recommends that clinicians routinely provide [the service] to eligible patients. (The USPSTF found at least fair evidence that [the service] improves important health outcomes and concludes that benefits outweigh harms.)

Recommendation: C

Language: The USPSTF makes no recommendation for or against routine provision of [the service]. (The USPSTF found at least fair evidence that [the service] can improve health outcomes but concludes that the balance of the benefits and harms is too close to justify a general recommendation.)

Recommendation: D

Language: The USPSTF recommends against routinely providing [the service] to asymptomatic patients. (The USPSTF found at least fair evidence that [the service] is ineffective or that harms outweigh benefits.)

Recommendation: I

Language: The USPSTF concludes that the evidence is insufficient to recommend for or against routinely providing [the service]. (Evidence that [the service] is effective is lacking, of poor quality, or conflicting and the balance of benefits and harms cannot be determined.)

USPSTF, United States Preventive Services Task Force

been adapted by the Physician Data Query (PDQ) comprehensive cancer data base of the National Cancer Institute, which provides a summary of evidence for treatment, screening, and prevention.[16] Table 22-7 outlines this approach to evaluating clinical evidence.

Applying the Evidence-based Approach for Clinical Decisions

Complex scenarios may arise when evaluating the evidence from both observational studies and clinical trials prior to making a clinical recommendation. For example, if several randomized trials of varying quality are done to address a particular research question, the results of these studies may not be consistent with each other. It also is possible that results from clinical trials may not reflect those from observational studies examining the same association. Lastly, in a number of clinical situations there is not enough good-quality data to assist in clinical decision making. "Real life" examples of each of these scenarios and the impact they have had on guideline recommendations are briefly reviewed in the following sections.

The recent renewal of the controversy over the degree of benefit from mammography screening is an example of the first scenario. At least seven randomized trials have been done, which vary in quality and design.[57,58] A review conducted by the Cochrane Collaboration concluded that

TABLE 22-7

 Evaluating the Evidence for Prevention and Screening Interventions: PDQ Guidelines

I. Description of the Evidence (The PDQ Editorial Board uses the same process for benefits and harms; the "evidence" referred to is the evidence relevant for answering the question of the magnitude of the health effects of widespread implementation.)
   A. Study design (Evidence from the best studies available; ranked from strongest to weakest)
      1. Evidence obtained from randomized controlled trials
      2. Evidence obtained from nonrandomized controlled trials
      3. Evidence obtained from cohort or case-control studies
      4. Evidence from ecologic and descriptive studies (e.g., international patterns studies, time series)
      5. Opinions of respected authorities based on clinical experience, descriptive studies, or reports of expert committees
   B. Internal Validity: "Quality" of Execution within the Study Design The Editorial Board uses design-specific criteria within each research design to assess the internal validity of the evidence. At present the Board uses the criteria developed by the U.S. Preventive Services Task Force (see Table 3 in [1]). These criteria may be modified over time as needed.
   C. Consistency (Coherence)/Volume of the Evidence
      1. One study (small vs. large number of participants; agree vs. disagree)
      2. Multiple studies (small vs. large number of participants; agree vs. disagree)
   D. Direction and magnitude of effects for health outcomes (both absolute and relative risks. As quantitative as possible; may vary for different populations).
      1. Small positive/negative magnitude (benefits/harms)
      2. Larger positive/negative magnitude (benefits/harms)
   E. External Validity
      1. Extent to which the intervention can be applied to usual practice with the same effects as in efficacy studies
      2. Effects among people in the general population, differences with study subjects
II. Assessment of the Evidence   The level of certainty (good, fair, poor) of our understanding of the direction and magnitude of the health effects (both benefits and harms) of widespread implementation.
   A. Example: Statement of Benefits
      "The overall evidence is [good/fair/poor] that use of intervention X [among population Y, where appropriate] leads to a reduction/increase in (a specific benefit)." In the Evidence of Benefit section, the actual evidence is detailed, including evidence and assessment of direction and magnitude of specific benefits.
   B. Example: Statement of Harms
      "The overall evidence is [good/fair/poor] that use of intervention X [among population Y] leads to a reduction/increase in (a specific harm)." In the Evidence of Harm section, the actual evidence is detailed, including evidence and assessment of the direction and magnitude of specific harms.

http:www.cancer.gov/cancerinfo/pdq

only two of these trials were of medium quality, two were seriously flawed and were excluded from further consideration, and the remainder were classified as poor-quality designs. The trials of medium-quality studies did not show a benefit of screening mammography in reducing breast cancer mortality.[57,58] However, the poor-quality trials were consistent with a reduction in breast cancer mortality. On review of these results a number of concerns about the available evidence were raised: (1)

the accuracy of cancer-specific mortality as an outcome; (2) the lack of information on potential harms from screening, which may include the overdiagnosis of breast neoplasms that are not clinically significant; and (3) the potential harms from treatment-related side effects, including cardiovascular disease associated with perhaps unnecessary (due to overdiagnosis of non–clinically significant tumors) radiation treatment.[59]

A simultaneous review of mammographic screening by the U.S. Preventive Task Force led to a change in their recommendations. Although breast cancer screening was recommended beginning at the age of 40 years, the grade of the recommendation was reduced from A to B due to questions about the quality of the screening studies.

The recommendation by the USPTF[60] now reads as follows:

> The U.S. Preventive Services Task Force (USPSTF) recommends screening mammography, with or without clinical breast examination (CBE), every 1–2 years for women aged 40 and older. (See "recommendation B," Table 22-6.)
>
> **Rationale:** The USPSTF found fair evidence that mammography screening every 12–33 months significantly reduces mortality from breast cancer. Evidence is strongest for women aged 50–69, the age group generally included in screening trials. For women aged 40–49, the evidence that screening mammography reduces mortality from breast cancer is weaker, and the absolute benefit of mammography is smaller, than it is for older women. Most, but not all, studies indicate a mortality benefit for women undergoing mammography at ages 40–49, but the delay in observed benefit in women younger than 50 makes it difficult to determine the incremental benefit of beginning screening at age 40 rather than at age 50.

The absolute benefit is smaller because the incidence of breast cancer is lower among women in their 40s than among older women. The USPSTF concluded that the evidence also can be generalized to women aged 70 and older (who face a higher absolute risk for breast cancer) if their life expectancy is not compromised by comorbid disease. The absolute probability of benefit from regular mammography increases along a continuum with age, whereas the likelihood of harms from screening (false-positive results and unnecessary anxiety, biopsies, and cost) diminish from ages 40 through 70. The balance of benefits and potential harms, therefore, grows more favorable as women age. The precise age at which the potential benefits of mammography justify the possible harms is a subjective choice. The USPSTF did not find sufficient evidence to specify the optimal screening interval for women aged 40 to 49.

The Canadian Task Force recommendation, updated in 2001, states "current evidence does not support the recommendation that screening mammography be included in or excluded from the periodic health examination of women aged 40–49 at average risk for breast cancer."[61] The grade is a "C," meaning there is "poor evidence regarding inclusion or exclusion of a condition in a PHE [periodic health examination] but recommendations may be made on other grounds." The recommendation by the Canadian Task Force updated in 1988, for women 50 to 69 years of age, states "there is good evidence for screening women 50–69 years by clinical examination and mammography. There is good evidence to recommend the clinical preventive action."[62]

This is an example of a situation where clinical guidelines differ from review of the same evidence. Neither randomized clinical trials nor analytical observation studies can totally avoid errors or bias in their design or analysis. The interpretation of the results of all types of studies requires careful consideration of both the quality of the studies and their results.

Comparisons between results from clinical trials and observational studies have been made for multiple clinical conditions with no evidence that observational studies were qualitatively different from clinical trials. The hierarchical approach to evidence-based medicine gives the greatest weight of evidence to randomized clinical trials. In this hierarchical approach, results from one poor-quality randomized clinical trial potentially can outweigh results from multiple good-quality analytical studies. This approach to weighing the available evidence has been questioned, however.[63,64] If results do differ across study designs, exploring the reasons for the disparity rather than concluding that it is simply due to design differences and potential biases may lead to a better understanding of the cause of the disparity. An example of disparity of results across clinical trials and observational studies is the association between dietary fruit, vegetable, and fiber intake, and the prevention of colon cancer.[65] Observational studies have supported a protective association between fiber, fruits, and vegetables and colon cancer.[21] Two interventional trials of the effect of dietary fiber (either by supplement or increasing dietary intake of fruits and vegetables) on the incidence of colon polyps, an intermediate endpoint for colon cancer, failed to show a benefit.[22,23] Whether short-term interventions employed in dietary or vitamin supplementation clinical trials can reflect the "real world" exposures examined in observational studies is questionable.[64] Differences in exposure windows and types of supplementation (e.g., food sources versus supplements) between intervention trials and observational studies may affect the interpretation of these disparate results and should be taken into consideration when making global recommendations.

One of the most difficult problems, and the most common, is making clinical decisions in the absence of evidence. An example of this scenario is the use of measurement of PSA concentrations for the early detection of prostate cancer. The USPSTF recommendation regarding screening for prostate cancer states that:

> ... the evidence is insufficient to recommend for or against routine screening for prostate cancer using prostate specific antigen (PSA) testing or digital rectal examination (DRE). (See recommendation I in Table 22-6.)
> *Rationale:* The USPSTF found good evidence that PSA screening can detect early-stage prostate cancer but mixed and inconclusive evidence that early

detection improves health outcomes. Screening is associated with important harms, including frequent false-positive results and unnecessary anxiety, biopsies, and potential complications of treatment of some cancers that may never have affected a patient's health. The USPSTF concludes that evidence is insufficient to determine whether the benefits outweigh the harms for a screened population.[66]

The Canadian Task Force[67] states "Exclusion is recommended on the basis of low positive predictive value and the known risk of adverse affects associated with therapies of unproven effectiveness." A D grade indicates that there is fair evidence to exclude routine screening with PSA from the periodic health examination of asymptomatic men over 50 years of age.

The Prostate Lung Colorectal Ovarian Cancer Screening Trial, begun in 1992, recruited over 74,000 men to evaluate the efficacy of PSA testing to reduce prostate cancer mortality, and has yet to report the results of its investigation.[19] This emphasizes the tremendous time and resources needed to generate the gold standard evidence from a randomized clinical trial. Prior to initiating the trial, clinical decisions to apply PSA testing as a screening test were made in the absence of evidence of benefit. The adoption of PSA screening in the clinical setting was reflected in the enormous short-term increase in the incidence of prostate cancer (see Fig. 22-2). The potential of overdiagnosis of clinically nonsignificant disease and resulting harm from treatment have been raised as important possible sources of harm.[16]

The rapid pace of technology and the introduction of tests with the potential for the early detection of cancer will require study designs that accurately and efficiently determine the impact of these tests on health outcomes. Demonstration of the clinical sensitivity and specificity of the test is important but not sufficient for determining clinical applicability of the test. The impact on health care management and health outcomes must be evaluated, because screening may result in harm as well as benefit. Rigorous design and conduct of observational study designs such as case-control and cohort studies in addition to clinical trials offer the potential to evaluate the effectiveness of screening and prevention interventions efficiently and accurately.

SUMMARY

In oncology, identifying prevention strategies and making decisions regarding their incorporation into clinical practice requires knowledge of the rates and risk factors for specific cancers, the benefits and limitations of both observational studies and clinical trials, the quality of the study, and the ability to weigh all the available evidence. The evidence-based approach provides a systematic method to weigh the evidence and develop clinical guidelines. Reliance solely on the hierarchical approach to weighing the evidence has limitations. A poorly done randomized clinical trial may provide less evidence than a well-performed observational study. In addition, it may not be feasible to conduct large-scale trials for prevention and screening interventions due to limited health care resources. Development of new design strategies along with reliance on well-conducted observational studies will be needed for efficient and effective evaluation of promising new strategies for their impact on health outcomes and aid in their translation to the clinical setting.

REFERENCES

1. Henderson BE: The cancer question: An overview of recent epidemiologic and retrospective data. Am J Obstet Gynecol 1989;161:1859–1864.
2. Pike MC, Peters RK, Cozen W, et al: Estrogen-progestin replacement therapy and endometrial cancer. J Natl Cancer Inst 1997;89: 1110–1116.
3. Herbst AL, Anderson D: Clear cell adenocarcinoma of the vagina and cervix secondary to intrauterine exposure to diethylstilbestrol. Semin Surg Oncol 1990;6:343–346.
4. Gordis L: Epidemiology. Philadelphia, WB Saunders, 1996.
5. Breslow L, Cumberland WG: Progress and objectives in cancer control. JAMA 1988;259:1690–1694.
6. Bailar JC 3rd, Gornik HL: Cancer undefeated. N Engl J Med 1997;336:1569–1574.
7. Bailar JC 3rd, Smith EM: Progress against cancer? N Engl J Med 1986;314:1226–1232.
8. Ries LAG, Eisner MP, Kosary CL, et al (eds): SEER Cancer Statistics Review, 1975–2000. Bethesda, MD: National Cancer Institute, 2003. Available at http://seer.cancer.gov/csr/1975_2000, 2003.
9. Gail MH, Brinton LA, Byar DP, Corle DK, Green SB, Schairer C, Mulvihill JJ: Projecting individualized probabilities of developing breast cancer for white females who are being examined annually. J Natl Cancer Inst 1989;81:1879–1886.
10. Kinsinger LS, Harris R, Woolf SH, Sox HC, Lohr KN: Summary of the evidence: Chemoprevention of breast cancer. Report of the U.S. Preventive Services Task Force, 3rd edition. Available at http:// www.ahrq.gov/clinic/3rduspstf/breastchemo/brstchemosum1.htm.
11. Parkin DM, Bray FI, Devesa SS: Cancer burden in the year 2000. The global picture. Eur J Cancer 2001;8:S4–S66.
12. The Centers for Disease Control and Prevention: Cancer registries: The foundation for cancer prevention and control. National Program for Cancer Registries. Division of Cancer Prevention & Control. 2003 Program Fact Sheet. Available at http://www.cdc.gov/cancer/npcr/register.htm.
13. North American Association of Central Cancer Registries. Available at www.naaccr.org.
14. Parkin DM, Whelan SL, Ferlay J, Teppo L, Thomas DB (eds): Cancer incidence in five continents, Vol. VIII. Geneva: World Health Organization, International Agency for Research on Cancer. Available at www.iarc.fr/.
15. World Health Organization. Available at http://www.who.int/en/.
16. PDQ Statement. Available at http://www.cancer.gov/cancerinfo/pdq/screening/prostate/healthprofessional.
17. Edwards BK, Howe HL, Ries LAG, et al: Annual report to the nation on the status of cancer, 1973–1999, featuring implications of age and aging on U.S. cancer burden. Cancer 2002;94:2766–2792.
18. Läärä E, Day NE, Hakama M: Trends in mortality from cervical cancer in the Nordic countries: association with organised screening programmes. Lancet 1987;1(8544):1247–1249.
19. Prorok PC, Andriole GL, Bresalier RS, et al: Design of the Prostate, Lung, Colorectal and Ovarian (PLCO) Cancer Screening Trial. Control Clin Trials 2000;6(Suppl):273S–309S.
20. Doll R, Peto R: The causes of cancer: quantitative estimates of avoidable risks of cancer in the United States today. J Natl Cancer Inst 1981;66:1191–1308.
21. Key TJ, Allen NE, Spencer EA, Travis RC: The effect of diet on risk of cancer. Lancet 2002;360(9336):861–868.
22. Schatzkin A, Lanza E, Corle D, et al: Lack of effect of a low-fat, high fiber diet on the recurrence of colorectal adenomas. Polyp Prevention Trial Study Group. N Engl J Med 2000;342:1149–1155.
23. Alberts DS, Martinez ME, Roe DJ, et al: Lack of effect of a high-fiber cereal supplement on the recurrence of colorectal adenomas. Phoenix Colon Cancer Prevention Physicians' Network. N Engl J Med 2000;342:1156–1162.
24. Schiffman MH, Castle P: Epidemiologic studies of a necessary causal risk factor: human papillomavirus infection and cervical neoplasia. J Natl Cancer Inst 2003;95:E2–PPE2.
25. El Serag HB: Hepatocellular carcinoma and hepatitis C in the United States. Hepatology 2002;36:S74–S83.
26. Geller SA: Hepatitis B and hepatitis C. Clin Liver Dis 2002;6:317–334.
27. Gallagher RP, Rivers JK, Lee TK, Bajdik CD, McLean DI, Coldman AJ: Broad-spectrum sunscreen use and the development of new nevi in white children: A randomized controlled trial. JAMA 2000;283:2955–2960.
28. Design of the Women's Health Initiative clinical trial and observational study. The Women's Health Initiative Study Group. Control Clin Trials 1998;19:61–109.
29. Schairer C, Lubin J, Troisi R, et al: Menopausal estrogen and estrogen-progestin replacement therapy and breast cancer risk. JAMA 2000;283:485–491.
30. Ross RK, Paganini-Hill A, Wan PC, et al: Effect of hormone replacement therapy on breast cancer risk: Estrogen versus estrogen plus progestin. J Natl Cancer Inst 2000;92:328–332.
31. Li CI, Malone KE, Porter PL, Weiss NS, Tang MT, Cushing-Haugen KL, Daling JR: Relationship between long durations and different regimens of hormone therapy and risk of breast cancer. JAMA 2003;289:3254–3263.
32. Collaborative Group on Hormonal Factors in Breast Cancer: Breast Cancer and Hormonal Contraceptives: Collaborative reanalysis of individual data on 53,297 women with breast cancer and 100,239 women without breast cancer from 54 epidemiological studies. Lancet 1996;347:1713–1727.
33. The Cancer and Steroid Hormone Study of the Centers for Disease Control and the National Institute of Child Health and Human Development: Combination oral contraceptive use and the risk of endometrial cancer. JAMA 1987;257:796–800.
34. The Cancer and Steroid Hormone Study of the Centers for Disease Control and the National Institute of Child Health and Human Development: The reduction in risk of ovarian cancer associated with oral contraceptive use. N Engl J Med 1987;316:650–655.
35. Marchbanks PA, McDonald JA, Wilson HG, et al: Oral contraceptives and the risk of breast cancer. N Engl J Med 2002;346:2025–2032.
36. Giardiello FM, Yang VW, Hylind LM, et al: Primary chemoprevention of familial adenomatous polyposis with sulindac. N Engl J Med 2002;346:1054–1059.
37. King MC, Wieand S, Hale K, et al: Tamoxifen and breast cancer incidence among women with inherited mutations in BRCA1 and BRCA2: National Surgical Adjuvant Breast and Bowel Project (NSABP-P1) Breast Cancer Prevention Trial. JAMA 2001;286: 2251–2256.
38. Helzlsouer KJ, Selmin O, Huang HY, et al: Association between glutathione S-transferase M1, P1, and T1 genetic polymorphisms and development of breast cancer. J Natl Cancer Inst 1998;90: 512–518.
39. Fenech M: Biomarkers of genetic damage for cancer epidemiology. Toxicology 2002;181–182:411–416.
40. Goode EL, Ulrich CM, Potter JD: Polymorphisms in DNA repair genes and associations with cancer risk. Cancer Epidemiol Biomarkers Prev 2002;11:1513–1530.
41. Prentice RL, Kakar F, Hursting S, et al: Aspects of the rationale for the Women's Health Trial. J Natl Cancer Inst 1988;80:802–814.
42. Jones DY, Schatzkin A, Green SB, et al: Dietary fat and breast cancer in the National Health and Nutrition Examination Survey I Epidemiologic Follow-up Study. J Natl Cancer Inst 1987;79:465–471.
43. Willett WC, Stampfer MJ, Colditz GA, Rosner BA, Hennekens CH, Speizer FE: Dietary fat and the risk of breast cancer. N Engl J Med 1987;316:22–28.
44. Last JM (ed): A Dictionary of Epidemiology, 4th ed. New York, Oxford University Press, 2001.
45. Schildkraut JM, Bastos E, Berchuck A: Relationship between lifetime ovulatory cycles and overexpression of mutant p53 in epithelial ovarian cancer. J Natl Cancer Inst 1997;89:932–938.

46. Szklo M, Nieto FJ (eds): Understanding lack of validity: Bias. In: Epidemiology: Beyond the Basics. Gaithersburg, MD, Aspen Publishers, 2000, pp 125–169.

47. Harris RP, Helfand M, Woolf SH, Lohr KN, Mulrow CD, Teutsch SM, Atkins D, for the Methods Word Group, third U.S. Preventive Services Task Force: Current methods of the U.S. Preventive Services Task Force: A review of the process. Am J Prev Med 2001;20(3S):21–35.

48. Clarke M, Oxman AD (eds): Cochrane Reviewers' Handbook 4.2.0 (updated March 2003). Available at http://www.cochrane.org/resources/handbook/index.htm.

49. Fisher B, Costantino JP, Wickerham DL, et al: Tamoxifen for prevention of breast cancer: report of the National Surgical Adjuvant Breast and Bowel Project P-1 Study. J Natl Cancer Inst 1998;90:1371–1388.

50. Hill AB: The environment and disease: Association or causation? Proc R Soc Med 1965;58:295–300.

51. Doll R: Proof of causality: deduction from epidemiological observation. Perspect Biol Med 2002;45:499–515.

52. U.S. Department of Health, Education and Welfare: Report of the Advisory Committee to the Surgeon General of the Public Health Service. 1964 Surgeon General Report: Reducing the Health Consequences of Smoking (Public Health Service Publication No. 1103.) Washington, DC, U.S. Government Printing Office, 1964.

53. Canadian Task Force on Preventive Health Care. Evidence-Based Clinical Prevention Available at http://www.ctfphc.org/index2.htm.

54. USPTF Guide to Clinical Preventive Services, 3rd ed, 2000–2003, Report of the U.S. Preventive Services Task Force. Available at http://www.ahrq.gov/clinic/cps3dix.htm.

55. Lawrence RS, Mickalide AD: Preventive services in clinical practice: Designing the periodic health examination. JAMA 1987;257: 2205–2207.

56. Sox HC Jr, Woolf SH: Evidence-based practice guidelines from the U.S. Preventive Services Task Force [editorial]. JAMA 1993;269: 2678.

57. Olsen O, Gotzsche PC: Cochrane review on screening for breast cancer with mammography. Lancet 2001;358(9290):1340–1342.

58. Olsen O, Gotzsche PC: Screening for breast cancer with mammography. Cochrane Database Syst Rev 2001;4:CD001877.

59. Early Breast Cancer Trialists' Collaborative Group: Favourable and unfavourable effects on long-term survival of radiotherapy for early breast cancer: an overview of the randomized trials. Lancet 2000;355:1757–1770.

60. Humphrey LL, Helfand M, Chan BKS, Woolf SH: Breast cancer screening. Summary of the evidence. Ann Intern Med 2002;137:344–346.

61. Ringash J, Canadian Task Force on Preventive Health Care: Preventive health care, 2001 update: Screening mammography among women aged 40–49 years at average risk of breast cancer. Canadian Medical Association Journal 2001;164:469–476.

62. Morrison BJ: Canadian Task Force on Preventive Health Care. Screening for breast cancer. Available at http://www.ctfphc.org/Tables/Ch65tab2.htm

63. Benson K, Hartz AJ: A comparison of observational studies and randomized, controlled trials. N Engl J Med 2000;342:1878–1886.

64. Concato J, Shah N, Horwitz R: Randomized, controlled trials, observational studies, and the hierarchy of research designs. N Engl J Med 2000;342:1887–1892.

65. Byers T: What can randomized controlled trials tell us about nutrition and cancer prevention? CA Cancer J Clin 1999;49: 353–361.

66. Prostate Cancer—Screening. U.S. Preventive Services Task Force, 3rd ed. Available at http://www.ahrq.gov/clinic/uspstf/uspsprca.htm.

67. Feightner JW: Screening for prostate cancer, in Canadian Task Force on the Periodic Health Examination. Canadian Guide to Clinical Preventive Health Care. Ottawa, Health Canada, 1994, pp 812–823.

CANCER PREVENTION, SCREENING, AND EARLY DETECTION

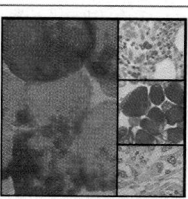

Frank L. Meyskens, Jr.

SUMMARY OF KEY POINTS

ETIOLOGY AND PATHOGENESIS

- Prevention of cancer is based on an understanding of the etiology and pathogenesis of the individual organ malignancies. The identification of at-risk individuals is based on familial/genetic and environmental influences.
- Smoking tobacco remains the number one cause of malignancy and accounts for about 30% of the mortality from cancer. The role of diet in cancer risk is substantial.
- Infections are an important component of cancer risk, and major etiologic agents for different organs include hepatitis B and C (hepatocellular), *Helicobacter pylori* (stomach), and human papillomavirus virus (cervix and some oral cancers).

SCREENING AND EARLY DETECTION

- Effective screening and early detection techniques for cancer include visual examination (skin, cervical, and oral cancers), cytology (cervical cancer), mammography (breast cancer), and fecal occult blood, sigmoidoscopy, and colonoscopy (colorectal cancers).
- Screening for prostate cancer by serum PSA measurement remains controversial, but the tide is turning toward acceptance of this approach.
- No successful method has been developed to screen for lung cancer.

CHEMOPREVENTION

- "Proof of principle" for the prevention of primary cancers has been established convincingly for breast cancer (tamoxifen) and hepatocellular carcinoma (vaccination against hepatitis virus B).
- Secondary aerodigestive cancers can be prevented with high-dose 13-cis retinoic acid but at the price of unacceptable toxicity.

- An increased incidence of secondary lung cancers in smokers supplemented with β-carotene or 13-cis retinoic acid demands particular caution in the development of chemoprevention agents.
- Prevention or regression of various intraepithelial neoplasias has been demonstrated: actinic keratoses (diclofenac), oral leukoplakia (retinoids), cervical intraepithelial neoplasms (topical retinoic acid), adenomatous polyps (calcium, celecoxib), and gastric dysplasia (anti-*Helicobacter pylori* therapy, antioxidants).
- Attempts to develop less toxic or low-dose combination interventions for all of the major cancers are being investigated.
- Useful resources for those interested in research in cancer prevention, screening, and early detection are provided.

BASIC CONCEPTS

Introduction

The guiding principles of this chapter and oncology should be that the best treatment of malignant disease is its prevention, and that the disease to be prevented is carcinogenesis, not cancer (Fig. 23-1).[1,2]

By the time a cancer is diagnosed, even with the advanced techniques now available, more than 90% of the biological life of the tumor is over, and the best chance to control the malignant process has been missed. The extensive advances in our understanding of carcinogenesis at the molecular level in the past decade, the rediscovery of intraepithelial neoplasia (IEN) as an early, recognizable precursor of many solid tumors that can be managed simply, and the well-defined successes of screening and early detection in reducing the morbidity and mortality from several major cancers, need to be brought to bear on the problem of malignancy in a concerted and widespread fashion, with clinical oncologists working closely with primary care physicians and subspecialists.[3] Because fewer than 50% of cancers are cured, once established, and because gains in treatment effectiveness have been increasingly incremental and expensive, early detection and prevention of cancer should be pursued aggressively as a means to reduce the burden of morbidity and mortality.[4]

Many major diseases of mankind have been controlled by the systematic application of prevention strategies, including morbidity and mortality from nutritional and infectious diseases and vehicular trauma.[1] Among chronic diseases, the incidence of cardiovascular disease has decreased markedly as smoking has declined, cholesterol and blood pressure have been lowered, and exercise has been encouraged. It is likely that these simple approaches have led to a greater overall benefit to health for the population than the effect of all intensive care units, but such direct comparisons are difficult to make. In general, appreciation of the role of prevention strategies in the overall management of cancer has been neglected by clinical oncologists, although health care planners and society as a whole are intensely interested in this topic.[5] Cancer prevention strategies can be considered at three different major levels: primary, secondary, and tertiary

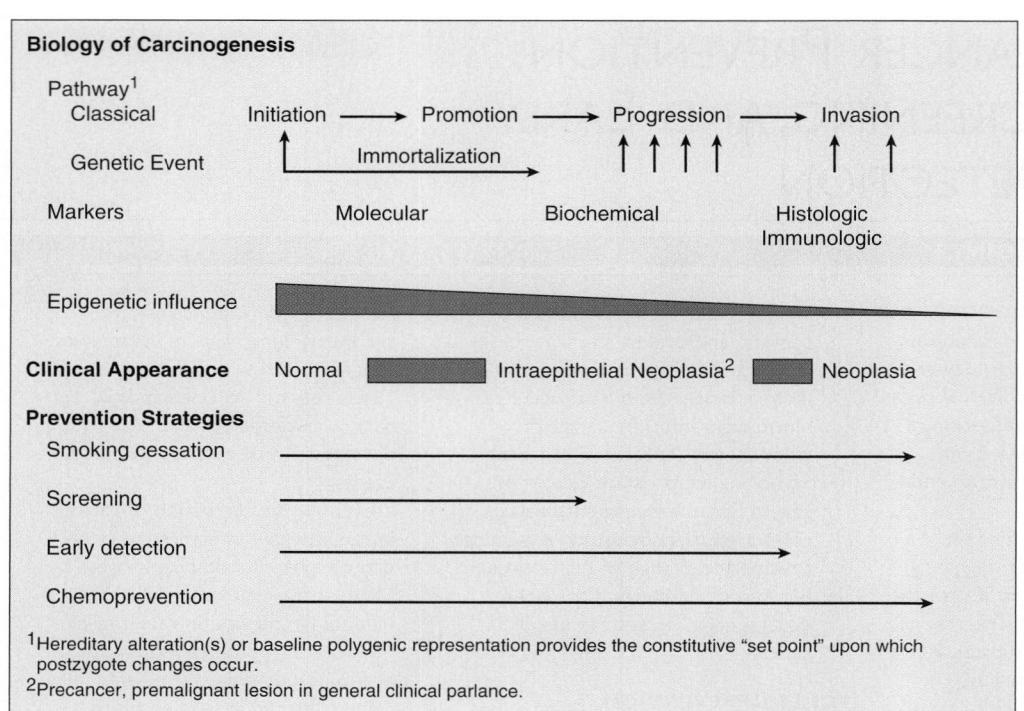

Figure 23-1. Integration of the biology of carcinogenesis and prevention.

(Table 23-1). This chapter will deal primarily with primary and secondary prevention and with tertiary prevention as represented by chemoprevention of second malignancies.

Normal, asymptomatic individuals are the population at which primary prevention is addressed. Major strategies for risk reduction include changes in diet, increased physical activity, tobacco awareness, decreased exposure to the sun, and reduced intake of alcohol. With the increasing identification of constitutive genetic alterations that predispose individuals to cancer, this group has been targeted for primary interventions such as prophylactic surgery.[6] Annual screening mammography in women older than 50 years of age and smoking cessation or chemoprevention in a group of asymptomatic smoking individuals are also examples of targeted primary prevention.

Secondary prevention is directed toward individuals with evidence of preneoplastic, clinically identifiable progression, but without frank malignancy. The phenomenon of IEN, also called preneoplasia or precancer, has become of widespread interest only recently (except with regard to cervical cancer), and management of these lesions has the potential to abrogate the disease process early. Many organ sites have preneoplastic counterparts that should be amenable to early intervention (Table 23-2). Representative examples of this type of secondary prevention include suppression or reversal of oral leukoplakia or Barrett's esophagus and inhibition of polyp formation or progression (Fig. 23-2).

Tertiary prevention involves decreasing the morbidity of established disease. Chemoprevention of second malignancies is a good example of tertiary prevention. The distinction between primary, secondary, and tertiary prevention can sometimes become blurred. Further, tertiary prevention and adjuvant therapies can share many of the same goals. From the viewpoint of the clinical oncologist, probably the best way to look at prevention is as one more therapeutic modality for the management of cancer, directed at its control in the earliest stages. The observation that the addition of a retinoid after bone marrow transplantation markedly enhances the survival of children with refractory neuroblastoma represents an

TABLE 23-1

Levels of Prevention in Cancer Management

	DEFINITION	EXAMPLE
Primary	Decrease risk for normal asymptomatic individuals	Screening* Smoking cessation Chemoprevention of breast cancer in asymptomatic women† Diet modification
Secondary	Decrease progression of preneoplastic processes	Reverse preneoplasia (CIN, leukoplakia) with chemoprevention‡ Early detection
Tertiary	Decrease morbidity of established disease	Chemoprevention of second malignancies

*Asymptomatic individuals; if symptomatic, then this would be an example of early detection.
†If women had prior breast cancer, this would be an example of tertiary prevention.
‡Almost all epithelial (solid tumor) cancers have a clinically identifiable precancerous stage known as intraepithelial neoplasia.

TABLE 23-2

Common Clinical Precursors (Intraepithelial Neoplasia) of Cancer

ORGAN SITE	PRECURSOR	METHOD OF DETECTION*
Oropharynx	Leukoplakia	Visual†
Skin	Actinic keratoses/moles	Visual†
Esophagus	Barrett's esophagus	Endoscopy
Colon	Adenoma (polyp)	Sigmoidoscopy, colonoscopy
Breast	LCIS, DCIS‡	Mammography, ultrasound, MRI
Cervix	Intraepithelial neoplasia	Colposcopy

*Cytology and/or biopsy is required in almost all cases before definitive therapy can be initiated.
†Elegant in situ optical spectroscopic methods are being developed to detect early preneoplastic changes, including enhancing the signals with fluorescent molecules.
‡Lobular and ductal carcinoma in situ.

informative synthesis of a quaternary treatment approach and a tertiary prevention modality.[7]

Avoidable Causes

An extensive analysis of the topic of avoidable causes of cancer was performed nearly 2 decades ago by Doll and Peto;[8] these investigators concluded that 50% to 70% of all human cancers were preventable. No new data has emerged that would alter that overall estimate, although some of the specifics have changed.[9] The major avoidable risk factors can be broadly separated into four areas: tobacco, infectious, chemical (including hormonal), and diet.

Tobacco smoke is far and away the most important carcinogen to which humans are exposed on a routine basis. The morbidity and mortality from tobacco smoke is huge and represents the major preventable cause of all diseases in American society, not just cancer. What is

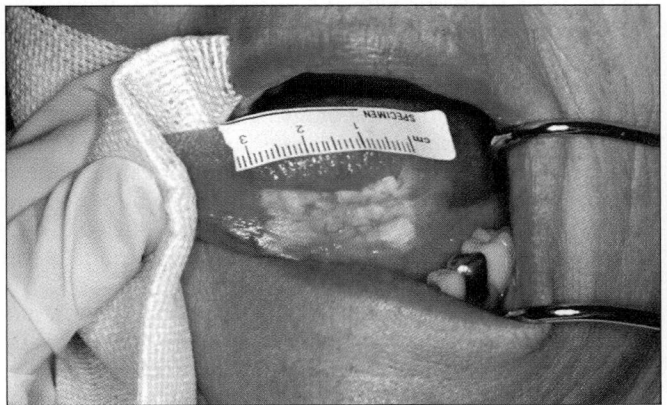

A

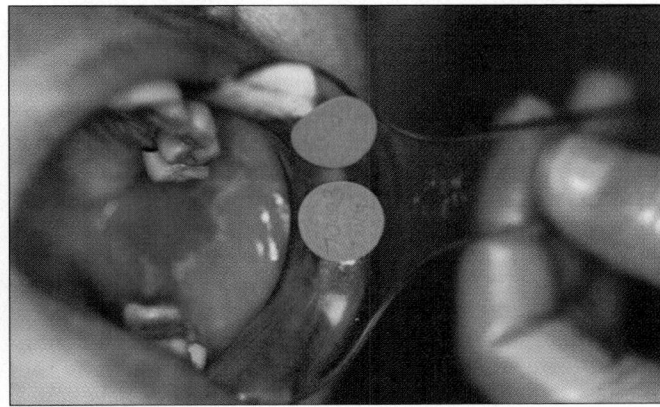

B

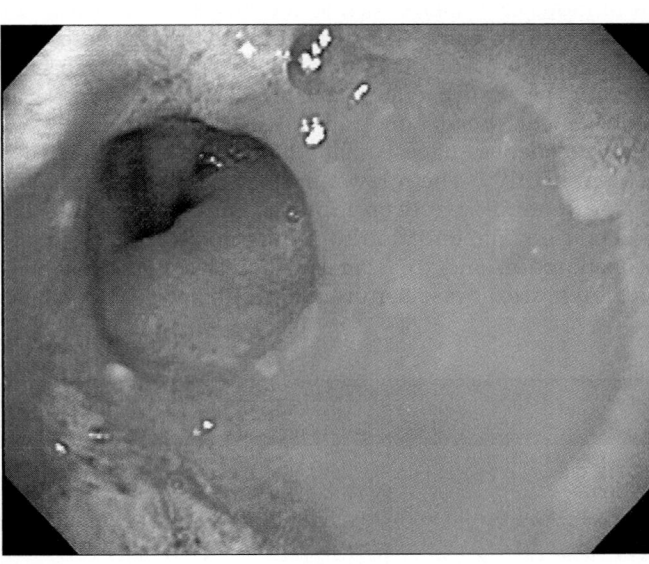

C

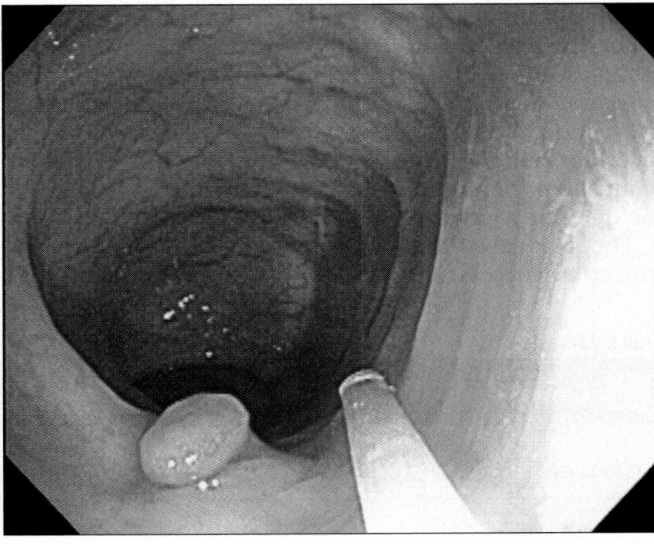

D

Figure 23-2. Examples of premalignant lesions. **A,** Leukoplakia. Whitish lesion on side of tongue. **B,** Erythroplakia. Reddish (dark area) lesion in otherwise normal-looking buccal cavity. **C,** Barrett's esophagus (pale area) with high-grade lesion (dark portion). **D,** Adenomatous polyp in proximal sigmoid colon.

MAJOR AVOIDABLE INFLUENCES ON CANCER DEVELOPMENT IN HUMANS

TOBACCO

Tobacco smoking has been linked causally with most lung and oropharyngeal cancers and is a significant contributor to the risk for esophageal, pancreatic, bladder, renal, and cervical cancers, as well as for acute myelogenous leukemia.

DIETARY

The role of diet is complex and unproven, but diets high in vegetables and fruits have been consistently protective.

INFECTIOUS

Human papilloma virus and hepatitis have been implicated, respectively, in the etiology of cervical, hepatic, and some oral cancers, as has the bacterium *Helicobacter pylori* in stomach cancer.

CHEMICAL CARCINOGENS

Some examples include aniline dyes (bladder), asbestos (mesothelium), hormones (breast, prostate, endometrium).

23-3). Hepatitis and human papilloma virus clearly play major roles in the development and evolution of hepatocellular and cervical carcinoma, respectively. Vaccines using various viral components as the target have recently been tested; results from these trials suggest that liver and cervical cancer are preventable.[19,20] In addition to the classical and long-recognized associations of the parasites *Clonorchiasis sinensis* to cholangiocarcinoma and *Schistosoma hematobium* to squamous cell carcinoma of the bladder, the bacterium *Helicobacter pylori* has now been accepted as an etiologic agent associated with gastric dysplasia, stomach cancer, and a rare type of lymphoma.[21,22] Early on, these diseases can be treated with antibiotics and the process reversed. Finally, it appears that viruses have a role in the evolution of some lymphomas (HTLV-1, Epstein-Barr). These recent findings all offer new approaches for primary and secondary prevention using standard and new microbiological and immunologic approaches.

A number of chemicals are known to play a role in cancer causation, perhaps the most widespread being aniline dyes (bladder cancer), asbestos (lung, mesothelioma) and hormones (breast, prostate). The role of endogenous and exogenous hormones in cancer causation is complex and is considered in detail in the sections on breast, prostate, and gynecologic organ sites.[23] Some of the most intensely debated issues in medicine relate to this area. For example, is the overall health benefit of hormone replacement therapy worthwhile? Recent results from the Women's Health Trial suggest not, although many argue that the short-term benefit on quality of life outweigh long term harm.[24,25]

The question of the specific role of dietary components in cancer prevention remains largely unanswered. Many comprehensive reviews on the topic are available, and the overall recommendation to eat an abundant amount of fruits and vegetables has not changed in 20 years.[26,27] Ambitious campaigns, such as the well-known "5-a-day for better health" campaign to encourage large-scale dietary changes continue.[28] The specific components responsible for the protective effects against cardiovascular disease and cancer remain unclear, however, although accumulating evidence suggests that folate might be an important component.[29,30] The roles of macronutrients, fat, and fiber in prevention have been topics of much discussion. The general recommendation to reduce total calories and fat consumption and to increase fiber is a good one with regard to cardiovascular disease prophylaxis, but whether

generally not appreciated is the wide carcinogenic range of molecular damage and the numerous organ sites affected by cigarette smoke.[10,11] In addition to the lungs, cigarette smoking contributes significant attributable risk to the development of cancers of the oropharynx (75%), bladder (50%), esophagus (50%), pancreas (25%), cervix (20%), kidney (15%), and bone marrow (10%). Cigarette smoke facilitates chromosomal instability and enhances transformation at all levels of cancer formation (initiation, promotion, progression), including adversely affecting the natural history of successfully resected early-stage lung cancer.[12,13] Although the incidence of cigarette smoking has fallen among males, in 1994 lung cancer surpassed breast cancer as the most common cause of death from cancer in females and continues to increase. Well-tested modules have been developed to assist health care workers, including physicians, in applying smoking prevention and cessation strategies.[14-17] Various forms of nicotine (gum, patch, inhalers, nasal sprays) and behavioral modulators (bupropion) have been effective in increasing the quit rate significantly at very low cost.[18]

The evidence for infectious involvement in human cancer has increased dramatically in the last decade (Table

TABLE 23-3

Cancers with an Infectious Etiology

CANCER	AGENT	MAJOR MODE OF TRANSMISSION	INTERVENTION
Hepatocellular carcinoma	Hepatitis virus	Maternal, oral	Vaccine
Gastric	*Helicobacter pylori*	Oral	Antibiotics
Cervix	Papilloma virus	Sexual	Vaccine

Several major cancers are of infectious etiology and can be eradicated by preventive intervention.

such a strategy affects cancer outcome remains unproven. Increasing epidemiologic data suggests that physical activity, basal metabolic index, and folate consumption could play critical roles, and a number of trials are underway to address these issues.[31,32]

There is growing evidence that changes in the insulin-like growth factor pathways play an important role in many aspects of lifestyle changes represented by a high basal metabolic index and its control.[33] With increasingly positive protective effects of physical exercise on cardiovascular disease being shown, there has been a renewed interest in the influence of physical exercise on malignant transformation and progression.[34] There has been a great deal of interest in micronutrients as preventive agents, but the results emanating from Supplementation in well-done randomized clinical trials to date have been disappointing.[26,35,36] Notable exceptions have included the report that Supplementation with a modest dose of vitamin A (25,000 IU per day) can decrease the appearance of cutaneous squamous cell cancer of the skin in individuals with prior actinic keratoses and two separate trials that Supplementation with a modest dose of calcium can decrease the subsequent prevalence of cancer polyps by 20%.[37-39]

Probably the most exciting diet-related development has been the identification of a wide range of potentially new and active chemoprevention compounds in food, such as protease inhibitors (soybeans), monoterpenes (citrus fruit oils), polyphenols (nuts), dithiolethiones (cruciferous vegetables), alliums (onion/garlic family), resveratrol (red wine); and many others.[40,41] The opportunity to genetically engineer foods to reduce the risk of heart disease and cancer is a topic of much scientific interest and commercial activity.[42] Nature created these molecules to deal with a hostile toxic environment, and figuring out how to use them for the prevention of cancer should be both scientifically interesting and clinically rewarding.

Screening and Early Detection

Strictly speaking, screening is limited to normal individuals. The science of screening identified many pitfalls in the design, analysis, and interpretation of such trials, including length and lead-time biases and many others.[43,44] Beyond the technical issues involved in study design, implementation, analysis, and interpretation, three other requirements must be met to demonstrate that a screening test is useful:

1. A test must be available that will detect cancer earlier than routine methods (e.g., clinical or self-examination).
2. There must be evidence that treatment at an earlier stage of disease will result in an improved outcome (decreased cause-specific morbidity or mortality).
3. There must be evidence of a total health benefit.[45] Increasing attention has been addressed to this issue, and the issue of disease-specific vs. all-cause mortality is an important one, particularly among older individuals.[46]

Fulfilling these requirements is difficult, and the issues specifically related to screening of different organ sites for precancers or cancers are discussed in those sections. Some generic comments are worthwhile, though. Enough evidence exists for a specific test for some organ sites that has been proven effective to recommend the routine adoption of screening (Table 23-4). Although the availability of cancer screening is generally increasing, usage is

TABLE 23-4

Effectiveness of Major Screening Approaches for Cancer*

ORGAN SITE	TEST	POSITIVE LEVEL OF EVIDENCE[†]	RECOMMENDED
Breast			
Over age 50	Mammography	Strong	Yes
Age 40–50	Mammography	Fairly strong	Yes
Cervix	Papanicolaou[‡]	Strong	Yes
Colorectal			
Over age 50	Occult fecal blood	Strong	Yes
	Sigmoidoscopy	Strong	Yes
	Colonoscopy[§]	Fairly strong	Yes
Lung	Chest roentgenogram	None[‖]	No
Melanoma	Skin examination	Moderate	Yes
Prostate	Prostate-specific antigen	Moderate	Yes[¶]

*Listed here are organ sites for which sufficient data exists to make a judgement. Although no specific trial evidence exists, routine physical examination of the skin, oral cavity, testicles, and ovary/uterus is worthwhile, as treatment success is closely related to stage at diagnosis and effective treatment is available in most cases.
†The concept of level of evidence is a valuable approach—a quantitative approach that is presented in detail in the PDQ section of the NCI Web site (http://cancernet. nci.nih.gov/clinpolq/screening). A randomized trial with survival as an endpoint is at the top of the hierarchy, while anecdotal evidence by experts is at the lowest.
‡Screening should begin with the onset of sexual activity.
§Evidence also exists that colonoscopy with excisional biopsy is an effective therapeutic maneuver but the cost of the procedure has precluded its general usage.
‖Several randomized trials of screening chest roentgenograms showed no effect on outcome. Spiral CT is currently being tested in a large national trial.
¶With careful follow-up and appropriate testing.

relatively low for some organ sites (e.g., colon) and among groups that lack health insurance or a usual source of care.[47] Many screening tests, however, are ineffective (e.g., routine chest roentgenograms in smokers being the most notable). The age of molecular diagnosis in screening is upon us and holds both promise and peril, but to date its use has not had a significant impact on the early diagnosis of clinically significant cancer.[48] A positive screening test might lead to aggressive intervention that could allow "cure" of the organ site disease but result in an overall increased morbidity or mortality that is not efficacious for a person's general health (e.g., radical prostatectomy for older individuals with a minimally increased PSA.) Finally, screening for currently incurable malignancies (e.g., pancreatic cancer) offers new ethical dilemmas. If we have little to offer therapeutically, do we want to know the risk? Maybe, maybe not. Perhaps earlier surgery might be able to affect the outcome in a few patients—for example, in families with early-onset pancreatic cancer.

Although early detection is, formally speaking, the evaluation of a symptomatic individual for cancer and therefore different from screening, many of the caveats regarding evaluation of this approach are the same. The increasing ability to identify high-risk populations, either by phenotypic criteria or by genetic analysis, also tends to lead to a blurring of the classic division between screening and early detection. With the rapid advances in molecular diagnostics, routine genetic typing of individuals at risk for major tumor types should not be too distant in the future, and quantitation of that risk (a concept we proposed quite some time ago)[49] and its evaluation at the time of detection present cause for real-world angst. Identification and referral of families at high risk for cancer susceptibility should be an increasing emphasis of clinical oncologists, but to date, participation by oncologists has been low.[5,50] At the very least, the ability to downshift the stage of a disease at the time of detection should eventually lead to improved survival as new treatment approaches emanate from causative understanding of a particular cancer. Proving this point, though, has been difficult for cancers of many organ sites.

The effectiveness of screening for the major types of cancer is summarized in Table 23-4 and is discussed in detail in the individual sections of this chapter. There are effective screening modalities for breast cancer, colorectal cancers, melanoma, and cervical cancers, whereas no compelling evidence exists for the value of screening for lung cancer. The effectiveness of PSA in screening for prostate cancer has been a subject of intense debate; we feel that the tide may be turning and that in the near future the evidence will support the routine use of PSA screening over age 50 with thoughtful management and follow-up of abnormal values.

Carcinogenesis and Chemoprevention

Carcinogenesis
Advances in our understanding of the biology of carcinogenesis (cancer formation) have sharpened our thoughts about screening and early detection and provided a guide to thinking about risk assessment

and chemoprevention.[51,52] Figure 23-1 serves as a useful general roadmap to reflect on these issues for all tumor types (see also O'Shaughnessy and colleagues[3] and Shureiqi and coworkers[53]). The classical model of carcinogenesis divides cancer evolution into three major epochs: initiation, promotion, and progression. This classification has served as a useful heuristic model for which considerable experimental evidence has been developed. In the past 10 years, the genetic paradigm for the development of cancer has been elegantly articulated and experimentally confirmed for some organ sites. A series of steps in response to separate molecular events at the genetic level is a useful platform from which to understand carcinogenesis in human epithelial tumors. Almost all human cancers examined in any detail have shown evidence of several acquired molecular abnormalities, although the "pathway" has been well defined only for colon and head and neck cancers.[54,55] The expression of these abnormalities has allowed the development of markers that could serve as indicators of cancer risk or disease progression or possibly as surrogate endpoints for chemoprevention agent testing.[3,56-58]

Utilization of markers of carcinogenesis to assess the status of the disease relative to diagnosis and treatment and for assessment of chemoprevention effect is an important and complex issue.[56,59,60] The continued development and validation of markers will be critical to the intelligent management of early-stage cancer.[61] What also has become clear is that environmental phenomena (e.g., hormones, diet, carcinogens) can influence the expression of genetic changes. At one extreme of the paradigm is retinoblastoma, in which loss of a single gene inevitably results in an ocular tumor at a young age; however, most common solid tumors in adults seem to have underlying polygenic contributions, which can be affected by a large range of exogenous factors, even when a deleterious mutation such as BRCA1 or BRCA2 is present.

Chemoprevention
The idea of the chemoprevention of human cancer has been with us for more than 2 decades, but only in the last few years have positive clinical trials been reported to support the preclinical data and their potential use in human beings.[62-65] Retinoids are a major group of compounds that have provided convincing "proof of principle" of chemoprevention in humans, but in general they have been too toxic for widespread use and have not been adopted widely.[66] The overall results of some of the key randomized chemoprevention trials are summarized in Table 23-5, which are discussed in more detail in the individual organ site sections. Major problems in developing chemoprevention as a modality for cancer management have been the length and size of the trials required to show changes in a definitive endpoint.[67,68] Consequently, only the National Cancer Institute and a few large research groups have been able to marshal the resources to develop broad-based chemoprevention efforts. Another significant issue in the design of early trials was that many large studies evolved primarily from epidemiologic observations, with little experimental data available. Because the implementation of large phase III

TABLE 23-5

Current Overall Status of Chemoprevention in Preventing Human Cancers*

ORGAN SITE	PRETRIAL LEVEL OF EVIDENCE	AGENT	STATUS OF CHEMO-PREVENTION	COMMENT
Breast	Strong	Tamoxifen	Effective	One large trial, very positive; two smaller trials showed no effect. Overall long-term health benefits need to be determined
Cervix[†]	Strong	Multiple	Ineffective to marginal	Numerous phase III trials of several compounds have not substantiated phase II trials except for topical transretinoid acid
Colon	Strong	Multiple	Mixed	Slight decrease (25%) in colon polyp recurrence by calcium or aspirin
Head and neck (secondary)	Moderately strong	13-cis retinoic acid	Effective but toxic	Follow-up trial at lower dose ineffective
Leukoplakia	Moderately strong	β-carotene	Promising	Single randomized trial needs confirmation
Tertiary	Strong	13-cis retinoic acid	Effective but toxic	Follow-up studies at lower doses in progress
Lung				
Primary	Strong	β-carotene	Ineffective	More lung cancers and increased higher overall mortality
Secondary (metaplasia)	Strong	Retinoids	Ineffective	Impressively negative
Prostate	Moderately strong	Finasteride	Accrual complete	Results indicate positive effects but are preliminary
		SELECT[‡]	Ongoing	Results in 2010
Skin	Strong	Retinoids	Effective in some cases	Seems to depend on stage of cancer development and strength of agent
		Diclofenac	Effective	Causes regression of actinic keratoses

*Details are discussed in individual sections.
[†]Cervix, effects on regression of cervical intraepithelial neoplasia.
[‡]Selenium and vitamin E. epidemiologic data from secondary analysis; experimental data moderate.

or IV chemoprevention trials is a 10 to 100 million dollar exercise, political influences on the funding process are substantial also.

An attempt to develop chemoprevention agents logically has been outlined, and systematic preclinical testing and evolution of sequential clinical trials are likely to avoid some of the mistakes of the past.[58,68,69] Several key elements are featured in this decision-analysis process:

- Preclinical in vitro and in vivo testing against a battery of molecular targets and cellular and animal models.
- Accurate identification of side effects and assessment of their importance.
- Evidence of modulation of anticipated biochemical or molecular markers in the relevant tissue in short-term human trials.
- A randomized 6- to 12-month study of multiple low doses of the candidate agent in a relevant patient/participant population, with careful identification of side effects, assessment of their importance, and evaluation of their biochemic, molecular, and/or histologic effects.

In this regard, we have performed a particularly informative series of studies in assessing topical transretinoic acid in cervical cancer prevention and difluoromethylornithine in colon cancer prevention,[70-74] while the M.D. Anderson group[61,75] has performed a series of important trials in aerodigestive cancers and the Arizona group has done the same for skin cancers.[76,77] Following this logical pathway of chemoprevention agent development assures that the probability of conducting a definitive phase III or IV study will be high and maximizes the chance for a successful outcome.

Although, to date, most agents have been developed based on epidemiologic or carcinogen models in animals, the increasing knowledge about the molecular basis of cancer progression in human tumors should result in the discovery and synthesis of highly specific drugs based on altered biochemical and signalling pathways.[69,78] The number of specific tumors for which prevention strategies could be reviewed is large. In this chapter, we review the major organ sites (aerodigestive, colon, breast, prostate) and those sites (skin, ovary, cervix) in which sufficient evidence exists to suggest that preventive strategies currently have a role in clinical oncology. We also offer a few comments on less studied cancers (stomach, liver) that are extremely common outside the United States and Europe. With the rapidly increasing scientific understanding of the biological basis for many tumor types and the recognition that screening, early detection, and chemoprevention should play a large role in the management of the carcinogenic process, we can anticipate that the list of therapeutic strategies for IEN and possibly earlier manifestations of cancer will grow rapidly over the next few years.

AERODIGESTIVE MALIGNANCIES

Introduction and Risk Reduction

Aerodigestive malignancies encompass a subset of cancers that include those that arise from the oral cavity, pharynx, esophagus, and lung.[75] These organ sites have been grouped together, as they share a mucosal epithelial field

Science of Clinical Oncology

1

that is directly subject to malignant transformation by the common toxin (tobacco), the major underlying etiologic agent for these malignancies. In addition to cigarette smoke, smokeless tobacco has also played, in recent years, an increasing contributory role in oral carcinogenesis, and oral cancer in the young adult has become increasingly common.[79] Alcohol also clearly plays a synergistic role with tobacco carcinogens in the development of oral and esophageal cancers, including second cancers.[80,81] Polymorphisms in the alcohol dehydrogenase gene involved with tobacco carcinogen metabolism could play an important role in determining risk for head and neck and tobacco-related malignancies.[82] The recent identification of human papilloma virus in more than 50% of oropharyngeal and nearly 100% of laryngeal tumors also could be playing a role.[83] Progress in understanding the biology of tobacco-associated carcinogenesis in the past few years has been rapid, and molecular models of head and neck and lung cancers have been characterized to a substantial degree.[55,84-86] What is clear from cytogenetic genomic hybridization and other studies is that although aerodigestive cancers share many similar changes early on (e.g., loss and gain of 3p and cyclin alterations), discrete subsets exist.[87] Because different genes are involved, this information should have a practical effect on the development of chemoprevention and other interventions (Table 23-6).

In 2002, more than 225,000 cancers developed in aerodigestive sites, and more 195,000 related deaths resulted in the United States[4] It is estimated that more than 500 million smokers now living will die of tobacco-related illnesses. As it is estimated that the etiology of more than 80% of aerodigestive cancers is tobacco-related, the cost to society of this legal carcinogen is extraordinarily high. The application of prevention strategies should have a favorable impact on decreasing morbidity and mortality from aerodigestive cancers; particularly important for the medical profession should be the adoption of proven, physician-facilitated smoking cessation methods.[14-18]

Screening and Early Detection

Oropharyngeal cancer occurs in a region of the body that is easily accessible to examination by a health care worker. The morbidity and mortality from oropharyngeal cancer is directly related to the stage at diagnosis, so effective screening and early detection should be worthwhile.[88] No definitive trial has been done, however, demonstrating that an early detection program can downshift stage at diagnosis of oropharyngeal cancer or reduce mortality in a screened population. Nevertheless, an inspection of the oral cavity should be part of every examination in high-risk patients (smokers) and can be made efficacious by careful inspection of the soft palate, tongue, and floor of the mouth, where 90% of all squamous cell cancers occur.[89,90] The preneoplastic lesions, leukoplakia and particularly erythroplakia, should be identified and, if necessary, biopsied, as they represent early observable signs of squamous cell carcinomas with different prognoses (see Fig. 23-2A and B). In appropriately screened populations of high-risk smokers and drinkers over age 40, a detection rate of oral cancers as high as 1 cancer in every 200 individuals examined has been achieved.[90] A successful screening program can be mounted using health caseworkers; for example, in Sri Lanka, where oral cancer is a common malignancy, a sensitivity of 58% was obtained for 660 patients with suspected cancers.[91]

Recent advances in optical biology also suggest that screening using autofluorescent techniques could allow detection of premalignant changes before the clinical appearance of disease.[92] The strong association of HPV with oral cancers in young, nonsmoking individuals[83] and the success of screening techniques in detecting cervical intraepithelial neoplasia (see the discussion that follows) suggest that oral screening for HPV should be adopted for those who are sexually active. Whether this group is the same population at risk for genital HPV has not been defined, but it would be reasonable to assume so.

Routine screening of esophageal cancer in the United States has not been attempted to a significant degree because it is relatively uncommon and therapeutic options are poor. In China and other Asian countries, however, the disease is much more common and found at high frequency in certain geographic locales. In these areas, screening and early detection using esophageal cytology are widely used, although the efficacy of these approaches has yet to be established.[93] Increased recognition of the metaplastic condition known as Barrett's esophagus (see Fig. 23-2C) has heightened interest in identifying these preneoplastic lesions in individuals with reflux, as treatment by acid suppression, laser therapy, and photodynamic therapy is at least partially successful.[94] Recent attempts to reverse or suppress these lesions with 13-cis-retinoic acid have been unsuccessful.[95]

Screening and early detection of lung cancer has not been an effective way to decrease morbidity or mortality. Four large randomized trials of screening chest roentgenograms in smokers have demonstrated no difference in

TABLE 23-6

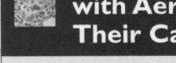

Biologic Abnormalities in Patients with Aerodigestive Malignancies and Their Cancers*

Predisposition

Molecular (DNA repair, telomerase)
Metabolic (p450, alcohol dehydrogenase)
Mutagen sensitivity profiles

Chromosomal Abnormalities

In the field
In the premalignancy
In the cancer

Altered Gene Expression that Predicts Responsiveness and Unresponsiveness

p53
RAR-β

*Most of the work has been done in patients with oral precancers and cancers; the degree to which these observations can be extrapolated to other aerodigestive cancer is speculative.

survival between the randomized groups.[96] Various new approaches, including spiral CT, sputum screening by quantitative microscopy, measurement of a variety of molecular changes during malignant progression, and use of fluorescent detection of lesions during bronchoscopy are being explored. To date, however, none of these approaches has yet proven useful over the long term nor decreased morbidity or mortality from lung cancer.

Chemoprevention

Epithelial cancers of the upper aerodigestive tract and lungs are the most extensively studied system for chemoprevention in humans, and the results are the most negative. The natural history of the disease process has been studied extensively and provides a rich platform from which to conduct chemoprevention trials. Field carcinogenesis by tobacco carcinogens with its associated epidemiologic risk and characterized molecular changes is a straightforward concept that has guided the development of chemoprevention studies in this area.[61,84] The recent identification of molecular, (e.g., DNA repair, telomerase), metabolic (e.g., p450, alcohol dehydrogenase), and mutagen sensitivity profiles that predispose to aerodigestive cancers, acquired chromosomal abnormalities in the field and in the cancers, and alterations of several molecular parameters that predict responsiveness and unresponsiveness, recently have provided useful detail from which to consider the next generation of rational chemoprevention trials.[61,97-102] The identification of a variety of molecular changes during head and neck cancer progression, in addition to readily identifiable histologic precursors, has provided a biologic base for understanding the interaction of carcinogenesis and chemoprevention of this disease (see Table 23-5). Recent studies of the molecular changes that accompany the progression of lung cancer—most notably the allelic-specific detection of chromosome 3 p at an early stage of lung cancer pathogenesis—also provides a useful paradigm and platform from which to develop well-considered chemoprevention approaches.[86]

To date, however, the results of primary, secondary, and tertiary chemoprevention trials of the lung have been disappointing (see Goodman[103] and McWilliams and Lam[104]). Two large placebo-controlled, multiagent randomized trials in heavy smokers (more than 47,000 participants) have been negative and showed no beneficial effect of retinol (vitamin A) or α-tocopherol (vitamin E).[105,106] More disturbingly, these two large, randomized trials indicate that current smokers Supplemented with oral β-carotene develop lung cancers at a rate 25% greater than the placebo group and also exhibit an increased overall mortality. These findings remain unexplained, although conceivably, the high concentration of β-carotene attained in the carcinogen-damaged lung might produce a form of β-carotene that functions as a pro-oxidant.[107,108] Other possibilities that might help explain the results regarding the adverse effect of β-carotene include:

- Lowering of the concentration of other micronutrients that might be protective.

- Stimulation of preneoplastic clones by enhancement of growth factor production.
- Complex genetic polymorphisms that lead to alteration of tobacco carcinogen metabolism.

Definitive secondary (metaplasia, atypia) and tertiary (second malignancy) chemoprevention trials that use a number of different retinoids and other compounds (folic acid, N-acetyl cysteine) have also yielded negative results.[103,104] Recently, anethole dithiolethione (an organosulfure compound) was shown in a randomized trial to reduce development of new bronchial dysplasia lesions and to slow progression of preexisting disease in current or former smokers.[109] This important finding needs confirmation.

Studies of secondary and tertiary chemoprevention of head and neck cancers have led to somewhat more encouraging results. Randomized trials have shown that isotretinoin causes regression of oral leukoplakia, although accompanied by substantial side effects.[110,111] Two randomized trials confirmed activity of β-carotene, although results from the later study were less convincing.[112,113] Several other, less toxic agents (retinol, 4-[hydroxyphenyl]-retinamide, and α-tocopherol) and selenium have also produced responses of premalignant lesions in phase II trials.[114] We have demonstrated substantial potential activity of bowman-birk inhibitor (a soybean-derived compound) against oral leukoplakia.[115] The results of randomized studies for these compounds have not yet been reported.

In a randomized phase III adjuvant trial of patients treated for head and neck cancer by local therapy, the synthetic retinoid 13-cis-retinoic acid (isotretinoin, accutane) at a high daily oral dose (50–100 mg/m^2) led to a reduction in the incidence of second primary tumors, a difference that was maintained for more than 5 years.[116,117] The rate of second primary tumors was affected greatly by tobacco smoking status, with the efficacy of chemoprevention decreasing sequentially in current and former smokers compared with non-smokers.[118] The side-effects in the 13-cis retinoic acid trial were substantial at this dosage level, however. These results with 13-cis retinoic acid were particularly significant in that a similarly designed randomized trial using another retinoid (etretinate) at a high dose showed no reduction of second primary tumors.[119] Therefore, the efficacy of low-dose isotretinoin (30 mg/day) to prevent second primary tumors after treatment of early-stage (I and II) head and neck cancer was tested in a randomized trial, with the hope that side effects could be decreased without losing efficacy. This strategy was unsuccessful and no difference in the apppearence of second malignancies in the placebo and treatment groups could be demonstrated (S. Lippman, personal communication).

Overall, these trials suggest that oral leukoplakia, but not bronchial metaplasia, can be reversed or suppressed by currently available chemopreventive agents. To date, "proof of principle" of chemoprevention in head and neck cancers has been achieved, but a great deal more positive information will need to be generated, and less toxic approaches or agents will need to be identified. Results from ongoing large-scale phase III trials, which include studies of low-dose retinoids to prevent second cancers in the upper aerodigestive tract and lungs, will need to be favorable before the strategy of chemoprevention can be adopted into standard medical practice for the management of aerodigestive cancers.

COLORECTAL CANCER

Introduction

Screening for and early detection of colorectal cancers results in 5-year survival rates of 90% for colon cancer and 80% for rectal cancer, providing that diagnosis and treatment occur before the lesions have spread beyond the bowel to regional lymph nodes or distant metastatic sites. Unfortunately, 65% of patients still present with higher-staged disease, leading to a lower overall 5-year survival rate of 50%.[4] In the United States, colon cancer is still responsible for more than 56,000 deaths per year, which is surpassed only by deaths secondary to lung cancer.[4] These statistics highlight the critical importance of identifying individuals at risk for the development of colorectal cancer and of screening and early detection in its management. This section will discuss various risk factors, both modifiable and unmodifiable, that increase susceptibility for the development of colorectal cancer and will review current screening guidelines. This information can be used to design more effective preventive strategies, which could employ genetic testing for individuals at risk and apply behavioral modification and chemoprevention.

Pathogenesis

Numerous epidemiologic, international, and experimental studies have evaluated various hereditary and environmental factors that could lead directly or indirectly to the development of colorectal cancers. It is believed that colon cancer is the result of a complex series of genetic and epigenetic events that occur when environmental factors interact with an individual's inherited or acquired susceptibility.[54,120] This interaction produces somatic mutations that accumulate over time and lead to neoplastic transformation of normal colonic epithelium into premalignant adenomatous polyps (see Fig. 23-2D) and ultimately into invasive disease. The natural history preceding the development of cancer can progress through several decades. Adenomatous polyps, especially the villous subtype, are the premalignant lesions in more than 90% of colorectal cancers. The risk of malignant degeneration depends on the size of the polyp (increasing greatly in those greater than 1–2 cm in size), duration of its presence, number present at the time of the initial examination, and the histological type.[121-122] Only adenomatous polyps seem to carry a premalignant risk; however, hyperplastic polyps are diagnosed more commonly in individuals with a smoking or drinking history, two predisposing factors for adenomatous polyp development.[123] The presence of hyperplastic polyps may warrant increased screening and prevention counseling, although further study of this issue is needed before definitive conclusions can be made.

Etiology

Heredity

Our understanding of the genetic and molecular alterations that precede the development of colorectal cancers has broadened and deepened over the past decade (Fig. 23-3).[124,125] This information has facilitated the identification of individuals who might benefit from early interventions with more vigilant screening, chemoprevention, or treatment. Based on studies of family histories, it is estimated that 20% to 30% of colorectal cancers have a significant hereditary component.[124] To date, however, genes associated with only two major

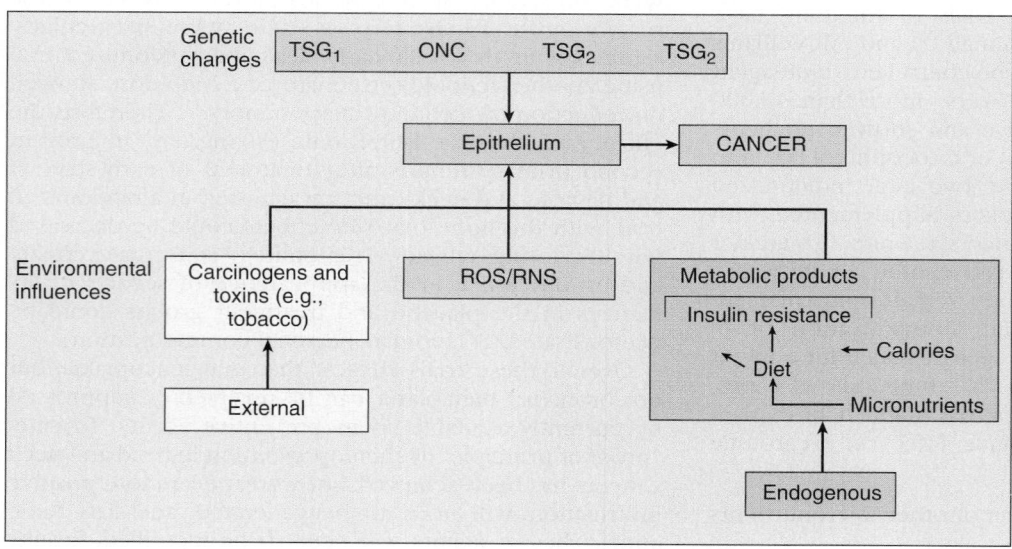

Figure 23-3. Colorectal cancer results from inherited genetic predisposition and acquired molecular alterations interacting with environmental and endogenous toxins that are themselves modified by gene products. TSG, tumor suppressor gene; ONC, oncogene; ROS/RNS, reactive oxygen and reactive nitrogen species form from normal metabolic processes (endogenous) and from exposure to carcinogens and toxins (external).

syndromes—familial adenomatosis polyposis (FAP) and hereditary nonpolyposis colon cancer (HNPCC)—have been identified clearly. Allelic deletions have been identified in patients diagnosed with these two autosomal dominant syndromes, FAP and HNPCC.[126-129] FAP comprises only 1% of colon cancer cases per year and is associated with a deletion of the APC gene on chromosome 5 (band q21). These patients develop thousands of adenomatous polyps that tend to be evenly distributed throughout the colon and rectum by the second or third decades of life. If surgical treatment by complete colectomy is not done, affected individuals are at high risk to develop colon cancer by the age of 40.[130,131] Recently, a highly specific mutation (T to A at nucleotide 3920) was found in 6% of Ashkenazi Jews, and about 28% of Ashkenazim have a family history of colorectal cancer.[132] This mutation created a small hypermutable region of the gene, thereby indirectly causing predisposition.

HNPCC is more common than FAP and makes up 5% to 10% of the cases of colon cancer diagnosed annually. Diagnosis requires that three or more relatives, representing at least two generations, be diagnosed with colorectal cancers before the age of 50.[133] One relative must be a first-degree relative of the proband patient. Patients tend to have cancers that arise in the proximal colon, and they also develop ovarian and endometrial cancers at a higher rate than the population at large. This syndrome is associated with defective DNA repair mechanisms, which lead to aberrant cell growth and tumor formation. These mutations occur on chromosomes 3 (hMLH1, 3p21) and 2 (hMSH2, 2p).[134-136] Based on extensive experimental and clinical data, Vogelstein and colleagues[54,126] hypothesized that a number of mutations occur and that it is the progressive accumulation of mutations that ultimately leads to invasive disease. This proposal has been substantiated extensively, and mutations associated with colorectal cancers have been identified involving proto-oncogenes, tumor suppressor genes, and certain key regulatory enzymes, such as cytochrome P450 and acetyltransferase.[125,137-142] Recent considerations suggest that colorectal cancers in adults develop through one of three different pathways (chromosomal instability, microsatellite instability, and CpG island methylator phenotype) and have different biologic behaviors.[120] The role of polymorphisms in metabolizing key molecules (including those present in the diet) is being examined closely and should provide a platform from which to understand gene-environment interactions. For example, polymorphisms in hepatic cytochrome P450 and acetyltransferase enzymes lead to rapid oxidation and acetylation of genotoxic compounds such as heterocyclic amines, which are present in processed foods.[142] Accelerated metabolism of these compounds increases an individual's risk of developing colorectal cancers threefold.

Diet

Although diet appears to play a significant role in colon carcinogenesis, the degree to which individual macronutrients and micronutrients contribute to the development of colorectal cancer has been elusive. In part, this difficulty stems from differences in design and methodology in studies that have been performed to evaluate this subject, including the type of dietary questionnaire administered, differences in cohorts such as age and ethnicity, confounding effects of other dietary components, selection and recall biases, sample size, and length of follow-up.

The majority of past evidence has demonstrated an increase in incidence and mortality rates from colorectal cancers in groups of people who consume a more "westernized" diet that is high in animal fat, total calories, and red meat but low in fiber and fruit and vegetable intake.[143,144] International and migrant studies have supported this observation. Recent studies, however, have indicated that the older evidence should be reconsidered. Large prospective cohort studies and several large randomized trials indicate that fiber does not appear to be protective nor fat contributory to colon cancer development.[145,146] In contrast, mechanistic considerations, metabolic studies, and epidemiologic studies suggest a strong protective effect of folate and an important role of insulin and insulin-like growth factors in colon cancer pathogenesis. Potter[120] and other researchers have done a particularly nice job in attempting to relate genetic changes, risk factors (including diet), and downstream molecules and pathogenesis.[147,148] The results of ongoing trials using folate Supplementation or dietary fat reduction should be of considerable interest.

Other Factors (Alcohol, Smoking, Exercise, Body Mass Index)

Primary prevention of colorectal cancer also requires that we understand factors other than diet that increase risk for colorectal carcinoma by initiating or promoting carcinogenesis. These include use of alcohol and tobacco sedentary lifestyle, and the metabolic changes that proceed from these.[27,147-149]

Many studies have demonstrated a relationship between alcohol use and colorectal cancer and adenoma formation.[150-155] It is still uncertain whether alcohol directly initiates DNA damage or acts as a promoter on cells that already have undergone preneoplastic changes. A low-methionine or low-folate diet might contribute to a situation leading to adenomas and colorectal cancer, as both methionine and folate are cofactors for DNA synthesis; lowered concentrations of these compounds leads to hypomethylation of DNA, which is a precursor to aneuploidy and loss of heterozygosity.[156] Various forms of a key enzyme, 5,10-methylenetetrahydrofolate reductase, which catalyzes the conversion of 5,10-methylenetetrahydrofolate to 5-methyltetrahydrofolate, have also been identified.[157] Some mutations of this enzyme increase its activity, whereas others decrease it. Low activity leads to decreased methionine synthesis and antagonizes methyl group metabolism in DNA synthesis.[157,158] This theory gained some support in the U.S. Male Health Professionals Study.[123] An association was found between high alcohol intake and methionine-deficient diets, after controlling for intakes of fat, red meat, fiber, level of physical activity, body mass index, and multivitamin and aspirin Supplementation. Alcohol might be particularly important for

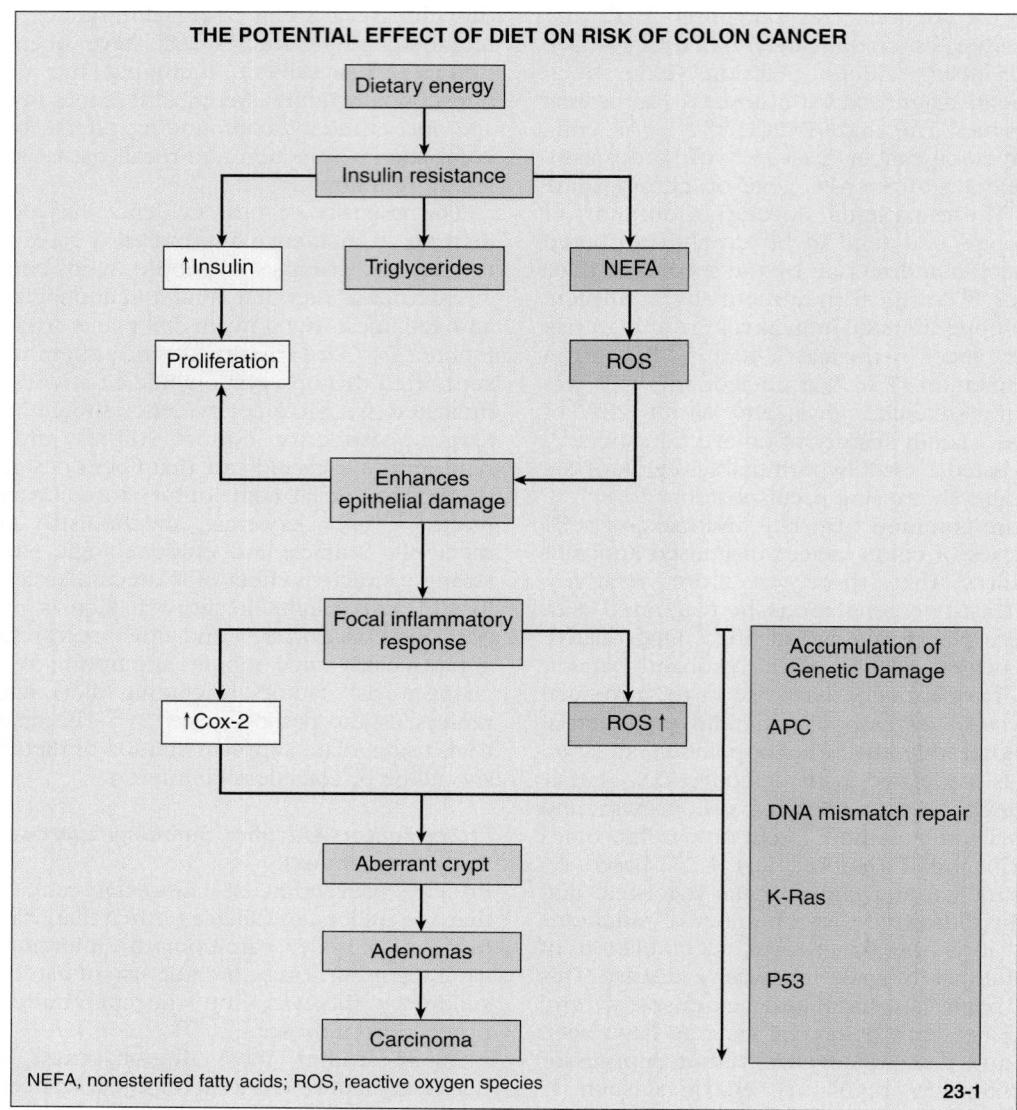

THE POTENTIAL EFFECT OF DIET ON RISK OF COLON CANCER

NEFA, nonesterified fatty acids; ROS, reactive oxygen species

23-1

progression of large adenomas to tumors.[159] Avoiding excess alcohol, while increasing dietary folate and methionine, seems like a reasonable approach to decreasing risk for colon cancer. Several large studies are underway to test whether Supplementation with folate can reduce adenomata development.

Cigarette smoking has been consistently associated with adenoma formation but less so with colon tumors, an observation that could be explained by the molecular nature of a subset of colon tumors in which microsatellite instability and/or p53-negative status is a prominent feature.[160,161] The Health Professionals Follow-up Cohort Study and the Nurse's Health Study observed more adenomas in individuals with a history of smoking than in those who did not smoke.[162,163] Analysis of the very large ACS Cancer Prevention II study indicates that 20% of colorectal cancers and 12% of deaths are associated with long-term cigarette smoking.[164]

Physical inactivity and high body mass index (BMI) also increase one's risk for colorectal cancers. A prospective study found a significant inverse association between leisure-time physical activity and incidence of colon cancer in participants of the Nurse's Health Study.[165] An inverse association was also observed between physical activity and the development of large (>1 cm) adenomas in the distal colon. In this same study, more adenomas were observed in individuals with a high BMI. Obesity, and in particular abdominal adiposity, has also been associated with an elevated risk for adenomatous polyps and colon cancer, but this has not been a universal finding. Increasing physical activity and maintaining lean body weight for the prevention of colorectal cancer probably has considerable merit for decreasing the incidence of polyps and colon cancer, as well as of other chronic diseases.

The mechanisms underlying these proposed effects are not clear, but a unifying hypothesis has been proposed recently and involves the sequential steps of consumption of excess dietary energy, development of insulin resistance, and increased circulating levels of insulin, triglycerides, and nonesterified fatty acids, which results in secondary colonic epithelial damage.[166] Recent epidemiologic evidence that associates insulin, IGF-1, and IGF-binding protein levels with colorectal cancers provides considerable support for this hypothesis.[167]

Screening and Early Detection

Population-based Data

A definitive amount of data has accumulated over the past few years indicating that colorectal cancer screening for persons at average risk is effective and reduces colorectal morbidity; agreement on the best screening modality remains unsettled, however.[168] Cost-saving analysis even supports the use of universal colonoscopy over the long term, notwithstanding the considerable practical challenges and total cost in achieving this goal. Probably everyone over 50 years of age needs to be screened. Yet surprisingly, less than 50% of individuals who should be screened are evaluated by fecal occult blood tests (FOBT), digital rectal exams (DRE), and/or sigmoidoscopy.[47,169]

Conflicting recommendations from government and private agencies contribute to the confusion. In general, all groups advocate screening in men and women beginning at the age of 50, as the incidence of colon cancer rises sharply between the ages of 50 and 55 and continues to double with each succeeding decade, reaching a peak by the age of 75. The American Cancer Society and the American College of Obstetricians and Gynecologists support yearly digital rectal exams beginning at age 40 and fecal occult blood tests performed yearly, once a person reaches 50 years of age. Sigmoidoscopy should occur every 3 to 5 years beginning at 50 years of age. Flexible sigmoidoscopy is superior to rigid sigmoidoscopy because it allows the examiner to visualize up to 60 cm of bowel mucosa and is easier on the patient.

There are numerous studies validating the use of DRE, FOBT, and sigmoidoscopy as effective screening tools, providing regular screening is performed (to detect lesions in this disease with a long preinvasive phase).[170-177] This is particularly important with the FOBT, as reported sensitivities are low and range between 22% and 92%. Sensitivity is higher when at least three tests are performed on different days and the samples are rehydrated with hydrogen peroxide. To decrease false negatives, which also increases the sensitivity of the test, patients should be instructed to avoid vitamin C and to eat a high-residue diet for several days prior to the test. The incidence of false positives is lowered when GI irritants (e.g., aspirin, oral iron, and meat products) are not consumed a few days prior to the FOBT. In general, screened, asymptomatic patients have a positive test 4% to 6% of the time. Only 5% to 10% of these individuals have colorectal cancers, and an additional 30% have benign polyps.[178,179] The positive predictive value is only about 20%, so a positive test can be costly, as follow-up requires evaluation by sigmoidoscopy or colonoscopy.[180] Randomized clinical trials have demonstrated a decrease in mortality by 15% to 33% with the regular use of serial FOBT, however.[174-176] Patients who received FOBT in conjunction with sigmoidoscopy in a Memorial Sloan Kettering Colon Cancer Trial had a significantly higher survival probability when compared with those who received sigmoidoscopy alone (70% vs 48%, respectively).[174] This is an impressive result.

Regular screening with sigmoidoscopy among patients over 50 years of age both reduces mortality from colorectal cancer and prolongs survival.[181-183] Studies need to be performed to clarify the optimal interval between screening and to develop recommendations for individuals at higher risk for adenomas or colorectal cancers. The early results of a "once-only" sigmoidoscopy at age 60, in which a high yield of adenomas was obtained, suggests that a less intense approach to screening could be a cost-effective strategy to prevent colon cancers.[184] Follow-up colonoscopy, however, suggested that a significant number of proximal adenomas were present. There is little doubt that screening colonoscopy is effective at identifying silent, large adenomas and colon cancers, but its cost effectiveness needs to be demonstrated; so must the optimal usage of fecal occult blood, sigmoidoscopy, and colonoscopy with regard to efficacy and cost (see Anderson and coworkers[185]). A particularly exciting new approach is the identification of colon cancer-specific mutations in fecal DNA.[186] A study of the adenomatous polyposis gene (APG), the initiating abnormality in most sporadic colon cancers, in the fecal DNA of normal individuals and patients with polyps shows considerable promise.[187] Although the specificity of this test was high (100%), the sensitivity was only 57%. However, integration of the test into the screening paradigm, (perhaps with FOBT) as a low-cost, general screen is an important goal. The DRE should be included in all examinations, as it enables evaluation of the distal rectum and prostate. Its sensitivity has decreased, however, with the temporal shift to more proximal lesions in the colon.[184] Other tests, including double-contrast barium enema, have not been evaluated completely as screening tests and are more expensive than DRE, F OBT, and sigmoidoscopy. We feel that these modalities should be reserved for those patients with positive screening tests.

High-Risk Individuals

Screening might need to be performed more frequently on certain individuals who are at increased risk for the development of adenomatous polyps or colorectal cancers. One particularly important group includes those who have had previous treatment for a primary colorectal cancer. Recent analysis indicates that evaluation of this high-risk group has been inadequate. Proctosigmoidoscopy or colonoscopy should begin at age 10 for first-degree relatives of individuals with FAP and at age 25 for individuals with a strong family history suggestive of HNPCC.[188,189] Genetic testing for the mutated APC gene in peripheral mononuclear cells of patients with early onset of adenomatous polyps or in first-degree relatives of FAP-affected individuals will help to determine who needs closer surveillance.[190] Counseling about diet, chemoprevention, and lifestyle factors can be provided for individuals who test positive for the mutated APC gene.

In addition, a colectomy should be considered if polyps are found.

Genetic testing for mutations in DNA repair genes should be performed on anyone whose family history is suggestive of HNPCC; counseling can then be provided for individuals who test positive.[129,191] A positive family history of colorectal cancer that does not meet criteria for FAP or HNPCC probably warrants earlier screening also, but guidelines have not been established definitively. A prospective study of approximately 120,000 men and women who underwent colonoscopy or sigmoidoscopy surveillance concluded that the age-adjusted relative risk for cancer was 1.72 with one first-degree relative with the disease, 2.75 with two first-degree relatives, and 5.37 with one first-degree relative who was under age 45 at the time of diagnosis.[192] It is estimated that up to 25% of patients with colon cancer have positive family histories. Baseline colonoscopies before 50 years of age seems reasonable among this group of patients with positive family histories.

Other high-risk conditions requiring close surveillance include individuals with a long-standing history of inflammatory bowel disease, a prior history of polypectomy or ureterosigmoidostomy, a personal history of ovarian, endometrial, or colon cancer, and finally anyone who has been treated for streptococcus bovis bacteremia.[188,193-195]

Other Health Factors

In considering health care resources, other issues that affect the development of colon cancer should be considered. The role of estrogen replacement on the development of colon cancer and on other health parameters in postmenopausal women is of great importance. The results of the Nurse's Health Study suggested that current estrogen replacement in postmenopausal women can reduce the risk of colon cancer (RR = 0.65); this effect disappeared after 5 years of no estrogen replacement.[196] When reproductive factors were examined among women who were diagnosed with colon cancer in this study, oral contraceptive pill use and later age of menarche were also associated with a decreased risk. In another study, women who delivered more than five children, especially if they had a positive family history of adenomas, were at increased risk for the development of adenomas.[197] In this study, however, no association was found with age at menarche, menopause, first birth, or oral contraceptive pill use. Despite this conflicting data about the role of various reproductive factors, ongoing multicenter clinical trials should help to clarify the relationship between estrogen and the development of colorectal cancers. Early results from the Women's Health Initiative Trial suggests a positive effect of hormone replacement therapy in reducing the incidence of colon cancer.[24]

The incidence of colorectal cancer is higher among men than among women (60.4 vs. 40.9/100,000/year, respectively) but increases in both sexes with age, with the majority of cancers being diagnosed after age 50.[4,198] Cancer of the bowel is also diagnosed more often in people from higher socioeconomic backgrounds; in industrialized nations, cancers are diagnosed more commonly in the distal colon. Countries that have a low incidence of colon cancer tend to have lesions in the proximal colon. The distribution of colorectal cancer within the bowel can also change the clinical presentation.[188] In general, patients with proximal lesions tend to suffer from chronic blood loss and the presence of iron deficiency anemia. Symptoms of abdominal pain, tenesmus, change in stool caliber, and hematoschezia are more likely to occur with lesions in the transverse colon, descending colon, sigmoid colon, and rectum.

Chemoprevention

Despite the enormous amount of epidemiologic observations and experimental data that support a protective role of many dietary constituents and other compounds against the development of adenomatous polyps and colorectal polyps, the results from definitive randomized trials have been modest, at best. Micronutrients—including vitamins C, E, and D, along with calcium, selenium, and β-carotene and nonsteroid anti-inflammatory agents (NSAIDS)—have been studied in a number of clinical trials. Greenberg and coworkers[199] completed a 4-year study of patients with resected polyps who received an antioxidant cocktail of vitamins E, C, and β-carotene.[199] There was no statistically significant difference in polyp formation between control subjects and treated subjects. A similar finding resulted from another 4-year study of patients with familial adenomatous polyposis for vitamins C and E but not for individuals who received wheat fiber Supplementation.[200] Among these patients, an inverse relationship was observed between the number of polyps visualized during colonoscopy and the patients who received fiber Supplementation vs. those who did not. The number of rectal crypt nuclei was decreased in patients in the Australian Polyp Prevention Project who received a diet Supplemented with only 25% fat and β-carotene compared with a diet consisting of 25% fat and wheat bran.[200] There was no statistically significant difference in polyp formation between the study groups, however. Therefore, β-carotene might either act at an earlier point of the carcinogenic process or is serving as a surrogate in epidemiologic studies for another compound.

In epidemiologic studies, an inverse relationship has also been reported between Supplementation with vitamin E, vitamin D, and calcium and colorectal cancers.[36] In addition, laboratory studies have shown that calcium can inhibit the growth of colonic epithelial cells and can neutralize carcinogens by forming insoluble soaps by binding to deconjugated bile acids or to certain fatty acids, hence reducing exposure to potentially toxic intraluminal compounds. Recently, a large randomized trial of more than 1000 individuals with a history of polyps showed that Supplementation with 1.5 g of calcium reduced new adenomatous polyp formation by 20%.[38] Another randomized trial showed that calcium Supplementation produced a modest but not significant reduction in the risk of adenoma recurrence.[39] A recent detailed analysis of the association between calcium intake and colon cancer risk in two large prospective cohorts observed a protective effect of calcium consistent with a threshold effect, suggesting that calcium intake beyond moderate levels may not be associated with a further risk reduction.[201] Additionally, in a double blind, randomized, placebo controlled trial of selenium Supplementation for skin cancer prevention, a secondary analysis showed that the number of colon, prostate and lung cancers were found to be reduced by 50% in the treatment arm.[202]

It is difficult to study the effects of micronutrient Supplementation on the formation of polyps and colorectal cancers given the inherent complexity of carcinogenesis. Understanding how various dietary components inhibit carcinogenesis will be instrumental in the development of novel dietary chemopreventive agents in the future. Factors such as type of micronutrient, dose, and duration of treatment, as well as cohort demographics (age and geographic location), and endpoints (polyp formation, or changes in the incidence and mortality of invasive cancer) are all important variables which can affect trial results. However despite these difficulties in study design, analysis, and interpretation, we should not dismiss the large amount of epidemiologic evidence and supportive experimental data demonstrating that the consumption of diets rich in fruits and vegetables, but low in fat, have a lower incidence of bowel cancer and cancer in general.[203-204] Results from the Women's Health Initiative Trial, the largest community-based clinical prevention and intervention trial ever conducted in the United States, will provide a great deal of information regarding the effects of dietary modification and calcium/vitamin D Supplementation on both colon and breast cancer development. Research from clinical trials should provide us with invaluable data on which to base dietary recommendations for the prevention of colorectal cancer.

There are also abundant scientific opportunities to explore the role of nondietary chemoprevention compounds in controlling colorectal cancer based on substantial studies of colon carcinogenesis (review).[205,206] Some of the more active nondietary compounds being studied include NSAIDS, and difluoromethylornithine (DFMO). Recent mechanistic studies indicate that induced epithelial regeneration and focal inflammation may be important early changes in the pathogenic process,[166,205] so that the use of nontoxic antiproliferative and anti-inflammatory agents as chemoprevention agents have a strong rationale.

DFMO has been found to be a potent inhibitor of carcinogenesis in experimental animal models by reducing the number and size of adenomas and carcinomas. This drug exerts its effects by irreversibly inhibiting ornithine decarboxylase, the first enzyme in the polyamine synthesis pathway. Suppressing intracellular pools of polyamines decreases cell growth and interferes with the process of carcinogenesis in essentially all animal models. We have reported the results of a long-term clinical trial, which serially measured the effects of different doses of DMFO on rectal mucosal polyamines over a 12-month time period and demonstrated consistent suppression without side-effects.[74] Demonstration of a dose of a chemopreventive agent that has a substantial biochemical effect without producing clinical side effects is an important goal. Currently, we are studying the prevention of adenomas in patients that have undergone polypectomies for adenomatous polyps. DMFO will be given in conjunction with sulindac over a 3-year period and its effect in reducing polyp recurrence is being studied in a randomized, placebo-controlled trial.

A considerable amount of experimental and epidemiologic evidence exists to support the use of NSAIDS to decrease the risk of colon cancer.[205,207-219] These compounds exert their antiproliferative effects on colonic cells by inhibiting prostaglandin synthesis by reversibly binding to cyclo-oxygenase as well as through a number of other newly discovered mechanisms.[220] Laboratory studies have consistently demonstrated that NSAIDS can inhibit chemically induced and transplanted tumors in rodents.[221-223] The interpretation of epidemiologic trials involving NSAIDS are challenging because of differences in design and methodology, including the particular agent chosen, the dose, frequency, and duration of use, and variable follow-up periods. Nevertheless, most case-control and cohort studies have demonstrated an association of a reduced risk of colon cancer with increased consumption of NSAIDS.

Analyses of subgroups of patients who routinely take these drugs—such as patients with rheumatoid arthritis (aspirin), inflammatory bowel disease (sulfazalazine), and FAP (sulindac) have reported a decrease in either adenomatous polyp formation or the development of colorectal cancer. A particularly important study was the Nurse's Health Study, which used three consecutive questionnaires to determine the rate of colorectal cancer among women who consumed aspirin and compared these rates to women who reported no aspirin use.[216] After at least a decade of regular aspirin use, at doses similar to those recommended for the prevention of cardiovascular disease, aspirin consumption was found to reduce the risk of colorectal cancer substantially. There has been a great deal of discussion regarding the relative efficacy and toxicity of nonspecific vs. cox-2-specific inhibitors.[224,225] Both celexcoxib and sulindac have been shown to cause regression of polyps in patients with FAP.[226,227] Sulindac was not effective in preventing the development of new polyps in these patients, however.[228] A large number of trials are currently being conducted to determine whether NSAIDS will be effective as cancer chemoprevention agents.[229]

The role of tertiary prevention in colorectal cancer has been little explored. As effective chemoprevention agents are developed, the group of patients who have been "cured" by standard therapy should become a focus of investigation, as the incidence of second primary colon cancers is high (about 25%).

Integration of Prevention Activities

A number of approaches exist to prevent the development of colorectal cancers. Successful primary prevention depends on public education and counseling about behavioral and dietary modifications that can be made to decrease an individual's risk, including increased physical activity and reduction of total calorie intake. In

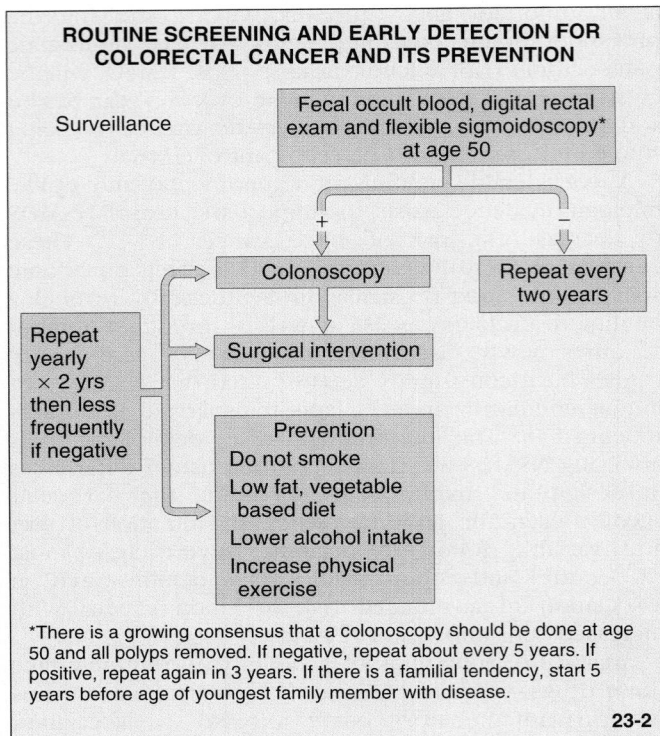

ROUTINE SCREENING AND EARLY DETECTION FOR COLORECTAL CANCER AND ITS PREVENTION

Surveillance

Fecal occult blood, digital rectal exam and flexible sigmoidoscopy* at age 50

+ → Colonoscopy

− → Repeat every two years

Colonoscopy → Surgical intervention

Repeat yearly × 2 yrs then less frequently if negative

Prevention
Do not smoke
Low fat, vegetable based diet
Lower alcohol intake
Increase physical exercise

*There is a growing consensus that a colonoscopy should be done at age 50 and all polyps removed. If negative, repeat about every 5 years. If positive, repeat again in 3 years. If there is a familial tendency, start 5 years before age of youngest family member with disease.

23-2

patients with adenomatous polyps, polypectomy is a useful preventive measure. Patients with FAP or HNPCC might require colectomies at a younger age to prevent development of cancer. New advances in genetic testing will help to select people who not only need closer surveillance but also might benefit from surgical treatment before cancer or premalignant polyps develop.

More vigilant screening in individuals at increased risk for the development of colorectal cancer is reasonable, but the appropriate screening tests, and the optimal interval between tests, require further clarification. More important, given that the majority of cancers occur in patients without a family history, is that everyone probably needs to be screened beginning at 50 years of age. Chemoprevention with DFMO, NSAIDS, and various micronutrients is still in experimental development but offers important alternatives for the future.

BREAST CANCER

Introduction

The morbidity and mortality from breast cancer remain high despite significant advances in our understanding and management over the last several decades. Therefore, prevention and early detection have become important challenges for the medical community. Several billion dollars could be saved annually if breast cancer were prevented and/or the disease were detected at an earlier stage. The widespread use of screening mammography, the increasing recognition that breast density is a major risk factor, the identification of high-risk individuals based on family history, the detection of deleterious mutations, and the "proof of principle" that tamoxifen can reduce the risk for a second breast cancer all anticipate more effective early management of this disease.

Etiology

Heredity

Primary prevention depends on our ability to identify individuals who are at increased risk for the development of breast cancer.[230] Although many risk factors can not be changed, knowledge of their presence can be used to identify high-risk individuals. Age, socioeconomic class, geographic location, race, and ages of menopause, menarche, and first birth are examples of risk factors that are difficult to change but important to know about. The incidence of breast cancer, like that of most cancers, increases with age. The majority of cases are diagnosed in women older than 40 years of age, with only 10% to 15% occurring in women less than 40 years old and fewer than 5% occurring among women younger than 35 years of age. Affluent women and individuals born in colder climates or in the Western hemisphere also tend to have a higher incidence of breast cancer. White women have more breast cancers than black, Asian, Hispanic, or native American women. It is of considerable interest that Hispanic and native American women have many of the same demographic variables (obesity, high fat, and low vegetable diet) that are associated with a high incidence of breast cancer in whites, but their incidence of breast cancer is nevertheless less than half that of whites.[231] By identifying who is at higher risk for breast cancer, health professionals can then counsel this subgroup of women and their families about the risks for breast disease and various ways to modify these risks, and they can encourage enrollment into clinical trials aimed at studying novel approaches for breast cancer risk reduction.

The most important step in trying to discern who is at risk is to take a detailed personal and family history extending back at least three generations.[232] Nearly 25% of women diagnosed with breast cancer have a family history of the disease.[232,233] Recent advances in our understanding of the molecular biology of breast cancer have led to the identification of specific mutations that might help identify women with a hereditary predisposition to developing breast cancer and might help predict who will respond to adjuvant therapy. Medical records, including pathology reports, should be obtained whenever possible to help complete an accurate pedigree. Recall bias is a significant problem when constructing pedigrees and can profoundly influence how we counsel patients; therefore, it is important to collect documentation whenever possible. Family histories need to be gathered from the maternal and paternal sides of the family. This latter step is often neglected and makes it impossible to counsel anyone in a meaningful way.

Although most cases of breast cancer are sporadic and a product of multiple genetic insults, approximately 5% are due to specific inherited germ-line mutations in the *BRCA1* and *BRCA2* tumor suppressor genes.[233-237] The estimated lifetime risk for breast cancer in *BRCA1* and

BRCA2 mutation carriers ranges from 55% to 85%, in comparison with the 13% lifetime risk for the general population.[237-239] Women with these mutations are also at increased risk for the development of a second breast cancer; *BRCA1* mutation carriers carry up to a 65% lifetime risk, and *BRCA2* carriers might share a similar risk.[239] Therefore, carriers of mutations in the *BRCA* genes and women with a personal or family history might benefit from prevention strategies and genetic counseling.

Genetic testing should be offered to individuals with a strong family history (breast or ovarian cancer in two or more generations), a history of multiple primaries (ovarian or breast, colon, endometrial), early age of onset of breast cancer (<35) or individuals of Ashkenazi Jewish descent, who carry a frequency of mutations in the *BRCA* genes estimated to be 2.2%.[237,238] Approximately one out of every 300 to 800 American women carries a *BRCA1* mutation; however, not every one of these women will develop breast cancer. This variable penetrance seen in *BRCA* mutation carriers highlights one of the dilemmas of genetic testing for *BRCA* gene abnormalities. Furthermore, a negative test might offer false reassurance, as it could represent a false negative. In addition, although a number of mutations in the *BRCA* genes have been sequenced, there are probably many more that we have not identified and for which we therefore cannot test. Practitioners should be aware of the uncertainty inherent in genetic testing for *BRCA* mutations and be prepared to counsel their patients accordingly.

Family history without a clearly defined genetic syndrome is also important in counseling patients about their risks for developing breast cancer.[240,241] A woman with a first-degree relative with premenopausal breast cancer carries anywhere between a 1.8- to 8.8-fold increased risk of developing a breast cancer in the future and is at high risk for harboring a deleterious mutation. This risk decreases to 1.2- to 4.0-fold in a woman who has a first-degree relative who developed breast cancer after menopause. Having a second-degree relative with breast cancer increases a woman's risk by approximately 1.5-fold.

Hormonal Factors

Women with a long lifetime exposure to estrogen are also more likely to develop breast cancer. The risk for breast

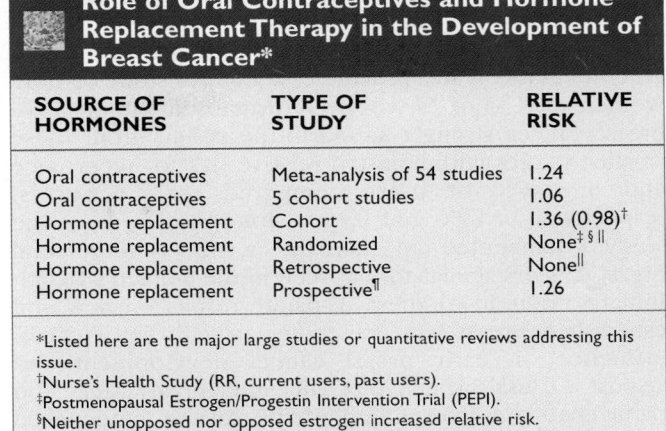

TABLE 23-7

Role of Oral Contraceptives and Hormone Replacement Therapy in the Development of Breast Cancer*

SOURCE OF HORMONES	TYPE OF STUDY	RELATIVE RISK
Oral contraceptives	Meta-analysis of 54 studies	1.24
Oral contraceptives	5 cohort studies	1.06
Hormone replacement	Cohort	1.36 (0.98)[†]
Hormone replacement	Randomized	None[‡ § ‖]
Hormone replacement	Retrospective	None[‖]
Hormone replacement	Prospective[¶]	1.26

*Listed here are the major large studies or quantitative reviews addressing this issue.
[†]Nurse's Health Study (RR, current users, past users).
[‡]Postmenopausal Estrogen/Progestin Intervention Trial (PEPI).
[§]Neither unopposed nor opposed estrogen increased relative risk.
[‖]Analyses were complex and "none" represents a summary opinion.
[¶]Women's Health Initiative, estrogen plus progestin in current users.

cancer increases by 20% if menarche occurs before the age of 12.[242] Furthermore, women who experience a late menopause, are nulliparous, or deliver their first child after 30 are also at increased risk. An induced abortion does not result in an increased risk of breast cancer.[243]

The subject of hormone replacement therapy and its role in the etiology and progression of breast cancer remains among the most intense in medicine (Table 23-7). Studies evaluating the role of hormone replacement in postmenopausal women have reported contradictory results, which is not surprising given that many of the studies evaluate different doses, preparations, follow-up times, and cohorts of different ages. The Nurse's Health study, which examined the relationship between breast cancer and hormone replacement among women aged 30 to 55 between 1976 and 1992, reported an increased relative risk of 1.36 among current users but not among past users (RR = .98).[244] Other studies have reported an increased risk among women who have taken synthetic as opposed to conjugated estrogens or who have taken 1.25 mg (RR = 2.0) rather than .625 mg per day or less of estrogen (RR = 1.08).[245,246] Conversely, the 3-year Postmenopausal Estrogen and Progesterone Intervention Trial did not find an increased risk of breast cancer in 875 healthy postmenopausal women aged 45 to 64.[247] A similar negative result had been found in an earlier study by Gambrell and associates,[248] who evaluated 5563 postmenopausal women for 37,236 patient-years. The recently reported results from the Women's Health Study, however, demonstrated an increased risk of invasive breast cancer (1.26) among those women taking estrogen plus progestin compared with placebo control subjects.[24] These findings have sparked an intense debate, with proponents of HRT advocating no change in prescribing habits and opponents vociferously advocating the opposite.

Other studies have evaluated survival differences in women who were taking estrogen when they were diagnosed with breast cancer and have found that these women actually experienced lower mortality rates than nonusers.[249,250] DiSaia and colleagues[250] observed there to

---

INDICATIONS FOR GENETIC TESTING IN BREAST CANCER*

A first-degree relative with breast cancer before age 40
Two or more relatives with breast or ovarian cancer at any age
Three or more relatives with breast, ovarian, or colon cancer at any age

———

*The indications for genetic testing in breast cancer and in other cancers is in rapid evolution as the true risks become better defined and as prevention (e.g., tamoxifen) and early detection (e.g., mammography, MRI) strategies mature.

be no difference in survival time or disease-free survival in a cohort of breast cancer survivors who received hormone replacement in comparison with a control group that was matched for stage, age, and node and receptor status. A recent large case control study of 2755 women aged 35 to 74 who were diagnosed with invasive breast cancer strongly supports the results from these smaller studies with adjusted relative risk for recurrence and mortality of users compared with nonusers, respectively, of 0.50 and 0.34.[251] Interestingly, this same study documented an increase in new contralateral breast cancers similar to that seen in the Women's Health Initiative trial. In to, these disparate results on new and established breast cancers argue strongly for a causal influence on early breast cancer development and against a causal influence of HRT after breast cancer on recurrence and mortality. Perhaps several randomized trials in Europe of HRT/estrogen replacement therapy (ERT) in menopausal women with a previous diagnosis of breast cancer will resolve the latter issue in a definitive manner.[252] A thoughtful discussion of the elements of informed consent surrounding the use of HRT for women with breast cancer is available.[253]

Estrogen has been implicated in promoting the growth of breast cancers. In contrast, the preponderance of evidence suggests that the risk for breast cancer from oral contraceptive use is very low or nonexistent (see Table 23-7). An overview of 54 epidemiological studies evaluating the role of oral contraceptives and breast cancer found the relative risk (RR) of current users to be 1.24 vs. no risk for women who had not taken them for 10 or more years.[254] Thomas[255] summarized the results of five cohort studies and found that the overall risk for ever-users to be 1.06. A recent exhaustive case control study involving 4575 women with breast cancer found no evidence for an increased risk (RR = 1.0) among either current or former users of oral contraceptives.[256] Neither initiation of oral contraceptive use at a young age nor the presence of a family history was associated with an increased risk for breast cancer. On the other hand, in a large, matched case-control study of *BRCA* mutation carriers use of oral contraceptives was associated with increased risk of breast cancer in *BRCA1* (OR = 1.20) but not in *BRCA2*.[257]

Oral contraceptives are used by more than 150 million women worldwide and offer a number of health benefits, including reduction in dysmennorrhea, fibrocystic breast changes, iron deficiency anemia, pelvic pain secondary to endometriosis, ectopic pregnancy, pelvic inflammatory disease, functional ovarian cyst formation, and the incidence of endometrial and ovarian cancers.[241] Patients should be counseled that there could be a slightly increased risk of developing breast cancer, although some believe that the apparent increase is due to surveillance bias, as physicians examine women taking oral contraceptive pills more frequently. Supporting this viewpoint is the observation that women with breast cancer who have taken oral contraceptives in the past do not experience lower survival rates when compared with women who have not taken them. Based on this data, current prescribing practices for oral contraceptives should not be changed, although the special case of *BCRA* mutation carriers needs to be assessed carefully on an individual basis.[257]

Other risk factors associated with breast cancer, such as proliferative fibrocystic changes in the breast, sedentary lifestyle, and diet, may be used to design preventive strategies for the high-risk woman. Overall, typical or atypical proliferative fibrocystic changes of the breast are associated with a two- to fourfold increased risk for the development of breast cancer.[258-261] Because the clinical significance varies depending upon the degree of hyperplasia and atypia present, the Cancer Committee of the College of American Pathologists has replaced the term *fibrocystic disease* with *fibrocystic changes*.[260] Possible treatment options for relieving symptoms related to fibrocystic changes include decreasing the consumption of foods rich in methylxanthines (e.g., chocolate, coffee, tea, and cola) or taking a Supplement such as vitamin E, or medications such as danocrine, bromocriptine, or tamoxifen. Although consumption of these drugs has been shown to decrease fibrocystic changes in the breast, studies have not been done to evaluate whether these changes actually decrease the increased risk of breast cancer.

Diet

Numerous studies have published contradictory results about the role of diet in the development of breast cancer. To date, there have been no randomized prospective studies performed to clarify the role of diet in the development of breast cancer; in this regard, the results from the Women's Health Initiative Study, in which women are randomized to low- and high-fat diets, will be of considerable importance.[205]

Many public health agencies advocate a low-fat, high-fiber diet to prevent breast cancer. The results from epidemiologic and experimental studies are not definitive, however.[261-275] Data linking diet to breast cancer comes largely from international and migration studies. First-generation Japanese American women and women who have recently migrated from Japan have risks for the development of breast cancer that approach those of native American women.[262] Differences are seen among women from various countries as well; for example, women in Great Britain have age-standardized mortality rates of approximately 28 per 100,000 versus those of Japanese women of 6 per 100,000.[263]

Women of tall stature or who have high body fat and mass have higher rates of breast cancer than other woman.[264-275] An increase in estrone and estradial as BMI increases has also been documented.[276] The recognition that a hormone (leptin) produced by fat cells vigorously stimulates the growth of normal and malignant breast cells could provide an important biologic link to the phenomenologic observation.[277] Some animal studies, however, have shown that caloric restriction in general, rather than a low-fat diet per se, decreases risk of breast cancer. This effect of caloric restriction could underlie the observation of why women who exercise have a lower risk of breast cancer. Another consideration is that women who exercise ovulate less frequently and therefore are not exposed to the higher levels of estrogen that normally occur in women who ovulate regularly.

Numerous epidemiologic studies suggest that alcohol has an effect on the development of invasive breast cancer. An extensive and detailed meta-analysis of the six largest prospective cohort studies addressing this issue showed that alcohol consumption was associated with a linear increase in breast cancer incidence for intakes less than 60 g/day (about two to five drinks).[278] The association was not modified by other factors, and higher alcoholic intakes (>60 gm/day) were not associated with further increased risk. Low dietary levels of selenium and antioxidants such as vitamins C, E, and β-carotene have been associated with breast cancer development and differences in survival.[279] β-carotene is the major provitamin A carotenoid and has differentiating and anti-proliferative effects on a variety of cells, including mammary carcinomas.[280] Levels of β-carotene have been analyzed in numerous studies and are lower in women with higher-staged breast cancer and breast cancer in general. A case control study from Europe, however, observed no differences in vitamin A or β-carotene levels between cases and control subjects.[281-283] Recent studies of soy intake in Singapore Chinese women are of great interest.[276,284] Soy intake was significantly associated with lowered plasma estrone and with more favorable mammographic patterns. Recently, there has been a great interest in gene-environment interactions and studies of micronutrients in relationship to metabolic pathways, and genetic polymorphisms are likely to be informative. Among women at high risk for breast cancer for other reasons (e.g., heredity), reducing alcohol consumption should be a straightforward way to reduce breast cancer risk.

Screening and Early Detection

Secondary prevention is aimed at detecting preinvasive lesions such as ductal carcinoma in situ (DCIS), lobular carcinoma in situ (LCIS), or early-staged breast cancers that have the potential to be cured with limited treatment. Screening tests include the self-breast examination, the clinical breast exam administered by health care professionals, and mammography. Successful implementation of widescale screening programs that incorporate these techniques, followed by treatment of detected lesions, is probably responsible for most of the decline in the overall death rate from breast cancer that occurred among American women from 1989 through 1993.[285] This decline continues and probably represents both the increased use of mammography and the effectiveness of systemic adjuvant therapy. Currently, 5-year survival rates for stage I breast cancers have increased to more than 90%.[4]

Although we encourage patients to perform monthly breast exams, a randomized trial indicates that this practice does not decrease overall mortality rates.[286,287] The most effective combination in decreasing the incidence of invasive disease is the clinical breast examination and mammography. The Breast Cancer Detection Demonstration Project showed that the sensitivity of the clinical breast exam and mammogram together was 70% to 80%, with increased sensitivity in older patients.[288,289] Although it is standard practice for a clinical breast examination to be performed annually, there has been a great deal of controversy surrounding the appropriate time to begin routine screening with mammograms. Randomized controlled trials of a large number of women on trials from several countries have unequivocally demonstrated a 40% decrease in mortality from breast cancer in women who have annual mammograms beginning at the age of 50.[290] Throughout the years, controversies have erupted regarding the magnitude of benefit from screening mammography. We continue to recommend the practice to women beginning at the age of 50 but encourage discussion of the risks and benefits associated with this procedure.

The opinion on routine screening in women between the ages of 40 and 49, however, is mixed.[291] Eight randomized controlled trials performed between 1963 and 1982 do not demonstrate a statistically significant difference in breast cancer mortality within 7 years after screening was initiated in women randomized to receive or not receive screening mammograms. A majority in a recent consensus panel used this information to state that there currently was not sufficient evidence to advocate routine screening mammography in women ages 40 to 49. Five of these trials, however, demonstrated a 16% decrease in mortality if follow-up continued for 10 years. There are many difficulties in interpreting these studies: They were not designed to screen women in their forties, but most women in these trials were in their late forties; the trials varied in length; some crossover occurred between patients in each group so that some women were screened who should not have been and vice versa; and there have been improvements in mammographic screening technology over time so that we might actually detect more lesions now and demonstrate a larger impact.[292-295] Because of these design flaws, coupled with the 16% decrease in mortality demonstrated in five of the trials, a minority report was issued advocating routine screening in the 40 to 49 age group.[291] As the minority report highlighted, the goal of mammography is to detect preinvasive lesions, and 15% to 20% of breast cancers are now diagnosed as DCIS or LCIS in younger women. The minority report correctly pointed out that the risk from radiation during mammography screening was overemphasized. The amount of radiation exposure to breast tissue per exam is approximately 0.06–0.45 cGy, which is negligible in comparison with the 7% baseline risk of developing breast cancer in a woman who is 35 years old. The U.S. Preventive Task Force has considered the issues carefully and recommends a screening mammography every 1 or 2 years for women aged 40 and older, a position we favor.[295] An important recent observation is that mammographic density is strongly associated with risk and is heritable.[296] This information should further target the premenopausal woman at higher risk for breast cancer; determination of the underlying genetic basis for breast density has now become of great interest, particularly as the use of a postemenopausal hormone therapy was strongly associated with an increase in mammographic density in the PEPI trial.[297]

New areas that are currently being evaluated for the enhancement of primary and secondary prevention strategies include the use of digital mammography, magnetic resonance imaging, optical scanning, ductal lavage for cytologies and molecular testing, nipple aspirates, and blood and urine assays for growth factors and auto-antibodies to oncoproteins and to tumor DNA. Validated biological markers of breast cancer risk and/or more sophisticated screening modalities might well increase our ability to detect lesions earlier in high-risk populations.

Chemoprevention

Three compounds—tamoxifen, raloxifene, and fenretinamide—have been advocated for the primary prevention of breast cancer. Tamoxifen, an estrogen antagonist in breast tissue, is currently being used as a therapeutic adjuvant to prevent recurrent breast cancer in all postmenopausal women with breast cancer and in premenopausal women who have estrogen receptor–positive breast cancer. Retrospective analysis of eight clinical trials found a significant reduction (35%) in the formation of contralateral breast cancers in those patients receiving tamoxifen.[298] Based on these results, a large, randomized trial to evaluate tamoxifen as a primary preventive agent in women without breast cancer was launched, and convincingly positive results were reported.[299] Women taking tamoxifen had 50% fewer breast cancers but had a higher incidence of uterine malignancies, deep venous thrombosis, and pulmonary emboli. All-cause mortality was similar to that of women in the general population; however, two other smaller randomized studies using tamoxifen to prevent breast cancer reported negative results.[300,301] A careful consideration of the potential value and harm of tamoxifen and other endocrine approaches to breast cancer chemoprevention has appeared recently.[302] Of considerable interest is the recent report that tamoxifen reduced second breast cancers in *BRCA2* but not in *BRCA1* carriers in the P-1 trial.[303] In this regard, a randomized trial of raloxifene (a selective estrogen receptor modulator) to prevent fractures in postmenopausal women has recently been reported.[304] In this trial, the risk of both breast and endometrial cancers was reduced significantly. At the current time, tamoxifen cannot be recommended routinely for women who are not at high risk for breast cancer,[302] and use of raloxifene as a preventative agent in any setting awaits the result of the large NSABP randomized trial comparing tamoxifen and raloxifene.

A chemoprevention trial evaluating the role of the synthetic vitamin A analog, 4-hydroxyphenyl-fenretinamide (4-HPR), showed a significant decrease in the development of contralateral breast cancers in women treated surgically for their primary cancers.[305] A follow-up study indicated that IGF-1 declined in women under age 50 who received fenretinide.[306] The role of 4-HPR in the prevention of breast cancer is complex and deserves further study, particularly as its toxicity is low. The pros and cons of chemoprevention for breast cancer have recently been reviewed, and the overall conclusion was reached that it cannot yet be recommended for general usage but

could be useful for reduction of risk among high-risk individuals.[307]

There are several other options for a woman who is at very high risk for breast cancer, including bilateral mastectomy or oophorectomy and lifestyle modification. Prophylactic bilateral mastectomies have been performed on some mutation carriers, but cases of breast cancer developing in the remaining breast tissue after subcutaneous and total mastectomies have been reported. In addition, such surgeries are dramatic procedures for a woman who has only a "probability" of developing breast cancer, and a decision analysis paradigm for these interventions has recently become available.[308] No long-term data exist on the effect of these surgeries in increasing the life expectancy of mutation carriers. Bilateral oophorectomy has been proposed as another option for premenopausal women who have completed their child bearing. Although castration has been shown to decrease the risk of breast cancer in young, nulliparous women, especially when it is performed before the age of 35, this remains a very controversial area in the management of breast disease. Secondary prevention can be accomplished by instructing these high-risk women about the importance of clinical breast examinations by a physician and screening mammograms, which should begin at a younger age, preferably at least 5 years earlier than the age at which the relative developed breast cancer.

PROSTATE CANCER

Introduction and Etiology

The age-adjusted incidence of prostate cancer rose slowly from 1965 to 1985 for unclear reasons. Parallel with aging of the baby-boomer population, the prevalence has also markedly increased since the general recommendation in the late 1980s by the American Cancer Society and the American Urological Association of yearly screening with prostate-specific antigen (PSA) after age 50. This recommendation led to the onset of widespread screening and a rapid increase in the incidence of prostate cancer that peaked in the early 1990s.[309]

A number of factors—age, familial/genetic, environmental, and hormonal—seem to contribute to the development of prostate cancer.[310,311] Prostate cancer exhibits a familial tendency that is currently not well defined, but at least one study suggests that 10% to 15% of cases could have a strong genetic component.[312] The loss of heterozygosity in some chromosomes in prostate cancer suggests that a gene related to some prostate cancers will be found.[313] Recently, the existence of a locus in chromosome 1 (band q 24) that predisposes men to develop early-onset prostate cancer has been verified, but a gene has not yet been isolated.[314]

The androgen dependence of prostate cancer led to the interesting hypothesis that variations in transcriptional activity by the androgen receptor regulated by CAG repeats could determine risk. Recent evidence, however, argues against such an association, although there could be specific underlying situations in which other genotype influences lead to such an effect.[315-317] Because these studies concentrate on identifying prostate cancer risk and most prostate cancers are not clinically significant, others have argued for identifying genotypes that are associated with clinically aggressive cancers that predict outcome (mortality). In this regard, the recent report documenting extensive mitochondrial mutations in primary prostate cancers might provide new insights into progression.[318]

Both epidemiologic and experimental data suggest that hormones, particularly testosterone, play a definitive role in the development of prostate cancer. In the rat model, testosterone induces prostate cancer, and in humans prostate cancer rarely occurs in castrated men.[319-321] Also, black men have a higher incidence of prostate cancer at all ages than white men, and Japanese men have the lowest incidence.[322-325] Whether this racial-ethnic variation in prostate cancer risk has a hormonal basis is still unclear, but a substantive amount of data supports this viewpoint.[324-326]

A high-fat diet and obesity could be associated with an increased risk of prostate cancer, but the studies to date have yielded inconsistent results.[327] One investigation suggests that the pre-adult hormonal milieu, as reflected in attained height and childhood obesity, could have a strong influence on prostate carcinogenesis.[328] Epidemiologic, animal model, and in vitro studies indicate that n-3 PUFA, lycopene, and selenium might also be important in the pathogenesis of prostate cancer.[329] Recently, GSTP1 has been proposed as a caretaker gene that serves to detoxify carcinogens associated with various lifestyle habits.[330]

Screening and Early Detection

The relative benefits and costs of screening for prostate cancer are currently among the most contentious issues in the medical community.[331-336] An excellent balanced editorial on this issue has appeared recently.[337] There are several major reasons why this controversy continues:

1. All available first-line techniques (digital rectal exam [DRE] and serum PSA) have high false-positive rates. This leads to a relatively low positive predictive value and the unnecessary workup of many normal individuals.
2. The natural history of prostatic intraepithelial neoplasia (PIN), the probable precursor of prostate cancer, is highly variable, and the natural history of the disease cannot currently be predicted reliably in any one particular case or by any specific biologic or pathologic marker.
3. The work-up of abnormal screening tests is invasive, requiring multiple biopsies of the prostate.
4. The treatment of prostate cancer produces significant morbidity and measurable mortality.
5. The false-negative rate is also high, which can produce a false level of assurance about the reliability of the screening tests.

These same five concerns regarding the use of PSA and DRE for screening also exist for their use for early

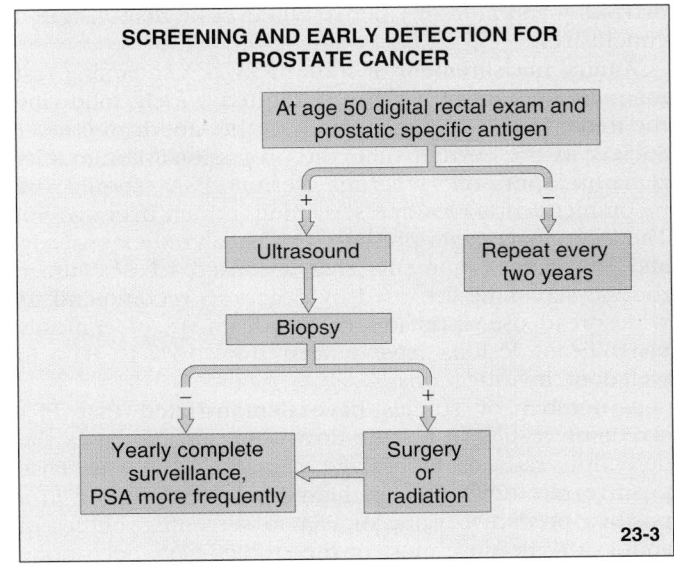

SCREENING AND EARLY DETECTION FOR PROSTATE CANCER

23-3

detection purposes, but the consequences are mitigated somewhat, as patients are by definition symptomatic on presentation.

The two most commonly used screening tests for prostate cancer are PSA and DRE, with transrectal ultrasound (TRUSP) reserved for patients with a positive PSA and/or DRE. Prior to the 1990s, yearly DRE after age 50 was the standard test used both for detection of prostate cancer and for screening. Although many primary care physicians use the DRE as part of a routine physical examination, assessment of its routine use indicates that DRE is performed in less than 50% of primary care encounters in which one would expect it to be done.[338]

A summary of the data indicates that the positive predictive value of DRE is relatively low (11%–26%), while the negative predictive value (85%–96%) is relatively high.[339] The most complete assessment to date evaluated 811 unselected serial patients from 50 to 80 years of age who underwent rectal examinations; 43 patients had a palpable nodule, and the positive predictive value of the 38 patients who underwent biopsy was 25%.[339] It is of great interest that 68% of the detected tumors were clinically localized, but only 30% were pathologically localized after radical prostatectomy. This data and other studies suggest that only about 20% to 25% of cases are localized at the time of a positive DRE; on the other hand, more than 25% of cases of prostate cancer are metastatic by the time a detectable palpable lump is detected on DRE.[339,340] Although the effectiveness of DRE is probably also significantly influenced by the skill of the examiner, it can easily be taught to health workers and is inexpensive and relatively nonmorbid and noninvasive. Its usage as a primary screening tool, however, has not been widely adopted, probably because of its inconvenience. Whether routine screening by DRE alone can reduce mortality from prostate cancer is unknown. With the emergence of serum PSA as the screening test of choice, it is unlikely that the specific value of DRE in reducing prostate cancer morbidity and mortality per se will ever be demonstrated conclusively.

Annual measurement of serum PSA as a screening test for prostate cancer has been adopted widely following the initial 1993 recommendation of the American Cancer Society. At the current time, the professional community remains split on whether serum PSA should be recommended for routine screening in men over age 50. The issues have been presented and analyzed extensively, and the same arguments that are used to discourage routine screening are used by others to recommend its widespread use. Estimates of overdiagnosis of clinically insignificant lesions have ranged from 15% to 84% in well-done investigations.[335,336]

A number of studies have demonstrated that PSA screening results in a stage downshift and increases the detection rate of early-stage cancers.[341-345] The false positive rate (25%–50%) is high, however, resulting in a positive predictive value of PSA in screening studies of about 30%. Because most of the studies have been done on symptomatic patients, the positive predictive values in a true screening effort are likely to be lower. In practical terms, this observation means that less than one-third of men with an elevated PSA will have biopsy-proven prostate cancer, and two-thirds will have a biopsy that is negative for prostate cancer. Even if biologically aggressive tumors (and this is unlikely in most cases) were being identified (see the discussion later in this chapter), a large number of men would undergo unnecessary prostate biopsies with the attendant fiscal cost and morbidity.

Because the value of a "normal" level of PSA (<4 ng/mL) is influenced by a number of physiologic parameters, there has been a great interest in enhancing the specificity of the test.[346] Techniques to improve the positive predictive value of PSA have included using age-adjusted reference ranges, PSA density (PSA level/size of prostate as measured by ultrasound), PSA velocity (change in PSA per unit of time), and ratio of bound to free PSA.[347-352] Although the validity of these strategies is currently unconfirmed, modeling has been important in determining the most effective use of tumor markers in other diseases, and it is likely that with enough time and information, the false-positive rate of PSA screening can be reduced. One way to reduce the false-positive rate is to combine PSA screening with DRE, and when appropriate, with TRUSP. A positive DRE increases the likelihood that a positive (i.e., abnormal) PSA is a true positive and therefore enhances the positive predictive value of the test. Further evaluations with TRUSP should further increase the positive predictive value.

The second major obstacle to the successful use of any screening modality for prostate cancer is that the biological aggressiveness of PIN and early prostate cancer is not identified with high reliability by serum PSA. Progressive prostate cancer is a serious disease with high morbidity and mortality; however, not all prostate cancers are serious, and indolent behavior is more common than not. For example, about 30% of men over age 50 have histologic evidence of prostate cancer at routine autopsy, suggesting a prevalence of prostate cancer of about 9 million.[353] As there are 40,000 deaths per year, about 1.2–1.5 million of these 9 million men, or about 15%, will eventually die of their disease. Thus, most prostate cancers in the population are latent and do not progress to clinical adversity; therefore, an aggressive workup of an elevated PSA should not be a reflex action.

A third major consideration in evaluating PSA as a useful screening test is that the subsequent workup and treatment have a significant complication rate. Follow-up testing of an elevated PSA requires a repeat PSA, DRE, TRUSP, and biopsy. These are relatively safe procedures, but about 0.1% to 0.4% of the 20% of screened men who undergo biopsy experience infection or bleeding, and almost all experience considerable anxiety while waiting for the results.[354-356] The potential complications of treatment can be quite serious and include impotence, incontinence, and death from radical prostatectomy. A recent summary of adverse outcomes of radical prostatectomy reported by a national probability sample of Medicare patients demonstrated a high rate of incontinence (from 2% using a catheter to 31% using pads), impotence (>50% without erection), surgical correction of strictures (20%), and a 0.6% 30-day postoperative mortality rate.[357] Radiation therapy is no less benign, but it carries a lower incidence of incontinence, a higher incidence of acute gastrointestinal complications, and a similar incidence of impotence.

A fourth major issue in PSA screening is the high false-negative rate. Numerous studies have demonstrated that many individuals (25%) with a normal PSA level have disease beyond the prostate.[358] Such results can lead to false reassurances and decreased follow-up when other factors suggest that a more aggressive work-up might be reasonable. Several studies suggest that a rising PSA, even in the normal range, is a cause for concern and reason enough to biopsy.[346,359,360]

Although serum measurement of PSA has been widely adopted in men over age 50 as a primary screening tool for prostate cancer, its value in improving the overall health of men has not been shown to date. The equally important issue of whether screening does more harm than good also remains unanswered, as the natural history of prostate cancer is so variable.[356,358] Decision analysis has been used to determine the benefits and risks of age- and quality-adjusted survival, but the results remain inconclusive.[361-364] Other studies suggest that screening might have the potential to decrease survival, particularly in the older individual.[364] There is, of course, no lack of critics of this viewpoint.[365,366] What information is needed to resolve this difficult and important issue? Perhaps only a series of randomized trials can lay this question to rest. Recently, the results of a randomized trial involving more than 40,000 men in the city of Quebec were reported, and those having a regular PSA had a 60% decrease in mortality from prostate cancer after 7 years.[367] The conduct and interpretation of this type of trial is complex, and the results of several other large screening studies will need to be available before definitive recommendations about the value of routine screening PSA can be made.[368-371] These targeted trials, however, will provide only a general guide regarding population-based screening using serum PSA in men over age 50 as an approach to identify potential prostate cancers. The current consensus by the U.S. Preventive Services Task Force is that the evidence is insufficient to recommend for or against routine screening for prostate cancer using PSA.[371]

An equally important issue is this: How do we identify and distinguish a biologically aggressive tumor in any one individual from those that will remain latent for the life of the individual? This is a very hard problem to study. Although the earliest features of prostate cancer pathogenesis remain obscure, recent studies of the biological features of intraepithelial hyperplasia of the prostate and of the "normal" prostate in individuals with a strong family history could shed some light on this issue.[371-374] Recent studies of the cytogenetic and molecular alterations in high-grade prostatic intraepithelial neoplasia (HGPIN) have indicated that LOH (loss of heterozygosity) is prominent and that certain oncogenes are expressed.[373,374] Defining the biological features of the preclinical phase of prostate cancer is critical to answer for innumerable reasons, not the least of which is to increase the effectiveness of PSA screening. In this regard, a large, randomized trial of men with T1b, T1c, or T2 prostate cancer demonstrated that radical prostatectomy was superior to "watchful waiting" in terms of disease-free survival but not in terms of overall survival.[375]

Chemoprevention

Although the development of rat prostate tumors has been studied for some time, this model system has been regarded as a poor one for carcinogenesis of the human prostate. The recent development of transgenic models that simulate the human disease represents an improvement in this regard.[376] Epithelial changes, including PIN, were identified in the human prostate long ago, although only recently have the biologic (and clinical) implications of these changes been recognized. The importance of these alterations, the recognition of the analogous evolution of the process to other epithelial cancers (e.g., cervical, oral), and its association with a wide spectrum of biologic abnormalities has moved PIN into the forefront as the likely, but clinically uncommon, preneoplastic precursor of prostate cancer.[376,377] An impressive array of studies measuring various biologic and molecular parameters in PIN have been done, and various biologic changes associated with the progression of prostate cancer have been identified. An array of different general changes have been identified, including loss of heterozygosity and changes in morphometry, differentiation, proliferation, apoptosis, and growth factors and their receptors. Many specific changes have been characterized, including DNA distribution, down-regulation of epidermal growth factor receptors, laminin a-2, and E-cadherin and up-regulation of bcl-2, p53, and selected matrix metalloproteinases and many others.[377,378]

What needs to be done now is to relate these biologic findings to the clinical aggressiveness of PIN and/or the eventual outcome of clinically relevant (nonindolent) prostate cancer. To be able to do so will help guide the difficult decisions after detection of an elevated serum PSA in biopsy samples during the screening and/or identification of PIN and during the early detection process. The diversity of acquired biologic abnormalities during prostate cancer development indicates a large number of potential targets for intervention with chemoprevention. Three major categories of chemoprevention agents are being currently considered: inhibitors of proliferation, hormonal modulators, and stimulators of differentiation.[371,379-381]

To date, two definitive randomized trials have been launched. The first phase III study is of the 5α-reductase inhibitor, finasteride, a compound currently approved for the treatment of benign prostatic hypertrophy.[381] The rationale for the usage of this drug for the chemoprevention of prostate cancer is based on its ability to inhibit the conversion of testosterone to its active form, which promotes the development of prostate cancer in animal systems. Accrual has been completed, and initial analysis of study results indicates a preventive benefit.[381A]

A second trial uses selenium and/or vitamin E. The rationale for the trial was based on secondary analyses of several large intervention trials in which prostate cancer was not the target, although recently some supportive experimental data also has become available.[382,383] Heavy smokers taking vitamin E as part of a large randomized trial to prevent lung cancer were found, incidentally, to have a markedly reduced incidence of prostate cancer.[384] In another study, a group of individuals at high risk for the development of skin cancer were randomized between selenium and a placebo.[202] Although there was no effect on skin cancer outcome, the incidence of several cancers, including prostate cancer, was markedly lower among participants taking selenium.[385] Although both of these observations are interesting, the generally negative experience with β-carotene as a chemoprevention agent, particularly in lung cancer (i.e., more cancers in active smokers taking the drug), mandates great caution in extrapolating the potential benefit of a compound from epidemiologic observations without extensive supporting experimental data. Accrual to this 2×2 factorial randomized trial (vitamin E, selenium) is ongoing, and results are anticipated in 2013. A large number of compounds are being investigated at the preclinical level. A few have advanced to the phase I/II clinical level. Studies of fenretinide failed to show an effect on relevant surrogate markers, while difluoromethylornithine was more successful.[372,386] Two other relatively unexplored areas of chemoprevention research in prostate cancer should also be mentioned: PIN and familial risk. Just as understanding the biology of PIN will affect our screening and early detection decisions, PIN should also serve as a useful marker in chemoprevention studies. Although the heterogeneity of lesions will make interpretation of effect of an intervention a challenge, PIN represents an important parameter for advancing our knowledge of early prostate cancer carcinogenesis and its modulation by candidate chemoprevention agents. A number of studies are in progress to use PIN as a screening tool for new chemoprevention agents. The roles of family studies and genetics in identifying individuals at high risk for prostate cancer are in their infancy, but epidemiologic studies support the notion that genetic risk plays a role, and clinical studies support the observation that early prostate cancer in some individuals is highly aggressive, while in others it is indolent. Linking these two parameters should identify a population of individuals in whom screening, early detection, and chemoprevention agents should be intensively directed.

Advances in the systemic therapy of advanced prostate cancer have been slow in coming. In a real sense, advances in the management of prostate cancer have been minimal since the introduction of hormonal therapy more than 50 years ago. It is likely that the widespread use of screening and early detection with an appropriate follow-up will reduce the morbidity and mortality from prostate cancer in a substantial way and that effective chemoprevention will be developed, as the major biological enhancer (androgens) of prostate cancer carcinogenesis is known.

SKIN CANCERS

Introduction

Each year, more than $2 billion is spent to treat patients diagnosed with skin cancers, the majority of which are malignant melanoma and basal and squamous cell carcinomas. These figures underestimate the true cost, as many of these cancers are treated in physicians' offices and are not reported to tumor registries. Furthermore, annual costs are expected to increase as the incidence and 5-year survival rates of these cancers continue to rise.[387,388] An aging population, depletion of the stratospheric ozone layer, and increased recreational exposure to ultraviolet radiation (UVR) represent some of the factors that contribute to the development of about 2 million cases of nonmelanoma (basal and squamous cell carcinomas) and 55,000 cases of melanoma diagnosed annually in the United States.[4] Understanding how these and other risk factors lead to alterations in key cellular processes like DNA synthesis and repair, oncogene activation, cell-cycle control, and apoptosis is the focus of intense research efforts aimed at designing novel preventive, diagnostic, and treatment strategies.[76,77] This section details the various primary, secondary, and tertiary preventive approaches for melanoma and nonmelanoma skin cancers. Incorporating these strategies into medical practice should decrease the incidence and mortality from skin cancer and should also decrease health care costs.

Etiology and Primary Prevention

Environmental

Successful primary prevention depends on the ability to identify individuals at risk for skin cancer and to use this information to educate both high-risk groups and the general population about various ways to reduce risk (Table 23-8). Many factors have been identified that increase an individual's risk for the development of both melanoma and basal and squamous cell cancers.[389-391] Exposure to UVR is a major risk factor.[392] Not only is cumulative UVR exposure important in the development

TABLE 23-8

Predisposition and Risk Factors for Skin Cancer

Nonmelanoma

Ultraviolet light (sun) exposure (cumulative)
Genetic
   Xeroderma pigmentosum
   Nevoid basal cell syndrome
Phenotypic
   Skin complexion
   Sunburn/tanning response
   Degree of freckling
Premalignant dermatoses
   Actinic (solar) keratoses
   Leukoplakia
   Chemical, thermal and scar keratoses
Chronic inflammation
Immunosuppression
Prior history of skin cancer

Melanoma

Ultraviolet light exposure (intermittent)
Genetic
   Melanocortin receptor variants
   Atypical or dysplastic nevi
   Dysplastic nevus syndrome
Phenotypic
   Less cutaneous pigmentation

of skin cancers, but it is apparent that acute, intermittent exposure to UVR is carcinogenic also.

The electromagnetic spectrum is composed of infrared, visible, and ultraviolet light. Ultraviolet light is responsible for causing the cellular and architectural changes in the epidermis and dermis, which lead to photo-aging and skin cancer.[392] Although the UVR spectrum is broad, UVR-B (290–320 nm) and UVR-A (320–400 nm) are the only wavelengths that routinely reach the earth's surface, as shorter wave lengths (UVR-C) are absorbed by the ozone layer. UVR-B is more potent than UVR-A in inducing neoplastic transformation in epidermal keratinocytes and melanocytes, which give rise to basal and squamous cell cancers and melanoma, respectively. UVR-A, however, has been found to penetrate the skin more deeply and is the predominant wavelength emitted from artificial lamps found in tanning salons.[392] More than 1 million adolescent and young women frequent these facilities daily and expose themselves to up to five times the amount of UVR that is emitted from the sun at any given time. The role of UVR-A radiation in the development of skin cancer will increase as this industry continues to grow.

The mechanism of action of UVR on the skin has been studied extensively.[393,394] Once photons penetrate through the stratum corneum, they are absorbed by cellular DNA and produce base substitutions in pyrimidines.[395,396] The substitution of thymidine for cytosine is pathognomonic for UVB-induced skin damage and is found in the tumor suppressor gene p53 in more than 90% of squamous cell skin cancers.[397-401] Basal cell cancers also contain p53 mutations.[402] Although UVR is regarded as contributing to the pathogenesis of melanoma, these types of mutations are uncommon, therefore raising the likelihood that the role of UVR is associative or complementary to the process. Normally, p53 acts to protect damaged cells by either inducing cell-cycle arrest (so that mutated DNA can be repaired or excised) or by inducing apoptosis.[403,404] UVR-induced p53 mutations disturb the cell cycle by inhibiting cyclin-dependent kinases, leading to uncontrolled cell proliferation. Cells with one mutated p53 allele can undergo clonal expansion and, if the other p53 allele is mutated, neoplastic transformation occurs. Therefore, UVR could both initiate and promote carcinogenesis.[404] Ultraviolet light might also have immunosupressive effects by interfering with the ability of Langerhans cells to process antigens.[405]

Other risk factors that increase one's susceptibility for the development of skin cancers include skin complexion and response to sunlight, degree of freckling, ethnicity, gender, age, geographic location, presence of premalignant skin lesions, medical history of exposure to ionizing radiation or PUVA, chronic skin irritation (ulcers, inflammation, or trauma), or a personal history of a germatodermatoses (xeroderma pigmentosum, nevoid basal cell carcinoma syndrome, and familial dysplastic nevus syndrome), lymphoreticular malignancy, granulomatous diseases, or other immunosuppressed states.

Health care providers should be aware of a number of premalignant dermatoses for the purpose of identifying patients who are at increased risk for the development of skin cancers. The most common lesion, actinic keratoses (solar keratoses), has been reported to undergo malignant transformation to squamous cell cancer in 12% of patients.[406] Histological evaluation of white patches occurring on mucous membranes, known as leukoplakia, is also important, as up to 20% could be dysplastic, with 3% to 6% becoming invasive cancers. Atypical and dysplastic nevi, large congenital nevi (>9 cm), and an increased number of moles are common precursor lesions of melanoma.[407] Chronic skin irritation from radiation (radiation dermatitis), chemicals (tar and arsenical keratoses), infrared light (thermal keratoses), and scars (scar keratoses) might also lead to malignant transformation. Any patient who is immunosuppressed (HIV diagnosis or transplant recipient) or who has a history of epidermo-dysplasia veruciformis or Bowen's disease (an intradermal carcinoma that often occurs on sun-exposed areas) should be considered for prevention protocols. Anyone who has a prior history of skin cancer is also at risk for a second primary cutaneous malignancy.[408-410] Patients diagnosed with thin melanomas (<75 mm in thickness; Breslow staging) were found to have a 4% chance of developing a second primary melanoma.[411-413] First-degree relatives of skin cancer patients also carry an increased risk.[408]

Heredity

A number of molecular abnormalities have been identified that could be responsible for the genetic instability preceding the development of invasive nonmelanoma skin cancers (Table 23-9). Defects in DNA repair genes, oncogenes, and tumor suppressor genes, as well as allelic losses in a number of chromosomes, have been described.[393,395] Mutations in the Ras oncogene have been

TABLE 23-9

Molecular Determinants of Carcinogenesis in Skin Cancer

Nonmelanoma

Mutated ras oncogenes (initiation)
Mutation in DNA repair genes (initiation)
Allelic loss in chromosomes 3p, 9p, 13y, 17p (promotion)

Melanoma

Allelic changes in chromosomes 9p, 15, 16
Progressive mutations
   Braf (immortalization)
   DNA repair genes (initiation)
   Cyclin-dependent kinases (progression)
   Ras oncogene (progression)

shown to initiate epidermal skin cancers.[414] Mutations in DNA repair genes (xeroderma pigmentosum, for example) bring about an inability to repair UVR damage to DNA efficiently, leading to the development of melanoma and epidermal skin cancers.[415,416] DNA repair capacity might be particularly important for individuals with other strong risk factors, such as low tanning ability and the presence of dysplastic nevi.[417] There are numerous examples of specific chromosomal abnormalities in nonmelanoma skin cancers. Allelic losses have been found in 9p, 13q, 17p, 17q, and 3p in squamous cell cancers and in 9q in basal cell cancers.[414] Recent studies of keratinocyte transformation have also focused on the UVR-mediated PI-3-kinase and p38 MAP kinase pathways.[418]

The genes and genetics of melanoma have recently been summarized.[419] One autosomal dominant syndrome that markedly increases an individual's lifetime risk for melanoma is familial dysplastic nevus syndrome. Melanoma in one or more first-degree relatives and the presence of a large number of moles (between 10 and 100) are required to diagnose this syndrome.[420] Rearrangements or deletions of genes have been found to occur in chromosomes 9 and 10 in patients with familial melanoma, atypical nevi, or early melanoma lesions. Two cyclin-dependent, kinase, tumor suppressor genes have been isolated on chromosome 9 (p15, p16). Mutations in this region lead to uncontrolled cell proliferation because the transition from G1 to S of the cell cycle is no longer inhibited.[421] The finding that the penetrance of one of these genes to frank melanoma is dependent on geographic variation emphasizes the role of environment in genetic expression[422] and the potential interaction of UVR and sunburn genotype.[423,424] Recently, certain polymorphisms in the melanocortin 1 receptor gene were shown to correlate with a reduced-response to melanotrophin, the major natural hormone that regulates cutaneous pigmentation.[425] Other studies suggest that loss of function mutations in the MCIR gene sensitizes human melanocytes to the DNA damaging effects of UV radiation, which could increase melanoma cancer risk.[426]

The recent identification of frequent raf B mutations in both melanomas and benign moles is also of great interest and suggests that this alteration could be the initial molecular change leading to immortalization.[427,428] Once

Science of Clinical Oncology

the significance of the genetic abnormalities in causing nonmelanoma and melanoma skin cancers is understood, we might be able to identify high-risk individuals who would benefit from prevention protocols and increased surveillance.

Preventive Measures

Numerous examples of primary preventive strategies exist. Protective clothing (hats, long sleeves, special FDA-approved fabrics), behavioral modification (avoid peak sun from 10:00 AM to 2:00 PM, avoid suntanning salons, and use appropriate shading), and liberal application of sunscreens are three such examples.[429,430] There are two types of sunscreens: blockers and reflectors. Blockers such as paraminobenzoic acid (PABA) absorb UVR-B only. Non-PABA blocker sunscreens absorb both UVR-A and UVR-B. Reflectors such as zinc oxide completely reflect UVR light. The SPF, or sun protective factor, is a measure of the comparison of the minimal erythema dose with and without sunscreen and should be at least 15. Finally, sunscreens should not wash off easily when bathing or sweating.

The current role of sunscreens in preventing skin cancer is the subject of considerable controversy.[431] Randomized trials have demonstrated that sunscreen use encourages prolonged sun exposure.[432,433] Another randomized study, however, has shown a protective effect of sunscreen use against the development of squamous cell cancer and nevi.[434,435] Based on these findings, we probably can conclude that regular sunscreen application needs to be combined with protective clothing to reduce the long-term risk for the development of melanoma and nonmelanoma skin cancers.[392]

In Australia, which has the highest incidence of skin cancers, other approaches that have been adopted include the passage of laws for employers to provide sun protection for employees, distribution of free sunscreens, tree planting campaigns, and public shade structures. In the United States, the Federal Trade Commission requires that protective eyewear be worn in tanning salons. In addition, signed informed consents and signs about health risks of UVR exposure in tanning salons are required.

USEFUL THINGS TO TELL YOUR PATIENTS ABOUT THE PREVENTION OF SKIN CANCER

Avoid sunburns (know your skin type—do you burn easily?)
Avoid tanning booths.
Use sunscreens with high SPF.
Stay covered up.*
Avoid outdoor recreation between 10 AM and 3 PM.
Minimize sunlight exposure.
Know your moles (and other skin lesions) and see a dermatologist promptly if they change or are new.

---

*A wet T shirt has an SPF of 0; several companies now make clothes that are specifically treated to give a high SPF.

Furthermore, in Texas an adult must accompany children attending tanning salons, and parental permission is mandatory for all minors. Attitude and behavioral modification of children (and their parents) informed by education and knowledge about sun exposure and skin damage/cancer is a reasonable goal and is most effective when started at a young age.[436,437]

Screening and Early Detection

The following are essential for effective screening:

- An understanding of the four characteristics of skin lesions that are suggestive of premalignant or malignant changes: asymmetry, border irregularity, color variegation, and diameter (6 mm or greater).
- Knowledge of important prognostic factors that should be recorded: anatomic location, ulceration, number of atypical lesions, presence of lymph nodes.
- Familiarity with the types and indications for the particular type of biopsy: shave biopsy, incisional biopsy, excisional bipsy, punch biopsy.
- Access to skilled pathologists who can comment on key histological criteria such as thickness (Breslow staging), margins, ulceration, regression, satellosis, angiolymphatic invasion, mitotic activity, precursor lesions, host response, and growth phase (radial vs. horizontal).

Screening for skin cancer, and in particular for melanoma, is supported by a number of criteria. Skin cancer is the most common cancer worldwide and is an important public health problem. Melanoma is second only to leukemia in terms of years of potential life lost, as it often affects younger people during the most productive periods of their lives.[437] Although basal and squamous cell cancers have a much better prognosis than melanoma, they cause considerable local disfigurement if not diagnosed and treated early. In addition, screening skin examinations are acceptable to both patients and health care providers. Premalignant cutaneous lesions tend to have a long latent phase, making early diagnosis and treatment possible with evidence that supports subsequent decreases in both incidence and mortality rates.[406]

Although no randomized, prospective studies evaluating the efficacy of screening for skin cancer have been conducted, nonrandomized studies support its practice. Thinner, melanoma lesions (stages I and II) are diagnosed more frequently with routine screening and intensive education programs. The Sydney Australia Melanoma Project demonstrated that widespread screening and education led to a decrease in the thickness of lesions from 2.5 mm to 0.8 mm, a decrease in the number of ulcerated lesions, an increase in the number of melanomas diagnosed in the radial rather than the vertical growth phase, and an increase in the 5-year survival rate to 94%.[438] A decrease in lesion thickness and an increase in the number of melanomas diagnosed were also confirmed in two other studies in Scotland and the United States.[438-440] Interestingly, a large skin cancer education and screening demonstration project found that 80% of study participants did not have a regular dermatologist; 50% saw their physician only because of the free skin examination; and 80% were receiving their first skin examination. Another interesting population-based, case-control study investigated whether skin self-examination would reduce the incidence of melanoma.[441,442] Although only 15% of participants in the study cohort practiced skin self-examination, they found that skin self-examination was associated with a reduced risk of melanoma in general and a reduced incidence of more advanced disease in melanoma patients. The authors concluded that mortality from melanoma might be reduced by as much as 63% if regular skin self-examinations were performed.

Challenges to effective screening examinations include the following:

- Lack of standardization of the examination and training that health care providers receive.
- Lack of accurate reporting to tumor registries (for melanoma; nonmelanoma skin cancers are not reported at all).
- Inability to motivate certain high-risk groups (e.g., white males) to come in for examination.
- An inability to screen adequately for the 1% to 2% of amelanotic cases of melanoma.

One step toward overcoming these challenges has been to designate the months of May and June as free skin cancer screening months in the United States in an attempt to attract more people for evaluation.

Chemoprevention

Nonmelanoma Skin Cancers

Clinical trials investigating the use of β-carotene, 13-cis retinoic acid, selenium, and NSAIDS have been performed on patients with a history of nonmelanoma skin cancers. Results using vitamin A derivatives have been mixed, which most likely reflects the complex biochemical and molecular mechanisms underlying the prodifferentiation or promaturation changes that these compounds produce. Three randomized clinical trials did not find a decrease in the recurrence rates of basal or squamous cell cancers in individuals at high risk for new skin cancers. Levine and colleagues[443] found no beneficial effect when using isotretinoin or retinol in high-risk subjects with at least four prior basal cell or squamous cell cancers. The Isotretinoin-Basal Cell Carcinoma Study Group also demonstrated that isotretoin did not prevent the recurrence of basal cell cancer in patients previously treated for basal cell cancer.[444] Finally β-carotene was not shown to prevent nonmelanoma cancers.[445] In contrast, in 2297 moderate-risk subjects with a history of actinic keratoses and at most two squamous or basal cell carcinomas, Supplementation with a moderate dose of retinol (25,000 IU daily) reduced the incidence of squamous cell (but not basal cell) cancers by 25%.[37] In addition, patients with xeroderma pigmentosum develop fewer new skin cancers after receiving high-dose isotretinoin.[446] It is clear from the conflicting data that more trials are needed before we can advocate routinely for or against a role of vitamin A derivatives in preventing skin cancers.

Negative results have also been produced in a large multicenter study involving selenium Supplementation.[202] In this double-blind, randomized, placebo-controlled study, 200 mcg of selenium daily did nor appear to prevent the development of future nonmelanoma skin cancers in patients with a history of basal or squamous cell skin cancer. A secondary analysis, however, showed that selenium decreased the overall mortality from some cancers, specifically colorectal, lung, and prostate.[447]

Finally, NSAIDs have been found to prevent the erythema that occurs 6 to 12 hours after acute sun exposure. In a large, randomized trial, topical application of the cox-1 inhibitor diclofenac was superior to placebo in clearing actinic keratoses lesions, and this formulation has now been approved for clinical use.[448] A small placebo-controlled study of 2-difluoromethyl-ornithine suggests that this compound might have comparable activity.[449] A comprehensive strategy for the development of chemoprevention drugs for nonmelanoma skin cancers has recently been described.[76,77]

Melanoma and Dysplastic Nevi

The effect of daily applications of topical β-all transretinoic acid (Retin-A, vitamin A acid, retinoic acid, tretinoin) was studied in three patients with biopsy-proven dysplastic nevus syndrome for 10 to 12 weeks.[450] Although minimal changes in the clinical appearance of the lesions were observed, striking histological changes were noted on biopsy after the treatment period; two lesions biopsied from two of the three patients were benign compound nevi and the third was similar but with minimal dysplastic change. These results suggested that retinoids might be effective chemopreventive agents in dysplastic nevus syndrome. There are alternative explanations for these results, including sampling artifact or regression of dysplastic changes from inflammation induced by the pretreatment biopsy. A recent study, however, in which transretinoic acid was applied to one side of the back in five patients with extensive dysplastic nevi, also demonstrated clinical and histologic regression of lesions on the treated side.[451] On the other hand, in a study of stage I and II patients at risk for relapse, study subjects were randomized to BCG alone or BCG plus retinol.[452] No difference in relapse-free survival was found between the two groups. A large randomized trial in a similar patient population compared a high dose of oral vitamin A to no treatment, and a similar result was obtained.[453] These studies indicate that retinol is not effective for patients who have already developed early-stage melanoma.

The development of chemoprevention agents for melanoma has progressed slowly, although advocacy of the inclusion of risk reduction endpoints into adjuvant trials is a good step forward.[454] The recent development of a transgenic model that simulates the human disease is also an important advance and should lead to a more systematic development of chemoprevention drugs.[455]

Tertiary Prevention

Lifetime surveillance of patients who have been diagnosed and treated for skin cancer is an important component of prevention. Many studies have shown that laboratory and radiological surveillance do not detect second primaries or recurrences beyond what is found on skin examination in patients with a history of melanoma. An NIH consensus statement published in 1992 recommended that patients with a history of melanoma receive skin and regional lymph node examinations every 6 months.[456,457] Particular attention should be paid to the scar of the previous excision site during these examinations. After 2 years of normal examinations, the interval between visits can be extended to 1 year. If an individual has any atypical moles, a positive family history for melanoma, or other poor prognostic factors, an evaluation (including cutaneous photography) every 3 to 6 months for the first 2 years (lengthening the interval between exams only if the atypical moles are stable) is recommended. No recent findings have affected these general recommendations. Newer biomarkers are being explored to detect melanoma earlier, but to date no validated successes have been reported.

Prevention of skin cancer depends on increasing the awareness of health care professionals and the public about the importance of early diagnosis and skin self-examinations. More research needs to be devoted to ways of motivating high-risk individuals to receive screening examinations. Public policy measures should be expanded and consideration given to other approaches, such as mandatory use of sunscreen and adequate clothing in daycare centers and public schools. The true measure of the various prevention strategies will come from studies of their ability to decrease both the incidence of and the mortality from skin cancers.

OVARIAN CANCER

Introduction

Ovarian cancer is the fourth leading cause of cancer mortality in women, after cancer of the lung, breast, and colorectum. Approximately 10% of ovarian cancers are associated with a BRCA mutation, while the remainder are sporadic.[458] The lifetime risk of developing ovarian cancer for the general population ranges between 1.4% and 1.6%.[459-461] Seventy percent of these women present with advanced-stage disease (spread beyond the pelvis or FIGO stage III/IV), which has led to a 40% overall 5-year survival rate with low 5-year survival rates for advanced-stage disease (stage III 5-year survival, 25.1%; stage IV 5-year survival, 11.1%).[462] Hence, most women who present with advanced disease die from their disease. Therefore, prevention of ovarian cancer is an important goal. Given that 90% of all ovarian cancers arise from the epithelial lining of the ovary rather than from the germ cells or sex-cord derivatives, preventive strategies outlined in the following pages pertain to the prevention of epithelial cancers.

Primary Prevention and Risk Reduction

Epigenetic Factors

A number of reproductive, environmental, and genetic factors could influence an individual's risk of developing

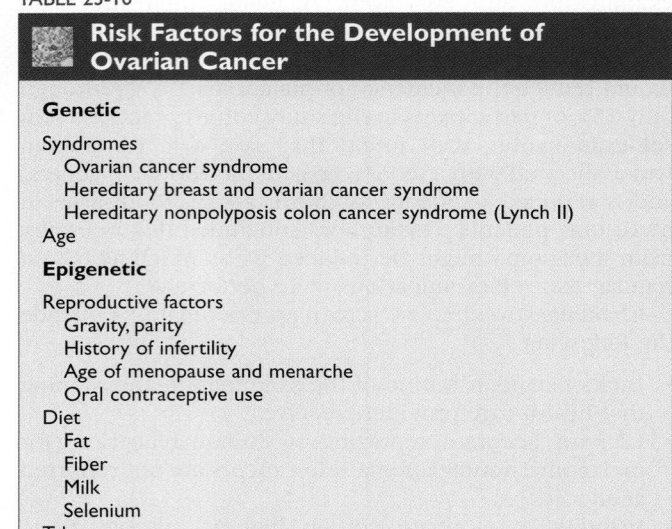

TABLE 23-10

Risk Factors for the Development of Ovarian Cancer

Genetic

Syndromes
    Ovarian cancer syndrome
    Hereditary breast and ovarian cancer syndrome
    Hereditary nonpolyposis colon cancer syndrome (Lynch II)
Age

Epigenetic

Reproductive factors
    Gravity, parity
    History of infertility
    Age of menopause and menarche
    Oral contraceptive use
Diet
    Fat
    Fiber
    Milk
    Selenium
Talc

ovarian cancer (Table 23-10). Advancing age is an important risk factor. Yancik[463] examined SEER data and data from the National Center for Health Statistics and found that more than 48% of all cases of ovarian cancer occurred among women greater than 65 years of age.

Important protective reproductive factors include increased number of pregnancies, oral contraceptive use, and breast-feeding. Whittemore and coworkers[464] reviewed data from 12 U.S. case-control studies conducted between 1956 and 1986 and determined that risk for the development of epithelial ovarian cancer was reduced with increasing number of pregnancies (regardless of the outcome), breast-feeding, and oral contraceptive use. Hankinson and associates[465] analyzed all epidemiologic studies of ovarian cancer and oral contraceptive use in the English literature published between 1970 and 1991 and found that the overall relative risk for the development of ovarian cancer among women who took oral contraceptive pills was 0.64, which is equivalent to a 36% reduction in risk in ever-users. The magnitude of risk reduction increased with duration of use, so that after 1 year of oral contraceptive use, a 10% to 12% risk reduction was observed. This increased to a 50% reduction after 5 years and held true for both nulliparous and multiparous women. No relationship between ovarian cancer risk and age of menarche, age of menopause, or duration of hormone replacement was shown. Conversely, increased risk was observed in nulliparous women who had a history of infertility. Critical analysis suggests that women with a history of infertility alone are at increased risk, and fertility drugs might not alter this risk further.[466]

A recent reanalysis of six large case-control studies involving 2768 incident cases demonstrated an overall OR of 0.66 in oral contraceptive users that continued to fall with duration of use; the effect was projected to persist for a lifetime after stopping.[467] Only a limited number of studies have examined the effect of hormone replacement therapy on ovarian cancer development. In the largest investigation reported to date, a cohort study of 44,241 participants in the Breast Cancer Detection and Demonstration Project (329 cases of ovarian cancer), estrogen-only use (but not combined estrogen-progesterone) was associated with a modest increased relative risk of ovarian cancer.[468]

Tubal ligation, and to a lesser degree hysterectomy, are associated with decreased risk of ovarian cancer. In a large prospective study of 121,700 nurses aged 30 to 55, a strong inverse relationship was found between tubal ligation and ovarian cancer, even after adjusting for age, parity, and oral contraceptive use (RR = 0.33). A statistically decreased risk after hysterectomy was also observed, but it was not as marked.[469]

A large prospective cohort study of 3,000,537 women (1511 deaths from ovarian cancer) showed that mortality rates from ovarian cancer were significantly increased in overweight and obese women who had never used hormone replacement therapy.[470] Other dietary factors, such as consumption of milk and selenium, might also modify an individual's risk for ovarian cancer, but the data is not convincing.

Finally, talc has been suggested as a possible factor leading to the development of ovarian cancer, as epithelial ovarian malignancy shares similarities with mesotheliomas, and talc is structurally similar to asbestos, a proven cause of mesotheliomas. Cramer and colleagues[471] first reported this association in 1982 when they assessed genital exposure to talc in 215 white females with epithelial ovarian cancer and 215 matched controls. They reported that 92 of the patients (48%) regularly used talc, either as a dusting powder on the perineum or on sanitary napkins, compared with 61 controls (28.4%). A relative risk of 1.92 was associated with these practices in the women with ovarian cancer. In a follow-up study, researchers determined that the risk for ovarian cancer was highest in women who applied talc directly to the perineum or undergarments on a daily basis for more than 10 years.[472]

Genetic Factors

Approximately 10% of all epithelial ovarian cancers are related to genetic mutations (hereditary, familial, other rare syndromes). Women considered to have a hereditary ovarian cancer syndrome must have at least two first-degree relatives with histologically confirmed ovarian cancer. These individuals carry an overall lifetime probability of developing ovarian cancer of approximately 50%. There are three "hereditary" autosomal dominant syndromes, which include the site-specific ovarian cancer syndrome, hereditary breast and ovarian cancer syndrome, and hereditary nonpolyposis colon cancer syndrome (HNPCC, Lynch II).[473] Together, these cancer syndromes account for 1% to 5% of the ovarian cancers that are diagnosed and generally occur 1 to 2 decades earlier than nonhereditary ovarian cancer.[474] The genetic linkage for the majority of the hereditary breast and ovarian cancer and the site-specific ovarian cancer syndromes has been found on the BRCA1 and BRCA2 loci on chromosome 17 (band q21). Specifically, the lifetime risk of developing ovarian cancers among BRCA1 and BRCA2 carriers is 15% to 60% and 15% to 28%, respectively.[475]

Women who report a family history of either a single first-degree relative and/or one or more non–first-degree relatives with ovarian cancer meet the definition of familial ovarian cancer syndrome. About 5% of diagnosed ovarian cancers fall into this category. Ovarian cancers can also occur as part of other rare, inherited, genetic syndromes such as Cowden's Disease or Li-Fraumeni Syndrome. Once individuals are identified with a familial or hereditary ovarian cancer syndrome, primary preventive strategies can be implemented, including oral contraceptive pill use, oophorectomy, and possibly dietary modification. Tubal ligations are not currently performed for the sole purpose of ovarian cancer prevention, as it is unlikely that this would be an effective prophylactic intervention.

Prophylactic oophorectomy is a subject of substantial controversy. It has been estimated that 700 prophylactic oophorectomies might need to be performed to prevent one case of ovarian cancer.[476] A person's age, medical history, reproductive plans, and proximity to menopause must be considered when trying to make an informed decision. In general, postmenopausal women or women older than 50 are encouraged to undergo this procedure, as the risk of ovarian cancer increases with age. Women who are younger than 50 but older than 40 years of age should be counseled on the risks and benefits associated with surgical menopause and subsequent hormone replacement, and on the risks of developing ovarian cancer based on their pedigree. There are two exceptions to these rules. One is the performance of prophylactic oophorectomies on women who are being operated on for a bowel cancer, as metastases are found in 25% of cases when the ovaries are carefully examined.[476,477] In addition, women with one of the three hereditary ovarian cancer syndromes should strongly consider oophorectomy at age 35 or at the completion of child bearing.[478] These women, however, should be counseled that they are still at increased risk for the development of intra-abdominal carcinomatosis, which is histologically similar to epithelial ovarian cancer but arises from the peritoneal lining. For example, Tobacman and coworkers[479] followed 28 women in 16 ovarian-cancer prone families; three women developed carcinomatosis between 9 months and 11 years after oophorectomy. Finally, carriers of germ-line mutations in BRCA1 and BRCA2 genes should be counseled about the option of prophylactic oophorectomy.[480] The recommendation is problematic, however, as there is heterogeneity in the type and number of mutations at the BRCA loci, which to date has made it difficult to quantify an individual's risk of developing ovarian cancer. Schrag and associates[481] performed an interesting decision analysis to determine the effect of prophylactic oophorectomy on life expectancy in women with BRCA1 and BRCA2 mutations. On average, a 30-year-old woman would increase her life expectancy from 0.3 to 1.7 years after undergoing bilateral oophorectomies. The analysis suggested that a woman could delay oophorectomy until she was 40 years of age with minimal loss of life expectancy.

Screening and Early Diagnosis

Early detection of ovarian cancer has not contributed to an overall improvement in survival of gynecologic malignancies.[482] Effective screening for a disease requires that the disease of interest has a premalignant phase, a long preclinical phase, stage-dependent outcome, curative treatments that are acceptable and readily available, and a cost-effective screening test that demonstrates good sensitivity, specificity, and positive predictive values. Unfortunately, the premalignant condition that progresses to invasive ovarian cancer has not been well defined. In addition, once invasive ovarian cancers develop, the preclinical phase is asymptomatic, with the result that most women present with advanced disease. Survival is not only stage dependent but also grade dependent. Primary treatment is surgical and in general is curative only if disease is confined to the ovaries. The available screening tests (pelvic ultrasound, serum CA-125 levels, and pelvic exams) are acceptable to patients and physicians but suffer from decreased specificity secondary to unacceptably high false-positive rates. Furthermore, the likelihood that an individual has ovarian cancer after a positive test (positive predictive value) is too low for available tests to be used for mass screening. In addition, screening might actually increase morbidity and mortality, as surgical exploration is the only way to diagnose ovarian cancer definitively. A decrease in mortality from ovarian cancer will occur only if we can detect early-stage disease reliably, which is not possible given available screening tests. Currently, there is insufficient evidence to support routine screening with transvaginal ultrasound and serial CA-125 serum measurements.[483]

Specific screening tests have been evaluated both individually and together in a variety of populations. Although the pelvic exam should be included in every annual physical examination, studies have shown that it is not extremely effective in diagnosing adnexal masses.[484] CA-125 is an antigenic determinant on a high-molecular-weight glycoprotein that is recognized by a monoclonal antibody (OC125).[485–489] It is expressed by 82% of ovarian carcinomas and in a percentage of other normal or pathological conditions including pelvic infections, endometriosis, pregnancy, menstruation, pancreatitis, renal failure, hepatitis, peritonitis, and congestive heart failure. Even in early-stage disease, however, CA-125 can detect only 50% of stage I disease and 60% of stage II disease.[489] Therefore, a normal CA-125 in the setting of an abnormal examina-

tion should not keep the physician from performing other diagnostic studies or surgical exploration. The real value of this tumor marker is in a premenopausal or postmenopausal woman who has a pelvic mass, particularly in the postoperative period, to measure response to treatment and progression of disease.

Ultrasonography by itself is easy to perform, but like CA-125 measurements, it is not an acceptable enough screening test to warrant its general use. Campbell and coworkers[490] performed abdominal scans on 5479 self-referred, asymptomatic women annually, and 15,977 scans and 326 laparotomies were performed for abnormal ultrasonographic findings. Five ovarian cancers were diagnosed, with three being of borderline histology. Therefore, 67 laparotomies had to be performed to diagnose one ovarian cancer, which is too high a false-positive rate to be acceptable. DePriest and Van Nagell and colleagues[491,492] performed transvaginal ultrasonography on 3220 asymptomatic postmenopausal women at the University of Kentucky. In this study, two stage I ovarian cancer and one stage IIIB ovarian cancer were diagnosed after 44 laparotomies. Although the use of transvaginal ultrasound in postmenopausal women yielded more favorable results (16 rather than 67 laparotomies to diagnose one ovarian cancer), the number of false positives was still too high. Currently, color flow imaging and measurements of pulsatility indexes are being coupled to transvaginal ultrasound to try to decrease the false-positive rate. Improvements in the ability to visualize both ovaries during a given examination might improve the accuracy of transvaginal ultrasound as a screening test. So might more accurate measurements of the morphological variations that exist between ovaries, among patients, and during different periods of the reproductive life cycle of a woman.[489] Numerous studies have combined pelvic examinations, CA-125 serum measurements, and transvaginal ultrasound.[493,494] Results from an ongoing NCI-supported multicenter trial evaluating the utility of transvaginal ultrasound and serial CA-125 measurements in 74,000 women who have been randomized to either annual pelvic exams with CA-125 measurements and pelvic ultrasounds or annual pelvic exams without CA-125 or ultrasound evaluation will help direct future screening practices. Until improvements in test characteristics of the various screening techniques can be accomplished, multimodality screening for ovarian cancer is recommended only for women with a hereditary ovarian cancer syndrome or *BRCA1* or *BRCA2* mutation, although no specific studies are available to support this practice.[459,494] Individuals with a strong family history that does not demonstrate an autosomal dominant inheritance pattern need to be evaluated on a case-by-case basis.

Chemoprevention

Chemoprevention studies for epithelial ovarian cancer have not been performed, although the data for oral contraceptive pills suggest strongly that these agents would be effective. In addition, DePalo and coworkers[495] completed a preliminary analysis of women with T1-T2 breast cancer who were randomized to oral 4-hydroxy-

---

PHILOSOPHY OF SCREENING AND EARLY DETECTION FOR OVARIAN CANCER

No good test for screening is currently available.
Concentrate on those patients with familial or heritable risk.
Transvaginal ultrasound and serum CA-125 are worth doing for selected patients.

fenretinamide or placebo. Six cases of ovarian cancer were diagnosed in the placebo group vs. none in the treated group (p = 0.02).[495] Long-term follow-up after the intervention phase has shown that no significant difference between the two groups was maintained once the intervention was stopped. Fenretinide and its derivatives continue to have considerable appeal, however, and further studies should clarify the role that this vitamin A derivative might play in the chemoprevention of ovarian cancer.[496]

In conclusion, a great deal of work remains to be done both in establishing the etiology of ovarian cancer and in developing strategies to prevent its occurrence and reoccurrence, but the opportunities seem great.[497]

CERVICAL CANCER

Introduction

Prevention of cervical cancer is one of medicine's greatest accomplishments. The recent demonstration of an effective vaccine against human papilloma virus (HPV), the major etiologic agent of cervical cancer, suggests that this disease eventually could become a worry of the past.[498] The U.S. annual mortality rate for cervical cancer has decreased from 26,000 deaths in 1941 to approximately 4000 deaths in 2002, which is impressive given the twofold increase in population in the United States during the second half of the 20th century.[4] Widespread usage of Papanicolaou smear screening is largely responsible for reduction of cervical cancer from the leading cause of cancer death in American women to an uncommon one. In fact, the incidence of cervical cancer has decreased by 70% since widespread screening began in the early 1940s.[499]

Unfortunately, these favorable statistics cannot be generalized to other countries or to certain subgroups within the United States. Cervical cancer is still the number one killer of women in underdeveloped nations, with 500,000 cases still being diagnosed worldwide every year. Recent statistics, published by the NIH as part of the SEER data, have suggested that the incidence of cervical cancer is on the rise again, and it is not clear what is responsible for this trend.[500] Whether this is due to a new subgroup of aggressive squamous intraepithelial preneoplastic lesions, an increase in adenocarcinoma, HIV, or some other factor is unknown. Currently, tremendous resources are being devoted to the development of strategies to identify and attract high-risk individuals to receive screening, to the education of the public and various health care providers about who is at risk and the frequency at which they should be screened, and to the evaluation of other screening alternatives to Supplement or even replace the conventional Pap smear, including sampling devices, liquid-based specimen collection systems, and automated instruments for rescreening cytologic smears read as negative.[501-504] In less well-developed countries, however, simple visual inspection of the cervix after acetic acid application could be the most effective approach in terms of both cost and lives saved.[505]

Primary Prevention and Risk Reduction

Numerous risk factors for preinvasive and invasive cervical disease have been identified, some of which are modifiable and others not (Table 23-11). Age, race, socioeconomic status, and degree of immunosuppression (HIV-positive individuals, transplant recipients) are difficult to change. Other factors, such as sexual and behavioral risk factors—including a high number of sexual partners for a woman or her partner; early age at first coitus, pregnancy, or marriage; history of sexually transmitted diseases; HPV infection; contraceptive choice; nutritional status; tobacco smoking; and frequency of Papanicolaou smear screening—might be modified more easily.

Cervical cancer is a sexually transmitted disease. Numerous studies and statistics have been published that lend definitive credence to this reality. Many of the epidemiologic and behavioral risk factors are direct and indirect surrogate markers for infection with HPV. The NIH has stated in a recent consensus statement that cervical cancer is largely preventable if young people modify their sexual behavior and decrease their exposure to HPV, which is the most important risk factor for the development of preinvasive and invasive cervical disease.[504,506-508] More than 100 types of this double-stranded DNA virus exist, with approximately 50 types found in the epithelial cells of the genital tract.[509] HPV is further subclassified into high-, intermediate-, and low-risk types. For example, HPV 16 and HPV 18 are high-risk types and have been found in many high-grade, preneoplastic and invasive cervical lesions. In contrast, HPV 6 and 11 are low-risk types and are generally found in condylomata accuminata (genital warts) or low-grade cervical lesions. Almost 90% of invasive cervical cancer specimens and more than 75% of high-grade cervical lesions have measurable HPV detected by available molecular biological techniques (hybridization or the polymerase chain reaction).[507,510,511]

The mechanism of action of HPV oncogenesis is related to their production of the E6 and E7 proteins that bind and inactivate tumor suppressor genes like p53 (E6) and Rb (E7) in cervical cells.[512] This, in turn, could lead to neoplastic transformation. HPV DNA has been found to integrate into host chromosomal DNA in many high-grade dysplastic and invasive cancer cervical specimens but not in the majority of low-grade cervical cancer precursor lesions. In the latter, the HPV DNA tends to exist in an

TABLE 23-11

Risk Factors for the Development of Cervical Cancer

Infection with the human papilloma virus (HPV)
Age, race, and socioeconomic status
Degree of immunosuppression (e.g., HIV positivity, transplant patients)
Sexual activity*
Tobacco smoking

*Sexual behavior is probably largely a surrogate for the risk of exposure to HPV.

unintegrated, circular form known as an episome. Although integration is an important step in malignant transformation, it is not essential, as some HPV DNA has been found in its episomal form in cervical cancer specimens.[513,514] Recent molecular epidemiologic studies suggest that different HPV 16 variants have different oncogenic potential, which could explain, in part, the wide geographic variation of cervical intraepithelial neoplasia (CIN) and cervical cancer in similarly infected populations.[515]

In general, women with cytological or histological evidence of HPV DNA should be counseled that they are at increased risk for the development of cervical disease, even though it is difficult to provide definitive risk assessments. One helpful study by Schiffman[516] that has helped to clarify this issue demonstrated that the presence of HPV in cervical cells was associated with a tenfold or greater risk for preinvasive cervical disease.[516] In addition, Koutsky and coworkers[20] performed two large prospective studies of women who had a normal Pap smear and found that those who tested HPV-positive had a 10- to 15-fold chance of developing a cytologic lesion compared with those who were HPV-negative.[20,517]

Clearly, not everyone with cytological evidence of HPV will progress to developing a preneoplastic cervical lesion, and even fewer progress to invasive disease.[518] Becker and associates[519] detected HPV DNA in 6% of women of reproductive age with healthy cervices. The presence of HPV DNA in women with normal Pap smears might be as high as 40%, however, and it is estimated that approximately 10 to 20 million women in the United States have detectable HPV DNA.[520-523] A very high percentage of women with low-grade squamous intraepithelial lesions (LSIL) were HPV-positive, and thus the mere presence of the virus offers little potential for HPV measurement to direct clinical management of women with this condition.[524] In conclusion, although numerous experimental, clinical, and epidemiological studies have established a definitive role for HPV in the development of cervical cancer, other factors such as age, contraceptive method, smoking history, degree of immunosupression, and nutritional status likely play a role in the progression and neoplastic transformation of HPV-infected cervical cells.

The grade of the cervical lesion also influences the risk of a cervical lesion progressing to invasive cancer. Many prospective studies have documented the percentage of the different grades of squamous intraepithelial lesions that will progress to higher-grade lesions.[525-528] Estimates indicate that it could take approximately 10 years, on average, for a preinvasive lesion to progress to an invasive cancer. Sixty percent of low-grade lesions spontaneously regress on their own without treatment, in comparison with 30% of high-grade cervical lesions. Ostor[528] critically reviewed the data and concluded that anywhere from 35% (CIN2) to 56% (CIN3) of high-grade lesions will persist. Therefore, the higher the grade of the lesion, the more likely it will either persist or progress. These wide ranges suggest that other factors play a significant role in determining the eventual outcome of premalignant cervical lesions.

The incidence of cervical cancer increases with age, with the mean age of diagnosis being 52.2 years and the peak incidences occurring between 35 to 39 and 60 to 64 years of age.[529] More than 25% of the diagnosed invasive cervical cancers and almost 50% of the women dying from this disease are women older than 65.[530] The National Health interview survey also found that women over 60 had not had a Pap smear in the last 3 years but had been seen as often as (if not more often than) younger women by their primary health care providers.[531] These data place older women in a high-risk category for the development of cervical cancer and challenge primary care providers to alter their practice style.

Differences in incidence and mortality rates of carcinoma in situ and cervical cancer have been reported across different ethnic groups. Although socioeconomic factors might be substantially responsible for the discrepancies, African Americans and Mexican Americans, especially if they do not speak English, are more commonly diagnosed with cervical cancer and ultimately will die more frequently than white women.[532] The age-adjusted incidence rates for blacks are 14 per 100,000, compared with 7.8 per 100,000 for white Americans.[533] Recent data reported by the NIH, however, revealed that the difference in incidence of cervical cancer between blacks and whites is disappearing, which suggests that efforts to target this high-risk group are succeeding.[504] This is not the case for Hispanics, as approximately 1.6 million Hispanic women remained unscreened in the United States.

Different methods of contraception might have different effects on the development of cervical disease. Barrier methods of contraception have been found to significantly decrease an individual's risk of developing cervical cancer (RR ~ 0.4).[534] Conversely, a weakly positive association has been observed between oral contraceptive use and the development of cervical disease.[535] It is difficult to conclude definitively that OCP use increases a person's risk for cervical disease because of important confounders such as sexual behavior and HPV infection.[536] There is, however, some evidence that OCP use could increase the risk of adenocarcinoma in young women.[537-539] Adenocarcinoma of the cervix and vagina also has been associated with a history of in utero exposure to DES.[540,541]

Evidence strongly implicates smoking as an independent risk factor in the development of cervical disease.[542] Brock and colleagues[543] found that smokers had a 4.5-fold increased risk of carcinoma in situ compared with matched controls. In a 10-year prospective study of cervical dysplasia, tobacco smoking was associated with a two- to fourfold increased risk of CIN3 and invasive cervical cancer in those women also infected with oncogenic HPV.[544] In addition, a significant dose-response relationship has been observed in women who smoked more or for longer periods of time.[542] Elevated levels of nicotine and continine have been found in the cervical mucous of smokers, which could alter local defense mechanisms (such as Langerhans cells) and/or be mutagenic themselves, leading to transformation of HPV-infected cervical cells.[545]

The relationship between immunosuppression and neoplasia is strong and has been documented in a number of ways. Studies of renal allograft patients have demonstrated a 4- to 16-fold increase in cervical dysplasia, a two- to ninefold increase in HPV infection, and a marked increase in synchronous cervical, vulvar, vaginal, and anal lesions.[546-548] The HIV epidemic has created a large population of immunosuppressed patients at risk for the development of cancer in general. In 1993, cervical cancer was added to Kaposi's sarcoma and non–Hodgkin's lymphoma as an AIDS-defining malignancy based on published reports by Miaman[549] and others describing the development of more aggressive cervical cancers in HIV infected women.[550,551] They observed that HIV-infected women, while still asymptomatic from their disease, presented with more advanced cancers, of higher grade, and at a younger age than what was expected in the immunocompetent population.

A number of other studies suggest an increased prevalence of cervical dysplasia in HIV-infected women with lesions that are more extensive, of higher grade, or found in multiple locations along the lower genital tract. Wright and coworkers[552] published an excellent cohort study that demonstrated a significant increase in the prevalence of preinvasive cervical disease. HIV-positive women attending an STD clinic in New York City had a 3.5-fold increased risk of cervical dysplasia over controls, after controlling for sexual behavior, HPV status, and smoking. An inverse relationship has been demonstrated between the development of cervical dysplasia and CD4 counts as well.[549] Cervical dysplasia recurred more frequently and sooner in women with CD4 counts that were lower than 500 than in those with CD4 counts greater than 500.

Screening and Early Detection

The Pap smear is medicine's most successful screening test.[503] Although it has never been subject to a randomized controlled clinical trial, this diagnostic test has been in widespread use since Drs. Traut and Papanicolaou published their findings in 1941.[553] International and regional surveys have documented decreases in both the incidence and mortality rates from cervical cancer among clinics that have widely adopted Pap smear screening. Scandinavian countries have reported reductions in mortality rates from cervical cancer by 30%–80%, depending on the country, the duration of the screening program, and frequency of screening (Iceland, 80% reduction; Finland, 50%; Sweden, 34%).[554] Canada and the United States also have experienced similar reductions in both incidence and mortality rates. The Pap smear is an effective screening test because it can detect disease early, which can subsequently be managed by available and effective treatments. In addition, the Pap smear is cost effective and acceptable to both physicians and patients. Currently, 50 million Pap smears are performed annually in the United States.

Despite the profound impact that the Pap test has had on decreasing the incidence of cervical cancer by facilitating early detection of preinvasive lesions, its validity has been questioned periodically. General misperceptions by the media, public regulatory agencies, plaintiffs, physicians, and the community at large exist regarding the role of this screening test.[555-557]

No screening test has a zero error rate, however, and the Pap smear is no exception. A great deal of media attention has focused on screening errors that have occurred in "Pap mills," where technicians were paid according to the number of slides they could screen.[503] Studies have reported that the false-negative rate ranges between 5% and 20% in good laboratories, suggesting that the overall sensitivity is approximately 80%. Many of the false-negative results are actually due to sampling errors rather than to screening or interpretation errors. In sampling errors, abnormal cells are either absent or unidentifiable because of inappropriate technique, unsatisfactory equipment, or difficult patient examination, making it hard to obtain a satisfactory sample. Interpretation errors occur when the health care provider fails to fill out the patient history on the cytology requisition or cytotechnologists are supervised inadequately.

Nevertheless, increased societal and political pressures have led to a number of steps to improve the accuracy of the Pap smear. The Clinical Laboratory Improvement Amendments (CLIA) was passed in 1988. This document defined the standards of cytology laboratory practice in the United States.[556] Three major changes in clinical practice that came from this document included mandatory rescreening of 10% of all negative Pap smears, review of all previous negative Pap smears within 5 years of a diagnosis of high-grade cervical dysplasia or invasive cancer, and limiting the number of slides that can be screened by a cytotechnician during an 8-hour work day to 100.

The Bethesda System was also developed in 1988 and then modified in 1991 to replace the cervical dysplasia or intraepithelial neoplasia (CIN) nomenclature used up to that time. For the most part, the Bethesda system has Supplemented rather than replaced the CIN designations.[557] It was designed to correlate cytology with histology, facilitate communication between the cytopathologist and the physician, facilitate research, and provide an international standard. Under this new classification system, low-grade squamous intraepithelial lesions include cytological changes consistent with HPV infection and CIN1. High-grade lesions include CIN2, CIN3, and carcinoma in situ. Two other categories are atypical glandular or squamous cells of undetermined significance. The National Cancer Institute has published interim guidelines that address the Bethesda System and the management of cytological abnormalities.[558]

New technologies to improve the accuracy of the Pap smear are emerging, but there are some concerns that these tests might be too costly for high-risk patients who need them the most (low-income, minority, or elderly women). If this new technology improves the sensitivity of testing sufficiently, however, there ultimately might be a positive cost-benefit effect through the prevention of cervical cancer. A detailed analysis of the costs and benefits of different strategies to screen for cervical cancer in less-developed countries has been presented.[559]

Compared with no well-organized screening, all strategies saved lives, at costs ranging from $121 to $6720 per life year saved (LYS), and they reduced mortality by up to 58%. The simple approach of VIA (visual inspection of the cervix after applying acetic acid) with appropriate follow-up was highly cost effective ($524 per LYS and 83% reduction in mortality) and could be a more reasonable approach in less well-developed countries or certain hard-to-reach populations in the United States.

Current screening guidelines of the American College of Gynecologists and the American Cancer Society include annual Pap smear and pelvic examinations for any woman who is sexually active and/or 18 or more years of age. After three consecutive normal Pap smears and examinations, a "low-risk" patient may increase the interval between screening from 1 year to 3 years. A high-risk individual is anyone who has had two or more sexual partners in her lifetime, intercourse prior to 20 years of age, a relationship with a male with multiple sexual partners, history of an abnormal Pap smear or gynecological cancer, or anyone who is immunosuppressed. Most American women should probably be considered high-risk and therefore should undergo yearly Pap smear screening until sexually inactive.

Conventional Pap smear screening has proven to be extremely effective. The success of this test and future screening modalities depends on realistic expectations about screening tests, continued quality assurance, improved sampling of cervical tissue, and the incorporation of newer technologies with a view to improving the accuracy of screening and interpretation of Pap smears. Successful implementation, however, needs to be cost effective and lead to further declines in the incidence and mortality from cervical cancer. The challenge of the next decade will be for cervical cancer screening to optimize the medical outcomes and economic costs in general and in special high-risk populations.[560]

Chemoprevention

The goal of chemoprevention of cervical disease is to prevent or delay the development of cervical cancer and its precursor lesions by interrupting or preventing the process of carcinogenesis at the cellular level, including vaccines.[560-564] Numerous clinical trials have been performed on cervices with biopsy-proven disease. The cervix is ideally suited for clinical studies that evaluate the process of carcinogenesis, because it is easily accessible for evaluation by Pap smear and colposcopy, and in general, abnormal cervical cells progress from low-grade lesions (HPV-positive cells and CIN1) to high-grade lesions (CIN2, CIN3, CIS) over an extended period of time.

A spectrum of intraepithelial changes occurs prior to the development of invasive cervical cancer, which are confined to the squamous epithelium above the basement membrane. In CIN, grade 1, abnormal cells rest just above the basement membrane. As the cells progress from CIN grade 1 to grade 2 and 3 disease, the abnormal cells occupy more of the thickness of the epithelium, and carcinoma in situ is a full-thickness lesion. Abnormal cells are identified by nuclear pleomorphism, loss of polarity,

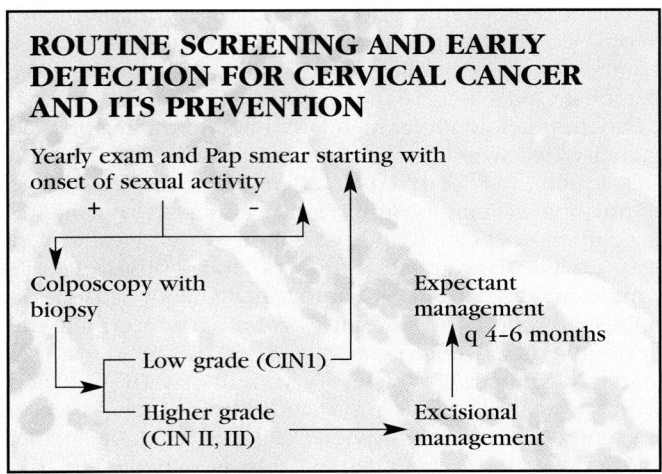

ROUTINE SCREENING AND EARLY DETECTION FOR CERVICAL CANCER AND ITS PREVENTION

presence of abnormal mitoses, and lack of differentiation as they progress from the basement membrane to the surface epithelium.

Numerous epidemiologic clinical studies have documented an association of low serum levels or diets low in vitamin C, vitamin A, and folic acid with an increased risk of cervical neoplasia and cancer.[565-570] For example, Liu and associates[570] published a case-control study of 257 women with colposcopically-proven cervical dysplasia and found that women with diets that were insufficient in vitamin A, ascorbate, riboflavin, and folate had a significantly higher risk of cervical dysplasia when compared with 133 controls.

A number of agents have been studied in chemoprevention trials of CIN. These include folate, vitamin A derivatives such as transretinoic acid (tRA), beta-carotene, and 4-hydroxyfenretinamide (4-HPR), and the polyamine synthesis inhibitor, difluoromethylornithine (DMFO). Folic acid is a coenzyme in DNA synthesis that plays a role in cell growth, proliferation, and differentiation. The compound was considered for chemoprevention trials after Whitehead and colleagues[571] observed that the cervical cells of women who took folic acid simultaneously with OCP had decreased megaloblastic features. Subsequently, Butterworth and coworkers[572] observed a significant association between low RBC folate levels (<660 nm/L) and the presence of cervical dysplasia. Butterworth and colleagues[573] then completed two studies in which study participants were randomized to 10 mg of folic acid daily or placebo. In the phase III study involving 235 women with CIN1 and CIN2 cervical disease, no difference in regression of the cervical lesions was evident in either group. The definitive phase III study was completed by Childers and associates,[574] who evaluated 331 women with biopsy-proven koilocytic atypia, CIN1- and CIN2-grade cervical disease.[574] After 6 months of follow-up, there was no significant difference in the regression of cervical disease between the placebo group and the group of women who took 5 mg of folic acid daily.

Vitamin A and its derivatives are important for growth, reproduction, vision, and epithelial cell differentiation.

This latter characteristic prompted intense research efforts directed at the chemoprevention of cervical intra-epithelial neoplasia, invasive cervical cancers, and other epithelial malignancies. After defining the prerequisite dose and toxicity profile of vitamin A acid (β-trans retinoic acid, tRA) a phase III clinical trial evaluated the role of this retinoid in the chemoprevention of high-grade cervical disease in 301 women.[70-72] Retinoic acid was applied topically to the cervix in a diaphragm-like device for 24 hours for 4 days every 4 months for 1 year. After 15 months of follow-up, significant regression of cervical lesions was observed in those women randomized to tRA for CIN2 disease but not CIN3 disease. In contrast, a randomized trial of 4-HPR for high-grade squamous intraepithelial lesions of the cervix yielded negative results, and there was a significant indication that CIN worsened in the treatment group.[575] Many women with cervical dysplasia are of reproductive age, and synthetic vitamin A derivatives are known to be teratogenic; this needs to be kept in mind when administering these compounds to young women. For now, use of natural or synthetic retinoids should occur only in the setting of a clinical trial. The natural vitamin A compound, betacarotene, has the advantage of not possessing the teratogenic toxicity profile of some of its synthetic counterparts; however, several large phase III studies of β-carotene Supplementation and CIN have been completed and have shown no effect on regression.[576,577]

Mitchell and colleagues,[578] at M.D. Anderson, are studying DMFO in women with biopsy-proven CIN3. The researchers recently published the results of a phase I study; the drug was well tolerated and significantly modulated the polyamine levels in cervical tissue. In addition, 50% of the patients experienced a complete or partial regression of their high-grade cervical lesions.[578]

In summary, chemoprevention of cervical disease has produced disappointing results. A beneficial effect of Supplementation with individual micronutrients has not been validated in randomized clinical trials. Nevertheless, we should not ignore the tremendous amount of nutritional epidemiological data that has been published, demonstrating the importance of diet in the prevention of cervical disease and of cancer in general. More laboratory studies are needed to understand the process of carcinogenesis that dysplastic epithelial cells undergo prior to the development of invasive disease. Such knowledge should serve as a useful guide to development of more effective agents, probably in concert with vaccines to HPV, which appear highly effective in the first reported trials.[20]

INTERNATIONALLY IMPORTANT CANCERS

Hepatocellular carcinoma (HCC) and stomach cancer are the number one and two causes of death from cancer worldwide.[579] With the increasing influx of Asian immigrants, these diseases have become more common in the United States as well. Over the past several years, important advances related to their control have become evident, and therefore a brief review of these findings is presented. Two excellent reviews have become available recently.[580,581] The major risk factor for HCC is exposure to hepatitis B or C virus.[580-583] Contributory risk factors include hepatoxins such as aflatoxin, excess alcohol exposure, and smoking, as well as male gender.[580,581,584] An impressive number of studies have demonstrated that vaccination can prevent the development of HCC caused by hepatitis B.[583,584-586] Likewise, interferon treatment appears effective in interrupting or slowing the processes that lead to HCC initiated by hepatitis C.[587,588]

Chemoprevention agents also appear to be effective in populations at risk for HCC due to HCV infection. A randomized trial of a cyclic retinoid has shown that this compound reduced development of a second primary HCC by one-third.[589,590] Several other agents also showed promise in less definitive trials, including glycyrrhizin (a licorice root extract) and activators of hepatoxin degradation, such as oltipraz.[581,590] The ability to detect circulating tumor nucleic acids in blood might allow earlier intervention in those at risk for HCC and other cancers.[591] Overall, advances in microbial oncology have led to a great deal of progress in understanding the etiologic basis of HCC and in developing strategies for its eradication and prevention.

Our basic understanding of the etiologic origin of stomach cancer has been affected greatly by a paradigm shift, and the recognition that *Helicobacter pylori* infection is central to gastric carcinogenesis in humans has been critical to the development of new prevention strategies.[592] Although individual susceptibility, lifestyle factors, and diet all play a role in the pathogenesis of gastric carcinoma, attributable risks for *H. pylori* range as high as 73%.[593,594] There now exists a full-fledged attempt to prevent gastric cancer by appropriate screening in high-risk populations followed by *H. pylori* eradication.[594,595] Epidemiologic data is supportive of a protective role for fruit and vegetable consumption, and a large, randomized trial of antioxidant Supplementation and anti-*H. pylori* therapy also appears promising.[596]

Rational approaches to the early detection and prevention of the microbial origin of HCC and stomach cancer are now established. Concerted public health efforts should lead to screening and their eradication.

USEFUL RESOURCES

For those interested in cancer prevention, particularly useful resources include the Journal of the National Cancer Institute and the Cancer Epidemiology Biomarkers and Prevention journal, and publications from the International Agency for Research on Cancer (www.iarc.fr/). This latter entity publishes a continuing series on early detection and prevention that represents an invaluable and critical analysis of current controversies. Useful Web sites include

The Division of Cancer Prevention, National Cancer Institute, National Institutes of Health (http://www3.cancer.gov/prevention/)

Chemoprevention—The Answer to Cancer? (http://ohioline.ag.ohio-state.edu/hyg-fact/5000/5051.html)
Harvard Center for Cancer Prevention, Harvard School of Public Health (www.hsph.harvard.edu/cancer/)
American Institute of Cancer Research (www.aicr.org/index.lasso)
International Society of Cancer Chemoprevention (www.iscac.org.)
Cancer Research Foundation of America (www.preventcancer.org)
National Foundation for Cancer Research (www.nfcr.org)

ACKNOWLEDGMENTS

The authors thank Sandy Schroeder for excellent administrative assistance in the preparation of this chapter. We thank Bill Armstrong and Ken Chang for the photographs in Figure 23-2. We also thank Janis DeJohn for preparing the section on useful resources and Daniel Pelot and Anne Simoneau for helpful comments on the manuscript. Preparation of this chapter was supported in part by P30CA62203 from the National Institutes of Health.

REFERENCES

1. Meyskens FL Jr: Strategies for prevention of cancer in humans. Oncology 1992;6:15–24.
2. Hong WK, Sporn MB: Recent advances in chemoprevention of cancer. Science 1997;278:1073–1077.
3. O'Shaughnessy JA, Kelloff GJ, Gordon GA, et al: Treatment and prevention of intraepithelial neoplasia; an important target for accelerated new agent development. Clin Can Res 2002;8:314–346.
4. Jemal A, Thomas A, Murray T, et al: Cancer Statistics (2002). CA Cancer J Clin 2002;52:23–47.
5. Young RC, Wilson CM: Cancer prevention: Past, present and future. Clin Can Res 2002;8:11–16.
6. Rebbeck TR, Lynch HT, Neuhausen SL, et al: Prophylactic oophorectomy in carriers of BRCA1 or BRCA2 mutations. N Engl J Med 2002;346:1616–1622.
7. Matthay KK, Villablanca JG, Seeger RC, et al: Treatment of high-risk neuroblastoma with intensive chemotherapy, radiotherapy, autologous bone marrow transplantation, and 13–cis–retinoic acid. Children's Cancer Group. N Engl J Med 1999;341:1165–1173.
8. Doll R, Peto R: The causes of cancer: Quantitative estimates of avoidable risks of cancer in the United States today. J Natl Cancer Inst 1981;66:1191–1308.
9. Willett WC: Diet, nutrition, and avoidable cancer. Environ Health Perspect 1995;103(Suppl 8):165–170.
10. Shields PG: Tobacco smoking, harm reduction, and biomarkers. J Natl Cancer Inst 2002;94:1435–1444.
11. Peto R, Lopez AD, Boreham J, et al: Mortality from tobacco in developed countries: Indirect estimation from national vital statistics. Lancet 1992;339:1268–1278.
12. Gaffney M, Altshuler B: Examination of the role of cigarette smoke in lung carcinogenesis using multistage models. J Natl Cancer Inst 1988;80:925–931.
13. Mulshine JL, Treston AM, Scott FM, et al: Lung cancer: Rational strategies for early detection and intervention. Oncology 1991;5:25–33.
14. Clinical opportunities for smoking intervention: A guide for the busy physician. Bethesda, MD, NIH publication No. 86, 1986, p 2178.
15. Skaar K, Tsoh J, Cinciripini P, et al: Current approaches in smoking cessation. Curr Opin Oncol 1996;8:434–440.
16. Skaar KL, Tsoh JY, McClure JB, et al: Smoking cessation. 1: An overview of research. Behav Med 1997;23:5–13.
17. Tsoh JY, McClure JB, Skaar KL, et al: Smoking cessation. 2: Components of effective intervention. Behav Med 1997;23:15–27.
18. Vainio H, Weidepuss E, Kleihunes P, et al: Smoking cessation in cancer prevention. Toxicology 2001;166:47–52.
19. Williams A: Reduction in the hepatitis B related burden of disease: Measuring the success of universal immunisation programs. Commun Dis Intell 2002;26:458–460.
20. Koutsky LA, Ault KA, Wheeler CM, et al: A controlled trial of a human papillomavirus type 16 vaccine. N Engl J Med 2002;347:1645–1651.
21. Huang JQ, Sridhar S, Chen Y, et al: Meta-analysis of the relationship between *Helicobacter pylori* seropositivity and gastric cancer. Gastroenterology 1998;114:1169–1179.
22. Goodwin CS: *Helicobacter pylori* gastritis, peptic ulcer, and gastric cancer: Clinical and molecular aspects. Clin Infect Dis 1997;25:1017–1019.
23. Feigelson HS, Henderson BE: Estrogens and breast cancer. Carcinogenesis 1996;17:2279–2284.
24. HRT Writing Group for the Women's Health Initiative Investigators. Risk and benefits of estrogen plus progestin in healthy postmenopausal women. Principal results from the Women's Health Initiative randomized controlled trial. JAMA 2002;288:321–333.
25. Kaplan B: Current attitudes toward hormone replacement therapy (HRT) prescribed during menopause. Clin Exp Obstet Gynecol 2002;29:167–171.
26. Greenwald P: Cancer prevention clinical trials. J Clin Oncol 2002;20(Suppl 18):14S-22S.
27. Willett WC: Diet and cancer: one view at the start of the millenium. Cancer Epi Biom Prev 2001;10:3–8.
28. Foerster SB, Kizer KW, Disogra LK, et al: California's 5 a day—for better health! campaign: An innovative population-based effort to effect large-scale dietary change. Am J Prev Med 1995;11:124–131.
29. Omenn GS: What accounts for the association of vegetables and fruits with lower incidence of cancers and coronary heart disease? Ann Epidemiol 1995;5:333–335.
30. Prinz-Langenohl R, Fohr I, Pietrzik K: Beneficial role for folate in the prevention of colorectal and breast cancer. Eur J Nutr 2001;40:98–105.
31. Holmes M, Pollack MN, Hankinson SE: Lifestyle correlates of plasma insulin-like growth factor-1 and insulin-like growth factor binding protein 3 concentration. Cancer Epi Biom Prev 2002;11:862–867.
32. Molloy AM, Scott JM: Folates and prevention of disease. Public Health Nutr 2001;4:601–609.
33. Friedenreich CM: Physical activity and cancer prevention: From observational to intervention research. Cancer Epi Biom Prev 2001;10:287–301.
34. Wannamethee AG, Shaper AG, Walker M: Physical activity and risk of cancer in middle-aged men. Br J Cancer 2001;85:1311–1316.
35. Ames BN, Wakimoto P: Are vitamins and mineral deficiencies a major cancer risk? Nature Rev Cancer 2002;2:694–704.
36. Meyskens FL Jr: Micronutrients. In DeVita V, Hellman S, Rosenberg S (eds): Cancer Principles and Practice, 5th edition. New York, Lippincott-Raven, 1997, pp 573–579.
37. Moon TE, Levine N, Cartmel B, et al: Effect of retinol in preventing squamous cell skin cancer in moderate-risk subjects: A randomized, double-blind, controlled trial. Southwest Skin Cancer Prevention Study Group. Cancer Epi Biom Prev 1997;6:949–956.
38. Baron JA, Beach M, Mandel JS, et al: Calcium Supplements for the prevention of colorectal adenomas. Calcium Polyp Prevention Study Group. N Engl J Med 1999;340(2):101–107.
39. Bonithon-Kopp C, Kronberg O, Giacosa A, et al: Calcium and fiber Supplementation in presentation of colorectal adenoma recurrence: A randomized intervention trial. Lancet 2000;14:1300–1306.
40. Tanaka T: Cancer chemoprevention by natural products. Oncol Reports 1994;1:1139–1146.
41. Mehta RG, Pezutu JM: Discovery of cancer preventive agents from natural products: From plants to prevention. Curr Oncol Rep 2002;4:478–486.
42. Knauf VC, Facciotti D: Genetic engineering of foods to reduce the risk of heart disease and cancer. Adv Exp Med Biol 1995;369:221–228.

43. Miller AB, Chamberlain J, Day NE, et al: Cancer Screening. Cambridge, Cambridge University Press, 1991.

44. Feinleib M, Zelen M: Some pitfalls in the evaluation of screening programs. Arch Environ Health 1969;19:412–415.

45. Black WC, Haggstrom DA, Welch HG: All-cause mortality in randomized trials of cancer screening. J Natl Cancer Inst 2002;94:167–173.

46. Woloshin S, Schwartz LM, Welch HG: Risk charts: putting cancer in context. J Natl Cancer Inst 2002;94:799–804.

47. Hiatt RA, Klabunde C, Breen N, Swan J, Ballard-Barbash R: Cancer screening practices from national health interview surveys: Past, present and future. J Natl Cancer Inst 2002;94:1837–1846.

48. Schatzkin A, Gail M: The promise and peril of surrogate endpoints in cancer research. Nature Rev Cancer 2002;21:19–27.

49. Lippman SM, Bassford TL, Meyskens FL: Quantitative assessment of cancer risk. Tex Med 1988;84:48–53.

50. Sweet KM, Bradley TL, Westman JA: Identification and referral of families at high risk for cancer susceptibility. J Clin Oncol 2002;20:528–537.

51. Barrett JC: Mechanisms of multistep carcinogenesis and carcinogen risk assessment. Environ Health Perspect 1993;100:9–20.

52. Bertram JS, Kolonel LN, Meyskens FL Jr: Rationale and strategies for chemoprevention of cancer in humans. Cancer Res 1987;47:3012–3031.

53. Shureiqi I, Reddy P, Brenner DE: Chemoprevention: General perspective. Critical Rev Hematol Oncol 2000;33:157–167.

54. Fearon ER, Vogelstein B: A genetic model for colorectal tumorigenesis. Cell 1990;61:759–767.

55. Sidransky D: Molecular genetics of head and neck cancer. Curr Opin Oncol 1995;7:229–233.

56. Sidransky D: Advances in cancer detection. Sci Am 1996;275:104–109.

57. Wong IHN, Lo YMD: New markers for cancer detection. Curr Oncol Rep 2002;4:471–477.

58. Kelloff GJ, Boone CW, Crowell JA, et al: Chemopreventive drug development: Perspectives and progress. Cancer Epi Biom Prev 1994;3:85–98.

59. Meyskens FL Jr: Biology and Intervention of the premalignant process. Cancer Bull 1992;43:475–480.

60. Meyskens FL Jr: Biomarkers, intermediate endpoints, and cancer prevention. J Natl Cancer Inst Monogr 1992;13:177–182.

61. Lee JJ, Hong WK, Hittelman WN, et al: Predicting cancer development in oral leukoplakia: Ten years of translational research. Clin Cancer Res 2000;6:1702–1710.

62. Sporn MB, Newton DL: Chemoprevention of cancer with retinoids. Fed Proc 1979;38:2528–2534.

63. Greenwald P: Chemoprevention of cancer. Sci Am 1996;275:96–99.

64. Lippman SM, Benner SE, Hong WK: Cancer chemoprevention. J Clin Oncol 1994;12:851–873.

65. Meyskens FL Jr: Chemoprevention of human cancer. A reasonable strategy? Recent Results Cancer Res 1998;151:113–121.

66. Sun SY, Lotan R: Retinoids and their receptors in cancer development and chemoprevention. Crit Rev Oncol Hematol 2002;41:41–55.

67. Meyskens FL Jr: Design of large and multiple agent chemoprevention trials. J Cell Biol 1998;34(Suppl):115–120.

68. Goodman GE: The clinical evaluation of cancer chemoprevention agents: Defining and contrasting phase I, II, and III objectives. Cancer Res 1992;52:2752s–2757s.

69. Kelloff GJ, Sigman CC, Hawk ET: Surrogate end-point biomarkers in chemopreventive drug development. In Miller AB, Bartsch H, Buffeta P, et al (eds): Biomarkers in Cancer Chemoprevention. Lyon, France, IARC Sci Publ No. 154, 2001, pp 13–26.

70. Meyskens FL Jr, Graham V, Chvapil M, et al: A phase I trial of beta-all-trans-retinoic acid delivered via a collagen sponge and a cervical cap for mild or moderate intraepithelial cervical neoplasia. J Natl Cancer Inst 1983;71:921–925.

71. Graham V, Surwit ES, Weiner S, et al: Phase II trial of beta-all-trans-retinoic acid for cervical intraepithelial neoplasia delivered via a collagen sponge and cervical cap. West J Med 1986;145:192–195.

72. Meyskens FL Jr, Surwit E, Moon TE, et al: Enhancement of regression of cervical intraepithelial neoplasia II (moderate dysplasia) with topically applied all-trans-retinoic acid: A randomized trial [see comments]. J Natl Cancer Inst 199;86:539–543.

73. Meyskens FL Jr, Gerner EW: Development of difluoromethylornithine (DFMO) as a chemoprevention agent. Clinical Can Res 1999;5:945–951.

74. Meyskens FL Jr, Gerner EW, Emerson S, et al: A randomized double-blind placebo-controlled phase IIb trial of difluoromethylornithine for colon cancer prevention. J Natl Cancer Inst 1998;90:1212–1218.

75. Kim ES, Hong WK, Khuri FR: Chemoprevention of aerodigestive tract cancers. Ann Rev Med 2002;53:223–243.

76. Stratton SP, Dorr RT, Alberts DS: The state-of-the-art in chemoprevention of skin cancer. Eur J Cancer 2000;36:1292–1297.

77. Stratton SP: Prevention of non-melanoma skin cancer. Curr Onco Rep 2001;4:295–301.

78. Kelloff GJ, Sigman CS, Johnson KM, et al: Perspectives on surrogate endpoints in the development of drugs that reduce the risk of cancer. Cancer Epi Biom Prev 2002;9:127–137.

79. Schantz SP, Yu GP: Head and neck cancer incidence trends in young Americans, 1973–1997, with a special analysis for tongue cancer. Arch Otolaryngol Head Neck Surg 2002;128:268–274.

80. Blot WJ, McLaughlin JK, Winn DM, et al: Smoking and drinking in relation to oral and pharyngeal cancer. Cancer Res 1988;48:3282–3287.

81. Day GL, Blot WJ, Shore RE, et al: Second cancers following oral and pharyngeal cancers: Role of tobacco and alcohol. J Natl Cancer Inst 1994;86:131–137.

82. Schwartz S, Doody DR, Fitzgibbons ED, et al: Oral squamous cell cancer risk in relation to alcohol consumption and alcohole dehydrogenase-3 genotypes. Cancer Epi Biom Prev 2001;10:1137–1144.

83. Mark J, Li AK, Glattre E, et al: Human papillomavirus infection as a risk factor for squamous cell carcinoma of the head and neck. N Eng J Med 2001;344:1125–1131.

84. Spitz MR, Wei Q, Li G, Wu X: Genetic susceptibility to tobacco carcinogenesis. Cancer Invest 1999;17:645–659.

85. Forastieve A, Koch W, Trotti A, et al: Head and neck cancer. N Eng J Med 2001;345:1890–1900.

86. Minna JD, Fong K, Zochbauer-Muller S, et al: Molecular Pathogenesis of lung cancer and potential translational applications. Cancer J 2002;8(Suppl):S41–S46.

87. Huang Q, Yu GP, McCormick SA, et al: Genetic differences detected by comparative genomic hybridization in head and neck carcinoma from different tumor sites: Construction of oncogenetic trees for tumor progression. Genes Chrom Cancer 2002;34:224–233.

88. Chiodo GT, Eigner T, Rosenstein DI: Oral cancer detection. The importance of routine screening for prolongation of survival. Postgrad Med 1986;80:231–236.

89. Krutchkoff DJ, Eisenberg E, Anderson C: Dysplasia of oral mucosa: A unified approach to proper evaluation. Mod Pathol 1991;4:113–119.

90. Mashberg A, Barsa P: Screening for oral and oropharyngeal squamous carcinomas. CA Cancer J Clin 1984;34:262–268.

91. Warnakulasuriya S, Pindborg JJ: Reliability of oral precancer screening by primary health care workers in Sri Lanka. Commun Dent Health 1990;7:73–79.

92. Hirsch FR, Prindiville SA, Miller YE, et al: Fluorescence versus white-light bronchoscopy for detection of preneoplastic lesions: a randomized study. J Natl Cancer Inst 2001;93:1885–1391.

93. Yang H, Berner H, Mei Q, et al: Cytologic screening for esophageal cancer in a high-risk population in Anyang County, China. Acta Cytol 2002;46:445–452.

94. Cameron AJ: Management of Barrett's esophagus. Mayo Clin Proc 1998;73:457–461.

95. Sampliner RE, Garewal HS: A Phase II trial of 13-cis-retinoic acid (Isotretinoin) in Barrett's esophogus. Gastroenterology 1988;94:A396.

96. Strauss GM: Measuring effectiveness of lung cancer screening: From consensus to controversy and back. Chest 1997;112:216S–228S.

97. Spitz MR, Lippman SM, Jiang H, et al: Mutagen sensitivity as a predictor of tumor recurrence in patients with cancer of the upper aerodigestive tract. J Natl Cancer Inst 1998;90:243-245.

98. Wei Q, Spitz MR: The role of DNA repair capacity in susceptibility to lung cancer: A review. Cancer Metast Rev 1997;16:295-307.

99. Arai T, Yasuda Y, Takaya T, et al: Application of telomerase activity for screening of primary lung cancer in broncho-alveolar lavage fluid. Oncol Rep 1998;5:405-408.

100. Lotan R, Xu XC, Lippman SM, et al: Suppression of retinoic acid receptor-beta in premalignant oral lesions and its up-regulation by isotretinoin. N Engl J Med 1995;332:1405-1410.

101. Lippman SM, Shin DM, Lee JJ, et al: p53 and retinoid chemoprevention of oral carcinogenesis. Cancer Res 1995;55:16-19.

102. Lippmann SM, Spitz MR: Lung cancer chemoprevention: An integrated approach. J Clin Oncol 2001;19:745-82s.

103. Goodman GE: Prevention of lung cancer. Thorax 2002;57:994-999.

104. McWilliams A, Lam S: New approaches to lung cancer prevention. Curr Oncol Rept 2002;4:487-494.

105. The α-tocopherol, β-Carotene Cancer Prevention Study Group: The effect of vitamin E and beta carotene on the incidence of lung cancer and other cancers in male smokers. N Engl J Med 1994;330:1029-1035.

106. Omenn GS, Goodman GE, Thornquist MD, et al: Effects of a combination of β-carotene and vitamin A on lung cancer and cardiovascular disease [see comments]. N Engl J Med 1996;334:1150-1155.

107. Burton GW, Ingold KU: β-Carotene: an unusual type of lipid antioxidant. Science 1984;224:569-573.

108. Wolf G: The effect of low and high doses of β-carotene and exposure to cigarette smoke on the lungs of ferrets. Nutr Rev 2002;60(3):88-90.

109. Lam S, MacAulay C, Riche JCG, et al: A randomized phase IIb trial of anethole dithiolethione in smokers with bronchial dysplasia. J Natl Cancer Inst 2002;94:1001-1009.

110. Hong WK, Endicott J, Itri LM, et al: 13-cis-retinoic acid in the treatment of oral leukoplakia. N Engl J Med 1986;315:1501-1505.

111. Lippman SM, Batsakis JG, Toth BB, et al: Comparison of low-dose isotretinoin with β carotene to prevent oral carcinogenesis [see comments]. N Engl J Med 1993;328:15-20.

112. Garewal HS, Meyskens FL Jr, Killen D, et al: Response of oral leukoplakia to β-carotene. J Clin Oncol 1990;8:1715-1720.

113. Mayne SJ, Cartmel B, Baum M, et al: Randomized trial of Supplemental β-carotene to prevent second head and neck cancer. Cancer Res 2001;61:1457-1463.

114. Armstrong WB, Meyskens FL Jr: Chemoprevention of head and neck cancer. Otolaryngol Head Neck Surg 2000;122(5):728-735.

115. Armstrong WB, Kennedy AR, Wan XS, et al: Clinical modulation of oral leukoplakia and protease activity by bowman-birk inhibitor concentrate in a phase IIa chemoprevention trial. Clin Cancer Res 2000;6:4684-4691.

116. Hong WK, Lippman SM, Itri LM, et al: Prevention of second primary tumors with isotretinoin in squamous-cell carcinoma of the head and neck [see comments]. N Engl J Med 1990;323:795-801.

117. Benner SE, Pajak TF, Lipman SM, et al: Prevention of second primary tumors with isotretinoin in patients with squamous cell carcinoma of the head and neck: Long-term follow-up. J Natl Cancer Inst 194;86:140-141.

118. Khuri FR, Kim E, Lee JJ: The impact of smoking status, disease stage, and index tumor site on second primary tumor incidence and tumor recurrence in the head and neck retinoid chemoprevention trial. Cancer Epi Biom Prev 2001;10:823-829.

119. Bolla M, Lefur R, Ton Van J, et al: Prevention of second primary tumours with etretinate in squamous cell carcinoma of the oral cavity and oropharynx. Results of a multicentric double-blind randomised study. Eur J Cancer 1994;30A:767-772.

120. Potter JD: Colorectal cancer: Molecules and populations. J Natl Cancer Inst 1999;91:916-932.

121. O'Brien MJ, Winawer SJ, Zauber AG, et al: The National Polyp Study. Patient and polyp characteristics associated with high-grade dysplasia in colorectal adenomas. Gastroenterology 1990;98:371-379.

122. Shinya H, Wolff WI: Morphology, anatomic distribution and cancer potential of colonic polyps. Ann Surg 1979;190:679-683.

123. Kearney J, Giovannucci E, Rimm EB, et al: Diet, alcohol, and smoking and the occurrence of hyperplastic polyps of the colon and rectum (United States). Cancer Causes Control 1995;6:45-56.

124. Calvert P, Frucht H: The genetics of colon cancer. Ann Int Med 2002;137:603-612.

125. Srivastava S, Verma M, Henson DE: Biomarkers for early detection of colon cancer. Clin Cancer Res 2001;7:1118-1126.

126. Vogelstein B, Fearon ER, Hamilton SR, et al: Genetic alterations during colorectal-tumor development. N Engl J Med 1988;319:525-532.

127. Solomon E, Voss R, Hall V, et al: Chromosome 5 allele loss in human colorectal carcinomas. Nature 1987;328:616-619.

128. Lynch HT, Smyrk TC, Watson P, et al: Genetics, natural history, tumor spectrum, and pathology of hereditary nonpolyposis colorectal cancer: An updated review. Gastroenterology 1993;104:1535-1549.

129. Lynch HT, Smyrk TC: Identifying hereditary nonpolyposis colorectal cancer [editorial; comment]. N Engl J Med 1998;338:1537-1538.

130. Erbe RW: Inherited gastrointestinal-polyposis syndromes. N Engl J Med 1976;294:1101-1104.

131. DeCosse JJ, Adams MB, Condon RE: Familial polyposis. Cancer 1977;39:267-273.

132. Laken SJ, Petersen GM, Gruber SB, et al: Familial colorectal cancer in Ashkenazim due to a hypermutable tract in APC. Nat Genet 1997;17:79.

133. Vasen HF, Mecklin JP, Khan PM, et al: The International Collaborative Group on Hereditary Non-Polyposis Colorectal Cancer (ICG-HNPCC). Dis Colon Rectum 1991;34:424-425.

134. Fishel R, Kolodner RD: Identification of mismatch repair genes and their role in the development of cancer. Curr Opin Genet Dev 1995;5:382-395.

135. Leach FS, Nicolaides NC, Papadopoulos N, et al: Mutations of a mutS homolog in hereditary nonpolyposis colorectal cancer. Cell 1993;75:1215-1225.

136. Fishel R, Lescoe MK, Rao MR, et al: The human mutator gene homolog MSH2 and its association with hereditary nonpolyposis colon cancer [published erratum appears in Cell 1994 Apr 8;77(1):167]. Cell 1993;75:1027-1038.

137. Goelz SE, Vogelstein B, Hamilton SR, et al: Hypomethylation of DNA from benign and malignant human colon neoplasms. Science 1985;228:187-190.

138. Forrester K, Almoguera C, Han K, et al: Detection of high incidence of K-ras oncogenes during human colon tumorigenesis. Nature 1987;327:298-303.

139. Baker SJ, Fearon ER, Nigro JM, et al: Chromosome 17 deletions and p53 gene mutations in colorectal carcinomas. Science 1989;244:217-221.

140. Kinzler KW, Nilbert MC, Su LK, et al: Identification of FAP locus genes from chromosome 5q21. Science 1991;253:661-665.

141. Kinzler KW, Nilbert MC, Vogelstein B, et al: Identification of a gene located at chromosome 5q21 that is mutated in colorectal cancers [see comments]. Science 1991;251:1366-1370.

142. Guengerich FP: Roles of cytochrome P-450 enzymes in chemical carcinogenesis and cancer chemotherapy. Cancer Res 1988;48:2946-2954.

143. Modan B: Role of diet in cancer etiology. Cancer 1977;40:1887-1891.

144. Weisburger JH, Wynder EL: Etiology of colorectal cancer with emphasis on mechanism of action and prevention. Import Adv Oncol 1987;197-220.

145. Alberts DS, Martinez ME, Roe DJ, et al: Lack of effect of a high-fiber cereal Supplement on the recurrence of colorectal adenomas. N Eng J Med 2000;20:1156-1162.

146. Schatzkin A, Lanza E, Corle D, et al: Lack of effect of a low-fat, high-fiber diet on the recurrence of colorectal adenomas. Polyp Prevention Trial Study Group. N Engl J Med 2000;342:1149-1155.

147. Levi F, Pasche C, LaVecchia C, Lucchini F, Franceschi S: Food groups and colorectal cancer risk. Br J Cancer 1999;79:1283-1287.

148. Matos E, Brandani A: Review on meat consumption and cancer in South America. Mutat Res 2002;30:506-507.

149. Adami HO, Day NE, Trichopolous, et al: Primary and secondary prevention in the reduction of cancer morbidity and mortality. Eur J Cancer 2001;37:5118–5127.
150. Erhardt JG, Kreichgauer HP, Meisner C, Bode JC, Bode C: Alcohol, cigarette smoking, dietary factors and the risk of colorectal adenomas and hyperplastic polyps—a case control study. Eur J Nutr 2002;41:35–43.
151. Almendingen K, Hofstad B, Vatn MH: Does intake of alcohol increase the risk of presence and growth of colorectal adenomas followed up in situ for three years? Scand J Gastroenterol 2002;37:80–87.
152. Bardou M, Montembault S, Giraud V, et al: Excessive alcohol consumption favours high risk polyp or colorectal cancer occurrence among patients with adenomas: A case control study. Gut 2002;50:38–42.
153. Matsuo K, Hamajima N, Hirai T, et al: Aldehyde dehydrogenase 2 (ALDH2) genotype affects rectal cancer susceptibility due to alcohol consumption. J Epidemiol 2002;12:70–76.
154. Almendingen K, Hofstad B, Vatn MH: Does intake of alcohol increase the risk and presence and growth of colorectal adenomas followed-up in situ for three years? Scand J Gastroenterol 2002;37:80–87.
155. Boutron MC, Faivre J, Dop MC, et al: Tobacco, alcohol and colorectal tumors: A multistep process. Am J Epi 1995;141:1035–1046.
156. La Vecchia C, Negri E, Pelucchi C, Franceschi S: Dietary folate and colorectal cancer. Int J Cancer 2002;102:545–547.
157. Mass J, Stampfer MJ, Giovannucci E, et al: Methylenetetrahydrofolate reductase polymorphism, dietary interactions, and risk of colorectal cancer. Cancer Res 1997;57:1098–1102.
158. Chen J, Giovannucci E, Kelsey K, et al: A methylenetetrahydrofolate reductase polymorphism and the risk of colorectal cancer. Cancer Res 1996;56:4862–4864.
159. Bardou M, Montembault S, Giraud V, et al: Excessive alcohol consumption favours high risk polyp or colorectal cancer occurrence among patients with adenomas: A case control study. Gut 2002;50:38–42.
160. Neugut AI, Terry MB: Cigarette smoking and microsatellite instability: Causal pathway or marker-defined subset of colon tumors. J Natl Cancer Inst 2000;92:1791–1795.
161. Slattery M, Curtin K, Anderson K, et al: Associations between cigarette smoking, lifestyle factors and microsatellite instability in colon tumors. J Natl Cancer Inst 2000;92:1831–1836.
162. Giovannucci E, Rimm EB, Stampfer MJ, et al: A prospective study of cigarette smoking and risk of colorectal adenoma and colorectal cancer in U.S. men. J Natl Cancer Inst 1994;86:183.
163. Giovannucci E, Colditz GA, Stampfer MJ, et al: A prospective study of cigarette smoking and risk of colorectal adenoma and colorectal cancer in U.S. women. J Natl Cancer Inst 1994;86:192.
164. Chao A, Thun MJ, Jacobs EJ, et al: Cigarette smoking and colorectal cancer mortality in the cancer prevention study II. J Natl Cancer Inst 2000;92:1888–1896.
165. Giovannucci E, Colditz GA, Stampfer MJ, et al: Physical activity, obesity, and risk of colorectal adenoma in women (United States). Cancer Causes Control 1996;7:253–263.
166. Bruce WR, Giacca A, Medline A: Possible mechanisms relating diet and risk of colon cancer. Cancer Epi Biom Prev 2000;9:1271–1279.
167. Sandhu MS, Dunger OB, Giovannuci FL: Insulin, insulin-like growth factor I(IGF-1), IGF binding proteins, their biologic interactions, and colorectal cancer. J Natl Cancer Inst 2002;94:972–980.
168. Pignone M, Rich M, Teutsch S, et al: Screening for colorectal cancer in adults at average risk: A summary of the evidence for the U.S. preventive services task force. Ann Int Med 2002;137:132–141.
169. Vernon SW: Participation in colorectal cancer screening: A review. J Natl Cancer Inst 1997;89:1406–1422.
170. Kewenter J, Bjork S, Haglind E, et al: Screening and rescreening for colorectal cancer. A controlled trial of fecal occult blood testing in 27,700 subjects. Cancer 1988;62:645–651.
171. Hardcastle JD, Thomas WM, Chamberlain J, et al: Randomised, controlled trial of faecal occult blood screening for colorectal cancer. Results for first 107.349 subjects. Lancet 1989;1:1160–1164.
172. Hardcastle JD, Chamberlain JO, Robinson MH, et al: Randomised controlled trial of faecal-occult-blood screening for colorectal cancer. Lancet 1996;348:1472–1477.
173. Kronborg O, Fenger C, Olsen J, et al: Randomised study of screening for colorectal cancer with faecal-occult-blood test [see comments]. Lancet 1996;348:1467–1471.
174. Winawer SJ, Flehinger BJ, Schottenfeld D, et al: Screening for colorectal cancer with fecal occult blood testing and sigmoidoscopy [see comments]. J Natl Cancer Inst 1993;85:1311–1318.
175. Mandel JS, Bond JH, Church TR, et al: Reducing mortality from colorectal cancer by screening for fecal occult blood. Minnesota Colon Cancer Control Study [published erratum appears in N Engl J Med 1993 Aug 26;329(9):672] [see comments]. N Engl J Med 1993;328:1365–1371.
176. Ederer F, Church TR, Mandel JS: Fecal occult blood screening in the Minnesota study: Role of chance detection of lesions [see comments]. J Natl Cancer Inst 1997;89:1423–1428.
177. Ransohoff DF, Lang CA: Screening for colorectal cancer with the fecal occult blood test: A background paper. American College of Physicians [see comments]. Ann Intern Med 1997;126:811–822.
178. Eddy DM: Screening for colorectal cancer [see comments]. Ann Intern Med 1990;113:373–384.
179. Allison JE, Feldman R, Tekawa IS: Hemoccult screening in detecting colorectal neoplasm: sensitivity, specificity, and predictive value. Long-term follow-up in a large group practice setting. Ann Intern Med 1990;112:328–333.
180. Barry MJ, Mulley AG, Richter JM: Effect of workup strategy on the cost-effectiveness of fecal occult blood screening for colorectal cancer. Gastroenterology 1987;93:301–310.
181. Gilbertsen VA: Proctosigmoidoscopy and polypectomy in reducing the incidence of rectal cancer. Cancer 1974;34(Suppl):936–939.
182. Selby JV, Friedman GD, Quesenberry CP, Jr., et al: A case-control study of screening sigmoidoscopy and mortality from colorectal cancer [see comments]. N Engl J Med 1992;326:653–657.
183. Newcomb PA, Norfleet RG, Storer BE, et al: Screening sigmoidoscopy and colorectal cancer mortality [see comments]. J Natl Cancer Inst 1992;84:1572–1575.
184. Segnan N, Senore C, Andreoni B, et al: Baseline findings of the Italian Multicenter Randomized Controlled Trial of "once-only sigmoidoscopy"—SCORE. J Natl Cancer Inst 2002;94:1763–1772.
185. Anderson WF, Guyton KZ, Hiatt RA, et al: Colorectal screening for persons at average cancer risk. J Natl Cancer Inst 2002;94:1126–1133.
186. Morin PJ, Volgelstein B, Kinzler KW: Apoptosis and APC in colorectal tumorigenesis. Proc Natl Acad Sci USA 1996;93:7950–7954.
187. Traverso G, Shuber A, Levin B, et al: Detection of APC mutations in fecal DNA from patients with colorectal tumors. N Engl J Med 2002;346:311–320.
188. Mayer RJ: Scientific American Medicine 12:VIII Gastrointestinal Cancer, 1998
189. Rustgi AK: Hereditary gastrointestinal polyposis and nonpolyposis syndromes. N Engl J Med 1994;331:1694–1702.
190. Powell SM, Petersen GM, Krush AJ, et al: Molecular diagnosis of familial adenomatous polyposis. N Engl J Med 1993;329:1982–1987.
191. Aaltonen LA, Salovaara R, Kristo P, et al: Incidence of hereditary nonpolyposis colorectal cancer and the feasibility of molecular screening for the disease [see comments]. N Engl J Med 1998;338:1481–1487.
192. Fuchs CS, Giovannucci EL, Colditz GA, et al: A prospective study of family history and the risk of colorectal cancer [see comments]. N Engl J Med 1994;331:1669–1674.
193. Nugent FW, Haggitt RC, Gilpin PA: Cancer surveillance in ulcerative colitis [see comments]. Gastroenterology 1991;100:1241–1248.
194. Husmann DA, Spence HM: Current status of tumor of the bowel following ureterosigmoidostomy: A review. J Urol 1990;144:607–610.
195. Klein RS, Catalano MT, Edberg SC, et al: Streptococcus bovis septicemia and carcinoma of the colon. Ann Intern Med 1979;91:560–562.

196. Grodstein F, Martinez ME, Platz EA, et al: Postmenopausal hormone use and risk for colorectal cancer and adenoma [see comments]. Ann Intern Med 1998;128:705-712.

197. Martinez ME, Grodstein F, Giovannucci E, et al: A prospective study of reproductive factors, oral contraceptive use, and risk of colorectal cancer. Cancer Epi Biom Prev 1997;6:1-5.

198. Beahrs OH: AJCC Manual for Staging of Cancer, 4th edition. Philadelphia, JB Lippincott, 1992, p76.

199. Greenberg ER, Baron JA, Tosteson TD, et al: A clinical trial of antioxidant vitamins to prevent colorectal adenoma. Polyp Prevention Study Group [see comments]. N Engl J Med 1994;331:141-147.

200. MacLennan R, Macrae F, Bain C, et al: Randomized trial of intake of fat, fiber, and beta carotene to prevent colorectal adenomas. The Australian Polyp Prevention Project [see comments]. J Natl Cancer Inst 1995;87:1760-1766.

201. Wu K, Willett WC, Fuchs CS, et al: Calcium intake and risk of colon cancer in men and women. J Natl Cancer Inst 2002;94:437-446.

202. Clark LC, Combs GF Jr., Turnbull BW, et al: Effects of selenium Supplementation for cancer prevention in patients with carcinoma of the skin. A randomized controlled trial. Nutritional Prevention of Cancer Study Group [see comments] [published erratum appears in JAMA 1997 May 21;277(19): 1520]. JAMA 1996;276:1957-1963.

203. Mason JB: Nutritional chemoprevention of colon cancer. Serum Gastrointest Dis 2002;13:143-153.

204. Lagiou P, Trichopoulou A, Trichopoulos D: Nutritional epidemiology of cancer: Accomplishments and prospects. Proc Nutr Soc 2002;61(2):217-220.

205. Marnett LJ, DuBois RN: COX-2: A target for colon cancer prevention. Annu Rev Pharmacol Toxicol 2002;42:55-80.

206. Alberts DS: Reducing the risk of colorectal cancer by intervening in the process of carcinogenesis: A status report. Cancer J 2002;8:208-221.

207. Kune GA, Kune S, Watson LF: Colorectal cancer risk, chronic illnesses, operations, and medications: Case control results from the Melbourne Colorectal Cancer Study. Cancer Res 1988;48: 4399-4404.

208. Rosenberg L, Palmer JR, Zauber AG, et al: A hypothesis: nonsteroidal anti-inflammatory drugs reduce the incidence of large-bowel cancer [see comments]. J Natl Cancer Inst 1991;83:355-358.

209. Logan RF, Little J, Hawtin PG, et al: Effect of aspirin and non-steroidal anti-inflammatory drugs on colorectal adenomas: Case-control study of subjects participating in the Nottingham faecal occult blood screening programme [see comments]. BMJ 1993;307:285-289.

210. Suh O, Mettlin C, Petrelli NJ: Aspirin use, cancer, and polyps of the large bowel. Cancer 1993;72:1171-1177.

211. Muscat JE, Stellman SD, Wynder EL: Nonsteroidal anti-inflammatory drugs and colorectal cancer [see comments]. Cancer 1994;74:1847-1854.

212. Pollard M, Luckert PH: Effect of indomethacin on intestinal tumors induced in rats by the acetate derivative of dimethylnitrosamine. Science 1981;214:558-559.

213. Thun MJ, Namboodiri MM, Heath CW Jr: Aspirin use and reduced risk of fatal colon cancer [see comments]. N Engl J Med 1991;325:1593-1596.

214. Thun MJ, Namboodiri MM, Calle EE, et al: Aspirin use and risk of fatal cancer. Cancer Res 1993;53:1322-1327.

215. Greenberg ER, Baron JA, Freeman DH Jr, et al: Reduced risk of large-bowel adenomas among aspirin users. The Polyp Prevention Study Group. J Natl Cancer Inst 1993;85:912-916.

216. Giovannucci E, Egan KM, Hunter DJ, et al: Aspirin and the risk of colorectal cancer in women. N Engl J Med 1995;333:609-614.

217. Paganini-Hill A, Chao A, Ross RK, et al: Aspirin use and chronic diseases: A cohort study of the elderly [see comments]. BMJ 1989;299:1247-1250.

218. Peleg II, Maibach HT, Brown SH, et al: Aspirin and nonsteroidal anti-inflammatory drug use and the risk of subsequent colorectal cancer [see comments]. Arch Intern Med 1994;154:394-399.

219. Schreinemachers DM, Everson RB: Aspirin use and lung, colon, and breast cancer incidence in a prospective study [see comments]. Epidemiology 1994;5:138-146.

220. Zhu J, Song X, Lin HP, et al: Using cyclooxygenase-2 inhibitors as molecular platforms to develop a new class of apoptosis-inducing agents. J Natl Cancer Inst 2002;94:1745-1757.

221. Lynch NR, Salomon JC: Tumor growth inhibition and potentiation of immunotherapy by indomethacin in mice. J Natl Cancer Inst 1979;62:117-121.

222. Farrell CL, Megyesi J, Del Maestro RF: Effect of ibuprofen on tumor growth in the C6 spheroid implantation glioma model. J Neurosurg 1988;68:925-930.

223. Moorghen M, Ince P, Finney KJ, et al: A protective effect of sulindac against chemically-induced primary colonic tumours in mice. J Pathol 1988;156:341-347.

224. Mccarthy D: Comparative toxicity of nonsteroidal anti-inflammatory compounds. Am J Med 1999;107:375-465.

225. Mukherjee D, Nissen SE, Topol EJ: Risk of cardiovascular events associated with selective COX-2 inhibitors. JAMA 2001;286: 954-959.

226. Steinbach G, Lynch PM, Phillips RKS, et al: The effect of celecoxib, a cyclooxygenase-2 inhibitor, in familial adenomatous polyposis. N Engl J Med 2000;342:1946-1952.

227. Girdiello FM, Hailton SR, Krush AJ, et al: Treatment of colonic and rectal adenomas with sulindac in familial adenomatous polyposis. N Engl J Med 1993;328:1313-1316.

228. Giardiello FM, Yang VW, Hylind LM, et al: Primary chemoprevention of familial adenomatous polyposis with sulindac. N Engl J Med 2002;346:1054-1059.

229. Hawk ET, Limburg J, Viner JL: Epidemiology and prevention of colorectal cancer. Surg Clin North Am 2002;82:905-941.

230. Madigan MP, Ziegler RG, Benichou J, et al: Proportion of breast cancer cases in the United States explained by well-established risk factors. J Natl Cancer Inst 1995;87:1681-1685.

231. Krieger N, Quesenberry C Jr, Peng T, et al: Social class, race/ethnicity and incidence of breast, cervix, colon, lung and prostate cancer among Asian, Black, Hispanic and White residents of the San Francisco Bay Area, 1988-1992. Cancer Causes Control 1999;10:525-537.

232. Easton DF, Bishop DT, Ford D, et al: Genetic linkage analysis in familial breast and ovarian cancer: Results from 214 families. The Breast Cancer Linkage Consortium. Am J Hum Genet 1993;52:678-701.

233. Couch FJ, DeShano ML, Blackwood MA, et al: BRCA1 mutations in women attending clinics that evaluate the risk of breast cancer. N Engl J Med 1997;336:1409-1415.

234. Hankey B, Brinton L, Kessler L, et al: SEER cancer statistics review 1973-1990. In Miller B, Reis L, Hankey B, et al (eds): National Institutes of Health Publication 93-2789. Bethesda, MD, National Institute of Health, 1993.

235. Struewing JP, Hartge P, Wacholder S, et al: The risk of cancer associated with specific mutations of BRCA1 and BRCA2 among Ashkenazi Jews [see comments]. N Engl J Med 1997;336: 1401-1408.

236. Ford D, Easton DF, Bishop DT, et al: Risks of cancer in BRCA1-mutation carriers. Breast Cancer Linkage Consortium. Lancet 1994;343:692-695.

237. Shattuck-Eidens D, Oliphant A, McClure M, et al: BRCA1 sequence analysis in women at high risk for susceptibility mutations. Risk factor analysis and implications for genetic testing [see comments]. JAMA 1997;278:1242-1250.

238. FitzGerald MG, MacDonald DJ, Krainer M, et al: Germ-line BRCA1 mutations in Jewish and non-Jewish women with early-onset breast cancer [see comments]. N Engl J Med 1996;334: 143-149.

239. Loman N, Johannson O, Kristoffersson U, et al: Family history of breast and ovarian cancers and BRCA1 and BRCA2 mutations in a population-based series of early-onset breast cancer. J Natl Cancer Inst 2001;93:1215-1223.

240. Anonymous: Statement of the American Society of Clinical Oncology: Genetic testing for cancer susceptibility, adopted on February 20, 1996. J Clin Oncol 1996;14:1730-1736; discussion 1737-1744.

241. DiSaia PJ, Creasman WT (eds): Clinical Gynecologic Oncology, 5th edition. St. Louis, MO, Mosby-year Book, 1997, p 403.

242. Brinton LA, Schairer C, Hoover RN, et al: Menstrual factors and risk of breast cancer. Cancer Invest 1988;6:245-254.

243. Rookus MA, van Leeuwen FE: Induced abortion and risk for breast cancer: Reporting (recall) bias in a Dutch case-control study [see comments]. J Natl Cancer Inst 1996;88:1759–1764.

244. Colditz GA, Hankinson SE, Hunter DJ, et al: The use of estrogens and progestins and the risk of breast cancer in postmenopausal women [see comments]. N Engl J Med 1995;332:1589–1593.

245. Bergkvist L, Adami HO, Persson I, et al: The risk of breast cancer after estrogen and estrogen-progestin replacement [see comments]. N Engl J Med 1989;321:293–297.

246. Dupont WD, Page DL: Menopausal estrogen replacement therapy and breast cancer [see comments]. Arch Intern Med 1991;151: 67–72.

247. Anonymous: Effects of estrogen or estrogen/progestin regimens on heart disease risk factors in postmenopausal women. The Postmenopausal Estrogen/Progestin Interventions (PEPI) Trial. The Writing Group for the PEPI Trial [see comments] JAMA 1995;273:199–208 [published erratum appears in JAMA 1995;274:1676].

248. Gambrell RD Jr, Maier RC, Sanders BI: Decreased incidence of breast cancer in postmenopausal estrogen-progestogen users. Obstet Gynecol 1983;62:435–443.

249. DiSaia PJ, Grosen EA, Odicino F, et al: Replacement therapy for breast cancer survivors. A pilot study. Cancer 1995;76:2075–2078.

250. DiSaia PJ, Grosen EA, Kurosaki T, et al: Hormone replacement therapy in breast cancer survivors: A cohort study [see comments]. Am J Obstet Gynecol 1996;174:1494–1498.

251. O'Meara ES, Rossing MA, Daling JR, et al: Hormone replacement therapy after a diagnosis of breast cancer in relation to recurrence and mortality. J Natl Cancer Inst 2001;93:754–762.

252. Pritchard KI: Hormone replacement therapy in women with a history of breast cancer. Oncologist 2001;6:353–362.

253. Chlebowski RT: Elements of informed consent for hormonal replacement therapy in patients with diagnosed breast cancer. J Clin Oncol 1999;17:130–142.

254. Anonymous: Breast cancer and hormonal contraceptives: Collaborative reanalysis of individual data on 53.297 women with breast cancer and 100.239 women without breast cancer from 54 epidemiologic studies. Collaborative Group on Hormonal Factors in Breast Cancer. Lancet 1996;347(9017):1713–1727.

255. Thomas DB: Update on breast cancer and oral contraceptives. Contracept Rept 1991;2:3.

256. Marchbanks PA, McDonald JA, Wilson MG, et al: Oral contraceptives and the risk of breast cancer. N Eng J Med 2002;346:2025–2032.

257. Narold SA, Dube M-P, Klijn J, et al: Oral contraceptives and the risk of breast cancer in BRCA1 and BRCA2 mutation carriers. J Natl Cancer Inst 2002;94:1773–1779.

258. Dupont WD, Parl FF, Hartmann WH, et al: Breast cancer risk associated with proliferative breast disease and atypical hyperplasia [see comments]. Cancer 1993;71:1258–1265.

259. Connolly JL, Schnitt SJ: Clinical and histologic aspects of proliferative and non-proliferative benign breast disease. J Cell Biochem Suppl 1993;17G:45–48.

260. Dupont WD, Page DL: Risk factors for breast cancer in women with proliferative breast disease. N Engl J Med 1985;312:146–151.

261. Rose DP, Boyar AP, Wynder EL: International comparisons of mortality rates for cancer of the breast, ovary, prostate, and colon, and per capita food consumption. Cancer 1986;58:2363–2371.

262. Buell P: Changing incidence of breast cancer in Japanese-American women. J Natl Cancer Inst 1973;51:1479–1483.

263. Adelstein AM, Staszewski J, Muir CS: Cancer mortality in 1970–1972 among Polish-born migrants to England and Wales. Br J Cancer 1979;40:464–475.

264. Knekt P, Albanes D, Seppanen R, et al: Dietary fat and risk of breast cancer. Am J Clin Nutr 1990;52:903–908.

265. Howe GR, Friedenreich CM, Jain M, et al: A cohort study of fat intake and risk of breast cancer [see comments]. J Natl Cancer Inst 1991;83:336–340.

266. Kushi LH, Sellers TA, Potter JD, et al: Dietary fat and postmenopausal breast cancer [see comments]. J Natl Cancer Inst 1992;84:1092–1099.

267. Willett WC, Hunter DJ, Stampfer MJ, et al: Dietary fat and fiber in relation to risk of breast cancer. An 8-year follow-up [see comments]. JAMA 1992;268:2037–2044.

268. Graham S, Zielezny M, Marshall J, et al: Diet in the epidemiology of postmenopausal breast cancer in the New York State Cohort [see comments]. Am J Epidemiol 1992;136:1327–1337.

269. Byrne C, Ursin G, Ziegler RG: A comparison of food habit and food frequency data as predictors of breast cancer in the NHANES I/NHEFS cohort. J Nutr 1996;126:2757–2764.

270. van den Brandt PA, Van't Veer P, Goldbohm RA, et al: A prospective cohort study on dietary fat and the risk of postmenopausal breast cancer. Cancer Res 1993;53:75–82.

271. Toniolo P, Riboli E, Shore RE, et al: Consumption of meat, animal products, protein, and fat and risk of breast cancer: A prospective cohort study in New York [see comments]. Epidemiology 1994;5:391–397.

272. Albanes D, Jones DY, Schatzkin A, et al: Adult stature and risk of cancer. Cancer Res 1988;48:1658–1662.

273. Albanes D, Taylor PR: International differences in body height and weight and their relationship to cancer incidence. Nutr Cancer 1990;14:69–77.

274. Albanes D: Caloric intake, body weight, and cancer: A review. Nutr Cancer 1987;9:199–217.

275. Kritchevsky D: Nutrition and breast cancer. Cancer 1990;66: 1321–1325.

276. Wu AH, Stanczyk FZ, Seow A, et al: Soy intake and other lifestyle determinants of serum estrogen levels among postmenopausal Chinese women in Singapore. Cancer Epi Biom Prev 2002;11: 844–851.

277. Hu X, Juneja SC, Maihle N, et al: Leptin—A growth factor in normal and malignant breast cells and for normal mammary gland development. J Natl Cancer Inst 2002;94:1704–1711.

278. Longnecker MP, Berlin JA, Orza MJ, et al: A meta-analysis of alcohol consumption in relation to risk of breast cancer. JAMA 1988;260: 652–656.

279. Byers T, Perry G: Dietary carotenes, vitamin C, and vitamin E as protective antioxidants in human cancers. Annu Rev Nutr 1992;12:139–159.

280. Fontana JA, Hobbs PD, Dawson MI: Inhibition of mammary carcinoma growth by retinoidal benzoic acid derivatives. Exp Cell Biol 1988;56:254–263.

281. Potischman N, McCulloch CE, Byers T, et al: Breast cancer and dietary and plasma concentrations of carotenoids and vitamin A. Am J Clin Nutr 1990;52:909–915.

282. Hakama M: Blood, biochemistry, and breast cancer. J Cancer Res Clin Oncol 1990;16:1199.

283. Gerber M, Cavallo F, Marubini E, et al: Liposoluble vitamins and lipid parameters in breast cancer. A joint study in northern Italy and southern France. Int J Cancer 1988;42:489–494.

284. Jakes RW, Duffy SW, Ng F-C, et al: Mammographic parachymal patterns and self-reported soy intake in Singapore Chinese women. Cancer Epi Biom Prev 2002;7:608–613.

285. National Cancer Institute, Cancer Facts, NCI Reports Improvement in Breast Cancer Death Rate. Bethesda, MD, National Cancer Institute, 1998.

286. Thomas DB, Gao DL, Ray RM, et al: Randomized trial of breast self-examination in Shangai; final results. J Natl Cancer Inst 2002;94:1445–1457.

287. Harris R, Kinsinger LS: Routine teaching breast self-examination is dead. What does this mean? JNCI 2002;94:1420–1421.

288. Byrne C, Smart CR, Chu KC, et al: Survival advantage differences by age. Evaluation of the extended follow-up of the Breast Cancer Detection Demonstration Project. Cancer 1994;74:301–310.

289. Morrison AS, Brisson J, Khalid N: Breast cancer incidence and mortality in the breast cancer detection demonstration project [published erratum appears in J Natl Cancer Inst 1989;81(19):1513]. J Natl Cancer Inst 1988;80:1540–1547.

290. Anonymous: Mammographic screening in asymptomatic women aged 40 years and older. Council on Scientific Affairs [see comments]. JAMA 1989;261:2535–2542.

291. National Institute of Health Consensus Development Statement 1997: Breast Cancer Screening for Women Ages 40–49. Bethesda, MD, 1997.

292. Tabar L, Fagerberg CJ, Gad A, et al: Reduction in mortality from breast cancer after mass screening with mammography. Randomised trial from the Breast Cancer Screening Working Group of the Swedish National Board of Health and Welfare. Lancet 1985;1:829–832.

293. Verbeek AL, Hendriks JH, Holland R, et al: Reduction of breast cancer mortality through mass screening with modern mammography. First results of the Nijmegen project, 1975–1981. Lancet 1984;1:1222–1224.

294. Smart CR: Highlights of the evidence of benefit for women aged 40–49 years from the 14-year follow-up of the Breast Cancer Detection Demonstration Project. Cancer 1994;74:296–300.

295. U.S. Prevention Task Force: Screening for breast cancer: Recommendation and rationale. Ann Int Med 2002;137:344–346.

296. Boyd NF, Dite GD, Stone J, et al: Heritability of mammographic density, a risk factor for breast cancer. N Eng J Med 2002;347:886–894.

297. Greendale GA, Reboussin BA, Slone S, et al: Postmenopausal hormone therapy and change in mammographic density. J Natl Cancer Inst 2003;95:30–37.

298. Nayfield SG, Karp JE, Ford LG, et al: Potential role of tamoxifen in prevention of breast cancer. J Natl Cancer Inst 1991;83:1450–1459.

299. Fisher B, Costantino JP, Wickerham DL, et al: Tamoxifen for prevention of breast cancer: Report of the National Surgical Adjuvant Breast and Bowel Project P-1 Study. J Natl Cancer Inst 1998;90(18):1371–1388.

300. Veronesi U, Maisonneuve P, Costa A, et al: Prevention of breast cancer with tamoxifen: Preliminary findings from the Italian randomised trial among hysterectomised women. Italian Tamoxifen Prevention Study [see comments]. Lancet 1998;352:93–97.

301. Powles T, Eeles R, Ashley S, et al: Interim analysis of the incidence of breast cancer in the Royal Marsden Hospital tamoxifen randomised chemoprevention trial [see comments]. Lancet 1998;352:98–101.

302. Powles TJ: Anti-oestrogenic prevention of breast cancer—The make or break point. Nature Rev Cancer 2002;2:787–794.

303. King MC, Wieand S, Hale K, et al: Tamoxifen and breast cancer incidence among women with inherited mutations in BRCA1 and BRCA2: National surgical adjuvant breast and bowel project (NSAPB-PI) breast cancer prevention trial. J Am Med Assoc 2001;286:2251–2256.

304. Cauley JA, Norton L, Lippmann ME, et al: Continued breast cancer risk reduction in postmenopausal women treated with raloxifene, 4 year results from the MORE trial. Multiple outcomes of raloxifene evaluation. Breast Cancer Res Treat 2001;65:125–134.

305. Veronesi U, De Palo G, Costa A, et al: Chemoprevention of breast cancer with fenretinide. IARC Sci Publ 1996;136:87–94.

306. Decensi A, Johansson H, Miceli R, et al: Long term effects of Fenretinide, a retinoic acid derivative, on the insulin-like growth factor system in women with early breast cancer. Cancer Epi Biom Prev 2001;10:1047–1053.

307. U.S. Preventive Services Task Force: Chemoprevention of breast cancer: Recommendations and rationale. Ann Int Med 2002;137:56–72.

308. Grann VR, Panageas KS, Whang W, et al: Decision analysis of prophylactic mastectomy and oophorectomy in BCRA1-positive or BCRA-2-positive patients. J Clin Oncol 1998;16:979.

309. Jacobsen SJ, Katusic SK, Bergstralh EJ, et al: Incidence of prostate cancer diagnosis in the eras before and after serum prostate-specific antigen testing [see comments]. JAMA 1995;274:1445–1449.

310. Pienta KJ, Esper PS: Risk factors for prostate cancer. Ann Intern Med 1993;118:793–803.

311. Rodriguez C, Calle EE, Miracle-McMahill HL, et al: Family history and risk of fatal prostate cancer. Epidemiology 1997;8:653–657.

312. Hemminki K, Czene K: Age specific and attributable risks of familial prostate carcinoma from the family-cancer database. Cancer 2002;6:1346–1353.

313. Karan D, Lin MF, Johansson SL, et al: Current status of the molecular genetics of human prostatic adenocaracinomas. Int J Cancer 2003;103:285–293.

314. Gronberg H, Isaacs SD, Smith JR, et al: Characteristics of prostate cancer in families potentially linked to the hereditary prostate cancer 1 (HPC1) locus. JAMA 1997;278:1251.

315. Gsur A, Preger M, Haidinger G, et al: Polymorphic CAG repeats in the androgen receptor gene, prostate-specific antigen polymorphism and prostate cancer risk. Carcinogenesis 2002;23:1647–1651.

316. Mir K, Edwards J, Paterson PJ, et al: The CAG trinucleotide repeat length in the androgen receptor does not predict the early onset of prostate cancer. BJU Int 2002;90:573–578.

317. Chen C, Lambarzi N, Weiss N, et al: Androgen receptor polymorphisms and the incidence of prostate cancer. Cancer Epi Biom Prev 2002;11:1033–1040.

318. Chen ZK, Gokden N, Greene GF, et al: Extensive somatic mitochondrial mutations in primary prostate cancer using laser capture microdissection. Cancer Res 2002;62:6470–6474.

319. Pollard M, Luckert PH, Schmidt MA: Induction of prostate adenocarcinomas in Lobund Wistar rats by testosterone. Prostate 1982;3:563–568.

320. Noble RL: The development of prostatic adenocarcinoma in Nb rats following prolonged sex hormone administration. Cancer Res 1977;37:1929–1933.

321. Hovenian MS, Demming CL: The heterologous growth of cancer of the human prostate. Surg Gynecol Obstet 1984;86:29–35.

322. Merrill RM, Weed DL, Feuer EJ: The lifetime risk of developing prostate cancer in white and black men. Cancer Epi Biom Prev 1997;6:763–768.

323. Demers RY, Swanson GM, Weiss LK, Kau TY: Increasing incidence of cancer of the prostate. The experience of black and white men in the Detroit metropolitan area. Arch Intern Med 1994;154:1211.

324. Ross RK, Coetzee GA, Reichardt J, et al: Does the racial-ethnic variation in prostate-cancer risk have a hormonal basis? Cancer 1995;75:1778–1782.

325. Ross RK, Bernstein L, Lobo RA, et al: 5-alpha-reductase activity and risk of prostate cancer among Japanese and US white and black males. Lancet 1992;339:887–889.

326. Vatten LJ, Ursin G, Ross RK, et al: Androgens in serum and the risk of prostate cancer: A nested case-control study from the Janus serum bank in Norway. Cancer Epi Biom Prev 1997;6:967–969.

327. Cohen LA. Nutrition and prostate cancer: a review. Ann NY Acad Sci 2002;963:148–155.

328. Giovannucci E, Rimm EB, Stampfer MJ, et al: Height, body weight, and risk of prostate cancer. Cancer Epi Biom Prev 1997;6:557–563.

329. Nelson WG, DeWeese TL, DeMarzo AM: The diet, prostate inflammation, and the development of prostate cancer. Cancer Metastasis Rev 2002;21:3–16.

330. Rebbeck TR: Inherited genotype and prostate cancer outcomes. Cancer Epi Biom Prev 2002;11:945–952.

331. Catalona WJ: Screening for prostate cancer [letter; comment]. JAMA 1995;273:1174.

332. Collins MM, Barry MJ: Controversies in prostate cancer screening. Analogies to the early lung cancer screening debate [see comments]. JAMA 1996;276:1976–1979.

333. Garnick MB, Fair WR: Prostate cancer: Emerging concepts. Part I [see comments]. Cancer 1992;69:1195–1200.

334. Etzione R, Penson DF, Legler JM, et al: Over diagnosis due to prostate-specific antigen screening: Lessons from U.S. Prostate Cancer incidence trends. J Natl Cancer Inst 2002;94:981–990.

335. McGregor M, Hanley JA, Boivin JF, et al: Screening for prostate cancer: Estimating the magnitude of overdetection. Can Med Assoc J 1998;159:1368–1372.

336. Yao SL, Lu-Yao G: Understanding and appreciating over diagnosis in the PSA era. J Natl Cancer Inst 2002;94:958–959.

337. Resnick MI: Editorial comment on screening for prostate cancer [Editorial]. In Ratliff TL, Catalona WJ, (eds): Genitourinary Cancer. Boston, Martinus, 1987, pp 94–99.

338. Stearns MW. Digital rectal examination. CA J Clinic 1974;24:100–103.

339. Chodak GW, Keller P, Schoenberg HW: Assessment of screening for prostate cancer using the digital rectal examination. J Urol 1989;141:1136–1138.

340. Thompson IM, Zeidman EJ: Presentation and clinical course of patients ultimately succumbing to carcinoma of the prostate. Scand J Urol Nephrol 1991;25:111–114.

341. Thompson IM, Seay TM: Will current clinical trials answer the most important questions about prostate adenocarcinoma? Oncology 1997;11:1109–1117.

342. Babaian RJ, Mettlin C, Kane R et al: The relationship of prostate-specific antigen to digital rectal examination and trans-rectal ultrasonagraphy: Findings of the American Cancer

Society National Prostate Cancer Detection project. Cancer 1992;69:1195–1200.

343. Brawer MK, Chetner MP, Beatie J, et al: Screening for prostatic carcinoma with prostate specific antigen. J Urol 1992;147:841–845.

344. Catalona WJ, Smith DS, Ratliff TL, et al: Detection of organ-confined prostate cancer is increased through prostate-specific antigen-based screening [see comments]. JAMA 1993;270:948–954.

345. Mettlin C, Murphy GP, Lee F, et al: Characteristics of prostate cancers detected in a multimodality early detection program. The Investigators of the American Cancer Society-National Prostate Cancer Detection Project. Cancer 1993;72:1701–1708.

346. Prestigiacomo AF, Stamey TA: Physiological variation of serum prostate specific antigen in the 4.0 to 10.0 ng/mL range in male volunteers [see comments]. J Urol 1996;155:1977–1980.

347. Bangma CH, Kranse R, Blijenberg BG, et al: The value of screening tests in the detection of prostate cancer. Part II: Retrospective analysis of free/total prostate-specific analysis ratio, age-specific reference ranges, and PSA density. Urology 1995;46:779–784.

348. Benson MC, Olsson CA: Prostate specific antigen and prostate specific antigen density. Roles in patient evaluation and management. Cancer 1994;74:1667–1673.

349. Carter HB, Pearson JD, Metter EJ, et al: Longitudinal evaluation of prostate-specific antigen levels in men with and without prostate disease [see comments]. JAMA 1992;267:2215–2220.

350. Carter HB, Pearson JD, Waclawiw Z, et al: Prostate-specific antigen variability in men without prostate cancer: Effect of sampling interval on prostate-specific antigen velocity. Urology 1995;45:591–596.

351. Oesterling JE, Jacobsen SJ, Chute CG, et al: Serum prostate-specific antigen in a community-based population of healthy men. Establishment of age-specific reference ranges [see comments]. JAMA 1993;270:860–864.

352. Catalona WJ, Richie JP, deKernion JB, et al: Comparison of prostate specific antigen concentration versus prostate specific antigen density in the early detection of prostate cancer: Receiver operating characteristic curves [see comments]. J Urol 1994;152:2031–2036.

353. Smith DS, Catalona WJ, Herschman JD: Longitudinal screening for prostate cancer with prostate-specific antigen [see comments]. JAMA 1996;276:1309–1315.

354. Woolf SH: Screening for prostate cancer with prostate-specific antigen. An examination of the evidence [see comments]. N Engl J Med 1995;333:1401–1405.

355. Chodak GW, Schoenberg HW: Early detection of prostate cancer by routine screening. JAMA 1984;252:3261–3264.

356. Johansson JE, Holmberg L, Johansson S, et al: Fifteen-year survival in prostate cancer. A prospective, population-based study in Sweden [see comments] [published erratum appears in JAMA 1997;278(3):206]. JAMA 1997;277:467–471.

357. Fowler FJ Jr, Barry MJ, Lu-Yao G, et al: Patient-reported complications and follow-up treatment after radical prostatectomy. The National Medicare Experience: 1988–1990 (updated June 1993). Urology 1993;42:622–629.

358. Lu-Yao GL, Yao SL: Population-based study of long-term survival in patients with clinically localised prostate cancer [see comments]. Lancet 1997;349:906–910.

359. Brawer MK, Chetner MP, Beatie J, et al: Screening for prostatic carcinoma with prostate specific antigen. J Urol 1992;147:841.

360. Carter HB, Pearson JD, Metter EJ, et al: Longitudinal evaluation of prostate-specific antigen levels in men with and without prosate disease. JAMA 1992;267:2215.

361. Mold JW, Holtgrave DR, Bisonni RS, et al: The evaluation and treatment of men with asymptomatic prostate nodules in primary care: A decision analysis [see comments]. J Fam Pract 1992;34:561–568.

362. Krahn MD, Mahoney JE, Eckman MH, et al: Screening for prostate cancer. A decision analytic view [see comments]. JAMA 1994;272:773–780.

363. Coley CM, Barry MJ, Flemming C, et al: Early detection of prostate cancer part II estimating the risks, benefits, and costs. Ann Intern Med. 1997;126:468–479.

364. Office of Technology Assessment: Costs and effectiveness of prostate cancer screening in elderly men. Washington, DC, Government Printing Office (OTA-BP-H-145), 1995.

365. Fleming C, Wasson JH, Albertsen PC, et al: A decision analysis of alternative treatment strategies for clinically localized prostate cancer. Prostate Patient Outcomes Research Team [see comments]. JAMA 1993;269:2650–2658.

366. Walsh PC: A decision analysis of alternative treatment strategies for clinically localized prostate cancer. J Urol 1993;150:1330–1332.

367. Diamond GP, Belange A, Bousseau G, et al: Decrease of prostate cancer screening first date from the Quebec prospective and randomized study. Am Soc Clin Oncol Proceedings: Plenary Session Ab#4, 1998.

368. Nijs HG, Tordoir DM, Schuurman JH, et al: Randomised trial of prostate cancer screening in The Netherlands: Assessment of acceptance and motives for attendance. J Med Screen 1997;4:102–106.

369. Schroder FH, Bangma CH: The European randomized study of screening for prostate cancer (ERSPC). Br J Urol 1997;79:68–71.

370. Gohagan JK, Prorok PC, Kramer BS, et al: Prostate cancer screening in the prostate, lung, colorectal, and ovarian cancer screening trial of the National Cancer Institute [see comments]. J Urol 1994;152:1905–1909.

371. Harris R, Lohr KN: Screening for prostate cancer: an update of the evidence for the U.S. Preventive Services Task Force. Ann Int Med 2002;137:917–929.

372. Simoneau AR, Gerner EW, Phung M, et al: α-difluoromethyl-ornithine and polyamine levels in the human prostate: Results of a phase IIa trial. J Natl Cancer Inst 2001;93:57–59.

373. Sakr W: High-grade prostate intraepithelial neoplasia: Additional links to a potentially more aggressive prostate cancer. J Natl Cancer Inst 1998;90:486–487.

374. Alcaraz A, Barranco MA, Corral JM, et al: High-grade prostate intraepithelial neoplasia shares cytogenetic alterations with invasive prostate cancer. Prostate 2001;47:29–35.

375. Holmberg L, Bill-Axelson A, Helgesen F, et al: A randomized trial comparing radical prostatectomy with watchful waiting in early prostate cancer. N Engl J Med 2002;347:781–789.

376. Bostwick DG, Rammani D, Qian J. Prostatic intraepithelial neoplasia animal models 2000. Prostate 2000;43:286–294.

377. Bostwick DG: High-grade prostatic intraepithelial neoplasia: The most likely precursor of prostate cancer. Cancer 1995;75:1823–1836.

378. Berner A, Danielsen HE, Pettersen EO, et al: DNA distribution in the prostate. Normal gland, benign and premalignant lesions, and subsequent adenocarcinomas. Anal Quant Cytol Histol 1993;15:247–252.

379. McConnell JD, Bruskewitz R, Walsh P, et al: The effect of finasteride on the risk of acute urinary retention and the need for surgical treatment among men with benign prostatic hyperplasia. Finasteride Long-Term Efficacy and Safety Study Group [see comments]. N Engl J Med 1998;338:557–563.

380. Karp JE, Chiarodo A, Brawley O, et al: Prostate cancer prevention: Investigational approaches and opportunities. Cancer Res 1996;56:5547–5556.

381. Aquilina JW, Lipsky JJ, Bostwick DG: Androgen deprivation as a strategy for prostate cancer chemoprevention. J Natl Cancer Inst 1997;89:689–696.

381A. Prevention of prostate cancer with finasteride. N Engl J Med 2003;349:1569–1572.

382. Lieberman RL, Nelson WG: New clinical trial strategies for prostate cancer prevention. Urology 2001;57(4A):1–247.

383. Venkateswasan V, Fleshner NE, Klotz LH: Modulation of cell proliferation and cell cycle regulators by vitamin E in human prostate carcinoma cell lines. J Urol 2002;168:1578–1582.

384. Heinonen O, Albanes D, Virtamo J, et al: Prostate cancer and Supplementation with α-tocopherol and β-carotene: Incidence and mortality in a controlled trial. J Natl Cancer Inst 1998;90:440–446.

385. Duffield-Lillico AJ, Reid ME, Turnbull BW, et al: Baseline characteristics and the effect of selenium Supplementation on cancer incidence in a randomized clinical trial: A summary report of the Nutritional Prevention of Cancer Trial. Cancer Epi Biom Prev 2002;11:630–639.

Science of Clinical Oncology

386. Sharp RM, Bello-DeOcamo D, Quader ST, Webber MM. N- (4-hydroxyphenyl) retinamide (4-HPR) decreases neoplastic properties of human prostate cells: An agent for prevention. Mutat Res 2001;496:163-170.

387. Glass AG, Hoover RN: The emerging epidemic of melanoma and squamous cell skin cancer [see comments]. JAMA 1989;262: 2097-2100.

388. Morbidity and Mortality Report Centers for Disease Control, Atlanta: Death rates of malignant melanoma among white men— United States, 1973-1988. Arch Dermatol 1992;128:451-452.

389. Kwa RE, Campana K, Moy RL: Biology of cutaneous squamous cell carcinoma [see comments]. J Am Acad Dermatol 1992;26:1-26.

390. Miller SJ: Biology of basal cell carcinoma (Part II). J Am Acad Dermatol 1991;24:161-175.

391. Setlow RB: The wavelengths in sunlight effective in producing skin cancer: A theoretical analysis. Proc Natl Acad Sci USA 1974;71:3363-3366.

392. Nola I, Kotrulja L: Skin photodamage and lifetime photoprotection. Acta Dermatovenerol Croat 2003;11:32-40.

393. Ananthaswamy HN, Pierceall WE: Molecular mechanisms of ultraviolet radiation carcinogenesis. Photochem Photobiol 1990;52:1119-1136.

394. DeGruijl FR: Photocarcinogenesis and UVA VSWB radiation skin. Pharmacol Skin Physiol 2002;15:316-320.

395. Ziegler A, Jonason AS, Leffell DJ, et al: Sunburn and p53 in the onset of skin cancer [see comments]. Nature 1994;372:773-776.

396. Taguchi M, Watanabe S, Yashima K, et al: Aberrations of the tumor suppressor p53 gene and p53 protein in solar keratosis in human skin. J Invest Dermatol 1994;103:500-503.

397. Brash DE, Rudolph JA, Simon JA, et al: A role for sunlight in skin cancer: UV-induced p53 mutations in squamous cell carcinoma. Proc Natl Acad Sci USA 1991;88:10124-10128.

398. Helander SD, Peters MS, Pittelkow MR: Expression of p53 protein in benign and malignant epidermal pathologic conditions [see comments]. J Am Acad Dermatol 1993;29:741-748.

399. Hutchinson F: Induction of tandem-base change mutations. Mutat Res 1994;309:11-15.

400. Oram Y, Orengo I, Baer SC, et al: p53 protein expression in squamous cell carcinomas from sun-exposed and non-sun-exposed sites. J Am Acad Dermatol 1994;31:417-422.

401. Brash DE, Ziegler A, Jonason AS, et al: Sunlight and sunburn in human skin cancer: p53, apoptosis, and tumor promotion. J Investig Dermatol Symp Proc 1996;1:136-142.

402. Ziegler A, Leffell DJ, Kunala S, et al: Mutation hotspots due to sunlight in the p53 gene of nonmelanoma skin cancers. Proc Natl Acad Sci USA 1993;90:4216-4220.

403. Selivanova G, Wiman KG: p53: A cell cycle regulator activated by DNA damage. Adv Cancer Res 1995;66:143-180.

404. Harris CC, Hollstein M: Clinical implications of the p53 tumor-suppressor gene [see comments]. N Engl J Med 1993;329: 1318-1327.

405. Kripke ML: Immunology and photocarcinogenesis. New light on an old problem. J Am Acad Dermatol 1986;14:149-155.

406. Sunlight, ultraviolet radiation and the skin. NIH Consensus Statement online, 1989;7:1

407. Tucker MA, Halpern A, Holly EA, et al: Clinically recognized dysplastic nevi. A central risk factor for cutaneous melanoma [see comments]. JAMA 1997;277:1439-1444.

408. Koh HK, Caruso A, Gage I, et al: Evaluation of melanoma/skin cancer screening in Massachusetts. Preliminary results. Cancer 1990;65:375-379.

409. Veronesi U, Cascinelli N, Bufalino R: Evaluation of the risk of multiple primaries in malignant cutaneous melanoma. Tumori 1976;62:127-130.

410. Karagas MR, Stukel TA, Greenberg ER, et al: Risk of subsequent basal cell carcinoma and squamous cell carcinoma of the skin among patients with prior skin cancer. Skin Cancer Prevention Study Group. JAMA 1992;267:3305-3310.

411. Lynch HT, Frichot BC, Lynch P, et al: Family studies of malignant melanoma and associated cancer. Surg Gynecol Obstet 1975;141:517-522.

412. Scheibner A, Milton GW, McCarthy WH, et al: Multiple primary melanoma—A review of 90 cases. Australas J Dermatol 1982;23:1-8.

413. Brobeil A, Rapaport D, Wells K, et al: Multiple primary melanomas: Implications for screening and follow-up programs for melanoma. Ann Surg Oncol 1997;4:19-23.

414. Quinn AG, Sikkink S, Rees JL: Basal cell carcinomas and squamous cell carcinomas of human skin show distinct patterns of chromosome loss. Cancer Res 1994;54:4756-4759.

415. Dumaz N, Drougard C, Sarasin A, et al: Specific UV-induced mutation spectrum in the p53 gene of skin tumors from DNA-repair-deficient xeroderma pigmentosum patients. Proc Natl Acad Sci USA 1993;90:10529-10533.

416. Sato M, Nishigori C, Zghal M, et al: Ultraviolet-specific mutations in p53 gene in skin tumors in xeroderma pigmentosum patients. Cancer Res 1993;53:2944-2946.

417. Landi MT, Baccarelli A, Tarone RE, et al: DNA repair, dysplastic nevi, sunlight sensitivity in the development of cutaneous malignant melanoma. J Natl Cancer Inst 2002;94:94-101.

418. Thompson EJ, Gupta A, Stratton MS, Bowden GT. Mechanism of action of a dominant negative c-jun mutant in inhibiting activator protein-1 activation. Mol Carcinog 2002;35(4):157-162.

419. Gibbs P, Brady BM, Robinson WA: The genes and genetics of malignant melanoma. J Cutan Med Surg 2002;6:229-235.

420. Elder DE, Green MH, Guerry D, et al: The dysplastic nevus syndrome: our definition. Am J Dermatopathol 1982;4:455-460.

421. Bishop DT, Demenais F, Goldstein AM, et al: Geographical variation in the penetrance of CDKN2A mutations for melanoma. J Natl Cancer Inst 2002;94:894-903.

422. Box NF, Duffy DL, Chen W, et al: MC1R Genotype modifies risk of melanoma in families segregating CDKN2A mutations. Am J Hum Genet 2001;69:765-773.

423. Van der Velden PA, Sandkujl LA, Bergman W, et al: Melnocortin-1 receptor variant R151C modifies melanoma risk in Dutch families with melanoma. Am J Hum Genet 2001;69:774-779.

424. Scott MC, Suzuki I, Abdel-Malek ZA: Regulation of the human melanocortin 1 receptor expression in epidermal melanocytes by paracrine and endocrine factors and by ultraviolet radiation. Pigment Cell Res 2002;15:433-439.

425. Sturm RA: Skin color and skin cancer—MCIR, the genetic link. Melanoma Res 2002;12:405-416.

426. Scott MG, Wakamatsu W, Ito S, et al: Human melanocortin 1 receptor variants, receptor function and melanocyte response to radiation. J Cell Science 2002;115:2349-2355.

427. Davies H, Bignell GR, Cox C, et al: Mutations of the BRAF in human cancer. Nature 2002;417:949-954.

428. Pollock PM, Harper UL, Hansen KS, et al: High frequency of BRAF mutations in nevi. Nat Genet 2003;33:19-20.

429. Menter JM, Hollins TD, Sayre RM, et al: Protection against UV photocarcinogenesis by fabric materials. J Am Acad Dermatol 1994;31:711-716.

430. Drolet BA, Connor MJ: Sunscreens and the prevention of ultraviolet radiation-induced skin cancer. J Dermatol Surg Oncol 1992;18:571-576.

431. Autier P: What is the role of currently available sunscreens in the prevention of melanoma? Photodermatol Photoimmunol Photomed 2001;17:239-240.

432. Autier P, Dove PF, Negrier S, et al: Sunscreen use and duration of sun-exposure: A double-blind, randomized trial. JNCI 1999;91: 1304-1309.

433. Autier P, Dove JF, Reis AC, et al: Sunscreen use and intentional exposure to ultraviolet light A and B radiation: A double blind randomized trial using personal dosimeters. Br J Cancer 2000;83:1243-1248.

434. Thompson SC, Jolley D, Marks R: Reduction of solar keratoses by regular sunscreen use [see comments]. N Engl J Med 1993;329: 1147-1151.

435. Autier P, Dove JF, Cattaruzza MS, et al: Sunscreen use, wearing clothes and number of nevi in 6 to 7 year old European children. European Organization for Research and Treatment of Cancer Melanoma Cooperative Group. JNCI 1998;90:1873-1880.

436. Ramstack JL, White SE, Hazelkorn KS, Meyskens FL Jr: Sunshine and skin cancer—A school-based skin cancer prevention project. J Cancer Education 1986;1(2):001-008.

437. Milne E, Johnston R, Cross D, Giles-Corti B, English D: Effect of a school-based sun-protection intervention on the development of melanocytic nevi in children. Am J Epidemiol 2002;155:739-745.

438. Balch CM, Soong SJ, Milton GW, et al: Changing trends in cutaneous melanoma over a quarter century in Alabama, USA, and New South Wales, Australia. Cancer 1983;52:1748-1753.

439. Freedberg KA, Geller AC, Miller DR, Lew RA, Koh HK: Screening for malignant melanoma: A cost-effectiveness analysis. J Am Acad Dermatol 1999;41:738-745.

440. MacKie RM, Hole D: Audit of public education campaign to encourage earlier detection of malignant melanoma. BMJ 1992;304:1012-1015.

441. Berwick M, Begg CB, Fine JA, et al: Screening for cutaneous melanoma by skin self-examination [see comments]. J Natl Cancer Inst 1996;88:17-23.

442. Elwood JM: Skin self-examination and melanoma [editorial; comment]. J Natl Cancer Inst 1996;88:3-5.

443. Levine N, Moon TE, Cartmel B, et al: Trial of retinol and isotretinoin in skin cancer prevention: A randomized, double-blind, controlled trial. Southwest Skin Cancer Prevention Study Group. Cancer Epi Biom Prev 1997;6:957-961.

444. Tangrea JA, Edwards BK, Taylor PR, et al: Long-term therapy with low-dose isotretinoin for prevention of basal cell carcinoma: A multicenter clinical trial. Isotretinoin-Basal Cell Carcinoma Study Group [see comments]. J Natl Cancer Inst 1992;84: 328-332.

445. Greenberg ER, Baron JA, Stukel TA, et al: A clinical trial of beta carotene to prevent basal-cell and squamous-cell cancers of the skin. The Skin Cancer Prevention Study Group [published erratum appears in N Engl J Med 1991;325:1324] [see comments]. N Engl J Med 1990;323:789-795.

446. Kraemer KH, DiGiovanna JJ, Moshell AN, et al: Prevention of skin cancer in xeroderma pigmentosum with the use of oral isotretinoin. N Engl J Med 1988;318:1633-1637.

447. Colditz GA: Selenium and cancer prevention. Promising results indicate further trials required [editorial; comment]. JAMA 1996;276:1984-1985.

448. Solarazone (diclofenac sodium) Gel USP, 2000.

449. Alberts DS, Dorr RT, Einspahn JG, et al: Chemoprevention of human actinic keratoses by topical 2-(Difluoromethyl)-dL-ornithine. Cancer Epi Biom Prev 2000;9:1281-1286.

450. Meyskens FL Jr., Edwards L, Levine NS: Role of topical tretinoin in melanoma and dysplastic nevi. J Am Acad Dermatol 1986;15: 822-825.

451. Halpern AC, Schuchter LM, Elder DE, et al: Effects of topical tretinoin on dysplastic nevi. J Clin Oncol 1994;12:1028-1035.

452. Meyskens FL Jr, Booth AF, Goff P, Moon TF: Randomized trial of BCG + Vitamin A for Stages I and II cutaneous malignant melanoma. In Salmon S (ed): Adjuvant Therapy of Cancer, vol 5. New York, Grune and Stratton, 1987, pp 665-669.

453. Meyskens FL Jr, Liu PY, Tuthill RJ, et al: Randomized trial of vitamin A versus observation as adjuvant therapy in high-risk primary malignant melanoma: A Southwest Oncology Group study. J Clin Oncol 1994;12:2060-2065.

454. Nathanson L. Risk reduction endpoints should be part of the design of adjuvant therapy clinical trials for patients with melanoma. Cancer 2001;91:881-988.

455. Lluvia-Prevatt M, Morreale J, Gregus J, et al: Effect of perillyl alcohol on melanoma in the T Pras mouse model. Cancer Epi Biom Prev 2002;11:573-579.

456. Mani S, Nair B, Poo WJ, et al: The role for close follow-up of melanoma patients with AJCC stages I-III: A preliminary analysis (Meeting abstract). Proc Annu Meet Am Soc Clin Oncol 1995;14:A1311.

457. Diagnosis and treatment of early melanoma. NIH Consensus Statement online 1992;1061:1-26.

458. Wenham RM, Lancaster JM, Berchuck A. Molecular aspects of ovarian cancer. Best Pract Res Clin Obst Gyn 2002;16:483-497.

459. Kerlikowske K, Brown JS, Grady DG: Should women with familial ovarian cancer undergo prophylactic oophorectomy? [see comments]. Obstet Gynecol 1992;80:700-707.

460. Carlson KJ, Skates SJ, Singer DE: Screening for ovarian cancer [see comments]. Ann Intern Med 1994;121:124-132.

461. Anonymous: Ovarian cancer: Screening, treatment, and followup. NIH Consensus Statement 1994;12:1-30.

462. Pecorelli S, Odicino F, Maisonneuve P, et al: Carcinoma of the ovary. J Epidemiol Biostat 1998;3:75-102.

463. Yancik R: Ovarian cancer. Age contrasts in incidence, histology, disease stage at diagnosis, and mortality. Cancer 1993;71:517-523.

464. Whittemore AS, Harris R, Itnyre J: Characteristics relating to ovarian cancer risk: Collaborative analysis of 12 US case-control studies. II. Invasive epithelial ovarian cancers in white women. Collaborative Ovarian Cancer Group [see comments]. Am J Epidemiol 1992;136:1184-1203.

465. Hankinson SE, Colditz GA, Hunter DJ, et al: A quantitative assessment of oral contraceptive use and risk of ovarian cancer. Obstet Gynecol 1992;80:708-714.

466. Bosetti C, Negri E, Trichopoulos D, et al: Long-term effects of oral contraceptives on ovarian cancer risk. Int J Cancer 2002;102:262-265.

467. Lacey JV: Menopausal hormone replacement therapy and risk of ovarian cancer. JAMA 2002;288:334-341.

468. Artini PG, Fasciani A, Cela V, et al: Fertility drugs and ovarian cancer. Gynecol Endocrinol 1997;11:59-68.

469. Hankinson SE, Hunter DJ, Colditz GA, et al: Tubal ligation, hysterectomy, and risk of ovarian cancer. A prospective study [see comments]. JAMA 1993;270:2813-2818.

470. Rodriguez C, Calle EE, Fakhrabadi D, et al: Body mass index, height and the risk of ovarian cancer mortality in a prospective cohort of postmenopausal women. Cancer Epi Biom Prev 2002;11: 822-828.

471. Cramer DW, Welch WR, Scully RE, Wojciechowski CA. Ovarian cancer and talc: A case-control study. Cancer 1982;50(2):372-376.

472. Harlow BL, Cramer DW, Bell DA, et al: Perineal exposure to talc and ovarian cancer risk. Obstet Gynecol 1992;80:19-26.

473. Pharoah PD, Ponder BA: The genetics of ovarian cancer. Best Pract Res Clin Obstet Gynaecol 2002;16(4):449-468.

474. Lynch HT, Watson P, Lynch JF, et al: Hereditary ovarian cancer. Heterogeneity in age at onset. Cancer 1993;71:573-581.

475. Matloff ET, Shappell H, Brierley K, et al: What would you do? Specialists' perspectives on cancer genetic testing, prophylactic surgery, and insurance discrimination. J Clin Oncol 2000;18:2484-2492.

476. American College of Obstetricians and Gynecologists: Prophylactic Oophorectomy. ACOG Technical Bulletin 111. Washington, DC, ACOG, 1987.

477. Barber HR: Ovarian cancer. CA Cancer J Clin 1986;36:149-184.

478. Struewing JP, Watson P, Easton DF, et al: Prophylactic oophorectomy in inherited breast/ovarian cancer families. J Natl Cancer Inst Monogr 1995;17:33-35.

479. Tobacman JK, Greene MH, Tucker MA, et al: Intra-abdominal carcinomatosis after prophylactic oophorectomy in ovarian-cancer-prone families. Lancet 1982;2:795-797.

480. Haber D: Prophylactic oophorectomy to reduce the risk of ovarian and breast cancer in carriers of BRCA mutations. N Eng J Med 2002;346:1660-1662.

481. Schrag D, Kuntz KM, Garber JE, et al: Decision analysis—Effects of prophylactic mastectomy and oophorectomy on life expectancy among women with BRCA1 or BRCA2 mutations [see comments] [published erratum appears in N Engl J Med 1997;337(6):434]. N Engl J Med 1997;336:1465-1471.

482. Averette HE, Steren A, Nguyen HN: Screening in gynecologic cancers. Cancer 1993;72:1043-1049.

483. American College of Obstetricians and Gynecologists: Cancer of the Ovary. ACOG Technical Bulletin 141. Washington, DC, ACOG, 1990.

484. Rulin MC, Preston AL: Adnexal masses in postmenopausal women. Obstet Gynecol 1987;70:578-581.

485. Bast RC Jr, Feeney M, Lazarus H, et al: Reactivity of a monoclonal antibody with human ovarian carcinoma. J Clin Invest 1981;68: 1331-1337.

486. Bast RC Jr, Klug TL, St John E, et al: A radioimmunoassay using a monoclonal antibody to monitor the course of epithelial ovarian cancer. N Engl J Med 1983;309:883-887.

487. Jacobs I, Bast RC Jr: The CA 125 tumour-associated antigen: A review of the literature. Hum Reprod 1989;4:1-12.

488. Niloff JM, Knapp RC, Schaetzl E, et al: CA125 antigen levels in obstetric and gynecologic patients. Obstet Gynecol 1984;64: 703-707.

489. Pittaway DE, Fayez JA: Serum CA-125 antigen levels increase during menses. Am J Obstet Gynecol 1987;156:75-76.

490. Campbell S, Bhan V, Royston P, et al: Transabdominal ultrasound screening for early ovarian cancer [see comments]. BMJ 1989;299:1363–1367.

491. Van Nagell JR Jr, DePriest PD, Puls LE, et al: Ovarian cancer screening in asymptomatic postmenopausal women by transvaginal sonography. Cancer 1991;68:458–462.

492. DePriest PD, Van Nagell JR Jr, Gallion HH, et al: Ovarian cancer screening in asymptomatic postmenopausal women. Gynecol Oncol 1993;51:205–209.

493. Jacobs I, Davies AP, Bridges J, et al: Prevalence screening for ovarian cancer in postmenopausal women by CA 125 measurement and ultrasonography [see comments]. BMJ 1993;306:1030–1034.

494. Schapira MM, Matchar DB, Young MJ: The effectiveness of ovarian cancer screening. A decision analysis model [see comments]. Ann Intern Med 1993;118:838–843.

495. DePalo G, Mariam L, Camerini T, et al: Effect of fenretinide on ovarian carcinoma occurrence. Gyn Oncol 2002;86:24–27.

496. Veronesi U, Decensi A: Retinoids for ovarian cancer prevention: Laboratory data sets the stage for thoughtful clinical trials. J Natl Cancer Inst 2001;93:486–489.

497. Barnes MN, Grizzle WE, Grubbs CJ, et al: Paradigms for primary prevention of ovarian carcinoma. CA Cancer J Clin 2002;52:216–225.

498. Crum CP: The beginning of the end for cervical cancer? N Engl J Med 2002;347:1703–1705.

499. SEER Cancer Statistics review 1973–1995. Bethesda, MD, National Cancer Institute.

500. Noller KL: Screening for vaginal cancer [editorial; comment]. N Engl J Med 1996;335:1599–1600.

501. Austin RM, McLendon WW: The Papanicolaou smear. Medicine's most successful cancer screening procedure is threatened [editorial] [see comments]. JAMA 1997;277:754–755.

502. Linder J: Automation of the Papanicolaou smear: A technology assessment perspective. Arch Pathol Lab Med 1997;121:282–286.

503. Koss LG: The Papanicolaou test for cervical cancer detection. A triumph and a tragedy [see comments]. JAMA 1989;261:737–743.

504. Cervical Cancer: NIH Consensus Statement. 1996;14(1):1–38.

505. Laara E, Day NE, Hakama M: Trends in mortality from cervical cancer in the Nordic countries: association with organised screening programmes. Lancet 1987;1:1247–1249.

506. Wright TC Jr, Richart RM: Role of human papillomavirus in the pathogenesis of genital tract warts and cancer. Gynecol Oncol 1990;37:151–164.

507. Schiffman MH, Bauer HM, Hoover RN, et al: Epidemiologic evidence showing that human papillomavirus infection causes most cervical intraepithelial neoplasia [see comments]. J Natl Cancer Inst 1993;85:958–964.

508. Reeves WC, Brinton LA, Garcia M, et al: Human papillomavirus infection and cervical cancer in Latin America. N Engl J Med 1989;320:1437–1441.

509. American College of Obstetricians and Gynecologists: Genital Human Papilloma Virus Infections, ACOG Technical Bulletin 193. Washington, DC, ACOG, 1994.

510. Munoz N, Bosch FX, de Sanjose S, et al: The role of HPV in the etiology of cervical cancer. Mutat Res 1994;305:293–301.

511. Cuzick J, Terry G, Ho L, et al: Human papillomavirus type 16 in cervical smears as predictor of high-grade cervical intraepithelial neoplasia [corrected] [published erratum appears in Lancet 1992;339(8802):1182] [see comments]. Lancet 1992;339:959–960.

512. Werness BA, Levine AJ, Howley PM: Association of human papillomavirus types 16 and 18 E6 proteins with p53. Science 1990;248:76–79.

513. Braun L, Mikumo R, Mark HF, et al: Analysis of the growth properties and physical state of the human papillomavirus type 16 genome in cell lines derived from primary cervical tumors. Am J Pathol 1993;143:832–844.

514. Cullen AP, Reid R, Campion M, et al: Analysis of the physical state of different human papillomavirus DNAs in intraepithelial and invasive cervical neoplasm. J Virol 1991;65:606–612.

515. Hildesheim A, Schiffman M, Bromley C, et al: Human papillomavirus type 16 variants and risk of cervical cancer. JNCI 2001;93:315–318.

516. Schiffman MH: Recent progress in defining the epidemiology of human papillomavirus infection and cervical neoplasia. J Natl Cancer Inst 1992;84:394–398.

517. Schlecht NF, Kulaga S, Robitaille J, et al: Persistent human papillomavirus infection as a predictor of cervical intraepithelial neoplasia. JAMA 2001;286:3106–3114.

518. Brinton LA: Epidemiology of cervical cancer—an overview. In Munoz N, Bosch FS, Shah K, Meheus A, et al (eds): The Epidemiology of Cervical Cancer and Human Papillomavirus. Lyon, France, FARC Scientific Publications, 1992, p 3.

519. Becker TM, Wheeler CM, McGough NS, et al: Cervical papillomavirus infection and cervical dysplasia in Hispanic, Native American, and non-Hispanic white women in New Mexico. Am J Public Health 1991;81:582–586.

520. Bauer HM, Hildesheim A, Schiffman MH, et al: Determinants of genital human papillomavirus infection in low-risk women in Portland, Oregon. Sex Transm Dis 1993;20:274–278.

521. Bauer HM, Ting Y, Greer CE, et al: Genital human papillomavirus infection in female university students as determined by a PCR-based method [see comments]. JAMA 1991;265:472–477.

522. Melkert PW, Hopman E, van den Brule AJ, et al: Prevalence of HPV in cytomorphologically normal cervical smears, as determined by the polymerase chain reaction, is age-dependent. Int J Cancer 1993;53:919–923.

523. Wheeler CM, Parmenter CA, Hunt WC, et al: Determinants of genital human papillomavirus infection among cytologically normal women attending the University of New Mexico student health center. Sex Transm Dis 1993;20:286–289.

524. ALTS Human papilloma testing for triage of women with cytological evidence of low-grade squamous intraepithelial lesions: Baseline data from a randomized trial. J Natl Cancer Inst 2000;92:397–402.

525. Koss LG, Stewart FW, Foote FW, et al: Some histological aspects of behavior of epidermal carcinoma in situ and related lesions of the uterine cervix. Cancer 1963;16:1160.

526. Green GH, Donovan JW: The natural history of cervical carcinoma in situ. J Obstet Gynaecol Br Commonw 1970;77:1–9.

527. McIndoe WA, McLean MR, Jones RW, et al: The invasive potential of carcinoma in situ of the cervix. Obstet Gynecol 1984;64:451–458.

528. Ostor AG: Natural history of cervical intraepithelial neoplasia: a critical review. Int J Gynecol Pathol 1993;12:186–192.

529. Boring CC, Squires TS, Tong T, et al: Cancer statistics, 1994. CA Cancer J Clin 1994;44:7–26.

530. Remington P, Lantz P, Phillips JL: Cervical cancer deaths among older women: Implications for prevention. Wis Med J 1990;89:32–34.

531. Surveillance Program, Division of Cancer Prevention and Control, National Cancer Institute, unpublished data, 1990.

532. Schairer C, Brinton LA, Devesa SS, et al: Racial differences in the risk of invasive squamous-cell cervical cancer. Cancer Causes Control 1991;2:283–290.

533. SEER, 1987–1991. Cancer Incidence in the United States. 10 Most Common Cancers by sex among whites and blacks, National Cancer Institute.

534. Hildesheim A, Brinton LA, Mallin K, et al: Barrier and spermicidal contraceptive methods and risk of invasive cervical cancer [see comments]. Epidemiology 1990;1:266–272.

535. Gram IT, Macaluso M, Stalsberg H: Oral contraceptive use and the incidence of cervical intraepithelial neoplasia [see comments]. Am J Obstet Gynecol 1992;167:40–44.

536. Brinton LA: Epidemiology of cervical cancer—Overview. IARC Sci Publ 1992;119:3–23.

537. Horowitz IR, Jacobson LP, Zucker PK, et al: Epidemiology of adenocarcinoma of the cervix. Gynecol Oncol 1988;31:25–31.

538. Davis JR, Moon LB: Increased incidence of adenocarcinoma of uterine cervix. Obstet Gynecol 1975;45:79–83.

539. Anton-Culver H, Bloss JD, Bringman D, et al: Comparison of adenocarcinoma and squamous cell carcinoma of the uterine cervix: A population-based epidemiologic study [see comments]. Am J Obstet Gynecol 1992;166:1507–1514.

540. Herbst AL, Cole P, Norusis MJ, et al: Epidemiologic aspects and factors related to survival in 384 Registry cases of clear cell adenocarcinoma of the vagina and cervix. Am J Obstet Gynecol 1979;135:876–886.

541. Herbst AL, Anderson D: Clear cell adenocarcinoma of the vagina and cervix secondary to intrauterine exposure to diethylstilbestrol. Semin Surg Oncol 1990;6:343-346.

542. Winkelstein W Jr: Smoking and cervical cancer—Current status: A review. Am J Epidemiol 1990;131:945-957.

543. Brock KE, MacLennan R, Brinton LA, et al: Smoking and infectious agents and risk of in situ cervical cancer in Sydney, Australia. Cancer Res 1989;49:4925-4928.

544. Castle PE, Wacholder S, Lorincz AT, et al: A prospective study of high-grade cervical neoplasia risk among human papillomavirus-infected women. J Natl Cancer Inst 2002;94:1406-1414.

545. Hellberg D, Nilsson S, Haley NJ, et al: Smoking and cervical intraepithelial neoplasia: Nicotine and cotinine in serum and cervical mucus in smokers and nonsmokers. Am J Obstet Gynecol 1988;158:910-913.

546. Penn I: Cancers of the anogenital region in renal transplant recipients. Analysis of 65 cases. Cancer 1986;58:611-616.

547. Halpert R, Fruchter RG, Sedlis A, et al: Human papillomavirus and lower genital neoplasia in renal transplant patients. Obstet Gynecol 1986;68:251-258.

548. Alloub MI, Barr BB, McLaren KM, et al: Human papillomavirus infection and cervical intraepithelial neoplasia in women with renal allografts. BMJ 1989;298:153-156.

549. Maiman M, Fruchter RG, Guy L, et al: Human immunodeficiency virus infection and invasive cervical carcinoma. Cancer 1993;71:402-406.

550. Rellihan MA, Dooley DP, Burke TW, et al: Rapidly progressing cervical cancer in a patient with human immunodeficiency virus infection. Gynecol Oncol 1990;36:435-438.

551. Schwartz LB, Carcangiu ML, Bradham L, et al: Rapidly progressive squamous cell carcinoma of the cervix coexisting with human immunodeficiency virus infection: Clinical opinion. Gynecol Oncol 1991;41:255-258.

552. Wright TC Jr, Ellerbrock TV, Chiasson MA, et al: Cervical intraepithelial neoplasia in women infected with human immunodeficiency virus: Prevalence, risk factors, and validity of Papanicolaou smears. New York Cervical Disease Study. Obstet Gynecol 1994;84:591-597.

553. Papanicolaou GN, Traut HF: The diagnostic value of vaginal smears in carcinoma of the uterus. Am J Obstet Gynecol 1941;42:193.

554. Laara E, Day NE, Hakama M: Trends in mortality from cervical cancer in the Nordic countries: Association with organised screening programmes. Lancet 1987;1:1247.

555. Kline TS: The Papanicolaou smear: A brief historical perspective and where we are today. Arch Pathol Lab Med 197;121:205.

556. Anonymous: Regulatory Closure of Cervical Cytology laboratories. MMWR 1997;46 (No.RR-17).

557. Anonymous: The 1988 Bethesda System for reporting cervical/vaginal cytological diagnoses. National Cancer Institute Workshop. JAMA 1989;262:931.

558. Kurman RJ, Henson DE, Herbst AL, et al: Interim guidelines for management of abnormal cervical cytology. The 1992 National Cancer Institute Workshop. JAMA 1994;271:1866.

559. Mandelblatt JS, Lawrence WF, Gaffikin L, et al: Costs and benefits of different strategies to screen for cervical cancer in less-developed countries. J Natl Cancer Inst 2002;94:1469-1483.

560. zur Hausen H: Papillomaviruses and cancer: from basic studies to clinical application. Nat Rev Cancer 2002;2(5):342-350.

561. Boone CW, Kelloff GJ, Steele VE: Natural history of intrepithelial neoplasia in humans with implications for cancer chemoprevention strategy. Cancer Res 1992;52:1651.

562. Greenwald P, Nixon DW, Malone WE, et al: Concepts in cancer chemoprevention research. Cancer 1990;65:1483.

563. Tindle RW: Immunomanipulative strategies for the control of human papillomavirus associated cervical disease. Immunol Res 1997;16:387-400.

564. Steller MA, Schiller JT: Human papillomavirus immunology and vaccine prospects. J Natl Cancer Inst Monogr 1996:21:145-148.

565. Palan PR, Mikhail MS, Basu J, et al: Plasma levels of antioxidant beta-carotene and α-tocopherol in uterine cervix dysplasia and cancer. Nutr Cancer 1991;15:13-20.

566. Butterworth CE Jr, Hatch KD, Soong SJ, et al: Oral folic acid Supplementation for cervical dysplasia: A clinical intervention trial. Am J Obstet Gynecol 1992;166:803.

567. Batieha AM, Armenian HK, Norkus EP, et al: Serum micronutrients and the subsequent risk of cervical cancer in a population-based nested case-control study. Cancer Epi Biom Prev 1993;2:335.

568. La Vecchia C, Decarli A, Fasoli M, et al: Dietary vitamin A and the risk of intraepithelial and invasive cervical neoplasia. Gynecol Oncol 1988;30:187.

569. Romney SL, Duttagupta C, Basu J, et al: Plasma vitamin C and uterine cervical dysplasia. Am J Obstet Gynecol 1985;151:976.

570. Liu T, Soong SJ, Wilson NP, et al: A case control study of nutritional factors and cervical dysplasia. Cancer Epi Biom Prev 1993;2:525.

571. Whitehead N, Reyner F, Lindenbaum J: Megaloblastic changes in the cervical epithelium: Association with oral contraceptive therapy and reversal with folic acid. JAMA 1973;226:1421.

572. Butterworth CE Jr, Hatch KD, Gore H, et al: Improvement in cervical dysplasia associated with folic acid therapy in users of oral contraceptives. Am J Clin Nutr 1982;35:73.

573. Butterworth CE Jr, Hatch KD, Macaluso M, et al: Folate deficiency and cervical dysplasia. JAMA 1992;267:528.

574. Childers JM, Chu J, Voigt LF, et al: Chemoprevention of cervical cancer with folic acid: A phase III Southwest Oncology Group Intergroup study. Cancer Epi Biom Prev 1995;4:155.

575. Follen M, Atkinson F, Schottenfeld D, et al: A randomized clinical trial of 4-hydroxphenlretinamide for high-grade squamous intraepithelial lesions of the cervix. Clin Cancer Res 2001;7:3356-3365.

576. Romney SL, Ho GY, Palan PR, et al: Effects of beta-carotene and other factors on outcome of cervical dysplasia and human papillomavirus infection. Gynecol Oncol 1997;65:483.

577. Keefe KA, Schell MJ, Brewer C, et al: A randomized, double-blind, Phase III trial using oral beta-carotene Supplementation for women with high-grade cervical intraeithelial neoplasia. Cancer Epi Biom Prev 2001;10:1029-1035.

578. Mitchell MF, Tortolero-Luna G, Lee JJ, et al: Phase I dose descalation trial of alpha-difluoromethylornithine in patients with grade 3 cervical intraepithelial neoplasia. Clin Cancer Res 1998;4:303.

579. Murray CJ, Lopez AD: Mortality by cause for eight regions of the world. Global Burden of Disease Study. Lancet 1997;349:1269-1276.

580. Monto A, Wright TL: The epidemiology and prevention of hepatocellular carcinoma. Serum Oncol 2001;28:441-449.

581. Guyton K, Kensler TW: Prevention of liver cancer. Curr Oncol Rept 2002;4:464-470.

582. Evans AA, Chen G, Ross EA, et al: Eight-year follow-up of the 90,000 person Haimen City cohort: I. Hepatocellular carcinoma mortality, risk factor and gender differences. Cancer Epi Biom Prev 2002;11:369-376.

583. Yoshizawa H: Hepatocellular carcinoma associated with hepatitis C virus infection in Japan: projection to other countries in the foreseeable future. Oncology 2002;62(Suppl 1):8-17.

584. Mori M, Hara M, Wada I, et al: Prospective study of hepatitis B and C viral infections, cigarette smoking, alcohol consumption, and other factors associated with hepatocellular carcinoma risk in Japan. Am J Epidemiol 2000;151:131-139.

585. Kao JH, Chen DS: Recent updates in hepatitis vaccination and the prevention of hepatocellular carcinoma. Int J Cancer 2002;97:269-271.

586. Chang MH, Shau WY, Chen CJ, et al: Hepatitis B vaccination and hepatocellular carcinoma rates in boys and girls. JAMA 2000;284:3040-3042.

587. Papatheodoridis GV, Papadimitropoulos VC, Hadziyannis SJ: Effect of interferon therapy on the development of hepatocellular carcinoma in patients with hepatitis C Virus-related cirrhosis: A meta-analysis. Aliment Pharmacol Ther 2001;15:689-698.

588. Camma C, Giunta M, Andreone P, Craxi A: Interferon and prevention of hepatocellular carcinoma in viral cirrhosis: An evidence based approach. J Hepatol 2001;34:593-602.

589. Muto Y, Moriwaki H, Ninomiya M, et al: Prevention of second primary tumors by an acrylic retinoid, polyprenoic acid, in patients with hepatocellular carcinoma. Hepatoma Prevention Study Group. N Eng J Med 1996;334:1561-1570.

590. Okuno M, Kojima S, Moriwaki H: Chemoprevention of hepatocellular carcinoma: Concept, progress and perspectives. J Gastroenterol Hepatol 2001;16:1329-1335.

Science of Clinical Oncology

591. Wong IHN, Lo YMD: New markers for cancer detection. Curr Oncol Rept 2002;4:471–477.

592. International Agency for Research on Cancer (IARC) Working Group: IARC Monographs on the evaluation of carcinogenic risks to humans: Schistosomes, liver flukes and *Helicobacter pylori*, vol 61. Lyon, France, IARC, 1994.

593. Pisani P, Parkin DM, Munoz N, Ferlay J: Cancer and infection: Estimates of the attributable fraction in 1990. Cancer Epi Biom Prev 1997;6:387–400.

594. Asghan RJ, Parsonnet J: *Helicobacter pylori* and risk for gastric adenocarcinoma. Semin Gastroint Dis 2001;12:203–208.

595. Schandl L, Malfertherine P, Evert MPA: Prevention of gastric cancer by *Heliobacter pylori* eradication. Digest Dis 2002;20: 18–22.

596. Correa P, Fontham ETH, Bravo JC, et al: Chemoprevention of gastric dysplasia: Randomized trial of antioxidant Supplements and anti-*Helicobacter pylori* therapy. J Natl Cancer Inst 2000;92:1881–1887.

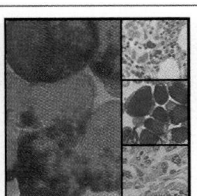

24

SMOKING CESSATION: CURRENT TREATMENTS AND FUTURE DIRECTIONS

Freda Patterson

Caryn Lerman

SUMMARY OF KEY POINTS

PREVALENCE AND IMPACT OF CIGARETTE SMOKING
- Almost one quarter (23.3%) of American adults currently smoke tobacco.
- Cigarette smoking accounts for over 1/3 of all cancer deaths.

NONPHARMACOLOGIC TREATMENTS
- 90% of smoking cessation treatment seekers will utilize nonpharmacologic methods.
- Modalities include educational materials, instructional videos, telephone hotlines, and varying intensities of behavioral counseling.
- Behavioral counseling includes elements such as nicotine fading, quit date contracting, trigger management, and relaxation techniques.
- Quit rates range from 4%–22%.

PHARMACOLOGIC TREATMENTS
- Nicotine gum, transdermal nicotine patch, nicotine nasal spray, and bupropion are the most widely used pharmacolgic treatments.
- Compared to placebo, nicotine replacement therapy and bupropion have been shown to double quit rates.
- Abstinence rates are higher when pharmacotherapy is combined with behavioral counseling.

INDIVIDUAL DIFFERENCES IN RESPONSE TO TREATMENT
- Females, African Americans, individuals with higher levels of negative affect or depression, and those with lower levels of social support respond less well to smoking cessation treatment (as demonstrated by lower quit rates and higher relapse rates).

SPECIAL POPULATIONS
- Cancer patients and pregnant women represent two groups for which specialized interventions can be highly effective.

INTRODUCTION

Cigarette smoking is the greatest preventable cause of cancer, accounting for more than one-third of all cancer deaths.[1] Despite decades of tobacco control efforts and widespread knowledge of the harmful effects of tobacco, a significant proportion of the world's population continues to smoke. In the United States, levels of smoking have leveled off in recent years, yet approximately 24% of American men and women are regular smokers (Table 24-1).[2] Clearly, to address this significant public health problem, new approaches to smoking prevention and treatment are needed.

TABLE 24-1

Rates of Current* Smoking in the United States, by Race and Gender for the Year 2000			
RACE	**MEN**	**WOMEN**	**TOTAL**
White, non Hispanic	25.9%	22.4%	24.1%
Black, non Hispanic	26.1%	20.9%	23.2%
Hispanic	24.0%	13.3%	18.6%
American Indian/Alaska native	29.1%	42.5%	36.0%
Asian	21.0%	7.6%	14.4%

*Smoked ≥100 cigarettes in their lifetimes and at time of interview, reported smoking every day or some days.
Source: CDC: Cigarette smoking among adults—United States, 2000. MMWR 2002;51:642–645.

In this chapter, we review what is known about the efficacy of smoking cessation treatment. We begin with a discussion of nonpharmacologic and pharmacologic approaches to smoking cessation (Table 24-2). In the following sections, we present data on demographic, psychological, and social factors influencing smoking cessation success and review smoking cessation in special populations, such as cancer patients and pregnant women. Finally, we briefly discuss potential future directions for smoking research, including interdisciplinary approaches that integrate perspectives from molecular genetics and behavioral science.

NONPHARMACOLOGIC TREATMENTS

Nonpharmacologic treatments, such as self-help materials and behavioral therapy, were the first available treatments for tobacco addiction.[3,4] Up to 90% of treatment-seeking smokers choose self-help treatments, including educational materials, instructional videos, telephone hotlines, and in some cases, brief advice from a health care provider.[3,5] Quit rates with these approaches are modest, ranging from 4% to 11%, with higher quit rates achieved by multimodal interventions.[6] For example, one study compared two single-mode interventions (self-help manual vs. tailored self-help manual) and two multiple-mode interventions (interactive computer reports plus tailored self-help manuals vs. personalized counselor calls plus interactive computer reports plus tailored manuals).

TABLE 24-2

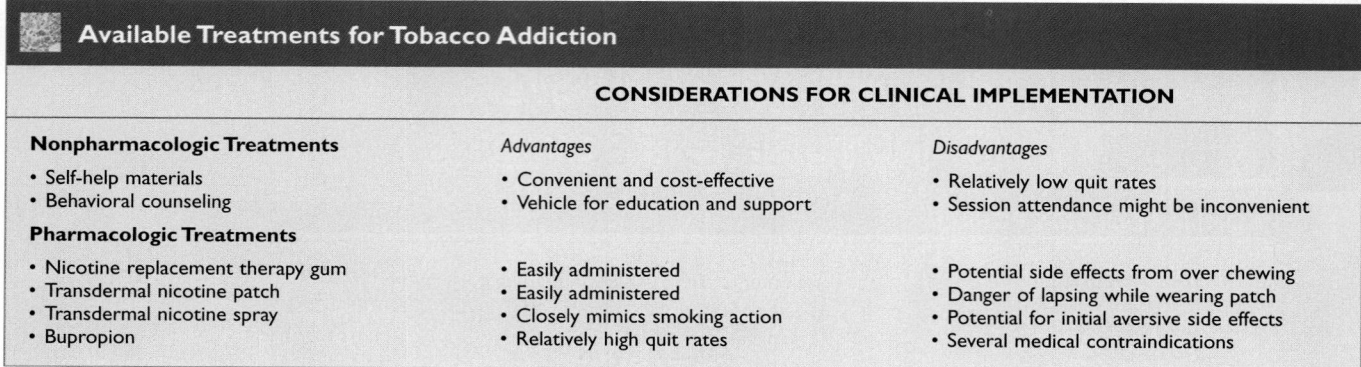

Results at six-month follow up showed that participants receiving either of the multimodal interventions were significantly more likely to be abstinent than the single-mode intervention groups.[7]

Behavioral therapy is widely regarded as a fundamental component of comprehensive smoking cessation interventions, either in an individual or group format. Elements such as nicotine fading, quit date contracting, trigger management, and relaxation techniques typically comprise behavioral counseling, producing quit rates of up to 20%.[8] An increased likelihood of quitting for some specific behavioral treatments has been reported.[4] Specifically, intratreatment social support (e.g., support from other group members; OR = 1.3), extratreatment social support (e.g., support from people outside of treatment; OR = 1.5), problem-solving (OR = 1.5), and rapid smoking (OR = 2.0) have been found to be more effective than control conditions.[4] On a larger scale, two national, behavioral-based smoking cessation programs that included behavioral and self-help treatment components (American Cancer Society and American Lung Association) yielded one-year sustained abstinence rates of 16% and 22%, respectively.[9]

A positive dose-response relationship between intervention intensity (i.e., number of modalities, length and number of contacts) and abstinence rates has been reported.[4] For example, a study that compared behavioral interventions of varying intensity (i.e., minimal vs. individual vs. group counseling) in smokers who were also administered transdermal nicotine reported a significant main effect for counseling condition.[10] Specifically, an overall continuous abstinence rate of 56% was reported for minimal counseling participants, 66% for individual participants, and 68% for group counseling participants.[10] Although marginal differences in abstinence rates between the individual and group counseling conditions were reported in this study, other studies have shown more substantial differences between these two conditions.[11] Further, review of smoking cessation counseling modalities concluded that individual counseling was marginally more effective than group counseling; however, the relative efficacy of these approaches warrants additional attention.[12]

PHARMACOLOGIC TREATMENT: NICOTINE REPLACEMENT THERAPY

The most commonly used nicotine replacement therapies include nicotine gum, transdermal nicotine patch, and nicotine nasal spray. The nicotine inhaler is used less widely. Additional replacement methods recently approved for use include the nicotine lozenge and nicotine water; however, efficacy data for these newer methods are not yet available. In this section, we review the data on the efficacy of nicotine gum, nicotine patch, and nicotine nasal spray.

Nicotine Gum

Nicotine gum in the 2 mg dose was the first over-the-counter, readily available treatment for smoking cessation.[13,14] Despite some adverse side effects, such as oral and gastric problems, jaw ache, and underdosing, nicotine

---

TREATMENT FOR SMOKING CESSATION

Treatment Seeking Smoker

Less intense; typically lower quit rates

Public Health Approaches
• Quit lines
• Media-based information
• Self-help/educational materials

Health Care Provider
• Offer/provision of NRT and/or bupropion
• Brief smoking cessation advice
• Possible referral to counselor or clinical trial

Formal Treatment
• Individual or group behavioral counseling
• Pharmacotherapy

More intense; typically higher quit rates

gum has been found to produce significantly higher quit rates compared with placebo.[15,16] In one of the first randomized, double-blind, controlled trials, results showed that participants who received nicotine gum (2 mg) were significantly more likely to be abstinent at the one- and six-month follow up assessments than placebo controls.[17] In an extensive review of 108 randomized clinical trials that incorporated at least a six-month follow-up assessment, participants using the gum were more than one-and-a-half times more likely (OR = 1.66) to remain abstinent at one year postquit date compared with participants using placebo.[16] The addition of smoking cessation counseling has been shown to boost the effectiveness of nicotine gum still further.[15]

The higher-dose 4 mg gum capsule has been shown to produce higher quit rates than the 2 mg gum capsule, particularly among highly dependent smokers.[18-20] For more dependent smokers, the 4 mg nicotine dose provides higher levels of nicotine replacement, which, in turn, could help to alleviate withdrawal symptoms and cigarette craving.[18,20-22] Tonnesen and colleagues (1988)[20] demonstrated that highly dependent smokers who received the 4 mg nicotine gum dose were 1.8 times more likely to be abstinent at six weeks postquit date than the highly dependent smokers who received the 2 mg dose. Similarly, among highly dependent smokers, abstinence rates were significantly higher for those receiving the 4 mg gum (63.2%) compared with the 2 mg (25%) and placebo gum (25%).[19] Although Garvey and colleagues (2000)[18] did not find a significant overall difference between the 4 mg and 2 mg gum dosage, their results did show that the 4 mg gum produced higher quit rates at one-year follow-up among highly dependent smokers than did the 2 mg dose.

Transdermal Nicotine Patch

The nicotine patch is one of the most widely used forms of nicotine replacement therapy, presumably because of its relatively few side effects and the ease with which it can be administered.[23,24] In a meta-analysis of 17 studies and more than 5000 participants (n = 5,098), quit rates among patch users were found to be more than double those for placebo at the end of treatment (27% vs. 13%, respectively) and at six-month follow-up (22% vs. 9%, respectively).[23] Several recent randomized, controlled trials have yielded similar results.[25-28]

An important clinical question that has received a great deal of scientific attention is whether higher patch doses are more effective for smokers with higher levels of nicotine dependence. This is based on the assumption that heavier smokers will not obtain sufficient nicotine replacement relative to their baseline levels from the standard 22 mg patch dose. To date, three studies have compared the higher 44 mg dose with the standard 22 mg dose.[10,29,30] One study reported higher abstinence rates among participants receiving 44 mg compared with 22 mg dose at four-month follow-up (39% vs. 24%, respectively); however, the difference was not statistically significant.[30] Another study found similar quit rates at six-month follow-up for smokers receiving the 44 mg and

22 mg doses.[10] In addition, 44 mg dose recipients in this study reported significantly increased rates of side effects (nausea, vomiting, erythema) compared with those receiving the 22 mg dose.[10] In contrast, another study reported a significant effect of patch dosage on abstinence rates at eight weeks postquit date; however, at one-year follow-up, differences in abstinence rates by patch dosage were no longer significant.[29] Thus, although the higher (44 mg) patch dose might produce higher quit rates than the standard 22 mg dose in the short term, evidence for enhanced efficacy over the long term is lacking.

Nicotine Spray

As a nicotine delivery device, nicotine nasal spray is considered to more closely mimic the delivery rate provided by cigarettes.[31] Whereas transdermal nicotine patch has been shown to reach a flat peak of plasma concentration within five to ten hours and nicotine gum peaks within 30 minutes, nicotine nasal spray reaches this peak within ten minutes.[32] However, side effects—such as burning sensation and watery eyes after use of the spray—have been reported to deter adherence to spray use, particularly during the first week of a quit attempt.[33] These effects typically dissipate after one week of treatment, as smokers develop tolerance to the spray's effects. Nicotine nasal spray has been reported in numerous randomized, controlled clinical trials to produce significantly higher abstinence rates than placebo spray.[31,34-36] At six- and twelve-month follow-up, abstinence rates of 29%–32% and 18%–27% have been reported, while placebo quit rates at the same time points have ranged from 10% to 18% and from 8% to 17%.[31,34-36]

Bupropion SR (Zyban)

Sustained release bupropion has emerged as an efficacious form of treatment for tobacco addiction and prevention of relapse.[4] The 300 mg dose of bupropion has been reported to outperform placebo and transdermal nicotine patch at both end of treatment and one-year follow-up.[37,38] Specifically, one-year quit rates of 30% were achieved by bupropion recipients, compared with 16% for those who received nicotine patch and 16% for those who received placebo.[37] A recent randomized controlled trial also reported bupropion to be effective for African American smokers, producing a quit rate of 36% at the end of treatment for participants taking bupropion compared with 19% for those receiving placebo.[39] Bupropion has also been demonstrated to reduce the relapse rate, especially among older smokers and those who gained little or no weight when quitting.[40]

Bupropion's precise mode of action has yet to be determined. There is some evidence to suggest that bupropion inhibits postsynaptic uptake of dopamine and norepinephrine.[41-43] Consistent with this hypothesis, a recent study reported that bupropion reduced negative affective states associated with abstinence.[44] There is also evidence that bupropion is a nicotinic receptor antagonist, leading to the hypothesis that treatment might reduce the reinforcing effects of smoking.[45] This putative mechanism has received some support in a recent study that compared the effects of an acute dose of bupropion vs. placebo in a sample of smokers who were not seeking treatment.[46] Smokers treated with a single dose of bupropion had significantly lower ratings of cigarette intensity than those treated with placebo, and there was a trend among those receiving bupropion for a reduction in ratings of smoking satisfaction. Interestingly, smokers receiving bupropion smoked significantly more cigarettes during an ad-lib smoking phase, leading to speculation that they were compensating for reduced rewarding effects of nicotine. Although bupropion's mode of action remains to be identified, its role as an efficacious smoking cessation treatment has been well established.

INDIVIDUAL DIFFERENCES IN CESSATION AND RESPONSE TO TREATMENT

Gender

Recent population data indicate that, although fewer women than men are current smokers (22.0% vs. 27.0%, respectively), the quit ratio (former smokers to current smokers) is consistently lower for women than for men (47% vs. 52%, respectively).[47,48] Because women who smoke are vulnerable to additional smoking-related diseases (e.g., breast and cervical cancers) and to risks related to pregnancy, oral contraception use, and menstrual function, understanding gender differences in smoking behavior and cessation is a high priority.[47]

Gender differences in smoking behaviors have been reported. Compared with men, women reportedly inhale less, take fewer puffs, and are less likely to smoke an entire cigarette.[47] In addition, women are more likely to switch from higher- to lower-nicotine cigarettes and have lower cotinine levels than men.[47]

Smoking cessation trials that have examined the efficacy of nicotine replacement therapies and behavioral smoking cessation counseling have demonstrated that women tend to underperform men in terms of both cessation and sustained abstinence.[49-51] In addition, relapse rates among women have been shown to be higher than among men.[52] On the other hand, one recent study that compared gender differences in response to bupropion indicated that quit rates for male and female participants were comparable, as was median time to relapse.[53] Thus, bupropion might reduce the reported gender disparity in smoking cessation outcomes.[50]

Several hypotheses have emerged to account for the gender differential response to cessation treatments. These include the following:

- Concern about postcessation weight gain[51,54]
- Reduced response by women to physical smoking cues (e.g., onset of withdrawal, craving) compared with "behavioral" smoking cues (e.g., smell of tobacco, coffee, situational prompts)[55,56]
- Reduced effect of NRT treatments (e.g., patch, spray, gum)[51]

- Elevated rates of depression (both clinical and subsyndromal)[57-60]

Race

Smoking prevalence data for American adults in the year 2000 indicate that approximately one-quarter of Caucasian (25.9%), African American (26.1%), and Hispanic (24.0%) adults currently smoke, while almost 29.1% of American Indian and 21.0% of Asians are current smokers.[2] As the largest racial groups in the United States are Caucasian (71.6%) and African American (12.3%), the majority of research studies on racial differences in smoking cessation have focused on these groups.[61]

Despite the comparable prevalence of smoking among Caucasian and African American groups, several notable differences exist in terms of smoking behaviors and cessation. African Americans have been reported to smoke approximately 35% fewer cigarettes than Caucasian smokers and tend to prefer mentholated, high-nicotine cigarettes.[62,63] Despite smoking fewer cigarettes, African Americans have a reduced ability to quit and maintain abstinence compared with Caucasians.[64] Although African American smokers are more likely than Caucasians to have quit for at least one day in the previous year (29.7% vs. 26.0%), they are less likely to achieve sustained tobacco abstinence (35.4% vs. 50.5%).[61] Two of the main reasons cited for this disparity have been the reduced likelihood of African Americans to solicit help (e.g., a smoking cessation group) or use NRT and the lack of cultural relevance of available smoking cessation interventions.[65,66]

Additional data suggest that African Americans are more heavily dependent on nicotine than Caucasians, even when number of cigarettes smoked per day is controlled.[67] African Americans are more likely to smoke higher nicotine/tar cigarettes, inhale more deeply, and puff more frequently.[63,68] This more efficient smoking topography might result in increased exposure to tobacco smoke toxins, higher levels of dependence, and greater susceptibility to disease and illness.[68] As a group, African Americans also metabolize nicotine more slowly than Caucasians; this slower mebabolism in turn could affect smoking patterns and nicotine dependence.[67-70]

Psychological Factors

Depression

Depression and its subsyndromal form (negative mood) have been shown to be more prevalent among smokers compared with nonsmokers and to impede smoking cessation and sustained abstinence. Between 31% and 61% of treatment-seeking smokers report a history of major depressive disorder (MDD), compared with 3.7%-6.7% rates of MDD in the general population.[71-73] Smokers with a history of MDD are less likely to quit successfully than smokers without such a history.[72]

There are several hypotheses as to why major depressive disorder is more prevalent among smokers and why smokers with this history are less likely to be able to quit. One theory is that depressed smokers might use nicotine to modulate negative affect.[74-76] Depressed smokers, compared with nondepressed smokers, are more likely to report smoking as a means to reduce negative affect and increase stimulation.[75] Treatment-seeking smokers with a history of major depressive disorder have also been reported to experience increased levels of depression and anger while quitting than those without a history of depression.[71] Heightened feelings of depression and negative affect after cessation have been found to prompt relapse.[77] Finally, smokers with higher levels of depression have been found to be more likely to have higher levels of nicotine dependence.[75] In turn, a higher level of nicotine dependence at baseline is predictive of continued smoking.[78]

The bulk of evidence clearly indicates that individuals with a history of major and subsyndromal depression are at heightened risk for continued smoking. Smoking cessation interventions targeted to smokers with a history of depression typically have included strategies for management of depressive symptoms and negative affect.[79-81] Hall and colleagues (1998)[81] found that 10 sessions of cognitive-behavioral therapy that included mood management techniques produced higher quit rates among participants with a history of MDD than those without a history of MDD. Similarly, another study that compared the efficacy of a cognitive behavioral treatment with a depression component with a standard smoking cessation intervention found that the cognitive behavioral treatment was more efficacious for participants with recurrent MDD.[80] These studies indicate the need for more intensive, tailored interventions for individuals who have a history of recurrent major depression.

Environmental Factors

Social Support

Social support has been found to facilitate smoking cessation among adults. In these studies, partner support has been defined by characteristics such as the following:

- Facilitating self-change
- Encouraging self-reward
- Minimizing stress by avoiding interpersonal conflict
- Taking over some of the smoker's responsibilities
- Offering problem solving advice
- Showing empathy
- Tolerating moodiness
- Showing concern for quitting

Such variables have been shown to account collectively for 74% of variance in quit rates[82] The Agency for Healthcare Research and Quality (AHQR) guidelines also endorse positive family and social support as being an efficacious intervention component.[4] A recent study that assessed the impact of adding a social support component to a community-based behavioral intervention showed that participants who brought a support person to group sessions were significantly more likely to be abstinent at three-, six-, and twelve-month assessments.[83]

In contrast, negative partner interactions have been found to predict lapse and relapse. Roski and colleagues (1996)[84] compared the effects of positive and negative partner support on cessation outcomes. Participants whose partners were less likely to offer negative support were more likely to sustain abstinence, while participants who lapsed were more likely to attempt to quit again if their partners offered positive support.[84] The authors suggest that positive partner support is more important in the early stages of quitting, whereas longer-term abstinence is facilitated by the absence of negative support.[84] This finding is supported by other studies.[85] The positive effects of social support are not limited to partners and spouses. Another study that utilized a "buddy system," in which participants used social support from another person (not necessarily a partner), have yielded quit rates more than twice that of the control intervention at four weeks follow-up (27% vs. 12%).[86]

Special Populations

Cancer Patients

Tobacco use is an important risk factor for the development of a variety of cancers, including cancers of the lung, head and neck, bladder, and cervix.[1,87] Continued smoking after cancer diagnosis has been shown to inhibit response to treatment, decrease quality of life, increase risk of recurrence, and reduce survival time.[87-90] Despite the benefits to be gained from cessation after diagnosis, a substantial proportion of cancer patients (30%–40%) continue to smoke.[91,92]

Considering the potential benefit to be gained from smoking cessation after cancer diagnosis, surprisingly little research has been devoted to promoting abstinence in this special population.[93] In addition, support for smoking cessation efforts in the clinical setting has been variable. In a national survey of oncology nurses, approximately one-third reported offering some form of smoking cessation treatment (e.g., counseling, providing cessation advice).[94] Lack of staff training, lack of time, and perceived lack of patient motivation were identified as some of the main barriers to more widely available smoking cessation treatment in the clinical oncology setting.[94]

In a review of smoking cessation among cancer patients, Pinto and colleagues found only four studies that assessed the efficacy of smoking cessation interventions specifically for cancer patients.[91,95-98] Griebel and colleagues (1998)[96] compared the efficacy of a minimal contact cessation intervention with a usual care condition among a sample of hospitalized cancer patients. The one-time, 20-minute minimal contact intervention included the following components:

- Education about the benefits of quitting
- Resources available for quitting
- Quitting and relapse prevention strategies[96]

At six weeks after intervention, almost one-quarter (21%) of the intervention group was abstinent compared with 14% of the usual care group.[96] Another study that compared a much more intensive intervention (six sessions of tailored, individual smoking cessation plus self-help booklets) with usual care yielded much higher quit rates than the Griebel study (63.8% vs. 76.8% at 12-month follow up). The intervention component, however, did not out perform the usual care condition.[95] Other studies have reported biochemically confirmed quit rates of 21%–75% at five- to six-week follow-up.[97,98]

The relatively high quit rates achieved by these interventions might be attributable to the highly salient nature of smoking cessation advice and counseling to cancer patients. One study, however, found that psychological factors such as higher levels of fatalistic beliefs and emotional distress were more prevalent among cancer patients who continued to smoke.[92] Thus, although cancer patients who continue to smoke might be receptive to smoking cessation interventions, the interaction of psychological factors (such as fatalistic beliefs) on their smoking behaviors could be a barrier to cessation. The benefits to be gained from cessation among this population warrant further examination of the factors that contribute to both continued smoking and prolonged abstinence.

Pregnant Women
Smoking among pregnant women represents a particular public health problem. Smoking can cause numerous adverse health complications for the fetus and newborn child, including the following:

- Intrauterine growth retardation
- Low birth weight
- Placenta previa
- Abrupto placentae
- Congenital malformations
- An increased risk for spontaneous abortion
- Premature births
- Neonatal and fetal mortality[47]

Despite these deleterious health effects, approximately 20%–30% of pregnant women continue to smoke for the duration of their pregnancy.[47,99-101]

Although up to 40% of pregnant women who smoke are reported to quit, usually unaided, prior to starting prenatal care (termed "spontaneous quitters"), the majority of these (60%–80%) will relapse by six months postpartum.[102,103] Pregnant women who do continue to smoke tend to be younger (15 to 24 years old), white, non Hispanic, unmarried, and unemployed, and they tend to have lower levels of education.[102,104] The main challenges facing tobacco control research in this area is how to promote cessation among pregnant women who do not quit spontaneously.

A variety of smoking cessation interventions for pregnant women has been tested. These include minimal contact smoking cessation interventions, delivered to pregnant women as part of their obstetric care, that include a brief counseling session and self-help materials. Such interventions have been reported to improve cessation rates by up to 30% in treated women compared with control groups.[105] Studies that have tested more intensive interventions (e.g., including longer, more frequent counseling sessions, mailings, telephone booster sessions) have produced a variety of results. In these studies, the more intensive intervention conditions have been shown variously to be more successful, equally successful, and even less successful than the minimal intervention or usual care conditions.[106-108] One possible reason for the lack of dose-response relationship between intervention intensity and cessation might be that pregnant women who do continue to smoke are more likely to be highly resistant to intervention.[108]

The option of using NRT as a treatment mode for pregnant smokers—especially highly resistant and dependent smokers—has been considered.[109] The recent "Clinical Practice Guideline for Treating Tobacco Use and Dependence" issued by the AHRQ states that NRT should be considered for pregnant women who are resistant to other forms of treatment, and when the health benefits of quitting will outweigh the risks incurred to the fetus by using NRT.[4] On the other hand, the lack of research on the safety, efficacy, and effectiveness of using NRT for treatment-resistant pregnant smokers currently limits the widespread use of this treatment option.

FUTURE DIRECTIONS

To make significant progress in reducing tobacco-related cancer mortality, a better understanding of the biobehavioral basis of nicotine addiction is clearly needed. Toward this end, several converging lines of evidence highlight the importance of elucidating the genetic underpinnings of nicotine dependence. Studies of twins have documented that as much as 70% of the variability in nicotine dependence is attributable to genetic factors (see Sullivan and Kendler[110]). As a result of advances in molecular biology and genomics technology, scientists are attempting to identify the specific genetic variants that could predispose to nicotine addiction and those genetic factors with protective effects. Although these early studies have been promising, the results to date are not yet conclusive (see Lerman and Berrettini[111]).

Research on the genetic determinants of smoking behavior might ultimately become valuable for tailoring smoking cessation to smokers' unique genetic profiles. For example, smokers who carry genetic polymorphisims associated with reduced domaminergic activity might experience greater benefit from nicotine nasal spray than patch because of the spray's greater rewarding effects. Alternatively smokers who have polymorphisms that reduce noradrenergic activity and who might be more prone to experience withdrawal symptoms, might have more success with the nicotine patch than with the nasal spray.

Investigations of polymorphic enzymes involved in drug metabolism are also key candidates for predicting response to pharmacotherapies for smoking cessation. For example, genetically determined individual differences in nicotine metabolism rate could alter both the biologically active dose of NRTs and the experience of side effects. Thus, genotyping of smokers in treatment could be valuable not only to select the optimal type of NRT, but also to optimize the dosage for a particular smoker.[112]

With regard to nonnicotine medication, ongoing studies are investigating the role of genetic factors in response to bupropion (Zyban) treatment. In a recent placebo-controlled trial of bupropion, smokers who have a decreased activity variant of CYP2B6 gene expressed greater increases in cravings for cigarettes following their target quit date and had higher lapse rates.[113] These effects were modified by a significant gender x–genotype x treatment interaction, suggesting that bupropion attenuated the effects of genotype among female smokers. Such information could be useful for identifying smokers who are most and least likely to benefit from bupropion and for tailoring treatment accordingly.

Research on the genetic and biobehavioral factors that influence response to smoking cessation treatment could significantly enhance our understanding of nicotine dependence and facilitate the design of new treatments for smoking cessation. Furthermore, by tailoring treatment to the individual smoker's needs, the efficacy of these treatments could be improved, and the hoped for reductions in tobacco-related cancer mortality might be realized.

REFERENCES

1. American Cancer Society: Cancer Facts and Figures, 2001, p 2.
2. CDC: Cigarette smoking among adults—United States, 2000. MMWR 2002;51:642-645.
3. Haxby DG: Treatment of nicotine dependence. Am J Health Syst Pharm 1995;52: 265-281.
4. Fiore MC, Bailey W, Cohen S: Treating tobacco use and dependence. Clinical practice guideline. Rockville, Md, US Department of Health and Human Services, Public Health Service, 2000.
5. Fiore MC, Novotny TE, Pierce JP, et al: Methods used to quit smoking in the United States. Do cessation programs help? JAMA 1990;263:2760-2765.
6. Curry SJ, McBride C, Grothaus LC, Louie D, Wagner EH: A randomized trial of self-help materials, personalized feedback, and telephone counseling with nonvolunteer smokers. J Consult Clin Psychol 1995;63:1005-1014.
7. Prochaska JO, DiClemente CC, Velicer WF, Rossi JS: Standardized, individualized, interactive, and personalized self-help programs for smoking cessation. Health Psychol, 1993;12:399-405.
8. Prochazka AV: New developments in smoking cessation. Chest 2000;117:169S-175S.
9. Lando HA, McGovern PG, Barrios FX, Etringer BD: Comparative evaluation of American Cancer Society and American Lung Association smoking cessation clinics. Am J Public Health 1990;80:554-559.
10. Jorenby DE, Smith SS, Fiore MC, et al: Varying nicotine patch dose and type of smoking cessation counseling. JAMA 1995;274: 1347-1352.
11. Fiore MC, Kenford SL, Jorenby DE, Wetter DW, Smith SS, Baker TB: Two studies of the clinical effectiveness of the nicotine patch with different counseling treatments. Chest 1994;105:524-533.
12. Stead LF, Lancaster T: Group behaviour therapy programmes for smoking cessation. Cochrane Database Syst Rev 2002;CD001007.
13. Rose JE: Nicotine addiction and treatment. Annu Rev Med 1996;47:493-507.
14. Silagy C, Mant D, Fowler G, Lodge M: Meta-analysis on efficacy of nicotine replacement therapies in smoking cessation. Lancet 1994;343:139-142.
15. Cepeda-Benito A: Meta-analytical review of the efficacy of nicotine chewing gum in smoking treatment programs. J Consult Clin Psychol 1993;61:822-830.
16. Silagy C, Lancaster T, Stead L, Mant D, Fowler G: Nicotine replacement therapy for smoking cessation. Cochrane Database Syst Rev 2002:(4)CD000146.
17. Hughes JR, Gust SW, Keenan RM, Fenwick JW, Healey ML: Nicotine vs, placebo gum in general medical practice. JAMA 1989;261: 1300-1305.
18. Garvey AJ, Kinnunen T, Nordstrom BL, et al: Effects of nicotine gum dose by level of nicotine dependence. Nicotine Tob Res 2000;2:53-63.
19. Sachs DP: Effectiveness of the 4-mg dose of nicotine polacrilex for the initial treatment of high-dependent smokers. Arch Intern Med 1995;155:1973-1980.
20. Tonnesen P, Fryd V, Hansen M, et al: Effect of nicotine chewing gum in combination with group counseling on the cessation of smoking. N Engl J Med 1988;318:15-18.
21. Niaura R, Goldstein MG, Abrams DB: Matching high- and low-dependence smokers to self-help treatment with or without nicotine replacement. Prev Med 1994;23:70-77.
22. Schneider NG, Jarvik ME: Time course of smoking withdrawal symptoms as a function of nicotine replacement. Psychopharmacology 1984;82:143-144.
23. Fiore MC, Smith SS, Jorenby DE, Baker TB: The effectiveness of the nicotine patch for smoking cessation. A meta-analysis. JAMA 1994;271:1940-1947.
24. West R, Hajek P, Nilsson F, Foulds J, May S, Meadows A: Individual differences in preferences for and responses to four nicotine replacement products. Psychopharmacology 2001;153:225-230.
25. Lewis SF, Piasecki TM, Fiore MC, Anderson JE, Baker TB: Transdermal nicotine replacement for hospitalized patients: a randomized clinical trial. Prev Med 1998;27:296-303.
26. Hurt RD, Dale LC, Fredrickson PA, et al: Nicotine patch therapy for smoking cessation combined with physician advice and nurse follow-up. One-year outcome and percentage of nicotine replacement. JAMA 1994;271:595-600.
27. Daughton DM, Fortmann SP, Glover ED, et al: The smoking cessation efficacy of varying doses of nicotine patch delivery systems 4 to 5 years post-quit day. Prev Med 1999;28:113-118.
28. Tonnesen P, Norregaard J, Simonsen K, Sawe U: A double-blind trial of a 16-hour transdermal nicotine patch in smoking cessation. N Engl J Med 1991;325:311-315.
29. Dale LC, Hurt RD, Offord KP, Lawson GM, Croghan IT, Schroeder DR: High-dose nicotine patch therapy. Percentage of replacement and smoking cessation. JAMA 1995;274:1353-1358.
30. Hughes JR, Lesmes GR, Hatsukami DK, et al: Are higher doses of nicotine replacement more effective for smoking cessation? Nicotine Tob Res 19991:169-174.
31. Schneider NG, Olmstead R, Mody FV, et al: Efficacy of a nicotine nasal spray in smoking cessation: A placebo-controlled, double-blind trial. Addiction 1995;90:1671-182.
32. Henningfield JE, Keenan RM: Nicotine delivery kinetics and abuse liability. J Consult Clin Psychol 1993;61:743-750.
33. Hurt R, Dale L, Croghan G, Croghan I, Gomez-Dahl L, Offord K: Nicotine nasal spray for smoking cessation: Pattern of use, side effects, relief of withdrawal symptoms, and cotinine levels. Mayo Clin Proc 1998;73:118-125.
34. Blondal T, Franzon M, Westin A: A double-blind randomized trial of nicotine nasal spray as an aid in smoking cessation. Eur Respir J 1997;10:1585-1590.
35. Hjalmarson A, Franzon M, Westin A, Wiklund O: Effect of nicotine nasal spray on smoking cessation. A randomized, placebo-controlled, double-blind study. Arch Intern Med 1994;154: 2567-2572.
36. Sutherland G, Russell MA, Stapleton J, Feyerabend C, Ferno O: Nasal nicotine spray: A rapid nicotine delivery system. Psychopharmacology 1992;108:512-518.
37. Jorenby DE, Leischow SJ, Nides MA, et al: A controlled trial of sustained-release bupropion, a nicotine patch, or both for smoking cessation. N Engl J Med 1999;340:685-691.
38. Hurt RD, Sachs DP, Glover ED, et al: A comparison of sustained-release bupropion and placebo for smoking cessation. N Engl J Med 1997;337:1195-1202.
39. Ahluwalia JS, Harris KJ, Catley D, Okuyemi KS, Mayo MS: Sustained-release bupropion for smoking cessation in African Americans: A randomized controlled trial. JAMA 2002;288: 468-474.
40. Hurt RD, Wolter TD, Rigotti N, et al: Bupropion for pharmacologic relapse prevention to smoking: Predictors of outcome. Addict Behav 2002;27:493-507.

Science of Clinical Oncology

41. Ascher JA, Cole JO, Colin JN, et al: Bupropion: A review of its mechanism of antidepressant activity. J Clin Psych 1995;56:395-401.

42. Cooper BR, Wang CM, Cox RF, Norton R, Shea V, Ferris RM: Evidence that the acute behavioral and electrophysiological effects of bupropion (Wellbutrin) are mediated by a noradrenergic mechanism. Neuropsychopharmacology 1994;11:133-141.

43. Sanchez C, Hyttel J: Comparison of the effects of antidepressants and their metabolites on reuptake of biogenic amines and on receptor binding. Cell Mol Neurobiol 1999;19:467-489.

44. Lerman C, Roth D, Kaufmann V, et al: Mediating mechanisms for the impact of bupropion in smoking cessation treatment. Drug Alcohol Depend 2002;67:219-223.

45. Slemmer JE, Martin BR, Damaj MI: Bupropion is a nicotinic antagonist. J Pharmacol Exp Ther 2000;295:321-327.

46. Cousins MS, Stamat HM, de Wit H: Acute doses of d-amphetamine and bupropion increase cigarette smoking. Psychopharmacology 2001;157:243-253.

47. US Department of Health and Human Services: Women and smoking: A report of the surgeon general. Rockville, Md, Public Health Service, Office of the Surgeon General, 2001.

48. Centers for Disease Control: Cigarette smoking among adults—United States, 1992, and changes in the definition of current cigarette smoking. MMWR 1994;43:342-346.

49. Wetter DW, Kenford SL, Smith SS, Fiore MC, Jorenby DE, Baker TB: Gender differences in smoking cessation. J Consult Clin Psychol 1999;67:555-562.

50. Ockene J: Smoking among women across the lifespan, prevalence, interventions and implications for cessation research. Ann Behav Med 1993;15:135-148.

51. Perkins KA: Smoking cessation in women. Special considerations. CNS Drugs 2001;15:391-411.

52. Gritz ER, Thompson B, Emmons K, Ockene JK, McLerran DF, Nielsen IR: Gender differences among smokers and quitters in the Working Well Trial. Prev Med 1998;27:553-561.

53. Gonzales D, Bjornson W, Durcan MJ, et al: Effects of gender on relapse prevention in smokers treated with bupropion SR. Am J Prev Med 2002;22:234-239.

54. Pirie PL, McBride CM, Hellerstedt W, et al: Smoking cessation in women concerned about weight. Am J Public Health 1992;82:1238-1243.

55. Perkins K, Grobe J, D'Amicao D, Fonte C, Wilson A, Stiller R: Low-dose nicotine nasal spray use and effects during initial smoking cessation. Exp Clin Psychopharmacol 1996;4:157-165.

56. Perkins KA, Gerlach D, Vender J, Grobe J, Meeker J, Hutchison S: Sex differences in the subjective and reinforcing effects of visual and olfactory cigarette smoke stimuli. Nicotine Tob Res 2001;3:141-150.

57. Abrams D, Monti P, Pinto R, Elder J, Brown R, Jacobus S: Psychosocial stress and coping in smokers who relapse or quit. Health Psychol 1987;6:289-303.

58. Borrelli B, Bock B, King T, Pinto B, Marcus BH: The impact of depression on smoking cessation in women. Am J Prev Med 1996;12:378-387.

59. Borrelli B, Niaura R, Keuthen NJ, et al: Development of major depressive disorder during smoking-cessation treatment. J Clin Psych 1996;57:534-538.

60. Glassman AH, Covey LS, Stetner F, Rivelli S: Smoking cessation and the course of major depression: A follow-up study. Lancet 2001;357:1929-1932.

61. US Department of Health and Human Services: Tobacco use among U.S. racial/ethnic minority groups. A report of the surgeon general. Executive summary. Atlanta, Centers for Disease Control, National Center for Chronic Disease Prevention and Health Promotion, Office on Smoking and Health, 1998.

62. Clark PI, Gautam S, Gerson LW: Effect of menthol cigarettes on biochemical markers of smoke exposure among black and white smokers. Chest 1996;110:1194-1198.

63. Ahijevych K, Gillespie J: Nicotine dependence and smoking topography among black and white women. Res Nurs Health 1997;20:505-514.

64. Pederson LL, Ahluwalia JS, Harris KJ, McGrady GA: Smoking cessation among African Americans: What we know and do not know about interventions and self-quitting. Prev Med 2000;31:23-38.

65. Piper ME, Fox BJ, Welsch SK, Fiore MC, Baker TB: Gender and racial/ethnic differences in tobacco-dependence treatment: A commentary and research recommendations. Nicotine Tob Res 2001;3:291-297.

66. Voorhees CC, Stillman FA, Swank RT, Heagerty PJ, Levine DM, Becker DM: Heart, body, and soul: Impact of church-based smoking cessation interventions on readiness to quit. Prev Med 1996;25:277-285.

67. Wagenknecht LE, Cutter GR, Haley NJ, et al: Racial differences in serum cotinine levels among smokers in the Coronary Artery Risk Development in (Young) Adults study. Am J Public Health 1990;80:1053-1056.

68. Benowitz NL: Smoking cessation trials targeted to racial and economic minority groups. JAMA 2002;288:497-499.

69. Perez-Stable EJ, Herrera B, Jacob P III, Benowitz NL: Nicotine metabolism and intake in black and white smokers. JAMA 1998;280:152-156.

70. Caraballo RS, Giovino GA, Pechacek TF, et al: Racial and ethnic differences in serum cotinine levels of cigarette smokers: Third National Health and Nutrition Examination Survey, 1988-1991. JAMA 1998;280:135-139.

71. Ginsberg D, Hall SM, Reus VI, Munoz RF: Mood and depression diagnosis in smoking cessation. Exp Clin Psychopharmacol 1995;3:389-395.

72. Glassman AH, Helzer JE, Covey LS, et al: Smoking, smoking cessation, and major depression. JAMA 1990;264:1546-1549.

73. Robins L, Helzer J, Weissman M, et al: Lifetime prevalence of specific psychiatric disorders in three sites. Arch Gen Psych, 1984;41:949-958.

74. Burgess ES, Brown RA, Kahler CW, et al: I. W. Patterns of change in depressive symptoms during smoking cessation: Who's at risk for relapse? J Consult Clin Psychol 2002;70:356-361.

75. Lerman C, Audrain J, Orleans CT, Boyd R, Gold K, Main D, Caporaso N: Investigation of mechanisms linking depressed mood to nicotine dependence. Addict Behav 1996;21:9-19.

76. Niaura R, Britt DM, Borrelli B, Shadel WG, Abrams DB, Goldstein MG: History and symptoms of depression among smokers during a self-initiated quit attempt. Nicotine Tob Res 1999;1:251-257.

77. Shiffman S, Paty JA, Gnys M, Kassel JA, Hickcox M: First lapses to smoking: Within-subjects analysis of real-time reports. J Consult Clin Psychol 1996;64:366-379.

78. Borrelli B, Hogan JW, Bock B, Pinto B, Roberts M, Marcus B: Predictors of quitting and dropout among women in a clinic-based smoking cessation program. Psychol Addict Behav 2002;16:22-27.

79. Hall SM, Munoz RF, Reus VI, et al: Mood management and nicotine gum in smoking treatment: A therapeutic contact and placebo-controlled study. J Consult Clin Psychol 1996;64:1003-1009.

80. Brown RA, Kahler CW, Niaura R, et al: Cognitive-behavioral treatment for depression in smoking cessation. J Consult Clin Psychol 2001;69:471-480.

81. Hall SM, Reus VI, Munoz RF, et al: Nortriptyline and cognitive-behavioral therapy in the treatment of cigarette smoking. Arch Gen Psych 1998;55:683-690.

82. Coppotelli HC, Orleans CT: Partner support and other determinants of smoking cessation maintenance among women. J Consult Clin Psychol 1985;53:455-460.

83. Carlson LE, Goodey E, Bennett MH, Taenzer P, Koopmans J: The addition of social support to a community-based large-group behavioral smoking cessation intervention: Improved cessation rates and gender differences. Addict Behav 2002;27:547-559.

84. Roski J, Schmid LA, Lando HA: Long-term associations of helpful and harmful spousal behaviors with smoking cessation. Addict Behav 1996;21:173-185.

85. Glasgow RE, Klesges RC, O'Neill HK: Programming social support for smoking modification: An extension and replication. Addict Behav 1986;11:453-457.

86. West R, Edwards M, Hajek P: A randomized controlled trial of a "buddy" systems to improve success at giving up smoking in general practice. Addiction 1998;93:1007-1011.

87. Cinciripini P, Gritz ER, Tsoh J, Skaar K: Smoking cessation and cancer prevention. In Holland J (ed): Psycho-oncology. New York, Oxford University Press, 1998, pp 27-44.

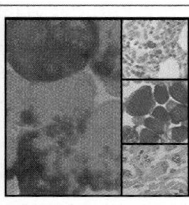

25

CHEMOTHERAPY

Michael C. Perry

Clay M. Anderson

Ross C. Donehower

SUMMARY OF KEY POINTS

HISTORY OF DRUG DISCOVERY

- The history of cancer chemotherapy and of the disciplines of medical oncology has been that of drug discovery.

CLINICAL USES OF CHEMOTHERAPY

- Adjuvant chemotherapy is the logical extension of the use of chemotherapy in patients who remain at high risk of recurrence after all clinically detectable disease has been eradicated.
- In specific cancers, the application of chemotherapy prior to any other anticancer therapy (neoadjuvant therapy) can provide improved survival and/or organ sparing and preservation of function.
- The most common use of cancer chemotherapy is in the management of advanced and metastatic disease. Although curative for several advanced cancers, chemotherapy is largely palliative for metastatic disease.

COMBINATION CHEMOTHERAPY

- Virtually all of the curative chemotherapy regimens developed for hematologic malignancies and for advanced solid tumors use combinations of active agents.
- A series of principles for the development of effctive combination regimens was developed in the 1970s and continues to be used today.
- Although the concept of using alternating non–cross-resistant chemotherapy regimens has a sound theoretical basis, this approach has not been established as a definitively superior means of delivering chemotherapy.

TUMOR CELL KINETICS AND THE USE OF CHEMOTHERAPY

- Mathematical models describing the interaction between tumor cell kinetics and response to chemotherapy have had a strong influence on development of clinical regimens.

THE CHEMOTHERAPEUTIC PROCESS

- The choice of chemotherapy for a specific patient must take into account physiologic age, performance status, nutritional status, prior therapy, pharmacogenetics, and comorbid conditions.

- The principles of drug selection include the pharmacologic characteristics of the individual agents, the route of administration, and the toxicity profile.
- Information regarding individual chemotherapeutic agents is presented according to drug class, mechanism of action, dosage forms, drug interactions, pharmacokinetics and metabolism, indications, and toxicity.

NEW DIRECTIONS IN DRUG DEVELOPMENT

- New categories of agents include differentiating agents, antiangiogenesis agents, signal transduction inhibitors, monoclonal antibodies, gene therapy, and vaccines.
- Computer modeling and combinatorial chemistry are powerful new tools for drug development.
- The roles of pharmacogenetics, pharmacokinetics, and pharmacodynamics are likely to become increasingly important in oncology.

INTRODUCTION

Although chemotherapy is a relatively recent addition to the therapeutic armamentarium for the treatment of patients with cancer, its role is expanding, and cytotoxic agents are used at some point during treatment for most patients with cancer. Historically, chemotherapy has been used principally as therapy for metastatic cancer after failed local therapies. Chemotherapy remains the treatment of choice for patients with metastatic cancer. The evolution of cancer therapy over the past several decades, however, has resulted in increased recognition of the important role that chemotherapy and radiation therapy can play in the management of apparently local-

ized and surgically resectable disease. This recognition has led to the development of other applications for systemic therapy designed to decrease postsurgical recurrences, when given as adjuvant therapy, or to allow more limited organ- and function-sparing surgical procedures to be done when chemotherapy is given preoperatively or concurrently with radiation therapy.

Perhaps more than any other disease, cancer requires close interaction among medical specialties. As our knowledge of how to combine surgery, radiation, and chemotherapy evolves optimally and as the efficacy and specificity of available chemotherapeutic agents improves, chemotherapy will play an even greater role in improving both the survival and quality of life for patients with cancer.

HISTORY OF DRUG DISCOVERY

Chemotherapy has its origins in the work of Paul Ehrlich, who coined the term in reference to the systemic treatment of both infectious diseases and neoplasia. Many of Ehrlich's concepts regarding the experimental evaluation of new therapies using murine or rat models have survived to the present day and have provided a number of important biologic insights that have been applied successfully to the clinical setting. Although the concept of treating cancers with drugs can be traced back several centuries, there were no examples of truly successful systemic cancer chemotherapy until the 1940s. Gilman and Philips[1] conducted the first clinical trial of nitrogen mustard in patients with malignant lymphomas at Yale University in 1942. The use of nitrogen mustard as a chemotherapeutic agent was suggested by the serendipitous findings of marrow and lymphoid hypoplasia in seamen exposed to mustard gas after the explosion of a ship containing material manufactured for use in chemical warfare in World War II.[2] This discovery supported previous evidence of a systemic lympholytic effect from alkylating agents of this type. The dramatic regressions of the lymphomas noted in this original study generated tremendous excitement for this new field of medicine, although enthusiasm was dampened by the fact that regrowth of tumor seemed inevitable. The results, initially published in 1946, could be said to mark the beginning of modern chemotherapy.

This same combination of "experiments of nature" and the observations of well-trained scientists has yielded a number of other important leads in the search for improved cancer therapy. These include, among others, the recognition by Farber and colleagues[3] of the importance of folates in cell growth in acute leukemia in children and the subsequent development of the first antifolate antimetabolites. This class of compounds produced perhaps the first examples of drug-induced cures of a metastatic cancer in gestational choriocarcinoma, and they remain in wide clinical use today.[4] For their recognition of the importance of nucleic acid synthesis to inhibition of cell growth and for the development of effective antipurine analogues for cancer and other diseases, Elion[5] and Hitchings were awarded the Nobel Prize in Medicine in 1988. Serendipity also has played a role in the recognition of the potential of vinca alkaloids, epipodophyllotoxins, and platinum coordination complexes as chemotherapy agents.[6,7] This scenario has been repeated with sufficient frequency that drug discovery programs such as that of the National Cancer Institute have made extensive use of the approach of mass screening of both natural products and synthetic compounds to identify lead compounds with potent antitumor activity and unique mechanisms of action.

Screening is key to the process of drug development because it narrows the enormous number of candidate drugs to a more manageable number for further study and possible clinical evaluation. Traditionally, this screening system has used transplantable murine tumors to search for evidence of biologic activity.[8] Although this system identified a series of compounds for clinical trial, there was continued uncertainty regarding the relevance of these murine cell lines to human cancers. The current screening system employs a panel of human cancer cell lines grown in culture that represent the major histologic subtypes and sites of origins of human cancer. It is also possible, and probably important, to include cell lines that express various drug resistance phenotypes, such as multidrug resistance (MDR), to evaluate new agents against tumor cells manifesting these potentially clinically important cellular characteristics. It also has been possible to automate the testing of candidate drugs in this system so that high-volume screening can be maintained.[9] Because this screening system uses human cancer cell lines, it is hoped that it will identify agents with unique promise against advanced solid tumors that would not be identified using other methods.

The history of cancer chemotherapy and of the discipline of medical oncology has been that of drug discovery. The pioneering discoveries of the early days of chemotherapy have allowed the development of a paradigm for drug discovery that persists, with modifications, to the present day. This organized approach to random screening of large numbers of compounds must be complemented in the drug development effort, however, by attempts to exploit new therapeutic targets identified in ongoing basic cancer research. When a putative target is identified based on its biologic significance in the cancer cell, this strategy suggests that the ability of potential therapeutic agents to interact with this target and to inhibit or modify its function should be evaluated as a primary screening procedure. This mechanism-based screening is often performed in simple cell-free systems in which the target and effector are isolated. Drugs identified as promising candidates by this mechanism-based approach to drug development also require the test systems that have been developed to validate their biologic activity in whole cells and experimental animal tumor models. Active new agents are needed for the treatment of all common human cancers. The ongoing work in drug development is crucial if our use of chemotherapy is to continue to improve and if its role in potentially curative therapy is to expand. A number of promising and novel strategies are being considered for clinical trials, including antiangiogenesis factors, drugs that affect intracellular signaling pathways, differentiating agents, agents that affect a cell's ability to undergo apoptosis, and gene-specific therapies such as antisense oligonucleotides and ribozymes. These approaches, and others which will undoubtedly follow, offer great promise for the future of cancer treatment.

CLINICAL USES OF CHEMOTHERAPY

Adjuvant Chemotherapy

Chemotherapy can be used in a number of ways in the treatment of cancer. The vast majority of cancer chemotherapy treatments are administered to patients with clinically obvious disease. The notable exception is

Science of Clinical Oncology

MANAGEMENT APPROACH

CANCERS TREATED EFFECTIVELY BY ADJUVANT CHEMOTHERAPY

Wilms' tumor
Osteosarcoma

Breast cancer
Colorectal cancer

adjuvant chemotherapy, which uses chemotherapy for patients who remain at high risk of recurrence after the primary tumor and all evidence of cancer have been surgically removed or treated definitively with radiation. Despite an apparently successful resection of primary breast, colon, or other primary cancers along with the regional lymph nodes, patients can be prospectively identified who are at high risk of recurrence of their disease. These criteria might differ for each tumor, but in general, the degree of local extension of the primary tumor, the presence of positive lymph nodes, and certain morphologic or biologic characteristics of the individual cancer cells are important determinants of that risk. The need for effective adjuvant therapy is strongly emphasized by the fact that chemotherapy usually fails to cure these cancers once recurrence has taken place. The theoretical advantage of treating patients with small total body tumor burden is very compelling, but, in fact, some patients who will receive chemotherapy have already been rendered disease free by the local therapy and would be cured without it.

The use of chemotherapy when the tumor burden is minimal avoids the problems of increasing tumor cell number, decreasing growth fraction, decreased vascular supply, hypoxia, tumor cell heterogeneity, and the likelihood of emergence of drug resistance, all of which occur with increasing frequency as tumors enlarge. Considerable experimental evidence suggests that cancers are most sensitive to chemotherapy during the early stages of growth. This increased sensitivity is believed to be the result of the high growth fraction and shorter cell cycle times, so that a given dose of drug might exert a greater therapeutic effect than in a larger, quiescent tumor.[10]

The selection of the specific chemotherapy regimen to be used as part of adjuvant chemotherapy for a particular cancer is based on objective response rates observed for patients with advanced cancers of the same type. These regimens should be selected carefully, as it is unrealistic to expect a chemotherapy regimen to be effective in preventing recurrences in the adjuvant setting

if the regimen does not have a substantial response rate in advanced disease. The selection of patients for adjuvant chemotherapy is based on the expected rate of recurrence for their initial clinical stage of cancer after local treatment alone. Initial demonstration of the efficacy of an adjuvant chemotherapy regimen requires comparison with a control group receiving no therapy beyond local management in a prospective clinical trial. Historical controls are notoriously unreliable in this regard and are not adequate to prove efficacy.

The typical endpoints of clinical chemotherapy—shrinkage of measurable tumor on physical examination or serial radiographic studies—are not available in this situation; in clinical trials of adjuvant therapy, relapse-free survival and overall survival are the principal measures of treatment effect. For an individual patient, there are no means to determine whether the adjuvant therapy and its resultant toxicity and expense have been beneficial or necessary.

This strategy of adjuvant therapy has been attempted in a wide variety of pediatric and adult tumors with some success and the principles of adjuvant therapy strategy are well established. In the cases of breast cancer and colon cancer, the number of lives saved by the adjuvant therapy approach is significant because of the large number of affected patients, despite the modest differences seen between treated and control patients with current treatment programs.

Neoadjuvant Chemotherapy

A second strategy that acknowledges the presence of micrometastatic disease at sites remote from the primary tumor at diagnosis is that of neoadjuvant chemotherapy.[11] As with adjuvant chemotherapy, treatment is directed at the possibility of systemic disease in patients with apparently localized disease, although in this instance chemotherapy is administered before surgery is performed. This approach has several potential advantages over conventional postoperative adjuvant chemotherapy.

MANAGEMENT APPROACH

PRINCIPLES OF ADJUVANT CHEMOTHERAPY

1. Effective chemotherapy must be available.
2. Known tumor should be removed by surgery.
3. Chemotherapy should be started as soon as possible postoperatively.
4. Chemotherapy should be given in maximally tolerated doses.
5. Chemotherapy should continue for a limited time period.
6. Chemotherapy should be intermittent, when possible, to minimize immunosuppression.

First, neoadjuvant or preoperative chemotherapy provides earlier exposure of potential micrometastases to chemotherapy than is achieved with the standard adjuvant approach. If the advantages of early chemotherapy treatment observed in the laboratory are exportable to the clinic, this should be an optimal approach to the treatment of micrometastases. Second, an objective response to chemotherapy in the primary lesion provides important in vivo evidence that the therapy being used has antitumor activity and suggests that the tumor at remote subclinical sites will be sensitive as well. By contrast, if the primary lesion does not respond, the likelihood of success of the initial chemotherapy regimen in eradicating micrometastases would seem to be greatly diminished. Monitoring the response thus provides an early opportunity to consider alternative chemotherapy approaches. This approach has perhaps best been described for osteosarcoma.[12] Third, significant regression of the primary tumor might allow local management to be tailored to the individual patient. For example, surgery might be technically easier because of the reduced tumor bulk, a more conservative surgical procedure could be considered, or radiation therapy might be administered in lieu of surgery.

The latter two approaches could permit organ sparing and function preservation for some patients. In some situations, preoperative chemotherapy is administered concurrently with radiation therapy, to improve local disease control and to treat systemic micrometastases. For cancer of the anal canal and bladder cancer, this approach has allowed organ-sparing procedures for a high percentage of patients. It has also served as highly effective preoperative therapy for esophageal cancer and squamous cell cancer of the head and neck.

The potential disadvantages of the neoadjuvant approach are also very real. First, chemotherapy is being used as initial therapy for a group of patients with cancers that are potentially curable by surgery alone in a small percentage of patients. If chemotherapy proves ineffective and the cancer becomes unresectable during treatment, great harm could be done. Second, the use of preoperative chemotherapy could obscure the true pathologic stage of the cancer by altering tumor size and margins and converting histologically positive nodes to negative. The inaccuracy of clinical staging for many cancers makes it difficult to be confident that a homogeneous group of patients has been treated, and this fact might confound interpretation of results of clinical trials. Third, if a dramatic clinical response results in the performance of an inappropriately conservative procedure or poor patient acceptance of the recommended procedure, and if the cancer then recurs, a significant disservice has been done to the patient.

Approximately seven types of cancers have been managed effectively using neoadjuvant chemotherapy. In all cases, this "effectiveness" might not imply improved survival. In some cases, organ sparing or function preservation is routinely possible and is ample justification for the use of this approach.

Management of Advanced and Metastatic Disease

The most common use of cancer chemotherapy is for the management of advanced or metastatic disease after failed local therapies, or in disease for which no alternative therapy has been found. This is perhaps the sternest test for chemotherapy, as tumor volume is significant and patients are often physically compromised by the effects of their disease. It is this clinical situation, however, in which the activity of new anticancer agents and combination chemotherapy regimens are initially evaluated. In treating patients with advanced cancer, it is possible both to determine the antitumor activity of the therapy on an individual patient basis and to define the response rate for the therapy accurately, by entering an appropriate number of patients with the same diagnosis and similar pretreatment characteristics in a clinical trial. The benefit of chemotherapy to patients can be inferred by the degree to which measurable or evaluable tumor responds to therapy.

Clearly, the most important measure of the efficacy of chemotherapy is the achievement of a complete response, defined as the disappearance of all radiographic and clinical evidence of measurable or evaluable tumor. It is the necessary first step to achieving a clinical cure. The achievement of a complete response results in a significant decrease in or disappearance of disease-related symptoms and generally translates into a meaningful prolongation of survival, even for patients who ultimately relapse. Therapy can be said to be curative only when the complete response is maintained after treatment is discontinued. The clinical importance of a complete response is therefore measured by the disease-free or relapse-free survival time. Partial responses are defined as a 50% decrease in cross-sectional area of measurable tumor masses and also can result in symptomatic benefit for patients, although survival is rarely significantly prolonged. Continued administration of the chemotherapy regimen is usually required to maintain the partial response. Unless the regimen is extremely well tolerated, the cumulative effects

---

MANAGEMENT APPROACH

CANCERS TREATED EFFECTIVELY BY NEOADJUVANT CHEMOTHERAPY

Soft tissue sarcoma
Osteosarcoma
Anal cancer

Bladder cancer
Larynx cancer
Esophageal cancer
Locally advanced breast cancer

MANAGEMENT APPROACH

CANCERS CURABLE OR OCCASIONALLY CURABLE WITH CHEMOTHERAPY ALONE

Cancers Curable with Chemotherapy Alone
Gestational choriocarcinoma
Hodgkin's disease
Germ cell cancer of the testis

Acute lymphoid leukemia
Non–Hodgkin's lymphoma (some subtypes)
Hairy cell leukemia (probable)

Cancers Occasionally Cured with Chemotherapy
Acute myeloid leukemia
Ovarian cancer
Small cell lung cancer

---

of chemotherapy might ultimately limit the benefit to the patient. The median duration of response among the complete and partial responders is often used as an endpoint in clinical trials of therapies.

Perhaps the greatest value to clinical investigators of documenting partial responses is in the evaluation of investigational new drugs, where preliminary evidence for antitumor activity of new drugs is often first observed. New agents that produce partial responses in patients with advanced cancer in phase I or II trials might warrant further evaluation at earlier stages of disease or in combination with other active agents. Patients who have stable disease while receiving therapy—that is, responses that do not meet the criteria for either an objective response or progressive disease—are reported in some clinical trials, although the scientific value of this measure in evaluating therapy can be legitimately questioned. For individual patients who experience extended periods of stable disease and symptomatic palliation on treatment after a period of rapid progression, the clinician (and patient) might consider the therapy of value and continue it on that basis. The importance of this endpoint could increase as novel agents that are not truly "cytotoxic," such as antimetastatic agents, differentiating agents, or agents that affect intracellular signaling, enter clinical trials. In these cases, it is possible that evidence of biologic effect may take a different form from that to which we have become accustomed with conventional cytotoxic agents.

Although objective responses, duration of survival, and cure rates have been our traditional chemotherapy endpoints, it has become increasingly clear that clinical researchers and clinicians caring for patients must consider other outcomes or endpoints also. These generally fall under the rubric of palliation of symptoms and improved quality of life.[13,14] Although these endpoints might be more subjective than the traditional ones, it is important that criteria for their evaluation be agreed on and that they be used routinely in clinical trials in which an improved cure rate is not a likely outcome. The palliative benefit to patients who do not have a curable disease is not well defined by our current criteria, and the addition of a semiquantitative means of assessing palliative benefit is critical.

Despite the obvious limitations of our current cytotoxic agents, chemotherapy is curative for several advanced human cancers. These diseases include gestational tropho-

blastic disease and several hematologic malignancies, but only one advanced solid tumor—germ cell cancer of the testis—can be said to be routinely curable with chemotherapy alone. Another group of cancers, such as small cell lung cancer and ovarian cancer, is occasionally cured with chemotherapy. The most common solid tumors, however—for example, cancers of the breast, lung, prostate, or gastrointestinal tract—when metastatic are not curable with current therapies. These diseases will provide the greatest challenge to the process of drug development and the practice of chemotherapy in the future and will continue to be the focus of active investigative efforts.

The reader is directed to the discussions of the management of individual cancers in Part III of this textbook, "Specific Malignancies." General principles regarding selection of chemotherapy and characteristics of specific drugs are discussed later in this chapter.

COMBINATION CHEMOTHERAPY

The optimal exploitation of the chemotherapy strategies discussed earlier requires the use of combination chemotherapy because, with rare exceptions, single agents do not cure cancer. Virtually all the curative chemotherapy regimens developed for hematologic malignancies or for the treatment of advanced solid tumors use combinations of active agents. Combination chemotherapy is also superior to the use of single agents in postsurgical adjuvant therapy and neoadjuvant therapy. The superior results achieved by combination chemotherapy can be explained in several ways. Resistance to any given single agent is almost always present, even in clinically responsive tumors, at diagnosis. Tumors that are initially "sensitive" to chemotherapy rapidly acquire resistance to single agents, either as a result of selection of a pre-existing clone of resistant tumor cells or due to an increased rate of mutation leading to drug resistance. Combination chemotherapy theoretically addresses both important phenomena by providing a broader range of coverage of initially resistant clones of cells and preventing or slowing the development of resistant clones.

A series of principles for the development of effective clinical combination chemotherapy programs has been recognized for a number of years and continues to be used in the design of new regimens.[15]

1. Only drugs that have demonstrated antitumor activity against the disease to be treated should be employed in combination. This principle seems self-evident but is not uniformly adhered to, particularly when a regimen is designed with the addition of a therapeutically inactive drug to promote biochemical synergy. Such regimens are rarely effective, and the strategy has been used infrequently.

2. Drugs to be used in the combination chemotherapy regimen should be administered at their optimal doses and schedules. If an agent has been shown to have a definable response rate when given at its maximum tolerated dose, it is unreasonable to expect a similar contribution to the overall response rate of a combination if the dose is reduced. This suggests that, when possible, the drugs chosen for inclusion in a combination should have nonoverlapping toxicities.

3. Drugs should be selected for inclusion in the combination that do not share the same mechanism of cytotoxicity or a common mechanism of cellular resistance. Practically speaking, this is often difficult to achieve, as several mechanisms of resistance often exist for an individual drug, some of which might be shared by chemically and mechanistically unrelated drugs (i.e., the well-defined multidrug resistance [MDR] phenotype).

4. The drug combination should be given in the shortest possible interval that allows for recovery of the normal tissue, which is the dose-limiting toxicity.

In the case of hematologic toxicity—in particular, neutropenia—it is often possible to maintain the dosing schedule and to shorten the period of granulocytopenia by the use of the hematopoietic growth factors granulocyte colony-stimulating factor (G-CSF) or granulocyte-macrophage colony-stimulating factor (GM-CSF).[16] In making the clinical decision regarding dosage modifications or the use of growth factors, the clinician should keep in mind the therapeutic goals of the therapy to be given. If the regimen has the potential for cure, every effort should be made to maintain the optimum dose and schedule. For treatment situations in which palliation is the realistic goal, dose reductions and lengthening of the interval between doses are appropriate options to be considered.

Cyclic Chemotherapy

Typically, combination chemotherapy regimens are given as repetitive cycles of a fixed drug combination. Although this approach has led to some success in hematologic malignancies and several solid tumors, it has not been the answer for advanced solid tumors. In an effort to improve the results with cyclic chemotherapy, the strategy has been modified to consider several hypotheses regarding possible limitations of this approach. The Goldie-Coldman hypothesis mathematically described the likelihood that drug-resistant cancer cells are present in a patient at diagnosis.[17] Goldie and Coldman proposed that tumor cells could acquire drug resistance before drug exposure on the basis of the spontaneous mutation rate intrinsic to the genetic instability of a particular tumor. The likelihood that resistant cells are present can be modeled as a function of tumor size or the number of tumor cells and the spontaneous mutation rate of the cells. The predicted frequency of spontaneous mutation of $1:10^{-5}$ to $1:10^{-6}$ divisions in proliferative tumor cells is consistent with in vitro studies of this phenomenon.[18] Although this discussion has focused on this phenomenon as a means by which cells might acquire drug resistance, it is equally plausible that the same type of genetic events could lead to an increase in vascular invasion and local spread or to an increased tendency to develop systemic metastases.[19] Preclinical studies have demonstrated clearly that the development of the metastatic potential can be the result of genetic instability.[20] The clinician can, therefore, be faced with a situation at initial diagnosis in which an apparently localized cancer has developed systemic metastases, and in which resistant tumor cells are already present even before therapy has been given. In this situation, it seems obvious that only combinations of active agents will have any significant effect.

The Goldie-Coldman hypothesis has several potential clinical ramifications that have been tested in prospective clinical trials. First, it suggests that the optimal strategy is to initiate chemotherapy when tumor size is still small. Second, as many effective drugs as possible should be used as early as possible in the chemotherapy regimen to prevent cells that are already resistant to one agent from developing further resistance to others in the combination. Optimally, all active drugs would be administered simultaneously, but clinical practicalities prevent this from being done. Finally, this hypothesis suggests that, if drugs cannot be used at full therapeutic doses because of overlapping toxicity or a pharmacologic interaction, they should be given in an alternating sequence that permits frequent exposure to each agent. These recommendations are not dramatically different from those general principles outlined previously.[15,20] The principal difference is

---

MANAGEMENT APPROACH

PRINCIPLES OF COMBINATION CHEMOTHERAPY

1. Only those agents proven effective should be used.
2. Each agent used should have a different mechanism of action.
3. Each drug should have a different spectrum of toxicity and (ideally) of resistance.
4. Each drug should be used at maximum dose.
5. Agents with similar dose-limiting toxicities can be combined safely only by reducing doses, resulting in decreased effects.
6. Drug combinations should be administered in the shortest interval between therapy cycles to allow for the recovery of normal tissue.

that the strategy is dictated by concern both for the drug resistance present at initiation of chemotherapy and for resistance that could develop during the application of therapy.

The primary clinical application of these principles has been in the development and use of alternating, non–cross-resistant chemotherapy regimens. This approach involves the use of multiple chemotherapy agents with different mechanisms of action that exhibit antitumor activity against the disease in question. The drugs are organized into two different combination chemotherapy regimens administered to patients on an alternating basis. The Goldie-Coldman hypothesis would suggest frequent alternation of these regimens (e.g., every second cycle), and this has been the general approach taken in prospective clinical trials that have examined this question. A more recent variation on this theme has been the development of hybrid regimens, in which elements of each regimen are administered during each cycle (e.g., on day 1 and day 8), rather than during every second cycle. This strategy has been most thoroughly evaluated in Hodgkin's disease (e.g., the MOPP [mechlorethamine, vincristine, procarbazine, prednisone]–ABV [doxorubicin, bleomycin, vinblastine] hybrid) and non–Hodgkin's lymphoma.[21,22] This strategy has been evaluated extensively to date in breast cancer, lymphomas, and small cell lung cancer (SCLC), among other diseases.

The available results have not provided definitive evidence of the value of this approach, as the use of alternating cycles of combination chemotherapy has not consistently proved to be more effective than full doses of a single chemotherapy regimen. The negative results to date do not completely invalidate the biologic plausibility of the hypothesis, however. In many cases, the alternating combinations used have been neither equally effective nor non–cross-resistant. In SCLC, several chemotherapy regimens are available that have roughly equal antitumor efficacies, and alternating chemotherapy regimens have been studied frequently in this disease. Early trials of this strategy in extensive SCLC demonstrated minimal survival benefit from the use of alternating chemotherapy regimens and a short prolongation of the duration of initial remission in some studies.[23-26] Other studies have suggested that the benefits of using more than one chemotherapy regimen in SCLC might be more apparent in limited-stage disease, where a survival advantage has been shown in several small studies.[27,28] In Hodgkin's disease, randomized trials of MOPP vs. ABVD (doxorubicin, bleomycin, vinblastine, dacarbazine) vs. MOPP alternated with ABVD have shown superiority of the alternating regimen and ABVD to MOPP alone in terms of both survival and complete remission.[29] A hybrid regimen of MOPP-ABVD has been shown to be superior to MOPP followed by ABVD.[30] In both cases, however, the testing of the hypothesis is clouded by the fact that, in these cooperative group studies, the MOPP regimen consistently required significant dosage reductions. In metastatic breast cancer, studies with a similar design have failed to demonstrate an advantage of alternating cycles of CMFVP (cyclophosphamide, methotrexate, 5-fluorouracil [5-FU], vincristine, prednisone) and VATH (vinblastine, doxorubi-

cin, thiotepa, halotensin) to either CAF (cyclophosphamide, doxorubicin, 5-FU) or VATH alone.[31] Collectively, these data suggest that the use of alternating non–cross-resistant chemotherapy regimens is an acceptable, but still not mandatory, alternative therapeutic strategy for these diseases. In some cases, the principal advantage might be to decrease the total doses of agents such as doxorubicin and cisplatin, which could have serious cumulative toxicities for those patients requiring prolonged chemotherapy.

TUMOR CELL KINETICS AND THE USE OF CHEMOTHERAPY

Alternative chemotherapy strategies are suggested by considering the possibility that the failure of chemotherapy to produce a cure in the in vivo situation might depend on factors other than the development of absolute biochemical or pharmacologic resistance. The heterogeneity of cancer cells includes their growth rate or cell cycle kinetic status and the biochemical characteristics of the cells that could determine drug resistance. Many of the concepts regarding cell growth that have helped guide the development of current chemotherapy were described by Skipper and Schabel[32,33] more than 30 years ago. Their model, based largely on work in murine leukemias, assumed that the growth rate of cancer cells in vivo is logarithmic. That is, growth rate and doubling time are constant and do not change with increasing or decreasing tumor size. These investigators also postulated a logarithmic-kill hypothesis for the killing of cancer cells by antineoplastic agents. This means that a given dose of drug will kill the same proportion of cells or decrease the number of cancer cells by the same number of logs, regardless of the tumor burden. Treatment failure in these authors' models was attributed to too great a tumor burden or to the fact that the dose of drug given did not result in a sufficiently large cell kill. This work established the essential relationship between tumor volume or cell number and curability of advanced cancers. These observations, coupled with the knowledge that more rapidly growing tumors are generally more sensitive to chemotherapy, suggested that the principal elements that determine the success of a chemotherapy regimen, in addition to biochemically mediated drug resistance, are tumor bulk, growth rate, and dosage of the chemotherapy regimen given.

Among the histologic types of cancer that have been studied, considerable differences in growth rates in the clinically observable range emerges.[34] Interestingly, the most chemosensitive tumors—such as germ cell cancer of the testis—tend to have the shortest doubling times and the fastest growth rate. Unresponsive cancers, such as colon cancer, appear to grow much more slowly. It has occasionally been possible to document clinically that human tumors grow exponentially for short periods, but most of the available data suggest that they generally do not grow with a constant doubling time.[35-39] In these cases, the data support a Gompertzian model of tumor growth and regression. In Gompertzian growth, the doubling time increases and the growth fraction of tumor decreases as the tumor becomes larger. Experimental models suggest that this observation is the result of decreased cell production rather than of increased cell loss in larger tumors.[40,41] A tumor theoretically responds to therapy depending on where it lies on the Gompertzian growth curve. In a patient with an advanced cancer and large tumor bulk, this model predicts a lower growth fraction and a lower fraction of cells killed by a given dose of therapy than would be the case with a smaller tumor. Alternatively, this concept of cell growth in human tumors supports the use of adjuvant therapy and the early institution of chemotherapy. When a small tumor burden is present, perhaps even clinically undetectable, the growth rate will be at its highest, and the fractional cell kill might be greatest for a given dose of chemotherapy. Experimental data strongly support the notion that the rate and extent of tumor reduction are related to the growth rate in a population of cells just prior to therapy.[42]

The Norton-Simon[42-44] model for the response of tumors to chemotherapy has used the concept of Gompertzian growth to explain clinically observed phenomena and to suggest treatment strategies. For example, Gompertzian growth kinetics have a major impact on the rate of tumor regrowth from residual cells that remain after chemotherapy that fails to achieve a cure.[43,44] The increased rate of tumor cell growth seen when tumors are small will minimize the differences in survival among patients with advanced disease who achieved complete vs. partial responses to systemic chemotherapy, because the residual tumor in the complete responders grows back faster.

The difficult problem that continues to confound the curative goal of cancer chemotherapy is the heterogeneity of the tumor cell population. The available models to help gain insight into the processes underlying this heterogeneity suggest that it exists at the biochemical and pharmacologic level (conferring absolute drug resistance) and at the cell cycle kinetic level (conferring relative drug resistance). All the available models favor the use of combination chemotherapy and the administration of doses of chemotherapy that are as intensive as possible. An important issue that remains is the optimal manner in which to treat a disease such as breast cancer, SCLC, or lymphoma, for which multiple agents that display some antitumor activity are available. The Goldie-Coldman hypothesis favors the use of all active drugs to be included in the treatment over the shortest time frame possible. This favors a strict alternating approach. The Norton-Simon approach advocates a crossover strategy by which each active regimen is used for a longer period of time (i.e., several cycles) before switching to the alternative regimen. Theoretically, this approach accomplishes two important goals. First, it maintains the most dose-intense administration of each regimen by giving it during every cycle rather than during alternate cycles. Second, it addresses the heterogeneous populations of cells, killing the most sensitive, rapidly growing cells first and then treating the slower growing, more resistant cells as efficiently as possible.

The concept of dose-dense chemotherapy received additional support with the recent publication of a Cancer and Leukemia Group B study in the adjuvant therapy of node-positive breast cancer.[45] A 2 × 2 factorial design was used, with patients randomized to receive concurrent adriamycin/cyclophosphamide followed by paclitaxel, each for four cycles, or sequential single agent adriamycin, cyclophosphamide, and paclitaxel, each for four cycles. Patients were also randomized to receive their therapy at 3-week (standard) or 2-week (dose-dense) intervals. Growth factor support was added to the 2-week schedule. Dose-dense treatment improved disease-free survival and overall survival compared with the 3-week cycles. There were no differences in terms of outcome between concurrent or sequential schedules.

The lack of difference between sequential and concurrent therapies raises fundamental questions about the conventional wisdom of combination therapies always being superior to sequential single agents. Although the results might be drug- and disease-specific, the data are consistent with the Norton-Simon predictions that dose density would improve therapeutic results and that giving drugs in sequence while maintaining dose density would maintain efficacy and reduce toxicity.[45]

These concepts have not been definitively tested clinically, and the available results do not totally support either approach. A direct comparison of alternating vs. sequential chemotherapy in the adjuvant chemotherapy of breast cancer was conducted using doxorubicin and the CMF (cyclophosphamide, methotrexate, and 5-FU) regimen.[45] In one arm of this study, patients received four courses of doxorubicin followed by eight courses of CMF; in the second arm, patients received two cycles of CMF alternating with one course of doxorubicin. This sequence was repeated four times, for a total of 12 cycles of chemotherapy. The total dose of all drugs was equal, but the patients in the first arm experienced significantly better disease-free and overall survival. In this case, the sequential approach was superior to the alternating schedule.

An intergroup trial involving patients with Hodgkin's disease came to a different conclusion.[30] In this study, a hybrid MOPP-ABV chemotherapy regimen was superior in terms of complete remission, failure-free survival, and overall survival, compared with the sequential use of MOPP followed by ABVD. Whether this study is a valid test of the concept or whether the results reflect the significant dose modifications in the MOPP arm remains unclear. In either case, these testable hypotheses need to be considered when future trials are designed. Obviously, the success of this approach depends on having a number of active agents and at least two active combinations of drugs. Unfortunately, these conditions are not present for many human cancers.

Despite the lack of agreement as to which of the tumor growth models is most useful in helping to design chemotherapy regimens, it is clear that they provide a structure with which to formulate questions and to test chemotherapy strategies. Refinement of the clinical approach to chemotherapy in the future will require attention to rigorously derived models of this type, in addition to the clinical empiricism that has often characterized the approach in the past.

THE CHEMOTHERAPEUTIC PROCESS

The choice of chemotherapy as the treatment modality for a given patient has significant implications and requires a detailed knowledge of the patient and his or her medical problems and social and emotional background, a general knowledge of chemotherapy, a specific knowledge of the program to be used, and the availability of laboratory and support services. The occasional therapist cannot expect to become an expert, any more than one can expect to become an accomplished chef simply by using a cookbook. Indicator lesions may be physical findings (e.g., lymphadenopathy, hepatomegaly, splenomegaly, subcutaneous nodules), radiologic abnormalities, or tumor markers in body fluids.

Patient Selection

Physiologic Age

Advanced age alone is seldom a valid criterion for excluding patients from chemotherapy. Nevertheless, age-related alterations (in addition to disease-related changes) in organ function suggest that aggressive (or even nonaggressive) programs could result in unacceptable toxicity. Examples of such changes include decreased bone marrow reserve with the possibility of enhanced myelosuppression, reduced renal function with the possibility of enhanced methotrexate or cisplatin toxicity, variable gastrointestinal (GI) absorption of oral chemotherapeutic agents, and altered drug metabolism by the liver, resulting in possible decreased effectiveness of chemotherapy.[46] Treatment decisions must also take into account the likelihood of benefit. The decision to treat acute granulocytic leukemia in an elderly patient, for whom toxicity is certain and the likelihood of benefit is small, is an example of a difficult situation.

Performance Score

Whether the Karnofsky or Zubrod scale is used, performance status or score (Table 25-1) correlates closely with survival in certain settings. This is most clearly expressed in non-SCLC, in which each decrement of 10% in the Karnofsky score results in a measurable decrease in survival. The implication is that patients with Zubrod performance scores of 3 or 4 or Karnofsky scores of less than 30% are usually not candidates for chemotherapy, unless the tumor is untreated and especially likely to respond.

TABLE 25-1

Patient Performance Score Using Zubrod and Karnofsky Scales

ZUBROD	KARNOFSKY (%)	DEFINITION
0	100	Asymptomatic
1	80–90	Symptomatic, fully ambulatory
2	60–70	Symptomatic, in bed <50% of day
3	40–50	Symptomatic, in bed >50% of day, but not bedridden
4	20–30	Bedridden

Nutrition

Although maintenance of usual body weight might be impossible in the setting of advanced malignancy, the ingestion of 1500 to 2000 calories daily is necessary to permit a satisfactory chance of tumor response. This is best accomplished through oral intake, if possible, using supplemental sources as necessary. If the patient cannot ingest enough calories, enteral or parenteral feeding should be considered.

Obesity

Chemotherapy in the massively obese patient carries a potential risk of overdosage if the patient's actual weight is used, whether dosing is on a milligram-per-kilogram basis or according to body surface area. There are no guidelines for this situation, and the pharmacokinetics of antineoplastic drugs in obese patients are poorly understood. It has been suggested that, when patients are to be treated with curative intent, they should receive full-dose intensity, using body surface area calculated on actual body weight or on ideal body weight, with dose escalations if tolerated.[47] Patients who are to receive palliative therapy can more safely be given doses based on ideal body weight.[48]

Prior Therapy

In breast cancer, in spite of positive estrogen/progesterone receptors, failure to respond to a hormonal manipulation decreases the likelihood of a response to subsequent hormonal treatment. Similarly, in virtually all malignancies, failure to respond to a first chemotherapy program lessens the probability of a response to second-line therapy, often because of the development of MDR.

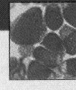

MANAGEMENT APPROACH

REQUIREMENTS FOR CHEMOTHERAPY

1. Biopsy-proven residual or metastatic disease*
2. Indicator lesion*
3. Satisfactory performance score and nutrition

4. Patient capable of informed consent
5. Minimal bone marrow, renal, and hepatic function (occasionally pulmonary or cardiac function important)
6. Available monitoring and support functions

*Exception: adjuvant chemotherapy

Organ Function

Altered end-organ function (bone marrow, renal, hepatic, cardiac, pulmonary) could eliminate the use of some chemotherapeutic agents entirely or require dose modification.[49] To avoid undue toxicity, it is essential to know the process of drug disposition and metabolism in this setting. Most oncologists find it useful to determine baseline bone marrow function by peripheral blood counts, hepatic and renal function by chemistry profiles, and (occasionally) cardiac function by echocardiography and gated pool cardiac scans, or pulmonary function by chest radiography and spirometry.

Coexisting Illnesses

Other nonneoplastic illnesses might modify the choice of chemotherapeutic agents, even if they do not eliminate the rationale of the use of chemotherapy. For instance, congestive heart failure rules out the possibility of the cardiotoxic drug doxorubicin, as severe chronic obstructive pulmonary disease should eliminate the use of the pulmonary toxin bleomycin. Similarly, diabetes might be aggravated by the use of corticosteroids.

Pharmacogenetics

The evolving field of pharmacogenetics has revealed that unexpectedly severe toxicity from 5-FU could be due to a deficiency of dihydropyrimidine dehydrogenase.[50] The prevalence of this enzyme deficiency in the general population is unknown, as is the impact of the heterozygous state on susceptibility to 5-FU toxicity. Similarly, determination of acetylator phenotype as defined by caffeine metabolism can accurately predict the extent of acetylation of amonafide, a DNA intercalating agent.[51] Determination of acetylation phenotype can thus be used to modify drug dosing to prevent excess toxicity.

Principles of Drug Selection

Single-agent therapy has largely been replaced by combination chemotherapy when cure is the goal of treatment. There are, however, circumstances in which single agents can be used with curative intent. These include methotrexate or dactinomycin in choriocarcinoma, and interferon, pentostatin, or cladribine (chlorodeoxyadenosine) in hairy cell leukemia.

Combination therapy is now the standard for the treatment of many disseminated or metastatic diseases and is curative in some.[52] Unfortunately, most of these diseases are relatively uncommon hematologic or pediatric malignancies, and the more common neoplasms of adults, such as cancers of the colon and rectum, lung, or breast, once metastatic, are seldom cured.

Chemohormonal therapy is the use of chemotherapeutic agents and hormonal agents, such as prednisone in the MOPP combination program, or prednisone with vincristine and daunorubicin in the treatment of acute lymphocytic leukemia (ALL). The inclusion of tamoxifen after cytoxan and doxorubicin in the chemotherapeutic program for breast cancer is another example. Biologic response modifiers, such as interferon (IFN) or interleukin-2 (IL-2), are used singly or in combination with chemotherapeutic agents.

Differentiating agents, the newest class of anticancer therapies, are currently represented by just one compound, all-trans-retinoic acid, which is effective in acute progranulocytic leukemia.

Route of administration has been usually a straightforward decision. Most chemotherapeutic agents are given intravenously, eliminating problems of compliance and absorption. Many of the hormonal agents and some chemotherapeutic agents, such as alkeran, chlorambucil, myleran, 6-mercaptopurine, and 6-thioguanine, are given by the oral route. More recently, oral etoposide and capcitibine, an oral form of 5-FU, have been added to the armamentarium of oral cytotoxic drugs. Absorption could be enhanced if these drugs are taken on an empty stomach. Methotrexate can be given orally, intravenously, intramuscularly, or intrathecally. IFN and IL-2 are usually given subcutaneously. Some chemotherapeutic agents can be instilled in body cavities to treat effusions, as in the example of bleomycin to treat pleural effusions. Continuous infusion therapy offers a potential advantage for cell cycle–specific drugs, such as antimetabolites, where prolonged exposure may increase cell kill. Cytosine arabinoside is most effective in the treatment of acute granulocytic leukemia, for example, when used as a continuous infusion over seven days.

Venous access must also be considered, and intravenous therapy might not be feasible if this cannot be established. Fortunately, the development of subcutaneously implanted venous access devices (central or peripheral), multilumen external catheters, and peripherally inserted catheters (PIC lines) has permitted the use of chemotherapy in many circumstances in which this was not possible previously.[53]

Drug programs, including dose, should be extracted from published articles and modified according to the patient's end-organ function (Table 25-2).

Dose Modification Guidelines

Drug doses are modified routinely for decreases in blood counts and for changes in renal or hepatic function. Individual protocols should be consulted for possible modifications. Table 25-2 outlines commonly used guidelines for dose reductions. The occurrence of certain toxicities, such as neurotoxicity from the vinca alkaloids or mucositis from methotrexate, is also used as an indication for reduction in dose or cessation of the drug.

Response Criteria

Complete response implies disappearance of all measurable or evaluable disease, signs, symptoms, and biochemical changes related to the tumor for at least 4 weeks, during which time no new lesions may appear. Partial response implies a reduction of greater than 50% in the sum of the products of the perpendicular diameters of all measurable lesions (compared with pretreatment measurements) lasting at least 4 weeks, during which no new lesions may appear and no existing lesion may enlarge. For hepatic lesions, a reduction of greater than 30% in the sum of the measured distances from the costal margin at the midclavicular line and at the xiphoid process to the edge of the liver is required. Stable disease is a less than 50% reduction or a less than 25% increase in the sum of the products of the two perpendicular diameters of all measured lesions, and the appearance of no new lesions for 8 weeks. Progression or relapse is

TABLE 25-2

Dose Modifications for Chemotherapy (% of Dose to Be Given)

HEMATOLOGIC TOXICITY

Platelet Count (/mm³)	Granulocytes/Total WBC			
	>2000/3500	1500–1999/3000–3499	1000–1499/2500–2999	<1000/2499
>100,000	100	75	50	0
50,000–99,000	50	50	50	0
<50,000	0	0	0	0

NEPHROTOXICITY

Drug	Creatinine Clearance			
	>60 mL/min	30–60 mL/min	10–30 mL/min	<10 mL/min
Bleomycin	NC	75	75	50
Cisplatin	NC	50	Omit	Omit
Cyclophosphamide	NC	NC	NC	50
Methotrexate	NC	50	Omit	Omit
Mithramycin	NC	75	75	50
Mitomycin	NC	75	75	50
Nitrosoureas	NC	Omit	Omit	Omit

HEPATOTOXICITY

Bilirubin (mg/dL)	SGOT (IU)	Drug				
		Adriamycin	Daunorubicin	Vinblastine + Vincristine + VP-16	Cyclophosphamide + Methotrexate	5-FU
<1.5	<60	100	100	100	100	100
1.5–3.0	60–180	75	75	50	100	100
3.1–5.0	>180	50	50	Omit	175	100
5.0		Omit	Omit	Omit	Omit	Omit

5-FU, 5-fluorouracil; NC, no change; SGOT, serum glutamic-oxaloacetic transaminase.

defined as an increase in the product of two perpendicular diameters of any measurable lesion by greater than 25% over the size present at entry into the study or, for patients who respond, over the size at time of maximum regression, or the appearance of new areas of malignant disease (usually excluding central nervous system [CNS] metastases). A two-step deterioration in performance status, greater than 10% loss of pretreatment weight, or increasing symptoms in and of themselves, do not constitute progression. Their appearance, however, should initiate a new evaluation for disease extent.

Follow-up

Adjuvant therapy is usually given for a set number of cycles, such as six cycles (or months) of chemotherapy after a modified radical mastectomy or lumpectomy for stage I or II breast cancer. For other situations, such as metastatic disease, it is common to re-evaluate the patient after two to three cycles (months) of therapy to determine its effectiveness. If therapy has clearly produced a response (using the criteria discussed previously) and is tolerable to the patient, it is usually continued for a set number of cycles or for two courses past a complete response (to eliminate any remaining microscopic tumor). If the disease has progressed during this interval, therapy

is discontinued, and a re-evaluation is undertaken. Stable disease after therapy represents the most difficult clinical situation encountered. If the therapy is tolerable to the patient in terms of side effects, then a mutual decision to continue is reasonable, realizing that eventually, progressive disease will be seen.

CHEMOTHERAPEUTIC AGENTS

The information regarding the agents listed in the charts that follow is taken from multiple sources, but the latest information from the manufacturer should be sought before initiating therapy.[48,54-59] Unless otherwise specified, all chemotherapeutic agents are capable of producing some degree of nausea and/or vomiting with administration, and myelosuppression, alopecia, and mucositis and/or diarrhea after treatment. Because most agents are also harmful to the gonads and fetus, these toxicities will not be spelled out. Administration of chemotherapy during pregnancy is warranted only in special circumstances and requires a particularly high level of expertise.[60] The increasing incidence of second malignancies as a late complication following successful chemotherapy should also be noted.

CHEMOTHERAPEUTIC AGENT	DRUG CLASS/MECHANISM OF ACTION	DOSAGE FORMS	DRUG INTERACTIONS	PHARMACOKINETICS/METABOLISM	TOXICITY	INDICATIONS	DOSING
Altretamine (Hexalen)—Hexamethylmelamine, HMM	Alkylating agent.	50-mg capsules.	Metabolism might be slowed by cimetidine or enhanced by phenobarbitol.	Well absorbed by mouth, metabolized in the liver. Elimination half-life 4–13 hours. Metabolites excreted in the urine.	Myelosuppression is dose limiting. Leukopenia, thrombocytopenia, nausea, and vomiting are common. Neurologic toxicity, including confusion, lethargy, weakness, and sensory changes, is common.	Food and Drug Administration (FDA) approved for refractory ovarian carcinoma.	4–12 mg/kg/day in divided doses for 3–6 weeks, or 150 mg/m^2/day for 14 days each cycle; higher doses have been used.
Amifostine (Ethyol)—WR-2721, Ethiofos	Cytoprotectant; free-radical scavenger.	500 mg of powder in vial.	Not known to decrease the effectiveness of any cytotoxic drug, but not yet adequately studied.	Poorly absorbed in the GI tract. After IV infusion, the drug is metabolized to inactive forms in the plasma. Metabolites are cleared in the urine.	Transient hypotension is dose limiting. Nausea, vomiting, and somnolence are common. Sneezing, hypocalcemia, and flushing can be seen.	FDA approved for pretreatment with cisplatin. Useful as a bone marrow, kidney, and nerve cyto-protectant. Useful with other alkylators. Also FDA approved as a radiation protectant to reduce xerostomia.	740 mg/m^2 IV infusion over 15 minutes given 15–30 minutes before the cytotoxic agent or radiation. Lower doses and subcutaneous administration have been used also.
Aminoglutethamide (Cytadren)	Aromatase inhibitor; blocks adrenal conversion of cholesterol to Δ_5-pregnenolone and peripheral conversion of androgens to estrogens.	250-mg tablets.	Aminoglutethamide must be given with hydrocortisone. Induces metabolism of warfarin, theophylline, digoxin, medroxy-progesterone, and dexamethasone.	Well absorbed by mouth, 25% plasma protein bound. Metabolized in the liver, elimination half-life of 7–9 hours. Excreted as unchanged drug and metabolites in the urine.	Adrenal insufficiency is universal and must be treated with corticosteroids. Other common toxicities include fatigue, lethargy, rash, fever, virilization, and hypercholesterolemia.	FDA approved for treatment of hormone-responsive breast cancer, and might be useful in prostate cancer and adrenal carcinoma.	250 mg PO qid with 40 mg of hydrocortisone daily in divided doses. Usually started at 250 mg bid and then increased after 2 weeks.
Amsacrine—AMSA, Acridinyl anisidide	Intercalating agent; topo-isomerase II inhibitor.	75-mg/1.5-mL vials in N,N-dimethyl-acetamide with 13.5 mL lactic acid diluent.	None noted.	Poorly available by oral route. Metabolized by the liver and excreted in bile and urine. Elimination half-life of 6–7 hours. Excretion is both biliary and urinary, as metabolites and unchanged drug.	Myelosuppression is dose limiting. Leukopenia, thrombocytopenia, transient elevation of liver function tests, and local venous irritation are common; nausea and vomiting and cardiac toxicity are seen; mucositis is rare.	Still investigational, used primarily for acute myelogenous leukemia (AML).	90–150 mg/m^2/day for 5 days; may be repeated after recovery of peripheral counts.
Anagrelide (Agrylin)	Inhibitor of platelet aggregation with an exploitable side effect of thrombo-cytopenia, for which the mechanism is unclear.	0.5-mg capsules.	Sucralfate could decrease absorption.	Good oral bioavailability; maximum plasma concentration occurs after 1 hour. The plasma half-life is 1.3 hours. The drug is metabolized extensively in the liver. Metabolites are excreted in the urine.	Other than thrombocytopenia, common toxicities include hypotension, headache, and palpitations. Rare toxicities include anemia, arrhythmias, angina pectoris, and congestive heart failure.	FDA approved for treatment of essential thrombocytosis as an orphan drug.	0.5 mg qid or 1 mg bid.

CHEMOTHERAPEUTIC AGENT	DRUG CLASS/ MECHANISM OF ACTION	DOSAGE FORMS	DRUG INTERACTIONS	PHARMACOKINETICS/ METABOLISM	TOXICITY	INDICATIONS	DOSING
Anastrazole (Arimidex)	Nonsteroidal aromatase inhibitor; blocks estrogen production selectively.	1-mg tablets.	None noted.	Well absorbed from the GI tract, with maximum plasma levels achieved within 2 hours. Terminal elimination half-life is 50 hours. The drug is extensively metabolized in the liver and is eliminated in the urine as metabolites and 10% unchanged drug. Despite hepatic and renal clearance being important, no adjustments are needed for abnormal function of these organs due to the wide therapeutic index of this drug.	The drug is very well tolerated. Asthenia, headache, and hot flashes occur in less than 15% of women. Diarrhea, abdominal pain, anorexia, nausea, and vomiting occur in 10% or fewer. Thrombophlebitis has been reported.	As adjuvant therapy of breast cancer and for treatment of postmenopausal women with breast carcinoma who have progressed on tamoxifen therapy.	1 mg PO q day. Higher doses are no more effective.
Arsenic Trioxide (Trisenox)	Novel arsenical differentiating agent.	Ampules containing 10 mg of drug in 10-mL solution.	None known.	Half-life of this compound is unknown. It is methylated in the liver and eliminated in the urine.	The "differentiation syndrome" is dose limiting and includes leukocytosis, fever, dyspnea, chest pain, tachycardia, hypoxia, and sometimes death. Corticosteroids seem to benefit this syndrome. QT prolongation is common. Common side effects include rash, pruritis, headache, arthralgias, anxiety, bleeding, nausea, and vomiting. Liver and renal toxicity are uncommon.	FDA approved for relapsed acute promyelocytic leukemia.	0.15 mg/kg/day in 100–250 mL of D5W until remission, not to exceed 60 doses, then up to 25 doses over five weeks for consolidation starting 3–6 weeks after achievement of remission.
l-Asparaginase (Elspar)—Colaspase	Naturally occurring enzyme derived from *Escherichia coli* or *Erwinia carotovora* that cleaves the amino acid asparagine, which is an essential amino acid required by rapidly proliferating cells.	10,000-IU vial of lyophilized cake.	None noted.	Not orally bioavailable. After IV or IM injection, the drug is metabolized intravascularly by proteolysis. Elimination half-life of 8–30 hours. No excretion is required.	Hypersensitivity can be life threatening, requiring anaphylaxis precautions and a 2-unit test dose. Coagulopathy is common and requires monitoring. Nausea, vomiting, abdominal cramps, anorexia, elevated liver function tests, and transient renal insufficiency are common. Lethargy, somnolence, fatigue, depression, and confusion are seen, as are pancreatitis and fever.	FDA approved for ALL; also used in AML, late-stage chronic myelogenous leukemia (CML), chronic lymphocytic leukemia (CLL), and non-Hodgkin's lymphomas.	After a 2-unit intradermal test dose, an IM dose of 6000 to 10,000 IU/m² every 3 days for nine doses, or 1000 IU/kg/day IV over 30 minutes for 10 days, has been used.

CHEMOTHERAPEUTIC AGENT	DRUG CLASS/ MECHANISM OF ACTION	DOSAGE FORMS	DRUG INTERACTIONS	PHARMACOKINETICS/ METABOLISM	TOXICITY	INDICATIONS	DOSING
PEG-Asparaginase (Oncaspar)— Pegaspargase	Naturally occurring enzyme, covalently linked to polyethylene glycol to reduce immunogenicity, slow metabolism, and prolong half-life. The enzyme cleaves the amino acid asparagine, which is an essential amino acid required by rapidly proliferating cells.	750 IU/mL in a 5-mL vial. No reconstitution or dilution necessary.	None noted. Can reduce effectiveness of methotrexate if given beforehand due to inhibition of cell division.	The drug is not absorbed by the GI tract. When given by IM injection, it has an elimination half-life of approximately 5 days and is not detected in urine or bile. Metabolized completely, clearance not dependent on renal or hepatic function.	Although less immunogenic that the non-PEGylated form, hypersensitivity and anaphylaxis still can occur. Toxicities similar to those of the non-PEGylated forms are seen, including elevated liver enzymes, coagulopathy, hypercholesterolemia, pancreatitis, hyperglycemia, fever, chills, anorexia, lethargy, confusion, headache, seizures, and azotemia.	FDA approved for treatment of ALL, and, like asparaginase, is also used for other leukemias and non-Hodgkin's lymphomas.	2500 IU/m² IM every 14 days with other chemotherapy agents for induction or maintenance.
Azacitadine— NSC-102816 (Investigational)	Antimetabolite, cytidine analog; incorporated into nucleic acids, causing interruption of or errors in transcription and replication of DNA.	100-mg vial of lyophilized powder.	None noted.	Not orally bioavailable. When administered by IV infusion, the drug is activated inside cells to the triphosphate form. It is deaminated in the liver. The elimination half-life is 3–6 hours. Parent drug and metabolites are excreted in the urine.	Myelosuppression is dose limiting. Leukopenia can be prolonged. Nausea and vomiting are common and can be severe. Diarrhea is common, stomatitis is rare. Hepatic enzyme elevation and liver function compromise are common. Transient azotemia is seen. Lethargy, confusion, and coma have been reported.	Investigational agent for AML.	150–300 mg/m²/day for 5 days every 3 weeks, or 150–200 mg/m² twice weekly for several weeks.
Azathioprine (Imuran)	Purine analogue antimetabolite, which is converted to 6-mercaptopurine in vivo.	50-mg tablets and 100-mg vials of lyophilized powder.	Azathioprine could inhibit the anticoagulant effects of warfarin. Allopurinol blocks the xanthine oxidase–mediated metabolism of azathioprine, requiring reduction of dose for those patients taking allopurinol. Angiotensin-converting enzyme inhibitors could exaggerate the myelo-suppressive effects of azathioprine.	Azathioprine has good oral bioavailability and is rapidly converted to mercaptopurine in the blood compartment. The parent drug and thiol metabolites have a half-life of about 5 hours, but the metabolism of active forms is very rapid, with virtually no azathioprine detectable in urine after a dose. Metabolism occurs in blood and liver. Inactive metabolites are excreted in the urine.	Myelosuppression is expected and dose limiting. Due to chronic dosing of this drug, the effects on leukocytes, platelets, and (to a lesser extent) red cells are slow in onset and usually reversible. A rare metabolic disorder called thiopurine methyltrasferase deficiency results in extreme sensitivity to this drug in affected persons. Nausea and vomiting are common but usually mild and transient during chronic therapy. Opportunistic infections are uncommon. Diarrhea, fever, myalgias, skin rashes, and interstitial pneumonitis are rare. Secondary malignancies have been reported. This drug should not be used during pregnancy or nursing.	FDA approved for renal transplant recipients and for rheumatoid arthritis. Also used in some hematologic malignancies.	Chronic dosing for the above indications is in the range of 1–3 mg/kg/day. Higher doses, using the intravenous formulation, are used in the immediate post-transplant period.

CHEMOTHERAPEUTIC AGENT	DRUG CLASS/ MECHANISM OF ACTION	DOSAGE FORMS	DRUG INTERACTIONS	PHARMACOKINETICS/ METABOLISM	TOXICITY	INDICATIONS	DOSING
Bacillus Calmette-Guérin (TICE BCG, TheraCys)— BCG	Immunostimulant/ vaccine; induces a cellular immune response at the site of instillation.	Freeze-dried powder in vials, 27 mg/vial, supplied with diluent.	Immunosuppressive drugs could block the reaction to BCG and also make the patient more prone to clinical infection from viable BCG organisms.	BCG is a live, attenuated bacteria culture, and as such, it does not enter the body in viable form in any quantity. Therefore, it has no detectable pharmacokinetic fate. In rare cases, however, a clinical infection can result from treatment, indicating invasion of the body at the site of administration into the systemic circulation.	Urinary symptoms predominate, including dysuria, hematuria, hesitancy, urgency, frequency, and secondary infection. Other toxicities include fever, chills, malaise, myalgias/arthralgias, anorexia, nausea, vomiting, and anemia. Clinical mycobacterial infection is rare, and generally is seen only in immuno-compromised patients.	Intravesical instillation is FDA approved for noninvasive bladder cancer after removal of papillary tumors. Also used for some experimental vaccine programs as an adjuvant to the vaccine.	81 mg per treatment, in 53 mL total volume, instructions as given previously. Given once weekly for 6 doses, and then at 3, 6, 12, 18, and 24 months after induction.
Bexarotene (Targretin)	Synthetic retinoid, differentiating agent.	75-mg capsules.	No formal studies done. Drugs that inhibit cytochrome P450 3A4 (e.g., keto-conazole, erythro-mycin, and gemfibrozil) expected to increase plasma levels and half-life of bexa-rotene. Known to decrease plasma levels of tamoxifen with concomitant administration.	Good oral bioavailability increased by a high-fat meal. Metabolized in the liver to oxidative metabolites by cytochrome P450 3A4, glucuronidated, eliminated in the bile.	Hyperlipidemia is dose-limiting and should be monitored while on therapy and treated as appropriate. Pruritis, leukopenia, diarrhea, fatigue, headache, and liver function test elevation can also be dose limiting. Rash, edema, fever, chills, and nausea are uncommon. Excessive bleeding and back or abdominal pain are rare.	FDA approved for treatment of cutaneous T-cell lymphoma (mycosis fungoides) refractory to at least one prior therapy.	300 mg/m² /day orally, dose adjusted for toxicity.
Bicalutamide (Casodex)	Nonsteroidal antiandrogen.	50-mg tablet.	Bicalutamide could enhance the anticoagulant effects of warfarin.	Bicalutamide is well absorbed after oral administration. It is highly protein bound. It undergoes conversion to inactive metabolites in the liver via oxidation and glucuronidation. It has a terminal half-life of several days. Parent drug and metabolites are excreted in the urine and feces.	Constitutional symptoms predominate, including hot flashes, decreased libido, depression, weight gain, edema, gynecomastia, early disease-site pain (flare reaction), and constipation. Nausea, vomiting, anorexia, diarrhea, and dizziness are uncommon. Dyspnea, anemia, fever, and rashes are rare.	FDA approved for stage D2 prostate cancer, in combination with a luteinizing hormone—releasing hormone (LHRH) agonist agent.	50 mg by mouth daily, in combination with an LHRH agonist agent.
Bleomycin (Blenoxane) —Bleo	Antitumor antibiotic; causes DNA strand breaks directly in normal and neoplastic cells.	Available as 15-U (15-mg) vials of lyophilized powder.	None noted.	Bleomycin is not orally bioavailable. After an IV infusion, it has an elimination half-life of 3–5 hours. Bleomycin is incompletely metabolized by intracellular aminopeptidases. Excreted in the kidney as unchanged drug and metabolites.	Pulmonary toxicity, including reversible and irreversible fibrosis, is dose limiting. Other common toxicities include fever, chills, rash, exfoliation, and anorexia. Nausea, vomiting, myelo-suppression, anaphylaxis, and mucositis are rare.	FDA approved for germ cell tumors, Hodgkin's disease, and squamous cell cancers. Used off-label for melanoma, ovarian cancer, and Kaposi's sarcoma. Also used as a sclerosing agent for malignant pleural or pericardial effusions.	After 1–6 hours of observation following a 2-unit IV test dose given over 15 minutes, the full dose can be given. The usual dose is 10–20 units/m² IV, IM, or SC one to two times per week or 15–20 units/ m² /day as a continuous infusion over 3–7 days. As a sclerosing agent, 60 units are generally used.

I

CHEMOTHERAPEUTIC AGENT	DRUG CLASS/ MECHANISM OF ACTION	DOSAGE FORMS	DRUG INTERACTIONS	PHARMACOKINETICS/ METABOLISM	TOXICITY	INDICATIONS	DOSING
Buserelin (Suprefact)— HOE 766	LHRH agonist; shuts off luteinizing hormone and follicle-stimulating hormone secretion, thereby resulting in chemical castration.	Available as vials for injection at 1 mg/mL and as an intranasal spray in a 10-mL canister.	Could cause pain flares in bone metastases if not given with a direct hormonal antagonist.	Intravascular and extravascular proteolysis.	Flare reactions as noted previously, which can be prevented. Castration symptoms such as hot flashes and decreased libido common. Other non-specific symptoms include headache, nausea, vomiting, diarrhea, constipation, weakness.	FDA approved for prostatic cancer.	500 µg SC tid for the first week, then 200 mg/day, or intranasally 800 mg tid followed by 400 mg tid.
Busulfan (Myleran)—BSF	Alkylating agent.	2-mg scored tablets (an IV form is not yet widely available).	None noted.	Excellent oral bioavailability, with peak levels in serum occurring at about 1 hour. Elimination half-life of 2.5 hours. Metabolized partially in liver. Parent drug and metabolites excreted in the urine.	Myelosuppression, partly chronic and cumulative, is dose limiting. Other common toxicities include nausea, vomiting, anorexia, mucositis, hyper-pigmentation, and elevated liver function tests (or veno-occlusive disease of the liver at transplant doses). Neurologic toxicity, including blurred vision, dizziness, and confusion, and interstitial lung disease are less common.	Regular-dose therapy in CML (FDA approved) and polycythemia vera. High-dose therapy in bone marrow transplant.	Regular dose: 4–8 mg/day. High dose: 8–16 mg/kg total dose.
Capecitibine (Xeloda)	Oral antimetabolite prodrug.	150-mg and 500-mg tablets.	Capecitibine increases the half-life, AUC, and prothrombin time effect of warfarin. Maalox, when given immediately after capecitibine, increases the oral bioavailability of capecitibine.	Readily absorbed by the GI tract, metabolized in vivo to fluorouracil in the liver by carboxylesterase and cytidine deaminase, and then in turn in the peripheral tissues and tumor tissue by thymidine phosphorylase. Capecitibine appears to produce higher levels of fluorouracil in tumor tissue than in normal tissues, probably because thymidine phosphorylase is expressed at higher levels in most tumor tissues.	Myelosuppression and palmar-plantar erythrodysesthesia are dose limiting. Diarrhea, fatigue, stomatitis, and hyperbilirubinemia are uncommon. Nausea, vomiting, and rash are rare.	FDA approved for metastatic breast cancer and metastatic colorectal cancer. Used also in head and neck squamous cell cancer.	The approved dose and schedule is 1250 mg/m² every 12 hours for 14 days every 21 days. Dose reductions are often required. Treatment delays are sometimes required. Other doses and schedules have been used.
Carboplatin (Paraplatin)— Carbo, CBDCA	Atypical alkyator; produces intra- and interstrand crosslinks in DNA via association bonds with the platinum molecule, leading to DNA strand breakage during replication.	Available as powder in glass vials, 50, 150, and 450 mg/vial	None noted.	Carboplatin is not orally bioavailable. It is rapidly cleared from the bloodstream after IV infusion, with a terminal half-life of 2.5 hours. It is cleared largely as unchanged drug by the kidneys.	Myelosuppression, especially thrombocytopenia, is dose limiting. Nausea and vomiting are mild. Renal and neuronal toxicity are rare.	FDA approved for ovarian cancer, and used extensively in testicular cancer; squamous cell cancers of the head, neck, and cervix; and lung cancer.	Dosing can be done on a per-meter-squared basis, or through several formulas that take into account renal function and desired level of thrombocytopenia (such as Calvert's formula). Typical doses with normal renal function are in the 300–500-mg/m² range as an IV infusion.

CHEMOTHERAPEUTIC AGENT	DRUG CLASS/MECHANISM OF ACTION	DOSAGE FORMS	DRUG INTERACTIONS	PHARMACOKINETICS/METABOLISM	TOXICITY	INDICATIONS	DOSING
Carmustine (BiCNU)—BCNU, Bischloronitrosourea	Alkylator agent in the nitrosourea class. Cell cycle–independent mechanism.	100-mg vial of carmustine powder and 3 mL vial of ethanol.	None noted.	Poorly available by the oral route. After an IV infusion, the drug is rapidly taken up by tissues, including the CNS. Extensively metabolized in the liver. The serum half-life is only 15 to 20 minutes. The parent drug and metabolites are cleared by the kidney.	Myelosuppression, which is slow in onset and cumulative, is dose limiting. Nausea and vomiting are common and can be severe. Hyperpigmentation and renal toxicity can be seen. Interstitial lung disease, including fibrosis, is rare but can occur with any dose. Transplant doses can cause severe liver toxicity and more frequent lung toxicity.	FDA approved for brain tumors, multiple myeloma, Hodgkin's disease, lymphoma. Also used for breast cancer, melanoma, stomach cancer, colon cancer, and liver cancer.	Single-agent dose is 150–200 mg/m² every 6 weeks. For transplant, the dose is as high as 600 mg/m², along with other drugs.
Carmustine Impregnated Wafer (Gliadel)—Polifeprosan 20 with Carmustine Implant	Novel delivery mechanism for classical nitrosurea alkylating agent.	Each individually packaged, sterile wafer contains 7.7 mg of carmustine.	No interactions known.	More than 70% of the copolymer degrades by 3 weeks. Gliadel wafers produce minimal systemic exposure to carmustine. The copolymer itself is biodegradable, but metabolites of the polymer have no known or expected pharmacologic implications.	Some toxicities at carmustine but less common due to local nature of therapy. Central nervous system toxicity possible.	FDA approved for adjuvant treatment of recurrent glioblastoma multiforme. Being tested in the setting of initial resection.	Up to eight wafers are placed in the resection cavity at the time of craniotomy and operative resection.
Chlorambucil (Leukeran)	Alkylating agent. Cell cycle independent.	2-mg tablets.	None noted.	Excellent oral bioavailability; maximum plasma level at 1 hour. Elimination half-life of 1 to 2 hours. Extensively metabolized in the liver to active and inactive metabolites, which are excreted via the kidneys.	Myelosuppression is dose limiting and universal, and it can be cumulative. Nausea, vomiting, and diarrhea are mild and uncommon. Sterility and alopecia occurs in a minority of patients. Pulmonary fibrosis and neurologic side effects are quite rare.	FDA approved for chronic lymphocytic leukemia (CLL) and low-grade lymphomas. Also used for Waldenström's macroglobulinemia, multiple myeloma, hairy cell leukemia, and rarely in some solid tumors.	16 mg/m²/day for 5 days every 4 weeks, or 0.4 mg/kg every 2 to 4 weeks, or 0.1–0.2 mg/kg/day for 3–6 weeks.
Cisplatin (Platinol)—cDDP, DDP, Cisplatinum, Cis-diamminedi-chloroplatinum (II)	Atypical alkylator; produces intra- and interstrand crosslinks in DNA via association bonds with the platinum molecule, leading to DNA strand breakage during replication.	Lyophilized powder in sealed vials of 10 mg and 50 mg, and as a 1-mg/mL solution in bottles of 50 mg and 100 mg.	None noted.	Poor oral bioavailability. After IV infusion, rapid distribution to tissues takes place, and the drug is more than 90% protein bound. Although the distribution half-life is less than 1 hour, the terminal half-life is 60–90 hours due to tissue retention. Not extensively metabolized. Elimination is via the kidneys.	Nephrotoxicity is dose limiting for an individual dose, while neurotoxicity, especially painful peripheral neuropathy, is dose limiting for cumulative doses. Myelosuppression is mild. Nausea and vomiting are common but manageable, and anorexia and diarrhea are common. Cumulative ototoxicity is also common. Chronic renal magnesium and potassium wasting is	Used for almost every class of solid tumor and lymphoma. FDA approved for testicular and ovarian cancers and transitional cell carcinoma.	Cisplatin can be given all in one IV infusion or daily as an IV infusion for several days for each cycle. Daily divided doses are somewhat better tolerated. The total dose per cycle ranges from 80 to 160 mg/m². Continuous infusion can also be used. Dose should be reduced for a creatinine clearance below

CHEMOTHERAPEUTIC AGENT	DRUG CLASS/ MECHANISM OF ACTION	DOSAGE FORMS	DRUG INTERACTIONS	PHARMACOKINETICS/ METABOLISM	TOXICITY	INDICATIONS	DOSING
					common and sometimes not reversible. Elevated liver transaminases can be seen, while alopecia and cardiac conduction abnormalities are rare.		60 mL/min. Adequate renal perfusion and urine output are critical for minimizing renal toxicity, and therefore prehydration and adequate post-treatment hydration are used, usually with normal saline with or without mannitol, potassium, and magnesium, along with the cisplatin. Cisplatin 100–200 mg/m^2 is also used intraperitoneally for ovarian cancer.
Cladribine (Leustatin)— Chlorodeoxy-adenosine, 2-CdA	Antimetabolite, purine analog; cytotoxic to dividing and nondividing cells via disruption of DNA function.	1-mg/mL solution in 20-mL vials.	None noted.	Not orally bioavailable. After IV administration, it has a distribution half-life of 36 minutes and an elimination half-life of 7 hours. Resistant to adenosine deaminase. Chemical conversion to the active form takes place intracellularly in all cells that have deoxycytidine kinase activity. Further information on metabolism and excretion is not available.	Renal toxicity is dose limiting, but at the typical doses used, myelosuppression is most prominent, including universal lymphopenia and common neutropenia and thrombocytopenia. Fever is common, while nausea and vomiting are rare and mild, and neurologic reactions are rare.	FDA approved for hairy cell leukemia. Also used in chronic and acute leukemias, lymphoma, and mycosis fungoides.	For hairy cell leukemia, the dose is 0.1 mg/kg/ day for 7 days as a continuous IV infusion, as a single treatment, or repeated once. Other doses have ranged from 0.1 to 0.3 mg/kg/day for 5 to 7 days. Can also be given subcutaneously.
Cyclophosphamide (Cytoxan, Neosar)— CTX, CPM, Cy	Prototypical alkylator drug. Cell cycle independent.	25-mg and 50-mg tablets for oral use, and vials of powder in 100-, 200-, 500-, 1000-, and 2000-mg sizes for IV administration.	None noted.	75% oral bioavailability; peak serum levels occur approximately 1 hour after administration. Activated by hepatic enzymes, and metabolized to inactive forms in the liver as well. Elimination half-life is 3–10 hours. Parent drug and metabolites are excreted in the urine.	Myelosuppression is dose limiting, with leukopenia being most significant. Nausea and vomiting are common, and can be chronic with oral administration. Hemorrhagic cystitis is uncommon with standard doses, but is common with doses over 2 g/m^2. Other toxicities of high-dose therapy include syndrome of inappropriate secretion of antidiuretic hormone, pulmonary fibrosis, and hemorrhagic myocarditis. Secondary malignancies are rare but well documented.	FDA approved for many malignancies and used for even more. Most commonly used for breast carcinoma, non-Hodgkin's lymphoma, ovarian carcinoma, and testicular cancer.	Doses range from 50 mg/m^2 for 14 days every 28 days, to standard IV doses of 600–2000 mg/m^2 once every 21 to 28 days, to transplant doses of 60 mg/kg IV for 2 days.

CHEMOTHERAPEUTIC AGENT	DRUG CLASS/ MECHANISM OF ACTION	DOSAGE FORMS	DRUG INTERACTIONS	PHARMACOKINETICS/ METABOLISM	TOXICITY	INDICATIONS	DOSING
Cytarabine (Cytosar-U)— AraC, Cytosine Arabinoside	Antimetabolite; incorporated into DNA during replication, leading to strand termination. This drug is S-phase specific.	Comes in 100-mg– 2000-mg vials of powdered drug.	None noted.	Parenteral bioavailability only. After an IV dose, it is distributed rapidly into tissues, where it is converted to AraC triphosphate and rapidly deaminated in the blood. It has an elimination half-life of 2–3 hours. Eliminated through the kidneys.	Myelosuppression, often severe and prolonged, is dose limiting. It affects all lineages. Nausea, vomiting, anorexia, mucositis, and diarrhea are common. Skin erythema with exfoliation is common. Keratitis and conjunctivitis are common. Hepatic inflammation and elevation of liver function tests are common. Flulike syndrome with fever is common. Neurologic toxicity, mostly central with ataxia being predominant, is common and usually mild, but it is dose dependent and could leave permanent dysfunction. It is more common with intrathecal administration. Pulmonary infiltrates after administration are uncommon but can be fatal. Cardiac complications are rare.	Acute myelogenous leukemia (AML), acute lymphoblastic lymphoma (ALL), and non-Hodgkin's lymphoma. Intrathecal use in acute leukemia.	Doses range from 100 mg/m²/day for 7 days as bolus or continuous infusion to 3 g/m² every 12 hours for 3 days. Doses less than 500 mg/m² are considered standard, while doses of 1 g/m² or more are considered high. The intrathecal dose is generally from 12 mg total dose up to 30 mg/m², given intermittently during systemic treatment.
Cytarabine, Liposomal (DepoCyt)	Novel liposomal preparation of an antimetabolite for extended exposure to cancer cells in the cerebrospinal fluid.	Vials containing 50 mg of drug in aqueous liposomal solution.	Minimal systemic exposure after intrathecal administration. Drug interactions not considered clinically important.	After intrathecal administration of liposomes, peak levels of cytarabine occur in the CSF at 5 hours, and half-life of cytarabine in the CSF is 100–200 hours. Cytarabine and metabolites eventually enter the plasma compartment, where they are eliminated in the urine.	Chemical arachnoiditis is common and dose limiting. Headache and back pain are the major clinical manifestations. Myelosuppression is common but usually mild. Fever, nausea, and vomiting are uncommon. Neurologic side effects are also uncommon.	FDA approved for treatment of lymphomatous meningitis. Appears to be active in leukemic meningitis and carcinomatous meningitis, but published experience is limited.	50 mg intrathecally via spinal needle or Ommaya reservoir over 1–5 minutes every 14 days for up to 9 doses and then every 28 days for up to 4 doses.
Dacarbazine (DTIC-Dome)—DTIC, DIC, Imidazole Carboxamide	Atypical alkylator; methylates guanine bases preferentially. Non-cell cycle dependent.	Vials of lyophylized drug containing 100, 200, or 1000 mg.	None noted.	Not orally bioavailable. After IV administration, the drug is activated by demethylation by microsomal enzymes in the liver and further metabolized to inactive forms. The elimination half-life is 3–5 hours. Active and inactive metabolites are largely excreted in the urine.	Myelosuppression is dose limiting. Nausea and vomiting are severe without aggressive antiemetic therapy. Fever is common and flulike syndrome is uncommon, as are diarrhea, stomatitis, alopecia, rash, or significant liver or renal toxicity.	FDA approved for the treatment of malignant melanoma and Hodgkin's disease, and also used for adult sarcomas and neuroblastoma.	Given by intravenous piggyback in doses of 375–1450 mg/m² every 2–3 weeks or 50–250 mg/m²/day for 5–10 days every 3–4 weeks.

CHEMOTHERAPEUTIC AGENT	DRUG CLASS/MECHANISM OF ACTION	DOSAGE FORMS	DRUG INTERACTIONS	PHARMACOKINETICS/METABOLISM	TOXICITY	INDICATIONS	DOSING
Dactinomycin (Cosmegen)—Actinomycin D, ACT-D	Antitumor antibiotic, inhibits transcription by complexing with DNA.	Available in vials of 0.5 mg of lyophilized drug.	None noted.	Poor oral bioavailability. After an IV dose, the drug is widely distributed except to the cerebrospinal fluid. It is metabolized in the liver. It has an elimination half-life of 30–40 hours. Dactinomycin and its metabolites are excreted in both bile and urine.	This drug is a moderate vesicant. Myelosuppression is dose limiting. Nausea, vomiting, skin erythema, acneiform lesions, and hyperpigmentation are common, while mucositis, diarrhea, and anorexia are uncommon. Hepatitis, ascites, fever, and hypocalcemia are rare.	FDA approved for Wilms' tumor, Ewing's sarcoma, rhabdomysarcoma, uterine carcinoma, germ cell tumors, and sarcoma botryoides, and also used for other sarcomas, melanoma, acute myeloid leukemia, ovarian cancer, and trophoblastic neoplasms.	1–2 mg/m² every 3 weeks or continuous infusions of 0.25–0.6 mg/m²/day for 5 days every 3–4 weeks.
Darbopoetin Alfa (Aranesp)	Erythropoietic growth factor, modified recombinant DNA peptide product.	Vials containing 25, 40, 60, 100, 150, 200, 300, and 500 mg of drug in 1 mL of either albumin or polysorbate aqueous solution.	No formal drug studies have been done. Exogenous testosterone and erythropoietin products used together could cause polycythemia.	After subcutaneous administration, absorption into the bloodstream is slow and dose limiting. Peak concentration occurs at approximately 30 hours, and half-life in the bloodstream is 30–90 hours. Metabolic fates and routes of elimination have not been studied formally.	Polycythemia can occur, and thus hemoglobin must be monitored during therapy. No other form of dose-limiting toxicity is known. Either hypertension or hypotension is common. Headache is uncommon. Cardiovascular events, including myocardial infarction, arrhythmia, or stroke, are uncommon but can be serious. Fever, edema, or pain is rare.	FDA approved for anemia caused by cancer chemotherapy for nonmyeloid malignancies and anemia associated with chronic renal insufficiency.	For anemia and renal insufficiency, the indicated dose is 0.45 mcg/kg SC or IV once weekly, titrated upward to achieve the target hemoglobin level of 12 g/dL. For anemic cancer patients receiving chemotherapy, the recommended dose is 2.25 mcg/kg SC once weekly, again with slow upward titration as needed to achieve a specific hemoglobin goal. Every other week and every 3 week doses are currently under evaluation.
Daunorubicin (Daunomycin, Cerubidine)—Rubidomycin	Anthracycline antitumor antibiotic, intercalating agent.	20-mg vials of powdered drug for reconstitution.	None noted.	Not orally bioavailable. After IV bolus, the drug is widely distributed and metabolized in the liver to active and inactive metabolites. The elimination of the parent drug is 18 hours, and that of the active metabolite daunorubicinol is about 25 hours. Elimination of parent drug and metabolites occurs via biliary and renal routes.	Daunorubicin is a vesicant. Precautions are necessary. Myelosuppression is dose limiting. Alopecia, nausea, vomiting, and stomatitis are common. Diarrhea, rash, elevated liver function tests, and transient arrhythmias are uncommon. Dose-related cardiomyopathy is uncommon below cumulative doses of 400–500 mg/m².	FDA approved for AML and ALL.	Given as a single IV injection daily for 1–5 days. Total dose per course up to 150 mg/m². A typical dose would be 45 mg/m²/day for 3 days.

CHEMOTHERAPEUTIC AGENT	DRUG CLASS/ MECHANISM OF ACTION	DOSAGE FORMS	DRUG INTERACTIONS	PHARMACOKINETICS/ METABOLISM	TOXICITY	INDICATIONS	DOSING
Daunorubicin, Liposomal (Daunosome)	Novel liposomal preparation of the anthracycline DNA intercalating agent daunorubicin, which modifies the pharmacokinetics and toxicities of the drug.	Single-use vials containing 50 mg of daunoru-bicin in an aqueous liposomal solution at a concentration of 2 mg/mL.	Significant interactions of liposomal daunorubicin and other drugs have not been observed.	Daunorubicin liposomes have a small volume of distribution after IV administration but are cleared rapidly from the plasma compartment into peripheral tissues with a half-life of about 4 hours. Low levels of metabolites are detected in the plasma, likely due to slow distribution of parent drug from the peripheral tissues to the liver for metabolism. Metabolic fates are as for the conventional drug.	In general, this agent has a milder side effect and toxicity profile than conventional daunorubicin. Myelosuppression is mild but still dose limiting. An acute syndrome of back pain, chest tightness, and flushing can occur uncommonly during administration, which can usually be treated symptomatically. Other cardiac side effects are rare. Skin rashes are rare. Nausea, vomiting, and alopecia are rare.	FDA approved for treatment of AIDS-associated Kaposi's sarcoma. Some experience in other solid tumors.	40 mg/m² IV infusion over 60 minutes every 2 weeks, with reduction and delay for significant myelosuppression.
Denileukin Diftitox (Ontak)	Recombinant DNA peptide fusion product combining interleukin-2 and a diphtheria toxin, allowing relative specificity of diphtheria toxin toward interleukin-2 receptor-expressing cells.	Vials of 300 µg in 2-mL frozen aqueous solution.	None known.	After IV administration, the plasma half-life of denileukin diftitox is about 80 minutes. Radiolabeling studies show that the drug accumulates in the vasculature, liver, and kidneys, but its specific metabolic fates are unknown. Antibodies against the drug have been shown to slow its clearance.	Denileukin diftitox has a broad range of toxicities similar to other peptide biological response modifiers, with hypotension and other manifestations of vascular leak syndrome being dose limiting. Fever, chills, edema, rash, fatigue, headache, nausea, vomiting, anorexia, and diarrhea are common. Dyspnea, cough, arthralgias, myalgias, and pharyngitis are uncommon. Infections associated with drug administration are common. Arrhythmias and significant neurologic, hepatic, or renal complications are rare.	FDA approved for recurrent cutaneous T-cell lymphoma (mycosis fungoides).	9 or 18 mcg/kg/day for 5 days as an IV infusion over at least 15 minutes, repeated every 21 days.
Dexamethasone (Decadron)—Dex, DXM	Corticosteroid that has pleiotrophic properties in various body tissues. Directly toxic to benign and malignant lymphocytes. Potent anti-inflammatory action.	Tablets ranging from 0.25 mg to 6 mg are available, as are an oral solution at 0.1 mg/mL and a solution for injection at 4–24 mg/mK.	Drugs that induce hepatic microsomal enzymes can enhance the metabolism of dexamethasone and decrease its effectiveness. This includes phenytoin, tegretol, and dilantin.	Well absorbed by the GI tract. Metabolized in the liver. Elimination half-life is 3–4 hours. Elimination of metabolites is primarily renal, with some biliary component.	Toxicities are shared with other corticosteroids and include leukocytosis, hyperglycemia, mood changes, euphoria, insomnia, increased appetite, weight gain, dyspepsia, exacerbation of peptic ulcer disease, cataracts, adrenal suppression, edema, and osteoporosis.	Used for many purposes in oncology and hematology patients, including treatment of multiple myeloma, CLL and ALL, non–Hodgkin's lymphoma, immune thrombocytopenic purpura, and hemolytic anemia. Also used to alleviate symptoms from brain or spinal cord metastases and other metastatic sites where edema and inflammation exist. Also used as an adjunctive antiemetic medication.	Oral and parenteral dosing are equivalent. Dosage for acute indications or active treatment involves total daily doses of 16–40 mg, sometimes with an initial "bolus" dose of up to 100 mg. Tapering treatments will decrease down to 1–2 mg/day. As an antiemetic, 10–20 mg is the standard dose.

CHEMOTHERAPEUTIC AGENT	DRUG CLASS/ MECHANISM OF ACTION	DOSAGE FORMS	DRUG INTERACTIONS	PHARMACOKINETICS/ METABOLISM	TOXICITY	INDICATIONS	DOSING
Dexrazoxane (Zinecard)— ADR-529, ICRF-187	Iron-chelating agent that serves as a free-radical scavenger/ cytoprotectant.	Lyophilized powder, 500 mg/vial, with diluent.	None noted.	The drug is not bioavailable by the oral route. After an IV dose, distribution in the body is widespread and rapid. Metabolism is predominantly hepatic. The terminal half-life is 3–4 hours. Parent drug and metabolites are excreted by the kidneys.	Dexrazoxone appears to worsen slightly the leukopenia induced by doxorubicin. Mild nausea and vomiting are common, fever, stomatitis, fatigue, anorexia, and hypotension are uncommon. Seizure, respiratory arrest, deep venous thrombosis, and significant liver toxicity are rare.	FDA approved as an "orphan drug" to prevent doxorubicin-induced cardiomyopathy.	Administered just prior to a dose of doxorubicin as a 15–30-minute infusion at a dose of 500–1000 mg/m².
Docetaxel (Taxotere)— RP-56976	Docetaxel is a semisynthetic taxane, a class of compounds that inhibit the mitotic spindle apparatus by stabilizing tubulin polymers, leading to death of mitotic cells.	20- and 80-mg vials at a concentration of 40 mg/mL in polysorbate 80 solvent.	Docetaxel given concurrently with cisplatin has been reported to increase the incidence and severity of peripheral neuropathy.	The drug has poor oral bioavailability. After a 1-hour infusion, docetaxel is widely distributed and has a triphasic elimination course, with a distribution half-life of 4 minutes, an elimination half-life of 1 hour, and a terminal half-life of 18 hours. Extent and byproducts of metabolism are not well known. The main excretion route is biliary.	Myelosuppression is universal and dose limiting. Alopecia is also universal. Edema and fluid accumulation, including pleural effusions and ascites, are common and can be dose limiting. Fluid accumulation is partially preventable with corticosteroid treatment before and after each cycle of docetaxel. Mild sensory or sensorimotor neuropathy is common. Mucositis and diarrhea are common and usually mild. Hypersensitivity reactions are uncommon and can be largely prevented through premedication with corticosteroids and antihistamines. Rash and elevated liver function tests are uncommon.	FDA approved for metastatic breast cancer and first- and second-line non–small cell lung cancer. Clinical experience increasing in ovarian cancer and other epithelial neoplasms.	The standard dose is 100 mg/m² IV over 1 hour every 3 weeks. Higher doses and other schedules have been used.
Doxorubicin (Adriamycin, Rubex)— Adria, Hydroxydaunorubicin	Anthracycline antitumor antibiotic, intercalating agent.	Available in vials of lyophilized powder containing 10 mg–150 mg of drug and as vials of 2-mg/mL solution in 10-mg–200-mg vials.	None noted.	The drug has poor oral bioavailability. After an IV dose, it is widely distributed in tissues and is 70% protein bound. It is metabolized in the liver to active and inactive forms. It has an elimination half-life of 18 hours or more. Most of the drug and metabolites are excreted through the biliary route.	Doxorubicin is a potent vesicant, and extravasation precautions are a must. Myelosuppression is universal and usually dose limiting with each individual cycle. Cardiotoxicity is common and can be dose limiting, though usually subclinical. Chronic, cumulative cardiomyopathy is expected when total dose exceeds 400–500 mg/m².	FDA approved for a variety of cancers, and used for many more. Most commonly used for breast carcinoma, adult sarcomas, pediatric solid tumors, Hodgkin's disease, non–Hodgkin's lymphomas, and ovarian cancer.	Standard doses range from 60 to 90 mg/m² IV as a bolus or continuous infusion over 48–72 hours every 3–4 weeks. Weekly and biweekly schedules are also used, with lower doses. Doses are usually reduced for elevated bilirubin levels.

CHEMOTHERAPEUTIC AGENT	DRUG CLASS/ MECHANISM OF ACTION	DOSAGE FORMS	DRUG INTERACTIONS	PHARMACOKINETICS/ METABOLISM	TOXICITY	INDICATIONS	DOSING
					This toxicity can be lessened by addition of dexrazoxone or by longer infusions. Acute cardiac effects, including arrhythmias, are seen less often and are unpredictable. Nausea and vomiting are common but manageable. Diarrhea and stomatitis are common but usually mild. Alopecia, rash, and hyper-pigmentation are common.		
Doxorubicin, Liposomal (Doxil)	Novel liposomal preparation of the anthracycline DNA intercalating agent doxorubicin.	Vials of 20 mg in 10 mL and 50 mg in 25 mL of doxorubicin in aqueous liposomal dispersion.	No formal drug interaction studies have been conducted. No important drug interactions have been reported.	The parent drug, doxorubicin, is metabolized in the liver and excreted primarily in the bile. Significant levels of the principal metabolite, doxorubicinol, have not been observed with the liposomal preparation, likely due to the slow distribution of free doxorubicin to the liver. The half-life of the liposomes in the plasma compartment is approximately 55 hours.	Myelosuppression is mild but dose limiting. Palmar and plantar erythrodys-esthesia is common and can occasionally be severe and dose limiting. Stomatitis and nausea are common but usually mild. Alopecia is uncommon. Acute infusion reactions including chest pain, back pain, dyspnea, and wheezing can occur uncommonly.	FDA approved for recurrent metastatic ovarian cancer and AIDS-related Kaposi's sarcoma. Also used commonly in metastatic breast cancer and multiple myeloma.	50 mg/m^2 IV infusion over 1 hour for ovarian cancer; 20 mg/m^2 IV infusion over 30 minutes for Kaposi's sarcoma.
Epirubicin (Ellence)	Anthracycline DNA intercalating agent.	Vials of 50 mg in 25 mL or 200 mg in 100 mL of aqueous solution.	Additive toxicities with other cytotoxic drugs should be expected. Cardiac toxicity of epirubicin can be enhanced when used with other drugs that can temporarily or permanently impair cardiac function. Cimetidine increases the AUC of epirubicin and should be stopped before starting epirubicin.	Epirubicin is metabolized primarily by the liver. The parent drug and metabolites are glucuronidated, and excreted in the bile much more than via renal clearance. Doses should be reduced for patients with mild to moderate hepatic dysfunction. Severe hepatic dysfunction is a contraindication for using epirubicin. Half-life of plasma levels is about 30–35 hours after IV administration.	Myelosuppression is universal and dose limiting. Alopecia is expected. This drug is a vesicant and precaution must be taken to avoid extravasation into soft tissue around veins. Nausea and vomiting are common but usually manageable. Stomatitis is common. Fatigue is common. Detectable cardiac dysfunction is uncommon to rare. Secondary leukemia is rare.	FDA approved for adjuvant therapy after optimal surgical treatment of localized breast cancer with involved axillary lymph nodes.	100–120 mg/m^2 by intravenous infusion every 3–4 weeks. Usually combined with cyclophosphamide and 5-fluorouracil.
Erythropoietin (Epogen, Procrit)— EPO, Eepoitin Alpha	Hematopoietic growth factor. Stimulates erythrocytic precursors.	Vials of 2000, 4000, and 10,000 units in solution.	Erythropoietin might temporarily decrease the effectiveness of heparin when the two drugs are given	This peptide must be given parenterally. After IV or subcutaneous dosing, it is detectable in plasma for 24 hours. It is distributed to a volume approximating	Hypertension is common but usually mild and not dose limiting. Injection site pain is common but mild. Flulike syndrome and diaphoresis are	The oncology indication is chemotherapy-induced anemia that is symptomatic. Also used for anemia of chronic renal failure and human	Starting doses of 150 U/kg SC three times per week were recommended, with increases up to 300 U/kg if there is

CHEMOTHERAPEUTIC AGENT	DRUG CLASS/ MECHANISM OF ACTION	DOSAGE FORMS	DRUG INTERACTIONS	PHARMACOKINETICS/ METABOLISM	TOXICITY	INDICATIONS	DOSING
			simultaneously. Oral aluminum–containing antacids could decrease the effectiveness of erythropoietin.	the total blood volume. It is degraded by proteolysis within the blood compartment. The half-life ranges from 4 to 27 hours. Onset of therapeutic effect takes at least 7 days. Excretion of intact peptide is negligible.	uncommon. Nausea and vomiting are rare. Seizures have been reported in dialysis patients receiving the drug. Iron deficiency anemia can occur after prolonged therapy, and concomitant iron administration can increase the effectiveness of erythropoietin. Hematocrit values should be monitored closely while on therapy to prevent polycythemia and hyperviscosity.	immunodeficiency virus (HIV)–associated anemia.	suboptimal effect after 6–8 weeks, although 40,000 units weekly with increases to 60,000 units is the most commonly used program.
Estramustine (Emcyt)	A conjugate of estrogen and an alkylating moiety, estramustine appears to work through estrogen-binding proteins to kill malignant cells through a nonalkylator mechanism, perhaps by inhibition of microtubules.	140-mg capsules.	None noted.	Well absorbed by mouth, subject to hepatic metabolism, with a terminal half-life of about 20 hours. Excretion route is not clearly delineated.	Nausea and vomiting are common and dose limiting but diminish over time. Headache, edema, decreased libido, and impotence are common. Gynecomastia and breast tenderness can be seen. Rash, alopecia, myelosuppression, hepatic toxicity, and thromboembolic events are rare.	FDA approved for the treatment of prostate cancer. Not used commonly for any other types of cancer.	The usual dose for prostate cancer is 15 mg/kg/day, which is typically given as 420 mg PO tid for most men.
Etoposide (Vespid)— VP-16, Epipodophyllotoxin; Also Available as Etoposide Phosphate (Etopophos)	Plant alkaloid; topoisomerase II inhibitor. Partially cell cycle dependent.	Etoposide comes in oral form as 50-mg capsules and in parenteral form as 100-mg multidose vials in solution at 20 mg/mL. Etoposide phosphate is available in 100-mg single-dose vials as lyophilized powder.	None noted.	Etoposide phosphate is rapidly converted to etoposide after IV infusion. Etoposide itself is extensively protein bound, metabolized in the liver, and has an elimination half-life of about 10 hours. About 50% of oral etoposide is absorbed via the GI tract, requiring oral doses to be twice as high as parenteral doses. Excreted both unchanged in the urine and as metabolites in the bile.	Myelosuppression, primarily leukopenia, is universal and dose limiting. Nausea and vomiting are common with PO administration but rare when the drug is given IV. Stomatitis and diarrhea are rare with normal doses but common with high doses. Alopecia is mild or absent. Hepatic toxicity and neuro-logic effects (peripheral neuropathy and CNS changes) are rare. Hypo-tension can occur with rapid administration of etoposide, but does not occur commonly when etoposide phosphate is infused over 5 minutes. Secondary AML has been reported after etoposide.	FDA approved for germ cell tumors and SCLC. Also used for lymphomas, AML, brain tumors, non-SCLC, and as high-dose therapy in the transplant setting for breast cancer, ovarian cancer, and lymphomas.	Etoposide can either be given over several days or at lower doses over many days. Typical doses are 50–120 mg/m²/day for 3–5 days given IV. Oral doses are generally twice the IV doses. A typical protracted oral course would be 50 mg/m²/day for 21 days given every 28 days. Transplant doses up to 1200 mg/m² over 1–3 days have been used.

CHEMOTHERAPEUTIC AGENT	DRUG CLASS/MECHANISM OF ACTION	DOSAGE FORMS	DRUG INTERACTIONS	PHARMACOKINETICS/METABOLISM	TOXICITY	INDICATIONS	DOSING
Exemestane (Aromasin)	Hormonal agent, steroidal aromatase inhibitor.	25-mg tablets.	In spite of the fact that exemestane is metabolized by cytochrome P450 3A4, ketoconazole does not affect its half-life or AUC, and no other drug-drug interactions have been identified.	After oral administration, approximately 40% of exemestane is absorbed from the gastrointestinal tract. Absorption is increased by a fatty meal. It is highly protein bound in the plasma. Exemestane is metabolized in the liver by cytochrome P450 3A4 and aldoketo-reductase. Metabolites are eliminated equally in urine and feces.	Though generally well-tolerated, exemestane is expected to cause or exacerbate hot flashes or intermittent flushing in some women. Fatigue and mild nausea are common. Vomiting, headache, and dyspnea are uncommon. It is teratogenic and should not be used in premenopausal women.	FDA approved for treatment of estrogen-responsive metastatic breast cancer in postmenopausal women who have progressed on prior hormonal therapy.	25 mg orally once daily after a meal.
Filgrastim (Neupogen)—G-CSF	Hematopoietic growth factor, relatively specific for the granulocyte lineage.	Available in single-use vials of 300 and 480 mg, in solution.	None noted.	After a bolus SC injection, peak plasma levels of filgrastim occur in 2–6 hours, while the elimination half-life is generally 7 hours or less. Metabolism is via proteolysis in the blood compartment. The intact molecule is largely absent from bile or urine.	Mild bone pain is common. Low-grade fever, myalgias, arthralgias, and transient hypotension are uncommon, as are hyperuricemia and transient elevations of lactate dehydrogenase and alkaline phosphatase. Leukocytosis leading to hypoxia or capillary leak syndrome has been reported. Anaphylaxis or allergic reaction is rare.	FDA approved for minimization of granulocytopenia after myelosuppressive chemotherapy. Also used to speed recovery of granulocytes in the setting of neutropenic fever after chemotherapy, for myelodysplastic syndromes, for congenital agranulo-cytosis, for cyclic neutropenia, and for mobilization of peripheral blood stem cells from patients or donors for transplant.	Starting dose is 5 mg/kg/day until neutrophil recovery (discontinue the drug after an absolute neutrophil count of 10,000 or greater has been achieved), although generally either the whole 300-mg or 480-mg vial is used. For post-transplant or high-dose chemotherapy applications, 10 mg/kg/day is the typical dose. There is no known maximum dose.
Floxuridine (FUDR)—FdUR, Fluorodeoxyuridine	Pyrimidine nucleotide analogue, antimetabolite. Cell cycle dependent.	Available in 500-mg vials of lyophilized powder.	Leucovorin will enhance the toxicity of floxuridine.	After infusion into the hepatic artery, the drug is phosphorylated to the active monophosphate form and incorporated into cells. Further hepatic metabolism to inactive forms is rapid. The elimination half-life is 30 minutes. Metabolites are cleared by the kidneys.	When given as a bolus, myelosuppression is dose limiting, while diarrhea and stomatitis are the dose-limiting toxicities of the more common protracted infusions. Other GI toxicities, all rare, include nausea, vomiting, anorexia, gastritis, cramping, enteritis, and duodenal ulcers. Liver toxicity, usually a cholestatic picture, is dose limiting with intrahepatic arterial infusions. Serious neurologic side effects, including ataxia and visual changes, are rare, as is fever.	FDA approved for regional (intra-arterial) treatment of GI adenocarcinomas metastatic to the liver. Sometimes used intravenously for the same tumors.	Protracted intra-arterial infusions are generally given at 0.1–0.6 mg/kg/day until grade III toxicity, sometimes according to a circadian schedule. IV doses range up to 60 mg/kg/week by various infusion schedules.

CHEMOTHERAPEUTIC AGENT	DRUG CLASS/ MECHANISM OF ACTION	DOSAGE FORMS	DRUG INTERACTIONS	PHARMACOKINETICS/ METABOLISM	TOXICITY	INDICATIONS	DOSING
Fludarabine (Fludara)— FAMP	Purine nucleotide analogue antimetabolite. Only partially cell cycle dependent.	Vials containing 50 mg each of lyophilized drug. Add 2 mL of sterile water to the vial to make a 25-mg/mL solution, and then dilute the desired dose further to a concentration of 0.04–1 mg/mL (depending on the infusion schedule).	None noted.	Fludarabine is available only by the parenteral route. After IV administration, the drug is metabolized to 2-fluoroaraA and distributed widely in tissues. It has an elimination half-life of 9–10 hours. The drug and metabolite are excreted primarily by the kidneys.	Neurotoxicity, including cortical blindness, confusion, somnolence, coma, and demyelinating lesions, is dose limiting, but the lower doses conventionally used rarely produce these side effects. At these doses, mild myelosuppression is the most common toxicity, with cumulative lymphopenia being the most clinically important. Nausea, vomiting, and other GI toxicities are rare. Alopecia and rash are also rare.	FDA approved for the treatment of CLL. Also used for low-grade lymphomas and for AML.	The standard regimen is 25 mg/m^2/day for 5 days by short IV infusion. Prolonged infusions have also been used.
5-Fluorouracil (Adrucil, Efudex)—5-FU	Pyrimidine antimetabolite; inhibitor of thymidylate synthase. Partially cell cycle dependent.	Available in solution in 0.5–5-g ampules or vials at a concentration of 50 mg/mL.	None noted.	Parenteral bioavailability only. After an intravenous dose, 80% of the drug is metabolized to the inactive dihydro-5-FU by dihydropyrimidine dehydrogenase in the liver. The rest of the drug is activated to fluorodeoxy-uridine monophosphate in the target cells. The elimination half-life is about 20 minutes. Excretion is via the kidneys.	GI toxicities, primarily mucositis for bolus injection and diarrhea for prolonged infusions, are dose limiting. Rare patients with dyhydropyrimidine dehydrogenase deficiency have excessive GI toxicity. Myelosuppression is generally less with continuous infusion schedules. Nausea and vomiting are uncommon and mild. Dermatitis and other cutaneous toxicities, including hand-foot syndrome, are common. Cerebellar ataxia and myocardial ischemia are rare.	FDA approved for colon, rectum, gastric, pancreas, and breast carcinomas, and used for a wide range of other neoplasms in combination regimens. Used for intrahepatic arterial infusion for liver metastases from GI tumors, and also used topically for various cutaneous neoplasms and disorders.	IV dosing schemes include weekly bolus, 5 days of bolus every 28 days, 4–5-day continuous infusions, or prolonged continuous infusions. Doses range from 300 to 3000 mg/m^2/day depending on the dosing scheme and schedule.
FluoxymesterOne (Halotestin, Oro-Testryl)	Synthetic steroidal androgen. Antagonizes estrogenic effects in estrogen-dependent target cells.	2-, 5-, and 10-mg tablets.	None noted.	The drug is available by the oral route, is metabolized in the liver, and has an elimination half-life of about 10 hours. Route of excretion is unknown.	Androgenic effects predominate. Hirsutism, amenorrhea, hoarseness, acne, and increased libido occur in women, while men might have gynecomastia. Mild edema is common. Liver abnormalities, including transaminitis, fatty change, cholestatic jaundice, and rarely carcinoma, are not uncommon. Polycythemia can occur.	FDA approved for the treatment of hormone-sensitive breast cancer and for hypogonadism in males.	The total daily dose for breast cancer is usually between 10 mg and 40 mg, divided into two or three doses daily.

CHEMOTHERAPEUTIC AGENT	DRUG CLASS/ MECHANISM OF ACTION	DOSAGE FORMS	DRUG INTERACTIONS	PHARMACOKINETICS/ METABOLISM	TOXICITY	INDICATIONS	DOSING
Flutamide (Eulexin)	Nonsteroidal antiandrogen.	125-mg capsules.	None noted.	Good oral bioavailability, with peak plasma levels after an oral dose at 1–2 hours. The drug is metabolized to active and inactive forms in the liver. The elimination half-life is 8–10 hours. Parent drug and metabolites are excreted in the urine.	Generally well tolerated. Gynecomastia, galactorrhea, and impotence are common. Nausea, vomiting, diarrhea, mild myelosuppression, myalgias, and elevated liver function tests are rare.	FDA approved for prostate carcinoma.	The standard dose is 250 mg PO tid. Often given in conjunction with an LHRH agonist such as leuprolide to create complete androgen blockade.
Gallium Nitrate (Ganite)	Heavy metal that antagonizes iron metabolism in tumor cells preferentially. Causes hypocalcemia by a similar mechanism.	500-mg vials (20-mL vials of a 25-mg/mL solution).	None noted.	This drug is not metabolized and has an elimination half-life of about 5 hours. Cleared unchanged in the urine.	Renal toxicity, including glomerular and tubular defects, is dose limiting but partly preventable with adequate hydration during therapy. Hypocalcemia is expected and common and can be dose limiting. Nausea, vomiting, diarrhea, and anorexia are not uncommon. Mild myelosuppression, rashes, hearing loss or tinnitus, visual disturbances, and transient neurologic symptoms are rare.	FDA approved for the treatment of malignancy-related hypercalcemia. Also used for advanced bladder carcinoma.	The standard dose and schedule is 300 mg/m²/ day for 7 days by continuous IV infusion in a volume of 1000 mL of normal saline.
Gemcitabine (Gemzar)	Antimetabolite. Gemcitabine is a nucleoside analogue that exhibits cell cycle–dependent and S-phase–specific cytotoxicity, likely due to inhibition of DNA synthesis.	Supplied as lyophilized powder in vials containing 200 and 1000 mg of drug.	None noted.	Gemcitabine has poor oral bioavailability. After IV infusion, the drug is distributed rapidly and has a half-life of less than 2 hours. It is metabolized throughout the body to inactive forms. Parent drug and metabolite are excreted principally by the kidneys.	Myelosuppression, including anemia, is mild but dose limiting. Nausea and vomiting are mild but common. Diarrhea and edema are sometimes seen. Elevated transaminases are common, as is fever during drug administration. Hematuria and proteinuria are uncommon. Acute dyspnea and rash are uncommon. Paresthesias and CNS depression are rare.	FDA approved for advanced pancreatic adenocarcinoma, NSCLC, and metastatic breast cancer; extensively used in bladder cancer also.	The usual dose in pancreatic cancer is 1000 mg/m² as an IV bolus weekly for up to 7 weeks, followed by a week of rest before another cycle is begun. Similar doses in combination with or without platinating agents are used for the other indications.
Gemtuzumab Ozogamicin (Mylotarg)	Novel toxin-conjugated monoclonal antibody directed at myeloid-lineage cells.	Amber single-use vials containing 5 mg of drug as a lyophilized powder.	No formal studies done and no important drug interactions yet noted. Other medications that cause myelo- suppression would	Gemtuzumab is given as a 2-hour IV infusion, after which the total calicheamycin (ozogamicin released from the antibody by hydrolysis) has a half-life of 45 hours for the first dose and 60 hours after	This peptide antibody linked to a toxin, given in a poor prognosis group of patients who are often medically fragile, can have marked acute toxicities. These include somewhat common	FDA approved for relapsed AML.	9 mg/m² as a 2-hour IV infusion given once up front and then again in 14 days.

CHEMOTHERAPEUTIC AGENT	DRUG CLASS/ MECHANISM OF ACTION	DOSAGE FORMS	DRUG INTERACTIONS	PHARMACOKINETICS/ METABOLISM	TOXICITY	INDICATIONS	DOSING
			be expected to worsen myelo-suppression caused by gemtuzumab.	the second dose. Metabolism of the toxin is hepatic. The elimination routes of the toxin and the antibody are unknown.	typical antibody infusion side effects including fever, chills, hypotension, dyspnea, and wheezing, and other uncommon toxicities including tachycardia, renal insufficiency, hepatic compromise (including hepatic venoocclusive disease), dizziness, headache, and rash. Leukopenia is expected and can be prolonged, causing a high risk of bacterial, fungal, and sometimes viral infections. Thrombocytopenia and anemia are common also. Nausea and vomiting and diarrhea are common. Serious coagulopathy or hemorrhage is rare.		
Goserelin Acetate (Zoladex)	LHRH that inhibits pituitary-gonadal axis function. This drug causes steroid hormone withdrawal from dependent tissues, including prostate cancer and breast cancer cells.	3.6-mg prefilled syringes.	None noted.	After the contents of the syringe are injected SC into adipose tissue, the depot of drug is slowly released over 28 days and peaks at 12–15 days. The elimination half-life is 4 hours, and the drug is not appreciably metabolized. Excretion is almost entirely by the urinary route.	Toxicity is mild. Endocrine side effects are most prominent and include hot flashes, diminished libido, impotence, gynecomastia, amenorrhea, and breakthrough vaginal bleeding. Other toxicities include flares of pain early during treatment in sites of disease, local tenderness at injection sites, headache, nausea, depression, and elevated cholesterol levels.	FDA approved for advanced prostate cancer, and used also in metastatic breast cancer.	3.6 mg SC usually in the abdomen, every 28 days.
Hydroxyurea (Hydrea)— Hydrocarbamide	Antimetabolite; inhibitor of ribonucleotide reductase, which converts nucleotides to the deoxyribose forms for DNA synthesis. Cell cycle dependent.	500-mg capsules.	None noted.	After oral administration, the drug is well absorbed, and drug levels peak in the blood 2 hours after a dose. The elimination half-life is 2–5 hours. Metabolism to inactive forms occurs in the liver. Renal excretion is the route of elimination.	Myelosuppression is common and dose limiting. Other toxicities include rash, headache, fever, and hyperuricemia. Nausea and vomiting are uncommon. Liver toxicity and serious neurologic toxicity are rare.	FDA approved for CML; commonly used for other myeloproliferative disorders, and also used occasionally for metastatic melanoma, refractory ovarian carcinoma, and squamous cell carcinoma of the cervix and head and neck.	For CML, the dose is 1000–3000 mg/day, while in solid tumors, the dose is either 80 mg/kg every third day or 1.25 g/m^2 every 8 hours once a week. For some doses once a week.

CHEMOTHERAPEUTIC AGENT	DRUG CLASS/ MECHANISM OF ACTION	DOSAGE FORMS	DRUG INTERACTIONS	PHARMACOKINETICS/ METABOLISM	TOXICITY	INDICATIONS	DOSING
Ibritumomab Tiuxetan— Yttrium-90 (Zevalin)	Monoclonal antibody directed to the B-cell surface antigen CD20 linked to beta-emitting radionuclide yttrium-90.	Kits for preparation of either the In-111 (used for predicting drug distribution) or Y-90 (used for therapy) form of the drug include a vial containing 3.2 mg of the antibody in saline solution along with three other vials for mixing. Y-90 is sent with the Y-90 kit. Rituxan and In-111 must be ordered separately.	None known. Formal studies have not been conducted.	Optimal irbitumomab/Y-90 binding and clinical effect requires pretreatment with unconjugated ibritumomab. The physical half-life of Y-90 is 64 hours, but the biological half-life of the agent in the body in terms of radio-activity detected is 30 hours. Metabolic and excretory fates of the radionuclide and antibody are not not known.	Ibritumomab/Y-90 should not be administered if the biodistribution of ibritumomab/In-111 is altered significantly. Antibody toxicities can include fever, chills, dyspnea, wheezing, urticaria, and rash. Radionuclide or total agent side effects include lymphopenia and myelosuppression of other cell lines, which can be prolonged. Infection risk is increased accordingly. Nausea, vomiting, and diarrhea are uncommon, as are arthralgias, myalgias, or neurologic side effects.	FDA approved for treatment of relapsed and/or transformed follicular B-cell lymphomas.	The first step of therapy is administration of a 250 mg/m² dose of rituximab, followed by a 1.6 mg/5 mCi dose of ibritumomab/In-111 as a 10-minute infusion. 9 days later, if biodistribution of the In-111-labeled product is normal, the same dose of rituximab is followed by a 1.6 mg/0.4 mCi per kg dose of ibritumomab/Y-90 as a 10-minute infusion.
Idarubicin (Idamycin)— 4-demethoxydaunorubicin	Anthracycline intercalating agent. Non-cell cycle dependent.	Lyophilized powder in vials of 5 mg and 10 mg.	None noted.	Idarubicin has poor oral bioavailability. After an IV dose, the drug is metabolized in the liver to active and inactive forms. The elimination half-life of the parent compound is 13–26 hours. Metabolites and some of the unchanged drug are almost exclusively excreted in bile.	Myelosuppression is common and generally dose limiting for each dose. The cumulative dose-limiting toxicity is cardiomyopathy, but idarubicin is less cardiotoxic than daunorubicin or doxorubicin. Nausea and vomiting are common but usually mild. Diarrhea and stomatitis are sometimes seen. Idarubicin is a weak vesicant or irritant.	FDA approved for the treatment of AML.	The standard dose as part of a "7 plus 3" regimen (with cytarabine) is 12 mg/m²/ day for 3 days for induction or re-induction/intensification. Other doses have been used.
Ifosfamide (Ifex)	Classic alkylating agent. Non-cell cycle dependent.	Available in 1-g and 3-g vials of powdered drug.	None noted.	After an intravenous dose, ifosfamide is activated by hepatic microsomal enzymes. It is then converted to inactive metabolites in the liver. The active form of the drug is the same as that for cyclophosphamide. The	Myelosuppression, hemorrhagic cystitis, and CNS toxicity are all fairly common and can be dose limiting. Hemorrhagic cystitis can largely be prevented by co-administration of the uroprotective agent mesna,	FDA approved for the treatment of recurrent germ cell tumors. Used for many other tumor types, including adult sarcomas, lymphoma, Hodgkin's disease, breast cancer, and ovarian cancer.	Ifosfamide is generally given IV over 3–5 days with a total dose of 8–12 g/m²/cycle, repeated every 3–4 weeks. It can be given as a short infusion each day or as a continuous infusion. Mesna is given

Science of Clinical Oncology

511

CHEMOTHERAPEUTIC AGENT	DRUG CLASS/ MECHANISM OF ACTION	DOSAGE FORMS	DRUG INTERACTIONS	PHARMACOKINETICS/ METABOLISM	TOXICITY	INDICATIONS	DOSING
				elimination half-life of the drug is 7–15 hours. The metabolites and some unchanged drug are excreted in the urine.	and nausea and vomiting are minimized with modern antiemetic regimens. The CNS toxicity, including lethargy, stupor, coma, myoclonus, and seizures, is usually mild and completely reversible. It is worse with impaired renal function. Renal dysfunction, usually reversible, is also seen with ifosfamide. Hepatic toxicity, diarrhea, and rash are rare.		IV concurrently, also by short infusion or continuous infusion. Hydration of greater than 3 L/day total, with saline or alkali solutions, is also recommended.
Imatinib Mesylate (Gleevec)	Specific receptor tyrosine kinase inhibitor, which selectively inhibits the tyrosine kinases of the bcr-abl, c-kit, and PDGF receptors.	100-mg capsules.	Imatinib plasma levels are enhanced by ketoconazole, and imatinib increases the plasma levels of other drugs that are metabolized by cytochrome P450 3A4. Inducers of this enzyme (e.g., phenytoin) would be expected to lower the plasma levels of imatinib.	Imatinib has good oral bioavailability, reaches peak serum levels in about 3 hours, and has an elimination half-life of 18 hours. It is metabolized in the liver by cytochrome P450 3A4 among other isoforms, with the demethylated metabolite showing similar activity to the parent drug. The parent drug and major metabolite are excreted primarily in the feces.	There is no definite dose-limiting toxicity of imatinib. Myelosuppression is significant in chronic myelogenous leukemia (CML) but mild in gastrointestinal stromal tumors. Hepatotoxicity is common but usually mild. Liver function tests should be monitored closely during therapy. Fluid retention is common but usually mild, as are nausea, vomiting, and diarrhea. Rash and fever are uncommon.	FDA approved for treatment of CML in the front-line setting, in accelerated phase, and in blast crisis. It is also approved for treatment of recurrent inoperable or metastatic gastrointestinal stromal tumors.	Total daily doses of 400–800 mg, once daily or divided.
Interferon-α (IntronA, Roferon), α-interferon, IFN-α	Biologic response modifier, antiviral, immuno-stimulant.	Available in vials of lyophilized powder or aqueous solution in quantities from 3 million to 50 million IU/vial.	None noted.	After parenteral administration, peak levels of IFN-α in the blood occur in 30 minutes to 8 hours depending on the route. The elimination half-life is 2–9 hours. IFN-α is catabolized throughout the body through proteolysis, but primarily in the renal tubules. Excretion of intact drug is minimal and not significantly affected by organ function.	Constitutional symptoms are predominant side effects and are dose limiting both in the short and long terms in lower-dose schedules. Acute side effects include fever, chills, nasal congestion, diarrhea, and malaise. Chronic side effects include fatigue, anorexia, weight loss, and depression. Neutropenia and thrombocytopenia, both of which are transient, are dose limiting at higher doses. Anemia also can occur, albeit with more chronic administration. Cardiac	FDA approved for non-malignant conditions and malignancies including melanoma, CML, hairy cell leukemia, Kaposi's sarcoma, and cutaneous T-cell lymphoma. Also used in multiple myeloma and low-grade lymphomas.	Dose depends on both the diagnosis and the brand or type of IFN-α. The doses for malignant conditions range from 2 million up to 30 million units/m^2 by the SC, IM, or IV route from three times per week to every day. Adjustments are made based on patient tolerance and laboratory parameters.

CHEMOTHERAPEUTIC AGENT	DRUG CLASS/MECHANISM OF ACTION	DOSAGE FORMS	DRUG INTERACTIONS	PHARMACOKINETICS/METABOLISM	TOXICITY	INDICATIONS	DOSING
					toxicity, including congestive heart failure and arrhythmias, is rare and almost always reversible. Serious CNS toxicity, including delerium and psychosis, or peripheral neuropathies are also rare and reversible. Hypocalcemia and hyperglycemia also can occur.		
Interleukin-2 (Proleukin)— Aldesleukin, IL-2	IL-2 is a glyco-protein cytokine, previously known as T-cell growth factor, that stimulates antigen-specific and nonspecific T-cell and other lymphocyte subsets and also triggers an inflammatory cytokine cascade. Its antineoplastic effects are dependent on an intact immune system.	Vials of lyophilized drug containing 18 million IU.	None noted.	IL-2 is available by the parenteral route only. It has an elimination half-life of 30–60 minutes. It is catabolized by proteolysis throughout the body. Negligible amounts of intact drug are found in urine or bile.	IL-2 has a wide range of moderate to severe toxicities that are both dose and schedule dependent. Toxicities tend to follow immediately after a bolus dose but accumulate gradually during a continuous infusion. Toxicities are higher for a given dose with continuous infusion compared with bolus dosing. Capillary leak syndrome, which is dose limiting for most IL-2 administration schedules, results in hypotension, edema, pulmonary congestion, renal insufficiency, arrhythmias, diarrhea, and possibly some of the CNS and hepatic toxicity seen with IL-2. Transient myelosuppression or more prolonged anemia occurs commonly, as do transient hyperbilirubinemia, elevation of transaminases, and electrolyte imbalances. Other constitutional symptoms that occur with IL-2 include fever, chills, malaise, arthralgia/myalgias, erythroderma, nasal congestion/rhinorrhea, and nausea/vomiting. Other serious and less common toxicities include lethargy or delerium, angina pectoris, congestive heart failure, frank respiratory failure, and infections, particularly gram-positive bacteremia.	FDA approved for high-dose bolus treatment of metastatic renal cell cancer and metastatic melanoma. Also used at lower doses for metastatic melanoma and for maintenance treatment of acute myeloid leukemia.	The FDA-approved dose for renal cell carcinoma and melanoma is a 600,000–720,000 IU/kg IV bolus every 8 hours for a maximum of 14 doses on days 1–5 and 11–15 every 6 weeks. Lower doses are used more commonly, especially continuous infusions of 3–18 million IU/m²/day for 96 hours. SC administration at similar daily doses also has been attempted with reasonable patient tolerance.

CHEMOTHERAPEUTIC AGENT	DRUG CLASS/ MECHANISM OF ACTION	DOSAGE FORMS	DRUG INTERACTIONS	PHARMACOKINETICS/ METABOLISM	TOXICITY	INDICATIONS	DOSING
Irinotecan (Camptosar)— CPT-11	A semisynthetic camptothecin, which functions as a topoisomerase I inhibitor. Partly cell cycle dependent.	Available in 100-mg vials as a 20-mg/mL aqueous solution.	None noted.	Irinotecan is only available by the parenteral route. After IV administration, the drug is converted partially from the active lactone form to the inactive carboxylate form through hydrolysis. The parent drug is metabolized in the intestine, liver, and plasma. The active metabolite of irinotecan, SN-38, also exists in the lactone and inactive carboxylate form in equilibrium in plasma. SN-38 is inactivated by glucuronidation in the liver. SN-38 is responsible for the majority of antitumor activity attributed to the parent drug. The elimination half-life of irinotecan is 8 hours, while the elimination half-life of SN-38 is about 12 hours. Excretion of parent drug and metabolites is largely via the bile.	Myelosuppression, primarily neutropenia, is common and dose limiting. Diarrhea is also common and can be dose limiting. Diarrhea can occur as part of a cholinergic syndrome, along with cramping, nausea, and vomiting, during or immediately after drug administration or for several days after drug administration. Anticholinergics and antidiarrheals will curtail the immediate diarrhea and other GI symptoms partially but are less effective in treating the delayed diarrhea. Flushing, rash, and alopecia are common. Significant hepatic, renal, neurologic, or pulmonary toxicities are rare.	Irinotecan is FDA approved for refractory or recurrent metastatic colon cancer, and it has now been used in other malignancies, including lung cancer, ovarian cancer, and lymphoma.	The recommended dosage for recurrent colon cancer is 125 mg/m^2 as a 90-minute IV infusion every week for 4 weeks, with this cycle repeated every 6 weeks. Other doses and schedules have been used.
Isotretinoin (Accutane)—13-cis- retinoic acid, 13-CRA	Isotretinoin is a retinoid derivative of vitamin A that binds to specific nuclear receptors and leads to changes in gene expression. This results in apoptosis or differentiation of many malignant or premalignant cell lines.	10-, 20-, and 40-mg capsules.	None noted.	Oral bioavailability is about 25%, and the drug is highly protein bound in plasma. It is metabolized in the liver and has an elimination half-life of 10–20 hours. Parent compound and metabolite are excreted in both the urine and feces.	Isotretinoin is teratogenic and should not be given to women of childbearing age without adequate contraception. Mucocutaneous side effects are common and dose limiting and include xerostomia, stomatitis, conjunctivitis, dry skin, pruritis, chelitis, rash, patchy alopecia, fragility of nails and skin, photosensitivity, and epistaxis. Other less common side effects include elevations in transaminases and bilirubin or frank hepatitis, hyperlipidemia, nausea, vomiting, anorexia, diarrhea, headache, fatigue, depression, and myalgias/ arthralgias. Anemia and pseudotumor cerebri are rare.	FDA approved for acne vulgaris. Has shown some effectiveness in chemoprevention of aerodigestive malignancies. Ongoing studies are testing its chemopreventative potential in other malignancies.	Daily oral doses of 0.5 to 4 mg/kg/day have been used in the chemoprevention trials, for durations of 2–6 months.

CHEMOTHERAPEUTIC AGENT	DRUG CLASS/MECHANISM OF ACTION	DOSAGE FORMS	DRUG INTERACTIONS	PHARMACOKINETICS/METABOLISM	TOXICITY	INDICATIONS	DOSING
Ketoconazole (Nizoral)	Oral antifungal agent that also acts as an androgen antagonist at high doses.	200-mg tablets.	Ketoconazole is a potent inhibitor of cytochrome P450 3A4. As such, it increases the potency of other drugs metabolized by that enzyme, isoform, including terfenadine, astemizole, cisapride, midazolam, triazolam, loratadine, and possibly cyclosporin, tacrolimus, methylprednisolone, and warfarin. Rifampin and isoniazid decrease the potency of ketoconazole. Ketoconazole has been reported to cause a disulfiram type reaction when used with alcohol.	Ketoconazole has good oral bioavailability. Its level peaks in the plasma in about 2 hours. It has a terminal half-life of about 8 hours. It is metabolized in the liver to several inactive metabolites. The metabolites are excreted in the bile.	This drug is not strictly an antineoplastic drug and is generally very well-tolerated. Nausea, vomiting, headache, dizziness, fever, chills, impotence, gynecomastia, leukopenia, hemolytic anemia, urticaria, and anaphylaxis are all rare. Hepatic toxicity is also rare. It has been fatal in unusual cases. Administration with terfenadine and astemizole has resulted in prolonged QT interval, arrhythmias, and deaths in rare cases. Other potential drug interactions are possible, as listed previously.	FDA approved for fungal infections, primarily yeast infections. Used in doses of up to 1200 mg a day for androgen-dependent or independent prostate cancer.	As described, used alone or in combination with chemotherapy, including doxorubicin.
Letrozole (Femara)	Nonsteroidal aromatase inhibitor.	2.5-mg tablets.	Studies have revealed no interactions between letrozole and warfarin or cimetidine. No other formal drug interaction studies have been done.	Letrozole has nearly 100% bioavailability, is metabolized in the liver, is glucuronidated, and is excreted by the kidneys. It has a terminal half-life of about 2 days. With daily administration, steady-state plasma levels are reached in 2–6 weeks.	This drug is generally well-tolerated. Muscle aches, nausea, hot flashes, and fatigue are uncommon, weight change, urticaria, and dyspepsia are rare.	FDA approved for treatment of metastatic estrogen-responsive breast cancer in post-menopausal patients.	2.5 mg orally once daily.
Leucovorin Calcium (Wellcovorin)—Citrovorum Factor, Folinic Acid, FA, LV	Tetrahydrofolate derivative and enzyme cofactor for thymidylate synthase and other purine and pyrimidine synthesis steps. Leucovorin bypasses the dihydrofolate reductase step, which is inhibited by methotrexate, and therefore can be used to "rescue"	Tablets in 5-mg to 25-mg sizes, powder for oral solution, and as vials of powdered drug in 3-mg–350-mg sizes.	Reduces the effectiveness and toxicity of dihydrofolate reductase inhibitors such as methotrexate.	Leucovorin has excellent bioavailability by the oral or parenteral route. It is oxidized in cofactor reactions throughout the body and is also partly metabolized. It has an elimination half-life of 2–4 hours. Excreted in the urine.	Leucovorin is generally very well tolerated. It occasionally causes stomach upset or nausea, rash, diarrhea, and headache. Allergic reactions have been reported.	Used for rescue of high-dose methotrexate therapy for a variety of neoplasms, and used as a potentiator of fluoropyrimidine therapy in gastrointestinal malignancies, particularly colorectal cancers.	For rescue from methotrexate, the usual dose is 10–25 mg/m² orally or IV every 6 hours starting up to 24 hours after the methotrexate, until methotrexate levels are less than 1×10^{-8} molar. When used to potentiate 5-FU, doses ranging from 20 to 500 mg/m², usually given IV, have been used, depending on the 5-FU dose.

CHEMOTHERAPEUTIC AGENT	DRUG CLASS/ MECHANISM OF ACTION	DOSAGE FORMS	DRUG INTERACTIONS	PHARMACOKINETICS/ METABOLISM	TOXICITY	INDICATIONS	DOSING
	normal cells from the toxicity of methotrexate after high doses are administered. In addition, leucovorin potentiates the toxicity of fluoropyrimidines such as fluorouracil by strengthening the association of the drug with its target enzyme, thymidylate synthase.						
Leuprolide Acetate (Leupron)—Leuprorelin Acetate	Gonadotropin-releasing hormone agonist, which serves paradoxically to shut down the pituitary release of gonadotropins with chronic exposure. This results in a dramatic decrease in gonadal estrogens and androgens, and growth inhibition of hormone-dependent neoplasms.	Available in vials for monthly administration (depot) containing 3.75 mg and 7.5 mg of powder, along with diluent and syringe. A multidose vial containing 2.8 mL of a 5-mg/mL solution along with syringes is also available for daily administration.	None noted.	Leuprolide is bioavailable by the parenteral route only. After an SC injection, about 90% of the drug is eventually absorbed. The depot form of the drug is absorbed slowly over days, while the injectable solution is absorbed over several hours. The elimination half-life of the drug, once in the serum, is 3 hours. Metabolism and excretion are not well delineated but are clinically unimportant.	Usually well tolerated, but side effects can affect many systems, including endocrine (hot flashes, impotence, gynecomastia, breast tenderness, diminished libido, amenorrhea, atrophic vaginitis, increased cholesterol); GI (nausea, constipation, anorexia, diarrhea); hepatic (elevation of transaminases); dermatologic (rash, changes in body hair composition, pruritis); and neuro-psychiatric (insomnia, depression, emotional lability, lethargy, memory loss). Significant cardiac toxicity is rare.	FDA approved for the treatment of hormone-dependent advanced prostate cancer. Also used for breast cancer and endometriosis.	The usual dose for prostate cancer is 7.5 mg of the depot form by SC injection once every month, or 1 mg of the injectable solution SC daily.
Lomustine (CeeNU)— CCNU	Nitrosourea alkylating agent. Cell cycle independent.	Available as 10-, 20-, and 100-mg capsules.	None noted.	Well absorbed after oral administration. Widely distributed in the body, including in the cerebrospinal fluid. Metabolized extensively in the liver to active metabolites. Elimination half-life is 72 hours. Metabolites are excreted in the urine.	Myelosuppression is dose limiting and tends to be cumulative. Nausea and vomiting are common but usually mild to moderate. Anorexia is also common but short lived. Pulmonary fibrosis can occur with long-term administration. Other toxicities, including CNS effects, hepatic or renal dysfunction, and secondary leukemia, are rare.	FDA approved for primary brain tumors and Hodgkin's disease. Also used in melanoma, multiple myeloma, other lymphomas, and breast cancer.	The recommended dose for brain tumors is 100–130 mg/m^2 orally every 6 weeks. Other doses and schedules have been used.

CHEMOTHERAPEUTIC AGENT	DRUG CLASS/ MECHANISM OF ACTION	DOSAGE FORMS	DRUG INTERACTIONS	PHARMACOKINETICS/ METABOLISM	TOXICITY	INDICATIONS	DOSING
Mechlorethamine (Mustargen)—Nitrogen Mustard, HN2	Classic alkylating agent. Cell cycle independent.	Vials of lyophilized powder containing 10 mg of drug.	None noted.	Mechlorethamine is not bioavailable orally. After an IV dose, the drug is rapidly deactivated in the blood by reaction with biomolecules. It has an elimination half-life of 15 minutes and has no significant organ metabolism. Virtually no excretion of the drug is detected in urine or stool.	This drug is a powerful vesicant, so optimal extravasation precautions and rapid infusion are a must. Tissue necrosis will occur if the drug extravasates, although sodium thiosulfate is a somewhat effective antidote. Vein discoloration and scarring are common. Nausea and vomiting are common, potentially severe, and often dose limiting. Myelosuppression is expected and also often dose limiting. Alopecia and infertility are often seen. Less common toxicities include anorexia, diarrhea, jaundice, tinnitus, and skin rash (common with topical treatment). Secondary leukemia and permanent hearing loss are rare.	FDA approved for a variety of hematologic malignancies and solid tumors, but generally used less in the last decade. Still used for Hodgkin's disease, and topically for cutaneous T-cell lymphoma.	The standard dose for Hodgkin's disease as part of the MOPP regimen is 6 mg/m^2 IV over 1–5 minutes on day 1 and day 8 of a 28-day cycle. The topical form is usually a 10-mg/60-mL solution or a 10-mg/dL ointment.
Medroxyprogesterone Acetate (Provera, Depo-Provera)	Steroidal progestational agent.	Available as tablets in sizes of 2.5, 5, and 10 mg, and as a suspension for depot injection as 100 or 400 mg/mL.	The metabolism of medroxy-progesterone acetate could be enhanced by aminoglutethamide, leading to decreased effect for a given dose.	This drug has good oral bioavailability. It is metabolized in the liver to inactive metabolites and has an elimination half-life of up to 60 hours. Parent drug and metabolites are excreted in the urine and bile.	Toxicities are mostly constitutional and not dose limiting. They include menstrual changes, ameorrhea, gynecomastia, hot flashes, edema, weight gain, fatigue, acne, hirsutism, anxiety, depression, sleep disturbance, and headache. Nausea, significant skin reactions or allergy, jaundice, and thrombo-phlebitis are uncommon.	FDA approved for treatment of advanced endometrial or renal cell carcinoma. Also used occasionally for breast or prostate cancer.	Loading doses of up to 1000 mg IM weekly and 400 mg IM every month have been used, while oral doses range from 100 to 300 mg/day. Much lower doses are used for gynecologic indications.
Megestrol Acetate (Megace)—Megestrol	Steroidal progestational agent.	20-mg and 40-mg tablets and 40-mg/mL oral solution.	None noted.	The drug is well absorbed by mouth, is metabolized in the liver to inactive compounds, and has an elimination half-life of 15–20 hours. Parent drug and metabolites are excreted in the urine.	Toxicities are similar to those of other progestins as noted previously. They include menstrual changes, hot flashes, edema, weight gain, fatigue, acne, hirsutism, anxiety, depression, sleep disturbance, and headache. Urinary frequency can occur also. Nausea, vomiting, diarrhea, skin rash or allergy, jaundice, and thrombophlebitis are uncommon.	FDA approved for treatment of breast and endometrial carcinoma. Also used for renal cell carcinoma and for appetite stimulation in HIV disease and cancer patients.	The standard dose for cancer treatment is 160 mg/day in divided doses or a single dose. The dose for appetite stimulation could be as high as 800 mg/day, which is where the concentrated oral solution is useful.

CHEMOTHERAPEUTIC AGENT	DRUG CLASS/ MECHANISM OF ACTION	DOSAGE FORMS	DRUG INTERACTIONS	PHARMACOKINETICS/ METABOLISM	TOXICITY	INDICATIONS	DOSING
Melphalan (Alkeran)— l-PAM, l-phenylalanine mustard, l-sarcolysin	Classical alkylating agent. Cell cycle independent.	2-mg tablets and vials for injection at 50 mg/ vial.	None noted.	Melphalan has unpredictable GI absorption, is highly protein bound, and is rapidly autometabolized by hydrolysis in the plasma. It has an elimination half-life of about 2 hours. Ten to 15 percent is excreted as unchanged drug in the urine.	Myelosuppression is expected and is dose limiting. Recovery can be prolonged, and effects can be cumulative. Large doses can cause significant nausea and vomiting. Diarrhea and stomatitis are uncommon. Vein reactions, including scarring, can occur, but this agent is not known as a vesicant. Other skin reactions are uncommon, as are pulmonary fibrosis, vasculitis, infertility, alopecia, and secondary leukemia.	Used primarily for multiple myeloma, but also FDA approved for ovarian carcinoma. Could also be useful in high-dose chemotherapy/ transplant settings and in regional perfusion of extremities for melanoma and sarcoma.	Doses for myeloma are typically in the range of 0.1 mg/kg/day for 2–3 weeks or up to 6 mg/m²/day for 5 days every 6 weeks. Transplant doses (IV or PO) range up to 140 mg/m² total. Doses for perfusion are either 0.45–0.9 mg/kg or dosed for a certain concentration in the perfusate.
Mercaptopurine (Purinethol)—6-MP, 6-mercaptopurine	Purine analogue antimetabolite; predominantly S-phase specific.	50-mg tablets. An IV formulation is investigational.	Allopurinol inhibits first-pass metabolism of mercaptopurine in the liver by xanthine oxidase, and therefore dose reduction is required if allopurinol is also being given.	6-MP has good oral bioavailability, undergoes extensive first-pass metabolism in the liver, and has an elimination half-life of about 7 hours. Intact drug and metabolites are excreted by the kidneys.	Myelosuppression is common and dose limiting. Nausea and vomiting occur occasionally but are usually mild. Diarrhea, anorexia, and stomatitis are less common. Headache and rash are uncommon. Fulminant hepatic toxicity is very rare, but lesser degrees of cholestasis and hepatitis are sometimes seen.	Mercaptopurine is FDA approved for treatment of acute lymphoblastic leukemia. It is occasionally used for other hematologic malignancies. There is an investigational IV formulation that does not yet have clinical indications.	The usual dose is 70–100 mg/m²/day for a defined period of days during induction or maintenance.
Mesna (Mesnex)— Mercaptoethane- sulfonate Sodium, Uromitexan	Thiol uroprotectant; binds to and inactivates acrolein, the highly reactive metabolite of cyclophosphamide and ifosfamide, helping to prevent hemorrhagic cystitis.	Available as aqueous solution at a concentration of 100 mg/mL.	Mesna does not decrease the effectiveness of cytotoxic drugs or radiation.	Mesna has an oral bioavailability of about 50% and is usually given IV. After an IV dose, mesna is converted in the plasma to dimesna, is filtered by the kidneys, and is converted back into mesna in the urine. It has an elimination half-life of 1 hour.	Mesna is usually very well tolerated. It has been described to occasionally cause nausea, vomiting, diarrhea, rash, fatigue, headache, hypotension, or arthralgias.	FDA approved for use as a uroprotectant when administering ifosfamide. Also effective for high-dose cyclophosphamide.	The usual daily dose of mesna is 60% of the daily mg amount of the ifosfamide, given by IV bolus before, 4 hours after, and 8 hours after the chemotherapy, or as a continuous infusion with a loading dose before the chemotherapy. Mesna may be continued for up to 24 hours after the chemotherapy has been completed.
Methotrexate (Mexate, Folex, Others)—MTX, Amethopterin	Antifolate antimetabolite; interferes with nucleotide	2.5-mg tablets, vials of powder	None noted.	Methotrexate has good oral bioavailability at low doses. After oral or IV dosing, it is distributed throughout the	Myelosuppression is expected and is usually dose limiting. Stomatitis and diarrhea are common.	FDA approved for a wide spectrum of malignant and nonmalignant diseases.	For malignant conditions, doses up to 100 mg/m² are considered low dose,

CHEMOTHERAPEUTIC AGENT	DRUG CLASS/ MECHANISM OF ACTION	DOSAGE FORMS	DRUG INTERACTIONS	PHARMACOKINETICS/ METABOLISM	TOXICITY	INDICATIONS	DOSING
	synthesis by inhibiting dihydrofolate reductase. Cell cycle dependent.	for injection of 20–1000 mg/ vial, and as a 2.5- and 25-mg/ mL aqueous solution for injection.		body water compartment. It will accumulate in "third-space" fluid compartments and exhibit prolonged toxicity, and therefore should be used with caution, if at all, in patients with significant pleural or peritoneal fluid. The drug is metabolized minimally in the liver and has an elimination half-life of about 3 hours, and even low concentrations of drug after most of the drug is eliminated can contribute to significant toxicity. Therefore, dosing based on renal function is critical. Excretion of this drug is entirely renal.	Nausea and vomiting are uncommon. Renal toxicity is uncommon and usually reversible, but can be severe. Many types of skin reactions can occur but are uncommon. Pulmonary fibrosis and hepatic fibrosis are rare. Encephalopathy is rare with moderate to low-dose therapy but is more common with high doses, intrathecal administration, or concomitant CNS radiation. It can be severe and permanent.	Most often used for acute leukemias, lymphomas, breast cancer, bladder cancer, squamous cell cancers, and sarcomas.	100–1000 mg/m² moderate dose, and over 1000 mg/m² high dose. Moderate and high doses require leucovorin rescue. Doses can be given weekly or at longer intervals. IV infusions can be 30 minutes or longer, including 24-hour continuous infusions. Methotrexate is also commonly given intrathecally, usually as a 12-mg dose in 10 mL of preservative-free saline.
Mitomycin C (Mutamycin)	Antitumor antibiotic; inhibits DNA and RNA synthesis.	Vials of powder in 5-, 20-, and 40-mg sizes.	None noted.	Poor oral bioavailability. After an IV dose, mitomycin C is rapidly metabolized to inactive forms in the liver, spleen, and kidneys, with an elimination half-life of about 1 hour. Parent drug and inactive metabolites are excreted in the urine.	Mitomycin C is a vesicant; extravasation precautions are a must. Myelo-suppression is expected and is dose limiting, with a white blood cell nadir at 4 weeks and full recovery at 6–7 weeks. Mild nausea, vomiting, anorexia, and fatigue are common. Uncommon toxicities include diarrhea, stomatitis, rash, fever, and renal insufficiency. Rare toxicities include veno-occlusive disease of the liver, hemolytic-uremic syndrome, and interstitial pneumonitis.	FDA approved for adenocarcinomas of the stomach and pancreas. Also used commonly in breast cancer and lung cancer.	The usual dose is 10–20 mg/m² IV over 2–5 minutes every 6–8 weeks.
Mitotane (Lysodren)— o,p'-DDD	Adrenal cortical cytotoxin.	500-mg tablets.	None noted.	This drug has moderate oral bioavailability, with a peak plasma level about 4 hours after an oral dose. Significant therapeutic effect is not seen until up to 4 weeks of continuous usage. Mitotane is metabolized in the liver and has a variable elimination half-life (due	Adrenal insufficiency is expected and must be abrogated with concomitant oral glucocorticoid usage (and sometimes mineralo-corticoids as well). Anorexia, nausea, vomiting, sedation, and lethargy are common. Hyper-cholesterolemia and	FDA approved for adrenocortical carcinoma.	The initial dose is usually 1 g/day in four divided doses, and this is increased up to 10 g/day as tolerated.

CHEMOTHERAPEUTIC AGENT	DRUG CLASS/MECHANISM OF ACTION	DOSAGE FORMS	DRUG INTERACTIONS	PHARMACOKINETICS/METABOLISM	TOXICITY	INDICATIONS	DOSING
				to storage of the drug in adipose tissue) of up to 160 hours. Mitotane is eliminated in the urine and bile.	elevation of liver function tests are also common. Rash is seen frequently but is usually mild. Myelosuppression, diarrhea, fever, wheezing, changes in blood pressure, and flushing are uncommon. Permanent CNS changes, retinopathy, nephrotoxicity, and hemorrhagic cystitis are rare.		
Mitoxantrone (Novantrone)—DHAD, Dihydroxyanthracenedione	Anthracycline antitumor antibiotic.	Vials of 2-mg/mL solution.	None noted.	Mitoxantrone has poor oral bioavailability. After an IV dose, it exhibits a large volume of distribution, undergoes metabolism in the liver, and has an elimination half-life of 24–37 hours. Mitoxantrone is eliminated through the bile.	Mitoxantrone is not a tissue vesicant. Myelosuppression, mostly limited to leukopenia, is expected and dose limiting. Nausea and vomiting are common but mild, stomatitis is common, and diarrhea and anorexia are less common. Elevated liver function tests are common, but significant hepatic toxicity is rare. Cardiotoxicity is uncommon and dose dependent. Pulmonary or neurologic toxicity is rare.	FDA approved for AML and prostate carcinoma. Also used for breast cancer, lymphoma, and hepatocellular carcinoma.	For AML, the typical dose is 10–12 mg/m²/day for 3 days by 30-minute infusion, along with AraC. For solid tumors, 12 mg/m² is given over 30 minutes every 3–4 weeks.
Nilutamide (Nilandron)	Orally administered nonsteroidal antiandrogen.	50-mg and 150-mg tablets.	Inhibits activity of several cytochrome P450 isoenzymes, and thus could increase the potency of several potentially toxic drugs such as warfarin, theophylline, and phenytoin. Caution and careful monitoring are advised during concomitant use of nilutamide with such medications.	Rapid and complete GI absorption has been demonstrated. Elimination half-life is about 45 hours. The drug is metabolized in the liver and eliminated in the urine.	Hot flashes, body hair loss, fatigue, loss of libido, and weight gain are common but usually mild. Loss of visual adaptation to the darkness is common but transient, and nausea and fever and dyspepsia are uncommon. Interstitial pneumonitis is rare.	FDA approved for treatment of metastatic prostate cancer.	The usual dose is 300 mg once daily for 30 days followed by 150 mg daily.
Octreotide, Octreotide Long-acting (Sandostatin, Sandostatin LA)—l-cysteinamide	Synthetic peptide analogue of somatostatin; inhibits other	Ampules containing 0.05, 0.1, and 0.5 mg in 1 mL of	Could interfere with insulin action, requiring increase in insulin dosage.	Not orally bioavailable, but absorbed rapidly after SC administration. Metabolized by hydrolysis throughout the body. No	GI side effects are dose limiting and include abdominal pain, vomiting, loose stool, occasional fat malabsorption, bloating,	FDA approved for carcinoid tumors causing carcinoid syndrome and for vasoactive peptide—	Doses from 50 mg twice a day to 1000 mg four times a day injected SC have been used. Continuous IV infusions

CHEMOTHERAPEUTIC AGENT	DRUG CLASS/ MECHANISM OF ACTION	DOSAGE FORMS	DRUG INTERACTIONS	PHARMACOKINETICS/ METABOLISM	TOXICITY	INDICATIONS	DOSING
	GI peptide actions, such as serotonin, insulin, glucagon, and gastrin	aqueous solution.		active metabolites. The half-life of elimination is about 1.5 hours. Intact drug is cleared via the kidneys.	and cholelithiasis. Elevations of liver function tests also can occur, but frank hepatitis is rare. Skin reactions, such as pain at the injection site or flushing, rash, or skin thinning, are sometimes seen. Constitutional symptoms, including rhinorrhea, xerostomia, sweating, throat discomfort, and vertigo, can be bothersome. Either hyper- or hypoglycemia can occur. Cardiac side effects, including angina, congestive heart failure, and hypo- or hypertension, are uncommon. Anxiety, depression, fatigue, and anorexia are uncommon, and seizures are rare.	secreting tumors. Also used for refractory diarrhea, either cancer related or treatment related, in cancer patients.	or administration of drug in total parenteral nutrition solutions has also been used.
Oprelvekin (Neumega) —interleukin-11, IL-11	Recombinant polypeptide cytokine molecule; multiple cellular actions, including stimulation of megakaryocyte proliferation and platelet production from megakaryocytes.	Vials containing 5 mg of lyophilized powder.	None noted.	Oprelvekin is available by parenteral routes only. With SC administration, it is absorbed into the circulation with a peak plasma concentration of 3 hours and has an elimination half-life of about 7 hours. This polypeptide agent is metabolized throughout the body by proteolysis. Excretion of drug is not substantial, due to degradation.	Headache, fever, malaise, dyspnea, rash, conjunctival irritation, fluid retention, and edema are common during administration, but not usually severe. Oral thrush, dizziness, diarrhea, pleural effusions, and transient anemia are uncommon. Paresthesias, ocular hemorrhage, atrial arrythmias, and exfoliative dermatitis are rare.	FDA approved for prevention of severe chemotherapy-related thrombocytopenia.	50 mg/kg/day SC injection until the postnadir platelet count is greater than 50,000/mm^3, starting 1 day after the completion of chemotherapy.
Oxaliplatin (Eloxatin)	New generation platinating agent. Disrupts DNA via intra- and interstrand crosslinks with two strong platinum association bonds in the molecule, which induces apoptosis beyond a certain level of DNA damage in malignant cells.	Clear glass single-use vials containing 50 mg or 100 mg of drug as a lyophilized powder.	No drug-drug interaction studies done and no interactions yet identified. Expected additive toxicities with other antineoplastic agents and neurotoxic drugs. Nephrotoxic drugs could slow clearance of oxaliplatin.	Oxaliplatin has poor oral bioavailibility. After IV administration, rapid distribution into tissues occurs, as well as rapid spontaneous conversion via hydrolysis into active drug and metabolites. The terminal half-life is long (>300 hours) but represents minimal plasma levels of the hydrolyzed drug. Elimination of platinum metabolites is via the kidneys.	Neurotoxicity, in the form of a transient neuropathy with each dose and a persistent, cumulative typical sensory poly-neuropathy, is very common and dose limiting. Myelosuppression is expected but mild and only sometimes dose limiting. Fatigue and nausea are common but mild. Diarrhea, stomatitis, edema, cough, hypersensitivity reactions, and extra-vasation injury are rare.	FDA approved for metastatic colorectal cancer in combination with 5-fluorouracil/ leucovorin. Has been used as a single agent in this disease and is being studied in other malignancies.	With 5-fluorouracil and leucovorin, the dose and schedule is 85 mg/m^2 IV every 2 weeks as a 2 hour infusion in 250–500 mL of D5W. As a single agent, the most studied doses are the same 2 week dose or 130 mg/m^2 IV every 3 weeks.

CHEMOTHERAPEUTIC AGENT	DRUG CLASS/ MECHANISM OF ACTION	DOSAGE FORMS	DRUG INTERACTIONS	PHARMACOKINETICS/ METABOLISM	TOXICITY	INDICATIONS	DOSING
Paclitaxel (Taxol, Onxol)	Naturally occuring taxane molecule; inhibits depolymerization of tubulin in the spindle apparatus, thereby inducing apoptosis in dividing cells.	Vials containing 30 mg and 100 mg of drug in nonaqueous solution.	Cisplatin administered before paclitaxel could enhance the myelosuppressive effect of paclitaxel. Coadministration of paclitaxel and doxorubicin could enhance the cardio-toxicity of doxorubicin.	Paclitaxel has poor oral bioavailability. After IV administration, the drug exhibits a large volume of distribution and undergoes metabolism in the liver. The elimination half-life is 15–50 hours. Excretion of drug and metabolites is predominantly via the bile.	Paclitaxel is an irritant or mild vesicant when extravasated into subcutaneous tissue. Myelosuppression, predominantly neutropenia, is expected and is dose limiting. Shorter infusions of the same dose produce less neutropenia. Mucositis is also very common, particularly with longer infusions. Peripheral neuropathy is common, usually mild, and increases with cumulative dose. Acute neuromyopathy is also common and occurs for several days after each dose. This syndrome could require opiate analgesics to control pain. Cardiovascular side effects, including hypertension, hypotension, premature contractions, and bradyarrhythmias, are common but rarely require intervention. Hyper-sensitivity reactions to paclitaxel, including urticaria, wheezing, chest pain, dyspnea, and hypotension, are common but are reduced in frequency and severity by premedication with corticosteroids and H_1 and H_2 histamine receptor blockers (recommended regimen is dexamethasone 20 mg PO 12 and 6 hours prior to paclitaxel and diphenhydramine 50 mg and cimetidine 300 mg IV 30 minutes prior to paclitaxel). Alopecia, usually complete, is expected. Other toxicities are uncommon and include nausea, vomiting, diarrhea, liver toxicity, and interstitial pneumonitis.	FDA approved for salvage therapy in ovarian cancer and for breast cancer in both the metastatic and adjuvant setting. Used also in lung cancer, head and neck cancers, and bladder cancer.	135–250 mg/m^2 IV over 3 hours or 24 hours every 3 weeks. Weekly schedules and longer infusions have also been used.

CHEMOTHERAPEUTIC AGENT	DRUG CLASS/ MECHANISM OF ACTION	DOSAGE FORMS	DRUG INTERACTIONS	PHARMACOKINETICS/ METABOLISM	TOXICITY	INDICATIONS	DOSING
Pamidronate (Aredia)— APD, Aminohydroxy- propylidene diphosphonate	Organic bisphosphonate; inhibitor of bone resorption by osteoclasts.	Vials of lyophilized powder containing 30 mg of drug.	None noted.	Pamidronate is available by the parenteral route only. After IV administration, the drug concentrates in the bone, spleen, and liver. Its metabolism is not well characterized. It has a terminal half-life of about 27 hours. Fifty percent of the parent drug is eliminated in the urine.	Pamidronate is usually quite well tolerated. Hypotension, syncope, tachycardia, and even atrial fibrillation have been reported uncommonly during the infusion. Hypocalcemia, hypophosphatemia, hypokalemia, and hypomagnesemia occur commonly but only rarely require intervention. Nausea, vomiting, and somnolence are rare.	FDA approved for malignancy-induced hypercalcemia. Can lead to pain relief and even tumor shrinkage of bone metastases in multiple myeloma, breast cancer, and prostate cancer.	60–90 mg/m² IV over 24 hours, although the clinical experience with infusions of 1–3 hours is extensive. Treatment may be repeated every 1–3 weeks. Peak effect occurs 3–7 days after a dose.
Pegfilgrastim (Neulasta)	Long-acting (PEGylated) recombinant DNA granulocytic growth factor polypeptide.	Syringes containing 6 mg of drug in 0.6 mL aqueous solution with a 27-gauge needle.	No formal drug interaction studies have been done.	PEGylation of filgrastim increases its half-life by decreasing renal clearance. After subcutaneous administration, the half-life is between 15 and 80 hours, with biologic activity lasting much longer.	Toxicity and side effect profile is essentially no different from that of filgrastim. Bone pain is common and usually mild and treatable but can be dose limiting. Nausea, fatigue, weakness, and diarrhea are rare. Very rare instances of adult respiratory distress syndrome, sickle cell crisis, splenic rupture, and severe allergic reaction have been seen with the parent drug, filgrastim.	FDA approved for prevention of severe granulocytopenia from cytotoxic chemotherapy for nonmyeloid malignancies.	6 mg SC after each chemotherapy cycle (generally used for a 3- or 4-week cycle duration).
Pentostatin (Nipent, Covidarabine)— 2'- deoxycoformycin, dCF	Purine analogue antimetabolite; inhibits adenosine deaminase. Partly cell cycle dependent.	Vials of lyophilized powder containing 0 mg of 1 drug.	None noted.	Only available as an IV preparation, pentostatin has an elimination half-life of about 5 hours and undergoes very little metabolism. The majority of a dose is eliminated in the urine as unchanged drug.	Myelosuppression is expected and dose limiting. Lymphopenia is severe and can lead to opportunistic infections. Anemia and thrombocytopenia are also common. Nausea and vomiting are common but mild. Fever and fatigue are also common. Anorexia, diarrhea, stomatitis, rash, elevated liver function tests, significant nephrotoxicity, and headache are uncommon. Hepatitis, acute tubular necrosis, and CNS alterations, including coma and seizures, are rare.	FDA approved for the treatment of hairy cell leukemia. Also used occasionally for non–Hodgkin's lymphoma and CLL.	The usual dose is 4 mg/m² IV bolus (with 1 to 2 L of IV hydration) every 2 weeks.

CHEMOTHERAPEUTIC AGENT	DRUG CLASS/ MECHANISM OF ACTION	DOSAGE FORMS	DRUG INTERACTIONS	PHARMACOKINETICS/ METABOLISM	TOXICITY	INDICATIONS	DOSING
Plicamycin (Mithracin)— Mithramycin	Antitumor antibiotic. Partly cell cycle dependent.	Supplied as lyophilized powder in vials containing 2.5 mg of drug.	None noted.	Available by the intravenous route only. After an IV dose, the drug is metabolized by the liver and has an elimination half-life of about 2 hours. Parent drug and metabolites are eliminated via the kidneys.	Plicamycin is a vesicant if extravasated into soft tissues. Hemorrhage, due to both thrombocytopenia and coagulopathy, is dose limiting. Other hematologic toxicities are uncommon. Nausea and vomiting are common but not severe. Stomatitis, diarrhea, and anorexia are less common. Rash is common, but severe cutaneous reactions, such as toxic epidermal necrolysis, are rare. Depletion of calcium, potassium, phosphate, and magnesium are expected but rarely require intervention. Renal toxicities, including proteinuria and azotemia, are uncommon. Elevated liver function tests and neurologic toxicity (including lethargy, weakness, anxiety, somnolence, and headache) are uncommon.	FDA approved for treatment of malignancy-induced hypercalcemia and also for treatment of germ cell tumors. Also has been used for CML in blast crisis.	The typical dose for germ cell tumors is 25–30 mg/kg/day IV infusion over 60 minutes for 8–10 days. For hypercalcemia, the same dose is given 1–3 times per week.
Prednisone (Deltasone, Others)	Corticosteroid.	Tablets in sizes from 1 mg to 50 mg and oral solution.	None noted.	Prednisone has good oral bioavailability and is metabolized extensively in the liver, primarily to the active form of the drug, prednisolone. It has an elimination half-life of approximately 4 hours. Liver disease can decrease conversion to the active form, requiring use of prednisolone instead of prednisone. Routes of excretion are not well delineated.	Toxicity is mostly in the form of constitutional symptoms, including mood changes (depressive, anxious, or euphoric), insomnia, indigestion, enhanced appetite, weight gain, acne, and cushingoid features. Other side effects may be more serious but are less common. Hyperglycemia and increased stomach acid predisposing to ulceration occur acutely, while osteopenia, cataracts, skin atrophy, and adrenal insufficiency occur with prolonged use.	FDA approved for a wide variety of malignant and nonmalignant conditions. Used in oncology for lymphoid malignancies, for palliative care, and for management of side effects/toxicities.	Lympholytic doses are generally in the range of 50–100 mg/m²/day for 5–14 days. Higher or lower doses are also used, depending on the indication.
Procarbazine (Matulane)— N-methylhydrazine	Alkylating agent. Cell cycle independent.	50-mg capsules.	This drug has monoamine oxidase inhibitory activity and therefore	Well absorbed by the oral route, reaching peak plasma levels in 1 hour, with good distribution to the	Myelosuppression is expected and dose limiting, but anemia is uncommon. Nausea and vomiting are	FDA approved for Hodgkin's disease, and might also be useful in non-Hodgkin's	In Hodgkin's disease regimens such as MOPP, the dose is 100 mg/m²/day for

CHEMOTHERAPEUTIC AGENT	DRUG CLASS/ MECHANISM OF ACTION	DOSAGE FORMS	DRUG INTERACTIONS	PHARMACOKINETICS/ METABOLISM	TOXICITY	INDICATIONS	DOSING
			should not be taken with certain types of food, including beer, wines, fermented cheese, chocolate, and fava beans, or with certain medications, including ethanol, decongestants, tricyclic antidepressants, antihypertensives, antihistamines, narcotics, barbiturates, phenothiazines, or other monoamine oxidase inhibitors.	cerebrospinal fluid. Procarbazine is metabolized by the liver and has an elimination half-life of about 1 hour. Largely excreted in the urine.	common and can be dose limiting as well. Rash, hives, and photosensitivity sometimes occur. Other side effects are uncommon and include anorexia, diarrhea, stomatitis, hypotension, tachycardia, syncope, flulike syndrome, interstitial pneumonitis, CNS excitation including seizures, and secondary malignancies.	lymphoma, multiple myeloma, brain tumors, melanoma, and lung cancer.	14 days during each cycle.
Rituximab (Rituxan)	Monoclonal antibody directed against the B-cell surface antigen CD20.	Sterile vials containing 100 and 500 mg of antibody in aqueous solution (10 mg/mL).	None noted.	Not available by the oral route, but when given IV, it is taken up by B lymphocytes and then degraded throughout the body by proteolysis, with a wide-ranging serum half-life of 11–105 hours (mean 60 hours) with the first dose. There is no appreciable excretion of this polypeptide.	Fever, chills, and malaise are common during administration, even with premedication with acetaminophen and diphenhydramine. Other infusion-related symptoms include nausea, vomiting, flushing, urticaria, angioedema, hypotension, dyspnea, bronchospasm, fatigue, headache, rhinitis, and pain at disease sites. These symptoms are generally self-limited, improve with slowing of the infusion, and resolve after infusion. Short-lived myelosuppression, abdominal pain, and myalgia are uncommon. Arrhythmias and angina pectoris are rare.	FDA approved for relapsed or refractory low-grade or follicular, CD20-positive, B-cell lymphomas.	The recommended dose is 375 mg/m² by IV infusion (starting at 50 mg/hour and increasing to 400 mg/hour maximum) weekly for 4 weeks. Higher doses, more doses, and longer courses are being used in other lymphoid malignancies.
Sargramostim (Leukine, Leukomax)— Granulocyte-Macrophage Colony-Stimulating Factor, GM-CSF	Cytokine; exhibits pleiotropic stimulatory effects on bone marrow progenitor cells.	Vials containing 250, 400, and 500 mg of lyophilized GM-CSF.	None noted.	Not available by the oral route, but has similar bioavailability when given IV or SC. Degraded throughout the body, predominantly in the liver and kidneys, with an elimination half-life of 2 hours. No appreciable excretion of this peptide occurs.	Constitutional symptoms, which tend to decrease over time, predominate at standard doses. Higher doses could cause capillary leak syndrome. Side effects include flushing, hypotension (or hypertension), dyspnea, fever, nausea, vomiting, fatigue, myalgias, bone pain, headache, and	FDA approved for the treatment of myelosuppression after ABMT. Could be useful to minimize myelosuppression after standard-dose chemotherapy, or to shorten the course of neutropenic fever. Immunostimulatory	250 µg/m²/day for 21 days or 5 µg/kg/day for 10–14 days.

CHEMOTHERAPEUTIC AGENT	DRUG CLASS/MECHANISM OF ACTION	DOSAGE FORMS	DRUG INTERACTIONS	PHARMACOKINETICS/METABOLISM	TOXICITY	INDICATIONS	DOSING
					skin rash. Thrombocytopenia can occur also. Fluid retention and edema rarely occur at standard doses. Progression of myelodysplastic syndrome has been documented in patients on GM-CSF.	properties of GM-CSF are still being investigated.	
Streptozocin (Zanosar)	Alkylating agent. Cell cycle independent.	Vials containing 1 g of lyophilized streptozocin.	None noted.	Streptozocin is only bioavailable by the IV route. It is metabolized primarily in the liver, and has an elimination half-life of less than 1 hour. Parent drug and metabolites are excreted in the urine.	GI side effects (nausea, vomiting, and cramping) or nephrotoxicity (glomerular and tubular damage) are common and potentially dose limiting. Myelosuppression is less often dose limiting. Elevated liver function tests can occur occasionally but are rarely clinically significant. Fever, delerium, and depression occur rarely. Streptozocin is an irritant if extravasated into perivenous soft tissue.	FDA approved for metastatic islet cell carcinoma, and could also be useful for advanced carcinoid tumor, pancreatic carcinoma, and Hodgkin's disease.	The usual dose is 500–1000 mg/m²/day by IV bolus for 5 days every 4 weeks.
Tamoxifen (Nolvedex)	Nonsteroidal antiestrogen; cytostatic effects on estrogen-dependent and nondependent malignant cells.	10- or 20-mg tablets.	None noted.	Tamoxifen has good oral bioavailability, is metabolized in the liver, and has an elimination half-life of about 7 days. Neither tamoxifen nor its major metabolite is found in the bile or urine.	Tamoxifen is usually very well tolerated. Constitutional symptoms are most prevalent and usually dose limiting. Hot flashes, sweating, mood changes, weight gain or loss, and stomach upset are most common. Nausea, vomiting, diarrhea, and constipation are less common. Menstrual changes, including significant vaginal bleeding, are uncommon. Venous thromboembolism, myelosuppression, and retinopathy are rare.	FDA approved for the treatment of breast cancer, generally in postmenopausal patients or those with estrogen receptor-positive tumors. The same dose has been approved for chemoprevention of breast cancer in high-risk individuals. Higher doses are used for melanoma and pancreatic cancer.	The standard dose for breast cancer is 10 mg PO bid (or 20 mg once a day).
Temozolomide (Temodar)	Atypical alkylator (semi-selective DNA methylator) drug sharing the same active metabolite as	Capsules containing 5, 20, 100, and 250 mg of temozolomide.	Coadministration with valproic acid results in decreased oral bioavailability of temozolomide by a minor amount. No other drug interactions have	Temozolomide has good bioavailability, enhanced by an empty stomach. After absorbtion into the blood stream, it is converted spontaneously to the active moiety MTIC. Peak plasma concentrations are	Myelosuppression is expected and dose limiting. It could be cumulative. Nausea is common but generally mild and treatable. Headache and fatigue are common. Rash or other cutaneous reactions are	FDA approved for treatment of recurrent high-grade astrocytomas. Used commonly for other gliomas and also for metastatic melanoma.	200 mg/m² PO on an empty stomach daily for 5 days on a 28-day cycle. Other doses and schedules have been used with similar clinical results.

CHEMOTHERAPEUTIC AGENT	DRUG CLASS/MECHANISM OF ACTION	DOSAGE FORMS	DRUG INTERACTIONS	PHARMACOKINETICS/METABOLISM	TOXICITY	INDICATIONS	DOSING
	dacarbazine, MTIC, but unlike dacarbazine is spontaneously converted to MTIC and also penetrates the blood-brain barrier effectively.		been identified.	occur in about 1 hour. The elimination half-life is about 1.8 hours. Parent drug, MTIC, and other metabolites are eliminated in the urine.	uncommon. Infections are common in this population, and probably some are caused by immuno-suppression known to occur with temozolomide.		
Teniposide (Vumon)—VM-26, PTG	Inhibitor of topoisomerase II; similar in action to etoposide.	Vials of 10-mg/mL solution containing 50 mg of drug.	Metabolism of teniposide is increased by inducers of liver microsomal enzymes, such as phenobarbital and carbamazepine.	Teniposide is available by the IV route only. It is extensively protein bound in the plasma and undergoes near-complete metabolism in the liver. It has an elimination half-life of 5 hours. Metabolites are excreted in the bile and urine.	Myelosuppression, predominently leukopenia, is universal and dose limiting. Otherwise usually well tolerated. Nausea, vomiting, diarrhea, stomatitis, and anorexia are uncommon. Alopecia is generally mild. Elevated liver function tests can occur but are not usually clinically significant. Allergic reactions, hypotension, fatigue, seizures, somnolence, fever, renal insufficiency, and secondary leukemia are all rare.	FDA approved for childhood ALL. Not used commonly for other malignancies, but does have activity against SCLC.	100 mg/m² once or twice weekly, or 20–60 mg/m²/day for 5 days as a slow IV infusion (at least 30 minutes).
Thalidomide (Thalomid)	Novel anti-angiogenic and immuno-modulating agent.	50-mg tablets.	Increases the sedative properties of barbiturates, chlorpromazine, and ethanol.	Although it has acceptable bioavailibility, thalidomide is slowly and incompletely absorbed from the GI tract. Metabolism appears to be via spontaneous hydrolysis, with an elimination half-life of about 6 hours. Exact quantification of elimination routes are unknown.	Historical teratogenicity has led to required strict evaluation and monitoring for those taking thalidomide, called the S.T.E.P.S. program. Strict procedures to prevent conception include barrier contraception for men, as the drug is present in semen of men who are taking it. Fatigue and peripheral neuropathy are the main toxicities and are dose limiting. Myelosuppression is uncommon and usually mild. Rash and headache are uncommon.	FDA approved for cutaneous leprosy. Used in oncology for multiple myeloma, renal cell carcinoma, metastatic melanoma, and malignant gliomas. It is also used as a treatment for cachexia due to its mild anabolic and appetite-stimulating properties.	Oncology doses range for 50 mg/day up to 1200 mg/day.
Thioguanine (Tabloid) —6-TG, Aminopurine-6-thiol hemihydrate	Purine analogue antimetabolite. Cell cycle dependent.	40-mg tablets.	None noted.	Thioguanine has modest but slow oral route absorption. It is almost completely metabolized in the liver and has an	Thioguanine is usually well tolerated. Leukopenia and thrombocytopenia are common and dose limiting. Nausea and vomiting,	FDA approved for AML in all phases of treatment. Could be useful in other leukemias. An injectable regimen.	The usual dose for leukemias is 2–3 mg/kg/day as part of an ongoing multidrug regimen.

CHEMOTHERAPEUTIC AGENT	DRUG CLASS/ MECHANISM OF ACTION	DOSAGE FORMS	DRUG INTERACTIONS	PHARMACOKINETICS/ METABOLISM	TOXICITY	INDICATIONS	DOSING
				elimination half-life of up to 11 hours. Metabolites are excreted in the urine.	stomatitis, diarrhea, rash, elevated liver function tests, hyperuricemia, and renal insufficiency are uncommon.	formulation does not yet have FDA approval.	
Thiotepa (TESPA)— Triethylenethiophospho-ramide, TSPA	Classical alkylating agent. Cell cycle independent.	Available as lyophilized powder in vials containing 15 mg of drug.	None noted.	With poor oral bioavailability, thiotepa is available by the parenteral route only. Extensive metabolism occurs in the liver, and the drug has an elimination half-life of 2–3 hours. Metabolites are excreted in urine.	Myelosuppression, predominantly leukopenia, is expected and dose limiting and could be cumulative. Nausea, vomiting, anorexia, stomatitis, and diarrhea are uncommon. Infertility, fever, angioedema, or urticaria is uncommon. Second malignancies such as acute leukemia are rare. With high-dose therapy and bone marrow rescue, stomatitis and cognitive impairment can be severe. Intravesical administration leads to predominantly urinary symptoms, including pain, hematuria, hemorrhagic cystitis, and rare ureteral obstruction.	FDA approved for the treatment of breast and ovarian carcinoma, as well as Hodgkin's disease and non–Hodgkin's lymphoma. Used for intravesical therapy of superficial bladder cancer, and also can be used for intracavitary and intrathecal administration. Used in the transplant setting for ovarian and breast carcinoma.	The usual dose is 12–16 mg/m² IV over 10 minutes every 1–4 weeks. In the transplant setting, doses up to 900 mg/m² have been used. The bladder instillation dose is 30–60 mg once weekly for 4 weeks. The intrathecal dose is 1–10 mg/m² 1–2 times per week.
Topotecan (Hycamtin)— Hycamptamine	Semisynthetic camptothecin molecule; an inhibitor of topoisomerase I, which is required by cells for both transcription and replication.	5-mg vials of lyophilized powder.	None noted.	No oral form of this drug is available. After IV administration, the drug is not extensively metabolized, and it has an elimination half-life of about 3 hours. A significant portion of the drug is excreted unchanged in the urine.	Myelosuppression, especially leukopenia, is expected and dose limiting. Thrombocytopenia and anemia are common but mild. Nausea, vomiting, and diarrhea are common but usually not severe. Headache, fever, fatigue, anorexia, malaise, and elevated liver function tests are also common. Hypertension, tachycardia, urticaria, renal insufficiency, hematuria, neuropathy, and mucositis are uncommon.	FDA approved for the treatment of refractory, relapsed ovarian carcinoma and for relapsed small cell lung cancer. Also used in myeloid leukemias.	The standard dose for ovarian cancer is 1.5 mg/m²/day for 5 days as a 30-minute infusion.
Toremifene (Fareston)	Nonsteroidal antiestrogen; cytostatic effects on estrogen-dependent and nondependent malignant cells.	60-mg tablets.	None noted.	Toremifene has good oral bioavailability and is bound extensively to plasma proteins. It is metabolized in the liver to active metabolites and has an elimination half-life of	Toremifene is usually very well tolerated. Hot flashes, nausea, sweating, dizziness, and fatigue are the most common side effects. Vomiting, diarrhea, anorexia, vaginal discharge, vaginal	FDA approved for the treatment of post-menopausal or estrogen receptor–positive metastatic breast cancer.	60 mg PO qid.

Science of Clinical Oncology

CHEMOTHERAPEUTIC AGENT	DRUG CLASS/MECHANISM OF ACTION	DOSAGE FORMS	DRUG INTERACTIONS	PHARMACOKINETICS/METABOLISM	TOXICITY	INDICATIONS	DOSING
				about 5 days. Parent drug and metabolites are excreted in the bile.	bleeding, and headache are less common. Venous thrombosis and pulmonary embolism are rare.		
Trastuzumab (Herceptin)	A genetically engineered humanized mouse monoclonal antibody directed against the her2/neu growth factor receptor overexpressed on many invasive breast carcinomas. Mechanism of action for clinical activity in breast cancer is unknown, but could be complement-mediated cell lysis, antibody-dependent cellular cytotoxicity, or induction of apoptosis.	Vials containing 440 mg of drug in aqueous solution.	None noted.	Binding studies show strong binding to cells over-expressing her2/neu molecules. Very little else is known regarding the distribution and metabolic fates of this molecule. The half-life should be very short, with minimal distribution outside the vascular compartment and minimal clearance by kidneys or liver (similar to other monoclonal antibodies and polypeptide agents).	Common toxicities include acute fever, chills, nausea, vomiting, and headache. Trastuzumab seems to worsen leukopenia, anemia, and diarrhea when given with chemotherapy compared with chemotherapy alone. Also, trastuzumab could have uncommon acute cardiotoxicity, which might add to the more common anthracycline-induced cardiotoxicity; therefore, the use of trastuzumab with doxorubicin is not indicated by the FDA.	FDA approved for her2/neu overexpressing metastatic or locally advanced breast cancer; has shown clinical benefit as a single agent and in conjunction with paclitaxel-based chemotherapy.	Loading dose of 250 mg or 4 mg/kg by intravenous infusion followed by weekly intravenous infusions of 100 mg or 2 mg/kg for up to 10 weeks (or longer).
Tretinoin (Vesanoid)—ATRA, All-trans-retinoic Acid	A naturally occurring retinoid; induces differentiation and apoptosis of malignant promyelocytes in acute promyelocytic leukemia.	10-mg capsules.	None noted.	This drug has good oral bioavailability and a very short elimination half-life of about 40 minutes. It induces its own metabolism in the liver, leading to decreased levels and clinical effect with continued administration. No appreciable excretion of the parent compound is evident.	Tretinoin is teratogenic, so women of childbearing age who take this drug must be on optimal contraceptive measures. Leukostasis and hemorrhage due to leukocytosis are dose limiting but uncommonly life threatening if the drug is stopped. "Retinoic acid syndrome," although not common, can be dose limiting and consists of fever, chest pain, dyspnea, hypoxia, pulmonary infiltrates, and pleural/pericardial effusions. It can be lethal but improves with cessation of the drug and is treatable with corticosteroids. Dry skin, exfoliation, xerostomia,	FDA-approved induction therapy for acute promyelocytic leukemia. Also of benefit in the maintenance phase of this disorder, and could have clinical activity in other hematologic malignancies.	For induction, the dose is 45 mg/m²/day PO for 30–90 days, depending on the clinical response.

CHEMOTHERAPEUTIC AGENT	DRUG CLASS/ MECHANISM OF ACTION	DOSAGE FORMS	DRUG INTERACTIONS	PHARMACOKINETICS/ METABOLISM	TOXICITY	INDICATIONS	DOSING
					and cheilitis are common. Elevations in liver function tests and hyperlipidemias are also common. Headache is often seen, but pseudotumor cerebri or other neurologic occurrences are uncommon.		
Vinblastine (Velban, Velsar, others)—VLB, Vincaleukoblastine	Vinca alkaloid; inhibitor of tubulin polymerization, and thereby mitosis. G_2-phase specific.	Vials of drug in solution (1 mg/mL), or lyophilized powder containing 10 mg of drug.	None noted.	Poor oral bioavailability. After an IV dose, the drug undergoes deacetylation in the liver to an active metabolite, followed by further metabolism. The elimination half-life is about 20 hours. Excretion is predominantly via the bile.	Vinblastine is a soft tissue vesicant, requiring extravasation precautions during administration. Myelosuppression, especially leukopenia, is expected and dose limiting. Anemia and thrombocytopenia are less common. Peripheral and autonomic neuropathies are less common than that observed with vincristine. Nausea and vomiting are uncommon, but constipation is more often seen. Acute reactions during administration, including dyspnea, wheezing, chest pain, tumor pain, and fever, are uncommon. Syndrome of inappropriate antidiuretic hormone secretion occurs rarely, as does angina pectoris.	FDA approved for multiple hematologic and solid neoplasms. Most often used for Hodgkin's disease, non–Hodgkin's lymphoma, germ cell tumors, and breast cancer.	Typical doses are between 6 and 10 mg/m^2 by IV push every 2–4 weeks, combined with other drugs. Can also be given as a continuous infusion over 96 hours at a dose of 1.7–2.0 mg/m^2/day.
Vincristine (Oncovin, Vincasar)— Leurocristine, VCR	Vinca alkaloid; inhibitor of tubulin polymerization, and thereby mitosis. G_2-phase specific.	Available as solution (1 mg/mL) in vials containing 1–5 mg of drug and in syringes containing 1 or 2 mg.	L-Asparaginase could decrease hepatic metabolism of vincristine.	Vincristine is bioavailable by the IV route only. It is metabolized by the liver. The elimination half-life is variable but usually greater than 10 hours. Parent drug and metabolites are excreted primarily in the bile.	Vincristine is a vesicant and should be administered with extravasation precautions. Neurotoxicity is dose limiting in the form of peripheral neuropathy, which is related to total cumulative dose. Autonomic neuropathy is less common, and CNS toxicity is rare. Myelo-suppression is mild. Nausea and vomiting are rare, but constipation is fairly common. Acute cardio-pulmonary or pain symptoms occurring during administration are uncommon. Transient elevation of liver function tests is sometimes seen.	FDA approved for Hodgkin's disease and other lymphomas, acute leukemias, rhabdomyo-sarcoma, neuroblastoma, and Wilms' tumor. Used for many other neoplasms as well.	The usual dose is 0.5 to 1.4 mg/m^2 IV push every 1–4 weeks. A continuous infusion of 0.5 mg/m^2/day over 96 hours has also been used.

CHEMOTHERAPEUTIC AGENT	DRUG CLASS/ MECHANISM OF ACTION	DOSAGE FORMS	DRUG INTERACTIONS	PHARMACOKINETICS/ METABOLISM	TOXICITY	INDICATIONS	DOSING
Vinorelbine (Navelbine)— 5'-noranhydrovinblastine, NVB	Semisynthetic vinca alkaloid; inhibitor of tubulin polymerization, and thereby mitosis. G_2-phase specific.	Available as vials of 10-mg/mL solution.	None noted.	This drug has fair oral bioavailability but is currently available only as an IV preparation. It is metabolized by the liver and has an elimination half-life of about 24 hours. Excretion is predominantly in the bile.	Vinorelbine is a mild vesicant, requiring extravasation precautions. Myelosuppression, mostly leukopenia, is expected and dose limiting. Significant nausea and vomiting are uncommon. Neurotoxicity in the form of neuropathy is less common and milder than that seen with vincristine. Tumor pain during administration has been reported. Acute reaction, such as dyspnea, chest pain, and wheezing have occurred during administration and might be prevented by premedication with corticosteroids.	FDA approved for the treatment of relapsed metastatic breast cancer and for NSCLC as a single agent or combined with a platinating agent.	The recommended dose is 30 mg/m² IV over 20 minutes every week, with dose adjustments based on leukocyte counts.
Zolendronic Acid (Zometa)	Bisphosphonate inhibitor of bone metastases.	Vials containing 4 mg of zolendronic acid in powder form.	No studies have identified interactions. Theoretical concerns include exacerbation of hypocalcemia if zolendronic acid is coadministered with aminoglycosides or thiazide diuretics. Also, zolendronic acid could exacerbate the renal effects of other nephrotoxic drugs.	Zolendronic acid is poorly absorbed by the GI tract and is thus given as an intravenous infusion. It is not metabolized and is excreted by the kidneys. It has a plasma terminal elimination half-life of about 150 hours.	Zolendronic acid is generally well-tolerated. The most common infusional side effect is fever, which is usually mild and treatable. Nausea and constipation are also common. Dyspnea, fatigue, diffuse pain, rash, and headache are uncommon. Renal insufficiency is uncommon and generally reversible after discontinuation of the drug, but it is more likely with higher doses than the approved and recommended 4-mg dose.	FDA approved for treatment of hypercalcemia of malignancy and for prevention of pathologic fractures in multiple myeloma and solid tumors with known bone metastases.	4 mg IV injection over 15 minutes once monthly.

NEW DIRECTIONS IN DRUG DEVELOPMENT

New Categories of Agents

Apart from traditional cytotoxic agents, which currently are still the predominant class of drugs used to treat cancer, several newer classes of agents and strategies are quickly entering the clinical arena. Several products of biotechnology, including the first monoclonal antibodies and recombinant cytokines or growth factors, are listed for clinical use in the preceding drug charts. In addition, some agents with unique mechanisms of action, including retinoids and the hypomethylating agent 5-azacytidine, are also in clinical use. Otherwise, these agents are for the most part still in development. They include differentiation agents, antiangiogenesis agents, signal transduction inhibitors, monoclonal antibodies, gene therapy strategies, and vaccines.

Differentiating Agents

Several classes of compounds have potent in vitro and in vivo differentiating effects on the malignant cell phenotype. This list includes the retinoids, vitamin D analogs, cyclo-oxygenase inhibitors, and the hypomethylating agent, deoxyazacytidine. Unfortunately, these agents generally do not eliminate the malignant clone or affect its genotype, and for this reason they might have only transient effects. Their role in chemoprevention is promising, as is their role in potentially affecting favorably the natural history of incurable malignancies. Interestingly, celecoxib has shown significant activity in reducing polyps in familial adenomatous polyposis and has been approved by the Food and Drug Administration (FDA) for this indication. It is being tested as prevention in more common settings of high risk for colon cancer.

Antiangiogenesis Agents

Solid tumors require an adequate blood supply to grow and metastasize. They must stimulate neovascularization to obtain oxygen, micronutrients, and growth factors and to eliminate waste products. Primary or metastatic tumors that do not facilitate their own blood supplies do not grow and can regress completely or remain dormant. Bulky tumors that outgrow their blood supplies undergo central necrosis. The molecular basis for tumor angiogenesis is being pieced together rapidly, and clinical implications are emerging. There are multiple new compounds in the oncology pharmaceutical pipeline that affect this process profoundly, but all have yet to demonstrate convincing clinical activity except for tumor necrosis factor-α, which has proven too toxic for clinical use. Agents in clinical trials currently include thalidomide, endostatin, and the anti-vascular endothelial growth factor antibody, bevicuzumab.

Signal Transduction Inhibitors

Basic oncology research has given us many important clues as to the molecules that drive the malignant phenotype. Although the basic defect is in the genome, the expression of that defect is manifested in how the cell interacts with its surrounding milieu, which can include other malignant cells, nearby normal cells, the extracellular matrix, and humoral factors. This interaction impacts the cell via surface membrane receptors and second messengers within the cell. These second messengers affect gene expression and cell phenotype via kinase cascades (signal transduction pathways) specific to the receptor/second messenger system that is activated. Within these receptor/second messenger systems, many oncogenes are mutated proteins that confer abnormal cellular responses to malignant cells. In recent years, many small and large molecule inhibitors of these cascades have been developed and tested for cytotoxic and cytostatic effects. Examples include genistein, limonene, and the farnesyl transferase inhibitors. The epithelial growth factor receptor-tyrosine kinase inhibitor gefitinib (Iressa, ZD1839) is another example of a new agent that has promise for routine use in relapsed–small cell lung cancer and (potentially) in other cancers.

Monoclonal Antibodies

Malignant cells are vulnerable to treatments directed at unique antigens expressed on their surface. Most of these treatments take the form of immunotherapy with vaccines or antibodies. Monoclonal antibodies are a special kind of antibody treatment, whereby a single immunoglobulin molecule or fragment specific to a given surface antigen is produced by an immortalized plasma cell clone in large quantities. The binding of this antibody to the surface of the malignant cell can lead to complement-mediated lysis, antibody-dependent cellular cytotoxicity, or signal transduction–mediated apoptosis. Attachment of a cytotoxin or radionuclide to the antibody adds another effector mechanism that can kill the target cell and surrounding cells. The monoclonal antibody can either be of murine origin or, through recombinant DNA techniques, can be made partly human (chimeric) or nearly completely human (humanized). Many of these molecules are in clinical trials, but only three unconjugated antibodies—rituximab for refractory B-cell lymphomas, alemtuzumab for CLL, and trastuzumab for recurrent breast cancer—and two conjugated antibodies—yttrium-90–linked irbituximab for B-cell lymphomas and ozogamicin-linked gemtuzumab for relapsed AML—have been approved by the FDA so far.

Gene Therapy

Treatment strategies incorporating specific ribonucleotide sequences come in many different varieties, such as antisense therapy (RNA), systemic viral vector transfection (RNA or DNA), DNA injection into tumors, and ex vivo transfected and selected tumor cells, immune cells, or bone marrow progenitors (DNA). Most of these techniques have demonstrated some effectiveness in animal models, and clinical trials are ongoing. No proof of efficacy has been shown, however, and the technical hurdles are still daunting.

Vaccines

Vaccine strategies to treat cancers have been used for more than 100 years. The principles of immune surveillance and tumor rejection have been well demonstrated in animal models and form the justification for human vaccine strategies. In the last 10 years, many human tumor antigens (and the humoral and cellular immune responses to them) have been characterized. To date, no convincing clinical evidence exists for sufficient efficacy of cancer vaccines, and the ability to correlate immune response to a vaccine and clinical effectiveness has been elusive. Recent advances in molecular immunology might hold the key to solving the puzzles of reinstating and measuring clinically relevent tumor immunogenicity. Several possibly effective cancer vaccines are currently in large Phase III trials, which could lead to FDA approval.

Computer Modeling and Combinatorial Chemistry

The pioneering discoveries of the early days of chemotherapy have permitted the development of a paradigm for drug discovery that persists, with modifications, to the present day. This organized approach to random screening of large numbers of compounds, however, must be complemented in the drug development effort by attempts to exploit new therapeutic targets identified in ongoing basic cancer research.

The molecular basis for antineoplastic therapy has been rapidly being unveiled since the 1990s. For many chemotherapy agents, the molecules responsible for drug transport, binding, effector mechanism, detoxification, and efflux out of cells are known. Therefore, new and better agents that result in tumor cell death and clinical response can be designed to exploit these known targets. This effort requires powerful computer programs, advanced chemistry techniques, three-dimensional modeling capabilities, and nucleotide sequences of all the relevant target protein genes. With these tools in place, one can create new small or large molecules or modify existing molecules by the addition or subtraction of functional groups, to direct the binding, specificity, inhibition, duration of action, and toxicity of these molecules based on chemical interactions with the target molecules. This process is called mechanistic drug development, and it uses computer modeling to predict the chemical composition of the new drugs, whether they be small-molecule inhibitors, peptides, proteins, or nucleotide sequences.

A related endeavor ongoing in the pharmaceutical industry and elsewhere is called combinatorial chemistry.[61-66] This process tests for binding interactions between new compounds or molecules and known targets that result in the desired cellular and clinical effect. The target is usually placed on a solid phase, and the candidate molecule is tested for binding to this solid phase. Once specific binding is documented, this compound is then tested for in vitro and in vivo biologic modulation (inhibition or stimulation) of the target molecule function. From there, standard testing of preclinical and clinical activity can be carried out with existing or new methods.

This ongoing work in drug development is crucial if our use of chemotherapy is to continue to improve and if its role in potentially curative therapy is to expand. Standard approaches and mechanistically based drug development will continue in parallel, and many new agents will undoubtedly follow, offering great promise for the future of cancer treatment.

Related fields in molecular oncology, called genomics and proteomics, also use powerful computer technology to analyze tumor samples for thousands of signals simultaneously on a single small slide, with DNA or cDNA made from mRNA in the case of genomics to look directly at genes or gene expression, and with protein fragments in the case of proteomics. Either technique allows the formulation of a pattern of phenotypic or genotypic expression of the cancer cell, from which patterns therapeutic targets can be discerned. This field is also moving forward rapidly and will become clinically relevant soon.

PHARMACOLOGIC APPROACHES

Drug Development

Although approximately 100 drugs are now in use to treat human cancers, the vast majority of cancers are not cured by chemotherapy. Since it no longer seems possible to identify one specific abnormality between cancerous and normal cells, additional agents with different modes of action must be sought. Although some chemotherapeutic agents (e.g., 5-fluorouracil) have been designed rationally, others (e.g., cisplatin) have been found by chance. The NCI is developing a chemical screening system that permits identification of a compound of interest—a lead compound—which can then be modified or enhanced, and the interaction of the compound with its target (enzyme, growth factor, or oncogene product) can be characterized. Appropriate bioassays are required for each lead agent as it is developed.

A significant fraction of our currently available chemotherapeutic agents are either natural products or derived from natural products, which often have complex structures that complicate synthesis efforts. Problems commonly arise in supply of starting material, the development of drug synthesis methods, and successful formulation of the drug so that it is absorbed and distributed appropriately. The problems of chemistry compound the difficulty in bringing drugs to clinical trials.

PHARMACOGENETICS

It is now clear that much of the variability in response to drugs is inherited. The genetically determined variability of drug response characterizes a research area known as pharmacogenetics. Individual variation in response to drugs is a significant clinical problem in several aspects. The identification of specific genes and gene products associated with various diseases might identify targets for new drugs. Identifying genes and allelic variants of genes that affect response to current drugs would be enormously valuable and would permit more precise prescribing guidelines and reduce adverse drug reactions. As an example, a clinically important polymorphism occurs in the enzyme thiopurine methytransferase (TPMT), which is responsible for metabolism of the antitumor agents,

6-thioguanine and 6-mercaptopurine. Children with inherited TPMT deficiency develop severe hematologic toxicity when exposed to such drugs, while those with high levels of the enzyme require higher doses to achieve the desired effect.[67] In the future, the development of new drugs for patients with specific genotypes would allow "drug stratification," with selection of specific drugs or doses based on pharmacogenetics.

PHARMACOKINETICS/ PHARMACODYNAMICS

Pharmacokinetics is the relationship between plasma concentration of a drug and time and is concerned with the drug's absorption, distribution, metabolism, and excretion. It is what the body does to the drug. The interpretation of pharmacokinetic data is usually based on assessment of total plasma clearance, either by measurement of the area under the plasma concentration-time curve (AUC) or of the steady-state plasma concentration during a constant infusion. A critical issue is intersubject variability in clearance; here, several factors come into play, including saturation of the major metabolic or excretory sites, protein binding, and body size. The evidence for the use of body surface area (BSA) in dosing oncology drugs is scarce, and other methods could be preferable.

Conversely, pharmacodynamics—the relationship between plasma concentration of the drug and its effects—is what the drug does to the body. Pharmacodynamics analyses have increasingly been incorporated into cancer drug development and complement pharmacokinetic studies, as pharmacodynamics, in conjunction with pharmacokinetics, permits a better prediction and understanding of effect, rather than evaluating plasma concentrations of unclear significance. To date, the influence of pharmacodynamics in oncology has been relatively limited, due to the tendency to use combination chemotherapy for most malignancies and to the considerable heterogeneity of the cancer population. Many oncology patients are older and have comorbidities that could affect pharmacokinetic-pharmacodynamic variability; hepatic metastases could alter drug metabolism; and there is often a significant lag time between the last measured plasma concentration and the first major therapeutic or toxic effect. The net result is that such studies are often not practical at the present time. This is a field of active investigation, however, and advances in this area might yield great benefits in tailoring treatment to the individual patient.

REFERENCES

1. Gilman A, Philips FS: The biological actions and therapeutic applications of b-chloroethyl amines and sulfides. Science 1946;103:409–415.
2. Infield GB: Disaster at Bari. New York, Macmillan, 1971.
3. Farber S, Diamond LK, Mercer RD, et al: Temporary remissions in acute leukemia in children produced by the folic acid antagonist, 4-aminopteroyl-glutamic acid. N Engl J Med 1948;238:787–793.
4. Hertz R, Lewis J, Lippsett M: Five years experience with the chemotherapy of metastatic choriocarcinoma and related trophoblastic tumors in women. Am J Obstet Gynecol 1961;82:631–640.
5. Elion GB: The purine path to chemotherapy. Science 1989;144:41–47.
6. Johnson IS, Armstrong JG, Gorman M, et al: The vinca alkaloids: A new class of oncolytic agents. Cancer Res 1963;23:1390–1427.
7. Rosenberg B, Van Camp L, Trosko JE, et al: Platinum compounds: A new class of potent antitumor agents. Nature 1969;222:385–386.
8. Driscoll JS: The preclinical new drug research program of the National Cancer Institute. Cancer Treat Rep 1984;68:63–76.
9. Shoemaker RH, Wolpert-DeFilippes MK, Kern DH, et al: Application of a human tumor colony forming assay to new drug screening. Cancer Res 1985;45:2145–2153.
10. Salmon SE: Kinetics of minimal residual disease. Recent Results Cancer Res 1979;67:1–15.
11. Frei E III, Clark JR, Miller D: The concept of neoadjuvant chemotherapy. In Salmon SE (ed): Adjuvant Therapy of Cancer, vol V. Orlando, Fl, Grune & Stratton, 1987, pp 67–75.
12. Rosen G, Caparos B, Huvos AG, et al: Preoperative chemotherapy for osteogenic sarcoma: Selection of post-operative adjuvant chemotherapy based on the response of the primary tumor to pre-operative chemotherapy. Cancer 1982;49:1221–1230.
13. Aaronson NK, Meyerowitz BE, Bard M, et al: Quality of life research in oncology. Past achievements and future priorities. Cancer 1991;67:839–843.
14. Gough IR, Dalgleish LI: What value is given to quality of life assessment by health professionals considering response to palliative chemotherapy for advanced cancer. Cancer 1991;68:220–225.
15. DeVita VT, Schein PS: The use of drugs in combination for the treatment of patients with cancer. Rationale and results. N Engl J Med 1973;288:998–1006.
16. American Society of Clinical Oncology recommendations for the use of hematopoietic colony-stimulating factors: Evidence-based, clinical practice guidelines. J Clin Oncol 1994;12:2471–2508.
17. Goldie JH, Coldman AJ: A mathematical model for relating the drug sensitivity of tumors to their spontaneous mutation rate. Cancer Treat Rep 1979;63:1727–1733.
18. Schimke RT: Gene amplification in cultured mammalian cells. Cell 1984;37:705–713.
19. Poste G, Fidler I: The pathogenesis of cancer metastases. Nature 1980;283:139–146.
20. DeVita VT, Young RC, Canellos GP: Combination vs. single agent chemotherapy: A review of the basis for selection of drug treatment of cancer. Cancer 1975;35:98–110.
21. Klimo P, Connors JM: MOPP/ABV hybrid program: Combination chemotherapy based on early introduction of seven effective drugs for advanced Hodgkin's disease. J Clin Oncol 1985;3:1174–1182.
22. Longo DL, DeVita VT, Duffey PL, et al: Superiority of ProMACE-CytaBOM over ProMACE + MOPP in the treatment of advanced diffuse aggressive lymphoma: Results of a prospective randomized trial. J Clin Oncol 1991;9:25–38.
23. Elliott JA, Österlind K, Hansen HH: Cyclic alternating non-cross-resistant chemotherapy in the management of small cell anaplastic carcinoma of the lung. Cancer Treat Rev 1984;11:103–113.
24. Österlind K, Sörenson S, Hansen HH, et al: Continuous versus alternating combination chemotherapy for advanced small cell carcinoma of the lung. Cancer Res 1983;43:6085–6089.
25. Daniels JR, Chak LY, Sikic BL, et al: Chemotherapy of small cell carcinoma of the lung: A randomized comparison of alternating and sequential combination chemotherapy programs. J Clin Oncol 1984;2:1192–1199.
26. Ettinger DS, Finkelstein DM, Abeloff MD, et al: A randomized comparison of standard chemotherapy versus alternating chemotherapy and maintenance versus no maintenance therapy for extensive stage small-cell lung cancer: A Phase III study of the Eastern Cooperative Oncology Group. J Clin Oncol 990;8:230–240.
27. Roth BJ, Johnson DH, Einhorn LH, et al: Randomized study of cyclophosphamide, doxorubicin, and vincristine versus etoposide and cisplatin versus alteration of these two regimens in extensive small-cell lung cancer: A Phase III trial of the Southeastern Cancer Study Group. J Clin Oncol 1992;10:282–291.

28. Fukuoka M, Furuse K, Saijo N, et al: Randomized trial of cyclophosphamide, doxorubicin, and vincristine versus cisplatin and etoposide versus alternation of these regimens in small-cell lung cancer. J Natl Cancer Inst 1991;83:855–861.

29. Canellos GP, Anderson JR, Propert KJ, et al: Chemotherapy of advanced Hodgkin's disease with MOPP, ABVD, or MOPP alternating with ABVD. N Engl J Med 1992;327:1478–1484.

30. Glick J, Young ML, Schilsky R, et al: MOPP/ABV hybrid chemotherapy for advanced Hodgkin's disease significantly improves failure-free and overall survival: the 8-year results of the intergroup trial. J Clin Oncol 1998;16:19–26, 2283 [comment].

31. Aisner J, Cirrincione C, Perloff M, et al: Combination chemotherapy for metastatic or recurrent carcinoma of the breasta randomized phase III trial comparing CAF versus VATH versus VATH alternating with CMFVP: Cancer and Leukemia Group B Study 8281. J Clin Oncol 1995;13:1443–1452.

32. Skipper HE, Schabel FM Jr, Wilcox WS: Experimental evaluation of potential anticancer agents. XII. On the criteria and kinetics associated with curability of experimental leukemia. Cancer Chemother Rep 1964;35:111.

33. Skipper HE: Laboratory models: The historical perspective. Cancer Treat Rep 1986;70:3–7.

34. Shackney SE, McCormack GW, Cuchural GJ: Growth rate patterns of solid tumors and their relation to responsiveness to therapy: An analytical review. Ann Intern Med 1978;89:107–121.

35. Collins VP, Loeffler K, Tivey H: Observations on growth rates of human tumors. Am J Roentgenol 1956;76:988–1000.

36. Tubiana M: Tumor cell proliferation kinetics and tumor growth rate. Acta Oncol 1989;28:113–121.

37. Sullivan PW, Salmon SE: Kinetics of tumor growth and regression in IgG multiple myeloma. J Clin Invest 1972;51:1697.

38. Spratt JS, Greenberg RA, Henser LS: Geometry, growth rates, and duration of cancer and carcinoma in situ of the breast before detection by screening. Cancer Res 1986;46:970–974.

39. DeMicheli R: Growth of testicular neoplasm lung metastases: Tumor specific relation between two Gompertzian parameters. Eur J Cancer 1980;16:1603–1608.

40. LaLa PK: Age-specific changes in the proliferation of Ehrlich ascites cells grown as solid tumors. Cancer Res 1972;32:628–636.

41. Watson JV: The cell proliferation kinetics of the EMT6/M/AC mouse tumor at four volumes during unperturbed growth in vivo. Cell & Tissue Kinet 1976;9:147–156.

42. Norton L, Simon R: Tumor size, sensitivity to therapy, and the design of treatment schedules. Cancer Treat Rep 1977;61:1307–1317.

43. Norton LA: A Gompertzian model of human breast cancer growth. Cancer Res 1988;48:7067–7071.

44. Norton L, Simon R: The Norton-Simon hypotheses revisited. Cancer Treat Rep 1986;70:163–169.

45. Citron ML, Berry DA, Cirrincione C, et al: Randomized trial of dose-dense versus conventionally scheduled and sequential versus concurrent combination chemotherapy as postoperative adjuvant treatment of node-positive primary breast cancer: First report of Intergroup Trial 9741/Cancer and Leukemia Group B Trial 9741. J Clin Oncol 2003;21:1431–1439.

46. Buzzoni R, Bonadonna G, Valagussa P, et al: Adjuvant chemotherapy with doxorubicin plus cyclophosphamide, methotrexate, and fluorouracil in the treatment of resectable breast cancer with more than three positive nodes. J Clin Oncol 1991;9:2134–2140.

47. Walsh SJ, Begg CB, Carbone PP: Cancer chemotherapy in the elderly. Semin Oncol 1989;16:66–75.

48. Baker DS, Grochow LB, Donehower RC. Should anticancer drug dose be adjusted in the obese patient? J Natl Cancer Inst 1995;87:333–334.

49. Smith TJ, Desch CE: Neutropenia-wise and pound-foolish: Safe and effective chemotherapy in massively obese patients. South Med J 1991;84:883–885.

50. Perry MC (ed): The Chemotherapy Sourcebook, 3rd ed. Philadelphia, Lippincott Williams & Wilkins, 2001.

51. Diasio RB, Beavers TL, Carpenter JT: Familial deficiency of dihydropyrimidine dehydrogenase: Biochemical basis for familial pyrimidinemia and severe 5-fluorouracil-induced toxicity. J Clin Invest 1988;81:47–51.

52. Ratain MJ, Mick R, Berezin F, et al: Paradoxical relationship between acetylator phenotype and amonafide toxicity. Clin Pharm Ther 1991;50:573–579.

53. Burris HA III: Combination chemotherapy. In Perry MC (ed): The Chemotherapy Sourcebook, 3rd ed. Philadelphia, Lippincott Williams & Wilkins, 2001, pp 69–73.

54. Groeger JS, Lucas AB, Coit DC: Venous access in the cancer patient. In De Vita VT Jr, Hellman S, Rosenberg SA (eds): PPO Updates, Principles and Practice of Oncology, vol 5. Philadelphia, JB Lippincott, 1991, pp 1–14.

55. AskRx Drug Information Program: Information Derived from the United States Pharmacopedial Dispensing Information, vol I (USP DI). Warrendale, Penna, Camdat Corporation, 1992.

56. Baltzer L, Berkery R (eds): Oncology Pocket Guide to Chemotherapy, 2nd ed. St. Louis, Mosby–Year Book, 1995.

57. Clinical Pharmacology Online, Version 1.13. Gold Standard Multimedia, Inc, October 14, 1997.

58. Fischer DS, Knobf MF, Durivage HJ (eds): The Cancer Chemotherapy Handbook, 4th ed. St. Louis, Mosby-Year Book, 1993.

59. Micromedex Computerized Clinical Information System, vol 94. Micromedex, Inc, 1997.

60. Physicians' Desk Reference, 57th ed. Montvale, NJ, Medical Economics, 2003.

61. Maghfoor I, Doll DC: Chemotherapy in pregnancy. In Perry MC (ed): The Chemotherapy Sourcebook, 3rd ed. Philadelphia, Lippincott Williams & Wilkins, 2001, pp 537–546.

62. Brown D: Future pathways for combinatorial chemistry. Mol Diversity 1997;2:217–222.

63. Combinatorial chemistry to develop new drugs. Cancer J Sci Am 1997;3:312–313.

64. Hruby VJ, Shenderovich M, Lam KS, Lebl M: Design considerations and computer modeling related to the development of molecular scaffolds and peptide mimetics for combinatorial chemistry. Mol Diversity 1996;2:46–56.

65. Kick EK, Roe DC, Skillman AG, et al: Structure-based design and combinatorial chemistry yield low nanomolar inhibitors of cathepsin D. Chem Biol 1997;4:297–307.

66. Plunkett MJ, Ellman JA: Combinatorial chemistry and new drugs. Sci Am 1997;276:68–73.

67. Lennard L, Lilleyman JS, Van Loon J, Weinshilboum RM: Genetic variation in response to 6-mercaptopurine for childhood acute lymphoblastic leukaemia. Lancet 1990;336:225–229.

Science of Clinical Oncology

THE BASICS OF RADIATION THERAPY

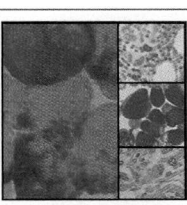

Ryan P. Smith

W. Gillies McKenna

SUMMARY OF KEY POINTS

HISTORICAL PERSPECTIVE

- The discovery of x-rays was made by Roentgen.
- Radioactivity was discovered by Becquerel, the Curies, and others.
- Advances in external beam radiation therapy, brachytherapy, and measurements are summarized.

RADIATION ONCOLOGY PHYSICS

- Several types of radiation are used clinically.
- Radiation can be produced by radioactive decay and by linear accelerators.
- Radiation can interact with matter via several mechanisms, the most important of which in radiation therapy is the Compton effect.
- Radiation used clinically today (megavoltage) has a skin-sparing effect, with a build-up region of dose followed by attenuation.

BIOLOGIC INTERACTIONS AND CONSIDERATIONS

- Radiation interacts with all biological materials, though the direct and indirect damage to DNA is believed to be the dominant form of radiation-induced damage.
- Radiation induces many molecular responses that induce cellular mechanisms for DNA damage repair, cell cycle arrests, and apoptosis.

- The most commonly used model of cell survival curves is the linear quadratic model, which uses α/β ratios.
- Cells repair sublethal and potentially lethal damage after exposure to radiation.
- The dose rate at which radiation is delivered is important to its effect on tissues.
- Radiation effect is modulated as cells progress through different stages of the cell cycle.
- Fractionation of radiation and altered fractionation schemes make use of tissues' varying responses to radiation to achieve higher therapeutic ratios.
- The response of cells to radiation is strongly oxygen dependent, expressed through the oxygen enhancement ratio.
- Radiosensitizers and radioprotectors can be given to enhance tumor cell killing or to protect normal tissues.

CLINICAL APPLICATION OF RADIOBIOLOGIC PRINCIPLES

- The goal of investigations into the aspects of radiation is to increase the therapeutic ratio.
- Radiation can have an effect on normal tissues, ranging from acute effects to late effects to carcinogenesis.

PROCESS IN RADIATION TREATMENT

- Successful treatment planning is imperative to the success of a radiation treatment course.
- Three-dimensional treatment planning and delivery have allowed for escalation of dose and sparing of normal tissues.
- Radiation is used as definitive treatment, as adjuvant or neoadjuvant treatment, as part of an organ-sparing therapy, and in palliation.

NEW MODALITIES IN RADIATION

- Intensity-modulated radiotherapy (IMRT) uses several noncoplanar radiation beam intensities to achieve a shaped dose distribution, increasing the therapeutic ratio.
- Neutron therapy has been investigated and shown to be efficacious for select patients.
- Because of its physical dose distribution, proton beam therapy is used to achieve extremely conformal radiation dose depositions, allowing for the treatment of tumors in close proximity to normal structures.

HISTORICAL PERSPECTIVE

In the closing years of the nineteenth century, many physicists were investigating the nature of electricity. It was known that if an electric potential was placed across two separated platinum electrodes, a spark would leap between them. The British physicist William Crookes, however, demonstrated that if the two electrodes were placed within a glass vessel that was then evacuated, as the vacuum increased the spark would at first be replaced by a glow that filled the whole vessel. As the vacuum was increased still further, a dark space would appear at the cathode electrode that would expand as the vacuum dropped until it filled the whole tube, and the walls of the vessel would then begin to fluoresce. On November 8, 1895, while passing electricity through a high-vacuum (Crookes) tube, Wilhelm Conrad Roentgen noted the fluorescence of a nearby piece of paper painted with barium platinocyanide. Because he had wrapped the Crookes tube in heavy opaque paper before beginning the experiment, he realized that this fluorescence of the paper could have been caused by a new, invisible type of ray that the tube was now emitting that was affecting both the shielded walls of the tube and the nearby piece of paper. Hence, the x-ray was discovered.[1,2]

Many scientists of that era were experimenting with Crookes tubes. During these experiments, many others likely observed the effects of x-rays but did not pursue an analysis of them. In fact, the first recorded x-ray exposure had been obtained five years earlier at the University of Pennsylvania by the physicist Arthur Willis Goodspeed, who was demonstrating a Crookes tube to his friend, the photographer W. N. Jennings.[3] A photographic plate was left nearby with two coins lying on it, which by tradition were the photographer's cab fare home. When the plate was later developed, it showed the image of the two coins (Fig. 26-1). Though Goodspeed and Jennings saved this exposure, they had no understanding of its meaning. It was not until five years later, when Roentgen noted the fluorescence of the plate during his experiment that anyone began to study these unknown "x"-rays. Roentgen studied the attenuation and the intensity of these x-rays and noted the inverse square law, which describes the loss of intensity of the x-rays with the inverse square of the distance between the tube and the plate.[4] He also noted that he could see the shadow of the bones in his hand when it was placed between the Crookes tube and the fluorescent paper. This led to the first human x-ray film on December 22, 1895, when he placed his wife's hand between the x-ray tube and a photographic plate (Fig. 26-2).

Roentgen first presented his findings on December 28, 1895 and sent the details of his experiments to physicists throughout the world.[4] Because the x-ray tube was a simple apparatus to replicate, many experiments on x-rays took place within a very short time. This quick, widespread experimentation rapidly produced advances in the new field. Within months of the discovery of x-rays, they were being used diagnostically in hospitals throughout the world. For example, the first medical x-rays at the University of Pennsylvania were taken in February of

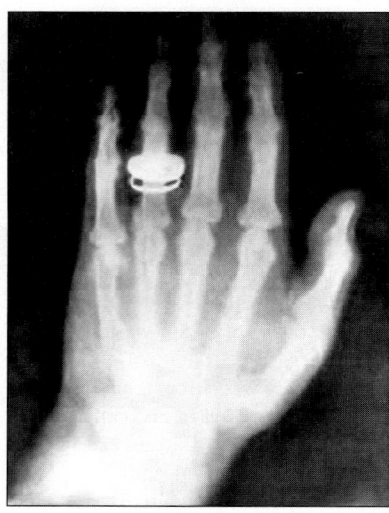

Figure 26-2. First radiograph, exposed by W.C. Roentgen, of his wife, Frau Roentgen, on December 22, 1895.

1896 (within three months of the discovery of the x-ray), and the University's first skiagrapher (painter of shadows), Charles Lester Leonard, was appointed the same year. Leonard later became one of the early x-ray "martyrs," losing his hands (and ultimately, his life) to radiation-induced skin cancer.

Radioactivity was discovered shortly after the x-ray and was equally important to the field of radiation oncology. Its discovery was linked indirectly to Roentgen's experiments. As the Crookes tubes produced x-rays, the walls of the tube would fluoresce. Other substances were also known to fluoresce spontaneously, and it was thought that these substances might also produce x-rays. This possibility was investigated by Henri Becquerel,[5] who observed the darkening of photographic plates by uranium salts. From this, he concluded that these same x-rays were emitted spontaneously and continuously from the uranium. He reported the results of his experiments with uranium to Pierre and Marie Curie, who coined the term *radioactivity* to describe it. They set out to isolate in purer form the radioactive substances within the uranium salts, and they reported the discovery of radium in 1898.[6]

Almost immediately, the biologic effects of ionizing radiation were recognized. Scientists and workers performing early experiments experienced significant radiation effects. Acutely, these were mainly erythema of the skin from exposure to the x-rays, with the carcinogenic properties of x-rays becoming evident later. Madame Curie herself died from aplastic anemia that was probably radiation induced. Becquerel reported radiation dermatitis on his own chest after carrying a sample of radium in his vest pocket.[7] Pierre Curie performed an experiment on himself, noting skin radiation changes and epilation after exposure to radium for only a few hours.[8] Reading of this, Alexander Graham Bell wrote to his friend, Dr Z. T Sowers, suggesting that if radium "sealed up in fine glass tube" were inserted "into the very heart" of a cancer, it might causer the tumor to regress.[9] Soon after learning of

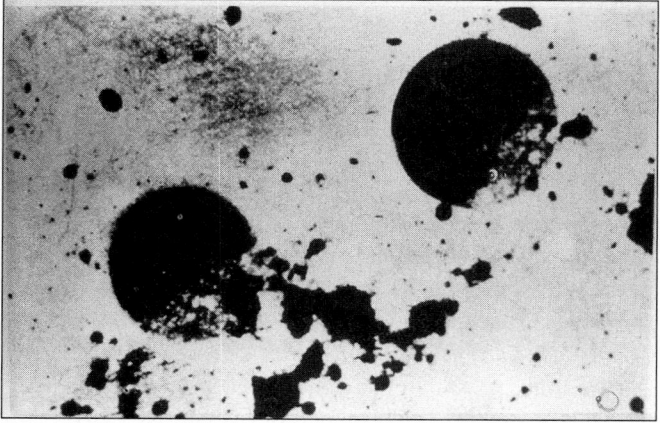

Figure 26-1. Image of the first x-ray developed, by accident, by Arthur W. Goodspeed and W.N. Jennings on February 22, 1890, at the University of Pennsylvania.

the radiation-induced erythema, physicians at St. Louis Hospital in Paris began treating patients with radiation. They found that tumors could be eradicated by radium exposure, thus beginning the use of ionizing radiation in the treatment of cancer.[8] The first cure with radiation, involving a patient with basal cell epithelioma, was reported in 1899.[10]

Hope that a cure for cancer lay in radiation therapy was soon replaced by skepticism when recurrences and toxicities were noted. The early treatments often involved very large single exposures aimed at the complete eradication of tumors.[11] These large exposures, together with the fact that the first x-ray machines were capable of producing only very low-energy x-rays with poor tissue penetration, resulted in extensive skin toxicities and other complications. Therefore, only superficial sites were originally treated by the direct application of radium, with impressive results.[12,13] Eventually, physicians started to insert radium directly into deep-seated tumors, effectively beginning the field of brachytherapy. Cervical cancer was first treated using this method, with dramatic responses noted.[14] Soon, other sites were treated, employing methods of dose calculations that are still used today.

External beam radiation therapy took longer to develop and might have been abandoned, had it not been for the work of Claude Regaud and Henri Coutard. They used smaller doses of radiation in several treatments delivered over several weeks.[11] Radiation oncology became a recognized medical field in 1922, when Coutard and Hautant reported their findings that advanced laryngeal cancer could be cured without severe toxicities using fractionated treatments.[15] By 1934, Coutard developed a fractionation scheme based on biologic experiments that remains the basis of fractionation today.[16]

Advances in measurements were also achieved when the skin erythema dose (the dose of x-rays required to give a light skin reaction) was replaced by the Roentgen in 1928.[17] The Roentgen, which was roughly the exposure received by placing one gram of radium at a distance of one yard for one hour, was a unit that expressed the radiation exposure and allowed for reproducible measurements and treatment dosages in different departments. It was calibrated by measuring the ionization of air using ionization chambers. With higher-energy beams, the size of the ionization chamber necessary to measure their effect becomes impossibly large. Thus, it was suitable only for low-energy x-rays and the Roentgen was replaced by a new unit, the rad.[18] The rad is the unit of absorbed dose and is a measure of the energy deposition per unit mass by all types of ionizing radiation. Biological effects in tissue exposed to ionizing radiation depend upon the energy deposited in the tissue rather than the amount of ionization that the radiation produces in air. The rad, an abbreviation for **r**adiation **a**bsorbed **d**ose, is not limited to x-rays or gamma rays and is not limited to exposure in air.

One rad is defined as the deposition of 100 ergs per gram of absorbing material. As a general rule, the absorbed dose in soft tissue from one Roentgen of intermediate-energy x-rays or gamma rays is roughly equivalent to one rad. The rad is now being replaced by the Gray (Gy),

which is defined as an absorbed energy 100 times greater than a rad (1 Gray = 100 rad = 1 joule/kg). This latter change is to make the unit of radiation consistent with the standard SI (Systeme International) units of measurement.

With time, ionizing radiation became more precise, and higher-energy machines capable of depositing dose at depth were invented. High-energy photons and electrons in the megavoltage range are now available, with accurate treatment planning and delivery. As the technology has progressed, radiation therapy has become increasingly sophisticated, with computer controls to deliver exact and modulated doses to depths and specific areas within the treatment field. Heavy particles—most notably neutrons and protons—are now being used, with even greater accuracy using greatly increased therapeutic ratios.

RADIATION ONCOLOGY PHYSICS

The field of radiation oncology uses energy in the form of radiation delivered to a target for cure or palliation. To understand radiation oncology, a full understanding of the particles and processes involved in the production and delivery of radiation must be attained. The following is an introduction to the physical properties of radiation that are fundamental to the clinical application of radiation to patients.

Types of Radiation

Electromagnetic radiation is energy that is transmitted at the speed of light through oscillating electric and magnetic fields. A photon has a wavelength λ, frequency ν, and energy $E=h\nu$, where h is Planck's constant (6.626×10^{-34} Joule seconds). The electromagnetic spectrum ranges from wavelengths of 10^5 m for AM radio waves to 10^{-12} m for x-rays and cosmic rays. Although electromagnetic radiation is conventionally described as waves, it is also valid to describe radiation in terms of photons, or particles with packets of energy. As energy varies inversely with wavelength, x-rays have a much greater energy than do radio waves. This high energy gives x-rays the property of being deeply penetrating, and hence able to be used therapeutically to treat deep-seated tumors.

Radiation used clinically consists of teletherapy, external beam radiation (from an outside source), and brachytherapy (using a source of radiation inserted or implanted into the patient). The electromagnetic radiation used in external beam radiation therapy consists of x-rays and gamma rays. They differ only in terms of their production, as gamma rays are produced within the nucleus from natural radioactive decay, and x-rays are produced outside of the nucleus. In practice, almost all x-rays are produced by machines (linear accelerators), and gamma rays used in radiation therapy are produced by the decay of radioactive substances. Radiation sources used in brachytherapy include radioactive nuclei that decay and emit positively charged alpha (α) particles, positively charged beta (β^+) particles, or negatively charged beta (β^-) particles along with a gamma ray. Clinically, α particles and β particles are absorbed locally, and except in rare cases, the gamma ray is responsible for the deposition of radiation dose.

The vast majority of forms of radiation used in the clinic today, whether external beam radiation or brachytherapy, are from x-rays, gamma rays, or electrons. These are termed to be low linear energy (LET) radiation and are distinguished from high linear energy transfer radiation, such as alpha particles or fast neutrons. Linear energy transfer is defined as the energy transferred per unit track length of the radiation, or how often a type of radiation will cause ionizations in the tissue it is traveling through. Low linear energy transfer radiation (x-rays, gamma rays, electrons) is sparsely ionizing and produces relatively few ionizations in the path by which it travels through tissues. This is in contrast to high linear energy transfer radiation such as neutrons, which produce many ionizations in its path and are thus referred to as densely ionizing (Fig. 26-3). This difference becomes important when discussing the effects of radiation on biologic tissues.

Radiation Production

Radiation Production by Radioactive Decay

The nucleus contains protons and neutrons that usually have stable configurations. When these configurations are not stable, they undergo spontaneous transformations to attempt to reach a more stable state. These disintegrations of isotopes into a more stable state are called radioactive decays, and the species that undergo these transformations are called radioactive. With these disintegrations, energy is released as a photon (gamma ray), which can be used for radiation therapy. The type of radioactive decay and type of particle emitted depend on the nuclear composition of the radioactive species. Regardless, the energy released as these decays occur is in the form of gamma rays, and it is these that are (usually) used clinically to deliver radiation dose.

The first radioactive species isolated was polonium, with radium discovered shortly thereafter; both species were discovered by the Curies.[6] Since that time, many other radioactive species have been discovered and produced artificially. A number of these are useful in treating cancer, again because of the photon that is emitted during the radioactive decay. Today, the main use of radioactive species is in brachytherapy, though Cobalt-60 units are also used for external beam treatment.

Radium was the most important implantation source for more than 50 years. There are many properties of radium that make it undesirable as a radioactive source, however. During its decay, radium produces radon gas, which is colorless and odorless but highly radioactive. Also, radium has a half-life (the time it takes for a radioactive substance to decay to half of its original strength) of 1600 years. These qualities make it an extremely significant hazard in the case of contamination. Hence, better isotopes were needed to replace radium (Table 26-1). Cesium-137 became the radioactive source used in most gynecologic brachytherapy implants. It has a somewhat lower energy gamma ray (i.e., it is less penetrating and thus easier to shield) and has no gaseous daughter nuclei. Also, its half-life is 30 years, so that a capsule of Cesium-137 can be used for many years before requiring replacement. Iridium-192 and iodine-125 are widely used for implantation throughout the body. They are supplied as small seeds or embedded into ribbon so that they can be placed directly into the tumor bed, regardless of the location. Palladium-103 or iodine-125 are used in prostate brachytherapy, one of the most common brachytherapy procedures, in which radioactive seeds are placed into the prostate gland. All three isotopes emit gamma rays of very low energy (i.e., less penetrating), making the radiation safe for the surrounding tissues and posing no risk of radiation exposure for people in the patient's environment. Strontium-90 is another radioactive isotope that has been used clinically. Strontium applicators have been used for many years for the treatment of pterigia, but more recently this is the isotope that is used in intravascular brachytherapy, which is used to prevent

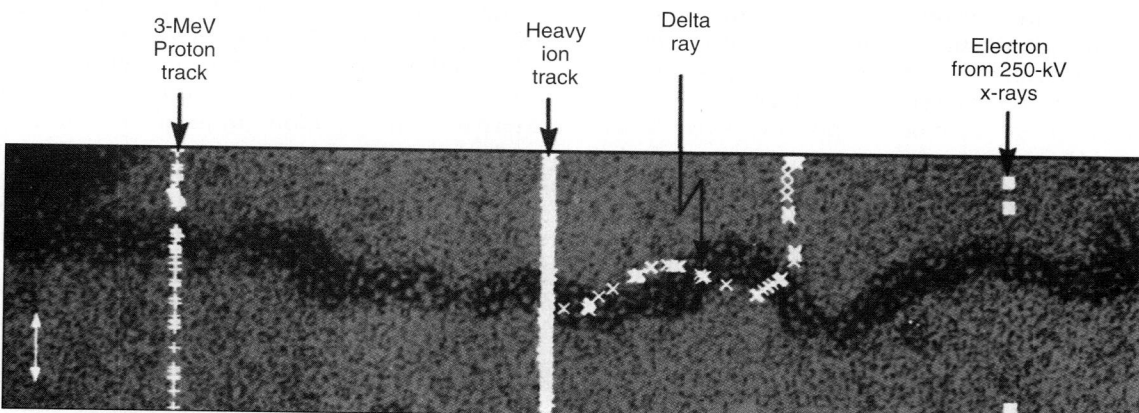

Figure 26-3. Computer simulations of sections of charged-particle tracks produced by different types of radiation passing through a strand of chromatin. Each cross represents a single ionization of either the chromatin or the surrounding medium. *Right track,* Low-linear energy transfer (LET) 100-keV electron, typical of those produced by 250-kVp x-rays. *Center track,* High-LET, high energy iron ion that produces a dense column of ionization; note the high-energy secondary delta ray coming out of the track. *Left track,* Medium-LET 3-MeV proton. The scale bar represents 50 nm. (From Cox JD, Ang KK [eds]: Radiation Oncology Rationale, Technique, Results, 8th ed. St. Louis, Mo, Mosby, 2003, p 44.)

TABLE 26-1

Therapeutic Isotopes

ISOTOPE	HALF-LIFE	AVERAGE ENERGY (KEV)
Photon		
^{226}Ra	1620 yr	830
^{137}Cs	30 yr	662
^{198}Au	2.7 days	412
^{192}Ir	73.8 days	370
^{125}I	60 days	28
^{103}Pd	16.97 days	21

ISOTOPE	HALF-LIFE	MAXIMUM ENERGY (KEV)
Beta		
^{32}P	14.3 days	1710
^{90}Sr/^{90}Y	28.5 yr/2.7 days	550/2280
^{188}W/^{188}Re	69.4 days/17 hr	350/2120
^{186}Re	3.8 days	1070
^{62}Zn/^{62}Cu	9.3 hr/9.7 min	660/2930
^{133}Xe	5.2 days	360
^{131}I	8.0 days	600
^{89}Sr	50.5 days	1495
^{166}Ho	26.8 hr	1850

keV, kiloelectron volt.
From Cox JD, Ang KK (eds): Radiation Oncology Rationale, Technique, Results, 8th ed. St. Louis, MO, Mosby, 2003, p.6

restenosis of coronary arteries. An important distinction is that the form of radiation used clinically with Strontium-90 is the actual β⁻ particle produced during its decay, not a gamma ray. The advantage of this is that it deposits its dose very superficially, sparing the outer wall of the arteries from receiving full doses of radiation.

Cobalt-60 is a very important radioisotope that is used in external beam radiotherapy (teletherapy). Cobalt machines were the first practical megavoltage machines and were pioneered by the Canadian physicist, H.E. Johns.[19] The radioactive decay of Cobalt-60 releases 1.2-Megavolt (MeV) gamma rays, which represents a major advance in external beam radiation treatment. The depth of penetration in tissue increases with increasing x-ray energy, but with x-ray energies up to 250 kilovolts (keV), the maximal dose is always deposited at the skin surface, and thus x-ray doses have always been limited by skin tolerance. This follows from the physics of x-ray interaction with matter, which is discussed in more detail in subsequent sections. At energies up to 250 keV, x-rays interact with matter via the photoelectric effect, whereby they interact with the tightly bound electrons close to the nucleus of an atom to cause ionization. This process begins to occur as soon as the photon interacts with matter (i.e., at the skin surface). Above 250 keV, a second form of interaction between x-rays and matter, called the Compton effect, begins to occur, and this becomes predominant in the megavoltage range. According to the Compton effect, x-rays interact with the loosely bound outer electrons, and there is a much greater probability that they will penetrate for some distance into tissue before such an interaction occurs. Thus, according to the Compton effect, the maximal dose is not at the skin surface but rather at some distance below the skin, leading to a "skin-sparing" effect. The medical community, knowing this, made a great push in the attempt to produce x-rays of high energy. St. Bartholomew's Hospital in London had a 1 MeV machine in the 1930s produced by an x-ray tube 30 feet long. Also in the 1930s, the physicist Robert van de Graaf devised a direct current electrostatic generator that could produce a 2 MeV beam. These machines, however, had low output and small field sizes and were mechanically unreliable. Cobalt-60 machines were simple in design and mechanically highly reliable, and they revolutionized the practice of radiotherapy. By their skin-sparing effect, doses of radiation required for treatment could be given safely for the first time without the desquamating skin toxicity that was the hallmark of kilovoltage radiotherapy. In time, Cobalt machines in the United States were largely replaced by linear accelerators, which have the advantage of producing more sharply defined beams of a variety of different energies and which can produce both electrons and x-rays. Linear accelerators can also be used with devices such as computer-controlled multileaf collimators, allowing much more precise dose delivery. Cobalt machines remain the workhorses of cancer treatment in much of the less developed world, however.

Radiation Production from Linear Accelerators
Most radiotherapy is delivered with beams of x-rays that were produced by directing highly accelerated electrons into a target. Two processes can produce x-rays when electrons are directed onto target atoms. The electrons can ionize these atoms by depositing sufficient energy so that an inner shell electron is ejected. The vacancy in the inner shell is filled by an outer-shell electron with the release of a photon called a characteristic x-ray. Characteristic x-rays are of low energy and of little utility in therapy. Another way of producing x-rays involves the interaction of an electron with the electromagnetic field of a nucleus. This interaction decelerates the electron, with the conservation of energy leading to the production of bremsstrahlung (braking energy) x-rays.

Before 1950, external beam radiation therapy was accomplished by accelerating electrons in a vacuum tube to hit a target, producing bremsstrahlung x-rays, with a maximum energy of about 300 keV. As just stated, these x-rays are low in energy compared to what is used today, with disadvantages of poor penetration and the deposition of dose maximally at the skin. The modern radiation therapy treatment machine is called a linear accelerator (Figs. 26-4 and 26-5). These machines use microwaves (with a frequency of ~3000 MHz) to accelerate electrons to very high energies. These electrons strike an x-ray target (usually tungsten) to produce a beam of (mainly bremsstrahlung) x-rays. This x-ray beam is flattened with a flattening filter, so that the beam is uniform throughout, and collimated by the collimator, so that the size of the beam can be selected. This high-energy beam is directed at the target volume within the patient, which is made up of the tumor and surrounding tissue that is to be treated.

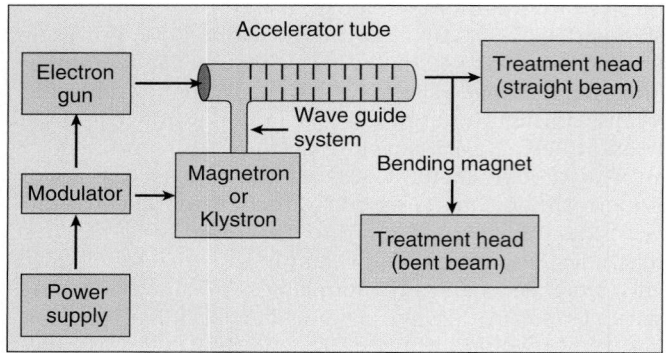

Figure 26-4. Block diagram of a typical medical linear accelerator. (From Leibel SA, Phillips TL [eds]: Textbook of Radiation Oncology. Philadelphia, WB Saunders, 1998, p 110.)

Another type of radiation that is used in therapeutic radiation and produced by linear accelerators is an electron beam. To produce an electron beam with a linear accelerator, instead of the accelerated electrons hitting a target to produce x-rays, the electrons strike a thin scattering foil, which spreads out the electron beam to an area large enough to be used for treatment. Electrons are used to treat areas of superficial depth in a patient.

Interaction of X-rays with Matter

After these high-energy x-rays are produced successfully, they can interact with matter via several different processes. Each interaction type has a probability, based on the composition of the matter and the energy of the x-rays. These interactions cause some photons (x-rays) to be removed from the forward-moving x-ray beam, causing an effect called attenuation, which is basically the loss of intensity and subsequent decrease in the deposition of dose as the beam reaches greater depths. The five possible interactions of x-rays with matter are:

1. Coherent scattering,
2. The photoelectric effect,
3. The Compton effect,
4. Pair production, and
5. Photodisintegration.

The most important of these interactions in radiation therapy are represented in Figure 26-6.

Coherent Scattering

Also called classic scattering, coherent scattering occurs when x-rays are of low energy. In coherent scattering, a photon is scattered from an electron with a resultant change in direction but no change in energy. The amount of coherent scattering that occurs in therapeutic (and even diagnostic) radiation is negligible. Also, because there is no transfer of energy, coherent scattering is of little importance in radiation therapy. Coherent scattering is important in processes such as x-ray crystallography.

Photoelectric Effect

The photoelectric effect was first described by Albert Einstein, and it was this contribution to physics, not his

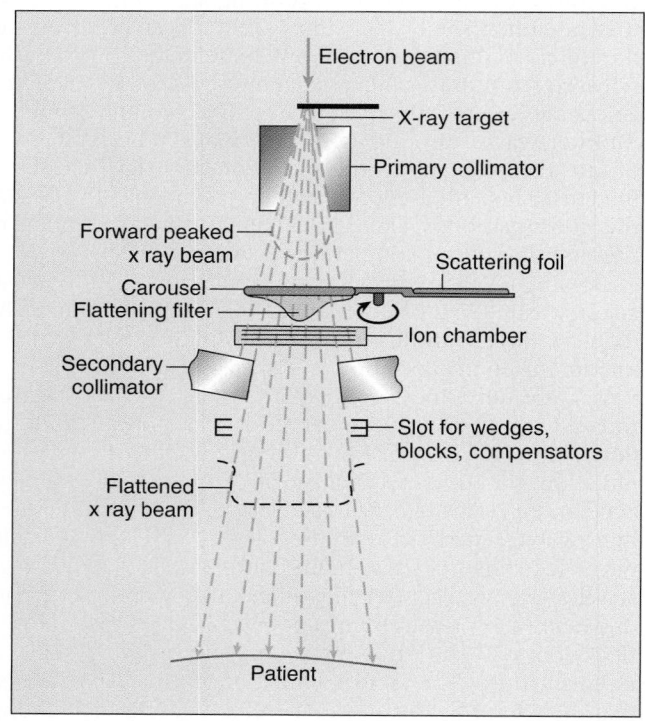

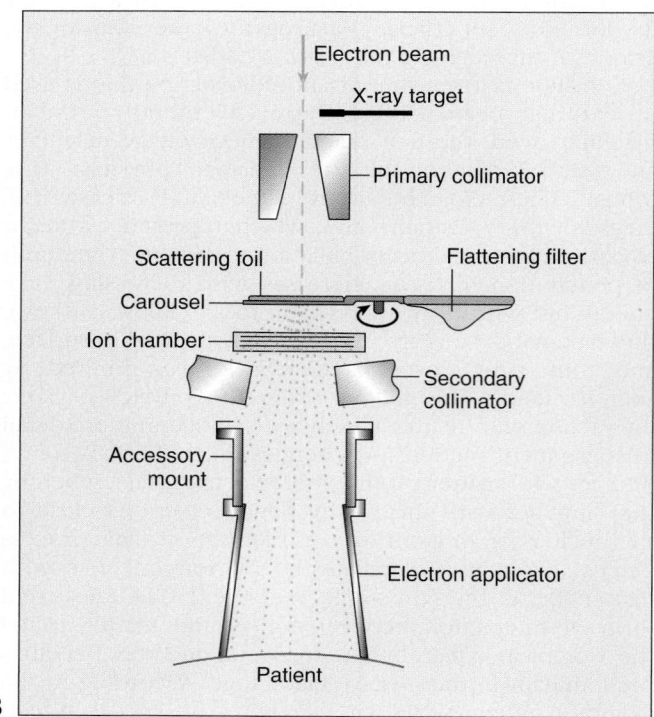

Figure 26-5. Schematic diagram showing the basic components of the treatment head of a modern linear accelerator. **A,** Components in place for x-ray therapy. **B,** Components in place for electron therapy. (From Leibel SA, Phillips TL [eds]: Textbook of Radiation Oncology. Philadelphia, WB Saunders, 1998, p 100.)

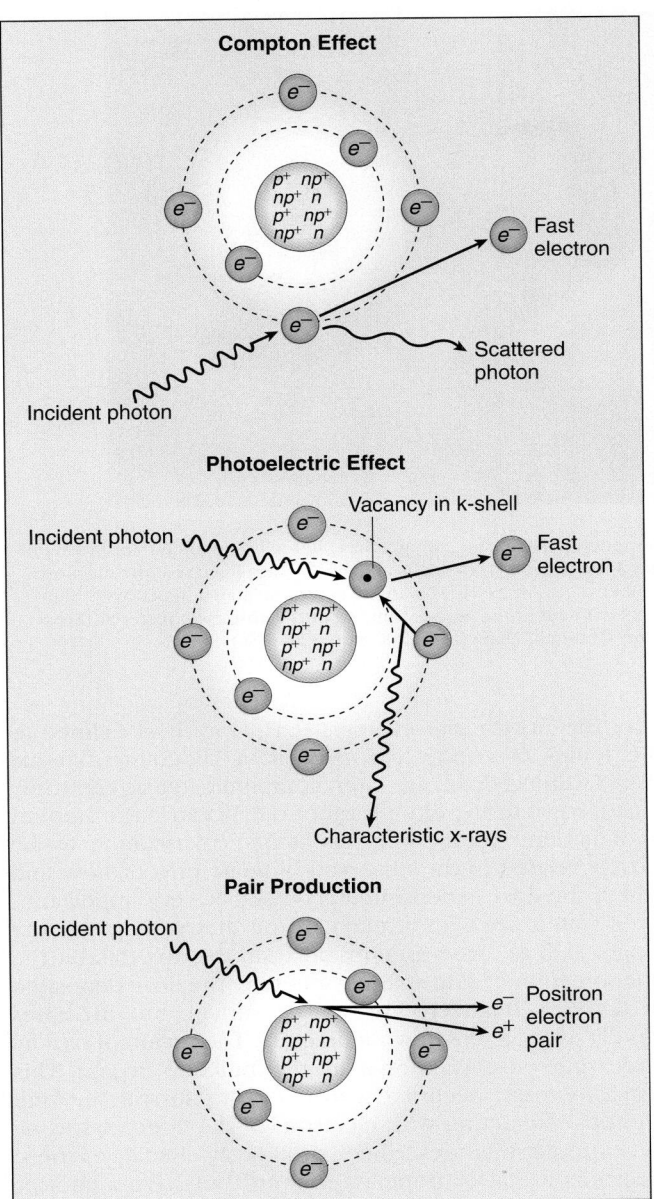

Figure 26-6. The first step in the absorption fof a photon of x-rays or gamma rays is the conversion of the energy of the photon into the kinetic energy of an electron or electron-positron pair. At higher energies, when the energy of the incident photon greatly exceeds the binding energy of the planetary electrons in the atoms of the absorber, the Compton process dominates. Part of the photon energy is given to the electron as kinetic energy, whereas the photon is deflected and has reduced energy.

At lower energies, when the binding energy of the planetary electrons of the atoms of the absorber is not small compared to the photon energy, the photoelectric effect is most important. The photon disappears completely as it interacts with a bound electron. The electron is ejected with kinetic energy equal to the photon energy, less the energy required to overcome the electron bond. The vacancy caused by the removal of the electron must be filled by an electron dropping from an outer orbit, giving rise to a photon of characteristic radiation.

At sufficiently high photon energies, the photon might interact with the powerful nuclear forces to produce an electron-positron pair. The first 1.02 MeV of photon energy is used to creat the rest mass of the pair, and the remainder is distributed equally between them as kinetic energy. (From Cox JD, Ang KK [eds]: Radiation Oncology Rationale, Technique, Results, 8th ed. St. Louis, MO, Mosby, 2003. p 5.)

discoveries regarding relativity, that led to Einstein's Nobel Prize in 1921. In the photoelectric effect, a photon interacts with a tightly bound inner shell electron of the target tissue. Complete absorption of the photon's energy occurs, with the ejection of the electron from the orbit. The probability of a photoelectric interaction is highly dependent on the atomic number (Z) of the material through which the photon is passing, and thus the photo-electric effect is very important in diagnostic radiology; it is the process that is the basis for the radiographic contrast between tissues (e.g., between bone [calcium and phosphorus] and fat [carbon and hydrogen]). The photoelectric effect is in most instances undesirable in radiation therapy. Typically, we do not want bony structures to be shielding underlying tumors. With higher-energy x-rays, such as are used in radiotherapy,

however, the contribution of the photoelectric effect is relatively small.

Compton Scattering

Compton scattering is the most important interaction in energies within the range used for radiation therapy. In Compton scattering, a photon transfers energy to an electron of the target tissue, causing the ejection of this electron. In contrast to the photoelectric effect, however, the energy of the photon is not completely absorbed, and instead is scattered at an angle relative to the forward direction of the original photon. This secondary photon interacts with tissue again and again, ionizing and depositing dose with each interaction. These interactions and subsequent ionizations are responsible for the biologic effects on tissues during radiation therapy.

Science of Clinical Oncology

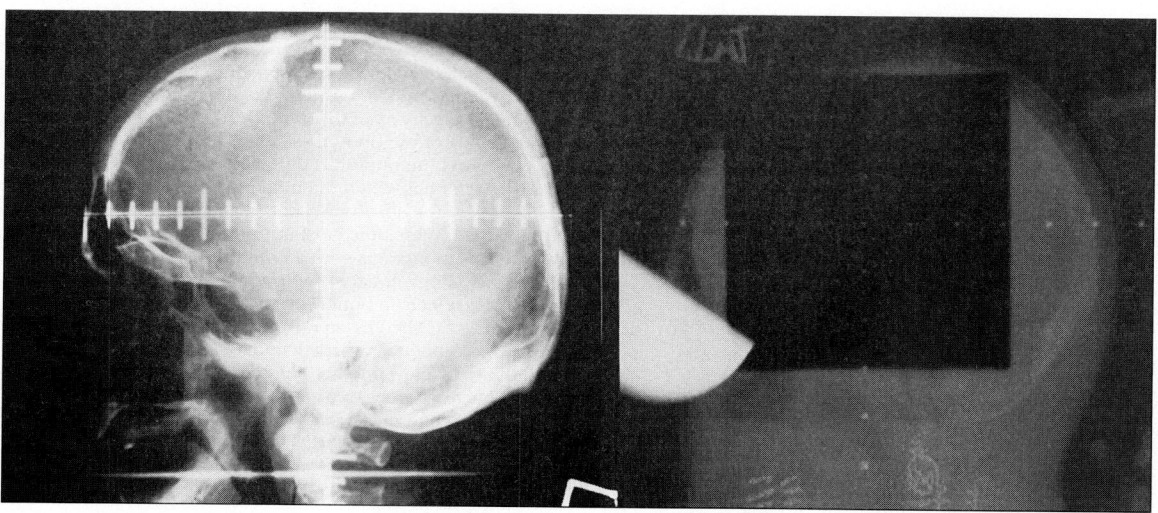

Figure 26-7. These two radiographs illustrate the attenutation differences of low-energy diagnostic radiographs (photoelectric interaction) vs. high-energy x-rays from a linear accelerator (Compton interaction). The skull radiograph on the left shows substantial bony detail because the diagnostic x-rays are preferentially attenuated by bone, which has much higher atomic number than soft tissue. The identical anatomic area filmed with high-energy x-rays shows little contrast in bone because Compton interactions are independent of the atomic number of the absorbing material. (From Lichter AS: Radiation therapy. In Abeloff M [ed]: Clinical Oncology, 2nd ed. London, Churchill Livingstone, 2000, pp 423–470.)

In contrast to the photoelectric effect, Compton interactions are independent of the atomic number of the tissue because these interactions tend to be with the loosely bound outer electrons in atoms, where the energy binding the electron to the atom is much less dependent on the atomic number (Z). This results in a fairly even probability of interaction (and hence, in a fairly even deposition of dose) throughout the different biologic tissues with which the x-rays would interact in a patient (Fig. 26-7).

Pair Production
Pair production occurs at high energies and is the interaction of a photon with a nucleus, with the spontaneous disappearance of the photon and the production of an electron and a positron (a positively charged electron). Pair production occurs at higher energies and becomes predominant in biologic tissues at about 25 MeV. This is above the range that is typically used in therapy, and for this reason it plays a small role in most cases.

Photodisintegration
At very high energies, x-rays can deposit so much dose into the nucleus of the target tissue that partial disintegration of the nucleus occurs, with emission of neutrons from the nucleus. Although this has little importance in the clinical interactions used in radiation therapy, the production of neutrons is important when planning shielding around high-energy linear accelerators for the sake of protecting patients and personnel from potentially carcinogenic low-dose radiation.

Deposition of Dose
The absorbed dose from an x-ray beam is the measure of the energy deposited by the beam and absorbed by the target. The unit of absorbed dose is the Gray (Gy), named after the British radiobiologist L.H. Gray. It is defined as the Joules of energy absorbed in a kilogram of tissue (J/kg). Clinical doses are often communicated as centiGray (cGy), equal to the older term of rad. Because the amount of radiation absorbed by the target is assumed to be closely related to the observed biologic effects, how and where the dose is deposited is obviously very important.

As stated previously, x-rays in the megavoltage energy range, such as those used in radiation therapy, exhibit the phenomenon of skin sparing, whereby the dose deposited in tissue is relatively low at the surface but increases rapidly over the first few millimeters. The region of rapidly increasing dose is known as the build-up region. This rapid increase occurs because of the forward-moving photons interacting with electrons of the target tissue via the interactions described previously. Because these electrons are also propelled forward but have a shorter course than the photons, there becomes an area at depth at which the number of electrons entering the plane of interaction from superficial interactions is exactly equal to the amount leaving the plane from interactions in that plane. This plane is termed the D_{max}, as it represents the maximum number of ionization events (Fig. 26-8). Past this point, as more interactions between the photon beam and tissue occur, fewer photons are available to travel forward and deposit dose at greater depths. This process is called attenuation. How quickly a photon beam is attenuated (i.e., how much dose it deposits at depth) is dependent on qualities both within the beam and within the target tissue. The most substantial effect on depth dose from the photon beam itself is the beam's energy (Fig. 26-9).

Linear accelerators typically produce beam energies ranging from 6 to18 MeV, and the dose at depth increases with beam energy. Therefore, an 18 MeV photon beam would deliver more dose to a given depth in a patient

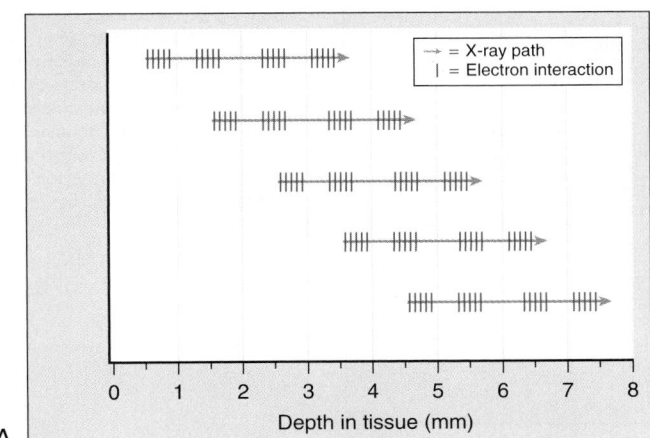

A

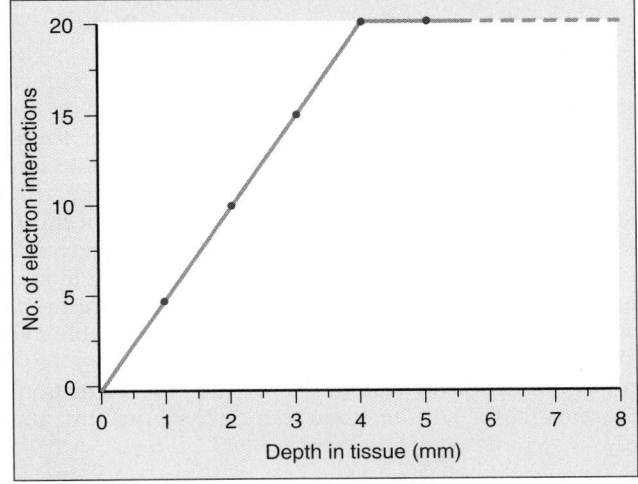

B

Figure 26-8. A, Simplified explanation of the phenomenon behind skin sparing. Assume that x-rays interact with tissue and liberate electrons that can have subsequent ionizations along their tracks. In this example, the electrons have a range of 4 mm and an average of five interactions (*red lines*) for each millimeter of tissue traversed. **B,** We can then count the number electron interactions and graph them. Note that the number of interactions increases with each millimeter of tissue until 4 mm of depth, where the number of interactions (20 in this case) reaches a maximum. If there were no attenuation of beam by tissue, this maximum number of interactions would continue to be observed at all depths. In reality, the intensity of the beam is attenuated by the tissue, and after the point of maximum dose, the number of interactions at greater depths will begin to decrease. (From Lichter AS: Radiation therapy. In Abeloff M [ed]: Clinical Oncology, 2nd ed. London, Churchill Livingstone, 2000, pp 423–470.)

than would a 6 MeV photon beam. An 18 MeV beam would also show more skin sparing (i.e., it would have a greater D_{max}). Another aspect that affects the depth dose is the size of the field of radiation used to treat the patient. With a larger field size, there is greater scattering of photons within the field during the interactions with electrons. This scatter effect leads to more interactions, which translates into a higher deposition of dose at depth. In other words, the dose at 10 cm depth within a patient from a photon beam that has a field size of 20 cm × 20 cm would be higher than the same photon beam with a field size of 5 cm × 5 cm. Many other factors go into the

calculation of dose delivered at varying depths in a patient, including scatter from the collimators in the machine, blocks to shield normal tissue, and wedges and compensators (which are used to shape the photon beam). Another main modifier in the target tissue that affects dose at depth is the density of the tissue being treated. Lung, for example, being less dense than soft tissue, allows more photon transmission. Additionally, the inverse square effect, first noted by Roentgen, must be taken into account. All of these factors must be taken into consideration when determining the dose being delivered to structures within the patient. Calculation of the dose given to a tumor or other volumes within a patient is thus complex, requiring much more knowledge than simply how much x-ray dose the machine is putting out.

As an energy source, electrons differ from photons in that electrons travel only a certain (short) distance within tissue. They are very light particles compared with the nuclei of the target tissue with which they interact. Hence, they lose a large fraction of their energy in a single process. This leads to much less skin sparing and the deposition of the majority of their dose in superficial tissues. Consequently, however, they are very useful for treatments in which the target of the radiation lies close to the surface of the patient, such as skin tumors (see Fig. 26-9).

BIOLOGIC INTERACTIONS AND CONSIDERATIONS

The basic understanding of the physical properties of a radiation beam must be coupled with an understanding of how radiation interacts with biologic tissues to cause damage. Through interactions with biologic tissue (mainly Compton interactions in the energies used in radiation therapy), radiation deposits energy as it travels through the patient. These interactions set secondary electrons in motion that go on to produce further ionizations. This ultimately results in the breaking of chemical bonds and damage to molecules and structures within the cell. If these broken bonds and subsequent damage occur to cells' critical structures, the most significant effect of the accumulation of radiation damage will be cell killing.

This process is obviously not as simple as just described. The deposition of radiation dose and the damage it induces is random and complex and depends on many aspects of both the radiation and the biologic tissue.

Interactions with Biologic Materials

Cell killing occurs when critical targets within the cell are damaged by radiation. Therefore, radiation that deposits dose near critical structures is more likely to incur a biologic effect. A number of biologic molecules or structures are potential targets for radiation damage, and there is still lively debate within the field as to whether there are multiple targets within the cell. Many circumstantial data indicate that DNA is the critical target for the biologic effects of radiation, although this specu-

Science of Clinical Oncology

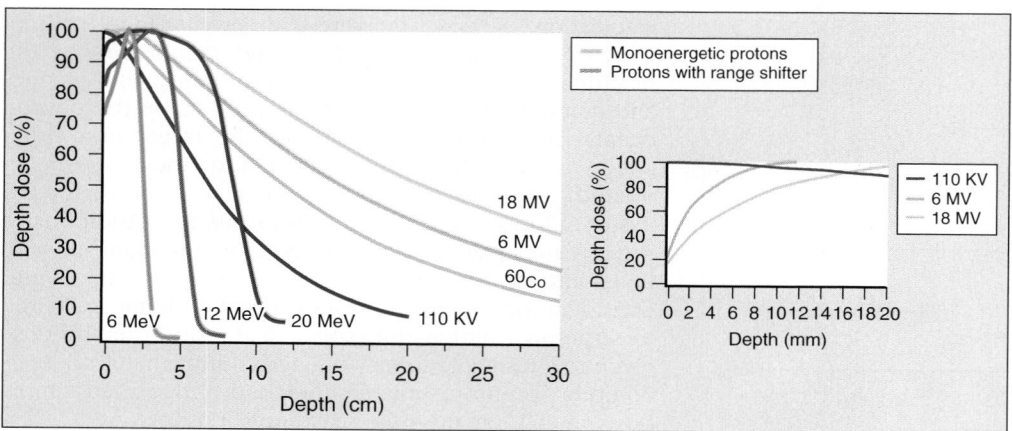

Figure 26-9. Percentage depth-dose curves for a variety of radiation types used in radiation therapy. These include x-rays and g-rays up to 18 MeV and various energies of electrons. The inset shows the pattern of absorption at shallow depths and provides a rationale for the skin-sparing effect.

lation remains without definitive proof. Measurement of DNA damage after radiation closely correlates with cell lethality.[20,21] Cells that are inhibited from repairing DNA damage or that are naturally deficient in DNA repair enzymes show a distinct radiosensitivity[22-24] Also, experiments in which the nucleus was irradiated selectively show that radiation caused cell death at a higher rate than did radiation of the cytoplasm.[25-27]

DNA damage can be termed direct or indirect (Fig. 26-10). If radiation is absorbed by the DNA itself, the atoms of the DNA can become ionized and damaged. This is termed the direct effect of radiation. Because the width of DNA is 1–4 nm and there is relatively little DNA in the cell, direct damage must be a relatively infrequent event.[28] More commonly, water molecules surrounding the DNA are ionized by the radiation. The ionization of water creates hydroxyl radicals, peroxide, hydrated electrons, and oxygen radicals. All of these species are highly reactive free radicals.[29] These radicals, in turn, interact with the DNA and cause damage. This is termed indirect damage. Eighty percent of a cell is composed of water, making indirect damage a much more common event.

Direct and indirect damage both work to cause broken bonds in the DNA backbone. These broken bonds can result in the loss of a base or of the entire nucleotide, or in complete breaking of one or both of the strands of DNA. Single-strand breaks are easily repaired using the opposite strand as a template. Therefore, single-strand breaks show little relation to cell killing, though they might result in mutation if the repair is incorrect. Double-strand breaks, on the other hand, are thought to be the most important lesion in DNA produced by radiation.[30] Double-strand breaks, as the name implies, results in the chromatin being snapped into two pieces. These double-strand breaks can result in mutations or, most important, in cell killing. Because x-rays are sparsely ionizing, there can be random stochastic processes in regions within the cell where ionization events are much more densely clustered than in other areas. The free radicals produced are also thought to be clustered in discrete areas. Therefore, the multiple broken bonds and resultant DNA damage that occurs could be highly localized. The term *locally multiply damaged site*, coined by John Ward,[31] or

the cluster hypothesis described by Goodhead[32] refers to this phenomenon, and Ward suggests that it is these clustered regions of DNA damage that lead to clinically significant effects.[31]

Most investigators believe that the dominant form of lethal radiation-induced DNA damage is the double-strand break, which ultimately results in mitotic death. In surviving irradiated cells, chromosomal aberrations such as nondisjunctions and micronuclei are detectable. Cells respond to double-strand DNA damage by invoking mechanisms that sense the damage and mechanisms that actually bring about repair. The earliest detectable event after exposure to ionizing radiation appears to be the phosphorylation of histone H2AX (i.e., the formation of "gamma-H2AX"), a reaction dependent on the ataxia

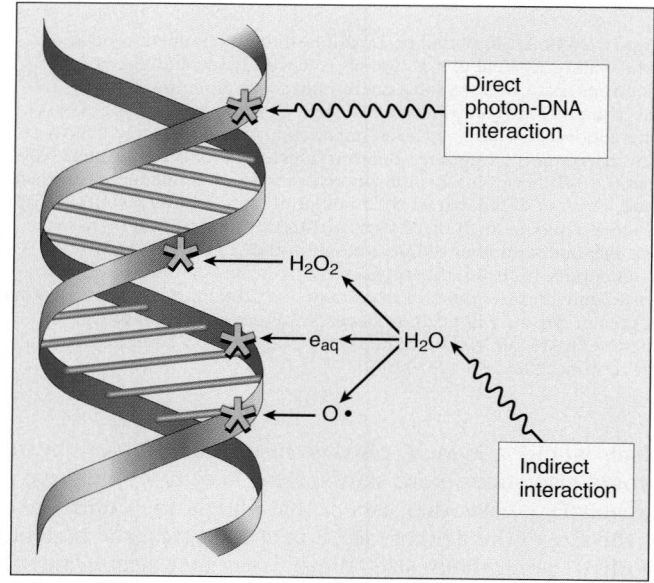

Figure 26-10. Two types of interactions are possible between x-rays and DNA. In the direct interaction, an x-ray interacts with the DNA molecule itself. This interaction is relatively rare. In the indirect interaction, x-rays ionize water and the reactive species that are created interact secondarily with DNA, causing damage and DNA strand breakage. (From Lichter AS: Radiation therapy. In Abeloff M [ed]: Clinical Oncology, 2nd ed. London, Churchill Livingstone, 2000, pp 423–470.)

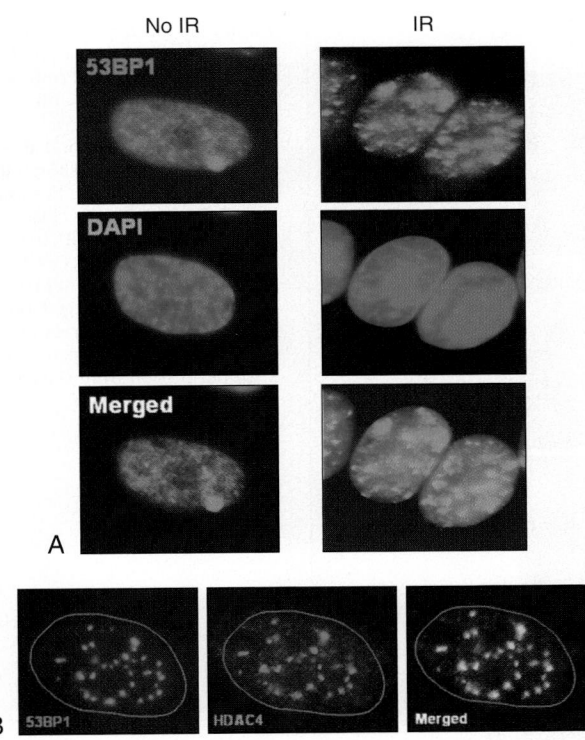

No IR   IR

53BP1

DAPI

Merged

A

B   53BP1   HDAC4   Merged

Figure 26-11. Ionizing radiation induces nuclear 53BP1 foci. **A,** 53BP1 protein localizes to nuclear foci at sites of double-strand DNA damage caused by ionizing radiation (IR). **B,** Recruitment of repair and chromatin remodeling factors at IR-induced 53BP1 foci. Bioactive proteins co-localize with 53BP1 at foci, including HDAC4 (shown), BRCA1, Rad50/NBS. (Used with permission from Gary Kao, MD, PhD, University of Pennsylvania.)

telangiectasia mutated (ATM) molecule.[33,34] This reaction is followed in turn by focal accumulation of 53BP1, a protein that appears to serve as a central mediator of a variety of critical pathways.[35] These include phosphorylating (and thereby conveying the DNA damage signal to) the tumor suppressor protein p53, phosphorylating ATM protein itself (thereby potentially amplifying the damage signal), recruiting proteins critical for repair (e.g., BRCA1 and HDAC4 [Fig. 26-11], and allowing the G2 cell cycle checkpoint (possibly through its interactions with the ATM).[36,37] These effects of 53BP1 therefore establish its importance in double-strand DNA damage sensing and repair, and potentially in tumor suppression as well.[38]

It is less clear how 53BP1 interfaces with or brings about the two main modes by which cells accomplish repair of double-strand DNA breaks, homologous repair (HR), and repair by nonhomologous endjoining (NHEJ). In HR, either the undamaged homologous chromosome or the sister chromatid of a replicated chromosome is used as the template to fill in missing DNA sequences in the damaged chromosome. Consequently, HR is most efficient in late S or G2 phase, when the sister chromatids have replicated but not yet separated. The requirement for a template to which the damaged chromosome is matched ensures that HR has great fidelity of repair. Human tumor cells commonly block in G2 after double-strand DNA damage, a time when repair activities are detectable

(Fig. 26-12). It is therefore plausible that the irradiation-induced G2 checkpoint allows more time for cells to accomplish HR and thereby survive radiation.[39]

In contrast to HR, repair by NHEJ is less cell-cycle dependent. In NHEJ, the blunt ends of chromosomes severed by radiation or other agents are directly rejoined. Although repair by NHEJ might in some ways be more efficient than by HR, NHEJ is considered highly mutagenic because the template-free rejoining of blunt ends lacks the specificity of HR. In NHEJ, it is possible for the ends of different chromosomes to be rejoined, giving rise to chromosomal aberrations or, potentially, to the expression of dangerous fusion proteins. It is therefore likely that mutagenesis associated with radiation is due in part to NHEJ.[40]

Radiation controls cancer cells through at least three main effects:

1. Inducing apoptosis.
2. Causing permanent cell cycle arrest or terminal differentiation.
3. Inducing cells to die of mitotic catastrophe.

Apoptosis is also known as "programmed cell death." The triggering of cell death is a process frequently seen in normal development, differentiation, immune responses, menstruation, neuronal development, and tissue turnover, and it also can be triggered by several noxious stimuli, including ionizing radiation. Radiation damage in this case triggers signaling cascades that invoke pre-existing mechanisms by which the cell self-destructs. Cells undergoing apoptosis show very characteristic features as they die, including dramatic blebbing and fragmentation of the nucleus.[41,42] Radiation with doses typically used in the clinic often induces apoptosis in lymphomas and other malignancies of hematopoetic origin. In contrast, apoptosis is far less commonly seen in tumors of epithelial origin, such as head and neck squamous cell cancers.[43] Tumors that commonly undergo apoptosis often have a brisk clinical response to radiation therapy.

Cell cycle arrest and terminal differentiation are also effective endpoints by which radiation exerts its effects. Cell cycle perturbations are seen characteristically after radiation exposure and were among the earliest observed biological effects of radiation.[44] Cells can show checkpoints or arrest in any phase of the cell cycle, although the best-described checkpoints with respect to radiation damage are the G1 and G2 checkpoints. Normal cells and those cancer cells that retain p53 function block in the G1 phase of the cell cycle. This is a p53-mediated event.[45-47] One of the earliest effects seen after radiation damage in cells with normal p53 function is a rise in the intracellular level of p53 due to protein stabilization and decreased protein turnover. This in turn leads to an induction of p21, a potent cyclin-dependent kinase inhibitor, leading to blockage of the cells in the G1 phase of the cell cycle.[48] This is only one of the many known functions of p53. It is also involved in the regulation of gene expression, apoptosis, and angiogenesis, among other important cellular processes.[49] The cell cycle arrest induced by p53 is frequently transient but in some cases can lead the cell to permanently exit the cell cycle and undergo

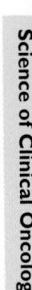

Science of Clinical Oncology

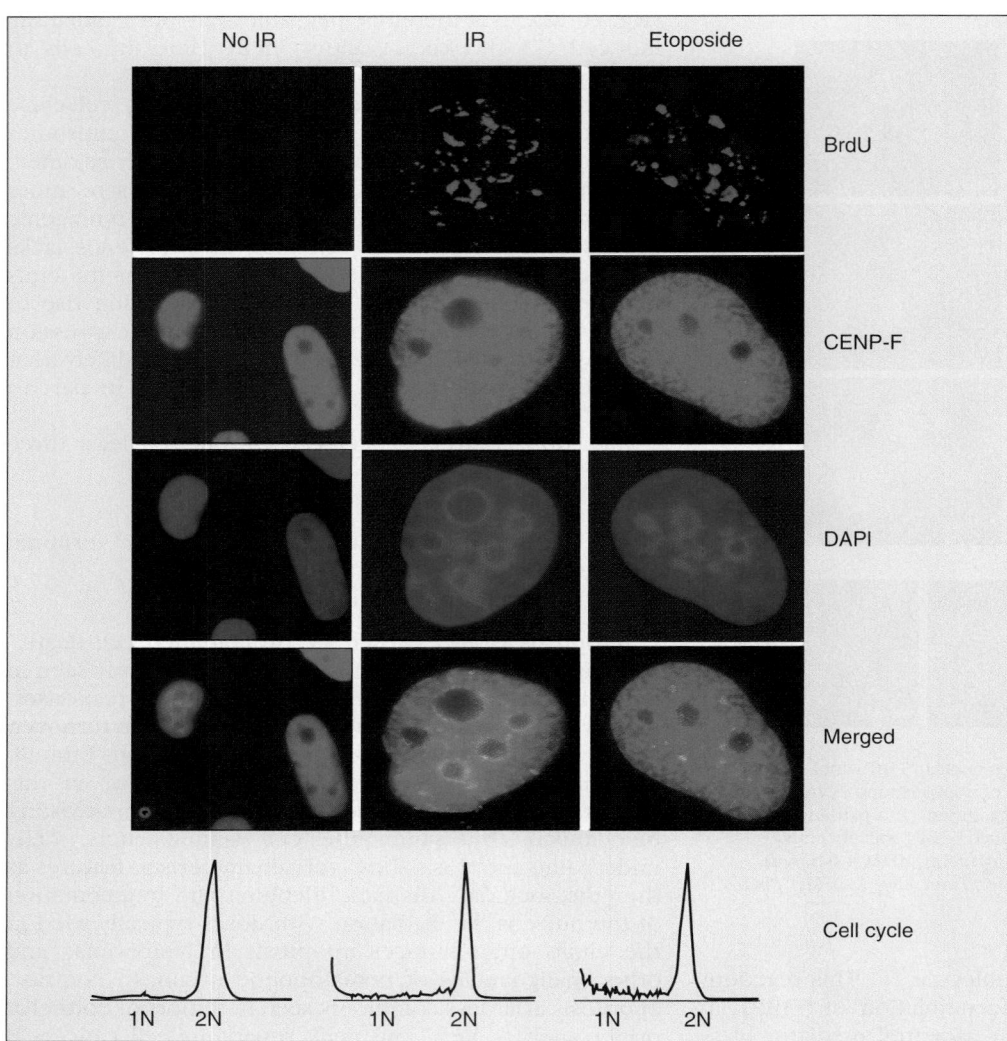

Figure 26-12. Repair activity in G2 cells after double strand DNA damage. Synchronized cells were mock-treated, treated with ionizing radiation (IR) or etoposide in S phase, and allowed to progress to G2 (as shown in the FACS profile in the bottom panel). During G2, the cells were pulse-labeled with BrdU, fixed, and then probed for BrdU, CENP-F (a marker of G2 cells), DAPI (stains DNA), or all three merged. BrdU uptake at discrete foci represents sites of active DNA repair. (Used with permission from Gary Kao, MD, PhD, University of Pennsylvania.)

a process that resembles terminal differentiation. The pathways invoked are consequently reminiscent of cellular senescence, in which cells also have lost the ability to cycle and proliferate.[50]

Many cancer cells—typically those with loss or mutation in the p53 protein pathway—have lost the ability to block in G1. These cells retain the ability to block in the G2 phase of the cell cycle. The G2 block is less well described at the molecular level than the G1 block but also involves effects that regulate the activity of cyclin-dependent kinases that are specific to the G2 phase of the cycle.[51] The G2 arrest is clearly related to cellular repair of radiation-induced DNA damage, in that cells that have lost the ability to arrest in G2 are exquisitely sensitive to DNA damage. Even in cells that re-enter the cycle after the G2 block, however, cell death can still be seen and can take several forms. Some cells fail in cytokinesis and form multinucleate giant cells. Some undergo mitotic catastrophe as they attempt to undergo mitosis. Others undergo delayed cell lysis that in some cases might be a delayed form of apoptosis.

Both tumor cells and normal tissues can differ in their sensitivity to radiation. In some cases, this is due to differential sensitivity to induction of apoptosis, but in others it is due to molecular mechanisms that are as yet poorly understood. A number of factors have been correlated with radioresistance, such as the presence of hypoxia, which could contribute to the poor prognosis of some tumors.[52,53] It has been hypothesized that oxygen helps "fix" damage induced by radiation in such a way that the radiation is more lethal to the cancer cells.[54] The specific molecular pathways involved in this phenomenon have not been fully elucidated, however. Most investigators agree that radiation primarily causes cell death by double-strand DNA damage; the inability of cancer cells to repair such damage results in their death. Although it is clear that cells that lack the ability to repair some forms of DNA damage are extremely sensitive to radiation damage, it is less clear that altered DNA repair capacity contributes to increased resistance to radiation.[23] Nevertheless, successfully identifying the proteins critically required to recognize and repair such DNA damage could provide potential targets for radiosensitizing cells. This remains a subject of active investigation.

Other factors that have been implicated in altered cellular sensitivity to radiation include a number of signal transduction pathways, including some that are known to be altered in tumors. Thus, for example, EGFR, Ras, and Raf have all been implicated in altered cellular sensitivity to radiation, and although the molecular mechanisms underlying their effects are still incompletely described, all are actively being targeted in clinical trials.[55-61] There is also great interest at this time in whether components of the tumor other than the tumor cells themselves might contribute to tumor sensitivity. In particular, in radiation oncology, as in other oncologic fields, there is great interest in knowing whether the vascular component contributes to tumor responses to radiation.[62]

Cell Survival Curves

One of the central ideas of radiation biology is that the loss of reproductive integrity in long-term survival assays is important to our understanding of the response of either a tumor or a normal tissue to radiation. When cells are exposed to lethal doses of radiation, they might not die immediately or within a few hours of treatment, or even sometimes within a single division of radiation. When cells have been observed by time-lapse cinematophotography after irradiation, it can be seen that some cells will survive and go on to form colonies, and some will die quickly, often by a process that resembles apoptosis, although this has not been shown definitively in many cases. Others will go through up to several rounds of abortive cell division before finally ceasing to divide and undergoing a variety of possible outcomes that might include terminal differentiation, formation of multinucleate giant cells, mitotic catastrophe, or delayed apoptosis.[63-67] Radiation biologists believe that it is the proportion of cells capable of forming a colony by sustained cell division that most fully predicts the effects of a dose of radiation. Cell survival curves have thus been very important in radiation biology to estimate survival of tumor cells within a population with increasing doses of radiation.

The first cell survival curves were demonstrated experimentally in the 1950s, when Puck and Marcus[68,69] plotted the survival of HeLa tumor line cells against increasing x-ray doses (Fig. 26-13). These curves are usually plotted with dose on a semilogarithmic scale. The most striking feature of these curves (for low linear energy transfer radiation) is that the effectiveness of killing per unit dose increases with increasing radiation dose. At low doses, the survival curve starts out as a shallow line, with the surviving fraction being an exponential function of dose. At higher doses, the curve increasingly bends, representing more cell killing per increase in unit dose of radiation. Eventually, at even higher doses, the curve might tend to straighten again. In contrast, high linear energy transfer radiation cell survival curves on a semilogarithmic plot are straight (albeit with a steeper slope) throughout, with survival always being an exponential function of dose. Survival curves contrasting low linear energy

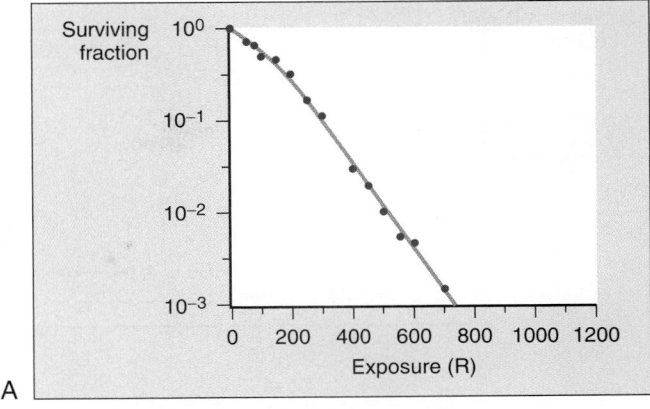

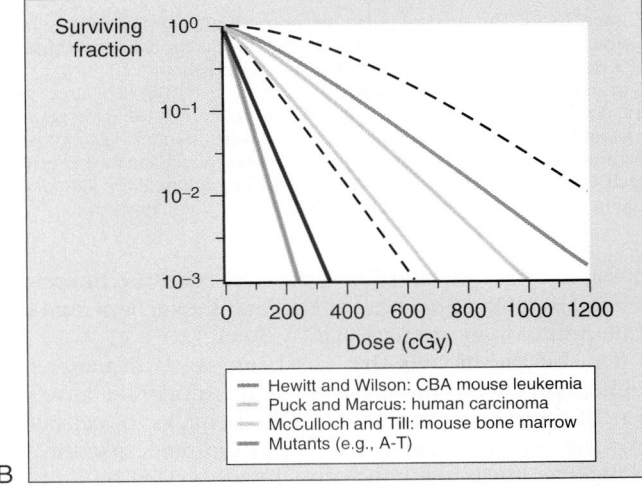

Figure 26-13. X-ray or gamma ray dose-survival curves for mammalian cells. **A,** The first such curve, reported in 1956 by Puck and Marcus. Note that the dose is expressed in roentgens (R), which, for the cells irradiated on the glass, must be multiplied by approximately 1.4 for the dose in cGy. **B,** A range of survival curves for other mammalian cells. The dashed lines encompass the range for "wild-type" cells of various origins. The steepest curves show a range typical of hypersensitive mutants, such as cells from patients with ataxia-telangiectasia (AT). (From Leibel SA, Phillips TL [eds]: Textbook of Radiation Oncology. Philadelphia, WB Saunders, 1998, p 4.)

transfer and high linear energy transfer radiation are shown in Figure 26-14.

A number of mathematical models have been devised to attempt to describe the shape of the cell survival curves that are observed experimentally, with an initial shallower slope and eventual bending (the "shoulder") and a final, steeper slope. These include target models, lethal and potentially lethal damage models, and repair saturation models. Some of these have been based on simple mathematical modeling without any real attempt to model known molecular events involved in cell killing, whereas others have been based on attempts to model some of the known molecular events (e.g., chromosome breaks or DNA repair) that are involved in cell killing. All of the models can describe the shape of the survival curve to a first approximation. None do so perfectly, and none take into account all the events and all of the possible mechanisms involved in cell death. In this text, it is not

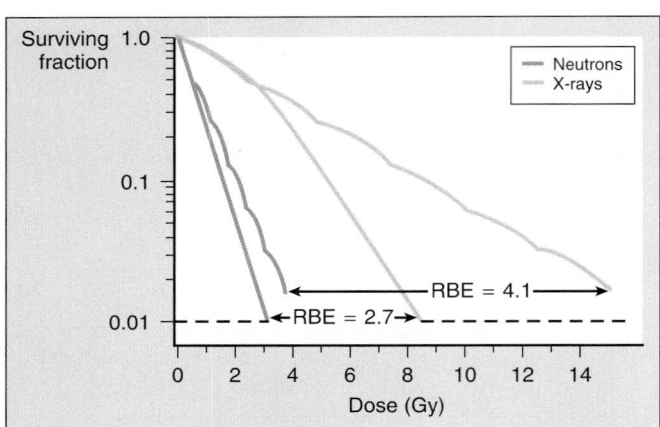

Figure 26-14. The survival curve for x-rays (low LET radiation) is characterized by a broad initial shoulder, whereas for neutrons (high LET radiation), the survival curve has little or no shoulder. Consequently, the relative biological effectiveness (RBE) gets larger as the dose gets smaller. When a dose is fractionated, the RBE is larger for a given level of cell killing than if the dose is given in a single exposure because the large shoulder of the x-ray dose-response curve is repeated each time. (From Cox JD, Ang KK [eds]: Radiation Oncology Rationale, Technique, Results, 8th ed. St. Louis, MO, Mosby, 2003, p 45.)

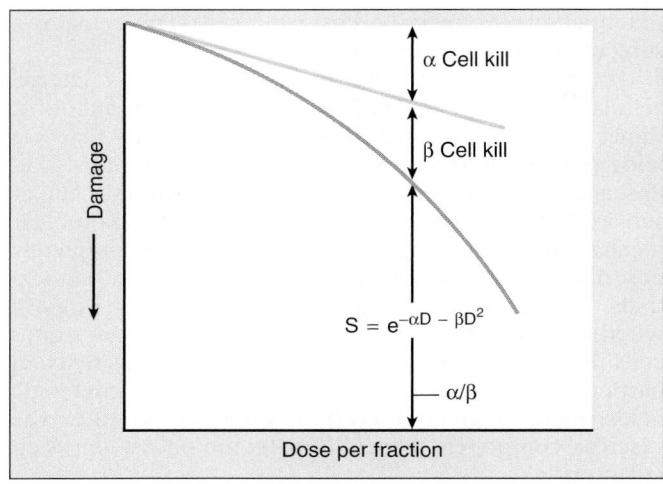

Figure 26-15. Dose response curves for mammalian cells are adequately fitted by the linear-quadratic relationship, at least over the range of doses of concern in radiation therapy. The form of the equation is

$$S = e^{-\alpha D - \beta D^2}$$

where S is the fraction of cells surviving a dose (D), and α and β are constants. Cell killing by the linear and quadratic term are equal when

$$\alpha D = \beta D^2.$$

This occurs when $D = \alpha/\beta$. (From Cox JD, Ang KK [eds]: Radiation Oncology Rationale, Technique, Results, 8th ed. St. Louis, MO, Mosby, 2003, p 14.)

possible to review all of these models, and the interested reader is referred to one of the many excellent texts of radiation biology, such as that by Steel.[70]

One of the models that has been most influential on clinical practice is the linear quadratic model because it is one of the models that best fits the behavior of cells after exposure to radiation doses within the range used in the clinic. The linear-quadratic model was devised by Kellerer and Rossi.[71] They proposed that radiation-induced cell killing resulted from two potential events, one of which has a linear relation to dose (exp[-αD]), the other having a quadratic relation to dose (exp[-βD²]). This was expressed mathematically by the "alpha-beta" equation, $S=e^{-(\alpha D + \beta D^2)}$, which was shown to fit most experimentally observed survival curves. S again represents survival of a cell population after a dose, D (Fig. 26-15). Chadwick and Leenhouts[72] proposed that this equation represented a molecular reality, suggesting that double-strand breaks in the DNA were the lethal lesions and that they could be produced by one energy deposition event (αD) or by two separate events, each involving a single strand of DNA (βD²), which then interacted. This is now thought to be unlikely because the probability of two tracks interacting within a single double helix is very small. Therefore, for the linear quadratic model, as for all the available models, the nature of the underlying lesions remains obscure. Additionally, this model does not take into account the important process of apoptosis. For many cell types, however, the linear-quadratic model is useful in describing dose responses for a population of cells.

Also derived from this expression is the α/β ratio, obtained by manipulating the equation just described. A point on the survival curve can be defined at which the components of cell killing can be seen to be equal to each other—that is, $\alpha D = \beta D^2$, or $D=\alpha/\beta$. In other words, for a cell population there exists a dose of radiation where

the linear (α) and quadratic (β) contributions to cell killing are equal. This dose is the dose equal to the ratio of α and β—the α/β ratio. The α/β ratio is specific to a cellular population and reflects the sensitivity of the cell to the two supposed types of damage. By this formulation, tissues that have an early response to radiation (skin, gut epithelium, and tumor cells) have a high α/β ratio. In other words, their survival curves stay straight for a longer period before the bend, with a higher contribution of single-event or α killing. Late-responding tissues such as spinal cord, kidney, and muscle, have survival curves that bend earlier, with resultant lower α/β ratios (Table 26-2). These late-responding tissues have "shoulders" on their survival curves within the range of doses commonly used in radiation therapy. This formulation led to the concept that altered fractionation schedules could be used to exploit this difference and treat tumor populations more effectively with respect to damage to late-responding tissues. This idea was the genesis for multiple clinical trials in the 1980s and 1990s. Some advances clearly came from this, such as the concomitant boost technique for head and neck cancer and the CHART (continuous hyperfractionated radiotherapy) regime for lung cancer.[73,74] Although interest in this continues in some areas, the increased difficulties of combining accelerated treatment regimes with concomitant chemotherapy has diminished the enthusiasm for this approach somewhat.

Cellular Repair

As noted previously, cells have complex mechanisms that are responsible for repairing radiation-induced damage.

TABLE 26-2

Ratio of Linear to Quadratic Terms from Multifraction Experiments

REACTION SITES	α:β (GY)
Early Reactions	
Skin	9–12
Jejunum	6–10
Colon	10–11
Testis	12–13
Callus	9–10
Late Reactions	
Spinal cord	1.7–4.9
Kidney	1.0–2.4
Lung	2.0–6.3
Bladder	3.1–7.0

From Cox JD, Ang KK (eds): Radiation Oncology Rationale, Technique, Results, 8th ed. St. Louis, MO, Mosby, 2003, p. 27.

The shoulder on the cell survival curve is thought to relate to the cell's ability to repair DNA damage. One of the clearest demonstrations of the cell's ability to repair radiation damage is the phenomenon called sublethal damage repair. It is observed that two doses of radiation given separated in time are less effective than the sum of the two doses given at a single time. The implication from this observation is that in the time interval between the first dose and the second dose, some of the damage from the first dose was repaired. Consistent with this conclusion is that the more closely the two doses are given in time, the more they resemble the effects of the large single dose, implying that the repair has measurable kinetics. Repair of sublethal damage was first demonstrated by Elkind and Sutton.[75,76] They noted that damage caused by radiation did not always produce cell killing and that this sublethal damage became lethal only when the

total amount of damage had accumulated to a sufficient level. Since then, sublethal damage has been demonstrated in virtually every biologic system tested, mainly through split-dose experiments (Fig. 26-16).[77-79] Remember that there is a correlation between cell killing and the production of asymmetric chromosomal aberrations (e.g., dicentrics and rings) from the interactions of double-strand breaks in the DNA. Therefore, sublethal damage repair can be interpreted as the repair of DNA damage that would have formed double-strand breaks by two separate hits (β killing). Because high linear energy transfer radiation interacts almost without exception by α killing, sublethal repair has very little importance in particle therapy.

By this formulation, cellular repair of DNA sublethal repair is evidenced by the existence of the shoulder on the cell survival curve. Cells show increased survival with split-dose radiation because the shoulder of the survival curve must be repeated with every fraction. In other words, the shoulder of the survival curve represents the accumulation and repair of sublethal damage. Cells that have a broad shoulder that start at low doses, with a resultant shallow initial slope, therefore, have a propensity for sublethal repair. These tissues, described previously as late-responding tissues with low α/β ratios, exhibit extensive sublethal repair and are spared preferentially by fractionation (Fig. 26-17).

A second type of cellular recovery after radiation, first described by Phillips and Tolmach,[80] is called potentially lethal damage repair. This represents radiation damage that might or might not lead to the killing of a cell, depending on the cell's condition and environment in the post-irradiation period. They noted that cells that are not proliferating, either by being out of the cell cycle due to contact inhibition or by being held in poor conditions that did not favor growth, showed less killing after irradiation than did the same cells dividing rapidly under optimal conditions. They postulated that resting cells had more

Figure 26-16. A, Increase in cell survival observed when a dose of radiation is delivered in two fractions separated by a time interval adequate for repair of sublethal damage. When the dose is split into two fractions, the shoulder must be expressed each time. **B,** The fraction of cells surviving a split dose increases as the time interval between the two dose fractions increases. As the time interval increases from zero to two hours, the increase in survival results from the repair of sublethal damage. In cells with a long cell cycle, or cells that are out of cycle, cell survival cannot be further increased by separating the dose by more than two or three hours. (From Cox JD, Ang KK [eds]: Radiation Oncology Rationale, Technique, Results, 8th ed. St. Louis, MO, Mosby, 2003, p 24.)

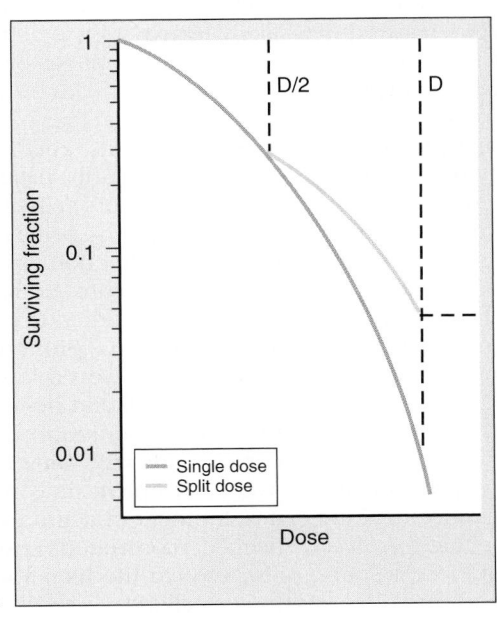

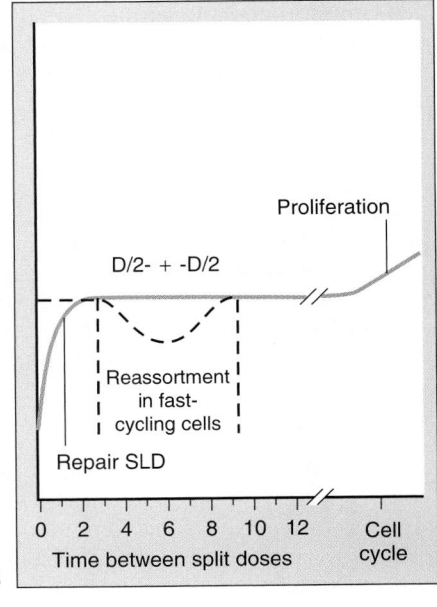

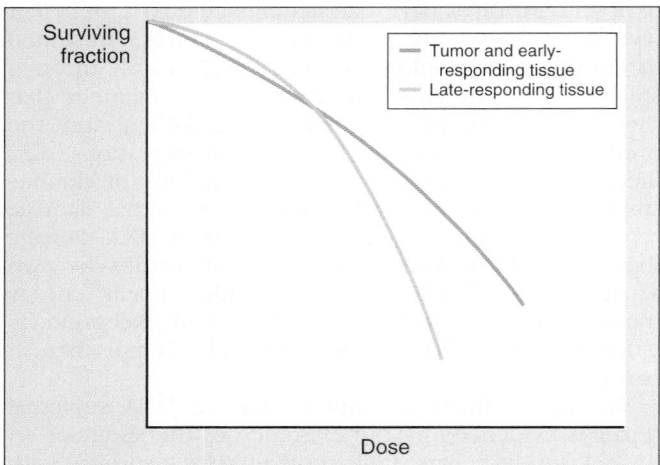

Figure 26-17. Illustrating the dose-response relationship for late-responding tissue is "curvier" than for early-responding tissue. The dose at which cell killing is equal by the linear and quadratic components is α:β. This is about 2 Gy for late-responding tissue and 8 to 10 Gy for early-responding tissue. (From Cox JD, Ang KK [eds]: Radiation Oncology Rationale, Technique, Results, 8th ed. St. Louis, MO, Mosby, 2003, p 27.)

time to repair DNA damage before re-entering the cell cycle than those cells that were dividing actively. Resting cells, then, exhibit more potentially lethal damage repair than dividing cells do. Because many cells in both the normal tissues and tumor might have entered the G0 phase of the cycle or be in regions where growth conditions are poor due to limited nutrient supply, potentially lethal damage repair might also contribute to resistance to therapy.

The extent of recovery from both sublethal damage and potentially lethal damage has been correlated with the repair of DNA and with the rejoining of chromosomal breaks.[81,82] Admittedly, no particular repair mechanism or chromosomal aberration has been associated with either process. Therefore, they could represent a continuum of the same process. Regardless, they both increase the survival of a cell population with fractionated radiation schedules. This can be manifested clinically by either an increase in normal tissue tolerance or a decrease in tumor control. The time that is required for sublethal/potentially lethal damage repair seems to be in the range of six hours. If doses are too closely spaced, unrepaired injury will accumulate between dose fractions, with the result that successive doses become more and more damaging.[83] This should all be kept in mind when designing a fractionated course of radiation. Although it could perhaps be beneficial in terms of tumor response, it might also be detrimental in terms of normal tissue sparing.

Dose Rate Effects

Due to sublethal damage repair, there is preferential sparing of late-responding tissues by fractionated radiation therapy. It should be kept in mind, however, that this is a relative sparing. In other words, as a radiation dose is split and delivered over more than one treatment, the killing

of the cells within the tumor also decreases, although not by as much as late-responding tissues. When determining cell survivals and the toxicity (both acute and late) of radiation therapy, other factors are involved also. The most prominent of these factors could be cell repopulation. As the total treatment time to deliver a dose of radiation lengthens, cells within a tissue have the ability to replenish, called repopulation. During a course of fractionated radiation therapy, the effect of sublethal repair and the effect of repopulation might be difficult to distinguish, though they both lead to diminished cell death with protraction of treatment times.

Dose rate effects apply to both inter-fraction repopulation and within a fraction of radiation. In studies by Fowler and colleagues[84] in experiments using pigskin, it was shown that as overall treatment time was lengthened, additional radiation was required to elicit the same effect. Because fraction size and fraction number were both kept constant, this finding was felt to reflect the contribution of repopulation to radiation's effect.

Dose rate effects have also been demonstrated within radiation fractions, first by Bedford and Hall.[85,86] They demonstrated that the survival of cells increased as dose rate decreased (from 7.3 Gy per minute to 0.1 Gy per hour). There also exists a dose rate below which reproduction of cells can continue in spite of radiation delivery.[87] This threshold varies with the tissue type, based on the sensitivity of the stem cells required to repopulate the cell population, the duration of the cell cycle, and the amount of adaptation that cells can undergo in response to radiation.[88]

The response to radiation injury and the survival of cells facing radiation are complex. Obviously, total radiation dose affects all tissues, with cell kill increasing as dose increases. There are many other factors that determine survival, however, many of which are still not known, although some generalizations can be gathered based on experiments involving varying dose levels, delivery schemes, and dose rates. Early-responding tissues such as skin, mucosa, bone marrow, and tumor cells, are likely to experience acute toxicities, which occur during the radiation course or shortly thereafter. These tissues have stem cells for repopulation, with maturation into functional cells. They exhibit a rapid cell turnover from these stem cells. The intensity of the toxicity in these tissues reflects the balance between cell killing and the regeneration of cells from surviving stem cells. This balance depends primarily on accumulation of radiation dose. Larger fraction sizes are a factor in determining the severity of acute toxicities, with larger fraction sizes resulting in higher toxicity than smaller fraction sizes. This is much less pronounced compared with late effects. Dose rate, however, has been shown to correlate with tumor cell kill and hence with the development of acute toxicity. In addition, a very important parameter that corresponds with tumor cell kill and acute toxicity is the overall treatment time. As treatment time is extended, the development of acute toxicities decreases. It has recently been demonstrated, however, that long treatment times also reduce the likelihood of cure by virtue of reduced tumor cell kill.

In contrast to acute toxicities in early-responding tissues, late effects occur in late-responding tissues, such as spinal cord, heart myocytes, kidney nephrons, etc. These are actually of more concern to a radiation oncologist, as they dictate end-organ damage from radiation. Provided that sufficient time between fractions is given to allow for the complete repair of sublethal damage, classic late effects have no dependence on overall treatment time. If the treatment course is intense enough to cause such severe acute toxicities as to reduce the stem cells of early-responding tissues below a threshold, however, the acute toxicity can progress to chronic tissue injury, termed consequential late effects. Late-responding tissues, though, are characterized by slow cellular turnover, with little repopulation during radiation treatments. Therefore, dose rate and overall treatment time play a minor role in the development of late toxicity. As stated previously, these tissues have a low α/β ratio, with the potential for significant sublethal damage repair between fractions. Hence, late-responding tissues are extremely sensitive to changes in dose per fraction.

Cell Cycle Effects

An important aspect that has not been mentioned is the modulation of radiation effect as cells progress through different stages of the cell cycle.[89-93] With tumor cells, which have a high growth fraction, this modulation could be of great importance. The radiosensitivity of cells changes as the cell progresses through the cell cycle, with cells in late G2 and mitosis being the most sensitive. Cells in mid-to-late S phase and early G2 phase are the most resistant to radiation. Moderate sensitivity exists for those cells in late G1 and early S phase, and cells in mid G1 are moderately resistant.

These differences in sensitivity allow for preferential killing of cells in those stages that are sensitive to radiation, with a subsequent relative accumulation of cells in the resistant S phase of the cell cycle. This translates into a relative radioresistance of the remaining cells to additional doses of radiation if reassortment into other phases of the cell cycle through natural progression of cell division does not occur (Fig. 26-18).

Radiation also disrupts progression through the cell cycle. Doses of radiation cause blocks in the G2-to-M-phase transition and in the G1-to-S-phase transition. These delays are governed by cell cycle "checkpoint" genes, which are responsive to DNA damage and transmit feedback addressing the readiness of the cell to progress to the next phase of the cell cycle. The radiation-induced G1 block is p53 dependent.[45,46] Because most tumors in adults are mutant or otherwise deficient in p53, the G2 block might be the more important block in tumor response to radiation. The G2 block is dose dependent, averaging one to two hours per Gy with increasing doses.[94] The G2 delay also varies in time depending on where the cell was in its cycle when it was irradiated. The delay is longest for cells irradiated in S and early G2 phase and shortest for cells irradiated in G1 phase.[94]

These variations in sensitivity with cell cycle changes could be related to the propensity of the DNA to be damaged or repaired in the various phases of the cell cycle. In late S and early G2 phases, repair of double-strand breaks by homologous repair is most efficient, compared with the G1 and early S phases (when a homologous chromosome is not available) and late G2 phase (when the chromatin is highly condensed and less accessible to repair.[95] Similarly, DNA is uncoiled at the beginning of the S phase, perhaps leading to increased susceptibility to radiation damage in this phase. Regardless of the reasoning behind preferential susceptibility with respect to the cell cycle, this observation again speaks to the importance of splitting the total radiation doses into fractions.

Fractionation

Schwarz first reported a biologic rationale for fractionated radiotherapy almost a century ago.[96] Regaud and Coutard[15,16] reported their clinical findings of fractionated therapy in the 1920s and 1930s. They found that with fractionation of the radiation dose, better tumor control could be attained for a given level of normal tissue toxicity. Subsequently, varying fractionation schedules have been proposed and tested throughout the world, all in the hope of achieving a greater therapeutic ratio of better cure per normal tissue toxicity.

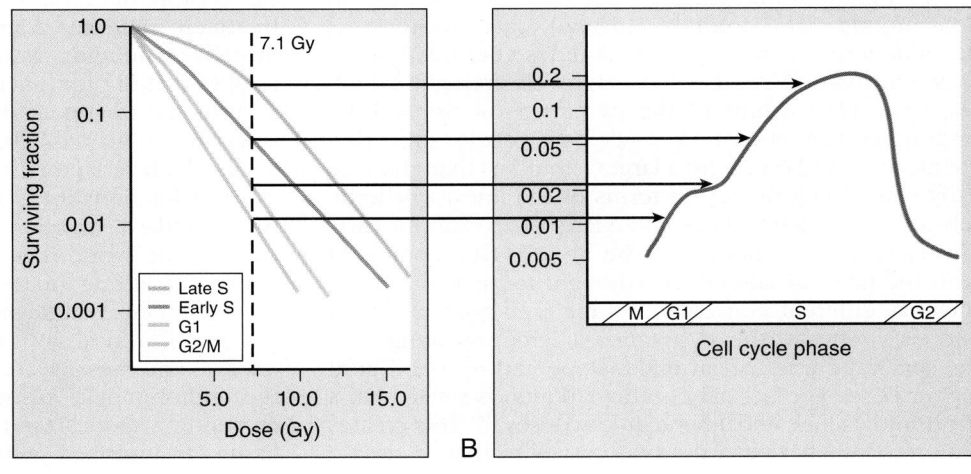

Figure 26-18. A, Cell survival curves for populations of Chinese hamster cells irradiated in different phases of the cell cycle. **B,** Graphic illustration of how these radiosensitivity differences translate into age response patterns.

Science of Clinical Oncology

The biologic basis of fractionation in radiation therapy has traditionally been understood in simple terms and makes use of the "four Rs of radiobiology"—**r**epair of sublethal damage, **r**eassortment of cells within the cell cycle, **r**epopulation, and **r**eoxygenation.

Dividing the total dose into a number of smaller fractions allows for normal tissue sparing because of the repair of sublethal damage between fractions. Fractionating the therapy also allows for reassortment of tumor cells into radiosensitive phases of the cell cycle, with reoxygenation of the tumor cells causing them to be more radiosensitive. If too much time is given between fractions, however, repopulation or proliferation of the tumor cells could occur.

Though this theory forms the basis for fractionated therapy, it is obviously much more complex than just described. Tumor populations and normal tissue represent a heterogeneous group of cells, all responding to radiation and the fractionation scheme differently. Some general characteristics can be applied, however. Some of this information has been described previously but deserves repeating.

Early-responding tissues include those tissues that are rapidly dividing and repopulating, such as the skin, mucous membranes, bone marrow, and tumor cells; these tissues are responsible for the acute toxicity seen with radiation therapy. The severity of acute toxicity reflects the rate of cell killing of early-responding tissues counteracted by regeneration by those tissues' surviving stem cells. This balance is based mainly on total treatment time. Prolonging overall treatment time spares the patient from the severity of acute toxicity, with short, intense treatment courses leading to severe acute toxicity. If the therapy is so intense that it does not allow a sufficient number of stem cells to survive, the acute toxicity can progress to consequential late effects.[97-99]

Late-responding tissues are responsible for the late toxicity from radiation therapy. These tissues, such as the spinal cord, connective tissue, and many organs, are composed mostly of terminally differentiated cells with no stem cell population. Therefore, there is usually no turnover of cells within a radiation treatment course, and no opportunity or need for regeneration to occur during treatment. Hence, the overall treatment time, in contrast to early-responding tissues, has little importance in determining late toxicity. Instead, late toxicity is dependent mainly on total dose and dose per fraction.

Again, these differences are seen by observing the dose-response relationships of the two types of tissue. Late-responding tissues have dose-response relationships that are more curved (i.e., with a larger shoulder) than those of early responding tissues. In terms of the linear quadratic relationship, this translates into a larger α/β ratio for early effects (generally thought to be at ~ 10 Gy), compared with the ratio for late effects (thought to be at ~ 2 Gy).[96] This has different consequences for each type of tissue. For early effects, the α/β ratio is large, meaning that the survival curve has an initial slope and no bend until higher doses. For late effects, the α/β ratio is small, with a short initial slope and a bend at low doses.[100] This creates a discrepancy between the two curves so that at certain doses, early-responding tissues (tumors included) will be killed preferentially compared with late-responding tissues (see Fig. 26-17). As fraction upon fraction of radiation is given at these doses, the killing of tumor cells is much greater than that of cells of normal organs, which are late responding. As can be seen, however, as fraction size increases, cells in late-responding tissues are killed in greater numbers. This explains the observation that late-responding tissues exhibit a much more marked change in survival with changes in dose per fraction. In other words, late-responding tissues are preferentially spared by dose fractionation.

Why the difference in these curves exists is not completely known, although there are some possible explanations. The first of these deals with cell cycle-specific sensitivity. Cells are sensitive to radiation during mitosis and G2 phase and resistant to radiation during S and early G1 or G0 phases. Though this resistance eventually is overcome with high doses, late-responding tissues have many quiescent cells, hence incurring radioresistance as these cells rest in G0. Tumor cells and early-responding cells, on the other hand, re-assort themselves into sensitive phases of the cell cycle, leading to radiosensitivity at smaller doses.

Another explanation of the differences in the dose curves deals with the repair of DNA damage. Late-responding tissues have a greater capacity for sublethal repair than do early responding tissues, hence the lower α/β ratio and the shallower survival curve at low doses. Though late-responding tissues have a higher repair capacity than early responding tissues, however, the repair kinetics themselves do not differ systematically between the two types of tissues.[101] Hence, there is a minimum limit of time between fractions, so repair in late tissues can be completed. If this is not allowed, drastic toxicity can result. This has been noted in studies that used fractionation schedules in which the interval between doses was less than 4.5 hours.[83,102,103] Though the explanation that these toxicities were due solely to incomplete repair has been questioned, most protocols now stipulate a six-hour interval between fractions to allow for complete repair to take place.

Provided that full recovery occurs between each fraction, most late radiation effects show no dependence on treatment course duration. In contrast, overall treatment time has a large effect on both acute toxicity in early-responding tissues and the cure of tumors. This implies that the tumors that show a decrease in curability with longer treatment times have a rapid regeneration in response to the cell killing that occurs with radiation.

All of these factors must be taken into consideration when a fractionation scheme is being designed. Though the "standard" fractionation schedule differs in many parts of the world, 1.8–2.0 Gy per day is considered the conventional fractionation schedule in the United States. Most regimens that deviate from this norm use more than one fraction in a day. This reduces both the size of the fraction and the total treatment time, to take advantage of the radiobiologic principles as they apply to early-responding tissues (and tumors) and to late-responding tissues as described previously.

Altered Fractionation Schemes

The standard of five fractions per week and 9–10 Gy of dose per week has evolved not as a biologically designed, optimal method of administration of radiation but rather from considerations such as the convenience of patients and staff, the availability of equipment, and financial concerns. Outside of the United States, the same nonmedical constraints have often dictated other fractionation regimens that usually employ fewer fractions over a shorter time period because of limited availability of high-energy treatment machines or trained radiation oncologists. In the 1990s, more attention was paid to attempts to alter the customary fractionation protocols toward schemes that would improve the biologic outcome from treatment, either through increased tumor sterilization or decreased normal tissue toxicity, or both. These attempts were undertaken because of the knowledge that the effects of radiation on acutely reacting tissues (e.g., skin and mucosa) are different from those on late-reacting tissues. Early-reacting tissues, which determine the patient's tolerance to treatment, are time dependent in their reactions. Because these tissues proliferate rapidly, prolonging the total time of therapy allows proliferation to take place and thus lessens the severity of the overall reaction. This is especially true about breaks (days off) from treatment, during which a mucosal or skin reaction can heal substantially in just a few days. Late-reacting tissues do not proliferate during a six- to seven-week course of treatment, and their reaction is thus not sensitive to overall treatment time. Late-reacting tissues are very sensitive to fraction size, however. It is now clear from a number of clinical studies that for the same total dose, late reactions are worse when large fractions are used compared with smaller ones.[104,105] This is understandable from the shape of the cell survival curves for early- and late-reacting tissue. Late-reacting tissues have low α/β ratios, and their survival curves bend at higher doses, causing a substantial difference in cell kill with large rather than small fractions. With little proliferation to make up the difference, the tissues become quite fraction-size dependent. If large fractions are used, the total dose must be lowered to achieve the same effect on long-term toxicity. Clinical examples of this effect are found most often in palliative regimens, in which 20 Gy in five fractions or 30 Gy in 10 fractions are given to spinal metastases and equate with 50 Gy in 25 fractions for spinal cord tolerance. Many Canadian and European centers give fewer numbers of larger fractions for curative treatment as well, reducing total dose for the sake of not amplifying late toxicity. If one considers how this might play out in a fractionated scheme, consider Figure 26-19. It becomes clear that a few large fractions preferentially damage late-reacting tissues, while larger numbers of smaller fractions preferentially spare them.

The other side of this coin is tumor proliferation. If many small fractions are used and the time it takes to deliver a course of radiation is protracted, tumor proliferation could negate any gains. When the aims are to both take advantage of the sparing of late tissue damage and avoid having treatment last for too many days,

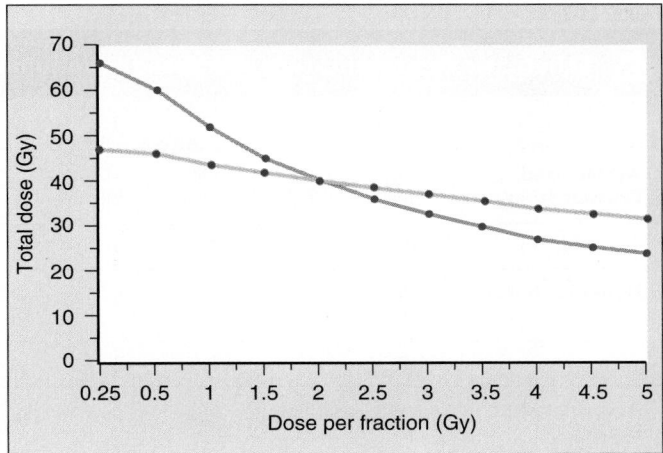

Figure 26-19. Influence of fraction size on complications in early- vs. late-reacting tissues. the α:β ratio for the early tissue (*blue curve*) was set at 10 in this example; the α:β ratio for the late tissue (*red curve*) was 2.5. The tissues were asssumed to have equal reactions to 40 Gy delivered at 2 Gy per fraction. Note that for equal reactions, the early-reacting tissue is far less dependent on fraction size. For large daily fractions, the late-reacting tissue will require substantial dose reduction to maintain equal clinical effects. Conversely, if fraction size is reduced, the late-reacting tissue will tolerate substantially higher doses of radiation. (From Lichter AS: Radiation therapy. In Abeloff M [ed]: Clinical Oncology, 2nd ed. London, Churchill Livingstone, 2000, pp 423–470.)

treatment has been given with multiple fractions per day. Several sample fractionation schemes are presented in Table 26-3. They can be categorized according to two basic strategies: hyperfractionation and accelerated fractionation.

With hyperfractionation, the fraction number is increased, and the dose per fraction is reduced. The total dose is larger, while the overall time is about the same as a conventional course (approximately seven weeks). This allows for the safe escalation of dose with respect to late normal tissue toxicity, as the fraction sizes are quite small. Accelerated tumor repopulation should not be excessive, as the overall time is unchanged. An example of hyperfractionation would be the treatment of head and neck cancer with 1.15 Gy twice daily (11.5 Gy per week). Thus, instead of a typical seven-week course of treatment delivering 63 Gy at standard fractionation, 80.5 Gy can be delivered during the same time period.[106] Several single-arm retrospective studies have reported results with hyperfractionated treatment of the head and neck that suggest benefit in terms of local control; an overview of the clinical experience with this technique also exists, showing overall increased local control.[107–110] A report of a large randomized trial in T2 and T3 oropharyngeal carcinoma showed a nearly 35% increase in local control in the hyperfractionated group, a finding that was statistically significant.[106] Other reports have not suggested such results, but overall the literature does suggest an advantage for hyperfractionation.[111,112]

In accelerated fractionation, the overall time of therapy is reduced, while the number of fractions, fraction size, and total dose might or might not be reduced. Here,

Science of Clinical Oncology

TABLE 26-3

Schematic Representation of Altered Fractionation Protocols

		WEEK 1	2	3	4				FX. NO.	FX. SIZE	TOTAL
Accelerated Fractionation*	am	‖‖	‖‖	‖‖	‖‖	I			42	1.6 Gy	67.2 Gy
	pm	‖‖	‖‖	‖‖	‖‖	I					

		WEEK 1	2	3	4	5	6	7	FX. NO.	FX. SIZE	TOTAL
Hyperfractionation	am	‖‖	‖‖	‖‖	‖‖	‖‖	‖‖	‖‖	70	1.15 Gy	80.5 Gy
	pm	‖‖	‖‖	‖‖	‖‖	‖‖	‖‖	‖‖			

		WEEK 1	2	3	4	5	6	7	FX. NO.	FX. SIZE	TOTAL
Accelerated Boost	am	‖‖	‖‖	‖‖	‖‖	‖‖	‖‖		40	1.8 Gy	69 Gy
	pm					‖‖	‖‖			1.5 Gy	

*Often includes break after two weeks to increase tolerance.

the advantage is that a reduction in overall time could counteract accelerated repopulation in the tumor. Late effects should be about the same, as the fraction size is standard (or reduced) and the total dose is not increased. An extreme example of accelerated fractionation is the British experience with 1.5 Gy three times daily for 12 consecutive days, giving 54 Gy in 36 treatments in about 1.5 weeks.[74] Another widely used scheme is the so-called "concomitant boost" schedule, in which the first 36 Gy is given in four weeks at 1.8 Gy per fraction, and while that larger field continues to a total of 54 Gy, a smaller boost field is added as a second daily treatment for the last two to three weeks, bringing the total dose to 72 Gy in six rather than eight weeks.[113] The results of a large randomized trial in head and neck patients showed an advantage to this technique in terms of local control, although to date no survival benefit has been seen.[73] One difficulty with hyperfractionated or accelerated schemes is the increased toxicity that can be seen in patients receiving concomitant chemotherapy, and combining chemotherapy and radiation is becoming increasingly common. Furthermore, these schemes—especially those that involve separation of doses in time—require the patient to come to clinic more than once daily, and hence they are highly inconvenient to the patient. Therefore, many clinicians feel that these strategies must show substantial benefit to be worthwhile. Nevertheless, the concomitant boost technique has become an established and accepted technique for patients with head and neck cancer, and research continues on other schemes worldwide.

Oxygen Effect

Many agents have been noted to modify the responses of cells and tissues to radiation. The best-known chemical modifier is oxygen. The response of cells to ionizing radiation is strongly oxygen dependent, with well oxygenated cells showing up to threefold greater sensitivity to the killing effects of ionizing radiation than the same cells under hypoxic conditions.[114] The effect of oxygen has been known for nearly a century, starting in 1912, when Swartz noted a reduction of radiation effect if blood flow to the exposed area was reduced.[115] Though many suspected the modifying properties of oxygen, the oxygen effect was first demonstrated quantitatively by Gray and Tomlinson in 1955.[116] This discovery had immediate implications, as it is well known that tumors have a much higher proportion of hypoxic cells than normal tissues do. Though many attempts have been made to circumvent this "built-in" radioresistance of tumor cells, tumor hypoxia continues to be a problem in therapeutic radiation oncology.

The oxygen enhancement ratio (OER) is the ratio of hypoxic to aerated doses needed to achieve the same biologic effect. For x-rays, the oxygen enhancement ratio is generally between 2 and 3, becoming more pronounced at higher doses (Fig. 26-20). In other words, the presence of oxygen in cells increases cell killing by radiation. The mechanism behind oxygen's radiosensitizing effect is thought to lie in the process of indirect damage, which is DNA damage resulting from the production of free radicals from water molecules. These free radicals break chemical bonds and produce chemical changes, initiating the chain of events that result in the expression of biological damage. After DNA damage from free radicals occurs, the damaged targets are generally quickly repaired by a reduction reaction involving reducing species such as thiols and intracellular glutathione, which restores the target to its original condition. Oxygen inhibits this repair of free radical-induced damage by forming irreversible peroxides in the injured biomolecules, thus "fixing" the radiation damage.

Consistent with this explanation of oxygen's effect is the fact that oxygen need not be present at the time of radiation for sensitization to occur, but it must be present shortly thereafter. Oxygen could be added after the radiation to sensitize cells, provided the delay is no longer than 5 ms.[117] Also consistent with this theory is the fact that high linear energy transfer radiation has a lower oxygen enhancement ratio than does low linear energy transfer radiation.

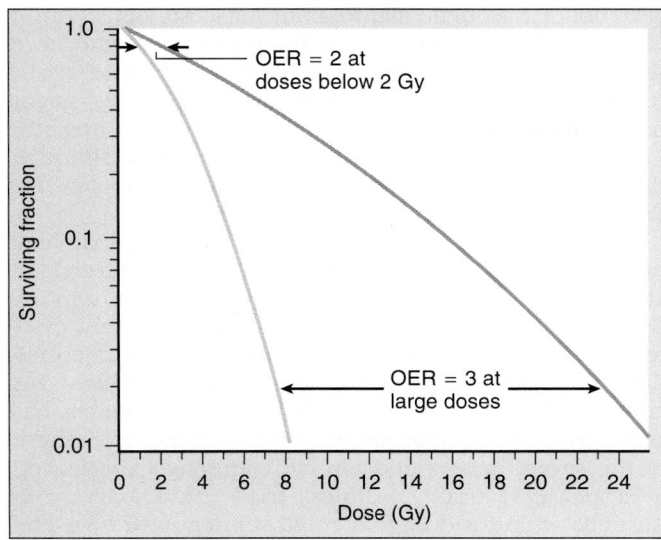

Figure 26-20. Cells irradiated in the presence of molecular oxygen are more sensitive to killing by x-rays than cells that are hypoxic (deficient in oxygen). The ratio of doses that produce the same level of biological damage in the absence of oxygen and in the presence of oxygen is known as the oxygen enhancement ratio (OER). At high doses, the OER has a value of about 3; its value seems to be smaller (close to 2) at doses below 2 Gy. (From Cox JD, Ang KK [eds]: Radiation Oncology Rationale, Technique, Results, 8th ed. St. Louis, Mo, Mosby, 2003, p 34.)

The concentration of oxygen required for this sensitization is small, as oxygen is a highly efficient radiosensitizer. Air has an oxygen concentration of approximately 155 mmHg. Hypoxic resistance occurs at concentrations between 0 mmHg and 20 mmHg. By the time a 20 mmHg concentration of oxygen is reached, the cell survival curve is similar to the curve obtained during fully oxygenated conditions. This is less than half of the partial pressure of oxygen normally found in tissues (approximately 40 mm Hg). A concentration as small as 5 mmHg results in a radiosensitivity halfway between hypoxic and fully oxygenated conditions. In practice, this means that hypoxia is not a major consideration for normal tissues; the minimum oxygen concentration to which most tissues will be exposed is at the level of venous blood (around 40–50 mmHg), well above the borderline for the oxygen sensitizing effect. Some normal tissues (e.g., cartilage or skin) might contain borderline hypoxic cells.[118]

Though the oxygen tension of normal tissues is similar to that of venous blood (40 mmHg), there is a heterogeneity of oxygen tension within the cells themselves. Some normal tissues contain a small percentage of cells that are borderline radiobiologically hypoxic. This percentage is amplified greatly in tumor tissues due to both chronic hypoxia and acute hypoxia. Chronic hypoxia (also termed diffusion-limited hypoxia) results from the propensity of tumors to outgrow their blood supplies. The distance to which oxygen could diffuse in respiring tissues was calculated by Tomlinson and Gray to be 100–180 μm.[116] Cells beyond this distance would be expected to be dead or dying (producing the observed areas of necrosis seen in tumors), but those on the fringe of this distance would make up a large hypoxic region of cells. Acute hypoxia, also known as perfusion-limited hypoxia, results from the transient closing of blood vessels within the tumors themselves. Other possible causes include changes in overall blood flow or decreases in red blood cell delivery. Like chronic hypoxia, acute hypoxia can create a substantial hypoxic population of cells within a tumor.[119]

These populations of hypoxic cells within tumors can cause significant limitations in the efficacy of radiation therapy. Cells within these hypoxic parameters retain properties of clonogenicity, yet they are protected from the effects of radiation because of the absence of oxygen to fix the radiation damage. Therefore, the presence of even a small population of hypoxic cells could limit (or even render impossible) overall success in radiation therapy in clinical situations.[120] This is an extremely important postulate, as it has been estimated that hypoxic fractions comprise up to 50% of tumors, with an average of 15% of all tumor cells being hypoxic (Fig. 26-21).[121]

Given that tumors contain hypoxic cells that greatly limit the success of radiation, how are clinical successes with radiation obtained? The answer might lie in the reoxygenation of tumor cells after radiation that has been observed in rodent tumors.[122-125] Reoxygenation occurs with both the chronic and acute mechanisms of hypoxia. In terms of chronic hypoxia, reoxygenation involves the shrinking of tumors during a course of radiation therapy. As cells die from exposure to radiation, surviving cells that previously were beyond the range of oxygen diffusion are brought closer to a blood supply and then reoxygenate. This process is fairly slow, taking place over a period of days, with dependence on the rate of tumor regression. Reoxygenation also occurs in terms of the mechanism responsible for acute hypoxia. Assuming that blood flow resumes in areas of acute hypoxia, reoxygenation might take place within minutes or hours.

The process of reoxygenation is thought to be important in the practice of radiation oncology and again suggests the importance of using a protracted, fractionated course of radiation therapy. If human tumors reoxgenate as efficiently as animal tumors do, using multiple fractions could be sufficient to deal with the

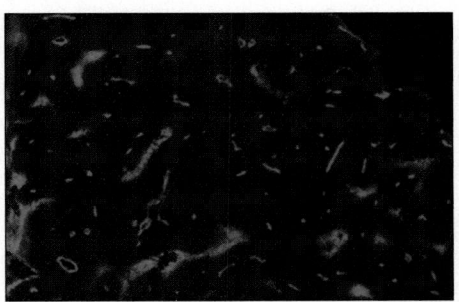

Figure 26-21. Microscopic photo of a leiomyosarcoma of the extremity stained with EF-5 displaying the heterogenicity of hypoxia within the tumor. Green color corresponds to capillaries within the tumor. Red areas correspond to areas of hypoxia, which are at a notable distance from the blood supply. (Used with permission from Sydney Evans, VMD, University of Pennsylvania.)

problem of hypoxic cell populations. On the other hand, attempts at increasing the partial pressures of oxygen in tumors and using oxygen-mimetic chemicals to increase the sensitivity of tumor cells to radiation have yielded mixed results. A number of new agents (e.g., EF5 [5-fluoro-etanidazole] and pimonidazole) are under active study to allow a more accurate assessment of the role of hypoxia in human tumors and cancer management.[126]

Radiosensitizers and Radioprotectors

The most common and most effective radiosensitizer is oxygen; however, there are obvious limitations to achieving levels of oxygen sufficient for sensitizing all tumor cells. To deal with the hypoxia problem, oxygen-mimetic compounds have been developed and tested (Fig. 26-22). These chemicals all have a similar electron affinity for the electrons produced by the ionization of biomolecules. The nitroimidazoles—including metronidazole, misonidazole, and etanidazole—all represent molecules with these characteristics. These compounds were all highly successful radiation sensitizers in animal model studies. Unfortunately, clinical trials have shown them to have limited efficacy.[118] There could be several reasons for this finding. As laboratory studies have continued to show encouraging results, diffusion into tissues seems to be the limiting quality in these compounds, just as it is for oxygen itself. In addition, severe side effects have been noted with some of these compounds at the drug concentrations required to produce a radiosensitizing effect, most notably peripheral neuropathy.[127,128] An additional problem is that in animal models (particularly rodent models), tumors grow rapidly and hence might have more hypoxia. Also, the tumors are

very uniform from animal to animal, making detection of effects more readily obtainable. Human tumors grow more slowly and are more heterogeneous. In clinical trials, therefore, the effect of the oxygen-mimetic drugs might have been diluted out by poor patient selection. Currently, no major trials are underway with these drugs, although this field could be revisited as methods improve for defining tumor oxygenation in human material.

Given the lack of efficacy seen with hypoxic cell radiosensitizers, other approaches have emerged to attack the hypoxia problem encountered in tumors. Tirapazamine is a compound that is activated to a cytotoxic molecule preferentially under hypoxic conditions.[53,129] Data suggest a synergistic effect when this compound is given with radiation. Clinical progress has been slow with tirapazamine, however, perhaps because of the severe nausea and muscle cramping experienced in a phase II trial.[130] Clinical trials are underway in Australia with this drug that could yet demonstrate useful efficacy.[131]

Compounds that interact with DNA might also act synergistically with radiation. In 1960, it was found that pyrimidines could be halogenated and incorporated into DNA because the van der Waal's radius of chlorine, bromine, or iodine was similar to the size of a methyl group side chain on uridine and because a halogenated uridine would be recognized by DNA polymerase. Therefore, halogenated pyrimidines (e.g., uridine with a bromine atom replacing the methyl group [BUDR] or an iodine replacing the methyl group [IUDR] could be substituted in DNA for a normal thymine.[132] DNA containing substituted halogenated pyrimidines is more susceptible to DNA double-strand breaks when exposed to UV or ionizing radiation.[133] Hence, cells are killed more effectively.[132,134] In clinical trials, these compounds have shown little efficacy.[135-137] It is thought that perhaps not enough of the halogenated pyrimidines are incorporated into the DNA, resulting in only minor radiosensitization.

Currently, the most widely used radiosensitizers are chemotherapeutic agents. Originally, the rationale for the combination of chemotherapy and radiation was to attack two different problems. Whereas radiation would address local control issues, chemotherapy was thought to rid the patient of micrometastases. Evidence of increased local control in patients receiving combined treatment, however, is now seen as evidence of chemotherapy's radiosensitizing effects, which have been demonstrated in many tumors. Examples include the use of mitomycin-C in anal cancer, taxanes in breast cancer, platinum agents in lung cancer, head and neck cancer, cervical cancer, and bladder cancer, and 5-FU in esophageal and pancreatic cancers (Table 26-4).[138-149] Though some of the improved outcome in these studies is obviously due to the elimination of micrometastases, improved local control from radiosensitization is likewise thought to be an important component.

Though the therapeutic ratio can be improved with radiosensitization, a benefit in terms of the relative sparing of normal tissues could also be attained using radioprotectors. The most abundant radioprotectors are those with sulfhydryl compounds, with cysteine first discovered

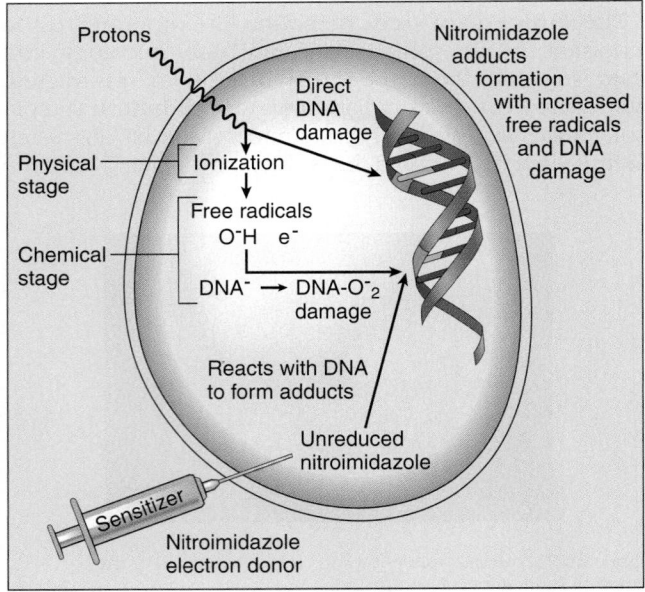

Figure 26-22. Hypoxic cell sensitizers increase DNA damage through free radical formation. (From Leibel SA, Phillips TL [eds]: Textbook of Radiation Oncology. Philadelphia, WB Saunders, 1998, p 44.)

TABLE 26-4

Chemotherapy Agents that Sensitize the Effects of Radiation

DRUG	PROPOSED MECHANISM OF ENHANCEMENT	CLINICAL USE
5-Fluorouracil	Inhibit thymidylate synthase causing ↓ DNA repair	Head and neck, gastrointestinal, bladder
Platinum	DNA cross-links; ↓ repair	Head and neck, gynecologic, bladder, lung
Gemcitabine	Inhibits ribonucleotide reductase, ↑ apoptesis	Pancreas, head and neck, lung
Paclitaxel	Microtubule stabilization	Lung, gynecologic malignancies, head and neck

to protect against the effects of radiation by Pratt and colleagues in 1948.[150] Since then, many other compounds have been found to be effective as radioprotectors, the most efficient of which has a free SH group separated from the rest of the molecule. The mechanisms of the radioprotection afforded by sulfhydryl-containing molecules include free radical scavenging and hydrogen donation to facilitate DNA repair (Fig. 26-23). The most common radioprotector in use clinically today is WR-2721 (amifostine), developed at the Walter Reed Institute of Research. It is converted to the active metabolite WR-1065 once in the cell and acts as a free radical scavenger.[151] Given intravenously or, more recently, subcutaneously, it has been demonstrated to be efficacious in reducing toxicity in head and neck cancers and lung cancer and is being tested in the treatment of several other malignancies.[152,153]

A question that is being addressed closely at this time is whether new classes of molecularly targeted agents

can be produced that will work with radiation as more specific sensitizers or protectors. We are entering a new era in cancer therapeutics. Instead of the traditional approach of nonspecifically and empirically testing cytotoxic agents on a wide variety of tumors, hoping that a suitable candidate might become apparent by serendipity, the new approach is to delineate the molecular mechanisms that promote tumor survival and then design drugs and treatment regimens that specifically target these mechanisms. This approach has resulted in spectacular successes in recent years. Drugs such as rituximab (Rituxan), trastuzumab (Herceptin), and imatinib mesylate (Gleevec) have capitalized on the knowledge that has emerged from the laboratory bench.[154-164] Each of these drugs represents a distinct departure from traditional chemotherapies and has been found to improve the efficacy of traditional chemotherapy dramatically. Each of these drugs has resulted in impressive improvements in the success of treatment and (most important) has significantly improved the survival rates of patients, often with reduced toxicity.

This targeted approach will continue to affect the practice of medical oncology, and it is likely that such an approach will also prove fruitful in finding strategies to enhance the efficacy of radiation therapy. A number of laboratories have dissected mechanisms and pathways that determine the cancer cell's ability to survive radiation treatment, providing targets that we should be able to exploit successfully. In fact, drugs that target some of these pathways (e.g., agents that target EGFR, Ras, and Cox-2) are already in development or in clinical trials in radiation oncology.[165,166] Some previously identified genes such as *ras* and *p53* have properties that are consistent with the idea that some of the mutational changes in tumor cells alter their response to conventional therapies. The hope is that over the next few years, not only will we better understand how these genes have their effects at the molecular level but we also might find other targets that can specifically be used to alter sensitivity to conventional treatment so that trial design with these agents can become rational rather than serendipitous. Potential targets include:

- Signal transduction pathways, for which targeting agents are already in clinical trials
- Pathways clearly involved in sensitivity to drugs and radiation, for which agents are not yet ready to proceed to human clinical trials but might soon be ready for animal trials

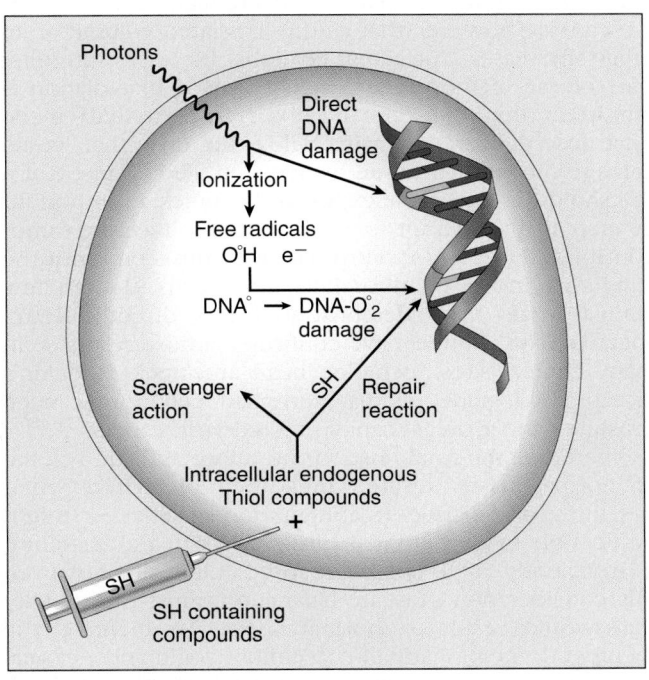

Figure 26-23. Chemical protectors: competition model. There is a dual action to chemical radioprotection: (1) thiols and sulfhydryl compounds act as repair compounds; (2) they compete with free radicals (scavenging effect). (From Leibel SA, Phillips TL [eds]: Textbook of Radiation Oncology. Philadelphia, WB Saunders, 1998, p 50.)

• Investigation of the molecular mechanisms involved in the most highly conserved (and thus likely the most important) cellular responses to cytotoxic stress

The hypothesis is that it is possible both to identify molecular targets in the cancer cell that modify the response of the cell to drugs or radiation and to define the molecular mechanisms that result in such altered sensitivity. There are a number of potentially interesting areas in which to search for these new targets. The "checkpoint theory" of Hartwell and Weinert [167,168] postulated that checkpoints are activated in response to cytotoxic damage to allow the cell to repair the damage or to progress down a pathway leading to apoptosis. Furthermore, many of the genes shown to be involved in checkpoint activation have been shown to be specifically mutated in cancer cells. [46,169-174] Therefore, analysis of cell cycle targets might be a ripe place to begin to search for strategies for developing specific radiation sensitizers. In the past five years, our knowledge of this area has evolved. Our current understanding of p53, for example, suggests that its roles in checkpoint control and activation of apoptosis are distinct from one another. [175] Furthermore, we now understand that cell survival pathways involving signal transduction might be distinct from those that activate checkpoints. We also have seen the initiation of clinical trials of new agents with radiation that clearly are based on potential molecular or biological targets.

Thus far, we have discussed classic radiobiologic principles backed by experimental evidence. These principles likely represent a simplistic view of cells' responses to radiation, however. In many cases, the mechanisms behind the experimental observations that are noted are not known, yet there are innumerable cellular responses to radiation. In the majority of these, the specifics require elucidation, but these cellular signals, transduction pathways, and molecular biologic phenomena are actively being investigated. This investigation could serve as the key to understanding the actual mechanisms behind cellular responses to radiation. The radiosensitizers developed previously might pale in comparison to the targeted therapies that could result from attacking signal transduction pathways and cell signaling proteins, thus leading to a more refined use of radiation therapy in clinical oncology.

CLINICAL APPLICATION OF RADIOBIOLOGIC PRINCIPLES

The goal of all investigations into the physical aspects and biologic principles behind radiation therapy is to attempt to increase the therapeutic index, which is defined as the tumor response for a fixed level of normal tissue damage. [176] Or to restate it another way, the goal is to increase tumor cell kill and hence tumor control while maintaining normal tissue toxicity within a tolerable range. Obviously, acute toxicity (encountered during treatment) is a concern and must be managed aggressively to ensure that the patient is able to complete the course of radiation therapy. When discussing normal tissue toxicity, however, late effects, which translate into end-organ damage, are usually considered the dose-limiting toxicity.

All organs have a threshold for normal tissue toxicity. These thresholds, though, often lack rigidity and are poorly defined, as they depend on the interaction of many factors. The most important factors in terms of normal tissue tolerance and toxicity are total dose delivered and the volume of the organ exposed to this dose. Calculating this relationship for normal tissue is not as simple as it is for tumors, however. When speaking in terms of tumor cure, the fraction of cells surviving determines the success of treatment, because a single surviving cell might suffice for regrowth of the tumor. For normal tissues, the tolerance is greatly dependent on the ability of stem cells to maintain a sufficient number of mature cells for proper organ function. This statement is an oversimplification, however, as the tolerance of an organ also depends on the structural organization of the organ, which some have termed functional subunits. [177,178] For example, consider the kidney and the spinal cord. If radiation permanently damages a number of nephrons, the end-organ function might not be affected as long as enough nephrons remain to maintain function. The functional subunits of the kidney, then, are said to be arranged in parallel. On the other hand, if one section of the spinal cord is damaged, the entire cord distal to the lesion will be disrupted. Organs such as the spinal cord, in which damage to one portion of the organ affects the function of the entire organ, have what is called serial functional subunits.

Functional subunits have yet to be identified for many organs, and the use of functional subunits to describe radiation tolerance of many organs remains a hypothesis. We can say, however, that as the irradiated volume of an organ increases, the complications increase. Although the volume of the organ that is exposed to radiation is important, this might not be observed as toxicity if the total dose delivered remains below the dose that would damage the normal tissue in question. The concept of a threshold for total dose exposure becomes an important concept as we attempt to escalate dose to increase tumor control. Clinical and in vitro data are consistent with the view that increased dose kills more cells, though few clinical trials have demonstrated this directly. Retrospective data, though, have confirmed a dose response in many clinical sites, including head and neck, Hodgkin's disease, high-grade glioma, non-small cell lung cancer, prostate cancer, breast cancer, and cervical cancer. [179-186]

Therefore, the total dose to the tumor and the volume of normal tissue treated must be considered when designing a radiation treatment course. Success might be possible in any tumor, regardless of size and histology, if sufficiently high doses are used. Clinically, however, this consideration must be balanced against the toxicity that would result to normal tissue. To increase the therapeutic ratio, many of the radiobiologic and physical principles of radiation have been used. These include all that have been described, including tumor localization, choosing the optimal energy and radiation modality, manipulating the dose rate, fractionation schemes, and the use of radiosensitizers and radioprotectors or targeted therapies. All are dependent on the accurate localization of the tumor and the accurate delivery of the radiation.

Effects of Radiation on Normal Tissue

The effects of radiation on normal tissue usually limit the doses of therapeutic radiation that can be administered safely.[187] For some clinical presentations—for example, a responsive tumor (e.g., lymphoma) located in radiation-tolerant tissues such as the low neck—cure is possible without a major risk of serious complications. In other situations—such as in the setting of advanced prostate cancer, where rectal complications can occur—cure is possible, but the risk of complications cannot be dismissed lightly. In still other situations—such as damage to normal brain tissue while treating high-grade gliomas—cure might not be possible without the risk of very severe sequelae. Finally, an increase in the control rate in many clinical situations might be possible only at the expense of more complications unless ways can be found to increase the tumor dose without substantially increasing the dose to surrounding normal tissues. The latter concept underlies the increased use of interstitial implantation techniques and the new field of three-dimensional conformal dose delivery, discussed later in this chapter.

It should be remembered that complication risk and cure trade off against one another. Complications are an inherent risk in any medical treatment, and one must weigh the risks of failure to control the tumor against the advantage of local control associated with a complication. There should also be an appreciation as to whether a complication can be managed with other types of treatment—for example, a colostomy for a rectal injury—or whether it is untreatable, as in the case of spinal cord transection. The context of the patient also enters into the decision concerning how much risk to take in any individual case. Advanced cervical cancer in a 40-year-old woman with small children to care for might be legitimately managed more aggressively than the same tumor in an 80-year-old woman with severe coronary artery disease and diabetes. For many established medical treatments, especially in life-threatening situations, a measurable risk of a fatal complication is accepted. So, too, should we recognize that appropriately applied radiation treatment will regrettably cause complications in some cases. The radiation oncologist should frankly discuss these possibilities with both the patient and the referring physician, allowing a joint understanding and a joint acceptance of risk. Understanding the effects of radiation on normal tissues is clearly critical to the proper use of this modality.

Acute Effects on Normal Tissues

The acute effects of radiation result from direct damage to parenchymal cells of organs that are sensitive to radiation. For purposes of discussion, an acute effect is defined as an effect seen during treatment and up to three months after the conclusion of therapy. A detailed discussion of this subject is beyond the scope of this chapter, but it has been reviewed elsewhere.[187,188] Table 26-5 summarizes the acute effects of radiation and their management.

Late Effects on Normal Tissues

Late effects are those that occur three months or longer after the end of therapy. Virtually any organ or tissue that is treated can express a syndrome of late radiation damage. The etiology of late damage is debated. Some believe that it is due to slow dropout of small vasculature, leading to organ cell loss, fibrosis, and eventual late organ failure.[189] Evidence for this viewpoint is supplied by morphologic studies of irradiated tissues where decreased vascularity can be observed in virtually every tissue type.[190] Others believe that late damage is due in large part to direct damage to parenchymal cells. This theory is plausible, as organs have widely differing sensitivities to radiation, but there is little evidence to suggest that blood vessels in one part of the body are more or less radiosensitive than in any other part. Thus, if vascular

TABLE 26-5

Acute Effects of Radiation		
ORGAN	**SYMPTOM**	**MANAGEMENT**
Systemic	Lethargy, fatigue	Symptomatic
Skin	Erythema, dry desquamation, pruritis, moist desquamation	Observation; topical steroids for pruritis; avoid occlusive dressings or clothing; drying agents for moist desquamation, Silvadine cream
Oral mucous membranes/teeth	Mucositis	Dental consultation pretreatment; rinse with sodium bicarbonate; fluoride treatment; viscous xylocaine and oral analgesics for pain; watch for and treat candidiasis
Esophagus	Esophagitis	Systemic analgesics; consider diagnosis of *Candida* esophagitis
Lung	Radiation pneumonitis	Observation in mild cases; prednisone in more serious cases
Liver	Radiation hepatitis	Symptomatic management
Small bowel	Cramping, diarrhea, nausea, and vomiting	Antidiarrheal agents; sulcralfate might protect; antiemetics; low-residue diet
Bladder	Frequency, urgency, dysuria	Urinary analgesics (e.g., pyridium) alpha$_1$-blocker (e.g. hytrin)
Rectum	Tenesmus	Symptomatic
Hematopoietic	Cytopenia	Transfusions; cytokines (e.g., erythropoietin, granulocyte colony-stimulating factor) are being studied

From Lichter AS: Radiation therapy. In Abeloff M (ed): Clinical Oncology, 2nd ed. London, Churchill Livingstone, 2000, pp 423–470.

Science of Clinical Oncology

TABLE 26-6

Estimated Organ Tolerance Doses in Radiation Therapy*

ORGAN	TOXICITY	TOLERANCE DOSE IN cGy (RANGE)[†]
Brain	Necrosis	5000–6000
Eye	Cataract	1000
	Keratitis	5000
	Retinal damage	4500–5000
Pituitary	Hypopituitarism	
Spinal cord	Paralysis	5000 (5-cm segment)
Skin	Necrosis	6000 (10 × 10 cm)
Salivary gland	Xerostomia	4000–5000
Thyroid	Hypothyroidism	4500
Lung	Pneumonitis	1750–2000
Heart	Peri-/paracarditis	4500
Esophagus	Stricture	5500–6000
Liver	Hepatitis	3000
Stomach	Ulcer/hemorrhage	5000
Kidney	Nephritis	2000–2500
Rectum	Ulcer/hemorrhage	6000
Ovary	Sterility/menopause	6000
Testis	Sterility	200
Bladder	Contracture	6500

*Dose to whole organ, unless noted.
[†]5% complication level at 200 cGy per fraction.
From Lichter AS: Radiation therapy. In Abeloff M (ed): Clinical Oncology, 2nd ed. London, Churchill Livingstone, 2000, pp 423–470.

damage were a final common pathway, then most organs should share similar radiation tolerance doses, and they do not.[191] In all likelihood, late damage represents a combination of vascular damage and direct organ cell depletion. For a more detailed discussion of late radiation effects, the reader is referred to some excellent reviews.[192,193] A summary of organ tolerances to radiation is presented in Table 26-6.

Carcinogenesis

Because radiation causes damage to DNA, and some of the damage is misrepaired, leading to cell death, it is not difficult to conceive that a radiation-damaged piece of DNA could be misrepaired with a small but nonlethal mistake. Alternatively, a base in the DNA strand could be damaged in a nonlethal way, but in a manner that alters the base sequence. Such a change in the sequence of DNA bases is called a mutation, and some mutations can lead to malignant transformation of the cell. Thus, radiation would be expected to be a carcinogen, and decades of research have confirmed this fact. Radiation is probably the most thoroughly studied carcinogen, and its ability to induce malignancy was first seen in the pioneers of clinical radiation research, many of whom lost fingers, hands, and lives to multiple aggressive skin cancers caused by repeated exposure to x-rays.[3] Over the years, a number of radiation-exposed populations have been studied, including radium watch dial painters and patients exposed to radiation for benign disease—for example, tuberculosis victims examined with multiple fluoroscopies over the course of many years, postpartum mastitis patients whose breasts were irradiated, ankylosing

spondylitis patients who received spinal irradiation, and children treated with radiation to reduce thymic enlargement.[194-198] One of the largest and most carefully studied populations has been the survivors of the atomic bomb explosions from Japan during World War II.[199,200] Today, our attention is drawn to the survivors of the Chernobyl nuclear accident in the former Soviet Union.[201,202]

Several principles of radiation-induced carcinogenesis have been deduced from these studies:

1. Radiation-induced cancer appears several years after exposure, often 5–10 years later for radiation-induced leukemias and 25–30 years later for solid malignancies.[203]

2. Leukemia is the most sensitive malignancy to radiation induction, with relative risks of 30 or more over the general population. The leukemias are seen at a peak of 6–8 years after exposure, after which they trail off.[204]

3. Not all cancers are sensitive to radiation induction. Whereas thyroid and breast cancer are induced readily, pancreatic and rectal carcinomas appear to have little sensitivity to radiation induction. There is no discernible pattern to organ sensitivity that has been deduced to date.[205]

4. Radiation induction of cancer is often age sensitive. For example, radiation of the breast during the teens and 20s can be quite dangerous, while irradiation after age 50 is rarely associated with breast cancer induction.[206,207]

5. The age distribution of radiation-induced cancers is similar to the naturally occurring incidence pattern. This finding suggests that radiation facilitates the appearance of malignancy rather than being entirely causative of the problem. Cancer is likely a multistep process, and a radiation exposure appears to fill in some of the required steps, while the remaining steps occur at the typical time course, yielding cancers with a characteristic age distribution.[208]

6. There is a unique relationship of dose to cancer induction. Cancers are induced with increased frequency as dose increases up to a point, after which increasing dose decreases the appearance of malignancy in both experimental and clinical situations (Fig. 26-24).[118,209] This is likely due to the amount of DNA damage being caused; at lower doses, cells can survive while sustaining nonlethal mutations, while at high doses, lethal mutations dominate. This finding implies that a high-dose therapeutic course of radiation should not induce large numbers of cancers in survivors. This appears to be the case, although it should be emphasized that cancer induction from radiation treatment can be and is seen.[209-211]

Although low doses of radiation can cause cancer, it is not known whether any dose is so low as not to be dangerous—that is, whether a threshold for adverse effects exists below which small doses of radiation have no biologic effect. Our information on radiation carcinogenesis comes from dosage data in the tens and hundreds of centigray (cGy). We have little or no data from doses in the 1- or 2-cGy range, and even fewer data in

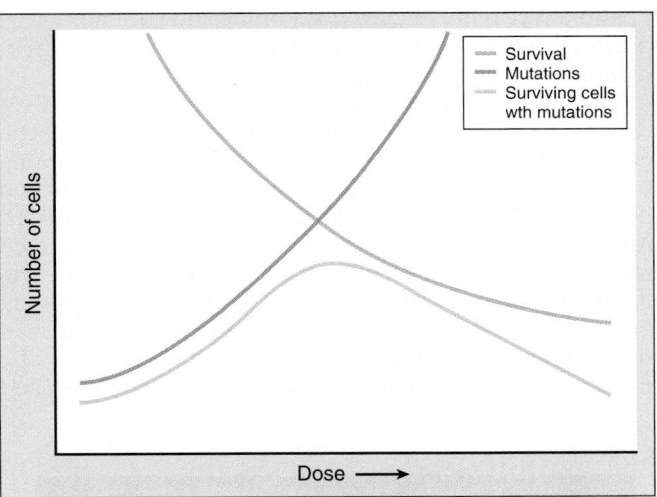

Figure 26-24. Relationship between dose and viable mutations. As the dose increases the number of mutations increases. As dose increases, however, survival of cells decrease. The composite, labeled "surviving cells with mutations," has a characteristic shape. Mutations increase up to a relatively low dose level and then begin to decrease. High-dose therapeutic radiation produces a very small number of secondary induced cancers. (From Lichter AS: Radiation therapy. In Abeloff M [ed]: Clinical Oncology, 2nd ed. London, Churchill Livingstone, 2000, pp 423–470.)

the tenths of cGy range, which are doses associated with many diagnostic x-ray exposures and with some population exposures relating to emissions from nuclear facilities, working with tracer doses of radionuclides, or visiting a patient with a radioactive implant in the hospital.[212] If such a safe threshold existed, it would make the public health aspects of radiation protection much less problematic. At present, a conservative approach to radiation exposure is followed, and it is assumed that any radiation exposure carries risk in a linear fashion. That is, we assume that if 100 cGy produces an effect, 1 cGy will produce one one-hundredth of that effect. Furthermore, population protection levels are calculated with an even more conservative concept of person-cGy, which implies that the same cancer risk will occur if one person is exposed to 1000 cGy that will occur if 1000 persons are each exposed to 1 cGy. From a biologic point of view, this type of calculation seems illogical, but it forms the basis of estimates for the amount of radiation to which the general population can be exposed with safety.[213] Overall, it is obviously prudent to eliminate as much unnecessary radiation exposure as possible. On the other hand, medically necessary radiation in the form of diagnostic or therapeutic radiation is many, many times more life saving compared to its risk, and thus it can easily be justified under even the most stringent estimates of carcinogenic risk of radiation.

PROCESS IN RADIATION TREATMENT

Radiation therapy is an important component of many patients' treatment regimens. It is often combined with surgery or chemotherapy for optimal treatment of the cancer. After evaluation of the patient has been done and the decision to use radiation has been made, perhaps the most important step in a radiation treatment course is the design of the radiation treatment itself.

Treatment Planning

Successful treatment planning is imperative to the success of a radiation treatment course. The goal is to identify the full extent of the tumor and areas of possible spread. Several considerations must be taken into account when considering this volume. These include the tumor histology, the extent of the gross disease, regions of microscopic spread but no gross disease, whether the treatment is being given postoperatively or in an undisturbed tumor bed, and the tolerances of adjacent structures. A plan must then be devised to treat this entire region to the dose desired for each region while keeping the volume of each normal tissue below its tolerance dose.

At one time, radiation treatment was performed by placing the patient directly on the treatment machine and setting up the fields for radiation treatment using surface anatomical landmarks. Although some radiation oncologists became highly skillful at this process and it is still occasionally used in emergency situations, it is obviously an uncertain process with many possibilities for error. In the modern era, the process of designing a radiation field starts with the simulation. In simulation, the treatment fields are designed for the patient before treatment is initiated. Simulation is used to determine the extent of disease and its relationship to other organs. The earliest simulators were fluoroscopy units designed to mimic the geometry of the treatment machines. The oncologist could thus obtain a "beam's eye view" of what would be included in the treatment field. Fluoroscopy was used to outline the boundaries of the field, with plain film x-rays being taken to include the general outline of the area to be treated. Though fluoroscopic simulators are still in use and efficacious, many three-dimensional (3-D) treatment planning systems to design conformal radiation treatment plans are now available to radiation oncologists. 3-D treatment planning systems use CT (or in some cases MRI or even PET) data to assist in setting up the radiation fields. This can be accomplished generally by three different methods:

1. The field can be set up by transferring CT data onto conventional simulation films.
2. CT images can be transferred to a computer-based treatment planning system. The fields are designed using the CT-based planning system, with verification done by taking films on a conventional simulator.
3. The third and most efficient method is to use a CT simulator to set up the radiation fields. The CT simulator combines the processes of obtaining CT images and field design into a single process. CT images of the patient are transferred directly to a computer system that allows the physician to outline the tumor volume and critical structures on individual CT slices. This, in effect, creates an accurate three-dimensional

recreation of both the patient's tumor that is to be treated and of normal tissues that are to be avoided during the delivery of radiation.

After the image data sets are obtained in any type of simulation, careful review of the clinical data must be done to delineate the tissue in need of treatment. This volume to be treated is defined as the target volume and is created by adding three components together. First, the gross tumor volume (GTV) is noted. This volume is expanded to create the clinical tumor volume (CTV) by accounting for the areas at risk for spread, such as adjacent tissues or draining lymphatic regions. The planning tumor volume (PTV) is reached by adding margin to correct for possible variability in daily positioning and patient motion during treatment. Some examples of 3-D treatment planning are shown in Figure 26-25.

The remainder of the planning process involves choosing the number of radiation beams required, the energy of these beams, and the angles and weighting of these beams needed to deliver the required radiation dose to the tumor with optimal sparing of normal tissues. After these beams are designed, digitally reconstructed radiographs are produced to reflect the designed treatment fields. The availability of 3-D treatment planning has allowed for greatly increased complexity of plans in the attempt to increase the therapeutic ratio via the designing of radiation fields, as the doses to the tumor and

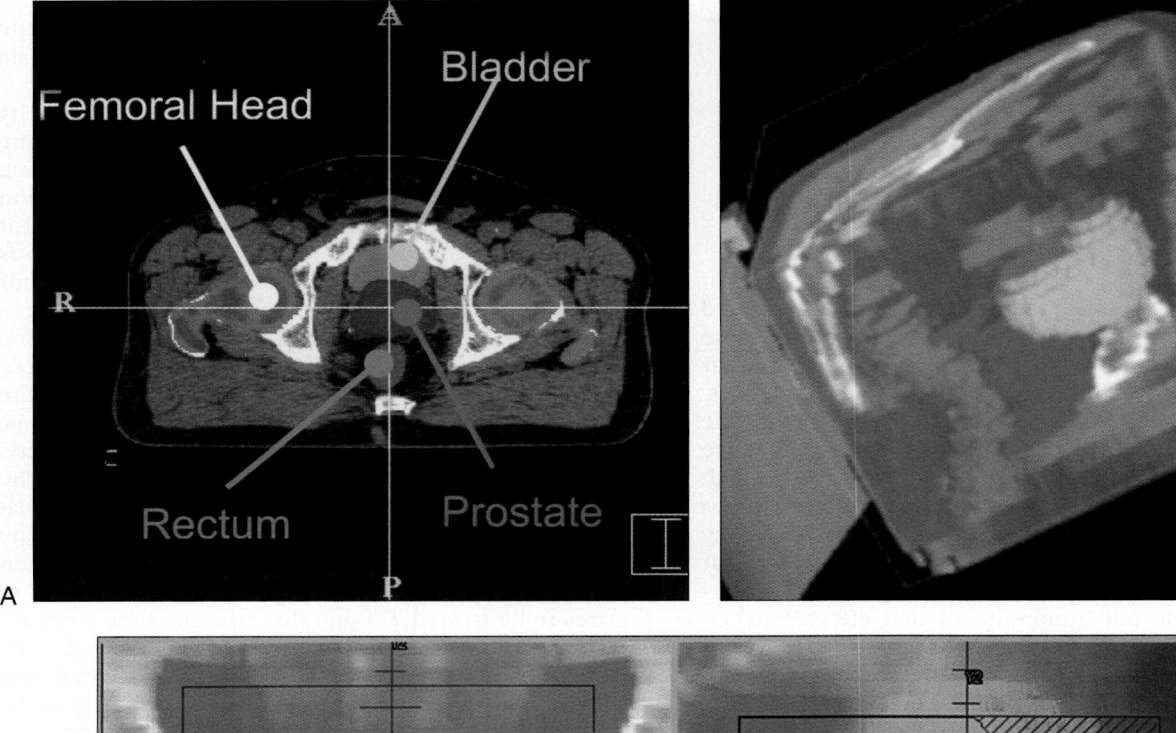

Figure 26-25. A, Transverse CT scan of a male pelvis with simulated organs shown. **B,** Three-dimensional surfaces of the prostate (green), rectum (blue), and bladder (yellow) reconstructed from outlines drawn on CT images. **C,** Digitally reconstructed radiographs (DRRs) of conventional anterior-posterior and lateral fields. Prostate is shown in red, seminal vesicles in blue, rectum in green, and bladder in yellow. (From Cox JD, Ang KK [eds]: Radiation Oncology Rationale, Technique, Results, 8th ed. St. Louis, MO, Mosby, 2003.)

normal organs can be evaluated accurately and three-dimensionally. This evaluation process allows assessment of the possible toxicity that could result from the radiation treatment via the evaluation of a dose volume histogram, which shows the dose delivered throughout the volume of the organ. Although it is never acceptable to treat an entire organ beyond its tolerance, there are circumstances when portions of an organ may be treated to close to or even beyond its tolerance. A consideration here is whether the organ in question is considered to have a serial or parallel structure. In an organ with a serial structure, failure of any component of the organ will cause failure of the entire organ. An example of this might be the spinal cord, where taking any segment of the cord beyond cord tolerance will cause failure of everything downstream. In a parallel organ, such as the lung or kidney, the patient might be able to tolerate loss of part of the organ's function, provided certain volume considerations are not exceeded (Fig. 26-26).

Normal tissues are shielded from the radiation beams in various ways. The first shields or blocks were simply hand-placed pieces of lead or depleted uranium that were inserted in the radiation field to shield the structures below them. When Powers invented a low-melting-point alloy of lead with similar beam attenuating properties, it became possible to create complex blocks that followed the divergent properties of the beam to more accurately

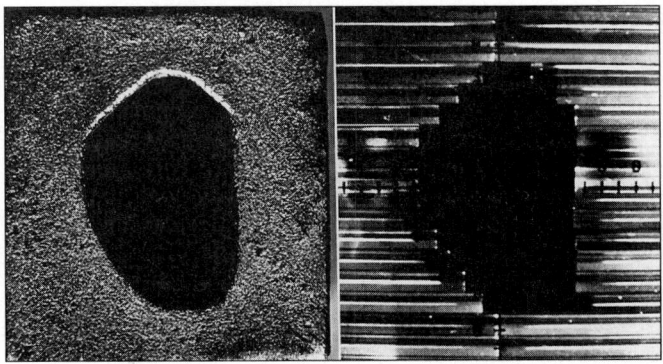

Figure 26-27. Traditionally, radiation fields have been shaped by pouring blocks from a low melting point lead alloy (*left*). The same shape can be created within seconds using a multileaf collimator (*right*). Multiple pairs of thin leaves are each driven by their own motor. The desired shape of the field is entered into a computer that drives the leaf motors and creates virtually any desired shape. (From Lichter AS: Radiation therapy. In Abeloff M [ed]: Clinical Oncology, 2nd ed. London, Churchill Livingstone, 2000, pp 423–470.)

shield organs defined on the simulation films.[214] Blocks were then custom made for each patient. A newer method of shielding is with the use of a multileaf collimator. The multileaf collimator system uses 1 cm or 0.5 cm "leaves" that are actually partitioned jaws of the collimator of the treatment machine. These leaves can be moved to block the radiation field to effectively shape the field as desired (Fig. 26-27).

Once treatment planning is completed, the patient begins the course of radiation therapy. The first step is to set up the patient to verify the simulation fields on the actual treatment machine. Each day, the patient is repositioned into the exact position in which the simulation and subsequent treatment planning were done. To aid in the repositioning, immobilization devices are often used, consisting of foam body casts or plastic head masks. These are made prior to simulation and are kept for use throughout the entire radiation course. Laser lights that converge on the exact isocenter (the point around which the treatment machine rotates) of the treatment machine are available within the treatment room and are used to assist in this repositioning. As 3-D techniques allow for greater refinement of treatment volumes and of the increasing complexity of plans, exact daily repositioning is absolutely imperative. A course of radiation can be any number of fractions, though in palliative cases it is usually between five and 15 fractions, with curative treatments often being between 25 and 40 fractions. Treatment is almost always delivered with five daily fractions per week, but accelerating treatment beyond this has shown some efficacy, although in some cases it has resulted in increased toxicity.[73,215,216]

Clinical Use of Radiation

Radiation is employed in oncologic care in several areas. It can be used as definitive treatment (with or without chemotherapy) where radiation is the sole curative

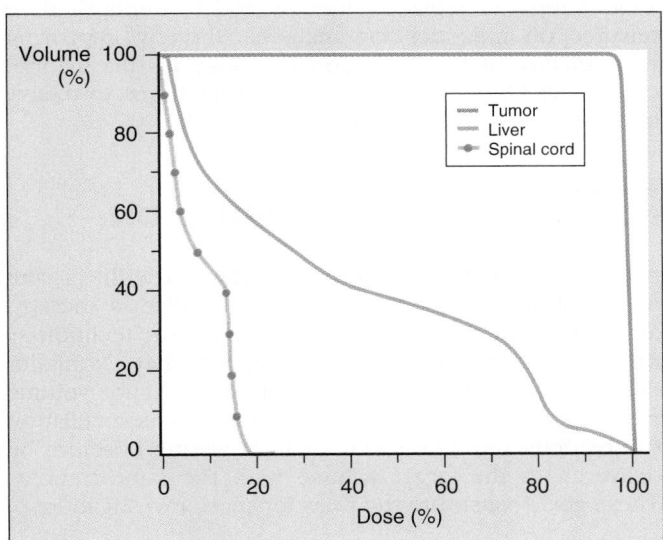

Figure 26-26. Dose-volume histogram. The percentage of the volume of a structure receiving a percentage dose level or more is illustrated in this cumulative histogram. For the tumor, 100% of the volume receives 100% of the dose, which is the desirable situation. For normal structures, lesser doses are given. In this example, 40% of the liver received 40% or more of the dose and 20% of the spinal cord received approximately 17% or more of the dose. A small portion of the liver received more than 90% of the prescribed dose, while no portion of the spinal cord received more than 20% of the prescribed dose. This plot is quite useful in presenting a large amount of complex three-dimensional dose-volum information in a fashion that can be assimilated quickly. (From Lichter AS: Radiation therapy. In Abeloff M [ed]: Clinical Oncology, 2nd ed. London, Churchill Livingstone, 2000, pp 423–470.)

modality. This definitive radiation therapy can often be used in place of a surgical procedure, hence resulting in organ preservation. Radiation can also be used adjuvantly or neoadjuvantly to increase the likelihood of local and regional control with surgical excision of a tumor, or to decrease the extent of the required surgical procedure, thus preserving a more functional outcome. Finally, radiation is the most common method employed to provide palliation of many symptoms related to tumor spread or growth. Obviously, a thorough discussion of radiation's use is beyond the scope of this chapter and will be given in the disease-specific chapters that follow, but an overview is provided here.

Definitive radiation therapy has been used for years to achieve cure in many types of cancers. Often, radiation is paired with concurrent chemotherapy. Using chemo-sensitization, radiation can have a synergistic effect on tumor cells, thus increasing the therapeutic index. This has had demonstrated benefits in head and neck cancer, small cell lung cancer, non–small cell lung cancer, cervical cancer, bladder cancer, anal cancer, pancreatic cancer, and esophageal cancer.[140-149,217-220]

Definitive radiation therapy has also been employed with conservative rather than radical surgery to result in organ preservation. This strategy has been demonstrated most prominently in the treatment of breast cancer. Whereas mastectomy was once the only potentially curative procedure, lumpectomy and adjuvant radiation therapy has been demonstrated to be equally effica-cious.[221] This same concept of local excision with adjuvant radiation has also been employed for extremity-sparing procedures in the treatment of soft-tissue sarcoma.[222] Radiation therapy has also been used in rectal cancer in selected patients to change the surgical procedure required from a colostomy-requiring operation to one that maintains normal sphincter function.[223,224] The use of radiation with surgery has converted many previously incurable patients with stage III and IV head and neck cancers into patients who can be treated with curative intent. Chemoradiation has also been used without any surgical procedure to preserve the larynx in patients with supraglottic and glottic cancers.[225,226]

Radiation therapy has also been used either before or after surgery to increase the rate of local control. Surgery has been used to increase cure in these instances by decreasing the tumor bulk that needs to be sterilized. The fewer logs of cells that need to be killed by radiation, the more efficacious radiation will be (Table 26-7). Radiation's effect after surgery is presumably exerted by eliminating the presence of microscopic disease in high-risk areas, such as in adjacent soft tissues or draining lymphatic regions. This concept applies in breast cancer, lung cancer, head and neck cancer, rectal cancer, pan-creatic cancer, esophageal cancer, sarcomas, endometrial cancer, central nervous system tumors, and prostate cancer.

Approximately 50% of all treatments in a typical radiation oncology clinic will be given with curative intent; the remainder will be palliative. Radiation is the main treatment modality for the relief of symptoms in

TABLE 26-7

Interrelationship of Biological Dose, Tumor Size, and Control by Irradiation

TOTAL DOSE (GY)*	HISTOLOGY	SIZE	CONTROL (%)
50	Squamous Adenocarcinoma	Subclinical ($<10^6$ cells)	95+
60	Squamous	<2 cm	85
		>4 cm	50
65	Squamous	2–4 cm	70
70	Squamous	2–4 cm	90
	Adenocarcinoma	>4 cm	60
75+	Squamous	>4 cm	90

*Approximation based on a minimum tumor dose of 2 Gy per fraction and five fractions per week.
From Cox JD, Ang KK (eds): Radiation Oncology Rationale, Technique, Results, 8th ed. St. Louis, MO, Mosby, 2003, p33.

patients with progressive and incurable cancers. It is often employed for hemostasis, relief of obstruction (airway, esophageal, etc.), and most important, for pain relief. Despite the remarkable advances in cancer treatment in the last decades, it remains true that up to 50% of patients diagnosed with cancer eventually will succumb to their disease. Some of the most gratifying experiences in radiation oncology come from the ability to relieve symptoms in patients with progressive cancer with a short course of radiation therapy and to diminish their reliance on narcotics for analgesia, thereby improving their quality of life. Radiation oncology in this manner epitomizes Osler's dictum, "To cure sometimes, to relieve often, to comfort always—this is our work."

NEW MODALITIES IN RADIATION

Advances are constantly being investigated with the aim of increasing the therapeutic ratio in radiation therapy. Many of the largest advances have been in the technology used to deliver radiation. The concept is that if a higher dose of radiation can be delivered to the tumor volume with respect to the surrounding normal tissues, radiation can be delivered with less toxicity or greater dose can be delivered to the target volume with the same toxicity. These goals constitute the basis for these investigations.

Intensity-Modulated Radiotherapy

Radiation oncology has striven to deliver the dose to the tumor ever more precisely and to diminish the dose to adjacent normal structures. The linear accelerator offered the ability to deliver shaped uniform beams from multiple angles as it rotated about the patient and represented a major step forward toward reaching this goal. The introduction of the multileaf collimator, whereby the machine itself (rather than an added beam-shaping device) shapes the beams, increased the efficiency of this process. Now, radiation oncologists and physicists are attempting to push this technology one step further. Because the leaves in a multileaf collimator are computer driven, it becomes possible to move the leaves continuously during treatment. Treatment thus becomes four-dimensional (in both time and space) rather than three-dimensional and allows for the selection of beams that are deliberately nonuniform, to deliver varying doses to varying parts of the treatment field. The CT simulator allows the patient to be simulated for treatment in virtual time rather than in real time, allowing the physician or a computer program under the physician's control to evaluate dozens (if not hundreds) of treatment plans to optimize the dose to the tumor. The beams chosen need no longer be coplanar in such a system. This technology forms the basis for what has become known as intensity-modulated radiation therapy. Intensity-modulated radiotherapy (IMRT) is based on the use of several noncoplanar radiation beam intensities incident on the patient to achieve a shaped, irregular dose distribution.[227,228] It represents the state-of-the-art in technological advancements in the field of radiation oncology in manipulation of dose distributions and represents an advance on 3-D conformal radiation treatments.

Radiation therapy treatment planning has been in the process of making dramatic changes since the advent of the computer age. Advances in computer hardware and programming have led to the development of three-dimensional radiation treatment planning and delivery systems.[229-231] The goal of 3-D conformal radiation therapy is to shape the area of high dose to the tumor volume while minimizing the dose to the surrounding tissues. The delivery of high dose to the tumor volume is accomplished using a set of fixed radiation beams, with normal tissue surrounding the tumor volume shielded from receiving the full dose of radiation. This shielding has classically been done with blocks made from cerrobend (a lead alloy), which stop the transmission of photons to those areas desired to be shielded. A newer method of shielding is with the use of the multileaf collimator (MLC), which is needed in IMRT.

The concept of conformal radiation is not new. The first report of conformal therapy was published in 1959.[232] Computerized treatment planning was also first reported in the 1950s.[233] The first real step in making the computer and the conformal planning clinically useful was the development of the beam's-eye view display.[234,235] The beam's-eye view display provides a view from the source of the radiation beam, resulting in a view similar to that achieved in a fluoroscopic simulator. This development, coupled with the CT scanner, led to the prospect of anatomy definition that had not been possible in radiation treatment planning and resulted in significant improvement in defining tumor volumes and critical structures.[236,237] In the late 1980s, 3-D radiation treatment planning systems began to be used clinically.[238-241] The additional advancements in 3-D treatment planning systems have led to its widespread use in many clinics.

Radiation delivery based on modulation of the beam has also been investigated for decades. The culmination

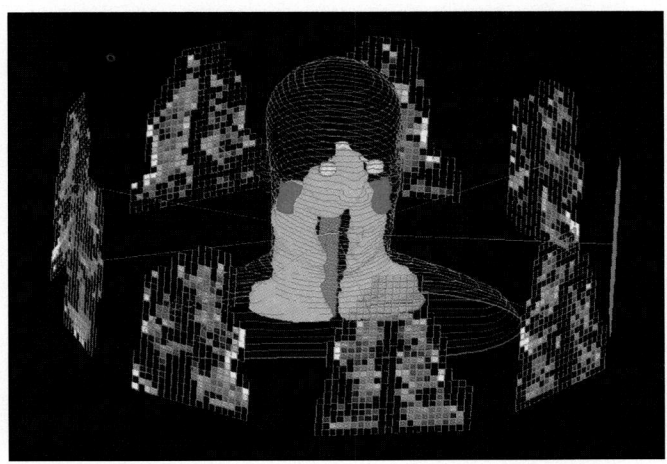

Figure 26-28. Advanced form of 3-D CRT–IMRT, which is based on the use of optimized nonuniform radiation beam intensities incident on the patient. Shown are a 3-D view of the patient, the PTV, spinal cord, parotid glands, and the nine intensity-modulated beams (with gray levels reflecting the intensity value) used to generate the IMRT dose distribution.

of these efforts has resulted in computer-controlled planning and delivery systems that have the ability to shape radiation doses like never before (Fig. 26-28). There are several IMRT delivery techniques, such as using photon and electron beams, including serial tomotherapy, and using a conventional multileaf collimator.[242-244] In tomotherapy, radiation is delivered in narrow slit beams, analogous to the techniques used for CT imaging systems.[244] Treatment is delivered to a narrow slice of the patient in an arc-type rotation. As the machine rotates around the patient, delivering radiation in an arcing manner, "beamlets" of varying intensity of radiation delivered are created by dynamic movement of the machine's multileaf collimator. In areas to which more dose is to be delivered, the leaves of the multileaf collimator are out of the field longer compared with those areas that require less deposition of dose. The end result of these interactions in serial adjoining axial slices is the conformal treatment that is desired. IMRT can also be done using static field techniques, where the beam moves to various fixed positions around the patient, but the multileaf collimator is used to vary the intensity of different parts of the beam during treatment of each field.

Obviously, these complex delivery systems must be coupled with elaborate treatment planning computers that are capable of complicated dose calculations. IMRT requires a method of designing and optimizing nonuniform beam intensity profiles for dose calculations. With these highly evolved treatments, the optimization of these plans would not be possible without the computer. An important concept that is used in IMRT is that of inverse planning, in contrast to the forward planning that is used in conventional 3-D conformal treatment planning. In forward treatment planning, the beam orientation, shape, size, modifiers, and so on, are defined first, followed by the calculation of dose that results from this design.

Changes to achieve better dose distribution are made by modifying the beam weighting, adding or subtracting beams, and so forth, until the desired dose distribution is achieved. In inverse treatment planning, the desired dose distribution is stated first, followed by computer optimization to adjust beam intensities to attempt to achieve that dose distribution. Optimization includes stating the dose that the tumor bed or areas at risk should receive, as well as limits of dose that normal tissues are able to receive. These parameters are based on maximizing the probability of tumor control and minimizing the toxicity profiles of the various normal tissues and organs. Because normal tissues have different tolerances, different organs will have different thresholds. After the computer optimizes the dose distribution, the physician may choose what is deemed to be an optimal plan.

With the technologically superior treatment planning and delivery system, IMRT can be used to deliver doses to irregularly shaped areas in a precise manner that was not possible previously (Fig. 26-29). This streategy is the latest method of increasing the therapeutic ratio of radiation treatment. To this point, there have been no reports of prospective randomized clinical studies using IMRT, a fac that obviously limits our knowledge of IMRT's effect on clinical outcome. Many clinical studies have verified the superior dose distributions, however, and have reported on small numbers of patients.

Many authors have completed treatment planning comparisons between IMRT plans and conventional treatment plans. These have been followed by publications that have emphasized clinical endpoints in patients treated with IMRT. The entire goal of IMRT is to increase

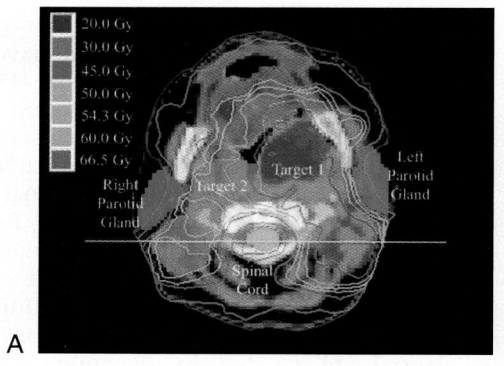

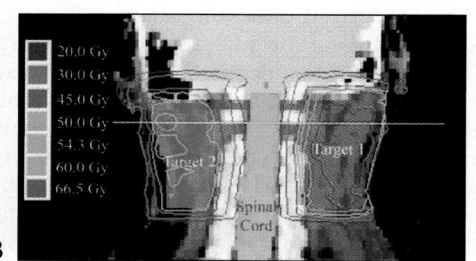

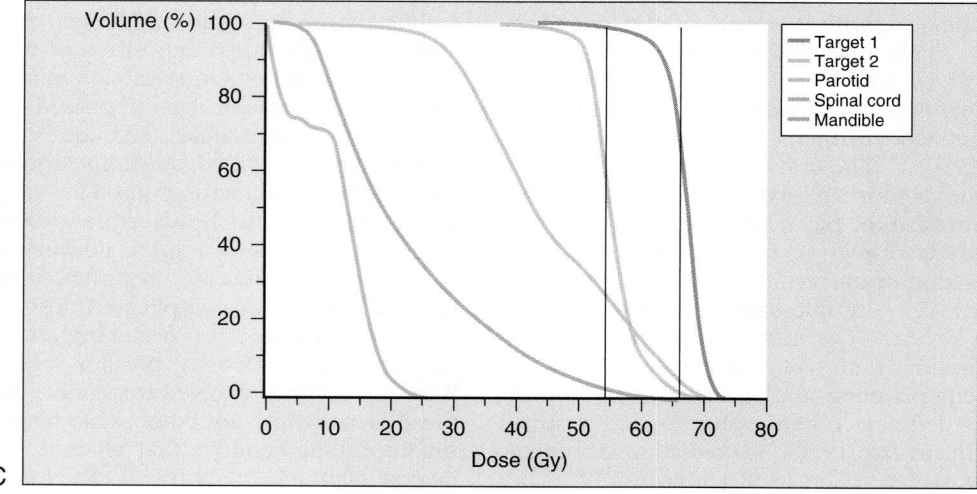

Figure 26-29. Typical head-and-neck IMRT treatment plan showing conformal avoidance of the spinal cord and parotid glands, while simultaneously delivering multiple-dose prescriptions (66.5 Gy and 54.3 Gy) to the two target volumes. **A,** Transverse cross-section. White line corresponds to the position of the coronal cross-section. **B,** Coronal cross-section. White line corresponds to the position of the transverse cross-section. **C,** DVHs of the target volumes and selected critical structures. Vertical bars indicate the prescription doses and highlight the increased dose heterogenity often encountered as a consequence of conformal avoidance.

the therapeutic ratio–delivering a higher tumor dose relative to normal tissues. Keeping this in mind, IMRT can be used to escalate the tumor volume to a higher dose while maintaining normal tissue toxicity at the same level. Among the sites and cancers investigated using IMRT to escalate total dose are non small cell lung cancer, intracranial tumors, and prostate cancer.[245-247] Alternatively, IMRT can be used to deliver conventional doses to the tumor bed, resulting in lower dose to normal tissues, with hopes of reducing toxicity. This strategy has been reported on in patients with breast cancer, head and neck cancer, mesothelioma, pancreatic cancer, and gynecologic cancers.[248-252] Many of these studies report favorable outcomes or dose distributions that conceivably would result in decreased toxicity, though no definitive study has conclusively demonstrated the clinical impact of IMRT. The dose distributions made possible by IMRT's planning and treatment delivery, however, show a significant potential for improvement in clinical outcomes.

IMRT is very much an evolving technique at this time and carries with it a number of potentially difficult problems that still need to be addressed. With IMRT, it is much more difficult than with 3-D conformal therapy to verify that treatment has been delivered correctly to the patient. If there is organ motion—and virtually every organ below the calvarium is in motion—then there is a possibility that the dose delivered differs significantly from the dose planned, as planning was done on static images. Finally, as more beams are added to the treatment and the daily treatment time increases, then although less normal tissue will be treated to tolerance doses, the volume of normal tissue that receives some dose of radiation in fact increases, as does the total-body dose of radiation. It remains to be seen how significant these problems will be to the development of this new technology.[253]

Particle Radiation Therapy

Particle beam therapy utilizes subatomic particles instead of x-rays or gamma rays to deliver the dose of radiation. The development and application of particle radiotherapy has been motivated by two main factors. One is the physical property that allows for precise dose localization and superior depth dose distribution with heavy charged particles such as protons. The other is the potential radiobiologic advantage of high linear energy transfer particles. High linear energy transfer radiation deposits more dose along its path than do conventional x-rays, which are low linear energy transfer radiation. This offers advantages for several potential reasons. First, high linear energy transfer radiation is more damaging to hypoxic cells. Second, there is less repair of damage induced by high linear energy transfer radiation. Also, damage from high linear energy transfer radiation is less cell cycle dependent.[118] These advantages have made neutron therapy, with its high linear energy transfer but depth dose characteristics resembling conventional x-rays, a potentially advantageous modality.

Neutron Therapy

Neutron radiotherapy was first begun in the late 1930s, to attempt to increase killing of hypoxic cells.[254] Because there was little understanding of the high linear energy transfer and resultant high relative biologic effectiveness (RBE) of neutrons, there were severe radiation sequelae with treatment.[255] It was not until the 1960s that clinical trials in neutron therapy were resumed, with adjustments in dose compensating for the high linear energy transfer and relative biologic effectiveness of neutrons.[256] Early trials failed to confirm the efficacy of neutron therapy, but because of the potential advantages of high linear energy transfer radiation, neutron therapy has been used widely in the attempt to control various tumors (Fig. 26-30). Approximately 30,000 patients have received neutron therapy worldwide, with mixed results.[257]

The most quoted site that was said to show an advantage for neutrons over conventional photons was in unresectable salivary gland carcinomas. Early single-institution studies indicated a therapeutic advantage of neutron therapy over photon therapy.[258] This prompted a phase III RTOG/MRC trial that showed a significant local control advantage of neutrons over photons (56% vs. 17%), but with no overall survival advantage due to distant metastases.[259] This advantage has also been shown more recently in major salivary gland tumors and also in minor salivary gland tumors.[260,261]

Neutron therapy has also been investigated in soft tissue sarcomas, osteogenic sarcomas, and chondrogenic sarcomas. These tumors are thought to be radioresistant to conventional x-rays and responsive to neutron therapy.[258] Phase II data and single-institutional data show the possibility of an advantage in unresectable sarcomas, though this has never been tested in a randomized clinical trial.[262,263]

Results of neutron therapy in head and neck cancer and in non-small cell lung cancer have not been as encouraging. Phase III data from head and neck neutron therapy trials indicate higher toxicity with no definite advantage in terms of local control, regional control, or survival with neutrons.[264-266] Similarly, studies done with neutrons in patients with non-small cell lung cancer are inconclusive with their results, showing no definite advantage with neutrons over conventional photons.[267-270]

There have been two randomized clinical trials comparing neutron therapy to photon therapy in patients with prostate cancer.[259,271] These studies show an advantage of neutrons in terms of locoregional control, with one study showing an overall survival advantage. Neither study showed an advantage in terms of disease-specific survival. Advocates of neutron therapy claimed that this represented a more efficacious treatment, while critics have challenged the results based on small sample size, contrasting outcomes when comparing with historical data, and high cost and limited availability of neutrons. This continues to represent an area of controversy.

Presently, there are no active clinical studies involving neutron therapy. It is used selectively in those tumors (e.g., salivary gland tumors, selected sarcomas) in which

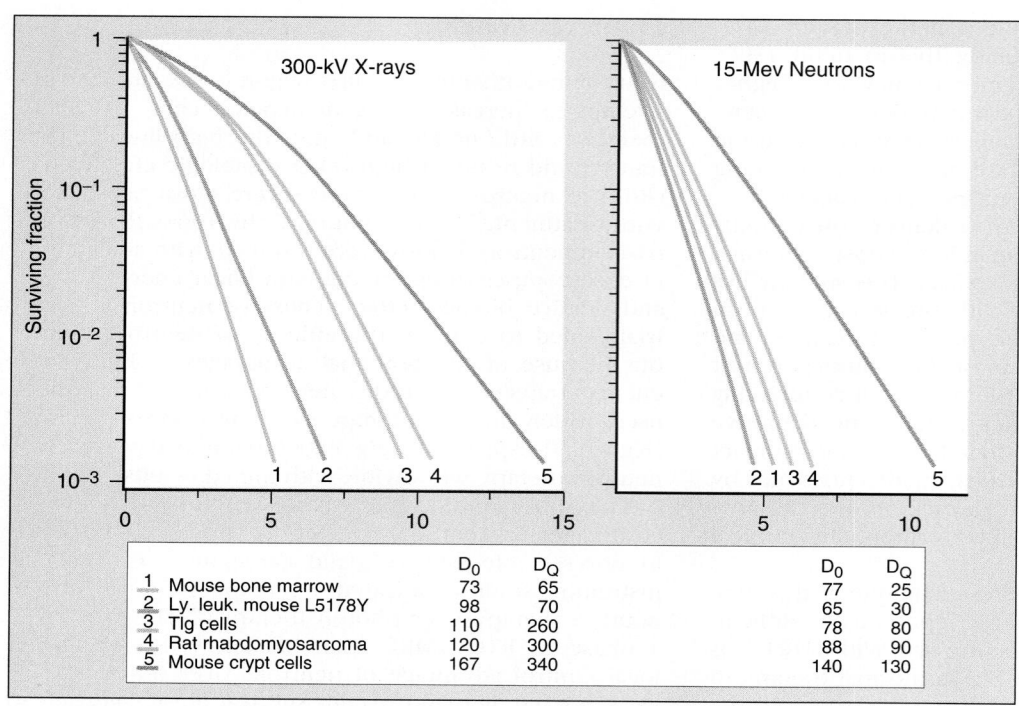

Figure 26-30. Survival curves for various types of clonogenic mammalian cells irradiated with 300-kV x-rays or 15-MeV d⁺ → T neutrons. *Curve 1,* Mouse hematopoietic stem cells. *Curve 2,* Mouse lymphocytic leukemia (Ly. leuk.) L5178Y cells. *Curve 3,* Tlg cultured cells of human kidney origin. *Curve 4,* Rat rhabdomyosarcoma cells. *Curve 5,* Mouse intestinal crypt stem cells. The variation in radiosensitivity between different cell lines is markedly less for neutrons than for x-rays. (From Cox JD, Ang KK [eds]: Radiation Oncology Rationale, Technique, Results, 8th ed. St. Louis, MO, Mosby, 2003, p 46.)

		D_0	D_Q	D_0	D_Q
1	Mouse bone marrow	73	65	77	25
2	Ly. leuk. mouse L5178Y	98	70	65	30
3	Tlg cells	110	260	78	80
4	Rat rhabdomyosarcoma	120	300	88	90
5	Mouse crypt cells	167	340	140	130

there is evidence for its effectiveness. Given reports of increased late toxicity and dose distributions that are far less optimal than charged particles such as protons, interest in neutron therapy is waning.[272]

Proton Therapy

Though protons have a slightly higher linear energy transfer than x-rays, they are not generally considered as high linear energy transfer particles. They achieve most of their advantage over x-rays in their physical dose distribution. When a heavy, charged particle, such as a proton, passes through tissue, the dose it deposits increases slowly with depth, then reaches a sharp increase at its maximum depth of penetration. This is called the Bragg peak (Fig. 26-31). The maximum depth of penetration can be adjusted by varying the energy of the proton beam or by adding or removing compensating material placed in the path of the beam. Frequently, in clinical use the Bragg peak is spread out in depth using specialized filters to achieve the dose deposition pattern desired, but still with the sharp dose fall-off at the deep edge of the beam. Using multiple beams or varying compensators, it is possible to design a 3-D dose deposition that is precisely confined to the tumor volume with minimal dose to the surrounding normal tissue.

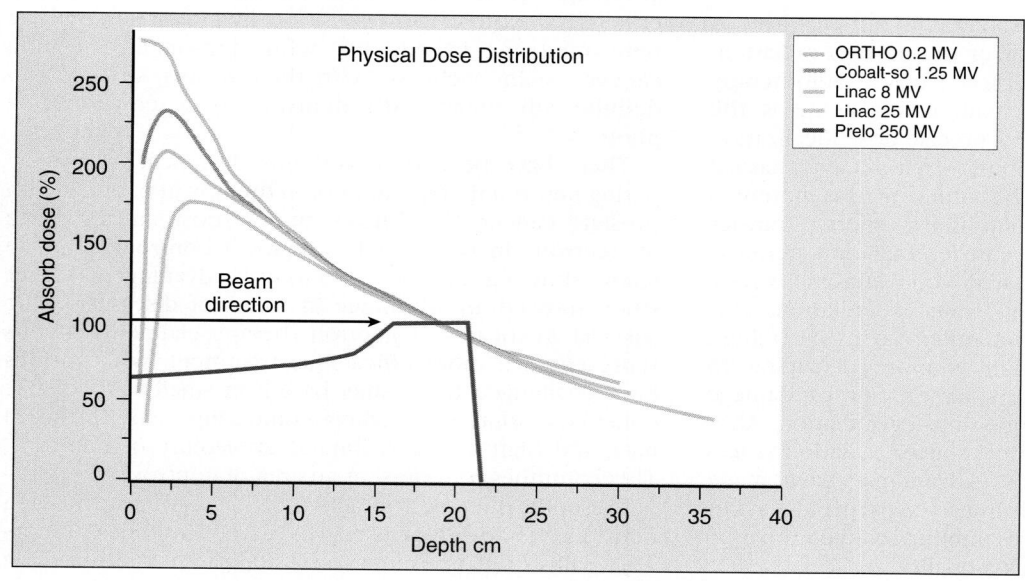

Figure 26-31. Depth-dose distributions for a proton beam compared with other photon beams. The dose for the proton beam is limited for the entrance tissues, reaches a peak at the desired depth, then displays an extremely sharp falloff.

The majority of patients treated with proton therapy have been patients whose tumors are in close proximity to critical structures. The precise dose deposition patterns made it possible to treat these tumors without crossing the threshold of toxicity of the normal structures (Fig. 26-32).

Patients with tumors of the skull base represent one site that fits into this category. The base of the skull is surrounded by critical structures—brain stem, optic chiasm, and cervical spinal cord, just to name a few. The two primary malignant tumors of the skull base are chordomas and chondrosarcomas. Both require fairly high doses of radiation if cure is to be achieved and often cannot be treated adequately with conventional radiation due to the low tolerance of normal structures. Using a combination of photons and protons, a local control rate approaching 70% has been reported.[273] Median tumor dose was 70 Gy-equivalent (physical dose × 1.1-the relative biologic effectiveness for protons), with low toxicities reported. Similar results have been published regarding local control of tumors of the cervical spine, a site obviously providing for difficulty in treatment without proton beam therapy, with a local control rate of 65%.[274]

Uveal melanoma is another malignancy that had been difficult to treat prior to the advent of proton beam therapy, secondary to toxicity to normal structures of the eye. Surgical enucleation was considered to be the treatment of choice. Proton therapy has become an alternative treatment for uveal melanomas. Massachusetts General Hospital has reported a 10- and 15-year actuarial local control rate of 95%, using 70 Gy-equivalent. Enucleation was avoided in the vast majority of patients, with only 2%–10% (depending on size of the primary tumor) requiring subsequent enucleation.[275,276] This high rate of control has also been reported by the group at the Paul Sherrer Institute in Switzerland, with a 10-year local control rate of 95%.[277] Again, subsequent enucleation rate was low (8%), with a 15-year overall eye retention rate of 84%.[278] With these outcome data, all patients could be considered for what is basically organ-sparing treatment in the form of proton beam therapy.

Tumors of the paranasal sinuses have also been treated using proton beam therapy, with the precision of proton beams allowing dose escalation up to 76 Gy-equivalent. Using a combination of photons and protons after partial resection or biopsy, local control rates for T3–T4 tumors have been reported up to 85%, again with low toxicity.[276,279]

More common tumors have also been treated with proton beam radiotherapy, with the high precision allowing for dose escalation in diseases that are difficult to control with conventional doses. Glioblastoma multiforme represents the epitome of these types of tumors, with progression after treatment and uniform fatality (usually from local recurrence) almost without exception. A phase II study of 23 patients was undertaken at the Massachusetts General Hospital, with dose escalation up to 90 Gy-equivalent using proton beams. Median survival was 20 months, with a three-year actuarial survival of 18%. Recurrence was seen in only one patient treated at the 90 Gy-equivalent dose level, but with radiation necrosis in seven of the 23 patients treated.[280]

Meningiomas are another type of CNS tumor that has been treated with protons. In a study of 46 patients with partially resected, biopsied, or recurrent meningiomas, a combination of photons and protons was used to deliver a median dose of 59 Gy-equivalent to the macroscopic tumor volume. Recurrence-free rate at five and 10 years was 100% and 88%, respectively. Eight patients, however, developed severe ophthalmologic, neurologic, or otologic long-term toxicity from radiotherapy.[281]

Prostate cancer is the only tumor in which dose escalation with protons has been tested against conventional radiation in a randomized trial.[282] Patients with T3–T4 prostate cancer who received 50.4 Gy via photons to a pelvic field were randomized to receive either an additional 16.8 Gy via photons or 25.2 Gy via protons. There was no overall difference in overall survival, disease-specific survival, or local control between the two groups. Additionally, there was an increase in toxicity in the proton arm, owing to the higher dose to the rectum.[283] This study was done in the 1970s, however, prior to the recognition of the importance of volume considerations to the toxicity of the rectum. Therefore, the rectum was not preferentially spared from radiation. Newer studies have demonstrated that in sparing the rectum during prostate irradiation, protons can be much more efficacious.[284] Protons are currently being tested in a randomized prospective fashion against 3-D conformal radiation in early prostate cancer patients, making use of more modern proton delivery techniques and providing better sparing of the rectum.

Proton therapy is also being studied actively in tumors with previous poor cure and control rates, such as hepatocellular carcinoma, non-small cell lung cancer, and stereotactic radiosurgery.[285-287]

Proton therapy is one of the most promising modalities that have resulted from technological advances in the field of radiation oncology. It represents the optimal therapeutic ratio available in terms of dose delivery. Therefore, although neutron therapy is falling out of favor in the radiation community, research into proton therapy dose planning and delivery continues to grow.

CONCLUSION

Radiation therapy has progressed a long way since the discovery of x-rays just over 100 years ago. The understanding of physical and biological principles behind radiation has led to great advancements in the field of radiation therapy. With the advent of computers and the possibility of 3-D treatment planning, the field has been advanced further, as the therapeutic index could be increased by dose escalation and more accurate shielding of normal tissues. Now, even greater advancements are underway with IMRT and the use of particle therapies such as protons. Clinical studies investigating these modalities and the development of radiosensitizers, and especially molecular biology-based targeted therapies, seem very likely to increase the efficacy of radiation in the years to come.

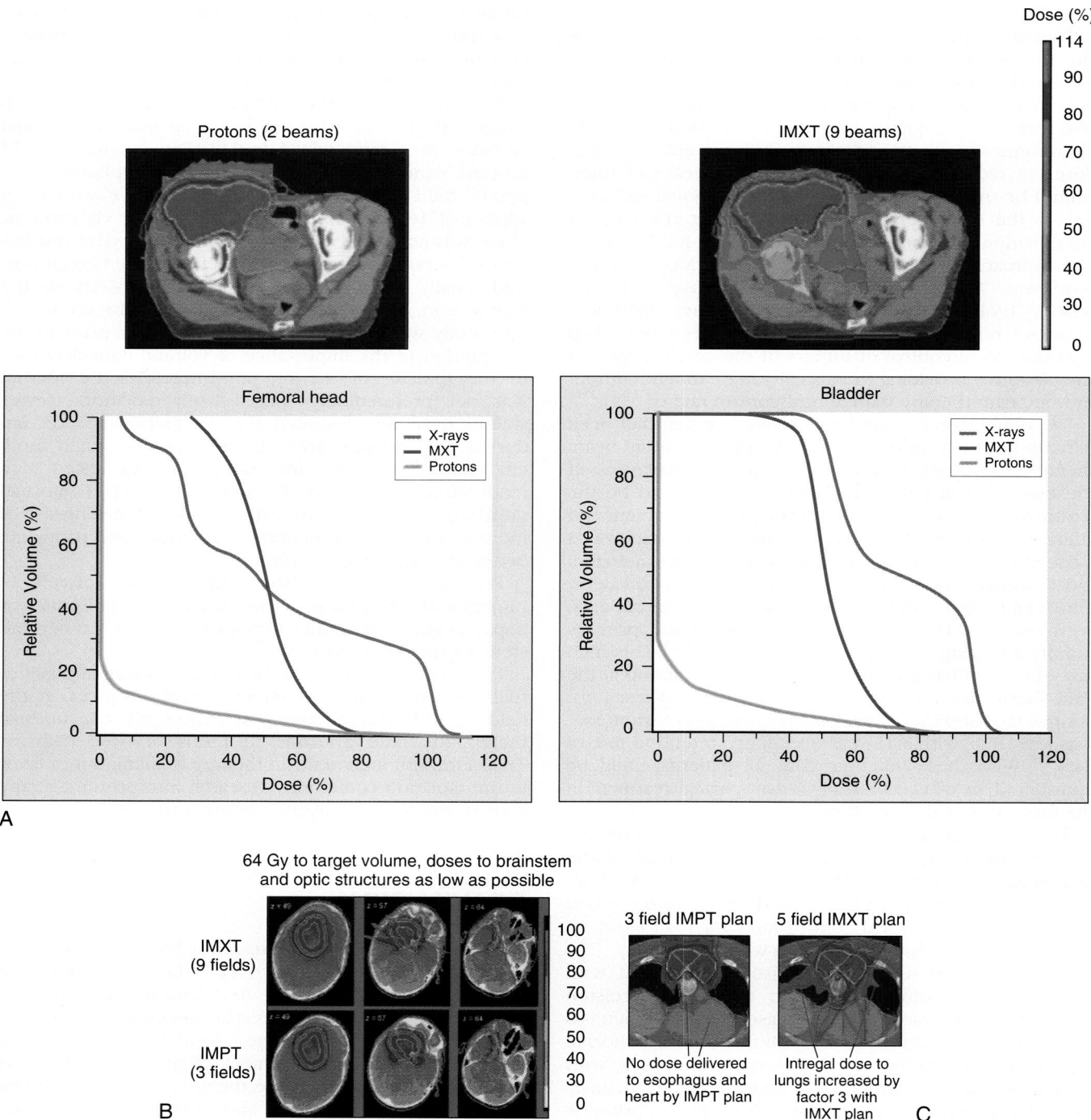

Figure 26-32. A, Proton beam arrangement compared with a complex IMRT plan of nine beams for treatment of a malignant melanoma. Note the full coverage of the target volume with sparing of normal tissues. **B,** Proton beam arrangement compared with an IMRT plan for treatment of a pediatric meningioma. **C,** Treatment of a thoracic paraspinal chordoma requiring contouring of the dose distribution around the spinal cord, while continuing to provide full coverage to the target volume-more easily attained with proton beams than with a complex IMRT plan. (Used with permission from Anthony Lomax, PhD, Paul Scherrer Institute, Switzerland.)

REFERENCES

1. Glasser O: Roentgen, 2nd ed. Springfield, Ill, Charles C. Thomas, 1958.
2. Rossi HH, Kellerer AM: Roentgen. Radiat Res 1995;144:124-128.
3. Brecher R, Brecher E: The Rays: A History of Radiology in the United States and Canada. Baltimore, Williams & Wilkins, 1969.
4. Roentgen, W: On a new kind of ray (translation). Br J Radiol 19331;4:32.
5. Myers WG: Becquerel's discovery of radioactivity in 1896. J Nucl Med 1976;17:579-582.
6. Curie P, Curie M, Bemont G: Sur une nouvelle substance fortement radioactive contenue dans la pechblende (note presented by M Becquerel). Compt Rend Acad Sci (Paris), 1898;127:1215.
7. del Regato J: The American Radium Society: Its diamond jubilee. Am J Clin Oncol 1991;14:93-100.
8. Giroud F: Marie Curie: A Life. New York, Holmes and Meier, 1986.
9. Brenner DJ: Radiation biology in brachytherapy. J Surg Oncol 1997;65:66-70.
10. Perez CA, Brady L (eds): Principles and Practice of Radiation Oncology, 3rd ed. Philadelphia, Lippincott Williams & Wilkins, 1997.
11. del Regato JA: Fractionation: a panoramic view. Int J Radiat Oncol Biol Phys 1990;19:1329-1331.
12. del Regato JA: Brachytherapy. Front Radiat Ther Oncol 1978;12:5.
13. Simpson F: Radium in the treatment of cancer and various other disease of the skin. JAMA 1916;67:1508.
14. Kelly H: Radium in the treatment of carcinoma of the cervix uteri and vagina. JAMA 1915;65:1874.
15. Coutard H: Roentgentherapy of epitheliomas of the tonsillar region, hypopharynx and larynx from 1920 to 1926. Am J Roentgenol 1932;28:313.
16. Coutard H: Principles of x-ray therapy of malignant diseases. Lancet 1934;2:1.
17. Houlthusen H: The present status of dosage measurements. Radiology 1928;10:292.
18. Johns HE, Cunningham J: The Physics of Radiology, 4th ed. Springfield, Ill, Charles C Thomas, 1983.
19. Johns HE: The physicist in cancer treatment and detection. Int J Radiat Oncol Biol Phys 1981;7:801-808.
20. Radford IR: Evidence for a general relationship between the induced level of DNA double-strand breakage and cell-killing after X-irradiation of mammalian cells. Int J Radiat Biol Relat Stud Phys Chem Med 1986;49:611-620.
21. Nunez MI, McMillan, TJ, Valenzuela MT, Ruiz de Almodovar JM, Pedraza V: Relationship between DNA damage, rejoining and cell killing by radiation in mammalian cells. Radiother Oncol 1996;39:155-165.
22. Lunec J: Introductory review: involvement of ADP-ribosylation in cellular recovery from some forms of DNA damage. Br J Cancer 1984;6(Suppl):13-18.
23. Dikomey E, Dahm-Daphi J, Brammer I, Martensen, R, Kaina B: Correlation between cellular radiosensitivity and non-repaired double-strand breaks studied in nine mammalian cell lines. Int J Radiat Biol 1998;73:269-278.
24. Kemp LM, Sedgwick SG, Jeggo P: A X-ray sensitive mutants of Chinese hamster ovary cells defective in double-strand break rejoining. Mutat Res 1984;132:189-196.
25. Munro TR: The relative radiosensitivity of the nucleus and cytoplasm of Chinese hamster fibroblasts. Radiat Res 1970;42:451-470.
26. Munro TR: The relative radiosensitivity of the nucleus and cytoplasm of Chinese hamster fibroblasts. Exp Cell Res 1960;20:613.
27. Walters R, Hofer K, Harris C: Radionuclide toxicity in cultured mammalian cells: Elucidation of the primary site of radiation damage. Ann Top Radiat Res Q 1977;12:389.
28. Brenner DJ, Ward JF: Constraints on energy deposition and target size of multiply damaged sites associated with DNA double-strand breaks. Int J Radiat Biol 1992;61:737-748.
29. Jonah CD: A short history of the radiation chemistry of water. Radiat Res 1995;144:141-147.
30. Powell S, McMillan TJ: DNA damage and repair following treatment with ionizing radiation. Radiother Oncol 1990;19:95-108.
31. Ward JF: Biochemistry of DNA lesions. Radiat Res 1985;8(Suppl):103-111.
32. Goodhead D: Physics of radiation action: Microscopic features that determine biological consequences. In Hagen U, Jung P, Streffer C (eds). 10th International Congress of Radiation Research, vol 2, Congress Lectures, Wurzburg, Germany, 1995, p 43.
33. Rogakou EP, Pilch DR, Orr AH, Ivanova VS, Bonner WM: DNA double-stranded breaks induce histone H2AX phosphorylation on serine 139. J Biol Chem 1998;273:5858-5868.
34. Burma S, Chen, BP, Murphy M, Kurimasa A, Chen, DJ: ATM phosphorylates histone H2AX in response to DNA double-strand breaks. J Biol Chem 2001;276:42462-42467.
35. Wang B, Matsuoka S, Carpenter PB, Elledge SJ: 53BP1, a mediator of the DNA damage checkpoint. Science 2002;298:1435-1438.
36. DiTullio RA Jr, Mochan TA, Venere M, et al: 53BP1 functions in an ATM-dependent checkpoint pathway that is constitutively activated in human cancer. Nat Cell Biol 2002;4:998-1002.
37. Kao GD, McKenna WG, Guenther MG, Muschel, RJ, Lazar MA, Yen, TJ: Histone deacetylase 4 interacts with 53BP1 to mediate the DNA damage response. J Cell Biol 2003;160:1017-1027.
38. Ward IM, Minn K, van Deursen J, Chen J: p53 Binding protein 53BP1 is required for DNA damage responses and tumor suppression in mice. Mol Cell Biol 2003;23:2556-2563.
39. Rothkamm K, Kruger I, Thompson LH, Lobrich M: Pathways of DNA double-strand break repair during the mammalian cell cycle. Mol Cell Biol 2003;23:5706-5715.
40. Pastink A, Eeken JC, Lohman PH: Genomic integrity and the repair of double-strand DNA breaks. Mutat Res 2001;480-481:37-50.
41. Kerr JFK, Wyllie AH, Currie AH: Apoptosis, a basic biological phenomenon with wider implications in tissue kinetics. Br J Cancer 1972;26:239-245.
42. Wyllie AH, Kerr JFR, Currie AR: Cell death: The significance of apoptosis. Intl Rev Cytol 1990;68:251-303.
43. Brown JM, Wouters BG: Apoptosis, p53, and tumor cell sensitivity to anticancer agents. Cancer Res 1999;59:1391-1399.
44. Howard A, Pelc SR: Synthesis of deoxyribonucleic acid in normal and irradiated cells and its relation to chromosome breakage. Heredity 1953;6(suppl.):261-273.
45. Kastan MB, Onyekwere O, Sidransky D, Vogelstein B, Craig RW: Participation of p53 protein in the cellular response to DNA damage. Can Res 1991;51:6304-6311.
46. Kastan MB, Zhan Q, El-Deiry WS, et al: A mammalian cell cycle checkpoint pathway utilizing p53 and GADD45 is defective in ataxia-telangiectasia. Cell 1992;71:587-597.
47. Kuerbitz SJ, Plunkett BS, Walsh WV, Kastan, MB: Wild-type p53 is a cell cycle checkpoint determinant following irradiation. Proc Natl Acad Sci USA 1992;89:7491-7495.
48. El-Deiry WS, Tokino T, Velculescu VE, et al: WAF1, a potential mediator of p53 tumor suppression. Cell 199375:817-825.
49. McDonald ER III, El-Deiry WS: Checkpoint genes in cancer. Ann Med 2001;33:113-122.
50. Hill RP, Rodemann HP, Hendry JH, Roberts SA, Anscher MS: Normal tissue radiobiology: From the laboratory to the clinic. Int J Radiat Oncol Biol Phys 2001;49:353-365.
51. Fletcher L, Cheng Y, Muschel, RJ: Abolishment of the Tyr-15 inhibitory phosphorylation site on cdc2 reduces the radiation-induced G(2) delay, revealing a potential checkpoint in early mitosis. Cancer Res 2002;62:241-250.
52. Adams GE, Hasan NM, Joiner MC: The Klaas Breur Lecture. Radiation, hypoxia and genetic stimulation: Implications for future therapies. Radiother Oncol 1997;44:101-109.
53. Brown JM, Giaccia AJ: Tumour hypoxia: The picture has changed in the 1990s. Int J Radiat Biol 1994;65:95-102.
54. Molls M, Stadler P, Becker A, Feldmann, HJ, Dunst J: Relevance of oxygen in radiation oncology. Mechanisms of action, correlation to low hemoglobin levels. Strahlenther Onkol 1998;174:13-16.
55. Harari PM, Huang SM: Radiation response modification following molecular inhibition of epidermal growth factor receptor signaling. Semin Radiat Oncol 2001;11:281-289.
56. McKenna WG, Weiss MC, Endlich B, Ling CC, Bakanauskas VJ, Kelsten ML, Muschel RJ: Synergistic effect of the v-myc oncogene with H-ras on radioresistance. Cancer Res 1990;50:97-102.

57. Kasid U, Pfeifer A, Weichselbaum RR, Dritschilo A, Mark GE: The raf oncogene is associated with a radiation-resistant human laryngeal cancer. Science 1987;237:1039-1041.

58. Kasid UN, Weichselbaum RR, Brennan T, Mark GE, Dritschilo A: Sensitivities of NIH/3T3-derived clonal cell lines to ionizing radiation: Significance for gene transfer studies. Cancer Res 1989;49:3396-3400.

59. Kasid U, Pfeifer A, Brennan T, et al: Effect of antisense c-raf-1 on tumorigenicity and radiation sensitivity of a human squamous carcinoma. Science 1989;243:1354-1356.

60. Kasid U, Weichselbaum R, Brennan T, Mark G, Dritschilo A: Sensitivities of NIH/3T3-derived clonal cell lines to ionizing radiation: Significance for gene transfer studies. Cancer Res 1989;49:3396-3400.

61. Kasid U, Pirollo K, Dritschilo A, Chang E: Oncogenic basis of radiation resistance. Adv Cancer Res 1993;61:195-233.

62. Garcia-Barros M, Paris F, Cordon-Cardo C, et al: Tumor response to radiotherapy regulated by endothelial cell apoptosis. Science 2003;300:1155-1159.

63. Chu K, Leonhardt EA, Trinh M, et al: Computerized video time-lapse (CVTL) analysis of cell death kinetics in human bladder carcinoma cells (EJ30) X-irradiated in different phases of the cell cycle. Radiat Res 2002;158:667-677.

64. Forrester HB, Albright N, Ling CC, Dewey WC: Computerized video time-lapse analysis of apoptosis of REC:Myc cells X-irradiated in different phases of the cell cycle. Radiat Res 2000;154:625-639.

65. Forrester HB, Vidair CA, Albright N, Ling CC, Dewey WC: Using computerized video time lapse for quantifying cell death of X-irradiated rat embryo cells transfected with c-myc or c-Ha-ras. Cancer Res 1999;59:931-939.

66. Guo M, Chen C, Vidair C, Marino S, Dewey WC, Ling CC: Characterization of radiation-induced apoptosis in rodent cell lines. Radiat Res 1997;147:295-303.

67. Vidair CA, Chen CH, Ling CC, Dewey WC: Apoptosis induced by X-irradiation of rec-myc cells is postmitotic and not predicted by the time after irradiation or behavior of sister cells. Cancer Res 1996;56:4116-4118.

68. Puck TT, Markus PI: The action of x-rays on mammalian cells. J Exp Med 1956;103:653-666.

69. Puck TT, Marcus PI, Cieciura SJ: Clonal growth of mammalian cells in vitro. Growth characteristics of colonies from single HeLa cells with and without a "feeder" layer. J Exp Med 1956;103:273-284.

70. Steel G: Basic Clinical Radiobiology, 3rd ed. London, Arnold, 2002.

71. Kellerer AM, Rossi HH: The theory of dual radiation action. Curr Top Radiat Res Q 1972;8:85.

72. Chadwick K, Leenhouts H: A molecular theory of cell survival. Phys Med Biol 1973;18:78.

73. Fu KK, Pajak TF, Trotti A, et al: A Radiation Therapy Oncology Group (RTOG) phase III randomized study to compare hyperfractionation and two variants of accelerated fractionation to standard fractionation radiotherapy for head and neck squamous cell carcinomas: First report of RTOG 9003. Int J Radiat Oncol Biol Phys 2000;48:7-16.

74. Saunders MI, Dische S, Grosch EJ, et al: Experience with CHART. Int J Radiat Oncol Biol Phys 1991;21:871-878.

75. Elkind M, Sutton H: X-ray damage and recovery in mammalian cells. Nature 1959;184:1293.

76. Elkind M, Sutton H: Radiation response of mammalian cells grown in culture. I. Repair of x-ray damage in surviving Chinese hamster cells. Radiation Res 1960;13:556.

77. Belli JA, Dicus GJ, Bonte FJ: Radiation response of mammalian tumor cells. I. Repair of sublethal damage in vivo. J Natl Cancer Inst 1967;38:673-682.

78. Belli JA, Shelton M: Potentially lethal radiation damage: repair by mammalian cells in culture. Science 1969;165:490-492.

79. Emery EW, Denekamp J, Ball MM, Field SB: Survival of mouse skin epithelial cells following single and divided doses of x-rays. Radiat Res 1970;41:450-466.

80. Phillips R, Tolmach L: Repair of potentially lethal damage in x-irradiated HeLa cells. Radiation Res 1966;29:413.

81. Nagasawa H, Little JB: Induction of chromosome aberrations and sister chromatid exchanges by X rays in density-inhibited cultures of mouse 10T1/2 cells. Radiat Res 1981;87:538-551.

82. Cornforth MN, Bedford JS: X-ray–induced breakage and rejoining of human interphase chromosomes. Science 1983;222:1141-1143.

83. Nguyen TD, Demange L, Froissart D, Panis X, Loirette M: Rapid hyperfractionated radiotherapy. Clinical results in 178 advanced squamous cell carcinomas of the head and neck. Cancer 1985;56:16-19.

84. Fowler J, Morgan R, Silvester J, et al: Experiments with fractionated x-ray treatment of the skin of pigs. I. Fractionation up to 28 days. Br J Radiol 1963;36:188.

85. Bedford JS, Hall E: Survival of HeLa cells cultured in vitro and exposed to protracted gamma irradiation. Br J Radiol 1964;39:896.

86. Hall E, Bedford JS: Dose rate: Its effect on the survival of HeLa cells irradiated with gamma-rays. Radiat Res 1964;22:305.

87. Lamerton L: Cell proliferation under continuous irradiation. Radiat Res 1966;27:119.

88. Lamerton L, Courtenay V: The steady state under continuous radiation. In: Dose Rate in Mammalian Radiation Biology, Conference 680410. Washington, DC, 1968, p 3.

89. Terasima T, Tolmach L: X-ray sensitivity and DAN synthesis in synchronous populations of HeLa cells. Science 1963;140:490.

90. Dewey WC, Stone LE, Miller HH, Giblak RE: Radiosensitization with 5-bromodeoxyuridine of Chinese hamster cells x-irradiated during different phases of the cell cycle. Radiat Res 1971;47:672-688.

91. Sinclair W, Morton R: Variations in x-ray response during the division cycle of partially synchronized Chinese hamster cells in culture. Nature 1963;199:1158.

92. Bedford JS, Mitchell JB: Dose-rate effects in synchronous mammalian cells in culture. Radiat Res 1973;54:316-327.

93. Mitchell JB, Bedford JS: Dose-rate effects in synchronous mammalian cells in culture. II. A comparison of the life cycle of HeLa cells during continuous irradiation or multiple-dose fractionation. Radiat Res 1977;71:547-560.

94. Terasima T, Tolmach L: Variations in several responses of HeLa cells to x-irradiation during the division cycle. Biophys J 1963;3:11.

95. Warters RL, Lyons BW: Variation in radiation-induced formation of DNA double-strand breaks as a function of chromatin structure. Radiat Res 1992;130:309-318.

96. Thames H, Hendry J: Fractionation in Radiotherapy. London, Taylor & Francis, 1987.

97. Peracchia G, Salti C: Radiotherapy with thrice-a-day fractionation in a short overall time: clinical experiences. Int J Radiat Oncol Biol Phys 1981;7:99-104.

98. Svoboda V: Accelerated fractionation: The Portsmouth experience 1971-1984. In: Varian's Fourth European Clinic Users Meeting. Zug, Switzerland, 1984, p 70.

99. van den Bogaert W, van der Schueren E, Horiot JC, et al: Early results of the EORTC randomized clinical trial on multiple fractions per day (MFD) and misonidazole in advanced head and neck cancer. Int J Radiat Oncol Biol Phys 1986;12587-591.

100. Withers HR, Peters LJ, Taylor JM, et al: Late normal tissue sequelae from radiation therapy for carcinoma of the tonsil: Patterns of fractionation study of radiobiology. Int J Radiat Oncol Biol Phys 1995;33:563-568.

101. Thames HD, Bentzen SM, Turesson I, Overgaard M, van den Bogaert W: Time-dose factors in radiotherapy: A review of the human data. Radiother Oncol 1990;19:219-235.

102. Marcial VA, Pajak TF, Chang C, Tupchong L, Stetz J: Hyperfractionated photon radiation therapy in the treatment of advanced squamous cell carcinoma of the oral cavity, pharynx, larynx, and sinuses, using radiation therapy as the only planned modality: (Preliminary report) by the Radiation Therapy Oncology Group (RTOG). Int J Radiat Oncol Biol Phys 1987;13:41-47.

103. Cox JD, Pajak TF, Marcial VA, et al: ASTRO plenary: interfraction interval is a major determinant of late effects, with hyperfractionated radiation therapy of carcinomas of upper respiratory and digestive tracts: results from Radiation Therapy Oncology Group protocol 8313. Int J Radiat Oncol Biol Phys 1991;20:1191-1195.

104. Fletcher GH: Hypofractionation: lessons from complications. Radiother Oncol 1991;20:10-15.

105. Cox JD: Large-dose fractionation (hypofractionation). Cancer 1985;55:2105-2111.
106. Horiot JC, Le Fur R, N'Guyen T, et al: Hyperfractionation versus conventional fractionation in oropharyngeal carcinoma: Final analysis of a randomized trial of the EORTC cooperative group of radiotherapy. Radiother Oncol 1992;25:231-241.
107. Wang CC: Accelerated hyperfractionation radiation therapy for carcinoma of the nasopharynx. Techniques and results. Cancer 1989;63:2461-2467.
108. Parsons JT, Mendenhall WM, Cassisi NJ, Isaacs JH, Jr., Million RR: Hyperfractionation for head and neck cancer. Int J Radiat Oncol Biol Phys 1988;14:649-658.
109. Pinto LH, Canary PC, Araujo CM, Bacelar SC, Souhami L: Prospective randomized trial comparing hyperfractionated versus conventional radiotherapy in stages III and IV oropharyngeal carcinoma. Int J Radiat Oncol Biol Phys 1991;21:557-562.
110. Baumann M, Bentzen SM, Ang KK: Hyperfractionated radiotherapy in head and neck cancer: A second look at the clinical data. Radiother Oncol 1998;46:127-130.
111. Stuschke M, Thames HD: Hyperfractionated radiotherapy of human tumors: Overview of the randomized clinical trials. Int J Radiat Oncol Biol Phys 1997;37:259-267.
112. Stuschke M, Thames H: Hyperfractionation: Where do we stand? Radiother Oncol 1998;46:131-133.
113. Ang KK, Peters LJ, Weber RS, et al: Concomitant boost radiotherapy schedules in the treatment of carcinoma of the oropharynx and nasopharynx. Int J Radiat Oncol Biol Phys 1990;19:1339-1345.
114. Steel G, Adama C, Peckham M: The Biological Basis of Radiotherapy. Amsterdam, Elsevier Science, 1983.
115. Kaplan HS: Historic milestones in radiobiology and radiation therapy. Semin Oncol 1979;6:479-489.
116. Tomlinson R, Gray L: The historical structure of some human lung cancers and the possible implications for radiotherapy. Br J Cancer 1955;9:539.
117. Howard-Flanders P, Moore D: The time interval after pulsed irradiation within which injury in bacteria can be modified by dissolved oxygen. I. ASearch for an effect of oxygen 0.02 seconds after pulsed irradiation. Radiat Res 1958;9:422-437.
118. Hall E: Radiobiology for the Radiologist, 5th ed. Philadelphia, JB Lippincott, 2000.
119. Kimura H, Braun RD, Ong ET, et al: Fluctuations in red cell flux in tumor microvessels can lead to transient hypoxia and reoxygenation in tumor parenchyma. Cancer Res 1996;56:5522-5528.
120. Fowler J, Morgan R, Wood C: Pretherapeutic experiments with the fast neutron beam from the Medical Research Council Cyclotron: I. The biological and physical advantages and problems of neutron therapy. Br J Radiol 1963;36:163.
121. Moulder JE, Rockwell S: Hypoxic fractions of solid tumors: experimental techniques, methods of analysis, and a survey of existing data. Int J Radiat Oncol Biol Phys 1984;10:695-712.
122. Van Putten LM, Kallman RF: Oxygenation status of a transplantable tumor during fractionated radiation therapy. J Natl Cancer Inst 1968;40:441-451.
123. Kallman RF: The phenomenon of reoxygenation and its implications for fractionated radiotherapy. Radiology 1972;105:135-142.
124. Chaplin DJ, Durand RE, Olive PL: Acute hypoxia in tumors: Implications for modifiers of radiation effects. Int J Radiat Oncol Biol Phys 1986;12:1279-1282.
125. Chaplin DJ, Olive PL, Durand RE: Intermittent blood flow in a murine tumor: Radiobiological effects. Cancer Res 1987;47:597-601.
126. Raleigh JA, Chou SC, Arteel GE, Horsman MR: Comparisons among pimonidazole binding, oxygen electrode measurements, and radiation response in C3H mouse tumors. Radiat Res 1999;151:580-589.
127. Dische S: Chemical sensitizers for hypoxic cells: A decade of experience in clinical radiotherapy. Radiother Oncol 1985;3:97-115.
128. Brown JM: Clinical trials of radiosensitizers: What should we expect? Int J Radiat Oncol Biol Phys 1984;10:425-429.
129. Brown JM: Exploiting tumour hypoxia and overcoming mutant p53 with tirapazamine. Br J Cancer 1998;77(Suppl 4):12-14.
130. Lee DJ, Trotti A, Spencer S, et al: Concurrent tirapazamine and radiotherapy for advanced head and neck carcinomas: A Phase II study. Int J Radiat Oncol Biol Phys 1998;42:811-815.
131. Rischin D, Peters L, Hicks R, et al: Phase I trial of concurrent tirapazamine, cisplatin, and radiotherapy in patients with advanced head and neck cancer. J Clin Oncol 2001;19:535-542.
132. Djordjevic B, Szybalski W: Genetics of human cell lines-incorporation of 5-bromo and 5-iododeoxyuridine into the deoxyribonucleic acid of human cells and its effect on radiation sensitivity. J Exp Med 1960;112:509.
133. Lawrence TS, Davis MA, Maybaum J, Stetson PL, Ensminger WD: The effect of single versus double-strand substitution on halogenated pyrimidine-induced radiosensitization and DNA strand breakage in human tumor cells. Radiat Res 1990;123:192-198.
134. Kinsella TJ, Mitchell JB, Russo A, Morstyn G, Glatstein E: The use of halogenated thymidine analogs as clinical radiosensitizers: Rationale, current status, and future prospects: non-hypoxic cell sensitizers. Int J Radiat Oncol Biol Phys 1984;10:1399-1406.
135. Kinsella TJ, Russo A, Mitchell JB, et al: A phase I study of intravenous iododeoxyuridine as a clinical radiosensitizer. Int J Radiat Oncol Biol Phys 1985;11:1941-1946.
136. Jackson D, Kinsella T, Rowland J, et al: Halogenated pyrimidines as radiosensitizers in the treatment of glioblastoma multiforme. Am J Clin Oncol 1987;10:437-443.
137. Phillips TL, Levin VA, Ahn DK, et al: Evaluation of bromodeoxyuridine in glioblastoma multiforme: A Northern California Cancer Center Phase II study. Int J Radiat Oncol Biol Phys 1991;21:709-714.
138. Bartelink H, Roelofsen F, Eschwege F, et al: Concomitant radiotherapy chemotherapy is superior to radiotherapy alone in the treatment of locally advanced anal cancer: Results of a phase III randomized trial of the European Organization for Research Treatment of Cancer Radiotherapy Gastrointestinal Cooperative Groups. J Clin Oncol 1997;15:2040-2049.
139. Bellon JR, Lindsley KL, Ellis GK, Gralow JR, Livingston RB, Austin Seymour MM: Concurrent radiation therapy paclitaxel or docetaxel chemotherapy in high-risk breast cancer. Int J Radiat Oncol Biol Phys 2000;48:393-397.
140. Curran W, Scott C, Langer C, et al: Long-term benefit is observed in a phase III comparison of sequential vs. concurrent chemo-radiation for patients with unresected stage III nsclc: RTOG 94-10. Proc Am Soc Clin Oncol 2003;22:621.
141. Brizel DM, Albers ME, Fisher SR, et al: Hyperfractionated irradiation with or without concurrent chemotherapy for locally advanced head neck cancer. N Engl J Med 1998;338:1798-1804.
142. Calais G, Alfonsi M, Bardet E, et al: Randomized trial of radiation therapy versus concomitant chemotherapy radiation therapy for advanced-stage oropharynx carcinoma. J Natl Cancer Inst 1999;91:2081-2086.
143. Adelstein DJ, Lavertu P, Saxton JP, et al: Mature results of a phase III randomized trial comparing concurrent chemoradiotherapy with radiation therapy alone in patients with stage III IV squamous cell carcinoma of the head and neck. Cancer 2000;88:876-883.
144. Morris M, Eifel PJ, Lu J, et al: Pelvic radiation with concurrent chemotherapy compared with pelvic para-aortic radiation for high-risk cervical cancer. N Engl J Med 1999;340:1137-1143.
145. Rose PG, Bundy BN, Watkins EB, et al: Concurrent cisplatin-based radiotherapy chemotherapy for locally advanced cervical cancer. N Engl J Med 1999;340:1144-1153.
146. Keys HM, Bundy BN, Stehman FB, et al: Cisplatin, radiation, adjuvant hysterectomy compared with radiation adjuvant hysterectomy for bulky stage IB cervical carcinoma. N Engl J Med 1999;340:1154-1161.
147. Shipley WU, Kaufman DS, Zehr E, et al: Selective bladder preservation by combined modality protocol treatment: Long-term outcomes of 190 patients with invasive bladder cancer. Urology 2002;60:62-67.
148. Herskovic A, Martz K, al-Sarraf M, et al: Combined chemotherapy radiotherapy compared with radiotherapy alone in patients with cancer of the esophagus. N Engl J Med 1992;326:1593-1598.

Science of Clinical Oncology

149. Moertel CG, Frytak S, Hahn RG, et al: Therapy of locally unresectable pancreatic carcinoma: A randomized comparison of high dose (6000 rads) radiation alone, moderate dose radiation (4000 rads + 5-fluorouracil), high dose radiation + 5-fluorouracil: The Gastrointestinal Tumor Study Group. Cancer 1981;48:1705-1710.

150. Pratt H, Tyree B, Straube R, Smith D: Cysteine protection against x-irradiation. Science 1949;110:213.

151. Vos O: Role of endogenous thiols in protection. Adv Space Res 1992;12:201-207.

152. Antonadou D, Pepelassi M, Synodinou M, Puglisi M, Throuvalas N: Prophylactic use of amifostine to prevent radiochemotherapy-induced mucositis xerostomia in head-and-neck cancer. Int J Radiat Oncol Biol Phys 2002;52:739-747.

153. Komaki R, Lee JS, Kaplan B, et al: Randomized phase III study of chemoradiation with or without amifostine for patients with favorable performance status inoperable stage II-III non-small cell lung cancer: Preliminary results. Semin Radiat Oncol 2002;12:46-49.

154. Coiffier B: Rituximab in combination with CHOP improves survival in elderly patients with aggressive non-Hodgkin's lymphoma. Semin Oncol 2002;29:18-22.

155. Czuczman MS, Fallon A, Mohr A, et al: HRituximab in combination with CHOP or fludarabine in low-grade lymphoma. Semin Oncol 2002;29:36-40.

156. Pastan I, Kreitman RJ: Immunotoxins in cancer therapy. Curr Opin Investig Drugs 2002;3:1089-1091.

157. Harries M, Smith I: The development clinical use of trastuzumab (Herceptin). Endocr Relat Cancer 2002;9:75-85.

158. Leyland-Jones B: Trastuzumab: Hopes realities. Lancet Oncol 2002;3:137-144.

159. Piccart-Gebhart MJ: Herceptin: The future in adjuvant breast cancer therapy. Anticancer Drugs 2001;12:S27-33.

160. Thomssen C: Trials of new combinations of Herceptin in metastatic breast cancer. Anticancer Drugs 2001;12:S19-25.

161. Workman P: New drug targets for genomic cancer therapy: Successes, limitations, opportunities, future challenges. Curr Cancer Drug Targets 2001;1:33-47.

162. Druker B: Signal transduction inhibition: results from phase I clinical trials in chronic myeloid leukemia. Semin Hematol 2001;38:9-14.

163. Druker BJ: STI571 (Gleevec) as a paradigm for cancer therapy. Trends Mol Med 2002;8:S14-18.

164. Schiffer CA: Signal transduction inhibition: Changing paradigms in cancer care. Semin Oncol 2001;28:34-39.

165. Robert F, Ezekiel MP, Spencer SA, et al: Phase I study of anti-epidermal growth factor receptor antibody cetuximab in combination with radiation therapy in patients with advanced head neck cancer. J Clin Oncol 2001;19:3234-3243.

166. Hahn SM, Bernhard EJ, Regine W, et al: A phase I trial of the farnesyltransferase inhibitor L-778,123 radiotherapy for locally advanced lung head neck cancer. Clin Cancer Res 2002;8:1065-1072.

167. Hartwell LH, Weinert TA: Checkpoints: Controls that ensure the order of cell cycle events. Science 1989;246:629-634.

168. Weinert TA: Dual cell cycle checkpoints sensitive to chromosome replication DNA damage in the budding yeast saccharomyces cerevisiae. Rad Res 1992;132:141-143.

169. Chiou S-K, Rao L, White E: Bcl-2 blocks p53-dependent apoptosis. Mol Cell Biol 1994;14:2556-2563.

170. Blank KR, Rudoltz MS, Kao GD, Muschel RJ, McKenna WG: The molecular regulation of apoptosis implications for radiation oncology. Intl J Radiat Biol 1997;71:455-466.

171. Ayene IS, Koch CJ, Krisch RE: Modification of radiation-induced strbreaks by glutathione: Comparison of single- and double-strand breaks in SV40 DNA. Radiat Res 1995;144:1-8.

172. Hollstein M, Sidransky D, Vogelstein B, Harris CC: p53 mutations in human cancers. Science 1991;253:49-53.

173. Bennett WP, el-Deiry WS, Rush WL, et al: p21waf1/cip1 transforming growth factor beta 1 protein expression correlate with survival in non-small cell lung cancer. Clin Cancer Res 1998;4:1499-1506.

174. El-Deiry WS, Kern SE, Pietenpol JA, Kinzler KW, Vogelstein B: Definition of a consensus binding site for p53. Nature Genet 1992;1:45-49.

175. Sun SY, Yue P, Wu GS, et al: Implication of p53 in growth arrest apoptosis induced by the synthetic retinoid CD437 in human lung cancer cells. Cancer Res 1999;59:2829-2833.

176. Goodman L, Gilman A: The pharmacological basis of therapeutics, vol 21. London, Macmillan, 1970.

177. Fajardo L: Patholgy of Radiation Injury. New York, Masson, 1982.

178. Withers HR, Taylor JM, Maciejewski B: Treatment volume tissue tolerance. Int J Radiat Oncol Biol Phys 1988;14:751-759.

179. Thames HD Jr, Peters LJ, Spanos W Jr, Fletcher GF: Dose response of squamous cell carcinomas of the upper respiratory digestive tracts. Br J Cancer 1980;41(Suppl):35-38.

180. Kaplan HS: Evidence for a tumoricidal dose level in the radiotherapy of Hodgkin's disease. Cancer Res 196;26:1221.

181. Bleehen NM, Stenning SP: A Medical Research Council trial of two radiotherapy doses in the treatment of grades 3 4 astrocytoma. The Medical Research Council Brain Tumour Working Party. Br J Cancer 1991;64:769-774.

182. Hazuka MB, Turrisi AT III, Lutz ST, et al: Results of high-dose thoracic irradiation incorporating beam's eye view display in non-small cell lung cancer: A retrospective multivariate analysis. Int J Radiat Oncol Biol Phys 1993;27:273-284.

183. Pollack A, Zagars GK, Starkschall G, et al: Prostate cancer radiation dose response: Results of the MD Anderson phase III randomized trial. Int J Radiat Oncol Biol Phys 2002;53:1097-1105.

184. Hanks GE, Martz KL, Diamond JJ: The effect of dose on local control of prostate cancer. Int J Radiat Oncol Biol Phys 1988;15:1299-1305.

185. Arriagada R, Mouriesse H, Sarrazin D, Clark RM, Deboer G: Radiotherapy alone in breast cancer. I. Analysis of tumor parameters, tumor dose local control: The experience of the Gustave-Roussy Institute the Princess Margaret Hospital. Int J Radiat Oncol Biol Phys 1985;11:1751-1757.

186. Perez CA, Breaux S, Madoc-Jones H, et al: Correlation between radiation dose tumor recurrence complications in carcinoma of the uterine cervix: stages I IIA. Int J Radiat Oncol Biol Phys 1979;5:373-382.

187. Schwade J, Lichter A: Management of acute effects of radiation therapy. In Carter S, Glatstein E, Livingston RB (eds): Principles of Cancer Treatment. New York, McGraw-Hill, 1982, p 212.

188. Kun L, Moulder J: General principles of radiation therapy. In Pizzo P, Poplack G (eds): Principles and Practice of Radiation Oncology, 2nd ed. Philadelphia, Lippincott, 1993, p 290.

189. Fajardo LF: Basic mechanisms and general morphology of radiation injury. Semin Roentgenol 1993;28:297-302.

190. Fajardo LF, Berthrong M: Vascular lesions following radiation. Pathol Annu 1988;23:297-330.

191. Withers H, Peters L, Kogelnik H: The pathobiology of late effects of irradiation. In Meyn R, Withers HR (eds): Radiation Biology in Cancer Research. New York, Raven Press, 1980, p 439.

192. Moss N: Moss' Radiation Oncology. St. Louis, Mo, CV Mosby, 1994.

193. Rubin P, Constine L, Williams J: Late effects of cancer treatment: Radiation drug toxicity. In Perez C, Brady L (eds): Principles and Practice of Radiation Oncology, 3rd ed. Philadelphia, Lippincott-Raven, 1998, p 155.

194. Stebbings JH, Lucas HF, Stehney AF: Mortality from cancers of major sites in female radium dial workers. Am J Ind Med 1984;5:435-459.

195. Boice JD Jr, Monson RR: Breast cancer in women after repeated fluoroscopic examinations of the chest. J Natl Cancer Inst 1977;59:823-832.

196. Shore RE, Hempelmann LH, Kowaluk E, et al: Breast neoplasms in women treated with x-rays for acute postpartum mastitis. J Natl Cancer Inst 1977;59:813-822.

197. Doll R: Radiation hazards: 25 years of collaborative research. Sylvanus Thompson memorial lecture, April 1980. Br J Radiol 1981;54:179-186.

198. Hempelmann LH, Pifer JW, Burke GJ, Terry R, Ames WR: Neoplasms in persons treated with x rays in infancy for thymic enlargement. A report of the third follow-up survey. J Natl Cancer Inst 1967;38:317-341.

199. Shimizu Y, Kato H, Schull WJ: Studies of the mortality of A-bomb survivors. 9. Mortality, 1950-1985: Part 2. Cancer mortality based on the recently revised doses (DS86). Radiat Res 1990;121:120-141.

200. Kato HM, Schull WJ: Studies of the mortality of A-bomb survivors. 7. Mortality 1950-1978: Part I. Cancer mortality. Radiat Res 1982;90:395-432.

201. Astakhova LN, Anspaugh LR, Beebe GW, et al: Chernobyl-related thyroid cancer in children of Belarus: A case-control study. Radiat Res 1998;150:349-356.

202. Weinberg AD, Kripalani S, McCarthy PL, Schull WJ: Caring for survivors of the Chernobyl disaster. What the clinician should know. JAMA 1995;274:408-412.

203. Little JB: Cellular, molecular, carcinogenic effects of radiation. Hematol Oncol Clin North Am 1993;7:337-352.

204. Miller G, Beebe G: Leukemia lymphoma myeloma. In Upton A, Albert R, Burns F, Shore RE (eds): Radiation Carcinogenesis. New York, Elsevier, 1986, p 245.

205. Kohn HI, Fry RJ: Radiation carcinogenesis. N Engl J Med 1984;310:504-511.

206. Land CE: Studies of cancer radiation dose among atomic bomb survivors. The example of breast cancer. JAMA 1995;274:402-407.

207. Boice JD Jr, Harvey EB, Blettner M, Stovall M, Flannery JT: Cancer in the contralateral breast after radiotherapy for breast cancer. N Engl J Med 1992;326:781-785.

208. Tubiana M: Effects of radiation on the human body. In Tubiana M (ed): Introduction to Radiobiology. London, Taylor & Francis, 1990, p 335.

209. Boice JD Jr, Engholm G, Kleinerman RA, et al: Radiation dose second cancer risk in patients treated for cancer of the cervix. Radiat Res 1988;116:3-55.

210. Hancock SL, Tucker MA, Hoppe RT: Breast cancer after treatment of Hodgkin's disease. J Natl Cancer Inst 1993;85:25-31.

211. Tucker MA, Jones PH, Boice JD Jr, et al: Therapeutic radiation at a young age is linked to secondary thyroid cancer. The Late Effects Study Group. Cancer Res 1991;51:2885-2888.

212. Direct estimates of cancer mortality due to low doses of ionising radiation: An international study. IARC Study Group on Cancer Risk among Nuclear Workers. Lancet 1994;344:1039.

213. Hendee WR: Estimation of radiation risks. BEIR V and its significance for medicine. JAMA 1992;268:620-624.

214. Korba A, Zivznuska FR, Purdy JA, Sorensen A, Powers WE: Pseudoblocks and portal localization. Radiology 1977;122:260-261.

215. Saunders M, Dische S, Barrett A, Harvey A, Gibson D, Parmar M: Continuous hyperfractionated accelerated radiotherapy (CHART) versus conventional radiotherapy in non-small-cell lung cancer: A randomised multicentre trial. CHART Steering Committee. Lancet 1997;350:161-165.

216. Kirkbride P, Hatton M, Lorigan P, Joyce P, Fisher P: Fatal pulmonary fibrosis associated with induction chemotherapy with carboplatin vinorelbine followed by CHART radiotherapy for locally advanced non-small cell lung cancer. Clin Oncol (R Coll Radiol), 2002;14:361-366.

217. Al-Sarraf M, LeBlanc M, Giri PG, et al: Chemoradiotherapy versus radiotherapy in patients with advanced nasopharyngeal cancer: Phase III randomized Intergroup study 0099. J Clin Oncol 1998;16:1310-1317.

218. Murray N, Coy P, Pater JL, et al: Importance of timing for thoracic irradiation in the combined modality treatment of limited-stage small-cell lung cancer. The National Cancer Institute of Canada Clinical Trials Group. J Clin Oncol 1993;11:336-344.

219. Perry MC, Herndon JE III, Eaton WL, Green MR: Thoracic radiation therapy added to chemotherapy for small-cell lung cancer: An update of Cancer Leukemia Group B Study 8083. J Clin Oncol 1998;16:2466-2467.

220. Epidermoid anal cancer: Results from the UKCCCR randomised trial of radiotherapy alone versus radiotherapy, 5-fluorouracil, mitomycin. UKCCCR Anal Cancer Trial Working Party. UK Co-ordinating Committee on Cancer Research. Lancet 1996;348:1049-1054.

221. Fisher B, Anderson S, Bryant J, et al: Twenty-year follow-up of a randomized trial comparing total mastectomy, lumpectomy, lumpectomy plus irradiation for the treatment of invasive breast cancer. N Engl J Med 2002;347:1233-1241.

222. Rosenberg SA, Tepper J, Glatstein E, et al: The treatment of soft-tissue sarcomas of the extremities: Prospective randomized evaluations of (1) limb-sparing surgery plus radiation therapy compared with amputation (2) the role of adjuvant chemotherapy. Ann Surg 1982;196:305-315.

223. Minsky BD, Cohen AM, Enker WE, Paty P: Sphincter preservation with preoperative radiation therapy coloanal anastomosis. Int J Radiat Oncol Biol Phys 1995;31:553-559.

224. Mohiuddin M, Regine WF, Marks GJ, Marks JW: High-dose preoperative radiation and the challenge of sphincter-preservation surgery for cancer of the distal 2 cm of the rectum. Int J Radiat Oncol Biol Phys 1998;40:569-574.

225. The Department of Veterans Affairs Laryngeal Cancer Study Group: Induction chemotherapy plus radiation compared with surgery plus radiation in patients with advanced laryngeal cancer. N Engl J Med 1991;324:1685-1690.

226. Maor M, Berkey B, Forastiere AA, et al: Larynx preservation tumor control in stage III IV laryngeal cancer: A three-arm randomized intergroup trial; RTOG 91-11. Proc Amer Soc Ther Rad Onc 2002;54:2.

227. Sternick E (ed): The Theory Practice of Intensity Modulated Radiation Therapy. Madison, Wisc, Advanced Medical Publishing, 1997.

228. Webb S: Intensity-Modulated Radiation Therapy. Bristol, England, Institute of Physics Publishing, 2000.

229. Mackie TR: Radiation therapy treatment optimization. Introduction. Semin Radiat Oncol 1999;9:1-3.

230. Purdy J, Starkschall G: A practical guide to 3-D planning conformal radiation therapy. Madison, Wisc, Advanced Medical Publishing, 1999.

231. Webb S: The physics of confromal therapy. Bristol, England, Institute of Physics Publishing, 1997.

232. Wright K, Primos B, Trump J, et al: Field shaping selective protection in megavolt radiation therapy. Radiology 1959;72:101.

233. Tsien K: The application of automatic computing machines to radiation treatment planning. Br J Radiol 1955;28:432.

234. Reinstein LE, McShan D, Webber BM, Glicksman AS: A computer-assisted three-dimensional treatment planning system. Radiology 1978;127:259-264.

235. McShan DL, Silverman A, Lanza DM, Reinstein LE, Glicksman AS: A computerized three-dimensional treatment planning system utilizing interactive colour graphics. Br J Radiol 1979;52:478-481.

236. Goitein M: Applications of computer tomography in radiotherapy treatment planning. In Orton C (ed): Progress in Medical Physics. New York, Plenum, 1982, p 195.

237. Ling C, Rogers C, Morton R (eds): Computed tomography in radiation therapy. New York, Plenum, 1982, p 195.

238. Fraass B, McShan D: 3-D treatment planning. I. Overview of a clinical planning system. In: 9th International Conference on the Use of Computers in Radiation Therapy, Schevenigen, The Netherlands, 1987.

239. Purdy J, Wong J, Harris W, et al: Three dimensional radiation treatment planning system. In: 9th International Conference on the Use of Computers in Radiation Therapy, Schevenigen, The Netherlands, 1987.

240. Sherouse G, Mosher C, Novins K, et al: Virtual simulation: Concept implementation. In: 9th International Conference on the Use of Computers in Radiation Therapy, Scheveningen, The Netherlands, 1987.

241. Mohan R, Barest G, Brewster LJ, et al: A comprehensive three-dimensional radiation treatment planning system. Int J Radiat Oncol Biol Phys 1988;15:481-495.

242. Brahme A: Design principles clinical possibilities with a new generation of radiation therapy equipment. A review. Acta Oncol 1987;26:403-412.

243. Mackie TR, Holmes T, Swerdloff S, et al: Tomotherapy: A new concept for the delivery of dynamic conformal radiotherapy. Med Phys 1993;20:1709-1719.

244. IMRT Collaborative Working Group Intensity-modulated radiotherapy: Current status issues of interest. Int J Radiat Oncol Biol Phys 2001;51:880-914.

245. Van Houtte P: New potentials of radiotherapy in non-small cell lung cancer: Stereotactic therapy IMRT. Curr Probl Cancer 2003;27:60-63.

246. Pirzkall A, Debus J, Haering P, et al: Intensity modulated radiotherapy (IMRT) for recurrent, residual, or untreated

skull-base meningiomas: Preliminary clinical experience. Int J Radiat Oncol Biol Phys 2003;55:362-372.

247. Zelefsky MJ, Fuks Z, Leibel SA: Intensity-modulated radiation therapy for prostate cancer. Semin Radiat Oncol 2002;12:229-237.

248. Hurkmans CW, Cho BC, Damen E, Zijp L, Mijnheer BJ: Reduction of cardiac lung complication probabilities after breast irradiation using conformal radiotherapy with or without intensity modulation. Radiother Oncol 2002;62:163-171.

249. Chao KS: Protection of salivary function by intensity-modulated radiation therapy in patients with head neck cancer. Semin Radiat Oncol 2002;12:20-25.

250. Ahamad A, Stevens CW, Smythe WR, et al: Intensity-modulated radiation therapy: A novel approach to the management of malignant pleural mesothelioma. Int J Radiat Oncol Biol Phys 2003;55:768-775.

251. Crane CH, Antolak JA, Rosen II, et al: Phase I study of concomitant gemcitabine IMRT for patients with unresectable adenocarcinoma of the pancreatic head. Int J Gastrointest Cancer 2001;30: 123-132.

252. Kavanagh BD, Schefter TE, Wu Q, et al: Clinical application of intensity-modulated radiotherapy for locally advanced cervical cancer. Semin Radiat Oncol 2002;12:260-271.

253. Glatstein E: Intensity-modulated radiation therapy: The inverse, the converse, the perverse. Semin Radiat Oncol 2002;12: 272-281.

254. Stone R: Neutron therapy specific ionization. AJR Am J Roentgenol 1948;59:771.

255. Brennan JT, Phillips TL: Evaluation of past experience with fast neutron teletherapy and its implications for future applications. Eur J Cancer 1971;7:219-225.

256. Catterall M: The treatment of advanced cancer by fast neutrons from the Medical Research Council's cyclotron at Hammersmith Hospital, London. Eur J Cancer 1974;10:343-347.

257. Gunderson L, Tepper J (eds): Clinical Radiation Oncology. Philadelphia, Churchill Livingstone, 2000.

258. Battermann JJ, Breur K, Hart GA, van Peperzeel HA: Observations on pulmonary metastases in patients after single doses multiple fractions of fast neutrons and cobalt-60 gamma rays. Eur J Cancer 1981;17:539-548.

259. Laramore GE, Krall JM, Thomas FJ, et al: Fast neutron radiotherapy for locally advanced prostate cancer. Final report of Radiation Therapy Oncology Group randomized clinical trial. Am J Clin Oncol 1993;16:164-167.

260. Douglas JG, Lee S, Laramore GE, Austin-Seymour M, Koh W, Griffin TW: Neutron radiotherapy for the treatment of locally advanced major salivary gland tumors. Head Neck 1999;21:255-263.

261. Douglas JG, Laramore GE, Austin-Seymour M, et al: Neutron radiotherapy for adenoid cystic carcinoma of minor salivary glands. Int J Radiat Oncol Biol Phys 1996;36:87-93.

262. Laramore GE, Griffith JT, Boespflug M, et al: Fast neutron radiotherapy for sarcomas of soft tissue, bone, cartilage. Am J Clin Oncol 1989;12:320-326.

263. Scharz R, Jrull A, Heyer D, et al: Neutron therapy in soft tissue sarcomas: A review of European results. Bull Cancer Radiother 1996;83S:110.

264. Griffin TW, Davis R, Hendrickson FR, Maor MH, Laramore GE: Fast neutron radiation therapy for unresectable squamous cell carcinomas of the head neck: The results of a randomized RTOG study. Int J Radiat Oncol Biol Phys 1984;10:2217-2221.

265. Griffin TW, Davis R, Laramore GE, et al: Mixed beam radiation therapy for unresectable squamous cell carcinomas of the head neck: The results of a randomized RTOG study. Int J Radiat Oncol Biol Phys 1984;10:2211-2215.

266. Maor MH, Errington RD, Caplan RJ, et al: Fast-neutron therapy in advanced head neck cancer: A collaborative international randomized trial. Int J Radiat Oncol Biol Phys 1995;32: 599-604.

267. Laramore GE, Bauer M, Griffin TW, et al: Fast neutron mixed beam radiotherapy for inoperable non-small cell carcinoma of the lung. Results of an RTOG randomized study. Am J Clin Oncol 1986;9:233-243.

268. Koh WJ, Krall JM, Peters LJ, et al: Neutron vs. photon radiation therapy for inoperable regional non-small cell lung cancer: Results of a multicenter randomized trial. Int J Radiat Oncol Biol Phys 1993;27:499-505.

269. Sawada K, Fukuma S, Seki Y, et al: Clinical experience in patients with Pancoast tumors treated by fast neutron radiotherapy. Gan No Rinsho 1983;A7:11.

270. Komaki R, Mountain CF, Holbert JM, et al: Superior sulcus tumors: Treatment selection results for 85 patients without metastasis (Mo) at presentation. Int J Radiat Oncol Biol Phys 1990;19:31-36.

271. Russell KJ, Caplan RJ, Laramore GE, et al: Photon versus fast neutron external beam radiotherapy in the treatment of locally advanced prostate cancer: Results of a randomized prospective trial. Int J Radiat Oncol Biol Phys 1994;28:47-54.

272. Cohen L, Saroja KR, Hendrickson FR, Lennox AJ, Hatcher MA, Kroc TK: Neutron irradiation of human pelvic tissues yields a steep dose-response function for late sequelae. Int J Radiat Oncol Biol Phys 1995;32:367-372.

273. Austin-Seymour M, Munzenrider J, Goitein M, et al: Fractionated proton radiation therapy of chordoma low-grade chondrosarcoma of the base of the skull. J Neurosurg 1989;70:13-17.

274. Fagundes MA, Hug EB, Liebsch NJ, Daly W, Efird J, Munzenrider JE: Radiation therapy for chordomas of the base of skull cervical spine: Patterns of failure outcome after relapse. Int J Radiat Oncol Biol Phys 1995;33:579-584.

275. Munzenrider JE, Verhey LJ, Gragoudas ES, et al: Conservative treatment of uveal melanoma: Local recurrence after proton beam therapy. Int J Radiat Oncol Biol Phys 1989;17:493-498.

276. Suit H: The Gray Lecture 2001: Coming technical advances in radiation oncology. Int J Radiat Oncol Biol Phys 2002;53:798-809.

277. Egger E, Schalenbourg A, Zografos L, et al: Maximizing local tumor control survival after proton beam radiotherapy of uveal melanoma. Int J Radiat Oncol Biol Phys 2001;51:138-147.

278. Egger E, Zografos L, Schalenbourg A, et al: Eye retention after proton beam radiotherapy for uveal melanoma. Int J Radiat Oncol Biol Phys 2003;55:867-880.

279. Fitzek MM, Thornton AF, Varvares M, et al: Neuroendocrine tumors of the sinonasal tract. Results of a prospective study incorporating chemotherapy, surgery, combined proton-photon radiotherapy. Cancer 2002;94:2623-2634.

280. Fitzek MM, Thornton AF, Rabinov JD, et al: Accelerated fractionated proton/photon irradiation to 90 cobalt gray equivalent for glioblastoma multiforme: Results of a phase II prospective trial. J Neurosurg 1999;91:251-260.

281. Wenkel E, Thornton AF, Finkelstein D, et al: Benign meningioma: Partially resected, biopsied, recurrent intracranial tumors treated with combined proton photon radiotherapy. Int J Radiat Oncol Biol Phys 2000;48:1363-1370.

282. Shipley WU, Verhey LJ, Munzenrider JE, et al: Advanced prostate cancer: The results of a randomized comparative trial of high dose irradiation boosting with conformal protons compared with conventional dose irradiation using photons alone. Int J Radiat Oncol Biol Phys 1995;32:3-12.

283. Benk VA, Adams JA, Shipley WU, et al: Late rectal bleeding following combined X-ray proton high dose irradiation for patients with stages T3-T4 prostate carcinoma. Int J Radiat Oncol Biol Phys 1993;26:551-557.

284. Yonemoto LT, Slater JD, Rossi CJ Jr, Antoine JE, Loredo L, Archambeau JO, et al: Combined proton photon conformal radiation therapy for locally advanced carcinoma of the prostate: Preliminary results of a phase I/II study. Int J Radiat Oncol Biol Phys 1997;37:21-29.

285. Tukuuye K, Matsui R, Sakie Y, et al: Results of proton therapy for hepatocellular carcinoma at the University of Tsukuba. In PTCOG, Tsukuba, Japan, 2001.

286. Bush DA, Slater JD, Bonnet R, et al: Proton-beam radiotherapy for early-stage lung cancer. Chest 1999;116:1313-1319.

287. Kliman B, Kjelberg R, Swisher B, et al: Proton beam therapy of acromegaly: A 20 year experience. In: Black P (ed): Secretory Tumors of the Pituitary Gland. New York, Raven Press, 1984, pp 295-307.

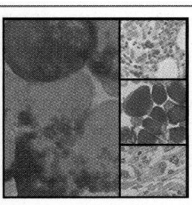

SURGICAL INTERVENTIONS IN CANCER

John E. Niederhuber

SUMMARY OF KEY POINTS

- Surgeon is part of a multidisciplinary team.
- Surgeon is frequently the "entry point" for patients who are newly diagnosed.
- Surgeon must have knowledge of the biology and natural history of the cancer to be treated.
- Surgeon must be technically experienced in diagnostic procedures and operative interventions.
- Surgeon must have appropriate

knowledge base in medical and radiation oncology.
- Patients treated in a multimodality setting have improved outcomes.
- Training of surgical oncologist must encompass:
  - etiology and genetic predispositions of cancer
  - prognostic factors and natural history of tumor
  - understanding of how to provide cost-effective treatment

- skills to develop, conduct, and manage clinical trials
- guidance of how to manage advanced disease
- guidance in how to offer compassionate support
- guidance in how to determine and evaluate outcomes
- Surgical oncologist should be an educational resource in the community.
- Surgical oncologist plays an important role in prevention and screening.

INTRODUCTION

Historically, surgery was the sole method used for treating cancer. However, with the introduction of ionizing radiation and the development of anticancer drugs, cancer therapy has rapidly progressed to involve the careful integration of an extensive array of therapeutic options in the treatment of both primary and recurrent tumors. As a result, the cancer surgeon no longer works alone, but is part of a multidisciplinary team involved in the treatment of most solid tumors.

As a member of this team, the surgeon is frequently the entry point for patients into the world of cancer care. It is the surgeon who most often establishes the diagnosis and staging of the primary cancer. This means that the responsibility for delivering the often devastating news to patients, educating patients and their families about the diagnosis and extent of disease, and informing them of the options for treatment frequently falls to the cancer surgeon. In this role, the cancer surgeon must have complete knowledge of the prognosis of the specific cancer and all options for potential therapy.

The surgeon must have a clear understanding of the biology of cancer and its natural history and also must be experienced in the technical procedures needed to accurately diagnose and appropriately resect primary cancers and, when indicated, locally recurrent and metastatic tumor. The cancer surgeon must also be prepared, in many cases, to function as the primary cancer care provider, or cancer-oriented "family physician," for the patient. The surgeon must provide for the patient a focus of treatment integration among the various cancer specialists. Cancer surgeons find that it is common for

patients to call or visit them for advice about all aspects of their treatment, which often leads to a lifelong relationship of continued care and follow-up.

HISTORICAL PERSPECTIVE

In medicine, professional and public acceptance of a subspecialty has historically depended largely on accomplishment. The development of the cancer surgeon subspecialty is no exception, and has been intimately tied to the history of surgery. In fact, surgical treatment of cancer has been significantly responsible for the role of surgery in modern medicine. The earliest discussion of surgical treatment of tumors appears in the E.S. *Papyrus* (ca. 1600 BC, but it is believed to be based on earlier writings dating back to 3000 BC).[1] The goal of the surgeon has always been to operate electively, without causing pain, and with a high rate of success. This has been especially true for cancer surgery.

The modern cancer surgeon must have an intimate knowledge not only of the fine technical art of surgery but of anatomy, pathology, biochemistry, genetics, physiology, pharmacology, bacteriology, and virology. The cancer surgeon must also possess an appropriate knowledge of general medicine as well as the cancer specialties of medical and radiation oncology. Many of the skills of the psychiatrist and psychologist are also required to assist patients and their families as they deal with the personal stresses brought on by cancer therapy, cancer progression, and end-of-life issues.

Before the introduction of anesthesia, surgery was primarily reserved for the treatment of abscesses and for managing trauma; the few operations performed for tumors were amputations. Not only did patients suffer excruciating pain in the absence of anesthesia, but also, before the advent of antisepsis, the death rate from infection was extraordinarily high. As a result, few patients were willing to undergo such intense pain electively, with so little chance of survival. The development of anesthesia and the introduction of antisepsis made elective surgical techniques for the treatment of cancer much more acceptable, and rapid developments in cancer surgery began to occur during the second half of the 19th century as tumor-specific elective surgeries were undertaken and refined.[2,3]

Cancer surgeons have historically provided significant leadership in the conduct of clinical trials. Most noteworthy have been the National Surgical Adjuvant Breast and Bowel Project (NSABP), initially under the direction of Bernard Fisher, and more recently, the American College of Surgeons Oncology Group (ACOS-OG), led by Samuel Wells. Surgeons have also been active participants in a number of other cooperative groups. The success of these surgeon-sponsored clinical trials placed surgeons as significant contributors to the clinical trials agenda of these groups, and showed the importance of surgical involvement in designing clinical trials and maintaining control of the quality of surgery when it was part of the study. This has proved especially important in evaluating studies of adjuvant therapy.

Anesthesia

Some of the first "clinical trials" of ether anesthesia took place in the parlor of Crawford Long, a dentist practicing in Georgia during the early 1840s. Long is said to have invited his friends over for "ether parties" to enjoy a temporary "loss of Southern inhibitions." Long witnessed that his friends lost not only their inhibitions, but also pain sensation. He is said to have used ether anesthesia in his dental practice as early as 1842. Unfortunately, Long's use of ether was not brought to the attention of the medical public.

John Collins Warren is responsible for two significant benchmarks in oncologic surgical history. He published the first American work on tumors in 1838, entitled "Surgical Observations on Tumors with Cases and Operations,"[4] and he was the surgeon in the first published account of the use of ether anesthesia for removal of a tongue cancer from Gilbert Abbott in 1846.[2] The anesthesia was administered by a dentist, William T. Morton, who had developed the technique. The operation involved excision of the submaxillary gland and part of the tongue.[5]

Antisepsis

Despite the advances made in anesthesia in the 1840s, sepsis remained a major barrier to successful surgery until Joseph Lister (subsequently Baron Lister), an accomplished surgeon, introduced the concept of bactericidal therapy with carbolic acid in 1867.[3] This was an outgrowth of Pasteur's theory that bacteria caused infection. Using carbolic acid as an antiseptic agent in conjunction

with heat sterilization of instruments, Lister dramatically decreased the rate of postoperative fatalities. He also developed absorbable ligatures and the drainage tube; both represent significant advances for surgical management of wounds and incisions.

Lister was indirectly responsible for the introduction of the first ready-to-use surgical dressings in 1886. Robert Wood Johnson heard an address in 1876 by James Lister; as a result, he developed sterile dressings wrapped in individual packages suitable for immediate use without the risk of contamination.

Although the value of Lister's contributions was not recognized by his senior colleagues, they were quickly adopted by his American follower, William Stewart Halsted,[6] the first professor of surgery at The Johns Hopkins Hospital. Halsted first introduced to the United States the meticulous techniques of tissue handling during surgery and the antiseptic methods proposed by Lister. Halsted, who had a major interest in cancer, was strongly supported in his work by his close friend and colleague at Hopkins, Sir William Osler. Osler was a student of abdominal malignancies, and the collaboration of these two great American physicians represents perhaps one of the earliest occurrences of the multidisciplinary approach to cancer treatment.

Development of Surgical Techniques

It took many centuries and a number of critical advances to elevate early surgeons to a level of acceptance in medicine and to a position of public value. Even so, most of the early knowledge of anatomy, microbiology, and physiology was amassed through the research efforts of surgeons. Initially, the surgeon's role in cases of cancer was to ablate growths using resection or cauterization. Resection and cauterization were limited to tumors of the extremities, breast, and other surface structures. Even simple amputations were accompanied by high rates of mortality secondary to infection before the advent of antisepsis. For example, the overall mortality rate for amputations was greater than 50%. There were, however, isolated reports of very low mortality rates after amputation using meticulous techniques to avoid hemorrhage and to minimize infection.[7]

Although the 19th century was a period devoted predominantly to descriptive anatomy and reports of a physiologic nature, this period also marked the first documentation of an industrial cancer, when Percivall Pott, in 1875, described the occurrence of cancer of the scrotum in chimney sweeps. Ephraim McDowell is credited with performing the first elective abdominal tumor resection in 1809, when he removed a gigantic ovarian mass weighing 22 pounds (9.98 kg). The patient survived to live another 30 years.

Eighteenth and 19th century surgeons were often the leaders of hospital reform; their ranks included such notables as the great English army surgeon, John Pringle; British surgeons William Farr, Edward Parkes, and John Simon; and New York surgeon Stephen Smith. They created less crowded patient conditions, improved ventilation, emphasized cleanliness as a way of improving hospital sanitation, and developed an environment that decreased the high mortality rate associated with surgery.

The period encompassing the late 19th century and early 20th century was exceptionally fertile for oncologic surgery. Albert Theodore Billroth performed the first gastrectomy, laryngectomy, and esophagectomy. Halsted, in addition to his contributions to antisepsis, also defined the principles of en bloc resection, as shown by the first radical mastectomy in 1890. Soon after the turn of the century, surgeons developed radical resections for specific organs. Hugh Young performed the first prostatectomy in 1904, and the first radical hysterectomy was performed by Ernst Wertheim in 1906. In 1908, W. Ernest Miles performed the first abdominoperineal resection of cancer of the rectum.

Surgery for cancer of the pancreas took a number of years to refine. The technique of pancreaticoduodenectomy was first successfully demonstrated by the German surgeon Kausch in 1912.[8] Originally, the operation was performed in two stages. A.O. Whipple, in 1935, performed three successful two-stage operations in the United States,[9] and is responsible for popularizing the procedure that became known as the "Whipple." In 1940, he performed a successful single-stage procedure.

These efforts, and those of countless others too numerous to be mentioned in this chapter, provided the foundation for modern cancer surgery (Table 27-1). The accomplishments of these and other pioneering physicians are particularly remarkable, viewed from a historical perspective, for, as Hippocrates said, "Life is short, the art long, opportunity fleeting, experiment treacherous, opportunity difficult."

The substantial advances in cancer surgery that are now taking place will clearly benefit patients with cancer during the 21st century. Although historically, the management of cancer involved surgery alone, today, only a handful of patients with cancer have only surgery as their treatment. Advances in multimodal therapy have changed the role of the surgeon; however, it is clear that the surgeon will continue to be the primary care provider for patients with cancer for many years to come.

MULTIDISCIPLINARY APPROACH

Cancer therapy is becoming increasingly complex, and today, most solid tumors, even very early cancers, are treated by more than one modality. This multidisciplinary approach to treatment requires the input and coordination of multiple specialists. To complicate matters even further, often more than one therapeutic option exists. This requires the specialists involved to agree on the treatment regimen to be followed.

Rapid advances in the science of oncology have had a major effect on the surgical treatment of patients with cancer as well as on surgical education and research. Increasing emphasis on multidisciplinary care raises the important question: Which physician specialty will be responsible for coordinating patient care in the future? Already, cancer care generally involves two or more modalities.

Medical oncologists have an increasingly prominent role in the care of the patient with cancer. Their responsibilities include administering and monitoring the patient's chemotherapy, hormone therapy, and in some instances, biologic therapy. Medical oncologists manage the toxicities of intravenous and oral anticancer therapy, and as a result, provide considerable supportive care, especially as new agents have been developed to better control nausea and fatigue.

The radiation oncologist provides an important modality of local and regional cancer therapy. Often, radiation therapy is used after surgery to improve local disease control rates, or even before surgery, to reduce tumor bulk or downstage the tumor. It is more and more common for radiation to be combined with simultaneous administration of chemotherapy or radiation sensitizer agents.

A report on increased survival outcomes for patients with ovarian cancer in Scotland led to an investigation of whether these differences were caused by prognostic factors or by the organization and delivery of cancer services. A retrospective study of 533 cases of ovarian

TABLE 27-1

Timeline of Surgical Benchmarks

DATE	SURGEON	PROCEDURE
1809	Ephraim McDowell	First elective abdominal surgery for excision of ovarian tumor
1846	John Collins Warren	Use of ether anesthesia for excision of submaxillary gland
1867	Joseph Lister	Introduction of antisepsis
1873	Theodor Billroth	Laryngectomy
1880s	Emil Theodor Kocher	Development of thyroid surgery
1890s	William Stewart Halsted	Radical mastectomy
1904	Hugh H. Young	Radical prostatectomy
1906	George Crile	Radical neck dissection
1906	Ernst Wertheim	Radical hysterectomy
1920s	William Stewart Halsted	First elective abdominal surgery for excision of ovarian tumor
	Harvey Cushing	Surgery for brain tumors
1935	A.O. Whipple	Pancreaticoduodenectomy

cancer registered in 1987 was performed. With adjustments for age, stage, pathology, degree of differentiation, and presence of ascites, survival improved with management by a multidisciplinary team at a joint clinic.[10]

An earlier study also confirmed the benefits of multimodal management. Patients with skeletal and soft tissue sarcomas of the extremity were treated with preoperative intra-arterial doxorubicin and radiation therapy, radical surgical resection, and postoperative chemotherapy or chemoimmunotherapy, resulting in the preservation of a functional extremity in 13 of 14 patients. Seven of eight patients with stage IIIA and IIIB soft tissue sarcomas that were managed with preoperative intra-arterial doxorubicin and radiation therapy followed by en bloc soft tissue resection and six patients with bone sarcomas that were managed with preoperative treatment followed by bone resection and replacement with cadaver bone allografts remained free of disease for 4 to 34 months. The results of the combined-modality approach were significantly better than those obtained in patients managed with surgical resection alone or with a combination of surgery and another single modality, in terms of both short-term recurrence-free survival and salvage of a functional extremity.[11]

There is a growing trend toward freestanding cancer care centers. The critical components of these centers are multidisciplinary cancer care, direct care and support services, a commitment to clinical trials, and a comprehensive program for quality assurance.[12] Comprehensive cancer centers affiliated with academic medical centers have an array of clinically focused investigations, including programs designed to test new therapies and research programs investigating the biology of cancer. These academic comprehensive cancer centers attract the elite of cancer clinician–scientists and basic scientists. As a result, patients receive better cancer care and greater support from experienced ancillary services. This translates into better quality of life as well as a longer life and greater hope for cure.

ROLE OF THE SURGICAL ONCOLOGIST

In recent years, a subspecialty of surgery known as surgical oncology has emerged to play an increasingly important role in the treatment of cancer (Table 27-2). There are many reasons for this evolution of subspecialization, but perhaps the most significant reasons are: (1) the increasing complexity of multidisciplinary cancer care; (2) the opportunities for clinical and laboratory investigation of cancer biology; (3) the rapid increase in the number of medical and radiation oncologists, which threatens to diminish significantly the traditional role of the surgeon in coordinating the management of cancer patients (even those with early disease); and (4) the expectation that surgeons have the latest information and newest treatment options.[13]

Today, the surgical oncologist is really a "cancer physician" who interacts with all other members of the cancer therapy team in a knowledgeable and confident manner. This new and important role requires a sound

TABLE 27-2

Role of the Surgical Oncologist

Consultant

Special training or skills
Tumor board

Organizer and Leader

Cancer programs
Cancer committee
Tumor registry
Oncology section

Educator

Cancer conferences
Teaching programs

Researcher

Clinical protocols

basis of knowledge about cancer biology (including cancer prevention and the biology of metastasis), imaging technologies, chemical and biologic therapy, and radiation therapy.

In an address before the American College of Surgeons, Murray Brennan of Memorial Sloan-Kettering Cancer Center in New York stated, "In defining what might be considered the role of the surgeon in cancer care, there are at least seven important areas that I believe need to have renewed emphasis."[14] Brennan used his experience with soft tissue sarcoma to illustrate the importance of the following performance objectives for the cancer surgeon: (1) understands etiology and genetic predisposition; (2) understands prognostic factors and natural history; (3) performs cost-effective treatment; (4) develops clinical trials; (5) guides advanced disease management; (6) guides compassionate support; and (7) evaluates outcome. Brennan's analysis of the cancer surgeon's role as a member of today's therapy team is an excellent real-life description of the responsibilities involved and the opportunities to provide real leadership in cancer care.

The surgical oncologist thus provides the leadership for cancer care, cancer research, and cancer teaching within the academic or hospital-based surgical community. This is an extremely important role, and it has become increasingly clear that programs that emphasize strong cancer leadership from surgical oncologists have developed solid research and clinical programs for patients seeking cancer treatment.

As part of the greater medical community, the surgical oncologist has the responsibility of introducing to the surgical community new information, new approaches to cancer diagnosis, and new approaches to therapy. The surgical oncologist is most often the one involved in the early stages of cancer diagnosis, an ideal position to provide significant institutional leadership in developing community interest in cancer prevention, including screening and early diagnosis.

In addition to local responsibilities, much ongoing work in national clinical trials depends heavily on surgical oncology leadership directed at establishing quality control of the surgical aspects of multidisciplinary protocols. The surgical oncologist is an important member of the design team and is critical to providing education to participating surgeons about standards of care, technical guidelines for the operative procedure, and collection of data. The surgeon member of the team is also essential for reviewing the staging data submitted by participating surgeons as well as information provided by quality control reports. When surgery is part of the therapy being evaluated in a clinical trial, it must be performed in a uniform manner by surgeons specifically trained and competent to deliver the procedure in a quality manner. This is especially obvious when evaluating outcomes of adjuvant therapy trials.

TRAINING IN SURGICAL ONCOLOGY

Historically, training in surgical oncology occurred at the small number of stand-alone cancer hospitals in the United States, primarily with the goal of preparing a select group of general surgeons to work as cancer specialists in university hospitals or at large medical centers.

During the 1970s, there was more interest in developing the subspecialty of surgical oncology within academic surgery training programs and in obtaining board certification, as had been done for other oncologic subspecialties. This effort by a number of prominent cancer surgeons encountered considerable difficulties in the ensuing years, and surgical oncology has yet to achieve recognition as a board-certified subspecialty.

There are many reasons for this. First and foremost is the fact that surgical cancer care in the community almost always falls to the general surgeon. Even in the university hospital setting, cancer surgery has not been the exclusive right of the surgical oncologist. The surgical oncologist, as a result, has always been viewed as somewhat redundant by general surgical colleagues.

To address some of these issues, a conference was held at the National Cancer Institute in 1979. It was the consensus of this conference that training in surgical oncology should involve a 2-year period after completion of a general surgery residency.[15] The committee charged a national organization, the Society of Surgical Oncology (SSO), with developing training guidelines and a review and approval process for identifying qualified training programs. Clearly, the hope of those involved was that expertise in surgical oncology could be increased in significant numbers and disseminated more broadly in the community practice arena, not just in academic centers. Further, it was hoped that the development of a number of university training programs would eventually lead to board certification. The curriculum that was eventually approved included a year of clinical surgery to ensure that the fellow was exposed to the technical aspects and clinical management of a sufficient number of patients with complex tumors and uncommon cancers. It was also stipulated that an additional 6 months of clinical training would be included and would include rotations in medical oncology, radiation oncology, and pathology. Those attending the conference believed that trainees should be educated in the basic and clinical sciences, including epidemiology, the biology of cancer, immunology, and carcinogenesis.[15]

The effort to enhance training in surgical oncology, broaden available training opportunities, and provide a measure of qualification or certification of competence have been supported and nurtured by the SSO, which was founded more than 50 years ago.[16] This society has become the leading academic oncologic society for surgeons around the world. In assuming this leadership role, the SSO has developed and disseminated optimal guidelines for the multidisciplinary care of patients with cancer, provided an important resource for continuing education through its annual meeting, initiated and supported a monthly journal (*The Annals of Surgical Oncology*), and has actively stimulated cancer research.[17] The society has willingly taken on the responsibility of evaluating and approving fellowship programs. It embraced the recommended guidelines proposed by the 1979 National Cancer Institute Committee, and in 1982, approved the first three training sites.[16] There are currently 14 approved programs, with approximately 70 positions available nationwide. A national matching system was developed, and an in-training national examination is given each year.

In 1992, the World Federation of Surgical Oncology Societies was inaugurated and immediately worked to develop "standards of education, training, and practice" in surgical oncology.[18,19] These guidelines were published and are summarized in Table 27-3. It is through efforts by the SSO and the World Federation of Surgical Oncology Societies that excellent training opportunities now exist for a significant number of general surgery graduates. Standardization of the process of review and accreditation ensures that more well-qualified cancer surgeons will be available to serve as experts in cancer care with multidisciplinary teams. The SSO deserves much praise and credit for its untiring and expert leadership in the training of future surgical oncologists.

TABLE 27-3

Guidelines for Training of Surgical Oncologists in Europe

- Receive training to a high level of technical competence and attain the clinical skills needed to manage common and complex cancers.
- Receive training in the evolving understanding of tumor biology, mechanisms of spread of disease, and other oncologic principles.
- Understand the principles, scope, and limitations of different modalities of radiation therapy.
- Be conversant with the theoretical and practical applications of cytotoxic chemotherapy.
- Be prepared to study and evaluate evidence from clinical trials and thereby be in a position to propose new avenues of research and study, both in the clinical setting and in the laboratory.
- Be trained to be discriminating in the application of modern technology in the investigation and treatment of malignant disease.
- Be involved, as a member of a team, in each step of the decision-making process in planning the strategy for the patient's care.

Adapted from O'Higgins N: Towards a high standard of surgical oncology throughout Europe. Eur J Cancer 1995;31A(Suppl 6):S22 © 1995 Elsevier Science, with permission.

Science of Clinical Oncology

CANCER MANAGEMENT

Prevention

The most effective weapon against cancer, of course, is prevention. In recent years, much of the debate about prevention has focused on the cost of delivering cancer prevention services. The level and quality of prevention services may be increased through a greater consensus about goals for cancer prevention, better organization to provide these services more efficiently to large populations, and improvement of health education. Social problems of unemployment, poverty, and limited medical coverage for a large number of people have significantly influenced access to services. The agenda for the future in cancer prevention should include fundamental research, intervention research, program delivery, patient access through free choice, and surveillance and monitoring.[20,21]

Certain conditions, often congenital or inherited genetic traits, are associated with the subsequent manifestation of cancer. In patients in whom these syndromes are known to be present and in whom cancers are likely to occur in nonvital organs, it may become necessary to remove the organ to prevent possible malignancy. In these instances, the surgeon has a responsibility to inform and educate the patient about the condition and to alert the family to the hereditary nature of the disorder and its possible occurrence in other family members. Table 27-4 outlines some common predisposing conditions and their corresponding malignancies.

For example, cryptorchidism is associated with a higher incidence of testicular cancer, which is often prevented by early prophylactic surgery. Patients with ulcerative colitis (with total and partial colonic involvement) are likely to have cancer of the colon if resection is not performed. Prophylactic surgery for patients with a family history of cancer (e.g., breast, ovarian, colon) is still a controversial issue, but recently, the identification of the *Ret* gene as the locus for familial medullary thyroid cancer has enabled surgeons to accurately predict at-risk individuals in the family, and to offer prophylactic thyroidectomy.[22] The

patient and surgeon must carefully balance the benefits and hazards of surgery with an understanding of the factors involved in determining increased risk.

Screening

The application of a screening test is a complex process, and multiple layers of evaluation are needed to prove test efficacy. Clearly, the screening test must be applied at the right time and to the appropriate population to be effective. Moreover, the screening test itself is merely designed to identify a possible condition that needs further in-depth evaluation. For the surgeon, the effectiveness and cost of screening are directly related to the strategies used to address positive test results.

For example, Lieberman[23] compiled data on colon cancer screening. Current screening with sigmoidoscopy and fecal occult blood testing is costly and is not likely to reduce colon cancer mortality rates by more than 50%. Ideal screening (both cost-effective and accurate) would reduce the number of patients screened by identifying high-risk patients and using a more sensitive test, such as colonoscopy, for verification of disease presence. Recent developments in molecular genetics may make this possible by identifying a set of genetic markers for risk stratification.[23]

The issue of cost-effectiveness and screening is currently a major concern among health care providers. Narrow-focused attempts at cost reduction could possibly discourage high-risk groups from participating in early-detection programs whose costs are not covered or provided for by health insurers, eliminating the benefit of early detection to both the patient and the health care system. Cost savings are possible with improved public health education about the appropriateness of early detection in the correct age groups with pertinent medical histories (Table 27-5).[24]

Diagnosis

Evaluation for surgical cure should be based on a histologically confirmed diagnosis of a treatable cancer confined to local or regional tissues. The diagnosis of cancer cannot be proved without a biopsy, and biopsy should be repeated if the diagnosis is questionable. There has been a remarkable advance in imaging technologies to improve the execution and outcome of selected biopsy procedures. Computed tomography (CT), ultrasonography, and magnetic resonance imaging are now frequently used to enhance needle guidance and placement. These techniques improve the accuracy and safety of needle placement along the target path, while avoiding injury to other structures. The use of three-dimensional stereotactic CT-guided biopsy is becoming increasingly widespread as a diagnostic tool. Stereotactic biopsy is appropriate for any lesion located in the brain stem, pons, or medulla.[25] This technology is also widely used to evaluate nonpalpable mammographically detected breast abnormalities. The use of these guidance techniques requires the surgeon to be familiar with the device and the approach.

TABLE 27-4

Common Predisposing Conditions and Associated Malignancies	
CONDITION	**ASSOCIATED MALIGNANCY**
Cryptorchid testis	Testicular
Chronic ulcerative colitis	Colon
Familial adenomatous polyposis	Colon and rectum
Hereditary nonpolyposis colon cancer	Colon and rectum
Family history of colon cancer	Colon and rectum
Multiple endocrine neoplasia (types II and III)	Medullary cancer of the thyroid
Leukoplakia	Squamous
Family history of breast cancer	Breast and ovary
Family history of ovarian cancer	Ovary and breast

TABLE 27-5

Ten Criteria for Cancer Screening Programs

1. Is the disease an important health problem?
   Probably yes
2. Is there effective therapy for patients with localized disease?
   Probably yes
3. Are treatment facilities for further diagnosis and treatment readily available?
   Probably yes
4. Is there an identifiable latent period or early symptomatic stage of the disease?
   Probably yes
5. Is there an effective screening technique?
   Probably yes
6. Are the tests acceptable to the screened population, particularly groups at increased risk for disease?
   Probably yes
7. Is the natural history of the disease, from its development to clinical manifestation, sufficiently known?
   Probably yes
8. Is there a generally acceptable strategy to identify patients who should receive treatment vs careful observation alone?
   Probably yes
9. Are the costs of screening acceptable?
   Probably yes
10. Does the treatment of early-stage disease have a favorable effect on prognosis?
    Probably yes

Adapted from Littrup PJ: Prostate cancer screening: Appropriate choices? Cancer 1994;74(Suppl):2016. © 1994 American Cancer Society, with permission.

It is very important for the surgeon to maintain a close relationship with the pathologist. If the patient has a pathologic diagnosis from an outside source, it is always necessary to have the diagnosis confirmed. It may even be necessary to obtain tissue blocks to prepare more slides, to perform more extensive cytologic marker studies, and occasionally, to perform additional biopsies to obtain a definitive diagnosis.

Four techniques are currently in use for obtaining tissue for diagnosis:

1. *Needle aspiration biopsy*. This approach involves aspirating tissue fragments through a needle guided into an area in which disease is suspected. It can usually be performed using local anesthesia or, possibly, no anesthesia. A recent study of the usefulness of CT-guided fine-needle aspiration in the diagnosis of malignancy in solid pulmonary nodules showed 76% sensitivity, 100% specificity, 100% positive predictive value, 52% negative predictive value, and 81% accuracy.[26] The disadvantage of aspiration biopsy is that it seldom yields a sufficient specimen for histologic diagnosis. As a result, there is always a margin of error in individual cell analysis, even with an exceptionally skilled cytologist. Cytology has the disadvantage of being unable to distinguish between invasive and noninvasive cancers, so a more detailed histologic diagnosis is usually necessary.
2. *Needle (core) biopsy*. This technique entails the retrieval of a small core of tissue, using a specially designed "core-cutting" needle. This specimen is usually sufficient for histologic diagnosis of most tumor types. Like aspiration biopsy, this technique is relatively cost-effective and can usually be performed using a local anesthetic.
3. *Incisional biopsy*. This technique involves surgical retrieval of a small segment of a larger tumor for diagnosis. The advantage of the procedure is that it yields enough histologic material to provide analysis of tumor markers. It is also often possible to perform this procedure in an outpatient setting using local anesthesia. Incisional biopsies are particularly useful in the diagnosis of sarcomas, large tumors, and unresectable tumors, and when the preferred treatment is nonsurgical. The disadvantages of incisional biopsy include possible sampling errors, the risk of trauma to the tumor, the possible risk of tumor spread, and the need for excisional biopsy if no cancer is diagnosed. Precise technique is essential.
4. *Excisional biopsy*. This technique is total removal of all suspicious tumor tissue, with little or no margin. The circumstances of the procedure dictate the use of local or general anesthesia. This procedure is the most definitive diagnostic tool of the four described. It provides adequate treatment for nonmalignant tumors and involves minimal trauma to the cancer. It is necessary to perform excisional biopsy if the results of incisional biopsy or core needle biopsy are inconclusive. One of the disadvantages is that it is generally limited to small tumors (e.g., lymph nodes, parotid tumors). It also involves a deeper area of dissection, which necessitates wider margins.

The proper placement of a biopsy incision is vital. Misplacement can compromise subsequent surgical procedures. The evidence concerning tumor spread from incisional and excisional biopsy is inconclusive. However, the surgeon should take extreme care to avoid using contaminated instruments on new tissue planes and to secure proper hemostasis of biopsy sites to avoid the spread of tumor along tissue planes.

The biopsy technique selected should be appropriate for the suspected lesion and should yield an adequate tissue sample for proper histologic diagnosis. Orientation of the specimen, if applicable, should be marked clearly and carefully by the surgeon, to facilitate proper histologic interpretation. Proper handling of excised tissue is the surgeon's responsibility.

Staging

Staging is the classification of the anatomic extent of cancer in an individual. Specific stage groups categorize cancers of particular anatomic sites. Staging is essential in the treatment process, and requires an understanding of the biology of cancer as well as the extent of disease.

The method of staging that is in general use is the tumor-node-metastasis (TNM) method developed by the International Union Against Cancer and the American Joint Committee on Cancer (Table 27-6). This convenient shorthand notation condenses lengthy descriptions into manageable classifications for comparison, treatment,

TABLE 27-6

TNM Classification System[27]

TNM System

Describes the anatomic extent of disease based on assessment of three components

T	Primary tumor size and extent
N	Regional lymph node involvement
M	Distant metastasis absent or present

Primary tumor (T)

TX	Primary tumor cannot be assessed
T0	No evidence of primary tumor
Tis	Carcinoma in situ
T1, T2	Increasing size or local extension
T3, T4	Increasing extent of primary tumor

Regional lymph nodes (N)

NX	Regional lymph nodes cannot be assessed
N0	No regional lymph node metastasis
N1, N2, N3	Increasing involvement of regional lymph nodes

Distant metastasis (M)

MX	Presence of distant metastasis cannot be assessed
M0	No distant metastasis
M1	Distant metastasis (may be further specified according to site of occurrence)

Histopathology

Qualitative assessment of category of tissue or cell type based on appearance

Histopathology grade (G)

GX	Grade cannot be assessed
G1	Well differentiated
G2	Moderately well differentiated
G3	Poorly differentiated
G4	Undifferentiated

Additional Descriptions

cTNM (or TNM)	Clinical, increasing size or local extension
pTNM	Pathologic
rTNM	Recurrence of tumor after disease-free interval
aTNM	First determined at autopsy

Stage Grouping

0	Tis, N0, M0
I	T1, N0, M0
IIA	T0, N0, M0
	T1, N1, M0
	T2, N0, M0
IIB	T2, N1, M0
	T3, N0

and prognosis. Other methods for grouping cancers have been shown to be less effective for providing adequate descriptions of the extent of disease, determining treatment options, and comparing treatment results.[27]

TREATMENT

Surgical Risk

Assessment of surgical risk is based on a number of factors. The physical status of the oncologic patient and the debilities that often accompany the disease process present specific challenges to the surgical team. Patients should undergo a complete evaluation before surgery, and any history of cardiac, pulmonary, hepatic, or renal disease should be documented. Emphasis should be placed on physiologic function rather than chronologic age. A study conducted at the Mayo Clinic in 1989 showed that patients 90 years of age and older tolerated the stress of a surgical procedure fairly well.[28] The physical status of the patients in the study was assessed using the American Society of Anesthesiologists Physical Status Classification (Table 27-7).

The performance scales most widely used by oncologic specialists are the Eastern Cooperative Oncology Group Performance Scale (ECOG-PS) and the Karnofsky Performance Status (KPS) rating. These performance scales are also useful to surgeons and anesthesiologists in determining operative risk. A comparison of the ECOG-PS and KPS ratings showed both methods to be valid prognostic indicators of functional status, but the ECOG-PS seemed slightly superior. If necessary, each can be converted to the other with sufficient accuracy.[29] These two classifications are outlined in Table 27-8.

Mortality caused by anesthetic complications is most often related to the physical status of the patient. Highly sophisticated techniques of anesthesia have increased the safety of major oncologic procedures. Many of these advances have their basis in modern cardiac surgery and transplantation, especially liver transplantation. The choice of anesthetic technique and agent should be appropriate for both the procedure and the patient. For example, surgery in the lower abdominal area, lower extremities, or pelvis may be performed with general or spinal anesthesia, depending on the patient's health status. The risk to the patient who has evidence of congestive heart failure would likely be increased by the use of general anesthesia as opposed to spinal anesthesia. However, patients with a history of ischemic heart disease may become agitated during a surgical procedure in which they are awake, thereby causing myocardial stress. The surgeon should work closely with the anesthesiologist to ensure proper selection of anesthetic application. Epidural-assisted general anesthesia is increasingly used for abdominal surgery, and provides an opportunity for improved pain management during postsurgical recovery.

TABLE 27-7

American Society of Anesthesiologists Physical Status Classification

CLASS	DESCRIPTION
I	Healthy patient
II	Mild systemic disease, no functional limitation
III	Severe systemic disease, definite functional limitation
IV	Severe systemic disease that is a constant threat to life
V	Moribund patient unlikely to survive 24 hours with or without operation

From Miller RD: Principles and Practice of Anesthesia, 2nd ed. New York, Churchill Livingstone, 1986, with permission.

TABLE 27-8

Eastern Cooperative Oncology Group Performance Scale (ECOG-PS) and Corresponding Karnofsky Rating

ECOG-PS GRADE	DESCRIPTION	KARNOFSKY RATING
0	Fully active, able to carry on all predisease activities without restriction	100
1	Restricted in physically strenuous activity, but ambulatory and able to carry out work of a light or sedentary nature (e.g., light housework, office work)	80–90
2	Ambulatory and capable of all self-care, but unable to carry out any work activities; up and about more than 50% of waking hours	60–70
3	Capable of only limited self-care; confined to bed or chair 50% or more of waking hours	40–50
4	Completely disabled; cannot carry on any self-care; totally confined to bed or chair	≤30

The oncologic patient is a particularly challenging surgical candidate. Operative mortality is usually defined as mortality that occurs within 30 days of a major operative procedure. The operative mortality statistics for oncologic patients can be deceptive. For example, patients who undergo a palliative procedure have a very high operative mortality rate, even if the surgery is successful. The cancer surgeon is ultimately responsible for ensuring that surgical intervention is safely undertaken, with an awareness of the possible risks and complications.

Surgery for Primary Cancer

At times, the cancer surgeon alone will be responsible for patient outcome, whereas at other times, a combination of therapeutic modalities may enhance the prospect of cure or quality of life. Surgery should always be extended or restricted with these considerations in mind. The cancer surgeon must think first as an oncologist and attempt to envision the entire course of a particular disease and its treatment. If surgery is indeed the best treatment option, then the surgeon may act on that conclusion.[30]

Appropriate treatment of primary cancer varies with the individual cancer type and the area involved. The cardinal principle of surgical cure is total removal of neoplastic tissue. This involves avoiding implantation of loose tumor cells; minimizing iatrogenic, lymphatic, and vascular dissemination of cancer cells; and obtaining a complete margin of normal tissue around the primary tumor (Table 27-9).

Surgical treatment is often combined with other modalities to improve outcome. To coordinate the appropriate care of the patient, the surgeon must fully understand the indications, risks, and benefits of using systemic and radiologic therapy, especially when the benefits of such modalities have been adequately studied in prospective clinical trials.

Surgery for Metastases

In many cases, patients in whom a single site of metastatic disease has been detected can undergo resection with a reasonable rate of success. Many patients with a limited number of metastases to sites such as the liver, brain, or lung can be cured by surgical resection. For example,

published experience indicates that resection of colorectal metastases to the liver should be performed when: (1) the number of liver tumors is less than four, (2) extrahepatic tumor is not demonstrable, and (3) a tumor-free margin of at least 10 mm can be obtained. The 5-year survival rate is 30% to 40% when all of these criteria are met.[31] Resection of pulmonary metastases in patients with soft tissue and bony sarcomas can cure as many as 30% of patients. The surgeon must consider a number of elements before undertaking surgery for metastatic disease. These include tumor histology, disease-free interval, tumor-doubling time, and the location, size, and extent of disease.

Cytoreductive Surgery

The results of experimental studies suggest that cytoreduction, or debulking of recurrent cancer, has important potential benefits. In the laboratory setting, reduction of the tumor increases the sensitivity of the remaining tumor to chemotherapy and radiation therapy by increasing the proportion of proliferating tumor cells, decreasing the number of therapeutic cycles necessary to eradicate the tumor, increasing cellular distribution of oxygen and nutrient within the tumor, and reducing the likelihood that resistant clones will develop.[32]

Evidence of human clinical benefit seems to be more limited. The benefits of cytoreduction are most dramatic when accompanied by effective chemotherapy or radiation; therefore, the value of cytoreduction has been acknowledged in pediatric solid tumors, lymphoma, and carcinoma of the ovary. Widespread application of cytoreduction, either alone or combined with other treatment modalities, lacks firm clinical support for common carcinomas.

TABLE 27-9

Adequate Margins of Resection

A complete margin of normal tissue around the primary lesion
Frozen sections used to evaluate tissue margins in instances of doubt
Complete removal of involved regional lymph nodes
Resection of involved adjacent organ
En bloc resection of biopsy tracts and tumor sinuses

Palliative Surgery

Palliative surgery is undertaken to relieve symptoms in the absence of cure. It is specifically designed to improve quality of life, and must be undertaken with this in mind. Examples of palliative surgery include relief of intestinal obstruction, removal of tumors to control pain or hemorrhage, and introduction of a feeding jejunostomy to permit adequate nutrition.

Reconstructive and Rehabilitative Surgery

Quality of life is an important consideration in the care of the patient with cancer. The cancer surgeon has the unique responsibility to attend to the patient's cosmetic as well as curative surgical needs. Breast reconstruction after mastectomy, transfer of tissue after head and neck surgery, and lysis of contractures or muscle transposition to restore muscular function after radiation therapy are examples of techniques that offer the patient with cancer a higher degree of comfort and improved quality of life.

Vascular Access

Placement of short-term and long-term indwelling central venous catheters has become a common surgical procedure performed on cancer patients. These catheters provide venous access for chemotherapeutic infusion and withdrawal of blood. A number of important developments in implantation technique and catheter design have decreased operative time and rendered this an almost exclusively outpatient procedure (see Chapter 52).

Surgery for Oncologic Emergencies

The patient with cancer presents a unique surgical risk. These patients are often neutropenic and thrombocytopenic, and have a high risk of hemorrhage and sepsis. The most common emergencies involve hemorrhage, perforation, intestinal obstruction, infection, or vital organ failure (see Chapter 53). When presented with an oncologic surgical emergency, the cancer surgeon must carefully assess the situation.

EDUCATION AND THE CANCER SURGEON

All surgical oncologists have an educational responsibility and teaching role that should extend to their hospital staff, students, residents, fellows, colleagues, and the community. The surgical oncologist should have the capacity to develop effective training programs, laboratory research programs, treatment guidelines, clinical trials, and protocols. The unique responsibility of being both a consultant in surgery and an oncologist falls to the cancer surgeon. In addition, surgical oncologists must teach other surgeons and surgical residents how to incorporate oncology principles into their practice.

A number of studies have shown a deficiency of cancer education for undergraduate medical students.[33,34] There is growing concern that the practice of cancer care by community surgeons will not succeed unless there are fundamental changes in surgical residency training programs and continuing education that more fully incorporate oncology principles.

In his presidential address to the SSO, Charles M. Balch outlined the education concerns most relevant to cancer surgeons: (1) developing more oncology educational materials, (2) increasing the educational effect on the training of surgical residents and medical students by strengthening liaisons with educational organizations in all oncologic disciplines, and (3) increasing the effect on continuing education by strengthening liaisons with national cancer organizations.[17]

David Sloan at the University of Kentucky, Lexington, has pointed out that faculty rarely observe residents interacting with patients with cancer, and surgical residents receive little formal education in oncology.[35,36] He and his group have studied the use of the Objective Structured Clinical Examination (OSCE) to evaluate individual resident performance and the effectiveness of educational programs designed to improve the oncologic clinical skills of general surgical residents.[36-38] They have correctly concluded that there is a pressing need for introducing a comprehensive performance-based educational program in oncology for surgical trainees. Sloan and colleagues have suggested and tested an intriguing modification of the OSCE for instruction, called the Structured Clinical Instruction Module. In a recent multi-institutional study, they showed its effectiveness in teaching clinical skills needed in the treatment of breast cancer.[39,40] It is clearly up to the surgical oncology faculty at each institution to initiate and direct such programs.

The surgical oncologist can provide leadership in academic institutions and provide the department with the credibility needed to be involved in decisions regarding resource allocation at the medical school as well as policy-making with regard to the institution's cancer program. Where programs in surgical oncology have been successful, they have had the appropriate critical intellectual mass and have been embraced enthusiastically by the department chair. As a result, the overall clinical, research, and educational programs of the department have all benefited.[41]

FUTURE DIRECTIONS

A major growth area in the surgical subspecialties is surgical oncology. Advances in cancer management demand an increasing supply of surgical oncology specialists who can fulfill a wide variety of functions in the rapidly changing environment of cancer care. Surgical oncologists must become increasingly knowledgeable about basic science, especially as it relates to the molecular and cellular processes of cancer development and metastases. With the completion of the human genome project, cancer surgeons, like their colleagues in medical oncology and radiation oncology, are entering a new era of molecular medicine.

Cancer, perhaps more than any major disease, will be at the forefront of discovery in this new era. Already we understand cancer as a disease that arises from changes within the DNA of specific tissue cells during their life span. These changes in the DNA of cells occur through deletions, amplifications, mutations, and translocations. They result in the production of growth-stimulating proteins or their receptors, a loss of proteins that normally act to control cell growth through regulation of the cell cycle or the normal apoptotic process of cell death, and DNA changes that result in a loss of ability to repair DNA when the process of DNA replication produces detrimental defects. The tremendous advances in genetics and cancer biology have spawned a new era of genomic and proteomic research.

Thus, the discipline of surgical oncology will be effected significantly in several ways. Perhaps the most notable of these will be derived from the intense efforts that are underway to understand the complete intracellular circuitry and the defects associated with various solid tumors. From this effort will come a new portfolio of validated molecular targets for therapeutic intervention and cancer prevention. These new agents promise to be easy to administer and significantly less toxic than the chemotherapy used today. The caveat, however, is that there will not be a single "magic bullet," and each patient's tumor must be carefully characterized to determine its specific potential therapeutic targets and matched to a rational regimen of unique molecularly targeted agents.

Almost certainly, the cancer surgeon will have an increasing role in the management of patients, from diagnosis through prevention of recurrence.[42] For the cancer surgeon, there will be a greater requirement to work in a multidisciplinary fashion in patient care. The cancer surgeon will need to play an increasing role in risk assessment, management of genetic screening, and cancer prevention. As a result, cancer surgeons must be well trained in the fundamentals of cancer biology, pharmacogenetics, and genetics. The cancer surgeon must possess experience and skills in the design and management of clinical trials, monitoring of adverse events, and statistical evaluation of end points. The types of cancer operations and the scope of surgical resection may also change as molecular techniques enhance oncologic treatment.[43]

The French writer Albert Camus said, "Real generosity toward the future lies in giving all to the present." Care of the patient with cancer is a complex process that requires devotion to the principle that each patient must be provided with the best treatment possible. Surgical oncology is a specialized core body of knowledge that is used to evaluate the best treatment and management options for each patient. The surgical oncologist attends to the future by providing leadership in education and research and forming meaningful partnerships with other oncologic disciplines to continue to provide the best possible patient care.

REFERENCES

1. Sigerist HE: A History of Medicine, vol. 1. Primitive and Archaic Medicine. New York, Oxford University Press, 1951.
2. Warren JC, Hayward G, Morton W: Surgical observations on tumors with cases and operations. Boston Med Surg J 1846;35:309.
3. Bishop WJ: The Early History of Surgery. London, Robert Hale, 1960.
4. Warren JC: Surgical observations on tumors with cases and operations. London, Churchill, 1838.
5. Hill GJ: Historic milestones in cancer surgery. Semin Oncol 1979;6:409.
6. Halsted WS: Surgical papers by William Stewart Halsted, vols. 1, 2. In Burket WC (ed): Baltimore, Johns Hopkins Press, 1924. (Reprinted in The Classics of Surgery Library, spec ed), Birmingham, AL, Gryphon Editions, 1984.
7. Wangensteen OH: Has medical history importance for surgeons? Surg Gynecol Obstet 1975;140:434.
8. Kausch W: Das carcinom der papilla duodenia und seine radikale entfernung. Beitrage Klin Chir 1912;78:439.
9. Whipple AO, Parsons WB, Mullins CR: Treatment of carcinoma of the ampulla of Vater. Ann Surg 1935;102:763.
10. Junor EJ, Hole DJ, Gillis CR: Management of ovarian cancer: Referral to a multidisciplinary team matters. Br J Cancer 1994;70:363.
11. Morton DL, Eilber FR, Townsend CM Jr, et al: Limb salvage from a multidisciplinary treatment approach for skeletal and soft tissue sarcomas of the extremity. Ann Surg 1976;184:268.
12. Lokich JJ, Silvers S, Brereton H, et al: Free-standing cancer centers: Rationale for improving cancer care delivery. Am J Clin Oncol 1989;12:402.
13. Balch CM, Bland KI, Brennan MF, et al: What is a surgical oncologist (editorial)? Ann Surg Oncol 1994;1:2.
14. Brennan MF: The surgeon as a leader in cancer care: Lessons learned from the study of soft tissue sarcoma. J Am Coll Surg 1996;182:520.
15. Schweitzer RJ, Edwards MH, Lawrence W Jr, et al: Training guidelines for surgical oncology. Cancer 1981;48:2336.
16. Hill GJ, Mohit-Tabatabai MA, Rush BF Jr: A decade of training in surgical oncology. J Surg Oncol 1995;58:1.
17. Balch CM: Surgical oncology in the 21st century: Presidential address. Arch Surg 1992;127:1272.
18. O'Higgins N: Towards a high standard of surgical oncology throughout Europe. Eur J Cancer 1995;31A(Suppl 6):S22.
19. Temple WJ, Morton DI, Mattheiem W, et al, for the World Federation of Surgical Oncology Societies: Surgical Oncology training programme guidelines. Eur J Surg Oncol 1996;22:538.
20. Engstrom PF: Cancer prevention and control priorities for the year 2000: A commentary. Cancer 1994;74(Suppl):1433.
21. Love RR: Cancer prevention through health promotion: Defining the role of physicians in public health. Cancer 1994;74(Suppl): 1418.
22. Wells SA Jr, Skinner MA: Prophylactic thyroidectomy, based on direct genetic testing, in patients at risk for the multiple endocrine

THE CANCER SURGEON

AS A CARE PROVIDER
Brings surgical skill and compassionate care to patients
Leads screening, prevention, and risk assessment programs
Facilitates molecular characterization of tumor and
  surrogate tissues
Coordinates multidisciplinary clinical care teams

AS A RESEARCHER
Facilitates laboratory research
Coordinates epidemiologic studies
Conducts clinical trials research
Develops novel approaches to education

AS A TEACHER
Ensures excellence in surgical care
Leads a multidisciplinary team to implement integrated
  oncology training

neoplasia type 2 syndromes. Exp Clin Endocrinol Diabetes 1998;106:29.

23. Lieberman D: Screening/early detection model for colorectal cancer: Why screen? Cancer 1994;74(Suppl):2023.

24. Littrup PJ: Prostate cancer screening: Appropriate choices? Cancer 1994;74(Suppl):2016.

25. Garcia-Rio F, Lobato SD, Pino JM, et al: Value of CT-guided fine needle aspiration in solitary pulmonary nodules with negative fiberoptic bronchoscopy. Acta Radiol 1994;35:478.

26. Koutrouvelis PG, Louie A, Lang E, et al: A three-dimensional stereotactic device for computed tomography-guided invasive diagnostic and therapeutic approaches. Invest Radiol 1993;28:845.

27. Rodary C, Flamont F, Donaldson SS: An attempt to use a common staging system in rhabdomyosarcoma: A report of an international workshop initiated by the International Society of Pediatric Oncology (SIOP). Med Pediatr Oncol 1989;17:210.

28. Hosking MP, Warner MA, Lobdell CM, et al: Outcomes of surgery in patients 90 years of age and older. JAMA 1989;261:1909.

29. Ferrigno D, Buccheri G: Karnofsky and ECOG performance status in lung cancer: Equivalence, construct validity, and predictive validity. Proc Annu Meet Am Soc Clin Oncol 1994;13(A1075):326.

30. Mattheiem W: 1939-1989: From oncologic surgery to surgical oncology (editorial). Eur J Surg Oncol 1989;15:471.

31. Tranberg K, Bengmark S: Metastatic tumours of the liver. In Blumgart LH (ed): Surgery of the Liver and Biliary Tract. Edinburgh, Churchill Livingstone, 1994, p 1388.

32. Wong RJ, DeCosse JJ: Cytoreductive surgery. Surg Gynecol Obstet 1990;170:276.

33. Smith WT, Tattersall MH, Irwig LM, Langlands AO: Undergraduate education about cancer. Eur J Cancer 1991;27:1448.

34. Sanidas EE, Aggelaki S, Xomeritaki H, et al: The influence of undergraduate medical cancer education on student' sensitivity towards cancer. J Cancer Educ 1993;8:19.

35. Sloan DA, Donnelly MB, Schwartz RW, et al: Assessing medical students' and surgery residents' clinical competence in problem solving in surgical oncology. Ann Surg Oncol 1994;1:204.

36. Sloan DA, Donnelly MB, Schwartz RW, et al: Measuring the ability of residents to manage oncologic problems. J Surg Oncol 1997;64:135.

37. Harden RM, Stevenson M, Downie WW, Wilson GM: Assessment of clinical competence using objective structured examination. Br Med J 1975;1:447.

38. Sloan DA, Donnelly MB, Johnson SB, et al: Use of an objective structured clinical examination (OSCE) to measure improvement in clinical competence during the surgical internship. Surgery 1993;114:343.

39. Sloan DA, Donnelly MB, Schwartz RW, et al: The multidisciplinary structured clinical instruction module as a vehicle for cancer education. Am J Surg 1997;173:220.

40. Sloan DA, Donnelly MB, Plymale MA, et al: Improving residents' clinical skills with the structured clinical instruction module for breast cancer: Results of a multiinstitutional study. Breast Cancer Education Working Group. Surgery 1997;122:324.

41. McKneally MF, Niederhuber JN, Roth JA, et al: Symposium on thoracic surgical oncology. Ann Thorac Surg 1990;50:500.

42. Niederhuber, JE: The things that matter most. Ann Surg Oncol 2002;9:709-716.

43. Arbeit JM: Molecules, cancer, and the surgeon: A review of molecular biology and its implications for surgical oncology. Ann Surg 1990;212:3.

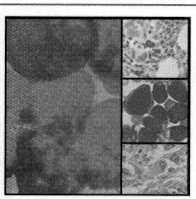

Julie M. Vose

BONE MARROW
TRANSPLANTATION

SUMMARY OF KEY POINTS

- Reestablishment of hematopoiesis and immune function after marrow ablative therapy can be accomplished with hematopoietic stem cells obtained from the bone marrow, peripheral blood, or fetal cord blood.
- The major complication of allogeneic transplants is graft-versus-host disease, whereas the limiting problem in autologous and syngeneic transplants is tumor recurrence.
- The use of allogeneic transplantation to treat malignancy is limited by lack of a donor (i.e., only one fourth to one third of Americans have a human leukocyte antigen [HLA]-matched sibling); the increasing incidence of severe graft-versus-host

disease with advancing age (i.e., few would routinely recommend the procedure after age 55 years); and the documentation for the graft-versus-malignancy effect for a limited number of cancers (i.e., hematopoietic and immune system malignancies and renal cell carcinoma).

- Mini- or nonmyeloablative allogeneic transplants use less-intensive preparative regimens aimed at the host T cells and not at the malignancy in an attempt to allow engraftment (i.e., and the subsequent immune attack on the cancer) while reducing the early toxicity and mortality. The ultimate impact on mortality and cancer-free

survival is unknown, with the most success to date in chronic myelogenous leukemia (CML), low-grade lymphoid malignancies, and renal cell carcinoma.

- Autologous transplantation has become standard therapy for relapsed Hodgkin's disease and chemotherapy-sensitive aggressive non-Hodgkin's lymphoma, consolidation of initial response in multiple myeloma, some pediatric malignancies, and refractory testicular cancer. It is frequently used in the primary therapy of high-risk aggressive non-Hodgkin's lymphoma and some acute leukemias, and in relapsed follicular lymphoma.

INTRODUCTION

Bone marrow transplantation (BMT) involves the intravenous infusion of hematopoietic progenitor cells to reestablish marrow function in a patient with a damaged or defective bone marrow. In most patients undergoing BMT, the marrow injury is from high-dose chemotherapy and/or radiation therapy administered as treatment for cancer. Although some have traced the origins of BMT to patients being fed bone marrow as a treatment for hematologic disorders at the end of the 19th century,[1] a more realistic starting point is a 1939 report of a patient who received 18 mL of intravenous marrow from his brother as a treatment for aplastic anemia.[2] The beginnings of modern BMT may be traced to work showing that rodents could be protected against lethal hematopoietic injury by the intravenous infusion of bone marrow.[3] The subsequent identification of transplantation antigens (i.e., the human leukocyte antigen [HLA] system in humans) and the development of cryobiology to permit reproducibly successful freezing and thawing of hematopoietic cells laid the groundwork for the difficult and time-consuming clinical trials that have brought allogeneic and autologous BMT to their present, albeit imperfect, states. Few areas in medicine so nicely illustrate the intimate

interactions of advances in laboratory and clinical science in the development of a new treatment.

The first successful allogeneic transplants were performed during the late 1960s, and this treatment approach gained gradual acceptance during the 1970s, primarily as a treatment for leukemia.[4] Autologous BMT was first successfully used for the cure of patients with lymphoma during the late 1970s[5] and became widely applied during the 1980s. The most common indication for allogeneic transplantation is acute leukemia and non-Hodgkin's lymphoma for autologous transplantation.

ALLOGENEIC AND SYNGENEIC BONE MARROW TRANSPLANTATION

Allogeneic BMT involves the transfer of hematopoietic progenitor cells between individuals. In the special case in which the donor and recipient are genetically identical, that is, identical twins, the correct term is *syngeneic transplantation*. To most physicians, the most difficult step in transplantation is deciding that their patient has a sufficiently poor outlook with alternative therapies that it is wise to accept the risk of a transplant. Allogeneic BMT has been successfully performed after the age of 60 years, but various transplant groups consider the oldest age for fully myeloablative transplant candidates to be 55 years or younger. Because survival rates decline with increasing age, in some situations, allogeneic BMT might be the treatment of choice for a certain group of patients with cancer only younger than a certain age. A major factor in the poorer results in older patients is a higher frequency of graft-versus-host disease (GVHD). However, the patient's general health also is important, and some transplant groups make decisions about treating a patient based on their estimation of the patient's physiologic age rather than his or her calendar age. More recently, a newer concept in allogeneic transplantation has been the nonmyeloablative transplant, in which a reduced-intensity regimen is given, allowing a less-toxic regimen to be used and a greater reliance on the "graft-versus-malignancy" effect for the therapy.[6,7]

For patients without a twin, an HLA-matched sibling donor is preferable for an allogeneic BMT. Because the genes for the HLA antigens are found on chromosome 6, one would expect HLA type to follow simple mendelian genetics (i.e., any two siblings would have a 1:4 chance of sharing the same HLA type). Except for an approximate 1% chance of crossing over (i.e., genetic material switched between chromosomes during meiosis), this is the case and the basis for HLA family typing. Because of the relatively small average size of American families, only 30% to 40% of Americans actually have an HLA-identical sibling. The following formula gives the chances for any particular person to have an HLA-matched sibling: Chances of having an HLA-matched sibling = $1 - (0.75)n$, where n is the number of potential sibling donors.

For patients not fortunate enough to have an HLA-matched sibling donor, but who might benefit from an allogeneic BMT, several solutions are available. These include the identification of an unrelated but closely HLA-matched person willing to donate bone marrow, availability of closely matched cord blood, or use of a less than perfectly matched related donor. An early report of the use of an HLA-matched unrelated marrow donor for a child with acute leukemia demonstrated that this approach could be successful.[8] Subsequent reports have demonstrated that results are better with closely HLA-matched donors[9] and that T-cell (i.e., the mediator of GVHD) depletion may ameliorate the severe GVHD often seen in this setting.[10] The extremely large number of possible HLA phenotypes (i.e., the theoretical number of possibilities is greater than the total world population) make finding an unrelated donor a difficult undertaking. Fortunately, certain HLA phenotypes occur more frequently than would be expected in persons with a similar genetic background. For example, it has been estimated that a registry of 200,000 persons of European ancestry would give another person of European ancestry a 40% to 50% chance of finding an HLA-matched donor.[11,12] The National Marrow Donor Program has been developed to facilitate unrelated BMT in the United States.[13] Because of the imprecision of traditional serologic studies, HLA typing at the molecular level by using oligonucleotide probes has been widely adopted in identifying unrelated donors.

An alternate approach is to identify related individuals who share some but not all HLA antigens.[14] Successful allogeneic BMT can be performed in this setting, although the risk of graft rejection and GVHD appears to be increased. Current results of transplantation with HLA-mismatched related donors suggest that mismatching gives fewer good results than with perfectly matched related donors, and the results become worse with higher degrees of mismatching.[14]

Once a donor has been identified, the next step is the use of high doses of chemotherapy and/or radiation therapy to accomplish three goals. The cytotoxic regimen is necessary to provide a sufficient degree of immunosuppression to avoid destruction of the allograft by residual immunologically active cells in the host and to destroy any residual cancer cells in the patient, and in some situations, the preparative regimen must provide "space" for the new marrow to grow. The choice of agents for a high-dose preparative regimen for BMT is somewhat limited. For example, dose escalation with doxorubicin is not practical because of its cardiotoxicity. Most preparative regimens for BMT use some combination of radiation therapy, alkylating agents, etoposide, and cytarabine. Even combinations of these agents used at high doses are not always truly myeloablative. With T-cell–depleted allogeneic transplants, some patients are eventually found to be mixed chimeras, indicating the survival of host hematopoietic stem cells.[15,16]

AUTOLOGOUS BONE MARROW TRANSPLANTATION

Autologous BMT involves re-establishing hematopoietic cell function in patients after high-dose therapy for cancer. The reinfused hematopoietic progenitor cells can come from the bone marrow or the peripheral blood (i.e., often referred to as peripheral stem cell transplantation). Autologous BMT differs from allogeneic BMT in a variety of ways (Table 28-1). Autologous BMT can be performed in older patients with comparative safety, probably because of the absence of GVHD as a major complication. If it becomes practical to remove hematopoietic stem cells from a patient, replace a defective gene, or add a missing one, and then transplant the altered cells, autologous BMT would be used as a part of genetic therapy for cancer.[17]

A major concern with autologous BMT is the reinfusion of viable tumor cells. Numerous methods, including in vitro treatment with chemotherapeutic agents or monoclonal antibodies plus complement, have been developed to remove contaminating tumor cells from the graft,[18,19] a process often referred to as *purging*, or to concentrate hematopoietic stem cells,[20,21] a process referred to as *positive selection*. Retrospective analyses have suggested that purging leads to a reduced relapse rate in patients with acute myeloid leukemia (AML)[18] and B-cell non-Hodgkin's lymphomas.[19] Tumor cells can be cultured from histologically negative bone marrow in some patients with lymphoma, leukemia, and breast cancer,[21-25] and patients with positive cultures have a poorer outlook. However, relapses often occur at sites of previously

TABLE 28-I

	ALLOGENEIC	AUTOLOGOUS
Comparison of Allogeneic and Autologous Bone Marrow Transplantation		
Oldest age to which applicable	40–55	60–70
Major problem in finding a donor	Finding a closely HLA-matched sibling or willing unrelated donor	Ability to collect sufficient numbers of hematopoietic progenitor cells uncontaminated by tumor cells
Most important complication	Graft-versus-host disease	Relapse of original disease
Anticancer effect of infused cells	Proved or suspected in a number of malignancies	Probably no—but data regarding cyclosporine-induced graft-versus-host effect or possible antilymphoma effect of peripheral stem cells are interesting
Most commonly treated cancers	Chronic myeloid leukemia, acute myeloid leukemia, acute lymphoid leukemia	Breast cancer, non-Hodgkin's lymphoma, Hodgkin's disease

HLA, human leukocyte antigen.
Adapted from Armitage JO: Bone marrow transplantation. N Engl J Med 1994;330:827, with permission.

known disease, raising the question of treatment resistance rather than reinfusion of tumor cells as the cause of relapse. This limits the ability of controlled clinical trials to answer the question definitively. This topic remains controversial and is not likely to be settled until gene-transfer experiments make it clear exactly which patients are likely to relapse because of tumor cells in the graft.[26] Using monoclonal antibodies such as rituximab before stem cell collection has also become a popular method of "in vivo" purging.[27]

MECHANICS OF BONE MARROW TRANSPLANTATION

Currently used methods for harvesting bone marrow are modifications of the technique reported by Thomas and Storb.[28] Marrow is usually harvested by repeated aspirations from the posterior iliac crest until an adequate number of cells has been removed. If sufficient cells cannot be obtained from the posterior iliac crest, marrow also can be harvested from the anterior iliac crest and sternum. The minimal number of nucleated marrow cells required for long-term repopulation in humans is not precisely known. In practice, the number of nucleated marrow cells harvested is usually 1 to 3 × 10^8/kg of recipient weight, depending on the diagnosis (i.e., higher for aplastic anemia), the type and intensity of pre-transplant conditioning, and whether the marrow graft will be modified in vitro. Marrow harvest is generally well tolerated.[29-31] Marrow is sometimes treated in vitro to remove unwanted cells before being returned to the patient. In allogeneic BMT with major ABO incompatibility between donor and recipient, it is necessary to remove the mature erythrocytes from the graft to avoid a hemolytic transfusion reaction.[32,33]

More recently, autologous transplantation also has been accomplished by concentrating circulating hematopoietic progenitor cells.[34] In general, at least 1 × 10^6 CD34+ cells are collected. The cells can be collected with no attempt to increase the number of circulating progenitor cells[35] during the recovery phase from exposure to chemotherapy,[36] after the administration of hematopoietic growth factors,[37] or by using both chemotherapy and growth factors.[37] It appears that cells collected during the administration of both granulocyte-macrophage (GM-CSF) or granulocyte colony-stimulating factor (G-CSF) lead to prompt and complete hematologic reconstitution.[37-39] Although it has been suggested that the speed of recovery is faster with blood cells than with marrow, a more significant factor in many cases might be the extent of primary cytotoxic therapy, with heavily pretreated patients recovering more slowly. The use of G-CSF seems to lead to an accelerated recovery of circulating neutrophils and platelets.[39] In patients being treated for lymphoma with autologous BMT, one retrospective study found better event-free survival in patients who had hematopoietic progenitors collected from the peripheral blood, rather than from the marrow.[40]

COMPLICATIONS OF BONE MARROW TRANSPLANTATION

In addition to the anticipated problems with severe prolonged myelosuppression, BMT is associated with several unique complications. These include some previously unappreciated disorders and others that provide new insights into previously recognized diseases.

Graft-Versus-Host Disease

GVHD describes an illness that generally appears after an allogeneic BMT, predominantly manifested by symptoms and signs referable to the skin, gastrointestinal system, and liver; the severity of the condition is graded based on the involvement of these organs[41] (Table 28-2). However, the most lethal complication is often the profound immune suppression that accompanies GVHD. The pathogenesis of this condition involves immunologically

TABLE 28-2

Classification of Patients with Acute Graft-versus-Host Disease

LEVEL/GRADE	SKIN	LIVER BILIRUBIN (mg/dL)	INTESTINAL TRACT (mL diarrhea/d)
Extent of Organ Injury			
Level			
1	Maculopapular rash <25% of body surface	2–3	>500
2	Maculopapular rash 25%–50% body surface	3–6	>1000
3	Generalized erythroderma	6–15	>1500
4	Generalized erythroderma with bullous formation and desquamation	>15	Severe abdominal pain, with or without ileus
Clinical Grading			
Grade			
I	1–2	0	0
II*	1–3	1	1
III	2–3	2–3	2–3
IV†	2–4	2–4	2–4

*Grade II or higher requires skin plus either liver or intestinal involvement or both.
†Requires extreme decrease in performance status.
Modified from Armitage JO: Bone marrow transplantation. N Engl J Med 1994;330:827, with permission.

competent cells in the graft-targeting antigens on the cells of the transplant recipient and producing the syndrome. It is uncertain why some organs (e.g., kidney) are usually spared from the process. In the rare situation in which GVHD follows an unirradiated blood transfusion in an immunologically impaired patient (e.g., someone receiving therapy for Hodgkin's disease), myeloid cells also are a target for destruction, and pancytopenia is typical. However, in a BMT recipient, the myeloid cells are part of the graft.

GVHD can be divided into two somewhat distinct clinical entities referred to as acute (i.e., occurring during the first 1 to 2 months after an allogeneic BMT) or chronic (i.e., developing at least 2 to 3 months after an allogeneic BMT). Patients undergoing allogeneic BMT typically undergo prophylactic treatment administered for acute GVHD. The most popular include cyclosporine, methotrexate, tacrolimus, corticosteroids, and T-cell depletion of the graft.[42-45] Even so, most adults develop some degree of acute GVHD after allogeneic BMT. Treatment for established severe acute GVHD includes high doses of corticosteroids, antithymocyte globulin, and monoclonal antibodies.[46-48]

Chronic GVHD shares certain clinical characteristics with other immunologic disorders such as scleroderma.[49] The strongest predictive factors in its development are the occurrence of acute GVHD and increasing patient age.[50,51] Left untreated, the condition is often fatal. Treatment using prednisone, cyclosporine, and/or thalidomide has improved the long-term outlook for these patients.[52,53] Major adverse prognostic factors for patients in whom chronic GVHD develops are thrombocytopenia, progressive presentation, and elevated bilirubin.[54,55]

Evidence that GVHD also is accompanied by a graft-versus-malignancy effect includes the lower relapse rate in leukemia patients in whom GVHD develops[56,57] and the higher leukemia relapse rate observed in patients who receive T-cell–depleted allografts or transplants

from identical twins in whom GVHD would not be expected.[45,58] However, separating the dangerous effects of GVHD from the presumed graft-versus-malignancy effect has not been simple. Routine infusions of donor buffy-coat cells lead only to a higher incidence of severe GVHD.[58,59] Attempts are ongoing to induce a graft-versus-malignancy effect in patients undergoing autologous BMT by the administration of cyclosporine to alter relative numbers of suppressor and effector lymphocytes.[60]

Graft Rejection

Marrow rejection represents, in most cases, destruction of the graft by immunologically active cells in the host. This complication is most frequent in patients with aplastic anemia who do not receive total body radiotherapy or in patients receiving mismatched or unrelated transplants.[61] Predisposing factors include previous blood transfusions, less-intensive high-dose preparative regimens, the use of methotrexate rather than cyclosporine to prevent GVHD, and the use of T-cell depletion to prevent GVHD.[61] Graft rejection is less likely when patients are given transplants before any transfusions of blood products,[62] but this is often not practical. Infusion of buffy-coat preparations from the marrow donor after the transplant has been demonstrated to reduce the frequency of graft rejection but to increase the frequency of severe GVHD.[63] The major approach to prevent graft rejection has been more immunosuppressive preparative regimens.[64,65] Incorporating antithymocyte globulin into the preparative regimen appears to lead to a marked reduction in the incidence of graft rejection.[66]

Pulmonary Complications

A cause of death after allogeneic BMT is a syndrome of fever, pulmonary infiltrates, hypoxia, and adult respiratory distress syndrome (ARDS) that is frequently referred to as post-BMT or idiopathic interstitial pneumonia.[67] The risks of cytomegalovirus (CMV) pneumonia have been decreased with the use of gancyclovir as a preemptive therapy when the CMV antigen is detected in the blood. Patients at highest risk are those with severe GVHD.[68] The use of CMV-negative blood products in patients who are CMV antibody negative at BMT,[69] administration of antibodies to CMV in the form of intravenous immunoglobulin (IVIG),[70,71] and the prophylactic administration of acyclovir[72] or gancyclovir[73] to patients at high risk have all reduced the incidence of this potentially lethal complication.

Although CMV pneumonitis is unusual in patients undergoing autologous BMT,[74] a possible complication in these patients is the occurrence in the first 3 to 4 weeks after marrow infusion of a syndrome of fever, pulmonary infiltrates, hypoxia, and development of ARDS without the identification of any definite causative agent.[75] In many patients, the most likely etiology is toxicity of the cytotoxic therapy. Because these patients often demonstrate increasing hemorrhage on repeated bronchial alveolar lavages, the phenomenon has been referred to as diffuse alveolar hemorrhage. This condition often responds to high doses of corticosteroids, and their early use has reduced the otherwise high mortality rate.[76]

Veno-occlusive Disease of the Liver

Veno-occlusive disease has been frequently reported after both allogeneic and autologous BMT. The diagnosis is made when two of the three major symptoms (i.e., jaundice, tender hepatomegaly, and ascites or unexplained weight gain) are present. In severely affected patients, progressive hepatic and often renal failure develop, and the condition is frequently fatal. Predisposing factors seem to be previous hepatic injury, higher than usual doses of chemotherapeutic agents, and transplantation from mismatched or unrelated donors.[77] Therapy has generally been unsatisfactory. Thrombolytic therapy has been reported to be successful in some cases.[78]

Other Complications

A great variety of other complications have been associated with BMT. These include the development of new diseases, such as diabetes mellitus, that seem to be transplanted with the new marrow in the recipient of an allogeneic transplant.[79] Disorders such as pancreatitis can occur as a complication of medications administered during the transplant process.[80] Neurologic complications include the development of Lhermitte's sign,[81] even without the use of radiation therapy in the transplant regimen, and Guillain-Barré syndrome.[82] Ocular complications of BMT include cataracts in patients who receive total body radiation therapy and post-transplant steroids.[83]

Acute cardiac complications of BMT can be manifested by rapidly progressive heart failure and death, presumably related to high doses of cyclophosphamide.[84] This complication seems to be related to altered cyclophosphamide metabolism.[85] More recently, sudden development of cardiac tamponade has been described in allogeneic

BMT in patients with thalassemia.[86] It also has become apparent that thrombotic and thromboembolic complications occur after BMT.[87] The latter complications seem to be due to altered levels of normal circulating anticoagulants.[88]

Hematologic complications of BMT include a variety of cytopenias. Autoimmune thrombocytopenia seems to respond to treatments similar to that patients who have not had a BMT.[89] Pure red-cell aplasia has been observed.[90] Pancytopenia has been recognized secondary to hypersplenism after allogeneic BMT.[91] Thrombotic thrombocytopenic purpura/hemolytic uremic syndrome has been associated with both allogeneic and autologous BMT.[92] The outcome has been poor, although some patients can respond to traditional therapy.

Endocrine complications after BMT have been related primarily to thyroid disease.[93] The most common long-term side effect is hypothyroidism, although we have seen hyperthyroidism occurring in patients after autologous BMT.

Bladder injury manifested as hemorrhagic cystitis is a well-recognized phenomenon occurring after any therapy using cyclophosphamide.[94] However, hemorrhagic cystitis in BMT patients occasionally appears to be associated with viral infections.[95] For most patients in whom cyclophosphamide seems to be the inciting agent, a variety of treatments have been used, including bladder irrigation and the administration of the sulfhydryl-containing compound sodium 2-mercaptoethane (mesna) to bind and inactivate cyclophosphamide metabolites. Randomized studies of the latter agent have demonstrated that it is at least as effective as other approaches at preventing hemorrhagic cystitis and has less toxicity.[96,97]

MALIGNANT DISEASES TREATED WITH BONE MARROW TRANSPLANTATION

Interpretation of the results of trials of BMT is always complicated by issues of patient selection. This can lead to underestimating the efficacy of BMT if it is used as a "last-gasp" salvage approach and overestimating its efficacy if only the least problematic cases are treated. Randomized trials, which would help resolve these issues, have been very difficult to conduct. Even if we have imperfect data, however, it is still necessary to make our best recommendation to our patients.

Acute Myeloid Leukemia

Some patients with AML can be cured with high-dose chemotherapy and/or radiotherapy and allogeneic BMT, even when treated for end-stage refractory leukemia.[98] Unfortunately, the cure rate in these cases is only approximately 10%. Long-term survival and an apparent cure rate of 20% to 40% have been achieved in patients treated in second or subsequent complete remission, and cure rates of 40% to 70% have been reported in patients given transplants in first complete remission.[99-101] Because some patients can be cured with standard chemotherapy regimens without BMT, and because cure rates of 20% to 30% have been reported for BMT in early first relapse,[102] withholding BMT until the first sign of treatment failure has been an increasingly popular strategy, particularly in older patients. Attempts to compare allogeneic with autologous BMT in patients with AML have generally led to the conclusion that autologous BMT is associated with a lower treatment-related mortality but a higher leukemia relapse rate.[103] In one large prospective trial, autologous BMT using unpurged marrow was compared with allogeneic BMT.[103] Relapses were more common in the autologous BMT patients (i.e., 60% vs 34%), and the overall survival 3 years after BMT was less (37% vs 66%). However, some evidence suggests that results with autologous BMT are better with purged bone marrow.[20]

Myelodysplastic Syndrome

This group of illnesses also goes by the names *dysmyelopoietic syndrome* and *preleukemia*. In young patients, these frequently lethal conditions occasionally develop. When an HLA-identical sibling can be identified, long-term disease-free survival and cure are possible with allogeneic BMT.[104,105] It should be remembered that short survival is associated primarily with dysmyelopoietic syndromes if an increased number of marrow blasts is present,[106] and perhaps BMT should be reserved for such patients and for those with unfavorable or complex cytogenetic abnormalities.

Acute Lymphoid Leukemia

The results of standard therapy in children are sufficiently good with intensive chemotherapy regimens that BMT as part of the primary therapy should probably be performed only in special situations, such as in patients with Philadelphia (Ph) chromosome–positive acute lymphoid leukemia (ALL), in which the cure rate with standard therapy is very low.[107] Children not cured with their primary chemotherapy regimen, particularly those who relapse early, are candidates for allogeneic BMT. Patients who relapse during the first 6 months after achieving an initial remission certainly do better with allogeneic BMT than with further chemotherapy, although with intensive salvage regimens, patients who relapse later might do equally well with either approach.[108]

The comparison of allogeneic and autologous BMT in children with ALL has shown a higher relapse rate with autologous BMT but a higher early death rate with allogeneic BMT and equivalent overall survival.[109] However, most physicians who perform BMT use allogeneic BMT if an HLA-matched sibling donor is available.

Allogeneic BMT done in first complete remission in adults has been reported to produce long-term disease-free survival in 40% to 70% of patients.[110,111] However, one retrospective comparison of two large databases suggested no advantage of autologous BMT over an effective chemotherapy regimen.[112] As with children, BMT is indicated in first remission for patients whose leukemia is Ph chromosome positive[107] and, probably, in second remission for patients with a short initial remission.

Chronic Myeloid Leukemia

When allogeneic BMT was shown to produce durable remissions in a small percentage of patients with the advanced or accelerated phase of this disease,[113] investigators attempted BMT in the early or stable chronic phase[113-115] and reported prolonged hematologic and cytogenetic remissions and an apparent cure rate of 49% to 72%. Allogeneic BMT from an HLA-matched sibling donor was previously the treatment of choice for patients of an appropriate age with stable-phase chronic myeloid leukemia (CML). However, with the introduction of imatinib (Gleevac), the use of allogeneic transplantation is now performed for those patients in whom Gleevac does induce a remission, or if the patients relapse after Gleevac.[116] Patients seem to do better when given transplants within the first year after diagnosis[113] and when they receive hydroxyurea rather than busulfan as their initial therapy for the leukemia. Both splenectomy and splenic radiation as a part of the preparation have frequently been performed, but neither has improved treatment results.[117] Some studies demonstrate that the use of interferon before transplant may have a potential effect on the outcome after transplantation.[118] Autologous BMT also has been performed in CML with interesting results.[119] Some patients can survive apparently leukemia free (i.e., Ph chromosome negative) for many years, despite the transplantation of Ph-containing cells. The explanation for this observation and the eventual outcome in these patients remain uncertain.

Chronic Lymphoid Leukemia

Chronic lymphoid leukemia (CLL) usually occurs in elderly people. However, when the disease develops in younger patients, allogeneic and autologous BMT have both been used.[120-121] Both approaches have produced leukemia-free survival in more than 50% of treated patients with brief follow-up. However, with further follow-up, those patients receiving an autologous transplant have demonstrated a high relapse rate.[122] It will take many years to document the curability of this disorder with BMT because of the long natural history of this usually indolent hematologic malignancy. More recently, the use of a nonmyeloablative approach to allogeneic transplantation for CLL and indolent lymphomas has become popular because of the decreased early toxicity.[6,7]

Multiple Myeloma

Both allogeneic and autologous BMT have been performed for multiple myeloma, because standard chemotherapy regimens rarely, if ever, cure the disease. The largest series of patients reported with allogeneic BMT found a 43% complete remission rate with 50% of complete responders alive and relapse free 48 months after transplant.[123] However, 20% of the patients died before engraftment, and 38% died of possible treatment-related complications.

Autologous BMT has frequently been performed for multiple myeloma.[124-126] The complete remission rate is lower than that with allogeneic BMT, but progression-free survivals at 1 year as high as 85% have been observed.[124] The treatment-related mortality rate with autologous BMT has been much less, averaging less than 10%. Patients with progressive resistant disease or those with a very high tumor burden have a poor result and probably should not be considered for this treatment. The preferred treatment for patients with multiple myeloma is now high-dose chemotherapy and an autologous transplant after induction chemotherapy at the time of diagnosis. The use of nonmyeloablative transplantation also may be beneficial in this patient population.

Non-Hodgkin's Lymphoma

Allogeneic, syngeneic, and autologous BMT have all been reported to yield long-term disease-free survival and an apparent cure for patients with intermediate and high-grade non-Hodgkin's lymphomas.[127-129] Patients with relapsed lymphoma are more likely to be cured when treated early in the course of the disease at the time that the tumor remains sensitive to chemotherapy[128] (Fig. 28-1). It is now apparent that patients who fail to achieve an initial complete remission, but who do not have other adverse prognostic factors, such as poor performance status or bulky disease, also can achieve long-term disease-free survival.[130] Because of the superior results achieved in patients treated earlier in the course of the disease, a number of investigators have incorporated high-dose therapy and autologous BMT into the primary treatment of patients with intermediate and high-grade

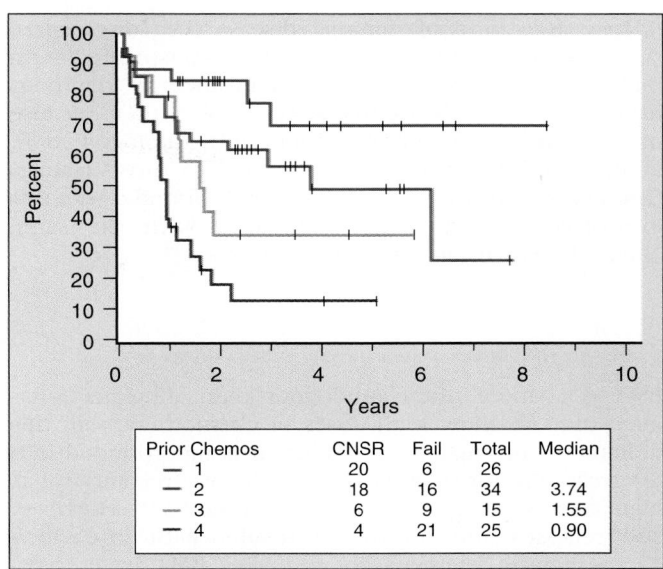

Prior Chemos	CNSR	Fail	Total	Median
— 1	20	6	26	
— 2	18	16	34	3.74
— 3	6	9	15	1.55
— 4	4	21	25	0.90

Figure 28-2. Curve represents failure-free survival after transplantation for follicular low-grade non-Hodgkin's lymphoma according to number of chemotherapy regimens patients received before transplantation. (Log-rank test, $P < .001$) (From Bierman PJ, Vose JM, Anderson JR, et al: High-dose therapy with autologous hematopoietic rescue for follicular low-grade non-Hodgkin's lymphoma. J Clin Oncol 1997;15:445, with permission.)

non-Hodgkin's lymphoma.[131-134] These results have been sufficiently encouraging (i.e., disease-free survival at 2 to 3 years of 60% to 90% in patients with poor prognostic factors) to indicate the need for controlled trials.

The use of BMT to treat patients with indolent non-Hodgkin's lymphomas is a more recent development. With either purged bone marrow or peripheral blood stem cells, disease-free survival of 40% to 60% has been seen in patients with relapsed follicular lymphoma, with median follow-up periods of approximately 3 years.[135-137] Bierman and colleagues[138] reported failure-free survivals of approximately 70% in patients given transplants only one chemotherapy failed (Fig. 28-2). However, the late relapses seen in this illness with conventional therapy make very long follow-up necessary to document the curative potential of this approach. The encouraging results seen in relapsed patients have led to early trials of the use of autologous BMT as part of primary therapy for patients with low-grade lymphoma.[139] Allogeneic transplantation for patients with recurrent indolent lymphoma have produced long-term disease-free survivals of 50% to 60%.[140,141] In addition, the use of nonmyeloablative transplantation for indolent lymphomas has become more popular.[142]

Hodgkin's Disease

High-dose therapy with autologous or allogeneic BMT has been widely performed in patients with recurrent Hodgkin's disease.[143,144] As in non-Hodgkin's lymphoma, patients have a superior result when treated soon after

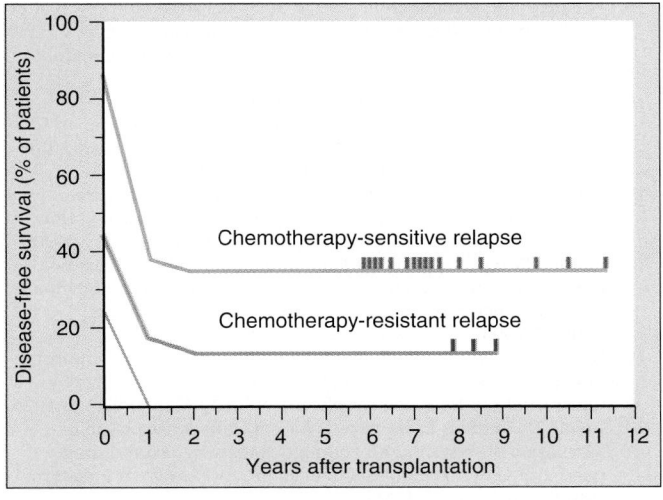

Figure 28-1. Curves represent the updated disease-free survival of 44 patients who underwent autologous bone marrow transplantation in sensitive relapse (*blue line*), 22 patients who received transplants in resistant relapse (*pink line*), and 34 patients who received transplants but never had a complete remission (*gray line*). Tic marks represent patients surviving in remission to that interval. (Data were provided by Dr. Thierry Philip from the Centre Léon-Bérard in Lyon, France, in Armitage JO: Bone marrow transplantation. N Engl J Med 1994;330:827, with permission.)

relapse at a time of minimal disease (i.e., disease-free survivals of 40% to 70%) than when transplanted with bulky disease after multiple chemotherapy regimens have failed (i.e., disease-free survival of <10%). Because of the lower treatment-related mortality, autologous BMT is preferred by most, but not all,[145,146] investigators. One controlled trial of autologous BMT found a superior event-free survival when compared with the same chemotherapy drugs given at lower doses.[145]

Neuroblastoma

BMT (i.e., more often autologous than allogeneic) has been used to allow high doses of chemotherapy in this difficult-to-cure malignancy. When it is incorporated into the treatment for stage IV disease, disease-free survival as high as 40% at 2 years has been seen.[147,148] However, late relapses and improving results with intensified chemotherapy regimens not requiring BMT have raised questions about the place of BMT in the treatment of this disorder. The data strongly suggest the need for randomized clinical trials.

Testicular Carcinoma

In patients with testicular carcinoma for whom platinum-based chemotherapy regimens fail to effect a cure, high-dose chemotherapy + autologous BMT has been used.[148,149] Disease-free survival at 2 years has been reported in 10% to 20% of these patients with far-advanced refractory disease. These results are similar to those reported in the treatment of lymphoma and suggest that results would be superior if the treatment were incorporated earlier during the course of the disease.

FUTURE OF BONE MARROW TRANSPLANTATION

Malignant diseases are likely to remain the major indication for BMT in the foreseeable future. The development of new drugs such as more effective chemotherapeutic agents and new generations of hematopoietic growth factors will undoubtedly alter the use of BMT. More effective chemotherapeutic agents may make transplantation unnecessary, and the reinfusion of hematopoietic stem cells may be made unnecessary in certain situations by more effective hematopoietic growth factors. Increasingly, better selections of patients, improved management of infections, and more rapid hematologic recovery through the use of hematopoietic growth factors will make BMT an outpatient undertaking. All these changes reduce cost. However, the major impediment to the wider application of BMT in patients who might benefit from the procedure is still likely to be economic. The place in America's developing health care policy for "high-tech" and expensive but sometimes effective therapies such as transplantation remains uncertain.

REFERENCES

1. Forkner CE: Leukemia and Allied Disorders. New York, Macmillan, 1938.
2. Osgood EE, Riddle MC, Mathews TJ: Aplastic anemia treated with daily transfusions and intravenous marrow: Case report. Ann Intern Med 1939;13:357.
3. Lorenz E, Uphoff DE, Reid TR, Shelton E: Modification of irradiation injury in mice and guinea pigs by bone marrow injections. J Natl Cancer Inst 1951;12:197.
4. Thomas ED, Storb R, Clift RA, et al: Bone marrow transplantation. N Engl J Med 1975;292:832, 895.
5. Appelbaum FR, Herzig GP, Ziegler JC, et al: Successful engraftment of cryopreserved autologous bone marrow in patients with malignant lymphoma. Blood 1978;52:85.
6. Chakraverty R, Peggs K, Chopra R, et al: Limiting transplantation-related mortality following unrelated donor stem cell transplantation by using a nonmyeloablative conditioning regimen. Blood 2002;99:1071.
7. Khouri I, Saliba RM, Giralt SA, et al: Nonablative allogeneic hematopoietic transplantation as adoptive immunotherapy for indolent lymphoma: Low incidence of toxicity, acute graft-versus-host disease, and treatment-related mortality. Blood 2001;98:3595.
8. Hansen JA, Clift RA, Thomas ED, et al: Transplantation of marrow from an unrelated donor to a patient with acute leukemia. N Engl J Med 1980;303:565.
9. Gingrich RD, Ginder GD, Goeken NE, et al: Allogeneic marrow grafting with partially mismatched, unrelated marrow donors. Blood 1988;71:1375.
10. Ash RC, Casper JT, Chitambar CR, et al: Successful allogeneic transplantation of T-cell-depleted bone marrow from closely HLA-matched unrelated donors. N Engl J Med 1990;322:485.
11. Gahrton G: Bone marrow transplantation with unrelated volunteer donors. Eur J Cancer 1991;27:1537.
12. Beatty PG, Dahlberg S, Mickelson EM, et al: Probability of finding HLA-matched unrelated marrow donors. Transplantation. 1988;45:714.
13. McCullough J, Hansen J: The National Marrow Donor Program: How it works; accomplishments to date. Oncology 1989;3:63.
14. Beatty PG, Clift RA, Mickelson EM, et al: Marrow transplantation from related donors other than HLA-identical siblings. N Engl J Med 1985;313:765.
15. Bertheas MR, Maraninchi D, Lafage M, et al: Partial chimerism after T-cell-depleted allogeneic bone marrow transplantation in leukemic HLA-matched patients: A cytogenetic documentation. Blood 1988;72:89.
16. Sondel PM, Hank JA, Trigg ME, et al: Transplantation of HLA-haploidentical T-cell-depleted marrow for leukemia: Autologous marrow recovery with specific immune sensitization to donor antigens. Exp Hematol 1986;14:278.
17. Van Bekkum DW, Bohre EPM, Houben PFJ, Knaan-Shanzer S: Regression of adjuvant-induced arthritis in rats following bone marrow transplantation. Proc Natl Acad Sci USA 1989;86:10090.
18. Gorin NE, Aegerter P, Auvert B, et al: Autologous bone marrow transplantation for acute myelocytic leukemia in first remission: A European survey of the role of marrow purging. Blood 1990;75:1606.
19. Gribben JG, Freedman AS, Neuberg D, et al: Immunologic purging of marrow assessed by PCR before autologous bone marrow transplantation for B-cell lymphoma. N Engl J Med 1991;325:1525.
20. Chang J, Coutinho L, Morgenstern G, et al: Reconstruction of haemopoietic system with autologous marrow taken during relapse of acute myeloblastic leukaemia and grown in long-term culture. Lancet 1986;1:294.
21. Shpall EJ, Stemmer SM, Johnston CF, et al: Purging of autologous bone marrow transplantation: The protection and selection of the hematopoietic progenitor cell. J Hematother 1992;1:45.
22. Philip I, Philip T, Favrot M, et al: Establishment of lymphomatous cell lines from bone marrow samples from patients with Burkitt's lymphoma. J Natl Cancer Inst 1984;73:835.
23. Sharp JG, Joshi SS, Armitage JO, et al: Significance of detection of occult non-Hodgkin's lymphoma in histologically uninvolved bone marrow by a culture technique. Blood 1992;79:1074.

24. Estrov Z, Grunbrger T, Dube ID, et al: Detection of residual acute lymphoblastic leukemia cells in cultures of bone marrow obtained during remission. N Engl J Med 1986;315:538.

25. Kemirkazik A, Kessinger A, Armitage JO, et al: Progenitor and lymphoma cells in blood stem cell harvests: Impact on survival following transplant. Bone Marrow Transplant 2001;28:207.

26. Brenner MK, Rill DR, Moen RC, et al: Gene-marking to trace origin of relapse after autologous bone-marrow transplantation. Lancet 1993;341:85.

27. Gianni AM, Magni M, Martelli M, et al: Long-term remission in mantle cell lymphoma following high-dose sequential chemotherapy and in vivo Rituximab-purged stem cell autografting (R-HDS regimen). Blood 2003;102:749.

28. Thomas ED, Storb R: Technique for human marrow grafting. Blood 1970;36:507.

29. Buckner CD, Clift RA, Sanders JE, et al: Marrow harvesting from normal donors. Blood 1984;64:630.

30. Bortin MM, Buckner CD: Major complications of marrow harvesting for transplantation. Exp Hematol 1983;11:916.

31. Kessinger A, Armitage JO: Harvesting marrow for autologous transplantation from patients with malignancies. Bone Marrow Transplant 1987;2:15.

32. Gale RP, Feig S, Ho W, et al: ABO blood group system and bone marrow transplantation. Blood 1977;50:185.

33. Jin N-R, Hill R, Segal G, et al: Preparation of red-blood-cell-depleted marrow for ABO-incompatible marrow transplantation by density-gradient separation using the IBM 2991 blood cell processor. Exp Hematol 1987;15:93.

34. Korbling M, Dorken B, Ho AD: Autologous transplantation of blood-derived hemopoietic stem cells after myeloblative therapy in a patient with Burkitt's lymphoma. Blood 1986;67:529.

35. Kessinger A, Armitage JO, Landmark JD: Autologous peripheral hematopoietic stem cell transplantation restores hematopoietic function following marrow ablative therapy. Blood 1988;71:723.

36. To LB, Shepperd KM, Haylock DN, et al: Single high doses of cyclophosphamide enable the collection of high numbers of hemopoietic stem cells from the peripheral blood. Exp Hematol 1990;18:442.

37. Gianni AM, Bregni M, Stem AC: Granulocyte-monocyte colony stimulating factor to harvest circulating hemopoietic stem cells for autotransplantation. Lancet 1989;1:580.

38. Elias AD, Ayash L, Anderson KC, et al: Mobilization of peripheral blood progenitor cells by chemotherapy and granulocyte-macrophage colony-stimulating factor for hematologic support after high-dose intensification for breast cancer. Blood 1992;79:3036.

39. Sheridan WP, Begley CG, Juttner CA: Effect of peripheral-blood progenitor cells mobilized by filgrastim (G-CSF) on platelet recovery after high-dose chemotherapy. Lancet 1992;339:640.

40. Vose JM, Anderson JR, Kessinger A, et al: High-dose chemotherapy and autologous hematopoietic stem cell transplantation for aggressive non-Hodgkin's lymphoma. J Clin Oncol 1993;11:1846.

41. Thomas ED, Storb R, Clift RA, et al: Bone-marrow transplantation. N Engl J Med 1975;292:895.

42. Storb R, Deeg HJ, Whitehead J, et al: Methotrexate and cyclosporine compared with cyclosporine alone for prophylaxis of acute graft versus host disease after marrow transplantation for leukemia. N Engl J Med 1986;324:729.

43. Ramsay NK, Kersey JH, Robison LL, et al: A randomized study of the prevention of acute graft-versus-host disease. N Engl J Med 1982;306:392.

44. Storb R, Deeg HJ, Pepe M, et al: Methotrexate and cyclosporine versus cyclosporine alone for prophylaxis of graft-versus-host disease in patients given HLA-identical marrow grafts for leukemia: Long-term follow-up of a controlled trial. Blood 1989;73:1729.

45. Mitsuyasu RT, Champlin RE, Gale RP, et al: Treatment of donor bone marrow with monoclonal anti-T-cell antibody and complement for the prevention of graft-versus-host disease. Ann Intern Med 1986;105:20.

46. Martin PJ, Schoch G, Fisher L, et al: A retrospective analysis of therapy for acute graft-versus-host disease: Initial treatment. Blood 1990;76:1464.

47. Kennedy MS, Deeg HJ, Storb R, et al: Treatment of acute graft-versus-host disease after allogeneic marrow transplantation: Randomized study comparing corticosteroids and cyclosporine. Am J Med 1985;78:978.

48. Herve P, Wijdenes J, Bergrat JP, et al: Treatment of corticosteroid resistant acute graft-versus-host disease by in vivo administration of anti-interleukin-2 receptor monoclonal antibody (B-B10). Blood 1990;75:1017.

49. Shulman HM, Sullivan KM, Weiden PL, et al: Chronic graft-versus-host syndrome in man: A long-term clinicopathologic study of 20 Seattle patients. Am J Med 1980;69:204.

50. Atkinson K, Horowitz MM, Gale RP, et al: Risk factors for chronic graft-versus-host disease after HLA-identical sibling bone marrow transplantation. Blood 1990;75:2459.

51. Storb R, Prentice RL, Sullivan KM, et al: Predictive factors in chronic graft-versus-host disease in patients with aplastic anemia treated by marrow transplantation from HLA-identical siblings. Ann Intern Med 1983;98:461.

52. Sullivan KM, Witherspoon RP, Storb R, et al: Alternating-day cyclosporine and prednisone for treatment of high-risk chronic graft-versus-host disease. Blood 1988;72:555.

53. Vogelsang GB, Farmer ER, Hess AD, et al: Thalidomide for the treatment of chronic graft-versus-host disease. N Engl J Med 1992;326:1055.

54. Sullivan KM, Witherspoon RP, Storb R, et al: Prednisone and azathioprine compared with prednisone and placebo for treatment of chronic graft-v-host disease: Prognostic influence of prolonged thrombocytopenia after allogeneic marrow transplantation. Blood 1988;72:546.

55. Wingard JR, Piantadosi S, Vogelsange GB, et al: Predictors of death from chronic graft-versus-host disease after bone marrow transplantation. Blood 1989;74:1428.

56. Weiden PL, Flournoy N, Thomas ED, et al: Antileukemic effect of graft-versus-host disease in human recipients of allogeneic-marrow grafts. N Engl J Med 1979;300:1068.

57. Weiden PL, Sullivan KM, Flournoy N, et al: Antileukemic effect of chronic graft-versus-host disease. N Engl J Med 1981;304:1529.

58. Horowitz MM, Gale RP, Sondel PM, et al: Graft-versus-leukemia reactions after bone marrow transplantation. Blood 1990;75:555.

59. Sullivan KM, Storb R, Duckner CD, et al: Graft-versus-host disease as adoptive immunotherapy in patients with advanced hematologic neoplasms. N Engl J Med 1989;320:828.

60. Yeager AM, Vogelsange GB, Jones RJ, et al: Induction of cutaneous graft-versus-host disease by administration of cyclosporine to patients undergoing autologous bone marrow transplantation for acute myeloid leukemia. Blood 1992;79:3031.

61. Champlin RE, Horowitz MM, van Bekkum DW, et al: Graft failure following bone marrow transplantation for severe aplastic anemia: Risk factors and treatment results. Blood 1989;73:606.

62. Anasetti C, Doney KC, Storb R, et al: Marrow transplantation for severe aplastic anemia: Long-term outcome in fifty "untransfused" patients. Ann Intern Med 1986;104:461.

63. Storb R, Doney KC, Thomas ED, et al: Marrow transplantation with or without donor buffy coat cells for 65 transfused aplastic anemia patients. Blood 1982;59:236.

64. McGlave PB, Haake R, Kim T, et al: Therapy of severe aplastic anemia in young adults and children with allogeneic bone marrow transplantation. Blood 1987;70:1325.

65. Champlin RE, Ho WG, Nimer SD, et al: Bone marrow transplantation for severe aplastic anemia: Effect of a preparative regimen of cyclophosphamide-low dose total lymphoid irradiation and post-transplant cyclosporine-methotrexate therapy. Transplantation 1990;49:720.

66. Storb R, Weiden PL, Sullivan KM, et al: Second marrow transplants in patients with aplastic anemia rejecting the first graft: Use of a conditioning regimen including cyclophosphamide and antithymocyte globulin. Blood 1987;70:116.

67. Wingard JR, Mellits ED, Sostrin MB, et al: Interstitial pneumonitis after allogeneic bone marrow transplantation: Nine-year experience at a single institution. Medicine (Baltimore) 1988;67:175.

68. Miller W, Flynn P, McCullough J, et al: Cytomegalovirus infection after bone marrow transplantation: An association with acute graft-v-host disease. Blood 1986;67:1162.

69. Bowden RA, Sayers M, Flournoy N, et al: Cytomegalovirus immune globulin and seronegative blood products to prevent primary cytomegalovirus infection after marrow transplantation. N Engl J Med 1986;314:1006.

70. Winston DJ, Ho WG, Lin C-H, et al: Intravenous immune globulin for prevention of cytomegalovirus infection and interstitial pneumonia after bone marrow transplantation. Ann Intern Med 1987;106:12.

71. Meyers JD, Leszcyzynski J, Zaia JA, et al: Prevention of cytomegalovirus infection by cytomegalovirus immune globulin after marrow transplantation. Ann Intern Med 1983;98:442.

72. Meyers JD, Reed ED, Shepp DH, et al: Acyclovir for prevention of cytomegalovirus infection and disease after allogeneic marrow transplantation. N Engl J Med 1988;318:70.

73. Goodrich JM, Mori M, Gleves CA, et al: Early treatment with ganciclovir to prevent cytomegalovirus disease after allogeneic bone marrow transplantation. N Engl J Med 1991;325:1601.

74. Wingard JR, Yen-Hung Chen D, Burns WH, et al: Cytomegalovirus infection after autologous bone marrow transplantation with comparison to infection after allogeneic bone marrow transplantation. Blood 1988;71:1432.

75. Robbins RA, Linder J, Stahl MG, et al: Diffuse alveolar hemorrhage in autologous bone marrow transplant recipients. Am J Med 1989;87:511.

76. Chao NJ, Duncan SR, Long GD, et al: Corticosteroid therapy for diffuse alveolar hemorrhage in autologous bone marrow transplant recipients. Ann Intern Med 1991;114:145.

77. Shulman HM, Hinterberger W: Hepatic veno-occlusive disease–liver toxicity syndrome after bone marrow transplantation. Bone Marrow Transplant 1992;10:197.

78. Bearman SI, Shuhart MC, Hinds MS, McDonald GB: Recombinant human tissue plasminogen activator for the treatment of established severe veno-occlusive disease of the liver after bone marrow transplantation. Blood 1992;80:2458.

79. Vialettes B, Maraninchi D, San Marco MP, et al: Autoimmune polyendocrine failure-type 1 (insulin-dependent) diabetes mellitus and hypothyroidism after allogeneic bone marrow transplantation. Diabetologia 1993;36:541.

80. Werlin SL, Casper J, Antoson D, Calabro C: Pancreatitis associated with bone marrow transplantation in children. Bone Marrow Transplant 1992;10:65.

81. Wen PY, Blanchard KL, Block CC, et al: Development of Lhermitte's sign after bone marrow transplantation. Cancer 1992;69:2262.

82. Eliashiv S, Brenner T, Abramsky O, et al: Acute inflammatory demyelinating polyneuropathy following bone marrow transplantation. Bone Marrow Transplant 1991;8:315.

83. Hamon MD, Gale RF, Macdonald ID, et al: Incidence of cataracts after single fraction total body irradiation: The role of steroids and graft versus host disease. Bone Marrow Transplant 1993;12:233.

84. Appelbaum FR, Strauchen JA, Graw RG: Acute lethal carditis caused by high-dose combination chemotherapy: A unique clinical and pathological entity. Lancet 1976;1:58.

85. Ayash LJ, Wright JE, Tretyakov O, et al: Cyclophosphamide pharmacokinetics: Correlation with cardiac toxicity and tumor response. J Clin Oncol 1992;10:995.

86. Angelucci E, Mariotti E, Lucarelli G, et al: Sudden cardiac tamponade after chemotherapy for marrow transplantation in thalassemia. Lancet 1992;339:287.

87. Patchell RA, White CL, Clark AW, et al: Nonbacterial thrombotic endocarditis in bone marrow transplant patients. Cancer 1985;55:631.

88. Gordon BG, Haire WD, Patton DF, et al: Thrombotic complications of BMT: association with protein C deficiency. Bone Marrow Transplant 1993;11:61.

89. Spruce W, Forman S, McMillan R, et al: Idiopathic thrombocytopenic purpura following bone marrow transplantation. Acta Haematol 1983;69:47.

90. Bierman PJ, Warkentin P, Hutchins MR, Klassen LW: Pure red cell aplasia following ABO mismatched marrow transplantation for chronic lymphocytic leukemia: Response to antithymocyte globulin. Leuk Lymphoma 1993;9:169.

91. Grigg AP, Berean K, Shore T, Phillips GL: Pancytopenia due to hypersplenism after allogeneic bone marrow transplantation. Bone Marrow Transplant 1992;10:177.

92. Silva VA, Frei-Lahr D, Brown RA, Herzig GP: Plasma exchange and vincristine in the treatment of hemolytic uremic syndrome/thrombotic thrombocytopenic purpura associated with bone marrow transplantation. J Clin Apheresis 1991;6:16.

93. Carlson K, Lonnerholm G, Smedmyr B, et al: Thyroid function after autologous bone marrow transplantation. Bone Marrow Transplant 1992;10:123.

94. Reynolds RD, Simerville JJ, O'Hara DD, et al: Hemorrhagic cystitis due to cyclophosphamide. J Urol 1969;101:45.

95. Arthur RR, Shah KV, Baust SJ, et al: Association of BK viruria with hemorrhagic cystitis in recipients of bone marrow transplants. N Engl J Med 1986;315:230.

96. Shepherd JD, Pringle LE, Barnett MJ, et al: Mesna versus hyperhydration for the prevention of cyclophosphamide-induced hemorrhagic cystitis in bone marrow transplantation. J Clin Oncol 1991;9:2016.

97. Vose JM, Reed EC, Pippert GC, et al: Mesna compared with continuous bladder irrigation as uroprotection during high-dose chemotherapy and transplantation: A randomized trial. J Clin Oncol 1993;11:1306.

98. Thomas ED, Buckner CD, Banaji M, et al: One hundred patients with acute leukemia treated by chemotherapy, total body irradiation, and allogeneic marrow transplantation. Blood 1977;49:511.

99. Thomas ED, Buckner CD, Clift RA, et al: Marrow transplantation for acute nonlymphoblastic leukemia in first remission. N Engl J Med 1979;301:597.

100. Blume KG, Beutler E, Bross KJ, et al: Bone-marrow ablation and allogeneic marrow transplantation in acute leukemia. N Engl J Med 1980;302:1041.

101. Santos GW, Tutschka PJ, Brookmeyer R, et al: Marrow transplantation for acute nonlymphocytic leukemia after treatment with busulfan and cyclophosphamide. N Engl J Med 1983;309P:1347.

102. Clift RA, Buckner CD, Applebaum FR, et al: Allogeneic marrow transplantation during untreated first relapse of acute myeloid leukemia. J Clin Oncol 1992;10:1723.

103. Lowenberg B, Verdonck LJ, Dekker AW, et al: Autologous bone marrow transplantation in acute myeloid leukemia in first remission: Results of a Dutch prospective study. J Clin Oncol 1990;8:287.

104. Appelbaum FR, Storb R, Rambert RE, et al: Treatment of preleukemic syndromes with marrow transplantation. Blood 1987;69:92.

105. O'Donnell MR, Nademanee AP, Snyder DS, et al: Bone marrow transplantation for myelodysplastic and myeloproliferative syndromes. J Clin Oncol 1987;5:1822.

106. Foucar K, Langdon RM, Armitage JO, et al: Myelodysplastic syndromes: A clinical and pathologic analysis of 109 cases. Cancer 1985;56:553.

107. Barrett AJ, Horowitz MM, Ash RC, et al: Bone marrow transplantation for Philadelphia chromosome-positive acute lymphoblastic leukemia. Blood 1992;79:3067.

108. Dopfer R, Henze G, Bender-Gotze C, et al: Allogeneic bone marrow transplantation for childhood acute lymphoblastic leukemia in second remission after intensive primary and relapse therapy according to the BFM- and CoAll-protocols: Results of the German cooperative study. Blood 1991;78:2780.

109. Kersey JH, Weisdorf D, Nesbit ME, et al: Comparison of autologous and allogeneic bone marrow transplantation for treatment of high-risk refractory acute lymphoblastic leukemia. N Engl J Med 1987;317:461.

110. Doney K, Buckner CD, Kopecky KJ, et al: Marrow transplantation for patients with acute lymphoblastic leukemia in first marrow remission. Bone Marrow Transplant 1987;2:355.

111. Chao NJ, Forman SJ, Schmidt GM, et al: Allogeneic bone marrow transplantation for high-risk acute lymphoblastic leukemia during first complete remission. Blood 1991;78:1923.

112. Horowitz MM, Messerer D, Hoelzer D, et al: Chemotherapy compared with bone marrow transplantation for adults with acute lymphoblastic leukemia in first remission. Ann Intern Med 1991;115:13.

113. Fefer A, Cheever MA, Thomas ED, et al: Disappearance of Ph¹-positive cells in four patients with chronic granulocytic leukemia

after chemotherapy, irradiation and marrow transplantation from an identical twin. N Engl J Med 1979;300:333.

114. Thomas ED, Clift RA, Fefer A, et al: Marrow transplantation for the treatment of chronic myelogenous leukemia. Ann Intern Med 1986;104:155.

115. Goldman JM, Apperley JF, Jones L, et al: Bone marrow transplantation for patients with chronic myeloid leukemia. N Engl J Med 1986;314:202.

116. Kantarjian HM, Cortes JE, O'Brien S, et al: Imatinib mesylate therapy in newly diagnosed patients with Philadelphia chromosome-positive chronic myelogenous leukemia: High incidence of early complete and major cytogenetic responses. Blood 2003;101:97.

117. Gratwohl A, Hermans J, Biezen AV, et al: No advantage for patients who receive splenic irradiation before bone marrow transplantation for chronic myeloid leukaemia: Results of a prospective randomized study. Bone Marrow Transplant 1992;10:147.

118. Talpaz M, Kantarjian HM, Kuzrock R, et al: Interferon-alpha produces sustained cytogenetic responses in chronic myelogenous leukemia. Ann Intern Med 1991;114:532.

119. Carella AM, Podesta M, Frassoni F, et al: Collection of "normal" blood repopulating cells during early hemopoietic recovery after intensive conventional chemotherapy in chronic myelogenous leukemia. Bone Marrow Transplant 1993;7:267.

120. Rabinowe SN, Soiffer RJ, Gribben JG, et al: Autologous and allogeneic bone marrow transplantation (BMT) for patients with Binet stage B and C B-cell chronic lymphocytic leukemia (B-CLL). Blood 1992;80:170a.

121. Khouri I, Thomas M, Andersson B, et al: Purged autologous bone marrow transplantation for chronic lymphocytic leukemia: Preliminary results. Blood 1992;80:66a.

122. Pavletic ZS, Bierman PJ, Vose JM, et al: High incidence of relapse after autologous stem cell transplantation for B-cell chronic lymphocytic leukemia or small lymphocytic lymphoma. Ann Oncol 1998;9:1023.

123. Gahrton G, Tura S, Ljungman P, et al: Allogeneic bone marrow transplantation in multiple myeloma. N Engl J Med 1991;325:1267.

124. Jagannath S, Vesole DH, Glenn L, et al: Low-risk intensive therapy for multiple myeloma with combined autologous bone marrow and blood stem cell support. Blood 1992;80:1666.

125. Reiffers J, Marit G, Boiron JM: Autologous blood stem cell transplantation in high-risk multiple myeloma. Br J Haematol 1989;72:296.

126. Anderson KC, Barut BA, Ritz J, et al: Monoclonal antibody-purged autologous bone marrow transplantation therapy for multiple myeloma. Blood 1991;77:712.

127. Phillips GL, Herzig RH, Lazarus HM, et al: Treatment of resistant malignant lymphoma with cyclophosphamide, total body irradiation, and transplantation of cryopreserved autologous marrow. N Engl J Med 1984;310:1557.

128. Philip T, Armitage JO, Spitzer G, et al: High-dose therapy and autologous bone marrow transplantation after failure of conventional chemotherapy in adults with intermediate-grade of high-grade non-Hodgkin's lymphoma. N Engl J Med 1987;316:1493.

129. Appelbaum FR, Sullivan KM, Buckner CD, et al: Treatment of malignant lymphoma in 100 patients with chemotherapy, total body irradiation, and marrow transplantation. J Clin Oncol 1987;5:1340.

130. Vose JM, Zhang MJ, Rowlings PA, et al: Autologous transplantation for diffuse aggressive non-Hodgkin's lymphoma in patients never achieving remission: A report from the autologous blood and marrow transplant registry (ABMTR). J Clin Oncol 2001;19:406.

131. Gulati SC, Shank B, Black P, et al: Autologous bone marrow transplantation for patients with poor-prognosis lymphoma. J Clin Oncol 1988;6:1303.

132. Haioun C, Lepage E, Gisselbrecht C, et al: Survival benefit of high-dose therapy in poor risk aggressive non-Hodgkin's lymphoma: Final analysis of the prospective LNH87-2 Protocol–A Groupe d'Etude des Lymphomes de l'Adulte Study. J Clin Oncol 2000;18:3025.

133. Santini G, Coser P, Chisesi T, et al: Autologous bone marrow transplantation for advanced stage adult lymphoblastic lymphoma in first complete remission: A pilot study of the Non-Hodgkin's Lymphoma Co-operative Study Group (NHLCSG). Bone Marrow Transplant 1989;4:399.

134. Nademanee A, Schmidt GM, O'Donnell MR, et al: High-dose chemoradiotherapy followed by autologous bone marrow transplantation as consolidation therapy during first complete remission in adult patients with poor-risk aggressive lymphoma: a pilot study. Blood 1992;80:1130.

135. Freedman AS, Ritz J, Neuberg D, et al: Autologous bone marrow transplantation in 69 patients with a history of low-grade B-cell non-Hodgkin's lymphoma. Blood 1991;77:2524.

136. Rohatiner AZS, Johnson PWM, Price CGA, et al: Myeloablative therapy with autologous bone marrow transplantation as consolidation therapy for recurrent follicular lymphoma. J Clin Oncol 1994;12:1177.

137. Bastion Y, Brice P, Haioun C, et al: Intensive therapy with peripheral blood progenitor cell transplantation in 60 patients with poor-prognosis follicular lymphoma. Blood 1995;86:3257.

138. Bierman PJ, Vose JM, Anderson JR, et al: High-dose therapy with autologous hematopoietic rescue for follicular low-grade non-Hodgkin's lymphoma. J Clin Oncol 1997;15:445.

139. Freedman AS, Gribben JG, Neuberg D, et al: High-dose therapy autologous bone marrow transplantation in patients with follicular lymphoma during first remission. Blood 1996;88:2780.

140. van Besien K, Sobocinski KA, Rowlings PA, et al: Allogeneic bone marrow transplantation for low-grade lymphoma. Blood 1998;92:1832.

141. Chopra R, Goldstone AH, Pearce R, et al: Autologous versus allogeneic bone marrow transplantation for non-Hodgkin's lymphoma: A case-controlled analysis of the European Bone Marrow Transplantation Group Registry. J Clin Oncol 1992;10:1690.

143. Carella AM, Congiu AM, Gaozza E, et al: High-dose chemotherapy with autologous bone marrow transplantation in 50 advanced resistant Hodgkin's disease patients: An Italian study group report. J Clin Oncol 1988;6:1411.

144. Armitage JO, Bierman PJ, Vose JM, et al: Autologous bone marrow transplantation for patients with relapsed Hodgkin's disease. Am J Med 1991;91:605.

145. Jones RJ, Piantadosi S, Mann RB, et al: High-dose cytotoxic therapy and bone marrow transplantation for relapsed Hodgkin's disease. J Clin Oncol 1990;8:527.

146. Linch DC, Winfield D, Goldstone AH, et al: Dose intensification with autologous bone-marrow transplantation in relapsed and resistant Hodgkin's disease: results of a BNLI randomized trial. Lancet 1993;341:1051.

147. Philip T, Zucker JM, Bernard JL, et al: Improved survival at 2 and 5 years in the LMCE1 unselected group of 72 children with stage IV neuroblastoma older than 1 year of age at diagnosis: Is cure possible in a small subgroup? J Clin Oncol 1991;9:1037.

148. Broun ER, Nichols CR, Kneebone P, et al: Long-term outcome of patients with relapsed and refractory germ cell tumors treated with high-dose chemotherapy and autologous bone marrow rescue. Ann Intern Med 1992;117:124.

149. Nichols CR, Andersen J, Lazarus HM, et al: High-dose carboplatin and etoposide with autologous bone marrow transplantation in refractory germ cell cancer: An Eastern Cooperative Oncology Group protocol. J Clin Oncol 1992;10:558.

Science of Clinical Oncology

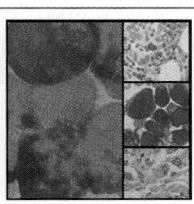

GENE THERAPY IN ONCOLOGY

James E. Talmadge

Kenneth H. Cowan

SUMMARY OF KEY POINTS

RECENT MAJOR IMPROVEMENTS IN GENE THERAPY
- Vector development.
- Vector targeting.
- Transgene expression.
- Approaches taken toward clinical development.

THERAPEUTIC PROMISE OF GENE THERAPY
- Implementation of the therapeutic promise of gene therapy has been limited by deficiencies associated with the current vectors.
- The ideal vector is one that can be targeted (either physically or via promoter expression) and is nontoxic, noninflammatory, and nonimmunogenic.
- The ideal vector should also have the potential to incorporate a large

transgene and result in high levels of both transduction and transgene expression.
- The duration of transgene expression and/or genomic integration needs to be regulatable.
- Recent clinical trials have implicated gene therapy in the death of at least one patient, resulting in the temporary suspension of clinical trials with adenovirus (Adv) vectors and the induction of leukemias in at least two and potentially three patients receiving retroviral vectors.

FIVE VECTOR ATTRIBUTES FOR FUTURE PROGRESS
- Improved efficiency of gene delivery—although many nonviral and viral vectors can induce high

gene delivery in cell lines, their potency in vivo has been poor.
- Specific targeting of cells or tissues to avoid expression of transgenes in healthy or unneeded tissues.
- Regulation of both transgene expression and duration of expression.
- Safety as a critical prerequisite.
- Low level of vector immunogenicity.

FUTURE DIRECTIONS OF GENE THERAPY
- The choice of disease and clinical implementation are critically important to the future development of gene therapy.
- Because of deficiencies in gene delivery and targeting, as well as expression levels, it is critical to pair the protocol with specific vector attributes.

INTRODUCTION

The development of deoxyribonucleic acid (DNA) assays and technologies has provided insight into the molecular basis of neoplasia. The detection of phenotypic and genotypic alterations in neoplastic diseases has increased optimism that molecular intervention might lead to improved clinical care for patients with cancer. In simple terms, gene therapy is the introduction of a nucleic acid sequence into a target cell, delivering the gene to a sufficient number of cells and with an effective level of gene expression. Both criteria require the use of a vector and, potentially, of a formulation to improve delivery. Although this approach is both simple and attractive, thus far gene therapy has promised much and delivered little because of the technical hurdles still to be overcome. A number of preclinical studies and clinical trials in cancer therapy have been undertaken to develop better gene transfer systems that are capable of modifying human tissues. The primary remaining challenges include improving the targeting of our existing vectors and increasing gene transduction efficiency. Overcoming these obstacles will facilitate the realization of targetable vectors and, given the systemic nature of most malignancies, will

help in the development of vectors that can be administered intravenously (IV). This chapter focuses on strategies to improve efficacy and on ongoing gene therapeutic strategies. We also will examine and discuss recent advances and indicate areas that require further development for clinical gene therapy to become a widely used treatment modality.

VECTORS

Viral Gene Transfer Vectors

Viral gene delivery has developed from a virus' innate ability to infect cells, which offers many intrinsic advantages:[1,2]

1. Specific cell-binding and cell-entry properties.
2. Efficient targeting of the transgene to the nucleus of the cell.
3. The ability to avoid intracellular degradation.

Most viral vectors involve the principle that an intact wild-type (wt) virus is modified for safe and effective gene transfer. In general, the more severely attenuated the viral vector is from the wt, the safer the virus is for use in gene therapy protocols and the poorer the yield obtained after propagation. Typically, two (or preferably, three) discontiguous partial or complete gene sequences are deleted to reduce the potential for homologous recombination. Deletion involves specific genes critical to viral replication that are modified or deleted, resulting in a recombinant viral vector that is "replication defective." The transgene to be delivered by the virus is typically inserted into the viral genome at the site created by the removal of viral replication genes. The transgene must be a smaller size to fit within the available space. This characteristic is critical, as the transgene cannot be packaged into an infectious particle if the new viral genome is too large. Many of the viruses that are used as vectors lack genes for replication in normal cells; therefore, the recombinant virus and its transgene must be grown in a packaging cell line that provides all of the complementary genes required for viral replication. The recombinant viral particles are purified as live infectious viruses and are replication incompetent in the absence of the packaging cell line. Alternatively, the packaging cell line can be used to infect (transduce) cells or tissues in vitro.

Retroviridae—Retrovirus

The Retroviridae is a large family of ribonucleic acid (RNA) viruses including Moloney-murine-lentivirus–related viruses (e.g., Moloney murine leukemia virus [MMLV]) and lentivirus (e.g., human immunodeficiency virus type 1 [HIV-1] and 2 [HIV-2]).[3] Their genomes consist of two identical positive-sense, single-stranded RNA molecules (~3.5 kb). The genomes are encased in a capsid along with the integrase and reverse transcriptase enzymes. Initially, retroviral vectors were the most widely used viral vectors, a distinction that has been replaced by Adv vectors in recent years. Retroviruses can transduce only those cells that are actively undergoing mitosis, which limits their utility with certain cell populations, especially hematopoietic stem cells (HSCs). Retroviral vectors provide good gene expression and are technically easy to produce, although the titers obtained are suboptimal. In addition, due to the potential for helper virus contamination, the production of retroviral vectors needs to be monitored.

Recombinant Moloney Murine Leukemia Virus (MMLV).

Most of the retroviral vectors that are used for gene therapy are based on MMLV. Vector replication is prevented by the deletion of the *gag*, *pol*, and *env* gene regions. The *gag* region encodes the capsid proteins; the *pol* region encodes reverse transcriptase and integrase; and the *env* region encodes proteins required for receptor recognition and envelope anchoring (Fig. 29-1). The genome includes long terminal repeats (LTRs) at either end, which play vital roles in initiating DNA synthesis and regulating transcription of the viral genes. The *gag*, *pol*, and *env* gene products are supplied by a complementary packaging cell line. When a retroviral vector plasmid is introduced into a packaging cell line, viral RNA is produced, packaged into virions, and secreted into the medium. Each resultant viral particle is able to integrate itself into the genome of the host cell but is unable to produce additional viral particles because it lacks the *gag*, *pol*, and *env* genes. The transduced DNA sequences are integrated stably into the chromosomal DNA of the target cells and in this way are transferred to cellular progeny of transduced cells. Perhaps the most exciting results obtained to date with retroviral vectors are documented in the studies of severe combined immune deficiency (SCID) discussed later in this review and the gene-marking studies of Malcolm Brenner and others.[4-7] In the later studies, it was shown that tumor cells within autologous

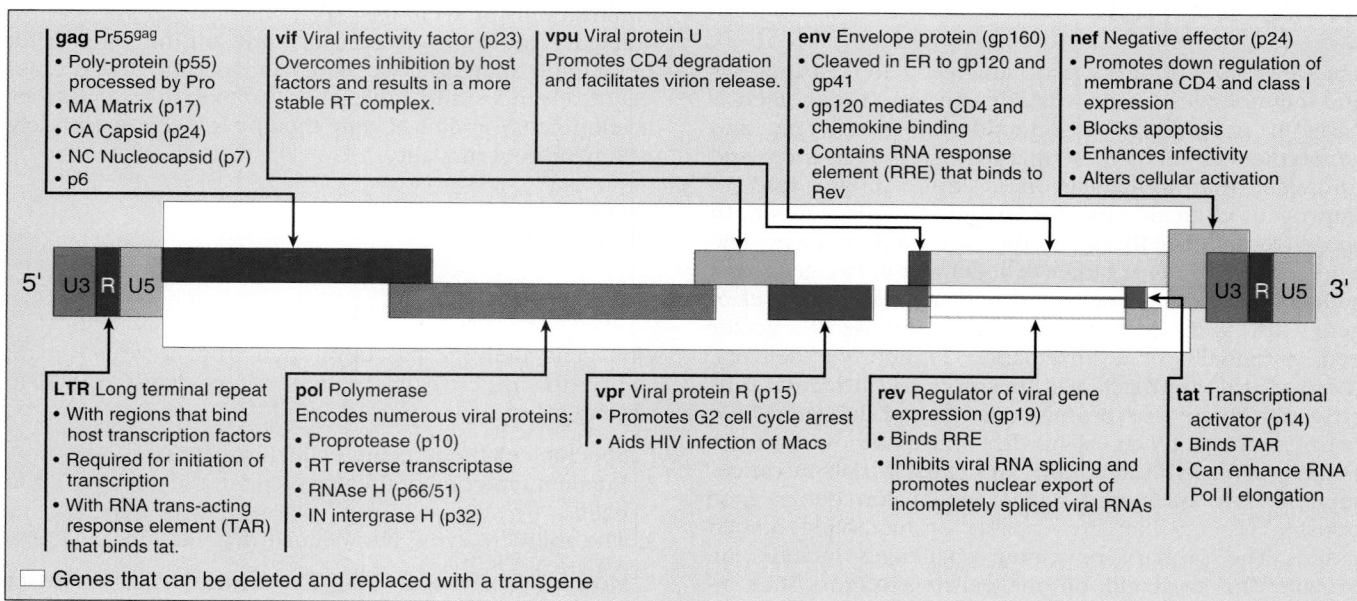

Figure 29-1. Retrovirus proviral genome and gene product functions. Overview of the 9-kb genome of the HIV provirus and a brief summary of the functions for the 9 genes encoding 15 proteins.

stem cell transplant products could be responsible for tumor relapse, at least for leukemia patients.

Recombinant Lentivirus. The most recently discovered members of the retrovirus family are the human and simian immunodeficiency viruses (HIVs and SIVs, respectively), which belong to a subclass of retroviruses known as lentiviruses.[8,9] The development of HIV gene therapy vectors has several potential advantages:

1. They can transduce actively dividing and nondividing cells.
2. Long-term, stable transgene expression occurs due to genetic integration.
3. These vectors have an inherent tropism for CD4 T cells, macrophages, and HSCs.

Genetic modifications, such as the introduction of vesicular stomatitis virus (VSV) G protein into the lentiviral envelope, can widen the tropism of this vector. Until it has been demonstrated that HIV-based vectors are safe, however, the use of these vectors for therapies targeting diseases other than HIV could be difficult to initiate clinically.[10] The in vitro efficiency of lentiviral vectors is at an acceptable level; however, in vivo expression is less efficient. Their clinical utility is dependent on the demonstration of efficiency within in vivo systems. In addition, there is a need to find protocols and/or procedures that can elevate the expression levels of the HIV virus in nondividing cells.[11,12]

Recombinant Adenovirus

Recombinant adenovirus (Adv) is a nonenveloped, icosahedral, double-stranded DNA virus with a capsid made up of 252 capsomeres (240 hexons and 12 pentons).[13] The large genome of Adv (36 kb) enables large genes to be inserted into an Adv-based vector. Transgenes in Adv vectors are not incorporated into the genome of transduced cells but rather remain as an extrachromosomal entity in the nucleus. First isolated from U.S. army recruits who had acute respiratory symptoms, Adv vectors have been found to be common human pathogens. To date, 49 serotypes have been characterized and associated with a variety of symptoms, ranging from a mild cold to acute febrile pharyngitis.[14] Replication-defective recombinant Adv vectors are currently the most commonly used viral vectors in clinical trials. Ad2 and Ad5 are used primarily for gene therapy applications. Recently, however, the Ad11 and Ad35 serotypes were shown to exhibit a unique tropism that includes HSCs, a finding that potentially widens their utility.[15-17]

The Adv vectors genome (Fig. 29-2) can be divided into two main regions, early (E) and late (L), according to the time at which their genes are expressed during virus replication. There are four regions of early genes that are termed *E1, E2, E3,* and *E4,* and one region of late genes comprising the five coding units termed *L1, L2, L3, L4,* and *L5.* The E1 region is essential for viral replication; therefore, recombinant Advs without the E1 region are considered replication defective. In a replication-defective Adv vector, the E1 region can be replaced with a transgene for expression. Further, removal of genetic material from the vector, such as the E3 and/or the E4 region, allows for larger genes to be inserted and reduces the viral immunogenicity.[18,19] Viruses without the E3 and E4 region are referred to as "gutless" and have decreased antigenicity.[20]

The E1 region of Adv vectors is subdivided into E1A and E1B. The E1A gene product is a viral transcription unit, which activates the expression of other Adv transcription units by binding to viral promoters. The E1B region codes for a 55-kD protein that interacts with the cellular p53 tumor suppressor protein and regulates the host cells' cycle progression supporting viral replication. E1B also binds to viral E4 proteins and to p53, which together act to depress host protein synthesis. The E2 region codes for viral DNA polymerase and the Adv single-stranded DNA-binding protein. The E3 region is not required for in vitro replication; however, it does offer the virus some protection against host defense mechanisms. The E4 region codes for proteins involved in:

- The regulation of viral and cellular protein expression
- The replication of viral DNA
- The switching off of host protein synthesis

The late genes (L1–L5) are expressed at the onset of viral DNA replication and code for structural polypeptides that are needed for virion assembly. This understanding

Figure 29-2. Adenovirus genome. The Adv genome is composed of early and late genes. The E1a gene encodes the initial viral transcription unit and must be deleted to prevent the recombinant virus from replicating. In most of the original Adv vectors, E1a and E1b are deleted. The second-generation vectors (known as gutless vectors) typically also have the E3 and/or E4 genes deleted. This deletion allows larger transgenes to be inserted into the Adv vector, and the deletion of E4 significantly reduces vector immunogenicity with the potential for a more prolonged transgene expression.

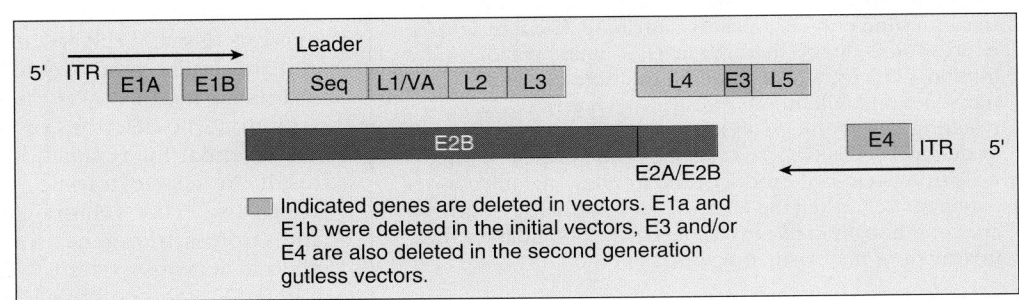

of viral replication has allowed the development of extremely elaborate, conditionally replicative Adv vectors capable of replication only in cancer cells.[21]

The transduction efficiency of Adv vectors is high compared with that of most other viral vectors. Because of the structural stability of the capsid polypeptides of Adv, viral particles can be purified and concentrated to a very high titer of ~1×10^{13} plaque-forming units (pfu)/mL. This is in contrast to retroviral titers, which achieve much lower titers (~1×10^7 pfu/mL) because of their envelopes' instability. Another distinguishing characteristic of Adv vectors is their lack of integration into the human genome. The Adv genome remains in the nucleus of the target cells as a nonreplicating extrachromosomal entity, thereby avoiding any potential for mutagenic effects caused by random integration into the host.

Potential shortcomings of Adv vectors include:

1. Transient expression, as the viral DNA does not integrate into the host.
2. Viral protein expression by the Adv vector after administration into a host.
3. A common pathogen and in vivo delivery could be hampered by the prior induction of host immunity.[1]

Because the period of Adv transgene expression is relatively short, this is a suboptimal vector if expression is desired for longer than 10 to 14 days. This short expression time is due mainly to the induction of a cytotoxic T-lymphocyte (CTL) response to viral polypeptides and, to some extent, to the transgene itself; especially if it is not expressed normally. Because the Adv genome does not integrate into the target cell, only one of the daughter cells (if the target cells are dividing) will contain the transgene. Manipulation of the immune response can result in longer expression, however. Adv gene delivery is ideally suited to those situations that require only a single period of transgene expression (for example, growth factor therapy), in which transient expression is desired. A second major

disadvantage of Adv vectors used in vivo is the immune response (CTL and antibody [Ab]), both endogenous and induced, which can preclude infection and cause the destruction of transduced cells, resulting in local tissue damage and inflammation. This shortcoming was demonstrated in the initial studies with intrabronchial delivery of Adv for the treatment of cystic fibrosis.[22,23] Host cells presenting peptides from Adv-encoded transgene products target the host cell for CTL-mediated destruction. A third major disadvantage of Adv vectors is that most humans are primed against at least one serotype, because Adv is a naturally occurring virus. Using the same serotype in a gene therapy context will likely result in a rapid and vigorous immune response, such that high levels of anti-Adv Ab occur in the sera within days of Adv vector administration. Another, similar problem is the potential secondary immune response induced by the readministration of a vector. It must be stressed that transgene expression can occur during a boost, although a shortened duration is observed. The augmentation of a CTL response by an Adv vector suggests the utility of Adv vectors as vaccine adjuvants.

Recombinant Adeno-associated Virus

Adeno-associated virus (AAV) vectors offer many of the same advantages as Adv vectors, including a wide host-cell range and a relatively high transduction efficiency.[24-26] AAV vectors stably integrate at specific sites in the host genome, and this phenomenon has the beneficial effect of a longer-lasting transgene expression. In addition, AAV vectors are stable and can infect a variety of dividing and nondividing cells, but they do not induce an immune response. AAV vectors cause little damage to target cells—unlike Adv, which can cause a high degree of cytopathogenicity. There is evidence, however, to suggest that AAV vectors are significantly less efficient than retroviral vectors at transducing primary cells, because most of their DNA remains extrachromosomal and does not integrate into the host genome. Furthermore, they cannot incorporate genes larger than 5 kb and must be screened closely for Adv contamination.

Recombinant Herpes Simplex Virus

Herpes simplex virus (HSV) vectors are developed primarily for protocols that target neuronal tissue.[27,28] Similar to Adv vectors, HSV vectors are maintained as an extrachromosomal DNA element in the nucleus of host cells but can establish long-lived asymptomatic infections in the sensory neurons of the peripheral and central nervous tissue.[29] HSV vectors also have a wide host range and are similar to Adv vectors in that they allow large gene inserts of up to 20 kb. These vectors are infective even with multiple deletions of immediate-early (IE) genes that are essential for replication, but these multiple deletions result in less cytotoxic vectors, thus reducing safety concerns.[30] HSV vectors can be produced at a high titer and express transgenes for a long period of time in the central nervous system.[31] The major concern associated with HSV is the potential for wt virus to replicate lytically

---

ADENOVIRAL VECTORS

Adenoviral (Adv) vectors have a number of positive and negative attributes. The positive attributes include the transduction of a wide profile of cellular phenotypes, including not only epithelial and carcinoma cells but also hematopoietic cells. Further, the use of Adv vectors results in a high frequency of transduction and high levels of transgene expression. A negative attribute of Adv vectors is transient expression, although for appropriate targets such transitory infection is a positive attribute. The transient expression is due to the high level of innate vector immunogenicity, which can limit multiple cycles of transduction and chronic transgene expression. The resulting Adv profile of activity is ideal for the transduction of dendritic cells (DCs) as vaccines, the purging of tumor cells from stem cell products, and intralesional injection of carcinomas. Further, the ability to develop Adv vectors that are conditionally replicative holds great potential for the treatment of neoplastic disease.

in the human brain, resulting in encephalitis. Other significant disadvantages with HSV vectors include:

1. Their requirement for additional engineering to increased efficiency.[30]
2. The transient expression associated with lytic infection and viral protein expression.
3. Their relatively low transduction efficiency.

Recombinant Vaccinia Virus

The origin of vaccinia virus (VV), the virus used for vaccination against smallpox, is not known, but it was probably derived from cowpox virus, variola virus, or a hybrid of the two.[32-35] Percutaneous VV vaccine administration results in protective cellular and humoral immune responses in greater than 95% of primary vaccinees. The recombinant VV vectors are highly attenuated, host-restricted, and non- or poorly replicating poxvirus strains (including the modified vaccinia Ankra [MVA] and canarypox or avipox vector [Alvac]) and thus do not create productive infections.[36-38] MVA is avirulent in normal and immunosuppressed animals and safe in humans.[39] Recent studies using transgenic mice provided a comparison of VV immunogenicity, including MVA and Western Reserve (WR). These studies demonstrated that MVA vaccines elicited CD8+ T-cell responses that are comparable to those induced by the replication-competent WR strain. Further, MVA vaccination was shown to be protective against a lethal respiratory challenge with the virulent WR strain.[40] The most frequent adverse complication of VV vaccination is inadvertent inoculation (usually autoinoculation) at other sites. Serious complications, which are more common among primary vaccinees and infants than among revaccinees and adults, include the following:

1. Generalized vaccinia in otherwise healthy individuals, which is generally self-limiting.
2. Eczema vaccinatum, which consists of disseminated cutaneous lesions in highly susceptible patients with eczema or other chronic skin diseases, which can be severe or even fatal.
3. Progressive vaccinia (vaccinia necrosum), which is a severe, potentially fatal illness seen in patients with immunodeficiency, whether congenital, acquired (e.g., via leukemia or lymphoma), iatrogenic (e.g., via chemotherapy or glucocorticoid treatment), or HIV-induced.
4. Postinfectious encephalitis, which is rare (three cases per million primary vaccinees), but can be fatal in 15% to 25% of cases and can leave 25% of patients with permanent neurologic sequelae.

Similar to Adv vectors, VV vectors are used for immune manipulation and as a vector for vaccines.[41] VV vectors have been employed worldwide to eradicate smallpox and, as discussed previously, provide a relatively safe live vaccine. Vaccinia vectors do not integrate into the genome of the host cell; however, they can accommodate large transgenes and are extremely immunogenic. VV vectors are used to immunize patients against tumor antigens (Ags) by cloning Ags and/or genes encoding proteins with adjuvant activity (e.g., cytokine or costimulating factor genes) into

the viral genome. Most transgenes are expressed at high levels in vivo, eliciting an Ag-specific response. Vector-induced immunity can limit the ability of the vaccinia transgenes to boost an immune response, however, which is an observation similar to that seen with Adv vectors. The current emphasis is on VV infection of dendritic cells (DCs) using a vector with an antigenic transgene.[41,42]

In association with the immunogenicity of VV vectors and their ability to deliver an antigenic transgene, they have been used clinically as a melanoma vaccine. In clinical studies by Wallack and colleagues,[43] a phase III trial of a vaccinia melanoma oncolysate, delivered as an active specific immunotherapy, was found to increase the disease-free or overall survival of patients with stage III melanoma in a surgical adjuvant setting. Other studies have used VV mutants that are conditionally replicative and can lyse cancer cells after viral replication. These vectors have been used in a strategy whereby insertional inactivation of the VV thymidine kinase (tk) gene was used to limit viral replication in cells with large intracellular nucleotide pools, such as tumor cells. In a similar approach, Mastrangelo and coworkers[44] inserted the gene for granulocyte macrophage-colony stimulating factor (GM-CSF) into the VV tk gene locus as a strategy to generate an oncolytic virus that induces antitumor immunity after infection of malignant melanoma. This vector is currently in a clinical trial of intralesional administration to patients with refractory, recurrent melanoma. In the first seven patients studied, two patients had a complete response, and three other patients had partial responses. Other oncolytic VV vectors have been engineered with cDNAs for cytokines such as interleukin 2 (IL-2) or with prodrug-activating enzymes such as cytosine deaminase (CD) to augment antineoplastic efficacy.[45,46]

The role of VV vectors as vaccines has focused predominantly on carcinoembryonic Ag (CEA) as the vaccine Ag. CEA is a glycoprotein self-Ag found on breast, lung, gastric, colon, and ovarian tumors. One such vector is a recombinant VV containing the CEA gene (rV-CEA).[47,48] In a phase I clinical trial, the safety of rV-CEA was demonstrated; however, no significant antineoplastic effects were observed.[49-51] Possible reasons for the lack of clinical efficacy in these trials include:

1. Prior exposure to the VV, leading to the development of anti-vaccinia immune responses after repeated vaccinations.
2. The advanced state of the patients' tumors.
3. A potentially compromised immune status of the patients.

A phase I rV-CEA study demonstrated that CEA-specific T-cell responses could be generated in humans after vaccination.[51] Another recombinant anti-CEA vaccine, Alvac-CEA, has been developed.[52,53] Similar to rV-CEA, Alvac-CEA contains the CEA gene, but unlike rV-CEA, it cannot replicate in mammalian cells. The safety of Alvac-CEA has been documented in a phase I trial in patients with advanced carcinomas.[54] A moderate but statistically significant increase in the number of CEA-specific CTL precursors was observed in seven of nine HLA-A2–positive patients treated with Alvac-CEA; however, objective

VACCINIA VIRAL VECTORS

Vaccinia viral (VV) vectors have a profile of activity analogous to that of adenoviral (Adv) vectors. That is, they can easily transduce a wide range of cells, resulting in transient expression, and have as a negative attribute a brief transgene expression due to the innate antigenicity of the vector. In contrast to Adv vectors, VV vectors almost inevitably lyse the transduced cell, rendering it potentially less attractive as a vector (especially for dendritic cell [DC] transduction) due to the shorter half-life of the transduced cell. Significant experience with the administration of both VV and Adv vectors as vaccines has provided a strong safety profile for both. In theory, the concomitant use of VV and Adv vectors makes possible cycles of vaccine delivery via transduced DCs, allowing a prime and boost immunization with DCs (which have a high frequency of transduction and levels of transgene expression) while reducing the concerns associated with the innate antigenicity of the viral vectors.

anticancer effects were not observed. Preclinical studies have suggested that the combination of rV-CEA and Alvac-CEA in a prime and boost protocol can induce a more vigorous T-cell response than either vaccine alone.[53] In a clinical prime and boost study, 18 patients with advanced tumors expressing CEA were randomized to receive either rV-CEA followed by three Alvac-CEA vaccinations, or Alvac-CEA (three times) followed by one rV-CEA vaccination. In this study, vaccination with rV-CEA followed by Alvac-CEA resulted in an increased frequency of Ag-specific interferon gamma (IFN-γ^+) cells by enzyme-linked immunospot assay (ELISPOT) relative to the reverse order of vaccination.[55]

Another method to enhance the responses to a vaccine is to incorporate a costimulatory signal. In the absence of a costimulatory signal, presentation of an Ag to T cells can result in anergy.[56] B7.1, which binds to CD28 on T cells, is one such costimulatory signal that results in the production of IL-2 and IFN-γ by T cells. In a vaccine study using VV vectors, 39 patients were treated with Alvac-CEA B7.1, which contains the gene for CEA.[57] In one study using the Alvac-CEA-B7.1 vaccine, patients with metastatic CEA-expressing adenocarcinomas received vaccine intradermally (ID) every 2 weeks for a total of four injections. In this phase I trial, 27% of the patients had disease stabilization after four vaccinations. Six of 31 patients with elevated serum CEA levels had a temporary decline in CEA. In addition, HLA-A2–positive patients demonstrated increased CEA-specific T-cell frequencies after three vaccinations.

Recombinant Alphavirus Vectors (Sindbis)

High-titer alphavirus vectors can induce for efficient gene delivery both in vitro and in vivo. Efficient central nervous system (CNS) infection via intranasal and vascular injections with virulent and avirulent replication-competent Semliki Forest virus (SFV) strains has been shown in animal models.[58-60] Replication-deficient alphavirus particles have a high local and transient transgene

expression in rodent brains. Further (and in contrast to Adv and VV vectors), repeated SFV injections are possible in the absence of an immunogenic response against SFV. Modifications to the envelope structure of Sindbis virus are possible, with resultant changes in host range and targeting. The favorable characteristics of alphavirus vectors include:

- Rapid production of high-titer virus.
- Broad host range.
- High RNA replication rate in the cytoplasm.
- High transgene expression levels.

Negative attributes include:

- Short-term expression.
- Strong cytotoxic effects on host cells.

Nonetheless, both these properties are advantageous for certain indicators, particularly vaccine production.

Nonviral Gene Transfer Vectors

Nonessential genes can be removed from viral vectors to allow room for transgene(s) to reduce inflammatory responses and to increase safety.[61,62] This process involves simplifying the virus, sometimes to an extreme. After undergoing such a process, a virus vector can be an artificial "vector shell" allowing the gene of interest to be expressed at high levels, in a highly regulated manner, and for a controlled period of time. Another approach to achieve the same result is to produce a vector that can introduce genetic material to the nucleus of cells.[61,63,64] This strategy has resulted in the development of several nonviral vector systems; however, the efficiency of "naked DNA" as a therapeutic is suboptimal without some form of carrier or formulation.

Direct DNA Injection/Transduction

One form of nonviral gene delivery is the use of purified DNA plasmids.[65] The transgene expression is low, however, unless hydrodynamic injection is employed.[66-68] The approach of naked DNA injection—typically intramuscular (IM)—is used with DNA vaccines and intratumoral injection. Despite the simplicity of this approach, transfection efficiency is low and results in limited expression. Various formulations, including lipid or pluronic formulations, and incorporation into nanoparticles or liposomes, have all been used to improve transduction efficacy and gene expression.[69-72]

Nonviral liposomal delivery systems can be injected intravenously with limited vector-associated toxicity, but with transgene expression, especially in the lungs.[73] Tumor targeting using tumor specific promoters, ligandation of receptors to the liposome surface, and pegylation of liposomes have all been studied.[74-82] Although some degree of tumor targeting has been observed using these delivery systems, the level of transgene expression is often depressed. Recent studies have revealed that liposome-DNA complexes can also elicit an inflammatory response when injected systemically, resulting in suppression of transgene expression.[83-88] Furthermore, failure to achieve increased or sustained gene expression after repeated

PLASMID VECTORS

The transduction efficiency of plasmid vectors is low, even with the use of formulations to improve transfection efficiency and increase transgene expression. Further, this approach appears to work better in vitro than in vivo. In contrast to viral vectors, plasmid vectors offer little innate antigenicity, although there have been reports of immune responses to bacterial genes. Positive attributes of plasmid vectors include the low level of innate immunogenicity and the potential for genomic integration. However, retroviral and (potentially) lentiviral vectors provide the same characteristics with higher levels of transgene expression and improved transduction efficiency relative to plasmids. Further, the improved transgene expression and transduction levels of retroviral and lentiviral vectors remain significantly lower than those of adenoviral and vaccinia vectors.

injections has been another major obstacle in the development of liposomes.[84,89] Recently, it was shown that cationic liposome (DOTAP:cholesterol or DOTAP:Chol)–DNA complexes can achieve effective levels of transgene expression in tumor-bearing lungs and, when injected intravenously, can achieve levels sufficient to cure immunocompetent mice with disseminated experimental metastases.[90] Further, repeated daily injections can result in a dose-dependent increase in transgene expression in tumor-bearing lungs.[91]

RNA Transduction

DNA is used primarily for transduction of DCs as a vaccine. Other Ag sources are also used with DCs, including peptides, recombinant or purified proteins, cellular extracts from tumor cells, apoptotic bodies, and DNA plasmid vectors. Nevertheless, the carrier of choice for loading DCs with tumor Ags is DNA or RNA.[92] Nucleic acid transfection leads to the display of multiple antigenic epitopes by both class I and II major histocompatibility complex (MHC) via the Ag-processing machinery of the patients' DCs, resulting in the display of the "most appropriate" peptides. This is in contrast to vaccine strategies based on synthetic peptides, which require the knowledge of the patient's unique peptide epitopes. Thus, nucleic acid transfection of DCs offers several advantages for both immunologic and practical considerations.

The bias for the use of DNA vectors includes an increased stability compared with RNA, the ability to produce plasmids in large quantities, and the ease with which the sequence can be modified to regulate expression.[93] In several respects, however, RNA vectors are also advantageous when compared with DNA transfection. RNA vector advantages include the ability to use total mRNA isolated from tumors to transfect DCs with no intervening cloning steps and the ability to express several or potentially all tumor-derived genes within DCs. Transfected RNA need only reach the cytoplasm of DCs, whereas DNA requires entry into the nucleus and

subsequent transcription. Further, it has been suggested that the low levels of antigenic epitope expression that occurs with RNA-transfected DCs could be advantageous, provided that expression levels are sufficient to generate a T-cell response.[92,93] When low levels of antigenic peptides are presented by DCs, only those T cells with high-affinity recognition are activated, thus skewing the response toward T cells that can better recognize the tumor cells. Conversely, when DCs present high levels of antigenic peptides, T cells of low affinity may be activated, thus masking or even preventing the activation of high-affinity T cells. This could result in T cells that kill cells with high Ag expression but cannot kill tumor cells, which typically express low Ag levels. Thus, RNA-transfected DCs might have greater efficacy for the activation of high-affinity T cells.[94]

Antisense

The principles of antisense technology are conceptually simple. Oligonucleotides are designed to hybridize to a defined target messenger RNA and to inhibit its translation into protein.[95-97] This approach was first employed in 1978 by Stephenson and Zamecnik[98] to inhibit the Rous sarcoma virus expression in chicken fibroblasts. Several antisense oligonucleotides are in clinical trials, and one has received Food and Drug Administration (FDA) approval for the treatment of cytomegalovirus retinitis.[98] Currently, an antisense to Bcl2 has been submitted for licensing by the FDA for the treatment of leukemia.[99] Although it is relatively easy to synthesize phosphodiester oligonucleotides, they cannot be used as drugs due to their sensitivity to nuclease degradation. To improve their resistance to nuclease digestion, different chemical modifications are used, including phosphorothioates, methylphosphonates, and phosphoramidates.[100,101] These modifications increase the stability of oligonucleotides, but they also alter the capacity to hybridize with RNA and reduce cellular internalization.

Small Interfering RNA

RNA interference is a recently discovered mechanism for silencing the transcription of mRNA. Small interfering RNA (siRNA) is generated by dicer, an endonuclease that cleaves long double-stranded RNA molecules into fragments of 21 to 23 basae pairs (bp) and are highly specific for the nucleotide sequence of its target mRNA siRNAs.[102,103] These siRNAs associate with helicase and nuclease molecules to form a large complex, termed *RNA-induced silencing complex*, which unwinds siRNA and directs precise, sequence-specific degradation of mRNA.

One potential application of this new RNA interference technology is functional genomics, where it can be used to dissect signaling pathways, identify genes important to development, and elucidate the function of novel genes in other biologic processes. Although RNA interference was discovered only recently, the field has exploded. It is now apparent that RNA interference is a highly conserved molecular mechanism that is used by eukaryotic organisms to control gene expression during development and to defend their genomes against invaders, such as transposons and RNA viruses.

Recently, it was shown that siRNA are active in vivo with resultant therapeutic activity.[104] In one study, systemic delivery of siRNAs was found to inhibit exogenous and endogenous gene expression in adult mice. Cationic liposome-based intravenous injection of a plasmid encoding the green fluorescent protein (GFP) with its cognate siRNA was found to inhibit GFP gene expression. Furthermore, an intraperitoneal (IP) injection of antitumor necrosis factor-alpha (TNF-α) siRNA has been found to inhibit lipopolysaccharide-induced TNF-α gene expression, whereas secretion of IL1-α was not inhibited. It is significant that the development of sepsis in mice after a lethal dose of lipopolysaccharide injection was substantially inhibited by pretreatment of the animals with anti-TNF-α siRNAs.

Liposomes and Virosomes

In their most basic form, liposomes consist of two lipid species: a cationic amphiphile and a neutral phospholipid.[91,105] Liposomes spontaneously bind to and condense DNA to form complexes that have a high affinity for the plasma membranes of cells, resulting in the uptake of liposomes to the cytoplasm by endocytosis. Many variations of this approach are used, resulting in varying levels of gene expression. Unfortunately, liposome-facilitated gene delivery is relatively ineffectual in vivo. More recently, some of the advantages of viral delivery vectors have been combined with the safety and "simplicity" of the liposome to produce fusigenic virosomes.[105] Virosomes are engineered by complexing the membrane fusion proteins with liposomes that have already encapsulated plasmid DNA. The inherent ability of the viral proteins in virosomes to fuse with cell membranes results in the efficient introduction of DNA to the target cell, providing improved gene expression. Viral vectors have limitations on the size of transgene that can be incorporated; in contrast, no such limit exists for virosome or liposome technology (at least in theory).

Ballistic Delivery (Gene Gun)

This physical method of gene delivery involves microcarriers (usually gold particles) coated with DNA and "fired" at high velocity using an explosive or gas-powered ballistic device called a gene gun.[106-108] Once the particles are inside the target cell, the DNA is slowly released from the microcarriers, resulting in gene transcription and translation. This application has been used extensively in vivo, but its clinical use is restricted to exposable surfaces or ex vivo transduction because the fired particles do not penetrate tissues deeply.[109]

Nanoparticles

Novel polymeric delivery systems (e.g., nanospheres), which can be administered in novel ways, are being developed.[110-112] These particles are potentially useful, as the smaller the size of the condensed DNA particles, the better the in vivo diffusion toward target cells and the trafficking within the cell. Individual plasmid molecules can be collapsed into a nanoparticle using detergents. For example, nanopartilce-based gene delivery was targeted to the neovasculature of mice using an intergrin-targeting ligand, resulting in tumor regression.[113]

GENE TARGETING

Targeted gene therapy of cancer can be achieved through:

- Targeted gene expression
- Vector targeting[13,114-116]

Although it is less important during ex vivo or intratumoral gene delivery, targeted gene therapy becomes crucial with systemic gene transfer. Impediments to gene therapy include the selectivity of existing vectors and the low efficiency of gene transfer. Overcoming these hurdles are critical to achieving vectors that can be targeted and injected intravenously—an important goal given the systemic nature of cancer.

Conditional Gene Targeting

Vector targeting is a goal for both viral and nonviral vectors.[13,114,115] The current emphasis is on tissue- or target-specific promoters, however. Transcriptional regulatory sequences are used, as they are responsible for protein production in carcinoma cells such as oncogene products. One example is the use of tissue-specific promoters to facilitate tumor-specific killing via expression of a suicide gene (such as the HSV-tk), followed by exposure to ganciclovir (GCV) or the expression of the CD gene and exposure to 5-fluorocytosine (5FC). In addition, transcriptional targeting is used to achieve conditionally targeted transgene expression.

Tissue-Specific Promoters

The production of proteins within a cell requires that the appropriate gene be transcribed into mRNA and then translated to protein.[114,117] This process is under multiple levels of control, with the regulation of transcription mediated by interactions between the enhancer/promoter region of the appropriate piece of DNA and the specific proteins or transcription factors that bind to this region. Activation or repression of promoters is achieved through interactions with specific transcription factors. Thus, some tissues might express specific proteins because the promoter for that gene is activated in that tissue alone. The success of transcriptional targeting is dependent on achieving a differential gene expression in cancer cells compared with normal cells. Transcriptional control of gene therapy is an important goal for two reasons:

1. Current gene-transfer vectors can be inefficient in gaining entry into the types of cells needing treatment.
2. Many therapeutic genes might be toxic if delivered to an unintended cellular target.

Criteria for selecting a promoter for use in a gene therapy protocol include consideration of the promoter's strength, its tissue specificity, and its size. Promoter candidates include regulatory elements that are already expressed by the malignant cell, tissue-specific promoters, or externally inducible sequences. Unfortunately, any of these candidate promoters can lack sufficient activity, specificity, or both. To address promoter potency, promoters and enhancers that retain cell-specific function are often linked to transactivators. Additional strategies to enhance promoter activity in malignant tissues include the use of cell-cycle elements, normal or abnormal tissue differentiation factors, hormones, cytokines, chemicals, or physical stimuli.

A convenient classification of candidate promoters for cancer gene therapy (Table 29-1) includes tumor-associated promoters, tissue-specific promoters, and inducible promoters. These are further discussed in the ensuing sections, as is the role of transcriptional regulation of replication-competent viruses. Specific examples are provided that are the most mature developmentally but should be viewed as representative. The most focused reviews and papers are referenced.

Tumor-Associated Promoters[118-120]

Telomerase. Telomerase, an RNA-dependent DNA polymerase that synthesizes new telomeric repeats at the end of chromosomes, is expressed in high levels in malignant tumors, stem cells, and germ cells, but not in normal

tissues. It is thought to be essential for the maintenance of the proliferative capacity of tumor cells, and for this reason it represents an attractive target for gene therapy. The human telomerase reverse transcriptase (hTERT) is regulated primarily at the transcriptional level, and its promoter has the potential for targeted cancer gene therapy.[121,122]

Tumor Vasculature. Another target for gene therapy is provided by the tumor's vasculature. The tumor vasculature has excellent accessibility to systemic delivery across all solid tumor types.[123] Indeed, high levels of vascular endothelial growth factor (VEGF), a growth stimulus for endothelial cells, have been correlated with a poor prognosis for specific tumor histotypes. VEGF activity is mediated by two high-affinity receptors: the tyrosine kinases VEGFR-1/flt-1 and VEGFR-2/flk-1. These ligand-stimulated tyrosine kinases are induced in a tumor stage-dependent manner during cancer progression and are expressed exclusively in tumor vascular endothelial

TABLE 29-1

Transcriptional Regulation for Cancer Gene Therapy

TRANSCRIPTIONAL MECHANISM	PROMOTER	TARGET TUMOR
Tissue Specificity	PSA, Kallikrein	Prostate
	Tyrosinase	Melanoma
	CEA	Hepatocellular carcinomas (HCC): breast, lung, and pancreatic cancers
	α-fetal protein (AFP)	HCC
	c-erb B2	Pancreas
	Amylase	Pancreas
	SP-B	Lung cancer
	Grp	Small cell lung carcinoma
	AVP	Small cell lung cancer
	Immunogloblin heavy chain	B lymphomas
	AP-2	Breast cancer
	α-lactalbumin	Breast cancer
	Osteocalcin	Osteosarcoma
	Prolactin	Prolactinoma
	Insulin	β-islet cells
	Whey acidic protein	Breast cancer
	Cirulatory leukoprotease inhibitor (CLPI)	Lung, colon, breast, bladder, oropharyngeal, ovarian, and endometrial carcinomas
	Glial fibrillary acidic protein	Brain astrocytes, glioma cells
	Albumin	Liver
	T-cell receptor	T lymphocytes
	Her 2/neu	Breast, pancreatic, and gastric carcinomas
	Myc-Max responsive element	Lung cancer
	MUC-1	Adenocarcinomas
Aberrant Tumor Biology	Telomerase	Urinary bladder and HCC
	FLK-1	Melanoma, fibrosarcoma, and breast tumor vessels
	E-selectin	Tumor vasculature
	VEGF	Lung cancer
	Hexokinase II	Lung cancer
	c-erb B2	Breast and pancreas tumors
	c-Myc	Small cell lung cancer
	L-plastin	Ovarian carcinoma
	SLPI	Lung and ovary tumors
Inducible Promoter	EGR-1	Glioma
	Hsp70	Prostate, breast, and melanomas
	Grp78	Fibrosarcoma
	MDR-1	Breast

cells.[124] This suggests that VEGF-receptors are promising targets for tumor endothelial cell-specific therapy.[123,125] Thus, the 939-bp Flk-1 promoter fragment and an enhancer element located in a 2.3-kb fragment upstream have been used to induce tumor endothelium-specific reporter gene expression in transgenic mice.[126] Targeting of the VEGF receptor/ligand system has been shown to be a useful approach with which to inhibit tumor growth and prolong survival in colon cancer.[125] The human preproendothelin-1 promoter has also been shown to have specificity for breast microvascular endothelial cells using a recombinant retroviral vector.[127]

Tumor-Specific Promoters

Prostate-Specific Antigen (PSA). PSA is expressed at a high level in the luminal epithelial cells of the prostate and is absent or expressed at low levels in other tissues. The PSA promoter is usually regulated by androgens, but it might retain its activity in an androgen-free environment. The minimal PSA promoter, however, is weak in both PSA-positive and PSA-negative cells and does not respond to androgenic stimuli. Nonetheless, the PSA promoter has been used to target the delivery of therapeutic genes to prostate tumors.[128-130]

Tyrosinase. Specificity for malignant melanoma may be conferred by the human tyrosinase promoter.[131-133] Driven by this promoter, in vitro and in vivo melanoma transduction by constructs results in selective transgene with the potential to induce tumor regression. Similarly, a construct consisting of the human tyrosinase promoter linked to two enhancer elements causes high-level, melanoma-specific expression of a reporter gene in transient transfection assays. The murine tyrosinase promoter-enhancer expression cassette expressed by an Adv vector maintains transcriptional specificity for pigment cell lineages, especially human melanoma cell lines.

Conditional Replication and Inducible Promoters.[134-136]

During evolution, various stress-response genes developed, and their promoters are now considered as gene therapy transcriptional regulation. Heat, hypoxia, glucose deprivation, irradiation, and chemotherapeutic agents upregulate stress response genes. Because of the relative weakness of tissue- and tumor-specific promoters, these inducible promoters are attractive as mediators of transient transgene activation. Promoters of these genes are also attractive for cancer gene therapy because they depend to a large extent on the biology of the tumor or are already induced by various therapeutic modalities.

Stress-Associated Genes. Genes that are upregulated during stress include the multidrug resistance gene-1 (MDR-1), human heat-shock protein (HSP), VEGF, irradiation-inducible Egr-1 (early growth response gene), and the tissue plasminogen activator (*tpa*) promoters. Irradiation-responsive promoter sequences have been identified for the *tpa* and Egr-1 genes.[137] The first irradiation-inducible promoter system used in combination with gene therapy involved the Egr-1 promoter driving either the radio-sensitizing cytokine TNF-α or tk. The HSP family is induced by a variety of environmental conditions, including heat, irradiation, photobeam irradiation, hypoxia, acidosis, hypoglycemia, and osmotic changes. These conditions can exist in poorly vascularized tumors and can trigger anticancer gene expression linked to the HSP70 promoter.[138] It is significant that HSP70 expression is upregulated in p53-deficient tumor cells, thereby providing transcriptional targeting.

Multidrug Resistance Genes (MDR-1). MDR-1 encodes a membrane effluxing glycoprotein, whose expression is induced by vincristine, actinomycin D, and doxorubicin. Its promoter is indirectly transactivated by these compounds and induces transcription and expression of therapeutic genes, such as TNF-α in tumors exposed to chemotherapy.[139] Chemotherapy can also induce another mechanism of drug-resistance, namely, activation of the glutathione detoxification system and apoptosis-controlling gene alterations (especially p53 and *bcl*-2). As the MDR-1 promoter contains heat-responsive elements, it is also activated by HSP. In addition to its promoter activity, MDR-1 can be transduced into hematopoitic stem cell to reduce the myelosuppressive effects of chemo- and radiotherapy.[140]

Dexamethasone.[141,142] A number of drug-related gene expression systems are available to control target gene transcription through the use of small-molecule–inducing compounds. Although the utility of such systems has been demonstrated in vitro and in transgenic mice, they are also targeting use in a therapeutic context.[143,144] Dexamethasone, a synthetic glucocorticoid, can selectively activate the p21 promoter in rat hepatoma cells via a glucocorticoid-responsive region between nucleotides 21481 and 21184.[145] This region does not contain a canonical glucocorticoid response element, but it confers specific dexamethasone responsiveness to heterologous prostate promoters.

Teracycline Response Elements. The Tet-controlled transcription system is made up of Tet-off and Tet-on transcriptional regulation, derived from the *E. coli* Tet-resistance operon.[146] The Tet-R system can be used to suppress or induce cytotoxic and reporter gene expression.[147,148] The latter selects gene expression to p53-deficient tumor cells. Similar to Tet-R, mifepristone is an orally bioavailable anti-progestin that can switch on gene expression in allosteric systems, whereby a chimeric transactivator activates a target gene.[149] This system can circumvent constitutive expression of transgenes in normal tissues by drug-specific and temporal regulation of the target gene. In addition, the replacement of the activation domain of the chimeric transactivator with a transcriptional repressor domain results in inducible repression of the transgene.[150]

Conditionally Replicative Viruses

Toxic or tumor suppressor gene expression from non-replicative vectors, as a single therapeutic, is inadequate to control solid tumor growth in humans.[151,152] Thus, replication-competent viruses (RCVs) have been developed and tested as therapeutic agents in cancer. Adv vectors are the most commonly used agents in this context, although retrovirus, reovirus, HSV, and VSV are all used for the treatment of malignancies.

The criteria governing the utility of RCV include infection efficacy, replication selectivity, viral dispersion from the injection site, and evasion of the host immune response. Augmented gene transfer efficiency has been reported for Adv vectors based on the Coxsackie Adv receptor (CAR)-independent cellular entry pathways.[153] Propagation of these vectors within tumor tissue remains a challenge, however. Recent improvements in our understanding of cancer biology have made possible the development of viral vectors with improved tumor-selective replication and the restriction of lytic effects to cancer cells. Dysregulation of the normal control over cell cycle and circumvention of physiologic apoptotic signals might allow tumor-selective replication of an engineered virus and, subsequently, direct oncolysis by viral cell killing.[154]

Conditionally Replicative Adenoviruses (CRAds).

CRAds are designed by the deletion of Adv natural genes encoding cell-cycle regulatory proteins and/or by placing a tissue-specific promoter to control a viral gene essential for viral replication. An example of a vector with a deleted Adv gene is the deletion of CRAd E1A (Table 29-2). This results in a loss of its conserved region 2, which precludes binding to the retinoblastoma gene (Rb) and eliminates the inhibitory effect of Rb on E2F. Consequently, the engineered Adv replicates selectively within cells in which the G1-S phase checkpoint is impaired (i.e., tumor cells).[155,156] Deletion of the Adv E1B 55 k protein was initially suggested to be selective for replication in p53-mutant cells, but this hypothesis has since been questioned.[157,158] Despite the mechanistic uncertainty, the E1B-deleted ONYX-015 virus selectively infects head and neck tumor cells and could show a clinical benefit in

patients with recurrent carcinomas.[159] Although ONYX-015 does not have a therapeutic transgene and relies on its lytic effect, this is the first clinical utility of a CRAd for cancer therapy. It should be noted that development of ONYX-015 was halted, primarily due to financial concerns. Recently, mutants of human Adv 5 (Ad5) with enhanced oncolytic activity have been isolated using a procedure termed *bioselection*. In this process, Ad5 is mutagenized and repeatedly passaged in a human colorectal cancer cell line. From such a cell line, mutants can be found that replicate more rapidly than wt Ad5 and that lyse cells up to a thousandfold more efficiently.[160] Another strategy for designing CRAds uses tissue-specific promoters to drive expression of E1A, thereby restricting viral replication to specific tissues or tumors.[161,162] The application of heterologous promoters in Adv vectors is difficult because their activity and specificity are often affected by viral enhancers and promoters. The E1A gene expressed from the alpha fetal protein (αFP) gene promoter induces relatively selective replication in hepatocellular carcinoma cells.[162] Control of Adv E1A expression under the minimal PSA enhancer/promoter has also been shown to confer prostate-specific oncolytic viral replication.[163] Recently, a re-engineered Adv vector with enhanced oncolytic efficacy was developed. This vector contained a novel regulatory circuit in which p53-dependent expression of an antagonist of the E2F transcription factor inhibits viral replication in normal cells. In tumor cells, however, the combination of the p53 pathway defects and deregulated E2F allows replication at near-wt levels. This Adv vector also has significantly enhanced efficacy for the treatment of human xenograft tumor models compared with the extensively studied E1B-deleted Adv vectors.[21]

CRAds for breast tumors have been created using the DF3/MUC1 promoter (which is abnormally activated in breast tumors) and are used to drive the expression of E1A. This CRAd selectively replicates in MUC1-positive cells and can inhibit the growth of human breast cancer xenografts.[164] Another approach is to target CRAd replication within estrogen receptor (ER)-positive tumors based on replacing the E1A and E4 promoters with a portion of the pS2 promoter containing two estrogen-responsive elements (EREs).[165] This promoter induces transcriptional activation of the E1A and E4 in response to estrogen in cells that express an ER. This CRAd is able to lyse ER-positive human breast cancer cell lines as efficiently as Adv, with decreased capacity to affect ER-negative cells.

Another strategy that has been reported recently employs the generation of a functional promoter/gene constellation only on Adv DNA replication, thereby providing selective transcriptional activation.[166] These strategies to discriminate between tumor and normal tissue are based on selective DNA replication of Adv vectors with the entire E1 gene in tumor cells deleted. An E1 deletion is considered to abolish Adv replication; however, human tumor cell lines apparently can support DNA replication of adenovirus with an E1 deletion. Inverted repeats (IRs) insert into the E1 region of AdE1 vectors can mediate genomic rearrangements, and bring a transgene into control of a promoter. Thus, formation of

TABLE 29-2

Transcriptional Regulation of Adv Replication	
GENETIC MODIFICATION	**BIOLOGICAL RESULT**
Deletion of E1A (AA 121-127)	Transformation deficiency
Deletion of E1B 55 K protein	Susceptibility to apoptosis
E1A control by the αFP promoter	E1A transcription limited to αFP⁺ cells
E1A control of the PSA promoter	E1A transcription limited to PSA⁺ cells
E1A control by the DF3/MUC1 promoter	E1A transcription limited to DF3/MUC1⁺ cells
E1A control by the pS2 promoter	E1A transcription limited to estrogen receptor⁺ cells
E1A control by the Sp-B promoter	E1A transcription limited to surfactant producing cells
E1 deletion	Selective DNA replication of Adv vectors in trans-complementing tumor cells

a functional expression cassette depends on viral DNA replication, which is expected to occur specifically in tumor cells.

Vector Targeting

Targeted, in vivo gene transfer is becoming a reality due to an improved understanding of influences that govern gene delivery.[13,17,114,115] Viral-based vectors are designed to avoid gene transfer through their native receptors and are redirected to tissue- and tumor-specific receptors. In most therapeutic applications, the vector is introduced into a mixed population of cells with the goal of delivering the therapeutic transgene to specific cells. Transduced stem cells can also be targeted to treat certain genetic diseases, improve tolerance to chemotherapy, or assist in tissue repair and remodeling. DCs can also be targeted for the development of improved vaccines. Finally, a systemically administered, targeted vector can potentially reach systemic disease. Nevertheless, these vectors require additional development, including clinical testing, reduced liabilities (including innate and acquired immune augmentation), and an improved understanding of the mechanisms that govern biodistribution and pharmacokinetics.

Ligand-directed targeting of gene vectors allows control of the site at which genes are expressed by imparting the capacity to distinguish between target and nontarget tissue(s). These ligand-directed targeting vectors achieve this capability through the addition of ligands to the vector that recognize receptors specific for a tissue or disease. This approach has met two goals:

1. Improved efficiency for the current gene-transfer vectors in transducing the targeted cells that need treatment.
2. Reduction in the toxicity due to delivery of therapeutic genes to unintended target cells.

Thus, ligand-directed targeting can potentially improve both the safety and the efficacy of gene transfer and make possible therapies that could not be envisioned with standard gene transfer vehicles.

Although targeting gene transfer to specific cells and tissues holds promise, it is a challenge for vector design. Regardless of the vector, three variables are critical to ligand-directed targeting. These include cellular specificity, physical barriers, and the host innate or acquired response, which could eliminate the vector from the circulation. Cellular specificity can be achieved by the use of ligands that recognize cell-specific receptors. For viral-based vectors, specificity requires a targeting element plus modification of the vector so that it no longer binds to its native cellular receptors. In the case of nonviral vectors, targeting requires modification of the vector to avoid nonspecific uptake. Apart from cellular specificity, physical barriers (e.g., the cellular matrix) can limit access of the vector to the target cell. Finally, avoiding elimination and neutralization of vectors by innate and acquired immunity is critical to gene transfer. This is critical, as Abs and serum proteins can directly inactivate the vector or direct it to the liver for rapid clearance, if the vector is given systemically.

Adenoviral Vectors

Our improved understanding of the attachment and entry processes of Adv vectors has facilitated the development of Adv-targeting vectors.[13,41,115] The nonenveloped subgroup C Adv vectors use at least two coat proteins to gain entry into cells. The knob portion of the fiber coat protein binds to the cellular receptor, coxsackievirus Adv receptor (CAR), and mediates virus attachment.[167,168] At the base of the fiber protein, the penton base coat protein contains an RGD motif that binds to integrins and facilitates vector uptake into the cell.[169] Compared with a vector with native receptor binding interactions intact, gene expression in the liver and other organs is substantially reduced after systemic administration of a vector containing mutations that ablate CAR and integrin binding.[170] This observation suggests that these receptor interactions are important for in vivo gene transfer. The loss of CAR and integrin binding also reduces gene transfer after direct injection. Further, it allows Adv vectors to be retargeted genetically.[17,171] Ablation of CAR binding alone does not significantly reduce liver gene transfer, which suggests that the standard two-step model of attachment via the CAR and entry by means of integrins does not apply to in vivo gene transfer to the liver, which instead likely involves kuffer cells.

Adv vectors have been retargeted by both genetic and nongenetic means. Peptides (including the fiber, penton base, and hexon) have been functionally incorporated into coat proteins, although few functional peptide ligands have been identified to date.[169,172-180] In addition to genetic modifications for retargeting viral vectors, ligation approaches have also been used with Adv vectors. Such approaches involve a bifunctional adaptor or bridging molecule that binds to the vector and to a target receptor. Such systems have demonstrated the feasibility of targeting conventional Adv vectors to more than 20 different receptors, including α_v integrins, endoglin, E-selectin, EpCAM, and folate receptors.[115] Specific targeting to the lung vasculature has also been demonstrated through a combination of receptor-based targeting via lung endothelial-specific receptor, angiotensin-converting enzyme (ACE), and promoter-based targeting through the endothelial-specific promoter, Flt-1.

Structural Modification of the Fiber Protein. One approach to Adv retargeting involves engineering of the knob domain of the fiber protein. In this domain, the introduction of heterologous cell targeting peptides requires consideration of the structural limitations of the fiber three-dimensional configuration. The fiber is synthesized as a monomer, which undergoes trimerization prior to its attachment to the penton base. Thus, any modification of the knob domain of the fiber must not impair trimer formation. In addition, the final quaternary configuration of the new fiber needs to make the incorporated ligand accessible to target cell receptor recognition and binding.

Recombinant Adv vectors have been constructed with a heparin/heparan sulphate-binding domain, consisting of polylysine residues added to the C-terminus of the fiber. Gene transfer to different mammalian cells has been obtained with a level of efficiency 10- to 300-fold higher compared with unmodified vector.[181] The main drawback with this approach is the lack of specificity, as most mammalian cells express heparin-containing cellular receptors. Genetic modification of the Adv fiber C-terminus is limited, as the addition of more than 25 to 30 amino acid (AA) residues renders the fiber trimer unstable and limits function.[182] The modification of Adv vectors by placing an RGD peptide in the HI loop rather than in the C-terminus of the fiber knob domain was reported recently.[173] This modification resulted in an increase in gene transfer to ovarian cancer cell lines (30- to 600-fold) and ovarian cancer cells (two- to threefold).

Modification of the Penton Base.

Retargeting of Adv vectors has also focused on the modification of the penton base, which mediates the second step of Adv infection (i.e., internalization). Recombinant Adv vectors have been generated in which the RGD motif in the penton base has been replaced by the FLAG peptide. Complexing this vector with a bispecific Ab—consisting of a monoclonal Ab to the FLAG epitope and a monoclonal Ab to integrins—was shown to target cells lacking the Adv fiber receptor, such as endothelial cells or human intestinal smooth muscle cells. Thus, the first two steps of Adv infection binding and internalization are both mediated by A_v integrins.[183] In addition, recombinant Adv vectors can be constructed of chimeric penton base proteins that recognize tissue-specific integrin receptors.[184]

Retroviral Vectors

Retroviral vectors were the first viral vectors to be targeted and the first to demonstrate the promise of vector targeting.[41,115] Since that time, the challenge has been to incorporate targeting ligands without compromising vector entry into target cells. There are now several approaches used to address this problem. One approach exploits pseudotyping, classically with the G-glycoprotein from the VSV, in which entry events are mediated through common membrane phospholipids.[185] Pseudotyped lentiviral and retroviral vectors have also been generated with glycoproteins from a variety of enveloped viruses, including Ebola virus, Marburg virus, rabies virus, LCMV, Mokola virus, human foamy virus, gibbon ape leukemia virus (GaLV), murine leukemia virus, influenza virus (HA), avian leukosis-sarcoma virus (ALSV-A), and respiratory syncytial virus.[186-195] Although these pseudotyped vectors vary in terms of degree of envelope shedding, efficiency of packaging, titer, and stability, they can be concentrated to high titers for in vivo comparisons of cellular tropisms.

Another vector modification involves the ligation of polypeptides at the N-terminal of env to extend the host range of ecotropic MLV. Examples include erythropoietin, heregulin, and CD4.[196-198] It should be stressed that coexpression of the wt *env* protein is necessary for infection to occur, possibly because incorporation of the engineered *env* protein in the virons can be facilitated by the oligomerization of both wt and chimeric *env* proteins. Another approach for engineering of the ecotropic MLV *env* protein involves the display of different polypeptide binding domains to the N-terminus of the ecotropic

Moloney MLV surface protein. Examples include the N-terminal moiety of the amphotropic MLV env, single chain Abs (ScAb) recognizing different cell surface receptors, heregulin, and epidermal growth factor (EGF).[199-205] In some of these studies, infection specificity was redefined, although with lower efficiencies than those obtained with viruses expressing wt amphotropic envelopes.[206,207]

Bifunctional bridging agents that recognize both the retrovirus and the targeted cell surface molecule provide evidence that retroviruses can enter cells via cell surface molecules that are not viral receptors. Such bridging agents have been used to infect human cells that are naturally resistant to ecotropic MLV-based vectors. The agents used usually consisted of an Ab to the MLV envelope protein connected to either another Ab or a growth factor that would bind to the appropriate receptor such as the EGFR, the insulin receptor, or MHC class I and class II molecules. Unfortunately, infection efficiencies for these agents are extremely low, emphasizing that binding of a retrovirus to a target other than the natural receptor cannot guarantee success.[208,209]

Nonviral Vectors

Nonviral vectors have no native receptor binding but do have a high incidence of nonspecific gene transfer from the high positive charge on many nonviral vectors.[62-64] Many nonviral vectors transduce lung vasculature, potentially due to vector-mediated red blood cell aggregation and arrest in the lung subsequent to intravenous administration. The solution to the problem of nonspecific delivery is to shield the vectors, either with hydrophilic polymers such as polyethylene glycol (PEG) or with a ligand to reduce the surface charge. This type of shielding is applied successfully to lipid-based systems and to cationic polymer-based systems (polyplex).

Ligand-directed liposomes have shown some success in targeting tumors. Coupling of a synthetic $\alpha_v\beta_3$-integrin ligand to cationic liposomes permits the selective delivery of a mutant *Raf* gene that causes apoptosis in angiogenic blood vessels within tumors. Systemic injection of the $\alpha_v\beta_3$-targeted liposome results in apoptosis of tumor-associated endothelium and the regression of primary and metastatic tumor(s). This accomplishment highlights the extension of this approach from in vitro to in vivo efficacy.[113]

Another promising advance is to coat polyethylenimine (PEI)-DNA polyplexes with a ligand, such as transferrin or transferrin plus PEG. Shielding by PEG or transferrin prevents nonspecific interactions with plasma proteins and erythrocytes but does not interfere with target cell interactions. When systemically administered in a sub-cutaneous tumor mouse model, the shielded complexes were shown to selectively transduce a well-vascularized, rapidly growing tumor. Although the specificity of this approach is high, the overall level of transduction is low.[210]

In all the studies to date that use nonviral approaches, the need for relatively high dosing levels (~100 µg/mouse) suggest that innate clearance mechanisms might need to be saturated before substantial gene transduction can occur. Other potential issues that remain include determining whether the high doses used in the animal studies can be manufactured and delivered successfully for human studies. Attaining further improvements in the efficiency of gene transfer and better defining the toxicity profiles associated with these vectors are also critical steps.

CLINICAL TRIAL THERAPEUTIC STRATEGIES

The development of gene therapy over the last decade has been on a roller-coaster ride that has yet to fulfill the promise of this exciting new research and therapeutic tool. Retroviral gene therapy has inarguably been shown to reverse congenic diseases. This was the first success for gene therapy, whereby a retroviral-based treatment was undertaken for infants suffering from X chromosome-linked SCID-X1. These studies provided the first demonstration of the potential for long-term treatment of hereditary diseases.[4] The success of this approach is due not only to gene therapy but also to improvements in our understanding of hematology and the availability of clinical-grade cytokines to support the transduction of adequate numbers of stem cells. These studies have resulted, however, in the concept of retroviral insertional carcinogenesis moving from a theoretic to a real concern in recent months. Two of the initial 11 children who received retroviral gene therapy for the treatment of SCID developed a leukemia-like condition.[211] Both of these cases, as well as a third in which leukemia has not yet developed, appear to be due to the insertion of the corrective gene near another gene called Lmo2, which helps to control cell growth and can contribute to cancer if turned on at the wrong time.[212] Nonetheless, the unique nature of this therapeutic strategy for patients who have no other viable therapeutic modality, and the responsiveness of the resultant leukemias to chemotherapy, suggest that it remains a justifiable therapeutic strategy for those patients who have no matching allotransplant donor. Clearly, this challenge is driving the development of alternative vectors and delivery vehicles to overcome this deficiency.

The second type of vector that has shown significant potential is the Adv vectors. In contrast to retroviral vectors, Adv vectors induce a transient gene expression and demonstrate both high transduction efficiency and high transgene expression; in addition, they can be grown to high titer for virus stocks.

Among the most important aspects associated with gene therapy are the potential to establish physiologic levels of transgene expression and the potential to regulate such expression. These advantages, coupled with the need for high levels of transduction efficiency, have resulted in the rapid development of Adv vectors. Further, the activity profile of these vectors (particularly transient gene expression) provides a focus for current clinical development strategies. Most notably, these protocols involve the induction of tumor apoptosis via systemic or interlesional injection of vectors with transgenes that induce apoptosis or result in the activation of cytotoxic drug precursors, such as TK or CD. In addition, Adv vectors

are being used to deliver Ags to Ag-presenting cells (e.g., DCs), resulting in the induction of an Ag-specific immune response and (theoretically at least) therapeutic activity.

Like retroviral vectors, Adv vectors have experienced "growing pains." Although the majority of the vectors used in current practice have been replication incompetent, the routes of administration and therapeutic targets have been variable and—in part because of this—various toxicity issues have developed. Studies using Adv-p53 vectors have shown clearly that these can be injected at doses up to approximately 7.5×10^{13} for IP administration, and 2.5×10^{13} viral particles has been identified as the maximum total dosage (MTD).[213] This same particle number, administered via the hepatic artery for the treatment of hepatic metastasis, has also been identified as the MTD.[214] Initially, Adv vectors were delivered based on PFU, a strategy found to be less rigorous quantatively when compared with a particle number strategy.[215] Yet, despite the known biodistribution and toxicity profile of Adv vectors—including Adv vectors delivered by vascular injection—one child with a non–life-threatening disease, ornithine transcarbamylase deficiency, was dosed with a high number of viral particles, resulting in his untimely demise.[216] The incident resulted in a regulatory hold on Adv for a period of time, which limited the use of Adv vectors. This toxicity problem has largely been overcome with increased clinical conservatism. Similarly, the immunologic reaction to the Adv vectors has been reduced by the use of second- or third-generation vectors (gutless), which have made a significant impact on safety, transgene expression, and duration of expression.[217] Indeed, Adv vectors have been used to deliver receptors for retroviral vectors to improve their transduction frequency.[218] Thus, retroviral and Adv vectors, in addition to "naked DNA" vectors, have predominated the clinic to date. Clearly, other agents are used, including AAV, alpha viruses, and herpes vectors, but to a lesser extent.

Several factors directly related to vectors have hampered the clinical progression of gene therapy. These include:

- Inefficient gene delivery, which is associated predominately with nonviral and retroviral vectors that have reasonable gene delivery efficacy in vitro but disappointing efficacy in vivo.
- A poor ability to target transgene expression to either cells or tissues of interest to avoid expression of toxic gene products in healthy or unintended target tissue.
- A short duration of expression due to poor replication and/or stability of episomal vectors and to inefficient or inappropriate integration of vectors into the host genome.
- Poor production of vectors at high titer, which is developmentally limiting in the cases of retroviral and gutless Adv vectors.
- Safety, which is a prerequisite for clinical gene therapy trials. Safety includes not only issues of direct toxicity but also the potential for homologous recombinant, which needs to be maintained at theoretically acceptable levels. Furthermore, targeted genomic integration has also recently been shown to be potentially critical.

Because of the challenges associated with targeting and transfection efficiency, the therapeutic strategies currently in use take advantage of the positive aspects of the vectors and limit their deficiencies. There are four overall approaches that reduce the challenges associated with the targeting and delivery of the transgene:

1. Hepatic arterial delivery of Adv p53 for the treatment of hepatic metastasis.[214,219,220]
2. Intratumoral administration of Adv vectors for head and neck tumors.[159,221,222]
3. Interlesional injection for the treatment of bladder cancer with Adv vectors.[223]
4. Intratumoral injection for the treatment of lung cancer.

The use of Adv vectors to purge hematopoietic stem cell products is also an exciting strategy that initially targeted breast cancer.[224-228] It has become a historical approach, however, with the reduction in transplantation for the treatment of metastatic breast cancer. These are the types of approaches that are needed for the successful development of gene therapeutics. The future of gutless vectors or vectors with improved targeting is bright, but at present such vectors introduce additional deficiencies such as low manufacturing titers.

The majority of gene therapy trials are focused on cancer, and in the United States slightly more than 400 protocols have been initiated for this indication. This represents approximately 63% of all clinical trials and the majority of clinical studies. The predominance of clinical vectors used are retroviral vectors, although Adv vectors are also being used extensively. The majority of therapeutic strategies are focused on immunotherapy, with the predominance of transgenes used being either cytokine or Ag. When one considers the timeline for most drug development, gene therapy is on target. Although there was considerable initial optimism, the reality is that a period of time and appropriate attention to toxicities, adverse events, and pharmacologic issues (including biodistribution and cell targeting) are required before success can be achieved. Great strides have been made as vector biology begins to catch up with improvements in vectors. It is our expectation that future successes (such as those found with SCID and retroviral vectors) can be expected, although future frustrations are also to be expected and appropriate conservatism must be maintained. One area that has a high potential for success is the utility of vectors such as VV and Adv to deliver Ags to DCs as a vaccine for the treatment of infectious diseases or tumors. Clearly, Adv and VV vectors have innate vector antigenicity, which is limiting these approaches and providing opportunities for "naked DNA" and formulated "naked DNA" for either vaccine priming or boosts. A successful clinical protocol will be achieved only if these liabilities are considered carefully, with appropriate attention to well-designed protocols that take advantage of the positive attributes of vectors and minimize their negative attributes. Within this review, we have attempted to stress the great strides have been made recently with targeting and to illustrate that the future is clearly bright.

ACKNOWLEDGMENTS

The authors wish to thank Ms. Kirsten Stites for her assistance with the preparation of the manuscript. This research was supported in part by the Nebraska Research Initiative Programs in Molecular Therapeutics (J. E. T.) and in Gene Therapy (J. E. T.).

REFERENCES

1. Lundstrom K: Latest development in viral vectors for gene therapy. Trends Biotechnol 2003;21:117–122.
2. Wickham TJ: Ligand-directed targeting of genes to the site of disease. Nat Med 2003;9:135–139.
3. McTaggart S, Al-Rubeai M: Retroviral vectos for human gene delivery. Biotechnology Advances 2002;20:1–31.
4. Cavazzana-Calvo M, Hacein-Bey S, de Saint BG, et al: Gene therapy of human severe combined immunodeficiency (SCID)-X1 disease. Science 2000;288:669–672.
5. Brenner MK, Rill DR, Moen RC, et al: Gene-marking to trace origin of relapse after autologous bone-marrow transplantation. Lancet 1993;341:85–86.
6. Rill DR, Moen RC, Buschle M, et al: An approach for the analysis of relapse and marrow reconstitution after autologous marrow transplantation using retrovirus-mediated gene transfer. Blood 1992;79:2694–2700.
7. Brenner MK, Heslop HE: Immunotherapy of leukemia. Leukemia 1992;6(Suppl 1):76–79.
8. Quinonez R, Sutton RE: Lentiviral vectors for gene delivery into cells. DNA Cell Biol 2002;21:937–951.
9. Negre D, Cosset FL: Vectors derived from simian immunodeficiency virus (SIV). Biochimie 2002;84:1161–1171.
10. Roy I: Ethical considerations in the use of lentiviral vectors for genetic transfer. Somat Cell Mol Genet 2001;26:175–191.
11. Watson DJ, Kobinger GP, Passini MA, Wilson JM, Wolfe JH: Targeted transduction patterns in the mouse brain by lentiviral vectors pseudotyped with VSV, Ebola, Mokola, LCMV, or MuLV envelope proteins. Mol Ther 2002;5:528–537.
12. Park F, Kay MA: Modified HIV-1 based lentiviral vectors have an effect on viral transduction efficiency and gene expression in vitro and in vivo. Mol Ther 2001;4:164–173.
13. Barnett BG, Crews CJ, Douglas JT: Targeted adenoviral vectors. Biochim Biophys Acta 2002;1575:1–14.
14. Shenk T. Adenoviridae. In Fields BN, Knipe DM, Howley PM (eds): Fields Virology. Philadelphia, Lippincott-Raven, 1996 pp 2111–2148.
15. Segerman A, Mei YF, Wadell G: Adenovirus types 11p and 35p show high binding efficiencies for committed hematopoietic cell lines and are infective to these cell lines. J Virol 2000;74:1457–1467.
16. Shayakhmetov DM, Papayannopoulou T, Stamatoyannopoulos G, Lieber A: Efficient gene transfer into human CD34(+) cells by a retargeted adenovirus vector. J Virol 2000;74:2567–2583.
17. Mizuguchi H, Hayakawa T: Adenovirus vectors containing chimeric type 5 and type 35 fiber proteins exhibit altered and expanded tropism and increase the size limit of foreign genes. Gene 2002;285:69–77.
18. Zou L, Zhou H, Pastore L, Yang K: Prolonged transgene expression mediated by a helper-dependent adenoviral vector (hdAd) in the central nervous system. Mol Ther 2000;2:105–113.
19. Grave L, Dreyer D, Dieterle A, et al: Differential influence of the E4 adenoviral genes on viral and cellular promoters. J Gene Med 2000;2:433–443.
20. Sakhuja K, Reddy PS, Ganesh S, et al: Optimization of the generation and propagation of gutless adenoviral vectors. Hum Gene Ther 2003;14:243–254.
21. Ramachandra M, Rahman A, Zou A, et al: Re-engineering adenovirus regulatory pathways to enhance oncolytic specificity and efficacy. Nat Biotechnol 2001;19:1035–1041.
22. Crystal RG, Jaffe A, Brody S, et al: A phase 1 study, in cystic fibrosis

patients, of the safety, toxicity, and biological efficacy of a single administration of a replication deficient, recombinant adenovirus carrying the cDNA of the normal cystic fibrosis transmembrane conductance regulator gene in the lung. Hum Gene Ther 1995;6:643–666.

23. Yei S, Mittereder N, Wert S, et al: In vivo evaluation of the safety of adenovirus-mediated transfer of the human cystic fibrosis transmembrane conductance regulator cDNA to the lung. Hum Gene Ther 1994;5:731–744.

24. Hauck B, Xiao W: Characterization of tissue tropism determinants of adeno-associated virus type 1. J Virol 2003;77:2768–2774.

25. Lai CM, Lai YK, Rakoczy PE: Adenovirus and adeno-associated virus vectors. DNA Cell Biol 2002;21:895–913.

26. Rabinowtz J, Samulski J: Adeno-associated virus expression systems for gene transfer. Curr Opin Biotechnol 1998;9:470–475.

27. Burton EA, Wechuck JB, Wendell SK, et al: Multiple applications for replication-defective herpes simplex virus vectors. Stem Cells 2001;19:358–377.

28. Goins WF, Sternberg LR, Croen KD, et al: A novel latency-active promoter is contained within the herpes simplex virus type 1 UL flanking repeats. J Virol 1994;68:2239–2252.

29. Hermens WT, Verhaagen J: Viral vectors, tools for gene transfer in the nervous system. Prog Neurobiol 1998;55:399–432.

30. Burton EA, Bai Q, Goins WF, Glorioso JC: Replication-defective genomic herpes simplex vectors: design and production. Curr Opin Biotechnol 2002;13:424–428.

31. Ozuer A, Wechuck JB, Goins WF, et al: Effect of genetic background and culture conditions on the production of herpesvirus-based gene therapy vectors. Biotechnol Bioeng 2002;77:685–692.

32. Mullen JT, Tanabe KK: Viral oncolysis. Oncologist 2002;7:106–119.

33. Dixon CW: Smallpox. Elsevier Science, 1962.

34. Fenner F, Henderson DA, Arita I, Jezek Z, Ladnyi ID: Smallpox and its eradication. Geneva, Switzerland, World Health Orgainization, 1988.

35. Henderson DA, Inglesby TV, Bartlett JG, et al: Smallpox as a biological weapon: Medical and public health management. Working Group on Civilian Biodefense. JAMA 1999;281:2127–2137.

36. Lee MS, Roos JM, McGuigan LC, et al: Molecular attenuation of vaccinia virus: Mutant generation and animal characterization. J Virol 1992;66:2617–2630.

37. Sutter G, Moss B: Novel vaccinia vector derived from the host range restricted and highly attenuated MVA strain of vaccinia virus. Dev Biol Stand 1995;84:195–200.

38. Moss B: Replicating and host-restricted non-replicating vaccinia virus vectors for vaccine development. Dev Biol Stand 1994;82:55–63.

39. Tartaglia J, Cox WI, Taylor J, et al: Highly attenuated poxvirus vectors. AIDS Res Hum Retroviruses 1992;8:1445–1447.

40. Drexler I, Staib C, Kastenmuller W, et al: Identification of vaccinia virus epitope-specific HLA-A*0201-restricted T cells and comparative analysis of smallpox vaccines. Proc Natl Acad Sci USA 2003;100:217–222.

41. Jenne L, Schuler G, Steinkasserer A: Viral vectors for dendritic cell-based immunotherapy. Trends Immunol 2001;22:102–107.

42. Jenne L, Thumann P, Steinkasserer A: Interaction of large DNA viruses with dendritic cells. Immunobiology 2001;204:639–648.

43. Wallack MK, Sivanandham M, Balch CM, et al: Surgical adjuvant active specific immunotherapy for patients with stage III melanoma: the final analysis of data from a phase III, randomized, double-blind, multicenter vaccinia melanoma oncolysate trial. J Am Coll Surg 1998;187:69–77.

44. Mastrangelo MJ, Maguire HC, Jr., Eisenlohr LC, et al: Intratumoral recombinant GM-CSF-encoding virus as gene therapy in patients with cutaneous melanoma. Cancer Gene Ther 1999;6:409–422.

45. Mukherjee S, Haenel T, Himbeck R, et al: Replication-restricted vaccinia as a cytokine gene therapy vector in cancer: Persistent transgene expression despite antibody generation. Cancer Gene Ther 2000;7:663–670.

46. McCart JA, Puhlmann M, Lee J, et al: Complex interactions between the replicating oncolytic effect and the enzyme/prodrug effect of vaccinia-mediated tumor regression. Gene Ther 2000;7:1217–1223.

47. Guadagni F, Roselli M, Cosimelli M, et al: Quantitative analysis of CEA expression in colorectal adenocarcinoma and serum: Lack of correlation. Int J Cancer 1997;72:949–954.

48. Kantor J, Irvine K, Abrams S, et al: Antitumor activity and immune responses induced by a recombinant carcinoembryonic antigen-vaccinia virus vaccine. J Natl Cancer Inst 1992;84:1084–1091.

49. Tsang KY, Zaremba S, Nieroda CA, et al: Generation of human cytotoxic T cells specific for human carcinoembryonic antigen epitopes from patients immunized with recombinant vaccinia-CEA vaccine. J Natl Cancer Inst 1995;87:982–990.

50. Kantor J, Irvine K, Abrams S, et al: Immunogenicity and safety of a recombinant vaccinia virus vaccine expressing the carcinoembryonic antigen gene in a nonhuman primate. Cancer Res 1992;52:6917–6925.

51. McAneny D, Ryan CA, Beazley RM, Kaufman HL: Results of a phase I trial of a recombinant vaccinia virus that expresses carcino-embryonic antigen in patients with advanced colorectal cancer. Ann Surg Oncol 1996;3:495–500.

52. Schlom J, Panicali D: Recombinant poxvirus vaccines. In Rosenberg SA (ed): Biologic Therapy of Cancer: Principles and Practice. Philadelphia, Lippincott Williams & Wilkins, 1999, pp 686–694.

53. Hodge JW, McLaughlin JP, Kantor JA, Schlom J: Diversified prime and boost protocols using recombinant vaccinia virus and recombinant non-replicating avian pox virus to enhance T-cell immunity and antitumor responses. Vaccine 1997;15:759–768.

54. Marshall JL, Hawkins MJ, Tsang KY, et al: Phase I study in cancer patients of a replication-defective avipox recombinant vaccine that expresses human carcinoembryonic antigen. J Clin Oncol 1999;17:332–337.

55. Marshall JL, Hoyer RJ, Toomey MA, et al: Phase I study in advanced cancer patients of a diversified prime-and-boost vaccination protocol using recombinant vaccinia virus and recombinant nonreplicating avipox virus to elicit anti-carcinoembryonic antigen immune responses. J Clin Oncol 2000;18:3964–3973.

56. Ward SG: CD28: A signalling perspective. Biochem J 1996;318 (Pt 2):361–377.

57. von Mehren M, Arlen P, Gulley J, et al: The influence of granulocyte macrophage colony-stimulating factor and prior chemotherapy on the immunological response to a vaccine (ALVAC-CEA B7.1) in patients with metastatic carcinoma. Clin Cancer Res 2001;7:1181–1191.

58. Lundstrom K: Alphaviruses as expression vectors. Curr Opin Biotechnol 1997;8:578–582.

59. Vaha-Koskela MJ, Tuittila MT, Nygardas PT, et al: A novel neurotropic expression vector based on the avirulent A7(74) strain of Semliki Forest virus. J Neurovirol 2003;9:1–15.

60. Keogh B, Atkins GJ, Mills KH, Sheahan BJ: Avirulent Semliki Forest virus replication and pathology in the central nervous system is enhanced in IL-12-defective and reduced in IL-4-defective mice: A role for Th1 cells in the protective immunity. J Neuroimmunol 2002;125:15–22.

61. Liu F, Huang L: Development of non-viral vectors for systemic gene delivery. J Control Release 2002;78:259–266.

62. Merdan T, Kopecek J, Kissel T: Prospects for cationic polymers in gene and oligonucleotide therapy against cancer. Adv Drug Deliv Rev 2002;54:715–758.

63. Schmidt-Wolf GD, Schmidt-Wolf IG: Non-viral and hybrid vectors in human gene therapy: An update. Trends Mol Med 2003;9:67–72.

64. Spack EG, Sorgi FL: Developing non-viral DNA delivery systems for cancer and infectious disease. Drug Discov Today 2001;6: 186–197.

65. Horn NA, Meek JA, Budahazi G, Marquet M: Cancer gene therapy using plasmid DNA: Purification of DNA for human clinical trials. Hum Gene Ther 1995;6:565–573.

66. Jiang J, Yamato E, Miyazaki J: Intravenous delivery of naked plasmid DNA for in vivo cytokine expression. Biochem Biophys Res Commun 2001;289:1088–1092.

67. Liu F, Song Y, Liu D: Hydrodynamics-based transfection in animals by systemic administration of plasmid DNA. Gene Ther 1999;6:1258–1266.

68. Zhang G, Budker V, Wolff JA: High levels of foreign gene expression in hepatocytes after tail vein injections of naked plasmid DNA. Hum Gene Ther 1999;10:1735–1737.

69. Fenske DB, MacLachlan I, Cullis PR: Stabilized plasmid-lipid particles: a systemic gene therapy vector. Methods Enzymol 2002;346:36–71.

70. Felgner PL, Gadek TR, Holm M, et al: Lipofection: a highly efficient, lipid-mediated DNA-transfection procedure. Proc Natl Acad Sci USA 1987;84:7413–7417.

71. Panyam J, Labhasetwar V: Biodegradable nanoparticles for drug and gene delivery to cells and tissue. Adv Drug Deliv Rev 2003;55:329–347.

72. Rolland AP: From genes to gene medicines: Recent advances in nonviral gene delivery. Crit Rev Ther Drug Carrier Syst 1998;15:143–198.

73. Templeton NS, Lasic DD, Frederik PM, et al: Improved DNA: Liposome complexes for increased systemic delivery and gene expression. Nat Biotechnol 1997;15:647–652.

74. Kurane S, Krauss JC, Watari E, et al: Targeted gene transfer for adenocarcinoma using a combination of tumor-specific antibody and tissue-specific promoter. Jpn J Cancer Res 1998;89:1212–1219.

75. Kunitomi M, Takayama E, Suzuki S, et al: Selective inhibition of hepatoma cells using diphtheria toxin A under the control of the promoter/enhancer region of the human alpha-fetoprotein gene. Jpn J Cancer Res 2000;91:343–350.

76. Chen J, Gamou S, Takayanagi A, et al: Targeted in vivo delivery of therapeutic gene into experimental squamous cell carcinomas using anti-epidermal growth factor receptor antibody: Immunogene approach. Hum Gene Ther 1998;9:2673–2681.

77. Park JW, Hong K, Carter P, et al: Development of anti-p185HER2 Immunoliposomes for cancer therapy. Proc Natl Acad Sci USA 1995;92:1327–1331.

78. Hara T, Aramaki Y, Takada S, Koike K, Tsuchiya S: Receptor-mediated transfer of pSV2CAT DNA to mouse liver cells using asialofetuin-labeled liposomes. Gene Ther 1995;2:784–788.

79. Lee RJ, Huang L: Folate-targeted, anionic liposome-entrapped polylysine-condensed DNA for tumor cell-specific gene transfer. J Biol Chem 1996;271:8481–8487.

80. Xu L, Pirollo KF, Chang EH: Transferrin-liposome-mediated p53 sensitization of squamous cell carcinoma of the head and neck to radiation in vitro. Hum Gene Ther 1997;8:467–475.

81. Woodle MC, Matthay KK, Newman MS, et al: Versatility in lipid compositions showing prolonged circulation with sterically stabilized liposomes. Biochim Biophys Acta 1992;1105:193–200.

82. Harrington KJ, Mohammadtaghi S, Uster PS, et al: Effective targeting of solid tumors in patients with locally advanced cancers by radiolabeled pegylated liposomes. Clin Cancer Res 2001;7:243–254.

83. Li S, Rizzo MA, Bhattacharya S, Huang L: Characterization of cationic lipid-protamine-DNA (LPD) complexes for intravenous gene delivery. Gene Ther 1998;5:930–937.

84. Li S, Wu SP, Whitmore M, et al: Effect of immune response on gene transfer to the lung via systemic administration of cationic lipidic vectors. Am J Physiol 1999;276:L796–L804.

85. Freimark BD, Blezinger HP, Florack VJ, et al: Cationic lipids enhance cytokine and cell influx levels in the lung following administration of plasmid: Cationic lipid complexes. J Immunol 1998;160:4580–4586.

86. Tan Y, Li S, Pitt BR, Huang L: The inhibitory role of CpG immunostimulatory motifs in cationic lipid vector-mediated transgene expression in vivo. Hum Gene Ther 1999;10:2153–2161.

87. Dow SW, Fradkin LG, Liggitt DH, et al: Lipid-DNA complexes induce potent activation of innate immune responses and antitumor activity when administered intravenously. J Immunol 1999;163:1552–1561.

88. Qin L, Ding Y, Pahud DR, et al: Promoter attenuation in gene therapy: interferon-gamma and tumor necrosis factor-alpha inhibit transgene expression. Hum Gene Ther 1997;8:2019–2029.

89. Song YK, Liu F, Chu S, Liu D: Characterization of cationic liposome-mediated gene transfer in vivo by intravenous administration. Hum Gene Ther 1997;8:1585–1594.

90. Ramesh R, Saeki T, Templeton NS, et al: Successful treatment of primary and disseminated human lung cancers by systemic delivery of tumor suppressor genes using an improved liposome vector. Mol Ther 2001;3:337–350.

91. Ito I, Began G, Mohiuddin I, et al: Increased uptake of liposomal-DNA complexes by lung metastases following intravenous administration. Mol Ther 2003;7:409.

92. Nair SK, Morse M, Boczkowski D, et al: Induction of tumor-specific cytotoxic T lymphocytes in cancer patients by autologous tumor RNA-transfected dendritic cells. Ann Surg 2002;235:540–549.

93. Mitchell DA, Nair SK: RNA-transfected dendritic cells in cancer immunotherapy. J Clin Invest 2000;106:1065–1069.

94. Mitchell DA, Nair SK: RNA-transfected dendritic cells in cancer immunotherapy. J Clin Invest 2000;106:1065–1069.

95. Francini G, Scardino A, Kosmatopoulos K, et al: High-affinity HLA-A(*)02.01 peptides from parathyroid hormone-related protein generate in vitro and in vivo antitumor CTL response without autoimmune side effects. J Immunol 2002;169:4840–4849.

96. Dias N, Stein CA: Potential roles of antisense oligonucleotides in cancer therapy. The example of Bcl-2 antisense oligonucleotides. Eur J Pharm Biopharm 2002;54:263–269.

97. Lebedeva I, Benimetskaya L, Stein CA, Vilenchik M: Cellular delivery of antisense oligonucleotides. Eur J Pharm Biopharm 2000;50:101–119.

98. Stephenson ML, Zamecnik PC: Inhibition of Rous sarcoma viral RNA translation by a specific oligodeoxyribonucleotide. Proc Natl Acad Sci USA 1978;75:285–288.

99. Orr RM: Technology evaluation: Fomivirsen, Isis Pharmaceuticals Inc/CIBA vision. Curr Opin Mol Ther 2001;3:288–294.

100. Vrana JA, Grant S, Dent P: Inhibition of the MAPK pathway abrogates BCL2-mediated survival of leukemia cells after exposure to low-dose ionizing radiation. Radiat Res 1999;151:559–569.

101. Stein CA: Two problems in antisense biotechnology: In vitro delivery and the design of antisense experiments. Biochim Biophys Acta 1999;1489:45–52.

102. Eckstein F: Side-effects and phosphorothioates. Nat Biotechnol 2002;20:549.

103. Kitabwalla M, Ruprecht RM: RNA interference—a new weapon against HIV and beyond. N Engl J Med 2002;347:1364–1367.

104. Leirdal M, Sioud M: Gene silencing in mammalian cells by preformed small RNA duplexes. Biochem Biophys Res Commun 2002;295:744–748.

105. Sorensen DR, Leirdal M, Sioud M: Gene silencing by systemic delivery of synthetic siRNAs in adult mice. J Mol Biol 2003;327:761–766.

106. Kunisawa J, Nakagawa S, Mayumi T: Pharmacotherapy by intracellular delivery of drugs using fusogenic liposomes: Application to vaccine development. Adv Drug Deliv Rev 2001;52:177–186.

107. Sohn RL, Murray MT, Schwarz K, et al: In-vivo particle mediated delivery of mRNA to mammalian tissues: Ballistic and biologic effects. Wound Repair Regen 2001;9:287–296.

108. Udvardi A, Kufferath I, Grutsch H, Zatloukal K, Volc-Platzer B: Uptake of exogenous DNA via the skin. J Mol Med 1999;77:744–750.

109. Yang NS, Burkholder J, Roberts B, Martinell B, McCabe D: In vivo and in vitro gene transfer to mammalian somatic cells by particle bombardment. Proc Natl Acad Sci USA 1990;87:9568–9572.

110. Wittig B, Marten A, Dorbic T, et al: Therapeutic vaccination against metastatic carcinoma by expression-modulated and immunomodified autologous tumor cells: A first clinical phase I/II trial. Hum Gene Ther 2001;12:267–278.

111. Vijayanathan V, Thomas T, Thomas TJ: DNA nanoparticles and development of DNA delivery vehicles for gene therapy. Biochemistry 2002;41:14085–14094.

112. Kirchweger G: Nanoparticles—the next big thing? Mol Ther 2002;6:301–302.

113. Lunsford L, McKeever U, Eckstein V, Hedley ML: Tissue distribution and persistence in mice of plasmid DNA encapsulated in a PLGA-based microsphere delivery vehicle. J Drug Target 2000;8:39–50.

114. Hood JD, Bednarski M, Frausto R, et al: Tumor regression by targeted gene delivery to the neovasculature. Science 2002;296:2404–2407.

115. Haviv YS, Curiel DT: Conditional gene targeting for cancer gene therapy. Adv Drug Deliv Rev 2001;53:135–154.

Science of Clinical Oncology

116. Galanis E, Vile R, Russell SJ: Delivery systems intended for in vivo gene therapy of cancer: Targeting and replication competent viral vectors. Crit Rev Oncol Hematol 2001;38:177–192.

117. Nakagawa S, Massie B, Hawley RG: Tetracycline-regulatable adenovirus vectors: Pharmacologic properties and clinical potential. Eur J Pharm Sci 2001;13:53–60.

118. Akporiaye ET, Hersh E: Clinical aspects of intratumoral gene therapy. Curr Opin Mol Ther 1999;1:443–453.

119. Kirch HC, Ruschen S, Brockmann D, et al: Tumor-specific activation of hTERT-derived promoters by tumor suppressive E1A-mutants involves recruitment of p300/CBP/HAT and suppression of HDAC-1 and defines a combined tumor targeting and suppression system. Oncogene 2002;21:7991–8000.

120. Pramudji C, Shimura S, Ebara S, et al: In situ prostate cancer gene therapy using a novel adenoviral vector regulated by the caveolin-1 promoter. Clin Cancer Res 2001;7:4272–4279.

121. Inga A, Monti P, Fronza G, Darden T, Resnick MA: p53 mutants exhibiting enhanced transcriptional activation and altered promoter selectivity are revealed using a sensitive, yeast-based functional assay. Oncogene 2001;20:501–513.

122. Takakura M, Kyo S, Kanaya T, et al: Cloning of human telomerase catalytic subunit (hTERT) gene promoter and identification of proximal core promoter sequences essential for transcriptional activation in immortalized and cancer cells. Cancer Res 1999;59:551–557.

123. Abdul-Ghani R, Ohana P, Matouk I, et al: Use of transcriptional regulatory sequences of telomerase (hTER and hTERT) for selective killing of cancer cells. Mol Ther 2000;2:539–544.

124. Xie B, Tam NN, Tsao SW, Wong YC: Co-expression of vascular endothelial growth factor (VEGF) and its receptors (flk-1 and flt-1) in hormone-induced mammary cancer in the Noble rat. Br J Cancer 1999;81:1335–1343.

125. Jaggar RT, Chan HY, Harris AL, Bicknell R: Endothelial cell-specific expression of tumor necrosis factor-alpha from the KDR or E-selectin promoters following retroviral delivery. Hum Gene Ther 1997;8:2239–2247.

126. Ellis LM, Takahashi Y, Liu W, Shaheen RM: Vascular endothelial growth factor in human colon cancer: Biology and therapeutic implications. Oncologist 2000;5(Suppl 1):11–15.

127. Heidenreich R, Kappel A, Breier G: Tumor endothelium-specific transgene expression directed by vascular endothelial growth factor-2 (Flk-1) promoter/enhancer sequences. Cancer Res 2000;60:6142–6147.

128. Jager U, Zhao Y, Porter CD: Endothelial cell-specific transcriptional targeting from a hybrid long terminal repeat retrovirus vector containing human prepro-endothelin-1 promoter sequences. J Virol 1999;73:9702–9709.

129. Shirakawa T, Gotoh A, Wada Y, et al: Tissue-specific promoters in gene therapy for the treatment of prostate cancer. Mol Urol 2000;4:73–82.

130. Lee SJ, Kim HS, Yu R, et al: Novel prostate-specific promoter derived from PSA and PSMA enhancers. Mol Ther 2002;6:415–421.

131. Yoshimura I, Ikegami S, Suzuki S, Tadakuma T, Hayakawa M: Adenovirus mediated prostate specific enzyme prodrug gene therapy using prostate specific antigen promoter enhanced by the Cre-loxP system. J Urol 2002;168:2659–2664.

132. Cao G, Zhang X, He X, Chen Q, Qi Z: A safe, effective in vivo gene therapy for melanoma using tyrosinase promoter-driven cytosine deaminase gene. In Vivo 1999;13:181–187.

133. Shi CX, Hitt M, Ng P, Graham FL: Superior tissue-specific expression from tyrosinase and prostate-specific antigen promoters/enhancers in helper-dependent compared with first-generation adenoviral vectors. Hum Gene Ther 2002;13:211–224.

134. Hart IR: Tissue specific promoters in targeting systemically delivered gene therapy. Semin Oncol 1996;23:154–158.

135. Szala S, Szary J, Cichon T, Sochanik A: Antiangiogenic gene therapy in inhibition of metastasis. Acta Biochim Pol 2002;49:313–321.

136. Patterson A, Harris AL: Molecular chemotherapy for breast cancer. Drugs Aging 1999;14:75–90.

137. Rossi FM, Blau HM: Recent advances in inducible gene expression systems. Curr Opin Biotechnol 1998;9:451–456.

138. Greco O, Marples B, Dachs GU, et al: Novel chimeric gene promoters responsive to hypoxia and ionizing radiation. Gene Ther 2002;9:1403–1411.

139. Lohr F, Huang Q, Hu K, Dewhirst MW, Li CY: Systemic vector leakage and transgene expression by intratumorally injected recombinant adenovirus vectors. Clin Cancer Res 2001;7:3625–3628.

140. Walther W, Stein U, Fichtner I, et al: Mdr1 promoter-driven tumor necrosis factor-alpha expression for a chemotherapy-controllable combined in vivo gene therapy and chemotherapy of tumors. Cancer Gene Ther 2000;7:893–900.

141. Moscow JA, Huang H, Carter C, et al: Engraftment of MDR1 and NeoR gene-transduced hematopoietic cells after breast cancer chemotherapy. Blood 1999;94:52–61.

142. Liu Y, Liggitt HD, Dow S, et al: Strain-based genetic differences regulate the efficiency of systemic gene delivery as well as expression. J Biol Chem 2002;277:4966–4972.

143. Shillitoe EJ, Noonan S: Strength and specificity of different gene promoters in oral cancer cells. Oral Oncol 2000;36:214–220.

144. Halaby IA, Lyden SP, Davies MG, et al: Glucocorticoid-regulated VEGF expression in ischemic skeletal muscle. Mol Ther 2002;5:300–306.

145. Pollock R, Clackson T: Dimerizer-regulated gene expression. Curr Opin Biotechnol 2002;13:459–467.

146. Cha HH, Cram EJ, Wang EC, et al: Glucocorticoids stimulate p21 gene expression by targeting multiple transcriptional elements within a steroid responsive region of the p21waf1/cip1 promoter in rat hepatoma cells. J Biol Chem 1998;273:1998–2007.

147. Schmeisser F, Donohue M, Weir JP: Tetracycline-regulated gene expression in replication-incompetent herpes simplex virus vectors. Hum Gene Ther 2002;13:2113–2124.

148. Imhof MO, Chatellard P, Mermod N: A regulatory network for the efficient control of transgene expression. J Gene Med 2000;2:107–116.

149. Zhu J, Gao B, Zhao J, Balmain A: Targeting gene expression to tumor cells with loss of wild-type p53 function. Cancer Gene Ther 2000;7:4–12.

150. Ngan ES, Schillinger K, DeMayo F, Tsai SY: The mifepristone-inducible gene regulatory system in mouse models of disease and gene therapy. Semin Cell Dev Biol 2002;13:143–149.

151. Burcin MM, BW OM, Tsai SY: A regulatory system for target gene expression. Front Biosci 1998;3:c1–c7.

152. Gomez-Navarro J, Curiel DT: Conditionally replicative adenoviral vectors for cancer gene therapy. Lancet Oncol 2000;1:148–158.

153. Takemoto S, Trovato R, Cereseto A, et al: p53 stabilization and functional impairment in the absence of genetic mutation or the alteration of the p14(ARF)-MDM2 loop in ex vivo and cultured adult T-cell leukemia/lymphoma cells. Blood 2000;95:3939–3944.

154. Krasnykh V, Dmitriev I, Navarro JG, et al: Advanced generation adenoviral vectors possess augmented gene transfer efficiency based upon coxsackie adenovirus receptor-independent cellular entry capacity. Cancer Res 2000;60:6784–6787.

155. van Beusechem VW, van den Doel PB, Grill J, Pinedo HM, Gerritsen WR: Conditionally replicative adenovirus expressing p53 exhibits enhanced oncolytic potency. Cancer Res 2002;62:6165–6171.

156. Suzuki K, Fueyo J, Krasnykh V, et al: A conditionally replicative adenovirus with enhanced infectivity shows improved oncolytic potency. Clin Cancer Res 2001;7:120–126.

157. Heise C, Hermiston T, Johnson L, et al: An adenovirus E1A mutant that demonstrates potent and selective systemic anti-tumoral efficacy. Nat Med 2000;6:1134–1139.

158. Bischoff JR, Kirn DH, Williams A, et al: An adenovirus mutant that replicates selectively in p53-deficient human tumor cells. Science 1996;274:373–376.

159. Edwards SJ, Dix BR, Myers CJ, et al: Evidence that replication of the antitumor adenovirus ONYX-015 is not controlled by the p53 and p14(ARF) tumor suppressor genes. J Virol 2002;76:2483–12490.

160. Nemunaitis J, O'Brien J: Head and neck cancer: gene therapy approaches. Part II: genes delivered. Expert Opin Biol Ther 2002;2:311–324.

161. Yan W, Kitzes G, Dormishian F, et al: Developing novel oncolytic adenoviruses through bioselection. J Virol 2003;77:2640–2650.

162. Yu DC, Sakamoto GT, Henderson DR: Identification of the transcriptional regulatory sequences of human kallikrein 2 and their use in the construction of calydon virus 764, an attenuated

replication competent adenovirus for prostate cancer therapy. Cancer Res 1999;59:1498–1504.

163. Hallenbeck PL, Chang YN, Hay C, et al: A novel tumor-specific replication-restricted adenoviral vector for gene therapy of hepatocellular carcinoma. Hum Gene Ther 1999;10:1721–1733.

164. Rodriguez R, Schuur ER, Lim HY, et al: Prostate attenuated replication competent adenovirus (ARCA) CN706: A selective cytotoxic for prostate-specific antigen-positive prostate cancer cells. Cancer Res 1997;57:2559–2563.

165. Kurihara T, Brough DE, Kovesdi I, Kufe DW: Selectivity of a replication-competent adenovirus for human breast carcinoma cells expressing the MUC1 antigen. J Clin Invest 2000;106:763–771.

166. Hernandez-Alcoceba R, Pihalja M, Wicha MS, Clarke MF: A novel, conditionally replicative adenovirus for the treatment of breast cancer that allows controlled replication of E1a-deleted adenoviral vectors. Hum Gene Ther 2000;11:2009–2024.

167. Steinwaerder DS, Carlson CA, Otto DL, et al: Tumor-specific gene expression in hepatic metastases by a replication- activated adenovirus vector. Nat Med 2001;7:240–243.

168. Bergelson JM, Cunningham JA, Droguett G, et al: Isolation of a common receptor for coxsackie B viruses and adenoviruses 2 and 5. Science 1997;275:1320–1323.

169. Tomko RP, Xu R, Philipson L: HCAR and MCAR: The human and mouse cellular receptors for subgroup C adenoviruses and group B coxsackieviruses. Proc Natl Acad Sci USA 1997;94:3352–3356.

170. Wickham TJ, Tzeng E, Shears LL, et al: Increased in vitro and in vivo gene transfer by adenovirus vectors containing chimeric fiber proteins. J Virol 1997;71:8221–8229.

171. Stecher H, Carlson CA, Shayakhmetov DM, Lieber A: Generation of adenovirus vectors devoid of all viral genes by recombination between inverted repeats. Methods Mol Med 2003;76:135–152.

172. Stecher H, Shayakhmetov DM, Stamatoyannopoulos G, Lieber A: A capsid-modified adenovirus vector devoid of all viral genes: Assessment of transduction and toxicity in human hematopoietic cells. Mol Ther 2001;4:36–44.

173. Krasnykh V, Dmitriev I, Mikheeva G, et al: Characterization of an adenovirus vector containing a heterologous peptide epitope in the HI loop of the fiber knob. J Virol 1998;72:1844–1852.

174. Dmitriev I, Krasnykh V, Miller CR, et al: An adenovirus vector with genetically modified fibers demonstrates expanded tropism via utilization of a coxsackievirus and adenovirus receptor-independent cell entry mechanism. J Virol 1998;72:9706–9713.

175. Yoshida Y, Sadata A, Zhang W, et al: Generation of fiber-mutant recombinant adenoviruses for gene therapy of malignant glioma. Hum Gene Ther 1998;9:2503–2515.

176. Bouri K, Feero WG, Myerburg MM, et al: Polylysine modification of adenoviral fiber protein enhances muscle cell transduction. Hum Gene Ther 1999;10:1633–1640.

177. Koizumi N, Mizuguchi H, Hosono T, et al: Efficient gene transfer by fiber-mutant adenoviral vectors containing RGD peptide. Biochem Biophys Acta 2001;1568:13–20.

178. Mizuguchi H, Kay MA: Efficient construction of a recombinant adenovirus vector by an improved in vitro ligation method. Hum Gene Ther 1998;9:2577–2583.

179. Mizuguchi H, Kay MA: A simple method for constructing E1- and E1/E4-deleted recombinant adenoviral vectors. Hum Gene Ther 1999;10:2013–2017.

180. Mizuguchi H, Xu Z, Ishii-Watabe A, Uchida E, Hayakawa T: IRES-dependent second gene expression is significantly lower than cap-dependent first gene expression in a bicistronic vector. Mol Ther 2000;1:376–382.

181. Mizuguchi H, Koizumi N, Hosono T, et al: A simplified system for constructing recombinant adenoviral vectors containing heterologous peptides in the HI loop of their fiber knob. Gene Ther 2001;8:730–735.

182. Wickham TJ, Roelvink PW, Brough DE, Kovesdi I: Adenovirus targeted to heparan-containing receptors increases its gene delivery efficiency to multiple cell types. Nat Biotechnol 1996;14:1570–1573.

183. Hong JS, Engler JA: Domains required for assembly of adenovirus type 2 fiber trimers. J Virol 1996;70:7071–7078.

184. Wickham TJ, Segal DM, Roelvink PW, et al: Targeted adenovirus gene transfer to endothelial and smooth muscle cells by using bispecific antibodies. J Virol 1996;70:6831–6838.

185. Bilbao G, Gomez-Navarro J, Curiel DT: Targeted adenoviral vectors for cancer gene therapy. Adv Exp Med Biol 1998;451:365–374.

186. Burns JC, Friedmann T, Driever W, Burrascano M, Yee JK: Vesicular stomatitis virus G glycoprotein pseudotyped retroviral vectors: Concentration to very high titer and efficient gene transfer into mammalian and nonmammalian cells. Proc Natl Acad Sci USA 1993;90:8033–8037.

187. Reiser J, Harmison G, Kluepfel-Stahl S, et al: Transduction of nondividing cells using pseudotyped defective high-titer HIV type 1 particles. Proc Natl Acad Sci USA 1996;93:15266–15271.

188. Mochizuki H, Schwartz JP, Tanaka K, Brady RO, Reiser J: High-titer human immunodeficiency virus type 1-based vector systems for gene delivery into nondividing cells. J Virol 1998;72:8873–8883.

189. Wool-Lewis RJ, Bates P: Characterization of Ebola virus entry by using pseudotyped viruses: Identification of receptor-deficient cell lines. J Virol 1998;72:3155–3160.

190. Mitrophanous K, Yoon S, Rohll J, et al: Stable gene transfer to the nervous system using a non-primate lentiviral vector. Gene Ther 1999;6:1808–1818.

191. Chan SY, Speck RF, Ma MC, Goldsmith MA: Distinct mechanisms of entry by envelope glycoproteins of Marburg and Ebola (Zaire) viruses. J Virol 2000;74:4933–4937.

192. Stitz J, Buchholz CJ, Engelstadter M, et al: Lentiviral vectors pseudotyped with envelope glycoproteins derived from gibbon ape leukemia virus and murine leukemia virus 10A1. Virology 2000;273:16–20.

193. Lewis BC, Chinnasamy N, Morgan RA, Varmus HE: Development of an avian leukosis-sarcoma virus subgroup A pseudotyped lentiviral vector. J Virol 2001;75:9339–9344.

194. Kobinger GP, Weiner DJ, Yu QC, Wilson JM: Filovirus-pseudotyped lentiviral vector can efficiently and stably transduce airway epithelia in vivo. Nat Biotechnol 2001;19:225–230.

195. Desmaris N, Bosch A, Salaun C, et al: Production and neurotropism of lentivirus vectors pseudotyped with lyssavirus envelope glycoproteins. Mol Ther 2001;4:149–156.

196. Beyer WR, Westphal M, Ostertag W, von Laer D: Oncoretrovirus and lentivirus vectors pseudotyped with lymphocytic choriomeningitis virus glycoprotein: generation, concentration, and broad host range. J Virol 2002;76:1488–1495.

197. Kasahara N, Dozy AM, Kan YW: Tissue-specific targeting of retroviral vectors through ligand-receptor interactions. Science 1994;266:1373–1376.

198. Han X, Kasahara N, Kan YW: Ligand-directed retroviral targeting of human breast cancer cells. Proc Natl Acad Sci USA 1995;92:9747–9751.

199. Matano T, Odawara T, Iwamoto A, Yoshikura H: Targeted infection of a retrovirus bearing a CD4-Env chimera into human cells expressing human immunodeficiency virus type 1. J Gen Virol 1995;76(Pt 12):3165–3169.

200. Cosset FL, Morling FJ, Takeuchi Y, et al: Retroviral retargeting by envelopes expressing an N-terminal binding domain. J Virol 1995;69:6314–6322.

201. Marin M, Noel D, Piechaczyk M: Towards efficient cell targeting by recombinant retroviruses. Mol Med Today 1997;3:396–403.

202. Russell SJ, Hawkins RE, Winter G: Retroviral vectors displaying functional antibody fragments. Nucleic Acids Res 1993;21:1081–1085.

203. Somia NV, Zoppe M, Verma IM: Generation of targeted retroviral vectors by using single-chain variable fragment: an approach to in vivo gene delivery. Proc Natl Acad Sci USA 1995;92:7570–7574.

204. Marin M, Noel D, Valsesia-Wittman S, et al: Targeted infection of human cells via major histocompatibility complex class I molecules by Moloney murine leukemia virus-derived viruses displaying single-chain antibody fragment-envelope fusion proteins. J Virol 1996;70:2957–2962.

205. Ager S, Nilson BH, Morling FJ, et al: Retroviral display of antibody fragments; interdomain spacing strongly influences vector infectivity. Hum Gene Ther 1996;7:2157–2164.

206. Schnierle BS, Moritz D, Jeschke M, Groner B: Expression of chimeric envelope proteins in helper cell lines and integration into Moloney murine leukemia virus particles. Gene Ther 1996;3:334–342.

207. Valsesia-Wittmann S, Drynda A, Deleage G, et al: Modifications in the binding domain of avian retrovirus envelope protein to

redirect the host range of retroviral vectors. J Virol 1994;68: 4609–4619.

208. Nilson BH, Morling FJ, Cosset FL, Russell SJ: Targeting of retroviral vectors through protease-substrate interactions. Gene Ther 1996;3:280–286.

209. Roux P, Jeanteur P, Piechaczyk M: A versatile and potentially general approach to the targeting of specific cell types by retroviruses: Application to the infection of human cells by means of major histocompatibility complex class I and class II antigens by mouse ecotropic murine leukemia virus-derived viruses. Proc Natl Acad Sci USA 1989;86:9079–9083.

210. Etienne-Julan M, Roux P, Carillo S, Jeanteur P, Piechaczyk M: The efficiency of cell targeting by recombinant retroviruses depends on the nature of the receptor and the composition of the artificial cell-virus linker. J Gen Virol 1992;73(Pt 12):3251–3255.

211. Ogris M, Brunner S, Schuller S, Kircheis R, Wagner E: PEGylated DNA/transferrin-PEI complexes: Reduced interaction with blood components, extended circulation in blood and potential for systemic gene delivery. Gene Ther 1999;6:595–605.

212. Check E: A tragic setback. Nature 2002;420:116–118.

213. Bowles C: Cancer risk clouds gene cures. New Scientist 2003;25:12.

214. Buller RE, Runnebaum IB, Karlan BY, et al: A phase I/II trial of rAd/p53 (SCH 58500) gene replacement in recurrent ovarian cancer. Cancer Gene Ther 2002;9:553–566.

215. Reid T, Warren R, Kirn D: Intravascular adenoviral agents in cancer patients: Lessons from clinical trials. Cancer Gene Ther 2002;9: 979–986.

216. Hutchins B, Sajjadi N, Seaver S, et al: Working toward an adenoviral vector testing standard. Molecular Therapy 2000;2:532.

217. Raper SE, Yudkoff M, Chirmule N, et al: A pilot study of in vivo liver-directed gene transfer with an adenoviral vector in partial ornithine transcarbamylase deficiency. Hum Gene Ther 2002;13:163–175.

218. Schiedner G, Morral N, Parks RJ, et al: Genomic DNA transfer with a high-capacity adenovirus vector results in improved in vivo gene expression and decreased toxicity. Nat Genet 1998;18: 180–183.

219. Nathwani AC, Persons DA, Stevenson SC, et al: Adenovirus-mediated expresssion of the murine ecotropic receptor facilitates transduction of human hematopoietic cells with an ecotropic retroviral vector. Gene Ther 1999;6:1456–1468.

220. Sung MW, Yeh HC, Thung SN, et al: Intratumoral adenovirus-mediated suicide gene transfer for hepatic metastases from colorectal adenocarcinoma: Results of a phase I clinical trial. Mol Ther 2001;4:182–191.

221. Warren RS, Kirn DH: Liver-directed viral therapy for cancer p53-targeted adenoviruses and beyond. Surg Oncol Clin N Am 2002;11:571–588, vi.

222. Nemunaitis J, Khuri F, Ganly I, et al: Phase II trial of intratumoral administration of ONYX-015, a replication-selective adenovirus, in patients with refractory head and neck cancer. J Clin Oncol 2001;19:289–298.

223. Villaret D, Glisson B, Kenady D, et al: A multicenter phase II study of tgDCC-E1A for the intratumoral treatment of patients with recurrent head and neck squamous cell carcinoma. Head Neck 2002;24:661–669.

224. Pagliaro LC: Gene therapy for bladder cancer. World J Urol 2000;18:148–151.

225. Kim M, Wright M, Deshane J, et al: A novel gene therapy strategy for elimination of prostate carcinoma cells from human bone marrow. Hum Gene Ther 1997;8:157–170.

226. Hirai M, Kelsey LS, Vaillancourt M, et al: Purging of human breast cancer cells from stem cell products with an adenovirus containing p53. Cancer Gene Ther 2000;7:197–206.

227. Hirai M, Kelsey L, Maneval DC, Vaillancourt MT, Talmadge JE: Adenovirus p53 purging for human breast cancer stem cell products. Acta Haematol 1999;101:97–105.

228. Watanabe T, Kuszynski C, Ino K, et al: Gene transfer into human bone marrow hematopoietic cells mediated by adenovirus vectors. Blood 1996;87:5032–5039.

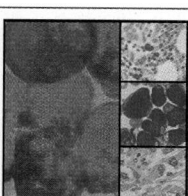

THE PRESENT AND FUTURE OF MOLECULARLY TARGETED THERAPY

Brian J. Druker

SUMMARY OF KEY POINTS

- "Molecularly targeted" refers to agents that target pathways that are activated in cancer cells, including those regulating growth, survival, and angiogenesis.
- Molecularly targeted agents should be separated into those that target genetically defined abnormalities in cancers and those that target pathways activated by these genetic defects.
- Agents that target early, causal genetic abnormalities in cancer, such as all-*trans*-retinoic acid (ATRA) for

- acute promyelocytic leukemia (APL) and imatinib for chronic myeloid leukemia (CML) and gastrointestinal stromal tumor (GIST), would be expected to yield high response rates, although resistance to single agents is likely.
- Responses to agents targeting pathways activated in cancer cells will be more difficult to predict, as this will depend on how important the target is to the survival of the cancer.

- Optimal testing of pathway-specific agents requires clinical trials that select patients based on genetic features of a tumor or evidence of pathway activation; includes measures of target modulation to assist in determining optimal doses and to assess the activity of an agent adequately; and develops novel endpoints that more accurately reflect the expected outcome of therapy.

INTRODUCTION

The term "molecularly targeted" has been used to refer to agents that target pathways that are activated in cancer cells, including those regulating growth, survival, and angiogenesis. With increased knowledge of these pathways, and buoyed by the success of agents such as imatinib (Gleevec), much optimism surrounds the field of molecularly targeted therapies. In contrast, modest results with agents such as gefitinib (Iressa) and bevacizumab (Avastin) have caused skepticism as to whether the field of molecularly targeted therapies will fulfill its promise. In this chapter, the current status of molecularly targeted therapies is explored and lessons learned from the development of several agents in this class are discussed. Most important, the term *molecularly targeted* is more precisely defined to separate agents that target genetically defined molecular defects in cancer [e.g., *BCR-ABL* (breakpoint cluster region-Abelson)] from those that target general pathways that are present in the establishment or maintenance of a cancer (e.g., cell-cycle components). This chapter does not comprehensively review all of the agents in clinical trials or development. Rather, examples of agents in each category are discussed to establish a framework for understanding this rapidly advancing and changing field.

AGENTS THAT TARGET GENETICALLY DEFINED ABNORMALITIES

Definition

The term "molecularly targeted" is a rather unfortunate choice of words, as it implies specificity. In reality, this term is completely nonspecific, as by definition all drugs, including all currently used chemotherapy agents, have molecular targets. It also is worth noting that the concept of molecularly targeted therapy is not new and was the basis for the development of many of the early chemotherapy drugs such as methotrexate, 5-fluorouracil, and L-asparaginase. These compounds were developed based on the assumption that biochemical differences exist between cancer cells and normal cells. As our understanding of the molecular basis of cancer has improved, agents that target specific genetically defined abnormalities in cancer cells have emerged. This class of compounds includes all-*trans*-retinoic acid (ATRA) for acute promyelocytic leukemia (APL), and imatinib (Gleevec) for chronic myeloid leukemia (CML) and gastrointestinal stromal tumor (GIST), as well as many others that are in clinical trials. This category includes only targets that have been genetically defined in human cancers. This could be through deletion, chromosomal translocation, or mutation. Overexpression or aberrant expression would not be an acceptable definition, unless it was genetically defined. For example, *MYC* expression in Burkitt's lymphoma, due to chromosomal translocation, would be genetically defined aberrant expression, whereas epidermal growth factor receptor (*EGFR*) overexpression in lung cancer, in the absence of a genetic lesion, would not be a genetically defined target. Numerous genetic defects have been identified in human cancers and are detailed in Sections 1 and 2 of this book. These genetic lesions have been broadly lumped into oncogenes and tumor suppressors and can be either somatic or germline. It is the thesis of this chapter that any genetically defined molecular abnormality would be a good target for antineoplastic therapy, and this is the focus of the initial portion of this chapter. This chapter does not review all of the known molecular genetic defects that have been identified in cancers; rather, several have been selected to exemplify the potential of this approach.

All-*Trans*-Retinoic Acid

The first example of clinical success of an agent that targets a molecular genetic defect in cancer was ATRA for APL. ATRA, however, was not developed for APL based on an understanding of the molecular pathogenesis of this disease. Rather, its clinical activity was determined empirically, before the molecular basis of this disorder was understood.[1,2] The majority of patients with APL have a (15;17) chromosomal translocation.[3] Cloning of the genes at the breakpoints of this translocation led to the discovery that the retinoic acid receptor α (*RARα*) was fused to the promyelocytic leukemia protein (PML).[4-7] This fusion protein interferes with *RARα* function and, in the absence of *RARα* activity, myeloid cells are blocked at the promyelocyte stage of development.[8] Treatment with pharmacologic doses of retinoic acid restores the function of the receptor, allowing normal cellular differentiation. In clinical trials, ATRA as a single agent achieves a 90% complete remission (CR) rate, but the majority of patients will relapse within 6 months, despite continuous therapy.[9] Even more remarkably, ATRA in combination with chemotherapy can cure more than 70% of patients with APL.[10]

Imatinib

Imatinib is a tyrosine kinase inhibitor that inhibits the activity of *ABL*, platelet-derived growth factor receptor (*PDGFR*) and *KIT*.[11] Given the known pathogenetic role of the *BCR-ABL* tyrosine kinase in CML and the preclinical activity of this agent in vitro and in vivo against *BCR-ABL*–expressing cells,[12] initial clinical trials were conducted in patients with CML.[13,14] The results of clinical trials with imatinib are reviewed in detail in Chapter 107. In brief, for newly diagnosed patients with chronic-phase CML, complete hematologic responses (CHRs) were obtained in 97% of patients, and complete cytogenetic responses in 76% of patients. With 18 months of follow-up, the rate of disease progression to accelerated or blast phase of the disease is 3.5%.[15] For patients in blast crisis who previously have not received imatinib, the hemato-

logic response rate is 52%, and the CR rate is 8%; however, 80% of patients relapsed within 1 year with single-agent imatinib.[16]

In several other cancers, imatinib has shown clinical benefits that are based on the profile of kinases inhibited by imatinib and an understanding of the genetic defects causing these malignancies (Table 30-1). For example, the recognition that *KIT* mutations were present in the majority of patients with GIST[17] led to clinical trials of imatinib in this indication. GISTs are mesenchymal neoplasms that can arise from any organ in the gastro-intestinal tract or from the mesentery or omentum. Bio-chemical evidence of *KIT* activation can be found in almost all GISTs, and in approximately 90% of cases, this activation is linked to somatic mutations of *KIT*, usually involving exon 9 or 11.[18] Further, evidence exists that *KIT* mutations occur early in the pathogenesis of this cancer.[18-20] In this previously chemotherapy-refractory malignancy, single-agent imatinib yielded a response rate of 53% to 65%, with another 19% to 36% of patients having disease stabilization.[21,22]

Imatinib also has shown significant activity in patients with acute lymphoblastic leukemia who are *BCR-ABL* positive,[23] patients with chronic myelomonocytic leukemia who have (5;12) translocations that fuse the *EVT6* (*TEL*) and *PDGFRB* genes, resulting in the activation of the *PDGFRB*,[24-26] and patients with dermatofibrosarcoma protuberans (DFSP).[27,28] DFSP is a low-grade sarcoma of the dermis that often recurs after surgical excision. These tumors are characterized by a (17;22) translocation involving the *COL1A1* and *PDGFB* genes, which leads to constitutive production of the growth factor *PDGFB* with consequent hyperactivation of the *PDGFRB*.[29]

As *KIT* and the *PDGFRs* are expressed in many common tumors and are reported to be activated by both autocrine and paracrine mechanisms, much interest has been shown in using imatinib broadly. As no other tumor has genetic evidence for involvement of these receptor systems, clinical trials with imatinib in these indications would be considered empirical clinical trials. Thus far,

TABLE 30-1

Diseases in Which Imatinib Has Shown Activity		
TARGET	**DISEASE**	**MECHANISM OF ACTIVATION**
ABL	CML	Chromosomal translocation t(9;22) – BCR-ABL
	ALL	Chromosomal translocation t(9;22) – BCR-ABL
KIT	GIST	Point mutation
PDGFRA	GIST	Point mutation
	HES	Intrachromosomal deletion FIPILI-PDGFRA
PDGFRB	CMML	Chromosomal translocation t(5;12) – EVT6-PDGFRB
	DFSP	Chromosomal translocation t(17;22) – colIAI-PDGFβ

ALL, acute lymphoblastic leukemia; CMML, chronic myelomonocytic leukemia; CML, chronic myeloid leukemia; DFSP, dermatofibrosarcoma protuberans; GIST, gastrointestinal stromal tumor; HES, hypereosinophilic syndrome.

single-agent activity of imatinib in tumors such as small cell lung cancer, breast, prostate, melanoma, and non-GIST sarcomas has been minimal.[30-34] One example in which empirical clinical trials of imatinib have been successful is hypereosinophilic syndrome (HES).[35] The dramatic empirical results of imatinib in HES prompted investigations of the molecular basis for the activity of imatinib in this disease. Two groups independently arrived at the conclusion that an intrachromosomal deletion on chromosome 4 resulted in a fusion between a gene of unknown function, *FIP1L1*, and a truncated *PDGFRA* in a large percentage of patients with this disorder.[36,37] The resulting FIP1L1-PRGFRA fusion protein is a constitutively activated tyrosine kinase that is imatinib-sensitive, thus accounting for the responsiveness of this disease to imatinib. Therefore imatinib has worked in diseases in which a genetic defect activates a target of imatinib, but imatinib has not worked in tumors in which a target of imatinib is expressed without genetic evidence of target activation, despite numerous reports of autocrine or paracrine activation of these targets. These data do not preclude the possibility that imatinib could be of benefit in these tumors in combination with other agents.

FLT3, RAF, and RAS Inhibitors

Although numerous molecular genetic defects in cancer have been identified, only a few agents in clinical trials target these abnormalities. *FLT3* mutations are among the most common molecular defects identified in patients with acute myeloid leukemia (AML), and the presence of this mutation imparts a poorer prognosis, regardless of the subtype of AML.[38-40] In approximately 20% of patients with AML and 3% of patients with myelodysplasia, *FLT3* contains an internal tandem duplication of the juxtamembrane domain.[39] More recently, another 7% of patients with AML and 3% with myelodysplasia were found to have a point mutation in the activation loop of the *FLT3* kinase domain.[38] These mutations lead to constitutive activation of the *FLT3* tyrosine kinase, and currently several inhibitors of the *FLT3* tyrosine kinase are in clinical trials. *FLT3* mutations in AML are likely late events as opposed to the *BCR-ABL* rearrangement in CML, *KIT* mutations in GIST, and *PML-RAR-α* in APL. Preliminary results from the clinical trials of *FLT3* inhibitors in AML patients with *FLT3* mutations show that these agents have clinical activity, but the durability of responses tends to be short.[41-43] Combination clinical trials with standard chemotherapy are planned or in progress.

Taking advantage of the human genome sequence and their ability to perform high-throughput sequencing, investigators at the Sanger Institute initiated a search for signal-transduction genes in the *RAS-RAF* pathway that are mutated in cancer. This effort paid off with the identification of a high frequency (59%) of *BRAF* mutations in melanoma.[44] Several groups confirmed this finding, and *BRAF* mutations also have been found in a high frequency of papillary thyroid carcinomas and in approximately 10% of colon carcinomas.[45-47] Interestingly, *RAS* and *RAF* mutations in these cancers are almost always mutually exclusive events,[45,47,48] providing genetic evidence that

these proteins are in the same pathway. *RAF* inhibitors are currently being evaluated in clinical trials.

RAS mutations are among the more common molecular genetic abnormalities in cancer. *RAS* mutations are present in more than 15% of all cancers, and in some cancers, such as pancreatic carcinoma, the frequency is as high as 90%.[49] Thus inhibitors of *RAS* function would likely be useful antineoplastic agents. RAS acts as a guanosine triphosphatase (GTPase), and this activity is essential for its function. Localization of *RAS* to the cytoplasmic face of membranes through a C-terminal lipid modification also is essential to *RAS* function. Thus far, it has not been possible to generate compounds that specifically inactivate the GTPase function of *RAS*. Instead, attention has focused on the lipid modification of *RAS* with inhibitors of the enzyme that transfers a farnesyl group to the C-terminus of *RAS*. Farnesyl transferase inhibitors (FTIs) are in phase II clinical trials, with only modest activity seen[50,51]; however, several problems are seen with these clinical trials. First, the most common forms of *RAS* mutated in human tumors, *K-* and *N-RAS*, also can be geranylgeranylated in the presence of FTIs, thus allowing membrane localization and activation of *RAS*, thereby circumventing the action of FTIs.[52,53] Second, numerous farnesylated proteins occur in a cell, and it is possible that these compounds do not work through one specific protein or that the critical target has not yet been identified. One potential target of FTIs is *RHOB*. FTIs alter the ratio of farnesylated to geranylgeranylated proteins, and the geranylgeranylated form of *RHOB* has growth-suppressive properties.[54] Whether this is the critical target of FTIs is not entirely clear.[53,55] Unfortunately, the lack of a thorough understanding of the mechanism of action of FTIs makes it difficult to predict where they would be best used. Despite the foregoing, *RAS* does remain a good target for anticancer therapy.

Targeting Other Genetic Defects

Given the number of genetic abnormalities identified in cancer, it is perhaps a bit surprising that no agents in clinical trials target these defects. Some of this could have to do with market size. For example, the anaplastic lymphoma kinase (*ALK*), which is activated by fusion to nucleophosmin (*NPM*) in anaplastic large cell lymphoma, and the rearranged during transfection (*RET*) tyrosine kinase in multiple endocrine neoplasia are well-defined genetic targets. As these are relatively uncommon disorders, compounds that specifically target these abnormalities would have small markets. The counter-argument to this is that these diseases would allow a rapid pathway to drug approval, and depending on the off-target activity of the compounds, they could be tested more broadly. This is similar to the pathway taken with imatinib. Its *ABL*-inhibitory activity allowed rapid Food and Drug Administration (FDA) approval in CML, and its activity against *KIT* and *PDGFR* has allowed rapid expansion to other disease indications.

Many of the genetic defects in cancers have not been targeted because many of them are loss-of-function mutations or deletions. For example, two of the most common mutations in cancer, *p53* and the retinoblastoma (*RB1*) gene, are in this category.[56] The optimal therapeutic strategy would be to replace the defective protein with a normal version, but several difficulties are found with this approach. The obvious difficulty is that this will require technologic developments that would allow gene replacement. Although this strategy should work in cases in which a gene and protein are deleted, in cases in which a malfunctioning protein might function as a dominant negative, it might be necessary to replace the defective gene and to target the abnormal allele.

In many cancers, mutations have occurred in transcription factors. For example, in acute leukemias, numerous fusion proteins that alter transcription factor function have been identified from analysis of the breakpoints of recurrent chromosomal translocations that characterize these cancers. Successful targeting of these proteins would require compounds that either inhibit or restore the DNA-binding ability of the mutated protein. Alternatively, as many of these proteins require dimerization for their function, compounds that inhibit the formation of active dimmers could be envisioned. To date, agents of this class have not been developed. Similarly, antiapoptotic proteins, such as BCL-2, function by binding to and inhibiting the function of proapoptotic proteins. Although small-molecule inhibitors that antagonize *BCL-2* function by disrupting its interactions with proapoptotic proteins have been tested in preclinical models,[57-59] these compounds have not yet reached the clinic. One way to circumvent these problems has been to downregulate protein expression by using antisense oligonucleotides. Antisense oligonucleotides to *BCL-2* are in clinical trials.[60] As follicular lymphomas have overexpression of *BCL-2* due to a translocation of the *BCL-2* gene into the immunoglobulin heavy-chain locus, this might be the ideal disease in which to test agents that antagonize *BCL-2* function or expression.

Another way to deal with the difficulties in developing drugs to target many of the noted genetic defects has been to take advantage of specific properties imparted to cancer cells by molecular genetic defects. For example, an adenovirus vector has been generated that replicates only in cells with defective *p53*.[61] Another class of agents is known as synthetic lethals. Synthetic lethal refers to the phenotype whereby inactivation of one gene allows a second gene to be inactivated and cause cell death, but inactivation of either gene alone has no effect on viability. For example, cells that have lost *pRB* and as a consequence have derepressed *E2F* are exquisitely sensitive to inhibitors of cyclin A/cyclin-dependent kinase-2 (*CDK2*) activity.[62] This latter category, targeting proteins or pathways that are downstream of defined genetic abnormalities, is discussed in greater detail later.

One of the advantages of classifying agents that target genetically defined lesions is that it allows a simple transition to targeted preventive strategies. Thus as genetic abnormalities are identified that contribute to cancer development, these abnormalities would also become good targets for preventive agents. Examples in this category include mismatch-repair genes implicated in colon cancer and the *BRCA1* and *BRCA2* genes. Many

of the same considerations discussed earlier for loss-of-function abnormalities apply to these genetic defects, but nonetheless, these would be ideal targets for molecular preventive interventions.

LESSONS LEARNED FROM CLINICAL TRIALS OF AGENTS TARGETING MOLECULAR GENETIC DEFECTS

In reviewing the lessons learned from agents that target genetically defined abnormalities, as few examples exist, extrapolations must be made with caution. Despite this, some consistent themes seem to be emerging.

Response Rates

The partial response rate to agents that target molecular genetic defects in cancer has been in excess of 50%, but CRs have been uncommon, particularly in advanced diseases such as GIST and CML blast crisis. It could be argued that the examples to date represent relatively simple malignancies such as leukemia and sarcomas. The agents used thus far either have targeted dominant growth-stimulatory pathways or have relieved a block to differentiation, and in most cases have targeted early, causative mutations as opposed to late genetic changes. It could be argued, however, that all malignancies will depend on this type of a genetic defect and that it is simply a matter of defining the genetic lesion in each malignancy. Each of these clinical trials targeted a relatively homogeneous population, that is, a population of patients whose tumors were genetically defined to be caused by the targeted defect. As the genetic definitions of tumors improve, the ability to match the right patient to the right drug by using these genetic definitions will vastly improve, and this should have an enormous impact on response rates and the ability to predict responses.

Resistance

Resistance to single agents, even those targeted to genetically defined abnormalities, has been common. The only exception to this has been chronic-phase patients with CML treated with imatinib.[15,63] In APL, resistance to ATRA is due to induction of metabolism of ATRA, upregulation of cellular retinoic acid–binding proteins, or mutations in the ligand-binding domain of the *RARα*.[64] In CML blast crisis and in the fraction of patients in chronic phase who respond to imatinib and then relapse, the most common mechanism of relapse has been point mutations in the *ABL* kinase domain that render the kinase variably insensitive to imatinib.[65,66] Similarly, in GIST, the most common mechanism of relapse has been mutations in *KIT* that are imatinib insensitive.[67] In contrast, *BCR-ABL*–independent mechanisms of resistance are more common than kinase-domain mutations in patients with CML in blast crisis who respond poorly to imatinib.[68]

Thus one of the themes emerging from studies of resistance is that the target for the drug remains important, even when resistance develops. A corollary to

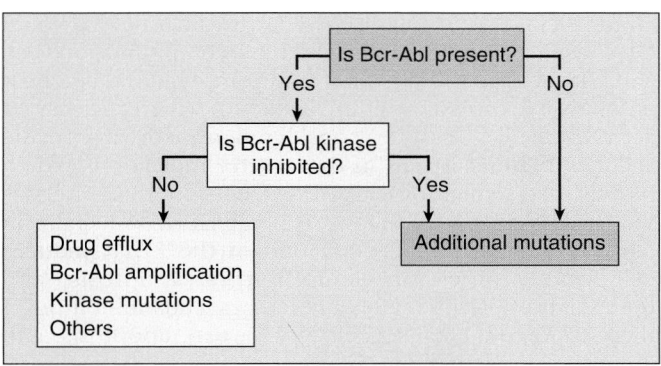

Figure 30-1. Distinguishing between potential mechanisms of relapse.

this is that clinical trials with these types of agents must incorporate assays to determine target modulation. This was well exemplified in the clinical trials of imatinib in CML. Initially, expression of the target should be the starting point for evaluation of relapse mechanisms, and in all patients who have relapsed, the *BCR-ABL* kinase remains present. A particularly useful categorization of imatinib resistance has been to determine whether persistent inhibition of the *BCR-ABL* kinase occurs (Fig. 30-1). Patients with persistent inhibition of the *BCR-ABL* kinase would be predicted to have additional molecular abnormalities besides *BCR-ABL* driving the growth and survival of the malignant clone. In contrast, patients with reactivation of the kinase would be postulated to have resistance mechanisms that either prevent imatinib from reaching the target or render the target insensitive to *BCR-ABL*. In the former category are mechanisms such as drug efflux or protein binding of imatinib. In the latter category are mutations of the *BCR-ABL* kinase that render *BCR-ABL* insensitive to imatinib and amplification of the BCR-ABL protein.

In the largest studies of resistance or relapse, the *BCR-ABL* kinase has been reactivated in the majority of patients who respond initially to imatinib and then relapse while continuing to receive therapy.[69] *BCR-ABL* kinase activity was analyzed by assessing tyrosine phosphorylation of CRKL, a direct substrate of the *BCR-ABL* kinase and the major tyrosine phosphorylated protein in CML patient samples.[13,69,70] In these studies, more than 50% and perhaps as many as 90% of patients with hematologic relapse have *BCR-ABL* point mutations in at least 13 different amino acids scattered throughout the *ABL* kinase domain.[65,68,71-74] Some other patients have amplification of *BCR-ABL* at the genomic or transcript level. In contrast, in patients with primary resistance (i.e., patients who do not respond to imatinib therapy), *BCR-ABL*–independent mechanisms are most common.[68] Similar types of studies could be envisioned for clinical trials of any targeted therapy.

Early Therapy

Another lesson learned in the clinical trials of imatinib is an old lesson for oncologists, and that is, the earlier in the course of a disease the treatment is administered,

the better the response. This is quite apparent from an examination of responses to imatinib in patients with CML in the chronic, accelerated, or blast phases, in which responses were significantly higher and more durable in patients with chronic-phase disease (Fig. 30-2). These data suggest that despite the presence of multiple mutations in advanced disease, the tumor remains sensitive to drugs that target a single, early causal mutation. However, the most important implication of this is that vastly improved techniques must be developed to diagnose cancers earlier in their course, when cancers are genetically much simpler and homogeneous. Even when used early, imatinib as a single agent has not entirely eradicated the disease. In newly diagnosed chronic-phase patients with CML, the majority of patients obtain a complete cytogenetic response with imatinib therapy.[15] This corresponds to an approximately two-log reduction in *BCR-ABL* levels by quantitative reverse transcriptase–polymerase chain reaction (RT-PCR) for *BCR-ABL*. However, fewer than 5% obtain a five-log or greater reduction in *BCR-ABL* levels,[75] which would correspond to undetectable levels of *BCR-ABL* transcripts or a molecular remission. Thus the majority of patients respond well but have molecular persistence of disease. An obvious concern exists that patients who do not achieve a molecular remission could relapse over time. It is not known whether the mechanisms of molecular persistence are the same as or different from the mechanisms of disease relapse; however, this raises the issue of whether single agents, even when used early in the course of a disease, will reliably be able to eradicate a cancer.

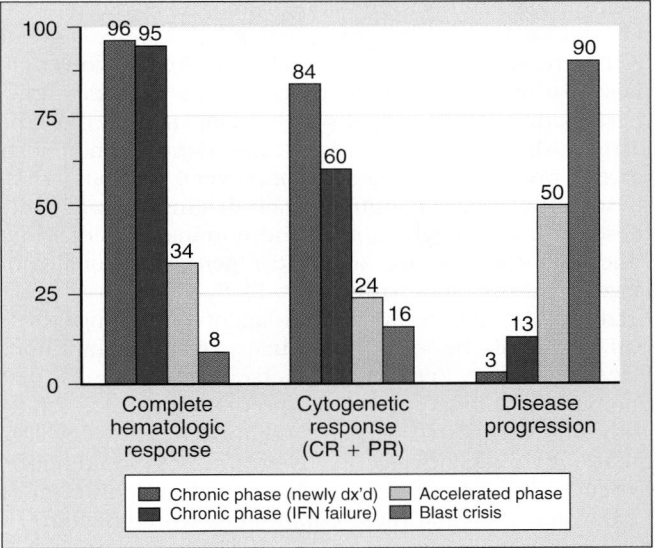

Figure 30-2. Phase II and III results of imatinib for chronic myeloid leukemia. The results shown are for newly diagnosed chronic-phase patients with a median follow-up of 18 months.[15] For the phase II studies in chronic-phase patients for whom interferon (IFN)-α therapy failed, accelerated-phase, and blast crisis patients, results are with a median follow-up of ≤30 months, and the rate of disease progression is at 24 months.[16,63,137] Complete response (CR) and partial response (PR) for cytogenetic responses include patients with Ph chromosome–positive metaphases of ≤35%.

Identification of Responding Patients and Patient Selection

In the clinical trials of imatinib in GIST, the majority of patients had activating *KIT* mutations in exon 11, and these patients had a partial response rate of close to 80%. In contrast, patients whose tumors expressed wild-type *KIT*, with no mutation, had a response rate of only 18%.[76] Thus *KIT* mutational status correlated with response. The implications of this finding are extremely important and again relate to identifying patients by using genetic definitions of tumor types. Thus in GIST, expression of *KIT* is not sufficient to predict responses; rather, a mutation in *KIT* is necessary for responses to be observed.

It also has been instructive to determine why 18% of patients with wild-type *KIT* expression respond to imatinib. Examination of tumors from patients with wild-type *KIT* expression showed that one third of these tumors had activating mutations of the *PDGFRA*.[77] These mutations occurred in two different exons. One set of mutations was imatinib sensitive, and this accounted for responses observed in patients whose tumors expressed wild-type *KIT*.[77] Thus careful evaluations of subsets of responding patients can yield important insights into disease pathogenesis and the mechanism of response to an agent.

AGENTS THAT TARGET PATHWAYS ACTIVATED IN CANCER CELLS

It has been postulated that cancer cells require activation of several pathways to manifest the malignant phenotype fully.[78] This includes stimulation of growth, allowing cell-cycle progression, suppression of apoptosis, recruitment of a blood supply, and reactivation of telomerase. Our ever-increasing knowledge of the proteins involved in these pathways has led to numerous agents that target these pathways. These pathway-specific targets must be distinguished from the genetically defined molecular targets previously discussed for several reasons. First, these pathways are common to all dividing cells. Second, these pathways might not be the dominant lesions in a cancer. In the absence of a clear genetic rationale for targeting a specific pathway, it likely is impossible to predict whether responses to agents targeting these pathways will be observed. Finally, many compounds targeting these pathways, such as angiogenesis or telomerase inhibitors, would be predicted to be cytostatic as opposed to cytocidal. This complicates the development of these agents, as objective responses would not be expected. This means either that novel endpoints must be developed or that these compounds would need to be used in combination with other agents for responses to be seen. Despite the foregoing, it should be noted that many agents in this category have already demonstrated clinical benefits and that any therapy that can improve response rates, quality of life, and survival of cancer patients is an important advance.

It should be readily apparent that a single compound could meet the definition of a genetically targeted agent and a pathway-specific agent, depending on the circumstances. Thus as discussed with imatinib, it would be considered a genetically targeted compound for CML and GIST, but for most solid tumors, in which a target for imatinib is expressed without genetic evidence of target activation, it would be considered a pathway-specific agent, and clinical trials in these latter indications would be at least semiempirical. Last, agents in this category will be classified according to their primary mechanism of action. For example, activation of the *EGFR* induces cell-cycle progression, inhibition of apoptosis, and upregulation of antiangiogenic factors. Thus inhibition of the *EGFR* could cause cell-cycle arrest, apoptosis, and inhibition of angiogenesis. As the primary and direct mechanism of action of the *EGFR* is to serve as a growth-factor receptor, it is classified as a growth-stimulatory agent. A target, such as *p53*, which has roles in cell-cycle progression, apoptosis, and maintenance of genetic stability could be included in any of these categories.

Growth-stimulatory Pathways

Drugs that target growth-stimulatory pathways in cancer include some of the most successful agents in cancer therapy. Specifically, this category includes agents that target the estrogen and androgen receptors, and these agents have yielded extremely high response rates in breast and prostate cancer. For example, responses to tamoxifen in estrogen receptor–positive metastatic breast cancer were nearly 50% in an era when tamoxifen was not routinely used in the adjuvant setting.[79] For agents that target the androgen receptor in prostate cancer, response rates are 60% to 85%. These high response rates are seen although activating mutations in either the estrogen or androgen receptors in breast or prostate cancer are uncommon. Thus it is clear that estrogen and androgen are critically important for the growth and survival of breast and prostate cells despite the lack of mutations in their receptors and the lack of evidence of constitutive activation of these growth pathways. In breast cancer patients, responses to tamoxifen in estrogen receptor–negative patients are uncommon.[79] Therefore it is possible to define a subgroup of patients with a high likelihood of responding to therapy based on target expression. Another important point about the use of antiestrogenic agents is that they have shown that a drug that is useful in advanced disease is also useful in earlier disease and as a preventive therapy.

The EGFR family is one of the most extensively studied growth-stimulatory pathways in cancer, and agents that target two members of this family, the *EGFR* (also known as *ErbB1* or *HER1*) and *HER2* (also known as *ErbB2* or *NEU*), have been FDA approved. In the case of the *EGFR*, extensive data report overexpression of this receptor in many cancers, although some glioblastomas and other cancers express a truncated and activated receptor.[80] For *HER2*, evidence exists of overexpression in breast cancer, and expression correlates with poorer survival.[81,82] Categorization of *HER2* as a target illustrates the complexity in trying to simplify definitions. The most common mechanism of *HER2* overexpression is gene amplification with increased gene copy number, which can be detected by fluorescent in situ hybridization (FISH).[82] This could potentially place *HER2* in the genetically defined category; however, it is not known whether this is a dominant defect in the development of breast cancer or whether other genes on chromosome 17 coordinately amplified with *HER2* also have a role in the disease.[83]

The approved agents that target the EGFR family members are gefitinib (Iressa), a small-molecular-weight tyrosine kinase inhibitor of the EGFR, and trastuzumab (Herceptin), a monoclonal antibody that targets *HER2*. Other small-molecule inhibitors of both receptors and monoclonal antibodies that target the EGFR (e.g., cetuximab) are in clinical trials.[80,84] In patients with non–small cell lung cancer (NSCLC), clinical trials with single-agent gefitinib and erlotinib (Tarceva), another small-molecular-weight EGFR inhibitor, have shown response rates in heavily pretreated patients in the 10% to 18% range.[80,85] With trastuzumab, in a similar heavily pretreated population of breast cancer patients, a 12% to 15% objective response rate was observed.[86,87] In the trastuzumab clinical trials, responses correlated with levels of receptor expression and were as high as 35% in previously untreated patients with the highest levels of *HER2* expression.[88] Thus patients with the highest likelihood of responding to trastuzumab can be identified prospectively. In contrast, *EGFR* expression has not correlated with responses to erlotinib.[89] Improved responses have been observed for combinations of trastuzumab with chemotherapy,[90] but this again has not been the case with gefitinib.[85] This could be because single-agent activity was so low that few responding patients were enrolled in the non–small cell lung cancer trials comparing gefitinib plus chemotherapy with chemotherapy alone.

In both of these cases, it is worth exploring why responses rates have not been higher (Fig. 30-3). As previously noted, expression might not be sufficient to predict response; rather, some measure of activation also would be necessary. In addition, it would be critical to determine whether the agent being tested modulates the target in the tumor. Unfortunately, in the clinical trials with gefitinib and trastuzumab, minimal data addressed

this issue. As such, it is possible that the target was not sufficiently modified in the tumor to induce a response. If a low response rate is observed, yet the target is known to be expressed and modulated by an agent, it could be that the target is not critical to the growth and survival of the cancer being tested. Of course, it could be possible that combinations with other agents or alternative endpoints would alter the interpretation of the results. Finally, one must consider that a subset of patients could respond well, and that identification of the mechanism underlying the response in these patients could yield insight into better patient selection.

It also is worth considering that the mechanism of action of gefitinib and trastuzumab is somewhat poorly defined. In the case of gefitinib, a small-molecular-weight tyrosine kinase inhibitor, minimal data have been published on the profile of kinases inhibited by this compound.[91] Thus it is possible that gefitinib targets an unknown kinase and that targeting of this kinase is responsible for the observed responses. With trastuzumab, the situation is a bit more complex, and possible mechanisms of action include (1) accelerated degradation of *HER2* leading to reduced cellular *HER2* expression; (2) inhibition of the activation of *HER2* by interference of the heterodimerization of *HER2* with other EGFR family members; and (3) targeting the immune system to cells overexpressing *HER2*.[92] As it is not clear what the relative contributions of these mechanisms are to the clinical efficacy of trastuzumab, it is not clear what should be measured as an endpoint to determine whether the target has been modulated by trastuzumab.

Targeting Signaling Proteins Downstream of Genetically Defined Molecular Abnormalities

This category includes numerous signaling proteins, of which a few examples include AKT and mTOR, acting downstream of *PTEN*; E2F and cyclinA/CDK2, acting downstream of *pRB*; or MEK and MAP kinases, acting downstream of *RAS* and *RAF*. Molecularly genetically defined targets previously discussed also might be contained in this category. For example, *RAS* is frequently mutated in human cancers, but it also is frequently activated by mutations occurring in upstream pathways, such as *BCR-ABL*, *KIT*, and others. The ability to predict how well agents in this category will work depends in part on how tightly linked the action of the molecular abnormality is to its downstream targets. It was previously noted that DFSP is caused by a chromosomal translocation that results in the constitutive production of the ligand for the *PDGFRB*. As all of the actions of this ligand are mediated through the *PDGFRB*, it is clear that targeting the *PDGFRB* with an inhibitor of its kinase activity should be a useful therapeutic strategy. In many other cases, however, signaling proteins initiate a cascade of events, and predicting the effects of targeting one of the downstream events would not be possible. Although this does not mean that this strategy would not work, it does imply that clinical trials will be more empirically based. Some of this empiricism can be dealt with in the same

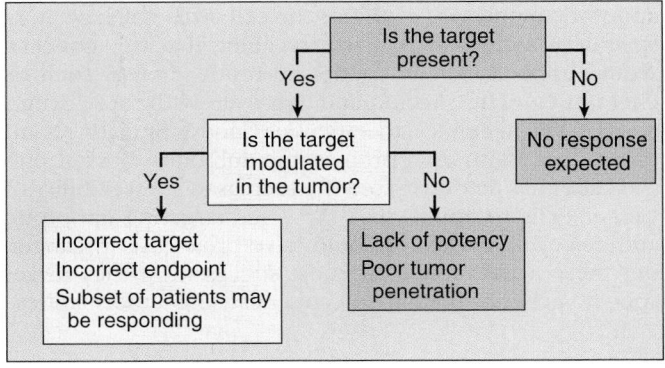

Figure 30-3. Evaluation of responses to targeted agents. This figure outlines the evaluation of a targeted therapy in clinical trials and how to interpret results if lower than expected responses are obtained.

manner as discussed for agents that target the genetically defined defects, that is, by selecting patients who are likely to respond in clinical trials. In this situation, this can be done by using the known link between the molecular defect and the target. For example, clinical trials with an mTOR inhibitor would best be performed in patients with activation of this protein, and patients whose tumors lack *PTEN* would be an ideal population.[93] Further, in vitro data demonstrate that cell lines that lack *PTEN* are extremely sensitive to mTOR inhibitors.[94,95] This concept of synthetic lethality was previously introduced in reference to the *pRB* pathway and inhibitors of cyclin A/CDK2.

Cell Cycle

It is clear from our knowledge of chemotherapeutic agents that targeting the cell cycle can be an effective anticancer strategy. With improved knowledge of the proteins and pathways that control cell-cycle progression, significant interest has been indicated in specifically targeting these pathways. Cell-cycle progression is carefully modulated by cyclins, cyclin-dependent kinases (CDKs), and cyclin-dependent kinase inhibitors (CKIs). A restriction point late in G_1 serves as a crucial transition point after which cells are committed to cell-cycle progression. The critical regulator of the G_1 restriction point is *pRB*.[56] *p53* function also is a critical integrator of signals at the G_1 restriction point; however, cells that lack *p53* also are blocked at the G_2 to mitosis transition.[96] Transcription factors, such as *MYC*, whose expression is induced by numerous growth factor pathways, also are crucial to facilitate cell-cycle progression. Last, during mitosis, numerous proteins have already been targets of anticancer agents, such as microtubules, and others are in development, such as inhibitors of kinesin, a protein required for chromosome segregation.

As previously noted, many of the proteins involved in the control of the cell cycle are dysregulated in human cancers and would be good targets for therapy. Several novel agents that target CDKs are in clinical trials.[97] One of the most advanced is flavoperidol, a broad-spectrum CDK inhibitor. Some activity of this agent has been seen in mantle cell lymphoma,[98] which is of particular interest, as the majority of mantle cell lymphomas overexpress cyclin D1 as a result of a chromosomal translocation.

An obvious issue with cell-cycle inhibitors is their specificity for cancer cells as opposed to normal cells, which could cause nonspecific toxicity. This also applies to agents that induce apoptosis and is discussed in the next section. Another issue has to do with redundancy of function. For example, CDK2 and cyclin E have been assumed to be indispensable for cell-cycle progression; however, targeted disruption of these genes was not embryonic lethal, nor were defects noted in continuously proliferating cells.[99,100] These data suggest that specific inhibitors of CDK2 might not lead to cell-cycle arrest unless CDK2 was the dominant pathway through which a cancer-causing mutation functioned. Disabling this pathway, however, in combination with agents that inhibit other cell-cycle pathways, could be an effective approach. Last, whether inhibitors of the cell cycle would cause cell-cycle arrest or induce apoptosis is not entirely clear, but this would have a substantial impact on choice of endpoints and optimal use for these agents.

Apoptosis

As the molecular mechanisms of cell death have been elucidated, numerous therapeutic targets in this pathway have been identified. The discovery of the cell-death pathways has also brought about an understanding that most cancer therapies work by inducing cell death. For most agents, however, this is a secondary effect. Thus accumulation of DNA damage from alkylating agents or radiation therapy leads to cell-cycle arrest and activation of cell-death pathways. The agents to be considered in this section are those that target specific proteins in the cell-death pathway. These include *BCL-2* family members, intracellular antiapoptotic proteins (IAPs), the tumor necrosis factor (TNF) family (TNF, *FAS* ligand, and TNF-related apoptosis-inducing ligand [TRAIL] and their receptors, and the caspases, as described in additional detail in Chapter 6. For cancer cells to survive, they must acquire resistance to apoptosis, and in some cancers, this is a causal event. This is the case in follicular lymphoma, which overexpresses *BCL-2* because of a chromosome translocation, thus making *BCL-2* an ideal target in this tumor. BCL-2 protein expression also is upregulated in many other cancers, and clinical trials with antisense *BCL-2* are currently in progress. Other agents in clinical trials include antibodies to TRAIL receptors that act as agonists, thus triggering apoptosis.[101,102]

One of the concerns about apoptosis-inducing agents and cell-cycle inhibitors is toxicity. This has not been the case for agents targeting growth factors, as most normal cells do not depend on a single growth factor for their survival. In contrast, tumors may develop "oncogene dependence" in which a single, dominant growth factor pathway becomes required for the growth and survival of the cancer. This has been one of the explanations advanced for both the success and lack of toxicity of agents targeting dominant growth factor pathways. With apoptosis-inducing agents, it also is possible that cells with activation of a dominant survival pathway would be susceptible to an agent that targets this pathway specifically. Of concern, however, is that any agent that activates apoptotic pathways or inhibits the cell cycle will have nonspecific toxicities. It is worth recalling that this concern would apply to many agents currently in use, such as chemotherapeutic agents, and that even with these drugs, it is possible to define a therapeutic window. Similarly, recent experience with the proteasome inhibitor bortezomib (Velcade) has demonstrated the increased susceptibility of cancer cells to apoptosis.[103,104] Thus targeting apoptotic and cell-cycle pathways could have broad use in cancer, but these agents might be most successful if they target specific genetically defined cancer-causing abnormalities.

Angiogenesis

All tumors require a blood supply, and a variety of therapies directed at interfering with the growth of new blood vessels are in development. The angiogenic pathway is described in detail in Chapter 9 and has stimulated enormous interest for anticancer therapeutics. In general, the activation of angiogenic pathways is secondary to the causal genetic abnormalities in a cancer, and only factors that directly affect blood vessel formation are considered in this section. One genetically defined mutation in a pathway that directly affects angiogenesis is mutation of the von Hippel-Lindau (*VHL*) gene. In patients with inherited mutations in this gene, benign and malignant tumors develop that histologically are characterized by hypervascularization.[105] Further, up to 80% of sporadic clear cell renal cell carcinomas have mutations in the *VHL* gene.[106,107] On a molecular level, loss of *VHL* function leads to upregulation of hypoxia-inducible factor a, with subsequent overproduction of vascular endothelial growth factor (VEGF).[108] VEGF stimulates the growth of endothelial cells and is a central factor in angiogenesis.

Based on this knowledge, a clinical trial of bevacizumab (Avastin), a monoclonal antibody that targets VEGF, was performed in patients with metastatic clear cell renal cell carcinoma. Patients receiving high-dose antibody therapy achieved a response rate of 10%. As compared with those treated with placebo, patients treated with the highest dose of antibody had prolongation of time to progression but no improvement in overall survival.[109] One of the problems with this study is that *VHL* mutations were not a requirement for enrollment, and the majority of patients did not have measurable plasma levels of VEGF. Bevacizumab also has been tested in combination with chemotherapy in patients with metastatic colon cancer, and a 4-month survival advantage was seen for patients randomized to the combination therapy arm.[110]

Other antiangiogenic agents are at earlier stages in clinical trials, but preliminary results show similarly modest results.[111-113] These modest results could be due to many factors including patient selection and selection of endpoints, particularly because angiogenesis inhibitors would be predicted to be cytostatic as opposed to cytotoxic agents. This could mean that longer treatment intervals or that combination with other agents will be needed to see clinical benefits. With these considerations in mind, surrogate markers, such as microvessel density, have been used to judge the effects of angiogenesis inhibitors; however, microvessel density has not correlated with response.[111] This could be due to lack of standardization of measurements, heterogeneity of tumors, and the pleiotropic effects of many of the antiangiogenesis agents in clinical trials. Alternate surrogate markers are being investigated and include measurement of proangiogenic proteins, imaging techniques, and measuring circulating endothelial cells that are recruited to form new blood vessels.[111,113,114]

Another area of promise in the angiogenesis field is the finding that the vasculature varies from organ to organ, and tumor blood vessels express markers that are not present in resting blood vessels of normal tissues.[115] These "vasculature signatures" might make it possible to target diagnostic and therapeutic agents to specific tumors or sites.[116,117]

Telomerase

The maintenance of telomeres, specialized structures at the ends of chromosomes, is essential for chromosome stability.[118] Chromosome ends progressively shorten with cell divisions, and without new synthesis of telomeres, cells would eventually undergo programmed cell death. Although telomerase is tightly repressed in most somatic cells, its expression is reactivated in most tumor cells. In a minority of tumors, telomere length is maintained by a recombination method.[78,119]

Telomerase is a unique reverse transcriptase consisting of an RNA subunit (telomerase RNA component, TERC) and a catalytic subunit (telomerase reverse transcriptase, TERT) that adds hexanucleotide repeats to the ends of telomeric DNA.[118] In addition, several regulatory proteins bind to the telomere.[120,121] As telomerase activity is limited to tumors and a few adult tissues with the capacity for self-renewal, telomerase has emerged as a target for therapy. Preclinical studies have targeted virtually all of the components of the telomerase pathway and demonstrate progressive telomere shortening with eventual growth arrest or apoptosis.[120] The translation of telomerase-targeting agents to the clinic will likely face many of the previously noted challenges for angiogenesis inhibitors. Specifically, tumor shrinkage would be expected only with lengthy treatment unless combined with other agents. Pharmacodynamic parameters might be useful endpoints, but would depend on the agent being tested and could include protein expression, telomerase activity, or telomere length.

Targeting Genetic Instability

Another common feature of cancer cells is genetic instability, and this could be an early event in many cancers. For example, up to 80% of in situ breast carcinomas are aneuploid.[122] As previously noted, *BRCA1*, *BRCA2*, and mismatch-repair genes are among several examples of germline mutations that increase mutational rates and predispose affected individuals to cancer. These and other abnormalities in this category would be obvious targets for molecular preventive strategies. As additional molecular determinants that lead to genetic instability are identified, targeting these abnormalities could be envisioned as an adjunct to other treatments to decrease the evolution of resistant clones. Genetic instability also is one of the consequences of inactivation of *p53*, and loss of *p53* function allows cells to divide despite DNA damage, thus contributing to resistance to chemotherapy and radiation therapy. Thus targeting *p53* or other similar activities that are permissive for cell replication in the presence of DNA damage could enhance or restore sensitivity to chemotherapy or radiation.

Agents That Target Cell-surface Markers on Cancer Cells

Other agents that have been called "molecularly targeted" are those that target cell-surface receptors. In this category are several agents targeting CD20 on B-cell malignancies, including rituximab (Rituxan),[123] and two radiolabeled CD20 conjugates, ibritumomab tiuxetan (Zevalin), a yttrium 90–labeled agent,[124] and iodine 131–labeled tositumomab (Bexxar).[125] Another immunoconjugate in this category is gemtuzumab ozogamicin (Mylotarg), a CD33 antibody linked to the cytotoxic agent calicheamicin for myeloid malignancies. These agents are discussed in greater detail in Chapter 31. Trastuzumab, cetuximab, and bevacizumab also are in this category and were discussed in the sections on targeting growth-factor pathways and angiogenesis. The specificity of action of agents in this category depends on the expression of the target on normal versus cancer cells. Clinical trials with rituximab have demonstrated that cross-linking of an antibody to a radioactive substance or chemical compound is not a necessity for clinical benefits to be observed. Potential mechanisms of action of rituximab include direct signaling of apoptosis, complement activation, and antibody-dependent cell-mediated cytotoxicity.[126]

DESIGN OF CLINICAL TRIALS WITH TARGETED AGENTS

Patient Selection

The development of targeted agents, whether targeted against genetically defined abnormalities or specific pathways, offers unique challenges for clinical trial design. As noted, patient selection can be critical to the success or failure of an agent. The importance of patient selection is illustrated in Figure 30-4, which shows a hypothetical set of clinical trials in which monotherapy with a targeted agent results in a 60% clinical response rate, but if and only if the target is present in the tumor. In the four examples shown in this figure, the target frequency varies from 90% to 10%, and the corresponding overall response rates vary from 54% to 6%. Without knowledge of the target frequency in a treated population, one might conclude that the trial with a 54% response rate was

	Target frequency	Target response rate	Observed response rate
100 patients	90% →	60% →	54%
100 patients	50% →	60% →	30%
100 patients	25% →	60% →	15%
100 patients	10% →	60% →	6%

Figure 30-4. Clinical outcome in a clinical trial of a molecularly targeted agent is determined by target frequency. In this set of hypothetical parallel clinical trials of the same agent, the response rate is 60% in patients whose tumor expresses the appropriate target. As the target frequency varies from 10% to 90% in the four trials, the overall clinical response ranges from 6% to 54%. In the absence of information concerning target frequency in the four trials, the results cannot be meaningfully compared and interpreted.

successful, but the trial with a 6% response rate was a failure. In both cases, however, the therapy was equally effective in patients who expressed the target (60% in both cases). Thus determination of target status in clinical specimens obtained from enrolled patients is crucial to the meaningful interpretation of clinical trial results. Indeed, the best results would most likely be obtained when patient eligibility for a trial is made contingent on target status. This example is the simplest possibility for clinical trial design; however, target expression might not always be sufficient to predict responses. Rather, some evidence for target activation could be required and only a subset of patients with target expression would respond. In these cases, combining expression of a target with the ability to determine its activation status would be necessary for optimal responses to be observed in clinical trials.

Dose Selection

The traditional endpoint of a phase I study for a new chemotherapy agent has been the determination of the maximally tolerated dose (MTD). This endpoint is justified on the assumption that "more is better" in terms of the clinical efficacy of traditional chemotherapy agents in treating cancer. With many targeted agents, however, MTDs have not been reached. Thus in phase I trials, the stopping dose would not necessarily be determined by toxicity, but rather by one of the following endpoints: (1) the dose that consistently achieves the target plasma level for maximum target modulation as predicted from preclinical studies; (2) direct confirmation of target modulation at test doses; and (3) failure to improve response rate with continued dose escalation. Of course, safety and tolerability continue to be critical components of any phase I trial.

Measurement of Pharmacodynamic Effects

Multiple methods exist for determining pharmacodynamic effects of a targeted agent. The most direct is biochemical measurement of target modulation in a tumor specimen. This could be straightforward in cases in which tumor cells can be obtained by skin biopsy or phlebotomy, but this approach creates difficulties in cases in which tumor specimens can be obtained only by more invasive procedure such as percutaneous biopsy. Other issues besides the feasibility of tumor procurement that could complicate the pharmacodynamic assessment of the effects of a targeted therapy include the heterogeneity of tumor tissue, the question of appropriate time points to obtain material, and the amount of tissue required to perform an assessment. Even in cases in which tumor specimens can be obtained readily, measurement of the status of the target might be technically difficult because of limitations in assay sensitivity. For example, in the case of CML, it has been difficult to derive direct measurement of *BCR-ABL* phosphorylation or kinase activity in neutrophils obtained from peripheral blood.[69]

Rather than directly assessing target modulation, it could be possible to use a surrogate marker. In the case of CML, the measurement of phospho-CRKL has proven to be useful in assessing the effectiveness of imatinib in inhibiting *BCR-ABL* activity in CML cells.[13,69] Likewise, some studies of EGFR inhibitors have measured EGFR phosphorylation or ERK activation or both in biopsies of normal skin as a surrogate for effects on the targeted EGFR-positive tumor cells.[127] Whether this is indicative of inhibition in the tumor, however, is not clear.

Another issue with the monitoring of pharmacodynamic endpoints has to do with the amount of target modulation required for a response to be seen. For example, with a kinase inhibitor, how much kinase inhibition is required for cell killing? In this regard, the timing of pharmacodynamic testing after administration of an agent could influence the results and interpretation of these tests.

Functional imaging might prove valuable for assessing an agent's activity. For example, positron emission tomography (PET) scans taken early during treatment of patients with GIST with imatinib are predictive of long-term response to imatinib.[128,129] As fluorodeoxyglucose (FDG)-PET scans measure metabolic activity of a tumor, this method might be useful only for agents that target dominant growth-stimulatory pathways. In the case of angiogenesis inhibitors, it could prove feasible to assess drug effect by measurement of vascular permeability by using dynamic magnetic resonance imaging (MRI) or other novel imaging techniques.[113,114]

Combination of Agents

Whether a cancer can be treated effectively with an agent that inhibits one of the pathways involved in cell growth or death could depend largely on the extent to which the growth of the tumor cells is dependent on the targeted protein. This principle can be illustrated by hypothetical tumor cells whose growth is dependent on protein A, protein B, or both protein A and B (Fig. 30-5). The growth of tumor cells that are dependent on a single protein would be inhibited by treatment with the appropriate agent. In contrast, no effect on proliferation would occur when cells dependent on protein A are treated with an agent that modulates the activity of protein B, or vice versa. In the case of tumor cells that are dependent on both protein A and B, therapy with an inhibitor against one of the proteins would reduce proliferation by only 50%. Complete inhibition of such cells could be achieved only when both proteins are inhibited. This model is based on actual experimental observations with factor-dependent human AML cells.[130] In some cancers, the situation could be even more complex, with tumor survival dependent on three or more proteins. In such cases, it could be necessary to target all of the proteins or to inhibit downstream effectors that are shared between all or most of the proteins.

This issue has significant implications for clinical trial design. In the foregoing model, a biologic effect does not necessarily equate with a clinical benefit. For example, in the case of a tumor that is co-dependent on protein A and B, treatment with an inhibitor specific to protein A would decrease proliferation by 50% (a biologic effect).

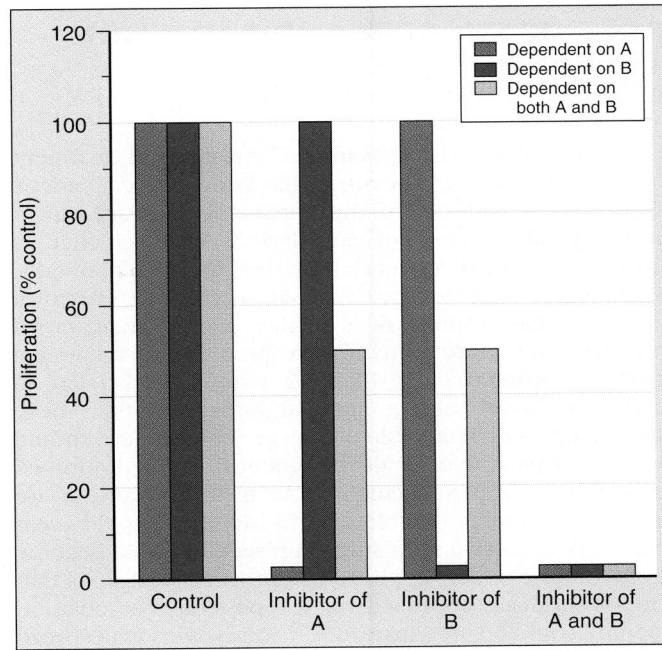

Figure 30-5. Effect of agents targeting protein A or protein B in tumors dependent on A and/or B for proliferation. The clinical effect of monotherapy with a given agent is determined by the dependence of the tumor cells on the targets modulated by that agent. In tumors dependent on more than one protein for survival, therapies must inhibit all of the critical proteins for maximal therapeutic effect.

Slowing the growth rate would not decrease the tumor size, however, and this result would be regarded as "progressive disease." If the endpoint of the clinical trial is an objective response rate, the agent would be dismissed as an ineffective therapy; however, endpoints such as delay in time to progression or prolongation of survival might reveal a therapeutic benefit. Additional studies combining an agent that targets protein A with other treatments (protein B inhibitor, cytotoxics, immune treatments, etc.) that could affect the other 50% of proliferation might result in improved clinical efficacy.

These issues demonstrate some of the difficulties faced in the development of targeted agents. Specifically, single agents might have minimal activity with standard endpoints for patients with advanced malignancies, and there could be a need to combine agents to see significant clinical activity. These issues could be particularly true in the clinical trials of angiogenesis inhibitors. Besides the need to consider alternative endpoints, it also is crucial to include measurement of target modulation before and during therapy. For example, if the targeted protein is not modulated in the tumor, this raises the possibility of poor tumor penetration or lack of potency of the agent. If, however, the protein is modulated and no measurable response is observed, this suggests that either the protein is not required for the growth and survival of the cancer and that an agent targeting this protein will not be clinically useful, or that an incorrect endpoint was selected to determine response.

ROLE OF SURGERY AND RADIATION THERAPY IN AN ERA OF MOLECULARLY TARGETED THERAPY

One of the most striking examples of successful treatment of a cancer in the 20th century has been cervical cancer. With widespread use of the Papanicolaou (Pap) smear and surgical resection of early lesions, the incidence of invasive cervical cancer has declined dramatically. Similarly, the increased use of colonoscopy with removal of polyps has resulted in a decline in the incidence of invasive colon carcinoma. The routine use of mammography in women older than 50 years has also led to increased breast cancer survival rates. Although these are examples of accessible organs or tissues, these should serve as a paradigm for development of vastly improved techniques for early detection. As most all cancers are much more highly curable in early stages, it would seem that early detection with surgical resection could become a much more widely applicable approach. For lesions that are not surgically approachable, it is possible that radiation therapy could be used instead. Obviously, with widespread use of early detection, it will be necessary to ensure that abnormalities that are detected are precancerous. As our definition of the molecular pathogenesis of early cancers improves, it also is possible that medical therapy could be used to prevent the progression of early abnormalities to cancer or be used to induce regressions of these early lesions without surgery or radiation.

As the molecular determinants of response to radiation become better defined, this knowledge also will be applied to enhancing tumor cell sensitivity to radiotherapy. Many targets that can enhance sensitivity to radiotherapy are in the previously discussed growth factor and angiogenesis pathways.[131,132] Additional targets for modulating radiosensitivity include DNA repair proteins.[131,133] As the cellular response to radiation is better defined, it might become possible to induce the expression of specific proteins that would then render the tumor susceptible to agents targeting the induced protein.[134,135] In effect, this would be a radiation-induced, synthetic lethal phenotype.

CONCLUSIONS AND FUTURE DIRECTIONS

Significant advances have been made in our understanding of the molecular abnormalities in cancer, and this information is now being translated into clinical reality. Remarkable successes have been seen with drugs that target genetically defined abnormalities in several cancers. The obvious goal would be to have a complete genetic profile of all cancers, with agents to target these abnormalities, and then selecting therapies would be entirely rational. Tumors with defined mutations would be treated specifically and effectively with agents that target these specific abnormalities. As methods for early diagnosis improve, it also should be possible to treat earlier in the course of the disease when cancers are more easily cured.[136] In addition, as a more thorough understanding is obtained of the genetic risks for cancer and how various genetic backgrounds interact with the environment, this should allow genetically targeted preventive strategies.

Before this goal can be achieved, much work must be done. In the meantime, numerous agents targeting pathways involved in the malignant process will be tested. In the absence of a clear genetic rationale for the use of these agents, clinical trials will have some degree of empiricism. Until we have a complete understanding of the genetics of all human tumors, the challenge for the cancer research community is to learn how to test these newer agents, how to integrate them with current therapies, and as much as possible, use the currently available information to guide clinical trials. This means designing clinical trials that more carefully select patients based on the genetic features of a tumor or evidence of pathway activation, including measures of target modulation in clinical trials to assist in determining optimal doses and to assess adequately the activity of an agent; developing novel endpoints that more accurately reflect the expected outcome of therapy; and learning how to combine agents more intelligently.

REFERENCES

1. Huang ME, Ye YC, Chen SR, et al: Use of all-*trans* retinoic acid in the treatment of acute promyelocytic leukemia. Blood 1988; 72:567.
2. Castaigne S, Chomienne C, Daniel MT, et al: All-*trans* retinoic acid as a differentiation therapy for acute promyelocytic leukemia, I: Clinical results. Blood 1990;76:1704.
3. Rowley JD, Golomb HM, Dougherty C: 15/17 translocation, a consistent chromosomal change in acute promyelocytic leukaemia. Lancet 1977;1:549.
4. de The H, Chomienne C, Lanotte M, et al: The t(15;17) translocation of acute promyelocytic leukaemia fuses the retinoic acid receptor alpha gene to a novel transcribed locus. Nature 1990;347:558.
5. Longo L, Pandolfi PP, Biondi A, et al: Rearrangements and aberrant expression of the retinoic acid receptor alpha gene in acute promyelocytic leukemias. J Exp Med 1990;172:1571.
6. Miller WH Jr, Warrell RP Jr, Frankel SR, et al: Novel retinoic acid receptor-alpha transcripts in acute promyelocytic leukemia responsive to all-trans-retinoic acid. J Natl Cancer Inst 1990;82:1932.
7. Kakizuka A, Miller WH Jr, Umesono K, et al: Chromosomal translocation t(15;17) in human acute promyelocytic leukemia fuses RAR alpha with a novel putative transcription factor, PML. Cell 1991;66:663.
8. Mistry AR, Pedersen EW, Solomon E, et al: The molecular pathogenesis of acute promyelocytic leukaemia: Implications for the clinical management of the disease. Blood Rev 2003;17:71.
9. Degos L, Wang ZY: All-trans-retinoic acid in acute promyelocytic leukemia. Oncogene 2001;20:7140.
10. Tallman MS, Nabhan C, Feusner JH, et al: Acute promyelocytic leukemia: Evolving therapeutic strategies. Blood 2002;99:759.
11. Buchdunger E, Matter A, Druker BJ: Bcr-Abl inhibition as a modality of CML therapeutics. Biochim Biophys Acta 2001;1551:M11.
12. Druker BJ, Tamura S, Buchdunger E, et al: Effects of a selective inhibitor of the ABL tyrosine kinase on the growth of BCR-ABL positive cells. Nature Med 1996;2:561.
13. Druker BJ, Talpaz M, Resta DJ, et al: Efficacy and safety of a specific inhibitor of the BCR-ABL tyrosine kinase in chronic myeloid leukemia. N Engl J Med 2001;344:1031.

14. Druker BJ, Sawyers CL, Kantarjian H, et al: Activity of a specific inhibitor of the BCR-ABL tyrosine kinase in the blast crisis of chronic myeloid leukemia and acute lymphoblastic leukemia with the Philadelphia chromosome. N Engl J Med 2001;344:1038.

15. O'Brien SG, Guilhot F, Larson RA, et al: Imatinib compared with interferon and low-dose cytarabine for newly diagnosed chronic-phase chronic myeloid leukemia. N Engl J Med 2003;348:994.

16. Sawyers CL, Hochhaus A, Feldman E, et al: Imatinib induces hematologic and cytogenetic responses in patients with chronic myeloid leukemia in myeloid blast crisis: Results of a phase II study. Blood 2002;99:3530.

17. Hirota S, Isozaki K, Moriyama Y, et al: Gain-of-function mutations of c-kit in human gastrointestinal stromal tumors. Science 1998; 279:577.

18. Rubin BP, Singer S, Tsao C, et al: KIT activation is a ubiquitous feature of gastrointestinal stromal tumors. Cancer Res 2001; 61:8118.

19. Heinrich MC, Rubin BP, Longley BJ, et al: Biology and genetic aspects of gastrointestinal stromal tumors: KIT activation and cytogenetic alterations. Hum Pathol 2002;33:484.

20. Corless CL, McGreevey L, Haley A, et al: KIT mutations are common in incidental gastrointestinal stromal tumors one centimeter or less in size. Am J Pathol 2002;160:1567.

21. Demetri GD, von Mehren M, Blanke CD, et al: Efficacy and safety of imatinib mesylate in advanced gastrointestinal stromal tumors. N Engl J Med 2002;347:472.

22. van Oosterom AT, Judson I, Verweij J, et al: Safety and efficacy of imatinib (STI571) in metastatic gastrointestinal stromal tumours: A phase I study. Lancet 2001;358:1421.

23. Ottmann OG, Druker BJ, Sawyers CL, et al: A phase 2 study of imatinib in patients with relapsed or refractory Philadelphia chromosome-positive acute lymphoid leukemias. Blood 2002;100:1965.

24. Golub TR, Barker GF, Lovett M, et al: Fusion of PDGF receptor beta to a novel ets-like gene, tel, in chronic myelomonocytic leukemia with t(5;12) chromosomal translocation. Cell 1994;77:307.

25. Apperley JF, Gardembas M, Melo JV, et al: Response to imatinib mesylate in patients with chronic myeloproliferative diseases with rearrangements of the platelet-derived growth factor receptor beta. N Engl J Med 2002;347:481.

26. Magnusson MK, Meade KE, Nakamura R, et al: Activity of STI571 in chronic myelomonocytic leukemia with a platelet-derived growth factor beta receptor fusion oncogene. Blood 2002;100:1088.

27. Maki RG, Awan RA, Dixon RH, et al: Differential sensitivity to imatinib of 2 patients with metastatic sarcoma arising from dermatofibrosarcoma protuberans. 2002;100:623.

28. Rubin BP, Schuetze SM, Eary JF, et al: Molecular targeting of platelet-derived growth factor b by imatinib mesylate in a patient with metastatic dermatofibrosarcoma protuberans. J Clin Oncol 2002;20:3586.

29. Simon MP, Pedeutour F, Sirvent N, et al: Deregulation of the platelet-derived growth factor b-chain gene via fusion with collagen gene COL1A1 in dermatofibrosarcoma protuberans and giant-cell fibroblastoma. 1997;15:95.

30. Johnson BE, Fischer T, Fischer B, et al: Phase II study of imatinib in patients with small cell lung cancer. Clin Cancer Res 2003;9:5880.

31. Modi S, Seidman A, Dickler M, et al: A phase II trial of STI571 in patients with metastatic breast cancer. Proc Am Soc Clin Oncol 2003;22:18a.

32. Rao KV, Goodin S, Capanna T, et al: A phase II trial of imatinib mesylate in patients with PSA progression after local therapy for prostate cancer. Proc Am Soc Clin Oncol 2003;22:409a.

33. Wyman K, Atkins MB, Hubbard F, et al: A phase II trial of imatinib mesylate at 800 mg daily in metastatic melanoma: Lack of clinical efficacy with significant toxicity. Proc Am Soc Clin Oncol 2003;22:713a.

34. Verweij J, van Oosterom A, Blay JY, et al: Imatinib mesylate (STI-571 Glivec, Gleevec) is an active agent for gastrointestinal stromal tumours, but does not yield responses in other soft-tissue sarcomas that are unselected for a molecular target: Results from an EORTC Soft Tissue and Bone Sarcoma Group phase II study. Eur J Cancer 2003;39:2006.

35. Gleich GJ, Leiferman KM, Pardanani A, et al: Treatment of hypereosinophilic syndrome with imatinib mesylate. Lancet 2002;359:1577.

36. Cools J, DeAngelo DJ, Gotlib J, et al: A tyrosine kinase created by fusion of the PDGFRA and FIP1L1 genes as a therapeutic target of imatinib in idiopathic hypereosinophilic syndrome. N Engl J Med 2003;348:1201.

37. Griffin JH, Leung J, Bruner RJ, et al: Discovery of a fusion kinase in EOL-1 cells and idiopathic hypereosinophilic syndrome. Proc Natl Acad Sci USA 2003;100:7830.

38. Yamamoto Y, Kiyoi H, Nakano Y, et al: Activating mutation of D835 within the activation loop of FLT3 in human hematologic malignancies. Blood 2001;97:2434.

39. Stirewalt DL, Kopecky KJ, Meshinchi S, et al: FLT3, RAS, and TP53 mutations in elderly patients with acute myeloid leukemia. Blood 2001;97:3589.

40. Meshinchi S, Woods WG, Stirewalt DL, et al: Prevalence and prognostic significance of Flt3 internal tandem duplication in pediatric acute myeloid leukemia. Blood 2001;97:89.

41. Smith BD, Levis M, Beran M, et al: Single agent CEP-701, a novel FLT3 inhibitor, shows initial response in patients with refractory acute myeloid leukemia. Proc Am Soc Clin Oncol 2003;22:194a.

42. Estey E, Fischer T, Giles F, et al: A randomized phase II trial of the tyrosine kinase inhibitor PKC412 in patients with acute myeloid leukemia (AML)/high-risk myelodysplastic syndromes (MDS) characterized by wild-type or mutated FLT3. Blood 2003;102:614a.

43. DeAngelo D, Stone RM, Bruner RJ, et al: Phase I clinical results with MLN-518, a novel FLT3 antagonist: Tolerability, pharmacokinetics, and pharmacodynamics. Blood 2003;102:65a.

44. Davies H, Bignell GR, Cox C, et al: Mutations of the BRAF gene in human cancer. Nature 2002;417:949.

45. Kimura ET, Nikiforova MN, Zhu Z, et al: High prevalence of BRAF mutations in thyroid cancer: Genetic evidence for constitutive activation of the RET/PTC-RAS-BRAF signaling pathway in papillary thyroid carcinoma. Cancer Res 2003;63:1454.

46. Cohen Y, Xing M, Mambo E, et al: BRAF mutation in papillary thyroid carcinoma. J Natl Cancer Inst 2003;95:625.

47. Brose MS, Volpe P, Feldman M, et al: BRAF and RAS mutations in human lung cancer and melanoma. Cancer Res 2002;62:6997.

48. Rajagopalan H, Bardelli A, Lengauer C, et al: Tumorigenesis: RAF/RAS oncogenes and mismatch-repair status. Nature 2002;418:934.

49. Rodenhuis S: ras and human tumors. Semin Cancer Biol 1992;3:241.

50. Caponigro F, Casale M, Bryce J: Farnesyl transferase inhibitors in clinical development. Expert Opin Invest Drugs 2003;12:943.

51. Head JE, Johnston SR: Protein farnesyltransferase inhibitors. Expert Opin Emerg Drugs 2003;8:163.

52. Prendergast GC, Rane N: Farnesyltransferase inhibitors: Mechanism and applications. Expert Opin Invest Drugs 2001;10:2105.

53. Sebti SM, Hamilton AD: Farnesyltransferase and geranylgeranyltransferase I inhibitors and cancer therapy: Lessons from mechanism and bench-to-bedside translational studies. Oncogene 2000;19:6584.

54. Du W, Lebowitz PF, Prendergast GC: Cell growth inhibition by farnesyltransferase inhibitors is mediated by gain of geranylgeranylated RhoB. Mol Cell Biol 1999;19:1831.

55. Cox AD, Der CJ: Farnesyltransferase inhibitors: Promises and realities. Curr Opin Pharmacol 2002;2:388.

56. Sherr CJ, McCormick F: The RB and p53 pathways in cancer. Cancer Cell 2002;2:103.

57. Wang JL, Liu D, Zhang ZJ, et al: Structure-based discovery of an organic compound that binds Bcl-2 protein and induces apoptosis of tumor cells. Proc Natl Acad Sci USA 2000;97:7124.

58. Tzung SP, Kim KM, Basanez G, et al: Antimycin A mimics a cell-death-inducing Bcl-2 homology domain 3. Nat Cell Biol 2001;3:183.

59. Degterev A, Lugovskoy A, Cardone M, et al: Identification of small-molecule inhibitors of interaction between the BH3 domain and Bcl-xL. Nat Cell Biol 2001;3:173.

60. Dias N, Stein CA: Potential roles of antisense oligonucleotides in cancer therapy: The example of Bcl-2 antisense oligonucleotides. Eur J Pharm Biopharm 2002;54:263.

61. McCormick F: Cancer-specific viruses and the development of ONYX-015. Cancer Biol Ther 2003;2:S157.

62. Chen YN, Sharma SK, Ramsey TM, et al: Selective killing of transformed cells by cyclin/cyclin-dependent kinase 2 antagonists. Proc Natl Acad Sci USA 1999;96:4325.

63. Kantarjian H, Sawyers C, Hochhaus A, et al: Hematologic and cytogenetic responses to imatinib mesylate in chronic myelogenous leukemia. N Engl J Med 2002;346:645.

64. Gallagher RE: Retinoic acid resistance in acute promyelocytic leukemia. Leukemia 2002;16:1940.

65. Shah NP, Nicoll JM, Nagar B, et al: Multiple BCR-ABL kinase domain mutations confer polyclonal resistance to the tyrosine kinase inhibitor imatinib (STI571) in chronic phase and blast crisis chronic myeloid leukemia. Cancer Cell 2002;2:117.

66. Corbin AS, La Rosée P, Stoffregen E, et al: Several Bcr-Abl kinase domain mutants associated with imatinib mesylate resistance remain sensitive to imatinib. Blood 2003;101:4611.

67. Fletcher JA, Corless CL, Dimitrijevic S, et al: Mechanisms of resistance to imatinib mesylate in advanced gastrointestinal stromal tumor. Proc Am Soc Clin Oncol 2003;22:815a.

68. Hochhaus A, Kreil S, Corbin AS, et al: Molecular and chromosomal mechanisms of resistance to imatinib (STI571) therapy. Leukemia 2002;16:2190.

69. Gorre ME, Mohammed M, Ellwood K, et al: Clinical resistance to STI-571 cancer therapy caused by BCR-ABL gene mutation or amplification. Science 2001;293:876.

70. Oda T, Heaney C, Hagopian J, et al: CRKL is the major tyrosine phosphorylated protein in neutrophils from patients with chronic myelogenous leukemia. J Biol Chem 1994;269:22925.

71. Branford S, Rudzki Z, Walsh S, et al: High frequency of point mutations clustered within the adenosine triphosphate-binding region of BCR/ABL in patients with chronic myeloid leukemia or Ph-positive acute lymphoblastic leukemia who develop imatinib (STI571) resistance. Blood 2002;99:3472.

72. Hofmann WK, Jones LC, Lemp NA, et al: Ph(+) acute lympho-blastic leukemia resistant to the tyrosine kinase inhibitor STI571 has a unique BCR-ABL gene mutation. Blood 2001;99:1860.

73. Roche-Lestienne C, Soenen-Cornu V, Grardel-Duflos N, et al: Several types of mutations of the Abl gene can be found in chronic myeloid leukemia patients resistant to STI571, and they can pre-exist to the onset of treatment. Blood 2002;100:1014.

74. von Bubnoff N, Schneller F, Peschel C, et al: BCR-ABL gene mutations in relation to clinical resistance of Philadelphia-chromosome-positive leukaemia to STI571: A prospective study. Lancet 2002;359:487.

75. Hughes TP, Kaeda J, Branford S, et al: Frequency of major molecular responses to imatinib or interferon alfa plus cytarabine in newly diagnosed chronic myeloid leukemia. N Engl J Med 2003;349:1423.

76. Heinrich MC, Corless CL, Demetri GD, et al: Kinase mutations and imatinib response in patients with metastatic gastrointestinal stromal tumor. J Clin Oncol 2003;21:4342.

77. Heinrich MC, Corless CL, Duensing A, et al: PDGFRA activating mutations in gastrointestinal stromal tumors. Science 2003;299:708.

78. Hanahan D, Weinberg RA: The hallmarks of cancer. Cell 2000;100:57.

79. Furr BJ, Jordan VC: The pharmacology and clinical uses of tamoxifen. Pharmacol Ther 1984;25:127.

80. Grunwald V, Hidalgo M: Developing inhibitors of the epidermal growth factor receptor for cancer treatment. J Natl Cancer Inst 2003;95:851.

81. Slamon DJ, Clark GM, Wong SG, et al: Human breast cancer: correlation of relapse and survival with amplification of the HER-2/neu oncogene. Science 1987;235:177.

82. Ross JS, Fletcher JA, Linette GP, et al: The Her-2/neu gene and protein in breast cancer 2003: Biomarker and target of therapy. Oncologist 2003;8:307.

83. Luoh SW: Amplification and expression of genes from the 17q11 approximately q12 amplicon in breast cancer cells. Cancer Genet Cytogenet 2002;136:43.

84. Baselga J, Hammond LA: HER-targeted tyrosine-kinase inhibitors. Oncology 2002;63(suppl 1):6.

85. Dancey JE, Freidlin B: Targeting epidermal growth factor receptor: Are we missing the mark? Lancet 2003;362:62.

86. Baselga J, Tripathy D, Mendelsohn J, et al: Phase II study of weekly intravenous recombinant humanized anti-p185HER2 monoclonal antibody in patients with HER2/neu-overexpressing metastatic breast cancer. J Clin Oncol 1996;14:737.

87. Cobleigh MA, Vogel CL, Tripathy D, et al: Multinational study of the efficacy and safety of humanized anti-HER2 monoclonal antibody in women who have HER2-overexpressing metastatic breast cancer that has progressed after chemotherapy for metastatic disease. J Clin Oncol 1999;17:2639.

88. Vogel CL, Cobleigh MA, Tripathy D, et al: Efficacy and safety of trastuzumab as a single agent in first-line treatment of HER2-overexpressing metastatic breast cancer. J Clin Oncol 2002;20:719.

89. Perez-Soler R, Chachoua A, Huberman M, et al: A phase II trial of the epidermal growth factor receptor (EGFR) tyrosine kinase inhibitor OSI-774, following platinum-based chemotherapy, in patients with advanced, EGFR-expressing non-small cell lung cancer. Proc Am Soc Clin Oncol 2001;19:310a.

90. Slamon DJ, Leyland-Jones B, Shak S, et al: Use of chemotherapy plus a monoclonal antibody against HER2 for metastatic breast cancer that overexpresses HER2. N Engl J Med 2001;344:783.

91. Ranson M, Hammond LA, Ferry D, et al: ZD1839, a selective oral epidermal growth factor receptor-tyrosine kinase inhibitor, is well tolerated and active in patients with solid, malignant tumors: Results of a phase I trial. J Clin Oncol 2002;20:2240.

92. Baselga J, Albanell J: Mechanism of action of anti-HER2 monoclonal antibodies. Ann Oncol 2001;12(suppl 1):S35.

93. Sawyers CL: Will mTOR inhibitors make it as cancer drugs? Cancer Cell 2003;4:343.

94. Neshat MS, Mellinghoff IK, Tran C, et al: Enhanced sensitivity of PTEN-deficient tumors to inhibition of FRAP/mTOR. Proc Natl Acad Sci USA 2001;98:10314.

95. Podsypanina K, Lee RT, Politis C, et al: An inhibitor of mTOR reduces neoplasia and normalizes p70/S6 kinase activity in Pten+/– mice. Proc Natl Acad Sci USA 2001;98:10320.

96. Vogelstein B, Lane D, Levine AJ: Surfing the p53 network. Nature 2000;408:307.

97. Sausville EA, Elsayed Y, Monga M, et al: Signal transduction–directed cancer treatments. Annu Rev Pharmacol Toxicol 2003;43:199.

98. Connors JM, Kouroukis C, Belch A, et al: Flavopiridol for mantle cell lymphoma: Moderate activity and frequent disease stabilization. Blood 2001;98:807a.

99. Geng Y, Yu Q, Sicinska E, et al: Cyclin E ablation in the mouse. Cell 2003;114:431.

100. Ortega S, Prieto I, Odajima J, et al: Cyclin-dependent kinase 2 is essential for meiosis but not for mitotic cell division in mice. Nat Genet 2003;35:25.

101. Hu W, Kavanagh JJ: Anticancer therapy targeting the apoptotic pathway. Lancet Oncol 2003;4:721.

102. Reed JC: Apoptosis-targeted therapies for cancer. Cancer Cell 2003;3:17.

103. Richardson PG, Barlogie B, Berenson J, et al: A phase 2 study of bortezomib in relapsed, refractory myeloma. N Engl J Med 2003;348:2609.

104. Mitchell BS: The proteasome, an emerging therapeutic target in cancer. N Engl J Med 2003;348:2597.

105. Lonser RR, Glenn GM, Walther M, et al: von Hippel-Lindau disease. Lancet 2003;361:2059.

106. Shuin T, Kondo K, Torigoe S, et al: Frequent somatic mutations and loss of heterozygosity of the von Hippel-Lindau tumor suppressor gene in primary human renal cell carcinomas. Cancer Res 1994;54:2852.

107. Kondo K, Yao M, Yoshida M, et al: Comprehensive mutational analysis of the VHL gene in sporadic renal cell carcinoma: relationship to clinicopathological parameters. Genes Chromosomes Cancer 2002;34:58.

108. Yang H, Kaelin WG Jr: Molecular pathogenesis of the von Hippel-Lindau hereditary cancer syndrome: Implications for oxygen sensing. Cell Growth Differ 2001;12:447.

109. Yang JC, Haworth L, Sherry RM, et al: A randomized trial of bevacizumab, an anti-vascular endothelial growth factor antibody, for metastatic renal cancer. N Engl J Med 2003;349:427.

110. Hurwitz H, Fehrenbacher L, Cartwright T, et al: Bevacizumab (a monoclonal antibody to the vascular endothelial growth factor) prolongs survival in first-line colorectal cancer (CRC): Results of a phase III trial of bevacizumab in combination with bolus IFL (irinotecan, 5-fluorouracil, leucovorin) as first-line therapy in patients with metastatic CRC [abstract 3646]. Proc Am Soc Clin Oncol 2003;22.

111. Kerbel R, Folkman J: Clinical translation of angiogenesis inhibitors. Nat Rev Cancer 2002;2:727.

112. Dredge K, Dalgleish AG, Marriott JB: Angiogenesis inhibitors in cancer therapy. Curr Opin Invest Drugs 2003;4:667.

113. Scappaticci FA: Mechanisms and future directions for angiogenesis-based cancer therapies. J Clin Oncol 2002; 20:3906.

114. Davis DW, McConkey DJ, Abbruzzese JL, et al: Surrogate markers in antiangiogenesis clinical trials. Br J Cancer 2003;89:8.

115. Ruoslahti E: Specialization of tumour vasculature. Nat Rev Cancer 2002;2:83.

116. Arap W, Pasqualini R, Ruoslahti E: Cancer treatment by targeted drug delivery to tumor vasculature in a mouse model. Science 1998;279:377.

117. Arap W, Haedicke W, Bernasconi M, et al: Targeting the prostate for destruction through a vascular address. Proc Natl Acad Sci USA 2002;99:1527.

118. McEachern MJ, Krauskopf A, Blackburn EH: Telomeres and their control. Annu Rev Genet 2000;34:331.

119. Shay JW, Wright WE: Telomerase: A target for cancer therapeutics. Cancer Cell 2002;2:257.

120. Saretzki G: Telomerase inhibition as cancer therapy. Cancer Lett 2003;194:209.

121. Hahn WC: Role of telomeres and telomerase in the pathogenesis of human cancer. J Clin Oncol 2003;21:2034.

122. Ottesen GL: Carcinoma in situ of the female breast: A clinico-pathological, immunohistological, and DNA ploidy study. APMIS Suppl 2003;108:1.

123. Avivi I, Robinson S, Goldstone A: Clinical use of rituximab in haematological malignancies. Br J Cancer 2003;89:1389.

124. Gordon LI, Witzig TE, Wiseman GA, et al: Yttrium 90 ibritumomab tiuxetan radioimmunotherapy for relapsed or refractory low-grade non-Hodgkin's lymphoma. Semin Oncol 2002; 29:87.

125. Zelenetz AD: A clinical and scientific overview of tositumomab and iodine I 131 tositumomab. Semin Oncol 2003;30:22.

126. Maloney DG, Smith B, Rose A: Rituximab: Mechanism of action and resistance. Semin Oncol 2002;29:2.

127. Albanell J, Rojo F, Averbuch S, et al: Pharmacodynamic studies of the epidermal growth factor receptor inhibitor ZD1839 in skin from cancer patients: Histopathologic and molecular consequences of receptor inhibition. J Clin Oncol 2002;20:110.

128. Van den Abbeele AD, Badawi RD: Use of positron emission tomography in oncology and its potential role to assess response to imatinib mesylate therapy in gastrointestinal stromal tumors (GISTs). Eur J Cancer 2002;38(suppl 5):S60.

129. Stroobants S, Goeminne J, Seegers M, et al: ^{18}FDG-Positron emission tomography for the early prediction of response in advanced soft tissue sarcoma treated with imatinib mesylate (Glivec). Eur J Cancer 2003;39:2012.

130. Heinrich MC, Blanke CD, Druker BJ, et al: Inhibition of KIT tyrosine kinase activity: A novel molecular approach to the treatment of KIT-positive malignancies. J Clin Oncol 2002;20:1692.

131. Ma BB, Bristow RG, Kim J, et al: Combined-modality treatment of solid tumors using radiotherapy and molecular targeted agents. J Clin Oncol 2003;21:2760.

132. Camphausen K, Menard C: Angiogenesis inhibitors and radiotherapy of primary tumours. Expert Opin Biol Ther 2002;2:477.

133. Sharan SK, Morimatsu M, Albrecht U, et al: Embryonic lethality and radiation hypersensitivity mediated by Rad51 in mice lacking Brca2. Nature 1997;386:804.

134. Quarmby S, Hunter RD, Kumar S: Irradiation induced expression of CD31, ICAM-1 and VCAM-1 in human microvascular endothelial cells. Anticancer Res 2000;20:3375.

135. Chakraborty M, Abrams SI, Camphausen K, et al: Irradiation of tumor cells up-regulates Fas and enhances CTL lytic activity and CTL adoptive immunotherapy. J Immunol 2003;170:6338.

136. Etzioni R, Urban N, Ramsey S, et al: The case for early detection. Nat Rev Cancer 2003;3:243.

137. Talpaz M, Silver RT, Druker BJ, et al: Imatinib induces durable hematologic and cytogenetic responses in patients with accelerated phase chronic myeloid leukemia: Results of a phase 2 study. Blood 2002;99:1928.

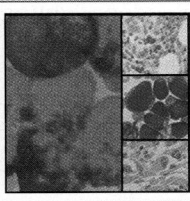

Theresa M. Busch

Stephen M. Hahn

PHOTODYNAMIC THERAPY

SUMMARY OF KEY POINTS

- Photodynamic therapy depends on the presence of a photosensitizer drug, laser light, and oxygen.
- Photodynamic therapy kills tumor cells through direct cellular cytotoxicity and/or through destruction of tumor vasculature.
- Photodynamic therapy is being actively evaluated as a treatment for a variety of malignant and premalignant conditions.
- Two photosensitizers are approved for oncologic use in the United States: porfimer sodium (Photofrin) and 5-aminolevulinic acid (Levulan).
- Porfimer sodium–mediated photodynamic therapy is approved

by the U.S. Food and Drug Administration for management of obstructing esophageal cancer, obstructing endobronchial lung cancer, microinvasive endobronchial lung cancer, and Barrett's esophagus.
- 5-Aminolevulinic acid is a topical photosensitizer that in combination with blue light has been approved for the management of actinic keratosis.
- Several photosensitizers are in clinical development. These new photosensitizers have the advantage of being pure compounds with reduced duration of photosensitivity.

- Photodynamic therapy shows great promise for the management of premalignant conditions, including Barrett's esophagus with high-grade dysplasia.
- Photodynamic therapy is being studied for the management of surface malignant lesions, including pleural spread of non–small cell lung cancer and peritoneal carcinomatosis.
- Interstitial photodynamic therapy has only recently been evaluated for management of locally recurrent prostate cancer, but in concept is an appealing approach to a difficult oncologic problem.

INTRODUCTION

Photodynamic therapy (PDT) is a locoregional cancer treatment modality used to treat a variety of malignant and premalignant conditions.[1,2] The therapeutic components of PDT are a drug (photosensitizer), usually administered systemically, and light of a wavelength specific to the absorption characteristics of the photosensitizer.[3] The photodynamic process is also dependent on the presence of oxygen.[4-9] The light used to activate a photosensitizer is nonionizing, a quality that differentiates it from therapeutic radiation (see Chapter 26). The dependence of PDT on the presence of both a photosensitizer and nonionizing radiation (light) increases the complexity of this treatment compared with other therapies for cancer, such as radiation therapy or chemotherapy. PDT also is complicated by an absolute dependence on oxygen. In therapeutic ionizing radiation, oxygen enhances responses but is not absolutely required.

Compared with conventional therapies, PDT has several advantages as a cancer treatment.[10] One of the major advantages of PDT is that the treatment effect can be limited to mucosal or serosal surfaces, so toxicity to underlying normal tissues is reduced. PDT is a superficial treatment because the light used to activate a photosensitizer is typically in the visible or near-infrared light range, which has limited depth of penetration in tissues. This shallow treatment effect of PDT is a potential advantage for management of superficial neoplasms, such

as skin cancer,[11-13] early cancer of the respiratory or digestive tract,[10] and malignant tumors that spread to serosal surfaces.[10,14-17] PDT for surface and superficial disease can be highly effective, as evidenced by the general success of PDT in the management of premalignant conditions.[18-24] Another advantage of PDT over other local therapies such as ionizing radiation and surgery is that treatment is generally noninvasive and usually can be administered more than one time. A third major advantage of PDT is that brachytherapy techniques used for local delivery of radiation by radiation oncologists can be adapted for delivery of light. Interstitial delivery of light may enable effective PDT for more deeply seated tumors.[25-27]

PDT must be used selectively in the clinic. PDT is not an appropriate treatment modality for many types of neoplasms. This would include cancers located in areas inaccessible to adequate light delivery and, most important, lesions for which locoregional therapy is not likely to affect the natural history of the cancer. The challenge for clinicians is to identify clinical situations in which delivery of light is feasible and in which PDT is likely to favorably affect the course of the cancer.

In North America, Europe, and Japan, PDT is accepted therapy for a number of malignancies. Researchers are investigating the use of PDT under experimental treatment protocols.[10] PDT with the photosensitizer porfimer sodium (Photofrin) has been approved by the U.S. Food and Drug Administration (FDA) for palliative management of obstructing esophageal cancer, palliative management of obstructing endobronchial lung cancer, definitive management of microinvasive endobronchial cancer, and treatment of Barrett's esophagus with high-grade dysplasia. PDT with 5-aminolevulinic acid (5-ALA; Levulan) has been approved by the FDA for the management of a premalignant skin condition, actinic keratosis. These drugs have been approved for other oncologic indications in Europe, Japan, and Canada.[1] PDT as monotherapy is being investigated as definitive or curative therapy for a number of malignant and premalignant conditions as well as an intraoperative adjuvant treatment to surgery.[14,15,28,29] The main advantage of using PDT as an adjuvant intraoperative therapy is that bulky tumors that cannot be completely eradicated with surgery may be sterilized after debulking by addition of PDT. In addition, adjuvant use of PDT may allow parenchyma-sparing operations, especially in the thorax.[30] Finally, PDT can be administered as a component of a multimodality approach that includes other cancer treatments such as radiation and chemotherapy.[10]

BASIC COMPONENTS OF PHOTODYNAMIC THERAPY

Investigation of PDT for cancer has been focused on attempting to understand the interaction of photosensitizer, light, and oxygen in tissues on a molecular, cellular, and tissue level.[5,31-33]

Photosensitizers

Photosensitizers are drugs usually administered intravenously in the outpatient setting several hours to days before light delivery (Table 31-1). Some drugs, such as 5-ALA, are administered topically. After systemic administration of the drug, patients are sensitive to visible light for periods ranging from 24 hours to 6 weeks, depending on the photosensitizer administered. Light sensitivity usually manifests as severe photosensitization.[34,35] Patients are advised to cover sun-exposed regions of the skin and to avoid direct sunlight or powerful indoor lighting. Lights used for ophthalmologic, dental, or operative procedures cause severe skin or mucosal reactions during the photosensitive period. Sunscreens that protect against UV light are not protective against cutaneous photosensitivity. Another photosensitivity reaction of clinical importance is burns of the nail beds from pulse oximeters used during operative or endoscopic procedures.[36] Pulse oximeters should be rotated to a different finger every 30 minutes to avoid this complication.

Many photosensitizers are porphyrins or porphyrin-like compounds.[1,3] Activation of a photosensitizer by light results in photoxidization reactions[37] whereby light of a specific wavelength excites the photosensitizer, which reacts either directly or indirectly with oxygen to produce singlet oxygen and other reactive oxygen species.[1,3] Singlet oxygen and other reactive oxygen species are thought to be responsible for the direct cytotoxicity caused by PDT.

Preclinical reports of photosensitizer concentration in tumor show selective retention of drug in tumors compared with some normal tissues.[38-41] The mechanism of selective retention of photosensitizers in experimental tumor systems has not been defined and may be related to the unique characteristics of tumors and their surrounding stroma compared with normal tissues.[1] Potential factors related to selective retention of photosensitizers include lipid content,[42] elevated numbers of low-density lipoprotein receptors,[43-46] abnormal tumor vasculature,[47,48] and decreased pH.[49]

Clinical data for photosensitizer concentration in human tumors have been published.[50-53] Ris et al.[50] reported that tumor biopsy specimens from patients with malignant mesothelioma showed up to 14 times the concentration of the photosensitizer meso-tetra-(hydroxyphenyl)-chlorin (mTHPC) as that found in normal tissues from the same patients. On the basis of in vivo measurements of porphyrin fluorescence, Peng et al.[51] reported greater accumulation of photosensitizer in basal cell carcinoma of the skin than in surrounding normal skin after topical application of lipophilic esters of 5-ALA. The presence of porphyrin fluorescence after topical application of 5-ALA

TABLE 31-1

Clinical Characteristics of Photosensitizers for Photodynamic Therapy				
PHOTOSENSITIZER	**EXCITATION WAVELENGTH**	**DURATION OF PHOTOSENSITIVITY**	**METHOD OF ADMINISTRATION**	**FDA-APPROVED ONCOLOGIC INDICATIONS**
Porfimer sodium (Photofrin)	630 nm	4–6 wk	Intravenous	1. Obstructing esophageal cancer 2. Obstructing lung cancer 3. Microinvasive endobronchial cancer
5-Aminolevulinic acid (Levulan)	Blue light	24 hr	Topical	Actinic keratosis
Meso-tetra-(hydroxyphenyl)-chlorin (mTHPC)	652 nm	15 days	Intravenous	
Motexafin lutetium	732 nm	3–24 hr	Intravenous	
SnET2	660–664 nm	2–3 wk	Intravenous	
N-Aspartylchlorin e6 (LS11)	664 nm		Intravenous	
2-[1-hexyloxy-ethyl]-2-devinyl pyropheophorbide-a (HPPH)	665 nm	24–48 hr	Intravenous	
Silicon phthalocyanine	672 nm	24 hr	Intravenous	

was found in patients with intraepithelial neoplasia of the cervix, and a relation was found between increased fluorescence in CIN and worsening grade of this lesion.[52] Results of one study suggested that tumor selectivity of photosensitizer uptake may not be present in some patients.[53] In biopsy specimens from the upper aerodigestive tracts of 30 patients, no selectivity of mTHPC uptake was found for tumor compared with surrounding normal mucosa. Selectivity of mTHPC uptake was found, however, in tumor compared with striated muscle and cartilage. Additional studies are needed to evaluate the distribution of photosensitizers in human cancer and normal tissue and to determine the factors associated with selective retention. If selective retention of photosensitizers in human tumors is a common feature of the pharmacodynamics of photosensitizer drugs, a better therapeutic index is expected for PDT than for other cancer treatments.

Porfimer sodium and 5-ALA are two photosensitizers approved by the FDA. Second-generation photosensitizers, including motexafin lutetium, mTHPC (Foscan), SnET2 (Purlytin), N-aspartyl chlorin e6 (LS11), silicon phthalocyanine (Pc4), and 2-[1-hexyloxy-ethyl]-2-devinyl pyropheophorbide-a (HPPH; Photochlor) are undergoing clinical evaluation as experimental agents.

Porfimer Sodium

Porfimer sodium is the first photosensitizer for clinical PDT that has been commercially available in the United States. Porfimer sodium is a purified version of hematoporphyrin derivative (HPD), a compound first used in clinical trials. HPD is a complex mixture of porphyrins, and porfimer sodium is a commercial preparation of HPD that has an enriched fraction of porphyrin oligomers and monomers.[3,54] Porfimer sodium is approved by the FDA for palliative management of obstructing esophageal cancer, palliative management of obstructing lung cancer, definitive management of microinvasive endobronchial cancer, and treatment of Barrett's esophagus with high-grade dysplasia. For these FDA-approved indications, it is recommended that porfimer sodium be activated by 630-nm light. The depth of PDT effect with porfimer sodium and 630-nm light is typically 2 to 5 mm. Shorter wavelengths of light have been used for conditions that require a shallower depth of damage.[14,15] For the FDA-approved indications, porfimer sodium is administered intravenously over 3 to 5 minutes 48 hours before light administration. Porphyrin is retained in skin; therefore a major side effect of porfimer sodium is cutaneous photosensitivity, which lasts approximately 4 to 6 weeks after administration. Approximately 20% to 25% of patients who receive porfimer sodium have sun sensitivity for as long as 3 months after treatment.

5-Aminolevulinic Acid

The photosensitizer 5-ALA is a precursor in the heme biosynthesis pathway.[1,55] Administration of 5-ALA, most commonly by oral or topical formulation, leads to production of endogenous porphyrin, protoporphyrin IX within cells. Induction of endogenous porphyrins by 5-ALA is greater in rapidly dividing cells and therefore may provide selectivity for tumors compared with normal tissues.[1,55] Topical 5-ALA is manufactured and distributed in the United States as Levulan. The combination of 5-ALA and blue light has been approved by the FDA for management of actinic keratosis. 5-ALA is applied only to the affected areas of skin, a method that avoids full-body cutaneous photosensitivity. 5-ALA has been administered orally in experimental clinical protocols,[2,55-57] but this route of administration has not been approved by the FDA. After an oral dose of 5-ALA, cutaneous photosensitivity occurs for approximately 24 hours. Nausea and increased values on liver function tests have been reported after oral administration of 5-ALA.[58] Other side effects include malaise, headache, and alopecia. Delivery of 630-nm, 532-nm, or 514-nm light typically is performed 4 to 6 hours after oral administration of 5-ALA. From a photobiologic perspective, the porphyrins produced by 5-ALA administration have a tissue effect similar to that of porfimer sodium.

Meso-tetra-(hydroxyphenyl)-chlorin

mTHPC (Foscan) is a second-generation chlorin photosensitizer approved in Europe for the palliative treatment of patients with squamous cell carcinoma of the head and neck that has not responded to other therapies. mTHPC is one of the most active photosensitizers available.[59,60] The high level of photosensitizer activity means that lower drug doses and smaller doses of light are needed for PDT with this drug than with other photosensitizers. The smaller light doses translate into shorter treatment times. For the approved European indication, mTHPC is administered intravenously at a dose of 0.15 mg/kg 96 hours before 652-nm light delivery. The depth of tissue effect with mTHPC-mediated PDT has been reported to be up to 1 cm.[28] The duration of cutaneous photosensitivity with mTHPC is approximately 15 days.

Motexafin Lutetium

Motexafin lutetium (Lutrin, lutetium texaphyrin, Lu-Tex) is another second-generation photosensitizer.[39,61] Motexafin lutetium is a pentadentate aromatic metalloporphyrin activated by 732-nm light. Absorption at this wavelength has the advantage of deeper penetration into tissues compared with the light used to activate other photosensitizers. In addition, because 732-nm light is in the near-infrared region, less light is absorbed by hemoglobin. This quality is clinically important because blood is less likely to interfere with delivery of 732-nm than with light of shorter wavelengths. Motexafin lutetium has not been approved for human use in the United States but is being studied for a variety of malignant diseases.[62] This photosensitizer is administered intravenously. Although the appropriate drug-light interval has not been completely established in clinical trials, it ranges from 3 to 24 hours. Motexafin lutetium has one of the highest reported tissue to normal tissue ratios of drug retention in preclinical studies.[39] One advantage of this compound compared with other photosensitizers is that the duration of cutaneous photosensitivity is 1 to 2 days. Sun sensitivity usually manifests as temporary burning, tingling, or numbness in sun-exposed regions.

SnET2

SnET2 (Purlytin) is a second-generation chlorin photo-sensitizer[63,64] being evaluated in clinical trials and has not been approved for routine human use in the United States. SnET2 is administered intravenously 24 hours before illumination with 660- to 664-nm light. Cutaneous photosensitivity is reported to last 2 to 3 weeks, although prolonged photosensitivity of one or more months has been reported in 10% to 15% of patients.[1]

LS11

LS11 is a chlorin-based photosensitizer (*N*-aspartyl chlorin e6; NPe6) that has been evaluated in a phase I PDT trial for management of recurrent adenocarcinoma of the breast, basal cell carcinoma, and squamous cell carcinoma.[65] LS11 is activated by 664-nm light and is associated with little cutaneous photosensitivity. A phase I/II trial of LS11 with a novel interstitial light-emitting diode illumination source developed by Light Sciences Corporation (Issaquah, Wash)[66] has been completed with patients with various malignant diseases. Plans for a phase II trial are underway.

HPPH

HPPH (2-[1-hexyloxy-ethyl]-2-devinyl pyropheophorbide-a; Photochlor) is a chlorin-based photosensitizer developed by researchers at Roswell Park Cancer Institute (Buffalo, NY). This agent is activated by 665-nm light[67] and is administered intravenously 24 to 48 hours before illumination. Current phase I/II trials of HPPH-mediated PDT include management of basal cell carcinoma and high-grade dysplasia in Barrett's esophagus and palliation of obstructive esophageal cancer. HPPH also is being studied for the management of lung cancer. Of a total of 19 treated patients, 12 patients experienced resolution of cutaneous photosensitivity within 72 hours after HPPH injection (3–6 mg/m²). Four patients had photosensitivity exceeding 72 hours. Three patients with photosensitivity 24 or 48 hours after injection were not evaluated at 72 hours.[68]

Silicon Phthalocyanine

Silicon phthalocyanine (Pc4) is a photosensitizer drug developed by Oleinick et al.[69-73] Pc4 is being evaluated clinically in a phase I trial at Case Western Reserve University. This photosensitizer is administered intravenously 24 hours before activation with 672-nm light. The duration of cutaneous photosensitivity is being determined in the phase I trial.

Light

The cytotoxicity caused by PDT depends on production of light of a specific wavelength to activate the photosensitizer. In general, the depth of tissue penetration of light increases with increased wavelength in the visible and near infrared range. The advantages of using higher wavelengths of light to activate a photosensitizer (such as those in the near-infrared range) include a greater depth of treatment effect and the ability to treat tissues with greater pigmentation.[12,40,74] Other factors that directly affect light penetration in tissues and influence the depth of PDT effect seen clinically include the geometry of the

tissues, the mode of light delivery (e.g., interstitial delivery versus external delivery), and the optical properties of the tissues.

Light dose or fluence for clinical PDT is expressed in joules per square centimeter (J/cm^2) or joules per centimeter (J/cm) and is a measure of light energy deposited. For the FDA-approved clinical indications, this value represents the light energy delivered by the laser. The total amount of light energy deposited in tissues is a combination of the incident light delivered by the laser and of light scattered by the tissues. The rate of light delivery or fluence rate is expressed in milliwatts per square centimeter (mW/cm^2) or milliwatts per centimeter (mW/cm). The light fluence delivered from the laser can be calculated by multiplying fluence rate (in W/cm^2 or W/cm) by total treatment time (in seconds). For example, a fluence rate of 0.5 W/cm (500 mW/cm) for 1000 seconds delivers an incident light dose of 500 J/cm. Clinical PDT treatments approved by the FDA are prescribed in terms of the incident light delivered from the laser (as described earlier) rather than the total dose of light that the tissues receive, which is a combination of scattered and incident light. Scattering of light by tissues leads to substantial differences in total dose.[75-77] Marijnissen et al.[77] performed a clinical study that demonstrated this point. Total light fluence including both incident and scattered light was measured in 16 patients undergoing whole-bladder-wall PDT with a fixed output of light from a laser (incident light). The true light fluence at the surface of the bladder was, on average, 4.8 times larger than the incident light dose. In individual patients, the true light fluence varied from 2.5 to 7.1 times the light fluence delivered from the laser. The use of incident fluence to prescribe PDT may therefore lead to large differences in light doses received by superficial tissues of individual patients. This outcome could lead to large differences in tumor and normal tissue responses to PDT. Dosimetry systems in which light detectors are used have been developed to measure both incident and scattered light.[28,78] These systems should allow clinicians to measure and therefore prescribe a consistent total light dose to the tissues.

In the clinic, light usually is produced with a laser. Dye lasers, which have traditionally been used to produce light for the clinic,[79] are useful because they can be tuned to produce a variety of wavelengths and thus are versatile sources of light for clinical PDT. Diode lasers produce a single wavelength of light; therefore for PDT a separate diode laser must be purchased for each drug-light combination.[80] If multiple photosensitizers are to be used in the clinic, multiple diode lasers or one tunable dye laser would be required. The advantages of diode lasers, however, are that they are compact, easy to use, and affordable. There does not appear to be any biologic or clinical difference between the laser light generated from a diode laser and that emitted from a dye laser. No difference in tissue or cellular effect of PDT has been described in comparisons of these two light-producing systems.[81]

Delivery of laser light for clinical use is accomplished with optical fibers coupled to lasers. A variety of fibers and applicators have been designed for clinical use

(Fig. 31-1).[79,82-84] Light delivery systems are designed to uniformly illuminate the desired site and to prevent thermal injury to the tissues. External illumination of surfaces such as skin can be achieved with flat-cut optical fibers or a microlens (Fig. 31-1A). Cylindrical diffusing fibers that emit light 360 degrees around the length of a fiber are commonly used through an endoscope or bronchoscope to manage cancers of the lung and esophagus (Fig. 31-1B). Cylindrical diffusing fibers are used for interstitial light delivery. Optical fibers enclosed in modified endotracheal tubes have been used in experimental protocols to deliver light intraoperatively (Fig. 31-1C).[82,85]

Oxygen

Oxygen is required for the cytotoxicity produced by PDT. Photosensitizers are activated by light to cause tissue damage in the presence of oxygen in a process called a *photoxidative reaction.*[1] Oxygen is a critical component of porphyrin-mediated PDT cytotoxicity, as demonstrated in vitro[86,87] and in vivo.[88,89]

Preexisting tumor hypoxia can affect the efficacy of PDT[89]; this effect is similar to the adverse effect of hypoxia on response to radiation therapy.[90-95] Furthermore, tissue oxygen is consumed during the PDT process as cytotoxic reactive oxygen species are formed.[96,97] The rate of this oxygen consumption can be controlled by the light conditions used for treatment. Illumination with lower fluence rates or fractionation of the light into short on and off times has been shown to significantly improve tumor oxygenation and treatment outcome in preclinical studies.[98,99] Such techniques, however, have limited application in the clinic because they necessitate lengthening the treatment time needed to deliver a prescribed dose.[100]

Despite data demonstrating an important role for oxygen in PDT, few clinical studies have systematically evaluated tumor hypoxia in patients undergoing PDT. In one study with patients receiving PDT for basal cell carcinoma, oxygenation of the nodules was measured with an Eppendorf needle electrode before and during PDT. It was found that PDT depleted oxygenation of some tumors.[6] In patients not receiving PDT, studies evaluating preexisting hypoxia in sarcoma, cervical cancer, and other tumors were performed with 2-nitroimidazole binding techniques[101-103] and an Eppendorf needle electrode.[104-108] Substantial heterogeneity in human tumor hypoxia within tumor types was observed, and a relation between hypoxia and treatment outcome was found.[90,105,106] These data support the need to evaluate tumor oxygenation in individual patients. Combination of PDT with treatments designed to improve tumor oxygenation, such as hyperbaric oxygen therapy, is being studied.[109-112]

MECHANISMS OF ACTION OF PHOTODYNAMIC THERAPY

Direct Cell Effects

PDT has direct cytotoxic effects on tumor and normal cells in vitro[81,113,114] and in vivo.[115,116] Cellular damage from PDT is a result of insult by reactive oxygen species,

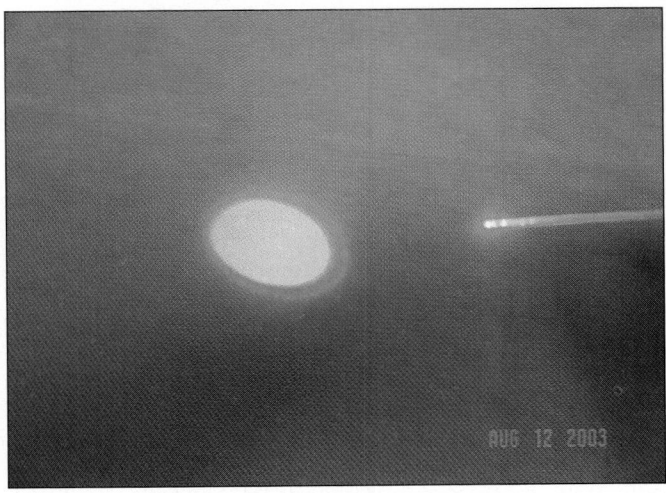

A

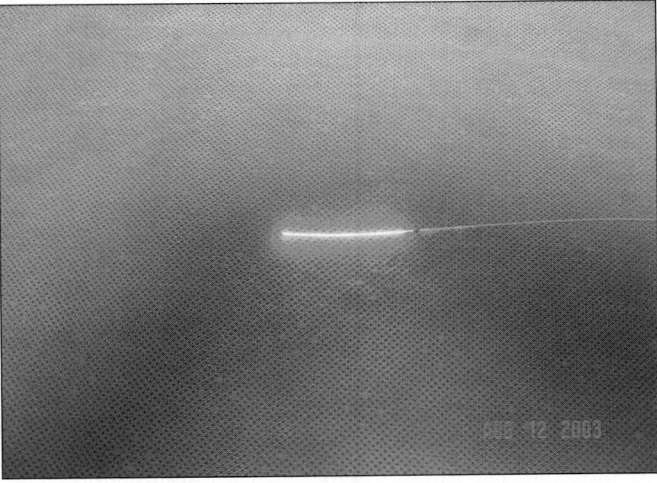

B

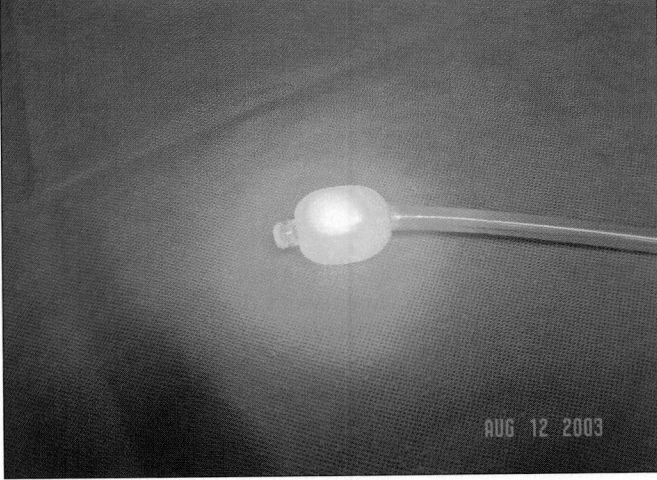

C

Figure 31-1. Fibers and applicators in clinical use.

Science of Clinical Oncology

which oxidize cell lipids and proteins.[117,118] The role of reactive oxygen species, especially singlet oxygen, in mediating direct tumor cell kill has been implicated by increases in clonogenicity when PDT is performed in the presence of inhibitors of reactive oxygen species.[119] In porfimer sodium–mediated PDT, membrane lipid peroxidation is detected immediately on initiation of light treatment,[120] and protection against lipid peroxidation leads to increases in cell viability.[121,122]

Subcellular localization of photosensitizer is important in determining the target of PDT damage. Photosensitizer localization is crucial because of the short lifetimes and correspondingly limited diffusion distances of the reactive intermediates involved in PDT photochemistry. The light-excited state of the photosensitizer tetrasulfonated aluminum phthalocyanine has a lifetime of 26 to 30 microseconds, whereas singlet oxygen has a lifetime of only 0.03 to 0.18 microseconds.[123] Accordingly, direct PDT damage is generally found at the subcellular site of photosensitizer localization.[124,125] Sites of photosensitizer localization include the mitochondria, Golgi apparatus, endoplasmic reticulum, lysosomes, and plasma and nuclear membranes.[125-127] Some photosensitizers may relocalize during PDT; for example, after low doses of light some phthalocyanine drugs appear to redistribute from the lysosomes to other areas of the cell.[128,129] In general, photosensitizers localize poorly to the nucleus, so PDT is associated with limited DNA damage and mutagenicity.[125,130]

The amount of direct tumor cell kill resulting from a particular in vivo PDT light dose can vary significantly depending on the photosensitizer and the fluence rate of illumination. Porfimer sodium–mediated PDT generally causes small amounts of direct tumor cell kill,[113,115,131] whereas other photosensitizers, such as aluminum phthalocyanine,[115] can cause significant cell kill during illumination. The fluence rate used for illumination can affect the amount of direct cytotoxicity through its effects on tumor oxygenation.[5,9,132] Because oxygen is a necessary substrate in the PDT reaction, less direct cytotoxicity is found in the presence of hypoxia.[8,87] Lower fluence rate, which preserves tumor oxygenation during PDT, or rapid fractionation of light, which enables tumor oxygenation to recover during brief pauses in illumination, both increase the amount of cytotoxicity during PDT.[131,133,134]

Vascular Effects

PDT-mediated photoxidization is not restricted to tumor cells. It can occur in normal tissues that have accumulated photosensitizer, such as vascular endothelial cells.[135] PDT insult to the vasculature can compromise tumor blood flow and lead to indirect PDT effects, such as nutritional starvation of tumor cells that escape direct cell kill. The importance of vascular damage to the PDT response was evidenced by abrogation of long-term tumor control when the vasculature in the skin immediately adjacent to or underlying an intradermal murine tumor was shielded from illumination.[136] In other studies, investigators measured significant reductions in tumor perfusion after PDT and correlated extent of vascular shutdown with tumor growth delay.[137] Vascular damage and accompanying ischemia due to PDT can cause substantial cell kill, as evidenced by a progressive decrease in clonogenicity of tumor cells removed at increasing times after PDT.[113,115,138]

Histologic changes in blood vessels after PDT include platelet aggregation, red blood cell agglutination, fibrin deposition and fibrinoid necrosis, and endothelial cell karyolysis and death.[139,140] The first evidence of cellular damage after PDT was found in the subendothelial zone, which provides structural support of the capillary wall.[141] This damage consisted of edema, fragmentation of collagen, and eventual complete destruction of the subendothelial zone.

The nature of the vascular response to PDT depends on the photosensitizer and its dosing. For example, vasoconstriction was observed after photosensitization with porfimer sodium and monosulfonated and tertiary butyl-substituted zinc phthalocyanine photosensitizers but not with disulfonated zinc phthalocyanines, LS11, or benzoporphyrin derivative.[140,142-144] Reduced blood flow associated with platelet aggregation and thrombus formation was found with benzoporphyrin derivative–, LS11-, and porfimer sodium–mediated PDT.[140,142,144] Increasing porfimer sodium doses from 5 mg/kg to 25 mg/kg was associated with corresponding increases in arteriole vasoconstriction and venule hyperpermeability during PDT.[142] Shortening the interval between LS11 administration and light delivery from 24 hours to 4 hours resulted in larger reductions in red blood cell column diameter within arterioles as a consequence of platelet aggregation.[144] Both fluence rate of illumination and total fluence delivered can affect vascular responses to PDT.[9,137] PDT effects on blood flow are dynamic. In some instances vascular perfusion decreases during treatment and then recovers, at least temporarily, after illumination.[9,142] Not surprisingly, ischemia-reperfusion injury can occur after PDT and may contribute to tumor response.[145]

Eicosanoids, including leukotrienes, thromboxanes, and prostaglandins, which mediate vascular effects such as dilation, constriction, leukocyte adhesion, and platelet aggregation, can be detected in PDT-treated cells and animals. They are produced by the action of cyclo-oxygenase or lipoxygenase on arachidonic acid released from photoxidized membranes. PDT-mediated release of prostaglandin E_2, prostaglandin F_{2a}, and prostacyclin has been detected in vitro.[146,147] In vivo, elevated serum levels of thromboxane B_2 and leukotriene B_4 have been found in PDT-treated rodents.[148] Single-dose inhibition of cyclo-oxygenase with indomethacin has abrogated PDT response,[148] as has inhibition of thromboxane.[149] In contrast, repeated administration of a specific cyclo-oxygenase-2 inhibitor, NS-398, over 20 days after PDT has been shown to significantly enhance tumor response. In this study, NS-398 reduced tumor expression of prostaglandin E_2 and vascular endothelial growth factor.[150] Other inhibitors of vascular endothelial growth factor have been found to enhance PDT response through antiangiogenic effects.[33]

The antivascular effects of PDT have been exploited in nononcologic applications. The photosensitizer benzoporphyrin derivative mono acid (verteporfin), in combination with 699-nm light is FDA approved for the management of age-related macular degeneration.[2] This disorder is the major cause of blindness among persons older than 50 years living in industrialized nations. Blindness from age-related macular degeneration is typically a result of choroidal neovascularization,[151] and PDT can be used to selectively occlude this neovasculature. PDT to 50 J/cm^2 at 15 minutes after intravenous verteporfin injection (6 mg/m^2) is generally applied multiple times over several years.[152]

Immunologic Effects

Results of animal studies have indicated that stimulation of the host immune system is required for definitive PDT responses. When PDT of EMT6 mammary sarcoma was performed in immunodeficient mice, a curative response was obtained, but this response was abrogated if the tumor was alternatively propagated in immunodeficient animals. Significantly, if the immunodeficient mice were reconstituted with bone marrow from immunocompetent animals, providing functional lymphocytes to the recipients, then a curative PDT response could be obtained in these recipients.[153]

The acute immune response to PDT is characterized by an inflammatory reaction and influx of host immune cells. Within minutes to hours after PDT, increases in tumor levels of neutrophils, monocytes, macrophages, and mast cells are detected.[154,155] This immune cell infiltrate initiates development of antitumor immunity (see later) and has direct tumoricidal effects. Macrophages isolated from PDT-treated tumors demonstrate more cytotoxicity against tumor cells than do macrophages isolated from control tumors.[154] Inactivation of macrophages leads to a significant reduction in the number of PDT cures,[156] whereas enhancement of macrophage activity markedly improves tumor response.[157] Mice deficient in mast cells, leukocytes, or components of complement exhibit a reduced phototoxic response.[158] Inhibition of PDT-created neutrophilia with antibody to granulocyte-macrophage colony-stimulating factor (G-CSF) greatly attenuates the efficacy of PDT.[159] Conversely, systemic treatment with G-CSF[160] or tumor-localized injection of cells producing granulocyte-macrophage colony-stimulating factor (GM-CSF)[161] leads to significant enhancement of the PDT tumor response. G-CSF treatment has been found to increase levels of circulating neutrophils,[160] and GM-CSF therapy has been found to increase the antitumor cytotoxicity of macrophages.[161]

The inflammatory response after PDT may prime the development of antitumor immunity. Tumor-associated macrophages or dendritic cells, which phagocytize PDT-inactivated tumor cells, are stimulated by the inflammatory process to act as antigen-presenting cells. Antigen presentation to helper T lymphocytes and subsequent activation of cytotoxic T cells leads to development of a tumor-specific adoptive immune response.[1] Numerous animal studies have been conducted to investigate the adaptive immune response to PDT. In one study, rats were resistant to a tumor challenge after previous curative PDT for a tumor of the same line in the same animal.[162] Furthermore, adoptive transfer of splenocytes from PDT-cured animals to new hosts protected the recipient animals from tumor challenge.[162] Tumor immunity also was acquired through animal inoculation with the lysate of in vitro PDT-treated tumor cells.[163] These lysates were found to stimulate maturation of dendritic cells, which may have made these cells more efficient at antigen presentation. In agreement with this suggestion, a significant increase in the cytotoxic activity of spleen cells was found in animals that received PDT-generated lysate.[163] In yet another study, the transferability of a curative outcome of PDT was investigated. Adoptive transfer of splenocytes from immunocompetent mice with tumors cured by PDT to immunodeficient mice incapable of a durable PDT response led to generation of PDT-created tumor cures in recipient mice.[164] Cytotoxic T lymphocytes and to a lesser extent helper T lymphocytes were identified as the immune cells responsible for transfer of the PDT outcome.[164]

Immunosuppression can accompany the inflammatory response after PDT. Immunosuppressive effects are evident in PDT-mediated inhibition of a contact hypersensitivity response to a topical hapten, such as dinitrofluorobenzene. Unresponsiveness to dinitrofluorobenzene can be mimicked in nonphotosensitized hosts through adoptive transfer of spleen or spleen and lymph cells from PDT-treated and dinitrofluorobenzene-sensitized animals.[165,166] A role for macrophages in PDT-created immunosuppression has been demonstrated,[157,166] and impairment of antigen presentation by Langerhans' cells has been found responsible for increased survival of allogenic mouse skin grafts.[167] The cytokine interleukin 10 (IL-10), which regulates cutaneous inflammatory responses, may[168] or may not[169,170] be involved in PDT-mediated inhibition of contact hypersensitivity, possibly depending on treatment factors such as the area (cutaneous versus transdermal) illuminated.[169]

Limited clinical investigation of PDT immune responses has been performed. After PDT for bladder cancer, increased levels of the cytokines IL-1β, IL-2, and tumor necrosis factor α were detected in urine, a finding that suggested at least a local immune response had occurred.[171] The presence of a systemic immune response after intraoperative PDT of the thoracic cavity has been suggested by increased serum cytokine levels of IL-1β, IL-6, IL-8, and IL-10,[172] but the contribution of surgery versus that of PDT is not yet elucidated. Possible involvement of cell-mediated immunity in the response of high-grade vulval intraepithelial lesions to PDT has been investigated with the finding of significantly more tumor infiltration by cytotoxic T lymphocytes in the lesions of women who responded to PDT compared with those who did not.[173]

Apoptotic versus Necrotic Cell Death

Mechanisms of cell death after PDT can include both apoptosis and necrosis. Apoptosis, or programmed cell death, is adenosine triphosphate dependent and characterized by distinct cellular processes, such as enzymatic cleavage of DNA, chromatin condensation, and cell shrinkage.[174] Necrosis, which is adenosine triphosphate independent, results from overwhelming insult to the tissue that leads to cell rupture and release of the contents of the cytoplasm.[174] The likelihood of cells' dying by an apoptotic as opposed to a necrotic mechanism is influenced by many factors, among them the photosensitizer and its subcellular localization, the light dose, and the tissue being treated. Photosensitizers that localize to the mitochondria are efficient inducers of apoptosis, whereas less or delayed apoptosis may be associated with drugs that localize to the plasma membrane.[175-177] Photosensitizers targeting lysosomes induce apoptosis in some instances[176,178] but not in others.[177] At high PDT doses the enzymes necessary for apoptosis may be destroyed, a process that leads to cell death by necrosis. Conversely, at doses too low to produce necrosis, apoptosis may lead to cell death.[179] Different cell types may also exhibit different sensitivities to PDT-created apoptosis.[180,181]

PDT-caused apoptosis frequently is characterized by loss of mitochondrial transmembrane potential, an increase in intracellular calcium, and translocation of cytochrome c from the mitochondria to the cytosol, where it binds to apoptosis activating factor 1 and activates caspases, which cause protein cleavage and ultimately DNA degradation.[179] These events may be associated with the opening of a channel in the mitochondrial inner membrane called the *permeability transition pore complex*. However, inactivation of this channel does not always block PDT-mediated apoptosis; thus the role of the permeability transition pore complex in PDT is controversial.[182] One component of the permeability transition pore complex that may be targeted by PDT is the peripheral benzodiazepine receptor. Some photosensitizers demonstrate an affinity for this receptor in a manner that correlates with their photosensitizing activity,[183,184] but this finding may be photosensitizer specific.[185,186] Although mitochondria are central to apoptotic signaling, photosensitizers localized to sites other than mitochondria can initiate apoptosis. Mechanisms for this process include cytochrome c release and induction of apoptosis as a result of release of calcium from PDT-damaged endoplasmic reticulum[187] or enzymatic cleavage of Bid, a proapoptotic protein, after PDT rupture of lysosomes.[179]

The role of the Bcl-2 family of proteins and the tumor suppressor p53 in PDT-created apoptosis has been investigated. The Bcl-2 family consists of many proteins that either promote, e.g., Bax and Bid, or inhibit, e.g., Bcl-2 and Bcl-xL, apoptosis. Overexpression of Bcl-2 or Bcl-xL has been associated with suppression of apoptosis after PDT with several photosensitizers.[188,189] This resistance to apoptosis has been found to be mediated by inhibition of caspase activity.[188,190] Some investigators have determined that overexpression of Bcl-2 can promote apoptosis if Bax also is overexpressed. Results of several investigations have suggested that the ratio of Bax to Bcl-2 affects apoptotic propensity.[191,192] PDT has been found to photodamage Bcl-2,[193,194] meaning PDT can directly affect the Bax:Bcl-2 ratio. In contrast to that found with Bcl-2 proteins, no consistent effect of p53 status on PDT response can be detected. Cells with wild-type p53 appear to be more sensitive to PDT than cells with deleted or mutated p53[195-197]; however, abrogation of p53 function

does not affect PDT sensitivity.[32] Furthermore, PDT can cause apoptosis in cell lines without functional p53.[196,197]

The presence of apoptosis after PDT in vivo has been documented in animal models as well as in clinical specimens. Animal studies have shown that PDT can cause apoptosis of tumor and normal cells,[198] including endothelial cells of the tumor-supporting vascular network.[199] As found in vitro, the extent and timing of apoptosis after PDT in vivo depend on a number of factors, including the photosensitizer used.[198,200] In clinical biopsies of actinic keratosis and nasopharyngeal carcinoma, increases in apoptosis were detected after PDT.[201,202] In 50% (4 of 8) of actinic keratosis samples positive for apoptosis 1 day after PDT, activation of caspase 3 also was detected.[201] In 75% (18 of 24) of nasopharyngeal carcinoma biopsies, upregulation of the proapoptotic protein Bak was found.[202] In other investigations, no association between pretreatment p53 status or Bcl-2 expression and PDT outcome was detected,[203] and no PDT-created changes in p53 expression, apoptotic index, caspase 3 activity, or Bcl-2 expression were found.[204] Still other investigators found increased Bcl-2 expression to be associated with a better response to PDT.[205] Although Bax expression was not investigated in these samples, it may have been the Bax:Bcl-2 ratio that was critical, because Bcl-2 is damaged by PDT.

CLINICAL USE OF PHOTODYNAMIC THERAPY

Approved Indications

Obstructing Esophageal Cancer

Esophageal cancer frequently is locally advanced and causes serious symptoms, most commonly dysphagia. Palliation of dysphagia is common in patients who have unresectable disease, who are unresponsive to chemotherapy or radiation, or who have recurrent disease.[206-208] Palliation can be achieved with brachytherapy,[209,210] external beam radiation,[207] balloon dilation,[208] metal stents,[211,212] or sclerosing agents.[213] PDT also is a potential palliative treatment of patients with obstructing esophageal cancer.

The effectiveness of PDT for palliating dysphagia in patients with obstructing esophageal cancer has been demonstrated in several studies.[214-217] Luketich et al.[217] administered porfimer sodium–mediated PDT to 77 patients with inoperable, obstructing, or bleeding esophageal carcinoma. Forty-eight hours after administration of 1.5 to 2.0 mg/kg porfimer sodium, 630-nm laser light was delivered. Four weeks after PDT, mean dysphagia scores improved in 91% of the patients. The mean dysphagia-free interval was 80 days, and the median survival was 5.9 months. Twenty-nine (38%) of the patients needed more than one treatment. The complication rate was low and included esophageal stricture, candidal esophagitis, pleural effusion, and cutaneous photosensitivity.[217] A multicenter randomized trial comparing porfimer sodium–mediated PDT with neodymium:yttrium-aluminum-garnet (Nd:YAG) laser therapy led to FDA approval of porfimer sodium–mediated PDT for this indication.[216] Two hundred thirty-six patients were enrolled in the study. Porfimer sodium, 2.0 mg/kg, was administered intravenously and followed by treatment in 40 to 50 hours with 630-nm light. In the PDT-treated group, 44% of patients had symptom improvement after 1 week, and 35% had improvement after 1 month, results similar to the those for the Nd:YAG-treated group. More objective tumor responses (complete response plus partial response) were observed in the PDT group (32% at 1 month for PDT versus 20% for Nd:YAG). Complete responses were more common in the PDT group: 9 complete responses with PDT versus 2 with Nd:YAG. There was a trend toward improved response to PDT in patients with tumors in the upper or lower third of the esophagus, in tumors larger than 10 cm, and in patients who had received previous therapy. The rate of adverse events (92%) was higher in the PDT group, although the rate of withdrawal from the study because of adverse events was similar for the two groups. The rates of severe adverse events were similar for the two groups, with the exception of esophageal perforation, which occurred at a higher rate in the Nd:YAG group than in the PDT group (7% versus 1%). The conclusions from this study were that PDT was as effective as Nd:YAG laser therapy for palliation of dysphagia and that the two treatments had similar levels of toxicity in patients with obstructing esophageal cancer.

Caution should be exercised when PDT is being considered in the care of a patient who has received previous external beam radiation combined with high-dose-rate brachytherapy. Sanfilippo et al.[218] reported life-threatening complications from porfimer sodium–mediated PDT in three patients with cancer of the upper aerodigestive tract. Two patients with esophageal cancer received combined chemotherapy and external beam radiation followed by intraluminal high-dose-rate brachytherapy. One patient with non–small cell lung cancer received external beam radiation therapy and intraluminal high-dose-rate brachytherapy. These patients were treated with porfimer sodium–mediated PDT for recurrent disease. Fistulas developed in both patients with esophageal cancer. The patient with non–small cell lung cancer experienced fatal, massive hemoptysis immediately after PDT. This complication was caused by necrotizing arteritis in the pulmonary artery. These case reports suggest that patients who have received treatment with both external beam radiation and intraluminal high-dose-rate brachytherapy are at higher risk of major complications from PDT. These toxicities were observed in patients who were previously treated with *both* external beam radiation therapy and high-dose-rate brachytherapy. We have found porfimer sodium–mediated PDT safe and effective for palliation of obstructing esophageal cancer in patients who have received previous external beam therapy alone.

PDT is effective palliative treatment of patients with obstructing esophageal cancer. In general, PDT for obstructing esophageal cancer is safe. One significant limitation is prolonged sun sensitivity associated with porfimer sodium–mediated PDT. It is reasonable, therefore, to consider other palliative measures, such as stent placement, before PDT. PDT can be used after stent placement in the care of patients who have tumor ingrowth after placement of expandable stents.[219]

Patient selection is an important factor in decisions about the use of PDT for obstructing esophageal cancer. Patients with tumors that have eroded into the tracheobronchial tree[220] or a major vessel,[218] patients with esophageal varices, and patients who have received the combination of previous external beam and high-dose-rate brachytherapy[218] are at high risk of major complications. PDT should be avoided in these patients.

The FDA-approved indications for porfimer sodium–mediated PDT are palliation of dysphagia associated with obstructing esophageal cancer or of partially obstructing esophageal cancer in patients who cannot be satisfactorily treated with Nd:YAG laser therapy. The FDA-approved regimen is intravenous injection of 2 mg/kg porfimer sodium 40 to 50 hours before 630-nm light delivery. The light is delivered with a cylindrical diffuser passed through the endoscope. A dose of 300 J/cm is delivered at a fluence rate of 400 mW/cm (total treatment time, 750 seconds). Patients may experience odynophagia, dysphagia, nausea, or vomiting after the initial light treatment. Transient atrial arrhythmias have also been reported.[221] A second light treatment may be given 96 to 120 hours after porfimer sodium administration.

Palliation of Obstructing Endobronchial Lung Cancer

Patients with obstructing endobronchial lung cancer have shortness of breath, fatigue, cough, and fever.[222] Many of these patients are not surgical candidates and need urgent palliative treatment. Treatment options include external beam radiation, brachytherapy, YAG laser ablation and stent placement, and PDT.[223-226]

In a study of porfimer sodium–mediated PDT in the care of patients with stage IIIa–IV lung cancer and an obstructing endobronchial lesion,[224] 100 patients were enrolled, 82% of whom had undergone previous chemotherapy or radiation therapy. Porfimer sodium, 2 mg/kg, was administered intravenously and followed 24 to 72 hours later with delivery of 630-nm light. Improvements in forced expiratory volume in 1 second (FEV_1) and forced vital capacity (FVC) were observed after PDT. Mean end luminal obstruction in these patients decreased from 86% to 18%. As expected for this patient population, median survival was poor at 5 months. A randomized trial comparing porfimer sodium–mediated PDT and Nd:YAG laser resection was performed with patients with lung cancer and luminal obstruction.[225] In that study, 31 patients were randomized to treatment with PDT (n = 14) or Nd:YAG laser resection (n = 17). Porfimer sodium, 2 mg/kg, was administered 40 to 50 hours before treatment with 630-nm light. Five patients in the PDT group needed a second treatment, as did one patient in the Nd:YAG group. Reduction in luminal obstruction was similar in the two groups, but the response was more durable in the PDT group. Symptom improvement was found with a decrease in dyspnea, hemoptysis, cough, and sputum production. Eighty-four percent of the patients had adverse events, although only one case of severe phototoxicity occurred.

Science of Clinical Oncology

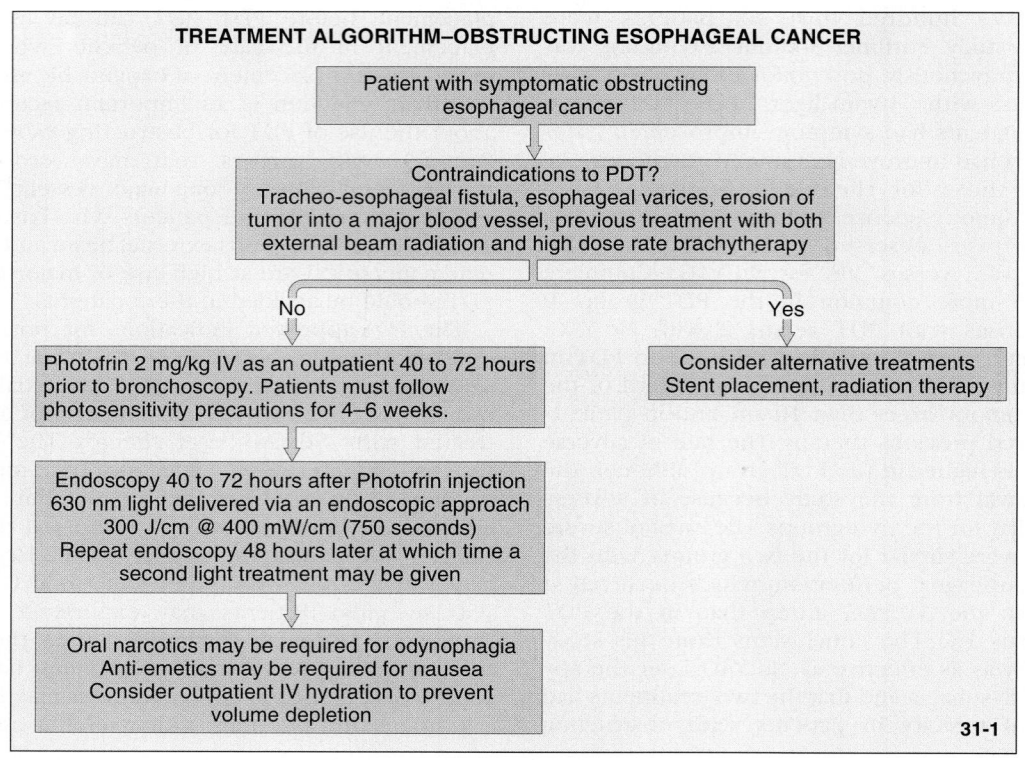

TREATMENT ALGORITHM—OBSTRUCTING ESOPHAGEAL CANCER

Patient with symptomatic obstructing esophageal cancer

Contraindications to PDT?
Tracheo-esophageal fistula, esophageal varices, erosion of tumor into a major blood vessel, previous treatment with both external beam radiation and high dose rate brachytherapy

No → Photofrin 2 mg/kg IV as an outpatient 40 to 72 hours prior to bronchoscopy. Patients must follow photosensitivity precautions for 4–6 weeks.

Yes → Consider alternative treatments Stent placement, radiation therapy

Endoscopy 40 to 72 hours after Photofrin injection 630 nm light delivered via an endoscopic approach 300 J/cm @ 400 mW/cm (750 seconds) Repeat endoscopy 48 hours later at which time a second light treatment may be given

Oral narcotics may be required for odynophagia Anti-emetics may be required for nausea Consider outpatient IV hydration to prevent volume depletion

31-1

The FDA has approved porfimer sodium–mediated PDT for the management of obstruction and palliation of symptoms in patients with completely or partially obstructing endobronchial lung cancer. The FDA-approved regimen is intravenous injection of 2 mg/kg porfimer sodium 40 to 50 hours before 630-nm light delivery. Light is delivered with a cylindrical diffuser through a bronchoscope. A dose of 200 J/cm is delivered at a fluence rate of 400 mW/cm (total treatment time, 500 seconds). Necrotic tissue often is found in the bronchial tree after light administration. It is wise to hospitalize patients with compromised pulmonary status after PDT to observe for worsening airway obstruction. If signs or symptoms of airway obstruction develop, administration of oxygen and corticosteroids should be considered. Early bronchoscopy is indicated for severe symptoms of obstruction. Bronchoscopy to debride the airway is otherwise required 48 to 72 hours after light delivery. A second light treatment may be given at that time.

PDT is efficacious in palliation of endobronchial obstruction, but serious complications, such as life-threatening hemoptysis have been reported.[218] Contraindications to bronchial PDT include tumor invasion of major vessels, tracheoesophageal fistula, and previous combined external beam radiation and high-dose-rate brachytherapy.[218]

Early-Stage Lung Cancer

Standard therapy for early-stage lung cancer is surgical resection.[227] Many patients, however, have poor lung function and are not candidates for surgery, and radiation therapy is an alternative to surgery. PDT is a good option for patients with microinvasive endobronchial lung cancer in whom surgery is not feasible. Most studies have shown that the efficacy of PDT for superficial endobronchial cancer is high and that the treatment is associated with manageable toxicity.

In a phase II study of porfimer sodium–mediated PDT for centrally located early-stage lung cancer,[228] light was delivered 48 hours after administration of 2 mg/kg porfimer sodium. Complete responses after PDT were observed in 90% of 42 evaluable patients; the median duration of complete response was 14 months. A short tumor length was the best predictor of complete response. It was hypothesized that the length of the tumor related to depth of tumor. Use of endobronchial ultrasound is under investigation to help better define depth of lesions and to improve selection of patients for PDT.[229] Results of a large study of PDT for early-stage lung cancer confirmed these encouraging results. Two hundred forty patients were enrolled in the trial.[230] Of the 95 patients with early-stage disease, 83% had a complete response after PDT.

The FDA has approved porfimer sodium–mediated PDT for the management of microinvasive endobronchial lung cancer in patients for whom surgery or radiation therapy is not indicated. The FDA-approved regimen is intravenous injection of 2 mg/kg porfimer sodium 40 to 50 hours before 630-nm light delivery. Light is delivered with a cylindrical diffuser through a bronchoscope. A dose of 200 J/cm is delivered at a fluence rate of 400 mW/cm (total treatment time, 500 seconds). A second bronchoscopy for debridement of necrotic tissue is performed 2 days after light treatment. A second light treatment may be given at that time. Hospitalization after PDT should

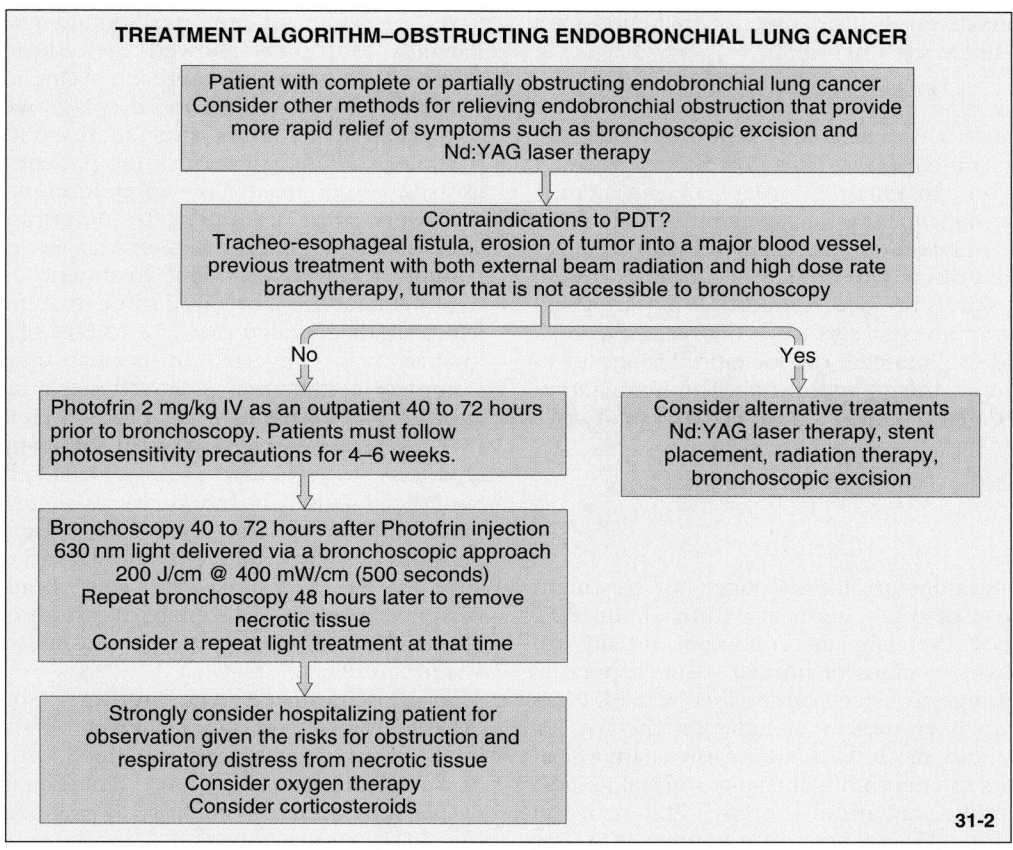

TREATMENT ALGORITHM–OBSTRUCTING ENDOBRONCHIAL LUNG CANCER

Patient with complete or partially obstructing endobronchial lung cancer
Consider other methods for relieving endobronchial obstruction that provide
more rapid relief of symptoms such as bronchoscopic excision and
Nd:YAG laser therapy

Contraindications to PDT?
Tracheo-esophageal fistula, erosion of tumor into a major blood vessel,
previous treatment with both external beam radiation and high dose rate
brachytherapy, tumor that is not accessible to bronchoscopy

No / Yes

Photofrin 2 mg/kg IV as an outpatient 40 to 72 hours
prior to bronchoscopy. Patients must follow
photosensitivity precautions for 4–6 weeks.

Consider alternative treatments
Nd:YAG laser therapy, stent
placement, radiation therapy,
bronchoscopic excision

Bronchoscopy 40 to 72 hours after Photofrin injection
630 nm light delivered via a bronchoscopic approach
200 J/cm @ 400 mW/cm (500 seconds)
Repeat bronchoscopy 48 hours later to remove
necrotic tissue
Consider a repeat light treatment at that time

Strongly consider hospitalizing patient for
observation given the risks for obstruction and
respiratory distress from necrotic tissue
Consider oxygen therapy
Consider corticosteroids

31-2

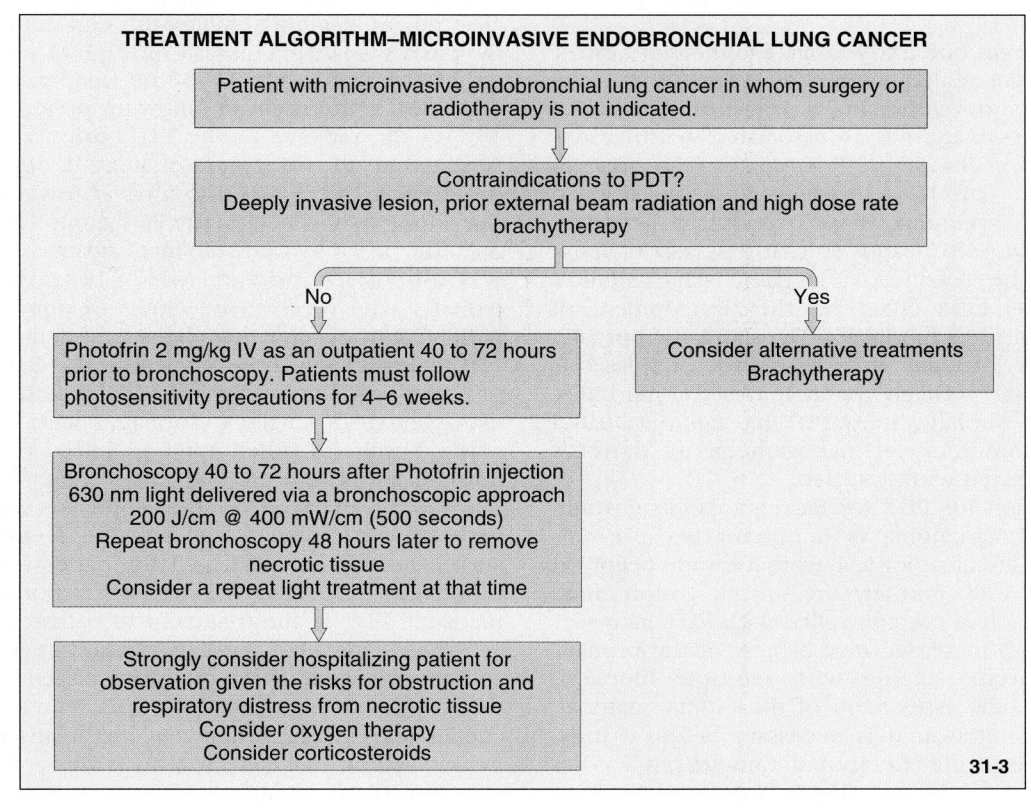

TREATMENT ALGORITHM–MICROINVASIVE ENDOBRONCHIAL LUNG CANCER

Patient with microinvasive endobronchial lung cancer in whom surgery or
radiotherapy is not indicated.

Contraindications to PDT?
Deeply invasive lesion, prior external beam radiation and high dose rate
brachytherapy

No / Yes

Photofrin 2 mg/kg IV as an outpatient 40 to 72 hours
prior to bronchoscopy. Patients must follow
photosensitivity precautions for 4–6 weeks.

Consider alternative treatments
Brachytherapy

Bronchoscopy 40 to 72 hours after Photofrin injection
630 nm light delivered via a bronchoscopic approach
200 J/cm @ 400 mW/cm (500 seconds)
Repeat bronchoscopy 48 hours later to remove
necrotic tissue
Consider a repeat light treatment at that time

Strongly consider hospitalizing patient for
observation given the risks for obstruction and
respiratory distress from necrotic tissue
Consider oxygen therapy
Consider corticosteroids

31-3

Science of Clinical Oncology

be strongly considered in the care of patients with compromised pulmonary function.

Actinic Keratosis

Actinic keratosis is a premalignant, superficial skin disorder caused by sun exposure. The FDA has approved a topical formulation containing 20% ALA (Levulan) administered with blue light for the management of nonhyperkeratotic actinic keratosis of the face or scalp. Levulan solution is applied directly to an actinic keratosis lesion, and perilesional skin is avoided. Application to periorbital tissue or to ocular or mucosal surfaces is not recommended. Blue light is used to illuminate one or more lesions 14 to 18 hours after topical drug application. The illumination time is 1000 seconds to deliver a dose of 10 J/cm^2.

Clinical Uses of Photodynamic Therapy under Active Investigation: Premalignant Conditions and Early Cancer

Premalignant conditions are ideally suited for treatment with PDT because of the superficial nature of the PDT effect on tissues.[10] Premalignant conditions usually are superficial, and wide regions of normal tissue, especially in the upper aerodigestive tract, can be involved. PDT has several advantages over surgery or radiation therapy for premalignant conditions: It is a noninvasive superficial therapy that limits the depth of damage to normal tissues. Furthermore, unlike radiation therapy, PDT can be administered more than once. In general, PDT for premalignant conditions of the upper aerodigestive tract is associated with high efficacy and low morbidity.

Barrett's Esophagus and Early-Stage Esophageal Cancer

Barrett's esophagus is a common clinical condition that is characterized by development of intestinal-type metaplasia in the esophagus. It is associated with gastroesophageal reflux disease.[231-234] Dysplasia can arise in association with Barrett's esophagus and can lead to development of carcinoma. Close observation is recommended in Barrett's esophagus so that dysplasia or frank carcinoma can be detected at an early stage. Medical management has little effect on the development of malignancy in Barrett's esophagus. The standard approach to treatment of patients with high-grade dysplasia is surgical resection.[235] Given the potential for morbidity associated with esophagectomy, PDT has been evaluated as potential nonoperative management of Barrett's esophagus associated with dysplasia.

Patient selection for PDT for Barrett's esophagus and early superficial carcinoma is important because this treatment is not effective for lesions that invade deeply in the esophageal wall. Furthermore, occult lymph node involvement, which is not controlled with PDT, increases in frequency with increased invasiveness of the primary tumor.[236,237] Careful staging with multiple biopsies, thorough pathologic assessment of the biopsy material, and endoscopic ultrasound is necessary before a treatment decision is made. Computed tomography of the chest and upper abdomen should be considered in evaluation of patients who have early carcinoma.

A large study of porfimer sodium–mediated PDT for Barrett's esophagus showed the efficacy and relative safety of this treatment approach.[22] One hundred patients with Barrett's esophagus and dysplasia were treated with 630-nm light 48 hours after administration of 2 mg/kg porfimer sodium. Thirteen of the patients had superficial invasive carcinoma. Follow-up endoscopy was performed 48 hours after treatment to determine whether an additional light delivery session was needed. Seventy-three patients received one light treatment, 22 received two treatments, and five received three treatments. Endoscopic examination revealed that 75% to 80% of treated Barrett's mucosa was converted to normal squamous mucosa. Complete elimination of Barrett's esophagus was found after PDT in 43 patients. Of these 43 patients, 8 received PDT alone, whereas 35 needed follow-up Nd:YAG laser ablation for residual areas of Barrett's esophagus. Superficial malignant lesions were eliminated in 10 of 13 patients. PDT was associated with acute, moderate chest pain and dysphagia that resolved in 3 to 5 days. Esophageal stricture was a common late complication of PDT for Barrett's esophagus. Esophageal strictures developed in 34 patients, and 11 patients needed multiple dilations for symptom relief.

In a randomized trial, porfimer sodium–mediated PDT combined with administration of the proton-pump inhibitor omeprazole was compared with administration of omeprazole alone for the management of high-grade dysplasia associated with Barrett's esophagus.[20] Patients in the PDT group received 2 mg/kg porfimer sodium followed 48 to 72 hours later by endoscopic laser therapy with 630-nm light.[20] A maximum of 3 courses of PDT were allowed. At 6-month follow-up endoscopy, high-grade dysplasia was ablated in 80% of the PDT plus omeprazole group compared with 40% of the omeprazole alone group ($P < .0001$). After a mean follow-up period of 12 months, 17% of the patients in the PDT group and 39% of the patients in the omeprazole alone group had disease progression. There was also a trend toward reduction in development of cancer in the PDT group (9% versus 19%). As in the previous study, the main adverse event from PDT was esophageal stricture, which developed in 12% of patients who received one light treatment and 38% of patients who received two light treatments.

The results of these clinical trials demonstrate that porfimer sodium–mediated PDT is effective for the management of Barrett's esophagus with high-grade dysplasia. Results of other, nonrandomized trials confirmed the effectiveness of PDT in this setting.[238-240] It is likely that superficial cancers of the esophagus will be detected with greater frequency given the aggressive endoscopic surveillance being instituted for patients with Barrett's esophagus. The FDA has approved porfimer sodium–mediated PDT in the treatment of patients with Barrett's esophagus and high-grade dysplasia. In general, porfimer sodium–mediated PDT is offered to patients with Barrett's esophagus and high-grade dysplasia who are not surgical candidates. It is important that physicians who use PDT in this setting make it clear to patients that surgery is standard treatment and that long-term data regarding the effectiveness of PDT are not yet available.

Carcinoma in Situ and Early Cancer of the Head and Neck

The rationale for considering PDT for premalignant lesions, carcinoma in situ of the head and neck, or early carcinoma is conceptually similar to that for considering PDT for microinvasive endobronchial carcinoma or Barrett's esophagus.[10] PDT in this setting is a noninvasive, superficial treatment that has shown efficacy and acceptable toxicity. PDT, however, is not FDA approved for these indications.

Several small studies have shown results with PDT for early head and neck cancer. In a study in which mTHPC was used to treat 27 patients with carcinoma in situ or microinvasive cancer, 83% of the patients treated had no evidence of recurrence after a median follow-up period of 15.3 months.[241] In four patients with T_1 or T_2 cancer, however, only one complete response was observed. Porfimer sodium also has been used in this clinical setting. Ten patients with diffuse field cancerization of the oral cavity were treated with porfimer sodium–mediated PDT.[24] All patients had diffuse areas of carcinoma in situ or superficial cancer of the oral cavity and oropharynx. Of the 10 patients treated, eight had complete responses in follow-up periods ranging from 6 months to 9 years. Another study of porfimer sodium–mediated PDT confirmed these results.[242]

PDT has been used to manage head and neck cancer beyond the oral cavity and oropharynx. Excellent results with HPD-mediated PDT were obtained in the care of patients with T_1 cancer of the larynx.[243] Thirty-two patients with carcinoma of the true vocal cord and no anterior commissure involvement were treated in the study. Complete responses occurred in 25 (78%) of 32 patients with a follow-up period of 12 to 48 months. In a series of 107 patients with cancer of the larynx, pharynx, and oral cavity, PDT was efficacious in the management of early cancer of the head and neck.[244-247] The patients were treated with 2 mg/kg porfimer sodium 48 hours before 630-nm light delivery. Of the patients with T_{is}/T_1 tumors of the larynx, 100% had a complete response to PDT with a 95% cure rate after a mean follow-up period of 37 to 44 months. Of patients with T_{is}/T_1 tumors of the oral cavity, 100% had a complete response rate with an 80% cure rate after a mean follow-up period of 40 months. Significant cutaneous phototoxicity due to unprotected light exposure developed in 2 of 107 patients. The degree of treatment-related pain was variable, but in all cases pain was adequately controlled with oral analgesics. PDT appears to be a promising modality for the management of premalignant lesions and early cancer of the head and neck. Active investigation of this modality is warranted.

Clinical Uses of Photodynamic Therapy under Active Investigation: Invasive and Advanced Cancer

Pleural Spread of Non–Small Cell Lung Cancer

There are other clinical situations in lung cancer in which PDT may have a role. Non–small cell lung cancer often spreads to the pleural surface and manifests as the presence of pleural effusion or studding of the pleura.

Malignant pleural spread of non–small cell lung cancer is a poor prognostic finding. Patients with this manifestation of the disease have a median survival period of 6 to 9 months, similar to that of patients with stage IV disease.[248-251] Chemotherapy has typically been the standard treatment of these patients. Surgery is generally not considered curative treatment of this group of patients.[250,252]

Radical surgery is not curative in patients with pleural spread of non–small cell lung cancer because microscopic pleural disease from the thoracic cavity is unlikely to be eradicated by resection. PDT is a superficial treatment that can be administered intraoperatively and is one possible method for managing residual microscopic disease after surgical resection. Pass and colleagues from the National Cancer Institute[16] first evaluated porfimer sodium–mediated PDT to the pleural surface in the care of patients with pleural malignant lesions, including non–small cell lung cancer, and performed a phase I study. The investigators determined the maximally tolerated dose of porfimer sodium–mediated PDT in the thoracic cavity after radical surgical resection and described serious complications, including intraoperative hemorrhage, bronchopleural fistula, and esophageal perforation.[253] The results of the study established that intrapleural PDT can be delivered safely in combination with radical surgery.

A phase II study was conducted of porfimer sodium–mediated PDT in the care of patients with non–small cell lung cancer that had spread to the pleura.[85] An attempt was made to incorporate pleural PDT into a multimodality approach including chemotherapy, radiation, and surgery. Sixteen patients, many with pathologic stage IIIA, T_4N_2 disease, were enrolled.[16] Most of the patients were treated with chemotherapy before surgical resection and with porfimer sodium–mediated PDT in the dose determined by Pass et al. Surgical procedures included segmentectomy, lobectomy, and pneumonectomy combined with resection of gross pleural disease. Laser light was administered intraoperatively. Postoperative radiation therapy was delivered to the mediastinum when indicated. Local control at 6 months was achieved in 10 patients, and the median survival period among all treated patients was 21.7 months. Complications included thrombocytopenia, cardiac arrhythmia, hypotension, azotemia, and elevated results of liver function tests. Two patients died postoperatively, one of acute respiratory distress syndrome and the other of sepsis. The survival and local control results were encouraging and support continued investigation of PDT in the management of non–small cell lung cancer with malignant pleural spread.

Mesothelioma

Malignant pleural mesothelioma is cancer of the pleural surface, for which there is no curative therapy. Patients with mesothelioma have a poor prognosis, the median survival period being 6 to 15 months.[254] Local failure is the predominant mode of recurrence of mesothelioma, and PDT has been investigated as an adjuvant to surgery for improvement of local control.[17,28-30,255,256] A phase II trial of porfimer sodium–mediated PDT was performed with patients with mesothelioma.[257] Patients were treated with porfimer sodium, maximal surgical debulking, and intraoperative delivery of 630-nm light. Patients who had stage III–IV disease (n = 24) had a median survival time of 10 months. No patient survived longer than 2 years. Patients with stage I and II disease (n = 13) had a median survival time of 36 months and a 61% 2-year overall survival rate. It was concluded that PDT was beneficial to patients with early-stage disease.

In a randomized phase III study[17] of porfimer sodium–mediated PDT for mesothelioma, 63 patients were enrolled, and all received preoperative immunochemotherapy consisting of tamoxifen, interferon α 2b, and cisplatin. Patients were randomized between PDT with surgery and surgery alone. Fifteen patients (24%) were taken off study because of inadequate debulking or because of disease progression before surgery. Complications occurred in 10 of 48 patients but did not differ between the two groups. One patient died of postoperative hemorrhage, and in each of the randomization groups, bronchopleural fistulas developed in 2 patients. No clinical benefit was found with the addition of PDT to surgery. The median recurrence-free survival time for patients in the PDT group was 8.5 months versus 7.7 months in the control group. The median survival time in the PDT group was 14.1 months versus 14.4 months in the control group.

The results of porfimer sodium–mediated PDT led to investigation of mTHPC-mediated PDT for mesothelioma. mTHPC-mediated PDT was used in two phase I studies.[29,30] In one study, 28 patients were treated, and several dose levels of drug were investigated. All patients underwent extrapleural pneumonectomy with intraoperative light delivery. Serious complications included myocardial infarction, bronchopleural fistula, esophageal fistula, diaphragmatic rupture, cardiac tamponade, spinal cord infarction, cutaneous photosensitivity, and empyema. Local control was achieved in 13 of 26 patients who received PDT, and the median survival time was 10 months. The investigators concluded that mTHPC-mediated PDT in combination with extrapleural pneumonectomy provided good local control but was associated with a high incidence of complications, which limited use of this treatment. A second phase I study showed mTHPC-mediated PDT was feasible and that it may have a role in combination with lung-sparing surgical procedures.[30] The results of these studies suggest that PDT has not proved superior to other adjuvant therapies or surgery alone in the treatment of patients with mesothelioma. Further study is necessary to determine the role of PDT in the management of this disease.

Advanced and Recurrent Head and Neck Cancer

PDT with a variety of photosensitizers has been investigated as sole treatment of patients with advanced carcinoma of the head and neck, but, in general, the results have been disappointing.[244,246,258] Although responses to treatment have been reported, recurrence is common. Therefore PDT used alone in the management of advanced or bulky cancer of the head and neck usually is considered palliative. The risk to benefit profile of the treatment should be considered with this factor in mind.

PDT may be useful, however, as palliative therapy for local recurrence of head and neck cancer after previous definitive therapy.[259] In this group of patients, the salvage rate with traditional therapies is poor. mTHPC has been approved in Europe for the management of locally recurrent head and neck cancer.

A different approach to treatment of patients with recurrent disease is PDT combined with surgical resection. The goal of this treatment is to use PDT to destroy any remaining cancer cells within the surgical bed. Biel[247] treated 10 patients with neck recurrences with intraoperative porfimer sodium–mediated PDT following resection. Recurrences developed in only three of the 10 patients treated in this manner.

Skin Cancer

PDT for cutaneous cancer (both primary and metastatic) and premalignant lesions has been extensively investigated, but the role of this therapy has not been defined, mostly because other therapies, such as surgery and radiation therapy, are associated with good outcome. 5-ALA–mediated PDT,[260-263] porfimer sodium–mediated PDT,[264] and mTHPC-mediated PDT[11] all have been reported to produce excellent outcome and good cosmetic results.

Intraperitoneal Malignant Tumors

Some cancers commonly spread to or originate in the serosal surfaces of the abdomen. These tumors include primary peritoneal cancer, ovarian cancer, sarcoma, gastrointestinal malignant tumors, and mesothelioma. This mode of cancer spread usually is incurable regardless of the site of origin. Traditional therapies such as surgery, radiation therapy, and chemotherapy can lead to tumor response, but local recurrence is the rule. PDT is potentially an ideal therapy for peritoneal carcinomatosis or sarcomatosis because of the superficial treatment effect.[10]

The results of a phase I study of surgery and intraperitoneal PDT (IP PDT) were encouraging, especially among patients with ovarian cancer.[15,82,265] A phase II trial of porfimer sodium–mediated IP PDT to determine the efficacy of this treatment in intraperitoneal malignant diseases is being conducted at the University of Pennsylvania.[266,267] Substantial toxicity has been reported, although final efficacy results have not been published. The use of PDT in the peritoneum, although conceptually appealing, is technically challenging given the large surface area that requires treatment and the underlying normal tissues.

Central Nervous System Tumors

Tumors of the central nervous system, especially malignant glioma, are associated with a high local failure rated despite treatment with standard surgery and radiation.[268,269] Intraoperative PDT has been investigated in the treatment of patients with these tumors as a means of reducing local failure after surgery. Muller and Wilson conducted two randomized multicenter trials of porfimer sodium–mediated PDT in the treatment of patients with primary and recurrent supratentorial glioma.[270-273] The authors concluded in preliminary studies that porfimer sodium–mediated PDT is safe in this setting and appeared to prolong survival in selected patients. Results of ongoing randomized trials should provide valuable information about the role of PDT in the management of central nervous system tumors.

Prostate Cancer

The treatment options for patients with early-stage prostate cancer include radical prostatectomy and radiation therapy (either external beam or seed implantation). Radical prostatectomy for disease in an early clinical stage results in 10-year survival rates of 60% to 70%.[274-276] External beam irradiation achieves similar results.[277,278] For patients with local recurrence of disease after radiation therapy, salvage options are limited. Treatments evaluated include radical prostatectomy,[279] cryosurgery,[280] and repetition of radiation therapy.[281] Unfortunately, these salvage procedures carry risk of morbidity, including rectal and urinary tract complications.[280,282,283] Safe and effective local salvage therapy for recurrent prostate cancer would be of interest.

PDT may have a role in the management of locally recurrent prostate cancer.[25,284-287] Adapting techniques from brachytherapy, preclinical studies have shown feasibility in canine models.[25,288] One study of mTHPC-mediated PDT[287] had encouraging results. Other trials with various photosensitizers are ongoing.

REFERENCES

1. Dougherty TJ, Gomer CJ, Henderson BW, et al: Photodynamic therapy [review]. J Natl Cancer Inst 1998;90:889–905.
2. Dougherty TJ: An update on photodynamic therapy applications. J Clin Laser Med Surg 2002;20:3–7.
3. Oleinick NL, Evans HH: The photobiology of photodynamic therapy: Cellular targets and mechanisms. Radiat Res 1998;150(5 suppl):S146–S156.
4. Busch TM, Hahn SM, Evans SM, Koch CJ: Depletion of tumor oxygenation during photodynamic therapy: Detection by the hypoxia marker EF3 [2-(2-nitroimidazol-1[H]-yl)-N-(3,3,3-trifluoropropyl)acetamide]. Cancer Res 2000;60:2636–2642.
5. Busch TM, Wileyto EP, Emanuele MJ, et al: Photodynamic therapy creates fluence rate-dependent gradients in the intratumoral spatial distribution of oxygen. Cancer Res 2002;62:7273–7279.
6. Henderson BW, Busch TM, Vaughan LA, et al: Photofrin photodynamic therapy can significantly deplete or preserve oxygenation in human basal cell carcinomas during treatment, depending on fluence rate. Cancer Res 2000;60:525–529.
7. Gomer CJ, Razum NJ: Acute skin response in albino mice following porphyrin photosensitization under oxic and anoxic conditions. Photochem Photobiol 1984;40:435–439.
8. Moan J, Sommer S: Oxygen dependence of the photosensitizing effect of hematoporphyrin derivative in NHIK 3025 cells. Cancer Res 1985;45:1608–1610.
9. Sitinik T, Hampton J, Henderson B: Reduction of tumour oxygenation during and after photodynamic therapy. Cancer Res 1998;77:1386–1394.
10. Hahn S, Glatstein E: The emergence of photodynamic therapy as a major modality in cancer treatment. Rev Contemp Pharmocother 1999;10:69–74.
11. Baas P, Saarnak AE, Oppelaar H, Neering H, Stewart FA: Photodynamic therapy with meta-tetrahydroxyphenylchlorin for basal cell carcinoma: A phase I/II study. Br J Dermatol 2001;145:75–78.
12. Karrer S, Szeimies RM, Hohenleutner U, Landthaler M: Role of lasers and photodynamic therapy in the treatment of cutaneous malignancy. Am J Clin Dermatol 2001;2:229–237.
13. Zeitouni NC, Shieh S, Oseroff AR: Laser and photodynamic therapy in the management of cutaneous malignancies. Clin Dermatol 2001;19:328–338.
14. Hahn SM, Fraker DL, Rubin SC, Kachur A, Yodh AG, Glatstein E: Intraperitoneal photodynamic therapy for peritoneal carcinomatosis and sarcomatosis. In Dougherty TJ (ed): Optical Methods for Tumor Treatment and Detection: Mechanisms and Techniques in Photodynamic Therapy IX. San Jose, Calif, SPIE—The International Society for Optical Engineering, 2000.
15. DeLaney TF, Sindelar WF, Tochner Z, et al: Phase I study of debulking surgery and photodynamic therapy for disseminated intraperitoneal tumors. Int J Radiat Oncol Biol Phys 1993;25:445–457.
16. Pass HI, DeLaney TF, Tochner Z, et al: Intrapleural photodynamic therapy: Results of a phase I trial. Ann Surg Oncol 1994;1:28–37.
17. Pass HI, Temeck BK, Kranda K, et al: Phase III randomized trial of surgery with or without intraoperative photodynamic therapy and postoperative immunochemotherapy for malignant pleural mesothelioma. Ann Surg Oncol 1997;4:628–633.
18. Wolfsen HC, Woodward TA, Raimondo M: Photodynamic therapy for dysplastic Barrett esophagus and early esophageal adenocarcinoma. Mayo Clin Proc 2002;77:1176–1181.
19. Wolfsen HC: Photodynamic therapy for mucosal esophageal adenocarcinoma and dysplastic Barrett's esophagus. Dig Dis 2002;20:5–17.
20. Overholt BF: A multicenter, partially blinded, randomised study of the efficacy of photodynamic therapy (PDT) using porfimer sodium (POR) for the ablation of high-grade dysplasia (HGD) in Barrett's esophagus (BE): Results of 6-month follow-up. Gastroenterology 2001;120(suppl):A-79.
21. Overholt BF, Panjehpour M: Photodynamic therapy for Barrett's esophagus. Gastrointest Endosc Clin N Am 1997;7:207–220.
22. Overholt BF, Panjehpour M, Haydek JM: Photodynamic therapy for Barrett's esophagus: Follow-up in 100 patients. Gastrointest Endosc 1999;49:1–7.
23. Hopper C: Photodynamic therapy: A clinical reality in the treatment of cancer. Lancet Oncol 2000;1:212–219.
24. Schweitzer VG, Photofrin-mediated photodynamic therapy for treatment of early stage oral cavity and laryngeal malignancies. Lasers Surg Med 2001;29:305–313.
25. Hsi RA, Kapatkin A, Strandberg J, et al: Photodynamic therapy in the canine prostate using motexafin lutetium. Clin Cancer Res 2001;7:651–660.
26. Fielding DI, Buonaccorsi GA, MacRobert AJ, et al: Fine-needle interstitial photodynamic therapy of the lung parenchyma: Photosensitizer distribution and morphologic effects of treatment. Chest 1999;115:502–510.
27. Fielding DI, Buonaccorsi G, Cowley G, et al: Interstitial laser photocoagulation and interstitial photodynamic therapy of normal lung parenchyma in the pig. Lasers Med Sci 2001;16:26–33.
28. Baas P, Murrer L, Zoetmulder FA, et al: Photodynamic therapy as adjuvant therapy in surgically treated pleural malignancies. Br J Cancer 1997;76 819–826.
29. Schouwink H, Rutgers ET, van der Sijp J, et al: Intraoperative photodynamic therapy after pleuropneumonectomy in patients with malignant pleural mesothelioma: Dose finding and toxicity results. Chest 2001;120:1167–1174.
30. Friedberg JS, Mick R, Stevenson J, et al: A phase I study of Foscan-mediated photodynamic therapy and surgery in patients with mesothelioma. Ann Thorac Surg 2003;75:952–959.
31. Gomer CJ, Luna M, Ferrario A, Wong S, Fisher AM, Rucker N: Cellular targets and molecular responses associated with photodynamic therapy. J Clin Laser Med Surg 1996;14:315–321.
32. Fisher AM, Ferrario A, Rucker N, Zhang S, Gomer CJ: Photodynamic therapy sensitivity is not altered in human tumor cells after abrogation of p53 function. Cancer Res 1999;59:331–335.
33. Ferrario A, von Tiehl KF, Rucker N, Schwarz MA, Gill PS, Gomer CJ: Antiangiogenic treatment enhances photodynamic therapy responsiveness in a mouse mammary carcinoma. Cancer Res 2000;60:4066–4069.

34. Dougherty TJ, Cooper MT, Mang TS: Cutaneous phototoxic occurrences in patients receiving Photofrin. Lasers Surg Med 1990;10:485–488.

35. Wolfsen HC, Ng CS: Cutaneous consequences of photodynamic therapy. Cutis 2002;69:140–142.

36. Radu A, Zellweger M, Grosjean P, Monnier P: Pulse oximeter as a cause of skin burn during photodynamic therapy. Endoscopy 1999;31:831–833.

37. Foote CS: Mechanisms of photooxygenation. Prog Clin Biol Res 1984;170:3–18.

38. Gomer C, Dougherty T: Determination of [3H]- and [14C] hematoporphyrin derivative distribution in malignant and normal tissue. Cancer Res 1979;39:146–151.

39. Young SW, Woodburn KW, Wright M, et al: Lutetium texaphyrin (PCI-0123): A near-infrared, water-soluble photosensitizer. Photochem Photobiol 1996;63:892–897.

40. Woodburn KW, Fan Q, Kessel D, Luo Y, Young SW: Photodynamic therapy of B16F10 murine melanoma with lutetium texaphyrin. J Invest Dermatol 1998;110:746–751.

41. Westerman P, Glanzmann T, Andrejevic S, et al: Long circulating half-life and high tumor selectivity of the photosensitizer meta-tetrahydroxyphenylchlorin conjugated to polyethylene glycol in nude mice grafted with a human colon carcinoma. Int J Cancer 1998;76:842–850.

42. Freitas I: Lipid accumulation: The common feature to photosensitizer-retaining normal and malignant tissues. J Photochem Photobiol B 1990;7:359–361.

43. Polo L, Valduga G, Jori G, Reddi E: Low-density lipoprotein receptors in the uptake of tumour photosensitizers by human and rat transformed fibroblasts. Int J Biochem Cell Biol 2002;34:10–23.

44. Hamblin MR, Newman EL: Photosensitizer targeting in photodynamic therapy. II. Conjugates of haematoporphyrin with serum lipoproteins. J Photochem Photobiol B 1994;26:147–157.

45. Korbelik M: Low density lipoprotein receptor pathway in the delivery of Photofrin: How much is it relevant for selective accumulation of the photosensitizer in tumors? J Photochem Photobiol B 1992;12:107–109.

46. Schmidt-Erfurth U, Diddens H, Birngruber R, Hasan T: Photodynamic targeting of human retinoblastoma cells using covalent low-density lipoprotein conjugates. Br J Cancer 1997;75:54–61.

47. Kurohane K, Tominaga A, Sato K, North JR, Namba Y, Oku N: Photodynamic therapy targeted to tumor-induced angiogenic vessels. Cancer Lett 2001;167:49–56.

48. Hamblin MR, Rajadhyaksha M, Momma T, Soukos NS, Hasan T: In vivo fluorescence imaging of the transport of charged chlorin e6 conjugates in a rat orthotopic prostate tumour. Br J Cancer 1999;81:261–268.

49. Bohmer RM, Morstyn G: Uptake of hematoporphyrin derivative by normal and malignant cells: Effect of serum, pH, temperature, and cell size. Cancer Res 1985;45:5328–5334.

50. Ris HB, Altermatt HJ, Inderbitzi R, et al: Photodynamic therapy with chlorins for diffuse malignant mesothelioma: Initial clinical results. Br J Cancer 1991;64:1116–1120.

51. Peng Q, Soler AM, Warloe T, Nesland JM, Giercksky KE: Selective distribution of porphyrins in skin thick basal cell carcinoma after topical application of methyl 5-aminolevulinate. J Photochem Photobiol B 2001;62:140–145.

52. Pahernik SA, Botzlar A, Hillemanns P, et al: Pharmacokinetics and selectivity of aminolevulinic acid-induced porphyrin synthesis in patients with cervical intra-epithelial neoplasia. Int J Cancer 1998;78:310–314.

53. Andrejevic Blant S, Grosjean P, Ballini JP, et al: Localization of tetra(m-hydroxyphenyl)chlorin (Foscan) in human healthy tissues and squamous cell carcinomas of the upper aero-digestive tract, the esophagus and the bronchi: A fluorescence microscopy study. J Photochem Photobiol B 2001;61:1–9.

54. Pandey RK, Dougherty TJ: Syntheses and photosensitizing activity of porphyrins joined with ester linkages. Cancer Res 1989;49:2042–2047.

55. Marcus SL, Sobel RS, Golub AL, Carroll RL, Lundahl S, Shulman DG: Photodynamic therapy (PDT) and photodiagnosis (PD) using endogenous photosensitization induced by 5-aminolevulinic acid (ALA): Current clinical and development status. J Clin Laser Med Surg 1996;14:59–66.

56. Ackroyd R, Brown NJ, Davis MF, Stephenson TJ, Stoddard CJ, Reed MW: Aminolevulinic acid-induced photodynamic therapy: Safe and effective ablation of dysplasia in Barrett's esophagus. Dis Esophagus 2000;13:18–22.

57. Kennedy JC, Marcus SL, Pottier RH: Photodynamic therapy (PDT) and photodiagnosis (PD) using endogenous photosensitization induced by 5-aminolevulinic acid (ALA): Mechanisms and clinical results. J Clin Laser Med Surg 1996;14:289–304.

58. Ackroyd R, Brown N, Vernon D, et al: 5-Aminolevulinic acid photosensitization of dysplastic Barrett's esophagus: A pharmacokinetic study. Photochem Photobiol 1999;70:656–662.

59. Ma L, Moan J, Berg K: Evaluation of a new photosensitizer, meso-tetra-hydroxyphenyl-chlorin, for use in photodynamic therapy: A comparison of its photobiological properties with those of two other photosensitizers. Int J Cancer 1994;57:883–888.

60. van Geel IP, Oppelaar H, Oussoren YG, van der Valk MA, Stewart FA: Photosensitizing efficacy of MTHPC-PDT compared to photofrin-PDT in the RIF1 mouse tumour and normal skin. Int J Cancer 1995;60:388–394.

61. Sessler JL, Miller RA: Texaphyrins: New drugs with diverse clinical applications in radiation and photodynamic therapy. Biochem Pharmacol 2000;59:733–739.

62. Ivy SP, Blatner G, Cheson BD: Clinical trials referral resource: Clinical trials with gadolinium-texaphyrin and lutetium-texaphyrin. Oncology (Huntingt) 1999;13:671, 674–676.

63. Mang TS, Allison R, Hewson G, Snider W, Moskowitz R: A phase II/III clinical study of tin ethyl etiopurpurin (Purlytin)-induced photodynamic therapy for the treatment of recurrent cutaneous metastatic breast cancer. Cancer J Sci Am 1998;4:378–384.

64. Kaplan MJ, Somers RG, Greenberg RH, Ackler J: Photodynamic therapy in the management of metastatic cutaneous adenocarcinomas: Case reports from phase 1/2 studies using tin ethyl etiopurpurin (SnET2). J Surg Oncol 1998;67:121–125.

65. Taber SW: Photodynamic therapy using mono-L-aspartyl chlorin e6 (Npe6) for the treatment of cutaneous disease: A Phase I clinical study. Clin Cancer Res 1998;4:2741–2746.

66. Chen J: New technology for deep light distribution in tissue for phototherapy. Cancer J 2002;8:154–163.

67. Bellnier DA, Henderson BW, Pandey RK, Potter WR, Dougherty TJ: Murine pharmacokinetics and antitumor efficacy of the photodynamic sensitizer 2-[1-hexyloxyethyl]-2-devinyl pyropheophorbide-a. J Photochem Photobiol B Biol 1993;20:55–61.

68. Bellnier DA: Population pharmacokinetics of the photodynamic therapy agent 2-[1-hexyloxyethyl]-2-devinyl pyropheophorbide-a in cancer patient. Cancer Res 2003;63:1806–1813.

69. Whitacre CM, Feyes DK, Satoh T, et al: Photodynamic therapy with the phthalocyanine photosensitizer Pc 4 of SW480 human colon cancer xenografts in athymic mice. Clin Cancer Res 2000;6:2021–2027.

70. Whitacre CM, Satoh TH, Xue L, Gordon NH, Oleinick NL: Photodynamic therapy of human breast cancer xenografts lacking caspase-3. Cancer Lett 2002;179:43–49.

71. Trivedi NS, Wang HW, Nieminen AL, Oleinick NL, Izatt JA: Quantitative analysis of Pc 4 localization in mouse lymphoma (LY-R) cells via double-label confocal fluorescence microscopy. Photochem Photobiol 2000;71:634–639.

72. Colussi VC, Feyes DK, Mulvihill JW, et al: Phthalocyanine 4 (Pc 4) photodynamic therapy of human OVCAR-3 tumor xenografts. Photochem Photobiol 1999;69:236–241.

73. Chiu S, Evans HH, Lam M, Nieminen A, Oleinick NL: Phthalocyanine 4 photodynamic therapy-induced apoptosis of mouse L5178Y-R cells results from a delayed but extensive release of cytochrome c from mitochondria. Cancer Lett 2001;165:51–58.

74. Koderhold G, Jindra R, Koren H, Alth G, Schenk G: Experiences of photodynamic therapy in dermatology. J Photochem Photobiol B 1996;36:221–223.

75. Star WM: Light dosimetry in vivo. Phys Med Biol 1997;42:763–787.

76. Marijnissen JP, Baas P, Beek JF, van Moll JH, van Zandwijk N, Star WM: Pilot study on light dosimetry for endobronchial photodynamic therapy. Photochem Photobiol 1993;58:92–99.

77. Marijnissen JP, Star WM, in 't Zandt HJ, D'Hallewin MA, Baert L: In situ light dosimetry during whole bladder wall photodynamic therapy: Clinical results and experimental verification. Phys Med Biol 1993;38:567–582.

78. Vulcan TG, Zhu TC, Rodriguez CE, et al: Comparison between isotropic and nonisotropic dosimetry systems during intraperitoneal photodynamic therapy. Lasers Surg Med 2000;26:292–301.

79. Pass HI: Photodynamic therapy in oncology: Mechanisms and clinical use. J Natl Cancer Inst 1993;85:443–456.

80. Ripley P: The physics of diode lasers. Lasers Med Sci 1996:8259–8267.

81. Hammer-Wilson MJ, Sun CH, Ghahramanlou M, Berns MW: In vitro and in vivo comparison of argon-pumped and diode lasers for photodynamic therapy using second-generation photosensitizers. Lasers Surg Med 1998;23:274–280.

82. Sindelar WF, DeLaney TF, Tochner Z, et al: Technique of photodynamic therapy for disseminated intraperitoneal malignant neoplasms: Phase I study. Arch Surg 1991;126:318–324.

83. Madsen SJ, Sun CH, Tromberg BJ, Hirschberg H: Development of a novel indwelling balloon applicator for optimizing light delivery in photodynamic therapy. Lasers Surg Med 2001;29:406–412.

84. van Veen P, Schouwink JH, Star WM, et al: Wedge-shaped applicator for additional light delivery and dosimetry in the diaphragmal sinus during photodynamic therapy for malignant pleural mesothelioma. Phys Med Biol 2001;46:1873–1883.

85. Freidberg JS, James M, Rosemarie M, et al: Multimodality treatment including pleural photodynamic therapy (PDT) for non-small cell lung cancer (NSCLC) patients with pleural carcinomatosis. In: Program/Proceedings of the 2001 Meeting of the American Society of Clinical Oncology, vol 20, abstract 1303. Alexandria, Va, ASCO, 2001, p 327a.

86. Mitchell J, McPherson S, DeGraff W, et al: Oxygen dependence of hematoporphyrin derivative-induced photoinactivation of Chinese hamster cells. Cancer Res 1985;45:2008–2011.

87. Chapman J, Stobbe CC, Arnfield MR, Santus R, Lee J, McPhee MS: Oxygen dependency of tumor cell killing in vitro by light-activated Photofrin II. Radiat Res 1991;126:73–79.

88. Henderson BW, Fingar VH: Relationship of tumor hypoxia and response to photodynamic treatment in an experimental mouse tumor. Cancer Res 1987;47:3110–3114.

89. Fingar VH, Wieman TJ, Park YJ, Henderson BW: Implications of a pre-existing tumor hypoxic fraction on photodynamic therapy. J Surg Res 1992;53:524–528.

90. Hockel M, Knoop C, Schlenger K, et al: Intratumoral pO2 predicts survival in advanced cancer of the uterine cervix. Radiother Oncol 1993;26:45–50.

91. Brizel DM, Dodge RK, Clough RW, Dewhirst MW: Oxygenation of head and neck cancer: Changes during radiotherapy and impact on treatment outcome. Radiother Oncol 1999;53:113–117.

92. Rofstad EK, Sundfor K, Lyng H, Trope CG: Hypoxia-induced treatment failure in advanced squamous cell carcinoma of the uterine cervix is primarily due to hypoxia-induced radiation resistance rather than hypoxia-induced metastasis. Br J Cancer 2000;83:354–359.

93. Vanselow B, Eble MJ, Rudat V, Wollensack P, Conradt C, Dietz A: Oxygenation of advanced head and neck cancer: Prognostic marker for the response to primary radiochemotherapy. Otolaryngol Head Neck Surg 2000;122:856–862.

94. Knocke TH, Weitmann HD, Feldmann HJ, Selzer E, Potter R: Intratumoral pO2-measurements as predictive assay in the treatment of carcinoma of the uterine cervix. Radiother Oncol 1999;53:99–104.

95. Brizel DM, Sibley GS, Prosnitz LR, Scher RL, Dewhirst MW: Tumor hypoxia adversely affects the prognosis of carcinoma of the head and neck. Int J Radiat Oncol Biol Phys 1997;38:285–289.

96. Tromberg BJ, Orenstein A, Kimel S, et al: In vivo tumor oxygen tension measurements for the evaluation of the efficiency of photodynamic therapy. Photochem Photobiol 1990;52:375–385.

97. Foster TH, Primavera MC, Marder VJ, Hilf R, Sporn LA: Photo-sensitized release of von Willebrand factor from cultured human endothelial cells. Cancer Res 1991;51:3261–3266.

98. Veenhuizen RB, Stewart FA: The importance of fluence rate in

99. van Geel IP, Oppelaar H, Marijnissen JP, Stewart FA: Influence of fractionation and fluence rate in photodynamic therapy with Photofrin or mTHPC. Radiat Res 1996;145:602–609.

100. Sitnik TM, Henderson BW: The effect of fluence rate on tumor and normal tissue responses to photodynamic therapy. Photochem Photobiol 1998;67:462–466.

101. Evans SM, Hahn SM, Magarelli DP, Koch CJ: Hypoxic heterogeneity in human tumors: EF5 binding, vasculature, necrosis, and proliferation. Am J Clin Oncol 2001;24:467–472.

102. Evans S, Hahn S, Pook DR, et al: Detection of hypoxia in human squamous cell carcinoma by EF5 binding. Cancer Res 2000;60:2018–2024.

103. Evans SM, Hahn SM, Magarelli DP, et al: Hypoxia in human intraperitoneal and extremity sarcomas. Int J Radiat Oncol Biol Phys 2001;49:587–596.

104. Hockel M, Vorndran B, Schlenger K, Baussmann E, Knapstein PG: Tumor oxygenation: A new predictive parameter in locally advanced cancer of the uterine cervix. Gynecol Oncol 1993;51:141–149.

105. Brizel DM, Rosner GL, Harrelson J, Prosnitz LR, Dewhirst MW: Pretreatment oxygenation profiles of human soft tissue sarcomas. Int J Radiat Oncol Biol Phys 1994;30:635–642.

106. Hockel M, Schlenger K, Aral B, Mitze M, Schaffer U, Vaupel P: Association between tumor hypoxia and malignant progression in advanced cancer of the uterine cervix. Cancer Res 1996;56:4509–4515.

107. Fyles A, Milosevic M, Wong R, et al: Oxygenation predicts radiation response and survival in patients with cervix cancer. Radiother Oncol 1998;48:149–156.

108. Movsas B, Chapman JD, Horwitz EM, et al: Hypoxic regions exist in human prostate carcinoma. Urology 1999;53:11–18.

109. Tomaselli F, Maier A, Sankin O, et al: Acute effects of combined photodynamic therapy and hyperbaric oxygenation in lung cancer: A clinical pilot study. Lasers Surg Med 2001;28:399–403.

110. Maier A, Anegg U, Fell B, et al: Effect of photodynamic therapy in a multimodal approach for advanced carcinoma of the gastroesophageal junction. Lasers Surg Med 2000;26:461–466.

111. Maier A, Anegg U, Fell B, et al: Hyperbaric oxygen and photodynamic therapy in the treatment of advanced carcinoma of the cardia and the esophagus. Lasers Surg Med 2000;26:308–315.

112. Maier A, Anegg U, Tomaselli F, et al: Does hyperbaric oxygen enhance the effect of photodynamic therapy in patients with advanced esophageal carcinoma? A clinical pilot study. Endoscopy 2000;32:42–48.

113. Henderson BW, Waldow SM, Mang TS, Potter WR, Malone PB, Dougherty TJ: Tumor destruction and kinetics of tumor cell death in two experimental mouse tumors following photodynamic therapy. Cancer Res 1985;45:572–576.

114. He J, Larkin HE, Li YS, et al: The synthesis, photophysical and photobiological properties and in vitro structure-activity relationships of a set of silicon phthalocyanine PDT photosensitizers. Photochem Photobiol 1997;65:581–586.

115. Chan WS, Brasseur N, La Madeleine C, van Lier JE: Evidence for different mechanisms of EMT-6 tumor necrosis by photodynamic therapy with disulfonated aluminum phthalocyanine or photofrin: Tumor cell survival and blood flow. Anticancer Res 1996;16:1887–1892.

116. Cincotta L, Foley JW, MacEachern T, Lampros E, Cincotta AH: Novel photodynamic effects of a benzophenothiazine on two different murine sarcomas. Cancer Res 1994;54:1249–1258.

117. Buettner GR, Kelley EE, Burns CP: Membrane lipid free radicals produced from L1210 murine leukemia cells by photofrin photosensitization: An electron paramagnetic resonance spin trapping study. Cancer Res 1993;53:3670–3673.

118. Gibson SL, Murant RS, Hilf R: Photosensitizing effects of hematoporphyrin derivative and photofrin II on the plasma membrane enzymes 5′-nucleotidase, Na+K+-ATPase, and Mg2+-ATPase in R3230AC mammary adenocarcinomas. Cancer Res 1988;48:3360–3366.

119. Henderson BW, Miller AC: Effects of scavengers of reactive oxygen and radical species on cell survival following photodynamic treatment in vitro: Comparison to ionizing radiation. Radiat Res 1986;108:196–205.

120. Kelley EE, Buettner GR, Burns CP: Production of lipid-derived free radicals in L1210 murine leukemia cells is an early oxidative event in the photodynamic action of Photofrin. Photochem Photobiol 1997;65:576-580.

121. Wang HP, Qian SY, Schafer FQ, Domann FE, Oberley LW, Buettner GR: Phospholipid hydroperoxide glutathione peroxidase protects against singlet oxygen-induced cell damage of photodynamic therapy. Free Radical Biol Med 2001;30:825-835.

122. Thomas JP, Girotti AW: Role of lipid peroxidation in hematoporphyrin derivative-sensitized photokilling of tumor cells: Protective effects of glutathione peroxidase. Cancer Res 1989;49:1682-1686.

123. Niedre M, Patterson MS, Wilson BC: Direct near-infrared luminescence detection of singlet oxygen generated by photodynamic therapy in cells in vitro and tissues in vivo. Photochem Photobiol 2002;75:382-391.

124. Teiten MH, Marchal S, D'Hallewin MA, Guillemin F, Bezdetnaya L: Primary photodamage sites and mitochondrial events after Foscan photosensitization of MCF-7 human breast cancer cells. Photochem Photobiol 2003;78:9-14.

125. Peng Q, Moan J, Nesland JM: Correlation of subcellular and intratumoral photosensitizer localization with ultrastructural features after photodynamic therapy. Ultrastruct Pathol 1996;20:109-129.

126. Teiten MH, Bezdetnaya L, Morliere P, Santus R, Guillemin F: Endoplasmic reticulum and Golgi apparatus are the preferential sites of Foscan localisation in cultured tumour cells. Br J Cancer 2003;88:146-152.

127. MacDonald IJ, Morgan J, Bellnier DA, et al: Subcellular localization patterns and their relationship to photodynamic activity of pyropheophorbide-a derivatives. Photochem Photobiol 1999;70:789-797.

128. Moan J, Berg K, Anholt H, Madslien K: Sulfonated aluminium phthalocyanines as sensitizers for photochemotherapy: Effects of small light doses on localization, dye fluorescence and photosensitivity in V79 cells. Int J Cancer 1994;58:865-870.

129. Ball DJ, Mayhew S, Wood SR, Griffiths J, Vernon DI, Brown SB: A comparative study of the cellular uptake and photodynamic efficacy of three novel zinc phthalocyanines of differing charge. Photochem Photobiol 1999;69:390-396.

130. MacDonald IJ, Dougherty TJ: Basic principles of photodynamic therapy. J Porphyrins Phthalocyanines 2001;5:105-129.

131. Sitnik TM, Henderson BW: Effects of fluence rate on cytotoxicity during photodynamic therapy. In SPIE Proceedings, 1997. San Jose, Calif, SPIE—The International Society for Optical Engineering, 1997, pp 95-102.

132. Coutier S, Bezdetnaya LN, Foster TH, Parache RM, Guillemin F: Effect of irradiation fluence rate on the efficacy of photodynamic therapy and tumor oxygenation in meta-tetra (hydroxyphenyl) chlorin (mTHPC)-sensitized HT29 xenografts in nude mice. Radiat Res 2002;158:339-345.

133. Iinuma S, Schomacker KT, Wagnieres G, et al: In vivo fluence rate and fractionation effects on tumor response and photobleaching: Photodynamic therapy with two photosensitizers in an orthotopic rat tumor model. Cancer Res 1999;59:6164-6170.

134. Foster TH, Hartley DF, Nichols MG, Hilf R: Fluence rate effects in photodynamic therapy of multicell tumor spheroids. Cancer Res 1993;53:1249-1254.

135. Chang CJ, Sun CH, Liaw LH, Berns MW, Nelson JS: In vitro and in vivo photosensitizing capabilities of 5-ALA versus photofrin in vascular endothelial cells. Lasers Surg Med 1999;24:178-186.

136. Fingar VH, Henderson BW: Drug and light dose dependence of photodynamic therapy: A study of tumor and normal tissue response. Photochem Photobiol 1987;46:837-841.

137. van Geel IP, Oppelaar H, Oussoren YG, Stewart FA: Changes in perfusion of mouse tumours after photodynamic therapy. Int J Cancer 1994;56:224-228.

138. van Geel IP, Oppelaar H, Oussoren YG, Schuitmaker JJ, Stewart FA: Mechanisms for optimising photodynamic therapy: Second-generation photosensitisers in combination with mitomycin C. Br J Cancer 1995;72:344-350.

139. Saito K, Mikuniya N, Aizawa K: Effects of photodynamic therapy using mono-L-aspartyl chlorin e6 on vessels and its contribution to the antitumor effect. Jpn J Cancer Res 2000;91:560-565.

140. Fingar VH, Kik PK, Haydon PS, et al: Analysis of acute vascular damage after photodynamic therapy using benzoporphyrin derivative (BPD). Br J Cancer 1999;79:1702-1708.

141. Nelson JS, Liaw LH, Orenstein A, Roberts WG, Berns MW: Mechanism of tumor destruction following photodynamic therapy with hematoporphyrin derivative, chlorin, and phthalocyanine. J Natl Cancer Inst 1988;80:1599-1605.

142. Fingar VH, Wieman TJ, Wiehle SA, Cerrito PB: The role of microvascular damage in photodynamic therapy: The effect of treatment on vessel constriction, permeability, and leukocyte adhesion. Cancer Res 1992;52:4914-4921.

143. Fingar VH, Wieman TJ, Karavolos PS, Doak KW, Ouellet R, van Lier JE: The effects of photodynamic therapy using differently substituted zinc phthalocyanines on vessel constriction, vessel leakage and tumor response. Photochem Photobiol 1993;58:251-258.

144. McMahon KS, Wieman TJ, Moore PH, Fingar VH: Effects of photodynamic therapy using mono-L-aspartyl chlorin e6 on vessel constriction, vessel leakage, and tumor response. Cancer Res 1994;54:5374-5379.

145. Korbelik M, Sun J, Zeng H: Ischaemia-reperfusion injury in photodynamic therapy–treated mouse tumours. Br J Cancer 2003;88:760-766.

146. Henderson BW, Donovan JM: Release of prostaglandin E2 from cells by photodynamic treatment in vitro. Cancer Res 1989;49:6896-6900.

147. Henderson BW, Owczarczak B, Sweeney J, Gessner T: Effects of photodynamic treatment of platelets or endothelial cells in vitro on platelet aggregation. Photochem Photobiol 1992;56:513-521.

148. Fingar VH, Wieman TJ, Doak KW: Mechanistic studies of PDT-induced vascular damage: Evidence that eicosanoids mediate this process. Int J Radiat Biol 1991;60:303-309.

149. Fingar VH, Siegel KA, Wieman TJ, Doak KW: The effects of thromboxane inhibitors on the microvascular and tumor response to photodynamic therapy. Photochem Photobiol 1993;58:393-399.

150. Ferrario A, Von Tiehl K, Wong S, Luna M, Gomer CJ: Cyclooxygenase-2 inhibitor treatment enhances photodynamic therapy-mediated tumor response. Cancer Res 2002;62:3956-3961.

151. Holz FG, Jorzik J, Schutt F, Flach U, Unnebrink K: Agreement among ophthalmologists in evaluating fluorescein angiograms in patients with neovascular age-related macular degeneration for photodynamic therapy eligibility (FLAP-study). Ophthalmology 2003;110:400-405.

152. Verteporfin in Photodynamic Therapy Study G: Verteporfin therapy of subfoveal choroidal neovascularization in age-related macular degeneration: Two-year results of a randomized clinical trial including lesions with occult with no classic choroidal neovascularization—verteporfin in photodynamic therapy report 2. Am J Ophthalmol 2001;131:541-560.

153. Korbelik M, Krosl G, Krosl J, Dougherty GJ: The role of host lymphoid populations in the response of mouse EMT6 tumor to photodynamic therapy. Cancer Res 1996;56:5647-5652.

154. Krosl G, Korbelik M, Dougherty GJ: Induction of immune cell infiltration into murine SCCVII tumour by photofrin-based photodynamic therapy. Br J Cancer 1995;71:549-555.

155. Gollnick SO, Liu X, Owczarczak B, Musser DA, Henderson BW: Altered expression of interleukin 6 and interleukin 10 as a result of photodynamic therapy in vivo. Cancer Res 1997;57:3904-3909.

156. Korbelik M, Cecic I: Contribution of myeloid and lymphoid host cells to the curative outcome of mouse sarcoma treatment by photodynamic therapy. Cancer Lett 1999;137:91-98.

157. Korbelik M, Naraparaju VR, Yamamoto N: Macrophage-directed immunotherapy as adjuvant to photodynamic therapy of cancer. Br J Cancer 1997;75:202-207.

158. Lim HW, Hagan M, Gigli I: Phototoxicity induced by hematoporphyrin derivative in C5-deficient, mast cell-deficient and leukopenic mice. Photochem Photobiol 1986;44:175-180.

159. de Vree WJ, Essers MC, Koster JF, Sluiter W: Role of interleukin 1 and granulocyte colony-stimulating factor in photofrin-based photodynamic therapy of rat rhabdomyosarcoma tumors. Cancer Res 1997;57:2555-2558.

160. de Vree WJ, Essers MC, de Bruijn HS, Star WM, Koster JF, Sluiter W: Evidence for an important role of neutrophils in the efficacy of photodynamic therapy in vivo. Cancer Res 1996;56:2908–2911.

161. Krosl G, Korbelik M, Krosl J, Dougherty GJ: Potentiation of photodynamic therapy–elicited antitumor response by localized treatment with granulocyte-macrophage colony-stimulating factor. Cancer Res 1996;56:3281–3286.

162. Chen WR, Singhal AK, Liu H, Nordquist RE: Antitumor immunity induced by laser immunotherapy and its adoptive transfer. Cancer Res 2001;61:459–461.

163. Gollnick SO, Vaughan L, Henderson BW: Generation of effective antitumor vaccines using photodynamic therapy. Cancer Res 2002;62:1604–1608.

164. Korbelik M, Dougherty GJ: Photodynamic therapy-mediated immune response against subcutaneous mouse tumors. Cancer Res 1999;59:1941–1946.

165. Elmets CA, Bowen KD: Immunological suppression in mice treated with hematoporphyrin derivative photoradiation. Cancer Res 1986;46:1608–1611.

166. Lynch DH, Haddad S, King VJ, Ott MJ, Straight RC, Jolles CJ: Systemic immunosuppression induced by photodynamic therapy (PDT) is adoptively transferred by macrophages. Photochem Photobiol 1989;49:453–458.

167. Obochi MO, Ratkay LG, Levy JG: Prolonged skin allograft survival after photodynamic therapy associated with modification of donor skin antigenicity. Transplantation 1997;63:810–817.

168. Simkin GO, Tao JS, Levy JG, Hunt DW: IL-6 contributes to the inhibition of contact hypersensitivity in mice treated with photodynamic therapy. J Immunol 2000;164:2457–2462.

169. Gollnick SO, Musser DA, Oseroff AR, Vaughan L, Owczarczak B, Henderson BW: IL-10 does not play a role in cutaneous Photofrin photodynamic therapy-induced suppression of the contact hypersensitivity response. Photochem Photobiol 2001;74:811–816.

170. Reddan JC, Anderson CY, Xu H, et al: Immunosuppressive effects of silicon phthalocyanine photodynamic therapy. Photochem Photobiol 1999;70:72–77.

171. Nseyo UO, Whalen RK, Duncan MR, Berman B, Lundahl SL: Urinary cytokines following photodynamic therapy for bladder cancer: A preliminary report. Urology 1990;36:167–171.

172. Yom SS, Busch TM, Friedberg JS, et al: Elevated serum cytokine levels in mesothelioma patients who have undergone pleurectomy or extrapleural pneumonectomy and adjuvant intraoperative photodynamic therapy. Photochem Photobiol 2003;78:75–81.

173. Abdel-Hady ES, Martin-Hirsch P, Duggan-Keen M, et al: Immunological and viral factors associated with the response of vulval intraepithelial neoplasia to photodynamic therapy. Cancer Res 2001;61:192–196.

174. Leist M, Nicotera P: The shape of cell death. Biochem Biophys Res Commun 1997;236:1–9.

175. Kessel D, Luo Y, Deng Y, Chang CK: The role of subcellular localization in initiation of apoptosis by photodynamic therapy. Photochem Photobiol 1997;65:422–426.

176. Luo Y, Chang CK, Kessel D: Rapid initiation of apoptosis by photodynamic therapy. Photochem Photobiol 1996;63:528–534.

177. Kessel D, Luo Y: Mitochondrial photodamage and PDT-induced apoptosis. J Photochem Photobiol B Biol 1998;42:89–95.

178. Woodburn KW, Fan Q, Miles DR, Kessel D, Luo Y, Young SW: Localization and efficacy analysis of the phototherapeutic lutetium texaphyrin (PCI-0123) in the murine EMT6 sarcoma model. Photochem Photobiol 1997;65:410–415.

179. Oleinick NL, Morris RL, Belichenko I: The role of apoptosis in response to photodynamic therapy: What, where, why, and how. Photochem Photobiol Sci 2002;1:1–21.

180. Wyld L, Reed MW, Brown NJ: Differential cell death response to photodynamic therapy is dependent on dose and cell type. Br J Cancer 2001;84:1384–1386.

181. Zhang J, Cao EH, Li JF, Zhang TC, Ma WJ: Photodynamic effects of hypocrellin A on three human malignant cell lines by inducing apoptotic cell death. J Photochem Photobiol B Biol 1998;43:106–111.

182. Moor AC: Signaling pathways in cell death and survival after photodynamic therapy. J Photochem Photobiol B Biol 2000;57:1–13.

183. Verma A, Facchina SL, Hirsch DJ, et al: Photodynamic tumor therapy: Mitochondrial benzodiazepine receptors as a therapeutic target. Mol Med 1998;4:40–45.

184. Dougherty TJ, Sumlin AB, Greco WR, Weishaupt KR, Vaughan LA, Pandey RK: The role of the peripheral benzodiazepine receptor in photodynamic activity of certain pyropheophorbide ether photosensitizers: Albumin site II as a surrogate marker for activity. Photochem Photobiol 2002;76:91–97.

185. Morris RL, Varnes ME, Kenney ME, et al: The peripheral benzodiazepine receptor in photodynamic therapy with the phthalocyanine photosensitizer Pc 4. Photochem Photobiol 2002;75:652–661.

186. Kessel D, Antolovich M, Smith KM: The role of the peripheral benzodiazepine receptor in the apoptotic response to photodynamic therapy. Photochem Photobiol 2001;74:346–349.

187. Granville DJ, Hunt DWC: Porphyrin-mediated photosensitization: Taking the apoptosis fast lane. Curr Opin Drug Discov Dev 2000;3:232–243.

188. Granville DJ, Jiang H, An MT, Levy JG, McManus BM, Hunt DW: Overexpression of Bcl-X(L) prevents caspase-3-mediated activation of DNA fragmentation factor (DFF) produced by treatment with the photochemotherapeutic agent BPD-MA. FEBS Letters 1998;422:151–154.

189. He J, Agarwal ML, Larkin HE, et al: The induction of partial resistance to photodynamic therapy by the protooncogene BCL-2. Photochem Photobiol 1996;64:845–852.

190. Granville DJ, Jiang H, An MT, Levy JG, McManus BM, Hunt DW: Bcl-2 overexpression blocks caspase activation and downstream apoptotic events instigated by photodynamic therapy. Br J Cancer 1999;79:95–100.

191. Kim HR, Luo Y, Li G, Kessel D: Enhanced apoptotic response to photodynamic therapy after bcl-2 transfection. Cancer Res 1999;59:3429–3432.

192. Srivastava M, Ahmad N, Gupta S, Mukhtar H: Involvement of Bcl-2 and Bax in photodynamic therapy-mediated apoptosis: Antisense Bcl-2 oligonucleotide sensitizes RIF 1 cells to photodynamic therapy apoptosis. J Biol Chem 2001;276:15481–15488.

193. Usuda J, Chiu SM, Murphy ES, Lam M, Nieminen AL, Oleinick NL: Domain-dependent photodamage to Bcl-2: A membrane anchorage region is needed to form the target of phthalocyanine photosensitization. J Biol Chem 2003;278:2021–2029.

194. Kessel D, Castelli M: Evidence that bcl-2 is the target of three photosensitizers that induce a rapid apoptotic response. Photochem Photobiol 2001;74:318–322.

195. Fisher AM, Rucker N, Wong S, Gomer CJ: Differential photosensitivity in wild-type and mutant p53 human colon carcinoma cell lines. J Photochem Photobiol B 1998;42:104–107.

196. Fisher AM, Danenberg K, Banerjee D, Bertino JR, Danenberg P, Gomer CJ: Increased photosensitivity in HL60 cells expressing wild-type p53. Photochem Photobiol 1997;66:265–270.

197. Tong Z, Singh G, Rainbow AJ: The role of the p53 tumor suppressor in the response of human cells to Photofrin-mediated photodynamic therapy. Photochem Photobiol 2000;71:201–210.

198. Lilge L, Portnoy M, Wilson BC: Apoptosis induced in vivo by photodynamic therapy in normal brain and intracranial tumour tissue. Br J Cancer 2000;83:1110–1117.

199. Engbrecht BW, Menon C, Kachur AV, Hahn SM, Fraker DL: Photofrin-mediated photodynamic therapy induces vascular occlusion and apoptosis in a human sarcoma xenograft model. Cancer Res 1999;59:4334–4342.

200. Zaidi SI, Oleinick NL, Zaim MT, Mukhtar H: Apoptosis during photodynamic therapy-induced ablation of RIF-1 tumors in C3H mice: Electron microscopic, histopathologic and biochemical evidence. Photochem Photobiol 1993;58:771–776.

201. Nakaseko H, Kobayashi M, Akita Y, Tamada Y, Matsumoto Y: Histological changes and involvement of apoptosis after photodynamic therapy for actinic keratoses. Br J Dermatol 2003;148:122–127.

202. Lai J, Tao Z, Xiao J, et al: Effect of photodynamic therapy (PDT) on the expression of pro-apoptotic protein Bak in nasopharyngeal carcinoma (NPC). Lasers Surg Med 2001;29:27–32.

203. Kawaguchi T, Yamamoto S, Naka N, et al: Immunohistochemical analysis of Bcl-2 protein in early squamous cell carcinoma of the bronchus treated with photodynamic therapy. Br J Cancer 2000;82:418–423.

204. McGarrity TJ, Peiffer LP, Granville DJ, et al: Apoptosis associated with esophageal adenocarcinoma: Influence of photodynamic therapy. Cancer Lett 2001;163:33–41.

205. Koukourakis MI, Corti L, Skarlatos J, et al: Clinical and experimental evidence of Bcl-2 involvement in the response to photodynamic therapy. Anticancer Res 2001;21:663–668.

206. Herskovic A, Martz K, al-Sarraf M, et al: Combined chemotherapy and radiotherapy compared with radiotherapy alone in patients with cancer of the esophagus. N Engl J Med 1992;326:1593–1598.

207. Cooper JS, Guo MD, Herskovic A, et al: Chemoradiotherapy of locally advanced esophageal cancer: Long-term follow-up of a prospective randomized trial (RTOG 85-01). Radiation Therapy Oncology Group. JAMA 1999;281:1623–1627.

208. Boyce HW Jr: Palliation of dysphagia of esophageal cancer by endoscopic lumen restoration techniques. Cancer Control 1999;6:73–83.

209. Gaspar LE, Nag S, Herskovic A, Mantravadi R, Speiser B: American Brachytherapy Society (ABS) consensus guidelines for brachytherapy of esophageal cancer. Clinical Research Committee, American Brachytherapy Society. Int J Radiat Oncol Biol Phys 1997;38:127–132.

210. Sur RK, Donde B, Levin VC, Mannell A: Fractionated high dose rate intraluminal brachytherapy in palliation of advanced esophageal cancer. Int J Radiat Oncol Biol Phys 1998;40:447–453.

211. Christie NA, Buenaventura PO, Fernando HC, et al: Results of expandable metal stents for malignant esophageal obstruction in 100 patients: Short-term and long-term follow-up. Ann Thorac Surg 2001;71:1797–1801.

212. Knyrim K, Wagner HJ, Bethge N, Keymling M, Vakil N: A controlled trial of an expansile metal stent for palliation of esophageal obstruction due to inoperable cancer. N Engl J Med 1993;329:1302–1307.

213. Payne-James JJ, Spiller RC, Misiewicz JJ, Silk DB: Use of ethanol-induced tumor necrosis to palliate dysphagia in patients with esophagogastric cancer. Gastrointest Endosc 1990;36:43–46.

214. Narayan S, Sivak MV Jr: Palliation of esophageal carcinoma: Laser and photodynamic therapy. Chest Surg Clin N Am 1994;4:347–367.

215. Lightdale CJ, Zimbalist E, Winawer SJ: Outpatient management of esophageal cancer with endoscopic Nd:YAG laser. Am J Gastroenterol 1987;82:46–50.

216. Lightdale CJ, Heier SK, Marcon NE, et al: Photodynamic therapy with porfimer sodium versus thermal ablation therapy with Nd:YAG laser for palliation of esophageal cancer: A multicenter randomized trial. Gastrointest Endosc 1995;42:507–512.

217. Luketich JD, Christie NA, Buenaventura PO, Weigel TL, Keenan RJ, Nguyen NT: Endoscopic photodynamic therapy for obstructing esophageal cancer: 77 cases over a 2-year period. Surg Endosc 2000;14:653–657.

218. Sanfilippo NJ, Hsi A, DeNittis AS, et al: Toxicity of photodynamic therapy after combined external beam radiotherapy and intraluminal brachytherapy for carcinoma of the upper aerodigestive tract. Lasers Surg Med 2001;28:278–281.

219. Scheider DM, Siemens M, Cirocco M, et al: Photodynamic therapy for the treatment of tumor ingrowth in expandable esophageal stents. Endoscopy 1997;29:271–274.

220. Maier A, Tomaselli F, Gebhard F, Rehak P, Smolle J, Smolle-Juttner FM: Palliation of advanced esophageal carcinoma by photodynamic therapy and irradiation. Ann Thorac Surg 2000;69:1006–1009.

221. Overholt BF, Panjehpour M, Ayres M: Photodynamic therapy for Barrett's esophagus: Cardiac effects. Lasers Surg Med 1997;21:317–320.

222. Lam S: Photodynamic therapy of lung cancer. Semin Oncol 1994;21(6 suppl 15):15–19.

223. LoCicero J 3rd, Metzdorff M, Almgren C: Photodynamic therapy in the palliation of late stage obstructing non-small cell lung cancer. Chest 1990;98:97–100.

224. Moghissi K, Dixon K, Stringer M, Freeman T, Thorpe A, Brown S: The place of bronchoscopic photodynamic therapy in advanced unresectable lung cancer: Experience of 100 cases. Eur J Cardiothorac Surg 1999;15:1–6.

225. Diaz-Jimenez JP, Martinez-Ballarin JE, Llunell A, Farrero E, Rodriguez A, Castro MJ: Efficacy and safety of photodynamic therapy versus Nd-YAG laser resection in NSCLC with airway obstruction. Eur Respir J 1999;14:800–805.

226. Maier A, Tomaselli F, Matzi V, et al: Comparison of 5-aminolaevulinic acid and porphyrin photosensitization for photodynamic therapy of malignant bronchial stenosis: A clinical pilot study. Lasers Surg Med 2002;30:12–17.

227. Martini N, Bains MS, Burt ME, et al: Incidence of local recurrence and second primary tumors in resected stage I lung cancer. J Thorac Cardiovasc Surg 1995;109:120–129.

228. Furuse K, Fukuoka M, Kato H, et al: A prospective phase II study on photodynamic therapy with photofrin II for centrally located early-stage lung cancer. The Japan Lung Cancer Photodynamic Therapy Study Group. J Clin Oncol 1993;11:1852–1867.

229. Miyazu Y, Miyazawa T, Kurimoto N, Iwamoto Y, Kanoh K, Kohno N: Endobronchial ultrasonography in the assessment of centrally located early-stage lung cancer before photodynamic therapy. Am J Respir Crit Care Med 2002;165:832–837.

230. Kato H, Okunaka T, Shimatani H: Photodynamic therapy for early stage bronchogenic carcinoma. J Clin Laser Med Surg 1996;14:235–238.

231. Webb DD: GERD warrants increased physician appreciation and improved treatment. Postgrad Med 2001;spec no:5–10.

232. Spechler SJ: Clinical practice: Barrett's esophagus. N Engl J Med 2002;346:836–842.

233. van Sandick JW, van Lanschot JJ, Tytgat GN, Offerhaus GJ, Obertop H: Barrett oesophagus and adenocarcinoma: An overview of epidemiologic, conceptual and clinical issues. Scand J Gastroenterol 2001;234(Suppl):51–60.

234. Ofman JJ: The relation between gastroesophageal reflux disease and esophageal and head and neck cancers: A critical appraisal of epidemiologic literature. Am J Med 2001;111(Suppl 8A):124S–129S.

235. Dent J: Approaches to oesophageal columnar metaplasia (Barrett's oesophagus). Scand J Gastroenterol 1989;168(Suppl):60–66.

236. Rice TW, Zuccaro G Jr, Adelstein DJ, Rybicki LA, Blackstone EH, Goldblum JR: Esophageal carcinoma: Depth of tumor invasion is predictive of regional lymph node status. Ann Thorac Surg 1998;65:787–794.

237. Sato F, Shimada Y, Li Z, Watanabe G, Maeda M, Imamura M: Lymph node micrometastasis and prognosis in patients with oesophageal squamous cell carcinoma. Br J Surg 2001;88:426–432.

238. Savary JF, Grosjean P, Monnier P, et al: Photodynamic therapy of early squamous cell carcinomas of the esophagus: A review of 31 cases. Endoscopy 1998;30:258–265.

239. Corti L, Skarlatos J, Boso C, et al: Outcome of patients receiving photodynamic therapy for early esophageal cancer. Int J Radiat Oncol Biol Phys 2000;47:419–424.

240. Panjehpour M, Overholt BF, Haydek JM, Lee SG: Results of photodynamic therapy for ablation of dysplasia and early cancer in Barrett's esophagus and effect of oral steroids on stricture formation. Am J Gastroenterol 2000;95:2177–2184.

241. Grosjean P, Savary JF, Mizeret J, et al: Photodynamic therapy for cancer of the upper aerodigestive tract using tetra(m-hydroxyphenyl)chlorin. J Clin Laser Med Surg 1996;14:281–287.

242. Grant WE, Hopper C, Speight PM, Macrobert AJ, Bown SG: Photodynamic therapy of malignant and premalignant lesions in patients with "field cancerization" of the oral cavity. J Laryngol Otol 1993;107:1140–1145.

243. Freche C, De Corbiere S: Use of photodynamic therapy in the treatment of vocal cord carcinoma. J Photochem Photobiol B 1990;6:291–296.

244. Biel MA: Photodynamic therapy of head and neck cancers. Semin Surg Oncol 1995;11:355–359.

245. Biel MA: Photodynamic therapy and the treatment of neoplastic diseases of the larynx. Laryngoscope 1994;104:399–403.

246. Biel MA: Photodynamic therapy and the treatment of head and neck neoplasia. Laryngoscope 1998;108:1259–1268.

247. Biel MA: Photodynamic therapy and the treatment of head and neck cancers. J Clin Laser Med Surg 1996;14:239–244.

248. Sugiura S, Ando Y, Minami H, Ando M, Sakai S, Shimokata K: Prognostic value of pleural effusion in patients with non-small cell lung cancer. Clin Cancer Res 1997;3:47–50.

249. Werner-Wasik M, Scott C, Cox JD, et al: Recursive partitioning analysis of 1999 Radiation Therapy Oncology Group (RTOG)

patients with locally-advanced non-small-cell lung cancer (LA-NSCLC): Identification of five groups with different survival. Int J Radiat Oncol Biol Phys 2000;48:1475–1482.

250. Sawabata N, Matsumura A, Motohiro A, et al: Malignant minor pleural effusion detected on thoracotomy for patients with non-small cell lung cancer: Is tumor resection beneficial for prognosis? Ann Thorac Surg 2002;73:412–415.

251. Fukuse T, Hirata T, Tanaka F, Wada H, et al: The prognostic significance of malignant pleural effusion at the time of thoracotomy in patients with non-small cell lung cancer. Lung Cancer 2001;34:75–81.

252. Yokoi K, Matsuguma H, Anraku M: Extrapleural pneumonectomy for lung cancer with carcinomatous pleuritis. J Thorac Cardiovasc Surg 2002;123:184–185.

253. Temeck BK, Pass HI: Esophagopleural fistula: A complication of photodynamic therapy. South Med J: 1995;88:271–274.

254. Antman K, Pass H, Schiff P: Benign and malignant mesothelioma. In DeVita VT, Rosenberg SA, Hellman S: Cancer: Principles and Practice of Oncology, 5th ed. Philadelphia, Lippincott-Raven, 1997, pp 1853–1878.

255. Takita H, Mang TS, Loewen GM, et al: Operation and intracavitary photodynamic therapy for malignant pleural mesothelioma: A phase II study. Ann Thorac Surg 1994;58:995–998.

256. Takita H, Dougherty TJ: Intracavitary photodynamic therapy for malignant pleural mesothelioma. Semin Surg Oncol 1995;11:368–371.

257. Moskal TL, Dougherty TJ, Urschel JD, et al: Operation and photodynamic therapy for pleural mesothelioma: 6-year follow-up. Ann Thorac Surg 1998;66:1128–1133.

258. Fan KF, Hopper C, Speight PM, Buonaccorsi GA, Bown SG: Photodynamic therapy using mTHPC for malignant disease in the oral cavity. Int J Cancer 1997;73:25–32.

259. Tong MC, van Hasselt CA, Woo JK: Preliminary results of photodynamic therapy for recurrent nasopharyngeal carcinoma. Eur Arch Otorhinolaryngol 1996;253:189–192.

260. Ormrod D, Jarvis B: Topical aminolevulinic acid HCl photodynamic therapy. Am J Clin Dermatol 2000;1:133–139.

261. Dijkstra AT, Majoie IM, van Dongen JW, van Weelden H, van Vloten WA: Photodynamic therapy with violet light and topical 6-aminolaevulinic acid in the treatment of actinic keratosis, Bowen's disease and basal cell carcinoma. J Eur Acad Dermatol Venereol 2001;15:550–554.

262. Wang I, Bendsoe N, Klinteberg CA, et al: Photodynamic therapy vs. cryosurgery of basal cell carcinomas: Results of a phase III clinical trial. Br J Dermatol 2001;144:832–840.

263. Jeffes EW, McCullough JL, Weinstein GD, Kaplan R, Glazer SD, Taylor JR: Photodynamic therapy of actinic keratosis with topical 5-aminolevulinic acid: A pilot dose-ranging study. Arch Dermatol 1997;133:727–732.

264. Gayl Schweitzer V: Photofrin-mediated photodynamic therapy for treatment of aggressive head and neck nonmelanomatous skin tumors in elderly patients. Laryngoscope 2001;111:1091–1098.

265. Sindelar W, FJ Sullivan, E Abraham, et al: Intraperitoneal photodynamic therapy shows efficacy in phase I trial. Proc Am Soc Clin Oncol 1995;14:447.

266. Bauer TW, Hahn SM, Spitz FR, Kachur A, Glatstein E, Fraker DL: Preliminary report of photodynamic therapy for intraperitoneal sarcomatosis. Ann Surg Oncol 2001;8:254–259.

267. Hendren SK, Hahn SM, Spitz FR, et al: Phase II trial of debulking surgery and photodynamic therapy for disseminated intraperitoneal tumors. Ann Surg Oncol 2001;8:65–71.

268. Garden AS, Maor MH, Yung WK, et al: Outcome and patterns of failure following limited-volume irradiation for malignant astrocytomas. Radiother Oncol 1991;20:99–110.

269. Sneed PK, Gutin PH, Larson DA, et al: Patterns of recurrence of glioblastoma multiforme after external irradiation followed by implant boost. Int J Radiat Oncol Biol Phys 1994;29:719–727.

270. Muller PJ, Wilson BC: Photodynamic therapy for recurrent supratentorial gliomas. Semin Surg Oncol 1995;11:346–354.

271. Muller PJ, Wilson BC: Photodynamic therapy for malignant newly diagnosed supratentorial gliomas. J Clin Laser Med Surg 1996;14:263–270.

272. Muller PJ, Wilson BC: Photodynamic therapy of malignant primary brain tumours: Clinical effects, post-operative ICP, and light penetration of the brain. Photochem Photobiol 1987;46:929–935.

273. Muller PJ, Wilson BC: Photodynamic therapy of malignant brain tumours. Can J Neurol Sci 1990;17:193–198.

274. Boxer RJ, Kaufman JJ, Goodwin WE: Radical prostatectomy for carcinoma of the prostate: 1951–1976—a review of 329 patients. J Urol 1977;117:208–213.

275. Middleton RG, Smith JA Jr, Melzer RB, Hamilton PE, et al: Patient survival and local recurrence rate following radical prostatectomy for prostatic carcinoma. J Urol 1986;136:422–424.

276. Veenema RJ, Gursel EO, Lattimer JK: Radical retropubic prostatectomy for cancer: A 20-year experience. J Urol 1977;117:330–331.

277. Bagshaw MA, Cox RS, Ray GR: Status of radiation treatment of prostate cancer at Stanford University. NCI Monogr 1988;(7):47–60.

278. Shipley WU, Prout GR Jr, Coachman NM, et al: Radiation therapy for localized prostate carcinoma: Experience at the Massachusetts General Hospital (1973–1981). NCI Monogr 1988;(7):67–73.

279. Tefilli MV, Gheiler EL, Tiguert R, et al: Salvage surgery or salvage radiotherapy for locally recurrent prostate cancer. Urology 1998;52:224–229.

280. Pisters LL, von Eschenbach AC, Scott SM, et al: The efficacy and complications of salvage cryotherapy of the prostate. J Urol 1997;157:921–925.

281. Grado GL, Collins JM, Kriegshauser JS, et al: Salvage brachytherapy for localized prostate cancer after radiotherapy failure. Urology 1999;53:2–10.

282. Lerner SE, Blute ML, Zincke H: Critical evaluation of salvage surgery for radio-recurrent/resistant prostate cancer. J Urol 1995;154:1103–1109.

283. Rogers E, Ohori M, Kassabian VS, Wheeler TM, Scardino PT: Salvage radical prostatectomy: Outcome measured by serum prostate specific antigen levels. J Urol 1995;153:104–110.

284. Chen Q, Chopp M, Dereski MO, et al: The effect of light fluence rate in photodynamic therapy of normal rat brain. Radiat Res 1992;132:120–123.

285. Chen Q, Huang Z, Luck D, et al: Preclinical studies in normal canine prostate of a novel palladium-bacteriopheophorbide (WST09) photosensitizer for photodynamic therapy of prostate cancers. Photochem Photobiol 2002;76:438–445.

286. Chang SC, Buonaccorsi G, MacRobert A, Bown SG, et al: Interstitial and transurethral photodynamic therapy of the canine prostate using meso-tetra-(m-hydroxyphenyl) chlorin. Int J Cancer 1996;67:555–562.

287. Nathan TR, Whitelaw DE, Chang SC, et al: Photodynamic therapy for prostate cancer recurrence after radiotherapy: A phase I study. J Urol 2002;168:1427–1432.

288. Chang SC, Buonaccorsi GA, MacRobert AJ, Bown SG: Interstitial photodynamic therapy in the canine prostate with disulfonated aluminum phthalocyanine and 5-aminolevulinic acid-induced protoporphyrin IX. Prostate 1997;32:89–98.

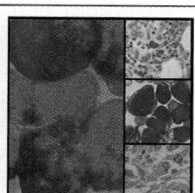

32

THERAPEUTIC ANTIBODIES AND IMMUNOLOGIC CONJUGATES

Nai-Kong V. Cheung

SUMMARY OF KEY POINTS

- Because of their tumor selectivity, monoclonal antibodies offer exceptional opportunities for targeted therapy.
- As naked antibodies, monoclonal antibodies kill tumors by receptor blockade and by actively inducing apoptosis.
- Tumor cytotoxicity is mediated in the presence of white cells by activating antibody-dependent cell-mediated cytotoxicity; and in the presence of serum, complement-mediated cytotoxicity.
- The effector functions of antibodies can be greatly enhanced as immunoconjugates, which include radioimmunoconjugates, immunocytokines, immunoliposomes, immunotoxins, immunoenzymes and cellular immunoconjugates.

- Naked antibodies can, on occasion, have overlapping toxicity profiles with chemotherapy and radiation therapies.
- Dose-limiting toxicities of immunoconjugates depend on the cytotoxic moiety (e.g., myelosuppression in radioimmunoconjugates) being used.
- It is generally believed that antibody therapy has been most successful in liquid tumors because these tumors are more accessible to intravenous antibodies.
- Antibodies are more likely to be beneficial at the time of minimal residual disease, especially when used in conjunction with standard therapy.
- The following antibodies have been licensed by the FDA for the applications stated:

- Tositumomab (Bexxar): non-Hodgkin's lymphoma (^{131}I, CD20)
- Alemtuzumab (Campath): chronic lymphocytic leukemia (CD52)
- Trastuzumab (Herceptin): breast cancer (HER2)
- Gemtuzumab ozogamicin (Mylotarg): acute myelogenous leukemia (calicheamicin, CD33)
- Rituximab (Rituxan): non-Hodgkin's lymphoma (CD20)
- Ibritumomab (Zevalin): non-Hodgkin's lymphoma (^{90}Y, CD20)
- In the coming decade, a number of monoclonal antibodies currently in various phases of clinical trial are likely to be added to the list. The prospects for further innovation in this emerging modality are highly favorable.

INTRODUCTION

The clinical development of antibody therapy was accelerated by the introduction of the hybridoma technique in 1975[1] and, more recently, the emergence of recombinant technology. Through these innovations, individual plasma cells can be immortalized, and cloning of heavy and light chain repertoires from animals and humans is now possible. In less than three decades, monoclonal antibodies (MAb) have evolved from bench research to inclusion in a rapidly increasing list of licensed pharmaceuticals. They have generated excitement on many frontiers and will likely play a pivotal role in the history of cancer medicine (Table 32-1). The clinical utility of MAb for in vitro diagnosis and ex vivo manipulation of blood or stem cells is well recognized. Their role in the treatment and prophylaxis of graft-versus-host disease[2,3] is detailed in Chapter 28. The use of B-cell idiotype[4] and antitumor anti-idiotypic antibodies as tumor vaccines[5] is described in Chapter 33. This chapter summarizes the application of therapeutic antitumor MAb and immunologic conjugates in cancer therapy.

EFFECTOR MECHANISMS OF MONOCLONAL ANTIBODIES

Antitumor monoclonal antibodies (MAb) can carry out highly effective tumoricidal functions both in vitro and in vivo (Fig. 32-1). These include signaling through receptor binding, antibody-dependent cell-mediated cytotoxicity (ADCC), and complement-dependent cytotoxicity (CDC).

Signaling by Receptor Cross-Linking and Receptor Blockade

Monoclonal antibodies are able to crosslink cell-surface receptors by using their antigen-combining sites. However, they vary in their ability to induce downstream effects. Anti-CD20 MAb induces apoptosis,[6,7] especially when the target antigen is highly cross-linked.[8] Similar observations have been made for anti-CD19 and anti-CD22 antibodies.[9] Upregulation of the pro-apoptotic Bax or repression of anti-apoptotic Bcl-x1 molecules probably is involved.[7] Alternatively, MAb can block receptor functions (e.g., EGF-R,[10] HER-2,[11] and VEGF-R[12]) by interfering with binding of the natural ligands.

661

TABLE 32-1

Antibody Therapy of Cancer: Historical Perspective

1901:	Nobel Prize for Emil Behring for work on serum therapy with Shibasaburo Kitasato
1908:	Nobel Prize for Paul Ehrlich for his work on passive immunization
1927:	Serotherapy of chronic myelogenous leukemia
1975:	Hybridoma technique of Hans Kohler and Caesar Milstein (winners of 1986 Nobel Prize)
1980:	MAb therapy of lymphoma
1986:	FDA approval of MAb as standard pharmaceuticals
1992:	Murine ^{111}In–anti-B72.3 for imaging colon and ovarian cancer
1997:	Chimeric anti-CD20 (rituximab) for B-cell lymphoma
1998:	Humanized anti-HER2 (trastuzumab) for breast cancer
1999:	Humanized anti-CD33 immunotoxin for acute myelogenous leukemia
2001:	Humanized anti-CD52 (alemtuzumab) for B-chronic lymphocytic leukemia
2002:	^{90}Y–anti-CD20 (Ibritumomab) for B-cell lymphoma
2003:	Murine ^{131}I–anti-CD20 (tositumomab) for B-cell lymphoma

Cytophilic MAb and ADCC

The cytophilic Fc region resides on the other end of the MAb molecule. There are three types of IgG (γ) Fc receptors (FcγR): FcγRI (CD64), FcγRII (CD32), and low-affinity FcγRIII (CD16) (Table 32-2).[13] All are trans-membrane glycoproteins except FcγRIIIB, which is anchored on neutrophils by glycosylphosphatidylinositol (GPI). Either as single-chain receptors (FcRα chain), or as complexes with γ or ζ chains, they transduce intracellular activation signals. The γ chain is also a component of FcRs for IgE and IgA, and the ζ chain is part of the T-cell antigen receptor/CD3 signaling complex. Most FcγRs are of the

activating type, where receptor engagement can induce phagocytosis, degranulation, antibody-dependent cell-mediated cytotoxicity, cytokine release, or regulation of antibody production. FcγRIIB contains inhibitory motifs in the cytoplasmic domain and mediates downregulation of these cellular functions. Additionally, a unique class of Fc receptor called FcRB (Brambell)/FcRn (neonatal) is found on endothelial cells and regulates antibody catabolism.[14] Recent correlation of FcγRIIIA polymorphism with clinical response to rituximab suggests that IgG affinity for Fc receptor can influence antitumor response in patients.[15,16] Human IgG1 also binds to the FcRn on endothelial cells, which protects immunoglobulins from lysosomal degradation, thereby prolonging the IgG half-life.[14] Besides IgG, both IgA1 and IgA2 can mediate efficient ADCC by binding to FcαR1 (CD89) on human neutrophils and monocytes/macrophages.[17]

Certain cancer cells such as colon carcinoma, lymphoma, leukemia, neuroblastoma, and melanoma are effectively killed by NK lymphocytes, granulocytes, and activated monocytes in vitro in the presence of specific MAb. Depending on the affinity of the MAb for the individual FcR, NK (FcγRII, FcγRIII), neutrophils (all 3 FcγR), or both can mediate efficient ADCC. Lym-1 (humanized IgG1 specific for HLA-DR on lymphoma) does not bind to FcγRIII, but exploits FcγRII for ADCC.[18] Similarly, ch14.18 (chimeric IgG1 specific for GD2 on neuroblastoma) depends on FcγRII in ADCC.[19] In contrast, 3F8 (murine IgG3 specific for GD2 on neuroblastoma) utilizes both FcγRII and FcγRIII for ADCC.[20] In addition to FcR, adhesion molecules are critical for MAb-mediated ADCC. These molecules include CR3 (CD11b/Cd18)[18-20] and CD66b[18] for neutrophil ADCC, and LFA-1 (CD11a/CD18) for lymphocyte ADCC.[21] Because cytokines can increase the expression of adhesion molecules, GM-CSF or

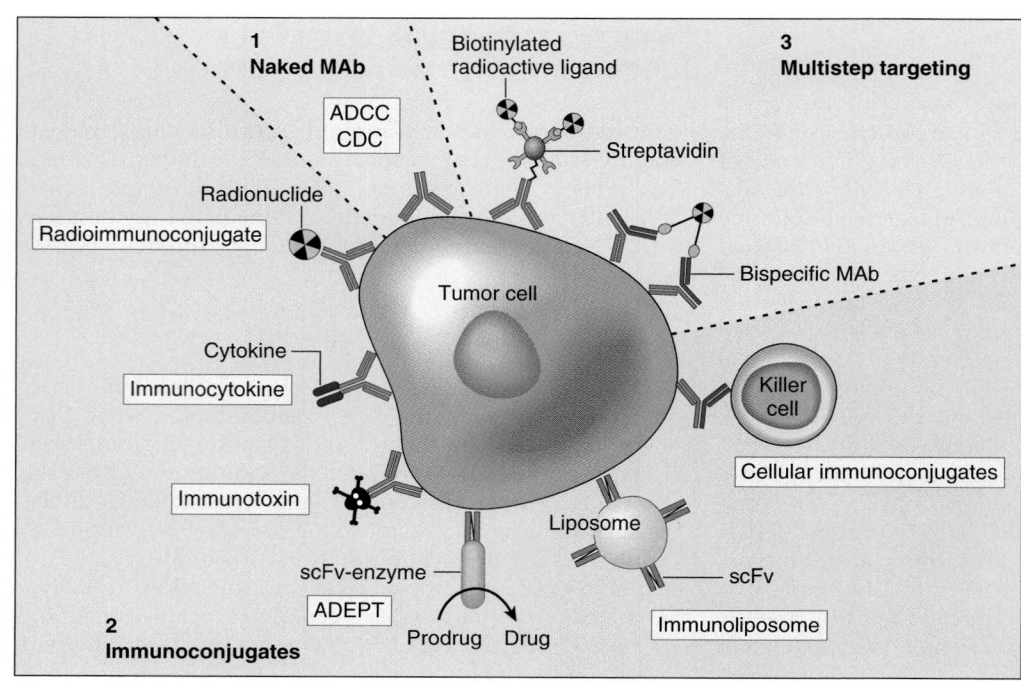

Figure 32-1. Effector mechanisms of monoclonal antibodies. ADEPT, antibody directed enzyme prodrug therapy; ADCC, antibody dependent cell-mediated cytotoxicity; CDC, complement dependent cytotoxicity; MAb, monoclonal antibody; scFv, single-chain Fv fragment. (Modified from Carter P: Improving the efficacy of antibody-based cancer therapies. Nat Rev Cancer 2001;1:118–129.)

TABLE 32-2

Properties of IgG Fc Receptors

FC RECEPTOR	FUNCTION	AFFINITY FOR hIgG	DISTRIBUTION ON WBC
CD64			
FcγRI	A	High	PMN, MONO, MΦ, DC
CD32			
FcγRIIA	A	Low*	PMN, MONO, MΦ, DC, NK
FcγRIIB	I	Low*	PMN, MONO, MΦ, B-cell
FcγRIIC	A	Low*	PMN, MONO, MΦ
CD16			
FcγRIIIA	A	Intermediate	MONO, MΦ, NK, DC
FcγRIIIB[†]	A	Low*	PMN

A, Activating; DC, dendritic cells; hIgG, human IgG; I, Inhibiting; MONO, monocytes; MΦ, macrophages; PMN, neutrophils; WBC, white blood cell.
*Prefers antibody-antigen complex.
[†]Glycosylphosphatidylinositol (GPI)-anchored.
From Ravetch and Bolland[13]; Kimberly et al.[16]; and Binstadt BA, Geha RS, Bonilla FA: IgG Fc receptor polymorphisms in human disease: Implications for intravenous immunoglobulin therapy. J Allergy Clin Immunol 2003;111:697–703.

IFN-γ has been used to activate granulocyte ADCC,[19,22-24] and IL-2 has been used similarly for lymphocyte ADCC.[25,26] Furthermore, because both GM-CSF and IL-2 expand the effector cell pools, they can have additional benefits in tumor therapy. Optimal combinations of MAb and cytokines in the appropriate clinical setting can bring favorable outcomes.[27-29]

Complement Activation

IgG initiates the classical complement cascade by binding C1q to its CH2 domain. Among human IgG subclasses, C1q is more avid for IgG1 and IgG3 over IgG2, and has no affinity for IgG4.[30] Some tumor cell lines (e.g., lymphoma and neuroblastoma) are sensitive to CDC. However, many are resistant to complement because of anticomplement surface proteins, including decay-accelerating factor (DAF, CD55),[31-33] homologous restriction factor (CD59),[31,34,35] and membrane cofactor protein (CD46).[32-34,36] The effect of complement activation extends beyond direct tumor lysis. Following complement activation, tumor-bound C3b is cleaved rapidly by plasma protease factor I to iC3b. Through CR3 (Mac-1 or alpha$_M$beta$_2$-integrin), and CR4 (CD11c/CD18, alpha$_X$beta$_2$-integrin) receptors on leukocytes, tumor cells are opsonized.[37] C3a and C5a, byproducts of complement activation, are potent mediators of inflammation[38] and are chemotactic for phagocytic leukocytes, drawing them to the tumor sites. C5a also can induce secondary cytokines to increase vascular permeability for both MAb and effector cells.

CLINICAL APPLICATION OF NAKED MAB (Table 32-3)

Lymphoma and Leukemia

In 1997, the anti-CD20 chimeric antibody rituximab became the first MAb approved by the US Food and Drug Administration (FDA) for the treatment of cancer. In a single-arm, multicenter study of 166 patients with relapsed or refractory, low-grade, or follicular non-Hodgkin's lymphoma (NHL), rituximab at a dose of

TABLE 32-3

Naked MAb for Cancer Therapy

ANTIBODY	ANTIGEN	ANTIBODY FORM	CANCER	EFFECTOR FUNCTION/MOLECULE	DRUG	STATUS
Alemtuzumab*	CD52	huIgG1	CLL, PLL	ADCC, CDC	Campath	Licensed
Trastuzumab[58]	HER2	huIgG1	Breast cancer	ADCC, CDC, receptor blockade	Herceptin	Licensed
Rituximab[108]	CD20	chIgG1	CLL	ADCC, CDC; interrupts signaling pathways	Rituxan	Licensed
3F8[29]	GD2	mIgG3	NB	ADCC, CDC		Phase II
ch14.18[62]	GD2	chIgG1	NB	ADCC, CDC		Phase II/III
Edrecolomab[68]	EpCAM	mIgG2a	Colorectal cancer	ADCC, CDC	Panorex	Phase III
Epratuzumab[46]	CD22	huIgG1	NHL	ADCC, CDC; interrupts signaling pathways		Phase III
IMC-C225 Cetuximab[74]	EGFR	chIgG1	Head and neck, colorectal cancer	ADCC, CDC; interrupts signaling pathways	Erbitux	Phase III
HuM195[48,49]	CD33	huIgG1	AML, MDS, APL	ADCC, CDC		Phase III
MAb-B43.13[72]	CA125	mIgG1	Ovarian cancer	Idiotype network	Ovarex	Phase III

ADCC, antibody–dependent cell-mediated cytotoxicity; ALL, acute lymphoblastic leukemia; AML, acute myelogenous leukemia; APL, acute promyelocytic leukemia; CDC, complement-dependent cytotoxicity; ch, chimeric; CLL, chronic lymphocytic leukemia; EpCAM, epithelial cellular adhesion molecule; EGFR, epidermal growth factor receptor; hu, humanized; Ig, immunoglobulin; Licensed, licensed by the FDA; MAb, monoclonal antibody; MDS, myelodysplastic syndrome; mu, murine; NB, neuroblastoma; NHL, non-Hodgkin's lymphoma; PLL, prolymphocytic leukemia.
From Osterborg A, Dyer MJ, Bunjes D, et al: Phase II multicenter study of human CD52 antibody in previously treated chronic lymphocytic leukemia. European Study Group of CAMPATH-1H Treatment in Chronic Lymphocytic Leukemia. J Clin Oncol 1997;15:1567–1574.

375 mg/m^2 four times weekly produced an overall response (OR) rate of 48%, complete response (CR) rate of 6%, and partial response (PR) rate of 42%. Median time to progression in responders was 13.1 months.[39] In this study, rituximab demonstrated activity in chemoresistant disease (29%) and in patients relapsing after anthracycline therapy (51%). The FDA-approved label later was expanded to include patients with bulky disease, retreatment of responders, and an extended treatment schedule of eight infusions.

For most patients, rituximab was well tolerated.[40] Severe adverse events thought to be secondary to complement activation often occurred with the first infusion,[41,42] especially if there were high numbers of circulating tumor cells. These infusion-related reactions usually appeared 30 to 120 minutes after MAb injection and typically were associated with severe cardiopulmonary events, with deaths (< 0.1%) occurring within 24 hours. B-cell depletion occurs in most patients, although the serum IgG level remains normal for 12 months or longer without increased incidence of infection.[39] Severe mucocutaneous reactions occur rarely (0.07%), resulting in some fatalities.

Because rituximab sensitizes drug-resistant B-cell lymphoma to etoposide, cisplatin, and doxorubicin,[43] it was tested in diffuse large B-cell NHL, where combination chemotherapy (cyclophosphamide, doxorubicin, vincristine, and prednisone [CHOP]) plus rituximab achieved 76% CR, progression-free survival (PFS) of 69% and overall survival (OS) of 83%, significantly better than the 60%, 49%, and 68%, respectively, with CHOP alone.[44] In a randomized trial of 399 elderly subjects with previously untreated diffuse large B-cell lymphoma, CHOP chemotherapy alone or CHOP plus rituximab produced OR of 63% and 76%, and OS at 2 years of 57% and 70%, respectively.[45] Other antibodies in active clinical trials include epratuzumab (huIgG1 anti-CD22) for NHL,[46] SGN-30 (chIgG1 anti-CD30) for Hodgkin's disease,[47] and HuM195 (huIgG1 anti-CD33) for myeloid leukemia.[48,49]

Campath-1H (Alemtuzumab), a humanized rat IgG1 anti-CD52 MAb, has activity against recurrent chronic lymphocytic leukemia and T-cell prolymphocytic leukemia.[50] In an international phase II study involving 21 centers (n = 93 patients), Campath-1H was administered at 30 mg, 3 times weekly for a maximum of 12 weeks, to patients with relapsed or refractory B-cell chronic lymphocytic leukemia who had previously failed fludarabine therapy. The OR was 33% (CR 2%, PR 31%). The median time to response and progression was 1.5 and 4.7 months, respectively, and median survival was 16 months. Grade 3 or 4 infections were reported in 26.9% of patients.[51] Based on this study, Campath-1H was approved by the FDA. Other clinical trials also have reported opportunistic infections, including bacterial sepsis and viral infections, as well as marrow aplasia following Campath-1H treatment.[50,52]

Solid Tumors

Trastuzumab (Herceptin) is a humanized MAb against the receptor tyrosine kinase ERBB2 (also known as HER2/NEU) on breast cancer cells. It can mediate a diverse spectrum of antitumor effector mechanisms. Besides CDC and ADCC, it can induce HER2 protein down regulation, prevent HER2-containing heterodimer formation, initiate G1 arrest, induce p27, prevent HER2 cleavage, and inhibit angiogenesis.[53] The application of trastuzumab in metastatic breast cancer achieved OR of 15% (3.6% CR, 11.7% PR, n = 222) with median response duration of 9.2 months and OS at 13 months.[54] Its efficacy in patients with recurrent or refractory ovarian cancer was limited by the low expression of HER-2 among these patients.[55] Based on its synergy with chemotherapy in vitro,[56,57] trastuzumab was tested in a large phase III trial of 469 patients, where its combination with chemotherapy produced a longer median response duration (9.1 vs 6.1 months), higher OR (50% vs 32%), and lower death rate at 1 year (22% vs 33%),[58] than chemotherapy alone. However, there was a significant increase in cardiotoxicity. Based on this trial, the FDA approved the use of trastuzumab and paclitaxel as a first-line treatment of HER2-overexpressing metastatic breast cancer. Further trials are underway to evaluate trastuzumab in combination with other forms of chemotherapy, including vinorelbine, docetaxel, anthracyclines, and platinum agents, especially in the adjuvant setting.[59]

Among the ganglioside antigens on neuroectodermal tumors, GD3 (MAb R24 for melanoma)[60] and GD2 (MAb 3F8 and ch14.18 for neuroblastoma)[29,61-63] have been tested clinically. GD2 is particularly relevant for the treatment of pediatric cancers since it is present on a variety of solid tumors in addition to neuroblastoma, including osteosarcoma, retinoblastoma, some soft tissue sarcomas, and brain tumors. Although the clinical effectiveness of anti-GD2 MAb was modest, response of microscopic marrow disease was consistent.[29,63] Clinical development of anti-GD2 MAb was due partly to its pain side effects, which have precluded dose escalation. At current doses, optimal application of anti-GD2 antibody is at the time of minimal residual disease.[64,65] An association of human antimouse antibody (HAMA) response and favorable patient outcome, plus the induction of Ab2 and Ab3 through the idiotype network, implicate the potential role of the host immune response in maintaining clinical remission.[66,67]

The use of naked MAb in the adjuvant setting to eradicate micrometastases also has been applied to colorectal cancer. The murine IgG$_{2a}$ 17-1A (Panorex), specific for EpCAM on malignant and normal epithelial cells, was administered in a randomized trial to 189 patients with Dukes' Stage C colorectal cancer metastatic to regional lymph nodes.[68] At 7 years of follow-up, overall mortality was reduced by 32% and recurrence rate by 23%. Although distant metastases were significantly reduced, local relapses were not. Anti-idiotype network and T-cell response against antibody-modified tumors have been proposed as potential antitumor mechanisms.[69-71] The correlation of improved survival and HAMA/idiotype network response also was reported for MAb B43.13 (anti-CA-125) in patients with ovarian cancer.[72] The roles of FcγR, dendritic cells and cross-priming of T cells following MAb treatment deserve further clinical investigation.[73] Cetuximab (chIgG1 anti-EGFR) is another antibody designed to induce receptor blockade, and is being

Figure 32-2. Immunogenicity of MAb. CH1, CH2, and CH3, constant region domains of an IgG heavy chain; scFv, single chain v fragment; VH, variable region of the heavy chain; VL, variable region of the light chain. Red; mouse; blue; human; green; recombinant protein to which scFv is genetically fused.

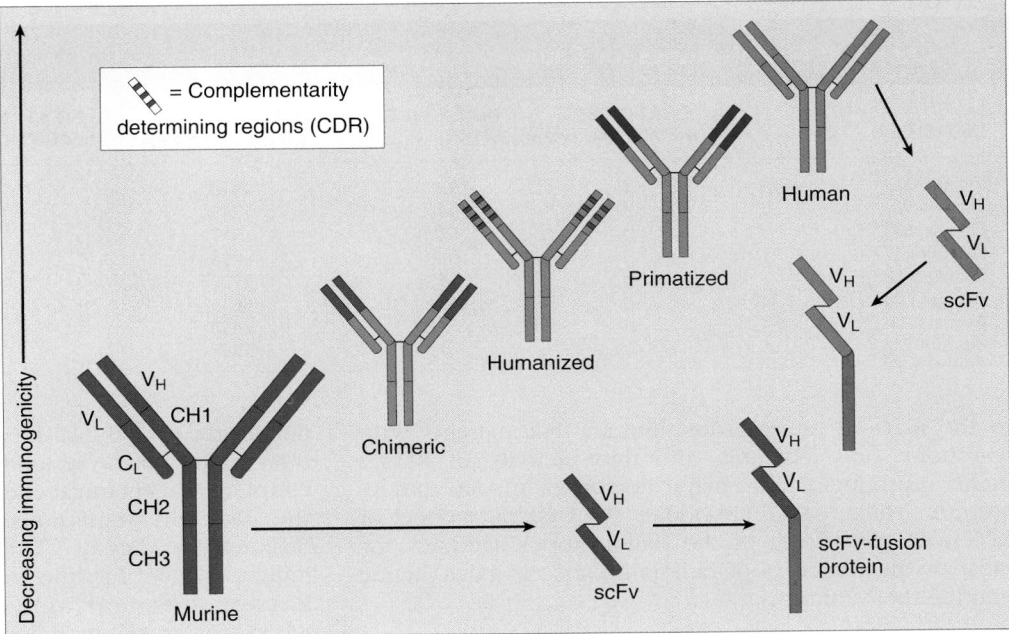

actively tested in Phase III trials in head and neck plus colorectal cancers.[74]

Complications and Contraindications

Toxicities of MAb are, in general, manageable and self-limited (Fig. 32-2). Common acute reactions include fever, chills, headache, nausea, fatigue, angioedema, urticaria, pruritus, blood pressure fluctuations, and bronchospasm. Lethal or irreversible side effects include cytokine release (antilymphocyte MAb) and complement activation (anti-CD20) syndromes,[41] immune suppression (anti-CD52),[50,52] and cardiotoxicity (anti-HER2).[58] A severe self-limited side effect is the pain syndrome from cross-reactivity of anti-GD2 MAb with peripheral pain fibers.[61,62] Murine MAb induce HAMA responses, which can alter the pharmacokinetic and pharmacodynamic properties of repeat MAb injections. Human antimouse antibody is directed primarily to the murine Fc portion of the antibody, although anti-idiotypic responses have been reported.[75] With chimeric, humanized, primatized, and human antibodies, immunogenicity is drastically reduced.[76-78] Clinical trials employing unmodified MAb as single agents in patients with malignancies generally have produced modest antitumor effects; NHL is an obvious exception.[39,79,80]

IMMUNOCONJUGATES

The clinical utility of naked MAb has been limited by both host (number and activity of effector cells, FcR polymorphism, and interference by inhibitory FcR) and tumor factors (antigen heterogeneity and complement regulatory proteins). Although the CDC and ADCC functions of naked MAb (see Fig. 32-1) can be improved by altering the

Fc protein structure[76] or by modifying Fc-glycosylation,[81,82] substantial gains in the clinical potentials of MAb have derived from research on immunoconjugates. These include (1) radioimmunoconjugates to deliver β- and α-emitters,[83] (2) immunocytokines to deliver cytokines to tumor sites while minimizing systemic toxicities,[84] (3) immunotoxins,[85] (4) antibody-directed enzyme prodrug therapy (ADEPT) to pretarget enzymes to tumor sites for prodrug activation so that high local concentrations of active drugs are released without triggering systemic toxicities,[86] (5) immunoliposomes to deliver drugs or toxins,[87] and (6) bispecific MAb (pretargeted to tumor or by ex vivo arming) to direct cells or ligands selectively to tumor.[88] More recently, a multistep targeting strategy has been developed to enhance tumor to normal tissue ratios (see Fig. 32-1).[89,90] The tumor is pretargeted using an antibody construct that has affinity for the tumor on one arm and for a radiolabeled hapten on the other arm. The radiolabeled hapten is administered after the antibody construct is cleared from circulation. Substantial improvements in the therapeutic index have been achieved.[83,91,92]

RADIOIMMUNOCONJUGATES[83]

MAb have the potential to target and ablate tumors in radioimmunotherapy (RIT). Radioimaging can map the biodistribution of MAb and quantify the relative amounts of MAb deposited in various tissues and organs, thus allowing more precise radiation dose estimates in therapeutic studies. With the advent of single photon emission computed tomography (SPECT) and positron emission tomography (PET), accurate dosimetry is more routine. In preclinical models ablation of established xenografts is possible,[93-95] although radiation damage

TABLE 32-4

Choice of Radioisotopes for Radioimmunotherapy

ISOTOPE	PARTICLE(S) EMITTED	HALF-LIFE (HRS)	MAXIMUM ENERGY (KEV)	MEAN RANGE OF α- OR β-PARTICLE EMISSION (MM)
Iodine 131 (^{131}I)	β, γ	193	610	0.8
Yttrium 90 (^{90}Y)	β	64	2280	2.7
Copper 67 (^{67}Cu)	β	62	577	1.8
Lutetium 177 (^{177}Lu)	β	161	496	1.5
Rhenium 188 (^{188}Re)	β, γ	17	2120	2.4
Actinium 225 (^{225}Ac)	α	240	5935	0.05–0.08
Astatine 211 (^{211}At)	α	7.2	7450	0.05–0.08
Bismuth 213 (^{213}Bi)	α	0.77	5982	0.05–0.08

to the marrow remains dose-limiting. For patients with lymphoma and leukemia, antitumor activity of RIT is highly reproducible, but major responses in solid tumors are rare. Unlike naked antibodies, the bystander effect of RIT from cross-firing of the radioisotopes accounts for most of the toxicities of radioimmunoconjugates, hence limiting their efficacy.

Choice of Radioisotopes for Radioimmunoconjugates (Table 32-4)

Most clinical applications of RIT utilize β-emitting radioimmunoconjugates. Beta particles have a relatively long range (0.8–5 mm) and low linear energy transfer (approximately 0.2 keV/μm). This long range results in the delivery of radiation not only to the antigen-positive, but also to antigen-negative tumor cells, as well as to the surrounding normal tissues. Thus, β-emitters can treat bulky diseases effectively, but are not optimal for the killing of single cells or micrometastasis. Most human studies of RIT have used iodine 131 (^{131}I), a long-lived β-particle emitter. Because of its γ-emission, it is also suitable for dosimetry studies. However, this γ-radiation poses a radiohazard at high treatment doses, necessitating patient isolation. In vivo dehalogenation can compromise tumor dose, with subsequent thyroid damage from the released iodide. Yttrium 90 (^{90}Y) is a pure β-emitter; its lack of γ-emissions allows outpatient treatment. However, ^{90}Y has limitations, including deposition in bone when

dissociated from the MAb complex. Unlike ^{131}I, which binds directly to tyrosine residues on the MAb, ^{90}Y requires the coupling of a chemical chelator to the MAb. Furthermore, the lack of γ-emissions means biodistribution and dosimetry studies of ^{90}Y necessitates trace-labeling with indium 111 (^{111}In), the biodistribution of which is not identical to that of ^{90}Y. Alpha particles are helium nuclei; when compared with β-particles, they have a shorter range (50–80 μm) and a higher linear energy transfer (approximately 100 keV/μm).[96] As few as one or two α-particles can destroy a target cell. Radioimmunotherapy using α-emitters should result in less nonspecific toxicity to normal bystanders as well as more efficient single cell killing. This is ideal for controlling minimal residual disease. α-particle-emitting isotopes such as astatine 211 and bismuth 213 have been tested in clinical trials. ^{213}Bi-HuM195 (anti-CD33) administered intravenously for AML,[97] and ^{211}At-8C16 administered intraventricularly or intrathecally for gliomas,[98] have been well tolerated and produce clinical responses. The relative lack of extramedullary toxicities should encourage further development of this targeting technique for micrometastases, or neoplasms on the surface of body compartments, such as ovarian cancer and leptomeningeal metastasis.[99]

Radiolabeled MAb for Lymphoma (Table 32-5)

In patient studies of RIT, sequestration of MAb in liver or spleen can compromise tumor delivery. To overcome uptake by the reticuloendothelial system, a large dose

TABLE 32-5

Radiolabeled MAb for Radioimmunotherapy

ANTIBODY	ANTIGEN	ANTIBODY FORM	CANCER	ISOTOPE	DRUG	STATUS
Tositumomab[103-107]	CD20	muIgG2a	NHL	^{131}I	Bexxar	Licensed
Ibritumomab[100-102]	CD20	muIgG1	NHL	^{90}Y	Zevalin	Licensed
hMN14 (Labetuzumab)[83]	CEA	huIgG	Colorectal	^{90}Y	CEA-Cide	Phase I/II
Epratuzumab[83]	CD22	huIgG	NHL	^{90}Y	LymphoCide	Phase III
Pemtumomab[83]	MUC-1	muIgG1	Ovarian	^{90}Y	Theragyn	Phase III

ADCC, antibody–dependent cell-mediated cytotoxicity; ALL, acute lymphoblastic leukemia; AML, acute myelogenous leukemia; APL, acute promyelocytic leukemia; CDC, complement-dependent cytotoxicity; ch, chimeric; CLL, chronic lymphocytic leukemia; EpCAM, epithelial cellular adhesion molecule; EGFR, epidermal growth factor receptor; hu, humanized; Ig, immunoglobulin; Licensed, licensed by the FDA; MAb, monoclonal antibody; MDS, myelodysplastic syndrome; mu, murine; NB, neuroblastoma; NHL, non-Hodgkin's lymphoma; PLL, prolymphocytic leukemia.
From Osterborg A, Dyer MJ, Bunjes D, et al: Phase II multicenter study of human CD52 antibody in previously treated chronic lymphocytic leukemia. European Study Group of CAMPATH-1H Treatment in Chronic Lymphocytic Leukemia. J Clin Oncol 1997;15:1567–1574.

of naked anti-CD20 antibody is needed to reduce liver uptake before RIT. In a three-component regimen (Zevalin), rituximab at 250 mg/m² at the rate of 100 mg/hr was first administered to clear peripheral blood B cells, followed within 4 hours by ^{111}In-ibritumomab tiuxetan and ^{90}Y-ibritumomab tiuxetan infusion. At 0.2 to 0.4 mCi/kg (7.4-15 MBq/kg) of ^{90}Y-ibritumomab, dosimetry data derived from four large trials showed median radiation absorbed doses of 7.4 Gy to spleen, 4.5 Gy to liver, 2.1 Gy to lung, 0.23 Gy to kidney, 0.62 Gy (blood-derived method) and 0.97 Gy (sacral image-derived method) to red marrow, and 0.57 Gy to total body, with a median effective blood half-life of 27 h.[100] Grade 4 neutropenia, thrombocytopenia, and anemia occurred in 30% to 35%, 10% to 14%, and 3% to 8% of patients, respectively. Myelodysplasia and acute myelogenous leukemia were reported in 1% of patients 8 to 34 months after treatment.[101] Serious grade 3 and 4 toxicities occurred in 3% of patients, and life-threatening events in 1% to 5%. Four weeks after therapy, no circulating B cells could be detected, and recovery began about 12 wks after therapy, usually to normal limits by 9 months. Serum IgG and IgA remained unchanged throughout, while IgM dropped below normal and recovered by 6 months. About 3.8% of patients developed HAMA or human antichimeric antibody (HACA). Among patients with relapsed or refractory NHL,[102] OR rate was 83% (37% CR and 40% PR). Median time to progression was 9.4 months. ^{131}I-tositumomab (Bexxar, anti-CD20) achieved 71% OR (34% CR) in a phase II trial (n = 59) of chemotherapy-refractory or relapsed patients with NHL. In 17% of patients HAMA was induced.[103] Using myeloablative doses of 280 to 785 mCi calculated to deliver 25 to 72 Gy to critical organs, 30 of 36 patients (83%) achieved durable CR, with OS of 68% and PFS of 42% (median follow-up, 42 months).[104,105] Hypothyroidism developed in 60% of patients 6 to 12 months after therapy, and secondary myelodysplastic syndrome (MDS)/AML was reported in 2% to more than 5%.[105,106] Similarly, myeloablative doses (10-31 Gy) of ^{131}I–anti-CD37 MAb produced 84% CR and 11% PR in patients with NHL, with eight patients in continual remission 46 to 95 months after therapy. Extramedullary toxicities were mild at doses less than 23 Gy, beyond which cardiopulmonary toxicity became dose-limiting.[107]

In a phase III randomized study, a single dose of 0.4 mCi/kg ^{90}Y-ibritumomab (n = 73) was more effective than rituximab, 375 mg/m²/week for 4 weeks in patients (n = 70) with relapsed or refractory low-grade, follicular, or transformed NHL.[108,109] This difference was statistically significant for OR (80% vs 56%), CR (30% vs 16%), and the probability of 6 months or more durable responses (64% vs 47%), respectively. Reversible myelosuppression was the primary toxicity noted with ^{90}Y-ibritumomab tiuxetan.[110] In other studies, increasing the dose or dose-intensity of rituximab has not produced a meaningful improvement in outcome.

Because the B-cell antigen CD22 is internalized, anti-CD22 antibody may be more effective when used in RIT than in its naked form. ^{131}I-LL2 MAb (anti-CD22) has antitumor activity against relapsed B-cell lymphoma.[111] In addition, unlike anti-CD20, good biodistribution was achieved with a humanized antibody (hLL2) without the need for preinjection of unlabeled antibody. Other internalizing antigens such as CD19[112] and HLA-DR10β[113] also are potential targets for RIT. Both low-dose and myeloablative doses of ^{131}I-Lym-1 had activity against NHL.[114] [67]Cu-Lym-1 was used for both imaging and therapy studies.[115] HAMA to Lym-1 was detected in 14% of patients and appeared to correlate with improved survival. HAMA-positive patients were living longer (median survival of 18 months) compared to the HAMA-negative group (9 months).[116] Other radiolabeled MAb, ^{131}I-anti-CR2,[117] ^{131}I-anti-CD37,[118] and ^{90}Y–anti-idiotype,[119] also have been used for the treatment of NHL with some success.

As part of marrow transplant conditioning, ^{131}I-tositumomab was combined with cyclophosphamide and etoposide in relapsed NHL; 83% OS and 68% PFS were achieved.[120] These results were favorable when compared to a historical control group given total body irradiation, where OS was 53% and PFS was 36%. In a separate study of relapsed mantle cell lymphoma, ^{131}I-tositumomab administered at doses to deliver 20 to 25 Gy to vital normal organs (median 510 mCi) was followed 10 days later with high-dose etoposide (30–60 mg/kg) plus cyclophosphamide (60-100 mg/kg), and infusion of cryopreserved autologous stem cells. Among the 11 evaluable patients, CR and OR were 91% and 100%, respectively. Overall survival at 3 years was estimated at 93%, and PFS at 61%.[121]

Rituximab is now part of the treatment strategies for most patients with NHL. However, most, if not all, patients eventually relapse and require further therapy. Retreatment of follicular or low-grade NHL with rituximab has an OR of 40% and CR of 11%, with a second response and time to progression that seem to be longer than with the initial antibody therapy. Both ^{131}I-tositumomab and ^{90}Y-ibritumomab tiuxetan have been shown to be effective in patients who relapse after or are resistant to rituximab.[122] The outcome for patients treated first with a radiolabeled antibody and then with an unconjugated antibody has not been evaluated. However, patients may not tolerate other therapy after failing RIT. A general approach in NHL is to use rituximab after chemotherapy failure, followed by RIT if rituximab fails.

Radiolabeled MAb for Leukemia[123]
Radiolabeled MAb targeted to lineage-specific antigens have been safely administered to patients with leukemia. ^{90}Y–anti-CD25 was active in acute T-cell leukemia (2 CR, 7 PR among 16 evaluable patients),[124] and myelosuppression was the main toxicity. ^{131}I-anti-CD33 (AML, MDS, myeloblastic CML),[125,126] ^{90}Y–anti-CD33,[123] ^{131}I-anti-CD45 (AML, ALL, MDS),[127] [188]Re-anti-CD66c (AML, ALL, CML),[128] all delivered significant radiation doses to the bone marrow and are particularly effective as part of a conditioning regimen for hematopoietic stem cell transplantation. Radioconjugates that emit α-particles ([213]Bi–anti-CD33 and [225]Ac–anti-CD33) may be better suited for the treatment of small-volume disease.[129,130]

Radioimmunotherapy of Solid Tumors (see Table 32-5)
The antitumor activity of RIT in solid tumors is less impressive. Intrathecal and intraventricular administration

for leptomeningeal carcinomatosis and intratumoral therapy of malignant brain tumors using [131]I-81C6 (anti-tenascin MAb) have produced objective responses and prolonged patient survival.[131,132] [211]At-81C6 is an example of α-particle therapy for minimal residual disease in malignant glioma.[133] Intravenous anti-GD2 [131]I-3F8 was tested in children with metastatic neuroblastoma (n = 24, 6–28 mCi/kg).[134] Responses were seen in both soft tissue masses and bone marrow. The use of myeloablative [131]I-3F8 (20 mCi/kg) to consolidate remission was tested in 35 patients (> 1 y of age) with newly diagnosed stage 4 neuroblastoma.[29] Extramedullary toxicities were limited to hypothyroidism, which occurred despite aggressive thyroid protection using potassium iodide, liothyronine (T3), and potassium perchlorate. [131]I-3F8 also was tested in RIT for GD2-positive leptomeningeal cancers in children and adults by intraventricular administration, with estimated radiation doses of 14.9 to 56 cGy/mCi to the cerebrospinal fluid and less than 2 cGy/mCi to blood and other organs outside the central nervous system.[135] A number of radiolabeled MAb have been tested in colorectal cancer with variable clinical benefit: ^{131}I-B72.3, ^{131}I–anti-CEA, ^{90}Y-CC49 (a second-generation murine B72.3 pancarcinoma antibody), ^{131}I-A33 or ^{131}I-CC49, at myeloablative doses (50 to 300 mCi/m²).[83] ^{131}I-hMN-14 (humanized anti-CEA IgG, 60 mCi/m²) has been administered to patients in remission or with small-volume colorectal metastasis; the potential for long-term benefit will have to await the results of formal randomized trials to be determined.[83]

Multistep Targeting

To improve tumor uptake and reduce systemic toxicity, a multistep procedure that pretargets the antibody before the binding of the cytotoxic ligand to the tumor has been employed successfully. Generally, a tumor-specific antibody is conjugated to a ligand binder, such as streptavidin or avidin (with high affinity for biotin) or ligand-specific antibody (binding to metal chelators such as diethylenetriamine pentaacetic acid [DTPA] or 1,4,7,10-tetraacetic acid [DOTA]).[89,136] In the first step, these antibody-streptavidin or F(ab')2-streptavidin conjugates (172–200 kd) are allowed to localize to tumors in vivo, and any excess is cleared from the blood. A small radiolabeled ligand (or its biotinylated form) is then injected intravenously. By virtue of the high-affinity interaction, the ligand penetrates tissues rapidly and is strongly taken up by the antibody conjugate at the tumor site. Unbound ligand is quickly excreted through the kidneys. Because of the short transit time of the toxic ligand (radionuclides or toxins), a substantial improvement in the therapeutic ratio is achievable without sacrificing the percent injected dose per gram in tumor. Multistep targeting of 200 mCi of ^{90}Y–DOTA is well-tolerated except for dose-limiting gastrointestinal toxicity thought to be related to MAb NT-LU-10 cross-reactivity with the gut.[137] A similar approach applied to NHL (using anti-CD20 MAb) also achieved tumor responses in both preclinical and Phase I/II studies.[138] A three-step approach, which uses biotinylated MAb, followed by avidin/streptavidin, and then by biotinylated radiometal chelate, has also been successful.[91,92] The bispecific antibody pretargeting system takes advantage of a bivalent hapten, which binds to the two arms of a tumor-localizing bispecific antibody.[83] These pretargeting concepts have the potential to be extended to other small ligands in addition to radioisotopes.

Immunocytokines

Cell-mediated cytotoxicity has been highly effective against tumors in vitro and in animal models. Immunocytokines[84,139] have shown remarkable success in activating and redirecting effectors to human tumors. Most of these studies have focused on NK, NKT or T cells,[84] and granulocytes.[19] Antibody-IL2 immunocytokine can eradicate metastatic murine neuroblastoma while inducing long-term antitumor immunity.[84,139] Following initial successes with IL2 immunocytokine, constructs containing other cytokines also have been tested with encouraging results.[84] These include IL12, tumor necrosis factor, and lymphotoxin. This emerging technology has been successfully applied to a number of antigens and tumor models, including GD2, human epithelial cell adhesion molecule (huEpCAM), CEA, EGF-R, HER2/neu, folate receptor, and B-cell idiotype. More recently, the combination of a plasmid DNA vaccine and IL-2 immunocytokine in the mouse model was shown to be more effective than when either was administered alone.[140] KS-IL2 (anticolorectal CA) and 14.18-IL2 (anti-GD2) both are in clinical trials; their toxicity profiles are generally acceptable, but clinical efficacy yet to be established.

Drug-Antibody Conjugates and ADEPT

To enhance the effector functions of MAbs, drugs have been conjugated to MAb for selective tumor delivery. Doxorubicin, melphalan, methotrexate, and vinca alkaloids conjugated to MAb have limited clinical success. BR96-doxorubicin directed at Lewis Y antigen has shown no clinical benefit in phase II trials in breast cancer[141] or gastric cancer.[142] Drugs and even DNA have been packaged in stealth (pegylated) liposomes coated with MAb or their fragments (e.g., scFv) for delivery to tumors.[143] However, slow extravasation of these liposomes into tissue space can be a limitation. Another novel approach, ADEPT, uses MAb to deliver a covalently conjugated enzyme to the tumor, which can then activate a nontoxic prodrug.[86,144] Despite preclinical successes, ADEPT has been difficult to translate into clinical benefit. Significant impediments to broadening its clinical implementation include immunogenicity of antibody-enzyme conjugate, as well as the presence of endogenous enzymes or endogenous substrates and endogenous inhibitors of these enzymes within tumors.

IMMUNOTOXINS

Ribosome-inactivating toxins can be potent cancer drugs. One major limitation is the lack of tumor selectivity.[145] Two-chain toxins (e.g., ricin and diphtheria toxin [DT]) utilize their B chain for cell-binding and their A chain for inhibition of protein synthesis; other toxins (e.g., *Pseudomonas* exotoxin [PE], pokeweed antiviral protein [PAP], gelonin) have a built-in site for cell attachment. When conjugated to MAb, they become immunotoxins. These toxins can be genetically modified for MAb conjugation and improved safety profile.[85] In recombinant toxins (e.g., PE40, PE38, or diphtheria toxin DAB$_{486}$), the cell-binding domains are replaced by scFv.[85,145]

Various monoclonal MAb have been conjugated to different toxins for clinical trials[145]: ricin toxin A-chain (RTA to anti-CD7, anti-CD22, and anti-CD25); DT (anti-IL2R); and PE (anti-CD25, anti-CD22, anti-Lewis Y, and anti-HER2). A common toxicity is the vascular leak syndrome, characterized by marked fluid overload, dyspnea, and sensorimotor neuropathies.[146] Deglycosylated RTA devoid of mannose and fucose has reduced hepatic sequestration, allowing longer serum half-life. An OR of 31% (2.6% CR, 29% PR) was achieved in patients with NHL following anti-CD22 deglycosylated RTA treatment.[147] Among 16 patients with cladribine-resistant hairy cell leukemia, anti-CD22-dsFv-PE (RFB4[dsFv]-PE38, BL22) induced 11 CR and 2 PR.[148] In addition to transient hypoalbuminemia and elevated aminotransferase levels, two patients had serious but reversible hemolytic uremic syndrome. Other highly toxic natural compounds also have been explored recently, for example, calicheamicins[149] and maytansinoids.[150] Gemtuzumab ozogamicin (Mylotarg) is an anti-CD33 antibody conjugated to calicheamicin. Acting like a prodrug, calicheamicin is released from the antibody following internalization, forming a diradical that induces double-strand DNA breaks. Gemtuzumab achieved a 30% response rate among refractory AML patients 60 years of age or older, with tolerable side effects, including fever, chills, and reversible neutropenia.[149] Anti-mucin MAb-calicheamicin conjugate has not been successful thus far.[151] With most immunotoxins, immunogenicity can be a major constraint. Whereas pegylation may reduce immunogenicity,[152] cytotoxic human proteins (e.g., human ribonuclease angiogenin) may circumvent this issue.[153]

Cellular Immunoconjugates with Bispecific Antibodies[88,154,155]

Tumor-selective MAb can be rendered cytophilic by conjugation with MAb specific for trigger molecules on T lymphocytes, NK cells, and granulocytes. These molecules include CD3, CD28, Fc receptors (CD64, CD16), and FcαRI (CD89).[88] One binding site of the bispecific antibody engages CD3 on T-cells; the other binding site determines tumor specificity e.g., B-NHL (CD19),[156] breast cancer (HER-2),[157] and Hodgkin's lymphoma (CD30).[158] Similar successes have been reported for the trigger molecule CD28 for ALL (CD19 and CD20)[159,160] and Hodgkin's disease.[161] Bispecific MAb targeted at FcγRI can redirect ADCC to specific tumors, including epithelial cancer (EGF-R),[162] and breast cancer (HER-2),[163] while those directed at FcγRIII have been successful against Hodgkin's disease (CD30)[164] and breast cancer (HER-2).[163] Because serum IgG competes for FcR, MAb made to recognize the FcR outside its Fc-binding site have been developed to circumvent this concern. Although bispecific MAb have potential in targeting small ligands (e.g., in multistep targeting), their clinical application in cellular immunoconjugates has been complicated by the generalized cytokine release from leukocytes and the inherent limitations of trafficking of effector cells into tumors.[154]

IMPROVING THE EFFICACY OF ANTIBODY-BASED CANCER THERAPIES[165]

To reduce the immunogenicity, MAb have been chimerized and humanized, or cloned from phage display libraries,[166] or produced in human IgG-transgenic or human transchromosomal mice (see Fig. 32-2). Chimeric MAb are made by joining the antigen-combining variable domains of a mouse MAb to human constant domains: mouse VL to human CL and mouse VH to human CH1–CH2–CH3.[46] In humanized MAb, the antigen-binding loops, known as complementarity-determining regions (CDRs) from a mouse MAb are grafted into a human IgG.[167] Human antibodies also can be derived from single-chain variable fragments (scFv) or Fab phage display libraries,[168] particularly useful for self-antigens.[169] Alternatively, human MAb can be made from hIgG-transgenic mice.[170]

Because Fc is necessary for antitumor effect, chimerizing mouse MAb with human γ1 and γ3 can improve ADCC and CDC functions. Similarly, removing FcγRIIB inhibitory receptor recognition also can enhance antitumor activity.[13] Point mutations in the Fc region increase affinity for activation receptor or decrease its affinity for the inhibitory receptor.[171] Glycosylation of IgG at Asn297 stabilizes the tertiary structure of the C$_H$2 domain, which is critical for effector function.[81] Glycosylation depends on the producer line, and increasing the bisected complex oligosaccharides in the Fc region has enhanced ADCC.[82] Complement-dependent cytotoxicity also can be improved by Fc region mutations to increase C1q binding.[172]

The antigen-binding affinity, molecular architecture, and oligomerization states of MAb can be reengineered to enhance tumor delivery and therapy.[173] For example, affinity can be increased using phage display libraries,[174] ribosome display,[175] DNA shuffling,[176] or yeast display combined with DNA shuffling.[177] However, because the "binding-site" barrier can impede tumor penetration if the MAb has high affinity,[178] the optimal MAb may indeed be a low-affinity IgG binding to a surface antigen expressed at high density (e.g., GD2 on neuroblastoma). In addition, the size of the MAb is critical. ScFv are small (25 kd) and rapidly cleared by the kidney. On the other hand, oligomers with MW in the range of 100 to 200 kd should be ideal for tumor targeting. Besides increasing avidity, oligomerization can increase antitumor activity through a multitude of mechanisms, including CDC/ADCC, induction of apoptosis, growth arrest, and synergy with chemotherapy or immunotoxins.[8] Using scFv as the building blocks, novel fusion proteins such as scFv-streptavidin can be highly effective platforms for multistep targeting.[179,180]

Science of Clinical Oncology

ALTERNATIVE TARGETS FOR ANTICANCER ANTIBODIES

Besides the ability to block receptors from interaction with their natural ligand, MAb can inhibit receptor dimerization or receptor interaction with coreceptors.[181] ErbB2 is a ligandless member of the ErbB receptor family that functions as a coreceptor with HER1/EGFR, HER3, and HER4. MAb 2C4 sterically hinders the recruitment of HER2into HER ligand complexes and inhibits in vitro and in vivo growth of breast and prostate tumors. The humanized antibody Omnitarg currently is in clinical trial. Most of the MAb targeting effort has been focused on individual tumor cells, but alternative strategies directed at tumor neovasculature[182] or tumor stroma[183] are promising approaches. MAb can be made to neutralize the angiogenic factor VEGF (e.g., bevacizumab [Avastin]),[184] or to block the VEGF-R2/KDR (e.g., IMC-1C11, chimeric anti-KDR).[185,186] Targeting tumor vasculature may have significant advantages over direct tumor targeting,[187] in that endothelial cells, unlike tumor cells, are less likely to acquire resistance. Another angiogenesis target is αVβ3 integrin, which initiates endothelial proliferation, migration, and matrix remodeling.[188] The chimeric IgG1 (MEDI-522), based on the preclinical antitumor activity of MAb specific for αVβ3,[189] currently is in clinical trial in patients with colorectal cancer.

CAN ONE SIZE FIT ALL?
Human tumors and their response to MAb-based therapies are heterogeneous. Although MAb share common structures and properties, the successful translation of their antitumor activity into survival benefit in patients requires a much better appreciation of the clinical biology of each individual tumor type, as well as an understanding of the fundamental biology of the antigens being targeted.

IS THERE AN OPTIMAL TIME TO USE MAb THERAPY?
It is likely that MAb therapy is most beneficial at the time of minimal residual disease (MRD). Accurate and sensitive measures of MRD will provide objective indicators of tumor response to help guide clinicians to apply this modality more effectively.

WHAT IS THE FUTURE ROLE OF ANTIBODY THERAPY IN TREATING CANCER?
As a rapidly expanding class of pharmaceuticals, MAb are now an important modality for cancer treatment. They have demonstrated antitumor activity in a broad spectrum of malignancies in the last two decades. The successful integration of MAb and immunoconjugates with other treatment modalities has the potential for achieving further improvements in symptom control and patient survival.

REFERENCES

1. Koehler G, Milstein C: Continuous culture of fused cells secreting antibody of pre-defined specificity. Nature 1975;256:495–496.
2. Jacobsohn DA: Novel therapeutics for the treatment of graft-versus-host disease. Expert Opin Investig Drugs 2002;11:1271–1280.
3. Hale G: Alemtuzumab in stem cell transplantation. Med Oncol 2002;19(suppl):S33–S47.
4. Levy R, Miller RA: Therapy of lymphoma directed at idiotypes. J Natl Cancer Inst Monogr 1990;(10)61–68.
5. Bhattacharya-Chatterjee M, Foon KA: Anti-idiotype antibody vaccine therapies of cancer. Cancer Treat Res 1998;94:51–68.
6. Shan D, Ledbetter JA, Press OW: Apoptosis of malignant human B cells by ligation of CD20 with monoclonal antibodies. Blood 1998;91:1644–1652.
7. Maloney DG, Smith B, Rose A: Rituximab: mechanism of action and resistance. Semin Oncol 2002;29:2–9.
8. Ghetie MA, Bright H, Vitetta ES: Homodimers but not monomers of Rituxan (chimeric anti-CD20) induce apoptosis in human B-lymphoma cells and synergize with a chemotherapeutic agent and an immunotoxin. Blood 2001;97:1392–1398.
9. Chaouchi N, Vazquez A, Galanaud P, Leprince C: B cell antigen receptor-mediated apoptosis. Importance of accessory molecules CD19 and CD22, and of surface IgM cross-linking. J Immunol 1995;154:3096–3104.
10. Mendelsohn J: Antibody-mediated EGF receptor blockade as an anticancer therapy: from the laboratory to the clinic. Cancer Immunol Immunother 2003;52:342–346.
11. Drebin JA, Link VC, Weinberg RA, Greene MI: Inhibition of tumor growth by a monoclonal antibody reactive with an oncogene-encoded tumor antigen. Proc Natl Acad Sci USA 1986;83:9129–9133.
12. Prewett M, Huber J, Li Y, et al: Antivascular endothelial growth factor receptor (fetal liver kinase 1) monoclonal antibody inhibits tumor angiogenesis and growth of several mouse and human tumors. Cancer Res 1999;59:5209–5218.
13. Ravetch JV, Bolland S: IgG Fc receptors. Annu Rev Immunol 2001;19:275–290.
14. Ghetie V, Ward ES: Multiple roles for the major histocompatibility complex class I-related receptor FcRn. Annu Rev Immunol 2000;18:739–766.
15. Cartron G, Dacheux L, Salles G, et al: Therapeutic activity of humanized anti-CD20 monoclonal antibody and polymorphism in IgG Fc receptor FcgammaRIIIa gene. Blood 2002;99:754–758.
16. Kimberly RP, Wu J, Gibson AW, et al: Diversity and duplicity: human FCgamma receptors in host defense and autoimmunity. Immunol Res 2002;26:177–189.
17. Dechant M, Vidarsson G, Stockmeyer B, et al: Chimeric IgA antibodies against HLA class II effectively trigger lymphoma cell killing. Blood 2002;100:4574–4580.
18. Ottonello L, Epstein AL, Dapino P, Barbera P, Morone P, Dallegri F: Monoclonal Lym-1 antibody-dependent cytolysis by neutrophils exposed to granulocyte-macrophage colony-stimulating factor: intervention of FcgammaRII (CD32), CD11b-CD18 integrins, and CD66b glycoproteins. Blood 1999;93:3505–3511.
19. Metelitsa LS, Gillies SD, Super M, Shimada H, Reynolds CP, Seeger RC: Antidisialoganglioside/granulocyte macrophage-colony-stimulating factor fusion protein facilitates neutrophil antibody-dependent cellular cytotoxicity and depends on FcgammaRII (CD32) and Mac-1 (CD11b/CD18) for enhanced effector cell adhesion and azurophil granule exocytosis. Blood 2002;99:4166–4173.
20. Kushner BH, Cheung NK: Absolute requirement of CD11/CD18 adhesion molecules, FcRII and the phosphatidylinositol-linked FcRIII for monoclonal antibody-mediated neutrophil antihuman tumor cytotoxicity. Blood 1992;79:1484–1490.
21. Edwards BS, Nolla HA, Hoffman RR: Resolution of adhesion- and activation-associated components of monoclonal antibody-dependent human NK cell-mediated cytotoxicity. Cell Immunol 1992;144:55–68.
22. Kushner BH, Cheung NK: GM-CSF enhances 3F8 monoclonal antibody-dependent cellular cytotoxicity against human melanoma and neuroblastoma. Blood 1989;73:1936–1941.

23. Vaickus L, Biddle W, Cemerlic D, Foon KA: Interferon gamma augments Lym-1-dependent, granulocyte-mediated tumor cell lysis. Blood 1990;75:2408–2416.

24. Masucci G, Ragnhammar P, Wersall P, Mellstedt H: Granulocyte-monocyte colony-stimulating-factor augments the interleukin-2-induced cytotoxic activity of human lymphocytes in the absence and presence of mouse or chimeric monoclonal antibodies (mAb 17-1A). Cancer Immunol Immunother 1990;31:231–235.

25. Munn DH, Cheung NK: Interleukin-2 enhancement of monoclonal antibody-mediated cellular cytotoxicity (ADCC) against human melanoma. Cancer Res 1987;47:6600–6605.

26. Sondel PM, Hank JA: Combination therapy with interleukin-2 and antitumor monoclonal antibodies. Cancer J Sci Am 1997;3(suppl 1):S121–S127.

27. Hjelm Skog A, Ragnhammar P, Fagerberg J, et al: Clinical effects of monoclonal antibody 17-1A combined with granulocyte/macrophage-colony-stimulating factor and interleukin-2 for treatment of patients with advanced colorectal carcinoma. Cancer Immunol Immunother 1999;48:463–470.

28. Kimby E: Beyond immunochemotherapy: combinations of rituximab with cytokines interferon-alpha2a and granulocyte colony stimulating factor. Semin Oncol 2002;29:7–10.

29. Cheung NK, Kushner BH, Kramer K: Monoclonal antibody-based therapy of neuroblastoma. Hematol Oncol Clin North Am 2001;15:853–866.

30. Tao MH, Smith RI, Morrison SL: Structural features of human immunoglobulin G that determine isotype-specific differences in complement activation. J Exp Med 1993;178:661–667.

31. Golay J, Zaffaroni L, Vaccari T, et al: Biologic response of B lymphoma cells to anti-CD20 monoclonal antibody rituximab in vitro: CD55 and CD59 regulate complement-mediated cell lysis. Blood 2000;95:3900–3908.

32. Gorter A, Meri S: Immune evasion of tumor cells using membrane-bound complement regulatory proteins. Immunol Today 1999;20:576–582.

33. Juhl H, Helmig F, Baltzer K, Kalthoff H, Henne-Bruns D, Kremer B: Frequent expression of complement resistance factors CD46, CD55, and CD59 on gastrointestinal cancer cells limits the therapeutic potential of monoclonal antibody 17-1A. J Surg Oncol 1997;64:222–230.

34. Niehans GA, Cherwitz DL, Staley NA, Knapp DJ, Dalmasso AP: Human carcinomas variably express the complement inhibitory proteins CD46 (membrane cofactor protein), CD55 (decay-accelerating factor), and CD59 (protectin). Am J Pathol 1996;149:129–142.

35. Chen S, Caragine T, Cheung NKV, Tomlinson S: CD59 expressed on a tumor cell surface modulates decay-accelerating factor expression and enhances tumor growth in a rat model of human neuroblastoma. Cancer Res 2000;60:3013–3018.

36. Jurianz K, Ziegler S, Garcia-Schuler H, et al: Complement resistance of tumor cells: basal and induced mechanisms. Mol Immunol 1999;36:929–939.

37. Ross GD, Vetvicka V, Yan J, Xia Y, Vetvickova J: Therapeutic intervention with complement and beta-glucan in cancer. Immunopharmacology 1999;42:61–74.

38. Hugli TE, Muller-Eberhard HJ: Anaphylatoxins: C3a and C5a. Adv Immunol 1978;26:1–53.

39. McLaughlin P, Grillo-Lopez AJ, Kink BK, et al: Rituximab chimeric anti-CD20 monoclonal antibody therapy for relapsed indolent lymphoma: half of patients respond to four-dose treatment program. J Clin Oncol 1998;16:2825–2833.

40. Grillo-Lopez AJ, Hedrick E, Rashford M, Benyunes M: Rituximab: ongoing and future clinical development. Semin Oncol 2002;29:105–112.

41. van der Kolk LE, Grillo-Lopez AJ, Baars JW, Hack CE, van Oers MH: Complement activation plays a key role in the side-effects of rituximab treatment. Br J Haematol 2001;115:807–811.

42. Byrd JC, Waselenko JK, Maneatis TJ, et al: Rituximab therapy in hematologic malignancy patients with circulating blood tumor cells: association with increased infusion-related side effects and rapid blood tumor clearance. J Clin Oncol 1999;17:791–795.

43. Demidem A, Lam T, Alas S, Hariharan K, Hanna N, Bonavida B: Chimeric anti-CD20 (IDEC-C2B8) monoclonal antibody sensitizes a B cell lymphoma cell line to cell killing by cytotoxic drugs. Cancer Biother Radiopharm 1997;12:177–186.

44. Coiffier B: Monoclonal antibodies combined to chemotherapy for the treatment of patients with lymphoma. Blood Rev 2003;17:25–31.

45. Coiffier B, Lepage E, Briere J, et al: CHOP chemotherapy plus rituximab compared with CHOP alone in elderly patients with diffuse large-B-cell lymphoma. N Engl J Med 2002;346:235–242.

46. Cesano A, Gayko U: CD22 as a target of passive immunotherapy. Semin Oncol 2003;30:253–257.

47. Wahl AF, Klussman K, Thompson JD, et al: The anti-CD30 monoclonal antibody SGN-30 promotes growth arrest and DNA fragmentation in vitro and affects antitumor activity in models of Hodgkin's disease. Cancer Res 2002;62:3736–3742.

48. Jurcic JG, DeBlasio T, Dumont L, Yao TJ, Scheinberg DA: Molecular remission induction with retinoic acid and anti-CD33 monoclonal antibody HuM195 in acute promyelocytic leukemia. Clin Cancer Res 2000;6:372–380.

49. Caron PC, Dumont L, Scheinberg DA: Supersaturating infusional humanized anti-CD33 monoclonal antibody HuM195 in myelogenous leukemia. Clin Cancer Res 1998;4:1421–1428.

50. Uppenkamp M, Engert A, Diehl V, Bunjes D, Huhn D, Brittinger G: Monoclonal antibody therapy with CAMPATH-1H in patients with relapsed high- and low-grade non-Hodgkin's lymphomas: a multicenter phase I/II study. Ann Hematol 2002;81:26–32.

51. Keating MJ, Flinn I, Jain V, et al: Therapeutic role of alemtuzumab (Campath-1H) in patients who have failed fludarabine: results of a large international study. Blood 2002;99:3554–3561.

52. Chakrabarti S, Mackinnon S, Chopra R, et al: High incidence of cytomegalovirus infection after nonmyeloablative stem cell transplantation: potential role of Campath-1H in delaying immune reconstitution. Blood 2002;99:4357–4363.

53. Baselga J, Albanell J: Mechanism of action of anti-HER2 monoclonal antibodies. Ann Oncol 2001;12(suppl):S35–S41.

54. Cobleigh MA, Vogel CL, Tripathy D, et al: Multinational study of the efficacy and safety of humanized anti-HER2 monoclonal antibody in women who have HER2-overexpressing metastatic breast cancer that has progressed after chemotherapy for metastatic disease. J Clin Oncol 1999;17:2639–2648.

55. Bookman MA, Darcy KM, Clarke-Pearson D, Boothby RA, Horowitz IR: Evaluation of monoclonal humanized anti-HER2 antibody, trastuzumab, in patients with recurrent or refractory ovarian or primary peritoneal carcinoma with overexpression of HER2: a phase II trial of the Gynecologic Oncology Group. J Clin Oncol 2003;21:283–290.

56. Pegram MD, Slamon DJ: Combination therapy with trastuzumab (Herceptin) and cisplatin for chemoresistant metastatic breast cancer: evidence for receptor-enhanced chemosensitivity. Semin Oncol 1999;26:89–95.

57. Baselga J, Norton L, Albanell J, Kim YM, Mendelsohn J: Recombinant humanized anti-HER2 antibody (Herceptin) enhances the antitumor activity of paclitaxel and doxorubicin against HER2/neu overexpressing human breast cancer xenografts. Cancer Res 1998;58:2825–2831.

58. Slamon DJ, Leyland-Jones B, Shak S, et al: Use of chemotherapy plus a monoclonal antibody against HER2 for metastatic breast cancer that overexpresses HER2. N Engl J Med 2001;344:783–792.

59. Smith I: Future directions in the adjuvant treatment of breast cancer: the role of trastuzumab. Ann Oncol 2001;12(suppl):S75–S79.

60. Houghton AN, Mintzer D, Cordon-Cardo C, et al: Mouse monoclonal antibody detecting GD3 ganglioside: a phase I trial in patients with malignant melanoma. Proc Natl Acad Sci USA 1985;82:1242–1246.

61. Cheung NK, Lazarus H, Miraldi FD, et al: Ganglioside GD2 specific monoclonal antibody 3F8—a phase I study in patients with neuroblastoma and malignant melanoma. J Clin Oncol 1987;5:1430–1440.

62. Yu A, Uttenreuther-Fischer M, Huang C-S, et al: Phase I trial of a human-mouse chimeric anti-disialoganglioside monoclonal antibody ch14.18 in patients with refractory neuroblastoma and osteosarcoma. J Clin Oncol 1998;16:2169–2180.

63. Kushner BH, Kramer K, Cheung NKV: Phase II trial of the anti-G(D2) monoclonal antibody 3F8 and granulocyte-macrophage colony-stimulating factor for neuroblastoma. J Clin Oncol 2001;19:4189–4194.

64. Cheung NK, Kushner BH, Yeh SD, Larson SM: 3F8 monoclonal antibody treatment of patients with stage 4 neuroblastoma: a phase II study. Int J Oncol 1998;12:1299–1306.

65. Cheung IY, Lo Piccolo MS, Kushner BH, Kramer K, Cheung NK: Quantitation of GD2 synthase mRNA by real-time reverse transcriptase polymerase chain reaction: clinical utility in evaluating adjuvant therapy in neuroblastoma. J Clin Oncol 2003;21:1087–1093.

66. Cheung NK, Cheung IY, Canete A, et al: Antibody response to murine anti-GD2 monoclonal antibodies: correlation with patient survival. Cancer Res 1994;54:2228–2233.

67. Cheung NK, Guo HF, Heller G, Cheung IY: Induction of Ab3 and Ab3′ antibody was associated with long-term survival after anti-G(D2) antibody therapy of stage 4 neuroblastoma. Clin Cancer Res 2000;6:2653–2660.

68. Riethmuller G, Holz E, Schlimok G, et al: Monoclonal antibody therapy for resected Dukes' C colorectal cancer: seven-year outcome of a multicenter randomized trial. J Clin Oncol 1998;16:1788–1794.

69. Lanzavecchia A, Abrignani S, Scheidegger D, Obrist R, Dorken B, Moldenhauer G: Antibodies as antigens. The use of mouse monoclonal antibodies to focus human T cells against selected targets. J Exp Med 1988;167:345–352.

70. Fagerberg J, Frodin JE, Ragnhammar P, Steinitz M, Wigzell H, Mellstedt H: Induction of an immune network cascade in cancer patients treated with monoclonal antibodies (ab1). II. Is induction of anti-idiotype reactive T cells (T3) of importance for tumor response to mAb therapy? Cancer Immunol Immunother 1994;38:149–159.

71. Herlyn D, Somasundaram R, Zaloudik J, et al: Anti-idiotype and recombinant antigen in immunotherapy of colorectal cancer. Cell Biophys 1994;24/25:143–153. MEDLINE

72. Berek JS, Schultes BC, Nicodemus CF: Biologic and immunologic therapies for ovarian cancer. J Clin Oncol 2003;21:168–174.

73. Amigorena S: Fc gamma receptors and cross-presentation in dendritic cells. J Exp Med 2002;195:F1–3, 2002

74. Needle MN: Safety experience with IMC-C225, an anti-epidermal growth factor receptor antibody. Semin Oncol 2002;29:55–60.

75. Hosono M, Endo K, Sakahara H, et al: Human/mouse chimeric antibodies show low reactivity with human anti-murine antibodies (HAMA). Br J Cancer 1992;65:197–200.

76. Morrison SL, Johnson MJ, Herzenberg LA, Oi VT: Chimeric human antibody molecules: mouse antigen-binding domains with human constant region domains. Proc Natl Acad Sci USA 1984;81:6851–6855.

77. Newman R, Alberts J, Anderson D, et al: "Primatization" of recombinant antibodies for immunotherapy of human diseases: a macaque/human chimeric antibody against human CD4. Biotechnology (N Y) 1992;10:1455–1460.

78. Queen C, Schneider WP, Selick HE, et al: A humanized antibody that binds to the interleukin 2 receptor. Proc Natl Acad Sci USA 1989;86:10029–10033.

79. Davis TA, Maloney DG, Czerwinski DK, Liles TM, Levy R: Anti-idiotype antibodies can induce long-term complete remissions in non-Hodgkin's lymphoma without eradicating the malignant clone. Blood 1998;92:1184–1190.

80. Lundin J, Osterborg A, Brittinger G, et al: CAMPATH-1H monoclonal antibody in therapy for previously treated low-grade Non-Hodgkin's lymphomas: a phase II multicenter study. J Clin Oncol 1998;16:3257–3263.

81. Wright A, Morrison SL: Effect of glycosylation on antibody function: implications for genetic engineering. Trends Biotechnol 1997;15:26–32.

82. Umana P, Jean-Mairet J, Moudry R, Amstutz H, Bailey JE: Engineered glycoforms of an antineuroblastoma IgG1 with optimized antibody-dependent cellular cytotoxic activity. Nat Biotechnol 1999;17:176–180.

83. Goldenberg DM: Advancing role of radiolabeled antibodies in the therapy of cancer. Cancer Immunol Immunother 2002;52:281–296.

84. Davis CA, Gillies SA: Immunocytokines: amplification of anti-cancer immunity. Cancer Immunol Immunother 2003;52:297–308.

85. Pastan I: Immunotoxins containing Pseudomonas exotoxin A: a short history. Cancer Immunol Immunother 2003;52:338–341.

86. Springer CJ, Niculescu-Duvaz II: Antibody-directed enzyme prodrug therapy (ADEPT): a review. Adv Drug Deliv Rev 1997;26:151–172.

87. Allen TM, Sapra P, Moase E, Moreira J, Iden D: Adventures in targeting. J Liposome Res 2002;12:5–12.

88. van Spriel AB, van Ojik HH, van De Winkel JG: Immunotherapeutic perspective for bispecific antibodies. Immunol Today 2000;21:391–397.

89. Boerman OC, van Schaijk FG, Oyen WJ, Corstens FH: Pretargeted radioimmunotherapy of cancer: progress step by step. J Nucl Med 2003;44:400–411.

90. Goldenberg DM, Chang CH, Sharkey RM, et al: Radio-immunotherapy: Is avidin-biotin pretargeting the preferred choice among pretargeting methods? Eur J Nucl Med Mol Imaging 2003;30:777–780.

91. Paganelli G, Bartolomei M, Ferrari M, et al: Pre-targeted locoregional radioimmunotherapy with 90Y-biotin in glioma patients: phase I study and preliminary therapeutic results. Cancer Biother Radiopharm 2001;16:227–235.

92. Cremonesi M, Ferrari M, Chinol M, et al: Three-step radioimmunotherapy with yttrium-90 biotin: dosimetry and pharmacokinetics in cancer patients. Eur J Nucl Med 1999;26:110–120.

93. Cheung NK, Landmeier B, Neely J, et al: Complete tumor ablation with iodine 131-radiolabeled disialoganglioside GD2-specific monoclonal antibody against human neuroblastoma xenografted in nude mice. J Natl Cancer Inst 1986;77:739–745.

94. Buchegger F, Pfister C, Fournier K, et al: Ablation of human colon carcinoma in nude mice by 131I-labeled monoclonal anti-carcinoembryonic antigen antibody F(ab′)2 fragments. J Clin Invest 1989;83:1449–1456.

95. Badger CC, Krohn KA, Shulman H, Flurnoy N, Bernstein ID: Experimental radioimmunotherapy of murine lymphoma with 131I-labeled anti T cell antibodies. Cancer Res 1986;46:6223–6228.

96. McDevitt MR, Sgouros G, Finn RD, et al: Radioimmunotherapy with alpha-emitting nuclides. Eur J Nucl Med 1998;25:1341–1351.

97. Sgouros G, Ballangrud AM, Jurcic JG, et al: Pharmacokinetics and dosimetry of an alpha-particle emitter labeled antibody: 213Bi-HuM 195 (anti-CD33) in patients with leukemia. J Nucl Med 1999;40:1935–1946.

98. Zalutsky MR, Zhao XG, Alston KL, Bigner D: High-level production of alpha-particle-emitting (211)At and preparation of (211)At-labeled antibodies for clinical use. J Nucl Med 2001;42:1508–1515.

99. Zalutsky MR, Vaidyanathan G: Astatine-211-labeled radiotherapeutics: an emerging approach to targeted alpha-particle radiotherapy. Curr Pharm Des 2000;6:1433–1455.

100. Wiseman GA, Kornmehl E, Leigh B, et al: Radiation dosimetry results and safety correlations from 90Y-ibritumomab tiuxetan radioimmunotherapy for relapsed or refractory non-Hodgkin's lymphoma: combined data from 4 clinical trials. J Nucl Med 2003;44:465–474.

101. Witzig TE, White CA, Gordon LI, et al: Safety of yttrium-90 ibritumomab tiuxetan radioimmunotherapy for relapsed low-grade, follicular, or transformed non-Hodgkin's lymphoma. J Clin Oncol 2003;21:1263–1270.

102. Wiseman GA, Gordon LI, Multani PS, et al: Ibritumomab tiuxetan radioimmunotherapy for patients with relapsed or refractory non-Hodgkin's lymphoma and mild thrombocytopenia: a phase II multicenter trial. Blood 2002;99:4336–4342.

103. Kaminski MS, Estes J, Zasadny KR, et al: Radioimmunotherapy with iodine (131)I tositumomab for relapsed or refractory B-cell non-Hodgkin's lymphoma: updated results and long-term follow-up of the University of Michigan experience. Blood 2000;96:1259–1266.

104. Johnson TA, Press OW: Therapy of B-cell lymphomas with monoclonal antibodies and radioimmunoconjugates: the Seattle experience. Ann Hematol 2000;79:175–182.

105. Liu SY, Eary JF, Petersdorf SH, et al: Follow-up of relapsed B-cell lymphoma patients treated with iodine-131-labeled anti-CD20 antibody and autologous stem-cell rescue. J Clin Oncol 1998;16:3270–3278.

106. Kaminski MS, Zelenetz AD, Press OW, et al: Pivotal study of iodine I 131 tositumomab for chemotherapy-refractory low-grade or transformed low-grade B-cell non-Hodgkin's lymphomas. J Clin Oncol 2001;19:3918–3928.

107. Press OW, Eary JF, Appelbaum FR, et al: Radiolabeled antibody therapy of B-cell lymphoma with autologous bone marrow support. N Engl J Med 1993;329:1219–1224.

108. O'Brien SM, Kantarjian H, Thomas DA, et al: Rituximab dose-escalation trial in chronic lymphocytic leukemia. J Clin Oncol 2001;19:2165–2170.

109. Byrd JC, Murphy T, Howard RS, et al: Rituximab using a thrice weekly dosing schedule in B-cell chronic lymphocytic leukemia and small lymphocytic lymphoma demonstrates clinical activity and acceptable toxicity. J Clin Oncol 2001;19:2153–2164.

110. Witzig TE, Gordon LI, Cabanillas F, et al: Randomized controlled trial of yttrium-90-labeled ibritumomab tiuxetan radioimmunotherapy versus rituximab immunotherapy for patients with relapsed or refractory low-grade, follicular, or transformed B-cell non-Hodgkin's lymphoma. J Clin Oncol 2002;20:2453–2463.

111. Juweid ME, Stadtmauer E, Hajjar G, et al: Pharmacokinetics, dosimetry, and initial therapeutic results with 131I- and (111)In-/90Y-labeled humanized LL2 anti-CD22 monoclonal antibody in patients with relapsed, refractory non-Hodgkin's lymphoma. Clin Cancer Res 1999;5:3292s–3303s.

112. Ma D, McDevitt MR, Barendswaard E, et al: Radioimmunotherapy for model B cell malignancies using 90Y-labeled anti-CD19 and anti-CD20 monoclonal antibodies. Leukemia 2002;16:60–66.

113. Lewis JP, Denardo GL, Denardo SJ: Radioimmunotherapy of lymphoma: a UC Davis experience. Hybridoma 1995;14:115–120.

114. DeNardo GL, DeNardo SJ, Goldstein DS, et al: Maximum-tolerated dose, toxicity, and efficacy of (131)I-Lym-1 antibody for fractionated radioimmunotherapy of non-Hodgkin's lymphoma. J Clin Oncol 1998;16:3246–3256.

115. DeNardo SJ, DeNardo GL, Kukis DL, et al: 67Cu-2IT-BAT-Lym-1 pharmacokinetics, radiation dosimetry, toxicity and tumor regression in patients with lymphoma. J Nucl Med 1999;40:302–310.

116. DeNardo GA, Bradt BA, Mirick GA, DeNardo SA: Human antiglobulin response to foreign antibodies: therapeutic benefit? Cancer Immunol Immunother 2003;52:309–316.

117. Scheinberg DA, Straus DJ, Yeh SD, et al: A phase I toxicity, pharmacology, and dosimetry trial of monoclonal antibody OKB7 in patients with non-Hodgkin's lymphoma: Effects of tumor burden and antigen expression. J Clin Oncol 1990;8:792–803.

118. Eary JF, Press OW, Badger CC, et al: Imaging and treatment of B-cell lymphoma. J Nucl Med 1990;31:1257–1268.

119. White CA, Halpern SE, Parker BA, et al: Radioimmunotherapy of relapsed B-cell lymphoma with yttrium 90 anti-idiotype monoclonal antibodies. Blood 1996;87:3640–3649.

120. Press OW, Eary JF, Gooley T, et al: A phase I/II trial of iodine-131-tositumomab (anti-CD20), etoposide, cyclo-phosphamide, and autologous stem cell transplantation for relapsed B-cell lymphomas. Blood 2000;96:2934–2942.

121. Gopal AK, Rajendran JG, Petersdorf SH, et al: High-dose chemo-radioimmunotherapy with autologous stem cell support for relapsed mantle cell lymphoma. Blood 2002;99:3158–3162.

122. Witzig TE, Flinn IW, Gordon LI, et al: Treatment with ibritumomab tiuxetan radioimmunotherapy in patients with rituximab-refractory follicular non-Hodgkin's lymphoma. J Clin Oncol 2002;20:3262–3269.

123. Burke JM, Jurcic JG, Scheinberg DA: Radioimmunotherapy for acute leukemia. Cancer Control 2002;9:106–113.

124. Waldmann TA, White JD, Carrasquillo JA, et al: Radio-immunotherapy of interleukin-2R alpha-expressing adult T-cell leukemia with Yttrium-90-labeled anti-Tac. Blood 1995;86:4063–4075.

125. Jurcic JG, Caron PC, Miller WH, Jr., et al: Sequential targeted therapy for relapsed acute promyelocytic leukemia with all-trans retinoic acid and anti-CD33 monoclonal antibody M195. Leukemia 1995;9:244–248.

126. Appelbaum FR, Matthews DC, Eary JF, et al: The use of radiolabeled anti-CD33 antibody to augment marrow irradiation prior to marrow transplantation for acute myelogenous leukemia. Transplantation 1992;54:829–833.

127. Matthews DC, Appelbaum FR, Eary JF, et al: Phase I study of (131)I-anti-CD45 antibody plus cyclophosphamide and total body irradiation for advanced acute leukemia and myelodysplastic syndrome. Blood 1999;94:1237–1247.

128. Bunjes D, Buchmann I, Duncker C, et al: Rhenium 188-labeled anti-CD66 (a, b, c, e) monoclonal antibody to intensify the conditioning regimen prior to stem cell transplantation for patients with high-risk acute myeloid leukemia or myelodysplastic syndrome: results of a phase I-II study. Blood 2001;98:565–572.

129. Jurcic JG, Larson SM, Sgouros G, et al: Targeted alpha particle immunotherapy for myeloid leukemia. Blood 2002;100:1233–1239.

130. McDevitt MR, Ma D, Lai LT, et al: Tumor therapy with targeted atomic nanogenerators. Science 2001;294:1537–1540.

131. Brown MT, Coleman RE, Friedman AH, et al: Intrathecal 131I-labeled antitenascin monoclonal antibody 81C6 treatment of patients with leptomeningeal neoplasms or primary brain tumor resection cavities with subarachnoid communication: phase I trial results. Clin Cancer Res 1996;2:963–972.

132. Reardon DA, Akabani G, Coleman RE, et al: Phase II trial of murine (131)I-labeled antitenascin monoclonal antibody 81C6 administered into surgically created resection cavities of patients with newly diagnosed malignant gliomas. J Clin Oncol 2002;20:1389–1397.

133. Zalutsky MR, Cokgor I, Akabani G, et al: Phase I trial of alpha-particle-emitting astatine-211 labeled chimeric anti-tenascin antibody in recurrent malignant glioma patients. Proc Am Assoc Cancer Res 2000;41:544. Abstract #3465.

134. Larson SM, Divgi C, Sgouros G, Cheung NKC, Scheinberg DA: Monoclonal antibodies: Basic principles—Radioisotope conjugates. In DeVita VT, Hellman S, Rosenberg SA (eds): Biologic Therapy of Cancer—Principles and Practice. Philadelphia, JB Lippincott 2000, pp 396–412.

135. Kramer K, Cheung NK, Humm JL, et al: Targeted radioimmunotherapy for leptomeningeal cancer using (131)I-3F8. Med Pediatr Oncol 2000;35:716–718.

136. Goldenberg DM: Targeted therapy of cancer with radiolabeled antibodies. J Nucl Med 2002;43:693–713.

137. Knox SJ, Goris ML, Tempero M, et al: Phase II trial of yttrium-90-DOTA-biotin pretargeted by NR-LU-10 antibody/streptavidin in patients with metastatic colon cancer. Clin Cancer Res 2000;6:406–414.

138. Weiden PL, Breitz HB, Press O, et al: Pretargeted radio-immunotherapy (PRIT) for treatment of non-Hodgkin's lymphoma (NHL): initial phase I/II study results. Cancer Biother Radiopharm 2000;15:15–29.

139. Lode HN, Reisfeld RA: Targeted cytokines for cancer immunotherapy. Immunol Res 2000;21:279–288.

140. Niethammer AG, Xiang R, Ruehlmann JM, et al: Targeted interleukin 2 therapy enhances protective immunity induced by an autologous oral DNA vaccine against murine melanoma. Cancer Res 2001;61:6178–6184.

141. Tolcher AW, Sugarman S, Gelmon KA, et al: Randomized phase II study of BR96-doxorubicin conjugate in patients with metastatic breast cancer. J Clin Oncol 1999;17:478–484.

142. Ajani JA, Kelsen DP, Haller D, Hargraves K, Healy D: A multi-institutional phase II study of BMS-182248-01 (BR96-doxorubicin conjugate) administered every 21 days in patients with advanced gastric adenocarcinoma. Cancer J 2000;6:78–81.

143. Park JW, Hong K, Kirpotin DB, Meyer O, Papahadjopoulos D, Benz CC: Anti-HER2 immunoliposomes for targeted therapy of human tumors. Cancer Lett 1997;118:153–160.

Science of Clinical Oncology

I

144. Syrigos KN, Epenetos AA: Antibody directed enzyme prodrug therapy (ADEPT): a review of the experimental and clinical considerations. Anticancer Res 1999;19:605–613.

145. Reiter Y: Recombinant immunotoxins in targeted cancer cell therapy. Adv Cancer Res 2001;81:93–124.

146. Longo DL, Duffey PL, Gribben JG, et al: Combination chemotherapy followed by an immunotoxin (anti-B4-blocked ricin) in patients with indolent lymphoma: results of a phase II study. Cancer J 2000;6:146–150.

147. Amlot PL, Stone MJ, Cunningham D, et al: A phase I study of an anti-CD22-deglycosylated ricin A chain immunotoxin in the treatment of B-cell lymphomas resistant to conventional therapy. Blood 1993;82:2624–2633.

148. Kreitman RJ, Wilson WH, Bergeron K, et al: Efficacy of the anti-CD22 recombinant immunotoxin BL22 in chemotherapy-resistant hairy-cell leukemia. N Engl J Med 2001;345:241–247.

149. Sievers EL, Larson RA, Stadtmauer EA, et al: Efficacy and safety of gemtuzumab ozogamicin in patients with CD33-positive acute myeloid leukemia in first relapse. J Clin Oncol 2001;19:3244–3254.

150. Liu C, Tadayoni BM, Bourret LA, et al: Eradication of large colon tumor xenografts by targeted delivery of maytanisinoids. Proc Natl Acad Sci USA 1996;93:8618–8623.

151. Pietersz GA, Wenjun L, Krauer K, Baker T, Wreschner D, McKenzie IF: Comparison of the biological properties of two anti-mucin-1 antibodies prepared for imaging and therapy. Cancer Immunol Immunother 1997;44:323–328.

152. Tsutsumi Y, Onda M, Nagata S, Lee B, Kreitman RJ, Pastan I: Site-specific chemical modification with polyethylene glycol of recombinant immunotoxin anti-Tac(Fv)-PE38 (LMB-2) improves antitumor activity and reduces animal toxicity and immunogenicity. Proc Natl Acad Sci USA 2000;97:8548–8553.

153. Suzuki M, Saxena SK, Boix E, et al: Engineering receptor-mediated cytotoxicity into human ribonucleases by steric blockade of inhibitor interaction. Nat Biotechnol 1999;17:265–270.

154. Friedrich SW, Lin SC, Stoll BR, Baxter LT: Antibody-directed effector cell therapy of tumors: analysis and optimization using a physiologically based pharmacokinetic model. Neoplasia 2002;4:449–463.

155. Scheffold C, Kornacker M, Scheffold YC, Contag CH, Negrin RS: Visualization of effective tumor targeting by CD8+ natural killer T cells redirected with bispecific antibody F(ab')(2)HER2xCD3. Cancer Res 2002;62:5785–5791.

156. Loffler A, Kufer P, Lutterbuse R, et al: A recombinant bispecific single-chain antibody, CD19 x CD3, induces rapid and high lymphoma-directed cytotoxicity by unstimulated T lymphocytes. Blood 2000;15:2098–2103.

157. Ohmi Y, Shiku H, Nishimura T: Tumor-specific targeting of T helper type 1 (Th1) cells by anti-CD3 x anti-c-ErbB-2 bispecific antibody. Cancer Immunol Immunother 1999;48:456–462.

158. Alas S, Emmanouilides C, Bonavida B: Inhibition of interleukin 10 by rituximab results in down-regulation of bcl-2 and sensitization of B-cell non-Hodgkin's lymphoma to apoptosis. Clin Cancer Res 2001;7:709–723.

159. Manzke O, Berthold F, Huebel K, Tesch H, Diehl V, Bohlen H: CD3xCD19 bispecific antibodies and CD28 bivalent antibodies enhance T-cell reactivity against autologous leukemic cells in pediatric B-ALL bone marrow. Int J Cancer 1999;80:715–722.

160. Brandl M, Grosse-Hovest L, Holler E, Kolb HJ, Jung G: Bispecific antibody fragments with CD20 X CD28 specificity allow effective autologous and allogeneic T-cell activation against malignant cells in peripheral blood and bone marrow cultures from patients with B-cell lineage leukemia and lymphoma. Exp Hematol 1999;27:1264–1270.

161. Bauer S, Renner C, Juwana JP, et al: Immunotherapy of human tumors with T-cell-activating bispecific antibodies: stimulation of cytotoxic pathways in vivo. Cancer Res 1999;59:1961–1965.

162. Curnow RT: Clinical experience with CD64-directed immunotherapy. An overview. Cancer Immunol Immunother 1997;45:210–215.

163. Stockmeyer B, Elsasser D, Dechant M, et al: Mechanisms of G-CSF-or GM-CSF-stimulated tumor cell killing by Fc receptor-directed bispecific antibodies. J Immunol Methods 2001;248:103–111.

164. Arndt MA, Krauss J, Kipriyanov SM, Pfreundschuh M, Little M: A bispecific diabody that mediates natural killer cell cytotoxicity against xenotransplanted huamn Hodgkin's tumors. Blood 1999;94:2562–2568.

165. Carter P: Improving the efficacy of antibody-based cancer therapies. Nat Rev Cancer 2001;1:118–129.

166. Heitner T, Moor A, Garrison JL, Marks C, Hasan T, Marks JD: Selection of cell binding and internalizing epidermal growth factor receptor antibodies from a phage display library. J Immunol Methods 2001;248:17–30.

167. Jones PT, Dear PH, Foote J, Neuberger MS, Winter G: Replacing the complementarity-determining regions in a human antibody with those from a mouse. Nature 1986;321:522–525.

168. Knappik A, Ge L, Honegger A, et al: Fully synthetic human combinatorial antibody libraries (HuCAL) based on modular consensus frameworks and CDRs randomized with trinucleotides. J Mol Biol 2000;296:57–86.

169. Griffiths AD, Malmqvist M, Marks JD, et al: Human anti-self antibodies with high specificity from phage display libraries. Embo J 1993;12:725–734.

170. Fishwild DM, O'Donnell SL, Bengoechea T, et al: High-avidity human IgG kappa monoclonal antibodies from a novel strain of minilocus transgenic mice. Nat Biotechnol 1996;14:845–851.

171. Shields RL, Namenuk AK, Hong K, et al: High resolution mapping of the binding site on human IgG1 for Fc gamma RI, Fc gamma RII, Fc gamma RIII, and FcRn and design of IgG1 variants with improved binding to the Fc gamma R. J Biol Chem 2001;276:6591–6604.

172. Idusogie EE, Wong PY, Presta LG, et al: Engineered antibodies with increased activity to recruit complement. J Immunol 2001;166:2571–2575.

173. Little M, Kipriyanov SM, Le Gall F, Moldenhaur G: Of mice and men: hybridoma and recombinant antibodies. Immunol Today 2000;21:364–370.

174. Schier R, McCall A, Adams GP, et al: Isolation of picomolar affinity anti-c-erbB-2 single-chain Fv by molecular evolution of the complementarity determining regions in the center of the antibody binding site. J Mol Biol 1996;263:551–567.

175. Hanes J, Schaffitzel C, Knappik A, Pluckthun A: Picomolar affinity antibodies from a fully synthetic naive library selected and evolved by ribosome display. Nat Biotechnol 2000;18:1287–1292.

176. Jermutus L, Honegger A, Schwesinger F, Hanes J, Pluckthun A: Tailoring in vitro evolution for protein affinity or stability. Proc Natl Acad Sci USA 2001;98:75–80.

177. Boder ET, Midelfort KS, Wittrup KD: Directed evolution of antibody fragments with monovalent femtomolar antigen-binding affinity. Proc Natl Acad Sci USA 2000;97:10701–10705.

178. Fujimori K, Covell DG, Fletcher JE, Weinstein JN: A modeling analysis of monoclonal antibody percolation through tumors: a binding-site barrier. J Nucl Med 1990;31:1191–1198.

179. Schultz J, Lin Y, Sanderson J, et al: A tetravalent single-chain antibody-streptavidin fusion protein for pretargeted lymphoma therapy. Cancer Res 2000;60:6663–6669.

180. Zhang M, Zhang Z, Garmestani K, et al: Pretarget radiotherapy with an anti-CD25 antibody-streptavidin fusion protein was effective in therapy of leukemia/lymphoma xenografts. Proc Natl Acad Sci USA 2003;100:1891–1895.

181. Agus DB, Akita RW, Fox WD, et al: Targeting ligand-activated ErbB2 signaling inhibits breast and prostate tumor growth. Cancer Cell 2002;2:127–137.

182. Halin C, Neri D: Antibody-based targeting of angiogenesis. Crit Rev Ther Drug Carrier Syst 2001;18:299–339.

183. Hofheinz RD, Al-Batran SE, Hartmann F, et al: Stromal antigen targeting by a humanised monoclonal antibody: an Early phase ii trial of sibrotuzumab in patients with metastatic colorectal cancer. Onkologie 2003;26:44–48.

184. Presta LG, Chen H, O'Connor SJ, et al: Humanization of an anti-vascular endothelial growth factor monoclonal antibody for the therapy of solid tumors and other disorders. Cancer Res 1997;57:4593–4599.

185. Zhu Z, Hattori K, Zhang H, et al: Inhibition of human leukemia in an animal model with human antibodies directed against vascular endothelial growth factor receptor 2. Correlation between

antibody affinity and biological activity. Leukemia 2003;17:604–611.

186. Posey JA, Ng TC, Yang B, et al: A phase I study of anti-kinase insert domain-containing receptor antibody, IMC-1C11, in patients with liver metastases from colorectal carcinoma. Clin Cancer Res 2003;9:1323–1332.

187. Huang X, Molema G, King S, Watkins L, Edgington TS, Thorpe PE: Tumor infarction in mice by antibody-directed targeting of tissue factor to tumor vasculature. Science 1997;275:547–550.

188. Brooks PC, Clark RA, Cheresh DA: Requirement of vascular integrin alpha v beta 3 for angiogenesis. Science 1994;264:569–571.

189. Gutheil JC, Campbell TN, Pierce PR, et al: Targeted antiangiogenic therapy for cancer using Vitaxin: a humanized monoclonal antibody to the integrin alphavbeta3. Clin Cancer Res 2000;6:3056–3061.

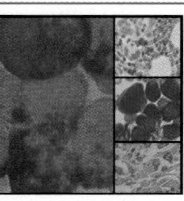

33

CANCER VACCINES

Michael C. Milone

Carl H. June

SUMMARY OF KEY POINTS

- Sensitive biomarker assays and genetic screening techniques can be used to recognize which patients are at risk of development of cancer and to identify early-stage premalignant lesions.
- Work with this cohort of patients is an ideal setting for testing of cancer vaccines.

- Modern vaccine approaches have made it possible to induce cellular immune responses against almost any human T-cell antigen.
- Development of improved adjuvants and the ability to overcome inhibitory signals enable induction autoimmunity in cancer patients.

- Oncologists may some day consider immunotherapy the fourth modality—in addition to surgery, radiation therapy, and chemotherapy—for treating patients with cancer.

INTRODUCTION

Effective immunity is a highly orchestrated event. It involves spatial and temporal cooperation of cells dispersed throughout an organism. Because of the grave consequences of failure of host defense, this critical physiologic system exhibits remarkable robustness and complexity. Although many of the key "players" in immunity were identified almost a century ago, decades of immunologic research and a revolution in molecular biology have only begun to reveal the organization and functioning of this complex system and to provide the tools for quantitative evaluation of tumor immunity (Table 33-1). With this knowledge comes the prospect of manipulating the immune response for a variety of therapeutic purposes.

Vaccination, the process of generating active immunity to a specified agent, and the entire field of immunology were born in 1796, when Edward Jenner made the seminal observation that smallpox infection could be prevented by inoculation with cowpox. Preventive vaccines for infectious disease have almost eliminated pathogens that once represented humankind's greatest obstacles to health and survival. Out of this tremendous success in public health emerges the scourge of cancer. According to epidemiologic data from 2001, cancer is the second leading cause of mortality in the United States, with more than 550,000 cancer-related deaths per year.[1] The goal of this chapter is to review how the immune system is being harnessed to control cancer. Although the immune system may not have been designed to handle this collection of diseases, exciting results indicate it is potentially capable of aiding in the difficult challenge.

ANTITUMOR IMMUNITY EXISTS

Paul Ehrlich first proposed the idea that the immune system suppresses most carcinomas. Fifty years later, Burnet and Thomas essentially simultaneously published the "cancer immunosurveillance" hypothesis, proposing that the immune system recognizes and aborts spontaneously arising transformed cells through acquisition of "new antigenic potentialities."[2,3] This hypothesis remained controversial for almost 40 years, because immuno-

TABLE 33-1

Major Advances in Tumor Immunology: 1990–2000

Identification of human tumor antigens
  Antigen disovery methods
  - SEREX[52]
  - Expression library screening with CTL lines[51,70],*
  Bioinformatic approaches to antigenic epitope identification
Development of highly sensitive methods for detecting antigen-specific T cells
  ELISPOT[†]
  MHC tetramer analysis[191]
Ability to isolate and culture dendritic cells ex vivo[137–139]

CTL, cytotoxic lymphocyte; ELISPOT, enzyme-linked immunospot assay; MHC, major histocompatibility complex; SEREX, expression library screening with serum from cancer patients.
*van der Bruggen P, Traversari C, Chomez P, et al: A gene encoding an antigen recognized by cytolytic T lymphocytes on a human melanoma. Science 1991;254:1643–1647.
†Czerkinsky CC, Nillson LA, Nygren H, Ouchterlony O, Tarkowski A: A solid-phase enzyme-linked immunospot (Elispot) assay for enumeration of specific antibody-secreting cells. J Immunol Methods 1983;65:109–121.

deficient mice were thought not to exhibit an increased incidence of tumors. However, results of more recent studies with both mice and humans have led to renewed interest in the cancer immunosurveillance theory. The array of knock-out mice available and a much greater understanding of immunity reveal that animals deficient in both innate and adaptive immunity have an increased incidence of spontaneous and induced tumors. This finding suggests an important role for the immune system in control of tumor formation.[4]

Although immunity is clearly important to tumor development in mice, these mechanisms do not necessarily operate in humans. Several lines of evidence, however, support a role for tumor immunosurveillance in humans. Tumors often are infiltrated by immune cells, such as tumor-infiltrating lymphocytes. The presence of these cells is associated with increased survival of patients with several tumor types.[5-10] Spontaneous development of devastating autoimmune complications, such as opsoclonus-myoclonus syndrome in persons with neuroblastoma,[11] paraneoplastic cerebellar degeneration in breast cancer,[12] and paraneoplastic encephalomyelitis/subacute sensory neuropathy in persons with small cell lung cancer,[13,14] lend further support to the immunogenic nature of many tumors. Finally, results of several long-term epidemiologic studies with immunodeficient persons (e.g., transplantation patients) have revealed significantly increased risk of tumor development, including those without known associations with oncogenic viruses.[4] The immunogenic nature of malignant cells is clear. How many tumors escape immune detection remains a highly studied area clearly important to successful cancer immunotherapy. However, increasing evidence that the immune system can recognize tumors reveals the potential for harnessing this system for prophylactic and therapeutic cancer vaccines.

OBSTACLES TO SUCCESSFUL CANCER IMMUNOTHERAPY

Despite the evident immunogenicity of tumors, the host immune system often tolerates them. Tumors evade immune detection and destruction by several mechanisms. Physical barriers such as the blood-brain barrier pose the first hurdle to immune effector cell recognition and destruction of tumors.[15] Establishment of an inhospitable tumor microenvironment (e.g., deprivation of the essential amino acid tryptophan by abundant indoleamine 2,3 dioxygenase) also may contribute to tumor escape from the immune system.[16]

Beyond physical barriers, tumors frequently downregulate or lose altogether the surface expression of target peptide in complex with major histocompatibility complex (MHC) antigens; therefore the tumors are not recognized by the T-cell antigen receptor. These changes occur through gene silencing or deletions of MHC class I genes, loss of other proteins essential for formation of the peptide/MHC complex,[17] or loss of nonessential antigens. Tumors have devised ways to subvert the immune system by acquisition of immunomodulatory proteins

that can delete or render effector T cells that recognize the tumor anergic.[18] Notable examples include tumor expression of RCAS (receptor-binding cancer antigen expressed on SiSo cells),[19] B7-H1 (also known as programmed death 1 ligand [PD-1L]),[20] and soluble NKG2D ligands,[21,22] which provide potent immunosuppressive signals to T and natural killer (NK) cells. Findings also suggest that tumors recruit antigen-specific T cells, such as CD4+CD25+ regulatory T cells, that actively suppress antitumor immune responses.[23,24] Overcoming this "tolerance" to a tumor is an important hurdle to effective cancer immunotherapy.

Beyond immune evasion, vaccination and other forms of immunotherapy are generally not administered to cancer patients until relatively late in disease, when tumors have reached large, clinically detectable sizes. Cancer patients are frequently debilitated by both growing cancer and concomitant chemotherapy and radiation treatment, limiting effectiveness of any vaccine. This practice is in striking contrast to administration of vaccines for most infectious diseases, whereby "healthy" persons are vaccinated before encounter with the infectious agent. The ability to harness an already compromised immune system is one of the greatest challenges to cancer immunotherapy, because patients with advanced disease usually are the subjects of phase I/II clinical trials.

NATURE OF EFFECTIVE ANTITUMOR IMMUNITY

Notwithstanding the aforementioned hurdles, numerous approaches to generating antitumor immunity in cancer patients have been explored. Several trials have documented the ability of the human immune system to respond to tumors that it previously ignored. Through clinical trials and the feverish pace of immunologic research in general, the nature of an effective immune response to human cancer is being unraveled.

The advent of successful monoclonal antibody therapy for malignant diseases such as lymphoma (anti-CD20, rituximab) and breast cancer (Her2-neu) has brought Erhlich's magic bullet hypothesis into the realm of reality.[25] Although humoral immunity alone appears useful, it is likely that an orchestrated humoral and cellular response will be even more effective. Evidence suggests that passive immunotherapy with monoclonal antibodies requires cellular immunity for full therapeutic effect.[26]

There are several reasons why generating cellular antitumor immunity is considered critical to any cancer vaccine. Antibody access to antigenic targets is limited essentially to those expressed on the surface of cancer cells. Many of the unique changes intrinsic to tumorigenesis occur in proteins that regulate the cell cycle, and most are not directly visible from outside the cell. In contrast, T cells target antigens derived from all subcellular compartments. Antigen recognition is thus limited mostly by the ability of tumor cells to process and present antigens on MHC molecules. The ability of T cells to "see" tumor cells is exemplified by a few of the many in vitro studies demonstrating T-cell killing of tumor cells in an

MHC-restricted, endogenous, antigen-specific manner.[22,27,28] Despite the abundance of in vitro and animal data indicating the importance of cellular immunity to antitumor immune responses,[29] few data exist regarding the effectiveness of this component of the immune system in eradicating tumors in humans. However, regression of tumors has been seen in association with adoptive transfer of CD8[+] cytotoxic T lymphocytes (CTLs) into melanoma patients. This finding supports a critical role of this component of the immune system in tumor immunotherapy.[30,31]

Increasing evidence also suggests that natural killer T (NKT) cells, a distinct subset of lymphocytes, which often use a restricted T-cell receptor (Vα24-Vβ11 in humans) regulate resistance to tumors.[22,32,33] Accumulating evidence indicates that NKT cells are involved in tumor immunosuppression and immunosurveillance.[34-37]

Although humoral and CD8[+] CTL responses are important, CD4[+] T cells also appear vital for antitumor immunity. CD4[+] T cells are indispensable for initiation of CTL responses to antigens encountered without potent inflammatory signals. Under these conditions, the CD4[+] T cells deliver activation signals to dendritic cells, "licensing" them for optimal activation of CTLs.[38] In addition, although CTL responses can be generated in the absence of CD4[+] T cells, there is evidence that CD4[+] T cells are essential to maintenance of a sustained, long-lasting CTL response.[39] Finally, macrophages may play a role in antitumor immune responses,[40] and CD4[+] T cells mediate important activating signals to these cells by production of cytokines, especially interferon γ.[41] Thus CD4[+] T-cell activation is likely to be a highly important component of any antitumor vaccination strategy.

Overall, the nature and composition of an effective antitumor immune response will likely depend on a variety of factors, including the origin, location, and stage of the tumor. The approach to tumor vaccination once was empiric. However, rapidly expanding knowledge of tumor–immune system interactions now allows more rational design of and it is hoped more effective tumor vaccines.

ANATOMY OF A CANCER VACCINE

The approach to cancer vaccination is quite different from the approach to vaccines against infectious agents. Pathogen-oriented vaccines generally are used to protect an individual against a "foreign" agent before contact with the agent. Immunity from many pathogens also largely depends on generation of potent humoral immune responses. Thus infectious disease vaccines in clinical use are generally more effective at stimulating antibody responses than they are at stimulating cellular immunity.

Unlike pathogens, cancers are derived from self antigens[42,43] and exhibit progressive growth despite an immune response. Cancer vaccination must overcome this tolerance. Notwithstanding these important differences, vaccines against infectious agents have taught us a great deal about generation of potent immunity in humans. Pathogen vaccines serve as the foundation for past and present cancer vaccines. Modifying these vaccine approaches and developing new approaches are essential for meeting the demands of this aggressive and often chronic disease.

Present dogma is that although cancer cells are antigenic, they are only poorly immunogenic. Therefore vaccines are generally composed of two components: one or more antigens that serve as targets of the immune response and an adjuvant that generates the signals necessary to render the cancer antigens immunogenic. Both aspects of the vaccine are critical to the nature of the ensuing immunity. However, cancer vaccine formulations differ greatly in source and nature of the tumor antigen and in adjuvants used. Researchers in the field of cancer immunology are working to elucidate the critical factors of both antigen and adjuvant.[15,44,45]

Choosing the Right Antigen: Toward Autoimmunity?

Antigens, the targets of the immune response, are critical to antitumor immunity. Tumor cells often have unique, tumor-specific macromolecules, such as the mutant oncogenic protein k-Ras[46] or the fusion protein derived from the *bcr-abl* translocation in CMLs.[47] Many other "normal" proteins or carbohydrates are aberrantly and/or preferentially expressed by tumor cells.[43] Even the vasculature associated with tumor-induced angiogenesis may serve as a target for tumor vaccines.[48,49] All of these modifications have the prospect of serving as targets of potentially effective antitumor immune responses.

Rapid discovery of tumor-associated antigens (TAAs) began with the screening method developed by Coulie and associates.[50] Using coculture with autologous tumors, these investigators established several in vitro CTL lines derived from patients with melanoma. These CTL lines were used to screen a library of melanoma genes expressed in antigen-loss variants of autologous tumor cells. With this method, the MAGE antigen was isolated as a candidate tumor rejection antigen in humans. Although this method of antigen detection has been extended to identification of many other TAAs, the necessity for cloning tumor-reactive T cells makes this screening process highly labor intensive. Zauderer and colleagues developed a much more efficient strategy for isolating MHC class I restricted tumor antigens.[51] Sahin and colleagues[52] developed a simpler method of expression library screening using serum from cancer patients Using this method (also known as SEREX), several tumor antigens targeted by the humoral immune system were identified with this method. Somewhat surprisingly, many antigens isolated as potent antibody targets also serve as CTL target antigens. Such antigens include the melanoma antigens MAGE and tyrosinase. In subsequent studies, the same group, using SEREX screening of esophageal carcinoma, identified the NY-ESO-1 protein, a cancer-testes type antigen (see later). The investigators confirmed the power of this serologic screening tool for detection of cellular as well as humoral TAAs.[53] These antigen discovery methods and others will likely yield many targets for use in cancer vaccination.

The list of TAAs is long. They can be classified into four general categories on the basis of specificity for tumor cells and their normal cell/tissue expression.[43] The most potent TAAs are not truly tumor antigens but are viral antigens expressed in virally induced tumors. The E6 and E7 oncoproteins of the human papillomaviruses (HPVs) are the best examples of this category.[54-56] Small changes such as amino acid substitutions or larger changes such as frameshift or gene fusion events can give rise to antigens that are immunologically distinct and recognizable in comparison with their normal protein counterparts.[57] These antigens represent a large portion of unique tumor antigens. Although not unique to tumors, several antigens may function as essentially tumor specific owing to extremely limited expression in normal tissues. The best characterized of these include the cancer-testes antigens of the MAGE, GAGE, and BAGE families.[42] These antigens are restricted in expression to only germ cells lacking classic MHC molecules and tumor cells. The least specific TAAs are those represented by the so-called differentiation antigens, proteins expressed by both tumor cells and the tissue from which the tumor is derived. Prototypic differentiation antigens are tyrosinase[58] or Melan-A,[59] which are normally expressed by healthy melanocytes in addition to malignant melanoma cells.

The best antigenic targets for cancer vaccination remain controversial.[60] The "tumor-specific" antigens arising as a consequence of mutation are attractive because of their specificity and resulting limited potential for autoimmune toxicity. These antigens, however, often are unique to the individual tumor. Vaccination against these antigens would necessitate individualized vaccines derived from tumor material that may frequently be extremely limited in supply. On the other hand, a tissue-specific antigen would have wider applicability, but this benefit may come at the price of greater autoimmune toxicity. Furthermore, significant thymic tolerance to differentiation antigens might also limit their ability to act as tumor rejection targets.

Despite the theoretical limitations of differentiation antigens, some patients with metastatic melanoma spontaneously experience the benign autoimmune "complication" of vitiligo. Development of vitiligo appears to portend improved prognosis among these patients.[61-64] T cells specific for MelanA/Mart1, tyrosinase, and gp100 melanocyte-specific antigens have been reported to mediate autoreactivity in vitiligo not associated with melanoma.[65] Some patients receiving high-dose interleukin 2 therapy for melanoma who respond to therapy also experience vitiligo. In striking contrast, this autoimmune toxicity rarely occurs among nonresponders.[66]

Although targets such as MART1 or tyrosinase are superb antigens for CTL-mediated immune responses against melanoma cells, they may not be the best antigenic targets for CD4[+] cells. The importance of CD4-T cell–mediated helper effects for sustained CTL responses necessitates identification of antigens capable of being processed and presented to CD4[+] T cells through MHC class II molecules. Detection of potent new MHC class II restricted antigens has lagged significantly behind research toward CTL epitopes. Some TAAs giving rise to CTL epitopes also appear to contain CD4 T-cell epitopes.[67-69] Identification of CD4[+] cell epitopes using new screening[70] and bioinformatics approaches is currently an area of intense investigation.

Successful immunotherapy for cancer will likely require generation of diverse immune responses. The fact that many of the most effective antigens are expressed by normal tissue raises important concerns for cancer immunotherapy. Although autoimmune destruction of melanocytes is of cosmetic concern but of little clinical significance, an autoimmune response to a tissue such as colon or lung could be life threatening. Thus autoimmunity is one of the most important potential toxicities of cancer vaccination.[44] Results of studies with an agonistic CTLA-4 antibody in patients with melanoma suggest autoimmunity may be a frequent complication of human tumor immunotherapy.[71,72] Careful monitoring for this complication is therefore an integral part of toxicity monitoring in all clinical cancer vaccine trials.

Sources of Antigen

Whole Tumor/Tumor Cell Lysates

The simplest source of tumor antigen is the tumor itself. Some of the earliest cancer vaccines relied on inoculation of crude preparations of autologous or allogeneic tumors into patients.[73,74] The main advantage of using tumor cells or their derivatives (e.g., lysates) of TAAs is available, including those yet to be identified. An important limitation of this vaccination strategy, however, is controlling the quality and purity of the vaccines. Without knowledge of the active component of these vaccines, it is difficult to compare batches of vaccine, especially those derived from autologous tumors that differ for every patient. In addition, the unknown nature of tumor antigens makes it difficult to develop in vitro assays for monitoring immune responses in vaccinated patients. Finally, although many, perhaps hundreds, of TAAs may be present in a tumor-derived vaccine preparation, these antigens are present in the context of thousands of self-antigens or alloantigens (in the case of allogeneic vaccines) that are irrelevant and perhaps even harmful.

Despite the many limitations, successful antitumor immune responses, both in vitro and in vivo, have been generated with these types of vaccines. Two phase II/III clinical trials of allogeneic, whole-cell,[75,76] and cell lysate–based[77,78] vaccines for melanoma have been conducted. Significant and specific delayed type hypersensitivity responses to the tumor occurred, and the whole-cell vaccine appeared to yield improvement. Nevertheless, randomized, controlled studies have yet to prove clinical benefit.

Several groups have attempted a more novel approach to whole tumor cell vaccination. RNA extracted from tumor cells can be used to load dendritic cells with tumor antigens.[79-81] The introduced messenger RNA is translated into protein, and the tumor-derived proteins are efficiently presented by way of the endogenous pathways of antigen presentation in the dendritic cells. Through amplification of tumor RNA, this method of antigen-loading may provide a limitless supply of well-defined tumor antigens.

Transfection into dendritic cells or other cells can provide a target for evaluation of immunity after vaccination. Additional manipulation of the RNA (depletion of RNA for irrelevant or suppressive proteins) may also yield advantages in vaccine specificity and potency and perhaps augment activity beyond that achieved with unmodified tumor extracts.

Defined-Antigen Vaccines

Although the whole tumor cell approaches are robust, they have several limitations besides their difficulty in standardization among vaccine batches. With the exception of allogeneic approaches, whole tumor cell vaccines depend on autologous tumor, which may not be readily available. Many of the procedures for formulating these vaccines are complicated to perform. Furthermore, even the simplest methods are relatively expensive to perform under practices that would be approved by the U.S. Food and Drug Administration (FDA). All of these features lead investigators in search of easier, less expensive, and more standardized ways to vaccinate.

Defined antigen vaccines have many advantages. Antigens can be produced abundantly through recombinant DNA technology or chemical synthesis. These vaccines are more readily manufactured under pharmaceutical conditions. Control over the quantity and quality of antigens also allows greater control over incorporation of the antigens into vaccines that may be essential to generation of consistently potent antitumor immune responses. Finally, optimal TAAs will be shared tumor antigens[82-84] and will therefore find applicability to a range of tumors and many different patients.

Antigenic peptides are commonly used as tumor antigens for incorporation into cancer vaccines. These molecules are synthesized relatively inexpensively and easily with current organic chemistry technology. The primary hurdle in peptide vaccine development is identifying the natural peptide epitopes of a particular antigen processed by tumor cells and recognized by T cells. This challenge has been met with many TAAs, such as tyrosinase and gp100 in melanoma. Both MHC class I and class II restricted peptides have been used.[85] With increased biochemical understanding of MHC molecules, bioinformatics algorithms have been developed that allow fairly reliable prediction of CTL epitopes encoded within a given protein that bind with high affinity to individual MHC class I molecules. This approach has been used to identify peptides from proteinase 3 and telomerase, and T cells recognizing these peptide epitopes exist naturally in vivo.[86,87]

Although there are many advantages to use of defined antigens in cancer vaccines, these antigens are not without their own set of disadvantages. The main limitation is the arduous task of identifying antigens important for tumor rejection. This procedure is complicated by the fact that antigen specificity is controlled by the MHC molecules expressed by an individual. Because significant heterogeneity exists in MHC expression, selection of antigens for use in vaccination must be individualized. Many vaccine trials are limited to patients who express the HLA A*201 allele, a common MHC gene that circum-

vents the need for testing of peptides that can be presented by many different HLA alleles.

In addition to difficulty identifying processed peptide epitopes of TAAs that can be chemically synthesized for use in a vaccine, peptide vaccination is also not as straightforward as expected. For example, studies have shown that vaccination with peptides spanning a defined, naturally antigenic region of the cancer-testis antigen, NY-ESO-1, can lead to significant induction of CTL responses. Surprising, however, is that most of this response is either low avidity or targeted toward "cryptic" epitopes derived from the original peptide, perhaps by proteolytic processing.[88] Most responding T cells, although peptide specific, are unable to recognize naturally presented antigen on tumor cells.

Defined antigen vaccines have tremendous advantages related to outcome monitoring and clinical production compared with whole tumor vaccines. Foremost, the capability of tetramer technology for precise quantification of antitumor responses has revolutionized postvaccination immune monitoring.[89] However, the narrow response to defined antigen vaccines will likely limit the clinical effectiveness of these vaccines in the face of tumors that mutate rapidly. Greater understanding of cancer biology and the proteins necessary to maintain a tumor's growth and survival will be essential for choosing the critical antigens for a particular tumor vaccine in the future.

Rebirth of Adjuvant

The nature of the antigen (e.g., protein, carbohydrate) is critical to an immune response, but the way in which an antigen is presented to the immune system is just as important. Generating immunity depends on the ability of the immune system to "see" an antigen as "nonself."[90,91] Antigen encountered without associated signals indicative of infectious nonself will largely remain unnoticed.[92,93] Many of these signals are inflammatory in nature. They mediate their T-cell immunostimulatory effects through activation of dendritic cells, a process that leads to their maturation into potent antigen-presenting cells (APCs). Changes induced in dendritic cells during an encounter with inflammatory signals include expression of CD80 and CD86. These molecules provide critical costimulatory signals to T cells necessary for full activation and differentiation into effective CTLs[94] or helper T cells.[95] T cells encountering antigenic receptor signals without these costimulatory signals generally become unresponsive T cells that subsequently fail to activate even when encountering antigen with proper costimulation at a later time.

Although used liberally, the term *adjuvant* generally refers to the delivery vehicle or associated signals delivered with one or more antigens. Given the importance of antigen presentation to the immune system in generating and shaping the subsequent immune response, the adjuvant is a vital component of any vaccine formulation. In some respects, the nature of the adjuvant may be more important than the antigen chosen, because even the best antigen will fail to protect without an appropriate adjuvant.[96]

Several properties of the adjuvant influence the outcome of vaccination. Adjuvants may serve as a depot for ensuring antigen persistence and sustained release of antigen. The ability of an adjuvant to attract and target APCs affects the amount of antigen required for generation of an immune response. Many adjuvants also promote activation and differentiation of APCs. Alterations in expression of various costimulatory molecules and cytokines by APCs subsequently affect the quality of the ensuing immune response, such that the nature of the adjuvant can influence the priming of naive T cells to differentiate into polarized cells that produce either inflammatory cytokines (e.g., interferon γ) or non-inflammatory cytokines (e.g., interleukin 4). Manipulation of these attributes of an adjuvant enable generation of a myriad of qualitatively and quantitatively different immune responses. The current hurdles for cancer vaccination are determining the nature of an effective antitumor immune response for a given tumor and selecting or developing the appropriate antigen/adjuvant system for achieving this response.

Development of adjuvants has received less attention than identification of antigens. Given the importance on the outcome of immune responses, renewed emphasis has been placed on adjuvant research. The growing regulatory environment in which most clinical studies are performed is a driving force toward adjuvant systems that are better defined chemically and functionally. An abundance of naturally derived and synthetic adjuvants are available. With the advent of ex vivo cellular manipulation and gene therapy, entirely new classes of adjuvants have become available.

Traditional Particulate Vaccines

One of the oldest and most widely used clinical adjuvants is aluminum salt. This adjuvant is formed by precipitation of aluminum hydroxide, aluminum phosphate, or alum into gel-like particles that bind to antigen. Other common adjuvants for infectious disease vaccines include oil-in-water and water-in-oil emulsions. These vaccines provide long-term persistence of antigens through a depot effect, and some, such as the aluminum salts, enhance endocytic uptake by APCs through particulate formation.[97]

Incorporation of immunomodulatory agents can enhance dendritic cell maturation and stimulate cytokines that improve efficacy and influence the nature of the ensuing immune response. Common agents incorporated into adjuvants include inflammatory agents such as muramyl dipeptide and their derivatives (e.g., Detox or Enhanzyn adjuvant system). These compounds include the active components of mycobacterial cell wall extracts, also found in Freund's adjuvant, which is frequently used in generating high-titer antibodies in animals. In addition, cytokines can be included directly in the adjuvant to achieve higher levels necessary for a desired effect. A limitation of many adjuvants is that they generate excellent antibody responses with little or no cellular immunity. Despite this shortcoming, the superb safety profile and low cost make these adjuvants popular choices.

Several particulate delivery systems have been developed that show promise for induction of greater cellular immunity in addition to humoral responses. Immuno-stimulating complexes (ISCOM) are an adjuvant system consisting of approximately 40-μm spherical liposome-like particles made from QuilA saponin mixed with cholesterol and phospholipid. In addition to potent antibody responses, immunostimulating complex vaccines prepared with purified proteins have been shown capable of generating potent and long-lived CTL responses to coadministered antigen.[98] Systems such as biodegradable nanoparticles and microparticles that form a stable system for efficient delivery of antigen and other immunomodulatory agents, such as granulocyte-macrophage colony-stimulating factor (GM-CSF), for attracting APCs have been developed. Although they yield both cellular and humoral immunity, these systems are significantly more difficult to prepare than traditional particulate adjuvants.[99]

Microorganisms as Adjuvants

Although cellular immunity can be induced with nonliving, particulate adjuvants, antigens that are delivered in the context of a "natural" infection produce significantly greater and long-lasting cell-mediated immunity. This result is due in part to the ability of the immune system to sense danger signals generated by infection.[100] The innate immune system has evolved numerous ways to detect microorganisms and ensure efficient delivery of infectious antigens to the antigen processing and presentation pathways of dendritic cells. This potent effect on generation of cellular immunity has been capitalized on through the use of a variety of bacteria and viruses as adjuvants for vaccines.[101-103]

The concept of using microorganisms to control cancer is hardly new. Clinical trials by Coley in the 19th century were the first documented attempts at the use of microorganisms for enhancing the immune response to heterologous tumor antigens.[104] In studies in the 1970s a variety of infectious agents were used to enhance tumor vaccine efficacy (so-called xenogenization).[105] Many components of bacteria have found utility in vaccines. Cell wall extracts from mycobacteria are widely used in adjuvant systems. Bacterial DNA is a potent activator of innate immunity through recognition of unmethylated cytosine-phosphate-guanosine (CpG)-containing DNA by the pattern-recognition receptor Toll-like receptor 9 (TLR-9).[106,107] Incorporation of CpG oligonucleotides into adjuvants has a potent effect on adjuvant activity.[108] In addition, this motif imparts immunogenicity to plasmid DNA, allowing effective use of naked DNA for vaccination.[109]

Several studies have explored the use of oncolytic viruses in therapy for cancer.[110,111] The basis of this therapy is thought to stem from the selective advantage of some viral strains for replication within tumor cells compared with normal cells. There are several indications that oncolytic viruses may have a role in cancer vaccines.[112-114]

Recombinant Microorganisms: The Twenty-First Century Vaccine?

Although synthetic adjuvants and extracts from bacteria serve as potent stimulators of immunity, these agents tend to promote strong humoral immunity but limited cellular responses. In an attempt to augment cellular immunity, many investigators have turned to recombinant microorganisms that stimulate potent cell-mediated immunity. Among these microorganisms are viruses and the intracellular pathogen *Listeria monocytogenes*. Because of tremendous advances in genetic engineering, it is a relatively simple undertaking to produce recombinant organisms that express TAAs.

For generation of significant cellular immunity, particularly CD8+ CTL activity, effective antigen delivery to the cytoplasm of cells is essential. Target peptides for MHC class I presentation are generally derived in the cytoplasm by protein degradation through the proteasome. Peptides are then transferred by the transporter associated with the antigen processing (TAP) system into the endoplasmic reticulum, where the peptides associate with MHC class I.[115] Because virus-encoded antigens are abundantly expressed in the cytoplasm of infected cells, viral antigens are efficiently processed and presented through this pathway. Recombinant viruses therefore are a superb vehicle for delivery of vaccine antigens into the MHC class I pathway of antigen presentation, and generation of the potent CD8 T-cell immune responses considered highly important for tumor immunity.

Viruses of several classes have been explored for use in vaccination. Poxviruses in particular have received attention because of their potent immunizing ability.[116,117] Extensive experience with smallpox vaccination has established the danger and safety of these viruses in vaccination of millions of persons. Recombinant DNA technology allows production of poxviruses that can be harnessed to generate potent immune responses to a myriad of antigens.

Before the genetic revolution, vaccinia virus (VV) was used in tumor immunotherapy as a nonspecific adjuvant in therapy for melanoma. Over the past decade, poxviruses encoding TAAs of all classes have been developed. Many studies have demonstrated the efficacy of these recombinant viruses in inducing strong cell-mediated immunity followed by eradication of tumors in mice.[118-120]

Although these results are promising, VV is a live, replicating virus. Smallpox vaccination was safely administered to healthy persons for prevention of disease. Poxvirus, however, can be deadly when administered to a person with compromised immune function. This danger has led to generation of modified VV that cannot replicate in human or most mammalian cells but appears to retain immunogenicity.[121-123] An additional problem that may interfere with use of recombinant VV (rVV) in vaccines is the prevalence of previous VV exposure for smallpox prevention. Whether this prior immunity limits subsequent vaccine efficacy is unclear. In addition to VV, recombinant avian poxviruses have been produced. These viruses are capable of generating protective immunity similar to that of VV, and they have been tested in humans with no significant toxicity.[124] This remarkable preclinical efficacy of VV has led to several human clinical trials of poxvirus vaccines.[125-128] Potent cellular immunity in humans has been demonstrated with these vaccines, and evidence of clinical efficacy is eagerly awaited.

In addition to recombinant viruses, bacteria have been genetically modified for use as live vaccines. *L. monocytogenes* is an intracellular bacterial pathogen that stimulates potent cell-mediated immunity. This strong immunostimulatory activity has been exploited for use in cancer vaccination, and several groups have demonstrated the ability of TAA-expressing *L. monocytogenes* to generate potent antitumor responses in tumor-bearing mice.[129-133] Gram-negative bacteria such as *Salmonella* and *Yersinia* organisms, mycobacteria, and even *Bacillis anthracis* have been developed for use in delivering vaccine antigens.[134]

The list of organisms that have been or might be exploited for use in vaccines is enormous. Each organism has unique immunologic properties that may be particularly useful for certain vaccines. Genetic modification of microorganisms offers the potential for generating potent and wide-ranging immune responses. This property may be essential for successful cancer vaccination for diverse tumor types.

Dendritic Cell Vaccines

One of the most important roles of any adjuvant is recruitment and delivery of an antigen to the cells that effectively process and present the antigen to T cells. A variety of cells have the ability to present antigens. Almost all cells process and present antigens through the MHC class I. However, this process rarely activates T cells, but rather leads to anergy from the lack of appropriate costimulation. B cells and macrophages have several costimulatory molecules that allow them to activate T cells. However, they primarily activate memory cells and are generally incapable of activating naive T cells. Dendritic cells were first described by Steinman and Cohn in the 1970s as cells with a "veiled" morphology that were potent stimulators of naive T cells with activity far superior to that of other APCs, such as B cells or macrophages.[135]

Although dendritic cells were originally identified in lymphoid tissues, immature dendritic cells exist anywhere the body interacts with the external environment, such as the skin and respiratory and gastrointestinal systems. These immature dendritic cells serve as sentinels in these locations, sampling their local milieu and awaiting the danger signals that stimulate maturation and migration of these cells. Many of the stimuli for maturation are derived from pathogens, such as lipopolysaccharide and viral double-stranded RNA. In addition, maturation can be induced by mechanical stress and inflammatory mediators such as interleukin 1 and TNF-α. On activation, these cells migrate to secondary lymphoid tissue, where they interact with and present antigens to both CD4+ and CD8+ T cells, leading to their activation. Although dendritic cell–T-cell interactions are a critical part of the antigen presentation performed by dendritic cells, dendritic cells also appear to interact with B cells, NK cells, and NKT cells.[136] All of these interactions help to initiate and ultimately shape the innate and acquired immune response to an antigen.

Generation of Dendritic Cells for Vaccines. The central role of dendritic cells in immunity has led to extensive exploration of these cells as an adjuvant for cancer

Science of Clinical Oncology

vaccines. Dendritic cells can be obtained for vaccine purposes by ex vivo differentiation of either monocytes[137,138] or CD34[+] progenitor cells.[139] Less commonly, dendritic cells are obtained by apheresis collection from donors after mobilization with growth factors such as GM-CSF and Flt3 ligand.[140] Although all of the methods for obtaining dendritic cells yield cells with potent ability to stimulate immune responses in vitro, there are likely to be qualitative and quantitative differences in dendritic cells derived from these methods for generation of effective immune responses in vivo. The dendritic cell–like cells derived by culture of monocytes or CD34[+] progenitors often are called *monocyte-derived dendritic cells* or *myeloid dendritic cells*. Whether these dendritic cells generated in vitro are the same cells as myeloid dendritic cells isolated from fresh blood remains controversial, and these cells may have distinct differences in immunogenicity.[141] Studies have revealed that in addition to myeloid dendritic cells, there are populations of cells that resemble myeloid dendritic cells morphologically or phenotypically but appear to have unique functional properties. These cells include the CD123[+] (interleukin 3R) plasmacytoid dendritic cells that produce abundant interferon α,[142] lymphoid CD8[+] dendritic cells in mice, and other dendritic cell populations that are much less defined in humans.[143] Although no method currently exists for reliable generation of these other dendritic cell populations in vitro, dendritic cells collected from blood after growth factor mobilization often contain varying proportions of these different dendritic cells.[144] The distinct effects of immunization with these dendritic cell populations remain to be elucidated.

The most commonly used method for ex vivo generation of dendritic cells entails use of monocytes cultured in the presence of GM-CSF and interleukin 4.[137,138] Other soluble mediators, such as prostaglandin E_2, and additional cytokines often are added to enhance differentiation and maturation of the dendritic cells.[145,146] No standardized method exists for generation of dendritic cells in vitro, and a great deal of variation in method exists among laboratories. Thus many vaccine trials differ greatly in purity, cell number, viability, and maturation of dendritic cells. These differences are likely to have important effects on the efficacy of vaccination. Standardization of dendritic cell preparation for vaccines will almost certainly be a critical issue for future clinical trials.

Antigen Loading onto Dendritic Cells. Antigens can be loaded onto dendritic cells with a multitude of methods. The methods vary depending on the source and nature of the antigen, the differentiation state of the dendritic cells, and the desired mode of presentation (i.e., MHC class I versus class II). Some of the methods are simple, and some are extremely complex, requiring technology not available to most laboratories.

The antigens used most frequently in dendritic cell–based cancer vaccines have been peptides. Loading of peptides onto the MHC molecules of dendritic cells is typically done by brief incubation of dendritic cells with peptides. The use of peptide-based vaccine, however, is limited to only individuals with particular HLA types, because binding to MHC molecules is highly specific. Moreover, ability to use a peptide is restricted only to proteins in which the naturally occurring immunodominant epitopes have been characterized.

For vaccination against unique TAAs when the appropriate epitopes are unknown, delivery of the antigen can be accomplished by one of several methods. Different approaches are required for optimal loading of MHC class I and class II molecules with antigens,[147-149] because endogenous proteins are primarily loaded onto the class I pathway. Exogenous proteins entering the endosomal pathway, however, are presented on class II molecules. Fusion of tumor cells with dendritic cells has been used to load dendritic cells with TAAs[150]; however this process is technically challenging because of the need for autologous tumor and dendritic cells. Transfection of RNA-encoding TAAs has been used to efficiently load MHC class I proteins,[151,152] an approach that is more practical because of ability to renew RNA libraries. Transfection with DNA is possible but requires cotransfection of foreign DNA sequences of unknown safety. Tumor antigens can be loaded onto dendritic cells directly from tumor cells because dendritic cells have a unique ability to take up apoptotic tumor cell debris and "cross-present" the acquired tumor antigens through MHC class I and II to T cells.[149,153,154] Tumor lysates and exosomes also have been used to load dendritic cells.[155]

Summary. Dendritic cell–based approaches represent one of the most exciting developments in cancer vaccines. There is little question that dendritic cell–based vaccines can initiate and augment an immune response to an antigen, whether it be a model antigen or a tumor antigen. Numerous methods of isolation, propagation, activation, and antigen loading of dendritic cells have been reported. A standardized method of vaccine delivery has not been determined. Undoubtedly, all of these features are sure to affect the clinical efficacy of a dendritic cell–based vaccine. Although development of new vaccine strategies is important, clinical trials that compare the various factors known to affect the outcome of use of dendritic cell vaccines are essential.

Novel Approaches to Generating Tumor Immunity

Vaccination in the Setting of Hematopoietic Stem Cell Transplantation

The alloimmune response is the most potent antitumor response.[156] Responses are most dramatic in hematologic malignant disease,[157] and there are increasing reports of major antitumor responses after allogeneic hematopoietic stem cell transplantation (SCT) in patients with solid tumors.[158,159] After allogeneic transplantation, a large number of T cells undergo activation in response to allogeneic antigens. The reduced-intensity conditioning in nonmyeloablative SCT allows treatment of elderly populations, who have a preponderance of solid tumors, with previously unavailable allogeneic transplantation.[160,161]

An attractive extension of this approach is immunization of donors with a recipient-derived tumor cell vaccine before donor cell harvest and transplantation. In a mouse model, Anderson and coworkers[162] immunized normal immunocompetent MHC-matched donors with a recipient-derived tumor cell vaccine to determine whether this treatment would substantially increase graft-versus-tumor (GVT) activity and extend survival of SCT recipients with preexisting micrometastatic tumor. The investigators found that pretransplantation immunization of allogeneic SCT donors with a recipient-derived whole tumor cell vaccine substantially increased GVT activity but also substantially exacerbated graft-versus-host disease (GVHD). In contrast, post-transplantation tumor vaccination of recipients against either fibrosarcoma or myeloid leukemia produced a substantial increase in GVT activity, which was capable of complete protection against tumor growth and of preventing growth of preexisting micrometastatic cancer cells. Furthermore, SCT recipients did not have signs of acute GVHD after tumor cell vaccination. This finding demonstrated that GVT activity could be augmented independently of GVHD.[163] In contrast to the toxicity associated with pretransplantation immunization of immunocompetent donors with whole tumor vaccines, results of studies in mice and humans have indicated safety and efficacy of donor immunization with defined antigens. In mice, C3H.SW donors were immunized against a tumor antigen before SCT, and CTLs were transferred along with bone marrow into irradiated MHC-matched, minor histocompatibility antigen–mismatched C57BL/6 recipients with established micrometastatic tumors. Donor immunization led to a significant increase in GVT activity, measured by reduced tumor growth and enhanced survival.[164]

In a study of nonmyeloablative SCT in mice, Luznik and associates[165] found that rejection of metastatic mammary tumors was independent of GVHD but absolutely dependent on the host immune system as well as alloresponsive T cells arising from the transplant. Nonmyeloablative SCT with donor lymphocyte infusion alone did not generate effective antitumor responses. Other investigators showed that tumor cell vaccines can induce potent tumor immunity after allogeneic transplantation.[166] The results of these studies therefore raise the possibility of combining cancer vaccination with allogeneic transplantation in novel vaccination strategies that may prove more efficacious than either modality alone.

Patients undergoing allogeneic transplantation and those receiving high-dose chemotherapy followed by autologous stem cell rescue remain lymphopenic and immunologically compromised for at least several months after therapy and perhaps for a year or more.[167] This immunosuppression may impair the ability of the immune system to respond to tumors. However, some of the changes that occur after transplantation may provide benefits to immunologic therapy, and these deserve exploration.

After transplantation or other treatments that render animals lymphopenic, mature, post-thymic lymphocytes undergo profound expansion that returns the lymphocyte pool to a normal resting size (so-called homeostatic proliferation).[168] Experimental evidence indicates that weak T-cell receptor interactions with self antigen displayed on MHC molecules (perhaps those involved in the original positive selection occurring in the thymus) play an important role in driving this homeostatic expansion.[169] Dummer and colleagues[170] hypothesized that it may be possible to break immunologic tolerance and generate antitumor immunity by taking advantage of these weakly autoreactive T cells undergoing homeostatic proliferation. These investigators demonstrated in a murine model that immunization during the period of lymphoid recovery following irradiation could lead to eradication of an otherwise lethal tumor. Whether this same phenomenon occurs in humans and contributes to the efficacy of high-dose chemotherapy followed by SCT remains to be examined. There are some indications that adoptively transferred T cells undergo homeostatic expansion after autologous SCT.[171] By taking advantage of homeostatic T-cell proliferation, vaccination of patients after transplantation may provide more robust responses than those that occurred with previous vaccination strategies.

Inhibition of Negative Signals

For several decades, results have indicated that subsets of T cells can suppress antitumor responses in animals.[172,173] Studies with patients with advanced malignant disease have shown that chemotherapy, especially cyclophosphamide, can augment antitumor immune responses to vaccines.[174-176] Results also have characterized the nature of suppressive T cells and have shown these cells are highly conserved in animals and humans.[177] Of interest to immunotherapists, these cells are recruited into the tumor microenvironment in patients with a variety of solid tumors.[23,24,178] Results of animal studies have shown that depletion of CD4+CD25+ regulatory T cells can lead to increased rejection of tumors.[179] The importance of these specific regulatory T cells in blocking immunologic rejection of tumors in humans remains to be elucidated.

Studies aimed at depletion of regulatory T cells combined with cancer vaccination are certainly warranted. Monoclonal antibodies that react with CD25 are typically used in animals to preferentially deplete CD25+ regulatory T cells. A similar method, perhaps with a humanized anti-CD25 monoclonal antibody, could be used in humans. Animal data suggest that CD4+CD25+ regulatory T cells are primarily formed in the thymus.[180,181] It is possible that their development and repopulation in recovering lymphopenic hosts may be impaired compared with other lymphocyte subsets. Thus combining vaccine therapy with autologous SCT may provide more effective antitumor immunity due to depletion effects on regulatory T-cell populations in addition to the potential effects of homeostatic proliferation.

Development of a lethal lymphoproliferative disorder of CD4 T cells in young CTLA-4–deficient mice[182,183] illuminates the pivotal role of the inhibitory signal provided by CTLA-4 for T-cell immune homeostasis. Transient CTLA-4 antibody blockade enhances antigen-specific T-cell responses with limited toxicities. Injection of anti–CTLA-4 antibodies stimulates rejection of moderately immunogenic murine tumors[184] and of intensified T-cell–mediated autoimmune encephalomyelitis.[185] Intriguing findings suggest that CTLA-4 antibody blockade increases tumor immunity in previously vaccinated cancer patients.[71,72] However, loss of tolerance may be a toxicity of this approach. Blockade of CTLA-4 induced grade III/IV auto-immune manifestations in 6 of 14 patients in one study.[72]

EVALUATION OF CANCER VACCINES

Cancer vaccines, although increasingly promising, are still experimental therapy. Even after more than 50 years of clinical research, only a single vaccine is currently FDA licensed in the United States for a cancer indication: hepatitis B virus vaccine for prevention of hepatocellular carcinoma. Nevertheless, a search of the National Cancer Institute PDQ database of U.S. clinical trials in July 2003 yielded 81 active phase I-III cancer vaccine trials. The number of vaccine strategies currently in clinical testing is almost as high as the number of trials. The variety of vaccines in preclinical testing surpasses those in clinical testing severalfold. Thus cancer vaccines are at present an active area of oncology and immunology research.

Vaccine Safety

One of the greatest concerns for any new therapy is safety. This is particularly true for cancer vaccines. Many of the adjuvants used in clinical practice are highly inflammatory compounds that carry real risk of local and systemic toxicity. Careful manufacturing under current Good Manufacturing Practices (cGMP) is essential. One of the requirements for successful cancer vaccination may be disruption of self-tolerance and subsequent serious autoimmunity (see earlier, Inhibition of Negative Signals). Thus, as in any new treatment, monitoring for these toxicities is a major goal of early-phase testing.

After several decades of clinical testing of cancer vaccines, thousands of patients have received vaccines with few serious adverse effects. Not unexpectedly with a vaccine, the most frequent complication is a flulike response of fever and chills that is accompanied by local inflammation at the site of vaccination and the occasional allergic reaction. Despite the report by Ludewig and coworkers[186] of serious autoimmunity in an animal tumor vaccine model, little clinically detectable autoimmunity has yet to be observed with cancer vaccines in humans, with the single exception of CTLA-4 blockade.[72] However, as vaccines become more effective at eliciting immunity, the potential for autoimmunity likely increases.[187] Thus close monitoring for this complication remains a critical part of vaccine trials.

Clinical Evaluation of Vaccine Efficacy

Evaluating cancer vaccines for clinical efficacy is difficult and expensive. Excellent discussions of immunologic endpoints and optimal trial design for therapeutic cancer vaccines have been published.[188,189] The best measurement of clinical outcome of any treatment is the ability of the treatment to alter progression of disease. Like other cancer therapies, cancer vaccines are generally evaluated for their effects on relapse-free survival, tumor regression (partial or complete), and overall survival. Considering the small number of subjects in most phase I/II vaccine trials, the lack of a control treatment group in phase I studies, and the reports in the literature of spontaneous tumor regression in cancer patients, it often is difficult to attribute, with any degree of certainty, observed tumor regression in these small studies to the effects of vaccination. The advanced disease present in most participants in early-phase studies also impedes the ability of investigators to observe treatment effects, especially those of a small magnitude.

Simon and colleagues[188] have argued that traditional phase II trials with patients with clinically measurable tumors often are not appropriate as initial trials of tumor vaccines. Vaccine trials are best conducted with patients who have intact immune systems, and for many types of cancer, this precludes enrollment of patients with measurable tumor burdens. With rare exception, tumor regression is not likely with most vaccines in patients with advanced metastatic disease. The likely scenario for tumor vaccines will be the care of patients at risk of cancer (prophylactic vaccines) or those with minimal disease (therapeutic vaccination). Thus traditional phase I designs based on escalation from a very low starting dose in patients with advanced cancer are not always necessary in cancer vaccine development. Early-stage trials should focus on vaccine immunogenicity endpoints while safety data are carefully collected.

Alternative Methods of Evaluating Vaccine Efficacy

Although the best way to assess the efficacy of a cancer vaccine may be through induction of tumor regression or alteration of the course of a tumor, incorporation of surrogate markers of vaccine efficacy into current and future trials should enhance the knowledge gained from these trials.[190]

One of the most important innovations in immunology research has been the development of MHC tetramer reagents.[191] These reagents are prepared by combining MHC class I (or class II), β2-microglobulin, and antigenic peptide in vitro. The soluble MHC class I molecule and β2-microglobulin form heterodimers that incorporate the antigenic peptide forming a structure identical to that found on cells. The MHC/peptide molecule is then tetramerized onto streptavidin labeled with a fluorescent molecule. Cells that express a T-cell receptor recognizing the MHC/peptide complex bind the tetramer reagent and are detectable with flow cytometry. This technology provides a highly sensitive method for detecting and enumerating antigen-specific T cells. It also allows other phenotypic and functional analyses of these T cells when combined with tools such as high-speed cell sorting[89] and automated ELISpot approaches.[189]

When the many new and powerful immune assessment techniques are combined, the composition, nature, and magnitude of an immune response induced by a cancer vaccine can be examined in far greater depth. When these data are considered in the context of new information regarding effective immunity, these surrogate markers of vaccine efficacy will undoubtedly bring cancer vaccine research into a new and exciting era.

STATE OF THE ART IN CANCER VACCINATION

Vaccine therapy is far from standard management of any malignant disease. However, melanoma, myeloma, lymphoma, cervical, and prostate cancers all have been the subjects of moderately successful phase II/III clinical trials. The results of a trial of an HPV vaccine for cervical cancer were striking.[192] Although HPV is an infectious disease vaccine, the success raises the real prospect of prevention of this serious malignant disease.

Melanoma

Melanoma has been the most frequent experimental target of clinical vaccine trials.[193] As a result, much of our current knowledge of TAAs, tumor immunogenicity, and antitumor immunity is derived from studies of this malignant tumor. Some experts argue that melanoma represents a uniquely immunogenic tumor, but this argument remains controversial. Poor responsiveness to conventional chemotherapy and radiation therapy, ability to readily identify pigmented metastatic growth, and perhaps a greater ease of tumor cell culture in vitro are likely contributing factors to the premier status of melanoma as a target of immunotherapy. Regardless of the reasons, the apparent immunogenicity of melanoma has led to several clinical vaccine trials, primarily in the adjuvant setting.

The earliest reported phase III study of a melanoma vaccine was reported by Livingston and associates.[194] This randomized, double-blind study examined the efficacy of a vaccine composed of GM2 ganglioside in bacille Calmette-Guérin (BCG)-containing adjuvant (later changed to QS1). The trial was based on the finding that tumor cells, including melanoma, selectively express GM2 gangliosides on the cell surface, producing a target for humoral immunity. The investigators enrolled 122 patients with American Joint Committee on Cancer stage III disease. Fifty-eight patients received the GM2-containing vaccine administered with BCG as adjuvant, and 64 received BCG alone. Although the investigators found no overall change in disease-free survival or overall survival rate, secondary analysis of patients in whom anti-GM2 antibodies developed demonstrated a significant increase of 17% in overall survival ($P = 0.02$) after a minimum follow-up period of 51 months.

Sondak and colleagues[78] examined the efficacy of an allogeneic vaccine produced by mixing two melanoma cell lysates with detoxified Freund's adjuvant (Melacine; Corixa, Seattle, Wash.). The study randomized 600 patients with $T_3N_0M_0$ disease to either vaccination or observation. The patients were followed for a median of 5.6 years with the primary study endpoints of relapse-free survival and overall survival. There was no evidence of improved disease-free survival among patients randomized to receive vaccine. A polyvalent, allogeneic, whole-cell vaccine comprising three allogeneic tumor cell lines is being tested in patients with advanced-stage melanoma (stage III or stage IV) in phase III clinical trials (CancerVax, Carlsbad, Calif.). The combination of therapeutic vaccination with CTLA-4 blockade also appears to have promise.[71] Many other studies of related vaccine strategies are under way.

Lymphoma and Leukemia

Some of the earliest attempts at tumor-specific vaccination were performed in patients with B-cell lymphoma. Lymphoma and myeloma have a unique characteristic among tumors in that each tumor expresses a unique tumor-specific antigen, the antigen receptor—immunoglobulin in the case of B-cell lymphoma. This tumor-specific molecule is derived from clonal rearrangement of the variable region that determines antigen specificity. This unique variable region, called the idiotype (Id), is immunogenic. In 1972 Lynch and coworkers[195] found the idiotype capable of inducing anti-Id antibody production and subsequent antitumor responses in a mouse transplantable-tumor model.

The first reported clinical study of lymphoma vaccine was conducted with patients with follicular lymphoma because of the relatively high expression of surface immunoglobulin in these tumors and because of relatively slow disease progression.[196,197] For a carrier protein the investigators used tumor-derived immunoglobulin conjugated to keyhole limpet hemocyanin (KLH). The immunogenic conjugate was mixed with an adjuvant and administered subcutaneously. Many of the patients developed anti-Id immune responses. Most of the responses were humoral (antibody) in nature and occurred mainly in patients with disease in complete remission at the time of vaccination. A smaller fraction (3 of 41 vaccinated patients) had cellular anti-Id responses as measured by in vitro cellular proliferation. Similar findings were reported in a smaller study by Barrios and associates.[198] In retrospect, these findings are not surprising given that immunization with soluble protein generally stimulates humoral type 2 immune responses. Despite the mostly humoral immunity generated in this study, a significant difference in progression-free survival was found for responders versus nonresponders (7.9 years versus 1.3 years, respectively) among subjects who received vaccination during the first remission. Subsequent studies showed that Id-conjugate vaccine in combination with GM-CSF[199] and Id-pulsed dendritic cells[200,201] can produce greater cellular immune responses in addition to prominent humoral responses, even in patients with evidence of disease at the time of treatment.

Although cellular rather than humoral immunity has been suggested as the important factor for clinical response,[199] anti-Id antibody has been shown to induce receptor phosphorylation in malignant lymphoma cells.[201] Whether some of the antitumor effects are mediated by anti-Id antibody in a manner similar to anti-CD20 monoclonal antibody remains to be elucidated. In a National Cancer Institute–sponsored, multicenter, randomized phase III trial (protocol NCI-00-C-0050) addressing the clinical effectiveness of Id vaccination for follicular lymphoma, Id/KLH+GM-CSF vaccination is being compared with carrier alone in combination with chemotherapy. Although a significant antilymphoma response is expected on the basis of very promising results of uncontrolled previous studies, the results of this phase III trial, if favorable, will provide much stronger evidence of the effectiveness of cancer vaccination.

Studies of vaccination against more aggressive lymphomas are at an earlier stage of clinical development than studies of follicular lymphoma.[201,202] This difference is partly related to the rapid progression of disease in patients with aggressive lymphoma and their reduced expression of Id antibody. This will likely be an area of more intense investigation given the lack of effective therapy and poor prognosis for diseases such as mantle cell lymphoma.

Several studies of vaccination against multiple myeloma with tumor-derived Id immunoglobulin similar to that for follicular lymphoma have been conducted. Unlike the relatively frequent, strong cellular and humoral immune responses detectable in lymphoma patients receiving Id vaccines, the anti-Id responses of myeloma patients are poor and infrequent.[203] This may be partly related to the more advanced disease or the previous therapy received by myeloma patients. Many patients in the reported studies received high-dose chemotherapy followed by autologous peripheral blood stem cell transplantation. This therapy appears to produce a state of immunodeficiency for several months after transplantation[167] and may affect ability to administer vaccine in the posttransplantation period. Furthermore, myeloma cells, unlike follicular lymphoma cells, are generally surface immunoglobulin negative, a condition that precludes myeloma cells as significant targets for antibody responses. Myeloma cells do appear to process and present idiotypic immunoglobulin through MHC class I, a finding that suggests cellular immune responses may be more important.[204,205] Several Id vaccines as well as whole cell vaccines are under investigation for this disease. The difficulty in demonstrating antimyeloma immune responses or clinical responses with current Id vaccines, however, illustrates some of the challenges to cancer vaccination. It also suggests that vaccines may have to be highly tailored toward the tumor being targeted.

A variety of vaccine approaches have been used for patients with acute and chronic leukemia.[206,207] The most promising TAAs identified are proteinase 3, a neutral serine protease overexpressed in chronic myelogenous leukemia and in many cases of acute myelocytic leukemia,[86,208] and WT1, the Wilms' tumor gene transcription factor, which is overexpressed in most cases of adult leukemia.[209]

Cervical Carcinoma

More than 450,000 new cases of cervical cancer are diagnosed annually worldwide.[210] More than 99% of these cases are associated with HPV infection, and HPV infection appears to be the principle initiating factor in most cases of cervical cancer.[211] HPV type 16, one of several "high-risk" strains, is implicated in more than one half of cases of cervical cancer.[212] Although infection initiates the neoplastic process, progression to invasive cervical carcinoma occurs over 5 to 10 years. Results of epidemiologic studies indicate that most HPV infections have only a short duration. Development of invasive carcinoma is associated with more persistent infections.[213] The immune system is thought to play an important role in control of HPV infection. Persistent infection leading to neoplasia appears more to be common and more rapid in immunosuppressed persons.[214]

The overwhelming association between HPV infection, particularly with the high-risk HPV type 16 strain, and cervical cancer has led to exploration of vaccination against HPV as a strategy to prevent cervical cancer. A double-blind, placebo-controlled trial of HPV type 16 vaccine had promising results. The vaccine consisted of virus-like particles generated by expression of the L1 capsid protein in yeast administered intramuscularly in an aluminum adjuvant. The vaccine was 100% efficacious at preventing persistent HPV-16 infection. In addition, nine cases of cervical intraepithelial neoplasia in 2392 women all occurred in the placebo group; no cases occurred in the vaccine group.

Although prevention of HPV infection may lead to a significant reduction in the incidence of cervical cancer, the potential for vaccination to alter the course of established malignant growth is far less clear. One advantage afforded in cervical cancer compared with other malignant lesions is expression of the oncogenic viral proteins E6 and E7, which are highly expressed by cells within neoplastic cervical lesions. Advanced-stage clinical trials are planned for a vaccine consisting of a fusion protein of E7 and a heat-shock protein as an adjuvant for patients with cervical dysplasia (Stressgen Biotechnologies, Victoria, BC, Canada). These virally produced TAAs are a superb target for immunization.

Prostate Carcinoma

A variety of therapeutic vaccine trials have been performed with patients with hormone refractory prostate cancer. Most trials are designed to stimulate immunity against antigens present only on prostate cells, such as prostate-specific antigen (PSA) and prostate-specific membrane antigen (PSMA). Autoimmune prostatitis is an expected consequence of many vaccine approaches to this disease, because it is a prototypic cancer of dispensable tissue.[44]

A phase I trial of the use of autologous prostate RNA transduced into autologous dendritic cells was successful at inducing tumor immunity in a substantial fraction of subjects.[151] On the basis of promising phase I/II results,[215] Dendreon Corp. sponsored a randomized, placebo-controlled phase III trial of autologous immature dendritic cells loaded with prostatic acid phosphatase in patients with hormone refractory prostate cancer (Provenage; Dendreon, Seattle, Wash.). Unfortunately, this trial did not reach statistical endpoints. However, ad hoc subgroup analysis showed significant clinical benefit for vaccination of men with a Gleason score of 7 or less. There was a more than twofold delay in both time to disease progression (hazard ratio, 2.2; $P = 0.002$) and time to development of disease-related pain (hazard ratio, 2.6; $P = 0.019$) compared with patients receiving placebo. Phase III follow-up trials are being conducted to further test this approach.

Cell-based vaccines consisting of irradiated allogeneic prostate cancer lines engineered to secrete GM-CSF have been administered with promising results.[216] A phase III trial is under development to further test this concept (GVAX; Cell Genesys, Foster City, Calif.).

Colorectal Carcinoma

Levamisole is a nonspecific adjuvant FDA approved for use in combination with the chemotherapeutic agent 5-fluorouracil in patients with stage C colorectal carcinoma. Edrecolomab (Panorex) is a monoclonal antibody directed against the 17-1A (Ep-CAM) antigen located on the cell surfaces of carcinoma. Edrecolomab is licensed for use in Germany for management of stage B and C colon cancer. An anti-Id monoclonal antibody to carcinoembryonic antigen (CEA), designated CeaVac, has been shown to induce humoral and cellular immunity to CEA in patients with colorectal cancer.[217] A phase III, randomized, placebo-controlled study of CeaVac in patients with metastatic colorectal cancer receiving chemotherapy with 5-fluorouracil and leucovorin was conducted by Titan Pharmaceuticals. Preliminary results from the study demonstrated a trend toward 2- to 3-month improvement in overall survival among patients receiving at least five doses of CeaVac versus placebo (modified intent-to-treat analysis). The investigators, however, found statistically significant improvement in the primary endpoint of survival in the evaluable overall efficacy population or the intent-to-treat population. A novel therapeutic vaccine approach with dendritic cells loaded with an altered peptide ligand for CEA resulted in induction of antitumor immunity and tumor regression in a small number of patients with advanced colon cancer.[94] The results are encouraging, and future vaccine trials may show clinical benefit in colorectal cancer.

REFERENCES

1. Arias E, Smith B: Deaths: Preliminary data for 2001. Natl Vital Stat Rep 2003;51:1–44.
2. Thomas L: In Lawrence H (ed): Cellular and Humoral Aspects of the Hypersensitive States. New York, Hoeber-Harper, 1959, pp 529–532.
3. Burnet FM: The concept of immunological surveillance. Prog Exp Tumor Res 1970;13:1–27.
4. Dunn GP, Bruce AT, Ikeda H, Old LJ, Schreiber RD: Cancer immuno-editing: From immunosurveillance to tumor escape. Nat Immunol 2002;3:991–998.
5. Nakano O, Sato M, Naito Y, et al: Proliferative activity of intra-tumoral CD8+ T-lymphocytes as a prognostic factor in human renal cell carcinoma: Clinicopathologic demonstration of antitumor immunity. Cancer Res 2001;61:5132–5136.
6. Marrogi AJ, Munshi A, Merogi AJ, et al: Study of tumor infiltrating lymphocytes and transforming growth factor-beta as prognostic factors in breast carcinoma. Int J Cancer 1997;74:492–501.
7. Zhang L, Conejo-Garcia JR, Katsaros D, et al: Intratumoral T cells, recurrence, and survival in epithelial ovarian cancer. N Engl J Med 2003;348:203–213.
8. Vesalainen S, Lipponen P, Talja M, Syrjanen K: Histological grade, perineural infiltration, tumour-infiltrating lymphocytes and apoptosis as determinants of long-term prognosis in prostatic adenocarcinoma. Eur J Cancer 1994;30A:1797–1803.
9. Halpern AC, Schuchter LM: Prognostic models in melanoma. Semin Oncol 1997;24(1 suppl 4):S2–S7.
10. Schumacher K, Haensch W, Roefzaad C, Schlag PM: Prognostic significance of activated CD8+ T cell infiltrations within esophageal carcinomas. Cancer Res 2001;61:3932–3936.
11. Rudnick E, Khakoo Y, Antunes NL, et al: Opsoclonus-myoclonus-ataxia syndrome in neuroblastoma: Clinical outcome and antineuronal antibodies—a report from the Children's Cancer Group Study. Med Pediatr Oncol 2001;36:612–622.
12. Albert ML, Darnell JC, Bender A, Francisco LM, Bhardwaj N, Darnell RB: Tumor-specific killer cells in paraneoplastic cerebellar degeneration. Nat Med 1998;4:1321–1324.
13. Dalmau J, Graus F, Rosenblum MK, Posner JB: Anti-Hu-associated paraneoplastic encephalomyelitis/sensory neuronopathy: A clinical study of 71 patients. Medicine (Baltimore) 1992;71:59–72.
14. Graus F, Keime-Guibert F, Rene R, et al: Anti-Hu-associated paraneoplastic encephalomyelitis: Analysis of 200 patients. Brain 2001;124:1138–1148.
15. Ochsenbein AF, Sierro S, Odermatt B, et al: Roles of tumour localization, second signals and cross priming in cytotoxic T-cell induction. Nature 2001;411:1058–1064.
16. Mellor AL, Munn DH: Tryptophan catabolism and T-cell tolerance: Immunosuppression by starvation? Immunol Today 1999;20:469–473.
17. Khong HT, Restifo NP: Natural selection of tumor variants in the generation of "tumor escape" phenotypes. Nat Immunol 2002;3:999–1005.
18. Ueda K, Toyokawa M, Nakamori H, et al: Immunosuppressive effect of serum in patients with ovarian carcinoma. Obstet Gynecol 1978;51:225–228.
19. Nakashima M, Sonoda K, Watanabe T: Inhibition of cell growth and induction of apoptotic cell death by the human tumor-associated antigen RCAS1. Nat Med 1999;5:938–942.
20. Dong H, Strome SE, Salomao DR, et al: Tumor-associated B7-H1 promotes T-cell apoptosis: A potential mechanism of immune evasion. Nat Med 2002;8:793–800.
21. Groh V, Wu J, Yee C, Spies T: Tumour-derived soluble MIC ligands impair expression of NKG2D and T-cell activation. Nature 2002;419:734–738.
22. Lurquin C, Van Pel A, Mariame B, et al: Structure of the gene of tum- transplantation antigen P91A: The mutated exon encodes a peptide recognized with Ld by cytolytic T cells. Cell 1989;58:293–303.
23. Woo EY, Yeh H, Chu CS, et al: Cutting edge: Regulatory T cells from lung cancer patients directly inhibit autologous T cell proliferation. J Immunol 2002;168:4272–4276.
24. Liyanage UK, Moore TT, Joo HG, et al: Prevalence of regulatory T cells is increased in peripheral blood and tumor microenvironment of patients with pancreas or breast adenocarcinoma. J Immunol 2002;169:2756–2761.
25. White CA, Weaver RL, Grillo-Lopez AJ: Antibody-targeted immunotherapy for treatment of malignancy. Annu Rev Med 2003;52:125–145.
26. Clynes RA, Towers TL, Presta LG, Ravetch JV: Inhibitory Fc receptors modulate in vivo cytoxicity against tumor targets. Nat Med 2000;6:443–446.
27. Fisk B, Blevins TL, Wharton JT, Ioannides CG: Identification of an immunodominant peptide of HER-2/neu protooncogene recognized by ovarian tumor-specific cytotoxic T lymphocyte lines. J Exp Med 1995;181:2109–2117.
28. Celis E, Tsai V, Crimi C, et al: Induction of anti-tumor cytotoxic T lymphocytes in normal humans using primary cultures and synthetic peptide epitopes. Proc Natl Acad Sci USA 1994;91:2105–2109.
29. Greenberg PD: Adoptive T cell therapy of tumors: Mechanisms operative in the recognition and elimination of tumor cells. Adv Immunol 1991;49:281–355.

30. Dudley ME, Wunderlich JR, Robbins PF, et al: Cancer regression and autoimmunity in patients after clonal repopulation with antitumor lymphocytes. Science 2002;298:850–854.

31. Yee C, Thompson JA, Byrd D, et al: Adoptive T cell therapy using antigen-specific CD8(+) T cell clones for the treatment of patients with metastatic melanoma: In vivo persistence, migration, and antitumor effect of transferred T cells. Proc Natl Acad Sci USA 2002;99:16168–16173.

32. Kawano T, Cui J, Koezuka Y, et al: Natural killer-like nonspecific tumor cell lysis mediated by specific ligand-activated Valpha14 NKT cells. Proc Natl Acad Sci USA 1998;95:5690–5693.

33. Metelitsa LS, Naidenko OV, Kant A, et al: Human NKT cells mediate antitumor cytotoxicity directly by recognizing target cell CD1d with bound ligand or indirectly by producing IL-2 to activate NK cells. J Immunol 2001;167:3114–3122.

34. Moodycliffe AM, Nghiem D, Clydesdale G, Ullrich SE: Immune suppression and skin cancer development: Regulation by NKT cells. Nat Immunol 2000;1:521–525.

35. Dhodapkar MV, Geller MD, Chang DH, et al: A reversible defect in natural killer T cell function characterizes the progression of premalignant to malignant multiple myeloma. J Exp Med 2003;197:1667–1676.

36. Tahir SM, Cheng O, Shaulov A, et al: Loss of IFN-gamma production by invariant NK T cells in advanced cancer. J Immunol 2001; 167:4046–4050.

37. Terabe M, Matsui S, Noben-Trauth N, et al: NKT cell-mediated repression of tumor immunosurveillance by IL-13 and the IL-4R-STAT6 pathway. Nat Immunol 2000;1:515–520.

38. Schoenberger SP, Toes RE, van der Voort EI, Offringa R, Melief CJ: T-cell help for cytotoxic T lymphocytes is mediated by CD40-CD40L interactions. Nature 1998;393:480–483.

39. Ho WY, Yee C, Greenberg PD: Adoptive therapy with CD8(+) T cells: It may get by with a little help from its friends. J Clin Invest 2002;110:1415–1417.

40. Bingle L, Brown NJ, Lewis CE: The role of tumour-associated macrophages in tumour progression: Implications for new anticancer therapies. J Pathol 2002;196:254–265.

41. Paulnock DM: Macrophage activation by T cells. Curr Opin Immunol 1992;4:344–349.

42. Boon T, van der Bruggen P: Human tumor antigens recognized by T lymphocytes. J Exp Med 1996;183:725–729.

43. Gilboa E: The makings of a tumor rejection antigen. Immunity 1999;11:263–270.

44. Pardoll DM: Inducing autoimmune disease to treat cancer. Proc Natl Acad Sci USA 1999;96:5340–5342.

45. Shankaran V, Ikeda H, Bruce AT, et al: IFNgamma and lymphocytes prevent primary tumour development and shape tumour immunogenicity. Nature 2001;410:1107–1111.

46. Linard B, Bezieau S, Benlalam H, et al: A ras-mutated peptide targeted by CTL infiltrating a human melanoma lesion. J Immunol 2002;168:4802–4808.

47. Wagner WM, Ouyang Q, Pawelec G: The abl/bcr gene product as a novel leukemia-specific antigen: Peptides spanning the fusion region of abl/bcr can be recognized by both CD4+ and CD8+ T lymphocytes. Cancer Immunol Immunother 2003;52:89–96.

48. Niethammer AG, Xiang R, Becker JC, et al: A DNA vaccine against VEGF receptor 2 prevents effective angiogenesis and inhibits tumor growth. Nat Med 2002;8:1369–1375.

49. Nair S, Boczkowski D, Moeller B, Dewhirst M, Vieweg J, Gilboa E: Synergy between tumor immunotherapy and antiangiogenic therapy. Blood 2003;102:964–971.

50. Coulie PG, Weynants P, Lehmann F, et al: Genes coding for tumor antigens recognized by human cytolytic T lymphocytes. J Immunother 1993;14:104–109.

51. Smith ES, Mandokhot A, Evans EE, et al: Lethality-based selection of recombinant genes in mammalian cells: Application to identifying tumor antigens. Nat Med 2001;7:967–972.

52. Sahin U, Tureci O, Schmitt H, et al: Human neoplasms elicit multiple specific immune responses in the autologous host. Proc Natl Acad Sci USA 1995;92:11810–11813.

53. Jager E, Chen YT, Drijfhout JW, et al: Simultaneous humoral and cellular immune response against cancer-testis antigen NY-ESO-1: Definition of human histocompatibility leukocyte antigen (HLA)-A2-binding peptide epitopes. J Exp Med 1998;187:265–270.

54. Durst M, Glitz D, Schneider A, zur Hausen H: Human papillomavirus type 16 (HPV 16) gene expression and DNA replication in cervical neoplasia: Analysis by in situ hybridization. Virology 1992;189:132–140.

55. Stoler MH, Rhodes CR, Whitbeck A, Wolinsky SM, Chow LT, Broker TR: Human papillomavirus type 16 and 18 gene expression in cervical neoplasias. Hum Pathol 1992;23:117–128.

56. Higgins GD, Phillips GE, Smith LA, Uzelin DM, Burrell CJ: High prevalence of human papillomavirus transcripts in all grades of cervical intraepithelial glandular neoplasia. Cancer 1992;70:136–146.

57. Disis ML, Cheever MA: Oncogenic proteins as tumor antigens. Curr Opin Immunol 1996;8:637–642.

58. Topalian S, Rivoltini L, Mancini M, et al: Human CD4+ T cells specifically recognize a shared melanoma-associated antigen encoded by the tyrosinase gene. Proc Natl Acad Sci USA 1994;91:9461–9465.

59. Kawakami Y, Eliyahu S, Delgado C, et al: Cloning of the gene coding for a shared human melanoma antigen recognized by autologous t cells infiltrating into tumor. Proc Natl Acad Sci USA 1994;91:3515–3519.

60. Berd D: Cancer vaccines: Reborn or just recycled? Semin Oncol 1998;25:605–610.

61. Cavallari V, Cannavo SP, Ussia AF, Moretti G, Albanese A: Vitiligo associated with metastatic malignant melanoma. Int J Dermatol 1996;35:738–740.

62. Cui J, Bystryn JC: Melanoma and vitiligo are associated with antibody responses to similar antigens on pigment cells. Arch Dermatol 1995;131:314–318.

63. Duhra P, Ilchyshyn A: Prolonged survival in metastatic malignant melanoma associated with vitiligo. Clin Exp Dermatol 1991;16: 303–305.

64. Nordlund JJ, Kirkwood JM, Forget BM, Milton G, Albert DM, Lerner AB: Vitiligo in patients with metastatic melanoma: A good prognostic sign. J Am Acad Dermatol 1983;9:689–696.

65. Lang KS, Caroli CC, Muhm A, et al: HLA-A2 restricted, melanocyte-specific CD8(+) T lymphocytes detected in vitiligo patients are related to disease activity and are predominantly directed against MelanA/MART1. J Invest Dermatol 2001;116:891–897.

66. Rosenberg SA, White DE: Vitiligo in patients with melanoma: Normal tissue antigens can be targets for cancer immunotherapy. J Immunother Emphasis Tumor Immunol 1996;19:81–84.

67. Consogno G, Manici S, Facchinetti V, et al: Identification of immunodominant regions among promiscuous HLA-DR-restricted CD4+ T-cell epitopes on the tumor antigen MAGE-3. Blood 2003;101:1038–1044.

68. Chaux P, Vantomme V, Stroobant V, et al: Identification of MAGE-3 epitopes presented by HLA-DR molecules to CD4+ T lymphocytes. J Exp Med 1999;189:767–778.

69. Zeng G, Touloukian CE, Wang X, Restifo NP, Rosenberg SA, Wang RF: Identification of CD4+ T cell epitopes from NY-ESO-1 presented by HLA-DR molecules. J Immunol 2000;165:1153–1159.

70. Wang RF, Wang X, Atwood AC, Topalian SL, Rosenberg SA: Cloning genes encoding MHC class II-restricted antigens: Mutated CDC27 as a tumor antigen. Science 1999;284:1351–1354.

71. Hodi FS, Mihm MC, Soiffer RJ, et al: Biologic activity of cytotoxic T lymphocyte-associated antigen 4 antibody blockade in previously vaccinated metastatic melanoma and ovarian carcinoma patients. Proc Natl Acad Sci USA 2003;100:4712–4717.

72. Phan GQ, Yang JC, Sherry RM, et al: Cancer regression and autoimmunity induced by cytotoxic T lymphocyte-associated antigen 4 blockade in patients with metastatic melanoma. Proc Natl Acad Sci USA 2003;100:8372–8377.

73. Nadler SH, Moore GE: Clinical immunologic study of malignant disease: Response to tumor transplants and transfer of leukocytes. Ann Surg 1966;164:482–490.

74. Mastrangelo MJ, Lattime EC, Maguire H Jr, Berd D: Whole cell vaccines. In Devita VT, Hellman S, Rosenberg SA (eds): Biologic Therapy of Cancer, 2nd ed. Philadelphia, JB Lippincott, 1999, pp 648–659.

75. Hsueh EC, Essner R, Foshag LJ, et al: Prolonged survival after complete resection of disseminated melanoma and active immunotherapy with a therapeutic cancer vaccine. J Clin Oncol 2002;20:4549–4554.

76. Morton DL, Hsueh EC, Essner R, et al: Prolonged survival of patients receiving active immunotherapy with Canvaxin therapeutic polyvalent vaccine after complete resection of melanoma metastatic to regional lymph nodes. Ann Surg 2002;236:438–448.

77. Sosman J, Unger J, Liu P, Flaherty L, et al: Adjuvant immunotherapy of resected, intermediate-thickness, node-negative melanoma with an allogeneic tumor vaccine: Impact of HLA class I antigen expression on outcome. J Clin Oncol 2002;20:2067–2075.

78. Sondak VK, Liu PY, Tuthill RJ, et al: Adjuvant immunotherapy of resected, intermediate-thickness, node-negative melanoma with an allogeneic tumor vaccine: Overall results of a randomized trial of the Southwest Oncology Group. J Clin Oncol 2002;20:2058–2066.

79. Nair SK, Morse M, Boczkowski D, et al: Induction of tumor-specific cytotoxic T lymphocytes in cancer patients by autologous tumor RNA-transfected dendritic cells. Ann Surg 2002;235:540–549.

80. Milazzo C, Reichardt VL, Muller MR, Grunebach F, Brossart P: Induction of myeloma-specific cytotoxic T cells using dendritic cells transfected with tumor-derived RNA. Blood 2003;101:977–982.

81. Grunebach F, Muller MR, Nencioni A, Brossart P: Delivery of tumor-derived RNA for the induction of cytotoxic T-lymphocytes. Gene Ther 2003;10:367–374.

82. Srivastava PK: Do human cancers express shared protective antigens? Or the necessity of remembrance of things past. Semin Immunol 1996;8:295–302.

83. Wang RF, Rosenberg SA: Human tumor antigens for cancer vaccine development. Immunol Rev 1999;170:85–100.

84. van der Bruggen P, Zhang Y, Chaux P, et al: Tumor-specific shared antigenic peptides recognized by human T cells. Immunol Rev 2002;188:51–64.

85. Phan GQ, Touloukian CE, Yang JC, et al: Immunization of patients with metastatic melanoma using both class I– and class II–restricted peptides from melanoma-associated antigens. J Immunother 2003;26:349–356.

86. Molldrem J, Dermime S, Parker K, et al: Targeted T-cell therapy for human leukemia: Cytotoxic T lymphocytes specific for a peptide derived from proteinase 3 preferentially lyse human myeloid leukemia cells. Blood 1996;88:2450–2457.

87. Vonderheide RH, Hahn WC, Schultze JL, Nadler LM: The telomerase catalytic subunit is a widely expressed tumor-associated antigen recognized by cytotoxic T lymphocytes. Immunity 1999;10:673–679.

88. Romero P, Valmori D, Pittet MJ, et al: Antigenicity and immunogenicity of Melan-A/MART-1 derived peptides as targets for tumor reactive CTL in human melanoma. Immunol Rev 2002;188:81–96.

89. Pittet MJ, Zippelius A, Speiser DE, et al: Ex vivo IFN-gamma secretion by circulating CD8 T lymphocytes: Implications of a novel approach for T cell monitoring in infectious and malignant diseases. J Immunol 2001;166:7634–7640.

90. Lafferty KJ, Warren HS, Woolnough JA, Talmage DW: Immunological induction of T lymphocytes: Role of antigen and the lymphocyte costimulator. Blood Cells 1978;4:395–406.

91. Mueller DL, Jenkins MK, Schwartz RH: Clonal expansion versus functional clonal inactivation: A costimulatory signalling pathway determines the outcome of T cell antigen receptor occupancy. Annu Rev Immunol 1989;7:445–480.

92. Matzinger P: The danger model: A renewed sense of self. Science 2002;296:301–305.

93. Janeway CA Jr, Medzhitov R: Innate immune recognition. Annu Rev Immunol 2002;20:197–216.

94. Fong L, Hou Y, Rivas A, et al: Altered peptide ligand vaccination with Flt3 ligand expanded dendritic cells for tumor immunotherapy. Proc Natl Acad Sci USA 2001;98:8809–8814.

95. June CH, Bluestone JA, Nadler LM, Thompson CB: The B7 and CD28 receptor families. Immunol Today 1994;15:321–331.

96. Plotkin SA, Mortimer EA: Vaccines, 2nd ed. Philadelphia, WB Saunders, 1994.

97. Cox JC, Coulter AR: Adjuvants: A classification and review of their modes of action. Vaccine 1997;15:248–256.

98. Takahashi H, Takeshita T, Morein B, Putney S, Germain RN, Berzofsky JA: Induction of CD8+ cytotoxic T cells by immunization with purified HIV-1 envelope protein in ISCOMs. Nature 1990;344:873–875.

99. McKeever U, Barman S, Hao T, et al: Protective immune responses elicited in mice by immunization with formulations of poly(lactide-co-glycolide) microparticles. Vaccine 2002;20:1524–1531.

100. Medzhitov R, Janeway CA Jr: How does the immune system distinguish self from nonself? Semin Immunol 2000;12:185–188.

101. Weiskirch LM, Paterson Y: Listeria monocytogenes: A potent vaccine vector for neoplastic and infectious disease. Immunol Rev 1997;158:159–169.

102. Xiang R, Lode HN, Chao TH, et al: An autologous oral DNA vaccine protects against murine melanoma. Proc Natl Acad Sci USA 2000;97:5492–5497.

103. Leitner WW, Hwang LN, deVeer MJ, et al: Alphavirus-based DNA vaccine breaks immunological tolerance by activating innate antiviral pathways. Nat Med 2003;9:33–39.

104. Coley WB: The treatment of malignant tumors by repeated inoculations of erysipelas: With a report of ten original cases. Am J Med Sci 1893;105:487–511.

105. Klein G, Klein E: Immune surveillance against virus-induced tumors and nonrejectability of spontaneous tumors: Contrasting consequences of host versus tumor evolution. Proc Natl Acad Sci USA 1977;74:2121–2125.

106. Hemmi H, Takeuchi O, Kawai T, et al: A Toll-like receptor recognizes bacterial DNA. Nature 2000;408:740–745.

107. Bauer S, Kirschning CJ, Hacker H, et al: Human TLR9 confers responsiveness to bacterial DNA via species-specific CpG motif recognition. Proc Natl Acad Sci USA 2001;98:9237–9242.

108. Krieg AM, Yi AK, Matson S, et al: CpG motifs in bacterial DNA trigger direct B-cell activation. Nature 1995;374:546–549.

109. Krieg AM, Yi AK, Schorr J, Davis HL: The role of CpG dinucleotides in DNA vaccines. Trends Microbiol 1998;6:23–27.

110. Heise C, Sampson-Johannes A, Williams A, McCormick F, Von Hoff DD, Kirn DH: ONYX-015, an E1B gene-attenuated adenovirus, causes tumor-specific cytolysis and antitumoral efficacy that can be augmented by standard chemotherapeutic agents. Nat Med 1997;3:639–645.

111. Coukos G, Courreges MC, Benencia F: Intraperitoneal oncolytic and tumor vaccination therapy with replication-competent recombinant virus: The herpes paradigm. Curr Gene Ther 2003;3:113–125.

112. Liu BL, Robinson M, Han ZQ, et al: ICP34.5 deleted herpes simplex virus with enhanced oncolytic, immune stimulating, and anti-tumour properties. Gene Ther 2003;10:292–303.

113. Toda M, Iizuka Y, Kawase T, Uyemura K, Kawakami Y: Immuno-viral therapy of brain tumors by combination of viral therapy with cancer vaccination using a replication-conditional HSV. Cancer Gene Ther 2002;9:356–364.

114. Todryk S, McLean C, Ali S, et al: Disabled infectious single-cycle herpes simplex virus as an oncolytic vector for immunotherapy of colorectal cancer. Hum Gene Ther 1999;10:2757–2768.

115. Reits EA, Vos JC, Gromme M, Neefjes J: The major substrates for TAP in vivo are derived from newly synthesized proteins. Nature 2000;404:774–778.

116. Paoletti E: Applications of pox virus vectors to vaccination: An update. Proc Natl Acad Sci USA 1996;93:11349–11353.

117. Kwak H, Horig H, Kaufman HL: Poxviruses as vectors for cancer immunotherapy. Curr Opin Drug Discov Devel 2003;6:161–168.

118. Meneguzzi G, Cerni C, Kieny MP, Lathe R: Immunization against human papillomavirus type 16 tumor cells with recombinant vaccinia viruses expressing E6 and E7. Virology 1991;181:62–69.

119. Roth J, Dittmer D, Rea D, Tartaglia J, Paoletti E, Levine AJ: p53 as a target for cancer vaccines: Recombinant canarypox virus vectors expressing p53 protect mice against lethal tumor cell challenge. Proc Natl Acad Sci USA 1996;93:4781–4786.

120. Overwijk WW, Tsung A, Irvine KR, et al: gp100/pmel 17 is a murine tumor rejection antigen: Induction of "self"-reactive, tumoricidal T cells using high-affinity, altered peptide ligand. J Exp Med 1998;188:277–286.

121. Holzer GW, Falkner FG: Construction of a vaccinia virus deficient in the essential DNA repair enzyme uracil DNA glycosylase by a complementing cell line. J Virol 1997;71:4997–5002.

122. Sutter G, Moss B: Nonreplicating vaccinia vector efficiently expresses recombinant genes. Proc Natl Acad Sci USA 1992;89:10847–10851.

123. Tartaglia J, Perkus ME, Taylor J, et al: NYVAC: A highly attenuated strain of vaccinia virus. Virology 1992;188:217–232.

124. Fries LF, Tartaglia J, Taylor J, et al: Human safety and immunogenicity of a canarypox-rabies glycoprotein recombinant vaccine: An alternative poxvirus vector system. Vaccine 1996;14:428–434.

125. Scholl SM, Balloul JM, Le Goc G, et al: Recombinant vaccinia virus encoding human MUC1 and IL2 as immunotherapy in patients with breast cancer. J Immunother 2000;23:570–580.

126. Sanda MG, Smith DC, Charles LG, et al: Recombinant vaccinia-PSA (Prostvac) can induce a prostate-specific immune response in androgen-modulated human prostate cancer. Urology 1999;53:260–266.

127. Marshall JL, Hoyer RJ, Toomey MA, et al: Phase I study in advanced cancer patients of a diversified prime-and-boost vaccination protocol using recombinant vaccinia virus and recombinant nonreplicating avipox virus to elicit anti-carcinoembryonic antigen immune responses. J Clin Oncol 2000;18:3964–3973.

128. Gulley J, Chen AP, Dahut W, et al: Phase I study of a vaccine using recombinant vaccinia virus expressing PSA (rV-PSA) in patients with metastatic androgen-independent prostate cancer. Prostate 2002;53:109–117.

129. Pan ZK, Weiskirch LM, Paterson Y: Regression of established B16F10 melanoma with a recombinant Listeria monocytogenes vaccine. Cancer Res 1999;59:5264–5269.

130. Jensen ER, Selvakumar R, Shen H, Ahmed R, Wettstein FO, Miller JF: Recombinant Listeria monocytogenes vaccination eliminates papillomavirus-induced tumors and prevents papilloma formation from viral DNA. J Virol 1997;71:8467–8474.

131. Paglia P, Arioli I, Frahm N, Chakraborty T, Colombo MP, Guzman CA: The defined attenuated Listeria monocytogenes delta mp12 mutant is an effective oral vaccine carrier to trigger a long-lasting immune response against a mouse fibrosarcoma. Eur J Immunol 1997;27:1570–1575.

132. Pan ZK, Ikonomidis G, Lazenby A, Pardoll D, Paterson Y: A recombinant Listeria monocytogenes vaccine expressing a model tumour antigen protects mice against lethal tumour cell challenge and causes regression of established tumours. Nat Med 1995;1:471–477.

133. Pan ZK, Ikonomidis G, Pardoll D, Paterson Y: Regression of established tumors in mice mediated by the oral administration of a recombinant Listeria monocytogenes vaccine. Cancer Res 1995;55:4776–4779.

134. Medina E, Guzman CA: Use of live bacterial vaccine vectors for antigen delivery: Potential and limitations. Vaccine 2001;19:1573–1580.

135. Steinman RM, Cohn ZA: Identification of a novel cell type in peripheral lymphoid organs of mice. II. Functional properties in vitro. J Exp Med 1974;139:380–397.

136. Fujii SI, Shimizu K, Smith C, Bonifaz L, Steinman RM: Activation of natural killer T Cells by alpha-galactosylceramide rapidly induces the full maturation of dendritic cells in vivo and thereby acts as an adjuvant for combined CD4 and CD8 T cell immunity to a coadministered protein. J Exp Med 2003;198:267–279.

137. Romani N, Gruner S, Brang D, et al: Proliferating dendritic cell progenitors in human blood. J Exp Med 1994;180:83–93.

138. Sallusto F, Lanzavecchia A: Efficient presentation of soluble antigen by cultured human dendritic cells is maintained by granulocyte/macrophage colony-stimulating factor plus interleukin 4 and downregulated by tumor necrosis factor alpha. J Exp Med 1994;179:1109–1118.

139. Caux C, Vanbervliet B, Massacrier C, et al: CD34+ hematopoietic progenitors from human cord blood differentiate along two independent dendritic cell pathways in response to GM-CSF+TNF alpha. J Exp Med 1996;184:695–706.

140. Gasparetto C, Gasparetto M, Morse M, et al: Mobilization of dendritic cells from patients with breast cancer into peripheral blood stem cell leukapheresis samples using Flt-3-ligand and G-CSF or GM-CSF: Cytokine 2002;18:8–19.

141. Osugi Y, Vuckovic S, Hart DNJ: Myeloid blood CD11c+ dendritic cells and monocyte-derived dendritic cells differ in their ability to stimulate T lymphocytes. Blood 2002;100:2858–2866.

142. Fitzgerald-Bocarsly P: Natural interferon-alpha producing cells: The plasmacytoid dendritic cells. Biotechniques 2002;(suppl):16–20,22,24.

143. Shortman K, Liu YJ: Mouse and human dendritic cell subtypes. Nat Rev Immunol 2002;2:151–161.

144. Jefford M, Schnurr M, Toy T, et al: Functional comparison of DC generated in vivo with Flt3 ligand or in vitro from blood monocytes: Differential regulation of function by specific classes of physiologic stimuli. Blood 2003;102:1753–1763.

145. Nestle FO, Alijagic S, Gilliet M, et al: Vaccination of melanoma patients with peptide- or tumor lysate-pulsed dendritic cells. Nat Med 1998;4:328–332.

146. Thurner B, Haendle I, Roder C, et al: Vaccination with Mage-3A1 peptide-pulsed mature, monocyte-derived dendritic cells expands specific cytotoxic T cells and induces regression of some metastases in advanced stage IV melanoma. J Exp Med 1999;190:1669–1678.

147. Zhou Y, Bosch ML, Salgaller ML: Current methods for loading dendritic cells with tumor antigen for the induction of antitumor immunity. J Immunother 2002;25:289–303.

148. Delamarre L, Holcombe H, Mellman I: Presentation of exogenous antigens on major histocompatibility complex (MHC) class I and MHC class II molecules is differentially regulated during dendritic cell maturation. J Exp Med 2003;198:111–122.

149. Pooley JL, Heath WR, Shortman K: Cutting edge: Intravenous soluble antigen is presented to CD4 T cells by CD8⁻ dendritic cells, but cross-presented to CD8 T cells by CD8⁺ dendritic cells. J Immunol 2001;166:5327–5330.

150. Gong J, Chen D, Kashiwaba M, Kufe D: Induction of antitumor activity by immunization with fusions of dendritic and carcinoma cells. Nat Med 1997;3:558–561.

151. Heiser A, Maurice MA, Yancey DR, et al: Induction of polyclonal prostate cancer-specific CTL using dendritic cells transfected with amplified tumor RNA. J Immunol 2001;166:2953–2960.

152. Nair SK, Heiser A, Boczkowski D, et al: Induction of cytotoxic T cell responses and tumor immunity against unrelated tumors using telomerase reverse transcriptase RNA transfected dendritic cells. Nat Med 2000;6:1011–1017.

153. Huang AY, Golumbek P, Ahmadzadeh M, Jaffee E, Pardoll D, Levitsky H: Role of bone marrow-derived cells in presenting MHC class I-restricted tumor antigens. Science 1994;264:961–965.

154. Olasz EB, Linton J, Katz SI: Soluble proteins and haptens on bone marrow-derived dendritic cells are presented to host CD4 T cells in an MHC-restricted manner. Int Immunol 2002;14:493–502.

155. Andre F, Schartz NE, Chaput N, et al: Tumor-derived exosomes: A new source of tumor rejection antigens. Vaccine 2002;20(suppl 4):A28–A31.

156. Weiden PL, Flournoy N, Thomas ED, et al: Antileukemic effect of graft-versus-host disease in human recipients of allogeneic-marrow grafts. N Engl J Med 1979;300:1068–1073.

157. Champlin R, Khouri I, Kornblau S, et al: Allogeneic hematopoietic transplantation as adoptive immunotherapy. Induction of graft-versus-malignancy as primary therapy. Hematol Oncol Clin North Am 1999;13:1041–1057.

158. Ueno NT, Rondon G, Mirza NQ, et al: Allogeneic peripheral-blood progenitor-cell transplantation for poor-risk patients with metastatic breast cancer. J Clin Oncol 1998;16:986–993.

159. Bay JO, Choufi B, Pomel C, et al: Potential allogeneic graft-versus-tumor effect in a patient with ovarian cancer. Bone Marrow Transplant 2000;25:681–682.

160. Childs RW, Clave E, Tisdale J, Plante M, Hensel N, Barrett J: Successful treatment of metastatic renal cell carcinoma with a nonmyeloablative allogeneic peripheral-blood progenitor-cell transplant: Evidence for a graft-versus-tumor effect. J Clin Oncol 1999;17:2044.

161. Feinstein L, Storb R: Nonmyeloablative hematopoietic cell transplantation. Curr Opin Oncol 2001;13:95–100.

162. Anderson LD Jr, Petropoulos D, Everse LA, Mullen CA: Enhancement of graft-versus-tumor activity and graft-versus-host disease by pretransplant immunization of allogeneic bone marrow donors with a recipient-derived tumor cell vaccine. Cancer Res 1999;59:1525–1530.

163. Anderson LD, Jr., Savary CA, Mullen CA: Immunization of allogeneic bone marrow transplant recipients with tumor cell

vaccines enhances graft-versus-tumor activity without exacerbating graft-versus-host disease. Blood 2000;95:2426-2433.

164. Anderson LD Jr, Mori S, Mann S, Savary CA, Mullen CA: Pretransplant tumor antigen-specific immunization of allogeneic bone marrow transplant donors enhances graft-versus-tumor activity without exacerbation of graft-versus-host disease. Cancer Res 2000;60:5797-5802.

165. Luznik L, Slansky JE, Jalla S, et al: Successful therapy of metastatic cancer using tumor vaccines in mixed allogeneic bone marrow chimeras. Blood 2003;101:1645-1652.

166. Teshima T, Mach N, Hill GR, et al: Tumor cell vaccine elicits potent antitumor immunity after allogeneic T-cell-depleted bone marrow transplantation. Cancer Res 2001;61:162-171.

167. Guillaume T, Rubinstein DB, Symann M: Immune reconstitution and immunotherapy after autologous hematopoietic stem cell transplantation. Blood 1998;92:1471-1490.

168. Marrack P, Bender J, Hildeman D, et al: Homeostasis of alpha beta TCR+ T cells. Nat Immunol 2000;1:107-111.

169. Surh CD, Sprent J: Homeostatic T cell proliferation: How far can T cells be activated to self-ligands? J Exp Med 2000;192:9F-14F.

170. Dummer W, Niethammer AG, Baccala R, et al: T cell homeostatic proliferation elicits effective antitumor autoimmunity. J Clin Invest 2002;110:185-192.

171. Laport GG, Levine BL, Stadtmauer EA, et al: Adoptive transfer of costimulated T cells induces lymphocytosis in patients with relapsed/refractory non-Hodgkin's lymphoma following CD34-selected hematopoietic cell transplantation. Blood 2003;102:2004-2013.

172. Berendt MJ, North RJ: T-cell-mediated suppression of anti-tumor immunity: An explanation for progressive growth of an immunogenic tumor. J Exp Med 1980;151:69-80.

173. North RJ: Cyclophosphamide-facilitated adoptive immunotherapy of an established tumor depends on elimination of tumor-induced suppressor T cells. J Exp Med 1982;155:1063-1074.

174. Berd D, Maguire HC Jr, Mastrangelo MJ: Induction of cell-mediated immunity to autologous melanoma cells and regression of metastases after treatment with a melanoma cell vaccine preceded by cyclophosphamide. Cancer Res 1986;46:2572-2577.

175. Berd D, Mastrangelo MJ, Engstrom PF, Paul A, Maguire H: Augmentation of the human immune response by cyclophosphamide. Cancer Res 1982;42:4862-4866.

176. Mastrangelo MJ, Berd D, Maguire H Jr: The immunoaugmenting effects of cancer chemotherapeutic agents. Semin Oncol 1986;13:186-194.

177. Chatenoud L, Salomon B, Bluestone JA: Suppressor T cells: They're back and critical for regulation of autoimmunity! Immunol Rev 2001;182:149-163.

178. Woo EY, Chu CS, Goletz TJ, et al: Regulatory CD4+CD25+ T cells in tumors from patients with early-stage non small cell lung cancer and late-stage ovarian cancer. Cancer Res 2001;61:4766-4772.

179. Sakaguchi S, Sakaguchi N, Shimizu J, et al: Immunologic tolerance maintained by CD25+ CD4+ regulatory T cells: Their common role in controlling autoimmunity, tumor immunity, and transplantation tolerance. Immunol Rev 2001;182:18-32.

180. Sullivan KE, McDonald-McGinn D, Zackai EH: CD4+ CD25+ T-cell production in healthy humans and in patients with thymic hypoplasia. Clin Diagn Lab Immunol 2002;9:1129-1131.

181. Jordan MS, Boesteanu A, Reed AJ, et al: Thymic selection of CD4+CD25+ regulatory T cells induced by an agonist self-peptide. Nat Immunol 2001;2:301-306.

182. Waterhouse P, Penninger JM, Timms E, et al: CTLA-4 deficiency causes lymphoproliferative disorder with early lethality. Science 1995;270:985-988.

183. Chambers CA, Sullivan TJ, Allison JP: Lymphoproliferation in CTLA-4-deficient mice is mediated by costimulation-dependent activation of CD4+ T cells. Immunity 1997;7:885-895.

184. Leach DR, Krummel MF, Allison JP: Enhancement of antitumor immunity by CTLA-4 blockade. Science 1996;271:1734-1736.

185. Perrin PJ, Davis TA, Maldonado JH, June CH, Racke MK: CTLA-4 blockade enhances clinical disease and cytokine production during experimental allergic encephalomyelitis. J Immunol 1996;157:1333-1336.

186. Ludewig B, Ochsenbein AF, Odermatt B, Paulin D, Hengartner H, Zinkernagel RM: Immunotherapy with dendritic cells directed

against tumor antigens shared with normal host cells results in severe autoimmune disease. J Exp Med 2000;191:795-804.

187. Gilboa E: The risk of autoimmunity associated with tumor immunotherapy. Nat Immunol 2001;2:789-792.

188. Simon RM, Steinberg SM, Hamilton M, et al: Clinical trial designs for the early clinical development of therapeutic cancer vaccines. J Clin Oncol 2001;19:1848-1854.

189. Asai T, Storkus WJ, Whiteside TL: Evaluation of the modified Elispot assay for gamma interferon production in cancer patients receiving antitumor vaccines. Clin Diagn Lab Immunol 2000;7:145-154.

190. Kalos M: Tumor antigen-specific T cells and cancer immunotherapy: Current issues and future prospects. Vaccine 2003;21:781-786.

191. Altman JD, Moss PA, Goulder PJ, et al: Phenotypic analysis of antigen-specific T lymphocytes. Science 1996;274:94-96.

192. Koutsky LA, Ault KA, Wheeler CM, et al: A controlled trial of a human papillomavirus type 16 vaccine. N Engl J Med 2002;347:1645-1651.

193. Kadison AS, Morton DL: Immunotherapy of malignant melanoma. Surg Clin North Am 2003;83:343-370.

194. Livingston PO, Wong GY, Adluri S, et al: Improved survival in stage III melanoma patients with GM2 antibodies: A randomized trial of adjuvant vaccination with GM2 ganglioside. J Clin Oncol 1994;12:1036-1044.

195. Lynch R, Graff R, Sirisinha S, Simms E, Eisen H: Myeloma proteins as tumor-specific transplantation antigens. Proc Natl Acad Sci USA 1972;69:1540-1544.

196. Kwak LW, Campbell MJ, Czerwinski DK, Hart S, Miller RA, Levy R: Induction of immune responses in patients with B-cell lymphoma against the surface-immunoglobulin idiotype expressed by their tumors. N Engl J Med 1992;327:1209-1215.

197. Hsu FJ, Caspar CB, Czerwinski DK, et al: Tumor-specific idiotype vaccines in the treatment of patients with B-cell lymphoma: Long term results of a clinical trial. Blood 1997;89:3129-3135.

198. Barrios Y, Cabrera R, Yanez R, et al: Anti-idiotypic vaccination in the treatment of low-grade B-cell lymphoma. Haematologica 2002;87:400-407.

199. Bendandi M, Gocke CD, Kobrin CB, et al: Complete molecular remissions induced by patient-specific vaccination plus granulocyte-monocyte colony-stimulating factor against lymphoma. Nat Med 1999;5:1171-1177.

200. Hsu FJ, Benike C, Fagnoni F, et al: Vaccination of patients with B-cell lymphoma using autologous antigen-pulsed dendritic cells. Nat Med 1996;2:52-58.

201. Timmerman JM, Czerwinski DK, Davis TA, et al: Idiotype-pulsed dendritic cell vaccination for B-cell lymphoma: Clinical and immune responses in 35 patients. Blood 2002;99:1517-1526.

202. Timmerman JM, Singh G, Hermanson G, et al: Immunogenicity of a plasmid DNA vaccine encoding chimeric idiotype in patients with B-cell lymphoma. Cancer Res 2002;62:5845-5852.

203. Ruffini PA, Neelapu SS, Kwak LW, Biragyn A: Idiotypic vaccination for B-cell malignancies as a model for therapeutic cancer vaccines: From prototype protein to second generation vaccines. Haematologica 2002;87:989-1001.

204. Li Y, Bendandi M, Deng Y, et al: Tumor-specific recognition of human myeloma cells by idiotype-induced CD8(+) T cells. Blood 2000;96:2828-2833.

205. Wen YJ, Barlogie B, Yi Q: Idiotype-specific cytotoxic T lymphocytes in multiple myeloma: Evidence for their capacity to lyse autologous primary tumor cells. Blood 2001;97:1750-1755.

206. Pinilla-Ibarz J, Cathcart K, Scheinberg DA: CML vaccines as a paradigm of the specific immunotherapy of cancer. Blood Rev 2000;14:111-120.

207. Molldrem J: Immune therapy of AML. Cytotherapy 2002;4:437-438.

208. Molldrem JJ, Kant S, Jiang W, Lu S: The basis of T-cell-mediated immunity to chronic myelogenous leukemia. Oncogene 2002;21:8668-8673.

209. Rosenfeld C, Cheever MA, Gaiger A: WT1 in acute leukemia, chronic myelogenous leukemia and myelodysplastic syndrome: Therapeutic potential of WT1 targeted therapies. Leukemia 2003;17:1301-1312.

210. Parkin DM, Bray FI, Devesa SS: Cancer burden in the year 2000: The global picture. Eur J Cancer 2001;37(suppl 8):S4-S66.

211. Walboomers JM, Jacobs MV, Manos MM, et al: Human papillomavirus is a necessary cause of invasive cervical cancer worldwide. J Pathol 1999;189:12-19.

212. Durst M, Gissmann L, Ikenberg H, zur Hausen H: A papillomavirus DNA from a cervical carcinoma and its prevalence in cancer biopsy samples from different geographic regions. Proc Natl Acad Sci USA 1983;80:3812-3815.

213. Ho GYF, Bierman R, Beardsley L, Chang CJ, Burk RD: Natural history of cervicovaginal papillomavirus infection in young women. N Engl J Med 1998;338:423-428.

214. Stanley MA: Immunobiology of papillomavirus infections. J Reprod Immunol 2001;52:45-59.

215. Small EJ, Fratesi P, Reese DM, et al: Immunotherapy of hormone-refractory prostate cancer with antigen-loaded dendritic cells. J Clin Oncol 2000;18:3894-3903.

216. Simons JW, Mikhak B, Chang JF, et al: Induction of immunity to prostate cancer antigens: Results of a clinical trial of vaccination with irradiated autologous prostate tumor cells engineered to secrete granulocyte-macrophage colony-stimulating factor using ex vivo gene transfer. Cancer Res 1999;59:5160-5168.

217. Foon KA, John WJ, Chakraborty M, et al: Clinical and immune responses in resected colon cancer patients treated with anti-idiotype monoclonal antibody vaccine that mimics the carcinoembryonic antigen. J Clin Oncol 1999;17:2889-2895.

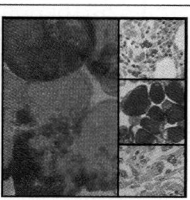

34

COMPLEMENTARY AND ALTERNATIVE MEDICINE

James M. Metz

Heather Jones

SUMMARY OF KEY POINTS

- Complementary and alternative medical therapies (CAM) are used by a significant number of cancer patients worldwide.
- Providing a nonthreatening environment for discussion of CAM will facilitate communication on this topic between physicians and patients.
- Many types of CAM may interact with conventional medications or cancer treatments and increase the toxicity or decrease the efficacy of these therapies.
- Some CAM has been shown to have side effects that mimic those of conventional cancer treatments.
- Physicians must warn patients about potential problems with CAM. They should also support those patients using those types of CAM that do not adversely effect cancer treatment.
- A number of complementary therapies may be effective for stress reduction and combating pain or nausea.
- Healthcare providers must familiarize themselves with the most common CAM treatments used by cancer patients so that informed discussions can occur.

INTRODUCTION

Complementary and alternative medicine (CAM) has infiltrated mainstream medical practices in recent years, driven mainly by patient desires to obtain these treatments. CAM therapies have gained increased exposure through television, magazines, books, and the Internet. Most medical professionals have limited relevant information and education on the subject and are unable to provide informed responses to questions about complementary and alternative methods. It is no longer acceptable to patients for physicians to label all of these alleged treatments as ludicrous and unfounded. It is also unacceptable for physicians to ignore the utilization of CAM, as numerous interactions with conventional medical therapies have been described in the scientific literature. Medical professionals must be able to converse intelligently about CAM with patients and learn not to ridicule those who use alternative and complementary techniques so long as they are safe. Physicians must also warn patients of dangers and hoaxes when appropriate.

Patients with cancer are prime consumers and targets for alternative medical therapies. Many feel that they are in a desperate and hopeless situation. Many simply want to gain back control over their lives, and use of CAM is an expression of this desire. Physicians must ask all patients under their care specifically about alternative and complementary medical practices that might be in use. Patients are more likely to discuss their adoption of these techniques openly when the physician provides a nonthreatening environment for discussion.

This chapter is a general introduction to the topic of CAM and will cover some of the more commonly used therapies. The goal is to provide relevant information on such therapies and improve physician/patient interactions whenever CAM treatments are discussed.

DEFINITION OF CAM

The terms *alternative medicine* and *alternative therapy* have become popular in recent years but do not accurately reflect or encompass the practices for which they are used. It is the generally accepted term that refers to a diverse assortment of philosophies, theories, and diagnostic, preventive, and therapeutic practices not generally viewed as arising from or belonging to the modern western medical paradigm.[1] Other popular terms are *complementary, unconventional,* and *integrative medicine;* all attempt to encompass the practice modalities not common to western medicine. The terms *complementary medicine* and *integrative medicine* are often used to acknowledge the blending of these nontraditional treatment modalities with more conventional views and therapeutic approaches. Some authors, on the other hand, prefer to define alternative medicine as treatment approaches not amenable to combination with conventional therapy.[2,3] Several other terms have been used to define this subject: unconventional, unorthodox, nontraditional, holistic, and nonwestern.[1]

The National Institutes of Health (NIH) Office of Alternative Medicine established a Panel on Definition and Description, charging it "to establish a definition of the field of complementary and alternative medicine (CAM) for purposes of identification and research; and to identify factors critical to thorough and unbiased description of CAM systems and practices that would be applicable to both quantitative and qualitative research."[4] The panel defined complementary and alternative medicine as follows: Complementary and alternative medicine (CAM) is a broad domain of healing resources that encompasses all health systems, modalities, and practices and their accompanying theories and beliefs, other than those intrinsic to the politically dominant health system of a particular society or culture in a given historical period. CAM includes all such practices and ideas self-defined by their users as preventing or treating illness or promoting health and well-being. Boundaries within CAM and between the CAM domain and the domain of the dominant system are not always sharp or fixed. Table 34-1 presents a list of CAM modalities defined by NIH.

USE OF CAM

The worldwide use of CAM varies by culture, religion, race, geographic location, and sex of the patient. Questionnaire studies have suggested that a large percentage of patients with cancer are using CAM. Estimates range from 9% to 64% depending on the definition of CAM and the cancer patient population studied.[5-10] There is evidence that the use of these treatments within the general United States population has increased during the past decade.[11] Also, studies suggest that many patients do not discuss the utilization of these treatments with their physicians.[8]

TABLE 34-1

CAM as Defined by the NIH

In 1992, the National Institutes of Health (NIH) convened a meeting to discuss the major areas of alternative medicine and to direct future research activities.[1]

As part of this meeting, the group defined the following seven fields of alternative therapy:

1. **Alternative systems of medical practice.** This field includes "folk" medicine and organized health care systems based on alternative practice. Examples include acupuncture, homeopathy, and naturopathy.
2. **Bioelectromagnetics.** Researchers in this field study how living organisms interact with electromagnetic fields. Magnetic field therapy is one example of bioelectromagnetics practice. It is most often used to treat osteoarthritis and nonunion bone fractures.
3. **Diet and nutrition.** This field includes the use of special diets to improve health. Examples include the macrobiotic diet and orthomolecular medicine.
4. **Herbal remedies.** This field includes the use of herbs and plants to promote and improve health. Herbal therapy is considered to be the most popular alternative therapy in the United States and is used for many conditions.
5. **Manual healing methods.** Practitioners use touch and manipulation to promote and improve health. Examples include chiropractic therapy, massage therapy, and therapeutic touch.
6. **Mind/body interventions.** This therapy uses the interconnectedness of mind and body to improve health. Examples include psychotherapy, meditation, guided imagery, hypnosis, biofeedback, and prayer. It is most commonly to treat nausea and vomiting (particularly for anesthesia or chemotherapy-induced hyperemesis gravidarum) and postoperative dental pain.
7. **Pharmacologic and biologic treatments.** This field includes treatment with drugs and vaccines not accepted by mainstream medicine. Examples include the use of shark cartilage, EDTA for chelation therapy (for coronary artery disease), and apiotherapy.

Risberg and colleagues[5] evaluated 252 patients with cancer in Norway and found that the cumulative risk of using CAM was 45% for patients under observation or cancer treatment. Females were much more likely than males to use these therapies. Liu and coworkers[6] evaluated 100 patients with advanced cancer receiving conventional cancer treatment in China. It was found that 64% were using some form of CAM, mainly herbal therapies. Begbie and associates[7] evaluated 319 patients with cancer in Australia and found that 22% used CAM treatments; 40% of the users did not discuss them with their physicians. Downer and colleagues[8] found that the 16% of 415 patients with cancer surveyed in England used CAM. The typical user of CAM tended to be younger, in the higher socioeconomic stratum, and female.

In the United States, the use of CAM is also prevalent. In a telephone survey of patients with cancer, 452 of 5047 patients (9%) admitted to using CAM techniques.[9] Mind/body interventions and dietary therapies were the most common. A study from the University of Pennsylvania showed that 40% of patients with cancer undergoing radiation therapy were using CAM. Only 7% of these patients, however, admitted to using these therapies during the standard history and physical examination.[11] Only after the addition of a few directed questions regarding CAM use did the majority of these patients reveal that they were using these therapies. Exercise and prayer were specifically excluded as CAM in this study. A recent study of patients with stage I–II breast cancer found that a complementary or alternative medical system was used by 57.3% of the patient population.[10] When exercise therapy was excluded from the analysis, 40% were using CAM. Younger age, increasing income, and higher educational level were predictors of such use. The definition of CAM can vary significantly among studies, which affects the percentage of utilization reported. Clearly, it is important to understand the precise definitions used in each study when comparisons are made.

There is very limited information available concerning the use of CAM therapies in the pediatric oncology population. An interview of the parents of 84 pediatric oncology patients in the Netherlands found that 26 of 84 children (31%) had used or were using CAM.[12] Of these children, 19 of 26 (73%) had suffered a relapse before using these techniques. Fernandez and coworkers[13] performed a study of pediatric oncology patients in British Columbia showing that 42% of the 366 respondents used some form of CAM treatment.

CANCER PREVENTION AND CAM

There is a growing body of literature relating to cancer prevention and CAM. More than 50% of U.S. adults use some type of vitamin, mineral, or other micronutrient supplement.[14] Several studies indicate that users of dietary supplements believe that supplements can prevent or treat chronic diseases, such as cancer and cardiovascular disease, despite limited scientific support for the efficacy of such use.[15-18] Information about micronutrient supple-

---

WHY PATIENTS USE COMPLEMENTARY AND ALTERNATIVE MEDICINE

The complex trend of public awareness of and use of complementary and alternative medicine (CAM) has grown extraordinarily in the past decade. This seemingly insatiable desire for ancient philosophies and approaches to medical care by the general public seems particularly odd because it comes at a time of extraordinary technological and therapeutic advances. A physician should understand what motivates a particular patient to seek CAM therapies before entering into a discussion with a patient—reaching this understanding can be quite challenging. The clinical literature for the most part has done an excellent job in documenting the incidence and patterns of CAM use but has often overlooked the more important question of why patients choose alternative modes of care. This motivation stems from a complex combination of social, cultural, philosophical, and personal factors that often differ among ethnic groups and disease types.

One reason for this phenomenon no doubt is the enormous increase in public access to worldwide information through the World Wide Web and extensive media coverage. Commercial advertising and continuous exposure through the lay press, ranging from tabloid publications to magazines, medical journals, and books, have vigorously promoted the concepts of disease prevention and healing by unconventional means, striking a responsive (and highly lucrative) chord in a truly global population.

Another reason for the popularity of CAM is the escalating cost of modern allopathic medical care. New technologies have been developed at a record pace, producing many medical, surgical, and diagnostic innovations, most of which are unquestionably improvements but which also are very costly. The expense and the resulting rationing of these new modalities by managed care programs in an attempt to reduce the costs of medical care have placed them out of reach for a considerable segment of the population. The outcome appears to be the creation of a strong public desire for a wide range of complementary and alternative modalities to prevent and treat the full scope of human illness.

Other reasons sited for CAM use have included an affinity for a holistic or natural approach to healing, the need to manage side effects, dissatisfaction with the mindset of physicians, and an overall failure of conventional therapies to meet patient needs. Additional insight can be gained by reviewing patient assessments of CAM providers. Patients often praise CAM providers for the ability to define an illness, the amount of time provided for patient visits, the involvement of the same provider over the course of treatment, and the attention to personality and personal experience. The satisfaction with treatments received often is not contingent on an improvement in the presenting complaint.

Many patients are more informed about complementary and alternative therapies than their physicians are, a situation that, in itself, should encourage physicians to learn more about CAM. CAM therapies offer patients "a participatory experience of empowerment, and authenticity, when illness threatens their sense of intactness and relationship to their world."* Understanding what motivates patients may better enable physicians to enter into a dialogue with them and encourage a positive physician-patient relationship.

*Pappus S, Perlman A: Complementary and alternative medicine: the importance of doctor-patient communication. Med Clin North Am 2002;86:1–10.

---

ments is becoming more common in the popular medical literature and is creating increased curiosity and awareness. The explosion of the micronutrient supplement market is compelling physicians to become aware of dietary supplements. Whether or not they are used in clinical practice is a decision for the individual physician. Given the increasing number of patients who are using micronutrient supplements, however, it is imperative that physicians have a good understanding of this topic.

Antioxidants

Fruits and vegetables appear to be protective against the major cancers.[19] Individuals who eat fruits and vegetables that are rich in carotenoids, and people with higher serum beta-carotene levels, have a lower risk of cancer, according to randomized trials in human populations.[20] The antioxidant vitamins (vitamin A and related compounds such as beta-carotene, as well as vitamins C and E) are prominent components of many fruits and vegetables. Conjecture regarding the micronutrients responsible for this beneficial effect has been extensive. The antioxidant vitamins function as scavengers for DNA-damaging, mutagenic oxygen free radicals.

Accumulating epidemiologic evidence suggests that a number of micronutrients might decrease the incidence of cancers of epithelial cell origin. These include vitamin A, vitamin C, vitamin E, and beta carotene. Dietary deficiency of vitamins A, C, and E has been implicated in the development of cancers of the lung, breast, oropharynx, stomach, bladder, prostate, and colon.[21-25] Squamous tissues deficient in vitamin A exhibit metaplastic differentiation that can be reversed by administration of vitamin A and related compounds.[26] There is evidence to suggest that diets rich in vitamin A and related compounds not only diminish the risk of certain cancers but also are protective against their development. Whereas vitamin C appears to inhibit the formation of carcinogenic nitrosamines that have been associated with the development of gastric cancer, vitamin E inhibits mutagenesis and cell transformation mainly through its antioxidant function.[27] Nonetheless, the role of vitamins C and E in neoplastic development remains particularly unclear. Although vitamins C and E function as antioxidants, there is little evidence to support any direct role for these vitamins in the inhibition or reversal of neoplastic growth and development.

Several recent studies of dietary supplementation highlight the importance of clinical trials in defining benefit.[28] Both the CARET (beta carotene and retinol) and the alpha-tocopherol beta carotene trials suggest that pharmacologic doses of beta carotene actually increase the risk of lung cancer among smokers or those with asbestos exposure.[29,30] A large, four-arm clinical trial of multiple dietary supplements in 30,000 subjects in Linxian, China, demonstrated no significant effect on cancer incidence; however, those subjects who received treatment with a combination of selenium, beta carotene, and alpha-tocopherol enjoyed statistically significant lower total and gastric cancer–specific mortality rates.[31]

Vitamin D, Calcium, and Selenium

Among the many minerals required for normal tissue development, calcium and selenium have received the most attention with regard to carcinogenesis. Both laboratory and preliminary clinical data suggest a role for calcium deficiency in the development of colon cancer. In epidemiologic studies, an inverse relationship has also been reported between vitamin E, vitamin D, and calcium supplementation and prostate cancer.[32] In addition, laboratory studies have shown that the active metabolite of vitamin D, 1,25-dihydroxyvitamin D (calcitriol), inhibits growth of both primary cultures of human prostate cancer cells and cancer cell lines; however, the mechanism by which the cells are growth inhibited has not been defined clearly.[33]

Recently, a large randomized trial of more than 1000 individuals with a history of polyps showed that supplementation with 1.5 g of calcium reduced new adenomatous polyp formation by 20%.[34]

The Nutritional Prevention of Cancer Study by Clark and associates[35] randomized 1312 patients to receive placebo or 200 μg of selenium per day and was designed to evaluate the effect of this supplement on the risk of developing new basal cell and squamous cell skin cancers. In the analysis of the primary outcomes, selenium supplementation had no effect on reducing the incidence of these skin cancers. After preliminary analyses showed a reduction in total carcinoma, however, the protocol was modified in 1990 to add total and cancer mortality and the incidence of lung, colon, rectal, and prostate cancers as secondary endpoints. Analysis of these endpoints revealed a preventive effect for cancers of the lung, prostate, colon, and rectum, but no reduction in risk of breast or bladder cancer.

Soybeans

Soy products are the primary food source for the isoflavone glycosides genistin and daidzin, which are metabolized by colonic microflora to the biologically active aglycones genistein and daidzein. These compounds, along with lignans, are generically named phytoestrogens and have structural similarities to estradiol. Evidence suggests that the consumption of diets rich in soybean products are associated with lower cancer mortality rates, particularly for cancers of the colon, breast, and prostate.[36-39]

The soy protein, the Bowman-Birk trypsin inhibitor (BBI), is also found in other beans and peas. BBI, now in clinical trials, has been shown to suppress carcinogenesis in laboratory animals and in in vitro transformation systems.[39]

It is difficult to study the effects of micronutrient supplementation on the formation of cancers given the inherent complexity of carcinogenesis. Information about the mechanisms of chemopreventive agents that inhibit carcinogenesis is still imperfect. Understanding how various dietary components inhibit carcinogenesis will be instrumental in the development of novel dietary chemopreventive agents in the future. Results from large trials like the Women's Health Initiative Trial and the Selenium and Vitamin E Cancer Prevention Trial (SELECT) will provide a great deal of information regarding the effects of dietary modification, calcium, selenium, and vitamin D and E supplementation on breast, prostate, and colon cancer.

CAM MODALITIES AND THEIR LEGISLATION AND REGULATION

The National Center for CAM

In 1990, Congress became aware of the rapidly developing interest in CAM in the United States. In 1991, the Office of Alternative Medicine (OAM) was established at the National Institutes of Health (NIH) but did not have formal status as a section or subsection. Initially, it was given an annual budget of approximately 2 million dollars. The budget was increased to 20 million dollars by 1997 (again, over considerable opposition in Congress), and the OAM has since been given increased status by being named the National Center for CAM, with an annual budget of 50 million dollars.[40] The charge of the National Center for CAM is to begin to appraise various CAM products as scientifically as possible through controlled studies. They have thus far been slow in reporting results, no doubt at least in part because of the complex nature of conducting meaningful double-blind, controlled studies with CAM products and therapies. Numerous studies, however, are now in various stages of completion through the National Center for CAM and many other facilities throughout the world. There are currently 13 institution-affiliated centers of research on CAM in the United States, and 75 medical schools in the United States are now teaching integrative medicine courses to their medical students.[40]

Herbal Medicine

Herbs have been used for medicinal purposes for thousands of years. Ancient Egyptians used herbs for the treatment of disease as early as 3000 B.C. Almost one quarter of the current pharmacopoeia is derived from botanicals. Digoxin is derived from foxglove, aspirin is derived from willow bark, narcotics are derived from the opium poppy, and birth control pills were developed from the Mexican yam. With the advent of modern medical science, people came to believe that synthetic ingredients were more effective than those found in nature, and the use of herbal remedies quickly diminished, especially in the United States. Current herbal preparations are sold mainly as nutritional products.[41]

Today, herbs are used widely in Europe and are again gaining popularity in the United States.[42] The most informative longitudinal data on use of herbal medicine stems from the two Harvard surveys.[42,43] The results indicated that between 1990 and 1997, the use of self-prescribed herbal medicines within the U.S. general population increased, from 2.5% in 1990 to 12.1% in 1997. During the same period, the proportion of individuals consulting practitioners of herbal medicine rose from 10.2% to 15.1%. These survey studies estimated that in 1997, the entire U.S. population spent approximately 5 billion dollars on herbal medicines. Most of this was out-of-pocket expenditure.[42-44]

Regulation of Herbals

The over-the-counter availability of herbal medicines fosters the notion that these medications are safe, and many casual users have inadequate knowledge about the use of these medications. Users often avoid discussing the use of these medications with their conventional care providers unless they are asked specifically about them.[11] These factors could set the stage for potential adverse drug reactions and interactions. Consumers in the United States are accustomed to products that have been tested and approved before sale. The Food and Drug Administration (FDA) functions to oversee the safety of foods, drugs, and medical devices sold in the United States.

Most herbal products in the United States are considered dietary supplements and for this reason are not regulated as medicines and are not required to meet the standards for drugs specified in the Federal Food, Drug, and Cosmetic Act. In 1994, the Dietary Supplement and Health Education Act (DSHEA) was passed. This legislation had profound effects on the regulation and marketing of herbal products in the United States. Herbs or other botanicals could be sold as dietary supplements and were not subjected to the rigorous regulations that applied to medicines.[45] Herbal products may be produced without the assurance of compliance standards for good manufacturing practices (although such standards are being developed), and they are marketed without prior approval of their efficacy and safety by the FDA. According to the DSHEA, the manufacturer of an herbal preparation is responsible for the truthfulness of claims made on the label and must have evidence that the claims are supported, yet the DSHEA neither provides a standard for the evidence needed nor requires submission of the evidence to the FDA. Under the DSHEA, the manufacturer is permitted to claim that the product affects the structure or function of the body, as long as there is no claim of efficacy for the prevention or treatment of a specific disease, and provided there is a disclaimer informing the user that the FDA has not evaluated the agent. Some of the claims on the labels of herbal products suggest that they can be used to treat disease, and supplementary materials, produced by parties other than the manufacturer, that overtly promote such use could be available where the herbal remedies are sold. According to the DSHEA, the manufacturer is responsible for controlling quality and safety, but if a concern about safety arises, the burden of proof lies not with the manufacturer but with the FDA, which must prove that the product is unsafe.[46,47]

Several European countries have implemented guidelines for licensing herbal remedies. In Germany, such products can be registered as medicines on the basis of information in approximately 300 monographs on herbs ("positive" monographs with concise information about terminology, composition, uses, contraindications, side effects, drug interactions, dosage, mode of administration, and actions, and "negative" monographs explaining insufficient benefits or unacceptable risks.[48]

The European Commission (which governs the European Union) recently publicized a draft directive on the licensing of traditional herbal preparations. If accepted, this proposal will require all members of the European Union to introduce a simplified procedure for these preparations so that they can receive a "traditional use" registration without the need to present data on efficacy from randomized trials.[47,49]

The simplified licensing approach allows a pre-marketing assessment of the quality and safety of a product and facilitates postmarketing surveillance and product recalls.[47]

Generally, herbal products are not evaluated by the strict preclinical toxicology and pharmacology guidelines that are in place for conventional drugs. Instead, the focus of the clinical trials is on the efficacy of the products. A number of herbal formulations are presently undergoing clinical trials. The FDA has established a hotline for information about herbal products and one for reporting adverse effects.[45]

Acupuncture

Acupuncture has been practiced in China for more than 5000 years. Around the same time, acupressure, which addresses similar points without needles, was developed in Japan. Acupuncture might be recommended by some for a variety of conditions, but abatement of pain or nausea and vomiting are of greatest interest for patients with cancer.

Acupuncturists use fine needles that vary in length from 0.5 cm to several centimeters. The needles, usually made of stainless steel or copper, are placed about 5 mm deep and are manipulated gently by hand. The needles can be stimulated with a weak electrical current or by heat. Many patients describe a tingling sensation and feel a sense of heaviness in the area where the needles are placed.

Much of the evidence in support of acupuncture is anecdotal. There have been studies suggesting that patients undergoing chemotherapy experience relief of nausea with acupuncture.[50,51] There also has been interest in evaluating acupuncture for radiation-induced mucositis in patients with head and neck cancer. Studies are also ongoing to evaluate the effectiveness of using acupuncture in reducing neuropathic pain after thoracotomy for lung cancer resection. There are also ongoing studies evaluating the use of acupuncture to relieve fatigue associated with radiation therapy treatments. Because of the widespread use of acupuncture and evolving scientific studies, an NIH panel of experts in 1997 issued a consensus statement for the use of acupuncture. According to this statement, clear evidence supports the effectiveness of acupuncture for the treatment of postoperative and chemotherapy-induced nausea and vomiting, nausea associated with pregnancy, and postoperative dental pain.[52]

Classical Oriental medical theory states that a life force called *qi* (pronounced "chi") is present in every organism and flows along interconnected meridians through the body, crossing at specific points. The meridians surface at various locations, representing the acupuncture points (these points are very similar to acupressure points). The opposing forces of *yin* and *yang* must be in balance before *qi* can get the body's vital functions to work normally; imbalance in these forces is the root cause of illness. Stimulating the acupoints restores the *yin-yang* balance and the flow of *qi*.

To date, scientists in the western world have found no evidence to support the existence of *qi*, *yin*, or *yang*. Bing and colleagues[53] found that stimulation of acupoints with needles activates the subnucleus reticularis dorsalis neurons that send projections to the dorsal horn of the spinal cord at all levels. The authors suggest that this anatomic structure might be involved in the modulation of pain. Grossman and Clement-Jones[54] postulated that the release of endorphins within the nervous system could reduce the perception of pain. Interestingly, it has also been shown that the acupoints have a similarity in location to some of the anatomic sites used for local and regional anesthesia.[55]

Acupuncture might benefit some patients with cancer. It is difficult to make broad recommendations on its applicability due to the paucity of clinical trials evaluating this alternative medical technique. Studies are in progress which, it is hoped, will shed additional light on the benefits of acupuncture.

Regulation of Acupuncture

Acupuncturists can be certified in two ways, depending on applicable state laws. They can complete a formal, full-time educational program that includes both classroom and clinical hours, or they can participate in an apprenticeship program. Acupuncturists must also complete a "Clean Needle Technique" approved course. Medical doctors with training in acupuncture also can obtain board certification. Certification for formally trained acupuncturists is through the National Certification Commission for Acupuncture and Oriental Medicine (NCCAOM). Medical doctors are certified through the American Academy of Medical Acupuncture and must possess a valid medical license. Currently, 37 of the 40 states that regulate acupuncturists require NCCAOM certification.

In response to petitions submitted by the acupuncture community, the FDA has reclassified acupuncture needles for general use from class III (the category in which clinical studies are required to establish safety and efficacy) to class II (a category that involves less stringent control by the FDA but does require good manufacturing and proper labeling). Manufacturers are required to label FDA needles for single use only. Acupuncture needles for clinical practice would be restricted to qualified practitioners as determined by state practice laws.[45]

Homeopathy

From the Greek words *homios* ("like") and *pathos* ("suffering"), homeopathy is a system of medicine whose first tenet is the principle of similars: A substance that can cause symptoms in a healthy person possibly can encourage self-healing in a person with an illness that presents with similar symptoms. This principle was developed into a practice of medicine in the eighteenth century by the renowned German physician Samuel Hahnemann. The theory of homeopathy is rooted in three of Hahnemann's principles:

1. The "law of similars," which states that a substance that can cause disease in a healthy person can cure similar symptoms in the diseased.
2. The principle of the "minimum dose," which states that by progressively diluting and succussing a substance, its curative properties are enhanced and its side effects minimized.
3. Prescribing for the individual, which advocates basing treatment not on the medical diagnosis but rather on a totality of symptoms that takes into account each patient's temperament, personality, and emotional and physical responses.[56]

The principles of homeopathy are not well understood by the public or the medical profession, yet medical consumers are using homeopathic treatments in increasing numbers. In the United States and Europe, the sale of homeopathic medicines increased by 20% to 30% annually in the 1980s and 1990s.[57] Two meta-analyses have been published suggesting that homeopathic remedies are more effective than placebo alone. Both studies conclude, however, that the current research and literature in the field does not meet the rigorous, scientific proof needed to establish efficacy of homeopathy for specific clinical conditions.[58,59] More research is needed before homeopathy can be declared clinically useful for any one condition.

Regulation of Homeopathy

Although in other countries homeopathic training and certification have been available for decades, the United States has not had full-time homeopathic schools or accredited professional education for more than 40 years.

Only three states (Arizona, Connecticut, and Nevada) license homeopaths. The scope of practice varies but includes the use of substances of animal, vegetable, or mineral origin given in microdoses and prepared according to homeopathic pharmacology. All three states use licensure as a means to authorize practice. These states require a DO or MD degree and certification in the study of homeopathy. Arizona and Nevada have independent examining boards. In Delaware and New Hampshire, the practice of homeopathy is regulated by the state although under no board. The Council of Homeopathic Education (CHE) has implemented a voluntary certification process that includes a written multiple-choice examination, an oral examination, a videotaped interview, and 10 case reports. A person can be admitted to examination only after completion of a required curriculum and clinical supervision. As of this date, this certification process has not been recognized by the U.S. government or by other medical boards.

The FDA is currently attempting to establish guidelines for the regulation of homeopathic products. The FDA takes the position that homeopathic remedies, which are used in the treatment of disease, are by definition drugs and should be regulated. In recent years, the FDA has exempted homeopathic products from the regular drug reviewing process if such drugs have been reviewed and approved by the Homeopathic Pharmacopeia of the United States (HPUS).[45]

Massage

Massage therapy has had a long and distinguished history, having been known to the ancient Chinese and Japanese and to the Greeks, Romans, and Egyptians. The "laying on of hands" was the primary form of healing throughout history in places such as ancient Greece, where Hippocrates wrote that the "physician must be experienced in many things, most especially in rubbing."[60] Massage therapy is considered a form of medical treatment in several countries—including China, Japan, Russia, and West Germany—where it is covered by national health insurance. In the United States, massage therapy still is considered a form of CAM. The popularity of massage therapy is growing. National and international massage therapy associations increased their membership by thousands of therapists during the 1990s.[61]

Regulation and Training for Massage

To become certified, massage therapists must complete a formal therapeutic massage bodywork program. They may also be considered for certification if they have training in anatomy, physiology, and kinesiology together with formal education and professional experience in bodywork and/or massage. Massage Provider Practice Acts for the regulation of massage exist in 22 states. Most statutes include directives for the treatment of soft tissue, muscle, or both. Techniques may include, but are not limited to, friction, beating, or percussion. Types of health conditions treated, depending on the practice act, include maintaining good health, improving muscle tone, and reducing stress. Board certification is through the National Certification Board for Therapeutic Massage and Bodywork and is required in 20 of the 29 states that regulate massage therapists.[45,61]

Naturopathic Medicine

Benedict Lust, a German physician, introduced naturopathy to the United States. He used the term *naturopathy* (from *natur,* to indicate nature, and *pathy* from homeopathy) to encompass all the natural approaches to healing. Several healing modalities have been added to the healing module to arrive at modern naturopathy. Naturopathic medicine is far from being a single scientific discipline. The basic principles are that healing comes from within more than from without and that medicine depends on the healing power of nature to cure. Naturopathy employs various natural means to empower the individual to reach the ability to self-heal. The basic tools include lifestyle modifications, nutrition, dietetics, herbs, breathing, education, and hydrotherapy. In addition, naturopaths may elect to use a variety of healing modalities, including acupuncture, botanicals, homeopathy, massage, and Oriental medicine. Naturopaths are the "generalists" of the alternative medicine world. The emphasis of their practice is on prevention, education, and health maintenance (Table 34-2).[62]

Regulation and Training for Naturopaths

Naturopathic physicians undergo a four-year training program that includes therapies such as homeopathy, clinical nutrition, manipulation, herbal medicine, and hydrotherapy. Naturopaths often may have additional training in Chinese medicine (acupuncture and herbs). Naturopaths are licensed in 12 states. The naturopathic certification exam is administered by the North American Board of Naturopathic Examiners. Each state defines the scope of practice differently, utilizing several adjunctive therapies including acupuncture, biofeedback, and nonprescriptive medications.[45,62]

Chiropractic

The word *chiropractic* is derived from two Greek words meaning "done by hand," and the term is defined as "the diagnosis, treatment and rehabilitation of conditions that affect the neuromuscular system."[63] Chiropractic care origins are in the manipulative health care modalities. It became an organized discipline approximately 100 years ago when Canadian Daniel David Palmer introduced it in the United States. A chiropractic system of health is based on two principles: a testable principle, which suggests that the structure and condition of the body influences how

---

TABLE 34-2

Six Basic Principles of Naturopathic Medicine[62]

THE BELIEF	THE RESULTANT PRINCIPLE
The belief that the body has the inherent ability to heal itself.	The healing power of nature.
The belief that health and disease result from the interaction of a person's physical, mental, emotional, genetic, environmental, and social components.	Treat the whole person.
The belief that one should treat the cause of disease, not merely the symptoms.	First, do no harm.
The belief that a physician's major role is to educate, empower, and motivate patients to take responsibility for their own health.	Identify and treat the cause.
	Prevention is the best cure.
	The physician is a teacher.

Science of Clinical Oncology

the body functions and heals; and the untestable principle, which indicates that the mind-body relationship is instrumental in maintaining health and affects the healing processes. Hence, the focus is on the body's ability to self-heal, on the nervous system's role in overall health, and on the interaction between body structure and the functioning of the nervous system. In the last decade, chiropractic care has gained measured acceptance and developed into a treatment and wellness modality that is practiced by 55,000 licensed practitioners and used by roughly 10% of the U.S. population. The majority of visits to chiropractors in the United States are for back pain. There are data that chiropractic treatment is as beneficial for low back pain as treatment given by primary care providers, orthopedists, and physical therapists.[63,64] The evidence for the use of chiropractic for other conditions is less compelling.

Regulation and Training of Chiropractors

Chiropractic care is licensed in all 50 states, with 45 states requiring insurers to include it in their plans. There is a large variation in the scope of practice; certain states restrict the practice to spinal manipulation, whereas others permit different procedures to be performed, such as acupuncture, electromyography, and laboratory diagnosis. The Council on Chiropractic Education (www.cce-usa.org) has accredited 17 colleges of chiropractic medicine in the United States. Chiropractors are licensed in 50 states and must pass either a state licensing examination or an examination given by the National Board of Chiropractic Examiners. Since 1974, chiropractic education has been established with a four-year curriculum monitored by the Council on Chiropractic Education (CCE). Admission requirements differ from school to school, although a minimum of two years of college education and specific science courses are required by all.[45,65]

Ayurveda

The word *ayurveda* derives from the Sanskrit *ayur,* meaning long life, and *veda,* knowledge. One of the world's oldest traditional healing systems, it has been documented and practiced in India for thousands of years. Ayurveda is a holistic system that deals with all aspects of life: the mind, body, and spirit. The ayurvedic practice is founded on the pooled wisdom of ancient Hindu saints and healers. Ancient ayurveda was meant essentially to promote health, rather than fight disease.

A basic theory states that everything in the material world is a sign of the unseen universe of energy or life force. The world was created from the unseen universe when the primordial sound created the five fundamental elements responsible for the material world: space, air, fire, water, and earth. These five elements manifest in the human physiology as three life energies called *doshas.* The three doshas are *vata* (space and air), *pitta* (fire and water), and *kapha* (water and earth). Each dosha, its subdivision, and underlying structures confer a particular characteristic and quality to each person. Health is a state of balance between the mind, body, and consciousness.

Several factors can disturb this balance, including congenital and genetic factors, natural tendencies, habits, seasonal factors, and internal and external traumas. The imbalance produced in the doshas disturbs the life force, producing the disease state.

Diagnosis is based on identifying the exact quality and nature of the imbalance and correcting it. This is accomplished through a detailed history, inspection, and examination. Radial pulse examination (three superficial and three deep pulses, bilaterally) and tongue, nail, and eye examinations, among others, are important parts of the ayurvedic diagnostic examination. Treatment consists of reestablishing the body's balance through a combination of interventions, which might include lifestyle changes, dietary modifications, meditation, yoga, breathing exercises, massage, aromatherapy, herbs, and detoxification.[66] Studies have documented the favorable effects of regular meditation on reducing cardiovascular risk factors and stress. Studies investigating the effects of ayurvedic herbal products on a wide variety of conditions including cancer, aging, and health promotion are ongoing.[67]

Regulation of and Training in Ayurveda

Ayurvedic medicine is the progenitor of several CAM disciplines. These include aromatherapy and massage. There is no national standardization of training and credentialing of ayurvedic practitioners, although a small number of states provide for certification. A wide variance of training and experience exists among practitioners.

THE CANCER PATIENT AND POPULAR CAM THERAPIES

The tendency of CAM disciplines to change and shift in popularity is not in response to new developments or randomized clinical trials but rather because particular therapies go in and out of vogue. Typically, a CAM therapy remains popular for a limited period of time, after which it is replaced by a new and usually nonvalidated CAM therapy. Popular CAM therapies that are currently used by patients with cancer are discussed next under the categories developed by the NIH.

Mind-Body Techniques

The effectiveness of meditation, biofeedback, and yoga in stress reduction and the control of particular physiologic reactions is well supported by accepted research. The belief that patients can use mental attributes and mind-body work to prevent or cure cancer has not been demonstrated in clinical studies.

Biofeedback

Biofeedback manipulates those physiologic responses that are normally controlled by the autonomic nervous system. A biofeedback therapist, of which there are more than 10,000 in the United States, can teach a patient how to control many involuntary functions. Some patients learn to control their heart rate, blood pressure, muscle tension, and emotions.

Monitoring electrodes are placed on the body or scalp by the biofeedback therapist. The electrodes are then connected to a computer or polygraph that emits a noise or signal indicating the intensity or level of the process to be controlled. The patient is then instructed to concentrate on influencing the signal. Specific mental exercises are carried out under the direction of the therapist. The patient is asked to visualize certain images that affect mood and might in time learn which mental exercises change the signals. After a number of sessions (usually 8 to 10), the patient might be able to affect certain of the autonomic processes.

Researchers at Vanderbilt University performed a randomized study to evaluate the effectiveness of a combination of biofeedback and relaxation training for the reduction of side effects of chemotherapy.[68] Biofeedback reduced some indices of physiologic arousal but did not modify the side effects of chemotherapy. Relaxation training, however, showed a decrease in nausea and anxiety during chemotherapy and a decrease in physiologic arousal after chemotherapy. The authors concluded that the major benefit of biofeedback was the relaxation training that accompanies the instruction, not the biofeedback alone.

The potential benefits from biofeedback therapy for the patient with cancer are relaxation and reduction of stress. These undoubtedly can improve the quality of life when successful and allow the patient with cancer to take an active role in his or her overall management. Biofeedback is a noninvasive procedure. Ten sessions with a biofeedback therapist cost approximately $500. There are no specific reports in the medical literature of side effects attributed to the use of biofeedback.

Guided Imagery

Guided imagery is a technique that relies heavily on the power of suggestion to create relaxing mental images. It is particularly useful for relieving stress and promoting serenity. Some patients find that it helps them cope with the diagnosis and the side effects of treatments more effectively.

The therapist instructs participants to visualize a specific image. Sometimes the participant is asked to visualize a mass of cancerous cells being attacked by the immune system, chemotherapy, or radiation therapy. Many patients use guided imagery audiotapes that provide instruction on meditation exercises, guided relaxation, and visualization techniques. Some patients use these tapes while they are receiving their chemotherapy or radiation therapy, or en route to receive treatment.

Syrjala and colleagues[69] evaluated relaxation and imagery training along with cognitive-behavioral coping skills for control of oral mucositis pain in patients receiving bone marrow transplantation. The authors found that patients who received relaxation and imagery training reported less pain than the control groups. There was no benefit to the addition of cognitive-behavioral skills, however.

The goal of guided imagery is to achieve total relaxation. Patients learn breathing exercises to help them attain an "inner calm," or they attempt to modify anxiety or pain by imagining a pleasurable scene or situation. Some patients with cancer find the method effective in promoting relaxation and relieving anxiety. It must be emphasized, however, that there is no reliable evidence that this technique affects disease progression or survival.

Guided imagery is a noninvasive therapy. Relaxation and guided imagery audiotapes cost approximately $10 to $20 and are available in local bookstores. Some patients prefer to visit a therapist for individualized training, which could be more expensive. There are no reports in the medical literature of side effects related to guided imagery.

Herbal Medicine and Biological Supplements

PC-SPES

PC-SPES (*PC* stands for prostate cancer, and *SPES* is derived from the Latin word for hope) is a patented preparation of eight herbs (Table 34-3).[70] PC-SPES is the only herbal medicine for prostate cancer that has been subjected to clinical trials.

Four clinical trials of PC-SPES have been carried out in the United States and Germany.[71-74] These trials have been single-arm, phase I/II designs in patients with prostate cancer and consistently have demonstrated prolonged decreases in PSA levels in most of those treated. The side effect profile of PC-SPES has been suggestive of an estrogenic effect (i.e., breast tenderness, decreased libido, impotence, venous thromboses), and components of PC-SPES contain known phytoestrogens.[72]

The largest and most recently reported study was a phase II trial of 70 patients with prostate cancer.[74] Each patient received 320 mg of dried extract orally, three times a day. All androgen-dependent patients experienced PSA declines of 80% or more, and 26 patients (81%) experienced PSA decreases to undetectable levels. At 15 months after start of treatment, only one patient had biochemical or objective progression. Over half the patients with androgen-independent disease had a PSA response, with a median duration of 18 weeks. Of the two androgen-dependent patients with positive bone scans at study entry, one patient had a scan that revealed complete resolution of the osseous lesions, and the second patient's scan showed improvement but did not yield normal results. One patient had measurable disease

TABLE 34-3

The Herbs in PC-SPES

Herb Name

Dendranthema morifolium Tzvel. (chrysanthemum)
Ganoderma lucidum
Glycyrrhiza glabra L.
Isatis indigotica
Panax pseudoginseng
Rabdosia rubescens
Saw palmetto
Scutellaria baicalensis Georgi (skullcap)

and experienced complete resolution of a bladder mass seen on pelvic CT scan, accompanied by a decline in PSA from 8.9 ng/mL to an undetectable level. PC-SPES was generally well tolerated. PC-SPES was associated with a number of endocrine side effects, including decreased libido, erectile dysfunction, gynecomastia or mastodynia, and hot flashes.

Despite these encouraging results, a survival benefit for PC-SPES has thus far not been demonstrated, and PC-SPES might possibly decrease PSA levels while masking increases in tumor growth. PC-SPES is associated with an increased risk of thromboembolic events.[75-77] Of enormous concern, PC-SPES was found to contain warfarin (and SPES, a more generic version for all cancers, to contain alprazolam), prompting the Food and Drug Administration to issue a recall of both products in February 2002.[78]

Hydrazine Sulfate

Cachexia remains a major problem in the treatment of patients with cancer who have advanced disease. There has been interest for a number of years in hydrazine sulfate for combating cachexia seen in patients with cancer. Gold[79] evaluated 84 patients with disseminated cancer and found that 59 of 84 (70%) improved subjectively, while 14 of 84 patients (17%) improved objectively when treated with hydrazine sulfate. It was concluded that the compound might favorably influence nutritional status and clinical outcome in patients with disseminated cancer.

Enthusiasm has been dampened by three prospective trials that have shown no benefit when hydrazine sulfate is added to standard treatment regimens. Loprinzi and colleagues[80,81] randomized 243 patients with non–small cell lung cancer and 127 patients with advanced colorectal cancer between hydrazine sulfate and a placebo and showed no benefit to hydrazine sulfate. Kosty and associates[82] randomized 291 patients with advanced non–small cell lung cancer to receive chemotherapy with or without hydrazine sulfate. No benefit was found with regard to pain control, cachexia, or survival in any of these studies. Hydrazine sulfate is not recommended for the treatment of any cancer-related symptoms, although it remains widely promoted on the Internet.

Shark Cartilage

Shark cartilage has gained increased popularity as an unconventional medical therapy for the treatment and prevention of cancer. Shark cartilage was initially promoted by William Lane, PhD, in his book *Sharks Don't Get Cancer* and the follow-up book, *Sharks Still Don't Get Cancer*. Sharks do develop tumors, however, including malignant tumors. They develop thyroid and central nervous system neoplasms, papillomas, oral cavity cancers, adenomas of the liver, chondromas, and odontomas.[83-85]

Shark cartilage is purported to contain angiogenesis inhibitors. A modest antiangiogenic effect has, in fact, been observed in vitro.[86] Shark cartilage is supplied in powder and capsule forms. It is usually taken orally but sometimes as an enema.

The television news program *60 Minutes* gave shark cartilage a huge boost a few years ago. The program reported a Cuban study of 29 patients with "terminal" cancer who were placed on shark cartilage; most "felt better" several weeks thereafter. "Feeling better" is not a reliable endpoint in a scientific study. The National Cancer Institute (NCI) performed a review of the study and concluded that the data were "incomplete and unimpressive."[87] *60 Minutes* allegedly refused to broadcast the findings of the NCI.

A small study on shark cartilage was reported at the American Society of Clinical Oncology in 1997.[88] Of the 58 patients with advanced cancer who were given shark cartilage for 12 weeks, not one objective complete response or partial response to shark cartilage was obtained. Only two patients reported significant improvement in the quality of life. There are currently ongoing rigorous studies of shark cartilage at a number of institutions, but no positive results have yet been published. It has been reported that shark cartilage can cause an elevation of liver function tests (LFTs) and frank hepatitis.[89] Patients on chemotherapy should be urged not to use shark cartilage enemas due to the risk of infection when patients are neutropenic.

Shark cartilage is relatively expensive. If it is taken as described by William Lane, the cost of the 16-week program is approximately $3000.

Mistletoe

Mistletoe (*Viscum album* L.) is one of the most commonly used CAM therapies in Europe.[5,90,91] The active compounds identified in mistletoe are lectins (glycoproteins) and viscotoxins (proteins). The lectin component has in vitro immunostimulant activity and has been shown to increase the number of peripheral blood lymphocytes. It has also demonstrated increased lymphocyte activity in patients with gliomas.[92-94] The viscotoxins have been shown to have direct cytotoxic activity against certain cancer cell lines.[95]

Mistletoe has been used primarily as an adjuvant to conventional cancer therapies to manage micrometastatic disease. Various mistletoe products have been evaluated in several randomized, controlled clinical trials. An analysis of 11 of the randomized trials of mistletoe published in 1994 found that although 10 of these studies reported improved survival in the mistletoe arm, many of these trials had deficiencies in 5 or more of the 10 criteria of good methodology. These methodological issues have led reviewers to question the validity of these studies and have promoted demands for further well-defined studies.[96]

Recently, two well-designed prospective randomized trials have reported negative results. The effect of adjuvant mistletoe lectin-1 standardized mistletoe preparation (Eurixor) treatment was tested in a prospective, randomized, clinical trial involving 477 patients with head and neck squamous cell carcinoma.[97] The European Organization for Research and Treatment of Cancer has completed a phase III randomized trial of adjuvant treatment with low-dose interferon-α vs. interferon-γ vs. mistletoe extract (Iscador M) vs. no further treatment after curative resection of high-risk stage I/IIB malignant melanoma. No benefit was seen in disease-free survival or overall survival for patients receiving either Eurixor or Iscador.[97,98]

Hoxsey Regimen and Essiac

The Hoxsey regimen, an herbal compound comprised of pokeroot, burdock root, barberry root, buckthorn bark, and stillingia root, was used first in 1924 by Harry Hoxsey. The recipe was passed down by his grandfather, a farmer who observed a horse cure itself of cancer by eating certain plants. Despite decades during which no supporting data have been forthcoming, the Hoxsey formula remains popular and in use among patients with cancer.[78]

Essiac is one of the most popular herbal medicines in North America and is a mixture of four herbs given by a Native American healer to Canadian nurse Renee Caisse. ("Essiac" is Caisse spelled backward.) Despite a lack of systematic research or documentation of its value, Essiac is promoted and purchased for all forms of cancer.[99]

Diet and Nutrition

Macrobiotic Diet

Various dietary regimens have been promoted for both the prevention and treatment of cancer. The macrobiotic diet was first described by George Ohsawa (1893–1966). He developed a diet consisting of 10 stages, with each stage more restrictive than the previous one. The final stage consisted of only rice and water. The American Medical Association and various governmental agencies have opposed the macrobiotic diet due to its restrictive nature. In fact, there were a number of reports of health problems and even deaths among those who have followed the diet.[100]

The macrobiotic diet has subsequently been modified and is regaining popularity in the United States, and generally consists of 50% to 60% whole grains, 20% to 25% vegetables, 5% to 10% beans and sea vegetables, and 5% soups. Some variations of the diet allow small amounts of fish. There can be alterations of the diet depending on the disease process.

The Kushi Institute is a strong proponent of the macrobiotic diet. Based in Massachusetts, it teaches the macrobiotic diet and lifestyle. Specific foods for the individual cancer patient are recommended. Numerous testimonials supporting the effectiveness of the macrobiotic diet are provided, but there have not been any controlled studies evaluating the Kushi Institute methods.

There have been a number of nutritional deficiencies reported in association with the macrobiotic diet. Breast milk from mothers who follow the macrobiotic diet contains less vitamin B_{12}, calcium, magnesium, and saturated fatty acids than the milk of mothers following "regular" diets.[101] Infants of mothers on the macrobiotic diet were found to have retarded growth, fat and muscle wasting, and slowed psychomotor development. Bone mineral content was evaluated in a study of adolescents who had followed a macrobiotic diet and compared with control patients without dietary restrictions.[102] It was reported that the bone mineral content was significantly lower in both boys and girls who had followed the macrobiotic diet. The authors suggest that this finding could have important implications for fracture risk in later life. Machiels and colleagues[103] reported a rare case of nutritional rickets in a young child due to the macrobiotic diet.

Megadose Vitamin C: A Closer Look

The use of vitamin C for the treatment of cancer has been publicized for many years. Many continue to claim efficacy without strong scientific data to back these claims. Linus Pauling, PhD, and Ewan Cameron, MD, claimed that high doses of vitamin C could significantly improve survival in patients with cancer. The claim was based on the known antioxidant properties of vitamin C and some epidemiologic evidence that populations with high dietary intake of the vitamin have decreased risk of some types of cancer. These scientists believed that much higher doses than the recommended daily intake of 60 mg/day of vitamin C were needed to prevent free radical damage within the body. Pauling and Cameron reported a study of 100 patients with terminal cancer treated with megadose vitamin C who had significantly improved survival when compared with historical controls.[104] It was recommended that patients with cancer take 10,000 mg of vitamin C daily based on their research.

The study was plagued by significant design issues. The patients with "terminal" cancer who were treated with vitamin C all came from Dr. Cameron's practice, while the historical controls were "terminal" patients who came from other sources in the area. It is conceivable that significant selection bias occurred between Dr. Cameron's patients given vitamin C and the patients of other physicians who were not offered any additional treatments.

Due to the exceptional reputation of Nobel Laureate Dr. Pauling, the Mayo Clinic performed a prospective randomized study to evaluate vitamin C. Creagan and coworkers[105] randomized 150 patients with advanced cancer to receive 10 g of vitamin C vs. a placebo. There was no difference in symptoms, performance status, appetite, or survival between the two groups. The authors concluded that high-dose vitamin C had no therapeutic benefit.

Dr. Pauling criticized the poor design of the Mayo Clinic study, claiming that the patients had poor performance status and too much prior treatment with chemotherapy. Based on his criticisms, a new trial was launched. Moertel and associates[106] randomized 100 patients with advanced colorectal cancer in a double-blind study to receive high-dose vitamin C (10 g daily) or a placebo. No patient received previous cytotoxic therapy, and all had good performance status. Again, vitamin C showed no advantage over placebo therapy with regard to disease progression, objective improvement in measurable disease, or survival. The authors concluded that high-dose vitamin C therapy is not effective against malignant disease regardless of whether the patient has had any prior chemotherapy.

Side effects of megadose vitamin C include diarrhea, renal stones, iron overload, and gastrointestinal dis-

TABLE 34-4

Examples of Potential Adverse Effects of Common CAM Modalities[107-119]

CAM	ADVERSE EFFECT
Ephedra species	Hypertension, tachycardia, stroke, seizures
St John's wort	Depression, nausea, hypersensitivity reactions
Laetrile	Emesis, headache, dizziness, obtundation, dermatitis
Antineoplastics	Somnolence, confusion
Ginseng	Sedative diarrhea, headache, hypertension, insomnia, nausea
Echinacea	Hypersensitivity reactions
Kelp	Hyperthyroidism
Saw palmetto	Urinary retention, headache, diarrhea, constipation, hypertension, nausea
Mistletoe	Local irritation, allergic reactions
Shark cartilage	Hepatitis, emesis, constipation
Ginkgo	Emesis, headache
Green tea	Insomnia, emesis, diarrhea, confusion
Hydrazine sulfate	Hepatorenal failure
Goldenseal (*Hydrastis canadensis*)	Uterine contractions

comfort. There are ardent supporters of megadose vitamin C despite the strong scientific evidence refuting its use in the treatment of cancer. Based on the current scientific literature, megadose vitamin C is not recommended for the prevention or treatment of cancer.

CAM AND TOXICITIES

There is a multitude of potential interactions between conventional cancer treatments and CAM therapies. Many of these are just beginning to be recognized by the medical establishment and reported in reputable scientific journals.[8-9] There is evidence that both renal

and hepatic function can be impaired by various CAM therapies.[10-15] Multiple biochemical pathways can be affected, including the lipoxygenase, cyclo-oxygenase, and cytochrome P-450 pathways.[11] These could affect drug concentrations in the body, resulting in increased toxicity and/or changes in effectiveness of chemotherapy and radiation therapy. Antioxidants could decrease the effectiveness of radiation therapy due to the scavenging of free radicals that can damage DNA and result in cell death.[16] Moreover, many of these therapies have their own side effects that can mimic those of conventional cancer treatments (Tables 34-4 and 34-5).[107-119] If the oncologist is not aware that a patient is using a particular CAM therapy and a patient develops a side effect, a conventional cancer treatment with established efficacy could be altered or discontinued.

Many forms of CAM are associated with no or minimal risk to a cancer patient; however, this is not true for all such therapies. It is well established that a variety of herbal medications can produce serious side effects. Quality control of these preparations can be a major concern. Issues include variability in biologic potency in different crops, the very realistic possibility of contamination (e.g., fungus, bacteria), and the use of the erroneous plant species.[120] Herbal remedies could contain lead, arsenic, mercury, tin, or zinc, which themselves can be toxic.[121]

Immunoaugmentative therapy (IAT) of Burton is based on balancing four protein components in the blood while strengthening the patients' immune system. The use of various organ extracts from cows and pigs is claimed to suppress tumors selectively and stimulate the immune defense cells.[122,123] No studies have shown clinical effectiveness of IAT; however, samples of infected material revealed evidence of hepatitis virus.[124]

The new toxic effects of a variety of herbal preparations continue to be reported. For example, kava kava, a widely publicized natural sleep medication, has been

TABLE 34-5

Potential Interactions between Herbal Medicines and Conventional Drugs[107-119]

HERB	DRUG	POTENTIAL INTERACTION
St. John's wort	Irinotecan, protease inhibitors, other drugs metabolized by CYP450	Reduced drug levels
	Cyclosporin	
	Oral contraceptives	
	Digoxin	
Hawthorn flower, Devil's claw, licorice	Digoxin	Alters the pharmacodynamics and monitoring of drug levels is prudent
Licorice	Potassium-sparing diuretics	Affects potassium levels
Kelp	Thyroxine	Iodine content of herb could interfere with thyroid replacement
Kava	Alprazolam	Additive sedative effects, coma
	Terazosin	
Evening primrose oil	Anticonvulsants	Lowered seizure threshold
Feverfew, garlic, ginseng, ginkgo, ginger, Dong quai	Warfarin	Altered bleeding time
Yohimbe bark	Centrally active antihypertensive agents	Yohimbine could antagonize guanabenz and methyldopa through its α_2-adrenoceptor antagonistic properties.
Ginseng	Phenelzine sulphate, estrogens, corticosteroids	Headache, tremulousness, manic episodes, additive effects

associated with severe liver dysfunction, leading to at least one case of hepatic failure and the requirement for a liver transplant.[112] Other herbal medications have also been shown to be associated with hepatotoxicity.[113]

Laetrile (amygdalin), derived from apricots and other fruit pits, is one of the oldest CAM medications and continues to be marketed to the public.[78] Amygdalin had been used for centuries; but, in the 1950s it was elevated to new heights under the trademark Laetrile. Proponents of Laetrile claimed that proper use of this substance could eradicate cancer entirely (www.worldwithoutcancer.com and www.sumeria.net/health/laetrile.html). Moertel and colleagues[115] carried out a phase II clinical trial, treating 178 previously untreated patients with cancer and of good performance status with Laetrile; vitamins A, C, E, and B complex; and other various minerals including pancreatic enzymes. Only one patient who had gastric carcinoma with cervical lymph node metastases had a possible short-lived partial 10-week response. All other showed no signs of response. There was no evidence of disease stabilization. Evaluation of toxicities revealed several patients with blood cyanide levels in the ranges known to kill animals and humans. Studies have demonstrated that this drug can produce symptoms of nausea, vomiting, headache, dizziness, and obtundation.[115,116,125]

To date, one of the gravest examples of the potential for harm associated with herbal medications is that of the development of renal failure and urothelial carcinoma in individuals who used the Chinese herb *Aristolochia fangchi*.[126,127] Due to a manufacturing error, this herb replaced another preparation (*Stephania tetrandra*) used in a weight-reducing pill. More than 40 individuals who took this pill developed progressive renal failure, and almost 50% were found to have urothelial cancer.[126]

Vitamin toxicities are uncommon but well defined. Megadoses of vitamin A can cause increased intracranial pressure and vomiting in children, and its chronic use in adults can lead potentially to hypercalcemia.[128] Vitamin B-complex overdose can lead to cardiovascular toxicity, including arrhythmias, edema, vasodilation, and allergic reactions. Megadoses of niacin can cause cardiac toxicity with arrhythmia, liver toxicity, and peptic ulceration. Long-term, high-dose toxicities include gouty arthritis, hyperglycemia, dry skin, and rashes. Vitamin B_6 in megadoses can cause peripheral neuropathies, with resulting numbness lasting for weeks. Vitamin C toxicities include the development of renal stones.[129] High-dose vitamin E therapy can interfere with blood coagulation by antagonizing vitamin K and inhibiting prothrombin production. A recent study of vitamin E demonstrated an increased number of strokes in the vitamin E treatment group compared with the control group.[130]

Acupuncture and chiropractic medicine are both generally quite safe; however, they too can be associated with irritating and more serious side effects.[131,132] Reported toxicities of acupuncture include transmission of infectious agents through needle insertion; broken, forgotten, or misapplied needles; pneumothorax; transient hypotension; minor bleeding; contact dermatitis; and pain.[131] There is always a small but finite risk of a cerebrovascular accident with cervical spinal manipulations.[132]

THE INTERNET AND CAM

The Internet has become a hotbed of CAM offerings and information over the past decade. The Internet was initially developed for the rapid exchange of information through government, industrial, and academic computers by the Advanced Research Project Agency of the U.S. Department of Defense (ARPANET) in the event of a nuclear war.[133,134] Since the public introduction of the Internet in 1994, there has been exponential growth of this computer resource. In August 2002, it was estimated that 64% of the United States population (177.6 million people) had access to the Internet.[135] This was increased from 56.5% of the population in October 2000.

Overall, there are limited data evaluating the use of the Internet by patients with cancer for obtaining information about CAM. In a study of 921 patients presenting to radiation oncology centers in the United States, it was found that 42% of patients presenting to an academic medical center and 25% presenting to a community medical center were using the Internet to find cancer-specific information.[136] Most other cancer-specific Internet use information comes from studies on patients with prostate cancer. A questionnaire study from England showed that 24% of patients with prostate cancer were using the Internet to obtain further health information.[137] A Canadian questionnaire study of patients with prostate cancer revealed that 35% of patients had used the Internet to obtain cancer-related information.[138] Another recent Canadian questionnaire study evaluated 191 patients with cancer regarding their reliance on the news media and the Internet as sources of medical information.[137] This showed that 50% used the Internet to obtain information and 7% used the Internet as their primary source of information. A study reporting on use of the Internet by 295 patients with prostate cancer in the United States showed that 32% were using the Internet to gather information.[139] Interestingly, 58% of these patients with prostate cancer used the Internet to search for information on CAM.

Many more patients are probably obtaining Internet-derived information from other people. Based on the user demographics of OncoLink (http://www.oncolink.upenn.edu), the cancer information resource from the University of Pennsylvania, many friends and family members are using the Internet to obtain cancer-related information (Table 34-6). Further confirmation of Internet use by friends and family comes from a questionnaire study by Vordermark and associates.[140] Of 139 German radiation oncology patients, 12% had used the Internet to obtain information about their cancer, but an additional 15% received Internet-derived information about their cancer from friends or family members. It is noteworthy that only 24% discussed the information obtained from the Internet with their physicians.

Yakren and colleagues[141] analyzed the use of media information, including the Internet, among patients with cancer and their companions at Memorial Sloan-Kettering Cancer Center. Of the 443 individuals who returned the completed surveys, it was found that 44% of the patients

TABLE 34-6

OncoLink Users

Cancer survivor	26%
Cancer patient	19%
Healthcare provider	20%
Friend or family of cancer patient	10%
Multiple combinations of above	17%
Unknown	6%

and 60% of the companions reported use of the Internet to obtain cancer-related information. This is very similar to the utilization rate of 41% found among patients at the University of Pennsylvania Cancer Center.[11]

The identification of good Internet sites can be difficult for the nonmedical person searching for information on complementary and alternative medicine. The general public requested 30% of all PubMed searches performed in 1999. A study by Bernstam and associates[142] evaluated the ability of a computer-literate lay user to perform multiple searches for various question types related to cancer on MEDLINE. A blinded investigator then rated the relevance of each search. The computer user was then given a custom interface to help with the searches through MEDLINE. Overall, there was significantly higher precision using the MEDLINE interface compared with unaided novice searching. This emphasizes the need for the medical community to help guide patients' search for medically relevant information on the Internet. Although this study does not specifically evaluate Web searches, these results could be generalizable to patients looking for information on the Web regarding CAM.

It can be a daunting task for the nonmedical person to evaluate the quality of Internet sites objectively, particularly those sites offering CAM. A recent study by RAND Health reported the quality of health information on the Internet.[143] A variety of health Web sites were evaluated, including 20 major Web sites for breast cancer information. It was found, on average, that two to four Web sites needed to be visited to find more than minimal coverage for at least 75% of the indicators for a topic. Although experts might be able to evaluate the quality and appropriate coverage of a topic quickly as in the RAND study, this can be very difficult for the patient. Meric and coworkers[144] found that popularity and traffic of breast cancer Web sites do not always correlate with quality. This observation again emphasizes the need for professionals to help guide the lay public to appropriate medical material on the Web.

Most health care providers have experienced patients entering the office for a medical visit with pages of CAM information printed from the Internet; however, there is only a limited number of studies actually documenting the use of the Internet to find information on CAM. Metz and colleagues[136] showed that 53% of patients with cancer using the Internet were interested in finding information about CAM. Most of these patients were doing so without the knowledge of their health care provider.

CAM therapies were purchased over the Internet by 12% of Internet users in this study, which did not specifically evaluate the type of therapy purchased. This emphasizes the need for physicians to become familiar with therapies offered over the Internet. Health care providers must discuss the use of these therapies with patients; particular discussions should emphasize the potential side effects and interactions with conventional cancer treatments.[11] Further studies are needed to directly assess the impact of CAM Web sites on patients with cancer.

A typical search on one of the Internet search engines (e.g., http://www.yahoo.com) for "alternative and complementary medicine" reveals more than 432,000 different Web site matches. Some of these sites provide credible information. Unfortunately, many are designed only to sell a specific product and give false or misleading information. It can be overwhelming for the average person without medical knowledge to sift through and understand the claims of many of these sites.

Some patients ask their health care providers for recommendations on evaluating Web sites offering CAM information. It is generally recommended to start with sites managed by major academic centers and the government, as these institutions maintain a level of quality outside of the Internet that is upheld on these Web sites. Also, it is important for patients to be wary of sites designed to sell a specific product or treatment. Table 34-7 provides some suggestions to guide patients when evaluating Internet sites. The list is not in any order of importance.

Table 34-8 recommends selected Web sites with reliable CAM information for the cancer patient and health care provider.

ALTERNATIVE MEDICINE CANCER CLINICS

Numerous cancer clinics promoting alternative medicine techniques have formed throughout the world. A complete enumeration is beyond the scope of this chapter, but none of them is known to have shown verifiable beneficial results when compared with conventional medical treatments. Case reports and testimonials abound, however. It is important that health care providers realize that these treatments are being promoted to their patients though the Internet, publications, and through word of mouth.

For example, Tijuana, Mexico, has long been a destination for patients seeking alternative medical therapies. At any one time, there are 50 to 70 alternative medicine clinics in operation at this location. It has been roughly estimated that 40,000 people travel to Tijuana annually in search of alternative treatments. Of these patients, 95% are from the United States. Many of these clinics operate in a hospital-type atmosphere, where the patients stay for a number of days or weeks for their therapy. A few clinics are strictly outpatient or day-treatment centers.

The therapies offered in these centers range from simple dietary management to complex operative treat-

TABLE 34-7

Evaluating Medical Web Sites

1. **Accuracy of information:** Sites posting information that is not referenced, or where authors and dates of content are not stated, should be avoided.

2. **Availability of editorial staff:** A Web resource should list its editorial staff and the credentials of the people behind the resource. Address and e-mail contact information should also be provided.

3. **Qualifications of editorial staff:** Many resources are run by people who are not qualified to provide medical advice. Fundamentally, there is nothing wrong with this, provided that their lack of qualification is clearly stated. The best information, however, is provided by health care professionals who are health care providers themselves. Much of what physicians, nurses, and other professionals are trained to do involves interacting with patients and providing information in the clearest, most appropriate manner.

4. **Freshness of content:** Sites with content that is updated regularly are likely to be ones that are best managed and most up-to-date.

5. **Disclosure of conflicts of interest:** Conflicts of interest should either be obvious or disclosed clearly to the users.

6. **Price of information:** So far, very few medical Web resources are charging for information. Although this could change in the future, open access to information with fees that are minimal should be the rule. If you are being charged for the information, make sure it is not information that others are providing for free.

7. **Confidentiality:** Most medical Web resources will not respond to direct medical inquiries by users. This is, in part, due to concerns over patient confidentiality and accuracy of information either sent to or received by the patient. It is important to make sure that sites requiring registration are not releasing contact data without permission.

8. **Reputation:** Resources known to be run by reputable institutions are more likely to provide more timely, accurate, and unbiased information.

9. **Look and feel:** Resources must balance between having an attractive resource and being able to provide the best possible information to users. Certainly, content rich in graphics is attractive, but if it is poorly organized, or if it takes an inordinate amount of time to download, it might not be serving its primary purpose.

10. **Navigation and searching:** Make sure that a site is well organized, easy to navigate, and has a good search engine.

Reproduced with permission from the editors at http://www.oncolink.upenn.edu.

TABLE 34-8

Selected Web Sites with reliable CAM information	
ORGANIZATION	**WORLD WIDE WEB ADDRESS**
American Botanical Council	www.herbalgram.org/
American Cancer Society	cancer.org
M.D. Anderson Cancer Center	www.mdanderson.org/departments/cimer/
Memorial Sloan-Kettering Cancer Center	www.mskcc.org/mskcc/html/11571.cfm
National Cancer Institute	www.cancer.gov/cancer_information/list.aspx?viewid=14821490-ee6c-4e7c-80b5-c4fb3cbbb07e
National Center for Complementary and Alternative Medicine	nccam.nih.gov/
Office of Complementary and Alternative Medicine	www3.cancer.gov/occam/
OncoLink (University of Pennsylvania Cancer Center)	oncolink.upenn.edu
Quackwatch	quackwatch.com

cells need more glucose and thus take up the chemotherapy more and there are no side effects."

Claims of benefit by these alternative medical centers have not been substantiated by the outside medical establishment. Based on the authors' own travels, however, some of these patients with hormone-responsive tumors (e.g., breast cancer and prostate cancer) are receiving hormonal therapies. Also, as mentioned previously, chemotherapy is sometimes offered along with the alternative treatments. This could account for some of the claims of response to these treatments.

These treatments are generally out-of-pocket medical expenditures, as they are not covered by medical insurance programs. Table 34-9 shows the estimated cost at some of the more popular centers offering alternative cancer treatments. Some of the prices do not include room and board. Many have added charges that might not be specified until the patient is seen and evaluated at the clinics. All require cash payment before treatment. Travel expenses are not included in the estimates.

CONCLUSIONS

Many patients with cancer and their friends and family members are searching for information regarding CAM. As health care providers, we must become educated on this topic so that we can guide our patients appropriately. CAM is here to stay, and we should support our patients when they are using complementary therapies that are safe. Health care providers must warn patients of potential or known interactions with conventional medications and treatments when appropriate. Clinical trials evaluating CAM should be developed and encouraged. CAM needs to be held to the same stringent criteria as conventional treatment modalities.

ments. Some of these treatments are innocuous, while others could be quite dangerous. For instance, some patients are offered insulin-induced hypoglycemic therapy (IHT). Patients are given insulin to drop the blood glucose level to less than 40 mg/dL, then infused with a glucose solution with a diluted chemotherapy solution. The rationale for this treatment is that the "starving cancer

TABLE 34-9

Popular Unconventional Cancer Therapy Clinics

CLINIC	LOCATION	TYPE OF THERAPY	DURATION OF TREATMENT	ESTIMATED COST
Kushi Institute	Brookline, MA	Macrobiotic diet	1 week	$1500*
Burzynski Clinic	Houston, TX	Antineoplastics	6 months	$50,000†
Immuno-Augmentive Centre	Bahamas	Immuno-Augmentive	3 months	$13,100‡
Hospital de Baja California del Sol	Tijuana	Gerson Method	1 month	$20,000§
Bio Medical Center	Tijuana	Hoxsey Herbal	Variable	$3800‖
Center for Cell Specific Therapy	Santo Domingo	Magnet Therapy	Variable	$20,000¶

*Based on published advertising on the Internet of $1495 for 1 week. Private counseling sessions are an additional $225 each.
‡Based on telephone quotation of intravenous therapy of $14,000 for the first month and $7200 for each additional month, with treatment averaging 6 months' duration. Oral formula is $6000 for the first month and $2000 for each additional month.
‡Published advertising fee schedule from the Immuo-Augmentive Centre of $7500 for the first four weeks and $700 per week thereafter for up to eight additional weeks. Supplies for home maintenance are $50 per week indefinitely.
§Based on published advertising on the Internet of $3990 per week for basic charges with a recommended stay of one month. "...Actual costs for any individual will become evident only during the course of treatment."
‖Based on telephone quotation of $3500 lifetime supply of Hoxsey Tonic, $300–$400 for blood work, and $25 consultation fee.
¶Based on brochure from the Center for Cell Specific Therapy. All patients are charged $20,000 regardless of the length of treatment.

REFERENCES

1. National Institutes of Health: Alternative Medicine: Expanding Medical Horizons. Washington, DC, U.S. Government Printing Office; 1992.
2. Cassileth BR: "Complementary" or "alternative"? It makes a difference in cancer care. Complement Ther Med 1999;7:35.
3. Schimpff SC: Complementary medicine. Curr Opin Oncol 1997;9:327.
4. Panel on Definition and Description: Defining and describing complementary and alternative medicine. CAM Research Methodology Conference, April 1995. Altern Ther 1997;3:49.
5. Risberg T, Lund E, Wist E, et al: Cancer patients use of nonproven therapy: A 5-year follow up study. J Clin Oncol 1998;16:6–12.
6. Liu JM, Chu HC, Chin YH, et al: Cross sectional study of use of alternative medicine in Chinese cancer patients. Jpn J Clin Oncol 1997;27:37–41.
7. Begbie SD, Kerestes ZL, Bell DR: Patterns of alternative medicine use by cancer patients. Med J Aust 1996;165:545–548.
8. Downer SM, Cody MM, McCluskey P, et al: Pursuit and practice of complementary therapies by cancer patients receiving conventional treatment. BMJ 1994;309:86–89.
9. Lerner IJ, Kennedy BJ: The prevalence of questionable methods of cancer treatment in the United States. CA Cancer J Clin 1992;42:181–191.
10. Burstein HJ, Gelber S, Guadagnoli E, et al: The use of complementary health stratagies by women with early stage breast cancer. Proc Am Soc Clin Oncol 1998;17:43a.
11. Metz JM, Jones H, Devine P, et al: Cancer patients use unconventional medical therapies far more frequently than standard history and physical examination suggest. Can J Sci Am 2001;7:149–154.
12. Grootenhuis MA, Last BF, de Graff-Nijkerk JH, et al: Use of alternative treatment in pediatric oncology. Cancer Nurs 1998;21:282–288.
13. Fernandez CV, Stutzer CA, MacWilliam L, et al: Alternative and complementary therapy use in pediatric oncology patients in British Columbia: Prevalence and reasons for use and nonuse. J Clin Oncol 1998;16:1279–1286.
14. Blendon RJ, DesRoches CM, Benson JM, Brodie M, Altman DE: Americans' views on the use and regulation of dietary supplements. Arch Intern Med 2001;161805–810.
15. Conner M, Kirk SF, Cade JE, Barrett JH: Why do women use dietary supplements? The use of the theory of planned behaviour to explore beliefs about their use. Soc Sci Med 2001;52:621–633.
16. Frank E, Bendich A, Denniston M: Use of vitamin-mineral supplements by female physicians in the United States. Am J Clin Nutr 2000;71:969–975.
17. Neuhouser ML, Patterson RE, Levy L: Motivations for using vitamin and mineral supplements. J Am Diet Assoc 1999;99:851–854.
18. Patterson RE, Neuhouser ML, White E, Hunt JR, Kristal AR: Cancer-related behavior of vitamin supplement users. Cancer Epidemiol Biomarkers Prev 1998;7:79–81.
19. World Cancer Research Fund and the American Institute for Cancer Research: Food, Nutrition and the Prevention of Cancer: A Global Perspective. Washington, DC, American Institute for Cancer Research, 1997.
20. Knekt P, Aromaa A, Maatela J, et al: Vitamin E and cancer prevention. Am J Clin Nutr 1991;53(Suppl):283–286.
21. Block G: Fruit, vegetables, and cancer prevention: A review of the epidemiological evidence. Nutr Cancer 1992;18:1–29.
22. Stahelin H, Gey K, Eichholzer M: Plasma anti-oxidant vitamins and subsequent cancer mortality in the 12-year follow-up of the prospective Basel study. Am J Epidemiol 1991;133:766–775.
23. Nomura AM, Stemmermann G, Heilbrun L: Serum vitamin levels and the risk of cancer of specific sites in men of Japanese ancestry in Hawaii. Cancer Res 1985;45:2369–2372.
24. Hennekens CH, Stampfer MJ, Willett W: Micronutrients and cancer chemoprevention. Cancer Detect Prev 1984;7:147–158.
25. Woutersen RA, Appel MJ, Van Garderen-Hoetmer A: Modulation of pancreatic carcinogenesis by antioxidants. Food Chem Toxicol 1999;37:981–984.
26. Hong WK, Lippman SM, Itri L: Prevention of second primary tumors with isotretinoin in squamous-cell carcinoma of the head and neck. N Engl J Med 1990;323:795–801.
27. Moore SR, Hill KA, Heinmoller PW, Halangoda A, Kunishige M, Buettner VL, et al: Spontaneous mutation frequency and pattern in big blue mice fed a vitamin E-supplemented diet. Environ Mol Mutagen 1999;34:195–200.
28. Lippman SM, Lee JJ, Sabichi AI: Cancer chemoprevention: Progress and promise. J Natl Cancer Inst 1998;90:1514–1528.
29. Alpha Tocopherol Beta Carotene Trial Group: The effect of vitamin E and beta-carotene on the incidence of lung cancer and other cancers in male smokers. N Engl J Med 1994;330:1029–1035.
30. Omenn GS, Goodman GE, Thornquist M, et al: The Beta-Carotene and Retinol Efficacy Trial (CARET) for chemoprevention of lung cancer in high-risk populations: Smokers and asbestos-exposed workers. Cancer Res 1994;54:2038–2043S.
31. Li JY, Taylor PR, Dawsey S, et al: Nutrition intervention trials in Linxian, China: Multiple vitamin/mineral supplementation, cancer incidence, and disease-specific mortality among adults with esophageal dysplasia. J Natl Cancer Inst 1994;86:1645–1649.
32. Crawford ED, Fair WR, Kelloff GJ, et al: Chemoprevention of prostate cancer: Guidelines for possible intervention strategies. J Cell Biochem 1992;16H(Suppl):140–145.
33. Blutt SE, Weigel NL: Vitamin D and prostate cancer. Proc Soc Exp Biol Med 1999;221:89–98.

34. Hyman J, Baron JA, Dain BJ, et al: Dietary and supplemental calcium and the recurrence of colorectal adenomas. Cancer Epidemiol Biomarkers Prev 1998;7:291.

35. Clark LC, Combs GF, Turnbull BW, et al: Effect of selenium supplementation for cancer prevention with carcinoma of the skin: A randomized controlled trial. JAMA 1996;276:1957–1963.

36. Setchell KDR, Cassidy A: Dietary isoflavones: Biological effects and relevance to human health. J Nutr 1999;129:758S–767S.

37. Messina MJ, Persky V, Setchell KDR: Soy intake and cancer risk: Review of the in vivo and in vitro data. Nutr Cancer 1994;21:113–131.

38. Messina MJ, Barnes S: The role of soy products in reducing risk of cancer. J Natl Cancer Inst 1991;83:541–546.

39. Kennedy AR: The evidence for soybean products as cancer preventive agents. J Nutr 1995;125:733S–743S.

40. Complementary and Alternative Medicine [entire issue]. JAMA 1998;280:1549–1640.

41. Ernst E, Pittler MH: Herbal medicine. Med Clin North Am 2002;86:149–161.

42. Eisenberg DM, Davis RB, Ettner SL, et al: Trends in alternative medicine use in the United States, 1990–1997. JAMA 1998;280(18):1569–1575.

43. Eisenberg DM, Kessler RC, Foster C, Norlock FE, Calkins DR, Delbanco TL: Unconventional medicine in the United States: Prevalence, costs, and patterns of use. N Engl J Med 1993;328(4):246–252.

44. Brevoort P: The booming US botanical market: A new overview. HerbalGram 1998;44:33–48.

45. Spence Cohen MJ: Complementary and Alternative Medicine: Legal Boundaries and Regulatory Perspectives. Baltimore, Johns Hopkins, 1998.

46. Ang-Lee MK, Moss J, Yuan CS: Herbal medicines and perioperative care. JAMA 2001;286:208–216.

47. De Smet PA: Herbal remedies. N Engl J Med 2002;347(25):2046–2056.

48. Blumenthal M (ed): The complete German Commission E monographs therapeutic guide to herbal medicines. Austin, Tex, American Botanical Council, 1998.

49. Licensing of medicines: Policy on herbal medicines. Herbal safety news. London, Medicines Control Agency, 2002. (Accessed November 22, 2002, at http://www.mca.gov.uk/ourwork/licensingmeds/herbalmeds/herbalsafety.htm).

50. Dundee JW, Ghaly RG, Fitzpatrick KT, et al: Acupuncture prophylaxis of cancer chemotherapy-induced sickness. J R Soc Med 1989;82:268–271.

51. Dundee JW, Yang J: Prolongation of the antiemetic action of P6 acupuncture by acupressure in patients having cancer chemotherapy. J R Soc Med 1990;83:360–362.

52. NIH Consensus Development Panel on Acupuncture: Acupuncture. JAMA 1998;280(17):1518–1524.

53. Bing Z, Villanueva L, LeBars D: Acupuncture-evoked responses of subnucleus reticularis dorsalis neurons in the rat medulla. Neuroscience 1991;44:693–703.

54. Grossman A, Clement-Jones V: Opiate receptors: Enkephalins and endorphins. Clin Endocrinol Metab 1983;12:31–56.

55. Matsumoto T, Lyu BS: Anatomical comparison between acupuncture and nerve block. Am Surg 1975;41:11–16.

56. Woodson CM, Shalts E: Homeopathy. Med Clin North Am 2002;86:47–62.

57. Eskinazi D: Homeopathy re-revisited. Arch Intern Med 1999;159:1981–1987.

58. Linde K, Clausius N, Ramirez G, et al: Are the clinical effects of homeopathy placebo effects? A meta-analysis of placebo-controlled trials. Lancet 1997;350(9081):834–843.

59. Linde K, Melchart D: Randomized controlled trials of individualized homeopathy: A state-of-the-art review. J Altern Complement Med 1998;4(4):371–388.

60. Ironson G, Field T, Scafidi F, et al: Massage therapy is associated with enhancement of the immune system's cytotoxic capacity. Int J Neurosci 1996;84:205–217.

61. Field T: Massage therapy. Med Clin North Am 2002;86:163–171.

62. Shealy CN, Thomas R (eds): The Complete Family Guide to Alternative Medicine. Rockport, Mass, Element Books, 1996.

63. Carey TS, Garrett J, Jackman A, McLaughlin C, Fryer J, Smucker DR: The outcomes and costs of care for acute low back pain among patients seen by primary care practitioners, chiropractors and orthopedic surgeons: The North Carolina back pain project. N Engl J Med 1995;333(14):913–917.

64. Cherkin DC, Deyo RA, Battie M, Street J, Barlow W: A comparison of physical therapy, chiropractic manipulation and provision of an educational booklet for the treatment of patients with low back pain. N Engl J Med 1998;339(15):1021–1029.

65. Cherkin D, Mootz R: Chiropractic in the United States: Training, practice and research. AHCPR, Pub. No. 98-N002, 1997.

66. Chopra A, Doiphode VV: Ayurvedic medicine: core concept, therapeutic principles, and current relevance. Med Clin North Am 2002;86:75–89.

67. Upadhyay RL: Prevention of diseases: An Ayurvedic approach. Indian J Med Sci 1998;52:119–124.

68. Burish TG, Jenkins RA: Effectiveness of biofeedback and relaxation training in reducing the side effects of cancer chemotherapy. Health Psychol 1992;11:17–23.

69. Syrjala KL, Donaldson, GW, Davis MW, et al: Relaxation and imagery and cognitive-behavioral training reduce pain during cancer treatment: A controlled clinical trial. Pain 1995;63:189–198.

70. Darzynkiewicz Z, Traganos F, Wu JM, Chen S: Chinese herbal mixture PC SPES in treatment of prostate cancer [review]. Int J Oncol 2000;17:729–736.

71. de la Taille A, Hayek OR, Buttyan R, Bagiella E, Burchardt M, Katz AE: Effects of a phytotherapeutic agent, PC-SPES, on prostate cancer: A preliminary investigation on human cell lines and patients. BJU Int 1999;84:845–850.

72. DiPaola RS, Zhang H, Lambert GH, Meeker R, Licitra E, Rafi MM, et al: Clinical and biologic activity of an estrogenic herbal combination (PC-SPES) in prostate cancer. [see comments] N Engl J Med 1998;339:785–791.

73. Pfeifer BL, Pirani JF, Hamann SR, Klippel KF: PC-SPES, a dietary supplement for the treatment of hormone-refractory prostate cancer. BJU Int 2000;85:481–485.

74. Small EJ, Frohlich MW, Bok R, Shinohara K, Grossfeld G, Kelly WK, et al: Prospective trial of the herbal supplement PC-SPES in patients with progressive prostate cancer. J Clin Oncol 2000;18:3595–3603.

75. Lock M, Loblaw DA, Choo R, et al: Disseminated intravascular coagulation and PC-SPES: A case report and literature review. Can J Urol 2001;8:1326–1329.

76. Schiff JD, Ziecheck WS, Choi B: Pulmonary embolus related to PC-SPES use in a patient with PSA recurrence after radical prostatectomy. Urology 2002;59:444.

77. Weinrobe MC, Montgomery B: Acquired bleeding diathesis in a patient taking PC-SPES. N Engl J Med 2001;345:1213–1214.

78. Cassileth BR, Vickers AJ: Complementary and alternative therapies. Urol Clin North Am 2002;30:369–376.

79. Gold J: Use of hydrazine sulfate in terminal and preterminal cancer patients: Results of investigational new drug (IND) study in 84 evaluable patients. Oncology 1975;32:1–10.

80. Loprinzi CL, Goldberg RM, Su JQ, et al: Placebo-controlled trial of hydrazine sulfate in patients with newly diagnosed non-small-cell lung cancer. J Clin Oncol 1994;12:1126–1129.

81. Loprinzi CL, et al: Randomized placebo controlled evaluation of hydrazine sulfate in patients with advanced colorectal cancer. J Clin Oncol 1994;12:1121–1125.

82. Kosty MP, Fleishman SB, Herndon JE, et al: Cisplatin, vinblastine, and hydrazine sulfate in advanced, non-small-cell lung cancer: A randomized placebo-controlled, double-blind phase III study of the Cancer and Leukemia Group B. J Clin Oncol 1994;12:1113–1120.

83. Wellings SR: Neoplasia and primitive vertebrate phylogeny: Echenoderms, prevertebrates, and fishes—A review. Natl Cancer Inst Monogr 1969;31:59–128.

84. Prieur DJ, Fenstermacher JD, Guarino AM: A choroid plexus papilloma in an elasmobranch (Squalus acanthias). J Natl Cancer Inst 1976;56:1207–1208.

85. Wolke RE, Murchelano RA: A case report of an epidermal papilloma in Mustelus canis. J Wildl Dis 1976;12:167–171.

86. Langer R, Lee A: Shark cartilage contains inhibitors of tumor angiogenesis. Science 1983;221:1185–1187.

87. Mathews J: Media feeds frenzy over shark cartilage as cancer treatment. J Natl Cancer Inst 1993;85:1190–1191.

88. Miller DR, Granick JL, Stark JJ, et al: Phase I/II trial of the safety and efficacy of shark cartilage in the treatment of advanced cancers. Proc Am Soc Clin Oncol 1997;16:49a.

89. Ashar B, Vargo E: Shark cartilage induced hepatitis. JAMA 1996;125:780–781.

90. Grothey A, Duppe J, Hasenburg A, Voigtmann R: Use of alternative medicine in oncology patients. Dtsch Med Wochenschr 1998;123: 923–929.

91. Munstedt K, Kirsch K, Milch W, Sachsse S, Vahrson H: Unconventional cancer therapy: Survey of patients with gynaecological malignancy. Arch Gynecol Obstet 1996;258:81–88.

92. Bocci V: Mistletoe (Viscum album) lectins as cytokine inducers and immunoadjuvant in tumor therapy: A review. J Biol Regul Homeost Agents 1993;7:1–6.

93. Mannel DN, Becker H, Gundt A, Kist A, Franz H: Induction of tumor necrosis factor expression by a lectin from Viscum album. Cancer Immunol Immunother 1991;33:177–182.

94. Lenartz D, Stoffel B, Menzel J, Beuth J: Immunoprotective activity of the galactoside-specific lectin from mistletoe after tumor destructive therapy in glioma patients. Anticancer Res 1996;16:3799–3802.

95. Jung ML, Baudino S, Ribereau-Gayon G, Beck JP: Characterization of cytotoxic proteins from mistletoe (Viscum album L.). Cancer Lett 1990;51:103–108.

96. Kleijnen J, Knipschildm P: Mistletoe treatment for cancer: Review of controlled trials in humans. Phytomedicine 1994;1:255–260.

97. Steuer-Vogt MK, Bonkowsky V, Ambrosch P, Scholz M, Neiss A, Strutz J, et al: The effect of an adjuvant mistletoe treatment programme in resected head and neck cancer patients: A randomised controlled clinical trial. Eur J Cancer 2001;37:23–31.

98. Eggermont AM, Keilholz U, Autier P, Ruiter DJ, Lehmann F, Lienard D: European Organization for Research and Treatment of Cancer Melanoma Group trial experience with more than 2,000 patients, evaluating adjuvant treatment with low or intermediate doses of interferon alpha-2b. [abstract] Eur J Cancer 1999;35:26.

99. Kaegi E: Unconventional therapies for cancer: 1. Essiac. The Task Force on Alternative Therapies of the Canadian Breast Cancer Research Initiative. Can Med Assoc J 1998;158:897–902.

100. Metz JM: Alternative medicine and the cancer patient: An overview. Med Pediat Oncology 2000;34:20–26.

101. Dagnelie PC, van Staveren WA: Macrobiotic nutrition and child health: Results of a population-based, mixed-longitudinal cohort study in the Netherlands. Am J Clin Nutr 1994;59:1187S–1196S.

102. Parsons TJ, van Dusseldorp M, van der Vliet M, et al: Reduced bone mass in Dutch adolescents fed a macrobiotic diet early in life. J Bone Miner Res 1997;12:1486–1494.

103. Machiels F, De Maeseneer M, Van Snick A, et al: A rare cause of rickets in a young child. J Belge Radiol 1995;78:276–277.

104. Cameron E, Pauling L: Supplemental ascorbate in the supportive treatment of cancer: Prolongation of survival times in terminal human cancer. Proc Natl Acad Sci USA 1976;73:3685–3689.

105. Creagan ET, Moertel CG, O'Fallen JR, et al: Failure of high-dose vitamin C (ascorbic acid) therapy to benefit patients with advanced cancer. A controlled trial. N Engl J Med 1979;301:687–690.

106. Moertel CG, Fleming TR, Creagan ET, et al: High-dose vitamin C versus placebo in the treatment of patients with advanced cancer who have had no prior chemotherapy. A randomized double-blind comparison. N Engl J Med 1985;312:137–141.

107. Green S: Immunoaugmentative therapy: An unproven cancer treatment. JAMA 1993;270:1719–1723.

108. Markman M: Safety issues in using complementary and alternative medicine. J Clin Oncol 2002;20:39–41.

109. Ernst E: The risk-benefit profile of commonly used herbal therapies: Ginkgo, St. John's wort, ginseng, Echinacea, saw palmetto, and kava. Ann Intern Med 2002;136:42–53.

110. Haller CA, Benowitz NL: Adverse cardiovascular and central nervous system events associated with dietary supplements containing ephedra alkaloids. N Engl J Med 2000;343:1833–1838.

111. Echinacea for prevention and treatment of upper respiratory infections. Med Lett Drugs Ther 2002;44:29–32.

112. Grossman L: The curious case of kava: Why did it take the FDA so long to finally sound the alarm? Time 2002;15a:58.

113. MacGregor FB, Abernethy VE, Dahabra S, et al: Hepatotoxicity of herbal remedies. BMJ 1989;299:1156–1157.

114. Hainer MI, Tsai N, Komura ST, et al: Fatal hepatorenal failure associated with hydrazine sulfate. Ann Intern Med 2000;133:877–880.

115. Moertel CG, Ames MM, Kovach JS, et al: A pharmacologic and toxicological study of amygdalin. JAMA 1981;245:591–594.

116. Moertel CG, Fleming TR, Rubin J, et al: A clinical trial of amygdalin (Laetrile) in the treatment of human cancer. N Engl J Med 1982;306(4):201–206.

117. Miller DR, Anderson GT, Stark JJ, et al: Phase I/II trial of the safety and efficacy of shark cartilage in the treatment of advanced cancer. J Clin Oncol 1998;16:3649–3655.

118. Parker MG: Shark cartilage-induced hepatitis. Ann Intern Med 1996;125:780–781.

119. Buckner JC, Malkin MG, Reed E, et al: Phase II study of antineoplastons A10 (NSC 648539) and AS2-1 (NSC 620261) in patients with recurrent glioma. Mayo Clin Proc 1999;74:137–145.

120. Murch SJ, KrishnaRaj S, Saxena PK: Phytopharmaceuticals: Problems, limitations, and solutions. Sci Rev Altern Med 2000;4:33–37.

121. Spencer D'Arcy PF: Adverse reaction and interactions with herbal medications. Adverse Drug React Toxicol Rev 1991;10:189.

122. Cassileth BR, Chapman CC: Alternative and complementary cancer therapies. Cancer Invest 1996;14(4):396.

123. Hauser SP: Unproven methods in cancer treatment. Curr Opin Oncol 1993;5(4):646.

124. U.S. Congress, Office of Technology Assessment: Colin immuno-augmentative therapy: Unconventional cancer treatment, pub No. OTH-H-405. Washington DC, U.S. Government Printing Office, 1990, pp 129–14735.

125. Lagnado L: Laetrile makes a comeback on the web: Long deemed illegal by the FDA, it's selling briskly again to desperate patients online. Wall Str J 2000;April 22:B1–B2.

126. Nortier JL, Martinez M-CM, Schmeiser HH, et al: Urothelial carcinoma associated with the use of a Chinese herb (Aristolochia fangchi). N Engl J Med 2000;342:1686–1692.

127. Lord GM, Cook T, Arlt VM, et al: Urothelial malignant disease and Chinese herbal nephropathy. Lancet 2001;358:1515–1516.

128. Spencer Frame B, et al: Hypercalcemia and skeletal effects in chronic hypovitaminosis A. Ann Intern Med 1974;80:44.

129. Spencer JW: Complementary/Alternative Medicine: An Evidence-based Approach. St. Louis, MO, Mosby, 1999.

130. Albanes D, et al: Effects of alpha-tocopherol and beta-carotene supplements on cancer incidence. Am J Clin Nut 1995;62(6 suppl):1427.

131. Kaptchuk TJ: Acupuncture: Theory, efficacy, and practice. Ann Intern Med 2002;136:374–383.

132. Meeker WC, Haldeman S: Chiropractic: A profession at the crossroads of mainstream and alternative medicine. Ann Intern Med 2002;136:216–227.

133. Hellawell GO, Turner KJ, Le Monnier KJ, et al: Urology and the Internet: An evaluation of Internet use by urology patients and of information available on urologic topics. BJU Int 2000;86:191–194.

134. Doyle DJ, Ruskin KJ, Engel TP: The Internet and medicine: Past, present, and future. Yale J Biol Med 1996;69:429–437.

135. Nielsen Net Ratings: Global Internet Usage. http://www.nielsennetratings.com/, 2002.

136. Metz JM, Devine P, DeNittis, et al: A multi-institutional study of Internet utilization by radiation oncology patients. Int J Radiation Oncology Biol Phys 2003;56:1201–1205.

137. McFarlane N, Parker JH, Denstedt JD: Urology and the Internet. Comtemp Urol 1999;11:38–40.

138. Chen X, Siu L: Impact of the media and the Internet on oncology: Survey of cancer patients and oncologists in Canada. J Clin Oncol 2001;19:4291–4297.

139. Smith RP, Devine P, Jones H, et al: Internet usage by prostate cancer patients undergoing radiation therapy. Urology 2003;62: 273–277.

140. Vordermark D, Kolbl O, Flentje M: The Internet as a source of medical information. Investigation in a mixed cohort of radiotherapy patients. Strahlenthe Onkol 2000;176:532–535.

141. Yakren S, Shi W, Thaler H, et al: Use of the Internet and other information resources among adult cancer patients and their companions [abstract]. Proc Amer Soc Clin Oncol 2001;20:1589.

142. Bernstam EV, Kamvar SD, Meric F, et al: Oncology patient interface to Medline [abstract]. Proc Amer Soc Clin Oncol 2001;20:974.

143. Berland GK, Elliott MN, Morales LS, et al: Health information on the Internet: Accessibility, quality, and readability in English and Spanish. JAMA 2001;285:2612–2621.

144. Meric F, Bernstam EV, Mirza NQ, et al: Breast cancer on the world-wide web: Determinants of web site popularity [abstract]. Proc Am Soc Clin Oncol 2001;20:1904.

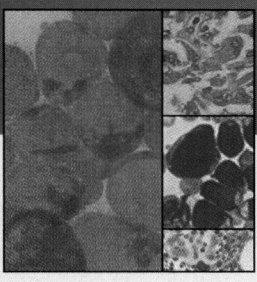

PART II

PROBLEMS COMMON TO CANCER AND ITS THERAPY

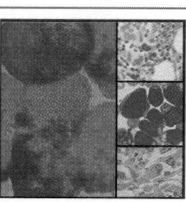

CANCER PAIN

Stuart A. Grossman

Suzanne Nesbit

SUMMARY OF KEY POINTS

INCIDENCE
Major Presenting Symptom of Malignancies
- Affects more than 30% of patients undergoing antineoplastic therapy
- Moderate to severe pain occurs in over 70% of patients during the later phases of their illness
- Significantly affects quality of life
- Frequently managed poorly

ETIOLOGY OF COMPLICATION
- Can be of nociceptive, neuropathic, or sympathetically maintained origin
- Due to direct tumor involvement (70%), evaluation or therapy (20%), or illness unrelated to the malignancy (<10%)

EVALUATION OF THE PATIENT
- Determining the etiology of pain is key to appropriate therapy
- Treat pain aggressively during evaluation
- Fully evaluate the pain using a careful history and physical examination, validated pain assessment scales, and selected laboratory tests

GRADING OF THE COMPLICATION
- Measurements of pain intensity using validated pain assessment scales
- Results should be recorded serially as an integral part of the medical record

TREATMENT
- 85% of patients can be well palliated using simple, inexpensive, "low-technology," oral analgesics
- Addition of appropriate adjuvant pain medications, alternate routes of opioid administration, antineoplastic therapy, nonpharmacologic approaches, neurostimulatory techniques, regional analgesia, and neuroablative procedures provides excellent palliation for nearly all patients with cancer pain

INCIDENCE

Facts

Pain is one of the most common and dreaded symptoms associated with cancer. It occurs in one-quarter to one-half of patients with newly diagnosed malignancies, in one-third of those undergoing treatment, and in more than three-quarters with advanced disease.[1,2] Overall, 75% of patients with cancer experience pain severe enough to require treatment with opioids during their illness.[3] Unrelieved pain directly affects patients' daily activities, quality of life, and psychological status. The importance of this symptom and the availability of excellent analgesic therapies make it imperative that health care providers be adept at the evaluation and treatment of cancer pain.

Etiology

Pain in patients with malignancies is a complex and often recurring process that occurs from many causes.[4] Ninety percent of pain in patients with cancer results from the tumor or its evaluation or therapy while less than 10% is due to unrelated illnesses.[3] In 70% of patients, pain develops from tumor invading or compressing soft tissue, bone, or neural structures. The common pain syndromes that result are listed in Table 35-1. The remaining 20% of cancer pain occurs from diagnostic and therapeutic procedures that these patients undergo in the process of

TABLE 35-1

Etiology of Pain in Cancer Patients

A. Direct Tumor Involvement (70%)
1. Invasion of bone
2. Invasion or compression of neural structures
3. Obstruction of hollow viscus or ductal system of solid viscus
4. Vascular obstruction or invasion
5. Mucous membrane ulceration or involvement

B. Cancer-Induced Syndromes (<10%)
1. Paraneoplastic syndromes
2. Pain associated with debility (i.e., bedsores, constipation, rectal or bladder spasm)
3. Other (i.e., postherpetic neuralgia)

C. Diagnostic or Therapeutic Procedures (20%)
1. Procedure-related pain (i.e., bone marrow aspiration or biopsy, lumbar puncture)
2. Acute postoperative pain or postsurgical syndromes (i.e., postmastectomy, postthoracotomy, postamputation syndromes)
3. Postradiation (i.e., injury to plexus or spinal cord, mucositis, enteritis)
4. Postchemotherapy (i.e., mucositis, peripheral neuropathy, aseptic necrosis)

D. Pain Unrelated to the Malignancy or Its Treatment (<10%)

From Grossman SA, Baumohl L: Evaluation and management of cancer pain. In Bone RC (ed): Current Practice of Medicine. Philadelphia, Current Practice, 1993, p 18.1.

evaluation and treatment.[5] Examples of these procedures include venipuncture, bone marrow aspiration and biopsy, endoscopy, lumbar puncture, invasive radiologic procedures, surgery, chemotherapy, and radiation therapy.

Surgery is a frequent cause of pain in patients with cancer and can consist of biopsy, removal, or debulking of a tumor or management of a complication of the tumor or its treatment, such as a small bowel obstruction. These procedures are associated with postoperative pain and injury to local nerves, which can produce neuromas and chronic pain syndromes that are severe and difficult to manage. Surgically induced nerve injuries are most commonly seen after breast cancer surgery, thoracotomy, radical neck dissection, and limb amputation.[6] Postmastectomy syndrome occurs in 4% to 10% of all women undergoing this type of breast cancer surgery.[7] It is most frequent in patients with postoperative complications or keloid formation and is characterized by a constricting, burning sensation in the posterior arm, axilla, and anterior chest. It can develop immediately after the procedure or months later and can be complicated by the secondary development of a frozen shoulder. Postthoracotomy syndrome occurs after nerve injury secondary to rib retraction and typically presents as an aching, burning sensation in the incisional area with local tenderness, sensory loss, and occasional autonomic changes. Injury to local nerves after a radical neck dissection can produce tightness and burning dysthesias in the area of sensory loss and acute, lancinating pain. The loss of neck musculature from this surgery can also result in a "droopy shoulder," thoracic outlet syndrome, and suprascapular nerve entrapment.[8]

Chemotherapy and radiation also produce significant pain in patients with cancer. Phlebitis, mucositis, hemorrhagic cystitis, and peripheral neuropathy are common complications of antineoplastic agents. Glucocorticoids, administered as a component of therapy, can cause aseptic necrosis of the hip, pseudorheumatism, and severe perineal pain when given rapidly in high doses. Examples of radiation-induced pain include mucositis, local skin reactions, enteritis, proctitis, fibrosis with nerve entrapment syndromes, and radiation myelopathy. Electric shock-like sensations that accompany flexion of the neck (Lhermittes syndrome) can last for months after radiation to the spinal cord. Painful peripheral nerve tumors can also follow radiation therapy, especially in patients with neurofibromatosis.

Patients with malignancies are also predisposed to painful infections. Common examples include pneumonia, urinary tract infection, wound infections, candida esophagitis, oral or genital herpes, and herpes zoster.

Current Status of Cancer Pain Management

Studies from hospices and from World Health Organization demonstration sites suggest that 85% of patients with cancer pain can be well palliated using oral opioids.[1,9,10] A wide array of effective options exist for the remaining 15% of patients. These include parenteral, transdermal, or intraspinal opioids, glucocorticoids, anti-inflammatory and adjuvant medications, antineoplastic therapies, and anesthetic and neurosurgical procedures.

Although proper use of available therapeutic approaches should result in excellent pain control in nearly 95% of patients with cancer pain, cancer pain remains grossly undertreated throughout the world.[11-13] In most countries, the unavailability of oral opioids is a major contributing factor.[14]

Even in countries such as the United States and the United Kingdom, where a wide range of opioid analgesics and routes of administration are available, studies suggest that cancer pain is undertreated.[15,16] A survey of oncologists highlights their reluctance to assess pain routinely and prescribe appropriate analgesics.[17] These findings have prompted the creation of cancer pain initiatives in most states and the development of cancer pain guidelines and algorithms by the American Society of Clinical Oncology, the Oncology Nursing Society, the American Pain Society, and the U.S. Public Health Service's Agency for Health Care Policy and Research.[18-22] In addition, to improve the overall management of pain in the United States, the Joint Commission on Accreditation of Healthcare Organizations has recently set new standards for pain management that are required for continued accreditation.[23]

Barriers to the Provision of Adequate Analgesia

Many reasons have been cited for the inadequate treatment of patients with cancer in developed nations who suffer pain (Table 35-2). Some relate directly to health care providers, including:

- Failure to appreciate the intensity of the pain their patients are experiencing
- Reluctance to evaluate the etiology of the pain
- Lack of training in pain management
- Excessive concern regarding the regulatory oversight of opioid prescribing

One major barrier to the provision of adequate analgesia in patients with cancer is the failure of health care providers to appreciate the intensity of patients' pain.

TABLE 35-2

 Major Reasons for Therapeutic Inadequacies in the Management of Cancer Pain

Patient Barriers

- Limited expectations regarding the ability to provide pain relief
- Excessive concern about addiction, tolerance, and toxicities of opioids
- Legitimate concern that more pain signifies progressive tumor

Health Care Provider Barriers

- Inaccurate perceptions of patient pain intensity
- Failure to determine the etiology of pain and apply specific therapy
- Lack of knowledge regarding opioid equivalencies and pharmacology
- Excessive concern about addiction, tolerance, and toxicities of opioids
- Excessive concern regarding the regulatory oversight of opioids

This occurs because pain is entirely subjective and can only be experienced and quantified by the patient. There are no pathopneumonic findings on physical examination, and laboratory studies can be normal. Assessment of pain is further complicated by the complexities surrounding death and dying and the fact that patients with chronic, severe pain might not appear or act uncomfortable. In one study examining health care provider perceptions of patient pain, pain intensity was quantitatively assessed using a visual analog scale in 103 consecutive patients admitted to the solid tumor service of a large cancer center.[24] Each patient's primary care nurse, house officer, and oncology fellow rated their perceptions of their patient's pain intensity using the same pain rating instrument as the patient. The results (Fig. 35-1) demonstrate a lack of correlation between the patient's and the health care provider's perception of patient pain. Furthermore, the concordance between patient and health care provider pain intensity scores was highest when patients had no pain and lowest when the patients were experiencing severe discomfort. Similar results have been obtained in studies of patients with cancer and their next of kin and in burn patients.[25,26]

There are many reasons why health care providers might be unaware of the pain their patients are experiencing. As pain is entirely subjective, its presence and intensity must be communicated to health care providers by patients. Patients, however, might not discuss their pain if they expect cancer to be painful or if they are concerned about opioid addiction, tolerance, or side effects or about diverting their physician's attention from treating the tumor.[27] In addition, they might be reluctant to admit to themselves or others that their pain has worsened, knowing that this could signify progression of the cancer. Health care providers also contribute to the lack of communication by neglecting to emphasize their interest or abilities in controlling pain and by failing to use validated pain assessment tools. Serial numeric pain ratings in the medical record will foster the necessary dialogue between patients and health care providers about pain management issues.[28]

These issues are greatly magnified in children, the elderly, or individuals with a history of drug abuse. Children have special difficulty in communicating pain intensity, and their unique pain management needs have been relatively neglected.[29,30] Special pain assessment tools are required, and the child's age and developmental level must be considered when planning assessment or interventions. Many elderly patients also find it difficult to communicate their discomfort to health care professionals, have multisystem disease, and are especially sensitive to the adverse effects of analgesics.[31] Those with cancer and a current or prior history of drug abuse often have difficulty finding health care providers who believe their reports of pain and who will provide the high doses of analgesics required in these opioid-tolerant individuals.[32]

Another barrier to the provision of adequate analgesia relates to the training of medical professionals. The principles of cancer pain management receive little attention in academic centers and relevant scientific societies. Medical school courses and textbooks typically focus on diseases rather than symptoms, and pain management issues are infrequently highlighted at ward rounds, educational conferences, or in the formal curriculum of those training to care for patients with cancer. These circumstances leave many health care professionals eager to concentrate on medical problems they feel competent to handle. In addition, the scarcity of research abstracts on cancer pain at the scientific meetings of physician oncologic societies reinforces the notion that pain control is a topic of limited importance.

The lack of training and emphasis on cancer pain management manifests in many ways, including physicians' lack of opioid prescribing skills, failure to evaluate the etiology of cancer pain, and excessive concerns regarding the regulatory oversight of opioid prescribing. In one study, 81 physician trainees, given a hypothetic patient case that included performing opioid conversions, 75% calculated a dose that was only one-third the correct dose, and only 5% calculated the dose correctly.[33] Another study of experienced oncology nurses indicated that they lack the capacity to recognize physician orders that could result in serious over- or underdosing of opioids.[34] These difficulties in calculating equi-analgesic doses have prompted the development of software to facilitate opioid conversions.[35]

Many physicians and nurses consider "cancer pain" a diagnostic entity that requires opioids, without a formal evaluation of the etiology of the pain. Although this approach can provide relief, it is often ineffective and can lead to indefensible medical practices. For example, progressive back pain in a patient with metastatic lung cancer can occur from a postobstructive pneumonia or tumor invasion of the esophagus, liver, spleen, pleura, pericardium, rib, vertebrae, intercostal nerves, brachial

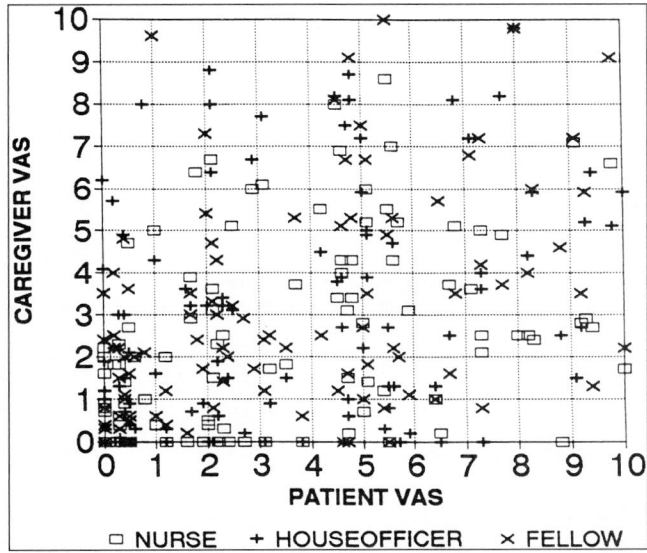

Figure 35-1. Correlation of health care provider and patient perceptions of patient pain. (From Grossman SA, Sheidler VR, Swedeen K, Mucenski J, Piantadosi S,: Correlation of patient and caregiver ratings of cancer pain. J Pain Symptom Manage 1991;6:53. © U.S. Cancer Pain Relief Committee.)

plexus, leptomeninges, or epidural space. Each of these diagnostic possibilities can be associated with a different therapeutic approach or sense of urgency. To provide opioids without evaluation would be a grave error in such a patient with an impending epidural cord compression. Furthermore, many common cancer pain syndromes might be better treated with therapies tailored to a patient's individual pain problem. These may include local radiation, nerve blocks, glucocorticioids, anticonvulsants, or surgery to maximize analgesia, minimize side effects, and improve quality of life.

Physicians, pharmacists, and nurses caring for patients with cancer must be willing to prescribe, dispense, and administer the opioids in doses required to alleviate their pain. Drug enforcement agencies often discourage opioid prescribing, however, in an attempt to reduce the illegal diversion of these drugs. Unfortunately, many health care professionals with limited knowledge and experience in the treatment of cancer pain react to the perceived threat of investigation by law enforcement agencies with

dramatic decreases in opioid prescribing.[36] This perception further contributes to the undertreatment of patients with cancer pain.

EVALUATION OF THE PATIENT WITH PAIN

A comprehensive assessment of cancer pain is the first important step toward optimal pain relief.[5,37] This evaluation should provide the clinician with sufficient information to carry out the following tasks:

1. Estimate the severity of pain.
2. Form a clinical impression regarding the etiology of the pain.
3. Determine the need for further diagnostic studies.
4. Formulate therapeutic recommendations that take into account the patient's overall medical and psychosocial status (Table 35-3).

TABLE 35-3

 Components of a Comprehensive Assessment of Cancer Pain

I.   Detailed History of Current Pain Problem

   A. Catalogue of pain (number and locations)
   B. Information for each pain
      1. Intensity (0–10)
      2. Locations and radiation
      3. Onset and changes over time
      4. Temporal pattern (constant, intermittent, etc.) and quality (burning, etc.)
      5. Exacerbating and relieving factors
      6. Associated neurologic or vasomotor abnormalities
      7. Other associated factors
      8. How the pain interferes with the patient's life
      9. Current therapeutic modalities (schedule, efficacy, side effects)
     10. Prior therapeutic modalities (schedule, efficacy, side effects)

II.   Oncologic History

   A. Histologic
   B. Presentation: Date, stage, sites of involvement
   C. Antineoplastic therapies: Dates, types, doses, toxicities, and response to each therapy
   D. Current sites of disease: Stable, responding, or progressive
   E. Patient expectations and goals

III. Medical History—May Be Affected by Pain Therapies

   A. Co-existing diseases
   B. Medications and allergies
   C. Substance abuse history
   D. Other constitutional symptoms (i.e., anorexia, fatigue, sedation and other changes in mental status, nausea, vomiting, dysphagia, dyspnea, constipation, urinary and sexual function, depression, dry mouth, ability to take medications by mouth, presence of a central venous catheter)

IV.   Personal and Social History

   A. Background: Age, educational, employment, marital, residential, religious, cultural, ethnic
   B. Current status: Functional status, caregivers and their health and availability, support system

V.   Physical Examination

VI.   Review of Additional Information

   A. Medical records, radiologic/laboratory studies
   B. Family members and physicians and/or nurses who know the patient and his illness

VII. Differential Diagnosis

VIII. Recommendations Regarding Work-Up and Therapy

IX.   Reassessment

From Grossman SA: Cancer pain assessment: A continual challenge: Supp Care Cancer 1994;2:105.

As with any serious medical condition, the assessment of cancer pain requires a detailed history, physical examination, and review of available records, laboratory data, and imaging studies. The special challenges associated with the assessment of cancer pain include the entirely subjective nature of pain, the complex multisystem involvement in patients with advanced malignancies, and the ever-changing clinical situation in this patient population.

A detailed pain history is the cornerstone of the assessment. This can be complex, as 75% of patients with advanced cancer have several concurrent painful sites, and nearly one-third have four or more separate pain problems.[38,39] Each distinct pain must be identified and characterized. Pertinent information should include its intensity, location, radiation, how and when it began, how it has changed over time, and what makes it better or worse. The quality of each pain, its temporal pattern, whether it is associated with neurologic or vasomotor abnormalities, how it interferes with the patient's life, and an account of the successes and failures of current and prior therapeutic modalities also provide valuable insight.

Many instruments have been developed to aid in pain assessment.[40-42] These attempts to characterize and quantify the quality and/or intensity of a patient's pain and represent the best available means to document the discomfort and to follow the results of therapy serially. Each instrument has its shortcomings, but several have been validated in patients with cancer pain and incorporated into clinical practice. Most contain a variant of the unidimensional visual analog scale (VAS) and a schematic representation of the body for the patient to indicate where their pain is located. The McGill Pain Questionnaire is comprehensive, but too awkward and time-consuming for most oncology patients in a clinical setting.[43-45] The Wisconsin Brief Pain Inventory, which can be completed in 15 minutes, provides information on the characteristics, severity, and location of the pain, its interference with normal life functions, and the efficacy of prior therapy. The Memorial Pain Assessment Card can be completed in less than one minute and features scales for the measurement of pain intensity and pain relief.[46] It is also designed to provide insight into global suffering or psychological distress. The Hopkins Pain Rating Instrument is a validated plastic version of the VAS which obviates the need for the paper, pencil, ruler, and measurements associated with the standard VAS.[47] This simplifies repeated pain intensity measurements, making it easier to reassess the efficacy of therapeutic endeavors on a continuing basis.[4]

A complete oncologic history is also essential, as 90% of cancer pain is related to the malignancy or cancer treatment.[49] The histology, presentation, stage, sites of involvement, and natural history and the history of surgery, radiation, chemotherapy, and hormonal treatments will help shape a therapeutic approach. In addition, it is important to note whether the malignancy is responding to therapy, stable, or progressing. A general medical history is also helpful, as pain treatments can affect coexisting medical problems, exacerbate constitutional symptoms, interact with other medications, or be contraindicated because of allergies. For example, a patient with painful bone metastases and severe peptic ulcer disease would not be an ideal candidate for potent anti-inflammatory agents. Opioids can be problematic in elderly males with severe benign prostatic hypertrophy or in patients with severe obstructive pulmonary disease and CO_2 retention. Likewise, knowledge that a patient tolerates food or fluids poorly by mouth, has an indwelling venous access device, or admits to substance abuse might influence decisions about the best way to control that patient's pain. The patient's age, functional status, social support, education, residence, health insurance, finances, and religious and cultural background might also figure prominently in planning therapy. A careful neurologic and physical examination also provides important clues as to the etiology of the pain.[50] Added insight can come from a review of available laboratory and imaging data, from medical records, and from discussions with family members and physicians who are familiar with the patient and his or her illness.

The history, physical examination, and review of other available data should provide the clinician with sufficient information to formulate a differential diagnosis for each of the patient's distinct pains and to make recommendations regarding the work-up and therapy for each. Based on this initial impression, analgesic therapy should be initiated. The nature of the treatment prescribed might depend on the clinician's judgment regarding the origin of the pain. Somatic, visceral, neuropathic, and sympathetically maintained pain are each approached somewhat differently (Table 35-4). Prompt institution of therapy reassures patients that their pain will receive immediate attention, ensures patient comfort for diagnostic studies, and can provide information on the accuracy of the clinician's assessment. Excellent pain relief suggests an accurate initial diagnosis and appropriate therapy, whereas suboptimal control might prompt a new treatment approach or a search for a different etiology of the pain.

One of the most difficult aspects of cancer pain management is that the patient's clinical situation is rarely static. The patient's underlying malignancy, antineoplastic therapy, and psychosocial status change continually during the course of the illness. As a result, the etiology and intensity of each new or worsening pain must be reassessed. The toxicities of the analgesics should also be evaluated periodically, as they can affect quality of life substantially. If significant toxicities are recognized, alternate approaches with a lower toxicity profile can be attempted.

THE MANAGEMENT OF CANCER PAIN

Nearly 85% of patients with cancer pain can achieve good control of their pain with conventional oral medications.[1-3,8,9] More aggressive or invasive therapies should provide pain relief to an additional 10% of patients, leaving only a small fraction of patients with cancer with inadequate relief.

TABLE 35-4

Classification of Cancer Pain

	CHARACTERISTICS	EXAMPLES	PRIMARY THERAPIES
Somatic	Constant, aching, gnawing, often well localized	Bone metastases	Treatment of tumor, anti-inflammatory agents, analgesics
Visceral	Constant, aching, often associated with nausea	Pancreatic cancer	Treatment of tumor, analgesics, nerve blocks
Neuropathic	Paroxysmal shock-like pain on top of a burning, constricting sensation	Plexopathy or postherpetic neuralgia	Treatment of tumor, analgesics, TENS, nerve blocks
Sympathetically maintained	Severe burning, squeezing, or constricting with local edema	Reflex sympathetic dystrophy	Sympathetic blockade, physiotherapy, adjuvant analgesics

TENS, transcutaneous electrical nerve stimulation.
From Grossman SA, Staats PS: The current management of pain in patients with cancer. Oncology (Huntingt) 1994;8:93.

Pharmacologic Therapy

Pharmacologic approaches are the most commonly used treatments for cancer pain, as they are effective, safe, and usually inexpensive.[3,51,52] These are classified as nonopioids, opioids, and adjuvant analgesics. The World Health Organization's analgesic ladder provides a framework for analgesic prescribing.[53,54] Aspirin, acetaminophen, or nonsteroidal anti-inflammatory agents (NSAIDs) are preferred for mild to moderate pain (Table 35-5). If these do not provide adequate analgesia, codeine, oxycodone, or hydrocodone will frequently provide excellent relief (Table 35-6). For persistent or severe pain, codeine (or its congener) is replaced by a potent opioid, such as morphine (Table 35-7). Drug substitution should be considered before an entire class of agents is abandoned, as patients frequently tolerate one NSAID or opioid better than another. In addition, patients with severe pain might need a strong opioid as initial therapy to ensure rapid pain relief.

The site of action of the nonopioids is primarily the peripheral nervous system. These agents are not associated with physical dependence, tolerance, or addiction, and they have a maximum dose associated with analgesia. Many are available in combination with a weak opioid. The anti-inflammatory component of aspirin and of the nonsteroidal anti-inflammatory agents (NSAIDs) is often useful for patients with somatic pain from bone metastasis, inflammation, or mechanical compression of tendons, muscles, pleura, and peritoneum, and for nonobstructive visceral pain.[55,56] Because some of these agents can affect platelet and renal function or act as antipyretics, they should be administered thoughtfully to patients receiving chemotherapy. The recent introduction of selective COX-2 inhibitors allows NSAIDs to be used with less risk of gastrointestinal bleeding and platelet dysfunction. Although these agents have not been studied formally in the treatment of cancer pain, they are being used secondary to their improved safety profile.[57] In addition, it is important to recognize that sustained high doses of acetaminophen can cause renal and hepatic damage, especially when combined with more than two ounces of alcohol per day or with other agents that cause liver damage or induce hepatic microsomes.

Most patients with moderate to severe pain rely primarily on opioid analgesics for the management of their cancer pain. The vast majority of patients can be managed with oral opioids. These are best given "around the clock" to keep pain under control. Although tolerance

TABLE 35-5

Dosing Data for Nonopioids

AGENT	DOSAGE
Acetaminophen	650 mg q4h
	975 mg q6h
Aspirin	650 mg q4h
	975 mg q6h
Carprofen	100 mg tid
Choline magnesium trisalicylate	1000–1500 mg tid
Choline salicylate	870 mg q3–4h
Diclofenac	50–75 mg q12–24h
Diflunisal	500 mg q12h
Etodolac	200–400 mg q6–8h
Fenoprofen	300–600 mg q6h
Flubiprofen	50–100 mg q12h
Ibuprofen	400–600 mg q6h
Indomethacin	25–50 mg q6–8h
Ketoprofen	25–60 mg q6–8h
Ketorolac tromethamine	PO: 10 mg q4–6h (maximum dose 40 mg/day)
	IM: 60 mg initially, then 30 mg q6h
	IV: 30 mg initially, then 15 mg q6h
	Duration of use not to exceed 5 days
Magnesium salicylate	650 mg q4h
Meclofenamate sodium	50–100 mg q6h
Mefenamic acid	250 mg q6h
Meloxicam	7.5–15 mg q24h
Nabumetone	500 mg q24h
Naproxen	250–275 mg q6–8h
Naproxen sodium	275 mg q6–8h
Piroxicam	10–20 mg q24h
Phenylbutazone	100 mg q8h
Sodium salicylate	325–650 mg q3–4h
Sulindac	150–200 mg q12–24g
Tolmetin	400–800 mg q8h
COX-2 inhibitors	
Celecoxib	100–200 mg q12h
Rofecoxib	12.5–25 mg q24h
Valdecoxib	10 mg q24h

TABLE 35-6

Opioids for Mild to Moderate Pain

DRUG	ROUTE	EQUIANALGESIC DOSE (mg)*	PEAK EFFECT (HOURS)	DURATION OF EFFECT (HOURS)	COMMENTS
Codeine	PO	200	0.5	3–6	Ceiling for analgesia reached at doses >240 mg/d orally.
	IV/IM	130	0.5	3–6	
Oxycodone	PO	30	0.5	3–6	No ceiling dose if given without fixed combinations; parenteral formulation not available.
Hydrocodone	PO	NA	0.5	4–6	Only available as fixed combination with acetaminophen or aspirin.
Propoxyphene	PO	NA	1.0	4–6	100 mg napsylate = 65 mg hydrochloride salt. Not recommended for treatment of cancer pain.

*Approximate potency relative to 10 mg of parenteral morphine.
Modified from Grossman SA, Gregory E: Cancer pain. In Kirkwood MT, Lotze MT, Yasko JM (eds): Current Cancer Therapeutics. Philadelphia, Current Medicine, 1994, p 290.

TABLE 35-7

Strong Opiates for Moderate to Severe Cancer Pain

DRUG	ROUTE	EQUIANALGESIC DOSE (mg)*	PEAK EFFECT (HOURS)	DURATION OF EFFECT (HOURS)	COMMENTS
Oxycodone	PO	30	0.5	3–6	No ceiling dose if given without fixed combinations; parenteral formulation not available.
	PO SR			12	
Morphine	PO	30–60	1.5–2.0	4–6	Many oral formulations for individual patient needs.
	PO (SR)	30–60	2.0–3.0	8–12	
	IV/IM	10	0.5–1.0	3–5	
Hydromorphone	PO	7.5	1.0–2.0	3–4	Good choice for SQ due to potency.
	PR	Unknown	Unknown	Unknown	
	IV/IM	1.5	0.5–1.0	3–4	
Meperidine	PO	300	1.0–2.0	3–6	Not preferred due to CNS toxic metabolite that accumulates in renal failure.
	IV/IM	75	0.5–1.0	2–3	
Levorphanol	PO	4.0	1.0–2.0	6–8	Long $T^{1/2}$ (11 hours) necessitates slow dose titration. Drug accumulation may occur.
	IV/IM	2.0	1.0–1.5	6–8	
Fentanyl	TD	0.1 (?)	72	12 or >	Short $T^{1/2}$ (<1 hour). TD dose titration difficult with depot in SQ adipose tissue. Transdermal fentanyl 25 mcg/hr approx = 45 mg/day oral morphine
	IV/IM	0.1	<1.0	0.5–1.0	
Methadone[†]	PO	20	?	4–6	Despite long $T^{1/2}$ (15–150+ hours), duration of analgesia is not prolonged; however drug accumulation can result in toxicities. Caution is warranted when converting to methadone in patients with high opioid tolerance.
	IV/IM	10	0.5–1.5	4–6	
Butorphanol	IN	2	1.0	3–4	Mixed agonist-antagonist may precipitate withdrawal in patient previously receiving a pure agonist, thus not generally recommended for cancer pain.
	IV/IM	2	0.5–1.0	3–4	

IN, intranasal; IV, intravenous; PO, oral; SQ, subcutaneous; TD, transdermal; (?), unknown.
*Approximate potency relative to 10 mg of parenteral morphine. *Caution:* Cross-tolerance between opioids is incomplete. Use caution when performing equianalgesic conversions. Titrate to clinical response.
[†]Ripamonti C, Groff L, Brunelli C, et al: Switching from morphine to oral methadone in treating cancer pain: What is the equianalgesic dose ratio? J Clin Oncol 1998;16:3216–3221; Moryl N, Santiago-Palma J, Kornick C, et al: Pitfalls of opioid rotation: Substituting another opioid for methadone in patients with cancer pain. Pain 2002;96:325–328; Bruera E, Neumann CM: Role of methadone in the management of pain in cancer patients. Oncology 1999;13:1275–1282; Pereira J, Lawlor P, Vigano E, et al: Equianalgesic dose ratios for opioids: A critical review of proposals for long term dosing. J Pain Symptom Manage 2001;22:672–687; Bruera E, Sweeny C: Methadone use in cancer patients with pain: A review. J Pall Med 2002;5:127–138.
Modified from Grossman SA, Gregory E: Cancer pain. In Kirkwood MT, Lotze MT, Yasko JM (eds): Current Cancer Therapeutics. Philadelphia, Current Medicine, 1994, p 290.

Problems Common to Cancer and Its Therapy

TABLE 35-8

Important Definitions in the Treatment of Cancer Pain

Physical Dependence

- A normal physiologic response to chronic opioid administration characterized by development of the abstinence syndrome on abrupt withdrawal of opioids.
- A potential problem in virtually all patients receiving moderate to high doses of opiates.

Tolerance

- A normal pharmacologic response to chronic opioid therapy characterized by the development of a relative resistance to analgesic and other effects of the drug.
- Overcome by increasing the dose administered.

Psychological Dependence (Addiction)

- Abnormal behavior pattern characterized by an all-consuming desire to obtain opioids for reasons other than pain relief. This often occurs at the expense of the patient's physical, social, and environmental well-being.
- Extraordinarily rare in patients with cancer pain.
- Not to be confused with "pseudo-addiction," which is behavior commonly seen in patients who are undertreated and in pain attempting to obtain appropriate analgesia.

Definitions Related to the Use of Opioids for the Treatment of Pain 2001. (Available at www.ampainsoc.org; www.asam.org)
Modified from Grossman SA, Gregory E: Cancer pain. In Kirkwood MT, Lotze MT, Yasko JM (eds): Current Cancer Therapeutics. Philadelphia, Current Medicine, 1994, p 290, with permission.

to these agents occurs, tumor progression is the most common reason for increasing opioid requirements. Tolerance can easily be overcome by raising opioid doses. Addiction is extremely rare in patients with cancer who are taking opioids for pain relief (Table 35-8). Most opioid side effects can be managed without excessive difficulty (Table 35-9). Constipation should be anticipated and treated prophylactically.

The opioids have their primary effect centrally, where they interfere with pain perception. They can be classified into three groups:

1. Morphine-like opioid agonists that bind competitively with μ and κ receptors (e.g., codeine, fentanyl, hydromorphone, morphine, oxycodone, and methadone)
2. Opioid antagonists that have no agonist receptor activity (e.g., naloxone)
3. Mixed agonists-antagonists (e.g., pentazocine and butorphanol) or partial agonists (e.g., buprenorphine).[58,59]

The mixed agonist-antagonist drugs have limited utility in cancer pain because of their side effect profiles and their propensity to induce opioid withdrawal in patients who have received opioid agonists. Tables 35-6 and 35-7 contain essential information on the opioids commonly used for mild and severe cancer pain.

Proper opioid prescribing is critical to patients with cancer, who often require high doses of opioids for long periods of time.[60]

Several classes of drugs that are used primarily for conditions other than pain have been found to be useful

TABLE 35-9

Management of Common Opioid Side Effects

SIDE EFFECT	MANAGEMENT	SPECIFIC AGENTS
Constipation	Begin bowel program when initiating therapy Combinations of agents may be useful	Stool softeners Irritants Bulk laxatives Lubricants Enemas
Nausea and vomiting	Treat with antiemetics, esp. phenothiazine and anticholinergic agents Switch to another opiate	Promethazine Prochlorperaxine Olanzapine 5HT$_3$ antagonists Scopolamine Hydroxyzine
Sedation	Use of stimulants	Dextroamphetamine Methylphenidate Modafinil
Pruritus	Treat with antihistamines Consider another opiate, avoiding morphine	Hydroxyzine Diphenhydramine
Myoclonus	Switch to another opiate or lower opiate dose Use of anxiolytics Avoid meperidine, especially in patients with impaired renal function	Benzodiazepines
Withdrawal symptoms	Taper dose by $^1/_2$ every other day when discontinuing	Clonidine

Modified from Grossman SA, Gregory E: Cancer pain. In Kirkwood MT, Lotze MT, Yasko JM (eds): Current Cancer Therapeutics. Philadelphia, Current Medicine, 1994, p 290, with permission; O'Mahony S, Coyle N, Payne R: Current management of opioid-related side effects. Oncology 2001;15:61–77; Cherny N, Ripamonti C, Pereira J, et al: Strategies to manage the adverse effects of oral morphine: An evidence-based report. J Clin Oncol 2001;19:2542–2554.

MANAGEMENT APPROACH

TENETS OF OPIOID PRESCRIBING

- Order opioids on a scheduled "around-the-clock" basis to optimize relief.
- Order an as-needed opioid to treat breakthrough or incident pain. For example, if a patient is taking morphine elixir, 100 mg orally every four hours, order an additional 25 to 50 mg of oral morphine elixir every two hours as needed for pain.
- Initiate a prophylactic bowel regimen at the same time opioids are prescribed. Patients usually require a combination of detergent and stimulant cathartics to treat opioid-induced constipation.
- Treat opioid-induced nausea and vomiting with aggressive anti-emetic management. This includes giving patients anti-emetics on an around-the-clock basis. Patients often become tolerant to this side effect several days after beginning opioids.
- Once baseline opioid requirements are determined, sustained-release opioid preparations can be used to reduce the number of pills taken each day.
- Teach the patient and family about the purpose and benefits of opioids to allay their fears about side effects and addiction. This instruction will improve patient compliance.

- Frequent assessment of pain relief is paramount during the opioid titration period. Titrate doses based on the patient's report of pain relief and/or the amount of as-needed opioid that has been required for patient comfort.
- Maximize the doses of one opioid before changing to another agent or route. Changes should be made primarily because of toxicities. For example, a patient taking 200 mg of controlled-release morphine every 12 hours and 200 mg of immediate release morphine daily for breakthrough pain should have the dose of controlled-release morphine increased to 300 mg every 12 hours if he or she is not experiencing significant opioid side effects. This approach is more likely to be beneficial than beginning titration with subcutaneous or intravenous morphine or oral hydromorphone.
- Refer to equi-analgesic tables when initiating or changing a patient's analgesic regimen (see Tables 35-6 and 35-7).
- Avoid chronic administration of intramuscular or rectal opioids.
- Do not use chronic administration of meperidine, which can be associated with the accumulation of normeperidine, a neurotoxic metabolite.

adjuvant analgesics in specific circumstances (Table 35-10).[61] Antidepressants and anticonvulsants can be effective in neuropathic pain. Psychostimulants can decrease opioid-induced sedation. Glucocorticoids are effective anti-inflammatory agents and are also used to reduce pain associated with brain edema and epidural metastases. Muscle relaxants, anxiolytic, antispasmodic, and neuroleptic agents also are employed for specific indications. Bisphosphanates reduce the incidence of skeletal complications, particularly in patients with myeloma and breast cancer.[62-64] Caution must be exercised in the use of adjuvant drugs that have sedative properties, as the dose of opioids should not be compromised by the toxicities of these secondary agents.

Although the vast majority of outpatients can be managed with oral opioids, alternative routes of analgesic administration are sometimes needed. Subcutaneous, intravenous, transdermal, transmucosal, or intraspinal opioids can be delivered by intermittent bolus, continuous infusion, or a combination of both, as is frequently the case with patient-controlled analgesia.[65,66] These alternative routes of administration should be considered when a patient has one of the following conditions:

- Intractable vomiting or bowel obstruction, making oral therapy impractical
- Ineffective pain relief despite titration to toxicity with several oral opioids
- Unacceptable toxicities to several oral opioids
- Such high opioid requirements that oral administration is impractical

The costs associated with these routes of opioid administration must be considered carefully (Table 35-11).[67] In addition, care must be taken to not to transform the home unnecessarily into a complex health care setting.

Subcutaneous opioid injections administered through a butterfly or subcutaneous needle on a fixed schedule are used commonly by hospices as an effective, less expensive alternative to continuous intravenous or subcutaneous infusions.[56,68] A transdermal system for opioid administration can be beneficial in some patients.[69,70] Although transdermal fentanyl provides patients with continuous drug delivery, it does not eliminate the need for an additional analgesics for breakthrough pain. The slow onset of action of fentanyl and the uncertainties associated in conversion from other opioids have led many to reserve transdermal fentanyl for patients with stable opioid requirements who do not have significant incidental pain.

Oral transmucosal fentanyl can be effective for patients with incident or breakthrough pain, for whom rapid onset and short duration of action are desired. This opioid is available in a sweetened lozenge on a handle. When placed into the mouth, a portion of the fentanyl is absorbed rapidly through the oral mucosa, while the remainder is swallowed and absorbed through the gastrointestinal tract.[71] The onset of analgesia can be as soon as five minutes. The optimal dose for this delivery system is found through titration and is not predicted by the around-the-clock dose of opioids.

Intraspinal opioids produce analgesia without blocking other sensory, motor, or sympathetic functions.[72,73] These

TABLE 35-10

Commonly Used Adjuvant Analgesics for Cancer Pain

DRUG CATEGORY	INDICATIONS	DRUGS	COMMON TOXICITIES	COMMENTS
Antidepressants	Neuropathic pain	Amitriptyline Nortriptyline Desipramine	Sedation, dry mouth, constipation, postural hypotension, urinary retention	Begin with low doses (10–25 mg); increase dose every few days; expect to see pain relief within several days, mood elevation within several weeks
Anticonvulsants	Neuropathic pain, myoclonic jerks	Phenytoin Carbamazepine Valproic acid Clonazepam Gabapentin	Drowsiness, dizziness, nausea, rash, bone marrow depression	Use loading dose with phenytoin; monitor platelets with carbamazepine
Psychostimulants	Opioid-induced sedation	Dextroamphetamine Methylphenidate Modafinil	Nervousness, irritability, insomnia, dizziness, dry mouth	Give early in the day to avoid insomnia; do not use if patient is already delirious or confused
Corticosteroids	Spinal cord compression, increased intracranial pressure, visceral distension	Decadron Methylprednisolone Prednisone	Gastritis, insomnia, fluid retention, hyperglycemia, proximal myopathy, increased appetite	
Muscle relaxants	Muscle spasm	Diazepam Baclofen Methocarbamol Cyclobenzaprine	Sedation, dizziness, nausea, weakness, confusion	
Benzodiazepines	Muscle spasm, myoclonus, anxiety, insomnia	Diazepam Lorazepam Alprozolam Midazalam Temazepam	Sedation, delirium, hypotension, headache, respiratory depression	Not analgesics; synergistic effect with opioids can cause respiratory depression
Antispasmodics	GI or bladder spasm	Diphenoxylate and atropine, loperamide, scopolamine patch, dicylomine	Sedation, dry mouth, constipation	
Neuroleptics	Delirium, agitation, nausea and vomiting, hiccoughs	Methotrimeprazine, haloperidol, prochlorperazine, chlorpromazine	Sedation, orthostatic hypotension, confusion, extrapyramidal reactions	Useful for symptoms other than pain; methotrimeprazine has analgesic properties
Bisphosphonates	Bone pain	Pamidronate Zoledronic acid	Hypocalcemia, fever, GI disturbances, anemia	Delays time to painful skeletal events; also used with analgesics for bone pain

GI, gastrointestinal.

TABLE 35-11

Opioid Analgesics: Routes of Administration and Associated Costs

ROUTE OF ADMINISTRATION	COMMENTS	COST CONSIDERATIONS*
Oral	Preferred route for cancer pain management.	$: D (immediate release products) $$: D (sustained release products)
Buccal/sublingual	Avoids 1st pass through the liver. Otherwise no advantage over oral and unavailable in U.S.	
Rectal	Available for morphine, oxymorphone, and hydromorphone. Dosing is considered equivalent to oral, but absorption may be erratic and incomplete.	$: D
Intranasal	Available for buprenorphine, but not evaluated for management of chronic pain.	$: D
Transdermal	Available for fentanyl. Absorption rates may be affected by subcutaneous fat stores, hypo- or hyperthermia, placement in a radiation port, and ambient temperature. Controversial conversion recommendations.	$$: D
Intramuscular	Contraindicated for management of chronic pain.	$$: D,S,RN
Subcutaneous	Bioavailability similar to IV. Infection, bleeding, and irritation at injection site may occur.	$$$: D,(P),S,Ph,RN,C
Intravenous	Indicated only when other routes have failed.	$$$: D,P,S,Ph,RN,(SF),C
Epidural/intrathecal	May be useful for avoiding systemic side effects of opiates. Usually not effective if systemic treatment has failed.	$$$$: D,P,S,Ph,RN,SF,C

*Costs: $, Overall cost ($, least expensive; $$$$, most expensive). Specific costs for each therapy include: D, drug; P, pump renal; S, supplies (tubing, filters, batteries, tape, heparin); Ph, pharmacy services; RN, nursing services; SF, surgical fee; C, risk of costly complications. ( ), might or might not be necessary for this route of delivery.
Modified from Grossman SA, Gregory E: Cancer pain. In Kirkwood MT, Lotze MT, Yasko JM (eds): Current Cancer Therapeutics. Philadelphia, Current Medicine, 1994, p 290.

can be delivered into the epidural space through a tunneled external catheter or to the subarachnoid space or lateral ventricles using a totally implanted pump. As the total daily dose of intraspinal opioid is one-tenth to one-hundredth of parenteral opioid, it is associated with fewer systemic toxicities. Chronic epidural or intrathecal opioids are invasive, expensive, and frequently ineffective in patients requiring high doses of systemic opioids. Tolerance, pruritus, urinary retention, and nausea and vomiting occur in up to 20% of patients receiving spinal opioids. Respiratory depression is unusual. The addition of low doses of anesthetic agents or agents such as clonidine to intrathecal and epidural opioids could add considerably to pain relief.[73,74] Intraspinal opioids are generally used after documentation of the failure of maximal doses of opioids through other routes.[75] They are indicated primarily for intractable pain in the lower part of the body, particularly when pain is bilateral or midline.

Antineoplastic Therapy

Antineoplastic therapy can provide analgesia if it reduces the size of lesions invading or compressing normal tissues. Radiation therapy is the treatment of choice for most patients with local pain from tumor progression. It is frequently administered to patients with symptomatic bone, brain, epidural, and plexus metastases.[76] Systemic radiopharmaceuticals such as strontium 89 and samarium-153-EDTMP are also used for the treatment of pain from bone metastases.[77,78] Chemotherapy can provide substantial pain relief in malignancies that respond to this therapeutic modality.[79] Surgery can be effective in relieving pain from intestinal obstruction, pathologic fractures, and obstructive hydrocephalus.[67]

Nonpharmacologic Therapy

Neurostimulatory techniques, such as transcutaneous electrical nerve stimulation (TENS), are safe, noninvasive, relatively inexpensive, and easily added to other analgesic approaches.[80] TENS could provide short-term benefits in patients with cancer, and a two- to four-week trial will often determine its clinical utility. Nonpharmacologic approaches such as progressive muscle relaxation, massage, use of heat or cold, guided imagery, biofeedback, and hypnosis are useful adjuncts to pain management.[81,82] Although psychotherapy is indicated for an associated depression, unrelieved pain can result in depression that is best treated with analgesic therapies.[83]

Invasive Therapy

Although most cancer pain can be well controlled using the techniques listed in the foregoing discussions, some pain remains refractory, and some patients have persistent adverse effects from opioids despite aggressive therapy with psychostimulants, antiemetics, and laxatives. The side effects can be severe enough that patients might refuse to take sufficient medication to relieve their pain. Adding adjuvant medications, changing to another opioid, or using continuous intravenous or subcutaneous infusions to reduce "peak" levels might be helpful. In selected patients, regional analgesia or neuroablative procedures might permit the doses of pharmacologic agents to be reduced substantially. These invasive approaches should be considered under the following conditions:

- If significant pain persists at doses of analgesics that are associated with intolerable side effects
- If excessive toxicities result from opioid analgesics
- If a careful assessment suggests that a low-risk procedure is likely to result in excellent analgesia

Regional Analgesia

Regional analgesia can be achieved with long-acting local anesthetics (such as bupivacaine) that provide pain relief for three to twelve hours, neurolytic agents (alcohol or phenol) that produce analgesia for weeks to months, or opioids injected into the epidural or subarachnoid space (Table 35-12).[84] Diagnostic blocks with local anesthetics are usually performed before neurolysis. This permits the anesthesiologist to determine the response to local

TABLE 35-12

Regional Anesthetic Techniques				
	TYPES OF BLOCKS	**EXAMPLES**	**INDICATIONS**	**COMMENTS**
Local anesthetic blocks	Diagnostic	Intercostal nerve block	Determine etiology of pain and the response and side effects following local therapies	Analgesic effect will last only hours
	Treatment of sympathetically maintained pain	Stellate ganglion block	Sympathetically maintained pain	Repeated blocks might be needed
	Trigger point injections	Trigger point injection	Myofascial pain syndrome	Repeated blocks might be needed
Neurolytic (alcohol or phenol) blocks	Peripheral	Intercostal nerve blocks	Chest wall tumor	Pain relief usually lasts several months
	Visceral	Celiac plexus block	Pancreatic cancer	Pain relief usually lasts several months
	Neuraxial	Epidural Intrathecal neurolysis	Pain localized to two or three dermatomes	Pain relief usually lasts several months

From Grossman SA, Staats PS: The current management of pain in patients with cancer. Oncology (Huntingt) 1994;8:93, with permission.

therapy and allows the patient to decide whether the "numbness" that replaces the pain is tolerable. If the pain can be relieved temporarily with local anesthetics, alcohol or phenol can be injected into the subarachnoid or epidural space to destroy nociceptive fibers in the dorsal rootlets, thus simulating a surgical rhizotomy. Although injections of these neurolytic agents are commonly called "permanent blocks," pain relief usually lasts several months. Neurolytic blocks can be particularly useful in the thoracic region, where they are associated with few motor complications. In the cervical and lumbar regions, nearly 20% of patients develop motor and/or sphincter dysfunction, which can be permanent. In patients with preexisting lower extremity paralysis, colostomy, or nephrostomy tubes, cases in which loss of motor or sphincter function might be less critical, lumbar neurolysis might be worthwhile. Other potential side effects of these procedures include hypotension, toxic reactions from accidental intravenous or subarachnoid administration, or pneumothorax after needle placement. Neurolysis is usually restricted to patients with a limited life expectancy, as it can produce a painful neuritis that becomes clinically apparent only months after the procedure.

Neurolytic blocks are employed in selected patients who have localized or regional pain. Percutaneous celiac plexus neurolysis is an outpatient procedure associated with few risks; it alleviates pain originating in the pancreas, stomach, gallbladder, or other upper abdominal viscera in most patients. One randomized, prospective, placebo-controlled trial comparing intraoperative celiac plexus injections of alcohol or saline in patients with advanced pancreatic cancer documents the efficacy of this procedure.[85] In other settings, it has been shown to decrease opioid requirements.[86] Although pain can recur months after a celiac block, subsequent blocks are often associated with excellent pain relief. Less commonly used neurolytic procedures include intercostal blocks (chest wall or rib pain), neuroaxial blocks (pain in two to three dermatomes), Gasserian ganglion neurolysis (pain in the anterior two-thirds of the head), and brachial plexus blocks (for patients with preexisting limb paralysis).

Neuroablative Procedures

Neuroablative procedures are performed infrequently on patients with cancer because of the success of more conservative approaches. The most commonly performed procedures are radio frequency ablation and the open unilateral anterolateral cordotomy, percutaneous cordotomy, and commissural myelotomy.[87,88] An open cordotomy is usually performed through a T2 or T3 laminectomy and produces excellent pain relief in the lower part of the body in 80% of patients. A 5% to 10% mortality rate and significant morbidity in an additional 15% of patients are reported for this procedure. Hemiparesis, urinary retention, sexual impotence, unmasking pain on the opposite side of the body, and late sensory abnormalities are not infrequent. Bilateral cordotomies are associated with higher complication rates. Percutaneous cordotomy is safer and provides excellent pain relief; however, pain recurs within three months in 50% of patients. A commissural myelotomy can be considered in selected

patients who experience bilateral pelvic and perineal pain. This involves a laminectomy and surgical division of the crossing fibers of the spinal cord. Although it can result in pain relief with sphincter sparing, few neurosurgeons have extensive expertise with this procedure.

DIFFICULT-TO-MANAGE PAIN PROBLEMS

Difficult-to-manage pain problems are most common in patients with any of the following conditions (Table 35-13):[89]

- Pain of neuropathic origin
- Episodic or incidental pain
- Impaired cognitive or communicative skills
- A history of substance abuse

Referral to an experienced multidisciplinary cancer pain team can be helpful if initial attempts to control pain in patients with these underlying problems are unsuccessful.

Patients with Pain of Neuropathic Origin

Any injury to the peripheral or central nervous system can cause neuropathic pain. This is often characterized by paroxysms of shock-like pain on top of a burning or constricting sensation. Neuropathic pain in patients with cancer commonly arises from tumor invading or compressing peripheral nerve, nerve plexus, or spinal cord. It can occur as a result of surgery, radiation, or chemotherapy as exemplified by postmastectomy and postthoracotomy syndromes, radiation-induced plexopathies, and chemotherapy-induced neuropathies.[90] Neuropathic pain also can accompany disorders that are unrelated to the tumor or its treatment, such as diabetes mellitus, nerve entrapment syndromes, and herpes zoster.

Providing adequate relief from neuropathic pain can be difficult even for the most experienced physicians.[89,91] Although this pain might improve on opioids, it appears to respond less well to these agents than does nociceptive pain. Optimal therapy for neuropathic pain often depends on opioids used in combination with a variety of nonopioid "adjuvant" analgesics (see Table 35-10). Tricyclic antidepressants have been studied most extensively in this situation and might work through the inhibition

TABLE 35-13

Difficult Problems in the Management of Cancer Pain

1. Impaired cognition
2. Limited ability to communicate
   A. Neurologic deficits
   B. Psychiatric illness
   C. Unable to communicate in the language of the health care providers
3. Past or present history of drug or alcohol abuse
4. Neuropathic pain
5. Incident or episodic pain (e.g., pleuritic, rectal, bladder, or esophageal pain)

of serotonin and norepinephrine. Although the most convincing efficacy data is with amitriptyline, this agent is associated with significant anticholinergic effects and sedation. Other drugs in this class with a more favorable toxicity profile include desipramine and nortriptyline.

Anticonvulsants are also helpful in the management of neuropathic pain, particularly if the pain has lancinating qualities.[61,92] The doses of these agents are similar to those used for the control of seizures. Care must be taken to avoid abrupt withdrawal, as this could induce seizures. Randomized controlled trials have demonstrated the efficacy and tolerability of gabapentin for the treatment of postherpetic neuralgia and painful diabetic neuropathy.[93,94] Other small studies suggest that it might help in the management of neuropathic pain secondary to cancer or its treatment.[95] This agent is well tolerated, no drug-drug interactions have been identified, and the average effective dose is 1800–3600 mg/day. Reports support the use of carbamazepine, valproic acid, and dilantin, although the myelosuppression associated with carbamazepine might compromise the ability to administer concurrent chemotherapy.[96] Clonazepam, a benzodiazapine, has also been used with some success.

Systemically administered local anesthetics have been used for the treatment of neuropathic pain.[61,97] Intravenous and subcutaneous lidocaine and oral mexiletine could decrease ectopic firing in neuromas, thereby reducing neuropathic pain. Anesthetic creams that produce few systemic side effects are also available. Capsaicin, a neurotoxin that selectively destroys nociceptors, is also manufactured as a topical preparation and provides relief in some patients. If oral agents and topical creams are ineffective, afferent input can be reduced with TENS or regional anesthetic techniques such as long-term epidural catheters or intrathecal pumps for the delivery of local anesthetics.[72,73,98] Neurolytic blocks, more invasive neurostimulatory techniques, or even neurosurgical procedures might be indicated in extreme situations.

Patients with Episodic or Incidental Pain

It is widely recognized that some patients experience transient, but severe, exacerbations of their pain. These can be difficult to treat and are often very troubling to the patient. These exacerbations can occur as a result of an inadequate analgesic regimen. For example, a patient who receives opioids every 6 hours and has good relief for only 4 hours needs a change in regimen to ensure that opioid levels will not fall below the analgesic threshold after 4 hours. This change is best accomplished by providing the agent more frequently or by administering sufficient doses of a sustained-release preparation. Episodic pain associated with voluntary or involuntary movements poses a more difficult therapeutic problem. Examples of these "incidental pains" are seen in patients with pelvic metastases or pathologic fractures who have severe pain with walking or sitting, patients with rib metastases who experience stabbing chest pain with movement or coughing, or patients with esophageal, rectal, or bladder lesions with pain on swallowing, defecation, or urination, respectively. Involuntary precipitants can include bowel

or ureteral distension. In a recent study of incident pain, nearly three-quarters was directly related to a neoplastic lesions, 20% resulted from of anti-neoplastic therapy, and the remainder was unrelated to the tumor or its treatment.[99]

Proper management of these patients requires a comprehensive assessment to determine the origin of the pain. Therapy directed at the underlying etiologic factors is most likely to provide pain relief. Relieving a bowel obstruction, repairing or splinting a fracture, treating a local metastatic lesion with radiation therapy, or performing a neurolytic block for a painful rib lesion provides better analgesia than opioids. The frequency and severity of incidental pain might also be reduced significantly by anti-inflammatory agents or corticosteroids in bone or nerve compression pain and by anticonvulsants or tricyclic antidepressants in neuropathic pain. In addition, agents that reduce the frequency of precipitating events should be employed. These include antitussives, laxatives, antiperistaltic drugs, or agents that reduce muscle spasms. Physiotherapy can be useful in musculoskeletal complications, and the cognitive and psychological approaches can be helpful to patients with these pains. Rarely, patients require invasive anesthetic or neurosurgical approaches for relief of these transient but severe pains. Local anesthetic injections might predict whether a patient is likely to respond to chemical neurolysis or a destructive neurosurgical procedure. Continuous epidural anesthetics and opioids might also be helpful in carefully selected patients.

Many of the approaches listed in the foregoing discussion might not be effective, or even possible or advisable, in the context of a patient's illness. In such situations, opioids remain the mainstay of therapy. The baseline dose of opioid can be escalated until pain relief or intolerable side effects occur. Although this approach might produce relief, patients are often excessively sedated during the intervals between the severe pains. Alternatively, patients might elect to take supplemental analgesics (usually short-acting opioids) 30 to 60 minutes before they know a precipitating event is likely to occur. If the pain is unpredictable, the additional medications are taken as soon as the pain begins. Parenteral opioids given by patient-controlled analgesia might be useful if the onset of action is too slow by the oral route.[100] The doses of these supplemental opioids must be determined from the patient's baseline opioid requirements. It is common to begin with 5% to 10% of the total daily opioid dose ordered every 2 to 3 hours as needed.

Patients with Impaired Cognitive or Communicative Function

The difficulties that physicians and nurses have determining the intensity of pain in patients with cancer have been described previously in this chapter. Problems in conveying pain intensity are greatly magnified in patients who cannot communicate with their health care providers or who are cognitively impaired. These deficits complicate the assessment of both pain intensity and pain relief. Some patients are unable to speak the language of the health care provider, while others have severe neurologic deficits, such as an expressive aphasia. As previously noted, children and the elderly have special difficulty communicating pain intensity. Patients with severe cognitive deficits present obvious problems in assessing an entirely subjective symptom. Delirious patients with cancer are often restless, moaning, and unable to convey the intensity, nature, or even location of their pain. These patients require a review of correctable factors contributing to the delirium. Neurologic events, infections, trauma, bladder distension, fecal impaction, hypoxia, or metabolic abnormalities are common. The patient's drug regimen should be simplified, and all agents with anticholinergic properties should be discontinued. If the patient is on an opioid, reducing the dose, switching agents, or using a continuous infusion or sustained-release preparation to avoid wide fluctuations in drug levels might result in improvement.

Patients with a History of Substance Abuse

The principles of cancer pain assessment and management in patients with a current or prior history of drug abuse are similar to those for any patient with cancer pain.[32] These individuals should not remain in pain as a result of this complicating medical problem. Patients with a history of drug abuse, however, often have difficulty finding physicians who believe their reports of pain and who will provide the high doses of analgesics required in these opioid-tolerant individuals. As a result, they can become angry, frustrated, and more persistent in their demands for opioids. This constellation of symptoms is also seen in patients who do not have a history of drug abuse but who have severe, untreated pain. Their preoccupation with obtaining analgesics is referred to as *pseudo-addiction* and tends to disappear rapidly with appropriate pain therapy.[101]

A frank discussion of major issues relating to the proper use of opioid analgesics for pain management with the patient, the patient's family, and the drug counselor is important. Contracts often help to ensure that all parties understand and agree to the same principles and plans for therapy. Oral agents are preferred, and local anesthetic options that could limit the need for opioids can be considered. Opioids, such as methadone, that are not highly desired "on the street" might be prescribed in lieu of morphine or hydromorphone.

CONCLUSION

Pain is common in patients with cancer and remains one of the most feared aspects of this illness, despite the excellent therapies that are available to provide pain relief. Cancer pain commonly results from tumor compressing or invading soft tissue, bone, or nerves or from diagnostic or therapeutic endeavors. The key to optimal pain management rests with a thorough assessment of the patient's pain. This involves a determination of pain intensity, an evaluation of the etiology of the pain, a carefully considered therapeutic plan, and repeated assessments of pain relief after therapeutic interventions. The vast majority of cancer pain can be well controlled with therapies readily available to most physicians. These include nonopioid analgesics, opioid analgesics, adjuvant medications, antineoplastic therapies, nonpharmacologic approaches, and noninvasive neurostimulatory techniques. Regional anesthetic or neurosurgical approaches should be considered for selected patients who continue to experience pain after an adequate trial of the foregoing therapies or who have unrelenting toxicities from these agents. They should also be considered for patients whose pain suggests that an inexpensive, low-risk procedure is likely to result in excellent analgesia. Examples of such cases include pancreatic cancer pain and thoracic pain in a dermatomal distribution. Referral to an experienced multidisciplinary pain team might be required in situations that are known to pose special challenges in pain management. These include patients with neuropathic pain, episodic or incident pain, impaired cognitive or communicative capabilities, or a history of substance abuse.

Cancer pain remains undertreated despite evidence that a careful assessment of cancer pain and the appropriate use of available therapies should result in excellent relief in nearly 95% of patients. Providing optimal cancer pain relief tests the skills and commitment of physicians, nurses, and pharmacists as the diagnostic, therapeutic, and social issues in these patients are complex and constantly changing. Meeting these challenges can be satisfying, as patients and family are grateful to find that pain can usually be alleviated. Furthermore, as noted in the American Society of Clinical Oncology's policy statement on cancer pain, "patients with cancer have a right to effective treatment of pain" and the "evaluation and treatment of cancer pain are an integral part" of each caregiver's responsibilities.[18]

REFERENCES

1. Twycross RC, Fairfield S: Pain in far-advanced cancer. Pain 1982;14:303–310.
2. Cleeland CS: The impact of pain on patients with cancer. Cancer 1984;54:2635–2641.
3. Foley KM: The treatment of cancer pain. N Engl J Med 1985;313:84–95.
4. Twycross R, Harcourt J, Bergl S: A survey of pain in patients with advanced cancer. J Pain Symptom Manage 1996;12:273–282.
5. Portnow J, Lim C, Grossman SA: Assessment of pain caused by invasive procedures in cancer patients. J NCCN 2003;3:435–439.
6. Cherny NI: Cancer pain: Principles of assessment and syndromes. In Berger AM, Portenoy RK, Weissman DE (eds): Principles and Practice of Supportive Oncology. Philadelphia, Lippincott Raven, 1998, pp 3–42.
7. Vecht CJ: Arm pain in the patient with breast cancer. J Pain Sympt Manage 1990;5:109–117.
8. Swift TR, Nichols FR: The droopy shoulder syndrome. Neurology 1984;34:212–215.
9. Stjernsward J, Teoh N: The scope of the cancer pain problem. Adv Pain Res Ther 1990;16:7–12.
10. Ventafridda V, Caraceni A, Gamba A: Field-testing of the WHO guidelines for cancer pain relief: Summary report of demonstration projects. Adv Pain Res Therapy 1990;16:451–465.
11. Grossman SA: Is pain undertreated in cancer patients? Adv Oncology 1993;9:9–12.

12. Grossman SA: Undertreatment of cancer pain: Barriers and remedies. Support Care Cancer 1993;1:74–78.

13. Joranson DE: Availability of opioids for cancer pain: Recent trends, assessment of system barriers, New World Health Organization guidelines, and the risk of diversion. J Pain Symptom Manage 1993;8:353–360.

14. Angarola RT: Availability and regulation of opioid analgesics. Adv Pain Res Therapy 1990;16:513–525.

15. Cleeland CS, Gonin R, Hatfield AK, et al: Pain and its treatment in outpatients with metastatic cancer. N Eng J Med 1994;330: 592–596.

16. Cleeland CS, Pandya KJ, Loehrer P, Gonin R, Baez L: Pain and treatment of pain in minority patients with cancer. The Eastern Cooperative Oncology Group Minority Outpatient Pain Study. Ann Intern Med 1997;127:813–816.

17. von Roenn JH, Cleeland CS, Gonin R, Hatfield AK, Pandya KJ: Physicians attitudes and practice in cancer pain management. A survey from the Eastern Cooperative Oncology Group. Ann Intern Med 1993;119:121–126.

18. Ad Hoc Committee on Cancer Pain: Cancer pain assessment and treatment curriculum guidelines. J Clin Oncol 1992;10: 1976–1982.

19. American Pain Society Quality of Care Committee: Quality improvement guidelines for the treatment of acute pain and cancer pain. JAMA 1995;274:1874–1880.

20. Spross JA, McGuire DB, Schmitt R: Oncology Nursing Society position paper on cancer pain. Oncol Nurs Forum 1990;17(4):595–614 (Part I); 17(5):751–7 (Part II); 17(6):825, 944–955 (Part III).

21. Jacox A, Carr DB, Payne R., et al: Management of cancer pain: Clinical practice guideline no. 9. AHCPR Publication No. 94–0592. Rockville, MD, Agency for Health Care Policy and Research, U.S. Dept of Health and Human Services, Public Health Service, 1994.

22. Grossman SA: Management of cancer pain: National Comprehensive Cancer Network guidelines. Oncology 1999;13:33–44.

23. Curtiss CP: JCAHO: Meeting the standards for pain management. Orthop Nurs 2001;20:27–30.

24. Grossman SA, Sheidler VR, Swedeen K, Mucenski J, Piantadosi S: Correlation of patient and caregiver ratings of cancer pain. J Pain Sympt Manage 1991;6:53–57.

25. O'Brien J, Francis A: The use of next-of-kin to estimate pain in cancer patients. Pain 1988;35:171–178.

26. Choiniere M, Melzack R, Girard N, Rondeau J, Paquin MJ: Comparisons between patients' and nurses' assessment of pain and medication efficacy in severe burn injuries. Pain 1990;40: 143–152.

27. Ward SE, Goldberg N, Miller-McCauley V, Mueller C, Nolan A: Patient-related barriers to management of cancer pain. Pain 1993;52:319–324.

28. Au E, Loprinzi CL, Dhodapkar M, et al: Regular use of a verbal pain scale improves the understanding of oncology inpatient pain intensity. J Clin Oncol 1994;12:2751–2755.

29. Schechter NL: Pain in children with cancer. Adv Pain Res Therapy 1990;16:57–72.

30. McGrath PA: Development of the World Health Organization guidelines on cancer pain relief and palliative care in children. J Pain Symptom Manage 1996;12:87–92.

31. Cleary JF, Carbone PP: Palliative medicine in the elderly. Cancer 1997;80:1335–1347.

32. Passik SD, Portenoy RK: Substance abuse issues in palliative care. In Berger AM, Portenoy RK, Weissman DE (eds): Principles and Practice of Supportive Oncology. Philadelphia, Lippincott Raven, pp 513–529.

33. Mortimer JE, Bartlett NJ: Assessment of knowledge about cancer pain management by physicians in training. J Pain Symptom Manage 1997;14:21–28.

34. Sheidler VR, McGuire DB, Gilbert MR, Grossman SA: Analgesic decision making skills of nurses. Oncol Nurs For 1992;19:1531–1534.

35. Grossman, SA, Nesbit S, Loscalzo M: Hopkins Opioid Program— Conversions for the PDA (Palm OS version), 2002. Available at www.hopkinskimmelcancercenter.org/specialtycenters/hop.cfm.

36. Sigler KA, Guernsey BG, Ingrim NB, et al: Effect of a triplicate prescription law on prescribing of schedule II drugs. Am J Hosp Pharm 1984;41:108–111.

37. Grossman SA: Cancer pain assessment: A continual challenge. Support Care Cancer 1994;2:105–110.

38. Cohen MZ, Easley MK, Ellis C, et al: Cancer pain management and the JCAHO's pain standards: An institutional challenge. J Pain Symptom Manage 2003;25:519–527.

39. Patrick DL, Ferketich SL, Frame PS, et al: National Institutes of Health State-of-the-Science Conference statement: Symptom management in cancer—Pain, depression, and fatigue, July 15–17, 2002. J NCI 2003;95:1110–1117.

40. Vallerand AH: Measurement issues in the comprehensive assessment of cancer pain. Semin Oncol Nurs 1997;13:16–24.

41. Paice JA, Cohen FL: Validity of a verbally administered numeric rating scale to measure cancer pain intensity. Cancer Nurs 1997;20:88–93.

42. Chibnal JT: Pain assessment in cognitively impaired and unimpaired older adults: A comparison of four scales. Pain 2001;92:173–186.

43. Melzack R: The McGill pain questionnaire: Major properties and scoring methods. Pain 1975;1:277–299.

44. Graham C, Bond SS, Gerkovich MM, Cook MR: Use of the McGill pain questionnaire in the assessment of cancer pain: Replicability and consistency. Pain 1980;8:377–387.

45. Kremer EF, Atkinson JH, Ignelzi RJ: Pain measurement: Affective dimensional measure of the McGill pain questionnaire with a cancer pain population. Pain 1982;12:153–163.

46. Fishman B, Pasternak S, Wallenstein S, Houde RW, Holland JC, Foley KM: The Memorial pain assessment card: A valid instrument for the evaluation of cancer pain. Cancer 1987;60:1151–1158.

47. Grossman SA, Sheidler VR, McGuire DB, Geer C, Santor D, Piantadosi S: A comparison of the Hopkins Pain Rating Instrument with standard visual analogue and verbal descriptor scales in patients with cancer pain. J Pain Symptom Manage 1992;7:196–203.

48. Rhodes DJ, Koshy R, Sheidler VR, Waterfield W, Wu A, Grossman SA: Feasibility of quantitative pain assessment in outpatient oncology practice. J Clin Oncol 2001;19:501–508.

49. Foley, KM: Pain syndromes in patients with cancer. In Bonica JJ, Ventafridda V (eds): Advances in Pain Research and Therapy, vol 2. New York, Raven Press, 1979, pp 59–75.

50. Portenoy RK: The physical examination in cancer pain assessment. Semin Oncol Nurs 197;13:25–29.

51. Cherny NI, Foley KM: Nonopioid and opioid analgesic pharmacotherapy of cancer pain. Hematol Oncol Clin North Am 1996;10:79–102.

52. Hanks G, Cherny N: Analgesic therapy. In Doyle D, Hanks G, MacDonald N (eds): Oxford Textbook of Palliative Medicine. Oxford, Oxford Medical Publications, 1998, pp 331–355.

53. Cancer Pain Relief and Palliative Care. Report of a WHO Expert Committee. WHO Technical Report Series, No. 804. Geneva, World Health Organization, 1990.

54. Zech DF, Lehmann KA, Hertel D, Grond S, Lynch J: Validation of World Health Organization Guidelines for cancer pain relief: A 10-year prospective study. Pain 1995;63:65–76.

55. Ventafridda V, Fochi V, DeConno D, Sganzerla E: Use of nonsteroidal anti-inflammatory drugs in the treatment of pain in cancer. Br J Clin Pharmacol 1980;10:3435–3465.

56. Eisenberg E, Berkey CS, Carr DB, Mosteller F, Chalmers TC: Efficacy and safety of nonsteroidal antiinflammatory drugs for cancer pain: A meta-analysis. J Clin Oncol 1994;12:2756–2765.

57. Rouff G, Lema M: Strategies in pain management: New and potential indications for COX-2 specific inhibitors J Pain Symptom Manage 2003;25S:S21–S31.

58. Jaffe JH, Martin WR: Opioid analgesics and antagonists. In Gilman AG, Rall TW, Nies AL, et al (eds): Goodman and Gilman's The Pharmacological Basis of Therapeutics, 8th ed. New York, Pergamon Press, 1990, pp 485–521.

59. Pasternak GW: Biochemistry and pharmacology of multiple mu opioid receptors. In Foley KM, Inturrisi CE (eds): Advances in Pain Research and Therapy, vol 8. New York, Raven Press, 1986, pp 337–344.

60. Max M, Payne R: Principles of Analgesic Use in the Treatment of Acute Pain and Cancer Pain, 4th ed. Glenview, IL, American Pain Society, 1999.

61. Portenoy RK: Adjuvant analgesics in pain management. In Doyle D, Hanks GWC, MacDonald N (eds): Oxford Textbook of Palliative Medicine, 2nd ed. Oxford, Oxford University Press, 1998, pp 361–390.

62. Body JJ, Piccart M, Coleman RE: Use of bisphosphonates in cancer patients. Cancer Treat Rev 1996;22:265–287.

63. Seaman J, Knight RD: Efficacy of pamidronate in reducing skeletal events in patients with advanced multiple myeloma. N Engl J Med 1996;334:488–493.

64. Hortobagyi GN, Theriault RL, Lipton A, et al: Long-term prevention of skeletal complications of metastatic breast cancer with pamidronate. J Clin Oncol 1998;16:2038–2044.

65. Nelson KA, Groh ES, Walsh D, et al: A prospective, within-patient, crossover study of continuous intravenous and subcutaneous morphine for chronic cancer pain. J Pain Symptom Manage 1997;13:262–267.

66. Paice JA, Williams AR: Intraspinal drugs for pain. In McGuire DB, Yarbro CH, Ferrell BR (eds): Cancer Pain Management, 2nd ed. Boston, Jones and Barlett, 1995, pp 131–158.

67. Ferrell BR: Cost issues surrounding the treatment of cancer related pain. J Pain Symp Manage 1994;9:221–234.

68. Crane RA: Intermittent subcutaneous infusion of opioids in hospice home care: An effective, economical, manageable option. Am J Hospice Pall Care, 1994;11:8–12.

69. Southam MA: Transdermal fentanyl therapy: System design, pharmacokinetics and efficacy. Anticancer Drugs 1995;6 S3:29–34.

70. Ahmedzai S, Brooks D: Transdermal fentanyl versus sustained-release oral morphine in cancer pain: preference, efficacy, and quality of life. The TTS-Fentanyl Comparative Trial Group. J Pain Symptom Manage 1997;13:254–261.

71. Streisand JB, Busch MA, Egan TD, Smith BG, Gay M, Pace NL: Dose proportionality and pharmacokinetics of oral transmucosal fentanyl citrate. Anesthesiology 1998;88:305–309.

72. Paice, JA, Magolan JM: Intraspinal drug delivery. Nurs Clin North Am 1991;26:477–498.

73. DuPen SL, Kharasch ED, Williams A, Miguel R, Allin D: Chronic epidural bupivicaine-opioid infusion in intractable cancer pain. Pain 1992;49:293–300.

74. Eisenach JC, DuPen S, Dubois M, et al: Epidural clonidine analgesia for intractable cancer pain. Pain 1995;61:391–399.

75. Smith TJ, Staats PS, Deer T, et al: Randomized clinical trial of an implantable drug delivery system compared with comprehensive medical management for refractory cancer pain: Impact on pain, drug-related toxicity, and survival. J Clin Oncol 2002;20:4040–4049.

76. Kagan AR: Radiation therapy in palliative cancer management. In Perez CA, Brady LW: Principles and Practice of Radiation Oncology. Philadelphia, JB Lippincott, 1992, pp 1495–1507.

77. Janjan NA: Radiation for bone metastases: Conventional techniques and the role of systemic radiopharmaceuticals. Cancer 1997;80(8S):1628–1645.

78. Silberstein EB, Eugene L, Saenger SR: Painful osteoblastic metastases: The role of nuclear medicine. Oncology (Huntingt) 2001;15:157–163.

79. MacDonald N: Role of medical and surgical oncology in the management of cancer pain. In Foley KM, Bonica JJ, Ventafridda V (eds): Advances in pain research and therapy (vol 16). New York, Raven Press, 1990, pp 27–44.

80. Grond S, Radbruch L, Meuser T, Sabatowski R, Lokk G, Lehman K: Assessment and treatment of neuropathic cancer pain following WHO guidelines. Pain 1999;79:15–20.

81. Loscalzo M: Psychological approaches to the management of pain in patients with advanced cancer. Hematol Oncol Clin North Am 1996;10:139–155.

82. Syrjala KL, Roth-Roemer SL: Nonpharmacologic approaches to pain. In Berger AM, Portenoy RK, Weissman DE (eds): Principles and Practice of Supportive Oncology. Philadelphia, Lippincott Raven, 1998, pp 77–91.

83. Massie MJ, Holland J: The cancer patient with pain: Psychiatric complications and their management. Med Clin North Am 1987;71:243–258.

84. Bonica JJ, Ventafridda V, Twycross RG (eds): Section E: Regional analgesia/anesthesia. In: The Management of Pain, 2nd ed. Malvern, Pa, Lea & Febiger, 1990, pp 1878–2039.

85. Lillemoe KD, Cameron JL, Kaufman HS, Yeo CJ, Pitt HA, Sauter PK: Chemical splanchnicectomy in patients with unresectable pancreatic cancer. Ann Surg 1993;217:447–455.

86. Mercadante S: Celiac plexus block versus analgesics in pancreatic cancer pain. Pain 1993;52:187–192.

87. Bonica JJ, Ventafridda V, Twycross RG (eds): Section F: Ablative neurosurgical operations. In: The Management of Pain, 2nd ed. Malvern, PA, Lea & Febiger, 1990, pp 2040–2103.

88. Stuart G, Cramond T: Role of percutaneous cervical cordotomy for pain of malignant origin. Med J Aust 1993;158:667–670.

89. Hanks G, Portenoy RK, MacDonald N, O'Neill WM: Difficult pain problems. In Doyle D, Hanks G, MacDonald N (eds): Oxford Textbook of Palliative Medicine, 2nd ed. Oxford, Oxford Medical Publications, 1998, pp 454–477.

90. Martin LA, Hagen NA: Neuropathic pain in cancer patients: Mechanisms, syndromes, and clinical controversies. J Pain Symptom Manage 1997;14:99–117.

91. Arner S, Meyerson BA: Lack of analgesic effects of opioids on neuropathic and idiopathic forms of pain. Pain 1988;33:11–23.

92. Rall TW, Schleifer LS: Drugs effective in the therapies of the epilepsies. In Gilman AG, Rall TW, Nies AL, et al (eds.): Goodman and Gilman's The Pharmacological Basis of Therapeutics, 8th ed. New York, Pergamon Press, 1990, pp 436–462.

93. Rowbotham M, Harden N, Stacey B, Bernstein P, Magnus-Miller L: Gabapentin for the treatment of postherpetic neuralgia: A randomized controlled trial. JAMA 1998;280:1837–1842.

94. Backonja M, Beydoun A, Edwards KR, et al: Gabapentin for the symptomatic treatment of painful neuropathy in patients with diabetes mellitus: A randomized controlled trial. JAMA 1998;280:1831–1836.

95. Bosnjak S, Jelic S, Susnjar S, Luki V: Gabapentin for relief of neuropathic pain related to anticancer treatment: A preliminary study. J Chemother 2002;14:214–219.

96. Beydoun A, Uthman BM, Sackellares JC: Gabapentin: Pharmacokinetics, efficacy, and safety. Clin Neuropharmacol 1995;18:469–481.

97. Glazer S, Portenoy RK: Systemic local anesthetics in pain control. J Pain Symptom Manage 1991;6:30–39.

98. Thompson JW, Filshie J: Transcutaneous electrical nerve stimulation and acupuncture. In Doyle D, Hanks GWC, MacDonald N (eds): Oxford Textbook of Palliative Medicine, 2nd ed. Oxford, Oxford University Press, 1998, pp 421–437.

99. Portenoy RK, Hagen NA: Breakthrough pain: Definition, prevalence, and characteristics. Pain 1990;41:273–282.

100. Ripamonti C, Bruera E: Current status of patient-controlled analgesia in cancer patients. Oncology 1997;11:373–380, 383–384; discussion 384–386.

101. Weissman DE, Haddox JD: Opioid pseudoaddiction: An iatrogenic syndrome. Pain 1989;36:363–366.

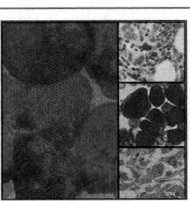

36

REHABILITATION OF THE PATIENT WITH CANCER

Patricia A. Ganz

Julienne E. Bower

SUMMARY OF KEY POINTS

REHABILITATION NEEDS OF THE PATIENT WITH CANCER

- Rehabilitation needs vary according to the phase of the disease, with physical needs being greatest in advanced cancer.
- Individual cancer sites have specific rehabilitation needs and understanding the physical and psychosocial sequelae of treatments is critical for both prevention of problems and specific rehabilitation interventions.
- Reproductive health concerns are common among patients of all ages with all types of cancer, although certain groups may be most concerned about issues of fertility, sterility, and menopause.
- Growing numbers of cancer survivors require careful attention to the late effects of cancer treatments and their medical and psychosocial consequences.

PSYCHOSOCIAL ISSUES

- Psychologic distress is extremely common after a cancer diagnosis; provision of education and support by the oncology team will help to alleviate fears and promote adjustment.
- Although most patients adjust well, some will have clinically significant symptoms of anxiety and depression that interfere with normal functioning and require treatment.
- All patients should be screened for emotional distress as part of their routine medical care, and organic causes of symptoms should be evaluated.
- Structured psychologic interventions are effective in reducing distress and improving quality of life; psychopharmacologic interventions may also be helpful for treating depression and anxiety disorders.

SEXUAL HEALTH AND FUNCTIONING

- Sexual problems are common in the general population and can be exacerbated by a diagnosis of cancer.
- Some cancer treatments (e.g., pelvic surgery, androgen deprivation) directly affect sexual functioning; other effects may be more subtle (e.g., pain and fatigue).
- The oncology team needs to be aware of the sexual effects of various treatments and be comfortable assessing whether a patient is having problems.
- Use of the PLISSIT model can be helpful in structuring assessment and interventions related to sexual problems.

INTRODUCTION

Three decades ago, at the inception of the National Cancer Act, the 5-year disease-free survival rate from cancer was in the 25% to 30% range, with a few cancer sites exceeding 50%. Cancer was still a stigmatized condition and few individuals openly spoke about their diagnosis or treatment experience. There was considerable debate about the appropriateness of telling patients about their cancer diagnosis, but with growing social and political movements emphasizing personal autonomy and informed consent, physicians more regularly told patients their diagnosis and began to involve them in treatment decisions. Treatments became increasingly complex, with multimodal therapies rather than surgery alone, and the National Cancer Institute's Clinical Trials Program expanded.

The situation today contrasts sharply with that in the past, with tremendous improvement in survival rates from cancer, including cures for many diseases.[1,2] Patients and survivors are actively involved in all aspects of their care,

with patient representatives serving as advisors to many scientific review bodies, professional organizations, and government agencies. Direct-to-consumer marketing of oncology products and treatments is widespread. Patients with cancer have high expectations of their treating oncology teams, and they are often willing to take more toxic treatments for even small differences in outcomes.[3] The longer survival rates and complex treatment regimens are not free of human costs, and thus in this chapter we focus on the rehabilitation needs of the patient with cancer in the early years of the twenty-first century. In this chapter we review the clinical epidemiology of rehabilitation needs in the patients with cancer, giving examples from common cancers and clinical situations. We discuss what is known about psychologic distress, depression, and anxiety in the setting of cancer; and we provide practical information about clinical interventions related to emotional and sexual health and functioning. Increasingly, attention to these issues is being integrated into the routine care of patients with cancer, and it is our hope that this chapter will facilitate greater understanding of these issues, as well as strategies for intervention when appropriate.

REHABILITATION NEEDS OF THE PATIENT WITH CANCER

Cancer occurs in more than 100 tissue sites in the body and thus can be very heterogeneous in its manifestations, biology, response to treatment, and time course. Nevertheless, it is still possible to define several distinct phases in the disease continuum that are experienced by the patient and lead to specific types of rehabilitation needs. By rehabilitation, we mean the systematic use of preventive interventions to address the physical, psychologic, and social needs that result from either the diagnosis or treatment of cancer. As the old adage says "An ounce of prevention is worth a pound of cure." However, in the management of cancer, we do not always recognize the opportunity to do preventive rehabilitation interventions, and so many times these occur after the fact. In this section, we describe common *phase-related* and *treatment-related* rehabilitation needs. Knowledge of common patterns of rehabilitation needs associated with phases and treatments can help the oncology health care team provide preventive interventions as appropriate (Table 36-1). Unique site-specific concerns are briefly discussed, along with other cross-cutting reproductive health effects and the late toxic effects of treatment.

Common Phase-Related Issues

At the time of *cancer diagnosis*, the physical rehabilitation needs of patients can range from none to many, depending on whether the cancer was diagnosed through screening (e.g., abnormal Papanicolaou test results, polyp on colonoscopy, abnormality on mammogram) or because of symptoms from advanced metastatic disease. Symptoms and the physical limitations that cancer causes are directly related to the extent of disease at diagnosis. In contrast, psychosocial distress is nearly universal at the time of diagnosis, and sometimes the patient with a screen-detected cancer will have more distress than patients with several months of clinical symptoms and more extensive disease. Shock, disbelief, and the need to face the uncertainties of treatment are common to all patients with newly diagnosed cancer. The impact on the family and the ability to continue work are also major considerations at this time.

During the time of *primary treatment*, asymptomatic individuals are likely to experience toxic effects from treatment (e.g., adjuvant therapy for breast or colorectal cancer), and their psychosocial concerns are likely to remain at a high level because of the ongoing stress of treatments. For patients with advanced malignancy, treatments may reduce disease-related symptoms but they also cause toxic effects. Patients with metastatic disease often mention the psychologic burden of continuous treatments, whereas patients with more time-limited treatments can focus on the eventual completion of therapy. For patients with early-stage cancer, going off treatment signals the end of treatment-related toxic effects, but it may still be many months before energy returns and hair regrows.[4] In addition, the psychologic distress associated with the end of treatments is often underestimated. Many patients worry about every new ache and pain being a symptom of recurrence, and their less frequent visits to the doctor mean that the professional reassurance and support that they had during treatment are not as available. Further, their family and friends may assume that everything is fine, even though the patient is now struggling with how to re-emerge into the nonpatient world and how to cope with the fears and uncertainties he or she has about the future. Much less research has been focused on this phase of recovery—the transition from patient to survivor.[5]

More research and clinical efforts are being devoted to the study of *long-term survivors* of cancer.[6,7] Among children with cancer, survival rates are extremely high, and there has been much interest in the long-term sequelae and late effects of cancer treatment, such as short stature, cognitive dysfunction, osteoporosis, cardiac dysfunction, fertility, and second malignancies.[8-19] There are also increasing numbers of adult cancer survivors (in excess of 8.9 million); and the most common types of cancer in survivors are breast, prostate, colorectal, and gynecologic cancers.[20] Further, an overwhelming number of cancer survivors are older than 65 years, raising concerns about the additive effects of past cancer treatments and the common comorbid conditions of aging.[21,22] In the past decade, there have been increasing numbers of studies that have examined the short-term and long-term rehabilitation needs and quality of life of these survivors.[6,7,23-34] Many of these studies suggest that these survivors have high levels of physical and emotional functioning, although they may be troubled with some symptoms or problems that remind them of the disease (e.g., body image concerns, sexual dysfunction, fatigue, and bladder or bowel problems).

TABLE 36-1

 Rehabilitation Concerns and Phase of the Disease

The Diagnostic Phase

Psychologic distress: shock, disbelief, depression
Symptoms and physical limitations from clinically advanced disease

Primary Treatment

Treatment toxic effects: nausea, vomiting, hair loss, fatigue
Psychologic distress: anxiety about whether treatments are working
Disruption in work and social activities

Transition to Cancer Survivor

Recovery from the physical toxic effects of treatment
Fear of recurrence
Return to normal work, social, and recreational activities

Long-term Survivorship

Late effects of treatment, including organ toxic effects
Second malignancies
Fertility/sterility; sexual dysfunction
Employment and insurance discrimination

Cancer Recurrence/Advanced Metastatic Disease

Physical symptoms from progressive disease
Psychologic distress, depressed mood
Preparing for death

Cancer recurrence is associated with a wide range of physical and psychosocial rehabilitation concerns.[35] Symptoms vary depending on the site of recurrence, but pain is a common problem at this time. This in turn can lead to fatigue, poor appetite, weight loss, and depressive symptoms, if the pain is not well-controlled. There are also major psychologic stresses associated with recurrence; and the patient, family, and health care providers may all experience a sense of failure, as well as the need to re-group and develop a new treatment strategy. Resumption of cytotoxic treatments or radiation therapy can add to the physical burden experienced by the patient at the time of recurrence.

Cancer Site-Specific Rehabilitation Concerns

Cancers at certain specific body sites have unique rehabilitation problems, and for this reason, involvement of a specialized rehabilitation team before and after surgery can be very helpful to the patient. Patients with *head and neck cancer* share a common set of problems in spite of a wide variety of specific cancer sites within this anatomic region. Surgery and radiotherapy are the mainstay of treatment; however, chemotherapy is being used more frequently in the neoadjuvant setting.[36,37] Most head and neck cancers are associated with tobacco and alcohol abuse by the patient.[38] Habitual use of tobacco and alcohol products are often associated with a variety of complex psychosocial problems related to addiction and lack of social support, and these factors may complicate treatment and rehabilitation.

Pretreatment dental evaluation is critical for patients receiving radiotherapy to the head and neck because post-treatment xerostomia can accelerate the development or progression of dental caries. Osteoradionecrosis can be a serious late complication of radiation treatment, with trauma to the irradiated bone hastening this process. Therefore all dental extractions should be completed before the initiation of radiation treatment, and careful oral hygiene should be maintained during and after radiation treatment. Compliance with oral hygiene regimens must be emphasized as a preventive strategy in this group of patients.

Maintenance of adequate nutrition is a problem for patients with cancers of the head and neck, because deglutition may be directly affected by the primary tumor or as a consequence of treatment. Liquid nutritional supplements play an important role in the rehabilitation of these patients, and enteral feedings may be required if oral intake is inadequate. Consultation with a dietitian is frequently helpful. Further, problems with speech, swallowing, and aspiration may be serious ongoing concerns for the patient with head and neck cancer.[39] The size and location of the tumor, as well as the treatment strategy, play an important role in the ultimate severity of these problems. Pretreatment counseling is important to assure patients that professionals will be available to address their needs in the post-treatment period. After treatment, patients should be evaluated by a speech-language pathologist to determine the extent of changes in speech, voice, and swallowing ability. Assessment of swallowing should include a videofluoroscopic examination of movement patterns of the structures in the oral cavity and pharynx. Speech and swallowing therapy should be initiated early, because several studies indicate that maximum improvement occurs at around 3 months after treatment ends.[39]

The accessory nerve is often severed as part of the radical neck dissection procedure, leading to denervation of the trapezius muscle. This can result in serious shoulder dysfunction, which has both physical and cosmetic effects.[40,41] The trapezius muscle plays a key role in upward rotation of the shoulder during abduction and flexion, and in addition, it is the major stabilizer of the scapula. The loss of this muscle's function can lead to shoulder malalignment and motor dysfunction, resulting in an inability to push, lift, or carry heavy objects. Shoulder range of motion can be limited and painful. Physical therapy interventions are available to address these problems and should be an integral part of the rehabilitation of these patients.[42] If motor dysfunction results from radical neck dissection, range of motion exercises, directed by a physical therapist, can facilitate the recovery process. Recent advances in surgery with nerve-sparing procedures have been associated with better functioning and quality of life.[43]

Cosmetic restoration of physical defects resulting from surgery to parts of the face or oropharynx (the nose, orbit, maxilla, or mandible) is an important problem for patients with head and neck cancer. Maxillofacial prosthodontists are the specialists who design the individualized prosthetic devices for these patients. These prostheses are used to restore both function and cosmesis. Without cosmetic rehabilitation, these patients may experience continued and worsening psychologic distress. Preparation of the maxillofacial prosthesis is a multistep process with pretreatment evaluation of the patient and several subsequent evaluations in the post-treatment period. Final prosthesis preparation does not occur until complete healing of the involved tissues has happened, which may be many months after diagnosis, surgery, and radiation treatment. In the interim, a temporary prosthesis is used. Patients are in considerable need of psychologic support during the period of adaptation to their physical loss, especially before completion of surgical reconstruction or prosthetic restoration.

Restoration of speech is an additional area of particular concern for patients with head and neck cancer. Tumors of the nose, mouth, pharynx, and larynx cause a variety of speech deficits. At the extreme is the patient with a total laryngectomy who will need training in esophageal speech or in using an electrolarynx or similar prosthetic sound-generating device. Patients who undergo partial or total glossectomy will also require speech therapy and may require prosthetic devices to assist in the speech rehabilitation process. The psychologic consequences of the loss of speech are legion and must be dealt with before surgery is performed, as well as in the post-operative period. Larynx-sparing procedures lead to better quality-of-life outcomes (less pain and depression), but this may not be directly related to preservation of speech.[44]

Laryngectomee support groups can be found in many communities and can serve as an invaluable resource for patients and their families.

Patients with *breast cancer* are another special population with unique rehabilitation needs. Because it is the most common cancer in women, breast cancer has been extensively evaluated in both the rehabilitation and psychosocial literature.[24,45-55] The primary treatment of breast cancer is associated with a high rate of both physical and psychologic problems.[54,55] The radical mastectomy (extensive surgery that includes removal of the pectoral muscles) has been replaced by the modified radical mastectomy (with or without reconstruction) and breast-conserving surgery. The axillary node dissection is the remaining cause of arm dysfunction in women receiving surgical treatment, and this may ultimately be replaced by the sentinel node dissection, currently being evaluated in large-scale phase III trials.[56-58] The major concern for women related to the management of the axilla is the risk of lymphedema.[59,60] Even with more limited breast surgery, patients still experience psychosocial and cosmetic rehabilitation problems.[53,61,62]

Regardless of whether breast conservation surgery or mastectomy is performed, physical problems after primary treatment are generally similar for the two groups of patients.[24,54,55] Frequent problems include fatigue, limited upper-extremity mobility, difficulty in lifting objects, arm weakness, difficulty doing household chores, and arm numbness. The literature suggests that there are few differences in quality of life, psychosocial adjustment, or performance status between patients who have undergone mastectomy and those who have had breast conservation surgery.[53,63-65] However, the patients who receive conservation surgery generally experience significantly fewer problems with clothing and body image. It is possible that the earlier diagnosis of very small tumors through mammographic screening, as well as increased use of sentinel lymph node biopsy, may be changing these observations. Recent data from our research group show significant differences in physical functioning for women treated with lumpectomy and sentinel node biopsy, compared with women treated with mastectomy, suggesting that for very small tumors, the morbidity from surgery is diminished compared with historic treatments.

With either type of breast cancer surgery, the axillary dissection increases the potential risk of lymphedema.[59] Radiotherapy, in combination with axillary dissection, contributes to the risk of lymphedema. Unfortunately, there are no evidence-based strategies for prevention or treatment of lymphedema,[59] and this is an important area for future investigation. It is commonly recommended that patients be cautioned about avoiding trauma or infection in the extremity with the axillary dissection, as well as avoiding venipuncture and blood pressure measurements in that arm; however, no hard data in support of lymphedema risk reduction are available for these latter recommendations. Nevertheless, they do make common sense. Prompt recognition of an infection and institution of antibiotic treatment may avert excessive edema as a response.

Today, breast cancer surgery is often done in the outpatient setting, and if women are hospitalized for surgery, they have very short stays. As a result, we find that women are frequently not educated about the possible development of lymphedema and the commonly recommended precautions. Unfortunately, once lymphedema is established, it is difficult to combat. Conservative management for mild edema includes elevation of the extremity, salt restriction, use of diuretics, and an exercise program. For more severe cases, intermittent pneumatic compression is useful for redistribution of fluid from the extremity. This can be maintained by use of a supportive garment or sleeve. For massive lymphedema that is refractory or with onset several years after the primary surgery, recurrence of the tumor in the axillary area should be ruled out by means of computed tomography or magnetic resonance imaging.

Restoration of physical appearance is very important for the woman who has had a mastectomy. The chest wall is usually quite tender in the immediate postoperative period, and therefore purchase of a permanent breast prosthesis should be deferred for several weeks. A temporary prosthesis made from soft and lightweight material (e.g., cotton, lamb's wool, or nylon stockings) can be pinned into the brassiere before a permanent prosthesis is purchased. An American Cancer Society Reach-to-Recovery volunteer will provide a temporary prosthesis when she visits the patient. In addition, the volunteer will often provide a list of stores in the local community that provide fitting and a selection of permanent prostheses. These permanent breast prostheses come in a wide variety of sizes, weights, and materials and also have a wide range of costs. Patients should be encouraged to examine a number of brands before purchasing one. Many specialty shops also provide a range of special garments (e.g., bathing suits, nightgowns) for use by women who have had mastectomies.

Surgical reconstruction of the breast should be offered to all women who choose or require a total mastectomy. The specific reconstructive procedure will depend on the type of primary surgery performed and the condition of the remaining tissue. The development of tissue expanders has aided in breast reconstruction for women whose overlying chest wall skin is relatively taut. Immediate reconstruction can be done at the time of the initial mastectomy by using a tissue expander, an implant, or an autologous tissue flap. Breast reconstruction often requires a number of surgical procedures, including reduction mammoplasty for the remaining breast, and not all women will choose to have additional surgery. Nevertheless, the option of reconstruction should be discussed with patients as part of the rehabilitation program.

Problems with sexuality and body image are frequently reported after breast cancer surgery.[23,54,66] It is important for the patient's partner to view the mastectomy scar early in the postoperative period, especially at the time the patient herself first sees the scar. In this way the couple can share in the loss and deal with the recovery together. There is less disruption in body image with breast-conserving surgery, yet even women who have had this type of surgery may feel uncomfortable with the changes in their bodies.[53] Chemotherapy treatments frequently lead to a decrease in sexual desire and impaired vaginal lubrication, with a resultant decline in the frequency of sexual intercourse.[23,25] These issues are discussed in more detail later in this chapter.

Prostate cancer is the most common cancer in men, and because of the widespread use of the prostatic specific antigen (PSA) test, many men are given the diagnosis when they are asymptomatic. This leads to considerable psychologic distress, especially associated with decision making about primary therapy. For localized disease, options may include radiation therapy, radical prostatectomy, or watchful waiting. Because the toxic effects of these approaches may vary considerably,[27,67,68] patients often experience a prolonged period of consultation and information seeking before they make a treatment decision. Major problems associated with surgery include incontinence and impotence, and rectal problems and impotence are associated with radiation.[67] Even though men may be prepared for these outcomes, for many men, the problems are very distressing when they occur. When androgen deprivation is added to the treatment of prostate cancer, additional problems include osteoporosis, loss of libido, and loss of body mass.[69,70] Issues related to sexual dysfunction are addressed later in this chapter.

Patients who require an *ostomy* as part of their cancer treatment also have special rehabilitation needs.[71] These include patients with rectal or sigmoid colon cancers and patients with a variety of pelvic tumors (bladder, cervix, uterus) for whom a urinary diversion is required. An enterostomal therapist should see the patient before surgery to provide information and reassurance about the ostomy, its function, and care. In addition, the therapist can aid the surgeon in identifying the best location for the stoma to ensure that it can be easily managed by the patient and so it will be adequately supported and be away from the belt line or body folds.

In the immediate postoperative period, the enterostomal therapist should begin direct teaching with the patient regarding the care of the stoma and the use of appliances. If the patient has difficulty adjusting to the stoma, the emotional response can impair the teaching process. The patient must be encouraged to view the stoma site and touch it to develop independence and self-confidence regarding self-care. Periodic home-care visits by an enterostomal therapist after the patient's discharge from the hospital will facilitate the recovery process and engender patient confidence in independent self-care. Meticulous skin care should be emphasized and monitored.

During the early postoperative period the patient and family members can benefit from peer support such as that available through the United Ostomy Association. A volunteer visitor with an ostomy can provide reassurance as a living example of an individual who has successfully adapted to life with a stoma. In addition, many local chapters of the organization have regular support groups and periodicals that are helpful. During the months after surgery, the patient should be encouraged to resume usual activities and work, including sexual activity. Sexual rehabilitation of the patient with an ostomy must address the physical loss of pelvic organs, as well as the presence of the stoma or appliance, and the psychologic impact of

the changes in personal bodily function related to elimination. Preoperative discussion of the sexual impact of treatment is extremely important for this population of patients.

Amputations for *bone* and *soft tissue cancers* lead to a wide range of physical and psychologic rehabilitation problems for patients receiving this treatment. The functional impairment relates to the location and extent of the primary tumor. Unlike amputations done for benign conditions, amputations for cancer are sometimes radical and include such procedures as a hemipelvectomy or forequarter amputation. A preoperative assessment should be performed to prepare the prostheses and to orient patients to the postoperative rehabilitation program. Crutch walking can be introduced at this time when balance is better and there is no pain. Rigid dressings are recommended in the postoperative period to decrease pain and the potential for phantom limb sensation. A physical therapy program should be initiated during the postoperative period to maintain strength and prevent contractures. The prosthesis cannot be used until stump shrinkage is complete, and at that time, the patient will need gait training and assistance in ambulation.

Advances in surgical treatments in the late 1970s and 1980s made it possible to perform limb-sparing surgical management of lower-extremity bone tumors. The reader is referred to a recent review article for discussion of the indications for amputation versus limb salvage surgery.[72] Other considerations in this patient population relate to the concomitant use of radiation and chemotherapy, making overall treatments more complex. Although survival rates are equivalent for amputation and limb salvage surgery, complications occur more often with limb salvage procedures.[72] Functional and health status outcomes have been assessed in the setting of preoperative and postoperative radiotherapy for extremity soft tissue sarcomas with a wide variety of standardized measures.[73-75] The timing of radiation therapy has minimal impact on the functioning of these patients; however, tumor characteristics (large resection, lower extremity) and wound complications have a detrimental effect on functioning after treatment.[75]

Bone and soft tissue cancers are primarily tumors of children, adolescents, and young adults. Patients at this life stage can be especially vulnerable to psychologic problems related to diagnosis and treatment. School is usually interrupted, particularly if the patient requires adjuvant chemotherapy. Recreational and social activities must be modified. Counseling should be offered to the patient and family to help them deal with the disruption caused by the cancer treatment and the long-term problems of physical and vocational rehabilitation.

Reproductive Health Concerns: Fertility, Sterility, and Menopause

Infertility as a consequence of cancer therapy is an important problem because more and more patients with cancer are expected to survive and be cured. Relatively little information is available about gonadal dysfunction and how it might be prevented. Several chemotherapy drugs (primarily alkylating agents) and radiation therapy are directly toxic to normal gonadal tissue and often, little can be done to eliminate the use of these treatments if cure is the goal of therapy. Potential infertility should be discussed with the patient before initiation of treatment. In a survey of 121 men who had undergone curative treatment for nonseminomatous testicular cancer, Schover and von Eschenbach[76] found that 56.9% reported that they produced no semen and that more than 20% had frequent anxiety related to infertility and lack of semen. Infertility is also a concern for survivors of Hodgkin's disease. Fobair and colleagues[29] found that 19% of 165 patients who wanted to have children after treatment for Hodgkin's disease were infertile.

Treatment planning for individuals likely to be cured of cancer must begin to take these findings into account. For men, it is possible to make use of sperm banking, although many men with newly diagnosed cancer may have azoospermia caused by the acute illness. However, in spite of the availability of sperm banking, it appears that it is infrequently offered to patients.[77,78] For women receiving radiation treatment for Hodgkin's disease, oophoropexy is recommended to decrease the dose of radiation to the ovaries, although this is less likely to be used today because of the decrease in use of staging laparotomy, as well as more limited radiation therapy ports. Avoidance of chemotherapy regimens that include alkylating agents can also decrease the likelihood of permanent amenorrhea. In women with breast cancer, amenorrhea from adjuvant chemotherapy is closely related to age at treatment, with rates increasing rapidly after the age of 40 years.[79]

Premature menopause in female patients with cancer can cause its own set of problems, leading to vasomotor symptoms, vaginal dryness, and sexual dysfunction, as well as weight gain and osteoporosis.[80-84] Estrogen supplementation is the most effective way to alleviate menopausal symptoms, and when not contraindicated, should be given for as short a time as possible because of the long-term adverse effects of this therapy.[85] Nonestrogen alternatives can be effectively used to manage these symptoms.[86,87] There is also a wide variety of medications that can be used to prevent osteoporosis and to lower lipid levels, if cardiovascular risk factors are a concern.

Late Toxic Effects from Treatments

Cancer survivors are at risk for a multitude of late effects from surgery, systemic chemotherapy, and radiation therapy. These are often organ-specific (e.g., bleomycin and pulmonary toxicity; doxorubicin and cardiac toxicity; nitrosourea and renal toxicity), and the true frequency of these toxic effects is unknown, given the limited data on late effects in survivors.[88] To the extent that this patient population will be expanding and that oncologists may no longer closely monitor patients beyond the first 5 years of treatment, it is probably advisable to make patients aware of the need for long-term follow-up and the potential toxic effects of different therapies. For example, young adult patients treated for Hodgkin's disease with mantle irradiation are at risk for premature coronary artery disease, and if they are women, breast cancer. Monitoring for these late effects should be a part of the preventive rehabilitation care for these survivors.

PSYCHOLOGIC DISTRESS, DEPRESSION, AND ANXIETY

Overview

Psychologic distress is extremely common after a cancer diagnosis. Cancer poses a significant threat to one's physical, emotional, social, financial, and existential well-being (Table 36-2). In response to these threats, patients may experience a variety of emotional reactions including shock, anger, disbelief, anxiety, and sadness. These are normal reactions that for most patients will resolve over time with appropriate education and support. However, some patients will experience more intense and prolonged distress that interferes with important aspects of their life and, potentially, their medical care. This level of distress is not normal or expected in patients with cancer and requires appropriate referral and treatment. The range of emotional responses is described in the following sections and includes normal reactions, adjustment disorders, major depression, and anxiety disorders. Psychologic and psychopharmacologic interventions used to treat these problems are also described.

Normal Responses

Receiving a cancer diagnosis is stressful and frightening for most individuals. Many believe that cancer is a death sentence and poses an immediate threat to their physical well-being. Cancer may also challenge basic assumptions about the world and the self, including one's sense of self-esteem, control over important outcomes, and feelings of meaningfulness and purpose in life.[89,90] Massie and Holland[91] describe a typical sequence of emotional responses to cancer diagnosis. Initially, patients may experience symptoms of shock, disbelief, denial, or despair as they struggle to accept and incorporate the reality of the diagnosis. This initial stage may be followed

TABLE 36-2

Spectrum of Psychologic Responses to Cancer

"Normal" responses	Feelings of shock, disbelief, fear, anger, sadness/grief
	Symptoms are transient, triggered by crisis or transition points including diagnosis, treatment onset, treatment completion, and recurrence.
Adjustment disorders	Exacerbation of "normal" response
	Symptoms interfere with social and occupational functioning.
Depression and anxiety disorders	Persistent feelings of depression and/or anxiety with cognitive and somatic symptoms
	Symptoms cause clinically significant impairment in social, occupational, or other areas of functioning.

by a period of turmoil and distress, characterized by symptoms of anxiety; sadness; ruminative thoughts; irritability; and difficulty sleeping, eating, and concentrating. These symptoms typically stabilize as patients adjust to new information, make decisions about treatment, and resume their normal activities. However, increases in symptoms may occur at other transition or crisis points, including treatment onset, treatment completion, and recurrence. Again, these symptoms typically subside as patients cope with the new situation.

Patients may also experience a variety of normal fears throughout the treatment course, including fears of disability, loss of roles, dependence or loss of control, loss of desirability, abandonment, and death. Grief is another normal response that may wax and wane as patients experience losses related to their diagnosis and treatment.[92] These symptoms are typically not persistent and do not cause serious impairments in patients' functioning.

Overall, most patients cope successfully with cancer diagnosis and treatment and experience good long-term psychologic adjustment. Within 1 to 2 years after diagnosis, patients who have completed treatment and are disease-free look essentially identical to healthy control subjects on measures of emotional well-being and overall quality of life.[23,26] Use of active, problem-focused coping, positive social support from family and friends, and having a general sense of optimism are all important in facilitating adjustment. Many patients describe positive changes in their lives related to their diagnosis, including positive changes in self-perception, interpersonal relationships, priorities, and goals.[93,94] They report feeling stronger, better able to cope with life's difficulties, and closer to their friends and relatives, with a heightened sense of the fragility and preciousness of life. For these individuals, cancer may have acted as a "wake up" call and led them to think seriously about the meaning and direction of their lives.

Adjustment Disorders

Although most patients are able to cope well with a cancer diagnosis, a significant number do experience more persistent or intrusive problems. Studies suggest that approximately 20% to 35% of patients with cancer experience clinically significant symptoms of depression or anxiety.[95] Many of these patients meet criteria for an adjustment disorder with anxious or depressed mood.[96] The essential feature of an adjustment disorder is the development of clinically significant emotional or behavioral symptoms in response to an identifiable psychosocial stressor.[97] Clinical significance is indicated either by marked distress that is in excess of what would be expected or by significant impairment in social or occupational functioning. The onset of symptoms occurs within 3 months of stressor onset and is resolved within 6 months after stressor termination. Among patients with cancer, an adjustment disorder typically involves an exacerbation of the "normal" responses described earlier. Patients who experience adjustment difficulties may show decreased performance at work and other tasks and temporary changes in social relationships. These disorders should be

taken seriously because they interfere with patients' quality of life and may affect compliance with treatment.

Demographic and physical risk factors for poor adjustment include younger age, greater physical impairment, symptom distress, and pain.[98] Psychologic risk factors include history of psychologic problems, avoidant coping, poor social support, pessimism, and inadequate communication with the health care team.[99-101] Patients who passively accept the cancer diagnosis, who deny or are fatalistic about the diagnosis, or who feel helpless and out of control are also at risk for adjustment problems.[98] These patients may also have some prior family association with cancer or a concurrent life event that overwhelms their typical coping resources and leads to an exaggerated emotional response.[91] Screening questions can be used to identify patients in distress or at risk for psychosocial problems. For example, "Do you have one person to talk to about your experience?" and "Would you say that you have experienced a lot of stressful or upsetting events over the last year?"[102] Those who report high levels of distress or who have many risk factors should be referred for psychologic evaluation and possible treatment.

Depression

Clinical depression is a serious illness that may go unrecognized in patients with cancer. Clinicians may be unfamiliar with the symptoms of depression, may mistake these symptoms for symptoms of the disease or effects of treatment, or may believe that depression is a normal reaction to a cancer diagnosis.[92] Although mild, transient symptoms of depression (e.g., feelings of sadness and irritability and changes in sleep, appetite, and concentration) are common after a cancer diagnosis, more prolonged and severe symptoms that interfere with patients' functioning require immediate attention. The importance of correctly diagnosing and treating depression is underlined by research showing that depression is associated with decreased compliance with medical care, lengthened hospital stays, and higher mortality rates in patients with chronic medical conditions.[103,104]

Estimates of the prevalence of depression in patients with cancer vary widely, from 1.5% to 50%, depending on the method of assessment and the patient population considered.[102,105] Overall, the average estimate is 15% to 25%[106-108] compared with a general population rate of approximately 6%. The highest rates of depression occur among hospitalized patients with significant levels of physical impairment. In addition, patients with pancreatic, lung, brain, and head and neck tumors have higher rates of depression.[95]

A major depressive episode is characterized by either depressed mood or markedly diminished interest or pleasure in normal activities, or both, for most of the day, nearly every day for a 2-week period. Other symptoms include significant weight loss or gain; insomnia or hypersomnia; psychomotor agitation or retardation; fatigue; feelings of worthlessness or excessive or inappropriate guilt; diminished ability to think or concentrate, or indecisiveness; and recurrent thoughts of death or recurrent suicidal ideation. To meet diagnostic criteria, the patient must experience at least four of these symptoms nearly every day for at least 2 weeks.[97] In addition, the symptoms must cause clinically significant distress or impairment in social, occupational, or other areas of functioning.

Detection of a depressive episode is complicated in patients with cancer because the somatic symptoms of depression (e.g., changes in sleep, energy, and appetite) may overlap with symptoms of medical illness. Psychologic symptoms may be more sensitive indicators of depression in this population, including pervasive hopelessness, helplessness, excessive guilt, worthlessness, feeling that life is without value, and prominent thoughts about death.[92] Grief reactions, or bereavement, can also overlap with symptoms of depression. Symptoms that may help to distinguish depression from bereavement include feelings of worthlessness, marked psychomotor retardation, and prolonged impairment, all of which are more closely associated with depression than grief.[105] Finally, delirium and dementia are very common in patients with advanced disease and can be mistaken for depression.[109]

Patients should be screened for depression during their regular medical visits. Although a clinical interview is required for formal diagnosis, screening can be accomplished by asking patients a few simple questions. Chochinov[92] reports that a single-item screening question—"Are you depressed most of the time?"—has high sensitivity and specificity for detecting depression among patients with cancer. Clinicians should also be aware of risk factors for depression (Table 36-3), which include a history of depression, history of drug or alcohol abuse, poorly controlled pain, and advanced disease with physical disability.[92,110] Other psychologic risk factors include social isolation, recent losses, pessimism, a disengaged or passive coping style, and a lack of perceived control.[105] Patients with any of these risk factors should be carefully watched for symptoms of depression throughout their treatment course.

Depression in patients with cancer may be related to organic causes, including direct effects of the disease or treatment on the central nervous system and metabolic or

TABLE 36-3

▓ **Factors That Influence Depression in Patients with Cancer**	
Risk Factors	History of depression
	History of alcoholism or substance abuse
	Poorly controlled pain
	Advanced stages of disease
	Social isolation; recent losses or stressors; pessimism; disengaged, passive, or avoidant coping; low perceived control
Biologic Influences	Direct effects of disease/treatment on CNS
	Metabolic, endocrine, or immune abnormalities secondary to disease/treatment
	Medications
	Corticosteroids
	Other anticancer medications

CNS, Central nervous system.

SCREENING AND TREATMENT OF PSYCHOLOGIC DISTRESS AND DEPRESSION

SCREENING/EVALUATION
Inquire about emotional distress at each patient visit; also evaluate risk factors for distress/depression.
Evaluate duration and intensity of symptoms and impairment of normal functioning.

SYMPTOMS OF DEPRESSION
Depressed mood and/or anhedonia
Changes in weight, sleep, energy, and concentration
Feelings of worthlessness, guilt, and hopelessness
Prominent thoughts about death

INTERVENTION
Provide all patients with education and support, including information about mental health services.
Provide referrals to patients at risk for distress/depression to structured group interventions or other psychosocial interventions.
Treat depression with psychotherapy and/or pharmacotherapy (e.g., selective serotonin reuptaake inhibitors, short-acting benzodiazepenes).

---

endocrine abnormalities that occur as a result of the disease or treatment, such as hypocalcemia and hypothyroidism. In addition, there is some evidence of immune abnormalities in depressed patients with cancer, specifically increases in proinflammatory cytokines.[111] These cytokines are known to cause depression-like symptoms in animal models[112] and may also play a role in depression seen in some patients with cancer. Finally, many of the medications used by patients with cancer may lead to depressive symptoms. These include steroids, interferon, interleukin-2, methyldopa, reserpine, barbiturates, propranolol, procarbazine, asparaginase, vinblastine, vincristine, and cyproterone.[92] It is important to accurately determine the cause of depression-like symptoms, if possible. In particular, organic causes of depression and those related to medication use and pain should be treated accordingly.

Anxiety

Symptoms of anxiety are very common in patients with cancer. One of the key features of anxiety is a subjective feeling of fear or dread about uncertain future outcomes, certainly a normal reaction to a cancer diagnosis. Anxiety is also characterized by physiologic symptoms, including increases in heart rate and respiration related to activation of the sympathetic nervous system. Behavioral symptoms of anxiety may include avoidance of or withdrawal from feared situations and activities. Anxiety can be triggered by psychologic aspects of the cancer experience or by physical, biologic, and medication-related causes, such as poorly controlled pain, abnormal metabolic states, or anxiety-producing medications. Anxiety reactions may also be related to pre-existing anxiety disorders, including phobias, panic disorder, and generalized anxiety disorder (characterized by persistent and excessive worry).[113]

Patients with cancer may also have acute stress disorders or post-traumatic stress disorder (PTSD) in response to cancer diagnosis and treatment. PTSD is an anxiety disorder that occurs after an extremely stressful or traumatic event, including diagnosis with a life-threatening illness such as cancer, which provokes feelings of intense fear, helplessness, or horror. Studies conducted with cancer survivors suggest that between 10% and 15% may meet criteria for PTSD within 5 years of diagnosis.[114,115] Risk factors include poor social support and occurrence of negative life events before cancer diagnosis.[115-117] In addition, poor physical health, fewer financial resources, and younger age have been associated with PTSD symptoms.[118,119]

The characteristic symptoms of PTSD are persistent re-experiencing of the event, persistent avoidance of stimuli associated with the event, numbing of general responsiveness, and persistent symptoms of increased arousal.[97] Symptoms of PTSD usually begin within 3 months of the trauma and must be present for more than 1 month and cause significant impairment in functioning. In acute stress disorder, symptoms occur within 1 month of the trauma and resolve within 4 weeks. There is some evidence that symptoms of PTSD decline over time; however, this disorder is associated with significant declines in quality of life[118] and merits attention and treatment in cancer survivors.

Interventions to Reduce Distress and Promote Well-Being

Receiving a cancer diagnosis imposes many demands on patients. They must learn about the medical aspects of their diagnosis, make decisions about treatment, and cope with the impact of the disease on their family, work, and long-term goals and well-being. All patients will benefit from education and support to help them manage this crisis period. Physicians can play a major role in facilitating patients' emotional adjustment by providing clear, understandable information about the disease in a caring and empathic manner. Patients with cancer who were seen by physicians who had been trained to communicate more clearly by using techniques such as simplification and repetition and to provide a supportive emotional context by conveying warmth, listening, and giving feedback reported fewer depressive symptoms and higher levels of satisfaction and control.[120] Giving patients a brief tour and orientation to the medical oncology clinic, providing written materials about clinic hours and procedures, and answering patients' questions have been associated with decreases in distress.[121] These findings underscore the importance of providing clear and thorough information to patients in a supportive environment.

Psychosocial interventions are also helpful in facilitating adjustment to cancer (Table 36-4). The general goals of most interventions are to provide information, reduce stress and distress, teach effective coping mechanisms, and provide support. Quantitative and narrative reviews demonstrate that psychologic interventions are associated

TABLE 36-4

Psychosocial Interventions to Reduce Distress and Promote Well-Being

Information and Reassurance from the Health Care Team

Specific Interventions

Individual counseling
Psychoeducational support groups
Journal writing exercises
Supportive-expressive therapy
Progressive muscle relaxation
Hypnosis

with clinically meaningful reductions in symptoms of emotional distress among patients with cancer, particularly symptoms of anxiety.[122-126] Beneficial effects on physical aspects of quality of life, including energy, pain, and physical functioning, have also been observed,.[127] There is some evidence that psychosocial interventions may be associated with positive changes in physiologic systems, including the endocrine[128] and immune systems,[129] and in physical health outcomes, including reduced medical visits for cancer-related problems[130] and longer survival.[131,132] However, these results have not been consistently observed.[133]

Positive changes have been seen with diverse psychosocial intervention methods, including education, cognitive-behavioral, and supportive-expressive treatments. Overall, structured treatments conducted by experienced and highly trained therapists are associated with better psychosocial outcomes.[125] Unstructured interventions without trained leaders, such as those providing only peer support and discussion, do not appear to be effective.[127] Group interventions are at least as effective as individual therapy[125]; however, some patients will not feel comfortable in the group setting and should be referred for individual treatment. Behavioral interventions appear to be particularly effective in reducing side effects of chemotherapy and acute treatment-related pain, especially hypnosis-like methods, progressive muscle relaxation, and guided imagery.[122,134]

Different types of treatment are also recommended for patients at different disease stages. Newly diagnosed patients, those in the early stages of treatment, and those with good prognoses may benefit most from short-term, targeted interventions focused on providing information about the disease and treatment and managing disease-related stress.[122] These interventions help patients cope with their cancer and may even enhance positive outcomes, such as increases in positive mood[127] and finding positive benefits in the cancer experience.[135] In contrast, patients with advanced-stage disease may benefit more from longer-term interventions emphasizing emotional expression and support, such as supportive-expressive group therapy.[136] These interventions are led by a trained therapist but focus more on daily coping, pain management, and existential issues related to a shortened life span.

The beneficial effects of psychosocial interventions depend in part on patients' pretreatment psychologic and physical status. Interventions are most effective for patients who are distressed,[125,126] have poor social support or few personal resources (e.g., low control, low self-esteem, and poor body image),[137] and those in pain.[133] Thus clinicians should be particularly diligent about referring patients who are experiencing (or at risk for) emotional or physical problems for psychosocial evaluation and treatment. However, all patients should be provided with information about mental health services, including both structured group interventions and individual therapists experienced with the unique medical and psychologic issues of patients with cancer.

Patients who are experiencing clinical levels of depression or anxiety will require more intensive and targeted treatment. For depressed patients, a combination of psychotherapy and pharmacotherapy may be most effective.[92] Both interpersonal and cognitive behavioral psychotherapy have been shown to be effective in treating depressed patients.[138] New classes of antidepressants, including selective serotonin reuptake inhibitors, have become the preferred class of antidepressants for treating clinically depressed patients with cancer because of their favorable side effect and toxicity profiles. These treatments may be effective even when the depression is clearly caused by cancer treatment, as in the case of interferon and interleukin-2.[139] Pharmacologic therapy may also be an important adjunct to behavioral interventions for patients with anxiety related to their cancer diagnosis and treatments. Short-acting benzodiazepines are useful in this setting. For patients with PTSD, specific types of behavioral therapy, such as stress inoculation training and exposure treatment, may be most effective.

SEXUAL HEALTH AND FUNCTIONING

Background and General Considerations

Among the many aspects of health and well-being, sexual health is seldom discussed by the patient and physician unless there are medically related symptoms (e.g., sexually transmitted diseases) or there is *severe* disruption of sexual functioning caused by physical or psychologic illness. Although we are sexual beings, sexual health is often taken for granted. Sexuality is considered a private matter and is not usually discussed in the physician's office. Thus most physicians have little experience discussing sexual health with their patients and are poorly prepared to address their sexual concerns.

Sexual health and functioning can be very important to the patient with cancer. Life-saving cancer treatments often affect physical and psychologic well-being and pose a serious threat to body image. Many surgical procedures have direct physical effects on the sex organs. While struggling to overcome their cancer, many patients will forgo normal sexual relations because of the severe fatigue and symptoms that decrease their sexual interest; however, during recovery from treatment, resumption of regular sexual activity is often a signal of return to health. At any point during the cancer experience, patients can benefit from the advice and counsel of their physicians on issues related to sexual health and functioning.

General Effects of Cancer Therapies and Their Effects on Sexual Health and Functioning

The normal human sexual response is exceedingly complex, and minor physical and psychologic changes may disrupt it. In addition, changes in level of sexual interest and activity occur normally as part of aging. These factors often exist in the background, preceding the diagnosis of cancer. Cancer and its treatments often cause severe physiologic, psychologic, personal, and interpersonal changes that affect sexual behavior. There are four major categories of sexual dysfunction—desire, arousal, orgasm, and pain—and different patterns of dysfunction may be associated with different treatments. Some of the most common problems are as follows:

- Chemotherapy can cause vaginal dryness and dyspareunia. Ovarian failure caused by chemotherapy leads to menopause, which can decrease the amount of vaginal lubrication.
- All treatments can cause fatigue, as a result of anemia or other toxic effects. Nausea and moderate to severe fatigue are reported by 90% of patients receiving chemotherapy. When "not feeling well," most people lose interest in sex.
- Bodily pain is a major problem, especially in advanced or recurrent cancer. Uncontrolled pain leads to psychologic distress and depression, which can affect sexual desire. In addition, opioid narcotics may have secondary effects on sexual functioning.
- Changes in body image and scarring as a result of surgery can decrease feelings of sexual attractiveness and desire, disrupting intimate relationships. The partner may not want to hurt the patient and will back off from lovemaking or any physical contact. The patient may think that the partner is not interested or is put off by the physical changes and thus will feel rejected. This problem can often be solved if the partner and the patient talk about what each is feeling and perceiving.
- Radiation to the pelvic region can cause shrinkage of tissues, irritation and drying of the vagina, pain, nausea, gastric distress, and serious fatigue. However, many of these conditions can be treated. In men, pelvic radiation can cause vascular damage that may lead to erectile dysfunction.
- Surgery in the pelvic area (e.g., bladder, rectum, prostate) can also involve dissection of nerves crucial to sexual arousal in men.
- Other body changes—a stoma, weight loss or gain, and hair loss—can affect body image and feelings of sexual attractiveness. In turn this can affect sexual functioning.
- Cancer treatments may cause changes in the sensitivity of sexual organs. If sensitivity is increased and the patient experiences pain, the ability to become aroused may change, which will have an effect on the sexual relationship.
- The effects of hormone therapy as a cancer treatment vary, depending on the specific treatments used. Tamoxifen, for example, often does not have a negative

effect on sexual function because, for some women, it works like an estrogen on the vaginal tissues. On the other hand, the androgen deprivation (e.g., orchiectomy, gonadotropin-releasing hormone analogs) used in prostate cancer treatment has a profound effect on a man's libido.

- The sexuality of men and women with cancer who are in the childbearing years can be affected by the possible loss of fertility or concerns about whether to conceive a child.

The Effect of Different Types of Cancer on Sexual Function

Treatment for breast cancer often produces the side effects of fatigue, diminished vaginal lubrication, nausea, and significant body changes including the loss of a breast from mastectomy. Early menopause is common.[79] The use of hormone replacement therapy is controversial in this population because of the concern that it will stimulate tumor growth. Tamoxifen can increase vaginal discharge in some women but otherwise does not have significant effects on sexual functioning.[140,141] In a large cross-sectional survey of North America, sexual functioning in women with a history of breast cancer was found to be similar to that of a group of age-matched menopausal women who had not had breast cancer.[23,142] However, breast cancer survivors who received adjuvant chemotherapy reported poorer sexual functioning than those who had not.[23,80,143] Body image is better for women who have had lumpectomy compared with those who have had mastectomy, but the type of surgery does not appear to affect sexual functioning.[61,143]

Findings from studies that assess sexuality in patients with testicular cancer are mixed, possibly because samples are made up of patients with different tumor types who received different treatments. A recent meta-analysis of 36 studies done between 1975 and 2000 showed that retrograde ejaculation was an important physical consequence of treatment but that it was unclear whether other sexual difficulties were disease- or treatment-related.[144] More sexual problems are reported in retrospective studies than in prospective studies. Rates of decreased sexual desire are moderately low for all treatment modalities and may improve with time. Occasional erectile problems are more common than permanent dysfunction, particularly in patients who received adjuvant radiation treatments. Problems with orgasm, particularly problems with intensity of orgasm and ejaculatory function, are the most common types of dysfunction documented. Problems in sexual functioning appear to be largely explained by ejaculatory dysfunction, which occurs more often in patients who received radiation therapy or retroperitoneal lymph node dissection in addition to orchiectomy. Despite disruption to physiologic sexual functioning, most men are sexually satisfied and only some report decreases in sexual activity.

In a recent cross-sectional evaluation of men who underwent orchiectomy, followed by infradiaphragmatic radiation, for stage I and II seminoma, body image and sexual functioning were examined.[145] In this study, the men's interest in sexual activity, erectile difficulties, and satisfaction with sexual life did not differ from those of age-matched healthy control subjects. However, 20% of the men expressed concerns about fertility and 52% reported body image changes.[145] In another study in which patients with testicular cancer were compared with men with Hodgkin's disease, similar rates of erectile dysfunction and concerns about fertility were observed.[28] In contrast to patients with seminoma, patients without seminoma treated with chemotherapy with or without retroperitoneal dissection report more difficulties with sexual functioning, especially related to the psychologic aspects of functioning (libido and arousal).[146] Recent studies regarding the use of sperm banking suggest that it is not widely used and that this is a major concern for patients.[77,78]

Erectile function is the aspect of functioning in men that is most disrupted after pelvic surgery, pelvic irradiation, or prostatectomy; and the majority of patients report some decrease in erectile ability[27,67,147] after these procedures. Moderate to high levels of disruption in orgasm and sexual activity are also common. Because prostate cancer is increasingly detected through screening, men may experience the side effects of treatment without significant clinical benefit from early detection.[148] A recent prospective follow-up study of men during the year after treatment demonstrated different outcomes from radiation and surgery, although there were substantial differences in age and comorbidity between the two treatment groups.[149] Substantial sexual dysfunctions may exist before these treatments as well.[150] Sildenafil has been used successfully in men who have experienced erectile dysfunction as a result of prostate cancer treatments.[151-153] Vacuum erection devices, intracorporal papaverine injections, or surgical implants may be considered for men who are unresponsive to oral therapy.[154,155] Androgen deprivation therapy, once used only for advanced disease, is now being used more often to treat localized prostate cancer or men with rising PSA levels and nonmeasurable disease. The effects of androgen deprivation on libido, energy, and body image are not insignificant.[70,156]

The majority of patients who have undergone cystectomy experience some problems with sexual functioning after treatment. Some men experience a decrease in sexual desire, but the most drastic impact is on erectile function, with most men reporting severe dysfunction. The proportion of erectile dysfunction has been reported to be lower when nerve-sparing procedures are performed. For women, there may be changes associated with decreased vaginal lubrication if they have estrogen deficiency,[157] and similar issues face both men and women if a stoma is created. Mansson and colleagues[158] administered a quality-of-life instrument to patients undergoing cystectomy and compared results for those who had continent cutaneous ileocecal diversion with those who had simple conduit diversion. Patients in both groups experienced equivalent declines in quality of life related to sexual problems, disturbed partner relationships, and emotional dysfunction.[158]

Most patients with lung cancer have advanced disease when they receive the diagnosis and thus often have severe physical symptoms. Shortness of breath, fatigue, and pain are important problems that can limit sexual activity in this group of patients.[159] Among long-term survivors, physical dysfunction and comorbidities can influence sexual interest and functioning.[6,159,160]

In patients with colorectal cancer, treatment may initially increase fatigue, and many patients may find that their bowel habits change. If they have surgery that leads to an ostomy, their feelings about their body image may become negative. In addition, some surgical procedures for colorectal cancer have the potential to damage the pelvic nerves, which may lead to erectile dysfunction in men. Overall, patients who undergo abdominoperineal resection report poorer sexual outcomes than patients who undergo low anterior resection.[161] Poor sexual outcomes in the former may be related to erectile dysfunction, bowel dysfunction, or the presence of a stoma.[162]

Among patients with *gynecologic cancers*, surgery and radiation can cause changes to the pelvis and sexual organs.[163-165] The vagina frequently becomes less elastic and shorter. Changes in vaginal sensation, shape, and lubrication are also common. Chemotherapy or surgery may result in early menopause, and some patients may not be able to receive hormone replacement therapy because of its potential to stimulate cancer growth (e.g., uterine adenocarcinoma).

Treatments for the leukemias and lymphomas are often quite toxic and can produce considerable fatigue and other side effects.[28-31] Although many of these diseases are curable, the chemotherapy and radiation may lead to toxicity in other organs, which can increase fatigue. The treatments often induce early menopause and lead to a need for hormone replacement therapy.[84]

Assessment and Intervention

A comprehensive assessment of severe sexual difficulties requires an interdisciplinary and multifaceted approach that is often beyond the scope of the oncology team; however, the majority of sexual problems can initially be assessed within the usual care setting. Some cancer centers and universities have expert sexual dysfunction clinics to which patients can be referred, and these might be used for the most difficult cases. In those settings, complex assessments of hormonal, physiologic, anatomic, psychologic, cognitive, behavioral, relational, and cultural factors are likely to be taken into account by clinicians who specialize in treating this problem. This will not be necessary for most patients with cancer, but it is useful to identify referral resources that can be used to evaluate complex cases. Several references are available for readers who wish to learn more about the prevalence of specific disorders and assessment procedures.[163,166-172]

Although a comprehensive assessment is unrealistic within the constraints of an oncology practice, a preliminary review of sexual difficulties is essential to providing optimal care to patients with cancer. Patients regularly report that they would like to discuss sexual issues with their physicians but feel reluctant to do so.[173,174] Therefore it is up to the medical team to broach the issue and open lines of communication. It is sometimes easiest to just ask

"How is your sex life going?" and then gauge the need for further inquiry based on the patient's response. If the patient says that everything is all right, then no further questioning may be necessary. However, the patient who is having difficulties and wants an opportunity to discuss the situation will usually be quite relieved that the question has been asked. Follow-up questions to the patient about each of the four categories of sexual dysfunction—desire, arousal, orgasm, and pain—as well as questions about sexual activity and satisfaction will generally provide sufficient information to determine the need for further testing or referral. One member of the oncology team (e.g., a nurse or social worker) might be identified as a primary resource for making sure every patient has an assessment of sexual concerns.

Counseling and Referral

After a member of the oncology team has raised the issue of sexuality and made a preliminary assessment of the reported problems, a decision must be made regarding the level and type of intervention that is needed. In some cases, the specific concerns that arise can be addressed directly by a member of the team who has expertise in sexuality and cancer. In addressing sexual problems of patients with cancer and their partners, the level of intervention should be matched to the intensity of the problems. There are four general levels of strategies, which Annon[175] has summarized by using the acronym PLISSIT. According to the PLISSIT model, the range of interventions includes giving permission, providing limited information, offering specific suggestions, and

---

STRATEGIES FOR ADDRESSING SEXUAL PROBLEMS: THE PLISSIT MODEL

P = PERMISSION GIVING
Invite patient and partner to raise concerns and ask
  questions about sexuality.
Encourage patient to communicate with partner about
  cancer and sexuality.
Normalize broad definition of sexuality.

LI = LIMITED INFORMATION
Provide information about sexual functioning, aging, and
  sexual problems related to the cancer experience.
Offer relevant written materials about cancer, sexuality, and
  community resources.
Describe options for psychosocial and medical
  interventions for enhancing sexual functioning.

SS = SPECIFIC SUGGESTIONS (TARGETED TO INDIVIDUAL PATIENT CONCERNS)
Discuss possibilities for increasing vaginal lubrication.
Offer recommendations for erectile aids.
Suggest positions for sexual activity to reduce discomfort.

IT = INTENSIVE THERAPY
Provide referral for individual, couples, or sex therapy, as
  needed.

conducting intensive therapy. The components of this model can be incorporated into the assessment and intervention process to help patients and their partners deal with sexual concerns and problems.

In terms of *permission giving*, one of the most important things a clinician can do is to raise the issue of sexuality with the patient and provide an opportunity to discuss any relevant concerns. Clinicians should be careful in these conversations to use a broad, inclusive, culturally sensitive definition of sexuality that is not limited to penile-vaginal intercourse. They should also be careful not to make assumptions about patients' sex lives (for example, assuming heterosexuality or assuming that the patient has a partner). In addition to broaching discussion of sexuality with the patient, the oncology team can help the patient by encouraging communication between the patient and his or her partner(s) about cancer and sexuality.

Providing patients and, when appropriate, their partners with *limited information* about sexual functioning, aging, and sexual problems related to the cancer experience can help to reduce the concerns that some patients have. Patients can also benefit from receiving written materials, such as those available from the National Cancer Institute and the American Cancer Society or other experts.[176] They may also benefit from learning about local resources for patients with cancer and cancer survivors.

For limited problems, *specific suggestions* or a brief course of sexual counseling may be sufficient. For example, for a woman with vaginal dryness, recommendation of a vaginal lubricant or moisturizer or prescription of vaginal estrogen might be extremely effective. Similarly, prescription of medication or an erectile aid can be very helpful for men with erectile dysfunction.

When information and relatively straightforward suggestions are insufficient, clinicians should make referrals for more *intensive therapy*. It is helpful to have available referrals for male and female therapists who have training in sex therapy and psychosocial oncology. Mental health professionals with special training will be able to conduct a comprehensive assessment and determine whether sex therapy, couples therapy, or individual therapy is needed. The oncology specialist often plays a pivotal role in ensuring the success of the treatment, even though the therapy is provided by another clinician. It is important to normalize the need for intervention by describing sexual problems in the context of rehabilitation from the cancer. Schover and colleagues[177] found that 63.5% of patients with cancer who received brief sexual counseling within a cancer center reported improvement. However, patients who were depressed or in conflicted marriages were least likely to benefit from counseling and probably need more specific attention to those underlying problems.

SUMMARY AND FUTURE DIRECTIONS

Contemporary cancer therapy is multimodal and involves many health care professionals as part of the treatment team. The increasing complexity of cancer therapies has

benefits and risks. The benefits include the chance for longer survival, cure, organ preservation, and improved quality of life. The risks include increased psychologic distress associated with treatment decision making, toxic effects of therapy, complicated treatment schedules, and disruption of everyday routines. Later effects may include organ toxicity, second malignancies, infertility, premature menopause, and significant sexual dysfunction. Although the oncology team usually has expertise in the medical and technical aspects of care, cancer rehabilitation issues are sometimes overlooked. With the growing number of childhood and adult cancer survivors, it is imperative that additional attention be given to the rehabilitation needs of cancer patients with cancer and cancer survivors.

We are fortunate that there is now a growing body of literature and an expanding national research program (e.g., National Cancer Institute, American Cancer Society) on the long-term consequences of cancer therapy. Most research done to date has been with convenience samples and observational cohorts. We expect that during the next decade, there will be increasing opportunities for prospective studies, especially within the National Cancer Institute's clinical trials cooperative groups, to define and describe the cancer rehabilitation outcomes associated with specific therapies. For example, how many women with breast cancer have amenorrhea during a particular adjuvant chemotherapy regimen or experience cognitive dysfunction with the same treatments? Can congestive heart failure in children treated for leukemia be prevented with cardioprotective agents? Can we prevent future breast cancer in teenage girls who receive mantle irradiation therapy for Hodgkin's disease? As these questions suggest, we now need to think about prevention of some of the rehabilitation problems experienced by cancer survivors. The oncology team will play a critical role in these efforts, and there is no better time than now to focus on understanding the rehabilitation concerns of the patient with cancer.

REFERENCES

1. Jemal A, Murray T, Samuels A, Ghafoor A, Ward E, Thun MJ: Cancer statistics, 2003. CA Cancer J Clin 2003;53:5–26.
2. Simmonds MA: Cancer statistics, 2003: Further decrease in mortality rate, increase in persons living with cancer. CA Cancer J Clin 2003;53:4.
3. Simes RJ, Coates AS: Patient preferences for adjuvant chemotherapy of early breast cancer: How much benefit is needed? J Natl Cancer Inst Monogr 2001;30:146–152.
4. Ahles TA, Silberfarb PM, Herndon J, et al: Psychologic and neuropsychologic functioning of patients with limited small-cell lung cancer treated with chemotherapy and radiation therapy with or without warfarin: A study by the Cancer and Leukemia Group B. J Clin Oncol 1998;16:1954–1960.
5. Mullan F: Seasons of survival: Reflections of a physician with cancer. N Engl J Med 1985;313:270–273.
6. Schag CA, Ganz PA, Wing DS, Sim MS, Lee JJ: Quality of life in adult survivors of lung, colon and prostate cancer. Qual Life Res 1994;3:127–141.
7. Gotay CC, Muraoka MY: Quality of life in long-term survivors of adult-onset cancers. J Natl Cancer Inst 1998;90:656–667.
8. Devney RB, Sklar CA, Nesbit ME, et al: Serial thyroid function measurements in children with Hodgkin disease. J Pediatr 1984;105:223–227.

9. Robison LL, Nesbit ME, Sather HN, Meadows AT, Ortega JA, Hammond GD: Height of children successfully treated for acute lymphoblastic leukemia: A report from the Late Effects Study Committee of Children's Cancer Study Group. Med Pediatr Oncol 1985;13:14-21.

10. Hamre MR, Robison LL, Nesbit ME, et al: Effects of radiation on ovarian function in long-term survivors of childhood acute lymphoblastic leukemia: A report from the Children's Cancer Study Group. J Clin Oncol 1987;5:1759-1765.

11. Bushhouse S, Ramsay NK, Pescovitz OH, Kim T, Robison LL: Growth in children following irradiation for bone marrow transplantation. Am J Pediatr Hematol Oncol 1989;11:134-140.

12. Katsanis E, Shapiro RS, Robison LL, et al: Thyroid dysfunction following bone marrow transplantation: Long-term follow-up of 80 pediatric patients. Bone Marrow Transplant 1990;5:335-340.

13. Tucker MA, Jones PH, Boice JD, et al: Therapeutic radiation at a young age is linked to secondary thyroid cancer. The Late Effects Study Group. Cancer Res 1991;51:2885-2888.

14. Robison LL: Survivors of childhood cancer and risk of a second tumor. J Natl Cancer Inst 1993;85:1102-1103.

15. Bhatia S, Ramsay NK, Bantle JP, Mertens A, Robison LL: Thyroid abnormalities after therapy for Hodgkin's disease in childhood. Oncologist 1996;1:62-67.

16. Bhatia S, Ramsay NK, Weisdorf D, Griffiths H, Robison LL: Bone mineral density in patients undergoing bone marrow transplantation for myeloid malignancies. Bone Marrow Transplant 1998;22:87-90.

17. Bhatia S, Meadows AT, Robison LL: Second cancers after pediatric Hodgkin's disease. J Clin Oncol 1998;16:2570-2572.

18. Green DM, Hyland A, Chung CS, Zevon MA, Hall BC: Cancer and cardiac mortality among 15-year survivors of cancer diagnosed during childhood or adolescence. J Clin Oncol 1999;17:3207-3215.

19. Green DM, Grigoriev YA, Nan B, et al: Congestive heart failure after treatment for Wilms' tumor: A report from the National Wilms' Tumor Study Group. J Clin Oncol 2001;19:1926-1934.

20. Estimated US Cancer Prevalence Counts: Who are our cancer survivors in the US? National Cancer Institute, Office of Cancer Survivorship Website. (Retrieved February 1, 2003, from http://www.dccps.nci.nih.gov/ocs/prevalence/index.html).

21. Yancik R, Ganz PA, Varricchio CG, Conley B: Perspectives on comorbidity and cancer in older patients: Approaches to expand the knowledge base. J Clin Oncol 2001;19:114-1151.

22. Yancik R, Wesley MN, Ries LA, Havlik RJ, Edwards BK, Yates JW: Effect of age and comorbidity in postmenopausal breast cancer patients aged 55 years and older. JAMA 2001;285:885-892.

23. Ganz PA, Rowland JH, Desmond K, Meyerowitz BE, Wyatt GE: Life after breast cancer: Understanding women's health-related quality of life and sexual functioning. J Clin Oncol 1998;16:501-514.

24. Ganz PA, Coscarelli A, Fred C, Kahn B, Polinsky ML, Petersen L: Breast cancer survivors: Psychosocial concerns and quality of life. Breast Cancer Res Treat 1996;38:183-199.

25. Ganz PA, Rowland JH, Meyerowitz BE, Desmond KA: Impact of different adjuvant therapy strategies on quality of life in breast cancer survivors. Recent Results Cancer Res 1998;152:396-411.

26. Ganz PA, Desmond KA, Leedham B, Rowland JH, Meyerowitz BE, Belin TR: Quality of life in long-term, disease-free survivors of breast cancer: A follow-up study. J Natl Cancer Inst 2002;94:39-49.

27. Litwin MS, Hays RD, Fink A, et al: Quality-of-life outcomes in men treated for localized prostate cancer. JAMA 1995;273:129-135.

28. Bloom JR, Fobair P, Gritz E, et al: Psychosocial outcomes of cancer: A comparative analysis of Hodgkin's disease and testicular cancer. J Clin Oncol 1993;11:979-988.

29. Fobair P, Hoppe RT, Bloom J, Cox R, Varghese A, Spiegel D: Psychosocial problems among survivors of Hodgkin's disease. J Clin Oncol 1986;4:805-814.

30. Kornblith AB, Anderson J, Cella DF, et al: Comparison of psychosocial adaptation and sexual function of survivors of advanced Hodgkin disease treated by MOPP, ABVD, or MOPP alternating with ABVD. Cancer 1992;70:2508-2516.

31. Kornblith AB, Herndon JE, Zuckerman E, et al: Comparison of psychosocial adaptation of advanced stage Hodgkin's disease and acute leukemia survivors. Cancer and Leukemia Group B. Ann Oncol 1998;9:297-306.

32. Kornblith AB, Anderson J, Cella DF, et al: Hodgkin disease survivors at increased risk for problems in psychosocial adaptation. The Cancer and Leukemia Group B. Cancer 1992;70:2214-2224.

33. Gritz ER, Wellisch DK, Wang HJ, Siau J, Landsverk JA, Cosgrove MD: Long-term effects of testicular cancer on sexual functioning in married couples. Cancer 1989;64:1560-1567.

34. Gritz ER, Carmack CL, de Moor C, et al: First year after head and neck cancer: Quality of life. J Clin Oncol 1999;17:352-360.

35. Frost MH, Suman VJ, Rummans TA, et al: Physical, psychological and social well-being of women with breast cancer: The influence of disease phase. Psychooncology 2000;9:221-231.

36. Dimery IW, Hong WK: Overview of combined modality therapies for head and neck cancer. J Natl Cancer Inst 1993;85:95-111.

37. Papadimitrakopoulou VA, Dimery IW, Lee JJ, Perez C, Hong WK, Lippman SM: Cisplatin, fluorouracil, and L-leucovorin induction chemotherapy for locally advanced head and neck cancer: The M.D. Anderson Cancer Center experience. Cancer J Sci Am 1997;3:92-99.

38. Gritz ER: Smoking and smoking cessation in cancer patients. Br J Addict 1991;86:549-554.

39. Logemann JA, Pauloski BR, Rademaker AW, Colangelo LA: Speech and swallowing rehabilitation for head and neck cancer patients. Oncology (Huntingt) 1997;11:651-656, 659.

40. Cheng PT, Hao SP, Lin YH, Yeh AR: Objective comparison of shoulder dysfunction after three neck dissection techniques. Ann Otol Rhinol Laryngol 2000;109:761-766.

41. El Ghani F, Van Den Brekel MW, De Goede CJ, Kuik J, Leemans CR, Smeele LE: Shoulder function and patient well-being after various types of neck dissections. Clin Otolaryngol 2002;27:403-408.

42. Dietz JH: Rehabilitation oncology. Somerset, NJ, John Wiley & Sons, 1981.

43. Terrell JE, Welsh DE, Bradford CR, et al: Pain, quality of life, and spinal accessory nerve status after neck dissection. Laryngoscope 2000;110:620-626.

44. Terrell JE, Fisher SG, Wolf GT: Long-term quality of life after treatment of laryngeal cancer. The Veterans Affairs Laryngeal Cancer Study Group. Arch Otolaryngol Head Neck Surg 1998;124:964-971.

45. Meyerowitz BE: Psychosocial correlates of breast cancer and its treatments. Psychol Bull 1980;87:108-131.

46. Meyerowitz BE, Sparks FC, Spears IK: Adjuvant chemotherapy for breast carcinoma: Psychosocial implications. Cancer 1979;43:1613-1618.

47. Meyerowitz BE, Watkins IK, Sparks FC: Psychosocial implications of adjuvant chemotherapy. A two-year follow-up. Cancer 1983;52:1541-1545.

48. Kemeny MM, Wellisch DK, Schain WS: Psychosocial outcome in a randomized surgical trial for treatment of primary breast cancer. Cancer 1988;62:1231-1237.

49. Schain WS, Fetting JH: Modified radical mastectomy versus breast conservation: Psychosocial considerations. Semin Oncol 1992;19:239-243.

50. Lewis FM, Bloom JR: Psychosocial adjustment to breast cancer: A review of selected literature. Int J Psychiatry Med 1978;9:1-17.

51. Spiegel D, Bloom JR: Pain in metastatic breast cancer. Cancer 1983;52:341-345.

52. Ganz PA, Hirji K, Sim MS, Schag CA, Fred C, Polinsky ML: Predicting psychosocial risk in patients with breast cancer. Med Care 1993;31:419-431.

53. Ganz PA, Schag AC, Lee JJ, Polinsky ML, Tan SJ: Breast conservation versus mastectomy. Is there a difference in psychological adjustment or quality of life in the year after surgery? Cancer 1992;69:1729-1738.

54. Schag CA, Ganz PA, Polinsky ML, Fred C, Hirji K, Petersen L: Characteristics of women at risk for psychosocial distress in the year after breast cancer. J Clin Oncol 1993;11:783-793.

55. Shimozuma K, Ganz PA, Petersen L, Hirji K: Quality of life in the first year after breast cancer surgery: Rehabilitation needs and patterns of recovery. Breast Cancer Res Treat 1999;56:45-57.

56. Whitworth P, McMasters KM, Tafra L, Edwards MJ: State-of-the-art lymph node staging for breast cancer in the year 2000. Am J Surg 2000;180:262-267.

57. Temple LKF, Baron R, Cody HS III, et al: Sensory morbidity after

sentinel lymph node biopsy and axillary dissection: A prospective study of 233 women. Ann Surg Oncol 2002;9:654-662.

58. Krag D: Why perform randomized clinical trials for sentinel node surgery for breast cancer? Am J Surg 2001;182:411-413.

59. Erickson VS, Pearson ML, Ganz PA, Adams J, Kahn KL: Arm edema in breast cancer patients. J Natl Cancer Inst 2001;93:96-111.

60. Ganz PA: The quality of life after breast cancer—solving the problem of lymphedema. N Engl J Med 1999;340:383-385.

61. Rowland JH, Desmond KA, Meyerowitz BE, Belin TR, Wyatt GE, Ganz PA: Role of breast reconstructive surgery in physical and emotional outcomes among breast cancer survivors. J Natl Cancer Inst 2000;92:1422-1429.

62. Fallowfield L: Offering choice of surgical treatment to women with breast cancer. Patient Educ Couns 1997;30:209-214.

63. Kiebert GM, de Haes JC, van de Velde CJ: The impact of breast-conserving treatment and mastectomy on the quality of life of early-stage breast cancer patients: A review. J Clin Oncol 1991;9:1059-1070.

64. Moyer A: Psychosocial outcomes of breast-conserving surgery versus mastectomy: A meta-analytic review [published erratum appears in Health Psychol 1997;16:442]. Health Psychol 1997;16:284-298.

65. Maunsell E, Brisson J, Deschenes L: Psychological distress after initial treatment of breast cancer. Assessment of potential risk factors. Cancer 1992;70:120-125.

66. Wolberg WH, Romsaas EP, Tanner MA, Malec JF: Psychosexual adaptation to breast cancer surgery. Cancer 1989;63:1645-1655.

67. Talcott JA, Rieker P, Clark JA, et al: Patient-reported symptoms after primary therapy for early prostate cancer: Results of a prospective cohort study. J Clin Oncol 1998;16:275-283.

68. Potosky AL, Legler J, Albertsen PC, et al: Health outcomes after prostatectomy or radiotherapy for prostate cancer: Results from the Prostate Cancer Outcomes Study. J Natl Cancer Inst 2000;92:1582-1592.

69. Potosky AL, Reeve BB, Clegg LX, et al: Quality of life following localized prostate cancer treated initially with androgen deprivation therapy or no therapy. J Natl Cancer Inst 2002;94:430-437.

70. Fowler FJ Jr, McNaughton CM, Walker CE, Elliott DB, Barry MJ: The impact of androgen deprivation on quality of life after radical prostatectomy for prostate carcinoma. Cancer 2002;95:287-295.

71. Hurny C, Holland J: Psychosocial sequelae of ostomies in cancer patients. CA Cancer J Clin 1985;35:170-183.

72. Nagarajan R, Neglia JP, Clohisy DR, Robison LL: Limb salvage and amputation in survivors of pediatric lower-extremity bone tumors: What are the long-term implications? J Clin Oncol 2002;20:4493-4501.

73. Davis AM, Bell RS, Badley EM, Yoshida K, Williams JI: Evaluating functional outcome in patients with lower extremity sarcoma. Clin Orthop 1999;358:90-100.

74. Davis AM, Sennik S, Griffin AM, et al: Predictors of functional outcomes following limb salvage surgery for lower-extremity soft tissue sarcoma. J Surg Oncol 2000;73:206-211.

75. Davis AM, O'Sullivan B, Bell RS, et al: Function and health status outcomes in a randomized trial comparing preoperative and postoperative radiotherapy in extremity soft tissue sarcoma. J Clin Oncol 2002;20:4472-4477.

76. Schover LR, von Eschenbach AC: Sexual and marital relationships after treatment for nonseminomatous testicular cancer. Urology 1985;25:251-255.

77. Schover LR, Brey K, Lichtin A, Lipshultz LI, Jeha S: Knowledge and experience regarding cancer, infertility, and sperm banking in younger male survivors. J Clin Oncol 2002;20:1880-1889.

78. Schover LR, Brey K, Lichtin A, Lipshultz LI, Jeha S: Oncologists' attitudes and practices regarding banking sperm before cancer treatment. J Clin Oncol 2002;20:1890-1897.

79. Goodwin PJ, Ennis M, Pritchard KI, Trudeau M, Hood N: Risk of menopause during the first year after breast cancer diagnosis. J Clin Oncol 1999;17:2365-2370.

80. Greendale GA, Petersen L, Zibecchi L, Ganz PA: Factors related to sexual function in postmenopausal women with a history of breast cancer. Menopause 2001;8:111-119.

81. Ganz PA: The role of hormones in breast carcinogenesis: Issues of relevance to female childhood cancer survivors. Med Pediatr Oncol 2001;36:514-518.

82. Ganz PA: Menopause and breast cancer: Symptoms, late effects, and their management. Semin Oncol 2001;28:74-283.

83. Ganz PA, Greendale GA: Menopause and breast cancer: Addressing the secondary health effects of adjuvant chemotherapy. J Clin Oncol 2001;19:3303-3305.

84. Syrjala KL, Roth-Roemer SL, Abrams JR, et al: Prevalence and predictors of sexual dysfunction in long-term survivors of marrow transplantation. J Clin Oncol 1998;16:3148-3157.

85. Risks and benefits of estrogen plus progestin in healthy postmenopausal women: Principal results from the Women's Health Initiative randomized controlled trial. JAMA 2002;288:321-333.

86. Ganz PA, Greendale GA, Petersen L, Zibecchi L, Kahn B, Belin TR: Managing menopausal symptoms in breast cancer survivors: Results of a randomized controlled trial. J Natl Cancer Inst 2000;92:1054-1064.

87. Loprinzi CL, Kugler JW, Sloan JA, et al: Venlafaxine in management of hot flashes in survivors of breast cancer: A randomised controlled trial. Lancet 2000;356:2059-2063.

88. Ganz PA: Late effects of cancer and its treatment. Semin Oncol Nurs 2001;17:241-248.

89. Janoff-Bulman R. Shattered assumptions: Towards a new psychology of trauma. New York, Free Press, 1992.

90. Taylor SE: Adjustment to threatening events: A theory of cognitive adaptation. Am Psychol 1983;38:1161-1173.

91. Massie MJ, Holland JC: Overview of normal reactions and the prevalence of psychiatric disorders. In Holland JC, Rowland JH (eds): Handbook of psychooncology. New York, Oxford University Press, 1989, pp 273-282.

92. Chochinov HM: Depression in cancer patients. Lancet Oncol 2001;2:499-505.

93. Cordova MJ, Cunningham LL, Carlson CR, Andrykowski MA: Posttraumatic growth following breast cancer: A controlled comparison study. Health Psychol 2001;20:176-185.

94. Tedeschi RG, Calhoun LG: Trauma and transformation: Growing in the aftermath of suffering. Thousand Oaks, Calif., Sage, 1995.

95. Zabora J, BrintzenhofeSzoc K, Curbow B, Hooker C, Piantadosi S: The prevalence of psychological distress by cancer site. Psychooncology 2001;10:19-28.

96. Derogatis LR, Morrow GR, Fetting J, et al: The prevalence of psychiatric disorders among cancer patients. JAMA 1983;249:751-757.

97. American Psychiatric Association: Diagnostic and statistical manual of mental disorders, 4th ed. Washington, DC, American Psychiatric Association, 1994.

98. van't Spijker A, Trijsburg RW, Duivenvoorden HJ: Psychological sequelae of cancer diagnosis: A meta-analytical review of 58 studies after 1980. Psychosom Med 1997;59:280-293.

99. Epping-Jordan JE, Compas BE, Osowiecki DM, et al: Psychological adjustment in breast cancer: Processes of emotional distress. Health Psychol 1999;18:315-326.

100. Lepore SJ, Helgeson VS: Social constraints, intrusive thoughts, and mental health after prostate cancer. J Soc Clin Psychol 1998;17:89-106.

101. Stanton AL: Cancer: Behavioral and psychosocial aspects. In Blechman EA, Brownell KD (eds): Behavioral medicine and women. New York, The Guilford Press, 1998, pp 588-594.

102. Sellick SM, Crooks DL: Depression and cancer: An appraisal of the literature for prevalence, detection, and practice guideline development for psychological interventions. Psychooncology 1999;8:315-333.

103. Stoudemire A, Thompson TL: Medication noncompliance: Systematic approaches to evaluation and intervention. Gen Hosp Psychiatry 1983;5:233-239.

104. Koenig HG, Shelp F, Goli V, Cohen HJ, Blazer DG: Survival and health care utilization in elderly medical inpatients with major depression. J Am Geriatr Soc 1989;37:599-606.

105. Newport DJ, Nemeroff CB: Assessment and treatment of depression in the cancer patient. J Psychosom Res 1998;45:215-237.

106. Massie MJ: Depressive disorders. In Holland JC, Rowland JH (eds): Handbook of Psychooncology. New York, Oxford University Press, 1989, pp 518-540.

Problems Common to Cancer and Its Therapy

107. McDaniel JS, Musselman DL, Porter MR, Reed DA, Nemeroff CB: Depression in patients with cancer. Diagnosis, biology, and treatment. Arch Gen Psychiatry 1995;52:89–99.

108. Breitbart W: Identifying patients at risk for, and treatment of major psychiatric complications of cancer. Support Care Cancer 1995;3:45–60.

109. Schwartz L, Lander M, Chochinov HM: Current management of depression in cancer patients. Oncology (Huntingt) 2002;16: 1102–1110.

110. Massie MJ. Depression. In Holland JC, Rowland JH (eds): Handbook of psychooncology. New York, Oxford University Press, 1989, pp 283–290.

111. Musselman DL, Miller AH, Porter MR, et al: Higher than normal plasma interleukin-6 concentrations in cancer patients with depression: Preliminary findings. Am J Psychiatry 2001;158:1252–1257.

112. Dantzer R, Bluthe RM, Kent S, Goodall G: Behavioral effects of cytokines: An insight into mechanisms of sickness behavior. Methods Neurosci 1993;17:130–150.

113. Massie MJ: Anxiety, panic and phobias. In Holland JC, Rowland JH (eds) Handbook of psychooncology. New York, Oxford University Press, 1989, pp 300–309.

114. Alter CL, Pelcovitz D, Axelrod A, et al: Identification of PTSD in cancer survivors. Psychosomatics 1996;37:137–143.

115. Andrykowski MA, Cordova MJ, Studts JL, Miller TW: Posttraumatic stress disorder after treatment for breast cancer: Prevalence of diagnosis and use of the PTSD Checklist-Civilian Version (PCL-C) as a screening instrument. J Consult Clin Psychol 1998;66:586–590.

116. DuHamel KN, Smith MY, Johnson Vickberg SM, et al: Trauma symptoms in bone marrow transplant survivors: The role of nonmedical life events. J Trauma Stress 2001;14:95–113.

117. Butler LD, Koopman C, Classen C, Spiegel D: Traumatic stress, life events, and emotional support in women with metastatic breast cancer: Cancer-related traumatic stress symptoms associated with past and current stressors. Health Psychol 1999;18:555–560.

118. Cordova MJ, Andrykowski MA, Kenady DE, McGrath PC, Sloan DA, Redd WH: Frequency and correlates of posttraumatic-stress-disorder-like symptoms after treatment for breast cancer. J Consult Clin Psychol 1995;63:981–986.

119. Tjemsland L, Soreide JA, Malt UF: Posttraumatic distress symptoms in operable breast cancer III: Status one year after surgery. Breast Cancer Res Treat 1998;47:141–151.

120. Rutter DR, Iconomou G, Quine L: Doctor-patient communication and outcome in cancer patients: An intervention. Psychol Health 1996;12:57–71.

121. McQuellon RP, Wells M, Hoffman S, et al: Reducing distress in cancer patients with an orientation program. Psychooncology 1998;7:207–217.

122. Fawzy FI, Fawzy NW, Arndt LA, Pasnau RO: Critical review of psychosocial interventions in cancer care. Arch Gen Psychiatry 1995;52:100–113.

123. Andersen BL: Psychological interventions for cancer patients to enhance the quality of life. J Consult Clin Psychol 1992;60:552–568.

124. Andersen BL: Biobehavioral outcomes following psychological interventions for cancer patients. J Consult Clin Psychol 2002;70:590–610.

125. Sheard T, Maguire P: The effect of psychological interventions on anxiety and depression in cancer patients: Results of two meta-analyses. Br J Cancer 1999;80:1770–1780.

126. Meyer TJ, Mark MM: Effects of psychosocial interventions with adult cancer patients: A meta-analysis of randomized experiments. Health Psychol 1995;14:101–108.

127. Helgeson VS, Cohen S, Schulz R, Yasko J: Education and peer discussion group interventions and adjustment to breast cancer. Arch Gen Psychiatry 1999;56:340–347.

128. Cruess DG, Antoni MH, McGregor BA, et al: Cognitive-behavioral stress management reduces serum cortisol by enhancing benefit finding among women being treated for early stage breast cancer. Psychosom Med 2000;62:304–308.

129. Fawzy FI, Kemeny ME, Fawzy NW, et al: A structured psychiatric intervention for cancer patients. II. Changes over time in immunological measures. Arch Gen Psychiatry 1990;47:729–735.

130. Stanton AL, Danoff-Burg S, Sworowski LA, et al: Randomized, controlled trial of written emotional expression and benefit finding in breast cancer patients. J Clin Oncol 2002;20:4160–4168.

131. Fawzy FI, Fawzy NW, Hyun CS, et al: Malignant melanoma. Effects of an early structured psychiatric intervention, coping, and affective state on recurrence and survival 6 years later. Arch Gen Psychiatry 1993;50:681–689.

132. Spiegel D, Bloom JR, Kraemer HC, Gottheil E: Effect of psychosocial treatment on survival of patients with metastatic breast cancer [see comments]. Lancet 1989;2:888–891.

133. Goodwin PJ, Leszcz M, Ennis M, et al: The effect of group psychosocial support on survival in metastatic breast cancer. N Engl J Med 2001;345:1719–1726.

134. Redd WH, Montgomery GH, DuHamel KN: Behavioral intervention for cancer treatment side effects. J Natl Cancer Inst 2001;93:810–823.

135. Antoni MH, Lehman JM, Kilbourn KM, et al: Cognitive-behavioral stress management intervention decreases the prevalence of depression and enhances benefit finding among women under treatment for early-stage breast cancer. Health Psychol 2001;20:20–32.

136. Spiegel D, Classen C: Group therapy for cancer patients: A research-based handbook of psychosocial care. New York, Basic Books, 2000.

137. Helgeson VS, Cohen S, Schulz R, Yasko J: Group support interventions for women with breast cancer: Who benefits from what? Health Psychol 2000;19:107–114.

138. Elkin I, Shea MT, Watkins JT, et al: National Institute of Mental Health Treatment of Depression Collaborative Research Program. General effectiveness of treatments. Arch Gen Psychiatry 1989;46:971–982.

139. Musselman DL, Lawson DH, Gumnick JF, et al: Paroxetine for the prevention of depression induced by high-dose interferon alfa. N Engl J Med 2001;344:961–966.

140. Day R, Ganz PA, Costantino JP, Cronin WM, Wickerham DL, Fisher B: Health-related quality of life and tamoxifen in breast cancer prevention: A report from the National Surgical Adjuvant Breast and Bowel Project P-1 Study. J Clin Oncol 1999;17: 2659–2669.

141. Fallowfield L, Fleissig A, Edwards R, et al: Tamoxifen for the prevention of breast cancer: Psychosocial impact on women participating in two randomized controlled trials. J Clin Oncol 2001;19:1885–1892.

142. Meyerowitz BE, Desmond KA, Rowland JH, Wyatt GE, Ganz PA: Sexuality following breast cancer. J Sex Marital Ther 1999;25:237–250.

143. Ganz PA, Desmond KA, Belin TR, Meyerowitz BE, Rowland JH: Predictors of sexual health in women after a breast cancer diagnosis. J Clin Oncol 1999;17:2371–2380.

144. Jonker-Pool G, van de Wiel HB, Hoekstra HJ, et al: Sexual functioning after treatment for testicular cancer—review and meta-analysis of 36 empirical studies between 1975–2000. Arch Sex Behav 2001;30:55–74.

145. Incrocci L, Hop WCJ, Wijnmaalen A, Slob AK: Treatment outcome, body image, and sexual functioning after orchiectomy and radiotherapy for stage I-II testicular seminoma. Int J Radiat Oncol Biol Phys 2002;53:1165–1173.

146. Jonker-Pool G, van Basten JP, Hoekstra HJ, et al: Sexual functioning after treatment for testicular cancer: Comparison of treatment modalities. Cancer 1997;80:454–464.

147. Schover LR, Fouladi RT, Warneke CL, et al: Defining sexual outcomes after treatment for localized prostate carcinoma. Cancer 2002;95:1773–1785.

148. Ganz PA, Litwin MS: Prostate cancer: The price of early detection. J Clin Oncol 2001;19:1587–1588.

149. Madalinska JB, Essink-Bot ML, de Koning HJ, Kirkels WJ, van der Maas PJ, Schroder FH: Health-related quality of life in patients with screen-detected versus clinically diagnosed prostate cancer preceding primary treatment. Prostate 2001;46:87–97.

150. Incrocci L, Madalinska JB, Essink-Bot ML, Van Putten WL, Koper PC, Schroder FH: Sexual functioning in patients with localized prostate cancer awaiting treatment. J Sex Marital Ther 2001;27:353–363.

151. Incrocci L, Koper PC, Hop WC, Slob AK: Sildenafil citrate (Viagra) and erectile dysfunction following external beam radiotherapy for prostate cancer: A randomized, double-blind, placebo-controlled, cross-over study. Int J Radiat Oncol Biol Phys 2001;51:1190-1195.

152. Schover LR, Fouladi RT, Warneke CL, et al: The use of treatments for erectile dysfunction among survivors of prostate carcinoma. Cancer 2002;95:2397-2407.

153. Zippe CD, Raina R, Thukral M, Lakin MM, Klein EA, Agarwal A: Management of erectile dysfunction following radical prostatectomy. Curr Urol Rep 2001;2:495-503.

154. Montorsi F, Salonia A, Zanoni M, Colombo R, Pompa P, Rigatti P: Counselling the patient with prostate cancer about treatment-related erectile dysfunction. Curr Opin Urol 2001;11:611-617.

155. Baniel J, Israilov S, Segenreich E, Livne PM: Comparative evaluation of treatments for erectile dysfunction in patients with prostate cancer after radical retropubic prostatectomy. BJU Int 2001;88:58-62.

156. Moinpour CM, Savage MJ, Troxel A, et al: Quality of life in advanced prostate cancer: Results of a randomized therapeutic trial. J Natl Cancer Inst 1998;90:1537-1544.

157. Schover LR, Fife M: Sexual counseling of patients undergoing radical surgery for pelvic or genital cancer. J Psychosoc Oncol 1985;3:21-41.

158. Mansson A, Johnson G, Mansson W: Quality of life after cystectomy. Comparison between patients with conduit and those with continent caecal reservoir urinary diversion. Br J Urol 1988;62:240-245.

159. Ganz PA, Schag CA, Lee JJ, Sim MS: The CARES: A generic measure of health-related quality of life for patients with cancer. Qual Life Res 1992;1:19-29.

160. Sarna L, Padilla G, Holmes C, Tashkin D, Brecht ML, Evangelista L: Quality of life of long-term survivors of non-small-cell lung cancer. J Clin Oncol 2002;20:2920-2929.

161. van Driel MF, Weymar Schultz WC, van de Wiel HB, Hahn DE, Mensink HJ: Female sexual functioning after radical surgical treatment of rectal and bladder cancer. Eur J Surg Oncol 1993;19:183-187.

162. Koukouras D, Spiliotis J, Scopa CD, et al: Radical consequence in the sexuality of male patients operated for colorectal carcinoma. Eur J Surg Oncol 1991;17:285-288.

163. Bergmark K, Avall-Lundqvist E, Dickman PW, Henningsohn L, Steineck G: Vaginal changes and sexuality in women with a history of cervical cancer. N Engl J Med 1999;340:1383-1389.

164. Andersen BL, Lachenbruch PA, Anderson B, deProsse C: Sexual dysfunction and signs of gynecologic cancer. Cancer 1986;57:1880-1886.

165. Andersen BL: Predicting sexual and psychologic morbidity and improving the quality of life for women with gynecologic cancer. Cancer 1993;71:1678-1690.

166. Laumann EO, Paik A, Rosen RC: Sexual dysfunction in the United States: Prevalence and predictors. JAMA 1999;281:537-544.

167. Laumann EO, Paik A, Rosen RC: The epidemiology of erectile dysfunction: Results from the National Health and Social Life Survey. Int J Impot Res 1999;11(suppl 1):S60-S64.

168. Wincze JP, Carey MP: Sexual dysfunction: A guide for assessment and treatment. New York, Guilford Press, 1991.

169. Andersen BL: Sexual functioning morbidity among cancer survivors. Current status and future research directions. Cancer 1985;55:1835-1842.

170. Andersen BL: How cancer affects sexual functioning. Oncology (Huntingt) 1990;4:81-88.

171. Schover LR, Jensen SB. Sexuality and chronic illness: A comprehensive approach. New York, Guilford Press, 1988.

172. Jensen SB, Schover LR: Brief sexual counseling for medical patients: A workshop for training professionals. J Sex Marital Ther 1988;14:13-28.

173. Loehr J, Verma S, Seguin R: Issues of sexuality in older women. J Womens Health 1997;6: 51-457.

174. Kaplan HS: A neglected issue: The sexual side effects of current treatments for breast cancer. J Sex Marital Ther 1992;18: 3-19.

175. Annon J: Behavioral treatment of sexual problems. Honolulu, Hawaii, Enabling Systems, 1974.

176. Schover LR: Sexuality and fertility after cancer. New York, John Wiley & Sons, Inc, 1997.

177. Schover LR, Evans RB, von Eschenbach AC: Sexual rehabilitation in a cancer center: Diagnosis and outcome in 384 consultations. Arch Sex Behav 1987;16:445-461.

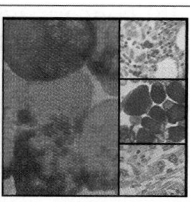

Rudranath Talukdar

Eduardo Bruera

CACHEXIA

SUMMARY OF KEY POINTS

- Cachexia is a syndrome defined by:
  - Weight loss of 5% from preillness weight
  - 5% weight loss over 2–6 months
  - Weight loss of 10% or greater equals moderate-to-severe malnutrition
- Determining actual weight loss may be confounded by presence of ascites or large pleural effusion).
- Cachexia is usually, but not always, associated with anorexia.
- Cachexia occurs in 80% of patients with advanced cancer and all occurrences are a combination of primary and secondary cachexia.
- Primary cancer cachexia is result of metabolic alterations:
  - An *increase* in energy expenditure
  - An *increase* in protein synthesis (acute phase proteins at expense of muscle proteins)
  - An *increase* in proteolysis, lipolysis, and glucose turnover

- A *decrease* in muscle proteins, lipogenesis, and ketone bodies
- Tumors produce proteolysis-inducing factor and lipid-mobilizing factor
- Autonomic dysfunction in advanced cancer causes gastroparesis, pseudo-obstruction, diarrhea, and constipation
- Secondary cancer cachexia is due to the presence of cancer and its treatment but is not directly caused by cancer. It is characterized by:
  - Impaired oral intake, impaired intestinal absorption, and excess loss of nutrients
- Secondary cachexia is the aspect of overall cachexia most amenable to treatment.
  - Aggravating factors are pain, constipation, dehydration, bowel obstruction, dysphagia, taste abnormalities, xerostomia, nausea, delirium, and infection

- Evaluation of cachexia can be accomplished by:
  - Serial weight determinations
  - Skin-fold thickness
  - Mid-arm circumference
  - Serum albumin
  - Bioelectrical impedance to measure total body fat, body mass, and body water
  - Determination of daily caloric intake
- Management of cachexia:
  - Nutritional therapy (oral, parenteral, and enteral via J-tube)
  - Pharmacologic therapy
  - Corticosteroids
  - Progestins
  - Antidopaminergic drugs
  - Others such as cyroheptadine, dronabinol, thalidomide, fish oil, androgens
  - Nonpharmacologic therapy
  - Counseling
  - Exercise

INTRODUCTION

Cachexia is a syndrome characterized by weight loss, lipolysis, muscle wasting, anorexia, chronic nausea, and asthenia, with resultant changes in body image.[1] Cachexia is usually but not always associated with anorexia, as shown in Figure 37-1. Its definition varies, but it is generally accepted as a weight loss of 5% from preillness weight or 25% weight loss over 2 to 6 months, and some clinicians believe that anorexia is a requirement for diagnosis.[2] It is increasingly referred to as the *anorexia-cachexia syndrome*.[3] It occurs in 80% of patients with advanced cancer, and the majority are afflicted with solid tumors such as breast cancer, but it also is prevalent in hematologic malignancies.[4,5]

The purpose of this chapter is to define the main causes of this syndrome and the multimodal options needed to treat it. Understanding cachexia and its causes will aid in its management and should increase the quality of life of the patients who have this distressing syndrome associated with cancer. Such knowledge will ease the burden for their families who suffer with them.

MECHANISM

The old hypothesis of cachexia, one that is still the prevalent dogma among the lay public and some medical professionals is one of a reductionist energy model. It can be described as analogous to a battery: the tumor uses up energy, acting as a drain, thereby not allowing the body to function at "full power" (Fig. 37-2).

Figure 37-1. The relation between cachexia and anorexia.

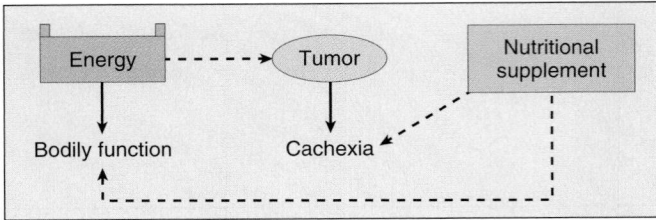

Figure 37-2. A reductionist energy model of cachexia.

The terminology we use to describe the syndrome is illustrative: "She/he is powerless to fight the disease." This view leads naturally to its corollary: if you add more power, then you can override the deterioration in bodily functions and "overpower" or "defeat" the cancer.

The mechanism of cancer-related cachexia can be divided for the purposes of discussion into two broad headings: Primary and Secondary.

Primary Cachexia

Primary cachexia and anorexia represent a metabolic syndrome, directly caused by the cancer, in which complex metabolic and neuroendocrine modifications occur in the context of an ongoing, altered, inflammatory state.[6,7] The metabolic alterations that occur can be listed as an *increase* in energy expenditure, protein synthesis (largely acute-phase proteins at the expense of muscle proteins), proteolysis, lipolysis, glucose turnover; and a *decrease* in muscle proteins, lipogenesis, and ketone bodies.

Pathogenesis of the Primary Cachexia-Anorexia Syndrome

In patients with this syndrome, the basal metabolic rate is increased, when corrected for lean body mass (LBM). The liver produces acute-phase proteins that play a role in the inflammatory and antitumor process but draw their energy from muscle breakdown. Glucose turnover is increased, and the anerobic pathway of glucose utilization (lactate pathway) is increased, while a relative glucose intolerance in muscle and insulin resistance develop. Hypertriglyceridemia is found in such patients from suppression of de novo lipogenesis and peripheral activation of lipolysis, whereas central (hepatic) lipogenesis is increased. Whole-body protein turnover is increased, and liver protein synthesis is directed toward increase in the production of acute-phase proteins and lower production of albumin. The overall turnover of branched-chain amino acids and alanine and glutamine in the muscle are increased.[8]

Feeding of the patient with cancer cachexia was found to increase acute-phase protein production without influencing the rate of albumin synthesis[9] and to increase muscle protein synthesis without changing proteolysis.[10] Food intake (appetite and hunger) are regulated by a complex process comprising sensory input, humoral signals,[11] and inhibitory or facilitory input from the brain, which has been trained in the cultural and psychosocial milieu.[8]

The vagus nerve mediates, in concert with the sympathetic system, the feeling of satiety from the liver and gastrointestinal (GI) tract. It also is affected by the antikinetic peptide, cholecystokinin, and it mediates the activity of ghrelin, a hormone that is adipogenic, orexigenic, and gastroprokinetic.[12] The effects of ghrelin were reported to be lost after vagotomy. Baseline plasma ghrelin level was elevated in patients with cachexia and lung cancer, and follow-up plasma ghrelin level increased in patients with anorexia after chemotherapy. Considering the positive energy effects induced by ghrelin, increased ghrelin may represent a compensatory mechanism under catabolic–anabolic imbalance in patients with cachexia and lung cancer.[13]

Other mediators such as neuropeptide Y, melanin-concentrating hormone, and endocannabinoids are orexigenic; neuropeptide Y is overexpressed in rats that have insulin-deficiency diabetes and are underfed. Endocannabinoid receptor type I (CB I) was involved in maintaining food intake.[14] CB I knockout mice eat less than wild-type mice, and CB I antagonist SR 141716A reduced food intake in wild-type but not in CB I knockout mice. Others, such as leptin and α-melanocyte–stimulating hormone, are anorexigenic. Leptin stimulates the catabolic and inhibits the anabolic pathways in the hypothalamus and the GI tract.[15] However, the effects of leptin on the cachexia syndrome are complex, and its levels tend to remain stable in patients with cancer. The suggestion is that decreasing fat stores inhibit leptin, whereas inflammation increases it.

Anabolic steroid hormones such as testosterone, nandrolone, oxandrolone, and fluoxymesterone have been shown to be reduced in men with acquired immunodeficiency syndrome (AIDS)-related cachexia, weight loss, and disease progression.[16-18] Studies in patients with cancer have shown a correlation between hypogonadism and weight loss. Three trials found that treatment with anabolic steroids had a minor effect on improving weight loss. Insulin-like growth factor–binding proteins (IGFBPs) have lower levels in later tumor stages.[19] This affects protein synthesis by increasing resistance to growth hormone (GH), such that the anabolic effects of GH on protein synthesis are diminished.

Cytokines play an important role in this mix. Tumor necrosis factor (TNF) has long been known to mimic the effects of cachexia and was first named "cachectin" after its role was suggested in kala-azar patients. As discussed later, thalidomide, an inhibitor of TNF, has been shown to increase the appetite and weight of patients with cachexia in some small series. Other proinflammatory cytokines include interleukin-1 (IL-1), IL-6, and interferon (INF)-gamma. However, cytokines work at a very local level, and serum concentrations do not reflect the completeness of their role in creating the syndrome that is cachexia.

Some factors are derived from tumors themselves. The proteolysis-inducing factor (PIF) appears to bind to skeletal muscle and liver cells and is correlated with weight loss.[20] The lipid-mobilizing factor (LMF) induces lipolysis and also is associated with weight loss.[21] Many studies reported isolation from many tumors a heterogeneous group of small peptides, generally labeled *toxohormones*, which cause various correlates of cachexia shortly after injection into mice.[22]

Autonomic dysfunction is common in advanced cancer patients, and that plays a part in the anorexia-cachexia syndrome through causing gastroparesis, pseudo-obstruction, diarrhea, and constipation.

Secondary Cachexia

Secondary cachexia is due to the cancer but not directly caused by it: the causes are impaired oral intake, impaired absorption, and excess loss, summarized in Table 37-1.

Clinically it is hard to distinguish the relative importance of any of these in any individual patient, and therefore, based on the clinical picture, a comprehensive program must be tailored for each patient. The relative impact of any of the secondary causes is a clinical judgment and calls forth the art of analysis by the physician. This is the part most amenable to treatment, as discussed later in this chapter.

Assessment of Anorexia and Cachexia

The assessment of secondary cachexia depends on the diagnosis of the many possible causes listed in Table 37-2. A systematic assessment of secondary cachexia is essential to determine the relative importance this plays in the overall clinical picture.

Common aggravating factors for anorexia-cachexia in advanced cancer are pain, constipation, bowel obstruction, dysphagia, taste abnormalities, xerostomia, nausea, delirium, and infection.

TABLE 37-1

Mechanism of Secondary Anorexia-Cachexia in Cancer Patients

Starvation and malnutrition
Impaired oral intake
Stomatitis, taste alterations, and zinc deficiency
Xerostomia, dehydration, autonomic failure, emesis
Severe constipation
Bowel obstruction
Severe pain, dyspnea, depression
Delirium
Social and financial problems
Impaired gastrointestinal absorption
Malabsorption
Exocrine pancreatic insufficiency
Chronic severe diarrhea
Significant protein loss
Frequent drainage of nutrient-rich ascitic or pleural fluid
Nephrotic syndrome
Other catabolic states
Chronic and acute infections
Treatment with proinflammatory cytokines
Chronic heart failure, chronic lung disease, or chronic renal failure
Other chronically uncontrolled diseases such as hypothyroidism, diabetes mellitus, cirrhosis
Loss of muscle mass
Prolonged bed-rest, deconditioning
Growth hormone deficiency, hypogonadism, aging, sarcopenia

Or a combination of all of the above.

TABLE 37-2

Symptom Assessment in Cachexia

Visual Analog Scale

Anorexia
Fatigue or asthenia
Chronic nausea
Perceived change of body image

Oral Intake

History of involuntarily reduced oral intake
Estimation of caloric intake

Body Composition

Weight and a recent history of involuntary weight loss
Clinical judgment of cachexia: subjective global assessment
Serum albumin
DEXA, estimation of body water
Anthropometric measurements such as mid-arm circumference, skin-fold thickness
Bio-impedance analysis

Function

Performance status
EFAT
FAACT
Dynamometer: grip strength, elbow flexor muscles, knee extensor muscles

Causes of Cachexia and Anorexia

See previous discussion and table of secondary and aggravating causes

Overall Condition of the Patient and the Family

Individual and familial impact of cachexia
Oncology situation, prognosis, antineoplastic treatments
Symptom distress from physical, psychosocial, and existential factors
Attitudes of the patient and family toward treatment goals and nutrition

DEXA, Dual energy x-ray absorptiometry; EFAT, Edmonton functional assessment tool; FAACT, Functional assessment of appetite cachexia therapy.

Bowel obstruction can have multiple causes, including extrinsic and internal occlusion from the tumor itself and functional obstruction from medications, usually opioids. Obstipation is a common and under-recognized problem in cancer patients and can lead to a vicious cycle of progressively increasing obstruction. Some cancers, such as ovarian cancers, are commonly associated with malignant bowel obstruction.

Dehydration also causes problems in multiple ways: by causing xerostomia and poor oral intake, by causing reduced intestinal fluids, and by reducing mentation. Other important, and often overlooked causes include decreased physical activity, impaired intestinal neuro-muscular function caused by opioids, calcium channel blockers, hypercalcemia, hypokalemia, anticholinergic drugs (e.g., tricyclic antidepressants), phenothiazines, serotonin (5-HT) antagonists, sympathomimetics such as clonidine, iron supplementation, antihistamines, hypothyroid state, autonomic failure, and plexopathy. A low zinc level in cancer patients has been associated with altered taste. Zinc supplementation improved this sensation.[23]

Clinical Evaluation of Cachexia

Weight loss is the main clinical finding in patients with cancer cachexia. A simple way of estimating the extent of weight loss is to calculate the percentage loss compared with the weight before the diagnosis of cancer. A weight loss of 10% or more is generally an indicator of moderate to severe malnutrition.[5] The presence of edema or fluid collection, such as ascites or large pleural effusions, can make interpretation of weight loss difficult. However, in the absence of these abnormalities, weight loss is a reliable sign of cachexia in cancer patients, mostly because this syndrome is a chronic feature.

Simple measurements taken at the bedside can help to characterize cachexia and the response to nutritional and pharmacologic interventions. The skin-fold thickness can be measured with simple calipers for the triceps, biceps, subscapular, and suprailiac regions. The mid-arm circumference can be used to calculate muscle circumference by a simple formula.[24] In some cases, laboratory tests can be used, such as albumin and rapid-turnover proteins including thyroxin-binding prealbumin and retinol-binding protein. However, tests for these short–half-life proteins are expensive and not very relevant to patients with cancer cachexia.

Bioelectrical impedance is a safe and rapid bedside technique that measures total body fat, body mass, and body water. Its main limitation is the lack of a standard norm in cancer patients.[25] However, it has accuracy for the prediction of body composition similar to that of the anthropometric tests.[25]

The assessment of caloric intake can be made at the bedside by a nutritionist or a trained nurse. It allows a better understanding of the contribution of decreased dietary intake to weight in a given patient. Methods such as dietary records, prospective records, and recall records have been used for the assessment of caloric intake.[25,26] However, limits exist to the use of recall records in the patients who have asthenia, depression, or cognitive failure. A simple method for prospective third-person assessment of food intake is the percentage calculation of food products consumed at each meal by the patient. Nurses or volunteers can perform this calculation by simple observation, and it correlates well with the actual weighing of the food.[27]

Anorexia is a major, if not the most important, target of nutritional and pharmacologic interventions. The intensity of this symptom can be reliably assessed with visual analogue scales, numeric scales, verbal descriptors, or subjective questionnaires, with items such as, "Do you feel your appetite has improved since starting the treatment?"[26] Anorexia is a multidimensional symptom, and it is generally the result of many factors such as those shown in Figure 37-3. In a given patient, the coexistence of multiple causes can be identified, some of them directly related to the presence of the tumor, and some of them to comorbid factors that are reversible, such as drugs, constipation, or depression, as illustrated in Figure 37-3.

It is crucial to emphasize that the division of the cachexia-anorexia syndrome into primary and secondary is important only to clarify the syndrome and for research purposes. Virtually all patients have a combination of

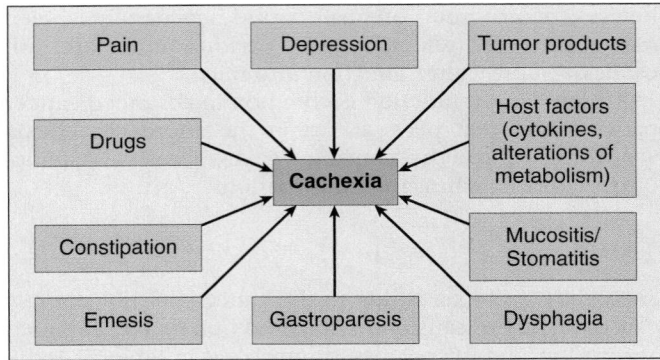

Figure 37-3. Coexistence of multiple causes of cachexia.

primary and secondary causes and must be managed as individuals.

MANAGEMENT

As seen from the preceding discussion, cachexia is a multidimensional construct, and a careful evaluation is essential to provide the therapy most likely to benefit the patient. Consideration must be given to the patient's physical, psychological, and social milieu. In such patients, often one is discussing options and coming to a joint decision with the family of the affected patient.

The few reversible causes of anorexia and cachexia are managed by their specialties (e.g., surgery for bowel obstruction vs a J-tube) and are outside the scope of this discussion (see Chapter 53). These must be assessed and treated and require close coordination between and among the various specialties taking care of the patient with cancer.

Obviously, the treatment of cancer cachexia is treating the cause (i.e., remove the tumor either mechanically or pharmacotherapeutically). This is often not an option; however, a targeted and selected group might benefit from systemic antineoplastic therapy to relieve or reduce their distress with anorexia and cachexia. For example, a patient with radiosensitive tumor compressing the bowel should have the benefit of radiation to relieve the distress.

For purposes of our discussion, management of cachexia and anorexia is divided into nutritional, pharmacologic, and nonpharmacologic, with the understanding that these modalities are interconnected and occur contemporaneously in nearly all patients (Table 37-3.)

Nutritional

For a long time, lack of nutrition was regarded as the cause for cachexia. From experience with kwashiorkor and protein-calorie malnutrition, it was thought that supplementing energy would solve the cachexia problem. During the decades of the 1980s and 1990s, valiant efforts were made to do just that. However, attempts to increase nutritional intake were not associated with an improvement in outcomes (survival, tumor response, reduction

TABLE 37-3

 Management of Cachexia

Nutritional

- Common misperception among patients and family that increased nutrition helps
- Small energy-dense meals best; fats, however, are hard to digest
- Attention to oral care
- Select patients with starvation component benefit from enteral and parenteral nutrition

Pharmacologic

- Corticosteroids: well proven to work for a short time in increasing appetite, weight, sense of well-being
- Progestins (medroxyprogesterone acetate) increase appetite, well-being, and weight (fat), and reduce fatigue
- Prokinetic agent: metoclopramide is effective in patients with chronic nausea or constipation, and those taking opioids
- Other agents with significant promise include thalidomide, oxandrolone, and, possibly, ghrelin. Limited value has been found with fish oil, Dronabinol, and cyproheptadine

Nonpharmacologic

- Counseling is very important, even critical, in reframing the concept of "starving to death"
- Exercise maintains lean body mass, especially in conjunction with agents such as androgens

---

QUESTIONS TO HELP IN ASSESSING THE BENEFIT OF NUTRITION

- Is the location or type of cancer causing a starvation component? Examples include patients with bowel obstruction, patients receiving radiation therapy in head and neck cancers, pre- and postsurgery patients, and patients treated with high-dose chemotherapy protocols. (One must not forget those patients kept without oral food [NPO] for one test after another for days while in the hospital!)
- Is reversible inflammation present? As discussed earlier, inflammation releases a cytokine soup with effects on cachexia
- What is the life expectancy of the patient? (Karnofsky and Eastern Cooperative Oncology Group [ECOG] scales; see Table 25-1)
- Is the patient dehydrated?
- What are the goals of the patient and his or her family? Is an adverse body image present? Realistic goals may include relief from hunger or modifying disrupted body image by increasing fat tissue
- Has dietary counseling been done? This has been reported to result in a temporary increase the caloric intake, around 450 kCal/day[34]

---

of cancer therapy–related toxicity, quality of life).[28-31] Feeding of the patient with cancer-related cachexia was reported to increase the synthesis of muscle proteins but did not influence proteolysis.[32] It accelerated acute-phase protein synthesis without influencing the rate of albumin synthesis.[33] Weight gain was associated primarily with an increase in LBM and more so with an increase in body water and fat. The American College of Physicians' guidelines for patients receiving chemotherapy discourages provision of routine parenteral nutrition. However, a subset of patients would benefit from nutritional supplementation. This subset consists of those in whom a starvation component of their cachexia is predominant (see secondary causes).

Small frequent meals and energy-dense snacks that are easy to eat are the best option for patients experiencing early satiety and reduced appetite.[35] Food should be served in pleasant surroundings, with small portions served on small plates so as not to overwhelm patients. Caregivers should avoid expressing concern over poor intake. Although fat is a high-energy source, food should not contain a lot of fat because it delays gastric emptying and may exacerbate nausea and vomiting. During end-stage disease, changes are found in taste perception and food sensitivities that result in reduced tolerance for extremes in temperature and flavor, and a reduced appetite for meat, thus leading to preferences for bland, starch-based foods. To increase intake, fluids or ice chips should be served between feedings rather than with them. Owing to compromised immune status, no raw eggs, uncooked meat, fish, or poultry should be served. Just as in medical treatment, the primary goal of nutritional support is to provide compassionate palliative care to the terminally ill patient by improving comfort and relief of symptoms.[36]

As the disease progresses, oral intake is likely to decrease to almost nothing. At that stage, adequate mouth care and small amounts of ice chips or sips of cold beverages may be adequate for some patients. For patients with symptoms related to dehydration, the use of hypodermoclysis can be very useful in maintaining adequate hydration at home at little cost and with minimal invasiveness.[37]

Consideration of enteral and parenteral nutrition should be made. If the bowel is available, it should be used. Enteral nutrition can have problems such as aspiration, diarrhea, constipation, fistulae, electrolyte abnormalities, hyperglycemia, feeding-tube malfunction, emesis, malabsorption, and infections. Parenteral nutrition may afford the patient the opportunity to go home and avoid hospitalization but must be weighed against infection risk, pneumothorax, electrolyte abnormality, repeated blood tests, venous thrombosis, malposition, blockage of access, and the severe cost burden. It may be difficult to withdraw parenteral nutrition once started because of family distress.

Pharmacologic Therapy

Corticosteroids

At least six double-blind randomized controlled trials have demonstrated the symptomatic effect of different types and doses of corticosteroids for cancer cachexia.[38] Most research has shown a limited effect of up to 4 weeks on symptoms such as appetite, food intake, sensation of well-being, and performance status. Most studies have not shown significant gain in body weight. The best type and dose of corticosteroids has not been established, but most investigators used doses of 20 to 40 mg prednisone or equivalent.[38] The mechanism of effect on appetite, energy, and well-being is unclear; it may be related to central euphoric activity, in addition to prostaglandin metabolites or the inhibition of cytokine release.[38] Despite the wide range of side effects and cautions recommended by some researchers, the use of corticosteroids in advanced cancer is becoming widely accepted. Owing to their short-lasting but significant symptomatic benefits, these drugs can be used in patients with short expected survival in whom weight gain is not a likely outcome.

Progestins

Trials of progestagens as therapy for hormone-responsive tumors found significant weight gain in patients with or without tumor response.[38] The findings prompted investigations of these drugs for treatment of cachexia. More than 12 randomized controlled trials found that megestrol acetate can improve appetite, caloric intake, and nutritional variables in patients with advanced cancer. Similar findings have been reported for patients with AIDS-related cachexia.[38] Megestrol acetate shows dose-related benefit (doses of 160 to 1600 mg) on appetite, caloric intake, weight gain (mostly fat), and sensation of well-being with an optimum dose of about 800 mg daily.[39] The adverse effects are probably related to dose and the number of tablets taken. Because this drug is expensive at high doses, a low starting dose is justifiable (300 to 480 mg daily) with titration upward according to clinical response. In patients who are expected to survive more than 4 weeks, a trial of megestrol acetate can be considered standard therapy for cachexia.

Recent studies of terminally ill patients have shown rapid (<1 week) symptomatic improvement (appetite, fatigue, and general well-being) with lower doses of megestrol (160 to 480 mg daily) compared with placebo, without any significant change in nutritional status.[40] These studies suggest that megestrol has beneficial symptomatic effects by mechanisms other than weight gain. Studies on medroxyprogesterone acetate also showed symptomatic and nutritional benefits.[41] The mechanism of action of these drugs remains to be clarified and may be related to glucocorticoid or anabolic activity, as well as to effects on cytokine release. Medroxyprogesterone acetate can induce appetite via stimulation of neuropeptide Y,[38] and it may inhibit the activity of some cytokines such as ILs 1 and 6 and TNF.[42] Both megestrol and medroxyprogesterone can induce thromboembolic complications; breakthrough bleeding, peripheral edema, hyperglycemia, hypertension, Cushing's syndrome, alopecia, adrenal suppression, and adrenal insufficiency, particularly if the drug is abruptly discontinued.[43] In most clinical trials, patients rarely need to stop these drugs because of side effects. However, one study of patients receiving anti-neoplastic therapy for non–small-cell lung cancer showed that megestrol might decrease survival and increase the rate of thromboembolic disease.[44]

Antidopaminergic Agents

Metoclopramide, an antidopaminergic drug with effective central antiemetic and gastric-emptying properties, is particularly effective for patients who complain of chronic nausea.[45] Autonomic failure and opioid therapy are among the conditions that predict a response to metoclopramide. In such patients, the use of regular oral or subcutaneous metoclopramide can result in significant improvement in appetite and food intake.[45]

Other Agents

Cyproheptadine, a 5-HT3 antagonist is used in Europe and Asia as an appetite stimulant but is quite sedating, thereby limiting its use in cancer patients.

Thalidomide is a mild anxiolytic and antiemetic and reduces the production of TNF-α. It was found to be useful in reducing the subjective symptoms of cachexia.[46] In an open-label study, patients taking thalidomide gained an average of 1.29 kg over a 2-week period after having lost weight in advanced esophageal cancer over the previous 2 weeks without thalidomide.[47] In a preliminary study of 37 evaluable patients, it was found that administration of thalidomide led to significant improvements in appetite, nausea, and sense of well-being.[48]

Dronabinol, a synthetic cannabinoid, is Food and Drug Administration (FDA) approved to treat nausea. Anecdotal evidence has suggested improvement in appetite, and it is widely used as a raw product outside medical practice. Limited evidence is found for appetite stimulation, however, with minor or no overall nutritional advantages in AIDS or cancer cachexia. The remaining indications are largely supported by anecdotal case reports and small uncontrolled case series.

The main limitation of cannabinoids has been the high frequency of adverse effects on the central nervous system. These consist mostly of perceptual abnormalities, including occasional hallucinations, dysphoria, abnormal thinking, depersonalization, and somnolence.[49,50] In addition, cannabinoids at higher doses have been associated with hypotension, ataxia, blurred vision, and dizziness. These effects appear to be mostly dose related and more severe in the elderly.

Uncontrolled studies have found that *fish oil*, in the form of eicosapentanoic acid (EPA) administered alone or as part of nutritional supplements,[51-53] is capable of stabilizing weight loss in some patients who have pancreatic cancer. Furthermore, a placebo-controlled study of 60 patients having generalized solid tumors who underwent fish oil treatment until death reported a survival advantage and increased performance status, and no changes in body weight or albumin level were observed; however, symptom distress was not assessed.[54] One recent randomized controlled trial found that fish oil without nutritional supplements did not significantly influence appetite, tiredness, nausea, well-being, caloric intake, nutritional status, or function after 2 weeks, compared with placebo in patients with advanced cancer and loss of both weight and appetite.[55] Another trial compared EPA, the active ingredient in fish oil, with or without megesterol acetate, and found no advantage over megesterol acetate alone.[56]

Androgens have received more attention recently, and some effects have been found. In two open-label, 4-month studies, 128 patients with human immuno-deficiency virus (HIV) and 131 with cancer received 20 mg of oxandrolone per day and also were educated about nutrition and exercise. Of those with cancer, 80%

maintained or gained weight; the average increase in lean tissue was 4 lbs. Patients with HIV gained an average of 4.6 lbs of lean tissue.[57]

Nandrolone, an injectable derivative of 19-nortestosterone, has had widespread off-label use among body builders. Its only current approved use is for anemia in patients with chronic renal failure. Several open-label studies and preliminary results of placebo-controlled studies suggest that nandrolone has the potential to be an effective therapy for lean tissue loss in patients with HIV-associated wasting. Weight gain up to 2 or more kilograms has been reported in studies of nandrolone (100 mg/week for 12 weeks) in borderline hypogonadal men with wasting,[58] and in eugonadal HIV-positive men with no history of weight loss that were given a considerably higher dose (600 mg/week for 12 weeks).[59] In this latter study, muscle mass and strength also increased significantly. In addition, subjects who were randomly assigned to undergo supervised progressive resistance exercise during nandrolone treatment had further increases in weight, LBM, and strength, suggesting that the protein anabolic effects of nandrolone can be augmented by concurrent resistance exercise.[59]

In another small study, patients randomized to nandrolone had significant decreases in total testosterone, sex-hormone–binding globulin, follicle-stimulating hormone, luteinizing hormone, and high-density lipoprotein (HDL) cholesterol levels, and increases in hemoglobin and hematocrit. Nandrolone had no significant effect on liver enzymes.[60]

Oxandrolone is an oral testosterone derivative approved by the FDA as a short-term treatment for weight loss incurred in conjunction with surgery, chronic infection, trauma, or prolonged use of corticosteroids. Oxandrolone treatment was associated with improvements in self-reported appetite and activity.[57] No toxicities were reported. Higher doses of oxandrolone have been studied in HIV-wasting, but no data are available on either safety or efficacy.

The effect of combining oxandrolone with testosterone and resistance exercise also has been studied.[61] A total of 24 eugonadal HIV-positive men with weight loss all received testosterone (100 mg/week) and underwent supervised progressive resistance exercise training for 8 weeks; in addition, they were randomly assigned to receive oxandrolone (20 mg/day) or placebo during this time. Increases in LBM (+6.9 vs +3.8 kg) and indices of strength were significantly greater in the group cotreated with oxandrolone, compared with changes in men who received testosterone and exercise only. As with pharmacologic testosterone and nandrolone, oxandrolone treatment produced significant decreases in HDL cholesterol.

Another oral agent, oxymetholone, promoted weight gain in HIV-positive patients (mean, +5.7 kg) when given in a dose of 50 mg 3 times daily in an open-label study.[62] The composition of weight gain was not measured. Self-reported appetite and quality of life also improved. More recently, preliminary data are available from a randomized, double-blind, placebo-controlled study in which 92 subjects received oxymetholone in total daily doses of 100 or 150 mg or placebo.[63] Both dosing levels of oxymetholone produced significant increases in weight and LBM (+3.7 and +2.7 kg for weight and LBM, respectively, in the group that received 100 mg/day). However, elevations in liver enzymes occurred in 14% of patients who received oxymetholone. The dose of 100 mg/day appeared to have equivalent efficacy, with less toxicity, than 150 mg/day. Oxymetholone is currently approved as a treatment for anemia, but not for wasting. This research from the HIV field may be applicable to cachexia in cancer patients, but that research has yet to be done.

Growth hormone stimulates muscle protein synthesis and wound healing in various catabolic states. Animal studies have shown that GH supplementation results in increased carcass weight, muscle weight, and muscle protein content in protein-fed, tumor-bearing animals.[64] In a randomized controlled trial in HIV patients, GH induced sustained weight gain, increased (LBM), loss of body fat, and increased strength, as measured by treadmill work over 12 weeks of treatment.[65] No such trial has been done in patients with cancer cachexia.

Some drugs have a following among the lay public, and for that reason, are mentioned here. Hydrazine sulfate was initially developed to inhibit gluconeogenesis. Pilot study reports of improved appetite and nutritional status prompted three large randomized placebo-controlled trials. None of these trials found any evidence of symptomatic improvement in terms of weight gain, but substantial side effects and deterioration in the quality-of-life scales were found in patients who were assigned hydrazine sulfate compared with those assigned placebo.[66–68] At present, therefore, no justification exists for further research on this drug. However, it continues to be widely used as an alternative therapy, both in North America and in Europe.

Insulin-like growth factor (IGF-I) was thought to be better than GH for sustaining weight gain; however, in metabolic studies, treatment with IGF-I did not consistently attain levels of nitrogen retention seen with GH, and its dosing was limited by the hypoglycemic effects of excess free IGF-I.[38]

Nonpharmacologic Therapy

Counseling of the patient and the family and loved ones is very important in assuring them that their fears and needs have a outlet to be expressed and acted on. In addition, it provides a venue to reframe the condition from that of "starving to death" to the more complex one of irreversible (usually) metabolic abnormalities and the futility of pushing nutrition. This reframing can decrease the distress in both patients and families and can maintain the social benefit of mealtimes.

Exercise, when possible, should be encouraged, as it reduces deconditioning and promotes maintenance of muscle mass. Patients should be encouraged to get out of their bed and hospital room to see the outside world. Physical therapy and occupational therapy are very important in maintaining muscle function, activities of daily living, and safety. Extensive psychosocial counseling for both the patient and their loved ones is needed as the

Cancer cachexia is a multidimensional syndrome caused by the interplay of a number of factors from the tumor and the body's response to the tumor, including humoral, nervous, and mechanical responses. The mainstay of treatment is treating the cancer, increasing appetite by treating constipation, using prokinetic agents such as metoclopramide, progestins such as medroxyprogesterone acetate, and androgens such as oxandrolone with a structured program of counseling. Increased nutritional intake by artificial means such as tube feedings and parenteral feedings is not generally associated with increased survival or better quality of life.

disease progresses, and the goals may need to be adapted. For example, going for a short trip in the car may no longer be an option, but sitting in the chair by the window might.

SUMMARY

The understanding of cachexia and anorexia has evolved over the last decade and has become a multidimensional and multicausal construct. Patients with cachexia will necessarily need to be assessed for all the complex reasons leading to cachexia and treated in a multimodal, multidisciplinary fashion to attain the maximal improvement in symptoms.

Basic research has shown and is showing the way in which tumors and host interact and pointing to therapeutic modalities. In the future, the role of newly characterized hormones such as ghrelin could become much more prominent, and others that made an initial splash, such as IGF, may fade.

Clinical research has shown the value of many drugs in alleviating symptoms, with prokinetic agents such as metoclopramide, steroids such as corticosteroids, medroxyprogesterone acetate, and the newer synthetic testosterone analogues such as oxandrolone. The effect of simple interventions such as relieving constipation also has been emphasized.

As discussed earlier, a thorough assessment of cachexia is necessary to attack the problem from multiple angles and not only from the point of view of reducing the tumor mass.

REFERENCES

1. Bruera E, Sweeney C: Cachexia and asthenia in cancer patients. Lancet Oncology 2000;1:138-147.
2. Strasser F, Bruera E: Cancer anorexia/cachexia syndrome: Epidemiology, pathogensis and assessment. In: Bruera E, Ripamonti C (eds): Gastrointestinal Symptoms in Advanced Cancer. Oxford, Oxford University Press, 2002, pp. 39-80.
3. Strasser F, Bruera E: Update on anorexia and cachexia. Hematol Oncol Clin North Am 2002;16(3):589-617.
4. Ma G, Bruera E (eds): Topics in Palliative Care, vol 2. New York, Oxford University Press, 1998.
5. Dunlop R, Bruera E: Anorexia-cachexia. In Higginson I, Bruera E (eds): Clinical Epidemiology of Cancer Cachexia. Oxford, Oxford University Press, 1996.
6. Tisdale MJ: Wasting in cancer. J Nutr 1999;129(suppl IS):243S-246S.
7. Jaskowiak NT, Alexander HR: The pathophysiology of cancer cachexia. In: Idoyle D, Hanks GWC, MacDonald N, (eds): Oxford Textbook of Palliative Medicine. 2nd ed. New York, Oxford University Press, 1998, pp 534-548.
8. Strasser F, Bruera E: Mechanism of cancer cachexia: Progress on disentangling a complex problem. Progress in Palliative Care 2002;10:161-166.
9. Barber MD, Fearon KC, McMillan DC, Slater C, Rose JA, Preston J: Liver export protein synthetic rates are increased by oral meal feeding in weight losing cancer patients. Am J Physiol Endocrinol Metab 2000;279:E707-E714.
10. Bozzetti F, Gavazzi C, Ferrari P, et al: Effect of total parenteral nutrition on the protein kinetics of patients with cancer cachexia. Tumori 2000;86:408-411.
11. Schwartz MW, Woods SC, Porte D Jr, et al: Central nervous system control of food intake. Nature 2000;404:661-671.
12. Nakazato M, Murakami N, Date Y, et al: A role for ghrelin in the central regulation of feeding. Nature 2001;409:194-198.
13. Shmizu Y, Nagaya N, Isobe T: Clin Cancer Res 2003;9:774-778.
14. Walsh D, Nelson KA, Mahmoud FA: Established and potential therapeutic applications of cannabinoids in oncology. Support Care Cancer. 2003;11:137-143.
15. Di Marzo V, Goparaju SK, Wang L, et al: Leptin-regulated endocannabinoids are involved in maintaining food intake. Nature 2001;410:822-825.
16. Simons JP, Schols AM, Burman WA, et al: Weight loss and low body cell mass in males with lung cancer: Relationship with systemic inflammation, acute phase response, resting energy expenditure and catabolic and anabolic hormones. Clin Sci (Lond) 1999;97:215-223.
17. Grinspoon S, Corcoran C, Lee K, et al: Loss of lean body and muscle mass correlates with androgen levels in hypogonadal men with acquired immunodeficiency syndrome and wasting. J Clin Endocrinol Metab 1996;81:4051-4058.
18. Dobs AS, Few WL III, Blackman MR, et al: Serum hormones in men with human immunodeficiency virus-associated wasting. J Clin Endocrinol Metab 1996;81:4108-4112.
19. Helle SI, Geisler S, Aas T, et al: Plasma insulin-like growth factor binding protein-3 proteolysis is increased in primary breast cancer. Br J Cancer 2001;85:183-186.
20. Todorov PT, Cariuk P, McDevitt T, et al: Characterization of a cancer cachectic factor. Nature 1966;379:739-742.
21. Islam-Ali B, Khan S, Price SA, et al: Modulation of adipocyte G-protein expression in cancer cachexia by lipid mobilizing factor (LMF). Br J Cancer 2001;85:758-763.
22. Rubin H: Cancer cachexia: Its correlations and causes. Proc Natl Acad Sci U S A. 2003;29:5384-5389. Epub 2003 Apr 17.
23. Ripamonti C, Zecca E, Brunelli C, et al: A randomized controlled trial to evaluate the effects of zinc sulfate on cancer patients with taste alterations caused by head and neck irradiation. Cancer 1998;82:1938-1945.
24. Conlisk EA, Haas JD, Martinez EJ, et al: Predicting body composition from anthropometry and bioimpedance. Am J Clin Nutr 1992;55:1051-1059.
25. Burman R, Chamberlain J: The assessment of the nutritional status, caloric intake, and appetite of patients with advanced cancer. In Bruera E, Higginson I (eds): Cachexia-Anorexia in Cancer Patients. Oxford, Oxford University Press, 1996, pp 83-93.
26. Persson C, Sjoden PO, Glimelius B: The Swedish version of the patient generated subjective global assessment of nutritional status: Gastrointestinal vs. urological cancers. Clin Nutr 1999;18:71-77.
27. Bruera E, Chadwicks S, Cowan L, et al: Caloric intake assessment in advanced cancer patients: A comparison of three methods. Cancer Treat Rep 1986;70:981-983.
28. Klein S, Kinney J, Jeejeebhoy K, et al: Nutrition support in clinical practice: Review of published data and recommendations for future research directions: Summary of a conference sponsored by the National Institutes of Health, American Society of Parenteral and Enteral Nutrition, and American Society for Clinical Nutrition. Am J Clin Nutr 1997;66:683-706.

29. Bozzetti F, Amadori D, Bruera E, et al: Guidelines on artificial nutrition versus hydration in terminal cancer patients: European Association for Palliative Care. Nutrition 1996;12:163-167.

30. Winter SM: Terminal nutrition: Framing the debate for the withdrawal of nutritional support in terminally ill patients [review]. Am J Med 2000;109:723-726.

31. Torelli GF, Campos AC, Meguid MM: Use of TPN in terminally ill cancer patients. Nutrition 1999;15:665-667.

32. Bozetti F, Gavarri C, Ferrari P, et al: Effect of total parenteral nutrition on the protein kinetics of patients with cancer cachexia. Tumori 2000;86:408-411.

33. Barber MD, Feron KC, McMillan DC, et al: Liver export protein synthetic rates are increased by oral meal feeding in weight losing cancer patients. Am J Physiol Endocrinol Metab 2000;279:E707-E714.

34. Ovesen L, Allingstrup L, Hannibal J, et al: Effect of dietary counseling on food intake, body weight, response rate, survival, and quality of life in cancer patients undergoing chemotherapy: A prospective randomized study. J Clin Oncol 1993;11:2043-2049.

35. Loprinzi CL, Goldberg RM, Goldberg JQ: Placebo-controlled trial of hydrazine sulfate in patients with newly diagnosed non-small-cell lung cancer. J Clin Oncol 1994;12:1126-1129.

36. Kosty MP, Fleishman SB, Herndon JE, et al: Cisplatin, vinblastine, and hydrazine sulfate in advanced non-small-cell lung cancer: A randomized placebo-controlled double-blind phase III study of the cancer and leukemia group B. J Clin Oncol 1994;12:1113-1120.

37. Bruera E, Legris MA, Kuehn N, et al: Hypodermoclysis for the administration of fluids and narcotic analgesics in patients with advanced cancer. J Pain Symptom Manage 1990;5:218-220.

38. Gagnon B, Bruera E: A review of the drug treatment of cachexia associated with cancer. Drugs 1998;55:675-688.

39. Loprinzi CL, Michalak JC, Schaid DJ, et al: Phase III evaluation of four doses of megestrol acetate as therapy for patients with cancer anorexia and/or cachexia. J Clin Oncol 1993;11:762-767.

40. Beller E, Tattersall M, Lumley T, et al: Improved quality of life with megestrol acetate in patients with endocrine-insensitive advanced cancer: A randomised placebo-controlled trial. Ann Oncol 1997;8:277-283.

41. Simons JP, Aaronson NK, Vansteenkiste JF, et al: Effects of medroxyprogesterone acetate on appetite, weight, and quality of life in advanced-stage non-hormone-sensitive cancer: A placebo-controlled multicenter study. J Clin Oncol 1996;14:1077-1084.

42. Mantovani G, Maccio A, Esu S, et al: Medroxyprogesterone acetate reduces the production of cytokines and serotonin involved in anorexia/cachexia and emesis by peripheral blood mononuclear cells of cancer patients. Biochem Soc Trans 1997;25:296(S).

43. Leinung MC, Liporace R, Miller CH: Induction of adrenal suppression by megestrol acetate in patients with AIDS. Ann Intern Med 1995;122:843-845.

44. Rowland KM, Loprinzi CL, Shaw EG, et al: Randomized double-blind placebo-controlled trial of cisplatin and etoposide plus megestrol acetate/placebo in extensive stage small cell lung cancer: A North America Cancer Treatment Group study. J Clin Oncol 1996;14:135-141.

45. Bruera E, MacEachern T, Spachynski K, et al: Comparison of the efficacy, safety and pharmacokinetics of controlled release and immediate release metoclopramide for the management of chronic nausea in patients with advanced cancer. Cancer 1994;74:3204-3211.

46. Khan SZ, Simpson EJ, Gle AT, et al: Esophageal cancer and cachexia: The effect of short-term treatment with thalidomide on weight loss and lean body mass. Aliment Pharmacol Ther 2003;17:677-682.

47. Khan ZH, Simpson EJ, Colt AT, et al: Esophageal cancer and cachexia: The effect of short-term treatment with thalidomide on weight loss and lean body mass. Aliment Pharmacol Ther 2003;17:677-682.

48. Bruera E, Neumann CM, Pituskin E, et al: Thalidomide in patients with cachexia due to terminal cancer. Preliminary report. Ann Oncol 1999;10:857-859.

49. Bagshaw MS, Hagen NA: Medical efficacy of cannabinoids and marijuana: A comprehensive review of the literature. J Palliat Care 2002;18:111-122.

50. Marhin BR: Identification of the endogenous cannabinoid system through integrative pharmacological approaches. J Pharmacol Exp Ther 2002;301:790-796.

51. Burns CP, Halabi S, Clamon GH, et al: Phase I clinical study of fish oil fatty acid capsules for patients with cancer cachexia: Cancer and Leukemia Group B Study 9473. Clin Cancer Res 1999;5:3942-3947.

52. Barber MD, Ross JA, Voss AC, et al: The effect of an oral nutritional supplement enriched with fish oil on weight-loss in patients with pancreatic cancer. Br J Cancer 1999;81:80-86.

53. Wigmore SJ, Barber MD, Ross JA, et al: Effect of oral eicosapentanoic acid on weight loss in patients with pancreatic cancer. Nutr Cancer 2000;36:177-184.

54. Gogos CA, Ginopoulos P, Salsa B, et al: Dietary omega-3 polyunsaturated fatty acids plus vitamin E restore immunodeficiency and prolong survival for severely ill patients with generalized malignancy: A randomized controlled trial. Cancer 1998;82:395-402.

55. Bruera E, Strasser F, et al: Effect of fish oil on appetite and other symptoms in patients with advanced cancer and anorexia/cachexia: A double-blind, placebo-controlled study. J Clin Oncol 2003;21:129-134.

56. An eicosapentainoic acid (EPA)-enriched supplement versus megestrol acetate (MA) versus both for patients with cancer-associated wasting: A collaborative effort from the North Central Cancer Treatment Group (NCCTG) and the National Cancer Institute of Canada. ASCO 2003, abstract 2987.

57. Boughton B: Drug increases lean tissue mass in patients with cancer Lancet Oncol 2003;4:135.

58. Strawford A, Barbieri T, Neese R, et al: Effects of nandrolone decanoate therapy in borderline hypogonadal men with HIV-associated weight loss. J Acquir Immune Defic Syndr 1999;20:137-146.

59. Sattler FR, Jaque SV, Schroeder ET, et al: Effects of pharmacological doses of nandrolone decanoate and progressive resistance training in immunodeficient patients infected with human immuno-deficiency virus. J Clin Endocrinol Metab 1999;84:1268-1276.

60. Mulligan K, Algren H, Schambelan M: Nandrolone decanoate in HIV+ men with wasting: A randomized, double-blind, placebo-controlled study. 4th International Conference Nutrition HIV Infection, Cannes, France, 2001, p 10.

61. Strawford A, Barbieri T, VanLoan M, et al: Resistance exercise and supraphysiologic androgen therapy in eugonadal men with HIV-related weight loss. JAMA 1999;281:1282-1290.

62. Hengge UR, Baumann M, Maleba R, et al: Oxymetholone promotes weight gain in patients with advanced human immunodeficiency virus (HIV-1) infection. Br J Nutr 1996;75:129-138.

63. Hengge UR, Stocks K, Faulkner S, et al: Randomized phase III trial of oxymetholone for the treatment of HIV wasting and lipodystrophy. Antivir Ther 2001;6 suppl 4:49.

64. Bartlett DL, Stein P, Torosian MH: Effect of growth hormone and protein intake on tumour growth and host cachexia. Surgery 1995;117:260-267.

65. Schambelan M, Mulligan K, Grunfeld C, et al: Recombinant human growth hormone in patients with HIV-associated wasting: A randomized, placebo-controlled trial. Ann Intern Med 1996;125:873-882.

66. Loprinzi CL, Kuross SA, O'Fallon JR, et al: Randomized placebo-controlled evaluation on hydrazine sulfate inpatients with advanced colorectal cancer. J Clin Oncol 1994;12:1121-1125.

67. Loprinzi CL, Goldberg RM, Su JQ: Placebo-controlled trial of hydrazine sulfate in patients with newly diagnosed non-small-cell lung cancer. J Clin Oncol 1994;12:1126-1129.

68. Kosty MP, Fleishman SB, Herndon JE, et al: Cisplatin, vinblastine, and hydrazine sulphate in advanced non-small-cell lung cancer: A randomized placebo-controlled double-blind phase III study of the Cancer and Leukaemia Group. Br J Clin Oncol 1994;12: 1113-1120.

Problems Common to Cancer and Its Therapy

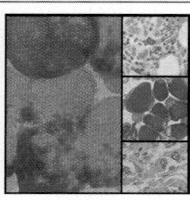

John D. Hainsworth

NAUSEA AND VOMITING

SUMMARY OF KEY POINTS

INCIDENCE

- Most common chemotherapy-associated toxicities
- More than 75 percent of patients receiving combination chemotherapy affected
- More frequent and severe with repetitive doses of chemotherapy
- Significant impact on quality of life and can influence patient compliance with treatment

ETIOLOGY OF COMPLICATION

- Acute nausea and vomiting mediated primarily by activation of serotonin

type 3 receptors in the gastrointestinal tract
- Mechanism of delayed nausea and vomiting (> 24 hours after chemotherapy) unknown

EVALUATION OF THE PATIENT

- Risk factors, including type of chemotherapy (drugs, doses, schedule), age, sex, and prior alcohol use, should be assessed before treatment

GRADING OF COMPLICATION

- Episodes of vomiting should be recorded (number, duration, time to

onset); severity of nausea can be graded using visual analog scale

TREATMENT

- Optimal treatment provides complete control of acute nausea and vomiting in most patients receiving highly emetogenic chemotherapy regimens; only 15% of patients have severe nausea and vomiting
- Delayed nausea and vomiting remain poorly controlled with current approaches

INTRODUCTION

Nausea and vomiting are common side effects associated with systemic chemotherapy. Although these complications of treatment are usually self-limiting and seldom life-threatening, the deleterious effects on nutritional status and quality of life can be substantial. The widespread use of combination chemotherapy regimens and the increased dose intensity of many standard treatments have increased the potential for severe chemotherapy-induced nausea and vomiting. In a patient survey conducted in 1983, nausea and vomiting were the two most feared chemotherapy-related side effects.[1]

The development of increasingly effective anti-emetic therapy during the past 20 years represents one of the most important advances in the supportive care of the patient with cancer. Until the early 1980s, the phenothiazines were the only drugs with proven anti-emetic efficacy for patients receiving chemotherapy. These drugs were no better than placebo therapy, however, in the management of cisplatin-induced nausea and vomiting.[2] Since that time, many additional agents have been developed, and the efficacy of therapy has improved so that most patients receiving cisplatin-based regimens for the first time can expect complete control of nausea and vomiting. Perhaps the best indication of the success of current anti-emetic therapy is reflected in results of a recent patient survey, according to which chemotherapy-induced emesis no longer ranks among the top ten feared side effects of chemotherapy.[3]

The identification of potent new anti-emetics has been made possible by an improved understanding of the physiology of the emetic reflex. Critical assessment of the optimal use of new agents for patients receiving chemotherapy has been facilitated by the development of reproducible methods of assessing nausea and vomiting, and by the conduct of carefully designed, randomized clinical trials.

PHYSIOLOGY OF THE VOMITING REFLEX

The pioneering work of Borison and Wang[4] more than 40 years ago provided the basis for understanding the vomiting reflex. In studies employing ablative techniques and electrical stimulation with microelectrodes (primarily in decerebrate cats), these investigators proposed the existence of two distinct sites in the brain stem believed to be critical for the control of emesis. The first of the sites, the so-called vomiting center, was thought to be located in the lateral reticular formation of the medulla. Electrical stimulation of this site triggered the vomiting reflex, while ablation prevented the vomiting induced by a variety of stimuli. The vomiting center was thought to be located adjacent to the other structures involved in the coordination of vomiting, including the respiratory, vasomotor, and salivary centers, and cranial nerves VIII and X. More recent studies have suggested that the "vomiting center" is actually not anatomically discrete, but that the initiation of the vomiting reflex is controlled by a complex system of networks located in the nucleus tractus solitarius.[5,6] The networks in this area control complex patterns of motor activity such as the vomiting reflex and are more accurately described as "central pattern generators."

The second important center identified by Borison and Wang was the chemoreceptor trigger zone (CTZ), located in the area postrema at the ventral aspect of the fourth ventricle. This center, located outside the blood-brain barrier, is exposed to various noxious agents borne in the blood or cerebrospinal fluid (CSF). Although electrical stimulation of the CTZ does not produce vomiting, intimate connections to the vomiting center permit stimulation of this center after exposure to bloodborne toxins. Ablation of the CTZ abolishes vomiting induced by these agents.

Although these concepts have been retained and are integral to the current understanding of the vomiting reflex, several other important components have also been recognized. Input from the gastrointestinal tract, predominantly through afferent vagal fibers, is critical in initiating the vomiting reflex after ingestion of noxious substances.[7] Incoming vagal afferents connect with the vomiting center directly; an intact CTZ is not essential when vomiting is initiated by this mechanism. It is now known that in addition to ingested substances, some bloodborne substances, including chemotherapeutic agents, can trigger the vomiting reflex through activation of the vagal afferent mechanism.

Two additional components of this complex system involve the vestibular apparatus and the higher brain stem and cortical structures. The vestibular system is involved primarily in initiating the vomiting reflex in motion sickness. Input from higher cortical centers appears to be critical in a variety of conditions, including anticipatory emesis seen for patients who have previously experienced chemotherapy-induced emesis. The various components of the vomiting reflex are illustrated diagrammatically in Figure 38-1, along with the clinical situations in which they are operative. Given the complexity of this system, it is not surprising that different pharmacologic approaches are necessary to control vomiting of different etiologies. It is also unlikely that a single anti-emetic agent effective in all types of nausea and vomiting will ever be identified.

Improved understanding of the neurochemistry of the emetic reflex has been important in developing anti-emetics with new mechanisms of action. The initial focus of such investigation was the area postrema, where receptors for a large number of neuroactive agents have been identified.[8-10] Many of these neurotransmitters (e.g., dopamine, histamine, acetylcholine, norepinephrine, substance P) are, in themselves, emetogenic agents. The development of pharmacologic agents that block specific sets of receptors has resulted in the identification of valuable anti-emetics, and it is likely that continued efforts in this area will be productive of additional valuable agents in the future.

In addition to neurotransmitters located in the CTZ, recent interest has focused on the role of various neuroactive substances in peripherally mediated emesis. Type 3 serotonin (5-HT$_3$) receptors have been identified in large quantities on vagal and splanchnic afferents within the gastrointestinal tract.[11] These peripheral receptors appear to be pivotal in the initiation of the acute nausea and vomiting caused by cisplatin and other strongly emetogenic chemotherapeutic agents; the development of specific 5-HT$_3$ receptor antagonists has provided an additional group of highly active anti-emetics.[12]

Although the mechanisms by which chemotherapeutic agents induce nausea and vomiting are not completely understood (and, in fact, might differ among various

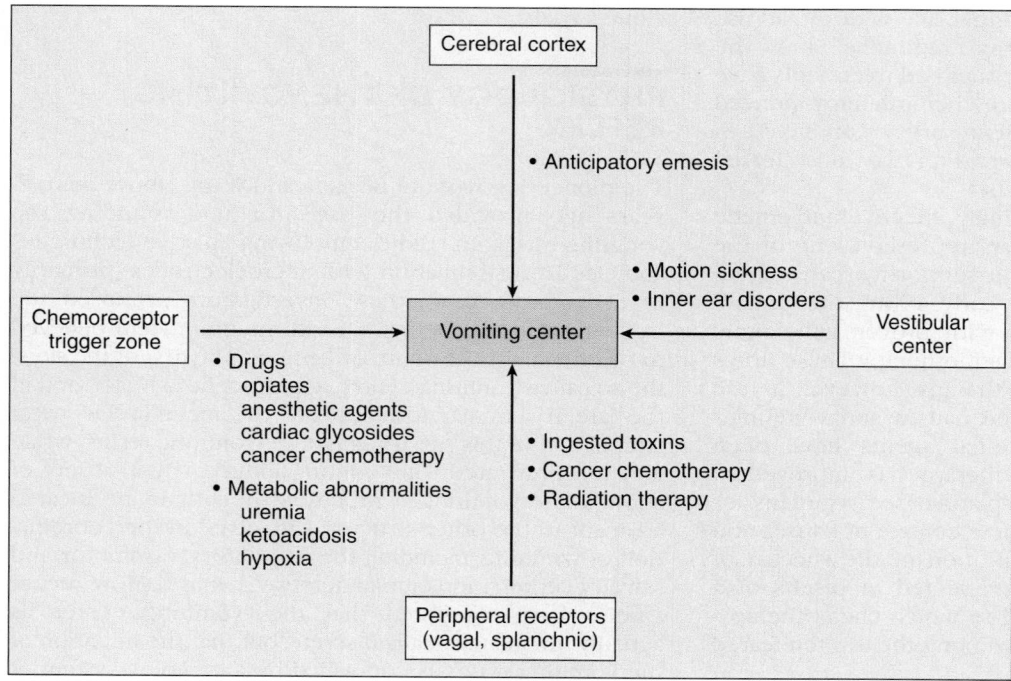

Figure 38-1. Schematic diagram of the various pathways for initiation of the vomiting reflex. Clinical syndromes mediated by each mechanism are illustrated.

agents), recent evidence implicates peripheral mechanisms in cisplatin-induced emesis. In animal models, cisplatin causes release of serotonin from small intestinal mucosa, presumably as a result of mucosal damage.[13,14] Increased urinary 5-hydroxyindoleacetic acid (5-HIAA) levels have been measured two hours after patients receive cisplatin, suggesting a similar release of serotonin.[15] The release of serotonin into the gastrointestinal tract probably induces emesis by binding to afferent vagal and splanchnic $5-HT_3$ receptors within the intestinal wall, thereby initiating vagal input to the vomiting center.[6]

CLINICAL FEATURES OF CHEMOTHERAPY-INDUCED EMESIS

Clinical Syndromes

Chemotherapy-induced nausea and vomiting can be subdivided into three distinct clinical syndromes, each having specific therapeutic implications. These syndromes and their clinical correlates are defined here; treatment approaches are considered later in the chapter. Because nausea and vomiting are common symptoms among patients with cancer, etiologies other than chemotherapy should also be considered. Among the diverse causes of nausea and vomiting among patients with cancer are intestinal obstruction, liver metastases, central nervous system involvement, and other medications (particularly narcotic analgesics). These etiologies should be considered especially when the time course or duration of nausea and vomiting is unusual for the known chemotherapy-induced syndromes.

Acute Nausea and Vomiting

Acute nausea and vomiting after the administration of chemotherapy occur within 24 hours after the chemotherapy dose. The nausea and vomiting during this phase are the most severe, hence the large majority of therapeutic interventions targeted for this phase. With most chemotherapeutic agents, acute nausea and vomiting begin one to two hours after intravenous administration. This delay in onset argues against a direct effect at the CTZ, which would be expected to produce emesis within minutes of intravenous drug administration. A peripherally mediated vomiting reflex, as described for cisplatin, offers a better explanation of the delayed onset of emesis. The onset of nausea and vomiting after the intravenous administration of cyclophosphamide is delayed even longer than with other agents, typically occurring nine to eighteen hours after administration of the drug.[16] The mechanism of cyclophosphamide-induced nausea and vomiting is unclear; the difference in the time of onset suggests that the mechanism might differ from that of other agents.

Delayed Nausea and Vomiting

Delayed nausea and vomiting occur 24 or more hours after chemotherapy administration. Although the severity is decreased in comparison with acute nausea and vomiting, the course can be more protracted, resulting in significant difficulties with hydration, nutrition, and performance status. Delayed emesis is most severe and frequent after administration of high-dose cisplatin; most patients treated with this drug experience some degree of delayed emesis, with onset most frequently 24 to 72 hours after chemotherapy.[17] In some patients, onset can occur as late as four to five days after treatment, persisting for several days. Patients who have poor control of acute nausea and vomiting are more likely to experience delayed nausea and vomiting as well; however, delayed emesis can occur among patients who have complete emetic control during the first 24 hours after administration of chemotherapy.

The pathophysiology of delayed emesis remains unclear, but it seems likely that this syndrome is mediated centrally by different neurotransmitters. $5-HT_3$-receptor antagonists, which are highly effective in the prevention of acute emesis, have limited activity in the treatment of delayed emesis. Conversely, the neurokinin-1 receptor antagonists, which block the action of substance P, have consistently shown activity against delayed emesis. Peripheral factors, including residual metabolites of chemotherapeutic agents or gastrointestinal mucosal damage, might also play a role.

Anticipatory Nausea and Vomiting

Anticipatory nausea and vomiting often occur among patients who have experienced poor control of emesis during previous courses of chemotherapy.[18,19] The onset can occur before or during chemotherapy administration. Because this is a conditioned response, certain associations with chemotherapy administration, such as the hospital environment or the oncologist's office, might trigger the onset of emesis.

Prognostic Factors

Multiple clinical factors that are important in determining the incidence and severity of chemotherapy-induced nausea and vomiting have been identified. These factors include the type of chemotherapy administered, certain patient characteristics, and the anti-emetic regimen employed (Table 38-1).

Chemotherapeutic Agents

The commonly used chemotherapeutic drugs are separated into five groups according to emetic potential in Table 32-2. Drugs in category 5 produce emesis in greater than 90% of patients, while drugs in category 1 produce emesis in fewer than 10%. The drugs that cause emesis most frequently also cause the most severe emesis. Emesis is most severe during the first eight hours after onset, but with strongly emetogenic drugs, patients are often ill throughout the 24-hour period after administration.

In general, the potential for acute nausea and vomiting increases with the dose of chemotherapy. Schedule of administration is also important with certain agents: Large intravenous bolus doses, or doses administered intravenously over a short period of time, are more likely to cause emesis than are smaller divided doses or continuous infusion.

TABLE 38-1

Determinants of Chemotherapy-Induced Nausea and Vomiting

Chemotherapy

Emetic potential of drug(s) used
Dose
Schedule of administration
Route of administration

Patient Characteristics

Age
Gender
Alcohol use
Emesis control during prior chemotherapy

Anti-emetics

Dose
Schedule
Combination regimens
Route of administration

The use of chemotherapeutic agents in combination increases the emetogenic potential of a treatment regimen. Based on the information in Table 38-2, Hesketh and colleagues[20] have proposed a model for predicting the emetogenic potential of a combination regimen (Table 38-3). As new combination regimens are introduced into clinical practice, application of this algorithm can result in optimum, cost-effective anti-emetic therapy.

Patient Characteristics

Several patient characteristics are important predictors of the development and severity of acute chemotherapy-induced nausea and vomiting. These factors are age, gender, history of alcohol intake, and history of previous chemotherapy.

Age. Data are conflicting regarding the effect of patient age on the severity of chemotherapy-induced nausea and vomiting. Increasing evidence, however, indicates that chemotherapy-induced emesis is more frequent in younger patients.[21,22] Before the introduction of the 5-HT$_3$-receptor antagonists, anti-emetic therapy was especially difficult among patients younger than 30 years due to the high incidence of acute dystonic reactions with the dopamine receptor antagonists (particularly high-dose metoclopramide).[23,24] These problems can be minimized or avoided completely with current regimens, however.

Gender. Anecdotal data have long suggested that women experience more frequent and severe chemotherapy-induced nausea and vomiting than do men. This conclusion has been disputed, as the cisplatin-based chemotherapy regimens administered to men and women in most anti-emetic studies have differed. Data from large prospective studies now indicate, however, that females do have more severe and frequent nausea and vomiting, even after controlling for chemotherapy regimen. In one such study, all patients received cisplatin-containing regimens and were treated with ondansetron; more

women receiving high-dose cisplatin with either 5-FU or etoposide for lung cancer or head and neck carcinomas had poor control of emesis than did men receiving these same regimens (49% vs. 29%, respectively).[22]

TABLE 38-2

Potential for Acute Nausea and Vomiting with Commonly Used Chemotherapeutic Agents

LEVEL	FREQUENCY OF EMESIS (%)	AGENT
5	> 90	Carmustine > 250 mg/m^2
		Cisplatin $\geq$ 50 mg/m^2
		Cyclophosphamide > 1,500 mg/m^2
		Dacarbazine
		Mechlorethamine
		Streptozocin
4	60–90	Carboplatin
		Carmustine $\leq$ 250 mg/m^2
		Cisplatin < 50 mg/m^2
		Cyclophosphamide > 750 mg/m^2 $\leq$ 1,500 mg/m^2
		Cytarabine > 1 g/m^2
		Doxorubicin > 60 mg/m^2
		Methotrexate > 1,000 mg/m^2
		Oxaliplatin
		Procarbazine (oral)
3	30–60	Cyclophosphamide $\leq$ 750 mg/m^2
		Cyclophosphamide (oral)
		Doxorubicin 20–60 mg/m^2
		Epirubicin $\leq$ 90 mg/m^2
		Hexamethylmelamine (oral)
		Idarubicin
		Ifosfamide
		Irinotecan
		Methotrexate 250–1000 mg/m^2
		Mitoxantrone
2	10–30	Docetaxel
		Etoposide
		5-Fluorouracil < 1,000 mg/m^2
		Gemcitabine
		Methotrexate > 50 mg/m^2 < 250 mg/m^2
		Mitomycin
		Paclitaxel
		Topotecan
1	< 10	Bleomycin
		Busulfan
		Capecitabine
		Chlorambucil (oral)
		2-Chlorodeoxyadenosine
		Fludarabine
		Gefitinib
		Hydroxyurea
		Imitanib
		Methotrexate $\leq$ 50 mg/m^2
		L-Phenylalanine mustard (oral)
		Liposomal doxorubicin
		Rituximab
		Thioguanine (oral)
		Trastuzumab
		Vinblastine
		Vincristine
		Vinorelbine

Adapted from Hesketh PJ, Kris MG, Grunberg SM: Proposal for classifying the acute emetogenicity of cancer chemotherapy. J Clin Oncol 1997;15:103–109.

TABLE 38-3

 Formula for Estimation of Emetogenic Potential of Combination Chemotherapy Regimens

- Use Table 38-2 to assign emetic level to each agent in the regimen
- Identify most emetogenic agent
- When considering the other components of the regimen, use the following rules:
  Level one agents do not contribute to emetogenicity
  Adding level 3 or 4 agents increases emetogenicity by one level/agent
  Adding level 2 agents (regardless of number) increases emetogenicity by one level greater than the most emetogenic agent

Examples of Algorithm Use

Regimen	Emetogenic level of agents in regimen	Emetogenic level of regimen
CMF	3 + 2 + 1	4
CAF	3 + 3 + 2	5
Paclitaxel/carboplatin	2 + 4	5
CVP	3 + 1 + 1	3

A, doxorubicin; C, cyclophosphamide; F, 5-fluorouracil; M, methotrexate; P, prednisone; V, vincristine.
Adapted from Hesketh PJ, Kris MG, Grunberg SM: Proposal for classifying the acute emetogenicity of cancer chemotherapy. J Clin Oncol 1997;15:103.

History of Alcohol Intake. Patients with a history of chronic alcohol intake (four to five mixed drinks per day) have more effective control of chemotherapy-induced nausea and vomiting when optimal anti-emetics are used.[25-27] In a prospective study of 52 patients receiving high-dose cisplatin along with combination anti-emetic therapy, 93% of those with a high alcohol intake experienced no emesis, as opposed to 61% of patients without this history.[25] It is important to emphasize, however, that the administration of highly emetogenic chemotherapy to these patients, in the absence of appropriate anti-emetic therapy, still results in a high incidence of severe acute nausea and vomiting. The mechanism of the alcohol effect is unclear; it is possible, however, that various receptor sites are less sensitive among patients with a history of alcohol intake and that blockade of these receptors is relatively easy with appropriate anti-emetics.

Previous Chemotherapy. Patients who have experienced poor control of emesis during previous chemotherapy are more likely to have unsatisfactory results with subsequent anti-emetics.[28,29] The development of an anticipatory component to the nausea and vomiting is certainly one factor; whether additional factors are also involved is unknown.

Conduct and Interpretation of Clinical Anti-emetic Trials
Because multiple patient characteristics and chemotherapy factors influence the incidence and severity of chemotherapy-associated nausea and vomiting, optimal design and interpretation of clinical trials with new anti-emetics or new combination regimens requires that these factors be taken into account. Definitive demonstration of

the superiority of an agent or regimen requires a large, randomized trial in which the comparison groups are matched with respect to the various patient characteristics and chemotherapy received. Patients should be receiving their initial dose of chemotherapy, in order to avoid the confounding effects of anticipatory emesis. Crossover trials are also difficult to interpret for this reason. Optimally, the treatment received should be double-blinded to avoid investigator or patient bias. As effective regimens now exist for all subgroups of patients, new treatments should be compared with existing treatments; the inclusion of a "no-treatment" or placebo arm in a randomized trial is inappropriate. The completion of this type of large controlled randomized trial has hastened the improvement of anti-emetic therapy and the rapid incorporation of new treatments into clinical practice.

When interpreting the results of anti-emetic trials, special attention should also be given to the definitions of therapeutic response and the methods used to assess efficacy. Most trials measure the number of emetic episodes as the primary efficacy parameter, as this is an objective measurement. Some trials also measure various secondary efficacy parameters, including nausea, food intake, and overall patient satisfaction with treatment. Even when emesis is used to measure efficacy, comparisons between trials must be made with caution, as definitions of response have varied also. "Complete response," in various studies, has been defined as "no vomiting," "no vomiting and only mild nausea," or "no vomiting and no nausea" during the 24 hours after chemotherapy. Clearly, response rates can vary substantially, depending on the definition used. Standardization of response assessment would greatly aid in the interpretation of future trials.

TREATMENT OF CHEMOTHERAPY-INDUCED NAUSEA AND VOMITING

Acute Nausea and Vomiting

Several families of drugs with anti-emetic activities have been identified. Table 38-4 lists the classes of anti-emetic agents in current use, in approximate order of anti-emetic potency. Only the 5-HT$_3$ receptor antagonists, the substituted benzamides, and the new class of neurokinin-1 receptor antagonists exhibit marked activity against highly emetogenic chemotherapy. As no single agent is ideal, combination anti-emetic regimens have been developed, which have further improved efficacy. Increased understanding of the mechanism of action of the various compounds has led to more rational development of combination regimens; in general, the most effective regimens employ agents with different mechanisms of action.

5-HT$_3$ Receptor Antagonists
The selective 5-HT$_3$ receptor antagonists are the most effective family of anti-emetics in the treatment of acute emesis. These agents block the serotonin type 3 receptors and are thought to exert their anti-emetic activity primarily

Problems Common to Cancer and Its Therapy

TABLE 38-4

Anti-emetic Agents

ANTI-EMETIC AGENT	MECHANISM OF ACTION	DOSE AND SCHEDULE FOR ACUTE NAUSEA AND VOMITING
5-HT$_3$ antagonists	5-HT$_3$ receptor blockade	
Ondansetron		8–32 mg IV (single dose)
Granisetron		10 µg/kg IV (single dose) or 2 mg PO
Dolasetron		1.8 mg/kg IV (single dose) or 200 mg PO
Substituted benzamides	Dopamine receptor blockade,	
Metoclopramide	5HT$_3$ receptor blockade	1–3 mg/kg IV q2h × 2–4 doses
Neurokinin-1 antagonists	NK-1 receptor blockade	Several compounds in development
Corticosteroids	Unknown	
Dexamethasone		10–20 mg IV or PO × 1 dose
Methylprednisolone		250–500 mg IV × 1 dose
Phenothiazines	Dopamine receptor blockade	
Prochlorperazine		10 mg PO q2–4h or 25 mg PR q4–6h or 10–20 mg IV q3–6h
Promethazine		25 mg PO or PR q4–6h
Thiethylperazine		10 mg PO q4–6h
Benzodiazepines	Anxiolytic, amnesic	
Lorazepam		1–2 mg IV q4h
Butyrophenones	Dopamine receptor blockade	
Haloperidol		1–3 mg IV or PO q2–6h
Droperidol		0.5–2 mg IV q4h
Cannabinoids	Central psychotropic action	
Dronabinol		5–10 mg PO q3–4h

through peripheral blockade in the small intestine (see the preceding discussion). Three agents in this class are currently commercially available in the United States: ondansetron, granisetron, and dolasetron. In randomized trials, all three of these drugs were superior to high-dose metoclopramide (the previous standard of therapy) in the prophylaxis of cisplatin-induced nausea and vomiting.[30-36]

Superiority to a variety of standard agents has also been demonstrated in the treatment of emesis produced by cyclophosphamide-based chemotherapy regimens.[37-41] Although randomized trials have not been performed with other emetogenic chemotherapeutic agents, the 5HT$_3$ receptor antagonists have demonstrated efficacy in preventing acute nausea and vomiting with all agents tested.

MANAGEMENT APPROACH

CHEMOTHERAPY-INDUCED NAUSEA AND VOMITING

Anti-emetic therapy for acute chemotherapy-induced nausea and vomiting should be based on the emetic potential of the chemotherapy regimen being used and should take into account individual patient risk factors (e.g., sex, age, history of alcohol use, previous emesis with chemotherapy). Excellent algorithms for the prediction of the likelihood of emesis with single chemotherapeutic agents or combination regimens have been developed. Patients receiving chemotherapy with moderate or high emetogenic potential should receive prophylaxis with a 5-HT$_3$ receptor antagonist plus dexamethasone. The three available 5-HT$_3$ receptor antagonists are equivalent in their clinical efficacy. Oral regimens are equivalent to intravenous regimens and are preferable for patients who tolerate oral medication.

Patients receiving mildly emetogenic therapy should receive dexamethasone (20 mg intravenously or orally); a 5-HT$_3$ receptor antagonist should be added with subsequent courses only if anti-emetic control is inadequate. Patients with breakthrough nausea and vomiting

should receive either prochlorperazine (10 mg orally or intravenously, or in 30 mg spansules) or lorazepam (1 mg intravenously every four hours). Additional doses of 5-HT$_3$ receptor antagonists or dexamethasone during the first 24 hours are usually ineffective.

Delayed nausea and vomiting occurs more than 24 hours after chemotherapy is administered and should be anticipated among patients receiving highly emetogenic regimens (particularly cisplatin, at least 100 mg/m^2, or cyclophosphamide). These patients should receive either:

1. Dexamethasone (8 mg orally twice daily for two days, then 4 mg twice daily for two days) plus metoclopramide (0.5 mg/kg orally four times daily for four days); or
2. Dexamethasone (same schedule) plus ondansetron (8 mg orally twice daily for four days). Dexamethasone alone is effective prophylaxis for patients with good control of acute emesis.

Patients with anticipatory nausea and vomiting should receive premedication with an anxiolytic agent (e.g., diazepam) two to three hours before chemotherapy.

TABLE 38-5

Maximally Effective Single Intravenous Doses of the 5-HT₃ Receptor Antagonists in Prophylaxis of Acute Chemotherapy-induced Emesis

	ONDANSETRON	GRANISETRON	DOLASETRON
Cisplatin-based regimens	32 mg*	10 µg/kg	1.8 mg/kg
Cyclophosphamide/doxorubicin regimens	24 mg*	10 µg/kg	1.8 mg/kg
Ineffective dose	Not determined with single dose	5 µg/kg	0.6 mg/kg (≥ 2.4 mg/kg schedule also inferior)

*Conflicting data exist; some randomized trials have shown 8 mg equivalent to 32 mg.

Early dose-finding studies with all three of these agents demonstrated a plateau in anti-emetic efficacy, above which no additional benefit was obtained with increasing dose.[42-45] These observations suggest that complete blockade of the 5-HT₃ receptors can be achieved with all three agents, after which administration of additional drug serves no further purpose. Based on this mechanism of action, it could be anticipated that all highly selective and efficient 5-HT₃ receptor antagonists would have similar anti-emetic efficacy. Indeed, the three commercially available drugs have now been compared extensively in various randomized, blinded clinical trials.[46-54] At maximally effective doses, the efficacy of ondansetron, granisetron, and dolasetron is equivalent. For patients receiving high-dose cisplatin therapy, use of appropriate doses of any one of these three agents results in complete control of emesis in 50–70% of patients during the first 24 hours after administration of chemotherapy. Complete control of emesis ranges from 70% to 80% among patients receiving moderately emetogenic regimens, usually cyclophosphamide-based.

The adverse events produced by the three available 5-HT₃ receptor antagonists are essentially identical. Mild to moderate headache is the most frequently observed toxicity and is produced by all three drugs in approximately 20% to 30% of patients. Other adverse events, including constipation and diarrhea, are mild and uncommon.

Dosing. Because of the relatively high cost of the 5-HT₃ receptor antagonists, use of the minimum effective dose is clinically important. Surprisingly, determination of this dose for the three available 5-HT₃ receptor antagonists has been somewhat difficult. For each agent, a single prophylactic dose is as effective as multiple doses during the first 24 hours. Therefore, the use of additional doses of these agents for "breakthrough" vomiting during this time is to be discouraged, and the writing of "as-needed" orders for these agents is never indicated.

In the prophylaxis of nausea and vomiting produced by high-dose cisplatin, conflicting data exist for the optimum ondansetron dose. A large randomized trial performed in the United States showed superior control with a 32-mg ondansetron dose vs. an 8-mg dose (48% vs. 35% complete control, respectively).[55] However, two similar randomized trials done in Europe showed no statistical differences between 8 mg and 32 mg of ondansetron.[56,57] With granisetron, dose-ranging studies have been fairly consistent, showing a decrease in activity when the dose falls below 10 µg/kg for patients receiving either highly or moderately emetogenic chemotherapy.[58,59] Escalating the dose of granisetron above 10 µg/kg is probably unnecessary, as a randomized trial showed no difference between 10 µg/kg and 40 µg/kg for patients receiving high-dose cisplatin therapy.[48] Dose ranging of dolasetron has also consistently demonstrated the efficacy of 1.8 mg/kg, with efficacy decreasing as doses fall below 0.6 mg/kg.[45,50] With this drug, some evidence exists that higher doses (2.4–5 mg/kg) might also be less effective.[60] Table 38-5 summarizes the optimal doses (i.e., the minimum fully effective doses) of each of the three available 5-HT₃ receptor antagonists in the prophylaxis of acute nausea and vomiting induced by both cisplatin-based regimens and cyclophosphamide-based regimens.

It is now clear that an ondansetron dose of 32 mg is not indicated except for patients receiving high-dose cisplatin. In a prospective trial, Hesketh et al.[61] demonstrated excellent anti-emetic control with 24 mg of ondansetron for patients receiving cyclophosphamide/doxorubicin-based chemtherapy, and with 8 mg of ondansetron for patients receiving moderately emetogenic regimens (e.g., cyclophosphamide, methotrexate, 5-fluorouracil [CMF]). The dosage of granisetron should not be lowered below 10 µg/kg, however, as inferior control has been demonstrated with lower doses.[45] With dolasetron, some latitude for dose reduction might exist, as similar results have been achieved with doses in the 1.2- to 1.8-mg/kg range in most studies.

Oral Administration. All three available 5-HT₃ receptor antagonists are bioavailable and well tolerated when administered orally. Because of the potential advantages of an oral anti-emetic regimen in terms of convenience and cost, oral vs. intravenous administration of these three agents has been evaluated in the prophylaxis of acute chemotherapy-induced nausea and vomiting. Randomized trials have demonstrated the equivalency of oral vs. intravenous administration of the 5-HT₃ receptor antagonists in the treatment of patients receiving either highly emetogenic or moderately emetogenic chemotherapy.[46,62-65] Optimal single oral doses of all three 5HT₃ receptor antagonists have been defined (Table 38-6).[66-69]

Neurokinin-1-Receptor Antagonists

The neurokinin-1 (NK-1) receptor is a recently identified component of the centrally mediated vomiting reflex. This receptor mediates the emetogenic action of substance P, a

TABLE 38-6

Recommended Anti-emetic Prophylaxis for Acute Chemotherapy-induced Nausea and Vomiting

EMETIC LEVEL OF CHEMOTHERAPY (CHANCE OF EMESIS)	ANTI-EMETIC REGIMEN	ADDITIONAL TREATMENT
5 (> 90%)	5-HT$_3$ + dexamethasone* (oral preferred)	Routine delayed emesis prophylaxis: metoclopramide/dexamethasone *or* 5-HT$_3$/dexamethasone Add prochlorperazine or lorazepam if incomplete control
4 (60–80%)	5-HT$_3$ + dexamethasone (oral preferred)	Routine prophylaxis for delayed emesis with dexamethasone alone. Add 5-HT$_3$ or metoclopramide if delayed nausea or emesis occurs
3 (30–60%)	5-HT$_3$ + dexamethasone (oral preferred)	
2 (10–30%)	Dexamethasone	Add 5-HT$_3$ during subsequent cycles if dexamethasone ineffective for acute nausea/vomiting
1 (< 10%)	None	Add dexamethasone if any nausea/vomiting occurs

5-HT$_3$ dosing:

Ondansetron	IV:	32 mg (class 5), 8–24 mg (class 4), 8 mg (class 3)
	O:	8 mg tid (or 24 mg single dose)
Granisetron	IV:	1 mg
	PO:	1–2 mg
Dolasetron	IV:	1.8 mg/kg
	PO:	200 mg

*Dexamethasone dosing: 20 mg PO or IV

tachykinin contained in vagal afferents innervating the area postrema and nucleus tractus solitarii in the brainstem.[10] Although no neurokinin-1 receptor antagonists have yet been approved for clinical use, several of these drugs are in the late stages of development and have already demonstrated efficacy in the treatment of both acute and delayed emesis.[70-73]

In a randomized, double-blind placebo-controlled trial, the efficacy of the NK-1 antagonist L754,030 was evaluated for patients receiving cisplatin-based chemotherapy.[71] All patients received prophylactic treatment with a standard granisetron/dexamethasone regimen; patients were randomized to three groups and received one of the following regimens:

1. L754,030 before cisplatin and daily on days one through five
2. L754,030 before cisplatin only
3. No L754,030

In this trial, the two groups receiving the NK-1 antagonist with granisetron/dexamethasone before cisplatin had better acute control of emesis than did those who received standard therapy (93% vs. 67% complete control, respectively). In addition, patients receiving L754,030 had reduced emesis during days two through five after administration of cisplatin (78% vs. 33% with no emesis). Similar beneficial effects on delayed emesis have been reported in other, smaller trials.[70,72,73] The combination of ondansetron/dexamethasone, however, was superior to the NK-1 antagonist MK869 plus dexamethasone in the acute control of emesis after cisplatin.[73] In all clinical trials to date, the NK-1 antagonists have been well tolerated, with no serious adverse events.

Therefore, it seems likely that this new category of anti-emetics will further improve the treatment of chemotherapy-induced emesis. Probable benefits include:

- Improvement in control of acute emesis, when added to a 5-HT3 receptor antagonist/dexamethasone combination, for patients receiving highly emetogenic chemotherapy
- Prevention of delayed emesis

The optimal combinations and the optimal duration of therapy with these agents remain to be defined.

Substituted Benzamides

Metoclopramide is the most frequently used drug in this class. It was the first drug to demonstrate substantial anti-emetic activity among patients treated with high doses of cisplatin. In a randomized study reported in 1981, patients receiving high doses of metoclopramide had significantly fewer episodes of emesis than patients given placebo (median, 1.0 vs. 10.5 emetic episodes; $P = 0.001$) or prochlorperazine (median, 1.5 vs. 12.0 emetic episodes; $P = 0.005$).[2] Additional studies confirmed that high doses of metoclopramide produced complete anti-emetic control in 20–38% of patients receiving high-dose cisplatin.[74-76] Metoclopramide is a dopamine receptor antagonist whose anti-emetic activity was initially attributed to this mechanism. It is now clear, however, that high doses of metoclopramide also block 5-HT$_3$ receptors, providing an additional mechanism of action.[77] Before the introduction of ondansetron, randomized trials indicated the superiority of high-dose metoclopramide over other agents, including haloperidol, droperidol, tetrahydrocannabinol, and dexamethasone.[74,78-80]

The major side effects of high-dose metoclopramide are extrapyramidal reactions caused by its dopamine receptor antagonism.[2,81] Acute dystonic reactions are the most dramatic adverse effects but are relatively uncommon in adults, occurring in only 2%–5% of cases. Akathisia, although less dramatic, is a more common problem and often persists for several hours. Both adverse effects are more common in young patients. In most adults, these side effects are not difficult to control or prevent. Intravenous diphenhydramine quickly ends an acute dystonic reaction, and the addition of lorazepam to metoclopramide-containing regimens greatly reduces the incidence of extrapyramidal reactions.[82]

From 1981 to 1991, high-dose metoclopramide was an integral component of anti-emetic therapy. Since then, however, 5-HT$_3$ receptor antagonists have been found to be more effective and less toxic agents and have largely replaced metoclopramide in the management of acute chemotherapy-induced emesis.

Corticosteroids

The anti-emetic mechanism of action of the corticosteroids is unclear. Unlike most other anti-emetics, there is no current evidence that neurotransmitter blockade is involved. The anti-emetic activity of the corticosteroids has been confirmed in several trials, predominantly for patients receiving moderately emetogenic chemotherapy.[83-86] Corticosteroids that have been used as anti-emetics include dexamethasone, methylprednisolone, and occasionally prednisone; no obvious differences in anti-emetic potency among these corticosteroids have been demonstrated. Because of their moderate anti-emetic activity, the corticosteroids are not ideal for single-agent use. They are very useful, however, when combined with other anti-emetics (see the discussion later in this chapter), presumably because they have a different mechanism of action.

The adverse effects of short courses of corticosteroid are mild and infrequent. Additional caution must be used in treating patients with diabetes mellitus or other conditions predisposing to difficulties with steroids. Occasional acute psychotic reactions have been observed.

Phenothiazines

The phenothiazines were the first family of agents to demonstrate substantial anti-emetic activity and are thought to act primarily as antidopaminergic agents. Several of these agents, including prochlorperazine, promethazine, and thiethylperazine, are still used frequently. In 1963, a randomized, double-blind, placebo-controlled trial documented the superiority of prochlorperazine and thiopropazate to placebo in the control of nausea and vomiting induced by fluorouracil.[87] Efficacy has also been documented against other moderately emetogenic chemotherapeutic agents.[88] These agents are ineffective against highly emetogenic chemotherapy, however, and should currently be used only in combination with other, more effective agents.[2] The side effects of the phenothiazines include sedation, akathisia, and, less commonly, acute dystonic reactions.

Benzodiazepines

Lorazepam is the only benzodiazepine that has found widespread use in anti-emetic therapy. Direct anti-emetic effects of lorazepam are minor; however, the sedative, anxiolytic, and amnesic effects have made this drug ideal for use in combination regimens.[89] Several trials have documented improved patient acceptance of lorazepam-containing combination regimens, even when the objective anti-emetic efficacy increased only slightly.[82,90] The use of intravenous lorazepam often causes marked sedation lasting several hours, which limits its use in the outpatient setting. In addition, some patients experience confusion, amnesia, and transient enuresis.

Butyrophenones

The butyrophenones, haloperidol and droperidol, have anti-emetic activity as a result of specific dopamine receptor blockade.[80,91,92] Both agents exhibit moderate anti-emetic efficacy, even against strongly emetogenic agents such as cisplatin; however, a randomized study comparing haloperidol and high-dose metoclopramide showed metoclopramide to be superior.[79] Common side effects of the butyrophenones include sedation, dystonic reactions, and akathisia; in addition, hypotension is occasionally encountered. Even before the introduction of the 5-HT$_3$ receptor antagonists, the butyrophenones were used sparingly, as they are less active than high-dose metoclopramide and have no advantage in toxicity profile. The availability of ondansetron has made these agents even less attractive; they should be considered a third-best choice for patients receiving cisplatin-containing regimens.

Cannabinoids

Anecdotal reports of reduced emesis among patients smoking marijuana during chemotherapy stimulated interest in the cannabinoids during the early 1980s. Several cannabinoids have been evaluated as anti-emetics; at present, dronabinol is the only commercially available agent in this class. This drug has anti-emetic activity for patients receiving moderately emetogenic chemotherapy; in this setting, it has been more effective than prochlorperazine.[93-95] The mechanism of action of the cannabinoids is incompletely defined; a central nervous system site of action has been postulated due to the marked psychoactive properties of these agents.

In spite of clear anti-emetic efficacy, the clinical use of cannabinoids has been limited due to their unfavorable toxicity profile in some patients. Frequent toxicities include dysphoria, hallucinations, vertigo, dry mouth, sedation, and disorientation. These side effects are more common in elderly patients. The cannabinoids should not be considered for first-line anti-emetic therapy, as more effective and better tolerated agents exist. They should be considered for the occasional patient with mild to moderate nausea and vomiting who has either poor tolerance or poor response to other anti-emetics.[96]

Combination Anti-emetic Therapy

Because none of the anti-emetic agents is ideal when used alone, a variety of combination regimens has been developed in an attempt to improve efficacy. In most combinations, drugs included have different mechanisms of action and are used at a dose and schedule that demonstrate optimal single-agent activity. The most successful combinations use drugs with nonoverlapping toxicities.

Problems Common to Cancer and Its Therapy

The corticosteroids have been most extensively evaluated as "second drugs" in combination regimens due to their ease of administration, minimal toxicity, and different mechanism of action. When combined with any of the available 5-HT$_3$ receptor antagonists, dexamethasone has consistently improved anti-emetic efficacy among patients receiving highly emetogenic or moderately emetogenic regimens.[97-101] In a recent meta-analysis of randomized trials comparing various regimens with or without dexamethasone, complete protection from emesis was increased by 16% when dexamethasone was added to a 5-HT$_3$ receptor antagonist.[102] Randomized studies also have shown that the addition of dexamethasone to high-dose metoclopramide improves anti-emetic efficacy.[103-105] The optimal dose and schedule of dexamethasone has not been formally evaluated; however, studies using a single intravenous dose of 20 mg before administration of chemotherapy have yielded results equivalent to those achieved with repetitive dexamethasone doses.

The efficacies of several other anti-emetics (e.g., prochlorperazine, chlorpromazine, haloperidol, nabilone) have also apparently been improved by adding a corticosteroid.[106-108] Most studies with these combinations, however, have not involved randomized comparisons to single agents, and the superiority of these combinations to dexamethasone alone is not clear. If these combinations are used, they should be reserved for prophylaxis for patients receiving regimens of mild to moderate emetogenic potential.

Limited data have been reported regarding triple drug combination anti-emetic therapy. Hesketh and associates[109] reported an 89% complete response rate when prochlorperazine (15-mg spansule 30 minutes before and 12 hours after treatment) was added to granisetron/dexamethasone for patients receiving high-dose cisplatin. Lebeau and colleagues[110] improved the efficacy of ondansetron/methylprednisolone by adding metopimazine (a phenothiazine) for patients receiving cisplatin who had previously been uncontrolled with the two-drug regimen. The addition of lorazepam to the combination of high-dose metoclopramide and dexamethasone has not resulted in consistent improvement in anti-emetic efficacy.[82,111,112] The lorazepam-containing regimens have been preferred by patients in these studies, however. This preference by patients receiving metoclopramide-containing regimens is not surprising, as the incidence of extrapyramidal side effects is reduced with the addition of lorazepam. On the other hand, the contribution of lorazepam to currently used 5-HT$_3$ receptor antagonist combinations is unclear, and sedation is consistently increased when lorazepam is added. In the future, the addition of an NK-1 receptor antagonist to a 5-HT$_3$ receptor antagonist/dexamethasone might improve both acute and delayed emesis control.[71]

Anticipatory Nausea and Vomiting

Because anticipatory nausea and vomiting are conditioned responses, effective control of chemotherapy-induced nausea and vomiting prevents the development of this reflex and is, therefore, the best strategy for preventing this problem.[18,19,113] Highly effective combination regimens using a 5-HT$_3$ receptor antagonist plus dexamethasone have greatly decreased the prevalence of this problem. For patients in whom anticipatory nausea and vomiting develop, treatment with anxiolytics such as the benzodiazepines is sometimes effective.[89] In addition, various nonpharmacologic approaches, including hypnosis and behavioral modification, have shown some benefit for these patients.[18,114,115]

Delayed Nausea and Vomiting

Compared with the excellent control of acute nausea and vomiting achieved for most patients, the treatment of delayed emesis is relatively ineffective. In a randomized study, Kris and colleagues[116] demonstrated that the combination of oral metoclopramide (0.5 mg/kg four times daily for four days) and dexamethasone (8 mg twice daily for two days, then four mg twice daily for two days) was superior to either placebo or dexamethasone alone in controlling delayed emesis after high-dose cisplatin. Fifty-two percent of patients receiving the two-drug combination had complete control of delayed vomiting, compared with 35% receiving dexamethasone alone and only 11% receiving placebo. These same investigators also documented substantial activity with a regimen containing prochlorperazine (30-mg spansules three times daily for two days, then 15 mg three times daily for two days) plus dexamethasone (8 mg twice daily for two days, then 4 mg twice daily for two days).[117]

Compared to their high degree of efficacy in the management of acute chemotherapy-induced nausea and vomiting, the contribution of the 5-HT$_3$ receptor antagonists to the management of delayed emesis is modest. As a single agent, ondansetron (8 mg orally twice daily, days two through six) demonstrated a significant benefit compared with placebo for patients receiving cisplatin-based chemotherapy.[118] Only 56% of patients, however, had major responses (fewer than three emetic episodes) on days two and three after administration of high-dose cisplatin. Randomized trials comparing the efficacy of dexamethasone alone vs. a 5HT$_3$-receptor antagonist/dexamethasone combination have yielded conflicting results.[119-122] For patients in whom emesis is well controlled during the first 24 hours, dexamethasone alone produces excellent results.[122] For patients who are either receiving highly emetogenic regimens or who experience nausea or emesis during the first 24 hours, combination treatment with either metoclopramide/dexamethasone or a 5-HT$_3$ receptor antagonist/dexamethasone is currently optimal. Complete control rates are only 50% to 60% with these combinations, however.

The anticipated introduction of the NK-1 receptor antagonists offers the potential for improved therapy of delayed nausea and vomiting. For patients receiving cisplatin-based chemotherapy, addition of L-754,030, an NK-1 receptor antagonist, to granisetron/dexamethasone improved the complete control of delayed emesis from 33% to 80%.[71] If these results are duplicated and are also obtained among patients receiving moderately emetogenic chemotherapy, the problem of delayed emesis will decrease substantially in the future.

Radiation-Induced Nausea and Vomiting

Radiation-induced nausea and vomiting are common with some types of radiation therapy and are related to the size of the radiation portal, the dose delivered, and the site of radiation. Radiation-induced emesis occurs acutely in more than 90% of patients receiving total-body irradiation. Among patients receiving conventional daily doses of radiotherapy (2 Gy/fraction), emesis develops within two to three weeks in about 50% of patients receiving an upper abdominal portal.[123] The mechanism of radiation-induced emesis remains unclear, but release of serotonin from the gastrointestinal enterochromaffin cells and subsequent involvement of the gastrointestinal 5-HT$_3$ receptors and vagal afferent fibers is most likely.

Most of the anti-emetic agents found active against chemotherapy-induced nausea and vomiting also have some activity against radiation-induced emesis; however, few randomized trials have been performed to identify an optimal regimen. Dexamethasone (2 mg orally three times daily) had efficacy compared with placebo during the first week of upper abdominal radiation therapy (complete emesis control 70% vs. 49%, respectively).[124] Daily oral ondansetron was more effective than metoclopramide for patients receiving upper abdomial radiation therapy and was more effective than placebo for patients receiving total-body irradiation.[125,126]

Given the postulated mechanism of radiation-induced emesis and the available clinical data, it seems likely that the 5-HT$_3$ receptor antagonists are the most active anti-emetic agents in this setting. Routine anti-emetic prophylaxis should accompany total-body irradiation. For patients receiving upper abdominal irradiation, in which the incidence of nausea and vomiting is lower, initial prophylaxis with phenothiazines or other less expensive agents might be a reasonable option. These patients should receive daily oral prophylaxis with a 5-HT$_3$ receptor antagonist, however, if nausea and vomiting is uncontrolled with other agents. Addition of dexamethasone might also be considered; however, the toxicity profile of daily dexamethasone during a four- to six-week course of radiation therapy has not been evaluated.

Summary of Recommendations for Combination Anti-emetic Therapy

Table 38-6 presents recommendations for optimal anti-emetic therapy for chemotherapy regimens based on their emetic potentials. The information presented in Tables 38-2 and 38-3 should be used to assign an emetic level to the chemotherapy agent or regimen being used. Patients receiving regimens with emetic level 3, 4, or 5 should receive a 5-HT$_3$ receptor antagonist plus dexamethasone for prophylaxis of acute nausea and vomiting. For patients who tolerate oral medication, oral anti-emetic combinations are preferable. If intravenous ondansetron is used, the dose should be adjusted based on the emetogenic potential of the chemotherapy regimen, as indicated in Table 38-6. Prophylaxis for delayed nausea and vomiting should be routine for all patients receiving regimens of emetic level 5 and for patients receiving cyclophosphamide-based regimens of emetic potential 4. Breakthrough nausea and vomiting should be managed by adding additional agents rather than by repeating doses of the agents used for prophylaxis.

Patients receiving regimens of low emetic potential (categories 1 and 2) do not require 5-HT$_3$ receptor antagonists and are usually managed effectively either with dexamethasone alone (category 2) or with no prophylactic anti-emetic therapy (category 1).

FUTURE DIRECTIONS

Major improvements in anti-emetic therapy during the past 15 years have resulted in complete protection from chemotherapy-induced nausea and vomiting in the majority of patients during the first 24 hours after administration of treatment. A minority of patients continues to have problems during the first 24 hours after treatment, and in most of these patients, breakthrough nausea and/or vomiting occurs more than 16 hours after administration of chemotherapy. Delayed nausea and vomiting remain the major unsolved problems in anti-emetic therapy, with 40% to 50% of patients continuing to experience some nausea and/or vomiting during days two through five after chemotherapy.

The evolution of standard chemotherapy for many types of cancer has had an impact on the anti-emetic therapy required. Two highly emetogenic chemotherapeutic agents, mechlorethamine and dacarbazine, are now uncommon in clinical practice. More importantly, the use of cisplatin has declined greatly during the last several years mostly due to its replacement by carboplatin, a drug with less emetogenic potential. Many of the more recent cytotoxic agents (e.g., paclitaxel, docetaxel, gemcitabine, topotecan, vinorelbine) are mildly emetogenic agents. Increasing use of these new drugs has also fortuitously enabled the more effective control of chemotherapy-induced emesis. Finally, it is likely that future targeted agents, many of which will be administered orally, will not be associated with nausea or vomiting in most patients. Recent experience with several of these agents, including rituximab, trastuzumab, and imitanib, confirms the low frequency of nausea, even in the absence of any prophylaxis.

Anticipated introduction of the NK-1 receptor antagonists in the near future offers promise for improvement in the management of delayed emesis. Continued well-designed clinical trials are necessary to define the most effective—and the most cost-effective—ways of incorporating these new agents into current anti-emetic regimens.

REFERENCES

1. Coates A, Abraham S, Kaye SB, et al: On the receiving end—Patient perception of the side effects of cancer chemotherapy. Eur J Cancer Clin Oncol 1983;19:203–208.

2. Gralla RJ, Itri LM, Pisko SE, et al: Anti-emetic efficacy of high dose metoclopramide: randomized trials with placebo and prochlorperazine in patients with chemotherapy-induced nausea and vomiting. N Engl J Med 1981;305:905–909.

3. Carelle N, Piotto E, Bellanger A, Germanaud J, Thuillier A, Khayat D: Changing patient perceptions of the side effects of cancer chemotherapy. Cancer 2002;95:155–163.

4. Borison HL, Wang SC: Physiology and pharmacology of vomiting. Pharmacol Rev 1953;5:193–230.

5. Miller AD, Wilson VJ: "Vomiting Center" reanalyzed: an electrical stimulation study. Brain Res 1983;270:154–158.

6. Carpenter DO: Neural mechanisms of emesis. Can J Physiol Pharmacol 1990;68:230–236.

7. Andrews PLR, Davis CJ, Bingham S, Davidson HI, Hawthorne J, Maskell L: The abdominal visceral innervation and the emetic reflex: pathways, pharmacology, and plasticity. Can J Physiol Pharmacol 1990;68:325–345.

8. Leslie RA: Neuroactive substances in the dorsal vagal complex of the medulla oblongata: Nucleus of the tractus solitarius, area postrema and dorsal motor nucleus of the vagus. Neurochem Int 1985;7:191–211.

9. Leslie RA, Shah Y, Thejomayen M, Murphy KM, Robertson HA: The neuropharmacology of emesis: The role of receptors in neuromodulation of nausea and vomiting. Can J Physiol Pharmacol 1990;68:279–288.

10. Ostuka M, Yoshioka K: Neurotransmitter functions of mammalian tachykinins. Physiol Rev 1993;73:229–308.

11. Fozard JR: Neuronal 5-HT receptors in the periphery. Neuropharmacology 1984;23:1473–1486.

12. Tyers MB: 5-HT$_3$ receptors. Ann N Y Acad Sci 1990;600:194–202.

13. Gunning SJ, Hagan RM, Tyers MB: Cisplatin induces biochemical and histological changes in the small intestine of the ferret [abstract]. Br J Pharmacol 1987;90:135P.

14. Endo T, Minami M, Monama Y, Saito H, Takeuchi M: Emesis-related biochemical and histopathological changes induced by cisplatin in the ferret. J Toxicol Sci 1990;15:235–244.

15. Cubeddu LX, Hoffman IS, Fuenmayor NT, Finn AL: Efficacy of ondansetron (GR38032F) and the role of serotonin in cisplatin-induced nausea and vomiting. N Engl J Med 1990;322:810–816.

16. Fetting JH, Grochow LB, Folstein MF, Ettinger DS, Colvin M: The course of nausea and vomiting after high-dose cyclophosphamide. Cancer Treat Rep 1982;66:1487–1493.

17. Kris MG, Gralla RJ, Clark RA, et al: Incidence, course, and severity of delayed nausea and vomiting following the administration of high-dose cisplatin. J Clin Oncol 1985;3:1379–1384.

18. Morrow GR: Prevalence and correlates of anticipatory nausea and vomiting in chemotherapy patients. J Natl Cancer Inst 1982;68:585–588.

19. Wilcox PM, Fetting JH, Nettesheim KM, Abeloff MD: Anticipatory vomiting in women receiving cyclophosphamide, methotrexate and 5-FU (CMF) adjuvant chemotherapy for breast carcinoma. Cancer Treat Rep 1982;66:1601–1604.

20. Hesketh PJ, Kris MG, Grunberg SM, et al: Proposal for classifying the acute emetogenicity of cancer chemotherapy. J Clin Oncol 1997;15:103–109.

21. Tonato M, Roila F, DelFavero A: Methodology of anti-emetic trials: a review. Ann Oncol 1991;2:107–114.

22. Hesketh PJ, Plagge P, Bryson JC: Single-dose ondansetron for prevention of acute cisplatin-induced emesis: analysis of efficacy and prognostic factors. In Branch AL, Grelot L, Miller AD, King GL (eds): Mechanisms and Control of Emesis. London, INSERM/John Libbey Eurotext, 1992, pp 235–243.

23. Kris MG, Tyson LB, Gralla RJ, Clark RA, Allen JC, Reilly LK: Extrapyramidal reactions with high-dose metoclopramide. N Engl J Med 1983;309:433–434.

24. Allen JC, Gralla RJ, Reilly L, Kellick M, Young C: Metoclopramide: dose-related toxicity and preliminary anti-emetic studies in children receiving cancer chemotherapy. J Clin Oncol 1985;3:1136–1141.

25. D'Acquisto RW, Tyson LB, Gralla RJ, et al: The influence of a chronic high alcohol intake on chemotherapy-induced nausea and vomiting {abstract}. Proc Am Soc Clin Oncol 1986;5:257.

26. Sullivan JR, Leyden MJ, Bell R: Decreased cisplatin-induced nausea and vomiting with alcohol ingestion. N Engl J Med 1983;309:796.

27. Hesketh PJ, Murphy WK, Lester EP, et al: GR 38032F (GRC507/75): A novel compound effective in the prevention of acute cisplatin-induced emesis. J Clin Oncol 1989;7:700–705.

28. Gralla RJ, Braun TJ, Squillante A: Metoclopramide: Initial clinical studies of high dosage regimens in cisplatin-induced emesis. In Poster E (ed): The Treatment of Nausea and Vomiting Induced by Cancer Chemotherapy. New York, Masson USA, 1981, pp 167–176.

29. Einhorn LH, Nagy C, Werner K, Finn AL: Ondansetron: a new antiemetic for patients receiving cisplatin chemotherapy. J Clin Oncol 1990;8:731–735.

30. Marty M, Pouillart P, Scholl S, et al: Comparison of the 5-hydroxytryptamine (serotonin) antagonist ondansetron (GR38032F) with high-dose metoclopramide in the control of cisplatin-induced emesis. N Engl J Med 1990;322:816–821.

31. DeMulder PHM, Seynaeve C, Vermorken JB, et al: Ondansetron compared with high-dose metoclopramide in prophylaxis of acute and delayed cisplatin-induced nausea and vomiting. Ann Intern Med 1990;113:834–840.

32. Hainsworth J, Harvey W, Pendergrass K, et al: A single-blind comparison of intravenous ondansetron, a selective serotonin antagonist, with intravenous metoclopramide in the prevention of nausea and vomiting associated with high-dose cisplatin chemotherapy. J Clin Oncol 1991;9:721–728.

33. Chevallier B, on behalf of the Granisetron Study Group: The control of acute cisplatin-induced emesis—A comparative study of granisetron and a combination regimen of high-dose metoclopramide and dexamethasone. Br J Cancer 1993;68:176–180.

34. Sledge GW, Einhorn L, Nagy C, House K: Phase III double-blind comparison of intravenous ondansetron and metoclopramide as anti-emetic therapy for patients receiving multiple-day cisplatin-based chemotherapy. Cancer 1992;70:2524–2528.

35. The Granisetron Study Group: The anti-emetic efficacy and safety of granisetron compared with metoclopramide plus dexamethasone in patients receiving fractionated chemotherapy over 5 days. J Cancer Res Clin Oncol 1993;119:555–559.

36. Chevallier B, Cappelaere P, Splinter T, et al: A double-blind, multicentre comparison of intravenous dolasetron mesylate and metoclopramide in the prevention of nausea and vomiting in caner patients receiving high-dose cisplatin chemotherapy. Support Care Cancer 1997;5:22–30.

37. Warr D, Willan A, Fine S, et al: Superiority of granisetron to dexamethasone plus prochlorperazine in the prevention of chemotherapy-induced emesis. J Natl Cancer Inst 1991;83:1169–1173.

38. Bonneterre J, Chavallier B, Metz R, et al: A randomized double-blind comparison of ondansetron and metoclopramide in the prophylaxis of emesis induced by cyclophosphamide, fluorouracil, and doxorubicin or epirubicin chemotherapy. J Clin Oncol 1990;8:1063–1069.

39. Marschner NW, Adler M, Nagel GA, Christmann D, Fenzl E, Upadhyaya B: Double-blind randomized trial of the anti-emetic efficacy and safety of ondansetron and metoclopramide in advanced breast cancer patients treated with epirubicin and cyclophosphamide. Eur J Cancer 1991;27:1137–1140.

40. Jones AL, Hill AS, Soukop M, et al: Comparison of dexamethasone and ondansetron in the prophylaxis of emesis induced by moderately emetogenic chemotherapy. Lancet 1991;338:483–487.

41. Marty M, on behalf of the Granisetron Study Group: A comparative study of the use of granisetron, a selective 5-HT$_3$ antagonist, versus a standard anti-emetic regimen of chlorpromazine plus dexamethasone in the treatment of cytostatic-induced emesis. Eur J Cancer 1990;26(Suppl 1):S28–S32.

42. Kris MG, Gralla RJ, Clark RA, Tyson LB: Dose-ranging evaluation of the serotonin antagonist GRC507/75 (GR38032F) when used as an anti-emetic in patients receiving anticancer chemotherapy. J Clin Oncol 1988;6:659–662.

43. Grunberg SM, Stevenson LL, Russell CA, McDermed JE: Dose ranging phase I study of the serotonin antagonist GR38032F for prevention of cisplatin-induced nausea and vomiting. J Clin Oncol 1989;7:1137–1141.

44. Riviere A, on behalf of the Granisetron Study Group: Dose finding study of granisetron in patients receiving high-dose cisplatin chemotherapy. Br J Cancer 1994;69:967–971.

45. Kris MG, Grunberg SM, Gralla RJ, et al: Dose-ranging evaluation of the serotonin antagonist dolasetron in patients receiving high-dose cisplatin. J Clin Oncol 1994;12:1045–1049.

46. Fauser AA, Duclos B, Chemaissani A, et al: Therapeutic equivalence of single oral doses of dolasetron mesylate and multiple doses of ondansetron for the prevention of emesis after moderately emetogenic chemotherapy. Eur J Cancer 1996;32A:1523–1529.

47. Martoni S, Angelelli B, Guaraldi M, Strocchi E, Pannuti F: Granisetron versus ondansetron in the prevention of cisplatinum-induced emesis: An open randomized cross-over study {abstract}. Proc Am Soc Clin Oncol 1994;13:431.

48. Navari R, Gandara D, Hesketh P, et al: Comparative clinical trial of granisetron and ondansetron in the prophylaxis of cisplatin-induced emesis. J Clin Oncol 1995;13:1242–1248.

49. Ruff P, Paska W, Goedhals L, et al: Ondansetron compared with granisetron in the prophylaxis of cisplain-induced acute emesis: A multicenter double-blind, randomized, parallel-group study. Oncology 1994;41:113–118.

50. Hesketh P, Navari R, Grote T, et al: Double-blind, randomized comparison of the anti-emetic efficacy of intravenous dolasetron mesylate and intravenous ondansetron in the prevention of acute cisplatin-induced emesis in patients with cancer. J Clin Oncol 1996;14:2242–2249.

51. Audhuy B, Cappelaere P, Martin M, et al: A double-blind, randomized comparison of the anti-emetic efficacy of two intravenous doses of dolasetron mesylate and granisetron in patients receiving high dose cisplatin chemotherapy. Eur J Cancer 1996;32A:807–813.

52. Bonneterre T, Hecquet B: Granisetron (IV) compared with ondansetron (IV plus oral) in the prevention of nausea and vomiting induced by moderately emetogenic chemotherapy: A cross-over study. Bull Cancer 1995;82:1038–1043.

53. Stewart A, McQuade B, Cronje JD, et al: Ondansetron compared with granisetron in the prophylaxis of cyclophosphamide-induced emesis in outpatients: A multicenter, double-blind, double-dummy, randomized, parallel-group study. Oncology 1995;52:202–210.

54. DelGiglio A, Soares HP, Caparroz C, Castro PC: Granisetron is equivalent to ondansetron for prophylaxis of chemotherapy-induced nausea and vomiting: Results of a meta-analysis of randomized controlled trials. Cancer 2000;89:2301–2308.

55. Beck TM, Hesketh PJ, Madajewicz S, et al: Stratified, randomized, double-blind comparison of intravenous ondansetron administered as a multiple-dose regimen versus two single-dose regimens in the prevention of cisplatin-induced nausea and vomiting. J Clin Oncol 1992;10:1969–1975.

56. Seynaeve C, Schuller J, Buser J, et al: Comparison of the anti-emetic efficacy of different doses of ondansetron, given as either a continuous infusion or a single intravenous dose, in acute cisplatin-induced emesis. A multicentre, double-blind, randomized, parallel group study. Br J Cancer 1992;66:192–197.

57. Marty M, d'Allens H: A single-daily dose of ondansetron is as effective as a continuous infusion in the prevention of cisplatin-induced nausea and vomiting. Ann Oncol 1990;1(Suppl 1):112–120.

58. Kamanabrov D: Intravenous granisetron–establishing the optimal dose. Eur J Cancer 1994;28A(Suppl 1):6–13.

59. Riviere A, on behalf of the Granisetron Study Group: Dose finding study of granisetron in patients receiving high-dose cisplatin chemotherapy. Br J Cancer 1994;69:967–971.

60. Lofters WS, Pater JL, Zee B, et al: Phase III double-blind comparison of dolasetron mesylate and ondansetron and an evaluation of the additive role of dexamethasone in the prevention of acute and delayed nausea and vomiting due to moderately emetogenic chemotherapy. J Clin Oncol 1997;15:2966–2973.

61. Hesketh PJ, Beck T, Uhlenhopp H, et al: Adjusting the dose of intravenous ondansetron plus dexamethasone to the emetogenic potential of the chemotherapy regimen. J Clin Oncol 1995;13:2117–2122.

62. Heron JF, Goedhals L, Jordaan JP, Cunningham J, Cedar E: Oral granisetron alone and in combination with dexamethasone: A double-blind randomized comparison against high-dose metoclopramide plus dexamethasone in prevention of cisplatin-induced emesis. Ann Oncol 1994;5:579–584.

63. Perez EA, Hesketh P, Sandbach J, et al: Comparison of single-dose oral granisetron versus intravenous ondansetron in the prevention of nausea and vomiting induced by moderately emetogenic chemotherapy: A multicenter, double-blind, randomized parallel study. J Clin Oncol 1998;16:754–760.

64. Gralla RJ, Navari RM, Hesketh PJ, et al: Single-dose oral granisetron has equivalent anti-emetic efficacy to intravenous ondansetron for highly emetogenic cisplatin-based chemotherapy. J Clin Oncol 1998;16:1568–1573.

65. Spector JI, Lester EP, Chevlen EM, et al: A comparison of oral ondansetron and intravenous granisetron for the prevention of nausea and emesis associated with cisplatin-based chemotherapy. Oncologist 1998;3:432–438.

66. Ettinger DS, Eisenberg PD, Fitts D, Friedman C, Wilson-Lynch K, Yocom K: A double-blind comparison of the efficacy of two dose regimens of oral granisetron in preventing acute emesis in patients receiving moderately emetogenic chemotherapy. Cancer 1996;78:144–151.

67. Rubenstein EB, Gralla RJ, Hainsworth JD, et al: Randomized, double-blind, dose-response trial across four oral doses of dolasetron for the prevention of acute emesis after moderately emetogenic chemotherapy. Cancer 1997;79:1216–1224.

68. Grote TH, Pineda LF, Figlin RA, et al: Oral dolasetron mesylate in patients receiving moderately emetogenic platinum-containing chemotherapy. Cancer J Sci Am 1997;3:45–51.

69. Hesketh PJ, Crews JR, Cohen R, Blackburn LM, Friedman CJ: Anti-emetic efficacy of single-dose oral granisetron (1mg vs 2mg) with moderately emetogenic chemotherapy. Cancer J 2000;6:157–161.

70. Kris MG, Radford JE, Pizzo BA, Inabinet R, Hesketh A, Hesketh PJ: Use of an NK-1 receptor antagonist to prevent delayed emesis after cisplatin. J Natl Cancer Inst 1997;89:817–818.

71. Navari RM, Reinhardt RR, Gralla RJ, et al: Reduction of cisplatin-induced emesis by a selective neurokinin-1-receptor antagonist. N Engl J Med 1999;340:190–195.

72. Hesketh PJ, Gralla RJ, Webb RT, Ueno W, et al: Randomized phase II study of the neurokinin-1-receptor antagonist CJ-11,974 in the control of cisplatin-induced emesis. J Clin Oncol 1999;17:338–343.

73. VanBelle S, Lichinitser MR, Navari RM, et al: Prevention of cisplatin-induced acute and delayed emesis by the selective neurokinin-1 antagonists, L-758,298 and MK-869. A randomized controlled trial. Cancer 2002;94:3032–3041.

74. Aapro MS, Plezia PM, Alberts DS, et al: Double-blind, crossover study of the anti-emetic efficacy of high-dose dexamethasone versus high-dose metoclopramide. J Clin Oncol 1984;2:466–471.

75. Kris MG, Gralla RJ, Tyson LB, et al: Improved control of cisplatin-induced emesis with high-dose metoclopramide and with combinations of metoclopramide, dexamethasone, and diphenhydramine. Results of consecutive trials in 255 patients. Cancer 1985;55:527–534.

76. Gordon CJ, Pazdur R, Ziccarelli A, Cummings G, Al-Sarraf M: Metoclopramide versus metoclopramide and lorazepam: Superiority of combined therapy in the control of cisplatin-induced emesis. Cancer 1989;63:578–582.

77. Fozard JR: 5-HT$_3$ receptors and cytotoxic drug-induced vomiting. Trends Pharmacol Sci 1987;8:44–60.

78. Gralla RJ, Tyson LB, Bordin LA, et al: Anti-emetic therapy: A review of recent studies and a report of a random assignment trial comparing metoclopramide with delta-9-tetrahydrocannabinol. Cancer Treat Rep 1984;68:163–172.

79. Grunberg SM, Gala KV, Lampenfeld M, et al: Comparsion of the anti-emetic effect of high-dose intravenous metoclopramide and high-dose intravenous haloperidol in a randomized double-blind crossover study. J Clin Oncol 1984;2:782–787.

80. Saller R, Hellenbrecht D: High doses of metoclopramide or droperidol in the prevention of cisplatin-induced emesis. Eur J Cancer Clin Oncol 1986;22:1199–1203.

81. Kris MG, Tyson LB, Gralla RJ, Clark RA, Allen JC, Reilly LK: Extrapyramidal reactions with high-dose metoclopramide. N Engl J Med 1983;309:433–434.

82. Kris MG, Gralla RJ, Clark RA, Tyson LB, Groshen S: Anti-emetic control and prevention of side effects of anticancer therapy with

lorazepam or diphenhydramine when used in combination with metoclopramide plus dexamethasone: A double-blind, randomized trial. Cancer 1987;60:2816–2822.

83. Chiara S, Campora E, Lionetto R, Bruzzi P, Rosso R: Methylprednisolone for the control of CMF-induced emesis. Am J Clin Oncol 1987;10:264–267.

84. Roila F, Tonato M, Basurto C, Minotti V, Ballatori E, Del Favero A: Double-blind controlled trial of the anti-emetic efficacy and toxicity of methylprednisolone (MP), metoclopramide (MTC) and domperidone (DMP) in breast cancer patients treated with I.V. CMF. Eur J Cancer Clin Oncol 1987;23:615–617.

85. Zaglama NE, Rosenblum SL, Sartiano GP, Brady M, Gonzalez MF, Valdivieso JG: Single, high-dose intravenous dexamethasone as an anti-emetic in cancer chemotherapy. Oncology 1986;43:27–32.

86. Cassileth PA, Lusk EJ, Torri S, Gerson SL: Anti-emetic efficacy of high-dose dexamethasone in induction therapy in acute nonlymphocytic leukemia. Ann Intern Med 1984;100:701–702.

87. Moertel CG, Reitemeier RJ, Gage RP: A controlled clinical evaluation of anti-emetic drugs. JAMA 1963;186:116–118.

88. Goldstein D, Levi JA, Woods RL, Russell J, Morgan J, Kerestes Z: Double-blind randomized cross-over trial of dexamethasone and prochlorperazine as anti-emetics for cancer chemotherapy. Oncology 1989;46:105–108.

89. Laszlo J, Clark RA, Hanson DC, Tyson L, Crumpler L, Gralla R: Lorazepam in cancer patients treated with cisplatin: A drug with antiemetic amnesic, and anxiolytic effects. J Clin Oncol 1985;3:864–869.

90. Bishop JF, Olver IN, Wolf MM, et al: Lorazepam: A randomized, double-blind, crossover study of a new anti-emetic in patients receiving cytotoxic chemotherapy and prochlorperazine. J Clin Oncol 1984;2:691–695.

91. Grossman B, Lessin LS, Cohen P: Droperidol prevents nausea and vomiting from cisplatinum. N Engl J Med 1979;301:47–49.

92. Neidhart J, Gayen M, Metz E: Haldol is an effective anti-emetic for platinum and mustard-induced vomiting when other agents fail. Proc Am Soc Clin Oncol 1980;21:365.

93. Sallan SE, Zinberg NE, Frei E III: Anti-emetic effect of delta-9-tetrahydrocannabinol in patients receiving cancer chemotherapy. N Engl J Med 1975;293:795–797.

94. Chang AE, Shiling DJ, Stillman RC, et al: Delta-9-tetrahydrocannabinol as an anti-emetic in patients receiving high-dose methotrexate: A prospective randomized evaluation. Ann Intern Med 1979;91:819–824.

95. Sallan SE, Cronin C, Zellen M, Zinberg NE: Antiemetics in patients receiving chemotherapy for cancer. A randomized comparison of delta-9-tetrahydrocannabinol and prochlorperazine. N Engl J Med 1980;302:135–138.

96. McCabe M, Smith FP, MacDonald JS, Wooley PV, Goldberg D, Schein PS: Efficacy of tetrahydrocannabinol in patients refractory to standard anti-emetic therapy. Invest New Drugs 1988;6:243–246.

97. Roila F, Tonato M, Cognetti F, et al: Prevention of cisplatin-induced emesis: A double-blind multicenter randomized crossover study comparing ondansetron and ondansetron plus dexamethasone. J Clin Oncol 1991;9:675–678.

98. Smith DB, Newlands ES, Spruyt OW, et al: Ondansetron (GR38032F) plus dexamethasone: Effective anti-emetic prophylaxis for patients receiving cytotoxic chemotherapy. Br J Cancer 1990;61:323–324.

99. Smyth JF, Coleman RE, Nicolson M, et al: Does dexamethasone enhance control of acute cisplatin-induced emesis by ondansetron? BMJ 1991;303:1423–1426.

100. Carmichael J, Hutchem A, Bessel E, et al: Comparison of granisetron alone and granisetron plus dexamethasone in the prophylaxis of cytotoxic induced emesis by chemotherapy. Br J Cancer 1994;70:1161–1164.

101. The Italian Group for Anti-emetic Research: Dexamethasone, granisetron, or both for the prevention of nausea and vomiting during chemotherapy for cancer. N Engl J Med 1995;332:1–5.

102. Ioannidis JPA, Hesketh PJ, Lau J: Contribution of dexamethasone to control of chemotherapy-induced nausea and vomiting: A meta-analysis of randomized evidence. J Clin Oncol 2000;18:3409–3422.

103. Strum SB, McDermed JE, Liponi DF: High-dose intravenous metoclopramide versus combination high-dose metoclopramide and intravenous dexamethasone in preventing cisplatin-induced nausea and emesis. A single-blind crossover comparison of anti-emetic efficacy. J Clin Oncol 1985;3:245–251.

104. Parikh PM, Charaak BS, Banavali SD, et al: A prospective, randomized double-blind trial comparing metoclopramide alone with metoclopramide plus dexamethasone in preventing emesis induced by high-dose cisplatin. Cancer 1988;62:2263–2266.

105. Grunberg SM, Akerley WL, Krailo MD, Johnson KB, Baker CR, Cariffe PA: Comparison of metoclopramide and metoclopramide plus dexamethasone for complete protection from cisplatinum-induced emesis. Cancer Invest 1986;4:379–385.

106. Gez E, Ben-Yosef R, Catane R, Brufman G, Biran S: Chloropromazine and dexamethasone in patients receiving cancer chemotherapy, particularly cisplatinum. A prospective randomized crossover study. Oncology 1989;49:150–154.

107. Silvey L, Carpenter JT, Wheeler RH, Lee J, Conolley C: A randomized comparison of haloperidol in preventing nausea and vomiting in patients receiving chemotherapy for breast cancer. J Clin Oncol 1988;6:1397–1400.

108. Niiranen A, Mattson K: Anti-emetic efficacy of nabilone and dexamethasone: A randomized study of patients with lung cancer receiving chemotherapy. Am J Clin Oncol 1987;10:325–328.

109. Hesketh PJ, Gandara DR, Hesketh AM, et al: Improved control of high-dose-cisplatin-induced acute emesis with the addition of prochlorperazine to granisetron/dexamethasone. Cancer J Sci Am 1997;3:180–183.

110. Lebeau B, Depierre A, Giovannini M, et al: The efficacy of a combination of ondansetron, methylprednisolone and metopimazine in patients previously uncontrolled with a dual anti-emetic treatment in cisplatin-based chemotherapy. Ann Oncol 1997;8:887–892.

111. Stephens SH, Silvey VL, Wheeler RH: A randomized, double-blind comparison of the anti-emetic effect of metoclopramide and lorazepam with or without dexamethasone in patients receiving high-dose cisplatin. Cancer 1990;66:443–446.

112. Sridhar KS, Donnelly E: Combination anti-emetics for cisplatin chemotherapy. Cancer 1988;61:1508–1517.

113. Cohen RE, Blanchard EB, Ruckdeschel JC, Smolen RD: Prevalence and correlates of post treatment and anticipatory nausea and vomiting in cancer chemotherapy. J Psychosom Res 1986;30:643–654.

114. Morrow GR, Morrell C: Behavioral treatment for the anticipatory nausea and vomiting induced by cancer chemotherapy. N Engl J Med 1982;307:1476–1480.

115. Burish TG, Lyles JN: Effectiveness of relaxation training in reducing adverse reaction to cancer chemotherapy. J Behav Med 1981;4:65–78.

116. Kris MG, Gralla RJ, Tyson LB, Clark RA, Cirrincione C, Groshen S: Controlling delayed vomiting: double-blind, randomized trial comparing placebo, dexamethasone alone, and metoclopramide + dexamethasone in patients receiving cisplatin. J Clin Oncol 1989;7:108–114.

117. Clark R, Kris M, Tyson L, Gralla RJ, O'Hehir M: Anti-emetic trials to control delayed vomiting following high-dose cisplatin {abstract}. Proc Am Soc Clin Oncol 1986;5:257.

118. Navari RM, Madajewicz S, Anderson N, et al: Oral ondansetron for the control of cisplatin-induced delayed emesis: A large, multicenter, double-blind, randomized comparative trial of ondansetron versus placebo. J Clin Oncol 1995;13:2408–2416.

119. Gridelli C, Immidio GP, Androsini G, et al: Ondansetron versus ondansetron plus dexamethasone in the prophylaxis of delayed emesis over three courses of cisplatin chemotherapy: Results of a double-blind, randomized study [abstract]. Proc Am Soc Clin Oncol 1996;15:545.

120. Pater JL, Lofters WS, Zee B, et al: The role of 5HT3 antagonists ondansetron and dolasetron in the control of delayed onset nausea and vomiting in patients receiving moderately emetogenic chemotherapy. Ann Oncol 1997;8:181–185.

121. Latreille J, Pater J, Johnston D, et al: Use of dexamethasone and granisetron in the control of delayed emesis for patients who receive highly emetogenic chemotherapy. J Clin Oncol 1998;16:1174–1178.

122. The Italian Group for Anti-emetic Research: Dexamethasone alone or in combination with ondansetron for the prevention of delayed nausea and vomiting induced by chemotherapy. N Engl J Med 2000;342:1554–1559.

123. Scarantino CW, Ornitz RD, Hoffman LG, Anderson RF Jr: Radiation-induced emesis: Effects of ondansetron. Semin Oncol 1992;19(Suppl 15):38–43.

124. Kirkbride P, Bezjak A, Pater J, et al: Dexamethasone for the prophylaxis of radiation-induced emesis: A National Cancer Institute of Canada Clinical Trials Group phase III study. J Clin Oncol 2000;18:1960–1966.

125. Priestman TJ, Roberts JT, Lucraft CH, et al: Results of a randomized, double-blind comparative study of ondansetron and metoclopramide in the prevention of nausea and vomiting following high-dose upper abdominal irradiation. Clin Oncol 1990;2:71–75.

126. Spitzer TR, Bryson JC, Cirenza E, et al: Randomized, double-blind, placebo-controlled evaluation of oral ondansetron in the prevention of nausea and vomiting associated with fractioned total body irradiation. J Clin Oncol 1994;12:2432–2438.

Problems Common to Cancer and Its Therapy

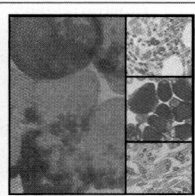

ORAL COMPLICATIONS

Charles L. Loprinzi

Dennis A. Gastineau

Robert L. Foote

SUMMARY OF KEY POINTS

INCIDENCE
- Mucositis is a major dose-limiting toxic effect from 5-fluorouracil (5-FU) and methotrexate.
- Mucositis is very common in patients receiving high doses of chemotherapy with bone marrow rescue.
- Radiation therapy to the oral cavity frequently causes a host of oral complications including mucositis, xerostomia, dental caries, tissue necrosis, and taste alterations.

ETIOLOGY OF COMPLICATIONS
- Direct injury to oral cavity tissue from cytotoxic chemotherapy or radiation therapy

- Secondary infections from treatment-induced myelosuppression
- Graft-versus-host disease (GVHD)

PROPHYLACTIC MEASURES
- Oral cryotherapy during administration of intravenous bolus 5-FU
- Pretreatment dental care, good oral hygiene, and possibly chlorhexidine rinses for patients receiving marrow-ablative chemotherapy
- Pretreatment dental care, good oral hygiene, and sophisticated treatment planning for patients receiving radiation therapy

TREATMENT
- Adequate systemic analgesic measures, including the use of narcotics, if necessary
- Antibiotics and/or antifungal medications in patients with evidence of infection
- Local analgesic methods including salt and baking soda solutions, viscous lidocaine, benzocaine, and other favorite "cocktails" (The efficacy of these measures has not been adequately evaluated to date.)

INTRODUCTION

The oral cavity is a common site for chemotherapy-induced and radiation-induced toxicity. This chapter discusses the etiology, incidence, prevention, and treatment of oral toxic effects of standard chemotherapy, intensive marrow-ablative chemotherapy, and radiation therapy.

CHEMOTHERAPY FOR SOLID TUMORS

Mucositis can be a major dose-limiting toxicity for anti-metabolite cytotoxic agents such as 5-fluorouracil (5-FU), capecitabine, methotrexate, and purine antagonists. Anti-tumor antibiotics (e.g., doxorubicin) and other cytotoxic agents (e.g., hydroxyurea and procarbazine) also cause mucositis occasionally. Mucositis is associated with considerable interpatient variability with no reliable means of predicting which new patients will experience chemotherapy-induced mucositis. Nonetheless, the intra-patient variability appears to be much less, necessitating reductions in drug doses in subsequent chemotherapy cycles for patients in whom severe mucositis develops.

The development of mucositis may be influenced by the drug administration schedule. When 5-FU is given in an intensive course for 5 consecutive days, oral mucositis is a common dose-limiting toxicity, and severe diarrhea is much less common.[1] On the contrary, when 5-FU is given once weekly or as a continuous low-dose intravenous infusion, diarrhea is a much more prominent toxic effect than mucositis.[2]

Combinations of drugs may potentiate mucositis. This is probably best illustrated by the potentiation of 5-FU from the addition of leucovorin factor.[1,2] Also, the combination of two mucositis-producing cytotoxic drugs (e.g., methotrexate and 5-FU) may lead to increased mucositis.

The precise mechanism by which cytotoxic drugs cause mucositis has not been clearly delineated. Presumably, causative agents damage rapidly reproducing mucosal epithelial cells, leading to mucosal inflammation and ulceration. The time course for the development of mucositis after a 5-day course of 5-FU–based chemotherapy is illustrated in Figure 39-1; the mucositis incidence peaks at 7 to 14 days after initiation of treatment with 5-FU.

It is unclear whether or not infection plays a role in the development of mucositis in patients receiving relatively standard chemotherapy for solid tumors (when patients do not have prolonged periods of profound myelosuppression). Further investigations may help delineate the role (or lack thereof) of viruses (e.g., reactivated herpes simplex), bacteria, and fungi in this process.

Prevention

Effective means of preventing mucositis would allow for an improved quality of life for patients receiving chemo-

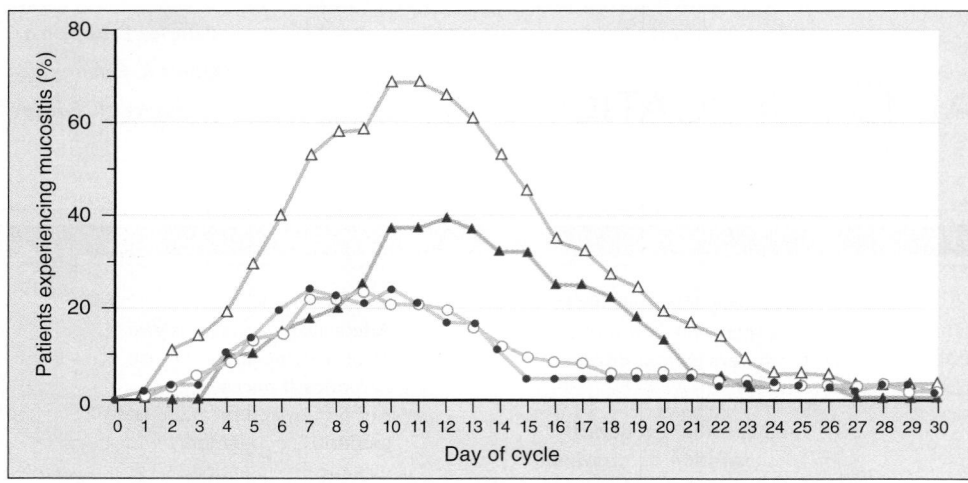

Figure 39-1. Illustrated data demonstrate percentages of patients with mucositis for 30 days after initiation of 5-fluorouracil–based chemotherapy. These data come from two sequential randomized trials[3,5]: one that compared 30 minutes of oral cryotherapy (▲) with a control group (△) and one that compared 30 minutes of cryotherapy (○) with 60 minutes of cryotherapy (●).

therapy. Theoretically, it might also improve the quantity of life by preventing dose reductions during subsequent chemotherapy cycles and permitting the administration of more dose-intensive treatment. In response to this clinical problem, many antidotes have been proposed for preventing 5-FU–induced mucositis.

One of these antidotes has stood the test of two controlled, crossover, randomized, clinical trials. On the basis of the relatively short half-life of intravenous 5-FU (5 to 20 minutes), and with the hope that temporary vasoconstriction of the oral mucosa would decrease 5-FU exposure, a prospective clinical trial was developed to study oral cryotherapy. Study patients receiving their first course of 5-FU–based chemotherapy were randomly assigned to receive oral cryotherapy or to serve as control subjects. The oral cryotherapy was administered by instructing patients to place ice chips in their mouths 5 minutes before each dose of 5-FU and to swish the ice around in their mouths continually, replenishing it so that the ice would be in their mouths for a total of 30 minutes. This study involved 95 patients and demonstrated a marked reduction (about 50% improvement) in stomatitis among the group assigned to cryotherapy[3] (see Fig. 39-1). Showing a healthy degree of skepticism regarding the findings from this first controlled trial, another group designed a trial to confirm or refute these findings. Using a similar trial design, they reported virtually identical findings, that is, that oral cryotherapy decreased oral mucositis by about 50%.[4] Another clinical trial, involving 179 patients, compared 30 versus 60 minutes of oral cryotherapy in a similar population of patients receiving 5-FU–based chemotherapy.[5] Although there was no substantial difference between the mucositis scores for these two groups, both groups had substantially less stomatitis than had been seen in the control arm of the initial cryotherapy trial (see Fig. 39-1). In all three trials, the oral cryotherapy was well tolerated. A recent Cochrane review[6] of mucositis indicated that oral cryotherapy was the only preventive therapy scientifically proven to be beneficial.

This therapy is administered by having the patient suck on crushed ice, starting 5 minutes prior to 5-FU administration and continuing this (replenishing the ice before it completely melts) for a total of 30 minutes. A randomized trial has determined that a longer duration of oral cryotherapy (60 minutes) does not provide any additional benefit.

This procedure would not be expected to be helpful for patients receiving 5-FU by continuous intravenous infusion or for those receiving methotrexate, based on prolonged times of serum drug concentrations in these situations. New data from pilot studies suggest that this oral cryotherapy might also be helpful in preventing edatrexate-induced mucositis, although this has not been confirmed by controlled clinical trials.

Based on this work, 30 minutes of oral cryotherapy should be standard for patients receiving 5-FU–based, intensive-course, 5-day chemotherapy. Obviously, this procedure would not be expected to be useful for patients receiving continuous 5-FU infusions. Nor would it be expected to work for methotrexate-induced mucositis, given the long half-life of methotrexate. Nonetheless, it is reasonable to recommend this oral cryotherapy procedure to patients who have had trouble with mucositis resulting from the intermittent administration of intravenous 5-FU as part of a combination chemotherapy

---

ORAL CRYOTHERAPY FOR PREVENTING 5-FLUOROURACIL–INDUCED MUCOSITIS

Two randomized clinical trials have decisively demonstrated that oral cryotherapy can inhibit the development of bolus 5-FU–induced mucositis. It is hypothesized that this works by causing local vasoconstriction during periods of peak 5-FU blood concentration, decreasing the delivery of 5-FU to the oral mucosa.

regimen (e.g.,CMF: cyclophosphamide [Cytoxan], methotrexate, and 5-FU; CAF: cyclophosphamide [Cytoxan], Adriamycin [doxorubicin], and 5-FU). In addition, nonrandomized investigations suggest that oral cryotherapy may decrease mucositis associated with trimetrexate, an antimetabolite that has a short half-life and can cause dose-limiting mucositis.[7-9]

Chamomile is a compound that has been touted as being useful for preventing and treating cytotoxic therapy–induced oral mucositis.[10] To appropriately study this possibility, the North Central Cancer Treatment Group (NCCTG) conducted a randomized, double-blind, placebo-controlled clinical trial to address whether chamomile would add to oral cryotherapy. Unfortunately, the results from this trial were convincingly negative.[11]

The amino acid glutamine appears to be essential for gut mucosal integrity, and data from pilot or otherwise small clinical trials have suggested that it may be useful for preventing or treating cytotoxic therapy–associated mucositis.[12-14] To address this possibility, investigators conducted two placebo-controlled clinical trials.[15,16] However, neither of these trials was able to suggest any benefit for this approach in patients receiving 5-FU–based chemotherapy.

Two other proposed antidotes have also failed to survive the rigors of randomized trials. The first of these involved the use of an allopurinol mouthwash. After positive reports from two small pilot studies,[17,18] this antidote became part of "standard clinical practice" at some institutions.[19,20] Nonetheless, a placebo-controlled, double-blind, randomized crossover clinical trial produced convincingly negative results.[21] These negative results have been independently supported by other investigators.[22] The second antidote involved the use of acyclovir; a relatively small placebo-controlled, randomized study involving 34 patients evaluated the prophylactic use of acyclovir for patients receiving mucositis-producing chemotherapy for head and neck cancers.[23] This trial failed to show any suggestion of benefit from acyclovir in this situation.

Other compounds that have been proposed for the prevention of chemotherapy-induced mucositis, although they have not been definitively evaluated, include vitamin E,[24] pentoxifylline, colony-stimulating factors,[25] keratinocyte growth factor,[26,27] and prostaglandin E_2.[28,29] In addition, there is suggestive evidence of a potential benefit from low-level laser therapy.[30-34] Further evaluation of this procedure is necessary before this can be recommended as a standard preventive approach.[35]

Treatment

Scant information is available regarding the effective treatment of chemotherapy-induced mucositis, despite a plethora of prescribed remedies. Frequently, a solution of salt and baking soda in water is used as a cleansing and soothing therapy. Also, benzocaine in a hydroxypropyl cellulose base, an agent that produces a protective physical barrier, has been reported to be helpful.[36] Local anesthetics such as viscous lidocaine are often used alone or as part of a cocktail (containing other drugs, e.g.,

> ## TREATMENT OF ESTABLISHED MUCOSITIS
>
> For patients with established mucositis, the first therapeutic measure used usually consists of having patients rinse their mouths every 2 to 4 hours with a salt and baking soda solution ($^1/_2$ tsp salt plus $^1/_2$ tsp baking soda in an 8-oz glass of warm water). This is often soothing (and thought to be cleansing) but has not been formally evaluated in any clinical trial.

magnesium hydroxide, diphenhydramine, and/or sucralfate). Results of a few pilot or small phase II trial studies have suggested that sucralfate could prevent mucositis or hasten the healing of stomatitis.[37-41] To address this possibility, the NCCTG conducted a double-blind, placebo-controlled, randomized clinical trial in patients with 5-FU–induced mucositis. In this trial, patients started the randomly determined treatment on the first day of mucosal irritation from 5-FU. Unfortunately, the results were convincingly negative.[42]

In addition, patients are counseled not to ingest spicy, coarse, hot, cold, or acidic foods or juices or medications or beverages containing alcohol, but rather to ingest soft, moist foods and nonalcoholic beverages.

For moderate or worse pain, local solutions (e.g., viscous lidocaine, magnesium hydroxide, and diphenhydramine) have been used alone or as components of "cocktails" to provide local anesthesia. These remedies, however, have not been adequately evaluated to date. Benzocaine in a hydroxypropyl cellulose base has been reported to be helpful for some patients and may be worth trying.

At times, chemotherapy-induced mucositis may be severe enough to require hospitalization. In this situation, narcotic analgesics may be needed for pain control and intravenous fluids may be necessary for hydration. Usually, the mucositis resolves after a few days of supportive care.

MARROW-ABLATIVE CHEMOTHERAPY

Bone marrow transplantation after high-dose chemotherapy and radiation therapy is being used in an increasing number of diseases and clinical settings. Essentially all antineoplastic therapy affects normal tissues, as well as malignant cells, and the increasing intensity of therapy requiring bone marrow rescue has increased toxic effects on other normal body tissues.[43] Both the intestinal tract and the bone marrow have rapidly dividing cells, and many treatments that are marrow ablative have major side effects on the intestinal tract. The oral cavity is a frequent site of these toxic side effects.

Oral complications are perhaps responsible for the greatest decline in quality of life early in the transplantation period. Symptoms include oral pain, difficulty in swallowing, and pain with swallowing. Signs include edema, erythema, vesicles, ulcers, and visible growth of organisms such as *Candida* species. The signs and symptoms often become so severe that the patient is unable to swallow saliva. In addition, nutrition may become compromised, requiring the institution of parenteral hyperalimentation. Interruption of the mucosal barrier may allow for the systemic spread of bacteria and other pathogens. Existing subclinical oral infections may blossom during major myelosuppression, thereby increasing the chance of sepsis.

During marrow-ablative chemotherapy and subsequent bone marrow transplantation, oral complications may result from myelosuppression, direct cytotoxic effects of chemotherapy on mucosal cells, or immunologic suppression or hyperreactivity. Major clinical problems resulting from myelosuppression include local infections such as tooth abscesses, cytomegalovirus infections, and herpes virus infections. Also, local hemorrhage can occur as a result of thrombocytopenia. Patients with severe mucositis are far more likely to experience bacteremia with *Streptococcus viridans* than are patients without mucositis.[44] Direct cytotoxic effects against mucosal cells are prominent with high-dose cyclophosphamide, anthracyclines, and etoposide, as well as with radiation therapy, all of which are commonly used in various marrow-ablative regimens. In addition, prophylaxis for graft-versus-host disease (GVHD) with methotrexate may increase mucosal ulceration. Immunologic perturbations may cause oral complications in the form of acute or chronic GVHD, as well as by diminishing the host's ability to react against microorganisms. Complications of chronic GVHD may result in xerostomia, increased dental caries, tooth loss, and sicca symptoms.

Pretreatment Evaluation

Before undergoing high-dose chemotherapy and bone marrow rescue, all patients should ideally have a comprehensive dental evaluation, including radiographs, to ensure that no occult oral infections exist that would blossom into major abscesses or sepsis when neutropenia develops. Extractions and endodontic procedures are ideally completed at least 7 to 14 days before the start of a high-dose conditioning regimen. Viral serologies should be obtained before transplantation to determine exposure to herpes simplex virus.

Monitoring of Mucositis

A formal evaluation of the oral cavity should occur daily. Examination of the mouth may be aided by the use of a Vaseline-coated tongue blade, because the mucosal surfaces are often dry and an uncoated wooden tongue blade may painfully adhere to mucosal surfaces. Administration of adequate pain medication before manipulation may allow a more complete evaluation. Proposed scoring systems provide reasonable descriptions of mucositis severity.[45,46] An awareness of the degree of mucositis will assist in pain control, investigation of fever, and the treatment of therapy-associated toxic effects.

The first evidence of mucositis is often pain and dysphagia. These symptoms usually occur before there are any signs of erythema or ulceration.[47] The frenulum and sublingual surfaces are frequently early sites of ulceration. Edema of the buccal mucosa is commonly seen, and the edema may sometimes extend to the tongue. In extremely severe mucositis, tongue edema may lead to impending airway obstruction.

Prevention and Treatment

With the onset of treatment, toothbrushing with a soft brush or sponge should be initiated. This care is designed to minimize the collection of debris in the mouth, which may serve as a culture medium for bacteria. Use of prophylactic chlorhexidine rinses (every 4 hours) is often recommended based on positive evidence generated from randomized clinical trials.[48,49] Oral acyclovir is indicated for patients with positive herpes simplex serology.[50] Prophylaxis of viral reactivation has dramatically decreased the morbidity associated with mucositis and transplantation.

Oral antifungal therapy is initiated either at the onset of mucositis or as an initial part of mouth care. Nystatin and clotrimazole solutions (or troches) are effective therapies for oral fungal infections. Fluconazole may also be useful if systemic antifungal therapy is used prophylactically. Local solutions do not usually provide added benefits. Steroids are rarely used when there is marked tongue edema with impending airway obstruction, and their value in this situation has not been clearly defined.

Acute GVHD, reactivation of herpes simplex, or both should be suspected when mucositis suddenly worsens 10 to 15 days after progenitor cell transfusion. The presence of copious diarrhea suggests acute GVHD. Severe gut GVHD requires treatment with systemic corticosteroids.

Cultures of lesions should be taken frequently to ensure sufficient specific coverage with antimicrobial therapy. Bacterial infections may be local or systemic, and the increased rate of sepsis associated with severe mucositis is striking. In the presence of severe mucositis, empiric antibiotics should include *Streptococcus viridans* coverage. Herpes simplex virus–complicated mucositis is often much more painful than mucositis from cytotoxic effects alone, and thus pain intensity can provide a clue to diagnosis in this situation.

The introduction of growth factors not only has affected the recovery of blood cells after high-dose chemotherapy but also appears to lessen some of the nonmarrow toxic effects of many chemotherapeutic regimens. Recombinant human granulocyte-macrophage colony-stimulating factor (GM-CSF) produces a lower incidence of bacteremia, which is thought to be due to a shorter course of neutropenia, as well as decreased alteration of the normal barrier function of the gastrointestinal tract.[51,52] Less mucositis is observed with growth factors, and this effect appears to be due to more than just a shorter period of granulocytopenia.[53] Further research is indicated to better understand the effects of growth factors on mucositis.

A diphenhydramine hydrochloride suspension may act as a local anesthetic. A lidocaine suspension can result in useful anesthesia, but it should be used with caution, because it can eliminate the gag reflex and increase the risk of aspiration. If local treatment measures do not provide effective pain relief, adequate coverage with parenteral narcotics is indicated. This may require parenteral morphine infusions of up to 15 mg/h. Addiction to narcotics triggered by administration during transplantation does not happen without a significant premorbid history, and concerns about addiction should rarely, if ever, interfere with adequate pain therapy.

RADIATION THERAPY

Mucositis

Etiology

The most troublesome acute reaction for patients receiving radiation therapy to the oral cavity is radiation-induced mucositis. Acute mucositis results from the loss of squamous epithelial cells owing to the sterilization of mucosal stem cells and the inhibition of transit cell proliferation. This leads to a gradual linear decrease in epithelial cell numbers. As radiation therapy continues, a steady state between mucosal cell killing and mucosal cell regeneration may occur because of an increased cell production rate from the surviving cells. Usually, however, cell regeneration cannot keep up with cell killing, and partial or complete denudation develops. This presents as patchy or confluent pseudomembranous mucositis. Healing eventually occurs when cells regenerate from the surviving mucosal stem cells. The loss of the epithelial barrier exacerbates insults from physical, chemical, and microbial agents. It has been reported that the oropharyngeal flora may contribute to radiation therapy–induced mucositis.[54-56] However, which flora are involved and which step in the mucositis process may be prevented by eliminating the offending flora remain unknown. One hypothesis is that endotoxins produced by gram-negative bacilli are potent mediators of the inflammatory process.

The oral cavity mucosa, having a relatively high turnover rate, changes early during a course of fractionated external-beam radiation therapy. With 200-cGy fractions per day, 5 days per week, mucosal erythema is typically noted within the first week or two of treatment. By approximately 2 to 3 weeks, the erythematous mucosa develops small whitish yellow patches called *patchy pseudomembranous mucositis*. These pseudomembranes represent collections of dead surface epithelial cells, fibrin, and polymorphonuclear leukocytes on a moist background. This acute reaction is typically accompanied by oral discomfort. In many patients, the patchy mucositis becomes confluent by the third or fourth week of radiation therapy and can be associated with significant pain.

The severity of mucositis is related to the daily dose of radiation therapy, the total cumulative dose, the volume of irradiated tissue, and the use of concurrent radiation-sensitizing and/or mucositis-inducing chemotherapeutic agents.[57-64] At fractions of 170- to 180-cGy daily, 5 days per week, the maximal reaction is typically intense erythema with occasional patchy mucositis. In this situation, the cell killing and repopulation of epithelial stem cells are in near equilibrium. If the daily dose is increased to 200 cGy or more, as in the case of altered fractionation schedules such as hyperfractionation (110 cGy to 150 cGy twice a day) or accelerated fractionation (160 cGy two or three times a day or concomitant boost with 180 cGy in the morning and 150 cGy in the afternoon), and the treatment volume is large (the entire oral cavity), cell killing will exceed the proliferative capacity of the epithelial stem cells, and almost all patients will have confluent mucositis by the third week of radiation therapy.[60,65-70] Mucositis first appears and is often most severe on the mucosa of the soft palate, tonsillar pillars, buccal mucosa, lateral border of the tongue, and pharyngeal walls. In contrast, mucositis less frequently involves the hard palate, gingival ridges, and the dorsum of the tongue during a course of radiation therapy or, alternatively, only after very high doses. In patients with metallic dental restorations, a prominent mucositis frequently develops on the adjacent buccal mucosa, and/or the lateral border of the adjacent tongue, or both as a result of backscattering of low-energy electrons.

Symptoms of oral discomfort are usually maximal 3 to 4 weeks into the course of radiation therapy. Thereafter, symptoms usually plateau and may even diminish in patients treated with radiation therapy alone, even though treatment is continued. After external-beam radiation therapy, the mucous membranes normally heal within 2 to 4 weeks, although an occasional patient may require several weeks or months. The latter is particularly true of patients treated with concurrent radiochemotherapy.

The mucositis produced by an interstitial radioactive implant typically appears 7 to 10 days after removal and is maximal approximately 2 weeks after removal. The mucositis generally heals by 6 weeks, unless the implanted volume was large, in which case, complete healing may require several months.[59]

Radiation-induced oral mucositis can result in intense pain, which may substantially limit adequate hydration and nutrition, prevent proper oral hygiene, serve as a portal for infection, and affect speech. All these effects can significantly interfere with the general well-being of the patient and may tempt the treating physician to interrupt the course of treatment to permit resolution of the acute symptoms. At times, the treatment may be discontinued altogether before delivery of a potentially curative dose of radiation therapy.

Rapidly accumulating clinical and radiobiologic evidence shows that the protraction of overall treatment time adversely influences the radiocurability of certain human tumors, particularly squamous cell carcinomas of the head and neck region.[71-76] In a retrospective study of nearly 500 patients with squamous cell carcinoma of the oral cavity and oropharynx, overall treatment time was found to significantly influence the probability of local tumor control.[72] The additional dose needed to compensate for a protracted course of radiation therapy has been attributed to an accelerated tumor clonogenic growth rate. Several retrospective studies and randomized clinical trials have demonstrated improved local control and survival when altered fractionation schemes that deliver conventional or higher doses of radiation therapy are used over a shorter-than-conventional period.[60,66-68,70,77-87] Therefore a break in radiation therapy because of mucositis may lead to treatment failure.

Prevention and Treatment

In light of the serious deleterious effects that radiation-induced oral mucositis may have on a patient's well-being and the potential loss of tumor control that may result from an interruption or prolongation of treatment because of mucositis, measures for preventing mucositis are being investigated. In one small trial the use of a benzydamine hydrochloride rinse for preventing radiation-induced mucositis was studied.[88] Benzydamine hydrochloride, a nonsteroidal drug, possesses analgesic, anesthetic, anti-inflammatory, and antimicrobial properties. Its action may be mediated by the prostaglandin system. Forty-three patients undergoing radiation therapy to the oropharyngeal region (4500 cGy in 15 fractions in 3 weeks or 6000 cGy in 25 fractions in 5 weeks) were randomly assigned (double-blind, placebo-controlled) to receive either benzydamine hydrochloride or a carrier base "placebo" consisting of 10% alcohol and artificial flavor and color. All 25 patients assigned to receive benzydamine hydrochloride were evaluable, but 6 of 18 patients who received placebo did not comply with the protocol and were thus removed from the study and not included in the statistical analysis. The total mucositis score was lower in the benzydamine group than in the placebo group ($P = .001$). The average area of mucositis during radiation therapy and the maximum mucositis score were also reported to be significantly less in the benzydamine group ($P = .05$). In addition, maximum size of ulceration ($P = .04$) and total area of ulceration ($P = .05$) were significantly less in the benzydamine group. Although not statistically significant, trends were seen in favor of the benzydamine group for less pain reported at rest ($P = .08$), less pain with eating ($P = .09$), greater pain reduction ($P = .07$), and improved anesthesia ($P = .10$). Thus this study provided preliminary evidence that benzydamine might be beneficial in patients undergoing radiation therapy to the oral cavity. However, the alcohol in the placebo control may have actually caused mucosal irritation and may thus have been responsible, in part, for patients in the placebo arm doing less well.

A larger, multicenter, randomized, double-blind, placebo-controlled clinical trial evaluating benzydamine hydrochloride for prophylaxis of radiation-induced oral mucositis demonstrated that that this agent was effective, safe, and well tolerated for prophylactic treatment of radiation-induced oral mucositis.[89] Patients were instructed to rinse for 2 minutes, four to eight times daily, before and during radiation therapy and for 2 weeks after completion of radiation therapy. Use of benzydamine was associated with significantly reduced erythema and ulceration and delayed use of systemic analgesics. Benzydamine was not effective for patients receiving accelerated radiation therapy. The authors of this study recommend routine prophylactic use of a benzydamine 0.15% oral rinse.

In another small trial, 25 patients receiving radiation therapy (6000 cGy in 30 fractions over 6 weeks or 5400 cGy in 18 fractions over 6 weeks) to the oral cavity were randomly assigned to use mouthwashes consisting of benzydamine or chlorhexidine, a broad-spectrum antimicrobial.[90] In this trial similar average pain scores, average mucositis grades, candidal carriage rates, and coliform bacteria carriage rates were reported in the two treatment groups. However, patients who received the chlorhexidine mouthwash tolerated that rinse better. Furthermore, fewer patients using chlorhexidine required a prolongation of radiation therapy because of oral symptoms. These authors concluded that chlorhexidine and benzydamine showed little difference in controlling overall pain and mucositis or the oral carriage of *Candida* species and coliform bacteria. Because patients better tolerated the chlorhexidine mouthwash, its use was preferred.

Several controlled clinical trials evaluated the combination of three relatively nonabsorbable antibiotics (tobramycin, polymyxin E, and amphotericin B) for patients undergoing radiation therapy to the oral cavity. In a prospective study, Spijkervet and associates[91] compared data from 15 patients receiving this antibiotic lozenge with data from 15 patients in each of two groups that had previously been randomly assigned to receive a chlorhexidine mouthwash or a placebo mouthwash. In all patients using the antibiotic lozenges, eradication of gram-negative bacilli was achieved within 3 weeks, whereas no effects on these flora were observed in the chlorhexidine or placebo groups ($P = .01$). The severity and extent of mucositis were also significantly reduced in the 15 patients receiving the antibiotic lozenge ($P = .05$). All patients in the antibiotic lozenge–treated group had erythema only, whereas 80% of the placebo- and chlorhexidine-treated patients had severe mucositis with extensive pseudomembranes, starting in the third week of a conventional radiation therapy protocol. No nasogastric tube feedings were required in the antibiotic lozenge–treated group, but 30% of patients in the chlorhexidine- and placebo-treated groups required tube feedings. Another small pilot study, performed by Mulkens and colleagues,[92] involved 25 patients. The maximum degree of mucositis noted was grade 2 (World Health Organization scoring system), and no treatment interruption or nasogastric tube feedings were required.

The results of a randomized, placebo-controlled, double-blind study have been reported by Symonds and colleagues.[93] A total of 275 patients were randomly allocated to suck a pastille containing amphotericin, polymyxin, and tobramycin four times daily ($n = 136$) or an identical-appearing placebo ($n = 139$). A large number of patients were inevaluable ($n = 54$), and there was a slight imbalance in the sites of disease. No statistically significant difference was found in the primary study end point (percentage of patients who had intermediate changes or pseudomembranes, 36% vs. 48%; $P = .48$). The comparison of the lowest recorded mucositis grade was statistically significantly different from the highest grade, favoring the active pastilles ($P = .009$) and indicating a beneficial effect, the magnitude of which was probably smaller than the trial was designed to detect. There were also reductions in mucositis distribution ($P = .002$), mucositis area (P = .028), dysphagia (P = .006), and weight loss (P = .009) in the active arm.

Members of the NCCTG also performed a randomized, placebo-controlled, study in which patients receiving radiation therapy to the oral cavity were randomly assigned to receive a placebo, a chlorhexidine mouthwash, or an antibiotic lozenge.[94,95] Fifty-eight patients received placebos (mouthwash or lozenge), 25 received a chlorhexidine mouthwash, and 54 received antibiotic lozenges. There was a trend for more mucositis, and there was substantially more toxicity in the chlorhexidine arm, so it was discontinued after a planned interim analysis. It appeared that the chlorhexidine mouthwash was actually detrimental. In addition, there were no substantial differences or trends in mucositis scores between the antibiotic lozenge and placebo arms as measured by health care providers. However, the mean patient-reported mucositis score and the duration of patient-reported grade 3 to 4 mucositis were both lower in patients assigned to the antibiotic lozenge arm (P = .02 and .007, respectively).

Wijers and co-workers,[96] from The Netherlands, conducted a placebo-controlled, double-blind, randomized study of radiation-induced mucositis reduction by selective elimination of oral flora with an oral paste. No statistically significant difference in objective or subjective mucositis scores was observed between the two study arms. The percentage of patients with positive cultures of aerobic gram-negative bacteria was significantly reduced in the antibiotic group. These results cast doubt on the hypothesis that these bacteria play an important role in the pathogenesis of mucositis.

El-Sayed and colleagues,[97] from Canada, also completed a multicenter, placebo-controlled, double-blind, prospective, randomized trial to evaluate the clinical efficacy of an antimicrobial lozenge containing bacitracin, clotrimazole, and gentamycin. One hundred thirty-seven patients were included. There were no statistically significant differences between the arms in median time to development of severe mucositis, extent of severe mucositis as measured by physicians, oral toxic effects as recorded by patients, or radiotherapy delays. The authors concluded that the lozenge did not have a significant impact on the severity of mucositis in patients treated with conventionally fractionated radiation therapy.[97]

In total, these trials do not provide convincing data of sufficient clinical magnitude to recommend use of antimicrobial mouthwashes (chlorhexidine or benzydamine), antibiotic lozenges, or paste as part of standard practice. For a critical review, the reader is referred to an article by Sutherland and Browman.[98]

The inability to control mucositis-related pain can be frustrating for both the patient and the treating physician. In a small trial, 18 patients were randomly assigned in a double-blind study to test the efficacy of (1) viscous lidocaine with 1% cocaine; (2) dyclonine hydrochloride 1.0%; (3) a mixture of kaolin-pectin solution, diphenhydramine, and saline; and (4) a placebo solution.[99] Four of the patients did not complete the study. No significant difference was found among the four solutions when pain relief and duration of relief were compared, but the power

to detect any statistical difference was poor because of the small number of patients. A randomized trial of morphine versus tricyclic antidepressants for treatment of radiation-induced mucositis pain in head and neck cancer showed that morphine produces greater pain relief than do tricyclic antidepressants.[100] Some patients, nonetheless, seemed to have sufficient pain control with tricyclic antidepressants alone. Thus tricyclic antidepressants may prove to be useful for patients with contraindications to opioid treatment. Tricyclic antidepressants were studied because of the similarities between mucositis pain and neuropathic pain. A mucosa-adhesive water-soluble polymer film containing topical anesthetics and antibiotics was evaluated for its abilities to alleviate pain caused by acute radiation-induced oral mucositis and to maintain good oral feeding and prevent secondary oral infections in an uncontrolled clinical trial.[101] Evensen and associates[102] found a sodium-sucrose octasulfate oral rinse to be ineffective in alleviating radiation-induced acute skin and mucosal reactions. Janjan and colleagues[103] reported improved pain management in patients undergoing radiation therapy for head and neck cancer with daily nursing intervention consisting of instructions on the use of mouthwashes and a three-step analgesic protocol consisting of acetaminophen, acetaminophen with codeine suspension, and liquid morphine for relief of mild, moderate, and severe pain. Patients were seen daily by a radiation oncology nurse who serially reviewed a 15-question pain survey completed by the 19 study patients before each radiation treatment. A physician promptly changed the prescribed analgesic regimen when the patient's symptoms changed. Marked differences in the control of pain related to radiation mucositis were observed in these patients as compared with patients from a prior study who used the same daily survey but had sporadic nursing intervention and no analgesic protocol. Patients who had daily nursing intervention reported fewer days of moderate and severe pain; had less pain throughout the day; and noted less disturbance in sleep, eating, and energy level. Weight loss of greater than 5 kg was noted in only 3 of 19 patients. Analgesics were used on 77% of treatment days and relieved all or most of the pain on 94% of these days. Thus daily review of a symptom survey by a radiation oncology nurse combined with a well-defined strategy for mouth care and analgesics appeared to improve pain management of radiation-induced oropharyngeal mucositis because of prompt attention to patient needs. Many narcotic pain medications come in a liquid formulation that is relatively easy to swallow or can be administered through a feeding tube. Fentanyl patches are also very effective for patients who cannot swallow.

New ways of preventing or minimizing radiation-induced mucositis are being evaluated. One such idea involves the use of a sucralfate suspension, an agent that appears to provide a protective barrier and may also have a cytoprotective effect. The latter may be mediated through prostaglandin release, resulting in increased mucosal blood flow, increased mucus production, increased mitotic activity, and a surface migration of cells.[37] However, results from small double-blind, placebo-controlled, randomized prospective trials are contradictory. Epstein and colleagues,[104] Carter and associates,[105] Makkonen and co-workers,[106] and Lievens and colleagues[107] found that prophylactic oral rinsing with sucralfate did not prevent radiation-induced oral ulcerative mucositis. Franzen and associates,[108] however, noted a significantly lower proportion of patients with severe mucosal reactions in their sucralfate group than in a placebo group. One report suggested that a combination of sucralfate and fluconazole may be effective in diminishing oral discomfort and pain associated with radiation and chemotherapy.[109] Lastly, two NCCTG trials evaluated sucralfate as an agent to prevent radiation-associated esophagitis and proctitis, with negative results from both studies.[110,111] Thus the randomized trials of sucralfate for therapy-induced mucositis do not establish a role for sucralfate in clinical practice.

In an evaluation of another intervention, Maciejewski and coworkers[112] reported that painting the buccal mucosa with a 2% silver nitrate solution for several days before radiation therapy stimulates normal mucosa repopulation during radiation therapy, producing a significantly less severe mucosal reaction and faster mucosal healing after completion of radiation therapy. Low-energy laser therapy may also activate epithelial healing. A phase III, randomized, placebo-controlled trial to evaluate the efficacy of low-energy helium-neon laser in the prevention of radiation-induced mucositis has been completed. This trial demonstrated significant reductions in severity and duration of oral mucositis associated with radiation therapy, even when combined with chemotherapy.[113] A double-blind, placebo-controlled, randomized trial of treatment with 40 mg of prednisone, beginning on day 8 of an accelerated course of radiation therapy, did not show a reduction in the intensity or duration of mucositis.[114] However, there was a trend favoring prednisone in terms of shorter treatment interruptions and a significant reduction in overall treatment time. These unique approaches to the problem of acute mucositis deserve further study.

Other preliminary studies have investigated the direct application of a prostaglandin E_2 gel,[115] the use of a combination of beclomethasone dipropionate and sodium alginate,[116] the use of oral glutamine,[117] and daily use of subcutaneous GM-CSF.[118] On the basis of preliminary data,[115] the Radiation Therapy Oncology Group (RTOG) completed a phase II study to evaluate the radioprotection of oral and pharyngeal mucosa by the prostaglandin E_1 analog, misoprostol, used as an oral rinse. The results are not yet available. Results of a small pilot randomized trial have suggested that oral glutamine may significantly reduce the duration and severity of oral mucositis during radiotherapy.[117] A 3-minute 30-mL oral rinse was used before meals and at bedtime, beginning on the first day of radiation therapy and ending on the last day. However, the less-than-convincing data associated with glutamine for chemotherapy-induced mucositis[15,16] raise doubt about whether glutamine is actually helpful. Results of pilot studies suggested that GM-CSF may be quite effective in the prevention and treatment of radiation-induced oral mucositis.[119,120] Saarilahti and colleagues[121] conducted

a randomized phase II study in 40 patients receiving conventional postoperative radiation therapy. Patients were randomly assigned to receive sucralfate or GM-CSF mouthwashes. Patients who received the GM-CSF mouthwash tended to have less severe oral mucositis ($P = .072$), significantly less mucosal pain ($P = .058$), and less need for opioids for pain relief ($P = .042$).[115] However, a prospective randomized clinical trial showed no evidence that subcutaneously administered GM-CSF reduced the severity of radiation-induced mucositis.[122] The RTOG is currently conducting a phase III study to test the efficacy and safety of GM-CSF in reducing the severity and duration of mucosal injury and pain associated with radiation therapy in patients with head and neck cancer. The GM-CSF will be administered subcutaneously. There is also interest in, and some early mouse mucosal data that would suggest that, keratinocyte growth factor may be efficacious in the prevention and treatment of radiation-induced mucositis.[123] A multicenter study of intravenous repifermin (keratinocyte growth factor 2) to reduce mucositis in patients with head and neck cancer receiving chemoradiotherapy is being developed.

The radioprotector amifostine has been evaluated as a means of preventing radiation-induced acute mucositis. One small ($n = 28$) randomized clinical trial reported that amifostine reduced the severity of acute mucositis ($P = .0001$).[124] A larger randomized trial ($n = 50$) reported that treatment duration (less frequent treatment interruptions) and the severity of acute mucositis were significantly reduced in the amifostine arm.[125] However, a larger phase III randomized trial ($n = 315$) failed to demonstrate a reduction in the incidence and severity of radiation-induced mucositis with amifostine.[126] Nausea, vomiting, hypotension, and allergic reactions were common side effects of this drug, with half the patients experiencing nausea, vomiting, or both. These side effects may be reduced by rapid intravenous push, optimal hydration of the patient, premedication with antiemetics, and subcutaneous administration. In total, present data are insufficient to recommend amifostine at the current dose and schedules to prevent mucositis associated with radiation therapy.[127]

One should not forget the role that sophisticated radiation therapy treatment planning can have in limiting the volume of normal tissues irradiated and thereby reducing the severity of normal tissue reactions. Kaanders and associates[128] recently reported that normal tissue reactions can be reduced in a substantial number of patients with head and neck cancer with the use of simple, custom-made, intraoral devices designed to exclude uninvolved tissues from the treatment portals or to provide shielding of tissues within the treatment area. Patients with primary cancers of the oral cavity, oropharynx, paranasal sinuses, and salivary glands are the best candidates for the use of such devices. These intraoral stents can be very useful in excluding the mucosa of the tongue and the floor of the mouth when hard palate, nasal cavity, and paranasal sinus malignancies are being treated. These same stents can be useful in excluding the palate mucosa during treatment of the tongue or floor of the mouth. Shielding stents made with a lead alloy were found to be useful in treatment of well-lateralized tumors of the oral cavity, parotid gland, lip, and skin of the cheek. These shielding stents can decrease the amount of radiation delivered to the contralateral mucosa. More frequent use of electron-beam and/or sophisticated three-dimensional conformal, multibeam, wedged-pair, or oblique treatment plans will also help exclude or minimize the radiation dose to uninvolved mucosa. Packing gauze between metallic dental restorations and mucosa of the lateral tongue and buccal area appears to be very beneficial in minimizing the dose from scattered radiation.

Given these data, what measures should be taken to prevent and treat mucositis in patients receiving radiation to the oral cavity? Standard practice often includes aggressive, good oral hygiene consisting of brushing teeth after each meal, using a soft toothbrush and baking soda toothpaste, and rinsing the mouth every 2 hours throughout the day with a half-strength hydrogen peroxide or alkaline saline solution. Patients should be instructed to avoid the use of irritating or abrasive substances such as commercial toothpastes and mouthwashes; tobacco; alcoholic beverages; extremely hot or cold drinks or foods; very spicy foods; acidic foods such as citrus fruits and their juices; and foods that are hard and coarse, such as pretzels, raw vegetables, potato chips, crackers, and hard bread. When discomfort develops, topical anesthetic agents can be used. As the pain progresses, use of systemic analgesics, including acetaminophen with codeine suspension or oral morphine sulfate elixir, may become necessary. Suspensions are preferred over elixirs, because they are formulated without alcohol. As suggested by Janjan and coworkers,[103] daily intervention by a radiation therapy nurse or physician with prompt increases in doses of systemic analgesics appears to result in improved pain control, improved sense of well-being, and less weight loss.

The mucosa of patients undergoing radiation therapy to the oral cavity should be examined at least once a week, and antibiotic or antifungal medications should be prescribed as infections are documented. Clotrimazole troches, one dissolved in the mouth five times a day for 14 days, generally work well for oral candidiasis. However, if significant mucositis or xerostomia has developed, it may be very difficult to dissolve lozenges in the oral cavity. In this situation, nystatin oral suspension or fluconazole in tablet or liquid form is often effective.

Xerostomia

The major salivary glands (parotid, submandibular, and sublingual) produce most of the salivary secretion (up to 80%). The rest of the saliva is produced by minor glands scattered throughout the oral cavity. It is estimated that the sublingual glands contribute only 2% to 5% of the salivary flow rate. Submandibular glands seem to be as important as or more important than parotid glands in the resting state, although parotid glands become the main contributors under stimulation.

When radiation therapy treatment fields include the major salivary glands, many patients will experience dryness of the oral mucosa during the first 1 or 2 weeks of treatment. Not only is the quantity of saliva reduced, but

its composition and physical properties are changed as well. Drastic reductions of baseline and reflex production of alkaline and watery secretions of serous acini often persist after the completion of radiation therapy. Without appropriate management, this problem can lead to progressive deterioration of the teeth, mucosa, gingiva, and mandible.

The acute radiation response of serous salivary glands has been shown to be due to interphase killing of serous cells. Chronic atrophy of these glands is attributed to the death of the reproductive stem cells and damage to the fibrovascular stroma.[129]

Marks and colleagues[130] have documented a progressive reduction in salivary flow rates, pH, and secretory immunoglobulin A (IgA) with increasing doses of radiation therapy. These investigators clearly demonstrated a dose response in terms of the late effect of radiation on parotid salivary flow. Nine of 10 parotid glands that received less than 1000 cGy continued to secrete measurable quantities of saliva after stimulation by sour grape drops. This was reduced to 4 of 8 after administration of 3000 cGy, 3 of 16 after 5000 cGy, and 0 of 24 after 7000 cGy. Franzen and associates[131] found that 15 of 16 patients receiving doses of less than 5200 cGy showed recovery of secretion beginning 2 months after treatment with continual improvement of the salivary flow for up to 18 months. Doses exceeding 6400 cGy caused irreversibly depressed parotid function in the majority of glands. Patients receiving doses of more than 6400 cGy to one gland had only slight dryness; however, patients with both glands irradiated showed severe problems with salivary flow and discomfort of dryness.[131] Mira and colleagues[132] showed that exclusion of more than 50% of both parotid glands from the direct radiation beam can prevent severe dryness when the rest of the major salivary glands are included in the field. Roesink and colleagues[133] found a linear correlation between postradiotherapy flow ratio and parotid gland dose and a strong volume dependency. They found no threshold dose and suggested that in radiation treatment planning, attempts should be made to achieve a mean parotid dose below 39 Gy (complication probability = 50%). They demonstrated some recovery of parotid function at 6 months and 1 year after radiation therapy.

Eisbruch and colleagues[134] suggested that a mean parotid gland dose of ≤26 Gy should be a planning goal if substantial sparing of the gland function is desired. Using the Normal Tissue Complication Probability model, they found that the dose/volume/function relationships in the parotid glands are characterized by dose and volume thresholds, steep dose/response/function relationships when the thresholds are reached, and a maximal volume dependence parameter. Chao and coworkers[135] observed a correlation between mean parotid dose and the fractional reduction of stimulated saliva output at 6 months after the completion of radiation therapy. They also noted that responses to quality-of-life questions on eating and speaking functions were significantly correlated with stimulated and unstimulated saliva flow at 6 months. Therefore sparing of the parotid glands should translate into objective and subjective improvement of xerostomia and quality of life in patients with head and neck cancer receiving radiation therapy. Eisbruch and colleagues[136] found that the degree of xerostomia was related to the degree of preradiation therapy xerostomia, the time since radiation therapy, and the mean dose to the major salivary glands (most notably the submandibular gland) and to the oral cavity. This would suggest that sparing of the oral mucosa with its minor salivary glands is an important goal in treatment planning to reduce the severity of radiation-induced xerostomia.

Mira and associates[132] also reported that patients with high pretreatment salivary flow rates experience less dryness after a particular dose of radiation therapy or treatment volume than patients with low pretreatment flow rates. These investigators found that the decrease in flow rate after radiation follows an exponential decay curve. A given dose of radiation therapy reduces flow by approximately the same percentage.[132] For example, a patient whose initial salivary flow rate is 0.2 mL/min would require reduction by only 50% to reach a minimal flow rate of 0.1 mL/min, whereas a patient whose flow rate is 1.0 mL/min would require a 90% reduction to reach the same minimal flow rate. The latter patient would require approximately three times as much radiation as the former patient to achieve a minimal flow rate. These same investigators showed that when almost all salivary tissue was irradiated, a dose of 3500 to 4000 cGy was capable of inducing minimal flow in patients with high initial flow rates and that 500 to 1500 cGy resulted in minimal flow rates in patients with low initial flow rates. Patients in whom minimal flow rates were induced during radiation therapy showed no recovery of flow for up to 17 months after treatment. Age also appears to be an important factor related to the degree of xerostomia after radiation therapy, because young patients are more likely than older patients to recover salivary flow.[59]

Prevention and Treatment of Xerostomia

Treatment of radiation-induced xerostomia includes the avoidance of any drugs that may also decrease the flow of saliva and contribute to the discomfort of xerostomia. These drugs may include anorectic agents, anticholinergics, antidepressants, antihistamines, antihypertensives, antipsychotics, antiparkinsonian agents, diuretics, caffeine, nicotine, hypnotics, and sedatives. Patients should be advised to take frequent sips of water and suck on ice chips. Because chewing stimulates the flow of saliva, patients with residual salivary function may be helped by eating foods such as carrots or celery or by chewing sugarless or xylitol-containing gum. Patients with xerostomia are highly susceptible to dental caries and should not use sugar-containing foods or acidic foods or beverages to stimulate salivary flow. Commercial nonprescription solutions used to lubricate the oral tissues may be the only effective treatment for patients without functioning salivary gland parenchyma or for those whose salivary glands do not respond to stimulation. Virtually all lubricants can provide some short-term relief for patients with xerostomia. Some studies have indicated that salivary substitutes containing carboxymethylcellulose or

---

> ## PREVENTION AND THERAPY OF RADIATION-INDUCED XEROSTOMIA
>
> Prevention of radiation-induced xerostomia has been actively studied in the recent past. Results from the use of pilocarpine in this situation have been mixed, with the largest placebo-controlled trial being negative. Amifostine, however, based on results of clinical trials, has been recently approved by the Food and Drug Administration in the adjuvant setting as an agent that can attenuate the development of xerostomia. Nonetheless, the inconvenience and toxicity of this drug therapy limit its use in some practices.

hydroxymethyl cellulose are more effective in relieving dryness than water- or glycerin-based solutions. Some patients prefer mucopolysaccharide solutions. Xialine, a xanthan gum–based saliva substitute, has been shown to be no better than placebo in decreasing the effects of xerostomia, although a trend was seen in favor of Xialine for improving problems with speech and senses.[137] Various reports have suggested that acupuncture can subjectively (patient-completed xerostomia inventories) and objectively (unstimulated and stimulated salivary flow rates) reduce symptoms of xerostomia and improve salivary flow rates.[138-140]

For the treatment of established radiation-induced xerostomia, the following are recommended:

- Pilocarpine: 5.0 mg, given orally three to four times a day, up to 10 mg three times a day maximum
- Artificial saliva (Mouthkote, Xerolube, Moistir, Salivert, Sage)
- Biotene products (gum, toothpaste, mouthwash)

Xerostomia primarily affects mastication and oral manipulation of dry, absorbent food material. Initiation and duration of the pharyngeal swallow do not appear to be affected.[141] Patients with severe xerostomia may be helped by eating soft, bland foods, especially cool or cold foods with a high liquid content such as ice cream, Popsicles, puddings, watermelon, and grapes. Solid foods can be made easier to swallow by adding gravies, sauces, melted butter, broths, mayonnaise, yogurt, or salad dressing. Dunking bread and other baked foods in milk, tea, or coffee will make them easier to swallow. Some patients may find a pureed diet or a full-liquid diet easier to swallow than solid foods. Addition of a liquid high-protein supplement will help ensure that patients are getting enough protein and calories. Hot, spicy, or acidic foods may be irritating and should be eaten with caution. Some patients find that a vaporizer or humidifier in the room or at the bedside helps alleviate the discomfort of xerostomia. Frequent oral rinses with an alkaline saline solution may help refresh the taste, moisten the mouth, and promote better hygiene.

Two large randomized, double-blind, placebo-controlled, multicenter clinical trials have documented the efficacy of oral pilocarpine (5.0 mg given orally three times a day) in relieving oral dryness; improving salivary flow, mouth comfort, and ability to speak; and reducing the need for oral comfort agents after head and neck irradiation. Adverse reactions are minimal, with the most common being mild to moderate sweating, which is dose-related. Best results may require continuous treatment for more than 8 weeks.[142-144] Most patients report significant relief of symptoms of xerostomia and improvement in quality of life that do not appear to be dependent on previous radiotherapy dose/volume parameters, suggesting that oral pilocarpine acts primarily by stimulating ectopic salivary glands and can be of benefit for a whole range of patients with xerostomia of varying severity.[145] Topical pilocarpine administration has shown results similar to those achieved with systemic treatment but with improved patient tolerance.[146] One small retrospective trial and one small double-blind, placebo-controlled, randomized trial suggest that pilocarpine (5.0 mg given orally four times a day), started the day before or on the same day as radiation therapy, given concurrently with radiation therapy and for 3 months after radiation therapy, results in a lower frequency of oral symptoms and xerostomia during treatment and afterward. It may not be necessary to continue the use after 3 months to maintain the benefit.[147,148] Nonetheless, a large placebo-controlled clinical trial conducted by the RTOG did not demonstrate any reduction in the incidence or severity of radiation-induced xerostomia with prophylactic use of pilocarpine 3 days before radiation therapy, during radiation therapy, and for 3 months after completion of radiation therapy.[8]

Amifostine appears to protect the salivary glands from the effects of radiation therapy and may prove to be helpful in preventing or minimizing the effects of xerostomia and loss of taste.[124-126] Buntzel and associates,[124] Brizel and co-workers,[126] and Antonadou and colleagues[125] have all reported significant reduction in the severity of acute and chronic radiation-induced xerostomia with prophylactic use of amifostine as determined by controlled clinical trials. There was no evidence that amifostine interfered with the antitumor effects of radiation therapy as measured by local or regional control and overall survival. Wasserman and associates[149] demonstrated that this reduction in xerostomia results in improvement in the ability to carry out normal functions with reduced discomfort as measured by a validated Patient Benefit Questionnaire. A small randomized trial demonstrated that amifostine may prevent deterioration of dental health.[150] The use of amifostine may be considered to decrease the incidence of acute and late xerostomia in patients undergoing fractionated radiation therapy in the head and neck region that includes the salivary glands.[127] Amifostine has been approved by the Food and Drug Administration for use in the postoperative adjuvant setting.

In selected patients with cancers in the oropharynx, hypopharynx, or larynx, it has been reported that surgical transfer of a submandibular gland into the submental space can be successfully accomplished.[151] If patients require postoperative radiation therapy, the submandibular gland can more readily be excluded from the irradiated volume, thus preserving some saliva production. This process requires validation by controlled clinical trials.

In the future, intensity modulated radiation therapy (IMRT) and altered radiation therapy fractionation schemes may lead to better preservation of salivary gland function. IMRT may be used to reduce the dose of radiation therapy to the major and minor salivary glands.[135,136] Leslie and Dische[152] evaluated the function of parotid glands in patients treated with three different radiation therapy schedules 9 or more months after completion of treatment. All patients received radiation therapy confined to one side of the head and neck region, so that the contralateral salivary gland could act as an internal control. Saliva was selectively collected from the parotid glands, and the stimulated flow rate and pH of the saliva were determined bilaterally. Twelve glands that had received conventionally fractionated radiotherapy to a dose of 60 to 66 Gy showed a mean percentage flow of 20% and a significant decrease in saliva pH. Six glands that had received continuous hyperfractionated accelerated radiation therapy showed mean percentage flows of 65% with only slight and nonsignificant decreases in saliva pH. These results suggest that treatment of squamous cell carcinoma of the head and neck with a continuous hyperfractionated and accelerated radiation therapy fractionation scheme can lead to improved function of the irradiated parotid gland. These results were attributed to the lower dose per fraction used, with subsequent greater repair of sublethal damage between treatment fractions.

Dental Caries

Patients undergoing radiation therapy to the oral cavity have an increased incidence of caries because of the lack of saliva to cleanse the teeth and changes in the quality of the saliva. This promotes oral cavity colonization with a more cariogenic flora. In addition, the discomfort associated with xerostomia and persistent mucositis may result in poor oral hygiene with infrequent brushing, flossing, and oral rinses. Some patients may also alter their diet to include sugar-containing drinks and soft foods to help alleviate the effects of xerostomia. Rampant caries can occur, involving all tooth surfaces (including the cervical portion) after just a few months of xerostomia.

Prevention and Treatment of Dental Caries

To prevent the development of dental caries (which may result in the need for extraction, soft tissue necrosis, bone exposure, and osteoradionecrosis) after a course of radiation therapy, all patients should undergo a thorough dental evaluation before treatment. Nonsalvageable teeth should be extracted, and an alveolotomy and primary wound closure should be performed, if indicated. A thorough dental prophylaxis should be performed, including scaling, root cleaning, curettage, and polishing. Restorative dental procedures including surgical endodontics should be performed for salvageable teeth. A preventive regimen should be initiated including plaque removal with the use of dental floss and thorough instructions for correct toothbrushing. Custom-made fluoride carriers should be fabricated, and a neutral 1.1% sodium fluoride gel should be applied to the teeth after breakfast and before bedtime for a period of 2 weeks, beginning as soon as possible after the initiation of radiation therapy. This may be reduced to one bedtime application for 1 month and then twice-weekly fluoride applications indefinitely. The dosage of the fluoride should be modified according to the patient's history of dental caries and oral hygiene performance. Patients should also use a calcium phosphate remineralizing rinse immediately after fluoride applications.

Edentulous patients should have their dentures evaluated, and ill-fitting dentures should be corrected. Patients should be discouraged from wearing their dentures until the mucosa is completely healed from the acute effects of radiation therapy (usually about 3 months).

After radiation therapy, patients should be seen every 3 months for frequent dental checkups. There is no concern regarding the additional x-ray exposure of dental films, because the dose is insignificant compared with the therapeutic dose given for the cancer therapy. All routine dental procedures can be performed without unusual precautions after a course of radiation therapy, except radical periodontal treatment and extractions, which may lead to osteoradionecrosis if not done with special care. When extractions are required after a course of radiation therapy, it is best to remove one tooth at a time with as little trauma to adjacent tissues as possible and to wait until healing is complete before proceeding to further extractions. Prophylactic antibiotic coverage should be started 1 day before extraction and continued until the site is completely healed. Some institutions favor the use of hyperbaric oxygen before extraction.[153] Primary closure of the wound should be carried out over a smooth bony surface, so that no sharp spicules or ridges are left beneath the mucosa. Postradiation therapy tooth extractions carried out in this manner have a good chance of complete healing without the development of necrosis.[154] When extreme root sensitivity occurs after radiation therapy, brushing fluoride onto the exposed root surface and using specially formulated commercially available toothpaste appears to decrease the sensitivity to some extent.

Soft Tissue and Bone Necrosis

The soft tissue necrosis of oral cavity mucosa that occurs after high doses of radiation therapy may be attributed to the obliteration of small blood vessels or severe mucositis with ulceration. Irradiated epithelium is thinner than normal and appears pale and atrophic. It also has telangiectatic vessels. The irradiated mucosa is more susceptible to mechanical injury and to the noxious effects of alcohol and tobacco. Soft tissue necrosis usually begins with breakdown of damaged mucosa, resulting in a small ulcer. Most soft tissue necroses will occur within 2 years after radiation therapy. Occurrence after 2 years is generally preceded by mucosal trauma. The risk of soft tissue necrosis is increased with larger fraction sizes, higher total doses, large volumes of irradiated mucosa, and the use of an interstitial implant.

Treatment of Necrosis

If recurrent cancer is not clinically suspected, biopsy should be avoided, because this may enlarge the area of necrosis. Topical anesthetics can relieve the discomfort associated with soft tissue necrosis and allow the patient to eat normally. Antibiotics often provide pain relief, particularly when the ulceration is deep and infected. It is essential that the patient discontinue the use of alcohol and tobacco. If the area of necrosis is traumatized by dentures, the dentures should not be worn until healing is complete.[59]

More than 90% of soft tissue necroses will heal with conservative treatment, although in some instances it may take many months. A small trial (consisting of 12 patients with 15 sites) of late radiation necrosis of the soft tissues has been conducted to evaluate the effect of pentoxifylline on a preliminary basis. The average duration of nonhealing before treatment with pentoxifylline was 30.5 weeks. With the institution of pentoxifylline (400 mg given orally three times a day), 13 of 15 necroses healed completely and 1 partially healed an average of 9 weeks after treatment was started. All patients had pain relief.[155] Additional case reports and small clinical trials have suggested that the combination of pentoxifylline, tocopherol, and clodronate may be beneficial in healing severe osteoradionecrosis, radiation-induced trismus, radiation-induced ulcerated fibrosis, soft tissue necrosis, and mucosal necrosis.[156-163] These results support further study of pentoxifylline in patients in whom soft tissue necrosis develops after a course of radiation therapy. The RTOG is currently evaluating the efficacy of pentoxifylline in healing irradiation-related soft tissue necrosis.

The mandible and maxilla will tolerate rather high doses of radiation therapy without serious problems, as long as the tissues overlying the bone remain intact. If soft tissue necrosis develops in the mucosa overlying the mandible or maxilla, the underlying bone may become exposed. This can lead to serious injury, resulting in bone necrosis (osteoradionecrosis). Compared with the maxilla, the gingiva of the mandible has a rather tenuous blood supply, placing the mandible at greater risk of exposure and necrosis. Most bone exposures will heal spontaneously after conservative treatment. At one institution, 86% of bone exposures healed after conservative treatment.[59] Small areas of bone exposure (<1 cm) generally heal spontaneously after a period of weeks to months. Larger areas of bone exposure may persist for a long period and may lead to bone necrosis, followed by sequestration. If exposed, necrotic bone may become infected. The necrotic process may then extend to involve adjacent bone for a considerable distance. Severe necrosis can then develop and lead to orocutaneous fistulae and pathologic fractures.

If the bone is rough or protrudes above the level of the gingiva, an oral surgeon may file it down to promote healing. Local debridement of moderate-size necrosis can be performed by an oral surgeon, if indicated. If the patient wears a denture, it should be withheld from use or relieved over the site of exposure. Pain is not a common symptom; if present, it can usually be controlled with analgesics. A local anesthetic can be applied with a cotton-tipped applicator, if needed, for pain control. Antibiotics frequently reduce infection and discomfort within a few days but should be continued for 2 to 3 weeks. Hyperbaric oxygen along with antibiotic therapy and local debridement may help promote healing.[59] Mandibular resection should be reserved as the last resort for the patient with intractable pain, recurrence of severe infections, fracture, or trismus.

Most bone problems develop within 3 to 12 months after radiation therapy, but some risk persists for many years, especially if the patient undergoes dental extractions. Necrosis is most likely to occur after extraction of mandibular teeth, although this is infrequent if special precautions are taken. The edentulous patient has a lower overall risk for bone necrosis compared with the dentulous patient.

Patients at highest risk for osteoradionecrosis appear to be those with tumors involving the gingiva or bone; those who continue to smoke or drink, or both, after radiation therapy; and those who receive high doses of radiation therapy, large treatment volumes, large fraction sizes, and/or interstitial implants.

Taste Alterations

Loss of taste occurs rapidly early in the course of radiation therapy to the oral cavity. Most patients report that the sense of taste is essentially nonexistent by the third or fourth week of treatment. After the completion of radiation therapy, most patients report some taste improvement within 1 to 2 months. Full recovery of taste usually requires 2 to 4 months. In some patients, taste never returns to normal, at least in part because of xerostomia. Although some have suggested that zinc therapy may be useful in improving taste acuity, no standard treatment can be recommended until further study is undertaken.[164] Currently, an NCCTG placebo-controlled, randomized trial is being carried out to determine the value of zinc for patients receiving radiation therapy to the oral cavity. Amifostine may protect against taste loss caused by irradiation.[124,126]

Trismus

Trismus may be caused by fibrosis of the muscles of mastication after high-dose radiation therapy to the oral cavity or oropharynx, surgical scarring, and/or advanced carcinomas involving the pterygoid and/or masseter musculature. The temporomandibular joint itself is relatively resistant to ankylosis caused by radiation therapy, but the risk of injury increases if the joint is invaded by tumor. The use of large daily treatment fractions also appears to increase the risk of trismus.

Prevention and Treatment of Trismus

High-energy x-ray beams and sophisticated multiple field techniques should be used whenever possible to reduce the dose of radiation therapy to the temporomandibular joint and to the muscles of mastication. Patients treated with both surgery and radiation therapy have a greater risk for trismus than patients treated with either modality alone. Patients at high risk for trismus and those in whom trismus has developed before treatment should perform jaw-stretching exercises daily in an attempt to increase the interarch or interincisor distance. A number of techniques are used, including commercially available jaw-stretching tools and less expensive stacked tongue blades, tapered corks, or clothespins. These devices are inserted between the teeth to increase the interincisor distance until slight pain is encountered. The exercises should be done for about 30 seconds every 2 hours. Additional tongue blades can be added or a thicker aspect of the cork can be placed between the teeth every few days to increase the interincisor distance and stretch the muscles of mastication.

Malignancy

The carcinogenic effect of ionizing radiation has long been recognized. The latent interval between radiation therapy and the development of cancer varies from several to many years. Kogelnik and colleagues[165] reviewed charts of 1163 patients treated for head and neck cancer at the M.D. Anderson Cancer Center who had survived a minimum of 5 years after treatment without having recurrent cancer. Follow-up for these patients ranged from 7.5 to 25.5 years. Patients were treated with surgery alone (337 patients) or radiation therapy with or without surgery (826 patients). The incidence of new cancers in the original disease site (1.8% vs. 2.7%), within the immediate vicinity of the original cancer (4.2% vs. 3.1%), or at sites remote from the primary tumor but still within the oral cavity or pharynx (4.7% vs. 5.7%) was very similar for patients treated with surgery alone versus patients treated with irradiation with or without surgery, respectively. It was concluded that moderate or high-dose radiation therapy did not produce any new squamous cell carcinomas of the mucous membranes. Similar findings were reported from the Fox Chase Cancer Center[166] and the University of California, Los Angeles.[167]

The rarity of radiation-induced sarcomas, the long latent period before their development, and the difficulty in obtaining reliable long-term follow-up data make the task of estimating the true risk of this problem difficult. However, most series include one or two cases of radiation-induced bone sarcoma per 1000 5-year survivors. If one were to assume malignant induction in 1 patient of every 500 long-term survivors, then with an estimated 5-year survival rate of 40% for all patients with head and neck cancer who received radiation therapy, it is calculated that 1 case would be induced per 1250 patients treated.[59] A review of the Mayo Clinic experience showed no difference in survival between patients with radiation-induced sarcomas of the mandible or maxilla and nonradiation-induced sarcomas of the same site (45% 5-year overall survival). Because some patients with radiation-induced osteogenic sarcomas of the mandible or maxilla can be cured, the risk of dying from a radiation-induced sarcoma after a course of radiation therapy is minimal and is very similar to the risk of death a patient accepts when undergoing general anesthesia and major head and neck cancer surgery.[168,169]

An association has also been noted between radiation therapy and thyroid tumors. The latent period is usually 10 to 30 years. Almost all reported cases have followed low doses of radiation therapy well below the doses used for squamous cell carcinomas of the oral cavity (<6 cGy to 1500 cGy). Doses greater than 2000 cGy are associated with a very low risk of induction of thyroid neoplasia compared with lower doses. This is likely because higher doses of radiation therapy either completely destroy follicular cells or at least render the surviving cells incapable of division. Not all thyroid neoplasms that develop after radiation therapy are malignant, and many of the malignant neoplasms that do develop (papillary and follicular carcinomas) are readily curable with surgery. Thus the risk of radiation-induced carcinoma should not be a major factor in determining treatment approaches for the typical patient with head and neck cancer.

Implementation of Prevention and Treatment of Radiation-Induced Oral Complications

Jansma and associates[170] recently surveyed all Dutch radiation therapy centers in which irradiation of patients with head and neck cancer is performed to determine which prevention and treatment regimens are used for oral sequelae resulting from head and neck radiotherapy. Survey questions included queries about screening, care before irradiation, care during radiation therapy, care during postradiation therapy, and the composition of the dental team who evaluated and treated the patients undergoing radiation therapy. Unfortunately, these investigators found a great diversity in the preventive approach to treatment of patients with head and neck cancer at Dutch radiotherapy institutes. Disturbing findings included a lack of well-defined guidelines in many centers, absence of a dental team at some centers, absence of an oral hygienist on some dental teams, and the observation that many patients were not referred to the dental team in a timely manner. Jansma and colleagues[171] recommend the development of a general protocol for the prevention of oral complications applicable at all head and neck cancer radiation therapy centers. Similar deficiencies are probably present at the head and neck cancer radiotherapy centers within the United States. It is strongly recommended that dedicated teams be assembled to administer aggressive care to patients receiving radiation therapy to the oral mucosa.[172] These teams should institute preventive measures and treat symptoms early in their course.

REFERENCES

1. Poon MA, O'Connell MJ, Moertel CG, et al: Biochemical modulation of fluorouracil: Evidence of significant improvement of survival and quality of life in patients with advanced colorectal carcinoma. J Clin Oncol 1989;7:1407–1418.
2. Petrelli NJ, Rustum YM, Bruckner H, Stablein D: The Roswell Park Memorial Institute and Gastrointestinal Tumor Study Group phase III experience with the modulation of 5-fluorouracil by leucovorin in metastatic colorectal adenocarcinoma. Adv Exp Med Biol 1988;244:143–155.
3. Mahood DJ, Dose AM, Loprinzi CL, et al: Inhibition of fluorouracil-induced stomatitis by oral cryotherapy. J Clin Oncol 1991;9:449–452.
4. Cascinu S, Fedeli A, Fedeli SL, Catalano G: Oral cooling (cryotherapy), an effective treatment for the prevention of 5-fluorouracil-induced stomatitis. Eur J Cancer B Oral Oncol 1994;30B:234–236.
5. Rocke LK, Loprinzi CL, Lee JK, et al: A randomized clinical trial of two different durations of oral cryotherapy for prevention of 5-fluorouracil-related stomatitis. Cancer 1993;72:2234–2238.
6. Clarkson JE, Worthington HV, Eden OB: Prevention of oral mucositis or oral candidiasis for patients with cancer receiving chemotherapy (excluding head and neck cancer). Cochrane Database Syst Rev 2000:CD000978.
7. Edelman MJ, Gandara DR, Perez EA, et al: Phase I trial of edatrexate plus carboplatin in advanced solid tumors: Amelioration of dose-limiting mucositis by ice chip cryotherapy. Invest New Drugs 1998;16:69–75.
8. Gandara DR, Edelman MJ, Crowley JJ, Lau DH, Livingston RB: (1997) Phase II trial of edatrexate plus carboplatin in metastatic non-small-cell lung cancer: A Southwest Oncology Group study. Cancer Chemother Pharmacol 1997;41:75–78.
9. Dreicer R, Propert KJ, Kuzel T, Kirkwood JM, O'Dwyer PJ, Loehrer PJ: A phase II trial of edatrexate in patients with advanced renal cell carcinoma. An Eastern Cooperative Oncology Group study. Am J Clin Oncol 1997;20:251–253.
10. Carl W, Emrich LS: Management of oral mucositis during local radiation and systemic chemotherapy: A study of 98 patients. J Prosthet Dent 1997;66:361–369.
11. Fidler P, Loprinzi CL, O'Fallon JR, et al: Prospective evaluation of a chamomile mouthwash for prevention of 5-FU-induced oral mucositis. Cancer 1996;77:522–525.
12. Klimberg VS, Souba WW, Dolson DJ, et al: Prophylactic glutamine protects the intestinal mucosa from radiation injury. Cancer 1990;66:62–68.
13. Klimberg VS, Salloum RM, Kasper M, et al: Oral glutamine accelerates healing of the small intestine and improves outcome after whole abdominal radiation. Arch Surg 1990;125:1040–1045.
14. Anderson PM, Subitz K: Oral glutamine suspension to ameliorate chemotherapy induced mucositis. ASPHO Proc 1993;2.
15. Jebb SA, Osborne RJ, Maughan TS, Mohideen N, Mack P, Mort D, et al: 5-Fluorouracil and folinic acid-induced mucositis: No effect of oral glutamine supplementation. Br J Cancer 1994;70:732–735.
16. Okuno SH, Woodhouse CO, Loprinzi CL, et al: Phase III controlled evaluation of glutamine for decreasing stomatitis in patients receiving fluorouracil (5-FU)-based chemotherapy. Am J Clin Oncol 1999;22:258–261.
17. Clark PI, Slevin ML: Allopurinol mouthwashes and 5-fluorouracil induced oral toxicity. Eur J Surg Oncol 1985;11:267–268.
18. Tsavaris N, Caragiauris P, Kosmidis P: Reduction of oral toxicity of 5-fluorouracil by allopurinol mouthwashes. Eur J Surg Oncol 1988;14;405–406.
19. Marini G, Simoncini E, Zaniboni A, Gorni F, Marpicati P, Zambruni A: 5-Fluorouracil and high-dose folinic acid as salvage treatment of advanced breast cancer: An update. Oncology 1987;44:336–340.
20. Fine S, Erlichman C, Kaizer L, et al: (1988) Phase II trial of 5FU + folinic acid (FA) as first line treatment for metastatic breast cancer. Proc Am Soc Clin Oncol 1988;8.
21. Loprinzi CL, Cianflone SG, Dose AM, et al: A controlled evaluation of an allopurinol mouthwash as prophylaxis against 5-fluorouracil-induced stomatitis. Cancer 1990;65:1879–1882.
22. Van der Vliet W, Erlichman C, Elhakim T: Allopurinol mouthwash for prevention of fluorouracil-induced stomatitis. Clin Pharm 1989;8:655–658.
23. Bubley GJ, Chapman B, Chapman SK, Crumpacker CS, Schnipper LE: Effect of acyclovir on radiation- and chemotherapy-induced mouth lesions. Antimicrob Agents Chemother 1989;33:862–865.
24. Wadleigh R, Redman R, Cohen M: Vitamin E in the treatment of chemotherapy-induced mucositis. Proc Am Soc Clin Oncol 1990;9.
25. Gabrilove JL, Jakubowski A, Scher H, et al: Effect of granulocyte colony-stimulating factor on neutropenia and associated morbidity due to chemotherapy for transitional-cell carcinoma of the urothelium. N Engl J Med 1988;318:1414–1422.

26. Farrell CL, Bready JV, Rex KL, et al: Keratinocyte growth factor protects mice from chemotherapy and radiation-induced gastrointestinal injury and mortality. Cancer Res 1998;58:933–939.

27. Dorr W, Noack R, Spekl K, Farrell CL: Modification of oral mucositis by keratinocyte growth factor: Single radiation exposure. Int J Radiat Biol 2001;77:341–347.

28. Matejka M, Nell A, Kment G, et al: Local benefit of prostaglandin E2 in radiochemotherapy-induced oral mucositis. Br J Oral Maxillofac Surg 1990;28:89–91.

29. Porteder H, Rausch E, Kment G, Watzek G, Matejka M, Sinzinger H: Local prostaglandin E2 in patients with oral malignancies undergoing chemo- and radiotherapy. J Craniomaxillofac Surg 1988;16:371–374.

30. Ciais G, Namer M, Schneider M, et al: [Laser therapy in the prevention and treatment of mucositis caused by anticancer chemotherapy]. Bull Cancer 1992;79:183–191.

31. Schubert M, Franquin JC, Niccoli-Filo W, Marcial F, Lloid M: Effects of low-energy laser on oral mucositis: A phase I/II pilot study. Cancer Res Week 1994;7.

32. Barasch A, Peterson DE, Tanzer JM, et al: Helium-neon laser effects on conditioning-induced oral mucositis in bone marrow transplantation patients. Cancer. 1995;76:2550–2556.

33. Cowen D, Tardieu C, Schubert M, et al: Low energy helium-neon laser in the prevention of oral mucositis in patients undergoing bone marrow transplant: Results of a double blind randomized trial. Int J Radiat Oncol Biol Phys 1997;38:697–703.

34. Migliorati C, Massumoto C, Edwardo F: Low-energy laser therapy in oral mucositis. J Oral Laser Applicat 2001;1:97–101.

35. Bianco JA, Appelbaum FR, Nemunaitis J, et al: Phase I-II trial of pentoxifylline for the prevention of transplant-related toxicities following bone marrow transplantation. Blood 1991;78:1205–1211.

36. LeVeque FG, Parzuchowski JB, Farinacci GC, et al: Clinical evaluation of MGI 209, an anesthetic, film-forming agent for relief from painful oral ulcers associated with chemotherapy. J Clin Oncol 1992;10:1963–1968.

37. Pfeiffer P, Madsen EL, Hansen O, May O: Effect of prophylactic sucralfate suspension on stomatitis induced by cancer chemotherapy. A randomized, double-blind cross-over study. Acta Oncol 1990;29:171–173.

38. Pfeiffer P, Hansen O, Madsen EL, May O: A prospective pilot study on the effect of sucralfate mouth-swishing in reducing stomatitis during radiotherapy of the oral cavity. Acta Oncol 1990;29:471–473.

39. Shenep JL, Kalwinsky DK, Hutson PR, et al: Efficacy of oral sucralfate suspension in prevention and treatment of chemotherapy-induced mucositis. J Pediatr 1988;113:758–763.

40. Ferraro JM, Mattern JQ II: Sucralfate suspension for stomatitis. Drug Intell Clin Pharm 1984;18:153.

41. Solomon MA: Oral sucralfate suspension for mucositis. N Engl J Med 1986;315:459–460.

42. Loprinzi CL, Ghosh C, Camoriano J, et al: Phase III controlled evaluation of sucralfate to alleviate stomatitis in patients receiving fluorouracil-based chemotherapy. J Clin Oncol 1997;15:1235–1238.

43. Raber-Durlacher JE, Abraham-Inpijn L, van Leeuwen EF, Lustig KH, van Winkelhoff AJ: The prevention of oral complications in bone-marrow transplantations by means of oral hygiene and dental intervention. Neth J Med 1989;34:98–108.

44. De Pauw BE, Donnelly JP, De Witte T, Novakova IR, Schattenberg A: Options and limitations of long-term oral ciprofloxacin as antibacterial prophylaxis in allogeneic bone marrow transplant recipients. Bone Marrow Transplant 1990;5:179–182.

45. Donnelly JP, Muus P, Schattenberg A, De Witte T, Horrevorts A, DePauw BE: A scheme for daily monitoring of oral mucositis in allogeneic BMT recipients. Bone Marrow Transplant 1992;9:409–413.

46. Weisdorf DJ, Bostrom B, Raether D, et al: Oropharyngeal mucositis complicating bone marrow transplantation: Prognostic factors and the effect of chlorhexidine mouth rinse. Bone Marrow Transplant 1989;4:89–95.

47. Kolbinson DA, Schubert MM, Flournoy N, Truelove EL: Early oral changes following bone marrow transplantation. Oral Surg Oral Med Oral Pathol 1988;66:130–138.

48. Ferretti GA, Ash RC, Brown AT, Parr MD, Romond EH, Lillich TT: Control of oral mucositis and candidiasis in marrow transplantation: A prospective, double-blind trial of chlorhexidine digluconate oral rinse. Bone Marrow Transplant 1988;3:483–493.

49. Ferretti GA, Raybould TP, Brown AT, et al: Chlorhexidine prophylaxis for chemotherapy- and radiotherapy-induced stomatitis: A randomized double-blind trial. Oral Surg Oral Med Oral Pathol 1990;69:331–338.

50. Engelhard D, Morag A, Or R, et al: Prevention of herpes simplex virus (HSV) infection in recipients of HLA-matched T-lymphocyte-depleted bone marrow allografts. Isr J Med Sci 1988;24:145–150.

51. Carrico CJ, Meakins JL, Marshall JC, Fry D, Maier RV: Multiple-organ-failure syndrome. Arch Surg 1986;121:196–208.

52. Brandt SJ, Peters WP, Atwater SK, et al: Effect of recombinant human granulocyte-macrophage colony-stimulating factor on hematopoietic reconstitution after high-dose chemotherapy and autologous bone marrow transplantation. N Engl J Med 1988;318:869–876.

53. Wardley AM, Jayson GC, Swindell R, et al: Prospective evaluation of oral mucositis in patients receiving myeloablative conditioning regimens and haemopoietic progenitor rescue. Br J Haematol 2000;110:292–299.

54. Al-Tikriti U, Martin MV, Bramley PA: A pilot study of the clinical effects of irradiation on the oral tissues. Br J Oral Maxillofac Surg 1984;22:77–86.

55. Bernhoft CH, Skaug N: Oral findings in irradiated edentulous patients. Int J Oral Surg 1985;14:416–427.

56. Wright WE, Haller JM, Harlow SA, Pizzo PA: An oral disease prevention program for patients receiving radiation and chemotherapy. J Am Dent Assoc 1985;110:43–47.

57. Sonis ST, Sonis AL, Lieberman A: Oral complications in patients receiving treatment for malignancies other than of the head and neck. J Am Dent Assoc 1978;97:468–472.

58. Engelmeier RL, King GE: Complications of head and neck radiation therapy and their management. J Prosthet Dent 1983;49:514–522.

59. Parsons JT: (1984) The effect of radiation on normal tissues of the head and neck. In Million RR, Cassisi NJ (eds): Management of head and neck cancer. A multidisciplinary approach. Philadelphia, JB Lippincott, pp 173–207.

60. Fu KK, Pajak TF, Trotti A, et al: A Radiation Therapy Oncology Group (RTOG) phase III randomized study to compare hyperfractionation and two variants of accelerated fractionation to standard fractionation radiotherapy for head and neck squamous cell carcinomas: First report of RTOG 9003. Int J Radiat Oncol Biol Phys 2000;48:7–16.

61. Calais G, Alfonsi M, Bardet, E, et al: Randomized trial of radiation therapy versus concomitant chemotherapy and radiation therapy for advanced-stage oropharynx carcinoma. J Natl Cancer Inst 1999;91:2081–2086.

62. Al-Sarraf M, LeBlanc M, Giri PG, et al: Chemoradiotherapy versus radiotherapy in patients with advanced nasopharyngeal cancer: Phase III randomized intergroup study 0099. J Clin Oncol 1998;16:1310–1317.

63. Wendt TG, Grabenbauer GG, Rodel CM, et al: Simultaneous radiochemotherapy versus radiotherapy alone in advanced head and neck cancer: A randomized multicenter study. J Clin Oncol 1998;16:1318–1324.

64. Zakotnik B, Smid L, Budihna M, et al: Concomitant radiotherapy with mitomycin C and bleomycin compared with radiotherapy alone in inoperable head and neck cancer: Final report. Int J Radiat Oncol Biol Phys 1998;41:1121–1127.

65. Bentzen SM, Saunders MI, Dische S, Bond SJ: Radiotherapy-related early morbidity in head and neck cancer: Quantitative clinical radiobiology as deduced from the CHART trial. Radiother Oncol 2001;60:123–135.

66. Horiot JC, Bontemps P, van den Bogaert W, et al: Accelerated fractionation (AF) compared to conventional fractionation (CF) improves loco-regional control in the radiotherapy of advanced head and neck cancers: Results of the EORTC 22851 randomized trial. Radiother Oncol 1997;44:111–121.

67. Staar S, Rudat V, Stuetzer H, et al: Intensified hyperfractionated accelerated radiotherapy limits the additional benefit of simultaneous chemotherapy—results of a multicentric

randomized German trial in advanced head-and-neck cancer. Int J Radiat Oncol Biol Phys 2001;50:1161–1171.

68. Skladowski K, Maciejewski B, Golen M, Pilecki B, Przeorek W, Tarnawski R: Randomized clinical trial on 7-day-continuous accelerated irradiation (CAIR) of head and neck cancer—report on 3-year tumour control and normal tissue toxicity. Radiother Oncol. 2000;55:101–110.

69. Poulsen MG, Denham JW, Peters LJ, et al: A randomised trial of accelerated and conventional radiotherapy for stage III and IV squamous carcinoma of the head and neck: A Trans-Tasman Radiation Oncology Group Study. Radiother Oncol 2001;60:113–122.

70. Horiot JC, Le Fur R, N'Guyen T, et al: Hyperfractionation versus conventional fractionation in oropharyngeal carcinoma: Final analysis of a randomized trial of the EORTC cooperative group of radiotherapy. Radiother Oncol 1992;25:231–241.

71. Peters LJ, Ang KK, Thames HD Jr: Accelerated fractionation in the radiation treatment of head and neck cancer. A critical comparison of different strategies. Acta Oncol 1988;27: 185–194.

72. Maciejewski B, Withers HR, Taylor JM, Hliniak A. Dose fractionation and regeneration in radiotherapy for cancer of the oral cavity and oropharynx: Tumor dose-response and repopulation. Int J Radiat Oncol Biol Phys 1989;16:831–843.

73. Withers HR, Taylor JM, Maciejewski B: (1988) The hazard of accelerated tumor clonogen repopulation during radiotherapy. Acta Oncol 1988;27:131–146.

74. Parsons JT, Bova FJ, Million RR: A re-evaluation of split-course technique for squamous cell carcinoma of the head and neck. Int J Radiat Oncol Biol Phys 1980;6:1645–1652.

75. Cox JD, Pajak TF, Marcial VA, et al: Interruptions adversely affect local control and survival with hyperfractionated radiation therapy of carcinomas of the upper respiratory and digestive tracts. New evidence for accelerated proliferation from Radiation Therapy Oncology Group Protocol 8313. Cancer 1992;69:2744–2748.

76. Pajak TF, Laramore GE, Marcial VA, et al: Elapsed treatment days—a critical item for radiotherapy quality control review in head and neck trials: RTOG report. Int J Radiat Oncol Biol Phys 1991;20:13–20.

77. Meoz RT, Fletcher GH, Peters LJ, Barkley HT Jr, Thames HD: (1984) Twice-daily fractionation schemes for advanced head and neck cancer. Int J Radiat Oncol Biol Phys 1984;10:831–836.

78. Wang CC, Blitzer PH, Suit HD: Twice-a-day radiation therapy for cancer of the head and neck. Cancer 1985;55:2100–2104.

79. Knee R, Fields RS, Peters LJ: Concomitant boost radiotherapy for advanced squamous cell carcinoma of the head and neck. Radiother Oncol 1985;4:1–7.

80. Wang CC: Local control of oropharyngeal carcinoma after two accelerated hyperfractionation radiation therapy schemes. Int J Radiat Oncol Biol Phys 1988;14:1143–1146.

81. Parsons JT, Mendenhall WM, Cassisi NJ, Isaacs JH Jr, Million RR: Hyperfractionation for head and neck cancer. Int J Radiat Oncol Biol Phys 1988;14:649–658.

82. Horiot JC, Le Fur R, N'Guyen T, et al: Hyperfractionated compared with conventional radiotherapy in oropharyngeal carcinoma: An EORTC randomized trial. Eur J Cancer 1990;26:779–780.

83. Datta R, Chandry AN, Gupta S: Twice-a-day versus once-a-day radiation therapy in head and neck cancer. Int J Radiat Oncol Biol Phys 1989;17:131–132.

84. Sanchiz F, Milla A, Torner J, et al: Single fraction per day versus two fractions per day versus radiochemotherapy in the treatment of head and neck cancer. Int J Radiat Oncol Biol Phys 1990;19: 1347–1350.

85. Pinto LH, Canary PC, Araujo CM, Bacelar SC, Souhami L: Prospective randomized trial comparing hyperfractionated versus conventional radiotherapy in stages III and IV oropharyngeal carcinoma. Int J Radiat Oncol Biol Phys 1991;21:557–562.

86. Saunders, MI, Dische S, Grosch EJ, et al: Experience with CHART. Int J Radiat Oncol Biol Phys 1991;21:871–878.

87. Ang KK, Peters LJ, Weber RS, et al: (1990) Concomitant boost radiotherapy schedules in the treatment of carcinoma of the oropharynx and nasopharynx. Int J Radiat Oncol Biol Phys 1990;19:1339–1345.

88. Epstein JB, Stevenson-Moore P, Jackson S, Mohamed JH, Spinelli JJ: Prevention of oral mucositis in radiation therapy: A controlled study with benzydamine hydrochloride rinse. Int J Radiat Oncol Biol Phys 1989;16:1571–1575.

89. Epstein JB, Silverman S Jr, Paggiarino DA, et al: Benzydamine HCl for prophylaxis of radiation-induced oral mucositis: Results from a multicenter, randomized, double-blind, placebo-controlled clinical trial. Cancer 2001;92:875–885.

90. Samaranayake LP, Robertson AG, MacFarlane TW, et al: The effect of chlorhexidine and benzydamine mouthwashes on mucositis induced by therapeutic irradiation. Clin Radiol 1988;39:291–294.

91. Spijkervet F, Vermey A, Panders A: Prevention of irradiation mucositis in head-neck cancer patients. Proc Am Soc Clin Oncol 1990;9.

92. Mulkens PJM, Karstens JH, Li L, Ammon J: A new approach for the reduction of irradiation-induced mucositis in patients with head and neck malignancies. Proc AM Soc Clin Oncol 1992;11.

93. Symonds RP, McIlroy P, Khorrami J, et al: The reduction of radiation mucositis by selective decontamination antibiotic pastilles: A placebo-controlled double-blind trial. Br J Cancer 1996;74:312–317.

94. Foote RL, Loprinzi CL, Frank AR, et al: Randomized trial of a chlorhexidine mouthwash for alleviation of radiation-induced mucositis. J Clin Oncol 1994;12:2630–2633.

95. Okuno SH, Foote RL, Loprinzi CL, et al: A randomized trial of a nonabsorbable antibiotic lozenge given to alleviate radiation-induced mucositis. Cancer 1997;79:2193–2199.

96. Wijers OB, Levendag PC, Harms ER, et al: Mucositis reduction by selective elimination of oral flora in irradiated cancers of the head and neck: A placebo-controlled double-blind randomized study. Int J Radiat Oncol Biol Phys 2001;50:343–352.

97. El-Sayed S, Nabid A, Shelley W, et al: Prophylaxis of radiation-associated mucositis in conventionally treated patients with head and neck cancer: A double-blind, phase III, randomized, controlled trial evaluating the clinical efficacy of an antimicrobial lozenge using a validated mucositis scoring system. J Clin Oncol 2002;20:3956–3963.

98. Sutherland SE, Browman GP: Prophylaxis of oral mucositis in irradiated head-and-neck cancer patients: A proposed classification scheme of interventions and meta-analysis of randomized controlled trials. Int J Radiat Oncol Biol Phys 2001;49:917–930.

99. Carnel SB, Blakeslee DB, Oswald SG, Barnes M: Treatment of radiation- and chemotherapy-induced stomatitis. Otolaryngol Head Neck Surg 1990;102:326–330.

100. Ehrnrooth E, Grau C, Zachariae R, Andersen J: Randomized trial of opioids versus tricyclic antidepressants for radiation-induced mucositis pain in head and neck cancer. Acta Oncol 2001;40:745–750.

101. Oguchi M, Shikama N, Sasaki S, et al: Mucosa-adhesive water-soluble polymer film for treatment of acute radiation-induced oral mucositis. Int J Radiat Oncol Biol Phys 1998;40: 1033–1037.

102. Evensen JF, Bjordal K, Jacobsen AB, Lokkevik E, Tausjo JE: Effects of Na-sucrose octasulfate on skin and mucosa reactions during radiotherapy of head and neck cancers—a randomized prospective study. Acta Oncol 2001;40:751–755.

103. Janjan NA, Weissman DE, Pahule A: Improved pain management with daily nursing intervention during radiation therapy for head and neck carcinoma. Int J Radiat Oncol Biol Phys 1992;23:647–652.

104. Epstein JB, Wong FL: The efficacy of sucralfate suspension in the prevention of oral mucositis due to radiation therapy. Int J Radiat Oncol Biol Phys 1994;28:693–698.

105. Carter DL, Herbert ME, Leopold KL, Brizel DM: Double blind randomized trial of sucralfate vs. placebo during a course of radical radiotherapy for head and neck squamous carcinoma. Int J Radiat Oncol Biol Phys 1997;39:234.

106. Makkonen TA, Bostrom P, Vilja P, Joensuu H: Sucralfate mouth washing in the prevention of radiation-induced mucositis: A placebo-controlled double-blind randomized study. Int J Radiat Oncol Biol Phys 1994;30:177–182.

107. Lievens Y, Haustermans K, Van den Weyngaert D, et al: Does sucralfate reduce the acute side-effects in head and neck cancer treated with radiotherapy? A double-blind randomized trial. Radiother Oncol 1998;47:149–153.

108. Franzen L, Henriksson R, Littbrand B, Zackrisson B: Effects of sucralfate on mucositis during and following radiotherapy of malignancies in the head and neck region. A double-blind placebo-controlled study. Acta Oncol. 1995;34:219-223.

109. Allison RR, Vongtama V, Vaughan J, Shin KH: Symptomatic acute mucositis can be minimized or prophylaxed by the combination of sucralfate and fluconazole. Cancer Invest 1995;13:16-22.

110. McGinnis WL, Loprinzi CL, Buskirk SJ, et al: Placebo-controlled trial of sucralfate for inhibiting radiation-induced esophagitis. J Clin Oncol 1997;15:1239-1243.

111. Kozelsky T, Martenson J, Sloan J, et al: Phase III double-blind study of glutamine versus placebo for the prevention of acute diarrhea in patients receiving pelvic radiation therapy. Proc Am Soc Clin Oncol 2001;20.

112. Maciejewski B, Zajusz A, Pilecki B, et al: Acute mucositis in the stimulated oral mucosa of patients during radiotherapy for head and neck cancer. Radiother Oncol 1991;22:7-11.

113. Bensadoun RJ, Franquin JC, Ciais G, et al: Low-energy He/Ne laser in the prevention of radiation-induced mucositis. A multicenter phase III randomized study in patients with head and neck cancer. Support Care Cancer 1999;7:244-252.

114. Leborgne JH, Leborgne F, Zubizarreta E, Ortega B, Mezzera J: Corticosteroids and radiation mucositis in head and neck cancer. A double-blind placebo-controlled randomized trial. Radiother Oncol 1998;47:145-148.

115. Staus-Rausch E, Porteder H, Sinzinger H: Treatment of oral mucositis caused by radiation and/or chemotherapy with PGE2 gel. Poster presented at the Second International Conference on Head and Neck Cancer, July/August, 1988, Boston.

116. Tamamura H, Tonami H, Higashi K: A new combination of mucosal protective drugs in patients with radiation-induced esophagitis. Int J Radiat Oncol Biol Phys 1990;19.

117. Huang EY, Leung SW, Wang CJ, et al: Oral glutamine to alleviate radiation-induced oral mucositis: A pilot randomized trial. Int J Radiat Oncol Biol Phys 2000;46:535-539.

118. Kannan V, Bapsy PP, Anantha N, et al: Efficacy and safety of granulocyte macrophage-colony stimulating factor (GM-CSF) on the frequency and severity of radiation mucositis in patients with head and neck carcinoma. Int J Radiat Oncol Biol Phys 1997;37:1005-1010.

119. Nicolatou O, Sotiropoulou-Lontou A, Skarlatos J, Kyprianou K, Kolitsi G, Dardoufas K: A pilot study of the effect of granulocyte-macrophage colony-stimulating factor on oral mucositis in head and neck cancer patients during X-radiation therapy: A preliminary report. Int J Radiat Oncol Biol Phys 1998;42:551-556.

120. Rovirosa A, Ferre J, Biete A: Granulocyte macrophage-colony-stimulating factor mouthwashes heal oral ulcers during head and neck radiotherapy. Int J Radiat Oncol Biol Phys 1998;41:747-754.

121. Saarilahti K, Kajanti M, Joensuu T, Kouri M, Joensuu H: Comparison of granulocyte-macrophage colony-stimulating factor and sucralfate mouthwashes in the prevention of radiation-induced mucositis: A double-blind prospective randomized phase III study. Int J Radiat Oncol Biol Phys 2002;54:479-485.

122. Makkonen TA, Minn H, Jekunen A, Vilja P, Tuominen J, Joensuu H: Granulocyte macrophage-colony stimulating factor (GM-CSF) and sucralfate in prevention of radiation-induced mucositis: A prospective randomized study. Int J Radiat Oncol Biol Phys 2000;46:525-534.

123. Dorr W, Spekl K, Farrell CL: Amelioration of acute oral mucositis by keratinocyte growth factor: Fractionated irradiation. Int J Radiat Oncol Biol Phys 2002;54:245-251.

124. Buntzel J, Kuttner K, Frohlich D, Glatzel M: Selective cytoprotection with amifostine in concurrent radiochemotherapy for head and neck cancer. Ann Oncol 1998;9:505-509.

125. Antonadou D, Pepelassi M, Synodinou M, Puglisi M, Throuvalas N: Prophylactic use of amifostine to prevent radiochemotherapy-induced mucositis and xerostomia in head-and-neck cancer. Int J Radiat Oncol Biol Phys 2002;52:739-747.

126. Brizel DM, Wasserman TH, Henke M, et al: Phase III randomized trial of amifostine as a radioprotector in head and neck cancer. J Clin Oncol 2000;18:3339-3345.

127. Schuchter LM, Hensley ML, Meropol NJ, Winer EP: 2002 Update of recommendations for the use of chemotherapy and radiotherapy protectants: Clinical practice guidelines of the American Society of Clinical Oncology. J Clin Oncol 2002;20:2895-2903.

128. Kaanders JH, Fleming TJ, Ang KK, Maor MH, Peters LJ: Devices valuable in head and neck radiotherapy. Int J Radiat Oncol Biol Phys 1992;23:639-645.

129. Stephens LC, Schultheiss TE, Price RE, Ang KK, Peters LJ: (1991) Radiation apoptosis of serous acinar cells of salivary and lacrimal glands. Cancer 1991;67: 1539-1543.

130. Marks JE, Davis CC, Gottsman VL, Purdy JE, Lee F: The effects of radiation of parotid salivary function. Int J Radiat Oncol Biol Phys 1981;7:1013-1019.

131. Franzen L, Funegard U, Ericson T, Henriksson R. Parotid gland function during and following radiotherapy of malignancies in the head and neck. A consecutive study of salivary flow and patient discomfort. Eur J Cancer 1992;28:457-462.

132. Mira JG, Wescott WB, Starcke EN, Shannon IL: Some factors influencing salivary function when treating with radiotherapy. Int J Radiat Oncol Biol Phys 1981;7:535-541.

133. Roesink JM, Moerland MA, Battermann JJ, Hordijk GJ, Terhaard CH: Quantitative dose-volume response analysis of changes in parotid gland function after radiotherapy in the head-and-neck region. Int J Radiat Oncol Biol Phys 2001;51:938-946.

134. Eisbruch A, Ten Haken RK, Kim HM, Marsh LH, Ship JA: Dose, volume, and function relationships in parotid salivary glands following conformal and intensity-modulated irradiation of head and neck cancer. Int J Radiat Oncol Biol Phys 1999;45:577-587.

135. Chao KS, Deasy JO, Markman J, et al: A prospective study of salivary function sparing in patients with head-and-neck cancers receiving intensity-modulated or three-dimensional radiation therapy: Initial results. Int J Radiat Oncol Biol Phys 2001;49:907-916.

136. Eisbruch A, Kim HM, Terrell JE, Marsh LH, Dawson LA, Ship JA: Xerostomia and its predictors following parotid-sparing irradiation of head-and-neck cancer. Int J Radiat Oncol Biol Phys 2001;50:695-704.

137. Jellema AP, Langendijk H, Bergenhenegouwen L, et al: (2001) The efficacy of Xialine in patients with xerostomia resulting from radiotherapy for head and neck cancer: A pilot-study. Radiother Oncol 2001;59:157-160.

138. Blom M, Lundeberg T: (2000) Long-term follow-up of patients treated with acupuncture for xerostomia and the influence of additional treatment. Oral Dis 2000;6:15-24.

139. Johnstone PA, Peng YP, May BC, Inouye WS, Niemtzow RC: Acupuncture for pilocarpine-resistant xerostomia following radiotherapy for head and neck malignancies. Int J Radiat Oncol Biol Phys 2001;50:353-357.

140. Johnstone PA, Niemtzow RC, Riffenburgh RH: Acupuncture for xerostomia: Clinical update. Cancer 2002;94:1151-1156.

141. Hamlet S, Faull J, Klein B, et al: Mastication and swallowing in patients with postirradiation xerostomia. Int J Radiat Oncol Biol Phys 1997;37:789-796.

142. LeVeque FG, Montgomery M, Potter D, et al: A multicenter, randomized, double-blind, placebo-controlled, dose-titration study of oral pilocarpine for treatment of radiation-induced xerostomia in head and neck cancer patients. J Clin Oncol 1993;11:1124-1131.

143. Johnson JT, Ferretti GA, Nethery WJ, Valdez IH, Fox PC, Ng D, et al: Oral pilocarpine for post-irradiation xerostomia in patients with head and neck cancer. N Engl J Med 1993;329:390-395.

144. Rieke JW, Hafermann MD, Johnson JT, et al: Oral pilocarpine for radiation-induced xerostomia: Integrated efficacy and safety results from two prospective randomized clinical trials. Int J Radiat Oncol Biol Phys 1995;31:661-669.

145. Horiot JC, Lipinski F, Schraub S: Can pilocarpine hydrochloride relieve xerostoma regardless of the destruction of major salivary glands? A prospective French cooperative study. Radiother Oncol 1996;40(Suppl 1).

146. Hamlar DD, Schuller DE, Gahbauer RA, et al: Determination of the efficacy of topical oral pilocarpine for postirradiation xerostomia in patients with head and neck carcinoma. Laryngoscope 1996;106:972-976.

147. Zimmerman RP, Mark RJ, Tran LM, Juillard GF: Concomitant pilocarpine during head and neck irradiation is associated with decreased posttreatment xerostomia. Int J Radiat Oncol Biol Phys 1997;37:571-575.

148. Valdez IH, Wolff A, Atkinson JC, Macynski AA, Fox PC: Use of pilocarpine during head and neck radiation therapy to reduce xerostomia and salivary dysfunction. Cancer 1993;71:1848–1851.

149. Wasserman T, Mackowiak JI, Brizel DM, et al: Effect of amifostine on patient assessed clinical benefit in irradiated head and neck cancer. Int J Radiat Oncol Biol Phys 2000;48:1035–1039.

150. Rudat V, Meyer J, Momm F, et al: Protective effect of amifostine on dental health after radiotherapy of the head and neck. Int J Radiat Oncol Biol Phys 2000;48:1339–1343.

151. Seikaly H, Jha N, McGaw T, Coulter L, Liu R, Oldring D: Submandibular gland transfer: A new method of preventing radiation-induced xerostomia. Laryngoscope 2001;111:347–352.

152. Leslie MD, Dische S: Parotid gland function following accelerated and conventionally fractionated radiotherapy. Radiother Oncol 1991;22:133–139.

153. Marx RE, Johnson RP, Kline SN: Prevention of osteoradionecrosis: A randomized prospective clinical trial of hyperbaric oxygen versus penicillin. J Am Dent Assoc 1985;111:49–54.

154. Levin AC: Dental management for the irradiated patient in management of head and neck cancer. A multidisciplinary approach. In Million RR, Cassisi NJ (eds): Management of head and neck cancer. A multidisciplinary approach. Philadelphia, JB Lippincott, 1984, pp 133–136.

155. Dion MW, Hussey DH, Doornbos JF, Vigliotti AP, Wen BC, Anderson B: Preliminary results of a pilot study of pentoxifylline in the treatment of late radiation soft tissue necrosis. Int J Radiat Oncol Biol Phys 1990;19:401–407.

156. Lefaix JL, Delanian S, Vozenin MC, Leplat JJ, Tricaud Y, Martin M: Striking regression of subcutaneous fibrosis induced by high doses of gamma rays using a combination of pentoxifylline and alpha-tocopherol: An experimental study. Int J Radiat Oncol Biol Phys 1999;43:839–847.

157. Delanian S, Lefaix JL: Complete healing of severe osteoradionecrosis with treatment combining pentoxifylline, tocopherol and clodronate. Br J Radiol 2002;75:467–469.

158. Chua DT, Lo C, Yuen J, Foo YC: A pilot study of pentoxifylline in the treatment of radiation-induced trismus. Am J Clin Oncol 2001;24:366–369.

159. Fischer M, Wohlrab J, Marsch W: Crux medicorum ulcerated radiation-induced fibrosis—successful therapy with pentoxifylline and vitamin E. Eur J Dermatol 2001;11:38–40.

160. Delanian S, Balla-Mekias S, Lefaix JL: Striking regression of chronic radiotherapy damage in a clinical trial of combined pentoxifylline and tocopherol. J Clin Oncol 1999;17:3283–3290.

161. Delanian S: Striking regression of radiation-induced fibrosis by a combination of pentoxifylline and tocopherol. Br J Radiol 1998;71:892–894.

162. Futran ND, Trotti A, Gwede C: Pentoxifylline in the treatment of radiation-related soft tissue injury: Preliminary observations. Laryngoscope 1997;107:391–395.

163. Gottlober P, Krahn G, Korting HC, Stock W, Peter RU: [The treatment of cutaneous radiation-induced fibrosis with pentoxifylline and vitamin E. An empirical report]. Strahlenther Onkol 1996;172:34–38.

164. Mossman KL, Henkin RI: Radiation-induced changes in taste acuity in cancer patients. Int J Radiat Oncol Biol Phys 1978;4:663–670.

165. Kogelnik HD, Fletcher GH, Jesse RH: Clinical course of patients with squamous cell carcinoma of the upper respiratory and digestive tracts with no evidence of disease 5 years after initial treatment. Radiology 1975;115:423–427.

166. Seydel HG: The risk of tumor induction in man following medical irradiation for malignant neoplasm. Cancer 1975;35:1641–1645.

167. Parker RG: Radiation-induced cancer as a factor in clinical decision making (the 1989 ASTRO Gold Medal address). Int J Radiat Oncol Biol Phys 1990;18:993–1000.

168. Ziffren SE: Comparison of mortality rates for various surgical operations according to age groups, 1951–1977. J Am Geriatr Soc 1979;27:433–438.

169. Vacanti CJ, VanHouten RJ, Hill RC: A statistical analysis of the relationship of physical status to postoperative mortality in 68,388 cases. Anesth Analg 1970;49:564–566.

170. Jansma J, Vissink A, Bouma J, Vermey A, Panders AK, Gravenmade EJ: A survey of prevention and treatment regimens for oral sequelae resulting from head and neck radiotherapy used in Dutch radiotherapy institutes. Int J Radiat Oncol Biol Phys 1992;24: 359–367.

171. Jansma J, Vissink A, Spijkervet FK, et al: Protocol for the prevention and treatment of oral sequelae resulting from head and neck radiation therapy. Cancer 1992;70:2171–2180.

172. National Institutes of Health Consensus Development Conference on Oral Complications of Cancer Therapies: Diagnosis, Prevention, and Treatment. Bethesda, Maryland, April 17–19, 1989. NCI Monogr 1989;1–184.

ALOPECIA AND CUTANEOUS COMPLICATIONS

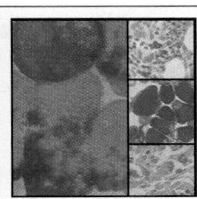

Leslie Robinson-Bostom

Teddy D. Pan

Charles J. McDonald

SUMMARY OF KEY POINTS

NONSPECIFIC REACTIONS

Alopecia

- Incidence
  - The most common of chemotherapy-related cutaneous toxicities.
  - Psychological trauma can lead to noncompliance with therapy.
- Etiology
  - Hair, by virtue of its highly profilerative matrix cells, is particularly susceptible to chemotherapy during anagen (growth phase).
  - There is considerable variation in cytotoxic effects on the hair matrix epithelium.
  - The degree of hair loss is related to specific drugs and to dosage, regimen, schedule, and route of administration.
- Evaluation of the patient
  - Anagen effluvium (loss of hair during growth phase) can begin 1 to 2 weeks after initiation of chemotherapy but is most noticeable after 1 to 2 months of continuous drug administration.
  - Alopecia is most pronounced on the scalp; eyebrows, eyelashes, beard, groin, and axillary areas are less susceptible, but alopecia in these areas can occur after many months of chemotherapy.
  - Telogen effluvium (loss of hair during resting phase) usually occurs about 3 to 6 months after chemotherapy and can also be induced by nonspecific physical and psychological stresses.
- Grading of the complication
  - Alopecia associated with chemotherapy is usually temporary.
  - Regrowth occurs 3 to 10 months after cessation of therapy.
  - Severity is dependent on the route, dose, and schedule of chemotherapy.

- Changes in color, texture, and other qualities of regrown hair are common.
- Prevention and treatment
  - Preparing the patient for the possible occurrence of alopecia, the use of educational materials that emphasize the temporary nature of the problem, and consultations regarding wigs are most important.
  - Scalp hypothermia could have increasing value as a preventative measure.
  - Some new and potentially effective agents and treatments are under investigation.

Cellulitis, Phlebitis, and Extravasation Necrosis

- Incidence
  - Cellulitis, phlebitis, and extravasation necrosis are among the most distressing complications of cancer chemotherapy.
  - These conditions are estimated to account for 2% to 5% of all adverse reactions from cancer chemotherapeutic agents.
  - They have been observed in 6.4% of a large group of patients using vascular access devices and in 6.5% of a group using standard peripheral venipuncture.
- Etiology of complications
  - Cytotoxic drugs irritate or escape through the lining of access veins during drug administration.
  - Local tissue injury is caused by infiltration of drug through surrounding tissue.
  - Drugs that bind to cellular DNA most frequently cause tissue necrosis.
  - Drugs that produce highly alkaline or highly acidic hypertonic solutions are also likely causes.
- Evaluation of the patient
  - Any patient who complains of acute burning pain or swelling

should be evaluated for these complications.
- The injection site should be inspected for swelling, erythema, and induration.
- Clusters of vesicles, large blisters, plaques, and ulceration precede extensive subcutaneous necrosis.
- Joint stiffness, limitation of motion, neuropathy, and causalgia are signs of extensive tissue involvement.
- Grading of the complication
  - A "venous flare" reaction, the least severe of the extravasation injuries, causes pruritus, tenderness, erythema, and edema overlying local access veins, but no tissue necrosis occurs.
  - Phlebitis occurs as a result of local vascular injury without extravasation.
  - Cellulitis occurs as a result of drug escaping from cutaneous vasculature causing minimal local inflammation.
  - Local tissue necrosis, the most severe reaction, results from a toxic drug escaping the cutaneous vasculature and dispersing throughout surrounding tissues.
- Treatment
  - Except for injury subsequent to the administration of mechlorethamine, the vinca alkaloids, and mitomycin C, treatment can be generalized.
  - Conservative nonsurgical treatment measures are effective for most lesions; however, surgical consultation should be sought immediately on suspecting extravasation injury.
  - Even with minimal treatment, phlebitis and cellulitis heal with few residual defects.
  - The infusion should be terminated, and if the line is not patent, it should be removed immediately.

SUMMARY OF KEY POINTS—*cont'd*

- Aspiration of the extravasated fluid should be attempted if the infusion line is patent.
- Elevation of the extremity for 48 hours or longer is important. Cooling of the extremity can be performed except after the alkylating agents mechlorethamine and mitomycin C (heat could be of some use after vinca alkaloid injury).
- If appropriate, antidotes such as sodium thiosulfate, dimethyl sulfoxide (DMSO), and hyaluronidase may be used through infusion or topical application; empiric use of antidotes should be avoided.
- Lesions that proceed to vesiculation, blister formation, and ulceration usually require surgical intervention.
- Persistent pain, swelling, and erythema are indications for surgical intervention, even in the absence of ulceration.

Palmar-Plantar Dysesthesia and Erythro-dysesthesia Syndrome (Acral Erythema)
- Incidence
  - The true incidence is unknown.
  - These conditions appear to occur commonly in clinical practice, the degree of severity being quite variable.
  - An incidence of 39% has been reported in a single study of administration of lomustine, doxorubicin, and cytosine arabinoside when used for patients with acute myeloid leukemia.
- Etiology of complication
  - Although 5-fluorouracil (5-FU) was implicated initially, a wide variety of chemotherapeutic

agents and combinations can cause these problems.
  - The concentration of drug accumulating at a site could be associated with the unique microscopic anatomic makeup of the skin of palms and soles.
  - Drug dosage appears to be related to disease severity.
- Evaluation of the patient
  - The onset of a tingling sensation in the hands and feet herald the onset of disease.
  - Burning, pain, and tenderness occur as the condition progresses.
  - Swelling and erythema of the palms are the first visible signs of disease. This is most noticeable over the thenar and hypothenar eminences.
  - Blisters occur in severe disease.
  - Desquamation occurs just before the sites heal.
- Grading of the complication
  - For most patients, symptoms are severe enough to cause termination of treatment.
  - For a few patients, signs and symptoms have been ignored and treatment has been continued.
- Treatment
  - Complete cessation of drug therapy and intensive topical care often clears the eruption without residual effect.
  - In a small number of patients, a reduction in drug dosage permits continuation of the treatment regimen.
  - Oral pyridoxine has been reported to allow continuation of treatment without worsening or recurrence of dysesthesia.
  - Rarely, therapists ignore signs and symptoms of dysesthesia and

continue chemotherapy while administering simple topical therapy.
  - The most effective topical therapy consists of frequent wet dressings and the application of midrange to potent corticosteroids.

Hyperpigmentation
- Incidence
  - Hyperpigmentation occurs in association with a wide variety of cytotoxic agents.
  - It can be generalized or localized.
  - Mucous membranes, hair, teeth, and nails also can be affected.
- Etiology
  - Hyperpigmentation caused by cancer chemotherapy is due to increased deposition of melanin in skin and mucous membranes.
  - Cytotoxic drugs have a direct stimulatory or toxic effect on melanocytes and also slow down the turnover and transit rate of epithelial cells.
- Evaluation of the patient
  - Differential diagnosis includes adrenal insufficiency, hemochromatosis, melasma, and noncytotoxic drug–induced pigmentation changes.
  - Specific cytotoxic drugs result in specific patterns of pigmentation.
- Treatment
  - Hyperpigmentation is primarily a cosmetic and psychological problem that generally does not interfere with continuation of therapy.
  - It resolves after cessation of therapy.
  - Sunscreens and avoidance of sun exposure could prevent accentuation of pigmentary changes.

INTRODUCTION

As with other pharmacologic agents used in the treatment of human disease, the administration of most cytotoxic or cancer chemotherapeutic agents can result in toxic side effects. And, as with other pharmacologic agents, toxicity is often manifested in the skin. Some toxic side effects occur at ordinary therapeutic drug dosages, while others occur as an extension of a therapeutic drug effect at higher dose levels. Toxic drug reactions in the skin can occur as idiosyncratic or allergic drug reactions.

Cancer chemotherapeutic drugs produce many common skin conditions, such as pruritus, urticaria, and angioedema. They also cause cutaneous reactions that are not shared by any other agent or class of agents—for example, the sclerotic effect that bleomycin can have on the skin.

A description of all the cutaneous reactions to cancer chemotherapeutic agents is beyond the scope of this book. Instead, we have elected to highlight a group of reactions that are fairly common and yet unique to cancer chemotherapy. Some reactions are associated with fairly severe sequelae and might direct the ultimate course of chemotherapy; others might appear severe upon occurrence but can be treated symptomatically, with no effect on the outcome of the treatment regimen.

For completeness, Table 40-1 lists most cancer treatment agents and the dermatologic conditions they can cause.

NONSPECIFIC REACTIONS

Alopecia

Of the myriad of drug-related cutaneous toxicities encountered by the cancer patient, alopecia is the most common.[1] Hair loss is an unfortunate side effect, because hair appearance often dictates a patient's self- and body image. Patients, especially females, receiving cancer chemotherapy often find alopecia psychologically and emotionally devastating. In fact, the occasional patient who is unable to cope with alopecia and the associated psychic trauma oftens opts to forego potentially curative treatments.[2]

Etiology

Systemic administration of a variety of cancer chemotherapeutic drugs can produce alopecia. Antineoplastic agents vary in their effects on hair matrix epithelium, hence their ability to induce alopecia. In addition, the degree of hair loss secondary to cancer chemotherapy is related to dosage, regimen, and route of administration. Chemotherapeutic drugs with a strong propensity to inducing alopecia include doxorubicin, daunorubicin, cyclophosphamide, and etoposide.[2-5]

Although low-dose and frequent-dosing regimens can involve a total drug dosage identical to that of high-dose infrequent dosing regimens, the incidence of alopecia associated with the low-dose regimen is often significantly lower.[6] In addition, novel dosage formulations of standard chemotherapeutic agents might ameliorate the extent of alopecia. Liposomes coupled with doxorubicin and mitoxantrone have been shown to decrease the extent of alopecia significantly.[7,8]

Clinical Manifestations

Drug-induced metabolic inhibition of hair follicle stem cells within the hair matrix results in a reduction of the number and size of epithelial cells contained within the hair shaft. This results in a partially constricted and weakened hair shaft that is susceptible to breakage even from trauma as minor as simple combing. Complete cessation of hair formation also can occur. Chemically damaged and mechanically manipulated hair is often more susceptible to this effect of chemotherapy.[9] Anagen effluvium (loss of hair during the growth phase of its cycle) can begin 1 to 2 weeks after a single dose of chemotherapy but will be most noticeable after 1 to 2 months of continuous drug administration. It also can occur as late as 2 to 3 weeks after chemotherapy.[9] Alopecia associated with anagen effluvium is most pronounced and widespread on the scalp, as this site normally contains 60% to 85% of its hairs in the proliferating anagen phase. Repeated drug doses given over the course of 1 to 2 months ultimately synchronize with each follicle's anagen phase; total inhibition of cell replication follows, and alopecia results. The eyebrows, eyelashes, beard, groin, and axillary hairs have fewer hair follicles in the anagen phase at any one time; consequently, repeated doses over many months are required to achieve significant alopecia in these areas. The onset of telogen effluvium (loss of hair during the resting phase of its cycle) occurs approximately 3 to 6 months after the start of chemotherapy.

Pathology

The normal scalp hair growth cycle consists of an anagen (growth) phase, a catagen (involution) phase, and a telogen (resting) phase. About 60% to 85% of scalp hairs are always in the anagen phase, 1% are in the catagen phase, and the remainder are in the telogen phase. Body hairs are not synchronized in such phases. During the anagen phase, rapidly dividing germinative cells within the matrix of scalp hair display a replication time approximating 24 hours. Thus, scalp hair, by virtue of its highly proliferative matrix cells, is particularly susceptible to growth inhibition of chemotherapeutic drugs. Inhibition (anagen effluvium) ranges from partial to total. Patients with fewer anagen hairs are less sensitive to anagen effluvium induced by chemotherapy.[9] Less commonly, certain drugs, such as recombinant interferon-α-2b (IFN-α2b), can induce the anagen hair into the dormant telogen phase, which is followed by a period of total epilation.[10] Telogen effluvium also can occur in response to the stress of chemotherapy or to an anemia associated with chemotherapy.

Differential Diagnosis

Most often, patients receiving cancer chemotherapy experience anagen effluvium; only a few might experience telogen effluvium. Alopecia induced by cancer chemotherapy is usually confined to the scalp and, although patchy at the start, generally progresses to total scalp involvement. Anagen effluvium alopecia usually persists throughout the period during which drug is given. Normally, hair returns shortly after drug administration ceases. There is always a temporal relationship to drug administration. Telogen effluvium usually occurs as anagen hairs are induced into the telogen state by psychic or bodily stress, high fever, nonmatrix toxic medication, or poor nutrition. Telogen effluvium is first noticeable about 3 to 6 months after insult and is temporary. Hair growth generally resumes, even as chemotherapy is continued.

Treatment and Outcome

It is important to remain cognizant of the potential psychological devastation that chemotherapy patients can

TABLE 40-1

Cutaneous Reactions to Agents Used in the Treatment of Cancer

DISEASE OR REACTION	DRUG	DISEASE OR REACTION	DRUG
Acrosclerosis	Bleomycin	Extravasation necrosis	Bleomycin
Actinic keratoses, inflamed (see Fig. 40-10)	Capecitabine		Carmustine
	Dacarbazine		Cisplatinum
	Dactinomycin		Dacarbazine
	Deoxycoformycin		Etoposide
	Doxorubicin		Fluorouracil
	Vincristine		Mechlorethamine
	5-Fluorouracil (cytarabine, doxorubicin, thioguanine combination)		Melphalan
			Paclitaxel
			Streptozocin
			Mithramycin
Alopecia	Bleomycin		Mitomycin (also delayed necrotic reactions)
	Busulfan		Taxol
	Carmustine (BCNU)	Cutaneous "flare" (must be differentiated from extravasation necrosis; excellent prognosis)	Doxorubicin
	Chlorambucil		Docetaxel
	Cyclophosphamide		Fluorouracil
	Cytarabine		Mitomycin
	Dacarbazine		Paclitaxel
	Dactinomycin	Dermatitis	
	Daunorubicin	Contact dermatitis (occurs principally with topical use)	
	Docetaxel		
	Doxorubicin	Allergic	Mechlorethamine
	Etoposide		Mitomycin
	Hydroxyurea	Contact systemic allergic erythema and desquamation	Chlorambucil
	5-Fluorouracil		Dactinomycin
	GM-CSF	De novo generalized eruption (erythematous macules; papules; scaling papules)	IL-2
	Idarubicin		IL-3
	Mechlorethamine		IFN-α
	Melphalan		IL-1β
	Methotrexate	Folliculitis also reported	IL-6
	Mitomycin	Pustular eruption reported	G-CSF
	Nitrosourea	Erythroderma	G-CSF
	Paclitaxel		TNF-α
	Procarbazine	Pustular contact dermatitis	IL-2
	TNF-α		5-Fluorouracil
	IFN-α	Papulosquamous lesions	Allopurinol
	IL-2	Exacerbation of psoriasis/de novo psoriasis	G-CSF
	Taxol/Taxotere		
	Thiotepa	Also localized to injection site Including erythrodermic psoriasis	IFN-α
	Vinblastine	Transient acantholytic dermatoses	IL-2
	Vincristine	Radiation enhancement	IL-4
Angioedema	Asparaginase		Bleomycin
	Cisplatin		Cisplatin
	Cyclophosphamide		Dactinomycin
	Vincristine		Doxorubicin
Blistering, localized	Bleomycin		Fluorouracil
Blistering, generalized	Vinblastine		Hydroxyurea
	IL-2 with concomitant antibiotics	Dermatomyositis-like eruption	Hydroxyurea
	G-CSF	Dysesthesia and erythrodysesthesia (acral erythema) (see Fig. 40-3)	Capecitabine
Bullous pyoderma gangrenosum	GM-CSF		Cyclophosphamide
Epidermolysis bullosa acquisita	IFN-α		Cytarabine
Paraneoplastic pemphigus	IL-2		Cisplatin
Pemphigus vulgaris			Daunorubicin
Linear IgA bullous dermatosis			Docetaxel
Cellulitis, phlebitis, and extravasation necrosis (see Fig. 40-2)	Dactinomycin		Daunorubicin
	Daunorubicin		Docetaxel
	Doxorubicin		Etoposide
Phlebitis	GM-CSF		Fluorouracil
	IL-3		5-Fluorodeoxyuridine
	IL-1α		Hydroxyurea
	IL-1β		
	Vinblastine		

TABLE 40-1

Cutaneous Reactions to Agents Used in the Treatment of Cancer—cont'd

DISEASE OR REACTION	DRUG	DISEASE OR REACTION	DRUG
Dysesthesia and erythrodysesthesia—cont'd	Lomustine	Neutrophilic eccrine hidradenitis—cont'd	Doxorubicin
	Methotrexate		Mitoxantrone
	6-Mercaptopurine		Procarbazine
	Mitomycin	Pemphigus vulgaris	IFN-β + IL-2
	Paclitaxel		IL-2
	Suramin	Pigmentation reactions	
	Taxotere	Depigmentation (noted during sequential chemoimmunotherapy for melanoma; correlated with tumor regression)	Carmustine
	Tegafur		Cisplatin
	Vinblastine		Dacarbazine, IL-2, IFN-α
	Vincristine		
Eccrine squamous syringometaplasia	Bleomycin	Hyperpigmentation	
	Cytarabine	Buccal mucosa	Busulfan
	Daunorubicin		Doxorubicin
	Doxorubicin	Diffuse	Bleomycin
	Mitoxantrone		Busulfan
	Suramin		Cyclophosphamide
Erythema, edema, and pain in ears	Cytarabine		Dactinomycin
Edema	IL-4		Daunorubicin
Erythema, edema, pain, pruritus, and burning: face, neck, and extremities	IL-2 administered with LAK or IFN-α		Doxorubicin
			Fluorouracil
Pruritus	G-CSF		Hydroxyurea
	IFN-α		Mechlorethamine
	IL-2	Hair	Fluorouracil
Erythema, hyperpigmentation: flagellate (see Fig. 40-4)	Bleomycin	Interphalangeal	Doxorubicin
			Fluorouracil
Erythema multiforme and TEN	Allopurinol (most frequently associated agent; TEN is often fatal)	Localized (vinca alkaloids)	Paclitaxel
			Plicamycin
		Nail	Bleomycin
	Cyclophosphamide		Busulfan
Folliculitis/acneiform	Bleomycin		Cisplatin
	Dactinomycin		Cyclophosphamide
Injection site reactions	G-CSF		Dacarbazine
	GM-CSF		Daunorubicin
	IL-3		Etoposide
	TNF-α		Methotrexate[68,70,71]
	IFN-α		Cisplatin
	IFN-λ	Occluded areas	Methotrexate
	SCF		Etoposide
Leg ulcers	Hydroxyurea		Ifosfamide
Lupus-like dermatitis	5-Fluorouracil		Nitrosourea
Lupus erythematosus–like rash, associated with clinical signs, symptoms, laboratory values of systemic disease	Interferon-α2a, 2b	Palms and soles	Thiotepa
			Cyclophosphamide
			Doxorubicin
			Ifosfamide
Nail dystrophy	Bleomycin		Bleomycin
	Cyclophosphamide		Cisplatin
	Daunorubicin	Photosensitivity	Fluorouracil
	Docetaxel		Mithramycin
	Doxorubicin		Thiotepa
	5-Fluorouracil		Dacarbazine
	Hydroxyurea		Fluorouracil
	Mitoxantrone		Flutamide
	Vinblastine	Radiation recall (see Fig. 40-5)	Bleomycin
	Vincristine		Cyclophosphamide
Neutrophilic eccrine hidradenitis	Bleomycin		Cytarabine
	Cisplatin		Dactinomycin
	Chlorambucil		Daunorubicin
	Cyclophosphamide		Doxorubicin
	Cytarabine		Etoposide
	Dacarbazine		Fluorouracil
	Dactinomycin		Hydroxyurea
	Daunorubicin		Lomustine

Continued

TABLE 40-1

Cutaneous Reactions to Agents Used in the Treatment of Cancer—*cont'd*

DISEASE OR REACTION	DRUG	DISEASE OR REACTION	DRUG
Radiation recall—*cont'd*	Melphalan	Ulceration	Hydroxyurea
	Mitomycin	Ulceration, digital	IFN-α
	Paclitaxel	Urticaria	Bleomycin
	Vinblastine	Localized to injection site	IL-3
	Tamoxifen	Generalized	GM-CSF
Reactivation of UV light–induced	Vinblastine	Vasculitis (cutaneous)	Busulfan
erythema	Methotrexate	Leukocytoclastic vasculitis	Cyclophosphamide
	Suramin		TNF-α
Sunburn recall	Methotrexate	Necrotizing vasculitis	G-CSF
Skin cancer (occurs principally	Methotrexate		GM-CSF
with topical use)	Mechlorethamine		Hydroxyurea
Sweet's syndrome	Busulfan		Methotrexate
	G-CSF		

G-CSF, granulocyte colony- stimulating factor; GM-CSF, granulocyte-macrophage colony-stimulating factor; IFN-α, interferon-α; IFN-β, interferon-β; IFN-λ, interferon-λ; IL-2, interleukin-2; IL-3, interleukin-3; IL-4, interleukin-4; IL-6, interleukin-6; IL-α, interleukin-Iα; IL-β, interleukin-β; LAK, lymphokine-activated killer; SCF, stem cell factor; TEN, toxic epidermal necrolysis; TNF-α, tumor necrosis factor-α.

experience with rapid loss of hair. Strategies to ameliorate the psychological effects include preparing patients mentally for such an event and reassuring them that this side effect is only temporary. Patients should receive useful information on scalp hair care and on the availability and acceptable appearance of wigs and other scalp covering.[11] In cooperation with the American Cancer Society, the Cosmetic Toiletries and Fragrances Association and groups of local beauticians have developed a highly successful image-building program called "Look Good, Feel Good." This program is available free of charge to cancer patients experiencing difficulty with alopecia and other cosmetic defects.

Prognosis

Alopecia associated with chemotherapy is temporary. Regrowth can be apparent 3 to 10 months after cessation of the offending medication. Regrowth of hair can occur during prolonged cycles of therapy.[12] Unfortunately, permanent alopecia has been reported infrequently with high-dose busulfan and bone marrow transplantation, and with high-dose chemotherapy with cyclophosphamide, thiotepa, and carboplatin.[13,14] Most patients experience some change in the character of their regrown hair. These changes, which include alterations in color, texture, and type of hair shaft, are often transient.[15]

Prevention

A variety of maneuvers have been employed in an attempt to protect patients from chemotherapy-induced alopecia. These have included physical modalities that temporarily decrease scalp blood flow and drug contact time with the hair follicle. This feat was first accomplished with an inflatable scalp tourniquet.[16] Variable results were achieved, and patient tolerance was not high. These poor results led to the development of scalp-cooling methods such as the MSC cold cap system, cooling fluid ring turbans, and cold air hoods that deliver cooling temperatures below 22°C that decrease both the metabolic rate of replicating matrix stem cells and blood flow to the follicle matrix.[9,17] Results using hypothermic devices has been encouraging.[18] Their efficacy is increased during use of a chemotherapeutic agent that has a short half-life (e.g., Adriamycin) and is given in low dose. Also, patients treated with rapidly administered combinations seem to benefit from scalp hypothermia.[15] Tumor metastases in the scalp have been reported after use of this technique (with a 0.25%–11% incidence).[9] Other side effects include headaches, dizziness, nausea, vomiting, aversion to ice, cold feeling, and heavy feeling on the head.[19] It has been suggested that hypothermia is contraindicated for patients with leukemia, lymphoma, or highly metastatic neoplasms. Hypothermia is also contraindicated for patients who have a tendency to develop migraine headaches.[9]

The use of dietary α-tocopherol, a free radical scavenger, has been shown to protect against Adriamycin-induced alopecia in the Angora rabbit.[20] Despite the positive report of an uncontrolled trial in which α-tocopherol protected against Adriamycin-induced alopecia in humans, controlled clinical studies have failed to confirm these findings.[21,22] Minoxidil 2% topical solution, marketed to treat male and female pattern alopecia, has not shown a beneficial effect in preventing alopecia during chemotherapy for gynecologic malignancies.[23] Folic acid can prevent alopecia when given with methotrexate.[9]

Protection from chemotherapy-induced alopecia with topically applied cyclosporin A and tacrolimus has been demonstrated in an animal model.[9,24] Imuvert has been shown to protect against alopecia induced by ara-C (cytarabine) and doxorubicin but not by cyclophosphamide. This protective effect is presumed to be mediated by interleukin-1 (IL-1).[25] AS101, a new immune modulator, has also been shown to prevent chemotherapy-induced alopecia.[9]

Electrotrichogenesis (ETG) or specific pulsed electrostatic fields have shown promising results in preventing chemotherapy-induced hair loss. A pilot study of 13 patients undergoing treatment with cyclophosphamide, methotrexate, and 5-fluorouracil for breast cancer showed good hair retention without attributable side effects.[26] M50054, 2,2'-methylenebis (1,3-cyclohexanedione), a novel inhibitor of apoptosis, might be an effective agent in the future for preventing or reducing chemotherapy-induced alopecia.[27]

Cellulitis, Phlebitis, and Extravasation Necrosis

It has been estimated that local skin toxicity, other than alopecia, accounts for 2% to 5% of all adverse reactions from antineoplastic drugs.[24] Dorr[28] states that "The extravasation of vesicant cancer chemotherapeutic agents remains one of the single most distressing complications that hematologists and oncologists face." Local tissue injury occurs when cytotoxic drugs irritate the lining of access veins during administration (phlebitis) or when a cytotoxic drug escapes the confines of the cutaneous vasculature and spreads throughout the surrounding tissues, causing a local inflammatory reaction (chemical cellulitis) or local tissue necrosis (extravasation necrosis). Cellulitis and necrosis can involve skin alone or can extend to subcutaneous tissue, muscle, fascia, and tendons. Extravasation frequently occurs during use of subcutaneous indwelling vascular access devices.[29] Brothers and colleagues[30] reported an extravasation incidence of 6.4% in a group of 300 patients using vascular access devices. By contrast, Barlock and coworkers[31] reported an extravasation incidence of 6.5% while using a standard peripheral venipuncture to administer doxorubicin.

Etiology

A wide variety of chemotherapeutic drugs have caused local cutaneous toxicity of varying severity. Clarification of the mechanism of local tissue injury after insult by chemotherapeutic agents awaits further investigation. It has been postulated that agents that produce highly alkaline, or acidic, hypertonic solutions are likely causes of local toxicity. Drugs that bind to DNA are considered the most frequent cause of soft-tissue necrosis subsequent to extravasation.[30] Necrotic tissue reactions can continue for weeks after withdrawal of the inciting agent, and reports of tissue reactions initially occurring weeks and months after exposure to a single agent support the concept of tissue binding as a likely cause of local necrotic reactions.[32] Other possible contributors to local tissue toxicity include local chemical irritant reactions and maturation arrest induced in proliferating cells secondary to normal biochemical actions of cancer chemotherapeutic drugs.

The list of agents associated with severe local tissue toxicity include the vinca alkaloids, vincristine and vinblastine; the alkylating agents, mechlorethamine and mitomycin C; the anthracyclines, doxorubicin and daunorubicin; and the antibiotic dactinomycin.[33-37] Other drugs less likely to cause severe local toxicity include 5-fluorouracil (5-FU), etoposide, bleomycin, cisplatin, mitoxantrone, paclitaxel, streptozocin, oxaliplatin, docetaxel, and doxil.[38-46]

Several cases of delayed local reactions and reactions after sunlight exposure have been attributed to mitomycin C.[47] A "recall" type of extravasation necrosis has also been associated with doxorubicin.[48] Delayed skin ulcers have been reported to appear within a prior mitomycin C infusion site after a second treatment given into a site on the opposite arm.[28]

Doxorubicin local tissue reactivity includes, in addition to necrosis and radiation "recall effect," a "venous flare" reaction.[48,49] The "venous flare" that occurs during infusion is characterized by a linear eruption in the skin overlying access veins of the forearm. Erythema, edema, induration, pruritus, and tenderness overlie the area of the injection site (Fig. 40-1). Superficial blisters and vesicles can appear. This reaction subsides without residual tissue damage within 48 hours after discontinuation of

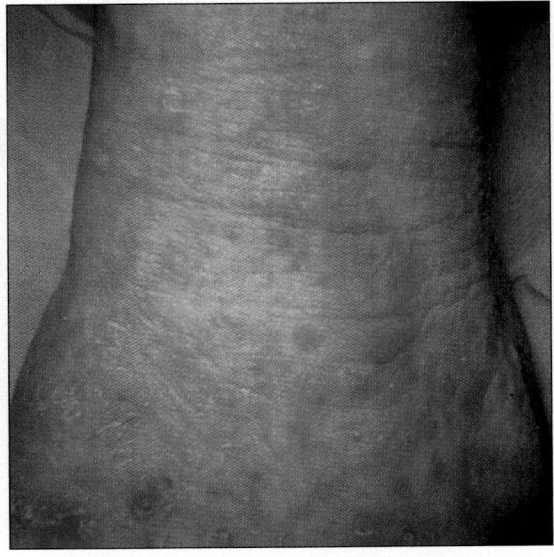

Figure 40-1. Venous flare reaction overlying access vein of the forearm.

the infusion. It has been estimated that venous flares occur in up to 3% of all Adriamycin infusions.[49]

Clinical Manifestations

During the infusion that leads to necrosis, patients often complain of acute burning pain and swelling, indicative of extravasated fluid collecting at the site. Within 7 days after the infusion, patients complain of pain, edema, erythema, and induration at the injection site. Severely involved untreated sites develop clusters of vesicles and large blisters, followed by ulceration or the development of a large plaque with a necrotic center, or both (Fig. 40-2). Underneath the plaque, or ulcer, extensive areas of necrosis might be found.

At the site of the ulcer or plaque, a hard black eschar ultimately forms. Peripheral to the eschar, erythema and swelling persist for weeks. Simultaneously with the involvement of subcuticular tissue, there are joint stiffness, limitation of motion, neuropathy, and causalgia in the affected parts.

Pathology

Bhawan and associates[50] and others reported early and late histologic changes in the skin of two patients with doxorubicin extravasation. In an earlier lesion, before eschar formation, marked epidermal hyperplasia is observed. Mitosis of many epidermal cells occurs. Individual necrotic keratinocytes are abundant. All other cell types show similar reactive responses. As expected, in a late lesion, beneath the area of ulcer formation, panepidermal, dermal, and subcutaneous tissue necrosis are seen. Lateral to the ulcer, there is marked epidermal hyperplasia. Fibroblasts and endothelial cells show signs of extreme reactivity. Lobular panniculitis best describes lesions of the subcutaneous fatty layers. Curiously, signs of inflammation are not usually described in old or new lesions.

Differential Diagnosis

Local tissue extravasation must be differentiated from the doxorubicin "venous flare" reaction, a self-limiting local reaction that occurs in the absence of extravasation. Radiation recall phenomenon can occur with infusions of

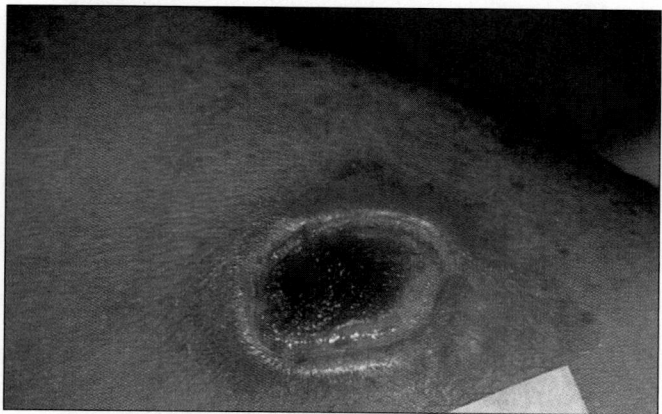

Figure 40-2. Extravasation injury, late-stage lesion with a central eschar, beneath which lies an extensive area of subcutaneous necrosis.

doxorubicin, mitomycin C, and 5-FU. These lesions tend to occur at remote sites of previous radiation dermatitis.

Treatment

Phlebitis and cellulitis tend to heal with minimum residual effects and with minimum treatment. These reactions are considered mild. There is considerable disagreement about the correct approach to management of severe local tissue toxicity.[29,51,52] Termination of the infusion is almost always followed by complete healing without residual defect in areas of phlebitis and cellulitis. Elevation and intermittent cooling of the affected part can accelerate the healing process. Rudolph and Larson[52] recommend treatment based on the agent causing extravasation: binding vs. nonbinding. Tsavaris and colleagues[51] report that conservative, nonsurgical measures are very effective for treating small (500 mm^2 or less), and medium-size (2000 mm^2 or less) areas of extravasation. In one study, 53 patients with acute tissue damage were managed with nonsurgical methods; all involved areas healed completely. Drugs studied were doxorubicin (eight patients), epirubicin (11 patients), mitoxantrone (five patients), vinblastine (five patients), and mitomycin C (three patients). Nonsurgical treatment was started immediately on recognition of an adverse event. The extravasated area was infiltrated with a hydrocortisone solution, 500 mg diluted in 10 mL normal saline, followed by daily applications of betamethasone and garamycin ointments. Topical applications were continued until healing was complete.

Dorr[28] and Rudolph and Larson[52] believe that there are very few indications for the use of local or systemic corticosteroids in the management of extravasations. This position is supported, in part, by the absence of histologic evidence of inflammation within areas of acute and chronic extravasation and by many experimental studies in animals that have failed to show a hydrocortisone effect on healing wounds.

The general use of other frequently recommended local antidotes is also frowned on by Dorr[28] and Rudolph and Larson.[52] At most extravasation sites, these investigators suggest avoiding the empiric use of sodium bicarbonate, sodium thiosulfate, heparin, calcium gluconate, magnesium sulfate, lidocaine, cimetidine, diphenhydramine, hyaluronidase, and a host of other chemical substances that are believed to inactivate drugs and reduce toxic effects on cells. In a number of experimental settings, Dorr and Rudolph and Larson believe that these substances have made necrosis and ulceration worse.

Recently, heparin fractions have been shown to prevent doxorubicin-induced extravasation necrosis in rats.[53] Suction and saline or vitamin C washout also reduce necrotic tissue size in doxorubicin-induced extravasation injury in rats.[54] There is general agreement among those managing local extravasations that the infusion should be terminated immediately if the patient complains of pain, burning, or stinging at the infusion site or if local swelling is observed. If the original infusion needle or catheter is patent, aspiration of extravasated fluid should be attempted. If extravasations occur during the administration of mechlorethamine or the vinca alkaloids, and after an attempt to aspirate has been made, the needle or catheter may remain in place for the infusion of one of several appropriate antidotes. If the line is not patent under any set of circumstances, it should be removed immediately.

Elevation of the involved extremity is recommended for at least 48 hours. Simultaneous local heat applications are recommended only if the vesicant is one of the vinca alkaloids.[33] Cooling of the extremity could be beneficial after other vesicant injury, except after administration of the alkylating agents mechlorethamine and mitomycin C.[55,56]

Several antidotes have been found useful after extravasation has occurred:

1. 0.17 M sodium thiosulfate through a patent intravenous line and 50% to 90% dimethyl sulfoxide (DMSO) applied topically after mechlorethamine and mitomycin C injury.
2. 59% to 90% DMSO solution applied topically after doxorubicin and other anthracyclines.
3. 150 U hyaluronidase injected into the site through a patent intravenous needle or catheter after vinca alkaloid and epidophyllotoxin injury.[29]

Dapsone for treatment of doxorubicin extravasation injury has been studied in the rat.[57] Timing and the ultimate use of surgical intervention are of utmost importance. Less than one third of all local extravasations proceed to blister and ulcer formation. Routine use of surgery is therefore not indicated. Persistent pain, swelling, and erythema are indications for surgical intervention even in the absence of ulceration and eschar formation. Severe blistering, ulceration, and persistent pain make surgical intervention mandatory. When surgery is employed, a wide excision of the surrounding tissue is necessary to remove all dead and necrotic tissue and any residual chemotherapeutic drug that might be fixed at the site.[58] Inordinate delay of surgery permits active drug to infiltrate and cause injury to tissues far beyond the original site of extravasation. In such cases, delay might ultimately cause the need for more extensive surgery ranging far beyond skin and subcutaneous tissues.

Surgical consultation should be sought immediately on suspecting extravasation injury. This is especially important when large lesions are suspected and when using the most active tissue vesicants. Persistent pain, erythema, and swelling, even in the absence of blister formation, require surgical consultation.

Outcome

Morbidity associated with extravasation injury is high, but mortality is nonexistent. The degree of discomfort experienced by some patients is severe enough to cause voluntary termination of treatments. Others become litigious, losing confidence in their therapist. The injury accompanying extravasation injury has no effect on disease status; thus there is no reason to stop treatment with a given agent. Unless extravasation occurs again, retreatment of the patient with the same agent is not associated with recurrence of necrosis.

Prevention

In every patient considered for treatment with a known vesicant, prevention of local tissue injury is paramount.

Prevention begins with selection of the infusion site. Sites to be avoided at all costs are the dorsal surfaces of the hands and the antecubital fossae, as well as extremities that have been sites of extensive ablative surgery. The preferred site of infusion is the proximal forearm that has not been surgically compromised, and where a large amount of subcutaneous tissue overlies vital structures. If tissue-poor areas such as the dorsal surface of the hand are used, a subcutaneous flexible indwelling catheter is preferred over the standard intravenous needle. When multiple infusions are anticipated over a prolonged period, placement of subcutaneous reservoirs with long indwelling lines should be considered. Nevertheless, even indwelling devices are not foolproof; an extravasation incidence of 6.4% has been reported.[30]

Drugs should always be administered through a free-flowing intravenous line. Any hint of obstruction within the line calls for immediate termination of the infusion and an attempt at correcting the problem. Every attempt should be made to administer a solution that is as dilute as possible over the shortest period of time, preventing injury from concentrated drug and eliminating lengthy exposure of tissues to a toxic agent.

Palmar-Plantar Dysesthesia and Erythrodysesthesia Syndrome (Acral Erythema)

An erythematous eruption of the palms and soles associated with the administration of mitotane was first reported in 1974 by Zuehlke.[59] Within a decade, numerous reports of a similar reaction occurring in a variety of patients and associated with multiple drugs began to appear.[60-71] The true incidence of this disease is unknown. Yet, on the basis of personal experience, the number of cases reported in the literature, and a reported incidence of 39% in a group of 72 adult patients treated for acute myeloid leukemia (AML) with the CHA regimen (lomustine, doxorubicin, cytosine arabinoside), one would suspect that erythrodysesthesia is fairly common in occurrence and is among the most frequently encountered cutaneous reactions to cancer chemotherapeutic agents.[63]

Etiology

Soon after Zuehlke's report in 1974,[59] other investigators reported observations of palmar-plantar erythrodysesthesia. Early reports described disease in patients with hematologic malignancies, followed shortly by reports describing the use of continuous infusions of 5-FU in a variety of solid tumors and the appearance of erythrodysesthesia.[61,70,71] Hence, 5-FU became widely accepted as the offending agent in nearly all cases of palmar-plantar erythrodysesthesia. A wide variety of chemotherapeutic agents and treatment regimens have also been associated—for example, cytosine arabinoside, doxorubicin, methotrexate, 6-mercaptopurine, hydroxyurea, etoposide, 5-fluoro-2'-deoxyuridine, and combinations of agents.[60,63-69] In addition, reports of acral erythema associated with the use of bolus 5-FU therapy for solid tumors have been published.[68,70,71] Recently, the new oral agent, capecitabine, has been reported to cause palmar-plantar erythrodysesthesia.[72] There appear to be no age, sex, or racial predilections for susceptibility to this phenomenon.

There is no known mechanism for the reaction pattern other than that it appears to be drug-dose dependent. It has been suggested (but is highly unlikely) that the unique anatomy of the skin of the palms and soles (i.e., a thicker stratum corneum than other sites), the absence of sebaceous glands on the palms and soles, and the presence of large numbers of active eccrine glands make it possible for large quantities of drug to accumulate in the stratum corneum or be excreted through the eccrine glands. Thus, these sites are bathed in toxic concentrations of drug, and local injury occurs.[68,73] A ^{99m}Tc-labeled acroaggregated albumin scan in a single patient with erythrodysesthesia did not reveal drug accumulation in hands and feet; it was concluded that this procedure eliminated shunting of drug and drug accumulation at the site as possible causes.[68] Other factors cited include increased temperature and increased extremity blood flow that could enhance direct drug toxicity in skin.[67]

Clinical Manifestations (Fig. 40-3A and 40-3B)
Weeks to months after beginning specific high-dose intravenous chemotherapy, dysesthesia and paresthesia, expressed as a tingling sensation in the hands and feet, herald the onset of the syndrome. Increasing discomfort—

consisting of burning sensations, pain, and tenderness while holding objects and while walking—signals progression of disease. Pain with swelling and erythema develop within 2 to 4 days of onset. Reddening begins over thenar and hypothenar eminences and spreads to involve the entire palm and sole. Blanching and erythema also occur on the interarticular spaces, and erythema appears in the periungual areas. Swelling and severe pain now occur even at rest. Eventually, many of the blanching areas become bullous. This is commonly seen with cytarabine therapy. Desquamation followed by healing of the palms and soles occurs within several weeks. In a few patients, erythematous scaling dermatoses develop on other body areas, together with nail disturbances, which include onycholysis. Recall-induced palmar-plantar erythrodysesthesia syndrome has been described with a variety of chemotherapy regimens.[74]

Pathology
Pathologic findings among nine patients have been described as nonspecific, showing mild focal spongiosis of the lower epidermis, mild to moderate epidermal atypia, mononuclear cell infiltration of the superficial dermis, and mild vasculitis of small vessels in two of the nine patients. Mild focal vacuolar degeneration of the basal cell layer has been described.[63] Immunofluorescent studies are negative.

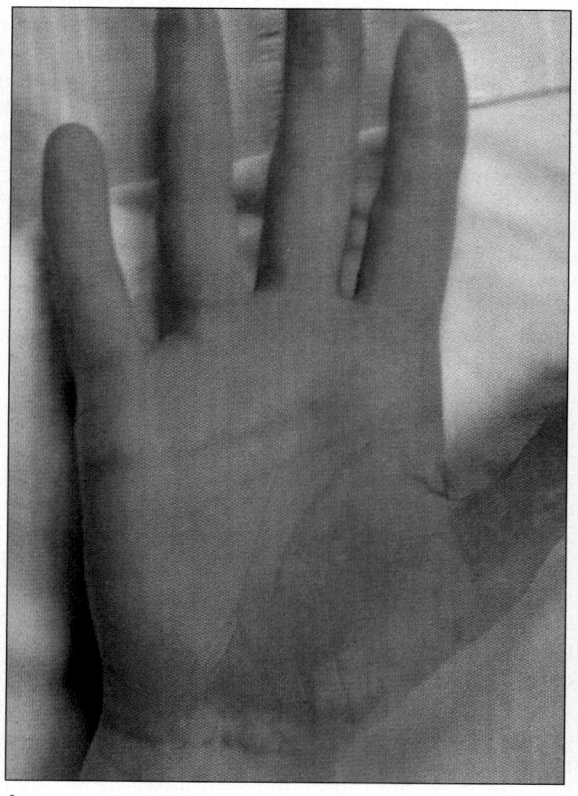

A

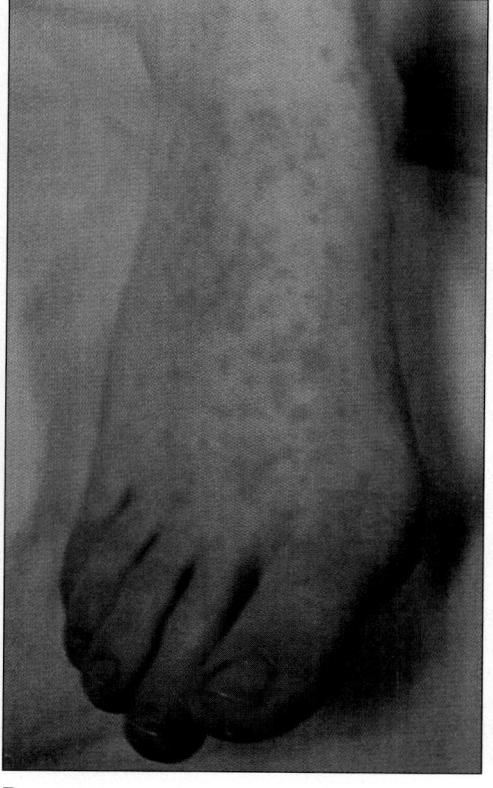

B

Figure 40-3. A, Palmar-plantar dysesthesia and erythrodysesthesia. Early manifestation with prominent erythema and edema. **B,** Late manifestation showing red papules, some of which are confluent over the dorsum of a red-to-purple foot.

Differential Diagnosis

Acral Erythema Associated with Acute Graft-versus-Host Disease. Although the most common cutaneous reaction associated with acute graft-versus-host disease (GVHD) is a generalized morbilliform eruption that progresses to blisters or skin necrosis, dermatitis of the palms and soles can occur as the earliest and only sign of the disease. Both dermatoses of GVHD usually occur within a period varying from 4 to 47 days after allogenic bone marrow transplantation, but the onset of palmar-plantar lesions may be delayed by up to 100 days.[75] Acute GVHD palmar-plantar erythema differs from palmar-plantar erythro-dysesthesia in that the process presents with reddening of the dorsal aspects of the fingers and within periungual skin. Diffuse erythema of the hands and feet soon follows. This feature is unlike the spotty erythema of erythrodysesthesia that begins on thenar and hypothenar areas. Pruritus and tenderness of the palms and soles characterize acute GVHD disease, as opposed to severe pain and swelling associated with the palmar-plantar dysesthesia syndrome. Other findings associated with acute GVHD and acral erythema include nausea, vomiting, intractable diarrhea, and a severe rise in serum bilirubin levels. Both diseases can occur concurrently.[73]

Acral Erythema Occurring in Severe Liver Disease. Acral erythema with severe liver disease is a chronic abnormality and is not generally associated with pain, blistering, or desquamation of the skin. Liver abnormalities are profound, with elevated serum enzymes and serum bilirubin.

Treatment

Treatment has been quite variable. In one subset of patients, complete cessation of chemotherapy was considered mandatory, followed by simple but intensive topical care consisting of frequent wet dressings and then applications of midrange potency corticosteroids. Often, this regimen is all that is required to clear the eruption. Pain, swelling, and blister formation clear within 1 week without residual effects. Many patients heal completely without therapeutic intervention.

In a second subset of patients, a moderate reduction in chemotherapy dosage and intensive topical care allow the therapist to continue with infusion chemotherapy.[65] A return to the original chemotherapy dosage is usually associated with recurrence of skin disease.

In a third subset of patients, cutaneous manifestations of the syndrome have been ignored, and treatment with the offending agent has been continued at pre-syndrome dose levels.[65] In this group of patients, Pagliuca and colleagues[65] state that only symptomatic treatment measures are required. Fabian and coworkers[76] and Vukelja and associates[77] have reported successful treatment of a group of patients using daily oral dosages of pyridoxine during 5-FU infusion therapy. Use of pyridoxine has permitted continued treatment with high-dose infusions of 5-FU without recurrence or worsening of the palmar-plantar dysesthesia syndrome, or without adverse effect on disease response to chemotherapy. The use of pyridoxine for prevention of dysesthesia is empiric.

Topical 99% DMSO has shown promising results for treatment of pegylated liposomal doxorubicin-induced palmar-plantar erthrodysesthesia.[78]

Outcome

Severe acral pain and blister formation can cause considerable morbidity and poor patient compliance. No matter how severe the process may appear, it has no effect on the patient's disease status. Except for the report by Pagliuca and coworkers,[65] most chemotherapists agree that acral dysesthesia is not life-threatening, yet it can cause sufficient discomfort to require withdrawal of drug or alteration in drug dosage. There is some indication that the use of pyridoxine could allow patients who have reacted to 5-FU to continue drug therapy at prereaction dosages.

Hyperpigmentation

A variety of patterns of hyperpigmentation have been described in association with cytotoxic agents. Cutaneous hyperpigmentation can be generalized or can occur in specific localized patterns. Mucous membranes, hair, teeth, and nails can also be affected by changes in pigmentation produced by cancer chemotherapy.

Etiology

Generalized hyperpigmentation has been described in association with busulfan, cyclophosphamide, bleomycin, 5-FU, mechlorethamine, hydroxyurea, daunorubicin, dactinomycin, doxorubicin, and procarbazine.[79-83] Localized patterns of skin hyperpigmentation occur after administration of cyclophosphamide, thiotepa, bleomycin, doxorubicin, daunorubicin, 5-FU, vinca alkaloids, plicamycin, and paclitaxel.[84-89] Mucosal pigmentation is seen after doxorubicin, 5-FU, cisplatin, and busulfan therapy.[87,90-92] Nail pigmentation is produced by cyclophosphamide, bleomycin, doxorubicin, daunorubicin, 5-FU, and hydroxyurea.[84,87,92-96] Alteration in hair pigmentation was described after methotrexate.[97] Cyclophosphamide could produce pigmentation of the teeth.[98]

Increased pigmentation from cancer chemotherapy is due to increased deposition of melanin in the skin and mucous membranes—a mechanism shown to occur when hyperpigmentation is produced by antimalarials, tetracyclines, or heavy metal therapy—and is not caused by an accumulation of drug or its byproducts. Melanin is a pigment-producing polymer, manufactured within the basal layer of the epidermis of skin, nails, and hair follicles by melanocytes. Melanocytes package the pigment into containers called melanosomes and distribute them to neighboring epithelial cells through tubular cytoplasmic extensions called dendritic processes. Alterations in baseline pigmentation can occur when there is an increase in melanin production, an increase in the size of melanosomes, or a change in the distribution of melanosomes within the epithelial cells of skin, nails, and hair. Cytotoxic agents might act to increase pigmentation by a direct stimulatory or toxic effect on melanocytes and also by slowing the turnover and transit rates of epithelial cells, thus allowing more time for the transfer of melanin to occur. Adrenocorticotropic hormone (ACTH) and melanocyte-stimulating hormone (MSH) are central nervous system–produced polypeptides that can stimulate overall pigmentation in humans. ACTH and MSH are known to produce generalized hyperpigmentation in Addison's disease after bilateral adrenalectomy for Cushing's disease and after parenteral administration. The role of these hormones in the normal regulation of human pigmentation is poorly understood, however. When serum ACTH and MSH levels have been studied in patients with pigmentary abnormalities who are receiving cytotoxic agents, no elevation of these hormones has been detected.[99,100]

Clinical Manifestations: Alkylating Agents

Busulfan. Busulfan can produce generalized brown hyperpigmentation that is accentuated on the face, trunk, and forearms. At times, this hyperpigmentation is accompanied by symptoms of fatigue, nausea, anorexia, and weight loss, resulting in a condition much like Addison's disease. In patients receiving busulfan, however, hyperpigmentation of mucous membranes and palmar creases is rarely observed, alopecia is absent, and there is no evidence of increased ACTH or MSH activity. Busulfan hyperpigmentation occurs in 5% to 15% of the treated individuals and resolves when the drug is discontinued.[79]

Carmustine. Carmustine (BCNU) has produced erythema followed by postinflammatory hyperpigmentation when it is spilled on the skin inadvertently, but parenteral use is not associated with pigmentary changes.[101]

Cyclophosphamide. Cyclophosphamide can cause generalized skin pigmentation (which could be photo-accentuated) in addition to localized pigmentation of the palms, soles, and nails.[84,95] Nail pigmentation can be diffuse or can present as horizontal or longitudinal dark bands. On cessation of therapy, this pigmentation usually resolves as the nail grows out. In one large series of patients treated with cyclophosphamide, the incidence of skin and nail pigmentation was less than 50%.[102] There is a single report of a child in whom a persistent brown line developed on the teeth as a result of cyclophosphamide therapy.[98]

Mechlorethamine. Used topically in the treatment of mycosis fungoides, mechlorethamine produces diffuse hyperpigmentation.[82] This problem can occur with or without clinical evidence of allergic or irritant contact dermatitis.

Melphalan. Melphalan has been reported to cause nail bed hyperpigmentation with longitudinal bands in a single patient with metastatic melanoma. This resolved after melphalan was discontinued.[103]

Thiotepa. Given intravenously in high doses, thiotepa has been reported to cause discreet areas of hyperpigmentation corresponding to sites occluded by adhesive patches or tape during chemotherapy. This effect might result from an enhanced local toxic effect of the drug, which is excreted in sweat.[85]

Clinical Manifestations: Antibiotics

Actinomycin. Persistent serpentine supravenous hyperpigmentation has been associated with actinomycin and vincristine chemotherapy.[104]

Bleomycin. Bleomycin causes several patterns of hyperpigmentation. A generalized darkening of the skin is described that includes the palmar creases and cuticles. Patchy pigmentation can occur at pressure points and might be delayed over the elbows, shoulders, and buttocks.[105] The most distinctive patterns consist of linear or "flagellate" streaks on the trunk that correspond to areas of pruritus and scratching (Fig. 40-4). Attempts to reproduce these lesions experimentally by rubbing the skin have met with variable success.[86,106] One series reported flagellate hyperpigmentation in one third of patients, with onset after 3 weeks of therapy and persistence of lesions for 5 months.[107] Horizontal brown nail banding has also been observed with bleomycin therapy.[108]

Dactinomycin. Intertriginous, trauma-induced, and diffuse hyperpigmentation have been associated with dactinomycin therapy.[109]

Daunorubicin. Closely related to doxorubicin, daunorubicin has also been reported to cause skin and nail pigmentation, but with less frequency. Transverse pigmented nail bands have been reported, in addition to polycyclic pigmentation of the scalp.[88,94]

Doxorubicin. Doxorubicin is associated with localized pigmentation of the palms and soles, dorsa of the hands, face, and interphalangeal and palmar creases.[87] Diffuse pigmentation also can occur.[95] Intraoral pigmentation occurs on the buccal mucosa and tongue.[87,90] Nail pigmentation can present as horizontal or longitudinal bands or in a diffuse manner.[87,93] These changes are more common among black patients.[93] MSH levels are not elevated in patients with doxorubicin-induced pigmentation.[99]

Figure 40-4. Bleomycin pigmentation. This is the most distinctive pattern of pigmentation following the administration of bleomycin. Erythematous, linear lesions often precede the appearance of increased pigmentation.

Clinical Manifestations: Mitotic Inhibitors

Etoposide. Hyperpigmentation occurs in occluded areas.[110]

Ifosfamide. Hyperpigmentation on the hands, feet, and occluded areas has been reported with ifosfamide.[111]

Mithramycin. Mithramycin has been associated with postinflammatory hyperpigmentation after intense flushing and facial edema.[112]

Paclitaxel. Localized hyperpigmentation occurs with paclitaxel therapy.

Procarbazine. Localized hyperpigmentation has also been reported with procarbazine.

Clinical Manifestations: Antimetabolites

5-Fluorouracil. 5-FU causes uniform pigmentation in sun-exposed areas in 2% to 5% of patients.[81] Localized hyperpigmentation also can occur at sites of radiation therapy.[113] Many localized patterns of pigmentation in nonirradiated areas have also been described. Serpentine supravenous hyperpigmentation occurs over veins used for repeated 5-FU infusions in the absence of phlebitis or thrombosis.[112] Serpentine pigmented streaks on the back and buttocks and reticulate pigmentation have also been reported.[114] Hyperpigmentation also can present in stria distensae.[115] Banded pigmentation over the small joints of the hands, diffuse pigmentation of the palms, and macular pigmentation of the palms and soles have been described.[111,116,117] Nail pigmentation can occur as transverse banding, and pigmentation of the oral mucosa can result after long-term therapy.[95,116]

Methotrexate. Methotrexate has been reported to cause horizontal dark banding of the hair after intermittent therapy, similar to the "flag sign" of kwashiorkor.[97]

Clinical Manifestations: Miscellaneous Drugs

Cisplatin. Cisplatin has been reported to produce a gingival band of pigmentation similar to a "lead line."[92] Hyperpigmentation at sites of pressure is common and is seen in up to 70% of patients.[95]

Hydroxyurea. Hydroxyurea caused generalized hyperpigmentation and scaling in 15% of 20 patients receiving long-term maintenance therapy. This was accompanied by partial alopecia, cutaneous and subcutaneous atrophy, and erythema of the face and hands.[83] Multiple longitudinal pigmented nail bands also have been observed.[96]

Pathology

Skin biopsies, when performed, have demonstrated a variety of alterations in both the amount of melanin present and its distribution within the epidermis. Melanin also can be seen in dermal macrophages. On occasion, the number of melanocytes might be increased; these cells might be larger than normal and might appear to have more dendritic processes.[118]

Differential Diagnosis

Diffuse generalized hyperpigmentation can be seen in Addison's disease or primary adrenal insufficiency, which could be caused by metastatic carcinomas or Hodgkin's lymphoma. Addison's disease is also characterized by constitutional symptoms of fatigue, anorexia, and malaise, which are found commonly among patients receiving cancer chemotherapy. Pigmentation in Addison's disease usually involves the oral mucosa and is accentuated in skin folds and creases, on the areolae and genitalia, and in sun-exposed areas. ACTH levels are elevated, and there is an abnormal response to ACTH stimulation in patients with Addison's disease. These laboratory findings are not present in patients with hyperpigmentation due to cytotoxic drugs.

Hemochromatosis, an iron storage disease, is characterized by diffuse bronze pigmentation, and the acquired form can present in patients who have received multiple blood transfusions. Hepatomegaly is usually present. Hyperpigmentation is primarily due to melanin, but hemosiderin deposition can be present in the skin also. Serum iron levels and saturation of transferrin are elevated in patients with hemochromatosis. Generalized hyperpigmentation along with melanin in the urine can occur in patients with advanced metastatic melanoma.

Melasma is an acquired macular brown pigmentation of the face that becomes more pronounced with sun exposure. It can be seen during pregnancy and in patients on oral contraceptive or phenytoin therapy. Multiple pigmented longitudinal nail bands can occur as a normal finding among dark-skinned individuals and can also be seen in metastatic melanoma.

Solitary pigmented longitudinal nail bands can be caused by benign melanocytic hyperplasia, lentigos, or junctional nevi in the nail matrix. A biopsy of the nail matrix should be performed in most cases to exclude subungual melanoma. Diffuse brown nail pigmentation can be caused by drugs other than cytotoxic agents, such as antimalarial agents, phenothiazines, tetracyclines, psoralens, and gold salts.

Treatment and Outcome

Hyperpigmentation secondary to cytotoxic agents is primarily a cosmetic problem and does not affect continuation of therapy. Some patients might suffer psychological distress but should be reassured that cutaneous hyperpigmentation, although persisting for several months, usually resolves after cessation of therapy. Nail pigmentation also resolves as the nails grow after discontinuation of therapy.

Prevention

Use of sunscreens and avoidance of excessive sun exposure might prevent further accentuation of pigmentary changes.

Nail Disorders

In addition to the pigmentary abnormalities already reviewed, cytotoxic drugs may otherwise disturb normal nail production to produce a variety of nail changes, including Beau's lines, transverse white bands, onycholysis, and brittle nails.

Etiology and Pathogenesis

Cytotoxic agents can have a direct toxic effect on the mitotically active cells of the nail matrix, which, as noted in the discussion on alopecias, can lead to cessation of growth with incomplete formation of the nail plate and the resultant formation of Beau's lines. Disruption of differentiation of nail keratinocytes can produce an abnormal nail plate. Measurements of the distance between Beau's lines and transverse white bands have demonstrated a temporal relationship between these nail abnormalities and drug administration.[119]

Signs and Symptoms

Beau's lines are transverse depressions of the nail plate produced when there is temporary cessation of nail growth. Typically, all nails are affected, but Beau's lines are most readily visible on the thumbs. They are commonly observed after short, intensive chemotherapy regimens.[119]

Multiple transverse white bands of all ten fingernails can result from combination chemotherapy featuring a variety of agents that include cyclophosphamide, doxorubicin, vincristine, prednisone, bleomycin, methotrexate, procarbazine, carmustine, semustine, and cisplatin.[120]

Onycholysis, or separation of the nail plate from the nailbed, has been reported among patients receiving 5-FU and bleomycin.[107,121] Doxorubicin also might cause onycholysis and in one case was associated with subungual blistering and blistering of the soles with subsequent callus formation.[122] Brittle nails have been reported secondary to the administration of 5-FU and hydroxyurea.[83,123]

Differential Diagnosis

Beau's lines can be seen after many febrile illnesses, after myocardial infarction, or with Raynaud's syndrome, zinc deficiency, or chronic dermatitis of the nail folds. Transverse white bands can sometimes be seen after an acute illness or after ingestion of arsenic, thallium, or fluoride. Onycholysis is common in psoriasis and is also seen in fungal infections of the nail and secondary to trauma.

RADIATION-ASSOCIATED REACTIONS

Two types of reactions have been associated with the use of chemotherapeutic drugs and ionizing radiation: radiation enhancement and radiation recall. The resulting reaction correlates with the specific drug given and with the sequence of administration.

Radiation Recall

Radiation recall is an acute inflammatory reaction that develops within an area of previous irradiation after

TABLE 40-2

Drugs Causing Radiation Recall Dermatitis	
DRUG	
5-Fluorouracil	Gemcitabine
Bleomycin	Hydroxycarbamide
Cytarabine	Hydroxyurea
Cyclophosphamide	Interferon-α-2b
Dacarbazine	Lomustine
Dactinomycin	Melphalan
Daunorubicin	Mercaptopurine
Docetaxel	Methotrexate
Doxorubicin	Oxaliplatin
Edatrexate	Paclitaxel
Etoposide	Tamoxifen

administration of a chemotherapeutic agent.[124] The reported involved organs include skin and mucous membranes, lungs, esophagus, gastrointestinal tract, central nervous system, bladder, and heart.[125,126]

Etiology

Multiple drugs have been reported to cause radiation recall and are listed in Table 40-2.[126-131] The most common drugs to cause this reaction are the cytotoxic antibiotics (dactinomycin, doxorubicin, daunorubicin, and bleomycin), the taxanes (paclitaxel, docetaxel), and methotrexate.[132]

Clinical Manifestations

Radiation recall can develop without clinically apparent antecedent radiation damage to the skin. Clinical manifestations usually develop within days after chemotherapy is given; however, the time interval between the initial radiotherapy and the resultant radiation recall can vary from several days to years.[133] Mild reactions appear as erythema and edema followed by dry desquamation, similar to first-degree burns (Fig. 40-5). More severe reactions are associated with moist desquamation, painful blistering, weeping, and in the most severe case, full skin necrosis and painful ulcerations. The severity of the cutaneous reaction appears to correlate with the time interval between radiation and chemotherapy, with the shortest time intervals resulting in more severe reactions.

Pathology

The pathogenesis of radiation recall is controversial. It has been proposed that lethal mutations passed on from surviving cells to their progeny might make them particularly susceptible to subsequent chemotherapy.[134] Recent data have shown that damage expressible as a lethal mutation is repairable; therefore the recall effect must be attributable to some other mechanism. It has been suggested that the tissue response in radiation recall is not the lymphocyte-mediated event that has been reported in an acquired immunodeficiency syndrome (AIDS) patient with significant immunosuppression (CD4

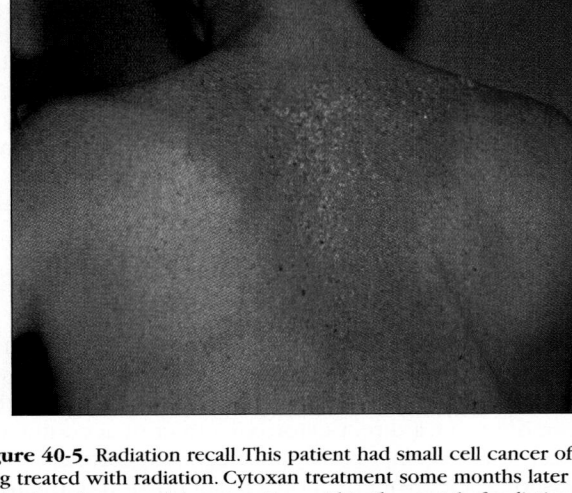

Figure 40-5. Radiation recall. This patient had small cell cancer of the lung treated with radiation. Cytoxan treatment some months later elicited erythema and desquamation within the portal of radiation. This lesion is now in the healing phase.

count, 30 cells/μL) after treatment with vinblastine.[135] The severity of the radiation recall reaction is related to the tissue at risk, type and dosage of drug, to the radiation dose utilized, and to the sequential relationship between the administration of radiation and the administration of the chemotherapeutic agent.[136]

Differential Diagnosis

Radiation recall reaction could be difficult to differentiate from cytostatic drug recall of acute inflammation caused by ultraviolet light B (UV-B) or other cutaneous irritants and infections. Areas that have experienced an acute or remote sunburn reaction due to UV-B or that have been sites of a previous irritation or infection can become further inflamed during the administration of a chemotherapeutic agent.

Treatment and Outcome

The milder cases of radiation recall, which are characterized by erythema, edema, and dry desquamation, are self-limiting. Patients are well advised to limit further irritation and injury to the affected areas. Cool compresses and lubricating creams or ointments provide symptomatic relief. In the more severe cases in which exudates and/or blister formation predominates, wet to dry compresses should be employed to promote drying. Upon cessation of exudate formation, moist wound healing strategies should be employed. Infected sites should be cultured and treated.

Radiation-induced necrotic ulcers are slow to heal. They are poor candidates for grafting because neovascularization and fibroblastic repair is limited. Strategies that attempt to both limit the amount of exudates and provide for moist wound healing should be employed. Topical corticosteroids have little effect on radiation recall.[137]

Radiation Enhancement

Certain chemotherapeutic drugs, termed *radiation sensitizers,* potentiate or enhance the effect of ionizing radiation. For radiation enhancement to occur, drug delivery must be concurrent with or follow within 3 weeks of radiation therapy.[138] Although radiation enhancement might be planned to increase tumor destruction, this technique often causes significant morbidity in noncancerous tissues.

Etiology

Radiation sensitizers (Table 40-3) include gemcitabine, interferon-α-2a, 13-cis-retinoic acid, doxorubicin, docetaxel, carboplatin, cisplatin, dactinomycin, methotrexate, 5-FU, bleomycin, and hydroxyurea.[139-143]

These drugs interfere with the repair processes that allow sublethally damaged cells to recover from radiation injury. The degree of reaction depends on the type of drug and dosage, the radiation dosage, and the time interval between the delivery of radiation and drug.

Clinical Manifestations

The clinical manifestations of radiation enhancement fall into one of three patterns:

1. A mild reaction consisting of erythema, edema, and dry desquamation.
2. A moderate reaction with moist desquamation, vesiculation, blister formation, and erosion.
3. Severe necrotic ulcerative reactions that could result in skin hypopigmentation.[144]

The affected sites are not limited to the radiation port but also involve contiguous skin.

Differential Diagnosis

Acute radiation-induced dermatitis could show clinical findings similar to those of radiation enhancement.

Treatment and Outcome

Prognosis and treatment are dependent on the severity of the reaction and are similar to those described in the section on radiation recall reactions.

Reactivation Dermatitis

Cytostatic drugs frequently reactivate acute inflammation and exacerbate preexisting eczema and other cutaneous

TABLE 40-3

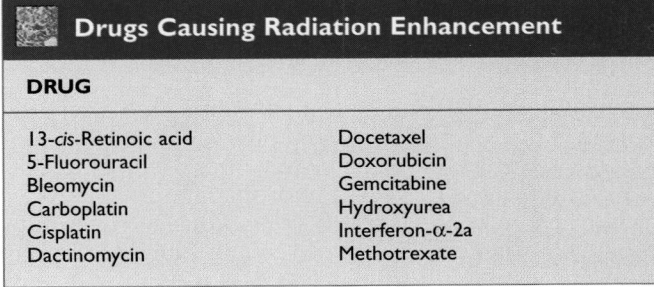

Drugs Causing Radiation Enhancement	
DRUG	
13-*cis*-Retinoic acid	Docetaxel
5-Fluorouracil	Doxorubicin
Bleomycin	Gemcitabine
Carboplatin	Hydroxyurea
Cisplatin	Interferon-α-2a
Dactinomycin	Methotrexate

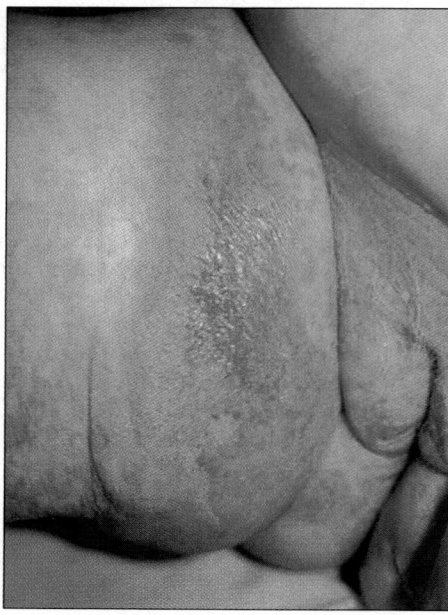

Figure 40-6. Reactivation dermatitis. This elderly diabetic female had a previous history of a *Candida* infection of the groin several years previously. Methotrexate administration on each of several occasions caused the development of a weeping erosive dermatitis.

diseases[145,146] (Fig. 40–6). IFN-α often exacerbates psoriasis and psoriatic arthritis.[147] It is postulated that because IFN-α is present in active psoriatic plaques and absent in normal skin, its administration might induce psoriasis.[148]

It is paradoxical that immunosuppressive agents can enhance cutaneous hypersensitivity reactions. Methotrexate blocks the induction of allergic contact dermatitis during the period of its administration, yet it can reactivate a positive patch test to 10% benzalkonium-chloride solution.[145] Cyclophosphamide-treated guinea pigs can experience an enhanced allergic contact dermatitis when challenged with dinitrocholorobenzene.[149] Burrows and associates[150] have described an adolescent with acute lymphoblastic leukemia treated with 6-mercaptopurine, cytosine arabinoside, vincristine, and methotrexate who experienced reactivation of previously treated scabies. Reactivation occurred after the course of methotrexate but not after administration of the other agents.

Although both topical and systemic administration of 5-FU can result in a seborrheic dermatitis-like eruption, this reaction does not appear to be reactivation, but rather a de novo cutaneous adverse effect.[151,152]

Neutrophilic Eccrine Hidradenitis

Neutrophilic eccrine hidradenitis is an acute dermatosis associated with the administration of multiple chemotherapeutic agents that include bleomycin, chlorambucil, cytarabine, daunorubicin, doxorubicin, mitoxantrone, vincristine, and topotecan.[153-160] Once considered rare and confined to adults receiving cytarabine for AML, it has been suggested more recently that the entity is more common than previously admitted. Not only has it been

observed in children undergoing systemic chemotherapy, but neutrophilic eccrine hidradenitis has also been reported in association with bacterial infections, AIDS, and a variety of other medications.[161,162] It has also been observed to occur in children and adults with a variety of cancers who are receiving a wide spectrum of systemic chemotherapeutic drugs. The clinical appearance is quite variable, yet the histopathologic picture remains characteristic.

Etiology

The primary histopathologic lesion in this disease is localized necrosis of the eccrine glands in the skin. Associated necrosis of apocrine glands has also been reported. The mechanism whereby necrosis is induced is unclear; however, a direct cytotoxic effect of accumulated drug on the eccrine coils has been suggested.[163] The reasons for a selective effect on a small portion of the total population of eccrine sweat glands is unknown. Lesions produced by the cytotoxic effect of an antimetabolite on rapidly dividing cells can be ruled out by the absence of an abundance of cells with mitoses within the epithelium of the secretory coil.[156] The histologic picture, which is quite characteristic, also tends to rule out hypersensitivity vasculitis as a cause. Necrosis caused by the accumulation of high concentrations of cytotoxic agents within the sweat glands cannot be excluded.

Clinical Manifestations

Affected patients present with a wide variety of cutaneous lesions. Tender erythematous to purpuric macules, papules, nodules, and plaques, some with dark central areas, suddenly appear on any body area during the administration of a cytotoxic agent. Lesions might appear within 2 to 3 days of starting chemotherapy or could go unnoticed until weeks after chemotherapy has started. Unusual presentations include periorbital edema with erythema and injection site reactions.[156-157] Usual manifestations include hyperpigmented plaques and painful edema of the ears.[155,158,164] Spiking fevers often accompany the onset of cutaneous lesions.

In many patients, skin lesions begin to resolve within 7 to 21 days after onset in spite of continuous chemotherapy administration. Likewise, new lesions can appear days and weeks after resolution of an original outcropping or might recur with the reinstitution of a course of chemotherapy. New papules, plaques, and nodules also might develop within sites previously occupied by the initial lesions.

Pathology

Histopathologic changes within affected skin sites are quite characteristic for this disease.[154,155,163] There is pronounced neutrophilic infiltration of the dermis about and focally within the eccrine glands, resulting in focal epithelial necrosis and basilar vacuolization of eccrine epithelial cells. Necrosis of apocrine glands also has been reported. Fitzpatrick and colleagues[159] note that the neutrophilic infiltrate is heaviest in those glands demonstrating vacuolar changes and less intense around those glands showing intense necrosis. Neutrophilic infiltration of the coiled duct and straight duct might or might not be observed. Some secretory coil epithelial cells show marked nuclear pyknosis and cytoplasmic eosinophilia. Mucinous degeneration of the eccrine gland adipose tissue cuff, along with an infiltrate of lymphocytes, eosinophils, and neutrophils, could be present, as could focal areas of hemorrhage within the dermis, mild to moderate spongiosis, and occasional vacuolization of the epidermis. In patients with active leukemia, abnormal or immature cells do not make up part of the infiltrate.[159]

Differential Diagnosis

Because neutrophilic eccrine hidradenitis is a fairly benign, self-limiting disease, it is imperative that it be differentiated clinically from other, more serious diseases that it might mimic. The variety of cutaneous lesions described in patients with neutrophilic eccrine hidradenitis could easily cause confusion with a fairly large number of clinical entities. Among these are leukemia cutis, cutaneous tumor metastases, erythema multiforme, vasculitis, drug hypersensitivity, sepsis (bacterial and fungal), Sweet's syndrome, and pyoderma gangrenosum. The localized nature of lesions associated with neutrophilic eccrine hidradenitis, and the temporal relationship of cutaneous lesions to the administration of chemotherapy, might aid clinically in differentiating neutrophilic eccrine hidradenitis from most diseases. Because the abnormal histopathologic picture presented by this disease is quite unique, histologic sampling of tissue is of importance.

The histologic differential diagnosis could include several entities involving necrosis of the eccrine gland, including bacterial sepsis with eccrine hidradenitis or other neutrophilic dermatoses; however, the well-trained pathologist, aided by the astute clinician, should make a definitive diagnosis possible.

Treatment and Outcome

Neutrophilic eccrine hidradenitis is a benign, self-limiting disease that generally requires no treatment. The disease does not appear to be influenced by chemotherapy protocols that include even high dosages of systemic corticosteroids. Within 7 to 10 days of origin, most lesions tend to resolve. Recurrent lesions appear to be less severe than preceding lesions and have been suppressed with concurrent dapsone administration.[164] In all patients described to date, healing occurs without residual scarring.

Prognosis

The prognosis for neutrophilic eccrine hidradenitis is excellent for total recovery without sequelae.

Syringosquamous Metaplasia

Although it can present as a histopathologic finding in association with various other cutaneous conditions, syringosquamous metaplasia (SSM) has become increasingly associated with a variety of chemotherapeutic agents and cancers.[165] It has been described in association with bleomycin, cytarabine, daunorubicin, doxorubicin, mitoxantrone, suramin, and docetaxel.[166,167]

Etiology

The exact etiology of SSM is unknown. It is presumed to be a reactive response of the eccrine duct epithelium to some type of offending agent or inflammatory process.

Clinical Manifestations

During or soon after the administration of chemotherapy, there is the onset of otherwise nondescript erythematous papules, plaques, or vesicles. These can be generalized or localized and have been reported to occur only in the intertriginous areas.[168,169]

Pathology

The characteristic histopathology consists of eosinophilic squamous metaplasia of the eccrine ducts within the dermis. Focal necrosis of the ductal epithelium has also been noted. The prominent neutrophilic infiltrate of neutrophilic eccrine hidradenitis is not present. These pathologic changes are not specific and have been described in other disorders unrelated to chemotherapy.[169]

Differential Diagnosis

The differential diagnosis is extensive and includes neutrophilic eccrine hidradenitis; bacterial, viral, or fungal infections; erythema multiforme, metastatic disease; and drug hypersensitivity. Histopathology is necessary to differentiate among these various entities.

Treatment and Outcome

The eruption is benign and resolves spontaneously after treatment is discontinued.

REACTIONS UNIQUE TO A SINGLE AGENT

Bleomycin Toxicity

Mucocutaneous reactions are the most common toxicities seen among patients treated with bleomycin. Alopecia, nail defects, hyperpigmentation, hyperkeratosis, and mucositis are most commonly encountered. Less common, but debilitating, are painful nodules and hyperkeratosis on the fingers; infiltrated violaceous plaques of the hands, feet, knees, and elbows; and skin ulcerations (Fig. 40-7). Bleomycin ulcerations can occur subsequent to vesiculations of the skin or can occur spontaneously without antecedent lesions. Ulcers that occur in vesiculated sites can be seen on any area of the body. Spontaneously occurring cutaneous ulcerations most often occur over bony prominences or over pressure areas of the body. A scleroderma-like syndrome involving the hands and feet is a unique cutaneous reaction, occurring with no other known chemotherapeutic agents (Fig. 40-8).[170]

Etiology

The precise cause of cutaneous sclerosis from treatment with bleomycin is unknown. Pulmonary fibrosis is a well-known effect that occurs in a very high percentage of patients after an average total dose of 300 to 400 mg of bleomycin. Total accumulative dosages associated with

Problems Common to Cancer and Its Therapy

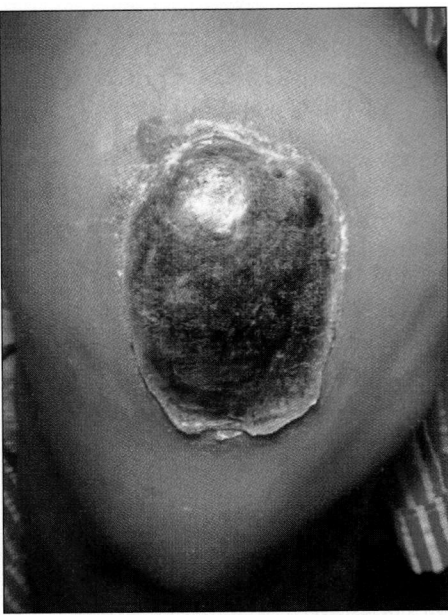

Figure 40-7. Bleomycin necrosis. These lesions can occur subsequent to vesiculation of the skin or spontaneously over bony prominences after the administration of bleomycin. This lesion is on the knee.

cutaneous sclerosis have not exceeded 100 mg. Bleomycin toxicities can also be correlated with high drug concentrations in organs showing toxicity.[171] Several studies have proposed multiple possible mechanisms of bleomycin-induced fibrosis. Bleomycin stimulates alveolar macrophages to release fibroblast growth factor[172] and upregulates transforming growth factor-β (TGF-β) messenger RNA (mRNA) expression, which is believed to play an integral role in collagen production and fibrosis in both cultured rat lung and human skin fibroblasts.[173,174] Bleomycin might also generate superoxide radicals, which are suggested to play an important role in inducing pulmonary fibrosis.[175] The onset of symptoms usually occurs within 6 months of an initial course of bleomycin.[170] Patients present with the rapid onset of bilateral edema and induration of the hand, forearm, feet, and lower extremity. Arthralgias, myalgias, and Raynaud's-like

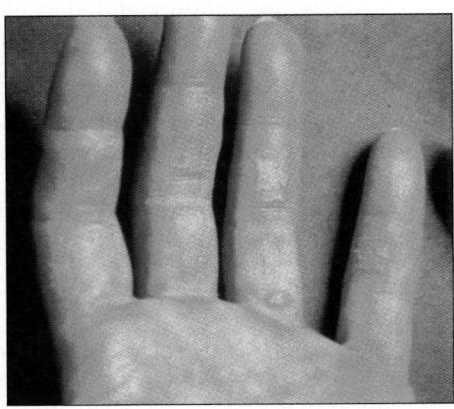

Figure 40-8. Bleomycin sclerosis. Slerotic papules and plaques are shown accompanied by intense hyperpigmentation of the body.

symptoms are associated with bleomycin toxicity. Sclerodactyly without cutaneous ulcerations, periungual erythema, or telangiectasias might be seen. All of these features might be seen in patients with systemic scleroderma.

Pathology
A positive antinuclear antibody, speckled pattern, can appear with the onset of cutaneous changes.[170] Other serologic changes characteristic of systemic scleroderma have not been reported. Pulmonary disease characteristic of systemic scleroderma is not usually found in concert with cutaneous sclerosis, probably because pulmonary toxicity occurs at much higher drug dosages (300 mg or greater).

Skin biopsy could show thinning and flattening of the epidermis. There is diffuse dermal sclerosis, with thickened eosinophilic collagen bundles extending from the superficial dermis to the subcutis. Eccrine ducts might be abnormally high in the dermis rather than at the dermal-subcutaneous junction. An inflammatory infiltrate is usually not prominent.

Differential Diagnosis
The cutaneous findings of sclerosis secondary to bleomycin administration closely resemble those found in idiopathic systemic scleroderma and occupational acroosteolysis secondary to exposure to polyvinyl chloride. A history of treatment with bleomycin distinguishes idiopathic from bleomycin-induced sclerosis.

Treatment and Outcome
Treatment consists of moderate dosages of systemic corticosteroids (i.e., 40–60 mg/day of prednisone). Dramatic resolution of sclerosis has been described after 1 month of treatment.[170] Other agents that have been used with varying degrees of success for systemic sclerosis or bleomycin-induced sclerosis include D-penicillamine, methotrexate, photopheresis, interferons, and cyclosporine.[176] Single-lung transplant has also been used for pulmonary fibrosis.[177] Outcome is variable in the untreated patient. Even the treated patient might show persistence of skin tightness in the distal phalanges.

Prevention
Patients receiving bleomycin therapy should be monitored frequently for the onset of adverse reactions, such as the acute onset of edema in the extremities. This occurs just before the onset of sclerosis. Just as the onset of pulmonary signs and symptoms is monitored when dosages exceed 400 mg, visible cutaneous changes should be looked for before the achievement of a dosage that exceeds 100 mg. Any patient experiencing cutaneous sclerosis should not be considered a candidate for further bleomycin treatment.

REACTIONS TO CYTOKINES

The advent of the use of cytokines in the treatment of cancer has led to a host of cutaneous reactions. The use of these powerful physiologic response modifiers in the setting of underlying malignancy, immunosuppression, other medications, and individual genetically determined host factors has precipitated a variety of both specific and nonspecific cutaneous responses. These reactions are summarized in Table 40-1. A detailed discussion of IL-2 is presented next.

Cutaneous Reactions to Interleukin-2

Recombinant human IL-2, or T-cell growth factor, is a glycoprotein that exhibits a wide variety of biologic effects on the immune system. It is finding increasing use in the treatment of advanced malignancies, including malignant melanoma, cutaneous T-cell lymphoma, renal cell carcinoma, advanced colorectal carcinoma, and advanced lymphoma.[178-186] IL-2 has been used after autologous bone marrow transplantation to prevent or reduce the high relapse rate of advanced hematologic malignancies.[187] In the clinical setting, IL-2 is often used in combination with other biologic response modifiers, including lymphokine-activated killer (LAK) cells and IFN-α.[183,187] IL-2 has also been complexed as a fusion toxin protein (Denileukin diftitox) for the treatment of cutaneous T-cell lymphoma.[189]

IL-2 alone and in combination with LAK and IFN-α has produced a wide variety of toxicities, including a characteristic cutaneous eruption. It is estimated that 50% to 100% of patients treated with IL-2 alone or in combination with other biologic response modifiers will experience some form of cutaneous eruption.[183,189]

Etiology

Within 48 to 72 hours after the start of an infusion of IL-2 alone or in combination with another cytokine, patients develop a skin eruption of varying severity. The precise etiology is unclear, except it appears that cutaneous reactions occur more often when high doses of IL-2 (100,000 μg/kg) rather than low doses (30,000 μg/kg) are used.[191] There is no difference in rate of occurrence, whether bolus or continuous infusions are administered. To date, no racial or sexual predominance has been observed. Nearly all patients treated with IL-2 develop a capillary leak syndrome, which, except for extensive edema, does not as yet appear to be entirely related to the development of cutaneous lesions. All patients receiving IL-2 therapy develop fever and chills. These symptoms tend to occur almost immediately with the initiation of treatment. A variety of ancillary medications are used during IL-2 induction therapy to reduce side effects associated with its administration. Among these are indomethacin, ranitidine, acetaminophen, and thiazide diuretics, any of which might induce skin eruptions in susceptible hosts. This is an unlikely possibility, as IL-2 skin eruptions often occur in the absence of ancillary drugs. Gaspari and coworkers[191] have studied IL-2 cutaneous reactions extensively and have concluded that there is immunohistochemical and histologic evidence to support the presence of a cell-mediated immune response during IL-2 therapy. Several other studies have implicated a possible role for nitric oxide, fas ligand and perforin,

and complement and other inflammatory mediators in affecting vascular permeability, resulting in a capillary leak syndrome.[192-195] It is likely that vascular leak syndrome occurs as a result of multiple mechanisms: cell-mediated damage, cytokine-mediated damage, inflammatory mediators, and modification of endothelial cell integrity and the extracellular matrix.[196,197]

Clinical Manifestations

Chills and fever along with transient cutaneous flushing occur during the first 24 to 48 hours of IL-2 administration. Forty-eight to 72 hours later, persistent erythema associated with itching and a burning sensation develop, first on the malar aspects of the face and then on the neck and chest. In a fewer number of patients, total body erythema (erythroderma) develops along with erythema and edema of the palms and soles (Fig. 40-9). If the use of IL-2 is combined with LAK cell infusions, it appears that the onset of the eruption might begin within 24 hours. Resolution of disease can occur within 2 to 3 days, when drug administration is stopped. Resolution is associated with continuing pruritus and desquamation of involved skin. Systemic manifestations of capillary leak syndrome are listed in Table 40-4.

There are at least three reports of erythema progressing to life-threatening bullous eruptions and toxic epidermal necrolysis-like lesions in three patients.[190,198] Staunton's[190] and Weiner's[198] groups believe that the histopathologic findings in each case separate these patients from those suffering the most frequently observed IL-2 reactions (Fig. 40-10). Erosions of the buccal mucosa, icterus,

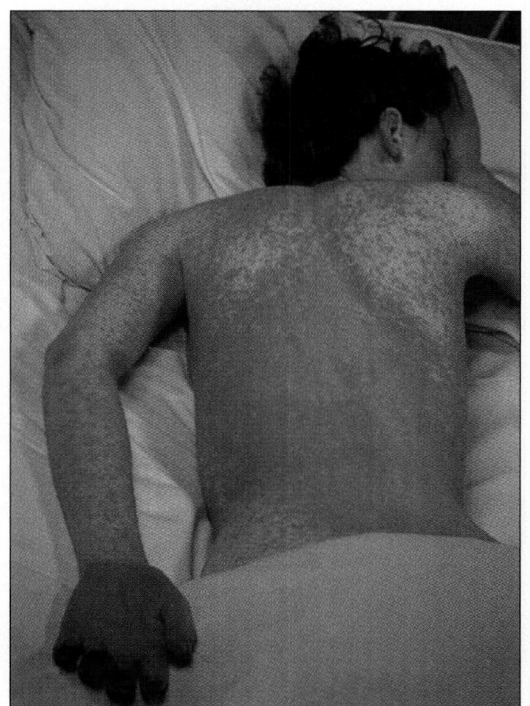

Figure 40-9. IL-2 cutaneous reaction. This patient's disease is characterized by intense facial redness, red swollen hands and feet, and a generalized macular eruption.

TABLE 40-4

Grades of Vascular Leak Syndrome

GRADE	CLINICAL MANIFESTATIONS
I	Minimal ankle-pitting edema
II	Ankle-pitting edema and a weight gain of less than 10 lb
III	Peripheral edema with a weight gain greater than 10 lb or pleural effusion with no pulmonary function deficit documented
IV	Anasarca; pleural effusion or ascites with pulmonary function deficit or pulmonary edema
V	Respiratory failure requiring mechanical ventilation in the setting of pulmonary edema or hypotension requiring pressor support

Sausville EA, Headlee D, Steler-Stevenson M, et al: Continuous infusion of the anti-CD22 immunotoxin, IgG-RFB4-SMPT-dgA, in patients with B-cell lymphoma: A phase I study. Blood 1995;85:3457–3465.

glossitis, and cutaneous erosions have also been described.[198] A persistent but not progressive vitiligo-like depigmentation has been described after IL-2 and IFN-λ, plus carmustine, cisplatin, and dacarbazine treatment of malignant melanoma.[199,200]

Pathology
Within the epidermis, foci of spongiosis, focal vacuolar basal cell degeneration, rare necrotic keratinocytes, and exocytosis of mononuclear cells are seen. In the dermis,

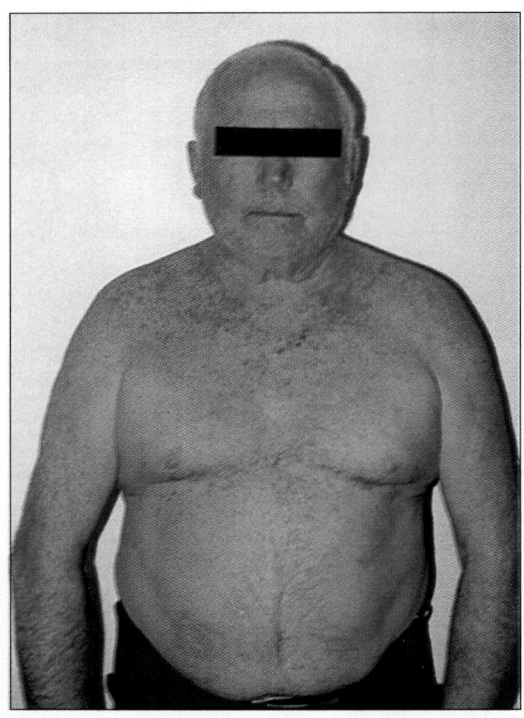

Figure 40-10. Inflamed actinic keratoses secondary to the administration of systemic 5-FU. This patient had extensively photodamaged skin showing "activation" of previously unrecognized actinic keratoses. Red scaling papules and cutaneous ulcerations predominate.

mild papillary edema, mild to moderate perivascular mononuclear cell infiltrates, and occasional engorgement of blood vessels occur.[190] These are nonspecific findings. Immunohistochemistry shows activated T cells within the epidermis and dermis with approximately equal numbers of class I and II reactive cells.

Differential Diagnosis
Viral and bacterial exanthems, drug or phototoxic reactions, toxic shock syndrome, staphylococcal scalded skin syndrome, toxic epidermal necrolysis, and acute graft-vs.-host reactions must be considered and ruled out with appropriate tests.

Treatment and Outcome
Cessation of treatment is followed 48 to 72 hours later with complete clearing of the skin and little or no residual effect except transitory hyperpigmentation.

Antihistamines given during drug administration and the application of emollients have shown some benefit in the relief of pruritus. The use of systemic glucocorticoids that could offer some immediate relief of symptoms is not indicated; glucocorticoids decrease IL-2 toxicity but might also reduce IL-2 efficacy.[201,202]

Gaspari and coworkers[191] graded cutaneous disease severity in 10 patients as follows:

- 1+: barely perceptible erythema.
- 2+: mild confluent erythema.
- 3+: severe erythema and edema of the skin.

Three patients who received 100,000 µg/kg of IL-2 experienced the highest mean severity score of 2.53 ± 0.37. Seven patients experienced a mean severity score of 1.18 ± 0.94. All patients, including those with severe blistering disease, experience complete skin clearing in 2 to 3 weeks if using good supportive skin care.

REFERENCES

1. Love RR, Leventhal H, Easterling DV, Nerenz DR: Side effects and emotional distress during chemotherapy. Cancer 1989;63:604.
2. Wiernik TH, Schmipff SC, Schiffer CA, et al: Randomized clinical comparison of daunorubicin (NSC-82151) along with a combination of daunorubicin (NSC-82151), cytosine arabinoside (NSC-63878) 6-thioguanine (NSC-752) and pyrimethamine (NSC-3061) for the treatment of acute nonlymphocytic leukemia. Cancer Treat Rep 1976;60:41
3. Benjamin RS: A practical approach to Adriamycin (NSC-123127) toxicology. Cancer Chemother Rep 1975;6:191.
4. Jessen RT, Straight M, Smith EB: Cutaneous and other complications of cyclophosphamide: A brief review. Rocky Mountain Med J 1978;75:204.
5. Estape J, Palombo H, Sanchez-Lloret J, et al: Chronic oral etoposide in non–small cell lung carcinoma. Eur J Cancer 1992;28A(4–5):835.
6. Umsawasdi T, Valdivieso M, Booser DJ, et al: Weekly doxorubicin versus doxorubicin every 3 weeks in cyclophosphamide, doxorubicin, and cisplatin chemotherapy for non–small cell lung cancer. Cancer 1989;64:1995.
7. Owen RR, Sells RA, Gilmore IT, et al: A phase I clinical evaluation of liposome-entrapped doxorubicin (Lip-Dox) in patients with primary and metastatic hepatic malignancy. Anticancer Drugs 1992;3:101.
8. Pestalozzi B, Schwendener R, Sauter C: Phase I/II study of

liposome-complexed mitoxantrone in patients with advanced breast cancer. Ann Oncol 1992;3:445.

9. Batchelor D: Hair and cancer chemotherapy: Consequences and nursing care—A literature study. Eur J Cancer Care 2001;10(3):147–163.

10. Brodin MB: Drug related alopecia. Dermatol Clin 1987;5:571.

11. Joss RA, Kiser J, Weston S, Brunner KW: Fighting alopecia in cancer chemotherapy. Recent Results Cancer Res 1988;106:117.

12. Hood AF: Cutaneous side effects of cancer chemotherapy. Med Clin North Am 1986;70:187.

13. Koppel RA, Boh EE: Cutaneous reactions to chemotherapeutic agents. Am J Med Sci 2001;321(5):327–335.

14. de Jonge ME, Mathot RA, Dalesio O, Huitema AD, Rodenhuis S, Beijnen JH: Relaionship between irreversible alopecia and exposure to cyclophosphamide, thiotepa and carboplatin (CTC) in high-dose chemotherapy. Bone Marrow Transplant 2002;30(9):593–597.

15. Robinson A, Jones W: Change in scalp hair after cancer chemotherapy. Eur J Cancer Clin Oncol 1989;25:155.

16. Hennessey JD: Alopecia and cytotoxic drugs. BMJ 1966;2:1138.

17. Christodoulou C, Klouvas G, Efstathiou E, et al: Effectiveness of the MSC cold cap system in the prevention of chemotherapy-induced alopecia. Oncology 2002;62(2):97–102.

18. Villani C, Inghirami, Pietrangeli D, et al: Prevention by hypothermic cap of antiblastic-induced alopecia. Eur J Gynaecol Oncol 1986;7:0392.

19. Dean JC, Griffith KS, Cetas TC: Scalp hypothermia: A comparison of ice packs and Kold Kap in the prevention of doxorubicin-induced alopecia. J Clin Oncol 1983;1:33.

20. Powis G, Kooistra KL: Doxorubicin-induced hair loss in the Angora rabbit: A study of treatments to protect against the hair loss. Cancer Chemother Pharmacol 1987;20:291.

21. Wood LA: Possible prevention of Adriamycin-induced alopecia by tocopherol [lettter]. N Engl J Med 1985;312:1060.

22. Martin JM, Diaz RE, Gonazales LJL, Sangro B: Failure of high dose tocopherol to prevent alopecia induced by doxorubicin. N Engl J Med 1986;315:894.

23. Granai CO, Fredrickson H, Gajewski W, et al: The use of minoxidil to attempt to prevent alopecia during chemotherapy for gynecologic malignancies. Eur J Gynaecol Oncol 1991;12:129.

24. Hussein AM, Stuart A, Peters WP: Protection against chemotherapy-induced alopecia by cyclosporin A in the newborn rat animal model. Dermatology 1995;190:192.

25. Hussein AM: Chemotherapy-induced alopecia: New developments. South Med J 1993;86:489.

26. Benjamin B, Ziginskas D, Harman J, Meakin T: Pulsed electrostatic fields (ETG) to reduce hair loss in women undergoing chemotherapy for breast carcinoma: A pilot study. Psycho-Oncology 2002;11(3):244–248.

27. Tsuda T, Ohmori Y, Muramatsu H, Hosaka Y, Takiguchi K, Saitoh F, et al: Inhibitory effect of M50054, a novel inhibitor of apoptosis, on anti-Fas-antibody-induced hepatitis and chemotherapy-induced alopecia. Eur J Pharmacol 2001;14;433(1):37–45.

28. Dorr RT: Antidotes to vesicant chemotherapy extravasations. Blood Rev 1990;4:41.

29. Ignoffo RJ, Friedman MA: Therapy of local toxicities caused by extravasation of cancer chemotherapeutic drugs. Cancer Treat Rev 1980;7:17.

30. Brothers TE, Niederhyber JE, Roberts JA, Ensminger WD: Experience with subcutaneous infusion ports in three hundred patients. Surg Gynecol Obstet 1988;166:295.

31. Barlock AL, Howser DM, Hubbard SM: Nursing management of Adriamycin extravasation. Am J Nurs 1979;137:94.

32. Luedke AW, Kennedy PJ, Rietschel RL: Histopathogenesis of skin and subcutaneous injury by Adriamycin. Plast Reconstruct Surg 1979;63:463.

33. Dorr RT, Alberts DS: Vinca alkaloid skin toxicity: Antidote and drug disposition studies in the mouse. J Natl Cancer Inst 1985;74:113.

34. Goodman LD, Wintrobe MM, Dameshek W, et al: Nitrogen mustard therapy. JAMA 1946;132:126.

35. Argenta LC, Manders EK: Mitomycin C extravasation injuries. Cancer 1983;51:1080.

36. Villani C, Pace S, Tomao S, et al: Skin necrosis due to antiblastics (procedures of prevention and therapy). Eur J Gynaecol Oncol 1986;7:58.

37. Frei E: The clinical use of actinomycin. Cancer Chemother Rep 1974;58:49.

38. Teta JB, O'Connor L: Local tissue damage from 5-fluorouracil extravasation. Oncol Nurs Forum 1984;11:77.

39. Dorr RT, Alberts DS: Skin ulceration potential without therapeutic anticancer activity for epipodophyllotoxin commercial diluents. Invest New Drugs 1983;1:151.

40. Preuss P, Partoff S: Cytostatic extravasations. Ann Plast Surg 1987;19:323.

41. Algarra SM, Dy C, Aparicio LA: Cutaneous necrosis after intra-arterial treatment with cisplatin. Cancer Treat Rep 1986;70:687.

42. Peters TM, Brijnen JA, Huinink WWB: Mitoxantrone extravasation injury. Cancer Treat Rep 1987;71:992.

43. Herrington JD, Figueroa JA: Severe necrosis due to paclitaxel extravasation. Pharmacotherapy 1997;17(1):163–165.

44. Baur M, Kienzer HR, Rath T, Dittrich C: Extravasation of oxaliplatin (eloxatin [R])—clinical course. Onkologie 2000;23(5):468–471.

45. Berghammer P, Pohnl R, Baur M, Dittrich C: Docetaxel extravasation. Support Care Cancer 2001;9(2):131–134.

46. Lokich J: Doxil extravasation injury: A case report. Ann Oncol 1999;10(6):735–736.

47. Fuller B, Lind M, Bonomi P: Mitomycin C extravasation exacerbated by sunlight. Ann Intern Med 1981;94:542.

48. Donaldson SS, Glick JM, Wilbur JR: Adriamycin activating a recall phenomenon after radiation therapy. Ann Intern Med 1974;81:407.

49. Vogelzang NJ: "Adriamycin flare": A skin reaction resembling extravasation. Cancer Treat Rep 1979;63:2067.

50. Bhawan J, Petry J, Rybak ME: Histologic changes induced in skin by extravasation of doxorubicin (Adriamycin). J Cutan Pathol 1989;16:158.

51. Tsavaris NB, Karagiaouris P, Tzannou I, et al: Conservative approach to the treatment of chemotherapy induced extravasation. Dermatol Surg Oncol 1990;16:519.

52. Rudolph R, Larson DL: Etiology and treatment of chemotherapeutic agent extravasation injuries: A review. J Clin Ocol 1987;5:1116.

53. Askar I, Erbas MK, Gurlek A: Effects of heparin fractions on the prevention of skin necrosis resulting from adriamycin extravasation: An experimental study. Ann Plast Surg 2002;49(3):297–301.

54. Yilmaz M, Demirdover C, Mola F: Treatment options in extravasation injury: An experimental study in rats. Plast Reconstr Surg 2002;109(7):2418–2423.

55. Dorr RI, Soble M, Alberts DS: Efficacy of sodium thiosulfate as a local antidote to mechlorethamine skin toxicity in the mouse. Cancer Chemother Pharmacol 1988;22:299.

56. Dorr RT, Soble M, Liddil JD, Keller JH: Mitomycin C skin toxicity studies in mice. Reduced ulceration and altered pharmacokinetics with topical dimethyl sulfoxide. J Clin Oncol 1986;4:1399.

57. Sommer NZ, Bayati S, Neumeister M, Brown RE: Dapsone for the treatment of doxorubicin extravasation injury in the rat. Plast Reconstr Surg 2002;109(6):2000–2005.

58. Loth TS, Eversmann WW Jr: Treatment methods for extravasations of chemotherapeutic agents: A comparative study. J Hand Surg 1986;11a:388.

59. Zuehlke RL: Erythematous eruption of the palms and soles associated with mitotane therapy. Dermatologica 1974;148:90.

60. Burgdorf WHC, Gilmore WA, Ganick RG: Peculiar acral erythema secondary to high dose chemotherapy for acute myelogenous leukemia. Ann Intern Med 1982;97:61.

61. Lokich JJ, Moore C: Chemotherapy-associated palmar plantar erythrodysesthesia syndrome. Ann Intern Med 1984;101:798.

62. Schey SA, Cooper J, Summerhays M: The "handfoot syndrome" occurring with chronic administration of etoposide. Eur J Haematol 1992;48:118.

63. Oksenhentler E. Landais P, Cordonnier C, et al: Erythema and systemic toxicity related to CHA induction therapy in acute myeloid leukemia. Eur J Cancer Clin Oncol 1989;25:1181.

64. Martins Da Chuna AC, Kappersberger K, Gardner H: Toxic skin reaction restricted to palms and soles after high-dose methotrexate. Pediatr Hematol Oncol 1991;8:277.

65. Pagliuca A, Kaczmarski R, Mufti GJ: Palmar-plantar erythema associated with combination chemotherapy. Postgrad Med J 1990;66:242.

66. Levine LE, Medenica MM, Lorincz AL, et al: Distinctive acral erythema occurring during therapy for severe myelogenous leukemia. Arch Dermatol 1985;121:102.

67. Cox GJ, Robertson DB: Toxic erythema of palms and soles associated with high-dose mercaptopurine chemotherapy. Arch Dermatol 1986;122:1413.

68. Neuss MN, Akwari OE, Stevenson DF: Painful palmar and plantar erythema associated with hepatic artery infusion of 5-fluoro-2'-deoxyuridine. J Natl Med Assoc 1987;76:669.

69. Silver FS, Espinoza LR, Hartman RC: Acral erythema and hydroxyurea. Ann Intern Med 1983;98:675.

70. Lokich JJ, Ahlgreen JD, Gullo JJ, et al: A prospective randomized comparison of continuous infusion fluorouracil with a conventional bolus schedule in metastatic colorectal carcinoma: A Mid-Atlantic Oncology Program Study. J Clin Oncol 1989;7:425.

71. Curran CF, Luce JK: Fluorouracil and palmar-plantar erythrodysesthesia. Ann Intern Med 1989;111:858.

72. Villalona-Calero MA, Blum JL, Jones SE, et al: A phase I and pharmacologic study of capecitabine and paclitaxel in breast cancer patients. Ann Oncol 2001;12:605–614.

73. Horwitz LJ, Dreizen S: Acral erythema induced by chemotherapy and graft-versus-host disease in adults with hematological malignancies. Cutis 1990;46:397.

74. Hui YF, Giles FJ, Cortes JE: Chemotherapy-induced palmar-plantar erythrodysesthesia syndrome—recall following different chemotherapy agents. Invest New Drugs 2002;20(1):49–53.

75. Crider K, Jansen J, Norins AL, et al: Chemotherapy induced acral erythema in patients receiving bone marrow transplantation. Arch Dermatol 1986;122:1023.

76. Fabian CJ, Molina R, Slavik M, et al: Pyridoxine therapy for palmar-plantar erythrodysesthesia associated with continuous 5-fluorouracil infusion. Invest New Drugs 1990;8:57.

77. Vukelja SJ, Lombardo FA, James WD, Weiss RB: Pyridoxine for the palmar-plantar erythrodysesthesia syndrome. Ann Intern Med 1989;111:688.

78. Lopez AM, Wallace L, Dorr RT, Koff M, Hersh EM, Alberts DS: Topical DMSO treatment for pegylated liposomal doxorubicin-induced palmar-plantar erythrodysesthesia. Cancer Chemother Pharmacol 1999;44(4):303–306.

79. Kyle RA, Schwartz RS, Oliner HL, et al: A syndrome resembling adrenal cortical insufficiency associated with long term busulfan (Myleran) therapy. Blood 1961;18:497.

80. Adrian RM, Hood AF, Skarin AT: Mucocutaneous reactions to antineoplastic agents. CA Cancer J Clin 1980;30:143.

81. Hrushevsky WJ: Unusual pigmentary changes associated with 5-fluorouracil therapy. Cutis 1980;26:181.

82. Van Scott EJ, Winters PL: Responses of mycosis fungoides to intensive external treatment with nitrogen mustard. Arch Dermatol 1970;102:507.

83. Kennedy BJ, Smith LR, Goltz RW: Skin changes secondary to hydroxyurea therapy. Arch Dermatol 1975;111:183.

84. Shah PC, Rao RKP, Patel AR: Cyclophosphamide-induced nail pigmentation. Br J Dermatol 1978;98:675.

85. Horn TD, Beveridge RA, Egorin MJ et al: Observations and proposed mechanism of N, N^1, N^{11}-triethylene thio-phosphormade (thiotepa)-induced hyperpigmentation. Arch Dermatol 1989;125:524.

86. Guillet G, Guillet MH: Cutaneous pigmented stripes and bleomycin treatment. Arch Dermatol 1986;122:381.

87. Rothberg H, Place CH, Steir O: Adriamycin (NS-123127) toxicity: Unusual melanotic reaction. Cancer Chemother Rep 1974;58:749.

88. Anderson LL, Thomas DE, Berger TG, et al: Cutaneous pigmentation after daunorubicin chemotherapy. J Am Acad Dermatol 1992;26:255.

89. Hrushevsky WJ: Serpentine supravenous 5-fluorouracil (NSC-19893) hyperpigmentation. Cancer Treat Rep 1976;60:639.

90. Rao SP, Potnis AV, Sobrinho TC, Brown AK: Pigmentation of the tongue after treatment with adriamycin. Cancer Treat Rep 1976;60:1402.

91. Bronner AK, Hood AF: Cutaneous complications of chemotherapeutic agents. J Am Acad Dermatol 1983;9:645.

92. Ettinger LJ, Freeman AL: The gingival platinum line: A new finding following cis-dichlorodiamine platinum (11) treatment. Cancer 1979;44:1882.

93. Morris D, Aisner J, Wiernik PH: Horizontal pigmented banding of the nails in association with adriamycin chemotherapy. Cancer Treat Rep 1977;61:499.

94. Demarinis M, Hendricks A, Stoltzner G: Nail pigmentation with daunorubicin therapy. Ann Intern Med 1978;89:516.

95. Levantine A, Almeyda J: Cutaneous reactions to cytostatic agents. Br J Dermatol 1978;98:675.

96. Vonnvouras S, Pakula AS, Shaw JM: Multiple pigmented nail bands during hydroxyurea therapy: An uncommon finding. J Am Acad Dermatol 1991;24:1015.

97. Wheeland RG, Burgdorf WHC, Humphrey GB: The flag sign of chemotherapy. Cancer 1983;51:1356.

98. Harrison BM, Wood CBS: Cyclophosphamide and pigmentation. BMJ 1972;1:352.

99. Kew MC, Mzamane D, Smith AG, et al: Melanocyte-stimulating hormone levels in doxorubicin-induced hyperpigmentation. Lancet 1977;1:811.

100. Harrold BP: Syndrome resembling Addison's disease following prolonged treatment with busulfan. BMJ 1966;1:462.

101. Frost P, DeVita VT: Pigmentation due to a new anti-tumor drug. Arch Dermatol 1966;94:265.

102. Solidoro A, Saenz R: Effects of cyclophosphamide (NSL-26271) on 127 patients with malignant lymphoma. Cancer Chemother Rep 1966;50:265.

103. Malacarne P, Zavagli G: Melphalan-induced melonychia striata. Arch Dermatol Res 1977;258:81.

104. Marcoux D, Anex R, Russo P: Persistent serpentine supraveous hyperpigmented eruption as an adverse reaction to chemotherapy combining actinomycin and vincristine. J Am Acad Dermatol 2000;43(3):540–546.

105. Blum RH, Carter SK, Agre K: A clinical review of bleomycin—a new antineoplastic agent. Cancer 1973;31:903.

106. Cohen IS, Mosher MB, O'Keefe EJ, et al: Cutaneous toxicity of bleomycin therapy. Arch Dermatol 1973;107:553.

107. Yagoda A, Mukerji B, Young C, et al: Bleomycin, an anti-tumor antibiotic: Clinical experience in 274 patients. Ann Intern Med 1972;77:861.

108. Shetty MR: Case of pigmented banding of the nail caused by bleomycin. Cancer Treat Rep 1977;61:501.

109. Coppes MJ, Jorgenson K, Arlette JP: Cutaneous toxicity following the administration of dactinomycin. Med Pediatr Oncol 1997;29:226–227.

110. Singal R, Tunnessen WW Jr, Wiley JM, Hood AF: Discrete pigmentation after chemotherapy. Pediatr Dermatol 1991;8:231–235.

111. Teresi ME, Murry DJ, Cornelius AS: Ifosfamide-induced hyperpigmentation. Cancer 1994;73(1):240–241.

112. Kennedy BJ: Metabolic and toxic effects of mithramycin during tumor therapy. Am J Med 1970;49:494.

113. Falkson G, Schulz EJ: Skin changes in patients treated with 5-fluorouracil. Br J Dermatol 1962;74:229.

114. Vukeljia SJ, Bonner MW, McCollough M, et al: Unusual serpentine hyperpigmentation associated with 5-fluorouracil: Case report and review of cutaneous manifestations associated with systemic 5-fluorouracil. J Am Acad Dermatol 1991;25:905.

115. Tsuji T, Sawabe M: Hyperpigmentation in striae distensae after bleomycin treatment. J Am Acad Dermatol 1993;28(3):503–505.

116. Reed WP, Morris DM: Maculopapular eruption resulting from systemic administration of 5-fluorouracil. Cutis 1984;33:381.

117. Perlin E, Ahlgren JD: Pigmentary effects from the protracted infusion of 5-fluorouracil. Int J Dermatol 1991;30:43.

118. Fitzpatrick JE, Hood AF: Histopathologic reactions to chemotherapeutic agents. Adv Dermatol 1988;3:161.

119. Singh M, Kaur S: Chemotherapy-induced multiple Beau's lines. Int J Dermatol 1986;25:590.

120. Shetty MR: White lines in the fingernails induced by combination chemotherapy. BMJ 1988;297:1635.

121. Katz ME, Hansen TW: Nail plate–nail bed separation: An unusual side effect of systemic fluorouracil administration. Arch Dermatol 1979;115:860.

122. Manalo FB, Marks A, Davis HL Jr: Doxorubicin toxicity: onycholysis, plantar callus formation, and peidermolysis. JAMA 1975;233:56.

123. Kennedy BJ, Theologides A: The role of 5-fluorouracil in malignant disease. Ann Intern Med 1961;55:719.

124. Sears ME: Erythema in areas of previous irradiation in patients treated with hydroxyurea. Cancer Chemother Rep 1964;40:31–32.

125. Young RC, Ozols RF, Meyers CE: The anthracycline antineoplastic drugs. N Engl J Med 1981; 305:139–153.

126. Jeter MD, Janne PA, Brooks S, et al: Gemcitabine-induced radiation recall. Int J Radiat Oncol Biol Phys 2002;53(2):394–400.

127. Kennedy RD, McAleer JJ: Radiation recall dermatitis in a patient treated with dacarbazine. Clin Oncol (R Coll Radiol) 2001;13(6): 470–472.

128. Morkas M, Fleming D, Hahl M: Challenges in oncology. Case 2. Radiation recall associated with docetaxel. J Clin Oncol 2002;20(3):867–869.

129. Thomas R, Stea B: Radiation recall dermatitis from high-dose interferon alfa-2b. J Clin Oncol 2002;20(1):355–357.

130. Chan RT, Au GK, Ho JW, Chu KW: Radiation recall with oxaliplatin: Report of a case and a review of the literature. Clin Oncol (R Coll Radiol) 2001;13(1):55–57.

131. Kharfan Dabaja MA, Morgensztern D, Markoe AM, Bartlett-Pandite L: Radiation recall dermatitis induced by methotrexate in a patient with Hodgkin's disease. Am J Clin Oncol 2001;24(2):211–213.

132. Yeo W, Johnson PJ: Radiation-recall skin disorders associated with the use of antineoplastic drugs. Am J Clin Dermatol 2000;1(2): 113–116.

133. Donaldson SS, Glick JM, Wilbur JR: Adriamycin activating a recall phenomenon after radiation therapy. Ann Intern Med 1974; 81:407–408.

134. Seymour CB, Mothersill C, Alper T: High yields of lethal mutations somatic mammalian cells that survive ionizing radiation. Int J Radiat Biol 1986;50:167.

135. Nemechek PM, Corder MC: Radiation recall associated with vinblastine in a patient treated for Kaposi sarcoma related to acquired immune deficiency syndrome. Cancer 1992;70(6):1605.

136. Wiatrak BJ, Myer CM: Radiation recall supraglottitis in a child. Am J Otolaryngol 1991;12:227.

137. Yarbro JW: Dermotoxicity. In Perry MC (ed): Toxicity of Chemotherapy. Orlando, Fla, Grune & Stratton, 1984.

138. Del Guidice SM, Gerstley JK: Sunlight-induced radiation recall. Int J Dermatol 1998;27:415.

139. Robinson BW, Shewach DS: Radiosensitization by gemcitabine in p53 wild-type and mutant MCF-7 breast carcinoma cell lines. Clin Cancer Res 2001;7(8):2581–2589.

140. Ryu S, Stein JP, Chung CT, et al: Enhanced apoptosis and radiosensitization by combined 13-cis-retinoic acid and interferon-alpha2a; role of RAR-beta gene. Int J Radiat Oncol Biol Phys 2001;51(3):785–790.

141. Amorino GP, Hamilton VM, Choy H: Enhancement of radiation effects by combined docetaxel and carboplatin treatment in vitro. Radiat Oncol Investig 1999;7(6):343–352.

142. Riggs CE, Bennett JP: Clinical pharmacology of individual antineoplastic agents. In Moossa AR, Schimpff SC, Robson MC (eds): Comprehensive Textbook of Oncology, vol 1. Baltimore, Williams & Wilkins, 1991, p 537.

143. Landren RC, Hussey DH, Barkley HT Jr, Samuels ML: Split-course irradiation plus hydroxyurea in inoperable bronchogenic carcinoma—a randomized study of 53 patients. Cancer 1974;34:1598.

144. DeSpain JD: Dermatologic toxicity. In Perry MC (ed): The Chemotherapy Source Book. Baltimore, Williams & Wilkins, 1992, p 531.

145. Moller H: Cytostatic drugs and inflammation. Lancet 1970;2:427.

146. Dunagin WG: Clinical toxicity of chemotherapeutic agents: Dermatologic toxicity. Semin Oncol 1982;9:139.

147. Pauluzzi P, Kokelj F, Perkan V, Pozzato G, Moretti M: Psoriasis exacerbation induced by interferon-alpha. Report of two cases. Acta Derm Venereol 1993;73(5):395.

148. Livden JK, Nilsen R, Bjerke JR, Matre R: In situ localization of interferons in psoriatic lesions. Arch Dermatol Res 1989;281(6):392–397.

149. Maguire HC Jr, Ettore VL: Enhancement of dinitrochlorobenzene (DNCB) contact sensitization by cyclophosphamide in the guinea pig. J Invest Dermatol 1967;48:39.

150. Burrows D, Bridges JM, Morris TCM: Reactivation of scabies rash by methotrexate. Br J Dermatol 1975;93:219.

151. Dudley K, Micetich K, Massa MC: Erythema with features of seborrheic dermatitis and lupus erythematosus associated with systemic 5-fluorouracil. Cutis 1987;39:64.

152. Dillaha CJ, Jansen GT, Honeycutt WM, Bradford AC: Selective cytotoxic effect of topical 5-fluorouracil. Arch Dermatol 1983;119(9):774–783.

153. Marini M, Wright D, Ropolo M, Abbruzzese M, Casas G: Neutrophilic eccrine hidradenitis secondary to topotecan. J Dermatolog Treat 2002;13(1):35–37.

154. Flynn TC, Harrist TJ, Murphy G, et al: Neutrophilic eccrine hidradenitis: A distinctive rash associated with cytarabine therapy and acute leukemia. J Am Acad Dermatol 1984;11:584.

155. Harrist TJ, Fine JD, Berman R, et al: Neutrophilic eccrine hidradenitis. Arch Dermatol 1982;118:263.

156. Bardenstein DS, Haluschak J, Gerson S, et al: Neutrophilic eccrine hidradenitis simulating orbital cellulites. Arch Ophthalmol 194;112:1460.

157. Aractingi S, Mallet V, Pinquier L, et al: Neutrophilic dermatoses during granulocytopenia. Arch Dermatol 1995;131:1141.

158. Scallan PJ, Kettler AH, Levy ML, et al: Neutrophilic eccrine hidradenitis. Evidence implicating bleomycin as a causative agent. Cancer 1988;62(12):2532.

159. Fitzpatrick JE, Bennion SD, Reed OM, et al: Neutrophilic eccrine hidradenitis associated with induction chemotherapy. J Cutan Pathol 1987;14:272.

160. Combemale P, Faisant M, Azoulay-Petit C, Dupin M, Kanitakis J: Neutrophilic eccrine hidradenitis secondary to infection with Serratia marcescens. Br J Dermatol 2000;142(4):784–788.

161. Krischer J, Rutschmann O, Roten SV, Harms M, Saurat JH, Pechere M: Neutrophil eccrine hidradenitis in a patient with AIDS. J Dermatol 1998;25(3):199–200.

162. Brehler R, Reimann S, Bonsmann G, Metze D: Neutrophilic hidradenitis induced by chemotherapy involves eccrine and apocrine glands. Am J Dermatopathol 1997;19(1):73–78.

163. Osttere LS, Wells J, Stevens HP, et al: Neutrophilic eccrine hidradenitis with an unusual presentation. Br J Dermatol 1993;128:696.

164. Shear NH, Knowles SR, Shapiro L, et al: Dapsone in prevention of recurrent neutrophilic eccrine hidradenitis. J Am Acad Dermatol 1996;35:819–822.

165. Bhawan J, Malhotra R: Syringosqumaous metaplasia: A distinctive eruption in patients receiving chemotherapy. Am J Dermatopathol 1990;12;1.

166. Karam A, Metges JP, Labat JP, et al: Squamous syringometaplasia associated with docetaxel. Br J Dermatol 2002;146(3):524–525.

167. Koppel RA, Boh EE: Cutaneous reactions to chemotherapeutic agents. Am J Med Sci 2001;321(5):327–335.

168. Wong P, Bangert JL, Levin N: A papulovesicular eruption in a man receiving chemotherapy for metastatic melanoma. Arch Dermatol 1993;129:233.

169. Valks R, Fraga J, Porras-Luque J, et al: Chemotherapy-induced eccrine squamous syringometaplasia. A distinctive eruption in patients receiving hematopoietic progenitor cells. Arch Dermatol 1997;133(7):873–878.

170. Kerr LD, Spiera H: Scleroderma in association with the use of bleomycin: A report of 3 cases. J Rheumatol 1992;19:294.

171. Luna MA, Bedrossan CWM, Lichtiger B, Salem PA: Interstitial pneumonitis associated with bleomycin therapy. Am J Clin Pathol 1972;58:501.

172. Denholm EM, Phan SH: the effects of bleomycin on alveolar macrophage growth factor secretion. Am J Pathol 1989;134: 355–363.

173. Clark JC, Starcher BC, Uitto J: Bleomycin-induced synthesis of type I procollagen by human lung skin fibroblasts in culture. Biochem Biophys Acta 1980;631:359–370.

174. Yamamoto T, Eckes B, Krieg T: Bleomycin increases steady-state levels of type I collagen, fibronectin and decorin gene expression in human skin fibroblasts. Arch Dermatol Res 2001;292:556–561.

Problems Common to Cancer and Its Therapy

175. Yamamoto T, Takagawa S, Katayama I, et al: Effect of superoxide dismutase on bleomycin-induced dermal sclerosis: Implications for the treatment of systemic sclerosis. J Invest Dermatol 1999;113(5):843–847.

176. Steen VD: Treatment of systemic sclerosis. Am J Clin Dermatol 2001;2(5):315–325.

177. Levine SM, Anzueto A, Peters JI, et al: Single lung transplantation in patients with systemic disease. Chest 1994;105(3):837–841.

178. Hamada I, Kato M, Okada K: Multi-cytokine therapy for advanced renal cell carcinoma: Determination of the minimal effective dose. Anticancer Res 2002;22(4):2429–2436.

179. Apisarnthanarax N, Talpur R, Duvic M: Treatment of cutaneous T cell lymphoma: Current status and future directions. Am J Clin Dermatol 2002;3(3):193–215.

180. Skubitz KM, Anderson PM: Inhalational interleukin-2 liposomes for pulmonary metastases: A phase I clinical trial. Anticancer Drugs 2000;11(7):555–563.

181. Farag SS, George SL, Lee EJ, et al: Postremission therapy with low-dose interleukin 2 with or without intermediate pulse dose interleukin 2 therapy is well tolerated in elderly patients with acute myeloid leukemia: Cancer and Leukemia Group B study 9420. Clin Cancer Res 2002;8(9):2812–2819.

182. Sobol RE, Shawler DL, Carson C, et al: Interleukin 2 gene therapy of colorectal carcinoma with autologous irradiated tumor cells and genetically engineered fibroblasts: A Phase I study. Clin Cancer Res 1999;5(9):2359–2365.

183. Mittleman A, Huberman M, Puccio C, et al: A phase I study of recombinant human interleukin-2 and alpha-interferon-2a in patients with renal cell cancer, colorectal cancer, and malignant melanoma. Cancer 1990;66:664.

184. Rosenberg SA, Mule JJ, Spiess PJ, et al: Regression of established pulmonary metastases and subcutaneous tumor mediated by the systemic administration of high-dose recombinant interleukin-2. J Exp Med 1985;161:1169.

185. Schwartzentruber DJ: Guidelines for the safe administration of high-dose interleukin-2. J Immunother 2001;24(4):287–293.

186. Allison MK, Jones SE, McGuffy P: Phase II trial of outpatient interleukin-2 in malignant lymphoma, chronic lymphocytic leukemia, and selected solid tumors. J Clin Oncol 1989;7:75.

187. Ozsahin H, Fluss J, McLin V, Wacker P, Miralbell R, Helg C: Rituximab with interleukin-2 after autologous bone marrow transplantation for acute lymphocytic leukemia in second remission. Med Pediatr Oncol 2002;38(4):300–301.

188. Hauschild A, Garbe C, Stolz W, et al: Dacarbazine and interferon alpha with or without interleukin 2 in metastatic melanoma: A randomized phase III multicentre trial of the Dermatologic Cooperative Oncology Group (DeCOG). Br J Cancer 2001;84(8):1036–1042.

189. Apisarnthanarax N, Talpur R, Duvic M: Treatment of cutaneous T cell lymphoma: Current status and future directions. Am J Clin Dermatol 2002;3(3):193–215.

190. Staunton MR, Scully MC, LeBoit PE, Aronson FR: Life-threatening bullous skin eruptions during interleukin-2 therapy. J Natl Cancer Inst 191;83:56.

191. Gaspari AA, Lotze MT, Rosenberg SA, et al: Dermatologic changes associated with interleukin-2 adminstration. JAMA 1987;258:1624.

192. Locker GJ, Kofler J, Stoiser B, et al: Relation of pro- and anti-inflammatory cytokines and the produciton of nitric oxide in patients receiving high-dose immunotherapy with interleukin-2. Eur Cytokine Netw 2000;11(3):391–396.

193. Lentsch AB, Miller FN, Edwards MJ: Mechanisms of leukocyte-mediated tissue injury induced by interleukin-2. Cancer Immunol Immunother 1999;47(5):243–248.

194. Rafi AQ, Zeytun A, Bradley MJ, et al: Evidence for the involvement of Fas ligand and perforin in the induction of vascular leak syndrome. J Immunol 1998;161(6):3077–3086.

195. Baluna R, Rizo J, Gordon BE, Ghetie V, Vitetta ES: Evidence for a structural motif in toxins and interleukin-2 that may be responsible for binding to endothelial cells and initiating vascular leak syndrome. Proc Natl Acad Sci USA 1999;96(7):3957–3962.

196. Rafi-Janajreh AQ, Chen D, Schmits R, et al: Evidence for the involvement of CD44 in endothelial cell injury and induction of vascular leak syndrome by IL-2. J Immunol 199;163(3):1619–1627.

197. Baluna R, Vitetta ES: Vascular leak syndrome: A side effect of immunotherapy. Immunopharmacology 1997;37(2–3):117–132.

198. Weiner JS, Tucker JA Jr, Wlather PJ: Interleukin-2 induced dermatotoxicity resembling toxic epidermal necrolysis. South Med J 1992;85:656.

199. Richards JM, Mehta N, Ramming K, Skosey P: Sequential chemoimmunotherapy in the therapy of metastatic melanoma. J Clin Oncol 1992;10:1338.

200. Rosenberg S, White D: Vitiligo in patients with melanoma: Normal tissue antigens can be targets for cancer immunotherapy. J Immunother Tumor Immunol 1996;19:81–84.

201. Vetto JT, Papa MZ, Lotze MT, et al: Reduction of toxicity of IL-2 and lymphokine activated killer cells in humans by the administration of corticosteroid. J Clin Oncol 1987;5:496.

202. Buzaid AC, Atkins M: Practical guidelines for the management of biochemotherapy-related toxicity in melanoma. Clin Canc Res 2001;7:2611–2619.

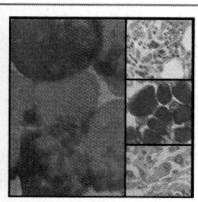

41

LYMPHEDEMA

Lance Everett Wyatt

Julian Joseph Pribaz

SUMMARY OF KEY POINTS

DEFINITION
- Lymphedema is the accumulation of protein-rich interstitial fluid within the skin and subcutaneous tissue.

ETIOLOGY AND CLASSIFICATION
- Primary lymphedema is thought to be a genetically determined disease with expression at or shortly after birth (*Milroy disease*), puberty (*lymphedema praecox*), or after 35 years of age (*lymphedema tarda*).
- Secondary lymphedema occurs as a result of a precipitating cause.

INCIDENCE
- The incidence of lymphedema is not known.
- The most common cause of secondary lymphedema worldwide is lymphatic filariasis.
- In Western countries, the most common cause is damage to or removal of lymph nodes by surgery, radiotherapy, tumor invasion, or the result of infection or inflammation.

DIAGNOSIS
- Diagnosis can be made in the majority of cases by history and physical examination; lymphoscintigraphy, computed tomography, and magnetic resonance imaging may occasionally be needed.
- Soft, pitting edema generally begins distally and progresses proximally over months to years.

GOALS OF TREATMENT
- There is no cure for lymphedema.
- Goals of therapy are to (1) reduce fluid production and accumulation; (2) reduce associated complications; and (3) improve limb function and appearance.

MEDICAL TREATMENT
- Skin care, extremity elevation, compressive garments, pneumatic compression pumps, noninvasive complex lymphedema therapy, and treatment of infection are the mainstays of medical therapy.

SURGICAL TREATMENT
- Surgery is a continuum of medical management and is performed for failure of medical management, gross extremity size and weight with impaired extremity function, severe skin changes, and recurrent lymphangitis (more than three episodes per year).
- Physiologic procedures attempt to restore lymphatic drainage.
- Excisional procedures remove lymph-producing as well as fibrosclerotic tissue and fat.

INTRODUCTION

Lymphedema is the accumulation of protein-rich interstitial fluid within the skin and subcutaneous tissue. Cases in which the etiology is unknown or which develop as a result of congenital lymphatic dysfunction are referred to as *primary lymphedema*. All forms of lymphedema that occur as a result of a precipitating cause are termed *secondary lymphedema*. No cure exists for lymphedema, so the aims of therapy are to reduce fluid production and accumulation, to reduce associated complications, and to improve limb function and appearance.

ETIOLOGY AND CLASSIFICATION

Liquid, macromolecules, and migrating cells traverse blood capillary endothelia, enter tissues, and are gradually absorbed into the lymphatic system. Lymph is transported by lymphatic capillaries (which are one cell thick without valves and located in interstitial tissues) into secondary lymphatics (few valves) and then into larger collecting vessels with multiple valves, which give them a beaded appearance. Lymph then traverses through lymph nodes and returns to the venous circulation via the thoracic duct. The lymphatic system is an open-ended, one-way, low-flow, low-pressure system in close contact with the extracellular matrix. Large lymphatic vessels have smooth muscle with intrinsic contractility, which serves as a critical pumping force that, in concert with skeletal muscle contraction, arterial pulsation compression, and negative intrathoracic pressure, transports lymph centrally toward the venous system. Lymphatic vessels form part of the immune system by transporting white blood cells within lymphoid organs (tonsils, thymus, spleen, Peyer's patches, and lymph nodes).

The most commonly used classification categorizes the etiology of lymphedema as *primary* or *secondary* to some inciting event. Primary lymphedema, which is thought to be due to aplasia or hypoplasia of the lymphatics, has long been thought to be a genetically determined disease with expression at or shortly after birth (*Milroy's disease*), puberty (*lymphedema praecox*), or after 35 years of age (*lymphedema tarda*). The time of onset may be related to the relative number of functioning lymphatics. It is generally thought that the fewer lymphatics, the earlier the onset. The molecular basis for congenital primary lymphedema (Milroy's disease) has been established as autosomal dominant with incomplete penetrance due to a mutation in the gene locus encoding for VEGFR3.[1,2] This condition may be diagnosed prenatally.[3]

Lymphedema praecox, the most common form of primary lymphedema, is responsible for as many as 94% of cases in large reported series. The uncertainties of this condition derive from its unusual, unexplained features: female predominance (ratio of females to males is estimated to be 10:1), development around the time of menarche, more common involvement of the left leg, and rare upper extremity involvement). Some have implicated the involvement of estrogenic hormones.[4] The edema typically is limited to the foot and calf. Lymphedema tarda, which develops later in life, accounts for fewer than 10% of cases of primary lymphedema. The precipitating cause often follows minor trauma or an inflammatory process (e.g., cellulitis) that can damage and possibly obstruct an already reduced number of lymphatics, tipping the balance in favor of lymphedema.

The most common cause of secondary lymphedema worldwide is lymphatic filariasis. In its most obvious manifestations, lymphatic filariasis, also known as elephantiasis, causes edema of the entire arm or leg; the genital regions (vulva, scrotum, breasts) also may be involved. Lymphatic filariasis is a significant cause of poverty in more than 80 countries in which it is endemic, primarily in Asia, Africa, the Western Pacific, and the Americas. Approximately 90% of these infections are caused by *Wuchereria bancrofti*, with most of the remainder by *Brugia malayi* and *B. timori*. The major vectors for *W. bancrofti* are *Culex*, *Aedes* species, and *Anopheles* mosquitoes. The World Health Organization estimates that at least 120 million people are infected, with approximately 40 million disabled as a result of this condition.

In Western countries, damage or removal of lymph nodes by surgery, radiotherapy, tumor invasion, or the result of infection or inflammation are the most common causes of secondary lymphedema. Upper extremity edema after axillary lymph node dissection is likely the most common cause of lymphedema in the United States.[5] The incidence of lymphedema of the arm after mastectomy ranges between 8% and 38%, depending on whether axillary lymph nodes are removed and whether radiation is used.[6] This number also varies because there is no standard definition of edema. Lymphedema of the lower extremity may occur after inguinal and pelvic lymph node dissection or irradiation, with a published frequency of 1% to 47%.[7,8]

Why do the vast majority of patients after surgery, regional node dissection, malignancy, radiotherapy, trauma, inflammation, and infection *not* develop lymphedema? The capacity for compensation by collateral flow and regeneration of damaged lymphatics may explain whether lymphedema develops. It is interesting to note that disrupted lymphatics are not reconnected during replantation or microsurgical free tissue transfer. Although temporary swelling of a replanted or transplanted part develops, the condition resolves without intervention. Radiocolloid lymphoscintigraphy with technetium-99m-antimony trisulfide colloid (Sb_2S_3) studies in patients without lymphedema have demonstrated spontaneous regeneration or reconnection of lymphatics after free tissue transfer.[9] These findings suggest that patients with this disease lack compensatory mechanisms necessary to prevent the development of lymphedema.

Lymphedema may be classified as either genetic or syndromic. Turner's syndrome, Noonan's syndrome, and Hennekam syndrome are examples of syndromic lymphedema. Lymphedema-distichiasis syndrome, cholestasis-lymphedema syndrome, all forms of primary, and most forms of secondary lymphedema may be classified as genetic lymphedema. Patients who manifest the disease at or shortly after birth may have a more severe form of lymphedema without sufficient compensatory mechanisms. The mildest forms of the condition may exist as a subclinical process with expression only after an inciting event.

PATHOPHYSIOLOGY

Lymphedema is confined to the subcutaneous compartment; the deep muscle regions appear to be clinically uninvolved. Extravasation of protein-rich fluid occurs when lymphatic transport capacity is reduced because of reduced numbers of functioning lymphatics or increased lymphatic load. This high-protein edema causes a shift in Starling's equilibrium, resulting in the accumulation of more fluid. In time, low oxygen tension, decreased macrophage function, and the presence of increasing amounts of protein-rich fluid give rise to a chronic inflammatory state and gradual tissue fibrosis. In chronic lymphedema, a hypertrophy of adipose tissue also occurs, but the mechanism for this has not been elucidated. The high-protein edema serves as a medium for bacteria, and episodes of infection so characteristic of the condition lead to additional lymphatic sclerosis and further lymphatic transport dysfunction (Table 41-1).

DIAGNOSIS

In the vast majority of patients, diagnosis can be made by history and physical examination. Edema generally begins distally and progresses proximally over months to years. Early in the course of lymphedema, the accumulation of protein-rich interstitial fluid results in a soft, pitting edema. With time, the chronic inflammatory state and accumulation of fat and gradual tissue fibrosis gives rise to a nonpitting edema. Skin changes may occur, but ulceration is infrequent. Patients may complain of fatigue or pressure in the extremity, but the complaint of pain should prompt the physician to search for an alternative cause. Lymphoscintigraphy with radiocolloids has been successful in delineating the anatomy of lymph vessels and in evaluating the dynamics of lymph flow. This technique has replaced lymphangiography, which may damage lymphatics and worsen lymphedema.[10] Lymphangiography is not recommended. Computed tomography and magnetic resonance imaging are useful to rule out malignancy.

TABLE 41-1

Pathophysiology of Lymphedema

- Reduced number of lymphatics below critical level
  Congenital lymphedema
  Surgical ablation
  Scar, radiation, infection
- Increased lymphatic load
  High-protein edema
  Increased osmotic pressure
  Inflammation
  Perilymphatic scarring
  Increased fatty deposition
- Progressive deterioration
  Increased volume
  Induration
  Fibrosis

The extent and degree of fibrosis correlates with the difficulty encountered with conservative management. Recurrent lymphangitis occurs as a result of lymph stasis, and stagnant lymph serves as a medium for bacteria. Lymph stasis, inflammation, fibrosis, and intermittent bouts of infection conspire to cause further destruction of remaining lymphatics, whose function is eventually compromised by fibrosclerotic changes. Edema from cardiac, renal, or hepatic insufficiency is distinguished from lymphedema by history and examination. Chronic venous insufficiency and postphlebitic syndrome are associated with aching discomfort and chronic pruritus.[11] Physical examination reveals hemosiderin deposits in the skin, dusky discoloration and venous engorgement with dependence, varicosities, and ulceration in advanced cases.

Myxedema of thyroid disease may be confused with lymphedema and develops when abnormal mucinous substances accumulate in the skin. Patients with myxedema present with roughening of the skin of the palms, soles, elbows, and knees. These patients also may have diminished sweat production, yellow-orange discoloration of the skin, thinning hair, and uneven nails. The process may be localized to the pretibial region in thyrotoxicosis[12] but is more generalized in hypothyroidism.

Lipedema is caused by the abnormal accumulation of fatty substances in the subcutaneous regions, typically between the pelvis and the ankle. The feet are spared, and the swelling is symmetric, bilateral, and often painful. The condition affects women or men with a feminizing disorder and arises within 1 to 2 years after the onset of puberty. Patients often have a propensity to bruising, possibly as a result of increased fragility of capillaries within the adipose tissue. Skin changes characteristic of lymphedema are not present, and consistent fat pads anterior to the lateral malleoli are found in patients with lipedema.[13]

In the United States, a frequent cause of lymphedema of both the upper and lower extremities is neoplastic disease. *Patients previously treated for neoplastic disease who develop new or worsening lymphedema must be*
evaluated for the recurrence of cancer. Malignant lymphedema often develops rapidly and results in intrinsic or extrinsic obstruction of lymph flow. Pain, generally absent in lymphedema, may be present[14] (Fig. 41-1).

Lymphangiosarcoma is an extremely rare tumor that initially appears as multiple blue-red subcutaneous nodules. In the upper extremity, it most frequently occurs in cases of chronic lymphedema after mastectomy (described by Stewart and Treves in 1948 and known as Stewart-Treves syndrome[15]). Lymphangiosarcoma seldom occurs in the lower extremity but may develop in the presence of lymphatic filariasis. The usual interval between mastectomy and the appearance of lymphedema is approximately 1 year; lymphangiosarcoma develops approximately 5 to 9 years after mastectomy. The reported incidence varies from between 0.07% and 0.45%.[16] Immunologic and electron microscopic studies suggest that these tumors arise from vascular endotheliocytes, despite the clinical appearance of arising from lymphatic vessels.

Why lymphangiosarcoma has a predilection for lymphedematous tissue is unknown. It has been shown that these tumors grow more consistently in lymphedematous as opposed to non–lymph-rich tissue. Some have speculated that the presence of a local immune deficiency creates a climate for malignant degeneration. Lymphangiosarcomas develop multicentrically and spread rapidly. These are extremely aggressive, highly malignant tumors; limb-sparing procedures are not recommended.

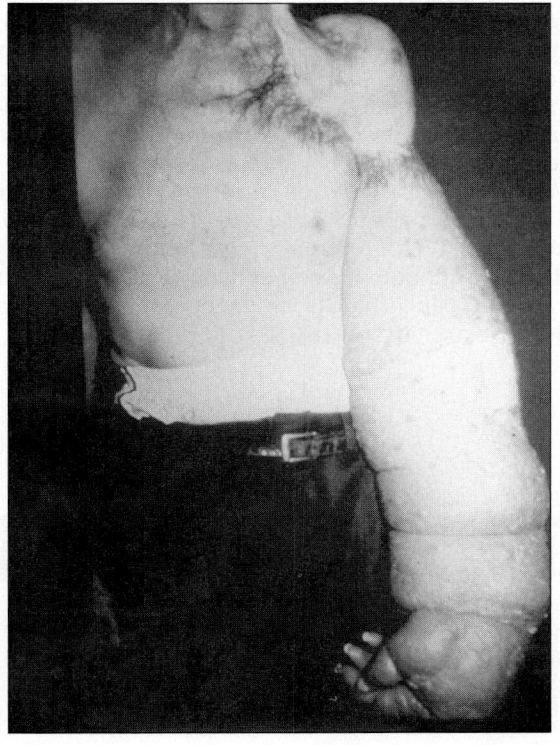

Figure 41-1. A 59-year-old man with gross end-stage obstructive lymphedema after recurrent squamous cell cancer excision and irradiation. The limb was functionless and was treated with amputation.

Amputation is the only hope for survival. Prognosis for patients with lymphangiosarcoma is extremely poor, with 5-year survival reported in between 8.5% and 13.6% despite aggressive treatment.[16]

MEDICAL MANAGEMENT

The aim of all forms of management is to restore the balance between the lymphatic load and the lymphatic transport capacity. A variety of available therapies may alter the course of disease. However, no treatment option is completely and permanently curative. The patient must understand the chronicity of the condition as well as the patient's important role in controlling the edema and preventing complications.

Limb girth should be assessed at the initial visit and at regular intervals thereafter to provide an accurate determination of the effect of therapy. Various methods allow assessment of limb volume, and all are prone to error in reproducibility. Measuring tapes may be used, and circumferential measurements should be obtained from standard, regional landmarks (antecubital fossa, etc.) (Table 41-2). The physician should recognize that measurements taken at various times of the day may yield different results; the girth of an extremity may increase throughout the day, as it is in a dependent position and subjected to the effects of gravity. Measurements of water volume displacement are more precise, but do not identify changes in a specific area of the limb (Fig. 41-2). Another useful modality to measure is the degree of limb tissue turgor; the degree of hardness or softness can be measured by an especially designed tonometer.[17] (Fig. 41-3). Patients should be serially followed up by physical examination, with any combination of the following: circumferential measurements, volume displacement, tonometry, serial photography, lymphoscintigraphy, and patient survey.

Weight reduction and extremity elevation are important measures that decrease edema. The patient must elevate the affected extremity at night. A sling may be used for the upper extremity, and elevating the foot of the bed on 4- to 6-inch blocks is recommended for edema of the lower extremity.

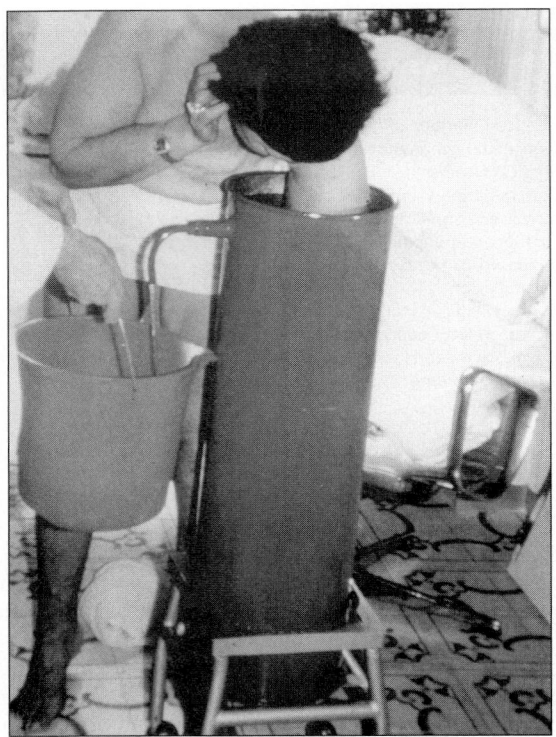

Figure 41-2. Tonometry measurement of the upper limb.

Custom-fitted elastic compressive garments (sleeves or stockings) are often worn during the day to maintain limb volume. The length of the garment should match the extent of disease. A comfortable fit is essential to ensure patient compliance.

Intermittent pneumatic compression with multi-chamber pumps removes excess fluid from the involved limb and may be helpful if used early in the course of disease, before the development of fibrosclerotic tissue changes. These devices apply a sequential pattern of compression to the extremity, permitting a physiologic

TABLE 41-2

Measurement of Lymphedema
• Linear: Girth   Hand (foot)   Wrist (ankle)   15 cm below elbow (knee)   Elbow (knee)   15 cm above elbow (knee)   • Volume   Water tank: volume displacement   • Tonometry

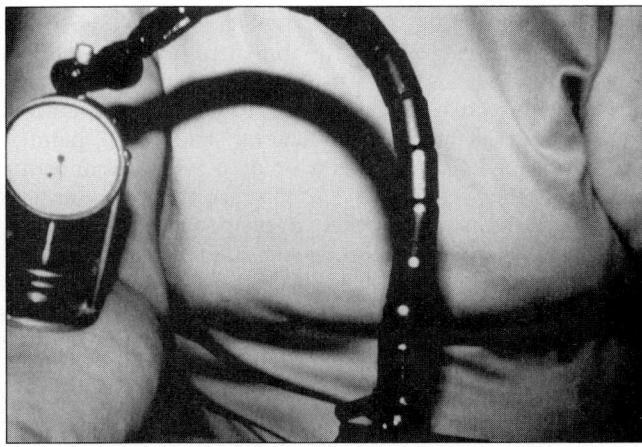

Figure 41-3. Volume measurement of the upper limb.

distal-to-proximal milking action of the lymphedematous limb.[18] Therapy is most effective if continued at regular intervals, and compressive garments should be worn between treatments. Cardiac failure, active infection, and deep venous thrombosis are contraindications to pump therapy.

Noninvasive complex lymphedema therapy (CLT), which consists of manual lymph drainage, compressive bandaging, and physical therapy exercises, may be used with promising results.[19] Complex lymphedema therapy facilitates lymph drainage by recruiting collateral vessels so that the lymphedematous area can be drained into normally functioning lymphatic systems. Recent series have demonstrated therapeutic responses in compliant patients.[20,21]

Basic skin care is essential in the prevention of infection and may assist in preventing associated skin changes, including dermatitis, hyperkeratosis, warty verrucosis, as well as breakdown of the epidermis and leakage of lymph fluid (lymphorrhea). Meticulous foot care for patients with lower extremity lymphedema with daily use of a low-pH, water-based lotion will help to prevent fungal infections of the web spaces. Topical antifungal therapy is recommended for localized fungal infections, but invasive infection may require systemic antifungal therapy.

Aggressive and prompt treatment of lymphangitis and cellulitis is recommended to prevent the development of sepsis. It is thought that each bout of sepsis causes further sclerosis of existing lymphatics. Systemic antibiotic therapy targeted toward staphylococcal and streptococcal species for 5 to 7 days, combined with bed rest and extremity elevation, is suggested. Approximately 15% to 25% of patients will have recurrent lymphangitis and cellulitis and these patients may require long-term prophylactic antibiotic therapy.

Benzopyrones have been advocated in the treatment of lymphedema.[22] 5,6-Benzo-α-pyrone (coumarin) is thought to have a stimulatory effect on macrophages and other elements of the immune system, enhancing proteolysis breaking down large complex tissue proteins into peptides, which can be absorbed by the venous system. Efficacy has been demonstrated in primary lymphedema as well as in lymphedema secondary to lymphatic filariasis.[23] These compounds are slow acting and used in mild cases of lymphedema; furthermore, orally administered coumarin may cause idiosyncratic hepatitis. Preliminary evidence suggests a possible role for dietary flavenoids[24] and dietary restriction of long-chain triglycerides[25]; more research is needed the better to clarify the efficacy of these therapeutic and dietary strategies.

Parasitic infections involving *W. bancrofti*, *B. malayi*, and *B. timori* are initially treated with albendazole and ivermectin or albendazole with diethylcarbamazine. Antihistamine and/or anti-inflammatory agents are used to control the allergic reactions to the dying parasite.

Laser therapy,[26] hyperthermia,[27] and intra-arterial injection of lymphocytes[28] are investigational treatments purported to play a role in the management of lymphedema. Further evidence is needed to clarify better the role of these modalities in the management of lymphedema (Table 41-3).

TABLE 41-3

Lymphedema: Medical Therapy

Meticulous skin care
Weight reduction
Limb elevation
Exercise
Custom-fitted elastic compressive garments
Pneumatic compressive pump
Noninvasive complex lymphedema therapy (CLT)
Treatment of infection

Diuretics (optional)
Heat (investigational)
Benzopyrones (investigational)
Dietary flavenoids (investigational)
Intra-arterial injection of lymphocytes (investigational)

SURGICAL MANAGEMENT

Numerous surgical procedures have been described for the treatment of lymphedema. None is curative, and quantitative, long-term data on outcome are sparse. Patients must view surgery as a continuum of management, and the physician must emphasize that surgery does not obviate the need for continued medical therapy.

It is estimated that approximately 10% of patients with lymphedema will need surgery.[29] Operative intervention has traditionally been recommended if medical therapy is ineffective in controlling lymphedema or preventing complications. Surgery also is recommended for impaired extremity function secondary to gross extremity size and weight, severe skin changes, and recurrent lymphangitis (more than three episodes per year) (Table 41-4).

All procedures aim to reduce lymph fluid accumulation, halt the progression of disease, improve limb function, reduce bulk and appearance, and facilitate conservative therapy. Physiologic procedures attempt to re-establish lymphatic drainage, whereas excisional procedures debulk the limb, removing both fibrosclerotic and normal, lymph-producing tissue and fat. This distinction is blurred, as many physiologically designed operations have excisional components; moreover, excisional procedures have an apparent physiological effect.[30] Combinations of excisional and physiological procedures also are commonly used to maximize the improvement in lymphedema (Table 41-5).

TABLE 41-4

Lymphedema: Surgical Indications

Failure of medical management
Excessive extremity size and weight, with functional impairment
Severe skin changes
Recurrent infection (more than three episodes of cellulitis or
    lymphangitis per year)

TABLE 41-5

Surgical Therapy

Physiologic

Lymphangioplasty
Omental transposition
Enteromesenteric bridge

Lymphaticovenous anastomoses
Lympholymphatic anastomoses

Excisional

Total skin and subcutaenous excision ("Charles procedure")
Buried dermal flap ("Thompson procedure")
Staged subcutaneous excision beneath flaps ("modified Homans' procedure")
Suction-assisted lipectomy

Physiologic Procedures

Physiologic procedures include lymphangioplasty,[29-36] pedicle flap procedures (omental transposition, entero-mesenteric bridge),[37-40] and microsurgical anastomosis (lymph nodal–venous, lymphaticovenous, lympholymphatic shunts).[41-48] Again, combinations of these techniques have proven to be helpful in reducing limb size.

Lymphatic Bridging

One of the earliest procedures for lymphedema was the subcutaneous implantation of silk threads (lymphangioplasty) advocated by Handley in 1908.[31] Many materials (rubber,[32] polythene,[33] polyvinylchloride[34]) have subsequently been used in the attempt to create drainage channels. This technique was abandoned because of the consistently high incidence of infection and extrusion of material.

Pedicle-flap procedures juxtapose lymphatic-rich flaps and lymphedematous tissue to induce lymphatic communication and provide drainage. Initially, tube pedicles with a random blood supply were fashioned in multiple stages by Gillies and Fraser[49] and Mowlem.[50] These resulted in considerable scarring and poor function. Clodius and colleagues[51] found that skin flaps with an axial blood supply also contained axial lymphatics and allowed spontaneous lymphatic connections. He reported using these flaps to improve brachial neuritis and upper extremity lymphedema simultaneously (Fig. 41-4). To date, as well as skin flaps, omentum and small bowel have been used as pedicle flaps. These operations require celiotomy; hernia, adhesion formation, and bowel obstruction have been reported with these procedures.

The omental-transposition operation depends on lymphatic connections developing between the omentum and lymphademator tissue (Fig. 41-5). This was first used by Dick[52] in 1935 in two cases of scrotal lymphedema. The omentum is rich in lymphatics and can easily reach the chest and axilla, but when it has to be lengthened to reach farther into the upper or lower limb, many of the lymphatics may be divided and thus not so useful. Goldsmith[38] reported long-term results but provided no

objective data on the extent of extremity size reduction. The complication rate was high, and there was no clarification as to how many patients were followed up beyond 3 years.

Hurst and associates[40] followed up for 2.5 to 7 years eight patients who underwent the enteromesenteric bridge procedure. This operation, physically limited to patients with proximal lymphatic obstruction at the level of the iliac or lower aortic nodes, also requires a celiotomy. Of patients in this series, 25% failed to improve and underwent a subsequent excisional procedure. Five patients were noted to improve clinically, but the authors provide no objective data.

Drainage into Deep Lymphatics

Thompson[53] proposed that a dermal wick of a lymphedematous tissue could be transposed deep to the muscle fascia, to allow bypass of lymph from superficial to deep lymphatics. Although he reported good results, this may have been due to the excisional procedures that accompanied the dermal wick.

Sawhney[54] studied this procedure with radioactive serum albumin, but was unable to demonstrate an increased uptake after dermal-wick procedures.

Microsurgical Procedures

Microsurgical procedures designed to reestablish lymphatic drainage to an affected extremity may be divided into three categories: (1) lymph nodal–venous shunts, (2) lymphaticovenous anastomoses (LVAs), and (3) lympholymphatic (L-L) anastomoses.

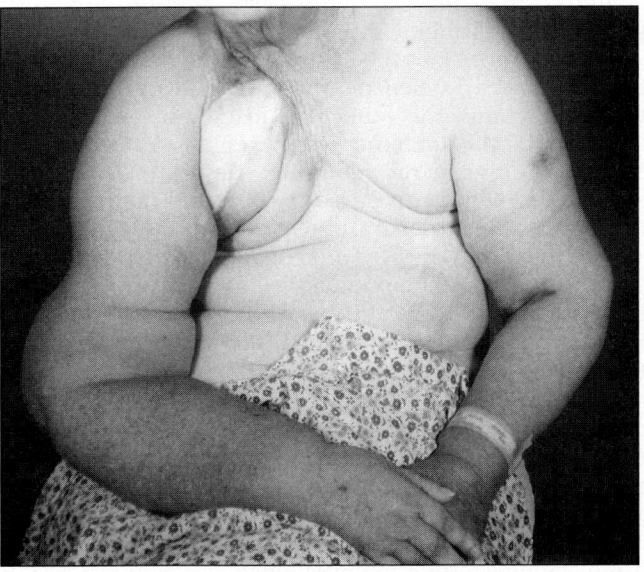

Figure 41-4. Patient with lymphedema and brachial plexus neuropathy after right radical mastectomy and irradiation for breast cancer. She was treated with excision of dense axially contracture, brachial plexus neurolysis, and latissimus dorsi myocutaneous flap to provide better coverage with well-vascularized tissue to the brachial plexus and also to help bridge obstructed upper limb lymphatics. Upper extremity volume decreased, and arm felt subjectively softer and less heavy for the patient.

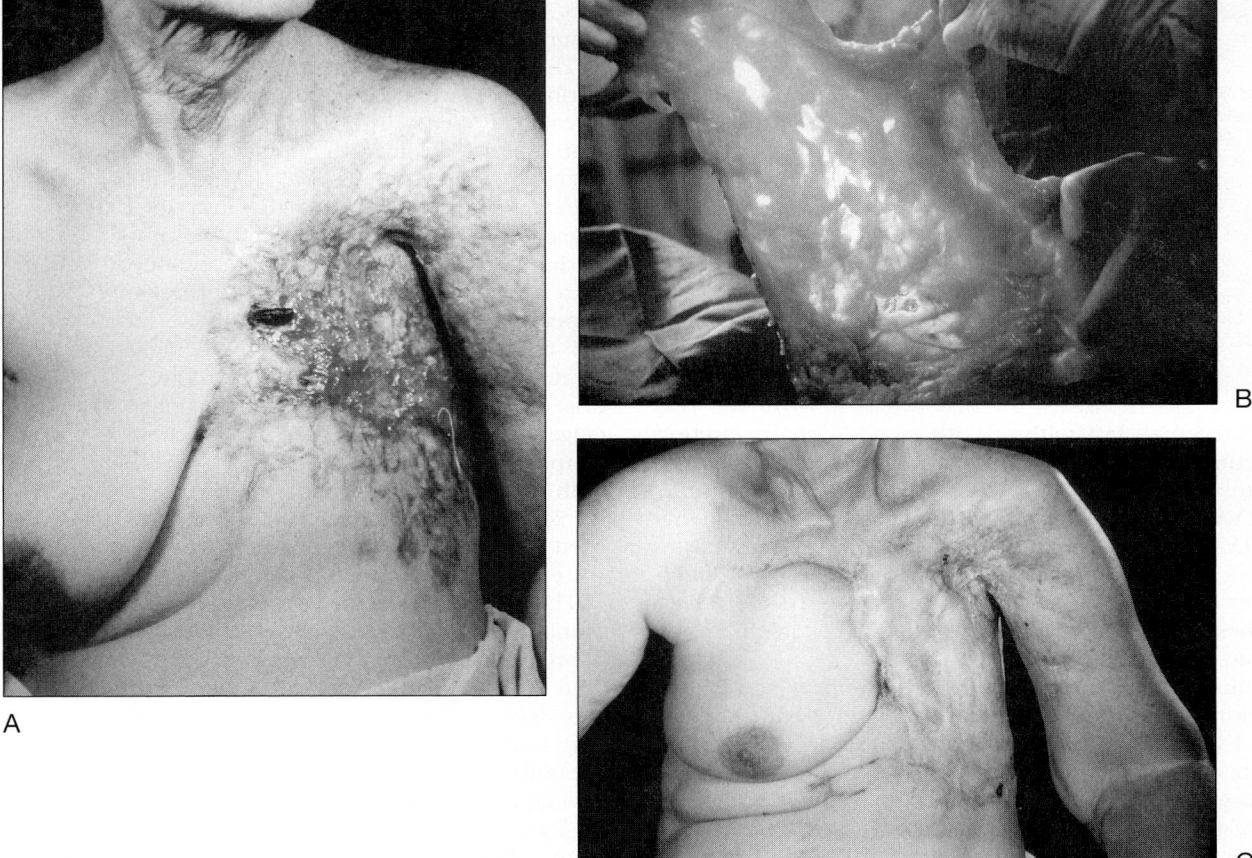

Figure 41-5. A, A 79-year-old woman with radiation necrosis of the left chest wall and axilla after radical mastectomy and irradiation with upper limb lymphedema. **B,** Omental flap is raised and pedicled on right gastroepiploic vessels. The chest wall and axilla were debrided; the omentum was transferred to cover both the chest wall and axilla and to serve as a bridge for lymphatic drainage. **C,** Nine months after radical debridement, omental flap, and skin graft to chest wall and axilla, with some improvement in upper limb lymphedema.

Lymph Nodal–Venous Shunts

Lymph nodal–venous shunts involve anastomosis of a transected lymph node to a neighboring vein. This was first described by Neilubowicz and Olszewski.[55] These procedures have been used for lymphedema involving the male and female genitalia, and these authors have reported good results in 50% of the patients. However, Calnan and co-workers[56] found that these lymph node–venous anastomoses remained patent for only a limited time in patients with lower extremity lymphedema, and by 3 months, they were all obstructed. Unfortunately, obstructive lymphedema usually results after lymphadenectomy, and thus lymph nodes are typically not available for use in this type of anastomosis.

Lymphaticovenous Anastomoses

Because lymph eventually drains into the venous system via the thoracic duct, in cases in which obstruction to flow occurs, it makes intuitive sense that it should be possible to bypass a lymphatic obstruction by allowing the lymph to enter the venous system more peripherally.

In obstructive lymphedema, lymphatic pressure is higher than venous pressure,[57] which should theoretically keep the LVA patent.

One of the pioneers of microlymphatic research for treatment of obstructive lymphedema was O'Brien, working at St. Vincent's Hospital in Melbourne, with whom the senior author trained and subsequently worked. In the first results, reported in 1976, an 83% patency of LVA was achieved in nonlymphedematous dogs. Considerable work was involved in creating a canine chronic lymphedema model, and once this was achieved, extensive research in LVA, free microvascular nodal transfers, and free microvascular omental transfers followed.[58-60]

Concurrent with this basic research, clinical studies on patients with obstructive lymphedema ensued. A 15-year study of 134 patients (116 female and 18 male patients) with established obstructive lymphedema from various causes and treated with LVA was reported in 1990.[44] Most patients (102) had lymphedema of the upper extremity, and 32, of the lower extremity. This group of patients were

TABLE 41-6

 St. Vincent's Lymphedema Experience

Surgery for obstructive lymphedema—154 patients (1974–1988)
134: LVA
  • 116 female, 18 male patients
  • Average age 52 yr
  • 102 upper limb, 32 lower limb
20: no suitable lymphatics

LVA, lymphaticovenous anastomosis.
Adapted from O'Brien et al: Long term results after microlympyhaticovenous anastomoses for treatment of obstructive lymphedema. Plast Reconstr Surg 1990;85:562.

all treated with LVA with or without additional reduction procedures. Of these patients, 90 were available for long-term follow-up (Tables 41-6 and 41-7): 52 patients had LVA only (mean, five anastomoses), and 38 patients had LVA plus segmental reduction (mean, 4.1 anastomoses). The results were graded both subjectively ("limb smaller and softer," "less weight," "more comfortable," "clothes fit better," etc.) and objectively with linear, volume, and tonometry measurements.

Subjectively, 73% and 78% reported improvement after LVA alone and LVA plus segmental reduction, respectively. Objectively, 42% had improvement after LVA alone, and 60% had improvement after LVA and reduction. Of the entire group, 58% reported fewer episodes of cellulitis. The results were generally better in the upper extremity compared with the lower extremity, a finding that other authors also reported.[48] Furthermore, of the patients that obtained postoperative improvement, none became worse later on. Of the remaining patients that did not

improve, 12% reported no change in lymphedema, and in 46%, the lymphedema became gradually worse, as is the natural history of untreated lymphedema.[44]

The technique used in this series of patients involved performing multiple LVA at multiple levels (wrist, medial forearm [upper calf], medial arm [leg]). In patients who would benefit from a segmental reduction, this was done laterally (upper lateral arm, lateral thigh). Patent blue dye was injected subdermally into the web spaces. A tourniquet was used, but the limb was not exsanguinated. With ×4 loupe magnification, the subcutaneous tissues were carefully dissected to isolate the lymphatics, which appeared as beaded, blue, thin, fragile vessels measuring 0.3 to 0.5 mm in diameter. Adjacent veins also were located or transposed from adjacent areas to lie near the dissected lymphatics. The lymphatics and veins were tagged with loose silk loops. The anastomosis of the lymphatic to the vein was performed in end-to-end fashion with the operating microscope and 11-0 nylon suture on a 75-μm needle. Approximately four to six sutures were used per anastomosis. As many anastomoses as possible were performed at multiple levels (Figs. 41-6 and 41-7).

This type of surgery is very demanding, but a significant number of patients obtain subjective improvement, and approximately half obtain measurable objective improvement. Critics of this type of surgery argue that no easy way exists of knowing how many LVAs stay patent in the long term.[46,48]

Similar results have been reported by Huang and colleagues,[57] who reported excellent and good results in 79% of patients, most of whom had obstructive lymphedema of the lower limb resulting from filariasis.[57] Both Huang and O'Brien have found that the results are better when the duration of the edema is shorter, and Huang, but not O'Brien, found that the number of anastomoses performed was significant, whereas O'Brien's group did not find the same correlation.

TABLE 41-7

St. Vincent's Lymphedema Experience

Long-Term Follow-up in 90 of 134 patients (1974–1988)

	LVA ONLY	LVA AND REDUCTION
Patients	52	38
No. of LVA (mean)	5	4.1
Mean vol. reduction	44% (10%–84%)	44% (10%–84%)
Subjective improvement	73%	78%
Objective improvement	42%	60%
Objective no change	12%	16%
Objective worse	46%	24%

58% Reduction cellulitis upper limb
  • Better results than lower limb
  • Hand better than forearm
  • All patients who improved initially continued to do so

LVA, lymphaticovenous anastomosis.
Adapted from O'Brien et al: Long term results after microlympyhaticovenous anastomoses for treatment of obstructive lymphedema. Plast Reconstr Surg 1990;85:562.

Lymphaticolymphatic Anastomosis

Lymphaticolymphatic (L-L) shunts bypass regional areas of lymphatic obstruction. Baumeister[61] first reported this technique in 1981 and later reported his results in 55 patients in 1990. He believes that L-L anastomoses are better than LVAs, as no increased back pressure is found, as can sometimes occur in higher venous pressure. He described the harvest of two to three lymphatic tracts from the anteromedial aspect of the thigh (adjacent to the saphenous vein).[61] In the lower extremity, these are pedicled from the normal limb to the lymphedematous limb, across the pubic area, and the lymphatics anastomosed to the dilated obstructed lymphatics on the involved side. For the upper extremity, the lymphatic grafts are harvested and transferred as free grafts to bridge the obstruction across the axilla with the proximal anastomoses into a lymphatic trunk in the neck. In his series of patients, Baumeister was able to show an 80% reduction in limb volume over a 3-year follow-up and also was able to demonstrate graft patency and improved transport index with lymphoscintigraphy. Better results were obtained in the upper limb[62] (Fig. 41-8).

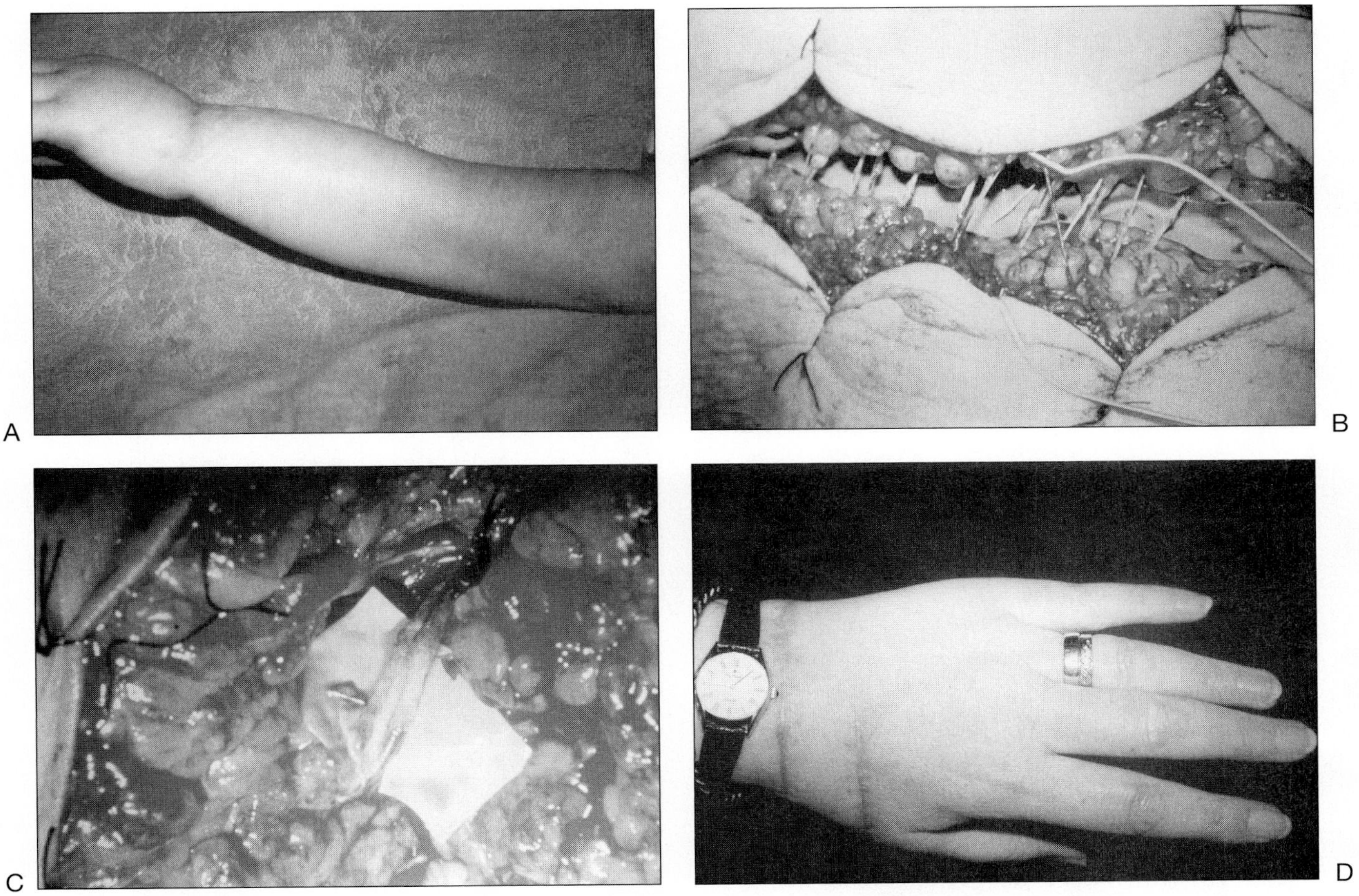

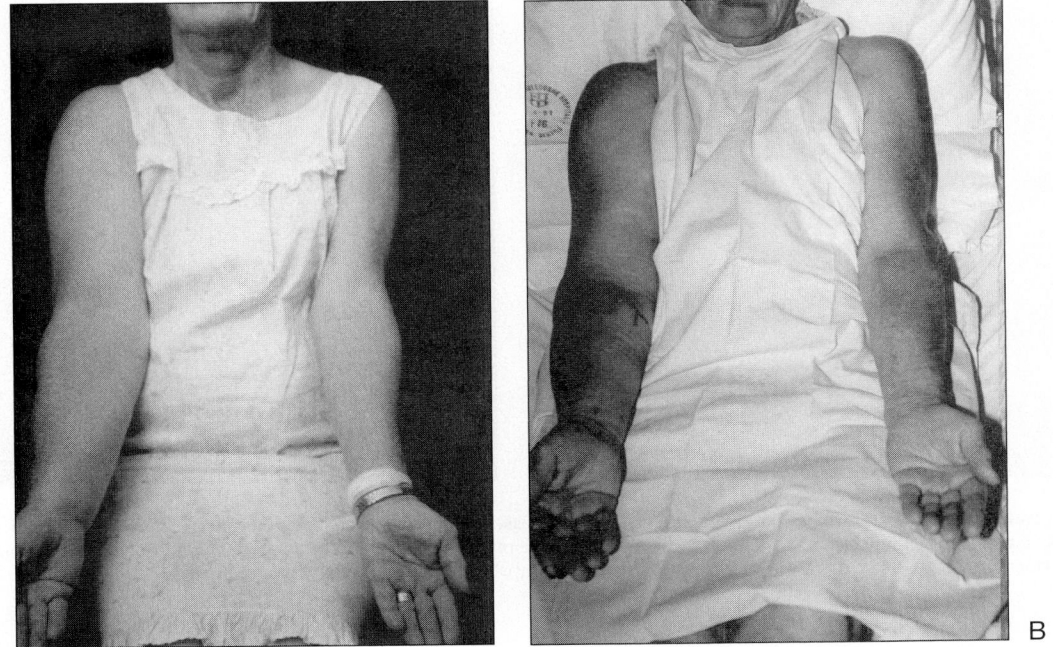

Figure 41-6. A, Patient with lymphedema of upper extremity affecting hand and forearm. **B,** Patent blue dye has been injected into web spaces and lymphatics, and veins dissected out at wrist, proximal forearm, and arm levels. **C,** Magnified view. Typical lymphaticovenous anastomoses completed. This patient had a total of six anastomoses at three levels. **D,** Three months after surgery, with complete resolution of the lymphedema; the patient was able to wear her rings.

Figure 41-7. A, Patient with lymphedema of right upper limb after mastectomy and irradiation. **B,** Six months after multiple-level lymphaticovenous anastomosis with smaller softer limb.

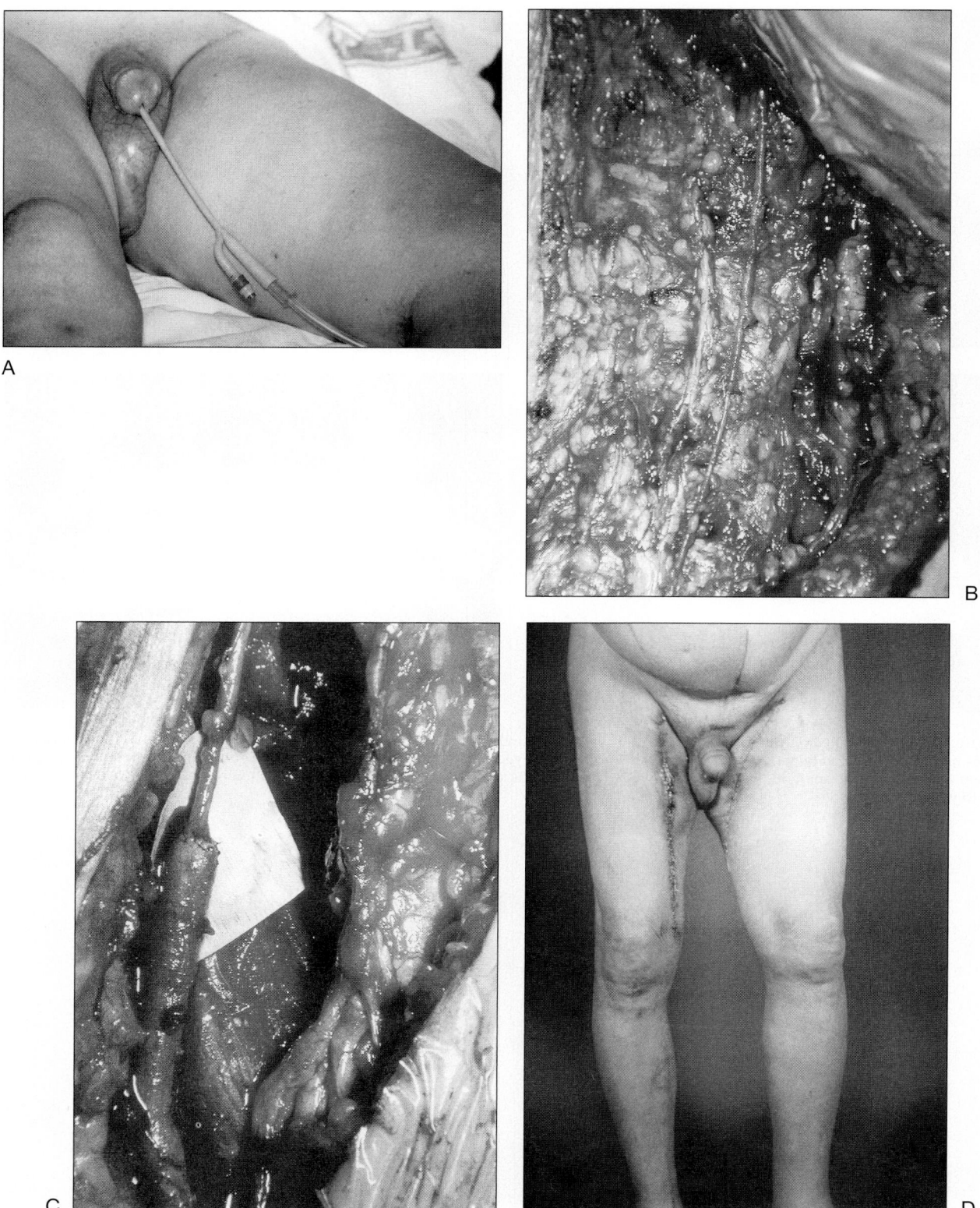

Figure 41-8. A, Patient with obstructive lymphedema of left legand increased venous pressures on manometry in saphenous vein. **B,** Dissection of right saphenous vein and surrounding lymphatics and pedicled across the pubic area to the left thigh (groin superior). **C,** Venous and lymphatic anastomoses performed. (groin superior). **D,** Two months after surgery: improvement in lymphedema in left leg.

Excisional Procedures

Excisional procedures include total skin and subcutaneous skin excision (erroneously referred to as the Charles procedure),[63-65] staged subcutaneous tissue excision (erroneously referred to as the Kondoleon operation),[66-71] and suction-assisted lipoplasty.[72-74] The buried dermal flap described by Thompson is an excisional procedure proposed to have a physiologic component.[75-78] Excisional procedures are suitable for both primary and secondary lymphedema.

Charles[63-65] described a surgical technique for the treatment of scrotal edema. The Charles procedure, however, has become an eponym for an operation in which the skin and subcutaneous compartment is completely excised and resurfaced with skin grafts.[63-65] Chronic ulceration, skin graft breakdown, and hypertrophic, unstable scarring have been consistently seen when split-thickness grafts are used.[64] Coverage with full-thickness grafts provides a more durable graft site, but graft breakdown and substantial scar formation also may occur.

Staged subcutaneous tissue excision was initially described by Sistrunk,[67] and modifications of the procedure have been reported by others, notably Homans.[68,69] This excisional approach removes significant amounts of skin and subcutaneous tissue, recognizing that the pathology of lymphedema is essentially limited to the superficial tissue compartment. The operation reduces the amount of subcutaneous tissue that produces lymph, and excisions of redundant skin also result in circumferential compression, which likely works in concert with muscular activity to facilitate the subdermal lymph drainage preserved within the flap. A recent study demonstrated long-lasting results for improvement in lower extremity lymphedema, regardless of cause, in a majority of patients treated.[70] This procedure has not been as effective for upper extremity lymphedema[63] (Figs. 41-9 and 41-10).

Although presented as a physiologically designed procedure, the buried dermal flap procedure described by Thompson[75] incorporates the excision of considerable amounts of tissue. In this procedure, the subcutaneous compartment is buried in the deep subfascial area in attempt to drain lymph. Radioactive iodinated human albumin clearance studies have been reported to support a physiologic improvement.[77] However, identical improvement in postoperative clearance was demonstrated in patients after skin and subcutaneous excision.[78] These findings could indicate that the reduction of the subcutaneous tissue improves overall function.

Suction-Assisted Lipectomy

Many authors have advocated the use of liposuction in both primary and secondary lymphedema to reduce the size of lymphatic extremities, as an alternative to segmental wedge excision, removing excess fluid and fat.[72-74] Most authors agree that patients who will benefit most from this procedure are those who have lymphedema of short duration and have yet to develop the fibrosclerotic changes associated with long-standing disease.

However, Brorson and colleagues[72,79,80] in Sweden have advocated a new concept in the management of upper extremity lymphedema in patients after mastectomy. Brorson has made a distinction between the presence of edema fluid and the increased fatty deposition that is seen in patients with chronic lymphedema. His hypothesis is that liposuction should address only the increased fatty deposit, and conservative methods should be used to treat the increased lymphatic fluid. He has rightly observed the very obvious fact that patients with chronic lymphedema have an increase in subcutaneous fatty deposition, a finding that has been greatly underappreciated by advocates of physiological-type approaches to the management of lymphedema. Brorson's strategy has been to reduce the edema first, using compression therapy until all the pitting edema has subsided, and then proceed to extensive circumferential liposuction with a specially designed cannula. His experience thus far has been in lymphedematous upper extremities in postmastectomy patients, and he has been able to achieve excellent long-term results with minimal complications. However, a mainstay of therapy after the surgery is ongoing controlled compression therapy, day and night, indefinitely. His studies have shown that the excess fat is permanently removed, and that there is no worsening of an already impaired lymph-transport system.[72,79,80]

Heat Treatment

The Chinese have been able to demonstrate that the use of local limb hyperthermia also is a useful adjunct for the treatment of lymphedema. In 1984, Zhang[81] reported a regimen of heating the involved limb to 6°C to 7°C above normal for 1 hour per day for 20 days. He used three to four courses that were 7 to 10 days apart. Between treatments, bandaging is used to compress the limb. He reported a reduction in limb volume in two thirds of patients and a sixfold decrease in incidence of cellulitis.

The continuing debate on the most efficacious medical and surgical approach underscores the need for intensified research. Management of patients with lymphedema suffers because of a lack of randomized, controlled prospective studies. Furthermore, no well-defined standards exist with respect to the definition of edema, documentation of results, and outcomes of therapy.

OUTCOMES

Little information exists on the economic outcome after surgery for lymphedema. This condition may manifest as recurrent infections, discomfort, functional impairment from increased extremity size and weight, musculoskeletal problems, psychosocial distress caused by cosmetic issues, and difficulty in carrying out activities of daily living.[82] However, patients should be informed that regional and Web-based support groups exist, and individuals with lymphedema who are compliant with management regimens can decrease in-hospital stays; many will enjoy a normal or near-normal quality of life.

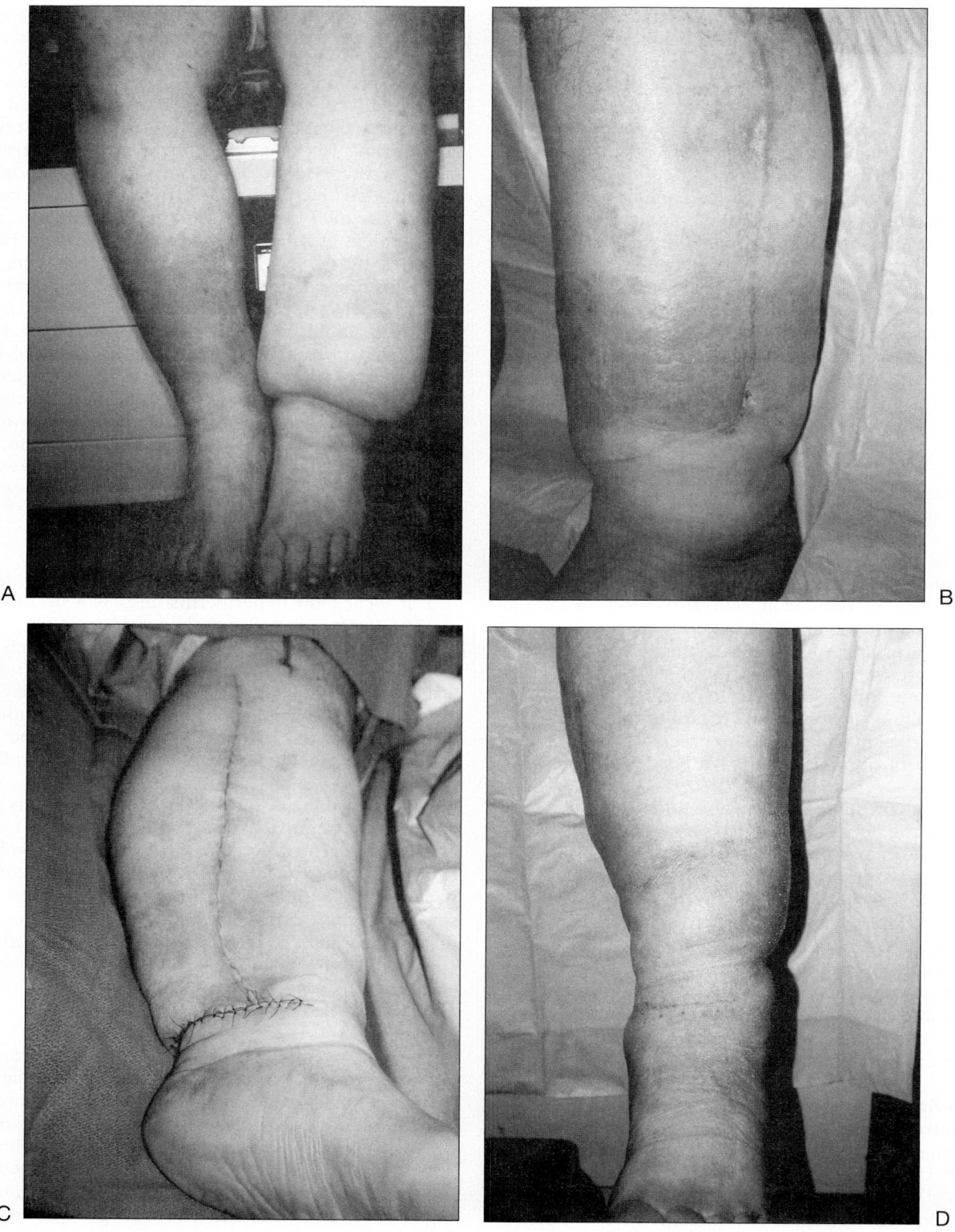

Figure 41-9. A, A 45-year-old patient with lymphedema tarda of left leg, with lymphedema worse laterally. **B,** At 17 months after first excision on lateral aspect of left leg before medical excision. **C,** Intraoperative view after medial wedge excisions. **D,** Four years after surgery with stable leg.

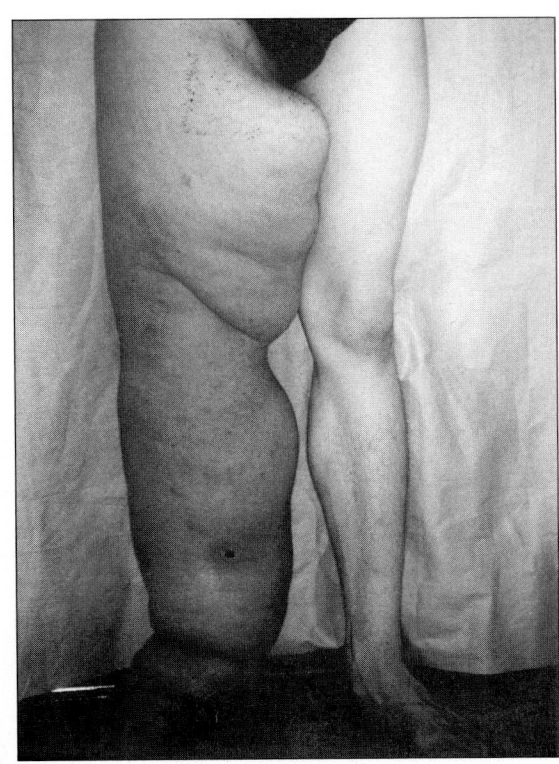

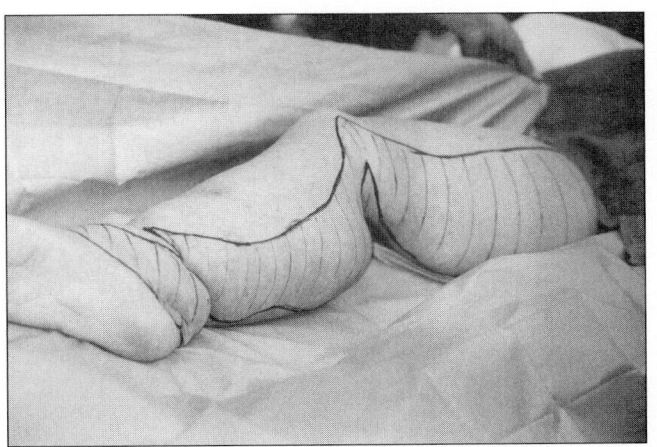

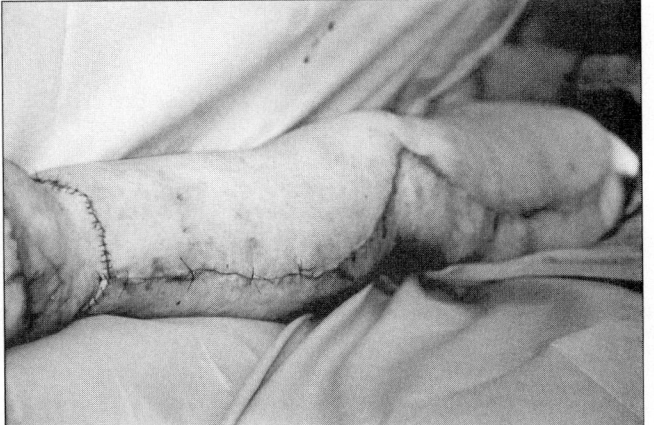

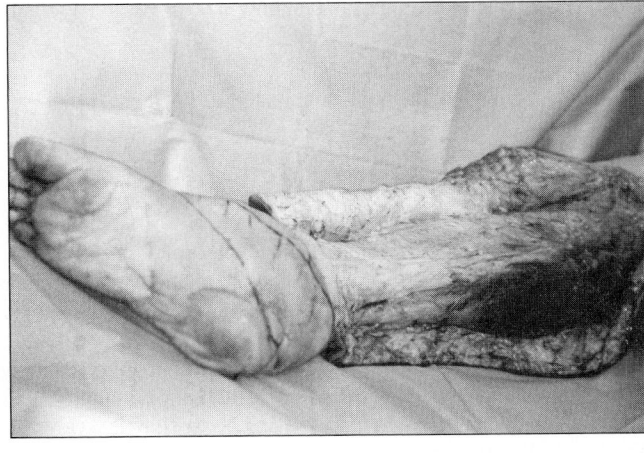

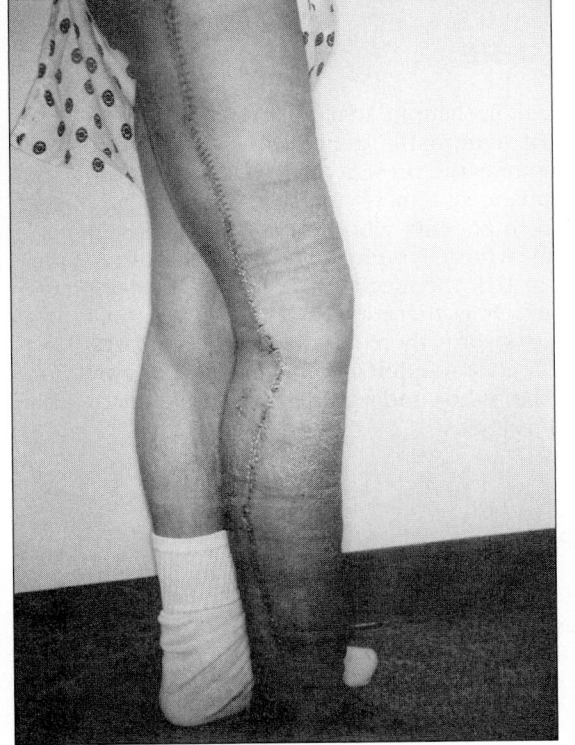

Figure 41-10. A, A 22-year-old man with gross primary lymphedema commencing in early puberty (lymphedema praecox). Patient unable to wear normal clothes. **B,** Extended medial wedge excision of the thigh, knee, calf, and ankle. **C,** Intraoperative view of filled leg after excision of lymphedematous tissue. **D,** Immediate intraoperative result. **E,** Three months after second-stage lateral wedge excision: lateral and anterior view.   *Continued*

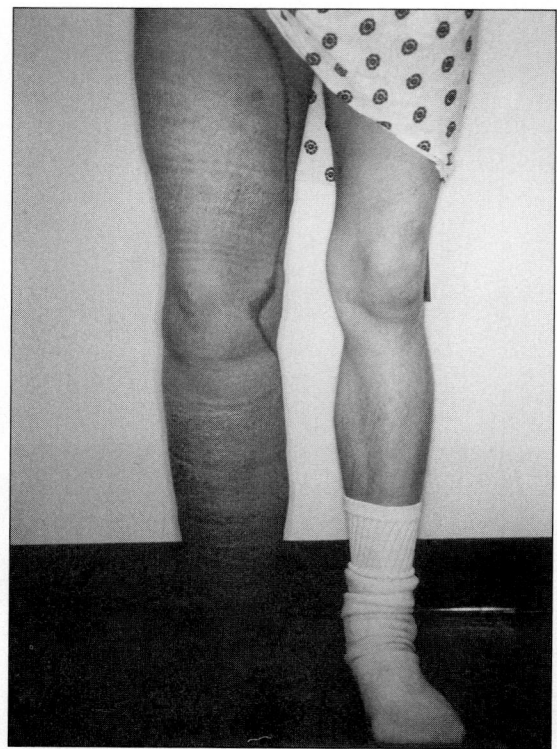
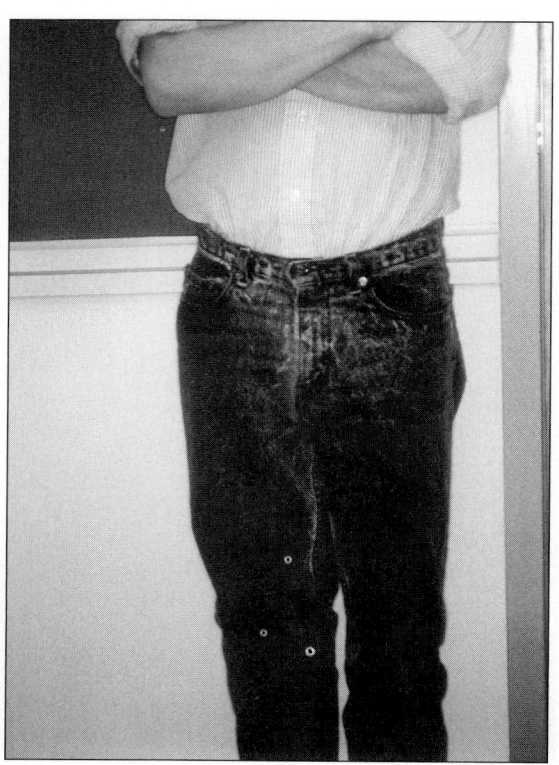

Figure 41-10, *cont'd.* **F,** Three months after second-stage lateral wedge excision: lateral and anterior view. **G,** Patient now able to wear normal clothes.

THE FUTURE

Those in whom lymphedema develops appear to be incapable of lymphatic generation or regeneration. Evidence suggests the presence of growth factors specific for the lymphatic system[83,84] and a capacity for lymphatic regeneration in patients who do not have lymphedema.[9] Do those in whom lymphedema develops after some inciting event lack the mechanisms needed for lymphatic vessel repair? Or is there a deficit in the response to a growth factor(s), or is there a lack of growth factor(s)? We submit that a genetic etiology explains why, in a fraction of individuals who undergo similar procedures, this condition develops.

SUMMARY

The large number of medical therapies and surgical procedures that have been described in the treatment of lymphedema emphasize the discouraging fact that this condition remains incurable by any means. The severity of symptoms may vary from mild extremity swelling to serious disabling or life-threatening complications such as recurrent infections and rarely, lymphangiosarcoma. Most patients are diagnosed by history and physical examination alone and may be managed conservatively. If this is unsuccessful, and the patient has primary lymphedema, then a reduction procedure is all that is available. Traditionally, this has involved staged resection of skin and subcutaneous tissue. However, liposuction is gaining popularity, especially in relatively early cases in which the quality of skin in good and little fibrosis is found. In patients with secondary or obstructive lymphedema that is not well controlled with conservative management, a physiological procedure, often using multiple modalities (e.g., pedicle flaps plus LVAs or LVAs with or without segmental reduction or liposuction) has been the authors' preferred method of treatment (Fig. 41-11). Regardless of treatment modality, patient cooperation is critical for successful outcome. Future efforts should focus on clarifying the genetic etiology of lymphedema, with hope that a better understanding of the basis of disease will lead to more effective treatment strategies.

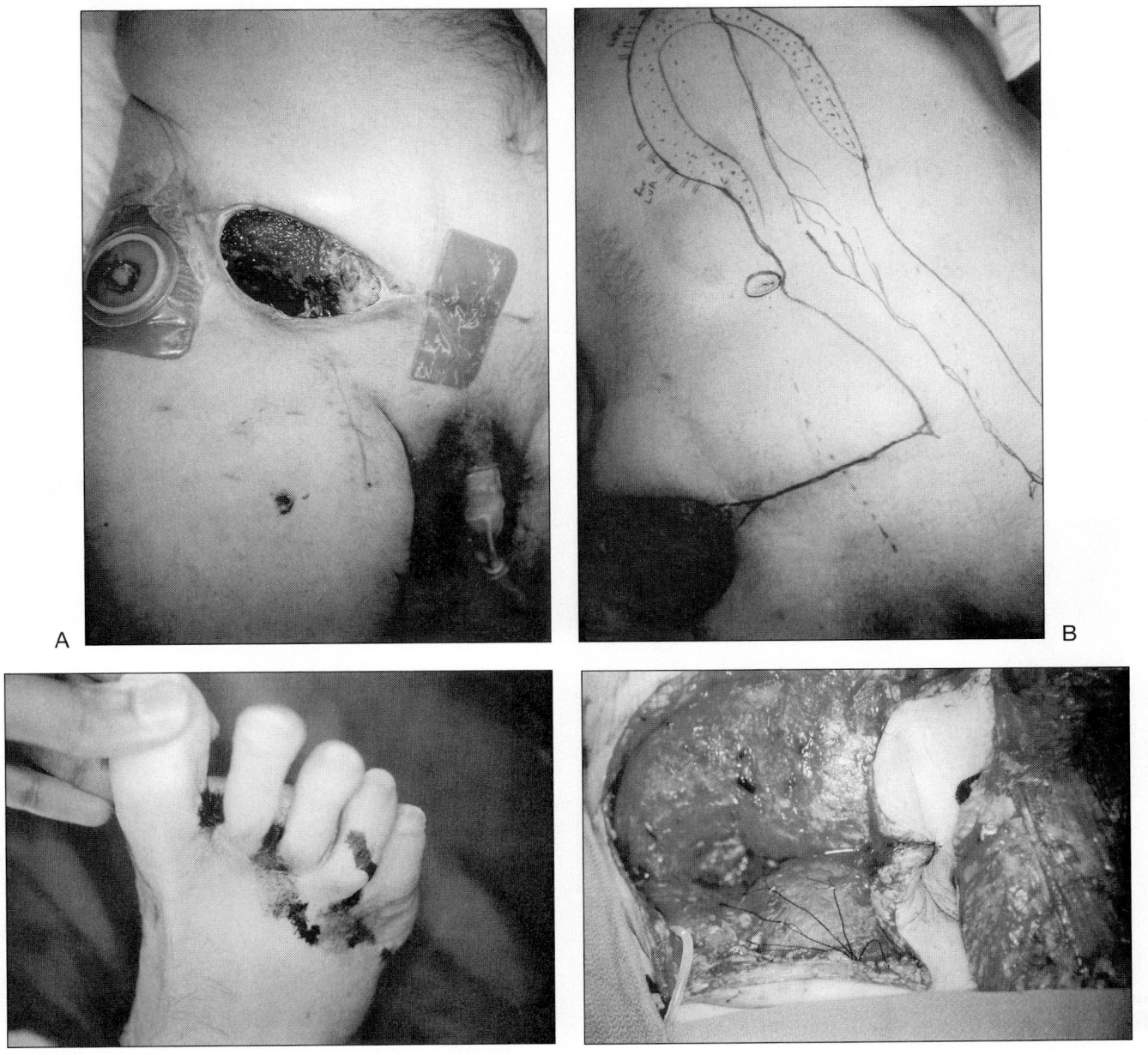

Figure 41-11. A, A 74-year-old patient with chronic wound draining lymphatic fluid in right hip area, after radical excision of chondrosarcoma and irradiation. The right leg is lymphedematous. **B,** Design of contralateral vertical rectus abdominis musculocutaneous (VRAM) flap (based on superficial and deep inferior epigastric vascular pedicle). The lymphatic drainage into left groin is intact. Plan to dissect out multiple small venous channels at upper aspect of flap for lymphaticovenous anastomoses (LVAs). **C,** Methyl blue dye injected intradermally into web spaces for foot. **D,** Multiple dilated lymphatics dissected out in upper right thigh, marked with silk loops.   *Continued*

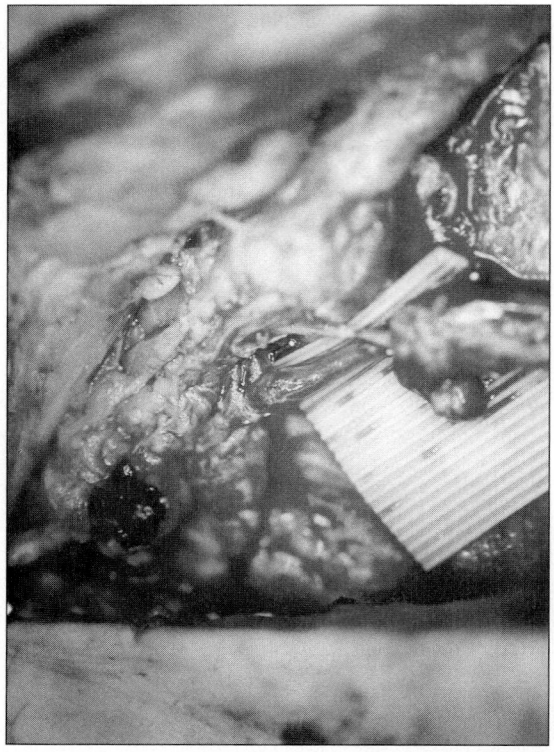

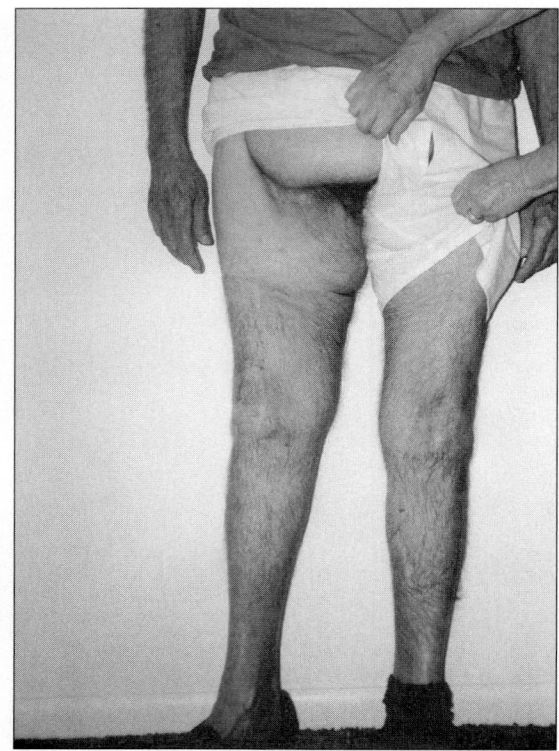

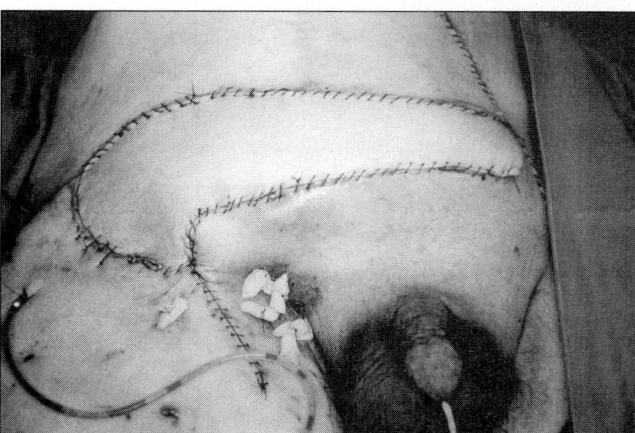

Figure 41-11, *cont'd*. E, The VRAM flap was transposed across the lower abdomen to the deficit in the right groin. Magnified view of two LVAs is shown. Four LVAs were performed from thigh lymphatics into small veins of distal (*top*) end of VRAM flap using 10-0 nylon suture. **F,** Immediate result after wound closure. **G,** Result at 11 months showing healed wound and reduced lymphedema.

REFERENCES

1. Karkkainen MJ, Ferrell RE, Lawrence EC, et al: Missense mutations interfere with VEGFR-3 signalling in primary lymphedema. Nat Genet 2000;25:153–159.
2. Irrthum A, Karkkainen MJ, Devriendt K, Alitalo K, Vikkula M: Congenital hereditary lymphedema caused by a mutation that inactivates VEGFR3 tyrosine kinase. Am J Hum Genet 2000;67:295–301.
3. Makhoul IR, Sujov P, Ghanem N, Bronshtein M: Prenatal diagnosis of Milroy's primary congenital lymphedema. Prenat Diagn 2002;22:823–826.
4. Wolfe JHN, Kinmonth JB: The prognosis of primary lymphedema of the lower limbs. Arch Surg 1981;116:1157–1160.
5. Segerstrom K, Bjerle P, Graffman S, Nystrom A: Factors that influence the incidence of brachial oedema after treatment of breast cancer. Scand J Plast Reconstr Surg Hand Surg 1992;26:223–227.
6. Kissin MW, Querci della Rovere G, Easton D, Westbury G: Risk of lymphoedema following the treatment of breast cancer. Br J Surg 1986;73:580–584.
7. Fiorica JV, Roberts WS, Greenberg H, Hoffman MS, La Polla JP, Cavanagh D: Morbidity and survival patterns in patients after radical hysterectomy and postoperative adjuvant pelvic radiotherapy. Gynecol Oncol 1990;36:343–347.
8. Werngren-Elgstrom M, Lidman D: Lymphoedema of the lower extremities after surgery and radiotherapy for cancer of the cervix. Scand J Plast Reconstr Surg Hand Surg 1994;28:289–293.
9. Slavin SA, Upton J, Kaplan WD, Van den Abbeele AD: An investigation of lymphatic function following free-tissue transfer. Plast Reconstr Surg 1997;99:730–741.

10. O'Brien BM, Das SK, Franklin JD, Morrison WA: Effect of lymphangiography on lymphedema. Plast Reconstr Surg 1981;68:922–926.

11. Bergan J, Yao J, Flinn W, McCarthy W: Surgical treatment of venous obstruction and insufficiency. J Vasc Surg 1986;3:174–181.

12. Bull RH, Coburn PR, Mortimer PS: Pretibial myxoedema: a manifestation of lymphoedema? Lancet 1993;341:403–404.

13. Rudkin GH, Miller TA: Lipedema: a clinical entity distinct from lymphedema. Plast Reconstr Surg 1994;94:841–847.

14. Scanlon E: James Ewing Lecture: The process of metastasis. Cancer 1985;55:1163–1166.

15. Stewart FW, Treves N: Lymphangiosarcoma in postmastectomy lymphedema. Cancer 1948;1:64–81.

16. Janse AJ, van Coevorden F, Peterse H, Keus RB, van Dongen JA: Lymphedema-induced lymphangiosarcoma. Eur J Surg Oncol 1995;21:155–158

17. Chen HC, O'Brien B, Pribaz JJ: The use of tonometry in the assessment of lymphedema. Br J Plast Surg 1988;41:399–402.

18. Pappas CJ, O'Donnell TF Jr: Long-term results of compression treatment for lymphedema. J Vasc Surg 1992;16:555–562.

19. Boris M, Weindorf S, Lasinski B, Boris G: Lymphedema reduction by noninvasive complex lymphedema therapy. Oncology 1994;8:95–106.

20. Ko DS, Lerner R, Klose G, Cosimi AB: Effective treatment of lymphedema of the extremities. Arch Surg 1998;133:452–458.

21. Szuba A, Cooke JP, Yousuf S, Rockson SG: Decongestive lymphatic therapy for patients with cancer-related or primary lymphedema. Am J Med 2000;109:296–300.

22. Casley-Smith JR, Morgan RG, Piller NB: Treatment of lymphedema of the arms and legs with 5,6-benzo-alpha-pyrone. N Engl J Med 1993;329:1158–1163.

23. Casley-Smith JR, Wang CT, Casley-Smith JR, Zi-hai C: Treatment of filarial lymphoedema and elephantiasis with 5,6-benzo-alpha-pyrone (coumarin). BMJ 1993;307:1037–1041.

24. Piller NB, Morgan RG, Casley-Smith JR: A double-blind, cross-over trial of O-(beta-hydroxyethyl)-rutosides (benzo-pyrones) in the treatment of lymphoedema of the arms and legs. Br J Plast Surg 1988;41:20–27.

25. Soria P, Cuesta A, Romero H, Martinez FJ, Sastre A: Dietary treatment of lymphedema by restriction of long-chain triglycerides. Angiology 1994;45:703–707.

26. Piller NB, Thelander A: Treatment of chronic postmastectomy lymphedema with low level laser therapy: a 2.5-year follow-up. Lymphology 1998;31:74–86.

27. Casley-Smith J, Casley-Smith J: Other physical therapy for lymphedema: pumps, heating, etc. In Casley-Smith J, Casley-Smith J (eds): Lymphedema. Adelaide, Lymphedema Association of Australia, 1991, p 155.

28. Ogawa Y, Yoshizumi M, Kitagawa T, et al: Investigation of the mechanism of lymphocyte injection therapy in treatment of lymphedema with special emphasis on cell adhesion molecule (L-selectin). Lymphology 1999;32:151–156.

29. Hafez HM, Wolfe JHN: Basic data underlying clinical decision making: Lymphedema. Ann Vasc Surg 1996;10:88–95.

30. Miller TA: Surgical management of lymphedema of the extremity. Ann Plast Surg 1978;1:184–187.

31. Handley WS: Lymphangioplasty: A new method for the relief of the brawny arm of breast cancer and for similar conditions of the lymphatic oedema: Preliminary note. Lancet 1908;1:783–785.

32. Walther C: Note sur une nouvelle methode de traitement de l'elephantiasis des membres. Bull Acad Natl Med 1918;3 (Ser. 79):195.

33. Hogeman KE: Artificial subcutaneous channels in draining lymphoedema. Acta Chir Scand 1955;100:154.

34. Jantet GA, Taylor GW, Kinmoth JB: Operations for primary lymphedema of the lower limb: Results after 1 to 9 years. J Cardiovasc Surg 1961;2:27–36.

35. Zeiman SA: Re-establishing lymph drainage for lymphedema of the extremities. J Int Coll Surg 1951;15:328–331.

36. Silver D, Puckett CL: Lymphangioplasty: A ten year evaluation. Surgery 1976;80:748–755.

37. Goldsmith HS, de los Santos R, Beattie EJ: Relief of chronic lymphedema by omental transposition. Ann Surg 1967;166:572–585.

38. Goldsmith HS: Long-term evaluation of omental transposition for chronic lymphedema. Ann Surg 1974;180:847–849.

39. Harii K: Clinical application of free omental flap transfer. Clin Plast Surg 1978;5:273–281.

40. Hurst PA, Stewart G, Kinmonth JB, Browse NL: Long-term results of the enteromesenteric bridge operation in the treatment of primary lymphedema. Br J Surg 1985;72:272–274.

41. Olszewski WL: The treatment of lymphedemas of the extremities with microsurgical lymphovenous anastomoses. Internatl Angiology 1988;7:312–321.

42. Baumeister RG, Siuda S: Treatment of lymphedema by microsurgical lymphatic grafting: What is proved? Plast Reconstr Surg 1990;85:64–74.

43. Rivero OR, Calnan JS, Reis ND, Taylor LM: Experimental peripheral lympho-venous communications. Br Plast Surg 1967;20:124–133.

44. O'Brien BMcC, Mellow CG, Khazanchi RK, Dvir E, Kumar V, Pederson WC: Long-term results after microlymphaticovenous anastomoses for the treatment of obstructive lymphedema. Plast Reconstr Surg 1990;85:562–572.

45. Olszewski WL: Lymphostasis: Pathophysiology, Diagnosis, and Treatment. Boca Raton, Fla, CRC Press, 1991.

46. Puckett CL, Jacobs GR, Hurvitz JS, Silver D: Evaluation of lymphovenous anastomoses in obstructive lymphedema. Plast Reconstr Surg 1980;66:116–120.

47. Weiss M, Baumeister RG, Tatsch K, Hahn K: Lymphoscintigraphy for noninvasive long-term follow-up of functional outcome in patients with autologous lymph vessel transplantation. Nuklearmedizin 1996;35:236–242.

48. Campisi C, Boccardo F, Alitta P, Tacchella M: Derivative lymphatic microsurgery: Indications, techniques, and results. Microsurgery 1995;16:463–468.

49. Gillies HD, Fraser FR: The lymphatic wick. Proc R Soc Med 1950;43:1054–1059.

50. Mowlem R: The treatment of lymphedema. Br J Plast Surg 1948;1:48–55.

51. Clodius L, Uhlschmid G, Hess K: Irradiation plexitis of the brachial plexus. Clin Plast Surg 1984;11:161–165.

52. Dick W: Uber die Lymphgefdsse des menschlichten Netzez, zugleich ein Beitrag zur Behandlung der Elephantiasis. Beitr Klin Chir 1935;162:296–314.

53. Thompson N: The surgical treatment of advanced post mastectomy lymphedema of the upper limb with later results of treatment by the buried dermal flap operation. Scand J Plast Surg 1969;3:54–60.

54. Sawhney CP: Evaluation of Thompson's buried dermal flap operation for lymphedema of the limbs: A clinical radioisotope study. Br J Plast Surg 1974;27:278–283.

55. Neilubowicz J, Olszewski W: Surgical lymphaticovenous shunts in patients with secondary lymphedema. Br J Surg 1968;55:440–442.

56. Calnan JS, Reis ND, Rivero OR, Copenhagen HJ, Mercurius-Taylor L: Natural history of lymph node to vein anastomosis. Br J Plast Surg 1967;20:134–145.

57. Huang GK, Hu R, Liu ZZ, Sherr YL, Lan TD, Pan GP: Microlymphaticovenous anastomosis in the treatment of lower limb obstructive lymphedema: Analysis of 91 cases. Plast Reconstr Surg 1985;76:671–685.

58. Chen HC, Pribaz JJ, O'Brien B, Knight KR, Morrison WA: Creation of distal canine limb lymphedema. Plast Reconstr Surg 1989;83:1022–1026.

59. Chen HC, O'Brien B, Rogers IW, Pribaz JJ, Eaton CJ: Lymph node transfer for the treatment of obstructive lymphedema in canine model. Br J Plast Surg 1990;43:578–586.

60. O'Brien B, Hickey MJ, Hurley JU, et al. Microsurgical transfer of the greater omentum in treatment of canine obstructive lymphedema. Br. J Plast Surg 190;43:440–446.

61. Baumeister RG, Siefert J, Wiebecke B, Hahn D: Experimental basis and first application of clinical lymph vessel transplantation of secondary lymphedema. World J Surg 1981;5:401–407.

62. Baumeister RG, Siuda S: Treatment of lymphedema by microsurgical lymphatic grafts: What is proved. Plast Reconstr Surg 1990;85:64–74.

63. Mavili ME, Naldoken S, Safak T: Modified Charles operation for primary fibrosclerotic lymphedema. Lymphology 1994;27:14–20.

64. Miller TA: Charles procedure for lymphedema: A warning. Am J Surg 1980;139:290–292.

65. Dellon AL, Hoopes JE: The Charles procedure for primary lymphedema: Long-term clinical results. Plast Reconstr Surg 1977;60:589–595.

66. Kondoleon E: Die operative Behandlung der elephantiastichen Oedema. Zentralbl Chir 1912;39:1022–1025.

67. Sistrunk WE: Further experiences with the Kondoleon operation for elephantiasis. JAMA 1918;71:800–806.

68. Homans J: The treatment of elephantiasis of the legs: A preliminary report. N Engl J Med 1936;215:1099–1104.

69. Auchincloss H: New operation for elephantiasis. Puerto Rico J Publ Health Trop Med 1930;6:149.

70. Miller TA, Wyatt LE, Rudkin, GH: Staged skin and subcutaneous excision for lymphedema: A favorable report of long-term results. Plast Reconstr Surg 1998;102:1486–1498.

71. Miller TA: Surgical approach to lymphedema of the arm after mastectomy. Am J Surg 1984;148:152–156.

72. Brorson H, Svensson H: Liposuction combined with controlled compression therapy reduces arm lymphedema more effectively than controlled compression therapy alone. Plast Reconstr Surg 1998;102:1058–1067.

73. Apesos J, Chami R: Functional applications of suction-assisted lipectomy: New treatment for old disorders. Aesthetic Plast Surg 1991;15:73–79.

74. O'Brien BMcC, Khazanchi RK, Kumar PAV, Dvir E, Pederson WC: Liposuction in the treatment of lymphedema: A preliminary report. Br J Plast Surg 1989;42:530–533.

75. Thompson N: Surgical treatment of chronic lymphoedema of the lower limb: With preliminary report of a new operation. Br Med J 1962;2:1566.

76. Thompson N: Buried dermal flap operation for chronic lymphedema of the extremities: Ten-year survey of results of 79 cases. Plast Reconstr Surg 1970;45:541–548.

77. Thompson N, Wee JTK: Twenty years experience of the buried dermis flap operation in the treatment of chronic lymphedema of the extremities. Chir Plast 1980;5:147–161.

78. Serville M: Surgical treatment of lymphedema: A report on 652 cases. Surgery 1987;101:485–495.

79. Brorson H: Liposuction gives complete reduction of chronic large arm lymphedema after breast cancer. Acta Oncol 2000;39:407–420.

80. Brorson H, Svensson H, Norrgren K, Thorsson O: Liposuction reduces arm lymphedema without significantly altering the already impaired lymph transport. Lymphology 1998;31:156–172.

81. Zhang TS, Huang WY, Han LY, Liu WY: Heat and bandage treatment of chronic lymphedema of the extremities. Chin Med J 1984; 97:567–577.

82. Brennan MJ, DePompolo RW, Garden F: Focused review: post-mastectomy lymphedema. Arch Phys Med Rehabil 1996;77:S74–S80.

83. Jeltsch M, Kaipainen A, Joukov V, et al: Hyperplasia of lymphatic in VEGF-C transgenic mice. Science 1997;276:1423–1425.

84. Kukk E, Lymboussaki A, Taira S, et al: VEGF-C receptor binding and pattern of expression with VEGF-3 suggests a role in lymphatic vascular development. Development 1996;122:3829–3837.

42

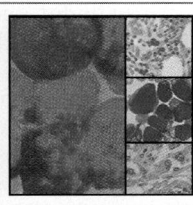

FATIGUE

SUMMARY OF KEY POINTS

INCIDENCE
- Fatigue may be a presenting symptom of malignancy or a signal of disease recurrence.
- Fatigue is the most prevalent symptom in patients with cancer.
- It affects more than 70% of patients receiving chemotherapy, radiation therapy, or biologic response modifier therapy.
- A significant level of fatigue occurs in more than 75% of patients with advanced cancer.
- Fatigue significantly reduces functional status.
- Fatigue significantly reduces quality of life.
- Fatigue in patients with cancer is often managed poorly.

ETIOLOGY OF COMPLICATIONS
- The etiology of fatigue is often multifactorial.
- Direct factors include the malignancy and cancer treatments.
- Contributing factors include pain, emotional distress, sleep disturbance, anemia, nutritional deficits, deconditioning, and comorbidities.
- Specific pathophysiologic mechanisms are unclear.

EVALUATION OF THE PATIENT
Screening should be done at initial visit, at regular intervals, and as clinically indicated.
Patients should be evaluated by means of focused history and physical examination, fatigue assessment,

selected laboratory tests, and assessment of contributing factors.

GRADING OF THE COMPLICATION
- Fatigue intensity should be measured with valid and reliable scales.
- Serial measurements should be recorded in the medical record for comparison.

TREATMENT
- Any identified contributing factors should be treated.
- Pharmacologic and nonpharmacologic should be added treatments according to patient's clinical status (e.g., active cancer treatment, disease-free follow-up, or palliative care at end of life).

INTRODUCTION

Definition

Fatigue in patients with cancer, often referred to as *cancer-related fatigue (CRF)*, has been defined by the National Comprehensive Cancer Network (NCCN) as a "persistent, subjective sense of tiredness related to cancer or cancer treatment that interferes with usual functioning."[1]

Fatigue is a universal human experience that, in healthy individuals, is regarded as a basic protective mechanism against the depletion of body reserves of adenosine triphosphate (ATP) and resulting exhaustion and possible tissue damage. Compared with the fatigue of healthy individuals, which resolves with adequate rest and sleep, the fatigue of patients with cancer often remains after a period of rest or sleep, is of greater magnitude and persistence, is more disruptive to activities of daily living, and has a more negative affective impact.[2] When patients with cancer were asked to describe their fatigue, responses revealed three major characteristics: physical sensations (59% of responses) such as weakness and decreased physical performance, affective sensations (29% of responses) such as sadness and diminished motivation, and cognitive effects such as difficult concentrating and decreased problem-solving ability (12% of responses).[2]

Cancer-related fatigue has been accepted as a diagnosis in the *International Statistical Classification of Diseases, 10th Revision–Clinical Modification* with the required criterion of "significant fatigue, diminished energy, or increased need to rest, disproportionate to any recent change in activity level" plus five or more criteria related to the impact of fatigue and present every day or nearly every day during 2 weeks of the previous month.[3] Although these criteria are promising in the diagnosis of CRF, they have been tested in only one study of cancer survivors in which prevalence of CRF was determined to be 17%.[3]

Incidence

CRF is the most prevalent unmanaged symptom reported by patients being treated for cancer, and it affects 70% to 100% of patients receiving cytotoxic chemotherapy, radiation therapy, stem cell or marrow transplantation, or treatment with biologic response modifiers.[4-8] Fatigue is a persistent, distressing symptom in 17% to 40% of patients who have completed treatment[3,9-11] and is a significant symptom in more than 75% of patients with metastatic disease.[12-14] The increasing prominence of CRF is related to both the increase in intensive multimodal cancer treatments, characterized by increased dose density and dose intensity, and better management of formerly predominant symptoms of pain, nausea, and vomiting. Patients report fatigue to be the most distressing symptom associated with cancer and its treatment, more distressing even than pain.[7,8]

Management of CRF is important for several reasons beyond its prevalence and the discomfort and distress it causes. First, high levels of fatigue affect functional status and the ability to tolerate cancer treatment. Recent research reports indicate that fatigue may have a profound effect on functional status,[15-17] and it is uncertain whether patients regain full functioning when treatment is over.[9] If fatigued patients cannot tolerate their cancer treatment or must choose between treatment and quality of life, control of their malignancy may be compromised.[6] In addition, high levels of fatigue affect patients' quality of life and interfere with their ability to engage in valued roles and activities.

DESCRIPTION OF FATIGUE

Etiology

Fatigue in patients with cancer is a complex and multi-factorial phenomenon that may have a variety of causes and contributing factors. The exact mechanisms involved in its pathophysiology are unknown.[18,19]

Fatigue may be caused by the malignancy itself or by cancer treatment and treatment-related anemia. Physiologic factors known to contribute to CRF are cachexia, deconditioning, and high levels of certain cytokines such as interleukin-1, interleukin-6, and tumor necrosis factor-α.[18] Psychosocial factors contributing to fatigue include anxiety, depression, and insomnia. Fatigue is also associated with high levels of other symptoms, especially pain.[20] In fact, fatigue commonly occurs in the context of multiple symptoms and in this context is highly correlated with decreased functional status.[15]

Patterns of Fatigue

Patients with cancer frequently report that fatigue begins with cancer treatment—or even during the stressful diagnostic process—continues during the course of active cancer treatment, and declines when treatment is over.[19] The fatigue may persist after treatment at a higher-than-baseline level, and a significant percentage of disease-free survivors report disruptive levels of fatigue for years after treatment. For example, in a survey of 1957 survivors of breast cancer, a third reported severe and persistent fatigue 3 years after diagnosis.[9]

Patterns of fatigue during the course of cancer treatments vary according to the type of treatment. Fatigue typically rises sharply after intravenous cytotoxic chemotherapy to a peak 48 to 72 hours later and drops to near-normal levels 3 weeks later, with a smaller peak occurring on days 10 to 14 with some regimens.[21-23] Studies have not shown substantial increases in fatigue during successive infusions.[24]

During radiation therapy for breast cancer, fatigue levels typically increase linearly over time to a maximum intensity during the fourth week of treatment and then plateau.[25,26] Levels of fatigue after radiation therapy return to normal in most patients within 3 weeks to 3 months[25,26] but are more likely to persist at high levels after chemotherapy. In a study of 322 patients with breast cancer in remission, post-treatment fatigue levels were highest in women who received chemotherapy in addition to radiation therapy and lowest in those who received radiation therapy only.[27]

EVALUATION

The National Comprehensive Cancer Network (NCCN) has developed guidelines for the evaluation and treatment of CRF on the basis of available research findings and clinical experience (see www.nccn.org for the most recent guidelines).[1] This multidisciplinary panel of experts in CRF developed an algorithm in which patients are screened regularly for fatigue by means of a brief screening instrument and are treated according to their level of fatigue and clinical status. The algorithm includes phases of screening, primary evaluation, intervention according to three levels of clinical status, and re-evaluation.

Progress in the management of CRF has been limited by several factors relating to screening. Patients are reluctant to report fatigue to health care professionals because they fear that their cancer therapy may be modified, doses may be reduced, or treatment may be stopped. Another reason patients give for not reporting CRF is that they believe it is a symptom to be endured (such as sleep problems or emotional distress), which they should be able to manage themselves. Many health care professionals are reluctant to screen for CRF because they are unaware of evidence-based treatments or because they are unaware of the distress and interference with function that accompany fatigue. The result is that fatigue in patients with cancer is underreported, underdiagnosed, and undertreated.

The guidelines recommend that screening for the presence and severity of fatigue occur at the patient's initial contact with an oncology care provider, at appropriate intervals (including the follow-up period after treatment ends), and as clinically indicated. If the patient reports the presence of fatigue during screening, the fatigue should be quantified for future comparison. Although a variety of valid and reliable research instruments are available to measure the multiple dimensions of fatigue,[28] many are lengthy and burdensome for patients with CRF. The guidelines recommend measuring the intensity of fatigue by using a brief clinical instrument such as the 0 to 10 rating scale commonly used to measure pain. On the 0 to 10 scale, 1 to 3 is generally considered to be a mild level of fatigue; 4 to 6, moderate; and 7 to 10, severe. Although moderate levels of fatigue may cause distress and a reduction in activity level, severe fatigue levels are accompanied by a marked decrease in the ability to work and perform other activities of daily living.[29,30]

If the patient reports no fatigue or a mild level, education should be provided regarding fatigue as a possible or common side effect of treatment, especially if the patient is embarking on a treatment regimen known to cause fatigue. A plan to reevaluate the fatigue level as cancer treatment proceeds is appropriate because fatigue levels commonly rise in later stages of treatment. Patients and family members who do not receive this information often interpret decreased energy as a lack of treatment effectiveness or even a progression of disease, and the fatigue becomes a major source of worry.

If the screening process reveals a moderate or severe level of fatigue (4 to 10 on the 0 to 10 scale), the clinician should perform a focused history and physical examination as part of the primary evaluation phase. This evaluation includes an assessment of the patient's current disease status to rule out recurrence or progression and a review of current medications. Many of the medications used during cancer treatment, such as antiemetics and narcotics, may interact to produce lethargy and fatigue. Other medications the patient may be taking for comorbidities, such as β-blockers for cardiac conditions, may contribute to worsening of fatigue.[1] The focused history should also include an in-depth fatigue assessment that evaluates the intensity and pattern of fatigue, the duration and changes over time, the exacerbating or alleviating factors, and interference with daily activities.[31]

An essential component of the focused history is an assessment of treatable factors that are known to commonly contribute to fatigue. The factors identified by the NCCN practice guidelines panel are pain, emotional distress, sleep disturbance, anemia, nutritional status, activity level, and comorbidities.[1] The guidelines recommend that these factors be assessed and treated as a first step in managing fatigue. Although these seven factors may not be the primary cause of the patient's fatigue, because these factors are known to increase the intensity, as well as the distress, of fatigue, treating these factors—if they are present—as an initial approach may reduce the fatigue to a tolerable level.

Numerous studies have shown that fatigue commonly clusters with pain, emotional distress, or sleep disturbance.[32-34] Depression, in particular, has been associated with fatigue,[35,36] but the two can be distinguished by their different patterns over the course of cancer treatment: depression decreases and fatigue increases.[37]

Anemia commonly occurs in patients with cancer as a result of the neoplastic process or myelosuppressive therapies. Hemoglobin levels below 9 g/dL are often accompanied by severe fatigue, and improvements in energy are measurable with anemia correction to hemoglobin levels of 12 to 13 g/dL.[38]

Nutritional deficits related to anorexia, nausea, vomiting, diarrhea, or mucositis can lead to impaired protein synthesis, weight loss, muscle wasting, cachexia, weakness, and fatigue in patients with cancer.[39] Appropriate treatment with supplementation and correction of fluid and electrolyte imbalances provides nutrients necessary for energy. Consultation with a nutrition expert may be appropriate.

Patients with moderate to severe fatigue should be assessed for changes in their ability to tolerate exercise and other daily activities. A decrease in regular activity frequently accompanies cancer diagnosis and treatment.

The resulting deconditioning can be ameliorated by a progressive increase in activity, which could decrease fatigue.

Noncancer comorbidities are important potential contributors to CRF. The status and current management of identified comorbidities should be evaluated, and more effective treatment should be instituted if the comorbidity is not optimally managed. Comorbidities that require evaluation include infections; cardiac, pulmonary, renal, hepatic, neurologic, and endocrine dysfunction; and hypothyroidism.[1]

If any of the seven contributing factors known to be associated with CRF are identified, they should be treated and the fatigue should be reevaluated. If the patient continues to have moderate to severe levels of fatigue, treatment with nonpharmacologic and pharmacologic clinical interventions should be instituted in accordance with the patient's clinical status (e.g., receiving active cancer treatment, receiving disease-free long-term follow-up, or receiving palliative care at end of life). In many instances, a combination of approaches must be used to successfully reduce the fatigue and restore optimum functioning.

CLINICAL INTERVENTIONS

Interventions for the clinical management of CRF include both specific and general approaches. When an etiologic or contributing factor for CRF, such as anemia or insomnia, can be identified, it should be treated by using clinical practice guidelines as an initial approach to fatigue management. Guidelines provide "best care" information based on current evidence to support treatment. However, in many patients with cancer, no cause for fatigue can be readily identified beyond the disease and cancer therapies. In this situation the approach to management is a general one.

Pharmacologic Therapy

Pharmacologic interventions include administration of erythropoietin alfa for chemotherapy-induced anemia, administration of medications for cause-specific treatments, such as antidepressants for depression and thyroid hormone replacement for hypothyroidism. Corticosteroids have been shown to increase feelings of well-being and energy levels in some patients with advanced cancer,[40] and psychostimulants have been used on a limited basis to increase energy and decrease fatigue.

Anemia is a common cause of CRF; it occurs in a majority of patients receiving myelosuppressive chemotherapy.[41] Three community-based, nonrandomized, open-label studies[42-44] and two double-blind randomized trials comparing erythropoietin alfa[45,46] with placebo have shown a beneficial effect on CRF, transfusion requirements, and quality of life. Erythropoietin alfa is effective in subcutaneous doses of 10,000 U three times a week or 40,000 U weekly.[44] Cleeland and colleagues[38] demonstrated that the incremental increase in the patient's quality of life was highest when the hemoglobin level

Problems Common to Cancer and Its Therapy

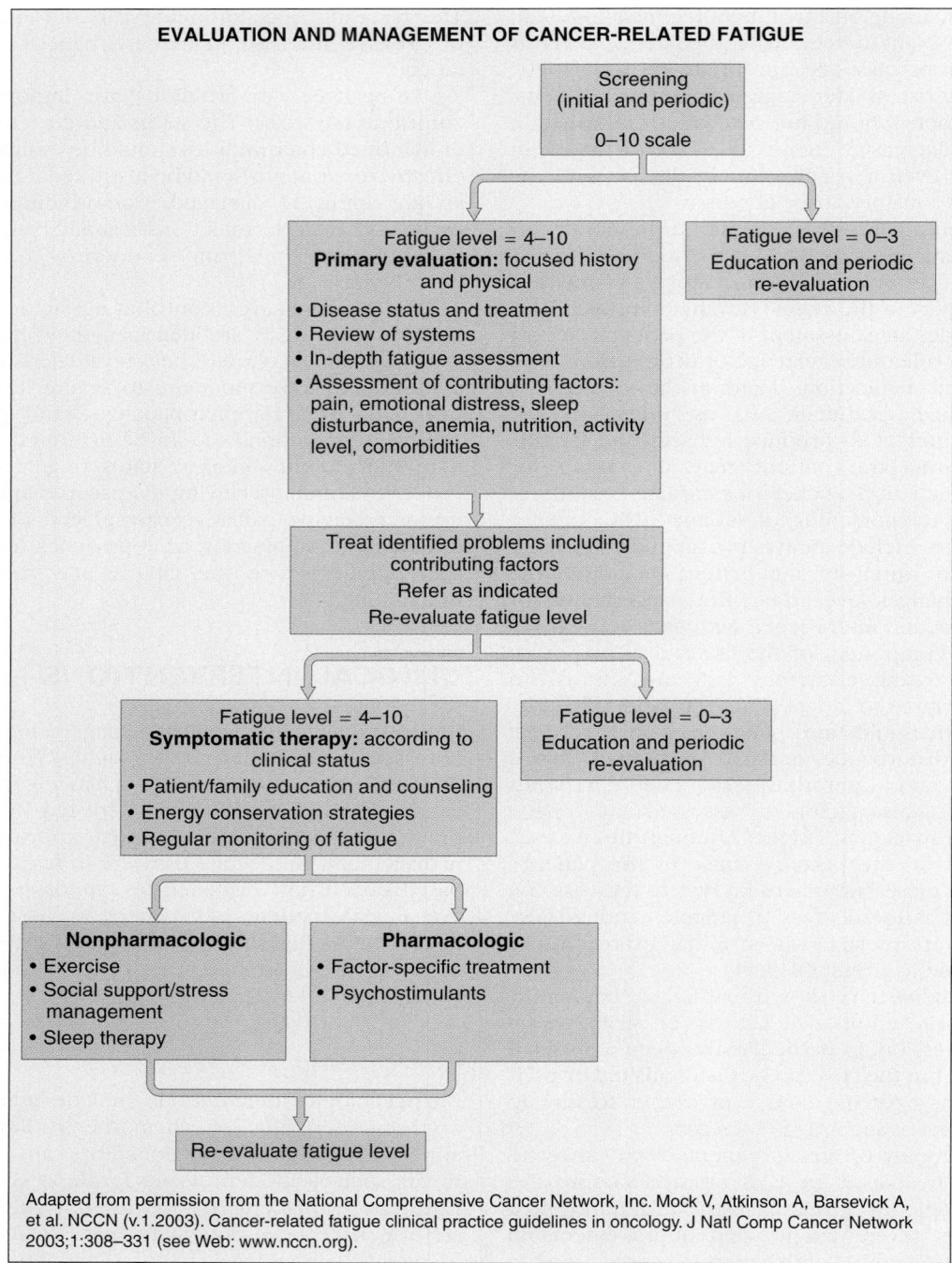

EVALUATION AND MANAGEMENT OF CANCER-RELATED FATIGUE

Screening
(initial and periodic)

0–10 scale

Fatigue level = 4–10
Primary evaluation: focused history and physical

- Disease status and treatment
- Review of systems
- In-depth fatigue assessment
- Assessment of contributing factors: pain, emotional distress, sleep disturbance, anemia, nutrition, activity level, comorbidities

Fatigue level = 0–3
Education and periodic re-evaluation

Treat identified problems including contributing factors
Refer as indicated
Re-evaluate fatigue level

Fatigue level = 4–10
Symptomatic therapy: according to clinical status

- Patient/family education and counseling
- Energy conservation strategies
- Regular monitoring of fatigue

Fatigue level = 0–3
Education and periodic re-evaluation

Nonpharmacologic
- Exercise
- Social support/stress management
- Sleep therapy

Pharmacologic
- Factor-specific treatment
- Psychostimulants

Re-evaluate fatigue level

Adapted from permission from the National Comprehensive Cancer Network, Inc. Mock V, Atkinson A, Barsevick A, et al. NCCN (v.1.2003). Cancer-related fatigue clinical practice guidelines in oncology. J Natl Comp Cancer Network 2003;1:308–331 (see Web: www.nccn.org).

rose from 11 to 12 g/dL. Two recent research reports[47,48] confirm the relationship between increases in hemoglobin during erythropoietin alfa treatment and quality-of-life improvements in patients with chemotherapy-related anemia. These studies provide good clinical evidence for reduction of CRF by returning the hemoglobin level in the patient with cancer and anemia to a more normal value. Published guidelines support treatment with erythropoietin alfa.[49,50] It is important to note that although most patients with anemia report significant fatigue and there is good evidence of fatigue reduction with anemia correction, the causes of CRF are multifactorial and many cancer patients with cancer and fatigue are not anemic.

Aside from the treatment with erythropoietin alfa, there are few controlled studies that have investigated pharmacologic therapy for CRF, although a few clinical reports have been published. Psychostimulants have been found to relieve fatigue in other chronic conditions such as multiple sclerosis[51] and human immunodeficiency virus infection,[52] but the data are limited regarding efficacy in CRF.

Methylphenidate has been found to be effective in reducing opiate-induced somnolence, acute depression, and cognitive dysfunction in the palliative care setting[53]; but only two studies have described use of methylphenidate as treatment for fatigue.[54,55] In both studies, successful reduction in fatigue levels was reported, but sample sizes were small (≤12) and study designs were flawed.

Pemoline, a central nervous system stimulant similar to methylphenidate, has shown some effectiveness in relief of fatigue in patients with multiple sclerosis (46% response) but has not been tested in patients with cancer.[56] In addition, serious liver problems have been reported in some patients receiving this drug. Modafinil has been used to treat narcolepsy, and some reports suggest that it may be helpful in managing CRF,[57] but no clinical trials have been conducted.

In summary, the evidence is strong for pharmacologic treatment for CRF in the case of erythropoietin alfa for correction of anemia, but evidence is insufficient to support use of psychostimulants. More research is needed before recommendations can be made regarding use of psychostimulants to manage CRF.

Nonpharmacologic Therapy

Nonpharmacologic interventions for CRF are notable in that they are effective, safe, and usually inexpensive; however, they have not been widely recognized for their efficacy, nor are they included as standard of care. Nonpharmacologic treatments include alterations in activity and rest—including exercise, sleep therapy, and energy conservation—and psychosocial support programs and coping strategies to reduce stress.

Strong evidence from clinical trials supports the efficacy of exercise to manage fatigue in patients with cancer (Table 42-1). The theory that supports exercise as a treatment for CRF suggests that the combined effects of cytotoxic treatments and reductions in physical activity during lengthy, often debilitating treatments lead to a decreased capacity for physical performance. Thus even ordinary activities are perceived as fatiguing. Regular exercise, even at a moderate level, can maintain and increase functional capacity and result in greater exercise tolerance as evidenced by increased cardiac output, reduced heart rate, and less fatigue as less energy is required to perform equivalent work. If the patient has severe deconditioning, advanced disease, or significant comorbidities, referral to a rehabilitation program supervised by a physical therapist or specialist in physical medicine or rehabilitation is indicated.

The cumulative evidence from studies of exercise in patients with cancer receiving active cancer treatment, as well as in survivors, demonstrates that this health-promoting activity has many positive benefits and few risks for patients with cancer. Table 42-1 displays the studies testing effects of exercise on CRF published in English-language journals since 1985. All of these investigations demonstrated significantly lower levels of fatigue in subjects who exercised when compared with control subjects. Furthermore, emotional distress and sleep disturbance were significantly lower in exercisers in the studies in which these outcomes were measured.

EXERCISE PRESCRIPTION FOR CANCER-RELATED FATIGUE

At the Sidney Kimmel Comprehensive Cancer Center at Johns Hopkins, we have evaluated a moderate symptom-limited walking exercise program to manage cancer-related fatigue in patients with solid tumors who are beginning outpatient treatment with adjuvant chemotherapy or radiation therapy. After initial testing with more than 100 patients with breast cancer, we have extended the program to include patients with prostate and colorectal cancer.

On screening during the cancer therapy planning visits, we identify patients who do not have metastatic disease or comorbidities that would contraindicate a regular walking program. In consultation with the patient's oncologist and an exercise physiologist, our oncology nurses teach the walking exercise program to consenting patients. Patients are given an individually tailored exercise prescription to follow throughout their cancer treatment. The initial prescription is to walk briskly for 15 to 20 minutes per day on 5 to 6 days of the week at a moderate intensity (target heart rate range of 60% to 80% of maximum heart rate), but the regimen is modified by the patient's age, physical condition, and planned cancer therapy. Each walking session begins and ends with 3 to 5 minutes at a slow pace as "warm-up" and "cool-down" to protect the heart. Patients progress, as tolerated, to a maximum of 30 minutes of walking on 5 to 6 days per week. Very debilitated or sedentary patients may need to begin by walking for 5- to 10-minute sessions twice daily until they can tolerate longer periods. We contact patients every 2 weeks to discuss their progress with the program and the side effects of cancer treatment. The exercise program is adjusted as indicated. Patients are taught how to exercise safely—including how to monitor pulse rate—and when to contact the oncology care team to report signs and symptoms (e.g., dizziness, chest pain). Patients are encouraged to walk with a family member or friend at a convenient location—neighborhood, shopping mall, or community exercise facility. The program is well accepted by patients, the cost is low, and walking is beneficial and safe. Our patients have experienced no adverse events that could be attributed to the exercise program.

The study sample sizes were small compared with most cancer treatment trials yet revealed very significant differences between groups; fatigue levels were found to be 40% to 50% lower in exercising subjects. Aerobic exercise interventions have consistently exhibited a powerful effect on CRF in these generally sedentary samples. All of the forms of exercise were aerobic and were primarily moderate home-based walking programs[17,23,58-61] with some laboratory treadmill or exercise bicycle interventions.[62-64] Research has indicated that patients do better in the home-based programs,[65] which are more convenient and cost-effective, although they lack the control of a supervised exercise regimen. Intensity of exercise varied in the studies but remained in a range known to achieve a training effect: 60% to 85% of maximum heart rate in sessions of about 30 minutes daily for 3 to 4 days a week.[66] In the 2001 report by Schwartz

TABLE 42-1

Effects of Exercise on Fatigue in Patients with Cancer

AUTHORS	SAMPLE	DESIGN	TYPE OF EXERCISE	RESULTS	LIMITATIONS / COMMENTS
MacVicar & Winningham, 1986	Patients with breast cancer CT/no staging data/ (N = 10); Nonpatients/ (N = 6)	Quasi-experimental, 3-group	Laboratory cycle ergometer 3x/wk for 10 wk 60%–85% HR max.	↑ Functional capacity ↓ Mood disturbance & fatigue in exercising patients (n = 6), as well as exercising nonpatients (n = 6). ↑ Mood disturbance in pt control subjects (n = 4).	Nonrandom group assignment. Small sample size.
Mock et al., 1994	Patients with breast cancer CT/stage I & II/N = 14	Experimental	Home-based walking 4-5x/ wk @ 30 min plus support group	↑ Walking ability in exercisers. ↓ Psychosocial distress compared with control subjects. ↓ Fatigue in exercisers.	Effects of exercise alone cannot be determined. Fatigue one-item VAS. Exercise was self-reported. Small sample size.
Mock et al., 1997	Patients with breast cancer RT/stage I & II/N = 46	RCCT	Home-based walking 4-5x/ wk @ 30 min.	↑ Walking ability in exercisers. ↓ Fatigue and other symptoms compared with control subjects.	Exercise was self-reported.
Dimeo et al., 1997	Mixed hematologic malignancies & solid tumors. Post-PBSCT survivors/N = 32	Quasi-experimental	Treadmill walking 80% HR max.	↑ Functional capacity in exercisers. ↓ Fatigue in exercisers by anecdote.	No fatigue measures.
Dimeo, Rumberger, & Keul, 1998	Mixed cancer survivors. Post-PBSCT/N = 5	I-Group, pretest/ post-test	Treadmill walking 80% HR max.	↑ Functional capacity & distance walked in exercisers. ↓ Fatigue by anecdote.	No fatigue measures. Small sample size.
Dimeo et al., 1999	Mixed hematologic malignancies & solid tumors PBSCT/N = 59	RCCT	Bed cycle ergometer 50% HR max.	↓ Fatigue and psych distress in exercisers.	No exercise outcomes reported.
Schwartz, 1999, 2000	Patients with breast cancer CT/stage I-III/N = 27	I-Group, pretest/ post-test	Home-based walking or patient choice 3x/wk	↑ Pretest to post-test walking ability. ↑ QOL & less fatigue in active exercisers vs noncompliers.	60% of subjects adhered to program. Single-group design.
Porock, 2000	Home hospice patients with advanced cancer N = 9	I-Group, pretest / post-test	Varied activities—walking, dancing, etc. for 2 wk	↑ Activity level in all. No ↑ in fatigue; trend of ↑ QOL & ↓ anxiety.	No control group. Small sample size.
Mock et al., 2001	Patients with breast cancer CT/RT/stage I-III/N = 50	RCCT	Home-based walking 4-5x/wk @ 30 min	↑ Walking ability in exercisers. ↓ Fatigue and other symptoms compared with controls.	Exercise was self-reported. 70% adherence in exercise group.
Schwartz et al., 2001	Patients with breast cancer CT/stage II/N = 61	I-Group, pretest/ post-test	Home-based walking or patient choice/8 wk 3-4x/wk @ 15-30 min	↑ Pretest to post-test walking ability. ↓ Fatigue in active exercisers.	61% of subjects adhered to program. Single-group design.
Mock et al., 2002	Patients with breast cancer CT/RT/stage I-III N = 111	RCCT	Home-based walking 4-5x/wk @ 30 min	↑ Walking ability in exercisers. ↓ Fatigue and other symptoms compared with controls.	Exercise was self-reported. 72% adherence in exercise group.
Schwartz, Thompson, & Masood, 2002	Patients with melanoma Interferon-α N = 12 plus 16 historical controls	Quasi-experimental	Patient selected 4x/wk @ 15 min plus methylphenidate 20 mg daily	↑ Functional ability. ↓ Fatigue and cognitive dysfunction in exercisers.	100% of subjects adhered to exercise: 67% adhered to methylphenidate. Small sample size.

CT, chemotherapy; HR, heart rate; PBSCT, peripheral blood stem cell transplant; QOL, quality of life; RCCT, randomized controlled clinical trial; RT, radiation therapy; VAS, visual analog scale.
Adapted with permission from National Comprehensive Cancer Network, Inc. Mock V, Atkinson A, Barsevick A, et al. NCCN (v. I.2003). Cancer-related fatigue clinical practice guidelines in oncology. J Natl Comp Cancer Network, 2003; I:308-331 (see Web: www.nccn.org).

and colleagues,[61] a dose-response pattern was demonstrated with fatigue levels inversely related to three increasing levels of exercise observed in the subjects. This suggests that a wide range of doses of exercise may be effective with no minimum effective dose yet established; therefore clinicians can be flexible in tailoring the exercise recommendation to accommodate the needs and conditions of individual patients. The Schwartz study also showed that patients who exercised more than 60 minutes per session were more likely to report increased levels of fatigue, suggesting that there is a maximum effective dose. Although no adverse events were reported in any of the studies, high-risk patients with serious comorbidities were excluded from participation.

The lengths of the exercise programs varied, but most began at the initiation of cancer treatment and continued until the end of adjuvant chemotherapy, radiation therapy, or hospital discharge after peripheral blood stem cell transplantation, demonstrating a beneficial effect on fatigue levels even during a 6-week program of radiation therapy for patients with breast cancer.[59]

Adherence to exercise programs is a challenge for both healthy and chronically ill populations. In the studies of patients with cancer, adherence ranged from 60% to 80% in the home-based programs to 100% in laboratory studies, a marked contrast to the 50% drop-out rate for healthy individuals who begin an exercise program.[67] Apparently patients with cancer are sensitized to the potential beneficial effects of health promotion activities.

The published exercise studies of patients with cancer have notable limitations. The majority of the studies were samples of female patients with breast cancer, and ethnic diversity and age ranges were limited. Thus the study results have limited generalizability to other cancer diagnoses, older individuals or children, and varied ethnic groups. Another limitation of the studies is that the exercise interventions were begun at a specific point in patients' cancer therapy—either the beginning or the end—regardless of their level of fatigue. There is limited information about the effectiveness and feasibility of initiating an exercise program for patients who already have high levels of fatigue and have difficulty performing activities of daily living. Only one small study (n = 5) involved patients referred to an exercise program because they had debilitating fatigue. Preventing CRF by initiating regular exercise early in the course of cancer treatment may be more effective than managing high levels of fatigue after it develops. Two review articles of exercise in patients with cancer have indicated that exercise facilitates rehabilitation and improves quality of life.[68,69] Other studies of exercise in patients with cancer have demonstrated improvements in functional capacity[65,70,71] and mood state.[72]

Rest and Sleep

Oncology care providers commonly recommend additional rest and sleep to patients with cancer who report distressing levels of CRF.[73] Patients who use additional rest and sleep to manage fatigue report that it helps, but does not relieve the symptom.[74] Several studies in which actigraphy was used to measure activity and sleep have demonstrated that patients with cancer spend increased time resting and sleeping but their pattern of sleep is often severely disrupted with awakenings nearly every hour.[22,75] Frequent night awakenings were accompanied by lower levels of daytime activity, more daytime napping, and high levels of fatigue.[76] The potential for deconditioning resulting from reductions in activity during lengthy cancer treatments may be an important contributing factor to CRF. Although sleep disturbances have been identified as a neglected problem in oncology,[77] the relationship between sleep problems and CRF has been inadequately explored. Only one pilot study in which a sleep intervention was tested has been published.[78]

Energy Conservation

Energy conservation is an intervention that utilizes planned management of personal energy resources to prevent their depletion. Strategies include priority setting, use of labor-saving devices, balancing periods of rest and activity, and delegating activities of lesser importance.[79] Energy conservation may be a particularly useful intervention for patients with advanced disease or those with significant weakness or debilitating fatigue. Although research is limited, results of a pilot study testing an energy conservation intervention has been published and indicates beneficial effects.[79]

Stress Reduction

Studies of psychosocial interventions aimed at stress reduction and improved coping have also demonstrated reductions in fatigue (Table 42-2). Since both depression and anxiety may be characterized by fatigue, it has been proposed that CRF is a response to the stress of cancer diagnosis and treatment through activation of the hypothalamic-pituitary-adrenal axis.[18] Since it is also evident that high levels of fatigue may lead to emotional distress when valued roles and activities are affected, the precise relationship between emotional distress and fatigue is not clearly understood.

The psychosocial interventions tested in the studies listed in Table 42-2 include support groups,[80,81] individual counseling,[82-84] a comprehensive coping strategy,[85] and stress management training.[86] The studies were randomized controlled clinical trials with adequate sample sizes and included a variety of cancer populations. All studies demonstrated significant effects of the intervention on fatigue levels. A limitation of the studies is that in nearly every case fatigue was a secondary end point measured by either a single item or a subscale of an instrument used to measure emotional distress.

Conclusion

Fatigue is the most prevalent symptom reported by patients with cancer and the source of much distress for them. Fatigue may have profound effects on functional status and quality of life. However, clinical evaluation and management of this disturbing side effect of cancer and

Problems Common to Cancer and Its Therapy

II

TABLE 42-2

Effects of Psychosocial Interventions on Fatigue in Patients with Cancer

AUTHORS	SAMPLE	DESIGN	INTERVENTION	RESULTS	COMMENTS
Spiegel, Bloom, & Yalom, 1981	Patients with breast cancer stage IV N = 86	RCCT	Support group weekly for 1 yr	↓ Anxiety, fatigue, confusion, & mood disturbance in experimental group	Fatigue measured by subscale on POMS
Forester, Kornfeld, & Fleiss, 1985	Patients with mixed cancer in RT N = 100	RCCT	Individual psychotherapy weekly for 10 wk	↓ Emotional & physical symptoms in experimental group	Fatigue measured by single item on the schedule of affective disorders & schizophrenia 25% dropped out of control group.
Fawzy et al., 1990	Patients with melanoma after surgery stage I & II N = 66	RCCT	Support group (incl education & stress management) weekly for 6 wk	↑ Coping & vigor in experimental group at 6 wk ↓ Fatigue, depression, & mood disturbance @ 6 months follow-up	Fatigue measured by subscale on POMS.
Fawzy, 1995	Patients with melanoma stage I & II N = 61	RCCT	Individual education & support by RN 3 hr	↓ Fatigue, anxiety, & mood disturbance in experimental group	Fatigue measured by subscale on POMS.
Gaston-Johansson et al., 2000	Patients with breast cancer with ABMT N = 110	RCCT	Comprehensive coping strategy program*	↓ Fatigue & nausea in experimental group.	Covariates controlled. Fatigue measured by VAS.
Given et al., 2002	Patients with mixed solid tumors & lymphoma in CT stage I–IV N = 113	RCCT	Tailored behavioral intervention in 10 contacts/ 18 wk	↓ Fatigue and pain ↑ Physical and social functioning in experimental group at 20 wk	Fatigue measured by the Symptom Experience Scale (measures "present" or "absent" only).
Jacobsen et al., 2002	Patients with mixed cancer in CT N = 411	RCCT, 3-group	Professionally administered stress management training or patient self-administered stress management training	Better physical functioning ↑ Vitality & better mental health in self-administered intervention compared with usual care or professional intervention	Fatigue measured as "vitality" on MOS SF-36.

*Preparatory information, cognitive restructuring, relaxation with imagery.
ABMT, autologous bone marrow transplantation; CT, chemotherapy; MOS SF-36, Medical Outcome Study Short Form–36; POMS, profile of mood state scale; RCCT, randomized controlled clinical trial; RT, radiation therapy; VAS, visual analog scale.
Adapted with permission from National Comprehensive Cancer Network, Inc. Mock V, Atkinson A, Barsevick A, et al. NCCN (v.1.2003). Cancer-related fatigue clinical practice guidelines in oncology. J Natl Comp Cancer Network, 2003;1:308–331 (see Web:www.nccn.org).

cancer treatment have been limited as a function of both patient and care provider barriers. Patients have been hesitant to report fatigue, and clinicians have been unaware of effective treatments.

Effective management of CRF begins with informed and supportive oncology care providers who perform initial and regular screening for fatigue and provide treatment as indicated by the patient's fatigue level. When patient fatigue levels are mild, education about fatigue is indicated. When fatigue levels are moderate or severe, the initial screening is expanded to include a focused evaluation of current disease and treatment status, review of body systems, and an in-depth fatigue assessment. The patient should be assessed for the presence of treatable contributing factors such as pain, emotional distress, sleep disturbance, anemia, nutritional deficits, decreased activity level, and unmanaged comorbidities. If any of these conditions are present, they should be treated as an initial step, and the fatigue should be re-evaluated. If none of these factors are present or if fatigue levels remain moderate or severe, fatigue management strategies should be considered as appropriate for the patient's clinical status.

Evidence-based interventions for managing CRF include correction of anemia, moderate exercise regimens, and psychosocial support programs. A combination approach may be needed, and referral to other members of the multidisciplinary team should be considered. Although CRF is common and expected, it can be managed and does not need to be distressful and disruptive to quality of life.

Several important gaps exist in our knowledge of fatigue and fatigue management. These are reflected in the recommendations for future research presented in Table 42-3. However, evidence-based practice guidelines are available to guide clinical care of patients with CRF, and health care professionals are increasingly aware of the importance of addressing this distressing symptom.

REFERENCES

1. Mock V, Atkinson A, Barsevick A, et al: Cancer-related fatigue clinical practice guidelines in oncology. J Natl Comp Cancer Network, 2003;1:308-331. Also available at http://www.nccn.org
2. Glaus A, Crow R, Hammond S: A qualitative study to explore the concept of fatigue/tiredness in cancer patients and in healthy individuals. Eur J Cancer Care 1996;5(suppl 2):8-23.
3. Cella D, Davis K, Breitbart W, Curt G: Cancer-related fatigue: Prevalence of proposed diagnostic criteria in a United States sample of cancer survivors. J Clin Oncol 2001;19:3385-3391.
4. Jacobsen PB, Hann DM, Azzarello LM, et al: Fatigue in women receiving adjuvant chemotherapy for breast cancer: Characteristics, course, and correlates. J Pain Symptom Manage 1999;18:233-242.
5. Sitzia J, Huggins L: Side effects of cyclophosphamide, methotrexate, 5-fluorouracil (CMF) chemotherapy for breast cancer. Cancer Pract 1998;6:13-21.
6. Malik UR, Makower DF, Wadler S: Interferon-mediated fatigue. Cancer 2001;9(suppl 6):1664-1668.
7. Curt G, Breitbart W, Cella D, et al: Impact of cancer-related fatigue on the lives of patients: New finding from the fatigue coalition. Oncologist 2000;5:353-360.
8. Vogelzang N, Breitbart W, Cella D, et al: Patient, caregiver, and oncologist perceptions of cancer-related fatigue: Results of a tri-part assessment survey. Semin Hematol 1997;34(suppl 2):4-12.
9. Bower J, Ganz P, Desmond K: Fatigue in breast cancer survivors: Occurrence, correlates, and impact on quality of life. J Clin Oncol 2000;18:743-753.
10. Broeckel JA, Jacobsen PB, Horton J, Balducci L, Lyman GH: Characteristics and correlates of fatigue after adjuvant chemotherapy for breast cancer. J Clin Oncol 1998;16:1689-1696.
11. Andrykowski MA, Curran SL, Lightner R: Off-treatment fatigue in breast cancer survivors: A controlled comparison. J Behav Med 1998;21:1-18.
12. Maughan TS, James RD, Kerr DJ, et al: Comparison of survival, palliation, and quality of life with three chemotherapy regimens in metastatic colorectal cancer: A multicentre randomized trial. Lancet 2000;359:1555-1563.
13. Walsh D, Donnelly S, Rybicki L: The symptoms of advanced cancer: Relationship to age, gender, and performance status in 1,000 patients. Support Care Cancer 2000;8:175-179.
14. Wolfe J, Grier HE, Klar N, et al: Symptoms and suffering at the end of life in children with cancer. N Engl J Med 2000;342:326-333.
15. Given B, Given C, Azzouz F, Stommel M: Physical functioning of elderly cancer patients prior to diagnosis and following initial treatment. Nurs Res 2001;50:222-232.
16. Nail L, Beck S, Lindau K: The nature of change using the functional performance index (FPI) with patients undergoing cancer treatment. Oncol Nurs Forum 2002;29:337 (abstract).
17. Mock V, McCorkle R, Ropka ME, Pickett M, Poniatowski B: Fatigue and physical functioning during breast cancer treatment. Oncol Nurs Forum 2002;29:338 (abstract).
18. Gutstein HB: The biologic basis of fatigue. Cancer 2001;92(suppl 1):1678-1683.
19. Morrow GR, Andrews PLR, Hickok JT, Roscoe JA, Matteson S: Fatigue associated with cancer and its treatment. Support Care Cancer 2002;10:389-398.
20. Blesch K, Paice J, Wickham R, et al: Correlates of fatigue in people with breast or lung cancer. Oncol Nurs Forum 1991;8:81-87.
21. Greene D, Nail LM, Fieler VK, Dudgeon D, Jones LS: A comparison of patient-reported side effects among three chemotherapy regimens for breast cancer patients. Cancer Pract 1998;6:143-152.
22. Berger AM: Patterns of fatigue and activity and rest during adjuvant breast cancer chemotherapy. Oncol Nurs Forum 1998;25:51-62.
23. Schwartz AL: Daily fatigue patterns and effect of exercise in women with breast cancer. Cancer Pract 2000;8:16-24.
24. Sadler IJ, Jacobsen PB: Progress in understanding fatigue associated with breast cancer treatment. Cancer Invest 2001;19:723-731.

TABLE 42-3

Recommendations for Future Cancer-related Fatigue Research

1. Additional intervention testing research, especially with pharmacotherapeutics, psychosocial interventions, sleep quality therapies, and conservation of energy approaches
2. Use of more rigorous research designs with larger sample sizes, control groups including healthy control subjects and attentional control subjects as appropriate, greater standardization of interventions to facilitate replication and increase internal validity
3. Targeting of more diverse populations of patients with cancer and selection of diverse samples—especially in regard to ethnicity, socioeconomic status, age, and type of cancer diagnosis
4. Exploration of fatigue interventions in recurrent disease and palliative care
5. Use of more objective instruments and outcomes to increase validity and reliability (e.g., actigraphy to measure activity and sleep, biochemical markers for fatigue)
6. Theory-based research with a focus on elucidating the mediating mechanisms for every intervention to facilitate our understanding of CRF
7. Investigation of secondary outcomes of fatigue interventions such as quality of life, return to work, use of health care resources, sleep quality, mood state, and survival

CRF, Cancer-related fatigue.

25. Irvine D, Vincent L, Graydon JE, et al: Fatigue in women with breast cancer receiving radiation therapy. Cancer Nurs 1998;21:127–135.

26. Greenberg DB, Sawicka J, Eisenthal S, Ross D: Fatigue syndrome due to localized radiation. J Pain Sympt Manage 1992;7:38–45.

27. Woo B, Dibble SL, Piper BF, Keating SB, Weiss MC: Differences in fatigue by treatment methods in women with breast cancer. Oncol Nurs Forum 1998;25:915–920.

28. Piper BF: Measuring fatigue. In Frank-Stromberg, M, Olsen SH (eds): Instruments for clinical health care research, 3rd ed. Sudbury, Mass, Jones & Bartlett 2004, pp 538–569.

29. Cleeland CS, Wang XS: Measuring and understanding fatigue. Oncology 1999;13:91–97.

30. Mendoza TR, Wang XS, Cleeland CS, et al: The rapid assessment of fatigue severity in cancer patients: Use of the Brief Fatigue Inventory. Cancer 1999;85:1186–1196.

31. Portenoy RK, Itri LM: Cancer-related fatigue: Guidelines for evaluation and management. Oncologist 1999;4:1–10.

32. Dodd MJ, Miaskowski C, Paul SM: Symptom clusters and their effect on the functional status of patients with cancer. Oncol Nurs Forum 2001;28:465–470.

33. Berger AM, Walker SN: An explanatory model of fatigue in women receiving adjuvant breast cancer chemotherapy. Nurs Res 2001;50:42–52.

34. State-of-the-Science Conference on Symptom Management in Cancer Pain, Depression, & Fatigue. Presented by the National Cancer Institute and with National Institutes of Health Office of Medical Applications of Research. Available at http://www.consensus.nih.gov

35. Hopwood P, Stephens RJ: Depression in patients with lung cancer: Prevalence and risk factors derived from quality-of-life data. J Clin Oncol 2000:18: 893–903.

36. Loge JH, Abramsen AF, Ekeberg O, et al: Fatigue and psychiatric morbidity among Hodgkin's disease survivors. J Pain Symptom Manage 2000;19:91–99.

37. Visser MR, Smets EM: Fatigue, depression and quality of life in cancer patients: How are they related? Support Care Cancer 1998;6:101–108.

38. Cleeland CS, Demetri GD, Glaspy J, et al: Identifying hemoglobin level for optimal quality of life: Results of an incremental analysis (abstract). Proc Am Soc Clin Oncol 1999;18:574.

39. Baracos VE: Management of muscle wasting in cancer-associated cachexia: Understanding gained from experimental studies. Cancer 2001;92(suppl 6):1669–1677.

40. Bruera E, Macmillan K, Kuehn N, et al: A controlled trial of megestrol acetate on appetite, caloric intake, nutritional status, and other symptoms in patients with advanced cancer. Cancer 1990;66:1279–1282.

41. Groopman J, Itri L: Chemotherapy-induced anemia in adults. J Nal Cancer Inst 1999;91:1616–1634.

42. Demetri G, Kris M, Wasde J, Degos L, Cella D: Quality-of-life benefit in chemotherapy patients treated with epoetin alfa is independent of disease response or tumor type: Results from a prospective community oncology study. J Clin Oncol 1998;16:3412–3425.

43. Glaspy J, Bukowski R, Steinberg D, Taylor C, Tchekmedyian S, Vadhan-Raj S: Impact of therapy with epoetin alfa on clinical outcomes in patients with nonmyeloid malignancies during cancer chemotherapy in community oncology practice. J Clin Oncol 1997;15:1218–1234.

44. Gabrilove JL, Cleeland CS, Livingston RB, Sarokham B, Winer E, Einhorn L: Clinical evaluation of once-weekly dosing of epoetin alfa in chemotherapy patients: Improvements in hemoglobin and quality of life are similar to three-times weekly dosing. J Clin Oncol 2001;19:2875–2882.

45. Österborg A, Brandberg Y, Molostova V, et al: Randomized double-blind, placebo-controlled trial of recombinant human erythropoietin, epoetin beta, in hematologic malignancies. J Clin Oncol 2002;20:2486–2494.

46. Littlewood TJ, Bajetta E, Nortier JWR, et al: Effects of epoetin alfa on hematologic parameters and quality of life in cancer patients receiving nonplatinum chemotherapy: Results of a randomized, double-blind, placebo-controlled trial. J Clin Oncol 2001;19:2865–2874.

47. Crawford J, Cella D, Cleeland CS, et al: Relationship between changes in hemoglobin level and quality of life during chemotherapy in anemic cancer patients receiving epoetin alfa therapy. Cancer 2002;95:888–895.

48. Fallowfield L, Gagnon D, Zagari M, et al: Multivariate regression analyses of data from a randomized, double-blind, placebo-controlled study confirm quality of life benefit of epoetin alfa in patients receiving non-platinum chemotherapy. Br J Cancer 2002;87:1341–1353.

49. Sabbatini P, Cella D, Chanan-Khan A, et al: Cancer and treatment-related anemia: Report of the National Comprehensive Cancer Network Practice Guidelines Anemia Panel (v.1.2002) (posted on Web at www.nccn.org).

50. Rizzo JD, Lichtin AE, Woolf SH, et al: Use of epoetin in patients with cancer: Evidence-based clinical practice guidelines of the American Society of Clinical Oncology and the American Society of Hematology. J Clin Oncol 2002;20:1–25.

51. Weinshenker BG, Penman M, Bass B, et al: A double-blind, randomized crossover trial of pemoline in fatigue associated with multiple sclerosis. Neurology 1992;42:1468–1471.

52. Breitbart W, Rosenfeld B, Kaim M, Funesti-Esch J: A randomized, double-blind, placebo-controlled trial of psychostimulants for the treatment of fatigue in ambulatory patients with human immunodeficiency virus disease. Arch Intern Med 2001;161:411–420.

53. Rozans M, Dreisbach A, Lertora JLL, Kahn MJ: Palliative uses of methylphenidate in patients with cancer: A review. J Clin Oncol 2002;20:335–339.

54. Sarhill N, Walsh D, Nelson KA, et al: Methylphenidate for fatigue in advanced cancer: A prospective open-label pilot study. Am J Hosp Palliat Care 2001;18:187–192.

55. Schwartz AL, Thompson JA, Masood N: Interferon-induced fatigue in patients with melanoma: A pilot study of exercise and methylphenidate. Oncology Nurs Forum August Online Exclusive 2002;291–317.

56. Homsi J, Walsh D, Nelson KA: Psychostimulants in supportive care. Supportive Care Cancer 2000;8:385–397.

57. Cox JM, Pappagallo M, Modafinil: A gift to portmanteau. Am J Hospice Palliative Care 2001;18:408–410.

58. Mock V, Burke MB, Sheehan PK, et al: A nursing rehabilitation program for women with breast cancer receiving adjuvant chemotherapy. Oncol Nurs Forum 1994;21:899–908.

59. Mock V, Dow KH, Meares C, et al: Effects of exercise on fatigue, physical functioning, and emotional distress during radiation therapy for breast cancer. Oncol Nurs Forum 1997;24:991–1000.

60. Mock V, Pickett M, Ropka M, et al: Fatigue and quality of life outcomes of exercise during cancer treatment. Cancer Practice 2001; 9:119–127.

61. Schwartz AL, Mori M, Gao R, Nail LM, King ME: Exercise reduces daily fatigue in women with breast cancer receiving chemotherapy. Med Sci Sports Exerc 2001;33:718–723.

62. Dimeo FC, Stieglitz R-D, Novelli-Fischer U, et al: Effects of physical activity on the fatigue and psychologic status of cancer patients during chemotherapy. Cancer 1999;85:2273–2277.

63. Dimeo FC, Tilmann MHM, Bertz H, et al: Aerobic exercise in the rehabilitation of cancer patients after high dose chemotherapy and autologous peripheral stem cell transplantation. Cancer 1997;79:1717–1722.

64. MacVicar SB, Winningham ML: Promoting the functional capacity of cancer patients. Cancer Bull 1986;38:235–239.

65. Segal R, Evans W, Johnson D: Structured exercise improves physical functioning in women with stages I and II breast cancer: Results of randomized controlled trial. J Clin Oncol 2001;19:657–665.

66. American College of Sports Medicine: ACSM's exercise management for persons with chronic diseases and disabilities. Champaign, Ill, Human Kinetics, 1997.

67. Dishman RK: Overview. In Dishman RK (ed): Exercise adherence. Champaign, Ill, Human Kinetics, 1998, 1–9.

68. Courneya KS, Friedenreich CM: Physical exercise and quality of life following cancer diagnosis: A literature review. Ann Behav Med 1999;21:171–179.

69. Pinto BM, Maruyam NC: Exercise in the rehabilitation of breast cancer survivors. Psychooncology 1999;8:191–206.

70. MacVicar MG, Winningham ML, Nickel JL: Effects of aerobic interval training on cancer patients' functional capacity. Nurs Res 1989;38:348–351.

71. Dimeo F, Fetscher S, Lange W, et al: Effects of aerobic exercise on the physical performance and incidence of treatment-related complications after high-dose chemotherapy. Blood 1997;90:3390–3394.

72. Segar ML, Katch VL, Roth RS, et al: The effect of aerobic exercise on self-esteem and depressive and anxiety symptoms among breast cancer survivors. Oncol Nurs Forum 1998;25:107–113.

73. Stone P, Ream E, Richardson A, et al: Cancer-related fatigue—a difference of opinion? Results of a multicentre survey of healthcare professionals, patients and caregivers. Eur J Cancer Care (Engl) 2003;12:20–27.

74. Graydon JE, Bubela N, Irvine D, Vincent L: Fatigue-reducing strategies used by patients receiving treatment for cancer. Cancer Nurs 1995;18:23–28.

75. Young-McCaughan S, Mays MZ, Arzola SM, et al: Change in exercise tolerance, activity and sleep patterns, and quality of life in patients with cancer participating in a structured exercise program. Oncol Nurs Forum 2003;30:1–12.

76. Berger AM, Farr L: The influence of daytime inactivity and nighttime restlessness on cancer-related fatigue. Oncol Nurs Forum 1999;26:1663–1671.

77. Savard J, Morin CM: Insomnia in the context of cancer: A review of a neglected problem. J Clin Oncol 2001;19:895–908.

78. Berger AM, Higginbotham P, VonEssen S, Kuhn B, Piper B, Agrawal S: Outcomes of a sleep intervention following adjuvant chemotherapy (abstract). Oncol Nurs Forum 2002;29:333.

79. Barsevick AM, Whitmer K, Sweeney C, Nail LM: A pilot study examining energy conservation for cancer treatment-related fatigue. Cancer Nurs 2002;25:333–341.

80. Fawzy FI, Cousins N, Fawzy NW, Kemeny M, Elashoff R, Morton D: A structured psychiatric intervention for cancer patients: I. Changes over time in methods of coping and affective disturbance. Arch Gen Psychiatry 1990;47:720–725.

81. Spiegel D, Bloom JR, Yalom ID: Group support for metastatic cancer patients: A randomized prospective outcome study. Arch Gen Psychiatry 1981;38:527–533.

82. Fawzy NW: A psychoeducational nursing intervention to enhance coping and affective state in newly diagnosed malignant melanoma patients. Cancer Nurs 1995;18:427–438.

83. Forester B, Kornfeld DS, Fleiss JL: Psychotherapy during radiotherapy: Effects on emotional and physical distress. Am J Psychiatry 1985;142:22–27.

84. Given B, Given CW, McCorkle R, et al: Pain and fatigue management: Results of a nursing randomized clinical trial. Oncoly Nurs Forum 2002;29:949–956.

85. Gaston-Johansson F, Fall-Dickson JM, Nanda J, et al: The effectiveness of the comprehensive coping strategy program on clinical outcomes in breast cancer autologous bone marrow transplantation. Cancer Nurs 2000;23:277–285.

86. Jacobsen PB, Meade CD, Stein KD, Chirikos TN, Small BJ, Ruckdeschel JC: Efficacy and costs of two forms of stress management training for cancer patients undergoing chemotherapy. J Clin Oncol 2002;20:2851–2862.

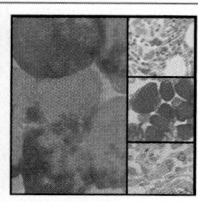

CARING FOR PATIENTS AT THE END OF LIFE

Janet L. Abrahm

SUMMARY OF KEY POINTS

- Physicians must be clear about prognosis, not overly optimistic.
- Patient decisions about resuscitation and entry into Phase I trials should be predicated on receiving accurate prognostic estimates.
- A sense of purpose can be maintained by patients who work on completing legacies, reconciliation, saying goodbye, and making plans for support or care of bereaved survivors.

DISTRESS

- Physical comfort is a prerequisite for exploring other sources of distress; consultation with anesthesia pain or palliative care specialists can be useful.
- Depression can be ameliorated even in the last weeks of life; delirium can be mistaken for pain and may exacerbate if treated with increases in opioid medication alone.
- Problematic relationships can create open wounds as painful as any physical injury.
- Families with young children are in special need of counseling and support.

- Ongoing losses (in physical attractiveness or physical or mental function, or of roles in family, community, or workplace) contribute to spiritual and existential distress. Life reviews and reconnection with sources of spiritual support, including religious rituals, can help.

HOSPICE CARE

- The gold standard of care at the end of life. Hospice teams are multidisciplinary (MD, RN, SW, chaplain, volunteers), but the referring physician remains in charge of the plan of care. Hospice programs provide care in the home, including all medications and durable medical equipment related to the terminal diagnosis. Patients need not be "Do Not Resuscitate" to enroll.
- Barriers to hospice referral include physician and patient reluctance to accept a terminal prognosis (i.e., less than six months), current inadequate reimbursement for palliative therapies, and physician, family and

patient misconceptions about entry criteria and services provided.

GRIEF AND BEREAVEMENT

- The intensity of a survivor's grief is based on the characteristics of the mourner, the nature of the death, and societal and cultural factors.
- Skillfully communicating the diagnosis and terminal prognosis, providing emotional, psychological, and spiritual support and physical comfort, helping families resolve outstanding issues, and making the death as peaceful as possible are all measures that diminish the suffering of the survivors.
- Survivors appreciate ongoing communication with the patient's physician. The formal bereavement program offered by hospice programs takes place during the first year after the patient's death. The program includes descriptions of typical manifestations of grieving and offers of counseling, support groups, and services of remembrance.

INTRODUCTION

When cure or even prolongation of life is no longer possible, oncologists have one last task remaining: to provide expert care to patients at the end of life and support for their families.[1] Despite physical comfort, patients can experience profound suffering from any of the following causes:

- Difficulty in maintaining personal dignity
- Losses of significant aspects of who they were at home, in the community, or in the workplace
- Lack of closure in important relationships
- Feelings of spiritual alienation
- Inability to discern the meaning in their lives[2]

When those problems are addressed, patients have the chance to attain transcendence, a sense that who and

what they have been will persist long after they have died.[3,4] Through collaborations with psychiatry, nursing, social work, and chaplaincy, oncology clinicians can promote physical comfort, social functioning, and psychological and spiritual well being.[5,6] We need never say, "There is nothing more I can do."

Patients rely on us to help them achieve a comfortable death that follows a time when goodbyes have been said, legacies have been established, and relationships have been brought to an acceptable closure. Their families need us to minimize the patient's suffering, obtain expert palliative care consultation when needed, and communicate clearly and often with them. Currently, however, such care is the exception rather than the rule.[7,8] This chapter provides an outline for oncology clinicians wishing to provide excellent care at the end of life and includes discussions of communication with patients and their families, approaches to ameliorating distress at the end of life, hospice care issues, manifestations of grief and bereavement, and suggestions for supporting bereaved survivors.

COMMUNICATION NEEDS OF PATIENTS AND FAMILIES

Timely, truthful, compassionate communication among patients who are dying, their families, and their physicians is needed to dispel fears (e.g., of unrelieved pain or of abandonment), to promote feelings of autonomy and control, to set goals of care, and to enable patients and families to be prepared for what is to come. The vast majority of them (80%–98%) want to be able to do the following:

- Name a proxy to make health care decisions.
- Know what to expect as their physical condition deteriorates.
- Put their financial affairs in order.
- Know that the doctor is comfortable talking about death and dying.
- Feel that the family and they themselves are prepared for their death.
- Have funeral arrangements in place.
- Have treatment preferences, especially about resuscitation, in writing.[9]

Families want to be able to say goodbye and be present when the death occurs, talk about their fears, and talk about the death with the clinicians.[10] Bereaved survivors are more likely to have a major depressive disorder if they feel that they have not been prepared for the death.[11] For them to be prepared, physicians must be clear about prognosis.

The cultural "norms" of medicine, however, favor optimism over accuracy in delivering prognosis.[12] Physicians might assume that patients would ask when they are ready for the information. There is no data, however, on how often patients with advanced refractory disease ask about their prognosis. Moreover, patients are known to be reticent to raise other important topics—such as uncontrolled pain or their wishes regarding resuscitation—with their physicians.[13,14] Physicians might also worry that giving a truthful prognosis will eliminate hope.

Through a truthful prognosis, however, patients with far-advanced disease can be helped to reframe what it is they are hoping for in the time that remains. Most patients hope for time to say goodbye and to bring closure to their lives. Even patients with far-advanced disease want to work on their legacies. Some dictate letters to be opened at significant events (graduations, weddings); others might want to narrate a scrapbook. Most want time at least for a personal, private review of who they were, what they did, and the difference they made.

Further, patients need to decide whether it still makes sense for them to be resuscitated. The likelihood of bad functional or cognitive outcomes affects their decisions, as does their understanding of their prognosis.[15] It is important, therefore, to tell a patient with widely metastatic cancer that resuscitation has very limited efficacy.[16-19] It is equally important to correct mistaken impressions of patients who really have only weeks or months to live. Patients who thought they had a greater than 10% chance of surviving six months, for example, usually want to be resuscitated. Only patients who thought they had a less than 10% chance of surviving for six months overwhelmingly choose comfort care and do not want to be resuscitated.[20]

Conversations about life-support preferences and those in which news of relapse or progression must be delivered take a significant emotional toll on the clinicians conducting them, especially those in busy practices in which each week many such talks are needed. Using straightforward communication strategies such as the S-P-I-K-E-S protocol can enhance the effectiveness of the communication both for the clinician and for the patient and family receiving the bad news.[21]

Communication needs of dying patients must also be culturally effective and extend to include psychosocial and spiritual needs, addressing loss, dignity, and the need for meaning.[4,5,22,23] Clinicians not experienced in such conversations might find it helpful to use the questions crafted by experts in this field (Table 43-1).[5,22-24]

DISTRESS

Dying patients might experience problems of a physical, psychological, social, or spiritual nature. These patients define quality of life at end of life as including

TABLE 43-1

Dignity Psychotherapy Question Protocol

Can you tell me a little about your life history, particularly those parts that you either remember most or think are the most important?

When did you feel most alive?

Are there specific things that you would want your family to know about you, and are there particular things you would want them to remember?

What are the most important roles (e.g., family, vocational, community service) you have played in life?

Why are they so important to you, and what do you think you accomplished in those roles?

What are your most important accomplishments, and what do you feel most proud of?

Are there particular things that you feel still need to be said to your loved ones, or things that you would want to take the time to say once again?

What are your hopes and dreams for your loved ones?

What have you learned about life that you would want to pass along to others?

What advice or words of guidance would you wish to pass along to your _____ (son, daughter, husband, wife, parents, other[s])?

Are there words, or perhaps even instructions, you would like to offer your family to provide them with comfort or solace?

In creating this permanent record, are there other things that you would like included?

Chochinov HM: Dignity-conserving care—A new model for palliative care: Helping the patient feel valued. JAMA 2002;287:2253.

physical comfort, a sense of control and dignity, relieving burden on their loved ones, strengthening and completing relationships with significant others, and avoiding prolongation of the dying process.[25] To provide quality care, therefore, oncologists need to collaborate with an interdisciplinary team such as that provided by palliative care and hospice programs. Palliative care practitioners are trained to address all dimensions of distress, including communication, decision making, management of complications of treatment and the disease, symptom control, psychosocial care of patients and their families, and care of the dying.[26]

Physical Causes

In the last days to week before death, a significant percentage of people exhibit or experience one or more of the following:

- Fatigue or pain (70%)
- Restlessness/agitation/delirium or noisy or moist breathing (60%)
- Urinary incontinence or retention (50%)
- Dyspnea (20%)
- Nausea and vomiting (10%)[27]

Most of the physical problems experienced by dying patients can be controlled using a limited number of medications given by the rectal, transdermal, or, if necessary, parenteral route (Table 43-2).

Pain Control

If oncologists use World Health Organization (WHO) guidelines for cancer pain relief, 50% of their patients near death will experience no pain, 25% will experience mild to moderate pain, and only 3% will experience severe pain.[28] Patients require close monitoring, and both opioids and nonopioid adjuvants are usually required. For patients unable to take pills, buccal, sublingual, transmucosal, or rectal opioids are usually effective.[29-31] There is no data on the absorption of transdermal opioids newly placed in patients near the end of life. Concentrated morphine or oxycodone oral solutions (20–40 mg/mL) can be given hourly or every two hours and are often satisfactory. Rectal administration of sustained-release opioid preparations are not FDA approved, but studies indicate that morphine absorption from a sustained-release preparation placed in the rectal vault is equivalent to that from oral administration.[32] If pain is a new problem and the patient is opioid-naive, institute therapy with 15–30 mg sustained-release morphine every 12 hours.

Adjuvants can also be given rectally or subcutaneously.[30] Patients previously benefiting from oral NSAIDs can receive rectal indomethacin; patients on a stable glucocorticoid dose for bone or nerve pain can receive subcutaneous dexamethasone. Rectal doxepin can replace oral tricyclic antidepressants.

Pain control must be maintained as death approaches. If the calculated opioid dose is too large to be delivered by sublingual, transdermal, or rectal routes, if pain relief

TABLE 43-2

Common Physical Problems in the Last Days of Life

PROBLEM	AGENT(S)	ROUTES, DOSES
Pain (continuous)	Morphine, hydromorphone	IV/SC infusion
	Fentanyl	Transdermal
	Morphine, oxycodone	SL oral concentrates
Pain (intermittent)	Morphine, oxycodone	SL oral concentrates
"Death rattle"	Scopolamine	Trans-derm Scop patch 1–3 q3d
	Hyoscyamine	0.125–0.25 mg SL tid–qid
Anxiety	Lorazepam	0.5–2 mg SL; q2h
	Clonazepam	0.5–2 mg bid po
Depression	Methylphenidate	2.5–5 mg PO qam or qam and noon
Delirium (mild)	Haloperidol	1–5 mg PO, SC, IV, PR q2–12h
	Chlorpromazine	12.5–50 mg PO, IV, PR q4–8h
	Olanzepine wafer	2.5–5 mg SL qhs or bid
Agitated delirium/or palliative sedation for refractory symptoms	Midazolam	0.4 mg–1 mg load; 0.4–1 mg/hr IV initial dose Rebolus and titrate as needed to target symptom/sign relief
	Pentobarbital	3 mg/kg IV load; 1–3 mg/kg/hr IV drip 120–200 mg PR q4h
	Lorazepam	0.5–1 mg/hour IV
	Propofol	2.5–5 µg/kg/minute IV
Dyspnea (anxiety)	Lorazepam	1 mg SL, PO q2h
Dyspnea (other)	Morphine	5–10 mg PO, IV or by nebulizer q2h
	Chlorpromazine	25–50 mg PO, PR q4–12h
Nausea	Combination of lorazepam, metoclopramide, dexamethasone or haloperidol	Compounded suppositories with desired agents (depending on presumed cause of nausea) q6hPR

IV, intravenous; PO, oral; PR, per rectum; SC, subcutaneous; SL, sublingual.
Data from Abrahm JL: A Physician's Guide to Pain and Symptom Management in Cancer Patients. Baltimore, Johns Hopkins University Press, 2000; and Cowan JD, Palmer TW: Practical guide to palliative sedation. Curr Oncol Rep 2002;4:242–249.

Problems Common to Cancer and Its Therapy

does not seem to be satisfactory using any of these routes, or if the routes are unacceptable to the patient or the caregiver, use a subcutaneous or intravenous opioid infusion.

Although pain relief is the goal in dying patients, the family is sometimes concerned that the opioid is "killing" the patient. If the respiratory rate of the patient declines, they might mistakenly think that the patient is over-sedated. Unlike patients who are in less advanced stages of their illness, the normal respiratory rate in terminal patients is about six to twelve breaths a minute. If the rate falls to fewer than six breaths per minute, reducing the dose of the opioid by 25% is usually effective; naloxone is almost never indicated in such situations.

Death Rattle

Pooling of secretions in the hypopharynx of dying patients causes the loud rasping sounds referred to as the "death rattle." Patients are usually unaware of these loud respirations, but they can be very distressing for families. Reposition the patient to a lateral recumbent position and, if needed, add hycosamine (0.125 mg three or four times daily sublingual [Levsin SL]) glycopyrrolate (SC 0.2 mg every four to eight hours or 0.6–1.2 mg per day by subcutaneous infusion) or scopolamine in a transdermal patch.[33]

Dyspnea

The prevalence of cancer-related dyspnea in dying patients is approximately 70%.[34] These patients benefit from the same symptomatic therapies recommended for patients with less advanced disease. Aggressive treatment of panic due to perceived breathlessness includes oral or parenteral morphine (5–10 mg orally), rectal or parenteral chlorpromazine, or parenteral midazolam for refractory panic.

Xerostomia

Although patients are unlikely to be thirsty or hungry, they might have dry mouths caused by opioids.[35] Rehydration is not indicated to relieve this symptom because there is no difference in the reports of thirst or dry mouth between dehydrated and normally hydrated dying patients, and no controlled studies have shown that rehydration is effective.[36] Providing parenteral hydration increases distress, causing nausea and vomiting from increased gastric secretions; dyspnea from ascites, upper airway secretions and pulmonary edema; and pain from ascites and peripheral edema.[35] Moistening the mouth with swabs, or offering sips of water, ice chips, or fruit-flavored ice, usually ameliorates the xerostomia.

Exsanguination

Massive hemoptysis, hematemesis, hematochezia, or exsanguination from a tumor eroding into a major vessel is rare but can be horrifying for professional caregivers, family members, or friends to observe. If the patient is likely to develop such a complication, ensure that there are dark-colored sheets, towels, and blankets available to mask the blood. Consider insertion of a peripherally inserted central catheter (PICC) line in patients who have no indwelling venous access device to ensure emergency intravenous access for patient sedation. Appropriate medications should be on hand, either on the hospital unit or in the home. If the patient is enrolled in a hospice program, the nurse can provide instruction for administering prefilled syringes of morphine, to be given intravenously when possible, or a benzodiazepine. Midazolam (Versed) can be given intramuscularly or intravenously; diazepam or lorazepam (e.g., Ativan) can be given rectally. When the event occurs, the patient is placed bleeding side down, in the Trendelenburg position if possible, and given midazolam for anxiety, and opioids if there is dyspnea or pain.

Psychological Causes

Anxiety

Anxiety in dying patients can arise from physical or psychological disorders.[37] Sepsis, hypoxia, metabolic abnormalities, withdrawal from opioids or benzodiazepines, drug reactions (e.g., akathesia from metoclopramide or paradoxical agitation from benzodiazepines), and uncontrolled pain all can present as anxiety. Patients with panic disorders, agitated depression, phobias, or adjustment disorders also can present with anxiety.

Nonspecific pharmacologic treatments usually include benzodiazepines (e.g., the short-acting lorazepam, 0.5–2 mg every two hours as needed, or long-acting clonazepam, 0.5–2 mg orally twice daily), selective serotonin reuptake inhibitors (SSRI) and, when there is evidence of delirium, neuroleptics (e.g., haloperidol, 1–5 mg orally or intravenously every two to twelve hours, or olanzepine, 2.5–5.0 mg at bedtime or twice daily). Opioids with or without benzodiazepines are useful for patients with dyspnea.[38] Nonpharmacologic treatments such as relaxation training, hypnosis, supportive psychotherapy, and counseling, are also very effective.[37]

Depression

Terminally ill patients who answer, "Yes", to the screening question, "Are you depressed?" are likely to be diagnosed as depressed in a more comprehensive evaluation.[39] To explore the subject further, clinicians can ask: How do you see your future? What do you imagine is ahead for yourself with this illness? What aspects of your life do you feel most proud of? Most troubled by?[40] The clinician can serve as a therapeutic agent by listening actively and by providing support for both the patient and the family. For depressed patients who have only a few weeks to live but can still take oral medications, methylphenidate (2.5–5 mg orally at 8 A.M. and noon, initial dosing) can provide rapid symptomatic improvement.[41]

Delirium

Delirium (hypoactive, hyperactive, or mixed) has been reported in up to 88% of dying patients.[42] Hypoactive delirium can be confused with depression, and agitated delirium can be confused with uncontrolled pain, especially in dying patients.[43,44] Patients with hypoactive delirium might appear withdrawn and sad, but careful mental status testing with tools such as the Folstein Mini-mental demonstrate significant cognitive impairment. Patients with agitated delirium might cry out, be restless, and pick at clothes or bed sheets. Patients with any type of delirium can experience insomnia and daytime somnolence, nightmares, agitation, irritability, distractibility, hypersensitivity to light and sound, anxiety, difficulty in concentrating or marshaling thoughts, fleeting illusions, hallucinations and delusions, emotional liability, attention deficits, and memory disturbances.[45] It is important, therefore, to treat the delirium even among patients without overt agitation.

The etiology of delirium among patients with advanced cancer is often multifactorial.[42] Medical causes include metabolic abnormalities (hypercalcemia, hyperglycemia, and uremia), malnutrition, dehydration, hypoxia, fever, infection, uncontrolled pain or hepatic failure, primary brain tumor, and brain metastases. Medications—especially opioids, NSAIDs, and high dose corticosteroids—often contribute to delirium. Substitution of another opioid might help reverse the delirium.[46] A comprehensive psychiatric evaluation (which can be done at home by appropriately trained clinicians) can differentiate delirium from anxiety, minor depression, anger, dementia, and psychosis.[45] Among patients who are very near the end of life, the burden of the evaluation might exceed the benefit of finding a specific, reversible cause. Empiric therapy that controls the delirium might suffice. Discussion with the patient's health care proxy can help clarify the best course of action. Treatment protocols for delirium are included in Table 43-2.

Agitation in the Dying Patient

Almost half of the patients who are actively dying of cancer show signs of restlessness and agitation. They might toss and turn, moan, have muscle twitching or spasm, and be awake only intermittently. Some are suffering from unresolved spiritual or social problems. The approach to assessment and treatment of agitated dying patients involves, sequentially, nonpharmacologic symptomatic therapy, an evaluation for reversible causes and treating those that are found, and empiric symptom management. Whenever a treatment resolves the agitation, it should be continued, and the patient should be reassessed. In rare cases, patients with agitation require sedation. The aggressiveness of the evaluation and the

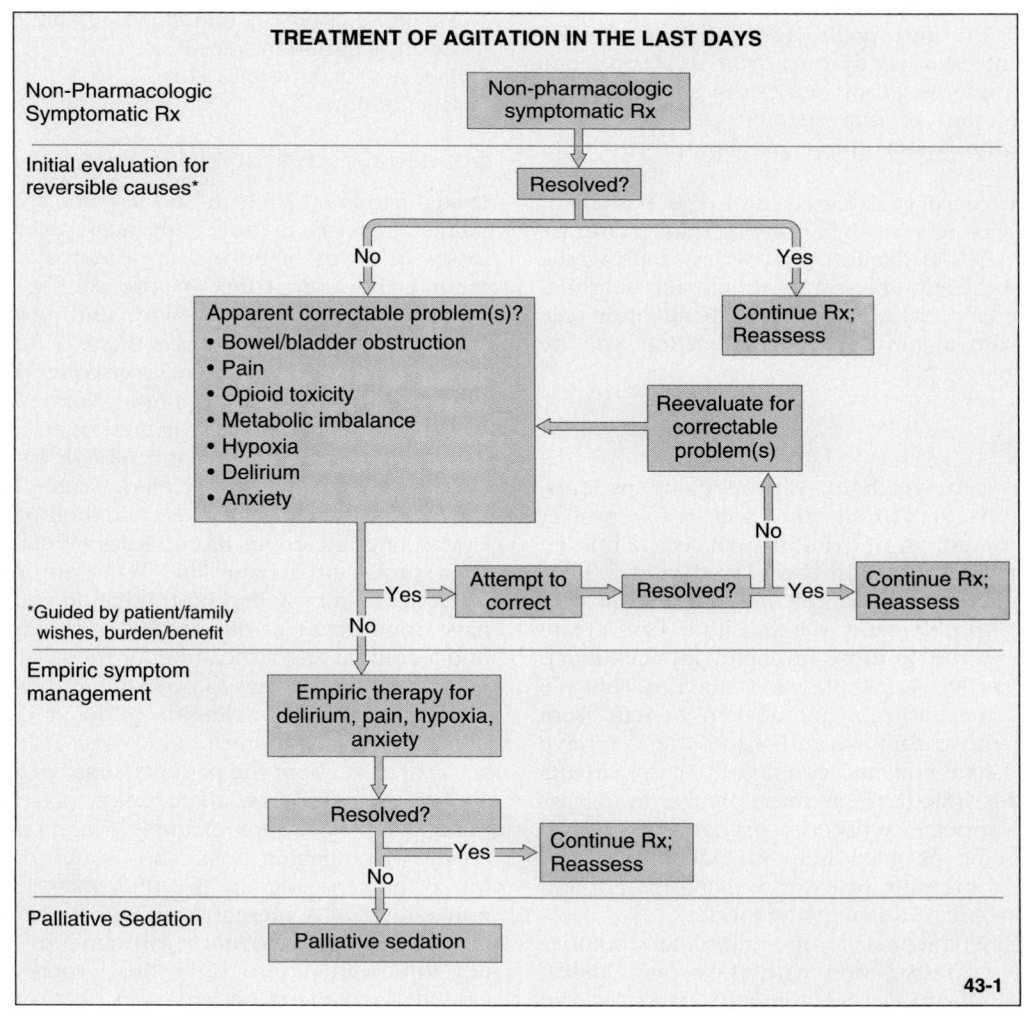

Problems Common to Cancer and Its Therapy

nature of the treatments given should be guided by the patient's goals and the burdens and benefits of each intervention. The site of care (hospital, nursing home, home) need not be the deciding factor on which palliative assessment and therapies to offer.

Many patients' agitation responds to nonspecific, nonpharmacologic measures, such as adjusting the lighting, decreasing extraneous noise in the room, playing favorite music, gently touching the patient, or having family and friends read to, pray with, or quietly talk with the patient. A visit from one of the hospital chaplains can be comforting. A visit from an estranged family member or friend, reassurance that loved ones are well cared for and are prepared for the patient's departure, and family permission to "let go" can have significant impact.

If these measures are not effective, the family and caregivers should weigh the burdens and benefits of searching for reversible causes. Those such as a full bladder, a fecal impaction, poorly cleared secretions, pain, or side effects from opioids or other medications are usually easy to detect and correct. Metabolic disturbances leading to delirium and pulmonary processes causing hypoxia or anxiety could require invasive maneuvers that do not seem appropriate. When a specific cause is found, decisions can be made regarding the burden and benefits of specific vs. symptomatic treatment. The patient's condition and goals, for example, dictate whether a patient who has dyspnea from a large pleural effusion should undergo a thoracentesis or simply receive opioids. If correction of one specific cause does not resolve the agitation, resume the search, as appropriate, for another one.

If no specific cause is detected, or if the search for specific causes is felt to be inappropriate, empiric therapies based on the likeliest process(es) causing the distress should be tried. Empiric treatment for delirium, pain, hypoxia, and anxiety often relieves the agitation (see Table 43-2). If the agitation persists, sedation will be required (see Table 43-2).

Social Causes

Family concerns can weigh heavily on dying patients. Practical concerns are often the easiest to resolve, although a major concern of dying patients is the burden they feel they are imposing on their loved ones.[25] They also want to strengthen and complete their relationships. For this reason, problematic relationships can create open wounds as painful as those from any physical injury. Dr. Ira Byock offers five simple phrases ("The Five Things") that encompass the subjects people can benefit from discussing with those they love: "Forgive me; I forgive you; thank you; I love you; and goodbye."[3] Many patients and families find it difficult to say these phrases or discuss these subjects. Social workers, psychologists, and psychiatrists can be of great help in facilitating these conversations and bringing peace to a dying patient and to the soon-to-be-bereaved family members.

Families of dying patients face an extraordinary number of challenges. They must cope with their own losses, organize and pay for home care, and care for the remainder of the family that is not ill. They are best helped by the following measures:

- Patient comfort
- Communication with health care providers
- Help with caregiving and meeting financial and social costs
- Maintaining stability
- Adapting to change
- Support for their grief and upcoming bereavement[47-49]

Oncology clinicians can help by simplifying medication regimens and planning for emergencies that can be foreseen.[50] See also "Addressing the Needs of Caregivers" for suggestions about how oncologists can address some of the family's needs. Social workers collaborate with the patient's primary oncology team to provide most of the support, explain the benefits of hospice and other needed services, and arrange family access to them.

Families with young children are in special need of counseling and support. Guidelines for clinicians who work with these parents and their children include six steps (which are described in detail in the reference provided):

1. Learn about the children.
2. Maximize the child's support system.
3. Facilitate honest communication about the illness.
4. Address common questions.
5. Prepare for hospital visits.
6. Say goodbye.[51]

Spiritual/Existential Causes

Dying patients also can suffer from spiritual and existential concerns. As cancer advances, patients face ongoing losses in terms of normal appearance and physical and mental function; roles in the family, community, or workplace; control, autonomy, and privacy.[2] Suffering arises when the illness robs them of something fundamental to who they are, and consequently, each person's sources of suffering are unique. For example, although loss of mobility might be irrelevant to someone whose major avocation is reading, it can be devastating to an avid golfer. Young patients particularly search for the meaning in their existence, their illness, and their premature deaths. Counseling, including life reviews (What have you been most proud of in your life? What surprised you most? What has made you happiest? What do you wish you could have done better or differently?) can help dying patients find a context and a meaning for their lives.

Some patients seem to be blaming themselves for their illness, even though scientific evidence does not support their belief. The concern could arise from a much larger sense of guilt about the patients' sense of failure to live the lives they should have lived. Other patients—those with uncontrolled pain, for example—might feel that God is testing or punishing them. They search their consciences for a transgression so dreadful that it deserved such punishment.[52] A mental health professional or chaplain might be able to provide reassurance or to help patients develop strategies to right the wrongs they feel they caused. Even dying patients can be provided hope: the

ADDRESSING THE NEEDS OF THE CAREGIVERS

During the last weeks to months of the patient's life, office visits become impractical. Regular contact by telephone, supplemented, when possible, by one or more home visits, retains the connection that patients and families need with their primary treatment team. Clinicians also can promote continuity and minimize feelings of abandonment by collaborating with the home care or hospice nurses and, as requested, with the social workers who are part of the home care team. Praising the family caregivers for the work they are doing, helping them anticipate upcoming problems and make contingency plans, and checking in with them at regular intervals promotes timely identification and, when possible, resolution of new problems.

Many family members and medical trainees have never seen anyone die an expected death outside an intensive care unit. The clinician familiar with the dying process can be a crucial source of information and comfort. For inpatients, the clinician works with the nursing team caring for the patient and also serves as an attentive observer striving to provide maximum comfort. I make at least two visits a day to stable patients to monitor their comfort through reports from nursing and family, to answer questions, and to educate professional and family caregivers as to what they should expect in the last days.

Patients who were formerly alert and communicative usually become less so. They are apparently still comforted by the touch and voices of those they love and might even emerge from what seemed to be an insensible state to greet a welcome newcomer. I tell families that to me, it is as though the patient lives in a house with many rooms, a mansion. As they come closer to dying, the patient moves farther and farther back in the house, and it is more and more effort for them to greet callers at the front of the house. But the callers are still welcome, as are their voices and conversation. I ask families to let patients know they have arrived, and then to add that patients should not feel obliged to speak to them. Patients can also be asked to provide a hand squeeze or other sign of recognition. With close family, I discuss the "Five Things" (see the section "Social Causes") and suggest that they find the time to share with the patient any of those sentiments they feel would be appropriate.

I reassure families that we know that dying patients are rarely hungry or thirsty, and that moistening the mouth is all that is needed. If necessary, I review the burdens of hydration (see the section on "Xerostomia"). I also explain about Cheyne-Stokes breathing and that it does not indicate that the patient is gasping for breath. I also ask them to feel free to let us know if the patient seems uncomfortable or develops noisy breathing, as we want to address any source of discomfort as rapidly as possible. I offer the services of chaplaincy, and I am also alert to whether a social worker would be helpful, if chaplains and social workers are not already involved. Many family members do not know that this kind of help is available to them in the hospital.

If the family has not done so already, I urge them to chose a funeral home and make all the necessary arrangements before the patient has actually died, to free themselves of that task when the death occurs. Families often ask how they will know that the patient is dying. I ask them to look for a marked decrease in urine output (in a foley bag, or diapers), cooling of the arms and legs, and new pallor or mottling of the skin. Some patients develop fecal incontinence as they die, so if hospice is not involved and the patient is at home, I alert the family to this possibility.

SUPPORTING THE WARD PERSONNEL AND THE HOUSESTAFF

To decrease potential feelings of guilt and anxiety, I review with all team members the history of the illness, the limits of the treatments that remain, the burdens of those treatments, and, when appropriate, the limits the patient has placed on further supportive measures. I also remind them that, despite our best efforts, patients still die, and that it is no one's fault. I also suggest things they can do that will enhance the patient's last days and that will further the healing process of the survivors.

During the hospitalizations that lead to death, and after the death itself, I try to dispel any misconceptions they have about their "fault" for the death and to praise the work they did to make the dying as comfortable as possible. This kind of support goes a long way toward enabling young physicians and ward staff to recover from the pain they experience when a patient dies, and to allow themselves to feel a sense of satisfaction for a job well done.

hope that in the absence of a cure, they will still be able to heal these wounds.

Religious rituals can be an important source of comfort and healing to dying patients and their families.[52] Even in a hospital setting, therefore, every effort should be made to identify and accommodate these spiritual practices. Appropriate hospital or community religious leaders should be welcomed as part of the patients' care team and should be assisted in performing the necessary rites after the patient dies.

Palliative Sedation for Refractory Symptoms

Sedation is considered when, despite expert evaluation and management, a patient who is near death continues to experience intolerable physical, psychological, or spiritual-existential distress.[53] Fewer than 5% of patients need palliative sedation; those who do most commonly suffer from refractory pain, cough, dyspnea, seizures, or delirium. The doses of opioid, benzodiazepine, or neuroleptic needed to control the symptom(s) sedate the patient. In other cases, the request for sedation for refractory symptoms arises when psychological or spiritual-existential concerns coexist with physical problems. Expert palliative care and pastoral consultation, evaluation by a psychiatrist, and discussions among the health care team, the patient, and the family members should be undertaken before palliative sedation is administered. Most often, all concerned reach a consensus on the need for and acceptability of sedation as a means of achieving symptom control. Obtaining formal informed consent, either from the patient or from the health care proxy, is recommended.

Medications used to produce the sedation that relieves the distressing symptom(s) include opioids, neuroleptics, intravenous benzodiazepines, and subcutaneous or intravenous barbiturates (see Table 43-2).[54] Intravenous hydration or enteral or parenteral nutrition can be provided if they meet the goals set by the patient and family. They are rarely used in imminently dying patients whether or not they are sedated, as these patients are rarely suffering from hunger or thirst.[35]

HOSPICE CARE

Hospice care can be an enormous source of comfort to families of dying patients and professional caregivers, particularly for those who have never witnessed a "natural" death. The team members have "been there," can explain what is likely to happen, and can provide expert symptom management during the last hours to days. Hospice care might also decrease the risk of death of surviving elderly widows.[55]

American patients, however, are generally very resistant to accepting a terminal prognosis.[56,57] To enroll in hospice, patients must acknowledge their six months prognosis, relinquish further curative therapy, and give informed consent. These requirements and common misconceptions about hospice care (Table 43-3) can be serious obstacles to enrollment in hospice programs.[32,58]

TABLE 43-3

Common Misconceptions about Hospice

- *Patients enrolling in hospice must choose not to be resuscitated.* Patients do not have to relinquish resuscitation to enroll in hospice. After they and their families fully understand the implications of the resuscitation, most patients elect not to be resuscitated.
- *Patients enrolled in hospice lose their primary physicians.* The referring attending physician continues to direct and approve all the patient's care.
- *Hospice patients cannot be hospitalized and remain enrolled in hospice.* Any hospice patient can be admitted to an acute, inpatient level of care to control a distressing symptom. Hospices can admit patients to contract beds in acute care hospitals or to their own inpatient facilities.
- *Hospice patients cannot participate in research projects while enrolled in hospice.* Hospice patients have the right to participate in research studies. Hospice ethics and research committees usually evaluate the burden vs. the benefit of the research on the patient, family, and hospice staff.
- *Hospice nursing personnel do not provide sophisticated care.* Hospice personnel provide expert palliative care that requires astute assessment and expert intervention tailored to the patient and family goals.
- *Patients can "use up" their hospice eligibility, so it is important not to enroll them too soon.* Patients are initially certified for three months of service, after which their physician and the hospice medical director are asked to recertify them indefinitely, at two-month intervals. Patients who chose to revoke the hospice benefit to seek life-prolonging therapies may chose to re-enroll if their goals change.
- *Patients must have a live-in caregiver to enroll in hospice.* With appropriate safeguards (e.g., "lock-boxes" to provide access in emergencies, and daily phone contact) hospice care can be safely provided to patients who "live alone."

Financial Considerations

The Hospice benefit (under Medicare) is a managed care, capitated reimbursement program that reimburses a hospice program a "per diem" rate based on the patient's level of care (approximately $130 per day for routine or respite care, approximately $500 per day for inpatient acute care.) In skilled nursing facilities, patients are receiving Medicare benefits for skilled care and cannot retain these and simultaneously enroll in the hospice Medicare benefit. Medicaid, private insurance, and health maintenance providers reimburse the hospice at various rates, and with the last, services must be approved through the plan's case manager. Aggressive palliation using chemotherapy or radiation is often prohibitively expensive for small to moderate-size hospices given this reimbursement schedule. Individual hospices must decide both which treatments are consistent with their philosophy and which they can afford. Most hospices must secure additional funding from grants and donations to provide the mandated services.

Further, the majority (80%) of the services a hospice program delivers must, by law, be to patients at home. Fewer than 1% of patients enrolled in hospice programs die in hospitals. Although the hospice program provides some help, the majority of the patient's care must be provided by family or friends or by privately paid professional caregivers. Some patients will not be able to stay at home, therefore, even with the maximum help hospice personnel and volunteers can offer.

Clinical Care Provided

Patients in hospice programs are cared for by medically directed, interdisciplinary teams that include the referring physician, the hospice medical director, a nursing director of patient services, office administrator, nurse, social worker, bereavement counselor, home health aide, chaplain, and volunteers. The core team also can request additional consultations from physicians, registered dietitians, or occupational, speech, or physical therapists (Table 43-4).

Levels of Care

Hospice programs provide a continuum of care, from home to the inpatient setting. Whereas most patients are cared for in their homes, all Medicare-certified hospices, as stated in the 1983 Federal Regulations, are required to provide four levels of care: *routine, continuous, inpatient,* and *respite.* They also provide *bereavement* care both to support family members experiencing "anticipatory grief" before the patient's death, and to communicate with and support the bereaved for the year after the death.

Routine care services are offered seven days a week, 24 hours a day. In addition to the patient's nurse, there is always an oncall registered nurse to provide phone support and make home visits when necessary. The registered nurse monitors the comfort of the patient and works with the referring physician to adjust the treatment regimen as needed. Occupational, speech, or physical

TABLE 43-4

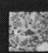

Medicare-mandated Hospice Services

Practitioners Available

Medical director, nurses, social workers, home health aides, chaplains, volunteers, administrative personnel, medical consultations, occupational therapy, physical therapy, speech therapy, bereavement counseling

Palliative Treatment of Terminal Illness

Prescription medications
Durable medical equipment and supplies
Oxygen
Radiation and chemotherapy
Laboratory and diagnostic procedures

Other Benefits

Transportation when medically necessary for changes in level of care
When needed, continuous care at home or in a skilled nursing facility or inpatient setting
Respite care (care in a nursing facility that provides a "respite" for the caregivers)

Medicare Hospice Regulations: 42 Codes of Federal Regulations, Part 418, 1993.

therapy and home health aides are provided as required. As death approaches, the patient's registered nurse reviews the dying process and provides the family or the inpatient or long-term care facility personnel with written materials that explain how they can determine that death is imminent. S/he also describes the signs and symptoms of dying, instructs them in emergency procedures, and is available for support while the patient dies.

Social workers offer support and family counseling and identify those who are at risk for a particularly painful bereavement period. They engage the patient and family in advance care and funeral planning and in completion of living wills and durable powers of attorney, provide applications for financial aid or waivers, and help identify financing for additional home health care. They assist patients in making plans for their survivors (e.g., guardianship for children), in completing life reviews, and, often work alongside the chaplain, to facilitate family reconciliation.

The team chaplain also offers home visits or coordinated care with the patient's own clergy. Chaplains are of help even to the nonreligious patients who have spiritual or existential sources of distress (e.g., loss of hope, loss of connection or of love, a need for forgiveness or to forgive, or a need to identify the meaning of their lives).

Volunteers, who are usually available two to four hours a week, help families in nonclinical areas. A hospice medical director works with the team and the patient's primary physician to optimize symptom management.

Continuous home care is provided for patients who require continuous symptom management and for whom the home care setting remains appropriate. Patients with, for example, unrelieved cough, dyspnea, pain, or delirium can receive 24-hour nursing services until the problem is brought under control. Home visits from a hospice medical director can also be provided.

If the patient's symptoms cannot be controlled at home, *inpatient care* is offered. Orders are written by inpatient unit personnel, and inpatient staff provide the care. The hospice team, however, continues to be responsible for the plan of care. Team members visit the patient as they would visit an outpatient, and the hospice medical director provides consultation as needed. The referring physician remains the primary physician and can bill for services under Medicare Part B.

Respite care is available generally for five days every month in a community skilled or intermediate nursing facility with which the hospice has a contract. The goal of the respite is either to provide a rest for the caregiver or to remove the patient to an adequate facility when the home is temporarily inadequate to meet the patient's care needs.

Medications/Treatments Provided

Hospice programs provide 95% of the cost of prescription drugs related to the terminal diagnosis and necessary for its palliative treatment (and many waive the other 5% if there is no insurance coverage). They also provide all durable medical equipment, supplies, and oxygen for needs related to the terminal diagnosis; laboratory and diagnostic procedures related to the terminal diagnosis; and transportation when this is medically necessary for changes in the patient's level of care (see Table 43-4).

GRIEF AND BEREAVEMENT

Survivor's grief is a "process of experiencing the psychological, behavioral, social, and physical reactions to the perception of loss," and it is distinguishable from the anxiety and depression that survivors might also be experiencing.[59,60] The intensity of a survivor's grief is based on the characteristics of the mourner himself or herself, the nature of the death, and societal and cultural factors. Rando[59] writes that being very attached to or very dependent on the deceased, having a great deal of ambivalence in one's feelings towards the deceased, a personal history of clinical depression, or difficulty with previous losses all can exacerbate the grief. Recent studies of psychiatric outpatients confirmed the association between attachment and dependence and severity of grief but also found that having more ambivalence predicted for less grief.[61] Sudden or accidental death, suicide, or homicide magnify the grief.[59] The perception of a violent death is associated with major depression in the survivors, but religious rituals, a good support system, and involvement with hospice programs for more than three days decrease depression.[62,63]

Each bereaved person's loss is unique, as are the experiences and manifestations of grief and mourning. Many people manifest typical symptoms of grief, some of which become less persistent as they rebuild their lives.[59,60,64,65] Recurrent intense symptoms typically occur at the anniversary of the death of the patient but can occur at unpredictable times, sparked by any type of reminder of the deceased. Although there are no rigid stages that bereaved survivors pass through, there are some typical manifestations of grief.

At the time of death, survivors appear numb, confused, or dazed, and usually express some form of denial as the reality of the death intensifies.[66] Behavior can range from uncontrolled shrieking to an unnerving calm.

In the weeks and months that follow, pain intensifies as the absence of the person who has died asserts itself repeatedly. Mourners yearn for the one who is dead and experience repeated pangs of intense grief; denial is replaced by disorganization, depression, disinterest, and despair.[65] Survivors commonly experience the feelings, behaviors, physical symptoms, spiritual concerns, and thoughts listed in "What You Can Expect When Someone Close to You Dies."

As the roles the deceased played in the marriage, the family, and the community become apparent to the survivors, they grieve each loss as they learn to cope with the increasing responsibilities. It is very difficult for people to move beyond loss if they never allow themselves to feel it in some way that is appropriate for them. Family obligations and unspoken strictures against demonstrations of grief can further impair a survivor's ability to experience the pain of the loss adequately. Putting those feelings away to deal with later or denying their existence only prolongs or inhibits the grieving process.

Often by a year or two after the loss, survivors accommodate to it.[59] They tacitly acknowledge the changes that must be made if they are ever to resume old relationships and responsibilities or to establish new ones and risk recurrent loss. Accommodation involves realizing that loving someone new need not mean betraying the memory of the person who has died.[59]

Some survivors, however, suffer from a distinct symptom complex called "complicated grief." Such patients are significantly functionally impaired and have extreme yearning for the deceased, together with feelings of "numbness, feeling that part of oneself has died, assuming symptoms of the deceased, disbelief, or bitterness" that persist for six months or longer after the death.[67] Such patients are at increased risk of medical and psychiatric illness.[68]

Interventions

Skillfully communicating the diagnosis and terminal prognosis, providing emotional, psychological, and spiritual support and physical comfort, helping families resolve outstanding issues, and making the death as

---

WHAT YOU CAN EXPECT WHEN SOMEONE CLOSE TO YOU DIES

Grief is often associated with feelings, thoughts, and physical symptoms, including:

Common Feelings/ Behaviors
- Fear or anxiety
- Anger or guilt
- Depression or despair
- Separation or longing
- Sudden wave of mental pain
- Confusion or inability to concentrate or make decisions
- Tearfulness or crying
- Sighing
- Restlessness
- Yearning
- Helplessness
- Relief
- Disbelief
- Hope

Spiritual
- Sense of the deceased's presence
- Faith may be strengthened, altered, or abandoned

Common Physical Symptoms
- Decreased or increased appetite
- Decreased energy; weakness of muscles
- Nausea and diarrhea
- Decrease or increase in sex drive
- Inability to sleep or sleeping too much
- Feeling something stuck in the throat
- Tightness in chest, breathlessness
- Increased sensitivity to noise
- Vivid dreams
- Dry mouth

Common Thoughts
- Preoccupation with "if only", "what if" and with memories
- "Who am I now?"

Most people find that their grief lasts anywhere from six months to two years. However, remember that each person is a unique individual and for some people, much more time is needed before the pain lessens.

WHAT YOU CAN DO
1. Allow yourself to feel the loss and to grieve over it.
2. Realize that your grief is unique.
3. Expect yourself to have some negative feelings.
4. Accept the help of others and let people know how they can help.
5. Give yourself time alone.
6. Exercise.
7. Read books about feelings of grief and the process of recovery.
8. Talk to others about your loss.
9. Attend community support groups.
10. **Most Important:** Understand that it is very likely that your pain will lessen.

WHAT IT IS BETTER NOT TO DO
1. Try not to make major changes.
2. Resist withdrawing from social activities.
3. Avoid excessive smoking or drinking.

WHEN YOU SHOULD CALL US
- If you have any questions or would like further information.
- If you feel that you would like professional counseling.
- If you need our help.

Abrahm, JL, Cooley, ME, Ricacho, L: Efficacy of an educational bereavement program for families of veterans with cancer. J Cancer Ed 1995;10:207–212.

SAMPLE OFFICE-BASED BEREAVEMENT PROGRAM[72]

AT THE TIME OF DEATH

Family members are often in a state of shock; their moods can swing widely from feeling numb to feeling distraught. This volatility can be frightening, so our staff explains that this reaction is normal and that they should not worry about controlling themselves.

If I am sad, I cry with the family; if family members need to talk things over, I ask leading questions that help them share their feelings. Most families want to review the circumstances of the death, to assure themselves that the patient did not suffer, and that everything that could have been done was done. I always try to find something for which I can praise them (e.g., their care of or their advocacy role for the patient) and add how lucky the patient was to have had them there when he or she needed them. If I cannot do this in person, I try to offer as much support as I could by telephone.

INITIAL FOLLOW-UP CALL

We next call the family within 24 to 48 hours of the death to offer our condolences and our help. During this call, we offer comfort and provide a listener for a reiteration of the story of the death and the meaning of it for the bereaved. If necessary, we again reinforced the normality of the wide emotional swings or other symptoms of acute grief that they might have been experiencing. We listen empathetically and indicate our continued support. We end the conversation by asking whether we can keep in touch, and we let them know we will call again in about a month. We also send a condolence letter. If the family was involved with hospice, we remind them that the hospice team is still available to them.

FOUR TO SIX WEEKS

About a month after we send the letter, we call again and offer to send a variety of materials we think would be helpful. These include a list of feelings and physical signs commonly experienced by those who are grieving and what to do or not to do about them (see "What You Can Expect When Someone Close to You Dies").

We also include a list of support groups in the family's area, including those hosted by the hospice, because talking about their loss with skilled bereavement counselors or others who have suffered the same losses can help their recovery. Groups such as Widow-to-Widow, or, for parents who have lost a child, Compassionate Friends or Candlelighters (www.candle.org) provide much needed help with rebuilding a life.

OTHER CONTACTS

Because this has been shown to be a time of most need for bereaved families, we call again at six months and repeat our offer of various materials. We also participate in the once- or twice-yearly memorial services held by our cancer center and by the hospices who cared for our patients and their families. And, because we anticipate recurrence of grief, we send a letter at the first anniversary of the person's death, and we send a "Holiday letter" a few weeks before Thanksgiving letting them know that they are still in our thoughts and would welcome a call.

Our staff finds the process very rewarding. I have noticed that as I speak to the survivors at longer and longer intervals and begin to remember the patients as they were before the terminal stages, it helps me achieve closure and makes it easier for me to move on.

---

peaceful as possible are all measures that diminish the suffering of the survivors. Survivors who feel unprepared for the patient's death have a higher risk of developing complicated grief.[69]

After the patient dies, survivors appreciate ongoing communication with the patient's physician.[67] When a formal bereavement program is offered, it usually takes place during the first year after the patient's death. After the formal program ends, the bereaved are welcome to continue to participate in any bereavement activities that have been meaningful to them (see "Sample Office-based Bereavement Program"). Survivors who experience severe grief symptoms or depression should be referred for formal assessment and consideration of pharmacologic treatment.[70,71] Unfortunately, although the depression often responds to standard therapy, there is no widely accepted effective therapy for the extreme grief symptoms.[67]

REFERENCES

1. American Society of Clinical Oncology: Cancer care during the last phase of life. J Clin Oncol 1998;16:1986.
2. Cassell E: The Nature of Suffering and the Goals of Medicine. New York, Oxford University Press, 1991.
3. Byock I: Dying Well: Peace and Possibilities at the End of Life. New York, Riverhead Books, 1997.
4. Block SD: Psychological considerations, growth and transcendance at the end of life. JAMA 2001;285:2898.
5. Stewart AL, Teno J, Patrick DL, Lynn J: The concept of quality of life of dying persons in the context of health care. J Pain Symptom Manage 1999;17:93.
6. Byock IR, Merriman MP: Measuring quality of life for patients with terminal illness: The Missoula-VITAS quality of life index. J Palliat Med 1998;12:231.
7. Means to a better end: A report on dying in America today. Last Acts, November 2002.
8. Foley KM, Gelband H (eds): Improving Palliative Care for Cancer: Summary and Recommendations. Washington DC, National Academy Press, 2001.
9. Steinhauser KE, Christakis NA, Clipp EC, McNeilly M, Grambow S, Parker J, et al: Preparing for the end of life: Preferences of patients, families, physicians, and other care providers, J Pain Sym Manage 2001;22:727.
10. Dawson NJ: Need satisfaction in terminal care settings. Soc Sci Med 1991;32:83.
11. Barry LC, Kasl SV, Prigerson HG: Psychiatric disorders among bereaved persons: The role of perceived circumstances of death and preparedness for death. Am J Geriatric Psych 2002;10:447.
12. Christakis N: Death foretold: Prophecy and prognosis in medical care. Chicago, University of Chicago Press, 1999.
13. Lamont E, Siegler M: Paradoxes in cancer patients' advance care planning. J Palliat Med 2000;3:27.
14. Gallup, GH: Spiritual beliefs and the dying process. A report on a

national survey conducted for the Nathan Cummings Foundation and Fetzer Institute. October 1997.

15. Fried TR, Bradley EH, Towle VR, Allore H: Understanding the treatment preferences of seriously ill patients. NEJM 2002;346:1061.

16. Ewer MS, Kish SK, Martin DG, Price KJ, Feeley TW: Characteristics of cardiac arrest in cancer patients as a predictor of survival after cardiopulmonary resuscitation. Cancer 2001;92:1905.

17. Rubenfeld GD, Crawford SW: Withdrawing life support from mechanically ventilated recipients of bone marrow transplants: A case for evidence-based guidelines. Ann Intern Med 1996;125:625.

18. Faber-Langendoen K: Resuscitation of patients with metastatic cancer. Is transient benefit still futile? [see comments]. Arch Intern Med 1991;151:235.

19. Schapira DV, Studnicki J, Bradham DD, Wolff P, Jarrett A: Intensive care, survival, and expense of treating critically ill cancer patients. JAMA 1993;269:783.

20. Weeks JC, Cook EF, O'Day SSJ, Peterson LM, Wenger N, Reding D, et al: Relationship between cancer patients' predictions of prognosis and their treatment preferences [see comments]. JAMA 1998;279: 1709.

21. Baile WF, Glober GA, Lenzi R, Beale EA, Kudelka AP: Discussing disease progression and end-of-life decisions. Oncology 1999;13:1021.

22. Crawley LM, Marshall PA, Lo B, Koenig BA: Strategies for culturally effective end-of-life care. Ann Intern Med 2002;136:673.

23. Chochinov HM: Dignity-conserving care—A new model for palliative care: Helping the patient feel valued. JAMA 2002;287: 2253.

24. Lo B, Ruston D, Kates LW, Arnold RM, Cohen C, Faber-Langendoen K, et al: Discussing religious and spiritual issues at the end of life: A practical guide for physicians. JAMA 2002;287:749.

25. Singer PA, Martin DK, Kelner M: Quality end-of-life care: patients' perspectives. JAMA 1999;281:163.

26. Foley KM, Gelband H: Improving Palliative Care for Cancer. Institute of Medicine and National Research Council, Washington, DC, National Academy Press, 2001.

27. Coyle N, Adelhardt J, Foley KM, Portenoy RK: Character of terminal illness in the advanced cancer patient: Pain and other symptoms during the last four weeks of life. J Pain Symptom Manage 1990;5:83.

28. Grond S, Zech D, Schug SA, Lynch J, Lehmann KA: Validation of World Health Organization guidelines for cancer pain relief during the last days and hours of life. J Pain Symptom Manage 1991;6:411.

29. Payne R, Coluzzi P, Hart L, Simmonds M, Lyss A, Rauck R, et al: Long-term safety of oral transmucosal fentanyl citrate for breakthrough cancer pain. J Pain Symptom Manage 2001;22:575.

30. Warren D: Practical use of rectal medication in palliative care. J Pain Symptom Manage 1996;11:378.

31. Carr D, Goudas L, Lawrence D, et al: Management of Cancer Symptoms: Pain, Depression, and Fatigue. Evidence Report/Technology assessment No. 61. Washington, DC. Agency for Healthcare Research and Quality. AHRQ Publication No. 02-E032, July 2002.

32. Kaiko Rf, Fitzmartin RD, Thomas GB, et al: The bioavailability of morphine in controlled-release 30 mg tablets. Pharmacotherapy 1992;12:107.

33. Rousseau PC: Non-pain symptom management in terminal care. Clin Geriatr Med 1996;12:313.

34. Reuben DB, Mor V: Dyspnea in terminally ill cancer patients. Chest 1986;89:234.

35. McCann RM, Hall WJ, Groth-Junker A: Comfort care for terminally ill patients; the appropriate use of nutrition and hydration. JAMA 1994;272:1263.

36. Ellershaw JE, Sutcliffe JM, Saunders CM: Dehydration and the dying patient. J Pain Symptom Manage 1995;10:192.

37. Breitbart W, Jaramillo JR, Chochinov HM: Palliative and Terminal care. In Holland JC (ed): Psycho-Oncology. Oxford, Oxford University Press, 1998, p 437.

38. Luce JM, Luce JA: Management of dyspnea in patients with far-advanced lung disease: "Once I lose it, it's kind of hard to catch it …". JAMA 2001;285:1331.

39. Chochinov HM, Wilson KG, Enns M, Lander S: "Are you depressed?" Screening for depression in the terminally ill. Am J Psychiatry 1997;154:674.

40. Block SD: Assessing and Managing Depression in the terminally ill patient. Ann Intern Med 2000;132:209.

41. Wallace AE, Kofoed LL, West AN: Double-blind, placebo-controlled trial of methylphenidate in older, depressed, medically ill patients. Am J Psychiatry 1995;152:929.

42. Lawlor PG, Gagnon B, Mancini IL, Pereira JL, Hanson J, Suarez-Almazor ME, et al: Occurrence, causes and outcomes of delirium in patients with advanced cancer: A prospective study. Arch Intern Med 2000;160:786.

43. Cassarett DJ, Inouye SK: Diagnosis and management of delirium near the end of life. Ann Intern Med 2001;135:32.

44. Coyle N, Breitbart W, Weaver S, et al: Delirium as a contributing factor to "crescendo pain": Three case reports. J Pain Symptom Manage 1994;9:44.

45. Breitbart W, Marotta R, Platt MM, et al: A double-blind trial of haloperidol, chlorpromazine, and lorazepam in the treatment of delirium in hospitalized AIDS patients. Am J Psychiatry 1996;153:231.

46. Indelicato RA, Portenoy RK: Opioid rotation in the management of refractory cancer pain. J Clin Oncol 2002;20:348.

47. Kristjanson L, Leis A, Koop PM, Carriere KC, Mueller B: Family members' care expectations, care perceptions, and satisfaction with advanced care: Results of a multi-site pilot study. J Palliat Care 1997;134:5.

48. Lederberg MS: The family of the cancer patient. In Holland JC (ed): Psycho-Oncology. Oxford, Oxford University Press, 1998, p 981.

49. Chochinov HM, Holland JC, Katz LY: Bereavement: A special issue in oncology. In Holland JC (ed): Psycho-Oncology. Oxford, Oxford University Press, 1998, p 1016.

50. Lynn J: Serving patients who may die soon and their families: The role of hospice and other services. JAMA 2001;285:925.

51. Rauch PK, Muriel AC, Cassem NH: Parents with cancer: Who's looking after the children. J Clin Onc 2002;20:4399.

52. Fitchett G, Handzo G: Spiritual assessment, screening, and intervention. In Holland JC (ed): Psycho-Oncology. Oxford, Oxford University Press, 1998, p 790.

53. Cherny NI, Portenoy RK: Sedation in the management of refractory symptoms: Guidelines for evaluation and treatment. J Palliat Care 1994;10:31.

54. Truog RD, Berde CB, Mitchell C, Grier HE: Barbiturates in the care of the terminally ill. N Engl J Med 1992;327:1678.

55. Christakis NA, Iwashyna TJ: The health impact of health care on families: A matched cohort study of hospice use by decedents, and mortality outcomes in surviving, widowed spouses. Soc Sci Med 2003;57:465.

56. Committee on Care at the End of Life, Institute of Medicine: The health care system and the dying patient. In Field MJ, Cassel CK (eds): Approaching Death, Improving Care at the End of Life. Washington, National Academy Press, 1997, p 47.

57. Callahan D: "Frustrated mastery: The cultural context of death in America." Western J Med 1995;163:226.

58. Kinzbrunner BM: Hospice: 15 years and beyond in the care of the dying. J Palliat Med 1998;1:127.

59. Rando TA: Treatment of Complicated Mourning, Champaign, Il: Research Press, 1993.

60. Prigerson HG, Bierhals AJ, Kasl SV, Reynolds CF III, Shear MK, Newsom JT, et al: Complicated grief as a disorder distinct from bereavement-related depression and anxiety: A replication study. Am J Psychiatry 1996;153:1484.

61. Piper WWE, Ogrodniczuk JS, Joyce AS, Mccallum M, Weideman R, Azim HF: Ambivalence and other relationship predictors of grief and depression in psychiatric outpatients. J Nerv Mental Dis 2001;189:781.

62. Barry LC, Kasl SV, Prigerson HG: Psychiatric disorders among bereaved persons: The role of perceived circumstances of death and preparedness for death. Am J Geriatric Psych 2002;10:447.

63. Bradley EH, Prigerson H, Carlson MDA, Cherlin E, Kasl SV, Johnson-Hurzeler R: Does length of hospice enrollment affect depression among surviving caregivers? in press

64. Worden JW: Bereavement. Sem Onc 1985;12:472.

65. Parkes CM: Bereavement. In Doyle D, Hanks GWC, Macdonald N (eds): Oxford Textbook of Palliative Medicine, 2nd ed. Oxford, Oxford University Press, 1997, p 995.

66. Lewis CS: A grief observed. New York, Bantam Seabury Press, 1963.
67. Prigerson HG, Jacobs SC: Caring for bereaved patients: "All the doctors just suddenly go." JAMA 2001;286:1369.
68. Jagger C, Sutton CJ: Death after marital bereavement: Is the risk increased? Statistics Med 1991;10:395.
69. Barry LC, Kasl SV, Prigerson HG: Psychiatric disorders among bereaved persons: The role of perceived circumstances of death and preparedness for death. Am J Geriatric Psych 2002;10:447.
70. Zisook S, Shuchter SR, Pedrelli P, Sable J, Deaciuc SC: Buproprion sustained release for bereavement: Results of an open trial. J Clin Psychiatry 2001;62:227.
71. Zygmont M, Prigerson HG, Houck PR, Miller MD, Shear MK, Jacobs S, et al: A post hoc comparison of paroxetine and nortriptyline for symptoms of traumatic grief. J Clin Psychiatry 1998;59:241.
72. Abrahm JL, Cooley ME, Ricacho L: Efficacy of an educational bereavement program for families of veterans with cancer. J Cancer Ed 1995;10:207–212.

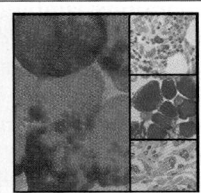

44

DISORDERS OF BLOOD CELL PRODUCTION IN CLINICAL ONCOLOGY

George D. Demetri

Kenneth C. Anderson

SUMMARY OF KEY POINTS

INCIDENCE

- The incidence of hematopoietic dysfunction is high (>90%) among cancer patients, with or without cytotoxic therapy.
- Anemia is the most common problem, red blood cell lineage nearly always being affected to some degree.
- Leukopenia is associated with cytotoxic treatment in 20% to 50% of patients with solid tumors.
- Clinically significant thrombocytopenia is far less common (<10% of cancer patients), although it is a common problem with high-dose chemotherapy and leukemia therapies.

ETIOLOGY OF THE COMPLICATION

- Marrow dysfunction usually is multifactorial.
- Host factors are nutritional deficiencies, decreased target cell number and function, decreased stem cell reserve, tumor suppression of hematopoiesis, and autoimmune syndromes.
- Iatrogenic factors are cytotoxic chemotherapy and radiation therapy.

EVALUATION OF THE PATIENT

- Determine the critical factors associated with hematopoietic dysfunction.
- Obtain the history and perform a physical examination and diagnostic laboratory studies.

- Assess the clinical significance of hematopoietic dysfunction.
- Assess the nature of the problem: acute versus chronic, mild versus severe, expected versus unexpected.
- Modify treatment plans accordingly.
- Treatment options may differ for endogenous and congenital versus acquired marrow failure.
- If the primary cause is a host factor, correct the problem if possible.
- If the primary cause is an iatrogenic factor, consider alterations of therapy as appropriate for patient and therapeutic goals (palliation versus cure).

TREATMENT OPTIONS FOR CORRECTION OF HEMATOPOIETIC DYSFUNCTION

- Pharmacologic dosing of hematopoietic cytokines.
- Prophylactic versus therapeutic intent.
- Mitigation of neutropenia with granulocyte colony-stimulating factor or granulocyte-macrophage colony-stimulating factor.
- Stimulation of erythropoiesis with erythropoietin.
- Stimulation of thrombopoiesis with interleukin 11 or newer thrombopoietins.
- Transfusional and cellular support for hematopoietic dysfunction.
- Red blood cell transfusions.
- Granulocyte transfusions.
- Platelet transfusions.
- Stem cell transplantation.
- Autologous versus allogeneic transfusion.

- Peripheral blood versus marrow-derived transfusion.
- Mobilized stem cells versus basal state hematopoiesis.
- Negative/positive selection versus bulk reinfusion.
- Immunohematologic considerations of transfusions.

TRANSFUSION-RELATED ISSUES AND COMPLICATIONS

- Transfusion-associated graft-versus-host disease is a risk for all patients, not just bone marrow transplant recipients.
- There is a rationale for 2500-cGy irradiation of blood components before transfusion.
- Transfusion carries risk of numerous infectious diseases, including hepatitis B and C, cytomegalovirus infection, and human immunodeficiency virus infection.

SPECIAL CONSIDERATIONS IN STEM CELL TRANSPLANTATION

- Blood component and cytokine support may differ in the specialized setting of intentional endogenous marrow failure induced by high-dose therapy and rescued with stem cell transplantation.
- Peripheral blood progenitor cells represent the latest technology in hematologic supportive care for mitigating the hematopoietic dysfunction associated with high-dose chemotherapy or chemoradiotherapy.

INTRODUCTION

The process by which the human body produces the formed elements of the blood is remarkably dynamic and prolific. As such, these hematopoietic processes in cancer patients may fail to function normally because of endo-genous problems or exogenous myelosuppressive insults. Given the physiologic importance of hematopoiesis, the consequences of such marrow failure states usually are grave if normal blood production is not resumed rapidly. Many types of hematopoietic dysfunction are encountered in the practice of clinical oncology and hematology. These range from rare congenital marrow failure syndromes, which are generally permanent, to acquired defects in hematopoietic proliferation or differentiation, which may be transient or permanent, and which are often iatrogenically related to therapy for cancer. This chapter identifies several of the more common hematopoietic dysfunction syndromes in patients with neoplastic disorders and discusses clinical management, including various types of blood component support as well as strategies for therapeutic intervention with recombinant human hematopoietic cytokines.

MECHANISMS OF MALIGNANCY-ASSOCIATED HEMATOPOIETIC DYSFUNCTION

Cancer and its treatment alter normal hematopoiesis by direct effects on hematopoietic stem cells or by indirect means, such as inhibition of production of and responsiveness to hematopoietic growth factors. In particular, the crucial microenvironmental interactions among bone marrow hematopoietic cells, microvascular endothelial cells, and connective tissue stromal cells can be disrupted by primary tumor in hematologic diseases intrinsic to marrow and by metastatic spread of tumor to the marrow from neoplasms originating in extramedullary sites. Hodgkin's disease, non-Hodgkin's lymphoma, malignant melanoma, neuroblastoma, Ewing's sarcoma, and carcinoma of the breast, prostate, lung, adrenal glands, thyroid, and kidney frequently involve the bone marrow of patients with advanced disease. Associated symptoms or radiographic abnormalities are commonly lacking. Leukoerythroblastic anemia, characterized by immature erythroid and myeloid elements in the peripheral blood, is occasionally a clinical indicator of tumor in the marrow.[1] Ultimately, diffuse involvement of marrow with tumor can lead to marrow fibrosis or necrosis, which may be associated with splenomegaly, thrombocytopenia, and extramedullary hematopoiesis with immature cells of all lineages in the peripheral blood.[2]

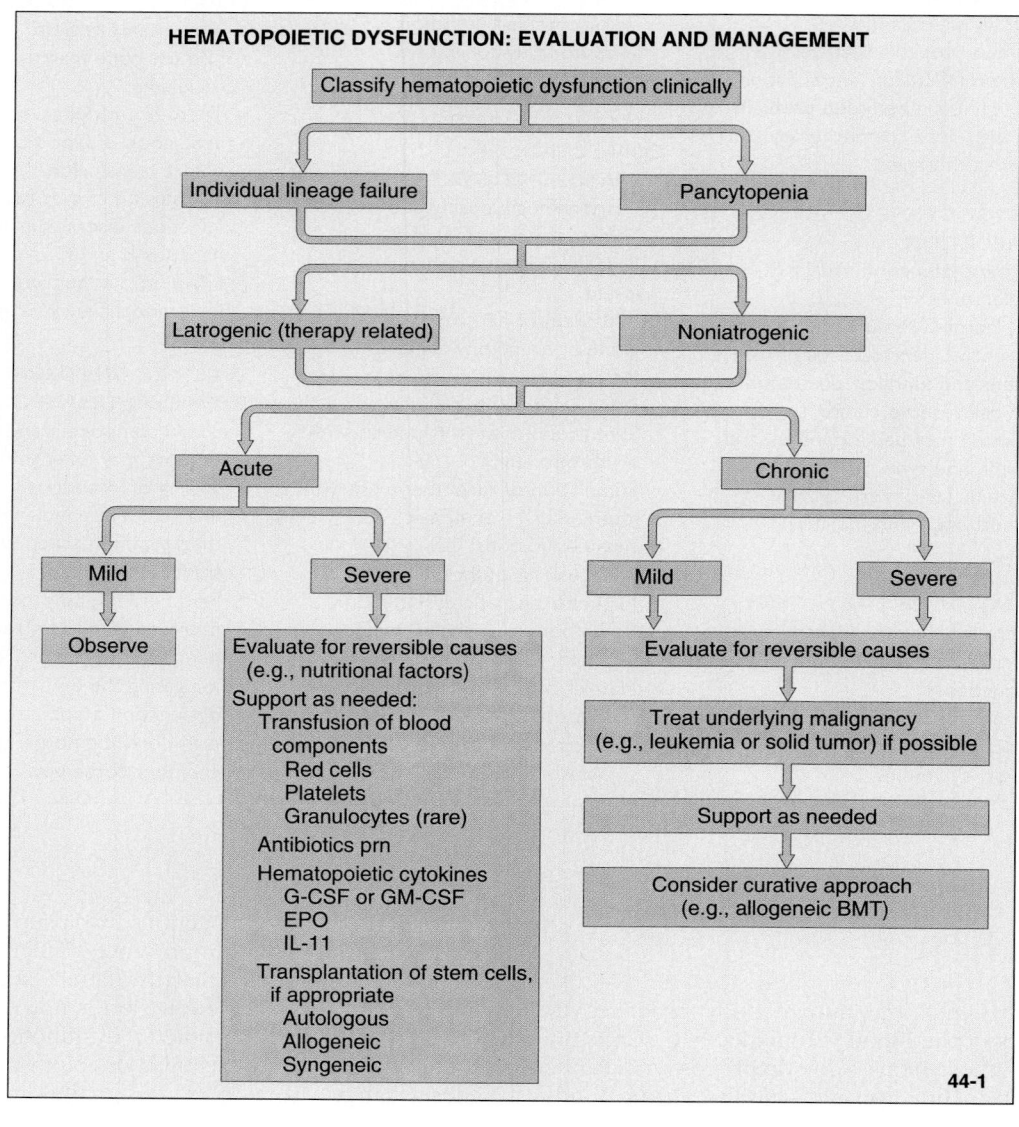

By far the most common cause of temporary hematopoietic dysfunction in patients with cancer is cytotoxic therapy for the malignant disease. The effects of cytotoxic therapy on marrow injury and recovery depend on several variables, including the following:

1. The cytotoxic drugs administered
2. The doses administered
3. The duration of therapy and amount of previous therapy (functional stem cell reserve)
4. The normal turnover rate of cells of different hematologic lineages

Bone marrow houses a storage compartment of proliferating cells at various stages of differentiation that can supply the peripheral blood with mature effector cells for 8 to 10 days after the pool of more primitive hematopoietic progenitor cells decreases its normal levels of division and maturation. Suppression of the peripheral blood count is therefore generally noticed a week or so after a toxic insult to the bone marrow. In patients to whom several of the most commonly used cytotoxic agents had been administered, leukopenia (and possibly thrombocytopenia) typically begins 7 to 10 days after drug treatment, nadir counts occurring on the 14th to 18th day. Recovery of counts is evident by the 21st day and generally reaches or exceeds the pretreatment baseline by the 28th day. The most active compartments of hematopoietic cell proliferation and differentiation are generally found within the lineage-committed progenitor cell subsets. True stem cells and extremely immature progenitor cells in the marrow usually exist in a noncycling quiescent state, which presumably protects them from excessive damage induced by common chemotherapeutic treatments (and the slings and arrows of daily environmental insults over a lifetime). The pharmacologic mechanism of a cytotoxic drug; the dose, route, and schedule of drug administration; drug metabolism; and the pattern of cell sensitivity influence the clinical presentation of drug-induced hematopoietic dysfunction. Cytotoxic drugs have actions at specific points in the cell cycle and often are classified on that basis. Hematopoietic stem cells may rebound after short-term exposure to a cell cycle–specific agent, whereas prolonged administration may result in permanent marrow dysfunction. For cell cycle–specific agents, such as cytosine arabinoside (ara-C) or methotrexate, recovery typically occurs rapidly (7–14 days), whereas non–cell cycle–specific agents (occasionally referred to as "stem cell poisons" or G_0-active agents) such as carmustine (BCNU) and busulfan cause a much more delayed nadir (e.g., at 4–5 weeks) and slow recovery (e.g., more than 6 weeks after drug administration). Moreover, a chronic deficit in marrow reserve occurs fairly quickly with sequential BCNU therapy but rarely, if ever, occurs after administration of cell cycle–specific agents such as ara-C. Bone marrow involvement with tumor can compromise physiologic reserves of true stem cells and more mature progenitor cells, shortening the time to peripheral leukopenia and thrombocytopenia and prolonging the time to hematologic recovery.

Radiation therapy also contributes to pancytopenia. Cells damaged by irradiation have limited divisional capacity before their progeny are rendered reproductively sterile; thus an irradiated cell may not appear to be damaged until it divides.[3] At the first postirradiation division, the cell (1) dies, (2) divides aberrantly and produces unusual forms, (3) is unable to divide yet remains physiologically functional, or (4) gives rise to one or more generations of genetically damaged progeny until the later cells become sterile. Because hematopoietic stem cells are thought to have very low capability of repair of sublethal irradiation damage, delivery of multiple small radiation fractions may mitigate toxicities in other normal tissues (e.g., lung, gastrointestinal tract) but does not spare bone marrow. During a course of fractionated irradiation, the ultimate effect on normal bone marrow depends on whether there has been proliferation in the irradiated field between the fractions or migration of cells from adjacent unirradiated sites. Finally, the effects of total-body irradiation qualitatively and quantitatively differ from those that occur with localized therapy. In particular, total-body irradiation profoundly suppresses both humoral and cellular immune function.[4]

DIFFERENTIAL DIAGNOSIS OF CANCER-ASSOCIATED HEMATOPOIETIC DYSFUNCTION

It is essential to keep in mind the numerous derangements in normal physiologic processes that can occur in the setting of cancer or cytotoxic treatment. Any of these derangements can contribute to pancytopenia. They include deficiencies or lack of bioavailability of nutritional factors, such as folate, iron, or other vitamins; abnormal regulatory mechanisms in hematopoiesis, such as cell-mediated suppression of hematopoiesis in aplastic anemia[5]; a blunted response to erythropoietin (EPO) with anemia in cancer patients[6]; and stimulation of thrombopoiesis associated with iron deficiency anemia. Marrow fibrosis and stromal damage can occur as part of a disease or as a reaction to therapy, thereby compromising bone marrow reserve and function. Immunologically mediated destruction of cells as well as factors such as splenomegaly can result in clinically significant cytopenia. Most important, occult bleeding must always be considered in the differential diagnosis of persistent anemia and refractory thrombocytopenia. These clinical examples emphasize the importance of careful assessment of the condition of cancer patients for clinically reversible causes of hematologic complications before these effects are attributed to the underlying neoplasm.

HEMATOPOIETIC DYSFUNCTION BY HEMATOLOGIC LINEAGE

Leukopenia

Leukopenia commonly is related to cancer and its treatment. In 1965, Hersh and colleagues[7] summarized the causes of death among patients with acute leukemia treated at the National Cancer Institute and found a marked decline in fatal hemorrhage (due to the availability of platelet transfusions) with a concomitant increase in occurrence of infections as a cause of death. A quantitative relation between circulating leukocytes and infection was established in the classic work by Bodey and associates.[8] In studies involving patients with leukemia undergoing myelosuppressive therapy, these investigators first described the proportional and quantitative relation between the probability of contracting an infection and both the severity and duration of leukopenia. The clinical risk of leukopenia, defined in early studies with patients with hematologic malignant diseases, has been widely extrapolated to include patients with solid tumors, who typically have much shorter-term chemotherapy-induced leukopenia. The clinical relevance of this extrapolation from patients with leukemia to those with solid tumors has never been subjected to rigorous prospective studies. The prognostic factors that determine an individual patient's risk of development of fever with neutropenia (or the risk of serious adverse outcome from a neutropenic period) remain very poorly understood. Talcott and colleagues[9,10] formulated models with which to predict outcome from clinical criteria at manifestation of fever and neutropenia, but the widespread validity of the models is still being tested. Nevertheless, most physicians reasonably view leukopenia (and neutropenia in particular) as a life-threatening clinical state that justifies medical intervention to minimize risks. In addition, the level of circulating neutrophils may have other indirect clinical effects (e.g., by forcing changes in chemotherapy administration and thereby indirectly leading to suboptimal antitumor efficacy of chemotherapy). Circulating neutrophil counts have traditionally been one of the clinical criteria used to determine whether a patient has recovered sufficiently from a previous cycle of cytotoxic chemotherapy and is ready to tolerate the next planned cycle, so as to avoid risk of excessive myelotoxicity. Thus inadequate neutrophil counts can delay chemotherapy administration or lead to the decision to reduce the chemotherapy dose. Although either decision may be reasonable, there may be situations in which delivery of a suboptimal chemotherapy dose or schedule would compromise clinical outcome. It often is quoted that suboptimal dosing of adjuvant chemotherapy has been shown to have an adverse effect on survival of node-positive breast cancer patients.[11] Although this effect has been found in large prospective trials of therapy for breast cancer, the clinical relevance of dose intensity (including both absolute chemotherapy dose delivered and dosing schedule) may have less importance in palliative treatment of patients with metastatic cancer. The importance of chemotherapy dose and schedule remains an area of active clinical investigation, and these questions are intimately tied to issues of hematopoietic supportive care.

Anemia

Anemia in patients with cancer or primary hematologic disorders ranges from mild to severe and often has multifactorial causes. Erythropoiesis in patients with early stages of cancer may be normal. Most commonly, both the incidence and the magnitude of anemia in patients with cancer increase as the disease progresses. Replacement of marrow hematopoietic elements by tumor is not essential for the development of anemia, even in patients with widely metastatic cancer. Malignancy-associated anemia is designated *anemia of chronic disease* only if the cellular pattern in the marrow is near normal, serum iron level and iron-binding capacity are low, the iron content of the marrow is normal or increased, and serum ferritin level is elevated.[12] The coexistence of a low plasma iron level with an adequate amount of storage iron helps differentiate anemia of chronic disease from iron deficiency anemia. Moreover, other causes of anemia, such as active hemolysis, uncontrolled bleeding, nutritional deficiency, and marrow replacement, must be ruled out. Finally, results of studies with chromium-labeled red blood cells (RBCs) suggest that RBC survival can be significantly shortened in certain patients with advanced cancer without classic clinical or laboratory evidence of hemolysis.[13] In some patients, such as those with histiocytic medullary reticulosis and Hodgkin's disease, erythrophagocytosis or hypersplenism may account for the decrease in RBC survival, but in others the cause of this phenomenon remains unclear.

Serum EPO levels have been reported to be inappropriately low for a given level of anemia in patients with cancer compared with a control population with anemia of benign causation.[6] Moreover, increases in EPO serum levels expected for a given degree of anemia can be further blunted by chemotherapy regimens with or without nephrotoxic agents such as cisplatin. The blunted ability of cancer patients to produce EPO is not absolute, because hypoxemia can induce a seemingly adequate EPO response. The specific molecular mechanisms regulating EPO-producing cells in the kidney and liver are unclear. It is possible that these EPO-producing cells are directly suppressed by the malignant growth itself or that the cells are functionally impaired by chemotherapy and radiation therapy. This phenomenon has been suggested as the cause of anemia associated with nephrotoxic chemotherapy (e.g., cisplatin), although direct erythroid marrow toxicity may play a role.[14,15] Because the endogenous EPO response to anemia is inappropriately low in patients with cancer,[16,17] management of anemia of cancer with pharmacologic dosing of recombinant human erythropoietic agents presents an appealingly rational therapeutic approach. This hypothesis has been tested extensively in prospective, placebo-controlled trials. The beneficial effects of providing supplemental erythropoietic cytokine support to cancer patients are discussed later.

Inappropriately low production of erythrocytes can be caused by inadequate EPO stimulation of progenitor cells committed to erythroid proliferation and differentiation pathways. However, endogenous signaling abnormalities in the target cell populations also can result in a similar anemic phenotype in the host. For example, patients with myelodysplastic syndrome (MDS) have evidence of inadequate cellular maturation despite the presence of large numbers of dysplastic erythroid progenitors in hypercellular marrow.

Immune hemolytic anemia occasionally is associated with neoplasms of the lymphocytic and reticuloendothelial systems. Anemia in such cases, usually moderate to severe, is associated with jaundice, splenomegaly, and increased urine and fecal urobilinogen excretion. RBC survival is decreased and the reticulocyte count increased, unless erythropoiesis is profoundly impaired. Hemolytic anemia may be due to warm-reacting immunoglobulin G (IgG) with a positive direct antiglobulin (Coombs') test result and positive reaction to antiserum specific for IgG on RBCs. This condition occurs most commonly in chronic lymphoid leukemia but also has been reported in patients with lymphoma, acute leukemia, myeloproliferative disorders, or carcinoma. IgM antibody can bind and cause agglutination in the cold. In either case, anemia occurs because of reticuloendothelial sequestration of RBCs coated with antibody or complement components (extravascular hemolysis). The combination of hemoglobinemia and hemoglobulinuria (due to extensive intravascular hemolysis) occurs very rarely and has been attributed to the presence of high titers of cold-reacting antibody.

Microangiopathic hemolytic anemia, characterized by RBC distortion and fragmentation on smear (schistocytes) and intravascular hemolysis with associated thrombocytopenia, is uncommon. When observed in oncology, however, microangiopathic hemolytic anemia usually is evident in patients with metastatic carcinoma (such as adenocarcinoma of the stomach, breast, prostate, lung, pancreas, gallbladder, or colon) or with advanced angiosarcoma.[18] Certain chemotherapeutic regimens may predispose a patient to this complication through mechanisms that remain obscure. Intravascular coagulation with low clotting factor level, fibrinolysis, increased level of fibrin degradation products, and increased fibrin catabolism may be present. RBC fragmentation may be due to deposition of fibrin within vessels, intravascular coagulation may be initiated by the release of thromboplastins by the tumor cells, or both mechanisms may be operative. Finally, anemia may be related to pure RBC aplasia without associated leukocyte or platelet marrow abnormalities, commonly associated with thymoma,[19] and rarely manifest itself in the setting of lymphoma or chronic lymphoid leukemia.

Thrombocytopenia

Thrombocytopenia in cancer patients usually is attributable to chemotherapy and radiation therapy, usually with high doses of treatment or following lengthy cumulative cytotoxic therapy over time. Impaired production of platelets because of a decrease or absence of megakaryocytes therefore is the most common cause of thrombocytopenia in patients with cancer. However, thrombocytopenia also can be caused by splenic sequestration in patients in whom splenomegaly is part of the primary neoplastic process. In this setting, increased numbers of megakaryocytes are evident, unless extensive marrow infiltration is present. Immune-mediated thrombocytopenia may be related to anti–human lymphocyte antigen (HLA) or anti–platelet-specific alloantibodies. Finally, thrombocytopenia may be related to disseminated

intravascular coagulation, especially in patients with acute myelocytic leukemia, lymphoma, or carcinoma of the lung, breast, gastrointestinal tract, or urogenital tract. In relative proportions, disseminated intravascular coagulation most commonly complicates acute promyelocytic leukemia owing to the presence of both thromboplastic material and fibrinolytic proteases in the promyelocytic subcellular components.[20]

Platelet function can be abnormal even if platelet count is normal. For example, platelet function can be abnormal in several chronic myeloproliferative disorders. Although most bleeding in patients with acute myeloid leukemia is related to thrombocytopenia, intrinsic abnormalities in platelet function have been described, including decreased platelet procoagulant activity and decreased aggregation and serotonin release responses to adenosine diphosphate, epinephrine, or collagen.[21] These defects may reflect the fact that megakaryocytes have originated from a leukemic stem cell. Platelet transfusions, coupled with treatment of the underlying disease, remain the mainstay of therapy for such platelet dysfunction syndromes. Platelet dysfunction also is evident in a fraction of patients with IgA myeloma or Waldenström's macroglobulinemia, multiple myeloma, and monoclonal gammopathy of undetermined significance.[22] In addition to thrombocytopenia, these factors may predispose to bleeding or hyperviscosity syndromes. These conditions also may be associated with acquired factor X deficiency in the setting of amyloidosis, a circulating heparin-like anticoagulant, fibrinolysis, and interference by myeloma protein with both fibrin polymerization and the function of other coagulation proteins. If any of these complicating syndromes is present, expeditious cytoreductive therapy for the underlying malignant disease is the intervention of choice, plasmapheresis being reserved for acute bleeding. Data from the National Cancer Institute in the early 1960s clearly demonstrated that leukemia patients died of hemorrhage during induction of remission with chemotherapy[7] and established the quantitative relation between platelet count and hemorrhage.[23] Although there is no argument that low circulating platelet count increases the risk of bleeding complications, a great deal of controversy has accompanied the question of the level of thrombocytopenia that merits prophylactic intervention. At many institutions, prophylactic platelet transfusions are given in the outpatient setting if the circulating platelet count decreases to less than 20,000 platelets/µL blood. Current practice patterns, however, are derived from extrapolation of the retrospective data derived from a very select subset of patients with malignant disease (i.e., leukemia patients undergoing remission induction therapy).[24] However, in two trials patients with leukemia were randomized to receive prophylactic platelet transfusions at levels of 10,000/µL or 20,000/µL. The investigators found that the lower threshold was safe and resulted in a lower number of platelet transfusions.[25-27] As is true of attempts to define the risk of circulating neutropenia in the absence of fever, the risk of circulating thrombocytopenia in the absence of bleeding remains a poorly defined clinical variable.[28] Nevertheless, thrombocytopenia can indirectly affect treatment of patients with malignant disease by causing postponement or dose reductions of planned cytotoxic drug regimens.

HEMATOPOIETIC CYTOKINES FOR IMPROVEMENT OF DYSFUNCTIONAL BLOOD CELL PRODUCTION IN CANCER PATIENTS

The cellular processes of hematopoiesis are regulated in part by humoral mediators variously known as hematopoietic growth factors or hematopoietic cytokines. Understanding of the biologic mechanisms of these soluble regulators of blood production has increased dramatically.[29-37] The availability of pure preparations of recombinant human hematopoietic cytokines for clinical use has prompted extensive study of these agents for amelioration of hematopoiesis in cancer patients. On the basis of these data, clinical practice guidelines have been developed for these agents to foster appropriate use, primarily driven by the cost of these recombinant drugs and the desire to optimize use of medical resources.[38-42]

For clinical applications, the development of hematopoietic cytokines has been based on preclinical evidence of stimulatory effects on specific hematopoietic cell lineages and processes. The clinical effects of a recombinant hematopoietic cytokine may diverge somewhat from the full spectrum of activity in laboratory models. For example, granulocyte-macrophage colony-stimulating factor (GM-CSF) is a true multilineage hematopoietic agent in vitro, stimulating cells in neutrophilic, eosinophilic, monocytic, erythroid, and megakaryocytic lineages.[43-45] However, the clinical activities of this molecule in vivo are found primarily in stimulation of the neutrophilic, eosinophilic, and monocytic lineage.[46] Although preclinical research is essential for understanding the basic biologic mechanisms of these cytokines, extrapolation to clinical application requires performance and judicious interpretation of well-designed clinical trials designed to evaluate efficacy and safety of recombinant agents in patients.

Treatment-Associated Neutropenia: Decreasing Risk and Improving Therapy with Hematopoietic Cytokines

The most common marrow failure state in patients with malignant disease is transient and iatrogenic: the myelosuppression that occurs as nonspecific toxicity associated with cytotoxic therapy for cancer. As part of this temporary marrow dysfunction, the neutrophil lineage usually is most severely impaired by the effect of most common chemotherapies. The true clinical effect of very transient (<5 days) neutropenia in patients with solid tumors remains limited in terms of risk of treatment-related mortality. However, treatment-related morbidity, in terms of hospitalization for fever with neutropenia, remains a rather common clinical event, especially with longer duration of neutropenia or with agents that cause mucositis and alter mucosal barriers to infection. For this reason, a great deal of clinical investigation has focused on the ability of hematopoietic cytokines to minimize the period of neutropenia and thus to alter the clinical outcome associated with myelosuppressive chemotherapy for cancer. The first hematopoietic cytokines with activity on the neutrophil lineage to be tested in the clinic were granulocyte colony-stimulating factor (G-CSF) and GM-CSF. Even in the earliest phase I clinical testing for toxicity, these agents proved remarkably effective in increasing circulating levels of leukocytes, particularly neutrophils.[36,47-49] Administration of pharmacologic doses of these recombinant molecules was well tolerated overall. Phase I testing of GM-CSF demonstrated dose-limiting toxicity (e.g., pleuropericarditis, capillary leak, venous thrombosis) associated with administration of very high daily doses of this agent. Clinical activity, however, was clearly documented at GM-CSF doses well below those associated with such severe adverse effects.[50] In contrast, phase I toxicity testing of G-CSF did not demonstrate dose-limiting toxicity, even at massive doses (e.g., >100 µg/kg/d).[47,51,52] Dose-escalation studies with G-CSF were halted because there seemed to be no reasonable medical indication for driving circulating neutrophil count to the exceedingly high levels (e.g., 80,000 neutrophils/µL blood) possible with safe and tolerable doses of this agent. Thus these agents proved appropriate clinical tools for use in adjunctive supportive care of patients with cancer.

Large-scale testing of G-CSF and GM-CSF proceeded extremely rapidly after initial toxicity testing in humans with few (if any) classic phase II clinical trials to confirm clinical efficacy, because clinical activities was already so evident in phase I studies. Large, multicenter, placebo-controlled, double-blind, randomized studies were performed to evaluate the clinical activity of both G-CSF and GM-CSF in minimizing the toxicity of myelosuppressive therapies. However, the primary clinical settings for randomized testing of these agents differed somewhat: G-CSF was tested as an adjunct to aggressive yet conventional-dose combination chemotherapy in patients with small cell lung cancer, whereas GM-CSF was tested as an adjunct to high-dose chemotherapy and radiation therapy with autologous bone marrow transplantation (BMT) for a heterogeneous population of patients with lymphoid malignant disease. Both agents were tested with "prophylactic intent"; the CSF was dosed immediately after the myelosuppressive insult, *before* the onset of infectious complications.

Several large, prospective, placebo-controlled studies have documented the clinical efficacy of G-CSF in mitigating myelosuppression in the neutrophilic lineage and in favorably influencing clinical outcome by decreasing the incidence of hospitalization for fever and neutropenia. One study in the United States[53] was conducted with a crossover design after the first cycle of chemotherapy. The design prohibited definitive interpretation of cumulative effects over multiple cycles (because most of the patients crossed over to open-label G-CSF by the end of the study). A similar study performed in Europe[54] did not have a crossover design. Both studies showed that prophylactic administration of G-CSF after aggressive dosing of conventional combination chemotherapy shortened the period of absolute neutropenia approximately 50% compared with results in the placebo control group. This result was associated with a significantly decreased incidence of hospitalization for fever with neutropenia.

To attain clinical benefits with G-CSF, patients have had to receive multiple daily subcutaneous injections after chemotherapy administration. More recently, the activity of G-CSF has been made more convenient in a pegylated version that has sustained biologic activity. This newer, pegylated version of G-CSF, known as pegfilgrastim, has been shown to have no significant differences from conventional G-CSF in terms of efficacy or side-effect profile when administered as a single injection after chemotherapy.[55-57]

GM-CSF has been tested as an agent for accelerating hematopoietic recovery from high-dose chemoradiotherapy with autologous BMT. Data from one large, randomized, prospective study demonstrated the ability of GM-CSF to accelerate neutrophil recovery compared with effects of a placebo, once the first signs of neutrophil recovery appeared in the periphery.[58] In application of these findings to other marrow dysfunction syndromes, this point is important: GM-CSF appeared to be unable to accelerate recovery of first signs of reconstitution of the mature neutrophil compartment, but GM-CSF significantly amplified the speed of reconstitution after some recovery had occurred. This phenomenon can be interpreted biologically as evidence that the target cells for GM-CSF are part of a committed progenitor cell pool that is ablated as part of the preparative cytotoxic regimen for autologous BMT. GM-CSF cannot influence the rate of repopulation of this committed progenitor cell pool. However, once some target cells are available, GM-CSF can drive those cells down proliferative and differentiative pathways, the result being acceleration of clinical single-lineage hematologic reconstitution. Compared with effects of placebo, no significant effects on platelet recovery were found. These findings were consistent with the lineage-restricted activity of GM-CSF found in other clinical trials. Certain clinical endpoints were significantly improved in this study: There was a 7-day decrease in the time to hospital discharge for GM-CSF–treated patients compared with placebo control patients. The effect on morbidity related to this highly myelosuppressive therapy was the major clinical outcome benefit. Whereas the foregoing studies evaluated prophylactic use of G-CSF or GM-CSF, another use might be treatment of patients with therapeutic intent only after an infectious episode has declared itself. Data from one multicenter trial suggested there may be limited clinical benefit to such an approach in certain patient subsets, but the overall benefit appeared to be less than if the hematopoietic cytokine had been used with prophylactic intent.[59] However, other studies have shown somewhat more activity,[60,61] and the therapeutic use of hematopoietic cytokines will require more thoughtful analysis before it can be ascertained which patients with fever and neutropenia may benefit the most from post hoc dosing.

These research findings document the ability to modulate the levels of neutrophils in clinically meaningful ways for patients undergoing myelosuppressive therapy. Application of these findings to the conventional practice of oncology remains a subject of great controversy.

The patient groups most likely to benefit from receiving adjunctive G-CSF or GM-CSF remain poorly defined. The cost of these agents is high, especially for drugs without primary antineoplastic activity whose primary role is reduction of treatment-related toxicity. Further research is necessary to define any possibility for survival benefit in patients treated with hematopoietic cytokines. Most investigators believe that any survival benefit will be related to the ability to deliver even higher, and more toxic, doses of cytotoxic therapy, but this hypothesis remains to be fully tested in appropriately designed clinical trials.

Another aspect of improving clinical outcome among patients is the potential for increasing the quality of life of patients undergoing myelosuppressive therapy. Cytokine support of myelosuppressive regimens may allow patients to tolerate these treatments with quantifiable increases in quality of life. This role of therapy remains speculative, however, and has not been studied prospectively. Only after the benefits of such treatments are defined can rational plans be made for appropriate use of these agents. Although expensive, judicious use of G-CSF or GM-CSF may prove cost-effective for a certain clinically important outcome.[62-64] Lengthy analyses of evidence supporting appropriate clinical settings for hematopoietic cytokine support of cancer patients have been developed by the American Society of Clinical Oncology.[38-42] These analyses have been disseminated to the oncology community as evidence-based clinical practice guidelines, and the recommendations are reviewed and updated annually. Changes in practice have been objectively observed since the original publication of these guidelines.[42]

Improving on Endogenous Erythropoietin: Pharmacologic Stimulation of Erythropoiesis in Cancer Patients

The causes of anemia in patients with cancer can be multifactorial, including bleeding, inadequate production, hemolysis, and nutritional deficiencies, among others. Tumor-bearing patients with anemia have been found to have relatively insufficient levels of native EPO compared with patients in whom anemia has occurred through a different mechanism.[6] Investigators have studied whether exogenous supplementation with a recombinant erythropoietic cytokine might ameliorate the anemia associated with cancer or cancer therapy. Whereas epoetin alfa (recombinant human EPO [rhEPO]) once was the only recombinant human cytokine that could stimulate erythropoiesis, an option now available is darbepoetin alfa (darbEPO).[65] Prospective, randomized, placebo-controlled studies have been performed with both of these molecules in a variety of anemic cancer patients, either untreated with cytotoxic therapy or undergoing treatment with a wide variety of cytotoxic regimens. These trials have generally shown a gradual increase (occurring after 3 to 4 weeks of erythropoietic hormone dosing) in hemoglobin levels in patients receiving pharmacologic dosing with rhEPO or darbEPO.[66-68] Interpretation of these studies is made difficult by the 2- to 4-week "lead time" before any beneficial effect was found in these patients, who were already anemic on entrance into the study.

Overall, however, delayed and moderate diminution was found in the transfusion requirements of these patients. These findings led the U.S. Food and Drug Administration (FDA) to approve the use of both rhEPO and darbEPO in the management of chemotherapy-associated anemia.[69,70] The efficacy results with rhEPO have been confirmed and expanded in large community-based practice studies to confirm effectiveness in more than 6000 cancer patients.[71-73] These single-armed "effectiveness studies" represent some of the larger studies in the oncology supportive care literature attempting to measure whether stimulation of erythropoiesis by EPO in anemic cancer patients might be more than simply a "transfusion substitute" strategy. In these trials, quantification of improvements in patient-assessed quality-of-life indicators, such as energy level, activity level, and overall sense of well-being, was performed. The results of these studies confirmed the findings from the initial placebo-controlled studies that patients who respond to rhEPO dosing with an increase in hemoglobin level report clinical benefits in quality-of-life measures.[71-73] In general, although erythropoiesis may be stimulated moderately by pharmacologic provision of exogenous rhEPO or darbEPO, much of the clinical value of treating cancer patients with these agents may revolve around the cost-effectiveness of these agents, given the relatively high cost of rhEPO and darbEPO owing to the large doses needed by cancer patients. It is important to recognize the complexities in these assessments, because varying measurements of quality of life and of the actual offsetting costs associated with blood transfusions may make erythropoietic therapy a reasonable and cost-effective alternative to transfusional support in selected patient subsets. Such clinical subsets remain poorly defined, however, and further research will be useful to identify the most appropriate clinical use of EPO in treating patients with cancer-associated and chemotherapy-induced anemic states.

Other clinical scenarios of hematopoietic dysfunction may exhibit anemia, either as the sole clinical manifestation or as part of a multilineage marrow failure state. For example, endogenous EPO levels may be low after autologous and allogeneic marrow transplantation.[74,75] Results of pilot studies have suggested that treatment with EPO in this setting may prove useful.[76,77]

Patients with MDS usually are anemic and frequently have elevated levels of endogenous EPO. Several small pilot trials have attempted to drive erythropoiesis more effectively by pharmacologic dosing of EPO and thereby achieve supraphysiologic levels of EPO.[13,78-83] Although generally small and nonrandomized, these clinical trials have consistently demonstrated clinical effects of EPO supplementation in a small subset of patients with MDS (approximately 25%). Although the prognostic factors that might be predictive of a response to EPO supplementation remain poorly understood, results of most trials suggest that patients with exceedingly high endogenous EPO levels (generally defined as >300 IU/μL blood) have a very low probability of responding to EPO. Interpretation of this literature is complicated by the varying criteria used by different investigative groups to define a positive "response" to EPO treatment. Nevertheless, undeniable and clinically significant benefits have been found in subsets of MDS patients, as have clear reductions in RBC transfusion requirements. A limited therapeutic trial of EPO supplementation in patients with anemia and transfusion requirements with relatively low endogenous EPO levels seems to be a reasonable approach. Again, the relatively high cost of this agent and the potential for a prolonged period of therapy (e.g., years in patients with low-risk MDS, such as refractory anemia) have made physicians and insurers wary of this therapeutic approach to chronic anemic disorders. Still, the risks of iron overload and other risks from prolonged transfusion requirements are costly and clinically significant, making the strategy of hematopoietic stimulation with EPO supplementation cost-effective in certain responding subsets. More research is required to evaluate this strategy in a more definitive manner.

Ameliorating Thrombocytopenia with Hematopoietic Cytokines: Challenges in Developing Clinically Useful Thrombopoietic Agents

Clinical investigation of hematopoietic cytokines to mitigate thrombocytopenia is far less advanced than the study of molecules that act on cells of the neutrophil or erythroid lineages. Platelet transfusional support remains the standard of acute care of patients with clinically significant thrombocytopenia. However, a single cytokine, recombinant human interleukin-11 (oprelvekin), has been approved by the FDA for prevention or management of chemotherapy-associated thrombocytopenia. Clinical development of other thrombopoietic cytokines has (until recently) represented an extremely competitive research field. In preclinical models, numerous molecules have shown thrombopoietic effects in vitro and in vivo.[84] Examples include interleukin-1 (IL-1), IL-3, IL-6, and IL-11 as well as leukemia inhibitory factor. In addition, use of the tools of recombinant DNA results in ability to cut and splice novel recombinant hybrid molecules that might exhibit thrombopoietic activity. One failed example of this was the PIXY 321 molecule (PIXYkine), a recombinant hybrid composed of the linked coding regions from the human GM-CSF and IL-3 genes.[85] Prospective, controlled, clinical trials of this molecule failed to show sufficient stimulation of platelet production to justify further use,[86] despite promising early reports of platelet stimulatory activity.[87] Other research groups have attempted to improve on nature further by developing cytokine receptor agonists mutated to increase the desired biologic activity. This strategy holds promise of decreasing unwanted cytokine-associated side effects (e.g., systemic inflammation or eosinophilia) while possibly increasing the desired effects (i.e., specific stimulation of thrombopoiesis). This mutational improvement of activity strategy has been combined with chimeric technology for development of novel fusion "synthokines."[88]

Clinical studies of thrombopoietins are complex in terms of clinically relevant endpoints. Because prophylactic platelet transfusions usually are given on the basis of a certain trigger point (often defined in practice as a circulating platelet count of 10,000 to 20,000 platelets/μL blood), the clinical outcome "platelet transfusion requirement" is a dependent variable based on a policy decision (i.e., which transfusion trigger is adopted).[89] In addition, the incidence of serious hemorrhagic consequences with current platelet transfusional support practices is so low that it prohibits a reasonably sized study from detecting any significant effect of a putative thrombopoietin. It will be interesting to evaluate this field as new molecules enter clinical testing, because the same problems that afflict neutrophil and erythroid cytokines (e.g., choosing which patients would most benefit from the agent and evaluation of appropriate and cost-effective use of expensive cytokines) will likely also relate to any cytokine with thrombopoietic activity. This issue may be even more relevant for a thrombopoietic cytokine than for cytokines in the other lineages. Data supporting dose-intensive chemotherapy that would be severe enough to affect platelet count are far weaker than those for chemotherapy that would lead to neutropenia or even anemia.

All clinical development projects of recombinant human IL-1, IL-3, PIXY321, IL-6, stem cell factor, and genetically engineered versions of thrombopoietin, such as megakaryocyte growth and development factor (MGDF) and promegapoietin, as thrombopoietic agents have essentially come to completion without leading to major clinical value. Although several of these molecules appear to have the clinical ability to induce a moderate increase in circulating platelet count, this development path is strewn with toxicity problems and insufficiently active molecules. Clinical testing of IL-1 has revealed the expectedly severe systemic toxicity of this inflammatory mediator.[90] Administration IL-3 and IL-6 is associated with some interpatient variability in response, and stimulation of increased platelet count does not occur until after several days of exogenous dosing.[91-97] Nevertheless, IL-3 has proved tolerable with constitutional dose-limiting toxicities that appear at doses higher than necessary to exhibit some clinical activity, analogous to that of GM-CSF. Large prospective studies have not demonstrated thrombopoietic efficacy of IL-3 or PIXY321 sufficient to affect clinical outcome in a meaningful manner.[86]

Recombinant human IL-11 has shown modest efficacy in preventing recurrent severe thrombocytopenia in the setting of aggressively dosed chemotherapy. This molecule (oprelvekin) achieved a milestone as the first cytokine approved by the FDA for stimulation of platelet production.[35,95,96]

Development of recombinant forms of human thrombopoietin, such as MGDF and promegapoietin, has been plagued by development of neutralizing antibodies in a small but important subset of patients. For MGDF, four cancer patients (among more than 800 patients exposed to MGDF) developed antibodies to the agent. Perhaps more worrisome, however, was development of neutralizing antibodies in 9 of 12 healthy persons who had received MGDF as part of a study evaluating the activity of this agent in healthy platelet donors. The effect was so dramatic that the biotechnology firm decided to immediately cease production and development of MGDF for clinical use.[98] Development of promegapoietin (a chimeric form of thrombopoietin and IL-3) also was stopped because of concerns about antibody development. Thus whereas recombinant human G-CSF and GM-CSF have been used safely in the care of thousands of cancer patients worldwide without serious danger of antibody development, there appears to be more reason for concern about antibody development against epitopes on the thrombopoietin molecule, at least administered by the subcutaneous route. This finding is unfortunate, because the activity and safety profile of recombinant human thrombopoietin appears particularly favorable.[99] One company continues to pursue clinical development of full-length recombinant human thrombopoietin. This research remains the last avenue for achieving clinical utility of this potent and primary regulator of human megakaryopoiesis.

STIMULATION OF HEMATOPOIETIC FUNCTION IN ENDOGENOUS MARROW FAILURE STATES WITH HEMATOPOIETIC CYTOKINES

Much of the clinical investigation in manipulating human hematopoietic function with pharmacologic doses of cytokines been conducted with patients who have relatively normal hematopoietic function that is temporarily perturbed by cytotoxic chemotherapy. Endogenous marrow failure syndromes represent another vehicle for testing the activity of hematopoietic agents. Myriad difficulties arise in these studies: Marrow failure syndromes are a heterogeneous group of congenital and acquired disorders with a wide spectrum of clinical manifestations and courses of disease. Making clinical sense out of such variability may prove a difficult task. Nevertheless, given the paucity of other effective therapeutic approaches for these disorders short of syngeneic or allogeneic BMT with curative intent, these syndromes will continue to be an area of investigative interest for delineating the effects of hematopoietic cytokines.

Congenital Marrow Failure Syndromes

Congenital marrow failure syndromes represent an unusual group of diseases that usually manifest in infants or children and result in lineage-restricted hematopoietic dysfunction or multilineage pancytopenia. Given the rarity of these disorders, large clinical trials designed to study uniform treatment approaches are difficult, if not impossible, to perform. The most persuasive data obtained on the ability of hematopoietic cytokines to modulate the clinical course of these disorders have been found among patients with severe congenital neutropenia (Kostmann's syndrome). In this disorder, peripheral neutropenia is found in association with presumptive myeloid maturation arrest in the late promyelocyte stage. An early pilot study documented the ability of one hematopoietic cytokine, G-CSF, to increase circulating neutrophil count in five patients and to maintain the level of neutrophils for a protracted period.[100] Clinical indications of benefit also were found in that patients had resolution of oral ulcers and a diminished incidence of infectious episodes compared with the period before administration of G-CSF. Contrasting data were obtained in a similar population of patients using GM-CSF. Four of five patients treated with GM-CSF did not have a peripheral neutrophil response, although all patients subsequently responded to G-CSF therapy.[101] These observations emphasize the important fact that the biologic activities of G-CSF and GM-CSF, while similar in many ways in vitro, may have important therapeutic differences in different clinical settings. Results of early pilot studies of G-CSF were confirmed in a large multicenter study involving patients with severe chronic neutropenic disorders. The results confirmed the ability of this cytokine to increase circulating neutrophil count and to diminish significantly the incidence of associated infectious events.[102]

Other congenital marrow failure states managed with hematopoietic cytokines have been studied. In five patients with Fanconi's anemia and neutropenia, GM-CSF administration resulted in increases in peripheral neutrophil counts in four of five patients, one patient having an erythroid response as well. No effect on platelets was found in this study. Diamond-Blackfan anemia is another clinical model in which hematopoietic cytokines have been studied. IL-3 administration was used in three small clinical pilot studies.[103-105] In two of the studies,[103,105] clinical responses were found in 3 of 6 and 4 of 17 patients, respectively. In the other trial,[104] none of 7 patients had a clinically significant response to exogenous IL-3 dosing. The reasons for this variability in response to IL-3 remain enigmatic. Therapy with cytokines for the management of amegakaryocytic thrombocytopenia has been described in a report of five patients with this rare disorder, which is characterized by isolated thrombocytopenia.[106] After use of IL-3 alone or IL-3 followed by GM-CSF, the investigators suggested that IL-3 increased thrombopoietic activity. GM-CSF did not appear to have any additional or synergistic effect on thrombopoiesis. Two of the five patients became platelet transfusion independent during prolonged maintenance therapy with IL-3. This phenomenon of delayed effects of cytokine treatment has been reported in other clinical situations and complicates interpretation of results of clinical cytokine trials. Many molecular mechanisms can be postulated to account for this effect, but further study is needed to characterize it fully.

Acquired Marrow Failure Syndromes

Chronic acquired marrow failure syndromes include MDS and myeloproliferative disorders. Both are stem cell disorders with functional blocks to normal differentiation pathways. Concern has been raised that cytokine treatment may accelerate emergence, survival, or proliferation of malignant leukemic clones and worsen the course of these diseases. In general, MDS has been more widely managed in investigational settings with hematopoietic

cytokines than have myeloproliferative disorders. Pharmacologic dosing with EPO may result in clinically meaningful responses in approximately 25% of patients with MDS and anemia. G-CSF has been tested in the care of neutropenic MDS patients and has been shown to increase neutrophil counts in most patients, often at doses lower than those used to support myelopoiesis in patients undergoing chemotherapy.[107,108] In addition, in a small pilot study with MDS patients, the combination of G-CSF and EPO appeared to retain activity on both the neutrophilic and the erythroid lineages.[109] GM-CSF also has shown activity in stimulation of myelopoiesis in MDS patients and patients with other marrow failure states.[110-114] In short, many pilot trials have shown the ability of cytokines to stimulate lineage-specific hematopoiesis in patients with impairment of blood production due to MDS. However, the actual clinical benefits have been poorly quantified and require further study. In some studies, cytokine therapy has been temporarily associated with leukemic transformation, particularly in patients with high blast counts in subsets of MDS at high risk of transformation, such as refractory anemia with an excess of blasts in transformation.[112] Whether these observations have been simple chance associations or causative ones remains uncertain. Larger scale, prospective studies are necessary to define fully the clinical risks and benefits of such therapeutic strategies. Large, prospective, randomized trials of G-CSF and GM-CSF have been performed with leukemia patients undergoing chemotherapy. In none of these trials did any increase in leukemic regrowth occur.[113] Much of the clinical problem for patients with endogenous acquired marrow failure involves platelet transfusion dependency. G-CSF, GM-CSF, and EPO cannot stimulate thrombopoiesis to any relevant degree in the clinic. Some cytokine trials have evaluated other agents as potential thrombopoietic stimuli. In particular, IL-3 has been tested in patients with bone marrow failure.[91-93] These studies showed a widely disparate response to IL-3, similar to the heterogeneity found when this agent was used in the management of congenital marrow failure states. In general, a multilineage hematopoietic response to IL-3 is possible, including increases in circulating neutrophils, eosinophils, monocytes, and, occasionally, reticulocytes and platelets. IL-3 effects appear to be dose related, and administration of high doses of IL-3 has been limited by constitutional side effects, including fever, fatigue, and headache. IL-6 has been tested in limited clinical evaluations for marrow failure. One study showed promising increases in circulating platelet count and megakaryocytic progenitor cells in MDS patients.[115] Remarkably little research has been conducted with primitive-acting agents, such as stem cell factor or thrombopoietin, because there are concerns that these agents might worsen the disease owing to stimulation of primitive neoplastic clones.

Hematologic manifestations of infection with human immunodeficiency virus (HIV) may include an acquired marrow failure state.[116,117] Cytokine trials with G-CSF,[118,119] GM-CSF,[120] and EPO,[121] alone or in combination, have shown that these agents can mitigate neutropenia and anemia to a great degree.

TRANSFUSIONAL SUPPORT OF MARROW DYSFUNCTION

Red Blood Cell Transfusion

Clinical Indications

In the past, it was hypothesized that maintenance of above-normal hemoglobin level in patients with cancer would allow uncommitted stem cells to differentiate preferentially into myeloid and thrombocytoid lineages. The result would be a shorter time to granulocyte and platelet recovery after chemotherapy.[122] This hypothesis is *not correct*. Transfusions of RBCs to cancer patients currently are given for the same medical indications generally used in other patient populations, mainly maintenance of oxygen delivery to tissues and hemodynamic homeostasis. Adequate oxygen-carrying capacity to maintain minimal acceptable cardiopulmonary function can be met by a hemoglobin concentration of 7 g/dL (a hematocrit of approximately 21%). At this low level of hemoglobin, intravascular volume is adequate for perfusion.[123] However, increasing amounts of data support the hypothesis that the functional status of patients at these "borderline" physiologic conditions is far from optimal.[71,72,124,125] In deciding whether to administer a transfusion to a specific patient, the physician should consider the patient's age, degree of anemia, intravascular volume, and presence of coexisting cardiac, pulmonary, or vascular conditions. To meet oxygen needs, some patients may need RBC transfusions at higher hemoglobin levels. In particular, hemoglobin level generally is maintained at 8 g/dL or higher in the setting of cancer and cancer therapy. Transfusing 1 unit of RBCs usually increases hemoglobin concentration 1 g/dL and hematocrit 2% to 3% in an average 70-kg adult. It usually is appropriate to transfuse at least 2 units of RBCs rather than a single unit. The problem remains that the effects of transfusion, although acutely relevant, are transient for many patients with cancer-related or chemotherapy-associated anemia. The effect of periodically declining hemoglobin levels on patient functional status is beginning to receive attention and is the subject of much research in the quality of life field.[71,72,125]

Red Blood Cell Products

In the United States, the number of homologous RBC transfusions has decreased since 1986, and there has been an associated increase in the use of autologous blood.[126] However, autologous donations have not been universally accepted in the care of patients with cancer or leukemia, owing to difficulty obtaining adequate supplies of autologous RBC components for patients who may already be predisposed to anemia. Another factor has been concern about the presence of circulating tumor cells in peripheral blood. Packed RBCs are prepared from 1 unit of whole blood by removal of plasma and are most commonly transfused for maintenance of adequate oxygen-carrying capacity. Whole blood rarely is transfused, except to restore volume in the setting of massive hemorrhage or to replete both RBCs and clotting factors in patients deficient in both. RBCs can be depleted of leukocytes by filtration, centrifugation, or washing to produce leukocyte-poor RBCs. Leukocyte-poor RBCs have been used to avoid febrile nonhemolytic transfusion reactions and alloimmunization. Use of this blood product is under evaluation for avoidance of cytomegalovirus (CMV) infection in transfusion recipients.[127] Washed RBCs are prepared by removal of additional plasma from packed RBCs and are used for avoidance of urticarial reactions to plasma proteins in transfusion recipients.[128] Febrile nonhemolytic and urticarial transfusion reactions complicate as many as 3% of transfusions.[129] A switch to provision of leukocyte-poor RBCs or washed RBCs alone may avoid febrile nonhemolytic and urticarial transfusion reactions, respectively. Washed RBCs may be useful in patients who are IgA deficient and who have anti-IgA antibodies, because these patients may have anaphylactic reactions after transfusion of blood or blood components containing IgA. Finally, frozen deglycerolized RBCs are both leukocyte and plasma poor. This product may be useful in patients with transfusion reactions to leukocytes or plasma and who are sufficiently depleted of leukocytes to prevent transfusion-related transmission of CMV.

Leukocyte Transfusion

Therapeutic granulocytes were first used nearly 30 years ago in leukemic patients with leukopenia and serious infection. The earliest trials that demonstrated the potential value of granulocyte transfusion were conducted with granulocytes harvested from patients with chronic granulocytic leukemia. The granulocyte transfusional products obtained from these patients with chronic granulocytic leukemia contained granulocyte cell dosages far in excess of those possible when healthy donors are used.[130] The importance of dose was defined: 10^{10} or fewer granulocytes were ineffective, whereas more than 10^{11} cells were effective. In an afebrile uninfected host, the half-life of granulocytes in the circulation is 6.7 hours (range, 4–10 hours), and the daily turnover rate is 230%. In the setting of fever or infection, or both, this turnover rate can be severalfold higher.[131] Parallel work with canine models showed that dogs deliberately made leukopenic by irradiation and given gram-negative bacteremia and pneumonia could be successfully treated with granulocyte transfusions.[132]

Five randomized, prospective clinical trials were conducted to investigate therapeutic leukocyte transfusion in the care of leukopenic patients with established infections.[131,133,134] Early studies showed benefit from leukocyte transfusions and defined several prognostic factors associated with clinical outcome: type of infecting organism, interval to bone marrow recovery, and dose of granulocytes transfused. Granulocyte transfusion was not beneficial in the most recent study,[134] in which recipients were not tested for antileukocyte antibodies, lower numbers of leukocytes were transfused, and a much better survival rate was found in the group treated with antibiotics alone. Because of improvement in efficacy of antibiotics in the 1980s and 1990s, therapeutic granulocytes now are used only rarely. An example is management of refractory gram-negative sepsis or visceral infection in a leukopenic patient who has reasonable expectation of marrow recovery. Even this finite clinical need may be decreased with use of recombinant myeloid growth factors (e.g., GM-CSF or G-CSF) to stimulate normal myeloid recovery and stimulate host cellular defense mechanisms.

Six randomized prospective trials of prophylactic leukocyte transfusion were conducted to determine whether these transfusions could prevent infection in leukopenic recipients.[131,133] Results of five of the studies indicated a protective effect of leukocyte transfusion, although the differences observed were significant in only two trials. Moreover, none of the studies demonstrated improvement in survival, because other adverse clinical effects, such as alloimmunization, transfusion reactions, CMV infection, and pulmonary infiltrates occurred more frequently in the group that received transfusions. The methods of these studies have been criticized because of inadequate donor-recipient matching and inadequate doses of granulocytes transfused. Nonetheless, at present, prophylactic granulocytes are not widely used in the supportive care of patients with cancer. Studies were conducted to evaluate the use of myeloid growth factors to stimulate increased yields of granulocyte harvests from healthy donors. The results showed that large numbers of mature granulocytes can be collected if healthy donors are primed with cytokines such as G-CSF.[135-137] Although these efforts rekindled interest in therapeutic granulocyte transfusion, indications for use of this treatment are rare because of the ability to stimulate recovery of host hematopoiesis with recombinant cytokines.[138-140]

Use of myeloid growth factors has been shown to increase the yield of granulocyte harvests from healthy donors. Massive numbers of mature granulocytes can be collected if healthy donors are primed with cytokines such as G-CSF.[135] Such research efforts may rekindle interest in therapeutic granulocyte transfusion.[138]

Technical Aspects of Obtaining Granulocytes for Transfusion

Granulocytes are harvested in a leukopheresis procedure with hydroxyethyl starch and sodium citrate. The process usually takes 90 minutes to remove adequate granulocytes (10^{10} or more) while RBCs are returned to the donor. These leukocytes are obtained from ABO-compatible donors. A leukoagglutination test using freshly obtained patient serum and donor white blood cells can be performed before transfusion to ensure compatibility and avoid leukoagglutinin-mediated pulmonary reactions in the recipient. Post-transfusion CMV interstitial pneumonitis is avoided through the use of only CMV-seronegative donors. Leukocytes are irradiated to prevent proliferation of T cells within the transfused product that could potentially engraft or induce GVH when transfused to an immunocompromised host.[141] Despite earlier allegations, patients receiving amphotericin therapy are not at increased risk of transfusion-related pulmonary reactions.[142]

Platelet Transfusion

Fresh whole blood was first transfused to thrombocytopenic patients in 1910. The result was a significant increase in platelet count, hemostasis, and improvement in bleeding time.[143] In the 1950s, platelets were first used for management of thrombocytopenia related to combination chemotherapy for leukemia.[144] In the 1960s investigation into the clinical sequelae of severe thrombocytopenia showed that platelet transfusional support could modify the course of hemorrhage in both pediatric and adult patients, the only difference being the doses required. In the 1970s, studies with children and adults confirmed the efficacy of platelet transfusion in prevention, rather than control, of hemorrhage.[145,146]

Few patients with cancer need platelet transfusions. Conversely, platelets are more commonly transfused to cancer patients than to patients with any other category of disease. The appropriate indications for transfusion of platelets were the subject of a National Institutes of Health consensus development conference[147] and remain a controversial subject.[89] To prevent hemorrhage 6 to 8 units of platelets (5.5×10^{10} platelets/unit) often are routinely transfused to cancer patients with platelet counts less than 10,000 to 20,000/µL. However, the implications of thrombocytopenia as a risk factor for hemorrhage and, therefore, the timing and dose of prophylactic platelets may vary in different clinical settings. For example, patients with thrombocytopenia due to acute myelocytic leukemia were reported to have increased bleeding with administration of up to 10,000/µL platelets. Patients with acute lymphoid leukemia, however, had similar risk of hemorrhage at up to 20,000/mL platelets.[148] Gmür and colleagues[149] reported that the threshold for prophylactic transfusion can be set at 5000/µL for leukemic patients without fever or bleeding and at 10,000/µL for patients with these clinical problems.[149] Two more recent randomized trials involving patients with leukemia compared 10,000/µL and 20,000/µL platelet counts as thresholds for prophylactic transfusion. The results showed the lower trigger was safe and resulted in a smaller number of platelet transfusions.[26,27] Young platelets are more efficient at controlling hemorrhage,[150] so the need for platelet transfusion is greater if the count is decreasing after chemotherapy, compared with a similar level during an increase from a nadir. Patients with chronic thrombocytopenia due to decreased platelet production (myelodysplastic disorders) may need transfusions. Patients with accelerated destruction but active production of platelets (idiopathic thrombocytopenic purpura), however, may not need routine platelet transfusions. Moreover, patients with chronic thrombocytopenia may tolerate lower absolute platelet counts without transfusion. In patients with abnormalities of platelet function, not absolute platelet count but number of functional platelets is important for prevention of bleeding. Bleeding time may aid in defining risk of bleeding. It is difficult to define an absolute platelet threshold for transfusion for all patients, and both timing and dose of prophylactic platelet transfusion must therefore be determined on a clinical basis.[89,151-154]

Use of Single- and Multiple-Donor Platelets for Transfusion

One unit of platelet concentrate is obtained from 1 unit of whole blood by centrifugation, and concentrates from multiple (six to eight) donors are pooled to produce a single component (random donor pooled concentrate) for transfusion. Individual platelet concentrates can be stored for up to 5 days before pooling and transfusion. The advent and refinement of apheresis techniques[155,156] have allowed harvesting of several units of platelets from and return of RBCs to a single donor. This method has greatly increased the feasibility of providing single-donor platelets and has not been shown to have clinically significant adverse effects on frequent donors. The development of closed sterile pheresis systems that minimize contact of platelets with air during collection, coupled with storage bags permeable to carbon dioxide, also allows storage of pheresis platelets before transfusion.

The chief advantage of multiple-donor platelet concentrate is availability, because the product is derived from conventional whole blood donations. Results of some studies suggest that alloimmunization can occur early in patients receiving multiple-donor platelets, that multiple-donor transfusions are then ineffective, and that restriction of the number of donors per transfusion may postpone development of refractoriness to random-donor platelet transfusion in thrombocytopenic patients.[157,158] A second potential advantage of use of single-donor platelets stems from the decreased risk of infection when the patient is exposed to fewer donors. Nonetheless, pooled random-donor platelets are routinely transfused initially, because platelet concentrates are a byproduct of whole-blood donations. Most single-donor platelet collections are used primarily to provide HLA-matched donors for alloimmunized recipients who have not responded to platelets from random donors. Although they are useful for avoiding transfusion-related CMV infection, single-donor platelets have not been used more generally to minimize alloimmunization or infection risk.

The effectiveness of platelet transfusion can be assessed by a laboratory value, the corrected increment in platelet count 1 hour or 10 to 15 minutes after transfusion,[159-161] bleeding time,[162] and observed clinical outcome after transfusion. Corrected platelet increment is defined as the increment in platelet count from the pretransfusion to the post-transfusion state corrected for number of units transfused and for body surface area of the recipient. A corrected increment of 15,000 to 20,000/µL is usual 18 to 24 hours after transfusion, provided fresh properly stored platelets have been transfused.[159] This value translates into an absolute increment at 1 hour of approximately 7000 to 11,000/µL for each unit of platelet concentrate administered to an average-sized person with a body surface area of 1.0 m^2. Bleeding time after transfusion serves as a measure of the number of functional platelets, particularly in patients known to have dysfunctional platelets. Techniques such as radiolabeling platelets can be used to diagnose and identify the site of accelerated platelet destruction, but the most important way to monitor the effectiveness of platelet transfusion is critical clinical assessment for the presence and extent of hemorrhage.

Factors Adversely Affecting the Efficacy of Transfused Platelets

If an appropriately low corrected platelet increment is detected soon after transfusion, the status of both the platelet product transfused and the recipient must be examined for possible explanations. Several factors involved in harvesting and storage of platelets before transfusion can lead to poor post-transfusion platelet survival: pH, number of contaminating leukocytes, concentration of platelets, plasma volume, temperature, time, and agitation during storage.[163] With the quality control measures currently in practice in most blood banks, it is uncommon to identify a problem in harvesting or donation that accounts for a poor post-transfusion increment.

If the survival of transfused platelets is compromised, several clinical conditions in the transfusion recipient may be responsible.[163,164] Patients with fever, infection, or both have increased consumption of platelets, even when there is no evidence of consumptive coagulopathy. Second, post-transfusion increments in platelet count may be less than expected owing to splenic sequestration, especially in the setting of splenomegaly.[165] Third, drug-induced platelet antibodies have been demonstrated that mediate immune destruction of platelets. Antibodies responsible for drug-induced thrombocytopenia may bind to platelets by their Fab regions rather than by attaching nonspecifically as immune complexes.[166] Platelet membrane glycoproteins GPIb and GPIIb/IIIa appear to be the preferred targets, although GPV also has been implicated.[167-173] Drug apparently binds to the platelet membrane, inducing a reversible structural change that provokes an antibody response. Drugs (e.g., methyldopa) may induce antibodies that mediate thrombocytopenia without direct drug-platelet interaction.[174] An alternative theory is that drugs such as penicillin bind covalently to the platelet membrane and induce hapten-dependent antibodies.[175] Finally, the survival of transfused platelets can be compromised if the recipient has antibodies against donor antigens of HLA-A and HLA-B loci, the ABH system, or platelet alloantigens.

Alloimmunization

Platelets bear HLA-A and HLA-B but lack HLA-C and HLA-DR antigens. There is a high correlation between development of lymphocytotoxic anti-HLA antibodies in the recipient and refractoriness to random-donor platelets.[176] Anti-HLA antibodies are most easily detectable with patient serum and a panel of lymphocytes representing known HLA specificities. The incidence and timing of production of anti-HLA antibodies after platelet transfusion remain controversial and may vary with the recipient population. Most studies document alloimmunization in 50% to 90% of patients who undergo multiple transfusions.[177] Some studies have shown that rate of alloimmunization increases with number of transfusions.[178] Others, however, have shown no relation between number of platelet transfusions given and rate of alloimmunization.[179] Moreover, a fraction of patients with cancer never become sensitized.[180,181] Nonetheless, it is crucial to test for anti-HLA antibodies whenever recipients become refractory to random-donor platelet transfusion, because response to random-donor platelet transfusion is poor in a sensitized host, and HLA-matched or family member platelets can be useful in this setting.[182-184]

Yankee and colleagues[182,183] first demonstrated that transfusion of platelets obtained from HLA-identical siblings or from unrelated donors matched at the HLA-A and HLA-B loci (grade A or B matches) could result in satisfactory post-transfusion increments in alloimmunized recipients refractory to random-donor platelet transfusion. Duquesnoy and associates[185] later found that donors with the same HLA antigens (grade B match) or HLA antigens cross-reactive with the patient's antigens (BX match) were equivalent. Evaluation of donors for the same or cross-reactive antigens became even more complex. For example, transfusion of platelets from donors lacking HLA-A2 who bear one or two (grade C match) or three of four (grade D match) antigens not present in the recipient may have favorable post-transfusion outcome in alloimmunized recipients. By contrast, transfusion of platelets from HLA-A2–positive donors who were HLA-A and HLA-B matches was unsuccessful.[186] Weak anti-HLA antibodies, which can cause platelet destruction in vivo, may not be detected by standard assays. Excellent platelet transfusion recoveries have been observed, however, despite a positive lymphocytotoxicity crossmatch.[176,185] Additional crossmatching techniques may be required in the 20% of sensitized patients who remain refractory even to HLA-matched platelets.

Recognition of the refractoriness associated with development of anti-HLA antibodies led to attempts to avoid or delay alloimmunization by modifying the platelets to be transfused. Because HLA antigens are expressed on leukocytes, investigators have attempted (1) to remove white blood cells from platelets before transfusion, (2) to use single-donor rather than multiple-donor platelets to minimize exposure to HLA antigens, and (3) to transfuse only HLA-matched or leukocyte-depleted HLA-matched platelets. Leukocyte-poor platelets have been prepared by additional centrifugation[187] or by the use of filters,[188-192] both of which deplete white blood cells by 2 to 3 logs with varying associated losses of platelets. In particular, exclusive transfusion of platelets with no more than 5×10^6 contaminating leukocytes did not induce formation of anti-HLA antibodies. By contrast, transfusion of similar numbers of non–leukocyte-depleted platelets did sensitize recipients. The use of single-donor platelets[157,158] or of ultraviolet (UV) irradiation of platelets[193-195] is being tested for prevention of alloimmunization. Results of the Trial to Reduce Alloimmunization to Platelets (TRAP) showed that administration of filtered single-donor apheresis platelets, filtered pooled random-donor platelet concentrates, and UV-B–irradiated pooled random-donor platelet concentrates all were effective strategies for reducing the incidence of platelet refractoriness in patients with newly diagnosed acute myeloid leukemia.[196] The timing of leukodepletion may be an important factor in determining the success of this method for preventing alloimmunization. The results of one animal study indicated that prestorage, but not poststorage, leukodepletion was effective in preventing alloimmunization.[197]

When sensitized recipients remain refractory to HLA-matched platelets, attempts have been made to perform additional crossmatching to identify more compatible platelet donors. These procedures include leukoagglutination, chromium-51 lysis, immunofluorescence, enzyme-linked immunoabsorbent assay (ELISA), assays of iodine-131–labeled platelet-associated IgG, and platelet aggregometry.[198,199] Such assays exhibit variable success in determining which platelets are effective in refractory patients, and no one assay or combination of methods has been universally accepted as predictive of response to transfusion.

Possible mechanisms for explaining unexpectedly suboptimal post-transfusion recovery among patients receiving HLA-matched ABO-compatible platelet transfusions include unrecognized HLA specificity, the presence of circulating immune complexes, and the presence of antibodies to platelet-specific antigens. Use of plasma exchange or intravenous immunoglobulin therapy before platelet transfusion in patients whose condition remains refractory to ABO-compatible HLA-matched platelets has been of mixed benefit.[200-202]

ABO Compatibility in Platelet Transfusion

The ABO blood group determinants, presumably absorbed from plasma, are present on platelets with a structure similar to that on erythrocytes.[203] Major antigens of the Rh, Duffy, Kidd, Kell, and Lutheran systems, in contrast, are not expressed on the surface of human platelets.[204] Clinical studies have shown that platelet transfusions can induce formation of isohemagglutinins owing to the presence of a small number of contaminating erythrocytes.[205] This finding suggests that ABO compatibility between donor and recipient may be important. However, results of in vitro studies have shown that exposure of group A and AB platelets to the appropriate anti-A and anti-AB alloantibodies and complement does not cause ultrastructural damage to the platelets or induce platelet aggregation.[206] This finding suggests that an ABO mismatch between donor and recipient is not an absolute contraindication to platelet transfusion.

The need for ABO compatibility between platelet donor and recipient has been directly examined in several studies. Some studies have shown a decreased recovery and survival of ABO-mismatched relative to ABO-compatible platelets.[207-209] Other studies have shown that platelet survival usually is only slightly influenced by ABO antibodies and not at all affected by Rho(D) antibodies in the recipient.[204,210] In a 1984 randomized trial of use of ABO-compatible versus ABO-incompatible platelets, the corrected increments after the first transfusion were equivalent, but higher increments were found after subsequent transfusion of ABO-compatible platelets in a subset of patients.[204] Finally, studies have shown that ABO-mismatched platelets may not be immunogenic in certain patients with cancer.[211]

ABO matching of donor and recipient is unimportant for most platelet transfusions. The fact that transfusions that are not group specific are considered safe and clinically effective greatly expands the availability of platelets for transfusion. However, in specific clinical settings, donor and recipient ABO compatibility may be important. For example, if HLA-matched but ABO-mismatched platelet transfusion does not result in a satisfactory increment after transfusion, HLA- and ABO-matched platelets may be of benefit.[212] Heal and colleagues[213] postulated that soluble plasma HLA-A and HLA-B and ABO antigens may contribute to destruction of donor and sometimes recipient platelets by an immune complex or another "innocent bystander" mechanism. Finally, very few hemolytic reactions have been caused by very high titers of isohemagglutinins in the plasma in transfused platelet concentrates directed at recipient erythrocytes.[214] This possibility rarely is a reason for providing only ABO-compatible platelets.

Platelet-Specific Antigens

A variety of alloantigen systems on platelets, including P1^A(ZW), P1^E, Ko, Bak, (LeK), and Pen,[215] have been described. Antibodies directed at these antigens can cause immune-mediated destruction of platelets in the presence or absence of anti-HLA antibodies. Sensitization to these antigens is rarely the cause of refractory thrombocytopenia in cancer patients.

One clinical sequela of interaction between antibodies and platelet alloantigens is post-transfusion purpura, which is caused by antibody directed at the PL^A1 antigen. In post-transfusion purpura, profound thrombocytopenia develops approximately 1 week after transfusion, primarily in women who have been immunized by earlier pregnancies or, less frequently, by a previous transfusion.[216] Almost all patients have been PL^A1-negative and have had anti-PL^A1 antibody in the plasma when thrombocytopenia has developed. Partial exchange transfusion, plasmapheresis, and high-dose intravenous immunoglobulin have been used to accelerate recovery from post-transfusion purpura.[217,218]

Immunohematologic Considerations and Immunosuppression

Transfusions can have immunosuppressive effects on recipients. In studies with animal models, investigators have found immune suppression and accelerated tumor growth in rats receiving allogeneic transfusion.[219] In humans, patients receiving multiple transfusions have decreased numbers of natural killer cells and increased numbers of circulating Ia^+ T cells. T4/T8 ratio also may be decreased.[220,221] The decrease in number of natural killer cells is directly related to the number of RBC units received and occurs only in patients who have received a transfusion within the past year.

Research has demonstrated increased renal graft survival in patients who had received blood from donors who shared at least one HLD-DR antigen.[222] Both increased cancer recurrence rates and an increased incidence of postoperative infection have been observed after transfusion.[223–225] Specifically, patients who did not receive transfusions fared better in 11 of 14 retrospective studies with a variety of stages and sites of colon cancer. When multivariate analysis was performed, transfusion was an independent unfavorable predictor of early recurrence or cancer-related death in 7 of 12 studies.

Patients receiving transfusions during surgery for colorectal cancer have been found to have higher rates of postoperative infection than those not receiving transfusions.[225] Evidence of an effect of transfusion on outcome of breast and prostate cancer is weak,[226,227] but data on renal and lung cancer suggest a deleterious effect of transfusion.[223] For example, in one study, the 5-year recurrence-free survival rate among patients with stage I non–oat cell lung cancer who received transfusions was 62%, whereas the rate among patients not receiving transfusions was 76%.[224] It is not yet possible, however, to be sure that factors other than transfusion, such as the biologic characteristics of the cancer and the degree of illness or immunosuppression of the patient, do not account for observed effects. Thus immunosuppression is another possible adverse effect of transfusion, further emphasizing the importance of justifying the medical and surgical indications for every transfusion. Although the mechanism of any transfusion-associated immunosuppressive effect in humans is unknown, cancer patients receiving only a small number of RBCs have had fewer recurrences and better survival than those receiving only whole blood or larger numbers of RBCs. These findings suggest that a factor present in whole blood (e.g., plasma) may be implicated.[225,228] Other studies are needed to define the precise relation between transfusion, immunosuppression of the recipient, and cancer recurrence. It is essential to emphasize that patients with cancer and marrow failure may be immunocompromised owing to the neoplastic disease, its treatment, or both. Thus the effects of transfusion on recipient immunity are of particular importance in this patient population.

Transfusion-Associated Graft-versus-Host Disease

Graft-versus-host disease (GVHD) is common after allogeneic BMT but is rarely recognized after transfusion or after transplantation of other organs. Transfusion-associated GVHD usually occurs in an immunosuppressed recipient (e.g., BMT recipients), but it also has been known to occur in more nearly immunocompetent recipients.[141,229,230] Clinical manifestations include fever, rash, anorexia, nausea, vomiting, and watery or bloody diarrhea, with or without elevated liver enzyme levels and hyperbilirubinemia. Because there are no pathognomonic features of GVHD, it is sometimes difficult to differentiate this syndrome from viral infection or drug eruption. Transfusion-associated GVHD usually is severe and, unlike the aftermath of allogeneic BMT, frequently results in pancytopenia secondary to marrow aplasia. Most reported cases of transfusion-associated GVHD have not responded to immunosuppressive therapy and have been fatal.

GVHD has occurred after transfusion of unirradiated blood components to at least 400 patients: patients with severe combined immunodeficiency, thymic hypoplasia, and Wiskott-Aldrich syndrome; premature newborns and those with erythroblastosis fetalis; patients with hematologic neoplasms, including Hodgkin's and non-Hodgkin's lymphoma, acute myeloid leukemia and acute lymphoid leukemia, chronic lymphoid leukemia, and aplastic anemia; patients with carcinoma and sarcoma, including neuroblastoma, glioblastoma, rhabdomyosarcoma, cervical carcinoma, small cell lung cancer, and germ cell tumor; patients recovering from cardiac surgery or cholecystectomy; and an apparently healthy 22-year-old woman.[229] This syndrome has developed after exchange and intrauterine transfusions and after transfusion of whole blood, plasma, RBCs, and platelets. Leukocytes harvested from healthy donors and from donors with chronic myelocytic leukemia have been transfused into patients with hematologic neoplasms and been implicated in transfusion-associated GVHD.

In 1986, a National Institutes of Health consensus development conference defined patients who have undergone BMT or those with other forms of immuno-deficiency as candidates for irradiated platelet concentrates to avoid GVHD.[147] Patients with leukemia or other cancers who may be immunosuppressed because of chemotherapy or radiation therapy or because of intrinsic immune dysfunction (e.g., Hodgkin's disease)[231] may be at risk of transfusion-associated GVHD. It had previously been assumed that among patients with Hodgkin's disease, combined radiation and chemotherapy were necessary as predisposing factors for development of transfusion-associated GVHD, but several cases of transfusion-associated GVHD have been documented in patients with Hodgkin's disease treated with chemotherapy alone.[232] Patients receiving high-dose chemotherapy followed by autologous BMT also are at risk of transfusion-associated GVHD.[233] Finally, immunocompetent patients who share an HLA haplotype with HLA homozygous blood donors also appear to be at risk of transfusion-associated GVHD.[230,234] Homozygosity for HLA type is more likely to occur among first-degree family members (parents, children, and siblings). It therefore has been recommended that cellular blood components from such donors be irradiated with at least 2500 cGy before transfusion.[235]

Strategies for Prevention of Transfusion-Associated Graft-versus-Host Disease

The only currently effective method of preventing transfusion-associated GVHD is γ irradiation of blood products before transfusion. Five hundred centigray of γ irradiation can abrogate the response of lymphocytes to allogeneic cells in mixed-lymphocyte culture, and 1500 cGy can reduce 90% the response to mitogen-induced stimulation.[236,237] Button and colleagues[238] examined the function of blood components after irradiation doses of 500 to 20,000 cGy and found that doses as high as 5000 cGy decreased mitogen stimulation 98.5% but did not compromise the function of cells other than lymphocytes. In that study, however, doses of 5000 cGy decreased by one third the yield of platelets after transfusion. Results of most studies suggest that irradiation at 1500 to 2000 cGy can reduce mitogen-responsive lymphocytes by 5 to 6 logs compared with unirradiated controls.[239] Doses of 1500 to 3500 cGy are currently used by most blood banks in the United States.[240] However, the observation that a small percentage of lymphocytes survive irradiation at these doses, coupled with a single reported case of apparent transfusion-associated GVHD in a BMT recipient who received only blood components

irradiated at 2000 cGy,[239] suggests that existing blood product irradiation guidelines may need reassessment. The current recommendation is to irradiate with 2500 cGy. Results of studies suggest no adverse effects of irradiation on storage of platelets,[241] but the clinical significance of potassium release on storage of irradiated RBCs has not been defined.[242]

A potential alternative method of prevention of transfusion-associated GVHD would be to deplete lymphocytes from blood products before transfusion. It has been found that the incidence and severity of GVHD after allogeneic BMT can be reduced if, before grafting, T cells are eliminated from the donor marrow by a variety of techniques.[243] In some techniques 2 to 3 logs of leukocytes are depleted from RBCs and platelets, so that leukocyte-poor RBCs and platelets contain 10^6 to 10^8 lymphocytes. However, because the number and precise T cells needed to mediate transfusion-associated GVHD remain undefined, it is unknown whether depletion of leukocytes with these techniques would decrease the risk of transfusion-associated GVHD.[244] A canine model has been used to demonstrate that UV rather than g irradiation of transfused leukocytes can abrogate GVHD in recipient animals.[245] In preliminary studies with human subjects, UV irradiation of blood components was used to minimize alloimmunization.[194,195]

Transfusion-Related Infectious Diseases

Hepatitis B

Although hepatitis B was formerly a common transfusion-related infection, the use of several generations of hepatitis B surface antigen assays to screen donors and the use of volunteer versus commercial donors has markedly reduced the incidence of hepatitis B transmitted by transfusion.[246-248] Since initiation of the use of antibody to hepatitis B core antigen (anti-HBcAg) as a surrogate test to screen potential donors for ability to transmit hepatitis C virus (HCV),[249,250] the incidence of transfusion-related hepatitis B has decreased even further.

Hepatitis C

Hepatitis C virus (formerly called non-A, non-B hepatitis) is the most common cause of transfusion-related hepatitis, but only 5% to 10% of patients with hepatitis C have a history of transfusion, and less than 5% report occupational exposure to blood.[250] Testing of donors at the time of each donation once was done to detect an elevated level of alanine aminotransferase (ALT) as well as anti-HBcAg, both of which are surrogate markers of a 20% chance of transmitting hepatitis C.[249,251] The advantage of screening is the possibility of reducing the number of cases of transfusion-related hepatitis C by one third. The disadvantage is that 70% to 80% of donors with anti-HBcAg or elevated ALT do not transmit HCV. Moreover, 1% to 3% and 4% to 8% of donors are deferred because of elevated ALT and anti-HBcAg, respectively.[250]

A single-stranded RNA togavirus has been described that appears to account for most cases of hepatitis C.[252] Infection with HCV may account for 80% of cases of chronic posttransfusion hepatitis C in Italy and Japan and

58% of cases in the United States.[253] In a specific assay for blood-borne HCV, a polypeptide synthesized by recombinant yeast clones of HCV is used to capture viral antibodies. In early testing, six of seven serum samples that transmitted HCV in chimpanzees were anti-HCV antibody–positive.[253] In humans, at least one donor in 9 of 10 cases of transfusion-related hepatitis C had antibodies to HCV. The pattern of immunologic response to HCV in humans has been characterized: Anti-HCV antibody persisted in 14 of 15 patients with chronic disease whose cases were followed for a mean of 6.9 years. By contrast, antibody disappeared after a mean of 4.1 years in three of five patients with acute resolving disease.[254] In some cases, anti-HCV antibody was not detectable until almost 6 months after transfusion. Because 33% of anti-HCV–seropositive donors have an elevated ALT level and 54% have antibody to HBcAg, it would appear that screening donors for antibody to HCV may help identify additional infectious donors and substantially reduce the incidence of transfusion-associated hepatitis C. Approximately 90% of blood donors with anti-HCV antibodies have infective virus in their blood.[255] Anti-HBcAg has been retained as a donor screening test, because the incidence of transfusion-related hepatitis B has decreased since institution of the test. The incidence of post-transfusion hepatitis C since implementation of these screening tests is 1 case per 103,000 units transfused.[256,257]

Cytomegalovirus
Cellular blood components transfused from CMV-seropositive donors to CMV-seronegative transplant recipients and neonates can cause CMV seroconversion and infection. In allogeneic BMT, transfusion with seronegative blood products (frozen deglycerolized RBCs and platelets drawn from CMV-seronegative donors) or treatment with immunoglobulin both appear to lessen the rate of CMV infection after allogeneic BMT when both donor and patient are seronegative but not when either is seropositive.[258,259] Use of both immunoglobulin and CMV-seronegative blood products appears to confer no additional benefit. CMV infection is strongly associated with acute GVHD[260,261] and may become less frequent owing to the development of effective prophylaxis for GVHD. In seropositive allogeneic BMT recipients, acyclovir therapy can lessen the incidence of CMV infection and related morbidity.[262] Although equivalent numbers of autologous and allogeneic BMT recipients seroconvert to or excrete CMV, recipients of autologous BMT rarely experience clinical sequelae.[260] Methods of CMV prophylaxis have therefore been reserved for allogeneic BMT when both donor and recipient are seronegative. They have not been used in autologous BMT. It should be noted, however, that in one study CMV pneumonia developed in 11 of 159 recipients of autologous BMT and was fatal in nine cases.

The traditional CMV-seronegative blood products are frozen deglycerolized RBCs and platelets harvested from CMV-seronegative donors. Filtered (leukocyte-poor) RBCs and platelets have been shown to decrease transfusion-acquired CMV infection in infants,[263] in patients undergoing treatment for acute leukemia,[264] and in recipients

of autologous[265] or allogeneic[266] BMT. The ability to use leukoreduced blood products to avoid transfusion-related CMV infection has markedly expanded the available donor pool and thereby the supply of noninfectious components.[267,268]

Bacterial Sepsis
Bacteria rarely survive in whole blood stored at 4°C. By contrast, platelets are stored at room temperature on an agitator and are a potential source of bacterial contamination, which can result in transfusion-related sepsis.[269-273] In vitro studies have shown that deliberate contamination of platelets with as few as 1 organism/mL on day 0 (gram-negative or gram-positive) can result in 10^8 organisms/mL or plateau phase growth after 48 to 72 hours of incubation. Storage of platelets for 5 days between harvest and transfusion is currently permitted; however, platelets should be used as soon as possible after harvest owing to considerations of in vitro function, in vivo recovery, and concern for bacterial contamination.

Thirteen cases, seven of them fatal, of post-transfusion *Yersinia enterocolitica* toxemia have been reported to the U.S. Centers for Disease Control and Prevention, since 1986.[274-276] Although minimizing the storage time of RBCs before transfusion or extending the screening process to exclude all potential donors with gastrointestinal symptoms or illness during the 4-week period before donation have been suggested as possible methods to minimize this problem, it is thought to be a rare event, and no formal guidelines have been established.

Human Immunodeficiency Virus and Acquired Immunodeficiency Syndrome
Of the reported cases of acquired immunodeficiency syndrome (AIDS), the largest risk groups remain homosexual or bisexual men (54.8%), intravenous drug abusers (23.1%), or both (5.3%).[277] Among transfusion recipients, 2.0% of AIDS cases occur in adults or adolescents and 0.1% of cases in children. These figures are meant not to minimize the importance of transfused blood as a vector for virus transmission but to place transfusion in perspective as a relatively infrequent risk factor.

With the recognition in 1983 that AIDS can be transmitted by transfusion,[278] several measures were implemented: (1) physicians were educated about the risks and benefits of transfusion; (2) autologous transfusion was recommended for elective surgery; and (3) questionnaires were used for anonymous self-deferment of high-risk donors. By mid-1983, pressure for directed donation from friends or family increased; however, directed donations are no safer than other donations. Since 1985, testing for antibodies to human immunodeficiency virus (HIV) has been done on all donors, and continuing efforts have been made to permit donors to confidentially advise blood collection centers to discard their blood, even after they have donated. Use of autologous blood, especially in elective surgery, is an important way to avoid infection and other risks of transfusion; however, autologous blood is not widely used in patients with cancer because of fear of contamination of tumor cells.

Problems Common to Cancer and Its Therapy

II

All homologous blood products are considered safe by the same standards: screening of the potential donor using questionnaire and ELISA screening for antibodies to HIV. The rate of true positivity, defined as ELISA reproducibly positive Western blot positive, in first-time blood donors is 0.04%.[279] A false-positive ELISA result can be attributable to other antibodies, such as antibodies to HLA and auto-antibodies. Some results have suggested that blood donors who are ELISA-defined repeatedly reactive Western blot indeterminate are rarely, if ever, infected with HIV-1 or HIV-2 but that a small percentage (0.04%) of HIV-infected persons continue to donate blood despite efforts to exclude them.[280,281] In the two years following implementation of ELISA screening in 1985, seven donors who tested ELISA-seronegative transmitted HIV by transfusion.[282] Donor recruiting and education techniques, coupled with testing, have a combined effectiveness of 99.9% in excluding infected persons before donation. Starting in 1988, the number of cases of transfusion-related AIDS leveled off, and the incidence should fall as the effects of screening measures are realized.[277]

A window period exists between exposure to HIV and production of antibody or seroconversion.[283] Although testing for HIV antigen may identify persons infected who have not seroconverted, such antigen testing cannot substitute for HIV antibody testing, because clearing of antigen can occur. In particular, production of antibody to p24 appears to correlate with disappearance of HIV antigen.[284] In studies of HIV-seropositive persons with hemophilia or members of high-risk groups, those who are HIV antigen positive have a more rapid onset of clinical sequelae of HIV infection.[285] Moreover, the presence of HIV antigen appears to correlate with heterosexual transmission of HIV infection.[286] With the use of donor questionnaires and screening for anti-HIV antibody, the risk of HIV transmission is 1 case in 493,000 transfusions.[255] This risk has been reduced even further with donor p24 antigen screening, which was introduced in the United States in 1996.[287] A survey of 500,000 blood donors conducted by the American Red Cross showed that testing for HIV antigen did not add to the efficacy of donor screening with anti-HIV antibody alone. HIV antigen therefore has not been recommended for routine use in the screening of blood donors. The current risk of transfusion-related HIV infection is 1 case per 225,000 units transfused.

Studies have traced the recipients of transfused products from donors who subsequently were identified as HIV antibody positive ("look-back" studies).[288,289] Most (90%) recipients of HIV-infected blood become seropositive; AIDS develops in approximately one half of recipients within 7 years, and the risk may be higher when AIDS develops in the donor soon after donation.[289] As is true of other infections occurring in immunocompromised hosts, HIV infection may be even more virulent in cancer patients.[290] Moreover, many of the clinical sequelae of HIV infection (e.g., pancytopenia) can be mistakenly attributed to the underlying cancer or its therapy.[116]

Human T-Lymphotrophic Virus Type 1

Human T-lymphocytic virus type 1 (HTLV-1) is associated with adult T-cell leukemia/lymphoma, tropical spastic paresis, and HTLV-1–associated myelopathy.[291] This virus clusters geographically in endemic areas, such as parts of Japan and the Caribbean. In the United States, the incidence of adult T-cell leukemia/lymphoma is similar to that in the Caribbean, because the U.S. cases occur among blacks or patients born outside the United States.[292] Most important, investigators have found antibodies to HTLV-1 in drug abusers from New York and shown that anti-HIV antibodies do not identify all persons infected with HTLV-1.[293] Minamoto and coworkers[294] documented anti–HTLV-1 antibodies in 6 of 211 patients with cancer who had undergone multiple transfusions. None of the HTLV-1–seropositive patients was HIV-1–seropositive; conversely, 18 patients were HIV-1–seropositive and HTLV-1–seronegative.

In Japan, deferment of blood donors with antibodies to HTLV-1 resulted in lowering of the HTLV-1 seroconversion rate in transfusion recipients from 53.6% to 0.9%.[295] In the United States, ELISA, immunoblot, and radioimmunoprecipitation screening of serum from 39,898 blood donors at eight blood centers in geographically distinct areas of the United States defined 10 donors (0.025%) as having anti–HTLV-1 antibodies.[296] In accord with FDA guidelines, all blood collection agencies in early 1989 initiated testing of all blood donors for anti–HTLV-1 antibodies at every donation. Persons with confirmed seropositivity are permanently deferred. High-risk groups who should not donate blood include patients with adult T-cell leukemia/lymphoma or tropical spastic paresis, persons from HTLV-1 endemic areas, female sexual partners of infected men, intravenous drug abusers, recipients of seropositive cellular blood products, and homosexual men. Studies in the United States documented that HTLV-1 has been transmitted by transfusion.[297,298] The current risk of HTLV-1 transmission is 1 case in 641,000 transfusions.[255]

Other Retroviruses

HTLV-2 was discovered in 1982 in a patient with hairy cell leukemia of T cells. No disease association (except for occasional cases of diverse malignant lymphoproliferative disease) or natural reservoir of infection (except drug abusers) has been found. Although there is serologic cross-reactivity between HTLV-1 and HTLV-2, type-specific identification of HTLVs can be achieved by polymerase chain reaction.[299] Of 28,000 samples repeatedly HIV-1 ELISA-positive in one study, 2% also were repeatedly HIV-2 ELISA-positive; however, none was truly HIV-2 infected.[300] Eighteen persons in the United States reported to the Centers for Disease Control and Prevention, all of whom had recently emigrated from West Africa, had had sexual contact with West Africans or had traveled to West Africa.[301] Although HTLV-2 has been reported to be transmitted by transfusion,[302-304] no positive results were found in 20 million Red Cross donations.[300] By June 1992, the FDA had determined that routine HIV-2 screening is necessary for blood and plasma donated for transfusion.

Parasitic Diseases

Because there are no practical laboratory screening tests for malaria, exclusion of donors who have traveled to or emigrated from endemic areas is the only effective measure for prevention of transfusion-related infection. Another parasite disease, babesiosis, can be transmitted by a symptom-free donor who has been bitten by a tick. This disease may be of particular importance to immuno-compromised or asplenic patients. Although transmission of syphilis by transfusion is possible, it requires that blood be drawn during the rather short period of spirochetemia and that the organisms remain viable at transfusion. Although performing a serologic test for syphilis does not prevent transmission of syphilis, because the result does not become positive until well after the brief period of infectivity, U.S. federal regulations require serologic screening of potential donors.

Another transfusion-related infection is Chagas' disease.[305] In Latin America, the risk of transmission is 13% to 23% for each unit of contaminated blood transfused. Most cases of Chagas' disease associated with transfusion are mild. Spontaneous resolution usually occurs, and patients enter an indeterminate phase with lifelong low-grade parasitemia, antibodies to parasite antigens, and absence of symptoms. Ten percent to 30% of persons with disease in the indeterminate phase eventually experience symptoms. In immunocompromised patients, Chagas' disease can take a more fulminant course. The diagnosis of acute infection is made by detection of parasites on a blood smear. The diagnosis of chronic infection is made by detection of serum antibodies. Neither test has the sensitivity or specificity necessary to be useful for screening blood donors. Potential blood donors emigrating from areas endemic for Chagas' disease are deferred.

Creutzfeldt-Jakob disease, an invariably fatal neurologic disease, has been associated with transfusion.[306] Donors in high-risk groups are deferred, and leukoreduction of blood products is recommended as a means of avoiding infection, because leukocytes are believed to be a vector of disease transmission.

MANAGEMENT OF HEMATOPOIETIC FAILURE STATES WITH BONE MARROW AND STEM CELL TRANSPLANTATION

Background

Transplantation with primitive stem and progenitor cells from bone marrow or peripheral blood harvests (BMT or peripheral blood stem cell transplantation [PBSCT]) is a technology that has evolved rapidly. In this chapter, PBSCT is subsumed under the more general term *bone marrow transplantation*. BMT is used to manage a spectrum of malignant and nonmalignant diseases.[307] High-dose chemotherapy or chemoradiotherapy may be considered to cause an acquired marrow failure state. Testing for HLA compatibility between donor and recipient combined with treatments to both minimize and control GVHD has resulted in widespread use of allogeneic BMT. The utility of BMT is on the rise owing to rapid expansion of the use of "minitransplants" or nonmyeloablative transplantation

procedures.[308,309] Only 40% of patients have histocompatible-related donors; however, allogeneic BMT from HLA-mismatched relatives or unrelated histocompatible donors had promising preliminary results.[310-312] Autologous BMT can result in long-term disease-free survival in a fraction of patients with multiple myeloma and lymphoma and has been extensively evaluated as therapy for other cancers.[313-317] The increase in the number of patients treated with these BMT approaches has allowed definition of efficacy and toxicity in various clinical settings and has facilitated delineation of hematologic engraftment and blood product requirements. The blood component laboratory plays a critical role in BMT by providing appropriate RBC, platelet, and blood component support and by processing or cryopreserving marrow.

Blood Component Support before Bone Marrow Transplantation

Because many patients undergoing BMT have received previous transfusions, sensitization to HLA antigens may have occurred. The effect of HLA sensitization on marrow engraftment is most evident in the setting of aplastic anemia: Reported graft rejection rates range from 25% to 60% among patients with aplastic anemia who have undergone multiple transfusions and received HLA-identical sibling marrow grafts.[318,319] The likelihood of sensitization to HLA antigens after transfusion varies among patient populations. In some studies sensitization appears to correlate with number of donor exposures.[320] When HLA-matched allogeneic BMT is to be performed, previous transfusions from family members, especially from the potential marrow donor, should be avoided because of risk of sensitization of the patient to both HLA and non-HLA antigens. Results of most studies also suggest that a patient's pretransplantation CMV status is predictive of the likelihood of infection after transplantation.[259] If the patient and donor are CMV seronegative, efforts should be made not to infect the patient by transfusion.

Blood Component Support after Bone Marrow Transplantation

Traditional BMT with high-dose chemotherapy or chemo-radiotherapy is followed by a period of pancytopenia lasting at least 2 to 4 weeks during which patients need multiple RBC and platelet transfusions. For example, patients with aplastic anemia undergoing allogeneic BMT received a median of 9 (range, 1–82) units of RBCs and 44 (range, 6–468) units of platelets, primarily during the first 4 weeks after grafting.[321] Several donor or patient factors can influence hematologic engraftment and necessitate blood product support after BMT.[319,322] In all recipients, engraftment may be compromised by disease or treatment-related effects on the marrow microenvironment. Reconstitution after allogeneic BMT may be relatively enhanced, because the donor marrow is healthy; however, the graft can be adversely affected by prophylaxis and management of GVHD. Moreover, in vitro T-cell depletion of donor marrow in some patients has

Problems Common to Cancer and Its Therapy

II

resulted in failure of engraftment and graft rejection. Autologous marrow can be intrinsically compromised by the underlying disease and by cytotoxic therapy received before marrow harvesting, by in vitro techniques used for removal of tumor cells, or by cryopreservation. In syngeneic BMT, donor marrow is histocompatible and healthy and is neither manipulated nor cryopreserved. However, the underlying disease and previous treatment of the recipient may, as is true in other types of BMT, compromise the marrow microenvironment and adversely affect engraftment. ABO incompatibility between marrow donor and recipient can be major, in which isohemagglutinin (antibody) in the recipient is directed against donor RBC antigens, or minor, in which isohemagglutinin in the donor is directed against recipient RBC antigens. Major ABO incompatibility is associated with risk of severe hemolytic reaction, graft rejection, or delayed engraftment.[322-324] Attempts to overcome major ABO incompatibility have included depletion of RBCs from the bone marrow graft before BMT or removal of iso-hemagglutinin from the recipient by large-volume plasma exchange, immunoabsorption, or both. Some investigators have supplemented these techniques with pre-BMT transfusion of donor-type blood or purified A or B substance to achieve complete adsorption of recipient isohemagglutinins. Although results suggest that major ABO-incompatible HLA-matched transplantation has resulted in no increase in patient mortality, incidence of rejection, delayed engraftment, or GVHD compared with ABO-compatible controls,[325] some reports suggest that RBC engraftment can be delayed in this setting.[326] The current standard practice in major ABO-incompatible HLA-matched BMT is to deplete RBCs from marrow before BMT, to anticipate possible delayed erythropoiesis and hemolysis after BMT, and to use methods of depleting recipient isohemagglutinins when present in high titer (at least 1:128).

Potential adverse outcome of minor ABO incompatibility between marrow donor and recipient includes rapid immune hemolysis at infusion of donor marrow owing to passive transfer of isohemagglutinin in the marrow plasma or delayed immune hemolysis caused by anti-RBC antibodies produced by the donor marrow.[322-324] There is no effect of minor ABO incompatibility on graft rejection, incidence and severity of GVHD, or patient survival. Although pre-BMT exchange transfusion of the recipient with RBCs of the donor's blood group has been used to prevent hemolysis caused by passive transfer of isohemagglutinin in the marrow product, this problem is rarely clinically significant and can more easily be avoided by removal of plasma from the marrow before infusion. Minor ABO incompatibility can result in adverse reactions due to production of anti-A or anti-B antibodies by donor marrow lymphocytes soon (1–3 weeks) after transplantation, particularly in patients receiving cyclosporine therapy or those receiving T-cell–depleted allografts.[327,328] In this setting, transfusions of group O or donor group RBCs are used to dilute the recipient RBCs; in some cases, exchange transfusion has been needed owing to very rapid engraftment of donor lymphocytes and production of anti-RBC antibodies.

Use of Hematopoietic Cytokines in Bone Marrow Transplantation

Hematopoietic cytokines such as GM-CSF and G-CSF have been shown to accelerate hematologic recovery in patients undergoing high-dose, putatively myeloablative, preparative regimens of chemotherapy or chemoradiotherapy with autologous bone marrow reinfusion.[58,329] Although the magnitude of this benefit may be debated, results of randomized trials of GM-CSF versus placebo have suggested that recovery of the neutrophil lineage occurs approximately 7 days earlier with supplemental GM-CSF than with placebo and that this more rapid recovery is associated with a shorter duration of hospital care after autologous BMT. Cost analyses have shown this to be a major determinant to delivering such high-dose therapies in a less expensive way, which should translate into increased cost-effectiveness based on assumptions of increased efficacy.[58] Use of hematopoietic cytokines is supported strongly by research findings, which are reflected in the clinical practice guidelines of the American Society of Clinical Oncology.[38-42]

Peripheral Blood Stem Cell Autotransplantation

One of the first clinical examples of the use of autologous PBSCs was collection and reinfusion of PBSCs from the chronic phase of chronic myelogenous leukemia in patients treated with high-dose cytotoxic therapy for subsequent accelerated or blastic-phase disease.[330] PBSCs engraft, as evidenced by return to the chronic phase. Some investigators have used reinfusion of PBSCs to achieve hematopoietic reconstitution after high-dose chemotherapy or total-body irradiation.[323,331-335] The potential advantages of use of PBSCs are as follows: (1) Leukapheresis is an outpatient procedure similar to platelet donation and avoids the need for hospitalization, multiple punctures, and general anesthesia in the harvest of bone marrow cells. (2) Adequate numbers of hematopoietic stem and progenitor cells can be collected from patients who have undergone hemipelvectomy or pelvic irradiation. (3) It may be possible to harvest adequate numbers of PBSCs from patients with tumor-involved marrow. Some data suggest that PBSCs may be less likely than bone marrow cell collections to contain occult micrometastatic tumor cell contamination.[336]

To obtain adequate numbers of PBSCs for cellular support of dose-intensive chemotherapy, an impracticably large number of phereses (e.g., on the order of 8 to 10 sessions) are necessary if patients with unperturbed hematopoiesis undergo harvesting in steady state. The number of phereses can be decreased if leukapheresis is done at the time of recovery after high-dose chemotherapy, especially with the additional stimulus of recombinant hematopoietic cytokines. It has been demonstrated with a variety of chemotherapy regimens for patients with cancer that the concentration of progenitor cells, such as granulocyte-macrophage colony-forming units (GM-CFUs) in the peripheral blood can increase as much as 20-fold over baseline level at the time of leukocyte recovery from chemotherapy.[337,338] Administration of certain hematopoietic cytokines alone has been shown to increase the concentration of progenitor cells in the circulation, primarily by mobilizing such cells from the marrow compartment into the blood.[339,340] The number of PBSCs can be further increased after chemotherapy by adjunctive therapy with cytokines such as G-CSF, GM-CSF, IL-3, or stem cell factor, so the total increase can be as much as 100 times the level of progenitor cells in the circulation compared with pretreatment baseline.[33,341]

Mobilization of PBSCs by cytokines such as G-CSF or GM-CSF, especially during the period of leukocyte recovery after chemotherapy, may facilitate collection of adequate numbers of PBSCs with fewer leukaphereses, thereby enhancing the ease and feasibility of using PBSCs in hematopoietic supportive care. Several investigators reported more rapid engraftment (compared with historical controls in whom autologous marrow alone had been reinfused) when both bone marrow and PBSCs were reinfused together[334,335,342,343] or when PBSCs alone[344] were used. In these historically controlled series, the clinical correlates were marked reduction in the number of RBC and platelet transfusions and a shortening of hospital stay. Further studies generally confirmed the excellent clinical activity of PBSC support of patients. Such complete and prompt hematologic recovery most likely will allow broader investigation of more intensive cytoreductive therapy as initial management of selected tumors with curative intent.

Regulation of Hematopoietic Stem Cell Processing

The use of hematopoietic stem cell (HSC) components to reconstitute hematopoiesis after myeloablative therapy is increasing in both the allogeneic as well as autologous setting. It is also becoming increasingly common for HSC components to be processed to purge malignant cells from autografts or deplete T lymphocytes from allografts as well as to isolate the specific cell populations essential for immune- and gene-mediated therapies. A variety of techniques have been developed to enrich or deplete cellular subsets by positive or negative selection, increasing both the duration and complexity of procedures performed in the cell-processing laboratory as well as requirements for quality control.

Principles of current good manufacturing practice and total quality management can be applied to HSC component processing. In 1991, the 14th edition of the American Association of Blood Banks *Standards for Blood Banks and Transfusion Services* was extended to include HSCs. In 1996, the American Association of Blood Banks published a separate *Standards for Hematopoietic Progenitor Cells* to expand and replace section Q of the *Standards for Blood Banks and Transfusion Services.*[345] These standards include sections concerning donor selection, component collection, processing, testing, labeling, storage, transportation, issue, infusion, and record keeping for hematopoietic progenitor cells, including autologous as well as allogeneic bone marrow, peripheral blood progenitor cells, and cord blood. Furthermore, the

Foundation for the Accreditation of Hematopoietic Cell Therapy (FAHCT) was formed in 1993 with programs for inspection and accreditation of hematopoietic cell collection and processing facilities as well as transplantation programs. The FAHCT standards represent a consensus document of several organizations working together in the field of clinical conduct of hematopoietic progenitor cell transplantation, including the International Society for Hematotherapy and Graft Engineering and the American Society for Blood and Marrow Transplantation.[346] The FDA reviewed the regulation of HSC components and in February 1997 issued a comprehensive draft document concerning an approach to regulation.[347]

FUTURE DIRECTIONS

It is clear that hematopoietic dysfunction in cancer patients represents a widely disparate group of clinical conditions. Understanding the pathophysiologic mechanisms of these conditions, whether endogenous or iatrogenic, is critical to development of a rational approach to diagnosis and therapy. These clinical scenarios present an important model of cellular proliferation and differentiation in humans. From this model a great deal may be learned with innovative translational research strategies. Basic scientific investigative work has resulted in clinically useful drugs that allow physicians to manipulate human hematopoiesis with recombinant cytokines. Use of such cytokines coupled with improved understanding of stem cell physiology and the differentiative and proliferative stimuli affecting progenitor cells may lead to novel therapeutic strategies for the care of patients with dysfunctional blood cell production associated with malignant disease.

REFERENCES

1. Weick JK, Hagedorn AB, Linman JW: Leukoerythroblastosis: Diagnostic and prognostic significance. Mayo Clin Proc 1974;49:111.
2. Kiraly JF, Wheby MS: Bone marrow necrosis. Am J Med 1976; 60:361.
3. Hellman S: Principles of radiotherapy. In DeVita VT, Hellman S, Rosenberg SA (eds): Cancer Principles and Practice of Oncology, 3rd ed. Philadelphia, JB Lippincott, 1989, p 267.
4. Lum LG: The kinetics of immune reconstitution after human marrow transplantation. Blood 1987;69:369.
5. Zoumbos NC, Gascon P, Djue J, et al: Circulating activated suppressor T lymphocytes in aplastic anemia. N Engl J Med 1985;312:257.
6. Miller CB, Jones RJ, Piantadose S, et al: Decreased erythropoietin response in patients with the anemia of cancer. N Engl J Med 1990;322:1689.
7. Hersh EM, Bodey GP, Niles BA, Freireich EJ: Causes of death in acute leukemia. A ten year study of 414 patients from 1954–1963. JAMA 1965;193:99.
8. Bodey GP, Buckley M, Sathe YS, Freireich EJ: Quantitative relationships between circulating leukocytes and infection in patients with acute leukemia. Ann Intern Med 1966;64:328.
9. Talcott J, Finberg R, Mayer R, Goldman L: The medical course of cancer patients with fever and neutropenia: Clinical identification of a low-risk subgroup at presentation. Arch Intern Med 1988;148:2561.

10. Talcott JA, Siegel RD, Finberg R, Goldman L: Risk assessment in cancer patients with fever and neutropenia: A prospective, two-center validation of a prediction rule. J Clin Oncol 1992;10:316.

11. Wood WC, Budman DR, Korzun AH, et al: Dose and dose intensity of adjuvant chemotherapy for stage II, node-positive breast carcinoma. N Engl J Med 1994;330:1253.

12. Lee GR: The anemia of chronic disease. Semin Hematol 1983;20:61.

13. Bowen D, Culligan D, Jacobs A: The treatment of anaemia in the myelodysplastic syndromes with recombinant human erythropoietin. Br J Haematol 1991;77:419.

14. Rothmann SA, Paul P, Weick JK, et al: Effect of cis-diamminedichloroplatinum on erythropoietin production and hematopoietic progenitor cells. Int J Cell Cloning 1985;3:415.

15. Smith DH, Guarneri CM, Whaling SM, Vokes EE: Erythropoietin response in cancer patients receiving cisplatin. Proc Am Assoc Cancer Res 1988;29:52.

16. Birgegard G, Wide L, Simonsson B: Marked erythropoietin increase before fall in Hb after treatment with cytostatic drugs suggest mechanism other than anaemia for stimulation. Br J Haematol 1989;72:462.

17. Piroso E, Erslev AJ, Caro J: Inappropriate increase in erythropoietin titers during chemotherapy. Am J Hematol 1989;32:248.

18. Brain MC, Azzapardi JG, Baker LRI, et al: Microangiopathic haemolytic anemia and mucin-forming adenocarcinoma. Br J Haematol 1970;18:183.

19. Hirst E, Robertson TI: The syndrome of thymoma and erythroblastopenic anemia. Medicine (Baltimore) 1967;46:225.

20. Gralnick HR, Abrell E: Studies of the procoagulant and fibrinolytic activity of promyelocytic leukemia. Br J Haematol 1973;24:89.

21. Cowan DH, Graham RR Jr, Baunock D: The platelet defect in leukemia, platelet ultrastructure, adenine nucleotide metabolism and the release reaction. J Clin Invest 1975;56:188.

22. Lackner H: Hemostatic abnormalities associated with dysproteinemias. Semin Hematol 1973;10:125.

23. Gaydos LA, Freireich EJ, Mantel N: The quantitative relation between platelet count and hemorrhage in patients with acute leukemia. N Engl J Med 1962;266:905.

24. Pisciotto PT, Benson K, Hume H, et al: Prophylactic versus therapeutic platelet transfusion practices in hematology/oncology patients. Transfusion 1995;35:498.

25. Rebulla P: Trigger for platelet transfusion. Vox Sang 2000;78(suppl 2):179–182.

26. Rebulla P, Finazzi G, Marangoni F, et al: The threshold for prophylactic platelet transfusions in adults with acute myeloid leukemia. N Engl J Med 1997;337:1870.

27. Wandt H, Frank M, Ehninger G, et al: Safety and cost effectiveness of a 10×10^9/L trigger for prophylactic platelet transfusions compared with the traditional 20×10^9/L trigger: A prospective comparative trial in 105 patients with acute myeloid leukemia. Blood 1998;91:3601.

28. Callow CR, Swindell R, Randall W, Chopra R: The frequency of bleeding complications in patients with haematological malignancy following the introduction of a stringent prophylactic platelet transfusion policy. Br J Haematol 2002;118:677–682.

29. Metcalf D: The granulocyte-macrophage colony-stimulating factors. Science 1985;229:16.

30. Morstyn G, Burgess AW: Hemopoietic growth factors: A review. Cancer Res 1988;48:5624.

31. Lieschke GJ, Burgess AW: Granulocyte colony-stimulating factor and granulocyte-macrophage colony-stimulating factor (parts I and II). N Engl J Med 1992;327:28, 99.

32. Demetri GD: Hematopoietic growth factors: Current knowledge, future prospects. Curr Probl Cancer 1992;16:179.

33. Broudy VC: Stem cell factor and hematopoiesis. Blood 1997;90:1345.

34. Samol J, Littlewood TJ: The efficacy of rHuEPO in cancer-related anaemia. Br J Haematol 2003;121:3–11.

35. Du X, Williams DA: Interleukin-11: Review of molecular, cell biology, and clinical use. Blood 1997;89:3897.

36. Welte K, Gabrilove J, Bronchud MH, et al: Filgrastim (r-metHuG-CSF): The first 10 years. Blood 1996;88:1907.

37. Kaushansky K, Drachman JG: The molecular and cellular biology of thrombopoietin: The primary regulator of platelet production. Oncogene 2002;21:3359–3367.

38. ASCO Ad Hoc Committee: American Society of Clinical Oncology recommendations for the use of hematopoietic colony-stimulating factors: Evidence-based, practice guidelines. J Clin Oncol 1994;12:2471.

39. ASCO Ad Hoc Committee: Update of recommendations for the use of hematopoietic colony-stimulating factors: Evidence-based, clinical practice guidelines. J Clin Oncol 1996;14:1957.

40. ASCO Ad Hoc Committee: 1997 Update of recommendations for the use of hematopoietic colony-stimulating factors: Evidence-based, clinical practice guidelines. J Clin Oncol 1997;15:3288.

41. Ozer H, Armitage JO, Bennett CL, et al: 2000 update of recommendations for the use of hematopoietic colony-stimulating factors: Evidence-based, clinical practice guidelines. American Society of Clinical Oncology Growth Factors Expert Panel. J Clin Oncol 2000;18:3558–3585.

42. Bennett CL, Weeks JA, Somerfield MR, Feinglass J, Smith TJ: Use of hematopoietic colony-stimulating factors: Comparison of the 1994 and 1997 American Society of Clinical Oncology surveys regarding ASCO clinical practice guidelines. Health Services Research Committee of the American Society of Clinical Oncology. J Clin Oncol 1999;17:3676–3681.

43. Sieff CA, Emerson SG, Donahue RE, et al: Human recombinant granulocyte-macrophage colony-stimulating factor: A multilineage hemopoietin. Science 1985;230:171.

44. Gasson JC, Weisbart RH, Kaufman SE, et al: Purified human granulocyte-macrophage colony-stimulating factor: Direct action on neutrophils. Science 1984;226:1339.

45. Gasson JC: Molecular physiology of granulocyte-macrophage colony-stimulating factor. Blood 1991;77:1131.

46. Demetri GD, Antman KHS: GM-CSF: Preclinical and clinical investigations. Semin Oncol 1992;19:362.

47. Gabrilove JL, Jakubowski A, Fain K, et al: Phase I study of granulocyte colony-stimulating factor in patients with transitional cell carcinoma of the urothelium. J Clin Invest 1988;82:1454.

48. Bronchud MH, Scarffe JH, Thatcher N, et al: Phase I/II study of recombinant human granulocyte colony-stimulating factor in patients receiving intensive chemotherapy for small cell lung cancer. Br J Cancer 1987;56:809.

49. Groopman JE, Mitsuyasu RT, DeLeo MJ, et al: Effect of recombinant human granulocyte-macrophage colony-stimulating factor on myelopoiesis in the acquired immunodeficiency syndrome. N Engl J Med 1987;317:593.

50. Antman K, Griffin J, Elias A, et al: Effect of recombinant human granulocyte-macrophage colony-stimulating factor on chemotherapy-induced myelosuppression. N Engl J Med 1988;319:593.

51. Morstyn G, Campbell L, Souza LM, et al: Effect of granulocyte colony stimulating factor on neutropenia induced by cytotoxic chemotherapy. Lancet 1988;1:667.

52. Gabrilove JL, Jakubowski A, Scher H, et al: Effect of granulocyte colony-stimulating factor on neutropenia and associated morbidity due to chemotherapy for transitional-cell carcinoma of the urothelium. N Engl J Med 1988;318:1414.

53. Crawford J, Ozer H, Stoller R, et al: Reduction by granulocyte colony-stimulating factor of fever and neutropenia induced by chemotherapy in patients with small-cell lung cancer. N Engl J Med 1991;325:164.

54. Trillet-Lenoir V, Green J, Manegold C, et al: Recombinant granulocyte colony stimulating factor reduces the infectious complications of cytotoxic chemotherapy. Eur J Cancer 1993;29A:319.

55. Johnston E, Crawford J, Blackwell S, et al: Randomized, dose-escalation study of SD/01 compared with daily filgrastim in patients receiving chemotherapy. J Clin Oncol 2000;18:2522–2528.

56. Holmes FA, O'Shaughnessy JA, Vukelja S, et al: Blinded, randomized, multicenter study to evaluate single administration pegfilgrastim once per cycle versus daily filgrastim as an adjunct to chemotherapy in patients with high-risk stage II or stage III/IV breast cancer. J Clin Oncol 2002;20:727–731.

57. Green MD, Koelbl H, Baselga J, et al: Randomized double-blind multicenter phase III study of fixed-dose single-administration pegfilgrastim versus daily filgrastim in patients receiving myelosuppressive chemotherapy. Ann Oncol 2003;14:29–35.

58. Nemunaitis J, Rabinowe SN, Singer JW, et al: Recombinant granulocyte-macrophage colony-stimulating factor after autologous bone marrow transplantation for lymphoid cancer. N Engl J Med 1991;324:1773.

59. Maher D, Green M, Bishop J, et al: Randomized, placebo-controlled trial of Filgrastim (r-metHuG-CSF) in patients with febrile neutropenia (FN) following chemotherapy [abstract]. Proc Am Soc Clin Oncol 1993;12:434.

60. Garcia-Carbonero R, Mayordomo JI, Tornamira MV, et al: Granulocyte colony-stimulating factor in the treatment of high-risk febrile neutropenia: A multicenter randomized trial. J Natl Cancer Inst 2001;93:31–38.

61. Garcia-Carbonero R, Paz-Ares L: Antibiotics and growth factors in the management of fever and neutropenia in cancer patients. Curr Opin Hematol 2002;9:215–221.

62. Gulati SC, Bennett CL: Granulocyte-macrophage colony-stimulating factor (GM-CSF) as adjunct therapy in relapsed Hodgkin disease. Ann Intern Med 1992;116:177.

63. Lyman GH, Lyman CG, Sanderson RA, Balducci L: Decision analysis of hematopoietic growth factor use in patients receiving cancer chemotherapy. J Natl Cancer Inst 1993;85:488.

64. Lyman GH, Balducci L: Update of the economic analyses of the use of the colony-stimulating factors. Curr Opin Hematol 1999;6:145–151.

65. Egrie JC, Browne JK: Development and characterization of darbepoetin alfa. Oncology (Huntingt) 2002;16(suppl 11): 13–22.

66. Abels RI: Use of recombinant human erythropoietin in the treatment of anemia in patients who have cancer. Semin Oncol 1992;19(suppl 8):29.

67. Abels R: Erythropoietin for anaemia in cancer patients. Eur J Cancer 1993;29A(suppl 2):S2.

68. Vansteenkiste J, Pirker R, Massuti B, et al: Double-blind, placebo-controlled, randomized phase III trial of darbepoetin alfa in lung cancer patients receiving chemotherapy. J Natl Cancer Inst 2002;94:1211–1220.

69. Ludwig H, Fritz E, Kotzmann H: Erythropoietin treatment of anemia associated with multiple myeloma. N Engl J Med 1990;322:1693.

70. Overbay DK, Manley HJ: Darbepoetin-alpha: A review of the literature. Pharmacotherapy 2002;22:889–897.

71. Glaspy J, Bukowski R, Steinberg D, et al: Impact of therapy with epoetin alfa on clinical outcomes in patients with nonmyeloid malignancies during cancer chemotherapy in community oncology practice. J Clin Oncol 1997;15:1218.

72. Demetri GD, Kris M, Wade J, et al: Quality-of-life benefit in chemotherapy patients treated with epoetin alfa is independent of disease response or tumor type: Results from a prospective community oncology study. J Clin Oncol 1998;16:3412.

73. Gabrilove JL, Cleeland CS, Livingston RB, Sarokhan B, Winer E, Einhorn LH: Clinical evaluation of once-weekly dosing of epoetin alfa in chemotherapy patients: Improvements in hemoglobin and quality of life are similar to three-times-weekly dosing. J Clin Oncol 2001;19:2875–2882.

74. Schapira L, Antin JH, Ransil BJ, et al: Serum erythropoietin levels in patients receiving intensive chemotherapy and radiotherapy. Blood 1990;76:2354.

75. Beguin Y, Clemons GK, Oris R, et al: Circulating erythropoietin levels after bone marrow transplantation: Inappropriate response to anemia in allogeneic transplants. Blood 1991;77:868.

76. Miller CB, Lazarus HM: Erythropoietin in stem cell transplantation. Bone Marrow Transplant 2001;27:1011–1016.

77. Baron F, Frere P, Beguin Y: Once weekly recombinant human erythropoietin therapy is very efficient after allogeneic peripheral blood stem cell transplantation when started soon after engraftment. Haematologica 2003;88:718–720.

78. Kurzrock R, Talpaz M, Estey E, et al: Erythropoietin treatment in patients with myelodysplastic syndrome and anemia. Leukemia 1990;5:985.

79. Stein RS, Abels RI, Krantz SB: Pharmacologic doses of recombinant human erythropoietin in the treatment of myelodysplastic syndromes. Blood 1991;78:1658.

80. Schouten HC, Vellenga E, Van Rhenen DJ, et al: Recombinant human erythropoietin in patients with myelodysplastic syndromes. Leukemia 1991;5:432.

81. Shepherd JD, Currie CJ, Sparling TG, et al: Erythropoietin therapy of myelodysplastic syndromes. Blood 1992;79:1891.

82. Rafanelli D, Grossi A, Longo G, et al: Recombinant human erythropoietin for treatment of myelodysplastic syndromes. Leukemia 1992;6:323.

83. Razzano M, Caslini C, Cortelazzo S, et al: Therapy with human recombinant erythropoietin in patients with myelodysplastic syndromes. Br J Haematol 1992;81:628.

84. Gordon MS, Hoffman R: Growth factors affecting human thrombopoiesis: Potential agents for the treatment of thrombocytopenia. Blood 1992;80:302.

85. Curtis BM, Williams DE, Broxmeyer HE, et al: Enhanced hematopoietic activity of a human granulocyte/macrophage colony-stimulating factor–interleukin-3 fusion protein. Proc Natl Acad Sci USA 1991;88:5809.

86. Vose JM, Pandite AN, Beveridge RA, et al: Granulocyte-macrophage colony-stimulating factor/interleukin-3 fusion protein versus granulocyte-macrophage colony-stimulating factor after autologous bone marrow transplantation for non-Hodgkin's lymphoma: Results of a randomized double-blind trial. J Clin Oncol 1997;15:1617.

87. Vadhan-Raj S, Broxmeyer HE, Andreeff M, et al: In vivo biologic effects of PIXY321, a synthetic hybrid protein of recombinant GM-CSF and IL-3 in cancer patients with normal hematopoiesis: A phase I study. Blood 1995;86:2098.

88. Feng Y, McKearn J: Improving on nature by engineering hematopoietic growth factors. In Wingard J, Demetri GD (eds): Clinical Applications of Hematopoietic Cytokines. New York, Kluwer, 1999.

89. Beutler E: Platelet transfusions: The 20,000/μl trigger. Blood 1993;81:1411.

90. Smith II JA, Longo DL, Alvord WG, et al: The effects of treatment with interleukin-1 on platelet recovery after high-dose carboplatin. N Engl J Med 1993;328:756.

91. Ganser A, Lindemann A, Seipelt G, et al: Effects of recombinant human interleukin-3 in patients with normal hematopoiesis and in patients with bone marrow failure. Blood 1990; 76:666.

92. Ganser A, Seipelt G, Lindemann A, et al: Effects of recombinant human interleukin-3 in patients with myelodysplastic syndromes. Blood 1990;76:455.

93. Kurzrock R, Talpaz M, Estrov Z, et al: Phase I study of recombinant human interleukin-3 in patients with bone marrow failure. J Clin Oncol 1991;9:1241.

94. Postmus PE, Gietema JA, Damsma O, et al: Effects of recombinant human interleukin-3 in patients with relapsed small-cell lung cancer treated with chemotherapy: A dose-finding study. J Clin Oncol 1992;10:1131.

95. Oprelvekin: Review of its pharmacology and therapeutic potential in chemotherapy-induced thrombocytopenia. BioDrugs 1998;2:159.

96. Tepler I, Elias L, Smith JW II, et al: A randomized placebo-controlled trial of recombinant human interleukin-11 in cancer patients with severe thrombocytopenia due to chemotherapy. Blood 1996;87:3607.

97. Demetri GD, Samuels B, Gordon M, et al: Recombinant human interleukin-6 (IL-6) increases circulating platelet counts and C-reactive protein levels in vivo: Initial results of a phase I trial in sarcoma patients with normal hemopoiesis. Blood 1992;80(suppl): 344.

98. Letter to investigators and patients. Thousand Oaks, CA, Amgen, October 1, 1998.

99. Kaushansky K: Thrombopoietin. N Engl J Med 1998;339:746.

100. Bonilla MA, Gillio AP, Ruggeiro M, et al: Effects of recombinant human granulocyte colony-stimulating factor on neutropenia in patients with congenital agranulocytosis. N Engl J Med 1989;320:1574.

101. Welte K, Zeidler C, Reiter A, et al: Differential effects of granulocyte-macrophage colony-stimulating factor and granulocyte colony-stimulating factor in children with severe congenital neutropenia. Blood 1990;75:1056.

102. Dale DC, Bonilla MA, Davis MW, et al: A randomized controlled phase III trial of recombinant human granulocyte colony-stimulating factor (filgrastim) for treatment of severe chronic neutropenia. Blood 1993;81:2496.

103. Dunbar CE, Smith DA, Kimball J, et al: Treatment of Diamond-Blackfan anemia with hematopoietic growth factors, granulocyte-macrophage colony-stimulating factor and interleukin-3: Sustained remission following IL-3. Br J Haematol 1991;79:316.

104. Olivieri NF, Berriman AM, Davis S, et al: Response to the hematopoietic growth factor IL-3 in patients with Diamond-Blackfan anemia. Blood 1991;78(suppl 1):153a.

105. Gillio AP, Faulkner L, Alter BP: Treatment of Diamond-Blackfan anemia with recombinant human IL-3. Blood 1993;82:744.

106. Guinan EC, Lee YS, Lopez KD, et al: Effects of interleukin-3 and granulocyte-macrophage colony stimulating factor on thrombo-poiesis in congenital amegakaryocytic thrombocytopenia. Blood 1993;81:1691.

107. Neben TY, Loebelenz J, Hayes L: Recombinant human interleukin-11 stimulates megakaryopoiesis and increases peripheral platelets in normal and splenectomized mice. Blood 1993;81:901.

108. Negrin RS, Haeuber DH, Nagler A, et al: Treatment of myelodysplastic syndromes with recombinant human granulocyte colony-stimulating factor: A phase I-II trial. Ann Intern Med 1989;113:976.

109. Negrin RS, Stein R, Vardiman J, et al: Treatment of the anemia of myelodysplastic syndromes using recombinant human granulocyte colony-stimulating factor in combination with erythropoietin. Blood 1993;82:737.

110. Vadhan-Raj S, Keating M, LeMaistre A, et al: Effects of recombinant human granulocyte-macrophage colony-stimulating factor in patients with myelodysplastic syndromes. N Engl J Med 1987;317:1545.

111. Vadhan-Raj S, Buescher S, LeMaistre A, et al: Stimulation of hematopoiesis in patients with bone marrow failure and in patients with malignancy by recombinant human granulocyte-macrophage colony-stimulating factor. Blood 1988;72:134.

112. Herrmann F, Lindemann A, Klein H, et al: Effect of recombinant human granulocyte-macrophage colony-stimulating factor in patients with myelodysplastic syndrome with excess blasts. Leukemia 1989;3:335.

113. Stone RM: Hematopoietic growth factors in acute leukemia. In Wingard J, Demetri GD (eds): Clinical Applications of Hematopoietic Cytokines. New York, Kluwer, 1999.

114. Schuster MW, Thompson JA, Larson R, et al: Randomized trial of subcutaneous granulocyte-macrophage colony-stimulating factor (GM-CSF) versus observation in patients (PTS) with myelodysplastic syndrome (MDS) or aplastic anemia (AA) [abstract]. Proc Am Soc Clin Oncol 1990;9:205.

115. Gordon MS, Neumanitis J, Hoffman R, et al: Phase I trial of subcutaneous (SC) recombinant human interleukin-6 (IL-6) in patients with myelodysplasia and thrombocytopenia [abstract]. Blood 1992;80(suppl 1):249a.

116. Zon LI, Groopman JE: Hematologic manifestations of the human immunodeficiency virus (HIV). Semin Hematol 1988;25:208.

117. Groopman JE, Feder D: Hematopoietic growth factors in AIDS. Semin Oncol 1992;19:408.

118. Miles SA, Mitsuyasu RT, Lee K, et al: Recombinant human granulocyte colony-stimulating factor increases circulating burst forming unit-erythron and red blood cell production in patients with severe human immunodeficiency virus infection. Blood 1990;75:2137.

119. Miles SA, Mitsuyasu R, Moreno J, et al: Combined therapy with recombinant granulocyte colony-stimulating factor and erythropoietin decreases hematologic toxicity from zidovudine. Blood 1991;77:2109.

120. Levine JD, Allan JD, Tessitore JH, et al: Recombinant human granulocyte-macrophage colony-stimulating factor ameliorates zidovudine-induced neutropenia in patients with acquired immunodeficiency syndrome (AIDS). Blood 1991;78:3148.

121. Fischl M, Galpin JE, Levine JD, et al: Recombinant human erythropoietin for patients with AIDS treated with zidovudine. N Engl J Med 1990;322:1488.

122. Smith PJ, Edert H: Evidence of stem cell competition in children with malignant disease. Lancet 1976;1:776.

123. Audet AM, Goodnough LT: Practice strategies for elective red blood cell transfusion. Ann Intern Med 1992;116:403.

124. Adamson JW, Eschbach JW: Erythropoietin for end-stage renal disease. N Engl J Med 1998;339:625.

125. Crawford J, Cella D, Cleeland CS, et al: Relationship between changes in hemoglobin level and quality of life during chemotherapy in anemic cancer patients receiving epoetin alfa therapy. Cancer 2002;95:888–895.

126. Mac N, Surgenor D: Collection and transfusion of blood in the United States, 1982–1988. N Engl J Med 1990;322:1646.

127. Snyder EL: Clinical use of white cell poor blood components. Transfusion 1989;29:568.

128. Goldfinger D, Lowe C: Prevention of adverse reactions to blood transfusion by the administration of saline washed red blood cells. Transfusion 1981;21:277.

129. Anderson KC, Gorgone BC, Wahlers E, et al: Preparation and clinical utility of leukocyte poor apheresis platelets. Transfusion Sci 1991;12:163.

130. Freireich EJ, Levin RH, Whang J, et al: The function and fate of transfused leukocytes from donors with chronic myelocytic leukemia in leukopenic recipients. Ann N Y Acad Sci 1964;113:1081.

131. Wright DG: Leukocyte transfusions: Thinking twice. Am J Med 1984;76:637.

132. Applebaum FR, Bowles CA, Makuch RW, Deisseroth AB: Granulocyte transfusion therapy of experimental *Pseudomonas* septicemia: Study of cell dose and collection technique. Blood 1978;52:323.

133. Clift RA, Buckner CD: Granulocyte transfusions. Am J Med 1984;76:631.

134. Winston DJ, Ho WG, Gale RP: Therapeutic granulocyte transfusions for documented infections: A controlled trial in ninety-five infectious granulocytopenic episodes. Ann Intern Med 1982;97:509.

135. Bensinger WI, Price TH, Dale DC: The effects of daily recombinant human granulocyte colony-stimulating factor administration on normal granulocyte donors undergoing leukapheresis. Blood 1993;81:1883.

136. Caspar CB, Seger RA, Berger J, Gmur J: Effective stimulation of donors for granulocyte transfusions with recombinant methionyl granulocyte colony-stimulating factor. Blood 1993;81:2866.

137. Adkins D, Ali S, Despotis G, et al: Granulocyte collection efficiency and yield are enhanced by the use of a higher interface offset during apheresis of donors given granulocyte-colony-stimulating factor. Transfusion 1998;38:557.

138. Strauss RG: Therapeutic granulocyte transfusions in 1993. Blood 1993;81:1675.

139. Saarinen UM, Hovi L, Vilinikka L, et al: Reemphasis on leukocyte transfusions: Induction of myeloid marrow recovery in critically ill neutropenic children with cancer. Vox Sang 1995;68:90.

140. Bhatia S, McCullough J, Perry EH, et al: Granulocyte transfusions: Efficacy in treating fungal infections in neutropenic patients following bone marrow transplantation. Transfusion 1994;34:226.

141. Anderson KC, Weinstein HC: Graft versus host disease after transfusion. N Engl J Med 1990;323:315.

142. Karp DD, Ervin TJ, Tuttle S, et al: Pulmonary complications during granulocyte transfusions: Incidence and clinical features. Vox Sang 1982;42:57.

143. Duke WW: The relation of blood platelets to hemorrhagic disease: Description of a method for determining the bleeding time and coagulation time and report of three cases of hemorrhagic disease relieved by transfusion. JAMA 1910;55:1185.

144. Farber S, Klein E: The nature and control of bleeding in acute leukemia and other thrombocytopenic states: A review of a 10 year program of research. Ann Paediatr Forum 1957;3:348.

145. Murphy S, Litwin S, Herring LM, et al: Indications for platelet transfusion in children with acute leukemia. Am J Hematol 1982;12:347.
146. Higby DJ: The prophylactic treatment of thrombocytopenic leukemic patients with platelets: A double blind study. Transfusion 1974;4:440.
147. Consensus Development Conference on Platelet Transfusion Therapy. JAMA 1987;258:1777.
148. Aderka D, Praff G, Santo M, et al: Bleeding due to thrombocytopenia in acute leukemias and reevaluation of the prophylactic platelet transfusion policy. Am J Med Sci 1986;291:147.
149. Gmür J, Burger J, Schanz Urs, et al: Safety of stringent prophylactic platelet transfusion policy for patients with acute leukaemia. Lancet 1991;338:1223.
150. Shulman NR, Watkins SP, Itscoitz SB, Students AB: Evidence that the spleen retains the youngest and hemostatically most effective platelets. Trans Assoc Am Physicians 1968;81:302.
151. Baer MR, Bloomfield CD: Controversies in transfusion medicine: Prophylactic platelet transfusion therapy—Pro. Transfusion 1992;32:377.
152. Patten E: Controversies in transfusion medicine: Prophylactic platelet transfusion revisited after 25 years—Con. Transfusion 1992;32:381.
153. Schiffer CA: Prophylactic platelet transfusion. Transfusion 1992;32:295.
154. Kretschmer V, Huss B, Dietrich G, et al: Determination of bleeding risk in thrombocytopenic patients receiving platelet substitution. Transfus Sci 1993;14:27.
155. Tullis JL, Eberle WG II, Baudanza P, Tinch R: Platelet-pheresis description of a new technique. Transfusion 1968;8:154.
156. Kurtz SR, McMican A, Carciero R, et al: Plateletpheresis experience with the Haemonetics blood processor 30, the IBM blood processor 2997 and the Fenwal CS-3000 blood processor. Vox Sang 1981;41:212.
157. Sintnicolaas K, Sizoo W, Haije WG, et al: Delayed alloimmunization by random single donor platelet transfusions: A randomized study to compare single donor and multiple donor platelet transfusions in cancer patients with thrombocytopenia. Lancet 1981;1:750.
158. Gmur J, Felten A von, Osterwalder B, et al: Delayed alloimmunization using random single donor platelet transfusions: A prospective study in thrombocytopenic patients with acute leukemia. Blood 1983;62:473.
159. Daly PA, Schiffer CA, Aisner J, Wiernik PH: Platelet transfusion therapy: One hour post-transfusion increments are valuable in predicting the need for HLA-matched preparations. JAMA 1980;243:435.
160. Gorgone BC, Andersen JW, Anderson KC, et al: Comparison of 15 min and 1H post-platelet counts in pediatric patients [abstract]. Transfusion 1986;26:555.
161. O'Connell B, Lee EJ, Shiffer CA, et al: The value of 10-minute post-transfusion platelet counts. Transfusion 1988;28:66.
162. Harker KA, Slichter SJ: The bleeding time as a screening test for evaluation of platelet function. N Engl J Med 1972;287:155.
163. Anderson KC: Hematologic complications. In Holland JF, Frei E III, Bast RC, et al (eds): Cancer Medicine. Philadelphia, Lea & Febiger, 1993, p 2294.
164. Bishop JF, McGrath K, Wolf MM, et al: Clinical factors influencing the efficacy of pooled platelet transfusions. Blood 1988;71:383.
165. Flatow FA, Freireich EJ: Effect of splenectomy on the response to platelet transfusion in three patients with aplastic anemia. N Engl J Med 1966;274:242.
166. Smith ME, Reid DM, Jones CE, et al: Binding of quinine- and quinidine-dependent drug antibodies to platelets is mediated by the Fab domain of the immunoglobulin G and is not Fc dependent. J Clin Invest 1987;79:912.
167. Kunicki TJ, Russel N, Nurden AT, et al: Further studies of the human platelet receptor for quinine- and quinidine-dependent antibodies. J Immunol 1981;126:398.
168. Berndt MC, Chong BH, Bull HA, et al: Molecular characterization of quinine/quinidine drug-dependent antibody platelet interaction using monoclonal antibodies. Blood 1985;66:1292.
169. Christie DJ, Mullen PC, Aster RH: Quinine- and quinidine-induced

170. Stricker RB, Shulman MA: Quinidine purpura: Evidence that glycoprotein V is a target platelet antigen. Blood 1986;67:1377.
171. Chong BH, Xiaoping D, Berndt MC, et al: Characterization of the binding domains on platelet glycoproteins Ib-X and IIB/IIIa complexes for the quinine/quinidine-dependent antibodies. Blood 1991;77:2190.
172. Fujisawa K, O'Toole TE, Tani P, et al: Autoantibodies to the presumptive cytoplasmic domain of platelet glycoprotein IIIa in patients with chronic immune thrombocytopenic purpura. Blood 1991;77:2207.
173. Kickler T, Kennedy SD, Braine HG: Alloimmunization to platelet-specific antigens on glycoproteins IIb-IIIa and Ib/Ix in multiply transfused thrombocytopenic patients. Transfusion 1990;30:622.
174. Shalev O, Brezis M: Methyldopa-induced thrombocytopenia in chronic lymphocytic-leukemia [letter]. N Engl J Med 1977;297:1471.
175. Murphy MF, Riordan T, Minchinton RM, et al: Demonstration of an immune-mediated mechanism of penicillin-induced neutropenia and thrombocytopenia. Br J Haematol 1983;55:155.
176. Herzig RH, Terasaki PI, Trapani RJ, et al: The relationship between donor-recipient lymphocytotoxicity and the transfusion response using HLA-matched platelet concentrates. Transfusion 1977;17:657.
177. Howard JE, Perkins HA: The natural history of alloimmunization to platelets. Transfusion 1978;18:496.
178. Van Eys J, Thomas D, Olivos B: Platelet use in pediatric oncology: A review of 393 transfusions. Transfusion 1978;18:169.
179. Dutcher JP, Schiffer CA, Aisner J, Wiernik PH: Alloimmunization following platelet transfusion: The absence of a dose-response relationship. Blood 1981;57:395.
180. Dutcher JP, Schiffer CA, Aisner J, Wiernik PH: Long-term follow-up of patients with leukemia receiving platelet transfusions: Identification of a large group of patients who do not become alloimmunized. Blood 1981;58:1007.
181. Holohan TV, Terasaki PI, Deisseroth AB: Suppression of transfusion-related alloimmunization in intensively treated cancer patients. Blood 1981;58:122.
182. Yankee RA, Grumet FC, Rogentine GN: Platelet transfusion therapy: The selection of compatible donors for refractory patients by lymphocyte HLA-typing. N Engl J Med 1969;281:1208.
183. Yankee RA, Graff KS, Dowling R, Henderson ES: Selection of unrelated compatible platelet donors by lymphocyte HL-A matching. N Engl J Med 1973;288:760.
184. Lohrmann HP, Bull MI, Decter JA, et al: Platelet transfusions from HL-A compatible unrelated donors to alloimmunized patients. Ann Intern Med 1974;80:9.
185. Duquesnoy RJ, Filip DJ, Rodey GE, et al: Successful transfusion of platelets "mismatched" for HLA antigens to alloimmunized thrombocytopenic patients. Am J Hematol 1977;2:219.
186. Duquesnoy RJ, Filip DJ, Aster RH: Influence of HLA-A2 on the effectiveness of platelet transfusions to alloimmunized thrombocytopenic patients. Blood 1977;50:407.
187. Schiffer CA, Patten E, Reilly J, Patel S: Effective leukocyte removal from platelet preparations by centrifugation in a new pooling bag. Transfusion 1987;27:162.
188. Murphy MF, Grint PCA, Hardiman AE, et al: Use of leukocyte-poor blood components and HLA-matched platelet donors to prevent HLA alloimmunization. Br J Haematol 1986;62:529.
189. Andreu G, Dewailly J, Leberre C, et al: Prevention of HLA immunization with leukocyte-poor packed red cells and platelet concentrates obtained by filtration. Blood 1988;72:964.
190. Sniecinski I, O'Donnell, Nowicki B, Hill LR: Prevention of refractoriness and HLA-alloimmunization using filtered blood products. Blood 1988;71:1402.
191. Van Marwijk Kooy M, Prooijen HC, Moes M, et al: Use of leukocyte-depleted platelet concentrates for the prevention of refractoriness and primary HLA alloimmunization: A prospective, randomized trial. Blood 1991;77:201.
192. Schiffer CA: Prevention of alloimmunization against platelets. Blood 1991;77:1.
193. Brand A, Claas FHJ, van Rood JJ: UV-irradiated platelets: Ready to use? Transfusion 1989;29:377.

194. Sherman L, Menitov J, Kagen LR, et al: Ultraviolet-B irradiation of platelets: A preliminary trial of efficacy. Transfusion 1992;32:402.

195. Andreu G, Boccaccio C, Lecrubier C, et al: Ultraviolet irradiation of platelet concentrates: Feasibility in transfusion practice. Transfusion 1990;30:401.

196. TRAP Study Group: Leukocyte reduction and ultraviolet B irradiation of platelets to prevent alloimmunization and refractoriness to platelet transfusions. N Engl J Med 1997;337:1861.

197. Blajchman MA, Bardossy L, Carmen RA, et al: An animal model of allogeneic donor platelet refractoriness: The effect of the time of leukodepletion. Blood 1992;79:1371.

198. Kickler TS, Braine H, Ness PM: The predictive value of crossmatching platelet transfusions for alloimmunized patients. Transfusion 1985;25:385.

199. Moroff G, Garratty G, Heal JM, et al: Selection of platelets for refractory patients by HLA matching and prospective crossmatching. Transfusion 1992;32:633.

200. Bensinger WI, Baker DA, Buckner CD, et al: Plasma exchange for platelet alloimmunization. Transplantation 1986;41:602.

201. Lee EJ, Norris D, Schiffer CA, et al: Intravenous immune globulin for patients alloimmunized to random donor platelet transfusion. Transfusion 1987;27:245.

202. Kickler T, Braine HG, Piantadosi S, et al: A randomized placebo controlled trial of intravenous gammaglobulin in alloimmunized thrombocytopenic patients. Blood 1990;75:313.

203. Murphy S: ABO blood groups and platelet transfusion. Transfusion 1988;28:401.

204. Dunstan RA, Simpson MB, Rosse WF: Erythrocyte antigens on human platelets: Absence of Rh, Duffy, Kell, Kidd and Lutheran antigens. Transfusion 1984;24:243.

205. McGinnis MH, Bronson WR, Freireich EJ, et al: Formation of red cell antibodies in response to platelet transfusions. Transfusion 1963;3:426.

206. Skinnider LF, Taylor D: The in vitro effect of anti-A and anti-AB alloantibodies on group A and AB platelets. Transfusion 1981;21:706.

207. Aster RH: Effect of anticoagulant and ABO incompatibility on recovery of transfused human platelets. Blood 1965;26:732.

208. Pfisterer H, Thierfelder S, Stich W: ABO Rh groups and platelet transfusion. Blut 1968;17:1.

209. Lee EJ, Schiffer CJ: ABO compatibility can influence the results of platelet transfusion: Results of a randomized trial. Transfusion 1989;29:384.

210. Duquesnoy RJ, Anderson AJ, Tomasulo PA, Aster RH: ABO compatibility and platelet transfusions of alloimmunized thrombocytopenic patients. Blood 1979;54:595.

211. Lichtiger B, Surgeon J, Rhorer S: Rh-incompatible platelet transfusion therapy in cancer patients. Vox Sang 1983;43:139.

212. Brand A, Sintnicolaas K, Class FHJ, Eernisse JG: ABH antibodies causing platelet transfusion refractoriness. Transfusion 1986;24:463.

213. Heal JM, Blumberg N, Masel D: An evaluation of crossmatching, HLA, and ABO matching for platelet transfusions to refractory patients. Blood 1987;70:23.

214. Pierce RN, Reich LM, Mayer K: Hemolysis following platelet transfusions from ABO-incompatible donors. Transfusion 1985;25:60.

215. Thompson CB, Jakubowski JA: The pathophysiology and clinical relevance of platelet heterogeneity. Blood 1988;72:1.

216. Abramson N, Eisenberg PD, Aster RH: Post-transfusion purpura: Immunological aspects and therapy. N Engl J Med 1974;291:1163.

217. Shulman NR, Aster RH, Leitner A, Hiller MC: A new syndrome of post transfusion purpura. J Clin Invest 1960;39:1928.

218. Cimo PL, Aster RH: Post-transfusion purpura: Successful treatment by exchange transfusion. N Engl J Med 1972;289:290.

219. Francis DMA, Shenton BK: Blood transfusion and tumour growth: Evidence from laboratory animals. Lancet 1981;2:871.

220. Gascon P, Zoumbos NC, Young NS: Immunologic abnormalities in patients receiving multiple blood transfusions. Ann Intern Med 1984;100:173.

221. Kaplan J, Sarnaik S, Gitlin J, Lusher J: Diminished helper/suppressor lymphocyte ratios and natural killer activity in recipients of repeated blood transfusions. Blood 1984;64:308.

222. Lagaaij EL, Hennemann IPH, Ruigro KM, et al: Effect of one HLA-DR antigen matched and completely HLA-DR-mismatched blood transfusions on survival of heart and kidney allografts. N Engl J Med 1989;321:701.

223. Blumberg N, Heal JM: Transfusion and host defenses against cancer recurrence and infection. Transfusion 1989;29:236.

224. Tartter PI, Burrows L, Kirschner P: Perioperative blood transfusion adversely affects prognosis after resection of stage I (subset NO) non-oat cell lung cancer. J Thorac Cardiovasc Surg 1984;88:659.

225. Tartter PI, Quintero S, Barron DM: Perioperative blood transfusion associated with infectious complications after colorectal cancer operations. Am J Surg 1986;152:479.

226. Kieckbusch ME, O'Fallon JR, Ahmann DL, Moore SB: Blood transfusion exposure does not influence survival in patients with carcinoma of the breast. Transfusion 29:500.

227. Ness PM, Walsh PC, Zahurak M, et al: Prostate cancer recurrence in radical surgery patients receiving autologous or homologous blood. Transfusion 1992;32:31.

228. Blumberg N, Chuang-Stein C, Heal JM: The relationship of blood transfusion, tumor staging, and cancer recurrence. Transfusion 1990;30:291.

229. Anderson KC: Clinical indications for blood component irradiation. In Baldwin ML, Jeffries L (eds): Irradiation of Blood Components. Bethesda, MD, American Association of Blood Banks, 1992, p 31.

230. Shivdasani RA, Haluska FG, Dock NL, et al: Graft-versus-host disease associated with transfusion of blood from unrelated HLA-homozygous donors. N Engl J Med 1993;328:766.

231. Twomey JJ, Rice L: Impact of Hodgkin's disease upon the immune system. Semin Oncol 1980;7:114.

232. Ekert H, Waters KD, Smith PJ: Treatment with MOPP or ChlVPP chemotherapy only for all stages of childhood Hodgkin's disease. J Clin Oncol 1988;6:1845.

233. Postmus PE, Mulder NH, Elema JD: Graft versus host disease after transfusions of non-irradiated blood cells in patients having received autologous bone marrow. Eur J Cancer Clin Oncol 1988;24:889.

234. Thaler M, Shamiss A, Orgad S, et al: The role of the blood from HLA-homozygous donors in fatal transfusion-associated graft-versus-host disease after open heart surgery. N Engl J Med 1989;321:25.

235. Moroff G, Luban NL: The irradiation of blood and blood components to prevent graft-versus-host disease: Technical issues and guidelines. Transfus Med Rev 1997;11:15–26.

236. Sprent J, Anderson RE, Miller JFAP: Radiosensitivity of T and B lymphocytes, II: Effect of radiation on response of T cells to alloantigens. Eur J Immunol 1974;4:204.

237. Valerius NH, Johansen KS, Nielson OS, et al: Effect of in vivo x-irradiation on lymphocyte and granulocyte function. Scand J Hematol 1981;27:9.

238. Button LN, DeWolf WC, Newburger PE, et al: The effects of irradiation on blood components. Transfusion 1981;21:419.

239. Drobyski W, Thibodeau S, Truitt R, et al: Third party mediated graft rejection and graft-versus-host disease after T cell depleted bone marrow transplantation, as demonstrated by hypervariable DNA probes and HLA-DR polymorphism. Blood 1989;74:2285.

240. Anderson KC, Goodnough LT, Pisciotto P, et al: Variation in blood component irradiation practice: Implications for prevention of transfusion associated graft versus host disease. Blood 1991;77:2096.

241. Read EJ, Kadis C, Carter CS, Leitman SF: Viability of platelets following storage in the irradiated state: A pair-controlled study. Transfusion 1988;28:446.

242. Davey RJ, McCoy NC, Yu M, et al: The effect of prestorage irradiation on posttransfusion red cell survival. Transfusion 1992;32:525.

243. Anderson KC, Nadler LM, Takvorian T, et al: Monoclonal antibodies: Their use in bone marrow transplantation. In Brown E (ed): Progress in Hematology. Orlando, FL, Grune & Stratton, 1987, p 137.

244. Akahoshi M: A case of transfusion-associated graft-versus-host disease not prevented by white cell-reduction filters. Transfusion 1992;32:169.

245. Deeg HJ, Graham TC, Gerhard Miller L, et al: Prevention of transfusion-induced graft-versus-host disease in dogs by ultraviolet irradiation. Blood 1989;74:2592.

246. Alter HJ, Holland PV, Purcell RH, et al: Post-transfusion hepatitis after exclusion of commercial and hepatitis B antigen-positive donors. Ann Intern Med 1972;77:691.

247. Public Health Service inter-agency guidelines for screening donors of blood, plasma, organs, tissues, and semen for evidence of hepatitis B and hepatitis C. Recomm Rep 1991;40:1.

248. Hoofnagle J: Post-transfusion hepatitis B. Transfusion 1990;30:384.

249. Stevens CE, Aach RD, Hollinger FB, et al: Hepatitis B virus antibody in blood donors and the occurrence of non-A, non-B hepatitis in transfusion recipients: An analysis of the transfusion-transmitted viruses study. Ann Intern Med 1984;101:733.

250. Kline WE, Bowman RJ, McCurdy KE, et al: Hepatitis B core antibody (anti-BHc) in blood donors in the United States: Implications for surrogate testing programs. Transfusion 1987;27:99.

251. Koziol DE, Holland PV, Alling DW, et al: Antibody to hepatitis B core antigen as a paradoxical marker for non-A, non-B hepatitis agents in donated blood. Ann Intern Med 1986;104:488.

252. Choo QL, Kuo G, Weiner A, et al: Isolation of a DNA clone derived from a blood borne non-A, non-B viral hepatitis genome. Science 1989;244:359.

253. Kuo G, Choo QL, Alter HJ, et al: An assay for circulating antibodies to a major etiologic virus of human non-A, non-B hepatitis. Science 1989;244:362.

254. Alter HJ, Purcell RH, Shih JW, et al: Detection of antibody to hepatitis C virus in prospectively followed transfusion recipients with acute and chronic non-A, non-B Hepatitis. N Engl J Med 1989;321:1294.

255. Esteban JI, González A, Hernández JM: Evaluation of antibodies to hepatitis C virus in a study of transfusion-associated hepatitis. N Engl J Med 1990;323:1107.

256. Schreiber GB, Busch MP, Kleinman SH, et al: The risk of transfusion-transmitted viral infections. N Engl J Med 1996;334:1685.

257. Donahue JG, Muñoz A, Ness PM, et al: The declining risk of post-transfusion hepatitis C virus infection. N Engl J Med 1992;327:369.

258. Winston DJ, Ho WG, Lin CH, et al: Intravenous immune globulin for prevention of cytomegalovirus infection and interstitial pneumonia after bone marrow transplantation. Ann Intern Med 1987;106:12.

259. Bowden RA, Sayers M, Flournoy N, et al: Cytomegalovirus immune globulin and seronegative blood products to prevent primary cytomegalovirus infection after marrow transplantation. N Engl J Med 1986;314:1006.

260. Wingard JR, Chen DYH, Burns WH, et al: Cytomegalovirus infection after autologous bone marrow transplantation with comparison to infection after allogeneic bone marrow transplantation. Blood 1988;71:1432.

261. Miller W, Flynn P, McCullough J, et al: Cytomegalovirus infection after bone marrow transplantation and association with acute graft-versus-host disease. Blood 1986;67:1162.

262. Meyers JD, Reed EC, Shepp DH, et al: Acyclovir for prevention of cytomegalovirus infection and disease after allogeneic marrow transplantation. N Engl J Med 1988;318:70.

263. Gilbert GL, Hayes K, Hudson IL, et al: Prevention of transfusion-acquired cytomegalovirus infection in infants by blood filtration to remove leucocytes. Lancet 1989;1:1228.

264. Murphy MF, Grint PCA, Hardiman AE, et al: Use of leukocyte-poor blood components to prevent primary cytomegalovirus (CMV) infections in patients with acute leukaemia. Br J Haematol 1989;70:253.

265. Bowden RA, Sayers M, Cays M, Slichter SJ: The role of blood product filtration in the prevention of transfusion associated cytomegalovirus (CMV) infection after marrow transplant. Transfusion 1989;29:595.

266. De Witte T, Schattenberg A, Van Dijk BA, et al: Prevention of primary cytomegalovirus infection after allogeneic bone marrow transplantation by using leukocyte-poor random blood products from cytomegalovirus-unscreened blood bank donors. Transplantation 1990;50:964.

267. Bowden RA, Slichter SJ, Sayers M, et al: A comparison of filtered leukocyte-reduced and cytomegalovirus (CMV) seronegative blood products for the prevention of transfusion-associated CMV infection after marrow transplant. Blood 1995;86:3599.

268. Sayers MH, Anderson KC, Goodnough LT, et al: Reducing the risk for transfusion-transmitted cytomegalovirus infection. Ann Intern Med 1992;116:55.

269. Anderson KC, Lew MA, Gorgone B, et al: Transfusion-related sepsis after prolonged platelet storage. Am J Med 1986;81:405.

270. Heal JM, Jones ME, Forey J, et al: Fatal *Salmonella* septicemia following platelet transfusion. Transfusion 1987;27:2.

271. Morrow JF, Braine HG, Kickler TS, et al: Septic reactions to platelet transfusions. JAMA 1991;266:555.

272. Goldman M, Blajchman MA: Blood product-associated bacterial sepsis. Transfus Med Rev 1991;V:73.

273. Barrett B, Andersen JW, Anderson KC: Strategies for the avoidance of bacterial contamination of blood components. Transfusion 1993;33:228.

274. Update: *Yersinia enterocolitica* bacteremia and endotoxin shock associated with red blood cell transfusions—United States, 1991. MMWR 1991;40:176.

275. Aber RC: Transfusion-associated *Yersinia enterocolitica*. Transfusion 1990;30:193.

276. Tipple MA, Bland LA, Murphy JJ, et al: Sepsis associated with transfusion of red cells contaminated with *Yersinia enterocolitica*. Transfusion 1990;30:207.

277. The HIV/AIDS epidemic: The first 10 years. Recomm Rep 1990;40:357.

278. Curran JW, Lawrence DN, Jaffe H, et al: Acquired immuno-deficiency syndrome (AIDS) associated with transfusions. N Engl J Med 1984;310:69.

279. Schorr JP, Berkowitz A, Cumming PD, et al: Prevalence of HTLV-III antibody in American blood donors. N Engl J Med 1985;313:384.

280. Jackson J, MacDonald KL, Caldwell J, et al: Absence of HIV infection in blood donors with indeterminate Western blot tests for antibody to HIV-1. N Engl J Med 1990;322:217.

281. Leitman SF, Klein HG, Melpolder JJ, et al: Clinical implications of routine tests for antibodies to human immunodeficiency virus in asymptomatic blood donors. N Engl J Med 1989;321:917.

282. Ward JW, Holmberg SD, Allen JR, et al: Transmission of human immunodeficiency virus (HIV) by blood transfusions screened as negative for HIV antibody. N Engl J Med 1988;318:473.

283. Marlink RG, Allan JS, McLane MF, et al: Low sensitivity of ELISA testing in early HIV infections. N Engl J Med 1986;315:1549.

284. Gaines H, von Sydow M, Sonnerborg A, et al: Antibody response in primary human immunodeficiency virus infection. Lancet 1987;1:1249.

285. Allain JP, Laurean Y, Paul DA, et al: Long term evaluation of HIV antigen and antibodies to p 24 and gp 41 in patients with hemophilia. N Engl J Med 1987;317:1114.

286. Laurean Y, Peynet J, Verroust F: HIV infection in sexual partners of HIV seropositive patients with hemophilia. N Engl J Med 1989;320:183.

287. Busch MP: Will human immunodeficiency virus p24 antigen screening increase the safety of the blood supply and, if so, at what cost? Transfusion 1995;35:536.

288. Ward JW, Bush TJ, Perkins HA, et al: The natural history of transfusion-associated infection with human immunodeficiency virus. N Engl J Med 1989;321:947.

289. Donegan E, Stuart M, Niland JC et al: Infection with human immunodeficiency virus type I (HIV-1) among recipients of antibody positive blood donations. Ann Intern Med 1990;113:733.

290. Anderson KC, Gorgone BA, Marlink R, et al: Transfusion acquired human immunodeficiency virus infection among immunocompromised hosts. Ann Intern Med 1986;105:519.

291. Blattner WA: Human T-lymphotrophic viruses and diseases of long latency. Ann Intern Med 1989;111:4.

292. Blayney DW, Blattner WA, Robert-Goroff M, Jaffe ES: The human T cell leukemia-lymphoma virus in the Southeastern United States. JAMA 1983;250:1048.

293. Robert-Guroff M, Weiss SH, Giron JA, et al: Prevalence of antibodies to HTLV-I, II, and III in intravenous drug abusers from AIDS endemic region. JAMA 1986;255:3133.

Problems Common to Cancer and Its Therapy

294. Minamoto GY, Gold JWM, Scheinberg DA, et al: Infection with human T-cell leukemia virus type I in patients with leukemia. N Engl J Med 1988;318:219.

295. Kamihira S, Nakasima S, Oyakawa Y, et al: Transmission of human T-cell lymphotrophic virus type 1 by blood transfusion before and after mass screening of sera from seropositive donors. Vox Sang 1987;52:43.

296. Williams AE, Fang CT, Slamon DJ, et al: Seroprevalence and epidemiological characteristics of HTLV-1 infection in U.S. blood donors. Science 1989;240:643–646.

297. Cohen ND, Munoz A, Reitz BA, et al: Transmission of retroviruses by transfusion of screened blood in patients undergoing cardiac surgery. N Engl J Med 1989;320:1171.

298. Gout O, Baulac C, Gessain A, et al: Rapid development of myelopathy after HTLV-1 infection acquired by transfusion during cardiac transplantation. N Engl J Med 1990;322:383.

299. Ehrlich GD, Glaser JB, LaVigne K, et al: Prevalence of human T-cell leukemia/lymphoma virus (HTLV) type II infection among high risk individuals: Type specific identification of HTLVs by polymerase chain reaction. Blood 1989;74:1658.

300. AABB Technical Bulletin. Bethesda, MD, American Association of Blood Banks, 1990, pp 90–96.

301. Surveillance of HIV-2 infection in blood donors—United States, 1987–1989. Recomm Rep 1990;39:829.

302. Shih JWK, Lee HH, Falchek M, et al: Transfusion-transmitted HTLV-I/II infection in patients undergoing open heart surgery. Blood 1990;75:546.

303. Donegan E, Busch MP, Galleshaw JA, et al: Transfusion of blood components from a donor with human T-lymphotropic virus type II (HTLV-II) infection. Ann Intern Med 1990;113:555.

304. Hjelle B, Mills R, Mertz G, Swenson S: Transmission of HTLV-II via blood transfusion. Vox Sang 1990;59:119.

305. Grant JH, Gold JWM, Wittner M, et al: Transfusion-associated acute Chagas disease acquired in the United States. Ann Intern Med 1989;111:849.

306. Whylie BR: Transfusion transmitted infection: Viral and exotic diseases. Anaesth Intens Care 1993;21:24.

307. Bortin MM, Rimm AA: Increasing utilization of bone marrow transplantation. Transplantation 1986;42:229.

308. Champlin R, Khouri I, Anderlini P, et al: Nonmyeloablative preparative regimens for allogeneic hematopoietic trans-plantation. Biology and current indications. Oncology (Huntingt) 2003;17:94–100.

309. Georges GE, Storb R: Review of "minitransplantation": Nonmyeloablative allogeneic hematopoietic stem cell transplantation. Int J Hematol 2003;77:3–14.

310. Beatty PG, Clift RA, Mickelson EM, et al: Marrow transplantation from related donors other than HLA-identical siblings. N Engl J Med 1985;313:765.

311. McGlave P, Scott E, Ramsey N, et al: Unrelated donor bone marrow transplantation therapy for patients with chronic myelogenous leukemia. Blood 1987;70:877.

312. Kernan NA, Bartsch G, Ash RC, et al: Analysis of 462 transplantations from unrelated donors facilitated by the National Marrow Donor Program. N Engl J Med 1993;328:593.

313. Armitage JO, Gale RP: Bone marrow transplantation in man: Report of an international cooperative study. Lancet 1 986;2:960.

314. Attal M, Harousseau JL, Stoppa AM, et al: A prospective, randomized trial of autologous bone marrow transplantation and chemotherapy in multiple myeloma. Intergroupe Francais du Myelome. N Engl J Med 1996;335:91–97.

315. Tallman MS, Gray R, Robert NJ, et al: Conventional adjuvant chemotherapy with or without high-dose chemotherapy and autologous stem-cell transplantation in high-risk breast cancer. N Engl J Med 2003;349:17–26.

316. Rodenhuis S, Bontenbal M, Beex LV, et al: High-dose chemotherapy with hematopoietic stem-cell rescue for high-risk breast cancer. N Engl J Med 2003;349:7–16.

317. Elfenbein GJ: Stem-cell transplantation for high-risk breast cancer. N Engl J Med 2003;349:80–82.

318. Storb R, Weiden PL: Transfusion problems associated with transplantation. Semin Hematol 1981;18:163.

319. Storb R, Prentice RL, Thomas ED: Marrow transplantation for treatment of aplastic anemia: An analysis of factors associated with graft rejection. N Engl J Med 1977;296:61.

320. Klingemann HG, Self S, Banaji M, et al: Refractoriness to random donor platelet transfusions in patients with aplastic anemia: A multivariate analysis of data from 264 cases. Br J Haematol 1987;66:115.

321. Wulff JC, Santner TJ, Storb R, et al: Transfusion requirements after HLA identical marrow transplantation in 82 patients with aplastic anemia. Vox Sang 1983;44:366.

322. Anderson KC: The role of the blood bank in hematopoietic stem cell transplantation. Transfusion 1992;32:272.

323. Anderson KC, Dzik W: Blood bank support in bone marrow and organ transplantation. In Benz EJ, Cohen HJ, Furie B, et al (eds): Hematology: Basic Principles and Practice. New York, Churchill Livingstone, 1991, p 1670.

324. Petz LD: Immunohematologic problems associated with bone marrow transplantation. Transfus Med Rev 1987;1:85.

325. Marmont AM, Domasio EE, Bacigalupo A, et al: A to O bone marrow transplantation in severe aplastic anemia: Dynamics of blood group conversion of early dyserythropoiesis in the engrafted marrow. Br J Haematol 1978;36:511.

326. Braine HG, Sensenbrenner LL, Wright SK, et al: Bone marrow transplantation with major ABO blood group incompatibility using erythrocyte depletion of marrow prior to infusion. Blood 1982;60:420.

327. Hows J, Beddow K, Gordon-Smith E: Donor-derived red blood cell antibodies and immune hemolysis after allogeneic bone marrow transplantation. Blood 1986;67:177.

328. Hazelhurst GR, Brenner MK, Wimperis JZ: Hemolysis after T-cell depleted bone marrow transplantation. Scand J Haematol 1986;37:1.

329. Brandt SJ, Peters WP, Atwater SK, et al: Effect of recombinant human granulocyte-macrophage colony-stimulating factor on hematopoietic reconstitution after high-dose chemotherapy and autologous bone marrow transplantation. N Engl J Med 1988;318:869.

330. Goldman JR, Catovsky D, Galton DAG: Reversal of blast cell crisis in CGL by transfusion of stored autologous buffy-coat cells. Lancet 1978;1:437.

331. Kessinger A, Armitage JO, Landmark JD, et al: Autologous peripheral hematopoietic stem cell transplantation restores hematopoietic function following marrow ablative therapy. Blood 1988;71:723.

332. Kessinger A, Armitage A, Landmark J, Weisenburger D: Reconstitution of human hematopoietic function with autologous cryopreserved circulating stem cells. Exp Hematol 1986;14:192.

333. Kessinger A, Armitage JO: The evolving role of autologous peripheral stem cell transplantation following high-dose therapy for malignancies. Blood 1991;77:211.

334. Gianni AM, Bregni M, Siena S, et al: Rapid and complete hematopoietic reconstitution following combined transplantation of autologous blood and bone marrow cells: A changing role for high dose chemoradiotherapy [abstract]. Hematol Oncol 1989;7:139.

335. Gianni AM, Siena S, Bregni M, et al: Granulocyte-macrophage colony-stimulating factor to harvest circulating haemopoietic stem cells for autotransplantation. Lancet 1989;2:580.

336. Douer D, Chaiwun B, Glaspy J, et al: Analysis of peripheral blood progenitor cell (PBPC) harvests for occult breast cancer micrometastases using a sensitive immunohistochemical method. Proc Am Soc Clin Oncol 1993;12:62.

337. Richman CM, Weiner RS, Yankee RA: Increase in circulating stem cells following chemotherapy in man. Blood 1976;47:1031.

338. To LB, Haylock DN, Kimber RJ, Juttner CA: High levels of circulating hematopoietic stem cells in very early remission from acute nonlymphocytic leukaemia and their collection and cryopreservation. Br J Haematol 1984;58:399.

339. Socinski MA, Cannistra SA, Elias A, et al: Granulocyte-macrophage colony-stimulating factor expands the circulating haemopoietic progenitor cell compartment in man. Lancet 1988;1:1194.

340. Duhrsen U, Villeval JL, Boyd J: Effects of recombinant human

granulocyte colony-stimulating factor of hematopoietic progenitor cells in cancer patients. Blood 1988;72:2074.

341. Herrmann F, Brugger W, Kanz L, Mertelsmann R: In vivo biology and therapeutic potential of hematopoietic growth factors and circulating progenitor cells. Semin Oncol 1992;19:422.

342. Sheridan WP, Begley CG, Juttner CA, et al: Effect of peripheral-blood progenitor cells mobilised by filgrastim (G-CSF) on platelet recovery after high-dose chemotherapy. Lancet 1992;339:640.

343. Mazanet R, Elias A, Hunt M, et al: Peripheral blood progenitor cells (PBPC)s added to bone marrow (BM) for hemopoietic rescue following high dose chemotherapy for solid tumors reduces morbidity and length of hospitalization [abstract]. Proc Am Soc Clin Oncol 1991;10:1140.

344. Elias AD, Ayash L, Anderson KC, et al: Mobilization of peripheral blood progenitor cells by chemotherapy and granulocyte-macrophage colony-stimulating factor for hematologic support after high-dose intensification for breast cancer. Blood 1992;79:3036.

345. Menitove JE: Standards for Hematopoietic Progenitor Cells. Bethesda, MD, American Association of Blood Banks Press, 1996.

346. Standards for hematopoietic progenitor cell collection, processing, and transplantation. Omaha, Neb, Foundation for the Accreditation of Hematopoietic Cell Therapy, 1996.

347. US Food and Drug Administration: Available at www.fda.gov/cber/tissue/rego.htm.

Problems Common to Cancer and Its Therapy

II

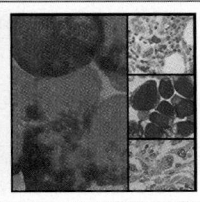

45

DIAGNOSIS, TREATMENT, AND PREVENTION OF CANCER-RELATED VENOUS THROMBOSIS

Steven R. Deitcher
Marcelo P. V. Gomes
William D. Haire

SUMMARY OF KEY POINTS

INTRODUCTION

EPIDEMIOLOGY OF CANCER-ASSOCIATED VENOUS THROMBOEMBOLISM

- Venous thrombosis has an incidence of approximately 15% in cancer patients.
- Venous thrombosis has been identified in up to 50% of cancer patients at autopsy.

NATURAL HISTORY OF CANCER-RELATED VENOUS THROMBOEMBOLISM

- Cancer patients with venous thrombosis at diagnosis have a worse prognosis.
- Cancer patients are more likely to have large, proximal, persistent, and recurrent venous thromboses.
- Venous thrombosis can complicate the management of any and all types of cancer.

CANCER-ASSOCIATED HYPERCOAGULABILITY

- Malignant tumors can cause venous stasis, vascular injury, procoagulant accumulation, natural anticoagulant deficiency, and impaired endogenous fibrinolysis.
- Plasma markers of coagulation activation do not predict development of thrombosis but may assist in prognosis determination.

CHALLENGES OF VENOUS THROMBOEMBOLISM DIAGNOSIS IN CANCER PATIENTS

- Cancer-associated venous thrombosis is likely underdiagnosed because of inadequate physician suspicion, underutilization of proper objective tests, and the asymptomatic nature of many thrombotic events.
- Clinical diagnosis alone lacks sensitivity and specificity for acute venous thrombosis.
- Diagnostic imaging studies like duplex ultrasound and lung

scintigraphy may provide more false-positive and false-negative results in cancer patients.

CHALLENGES OF VENOUS THROMBOEMBOLISM TREATMENT IN CANCER PATIENTS

- Cancer patients may not respond to nor benefit from standard approaches to venous thrombosis management as do patients without cancer.
- Tendencies toward thrombocytopenia, osteopenia, malnutrition, brain metastasis, hepatic metastasis, and bleeding all complicate thrombosis care in cancer patients.
- Cancer patients are more likely to manifest heparin resistance and warfarin failure and to have limited venous access to support therapeutic anticoagulant monitoring.

CANCER PATIENT RESPONSE TO LOW-MOLECULAR-WEIGHT HEPARINS

- Low-molecular-weight heparins are safe and effective for the short- and long-term management of venous thrombosis in cancer patients.
- Low-molecular-weight heparins are associated with lower recurrent thrombosis rates than is oral warfarin during up to 6 months of anticoagulation therapy.
- Low-molecular-weight heparins may affect survival in subgroups of cancer patients with and without venous thrombosis.

LOWER-EXTREMITY DEEP VENOUS THROMBOSIS MANAGEMENT

- Diagnosis should be sought by using duplex ultrasound with magnetic resonance venography, computed tomography, and venography reserved for confirmation.
- D-dimer testing is likely less sensitive and less specific in cancer patients.

- Low-molecular-weight heparins are likely to be the best drugs to minimize recurrence rates without significantly increasing bleeding complication rates.
- It is prudent to continue anticoagulation for a minimum of 6 months and until all cytotoxic therapy has been completed and no evidence of active cancer is found.

UPPER-EXTREMITY DEEP VENOUS THROMBOSIS MANAGEMENT

- Duplex ultrasound and venography are the mainstay of upper extremity thrombosis diagnosis.
- Upper extremity thrombosis should be treated like lower extremity thrombosis, with the exception of catheter-related thrombosis, which may require catheter removal.

PULMONARY EMBOLISM MANAGEMENT

- Helical computed tomography (CT) and lung scintigraphy are both means of objectively diagnosing pulmonary embolism. Helical CT is preferred when the chest radiograph is not normal.
- Pulmonary embolism should be treated in a similar fashion and based on the same principles as lower extremity deep venous thrombosis.
- The risks of thrombolysis should be reserved for patients with hemodynamically unstable pulmonary embolism.

INFERIOR VENA CAVA AND INTRA-ABDOMINAL DEEP VENOUS THROMBOSIS MANAGEMENT

- Magnetic resonance and contrast venography are the preferred methods for diagnosis.
- Incidental findings of intra-abdominal vein thrombosis on standard CT scans should be confirmed by a more approriate diagnostic method.

891

SUMMARY OF KEY POINTS, continued

- Treatment should be the same as for lower extremity deep venous thrombosis.

SUPERFICIAL THROMBOPHLEBITIS MANAGEMENT

- Superficial venous thrombosis may herald the diagnosis of cancer and should be treated with local measures such as warm compresses and analgesics.
- Patients with superficial thrombophlebitis may harbor asymptomatic deep venous thrombosis, so screening duplex ultrasound is recommended.

INFERIOR VENA CAVA FILTERS

- Inferior vena cava filters should be reserved for patients with acute lower extremity or pelvic thrombosis who have a contraindication to anticoagulation or documented anticoagulation failure.
- Inferior vena cava filters may reduce the incidence of all pulmonary embolism in the short run after diagnosis of a deep vein thrombosis, but also increase the risk of recurrent deep vein thrombosis in the long run.

VENOUS THROMBOSIS PREVENTION IN THE CANCER PATIENT

- Greater attention to prevention would reduce our need to provide thrombosis treatment to this challenging population of at-risk patients.
- Pharmacologic prophylaxis is safe and effective in a wide range of surgical and medical oncology patients and settings.

FUTURE PROSPECTS

INTRODUCTION

Venous thromboembolic disease (VTE), including deep venous thrombosis (DVT) and pulmonary embolism (PE), is a common but often underdiagnosed and under-appreciated clinical problem in oncology that results in significant patient morbidity and mortality. Timely and accurate diagnosis of VTE is imperative because of the unacceptable outcomes associated with a misdiagnosis. VTE diagnosis based on clinical grounds alone is un-reliable, so physicians should select an appropriate objective diagnostic test to confirm or refute their clinical suspicions. Compression duplex ultrasound remains the first-line imaging test for both suspected upper and lower extremity DVT. Magnetic resonance venography (MRV) is a valid alternative when ultrasound is inconclusive. Helical (spiral) computed tomography (CT) and ventilation-perfusion (V/Q) lung scintigraphy remain the first-line imaging modalities for suspected acute PE. Spiral CT is preferred in cases of obvious pulmonary or pleural-based disease. Indeterminate initial studies should prompt performance of additional tests, possibly including the "gold standard," contrast venography and pulmonary angiography. Evidence to date suggests that D-dimer assays may be unreliable in excluding VTE in cancer patients.

Standard VTE treatment practices including the use of intravenous unfractionated heparin (UFH) for initial anticoagulation, oral warfarin for chronic anticoagulation, and the prescription of only 3 to 6 months of total therapy may not be optimal in the setting of active cancer and ongoing anticancer therapy. Challenges of VTE management in cancer patients include heparin resistance due to excess circulating acute-phase proteins, increased recurrence rates during and after standard-intensity warfarin therapy, limited venous access to support therapeutic monitoring, and anticoagulation intensity–independent increased bleeding rates during anticoagulation. Bleeding during anticoagulation is of particular concern in patients with disease- or chemotherapy-related thrombocytopenia, central nervous system (CNS) involvement with cancer, and recent invasive procedures. Low-molecular-weight heparins (LMWHs) have been shown to be at least as effective and safe for initial anticoagulation compared with UFH in persons with acute VTE and have gained popularity in the setting of VTE in cancer. LMWHs have the advantage of less nonspecific protein binding, subcutaneous weight-based dosing without the need for monitoring in most cases, and probably less heparin-induced thrombocytopenia. Recent trials demonstrated efficacy superiority of select LMWHs in place of oral warfarin for long-term anticoagulation in the cancer patient.

The challenges of proper VTE diagnosis and treatment in the cancer patient are best averted by expanded use of VTE-prevention modalities. Trials have shown that medically ill patients have a high risk of VTE similar to that of high-risk surgical patients. LMWHs have emerged as the premier pharmacologic agents for VTE prevention. Extended prophylaxis beyond acute-care hospitalization has a role in minimizing the total risk of VTE development. Newer agents may improve the efficacy, safety, and convenience of LMWH-based prophylaxis.

This chapter addresses the diagnosis, treatment, and prevention of VTE specifically in the cancer patient population. The potential for anticoagulant therapy to enhance cancer patient survival and the role of anti-coagulants-in-development to affect cancer patient care also are addressed.

EPIDEMIOLOGY OF CANCER-ASSOCIATED VENOUS THROMBOEMBOLISM

The incidence of clinically apparent (i.e., symptomatic) VTE in cancer patients has been reported to be approximately 15%, with reported incidence rates ranging from 3.8% to 30.7%.[1,2] This is in comparison to an age-adjusted VTE incidence of 2.5% in the general population.[3] The wide range of reported incidence rates likely reflects differences in patient tumor histology, investigator level of VTE clinical suspicion, and VTE confirmation methods. Nonetheless, studies have uniformly demonstrated a higher incidence of VTE in patients with cancer of a specific organ compared with those with benign diseases of the same organ. In a Scandinavian retrospective study of more than 63,000 patients hospitalized for acute VTE, 18% had been diagnosed with cancer before the VTE.[4] A large Medicare registration study revealed that cancer patients were diagnosed with VTE at the time of initial hospitalization at a higher rate than were patients admitted for nonmalignant disorders.[5]

The risk of postoperative DVT in cancer patients after general surgery is as high as 36% and exceeds that of noncancer surgical patients by 1.5- to 3.6-fold.[6-8] VTE detection rates as high as 50% in autopsy series have been reported but may still not represent the true magnitude of VTE-related illness in cancer.[9] Limiting factors in the proper antemortem detection of VTE in cancer patients include an inadequate index of suspicion by many clinicians and idiosyncrasies of VTE diagnostic modalities, as described later.[10] The former is exacerbated by the fact that VTE is often asymptomatic, and even when symptoms are present, they are often nonspecific or mistakenly attributed to the underlying malignancy itself.

NATURAL HISTORY OF CANCER-RELATED VENOUS THROMBOEMBOLISM

Thrombosis may be a presenting feature of occult malignancy, a life-threatening component of early or advanced cancer, and a complication of anticancer therapy itself. Patients with cancer diagnosed at the time of acute VTE detection have a greater likelihood of distant metastases at the time of diagnosis compared with individuals without concomitant VTE [44% vs. 35.1%; prevalence ratio, 1.26; 95% confidence interval (CI), 1.13–1.40] and significantly lower 1-year survival rates (12% vs. 36%; $P < .001$).[4] VTE presentations in the cancer patient include symptomatic DVT, PE, superficial thrombophlebitis, central venous access device–associated thrombosis, arterial thrombosis, and nonbacterial thrombotic endocarditis. Asymptomatic VTE, although often viewed as clinically insignificant, can evolve into symptomatic VTE, and both may be particularly deleterious in the cancer patient by promoting vascular endothelial growth factor (VEGF) expression.[11] VTE is likely to be a common proximate cause of death in patients with solid tumors.

The natural history of VTE in the cancer patient differs significantly from that in the noncancer patient. Cancer patients are more likely than noncancer patients to present with proximal DVT.[12] Cancer patients have been shown to present with a greater initial thrombus burden, to experience greater clinical deterioration despite anticoagulant therapy, and to have less venographic improvement in response to standard treatment when compared with noncancer patients.[12]

The perception by many physicians has been that cancer patients have a greater propensity toward recurrent VTE, both during and after completion of a course of antithrombotic therapy.[13] Recent studies have substantiated the high risk of recurrence. A population-based retrospective study of 404 individuals showed that persons with cancer have a twofold to threefold increased risk of recurrent VTE.[14] Antineoplastic therapy further accentuated the risk of recurrence in the cancer patient population. The 5-year cumulative incidence of recurrent VTE was 21.5% in a prospective cohort study of 738 consecutive patients with a first or second DVT.[15] The relative risk of recurrence was 1.97 in patients with cancer. Another prospective study reported an overall VTE recurrence rate of 10.3% in 58 patients with cancer compared with 4.7% in 297 patients without cancer.[16,17] The fact that cancer patients had a higher recurrence rate while reportedly "therapeutically" given anticoagulated suggests that the usual target international normalized ratio (INR) range of 2.0 to 3.0 may not be therapeutic at all. Prandoni and colleagues[18] recently reported a 20.7% (95% CI, 15.6–25.8) 12-month incidence of recurrent VTE in cancer patients with VTE compared with a 6.8% (95% CI, 3.9–9.7) 12-month incidence of recurrence in noncancer patients with VTE. The greatest risk of recurrent VTE was observed in patients with genitourinary tract, gastrointestinal tract, and lung cancers, and predominantly during the first month of anticoagulation.[18] Bona and associates[19,20] provided a contradictory point of view by reporting similar VTE recurrence rates of 0.013 events per patient-month of treatment in 104 cancer patients compared with 0.002 events per patient-month in 208 noncancer patients.

A recent analysis of malignancy status–specific and INR range–specific VTE recurrence rates revealed that patients with VTE and malignancy ($n = 261$) have an overall thromboembolism recurrence rate of 27.1 events per 100 patient years compared with 9 recurrent events per 100 patient years in individuals with VTE and no malignancy.[21] In both patient populations, the rate of VTE recurrence was greatest during periods when the INR was 2.0 or less (the lower boundary of the target INR range). Patients without cancer had 15.9 recurrent events per 100 patient years during such periods of suboptimal warfarin anticoagulation, whereas patients with underlying malignancy had a VTE recurrence rate of 54 events per 100 patient years during similar periods of inadequate anticoagulation. Thus it can be surmised that cancer patients are exquisitely sensitive to periods during which the INR is less than a target level of 2.0 to 3.0.

Venous thrombosis has been traditionally associated with aerodigestive tract adenocarcinomas involving the pancreas, stomach, and lungs. A closer look at DVT and PE incidence rates for different tumor histologic types, though, reveals that ovarian carcinoma, primary brain tumors, and lymphomas are among the four tumor types with the highest VTE rates.[5] This is of particular interest, considering that hematologic malignancies such as lymphoma have traditionally been viewed as coagulation-inert histologic types, and management of malignancy-associated VTE has traditionally been viewed as the sole domain of the solid tumor medical oncologist. Thrombosis can affect the clinical course of all histologic types, of all stages, of all grades, and during any and all treatments.

CANCER-ASSOCIATED HYPERCOAGULABILITY

Different tumors, of different extent, in different patients, with different comorbidities, and different inherited hypercoagulable states, likely promote the development of VTE by different combinations of tumor-associated and non–tumor-associated procoagulant mechanisms (Table 45-1). Solid tumor–mediated extrinsic vascular compression and invasion can obstruct venous return, resulting in blood flow stasis, endothelial cell injury, and coagulation activation.[1,22,23] Tumor cells can directly promote thrombin generation by producing tissue factor, expressing the coagulation factor X activator known as cancer procoagulant, and by displaying surface sialic acid residues that can support nonenzymatic factor X activation.[24-27] Tumor cells also can indirectly promote thrombin generation by eliciting tissue factor expression by monocytes and endothelial cells.[25] Selected tumors may mediate an accentuation of platelet activation and accumulation, whereas other tumor cells may express surface phospholipid species such as phosphatidyl serine, which can support prothrombin and factor X activation.[25]

Malignancy-associated inflammation can result in increased concentrations of acute-phase proteins such as factor VIII, fibrinogen, and von Willebrand factor.[28] Whether in the setting of active malignancy or in otherwise normal patients, elevations of these acute-phase proteins are associated with an increased risk of thrombosis.[29] Tumor-associated increases in plasminogen activator inhibitor-1 (PAI-1) can result in impaired endogenous fibrinolysis.[30] Malignancy-associated acquired deficiencies of natural anticoagulant proteins like protein S have been described.[31] Fareed and coworkers[32] performed baseline profiling of cancer patients with acute VTE and found elevated levels of factor VIII, von Willebrand factor, PAI-1, and the dilute Russell viper venom time (a specific lupus anticoagulant assay) in 35%, 97%, 42%, and 65% of patients, respectively. Deficiency of protein C, protein S, and antithrombin were found in 33%, 57%, and 8% of patients, respectively.[32] This study underscored the multifactorial pathogenesis of cancer-associated thrombosis. The variation between different cancer patients with regard to their hypercoagulable tendencies makes specific prognostic testing for cancer-associated thrombosis challenging and of limited clinical usefulness.

Although coagulation-marker testing may fall short of being able to predict which cancer patients are most apt to develop VTE, such testing may assist in prognosis determination. Beer and colleagues[33] performed a prospective evaluation of the predictive value of coagulation-activation markers for survival in cancer patients. They quantified thrombin-antithrombin complex (TAT), prothrombin fragment 1+2 (F1+2), D-dimer, fibrin monomer, and fibrinopeptide A (FPA). In general, patients with active malignancy, those with active adenocarcinoma, those with extensive disease, and those who died during follow-up (mean, 17 months) had significantly higher marker levels. A comparison of first and fourth quartiles in active cancer patients revealed significant odds ratios of death for fibrin monomer, TAT, D-dimer, F1+2, and FPA of 4.1, 2.8, 2.7, 2.4, and 2.4, respectively.[33]

Non–tumor-derived VTE risk factors in the cancer patient include central venous catheters and antineoplastic agents themselves. Central venous catheters are the major risk factor for upper extremity DVTs in the cancer patient population and can precipitate superior vena cava (SVC) thrombosis and SVC syndrome.[34-39] These DVTs may result in PE, cause catheter dysfunction, and serve as a nidus for catheter-related infection.[40] Antineoplastic agents themselves, including cytotoxic chemotherapy, selective estrogen-receptor modulators, antiangiogenic agents, and especially combinations of these drugs, are associated with an increased risk of VTE.[23,41-45] Thalidomide, an immunomodulating and antiangiogenic agent, has been linked to VTE in patients with multiple myeloma, especially when combined with anthracycline antineoplastic drugs.[46,47] Theorized mechanisms of antineoplastic agent-induced hypercoagulability are varied and not completely elucidated. Medical complications of cancer and its therapy (including congestive heart failure, major infection, pathologic fractures, extended immobility, and preexistent VTE) can exacerbate the tendency to venous thrombosis. Common inherited risk factors for VTE such as factor V Leiden and prothrombin G20210A have not been found to be more prevalent in cancer patients with thrombosis than in the general population.[48]

TABLE 45-1

 Venous Thromboembolic Event Risk Factors in Cancer Patients

Tumor-Associated Procoagulant Mechanisms in the Cancer Patient

Extrinsic vascular compression and invasion
Tissue factor production
Cancer procoagulant production
Sialic acid residue support of nonenzymatic factor X activation
Promotion of tissue factor production by monocytes and endothelial cells
Accentuated platelet activation and accumulation
Expression of phosphatidyl serine, which supports prothrombinase and tenase activity
Inflammation-mediated increases in factor VIII, fibrinogen, and von Willebrand factor
Impaired endogenous fibrinolysis due to excess levels of plasminogen activator-inhibitor 1
Acquired deficiencies of natural anticoagulants

Nontumor-Associated Procoagulant Mechanisms in the Cancer Patient

Central venous access devices
Antineoplastic agent–induced platelet activation and endothelial cell damage
Anthracycline-induced congestive heart failure
Immobility

CHALLENGES OF VENOUS THROMBOEMBOLISM DIAGNOSIS IN CANCER PATIENTS

Selection of the most appropriate and effective treatment for a patient's cancer is dependent on a timely and accurate assessment of tumor histology, disease stage, and patient performance status. In similar fashion, prescription of the most appropriate and effective treatment for a cancer patient's disease- or treatment-associated VTE is dependent on a timely and accurate diagnosis. Failure to surpass a minimum threshold of anticoagulant intensity [activated partial thromboplastin time (aPTT) >1.5 times control for intravenous UFH] within 24 hours of acute DVT diagnosis is associated with a markedly increased risk of late thrombosis recurrence.[49] It thus makes sense that patients with acute DVT in whom a proper diagnosis is significantly delayed should have similar suboptimal outcomes. Classification of venous thromboses as superficial versus deep and distal versus proximal, differentiation between acute and remote thrombotic events, and distinction between a venous filling defect and extrinsic vessel compression are required to ensure that patients are appropriately treated.

It has long been recognized that the diagnosis of DVT and PE made on clinical grounds alone is notoriously unreliable.[50,51] The severity of limb edema and pain is often unrelated to the location and extent of DVT, whereas the symptoms of PE vary depending on the degree and extent of vessel occlusion, as well as on a patient's cardiopulmonary reserve. The classically described Homans' sign (calf discomfort triggered by passive dorsiflexion of the foot) has been found in only 8% to 60% of symptomatic patients with confirmed DVT, and in up to 40% of symptomatic individuals without DVT.[52-55] Half of the patients with clinically suspected DVT do not have the diagnosis confirmed by objective testing.[50-53] Data from the Prospective Investigation of PE Diagnosis (PIOPED) Study revealed that dyspnea, pleuritic chest pain, cough, and lower extremity edema, among other symptoms, were present in similar frequencies (30% to 70%) among patients with or without angiographically confirmed PE.[56] In cancer patients, the clinical diagnosis of DVT or PE is unlikely to be more accurate and may be even less accurate.

VTE is often asymptomatic or minimally symptomatic, and, even when symptoms are present, they are nonspecific and can be easily attributable to the underlying malignancy. Surveys have shown that constitutional symptoms such as weakness and fatigue occur in 50% to 70% of patients in hospice or palliative care,[57,58] whereas dyspnea and cough occur in 25% to 50% of such patients and in more than 40% of patients with advanced cancer, respectively.[58-62] The incidence of upper extremity (UE) edema due to lymphedema in women after axillary lymph node dissection and/or radiotherapy for breast cancer has been reported to range from 6% to 30%.[63] In a series of more than 2000 palliative care patients with different types of pain syndromes, 22% and 11% had lower extremity (LE) and UE pain, respectively.[64] None of these

symptoms is unique to a particular disorder, and the etiology may be related to the underlying malignancy itself, a venous thrombotic complication, or both. Likewise, worsening dyspnea in a patient with primary or metastatic lung cancer; limb edema in a patient with bulky pelvic, axillary, or mediastinal tumor or adenopathy; and abdominal pain after colectomy or abdominal hysterectomy in patients with colon cancer or uterine cancer are a few examples in which VTE may mimic, be confused with, or be coexistent with the underlying disease. Therefore awareness that VTE is a common complication of cancer and possession of a high index of suspicion are necessary to avoid missing a diagnosis of DVT or PE.

Compared with noncancer patients, those with cancer have a greater risk of bleeding while receiving oral anticoagulant therapy and a threefold to sixfold higher rate of recurrent VTE.[18,21] Therefore the diagnosis of DVT and PE should not be made on clinical grounds alone, and objective diagnostic confirmation is mandatory. Failure to make a timely diagnosis of VTE may result in significant morbidity and mortality because of recurrent VTE, whereas empirical anticoagulation therapy without a confirmed diagnosis may expose the cancer patient to unnecessary and potentially avoidable risk in the absence of any tangible benefit. With the exception of cases of superficial thrombophlebitis, any signs and symptoms suggestive of VTE should be used not as diagnostic endpoints, but simply as a compelling reason to pursue further testing.

Although the methods used to confirm the diagnosis of DVT or PE in noncancer and cancer patients are the same, particular features of the underlying malignant disease may, in some circumstances, reduce the accuracy of those diagnostic methods. The presence of direct tumor invasion of blood vessels or extrinsic venous compression by a bulky tumor or adenopathy, as well as rare primary vascular tumors, may all lead to false-positive diagnoses of DVT. Likewise, primary pulmonary artery tumors and compression of a pulmonary artery or vein by tumor or adenopathy may result in impaired regional pulmonary perfusion. This may be interpreted as "high probability" or "indeterminate" for PE on V/Q lung scanning (V/Q scan), or lead to interpretative pitfalls on helical (spiral) CT. Prior radiation therapy to the chest wall also may lead to false-positive perfusion defects on V/Q scan, whereas fluctuating platelet counts may impair the ability of nuclear scintigraphy methods to detect LE-DVT. Moreover, increased baseline D-dimer levels in some cancer patients and impaired endogenous fibrinolysis in others may at least in part explain the limitation of D-dimer assays in excluding VTE in this population. Thus an understanding of the limitations inherent to the various diagnostic modalities and of the circumstances in which these modalities may result in false-positive and false-negative diagnosis are of the utmost importance. Because the cancer population may be subject to a higher rate of nondiagnostic, false-positive, and false-negative noninvasive tests than patients without cancer, it is possible that many cancer patients will require more than one diagnostic test to prove or rule out conclusively a diagnosis of DVT or PE.

Historically, the diagnostic approach to DVT and PE has shifted from purely clinical (insensitive and nonspecific) and angiography based (invasive) to being dependent primarily on noninvasive or minimally invasive imaging techniques. These newer methods are less accurate to detect calf, pelvic, and intra-abdominal DVT, as well as PE in the subsegmental branches of the pulmonary artery. As a consequence, a number of clinical management models have been reported and validated.[65-68] These models combine clinical assessment (pretest probability of DVT or PE) with noninvasive imaging tests and D-dimer assays, with the goal of reducing the need for repeated or invasive confirmatory tests but without compromising patient safety. The majority of patients included in these studies had a low-to-moderate pretest VTE risk, and the combination of a low pretest risk with a negative imaging test and a negative D-dimer has been shown to exclude DVT or PE safely.[65-68] However, in these studies, patients with high pretest clinical probability of VTE and a negative or indeterminate initial test result almost invariably went on to undergo additional testing, including invasive studies.

Given the high incidence of VTE and the impact of such a diagnosis on cancer patients, it is our opinion that all patients with active cancer should be considered as having a "high pretest probability" or "high clinical suspicion" in models that rely on pretest clinical assessment. In addition, management models that include currently available D-dimer assays as part of the risk assessment should not be used to aid in the diagnosis of VTE in the cancer population for reasons discussed later in this chapter.

CHALLENGES OF VENOUS THROMBOEMBOLISM TREATMENT IN CANCER PATIENTS

DVT and PE warrant prompt institution of antithrombotic therapy to prevent thrombus propagation, embolization, and recurrence effectively; to ameliorate patient symptoms; and to allow thrombus organization, plasmin-mediated lysis, and restoration of venous patency.[69] Specific therapy and duration of therapy in the cancer patient depend on thrombus location (i.e., iliofemoral DVT vs. calf DVT), thrombus extent (i.e., massive PE vs. subsegmental PE), underlying thrombosis "trigger" (i.e., major abdominal surgery vs. thalidomide-based therapy for multiple myeloma), and patient comorbidities (e.g., self-limited thrombocytopenia and hemorrhagic brain metastases). Despite the special attention afforded the cancer patient with regard to other disease-related complications such as hypercalcemia, nausea, fatigue, and pain, the recommended and most commonly used treatment of VTE in patients with active cancer is not significantly different from the regimens prescribed to VTE patients without malignancy.[70] Ideally, unique features of individual cancer patients, the natural history of VTE in cancer patients, and cancer patient response to various anticoagulant agents should be noted and should affect our approach to VTE treatment in this group.

Heparin Resistance

Cancer patients, like others with acute illness and inflammatory processes, have a propensity toward heparin resistance. "True" heparin resistance causes inadequate anticoagulant and antithrombotic responses from what would otherwise be perceived as an adequate dose of heparin. Some have deemed a requirement of more than 35,000 units of heparin per 24-hour period, regardless of patient weight, to reflect this form of heparin resistance.[71] With true heparin resistance, both a measurement of anticoagulant activity like the aPTT and a measurement of antithrombotic activity like the anti–factor Xa activity assay demonstrate inadequate degrees of heparin activity. True heparin resistance most likely results from the nonspecific binding of heparin to mononuclear white cells, vascular endothelial cells, and acute-phase protein such as histidine-rich glycoprotein, vitronectin, and platelet factor 4, resulting in an inadequate quantity of free or antithrombin-bound heparin.[72] Another potential cause of heparin resistance in the cancer patient is disseminated intravascular coagulation (DIC)-associated antithrombin deficiency.

Cancer patients can also manifest an "apparent" heparin resistance characterized by dissociation between the aPTT and heparin assays.[71] In these patients, the aPTT may be normal or near normal, while the antifactor Xa activity assay reveals a heparin activity level within the therapeutic range of 0.3 and 0.7 IU/mL. Simply escalating the dose of heparin to achieve the desired aPTT without checking a heparin assay may result in a pronounced bleeding risk. Dissociation between the aPTT and heparin concentration likely reflects elevated levels of factor VIII that can shorten the in vitro aPTT without affecting the antithrombotic actions of the drug.

Warfarin Failure

Warfarin failure is the term often used to describe the development of an objectively documented recurrent VTE, despite an apparently stable INR between 2.0 and 3.0. Such an event suggests that this degree of anticoagulation was insufficient to neutralize the sum of hypercoagulable stimuli in a given individual. Warfarin failure must be distinguished from early thrombus extension during the initial period of acute parenteral anticoagulation. Underlying cancer, because of its potent prothrombotic nature, is often suspected in the setting of warfarin failure. Patients with VTE and known cancer are at an increased risk for recurrent thrombosis compared with noncancer patients.[12,14,15,18,21,73] This may reflect cancer-associated hypercoagulability in excess of warfarin-induced anticoagulation or reflect less ability to keep cancer patients within the target INR range. Cancer patients have been shown to spend less time (43.3%) within the target INR of 2.0 to 3.0 than do control noncancer patients (56.9%) during standard warfarin anticoagulation.[19] It is likely that cancer patients spend approximately 30% of their time with an INR 2.0 or less and 30% of the time with 3.0 or more. The remaining time is probably spent "in transit" between these out-of-target extremes. As has been shown by Hutten and associates,[21] cancer patients are at a particularly high risk for recurrent VTE when the INR is 2.0 or less. An increased frequency of therapeutic monitoring does not necessarily improve outcome in cancer patients with VTE.[17,19,20]

Malnutrition

Cancer patients can experience periods of excess catabolism, anorexia, corticosteroid-induced appetite stimulation, antimicrobial therapy, parenteral nutrition, and compromised hepatic function.[74] Each can affect either vitamin K supply or metabolism, and thus vitamin K antagonist (i.e., warfarin) therapy. These often unpredictable aspects of the cancer patient may contribute to the greater degree of INR instability during oral warfarin therapy. An increasing number of cancer patients are relying on over-the-counter dietary supplements and herbal preparations to compensate for malnutrition, alleviate symptoms, and complement traditional anticancer therapy. Unfortunately, these preparations may contain vitamin K, vitamin K analogs, or compounds known to affect warfarin anticoagulation (e.g., *Ginkgo biloba*). Reliance on acetaminophen-containing narcotic and non-narcotic analgesics also can affect the toxicity of oral warfarin.[75,76]

Thrombocytopenia

Thrombocytopenia in the cancer patient can develop for a multitude of underlying reasons. Some patients have decreased platelet production secondary to myelosuppressive chemotherapy or marrow infiltration by tumor. Others have peripheral consumption of platelets due to hypersplenism associated with Hodgkin's disease and lymphoproliferative disorders or congestive splenomegaly due to thrombosis and/or portal hypertension associated with extensive hepatic metastases. Other patients experience peripheral platelet destruction due to autoimmune clearance associated with low-grade non-Hodgkin's lymphomas and chronic lymphocytic leukemia, whereas others have consumption due to DIC. Thrombocytopenia that develops during heparin administration for VTE prevention or treatment should be considered heparin-induced thrombocytopenia (HIT) until proven otherwise.[77] Detection of HIT in patients with preexistent cancer-associated thrombocytopenia can be difficult. Because cancer patients may possess antiheparin: platelet factor 4 antibodies even in the absence of clinical HIT (personal communication, Dr. Jawed Fareed), testing should be reserved for the patient with new thrombocytopenia that develops during or shortly after a heparin exposure and without another possible explanation.

The safety of administering systemic anticoagulation for any duration of time in patients with thrombocytopenia is likely dependent on the etiology and degree of thrombocytopenia, the presence or absence of concomitant platelet hypofunction, the location of primary and metastatic tumors, platelet transfusion responsiveness, and the anticipated duration of thrombocytopenia. No exact cutoff value has been established below which it is uniformly unsafe to administer heparin, LMWH, or oral anticoagulation. The fact that diverse cutoff values of 20,000/μL, 50,000/μL, and 100,000/μL are often used reflects a lack of physician consensus about the bleeding risk associated with thrombocytopenia and a wide range of comfort levels with anticoagulation in this setting. Recent cancer-associated VTE treatment trials comparing long-term dalteparin and enoxaparin with standard warfarin anticoagulation used minimum platelet counts of 75,000/μL and 50,000/μL, respectively, as study inclusion criteria.[78,79]

Bleeding Tendencies

Contemporary evidence on the risk of anticoagulation-related hemorrhage in cancer patients remains conflicting, with primarily retrospective studies supporting a greater bleeding risk in cancer patients and mainly prospective cohort studies suggesting that the risk is no greater than that in noncancer patients. The true risk most likely depends on the temporal relation between anticoagulation and major invasive and surgical procedures, concomitant thrombocytopenia or antiplatelet medication consumption, as well as the location and vascularity of cancerous lesions. Erosive, friable endobronchial, gastrointestinal, and genitourinary lesions are more likely prone to bleed during anticoagulation than at baseline. As in the noncancer population, older cancer patients and those with anemia, diabetes, recent myocardial infarction, renal insufficiency, history of stroke, and history of gastrointestinal bleeding are most likely at a greater risk for warfarin-associated bleeding.[80,81]

A large, retrospective, population-based study from the Mayo Clinic demonstrated that malignancy was associated with major bleeding with a relative hazard ratio of 4.26 (95% CI, 1.61–11.33) in univariate analysis and 4.07 (95% CI, 1.53–10.87) in multivariate analysis.[82] A recent retrospective analysis of 1303 patients enrolled in two large randomized, prospective trials comparing intravenous UFH with subcutaneous LMWH for initial VTE management also demonstrated a greater likelihood of major bleeding in patients with VTE and cancer.[21] The incidence of bleeding was 4.2, 2.1, and 13.3 events per 100 patient years in all patients, noncancer patients ($n = 1039$), and cancer patients ($n = 264$), respectively. The bleeding rate correlated with anticoagulation intensity in the noncancer patients but was independent of INR level in the cancer patient group. The major limitation of this study was the small total number of major bleeding events ($n = 12$). One small, prospective study revealed an odds ratio of 2.4 for bleeding in cancer patients with VTE compared with noncancer patients with VTE.[83] A recently published study revealed that the 12-month cumulative incidence of major bleeding in cancer patients treated for symptomatic DVT was 12.4% (95% CI, 6.5–18.2) compared with 4.9% (95% CI, 2.5–4.1) in treated noncancer patients ($P = .015$).[18]

Two other prospective studies have shown that the overall and major bleeding rates noted in DVT patients with and without cancer were not significantly different. Prandoni and coworkers[16,17] reported major bleeding rates of 3.4% and 3.0%, respectively, in VTE patients with and without cancer during the first 3 months of oral anticoagulation. Overall bleeding rates in the same groups were 8.6% and 9.8%, respectively. Bona and colleagues[19,20] reported major bleeding rates of 0.004 and 0.003 events per patient-month of therapy in patients with and without cancer, respectively.

A recently published analysis and the largest study to date suggests that the risk of major bleeding in cancer patients receiving oral warfarin after acute VTE is increased approximately sixfold and independent of the INR intensity.[21]

Osteopenia and Lytic Skeletal Lesions

Cancer patients, and those affected by multiple myeloma and breast carcinoma in particular, are often plagued by osteopenia, lytic skeletal lesions, and pathologic fractures. Immobility as a result of chronic bone pain and fractures may promote DVT. Prolonged administration of UFH can result in osteopenia and osteoporosis in up to 30% of noncancer patients, is associated with a 1% to 2% incidence of vertebral fracture, and certainly has the potential to exacerbate cancer-associated bone loss.[84-86] Experimental models have demonstrated simultaneous increases in osteoclast activity and decreased osteoblast activity in response to UFH exposure. Less osteoclast activation is observed in response to LMWH exposure.[87-89]

Primary and Metastatic Central Nervous System Tumors

Patients with primary brain tumors and metastatic CNS lesions are at an increased risk for developing VTE and are viewed by many as having an absolute contraindication to systemic anticoagulation.[90] CNS hemorrhage is of particular concern in patients with highly vascular brain metastases, such as those from choriocarcinoma, melanoma, and renal cell carcinoma. VTE in these cancer patients may prompt the placement of an IVC filter instead of systemic anticoagulation. Controlled CNS metastases (i.e., after radiation therapy) are often viewed as less prone to bleed. Available limited data from several series suggest that the risk of spontaneous intracranial bleeding in patients with primary brain tumors (mainly glioblastoma multiforme) and CNS metastases may not be greater in those who receive anticoagulant therapy compared with those not receiving anticoagulant therapy.[91-96] A major limitation of these reports is that most studied patients received prophylactic, and not treatment, intensity of UFH or warfarin. Careful dosing and frequent therapeutic monitoring are imperative, especially in patients receiving concomitant phenytoin therapy.

Analysis of subgroups enrolled in the first prospective, controlled VTE treatment trials to enroll patients with CNS malignancies we hope will provide needed insight into this management dilemma.[78,79] In one of these trials, six patients with primary CNS cancer, CNS lymphoma, or CNS metastases were treated per protocol without developing minor or major bleeding or a recurrent VTE.[79,97]

Limited or Compromised Venous Access to Support Therapeutic Monitoring

Initial management of acute VTE with continuous infusion UFH requires short-term but consistent intravenous access and frequent phlebotomy for therapeutic monitoring. With regard to oral warfarin, a narrow therapeutic index and wide intra- and interindividual variations in degree of anticoagulation achieved with a particular dose warrant frequent therapeutic monitoring and dose adjustment. Both UFH and warfarin therapeutic monitoring are associated with cost, patient inconvenience, and patient discomfort. Because of fluctuations in nutritional status and unpredictable fluctuations in the INR in cancer patients, frequent INR monitoring (once to twice weekly) may be required. The need for frequent phlebotomy and intravenous-access insertion can result in a cancer patient's having limited to no usable peripheral veins. Venous sampling via central venous catheter for therapeutic monitoring may result in false prolongations of the aPTT and prothrombin time due to sample contamination.

Persistent Hypercoagulability

Active residual cancer, of any extent, and active anticancer therapy of any form represent persistent hypercoagulable states. The magnitude of the prothrombotic stimulus may actually intensify with time as disease burden and metastases mount. As in other persistent hypercoagulable states, including congenital deficiencies of natural anticoagulants and chronic antiphospholipid antibodies, active malignancy and ongoing therapy should prompt an extended duration of anticoagulant therapy.

CANCER PATIENT RESPONSE TO LOW-MOLECULAR-WEIGHT HEPARINS

Several prospective, randomized, controlled trials have demonstrated the efficacy and safety equivalency of intravenous, aPTT-adjusted, UFH and subcutaneous, weight-based LMWH for the treatment of acute LE-DVT.[98-102] The major advantage of subcutaneous LMWH is that it can be self-administered at home, without the need for therapeutic monitoring.[103] This translates into a significant reduction in mean hospital length of stay compared with UFH initial therapy (1.1 vs. 6.5 days). Patients may be begun on LMWH in the hospital and then discharged in an "accelerated" fashion to continue the bridging to oral warfarin or may be treated exclusively in the outpatient setting. A reduction in length or avoidance of hospitalization may be of particular importance in immunocompromised cancer patients who are prone to nosocomial infections. LMWH treatment does require once- or twice-daily subcutaneous injection but does not require phlebotomy for therapeutic monitoring in the majority of patients. Cancer patients may be even more adept and accepting of subcutaneous injections than are noncancer patients because of experience with self-administered hematopoietic growth factor therapy.

LMWHs are associated with less HIT than is UFH, especially in heparin-naive patients.[104] This makes LMWHs particularly attractive for VTE prevention and treatment in cancer patients with disease- and chemotherapy-related thrombocytopenia in whom HIT detection may be hindered by preexistent low platelet counts. LMWHs are associated with less osteopenia in animal models and may offer a theoretical treatment advantage in cancer patients with osteolytic lesions.[88,89] Osteoporosis, though, has been reported with long-term LMWH use, and an increase in spontaneous fracture has been described during long-term LMWH exposure in pregnant women.[84-86]

LMWHs display less nonspecific binding to acute-phase plasma proteins, platelets, mononuclear leukocytes, and endothelial cells.[102] Active cancer patients treated with LMWHs are thus, theoretically, less likely to experience true heparin resistance. LMWHs also have been shown to promote a small but significantly greater degree of thrombus regression and restoration of venous patency than does UFH.[12] Disadvantages of LMWHs include the inability to be completely reversed by protamine sulfate in the event of bleeding or unanticipated surgery.[103] LMWH accumulation in patients with severe (creatinine clearance, <30 mL/minute) renal insufficiency precludes its predictable use in cancer patients with renal failure.

Two early meta-analyses of randomized controlled clinical trials comparing LMWHs with UFH in patients with acute DVT demonstrated a reduction in short-term mortality in cancer patients treated with LMWH (relative risks, 0.44 and 0.33, respectively).[105,106] More recent meta-analyses demonstrated an overall survival advantage in VTE patients treated with LMWHs compared with UFH.[107,108] Much of this observed advantage was derived from a single trial comparing tinzaparin with UFH.[100,109] A total of 97 cancer patients were included in the analysis, 47 of whom received tinzaparin. Death rates at 3 months were 10.6% in those randomized to tinzaparin and 28% in those who received UFH ($P = .041$).[100] Proposed mechanisms for the survival advantage include tumor growth retardation, metastasis prevention, tumor neovascularization inhibition, and fatal VTE prevention.[110,111] If real, the survival advantage associated with LMWH is likely due to a combination of effects. Properly powered prospective randomized trials are needed to confirm the meta-analysis and preclinical experimental observations.

Kakkar and associates[112] reported on a randomized, placebo-controlled trial of dalteparin, 5000 anti-Xa units daily, in patients with advanced solid tumor malignancy, without evidence of underlying thrombosis, with the primary objective of determining effect on survival at 1 year. The Kaplan-Meier survival estimates at 1, 2, and 3 years after randomization were 42%, 19%, and 13%, respectively, for placebo, and 45%, 27%, and 21% for the dalteparin group ($P = .29$). Although no significant early impact was seen on survival, a post hoc analysis of those surviving more than 17 months demonstrated survival estimates at 2 and 3 years after randomization of 56% and 37%, respectively, for placebo, versus 77% and 59% for dalteparin ($P = .04$).[112] A recent analysis of the impact of dalteparin on survival in patients with thromboembolism reported no difference in mortality at 12 months between those treated for 6 months with dalteparin and those treated with oral warfarin (56% vs. 58%).[113] A post hoc subgroup analysis suggested that long-term treatment–intensity dalteparin may reduce mortality in cancer patients with nonmetastatic disease and acute VTE compared with oral anticoagulation with warfarin (20% vs. 35%).

LMWH preparations differ in manufacturing methods, mean molecular weight, molecular weight distribution, effect on tissue factor pathway inhibitor expression, and possibly clinical effect. In part, for these reasons, LMWHs should not be viewed as interchangeable, and favorable data on one preparation do not necessarily apply to any other.

LOWER-EXTREMITY DEEP VENOUS THROMBOSIS MANAGEMENT

Diagnosis of Lower Extremity Deep Venous Thrombosis in Cancer Patients

The LE deep venous segments that can be affected by thrombosis include, in ascending order from the ankle, the paired calf veins (posterior tibial, anterior tibial, peroneal, gastrocnemius, and soleal), the popliteal, superficial femoral, deep femoral (profunda femoral), common femoral, and external and common iliac veins. The superficial and the deep femoral veins converge to form the common femoral vein in the proximal thigh. Despite its terminology, the superficial femoral vein is actually a deep vein and *not* a superficial vein; isolated superficial femoral vein thrombosis should thus be treated as a DVT and not viewed as a superficial thrombophlebitis. Currently available diagnostic methods for the objective diagnosis and exclusion of lower-extremity DVT include several imaging techniques and biochemical assays (Table 45-2). Although contrast venography remains the gold-standard method for lower-extremity DVT diagnosis, duplex ultrasound is the most appropriate initial diagnostic test due to the combination of accuracy, noninvasiveness, short examination time, portability of newer equipment, and lower cost.

Contrast Venography

Contrast venography has the ability to outline the deep venous system after the injection of radiopaque contrast

TABLE 45-2

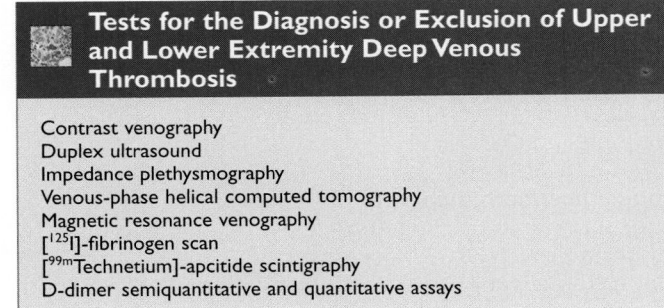

Tests for the Diagnosis or Exclusion of Upper and Lower Extremity Deep Venous Thrombosis

Contrast venography
Duplex ultrasound
Impedance plethysmography
Venous-phase helical computed tomography
Magnetic resonance venography
[^{125}I]-fibrinogen scan
[^{99m}Technetium]-apcitide scintigraphy
D-dimer semiquantitative and quantitative assays

medium into a dorsal foot vein. A central deep venous access (e.g., popliteal or common femoral vein) is usually necessary for adequate opacification of the pelvic (iliac) veins.[50,51] Available contrast agents include ionic and non-ionic iodinated aromatic-acid salts of varying osmolality and CO_2. CO_2 may provide an uneven intravascular distribution but is not nephrotoxic and is quite inexpensive to use. The presence of a constant intraluminal filling defect in at least two distinct projections is the most reliable diagnostic criterion for acute DVT.[50,114] Nonfilling of one or more venous segments proximal to the site of injection, abrupt termination of the column of contrast at a constant site, and the presence of flow in collateral veins are indirect signs that can be caused by artifacts. Artifacts may result from improper contrast administration and flow artifacts, particularly at the common femoral vein level, when nonopacified blood from the deep femoral vein mixes with opacified blood from the superficial femoral vein.[50,51]

The greatest limitations of venography are primarily related to its invasiveness and need for intravenous injection of contrast medium. The procedure also requires meticulous technique as well as experienced radiologists to avoid misinterpretation of inadequate studies.[51,115] Unsuccessful venograms have been reported in 2% to 20% of examinations, because of either inadequate technique with failure to outline a venous segment properly or inability to perform the test,[114-116] and interobserver disagreement ranges from 4% to 21%.[114] Although the deep femoral (profunda) vein is visualized only 50% of the time, isolated deep femoral vein DVT appears to be very rare.[50,117] Indeterminate findings also may result from the lack of visualization of the calf veins, which may occur because of nonfilling of the calf veins either because of improper test technique or occlusive DVT.[50,118,119] Other limitations include the fact that examinations cannot be performed at the bedside and are restricted to the limb where venous access has been gained.[120]

Complications of contrast venography include post-procedure DVT in approximately 2% to 10% of examinations[50,51,53,116,121] and superficial thrombophlebitis at the site of contrast injection.[50,51,116] Rare complications include tissue necrosis due to extravasation of contrast during injection and hypersensitivity reactions.[50,51,116]

Nonfilling of the iliac veins during contrast venography in cancer patients with known or suspected pelvic masses neither rules in nor rules out DVT. Such finding may be due to DVT, extrinsic venous compression by tumor, or both. In one study, 51% of all high-grade non–Hodgkin's lymphoma patients who were diagnosed with VTE also had concomitant pelvic venous compression by bulky lymphadenopathy.[22] In this situation of nonvisualization of the pelvic veins, an alternative imaging method, such as CT or magnetic resonance imaging (MRI), should be considered to assess for the presence of extrinsic vascular compression.[10]

Impedance Plethysmography

Impedance plethysmography (IPG) was a commonly used noninvasive, VTE diagnostic modality, particularly before the advent of duplex ultrasound.[50,51] The method consists of detecting changes in the electrical resistance (impedance) that result from blood-volume changes in the calf produced by abrupt deflation of a pneumatic thigh cuff inflated to a pressure of 50 mm Hg.[50,51]

IPG sensitivity for the diagnosis of proximal (i.e., above-the-knee) DVT has ranged from 60% to 95%,[51,122,123] but IPG is insensitive for the detection of calf DVT.[50,51,123] Most important, IPG does not differentiate between DVT and nonthrombotic venous occlusion.[50] False-positive examinations can result from conditions that increase central venous pressure (e.g., congestive heart failure, SVC syndrome, cor pulmonale), increase intra-abdominal pressure (e.g., pelvic mass, pregnancy), increase LE venous pressure (e.g., extrinsic compression of a vein by tumor or bulky adenopathy), or decrease venous return from the legs (e.g., previous DVTs).[50,51,123,124] False-negative results occur in the setting of calf DVT, nonocclusive DVTs, and improper technique.[50,51,123] Cancer patients are commonly afflicted by a number of the known conditions that result in false-positive or false-negative IPG results.[124] Not surprisingly, IPG has been shown to be insensitive (sensitivity of 71%) for the detection of proximal lower-extremity DVT in cancer patients,[124] and thus should be avoided.

Duplex Ultrasound

A venous duplex ultrasound study combines real-time B-mode ultrasound with pulsed-color Doppler flow imaging. The former provides direct visualization of the vessels and surrounding tissues, whereas the latter detects blood flow when the emitted ultrasound energy is reflected by red blood cells and sensed at a different frequency (Doppler shift).[10] The lower extremity deep venous segments that can routinely be examined by duplex ultrasound include the very distal external iliac, common femoral, superficial femoral, popliteal, and calf veins.

The diagnosis of DVT with duplex ultrasound relies on a combination of the following findings: vein non-compressibility, vein dilatation, visualization of echogenic intraluminal material, and lack of spontaneous and augmented blood flow.[115,125] The most widely used and reliable, validated criterion is lack of vein wall compressibility on B-mode ultrasound.[125-127] The other criteria are relatively inaccurate when applied individually.[126,128] Most important, however, the use of these criteria in combination does appear to increase the accuracy of the examination.[128]

Although the sensitivity and specificity of compression duplex ultrasound for acute femoropopliteal DVT have been reported to be quite high in symptomatic patients (92% to 100% and 94% to 100%, respectively),[115,125-129] it lacks adequate sensitivity when used for screening of asymptomatic individuals.[115] In addition, duplex ultrasound has been reported to lack adequate sensitivity (36% to 95%) for the detection of calf DVT, despite comparable specificity (89% to 100%).[115,118,125,126,130] A number of conditions may impair the ability of duplex ultrasound to detect calf vein thrombi, such as edema, large calf size, and the presence of open wounds, surgical bandages, or even large collateral veins, all of which lead to a high rate (10% to 40%) of inadequate examinations that impair interpretation.[130,131] This technical inadequacy is the likely explanation for the lower sensitivity of duplex ultrasound to detect calf DVT. Two studies comparing the sensitivities of all (adequate plus inadequate) calf examinations versus adequate-only examinations have shown sensitivities that increased from 73% and 85% to 95% and 99%, respectively.[132,133] In addition, the use of color Doppler has been shown to facilitate the localization and visualization of the calf veins, yielding fewer indeterminate examinations than venography in patients with isolated calf DVT.[118,134] Lack of color Doppler examination may explain the lower accuracy in early studies. Visualization of the calf veins by duplex ultrasound also has been enhanced by the use of an intravenous contrast agent, which in a small series led to reduction in the number of inadequate calf vein examinations from 55% to 20%.[135] Contrast ultrasound has the potential to improve the accuracy of this diagnostic modality even further.

The advantages of duplex ultrasound include the fact that it is noninvasive, and bilateral examinations can be performed in a timely fashion. Unlike venography, duplex ultrasound may also increase the overall diagnostic yield of calf examinations because of its ability to detect extravascular pathology, such as hematomas and Baker's cysts.[115,125,129,132,134]

Pitfalls of duplex ultrasound include the risk of false-positive incompressibility of the distal superficial femoral vein at the level of Hunter's (femoral) canal; the risk of setting the color gain inappropriately high, leading to "color-blossoming" that may obscure nonocclusive DVTs; and the potential to miss a DVT diagnosis in patients with duplicate venous systems or with the rare cases of isolated deep femoral DVTs.[115,118,125,129,136,137]

An important limitation of duplex ultrasound is the inability to perform compression maneuvers adequately in the veins above the inguinal ligament (common iliac and proximal external iliac veins). The lowest accuracy of duplex ultrasound was reported by a study that attempted to visualize and interpret iliac vein compression maneuvers routinely.[128] Although these venous segments may be visualized and interrogated for the presence of spontaneous blood flow and normal respiratory phasicity, these criteria are insensitive because normal flow may be present in cases of nonocclusive DVT. Only the distal 3 cm of the external iliac veins could be adequately visualized by one study,[130,138] with partial visualization of the external and common iliac veins being accomplished in 79% and 47% of the examinations, respectively.[136] Therefore a negative LE duplex ultrasound does not rule out iliac vein thrombosis, whereas attempts to diagnose iliac vein DVT by compression ultrasound alone may lead to a number of false-positive DVT diagnoses.[128,139] Conversely, the use of Doppler flow imaging may assist in the diagnosis of pelvic vein DVT or extrinsic compression: In a study of 37 cancer patients with leg edema and negative compression ultrasound, a 100% correlation was found between a monophasic waveform in the common femoral vein by spectral Doppler and the presence of either more proximal, not directly visualized DVT, or extrinsic pelvic venous compression by a mass.[140] However, this finding does not differentiate iliac DVT from extrinsic venous compression by tumor.

A controversial issue is the need for bilateral LE duplex ultrasound in patients with unilateral LE symptoms. Six studies have shown rates of isolated DVT in the asymptomatic, contralateral leg ranging from 0% to 5%, with another 2% to 22% of patients having bilateral DVT despite unilateral symptoms.[141-146] One study performed exclusively in cancer patients found that 1% of patients had DVT in the asymptomatic contralateral leg, whereas an additional 7% had bilateral DVT.[142] A further study that used bilateral duplex ultrasound examinations in patients with unilateral symptoms found that eight (53%) patients who had DVT in the asymptomatic limb had active cancer, and in seven of those eight patients, symptoms developed in the previously asymptomatic limb during the first month of anticoagulation therapy.[144] Of these seven, four were diagnosed with a new DVT in a previously unaffected venous segment, but three were found not to have a new DVT, illustrating the relevance of detecting symptomless DVT in the cancer population.[144] Lack of documentation of acute DVT in an asymptomatic limb could negatively affect patient management by leading to a false diagnosis of recurrent VTE and "warfarin failure" in future duplex ultrasound examinations. Thus a cancer patient should always undergo bilateral duplex ultrasound examinations for suspected LE-DVT, even if the symptoms are unilateral.[10]

Another limitation of duplex ultrasound is that the accuracy of compression maneuvers to detect recurrent DVT is uncertain. The ability to distinguish acute from remote (chronic) DVT is hampered by the fact that 50% of patients with prior LE-DVT will have some degree of residual vein obstruction.[147,148] Old, organized thrombi may appear hyperechoic and heterogeneous sonographically, but this may not help to differentiate acute from remote DVT.[125] Unless the new DVT is found in a previously normal venous segment, compression ultrasound may be unreliable.[125,148] Although serial duplex ultrasound evaluation of vein diameters and comparison with prior ultrasound measurements has been proposed as an alternative means of diagnosing recurrent DVT (with an incremental increase in vein diameter being attributed to recent DVT),[149,150] this method has not been validated by a large-scale prospective comparison with contrast venography. It also is unclear whether the same protocol would be as useful in cancer as in noncancer patients.

Contrast-Enhanced Computed Tomography
CT has not been validated as a method for DVT diagnosis (i.e., no accuracy studies have been performed comparing it with the gold-standard contrast venography, no interobserver variability has been formally assessed, and no validation (outcome) studies have been performed).[151-153] Thus it should not be routinely used for this purpose. However, because cancer patients frequently undergo body CT as a component of initial tumor staging, assessment of cancer recurrence and surveillance, or as a workup for persistent fever, physicians are frequently faced with the dilemma of an incidental finding of filling defects involving the pelvic veins or common femoral veins. In this situation, it is imperative that the diagnosis

be confirmed by a validated method, such as duplex ultrasound or contrast venography.[10]

The use of combined helical CT pulmonary angiography with CT venography (venous phase CT) of the pelvis and proximal legs has been studied as a means to detect DVT in patients with suspected PE.[117,154-156] The examination starts 2 to 4 minutes after contrast is injected for helical CT of the chest, and images are obtained either at 4- to 5-cm intervals or contiguously from the diaphragm to the ankles.[117] Criteria for acute DVT include visualization of a filling defect in an opacified vein, a nonopacified segment between normally opacified proximal and distal segments, venous dilatation (when compared with the contralateral side), and venous wall ring enhancement.[117,154-156] The sensitivity and specificity range from 71% to 100% and 87% to 100%, respectively, when compared with duplex ultrasound.[117,154-156]

Advantages of helical CT venography include its ability to visualize the IVC, portal, ovarian, and renal veins, as well as the soft tissues, to detect the presence or absence of intra-abdominal DVT and concomitant extrinsic venous compression.[117,157] No formal studies have been performed to assess the usefulness of this modality in differentiating acute from chronic DVT, although possible signs of chronicity include venous wall calcification and "shrunken" vessels.[117,156] A disadvantage of helical CT venography is that it requires the use of iodinated contrast, and if contiguous image acquisition is used, the effective radiation dose is exponentially increased. This has led some to state that the use of this technique should be limited in individuals younger than 30 years.[153,158]

False-positive DVT diagnoses have occurred because of flow artifacts, particularly at the level of the calf and pelvic veins, and also because of muscle hematomas and abscesses.[154,157] False-negative findings have occurred in cases of extensive bilateral DVTs, in which no normal vein enhancement in either limb is seen, so no contralateral normal vein is present for comparison, and a case of a thrombosed left-sided IVC that was misinterpreted as necrotic lymph nodes.[157,159]

Although observational and accuracy studies of helical CT venography do exist, no comparisons with venography and no clinical outcome studies have been performed. The appropriateness of this technique in cancer clinical practice is unclear at this time. PIOPED II is a large prospective study that will include performance of spiral CT venography in every patient who undergoes spiral CT to diagnose PE.[160]

Magnetic Resonance Venography

Magnetic resonance angiography (MRA) to evaluate the venous system (MRV) can be performed with time-of-flight (TOF) and phase-contrast techniques. The most commonly used is an axial, two-dimensional (2D) TOF technique based on standard 2D gradient-echo imaging, with or without gadolinium enhancement.[161] The observed signs of acute DVT as seen by MRV include total obstruction of the vein and venous dilatation, as well as the presence of a rim of increased signal intensity surrounding the thrombus.[162,163] Although one study suggested that the pattern of rim enhancement was useful

in differentiating acute from chronic DVT, no correlation with contrast venography was performed.[164]

MRV has been shown to be as accurate as duplex ultrasound for diagnosing LE-DVT in three prospective studies that compared the two methods with contrast venography (100% sensitivity, 95% to 100% specificity).[162,163,165,166] False-positive diagnoses occurred in patients with extrinsic compression of the iliac veins.[162] The method is less accurate when evaluating for calf DVT.[167]

Advantages of MRV include the lack of need for intravenous iodinated contrast and the ability to assess for the presence of extrinsic venous compression when combined with soft tissue–weighted MRI, and the fact that, unlike duplex ultrasound, MRV can routinely visualize the pelvic veins.[168] Disadvantages include cost and lack of wide availability.[169]

Nuclear Scintigraphy

Activated platelets expressing glycoprotein IIb/IIIa (GP IIb/IIIa) that become incorporated into acute evolving venous thromboses serve as the physiologic target for [99mtechnetium]-apcitide (AcuTect) in the diagnosis of LE-DVT. A phase III prospective clinical trial in 280 patients who underwent both [99mTc]-apcitide scintigraphy and contrast venography demonstrated an overall sensitivity and specificity of 76% and 73%, respectively, for imaging acute LE-DVT.[170] Higher sensitivity and specificity (91% and 84%, respectively) were seen in patients with their first DVT event and signs and symptoms of less than 3 days' duration, and false-negative diagnoses occurred more frequently in patients with calf DVT.[170] Because [99mTc]-apcitide is a functional rather than anatomic diagnostic imaging method, it has the theoretical potential to discern acute from chronic (without activated platelets) thrombus. In cancer patients, thrombocytopenia of any etiology and tumor-associated platelet activation likely limit the usefulness of this technique for the diagnosis of acute LE-DVT.

[125I]-Fibrinogen leg scanning was used mostly in the 1970s and early 1980s for the diagnosis of acute LE-DVT.[50,51] It was highly sensitive (90%) for calf DVT but insensitive (60% to 80%) for DVT involving the proximal veins because the isotope is a relatively low gamma emitter and because the bladder frequently contained radioactive urine.[51] The use of this method has largely been abandoned because of its attendant risk of transmissible viral diseases and the wide availability of duplex ultrasound. In addition, [125I]-fibrinogen leg scanning was never used alone for the diagnosis of acute DVT because it can take up to 72 hours to become positive.[51] Other radiolabeled peptides under investigation for DVT diagnosis include [99mTc]-DMP 444 and [99mTc]-FDB (fibrin domain of fibronectin).[171] A radiolabeled antibody targeted against the DD domain of fibrin also is under development.

D-dimer

D-dimer is a cross-linked degradation product resulting from the plasmin-mediated lysis of cross-linked fibrin. Three readily available techniques are used to assay D-dimer: enzyme-linked immunosorbent assays (ELISA), plasma-based latex agglutination, and whole-blood hemagglutination (WBA) assays. Qualitative latex agglutination assays are relatively inexpensive to perform, widely available, and rapidly performed, but are not sufficiently sensitive to exclude VTE.[172] Both ELISA and WBA assays have been prospectively studied in clinical management trials and found to have high negative predictive values in outpatients with suspected VTE.[173,174] These studies suggest that lack of D-dimer elevation combined with a negative noninvasive imaging test reliably excludes LE-DVT, but D-dimer elevation alone neither rules in nor rules out thrombosis. In general, these D-dimer assays are excellent screening tests for VTE, but the negative predictive value of the WBA D-dimer assay has been shown to be lower in cancer patients (78.9%) than in those without cancer (96.5%).[175] Thus it is not as useful for excluding VTE in cancer patients. Conversely, false-negative D-dimer results have been described in cancer patients with PE and baseline impaired endogenous fibrinolysis due to excessive levels of plasma PAI-1.[30] More recently, however, both a subgroup analysis of a retrospective cohort study and a prospective cohort study showed that the negative predictive value of a new latex agglutination assay remained high and reliably excluded DVT in cancer patients.[176,177] However, confidence intervals in the latter study were somewhat wide; thus additional studies are needed to determine whether the D-dimer assay is truly reliable in excluding DVT in the cancer population.[177] Until conclusive evidence from larger studies is available, we believe that D-dimer assays should not be used to exclude VTE in cancer patients.

Lower-Extremity Deep Venous Thrombosis

Patients with clinically suspected LE-DVT or an incidental finding of DVT on CT should be initially evaluated with duplex ultrasound. A nondiagnostic ultrasound examination should prompt further evaluation with contrast venography. If the patient is known to have a pelvic mass and has either no opacification of the pelvic veins by venography or a monophasic Doppler signal during sonographic interrogation of the common femoral vein, MRV or CT should also be considered to rule out concomitant extrinsic venous compression. Given the high rate of VTE recurrence and "warfarin failure" in cancer patients, it is advisable to pursue contrast venography in cases of suspected DVT recurrence in which the duplex ultrasound does not detect a new DVT in a previously normal segment. Unfortunately, however, venography also has limitations in diagnosing recurrent DVT involving previously involved venous segments, and neither MRV nor CT has been validated or conclusively shown to differentiate acute from chronic DVT reliably.

Treatment of Lower-Extremity Deep Venous Thrombosis in Cancer Patients

General guidelines for VTE management have been published elsewhere.[69,178] Specific, evidence-based guidelines for VTE management in the cancer population are lacking. Analysis of recently completed and ongoing clinical trials may provide the basis for future detailed guidelines. In the meantime, cancer patients with VTE should be treated in a manner that takes the previously described unique features, subgroup analyses of prospec-

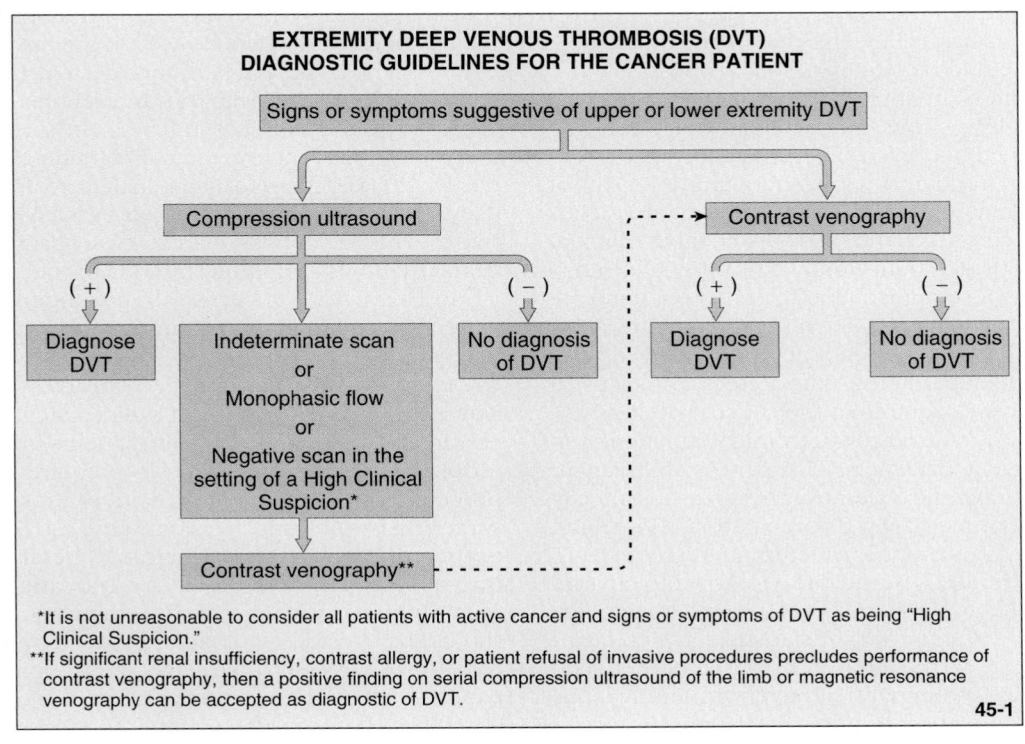

EXTREMITY DEEP VENOUS THROMBOSIS (DVT) DIAGNOSTIC GUIDELINES FOR THE CANCER PATIENT

Signs or symptoms suggestive of upper or lower extremity DVT

Compression ultrasound

(+) Diagnose DVT

Indeterminate scan or Monophasic flow or Negative scan in the setting of a High Clinical Suspicion*

(−) No diagnosis of DVT

Contrast venography

(+) Diagnose DVT

(−) No diagnosis of DVT

Contrast venography**

*It is not unreasonable to consider all patients with active cancer and signs or symptoms of DVT as being "High Clinical Suspicion."
**If significant renal insufficiency, contrast allergy, or patient refusal of invasive procedures precludes performance of contrast venography, then a positive finding on serial compression ultrasound of the limb or magnetic resonance venography can be accepted as diagnostic of DVT.

45-1

DEEP VENOUS THROMBOSIS ANTICOAGULANT TREATMENT IN THE CANCER PATIENT

INITIAL PHASE ANTICOAGULANT
- Acute treatment with a parenteral agent (unfractionated heparin or low-molecular-weight heparin) in the inpatient or outpatient setting
- Intravenous unfractioned heparin should initially be dosed based on patient weight and adjusted to achieve an activated partial thromboplastin time that corresponds to an anti-factor Xa activity level of 0.3–0.7 U/mL
- Subcutaneous low-molecular-weight heparins should be dosed based on patient weight, avoided in persons with calculated or actual creatinine clearance rates less than 30 mL/min, and not monitored in the majority of cases
- When using enoxaparin sodium for initial phase anticoagulation, we prefer to use 1 mg/kg twice daily, instead of 1.5 mg/kg once daily
- We prefer using a low-molecular-weight heparin rather than unfractionated heparin in order to facilitate outpatient management and because of evidence suggesting a possible survival advantage

SUBACUTE PHASE ANTICOAGULANT
Up to 6 months
- Subacute management can consist of oral warfarin with a target international normalized ratio (INR) between 2.0 and 3.0 or once daily subcutaneous low-molecular-weight heparin without therapeutic monitoring
- Warfarin therapy requires a minimum of 4 days overlap with the parenteral agent used for initial phase anticoagulant and can be difficult to maintain between an INR of 2.0 and 3.0 because of variable nutrition, concomitant medications, and hepatic dysfunction
- We favor low-molecular-weight heparin because of excellent patient compliance, reduced on-treatment thrombosis recurrence rates, and a possible survival advantage

CHRONIC PHASE ANTICOAGULANT
Beyond 6 months
- Patients with persistent hypercoagulability from their malignancy, anticancer therapy, antiphospholipid antibody, or underlying inherited prothrombotic state such as deficiency of a natural anticoagulant have their subacute phase therapy extended until the persistent hypercoagulable state has resolved or completed
- Attenuated intensity therapy with warfarin (INR 1.5 to 2.0) and low-molecular-weight heparin (primary prophylaxis intensity) are not recommended for patients with active malignancy and those receiving anti-cancer therapy

tive, randomized VTE treatment trials, and recently completed LMWH trials into account.

Initial Anticoagulation Therapy

The mainstay of pharmacologic therapy for VTE in all patients remains anticoagulation. Initial (acute phase) therapy typically consists of parenteral UFH or LMWH for a minimum of 4 days and until a stable, target intensity of warfarin treatment has been achieved.[178] Treatment with UFH or LMWH should be begun as soon as possible after VTE diagnosis unless an absolute contraindication exists. Whenever possible, therapy should actually begin as soon as VTE is suspected and even before diagnostic tests are obtained. A delay in achieving a therapeutic intensity of initial parenteral therapy may negatively affect a patient's long-term VTE recurrence rate.[49,179,180] Weight-based initial dosing of UFH (80-U/kg bolus followed by 18 U/kg/hour) with subsequent dose adjustments based on a standardized nomogram facilitates achieving a therapeutic aPTT within 24 hours of treatment commencement.[181] Because of problems with heparin resistance, greater than usual doses of UFH may be required in the cancer patient.

LMWH may be preferred for both initial inpatient and outpatient treatment of acute VTE in the stable cancer patient for the safety, efficacy, and survival reasons already discussed. The optimal LMWH preparation, dose, and dosing frequency remain to be determined. Acute DVT treatment safety and efficacy data exist for enoxaparin, 1.5 mg/kg once daily, and enoxaparin, 1.0 mg/kg twice daily, in cancer patients.[182] No statistically significant difference in VTE recurrence rate was observed between patients randomized to initial treatment with intravenous UFH, once-daily enoxaparin, and twice-daily enoxaparin.

Of the 47 cancer patients randomized to the twice-daily dosing (total daily dose of 2.0 mg/kg), 3 (6.4%), recurrent VTE developed compared with 6 (12.2%) of the 49 cancer patients allocated to once-daily dosing (total daily dose of 1.5 mg/kg).[182] This trend has led many physicians to advocate twice-daily dosing of enoxaparin for initial VTE treatment in cancer patients. The observed difference probably reflects the difference in total daily dose rather than an inherent inadequacy of once-daily dosing. This fact is important to note when considering the use of once-daily LMWHs like tinzaparin and dalteparin. Tinzaparin, 175 IU/kg once daily, has an excellent safety and efficacy track record in cancer patients.[100] Dalteparin is given at a dose of 200 IU/kg up to a maximal dose of 18,000 IU once daily. Whether these or higher total daily doses of these two agents given as divided twice-daily injections in cancer patients would be superior to the standard dosing is not known. Concerns about underdosing cancer patients weighing more than 90 kg with standard-dose dalteparin may be justified.

Despite the excellent safety profiles of LMWHs in cancer and noncancer patients alike, initial inpatient UFH treatment may be preferred in patients at very high risk for bleeding and in those likely to require urgent invasive procedures. Such patients include those with recent surgery, gastrointestinal lesions, any past gastrointestinal or neuraxial bleeding, significant anemia, and marked thrombocytopenia. At present, cancer patients with severe renal dysfunction and most weighing more than 120 kg should be treated with adjusted-dose, monitored UFH. Based on a recent pharmacokinetic analysis in obese patients up to 165 kg, tinzaparin appears to be able to be dosed based on actual weight without dose adjustment.[183]

Patients with nonhemorrhagic CNS primary tumors or metastatic CNS lesions and VTE should be considered for anticoagulation, preferably begun in the hospital. The randomized study of enoxaparin sodium alone versus initial enoxaparin sodium followed by warfarin for a 180-day period as secondary prevention of venous thromboembolic events in patients with active malignancy (ONCENOX) trial enrolled six patients with confirmed CNS malignancy, all of whom were treated exclusively in the outpatient setting, and in none of whom did recurrent VTE or bleeding complications develop.[97] Patients with hemorrhagic CNS lesions are probably best treated with IVC filter placement.

Subcutaneous fondaparinux, 7.5 mg once daily, has been shown to be as safe and effective as subcutaneous enoxaparin for the initial treatment of patients with acute DVT and adjusted-dose intravenous UFH for the initial treatment of patients with acute PE.[184] Specific data in patients with active cancer and VTE have not been published. Ximelagatran, an oral direct thrombin inhibitor, holds promise as an anticoagulant for the initial, subacute, and chronic long-term treatment of acute VTE. Ximelagatran offers the convenience of fixed dosing without the need for therapeutic monitoring or subcutaneous injections. A potential pitfall of this agent that may be of particular concern in cancer patients is reversible liver function test elevation in roughly 6% of treated patients.

Chronic Anticoagulation Therapy

Chronic-phase anticoagulation for VTE has traditionally consisted of oral warfarin dosed to achieve an INR between 2.0 and 3.0.[75] Cancer patients with lupus anticoagulants and baseline elevated prothrombin times may require alternative warfarin therapeutic monitoring in place of the INR.[185] Chromagenic factor X activity assays or assessment of individual vitamin K–dependent factor activity levels on dilute plasma samples are acceptable alternatives. Warfarin therapy can be started as soon as a therapeutic-intensity aPTT has been achieved with UFH or an initial weight-based dose of LMWH has been given. Bolus dosing of warfarin does not help achieve a stable, target INR faster and may actually delay achievement of a stable INR and prolong hospitalization.[186] Initial dosing with 2.5 to 7.5 mg per day (based on patient weight and nutritional status) seems prudent. Frequent (weekly) INR monitoring may not actually facilitate a more stable INR in cancer patients but still seems prudent.[187] Warfarin therapy *alone* is contraindicated in the setting of acute thrombosis because of the inherent delay in achieving therapeutic anticoagulation and the theoretical transient exacerbation of hypercoagulability caused by a rapid reduction in protein C functional activity.[188] This warfarin-induced paradoxical hypercoagulability may contribute to warfarin-induced limb gangrene in patients with HIT and to warfarin-induced skin necrosis and may be particularly troublesome in patients with hypercoagulability of malignancy.

Warfarin Failure

Patients in whom objectively confirmed recurrent VTE develops during periods of subtarget INR (≤2.0) should be restarted on treatment-intensity UFH or LMWH until a stable INR between 2.0 and 3.0 is achieved. Patients in whom objectively confirmed recurrent VTE develops despite an INR between 2.0 and 3.0 (warfarin failure) can either be treated with UFH or LMWH until a higher intensity of oral anticoagulation (INR, 3.0 to 4.0) is attained or switched to primary long-term therapy with LMWH.[73,189] LMWH therapy is gaining popularity in patients with warfarin failure because of the challenges of warfarin therapy regulation at any target intensity and data from early randomized trials suggest efficacy and safety comparability to warfarin.[190-192] The optimal long-term anticoagulation dose of any LMWH is not known and may be less than the dose used during initial VTE treatment. The ONCENOX trial evaluated the feasibility, safety, and efficacy of long-term enoxaparin at 1.5 mg/kg once daily and 1.0 mg/kg once daily based on this supposition.[79]

Long-term Anticoagulation Therapy with Low-molecular-weight Heparin

Each of the three commercially available LMWHs in the United States has been recently studied as a substitute for oral warfarin in the management of cancer patients with acute VTE (Table 45-3).[78,79,193,194] In the randomized trial of long-term dalteparin LMWH versus oral anticoagulant therapy in cancer patients with VTE (CLOT), 8.0% of LMWH-treated patients experienced recurrent VTE during 6 months of treatment compared with 15.8% of those treated with warfarin (target INR, 2.5).[78] In the ONCENOX trial, in 3.3% of the patients treated for 180 days with one of the two once-daily doses of enoxaparin, recurrent VTE developed, compared with 6.7% of those treated with warfarin (target INR, 2.0 to 3.0).[79] In the comparison of LMWH and warfarin for the secondary prevention of VTE in patients with cancer (CANTHANOX) trial, in 3.0% of the patients treated for 3 months with enoxaparin, 1.5 mg/kg once daily, recurrent VTE developed, compared with 4.2% of those treated with oral warfarin.[194] In the cancer subgroup of the randomized trial evaluating long-term LMWH therapy for 3 months versus intravenous heparin followed by warfarin sodium (LITE), in 5.9% of those treated with tinzaparin, recurrent VTE developed, compared with 10.5% of those treated with heparin followed by warfarin.[193] Major bleeding rates were not statistically different between the treatment groups in

TABLE 45-3

Long-term Low-molecular-weight Heparin Therapy in Cancer-associated Venous Thromboembolic Events		
	VTE RECURRENCE RATE (%)	
	LMWH	**WARFARIN**
CLOT (dalteparin)[78]	27/336 (8.0)	53/336 (15.8)
LITE (tinzaparin)[193]	6/101 (5.9)	11/105 (10.5)
CANTHANOX (enoxaparin)[194]	2/67 (3.0)	3/71 (4.2)
ONCENOX (enoxaparin)[79]	2/61 (3.3)	2/30 (6.7)
TOTAL	37/565 (6.5)	69/542 (12.7)

these clinical trials. These studies support the use of once-daily subcutaneous LMWH in place of oral warfarin in cancer patients with acute VTE to minimize recurrent VTE rates.

Duration of Anticoagulation

With regard to the optimal duration of anticoagulation in patients with VTE in the setting of cancer, it seems prudent to treat for a minimum of 6 months and at least until all cancer therapy has been completed and the patient has been deemed to have no residual malignancy.[195-197] Residual malignancy constitutes a persistent hypercoagulable state, which typically warrants long-term anticoagulant treatment. Warfarin therapy itself has been shown to improve survival in patients with extensive-stage small cell lung carcinoma and a longer duration of oral anticoagulation (6 months vs. 6 weeks) after acute VTE has been shown to reduce the risk of developing genitourinary tract cancers.[198,199]

The recently published study of long-term, low-intensity warfarin therapy for the prevention of recurrent VTE (PREVENT) demonstrated a 64% reduction in recurrent VTE without increased risk of major bleeding compared with placebo when warfarin with a target INR of 1.5 to 2.0 is prescribed to patients after completion of a standard course of anticoagulation for idiopathic VTE.[200] This study specifically excluded patients with known active malignancy and thus should not be applied to this population.

UPPER-EXTREMITY DEEP VENOUS THROMBOSIS MANAGEMENT

Diagnosis of Upper-Extremity Deep Venous Thrombosis in Cancer Patients

The UE deep venous segments that can be affected by thrombosis include, in ascending order from the elbow, the brachial, axillary, subclavian, and brachiocephalic veins, as well as the SVC. Similar to LE-DVT, the prevalence of confirmed DVT is less than 50% among symptomatic patients suspected of having UE-DVT.[39] Therefore diagnostic confirmation by an imaging method is mandatory. In general, the same modalities used for the diagnostic approach of LE-DVT apply for patients with suspected UE-DVT. However, no formal studies of helical CT venography, nuclear scintigraphy, or impedance plethysmography have been performed to diagnose DVT in the upper extremities, and, as previously discussed, D-dimer assays should not be considered reliable for the exclusion of DVT in a patient with cancer.

Contrast Venography

A number of anatomic variants and the converging nature of the central venous anatomy in the UE can lead to flow turbulence artifacts that may complicate the interpretation of UE venography.[201] In addition, because the technique is usually performed by contrast injection in an antecubital vein, it does not visualize the internal jugular veins, which can be easily visualized by duplex ultrasound. Similar to its applicability in the lower extremities, the single most reliable criterion for acute DVT is the presence of a constant, intraluminal filling defect in at least two different projection views. The complications related to the use of contrast medium are infrequent and similar to those described for LE-DVT. However, no data are available on the incidence of DVT after venography in the UEs.

Duplex Ultrasound

The internal jugular, subclavian, axillary, and brachial veins can be routinely visualized in the neck and arms. However, the medial two thirds of the subclavian veins are not easily compressible because of their anatomic location behind the clavicles.[202] In addition, it is not technically feasible to perform compression maneuvers at the level of the brachiocephalic veins and the SVC; in fact, the right brachiocephalic vein and the SVC are usually not visualized by ultrasound examination. Even if these segments of the subclavian veins and left brachiocephalic veins are visualized, duplex ultrasound has not been validated for the detection or exclusion of DVT in these locations because the diagnosis cannot be established by the compression method. Rather, DVT in those locations is suggested by indirect Doppler-flow criteria such as lack of diameter change with inspiration and incomplete color filling of the lumen, and by the presence of echogenic material on B-mode ultrasound imaging.[202]

The sensitivity and specificity of duplex ultrasound for the diagnosis of acute symptomatic axillosubclavian DVT range from 96% to 100% and 94% to 100%, respectively.[39,203-205] Studies of the accuracy associated with other sonographic criteria than vein compressibility have been found to possess a lower sensitivity of 50% to 73%.[203,206] The presence of an indwelling catheter in aUE vein has been shown not to alter significantly the Doppler-flow dynamics compared with the contralateral vein that does not have a catheter in place.[207] Nevertheless, duplex ultrasound appears to be unreliable as a screening method to diagnose asymptomatic, catheter-related UE-DVT.[208]

Other Imaging Modalities

Neither contrast-enhanced CT nor MRV has been validated in evaluating the UEs, including the SVC. CT is not an ideal method because the convergence of the central veins in the upper chest is frequently associated with flow artifacts.[209] Thus the diagnosis of any suspected SVC or innominate DVT found by CT should ideally be confirmed by contrast venography. No studies have reported on the use of helical CT venography for central chest veins.

Two early studies (28 and 25 arms examined, respectively) correlating MRV with contrast venography for the diagnosis of acute axillary-subclavian DVT found a sensitivity and specificity of 80% and 100%, respectively.[210,211] However, in one study, the sensitivity for nonocclusive DVT was quite low (20%) compared with the one for occlusive DVT (80%).[210] Nevertheless, MRV appears to be very accurate in detecting conditions that may be associated with UE or central chest vein extrinsic compression or stenosis.[201,212,213] Two studies in selected patients with UE central venous abnormalities showed 100% correlation between 3D, gadolinium-enhanced MRV and contrast venography for detecting SVC and brachiocephalic vein stenosis or compression.[201,213]

Treatment of Upper Extremity Deep Venous Thrombosis in Cancer Patients

Central venous catheter–associated DVT has been described in up to 56% of patients with indwelling catheters.[214] These "UE" DVTs may result in SVC thrombosis, SVC syndrome, and PE. The true risk of PE from central venous catheter–associated thromboses is often debated. Prandoni and coworkers[39] and Bernardi reported a 36% rate of PE complicating UE DVT; Monreal and colleagues[215] reported a 16% rate of PE in this setting. Ault and Artal,[216] in contrast, suggested that PE is uncommon in patients with central venous catheters based on a lack of any PE in 33 of their patients with DVT due to peripherally placed central catheters. In patients with symptomatic central venous catheter–related DVT and a functional catheter, line removal is often unnecessary. Anticoagulation management following the same guidelines as for LE-DVT in the cancer patient is recommended. Continuation of anticoagulation for the life of the catheter seems reasonable. This management approach allows uninterrupted cancer treatment and prevents the need for additional vascular-access surgery. Central venous catheter–related DVT in conjunction with a dysfunctional catheter usually warrants anticoagulation and line removal. Thrombolytic therapy followed by anticoagulation may alleviate thrombosis-related symptoms more quickly and completely than anticoagulation alone.[37,217] Randomized trials comparing thrombolysis with anticoagulation for central venous catheter–associated DVTs are lacking.

PULMONARY EMBOLISM MANAGEMENT

Diagnosis of Pulmonary Embolism in Cancer Patients

Currently available tests for the diagnostic confirmation or exclusion of PE include various imaging methods and blood-based biochemical assays (Table 45-4). Although many believe that pulmonary angiography is no more accurate than helical CT, pulmonary angiography remains the gold-standard diagnostic test for PE. However, helical CT and V/Q lung scanning are the most appropriate initial tests because they are noninvasive and widely available.

TABLE 45-4

Tests for the Objective Diagnosis or Exclusion of Pulmonary Embolism

Pulmonary angiography
Ventilation-perfusion lung scintigraphy
Helical (spiral) computed tomography
Magnetic resonance angiography
D-dimer semiquantitative and quantitative assays

Pulmonary Angiography

Pulmonary angiography is typically performed via common femoral vein access (or internal jugular or brachial vein) and can include selective catheterization of either or both the right and left main pulmonary arteries. The pulmonary vascular tree is then visualized after an injection of iodinated contrast medium.[218]

Based on clinical-outcome studies, the sensitivity and specificity of pulmonary angiography have been estimated to be 98% and 97%, respectively.[219,220] The specificity of pulmonary angiography approaches 100% when a filling defect or abrupt "cut-off" of a pulmonary artery branch is present.[220,221] Ancillary findings that may be present but are not specific for PE include abnormal distribution of flow to the different lobes, delayed venous return, and partially opacified, tortuous vessels.[218,221] The accuracy of the test is not influenced by the presence of chronic obstructive pulmonary disease (COPD).[221] In the PIOPED study, interobserver disagreement occurred more often for the exclusion of PE (17%) than for PE confirmation (8%) by pulmonary angiography.[222] Experts agreed 98%, 90%, and 66% of the time on the presence of lobar, segmental, and subsegmental PE, respectively.[220]

Complications reported with pulmonary angiography include minor and major complications as well as death. These three endpoints were observed in 5%, 1% and 0.5%, respectively, in 1111 patients who underwent pulmonary angiography in the PIOPED study.[220] A review of more than 7000 patients undergoing pulmonary angiography revealed a 0.1% death rate with the procedure.[223]

Ventilation/Perfusion Lung Scintigraphy

V/Q lung scanning combines ventilation and perfusion nuclear medicine imaging techniques. The ventilation (V) study involves the inhalation of a radioactive gas (e.g., xenon), which provides an image of all ventilated portions of the lung. The perfusion (Q) study consists of an intravenous injection of [^{99m}Tc]-labeled macroaggregated human serum albumin particles with the patient in supine position, and the particles become trapped in approximately 0.1% of the pulmonary capillary bed.[221] Any obstruction to arterial flow is viewed as an area of hypoperfusion and called a "perfusion defect" on gamma-camera images. The presence of multiple segmental perfusion defects increases the test specificity for PE.[221] Based on the presence and extent of matched (absence of both perfusion and ventilation) and unmatched (absence of perfusion but preserved ventilation) defects, the V/Q scan can be interpreted by using PIOPED published criteria as either normal or low probability, intermediate probability, or high probability for PE.[222,224]

Because they provide indirect evidence of PE, V/Q scans are most clinically useful when considered in combination with an assessment of pretest clinical suspicion.[222] Based on PIOPED data, a normal V/Q scan essentially rules out clinically significant PE, and a high-probability V/Q scan alone has a high positive predictive value (88%) for PE, with 96% of patients with high pretest clinical suspicion and a high-probability V/Q scan having PE documented by pulmonary angiography.[222] Only 4% of patients with both low-probability V/Q scan and low

Problems Common to Cancer and Its Therapy

clinical suspicion had PE on angiography.[222] Low- and intermediate-probability scans are now considered together as being "indeterminate" scans.

A plain chest radiograph is necessary before interpretation of a V/Q scan. Pleural effusions, bullous disease, pulmonary infiltrates or masses, and atelectasis have been associated with a higher frequency of indeterminate-probability scans and with a lower positive predictive value of high-probability findings.[221]

V/Q scan has the advantage of not using iodinated contrast. Its greatest limitation as a diagnostic tool for PE is that it provides a definitive result in a minority of patients. In the PIOPED series, only 13% had a normal study, and 14% had a high-probability scan.[222] Therefore it can be expected that as many as 73% of all patients undergoing a V/Q scan will have a nondiagnostic, indeterminate scan that warrants further testing such as pulmonary angiography to confirm or exclude PE. In addition, it has been demonstrated that the rates of nondiagnostic V/Q scan findings increase significantly from 21% to 63% in patients without COPD to 46% to 91% in those with COPD,[225,226] and from 9% in patients with normal chest radiographs to 48% in patients with abnormal chest radiographs.[227]

Pitfalls in the interpretation of V/Q scintigraphy may represent a significant problem in the cancer population, particularly when primary or secondary (metastatic) pulmonary involvement is present. Patients with a history of PE may have a high-probability V/Q scan that does not reflect a new, acute event but rather the remnants of old PE.[221,222] False high-probability scans may occur as a consequence of an abnormal perfusion scan due to pulmonary artery invasion or compression, regional hypoventilation secondary to bronchial compromise, pulmonary vein obstruction by hilar masses or adenopathy, and pulmonary leukostasis, which have been described in lymphoma, osteosarcoma, neuroblastoma, lymphangitic carcinomatosis, lung carcinoma, carcinoid, left atrial leiomyosarcoma, metastatic renal cell carcinoma, pulmonary artery sarcomas, and acute myelogenous leukemia.[228-251] Areas of V/Q mismatch also have been described as a result of prior radiation therapy to the chest in patients with breast and lung carcinoma.[252-255]

Helical (Spiral) Computed Tomography Angiography

Contrast-enhanced spiral CT is performed by scanning a distance of 10 to 12 cm from the aortic arch to 2 cm below the inferior pulmonary veins during a single 30-second breath hold while the pulmonary vasculature is opacified by the automated injection of iodinated contrast medium.[256] Technical parameters such as collimation, rate and timing of contrast administration and scanning delay, as well as breathing, motion artifacts, and even central venous catheters can influence the timing and quality of opacification of the pulmonary arteries, thus having the potential to compromise the quality of the study.[221,256-258] The rate of studies inadequate for interpretation ranges from 2% to 13%.[225,256,259-263]

Spiral CT has an overall sensitivity of 53% to 100% and specificity of 78% to 100% for the diagnosis of PE.[259-268] These rates approach 95% to 100% for the central and segmental pulmonary arterial branches, but are lower (sensitivity, 53% to 63%) for PE involving the subsegmental branches. The accuracy of helical CT is highly influenced by, and dependent on, the equipment being used. Earlier CT scanners included 5-mm collimation that resulted in an effective section thickness of 6.57 mm and imaging reconstruction at 3-mm intervals.[256,269,270] Many currently available CT scanners include 2-mm to 3-mm collimation, resulting in effective section thickness of 2 mm to 4 mm and improved visualization of the subsegmental arterial bed.[256,269-271] The newest-generation multislice CT scanners allow subsecond scanning with 1.25-mm collimation, 1.25-mm section thickness, and image reconstruction at 0.6-mm intervals.[256,269,270] Although these modern scanners also have been shown to improve visualization of subsegmental arteries significantly, two recent studies disagreed on whether this improved visualization led to higher detection rates of subsegmental PE.[272,273] In addition, the use of workstations for image viewing and primary interpretation has been shown to increase the detection of PE by 25% in comparison to hard-copy image viewing.[274]

Studies with the highest frequency of isolated subsegmental PE, hence lowest spiral CT sensitivity, have been reported in patients who also had a nondiagnostic V/Q scans,[266] and studies have shown that the prevalence of subsegmental PE ranges from 6% to 36%.[265,266,275] Whether subsegmental PE is clinically relevant and should definitively be detected remains a controversial matter. A total of six prospective management studies have been performed with spiral CT in patients with indeterminate V/Q-scan findings.[276-281] In five of these studies, patients with a negative helical CT also underwent LE duplex ultrasound, with anticoagulation being held after a negative result.[276-279,281] Follow-up periods ranged from 3 to 6 months, and rates of recurrent VTE ranged from 2% to 4%.[276-279,281] The only study that withheld anticoagulation on the basis of a negative helical CT alone reported a 1% rate of VTE recurrence in patients with low pretest probability for PE.[280] Because these studies did not rely on a negative CT alone before withholding anticoagulation, and because the sensitivity of helical CT is low in patients with nondiagnostic V/Q scans,[152,259,265,266] the current evidence is insufficient to rely on a negative helical CT alone to justify withholding anticoagulation and even to support the hypothesis that subsegmental PE is not clinically significant.[152,270,279,280,282,283]

The major advantages of spiral CT include the rapid nature of data acquisition and the lower percentage of nondiagnostic studies due to its ability to evaluate vascular as well as nonvascular intrathoracic structures simultaneously and provide an alternative diagnosis that either suggests or supports the final clinical diagnosis in 26% to 67% of examinations.[260,262,265,279,281] Although some have suggested that the presence of such alternative diagnoses adequately excludes PE, other studies have shown that the frequency of alternative diagnoses was the same in patients with and without confirmed PE.[284] Therefore even the presence of an alternative explanation to the patient's symptoms does not necessarily imply that it is safe to withhold anticoagulation, and pursuit of pulmonary angiography may still be appropriate in such patients.

Magnetic Resonance Angiography

MRA is a promising technique in patients with suspected PE, particularly with the use of 3D, gadolinium-enhanced imaging.[161,221,285] The sensitivity and specificity of MRA for the detection of PE are 50% to 100% and 95%, respectively.[151,285,286] The sensitivity is less than 50% for subsegmental PE,[285,286] and overall accuracy is highly dependent on the technique and experience of the interpreting physicians.[286] In cases of suspected pulmonary artery sarcoma, MRI appears to be more useful than CT because the presence of gadolinium enhancement suggests tumor instead of thrombus.[247]

Echocardiography

The sensitivity and specificity of the transesophageal echocardiogram for the detection of central pulmonary artery PE range from 76% to 97% and 77% to 100%, respectively, when compared with helical CT.[287-289] However, the sensitivity for peripheral PE is lower.[288] Echocardiography currently appears to be most useful when assessing patients who are hemodynamically unstable, are unable to undergo helical CT or V/Q scan, and need to have a work-up initiated at the bedside.

Pulmonary Embolism

When a cancer patient is suspected of having PE, a chest radiograph (CXR) should be performed to exclude other conditions that may require immediate intervention such as a central line–related tension pneumothorax, pulmonary hemorrhage, and malignant pleural effusion. However, the CXR should not be used as a means of supporting or refuting the need for specific diagnostic testing for PE. Helical CT is probably best indicated when the CXR is abnormal, and in individuals with known pulmonary disease. Alternatively, if the CXR is normal, a V/Q-scan approach also is appropriate, but it is important

that physicians clearly establish and document their pretest clinical suspicion of PE. Otherwise, PIOPED probability criteria may not be applicable. Regardless of the initial diagnostic approach, an indeterminate or negative initial test result should be followed by a duplex ultrasound of the legs and possibly of the arms as well, particularly in patients with symptoms of pain and swelling or who have an indwelling catheter. A positive duplex ultrasound does not confirm PE, but detection of acute DVT will prompt and justify systemic anticoagulation.

In the cancer patient suspected of having PE, the combination of a nondiagnostic helical CT or V/Q scan with the absence of acute DVT by duplex ultrasound warrants the performance of pulmonary angiography. In this clinical setting, the risks of pulmonary angiography are sufficiently low and are outweighed by the benefits. Pulmonary angiography also is indicated in the setting of a normal spiral CT alone, particularly with a high pretest suspicion.

Treatment of Pulmonary Embolism in Cancer Patients

Most cancer patients with symptomatic PE should be treated with anticoagulation by following the same guidelines for treatment that are applied to DVT.[72,102,290] Initial inpatient intravenous UFH is recommended in symptomatic patients with extensive PE. Some patients, including cancer patients, with PE may derive benefit from thrombolytic therapy to degrade actively the thrombus obstructing the pulmonary vasculature. Clear indications for PE thrombolysis are debated.[291,292] Thrombolysis has been demonstrated to improve survival in patients with massive PE plus shock and is probably indicated in these patients regardless of cancer status. When compared with anticoagulation alone, thrombolytic therapy results

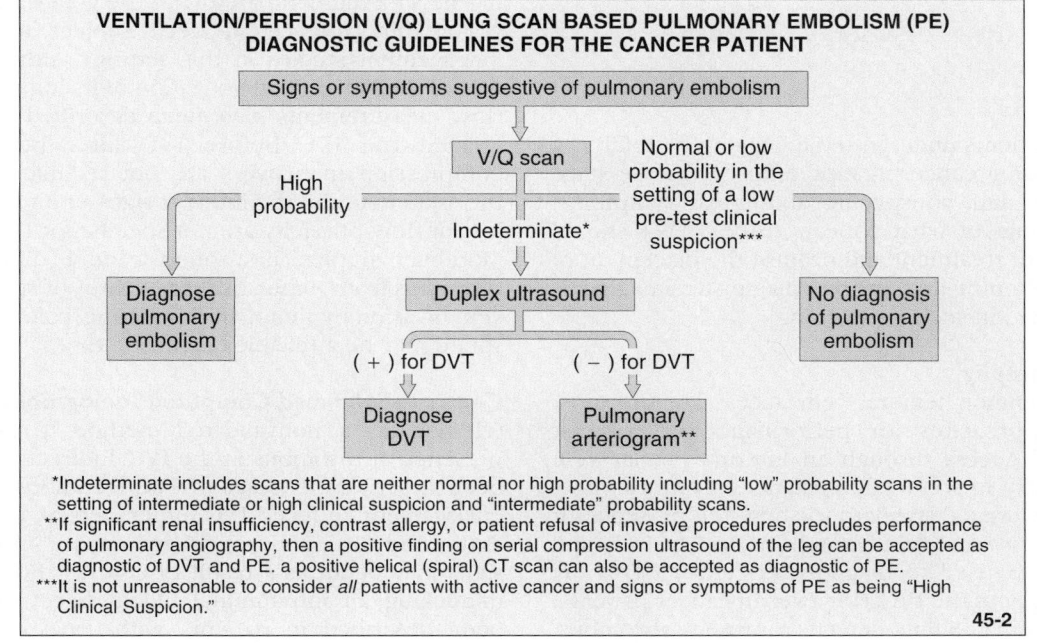

VENTILATION/PERFUSION (V/Q) LUNG SCAN BASED PULMONARY EMBOLISM (PE) DIAGNOSTIC GUIDELINES FOR THE CANCER PATIENT

Signs or symptoms suggestive of pulmonary embolism → V/Q scan

- High probability → Diagnose pulmonary embolism
- Indeterminate* → Duplex ultrasound
  - (+) for DVT → Diagnose DVT
  - (–) for DVT → Pulmonary arteriogram**
- Normal or low probability in the setting of a low pre-test clinical suspicion*** → No diagnosis of pulmonary embolism

*Indeterminate includes scans that are neither normal nor high probability including "low" probability scans in the setting of intermediate or high clinical suspicion and "intermediate" probability scans.
**If significant renal insufficiency, contrast allergy, or patient refusal of invasive procedures precludes performance of pulmonary angiography, then a positive finding on serial compression ultrasound of the leg can be accepted as diagnostic of DVT and PE. a positive helical (spiral) CT scan can also be accepted as diagnostic of PE.
***It is not unreasonable to consider *all* patients with active cancer and signs or symptoms of PE as being "High Clinical Suspicion."

45-2

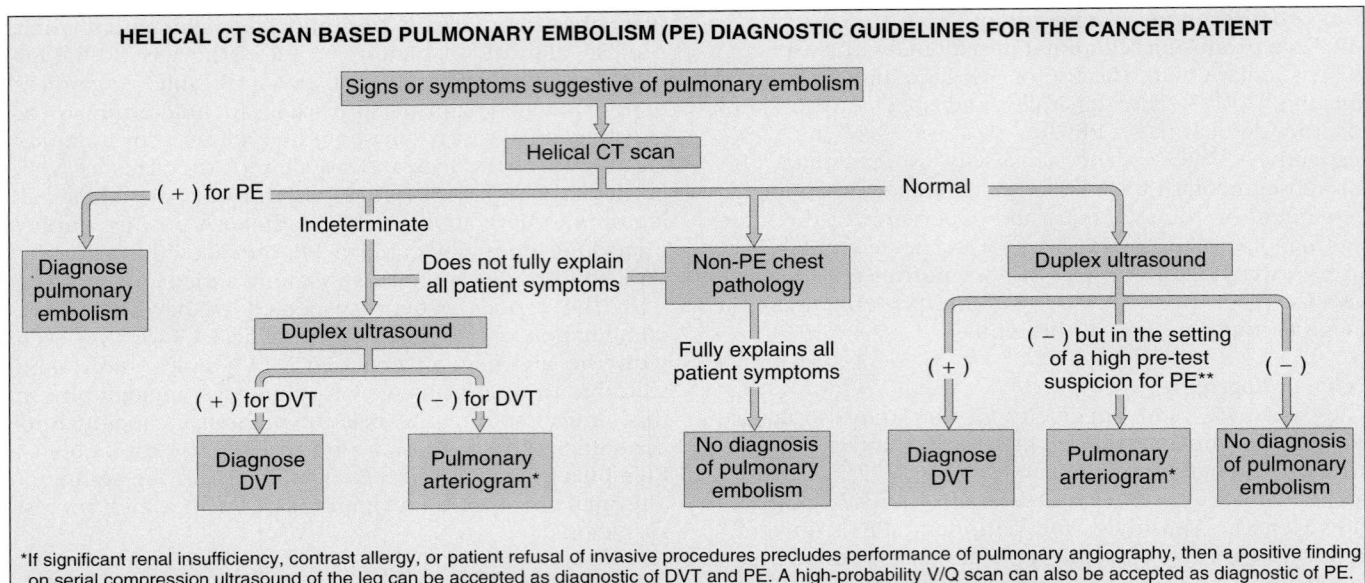

HELICAL CT SCAN BASED PULMONARY EMBOLISM (PE) DIAGNOSTIC GUIDELINES FOR THE CANCER PATIENT

*If significant renal insufficiency, contrast allergy, or patient refusal of invasive procedures precludes performance of pulmonary angiography, then a positive finding on serial compression ultrasound of the leg can be accepted as diagnostic of DVT and PE. A high-probability V/Q scan can also be accepted as diagnostic of PE.
**It is not unreasonable to consider *all* patients with active cancer and signs or symptoms of PE as being "High Clinical Suspicion."

45-3

in more rapid thrombus lysis, an early improvement in pulmonary blood flow, and improvement of right ventricular function.[293] However, these improvements in cardiopulmonary function alone have not resulted in decreased mortality in stable patients without significant hemodynamic compromise. Thrombolysis is contraindicated in any cancer patient with significant transfusion-refractory thrombocytopenia, active bleeding, and CNS lesions.[294]

INFERIOR VENA CAVA AND INTRA-ABDOMINAL DEEP VEIN THROMBOSIS MANAGEMENT

Diagnosis of Inferior Vena Cava and Intra-abdominal Deep Vein Thrombosis in Cancer Patients

Many cancer patients undergo serial imaging with CT as a means of assessing cancer-therapy efficacy, disease stage or progression, and nonspecific abdominal symptoms. Incidental findings of what appears to be a DVT should not affect patient treatment and prompt the placement of an IVC filter. Prompt and proper diagnostic imaging is especially needed in such a situation.

Contrast Venography
Popliteal or common femoral vein access are the most appropriate approaches for performance of contrast cavography.[50,51] Access through an internal jugular vein may be necessary in some circumstances. Contrast venography is the reference standard to show the presence or absence of IVC or renal vein thrombosis conclusively, and the same criteria used to diagnose LE- and UE-DVT by venography apply to the IVC. However, in cancer patients, not all intraluminal filling defects represent thrombus,

and the distinction between intravascular tumor and thrombus may require further investigation with CT or MRI and, in some selected cases, with transvenous catheter-guided biopsy. Likewise, if the column of contrast does not opacify the IVC, CT or MRI is indicated to assess for the presence of extrinsic compression or invasion by tumor. The diagnosis of portal, mesenteric, or ovarian vein thromboses by venography is more challenging because of limited ability to perform selective contrast injections.

Duplex Ultrasound
No studies have validated the use of duplex ultrasound for the detection of IVC thrombosis (i.e., duplex ultrasound has never been compared with the gold-standard contrast venography, nor has it been subject to accuracy or management studies in this setting). Although visualization of the IVC and interrogation of its lumen for Doppler-flow measurements have been described in studies that imaged the IVC before IVC filter placement,[295-298] compression maneuvers are not technically feasible in the abdomen, and the indirect signs of impaired flow and loss of flow phasicity are not specific for IVC thrombosis. Moreover, duplex ultrasound cannot differentiate IVC thrombus from tumor, except in cases of suspected portal vein invasion by tumor. In this setting, color-Doppler ultrasound may be a reliable diagnostic tool.[299]

Contrast-Enhanced Computed Tomography
CT remains a nonvalidated method to assess for the presence of thrombus in the IVC. Indirect signs that have been described in cases of IVC thrombosis include IVC enlargement, reduced IVC lumen density compared with that of the aorta, and rim enhancement.[300] However, these signs may occur as a result of contrast flow phenomena mimicking an intraluminal filling defect and also have been described in patients with renal cell or adrenal

cortical carcinoma extending into the renal veins and IVC, producing a "tumor thrombus."[300-304] Although spiral CT venography has been shown to visualize the intra-abdominal veins accurately,[116] no formal studies have been published. Any incidental finding of an IVC or renal vein "filling defect" by CT should ideally be confirmed by venography and not prompt the initial placement of an IVC filter.

The previously mentioned features also are used in the diagnosis of portal and mesenteric vein thrombosis by CT.[305,306] These signs are of little value in a patient with a history of portal vein thrombosis who is suspected to have a recurrent event. Although the true sensitivity of contrast-enhanced CT in diagnosing portal vein thrombosis is unknown, its specificity has been suggested to be quite high.[305] The presence of cavernous transformation—a "mass-like" network of collateral veins—is suggestive of remote portal vein thrombosis.[305,306]

Only one retrospective case series pertaining to the diagnostic imaging of ovarian vein thrombosis in cancer patients has been published.[307] In this small study, none of the six patients with ovarian DVT had the related CT findings of uterine enlargement and other pelvic masses typically described in larger series of patients with puerperal ovarian DVT.[307] Similar to portal DVT, these indirect CT signs are not useful in a patient with a history of ovarian vein thrombosis, because at least half of the patients will not have normalization of the original CT findings after 3 months to 2 years after the index event.[308]

Magnetic Resonance Venography

MRV is currently considered the diagnostic method of choice for diagnosing IVC, renal, and portal vein thrombosis, particularly when spin-echo and cine MRI techniques are used in combination.[161,169] In a small series of 26 patients with puerperal ovarian DVT, MRV had 100% sensitivity and specificity.[308] Spin-echo MRI may help differentiate acute from chronic thrombus based on differences in patterns of signal intensity.[161,310]

Artifacts created by flow phenomena may cause signal voids at the junction of the renal vein and the IVC because this is an area of slow and convergent blood flow. This may lead to a false-positive diagnosis of IVC thrombosis.[311] MRI also is limited in distinguishing true portal DVT from tumor invasion of the portal vein unless an adjacent mass is seen.[161]

The rare IVC leiomyosarcoma appears to be equally demonstrated by CT or MRI, although MRI is superior because it seems to be capable of differentiating tumor (homogeneous, intermediate signal intensity on T_1-weighted images, and high signal intensity on T_2-weighted images) from thrombus (hyperintense on T_1- and T_2-weighted images).[312-314]

Treatment of Inferior Vena Cava and Intra-abdominal Deep Venous Thrombosis in Cancer Patients

No specific guidelines exist for the treatment of IVC and other intraabdominal DVT in the cancer patient or noncancer patient. Whether to use standard anticoagulant therapy as is used for proximal LE-DVT or catheter-directed thrombolytic therapy depends on the extent of thrombosis, patient symptoms, and patient bleeding risk. Patients with acute, complete IVC occlusion may develop significant bilateral LE swelling and pain and are at risk for phlegmasia cerulean dolens (venous limb gangrene). Such patients may benefit most from pharmacologic or mechanical thrombolysis. Long-term anticoagulation is likely warranted.

SUPERFICIAL THROMBOPHLEBITIS MANAGEMENT

Diagnosis of Superficial Thrombophlebitis in Cancer Patients

Superficial venous thrombophlebitis (SVT) is the only manifestation of venous thromboembolic disease that does not require objective diagnostic imaging. The diagnosis can be made clinically by the detection of a palpable tender cord in the course of a superficial vein; the induration of the vein is usually associated with erythema of the overlying skin.[315] The clinical differential diagnosis includes sarcoidal granulomas, Kaposi's sarcoma, and lymphangitis.[315]

Duplex ultrasound should be considered to rule out concomitant DVT, particularly when the greater or lesser saphenous veins are involved. The most common location for progression from SVT to DVT to occur is at the junction between the greater saphenous vein (a superficial leg vein) and the common femoral vein (a proximal deep leg vein). Proximity of an SVT to the junction between the involved superficial vein and its connection to the deep venous system does not seem to affect the likelihood of PE. The rates of DVT in patients with clinical signs and symptoms of isolated SVT have been reported to range from 6% to 57%,[316-320] and the rates of symptomatic PE have been reported to range from 4% to 10%.[316,317,321]

Trousseau's syndrome or migratory thrombophlebitis was initially described in patients with mucin-secreting carcinoma of the gastrointestinal tract.[315] It is unclear whether the "thrombophlebitis" in many of the reported cases was manifested as SVT or DVT. The SVT related to Trousseau's syndrome typically was first seen as multiple tender nodules, which progressed to form palpable cords, usually involving the bilateral LEs and, on occasion, the UE veins and the abdominal wall veins as well.[315,322]

Treatment of Superficial Thrombophlebitis in Cancer Patients

Typically, nonsteroidal anti-inflammatory drugs and warm compresses are adequate treatment for SVT symptom control. When the deep system is involved or symptomatic pulmonary embolism is diagnosed, standard anticoagulant therapy is indicated. Because of the reported high rate of progression from SVT to DVT, many physicians treat SVT with anticoagulants for a variable time. Anticoagulants like UFH and LMWH may help relieve symptoms related to vessel inflammation but are probably best reserved for individuals with recurrent SVT or documented DVT. Serial ultrasound to detect meaningful SVT progression seems prudent in selected cases such as those with SVT already at the saphenofemoral junction.

INFERIOR VENA CAVA FILTERS

IVC filters are often placed in cancer patients with acute VTE, especially in the settings of thrombocytopenia, active bleeding, and CNS malignancy.[323-325] Limitations to IVC filters include technical difficulties during insertion, insertion-site hemorrhage or thrombosis, caval thrombosis and obstruction below the filter, filter change of position (migration or tilting), caval erosion and perforation, and filter failure.[326,327] IVC filters obviously play no role in the management of UE-DVT. SVC filter placement has been shown to be technically feasible, but outcomes data are lacking.[328] A recent study published by Decousus and associates[329] addressed the impact of IVC filter placement on PE prevention and DVT recurrence rate. All patients had proximal DVT, and all received anticoagulation. Placement of an IVC filter conferred a significant benefit in preventing PE within the first 12 days after DVT, with PE developing in 4.8% of patients without filters compared with 1.1% with filters ($P = .03$). At 2 years' follow-up, however, the benefit was no longer statistically significant with regard to symptomatic PE prevention. Moreover, at 2 years, those patients with prophylactic filter placement had a higher risk of DVT recurrence than did those who did not have a filter placed (20.8% vs. 11.6%; $P = .02$).[329] These findings underscore the need for caution in placing filters, especially when patients are receiving cancer treatment with a curative intent, and long-term survival is contemplated. When a filter is placed because of a transient contraindication to anticoagulation, appropriate pharmacologic therapy should be commenced once the contraindication has passed.

VENOUS THROMBOSIS PREVENTION IN THE CANCER PATIENT

The relation between cancer and clinical thrombosis has been recognized for more than 150 years. The concept of and an appreciation of thromboprophylaxis have been widely accepted, primarily in the surgical setting, for more than 25 years. However, only in the last decade has the widespread application of thromboprophylaxis to patients with cancer begun to receive significant attention from the medical community. One of the observations driving this level of interest is the expanding body of data suggesting that the connection between thrombosis and cancer may well be a "two-way street."

In the not-too-distant past, the prevailing opinion was that cancer caused thrombosis and that, although it was a regrettable complication, thrombosis did not significantly affect the overall clinical course of the patient with cancer. The interactions between cancer and thrombosis may not be as simple as that. Take the time-honored observation that in an inordinate number of patients with

idiopathic VTE, cancer develops in the subsequent several months[330]; extend the follow-up for several years, and one finds that the rate of malignancy continues to increase inordinately in this population for at least 6 years, with no evidence of a plateau developing in the curve.[331] Although it is conceivable that some aspect of an occult malignancy (even one that does not become clinically apparent for 6 years) promotes thrombosis, it is equally conceivable that some pathophysiologic element related to the thrombosis, itself, may promote the development or progression of the cancer. If this were true, then it would logically follow that alterations in the biology of thrombosis might alter the likelihood of subsequent malignancy.

Data from randomized clinical trials support this hypothesis. Patients who receive oral warfarin secondary prophylaxis for 6 months after an idiopathic VTE have a lower rate of subsequent malignancy over the ensuing 6 years than do patients randomized to receive only 6 weeks of anticoagulation.[331] Not only does it appear that thrombosis may, through mechanisms unknown, predispose to the development of cancer, but the presence of thrombosis[332] or even evidence of activation of coagulation without overt thrombosis[33] also is associated with more aggressive behavior of the associated malignancies. This body of data, taken to its logical conclusion, allows the development of a hypothesis that thromboprophylaxis could be used for both primary prevention of and treatment of some forms of cancer. Add to this the facts that standard anticoagulation treatment of acute VTE is less efficacious and more toxic in cancer patients compared with noncancer patients (see previous sections) and that the risk of death from PE may be higher in cancer patients than in noncancer patients,[333,334] and it becomes clear that prevention of thrombosis is clinically important in patients with cancer. To date, the available data on thromboprophylaxis specifically in cancer patients is derived mainly from studies whose major endpoints included the incidence of any (primarily asymptomatic) DVT rather than more meaningful endpoints such as disease progression, fatal PE, and survival. However, with meta-analysis, heparin thromboprophylaxis that was successful in preventing asymptomatic DVT in patients without cancer has been shown to prevent both symptomatic DVT and fatal PE.[335] Therefore it is reasonable to infer that any intervention that prevents asymptomatic DVT also prevents clinically significant thromboembolic disease in patients with cancer. Data discussed earlier also raise the possibility that thromboprophylaxis in the cancer patient may modify the course of the malignancy in a favorable manner. Consequently, comments contained in the remainder of this section are based on the assumption that thromboprophylaxis (operationally defined as any intervention that prevents asymptomatic DVT) is clinically useful and should be used in cancer patients in several common, clinically defined situations.

Thromboprophylaxis in Surgical Oncology

Most studies of surgical thromboprophylaxis, such as those focusing on elective joint replacement, have not differentiated between patients with and without underlying malignancy. Consequently, the quantitative risk added by the presence of cancer to each and every type of surgical procedure is unknown. Despite this, any patient older than 40 years undergoing any major surgery in the setting of active or prior cancer has been categorized by the American College of Chest Physicians Consensus Conference on Antithrombotic Therapy as being in the "highest risk" group of patients, with an estimated risk of proximal DVT of 10% to 20% and fatal PE of 0.2% to 5.0% without thromboprophylaxis.[336]

Two basic methods of thromboprophylaxis have been widely studied in surgical patients: mechanical and pharmacologic. For practical purposes in surgical oncology, mechanical forms of prophylaxis are limited to external pneumatic compression (EPC) boots, whereas pharmacologic methods are limited to heparin derivatives.

EPC has been found to provide a modest degree of efficacy in surgical oncology, with ultrasound-defined failure rates varying from 1% in gynecologic oncology patients[337] to 14% in cancer patients undergoing orthopedic procedures.[338] Assuming they are applied correctly 100% of the time, EPC boots are a cost-effective form of prophylaxis during and after high-risk gynecologic oncology procedures.[339] Unfortunately, the assumption of proper application of EPC devices 100% of the time is generally incorrect in practice, with rates of 33% being more common.[340] In evaluation of the efficacy of EPC in gynecologic surgery, the presence of cancer has been found to be an independent risk factor for failure, with a relative risk of DVT of 4.9 compared with noncancer patients.[341] EPC as the sole method of prophylaxis is not recommended for the "highest risk" patients[336] and should not be relied on for most surgical procedures performed on cancer patients.

Heparins form the mainstay of pharmacologic methods of thromboprophylaxis, although other medications, most notably the oral direct thrombin inhibitor ximelagatran, may begin to play a major role in the near future.[342] The efficacy of UFH and its derivatives has been studied primarily in noncancer patients undergoing surgery. The first major investigation of the efficacy of heparin in curative cancer surgery was a prospective, randomized, double-blind study comparing subcutaneous UFH, 5000 units 3 times daily, with subcutaneous enoxaparin, 40 mg once daily, begun 2 hours before surgery.[343] Contrast venography within 24 hours of the last drug injection (10 ± 2 days) was scheduled to be performed in all patients. Of 1116 randomized patients, 319 UFH-treated patients and 312 enoxaparin-treated patients were evaluable. Total VTE, symptomatic DVT, and any DVT were detected in 18.2%, 1.9%, and 17.6% of the UFH-treated patients and in 14.7%, 1.3%, and 14.4% of the enoxaparin-treated group. These rates of thrombosis are more than twice that generally seen in noncancer patients undergoing general surgery receiving the same medications and evaluated with the same endpoints.[336] As the data demonstrate, most detected thromboses were asymptomatic (any DVT minus symptomatic DVT). To deal with the high failure rate of pharmacologic thromboprophylaxis in this group of patients, two different, and not mutually exclusive,

approaches could be taken: (1) find a way to improve in-hospital efficacy, and/or (2) find a way to prevent these asymptomatic thrombi from propagating and posing a risk of death after hospital discharge. The first approach might be accomplished by combining mechanical and pharmacologic methods of prophylaxis. This approach has been shown to be valid in noncancer patients by using EPC and graduated-compression stockings combined with UFH or LMWH[344,345] and has shown promise in patients undergoing craniotomy for brain tumors.[346] The second approach might be accomplished by extending the duration of thromboprophylaxis sufficiently long that the asymptomatic thromboses fail to propagate, fail to embolize, and successfully undergo spontaneous thrombolysis. This approach has been recently found to be valid as well.

A similar group of patients undergoing planned curative open surgery for abdominal or pelvic cancer were all given enoxaparin, 40 mg once daily for 6 to 10 days, and subsequently randomized to 21 additional days of enoxaparin at the same dose or 21 days of placebo.[347] Bilateral venography was performed between days 25 and 31 after surgery, and patients were clinically followed up for a total of 3 months after surgery. A total of 501 patients were randomized with 332 patients included in the efficacy analysis. The group randomized to enoxaparin had a 4.8% rate of any DVT at 4 weeks compared with 12.0% in the placebo group (P = .02). The majority of detected DVTs were asymptomatic and involved calf veins. Approximately 1.5% of patients in both groups had clinically apparent VTE in the 2 months of follow-up with no prophylaxis (an annualized rate of 9%, roughly 90 times that of the normal population).[347] Taken in total, these data suggest that the following scheme should be strongly considered for all cancer patients undergoing major surgery:

- All should be given combined EPC and prophylactic-intensity LMWH during hospitalization (unless contraindicated by renal insufficiency or a history of heparin-induced thrombocytopenia)
- All should be given LMWH in prophylactic doses for 3 weeks after hospitalization (with the same caveats)
- Extended thromboprophylaxis with prophylactic doses of LMWH or warfarin should be given for those with continuing risk factors for VTE, such as chemotherapy, infection, paralysis, and use of central venous catheters

Prevention of Central Venous Access Device–Associated Thrombosis

The quantitative scope of the problem of central venous catheter–related UE, internal jugular, and thoracic vein thrombosis depends on the method of detection. The incidence ranges from 2.4% to 35% if only symptomatic events are considered[348-357] and from 36% to 66% if surveillance venography is used to detect all thromboses.[348,349,358,359] By consensus, a "high risk" of DVT is present when the frequency of proximal vein thrombosis is between 4% and 8%.[336] This places cancer patients with central venous catheters at "high risk" of thrombosis. These thrombi are not benign, having at least a 25% incidence of asymptomatic PE.[360] Given that PE is a significant cause of death among cancer patients, central venous catheter–related DVT must be considered a potentially lethal problem.

In addition to their shared relation with PE, central venous catheter–related DVTs also pose clinical problems different from those seen with LE-DVT. As with leg-vein DVT, not all central venous catheter–related thromboses undergo complete physiologic thrombolysis. An unknown fraction undergo organization and remain as a permanent obstruction to the involved veins. These organized thrombi prevent insertion of subsequent catheters at that vascular site, such as at the time of tumor relapse, from 14% to 30% of the time.[358,361] Central venous catheter–related thrombi also can be a nidus for infection. The risk of sepsis in patients with central venous catheter–related DVT is 2.62 times that of patients with catheters but without thrombosis.[362]

By consensus, the "gold standard" for determining efficacy of any method of thromboprophylaxis is the randomized clinical trial using contrast venography–documented thrombosis as an endpoint.[336] Studies using purely clinical endpoints are generally not used in this context. Both fixed-dose warfarin (1 mg daily, beginning 3 days before catheter placement) and fixed-dose subcutaneous LMWH (dalteparin, 2500 units daily, and nadroparin, 2850 units daily) have been studied by using surveillance venography and found to be effective.[348,360,363] Reported rates of thrombosis in the active therapy groups were in the 6% to 10% range. In large studies monitoring for symptomatic venous thrombosis, fixed-dose warfarin was effective compared with placebo, reducing the incidence from 13% to 4.3%.[351] A smaller and probably underpowered study using clinical endpoints failed to find efficacy with this dose of warfarin.[364] None of the studies has shown toxicity with these methods of prophylaxis, although while receiving antibiotic therapy, patients taking fixed-dose of warfarin often had sufficiently long prothrombin times that a bleeding risk was probable.[349] During times of acute illness, especially when using antibiotics, prothrombin time monitoring is recommended in patients receiving the dose of 1 mg/day warfarin.

In addition to prevention of thrombosis, these methods of prophylaxis have been estimated to reduce the incidence of bacteremia and sepsis, with a relative risk of 0.26 compared with no prophylaxis.[365] Because of the high risk of thrombosis and the demonstrated efficacy, expert consensus has recommended use of either 1 mg of warfarin daily or prophylactic doses of LMWH in patients with central venous catheters.[336] Despite the data and expert recommendations, thromboprophylaxis is still not widely used.[366] This is an area with significant room for improvement in clinical practice.

Prevention of Central Venous Access Device–Associated Thrombotic Occlusion

Very little work has been directed at finding methods of prevention of central venous catheter thrombotic occlusion. Thrombotic occlusion can manifest as the inability to infuse, inability to withdraw, or a combination of the two, known as total occlusion. The methods used to prevent central venous catheter–associated DVT have not been evaluated for efficacy in prevention of catheter obstruction. Although it is widely held that "heparin flushing" and "meticulous catheter care" prevent this problem, no experimental data support this contention. Indeed, retrospective data suggest that heparin flushing does not prevent thrombotic catheter occlusion.[367] Heparin flushing of catheters does, however, have demonstrable toxicity in the form of HIT and thrombosis.[368] Fortunately, for those patients experiencing thrombotic catheter obstruction, a readily available and highly effective therapy is available. Thrombolytic therapy with low-dose recombinant tissue-type plasminogen activator instilled into the obstructed catheter has roughly a 90% likelihood of restoring catheter function at 4 hours. Consequently, in the face of limited data on efficacy, infrequent but potentially severe toxicity, and highly effective salvage therapy, routine flushing of catheters with UFH to prevent occlusion cannot be recommended. Flushing of catheters with normal saline after each use is suggested as a preferable alternative to heparin flushing.

The only parameter that has been found to affect rates of thrombotic catheter occlusion is the anatomic location of the catheter tip. Catheters whose tips have been placed in the innominate vein have an inordinate incidence of thrombosis,[369] especially compared with those whose tips are in the lower portion of the SVC or right atrium.[370] Use of intraoperative guide-wire measurement or alternative techniques to assure that the catheter tip is placed in the lowest third of the SVC is recommended.

Thromboprophylaxis during Chemotherapy

Chemotherapy is an independent risk factor for both VTE[371,372] and death within 1 week of VTE,[335] above and beyond that conferred by the presence of cancer alone. Unfortunately, the absolute risk of VTE conferred has been studied only in a relative few of the many chemotherapy regimens used to treat the wide spectrum of known malignant diseases. The absolute risk of VTE varies from 1.3% per year with tamoxifen only to 7.9% per year with tamoxifen combined with CMF (cyclophosphamide, methotrexate, and 5-fluorouracil) as adjuvant therapy for breast cancer[45] to as much as 43% during shorter-duration therapy of a variety of malignancies with thalidomide-containing regimens.[47,373] The 0.1% per year risk in the general population pales in comparison to these rates of VTE.

Despite the growing recognition of chemotherapy as a risk for VTE, little has been done to evaluate the role of primary thromboprophylaxis. The only trial to evaluate prophylaxis formally in the setting of systemic therapy for randomized breast cancer patients on active therapy with either warfarin, 1 mg daily for the first 6 months, followed by adjusted-dose warfarin to achieve an INR between 1.5 and 1.9 or placebo. The study compared the rates of clinically detected VTE over a mean of 6 months.[374] Active therapy reduced the incidence of VTE from 4.4% to 0.7%, with no differences in the rates of major bleeding complications. This intervention did not increase the costs of medical care for these patients.[375] Secondary prophylaxis (prevention of recurrence after the initial episode of VTE) by using warfarin in therapeutic doses has been effective in a limited number of patients taking thalidomide,[47] suggesting that standard methods of thromboprophylaxis may be effective in a spectrum of chemotherapy regimens. In short, this phenomenon of chemotherapy-related VTE has not been given the attention it deserves, given the potential scope of the problem. Despite this, because of the low toxicities of current thromboprophylactic measures, it seems reasonable to recommend either warfarin in doses to prolong the INR to 1.5 to 1.9 or prophylactic doses of LMWH for patients receiving chemotherapy regimens associated with a meaningful increased risk of VTE.

Thromboprophylaxis for the Hospitalized Cancer Patient

Being sufficiently ill to require hospitalization for any reason is associated with a 100-fold increase in the risk of VTE[376] and an 18-fold increase in the risk of death within 1 week of VTE[335] compared with community residents. Patients hospitalized for medical illness account for almost 23% of all cases of VTE.[372] Hospitalization for medical illness complicating cancer further increases the risk of VTE.[372,377] Patients with cancer hospitalized for non-surgical illness account for almost 30% of all cases of VTE,[371] making this population a prime target for the use of thromboprophylaxis.

Thromboprophylaxis has not been studied specifically in medically ill cancer patients. Inferences must be made from studies of a wide spectrum of patients with medical illnesses, some of whom have cancer. In this population, meta-analysis has shown that thromboprophylaxis with UFH or LMWH is associated with a more than 50% reduction in symptomatic DVT and PE without an increase in bleeding complications.[378] The first and only prospective, randomized, controlled trial of thromboprophylaxis in this group of patients using the gold standard of contrast venography endpoint randomized 866 patients (14% of whom had cancer) to receive either placebo or one of two doses of enoxaparin (20 mg daily or 40 mg daily) during their hospitalization.[379] At the time of discharge, DVT had developed in approximately 15% in the placebo group and the group randomized to receive 20 mg of enoxaparin daily but only in 5.5% in the group randomized to receive 40 mg of enoxaparin daily, a risk reduction of more than 60% that was highly statistically significant. This population of medically ill patients was at high risk of bleeding complications. As a group, 1.3% experienced major hemorrhage during their hospitalization (a median of 7 days). The use of enoxaparin was not associated with an increase in this basal rate of major hemorrhage. This therapy was associated with a small increase in the cost of hospitalization but may actually be cost effective if one considers the savings from not having to treat as many new VTEs.[380] These data strongly suggest that all hospitalized cancer patients receive thromboprophylaxis with an LMWH (preferably 40 mg of enoxaparin daily)

unless contraindicated by either severe renal insufficiency or a history of HIT.

Chemotherapy-related thrombocytopenia, intracranial malignancy, and gastrointestinal lesions have been perceived by some physicians as contraindications to the use of prophylactic doses of LMWH. Whereas no data formally evaluate the safety of prophylactic LMWH in these high-risk situations, inferences can be made from several sources. Patients undergoing elective neuro-surgery, including surgery for intracranial malignancy, have an incidence of bleeding similar to that of hospitalized medical patients (approximately 2% to 3%).[346,381] This rate of bleeding was not increased with the use of 40 mg of enoxaparin daily.[381] Patients undergoing curative abdominal and pelvic surgery for cancer do not have an increased rate of bleeding complications with the use of this dose of enoxaparin.[343] From these data, it appears that the use of prophylactic doses of LMWH is unlikely to pose an additive risk of bleeding over that inherent with the underlying disease. Consequently, unless the extent of the intracranial or gastrointestinal disease or the degree and duration of thrombocytopenia is great, these comorbidities pose only a relative, and probably small, contraindication to the use of pharmacologic thromboprophylaxis. In situations in which this type of prophylaxis is perceived to be contraindicated, use of EPC and/or periodic ultrasound surveillance[382] is strongly recommended.

In the previously mentioned thromboprophylaxis trial,[379] all patients were monitored for the development of symptomatic VTE for 3 months after discharge. In approximately 1% of the patients, symptomatic DVT or PE developed during this time: roughly 40 times the incidence of VTE in the general population. This incidence is similar to that seen in the 3-month follow-up of patients undergoing curative surgery for cancer,[347] where prolonged use of enoxaparin after discharge has been shown to be safe and effective in prevention of DVT. These data suggest that the risk of VTE does not end as the patient passes out through the doors of the hospital, but continues for a protracted period. Extended thromboprophylaxis, as used in cancer surgery, should be strongly considered, especially in patients whose in-hospital cancer therapy has not been completely curative.

FUTURE PROSPECTS

As more and more oncologists become aware of the importance and challenges of clinical thrombosis in patients with malignancy, we will likely see more attention paid to earlier venous thrombosis diagnosis, optimization of acute and chronic venous thrombosis management, and greater compliance with thromboprophylaxis recommendations. We hope venous thrombosis will be viewed less as simply a nuisance during the care of cancer patients and more as a major source of patient morbidity, treatment delay, and mortality.

Continued improvements in duplex ultrasound, CT, and MRI are expected. The ability to "scan" the pulmonary vasculature, abdominal vasculature, pelvic veins, and lower extremities with one contrast injection and one imaging session will likely be perfected. This will provide a more comprehensive approach to thrombosis confirmation and limit intravenous contrast exposure. Nuclear medicine scans capable of whole-body thrombus imaging are on the horizon and may even assist with the detection of occult malignancy in patients with an initial idiopathic VTE. Integration of diagnostic algorithms into one's oncology practice may assist the busy clinician with decision making in the setting of suspected DVT and PE.

We foresee continued interest in developing improved strategies to treat VTE specifically in the cancer patient. Further reduction in both thrombosis recurrence rates and bleeding rates is needed. Prospective clinical trials are needed to support the long-term anticoagulation of the cancer patient with thrombosis. In particular, optimal management of the women with thrombosis and the need for years of adjuvant hormonal therapy for breast cancer must be clarified. Despite excellent compliance with daily subcutaneous LMWH for up to 6 months of VTE therapy, newer oral anticoagulants may make long-term anticoagulation more palatable to all patient populations. Ximelagatran, an oral direct thrombin inhibitor, has been shown to be effective for the treatment of VTE in phase III trials and may be approved for use in chronic atrial fibrillation in the near future. Consistent reports of reversible liver function test abnormalities in up to 6% to 10% of treated patients may limit use in cancer patients prone to liver metastases and those receiving hepatically metabolized chemotherapeutic agents. Further research into the anticancer and survival-prolongation properties of selected anticoagulants may identify a particular agent or class of agents as being ideal in cancer patients, in general, or in those with specific responsive tumor histologies.

Prevention will continue to be of paramount importance. It is always easier and less potentially toxic to prevent thromboses with low doses of anticoagulation than to treat life-threatening thromboses with longer courses of higher doses of the same drugs. Ongoing research attempting to link thrombisis with accelerated tumor neovascularization, growth, and metastases may highlight the importance and value of aggressive primary thrombosis prevention in all cancer patients. Time and significant research efforts will tell.

REFERENCES

1. Prandoni P, Piccioli A, Girolami A: Cancer and venous thromboembolism: An overview. Haematologica 1999;84:437–445.
2. Brill-Edwards P, Ginsberg JS, Johnston M, Hirsh J: Establishing a therapeutic range for heparin therapy. Ann Intern Med 1993;119:104–109.
3. Hansson PO, Welin L, Tibblin G, et al: Deep vein thrombosis and pulmonary embolism in the general population: "The Study of Men Born in 1913." Arch Intern Med 1997;157:1665–1670.
4. Sorensen HT, Mellemkjaer L, Steffensen FH, Olsen JH, Nielsen GL: The risk of a diagnosis of cancer after primary deep venous thrombosis or pulmonary embolism. N Engl J Med 1998;338:1169–1173.
5. Levitan N, Dowlati A, Remick SC, et al: Rates of initial and recurrent thromboembolic disease among patients with malignancy versus those without malignancy: Risk analysis using Medicare claims data. Medicine 1999;78:285–291.
6. Kakkar VV, Howe CT, Nicolaides AN, Renney JT, Clarke MB: Deep vein thrombosis of the leg: Is there a "high risk" group? Am J Surg 1970;120:527–530.
7. Walsh JJ, Bonnar J, Wright FW: A study of pulmonary embolism and deep leg vein thrombosis after major gynaecological surgery using labeled fibrinogen-phlebography and lung scanning. J Obstet Gynaecol Br Commonw 1974;81:311–316.
8. Piccioli A, Prandoni P, Ewenstein BM, Goldhaber SZ: Cancer and venous thromboembolism. Am Heart J 1996;132:850–855.
9. Luzzatto G, Schafer AI: The prothrombotic state in cancer. Semin Oncol 1990;17:147–159.
10. Gomes MPV, Deitcher SR: Diagnosis of venous thromboembolic disease in cancer patients. Oncology (Huntingt) 2003;17:126–135, 139.
11. Deitcher SR, Goldman CK, Ruiter K: Vascular endothelial growth factor (VEGF) levels in patients with idiopathic acute proximal deep venous thrombosis. Thromb Haemost 86(suppl):1517.
12. Breddin HK, Hach-Wunderle V, Nakov R, Kakkar VV: Effects of a low-molecular-weight heparin on thrombus regression and recurrent thromboembolism in patients with deep-vein thrombosis. N Engl J Med 2001;344:626–631.
13. Krauth D, Holden A, Knapic N, Liepman M, Ansell J: Safety and efficacy of long-term oral anticoagulation in cancer patients. Cancer 1987;59:983–985.
14. Heit JA, Mohr DN, Silverstein MD, Petterson TM, O'Fallon WM, Melton LJ: Predictors of recurrence after deep vein thrombosis and pulmonary embolism: A population-based cohort study. Arch Intern Med 2000;160:761–768.
15. Hansson PO, Sorbo J, Eriksson H: Recurrent venous thromboembolism after deep vein thrombosis incidence and risk factors. Arch Intern Med 2000;160:769–774.
16. Prandoni P, Lensing AW, Cogo A, et al: The long term clinical course of acute deep venous thrombosis. Ann Intern Med 1996;125:1–7.
17. Prandoni P: Antithrombotic strategies in patients with cancer. Thromb Haemost 1997;78:141–144.
18. Prandoni P, Lensing AW, Piccioli A, et al: Recurrent venous thromboembolism and bleeding complications during anticoagulant treatment in patients with cancer and venous thrombosis. Blood 2002;100:3484–3488.
19. Bona RD, Sivjee KY, Hickey AD, Wallace SB, Wajcs SB: The efficacy and safety of oral anticoagulation in patients with cancer. Thromb Haemost 1995;74:1055–1058.
20. Bona RD, Hickey AD, Wallace DM: Efficacy and safety of oral anticoagulation in patients with cancer. Thromb Haemost 1997;78:137–140.
21. Hutten BA, Prins MH, Gent M, Ginsberg J, Tijssen JGP, Buller HR: Incidence of recurrent thromboembolic and bleeding complications among patients with venous thromboembolism in relation to both malignancy and achieve international normalized ratio: A retrospective analysis. J Clin Oncol 2000;8:3078–3083.
22. Ottinger H, Belka C, Kozole G, et al: Deep venous thrombosis and pulmonary embolism in high-grade non Hodgkin's lymphoma: Incidence, causes and prognostic relevance. Eur J Haematol 1995;54:186–194.
23. Levine MN: Prevention of thrombotic disorders in cancer patients undergoing chemotherapy. Thromb Haemost 1997;78:133–136.
24. Edwards RL, Silver J, Rickles FR: Human tumor procoagulants: Registry of the Subcommittee on Haemostasis and Malignancy of the Scientific and Standardization Committee, International Society on Thrombosis and Haemostasis. Thromb Haemost 1993;69:205–213.
25. Falanga A, Donati MB: Pathogenesis of thrombosis in patients with malignancy. Int J Hematol 2001;73:137–144.
26. Gordon S: Cancer cell procoagulants and their implications. Hematol Oncol Clin North Am 1992;6:1359–1374.
27. Rickles FR, Hair GA, Zeff RA, Lee E, Bona RD: Tissue factor expression in human leukocytes and tumor cells. Thromb Haemost 1995;74:391–395.
28. Bevilacqua MP, Pober JS, Majeau GR, Fiers W, Cotran RS, Gimbrone MA: Recombinant tumor necrosis factor induces procoagulant activity in cultured human vascular endothelium: Characterization and comparison with the actions of interleukin-1. Proc Natl Acad Sci USA 1996;83:4533–4537.

29. Deitcher SR, Carman TL, Sheikj M, Gomes M: Hypercoagulable syndromes: Evaluation and management strategies in acute limb ischemia. Semin Vasc Surg 2001;14:74-85.

30. Deitcher SR, Lucore C, Eisenberg PR: Impaired resolution of a massive pulmonary embolus associated with an impaired fibrinolytic response. Am J Med 1994;96:483-484.

31. Deitcher SR, Erban JK, Limentani SA: Acquired free protein S deficiency asociated with multiple myeloma. Am J Hematol 1996;51:319-323.

32. Fareed J, Hoppensteadt D, Lietz H, Tobu M, Cort S, Deitcher S: Multifactorial etiology of cancer associated venous thrombosis: Results from the baseline profiling of cancer patients recruited in a study for the secondary prevention of venous thrombosis with a low molecular weight heparin (ONCENOX). Proc Am Soc Clin Oncol 2002;22:741(abstr 2979)

33. Beer JH, Haeberli A, Vogt A, et al: Coagulation markers predict survival in cancer patients. Thromb Haemost 2002;88:745-749.

34. Anderson AJ, Krasnow SH, Boyer MW, et al: Thrombosis: The major Hickman catheter complication in patients with solid tumor. Chest 1989;95:71-75.

35. Bona RD: Thrombotic complication of central catheters in cancer patients. Semin Thromb Hemost 1999;25:147-157.

36. Gould JR, Carloss HW, Skinner WL: Groshong catheter-associated subclavian venous thrombosis. Am J Med 1993;95:419-423.

37. Kee ST, Kinoshita L, Razavi MK, Nyman CP, Semba CP, Dake MD: Superior vena cava syndrome: Treatment with catheter-directed thrombolysis and endovascular stent placement. Radiology 1998;206:187-193.

38. Patel V, Igwebe T, Mast H, Karetzky MS: Superior vena cava syndrome; current concepts of management. N Engl J Med 1995;92:245-248.

39. Prandoni P, Polistena P, Bernardi E, et al: Upper extremity deep vein thrombosis: Risk factors, diagnosis, and complications. Arch Intern Med 1997;157:57-62.

40. Raad II, Luna M, Khalil SA, Costerton JW, Lam C, Bodey GP: The relationship between the thrombotic and infectious complications of central venous catheters. JAMA 1994;271:1014-1016.

41. Goodnough LT, Saito H, Manni A, Jones PK, Pearson OH: Increased incidence of thromboembolism in stage-4 breast cancer patients treated with a five-drug chemotherapy regimen: A study of 159 patients. Cancer 1984;54:1264-1268.

42. Gail MH, Costantino JP, Bryant J, et al: Weighing the risks and benefits of tamoxifen treatment for preventing breast cancer. J Natl Cancer Inst 1999;91:1829-1846.

43. Saphner T, Tormey DC, Gray R: Venous and arterial thrombosis in patients who received adjuvant therapy for breast cancer. J Clin Oncol 1991;9:286-294.

44. Levine MN, Gent M, Hirsh J, et al: The thrombogenic effect of anticancer drug therapy in women with stage-2 breast cancer. N Engl J Med 1988;318:404-407.

45. Pritchard KI, Paterson AH, Paul NA, Zee B, Fine S, Pater J: Increased thromboembolic complications with concurrent tamoxifen and chemotherapy in a randomized trial of adjuvant therapy for women with breast cancer: National Cancer Institute of Canada Clinical Trials Group Breast Cancer Site Group. J Clin Oncol 1996;14:2731-2737.

46. Zangari M, Siegel E, Anaissie E, et al: Risk factors for deep vein thrombosis in a large group of myeloma patients treated with thalidomide: The Arkansas Experience. Blood 2001;98:161a.

47. Zangari M, Anaissie E, Barlogie B, et al: Increased risk of deep-vein thrombosis in patients with multiple myeloma receiving thalidomide and chemotherapy. Blood 2001;98:1614-1615.

48. Hoppensteadt D, Fareed J, Lietz H, Tobu M, Cort S, Deitcher S: Malignancy related thrombotic state is independent of defects in factor V Leiden, prothrombin 20210 and MTHFR: Results from the initial profiling of cancer patients enrolled in the ONCENOX trial. Proc Am Soc Clin Oncol 2003;22:861(abst 3461).

49. Hull RD, Raskob GE, Brant RF, et al: The importance of initial heparin treatment on long-term clinical outcomes of antithrombotic therapy: the emerging theme of delayed recurrence. Arch Intern Med 1997;157:2317-2321.

50. Gallus AS, Hirsh J, Hull R, van Aken WG: Diagnosis of venous thromboembolism. Semin Thromb Hemost 1976;2:203-231.

51. Hull R, Raskob G, Leclerc J, et al: The diagnosis of clinically suspected venous thrombosis. Clin Chest Med 1984;5:439-456.

52. Sandler DA, Martin JF: Liquid crystal thermography as a screening test for deep-vein thrombosis. Lancet 1985;1:665-667.

53. Hull R, Hirsh J, Sackett DL, et al: Clinical validity of a negative venogram in patients with clinically suspected venous thrombosis. Circulation 1981;64:622-625.

54. Cranley JJ, Canos AJ, Sull WJ: The diagnosis of deep venous thrombosis: Fallibility of clinical symptoms and signs. Arch Surg 1976;111:34-36.

55. Haeger K: Problems of acute deep venous thrombosis, I: The interpretation of signs and symptoms. Angiology 1969;20:219-223.

56. Stein PD, Terrin ML, Hales CA, et al: Clincal, laboratory, roentgenographic, and electrocardiographic findings in patients with acute pulmonary embolism and no pre-existing cardiac or pulmonary disease. Chest 1991;100:598-603.

57. Bruera E, Macmillan K, Pither J, MacDonald RN: Effects of morphine on the dyspnea of terminal cancer patients. J Pain Sympt Manag 1990;5:341-344.

58. Donnely S, Walsh D, Rybicki L: The symptoms of advanced cancer: Identification of clinical and research priorities by assessment of prevalence and severity. J Palliat Care 1995;11:27-32.

59. Bruera E, MacEachern T, Ripamonti C, Hanson J: Subcutaneous morphine for dyspnea in cancer patients. Ann Intern Med 1993;119:906-907.

60. Cowcher K, Hanks GW: Long-term management of respiratory symptoms in advanced cancer. J Pain Sympt Manag 1990;5:320-330.

61. Coyle N, Adelhardt J, Foley KM, Portenoy RK: Character of terminal illness in the advanced cancer patient: Pain and other symptoms during the last four weeks of life. J Pain Sympt Manag 1990;5:83-93.

62. Connill C, Verger E, Henríquez I, et al: Symptom prevalence in the last week of life. J Pain Sympt Manag 1997;14:328-331.

63. Petrek JA, Heelan MC: Incidence of breast carcinoma-related lymphedema. Cancer 1998;83:2776-2781.

64. Zech DFJ, Grond S, Lynch J, Hertel D, Lehmann KA: Validation of World Health Organization guidelines for cancer pain relief: A 10-year prospective study. Pain 1995;63:65-76.

65. Wells PS, Anderson DR, Ginsberg J: Assessment of deep vein thrombosis or pulmonary embolism by the combined use of clinical model and noninvasive diagnostic tests. Semin Thromb Hemost 2000;26:643-656.

66. Michiels JJ, Freyburger G, van der Graaf F, Janssen M, Oortwijn W, van Beek EJR: Strategies for the safe and effective exclusion and diagnosis of deep vein thrombosis by the sequential use of clinical score, D-dimer testing, and compression ultrasonography. Semin Thromb Hemost 2000;26:657-667.

67. Musset D, Parent F, Meyer G, et al: Diagnostic strategy for patients with suspected pulmonary embolism: A prospective multicentre outcome study. Lancet 2002;360:1914-1920.

68. Kraaijenhagen RA, Piovella F, Bernardi E, et al: Simplification of the diagnostic management of suspected deep vein thrombosis. Arch Intern Med 2002;162:907-911.

69. Deitcher SR, Carman TL: Deep venous thrombosis and pulmonary embolism. Curr Treat Options Cardiovasc Med 2002;4:223-238.

70. Scates SM: Diagnosis and treatment of cancer-related thrombosis. Hematol Oncol Clin North Am 1992;6:1329-1339.

71. Levine MN, Hirsh J, Gent M, et al: A randomized trial comparing activated thromboplastin time with heparin assay in patients with acute venous thromboembolism requiring large daily doses of heparin. Arch Intern Med 1994;154:49-56.

72. Hirsh J, Warkentin TW, Shaughnessy SG, et al: Heparin and low-molecular-weight heparin; mechanisms of action pharmacokinetics, dosing considerations, monitoring, efficacy, and safety. Chest 2001;119(suppl):64S-94S.

73. Chan A, Woodruff RK: Complications and failure of anticoagulation therapy in treatment of venous thromboembolism in patients with disseminated malignancy. Aust N Z J Med 1992;22:119-122.

74. Deitcher SR: Interpretation of the international normalized ratio in patients with liver disease. Lancet 2002;359:47-48.

75. Hirsh J, Dalen JE, Anderson D, et al: Oral anticoagulants:

Mechanism of action, clinical effectiveness, and optimal therapeutic range. Chest 2001;119(suppl):8S–21S.

76. Wells PS, Holbrook AM, Crowther NR, et al: The interaction of warfarin with drugs and food: A critical review of the literature. Ann Intern Med 1994;121:676–683.

77. Deitcher SR, Carman TL: Heparin induced thrombocytopenia: Natural history, diagnosis, and management. Vasc Med 2001;6:113–119.

78. Lee AY, Levine MN, Baker RI, et al: Randomized comparison of low-molecular-weight heparin versus oral anticoagulant therapy for the prevention of recurrent venous thromboembolism in patients with cancer. N Engl J Med 2003;349:146–153.

79. Deitcher SR, Kessler CM, Merli G, Rigas J, Lyons RM, Cort S: Secondary prevention of venous thromboembolic events in patients with active malignancy: A randomized study of enoxaparin sodium alone versus initial enoxaparin sodium followed by warfarin for a 180-day period. Proc Am Soc Clin Oncol 2003;22:761(abst 3060).

80. Beyth RJ, Quinn LM, Landefeld S: Prospective evaluation of an index for predicting the risk of major bleeding risk outpatients treated with warfarin. Am J Med 1998;105:91–99.

81. Levine MN, Raskob G, Landefeld S, Kearon C: Hemorrhagic complications of anticoagulant treatment. Chest 119(suppl):108S–121S.

82. Gitter MJ, Jaeger TM, Petterson TM, Gersh MD, Silverstein MD: Bleeding and thromboembolism during anticoagulant therapy: A population-based study in Rochester, Minnesota. Mayo Clin Proc 1995;70:725–733.

83. Wester JPJ, de Valk HW, Nieuwenhuis HK, et al: Risk factors for bleeding during treatment of acute venous thromboembolism. Thromb Haemost 1996;76:682–688.

84. Melissari E, Parker CJ, Wilson NV, et al: Use of low molecular weight heparin in pregnancy. Thromb Haemost 1992;68:652–656.

85. Sanson B-J, Lensing AW, Prins MH, et al: Safety of low-molecular-weight heparin in pregnancy: A systematic review. Thromb Haemost 1999;81:668–672.

86. Nelson-Piercy C, Letsky EA, de Swiet M: Low-molecular-weight heparin for obstetric thromboprophylaxis: Experience of sixty-nine pregnancies in sixty-one women at high risk. Am J Obstet Gynecol 1997;176:1062–1068.

87. Shaughnessy SG, Young E, Deschamps P, Hirsh J: The effects of low molecular weight and standard heparin on calcium loss from fetal rat calvaria. Blood 1995;86:1368–1373.

88. Muir JM, Hirsh J, Weitz JI, Andrew M, Young E, Shaughnessy SG: A histomorphometric comparison of the effects of heparin and low molecular weight heparin on cancellous bone in rats. Blood 1997;89:3236–3242.

89. Bhandari M, Hirsh J, Weitz J, et al: The effects of standard and low molecular weight heparin on bone nodule formation in vitro. Thromb Haemost 1998;80:413–417.

90. Carman TL, Kanner AA, Barnett GH, Deitcher SR: Neurosurgery thromboprophylaxis following tumor surgery: A survey. South Med J 2003;96:17–22.

91. Altschuler E, Moosa H, Selker RG, Vertosick FT: The risk and efficacy of anticoagulant therapy in the treatment of thromboembolic complications in patients with primary malignant brain tumors. Neurosurgery 1990;27:74–77.

92. Choucair AK, Silver P, Levin VA: Risk of intracranial hemorrhage in glioma patients receiving anticoagulant therapy for venous thromboembolism. J Neurosurg 1987;66:357–358.

93. Norris LK, Grossman SA: Treatment of thromboembolic complications in patients with brain tumors. J Neurooncol 1994;22:127–137.

94. Olin JW, Young JR, Graor RA, Ruschhaupt EG, Beven EG, Bay JW: Treatment of deep vein thrombosis and pulmonary emboli in patients with primary and metastatic brain tumors. Arch Intern Med 1987;147:2177–2179.

95. Ruff RL, Posner JB: Incidence and treatment of peripheral venous thrombosis in patients with glioma. Ann Neurol 1983;13:334–336.

96. Schiff D, DeAngelis LM: Therapy of venous thromboembolism in patients with brain metastases. Cancer 1994;73:493–498.

97. Kessler CM, Deitcher SR, Merli G, Rigas J, Lyons RM, Cort S: Low molecular weight heparin (enoxaparin) provides safe and effective antithrombotic therapy in active primary brain malignancies. Proc Am Soc Clin Oncol 2003;22:741(abst 2980).

98. Levine M, Gent M, Hirsch J, et al: A comparison of low-molecular-weight heparin administered primarily at home with unfractionated heparin administered in the hospital for proximal deep-vein thrombosis. N Engl J Med 1996;334:677–681.

99. Koopman MM, Prandoni P, Piovella F, et al: Treatment of venous thrombosis with intravenous unfractionated heparin administered in the hospital as compared with subcutaneous low-molecular-weight heparin administered at home. N Engl J Med 1996;334:682–687.

100. Hull RD, Raskob GL, Pineo GF, et al: Subcutaneous low-molecular-weight heparin compared with continuous intravenous heparin in the treatment of proximal vein thrombosis. N Engl J Med 1992;326:975–982.

101. Lindmarker P, Holmstrom M, Granqvist S, et al: Comparison of once-daily subcutaneous Fragmin with continuous intravenous unfractionated heparin in the treatment of deep vein thrombosis. Thromb Haemost 1994;72:186–190.

102. The Columbus Investigators. Low-molecular-weight heparin in the treatment of patients with venous thromboembolism. N Engl J Med 1997;337:657–662.

103. Weitz JI: Low molecular weight heparins. N Engl J Med 1995;337:688–698.

104. Warkentin TE, Levine MN, Hirsh J, et al: Heparin-induced thrombocytopenia in patients treated with low-molecular-weight heparin or unfractionated heparin. N Engl J Med 1995;332:1330–1335.

105. Lensing AW, Prins MH, Davidson BL, Hirsh J: Treatment of deep venous thrombosis with low molecular weight heparins: A meta-analysis. Arch Intern Med 1995;155:601–607.

106. Siragusa S, Cosmi B, Piovella, Hirsh J, Ginsberg JS: Low molecular weight heparins and unfractionated heparin in the treatment of patient with acute venous thromboembolism; results of a meta-analysis. Am J Med 1996;100:269–277.

107. Gould MK, Dembitzer AD, Doyle RL, Hastie TJ, Garber AM: Low-molecular-weight heparins compared with unfractionated heparin for treatment of acute deep venous thrombosis: A meta-analysis of randomized, controlled trails. Ann Intern Med 1999;130:800–809.

108. Dolovich LR, Ginsberg JS, Douketis JD, Holbrook AM, Cheah G: A meta-analysis comparing low-molecular-weight heparins with unfractionated heparin in the treatment of venous thromboembolism: Examining some unanswered questions regarding location of treatment, product type, and dosing frequency. Arch Intern Med 2000;160:181–188.

109. Green D, Hull RD, Brant R, Pineo GF: Lower mortality in cancer patients treated with low-molecular-weight versus standard heparin. Lancet 1992;339:1476.

110. Folkman J, Langer R, Linhardt RJ, Haudenschild C, Taylor S: Angiogenesis inhibition and tumour regression caused by heparin or heparin fragment in the presence of cortisone. Science 1983;221:719–725.

111. Norrby K: Heparin and angiogenesis: A low-molecular-weight fraction inhibits and a high-molecular-weight fraction stimulates angiogenesis systematically. Haemostasis 1993;23(suppl):141–149.

112. Kakkar AK, Kadziola Z, Williamson RCN, Levine MN, Low V, Lemoine NR: Low molecular weight heparin therapy and survival in advanced cancer. Blood 2002;100:148a(abst 557).

113. Lee AY, Julian JA, Levine MN, et al: Impact of dalteparin low-molecular-weight heparin (LMWH) on survival: Results of a randomized trial in cancer patients with venous thromboembolism (VTE). Proc Am Soc Clin Oncol 2003;22:211(abst 846).

114. Lensing AWA, Buller HR, Prandoni P, et al: Contrast venography, the gold standard for the diagnosis of deep vein thrombosis: Improvement in observer agreement. Thromb Haemost 1992;67:8–12.

115. Fraser JD, Anderson DR: Deep venous thrombosis: recent advances and optimal investigation with US. Radiology 1999;211:9–24.

116. Brown DB, Singh H, Cardella JF, et al: Quality improvement guidelines for diagnostic infusion venography. J Vasc Interv Radiol 2002;13:449–452.

117. Katz DS, Loud PA, Bruce D, et al: Combined CT venography and

pulmonary angiography: A comprehensive review. Radiographics 2002;22:S3–S24.

118. Atri M, Herba MJ, Reinhold C, et al: Accuracy of sonography in the evaluation of calf deep vein thrombosis in both postoperative surveillance and symptomatic patients. AJR Am J Roentgenol 1996;166:1361–1367.

119. Björgell O, Nilsson PE, Jarenros H: Isolated nonfilling of contrast in deep leg vein segments seen on phlebography, and a comparison with color Doppler ultrasound, to assess the incidence of deep leg vein thrombosis. Angiology 2000;51:451–461.

120. Cronan JJ, Murphy TP: A comprehensive review of vascular ultrasound for intensivists. J Intens Care Med 1993;8:188–201.

121. Albrechtsson U, Olsson C-G: Thrombotic side-effects of lower-limb phlebography. Lancet 1976;1:723–724.

122. Anderson DR, Lensing AWA, Wells PS, Levine MN, Weitz JI, Hirsh J: Limitations of impedance plethysmography in the diagnosis of clinically suspected deep-vein thrombosis. Ann Intern Med 1993;118:25–30.

123. Kristo DA, Perry ME, Kollef MH: Comparison of venography, duplex imaging, and bilateral impedance plethysmography for diagnosis of lower extremity deep vein thrombosis. South Med J 1994;87:55–60.

124. Keefe DL, Roistacher N, Pierri MK: Evaluation of suspected deep venous thrombosis in oncologic patients. Angiology 1994;45:771–775.

125. Dauzat M, Laroche JP, Deklunder G, et al: Diagnosis of acute lower limb deep venous thrombosis with ultrasound: trends and controversies. J Clin Ultrasound 1997;25:343–358.

126. Lensing AWA, Prandoni P, Brandjes D, et al: Detection of deep-vein thrombosis by real-time B-mode ultrasonography. N Engl J Med 1989;320:342–345.

127. Cogo A, Lensoing AWA, Prandoni P, Büller HR, Girolami A, ten Cate JW: Comparison of real-time B-mode ultrasonography and Doppler ultrasound with contrast venography in the diagnosis of venous thrombosis in symptomatic outpatients. Thromb Haemost 1993;70:404–407.

128. Killewich LA, Bedford GR, Beach KW, Strandness DE Jr: Diagnosis of deep venous thrombosis: A prospective study comparing duplex scanning to contrast venography. Circulation 1989;79:810–814.

129. White RH, McGahan JP, Daschbach MM, Hartling RP: Diagnosis of deep vein thrombosis using duplex ultrasound. Ann Intern Med 1989;111:297–304.

130. Rose SC, Zwiebel WJ, Nelson BD, et al: Symptomatic lower extremity deep venous thrombosis: Accuracy, limitations, and role of color duplex flow imaging in diagnosis. Radiology 1990;175:639–644.

131. Simons GR, Skibo LK, Polak JF, Creager MA, Klapec-Fay JM, Goldhaber SZ: Utility of leg ultrasonography in suspected symptomatic isolated calf deep venous thrombosis. Am J Med 1995;99:43–47.

132. Vogel P, Laing FC, Jeffrey RB Jr, Wing VW: Deep venous thrombosis of the lower- extremity: US evaluation. Radiology 1987;163:747–751.

133. Miller N, Satin R, Tousignant L, Sheiner NM: A prospective study comparing duplex scan and venography for diagnosis of lower-extremity deep vein thrombosis. Cardiovasc Surg 1996;4:505–508.

134. Bradley MJ, Spencer PA, Alexander L, Milner GR: Colour flow mapping in the diagnosis of the calf vein thrombosis. Clin Radiol 1993;47:399–402.

135. Bucek RA, Kos T, Schober E, et al: Ultrasound with Levovist in the diagnosis of suspected calf vein thrombosis. Ultrasound Med Biol 2001;27:455–460.

136. Wright DJ, Shepard AD, McPharlin M, Ernst CB: Pitfalls in lower extremity venous duplex scanning. J Vasc Surg 1990;11:675–679.

137. Hoffman LV, Bluemke DA, Fishman EK. Thrombosis of the deep femoral vein: A potential pitfall of color flow duplex Doppler ultrasonography. South Med J 1997;90:1244–1247.

138. Messina LM, Sarpa MS, Smith MA, Greenfield LJ: Clinical significance of routine imaging of iliac and calf veins by color flow duplex scanning in patients suspected of having acute lower extremity deep venous thrombosis. Surgery 1993;114:921–927.

139. De Maeseneer MG, Tielliu IF, Tjalma WA, Van Schil PE: Lack of compressibility of the common femoral vein: Unequivocal sign of proximal deep venous thrombosis on duplex ultrasound? Cardiovasc Surg 2000;8:289–291.

140. Bach AM, Hann LE: When the common femoral vein is revealed as flattened on spectral Doppler sonography: Is it a reliable sign for diagnosis of proximal venous obstruction? AJR Am J Roentgenol 1997;168:733–736.

141. Garcia ND, Morasch MD, Ebaugh JL, et al: Is bilateral ultrasound scanning of the legs necessary for patients with unilateral symptoms of deep vein thrombosis? J Vasc Surg 2001;34:792–797.

142. Giess CS, Bach AM, Hann LE: Lower extremity venous sonography in the high-risk cancer population: One leg or two? AJR Am J Roentgenol 2001;176:1049–1052.

143. Miller N, Obrand D, Tousignant L, Gascon I, Rossignol M: Venous duplex scanning for unilateral symptoms: When do we need a contralateral evaluation? Eur J Vasc Endovasc Surg 1998;15:18–23.

144. Prandoni P, Lensing AWA, Piccioli A, Bagatella P, Girolami A: Ultrasonography of contralateral vein in patients with unilateral deep-vein thrombosis. Lancet 1998;352:786.

145. Naidich JB, Torre JR, Pellerito JS, et al: Suspected deep venous thrombosis: is US of both legs necessary? Radiology 1996;200:429–431.

146. Strothman G, Blebea J, Fowl RJ, Rosenthal G: Contralateral duplex scanning for deep venous thrombosis is unnecessary in patients with symptoms. J Vasc Surg 1995;22:543–547.

147. Heijboer H, Jongbloets LMM, Buller HR, et al: Clinical utility of real-time compression ultrasonography for diagnostic management of patients with recurrent venous thrombosis. Acta Radiol 1992;33:297–300.

148. Cronan JJ: Recurrent deep venous thrombosis: Limitations of US. Radiology 1989;170:739–742.

149. Prandoni P, Cogo A, Bernardi E, et al: A simple ultrasound approach for the detection of recurrent proximal-vein thrombosis. Circulation 1993;88:1730–1735.

150. Prandoni P, Lensing AWA, Berbardi E, Villalta S, Bagatella P, Girolami A, for the DERECUS Investigators Group: The diagnostic value of compression ultrasonography in patients with suspected recurrent deep vein thrombosis. Thromb Haemost 2002;88:402–406.

151. Anonymous. The diagnostic approach to acute venous thromboembolism: Clinical practice guidelines by the American Thoracic Society. Am J Respir Crit Care Med 1999;160:1043.

152. Bates SM, Ginsberg JS: Helical computed tomography and the diagnosis of pulmonary embolism. Ann Intern Med 2000;132:240–242.

153. Mayo JR, Ketai LH: Combined CT venography and pulmonary angiography. Radiographics 2002;22:S20–S22.

154. Garg K, Kemp JL, Wojcik D, et al: Thromboembolic disease: Comparison of combined CT pulmonary angiography and venography with bilateral leg sonography in 70 patients. AJR Am J Roentgenol 2000;175:997–1001.

155. Loud PA, Katz DS, Klippenstein DL, Shah RD, Grossman ZD: Combined CT venography and pulmonary angiography in suspected thromboembolic disease: Diagnostic accuracy for deep venous evaluation. AJR Am J Roentgenel 2000;174:61–65.

156. Peterson DA, Kazerooni EA, Wakefield TW, et al: Computed tomographic venography is specific but not sensitive for diagnosis of acute lower-extremity deep venous thrombosis in patients with suspected pulmonary embolism. J Vasc Surg 2001;34:798–804.

157. Ghaye B, Szapiro D, Willems V, Dondelinger RF: Pitfalls in CT venography of lower limbs and abdominal veins. AJR Am J Roentgenol 2002;178:1465–1471.

158. Rademaker J, Griesshaber V, HIdajat N, Oestmann JW, Felix R: Combined CT pulmonary angiography and venography for diagnosis of pulmonary embolism and deep vein thrombosis: Radiation dose. J Thorac Imaging 2001;16:297–299.

159. Duwe KM, Shiau M, Budorick NE, Austin JHM, Berkmen YM: Evaluation of the lower extremity veins in patients with suspected pulmonary embolism: A prospective comparison of helical CT venography and sonography. AJR Am J Roentgenol 2000;175:1725–1731.

160. Gottschalk A, Stein PD, Goodman LR, Sostman HD: Overview of prospective investigation of pulmonary embolism diagnosis (PIOPED), II. Semin Nuclear Med 2002;32:173–182.

161. Link KM, Lesko NM: Magnetic resonance angiography: Great vessels and abdomen. In Stark DD, Bradley WG Jr (eds): Magnetic resonance imaging. St. Louis, Mosby, 1999, pp 373–383.

162. Carpenter JP, Holland GA, Baum RA: Magnetic resonance venography for the detection of deep venous thrombosis: Comparison with contrast venography and duplex Doppler ultrasonography. J Vasc Surg 1993;18:734–741.

163. Dupas B, El Kouri D, Curtet C, et al: Angiomagnetic resonance imaging of iliofemorocaval venous thrombosis. Lancet 1995;346:17–19.

164. Froehlich JB, Prince MR, Greenfield LJ, Downing J, Shah NL, Wakefield TW: "Bull's-eye" sign on gadolinium-enhanced magnetic resonance venography determines thrombus presence and age: A preliminary study. J Vasc Surg 1997;26:809–816.

165. Laissy JP, Cinqualbre A, Loshkajian A, et al: Assessment of deep venous thrombosis in the lower limbs and pelvis: MR venography versus duplex Doppler sonography. AJR Am J Roentgenol 1996;167:971–975.

166. Evans AJ, Sostman HD, Knelson MH, et al: Detection of deep venous thrombosis: Prospective comparison of MR imaging with contrast venography. AJR Am J Roentgenol 1993;161:131–139.

167. Sica GT, Pugach ME, Koniaris LS, et al: Isolated calf vein thrombosis: Comparison of MR venography and conventional venography after initial sonography in symptomatic patients. Acad Radiol 2001;8:856–863.

168. Spritzer CE, Norconk JJ Jr, Sostman HD, Coleman RE: Detection of deep venous thrombosis by magnetic resonance imaging. Chest 1993;104:54–60.

169. Hartnell GG. Imaging in blood stasis: The role of imaging techniques in defining the causes, presence, and effects of blood stasis. Hematol Oncol Clin North Am 2000;14:299–323.

170. Taillefer R, Edell S, Innes G, et al: Acute thromboscintigraphy with 99mTc-apcitide: Results of the phase 3 multicenter clinical trial comparing 99mTc-apcitide scintigraphy with contrast venography for imaging acute DVT. J Nucl Med 2000;41:1214–1223.

171. Taillefer R: Radiolabeled peptides in the detection of deep venous thrombosis. Semin Nucl Med 2001;31:102–123.

172. Brill-Edwards P, Lee A: D-dimer testing in the diagnosis of acute venous thromboembolism. Thromb Haemost 1999;82:688–694.

173. Ginsberg JS, Kearon C, Douketis J, et al: The use of D-dimer testing and impedance plethysmographic examination in patients with clinical indications of deep vein thrombosis. Arch Intern Med 1997;157:1077–1081.

174. Bernardi E, Prandoni P, Lensing AW, et al: D-dimer testing as an adjunct to ultrasonography in patients with clinically suspected deep vein thrombosis: Prospective cohort study: The Multicenter Italian D-dimer Ultrasound Study Investigators Group. Br Med J 1998;317:1037–1040.

175. Lee AYY, Julian JA, Levine MN, et al: Clinical utility of a rapid whole-blood D-dimer assay in patients with cancer who present with suspected acute deep venous thrombosis. Ann Intern Med 1999;131:417–423.

176. Bates SM, Grand'Maison A, Johnston M, et al: A latex D-dimer reliably excludes venous thromboembolism. Arch Intern Med 2001;161:447–453.

177. Bates SM, Kearon C, Crowther M, et al: A diagnostic strategy involving a quantitative latex D-dimer assay reliably excludes deep venous thrombosis. Ann Intern Med 2003;138:787–794.

178. Hyers TM, Agnelli A, Hull RD, et al: Antithrombotic therapy for venous thromboembolic disease. Chest 2001;119(suppl):176S–193S.

179. Anand SS, Bates S, Ginsberg JS, et al: Recurrent venous thrombosis and heparin therapy: An evaluation of the importance of early activated partial thromboplastin times. Arch Intern Med 1999;159:2029–2032.

180. Hull RD, Raskob GE, Brant RF, Pineo GF, Valentine KA: Relation between the time to achieve the lower limit of the aPTT therapeutic range and recurrent venous thromboembolism during heparin treatment for deep vein thrombosis. Arch Intern Med 1997;157:2562–2568.

181. Raschke RA, Reilly BM, Guidry JR, et al: The weight-based heparin dosing nomogram compared with a standard care nomogram: A randomized, controlled trial. Ann Intern Med 1993;119:874–881.

182. Merli G, Spiro TE, Olsson C-G, et al: Subcutaneous enoxaparin once or twice daily compared with intravenous unfractionated heparin for treatment of venous thromboembolic disease. Ann Intern Med 2001;134:191–202.

183. Hainer JW, Barrett JS, Assaid CA, et al: Dosing in heavy-weight/obese patients with the LMWH, tinzaparin: A pharmacodynamic study. Thromb Haemost 2002;87:817–823.

184. The Matisse Investigators: Fondaparinux (Arixtra) in comparison to (low molecular weight) heparin for the initial treatment of symptomatic deep venous thrombosis or pulmonary embolism: The Matisse Clinical Outcome Studies. Blood 2002;100:abst 302.

185. Moll S, Ortel TL: Monitoring warfarin therapy in patients with lupus anticoagulants. Ann Intern Med 1997;127:177–185.

186. Harrison L, Johnston M, Massicotte MP, Crowther M, Moffat K, Hirsh J: Comparison of 5-mg and 10-mg loading doses in initiation of warfarin therapy. Ann Intern Med 1997;126:133–136.

187. Fihn SD, McDonell M, Martin D, et al: Risk factors for complications of chronic anticoagulation. Ann Intern Med 1993;118:511–520.

188. Choueiri T, Deitcher SR: Why shouldn't we solely use warfarin to treat acute venous thrombosis? Cleve Clin J Med 2002;69:546–548.

189. Monreal M, Lafoz E, Olive A, del Rio L, Vedia C: Comparison of subcutaneous unfractionated heparin with a low molecular weight heparin (Fragmin) in patients with venous thromboembolism and contraindications to coumarin. Thromb Haemost 1994;71:7–11.

190. Pini M, Aiello S, Manotti C, et al: Low molecular weight heparin versus warfarin in the prevention of recurrences after deep vein thrombosis. Thromb Haemost 1994;72:191–197.

191. Das SK, Cohen AT, Edmondson RA, Melissari E, Kakkar VV: Low-molecular-weight heparin versus warfarin for prevention of recurrent venous thromboembolism: A randomized trial. World J Surg 1996;20:521–527.

192. Loaciuk S, Bielska-Falda H, Noszczyk W, et al: Low molecular weight heparin versus acenocoumarol in the secondary prophylaxis of deep vein thrombosis. Thromb Haemost 1999;81:26–31.

193. Hull RD, Pineo GF, Mah AF, Brant RF: A randomized trial evaluating long-term low-molecular-weight heparin therapy for three months versus intravenous heparin followed by warfarin sodium. Blood 2002;100:148a(abst 556).

194. Gruel Y, Meyer G, Marjanovic Z, et al: Canthanox, a randomized controlled study comparing low molecular weight heparin and warfarin for the prevention of recurrent venous thromboembolism in patients with cancer. Blood 2001;98:707a.

195. Schulman S, Rhedin AS, Lindmarker P, et al: A comparison of six weeks with six months of oral anticoagulant therapy after a first episode of venous thromboembolism. N Engl J Med 1995;332:1661–1665.

196. Kearon C, Gent M, Hirsh J, et al: A comparison of three months of anticoagulation with extended anticoagulation for a first episode of idiopathic venous thromboembolism. N Engl J Med 1999;340:901–907.

197. Schulman S, Granqvist S, Holström M, et al: The duration of oral anticoagulant therapy after a second episode of venous thromboembolism. N Engl J Med 1997;336:393–398.

198. Zacharski LR, Henderson WG, Rickles FR, et al: Effect of warfarin on survival in small cell carcinoma of the lung: Veterans Administration Study No. 75. JAMA 1981;245:831–835.

199. Schulman S, Lindmarker P: Incidence of cancer after prophylaxis with warfarin against recurrent venous thromboembolism: Duration of anticoagulation trial. N Engl J Med 2000;342:1953–1958.

200. Ridker PM, Goldhaber SZ, Danielson E, et al: Long-term, low-intensity warfarin therapy for the prevention of recurrent venous thromboembolism. N Engl J Med 2003;348:1425–1434.

201. Thornton MJ, Ryan R, Varghese JC, et al: A three-dimensional gadolinium-enhanced MR venography technique for imaging central veins. AJR Am J Roentgenol 1999;173:999–1003.

202. Weissleder R, Elizondo G, Stark DD: Sonographic diagnosis of subclavian and internal jugular vein thrombosis. J Ultrasound Med 1987;6:577–587.

203. Baarslag H-J, van Beek EJR, Koopman MMW, Reekers JA: Prospective study of color duplex ultrasound compared with contrast venography in patients suspected of having deep venous thrombosis of the upper extremities. Ann Intern Med 2002;136:865-872.

204. Mustafa BO, Rathbun SW, Whitsett TL, Raskob GE: Sensitivity and specificity of ultrasonography in the diagnosis of upper extremity deep vein thrombosis: A systematic review. Arch Intern Med 2002;162:401-404.

205. Baxter GM, Kincaid W, Jeffrey RF, Millar GM, Porteous C, Morley P: Comparison of color Doppler ultrasound with venography in the diagnosis of axillary and subclavian deep vein thrombosis. Br J Radiol 1991;64:777-781.

206. Knudson GJ, Wiedemeyer DA, Erickson SJ, et al: Color Doppler sonographic imaging in the assessment of upper-extremity deep venous thrombosis. AJR Am J Roentgenol 1990;154:399-403.

207. Burbidge SJ, Finlay DE, Letourneau JG, Longley DG: Effects of central venous catheter placement on upper extremity duplex US findings. J Vasc Interv Radiol 1993;4:399-404.

208. Haire WD, Lynch TG, Lund GB, Lieberman RP, Edney JA: Limitations of magnetic resonance imaging and ultrasound-directed (duplex) scanning in the diagnosis of subclavian vein thrombosis. J Vasc Surg 1991;13:391-397.

209. Moncada R, Cardella R, Demos TC, et al: Evaluation of superior vena cava syndrome by axial CT and CT phlebography. AJR Am J Roentgenol 1984;143:731-736.

210. Haire WD, Lynch TG, Lieberman RP, et al: Utility of duplex ultrasound in the diagnosis of symptomatic catheter-induced subclavian venous thrombosis. J Ultrasound Med 1991;10:493-496.

211. Hansen ME, Spritzer CE, Sostman HD: Assessing the patency of mediastinal and thoracic inlet veins: Value of MR imaging. Am J Radiol 1990;155:1177-1182.

212. Finn JP, Edelman RR, Zisk J, et al: Central venous occlusion: MR angiography. Radiology 1993;187:245-251.

213. Hartnell GG, Hughes LA, Finn JP, et al: Magnetic resonance angiography of the central chest veins: A new gold-standard? Chest 1995;107:1053-1057.

214. Balestreri L, De Cicco M, Matovic M, Coran F, Morassut S: Central venous catheter-related thrombosis in clinically asymptomatic oncology patients: A phlebographic study. Eur J Radiol 1995;20:108-111.

215. Monreal M, Raventos A, Lerma R, et al: Pulmonary embolism in patients with upper extremity DVT associated to venous central lines—a prospective study. Thromb Haemost 1994;72:548-550.

216. Ault M, Artal R. Upper extremity DVT: What is the risk? Arch Intern Med 1998;158:1950-1952.

217. Fraschini G, Jadeja J, Lawson M, Holmes FA, Carrasco HC, Wallace S: Local infusion of urokinase for the lysis of thrombosis associated with permanent central venous catheters in cancer patients. J Clin Oncol 1987;5:672-678.

218. Goodman PC: Pulmonary angiography. Clin Chest Med 1984;5:465-477.

219. van Erkel AR, van Rossum AB, Bloem JL, Kievit J, Pattynama PMT: Spiral CT angiography for suspected pulmonary embolism: A cost-effectiveness analysis. Radiology 1996;201:29-36.

220. Stein PD, Athanasoulis C, Alavi A, et al: Complications and validity of pulmonary angiography in acute pulmonary embolism. Circulation 1992;85:462-468.

221. Gotway MB, Edinburgh KJ, Feldstein VA, et al: Imaging evaluation of suspected pulmonary embolism. Curr Probl Diag Radiol 1999;28:132-184.

222. The Prospective Investigation of Pulmonary Embolism Diagnosis (PIOPED) Investigators: Value of the ventilation/perfusion scan in acute pulmonary embolism. JAMA 1990;263:2753-2759.

223. Smith TP: Pulmonary embolism: What's wrong with this diagnosis? AJR Am J Roentgenol 2000;174:1489-1497.

224. Gottschalk A, Sostman HD, Coleman RE, et al: Ventilation-perfusion scintigraphy in the PIOPED study, Part II: Evaluation of the scintigraphic criteria and interpretations. J Nucl Med 1993;34:1119-1124.

225. Hartmann IJC, Hagen PJ, Melissant CF, Postmus PE, Prins MH, on behalf of the ANTELOPE Study Group: Diagnosing acute pulmonary embolism: Effect of chronic obstructive pulmonary disease on the performance of D-dimer testing, ventilation/perfusion scintigraphy, spiral computed tomographic angiography, and conventional angiography. Am J Respir Crit Care Med 2000;162:2232-2237.

226. Lesser BA, Leeper KV, Stein PD, et al: The diagnosis of acute pulmonary embolism in patients with chronic obstructive pulmonary disease. Chest 1992;102:17-22.

227. Forbes KPN, Reid JH, Murchison JT: Do preliminary chest X-ray findings define the optimum role of pulmonary scintigraphy in suspected pulmonary embolism? Clin Radiol 2001;56:397-400.

228. Shields JJ, Cho KJ, Geisinger KR: Pulmonary artery constriction by mediastinal lymphoma simulating pulmonary embolus. AJR Am J Roentgenol 1980;135:147-150.

229. Chow B, Wittram C, Lee VW: Unilateral absence of pulmonary perfusion mimicking pulmonary embolism. AJR Am J Roentgenol 2001;176:712.

230. Stinson JM, Goodwin RA Jr: Pulmonary vein obstruction by bronchogenic carcinoma. South Med J 1976;69:1482-1483.

231. Nguyen KT, Sanfilippo AJ, Rosen WS, Cheeseman FD: Primary left atrial leiomyosarcoma simulating pulmonary thromboembolism. Can Assoc Radiol J 1994;45:48-51.

232. Li DK, Seltzer SE, McNeil BJ: V/Q mismatches unassociated with pulmonary embolism: case report and review of the literature. J Nucl Med 1978;19:1331-1333.

233. Veatch MD, Lewin JM, O'Brien RF, Crausman RS: Small cell carcinoma as the cause for a nondiagnostic V/Q lung scan. Am J Emerg Med 1996;14:183-185.

234. Vassallo CL, Gee JBL, Wholey MH, Vester JW: Lung scanning in hilar bronchogenic carcinoma. Am Rev Respir Dis 1968;97:851-857.

235. Green N, Swanson L, Kern W, Irwin L, Berne CJ: Lymphangitic carcinomatosis: Lung scan abnormalities. J Nucl Med 1976;17:258-260.

236. Achong DM. Ventilation-perfusion mismatch caused by extrinsic compression of the pulmonary artery: Correlative imaging. Clin Nucl Med 1994;19:61-63.

237. White RI, James AE Jr, Wagner HN: The significance of unilateral absence of pulmonary artery perfusion by lung scanning. AJR Am J Roentgenol 1971;111:501-509.

238. Gandhi V, Shapiro JM: Unilateral absent pulmonary perfusion due to bronchogenic carcinoma. South Med J 1998;91:392-394.

239. Seal EC, Rutter HR, Horrigan MC, Britton MG: Left atrial tumour mimicking pulmonary embolism. Respir Med 1997;91:562-564.

240. Palevsky HI, Cone L: A case of "false-positive" high probability ventilation-perfusion lung scan due to tuberculous mediastinal adenopathy with a discussion of other causes of "false-positive" high probability ventilation-perfusion lung scans. J Nucl Med 1991;32:512-517.

241. Ogawa Y, Ahizawa K, Hashmi R, Takemoto Y, Hayashi K: Regional ventilation-perfusion mismatch in interstitial pneumonia: Correlation between scintigraphy and CT. Clin Nucl Med 1997;22:166-171.

242. Martino J, Allende J, Herrero A, et al: Nonembolic high-probability perfusion lung scan for pulmonary thromboembolism. Am J Emerg Med 1994;12:664-666.

243. Mendelson DS, Train JS, Goldsmith SJ, et al: Ventilation-perfusion mismatch due to obstruction of pulmonary vein. J Nucl Med 1981;2:1062-1063.

244. Sutter CW, Stadalnik RC: Unilateral absence or near absence of pulmonary perfusion on lung scanning. Semin Nucl Med 1995;25:72-74.

245. Velchik MG, Tobin M, McCarthy K: Nonthromboembolic causes of high-probability lung scans. Am J Physiol Imaging 1989;4:32-38.

246. Delany SG, Doyle TCA, Bunton RW, Hung NA, Joblin LU, Taylor DR: Pulmonary artery sarcoma mimicking pulmonary embolism. Chest 1993;103:1631-1633.

247. Cox JE, Chiles C, Aquino SL, et al: Pulmonary artery sarcomas: A review of clinical and radiologic features. J Comput Assist Tomogr 1997;21:750-755.

248. Krüger I, Borowski A, Horst M, de Vivie ER, Theissen P, Gross-Fengels W: Symptoms, diagnosis, and therapy of primary sarcomas of the pulmonary artery. Thorac Cardiovasc Surg 1990;38:91-95.

249. Madu EC, Taylor DC, Durzinsky DS, Fraker TD: Primary intimal

sarcoma of the pulmonary trunk simulating pulmonary embolism. Am Heart J 1993;125:1790–1792.

250. Olsson HE, Spitzer RM, Ernston WF: Primary and secondary pulmonary artery neoplasia mimicking acute pulmonary embolism. Radiology 1976;118:49–53.

251. Kaminsky DA, Hurwitz CG, Olmstead JI: Pulmonary leukostasis mimicking pulmonary embolism. Leuk Res 1999;24:175–178.

252. Slavin JD, Friedman NC, Spencer RP: Radiation effects on pulmonary ventilation and perfusion. Clin Nucl Med 1993;18: 81–82.

253. Groth S, Johansen H, Sørensen PG, Rossing N: The effect of thoracic irradiation for cancer of the breast on ventilation, perfusion and pulmonary permeability. Acta Oncol 1989;28:671–678.

254. Chin BB, Welsh JS, Kleinberg L, et al: Nonsegmental ventilation-perfusion scintigraphy mismatch after radiation therapy. Clin Nucl Med 1999;24:54–56.

255. Bateman NT, Croft DN: False-positive lung scans and radiotherapy. BMJ 1976;1:807–808.

256. Remy-Jardin M, Remy J: Spiral CT angiography of the pulmonary circulation. Radiology 1999;212:615–636.

257. Gotway MB, Patel RA, Webb WR: Helical CT for the evaluation of suspected acute pulmonary embolism: Diagnostic pitfalls. J Comput Assist Tomogr 2000;24:267–273.

258. Hartmann IJC, Lo RTH, Bakker J, de Monyé W, van Waes PFGM, Pattynama PMT: Optimal scan delay in spiral CT for the diagnosis of acute pulmonary embolism. J Comput Assist Tomogr 2002;26:21–25.

259. van Rossum AB, Treurniet FEE, Kieft GJ, Smith SJ, Schepers-Bok R: Role of spiral volumetric computed tomographic scanning in the assessment of patients with clinical suspicion of pulmonary embolism and abnormal ventilation/perfusion scan. Thorax 1996;51:23–28.

260. Mayo JR, Remy-Jardin M, Müller NL, et al: Pulmonary embolism: Prospective comparison of spiral CT with ventilation-perfusion scintigraphiy. Radiology 1997;205:447–452.

261. Garg K, Welsh CH, Feyerabend AJ, et al: Pulmonary embolism: Diagnosis with spiral CT and ventilation-perfusion scanning: Correlation with pulmonary angiographic results or clinical outcome. Radiology 1998;208:201–208.

262. Kim KI, Müller NL, Mayo JR: Clinically suspected pulmonary embolism: Utility of spiral CT. Radiology 1999;210:693–697.

263. Qanadli SD, Hajjam ME, Mesurolle B, et al: Pulmonary embolism detection: Prospective evaluation of dual-section helical CT versus selective pulmonary arteriography in 157 patients. Radiology 2000;217:447–455.

264. Remy-Jardin M, Remy J, Wattinne L, Giraud F: Central pulmonary thromboembolism: Diagnosis with spiral volumetric CT with single-breath-hold technique: Comparison with pulmonary angiography. Radiology 1992;185:381–387.

265. van Rossum AB, Pattynama PMT, Ton ERTA, et al: Pulmonary embolism: Validation of spiral CT angiography in 149 patients. Radiology 1996;201:467–470.

266. Goodman LR, Curtin JJ, Mewissen MW, et al: Detection of pulmonary embolism in patients with unresolved clinical and scintigraphic diagnosis: Helical CT versus angiography. AJR Am J Roentgenol 1995;164:1369–1374.

267. Drucker EA, Rivitz SM, Shepard J-AO, et al: Acute pulmonary embolism: Assessment of helical CT for diagnosis. Radiology 1998;209:235–241.

268. Perrier A, Howarth N, Didier D, et al: Performance of helical computed tomography in unselected outpatients with suspected pulmonary embolism. Ann Intern Med 2001;135:88–97.

269. Garg K: CT of pulmonary thromboembolic disease. Radiol Clin North Am 2002;40:111–122.

270. de Monyé W, Pattynama PMT: Contrast-enhanced spiral computed tomography of the pulmonary arteries: An overview. Semin Thromb Hemost 2001;27:33–39.

271. Remy-Jardin M, Baghaie F, Bonnel F, Masson P, Duhamel A, Remy J: Thoracic helical CT: Influence of subsecond scan time and thin collimation evaluation of peripheral pulmonary arteries. Eur Radiol 2000;10:1297–1303.

272. Remy-Jardin M, Tillie-Leblond I, Szapiro D, et al: CT angiography of pulmonary embolism in patients with underlying respiratory disease: Impact of multislice CT on image quality and negative predictive value. Eur Radiol 2002;12:1971–1978.

273. Schoepf UJ, Holzknecht N, Helmberger TK, et al: Subsegmental pulmonary emboli: Improved detection with thin-collimation multi-detector row spiral CT. Radiology 2002;222:483–490.

274. Gosselin MV, Rubin GD, Leung AN, Huang J, Rizk NW: Unsuspected pulmonary embolism: Prospective detection on routine helical CT scans. Radiology 1998;208:209–215.

275. Stein PD, Henry JW: Prevalence of acute pulmonary embolism in central and subsegmental pulmonary arteries and relation to probability interpretation of ventilation/perfusion lung scans. Chest 1997;111:1246–1248.

276. Ferretti GR, Bosson J-L, Buffaz P-D, et al: Acute pulmonary embolism: Role of helical CT in 164 patients with intermediate probability at ventilation-perfusion scintigraphy and normal results at duplex US of the legs. Radiology 1997;205:453–458.

277. Blachere H, Latrabe V, Montaudon M, et al: Pulmonary embolism revealed on helical CT angiography: Comparison with ventilation-perfusion radionuclide lung scanning. AJR Am J Roentgenol 2000;174:1041–1047.

278. Ost D, Rozenshtein A, Saffran L, Snider A: The negative predictive value of spiral computed tomography for the diagnosis of pulmonary embolism in patients with nondiagnostic ventilation-perfusion scans. Am J Med 2001;110:16–21.

279. Tillie-Leblond I, Mastora I, Radenne F, et al: Risk of pulmonary embolism after a negative spiral CT angiogram in patients with pulmonary disease: 1-year clinical follow-up study. Radiology 2002;223:461–467.

280. Nilsson T, Olausson A, Johnsson H, Nyman U, Aspelin P: Negative spiral CT in acute pulmonary embolism. Acta Radiol 2002;43: 486–491.

281. van Strijen MJL, de Monyé W, Schiereck J, et al: Single-detector helical computed tomography as the primary diagnostic test in suspected pulmonary embolism: A multicenter clinical management study of 510 patients. Ann Intern Med 2003;138:307–314.

282. van Beek EJR, Brouwers EMJ, Song B, Bongaerts AHH, Oudkerk M: Lung scintigraphy and helical computed tomography for the diagnosis of pulmonary embolism: A meta-analysis. Clin Appl Thromb Hemost 2001;7:87–92.

283. Rathbun SW, Raskob GE, Whisett TL: Sensitivity and specificity of helical computed tomography in the diagnosis of pulmonary embolism: A systematic review. Ann Intern Med 2000;132:227–232.

284. Shah AA, Davis SD, Gamsu G, Intriere L: Parenchymal and pleural findings in patients with and patients without acute pulmonary embolism detected at spiral CT. Radiology 1999;211:147–153.

285. Meaney JFM, Weg JG, Chenevert TL, et al: Diagnosis of pulmonary embolism with magnetic resonance angiography. N Engl J Med 1997;336:1422–1427.

286. Oudkerk M, van Beek EJR, van Ooijen PMA, et al: Comparison of contrast-enhanced magnetic resonance angiography and conventional pulmonary angiography for the diagnosis of pulmonary embolism: A prospective study. Lancet 2002;359:1643–1647.

287. Wittlich N, Erbel R, Eichler A, et al: Detection of central pulmonary artery thromboemboli by transesophageal echocardiography in patients with severe pulmonary embolism. J Am Soc Echocardiogr 1992;5:515–524.

288. Steiner P, Lund GK, Debatin JF, et al: Acute pulmonary embolism: Value of transthoracic and transesophageal echocardiography in comparison with helical CT. AJR Am J Roentgenol 1996;167:931–936.

289. Pruszczyk P, Torbicki A, Kuch-Wocial A, Szulc M, Pacho R: Diagnostic value of transesophageal echocardiography in suspected haemodynamically significant pulmonary embolism. Heart 2001;85:628–634.

290. Simonneau G, Sors H, Charbonnier B, et al: A comparison of low-molecular-weight heparin with unfractionated heparin for acute pulmonary embolism. N Engl J Med 1997;337:663–669.

291. Goldhaber SZ: Thrombolysis in pulmonary embolism: A debatable indication. Thromb Haemost 2001;86:444–451.

292. Arcasoy SM, Kreit JW: Thrombolytic therapy of pulmonary

embolism: A comprehensive review of current evidence. Chest 1999;115:1695-1707.

293. Konstantinides S, Tiede N, Geibel A, Olschewski M, Just H, Kasper W: Comparison of alteplase versus heparin for resolution of major pulmonary embolism. Am J Cardiol 1998;82:966-970.

294. Kanter DS, Mikkola KM, Patel SR, Parker SZ, Golhaber SZ: Thrombolytic therapy for pulmonary embolism: Frequency of intracranial hemorrhage and associated risk factors. Chest 1997;111:1241-1245.

295. Kazmers A, Groehn H, Meeker C: Duplex examination of the inferior vena cava. Am Surg 2000;66:986-989.

296. Friedland M, Kazmers A, Kline R, et al: Vena cava duplex imaging before caval interruption. J Vasc Surg 1996;24:608-613.

297. Conners MS, Becker S, Guzman RJ, et al: Duplex scan-directed placement of inferior vena cava filters: A five-year institutional experience. J Vasc Surg 2002;35:286-291.

298. Liu G-C, Angtuaco TL, Ferris Ej, Shah HR, Reifsteck JE, Hashfield DL: Inferior vena caval filters: Noninvasive evaluation. Radiology 1986;160:521-524.

299. Ricci P, Cantisani V, Biancari F, et al: Contrast-enhanced color Doppler US in malignant portal vein thrombosis. Acta Radiol 2000;41:470-473.

300. van Breda A, Rubin BE, Druy EM: Detection of inferior vena cava abnormalities by computed tomography. J Comput Assist Tomogr 1979;3:164-169.

301. Stanley JH, Sanchez F, Vujic I, Schabel SI: Failure to visualize the abdominal portion of the inferior vena cava with computed tomography: A clue to underlying abdominal pathology. Br J Radiol 1986;59:1163-1166.

302. Marks WM, Korobkin M, Callen PW, Kaiser JA: CT diagnosis of tumor thrombosis of the renal vein and inferior vena cava. Am J Roentgenol 1978;131:843-846.

303. Glazer GM, Callen PW, Parker JJ: CT diagnosis of tumor thrombus in the inferior vena cava: Avoiding the false-positive diagnosis. Am J Roentgenol 1981;137:1265-1267.

304. Didier D, Racle A, Etievent JP, Weill F: Tumor thrombus of the inferior vena cava secondary to malignant abdominal neoplasms: US and CT evaluation. Radiology 1987;162:83-89.

305. Marn CS, Francis IR: CT of portal venous occlusion. Am J Roentgenol 1992;159:717-726.

306. Valla D-C, Condat B: Portal vein thrombosis in adults: Pathophysiology, pathogenesis and management. J Hepatol 2000;32:865-871.

307. Jacoby WT, Cohan RH, Baker ME, et al: Ovarian vein thrombosis in oncology patients: CT detection and clinical significance. Am J Roentgenol 1990;155:291-294.

308. Yassa NA, Ryst E: Ovarian vein thrombosis: A common incidental finding in patients who have undergone total abdominal hysterectomy and bilateral salpingo-oophorectomy with retroperitoneal lymph node dissection. Am J Roentgenol 1999;172:45-47.

309. Kubik-Huch RA, Hebisch G, Huch R, Hilfiker P, Debatin JF, Krestin GP: Role of duplex color Doppler ultrasound, computed tomography, and MR angiography in the diagnosis of septic puerperal ovarian vein thrombosis. Abdom Imaging 1999;24:85-91.

310. Soler R, Rodriguez E, Lopez MF, et al: MR imaging in inferior vena cava thrombosis. Eur J Radiol 1995;119:101-107.

311. Cheng HC, Chu WC, Chai JW: Convergent flow phenomenon mimics the appearance of venous thrombosis in gradient-echo images with or without the presence of a contrast agent. Magn Reson Imaging 1997;15:863-867.

312. Blum U, Wildanger G, Windfuhr M, et al: Preoperative CT and MR imaging of inferior vena cava leiomyosarcoma. Eur J Radiol 1995;20:23-27.

313. Roy C, Beaujeux R, Mutter D: Leimyosarcoma of the femoral vein: imaging findings. AJR Am J Roentgenol 1993;160:1125-1126.

314. van Zanten TEG, Golding RP: CT and MR demonstration of leiomyosarcoma of inferior vena cava. J Comput Assist Tomogr 1987;11:670-674.

315. Samlaska CP, James WD: Superficial thrombophlebitis, II: Secondary hypercoagulable states. J Am Acad Dermatol 1990;23:1-18.

316. Kalodiki E, Nicolaides AN: Superficial thrombophlebitis and low-molecular-weight heparins. Angiology 2002;53:659-663.

317. Lutter KS, Kerr TM, Roedersheimer LR, Lohr JM, Sampson MG, Cranley JJ: Superficial thrombophlebitis diagnosed by duplex scanning. Surgery 1991;110:42-46.

318. Jorgensen JO, Hanel KC, Morgan AM, Hunt JM: The incidence of deep venous thrombosis in patients with superficial thrombophlebitis of the lower limbs. J Vasc Surg 1993;18:70-73.

319. Chengelis DL, Bendick PJ, Glover JL, Brown OW, Ranval TJ: Progression of superficial venous thrombosis to deep vein thrombosis. J Vasc Surg 1996;24:745-749.

320. Bouanameaux H, Reber-Wasem M-A: Superficial thrombophlebitis and deep vein thrombosis: A controversial association. Arch Intern Med 1997;157:1822-1824.

321. Blumemberg RM, Barton E, Gelfand ML, Skudder P, Brennan J: Occult deep venous thrombosis complicating superficial thrombophlebitis. J Vasc Surg 1998;27:338-343.

322. Martins EBG, Fleming KA, Garrido MC, Hine KR, Chapman RWG: Superficial thrombophlebitis, dysplasia, and cholangiocarcinoma in primary sclerosing cholangitis. Gastroenterology 1994;107:537-542.

323. Schwarz RE, Marrero AM, Conlon KC, Burt M: Inferior vena cava filters in cancer patients: Indications and outcomes. J Clin Oncol 1996;14:652-657.

324. Ihnat DM, Mills JL, Hughes JD, Gentile AT, Berman SS, Westerband A: Treatment of patients with venous thromboembolism and malignant disease: Should vena cava filter placement be routine? J Vasc Surg 1998;28:800-807.

325. Streift MB: Vena cava filters: A comprehensive review. Blood 2000;95:3669-3677.

326. Athanasoulis CA, Kaufman JA, Halpern EF, Waltman AC, Geller SC, Fan CM: Inferior vena caval filters: A review of a 26-year single-centre clinical experience. Radiology 2000;21:54-66.

327. Millward SF, Peterson RA, Moher D, et al: LGM (Vena Tech) vena caval filter: Experience at a single institution. J Vasc Interv Radiol 1994;5:351-356.

328. Spence LD, Gironta MG, Malde HM, et al: Acute upper extremity deep venous thrombosis: Safety and effectiveness of superior vena caval filters. Radiology 1999;210:53-58.

329. Decousus H, Leizorovicz A, Parent F, et al: A clinical trial of vena caval filters in the prevention of pulmonary embolism in patients with proximal deep-vein thrombosis. N Engl J Med 1998;338:409-415.

330. Prandoni P, Lensing AW, Buller HR, et al: Deep-vein thrombosis and the incidence of subsequent symptomatic cancer. N Engl J Med 1992;327:1128-1133.

331. Schulman S, Lindmarker P: Incidence of cancer after prophylaxis with warfarin against recurrent venous thromboembolism. N Engl J Med 2000;342:1953-1958.

332. Sørensen HT, Mellemkjær L, Olsen JH, et al: Prognosis of cancers associated with venous thromboembolism. N Engl J Med 2000;343:1846-1850.

333. Shen VS, Pollak EW: Fatal pulmonary embolism in cancer patients: Is heparin prophylaxis justified? South Med J 1980;73:841-843.

334. Heit JA, Silverstein MD, Mohr DN, et al: The epidemiology of venous thromboembolism in the community. Thromb Haemost 2001;86:452-463.

335. Collins R, Scrimgeour A, Yusuf S, et al: Reduction in fatal pulmonary embolism and venous thrombosis by perioperative administration of subcutaneous heparin: Overview of results of randomized trials in general, orthopedic, and urologic surgery. N Engl J Med 1988;318:1162-1173.

336. Geerts WH, Heit JA, Clagett GP, et al: Prevention of venous thromboembolism. Chest 2001;119:132S-175S.

337. Maxwell GL, Synan I, Dodge R, et al: Pneumatic compression vs low molecular weight heparin in gynecologic oncology surgery: A randomized trial. Obstet Gynecol 2001;98:989-995.

338. Lin PP, Graham D, Hann LE, et al: Deep venous thrombosis after orthopedic surgery in adult cancer patients. J Surg Oncol 1998;68:41-47.

339. Maxwell GL, Myers ER, Clarke-Pearson DL: Cost-effectiveness of deep venous thrombosis prophylaxis in gynecologic oncology surgery. Obstet Gynecol 2000;95:206-214.

340. Comerota AJ, Katz ML, White JV: Why does prophylaxis with external pneumatic compression for deep vein thrombosis fail? Am J Surg 1992;164:265-268.

341. Clarke-Pearson DL, Dodge RK, Synan I, et al: Venous thromboembolism prophylaxis: Patients at high risk to fail intermittent pneumatic compression. Obstet Gynecol 2003;101:157–163.

342. Eriksson BI, Bergqvist D, Kalebo P, et al: Ximelagatran and melagatran compared with dalteparin for prevention of venous thromboembolism after total hip or knee replacement: The METHRO II randomized trial. Lancet 2002;360:1441–1447.

343. ENOXACAN Study Group: Efficacy and safety of enoxaparin vs unfractionated heparin for prevention of deep vein thrombosis in elective cancer surgery: A double-blind randomized multicentre trial with venographic assessment. Br J Surg 1997;84:1099–1103.

344. Ramos R, Salem BI, De Pawlikowski MP, et al: The efficacy of pneumatic compression stockings in the prevention of pulmonary embolism after cardiac surgery. Chest 1996;109:82–85.

345. Agnelli G, Piovella F, Buoncristiani P, et al: Enoxaparin plus compression stockings compared with compression stockings alone in the prevention of venous thromboembolism after elective neurosurgery. N Engl J Med 1998;339:80–85.

346. Goldhaber SZ, Dunn K, Gerhard-Herman M, et al: Low rate of venous thromboembolism after craniotomy for brain tumor using multimodality prophylaxis. Chest 2002;122:1933–1937.

347. Bergqvist D, Agnelli G, Cohen AT, et al: Duration of prophylaxis against venous thromboembolism with enoxaparin after surgery for cancer. N Engl J Med 2002;346:975–980.

348. Bern MM, Lokich JJ, Wallach SR, et al: Very low doses of warfarin can prevent thrombosis in central venous catheters. Ann Intern Med 1990;112:423–428.

349. De Cicco M, Matovic M, Balestreri L, et al: Central venous thrombosis: An early and frequent complication in cancer patients bearing long-term Silastic catheter. A prospective study. Thromb Res 1997;86:101–113.

350. Boraks P, Seale J, Price J, et al: Prevention of central venous catheter associated thrombosis using minidose warfarin in patients with haematological malignancies. Br J Haematol 1998;101:483–486.

351. Trerotola SO, Kuhn-Fulton J, Johnson MS, et al: Tunneled infusion catheters: Increased incidence of symptomatic venous thrombosis after subclavian vs internal jugular venous access. Radiology 2000;217:89–93.

352. Frank DA, Meuse J, Hirsch D, et al: The treatment and outcome of cancer patients with thromboses on central venous catheters. J Thromb Thrombol 2000;10:271–275.

353. Minassian VA, Sood AK, Lowe P, et al: Long-term central venous access in gynecologic cancer patients. J Am Coll Surg 2000;191:403–409.

354. Eastman ME, Khorsand M, Maki DG, et al: Central venous device-related infection and thrombosis in patients treated with moderate dose continuous-infusion interleukin-2. Cancer 2001;91:806–814.

355. Kuriakose P, Colon-Otero G, Paz-Fumagalli R: Risk of deep venous thrombosis associated with chest vs arm central venous subcutaneous port catheters: A 5-year single-institution retrospective study. J Vasc Interv Radiol 2002;13:179–184.

356. Soo RA, Gosbell IB, Gallo JH, et al: Hickman catheter complications in a haematology unit, 1996–1998. Intern Med J 2002;32:100–103.

357. Fijnheer R, Paijmans B, Verdonck LF, et al: Factor V Leiden in central venous catheter-associated thrombosis. Br J Haematol 2002;118:267–270.

358. Horne MK, May DJ, Alexander R, et al: Venographic surveillance of tunneled venous access devices in adult oncology patients. Ann Surg Oncol 1995;2:174–178.

359. Monreal M, Alastrue A, Rull M, et al: Upper extremity deep venous thrombosis in cancer patients with venous access devices: Prophylaxis with a low molecular weight heparin (Fragmin). Thromb Haemost 1996;75:251–253.

360. Monreal M, Lafoz E, Ruiz J, et al: Upper-extremity deep venous thrombosis and pulmonary embolism: A prospective study. Chest 1991;99:280–283.

361. Haire WD, Lynch TG, Lieberman RP, et al: Duplex scans before subclavian vein catheterization predict unsuccessful catheter placement. Arch Surg 1992;127:229–230.

362. Timsit JF, Farkas JC, Boyer JM, et al: Central vein catheter-related thrombosis in intensive care patients: incidence, risk factors and relationship with catheter-related sepsis. Chest 1998;114:207–213.

363. Mismetti P, Mille D, Laporte S, et al: Low-molecular-weight heparin (nadroparin) and very low doses of warfarin in the prevention of upper extremity thrombosis in cancer patients with indwelling long-term central venous catheters: A pilot randomized trial. Haematologica 2003;88:67–73.

364. Heaton DC, Han DY, Inder A: Minidose (1 mg) warfarin as prophylaxis for central vein catheter thrombosis. Intern Med J 2002;32:84–88.

365. Randolph AG, Cook DJ, Gonzales CA, et al: Benefit of heparin in central venous and pulmonary artery catheters: A meta-analysis of randomized controlled trials. Chest 1998;113:165–171.

366. Carr KM, Rabinowitz I: Physician compliance with warfarin prophylaxis for central venous catheters in patients with solid tumors. J Clin Oncol 2000;18:3665.

367. Stephens LC, Haire WD, Tarantolo S, et al: Normal saline vs heparin flush for maintaining central venous catheter patency during apheresis collection of peripheral blood stem cells (PBSC). Transfus Sci 1997;18:187–193.

368. Tezcan AZ, Tezcan H, Gastineau DA, et al: Case report: Heparin-induced thrombocytopenia after bone marrow transplantation: Report of two cases. Bone Marrow Transplant 1994;14:487–490.

369. Haire WD, Edney JA, Landmark JD, et al: Thrombotic complications of subclavian apheresis catheters in cancer patients: Prevention with heparin infusion. J Clin Apheresis 5:1990;188–191.

370. Stanislav GV, Fitzgibbons RJ, Bailey RT, et al: Reliability of implantable central venous access devices in patients with cancer. Arch Surg 1987;122:1280–1283.

371. Heit JA, Silverstein MD, Mohr DN, et al: Risk factors for deep vein thrombosis and pulmonary embolism. Arch Intern Med 2000;160: 809–815.

372. Heit JA, O'Fallon WM, Petterson TM, et al: Relative impact of risk factors for deep vein thrombosis and pulmonary embolism. Arch Intern Med 2002;162:1245–1248.

373. Desai AA, Vogelzang NJ, Rini BI, et al: A high rate of venous thromboembolism in a multi-institutional phase II trial of weekly intravenous gemcitabine with continuous infusion fluorouracil and daily thalidomide in patients with metastatic renal cell carcinoma. Cancer 2002;95:1629–1636.

374. Levine M, Hirsh J, Gent M, et al: Double-blind randomised trial of very-low-dose warfarin for prevention of thromboembolism in stage IV breast cancer. Lancet 1994;343:886–889.

375. Rajan R, Gafni A, Levine M, et al: Very low-dose warfarin prophylaxis to prevent thromboembolism in women with metastatic breast cancer receiving chemotherapy in economic evaluation. J Clin Oncol 1995;13:42–46.

376. Heit JA, Melton LJ, Lohse CM, et al: Incidence of venous thromboembolism in hospitalized patients vs community residents. Mayo Clin Proc 2001;76:1102–1110.

377. Samama MM, for the Sirius Study Group: An epidemiologic study of risk factors for deep vein thrombosis in medical outpatients. Arch Intern Med 2000;160:3415–3420.

378. Mismetti P, Laporte-Simitsidis S, Tardy B, et al: Prevention of venous thromboembolism in internal medicine with unfractionated or low-molecular-weight heparins: A meta-analysis of randomised clinical trials. Thromb Haemost 2000;83:14–19.

379. Samama MM, Cohen AT, Darmon J-Y, et al: A comparison of enoxaparin with placebo for the prevention of venous thromboembolism in acutely ill medical patients. N Engl J Med 1999;341:793–800.

380. de Lissovoy G, Subedi P: Economic evaluation of enoxaparin as prophylaxis against venous thromboembolism in seriously ill medical patients: A US perspective. Am J Manag Care 2002;8:1082–1088.

381. Agnelli G, Piovella F, Buoncristiani P, et al: Enoxaparin plus compression stockings compared with compression stockings alone in the prevention of venous thromboembolism after elective neurosurgery. N Engl J Med 1998;339:80–85.

382. Estrada CA, McElligott J, Dolezal JM, et al: Asymptomatic patients at high risk for deep venous thrombosis who receive inadequate prophylaxis should be screened. South Med J 1999;92:1145–1150.

46

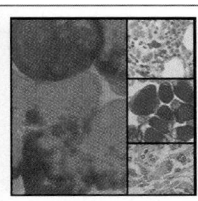

FEVER IN THE NEUTROPENIC CANCER PATIENT

Alison G. Freifeld

Andre Kalil

Edward Rubenstein

SUMMARY OF KEY POINTS

INCIDENCE

- Neutropenia is a frequent occurrence in cancer patients due to the underlying disease or its therapy.
- The frequency of infectious complications is related to the degree and duration of neutropenia.
- Infection (either clinically or microbiologically defined) can be documented in about 40% of febrile episodes, and the remaining episodes are of unknown etiology. In either case, empirical antibiotic therapy is essential.

PATHOGENS

- The most common infecting organisms are gram-positive cocci, especially coagulase-negative staphylococci, viridans streptococci, and *Staphylococcus aureus*; the predominant gram-negative pathogens are *Escherichia coli*, *Klebsiella* spp., and *Pseudomonas aeruginosa*.

- Fungal infections are not uncommon in bone marrow transplant and leukemia patients and are usually caused by *Candida* spp. or *Aspergillus* spp. *Candida albicans* infections are infrequent in the setting of fluconazole prophylaxis, but non-*C. albicans* are increasing in incidence.

TREATMENT

- Cultures should be collected and antibiotic therapy should be instituted promptly.
- Antibiotic regimen should be active against the common gram-positive cocci and gram-negative bacilli (including *P. aeruginosa*) and may include monotherapy or combinations of antibiotics. However, vancomycin should be strictly reserved for specific indications.
- Low-risk patients (no medical comorbidities) may be treated as outpatients with oral ciprofloxacin plus amoxicillin-clavulanate.

- Predominant pathogens within the hospital and their antibiotic-susceptibility patterns should influence antibiotic selection.
- If the patient has persistent fever after 3 to 4 days, and the infecting organism has not been identified, therapy may be modified if the patient is unstable or new clinical or microbiologic data dictate a change.
- Often it is necessary to institute antifungal therapy on an empirical basis after day 5 to 7 of broad-spectrum antibiotics if the patient is still febrile.
- Treatment of fungal infections is seldom successful unless the neutropenia resolves.
- Colony-stimulating factors and white blood cell transfusions may be considered in some neutropenic patients with a documented infection who are not responding to antimicrobial therapy.

INTRODUCTION

Neutropenia is a common and predictable consequence of many cytotoxic cancer therapies and a frequent complication of malignancies that impair bone marrow function. Neutrophilic granulocytes are a critical component of host defenses, primarily against bacterial and fungal pathogens. They mediate many inflammatory responses toward invading organisms to contain and eliminate infections. Accordingly, a deficit of neutrophils (i.e., neutropenia) is associated with an increase in susceptibility to infections as well as an attenuation of inflammatory responses to infections. Clinical signs and symptoms of inflammation may be muted, even in the setting of active infection in the neutropenic patient. Infection unopposed by innate neutrophil responses can progress rapidly and relentlessly, leading to high levels of morbidity and mortality. Oncologists must be aware of this risk and approach neutropenic cancer patients with care and vigilance.[1]

This chapter focuses on infections during the early phases of chemotherapy-induced neutropenia, primarily in relatively lower risk patients (i.e., those who have solid tumors or who are undergoing autologous stem cell transplant). Patients with acute leukemia or those undergoing allogeneic stem cell transplant are at higher risk for serious infections, and the spectrum of infections in those patients is expanded, as described in Chapter 47.

NEUTROPENIA AS A RISK FACTOR FOR INFECTION

The association between neutropenia and increased infection risk was initially demonstrated by Bodey and colleagues[2] in 1966 in a study of leukemic patients undergoing cytotoxic therapy. The data show that the frequency of infectious complications is inversely related to the degree and duration of neutropenia (Fig. 46-1). Infection risk starts to increase when the neutrophil

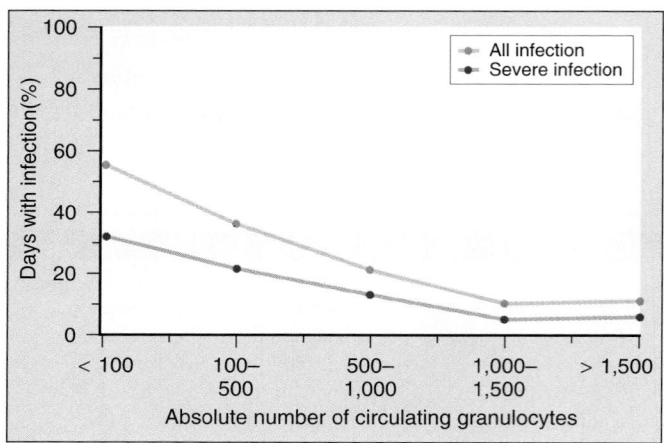

Figure 46-1. Relation between neutrophil count and infection in patients with acute leukemia.

count decreases to less than 1000 cells/mm^3 and increases dramatically when it is less than 500 cells/mm^3. Fewer than half of the neutropenic patients who become febrile will have an identified or occult infection. In roughly 10% to 20% or more of patients with neutrophil counts less than 100 cells/mm^3, a bloodstream infection will develop. The remainder of patients with fever and neutropenia have a "fever of undetermined origin" (FUO), with no identifiable source despite examination and cultures.[1-3]

The duration of neutropenia also is an important determinant of both infection risk and infection type. Brief durations of neutropenia, particularly those lasting less than 7 days, are associated with a rapid and favorable response to empirical antibiotic therapy.[4] A neutrophil count persistently less than 500 cells/mm^3 for more than 10 days is considered to represent a "high risk" state. Such patients are not only at high risk of developing an infection, but they also are at greater risk for infection-related morbidity and mortality as a consequence of prolonged neutropenia. Prolonged and profound neutropenia is a particular risk for acquiring invasive fungal disease such as *Aspergillus*, a frequently fatal invasive mold infection. The pathogens responsible for initial infections, early in the course of fever and neutropenia, are primarily bacteria and viruses, whereas antibiotic-resistant bacteria, yeast, fungi, and viruses are common causes of subsequent infections. Deaths are usually due to these subsequent infections. Mortality due to initial infections is relatively rare.[5,6]

In addition to cytotoxic chemotherapy, other cases of neutrophil deficiency may be due to bone marrow incompetence as a result of myelodysplastic syndrome or to crowding out of normal granulocytic precursors by tumor cells. "Functional neutropenia" due to impaired neutrophil microbicidal activity may arise as a consequence of underlying disease such as leukemia or therapies such as steroids. Ineffective neutrophil killing leaves the patient highly vulnerable to infection despite seemingly normal peripheral white blood cell counts.

OTHER RISK FACTORS FOR INFECTION

Disruption of integumentary, mucosal, and mucociliary barriers by cytotoxic therapies provides opportunities for invasion by colonizing bacteria on the skin, gastrointestinal (GI) tract, or mucous membranes (Table 46-1). Shifts in normal colonizing microbial flora at these sites occur as a result of chemotherapy, antibiotic use, and nosocomial exposures, leading to increased colonization with gram-negative and/or antibiotic-resistant pathogens. Indwelling catheters pose a significant breach in host defense, permitting access of skin flora and other pathogens directly into blood or subcutaneous tissue. Tumor growth can disrupt normal anatomic structures, whereas cancer surgery may result in anatomic alterations and wounds, providing local sites of pathogen entry. Underlying diseases and cancer therapies also play important roles in infection risk. For example, hypogammaglobulinemia often complicates chronic lymphocytic leukemia (CLL) or multiple myeloma, so that patients are at increased risk for severe pneumococcal infections, *Haemophilus influenzae* or *Neisseria meningitides*. In contrast to patients with solid tumors, those with acute leukemias are more likely to have overwhelming sepsis or invasive fungal infections because of prolonged periods of profound neutropenia. Patients with acute lymphocytic leukemia, Hodgkin's disease, or non-Hodkin's lymphoma (NHL) typically have defects in cell-mediated immunity that predispose them to *Pneumocystis carinii* pneumonia, cryptococcal disease, or infections with intracellular organisms such as *Salmonella* or *Listeria*. Steroid therapy induces a broad immunosuppressive effect, including impaired chemotaxis and killing by neutrophils, impaired T-cell function, and alterations in skin and mucosal barriers. Long-term and/or high-dose steroid therapy is a significant risk factor for invasive fungal infections, in particular (i.e., aspergillus and cryptococcus) as well as *P. carinii* (usually seen with a steroid taper), bacterial infections, and *Mycobacterium tuberculosis* reactivations. High-dose cytosine arabinoside therapy causes mucositis that may predispose to life-threatening streptococcal bacteremias. Fludarabine and pentostatin cause prolonged suppression of CD4

TABLE 46-1

Additional Factors Influencing the Risk of Infection in Neutropenic Patients
Intravenous devices
Mucositis
Lymphopenia
Chemotherapeutic regimen
Adrenal corticosteroid therapy
Tissue damage
Bone marrow transplantation
Acute leukemia
Antimicrobial prophylaxis
Colonization
Environmental sources
Seasonal exposures

lymphocytes and attendant susceptibility to infections with *Listeria*, *P. carinii* and herpesvirus.[6]

SOURCES OF INFECTION

Colonization by pathogenic bacteria, fungi, or viruses is generally a prerequisite for infection. Accordingly, endogenous bacterial and fungal flora and latent herpesvirus infections account for the majority of initial infections in the neutropenic cancer patient.[7] These include skin colonizers such as *Staphylococcus aureus* and coagulase-negative staphylococci, viridans streptococci, and herpes simplex from the oropharynx, and gram-positive bacteria as well as enteric gram-negative bacteria from the gut. *Candida albicans* infections are often derived from the skin or the GI or female genital tracts. Latent infections that may reactivate during immunosuppression include herpes simplex, varicella zoster, Epstein-Barr virus, and cytomegalovirus (CMV), as well as hepatitis B or C viruses, *M. tuberculosis*, and *Toxoplasma gondii*. Contaminated blood products, hospital equipment, water sources, and nosocomial spread of organisms from health care workers represent less common albeit significant sources of infection in immunocompromised cancer patients. Common nosocomially spread infections include *Clostridium difficile*, respiratory viruses, vancomycin-resistant Enterococci, and other multiresistant bacteria. Water sources such as faucets and shower heads have been implicated in the spread of *Legionella*. Outbreaks of infection related to intravenous solutions have been well documented with *Klebsiella* and *Enterobacter*.[8] Foods can be a potential infection source, particularly unwashed fruits and vegetables. Neutropenic patients are generally advised to avoid raw foods of this type unless measures are taken to peel or thoroughly wash them. Potted plants, mulch, excavation, and building or renovation sites have been identified as sources of *Aspergillus* spp. and other molds that may cause disease.[9,10]

SPECIFIC SITES OF INFECTION

Bacteremia

Bloodstream infections occur in about 20% of febrile patients with neutrophil counts of less than 100/mm³.[1–4] The risk of bacteremia is related to the depth of neutropenia, the presence of an indwelling catheter, or any tissue sites of infection. The majority of bacteremias are due to gram-positive organisms, with coagulase-negative staphylococci and streptococci predominating. Gram-negative pathogens, including *Escherichia coli*, *Enterobacter*, *Klebsiella*, and *Pseudomonas aeruginosa* are important, albeit less frequent pathogens (Table 46-2).

A classification system for bacteremias in febrile neutropenic patients has been developed, based on size and presence of associated tissue involvement.[11] Complex bacteremias were those associated with deep-tissue infections of the lung, the liver and spleen, the kidney, the

colon, bone and joints, veins and heart, meninges, soft tissues with necrosis, or skin/soft tissue/wound/cellulitis >5 cm. Simple bacteremias were associated with less tissue involvement (bacteruria, otitis, pharyngitis, soft tissue <5 cm). The prognostic significance of complex infection associated with bacteremia on survival was dramatic. At 21 days, 20% of patients with complex infections were dead compared with only 5% of patients with simple bacteremias ($P < .0001$). Profoundly neutropenic patients with simple bacteremias had a much higher response rate to antibiotics compared with patients with complex bacteremias (94% vs 70%; $P < .0001$). The median time to defervescence for patients with simple bacteremias was half that observed for patients with complex bacteremias (2.5 days vs 5.3 days; $P < .0001$).

Skin

Primary infections of the skin and soft tissue are commonly associated with fever in the patient with neutropenia. The differential diagnosis in febrile neutropenic patients includes infections that are localized to skin or disseminated from a bacterial source. Erythema gangrenosum is a localized necrotic skin lesion that portends a bloodstream infection, especially due to *P. aeruginosa*. Other causes of rash include the underlying disease itself and hypersensitivity reactions to drug therapy. Wolfson and associates[12] developed a helpful classification based on pathophysiology of skin lesions in the compromised host. Infections are grouped into four areas: (1) those typical of normal hosts (but with a greater propensity for serious disease in the compromised host; e.g., *S. aureus* and *Staphylococcus pyogenes*); (2) those

TABLE 46-2

Organisms Causing Infection in Neutropenic Patients

COMMON	UNCOMMON
Gram-Positive	
Staphylococcus epidermidis	*Enterococcus*
Staphylococcus aureus	*Corynebacterium jeikeium*
Staphylococcus viridans	*Bacillys* spp.
	Stomatococcus mucilaginosus
	Clostridium spp.
Gram-Negative	
Escherichia coli	*Stenotrophomonas maltophilia*
Klebsiella spp.	*Capnocytophaga* sp.
Pseudomonas aeruginosa	*Acinetobacter* sp.
Enterobacter spp.	
Serratia marcescens	
Fungi	
Candida spp.	*Mucorales*
Aspergillus spp.	*Fusarium* spp.
	Trichosporon beigelii
	Blastoschizomyces capitatus
Viruses	
Herpes simplex	Cytomegalovirus
Respiratory syncytial virus	Influenza

Problems Common to Cancer and Its Therapy

II

with extensive cutaneous involvement by pathogens that normally cause minor disease (e.g., varicella-zoster, herpes simplex, *Candida*, and *Malassezia*); (3) those from a cutaneous source with an opportunistic pathogen (e.g., atypical mycobacteria and *Aspergillus*); and (4) those from a noncutaneous source (*P. aeruginosa*, *S. aureus*, *Aeromonas hydrophila*, *Vibrio* spp., *C. septicum*, *Klebsiella pneumoniae*, *Histoplasma capsulatum*, and *C. immitis*).

The typical signs of cellulites, including erythema, warmth, tenderness, and swelling, may be present, but purulent drainage and abscess formation rarely occur during neutropenia. Secondary aspiration of the lesion is seldom possible. A skin biopsy for culture and histopathologic examination may be useful in these circumstances, although it must be balanced by anticipated poor wound healing subsequently. When a systemic bacterial infection or an endemic mycosis is suspected, blood cultures and specific serologic tests may increase the yield of a diagnosis.

Lungs

The lungs are the site of infection with the greatest associated morbidity and mortality, even when a specific pathogen is not identified. About 25% of all febrile episodes in the neutropenic patient and 50% of documented infections are pneumonias.[13] Auscultatory abnormalities in the chest may be minimal or nonexistent, and the chest radiograph examination is normal at the onset of symptoms in 30% of neutropenic patients.[14] A computed tomography (CT) scan of the chest may further define the pulmonary process. Neutropenia will decrease the diagnostic advantage normally provided by the sputum examination, because purulent sputum production is rare in this setting. Bronchoalveolar lavage (BAL) may increase the diagnostic yield, especially for *P. carinii*, viruses, and bacteria. The yield for molds such as *Aspergillus* with this procedure has been mostly in the range of 50% for suspected cases, so a negative BAL does not necessarily rule out an invasive fungal process. However, the use of polymerase chain reaction (PCR) techniques in BAL may increase these yields.[15] A diagnostic serum technique based on the detection of galactomannan, a cell-wall component of *Aspergillus*, has recently been evaluated.[16] However, the exact role of this test must be further defined in large prospective studies. If the clinical picture, radiography, and BAL are nondiagnostic, a thoracoscopic lung biopsy should be considered if the patient's platelet count is adequate.

Numerous infectious and noninfectious causes of pulmonary infiltrates are found in the cancer patient with fever and neutropenia.[13] Noninfectious causes include the underlying disease itself, radiation therapy, drug toxicity, pulmonary hemorrhage, and leukostasis. Infectious involvement of the lungs may be caused by bacteria (*Pneumococcus*; Enterobacteriaceae; pseudomonads; *Legionella* spp.), fungi (*Candida*; *Aspergillus*; *Fusarium* spp.), viruses [influenza; parainfluenza; respiratory syncytial virus (RSV); CMV; herpes simplex virus (HSV)] and Protozoa (*Toxoplasma*; *Cryptococcus*; *Strongyloides*).

The empirical antimicrobial regimen for pneumonia should be designed based on the patient's clinical condition, chest radiograph, and CT appearance. Focal lesions are suggestive of bacterial etiology and should be treated accordingly with broad-spectrum antibiotics. Nodular lesions are suggestive of mold infection such as *Aspergillus*. The superiority of voriconazole over amphotericin B for the treatment of proven or probable aspergillosis was recently demonstrated in a large clinical trial, so most experts consider voriconazole the initial therapy of choice for this infections.[17] A diffuse interstitial picture is suggestive of atypical pneumonia, such as *Legionella* and *Mycoplasma*, or opportunistic infections such as *P. carinii* and CMV. Atypical pneumonias are treated with fluoroquinolones (except ciprofloxacin) or a macrolide. *P. carinii* standard treatment is with trimethoprim/sulfamethoxazole (TMP/SMZ) at high doses (20 mg/kg/day). CMV pneumonia requires treatment with intravenous (IV) ganciclovir. Intravenous immunoglobulin appears to play an important role as an adjuvant treatment for CMV pneumonia.[18]

Vascular Access Devices

Patients with cancer commonly require indwelling venous access devices (VADs) for the administration of chemotherapy, blood products, and parenteral nutrition, as well as for withdrawal of blood for therapy monitoring and microbiologic evaluation. Infection is a common complication of indwelling catheters. The risk of infection varies with the device used, duration of placement, and extent of the patient's immunosuppression. Local signs and symptoms, such as erythema and tenderness, are unreliable indicators of catheter infection even in the immunocompetent patient. However, the evolution of these signs over time is suggestive of infection. VAD infections are categorized as entry-site infections, tunnel or pocket infections, and catheter-associated bloodstream infections.

Entry-site infections can be treated effectively with appropriate antimicrobial therapy without the need for catheter removal. Tunnel and pocket infections require catheter removal, as well as the immediate initiation of an empirical antimicrobial therapy that includes vancomycin to cover *S. aureus*, until culture results are available.

It is often difficult to determine whether a bloodstream infection is related to the VAD, because frequently no evidence of local catheter inflammation is seen. Most catheter-related infections will respond to antimicrobial therapy alone without catheter removal, with certain exceptions. Catheter removal is advisable for patients with bloodstream infections caused by fungi (yeasts and molds) and nontuberculous *Mycobacteria* (*M. chelonae*, *M. fortuitum*, *M. abscessus*). For other bacteria, the decision concerning the need for catheter removal will depend on the severity of the clinical picture, the degree of immunosuppression, and the availability of a new vascular access in a given patient. It is notable that certain catheter infections such as those due to *Bacillus* organisms, *Corynebacterium jeikeium*, *S. aureus*, *P. aeruginosa*, *Stenotrophomonas maltophilia*, and vancomycin-resistant *Enterococcus* may be considered to be treated by the combination of catheter removal and antibiotics. *Staphylococcus aureus* may cause endocarditis, and the value of the transesophageal echocardiography in the setting of any *S. aureus* bloodstream infections has been well demonstrated to determine duration of therapy.[19] In general, if blood cultures remain positive despite antimicrobial therapy for more than 48 hours, or if the patient is clinically unstable, the catheter should be removed independent of the etiology.

Upper Gastrointestinal Tract

Mucositis of the oral cavity and alimentary mucosa results from many cytotoxic therapies for cancer. Disruption of the gastrointestinal mucosa causes erosions and inflammation that can provide a portal of entry for colonizing organisms. It may be difficult to discriminate between drug-induced and infection-induced mucositis. Esophageal symptoms of odynophagia, dysphagia, and retrosternal or epigastric discomfort do not point to a specific etiology. The most common organisms causing local infection are herpes simplex virus and *Candida* spp., although gram-negative and anaerobic bacteria also may be causative organisms. The treatment of presumed esophagitis is often based on the empirical administration of antacids and/or systemic antifungal or antiviral therapy. For patients who do not respond to empirical therapy with these agents, careful upper endoscopy may be considered to obtain a more precise diagnosis based on direct visualization of the lesions as well as on tissue collection for histopathologic and microbiologic examination. Esophageal endoscopy may be associated with substantial morbidity in patients who are profoundly neutropenic and/or thrombocytopenic, and it is often advisable to wait until counts recover before proceeding.

Lower Gastrointestinal Tract

Enteritis clinically manifested by diarrhea may occur in the patient with fever and neutropenia. Similar to the involvement of the upper GI tract, the differentiation between noninfectious causes, such as drug-induced mucositis and infection-induced mucositis, may be difficult. *C. difficile* enteritis has mainly been associated with previous antibiotic therapy, but occasionally with cancer chemotherapy.[20] If a *C. difficile* toxin screen is positive, therapy with oral metronidazole should be implemented. Other bacterial causes of diarrhea are uncommon in cancer patients unless exposure to such pathogens has occurred. CMV can cause protracted and/or hemorrhagic diarrhea, especially in infected children.

Typhlitis (also known as *neutropenic enterocolitis*) is a unique and potentially life-threatening syndrome in the febrile neutropenic patient, particularly in those with leukemia or who have had intensive cytotoxic therapy. It commonly appears with abdominal pain, especially in the right lower quadrant, and often with attendant rebound tenderness, decreased bowel sounds, fever, and diarrhea. Typhlitis may be limited to the cecum, but can involve the entire intestine. CT scanning is the diagnostic study of choice and usually demonstrates thickening of the bowel wall.[21] *C. septicum*, *P. aeruginosa*, enteric gram-negatives, and anaerobes are the most common pathogens associated with this syndrome. *C. difficile* is occasionally associated with typhlitis, so metronidazole should be included in the initial antibiotic treatment regimen for this condition. Severe sepsis, bowel perforation, and hemorrhage may accompany or follow typhlitis. Therapy consists of nasogastric suction, bowel rest, IV fluid, and broad-spectrum antibiotics to cover the gram-negatives and anaerobes cited earlier. In approximately 5% of patients with typhlitis, complications develop requiring surgical intervention, including uncontrolled sepsis, lower GI bleeding, or perforation.[22]

Perirectal infection occurs primarily in patients with acute leukemia and especially among those with monocytic and myelomonocytic leukemia, although it is relatively uncommon. The usual symptoms are fever, pain on defecation, and persistent rectal discomfort. Although anaerobes are thought to play a role in these infections, the associated bacteremias are most likely caused by *P. aeruginosa*, *E. coli*, and other enteric gram-negative bacteria. Therapy consists of broad-spectrum antibiotics, warm compresses, and stool softeners. Although few abscesses develop in the absence of neutrophils, some patients will benefit from surgical incision and drainage.

Sinuses

Cytotoxic therapy disrupts the natural cleansing mechanisms in the nasal passages and increases sinus colonization with pathogenic bacteria. The symptoms of sinus infection may be milder than those in the normal patient because of impaired inflammatory response. A limited sinus CT scan is highly sensitive for the diagnosis of acute sinusitis and may help to distinguish bacterial from viral or fungal etiology. Bony erosion on the CT scan strongly suggests invasive fungal infection and should prompt immediate evaluation by a specialist in ear, nose, and throat surgery. Suspected bacterial sinusitis should be treated with appropriate broad-spectrum antibiotics. If a mold infection such as *Aspergillus* is suspected, a sinus biopsy should be performed for culture and histopathologic examination, and treatment with antifungal therapy directed toward filamentous fungi such as amphotericin B or voriconazole should be initiated.

MAJOR PATHOGENS

The range of identified initial infecting pathogens is fairly limited. In past decades from the 1960s to the 1980s, gram-negative organisms originating from bowel colonization were the predominating cause of microbiologically documented infections in neutropenic patients.[1-5] The association of gram-negative infections, particularly *P. aeruginosa*, with septic shock and severe pneumonia in this setting is the reason that a potent antipseudomonal antibiotic is at the core of most empirical therapy regimens developed then. Gram-positive organisms have since become the most common pathogens isolated from neutropenic patients with fever. This trend over the last 20 years indicates that gram-positive bacteria accounted for 60% to 70% of documented bloodstream infections (see Fig. 46-1).[23] Coagulase-negative staphylococci, viridans streptococci, and enterococci predominate, although *S. aureus* also is a common serious pathogen. Gastrointestinal flora, including *E. coli, Klebsiella* spp., and *P. aeruginosa* are the most common gram-negative pathogens. HSV and respiratory viruses including RSV, parainfluenza, and influenza A and B also are frequent initial pathogens. Deaths resulting from initial infections remain uncommon, generally in the 5% to 10% range. Subsequent infections isolated later in the course of fever and neutropenia are caused by organisms that are often the most difficult to diagnose, most resistant to treatment, and associated with the highest rates of major morbidity and mortality.

Staphylococcus epidermidis

S. epidermidis currently is the most common cause of bacteremia among patients receiving immunosuppressive cancer therapy.[24] The increased frequency of these infections is related to both the widespread use of intravascular catheters, especially long-term indwelling catheters, and the use of prophylactic antibiotic regimens that are inactive against these organisms. *S. epidermidis* commonly colonizes bowel and skin surfaces and is a frequent contaminant, but it may be a prominent source of morbidity, particularly in relation to catheter infections. Because *S. epidermidis* is a common contaminant, a single positive blood culture for this organism may not be considered to represent a true infection. The diagnosis is made if two or more blood cultures (appropriately obtained) are positive for *S. epidermidis* and the clinical picture is compatible. If these criteria are fulfilled, the patient is considered to have a documented infection due to this organism. Because the vast majority of *S. epidermidis* is methicillin resistant, vancomycin is the drug of choice.[23]

Staphylococcus aureus

S. aureus infections may account for up to one fourth of all infections and 10% to 15% of all bloodstream infections in patients with malignancy and neutropenia.[23] The clinical picture is variable and depends on the site of infection. As in the immunocompetent patient, *S. aureus* may cause bacteremia and may seed distant sites to cause pneumonia, endocarditis, or osteomyelitis. Because of the typical virulence of this organism, the neutropenic patient should be treated as early as possible with the most potent antistaphylococcal therapy available, depending on the resistance patterns seen at a given institution. Even a single positive blood culture for *S. aureus* is enough to institute at least 2 weeks of antibiotics. While sensitivities are pending, vancomycin is the drug of choice. Linezolid, a new antibiotic with potent gram-positive activity, has recently been approved for nosocomial pneumonia and complicated skin infections caused by methicillin-susceptible and -resistant strains of *S. aureus*. Resistance to linezolid has already been reported to occur during therapy, however, in rare instances.[24]

Streptococcus viridans

The frequency of viridans streptococcal bacteremia (also called "alpha" streptococci in many microbiology laboratories) in the febrile neutropenic patient has increased over the last three decades.[25] Once thought to be only a contaminant, it is now clear that viridans streptococcal bacteremia accounts for significant morbidity and mortality in the neutropenic patient. Up to one fourth of the patients with alpha streptococcal bacteremia may have a fulminant picture of septic shock characterized by hypotension, rash, and palmar desquamation, and in 10%, adult respiratory distress syndrome develops. Endocarditis occurs rarely in the neutropenic patient. β-Lactam antibiotics plus an aminoglycoside are the usual therapy of choice. However, if *Streptociccus mitis* is known or suspected in a neutropenic patient, the addition of vancomycin is recommended, because the majority of *S. mitis* are β-lactam resistant. Risk factors associated with viridans streptococcal bacteremias include high-dose cytosine arabinoside treatment, profound neutropenia, prophylactic administration of TMP/SMZ or a fluoroquinolone, use of antacids or H_2-receptor antagonists, presence of mucositis, large radiation dose to the oral cavity, HSV infections, and the presence of an indwelling venous catheter. Despite the use of levofloxacin prophylaxis, breakthrough viridans streptococcal bacteremia due to fluoroquinolone-resistant strains has been well documented.[26]

Bacillus Species

Most of the infections are caused by *Bacillus cereus* and *Bacillus subtilis* involve the skin at the catheter site or sites of trauma.[27] Impetiginous necrotic lesions, ulcerations, and rapidly spreading gas gangrene have been reported in severely neutropenic patients.[28] However, similar to the *S. epidermidis* dilemma, the isolation of this organism from a single blood culture does not always indicate infection. It is important to correlate the clinical picture with two or more positive blood cultures to improve the diagnostic yield. Catheter-related bacteremias usually require catheter removal for the resolution of infection. Prompt recognition of this pathogen is important because *B. cereus* is resistant to most β-lactam antibiotics, but is susceptible to imipenem, vancomycin, and aminoglycosides.

Pseudomonas aeruginosa

Although the frequency of gram-negative infections has decreased among neutropenic patients in recent years, *P. aeruginosa* remains a serious threat. Sepsis is the most common presenting picture, but this organism can cause pneumonia, severe otitis externa, sinusitis, mastoiditis, endophthalmitis, and meningitis. Erythema gangrenosum skin lesions may be an important distinguishing feature of *Pseudomonas* bacteremia. The lesions are small, round, indurated nodules found in the groin, perianal area, extremities, and axillary areas that often begin as vesicles and progress to hemorrhage, necrosis, and ulceration.

An antipseudomonal β-lactam is the mainstay of treatment, and many experts would consider adding an aminoglycoside for synergy. However, if the patient with *Pseudomonas* infection is severely ill, combination therapy with maximal doses is recommended. Mortality remains high despite advances in therapy, ranging from one third to two thirds of the cases.[29] Unfavorable outcome is associated with absolute granulocyte count of less than 100 cells/mm[3], persistent neutropenia, septic shock, renal failure, and metastatic foci of infection.[30]

Candida

The spectrum of disease caused by *Candida* spp. ranges from mild mucocutaneous lesions (e.g., thrush) to disseminated deep-tissue involvement (e.g., hepatosplenic candidiasis). All forms of invasive candidiasis probably follow an episode of candidemia. However, not all candidemias are clinically or microbiologically detected, and end-organ disease may be the first manifestation of invasive candidiasis. Fewer than half of those with invasive disease have a prior positive blood culture for *Candida*.[31]

Neutropenia, the presence of an indwelling venous catheter, and chemotherapy-associated GI mucosal injury are important risk factors for invasive candidiasis, rendering cancer patients at especially high risk. *Candida*-related mortality rates of 33% to 75% are reported in cancer patients.[32] Because of the difficulty in diagnosing this infection and the associated high mortality, any blood culture found to grow even a single colony of *Candida* must be regarded as a sign of true infection, and the patient should receive therapy. Clinical signs of candidemia may range from fever alone to fulminant sepsis. About 15% of neutropenic patients will have pustular skin lesions. *C. albicans* accounts for about half of the cases, but non-*albicans* species, especially *C. glabrata* and *C. krusei*, are increasing in incidence. Notably, these species are somewhat resistant or fully resistant to fluconazole, respectively.

Amphotericin B or its lipid formulations remain the treatment of choice for candidemia or deep-tissue invasive disease in neutropenic patients. Fluconazole or caspofungin are acceptable alternatives for sensitive species in non-neutropenic patients. Indeed, a recent randomized trial found caspofungin to be superior to amphotericin B in the treatment of non-neutropenic patients with invasive candidiasis.[33] Caspofungin is approved for candidemia in non-neutropenic patients as well as for peritonitis, intra-abdominal abscess, and pleural space infections due to *Candida*. However, a paucity of data in neutropenic patients does not allow its current recommendation in that setting.

Catheter-related candidemia should be treated with antifungal therapy, and the catheter should be removed in most cases.[34] For a patient who has candidemia and a nontunneled central venous catheter infection, initial management should include an attempt to exchange the catheter. For a patient who has candidemia and a tunneled central venous catheter infection, the decision about its removal should be based on the likelihood of catheter-related candidemia. Factors indicating catheter-related candidemia include (1) isolation of *Candida parapsilosis* from blood samples; (2) quantitative blood cultures showing fivefold the number of colonies isolated from blood drawn through the catheter, compared with blood drawn from a peripheral vein; (3) differential time to positivity (>2 hours) for blood samples drawn from a percutaneous site, compared with those drawn through the catheter; (4) candidemia in a patient who is receiving hyperalimentation through the catheter; and (5) persistent candidemia while receiving systemic antifungal therapy.[35] Catheter removal is strongly encouraged under any of these circumstances.

Hepatosplenic Candidiasis

Hepatosplenic candidiasis is a form of chronic disseminated candidiasis that almost exclusively affects patients undergoing leukemia induction or stem cell transplantation.[36] It generally manifests only on recovery from neutropenia, as persistent fevers unresponsive to antibacterial agents. Patients may have right upper quadrant tenderness and a variety of other GI symptoms. Consistent laboratory findings include marked elevation of alkaline phosphatase, with normal or mildly elevated bilirubin and transaminases, and a rebound leukocytosis after neutrophil recovery. Blood cultures are almost always negative for fungal growth, as are liver biopsies. Suspicion of hepatosplenic candidiasis is confirmed by the presence of multiple well-defined lesions in the liver and/or spleen, and occasionally in the kidneys on CT scan or ultrasound. Characteristic lesions also may be seen on ultrasound or magnetic resonance imaging (MRI). Liver biopsy and histopathology may be performed to confirm the diagnosis. A prolonged course of therapy, initially with amphotericin B or a lipid formulation, and then with fluconazole for a number of months, has been advocated. For patients with acute leukemia and hepatosplenic candidiasis, repeated cycles of chemotherapy may be given once the infection is stabilized, and the antifungals are continued through the courses of cytotoxic therapy.

Aspergillus

Aspergillus is uncommon among patients receiving routine chemotherapy for solid tumors. It is most often seen in high-risk patients with prolonged neutropenia, prolonged high-dose steroid therapy, and/or graft-versus-host disease. The two most common sites of primary invasive disease are the lungs and the sinuses. Approximately one third of patients with acute invasive pulmonary aspergillosis have no attributable symptoms or signs initially, and the suspicion may arise just from surveillance image studies.[37] Sometimes the only evidence of infection is prolonged fever with nodular or other atypical pulmonary infiltrates that fail to respond to antibacterial therapy.

Dry cough, low-grade fever, and pleuritic or nonspecific chest pain are characteristic presenting symptoms. Hemoptysis and pneumothorax are rare presenting features. Plain radiographs may be completely normal early in the picture or may show the classic wedge-shaped pleural-based densities or cavities later in the disease process. CT scan findings appear to be more sensitive and specific than plain chest radiographs, especially early in the picture. A chest CT may show the "halo sign" (an area of low attenuation surrounding a nodular lung lesion caused by blood or edema) initially and later, the "crescent sign" (an air crescent near the periphery of a lung nodule, caused by contraction of infarcted tissue). Although these CT abnormalities are not diagnostic of invasive aspergillosis, they are highly suggestive of this infection in the high-risk patient. BAL may be very helpful if septate hyphae with acute-angle branching are seen on Gomori methenamine silver or periodic acid–Schiff stains. However, the definitive diagnosis of invasive disease requires both culture and histopathologic evidence of *Aspergillus*. Enzyme-linked immunosorbent assay (ELISA), enzyme immunoassay (EIA), and immunoblot assays have been recently developed to detect *Aspergillus* galactomannan in urine, sera, cerebrospinal fluid, and BAL, but the utility of these tests is unclear.[38] If suspicion exists of invasive pulmonary aspergillosis in an immunocompromised patient, antifungal therapy directed against *Aspergillus* should be promptly started, even before the final confirmation of infection. Voriconazole is the current drug of choice for invasive aspergillosis based on recent results from a large phase III trial, in which it proved superior to amphotericin B with regard to disease responses and survival after 12 weeks of therapy.[17] Secondary therapies include amphotericin B and its lipid formulations and liquid itraconazole. Caspofungin is approved for invasive aspergillosis refractory to or in patients intolerant of other therapies (i.e., amphotericin B, lipid formulations of amphotericin B, and/or itraconazole). Combination therapy may be used in cases that are refractory to monotherapy on the basis of theoretical and in vitro evidence of synergy between caspofungin and azoles or amphotericin.[39,40] However, no specific recommendations can be made now because of the lack of clinical data supporting or rejecting this approach. Severe hemoptysis or lesions impinging on the great vessels or major airways may require surgical treatment.

The initial symptoms of invasive *Aspergillus* sinusitis such as fever, cough, headache, and occasional epistaxis may not be clinically differentiated from bacterial sinusitis. A black eschar on the nose, nasal septum, or palate strongly suggests a fungal etiology. As infection progresses, destruction of sinuses and periorbital tissues occurs. The organism may erode through the base of the skull and cause cerebral infarction or extensive destruction of the palate. Pulmonary and sinus aspergillosis may occur simultaneously. CT scan and/or MRI of the sinuses are the diagnostic tests of choice and help to delineate the extent of the disease. Bony erosion on CT scan of sinuses in a neutropenic patient is highly suggestive of aspergillosis. Culture and histopathologic examination are required for the definitive diagnosis, but therapy should be promptly started with the slightest suspicion of invasive *Aspergillus* sinusitis. Amphotericin B has been the most commonly used therapy, although voriconazole is now considered the drug of choice for invasive *Aspergillus* sinusitis. Endoscopic surgery for ethmoid sinus disease and debridement may be used as an adjunctive therapy when orbital, facial, or intracranial involvement is present.

APPROACH TO FEVER IN THE NEUTROPENIC PATIENT

Fever is often the only reliable sign of significant underlying infection in the neutropenic patient. No specific clinical features or patterns of fever can accurately distinguish between fever due to an infection versus that due to a noninfectious cause.[1] Therefore all febrile neutropenic patients should receive empirical broad-spectrum antibiotics, ideally within 1 hour of presentation. Although a clinically or microbiologically documented source of fever is not found in most patients with fever and neutropenia, the rapid initiation of empirical antibiotics remains an important standard of care for all patients in this setting.

Definitions

The precise definitions of fever and neutropenia vary slightly from one center to another. Guidelines developed by the Infectious Disease Society of America (IDSA) and U.S. Food and Drug Administration for evaluating antimicrobial therapy for fever and neutropenia are widely used, however.[41]

Fever is considered to be single temperature measurement of 38.3°C (101°F) or greater, in the absence of other obvious causes. A temperature of 38°C or greater for an hour or more is considered a "febrile state" that also requires prompt evaluation and intervention in the setting of neutropenia. Rarely, a neutropenic patient who is afebrile may have signs or symptoms of infection (i.e., abdominal pain, severe mucositis, perirectal pain) and should be considered to have an active infection. The concomitant administration of corticosteroids may also initially blunt the fever response. Afebrile neutropenic patients who show signs or symptoms suggestive of an infection should have empirical antibiotics started immediately because of their increased risk for serious invasive infections.[41] (see later).

Neutropenia is defined as an absolute neutrophil count (ANC) less than 1000 cells/mm^3 in some centers, but more often is designated by a neutrophil counts of less than 500 cells/mm^3, which is a level associated with a much higher risk for infection. For practical purposes, an ANC of less than 500 cells/mm^3, or a count that is anticipated to fall below that level within 48 hours, constitutes a state of neutropenia.

Initial Evaluation

The initial evaluation should be directed toward determining the possible sites of infection and causative organisms and assessing the patient's level of risk for infection-related complications. A thorough site-specific review of systems is essential. Pertinent history includes recent antibiotic therapy, recent surgery or other invasive procedures such as biopsies or catheter placement, as well as possible exposure to infections from close contacts and household members, foods, animals, or travel.

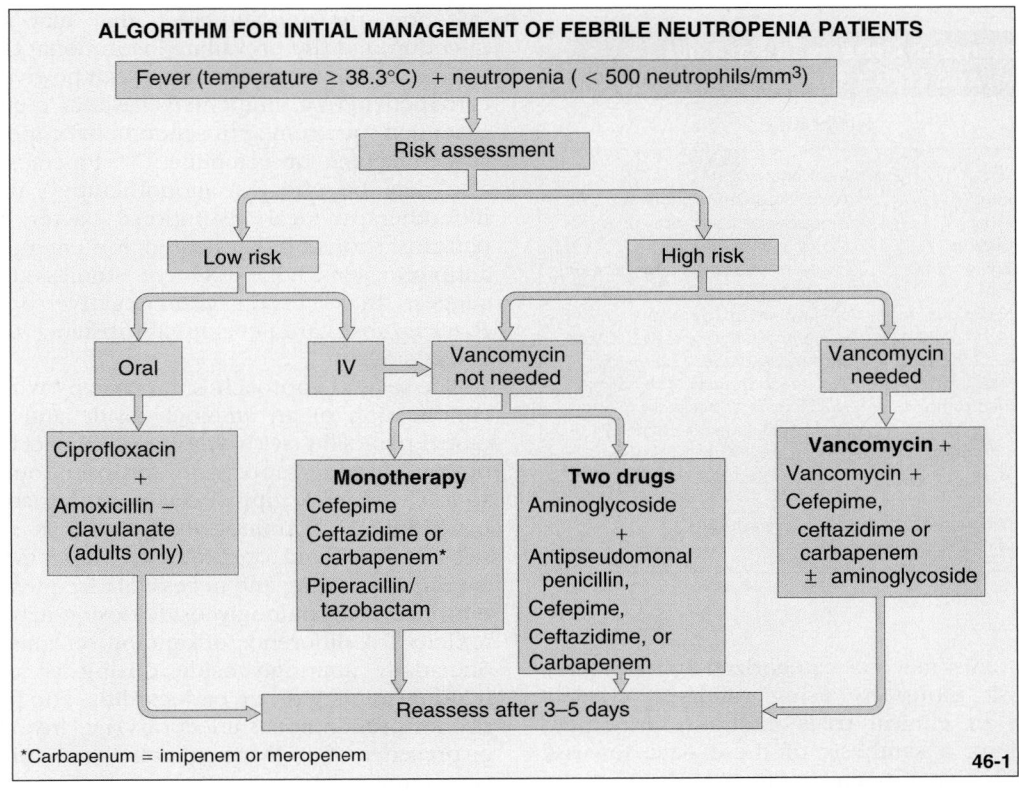

ALGORITHM FOR INITIAL MANAGEMENT OF FEBRILE NEUTROPENIA PATIENTS

Fever (temperature ≥ 38.3°C) + neutropenia (< 500 neutrophils/mm³)

Risk assessment

Low risk / High risk

Oral | IV | Vancomycin not needed | Vancomycin needed

Ciprofloxacin + Amoxicillin – clavulanate (adults only)

Monotherapy
Cefepime
Ceftazidime or carbapenem*
Piperacillin/ tazobactam

Two drugs
Aminoglycoside + Antipseudomonal penicillin, Cefepime, Ceftazidime, or Carbapenem

Vancomycin +
Vancomycin + Cefepime, ceftazidime or carbapenem ± aminoglycoside

Reassess after 3–5 days

*Carbapenum = imipenem or meropenem

46-1

The physical examination should focus on common potential sites of infection, again keeping in mind that the manifestations of infection are muted in the absence of inflammatory cells. Careful examination of the oropharynx may reveal ulcers, or plaquelike lesions may be due to herpes or thrush, and appropriate tests should be sent to evaluate them. Catheter sites require careful assessment for erythema, tenderness, or discharge. Bacterial cellulitis of the skin or perirectum may have minimal induration and erythema; pimples or pustules are uncommon without neutrophils to create pus. Similarly, few respiratory symptoms may be found, and auscultation of the lungs may reveal few adventitial sounds there, but an infiltrate may be seen on radiograph.[42] A urinary tract infection may not be associated with dysuria. GI tract mucositis due to cytotoxic chemotherapy can lead to sore throat, oral ulcers, and/or diarrhea that are indistinguishable from symptoms of infection. Abdominal pain in neutropenic patients may signify a wide variety of problems, including intestinal tumor necrosis or neutropenic enterocolitis, both of which can result in intra-abdominal catastrophe or sepsis.

Initial laboratory evaluation should include a complete blood count and differential white cell count to determine the degree of neutropenia, liver and renal function tests, oxygen saturation, and urinalysis. Chest radiographs should be performed if signs and symptoms suggest a pulmonary process, but they may have minimal findings initially in neutropenic patients with pneumonia.

Two blood culture samples, each consisting of 20 to 40 mL of blood, should be obtained from febrile, neutropenic patients.[41] The volume of blood taken for culture enhances the chances of recovering a pathogen.[43] The utility of taking blood from both a vascular catheter and a peripheral vein is controversial. Although dual-site cultures may help determine whether the catheter is a source of infection, a recent meta-analysis revealed little clinical value in culturing two separate sites.[44] Accordingly, some experts recommend that only catheter-derived blood cultures (two sets) are necessary. Quantitative blood cultures are not routinely used because of their expense.

Cultures of any suggestive sites of infection should be performed: diarrheal stools should be tested for the presence of *C. difficile* toxin, viral cultures sent of suspected oral or perineal lesions for HSV, and nasal wash or swab cultures for respiratory viruses obtained in patients with suggestive symptoms during the winter season.

Risk Assessment

Risk assessment should be performed as part of the initial evaluation (Table 46-3). Risk assessment attempts to predict the probability that a patient will experience serious complications during a febrile episode, and also helps determine whether the patient who is at low risk for serious complications could safely receive treatment outside of the traditional hospital setting and receive initial empirical therapy with oral antibiotics. Clinical-prediction rules and many prospective clinical trials have shown that risk categorization can predict outcomes, including complications and mortality, during the febrile

TABLE 46-3

Risk-Assessment Criteria in Patients with Fever and Neutropenia

LOW RISK	HIGH RISK
• Outpatient • No associated acute comorbid illness that independently indicates inpatient treatment or close observation • Good performance status (ECoG 0–1) • Serum creatinine, ≤2.0 mg/dL; liver function tests, ≤3× normal • Nontransplant, solid tumor, or lymphoma patient • Anticipated total duration of neutropenia, <7 days	• Inpatients • Associated comorbid illness that requires hospitalization, or is clinically unstable (i.e., hypotension, dehydration, altered mental status, abdominal pain, pneumonia, or hypoxia) • Uncontrolled/progressive cancer • Serum creatinine, >2.0 mg/dL, liver function tests, >3× normal • HSCT or BMT recipient • Prolonged severe neutropenia anticipated: ≤100 cells/μL for ≥7 days

BMT, bone marrow transplant; ECoG, electrocorticography; HSCT, hematopoietic stem cell transplant.

episode.[45-57] Patients may be categorized into either a high- or low-risk group by using validated clinical-prediction rules or clinical trials methods for patient eligibility. Based on a synthesis of these data, low-risk patients generally have been defined as having the following characteristics:

• Outpatient status at onset of fever during neutropenia
• Solid tumor or hematologic malignancy with no history of fungal infection
• No comorbid illnesses at presentation (e.g., hypotension, dehydration, altered mental status, respiratory/renal/hepatic insufficiency, uncontrolled pain)
• Anticipated duration of neutropenia less than 10 days
• Age 60 years or younger

High-risk patients are those with one or more of the following:

• Uncontrolled underlying cancer
• Inpatient status at presentation with fever and neutropenia
• A comorbid medical illness at presentation
• Long duration of neutropenia anticipated (more than 10 days)

Empirical Antibiotic Therapy: General Principles

Numerous clinical trials over the last three decades have failed to demonstrate the clear superiority of one empirical antibiotic therapy regimen over all others. However, effective and reliable regimens are characteristically bactericidal for gram-negative pathogens, particularly *P. aeruginosa*, even in the absence of neutrophils. Several antibiotic approaches are acceptable, but it is important to note that the final choice of a specific regimen will depend on the patient's risk factors for

infection, the specific sites that may be sources of infection, and the prevailing institutional flora.[58]

First, antibiotic monotherapy can be given with either a carbapenem (e.g., imipenem-cilastatin, meropenem) or an extended-spectrum antipseudomonal cephalosporin, such as ceftazidime or cefepime.[59-62] Piperacillin/tazobactam also may be effective monotherapy.[63] Before initiating monotherapy, local institutional bacterial susceptibility patterns should be evaluated for emerging changes in antibiotic sensitivities. Recent studies at some centers suggest that certain gram-negative organisms (e.g., *P. aeruginosa*) are developing resistance to cefepime and ceftazidime.[64]

The second approach is duotherapy with either (1) the combination of an aminoglycoside and an antipseudomonal penicillin (with or without a β-lactamase inhibitor) or an extended-spectrum antipseudomonal cephalosporin[65-67]; or (2) ciprofloxacin plus an antipseudomonal penicillin.[45-47,68] Aminoglycoside use is associated with risks of renal and otic toxicity. These toxicities require careful monitoring and necessitate frequent reassessment, but once-a-day aminoglycoside dosing may diminish renal toxicity.[67] A difference of opinion remains as to whether once-daily aminoglycoside dosing is appropriate for treating meningitis or endocarditis. For patients at high risk for pseudomonas infections (i.e., history of infections or presence of ecthyma gangrenosum), initial duotherapy is recommended.

Double β-lactam antibiotic combinations using a combination of an extended-spectrum cephalosporin, antipseudomonal penicillin, and/or monobactams (e.g., aztreonam) also have been effective as initial antibiotic

PRINCIPLES OF INITIAL EMPIRICAL ANTIBIOTIC SELECTION

Empirical antibiotic therapy should be started promptly in patients. It is possible to treat most infections successfully with a single broad-spectrum β-lactam antibiotic or a combination of a β-lactam plus an aminoglycoside.

Aminoglycosides are as effective and no more toxic when administered in a single dose as when given in divided doses. Patients receiving other ototoxic or nephrotoxic agents are at greater risk of aminoglycoside toxicity, irrespective of the dosage schedule.

Aminoglycosides alone are ineffective for therapy of infections in neutropenic patients and must be given in combination with an appropriate β-lactam antibiotic.

Not all β-lactam antibiotics are equally efficacious.

Antibiotic selection must take into consideration the predominant pathogens and antibiotic sensitivity patterns within the hospital.

Once the patient's infection is definitely responding clinically, an oral regimen may be substituted for intravenous therapy.

Patients with persistent fever should be considered for empirical antifungal therapy, but the patient must be examined carefully for other possible causes.

Selected febrile neutropenic patients can be treated with oral antimicrobial agents in an outpatient setting.

TABLE 46-4

Vancomycin Use in Appropriate or Acceptable

Vancomycin should be considered as initial therapy only in patients at high risk of serious gram-positive pathogen infection. Because of the increased risk of gram-positive infections and the emergence of vancomycin-resistant organisms, empirical vancomycin should be avoided except for serious infections associated with the following clinical situations:

- Clinically apparent, serious, catheter-related infection
- Substantial mucosal damage and high risk for infection with penicillin-resistant viridans streptococci (especially patients with preceding prophylaxis with quinolone antibiotics or trimethoprim/sulfamethoxazole)
- Blood culture positive for gram-positive bacterium before final identification and susceptibility testing
- Known colonization with penicillin/cephalosporin-resistant pneumococci or methicillin-resistant *Staphylococcus aureus*
- Hypotension or septic shock without an identified pathogen

Vancomycin should be discontinued in 2–3 days after starting if a resistant gram-positive infection is not identified.

From CDC Guidelines, 1995

therapy.[69] Some experts advise caution in using double β-lactam combinations because of the potential for gram-negative bacillary resistance or an increase in fungal superinfections.[41]

The third recommended approach is the use of vancomycin along with one of the aforementioned antibiotic regimens, but only for specific indications (Table 46-4). Support for the judicious use of vancomycin has developed because of the emergence of β-lactam–resistant gram-positive pathogens, such as *S. aureus*, coagulase-negative staphylococci, viridans streptococci, enterococci, and *C. jeikeium*.

Initial Empiric Antibiotic Therapy in Low-Risk Patients

For patients who are determined to be at low risk for developing infection-related complications during the course of neutropenia, oral ciprofloxacin *plus* amoxicillin/clavulanate (or clindamycin for patients who are allergic to penicillin) is an effective alternative to intravenous monotherapy, based on several large randomized studies.[45-47] Several small studies investigated the efficacy of high-dose ciprofloxacin or ofloxacin for empirical oral monotherapy, but the evidence does not currently support the routine use of these fluoroquinolones for monotherapy in low-risk patients with fever and neutropenia.[48,49,70,71] Ciprofloxacin as a single agent does not provide adequate coverage for certain gram-positive organisms (e.g., *S. aureus*, alpha streptococci), and therefore should never be used without an additional antibiotic directed toward those pathogens.

Empirical Vancomycin Therapy

A considerable debate is found about the use of empirical vancomycin in patients with fever and neutropenia. The clinical concern has been that a small portion of infections caused by gram-positive pathogens can be fulminant and lead to rapid death in patients who are not treated promptly with appropriate antibiotics. However, a large, prospective, randomized trial from the European Organization for Research and Treatment of Cancer failed to show true clinical advantages for empirical vancomycin in adults.[72] This study reported that empirical vancomycin decreased the number of days the patients had fever but did not improve survival. The major concern surrounding the uncontrolled use of vancomycin has been the emergence of vancomycin-resistant organisms, especially enterococci. The increase in vancomycin resistance generally has been associated with excessive use of vancomycin among hospitalized patients. The Hospital Infection Control Practices Advisory Committee of the Centers for Disease Control and Prevention has issued guidelines for the appropriate use of vancomycin that are aimed at preventing the spread of vancomycin resistance.[73] Vancomycin addition should be considered only in patients at high risk for serious gram-positive infection. Specific clinical situations that may justify initial use of vancomycin therapy in the febrile neutropenic cancer patient population are as follows (see Table 46-4):

- Serious, clinically apparent, catheter-related infections are documented. Many of these infections are caused by coagulase-negative staphylococcal isolates, which have high-level β-lactam antibiotic resistance.[74]
- Substantial mucosal damage is found with high risk for infection with penicillin-resistant viridans streptococci. Notably, 18% to 29% of viridans streptococci isolated will be β-lactam resistant.[75] High-dose cytarabine or intensive therapy that damages oropharyngeal mucosal barriers has been associated with an increased risk of such viridans streptococcal infections.[25]
- The patient's blood cultures are positive for gram-positive bacteria before final identification and susceptibility testing.
- Known colonization is present with β-lactam–resistant pneumococci or methicillin-resistant *S. aureus*.
- The patient received previous prophylaxis with ciprofloxacin or TMP/SMZ. Both of these agents have been associated with an increased risk of gram-positive infections.[25,26,75] The broad-spectrum, gram-negative, bacillary coverage and limited gram-positive pathogen activity of these drugs allow colonization and subsequent infection with such organisms. The newer fluoroquinolones with enhanced gram-positive activity (e.g., levofloxacin, moxifloxacin, gatifloxacin) may be more effective in preventing gram-positive infections, although severe viridans streptococcal infections have been noted to break through levofloxacin prophylaxis.
- Hypotension or septic shock develops in the patient without an identified pathogen.

Empirical vancomycin could be considered in any of these situations, but the therapy should be reassessed within 2 to 3 days of initiation. If a resistant gram-positive pathogen cannot be identified, empirical vancomycin therapy should then be discontinued.[73]

Initial Empirical Therapy for Patients Who Are Clinically Unstable

Because of the high mortality rate in patients with fever and neutropenia seen with the systemic inflammatory response syndrome, initial triple-drug therapy with a carbapenem, an aminoglycoside, and vancomycin is recommended for these patients. Patients who have hypotension when with fever and neutropenia, or those who have a history of *P. aeruginosa* colonization or invasive disease, should receive dual therapy with an antipseudomonal β-lactam (cephalosporin or penicillin) plus an aminoglycoside or ciprofloxacin.

Follow-up

Daily evaluation by a health care professional who is experienced in treating patients with fever and neutropenia is essential. The daily examination should focus on a site-specific assessment, and an infectious disease consultation should be considered for all complicated cases or progressive infections. At least 3 to 4 days of antibiotic treatment is usually required to determine the efficacy of the initial regimen. It is important to remember that the time to defervescence for febrile cancer patients with neutropenia who receive appropriate initial antibiotic therapy ranges from 2 to 7 days.[1,65] This rate of fever response should be considered when clinicians are assessing the need to adjust initial antibiotics.

Although slow defervescence of fever is anticipated, it still often complicates decisions regarding the need for repeated blood cultures. Whereas some experts recommend daily blood cultures until the patient becomes afebrile, increasing evidence suggests that daily blood cultures are unnecessary in neutropenic patients with persistent fever.[76] Current bacterial blood culture systems, such as the BACTEC continuous-monitoring culture system, can detect 90% to 100% of bacterial pathogens within 48 hours of culture. For this reason, ordering additional cultures before obtaining the results from the initial series should be discouraged, unless the patient is failing to show clinical response. Daily review of previously obtained cultures is critical, and it is recommended that clearance of bloodstream bacterial or fungal infections be documented with follow-up cultures.

The most important determinants of the duration of antimicrobial therapy are documentation of infection and the patient's neutrophil count. This observation has led some specialists to recommend continuation of antibiotics until there are signs of hematologic recovery.[77] However, others argue that continuing antibiotics may increase the risk of drug toxicity, prolong hospitalization, and increase the risk of subsequent infection with fungi or resistant bacteria.

Subsequent Modifications of Empirical Antibiotics

No empirical antibiotic regimen initially administered for fever and neutropenia can be expected to cover all possible infections that may occur during the course of neutropenia; therefore modifications of the initial regimen are sometimes required. Patients with a fever persisting beyond 4 days of initial antimicrobial therapy and without an identifiable site or source of infection should undergo reassessment of their antimicrobial therapy. The need for a change in therapy should be based on the patient's clinical status, results of examination and cultures, and likelihood of early marrow recovery. Although fever resolution may be slow, persistent fever may suggest a nonbacterial infection, a bacterial infection that is resistant to empirical antibiotics, the emergence of a secondary infection, a closed-space infection, inadequate antimicrobial serum levels, or drug fever. These patients may be quite complicated, and, in rare circumstances, serial antimicrobial changes will be necessary. However, frequent and arbitrary antibiotic changes for persistent fever, in an otherwise stable patient, are discouraged. An infectious disease consultation for these patients is strongly recommended. The clinically stable patient with persistent fever may be safely watched without altering the initial antimicrobial therapy. Vancomycin that may have been started earlier should be discontinued if the patient does not meet the criteria for its use. If the fever persists beyond 5 to 7 days, a change in antibiotic regimen or initiation of empirical antifungal therapy should be strongly considered.[1,41] For patients with a documented infection, it is important to note that tissue-based infections such as pneumonia may take longer to respond to antimicrobial therapy.

For the patient who is persistently febrile and clinically unstable, a change in antibacterial antibiotics may be needed. The addition of increased gram-negative bacillary coverage is often recommended. The addition of vancomycin should be considered if the patient's clinical situation justifies its use, as per Table 46-4. If fever persists or is recrudescent beyond 5 to 7 days of empirical antibiotic therapy, antifungal therapy should be initiated empirically because the risk of invasive fungal disease increases with prolonged neutropenia.[1,41]

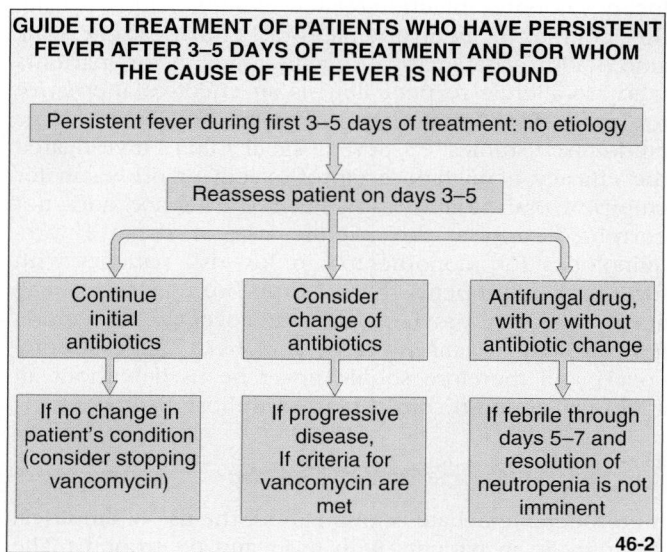

GUIDE TO TREATMENT OF PATIENTS WHO HAVE PERSISTENT FEVER AFTER 3–5 DAYS OF TREATMENT AND FOR WHOM THE CAUSE OF THE FEVER IS NOT FOUND

Persistent fever during first 3–5 days of treatment: no etiology

Reassess patient on days 3–5

Continue initial antibiotics	Consider change of antibiotics	Antifungal drug, with or without antibiotic change
If no change in patient's condition (consider stopping vancomycin)	If progressive disease, If criteria for vancomycin are met	If febrile through days 5–7 and resolution of neutropenia is not imminent

46-2

Empirical Antifungal Therapy

Although amphotericin B has been the standard empirical antifungal agent used for patients with prolonged or recrudescent fever during neutropenia (e.g., after 5 to 7 days of broad-spectrum antibiotics), itraconazole has recently been demonstrated to have efficacy in this setting as well.[78] However, the Food and Drug Administration recently issued a warning about the potential for patients receiving itraconazole to develop liver or heart failure.[79] It appears that the duration of therapy is important, with the incidence of adverse effects increased among patients who receive prolonged courses of therapy. The committee recommends caution in using itraconazole as empirical antifungal therapy in patients with cancer in whom fever and neutropenia develop.

A recently published randomized comparison of voriconazole and liposomal amphotericin B for empirical antifungal therapy in patients with neutropenia and persistent fever showed that both agents were generally effective, but the results failed to fulfill the protocol-defined criteria for noninferiority of voriconazole versus the amphotericin preparation. However, breakthrough fungal infections were less frequent in patients receiving voriconazole.[80]

Duration of Antibiotic Therapy

It is recommended that empirical antibiotics continue until recovery to more than 500 neutrophilic cells/mm³ or an ANC more than 100 cells/mm³ for more than 2 days, as long as the neutrophil count is likely to continue to increase (patients are often taking a growth factor). This recommendation assumes that the patient is clinically well and afebrile for at least 24 hours before antibiotic discontinuation. Some experts recommend a minimum of at least 4 days of antibiotics, even if ANC recovery is more rapid.[1,41]

Patients who become afebrile but remain persistently neutropenic (<500 neutrophilic cells/mm³) should receive a more prolonged course of antibiotic therapy. Most experts recommend a 10- to 14-day course of treatment. Treatment for such patients should not be discontinued until the patient has been afebrile for at least 5 to 7 days.

Documented infections should be treated for a minimum duration of 7 to 14 days with an antibiotic regimen that is narrowed and directed toward any organisms that have been documented microbiologically. Most experts prefer to continue antibiotics at least until the ANC returns to more than 500 cells/mm³. A longer course is given if clinically necessary, regardless of neutrophil recovery.[1,41]

PROPHYLAXIS

Antibacterial Prophylaxis

In general, the use of antibacterial prophylaxis is not recommended for cancer patients who are undergoing routine chemotherapy. No substantive data indicate that antibiotic prophylaxis reduces infection or mortality in this patient population. However, it appears that patients at higher risk (e.g., leukemic or stem cell transplant patients) may benefit from prophylactic antibiotics. Different antibacterial prophylaxis strategies have been studied, most commonly selective GI decontamination with nonabsorbable antibiotics or systemic prophylaxis with absorbable agents. However, the interpretation of numerous trials is complicated because of different study designs, lack of controlled groups, heterogeneous patient populations, and failure to monitor properly the compliance with prophylaxis.[81-87]

TMP-SMZ prophylaxis has been associated with lower infection rates, especially among patients who had neutropenia longer than 2 weeks after reinduction of cytotoxic therapy for leukemia.[82,88] However, the use of prophylaxis also has been associated with higher rates of fungal overgrowth, and it has not had any impact on overall patient mortality.[88] Furthermore, myelosuppression and the development of drug-resistant bacteria may occur with the use of TMP-SMZ. Fluoroquinolones, such as ciprofloxacin and levofloxacin, have been associated with prevention of febrile episodes of infectious origin, especially gram-negative bacillary infections in high-risk populations.[86] However, fluoroquinolone prophylaxis has had no effect on the rate of gram-positive and fungal infections and no consistent effect on overall mortality in numerous studies. Moreover, bacteremia with methicillin-resistant *S. aureus* and the emergence of quinolone-resistant gram-negative bacilli may occur more frequently in neutropenic patients who receive fluoroquinolone prophylaxis.[88,89] Thus the IDSA recommends, "these antibiotics should not be used as prophylaxis routinely in medical centers in which resistance has already been observed or if parenteral quinolones are part of the empirical therapy for febrile episodes in neutropenic patients."[41] Most experts reserve fluoroquinolone prophylaxis for patients undergoing leukemia induction therapy or stem cell transplant. Little experience has accrued with the newer fluoroquinolones, such as moxifloxacin or gatifloxacin, for this purpose because they lack potent antipseudomonal activity that is thought to be a prerequisite for prophylaxis in neutropenic patients.

Antifungal Prophylaxis

Azole prophylaxis is not used routinely for patients undergoing less-intensive cytoxic therapies, such as chemotherapy for solid tumors, because the risk of invasive infections due to *Candida* and *Aspergillus* are relatively low. However, as with antibacterial prophylaxis, azole prophylaxis is beneficial in higher risk patients. Fluconazole or itraconazole prophylaxis has been shown to reduce the frequency of both superficial and systemic *Candida* infections in patients who undergo stem cell transplantation.[90-92] It is important to note that fluconazole has no activity against *C. krusei* and only dose-dependent activity against *C. glabrata*, so it may not reliably cover these organisms. The routine use of this drug for prophylaxis may shift the fungal colonization pattern in a given institution toward more azole-resistant species.[93] Furthermore, fluconazole has no antifungal activity against molds such as *Aspergillus*, so it cannot be relied on to prevent invasive disease due to these organisms.

Antiviral Prophylaxis

Disseminated CMV and HSV infections are not common causes of fever in neutropenic patients. Reactivation of HSV infection may occur after chemotherapy. HSV reactivations are associated with increased mucosal damage, resulting in increasing pain, limitation of the patient's ability to maintain oral hydration and nutrition, and an increased risk of bacterial and fungal superinfections. Therefore HSV prophylaxis with acyclovir, valacyclovir, or famciclovir may be considered in patients who have had an outbreak during a prior chemotherapy cycle or in those who are undergoing intensive chemotherapies and are seropositive for HSV.

ADJUNCTIVE THERAPIES

Hematopoietic Growth Factors

Prophylactic use of hemopoietic growth factors is common in the setting of intensive chemotherapy regimens such as stem cell transplant. However, treatment of fever or infection with growth factors is not standard practice, as no benefit has been demonstrated. Several randomized controlled trials have been performed with growth factors as an adjunctive therapy to antimicrobials in the febrile patient with neutropenia.[94-97] The only consistent finding among most of the studies has been a minor decrease in the duration of neutropenia. No consistent impact on morbidity (duration of fever and use of antimicrobial) or mortality has been observed. Both the IDSA[41] and the American Society of Clinical Oncology[98] guidelines do not recommend the routine use of growth factors to treat febrile neutropenic patients. However, therapy with colony-stimulating factors could be considered for the patient who remains severely neutropenic and has a serious infection such as bacterial sepsis, pneumonia, severe cellulites or sinusitis, systemic fungal infections, hypotensive episodes, and multiorgan dysfunction secondary to sepsis.

Granulocyte Transfusions

Even though the use of granulocyte transfusion may potentially increase the response to antimicrobial therapy, benefits may be tempered by significant toxicities such as the transmission of CMV, alloimmunization associated with fever, graft-versus-host reactions if granulocytes are not irradiated, and progressive platelet refractoriness. Therefore the few situations in which this therapy may be potentially considered are the bacterial and fungal infection that can not be controlled with optimal antimicrobial therapy and/or granulocyte–colony-stimulating factor.[99-101]

REFERENCES

1. Pizzo PA: Management of fever in patients with cancer and treatment-induced neutropenia. N Engl J Med 1993;32:1323-1332.
2. Bodey GP, Buckley M, Sathe YS, Freireich EJ: Quantitative relationships between circulating leukocytes and infection in patients with acute leukemia. Ann Intern Med 1966;64:328-340.
3. Schimpff SC: Empiric antibiotic therapy for granulocytopenic cancer patients. Am J Med 1986;80:13-20.
4. Pizzo PA, Robichaud KJ, Wesley R, Commers JR: Fever in the pediatric and young adult patient with cancer. A prospective study of 1001 episodes. Medicine (Baltimore) 1982;61:153-165.
5. Wade JC: Management of infection in patients with acute leukemia. Hematol Oncol Clin North Am 1993;7:293-315.
6. O'Brien S, Kantarjian H, Beran M, et al: Results of fludarabine and prednisone therapy in 264 patients with chronic lymphocytic leukemia with multivariate analysis-derived prognostic model for response to treatment. Blood 1993;82:1695-1700.
7. Schimpff SC, Young VM, Greene WH, et al: Origin of infection in acute nonlymphocytic leukemia. Significance of hospital acquisition of potential pathogens. Ann Intern Med 1972;77:707-714.
8. Chodoff A, Pettis AM, Schoonmaker D, Shelly MA: Polymicrobial gram-negative bacteremia associated with saline solution flush used with a needleless intravenous system. Am J Infect Control 1995;23:357-363.
9. Moe G: Low microbial diets for patients with granulocytopenia. In As B (ed.): Nutrition Management of the Cancer Patient. Rockville, MD, Aspen, 1990, pp 125-134.
10. Anonymous: Guidelines for preventing opportunistic infections among hemtopoietic stem cell transpalnt recipients. MMWR 2000;49:1-128.
11. Elting LS, Rubenstein EB, Rolston KV, Bodey GP: Outcomes of bacteremia in patients with cancer and neutropenia: observations from two decades of epidemiological and clinical trials. Clin Infect Dis 1997;25:247-259.
12. Wolfson JS, Sober AJ, Rubin RH: Dermatologic manifestations of infection in the compromised host. Annu Rev Med 1983;34:205-217.
13. Whimbey E, Goodrich J, Bodey GP: Pneumonia in cancer patients. Cancer Treat Res 1995;79:185-210.
14. Valdivieso M, Gil-Extremera B, Zornoza J, Rodriquez V, Bodey GP: Gram-negative bacillary pneumonia in the compromised host. Medicine (Baltimore) 1977;56:241-254.
15. Raad I, Hanna H, Huaringa A, et al: Diagnosis of invasive pulmonary aspergillosis using polymerase chain reaction-based detection of aspergillus in BAL. Chest 2002;121:1171-1176.
16. Herbrecht R, Letscher-Bru V, Oprea C, et al: Aspergillus galactomannan detection in the diagnosis of invasive aspergillosis in cancer patients. J Clin Oncol 2002;20:1898-1906.
17. Herbrecht R, Denning DW, Patterson TF, et al: Voriconazole versus amphotericin B for primary therapy of invasive aspergillosis. N Engl J Med 2002;347:408-415.
18. Reed EC, Bowden RA, Dandliker PS, Lilleby KE, Meyers JD: Treatment of cytomegalovirus pneumonia with ganciclovir and intravenous cytomegalovirus immunoglobulin in patients with bone marrow transplants. Ann Intern Med 1988;109:783-788.
19. Rosen AB, Fowler VG Jr, Corey GR, et al: Cost-effectiveness of transesophageal echocardiography to determine the duration of therapy for intravascular catheter-associated Staphylococcus aureus bacteremia. *Ann Intern Med*. 1999;130:810-820.
20. Bartlett JG: Clostridium difficile-associated Enteric Disease. Curr Infect Dis Rep 2002;4:477-483.
21. Kirkpatrick ID, Greenberg HM: Gastrointestinal complications in the neutropenic patient: characterization and differentiation with abdominal CT. Radiology 2003;226:668-674.
22. Song HK, Kreisel D, Canter R, et al: Changing presentation and management of neutropenic enterocolitis. Arch Surg 1998;133:979-982.
23. Wisplinghoff HS, RP Wenzel, Edmond MB: Current trends in the epidemiology of nosocomial bloodstream infections in patients with hematological malignancies and solid neoplasms in hospitals in the United States. Clin Infect Dis 2003;36:1103-1110.

24. Tsiodras S, Gold HS, Sakoulas G, et al: Linezolid resistance in a clinical isolate of Staphylococcus aureus. Lancet 2001;358: 207-208.

25. Tunkel AR, Sepkowitz KA: Infections caused by viridans streptococci in patients with neutropenia. Clin Infect Dis 2002;34:1524-1529.

26. Razonable RR, Litzow MR, Khaliq Y, et al: Bacteremia due to viridans group Streptococci with diminished susceptibility to Levofloxacin among neutropenic patients receiving levofloxacin prophylaxis. Clin Infect Dis 2002;34:1469-1474.

27. Banerjee C, Bustamante CI, Wharton R, Talley E, Wade JC: Bacillus infections in patients with cancer. Arch Intern Med 1988;148: 1769-1774.

28. Bodey GP: Dermatologic manifestations of infections in neutropenic patients. Infect Dis Clin North Am 1994;8:655-675.

29. Maschmeyer G, Braveny I: Review of the incidence and prognosis of Pseudomonas aeruginosa infections in cancer patients in the 1990s. Eur J Clin Microbiol Infect Dis 2000;19:915-925.

30. Mallolas J, Gatell JM, Miro JM, Marco F, Soriano E: Epidemiologic characteristics and factors influencing the outcome of Pseudomonas aeruginosa bacteremia. Rev Infect Dis 1990;12: 718-719.

31. Swerdloff JN, Filler SG, Edwards JE Jr: Severe candidal infections in neutropenic patients. Clin Infect Dis 1993;17(Suppl 2): S457-S467.

32. Uzun O, Anaissie EJ: Predictors of outcome in cancer patients with candidemia. Ann Oncol 2000;11:1517-1521.

33. Mora-Duarte J, Betts R, Rotstein C, et al: Comparison of caspo-fungin and amphotericin B for invasive candidiasis. N Engl J Med 2002;347:2020-2029.

34. Rex JH, Walsh TJ, Sobel JD, et al: Practice guidelines for the treatment of candidiasis. Infectious Diseases Society of America. Clin Infect Dis 2000;30:662-678.

35. Mermel LA, Farr BM, Sherertz RJ, et al: Guidelines for the management of intravascular catheter-related infections. Clin Infect Dis 2001;32:1249-1272.

36. Kontoyiannis DP, Luna MA, Samuels BI, Bodey GP: Hepatosplenic candidiasis. A manifestation of chronic disseminated candidiasis. Infect Dis Clin North Am 2000;14:721-739.

37. Stevens DA, Kan VL, Judson MA, et al: Practice guidelines for diseases caused by Aspergillus. Infectious Diseases Society of America. Clin Infect Dis 2000;30:696-709.

38. Alexander BD: Diagnosis of fungal infection: new technologies for the mycology laboratory. Transpl Infect Dis 2002;4(Suppl 3): 32-37.

39. Arikan S, Lozano-Chiu M, Paetznick V, Rex JH: In vitro synergy of caspofungin and amphotericin B against Aspergillus and Fusarium spp. Antimicrob Agents Chemother 2002;46:245-247.

40. Perea S, Gonzalez G, Fothergill AW, et al: In vitro interaction of caspofungin acetate with voriconazole against clinical isolates of Aspergillus spp. Antimicrob Agents Chemother 2002;46: 3039-3041.

41. Hughes WT, Armstrong D, Bodey GP, et al: 2002 guidelines for the use of antimicrobial agents in neutropenic patients with cancer. Clin Infect Dis 2002;34:730-751.

42. Donowitz GR, Harman C, Pope T, Stewart FM: The role of the chest roentgenogram in febrile neutropenic patients. Arch Intern Med 1991;151:701-704.

43. Mermel LA, Maki DG: Detection of bacteremia in adults: consequences of culturing an inadequate volume of blood. Ann Intern Med 1993;119:270-272.

44. Siegman-Igra Y, Anglim AM, Shapiro DE, et al: Diagnosis of vascular catheter-related bloodstream infection: a meta-analysis. J Clin Microbiol 1997;35:928-936.

45. Freifeld A, Marchigiani D, Walsh T, et al: A double-blind comparison of empirical oral and intravenous antibiotic therapy for low-risk febrile patients with neutropenia during cancer chemotherapy. N Engl J Med 1999;341:305-311.

46. Rubenstein EB, Rolston K, Benjamin RS, et al: Outpatient treatment of febrile episodes in low-risk neutropenic patients with cancer. Cancer 1993;71:3640-3646.

47. Kern WV, Cometta A, De Bock R, et al: Oral versus intravenous empirical antimicrobial therapy for fever in patients with granulocytopenia who are receiving cancer chemotherapy. International Antimicrobial Therapy Cooperative Group of the European Organization for Research and Treatment of Cancer. N Engl J Med 1999;341:312-318.

48. Malik IA, Abbas Z, Karim M: Randomised comparison of oral ofloxacin alone with combination of parenteral antibiotics in neutropenic febrile patients. Lancet 1992;339:1092-1096.

49. Hidalgo M, Hornedo J, Lumbreras C, et al: Outpatient therapy with oral ofloxacin for patients with low risk neutropenia and fever: a prospective, randomized clinical trial. Cancer 1999;85:213-219.

50. Talcott JA, Siegel RD, Finberg R, Goldman L: Risk assessment in cancer patients with fever and neutropenia: a prospective, two-center validation of a prediction rule. J Clin Oncol 1992;10: 316-322.

51. Talcott JA, Finberg R, Mayer RJ, Goldman L: The medical course of cancer patients with fever and neutropenia. Clinical identification of a low-risk subgroup at presentation. Arch Intern Med 1988; 148:2561-2568.

52. Klastersky J, Paesmans M, Rubenstein EB, et al: The Multinational Association for Supportive Care in Cancer risk index: A multinational scoring system for identifying low-risk febrile neutropenic cancer patients. J Clin Oncol 2000;18:3038-3051.

53. Feld R, Paesmans M, Freifeld AG, et al: Methodology for clinical trials involving patients with cancer who have febrile neutropenia: updated guidelines of the Immunocompromised Host Society/Multinational Association for Supportive Care in Cancer, with emphasis on outpatient studies. Clin Infect Dis 2002;35:1463-1468.

54. Malik IA, Khan WA, Karim M, Aziz Z, Khan MA: Feasibility of outpatient management of fever in cancer patients with low-risk neutropenia: results of a prospective randomized trial. Am J Med 1995;98:224-231.

55. Elting LS, Rubenstein EB, Rolston K, et al: Time to clinical response: an outcome of antibiotic therapy of febrile neutropenia with implications for quality and cost of care. J Clin Oncol 2000;18:3699-3706.

56. Mustafa MM, Aquino VM, Pappo A, Tkaczewski I, Buchanan GR: A pilot study of outpatient management of febrile neutropenic children with cancer at low risk of bacteremia. J Pediatr 1996;128:847-849.

57. Karthaus M, Wolf HH, Kampfe D, et al: Ceftriaxone monotherapy in the treatment of low-risk febrile neutropenia. Chemotherapy 1998;44:343-354.

58. Rubin M, Hathorn JW, Pizzo PA: Controversies in the management of febrile neutropenic cancer patients. Cancer Invest 1988;6:167-184.

59. Ramphal R, Gucalp R, Rotstein C, Cimino M, Oblon D: Clinical experience with single agent and combination regimens in the management of infection in the febrile neutropenic patient. Am J Med 1996;100:S83-S89.

60. De Pauw BE, Deresinski SC, Feld R, Lane-Allman EF, Donnelly JP: Ceftazidime compared with piperacillin and tobramycin for the empiric treatment of fever in neutropenic patients with cancer. A multicenter randomized trial. The Intercontinental Antimicrobial Study Group. Ann Intern Med 1994;120:834-844.

61. Freifeld AG, Walsh T, Marshall D, et al: Monotherapy for fever and neutropenia in cancer patients: a randomized comparison of ceftazidime versus imipenem. J Clin Oncol 1995;13:165-176.

62. Cometta A, Calandra T, Gaya H, et al: Monotherapy with meropenem versus combination therapy with ceftazidime plus amikacin as empiric therapy for fever in granulocytopenic patients with cancer. The International Antimicrobial Therapy Cooperative Group of the European Organization for Research and Treatment of Cancer and the Gruppo Italiano Malattie Ematologiche Maligne dell'Adulto Infection Program. Antimicrob Agents Chemother 1996;40:1108-1115.

63. Del Favero A, Menichetti F, Martino P, et al: A multicenter, double-blind, placebo-controlled trial comparing piperacillin-tazobactam with and without amikacin as empiric therapy for febrile neutropenia. Clin Infect Dis 2001;33:1295-1301.

64. Jacobson K, Rolston K, Elting L, et al: Susceptibility surveillance among gram-negative bacilli at a cancer center. Chemotherapy 1999;45:325-334.

65. Cometta A, Zinner S, de Bock R, et al: Piperacillin-tazobactam plus amikacin versus ceftazidime plus amikacin as empiric therapy for

fever in granulocytopenic patients with cancer. The International Antimicrobial Therapy Cooperative Group of the European Organization for Research and Treatment of Cancer. Antimicrob Agents Chemother 1995;39:445-452.

66. Cordonnier C, Herbrecht R, Pico JL, et al: Cefepime/amikacin versus ceftazidime/amikacin as empirical therapy for febrile episodes in neutropenic patients: A comparative study. The French Cefepime Study Group. Clin Infect Dis 1997;24:41-51.

67. Leoni F, Ciolli S, Pascarella A, et al: Ceftriaxone plus conventional or single-daily dose amikacin versus ceftazidime/amikacin as empiric therapy in febrile neutropenic patients. Chemotherapy 1993;39:147-152.

68. Flaherty JP, Waitley D, Edlin B, et al: Multicenter, randomized trial of ciprofloxacin plus azlocillin versus ceftazidime plus amikacin for empiric treatment of febrile neutropenic patients. Am J Med 1989;87:S278-S282.

69. Winston DJ, Ho WG, Bruckner DA, Champlin RE: Beta-lactam antibiotic therapy in febrile granulocytopenic patients. A randomized trial comparing cefoperazone plus piperacillin, ceftazidime plus piperacillin, and imipenem alone. Ann Intern Med 1991;115:849-859.

70. Giamarellou H, Bassaris HP, Petrikkos G, et al: Monotherapy with intravenous followed by oral high-dose ciprofloxacin versus combination therapy with ceftazidime plus amikacin as initial empiric therapy for granulocytopenic patients with fever. Antimicrob Agents Chemother 2000;44:3264-3271.

71. Aquino VM, Herrera L, Sandler ES, Buchanan GR: Feasibility of oral ciprofloxacin for the outpatient management of febrile neutropenia in selected children with cancer. Cancer 2000;88:1710-1714.

72. EORTC International Antimicrobial Therapy Cooperative Group, National Cancer Institute of Canada: Vancomycin added to empirical combination antibiotic therapy for fever in granulocytopenic cancer patients. J Infect Dis 1991;163:951-958.

73. Hospital Infection Control Practices Advisory Committee (HICPAC): Recommendations for preventing the spread of vancomycin resistance. MMWR Recomm Rep 1995;44(RR-12):1-13.

74. Wade JC, Schimpff SC, Newman KA, Wiernik PH: Staphylococcus epidermidis: An increasing cause of infection in patients with granulocytopenia. Ann Intern Med 1982;97:503-508.

75. International Antimicrobial Therapy Cooperative Group of the European Organization for Research and Treatment of Cancer: Reduction of fever and streptococcal bacteremia in granulocyto-penic patients with cancer. A trial of oral penicillin V or placebo combined with pefloxacin. JAMA 1994;272:1183-1189.

76. Serody JS, Berrey MM, Albritton K, et al: Utility of obtaining blood cultures in febrile neutropenic patients undergoing bone marrow transplantation. Bone Marrow Transplant 2000;26:533-588.

77. Pizzo PA, Robichaud KJ, Gill FA, et al: Duration of empiric antibiotic therapy in granulocytopenic patients with cancer. Am J Med 1979;67:194-200.

78. Boogaerts M, Winston DJ, Bow EJ, et al: Intravenous and oral itraconazole versus intravenous amphotericin B deoxycholate as empirical antifungal therapy for persistent fever in neutropenic patients with cancer who are receiving broad-spectrum antibacterial therapy. A randomized, controlled trial. Ann Intern Med 2001;135:412-422.

79. Itraconazole, terbinafine possibly linked to liver failure. Am J Health Syst Pharm 2001;58:1076.

80. Walsh TJ, Pappas P, Winston DJ, et al: Voriconazole compared with liposomal amphotericin B for empirical antifungal therapy in patients with neutropenia and persistent fever. N Engl J Med 2002;346:225-234.

81. Bow EJ, Loewen R, Vaughan D: Reduced requirement for antibiotic therapy targeting gram-negative organisms in febrile, neutropenic patients with cancer who are receiving antibacterial chemoprophylaxis with oral quinolones. Clin Infect Dis 1995;20:907-912.

82. Ward TT, Thomas RG, Fye CL, et al: Trimethoprim-sulfamethoxazole prophylaxis in granulocytopenic patients with acute leukemia: evaluation of serum antibiotic levels in a randomized, double-blind, placebo-controlled Department of Veterans Affairs Cooperative Study. Clin Infect Dis 1993;17:323-332.

83. Kerr KG, Armitage HT, McWhinney PH: Activity of quinolones against viridans group streptococci isolated from blood cultures of patients with haematological malignancy. Support Care Cancer 1999;7:28-30.

84. Martino R, Subira M, Altes A, et al: Effect of discontinuing prophylaxis with norfloxacin in patients with hematologic malignancies and severe neutropenia. A matched case-control study of the effect on infectious morbidity. Acta Haematol 1998;99:206-211.

85. Hughes WT, Rivera GK, Schell MJ, Thornton D, Lott L: Successful intermittent chemoprophylaxis for Pneumocystis carinii pneumonitis. N Engl J Med 1987;316:1627-1632.

86. Kern W, Kurrle E: Ofloxacin versus trimethoprim-sulfamethoxazole for prevention of infection in patients with acute leukemia and granulocytopenia. Infection 1991;19:73-80.

87. Gomez-Martin C, Sola C, Hornedo J, et al: Rifampin does not improve the efficacy of quinolone antibacterial prophylaxis in neutropenic cancer patients: results of a randomized clinical trial. J Clin Oncol 2000;18:2126-2134.

88. Horvathova Z, Spanik S, Sufliarsky J, et al: Bacteremia due to methicillin-resistant staphylococci occurs more frequently in neutropenic patients who received antimicrobial prophylaxis and is associated with higher mortality in comparison to methicillin-sensitive bacteremia. Int J Antimicrob Agents 1998;10:55-58.

89. Gomez L, Garau J, Estrada C, et al: Ciprofloxacin prophylaxis in patients with acute leukemia and granulocytopenia in an area with a high prevalence of ciprofloxacin-resistant Escherichia coli. Cancer 2003;97:419-424.

90. Goodman JL, Winston DJ, Greenfield RA, et al: A controlled trial of fluconazole to prevent fungal infections in patients undergoing bone marrow transplantation. N Engl J Med 1992;326:845-851.

91. Ellis ME, Clink H, Ernst P, et al: Controlled study of fluconazole in the prevention of fungal infections in neutropenic patients with haematological malignancies and bone marrow transplant recipients. Eur J Clin Microbiol Infect Dis 1994;13:3-11.

92. Marr KA, Seidel K, White TC, Bowden RA: Candidemia in allogeneic blood and marrow transplant recipients: evolution of risk factors after the adoption of prophylactic fluconazole. J Infect Dis 2000;181:309-316.

93. Wingard JR, Merz WG, Rinaldi MG, et al: Increase in *Candida krusei* infection among patients with bone marrow transplantation and neutropenia treated prophylactically with fluconazole. N Engl J Med 1991;324:1274-1277.

94. Hartmann LC, Tschetter LK, Habermann TM, et al: Granulocyte colony-stimulating factor in severe chemotherapy-induced afebrile neutropenia. N Engl J Med 1997;336:1776-1780.

95. Ravaud A, Chevreau C, Cany L, et al: Granulocyte-macrophage colony-stimulating factor in patients with neutropenic fever is potent after low-risk but not after high-risk neutropenic chemotherapy regimens: results of a randomized phase III trial. J Clin Oncol 1998;16:2930-2936.

96. Vellenga E, Uyl-de Groot CA, de Wit R, et al: Randomized placebo-controlled trial of granulocyte-macrophage colony-stimulating factor in patients with chemotherapy-related febrile neutropenia. J Clin Oncol 1996;14:619-627.

97. Freifeld APP: Colony stimulating factors and neutropenia: intersection of data and clinical relevance. J Natl Cancer Inst 1995;87:7811-7812.

98. Ozer H: American Society of Clinical Oncology guidelines for the use of hematopoietic colony-stimulating factors. Curr Opin Hematol 1996;3:3-10.

99. Peters C, Minkov M, Matthes-Martin S, et al: Leucocyte transfusions from rhG-CSF or prednisolone stimulated donors for treatment of severe infections in immunocompromised neutropenic patients. Br J Haematol 1999;106(3):689-696.

100. Illerhaus G, Wirth K, Dwenger A, et al: Treatment and prophylaxis of severe infections in neutropenic patients by granulocyte transfusions. Ann Hematol 2002;81:273-281.

101. Cesaro S, Chinello P, De Silvestro G, et al: Granulocyte transfusions from G-CSF-stimulated donors for the treatment of severe infections in neutropenic pediatric patients with onco-hematological diseases. Support Care Cancer 2003;11:101-106.

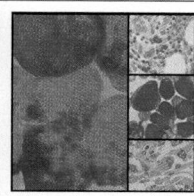

47

INFECTION IN THE SEVERELY IMMUNOCOMPROMISED PATIENT

Jo-Anne H. van Burik

Alison G. Freifeld

SUMMARY OF KEY POINTS

- Patients undergoing allogeneic stem cell transplant or therapy for acute leukemia are considered at "high risk" for infectious complications.
- Risk periods for infections after stem cell transplant (pre-engraftment or neutropenic period, usually first 10 to 20 days; early post-transplant, through day 100; and late post-transplant, after day 100) are associated with specific infection risks.
- Pretransplant serostatus for herpesviruses such as herpes simplex virus and cytomegalovirus are important to determine prophylactic measures.
- Antibiotic prophylaxis is controversial for transplant and leukemia patients. Fluoroquinolones are commonly used and have been shown to decrease gram-negative infections, but no consistent

decrease in mortality has been demonstrated.
- Fluconazole prophylaxis is a currently accepted strategy for reducing the incidence of invasive *Candida* infections in high-risk patients; however, fluconazole has no activity against *Aspergillus* and other molds, so newer agents are being evaluated.
- Fever during neutropenia requires immediate evaluation, appropriate cultures, and prompt initiation of empirical broad-spectrum antibacterial therapy with a defined regimen that covers *Pseudomonas aeruginosa*, enteric gram-negative organisms, as well as common institutional pathogens.
- Pulmonary infiltrates should be evaluated with bronchoscopy, in general, and a high suspicion should be maintained for mold

infections or those due to resistant bacteria.
- Post-transplant infections up to day 100 commonly include cytomegalovirus reactivation disease, *Pneumocystis* (in patients not taking prophylaxis), invasive sinopulmonary mold (e.g., *Aspergillus*) infections, and reactivations of varicella-zoster virus.
- Delayed infections after transplant typically include those due to encapsulated organisms such as *Streptococcus pneumoniae*, *Neisseria meningitides*, and *Haemophilus influenzae*. Vaccination against these and other pathogens should be undertaken starting at 1 year after transplant; live virus vaccines (varicella-zoster virus and mumps/ measles/rubella) should not be given until 2 years after transplant.

INTRODUCTION

Prevention, diagnosis, and management strategies for infections that develop in the immunocompromised cancer patient are based on the type and degree of immune compromise. When infection is suspected because fever occurs during neutropenia, the severely immunocompromised cancer patient is managed with the same general method outlined in Chapter 46. This chapter focuses on infections occurring in the hematopoietic stem cell transplant recipient and also includes those who are severely immunocompromised by acute leukemia and its therapies. These patients (transplant and acute leukemia) generally differ from those with solid tumors in that the chemotherapies to which they are exposed often result in a more profound and prolonged set of immune deficits. In addition, patients with leukemia often have immune compromise such as the profound functional neutropenia that accompanies acute myelogenous leukemia or the T-cell impairments associated with acute lymphocytic leukemia. Accordingly, they are susceptible to a more invasive, potentially life-threatening array of infections. Oncologists must be aware of current standards for the

prevention and treatment of common infectious complications in these high-risk patients.

RISK PERIODS DURING MYELOABLATIVE HEMATOPOIETIC STEM CELL TRANSPLANT

Three predictable periods of immune compromise occur during the course of both allogeneic and autologous transplantation (Fig. 47-1).[1-3] The pre-engraftment phase encompasses the first month or so after transplant and includes the period of neutropenia after conditioning. Periods of neutropenia for both allogeneic and autologous transplant are now typically in the 10- to 14-day range with the routine use of colony-stimulating factors, and prolonged neutropenia is no longer the rule. Nonetheless, neutropenia remains the main infection risk during this initial phase, along with disruption of mucocutaneous barriers by treatment-related mucositis and by the presence of indwelling venous catheters. Bacterial infections derived from normal skin and gastrointestinal (GI) tract flora, including coagulase-negative staphylococci and enteric gram-negative bacilli, are the most common

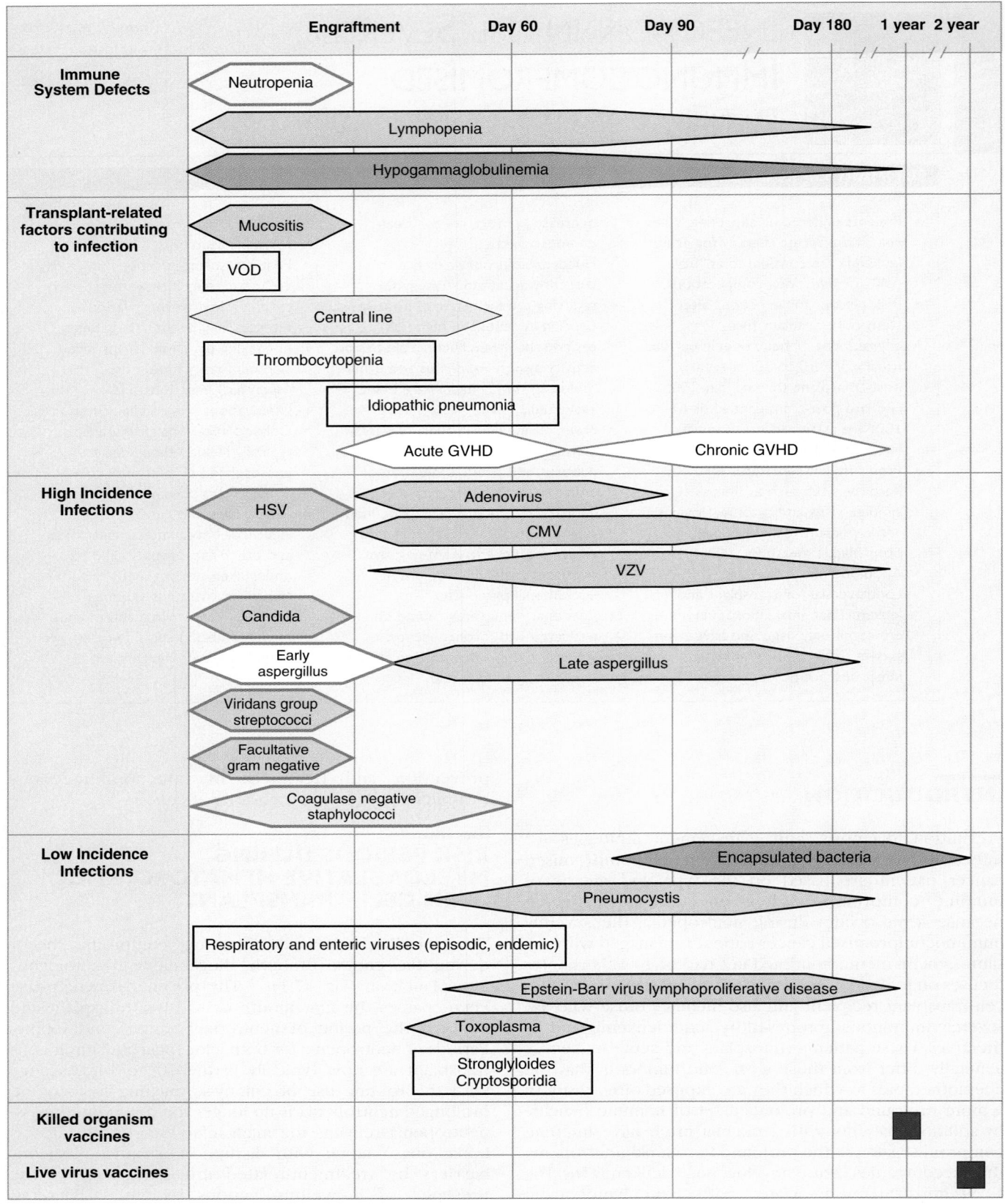

Figure 47-1. Phases of predictable immune suppression with their opportunistic infections among allogeneic hematopoietic stem cell transplant recipients.

causes of first fever during neutropenia, when an etiology is identified. Herpes simplex virus (HSV) and invasive candidiasis also are fairly prevalent early infections, with invasive molds such as *Aspergillus* being more frequent after prolonged periods (>3 weeks) of neutropenia.

The second phase is the postengraftment period from approximately day 30 to day 100 after transplant. This phase is characterized by impairments of cell-mediated immunity for both transplant types, with reactivations of herpesviruses being common if prophylaxis is not given. In the allogenic setting, and particularly in those with some degree of graft-versus-host disease, silent blood-stream cytomegalovirus (CMV) reactivations are more frequent and can progress to tissue-invasive disease including pneumonitis, hepatitis, and colitis. *Pneumocystis* and *Aspergillus* are more likely to occur during the postengraftment phase, especially if the patient is on steroid therapy.

The late post-transplant phase is considered the time after day 100. In autologous transplant recipients, significant immune reconstitution generally develops in the first 6 to 12 months with, accordingly, a low rate of late opportunistic infections thereafter. However, allogeneic recipients may have prolonged immune dysregulation over the first year or more, especially those with active acute and chronic graft-versus-host disease. These patients are at risk for herpesvirus reactivations, including CMV and varicella-zoster virus (VZV), as well as Epstein-Barr virus (EBV)-related post-transplant lymphoproliferative disorder (PTLD), infections due to encapsulated bacteria (*Streptococcus pneumoniae, Haemophilus influenzae,* and *Neisseria meningitidis*), and pneumonitis from respiratory viruses such as influenza, parainfluenza, and respiratory syncytial virus (RSV).

With the recognition that each phase of post-transplant immunosuppression is associated with certain common infections, prophylactic regimens to prevent these bacterial, viral, and fungal diseases have evolved over the last few decades. The clinical presentations of major infections and their treatment algorithms are presented herein, along with the preventive measures and standard environmental precautions used to address them.

MEASURES TAKEN BEFORE TRANSPLANT TO PREVENT INFECTION IN TRANSPLANT RECIPIENTS

Antimicrobial prophylaxis regimens are directed toward infections that occur commonly or with high morbidity and/or mortality.[4] However, if excessive risk, such as high toxicity or prohibitive cost, is associated with the preventive regimen, the benefit may be forfeited. Algorithms for these prophylactic regimens constantly are refined as changes occur in epidemiology, diagnostic methods, or new treatment agents for infections. Nonetheless, infections still occur when diagnostic methods are not sensitive enough or when the infecting agents are able to break through prophylactic antimicrobials.

Measures taken to prevent infection in the pre-engraftment transplant patient that are different from those taken for the neutropenic patient described in Chapter 46 include pretransplant serostatus blood work, review of common-sense measures that will assist in the prevention of infection, and environmental and pharmacologic measures to prevent infection.

Pretransplant Serostatus Blood Work

When transplantation started in the late 1960s/early 1970s, the serostatus of herpesviruses (HSV, VZV, CMV, and EBV) that could exist latently in the body was checked before transplant to determine if the patient was at risk for reactivation. Current testing of the donor and recipient before the transplant preparative regimen begins includes latent viruses [herpesvirus antibodies, as well as hepatitis panels, and human T-cell lymphotrophic virus antibodies (HTLV I/II), and human immunodeficiency virus (HIV)], and syphilis.

The only test result that could lead to immediate cancellation of the transplant would be a positive HIV test in a patient not known to be seropositive. If the screening test for HIV is positive from either the donor or recipient, a Western blot study should be completed to confirm the result before informing the individual of the screening test result. Otherwise unnecessary stress will result when there is a chance that the screening test was a false positive. Any time a positive HIV test result is conveyed to a patient, appropriate counseling must be provided.[5]

Several serostatus test results, if positive, would not cancel the transplant but would lead to a different action plan.[6] If the indirect screening test for syphilis, such as the rapid plasma reagin (RPR) or VDRL, returns positive and is confirmed by a direct test, the fluorescent treponemal antibody test, then the patient should receive high-dose penicillin prophylaxis for 10 days after transplantation product infusion, followed by another 11 days of viridans group *Streptococcus* prophylaxis.

If the antibody test for HSV indicates prior infection, or if the patient can provide a clinical history of HSV infection (such as mucosal sores), latent HSV infection exists and has the potential to reactivate during periods of combined T-cell immune suppression and neutropenia. This patient will require a medication targeted to HSV (such as acyclovir at 5 mg/kg every 8 hours or oral valacyclovir 500 mg q12 hrs) for the neutropenic phase of transplant.[7-10] A patient undergoing induction therapy for acute leukemia will not usually have a serologic antibody test for HSV before chemotherapy, but may reactivate latent HSV, especially if neutropenia is prolonged. HSV lesions can appear as black scabs on the outside of the lips, white/yellow-based ulcers when found on oral mucosa, or as an usually severe exacerbation of mucositis. If reactivation does occur, many clinicians will use antiviral prophylaxis with subsequent cycles of chemotherapy.[11]

Hepatitis B (core antibody, surface antibody, and surface antigen) and C serologies are tested in donor and recipient before transplant. Hepatic dysfunction from either hepatitis B or C after transplant can lead to life-threatening liver complications.[12-14] Short-term complications are usually due to hepatitis B, whereas cirrhosis developing over a period of years is due to hepatitis C.[15]

A hepatitis-infected individual can be used as a donor if no alternative donor is available or if the intended recipient is already seropositive. The risk of transmission is small when a hepatitis B–positive donor has an undetectable viral load. Transmission can be reduced by treating donors who have detectable viral loads and by transfer of immunity from donor to recipient.[12] A surface antigen–positive hepatitis B donor with a high viral load or a donor with high hepatitis C viral load should be treated with appropriate antivirals to reduce viral loads before transplant.[16,17]

If the transplant recipient has serologic evidence of prior infection with hepatitis B or C, viral-load levels of these viruses should be checked before and monitored after transplant, in conjunction with gastroenterology consultation. Those with high circulating hepatitis B viral loads should receive lamivudine.[16,18] Hepatitis C is currently treated with pegylated (PEG)-interferon and ribavirin, with acceptable safety profiles and cure of more than 50% of treated patients.[19] Careful follow-up of recipients with detectable viral loads is recommended.[18]

Regarding hepatitis C, no evident correlation exists between hepatitis C genotype and type or severity of liver disease after transplantation.[20]

If the patient is CMV seropositive before transplant, the patient should be followed up with a weekly diagnostic monitoring test,[21,22] such as pp65 antigenemia[23] or polymerase chain reaction (PCR)[24] that is used at a given institution. Weekly CMV testing continues for 10 to 20 weeks after transplant. No monitoring typically occurs during neutropenia because a detectable circulating white count is usually necessary for CMV to reactivate. If the recipient is CMV seronegative before transplant and the donor is seropositive, the same monitoring algorithm as for the CMV-seropositive recipient is followed.

If both the recipient and donor are CMV seronegative, seroconversion with blood products is possible. Accordingly, CMV-seronegative or filtered blood products should be used.[25,26] Weekly CMV monitoring can then be performed for a minimum of 6 to 10 weeks thereafter.

Serology for human herpesvirus type 6 (HHV-6) is not generally tested before transplant,[27] although more than 95% of adults are seropositive for this virus. The transplant patient at risk for reactivating HHV-6 is typically one who is not receiving herpesvirus antiviral prophylaxis during the transplant procedure, so a high index of suspicion should be maintained if such patients develop features that might be attributable to HHV-6, such as pneumonitis or encephalitis with fever.[28]

Antibody tests that are checked variably among local institutions include VZV, EBV, and *Toxoplasma*. A history of chickenpox is an adequate surrogate for performing the VZV antibody test. As an alternative to ordering a varicella serology on every patient, the test could be ordered only for those with no history of varicella infection or vaccination.

Knowing the serostatus of VZV is not so important as knowing the serostatus of CMV because, generally, acyclovir used to prevent reactivation of the HSV and CMV during neutropenia also will prevent VZV for the majority of transplant recipients. Within a few months after transplant, acyclovir prophylaxis is usually discontinued. Characteristic lesions in a dermatomal distribution readily are recognized as VZV reactivations (zoster), and zoster is easily treated in most cases.[29,30] However, the VZV serostatus does become important if, at some time after transplant, the patient is exposed to a person with active or incubating chickenpox. Seronegative VZV patients should receive varicella-zoster immune globulin (VZIG) prophylaxis within 96 hours of significant exposure.[3]

Knowing the EBV serostatus before transplant is not mandatory because 95% of patients can be assumed to be seropositive. EBV reactivation is in the differential diagnosis of any space-occupying mass after transplantation, but this usually comes into play many months after the neutropenic phase of transplant.[31] Now that there is a new diagnostic assay (quantitative EBV viral load) and new treatment possibilities (that remain to be proven, such as anti-CD20), EBV algorithms appear to be switching back to ordering an EBV viral capsid antigen immunoglobulin G (IgG) level before transplant, so that providers know which patients to target with quantitative viral load studies.[32] However, many unknowns still exist regarding this continuously changing algorithm: which quantitative assay to use, how frequently to monitor, and what threshold of a detectable viral load to use to begin treatment (or wait until there is post-transplant lymphoproliferative disease?).

Historically, 15% of patients receiving transplants in the United States are seropositive for *Toxoplasma*, but this percentage may be higher for European centers.[33] The risk of reactivation among seropositive patients is 2%, for an overall incidence of fewer than 1% of transplant recipients.[33,34] Because the incidence is so low, it is difficult to determine whether any medications used to treat the infection (e.g., high-dose sulfa) would be effective for prophylaxis (e.g., low-dose sulfa). It is likely that low-dose sulfa-based regimens such as those used to prevent *Pneumocystis* pneumonia also are effective in preventing *Toxoplasma*.[34,35]

Review of Commonsense Measures That Will Assist in the Prevention of Infection

Common sense measures that should be discussed before transplant concern diet, travel, crowds, and pets.[36] Additionally, a history of family or social exposure to tuberculosis should be used to guide whether a Mantoux test should be applied before transplantation.

Diet should be reviewed so that both the provider and patient recognize whether the patient is taking any restricted foods or herbal supplements.[36] Patients may not realize that providers group these supplements with medications, and that most herbal supplements will have to be discontinued on transplantation.[37] Ground-meat products must be cooked thoroughly so that bacteria distributed onto meat in the grinding process are killed. Any fruits or vegetables that cannot be peeled must be washed. Salad bars are associated with occasional transmission of infections. Food products that inherently contain infectious organisms should be avoided, including undercooked eggs. For example, miso paste for soup[38] is known to have *Aspergillus* organisms recovered when cultured. Blue cheeses have molds spiked into the cheese wheel as they are curing, and soft cheeses carry the potential risk of *Listeria* infection, as do unpasteurized dairy products. Yogurt contains *Lactobacillus*, which has been found to cause lung infection rarely, possibly after aspiration events.[39]

No particular restrictions apply to travel, but strategies to minimize transmission of infectious diseases have been summarized.[36] Some social situations, such as sitting in a crowded movie theater or classroom, increase the risk of acquiring a viral illness. Turning away from individuals who are coughing or sneezing, or even quickly donning a mask, may be helpful in preventing transmission of infection in this situation. Patients should be instructed to practice appropriate infection prevention by hand-washing as soon as possible after being close to someone with a cold. Given recent outbreaks of Noroviruses (Norwalk-like viruses) involving cruise ships and other types of outbreaks (e.g., *Staphylococcus*) commonly associated with the close living quarters of this type of vacation, cruise ships should not be high on the list for vacation choices.[40,41]

Healthy dogs and cats are considered acceptable pets. However, the immunosuppressed patient should not be responsible for scooping cat litter because of potential *Toxoplasma* cyst exposure. Similarly, the patients should not play in sandboxes, because these areas are concentrated sites that outdoor cats may consider to be litter boxes. Because reptiles of many sorts have been reported to be infected with *Salmonella*, patients should not touch these animals or the inside or outside of their aquarium homes. The heated water of tropical fish tanks may carry *Mycobacterium marinum*. *Cryptococcus* and *Chlamydia psittaci* can be transmitted from large pet birds.

Environmental Measures to Prevent Infection

Handwashing or, preferably, the use of alcohol-based hand-rub disinfectant is the mainstay of infection prevention in the hospital or clinic.[42] Persons entering the patient room to perform examination or touch the patient (including visitors as well as health care workers) should wash or disinfect their hands outside the room.[43] During respiratory virus season, infection control will often add extra signs to doorways and other places on the wards to remind visitors of the importance of handwashing. Staff and visitors without control of body secretions should not be permitted to have direct patient contact. However, routine use of gown, gloves, and/or masks is not required in the presence of a neutropenic patient.

Some infectious situations will lead to special isolation procedures.[43] Contact isolation (gloves, gowns) is used for patients with adenovirus, methicillin-resistant *Staphylococcus aureus* or *Clostridium difficile* infection. Droplet precautions are added to contact precautions for respiratory virus or varicella infection. Carriers of vancomycin-resistant enterococcus are placed in contact isolation until they meet federally determined criteria for discontinuation of isolation, including negative culture from the

original site of positive culture, if the site is still available for culture (as in wound or urine, etc.), plus three consecutive negative rectal swabs taken at least 1 week apart.[44]

High-efficiency particulate air (HEPA) filtration has replaced laminar air flow (LAF) as the means of prevention of infection through ventilation in most transplant centers.[43] With at least 12 air exchanges per hour, HEPA filters are capable of removing particles larger than 0.2 μm in diameter, such as mold spores. In addition, it is recommended that room-air pressure be maintained continuously above that of the corridor (i.e., positive-pressure environment). These environmental measures are recommended for allogeneic transplant recipients; it does not appear that autologous transplant recipients require this level of protection. For individual patients, such as those who will receive T-cell–depleted transplants, the transplant might be "upgraded" to an LAF environment. However, not all centers continue to maintain LAF patient rooms, and the use of these facilities remains controversial.[43]

Patients might ask if portable HEPA filters should be purchased for the home or apartment that will be occupied after hospitalization is over. In the broadest sense, this extra measure can be used on an individual basis, but if portable HEPA filters are used, then they should be obtained for each of the rooms that the patient will occupy during the day and night, and each unit should be sized for the individual room.

Prophylactic Antimicrobial Agents

Many fevers in the pre-engraftment phase of transplantation, or the prolonged neutropenia after induction leukemia therapy, are due to bacterial infections, so broad-spectrum antibacterial prophylaxis is often used during this risk period, especially in the allogeneic setting. No consensus has been reached about the routine use of prophylactic antibiotics for autologous transplant recipients or leukemia patients.[45,46] The exact antibiotic agents used vary from center to center and sometimes from protocol to protocol within an individual institution, while some choose to not use prophylaxis at all. Fluoroquinolones are commonly used prophylactic agents in allogeneic transplant, as they have been shown to decrease gram-negative infections. However, the impact of fluoroquinolone prophylaxis on overall or even infection-specific mortality has not been consistent among randomized studies. Furthermore, reports of severe viridans group *Streptococcus* (α-streptococcal) breakthroughs, with high morbidity and mortality rates, and fluoroquinolone-resistant gram-negative infections have recently limited enthusiasm for this type of prophylaxis in some centers.[47,48]

Mucositis, or breakdown of mucosal barriers, is common during this period, and the damaged oral cavity is often the source of bacterial or fungal bloodstream infections.[49,50] Such patients should receive antibiotic prophylaxis for alpha-streptococcal infections until day 21 after transplantation.[51,52] Concerns about α-streptococcal bacteremia escaping fluoroquinolone prophylaxis have led to the addition of a penicillin, macrolide, vancomycin,

Problems Common to Cancer and Its Therapy

or cephalosporin to the prophylactic regimen in some centers. Studies indicate that such additions do decrease documented gram-positive infections without altering the incidence of fever during neutropenia, or the rate of mortality.[53]

Central venous catheter placement through the skin, a normally formidable barrier to infection, may lead to bloodstream infection. Colonizing gram-positive skin organisms may gain access to the bloodstream despite sterile, operative placement of these catheters and antisepsis cleansing procedures around them.[54] However, because the gram-positive bacteremias are typically not life-threatening in the same fashion as are gram-negative bacteremias, direct prophylactic coverage is not necessary for central venous catheter placement.[55-57] During workup of a new fever in a patient with an indwelling catheter or port, some centers will add vancomycin for several days until blood cultures demonstrate no gram-positive bacteremia. However, because gram-negative catheter infections may have more serious hemodynamic consequences, we advocate empirical treatment only with a third- or fourth-generation cephalosporin for patients with non-neutropenic new fever and an indwelling venous catheter (no vancomycin routinely in a stable patient).

Candida species that colonize the mouth and gut proliferate with a higher burden of organisms when antibacterial agents, such as those used for prophylaxis, suppress the coexisting bacterial flora population. Fluconazole prophylaxis has been clearly demonstrated to prevent candidemia and hepatosplenic candidiasis among allogeneic transplant recipients.[58-60] However, fluconazole does not have activity against yeasts such as *C. glabrata* and *C. krusei*, or molds such as *Fusarium*, *Aspergillus*, and the *Zygomycetes*. Therefore standard fluconazole prophylaxis may change as new antifungal agents and/or diagnostic tests are validated. Candidemia occurs in 4% to 7% of transplant recipients who receive fluconazole prophylaxis, although the majority of these breakthrough isolates are either resistant *C. albicans* or the intrinisically insensitive species such as *C. glabrata* or *C. krusei*.[61,62]

Pulmonary and sinus infections from inhaled molds occur at the low rate of less than 3% before engraftment because of the environmental measures taken for air filtration.[58,59] Furthermore, the routine use of colony-stimulating factors has reduced the typical duration of neutropenia associated with transplantation, thus eliminating a major risk factor for invasive mold infections. Most invasive mold infections now occur later in the post-transplant period, and they are frequently associated with steroid use for graft-versus-host disease.

DIAGNOSIS OF INFECTION AND MANAGEMENT OF FEVER IN THE PREENGRAFTMENT HEMATOPOIETIC STEM CELL TRANSPLANT RECIPIENT OR LEUKEMIA PATIENT

Most aspects of epidemiology, diagnosis, and treatment of fever in the neutropenic host have been outlined in Chapter 46. This section discusses the predictable infections that can occur in the transplant or leukemia patient with profound neutropenia/lymphopenia. Many of these infections are analogous to those in oncology patients undergoing intensive chemotherapy regimens. In the allogeneic transplant setting, this pre-engraftment period extends from the onset of neutropenia until donor neutrophils have engrafted.

Fever

Despite specific antimicrobial prophylaxis measures directed against common pathogens, many fevers will occur among most pre-engraftment transplant recipients. Fever can be divided into three sets of differentials: infectious fever with an obvious source, infectious fever without an obvious source, and noninfectious fever. Risk-factor assessment should include knowledge of the temporal relation to blood-product infusions, recent exposures (e.g., contagious people, pets, foods, locations), height of the fever, whether the fever is accompanied by chills, rigors, or diaphoresis, and response to antipyretics. Symptom assessment should include headache, sinus drainage, sore throat, ear pain, cough, sputum production, shortness of breath, abdominal pain, diarrhea, and dysuria. However, many of these symptoms may be muted or absent during neutropenia, despite the presence of active infection.

Daily examination of any severely immunocompromised patient should be directed to include vital signs, mental status, oral cavity, indwelling catheter exit site, skin, lungs, heart, and abdomen. When fever is present, the examination should be expanded to include the sinuses (especially if there were any recent nasal manipulations), neurologic system, genitourinary system, and the perianal area looking for tenderness (neutropenic patient) or abscess (patient with neutrophils), particularly in the patient with acute leukemia.[63] The physical examination is helpful in determining the etiology of fever among cancer patients, because certain infections occur predictably among severely immunocompromised patients: mucositis, line infections, sinusitis, and pneumonia.

The initial workup of fever, regardless of whether an infectious or noninfectious source is suspected, includes two sets of blood cultures, culture of symptom-related sites even if there is no obvious source [e.g., sputum, urine, with or without stool, with or without cerebrospinal fluid (CSF)], review of medication list for potential contributors to drug fever, review of recent transfusions, chest radiograph, and scan of any symptom-related body systems. Many times two sets of blood cultures will be drawn through an existing indwelling line without being drawn from a peripheral site concurrently. Indications to draw a peripheral culture include new outpatient fever, a new heart murmur, and recent access of an older line. The empirical management of fever during the pre-engraftment (neutropenic) phase of transplant is essentially the same as that outlined in Chapter 46 for lower-risk patients. Empirical antibiotics for first fever generally consist of a potent anti-*Pseudomonas* agent or combination. The specific regimen is highly institution dependent. It is notable, however, that many transplant patients have significant oral mucositis and are receiving fluoroquinolone prophylaxis, and these are two important risk factors for the development of viridans-group streptococcal bacteremia. Accordingly, vancomycin may be added to the initial empirical regimen in these selected cases until preliminary blood culture results are available, usually within 72 hours of starting the drug. At that point, if cultures demonstrate no gram-positive organisms, vancomycin should be stopped. The effects of newer fluoroquinolones with more potent gram-positive activity may obviate the need for additional coverage, but no studies have yet addressed this question.

Fever Without an Obvious Infectious Source

More than half of all new fevers in neutropenic patients are without a known etiology. Nonetheless, empirical antibiotic therapy is mandatory, as an occult infection may be the cause of the fever. If no obvious source of infection is found in a pre-engraftment transplant patient receiving standard antimicrobial prophylaxis, then further systematic review of the patient is required. Most pre-engraftment allogeneic transplant patients and many acute leukemic patients will already be receiving acyclovir prophylaxis if they are HSV seropositive, and an azole for fungal prophylaxis. Once fever develops in these high-risk patients, broad spectrum empirical antibiotics generally replace the prophylactic antibiotic in an effort to cover predictable invasive bacterial pathogens. Even if no obvious infection source is found, it takes an average of 3 or 4 days for neutropenic patients to defervesce after empirical therapy has been started.[64] If fever persists, daily assessments are required to determine if signs and symptoms have developed that would lead to modifications of the initial empirical antibiotic regimen and/or to the ongoing prophylactic agents. For example, the presence of erythema, tenderness, or discharge at the catheter exit site will prompt addition of vancomycin, as will the development of severe mucositis. Oral or esophageal mucositis should also initiate an investigation for HSV reactivation and the addition of acyclovir, if it is not already being given.

Patients who remain febrile through day 5 to 7 after starting empirical antibiotics are candidates for empirical antifungal therapy with a drug that is active against *Aspergillus*. Because fluconazole has no activity against molds, fluconazole prophylaxis should be discontinued in favor of a drug such as amphotericin B, a lipid amphotericin formulation, voriconazole, or even itraconazole, to cover the possibility of occult mold infection. Table 47-1 provides a guide to situations in which antimicrobial modifications should be considered.

The basic differential diagnosis of noninfectious fever in the patient with cancer includes malignancy (evolution of hematologic malignancy, solid tumors including PTLDs, and liver metastases), transfusion of blood products, drug fever, autoimmune phenomena, and endocrine disorders (such as malignant hyperthermia). Transfusion-related fever and drug fever are probably the most commonly encountered causes of noninfectious fever in oncologic practice. Transfusion-related fever is typically brief and self-limited. Although the cause of fever may not ever be identified, most authorities recommend continuing empirical antibiotics until recovery of the absolute neutrophil count (ANC) to more than 500 cells/mm^3.

Drug Fever

A drug may induce fever by increasing metabolism, mimicking endogenous pyrogens, evoking a cellular or humoral immune response, interfering with heat dissipation peripherally, or damaging tissue. Drug-induced fevers typically begin 7 to 10 days after drug administration is initiated. They are often low-grade, persist for as long as the drug is continued, cause eosinophilia in up to one fifth of cases, and may be associated with rash. Fever will disappear soon after stopping an offending drug, usually over the course of 2 to 3 days or approximately seven half-lives of the drug. Certain drugs have a higher tendency to be associated with drug fever than do others, such as β-lactams, sulfonamides, vancomycin,[65] mycophenolate mofetil,[66] hydroxyurea,[67] and azathioprine.

Pulmonary Infiltrates

The pattern of pulmonary infiltrates seen on chest radiograph may give clues as to specific infectious and noninfectious etiologies (Table 47-2).[68,69] Although chest radiography is a good initial screen, computed tomography (CT) of the chest often provides more useful information in terms of characterizing the nature of the infiltrate and assisting the pulmonologist in determining where to direct the bronchoscope for highest yield. Bronchoscopy is generally the initial course of action when dealing with pulmonary infiltrates. In the neutropenic patient with new infiltrates, the diagnostic yield of bronchoscopy with lavage has been reported to be as high as 65%, even among patients receiving broad-spectrum antibiotics and antifungal coverage.[70] While awaiting culture results, coverage with a broad regimen that includes activity against *Legionella* as well as serious gram-negative pathogens such as *Pseudomonas*, is appropriate.

Anaerobic Infections

Typhlitis, or neutropenic enterocolitis, and retropharyngeal abscess are two relatively common anaerobic infections that may occur during neutropenia. Both of these infections occur at sites where biopsy generally is contraindicated. Typhlitis is preceded by fever, abdominal pain, and right lower quadrant tenderness that may be associated with rebound. CT scan of the abdomen will show right-sided colonic inflammation with thickening of the mucosa and, occasionally, pneumatosis coli.[50,71,72] Excessive soft tissue swelling of the neck during mucositis can be described as a Ludwig's angina variant. Anaerobic and antifungal antimicrobial agents should be added for either of these clinical findings.

TABLE 47-1

Approach to Management of Fever and Infection in the High-Risk Cancer Patient (Hematopoietic Stem Cell Transplant or Acute Leukemia)

HISTORY AND PHYSICAL FINDINGS	MODIFICATIONS OF ANTIMICROBIAL COVERAGE OR DIAGNOSTIC TEST INDICATED
Fever during neutropenia	Begin empirical antibiotics regimen (see text, Chapter 46).
	If on antibiotic prophylaxis, then empirical therapy must be of a different class from the prophylaxis (i.e., if patient is on a fluoroquinolone prophylaxis, then switch to a β-lactam–based regimen)
Hypotension, signs of sepsis	Broad antimicrobial coverage with triple antibiotics (e.g., carbapenem, vancomycin, plus aminoglycoside)
	If cultures negative for gram-positive organisms, consider discontinuing vancomycin after 3 days
Fever that is persistent or recrudescent on or after day 5 of broad-spectrum empirical antibiotic regimen	Empirical antifungal therapy: Add amphotericin B product or voriconazole
Severe oral or esophageal mucositis	Send viral (HSV) culture
	Add antiviral coverage (if not already being given)
	Consider antiviral resistance to prophylaxis if esophagitis is late in course of neutropenia
	Add antifungal agent for possible *Candida* esophagitis
	Switch streptococcal coverage to vancomycin
	Esophagoscopy may be indicated
Catheter exit site or tunnel erythema, tenderness, or discharge or cellulitis at any site	Culture any discharge
	Add vancomycin
	For tunnel infection (erythema and tenderness 3 cm above exit site), catheter removal and surgical debridement are generally required
Possible anaerobic infection:	Add metronidazole to broad-spectrum antibiotics
Abdominal pain, especially right lower quadrant, suggestive of neutropenic enterocolitis	CT scan of affected area
	Supportive care: Avoid surgical intervention if possible in a neutropenic patient
Oropharyngeal/neck soft tissue swelling	
New pulmonary infiltrate	Bronchoscopy (with or without biopsy) is the preferred method for evaluating new infiltrates in the high-risk patient
	Nodular: add mold coverage with voriconazole or amphotericin B
	Alveolar: broaden gram-negative coverage and add *Legionella* coverage (quinolone or macrolide)
	Interstitial: send diagnostic studies for both respiratory viruses and herpesviruses, particularly CMV
	Review patient history for risk factors for tuberculosis or endemic fungi
Upper respiratory symptoms of coryza, congestion during fall/winter	Nasal wash or swab for respiratory viruses culture and rapid antigen tests for RSV and influenza
Hemorrhagic cystitis	Urine viral culture and BK virus PCR

CMV, cytomegalovirus; CT, computed tomography; HSV, herpes simplex virus; PCR, polymerase chain reaction; RSV, respiratory syncytial virus.

Invasive Molds

Early invasive aspergillosis can be rapidly fatal over several days during the pre-engraftment phase of transplant. Patients usually receive fluconazole prophylaxis, which has no activity against molds. Mortality in transplant recipients with active mold infection is greater than 80%.[73] Unfortunately, amphotericin products are often toxic when used at the high doses required to treat mold infections, and are therefore likely to increase the morbidity of the transplant. Recently micafungin, a new, safe echinocandin antifungal, with activity against *Aspergillus* and other molds, was shown to be effective in preventing aspergillosis in a randomized study.[74]

Earlier recognition of invasive mold infections (before CT-scan abnormalities are seen) would also potentially improve outcome. A promising diagnostic assay, the *Aspergillus* galactomannan test, is undergoing validation testing in clinical trials to determine whether knowledge of results can change use of empirical therapy to treat febrile patients at high risk of invasive aspergillosis.[75,76]

The presence of circulating galactomannan has been shown to indicate invasive aspergillosis 2 to 3 weeks before the onset of infection in some trials. Biweekly monitoring for galactomannan during high-risk periods after transplant, and whenever an unexplained fever appears, may potentially allow initiation of preemptive therapy before life-threatening infection ensues. Certainly the algorithm for fungal prophylaxis will continue to be refined as new antifungal agents are demonstrated to be safe and effective, and new diagnostics become available.

Viral Infections

Herpes simplex has traditionally been the most commonly isolated virus during the pre-engraftment phase of transplant, but since the widespread use of acyclovir prophylaxis,[7] this infection is now infrequently seen. Institutions uniformly use acyclovir to prevent reactivation of HSV before engraftment, when it will also prevent VZV reactivations.[7] CMV infections are not typically

TABLE 47-2

Pulmonary Infiltrates and Their Association with Specific Infectious and Noninfectious Etiologies

RADIOLOGIC SIGN	DIFFERENTIAL
Interstitial infiltrates	Pulmonary edema
	Diffuse alveolar damage
	Idiopathic pneumonia syndrome
	Respiratory viruses: RSV, parainfluenza, influenza, adenovirus, enterovirus
	Herpesviruses: CMV, HSV, VZV, HHV-6
	Pneumocystis pneumonia
Focal airspace disease	Bacterial pneumonia
	Fungal pneumonia
Nodules	Fungal pneumonia (aspergillosis)
	Nocardia
	Legionella
	Septic bacterial emboli
	Mycobacterial infection (with cavitation)
	EBV LPD
	Relapsed malignancy
	Pulmonary embolism (pleural based)
Halo sign or air-crescent sign	Aspergillosis

CMV, cytomegalovirus; EBV, Epstein-Barr virus; HHV, human herpes virus; HSV, herpes simplex virus; LPD, lymphoproliferative disorder; RSV, respiratory syncytial virus; VZV, varicella-zoster virus.

seen in the pre-engraftment phase but occur later in the transplant course, after several months have passed. However, when clinically significant CMV infection does occur during neutropenia, it is important to note that the antigenemia test cannot be used for either diagnosis or monitoring of response to therapy, because white cells are required for this test to be interpretable.[77,78]

DIAGNOSIS OF INFECTION IN THE HEMATOPOIETIC STEM CELL TRANSPLANT RECIPIENT AFTER ENGRAFTMENT

Once the donor neutrophil line has engrafted, infections that occur thereafter are often related to a lack of T-cell–mediated immunity. Historically these infections have been recognized as occurring between days 30 to 100 and after day 100 after transplant However, because prophylactic strategies over the last decade have focused heavily on the infections that occurred between engraftment and day 100, many of the infections that would previously have been categorized as occurring only before day 100 now occur later, once prophylaxis stops. Therefore this section does not distinguish these infections by time after transplant.

Outpatient transplant recipients inhale mold spores and *Pneumocystis* cysts from the environment daily, so common exogenously acquired infections include *Pneumocystis jiroveci* (previously *carinii*) pneumonia (PCP)[79] and aspergillosis.

Common reactivation infections include EBV, VZV, and CMV. The majority of EBV reactivations are subclinical and require no therapy. In addition, quantitative EBV viral load diagnostic testing is relatively new and not standardized across institutions, so the algorithms for monitoring and initiation of treatment are vague.[32,80]

Varicella Zoster Virus

Transplant recipients susceptible to primary VZV infection include those who are seronegative, or who have no VZV history of chickenpox or zoster but who have a recent significant exposure. For these patients, VZIG should be provided within 96 hours of a significant exposure. Patients with positive serology can become clinically reinfected after a strong exposure and should be provided with acyclovir prophylaxis if not already receiving it at the time of exposure. VZV reactivations from latency (zoster) are usually recognized by their characteristic dermatomal distribution. Multiple episodes of zoster are possible.

The diagnosis is definitively made by scraping the base of an unroofed lesion and sending the cellular material for culture and/or direct fluorescent antibody staining for VZV.[81] Uncommon presentations of VZV disease include hemorrhagic pneumonia, hepatitis (may occur without skin lesions, manifested by very high liver enzyme elevations),[82-84] central nervous system (CNS) disease,[85] thrombocytopenia, and retinal necrosis.[86] For transplant recipients who have been treated for a zoster episode, some centers provide additional acyclovir prophylaxis until 1 year after transplant.

Cytomegalovirus

The majority of transplant recipients will initially manifest CMV reactivation silently, this is typically detected by the weekly monitoring test. Seeding of end organs with severe illness can occur if subclinical reactivations are not treated. The pulmonary tree is the most common site of CMV-induced pathology, although the GI tract, marrow (low counts), liver (increasing enzyme tests), brain, and retina also may be involved. The diagnosis of end-organ manifestations is made by recovery of CMV from the affected clinical site combined with a compatible clinical picture of infection. The gold-standard method of diagnosis is tissue biopsy showing CMV inclusions, combined with recovery of CMV in culture. Because tube culture on a fibroblast monolayer may take 3 weeks for cytopathic effect to become apparent, more rapid virologic methods include shell vial culture testing, immunohistochemical staining, and PCR.

Universal CMV prophylaxis with ganciclovir is not generally used because it prolongs potentially unnecessary exposure to this marrow-toxic drug. Instead, many patients are treated "preemptively" with ganciclovir or oral valganciclovir when the weekly CMV PCR viral load or pp65 antigenemia monitoring test meets the institutional positive threshold. Even with this pre-emptive strategy, ganciclovir appears simply to shift the timing of CMV reactivations to later (after day 100) in the postengraftment course, after it is discontinued in those transplant recipients at higher risk.[23] Initial antigenemia levels do not predict the severity of CMV disease.[87]

Pneumocystis

Prophylaxis options for *Pneumocystis* include trimethoprim/sulfamethoxazole, aerosol pentamidine, full-dose dapsone,[88] and atovaquone.[89] Since prophylaxis is routine, the incidence of PCP is quite low. The most common presenting symptoms are dyspnea, cough, and fever. Diagnosis requires demonstration of the organism in stained respiratory specimens (sputum, bronchoalveolar lavage). Disease probably occurs as both primary infection and activation of latent infection. Most cases manifest between days 40 and 80 after transplant,[90] but have been reported as early as day 12[91] and as late as month 42.[92] Once the lymphocyte arm of the white cell line is more fully reconstituted, *Pneumocystis* infections do not occur with any regularity. Prophylaxis is generally discontinued 2 years after transplant, or longer if immunosuppression is ongoing.

Invasive Mold Infections

Because fluconazole is effective in preventing early death from *Candida* yeast infections, longer-lived patients now acquire infections from fluconazole-resistant *Candida* and invasive molds. This was demonstrated in a study of transplant autopsy subjects, in which fluconazole prophylaxis was associated with a significantly lower frequency of candidal infections, 8% versus 27% in those receiving placebo.[93] The number of transplant patients with mold infections was higher among those who had received prophylactic fluconazole, 29% versus 18%.[93]

Mold spores may begin a localized infection that, after several months of immunosuppressive therapy for graft-versus-host disease, germinates into an infection with an overwhelming organism burden. *Aspergillus* is the most common mold in engrafted recipients, with *Fusarium*, *Scedosporium*, and the *Zygomycetes* occurring less often. However, the pulmonary and sinus manifestations of these different molds may mimic those of *Aspergillus*. Radiographic findings of pulmonary disease may include segmental and multilobar consolidation, perihilar infiltrates, multiple small nodules, peripheral wedge-shaped nodular masses, pleural effusions, cavitating lesions with an internal crescent of air, and nodules with a surrounding halo of ground glass.

Attempts at fungal isolation are often unrewarding. Blood cultures are invariably negative in *Aspergillus* infection, and bronchoscopy confirms the diagnosis in fewer than 50% of cases.[94,95] A high index of suspicion is essential to turn subtle initial clinical symptoms and signs into an early diagnosis. *Aspergillus* is a major contributor to mortality, and the need continues for better rapid and microbe-specific diagnostic and therapeutic options.

The vast majority of mold infections occur in the lung, whereas fewer disseminate to sinuses, skin, or abdominal organs.[73,96] *Fusarium* is notable for causing tender, red skin nodules and positive blood cultures for mold in about half of cases. Infection with any of the *Zygomycetes*

organisms (*Mucor*, *Rhizopus*, *Rhizomucor*) have a later onset of disease (after day 90) and a longer median duration of survival. Sinus disease with erosion through tissue planes is a feature of *Zygomycetes* infections. The mortality rate is around 80% for transplant patients with proven infection. Sixty percent of those colonized will progress to invasive infection.[73]

DELAYED INFECTIONS AFTER HEMATOPOIETIC STEM CELL TRANSPLANT

Encapsulated Organism Prophylaxis

Penicillin prophylaxis has decreased the incidence of infection-related morbidity and mortality from the polysaccharide encapsulated bacteria (*S. pneumoniae*, *H. influenzae* type b, and *N. meningitidis*) significantly. A few cases of penicillin-resistant pneumococcal infections have been reported, prompting a change in prophylaxis from penicillin to a quinolone.[97,98] Prophylaxis is generally discontinued around 1 or 2 years after transplant, or later if immunosuppression is ongoing at the 2-year point. Once the patient is ready for vaccinations, conjugate pneumococcal and *H. influenzae* type b vaccines are given.

Vaccination

Recipients of transplant frequently lose antibody response to viral and bacterial pathogens previously targeted by childhood vaccination. Although practice varies among transplant centers, killed-organism vaccines are often given around 1 year after transplant, and live-virus vaccines, after about 2 years (Table 47-3). The efficacy of vaccination is influenced by the time elapsed since transplantation, the nature of the hematopoietic graft, the presence of graft-versus-host disease, and the use of serial immunization.[99] Despite this evidence, a national survey of transplant immunization practices revealed that vaccines were underused and schedules for revaccination varied.[100] Currently all transplant recipients should be immunized on the same schedule regardless of stem cell source.[101]

INFECTIONS AFTER NONMYELOABLATIVE HEMATOPOIETIC STEM CELL TRANSPLANT

Nonmyeloablative transplant is associated with shorter periods of severe neutropenia, fewer episodes of bacteremia in the first 30 days, and a trend toward fewer episodes of bacteremia during the first 100 days after the transplant.[102] However, this type of transplant procedure may be associated with severe graft-versus-host disease, high-dose corticosteroid use, and relapsed or refractory disease. It is not surprising that the overall incidence of CMV disease and invasive fungal infections is similar to

TABLE 47-3

Vaccine Schedule After Hematopoietic Stem Cell Transplant

VACCINE	12 MO	14 MO	24 MO
Inactivated-organism Vaccines, Begin Reimmunization with 1-Year Anniversary Visit			
Diphtheria, tetanus, pertussis	X	X	X
Haemophilus influenzae type B conjugate	X	X	X
Hepatitis B	X	X	X
Pneumococcal 23-valent	X		Optional
Inactivated polio	X	X	X
Influenza	seasonal if >6 months following HSCT		
Live-virus Vaccines, Reimmunize with 2-Year Anniversary Visit if No Active Graft-versus-Host Disease or Immunosuppressive Therapy			
Mumps/measles/rubella			X
Varicella			X

that of conventional transplant by the end of the first year after transplantation.[103,104] Therefore nonmyeloablative transplant recipients should receive surveillance for CMV and fungal infections beyond day 100, and preemptive or prophylactic treatment similar to that of myeloablative transplant recipients between day 100 and 1 year after the procedure.

TREATMENT GUIDELINES FOR THE COMMON INFECTIONS

Bacteria

Once a gram-positive bacterial infection is identified, vancomycin therapy is used empirically until the susceptibility profile is available, at which point, the regimen is tailored to a single agent. If the patient is known to be colonized with vancomycin-resistant enterococcus (VRE) and the Gram stain indicates gram-positive organisms that are chaining, empirical VRE therapy is appropriate until the organism is identified and the susceptibility profile is available.

Once a gram-negative infection is identified, empirical therapy that includes *Pseudomonas* coverage is continued until the susceptibility profile is available. For many infections, the regimen can then be tailored to a single agent. If the organism is known to have an inducible β-lactamase enzyme (e.g., *Enterobacter*), therapy is tailored to two agents with two different mechanisms of action, such as a carbapenem plus a fluoroquinolone. For bloodstream infections due to bacteria or yeast, blood cultures should be followed up daily for several days to determine the date of last positive culture. Removal of central venous catheters may be required for some but not all infections.[61,105] At the end of a 14-day treatment course beyond the last positive culture, the patient should be returned to a gram-negative prophylaxis regimen if still neutropenic.

Anaerobic antimicrobial agents such as metronidazole or clindamycin, a carbapenem, or antianaerobic penicillin, should be added for typhlitis, enlargement of the neck soft tissue (Ludwig's angina-variant), or culture-documented anaerobic infection. Metronidazole is recommended in the setting of typhlitis because *C. difficile* may be a causative agent. Antifungal agents also should be part of the treatment regimen for typhlitis.[106-108]

Infrequently, tuberculous and nontuberculous mycobacteria are responsible for infections in the bloodstream, catheters, or pulmonary tree.[109,110] Organism identification and drug sensitivities may take several weeks to return. Mycobacterial pneumonias can be empirically treated as tuberculosis if the patient has risk factors for tuberculosis. For those patients without risk factors for tuberculosis, recovery of acidfast bacilli should prompt empirical therapy for atypical mycobacteria, usually with clarithromycin and either a quinolone or ethambutol, until specific susceptibility information returns. Tailored therapy often continues for 3 to 6 months.

Viruses

Herpes simplex reactivation infections are treated with lower doses of acyclovir (e.g., 5 mg/kg IV every 8 hours) or similar drugs, whereas VZV infections are treated with higher doses (e.g., acyclovir 10 mg/kg IV every 8 hours or oral valacyclovir 500 mg every 8 hours). Because many of these patients have not been exposed to acyclovir for any length of time before transplant (the exception will be patients previously treated with recurrent courses of acyclovir for frequent outbreaks of genital herpes), little reason exists to expect viral isolates with resistance to acyclovir. However, HSV infections that break through acyclovir prophylaxis should be considered acyclovir resistant until viral sensitivity testing can be performed, and consideration should be given to initiating treatment with foscarnet or cidofovir. Reports of acyclovir-resistant varicella are extremely rare.[111]

CMV treatment is initiated with induction doses of the antiviral agent for at least 2 weeks, followed by approximately 6 weeks of maintenance dosing, which is one half the induction dose. Ganciclovir is generally used for the initial antiviral course (5 mg/kg IV every 12 hours induction dose; 5 mg/kg IV once daily maintenance dose) when end-organ disease is documented, although some centers are increasingly using oral valganciclovir to treat asymptomatic increases in antigenemia or viral load (i.e., preemptive therapy). The duration of induction (1 to 3 weeks) varies by institution. An increasing viral load, when checked weekly during the first 1 to 2 months of antigenemia therapy, signals the need for continued induction dosing or reinduction dosing.[112]

When the end-organ manifestation of CMV is pneumonitis, intravenous immune globulin (IVIG) is added on an every-other-day basis for the duration of induction.[113,114] When CMV manifests in an end organ other than the lungs, the use of IVIG is not so clearly delineated. For other end-organ manifestations of CMV disease, IVIG can be added if the patient's total IgG level is below 400 mg/dL. No clear advantage favors CMV hyperimmune globulin over IVIG.[115]

HHV-6 has 60% DNA homology with CMV, and treatment of documented infection is usually initiated with induction doses of foscarnet or ganciclovir. Responses to antiviral therapy are not universal, and benefits of foscarnet versus ganciclovir have not been determined.[28]

Respiratory virus infections are seasonal, except for parainfluenza.[68,69] A frequent pathogen with clinical significance is respiratory syncytial virus (RSV), although influenza, adenovirus, enteroviruses, the herpesviruses (including HHV-6), and rhinovirus also produce diffuse interstitial infiltrates. Documented infection leads to the initiation of contact and droplet isolation precautions. Treatment for RSV may include aerosolized ribavirin, IVIG, and in some cases, anti-RSV monoclonal antibody therapy.

Cidofovir is an antiviral with a broad range of activity but which can be associated with significant renal toxicity. However, when combined with aggressive supportive measures, cidofovir is considered an adjunct in treating several of the viruses associated with hemorrhagic cystitis (i.e., BK virus)[116,117] and disseminated adenovirus infections.[118]

Fungi

The majority of yeast infections are due to *Candida*. Information regarding specifics of the infection usually come in three steps: identification that a "yeast" is involved, followed several days later by the *Candida* species, followed again several days to a week later by drug susceptibilities of individual isolate (if routinely available at the institution). With the approval of several new antifungal agents in recent years (mold-active azoles such as voriconazole and the echinocandins such as caspofungin or micafungin), empirical treatment of a "yeast" should include coverage for a non-*albicans Candida* species until identification of the species is made. In past years, such coverage usually meant the use of systemic amphotericin β or one of its lipid derivatives,

but now can also include one of the echinocandins or an advanced-generation azole. The use of echinocandins for *Candida* infections should, however, be limited to non-neutropenic patients.

Mold infections will commonly localize to the lungs, brain, and skin. Most molds will be susceptible to amphotericin, voriconazole, itraconazole, or an echinocandin. Results of a recent randomized trial indicate that primary therapy of invasive aspergillosis does not need to be initiated with amphotericin, the gold-standard antifungal agent since the 1960s. Rather, voriconazole, a broad-spectrum triazole that is active against *Aspergillus* species, demonstrated successful outcomes in 53% of voriconazole-treated patients compared to only 32% of amphotericin-treated patients (followed by other licensed antifungal therapy). The survival rate at 12 weeks was 71% in the voriconazole group versus 58% in the amphotericin group. Although transient visual disturbances are common with voriconazole, it can now be considered the standard approach to initial treatment of invasive aspergillosis.[119]

Long-term treatment with itraconazole is limited to those patients in whom acceptable serum levels of the drug can be documented. Echinocandin agents may be fungistatic, rather than fungicidal, in the case of mold infections, because their interruption of cell-wall synthesis is limited to areas of growing hyphal tips. At present, caspofungin is approved only for salvage therapy ("second line") of aspergillosis.

Treatment of CNS mold infections (other than *Zygomycetes*) should include voriconazole, which (on the basis of a small number of samples) attains CSF levels approximately 50% those of plasma or CNS tissue levels approximately 200% those of plasma. The alternative treatment for CNS mold infection (intraventricular amphotericin accompanied by systemic amphotericin) is very toxic and rarely used. Molds that are often resistant to amphotericin but may be susceptible to voriconazole include *Fusarium, Scedosporium/Pseudallescheria*, and *Trichosporon*.

Zygomycetes are uniquely susceptible to amphotericin products, although some anecdotal and in vitro evidence indicates that an investigational azole, posaconazole, is effective. Surgical debridement is an important adjunct to the treatment of zygomycoses.[120]

REFERENCES

1. Leather HL, Wingard JR: Infections following hematopoietic stem cell transplantation. Infect Dis Clin North Am 2001;15:483–520.
2. van Burik JA, Weisdorf DJ: Infections in recipients of blood and marrow transplantation. Hematol Oncol Clin North Am 1999;13:1065–1089.
3. Guidelines for preventing opportunistic infections among hematopoietic stem cell transplant recipients. MMWR Recomm Rep 2000;49:1–125.
4. Sullivan KM, Dykewicz CA, Longworth DL, et al: Preventing opportunistic infections after hematopoietic stem cell transplantation: The Centers for Disease Control and Prevention, Infectious Diseases Society of America, and American Society for Blood and Marrow Transplantation Practice Guidelines and beyond. Hematology (Am Soc Hematol Educ Program) 2001;1:392–421.
5. Centers for Disease Control and Prevention. Revised guidelines

for HIV counseling, testing, and referral. MMWR Recomm Rep 2001;50:1-57.

6. Gibel LJ, Sterling W, Hoy W, Harford A: Is serological evidence of infection with syphilis a contraindication to kidney donation? Case report and review of the literature. J Urol 1987;138: 1226-1227.

7. Wade JC, Newton B, Flournoy N, Meyers JD: Oral acyclovir for prevention of herpes simplex virus reactivation after marrow transplantation. Ann Intern Med 1984;100:823-828.

8. Liesveld JL, Abboud CN, Ifthikharuddin JJ, et al: Oral valacyclovir versus intravenous acyclovir in preventing herpes simplex virus infections in autologous stem cell transplant recipients. Biol Blood Marrow Transplant 2002;8:662-665.

9. Dignani MC, Mykietiuk A, Michelet M, et al: Valacyclovir prophylaxis for the prevention of herpes simplex virus reactivation in recipients of progenitor cells transplantation. Bone Marrow Transplant 2002;29:263-267.

10. Epstein JB, Ransier A, Sherlock CH, Spinelli JJ, Reece D: Acyclovir prophylaxis of oral herpes virus during bone marrow transplantation. Eur J Cancer B Oral Oncol 1996;32B:158-162.

11. Warkentin DI, Epstein JB, Campbell LM, et al: Valacyclovir versus acyclovir for HSV prophylaxis in neutropenic patients. Ann Pharmacother 2002;36:1525-1531.

12. Arai S, Lee LA, Vogelsang GB: A systematic approach to hepatic complications in hematopoietic stem cell transplantation. J Hematother Stem Cell Res 2002;11:215-229.

13. Strasser SI, McDonald GB: Hepatitis viruses and hematopoietic cell transplantation: a guide to patient and donor management. Blood 1999;93:1127-1136.

14. Locasciulli A, Bruno B, Alessandrino EP, et al: Hepatitis reactivation and liver failure in haematopoietic stem cell transplants for hepatitis B virus (HBV)/hepatitis C virus (HCV) positive recipients: a retrospective study by the Italian group for blood and marrow transplantation. Bone Marrow Transplant 2003;31:295-300.

15. Strasser SI, Sullivan KM, Myerson D, et al: Cirrhosis of the liver in long-term marrow transplant survivors. Blood 1999;93: 3259-3266.

16. Lau GK, He ML, Fong DY, et al: Preemptive use of lamivudine reduces hepatitis B exacerbation after allogeneic hematopoietic cell transplantation. Hepatology 2002;36:702-709.

17. Vance EA, Soiffer RJ, McDonald GB, Myerson D, Fingeroth J, Ritz J: Prevention of transmission of hepatitis C virus in bone marrow transplantation by treating the donor with alpha-interferon. Transplantation 1996;62:1358-1360.

18. Lau GK, Leung YH, Fong DY, et al: High hepatitis B virus (HBV) DNA viral load as the most important risk factor for HBV reactivation in patients positive for HBV surface antigen undergoing autologous hematopoietic cell transplantation. Blood 2002;99:2324-2330.

19. Foster GR: Pegylated interferon with ribavirin therapy for chronic infection with the hepatitis C virus. Expert Opin Pharmacother 2003;4:685-691.

20. Locasciulli A, Testa M, Pontisso P, et al: Hepatitis C virus genotypes and liver disease in patients undergoing allogeneic bone marrow transplantation. Bone Marrow Transplant 1997;19:237-240.

21. Boeckh M, Gallez-Hawkins GM, Myerson D, Zaia JA, Bowden RA: Plasma polymerase chain reaction for cytomegalovirus DNA after allogeneic marrow transplantation: comparison with polymerase chain reaction using peripheral blood leukocytes, pp65 antigenemia, and viral culture. Transplantation 1997;64:108-113.

22. Yakushiji K, Gondo H, Kamezaki K, et al: Monitoring of cytomegalovirus reactivation after allogeneic stem cell transplantation: comparison of an antigenemia assay and quantitative real-time polymerase chain reaction. Bone Marrow Transplant 2002;29:599-606.

23. Boeckh M, Gooley TA, Myerson D, Cunningham T, Schoch G, Bowden RA: Cytomegalovirus pp65 antigenemia-guided early treatment with ganciclovir versus ganciclovir at engraftment after allogeneic marrow transplantation: a randomized double-blind study. Blood 1996;88:4063-4071.

24. Kaiser L, Perrin L, Chapuis B, et al: Improved monitoring of cytomegalovirus infection after allogeneic hematopoietic stem

25. Ljungman P, Larsson K, Kumlien G, et al: Leukocyte depleted, unscreened blood products give a low risk for CMV infection and disease in CMV seronegative allogeneic stem cell transplant recipients with seronegative stem cell donors. Scand J Infect Dis 2002;34:347-350.

26. Bowden RA, Slichter SJ, Sayers M, et al: A comparison of filtered leukocyte-reduced and cytomegalovirus seronegative blood products for the prevention of transfusion-associated CMV infection after marrow transplant. Blood 1995;86:3598-3603.

27. Boutolleau D, Fernandez C, Andre E, et al: Human herpesvirus (HHV)-6 and HHV-7: Two closely related viruses with different infection profiles in stem cell transplantation recipients. J Infect Dis 2003;187:179-186.

28. Zerr DM, Gupta D, Huang ML, Carter R, Corey L: Effect of antivirals on human herpesvirus 6 replication in hematopoietic stem cell transplant recipients. Clin Infect Dis 2002;34:309-317.

29. Arvin AM: Varicella-Zoster virus: Pathogenesis, immunity, and clinical management in hematopoietic cell transplant recipients. Biol Blood Marrow Transplant 2000;6:219-230.

30. Steer CB, Szer J, Sasadeusz J, Matthews JP, Beresford JA, Grigg A: Varicella-zoster infection after allogeneic bone marrow transplantation: Incidence, risk factors and prevention with low-dose aciclovir and ganciclovir. Bone Marrow Transplant 2000;25:657-664.

31. Loren AW, Porter DL, Stadtmauer EA, Tsai DE: Post-transplant lymphoproliferative disorder: a review. Bone Marrow Transplant 2003;31:145-155.

32. van Esser JW, Niesters HG, van der Holt B, et al: Prevention of Epstein-Barr virus-lymphoproliferative disease by molecular monitoring and preemptive rituximab in high-risk patients after allogeneic stem cell transplantation. Blood 2002;99:4364-4369.

33. Slavin MA, Meyers JD, Remington JS, Hackman RC: *Toxoplasma gondii* infection in marrow transplant recipients: A 20 year experience. Bone Marrow Transplant 1994;13:549-557.

34. Martino R, Maertens J, Bretagne S, et al: Toxoplasmosis after hematopoietic stem cell transplantation. Clin Infect Dis 2000;31:1188-1195.

35. Fishman JA: Prevention of infection caused by *Pneumocystis carinii* in transplant recipients. Clin Infect Dis 2001;33: 1397-1405.

36. Dykewicz CA: Summary of the guidelines for preventing opportunistic infections among hematopoietic stem cell transplant recipients. Clin Infect Dis 2001;33:139-144.

37. Oliver MR, Van Voorhis WC, Boeckh M, Mattson D, Bowden RA: Hepatic mucormycosis in a bone marrow transplant recipient who ingested naturopathic medicine. Clin Infect Dis 1996;22:521-524.

38. Kino T, Chihara J, Mitsuyasu K, et al: A case of allergic bronchopulmonary aspergillosis caused by *Aspergillus oryzae* which is used for brewing bean paste (miso) and soy sauce (shoyu). Nihon Kyobu Shikkan Gakkai Zasshi (article in Japanese) 1982;20:467-475.

39. MacGregor G, Smith AJ, Thakker B, Kinsella J: Yoghurt biotherapy: Contraindicated in immunosuppressed patients? Postgrad Med J 2002;78:366-367.

40. Outbreaks of gastroenteritis associated with noroviruses on cruise ships—United States, 2002. MMWR Morb Mortal Wkly Rep 2002;51:1112-1115.

41. Minooee A, Rickman LS: Infectious diseases on cruise ships. Clin Infect Dis 1999;29:737-743, quiz 744.

42. Boyce JM, Pittet D: Guideline for Hand Hygiene in Health-Care Settings: Recommendations of the Healthcare Infection Control Practices Advisory Committee and the HICPAC/SHEA/APIC/IDSA Hand Hygiene Task Force. Infect Control Hosp Epidemiol 2002;23:S3-S40.

43. Dykewicz CA: Hospital infection control in hematopoietic stem cell transplant recipients. Emerg Infect Dis 2001;7:263-267.

44. Recommendations of the Hospital Infection Control Practices Advisory Committee (HICPAC): Recommendations for preventing the spread of vancomycin resistance. MMWR Recomm Rep 1995;44:1-13.

45. Sepkowitz KA: Antibiotic prophylaxis in patients receiving

hematopoietic stem cell transplant. Bone Marrow Transplant 2002;29:367–371.

46. Hughes WT, Armstrong D, Bodey GP, et al: 1997 guidelines for the use of antimicrobial agents in neutropenic patients with unexplained fever. Clin Infect Dis 1997;25:551–573.

47. Persson L, Vikerfors T, Sjoberg L, Engervall P, Tidefelt U: Increased incidence of bacteraemia due to viridans streptococci in an unselected population of patients with acute myeloid leukaemia. Scand J Infect Dis 2000;32:615–621.

48. Razonable RR, Litzow MR, Khaliq Y, Piper KE, Rouse MS, Patel R: Bacteremia due to viridans group streptococci with diminished susceptibility to levofloxacin among neutropenic patients receiving levofloxacin prophylaxis. Clin Infect Dis 2002;34:1469–1474.

49. Filicko J, Lazarus HM, Flomenberg N: Mucosal injury in patients undergoing hematopoietic progenitor cell transplantation: new approaches to prophylaxis and treatment. Bone Marrow Transplant 2003;31:1–10.

50. Blijlevens NM, Donnelly JP, De Pauw BE: Mucosal barrier injury: Biology, pathology, clinical counterparts and consequences of intensive treatment for haematological malignancy: an overview. Bone Marrow Transplant 2000;25:1269–1278.

51. Collin BA, Leather HL, Wingard JR, Ramphal R: Evolution, incidence, and susceptibility of bacterial bloodstream isolates from 519 bone marrow transplant patients. Clin Infect Dis 2001;33:947–953.

52. Steiner M, Villablanca J, Kersey J, et al: Viridans streptococcal shock in bone marrow transplantation patients. Am J Hematol 1993;42:354–358.

53. Tunkel AR, Sepkowitz KA: Infections caused by viridans streptococci in patients with neutropenia. Clin Infect Dis 2002;34:1524–1529.

54. Elishoov H, Or R, Strauss N, Engelhard D: Nosocomial colonization, septicemia, and Hickman/Broviac catheter-related infections in bone marrow transplant recipients. A 5-year prospective study. Medicine (Baltimore) 1998;77:83–101.

55. Koya R, Andersen J, Fernandez H, et al: Analysis of the value of empiric vancomycin administration in febrile neutropenia occurring after autologous peripheral blood stem cell transplants. Bone Marrow Transplant 1998;21:923–926.

56. Schots R, Trullemans F, Van Riet I, et al: The clinical impact of early gram-positive bacteremia and the use of vancomycin after allogeneic bone marrow transplantation. Transplantation 2000;69:1511–1514.

57. Arns da Cunha C, Weisdorf D, Shu XO, DeFor T, Pastor JD, 3rd, Johnson JR: Early gram-positive bacteremia in BMT recipients: impact of three different approaches to antimicrobial prophylaxis. Bone Marrow Transplantation 1998;21:173–180.

58. Goodman JL, Winston DJ, Greenfield RA, et al: A controlled trial of fluconazole to prevent fungal infections in patients undergoing bone marrow transplantation. New England Journal of Medicine 1992;326:845–851.

59. Slavin MA, Osborne B, Adams R, et al: Efficacy and safety of fluconazole prophylaxis for fungal infections after marrow transplantation-a prospective, randomized, double-blind study. Journal of Infectious Diseases 1995;171:1545–1552.

60. MacMillan ML, Goodman JL, DeFor TE, Weisdorf DJ: Fluconazole to prevent yeast infections in bone marrow transplantation patients: a randomized trial of high versus reduced dose, and determination of the value of maintenance therapy. Am J Med 2002;112:369–379.

61. Safdar A, van Rhee F, Henslee-Downey JP, Singhal S, Mehta J: *Candida glabrata* and *Candida krusei* fungemia after high-risk allogeneic marrow transplantation: No adverse effect of low-dose fluconazole prophylaxis on incidence and outcome. Bone Marrow Transplant 2001;28:873–878.

62. Marr KA, Seidel K, White TC, Bowden RA: Candidemia in allogeneic blood and marrow transplant recipients: evolution of risk factors after the adoption of prophylactic fluconazole. J Infect Dis 2000;181:309–316.

63. Marena C, Zecca M, Carenini ML, et al: Incidence of, and risk factors for, nosocomial infections among hematopoietic stem cell transplantation recipients, with impact on procedure-related mortality. Infect Control Hosp Epidemiol 2001;22:510–517.

64. Freifeld A, Marchigiani D, Walsh T, et al: A double-blind comparison of empirical oral and intravenous antibiotic therapy for low-risk febrile patients with neutropenia during cancer chemotherapy. N Engl J Med 1999;341:305–311.

65. Smith PF, Taylor CT: Vancomycin-induced neutropenia associated with fever: similarities between two immune-mediated drug reactions. Pharmacotherapy 1999;19:240–244.

66. Chueh SC, Hong JC, Huang CY, Lai MK: Drug fever caused by mycophenolate mofetil in a renal transplant recipient—a case report. Transplant Proc 2000;32:1925–1926.

67. van der Klooster JM, Sucec PM, Stiegelis WF, Hagenbeek A: Fever caused by hydroxyurea: a report of three cases and review of the literature. Neth J Med 1997;51:114–118.

68. Veys P, Owens C: Respiratory infections following haemopoietic stem cell transplantation in children. Br Med Bull 2002;61:151–174.

69. Martino R, Ramila E, Rabella N, et al: Respiratory virus infections in adults with hematologic malignancies: A prospective study. Clin Infect Dis 2003;36:1–8.

70. Hohenadel IA, Kiworr M, Genitsariotis R, Zeidler D, Lorenz J: Role of bronchoalveolar lavage in immunocompromised patients with pneumonia treated with a broad spectrum antibiotic and antifungal regimen. Thorax 2001;56:115–120.

71. Boggio L, Pooley R, Roth SI, Winter JN: Typhlitis complicating autologous blood stem cell transplantation for breast cancer. Bone Marrow Transplant 2000;25:321–326.

72. Schaller RT Jr, Schaller JF: The acute abdomen in the immunologically compromised child. J Pediatr Surg 1983;18:937–944.

73. Wald A, Leisenring W, van Burik JA, Bowden RA: Epidemiology of *Aspergillus* infections in a large cohort of patients undergoing bone marrow transplantation. J Infect Dis 1997;175:1459–1466.

74. van Burik J-A, Ratanatharathorn V, Lipton J, Miller C, Bunin N, Walsh T: Randomized, double-blind trial of micafungin versus fluconazole for prophylaxis of invasive fungal infections in patients undergoing hematopoietic stem cell transplant, ICAAC, San Diego, California, September 27–30, 2002.

75. Maertens J, Verhaegen J, Lagrou K, Van Eldere J, Boogaerts M: Screening for circulating galactomannan as a noninvasive diagnostic tool for invasive aspergillosis in prolonged neutropenic patients and stem cell transplantation recipients: a prospective validation. Blood 2001;97:1604–1610.

76. Maertens J, Van Eldere J, Verhaegen J, Verbeken E, Verschakelen J, Boogaerts M: Use of circulating galactomannan screening for early diagnosis of invasive aspergillosis in allogeneic stem cell transplant recipients. J Infect Dis 2002;186:1297–1306.

77. Limaye AP, Huang ML, Leisenring W, Stensland L, Corey L, Boeckh M: Cytomegalovirus (CMV) DNA load in plasma for the diagnosis of CMV disease before engraftment in hematopoietic stem-cell transplant recipients. J Infect Dis 2001;183:377–382.

78. Limaye AP, Bowden RA, Myerson D, Boeckh M: Cytomegalovirus disease occurring before engraftment in marrow transplant recipients. Clin Infect Dis 1997;24:830–835.

79. Stringer JR, Beard CB, Miller RF, Wakefield AE: A new name (*Pneumocystis jiroveci*) for Pneumocystis from humans. Emerg Infect Dis 2002;8:891–896.

80. van Esser JW, van der Holt B, Meijer E, et al: Epstein-Barr virus (EBV) reactivation is a frequent event after allogeneic stem cell transplantation (SCT) and quantitatively predicts EBV-lymphoproliferative disease following T-cell–depleted SCT. Blood 2001;98:972–978.

81. de Jong MD, Weel JF, van Oers MH, Boom R, Wertheim-van Dillen PM: Molecular diagnosis of visceral herpes zoster. Lancet 2001;357:2101–2102.

82. David DS, Tegtmeier BR, O'Donnell MR, Paz IB, McCarty TM: Visceral varicella-zoster after bone marrow transplantation: report of a case series and review of the literature. Am J Gastroenterol 1998;93:810–813.

83. Schiller GJ, Nimer SD, Gajewski JL, Golde DW: Abdominal presentation of varicella zoster infection in recipients of allogeneic bone marrow transplantation. Bone Marrow Transplant 1991;7:489–491.

84. Verdonck LF, Cornelissen JJ, Dekker AW, Rozenberg-Arska M: Acute

abdominal pain as a presenting symptom of varicella zoster virus infection in recipients of bone marrow transplants. Clin Infect Dis 1993;16:190–191.

85. Tenenbaum T, Kramm CM, Laws HJ, Nurnberger W, Lenard HG, Gobel U: Pre-eruptive varicella zoster virus encephalitis in two children after haematopoietic stem cell transplantation. Med Pediatr Oncol 2002;38:288–289.

86. Austin R: Clinical review. Progressive outer retinal necrosis syndrome: A comprehensive review of its clinical presentation, relationship to immune system status, and management. Clinical Eye and Vision Care 2000;12:119–129.

87. Nichols WG, Corey L, Gooley T, et al: Rising pp65 antigenemia during preemptive anticytomegalovirus therapy after allogeneic hematopoietic stem cell transplantation: Risk factors, correlation with DNA load, and outcomes. Blood 2001;97:867–874.

88. Souza JP, Boeckh M, Gooley TA, Flowers ME, Crawford SW: High rates of *Pneumocystis carinii* pneumonia in allogeneic blood and marrow transplant recipients receiving dapsone prophylaxis. Clin Infect Dis 1999;29:1467–1471.

89. Colby C, McAfee S, Sackstein R, Finkelstein D, Fishman J, Spitzer T: A prospective randomized trial comparing the toxicity and safety of atovaquone with trimethoprim/sulfamethoxazole as *Pneumocystis carinii* pneumonia prophylaxis following autologous peripheral blood stem cell transplantation. Bone Marrow Transplant 1999;24:897–902.

90. Tuan IZ, Dennison D, Weisdorf DJ: *Pneumocystis carinii* pneumonitis following bone marrow transplantation. Bone Marrow Transplant 1992;10:267–272.

91. Saito T, Seo S, Kanda Y, et al: Early onset *Pneumocystis carinii* pneumonia after allogeneic peripheral blood stem cell transplantation. Am J Hematol 2001;67:206–209.

92. Lyytikainen O, Ruutu T, Volin L, et al: Late onset *Pneumocystis carinii* pneumonia following allogeneic bone marrow transplantation. Bone Marrow Transplant 1996;17:1057–1059.

93. van Burik J-A, Leisenring W, Myerson D, et al: The effect of prophylactic fluconazole on the clinical spectrum of fungal diseases in bone marrow transplant recipients with special attention to hepatic candidiasis: an autopsy study of 355 patients. Medicine (Baltimore) 1998;77:246–254.

94. Albelda SM, Talbot GH, Gerson SL, Miller WT, Cassileth PA: Role of fiberoptic bronchoscopy in the diagnosis of invasive pulmonary aspergillosis in patients with acute leukemia. Am J Med 1984;76:1027–1034.

95. Reichenberger F, Habicht J, Matt P, et al: Diagnostic yield of bronchoscopy in histologically proven invasive pulmonary aspergillosis. Bone Marrow Transplant 1999;24:1195–1199.

96. Marr KA, Carter RA, Crippa F, Wald A, Corey L: Epidemiology and outcome of mould infections in hematopoietic stem cell transplant recipients. Clin Infect Dis 2002;34:909–917.

97. Tauro S, Dobie D, Richardson G, Hastings M, Mahendra P: Recurrent penicillin-resistant pneumococcal sepsis after matched unrelated donor transplantation for refractory T cell lymphoma. Bone Marrow Transplant 2000;26:1017–1019.

98. Schutze GE, Mason EO Jr, Wald ER, et al: Pneumococcal infections in children after transplantation. Clin Infect Dis 2001;33:16–21.

99. Singhal S, Mehta J: Reimmunization after blood or marrow stem cell transplantation. Bone Marrow Transplant 1999;23:637–646.

100. Henning KJ, White MH, Sepkowitz KA, Armstrong D: A national survey of immunization practices following allogeneic bone marrow transplantation. JAMA 1997;277:1148–1151.

101. Gandhi MK, Egner W, Sizer L, et al: Antibody responses to vaccinations given within the first two years after transplant are similar between autologous peripheral blood stem cell and bone marrow transplant recipients. Bone Marrow Transplant 2001;28:775–781.

102. Junghanss C, Marr KA, Carter RA, et al: Incidence and outcome of bacterial and fungal infections following nonmyeloablative compared with myeloablative allogeneic hematopoietic stem cell transplantation: A matched control study. Biol Blood Marrow Transplant 2002;8:512–520.

103. Hagen EA, Stern H, Porter D, et al: High rate of invasive fungal infections following nonmyeloablative allogeneic transplantation. Clin Infect Dis 2003;36:9–15.

104. Junghanss C, Boeckh M, Carter RA, et al: Incidence and outcome of cytomegalovirus infections following nonmyeloablative compared with myeloablative allogeneic stem cell transplantation, a matched control study. Blood 2002;99: 1978–1985.

105. Bodey GP, Mardani M, Hanna HA, et al: The epidemiology of *Candida glabrata* and *Candida albicans* fungemia in immunocompromised patients with cancer. Am J Med 2002;112:380–385.

106. Otaibi AA, Barker C, Anderson R, Sigalet DL: Neutropenic enterocolitis (typhlitis) after pediatric bone marrow transplant. J Pediatr Surg 2002;37:770–772.

107. Sloas MM, Flynn PM, Kaste SC, Patrick CC: Typhlitis in children with cancer: A 30-year experience. Clin Infect Dis 1993;17:484–490.

108. Katz JA, Wagner ML, Gresik MV, Mahoney DH Jr, Fernbach DJ: Typhlitis. An 18-year experience and postmortem review. Cancer 1990;65:1041–1047.

109. Roy V, Weisdorf D: Mycobacterial infections following bone marrow transplantation: A 20 year retrospective review. Bone Marrow Transplantation 1997;19:467–470.

110. Gaviria JM, Garcia PJ, Garrido SM, Corey L, Boeckh M: Nontuberculous mycobacterial infections in hematopoietic stem cell transplant recipients: Characteristics of respiratory and catheter-related infections. Biol Blood Marrow Transplant 2000;6:361–369.

111. Reusser P, Cordonnier C, Einsele H, et al: European survey of herpesvirus resistance to antiviral drugs in bone marrow transplant recipients. Infectious Diseases Working Party of the European Group for Blood and Marrow Transplantation. Bone Marrow Transplant 1996;17:813–817.

112. Nichols WG, Boeckh M: Rising cytomegalovirus antigenemia on preemptive therapy: practical aspects. Blood 2001;98:1629.

113. Reed EC, Bowden RA, Dandliker PS, Lilleby KE, Meyers JD: Treatment of cytomegalovirus pneumonia with ganciclovir and intravenous cytomegalovirus immunoglobulin in patients with bone marrow transplants. Ann Intern Med 1988;109:783–788.

114. Emanuel D, Cunningham I, Jules-Elysee K: Cytomegalovirus pneumonia after bone marrow transplantation successfully treated with the combination of ganciclovir and high-dose intravenous immunoglobulin. Ann Intern Med 1988;109:777–782.

115. van Burik JA, Lawatsch EJ, DeFor TE, Weisdorf DJ: Cytomegalovirus enteritis among hematopoietic stem cell transplant recipients. Biol Blood Marrow Transplant 2001;7:674–679.

116. Gonzalez-Fraile MI, Canizo C, Caballero D, et al: Cidofovir treatment of human polyomavirus-associated acute haemorrhagic cystitis. Transpl Infect Dis 2001;3:44–46.

117. Held TK, Biel SS, Nitsche A, et al: Treatment of BK virus-associated hemorrhagic cystitis and simultaneous CMV reactivation with cidofovir. Bone Marrow Transplant 2000;26:347–350.

118. Ljungman P, Ribaud P, Eyrich M, et al: Cidofovir for adenovirus infections after allogeneic hematopoietic stem cell transplantation: a survey by the Infectious Diseases Working Party of the European Group for Blood and Marrow Transplantation. Bone Marrow Transplant 2003;31:481–486.

119. Herbrecht R, Denning DW, Patterson TF, et al: Voriconazole versus amphotericin B for primary therapy of invasive aspergillosis. N Engl J Med 2002;347:408–415.

120. Freifeld AG, Iwen P: Zygomycosis. In Kauffmann CA (ed): Seminars in Respiration and Critical Care Medicine, 2004 (in press).

Problems Common to Cancer and Its Therapy

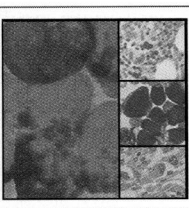

HYPERCALCEMIA

A. Ross Morton

Allan Lipton

SUMMARY OF KEY POINTS

INCIDENCE
- Hypercalcemia is the major metabolic abnormality associated with malignant disease.
- It occurs in approximately 10% of patients with cancer.
- It has a specific predilection for squamous carcinoma of the bronchus, carcinoma of the breast, and multiple myeloma.
- It is frequently recognized late and managed poorly.

ETIOLOGY OF COMPLICATION
- Parathyroid hormone-related protein (PTHrP) produces hormonal and paracrine effects.
- Factors released by or in response to metastases in bone (receptor activator of nuclear factor-κB ligand [RANKL], transforming growth factor-α [TGF-α], tumor necrosis factor [TNF], interleukin-1 [IL-1]) cause paracrine effects.

- Final common pathway is osteoclastic bone resorption.
- It is aggravated by renal functional abnormalities or renal effects of PTHrP, or both.

EVALUATION OF THE PATIENT
- Determination of the stage of disease and subsequent antineoplastic options provides a logical approach to management.
- Patient symptomatology is more relevant than the absolute calcium level.
- The total calcium concentration must be corrected for serum albumin concentration.
- Close attention to volume status and renal function are mandatory.
- Causes of hypercalcemia other than malignancy should be considered.

GRADING OF THE COMPLICATION
- Patients with symptoms due to their hypercalcemia should be treated as severely affected irrespective of the absolute calcium level.
- A corrected serum calcium of less than 3.0 mmol/L is considered mild, 3.0–3.5 mmol/L is moderate, and greater than 3.5 mmol/L is severe.

TREATMENT
- Antitumor therapy should be employed for best long-term results.
- Consideration should be given to active palliation in the face of advanced disease when antitumor options are exhausted.
- Extracellular fluid volume should be expanded to induce a calciuresis.
- Antiresorptive therapy (bisphosphonates with or without calcitonin) should be considered as first-line therapy.

INTRODUCTION

Hypercalcemia is one of the most common metabolic complications of malignancy. Even though it occurs in approximately 8% to 10% of patients with malignant disease, the diagnosis is frequently delayed. A knowledge of the tumor types associated with hypercalcemia, the mechanisms generating the hypercalcemia, and the symptom constellation will lead to prompt diagnosis, timely and appropriate intervention, and amelioration of morbidity.

Hypercalcemia in association with malignant disease was first reported by Zondek and colleagues in 1924,[1] and the first review of a large series was by Gutman and colleagues in 1936.[2] Since then, the syndrome has become increasingly well recognized and characterized. The frequency with which hypercalcemia occurs varies considerably with tumor type (Tables 48-1 and 48-2), but it is most commonly seen in association with squamous carcinoma of the bronchus, carcinoma of the breast, and multiple myeloma.[3–5] It is of considerable interest that some tumors that frequently metastasize to bone—for example, small cell carcinoma of the lung, carcinoma of the prostate, and some other common tumors, such as adenocarcinoma of the colon and stomach—are rarely associated with hypercalcemia.

TABLE 48-1

Tumor Types Associated with Hypercalcemia	
TUMOR TYPE	**HYPERCALCEMIC CASES (%)**
Lung	35
Breast	25
Hematologic (myeloma, lymphoma)	14
Genitourinary	6
Other/unknown	20

Modified from Mundy GR, Martin TJ: The hypercalcemia of malignancy: Pathogenesis and management. Metabolism 1982;31:1247.

TABLE 48-2

Frequency of Hypercalcemia Associated with Specific Tumor Types

TUMOR TYPE	FREQUENCY (%)
Multiple myeloma	33
Carcinoma of the breast	10
Carcinoma of the bronchus	6
Other	1–6

Data from Fisken RA, Heath DA, Bold AM: Hypercalcaemia hospital survey. Q J Med 1980;196:405 and Coleman RE, Rubens RD: The clinical course of bone metastases from breast cancer. Br J Cancer 1987;55:61.

ETIOLOGY

Before we discuss the possible etiologies of hypercalcemia in malignant disease, a short review of normal calcium homeostasis is appropriate. The adult human body contains approximately 1 kg of calcium, of which all but 10 g is lodged in bone. Most of the extraosseus calcium is found in the extracellular fluid, but the minute concentrations present in cells (10^{-8} to 10^{-7} M) are vital to normal cellular function and control. The total body calcium is dependent on the balance between calcium intake and calcium loss. Figure 48-1 demonstrates the normal calcium metabolism.[6] The normal dietary calcium intake is approximately 1 g per day (25 mmol). Absorption of dietary calcium is incomplete (25%–50%), and in healthy individuals it is approximately 300 mg (7.5 mmol per day). Bone represents an enormous reservoir of calcium, yet autoradiographic studies have demonstrated that very little transfer of calcium (on the order of 500 mg [12.5 mmol per day]) occurs between bone and the plasma in health.[7] When net calcium balance is zero, the body is required to excrete approximately 150 mg (3.75 mmol) of calcium daily. The kidney filters large amounts (10 g [250 mmol]) of calcium daily. Of this amount, 65% is reabsorbed in the proximal convoluted tubule, 25% in the ascending limb of the loop of Henle, and a variable amount in the distal convoluted tubule. Calcium reabsorption in the proximal tubule is independent of hormonal control but is closely linked to the reabsorption of sodium, a phenomenon that has important consequences in and implications for the treatment of hypercalcemia. Calcium reabsorption from the distal tubule is enhanced in the presence of parathyroid hormone (PTH), and it is at this site that the fine-tuning of calcium homeostasis occurs. The maximal reabsorptive capacity of the kidneys is limited to about 600 mg per day (15 mmol per day); thus, bone resorption can increase by approximately 150% over bone formation before the renal clearance mechanisms are overwhelmed.

The total plasma calcium consists of free plasma calcium (which amounts to approximately 50% of the total) and calcium bound to albumin (and occasionally to other proteins, including paraproteins), which varies with the level of plasma proteins but accounts for approximately 40% of the total. The remaining 10% is complexed with ions such as bicarbonate and citrate (Fig. 48-2). In physiologic terms, the plasma free (or "ionized") calcium carries the greatest significance. Direct measurement of the plasma free calcium is possible using ion-selective electrodes, but for the most part, total plasma calcium is measured. Because there is a reasonable correlation between serum albumin and serum calcium, algorithms have been suggested to "correct" the total plasma calcium for albumin concentration. Although no algorithm is 100% specific or sensitive for the detection of all true cases of hypercalcemia, the following equation has the merits of accuracy and simplicity.[8,9]

Ca (corrected) = Ca (measured) + {0.8 × (4 – albumin concentration)}
Conventional units
Ca (corrected) = Ca (measured) + {0.02 × (40 – albumin concentration)}
SI units

Calcium homeostasis is regulated through three hormone systems: PTH, calcitonin, and 1,25-$(OH)_2D_3$ (the main active metabolite of the vitamin D complex of sterols). These hormones bring about their effects by altering calcium absorption from the gastrointestinal tract (1,25-$(OH)_2D_3$), calcium resorption from bone (PTH and calcitonin), and calcium reabsorption in the kidney (PTH, 1,25-$(OH)_2D_3$, and possibly calcitonin). Furthermore, 1,25-$(OH)_2D_3$ metabolism is sensitive to changes in PTH levels and vice versa.

PTH is the main circulating stimulator of increased calcium mobilization from bone. Circulating parathyroid hormone is a polypeptide containing 84 amino acid residues; however, all of the bioactivity of the hormone appears to be contained in the initial 34 amino acid residues.[10]

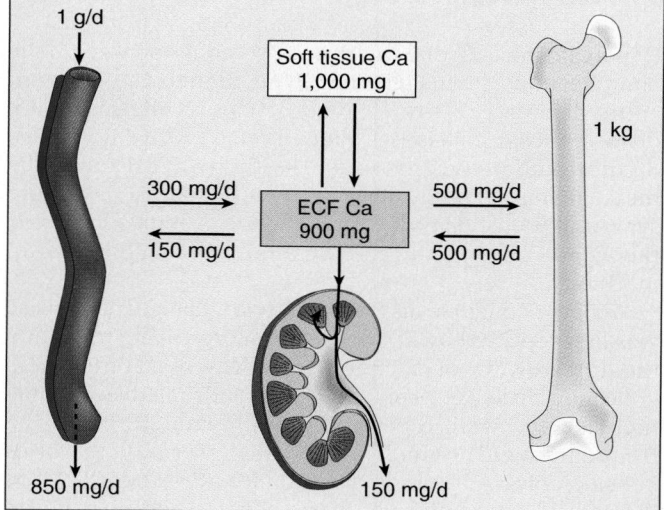

Figure 48-1. Normal calcium homeostasis. ECF, extracellular fluid. (From Mundy GR: Calcium Homeostasis: Hypercalcemia and Hypocalcemia. London, Martin Dunitz, 1990, p 2, with permission.)

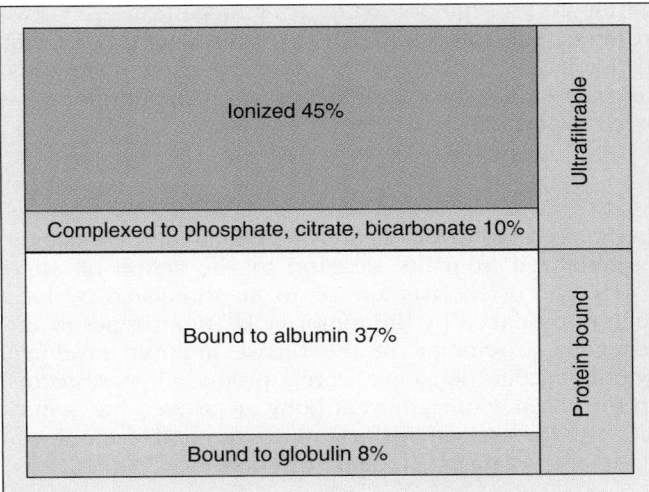

Figure 48-2. The constituents of total calcium within the serum.

The physiologic antagonist to PTH is calcitonin, a 32–amino acid polypeptide hormone secreted by the C cells of the thyroid gland. It causes rapid suppression of osteoclast activity and thus enhances net calcium absorption into bone. Its effects are short lived in the presence of continued infusion, presumably due to downregulation of receptors.[11] Although it is usual to consider calcitonin purely in terms of its effects on plasma calcium levels, these are unlikely to represent its true physiologic role, as in both the absence of calcitonin (following total thyroidectomy) and in the presence of large circulating amounts (seen in medullary carcinoma of the thyroid), gross disturbance of calcium balance is extremely rare.

Based on an understanding of normal calcium homeostasis, it can be seen that there are three potential mechanisms that can cause hypercalcemia of malignancy. Calcium can be mobilized from bone in quantities sufficient to overwhelm the renal excretory mechanism; renal reabsorption of calcium can be inappropriately increased (or excretion can be decreased); and gastrointestinal absorption of calcium can be enhanced.

It has been convenient to ascribe abnormal patterns of calcium transport to different tumor types. Squamous carcinoma of the bronchus can be associated with hypercalcemia in the absence of bony metastases, suggesting a humoral factor in the genesis of the hypercalcemia. Multiple myeloma is associated with local bone destruction and, frequently, with abnormalities of renal function. Carcinoma of the breast causes excessive calcium mobilization from bone in the presence of multiple osseous metastases.

The techniques of molecular biology have produced a wealth of information in recent years that tends to merge these mechanisms while providing insight into the mechanisms of hypercalcemia and suggesting logical therapeutic interventions.

TYPES OF HYPERCALCEMIA OF MALIGNANCY

Humoral Hypercalcemia

In 1980, Stewart and colleagues[12] described a series of 50 patients with hypercalcemia and malignant disease. In their extensive metabolic evaluation, they were able to characterize the patients into two groups dependent on their excretion of nephrogenous cyclic AMP (NcAMP). Patients with high NcAMP shared other features with primary hyperparathyroidism, including a lowered renal phosphate threshold. There were, however, significant differences between these groups in terms of fasting urinary calcium excretion, 1,25-dihydroxyvitamin D concentrations, and immunoreactive PTH levels. They concluded that urinary NcAMP was a useful marker for identifying hypercalcemia of malignancy associated with a humoral factor—so-called humoral hypercalcemia of malignancy (HHM)—but that this factor was not native PTH.

Parathyroid Hormone-related Protein

In 1941, in a clinicopathologic conference published in the *New England Journal of Medicine*,[13] a patient with renal cell carcinoma and a low bony metastatic burden who had hypercalcemia and hypophosphatemia was described. Fuller Albright noted that the hypercalcemia was out of keeping with the extent of the disease, and that the combination of hypercalcemia and hypophosphatemia was more reminiscent of hyperparathyroidism (indeed, the patient had had a surgical exploration of the neck). Although Albright was unable to demonstrate PTH in a biopsy of the tumor in his patient, this observation, and subsequent similar case reports, led to the concept of pseudohyperparathyroidism, or ectopic PTH secretion by tumors.

In 1966, Lafferty[14] collected 50 cases of hypercalcemia from the literature. These cases were selected for the absence of radiographic or postmortem findings of skeletal metastases (30 patients), a significant fall in serum calcium after tumor resection (20 patients), and the positive identification of immunoreactive PTH material in tumor extracts (seven patients). The tumor types described in his review (Table 48-3) remain those most frequently associated with HHM.

Advances in molecular biology, in association with the failure to detect circulating immunoreactive PTH using more reliable assays, cast increasing doubt on the role of native PTH in HHM. In 1983, Simpson and colleagues,[15] using complementary DNA probes to PTH messenger RNA (mRNA), failed to demonstrate the production of PTH mRNA in many of the tumors considered as prime candidates for ectopic PTH secretion.

In 1987, Burtis and colleagues,[16] Moseley and colleagues,[17] and Strewler and colleagues[18] published descriptions of a polypeptide hormone isolated from tumors that are associated with the hypercalcemia of malignancy. The primary structure of these peptides shows considerable N-terminal homology with native

TABLE 48-3

Tumor Types Associated with Humoral Hypercalcemia of Malignancy

TUMOR TYPE	PERCENTAGE
Bronchial squamous carcinoma	28
Renal carcinoma	30
Urothelial carcinoma	8
Squamous carcinoma*	8
Other	26

*Squamous carcinoma at sites other than bronchus.
Data from Lafferty FW: Pseudohyperparathyroidism. Medicine 1966;45:247.

PTH (Fig. 48-3) and has led to the terminology *para-thyroid hormone-related protein* (PTHrP). To ascribe responsibility for the genesis of HHM to this group of peptides, a number of conditions have had to be met. It is not sufficient to find the peptide within the tumor histochemically nor to confirm its in vitro production in tissue culture. It must be clear that the substance is being secreted by the tumor and is present in a biologically active form in the serum. Furthermore, ablation of the tumor (surgically, radiotherapeutically, or chemotherapeutically) must be associated with a fall in the level of the factor and a normalization of the calcium. Using athymic mice bearing a human tumor responsible for HHM, Kukreja and colleagues[19] observed the development of hypercalcemia, hypophosphatemia, and enhanced production of NcAMP. The researchers then infused an antiserum directed against synthetic human PTHrP and were able to reverse these biochemical abnormalities in the mice. These experiments provided strong supportive evidence for a cause-and-effect relationship between PTHrP and HHM.

In a study of 65 patients with hypercalcemia and malignant disease, Budayr and coworkers[20] found elevated circulating levels of PTHrP in 55% of cases. It has also been suggested that there might be a role for measuring PTHrP in the investigation of hypercalcemia now that commercial assays are available. Indeed, Ratcliffe and associates[21] identified elevated levels of PTHrP in 10 of 46 individuals prior to the diagnosis of their malignancies,

although the tumors were truly occult in only two patients. The role of PTHrP in hypercalcemia of malignancy has been the subject of an extensive review, and information on the physiologic role of this hormone has been reviewed by Strewler.[22,23]

Local Osteolytic Hypercalcemia

In the presence of a large bony metastatic burden, calcium is mobilized from the skeleton by the action of osteoclasts. The osteoclasts appear to be stimulated by local factors produced by the tumor cells. Tumor types in this category (carcinoma of the breast, multiple myeloma, lymphoma, and leukemia) rarely produce hypercalcemia in the absence of significant bony metastases, but it must be remembered that local and humoral factors can interact to aggravate bone destruction.

Multiple Myeloma

Bone resorption, osteopenia, and hypercalcemia are characteristic features of patients with multiple myeloma (MM). The neoplastic cells are in close proximity to bone by the very nature of the condition. Mundy and colleagues[24] demonstrated that supernatants from myeloma cells in tissue culture generated osteoclast activating factors (OAFs) that could induce the mobilization of ^{45}Ca from fetal rat long bones. Furthermore, they provided histologic evidence that the bone resorption was being undertaken by osteoclasts in close association with myeloma cells. The nature of the OAFs in MM has been an issue of some controversy. Dewhirst and associates[25] purified and partially sequenced OAFs from stimulated normal peripheral blood mononuclear cells and found identity with IL-1β. Garrett and coworkers[26] described excessive production and secretion of lymphotoxin (TNF-β) by several cultured myeloma cell lines, in the absence of identifiable mRNA for IL-1.

More recently, it has become apparent that IL-6 has an important role to play in the development and maintenance of the myeloma phenotype.[27] IL-6 has been reported to have bone resorbing activity in some in vitro models, but not in others.[28,29] It does, however, appear to potentiate the actions of other cytokines (including IL-1 and TNF) and thus is likely to contribute significantly to the hypercalcemia of this condition. Indeed, a correlation has been drawn between serum levels of IL-6 and osteolysis in patients with MM. Other potential candidates for the enhanced bone resorption found in myeloma include the granulocyte-macrophage and monocyte colony-stimulating factors, which enhance the generation of new osteoclasts.

The picture of hypercalcemia in MM is further complicated by the various renal deficits that are a feature of at least 20% of patients with this condition. The major impact is a reduction in glomerular filtration rate, which decreases the kidneys' ability to excrete a calcium load.

Carcinoma of the Breast

It is generally considered that hypercalcemia is rare in patients with carcinoma of the breast in the absence of widespread osseous metastases. Bony destruction is again

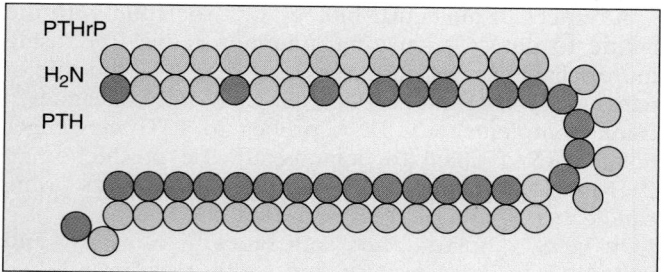

Figure 48-3. Sequence homology between PTHrP (1–34) and PTH (1–34). Blue circles indicate identical amino acids between the polypeptides; purple and yellow circles indicate that the corresponding amino acids are not identical.

mediated by stimulated osteoclasts. It has been suggested that breast cancer cells themselves might be capable of resorbing bone, but this does not appear to be a major mechanism.[30] Breast cancer cells are able to produce a number of factors that could act at a local level to enhance osteolysis. TGF-α is a polypeptide growth factor that acts by stimulating the epidermal growth factor (EGF) receptor. Breast cancer cells in culture produce TGF-α activity, which appears to be estrogen sensitive.[31] When injected into mice, TGF-α produced a mild hypercalcemia (10% above that of control subjects), but a dose-response ceiling was observed with single injections.[32] Both TGF-α and EGF can be found immunopathologically in breast cancer cells, and their local release in bone could be predicted to enhance osteoclastic activation and bone resorption.

Prostaglandins, particularly of the E series, have long been known to stimulate bone resorption.[33] Their roles in breast cancer and in hypercalcemia in general are of specific interest because of the ready availability of inhibitors of their synthesis. An early report by Galasko and Bennett[34] indicated that the recruitment of osteoclasts and bone destruction stimulated by implants of the VX$_2$ carcinoma in rabbits could be mitigated by the oral administration of the cyclo-oxygenase inhibitor indomethacin. Similarly, Powles and associates[35] demonstrated that aspirin and indomethacin could prevent the development of osteolytic bone metastases and hypercalcemia in rats bearing the Walker carcinosarcoma. Unfortunately, the use of prostaglandin synthesis inhibitors has not been effective in influencing the course of metastatic bone disease in patients with breast cancer.

Despite these statements, it is also clear that not all cases of hypercalcemia in carcinoma of the breast are wholly dependent on metastatic disease. Percival and colleagues[36] investigated the mechanism of hypercalcemia in 22 patients with breast cancer. They estimated that, although 46% of the increase in calcium concentration could be accounted for by increased bone turnover, a further 40% could be accounted for only by increased tubular reabsorption of calcium. These data were obtained in the face of euvolemia and suggested that a renal mechanism other than a reduction in glomerular filtration rate was important. Thus, it is not surprising to find that one of the original tumor types from which PTHrP was isolated was breast cancer.[17] In a study of 98 women with varying degrees of breast cancer, Bundred and coworkers[37] noted elevated PTHrP levels in 12 of 13 hypercalcemic patients. Furthermore, tumor staining for PTHrP was positive in 22 of 25 patients who had bone metastases and later developed hypercalcemia. Data also indicate that production of PTHrP by malignant cells can confer on those cells a predilection for metastasizing to bony sites.[38]

Receptor Activator of Nuclear Factor-κB Ligand and Osteoprotegerin in Local Osteolytic Hypercalcemia

The identification of the cytokine system involving the receptor activator of nuclear factor-κB ligand (RANKL), the target of this polypeptide (receptor activator of nuclear factor-κB-RANK), and the controlling inhibitor osteoprotegerin (OPG) that acts as a soluble decoy receptor, has represented a major breakthrough in the understanding of local control of bone cell biology. An excellent review has been published by Hofbauer.[39] Essentially, RANKL, produced by osteoblasts, is responsible for osteoclast differentiation and function. Infusion of RANKL causes severe hypercalcemia and osteoporosis in animal models.[40] A number of tumor models for the production of hypercalcemia by expression of RANKL have been postulated. These include the local stimulation of RANKL by breast cancer cells via PTHrP and the direct secretion of RANKL by myeloma cells.[41,42] Given the blocking effect of OPG on RANKL, a new therapeutic opportunity for the treatment of hypercalcemia could be realized.

Vitamin D–linked Hypercalcemia

In the majority of patients with hypercalcemia, levels of 1,25-dihydroxyvitamin D$_3$, the active metabolite of vitamin D, are suppressed. Normal vitamin D metabolism is closely controlled at the stage of 1α-hydroxylation of 25-hydroxyvitamin D$_3$ in the proximal convoluted tubules of the kidney. The renal tubular 1α-hydroxylase is stimulated by increased levels of PTH and hypophosphatemia, inhibited by hyperphosphatemia, and decreased in activity as PTH levels fall. Since 1981, it has been known that extrarenal, substrate-dependent 1α-hydroxylation can occur in patients with sarcoidosis.[43] The site of the ectopic 1α-hydroxylation appears to be in the macrophages associated with the granulomata.

Abnormal vitamin D metabolism, characterized by a substrate-dependent conversion of 25-hydroxyvitamin D$_3$ to 1,25-dihydroxyvitamin D$_3$ in association with hypercalcemia, was described in 1985 by Davies and colleagues[44] in a patient with Hodgkin's disease. Hypercalcemia has been regarded as an uncommon complication of hematologic malignancies other than myeloma. Only four cases of hypercalcemia were reported by Canellos[45] from a series of 217 patients with advanced lymphoma. Scattered case reports of hypercalcemia and abnormally elevated 1,25-(OH)$_2$D$_3$ have appeared in the literature.[46,47] It has become apparent that as many as 50% or more of patients with adult T-cell lymphoma might have hypercalcemia. Recent evidence suggests that the mechanism of hypercalcemia in adult T-cell lymphoma is due to overexpression of RANKL in the malignant T-cells, inducing excessive osteoclast formation and activity.[48,49] Adams and associates[48] identified 15 lymphoma patients with hypercalcemia over an 11-year period. Seven patients had elevated 1,25-dihydroxyvitamin D$_3$ levels, and one further patient had a level in the midnormal range. One of four patients with acquired immunodeficiency syndrome (AIDS)-associated lymphoma had an elevated 1,25-(OH)$_2$D$_3$ level. Although this and other studies provide some evidence that abnormal vitamin D metabolism could be responsible for some of the cases of hypercalcemia in lymphomas, clearly not all cases can be explained by this mechanism.

In a study of 76 patients with hematologic malignancies and hypercalcemia, Kremer and colleagues[50] noted elevation of PTHrP levels in individuals with non-

Hodgkin's lymphoma and in advanced Hodgkin's disease. In many of these patients, $1,25\text{-}(OH)_2D_3$ levels were suppressed.

Special Cases

Pseudohypercalcemia

The phenomenon of psuedohypercalcemia is a rare condition in which excess calcium bound to nonalbumin plasma proteins results in an elevated total serum calcium concentration. These proteins are usually monoclonal proteins associated with multiple myeloma and benign monoclonal gammopathy.[51] The ionized calcium concentration is normal under these circumstances, but correction formulae using albumin give falsely abnormal results.

Multiple Endocrine Neoplasia

The multiple endocrine neoplasia (MEN) syndromes are a fascinating group of disorders associated with hyperfunction of two or more endocrine glands. The association of these syndromes with hypercalcemia has been the topic of a major review.[52]

Hyperparathyroidism or parathyroid hyperplasia is a feature of both MEN-1 and MEN-2. Hypercalcemia is usually mild and frequently asymptomatic. The role of parathyroidectomy is unclear in MEN-1 and MEN-2B, but the association with medullary carcinoma of the thyroid in MEN-2A means that it will more frequently be undertaken in this condition.

Tamoxifen-linked Hypercalcemia

Hypercalcemia in association with the use of estrogen or antiestrogen therapy for carcinoma of the breast has been recognized for more than 50 years. The severity of the hypercalcemia is variable, but it can be fatal. The mechanism by which tamoxifen and similar agents cause hypercalcemia is unclear. Cell culture studies suggest that prostaglandins could be the main mediators of the response.[53] A role for prostaglandins would be compatible with the clinical picture of a tamoxifen "flare," which, in addition to the hypercalcemia, is frequently associated with bone pain.

EVALUATION OF THE PATIENT

That malignancy is the cause of hypercalcemia is usually not hard to establish. Nonetheless, careful consideration of other causes of hypercalcemia is warranted for all patients. The differential diagnosis of isolated hypercalcemia is a long one (Table 48-4). It is worth noting, however, that immobilization is common in patients with cancer, that primary hyperparathyroidism is not a rare disease, and that the iatrogenic causes of hypercalcemia are easily remedied.

Clinical Findings

The syndrome of hypercalcemia of malignancy is often overlooked because many of the symptoms are

TABLE 48-4

Causes of Hypercalcemia (Other Than Malignant Disease)

TYPE	CAUSE
Endocrine	Hyperparathyroidism
	Hyperthyroidism
	Addison's disease
Iatrogenic	Immobilization
	Vitamins A and D
	Thiazide diuretics
	Lithium
Other	Paget's disease of bone
	Granulomatous disease

nonspecific or vague and are ascribed to the underlying malignant process or to its therapy. The symptoms of hypercalcemia are protean. Only parts of the old dictum of "stones, bones, abdominal groans, and psychic moans" used in the description of the symptoms due to primary hyperparathyroidism hold true.

Gastrointestinal symptoms are present in nearly all affected individuals. Nausea, anorexia, and vomiting are early symptoms, but they can easily be confused with the side effects of tumor treatment or with symptoms produced directly by the tumor itself. By inducing dehydration and hence aggravating the hypercalcemia, these complications set up a vicious cycle. Constipation is common, and complete ileus can occur at severely raised calcium levels. Cramping abdominal pains, such as those seen in primary hyperparathyroidism, are encountered occasionally, but acute pancreatitis or peptic ulceration complicating the hypercalcemia of malignancy is extremely rare.

The major effect of hypercalcemia on the kidney is to impair renal concentrating ability. Urine, dilute compared with plasma, is excreted in large volume. As the hypercalcemia and the polyuria persist, volume depletion ensues, with a resultant fall in the glomerular filtration rate. Further impairment of the kidney's ability to handle the abnormal calcium load occurs, and the hypercalcemia is aggravated. Tubular damage continues and manifests as acquired renal tubular acidosis, glycosuria, and aminoaciduria. An important consequence of the tubular malfunction is a natriuresis. This results in a sodium loss that aggravates the hypercalcemia, as the mechanisms for conserving sodium and calcium within the kidney are similar. A syndrome akin to nephrogenic diabetes insipidus occurs, and polydipsia is, therefore, an early feature. Unfortunately, the gastrointestinal symptoms of anorexia and vomiting overcome the thirst, and intense dehydration can occur. Nephrocalcinosis and nephrolithiasis require hypercalcemia of a prolonged duration and are therefore atypical of the syndrome.

Neuropsychiatric symptoms of apathy, depression, and fatigue are frequently overlooked and ascribed to the underlying neoplasm. Muscle weakness itself can be profound and can confine the patient to bed. This immobility leads to further calcium mobilization and enhances the hypercalcemia. As hypercalcemia continues to worsen, confusion and finally coma supervene. Focal neurologic symptoms, including ataxia, which resolve on normalization of the serum calcium, also can occur but are rare.

Pruritis is a well recognized, if infrequent, complication of hypercalcemia, as are various irritating eye symptoms. Their frequency in malignant hypercalcemia is less than in primary hyperparathyroidism.

Bone pain is a frequent symptom of both malignant disease and hypercalcemia. Clearly, this might in part be related to the presence of metastases within bone causing areas of increased intramedullary pressure, ischemia, or microfractures, but the symptom is also present in the absence of demonstrable metastatic disease.

The syndrome of hypercalcemia of malignancy, therefore, presents insidiously, with anorexia, fatigue, apathy, and polyuria, but it can progress rapidly to obtundation and death.

Laboratory Investigations

From a practical point of view, a few well-chosen, simple investigations are all that are required to aid in the diagnosis, therapy, and monitoring of patients. From the academic point of view, these and less readily available investigations can enhance the understanding of the hypercalcemic process in any given individual.

A complete blood count and estimation of the platelet count are required. Measurements of serum electrolytes, blood urea nitrogen, and creatinine are mandatory. Because of the importance of protein binding on the "free" calcium concentration, serum albumin should always be measured with the serum calcium, and a correction formula (such as the one given previously) should be employed. In asymptomatic patients with hypercalcemia and multiple myeloma, a serum ionized calcium should be obtained.

Renal function and the response of the serum calcium to therapy should be monitored daily until the calcium concentration normalizes, and weekly thereafter unless circumstances necessitate more frequent investigation.

Biochemical clues to the presence of HHM due to PTHrP include hypophosphatemia, hyperchloremia, and a mild metabolic alkalosis, although these could not be considered diagnostic. Urinary excretion of calcium is high, as is urinary cyclic adenosine monophosphate (cAMP). The renal phosphate threshold is low, indicating a renal phosphate leak, and significant hypophosphatemia can result following treatment of the hypercalcemia.

Serum immunoreactive PTH is low or undetectable unless the primary site of malignancy is the parathyroid gland itself. Vitamin D metabolites are also frequently low in most cases of hypercalcemia, despite the fact that PTHrP is capable of stimulating renal 1α-hydroxylase. Measures of osteoblastic function, such as alkaline phosphatase and bone gla-protein (osteocalcin), have little to offer in the diagnosis or management of hypercalcemia.

Radiographs and isotope bone scans might be pertinent for prognostication and follow-up but do not help delineate the cause of the hypercalcemia, nor are they useful in predicting the response to therapy.

GRADING THE COMPLICATION

Although it is possible to grade hypercalcemia according to mild, moderate, and severe categories on the basis of a biochemical value, it is important to note that the development and severity of symptoms do not appear to be strictly related to the serum calcium level. As a general rule, patients with symptoms readily related to hypercalcemia should be treated as severe cases, regardless of the objective degree of elevation of the calcium level. A frequently made but poorly understood observation is that patients with tumor-induced hypercalcemia often have greater symptomatology for any given rise in calcium level compared with patients with primary hyperparathyroidism. Our approach to the treatment of hypercalcemia of malignancy is based on the following classification of hypercalcemia. It is worth noting that many factors other than the serum calcium level affect the logical choice for therapy.

Mild Hypercalcemia

Patients in this group are asymptomatic and have a serum calcium level of less than 3.0 mmol/L. The abnormality is frequently detected as part of the routine biochemical work-up in patients with tumor types known to predispose to hypercalcemia. These individuals, therefore, are usually outpatients. Although urgent management of the hypercalcemia is not indicated, several considerations must be borne in mind. The natural history of tumor-induced hypercalcemia is for the condition to worsen. A re-evaluation of the current antineoplastic regimen and response to treatment is warranted, as the development of hypercalcemia might be an early indication of a diminishing response to therapy. The development of any intercurrent insult to the kidneys is likely to precipitate more severe hypercalcemia. Intercurrent insult includes both any situation in which volume depletion could occur, and the introduction of nephrotoxic agents, such as nonsteroidal anti-inflammatory agents.

Moderate Hypercalcemia

In asymptomatic patients with a serum calcium of 3.0 to 3.5 mmol/L, the situation is more serious. Although this level of calcium might not be life threatening, little is required to tip the scales toward a more serious problem.

Severe Hypercalcemia

All patients with symptoms attributable to hypercalcemia should be treated as an acute medical emergency. Furthermore, patients with a serum calcium concentration (corrected for albumin) greater than 3.5 mmol/L require urgent treatment.

TREATMENT

The serum calcium concentration can be reduced in almost all patients with tumor-induced hypercalcemia.

A variety of antihypercalcemic regimens remains in common use, although the wide therapeutic index and high success rates of the newer bisphosphonates has resulted in their use as first-line management in the majority of cases. Although it has been possible to target osteoclast-mediated bone resorption in a fairly specific way, the same cannot be said for enhanced renal tubular calcium reabsorption or gastrointestinal calcium absorption.

Selection of therapy should be geared to a knowledge of the individual tumor type (and hence, to the likely mechanism underlying the hypercalcemia) and to the states of the patient's renal function and bone marrow reserve. Any specific antineoplastic therapy that can be used, be it surgical, radiotherapeutic, or chemotherapeutic, will be a powerful adjuvant to antihypercalcemic therapy.

Ethical Considerations

The first decision is whether or not to treat this complication. Unless specific antitumor therapy is available, the majority of patients who develop hypercalcemia of malignancy are in the last few weeks of their lives (Fig. 48-4). Thus, it can be argued that treatment is not indicated for all cases of hypercalcemia associated with malignancy. For some, however, the use of an effective, safe treatment to ameliorate the substantial morbidity of hypercalcemia and to allow patients to return home is clearly warranted.

General Considerations

The best treatment is one directed specifically and effectively at the underlying malignant disease. Early mobilization is a laudable but often unachievable goal in patients with advanced malignant disease. Thiazide diuretics should be avoided because they promote renal tubular calcium reabsorption.

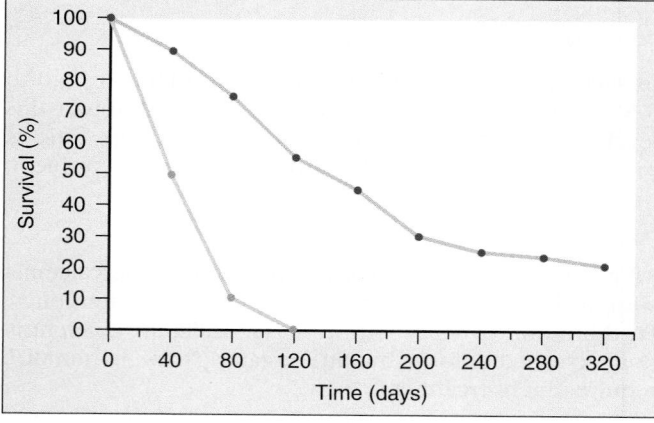

Figure 48-4. Survival curves for patients with cancer and hypercalcemia. *Red circles*, specific anticancer therapy; *yellow circles*, no anticancer therapy. (From Ralston SH, Gallacher SJ, Patel U, et al: Cancer-associated hypercalcemia: morbidity and mortality. Ann Intern Med 1990;112:499.)

Although dietary restriction of calcium seems intuitively appropriate, gastrointestinal calcium absorption is low in most cases of hypercalcemia associated with malignant disease. A notable exception is among patients whose tumors are associated with a substrate-dependent 1α-hydroxylase, which allows continued production of calcitriol. Patients taking supplemental vitamin D and vitamin A (β-carotene) should be advised of the hypercalcemic effects of these agents.

Extracellular Fluid Volume Expansion

Most patients with hypercalcemia of malignancy have significant depletions of fluid volume (on the order of 5 to 10 L) due to the combined effects of anorexia, vomiting, and nephrogenic diabetes insipidus. In this state, the glomerular filtration rate is reduced, and the response by the proximal convoluted tubule is to increase sodium retention. Concomitantly, proximal tubular resorption of calcium is also increased. The aim of fluid replacement in these circumstances should be to induce a state of mild fluid overload. Restoration of a normal circulating blood volume restores the glomerular filtration rate and increases the fractional excretion of calcium. Further salt loading, on the other hand, induces natriuresis and concomitant calciuresis. Care must be taken to avoid severe congestive cardiac failure in elderly patients or in patients with poor cardiac reserve. Because of the hypoalbuminemia that frequently accompanies advanced malignant disease, dependent edema is to be expected during volume expansion. Care must also be taken to ensure an adequate intake of free water. In the presence of severe hypercalcemia, a resistance to the distal tubular actions of antidiuretic hormone may predispose obtunded patients to significant hypernatremia. After restoration of euvolemia, a maintenance infusion of 3 L/d of 0.9% saline solution will induce continued natriuresis. Patients should be encouraged to drink freely. During such aggressive fluid management, other electrolyte abnormalities are likely to be uncovered or precipitated. Despite impaired renal function, both hypokalemia and hypomagnesemia are frequent findings, and appropriate supplementation could be required.

Although serum calcium can be expected to fall while a patient is on this regimen, restoration of normocalcemia is unlikely (Fig. 48-5). Failure to restore normal fluid balance, however, will greatly detract from the success of subsequent therapeutic measures.

Calciuretic Therapy

Aside from the calciuretic effects of saline overload, two other agents are commonly employed to induce renal calcium wasting: furosemide and calcitonin.

Furosemide

Furosemide is a diuretic agent whose main site of action is in the thick ascending limb of the loop of Henle (thus making this agent a *loop diuretic*), where it completely and reversibly inhibits the $Na^+/K^+/2Cl^-$ cotransporter. In the euvolemic and volume-expanded state, the fractional

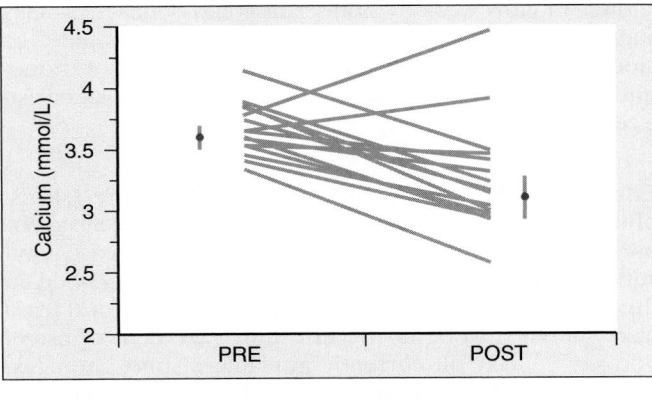

Figure 48-5. Effect of rehydration on 16 hypercalcemic patients. (Data from Hosking DJ, Cowley A, Bucknall A: Rehydration in the treatment of severe hypercalcemia. Q J Med 1981;200:473.)

excretion of calcium can be increased by up to 30% by loop diuretics. If a patient is volume depleted, however, enhanced proximal tubular sodium and calcium resorption can obviate this response. Thus, the potential exists for loop diuretics to aggravate hypercalcemia if adequate attention is not paid to fluid volume status. In the initial report of the effectiveness of this treatment, the regimen involved the administration of doses of furosemide in the region of 100 mg every two hours.[54] Therapy this aggressive would require the facilities of an intensive care unit to ensure adequate fluid monitoring. Although substantial falls in the serum calcium can be achieved, a rationale for the use of this treatment for other than acute situations is lacking, in that the primary cause of the hypercalcemia—increased bone resorption—is not affected. Given the risks of severe electrolyte disturbances and the availability of potent antiresorptive medication, the use of loop diuretics should be reserved primarily for situations of fluid overload, rather than used as antihypercalcemic agents.

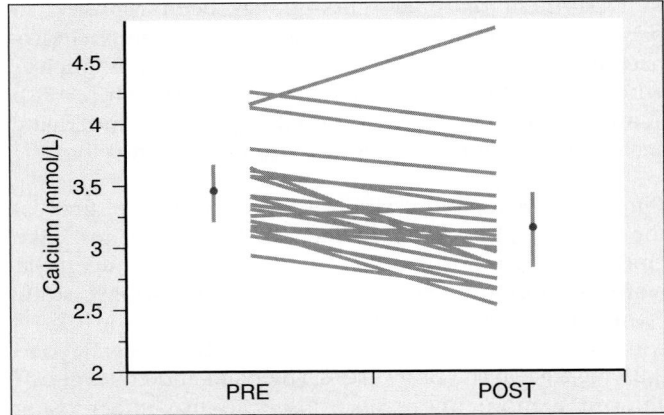

Figure 48-6. Effect of calcitonin (100 U daily) in 21 hypercalcemic patients. (Data from Hosking DJ, Gilson D: Comparison of the renal and skeletal actions of calcitonin in the treatment of severe hypercalcemia of malignancy. Q J Med 1984;211:359.)

Calcitonin

The renal actions of calcitonin are complex. The calciuretic effect appears to be due to inhibition of calcium reabsorption in the distal tubules. This, in turn, is dependent on an adequate delivery of calcium to the distal nephron, a situation that is compromised by the extracellular fluid volume depletion in hypercalcemia. This renal tubular effect is rapid, however, and in a study by Hosking and Gilson,[55] it accounted for a mean fall of 0.35 ± 0.057 mmol/L in 11 patients who responded well (Fig. 48-6). Administration of calcitonin can be of great value as an adjunct to more potent antiresorptive therapies.

Antiresorptive Therapy

Given that bone resorption is increased in the majority of cases of hypercalcemia of malignancy, the best treatment after that designed to combat the tumor itself is one directed at bone resorption. The osteoclasts represent the final common pathway for bone resorption in both humoral and local osteolytic hypercalcemia. The following agents, which inhibit osteoclast function, not surprisingly are highly effective antihypercalcemia treatment.

Bisphosphonates

The bisphosphonates are a class of compounds—structural analogues to pyrophosphate (PP_i)—in which the P-O-P bond is replaced by a P-C-P bond stable to enzymatic cleavage. Figure 48-7 shows the structure of some of the available bisphosphonates compared with the structure of PP_i.

Pharmacokinetic and pharmacodynamic studies of bisphosphonates indicate that these compounds are absorbed poorly from the gastrointestinal tract after oral administration. Studies in healthy adult male volunteers have shown that gastrointestinal absorption is on the order of 1% to 3% but varies between individuals.[56,57] Diet has a profound effect on gastrointestinal absorption, reducing the effective bioavailability of the drug to zero if it is taken with food.[58] Once absorbed, it appears that approximately 50% of the compound is excreted unchanged in the urine, the rest being sequestered in bone and soft tissue, where its half-life (in rats) is four months.[59,60] From the experiments of Jung and colleagues,[61] it appears that bone mineral has a very high affinity for bisphosphonates. Although the bulk of any absorbed bisphosphonate is relocated rapidly to bone, this is nonhomogeneous and varies with the state of bone activity. Indeed, this principle is made use of for isotope bone scanning using ^{99m}Tc-labeled bisphosphonates. Furthermore, it is likely that the release of bisphosphonate will be enhanced in areas of rapid bone turnover, leading to an unpredictable recirculation of the drug.[62]

The precise mechanism of action of these compounds is unclear. Evidence for a marked physicochemical effect of bisphosphonates came from work by Robertson and colleagues,[63] who demonstrated that compounds such as PP_i and bisphosphonates had major effects on the ionic makeup of the hydration layer usually surrounding hydroxyapatite crystals in suspension. This interaction

Problems Common to Cancer and Its Therapy

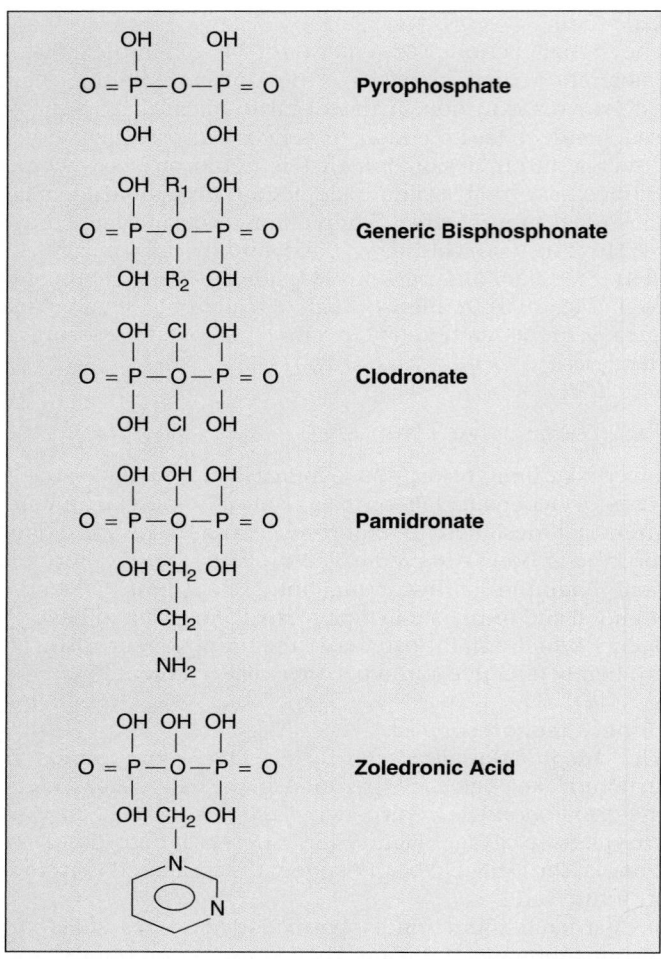

Figure 48-7. Structural formulae of commonly studied bisphosphonates in relation to the generic bisphosphonate and to pyrophosphate.

alters the calcium phosphate product both at the surface of the crystal and in the immediate vicinity, thus inhibiting further crystal development and dissolution.

Lysosomal enzyme systems in osteoclasts have been implicated in the process of bone resorption, and it is possible that inhibition of these enzymes—notably the acid hydrolases but also the enzymes responsible for energy production and protein synthesis by bisphosphonates—could account in some way for their effects.[64-66]

In an extensive coverage of the cellular morphologic changes induced by bisphosphonates, Plasmans and associates[67] investigated changes in osteocyte, osteoblast, and osteoclast morphology induced by etidronate in a model of heterotopic bone formation. They discovered that the normal ruffled border of the osteoclasts appeared to shrink, and from this observation they coined the term *frustrated osteoclasts*. Furthermore, transient abnormal calcium storage in the mitochondria of osteoblasts was noted, and the osteocytes appeared to be stimulated into greater activity, with enhancement of subcellular organelles. Although in many in vivo studies no evidence for a failure in the development of osteoclasts had been

shown, in vitro work by Boonekamp and colleagues[68] has suggested that pamidronate (but not etidronate or clodronate) was able to inhibit the accession of mononuclear osteoclast precursors to a previously osteoclast-free system.

Etidronate. Etidronate (1-hydroxy-ethylidene-1,1-bisphosphonate) was the first bisphosphonate licensed for use in the management of metabolic bone disease. Oral administration of this agent became well established in the treatment of Paget's disease of bone, and clinical trials have shown it to be of use in the management of osteoporosis.[69,70] Like all currently available bisphosphonates, etidronate suffers from poor and unpredictable oral bioavailability. The hypocalcemic response to intravenous etidronate is not as marked as with newer bisphosphonates. A conservative estimate suggests that normocalcemia can be restored for approximately 40% of patients. Evidence for a sequential beneficial effect of oral etidronate following normalization of serum calcium exists but is poor (see "Long-Term Treatment" later in this chapter). Etidronate differs from other bisphosphonates studied in that its use is frequently associated with hyperphosphatemia.

Clodronate. The use of intravenous clodronate (dichloromethylene bisphosphonate) for the control of the hypercalcemia of malignancy was investigated by several groups in the United States and Europe in the early 1980s. The appearance of three cases of acute leukemia in 664 patients led to the temporary withdrawal from use of this agent pending analysis of the likelihood of leukemia being a true side effect.[71] Thereafter, much of the investigation of this agent has been limited to groups in Europe and, more recently, Canada, where clodronate has approval for use as an antihypercalcemic agent.

Clodronate is a highly effective agent in restoring normocalcemia. Oral clodronate also appears able to induce a normocalcemic response, but in the clinical situation of the acute management of hypercalcemia, the intravenous route is preferable.[72]

Impairment of renal function has been reported in patients receiving rapid infusions of intravenous clodronate in the setting of multiple myeloma.[73] It is unclear whether a direct cause-and-effect relationship with administration of clodronate holds, given the underlying renal complications in patients with multiple myeloma.

Pamidronate. Pamidronate disodium was the first of the aminobisphosphonates licensed for clinical use. Like clodronate, pamidronate is a very effective agent at restoring normocalcemia.[74] An early dose-response study from Europe carried out by Body and colleagues in 1987[75] showed little advantage to increasing the dose beyond 0.25 mg/kg. On the other hand, Thiébaud and colleagues[76] showed a more impressive dose-response effect using single intravenous infusions of pamidronate (30–90 mg) in terms of both restoration of normocalcemia and duration of the normocalcemic response. This finding was confirmed in a large multicenter trial in the United

States.[77] In the early studies, pamidronate was given in divided doses over a period of several days. It is possible, however, to achieve the same effect with single-dose therapy.[78] Dodwell and colleagues[79] have studied more rapid infusion rates and have shown that the drug can be given safely and efficaciously over a two-hour period.

Zoledronic Acid. Zoledronic acid is a highly potent bisphosphonate containing a heterocyclic imidazole group. Preclinical studies indicated that it was many times more active than pamidronate, and a dose finding study indicated that the effective dose was on the order of 0.02–0.04 mg/kg.[80] Studies using 4 mg and 8 mg infusions of zoledronic acid indicate the efficacy to be on the order of 80%–90% in restoring normocalcemia, but concern over the possible development of renal dysfunction at the higher dose has led to the recommendation that the starting dose of zoledronic acid be 4 mg.[81] A major advantage of this agent is the short infusion times required (5–10 minutes in initial studies), which simplifies outpatient treatment significantly.

Comparative Studies Involving Bisphosphonates. Ralston and colleagues[82] compared the hypocalcemic effect of pamidronate disodium with that of mithramycin and a combination of corticosteroids and calcitonin. They demonstrated that pamidronate induced a more effective fall in serum calcium than either mithramycin or the combination of corticosteroids and calcitonin, although the time to the onset of the effect was longer. Thürlimann and colleagues[83] performed a comparative, randomized, crossover study to compare the hypocalcemic effects of a single intravenous dose of 60 mg pamidronate with 20 µg/kg mithramycin. There were no primary failures in the pamidronate-treated group (11 of 11), but six of 14 patients in the mithramycin-treated group failed to achieve normocalcemia. When those patients, along with two others from this group who had become hypercalcemic again, were treated with pamidronate, all eight became normocalcemic.

A comparative study involving the three commonly available bisphosphonates in Europe demonstrated that a single intravenous infusion of 30 mg pamidronate induced a more rapid and more pronounced fall in serum calcium than 600 mg of clodronate given as a single intravenous dose or 7.5 mg/kg etidronate given intravenously for three days.[84] A multicenter U.S. study comparing the hypocalcemic effects of etidronate and pamidronate confirmed the superiority of the latter bisphosphonate.[85]

A pooled analysis of two studies involving 287 patients demonstrated a significantly better response rate for zoledronic acid (4 mg and 8 mg) compared with pamidronate (90 mg).[86] The complete response rate for both zoledronic acid doses (defined as normocalcemia at day 10) was similar (88.4% for patients given 4 mg; 86.7% for patients given 8 mg), whereas the response rate for pamidronate was 69.7%. Although these studies confirmed the superiority of zoledronic acid to pamidronate in the sample population, it should be noted that the response rate to pamidronate was lower than has been reported in previous trials.

Effect of Tumor Type on Response to Bisphosphonates. Although the primary mechanism in the generation and maintenance of hypercalcemia in malignant disease is enhanced bone resorption, tumor types differ significantly in the way they bring this about. Morton and coworkers[74] could detect no statistically significant difference between hypercalcemic patients with squamous carcinoma of the bronchus ($n = 12$), carcinoma of the breast ($n = 6$), or multiple myeloma ($n = 5$) in their response to 60 mg pamidronate. More recently, it has been suggested that a low renal phosphate threshold (indicative of the effects of PTHrP) may be used to indicate the likelihood of a poor response to treatment,[87] and Dodwell and colleagues[88] have demonstrated a statistically significant relationship between the circulating PTHrP concentration and the time to normalization of hypercalcemia.

Duration of Response to Bisphosphonate Therapy. The duration of response to bisphosphonates is difficult to determine and varies considerably between individuals. Elucidation of the duration of response is also compounded by the high mortality in this group of patients due to their tumors and by the introduction of specific and effective antineoplastic therapy for patients with cancer of the breast and multiple myeloma. In the patients treated by Morton and colleagues,[74] only 11 of 30 patients (37%) survived longer than one month following the onset of their hypercalcemia. In this study, the median time to recurrence of hypercalcemia was approximately three weeks. The same median duration of normocalcemia was also found by Harinck and Bijvoet[89]; however, a longer duration of 35 days was reported by Thiébaud and colleagues.[76] Median time to relapse in the studies comparing zoledronic acid with pamidronate was 30-40 days with zoledronic acid and 17 days with pamidronate.[86] Unfortunately, it is not possible to predict the length of time that any specific patient will remain normocalcemic.

Side Effects of Bisphosphonates. In general, bisphosphonate therapy is well tolerated. Low-grade pyrexia is noted in 10%–15% of patients. The use of rapid intravenous infusions of clodronate and etidronate has been associated with deterioration in renal function in patients with previously diminished renal reserves. The observation of more frequent renal abnormalities in patients receiving 8 mg zoledronic acid has led to the recommendation that 4 mg be the starting dose. Hyperphosphatemia is noted with etidronate therapy, but hypophosphatemia is seen with clodronate and pamidronate treatment. The mechanisms of phosphate imbalance are unclear, although etidronate appears to have a specific effect on renal phosphate handling.[90] Prolonged use of etidronate has been associated with a fracturing osteomalacia in patients with Paget's disease of bone, but this is of little relevance in hypercalcemic individuals. Oral bisphosphonates are associated with gastrointestinal intolerance and are probably best avoided in the acute situation.

Other Bisphosphonates. Alendronate disodium is a potent aminobisphosphonate that is being used in an oral form in the management of osteoporosis. A dose-response study demonstrated that alendronate 10 mg intravenously over a two-hour period restored normal calcium levels in 90% of patients.[91] No long-term studies with oral alendronate in hypercalcemic patients are available.

Ibandronate is a bisphosphonate that is approximately 50 times more potent than pamidronate in animal models of bone resorption. A dose-response study of this agent showed that an intravenous dose of 6 mg was highly effective at restoring normal calcium levels.[92]

Plicamycin (Mithramycin)

This bacteriostatic antibiotic agent was used in the late 1960s for the treatment of germ cell tumors.[93] A side effect of this agent in normocalcemic individuals was hypocalcemia. The mechanism of the hypocalcemia is unclear, although in vitro studies suggest that a direct toxic effect on osteoclasts is responsible.[94] Despite a long list of side effects that include marrow, hepatic, and renal toxicity, plicamycin remains a widely used agent for the management of hypercalcemia. Plicamycin is effective at restoring normocalcemia in approximately 80% of patients, and many consider the toxic effects to be overstated, as the antihypercalcemic effect is seen at doses 10 times lower than those used in the original antineoplastic regimens. A standard infusion of 25 μg/kg over a period of four to six hours is most often used. Longer duration of infusion can reduce the nausea caused by this agent but adds to the risk of extravasation and local irritation. The hypocalcemic effect is seen within the first 24 hours, but the duration of response is unpredictable.

One serious reported drawback with plicamycin is the development of severe, rapid, rebound hypercalcemia that occurs in an unpredictable fashion.[95] Furthermore, most of the toxic effects of plicamycin are cumulative. Thus, its use in the long-term management of hypercalcemia is limited.

Although the safer (and more effective) amino-bisphosphonates have replaced plicamycin as first-line antiresorptive therapy, this agent might be of use for the infrequent case in which hypercalcemia proves resistant.

Calcitonin

Because calcitonin has both calciuretic and antiresorptive actions, it would appear that this would be the ideal antihypercalcemic agent. The antiresorptive effects of calcitonin are related directly to osteoclast toxicity, and possibly, to inhibition of new osteoclast recruitment. When used as a single agent, the hypocalcemic effect of calcitonin is modest at best, and resistance to the effects of calcitonin develops rapidly.

Nonetheless, a major role for calcitonin in combination with powerful antiresorptive agents is emerging. Fatemi and associates[96] reported an enhanced and more rapid hypocalcemic effect with the combination of etidronate and calcitonin, as had Ralston and colleagues[97] with pamidronate and calcitonin.

Although calcitonin originally was recommended for subcutaneous use, newer routes of delivery, including suppositories and nasal sprays, have been developed with varying levels of efficacy.

In cases of life-threatening hypercalcemia, or when neurologic symptoms are a major feature, we recommend the use of 8 MRC (Medical Research Council) units/kg given intramuscularly every six hours for one or two days in association with an intravenous bisphosphonate. This regimen has the advantage of combining the rapid calciuretic effect of calcitonin with the powerful, prolonged antiresorptive effect of the bisphosphonate.[98]

Gallium Nitrate

Hypocalcemia was noted as a side effect of therapy among patients receiving gallium nitrate for the management of lymphoma.[99] Thereafter, its effectiveness was confirmed by Warrell and colleagues[100] in open-labeled studies and in a randomized, double-blind comparative study with calcitonin.[101] The mechanism of action of gallium is unknown, although it is clear that urinary calcium excretion is reduced. By implication, bone resorption is reduced, although no histologic changes were noted in explants of fetal long bones exposed to this agent.

Gallium nitrate requires intravenous administration. The best investigated regimens involve sequential five-day infusions of 200 mg/m²/day. At this dose, the drug is relatively free of side effects, although caution is required if other nephrotoxic agents (e.g., aminoglycosides) are being used.

Prostaglandin Synthesis Inhibitors

As discussed previously, prostaglandins (notably prostaglandin E_2) have potent bone resorbing effects in relationship to certain tumor types. Thus it was hoped that a significant subset of patients might be found who would respond to prostaglandin synthesis inhibitors such as indomethacin. Although well characterized case reports have shown a good response to these agents, in general they are ineffective for the treatment of tumor-induced hypercalcemia.[102] Seyberth and coworkers[103] attempted to characterize those patients who might be responsive in terms of their biochemical parameters. As one might expect intuitively, those patients with a high urinary excretion of prostaglandin E_2 metabolites showed the best response. In general, however, no reliance can be placed on prostaglandin synthesis inhibitors in this clinical setting.

Other Therapies

Corticosteroids

Glucocorticoids are commonly employed in the management of tumor-induced hypercalcemia despite significant evidence that their usefulness is limited. The mechanism of any hypocalcemic effect produced by these agents is unclear. In patients with multiple myeloma and lymphoid malignancies, glucocorticosteroids form part of the antineoplastic regimen (e.g., melphalan and prednisone, VAD [vincristine, doxorubicin, and dexamethasone], MOPP [mechlorethamine, vincristine, procarbazine, and prednisone], CHOP [cyclophosphamide, doxorubicin, vincristine, and prednisone]) because of their known cytotoxic effect on lymphoid tissue. Furthermore, because glucocorticosteroids block absorption of calcium from the gut, they can be expected to be useful for patients with vitamin D–mediated hypercalcemia where gastrointestinal absorption of calcium is enhanced.

In patients with solid tumors, corticosteroids are not usually effective and have no role in the management of hypercalcemia.[104]

Phosphate

The use of intravenous phosphate to complex calcium and induce precipitation in the extracellular fluid and soft tissue can no longer the supported.[105] Oral phosphate, however, is less toxic and may be tried for the long-term management of hypercalcemia. The dose-limiting side effect of the oral agent is diarrhea. Although oral phosphate acts primarily as a gastrointestinal calcium chelator, it also might have some inhibitory effects on osteoclast function.

Dialysis

Hemodialysis using a dialysate bath free of calcium can be used in the emergency treatment of hypercalcemia.

Potential Future Therapies

Osteoprotegerin

Osteoprotegerin (OPG) is a soluble receptor belonging to the tumor necrosis factor receptor superfamily. In terms of bone metabolism, it is thought to act as a modulator of osteoclast differentation and function by acting as an inhibitory (or decoy) receptor for the polypeptide receptor activator of nuclear factor-κB ligand (RANKL). RANKL is also known as osteoclast differentiation factor (ODF) and as TNF-related activation-induced cytokine (TRANCE). (For a review, see reference 39). OPG has been shown to reverse hypercalcemia induced by a number of factors, including IL-1, TNF-α, PTH, PTHrP and 1,25(OH)$_2$D$_3$, and in a mouse model of humoral hypercalcemia of malignancy.[106,107] The results of Phase I and II human studies are awaited with interest.

Antibodies to PTHrP

Infusion of antibodies directed against PTHrP has long been known to reverse hypercalcemia in murine models.[21] Results of Phase I and II human studies with these agents are also awaited with interest.

Long-Term Treatment

For patients for whom no antitumor therapy is available, long-term survival is unusual. By implication, there are few good long-term studies on the management of hypercalcemia, and most results are anecdotal. Individualization of therapy is the rule. Patients should be advised to drink an adequate volume of fluid (2 to 3 L daily) and to maintain their mobility as long as possible. They should be reminded of the symptoms of hypercalcemia and urged to report for treatment early should those symptoms arise. Table 48-5 shows suggested maintenance treatments for the hypercalcemia of malignancy.

The importance of palliative care cannot be overemphasized in the management of these unfortunate individuals.

TABLE 48-5

Options for Long-term Management of Hypercalcemia of Malignancy

AGENT	DOSE	FREQUENCY*
Intravenous zoledronic acid	4 mg over 15 min	Every 2–3 weeks
Intravenous pamidronate[†]	60–90 mg over 2–4 h	Every 2–3 weeks
Oral pamidronate[‡]	200–1,200 mg	Daily
Oral clodronate[§]	3,200 mg	Daily
Oral etidronate[¶,‖]	20 mg/kg	Daily
Oral phosphate	2–3 g	Daily
Corticosteroids	Variable	Daily
Multiple myeloma		
Carcinoma of the breast		
NSAIDs	Variable	Daily

NSAIDs, nonsteroidal anti-inflammatory drugs.
*Suggested frequencies and doses may be altered to suit individual patients.
[†]Dodwell DJ, Howell A, Morton AR, et al: Infusion rate and pharmacokinetics of intravenous pamidronate in the treatment of tumour-induced hypercalcemia. Postgrad Med J 1992;68:434.
[‡]Thiébaud D, Portmann L, Jaeger PH, et al: Oral versus intravenous AHPrBP (APD) in the treatment of hypercalcemia of malignancy. Bone 1986;7:247.
[§]Chapuy MC, Meunier PJ, Alexandre CM, Vignon EP: Effects of disodium dichloromethylene diphosphonate on hypercalcemia produced by bone metastases. J Clin Invest 1980;65:1243.
[¶]Ringenberg QS, Ritch PS: Efficacy of oral administration of disodium etidronate in maintaining normal serum calcium levels in previously hypercalcemia cancer patients. Clin Ther 1987;9:318.
[‖]Hasling C, Charles P, Mosekilde L: Etidronate disodium in the management of malignancy-related hypercalcemia. Am J Med 1987;82:51.

A logical therapeutic regimen for the acute management of tumor-induced hypercalcemia is shown in "Management of Hypercalcemia of Malignancy." This regimen represents one approach to this problem. Other equally valid regimens are possible, and individualization of regimens is mandatory for long-term therapy.

MANAGEMENT OF HYPERCALCEMIA OF MALIGNANCY

The most effective way to control the hypercalcemia of malignant disease is by therapy aimed at eradicating or reducing the tumor burden. Chemotherapy, radiation therapy, and surgical therapy all have roles to play. In the absence of effective antitumor therapy, the patient's general condition and immediate prognosis should be used to guide the decision to embark on aggressive antihypercalcemic therapy, active palliation, or both. The introduction of agents with high efficacy and few side effects has broadened the oncologist's options.

Our practice is to discuss treatment options with the patients and their families, emphasizing that the drugs used to control the hypercalcemia have little or no impact on the progression of the underlying cancer but will help the symptoms of the hypercalcemia. Volume expansion with 0.9% saline is begun immediately. The rate is determined by the state of hydration of the individual patient as assessed by the clinician. An infusion of intravenous bisphosphonate (zoledronic acid or pamidronate) is begun at the same time as saline volume expansion. In the presence of severe hypercalcemia and

Continued

MANAGEMENT OF HYPERCALCEMIA OF MALIGNANCY—*cont'd*

neurologic symptomatology, calcitonin 8 MRC units/kg intramuscularly every six hours is used in conjunction with the bisphosphonate.

Biochemical response is rapid. The serum calcium can be expected to fall after 24 hours. Most patients reach a nadir calcium value in five to seven days. We maintain natriuresis by continuing the saline infusion until normocalcemia is reached. Volume overload, as evidenced by an elevation of the jugular venous pressure, the development of a fourth heart sound, pulmonary congestion, or peripheral edema, is treated with furosemide, which has the added benefit of inducing calciuresis. Care is taken to avoid volume depletion during use of the diuretic. Close attention is paid to renal function and electrolyte balance, as hypokalemia, hypomagnesemia, and hypophosphatemia are common sequelae of this treatment approach. Failure to respond to bisphosphonate therapy is a poor prognostic feature, but alternative antiresorptive therapy can be attempted (gallium nitrate, plicamycin).

In the absence of effective antitumor therapy, hypercalcemia is almost certain to recur if the patient survives long enough. The duration of normocalcemia is variable, and further antihypercalcemic therapy must be individualized. Patients are advised to maintain a high fluid intake (3 L daily). Corrected calcium concentration is determined weekly. We retreat patients when the corrected serum calcium exceeds 2.7 mmol/L and at regular intervals thereafter. Retreatment is performed on an outpatient basis when possible. The dose of bisphosphonate is based on the last dose that reversed the hypercalcemia.

Often the malignant process is at such an advanced stage that death occurs within a few weeks of the development of hypercalcemia. Because of this, we involve palliative care early in the management of hypercalcemic patients.

REFERENCES

1. Zondek H, Petow H, Seibert W: Die Bedeutung der Calciumbestimmung im Blute für die Diagnose der Niereninsuffizienz. Z Klin Med 1924;99:129.
2. Gutman AB, Tyson LT, Gutman BE: Serum calcium, inorganic phosphorus and phosphatase activity in hyperparthyoidism, Paget's disease, multiple myeloma and neoplastic disease of bone. Arch Intern Med 1936;57:379.
3. Mundy GR, Martin TJ: The hypercalcemia of malignancy: Pathogenesis and management. Metabolism 1982;31:1247.
4. Fisken RA, Heath DA, Bold AM: Hypercalcaemia—A hospital survey. Q J Med 1980;196:405.
5. Coleman RE, Rubens RD: The clinical course of bone metastases from breast cancer. Br J Cancer 1987;55:61.
6. Mundy GR: Calcium Homeostasis: Hypercalcemia and Hypocalcemia. London, Martin Dunitz, 1990, p 2.
7. Parfitt AM: Equilibrium and disequilibrium hypercalcaemia: New light on an old concept. Metabolic Bone Dis Rel Res 1979;1:279.
8. Payne RB, Little AJ, Williams RB, Milner JR: Interpretation of serum calcium in patients with abnormal serum proteins. Br Med J 1973;4:643.
9. Morton AR, Hercz G: Hypercalcemia in dialysis patients: Comparison of diagnostic methods. Dialysis Transplant 1991;20:661.
10. Potts JT Jr, Kronenberg HM, Rosenblatt M: Parathyroid hormone: Chemistry, biosynthesis and mode of action. Adv Protein Chem 1982;35:323.
11. Tashjian AH Jr, Wright DR, Ivey JL, Pont A: Calcitonin binding sites in bone: Relationship to biological response and "escape." Recent Prog Horm Res 1978;34:285.
12. Stewart AF, Horst R, Deftos LJ, et al: Biochemical evaluation of patients with cancer-associated hypercalcemia. N Engl J Med 1980;303:1377.
13. Albright F: Case records of the Massachusetts General Hospital, No 27461. N Engl J Med 1941;225:789.
14. Lafferty FW: Pseudohyperparathyroidism. Medicine 1966;45:247.
15. Simpson EL, Mundy GR, D'Souza SM, et al: Absence of parathyroid hormone messenger RNA in nonparathyroid tumors associated with hypercalcemia. N Engl J Med 1983;309:325.
16. Burtis WJ, Wu T, Bunch C, et al: Identification of a novel 17,000-dalton parathyroid hormone-like adenylate cyclase-stimulating protein from a tumor associated with humoral hypercalcemia of malignancy. J Biol Chem 1987;62:7151.
17. Moseley JM, Kubota M, Diefenbach-Jagger H, et al: Parathyroid hormone-related protein purified from a human lung cancer cell line. Med Sci 1987;84:5048.
18. Strewler GJ, Stern PH, Jacobs JW, et al: Parathyroid hormone like protein from human renal carcinoma cells. J Clin Invest 1987;80:1803.
19. Kukreja SC, Shevrin DH, Wimbiscus SA, et al: Antibodies to parathroid hormone-related protein lower serum calcium in athymic mouse models of malignancy-associated hypercalcemia due to human tumors. J Clin Invest 1988;82:1798.
20. Budayr AA, Nissenson RA, Klein RF, et al: Increased serum levels of a parathyroid hormone-like protein in malignancy-associated hypercalcemia. Ann Intern Med 1989;111:807.
21. Ratcliffe WA, Hutchesson ACJ, Bundred NJ, Ratcliffe JG: Role of assays for parathyroid-hormone-related protein in investigation of hypercalcaemia. Lancet 1992;339:164.
22. Goltzman D, Henderson JE: Parathyroid hormone-related peptide and hypercalcemia of malignancy. In Arnold A (ed): Endocrine Neoplasms. Kluwer Academic Publishers, 1997.
23. Strewler GJ: The physiology of parathyroid hormone-related protein. N Engl J Med 2000;342:177.
24. Mundy GR, Raisz LG, Cooper RA, et al: Evidence for the secretion of an osteoclast stimulating factor in myeloma. N Engl J Med 1974;291(20):1041.
25. Dewhirst FE, Stashenko PP, Mole JE, Tsurumachi T: Purification and partial sequence of human osteoclast-activating factor: Identity with interleukin 1β. J Immunol 1985;135:2562.
26. Garrett R, Durie BGM, Nedwin GE, et al: Production of lymphotoxin, a bone-resorbing cytokine, by cultured human myeloma cells. N Engl J Med 1987;317:526.
27. Klein B, Bataille R: Cytokine network in human multiple myeloma. Hematol Oncol Clin North Am 1992;6:273.
28. Al-Humidan A, Ralston SH, Hughes DE, et al: Interleukin 6 does not stimulate bone resorption in neonatal mouse calvariae. J Bone Miner Res 1991;6:3.
29. Ishimi Y, Miyaura C, Jin CH, et al: IL-6 is produced by osteoblasts and induces bone resorption. J Immunol 1990;145:3297.
30. Galasko CSB: Mechanisms of bone destruction in the development of skeletal metastases. Nature 1976;263:507.
31. Perroteau I, Salomon D, DeBortoli M, et al: Immunological detection and quantitation of alpha transforming growth factors in human breast carcinoma cells. Breast Cancer Res Treat 1986;7:201.
32. Tashjian A Jr, Voelkel EF, Lloyd W, et al: Actions of growth factors on plasma calcium. J Clin Invest 1986;78:1405.
33. Klein DC, Raisz LG: Prostaglandins: Stimulation of bone resorption in tissue culture. Endocrinology 1970;86:1436.
34. Galasko CSB, Bennett A: Relationship of bone destruction in skeletal metastases to osteoclast activation and prostaglandins. Nature 1976;263:508.
35. Powles TJ, Clark A, Easty DM, et al: The inhibition by aspirin and indomethacin of osteolytic tumour deposits and hypercalcaemia

in rats with Walker tumour, and its possible application to human breast cancer. Br J Cancer 1973;28:316.

36. Percival RC, Yates AJP, Gray RES, et al: Mechanisms of malignant hypercalcemia in carcinoma of the breast. Br Med J 1985;291:776.

37. Bundred NJ, Ratcliffe WA, Walker RA, et al: Parathyroid hormone related protein and hypercalcaemia in breast cancer. Br Med J 1991;303:1506.

38. Guise TA, Yin JJ, Taylor SD, et al: Evidence for a causal role of parathyroid hormone-related protein in the pathogenesis of human breast cancer-mediated osteolysis. J Clin Invest 1996;98:1544.

39. Hofbauer LC, Heufelder AE. Role of receptor activator of nuclear factor-κB ligand and osteoprotegerin in bone cell biology. J Mol Med 2001;79:243.

40. Lacey DL, Timms E, Tan H-L, et al: Osteoprotegerin (OPG) ligand is a cytokine that regulates osteoclast differentiation and activation. Cell 1998;93:165.

41. Chikatsu N, Takeuchi Y, Tamura Y, et al: Interactions between cancer and bone marrow cells induce osteoclast differentiation factor expression and osteoclast-like cell formation in vitro. Biochem Biophys Res Commun 2000;267:632.

42. Westin JS, Ljunghall S, Nilsson K, Ljunggren O. Human multile myeloma cell lines express mRNA for osteoclast differentiation factor. J Bone Miner Res 1999;14(Suppl 1):F063.

43. Barbour GL, Coburn JW, Slatopolsky E, et al: Hypercalcemia in an anephric patient with sarcoidosis: Evidence for extrarenal generation of 1,25-dihydroxyvitamin D. N Engl J Med 1981;305:440.

44. Davies M, Mawer EB, Hayes ME, Lumb GA: Abnormal vitamin D metabolism in Hodgkin's lymphoma. Lancet 1985;i:1186.

45. Canellos GP: Hypercalcemia in malignant lymphoma and leukemia. Ann N Y Acad Sci 1974;230:240.

46. Breslau NA, McGuire JL, Zerwekh JE, et al: Hypercalcemia associated with increased serum calcitriol levels in three patients with lymphoma. Ann Intern Med 1984;100:1.

47. Rosenthal N, Insogna KL, Godsall WJ, et al: Elevations in circulating 1,25-dihydroxyvitamin D in three patients with lymphoma-associated hypercalcemia. J Clin Endocrinol Metab 1985;60:29.

48. Adams JS, Fernandez M, Gacad MA, et al: Vitamin D metabolite–mediated hypercalcemia and hypercalciuria patients with AIDS- and non-AIDS-associated lymphoma. Blood 1989;73:235.

49. Nosaka K, Miyamoto T, Sakai T, Mitsuya H, Suda T, Matsuoka M: Mechanism of hypercalcemia in adult T-cell leukemia: Over-expression of receptor activator of nuclear factor kappaB ligand on adult T-cell leukemia cells. Blood 2002;99:634.

50. Kremer R, Shustik C, Tabak T, et al: Parathyroid-hormone related peptide in hematologic malignancies. Am J Med 1996;100:406.

51. Merlini G, Fitzpatrick LA, Siris ES, et al: A human myeloma immunoglobulin G binding four moles of calcium associated with asymptomatic hypercalcemia. J Clin Immunol 1984;4:185.

52. Fitzpatrick LAP: Hypercalcemia in the multiple endocrine neoplasia syndromes. Endocrinol Metab Clin North Am 1989;18:741.

53. Valentin-Opran A, Eilon G, Saez S, Mundy GR: Estrogens and antiestrogens stimulate release of bone resorbing activity by cultured human breast cancer cells. J Clin Invest 1985;75:726.

54. Ralston SH, Gallacher SJ, Patel U, et al: Cancer-associated hypercalcemia: Morbidity and mortality. Ann Intern Med 1990;112:499.

55. Hosking DJ, Gilson D: Comparison of the renal and skeletal actions of calcitonin in the treatment of severe hypercalcemia of malignancy. Q J Med 1984;211:359.

56. Recker RR, Saville PD: Intestinal absorption of disodium ethane 1-hydroxy-1, 1-diphosphonate (disodium etidronate) using a deconvolution technique. Toxicol Appl Pharmacol 1973;24:580.

57. Dittert LW: Pharmacokinetic prediction of tissue residues. J Toxicol Environ Health 1977;2:735.

58. Fogelman I, Smith L, Mazess R, et al: Absorption of oral diphosphonate in normal subjects. Clin Endocrinol 1986;24:57.

59. Michael WR, King WR, Wakim JM: Metabolism of disodium ethane-1-hydroxy-1,1-diphosphonate (disodium etidronate) in the rat, rabbit, dog and monkey. Toxicol Appl Pharmacol 1972;21:503.

60. Francis MD, Martodam RR: Chemical, biochemical and medicinal properties of the diphosphonates. In Hilderbrand RL (ed): The Role of Phosphonates in Living Systems. Boca Raton, Fl, CRC Press, 1983.

61. Jung A, Bisaz S, Fleisch H: The binding of pyrophosphate and two diphosphonates on hydroxyapatite crystals. Calcif Tissue Res 1973;11:269.

62. Russell JE, Termine JD, Avioli LV: Experimental renal osteodystrophy: the response to 25-hydroxycholecalciferol and dichloromethylene diphosphonate therapy. J Clin Invest 1975;56:548.

63. Robertson WG, Morgan DB, Fleisch H, Francis MD: The effects of diphosphonates on the exchangeable and non-exchangeable calcium and phosphate of hydroxyapatite. Biochim Biophys Acta 1972;261:517.

64. Vaes G: On the mechanism of bone resorption. J Cell Biol 1968;39:676.

65. Felix R, Russell RGG, Fleisch H: The effects of several diphosphonates on acid phosphohydrolases and other lysosomal enzymes. Biochim Biophys Acta 1976;429:429.

66. Lerner U, Larsson A: Effects of four bisphosphonates on bone resorption, lysosomal enzyme release, protein synthesis and mitotic activities in mouse calvarial bone in vitro. Bone 1987;8:179.

67. Plasmans CMT, Jap PHK, Kujipers W, Slooff TJJH: Influence of diphosphonate on the cellular aspect of young bone tissue. Calcif Tissue Int 1980;32:247.

68. Boonekamp PM, van der Wee-Pals LJA, van Wijk-van Lennep MML, et al: Two modes of action of bisphosphonates on osteoclastic resorption of mineralized matrix. Bone Miner 1986;1:27.

69. Storm T, Thamsborg G, Steiniche T, et al: Effect of intermittent cyclical etidronate therapy on bone mass and fracture rate in women with postmenopausal osteoporosis. N Engl J Med 1990;322:1265.

70. Watts NB, Harris ST, Genant HK, et al: Intermittent cyclical etidronate treatment of postmenopausal osteoporosis. N Engl J Med 1990;323:73.

71. Witte RS, Koeller J, Davis TE, et al: A randomized study in the treatment of cancer-related hypercalcemia. Arch Intern Med 1987;147:937.

72. Chapuy MC, Meunier PJ, Alexandre CM, Vignon EP: Effects of disodium dichloromethylene diphosphonate on hypercalcemia produced by bone metastases. J Clin Invest 1980;65:1243.

73. Bounameaux HM, Schifferli J, Montani JP, Chatelanat F: Renal failure associated with intravenous diphosphonates. Lancet 1983;i:471.

74. Morton AR, Cantrill JA, Craig AE, et al: Single dose versus daily intravenous aminohydroxypropylidene biphosphonate (APD) for the hypercalcaemia of malignancy. Br Med J 1988;296:811.

75. Body JJ, Pot M, Borkowski A, Sculier JP, Klastersky J: Dose/response study of aminohydroxypropylidene bisphosphonate in tumor-associated hypercalcemia. Am J Med 1987;82:957.

76. Thiébaud D, Jaeger PH, Jacquet AF, Burckhardt P: Dose-response in the treatment of hypercalcemia of malignancy by a single infusion of the bisphosphonate AHPrBP. J Clin Oncol 1988;6:762.

77. Nussbaum SR, Mallette L, Gagel R, et al: Pamidronate (APD) treatment of hypercalcaemia associated with malignancy— Preliminary report of a multicenter double-blind trial. In Rubens RD (ed): The Management of Bone Metastases and Hypercalcaemia by Osteoclast Inhibition. Bern, Hogrefe and Huber, 1990, p 44.

78. Cantwell BMJ, Harris AL: Effect of single high dose infusions of aminohydroxypropylidene diphosphonate on hypercalcaemia caused by cancer. Br Med J 1987;294:467.

79. Dodwell DJ, Howell A, Morton AR, et al: Infusion rate and pharmacokinetics of intravenous pamidronate in the treatment of tumour-induced hypercalcaemia. Postgrad Med J 1992;68:434.

80. Body JJ, Lortholary A, Romieu G, et al: A dose finding study of zoledronate in hypercalcemia patients. J Bone Miner Res 1999;14:1557.

81. Major PP, Coleman RE: Zoledronic acid in the treatment of hypercalcemia of malignancy: Results of the international clinical development program. Semin Oncol 2001;28(Suppl 6):17.

82. Ralston SH, Dryburgh FJ, Cowan RA, et al: Comparison of

aminohydroxypropylidene diphosphonate, mithramycin, and corticosteroids/calcitonin in treatment of cancer-associated hypercalcaemia. Lancet 1985;ii:907.

83. Thürlimann B, Waldburger R, Senn HJ, Thiebaud D: Plicamycin and pamidronate in symptomatic tumor-related hypercalcemia: A prospective randomized crossover trial. Ann Oncol 1992;3:619.

84. Ralston SH, Gallacher SJ, Patel U, et al: Comparison of three intravenous bisphosphonates in cancer-associated hypercalcemia. Lancet 1989;ii:1180.

85. Gucalp R, Ritch P, Wiernik PH, et al: Comparative study of pamidronate disodium and etidronate disodium in the treatment of cancer-related hypercalcemia. J Clin Oncol 1992;10:134.

86. Major PP, Lortholary A, Hon J, et al: Zoledronic acid is superior to pamidronate in the treatment of hypercalcemia of malignancy—A pooled analysis of two randomized, controlled clinical trials. J Clin Oncol 2001;19:558.

87. Gurney H, Kefford R, Stuart-Harris R: Renal phosphate threshold and response to pamidronate in humoral hypercalcaemia of malignancy. Lancet 1989;ii:241.

88. Dodwell DJ, Abbas SK, Morton AR, Howell A: Parathyroid hormone-related protein(50–69) and response to pamidronate therapy for tumour-induced hypercalcaemia. Eur J Cancer 1991;27:1629.

89. Harinck HIJ, Bijvoet OLM: Clinical aspects of the treatment of tumour-induced hypercalcaemia with APD. Disodium pamidronate (APD) in the treatment of malignancy-related disorders. In Burckhardt P (ed): Disodium Pamidronate (APD) in the Treatment of Malignancy-Related Disorders. Bern, Hans Huber, 1989, p 64.

90. McCloskey EV, Yates AJP, Gray RES, et al: Diphosphonates and phosphate homeostasis in man. Clin Sci 1988;74:607.

91. Nussbaum SR, Warrel RP Jr, Rude R, et al: Dose-response study of alendronate sodium for the treatment of cancer-associated hypercalcemia. J Clin Oncol 1993;11:1618.

92. Ralston SH, Thiébaud D, Herrmann Z, et al: Dose-response study of ibandronate in the treatment of cancer-associated hypercalcemia. Br J Cancer 1997;75:295.

93. Brown JH, Kennedy BJ: Mithramycin in the treatment of disseminated testicular neoplasms. N Engl J Med 1965;272:111.

94. Minkin C: Inhibition of parathyroid hormone stimulated bone resorption in vitro by the antibiotic mithramycin. Calcif Tissue Res 1973;13:249.

95. Perlia CP, Gubisch NJ, Wolter J, et al: Mithramycin treatment of hypercalcemia. Cancer 1970;25:389.

96. Fatemi S, Singer FR, Rude RK: Effect of salmon calcitonin and etidronate on hypercalcemia of malignancy. Calcif Tissue Int 1992;50:107.

97. Ralston SH, Alzaid AA, Gardner MD, Boyle IT: Treatment of cancer associated hypercalcaemia with combined aminohydroxypropylidene diphosphonate and calcitonin. Br Med J 1986;292:1549.

98. Luce K, O'Donnell DE, Morton AR: A combination of calcitonin and bisphosphonate for the emergency treatment of severe tumor-induced hypercalcemia. Calcif Tissue Int 1993;52:70.

99. Krakoff IH, Newman RA, Goldberg RS: Clinical toxicologic and pharmacologic studies of gallium nitrate. Cancer 1979;44:1722.

100. Warrell RP, Bockman RS, Coonley CJ, et al: Gallium nitrate inhibits calcium resorption from bone and is effective treatment for cancer-related hypercalcemia. J Clin Invest 1984;73:1487.

101. Warrell RP, Israel R, Frisone M, et al: Gallium nitrate for acute treatment of cancer-related hypercalcemia. Ann Intern Med 1988;108:669.

102. Seyberth HW, Segre GV, Morgan JL, et al: Prostaglandins as mediators of hypercalcemia associated with certain types of cancer. N Engl J Med 1975;293:1279.

103. Seyberth HW, Segre GV, Hamet P, et al: Characterization of the group of patients with the hypercalcemia of cancer who respond to treatment with prostaglandin synthesis inhibitors. Trans Assoc Am Physicians 1976;89:92.

104. Percival RC, Yates AJP, Gray RES, et al: Role of glucocorticoids in management of malignant hypercalcemia. Br Med J 1984;289:287.

105. Carey RW, Schmitt GW, Kopald HH, Kantrowitz PA: Massive extraskeletal calcification during phosphate treatment of hypercalcemia. Arch Intern Med 1968;122:150.

106. Morony S, Capparelli C, Lee R, et al: A chimeric form of osteoprotegerin inhibits hypercalcemia and bone resorption induced by IL-1beta, TNF-alpha, PTH, PTHrP, and 1,25(OH)$_2$D$_3$. J Bone Miner Res 1999;14:1478.

107. Capparelli C, Kostenuik PJ, Morony S, et al: Osteoprotegerin prevents and reverses hypercalcemia in a murine model of humoral hypercalcemia of malignancy. Cancer Res 2000;60:783.

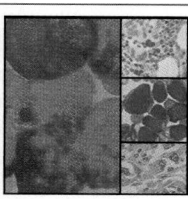

Richard L. Heideman

Nancy H. Heideman

49

HYPONATREMIA

SUMMARY OF KEY POINTS

INCIDENCE
- Hyponatremia is a common problem in many malignancies.
- It occurs in at least 5% of hospitalized patients.
- Hyponatremia is present in 10%–30% of patients with small cell lung cancer.

ETIOLOGY
- Hyponatremia has multiple causes; primary extrarenal sodium loss associated with diarrhea, vomiting, or hemorrhage is the most common.
- The syndrome of inappropriate antidiuretic hormone (SIADH) is associated with several malignancies, particularly small cell lung cancer.
- Pseudohyponatremia is associated with hyperglycemia, hyperproteinemia, or hyperlipidemia.
- Water overload at surgery, low

sodium intravenous fluids, or polydipsia are other causes.
- Additional causes include edematous states such as malignant peritonitis, heart failure, hepatic tumor, or cirrhosis.
- Thyroid and adrenal deficiencies can result in hyponatremia.
- Renal sodium loss can be mediated by diuretics or natriuretic peptides (particularly with central nervous system injury).

EVALUATION OF THE PATIENT
- Start by accessing plasma osmolality and ECF volume.
- SIADH is a common cause but must be a diagnosis of exclusion.

GRADING OF THE COMPLICATION
- Many patients are asymptomatic.
- Sodium concentrations below 125 mEq/L and those developing

rapidly are most likely to be symptomatic.
- Symptomatic hyponatremia is a medical emergency.

TREATMENT
- Isotonic saline (0.9%) is an appropriate fluid for most patients.
- Correction of sodium should occur slowly and at a rate that approximates its development; 10–12 mEq/L over the first 24 hours is considered safe.
- Overly rapid correction is associated with severe neurologic morbidity.
- Hypertonic saline is appropriate only in symptomatic patients with very low sodium; discontinue once serum sodium becomes 120–125 mEq/L.
- Water restriction is the primary approach to SIADH.

INTRODUCTION

Hyponatremia is among the most common electrolyte disturbances faced in clinical medicine. As published in the 1980s, an incidence of 2.5% among hospitalized patients could be an underestimation of the true frequency of this problem.[1] If one defines hyponatremia as a serum sodium concentration of less than 135 mEq/L, then a report showing that sodium concentration among 5000 hospitalized patients is skewed toward the lower end of the range, 134 ± 6 mEq/L, supports a view that hyponatremia often goes unnoticed and unreported in many patients.[2] This is particularly sobering in light of the substantial morbidity and mortality that can be associated with hyponatremia. Among patients with cancer, clinical experience suggests that the overall incidence of hyponatremia is perhaps even higher than in other populations. Many individual histologic entities and specific disease sites (brain, lung, mediastinum) are predisposed to the development of hyponatremia. For example, the incidence of hyponatremia among patients with small cell carcinoma of the lung is as high as 30% (resulting from ectopic argenine vasopressin production

by tumor). This chapter will focus on the physiology of sodium and water balance and on the therapeutic approach to the most common causes of hyponatremia.

Sodium (Na+) is the dominant ion of the extracellular fluid and thus the prime contributor to osmolality. Sodium and water balance are tightly linked, and disturbances of one are also generally reflected in the other. This balance is the result of multiple homeostatic feedback loops that revolve around protection of intravascular volume. Components of this integrated homeostatic system include the hypothalamic osmoreceptors, the adrenals (via the renin-angiotensin-aldosterone cascade), the cardiac, glomerular, and carotid baroreceptors, and changes in renal tubular permeability to water and sodium in response to ADH and natriuretic peptides. Thus, there could be multiple paths to hyponatremia.

Definitions

Hyponatremia and hypernatremia are conditions of altered tonicity. To put the physiology of the problem into proper perspective, it is important to understand the difference between osmolality and tonicity. Osmolality is the concentration of all particles in a fluid. Particles are either "effective" or "ineffective" osmoles. Ineffective osmoles are solutes that can cross the cell membrane freely and distribute equally in the intracellular fluid (ICF) and extracellular fluid (ECF) yet produce no net movement of water. Examples of physiologically ineffective osmoles include urea and ethanol; their addition to the ECF produces no change in osmolality, as they equilibrate rapidly with the ICF.

Solutes that do not cross the membrane freely or that are kept predominantly to one side by a transporter are referred to as effective osmoles. Only effective osmoles contribute to tonicity. In the physiologic setting, sodium is the major effective osmolar solute. It is relatively restricted to the ECF and is thus the major determinant of ECF tonicity. Other examples of physiologically effective osmoles are glucose and mannitol, two large molecules that are also relatively restricted to the ECF. Potassium and a host of organic compounds that are dominantly restricted to the intracellular milieu are the major osmolar solutes of the ICF and the major determinants of ICF tonicity. Despite the differences in tonicity of these compartments, the osmolality of the ECF and ICF are quite similar as a result of water movement. This does not mean, however, that the volume of the ECF and ICF are the same. The distribution of water in these two spaces is not at all similar; 60%–75% of total body water resides within the ICF and the remainder in the ECF. Within the ECF, approximately 65% is apportioned to plasma, and the rest is interstitial fluid between cells.

OSMOLAR HOMEOSTASIS: THE CONTROL OF WATER AND SODIUM

From the perspective of sodium, the job of the osmoregulatory system is to prevent either hyper- or hyponatremia and the secondary movement of water that can change cell volume and disrupt function. Under normal circumstances, plasma osmolality is kept within a relatively constant osmolar range of 275–290 mOsmol/kg. The maintenance of this narrow range is primarily the result of argnine vasopressin (ADH or antidiuretic hormone), thirst, and renal function.

ADH provides the most sensitive control mechanism. Changes in serum osmolality of as little as 1%–2% can be sensed by the hypothalamic osmoreceptors and can trigger ADH secretion from the posterior pituitary.[1,3-5] At the renal level, ADH acts on receptors in the collecting ducts to initiate a passive reabsorption of water. The threshold for ADH release occurs at a plasma osmolality of 280–290 mOsmol/kg; below 280 mOsmol/kg, the secretion of ADH is suppressed.[4,5] Although there is a roughly linear rise in ADH with osmolality, a plateau in its effect occurs at an osmolality of 295 or greater. Thus, there is a limit to the ability of ADH to reduce hypertonicity.

Another group of osmoreceptors located in the anterior hypothalamus stimulate thirst. Thirst is recruited to aid in osmolar balance at or near the serum osmolality at which ADH begins to show its plateau in effect. Thirst can also be recruited by changes in plasma volume sensed by carotid and cardiac baroreceptors, although they are much less sensitive than osmoreceptors with respect to this ability.

Carotid baroreceptors responding to a decrease in effective blood volume can stimulate ADH release also.[4] The sensitivity of this system is significantly less than that of the hypothalamic osmoreceptors, and a change in vascular volume of 8%–10% or more is required to initiate this nonosmotic stimulus for ADH release. In contrast to the more linear control of ADH by the hypothalamus, the relationship between volume depletion and baroreceptor-mediated ADH release is exponential once the threshold is exceeded.[4] Thus, in clinical situations characterized by decreased effective circulating volume (e.g., in anthracycline-induced congestive heart failure or third space fluid accumulations from malignant ascites or hepatic cirrhosis), nonosmotic baroreceptor-mediated stimulation of ADH can override the osmotic suppression of ADH release that would otherwise be expected as a result of the expanded hypotonic ECF space.[6] The net result can be a spiraling decrease in sodium as more water is retained, and effective volume continues to decline even further.

Although most osmoregulation is affected by water as just described, sodium also has an active regulatory mechanism. Reabsorption of sodium in the renal tubule is the dominant mechanism of regulation; under normal conditions, about 70% of filtered sodium is reabsorbed. Active excretion of sodium also occurs and is mediated through the actions of a group of related natriuretic peptides that inhibit sodium reabsorption.[7-9] The best described of these, atrial natriuretic peptide (ANP), is released from cells in the atrial chambers of the heart and in response to central volume overload. Others appear to be released with central nervous system injury. Although there remains much to be learned about the multiple and complex physiologic effects of these peptides, their actions in medullary collecting tubules and their inhibitory effect on the rennin-angiotensin-aldosterone system result in a sodium diuresis.

Cellular Adaptations to Hyponatremia

In response to hypotonic conditions, water moves from the ECF into the ICF and causes an expansion of cell volume. If this remains unopposed, cell lysis would eventually occur. On a day-to-day basis, the Na+, K+ ATPase pump in the cell membrane maintains cell volume by pumping out the small amounts of sodium that "leak" into cells in exchange for potassium. In the setting of acute hypotonicity, additional mechanisms must come into play; cells adjust initially by losing sodium, potassium, and chloride across stretch-activated membrane channels. However, this process reaches its limit of compensation within several hours. In the setting of more slowly developing or chronic hypotonic states, loss of intracellular organic osmoles such as free amino acids, inositol, glutamate, and creatinine are part of the compensation process.[10-13] In the reverse setting of hypertonicity, adaptations include upward adjustments in the concentration of these intracellular organic osmoles. Because change in the concentrations of organic osmoles requires several days to be complete, these adaptations are not effective in acute events affecting tonicity.

The brain is particularly sensitive to changes in tonicity. Hypotonic stresses that lead to cell swelling are tolerated poorly in the central nervous system because of the constraints that the skull places on increased volume. The most feared change is increased intracranial pressure; coma and death can occur with as little as a 10% increase in brain volume.[14] Another debilitating and potentially lethal complication is the osmotic demyelination syndrome. This is an uncommon but devastating result of an overly rapid correction of hyponatremia, which leads to demyelination in the pons and exrapontine white matter.[15-17] Thus, both the initiating process and the intervention can be associated with significant morbidity and mortality.

HYPONATREMIC STATES

Hyponatremia is defined as a serum sodium less than 135 mEq/L. It is a manifestation of many and varied disordered states, and the management of each can vary. Although hyponatremia is seen most frequently in association with a low plasma osmolality (hypotonic hyponatremia), it also can occur in settings of high or low osmolality. Similarly, hyponatremia can also be associated with normal, increased, or decreased ECF. Identification of the likely etiology and proper approach to hyponatremia begins with evaluating plasma osmolality and ECF volume. In the sections that follow, hyponatremia is characterized and and addressed by these parameters. A graphic representation of many hyponatremic states is shown in Figure 49-1.

Pseudohyponatremia

From the clinical point of view, the first priority is to determine whether the observed hyponatremia is truly a hypotonic process or a pseudohyponatremia. There are two situations in which low sodium occurs without hypotonicity and in which sodium can be fictitiously low. These conditions result from the presence of substances that alter the volume of plasma water in which sodium is measured.

Pseudohyponatremia is common in the setting of the high serum osmolality associated with hyperglycemia or the use of some other restricted solute. These situations cause a shift of water from the ICF to the ECF, resulting in sodium dilution and hypertonic plasma. As a general rule, each 100 mg/dL increase in glucose reduces serum sodium by 1.6 mEq/L. The presence of some other non-glucose, active substance (e.g., manitol) is identified by finding a 10-point or greater difference in the measured vs. the calculated osmoloality. This "osmolar gap" can also be increased in azotemia and in ethanol and methanol intoxications. Although the plasma osmolality is increased by the addition of these molecules, the true sodium is normal.

Pseudohyponatremia also can occur in the setting of a normal plasma osmolality, as a result of an increase in relatively high molecular weight substances, such as occurs with Bence-Jones proteins in multiple myeloma or in hyperlipidemia. In these situations, the volume of plasma in which sodium is measured is expanded, and the volume of plasma water is correspondingly diminished. Thus, if sodium is normalized to the volume of sampled plasma, it will be reported as artificially low. On the other hand, if sodium is measured using an ion-selective electrode that measures sodium only in the aqueous phase of plasma, its concentration will be reported as normal. Thus, it is important to know how a given lab determines sodium concentration.

Patients with pseudohyponatremia are not at risk for complications of low sodium and do not require sodium correction; their true plasma sodium and osmolality are normal.

Hypotonic Hyponatremia

Hyponatremia in the setting of hypotonic plasma (hypotonic hyponatremia) is the most common type of low serum sodium.[1,3,19] It represents a process in which there is an excess of water in relation to sodium either as a result of sodium loss or water gain. Several potential causes of this problem are outlined in the ensuing discussion and summarized in Table 49-1. Most such situations are also characterized by the relative inability to excrete water. Although many patients might be asymptomatic, it is important to recognize and react appropriately to hyponatremia, particularly those cases that develop rapidly. Failure to do so can lead to serious and potentially deadly neurologic sequelae.

Hypovolemia

Hyponatremia developing in the setting of either decreased ECF or hypovolemia is a result of both sodium loss and water loss. As adaptations to volume loss occur, however, a relative excess of water over sodium develops.

The most common causes of decreased ECF are a result of extrarenal fluid losses such as diarrhea, vomiting, or third space sequestrations of body fluid, as in malignant peritonitis. The net effect of these problems is the stimulation of ADH secretion and thirst in an effort to enhance water retention and restore ECF volume. The decreased circulating volume, renal hypoperfusion, and ADH-mediated water retention combine to impair renal water excretion and produce dilutional hyponatremia. The

---

CALCULATED PLASMA OSMOLALITY (mOsm/kg)

$$2 \times ([Na] + [K] + BUN/2.8 + glucose/18.$$

Note that measure osmolality is generally 10 mOsm/kg higher than calculated osmolality because of the effect of minor solutes such as magnesium, calcium, protein, phosphates, and amino acids. Normal osmolality is 287 ± 4, with a normal range extending from 280 to 290 mOsm/kg.

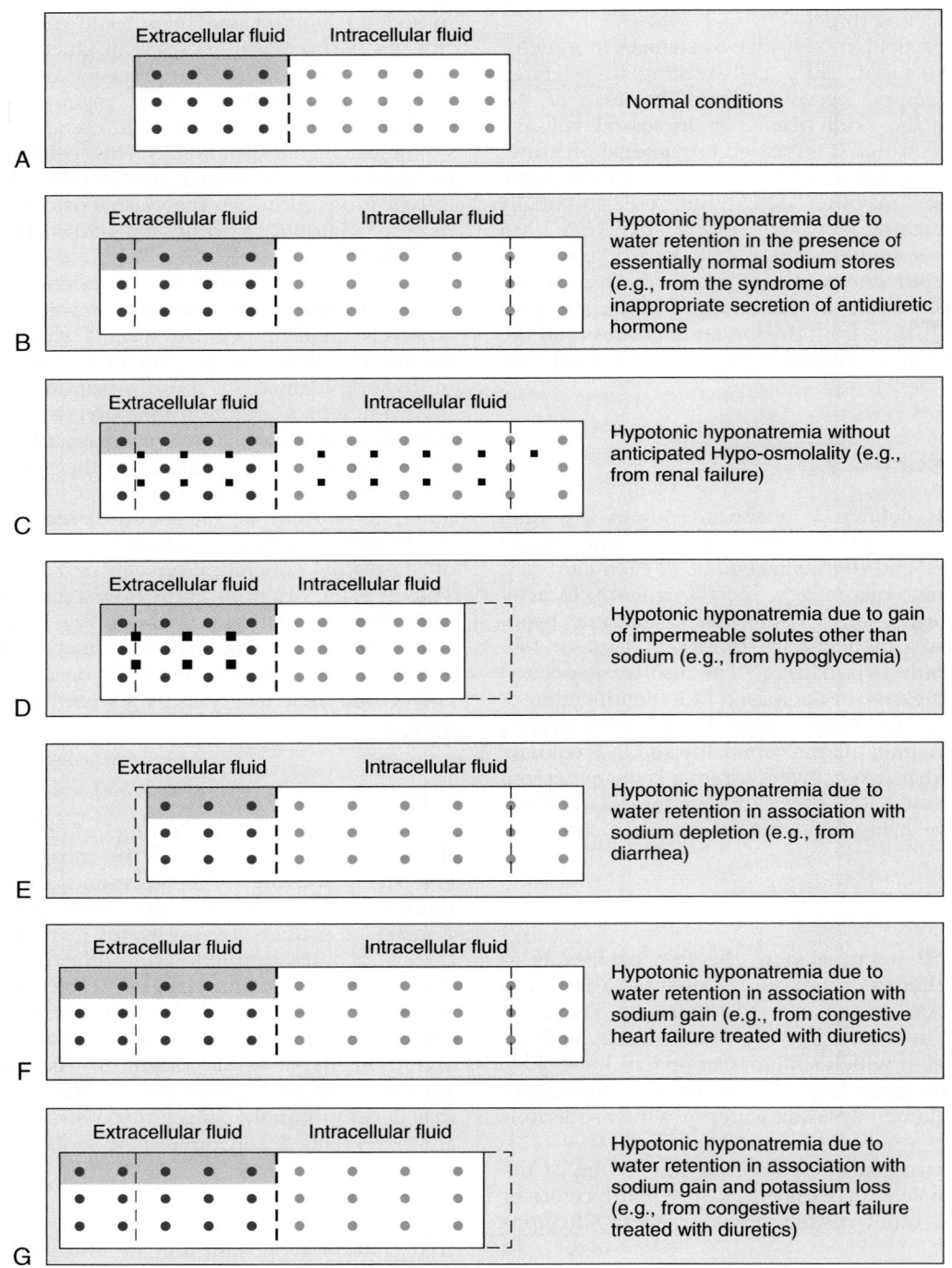

Figure 49-1. Extracellular-fluid and intracellular-fluid compartments under normal conditions and during states of hyponatremia. **A,** Normally the extracellular-fluid and intracellular-fluid make up 40% and 60% of total body water, respectively. **B,** With the syndrome of inappropriate secretion of antidiuretic hormone, the volumes of extracellular fluid and intracellular fluid expand (although a small element of sodium and potassium loss, not shown, occurs during inception of the syndrome). **C,** Water retention can lead to hypotonic hyponatremia with the anticipated hypo-osmolality in patients who have accumulated ineffective osmoles, such as urea. **D,** A shift of water from the intracellular-fluid compartment to the extracellular-fluid compartment, driven by solutes confined in the excellular fluid, results in hypertonic (translocation) hyponatremia. **E,** Sodium depletion (and secondary water retention) usually contracts the volume of extracellular fluid but expands the intracellular-fluid compartment. At times, water retention can be sufficient to restore the volume of extracellular fluid to normal or even above normal levels. **F,** Hypotonic hyponatremia in sodium retentive states involves expansion of both compartments, but predominantly the extracellular-fluid compartment. **G,** Gain of sodium and loss of potassium in association with a defect of water excretion, as they occur in congestive heart failure treated with diuretics, lead to expansion of the extracellular-fluid compartment but contraction of the intracellular-fluid compartment. In each panel: *red circles,* sodium; *yellow circles,* potassium; *large squares,* impermeable solutes other than sodium; *small squares,* permeable solutes; *broken line,* cell membrane; *shading,* intravascular volume.

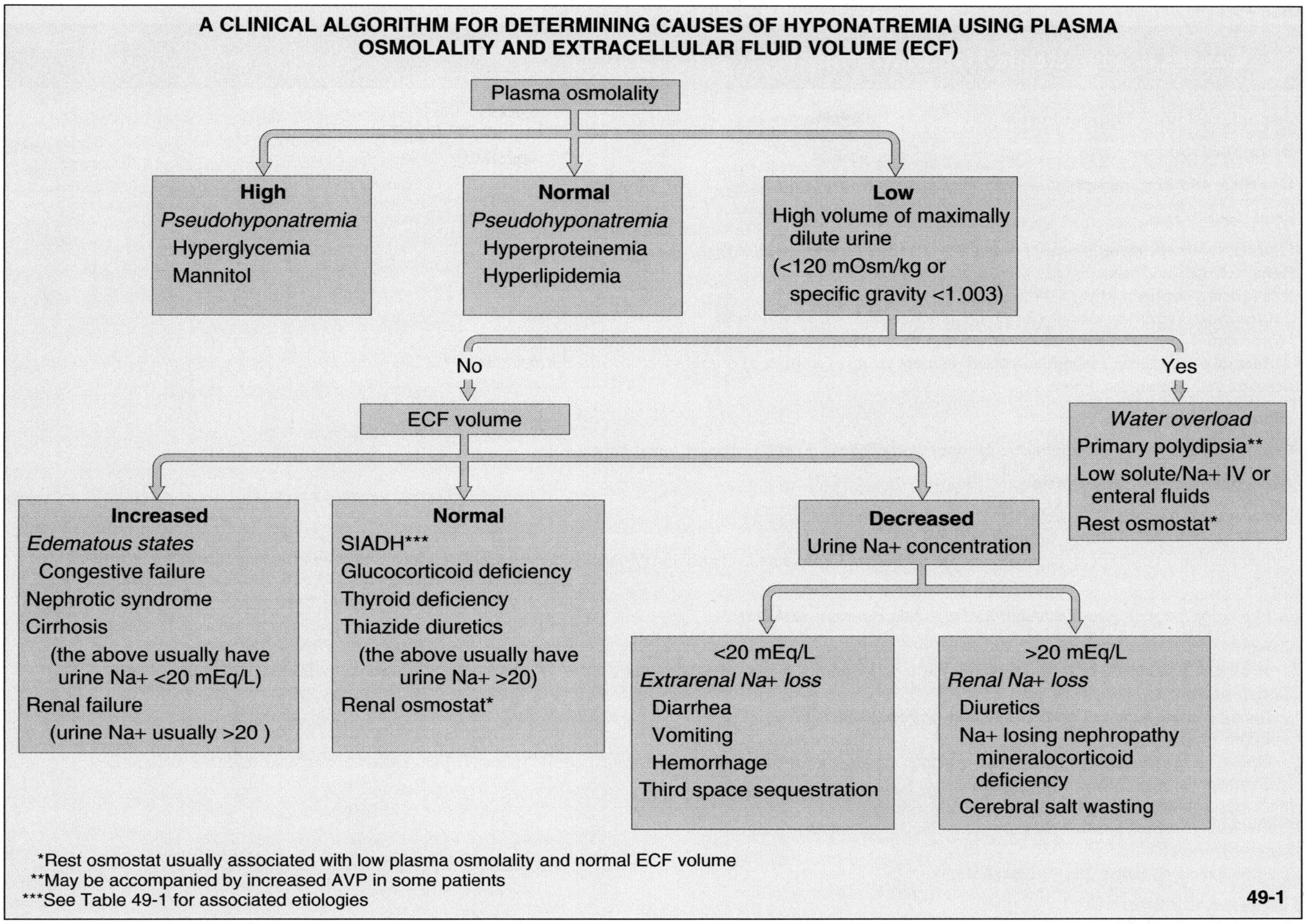

A CLINICAL ALGORITHM FOR DETERMINING CAUSES OF HYPONATREMIA USING PLASMA OSMOLALITY AND EXTRACELLULAR FLUID VOLUME (ECF)

Plasma osmolality

High
Pseudohyponatremia
Hyperglycemia
Mannitol

Normal
Pseudohyponatremia
Hyperproteinemia
Hyperlipidemia

Low
High volume of maximally dilute urine
(<120 mOsm/kg or specific gravity <1.003)

No

Yes

ECF volume

Water overload
Primary polydipsia**
Low solute/Na+ IV or enteral fluids
Rest osmostat*

Increased
Edematous states
Congestive failure
Nephrotic syndrome
Cirrhosis
(the above usually have urine Na+ <20 mEq/L)
Renal failure
(urine Na+ usually >20)

Normal
SIADH***
Glucocorticoid deficiency
Thyroid deficiency
Thiazide diuretics
(the above usually have urine Na+ >20)
Renal osmostat*

Decreased
Urine Na+ concentration

<20 mEq/L
Extrarenal Na+ loss
Diarrhea
Vomiting
Hemorrhage
Third space sequestration

>20 mEq/L
Renal Na+ loss
Diuretics
Na+ losing nephropathy
mineralocorticoid deficiency
Cerebral salt wasting

*Rest osmostat usually associated with low plasma osmolality and normal ECF volume
**May be accompanied by increased AVP in some patients
***See Table 49-1 for associated etiologies

49-1

hyponatremia could be made worse by the concomitant depletion of potassium in severe diarrhea or vomiting and by the secondary migration of sodium into cells to compensate. Because the major pathology in these situations is nonrenal, these patients should have a low urine sodium excretion. As a rule of thumb, a urine sodium of less than 20 mEq/L suggests renal sodium conservation. The management of these patients is primarily saline volume expansion. Potassium may be added as necessary.

Hyponatremia associated with the use of thiazide diuretics is a result of sodium, potassium, and volume depletion. Secondary water retention can occur as a result of ADH response to volume loss. Urine sodium is characteristically elevated (>20 mEq/L) in these patients, reflecting increased renal sodium loss. This form of hyponatremia is characterized by hypovolemia or euvolemia with little decrease in effective plasma volume. In contrast, the loop diuretics (e.g., furosemide) cause significant hyponatremia only rarely. This is a result of their inhibition of sodium re-uptake and reduced renal interstitial tonicity that limits passive water reabsorption. The management of these patients involves cessation of diuretic medication and volume expansion with saline.

Another cause of hypotonic hyponatremia is salt wasting associated with renal dysfunction.[1,18,19] This can occur as a result of obstructive uropathy from abdominal and retroperitoneal tumors, loss of renal structure as in polycystic disease, or tubular epithelial damage associated with interstitial nephritis. The latter can occur as a result of several chemotherapeutic agents (especially cisplatin, aminoglycosides, or amphotericin) or of infection, all of which can limit sodium reabsorption and diminish free water excretion. As expected, urine sodium is high (>20 mEq/L) in these situations. The management of these situations relies on addressing the underlying problem and on replacing volume with saline.

Hypervolemia

In the disease states listed in this discussion, hyponatremia develops despite the fact that total body sodium is generally increased. This is a result of physiologic adaptations s to disease that cause an even larger increase in total body water (particularly in the ECF), thus driving sodium down.

Congestive heart failure, ascites associated with malignant peritonitis or cirrhosis, and nephrotic syndrome

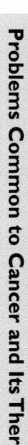

Problems Common to Cancer and Its Therapy

TABLE 49-1

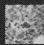 **Causes of Hypotonic Hyponatremia**

Associated with Hypovolemia

Extra Renal Sodium Loss:

Diarrhea, vomiting, hemorrhage, fluid sequestration (third space), excessive sweating.

Renal Sodium Loss:

Diuretics, *osmotic diuresis (use of mannitol with cisplatin over multiple days)*
Renal tubular acidosis
Salt loosing nephropathy
   Interstitial nephritis, urinary tract obstruction, Bartter's syndrome
Hormonal
   Adrenal insufficiency (mineralocorticoid deficiency; most common as a late effect of cranial irradiation)
Cerebral salt wasting syndrome

Edematous States:

Congestive heart failure, nephrotic syndrome, *malignant ascites*, cirrhosis, renal failure

Associated with Euvolemia

Distal tubule diuretics
Loop diuretics (furosemide, ethacrynic acid)
Hypothyroidism (early effect of cranial and/or craniospinal irradiation) adrenal insufficiency (glucocorticoid deficiency; most commonly a late effect of cranial irradiation)

Syndrome of Inappropriate Secretion of Antidiuretic Hormone (SIADH)

Cancer
   Small cell carcinoma of lung, Hodgkins disease, leukemia, lymphoma, adenocarcinoma of pancreas and duodenum, breast, and many others
CNS lesions
   Tumor, stroke, subarachnoid bleed, hemorrhage, infection
Selected drugs
   Opiates, phenothiazines, vincristine, cyclophosphamide, Ifosfamide, cisplatin, carbamazipine, tricyclics, NSAIDS, selective serotonin reuptake inhibitors,
   desmopressin, nicotine, chloropropamide
Increased intrathoracic pressure
   Mediastinal tumor, positive pressure ventilation, pneumonia
Reset osmostat*
Trauma, *pain, and stress (postoperative state)*
AIDS

Associated with Hypervolemia

Primary polydipsia[†]
Excessive dilute or sodium free irrigants during surgery
Tap water enemas

Common cancer-associated causes are italicized.
* Normal volume accompanied by low plasma osmolality.
[†] May also be accompanied by decreased water excretion as a result of AVP stimulation.

are edematous states with increased ECF. Despite the edema, however, these diseases are usually associated with decreased effective circulating volume that stimulates a response much like the conditions with primary ECF depletion noted earlier.[1,18,20,21] Both ADH secretion and thirst lead to volume expansion, and there is relatively impaired renal water excretion from both ADH and diminished effective renal perfusion. It is noteworthy that in these diseases, carotid baroreceptor response to decreased effective volume is often the dominant stimulus for ADH release.[6] The management of this situation is centered on improving effective circulating volume by addressing the underlying problem and restricting both sodium and water.

Hypotonic hyponatremia occurring in the setting of volume expansion can also develop in patients with renal failure.[1,18,19] Accumulation of ineffective osmols (e.g.,

urea) leads to increased osmolality in both the ICF and ECF, with consequent water retention and an increase in the volume of both compartments. Thus, a dilutional hyponatremia occurs in the setting of increased ECF. Urea is an ineffective osmole that crosses membranes easily and contributes to osmolality in both the intra- and extravascular spaces; thus, plasma osmolality can be normal despite the expanded ECF. As with the edematous states described previously, management is centered on treatment of the primary disease (dialysis) and on restriction of both sodium and water.

Hyponatremia as a result of excessive water intake, such as psychogenic polydipsia or low-sodium intravenous or enteral fluids, are examples of hypotonic hyponatremia in the setting of increased ECF.[18,19,21,22] Although renal water excretion is usually normal in these patients, the volume of water intake overwhelms the normal ability of the kidney to excrete the maximum of 26L/1.73 M2 per day of free water. A moderate to significantly increased ECF usually accompanies these problems. Characteristic of these states is the excretion of large volumes of maximally dilute urine, indicating intact renal function. Depending on how rapidly the problem has evolved, the degree of hyponatremia, and the presence of symptoms, treatment is aimed at net water loss or sodium replacement.

Isovolemia

Patients who develop hyponatremia in the setting of normal or near-normal ECF volume generally have a modest increase in water relative to sodium. This condition generally signals the syndrome of inappropriate antidiuretic hormone secretion (SIADH).[4,18,19,21,22] It is noteworthy, however, that increased ADH by itself is generally insufficient to cause significant hyponatremia; water intake is necessary for the dilutional effect to occur. Although SIADH is often classified as an isovolemic hyponatremia because of the lack of edema and overt signs of volume expansion, most patients have expansion of their ECF manifested by diminished urine output and weight gain.[8] Despite the hyponatremia, an ANP-mediated natriuresis occurs in response to the volume expansion. This, and the diminished sodium reabsorption associated with volume expansion, further decrease plasma sodium and limit the formation of edema. Eventually, a new equilibrium between sodium intake and excretion occurs, such that intake and output are matched.[4] Thus, attempts to correct SIADH with the addition of sodium alone are rarely successful; water restriction remains the primary method of management in asymptomatic patients.[8] SIADH is a diagnosis of exclusion. To make the diagnosis, the following criteria should be met:

- Other causes of hyponatremic hyponatremia, particularly hormone deficiencies (e.g., thyroid and adrenal) and a reset osmostat are absent (see related topics covered later in this chapter).
- The patient should be clinically isovolemic or only mildly hypervolemic. The presence of edema or clinical volume overload is not compatible with SIADH.
- The plasma osmolality should be 280 mOsm/kg or less. Higher osmolality does not support the "inappropriate" nature of ADH secretion.
- Urine osmolality must be greater than plasma (500 mOsm or greater) and urine sodium must be in excess of 20–30 mEq/L; concentrations of 40 mEq/L or greater are not uncommon.

SIADH is associated with a wide variety of clinical settings (see Table 49-1).[8,18,20,21] The most common cause of SIADH in clinical oncology is the ectopic production of ADH by tumor. Although small cell anaplastic carcinoma of the lung is the most frequent cause, several other neoplasms also can be associated with the problem (see Table 49-1).[1,2] Even though serum ADH is increased in up to 40% of patients with small cell lung carcinoma, the clinical manifestations occur in only 10% of such patients. The latter have latent SIADH, which might become evident only in the setting of water loading. It should be noted that ectopic ADH secretion is not steady, nor is it usually at a level that approaches the maximal release by the hypothalamus. Thus, an episode of volume depletion still can produce nonosmotic ADH release.

A number of pharmaceutical products, including several antineoplastic compounds, are also associated with SIADH. Most notable among these is vincristine, which has been associated with acute and severe SIADH. The problem generally develops two to three days after vincristine administration, is associated with increased ADH levels, and can persist for days to weeks. High-dose (2 gm/M2) cyclophosphamide is also capable of inducing SIADH through a mechanism thought to be related to direct renal tubular effects and possible enhancement of ADH activity.[18,22] In contrast to hyponatremia due to vincristine, the hyponatremia associated with cyclophosphamide occurs within several hours of administration, and there is no increase in ADH secretion. Curiously, we have not identified SIADH associated with the use of ifosfamide, which is structurally similar to cyclophosphamide. Ifosfamide has, however, been associated with significant renal toxicity and a Fanconi-like tubulopathy characterized by the wasting of multiple electrolytes, glucose, and protein. The platinating agents, cisplatin and (less commonly) carboplatin have also been associated with hyponatremia, although the mechanism of these agents could be related in part to direct renal toxicity and not to SIADH. A number of other drugs listed in Table 49-1 also can cause SIADH.

The management of SIADH depends on how rapidly the problem has evolved and the degree of hyponatremia; it must include treatment aimed at the underlying disease process. In the asymptomatic patient with SIADH who has a serum sodium greater than 125 mEq/L, water restriction is the primary mode of management. The use of furosemide is appropriate for patients who do not respond well to fluid restriction alone. In the symptomatic patient, partial correction with 3% hypertonic saline and furosemide is indicated (see ensuing discussion).[2,4,18,20] Even in these cases, however, treatment must eventually rely on water restriction.

Cerebral salt wasting (CSW) is a cause of hyponatremia associated with intracranial disease or injury.[8,23,24] It is important to differentiate this process from SIADH, which it can resemble closely and for which it is often mistaken. The approaches to treatment for CSW and SIADH are quite different from one another. CSW is mediated by very different but not yet fully defined physiologic circumstances. It is characteristically associated with volume depletion rather than with the isovolemic or modestly expanded state of SIADH. At a basic level, primary central nervous system (CNS) tumors, subarachnoid hemorrhage, and increased intracranial pressure all appear to be associated with the release of natriuretic peptides from brain, cardiac foci, or both, causing a sodium diuresis and ECF volume loss. Water restriction, the typical approach to SIADH, is contraindicated in CSW, which requires both volume and sodium replacement.[8,20,25]

Reset Osmostat

Resetting of the hypothalamic osmostat also can cause hyponatremia.[20,26-28] This condition is generally associated with chronic hyponatremia and has been seen in a variety of malignancies and in cachexia, malnutrition, and pregnancy. A common setting is in patients with hypothalamic tumors or hypothalamic injury from trauma or surgery. Although it is incompletely understood, the mechanism appears to be one in which the set point for ADH release is adjusted downward. Such individuals might have stable plasma sodium concentrations in the range of 125 to 135 mEq/L and are generally asymptomatic. Treatment is unnecessary and even if attempted is generally unsuccessful, as thirst and ADH maintain sodium at the new set point. By itself, this is a relatively benign problem unassociated with neurologic sequelae. In association with other central water and sodium problems, however (e.g., diabetes insipidus or loss of thirst that could accompany hypothalamic/pituitary tumor or injury), a reset osmostat can become a challenge.

HYPONATREMIA IN ASSOCIATION WITH HORMONE DEFICIENCIES

Hyponatremia also can occur in the setting of a number of primary or secondary hormone deficiencies, such as hypothroidism or hypocortisolism.[1,9,20,29] Although these are generally associated with a euvolemic state, hypervolemia may occur also. It is important to keep the hyponatremia associated with these deficiencies in mind, as they can be slow to evolve after organ injury and can easily be mistaken for SIADH.

Although the mechanism of hyponatremia in hypothyroidism is not fully understood, the relatively low cardiac output, a decrease in renal perfusion, impaired water excretion, and ADH secretion all appear to be involved. Patients with milder forms of hypothroidism might be euvolemic and have only modestly decreased sodium. In advanced disease, however, the increase in ADH secretion can be mediated by a carotid baroreceptor stimulus in response to the perception of reduced volume. Settings commonly associated with hypothroidism occur in those patients who have received head and neck or craniospinal irradiation. It can take one to two years for clinically evident hypothyroidism to develop after such events. The treatment of this problem relies largely on thyroid replacement. In patients with advanced disease, temporary sodium and water restriction might also be helpful.

In the setting of adrenal insufficiency, hyponatremia can be a result of mineralocorticoid deficiency, glucocorticoid deficiency, or both. The mechanisms of hyponatremia in these two settings are entirely independent of each other. Primary and metastatic tumors to the adrenal can reduce both hormones. Isolated glucocorticoid deficiency can occur as a result of hypothalamic or pituitary tumors, surgery, or CNS radiation therapy. Central ACTH regulation is relatively radioresistant and generally requires doses exceeding 50 Gy before damage occurs. Even then, there can be a long latency. Glucocorticoid deficiency is generally characterized by hyponatremia in the setting of normal or modestly expanded ECF. Cortisol is necessary for maximum urinary dilution free water excretion. A deficiency results in water retention from increased water permeability in the renal collecting tubules. This action seems to be independent of ADH, as patients with panhypopituitism who are given cortisol replacement soon exhibit diabetes insipidus. In the setting of an otherwise intact hypothalamic/pituitatry axis, cortisol deficiency is also associated with some increase in ADH secretion. Thus, management might require not only cortisol replacement but also desmopressin acetate (DDAVP) to control the diabetes insipidus that cortisol has "unmasked."

In mineralocorticoid deficiency, the renin-angiotensin system is compromised, and there is generally a contraction of effective circulating volume because of diminished capacity by the kidney to reabsorb sodium. In response to diminished volume, baroreceptor-mediated ADH release and water retention can drive sodium lower.

SYMPTOMS AND MANAGEMENT OF HYPONATREMIA

Most patients with hyponatremia are relatively asymptomatic, and treatment can be aimed at the underlying disease. Symptomatic hyponatremia should be considered a medical emergency. In the absence of infections and issues related to tumors, congestive failure, and the other edematous states, the symptoms associated with hyponatremia depend on the depth of the sodium concentration and the rapidity of its onset. When hyponatremia develops within a matter of several hours as a result of acute hypotonic volume load, neurologic findings related to evolving cerebral edema dominate. Those patients in whom hyponatremia develops over an extended period (48 hours or greater) might have only mild lethargy, muscular symptoms, and anorexia even though their serum sodium might be the same or even lower than that of patients who develop the problem acutely.

Mild symptoms characterized by vomiting, malaise, and even agitation are usually seen in patients with sodium concentrations above 125 mEq/L. As sodium falls further, muscle cramps and weakness, as well as neurologic symptoms including lethargy, headache, and confusion can occur. Sodium levels below 120 mEq/L are associated with seizures and coma.

In all but the unequivocal acute volume overload state and patients with neurologic signs, it is wise to assume that hyponatremia is a chronic process that has developed over several days or more. The rationale for this assumption is that chronic hyponatremia must be corrected slowly. Too rapid a correction is associated with severe, life-threatening central nervous system complications from osmotic demyelination syndrome.

Osmotic demyelination is related to an overly aggressive sodium correction. Rapid but relatively modest degrees of sodium correction can cause ECF to appear hypertonic to the cell (even though sodium is still low).

A number of risk factors associated with this problem have been identified. Among these are patients with alcoholism, malnutrition, hepatic disease, and chronic illness. The most important risk factor is a correction at a rate that exceeds 12 mEq/L in 24 hours and 18-24 mEq/L in 48 hours.[1,2,4,16,18,21] It should be noted that there is typically a delay of two to four days (and sometimes as long as six days) before the signs of brain injury and demyelination occur. Thus, it is possible to see patients improve initially but have a subsequent neurologic decline some days after the start of correction. Patients with acute hyponatremia have significantly less risk of developing this problem than do those with chronic hyponatremia.[16]

Treatment of Asymptomatic Hyponatremia

Hypovolemic hyponatremia is generally associated with the symptoms of volume depletion, and these patients are not at risk for the neurologic complications related to cerebral edema that acompany acute hyponatremia. They might, however, be subject to osmotic demyelinating syndrome associated with rapid sodium correction. The management of patients with mild hypovolemic hyponatremia from chronic renal sodium loss or overuse of diuretics is best performed by giving isotonic (0.9%) saline or, if tolerated, oral salt tablets. A rate of correction aimed at no more than 12 mEq/L per day over a period of two to three days is generally sufficient.

In the isovolemic hyponatremias that commonly result from SIADH, treating the underlying disease, stopping any potentially offending drugs, and water restriction are the methods of choice. Rigorous restriction of free water to as little as 30%-70% of maintenance needs might be necessary and could take two to three days to become effective. The often attempted use of isotonic saline at a lower than maintenance rate is a doomed strategy because an isotonic load is excreted quickly with little or no net change in serum sodium. In patients who do not tolerate or who are noncompliant with water restriction or in whom furosemide is contraindicated or ineffective, the use of democycline could be appropriate. A dose of 300-600 mg twice daily will induce a nephrogenic diabetes insipidus-like state with increased free water excretion. Lithium carbonate can produce the same result but is generally not well tolerated because of the dose required.[30-32]

In relatively asymptomatic hypervolemic hyponatremic patients, modest fluid restriction, sodium restriction, and the use of a loop diuretic to promote renal free water excretion are appropriate measures. These measures will be ineffective, however, without management aimed at the underlying edematous disease state.

Treatment of Acute Symptomatic Hyponatremia

Acute hyponatremia—most frequently the result of volume overload with hypotonic fluids—generally manifests by the presence of some neurologic findings as a result of evolving cerebral edema. These patients generally have a serum sodium below 120 mEq/L. The goal

---

> ### SODIUM DEFICIT
>
> [desired Na - measured Na] × 0.6 body weight (kg) = mEq of Na^+ needed.

---

of treatment for these patients should be to raise the serum sodium sufficiently to stop any seizure activity and to correct cerebral edema. Experience suggests that changes in serum sodium of as little as 5% can diminish cerebral edema, and increases of as little as 3-6 mEq/L can stop most seizures.[33-35] With this in mind, a rate of correction of about 1-1.5 mEq/hr during the first four to six hours is often sufficient to manage the acute neurologic problems. Anticonvulsants might be necessary for those with seizures. Using the formulas for correcting sodium deficit and knowing the sodium content of different intravenous solutions, the rate and type of fluid administration can be calculated easily. This initial correction might employ the use of 3% hypertonic saline. Acute, symptomatic hyponatremia is the only condition in which the use of a hypertonic saline solution is unequivocally an appropriate intervention. Although patients with acute hyponatremia have a lower risk of osmotic demyelination than those who develop low sodium on a more chronic basis (>48 hours), the use of hypertonic saline should be limited to achieving an initial increase of 3-6 mEq/L or a serum sodium of 120-125 mEq/L. After the initial period of correction, the rate of sodium rise should be limited to 0.5 mEq/L using 0.9% (isotonic) saline. Correction rates of 10-12 mEq/L during the first 24-hour period and 18 mEq/L over the first 48 hours are safe.[2,4,18,21]

The addition of furosemide during the initial correction period has been advocated as a method of encouraging free water excretion by the kidney. Furosemide diminishes interstitial renal medullary tonicity, impairs urinary concentrating ability, and leads to a hypotonic urine with a concentration of about 0.45% saline (75 mEq/L). Although this often appears to be helpful, it should probably be limited to a single dose, thus minimizing too rapid a correction. Furosemide is particularly useful in a frail patient with diminished cardiac reserve, in whom the use of hypertonic saline could incite congestive failure. Furosemide should not be used in hypovolemic patients.

Management of Chronic Hyponatremia/SIADH

The management of these patients relies on treating the underlying disease. Examples include the treatment of

---

> ### SODIUM CONTENT OF COMMON INTRAVENOUS SOLUTIONS
>
> | Solution | Na^+ (mEq/L) | Na^+ (mEq/cc) |
> |---|---|---|
> | 3% saline | 513 | 0.513 |
> | 0.9% saline | 154 | 0.154 |
> | Ringers lactate | 130 | 0.130 |

malignancies, hormone replacement, removal of drugs associated with SIADH, providing adequate sodium (and water) needs for patients receiving enteral feeding, and compensating for disordered thirst. Preventive measures, such as the preference for the use of isotonic saline in "at risk" patients (malignancy, chemotherapy, positive pressure ventilation, and other states noted in Table 49-1) who require hydration, are equally important. It is important to remember that correction of chronic hyponatremia must be executed slowly to avoid the potential of osmotic demyelination. Asymptomatic patients who have slowly developed sodium concentrations as low as 105–110 mEq/L have been corrected successfully using an initial rate of 0.5 mEq/L/hour or less to bring them to serum levels of 120 mEq/L. After this, the rate of correction may be liberalized, keeping in mind the risk factors for demyelination noted earlier. Although it is permissible to initiate treatment with 3% saline solutions in these severely hyponatremic patients, the need to do so and the potential risks of too rapid a correction in a relatively asymptomatic patient suggest isotonic saline as a safer alternative. For unstable patients and those with neurologic symptoms, the approach to treatment should be similar to that noted earlier for acute symptomatic hyponatremia, but at a slower pace; a planned initial rise in sodium of 4–6 mEq/L over 12 hours, followed by a more gradual correction at a rate not to exceed 12 mEq/L during the first 24 hours, is considered safe (including the initial 4–6 mEq/L correction). During the second 24 hours, the rate of correction should be even more gradual than for the acutely symptomatic patient. A rate of 0.5 mEq/L or less, with the plan of limiting sodium rise to no more that 18 mEq/L over the initial 48 hours, is appropriate. Some authors suggest an even slower rate of correction, limiting sodium rise to no more than 8 mEq/L in any 24-hour period.[18] Furosemide may be used during the initial correction phase but should probably be limited to a single dose to minimize too rapid a correction, particularly in the setting of hypertonic saline use.

A more challenging situation is that of a patient with severe hyponatremia associated with a malignancy. Such patients should have at least a partial correction to a sodium above 125 mEq/L (and preferably above 130 mEq/L) before proceeding with chemotherapy and hydration. Even then, they remain at risk for recurrence and must be monitored carefully as treatment and tumor lysis begin.

A caution is that the correction of a hypovolemic hyponatremia associated with excessive use of thiazide diuretics might occur more rapidly than anticipated. As volume is replaced, these patients might quickly regain the ability to excrete a hypotonic urine that could cause an unintended acceleration of sodium correction. Likewise, other hypovolemic patients are at risk for rapid correction. As their volumes are expanded and the nonosmotic stimulus of ADH decreases, accelerated sodium correction can occur. Again, the use of isotonic rather than hypertonic saline for correction, as well as frequent evaluations of volume and sodium status, limit the potential for too rapid a rate of correction.

EXAMPLE CASES

Postoperative Symptomatic Hyponatremia

A 56-year-old woman who is now 48 hours after an uncomplicated resection of a breast tumor is reported by her family to be more lethargic and somewhat confused compared with the day before. She has a tonic-clonic seizure that is controlled rapidly with lorazepam. Serum chemistries reveal a sodium of 115 mEq/L, a potassium of 3.3 mEq/L, and a serum osmolality of 245 mOsm/kg. Her urine osmolality is 125 mEq/L, and urine sodium is 20 mEq/L. On examination, she has a heart rate of 90, is normotensive, and has no peripheral edema. Her preoperative weight is 65 kg. Based on the foregoing data, a likely diagnosis is hypotonic hyponatremia in what appears to be a euvolemic patient. The differential diagnosis includes SIADH from the pain and stress of surgery and/or from the use of morphine for postoperative discomfort, or dilutional hyponatremia from hypotonic volume overload. SIADH would be expected to be associated with a more concentrated urine and a urine sodium well in excess of 20 mEq/L. Her record indicates that she received 2.5 L of D5W during surgery. Additionally, it is noted that she has had several glasses of water over the last 12 hours, the exact amount unknown. The highly dilute urine, the relatively low urine sodium in the setting of a low serum osmolality, and her history are characteristic of acute hypotonic fluid overload. Because the patient is symptomatic, the initial plan should be to increase her serum sodium by 3–6 mEq/L over the course of 3–6 hours. Based on her weight and gender, the appropriate factor for determining the volume of ECF in need of correction is 0.5, thus giving a volume of 32.5 L (0.5 × 65 kg). An initial correction of 5 mEq/L over the course of 6 hours is planned using 3% saline. The total amount of sodium needed is 163 mEq (32.5 kg × 5 mEq/L). Given over 6 hours, this equates to 27 mEq per hour. Using 3% saline, which contains 0.513 mEq/cc of sodium, her hourly fluid rate becomes:

$$\frac{27 \text{ mEq Na}}{0.513 \text{ mEq Na/cc 3\% saline}} = 53 \text{ cc/hr for six hours}$$

If furosemide is given at the start of the initial correction, the time to correction might be somewhat longer as a result of both free water and sodium loss (Furosemide produces a roughly 0.45% saline diuresis). Thus, sodium should be monitored every two hours, and the infusion rate should be adjusted accordingly.

At the end of the initial six hours, the serum sodium is 119 mEq/L, and there have been no further seizures. The

---

CALCULATING THE RATE OF FLUID ADMINISTRATION

$$\frac{\text{Na}^+ \text{ Deficit}}{\text{Na}^+ \text{ mEq/L}} = \text{rate (cc/hr)}$$

patient remains unresponsive, however. Based on this, an additional 5 mEq/L sodium correction is planned. Even though patients with acute volume overload are not at high risk for osmotic demyelination associated with rapid correction, it is wise to assume that the problem occurred slowly to minimize the potential for development of this condition. Thus, the second-phase correction should be done at a much slower rate of 0.5 mEq/L/hour, with the goal of not exceeding a total correction of more than 12 mEq/L over the first 24 hours. Another 163 mEq of sodium will be required (32.5 kg × 5 mEq/L) over the next 18 hours. As the patient is still unresponsive, it is appropriate to use 3% saline for correction. The hourly rate of correction now changes to 163 mEq/18 hours, or 9 mEq/hour. Using 3% saline, this becomes:

$$\frac{9 \text{ mEq Na}}{0.513 \text{mEq Na/cc 3\% saline}} = 17 \text{ cc/hr for 12 hours}$$

At the end of 24 hours, the patient's serum sodium is 125 mEq/L, and she is somewhat lethargic but arousable. At this point, it is appropriate to switch to isotonic saline (0.9%) for further correction. The goal is now to continue correction, limiting the total amount of correction in the first 48 hours to 18 mEq/L. Thus, an additional 8 mEq/L of sodium will be given over the second 24-hour period, for a total of 260 mEq of sodium (8 mEq/L × 32.5 L) or 11 mEq/hr. Using isotonic saline, the rate becomes:

$$\frac{11 \text{mEq}}{0.154 \text{ mEq/cc/0.9\% saline}} = 70 \text{ cc/hr} \times 24 \text{ hours}.$$

At the end of the first 48 hours, the patient's serum sodium is 132 mEq/L, and she is alert and responsive. Further correction with 0.9% saline at a rate of no more than 0.5 mEq/L/hour over the next 12–24 hours will result in a normal sodium having been achieved over a period of time long enough and at a slow enough rate to minimize the potential for CNS demyelination.

Hypotonic Hyponatremia Associated with Euvolemia

A 72-year-old man with recently diagnosed small cell lung carcinoma is noted to have become increasingly confused and lethargic over the last 72 hours. He has not yet started chemotherapy. Of note, he has been on replacement therapy for hyperthyroidism for several years. His wife isn't sure whether he has been taking his thyroid replacement over the last several days. Laboratory evaluation reveals a serum sodium of 112 mEq/L, potassium at 3.6 mEq/L, and an osmolality of 225 mOsm/kg. The urine osmolality is 590 mOsm/kg. His blood pressure and heart rate are normal, and there is no evidence of edema, suggesting that he is euvolemic. His urine sodium is 50 mEq/L. His weight is 66 kg. Although the temptation to make the diagnosis of tumor-related SIADH is strong, this must be a diagnosis of exclusion. Other possible causes of euvolemic hypotonic hyponatremia include overuse of a diuretic and glucocorticoid or thyroid deficiency (see Fig. 49-1). He has not been on any diuretics, and cortisol deficiency seems remote because his

potassium is normal and he has been an otherwise healthy, active man except for recent events. Although known to have primary hypothyroidism, it is unlikely that missing two to three days of replacement therapy would put him at risk for hyponatremia. Thus, tumor-related SIADH is the most likely diagnosis. He is given one liter of normal saline (0.9%), and two hours later his serum sodium is 110 mEq/L and his urine osmolality remains at 590 mOsm/kg. Although this might initially be surprising, recall that patients with SIADH have a relatively fixed urine osmolality due to tonic ADH secretion, and they retain the ability to excrete sodium despite their hyponatremia. Thus, the net effect of isotonic saline was to produce further dilution of serum sodium, as a concentrated sodium-containing urine is excreted, leaving a relative free water gain.

The approach to this symptomatic patient involves raising his sodium to a level of 120 mEq/L and then restricting free water. The goal is to provide an initial sodium increase of 3–6 mEq/L. Knowing that the hyponatremia has developed over a period of at least 72 hours based on the patient's history, the rate of correction should be similar to minimize the potential for osmotic demyelination, for which he is at significant risk. Based on this information, the goal is an increase in serum sodium of no more than 10–12 mEq/L over the first 24 hours at a rate of no more than 0.5 mEq/L/hour. Because he is an elderly man, the factor for determining his total body water is 0.5, thus making his total ECF volume 23 L (0.5 × 66 kg). Although the use of isotonic saline is often a better plan for correcting patients who have developed their hyponatremia chronically, 3% saline is acceptable for this patient because he is symptomatic.

Raising his sodium by 10 mEq/L to 120 mEq/L over the next 24 hours requires 10 mEq/L of sodium by 23 L, for a total of 230 mEq of sodium.

$$\frac{230 \text{ mEq}}{0.51 \text{ mEq/mL/3\% saline}} = \frac{450 \text{ mL of 3\% saline}}{\text{at 19 mL/hr}}$$

This correction rate is only 0.4 mEq/L/hr and within the guidelines for minimizing the risk of osmotic demyelination discussed earlier in the chapter. Also, keep in mind that the rate of correction should be limited to 18 mEq/L within the first 48 hours. If furosemide is used at the start of the initial correction, the rate of correction might even be somewhat slower, as noted in the previous case example. At 24 hours, the patient's serum sodium is 119 mEq/L; he is lethargic but arousable and less confused, and the objective of bringing his sodium close to 120 mEq/L has been achieved. If he had not been clinically improved, it might have been prudent to increase his sodium another 5 mEq/L over the next 12 hours, to about 125 mEq/L. At this point, with an improved patient and a sodium of 119 mEq/L, it is appropriate to began water restriction, limiting water and anything that becomes water at body temperature (e.g., gelatin and ice cream) to 1 L/day. Over the next 48–72 hours, one should expect to see his sodium increase to 130 mEq/L or more. At this point, it is appropriate to began management of his tumor.

Hyponatremia with Diminished ECF

A 12-year-old, 50 kg male underwent resection of a large temporal lobe tumor 48 hours previously; the tumor has been associated with significantly increased intracranial pressure. He is irritable but lucid, complaining of leg cramps; he has a moderate hypotension of 100/60 and a moderate sinus tacchycardia of 120 beats per minute and has developed significantly increased urine output of 6 mL/kg/hr over the last 12 hours. Serum chemistries reveal a sodium of 124 mEq/L, potassium of 4.5 mEq/L, BUN of 17, and creatinine of 1.2. His serum osmolality is 300 mOsm/kg, urine osmolality is 350 mOsm/L, and urine sodium is 155 mEq/L. Review of his record shows that the received 0.5 gm/kg dose of mannitol before surgery and 1 L of normal saline during surgery. Over the last 24 hours, he has been drinking ad lib and appears to have increased thirst. His exam suggests some degree of hypovolemia, and the elevated urine sodium is compatible with either a primary salt wasting process or SIADH. The urine sodium and moderate urine concentration are not consistent with diabetes insipidus. The latter is unlikely given his increased serum osmolality, excessive urine output, and signs of hypovolemia. A hypovolemic hyponatremia characterized by excessive renal sodium loss in a neurosurgical setting is characteristic of cerebral salt wasting.

Recognizing that the serum sodium has probably developed acutely and is likely to quickly drop even further given the amount of sodium he is excreting and the fact that he is developing some mild symptoms (irritability and muscle cramps), the decision is to make a partial correction of his sodium to diminish the potential of more severe symptoms. At the same time, his hypovolemia must be treated, and his ongoing losses must be replaced. The plasma volume for this adolescent male is 30 L (0.6 × 50 kg). Because the sodium loss has been rapid, the decision is taken to raise his sodium by 4 mEq/L over six hours. Thus, a total of 120 mEq of sodium over six hours will be needed at a rate of 20 mEq/hour using 3% saline.

$$\frac{20 \text{ mEq Na}}{0.513 \text{ mEq Na/cc 3\% saline}} = 39 \text{ cc/hr}$$

Simultaneously, it is necessary to replace his urine output, volume for volume, with isotonic saline. To this it is necessary to add an amount calculated to represent his current volume deficit with the intent of correcting it over 24 hours. After 24 hours, the patient appears euvolemic with a normal blood pressure and heart rate. Having replaced his volume deficit, it is now prudent to decrease the rate of isotonic saline correction to match urine output. The natriuresis continues for several days, but isotonic saline keeps the serum sodium at 138 mEq/L. At this point, the patient is stable, is able to drink, and appears to have a normal thirst. He can be discharged on oral NaCl supplements approximating his renal sodium loss. Two weeks later, he appears well, and his urine output has diminished to 3 mL/kg/day. He is on a normal diet, and urine osmolality has increased to 550 mEq/L with 50 mEq/L of sodium. The serum sodium is 138 mEq/L. At this point, sodium chloride supplements are stopped, and the patient's serum sodium remains normal.

REFERENCES

1. McDonald GA, Dubose TD Jr: Hyponatremia in the cancer patient. Oncology 193;7:55–64, 1993.
2. Miller M: Endocrine and metabolic dysfunction syndromes in the critically ill. Crit Care Clin 2001;17:11–23.
3. Roberston GL: Physiology of ADH secretion. Kidney Int 1987;32: 520.
4. Haycock GB: The syndrome of inappropriate secetion of antiduretic hormone. Pediatr Nephrol 1995;9:375–381.
5. Gines P: Vasopressin in pathophysiological states. Semin Nephrol 1994;14:384.
6. Schrier RW: Body fluid volume regulation in health and disease: A unifying hypothesis. Ann Int Med 1990;113:155–159.
7. Epstein FH: Natriuretic peptides. New Engl J Med 1998;339: 321–328.
8. Palmer BF: Hyponatremia in a neurosurgical patient: Syndrome of inappropriate antidiuretic hormone secretion versus cerebral salt wasting. Nephrol Dial Transplant 2000;15:262–268.
9. Kokko JP: Fluids and Electrolytes. In Goldman L, and Bennett JC (eds): Cecil Textbook of Medicine. Philadelphia, WB Saunders, 2000, pp 540–571.
10. Law RO: Amino acids as volume regulatory osmolytes in mammalian cells. Comp Biochem Physiol 1991;99:263.
11. Lien YH, Shapiro JI, Chan L: Study of brain electrolytes and organic osmolytes during correction of chronic hyponatremia: Implication for pathogenesis of central pontine myelinolysis. J Clin Invest 1991;88:303.
12. Verbalis JG, Gullans SR: Hyponatremia causes large sustained reduction in brain content of multiple orangic osmolytes in the rat. Brain Res 1991;567:274.
13. Trachtman H: Cell volume regulation: A review of cerebral adaptive mechanisms and implications for clinical treatment of osmolal disturbances: II. Pediatr Nephrol 1992;6:104.
14. Sterns RH: The management of symptomatic hyponatremia. Semin Nephrol 1990;10:503.
15. Brunner JE, Redmond JM, Haggar AM, et al: Central pontine myelinolysis and pontine lesions after rapid correction of hyponatremia: A prospective magnetic resonance imaging study. Ann Neurol 1990;27:61–66.
16. Sterns RH, Cappuccio JD, Silver SM, et al: Neurologic sequelae after treatment of severe hyponatremia: A multicenter perspective. J Am Soc Nephrol 1994;8:1522–1530.
17. Laureno R, Karp BI: Myelinolysis after correction of hyponatremia. Ann Int Med 1997;126:57–62.
18. Adrogue HJ, Madias NE: Hyponatremia. New Engl J Med 2000;342:1581–1589.
19. Rose BD, Post TW: Clinical Physiology of Acid-base and Electrolyte Disorders, 5th ed. New York, McGraw-Hill, 2001, pp 707–711.
20. Milonis HJ, Liamis GL, Elisaf MS: The hyponatremic patient: A systematic approach to laboratory diagnosis. CMAJ 2002;166:1056–1062.
21. Avnr ED: Clinical disorders of water metabolism: Hyponatremia and hypernatremia. Pediatr Ann 1995;24:23–30.
22. Kapoor M, Chan GZ: Fluid and electrolyte abnormalities. Crit Care Clin 2001;17:503–529.
23. Kappy MS, Ganong CA: Cerebral salt wasting in children: The role of atrial natriuretic hormone. Adv Pediatr 1996;43:271–308.
24. Al-Mufti H, Arieff AI: Hyponatremia due to cerebral salt-wasting syndrome. Am J Med 1984;77:740–746.
25. Harrigan MR: Cerebral salt wasting syndrome: A review. Neurosurgery 1996;38:152–160.
26. Elisaf MS, Konstantinides A, Siamopoulos KC: Chronic hyponatremia due to reset osmostat in a patient with colon cancer. Am J Nephrol 1996;16:349–351.
27. Elisaf MS, Milionis HJ, Siamopoulos KC: Chronic hyponatremia secondary to reset osmostat in a patient with advanced ovarian cancer. J Exp Clin Cancer Res 1996;15:313–314.
28. Lipschutz JH, Arieff AI: Reset osmostat in a healthy patient. Ann Int Med 1994;120:574–576.
29. Hanna FW, Scanlon MF: Hyponatremia, hypothroidism and the role of arginine-vasopressin. Lancet 1997;350:755–756.

30. White MG: Treatment of the syndrome of inappropriate secretion of antidiuretic hormone with lithium carbonate. New Engl J Med 1975;292:390.
31. Cherill DA: Demeclocycline treatment in the syndrome of antidiuretic hormone secretion. Ann Int Med 1975;83:654.
32. Forrest JN: Superiority of demeclocycline over lithium in the treatment of chronic syndrome of inappropriate secretion of antidiuretic hormone. New Engl J Med 1978;298:173.
33. Sterns RH, Narins RG: Hypernatremia and hyponatremia: Pathophysiology, diagnosis and therapy. In Androgue HJ (ed): Contemporary Management in Critical Care, vol 1, no 2: Acid-base and Electrolyete Disorders. New York, Churchill Livingstone, 1991, pp 161-191.
34. Sterns RH: The treatment of hyponatremia: First, do no harm. Am J Med 1990;88:557-560.
35. Sarnaik A, Meert K, Hackbarth R, et al: Management of hyponatremic seizures in children with hypertonic saline: A safe and effective strategy. Crit Care Med 1991;19:758-762.

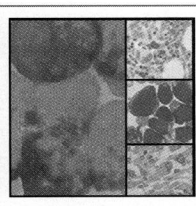

50

TUMOR LYSIS SYNDROME

Michael R. Bishop

Mitchell S. Cairo

Peter F. Coccia

SUMMARY OF KEY POINTS

INCIDENCE AND EPIDEMIOLOGY

- The exact incidence of tumor lysis syndrome is unknown; incidence in high-grade non-Hodgkin's lymphoma is approximately 40%.
- Tumor lysis syndrome is most commonly associated with acute lymphocytic leukemia and "high-grade" non-Hodgkin's lymphoma; however, it has been observed in a variety of hematologic and solid malignancies.
- Tumor lysis syndrome has been observed with the administration of chemotherapy, corticosteroids, radiation, hormonal agents, and biologic response modifiers. Tumor lysis syndrome can occur spontaneously before the initiation of therapy.

ETIOLOGY

- Tumor lysis syndrome results from the rapid release of intracellular ions

and metabolites from malignant cells after the initiation of cytotoxic therapy.
- The body's inability to handle the increased concentrations of ions and metabolites results in the characteristic metabolic abnormalities associated with tumor lysis syndrome, including hyperuricemia, hyperphosphatemia, hypocalcemia, and uremia.
- The metabolic disturbances associated with tumor lysis syndrome can lead to life-threatening complications including arrhythmias and acute renal failure.

EVALUATION OF THE PATIENT

- Patients with tumors with a high proliferative rate and sensitivity to cytotoxic therapy, large tumor masses, preexisting renal insufficiency, and high serum lactate dehydrogenase levels are at highest

risk for the development of tumor lysis syndrome.

MANAGEMENT AND TREATMENT

- Recognition of patients at risk for the development of tumor lysis syndrome is the most important management issue.
- Establishing central venous access and administration of intravenous fluids and allopurinol or rasburicase should begin before the initiation of tumor therapy.
- Alkalinization of urine with sodium bicarbonate or acetazolamide is controversial.
- Prompt initiation of hemodialysis may aid in the reversal of severe complications associated with tumor lysis syndrome.

INTRODUCTION

Tumor lysis syndrome is a spectrum of metabolic derangements that occur from tumor breakdown usually associated with the initiation of cytotoxic therapy of malignancy in both children and adults. The syndrome is characterized by numerous metabolic abnormalities including hyperuricemia, hyperphosphatemia, hypocalcemia, and uremia; and it frequently leads to acute renal failure.[1-5] Tumor lysis syndrome results from the rapid destruction of malignant cells and the release of their intracellular contents into the extracellular space after the initiation of therapy. The abrupt release of intracellular ions, nucleic acids, proteins, and their metabolites can overwhelm the body's normal homeostatic mechanisms and cause severe metabolic disturbances that require clinical intervention.

Tumor lysis syndrome has been primarily observed in acute lymphocytic leukemia and high-grade non-Hodgkin's lymphomas, in particular Burkitt's lymphoma.[2,4-6] However, tumor lysis syndrome has also been recognized in a variety of other malignancies, both hematologic and solid

(Table 50-1). These malignancies share the characteristics of a high proliferative rate and a relative sensitivity to cytotoxic therapy.[2,4,7] Other hematologic malignancies associated with tumor lysis syndrome include acute myeloid leukemia, chronic lymphocytic leukemia, chronic myeloid leukemia, and low-grade and intermediate-grade non-Hodgkin's lymphomas.[8-13] Tumor lysis syndrome has also been reported to occur in a number of solid tumors such as breast cancer, testicular cancer, medulloblastoma, and small cell carcinoma of the lung.[14-18]

The overall incidence of tumor lysis syndrome is unknown because it has only been closely studied in high-grade non-Hodgkin's lymphomas.[4,5] In a retrospective study of 102 patients with high-grade non-Hodgkin's lymphoma, the incidence of tumor lysis syndrome was reported to be 42% as determined by serial laboratory testing.[5] The incidence of clinically significant tumor lysis syndrome was only 6% in the same group of patients.

The development of tumor lysis syndrome is not limited to the administration of chemotherapy alone. Reports of tumor lysis syndrome have been associated with the administration of radiation therapy, corticosteroids, hormonal agents, biologic response modifiers,

TABLE 50-1

Malignancies That Have Been Associated with Tumor Lysis Syndrome

HEMATOLOGIC MALIGNANCIES	SOLID TUMORS
Acute lymphocytic leukemia	Breast cancer
Acute myeloid leukemia	Germ cell/testicular cancer
Chronic lymphocytic leukemia	Medulloblastoma
Prolymphocytic leukemia	Merkel cell carcinoma
Chronic myelogenous leukemia	Lung cancer
(blast crisis)	Non-small cell lung cancer
Non-Hodgkin's lymphoma	Small cell
Follicular	Melanoma
Diffuse large cell	Choriocarcinoma
Burkitt's	Hepatocellular carcinoma
T-cell	Thymoma
Hodgkin's disease	Teratoma
Plasma cell disorders	Gastric cancer
Multiple myeloma	Vulvar carcinoma
Amyloidosis	Colorectal cancer
Plasmacytoma	Neuroblastoma
Myeloproliferative disorders	Langerhans cell histiocytosis
Myelofibrosis	

monoclonal antibodies, and more recently, the low-molecular-weight inhibitor, imatinib mesylate, better known as Gleevec.[19-24] Tumor lysis syndrome is not limited to systemic administration of agents; it has been observed with intrathecal administration of chemotherapy and with chemo-embolization. Some more unusual clinical situations in which tumor lysis syndrome has been observed include fever, pregnancy, and general anesthesia. It is extremely important clinically to note that tumor lysis syndrome can occur spontaneously, before the initiation of any intervention.

The identification of patients at risk for the development of tumor lysis syndrome is the most important aspect of management so that prophylactic measures may be initiated before the initiation of therapy. Most of the complications can be readily managed when they are recognized early; however, delay in recognition and initiation of treatment of tumor lysis syndrome can be life-threatening.[25-27]

PATHOPHYSIOLOGY

The majority of agents that are used in the treatment of malignancies are dependent on the proliferative rate of malignant cells for their activity.[28] In tumors with a high proliferative rate, a relatively large mass, and a high sensitivity to cytotoxic agents, the initiation of therapy often results in the rapid release of intracellular anions, cations, and the metabolic products of proteins and nucleic acids into the bloodstream. The increased concentrations of uric acid, calcium, phosphates, potassium, and urea can overwhelm the body's natural mechanisms to maintain normal levels and result in the clinical spectrum associated with tumor lysis syndrome.

Hyperuricemia and its associated complications are the most common clinical complications of tumor lysis syndrome, and more importantly, predispose to many of the other clinical manifestations. Hyperuricemia results from rapid release and catabolism of intracellular nucleic acids.[29] Purine nucleic acids are catabolized to hypoxanthine, then xanthine, and finally uric acid by xanthine oxidase. Uric acid clearance is renal, and in normal circumstances approximately 500 mg of uric acid is excreted through the kidneys each day.[30] Uric acid has a pKa of 5.4 to 5.7 and is poorly soluble in water. At normal concentrations and at physiologic blood pH, more than 99% of uric acid is in the ionized form.[30,31] The concentration of uric acid has been noted to be elevated in patients with acute leukemias and lymphomas even before the initiation of therapy.[32] The high concentrations of uric acid increase the risk for uric acid crystal precipitation in the renal collecting ducts and distal tubules, which are sites of urinary acidification.[33] General clinical manifestations of hyperuricemia include nausea, vomiting, diarrhea, and anorexia. Uric acid crystal precipitation within renal tubules results in a decline in glomerular filtration and the subsequent development of acute renal failure. The risk of acute renal failure caused by uric acid precipitation may be increased by dehydration, which is often present at the time of diagnosis; ureteral obstruction by tumor; a history of renal insufficiency; and the possible need for nephrotoxic antibiotics, such as aminoglycosides, in patients with active infections. If the hyperuricemia results in acute obstructive uropathy, other clinical manifestations may include hematuria, flank pain, hypertension, azotemia acidosis, edema, oliguria, anuria, lethargy, and somnolence.

Hyperphosphatemia results from the rapid release of intracellular phosphorous from malignant cells, which may contain as much as four times the amount of organic and inorganic phosphates as that of normal cells.[2,34] Initially, the kidneys are able to respond to the increased concentration of phosphorous from tumor lysis by increased urinary excretion and decreased tubular absorption of phosphorous. Eventually, however, the tubular transport mechanism becomes saturated and is unable to maintain normal serum phosphorous levels. The development of hyperphosphatemia may be further exacerbated by acute renal insufficiency associated with uric acid precipitation, resulting in obstructive uropathy or other complications of tumor therapy. Hyperphosphatemia can lead to the development of acute renal failure after precipitation with calcium in renal tubules during tumor lysis syndrome.[35,36] Hyperphosphatemia may be associated with nausea, vomiting, diarrhea, lethargy, and seizures. More importantly, hyperphosphatemia may result in tissue precipitation of calcium-phosphate crystals, resulting in hypocalcemia, metastatic calcification, intrarenal calcification, nephrocalcinosis, nephrolithiasis, and additional acute obstructive uropathy. The serum concentration of calcium rapidly decreases as precipitation with phosphate occurs. Hypocalcemia is one of the most critical clinical manifestations of tumor lysis syndrome and has been associated with the development of severe muscle cramping, tetany, and cardiac arrhythmias. In addition to the kidneys, other tissues such as muscle may be sites of precipitation of calcium and phosphorous.[35]

Hyperkalemia may also be a life-threatening consequence of tumor lysis syndrome.[25,26] Hyperkalemia results from the kidneys' inability to clear the massive load of intracellular potassium released by lysed tumor cells. General clinical manifestations of hyperkalemia may include nausea, anorexia, vomiting, and diarrhea. More specific complications include neuromuscular and cardiac abnormalities. Neuromuscular signs and symptoms may include muscle weakness, cramps, paresthesias, and possible paralysis. Cardiac manifestations may include asystole, ventricular tachycardia or fibrillation, syncope, and possible sudden death.[25,26]

Increases in blood urea nitrogen and creatinine levels occur as a result of renal impairment associated with acute uric acid crystal nephropathy, calcium-phosphate and nephrocalcinosis, or a combination of the two, leading to an acute obstructive uropathy syndrome. A correlation with the pretreatment serum lactate dehydrogenase (LDH) level and the development of azotemia has been reported, and the blood urea nitrogen level will generally rise in parallel with the rise in the serum phosphorous level.[2,5] Acute clinical manifestations may include uremia resulting in nausea, vomiting, and lethargy; oliguria or anuria leading to fluid retention; edema, hypertension, congestive heart failure, metabolic disturbances, and exacerbations of hyperphosphatemia and/or hyperkalemia (see previous discussion); flank or back pain; hematuria; and severe acidosis. Extreme elevations in blood urea nitrogen levels can result in a platelet function defect, cellular immunodeficiency, and inflammatory pericarditis.[37,38] Furthermore, acute obstructive uropathy may precipitate acute renal failure (anuria), confusion, somnolence, seizures, and/or coma.

TREATMENT

The management of tumor lysis syndrome may be divided into preventative and immediate treatments (Table 50-2). The ability to prevent tumor lysis syndrome is highly dependent on the immediate recognition of patients at

TABLE 50-2

Initial Management of Patients at Risk for Tumor Lysis Syndrome

1. Identification of the patient at risk (see Table 50-3).
2. Admit to intensive care or oncology unit.
3. Establish adequate venous access.
4. Delay tumor therapy, if possible.
5. Perform baseline electrocardiogram and continuous cardiac monitoring.
6. Determine baseline and serial serum LDH, uric acid, Na$^+$, K$^+$, creatinine, BUN, phosphorous, and Ca^{++} levels.
7. Provide intravenous hydration with hypotonic or isotonic saline solution at 2500 to 3000 mL/m^2/24 hours.
8. Give allopurinol, 300 to 400 mg/m^2 orally, or rasburicase, 0.20 mg/kg/day intravenously, over 30 minutes for 3 to 7 days.
9. Urinary alkalinization (optional):
   a. Sodium bicarbonate 50 to 100 mEq/L of intravenous fluids
   or
   b. Acetazolamide 150 to 500 mg/m^2

TABLE 50-3

Clinical Characteristics of Patients at High Risk for Tumor Lysis Syndrome

Tumors with a high proliferative rate (e.g., acute lymphocytic leukemia and high-grade non-Hodgkin's lymphoma) and sensitivity to cytotoxic agents
Large tumor masses
Renal insufficiency and obstructive uropathy
Elevated serum lactate dehydrogenase or uric acid level
Dehydration

risk for its development (Table 50-3). Patients at high risk include those with a tumor with a high proliferative rate, large tumor masses, preexisting renal insufficiency, and elevated levels of phosphorous, uric acid, or both before the initiation of therapy.[4,5,39] The elevation of the serum LDH level before the initiation of therapy has also been associated with the recognition of patients at risk for tumor lysis syndrome.[4,5] Tumor therapy should be delayed in patients at high risk for development of tumor lysis syndrome until prophylactic measures can be initiated. Unfortunately, a delay in therapy is not possible for many patients because of the aggressive nature of their underlying malignancy. In this clinical situation, a decision must be made regarding the relative risks in the delay of tumor therapy versus the risk of development or exacerbation of tumor lysis syndrome and its associated complications including acute renal failure. Regardless of time constraints, the patient should have reliable venous access and be treated in an intensive care or oncology unit with personnel who are trained and familiar with the complications associated with tumor lysis syndrome. The unit should have, at a minimum, the capability of continuous cardiac monitoring and preferably the capacity for hemodialysis.

The patient's vital signs, weight, urinary output, and fluid intake need to be carefully monitored. Serum creatinine, blood urea nitrogen, sodium, potassium, calcium, phosphorous, LDH and uric acid levels should be determined before therapy and every 6 to 8 hours for the first 48 to 72 hours after the initiation of tumor therapy. The LDH level serves as an excellent marker for tumor proliferation and response to therapy. Patients should have a baseline electrocardiogram and continuous cardiac monitoring until the completion of treatment. Ideally, all patients should receive intravenous hydration 24 to 48 hours before the initiation of tumor therapy.[3,5,39]

Intravenous hydration, preferably with a hypotonic or isotonic saline solution at 2500 to 3000 mL/m^2/24 hours, should begin 24 to 48 hours before the initiation of therapy and continue for 48 to 72 hours after completion of chemotherapy. Care must be taken to prevent severe hyponatremia, especially when hypocalcemia is present, because the risk of seizures is increased.[3] A hypotonic saline solution should be used when the urinary sodium concentration is less than 150 mEq/L to reduce the risk of uric acid supersaturation.[40] The rate and amount of fluid is dependent on each patient's cardiovascular function. Administration of mannitol may be considered if a sufficient diuresis cannot be achieved with intravenous

AN APPROACH TO THE MANAGEMENT AND TREATMENT OF TUMOR LYSIS SYNDROME

	Decreased Urinary Output (<50 mL/h)	Hyperkalemia	Uremia	Hypocalcemia	Hyperuricemia	Hyperphosphatemia
Primary intervention	Mannitol challenge	K+ binding resin		Cautious replacement	Allopurinol or rasburicase	Aluminum hydroxide (200–500 mg/kg)
Clinical manifestation	Renal insufficiency or fluid overload	Arrhythmia	Pericarditis or platelet dysfunction	Arrhythmia or tetany	Renal insufficiency	Renal insufficiency
Secondary intervention	Hemodialysis	Treat arrhythmia	Hemodialysis	Treat arrhythmia	Hemodialysis	Hemodialysis

hydration alone.[3,41] A test dose of 200 to 500 mg/kg may be given intravenously and discontinued if an appropriate increase in urine output is not observed. Careful attention must be given to the administration of both intravenous fluids and mannitol to avoid fluid overload and the potential for congestive heart failure.

In addition, it is necessary to administer a hypouricemic agent, either allopurinol or rasburicase, before the initiation of therapy. Allopurinol is a potent inhibitor of xanthine oxidase and blocks the conversion of hypoxanthine and xanthine to uric acid.[42] Although allopurinol prevents new uric acid formation, it does not reduce the amount of uric acid already present. Thus allopurinol requires administration for 2 to 3 days before the serum uric acid level begins to fall and therefore needs to be initiated 2 to 3 days before the initiation of cytotoxic therapy. Allopurinol is generally given at a dose of at least 600 mg/day.[43] Allopurinol is known to interfere with the degradation of 6-mercaptopurine, 6-thioguanine, and azathioprine through inhibition of the p450 pathway; and the dose of allopurinol should be reduced 50% to 75% in patients receiving these chemotherapeutic agents.[44] Allopurinol should be used with caution in patients with underlying renal insufficiency because it can cause a syndrome consisting of rash, hepatitis, eosinophilia, and worsening renal function.[45] A previous limitation of allopurinol has been the requirement for administration by the oral route. Some critically ill patients or young infants may be unable to tolerate oral medications during the prevention or treatment of tumor lysis syndrome. An intravenous preparation of allopurinol is now available.[46]

An alternative to inhibiting uric acid formation by competitively inhibiting xanthine oxidase is to promote the catabolism of uric acid to allantoin by uric acid oxidase. Allantoin is 5 to 10 times more soluble in the urine than uric acid.[47] Urate oxidase is an endogenous enzyme commonly found in many mammalian species, but unfortunately, not in humans. Urate oxidase, extracted from *Aspergillus flavus*, has been demonstrated to significantly reduce uric acid levels in patients at high risk for tumor lysis syndrome.[48] Recently, the gene coding for urate oxidase was isolated and expressed in yeast to yield large quantities of the pure recombinant form of urate oxidase (rasburicase). In a multicenter trial, 52 pediatric patients with hematologic malignancy at high risk for

tumor lysis syndrome were randomly assigned to receive allopurinol or rasburicase.[49] Uric acid levels significantly decreased by 85% with rasburicase as compared with 12% with allopurinol within 4 hours of drug administration. Rasburicase should be avoided in patients with glucose-6-phosphate dehydrogenase deficiency.

The alkalinization of urine is a controversial area because of the concern about increasing the risk of calcium phosphate precipitation and decreasing the serum concentration of ionized calcium.[5] Systemic alkalosis increases calcium binding to proteins and subsequently decreases the ionized calcium concentration. The rationale behind urinary alkalinization is to raise the urinary pH to decrease the incidence of uric acid precipitation. Fifty to 100 milliequivalents of sodium bicarbonate may be added to each liter of intravenous fluids to obtain an isotonic solution.[3,4] Attempts are made to maintain urinary pH ≥ 7.0. Alkalinization of the urine may be successful in preventing uric acid precipitation but may be unsuccessful in preventing the precipitation of xanthine, which has a pKa of 7.4.[43] Acetazolamide, a carbonic anhydrase inhibitor, may also be used for urinary alkalinization. Acetazolamide is generally administered at a dose of 150 to 500 mg/m^2/day. Acetazolamide is contraindicated in patients with systemic acidosis because it inhibits the renal excretion of hydrogen ions.[1,3]

When time permits, attempts should be made to correct fluid overload or depletion and electrolyte and acid-base abnormalities and to establish adequate urinary output before the initiation of therapy. Caution should be used in calcium replacement for symptomatic hypocalcemia because it may further exacerbate calcium phosphate precipitation.[50] Hyperkalemia should be treated expediently with standard measures such as the administration of sodium polystyrene sulfonate, a potassium-binding resin, at a dose of 15 to 60 g/day given orally. There should be little hesitation about initiating hemodialysis to correct this electrolyte abnormality. Aluminum hydroxide, given orally or through a nasogastric tube at a dose of 15 mL (50 to 150 mg/kg/24 hours) every 4 to 6 hours, should be used to treat hyperphosphatemia. The incidence of tumor lysis syndrome declines after the first 48 to 72 hours of treatment, and a decline in the serum LDH level serves as an excellent marker for a decrease in tumor lysis. However, close monitoring of the patient should continue until treatment is completed.[1,4,5] Treatment of asymptomatic hypocalcemia is generally not recommended. In patients with symptomatic hypocalcemia, intravenous calcium gluconate (50 to 100 mg/kg per dose) may be administered to correct the clinical symptoms; however, this may increase the risk of calcium phosphorus deposition and acute obstructive uropathy.

For patients who have acute renal failure, significant uremia, or severe electrolyte abnormalities associated with tumor lysis syndrome, the general consensus is that hemodialysis should be initiated as soon as possible.[51] Continuous hemofiltration has been used to correct fluid overload and electrolyte abnormalities associated with tumor lysis syndrome in children.[52] The failure to promptly initiate hemodialysis for acute renal failure may turn a potentially reversible clinical situation into an irreversible one.

SUMMARY

Successful management and treatment of tumor lysis syndrome is highly dependent on the prompt identification of clinical and laboratory characteristics, signs, and symptoms of patients at risk. The initiation of prophylactic measures, especially hydration and administration of allopurinol, and the early recognition and treatment of metabolic abnormalities result in the successful avoidance of the severe and life-threatening complications associated with tumor lysis syndrome.

REFERENCES

1. Frei E III, Bentzel CJ, Rieselbach R, Block JB: Renal complications of neoplastic disease. J Chron Dis 1963;16:757.
2. Zusman J, Brown DM, Nesbit ME: Hyperphosphatemia, hyperphosphaturia, and hypocalcemia in acute lymphoblastic leukemia. N Engl J Med 1973;289:1335.
3. Lynch RE, Kjellstrand CM, Coccia PF: Renal and metabolic complications of childhood non-Hodgkin's lymphoma. Semin Oncol 1977;4:325.
4. Cohen LF, Balow JE, Magrath IT, Poplack DG, Ziegler JL: Acute tumor lysis syndrome: A review of 37 patients with Burkitt's lymphoma. Am J Med 1980;68:486.
5. Hande KR, Garrow GC: Acute tumor lysis syndrome in patients with high-grade non-Hodgkin's lymphoma. Am J Med 1993; 94:133.
6. Brereton HD, Anderson T, Johnson RE, Schein PS: Hyperphosphatemia and hypocalcemia in Burkitt's lymphoma: Complications of chemotherapy. Arch Intern Med 1975;135:307.
7. Arseneau JC, Canellos GP, Banks PM, Beard CW, Gralnick HR, DeVita VT Jr: American Burkitt's lymphoma: A clinicopathologic study of 30 cases. I. Clinical factors relating to prolonged survival. Am J Med 1975;58:314.
8. O'Reagan S, Carson S, Chesney RW, Drummond KN: Electrolyte and acid-base disturbances in the management of leukemia. Blood 1977;49:345.
9. Gomez GA, Han T: Acute tumor lysis syndrome in prolymphocytic leukemia. Arch Intern Med 1987;147:375.
10. Cervantes F, Ribera JM, Granena A, Montserrat E, Rozman C: Tumour lysis syndrome with hypocalcemia in accelerated chronic granulocytic leukemia. Acta Haematol 1982;68:157.
11. Przepiorka D, Gonzales-Chambers R: Acute tumor lysis in a patient with chronic myelogenous leukemia in blast crisis: Role of high-dose ara-C. Bone Marrow Transplant 1984;6:281.
12. Boccia RV, Longo DL, Lieber ML, Jaffe ES, Fisher RI: Multiple recurrences of acute tumor lysis syndrome in an indolent non-Hodgkin's lymphoma. Cancer 1985;56:2295.
13. Sparano J, Ramirez M, Wiernik PH: Increasing recognition of corticosteroid induced tumor lysis syndrome in non-Hodgkin's lymphoma. Cancer 1990;65:1072.
14. Stark ME, Morgan MC, Dyer CD, Coonley CJ: Fatal tumor lysis syndrome with metastatic breast carcinoma. Cancer 1989;64:738.
15. Barton JC: Tumor lysis syndrome in nonhematopoietic neoplasms. Cancer 1989;64:738.
16. Tomlinson GC, Solberg LA: Acute tumor lysis syndrome with metastatic medulloblastoma: A case report. Cancer 1984;53:1783.
17. Dirix LY, Prove A, Bequart D, Wouters E, Vermeulen P, VanOosterom A: Tumor lysis syndrome in a patient with metastatic Merkel cell carcinoma. Cancer 1991;67:2207.
18. Kalemkerian GP, Darwish B, Varterasian ML: Tumor lysis syndrome in small cell carcinoma and other solid tumors. Am J Med 1997;103:363.
19. Lehr H, Oppenheimer GD: Anuria following radiation therapy in leukemia. JAMA 1950;143:806.
20. Cech P, Block JB, Cone IA, Stone R: Tumor lysis syndrome after tamoxifen flare. N Engl J Med 1986;315:263.
21. Fer MF, Bottino GC, Sherwin SA, et al: Atypical tumor lysis syndrome in a patient with T cell lymphoma treated with recombinant leukocyte interferon. Am J Med 1984;77:953.
22. Simmons ED, Somberg KA: Acute tumor lysis syndrome after intrathecal methotrexate administration. Cancer 1991;67:2062.
23. Jensen M, Winkler U, Manzke O, Diehl V, Engert A: Rapid tumor lysis in a patient with B-cell chronic lymphocytic leukemia and lymphocytosis treated with an anti-CD20 monoclonal antibody (IDEC-C2B8, rituximab). Ann Hematol 1998;77:89.
24. Dann EJ, Fineman R, Rowe JM: Tumor lysis syndrome after STI571 in Philadelphia chromosome-positive acute lymphoblastic leukemia. J Clin Oncol 2002;20:354.
25. Arseneau JC, Bagley CM, Anderson T: Hyperkalemia, a sequel to chemotherapy of Burkitt's lymphoma. Lancet 1973;1:10.
26. Wilson D, Stewart A, Szwed J, Einhorn LH: Cardiac arrest due to hyperkalemia following therapy for acute lymphoblastic leukemia. Cancer 1977;39:2290.
27. Cohen LF, Balow JE, Magrath IT, Poplack DG, Ziegler JL: Acute tumor lysis syndrome. Am J Med 1980;68:486.
28. Tannock I: Cell kinetics and chemotherapy: A critical review. Cancer Treat Rep 1978;62:1117.
29. Seegmiller JE, Laster L, Howell RR: Biochemistry of uric acid and its relationship to gout. N Engl J Med 1963;268:712.
30. Klinenberg JR, Goldfinger S, Seegmiller JE: The effectiveness of the xanthine oxidase inhibitor allopurinol in the treatment of gout. Ann Intern Med 1965;62:638.
31. Gutman AB, Yu TF: Uric acid nephrolithiasis. Am J Med 1968;45:756.
32. Rieselbach RE, Bentzel CJ, Cotlove E, Frei E III, Freireich EJ: Uric acid excretion and renal function in the acute hyperuricemia of leukemia. Am J Med 1964;37:872.
33. Conger JD, Falk SA: Intrarenal dynamics in the pathogenesis and prevention of acute urate nephropathy. J Clin Invest 1977;59:786.
34. Rigas DA, Duerst ML, Jump ME: The nucleic acids and other phosphorous compounds of human leukemic leukocytes: relation to cell maturity. J Lab Clin Med 1956;48:356.
35. Boles JM, Dutel JL, Briere J, et al: Acute renal failure caused by extreme hyperphosphatemia after chemotherapy of an acute lymphoblastic leukemia. Cancer 1984;53:2425.
36. Ettinger DS, Harker WG, Gerry HW, Sanders RC, Saral R: Hyperphosphatemia, hypocalcemia, and transient renal failure: results of cytotoxic treatment of acute lymphoblastic leukemia. JAMA 1978;239:2472.
37. Rabiner SF: Uremic bleeding. Prog Hemost Thromb 1972;1:233.
38. Newberry WM, Sanford JP: Defective cellular immunity in renal failure: Depression of reactivity of lymphocytes to phytohemagglutinin by renal failure serum. J Clin Invest 1971;50:1262.
39. Schilsky RL: Renal and metabolic toxicities of cancer chemotherapy. Semin Oncol 1982;9:75.
40. Pak CYC, Waters O, Arnold L, Holt K, Cox C, Barilla D: Mechanism for calcium urolithiasis among patients with hyperuricosuria. J Clin Invest 1977;59:526.

41. Barry KG, Hunter RH, Davis TE, Crosby WH: Acute uric acid nephropathy. Arch Intern Med 1963;111:452.

42. Spector T: Inhibition of urate production by allopurinol. Biochem Pharmacol 1977;26:355.

43. Hande KR, Hixson CV, Chabner BA: Postchemotherapy purine excretion in lymphoma patients receiving allopurinol. Cancer Res 1981;41:2273.

44. Rundles RW, Wyngaarden JB, Hitchings GH, et al: Effects of a xanthine oxidase inhibitor on thiopurine metabolism, hyperuricemia and gout. Trans Assoc Am Physicians 1963;76:126.

45. Hande KR, Noone RM, Stone WJ: Severe allopurinol toxicity: Description and guidelines for prevention in patients with renal insufficiency. Am J Med 1984;76:47.

46. Smalley RV, Guaspari A, Haase-Statz S, Anderson SA, Cederberg D, Hohneker JA: Allopurinol: Intravenous use for prevention and treatment of hyperuricemia. J Clin Oncol 2000;18:1758.

47. Brogard JM, Coumaros D, Franckhauser J, Stahl A, Stahl J: Enzymatic uricolysis: A study of the effect of a fungal urate-oxydase. Rev Eur Etud Clin Biol 1972;17:890.

48. Pui CH, Relling MV, Lascombes F, et al: Urate oxidase in prevention and treatment of hyperuricemia associated with lymphoid malignancies. Leukemia 1997;11:1813.

49. Goldman SC, Holcenberg JS, Finklestein JZ, et al: A randomized comparison between rasburicase and allopurinol in children with lymphoma or leukemia at high risk for tumor lysis. Blood 2001;97:2998.

50. Goldsmith RS, Ingbar SH: Inorganic phosphate treatment of hypercalcemia of diverse etiologies. N Engl J Med 1966;274:1.

51. Steinberg SM, Galen MA, Lazarus M, Lazarus JM, Hampers CL, Merrill SP: Hemodialysis for acute anuria uric acid nephropathy. Am J Dis Child 1975;129:956.

52. Bishof NA, Welch TR, Strife F, Ryckman FC: Continuous hemodiafiltration in children. Pediatrics 1990;85:819.

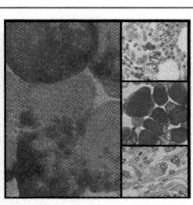

51

PARANEOPLASTIC NEUROLOGIC SYNDROMES

Josep Dalmau

Myrna R. Rosenfeld

SUMMARY OF KEY POINTS

- Paraneoplastic neurologic syndromes include an extensive group of disorders that can affect any part of the central or peripheral nervous system.
- There is evidence that many paraneoplastic neurologic syndromes have an immunopathogenesis and are mediated by immunologic responses triggered by the presence of a cancer.
- Antibodies directly mediate some paraneoplastic disorders of the neuromuscular junction and

peripheral nervous system, such as myasthenia gravis, the Lambert-Eaton myasthenic syndrome, and neuromyotonia. For these disorders and a few paraneoplastic neurologic syndromes of the central nervous system, immunotherapy may result in neurologic improvement.
- For paraneoplastic neurologic syndromes of the central nervous system, the response to any type of therapy is, in general, disappointing, and the main concern should be to rule out other diagnostic

possibilities or uncover the presence of the associated neoplasm.
- Treatment of paraneoplastic neurologic syndromes should be aimed at the tumor, because stabilization and (less often) improvement of neurologic symptoms after tumor treatment have been reported for almost all syndromes. In a few cases, treatment with immunosuppression may have some effect on the paraneoplastic neurologic syndrome.

INTRODUCTION

Clinically significant paraneoplastic neurologic syndromes occur in fewer than 1% of all cancer patients. Paraneoplastic syndromes may affect any part of the neuraxis. In some, a single cell type, such as the Purkinje cells in paraneoplastic cerebellar degeneration (PCD), is predominantly involved; in others, however, any neuron of the central or peripheral nervous system may be affected, as in paraneoplastic encephalomyelitis (PEM) and sensory neuropathy (PSN).[1,2] Because of this variable distribution of pathological involvement, patients with these disorders may present with symptoms of unifocal or multifocal involvement of the nervous system.

The cause of most paraneoplastic neurologic syndromes is unknown, but most are thought to have an immunopathogenesis. One hypothesis is that the expression of neuronal antigens by the tumor triggers an immune response against the tumor, and that immune response affects the nervous system. An immune-mediated pathogenesis has been demonstrated for the Lambert-Eaton myasthenic syndrome (LEMS).[3,4] Patients with LEMS have serum antibodies against voltage-gated calcium channels that are expressed by the tumor, which usually is a small cell lung cancer (SCLC). These antibodies block the entry of calcium necessary for the release of quanta of acetylcholine and result in neuromuscular weakness. Removal of the serum antibodies results in improvement of symptoms. In paraneoplastic myasthenia gravis (MG), a thymoma triggers an immune response against the acetylcholine receptor at the postsynaptic level of the

neuromuscular junction, resulting in weakness and fatigability.[5] A similar antibody-mediated mechanism directed against voltage-gated K+ channels has been reported in paraneoplastic neuromyotonia.[6] Antibodies directed to mGluR1 and voltage-gated calcium channels may be pathogenic in a small subgroup of patient with paraneoplastic cerebellar degeneration.[7,8] Autonomic dysfunction, sometimes associated with cancer, may result from immunity to the nicotinic acetylcholine receptor.[9]

Aside from these syndromes and cancer- and melanoma-associated retinopathy, the immune origin of other paraneoplastic neurologic disorders has not been proved but is supported by several findings. Patients with these disorders have high titers of antibodies that react with antigens restricted to the nervous system and tumor.[10,11] The antibodies are specific markers of characteristic syndromes and tumors and are produced intrathecally.[12,13] Similar antibodies are not found in other inflammatory disorders of the central nervous system associated with neuronal destruction, or with tumors that do not express the specific antigen. Finally, for some paraneoplastic syndromes of the central nervous system there is circumstantial evidence suggesting that T-cell mediated mechanisms play a major pathogenic role. Autopsies of patients with paraneoplastic syndromes of the central nervous system show intense inflammatory infiltrates of mononuclear cells, including CD4+ and CD8+, which predominate in the areas of the nervous system that are symptomatic.[13,14] The mechanism whereby CD4+ or CD8+ cytotoxic T-cells recognize antigens expressed in neurons that normally lack expression of the antigen-presenting major histocompatibility complex (MHC) class I and II molecules is unknown.

Identification of the paraneoplastic origin of a patient's symptoms is important, because in more than two thirds of patients the neurologic symptoms develop before the cancer is detected. Keeping in mind that similar disorders may occur without cancer, diagnosis of a paraneoplastic origin for a disorder depends heavily on the index of suspicion.

This is based in part on the syndrome, because some syndromes are more likely than others to have a paraneoplastic origin. For example, the likelihood that LEMS or subacute cerebellar degeneration in a middle-aged or elderly patient is paraneoplastic is probably more than 50%.[15,16] In contrast, subacute sensory neuropathy or dermatomyositis are probably paraneoplastic in origin in less than 20% of patients.[17,18] In most paraneoplastic syndromes, symptoms develop acutely or subacutely and may resemble a viral process. Symptoms evolve over weeks or months and then stabilize, differentiating them from the more chronic and progressive degenerative diseases of middle age and adulthood.

The finding that some paraneoplastic neurologic syndromes of the central or peripheral nervous system are associated with specific antineuronal antibodies has had a major impact on our ability to diagnose and manage these disorders.[19] These antibodies serve as markers of the paraneoplastic origin of neurologic symptoms and as markers for the presence of specific types of tumors (Table 51-1).

TABLE 51-1

Immune Associations in Paraneoplastic Neurologic Disorders

ANTIBODY	SYNDROME	TUMOR
Anti-Hu	PEM/PSN	SCLC
Anti-Yo	PCD	Ovary, breast
Anti-Ma	Brainstem encephalitis/PCD	Several
Anti-Ma2	Limbic/brainstem encephalitis	Testicular
Anti-Ri	Opsoclonus-ataxia	Breast, gynecologic
Anti-Tr	PCD	Hodgkin's lymphoma
Anti-amphiphysin	Stiff-man syndrome	Breast, SCLC
Anti-CV2/CRMP5	PEM/PCD	SCLC, several
Anti-recoverin	Paraneoplastic retinopathy	SCLC

PCD, paraneoplastic cerebellar degeneration; PEM, paraneoplastic encephalomyelitis; PSN, paraneoplastic sensory neuropathy; SCLC, small cell lung cancer.

PARANEOPLASTIC SYNDROMES OF THE CENTRAL NERVOUS SYSTEM

Paraneoplastic Encephalomyelitis

Patients with paraneoplastic encephalomyelitis (PEM) develop symptoms of multifocal involvement of the nervous system resulting in several syndromes that may occur in isolation or in various combinations.[16] These

---

DIAGNOSIS OF PARANEOPLASTIC NEUROLOGIC SYNDROMES

Diagnosis of a paraneoplastic neurologic syndrome is relatively straightforward in patients who develop symptoms of a well-defined syndrome that typically is associated with cancer. The specificity of paraneoplastic antineuronal antibodies for paraneoplastic neurologic syndromes or some types of cancer makes them useful diagnostic tools. In the right clinical context, therefore, the detection of a paraneoplastic antibody in the serum or cerebrospinal fluid helps to establish the diagnosis and focus the search on the neoplasm. If the detected antibody is one that is not usually associated with the patient's neurologic syndrome, other etiologies for the neurologic dysfunction should be considered. Similarly, if the detected cancer is not the histologic type typically found in association with the patient's antibody (e.g., anti-Yo with lung cancer rather than breast or ovarian cancer), the presence of a second neoplasm should be suspected. A search for another neoplasm is definitely indicated if the tumor cells do not express the target antigen of the paraneoplastic antibody. If paraneoplastic antibodies are present but a cancer is not discovered, it should be assumed that the patient is harboring an occult neoplasm unless proven otherwise. Body positron emission tomographic (PET) scans may detect tumors that escape detection by other standard imaging methods. In patients with a history of cancer or who have recently gone into tumor remission, the development of a paraneoplastic neurologic syndrome often heralds tumor recurrence.

The diagnosis of paraneoplastic neurologic syndromes is more difficult to establish in patients who develop symptoms that are less characteristic (e.g., brainstem dysfunction, myelopathy), especially if no antibodies are found in the serum or cerebrospinal fluid. In such a case, and if other non–cancer-associated etiologies have been ruled out, analysis for serologic markers of cancer (e.g., CEA, CA-125, CA-15-3, PSA) may provide evidence for the presence of cancer. Immunoelectrophoresis may disclose M-proteins in serum or urine, suggesting a plasma cell dyscrasia. A skeletal survey to rule out lytic or osteosclerotic myeloma should be considered for patients with peripheral neuropathy associated with a monoclonal gammopathy. Computed tomographic imaging of the chest is the study of choice to demonstrate a suspected lung cancer. Due to the common association of breast and gynecologic cancers with paraneoplastic disorders, a mammogram and pelvic CT scan or ultrasound should be done in any woman with a suspected paraneoplastic neurologic syndrome. Men with symptoms of limbic and brainstem encephalitis should be examined with testicular ultrasound. Whole-body PET scans are useful when other tests are negative. The best approach for treating paraneoplastic neurologic syndromes is to discover and treat the tumor promptly and provide supportive care for the neurologic deficits with symptomatic treatment and physical therapy.

APPROACH TO THE PATIENT WITH A SUSPECTED PND OR THE CNS

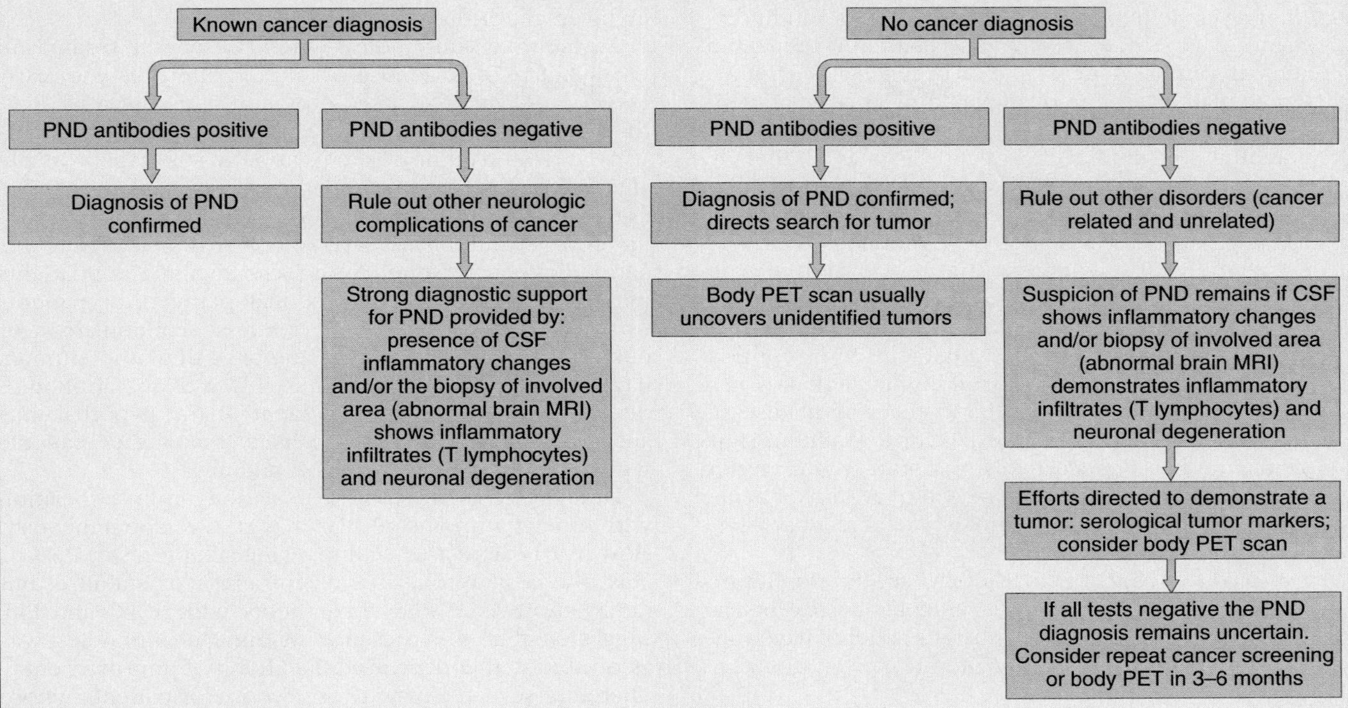

Known cancer diagnosis

- PND antibodies positive
  - Diagnosis of PND confirmed

- PND antibodies negative
  - Rule out other neurologic complications of cancer
  - Strong diagnostic support for PND provided by: presence of CSF inflammatory changes and/or the biopsy of involved area (abnormal brain MRI) shows inflammatory infiltrates (T lymphocytes) and neuronal degeneration

No cancer diagnosis

- PND antibodies positive
  - Diagnosis of PND confirmed; directs search for tumor
  - Body PET scan usually uncovers unidentified tumors

- PND antibodies negative
  - Rule out other disorders (cancer related and unrelated)
  - Suspicion of PND remains if CSF shows inflammatory changes and/or biopsy of involved area (abnormal brain MRI) demonstrates inflammatory infiltrates (T lymphocytes) and neuronal degeneration
  - Efforts directed to demonstrate a tumor: serological tumor markers; consider body PET scan
  - If all tests negative the PND diagnosis remains uncertain. Consider repeat cancer screening or body PET in 3–6 months

51-1

---

include limbic encephalitis, cerebellar degeneration, brainstem encephalitis, myelitis, and sensory and autonomic neuropathies.

Paraneoplastic encephalomyelitis has been described in association with many tumors, but in 70% of patients the underlying tumor is a SCLC. Most tumors are diagnosed within the first 2 years of neurologic presentation. Most patients with PEM and SCLC have high titers of anti-Hu antibodies in their serum and cerebrospinal fluid (CSF), as do some patients with PEM associated with other types cancer.[11,20]

The onset of symptoms is subacute. Sensory neuropathy is the most common initial manifestation, followed by brainstem and limbic encephalopathy.[2,21,22] In general, there is a relentless progression; less frequently, progression of symptoms is intermittent until stabilization. Spontaneous improvement is rare but has been described in patients with limbic encephalitis.[23] For most patients the neurologic deficits are severe and incapacitating. Respiratory or autonomic failure due to neurologic dysfunction is a common cause of death.[2]

About one third of patients with PEM develop symptoms of cerebellar or brainstem dysfunction.[11,22,24,25] Motor weakness, muscle atrophy, and fasciculations are found in 20% of patients with PEM.[2] When spinal cord involvement predominates, a diagnosis of subacute motor neuron dysfunction or atypical motor neuron disease may be considered until other areas of the nervous system become involved.[26,27] Autonomic dysfunction affects about 30% of patients. Symptoms include orthostatic hypotension, gastrointestinal paresis, and pseudo-obstruction.[28,29] Hypothermia, hypoventilation, sleep apnea, and cardiac arrhythmias may be the cause of sudden death in these patients.

About 75% of patients with anti-Hu associated PEM develop an asymmetric pansensory neuropathy known as paraneoplastic sensory neuronopathy (PSN).[2,22] Often associated with painful dysesthesias, PSN results from inflammation of the dorsal root ganglia and neuronal degeneration. For patients in whom motor weakness and a sensory neuropathy develop subacutely, the initial diagnosis may be of acute inflammatory polyneuritis (Guillain-Barré syndrome).[30]

Paraneoplastic Limbic Encephalitis

Symptoms of paraneoplastic limbic encephalitis (PLE) may develop alone but more commonly are found in association with brainstem dysfunction, cerebellar symptoms, or PSN (see the section on PEM).[2] The most common underlying tumor is SCLC, followed by testicular cancer. Regardless of the tumor type, the neurologic dysfunction usually precedes the diagnosis of cancer.

The most characteristic finding is short-term memory deficits with relative preservation of other cognitive functions.[31,32] Memory deficits often become evident after several weeks of depression, personality changes, irritability, and seizures. Partial complex temporal lobe

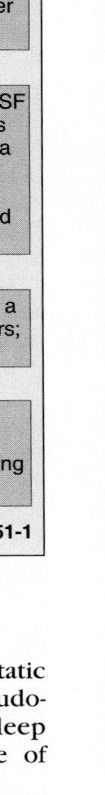

Problems Common to Cancer and Its Therapy

seizures, with or without motor involvement of the face and extremities, are common. Some patients develop signs of diencephalic-hypothalamic dysfunction, including drowsiness, hyperthermia, hyperphagia, and, less often, pituitary hormonal deficits. The disorder may resemble a viral encephalitis or a rapidly developing dementia due to a primary neurodegenerative disorder.

Paraneoplastic limbic encephalitis is one of the few paraneoplastic neurologic disorders in which neuro-imaging may be useful. Typical MRI findings include unilateral or bilateral mesial temporal lobe abnormalities best seen on T2-weighted and fluid attenuation inversion recovery (FLAIR) images (Fig. 51-1).[23,33,34] On T1 sequences, the temporal-limbic regions may be hypo-intense and sometimes may enhance with contrast injection. Patients with herpes simplex encephalitis may have similar MRI findings in the early stages of the disease. However, these patients usually develop prominent signs of edema and mass effect involving one or both inferior-medial temporal lobes, inferior frontal lobes, and cingulate gyrus, often associated with gyral enhancement and signs of hemorrhage.[35,36]

The major findings on pathology are in the hippo-campus, parahippocampal gyrus, cingular cortex, insular cortex, and diencephalon.[32] Almost all patients have mild abnormalities in other areas of the nervous system in a pattern of distribution resembling PEM, suggesting that PLE should be regarded as PEM with predominant involvement of the limbic structures.

Antineuronal antibodies, when present in serum and CSF, facilitate the diagnosis of PLE and often allow for early detection of the associated tumor. In patients with SCLC, the anti-Hu antibody is present in about 50% of cases with predominant or isolated symptoms of limbic enceph-alitis.[37] A few patients have been reported with limbic encephalitis and anti-CV2 antibodies. In these patients the underlying tumors are SCLC and thymoma.[38] Anti-Ma2 antibodies may be found in the serum and CSF of patients with limbic or brainstem encephalopathy; these patients usually have testicular cancer (either seminomatous or nonseminomatous germ cell tumors), but other tumors have been reported.[13] Patients with anti-Ma2 antibodies often have additional involvement of the hypothalamus and brainstem and are more likely than other patients with PLE to have abnormal MRI findings.[39]

Limbic encephalopathy, in isolation or in association with other symptoms of PEM, may resolve spontaneously. However, if there are accompanying symptoms of PEM or PSN, these symptoms usually progress or stabilize, but rarely improve. A study of patients with SCLC and PLE suggested that the presence of anti-Hu antibodies was associated with a decreased likelihood of improvement.[37] There are several isolated case reports of patients whose limbic encephalopathy improved after treatment of the tumor.[13,40,41] In some patients the early use of cortico-steroids seemed to be partially effective.

Paraneoplastic Cerebellar Degeneration

Paraneoplastic cerebellar degeneration (PCD) is charac-terized by the subacute development of rapidly pro-gressive cerebellar dysfunction that stabilizes after a few months, leaving the patient severely disabled.[25] Postmortem studies demonstrate nearly or total loss of Purkinje cells with relative preservation of other cerebellar neurons and Bergmann astrogliosis (Fig. 51-2). Almost every type of tumor has been reported in association with PCD; the most common neoplasms are gynecologic tumors, breast and lung cancers, and lymphomas.[42] In about 60% of patients the neurologic symptoms precede the detection of the tumor.

Presenting symptoms of PCD include dizziness, visual problems, nausea, vomiting, and dysarthria. Within days or even hours the patient develops ataxia of gait and extremities, usually accompanied by dysphagia. Some patients with PCD who have gynecologic or breast tumors have serum and CSF antibodies called anti-Yo that react with 34 and 62-kDa proteins expressed by Purkinje cells and the underlying tumor.[43] Other patients develop PCD that is not associated with anti-Yo antibodies. Some of these patients have PCD in association with Hodgkin disease, in which case the antibody anti-Tr usually is found (Fig. 51-3).[44]

For patients with SCLC, paraneoplastic cerebellar degeneration may develop in association with LEMS.[42,45] Symptoms of LEMS often are treatable, so suspicion that it may be present should prompt an appropriate investi-

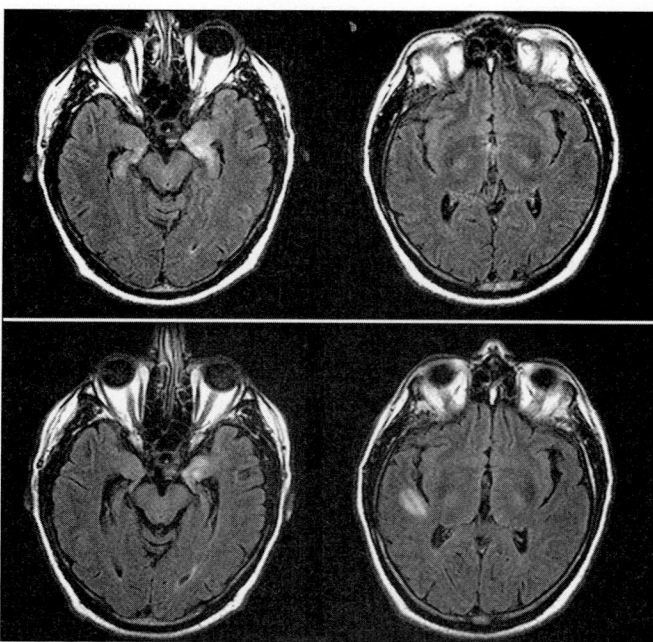

Figure 51-1. Abnormalities seen on magnetic resonance imaging (MRI). Fluid-attenuated inversion recovery (FLAIR) sequences from two MRI studies performed on a patient with paraneoplastic limbic encephalitis associated with a papillary thyroid carcinoma that was confined to the thyroid gland. The top panels show bilateral hyperintensity of the medial aspect of the temporal lobes (hippocampi), with the left greater than the right. Another MRI scan obtained 6 months later (*lower panels*) shows atrophy of the hippocampi and new signal abnormality in the right posterior insular region. The patient had severe short-term memory loss, with no significant changes between the two MRI studies.

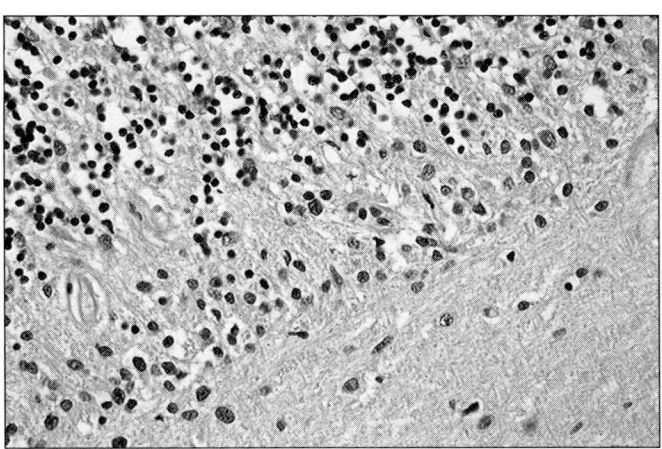

Figure 51-2. Section of cerebellum from a patient with adenocarcinoma of the ovary and paraneoplastic cerebellar degeneration associated with anti-Yo antibodies. Bergmann gliosis is seen, and Purkinje cells, which normally are located between the granular cell layer (*top left*) and the molecular cell layer (*bottom right*), are absent.

gation with electrophysiologic testing or measurement of antibodies directed against P/Q-type voltage-gated calcium channels. Recent studies demonstrate that these antibodies also may be present in some patients with SCLC and PCD who do not have symptoms of LEMS.[8]

A distinctive clinical syndrome that occurs predominantly in women is characterized by the subacute onset of ataxia and opsoclonus.[46] The ataxia occurs predominantly in the trunk, causing severe gait difficulty and frequent falls. In half of these patients neurologic symptoms develop before the diagnosis of the tumor, which usually is found to be a breast cancer. The serum

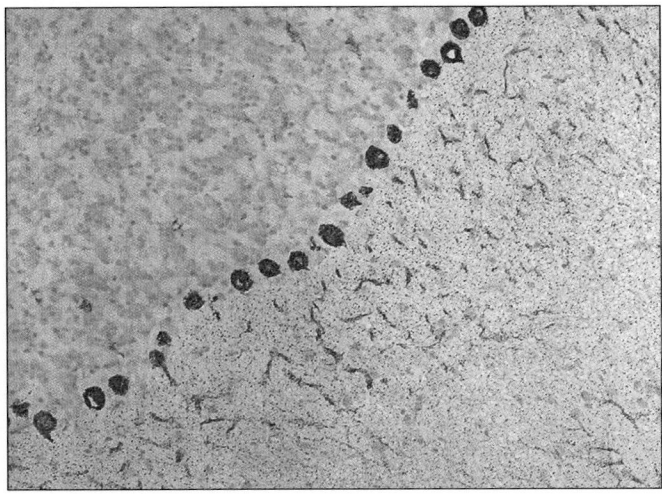

Figure 51-3. Detection of an anticerebellar antibody (anti-Tr) in the serum of a patient with paraneoplastic cerebellar degeneration. A frozen section of rat cerebellum incubated with the serum of the patient shows a characteristic dot-like reactivity with the cytoplasm of Purkinje cells and molecular layer of the cerebellum. This antibody, anti-Tr, is a specific marker of paraneoplastic cerebellar degeneration associated with Hodgkin lymphoma.

and CSF of these patients contain an antibody called anti-Ri, which is expressed by neurons and the associated tumor.[46,47]

Patients with SCLC can develop PCD with and without anti-Hu antibodies. When anti-Hu antibodies are present, the PCD is a component of the syndrome of PEM.[2,22] These patients eventually develop signs and symptoms of multifocal neurologic disease.

A subgroup of patients develops PCD in the setting of brainstem dysfunction. These patients have serum and spinal fluid antibodies against Ma1 and Ma2 proteins expressed in neurons and spermatogenic cells of testis. These patients have a variety of associated cancers, including lung, breast, parotid, and colon.[48]

Necrotizing Myelopathy

Necrotizing myelopathy is a rare syndrome that has been described in association with various carcinomas and lymphoma.[49,50] The symptomatology and pathology are identical to those of viral myelitis due to herpes simplex virus type 2. Patients present with the acute or subacute onset of ascending spinal cord dysfunction resulting in a flaccid, areflexic paraplegia.[51] This may be preceded or accompanied by back or radicular pain. Symptoms progress over days to weeks, with death often resulting from respiratory failure. No treatment has been shown to be effective.

Examination of the CSF may reveal a mild pleocytosis with elevated proteins but often it is acellular.[52] Myelography may be normal or show swelling of the spinal cord. In one study, the MRI scan of a patient with non-SCLC and a biopsy consistent with necrotizing myelopathy demonstrated increased T2 signal and patchy contrast enhancement in the mid- to upper thoracic cord.[53]

The diagnosis of necrotizing myelopathy requires the exclusion of other potentially treatable causes of spinal cord dysfunction, such as metastatic cord compression, leptomeningeal metastasis, and intramedullary cord metastasis. Postradiation myelopathy also should be considered, but can be distinguished by the history and a longer, insidious onset with slow progression over months to years.[16]

Motor Neuron Syndromes

The concept of paraneoplastic motor neuron dysfunction is based on reports of patients with typical amyotrophic lateral sclerosis (ALS) who improved after treatment of the underlying tumor, suggesting a relation that is more than coincidental.[54,55] In patients with cancer and symptoms of motor neuron disease, the most common neoplasms are carcinoma of the lung, breast, and lymphoma. For these patients the neurologic syndrome and laboratory studies are similar to those typically seen in patients with ALS.

Patients with PEM may develop symptoms resembling those of motor neuron disease.[2,26] These patients almost always develop signs of involvement of other areas of the nervous system, which, along with the presence of the anti-Hu antibody, helps to rule out typical ALS.

Patients with both Hodgkin and non-Hodgkin lymphoma may develop a subacute lower motor neuronopathy.[56-58] Typically, these patients have a subacute, progressive, painless, and asymmetrical involvement of the extremities with the legs more affected than the arms. In contrast to typical ALS, fasciculations are rare, bulbar muscles usually are spared, and upper motor neuron signs are absent. The CSF is normal or shows mildly increased proteins, and electrophysiologic studies demonstrate denervation with normal or mild slowing of motor nerve conduction velocities. Neurologic stabilization or spontaneous improvement may occur. Paraneoplastic subacute lower motor neuronopathy must be distinguished from the lower motor neuron dysfunction that patients may develop after radiation therapy of the spinal cord.[59]

Muscle Rigidity, Stiff-man Syndrome, and Neuromyotonia

Paraneoplastic muscle rigidity and stiffness are associated with neuromyotonia, encephalomyelitis, and stiff-man syndrome. Neuromyotonia is characterized by muscle stiffness, myokymia, and delayed muscle relaxation. It often is found in association with a sensorimotor polyneuropathy and has been described most often in patients with thymoma and SCLC.[60,61] An autoimmune etiology for neuromyotonia is supported by the presence of serum antibodies that interfere with the function of voltage-gated potassium ion channels.[62] Electrophysiologic studies reveal large numbers of bizarre, high-frequency motor unit discharges during voluntary contraction that persist during relaxation. This is in contrast to patients with stiff-man syndrome, who have continuous but relatively normal motor unit activity.[63] Treatment with phenytoin, carbamazepine, or plasma exchange may be effective in some patients.

The stiff-man syndrome is an unusual disorder characterized by progressive muscle stiffness, aching, muscle spasms, and rigidity. The stiffness develops over months and is most prominent in the paraspinal muscles and lower limbs. The muscle spasms are painful and are triggered by a variety of stimuli. They are severe enough to produce limb deformities and fractures.[64] There are no other associated neurologic abnormalities; CSF may show oligoclonal bands and increased IgG index, and neuroradiologic studies are usually normal. The tumors most commonly involved include breast cancer, SCLC, and thymoma. A subset of patients with paraneoplastic stiff-man syndrome and breast cancer or SCLC have antibodies that react with amphiphysin, a neuronal synaptic protein.[64-66] When stiff-man syndrome occurs in patients who do not have cancer, the disorder is associated with antibodies against glutamic acid decarboxylase (GAD).[67,68] These patients usually develop diabetes and other endocrine deficits. Treatment of the tumor with corticosteroids or intravenous immunoglobulin (IVIg) may lead to improvement.

A rare disorder seen in patients with cancer is progressive encephalomyelitis with rigidity.[69] This most often is associated with SCLC. Patients with this disorder usually develop brainstem dysfunction, rigidity, and spinal myoclonus due to widespread dysfunction of the central nervous system. The cervical portion of the spinal cord is most commonly affected.[70]

Paraneoplastic Opsoclonus-Myoclonus

Opsoclonus is a disorder of ocular motility characterized by the presence of spontaneous, arrhythmic, large-amplitude conjugate saccades occurring in all directions of gaze without a saccadic interval.[71] In cancer patients, opsoclonus can have a paraneoplastic origin, in which case it often is associated with myoclonus of the head, trunk, or extremities (paraneoplastic opsoclonus-myoclonus). The differential diagnosis includes viral, toxic, metabolic, and vascular disorders.

In children, paraneoplastic opsoclonus-myoclonus is a well known complication of neuroblastoma.[72,73] In half of these patients, the opsoclonus is detected before the neuroblastoma is diagnosed, but it may develop after the tumor is diagnosed, during remission, or at recurrence. The onset is subacute with frequent fluctuations of symptoms; in some patients symptoms may resolve spontaneously. Treatment with steroids or adrenocorticotropic hormone (ACTH), or treatment of the tumor, results in improvement in one half to two thirds of patients.[74] Despite an initial response, however, about 60% of patients are left with permanent neurologic deficits, including language and cognitive dysfunction.[75]

Paraneoplastic opsoclonus-myoclonus also has been described in adult patients with cancer. Most of these patients have an underlying SCLC, although there are individual case reports associated with other tumors including carcinomas of the uterus, fallopian tube, breast, bladder, thyroid, and thymus; chondrosarcoma; and Hodgkin disease.[71,76-78] A small number of cases of women with breast cancer, anti-Ri antibodies, and opsoclonus have been reported.[46,79] Patients with anti-Ri antibodies often have other symptoms suggesting a more diffuse involvement of the brainstem, whereas patients without anti-Ri antibodies tend to have limb or truncal myoclonus and encephalopathy.

Compared to the idiopathic form of opsoclonus-myoclonus, from which patients often recover, paraneoplastic opsoclonus-myoclonus in adults has a more severe clinical course, even when treated aggressively with IVIg or corticosteroids. For those patients who develop an associated encephalopathy, one series noted improved outcomes in those patients whose tumors (usually SCLC) were promptly identified and treated.[80] At present, there are no immunologic markers to identify the adult patients with paraneoplastic opsoclonus-myoclonus. A recent study found a high incidence of autoimmune responses to a variety of neuronal autoantigens but did not identify a specific antibody marker.[81]

Paraneoplastic Syndromes of the Visual System

In patients with cancer, visual symptoms and blindness usually are related to metastatic infiltration of the optic nerves by tumor and neurotoxicity from chemotherapy and radiation therapy.[82-85] Paraneoplastic visual syndromes can result from retinopathy and optic neuritis. Paraneoplastic optic neuritis is very rare. It may develop in isolation, but usually it is associated with PEM.[86] The onset is subacute with painless bilateral visual loss.[87,88]

The paraneoplastic retinopathies are a heterogeneous group of syndromes including cancer- and melanoma-associated retinopathy. These two syndromes have specific clinical, electrophysiologic, and pathological characteristics and distinct immunologic associations. Patients with cancer-associated retinopathy develop acute or subacute visual loss due to degeneration of the retinal photoreceptor or ganglion cells.[89,90] The onset usually is unilateral, but progresses to become bilateral over days or weeks. Initial symptoms include photosensitivity, light-induced glare, color vision deficits, intermittent visual obscurations, and central or ring-like scotomas. For most patients the underlying tumor is a SCLC, but there have been a few case reports associated with breast or gynecologic cancers. Visual symptoms usually are detected before the tumor is diagnosed. Visual evoked responses usually are normal, but electroretinograms demonstrate reduced or flat responses to photopic and scotopic stimuli suggesting dysfunction of cones and rods. Examination of the CSF may reveal a mild pleocytosis, and neuroimaging studies are normal.

The serum of some patients with paraneoplastic retinopathy contains antibodies that react with antigens expressed by photoreceptors and ganglion cells. The most common antibody is against recoverin, a 23-kd photoreceptor calcium binding protein,[91] and the presence of anti-recoverin antibodies almost always indicates that the associated tumor is a SCLC.[92] These antibodies cause apoptotic retinal cell death, suggesting a direct pathogenic role.[93] Other antigens that are targets of immune responses in some patients include tubby-like protein 1 and the photoreceptor-specific nuclear receptor (PNR).[94,95] Although the role of the latter antibodies in the pathogenesis of the retinopathy is unknown, mutations of the PNR gene have been identified in a cohort of patients with enhanced s-cone syndrome, a disorder of retinal cell development that progresses to retinal degeneration.[96,97] This suggests a mechanism whereby antibodies interfere with autoantigen function, resulting in retinal cell death.

Melanoma-associated retinopathy (MAR) has been described in patients with metastatic cutaneous melanoma. These patients present with acute visual loss years or months after the diagnosis of the metastatic disease.[98,99] These patients have serum antibodies that target unidentified proteins localized in the bipolar cells of the retina.[100,101] The electroretinogram shows selective loss of the photopic "b" wave with relative preservation of the "a" and "d" wave forms. Intraocular injection of serum from patients with MAR reproduces the retinal abnormalities, demonstrating that the antibodies are pathogenic.[99]

For both paraneoplastic retinopathy and MAR, the visual loss usually is irreversible. Treatment with immunosuppression, plasma exchange, or steroids usually is ineffective, but in rare cases it may result in symptom stabilization.[102,103]

PARANEOPLASTIC SYNDROMES OF THE PERIPHERAL NERVOUS SYSTEM

Paraneoplastic Sensory Neuronopathy

Paraneoplastic sensory neuronopathy (PSN) resulting from dorsal root ganglia dysfunction may develop in isolation but most often is a fragment of PEM. Patients typically develop asymmetric pain and paresthesias that can mimic radiculopathy or multineuropathy.[104] Symptoms usually progress over weeks or months to involve other extremities and sometimes the trunk.[2] Cranial nerves may be affected, resulting in loss of taste, facial numbness, and sensorineural deafness. Eventually there is severe involvement of all modalities of sensation, resulting in pseudoathetotic movements of the hands, a debilitating sensory gait ataxia, and neuropathic pain that are difficult to control.

In more than 80% of patients with PSN the associated tumor is SCLC. Sensory symptoms usually precede the diagnosis of the tumor. Electrophysiologic studies confirm the isolated or predominant involvement of the sensory pathways, but in some patients motor conduction velocities may be affected.[105] These patients show evidence of both demyelination and axonal degeneration in association with loss of neurons in the dorsal root ganglia.

Patients who develop PSN as a component of paraneoplastic encephalomyelitis often have anti-Hu antibodies, and the associated cancer is almost always a SCLC (Fig. 51-4).[2,22] For those patients with PSN without anti-Hu antibodies, associated cancers include SCLC, non-SCLC lung tumors and breast cancer. Except for the detection of anti-Hu antibodies in patients with SCLC, laboratory studies of patients with PSN are nonrevealing. The CSF may show increased proteins and a mononuclear pleocytosis.

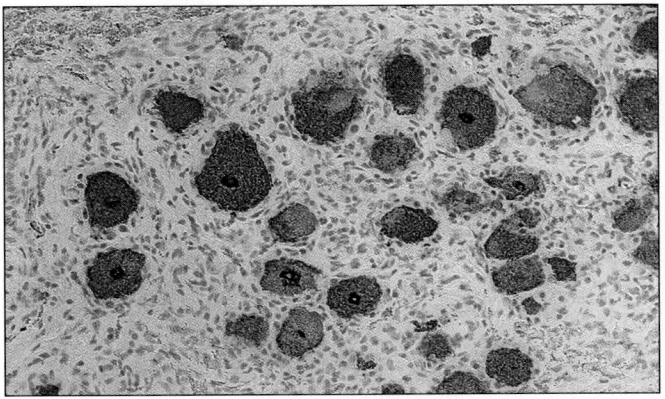

Figure 51-4. Detection of an antineuronal antibody (anti-Hu) in the serum of a patient with paraneoplastic sensory neuronopathy. A frozen section of rat dorsal root ganglion incubated with the serum of the patient shows intense immunolabeling of the neurons, with reactivity predominantly involving the nuclei. This antibody, anti-Hu, usually is associated with paraneoplastic sensory neuronopathy (or dorsal-root ganglionitis) and encephalomyelitis. Patients with anti-Hu antibodies usually harbor a small cell lung cancer.

Sensorimotor Neuropathies

Many patients with cancer, particularly those with advanced disease and significant weight loss, develop signs and symptoms of peripheral neuropathy. In most patients an identifiable cause such as a nutritional deficit, hepatic or renal failure, the use of chemotherapeutic agents, or leptomeningeal metastases can be found. Mononeuropathies and plexopathies in cancer patients most often are secondary to compression of nerves by tumor or hemorrhage and infarction secondary to leukemic infiltration.[106,107] A paraneoplastic brachial neuritis may occur with increased frequency in patients with Hodgkin disease.[108,109] The clinical presentation is similar to that of brachial neuritis observed in patients without cancer, with the initial pain complaints followed by the development of paresthesias and weakness.

A subacute or chronic sensorimotor neuropathy may occur with any malignancy but most commonly is associated with lung cancers.[106,110] The onset usually follows the cancer diagnosis, but it may precede it by several months or years. Lower extremities are involved predominantly, with symptoms spreading proximally over the course of the disease with rare involvement of cranial nerves. Weakness develops late, and most patients have slowly progressive disease.

An acute rapidly progressive sensorimotor polyneuropathy can be seen in association with Hodgkin lymphoma.[111] The syndrome is clinically indistinguishable from Guillain-Barré syndrome (GBS). A similar syndrome has been reported in patients with solid tumors. These patients have the same response to plasma exchange and IVIg as those with idiopathic GBS, and a few patients develop a relapsing and remitting course.

Approximately 10% of patients with multiple myeloma develop a clinically significant neuropathy. The neuropathy, most often sensorimotor, commonly precedes the diagnosis of the myeloma and is slowly progressive.[112] Treatment of the myeloma usually does not alter the course of the neuropathy. Other causes of peripheral nerve or nerve root involvement include deposits of amyloid and root compression by spine metastases. Osteosclerotic myeloma represents about 3% of all cases of myeloma. More than 50% of these patients develop a predominantly motor paraneoplastic peripheral neuropathy that often is the initial presentation of the myeloma.[113] The clinical picture is similar to that of chronic inflammatory demyelinating polyneuropathy.[114] Resection or radiation of the sclerotic lesions often results in neurologic improvement.[112]

Ten percent of patients with Waldenström macroglobulinemia develop a peripheral neuropathy with predominant sensory involvement. In some, the monoclonal IgM has activity against myelin-associated glycoprotein or gangliosides.[115]

The POEMS syndrome (polyneuropathy, organomegaly, endocrinopathy, monoclonal proteinemia, and skin changes) is a rare disorder that can develop in association with any form of myeloma but occurs most often with osteosclerotic myeloma.[114,116,117] Patients develop a severe, symmetric, sensorimotor neuropathy that is associated with muscle atrophy.

Vasculitic Neuropathy

Paraneoplastic vasculitis may be systemic or confined to nerve and muscle. When systemic, the small vessels of the skin commonly are affected. The most frequently associated tumors are lymphomas and leukemias.[118,119] A paraneoplastic microvasculitis of the muscle and nerve without systemic vasculitis has been reported in older patients with solid tumors, particularly carcinoma of the prostate, kidney, lung, endometrium, and lymphoma.[120] These patients develop symptoms of symmetric or asymmetric painful sensorimotor neuropathy. As a result of the muscle vasculitis, patients can develop proximal muscle weakness. The diagnosis is suggested by the presence of elevated proteins in CSF and an elevated erythrocyte sedimentation rate and confirmed by biopsy of nerve and muscle. This disorder may respond to steroids and cyclophosphamide or other types of immunosuppression.

Autonomic Neuropathy

Paraneoplastic autonomic neuropathy usually occurs as a component of other disorders, such as LEMS and PEM, but may rarely occur as the predominant symptom.[2] These patients can develop several life-threatening complications, such as gastrointestinal paresis with pseudo-obstruction, cardiac dysrhythmias, and postural hypotension. Additional symptoms include dry mouth, erectile dysfunction, anhidrosis, and sphincter dysfunction. Paraneoplastic autonomic neuropathy has been reported in association with several tumors, including SCLC, cancer of the pancreas, cancer of the testis, carcinoid tumors, and lymphoma. When the autonomic dysfunction is a component of PEM, serum anti-Hu and anti-CV2/CRMP5 antibodies may be positive. Serum antibodies to ganglionic acetylcholine receptors have been reported, but they also occur without a cancer association.[121]

PARANEOPLASTIC SYNDROMES OF THE NEUROMUSCULAR JUNCTION

Myasthenia Gravis

Myasthenia gravis (MG) results from an immune response directed against the acetylcholine receptor at the neuromuscular junction. Thymic abnormalities are reported to occur in approximately 75% of patients with MG. Of these, 15% have microscopic or gross evidence of thymoma and 85% have evidence of thymic hyperplasia. Most patients develop weakness of the extremities and the ocular and bulbar muscles, but a few patients have pure ocular involvement.[5,122] The most common presenting signs are ptosis and intermittent diplopia. Proximal muscles tend to be more affected than distal muscles, and muscle atrophy is rare. Deep tendon reflexes are preserved. Pain usually is not reported, although some patients complain of paresthesias. Aspiration secondary to dysphagia and ventilatory paralysis secondary to respiratory muscle involvement may be causes of death.[123]

The initial approach to treatment should be directed at the underlying tumor. Additional therapeutic strategies, including symptomatic treatment (e.g., anticholinesterase drugs), immunomodulation (e.g., plasma exchange, IVIg), and immunosuppression (e.g., steroids, azathioprine, and others) are similar for patients with and without cancer.

Lambert-Eaton Myasthenic Syndrome

The Lambert-Eaton myasthenic syndrome (LEMS) is a disorder of the neuromuscular junction in which the presence of autoantibodies against P/Q type voltage-gated calcium channels results in a defect in the presynaptic quantal release of acetylcholine.[4,124,125] Approximately 60% of patients with LEMS have an associated SCLC.[15] In most patients, the neurologic symptoms develop before (70%) or at the same time (25%) that the tumor diagnosis is made.[126]

Patients present with lower extremity weakness, increased fatigability, and difficulties walking, rising from a chair, or climbing stairs. Some patients report a brief increase in muscle strength following a period of activity. Nerve conduction studies show a very low amplitude compound muscle action potential that increases progressively (>200%) in response to fast rates (20–50 Hz) of repetitive stimulation or after a short period of maximum voluntary contraction (Fig. 51-5). Detection of antibodies against the P/Q type voltage gated calcium channel currently is used as a serologic test for LEMS.[124]

At least 50% of patients have evidence of autonomic dysfunction such as dry mouth, impotence, constipation, or impaired sweating.[15,127,128] Mild and usually transient cranial nerve dysfunction occurs in the majority of patients.[129] Although rare, respiratory muscle weakness may occur, even to the point of requiring assisted ventilation. In contrast to MG, where the deep tendon reflexes are usually spared, in LEMS they are reduced or absent, especially in the lower extremities. In some patients, LEMS may develop in association with PCD or PEM.[8,42]

When LEMS is associated with cancer, most patients will experience neurologic improvement with combined cancer treatment and therapy directed toward the LEMS.

The latter includes medications that increase the presynaptic release of acetylcholine and immunomodulation. The use of 3,4-diaminopyridine results in moderate to marked neurologic improvement in 80% of patients.[130] If 3,4-diaminopyridine is not available, a combination of pyridostigmine and guanidine may be beneficial.[131] Plasma exchange and IVIg are useful for treating patients with severe weakness.[132] Neurologic improvement occurs within days or weeks but is transient. For patients who are refractory to these treatments, long-term immunosuppression with prednisone or azathioprine may be effective. Patients whose neurologic symptoms relapse should be evaluated for tumor recurrence.

PARANEOPLASTIC MYOPATHIC SYNDROMES

Polymyositis-Dermatomyositis

About 9% of patients with polymyositis develop cancer. Because the neoplasm often is diagnosed several years before or after the diagnosis of the polymyositis, this connection may represent a coincidental occurrence and casts doubt on the role of cancer in the pathogenesis of the neurologic disorder.[17] In contrast, 15% of patients with dermatomyositis develop cancer, and in most patients the tumor is diagnosed by the time the myopathic symptoms develop.[17] Cancers of the breast, lung, ovary, and stomach are the most commonly associated tumors.

Clinical symptoms are similar for patients with and without cancer.[133] Patients with dermatomyositis may present with a reddish or purplish skin rash that often precedes the onset of proximal muscle weakness. Serum creatine kinase levels are usually but not always elevated. Respiratory muscle weakness may lead to ventilatory failure and contribute to death. Other symptoms include arthralgias and muscle contractures, myocardial inflammation leading to congestive heart failure, and interstitial lung disease.[134] Reflexes and sensory exam are usually normal.

Several autoantibodies have been identified in patients with polymyositis and dermatomyositis. Jo-1 antibodies are identified in a group of patients with either disorder

Figure 51-5. Electrophysiologic study of a patient with small cell lung cancer and the Lambert-Eaton myasthenic syndrome. **A,** Facilitation of the compound motor action potential (CMAP) seen after 10 seconds of maximal voluntary contraction. **B,** Progressive increase of the CMAP amplitude with high-frequency repetitive stimulation. These are the classic electrophysiologic findings in patients with LEMS.

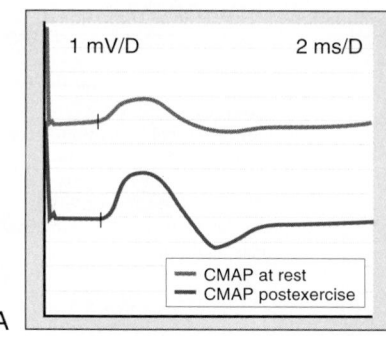

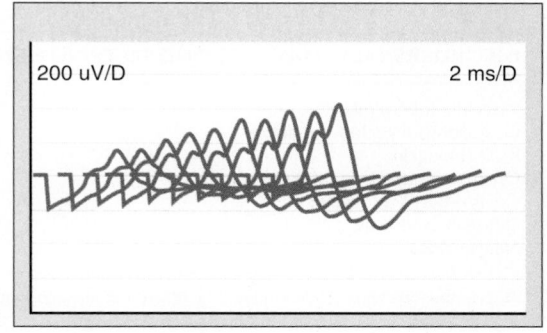

and are associated with interstitial lung disease.[135,136] Antinuclear antibodies typical of other connective tissue diseases also can be detected.[137] There are no specific markers indicative of the paraneoplastic origin of dermatomyositis. Dermatomyositis and polymyositis usually respond to corticosteroids and other types of immunosuppression (e.g., azathioprine). High-dose IVIg has proven to be effective for dermatomyositis.

Acute Necrotizing Myopathy

Acute necrotizing myopathy has been described in patients with cancer of the lung, bladder, breast, and gastrointestinal tract.[138] Patients present with symmetric weakness of the extremities associated with pain and a marked increase of serum muscle enzymes. Symptoms progress rapidly to involve pharyngeal and respiratory muscles, often resulting in death. The electrophysiologic studies are consistent with myopathy, and pathology studies demonstrate extensive muscle necrosis with little or no inflammatory infiltrates. It has been suggested that acute necrotizing myopathy represents a severe and more rapid form of polymyositis, but this remains unproven.[139]

TREATMENT AND PROGNOSIS

In general, the neurologic paraneoplastic syndromes of the central nervous system have a subacute, progressive course that in weeks or months results in severe deficits or death.[2,43] Spontaneous improvement has been observed in some patients with opsoclonus-myoclonus, mostly children with neuroblastoma,[140] PCD associated with Hodgkin disease,[44,141] subacute motor neuronopathy,[57] and sensorimotor neuropathies that usually fulfill the criteria of acute or chronic Guillain-Barré syndrome.[111,142,143] Progression to severe disability is seen less

often in the neuromuscular disorders that develop after the diagnosis of the tumor, such as some sensorimotor neuropathies. A few patients with anti-Hu–associated sensory neuronopathy, and patients with PCD, particularly those without anti-Yo antibodies, may have a mild, indolent clinical course or even stabilize with only moderate neurologic deficits.[42,144] A classification of the paraneoplastic neurologic disorders by expected treatment response is given in Table 51-2.

Improvement of neurologic symptoms after tumor treatment has been reported for almost all the paraneoplastic syndromes.[145] However, the actual impact of antineoplastic therapy on the paraneoplastic symptoms is difficult to assess. This difficulty is due in part to the low incidence of neurologic paraneoplastic syndromes and the lack of effective treatment for some neoplasms. The rapid and apparently irreversible neuronal damage that is characteristic of many paraneoplastic symptoms may allow potentially effective treatments to arrest, but not revert, the neurological symptoms. Despite these limitations in assessment, some patients with limbic encephalitis have neurologic improvement, which appears to relate to tumor treatment.[23]

For those paraneoplastic disorders of the peripheral nervous system associated with pathogenic antibodies (e.g., MG, LEMS, neuromyotonia), removal of the antibodies,[146] treatment of the tumor (removing the source of antigen), or immunosuppression often is effective.[147] For other paraneoplastic disorders, the symptoms sometimes evolve independently of the course of the tumor. An exception is osteosclerotic myeloma, in which treatment of the myeloma can result in dramatic improvement of an associated sensorimotor neuropathy.[148-150]

Immunosuppressive treatments including corticosteroids, IVIg, and plasma exchange have been used in paraneoplastic syndromes that appear to result from immune-mediated mechanisms.[145,151] These include

TABLE 51-2

Treatment Response of Paraneoplastic Disorders

DISORDERS THAT USUALLY RESPOND TO TREATMENT	TREATMENT
Myasthenia gravis	Tumor, plasmapheresis, IVIg, immunosuppression
Lambert-Eaton myasthenic syndrome	Tumor, plasmapheresis, IVIg, 3,4 diaminopyridine
Dermatomyositis	Steroids, IVIg, immunosuppression
Opsoclonus/myoclonus (pediatric)	Tumor, corticosteroids, ACTH
Carcinoid myopathy	Tumor, cyproheptadine
Neuropathy (osteosclerotic myeloma)	Tumor, radiation
DISORDERS THAT MAY RESPOND TO TREATMENT	
Vasculitis (nerve/muscle)	Steroids
Opsoclonus/myoclonus (adults)	Tumor, steroids, protein A column, clonazepam, diazepam, baclofen
PCD (Hodgkin)	Tumor
Opsoclonus/ataxia (anti-Ri–associated)	Steroids, plasmapheresis
Guillain-Barré (Hodgkin)	Tumor, plasmapheresis, IVIg
Stiff-man syndrome	Tumor, steroids, diazepam, baclofen, IVIg
Neuromyotonia	Plasmapheresis

ACTH, adrenocorticotropic hormone; IVIg, intravenous immunoglobulin demyelinating sensorimotor neuropathies, vasculitic neuropathy[152] and dermatomyositis.[153,154] In these disorders, clinical improvement can be expected after treatment because the area of the nervous system involved is not irreversibly damaged. Large series examining plasma exchange and IVIg in paraneoplastic disorders of the CNS have not shown any significant benefit.[155,156] There are however, individual case reports of improvements.[80,157-159]

REFERENCES

1. Verschuuren J, Chuang L, Rosenblum MK, et al: Inflammatory infiltrates and complete absence of Purkinje cells in anti-Yo-associated paraneoplastic cerebellar degeneration. Acta Neuropathol (Berl) 1996;91:519-525.
2. Dalmau J, Graus F, Rosenblum MK, Posner JB: Anti-Hu-associated paraneoplastic encephalomyelitis/sensory neuronopathy. A clinical study of 71 patients. Medicine 1992;71:59-72.
3. Fukunaga H, Engel AG, Lang B, et al: Passive transfer of Lambert-Eaton myasthenic syndrome with IgG from man to mouse depletes the presynaptic membrane active zones. Proc Natl Acad Sci USA 1983;80:7636-7640.
4. Lang B, Newsom-Davis J, Wray D, et al: Autoimmune aetiology for myasthenic (Eaton-Lambert) syndrome. Lancet 1981;2:224-226.
5. Drachman DB: Myasthenia gravis. N Engl J Med 1994;330: 1797-1810.
6. Hart IK, Waters C, Vincent A, et al: Autoantibodies detected to expressed K+ channels are implicated in neuromyotonia. Ann Neurol 1997;41:238-246.
7. Sillevis SP, Kinoshita A, De Leeuw B, et al: Paraneoplastic cerebellar ataxia due to autoantibodies against a glutamate receptor. N Engl J Med 2000;342:21-27.
8. Fukuda T, Motomura M, Nakao Y, et al: Reduction of P/Q-type calcium channels in the postmortem cerebellum of paraneoplastic cerebellar degeneration with Lambert-Eaton myasthenic syndrome. Ann Neurol 2003;53:21-28.
9. Lennon VA, Ermilov LG, Szurszewski JH, Vernino S: Immunization with neuronal nicotinic acetylcholine receptor induces neurological autoimmune disease. J Clin Invest 2003;111: 907-913.
10. Furneaux HM, Rosenblum MK, Dalmau J, et al: Selective expression of Purkinje-cell antigens in tumor tissue from patients with paraneoplastic cerebellar degeneration. N Engl J Med 1990;322:1844-1851.
11. Dalmau J, Furneaux HM, Gralla RJ, et al: Detection of the anti-Hu antibody in the serum of patients with small cell lung cancer— a quantitative western blot analysis. Ann Neurol 1990;27:544-552.
12. Furneaux HM, Reich L, Posner JB: Autoantibody synthesis in the central nervous system of patients with paraneoplastic syndromes. Neurology 1990;40:1085-1091.
13. Voltz R, Gultekin SH, Rosenfeld MR, et al: A serologic marker of paraneoplastic limbic and brain-stem encephalitis in patients with testicular cancer N Engl J Med 1999;340:1788-1795.
14. Jean WC, Dalmau J, Ho A, Posner JB: Analysis of the IgG subclass distribution and inflammatory infiltrates in patients with anti-Hu-associated paraneoplastic encephalomyelitis. Neurology 1994;44:140-147.
15. O'Neill JH, Murray NM, Newsom-Davis J: The Lambert-Eaton myasthenic syndrome. A review of 50 cases. Brain 1988;111: 577-596.
16. Posner JB: Neurologic Complications of Cancer. Philadelphia: FA Davis, 1995.
17. Sigurgeirsson B, Lindelof B, Edhag O, Allander E: Risk of cancer in patients with dermatomyositis or polymyositis. A population-based study. N Engl J Med 1992;326:363-367.
18. Hochberg MC, Feldman D, Stevens MB: Adult onset polymyositis/dermatomyositis: an analysis of clinical and laboratory features and survival in 76 patients with a review of the literature. Semin Arthritis Rheum 1986;15:168-178.
19. Dalmau JO, Posner JB: Paraneoplastic syndromes affecting the nervous system. Semin Oncol 1997;24:318-328.
20. Graus F, Cordon-Cardo C, Posner JB: Neuronal antinuclear antibody in sensory neuronopathy from lung cancer. Neurology 1985;35:538-543.
21. Lucchinetti CF, Kimmel DW, Lennon VA: Paraneoplastic and oncologic profiles of patients seropositive for type 1 antineuronal nuclear autoantibodies. Neurology 1998;50:652-657.
22. Graus F, Keime-Guibert F, Rene R, et al: Anti-Hu-associated paraneoplastic encephalomyelitis: analysis of 200 patients. Brain 2001;124:1138-1148.
23. Gultekin SH, Rosenfeld MR, Voltz R, et al: Paraneoplastic limbic encephalitis: neurological symptoms, immunological findings, and tumor association in 50 patients. Brain 2000;123:1481-1494.
24. Henson RA, Hoffman HL, Urich H: Encephalomyelitis with carcinoma. Brain 1965;88:449-464.
25. Henson RA, Urich HE: Cancer and the Nervous System: The Neurological Manifestations of Systemic Malignant Disease. London: Blackwell Scientific, 1982.
26. Forsyth PA, Dalmau J, Graus F, et al: Motor neuron syndromes in cancer patients. Ann Neurol 1997;41:722-730.
27. Verma A, Berger JR, Snodgrass S, Petito C: Motor neuron disease: a paraneoplastic process associated with anti-Hu antibody and small-cell lung carcinoma. Ann Neurol 1996;40:112-116.
28. Veilleux M, Bernier JP, Lamarche JB: Paraneoplastic encephalomyelitis and subacute dysautonomia due to an occult atypical carcinoid tumour of the lung. Can J Neurol Sci 1990;17:324-328.
29. Lennon VA, Sas DF, Busk MF, et al: Enteric neuronal autoantibodies in pseudoobstruction with small- cell lung carcinoma. Gastroenterology 1991;100:137-142.
30. Graus F, Elkon KB, Lioberes P, et al: Neuronal antinuclear antibody (anti-Hu) in paraneoplastic encephalomyelitis simulating acute polyneuritis. Acta Neurol Scand 1987;75:249-252.
31. Corsellis JA, Goldberg GJ, Norton AR: "Limbic encephalitis" and its association with carcinoma. Brain 1968;91:481-496.
32. Bakheit AM, Kennedy PG, Behan PO: Paraneoplastic limbic encephalitis: clinico-pathological correlations. J Neurol Neurosurg Psychiatr 1990;53:1084-1088.
33. Dirr LY, Elster AD, Donofrio PD, Smith M: Evolution of brain MRI abnormalities in limbic encephalitis. Neurology 1990;40: 1304-1306.
34. Lacomis D, Khosbin S, Schich RM: MR imaging of paraneoplastic limbic encephalitis. J Comput Assist Tomogr 1990;14:115-117.
35. Demaerel P, Wilms G, Robberecht W, et al: MRI of herpes simplex encephalitis. Neuroradiology 1992;34:490-493.
36. Kapur N, Barker S, Burrows EH, et al: Herpes simplex encephalitis: long term magnetic resonance imaging and neuropsychological profile. J Neurol Neurosurg Psychiatry 1994;57:1334-1342.
37. Alamowitch S, Graus F, Uchuya M, et al: Limbic encephalitis and small cell lung cancer—clinical and immunological features. Brain 1997;120:923-928.
38. Honnorat J, Antoine JC, Derrington E, et al: Antibodies to a subpopulation of glial cells and a 66 kDa developmental protein in patients with paraneoplastic neurological syndromes. J Neurol Neurosurg Psychiatry 1996;61:270-278.
39. Rosenfeld MR, Eichen J, Wade D, et al: Molecular and clinical diversity in paraneoplastic immunity to Ma proteins. Ann Neurology 2001;50:339-348.
40. Markham M, Abeloff MD: Small-cell lung cancer and limbic encephalitis. Letter to the editor. Ann Intern Med 1982;96:785.
41. Pfliegler G, Posan E, Glaub D, et al: Hodgkin's disease and memory loss: another case of the Ophelia syndrome. Br J Haematol 1990;74:232.
42. Mason WP, Graus F, Lang B, et al: Small-cell lung cancer, paraneoplastic cerebellar degeneration and the Lambert-Eaton myasthenic syndrome. Brain 1997;120:1279-1300.
43. Peterson K, Rosenblum MK, Kotanides H, Posner JB: Paraneoplastic cerebellar degeneration. I. A clinical analysis of 55 anti-Yo antibody-positive patients. Neurology 1992;42:1931-1937.
44. Graus F, Dalmau J, Valldeoriola F, et al: Immunological characterization of a neuronal antibody (anti-Tr) associated with paraneoplastic cerebellar degeneration and Hodgkin's disease. J Neuroimmunol 1997;74:55-61.
45. Clouston PD, Saper CB, Arbizu T, et al: Paraneoplastic cerebellar degeneration. III. Cerebellar degeneration, cancer, and the

Lambert-Eaton myasthenic syndrome. Neurology 1992;42:
1944-1950.

46. Luque FA, Furneaux HM, Ferziger R, et al: Anti-Ri: an antibody
associated with paraneoplastic opsoclonus and breast cancer. Ann
Neurol 1991;29:241-251.

47. Sutton IJ, Barnett MH, Watson JD, et al: Paraneoplastic brainstem
encephalitis and anti-Ri antibodies. J Neurol 2002;249:1597-1598.

48. Dalmau J, Gultekin SH, Voltz R, et al: Ma1, a novel neuronal and
testis specific protein, is recognized by the serum of patients with
paraneoplastic neurologic disorders. Brain 1999;122:27-39.

49. Grisold W, Lutz D, Wolf D: Necrotizing myelopathy associated with
acute lymphoblastic leukemia. Case report and review of
literature. Acta Neuropathol (Berl) 1980;49:231-235.

50. Ojeda VJ: Necrotizing myelopathy associated with malignancy. A
clinicopathologic study of two cases and literature review. Cancer
1984;53:1115-1123.

51. Mancall EL, Rosales RK: Necrotizing myelopathy associated with
visceral carcinoma. Brain 1964;87:639-656.

52. Handforth A, Nag S, Sharp D, Robertson DM: Paraneoplastic
subacute necrotic myelopathy. Can J Neurol Sci 1983;10:
204-207.

53. Glantz MJ, Biran H, Myers ME, et al: The radiographic diagnosis
and treatment of paraneoplastic central nervous system disease.
Cancer 1994;73:168-175.

54. Rosenfeld MR, Posner JB: Paraneoplastic motor neuron disease.
Adv Neurology 1991;56:445-459.

55. Gordon PH, Rowland LP, Younger DS, et al: Lymphoproliferative
disorders and motor neuron disease: an update. Neurology
1997;48:1671-1678.

56. Rowland LP, Schneck SA: Neuromuscular disorders associated
with malignant neoplastic disease. J Chron Dis 1963;16:777-795.

57. Schold SC, Cho ES, Somasundaram M, Posner JB: Subacute motor
neuronopathy: a remote effect of lymphoma. Ann Neurol
1979;5:271-287.

58. Walton JN, Tomlinson BE, Pearce GW: Subacute "poliomyelitis" and
Hodgkin's disease. J Neurol Sci 1968;6:435-445.

59. Sadowsky CH, Sachs E Jr, Ochoa J: Postradiation motor neuron
syndrome. Arch Neurol 1976;33:786-787.

60. Walsh JC: Neuromyotonia: an unusual presentation of
intrathoracic malignancy. J Neurol Neurosurg Psychiatry
1976;39:1086-1091.

61. Garcia-Merino A, Cabello A, Mora JS, Liano H: Continuous muscle
fiber activity, peripheral neuropathy, and thymoma. Ann Neurol
1991;29:215-218.

62. Shillito P, Molenaar PC, Vincent A, et al: Acquired neuromyotonia:
evidence for autoantibodies directed against K+ channels of
peripheral nerves. Ann Neurol 1995;38:714-722.

63. Kasperek S, Zebrowski S: Stiff-man syndrome and encephalomyelitis. Report of a case. Arch Neurol 1971;24:22-30.

64. Folli F, Solimena M, Cofiell R, et al: Autoantibodies to a 128-kd
synaptic protein in three women with the stiff-man syndrome
and breast cancer. N Engl J Med 1993;328:546-551.

65. David C, Solimena M, De Camilli P: Autoimmunity in stiff-man
syndrome with breast cancer is targeted to the C-terminal region
of human amphiphysin, a protein similar to the yeast proteins,
Rvs167 and Rvs161. FEBS Letters 1994;351:73-79.

66. De Camilli P, Thomas A, Cofiell R, et al: The synaptic vesicle-
associated protein amphiphysin is the 128- kD autoantigen of
stiff-man syndrome with breast cancer. J Exp Med
1993;178:2219-2223.

67. Solimena M, Folli F, Aparisi R, et al: Autoantibodies to GABA-ergic
neurons and pancreatic beta cells in stiff-man syndrome. N Engl J
Med 1990;322:1555-1560.

68. Vincent A, Grimaldi LM, Martino G, et al: Antibodies to 125I-
glutamic acid decarboxylase in patients with stiff man syndrome.
J Neurol Neurosurg Psychiatry 1997;62:395-397.

69. Whitely AM, Swash M, Urich H: Progressive encephalomyelitis
with rigidity. Brain 1976;99:27-42.

70. Roobol TH, Kazzaz BA, Vecht CJ: Segmental rigidity and spinal
myoclonus as a paraneoplastic syndrome. J Neurol Neurosurg
Psychiatry 1987;50:628-631.

71. Dropcho E, Payne R: Paraneoplastic opsoclonus-myoclonus.
Association with medullary thyroid carcinoma and review of the
literature. Arch Neurol 1986;43:410-415.

72. Dyken P, Kolar O: Dancing eyes, dancing feet: infantile poly-
myoclonia. Brain 1968;91:305-320.

73. Pranzatelli MR: The immunopharmacology of the opsoclonus-
myoclonus syndrome. Clin Neuropharmacol 1996;19:1-47.

74. Dropcho EJ, Kline LB, Riser J: Antineuronal (anti-Ri) antibodies in a
patient with steroid-responsive opsoclonus-myoclonus. Neurology
1993;43:207-211.

75. Russo C, Cohn SL, Petruzzi MJ, de Alarcon PA: Long-term
neurologic outcome in children with opsoclonus-myoclonus
associated with neuroblastoma: a report from the Pediatric
Oncology Group. Med Pediatr Oncol 1997;28:284-288.

76. Kay CL, Davies-Jones GAB, Singal R, Winfield DA: Paraneoplastic
opsoclonus-myoclonus in Hodgkin's disease. J Neurol Neurosurg
Psychiatry 1993;56:831-832.

77. Ridley A, Kennard C, Scholtz CL, et al: Omnipause neurons in two
cases of opsoclonus associated with oat cell carcinoma of the
lung. Brain 1987;110:1699-1709.

78. Scholz J, Vieregge P, Ruff C: Paraneoplastic opsoclonus-myoclonus
syndrome in metastatic ovarian carcinoma. J Neurol Neurosurg
Psychiatry 1994;57:763-764.

79. Budde-Steffen C, Anderson NE, Rosenblum MK, et al: An
antineuronal autoantibody in paraneoplastic opsoclonus. Ann
Neurol 1988;23:528-531.

80. Bataller L, Graus F, Saiz A, Vilchez JJ: Clinical outcome in adult
onset idiopathic or paraneoplastic opsoclonus-myoclonus. Brain
2001;124:437-443.

81. Bataller L, Rosenfeld MR, Graus F, et al: Autoantigen diversity in the
opsoclonus-myoclonus syndrome. Ann Neurol 2003;53:347-353.

82. Coppeto JR, Monteiro M, Cannarozzi DB: Optic neuropathy
associated with chronic lymphomatous meningitis. J Clin
Neuroophthalmol 1988;8:39-45.

83. Al-Tweigeri T, Magliocco AM, DeCoteau JF: Cortical blindness as a
manifestation of hypomagnesemia secondary to cisplatin therapy:
case report and review of literature. Gynecol Oncol 1999;72:
120-122.

84. Sakai C, Takagi T, Wakatsuki S: Primary meningeal lymphoma
presenting solely with blindness: a report of an autopsy case. Int J
Hematol 1996;63:325-329.

85. Pomeranz HD, Henson JW, Lessell S: Radiation-associated cerebral
blindness. Am J Ophthalmol 1998;126:609-611.

86. Akihiko O, Inoue T, Fukuda N, et al: A case with paraneoplastic
optic neuropathy presenting bitemporal hemianopsia.
Neuroopthalmol 1991;11:325-328.

87. Pillay N, Gilbert JJ, Ebers GC, et al: Internuclear ophthalmoplegia
and "optic neuritis": paraneoplastic effects of bronchial
carcinoma. Neurology 1984;34:788-791.

88. Hoogenraad TU, Sanders E, Tan K: Paraneoplastic optic neuritis
and encephalomyelitis, report of a case. Neuroophthalmol
1989;9:247-250.

89. Jacobson DM, Thirkill CE, Tipping SJ: A clinical triad to diagnose
paraneoplastic retinopathy. Ann Neurol 1990;28:162-167.

90. Jacobson DM, Thirkill CE: Paraneoplastic cone dysfunction: an
unusual visual remote effect of cancer. Arch Ophthalmol
1995;113:1580-1582.

91. Adamus G, Guy J, Schmied JL, et al: Role of anti-recoverin
autoantibodies in cancer-associated retinopathy. Invest
Ophthalmol Vis Sci 1993;34:2626-2633.

92. Polans AS, Burton MD, Haley TL, et al: Recoverin, but not visinin, is
an autoantigen in the human retina identified with a cancer-
associated retinopathy. Invest Ophthalmol Vis Sci 1993;34:81-90.

93. Shiraga S, Adamus G: Mechanism of CAR syndrome: anti-recoverin
antibodies are the inducers of retinal cell apoptotic death via the
caspase 9- and caspase 3-dependent pathway. J Neuroimmunol
2002;132:72-82.

94. Kikuchi T, Arai J, Shibuki H, et al: Tubby-like protein 1 as an
autoantigen in cancer-associated retinopathy. J Neuroimmunol
2000;103:26-33.

95. Eichen JG, Dalmau J, Demopoulos A, et al: The photoreceptor
cell-specific nuclear receptor is an autoantigen of paraneoplastic
retinopathy. J Neuroophthalmol 2001;21:168-172.

96. Marmor MF, Jacobson SG, Foerster MH, et al: Diagnostic clinical
findings of a new syndrome with night blindness, maculopathy,
and enhanced S cone sensitivity. Am J Ophthalmol 1990;110:
124-134.

97. Haider NB, Jacobson SG, Cideciyan AV, et al: Mutation of a nuclear receptor gene, NR2E3, causes enhanced S cone syndrome, a disorder of retinal cell fate. Nat Genet 2000;24:127–131.

98. Singh AD, Milam AH, Shields CL, et al: Melanoma-associated retinopathy. Am J Ophthalmol 1995;119:369–370.

99. Lei B, Bush RA, Milam AH, Sieving PA: Human melanoma-associated retinopathy (MAR) antibodies alter the retinal ON-response of the monkey ERG in vivo. Invest Ophthalmol Vis Sci 2000;41:262–266.

100. Weinstein JM, Kelman SE, Bresnick GH, Kornguth SE: Paraneoplastic retinopathy associated with antiretinal bipolar cell antibodies in cutaneous malignant melanoma. Ophthalmology 1994;101:1236–1243.

101. Milam AH, Saari CJ, Jacobson SG, et al: Autoantibodies against retinal bipolar cells in cutaneous melanoma-associated retinopathy. Invest Ophthalmol Visual Sci 1993;34:91–100.

102. Keltner JL, Thirkill CE: Cancer-associated retinopathy vs recoverin-associated retinopathy. Am J Ophthalmol 1998;126:296–302.

103. Keltner JL, Thirkill CE, Tyler NK, et al: Management and monitoring of cancer-associated retinopathy. Arch Ophthalmol 1992;110:48–53.

104. Chalk CH, Windebank AJ, Kimmel DW, McManis PG: The distinctive clinical features of paraneoplastic sensory neuronopathy. Can J Neurol Sci 1992;19:346–351.

105. Camdessanche JP, Antoine JC, Honnorat J, et al: Paraneoplastic peripheral neuropathy associated with anti-Hu antibodies. A clinical and electrophysiological study of 20 patients. Brain 2002;125:166–175.

106. Vital C, Vital A, Julien J, et al: Peripheral neuropathies and lymphoma without monoclonal gammopathy: a new classification. J Neurol 1990;237:177–185.

107. Haberland C, Cipriani M, Kucuk O, et al: Fulminant leukemic polyradiculoneuropathy in a case of B-cell prolymphocytic leukemia. Cancer 1987;60:1454–1458.

108. Pezzimenti JF, Bruckner HW, DeConti RC: Paralytic brachial neuritis in Hodgkin's disease. Cancer 1973;31:626–632.

109. Lachance DH, O'Neill BP, Harper CM Jr, et al: Paraneoplastic brachial plexopathy in a patient with Hodgkin's disease. Mayo Clin Proc 1991;66:97–101.

110. Antoine JC, Mosnier JF, Absi L, et al: Carcinoma associated paraneoplastic peripheral neuropathies in patients with and without anti-onconeural antibodies. J Neurol Neurosurg Psychiatry 1999;67:7–14.

111. Lisak RP, Mitchell M, Zweiman B, et al: Guillain-Barré syndrome and Hodgkin's disease: three cases with immunological studies. Ann Neurol 1977;1:72–78.

112. Kelly JJ Jr, Kyle RA, Miles JM, et al: The spectrum of peripheral neuropathy in myeloma. Neurology 1981;31:24–31.

113. Dellagi K, Dupouey P, Brouet JC, et al: Waldenstrom's macroglobulinemia and peripheral neuropathy: a clinical and immunologic study of 25 patients. Blood 1983;62:280–285.

114. Nakanishi T, Sobue I, Toyokura Y, et al: The Crow-Fukase syndrome: a study of 102 cases in Japan. Neurology 1984;34:712–720.

115. Cruz M, Jiang Y-P, Ernerudh J, et al: Antibodies to myelin-associated glycoprotein are found in cerebrospinal fluid in polyneuropathy associated with monoclonal serum IgM. Arch Neurol 1991;48:66–70.

116. Milanov I, Georgiev D: Polyneuropathy, organomegaly, endocrinopathy, monoclonal gammopathy and skin changes (POEMS) syndrome. Can J Neurol Sci 1994;21:60–63.

117. Miralles GD, O'Fallon JR, Talley NJ: Plasma-cell dyscrasia with polyneuropathy. The spectrum of POEMS syndrome. N Engl J Med 1992;327:1919–1923.

118. Hayem G, Gomez MJ, Grossin M, et al: Systemic vasculitis and epithelioma. A report of three cases with a literature review. Rev Rhum Engl Ed 1997;64:816–824.

119. Sanchez-Guerrero J, Gutierrez-Urena S, Vidaller A, et al: Vasculitis as a paraneoplastic syndrome. Report of 11 cases and review of the literature. J Rheumatol 1990;17:1458–1462.

120. Oh SJ: Paraneoplastic vasculitis of the peripheral nervous system. Neurol Clin 1997;15:849–863.

121. Vernino S, Adamski J, Kryzer TJ, et al: Neuronal nicotinic ACh receptor antibody in subacute autonomic neuropathy and cancer-related syndromes. Neurology 1998;50:1806–1813.

122. McQuillen MP: Ocular myasthenia gravis. Arch Neurol 1997;54:229.

123. Quera-Salva MA, Guilleminault C, Chevret S, et al: Breathing disorders during sleep in myasthenia gravis. Ann Neurol 1992;31:86–92.

124. Motomura M, Johnston I, Lang B, et al: An improved diagnostic assay for Lambert-Eaton myasthenic syndrome. J Neurol Neurosurg Psychiatry 1995;58:85–87.

125. Elmqvist D, Lambert EH: Detailed analysis of neuromuscular transmission in a patient with the myasthenic syndrome sometimes associated with bronchogenic carcinoma. Mayo Clin Proc 1968;43:689–713.

126. Sanders DB: Lambert-Eaton myasthenic syndrome: clinical diagnosis, immune- mediated mechanisms, and update on therapies. Ann Neurol 1995;37:S63–S73.

127. O'Suilleabhain P, Low PA, Lennon VA: Autonomic dysfunction in the Lambert-Eaton myasthenic syndrome: serologic and clinical correlates. Neurology 1998;50:88–93.

128. Riva M, Brioschi AM, Marazzi R, et al: Immunological and endocrinological abnormalities in paraneoplastic disorders with involvement of the autonomic nervous system. Ital J Neurol Sci 1997;18:157–161.

129. Clark CV, Newsom-Davis J, Sanders MD: Ocular autonomic nerve function in Lambert-Eaton myasthenic syndrome. Eye 1990;4:473–481.

130. Lundh H, Nilsson O, Rosen I, Johansson S: Practical aspects of 3,4-diaminopyridine treatment of the Lambert-Eaton myasthenic syndrome. Acta Neurol Scand 1993;88:136–140.

131. Oh SJ, Kim DS, Head TC, Claussen GC: Low-dose guanidine and pyridostigmine: Relatively safe and effective long-term symptomatic therapy in Lambert-Eaton myasthenic syndrome. Muscle Nerve 1997;20:1146–1152.

132. Bain PG, Motomura M, Newsom-Davis J, et al: Effects of intravenous immunoglobulin on muscle weakness and calcium-channel autoantibodies in the Lambert-Eaton myasthenic syndrome. Neurology 1996;47, 678–683.

133. Griggs RC, Mendell JR, Miller RG: Inflammatory myopathies. I. Evaluation and Treatment of Myopathies. Philadelphia, FA Davis, 1995, pp 154–210.

134. Poveda GF, Merino JL, Mate I, et al: Polymyositis associated with anti-Jo1 antibodies: severe cardiac involvement as initial manifestation. Am J Med 1993;94:110–111.

135. Marie I, Hatron PY, Hachulla E, et al: Pulmonary involvement in polymyositis and in dermatomyositis. J Rheumatol 1998;25:1336–1343.

136. Dalakas MC: Immunopathogenesis of inflammatory myopathies. Ann Neurol 1995;37:S74–S75.

137. Hietarinta M, Meyer O, Haim T, et al: Antinuclear and antinucleolar antibodies in patients with scleroderma- polymyositis overlap syndrome. Br J Rheumatol 1996;35:1326–1327.

138. Levin MI, Mozaffar T, Al Lozi MT, Pestronk A: Paraneoplastic necrotizing myopathy: clinical and pathological features. Neurology 1998;50:764–767.

139. Vosskamper M, Korf B, Franke F, Schachenmayr W: Paraneoplastic necrotizing myopathy: a rare disorder to be differentiated from polymyositis. J Neurol 1989;236:489–492.

140. Lott I, Kinsbourne M: Myoclonic encephalopathy of infants. Adv Neurol 1986;43:127–136.

141. Hammack J, Kotanides H, Rosenblum MK, Posner JB: Paraneoplastic cerebellar degeneration. II. Clinical and immunologic findings in 21 patients with Hodgkin's disease. Neurology 1992;42:1938–1943.

142. Croft PB, Urich H, Wilkinson M: Peripheral neuropathy of sensorimotor type associated with malignant disease. Brain 1967;90:31–66.

143. Hussein KK, Shaw MT, Oleinick SR: Autoimmune thrombocytopenia and peripheral neuropathy heralding Hodgkin's disease. South Med J 1975;68:1414–1416.

144. Graus F, Bonaventura I, Uchuya M, et al: Indolent anti-Hu-associated paraneoplastic sensory neuropathy. Neurology 1994;44:2258–2261.

145. Rosenfeld MR, Dalmau J: Current therapies for paraneoplastic neurologic syndromes. Curr Treat Options Neurol 2003;5:69–77.

Problems Common to Cancer and Its Therapy

146. Newsom-Davis J, Murray NM: Plasma exchange and immunosuppressive drug treatment in the Lambert-Eaton myasthenic syndrome. Neurology 1984;34:480–485.

147. Chalk CH, Murray NM, Newsom-Davis J, et al: Response of the Lambert-Eaton myasthenic syndrome to treatment of associated small-cell lung carcinoma. Neurology 1990;40:1552–1556.

148. Benito-Leon J, Lopez-Rios F, Rodriguez-Martin FJ, et al: Rapidly deteriorating polyneuropathy associated with osteosclerotic myeloma responsive to intravenous immunoglobulin and radiotherapy. J Neurol Sci 1998;158:113–117.

149. Rotta FT, Bradley WG: Marked improvement of severe polyneuropathy associated with multifocal osteosclerotic myeloma following surgery, radiation, and chemotherapy. Muscle Nerve 1997;20:1035–1037.

150. Parra R, Fernandez JM, Garcia-Bragado F, et al: Successful treatment of peripheral neuropathy with chemotherapy in osteosclerotic myeloma. J Neurol 1987;234:261–263.

151. Graus F, Delattre J-Y: Immune modulation of paraneoplastic neurologic disorders. Clin Neurol Neurosurg 1995;97:112–116.

152. Oh SJ, Slaughter R, Harrell L: Paraneoplastic vasculitic neuropathy: a treatable neuropathy. Muscle Nerve 1991;14:152–156.

153. Dalakas MC: Polymyositis, dermatomyositis, and inclusion-body myositis. N Engl J Med 1991;325:1487–1498.

154. Dalakas MC, Illa I, Dambrosia JM, et al: A controlled trial of high-dose intravenous immune globulin infusions as treatment for dermatomyositis. N Engl J Med 1993;329:1993–2000.

155. Graus F, Vega F, Delattre J-Y, et al: Plasmapheresis and antineoplastic treatment in CNS paraneoplastic syndromes with antineuronal autoantibodies. Neurology 1992;42:536–540.

156. Uchuya M, Graus F, Vega F, et al: Intravenous immunoglobulin treatment in paraneoplastic neurological syndromes with antineuronal autoantibodies. J Neurol Neurosurg Psychiatry 1996;60:388–392.

157. Cher LM, Hochberg FH, Teruya J, et al: Therapy for paraneoplastic neurologic syndromes in six patients with protein A column immunoadsorption. Cancer 1995;75:1678.

158. Cocconi G, Ceci G, Juvarra G: Successful treatment of subacute cerebellar degeneration in ovarian carcinoma with plasmapheresis. A case report. Cancer 1985;56:2318.

159. Counsell CE, McLeod M, Grant R: Reversal of subacute paraneoplastic cerebellar syndrome with intravenous immunoglobulin. Neurology 1994;44:1184.

ESTABLISHING AND MAINTAINING VASCULAR ACCESS

John C. Mansour

John E. Niederhuber

SUMMARY OF KEY POINTS

- More than 500,000 vascular access devices are used in the United States each year.
- Catheter tip in SVC or IVC provides large lumen and high flow.
- Types of central access systems:
  - Traditional central line for short-term use
  - Tunneled central lines for long-term use
  - Surgically implanted infusion ports
  - Peripherally inserted central catheters (PICC lines)
- Three questions to ask when selecting a catheter system:
  - What device best meets the patient's therapy needs?
  - How is the device most safely inserted and maintained?

- What are the likely immediate and long-term complication risks in this patient?
- Vascular access devices can be placed using a number of anatomic sites to access SVC or IVC: subclavian vein, internal jugular vein, external jugular vein, and femoral vein.
- Insertion can occur via Seldinger technique (closed) or by operative exposure of vein (open) technique.
- Complications include vascular laceration, arterial puncture, pneumothorax (2%), hemothorax, and air embolus (overall placement complications should be <5%).
- Long-term complications include catheter exit site or tract infection,

catheter-associated sepsis, cardiac arrhythmias, catheter colonization, catheter thrombus (~30%), fibrin sheath, extravasation, occluded catheter, and shearing of catheter.
- Factors increasing risk of catheter-associated infection:
  - Prolonged duration of indwelling time
  - Multiple-lumen catheters
  - Femoral or internal jugular vein locations
  - Non–catheter-related bacteremia (neutropenic patient)
  - Number of times the system is accessed
  - Difficult catheter placement
  - Poor technique in catheter or port-site care

INTRODUCTION

During the course of their disease, most patients with cancer require intravenous chemotherapy, frequent blood sampling, transfusion of blood products, and occasionally, total parenteral nutrition. Many of these intravenously administered therapies—especially the chemotherapies—are inflammatory to small peripheral veins. As anticancer therapies have become more complex, the need for vascular access during active treatment has become essential. Over the past three decades, techniques for obtaining and maintaining central vascular access have been developed and refined, and as a result, many different devices and techniques are available for use in the patient with cancer. Managing the treatment of patients with cancer requires a thorough familiarity with the special use of vascular access devices. This chapter provides a review of the pros and cons of various devices, insertion methods, and catheter maintenance techniques.

Although it would be ideal to base vascular access decisions on solid clinical information, few randomized controlled trials have examined the clinical controversies involved with chronic vascular access for the patient with cancer. In addition, many of the larger studies regarding central vascular access were performed in the inpatient intensive care unit (ICU) setting. Comparing this patient group to patients with cancer who are receiving chemotherapy or weekly blood draws on an outpatient basis could lead to inaccurate conclusions. It is important, however, to review the available randomized trials, a number of carefully performed retrospective analyses, and pertinent ICU literature to address some of the questions concerning vascular access for the patient with cancer.

When managing a patient who requires vascular access for treatment of a malignancy, there are three important questions. The first question is: What device will best meet this patient's therapeutic needs? Patients might require access for delivery of chemotherapy, parenteral nutrition, and frequent blood draws. They might also have medical comorbidities that influence the choice of device. Fortunately, many different devices and anatomic insertion locations are available.

The second question is: How can we most safely insert and maintain central venous access? Learning to place and maintain central lines requires a thorough knowledge of cardinal vein anatomy. Lines placed without difficulty have a lower risk of failing in the long term.

The final question is: What are the immediate and long-term complications of vascular access procedures that are unique to the oncology patient population? It is imperative that the responsible physician be trained to recognize and manage complications arising from these nearly ubiquitous devices.

CHOOSING THE RIGHT DEVICE

Clinical oncologists use the vascular access devices discussed in this chapter to aspirate blood and infuse agents into central veins. The reason to access the central system instead of peripheral veins revolves around the increased blood flow of these large veins, examples of which include the superior vena cava (SVC) and inferior vena cava (IVC). Many chemotherapeutics and parenteral nutrition formulations act as vesicants to the venous intima, causing inflammation and thrombosis of smaller veins. By infusing this type of product into the higher-flow, less thrombogenic cardinal veins, the durability and safety of vascular access can be extended and patient comfort can be enhanced significantly.

Percutaneous Central Lines

Traditional central lines are placed using the Seldinger technique described in detail later in this chapter. The subclavian vein, internal jugular vein, or femoral vein is cannulated percutaneously, and the catheter is placed using guidewire assistance. There is a very short distance between the skin and the catheter's entry point into the vein. Theoretically, this proximity to skin flora increases the risk of subsequent central line infection.

These central lines are in common use throughout most hospitals for oncology patients, for critically ill patients who require central access, or for any patients who require infusions that are poorly tolerated via peripheral intravenous access. Such central lines provide excellent short-term access to the central venous system. In general, percutaneous central lines are considered only for short-term use, and after the first seven to ten days, percutaneous central lines have a markedly higher incidence of infection despite optimal skin entrance site dressing techniques. Obviously, prolonged patient neutro-penia and episodes of bacteremia could result in shorter life spans of such catheters.

Patients could benefit from these traditional central venous catheters if they require a relatively short course of infusion or if they need a bridge to placement of a more long-term catheter. Meticulous sterile dressing changes are an absolute necessity for outpatients who need short-term therapy via these lines. Patients without the resources or dexterity to care for percutaneous central lines are at a prohibitively increased risk of line infection, bacteremia, or thrombotic event and should be provided with a long-term form of central access. Certain comorbid conditions (e.g., burns, open wounds near the line site, or tracheostomy) preclude placement of this type of vascular access.

Surgically Tunneled Central Lines

Most oncology patients need a long-term form of central venous access rather than a traditional central line. Surgically tunneled central lines were developed to increase the distance between the skin entrance site and the puncture of the vein. The hypothesis was that by increasing this distance, the life span of the central access would be increased by decreasing the incidence of infection and thrombosis. Tunneled central lines are commonly referred to by the name of the first brand marketed, Hickman. Other examples include Broviac, Quinton, and Groshong (Fig. 52-1). These polymeric silicone rubber venous access catheters are placed via a subcutaneous tunnel that is described in detail later in this chapter. Clinical studies have supported the hypothesis that increasing the distance between the catheter exit site in the skin and the hole in the vein decreases the incidence of externally derived infection.[1,2] Studies suggest that the incidence of bloodstream infections associated with tunneled catheters is approximately 1 to 2 per 1000 catheter days.[3] The frequency of bacteremia

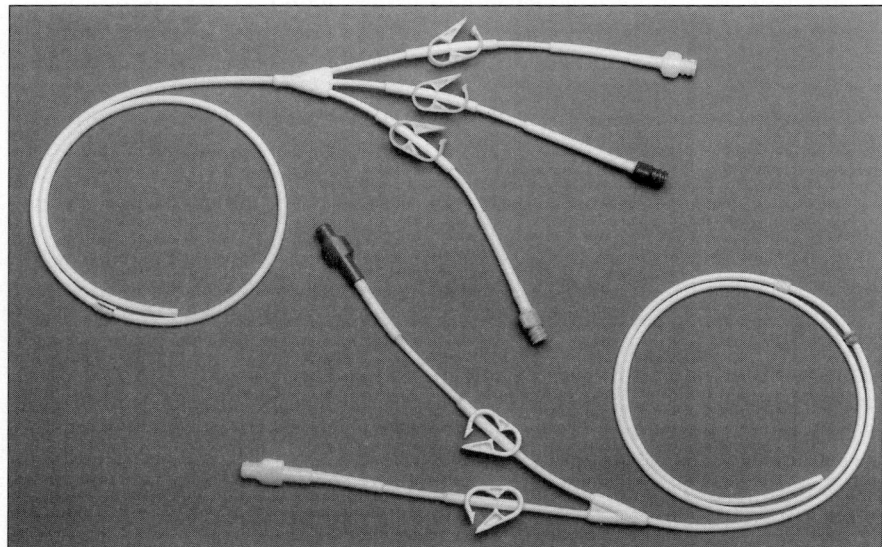

Figure 52-1. Examples of standard double- and triple-lumen Hickman catheters. The double-lumen catheter has both the standard Dacron cuff and an additional antibacterial barrier cuff.

among nontunneled catheters has been reported at between 1.0 and 13.0 per 1000 catheter days.[4]

A Dacron cuff 3–4 cm from the exit site encourages scar formation to fix the catheter in place. This exaggerated scarring eliminates the need for long-term sutures holding the catheter in place to the skin. Avoiding these fixation sutures can decrease the incidence of stitch reactivity and associated localized skin infections.

By tunneling the central line, clinicians frequently can extend the lifespan of these catheters to six months. One drawback of this type of central access device is the inconvenience of placing and removing the lines. In most instances, surgeons insert these lines in the operating room under local anesthetic and intravenous sedation. Therefore, these procedures require coordination of the patient, the surgeon, the anesthesia staff, and the operating room staff. They are also more uncomfortable to remove than nontunneled lines due to the Dacron cuff scar reaction. Removal requires intravenous sedation and local anesthesia but can be accomplished outside of the operating room.

Surgically Implanted Infusion Ports

Implantable ports consist of a small injection reservoir with a self-sealing membrane; they are placed entirely beneath the skin. There is no external catheter. An internal catheter runs from the reservoir into the subclavian or internal jugular vein to provide central access. The internal catheter is essentially identical to those used for tunneled central lines. A noncoring (Huber) needle can pass directly through the skin into the reservoir for infusion or aspiration.[5] The self-sealing rubber cap on the reservoir prevents leakage from the reservoir after withdrawal of the Huber needle. The gauge of the noncoring needle— not the catheter—typically limits flow through the port system (Fig. 52-2). The ports can also be used for continuous drug infusion, as shown in Figure 52-3.

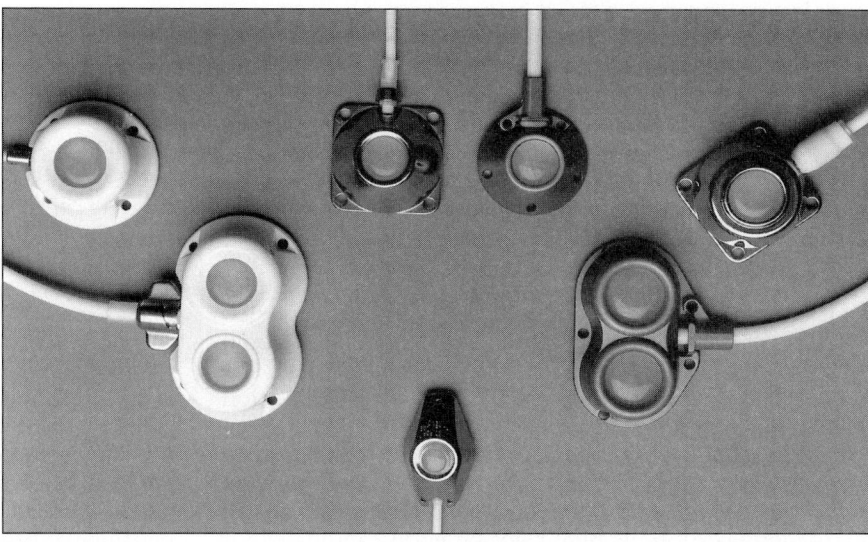

A

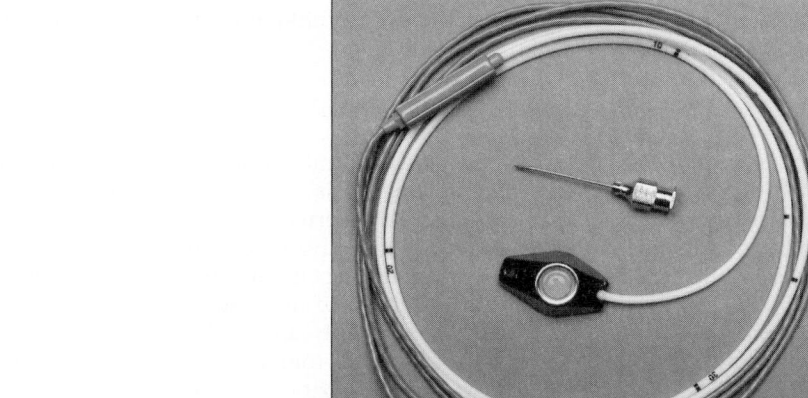

B

Figure 52-2. A, Examples of a number of different implantable infusion devices: Low-profile titanium ports (*top center*); peripheral access port used in the arm (*bottom center*); single and dual polysulfone-titanium ports (*left*); single- and double-lumen standard profile ports (*right*). **B,** Peripheral access catheter for placement of small port in forearm. This system utilizes fluoro-free thermosensor (gray wire) initially inside white silicon catheter. An external wand over the chest determines site of catheter tip placement.

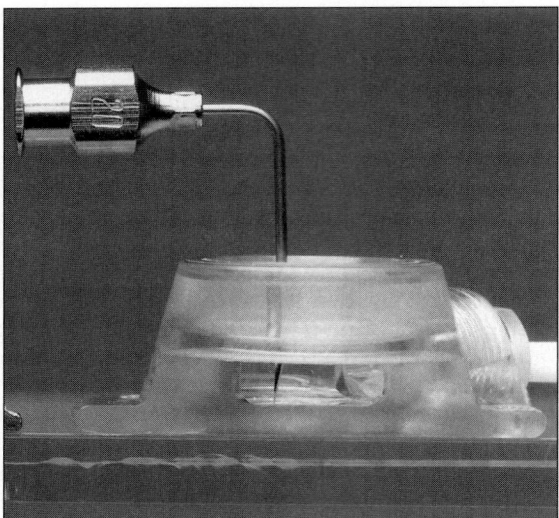

Figure 52-3. Demonstration of placement of deflected point (Huber) needle in port. Lower portion of port has been cut away to show needle tip in reservoir. This example of bent needle shows how needle can be taped and secured at skin surface for protracted infusion using an external pump.

The theoretical concern that bacteria more easily traverse the short distance between the skin and the "neo-vein" or reservoir and cause increased rates of infection does not prove true.[6-12] Sterile technique and site care lead to an infection risk comparable to that of tunneled catheters. With adequate care, the rate of infection could be four- to fivefold less than for tunneled catheters.[3] The low rates of infection and extravasation make infusion ports ideally suited for patients with cancer who need long-term single-lumen access and a low-maintenance catheter. Experience has shown, however, that patients with prolonged periods of neutropenia or significant risk of cutaneous eruptions might not be good candidates for port devices. The visible lump of the port could bother extremely thin patients; however, the port is hidden from plain view in most people.

Long-Line Central Access

Also known as peripherally inserted central catheters (PICC lines), this vascular access device is becoming increasingly popular. The catheter is inserted into a brachial, cephalic, or antecubital vein and advanced into the subclavian vein or higher. Successful placement rates of 75% might be improved by the addition of ultrasound guidance.[13] These lines can be placed simply and easily in the outpatient office setting and are well tolerated by patients with minimal risk. Many oncology patients have poor arm veins after multiple peripheral infusions and are therefore poor candidates for this technique. The 50% risk of catheter-related thrombosis is the greatest drawback to more widespread use of PICC lines in oncology patients. This problem is secondary to the presence of a long length of catheter within the vein and to the catheter tip

in the relatively low flow subclavian vein. Advancing the catheter tip into the SVC can reduce the incidence of thrombosis by more than half.[14] Accurate placement of the catheter tip in the SVC can be nearly impossible in light of the large displacement of the catheter tip (up to 8 cm) with normal arm range of motion.[15]

INSERTING VASCULAR ACCESS DEVICES

Providing patients with cancer with appropriate vascular access requires not only a thorough knowledge of available devices but also technical expertise in the procedures for placing these catheters. Although these procedures are sometimes viewed as routine, the risks of poor technique can be devastating for the patient. Before undertaking the procedure, one should carefully consider everything from choosing the site of insertion to selecting the dressing used at the end of the procedure (Table 52-1).

Choosing Insertion Location

Vascular access devices can be placed using a number of different access points, including the internal jugular, subclavian, external jugular, and femoral veins. There even have been reports of placement of a Hickman catheter into the azygous vein using a percutaneous translumbar approach.[16] The vast majority of catheters used for long-term vascular access in patients with cancer are placed in the internal jugular and subclavian veins. We will limit this discussion to these most common access sites.

The most frequent site for insertion of vascular access devices in the oncology population is the subclavian vein. It is important to understand that the anatomy of this location can be altered by clavicular fracture or previous median sternotomy, and for a patient with such a history, an alternate site should be considered. Even for patients with standard venous anatomy, the acute angle at the confluence of the subclavian and internal jugular veins at the brachiocephalic vein can complicate the passing of the guidewire into the SVC. There is a higher incidence of pneumothorax, hemothorax, and catheter malposition among inexperienced operators, and a higher incidence of vein stenosis with subclavian vein placement compared with internal jugular placement.[17-19] A subclavian artery puncture during line placement can be difficult to control due to the position of the artery posterior to the clavicle. A catheter placed on the anterior chest wall is more comfortable and easier to cover with clothing, however, than a line in the neck. Additionally, some authors have concluded that with lines in place for more than four days, the risk of line infection is less for subclavian catheters than for internal jugular catheters.[17,18]

In many ways, the internal jugular vein is the ideal location with regard to ease of placement of a central catheter. The path of the guidewire during placement is straight, thereby limiting many guidewire complications and catheter malposition. In the event of carotid artery puncture, arterial bleeding can be controlled safely with the application of direct pressure. This advantage is especially important in the thrombocytopenic patient. The incidence of central venous occlusion is decreased, which could be important for patients who are likely to need an arteriovenous fistula for hemodialysis in the future. Unfortunately, patients often complain of pain with neck and shoulder movements after placement of an internal jugular catheter.

Preparing to Place the Vascular Access Device

Adequate preparation for placing a central venous catheter for oncology patients includes several steps before the actual line insertion. The surgeon must make several decisions that can limit the incidence of both immediate and delayed complications and ensure optimal line function.

Studies suggest that providing a single dose of prophylactic antibiotic to cover common skin flora before inserting the vascular access device reduces central line infection. It is difficult, however, to determine how this small benefit affects antibiotic resistance and subsequent infections. Using central venous catheters impregnated with antibiotics could be more effective in dealing with infectious complications and will be discussed later in this chapter.[20,21]

Clearly, it is essential to perform these procedures in as sterile an environment as possible, and most catheters are placed in the operating suite. At the very least, a sterile surgical field with mask, gown, cap, gloves, and a large sterile drape should be used to minimize the risk of line infection.[22] The skin of the entire anterior neck and chest should be prepared with chlorhexidine, which is superior to povidone-iodine or alcohol in limiting line infections.[23-26]

The choice to use ultrasound guidance to identify the vein during cannulation should be addressed before beginning the procedure. Less experienced operators will likely benefit from the use of ultrasound guidance as an adjunct to the anatomic landmarks technique.[27,28] Ultrasound can decrease the incidence of arterial puncture and placement failure. Although a few reports in the literature exist regarding the advantage of these techniques, such superiority is generally judged when compared with unacceptably high rates of complications using the blind approach as the control group.

Another question to be answered before beginning the procedure is somewhat controversial. The operator must decide where to position the catheter tip within the central vein. Clearly, catheters positioned with the tip in the right atrium will function longer as a source for aspirating blood samples than those with the tip positioned in the SVC.[29,30] A case review of thrombosed catheters documents that the position of the tip of the catheter at the time of thrombosis seems to be the most important contributing factor.[31-36] The closer the catheter tip is to the right atrium, the lower the frequency of thrombosis and infection. The higher the tip of the catheter is positioned above the atrium, the greater the incidence of catheter thrombosis. The risk of a catheter tip in the right atrial position is primarily that of cardiac arrhythmias when the tip is in the lower half of the atrium near the tricuspid valve. An additional risk of right atrial catheter placement is right atrial thrombus or right atrial erosion.[37] These risks have led the Food and Drug Administration to publicly warn operators to avoid placement of the catheter tip within the right atrium. Instead, the catheter tip should sit at the junction of the SVC and the right atrium. Placement of the catheter tip higher in the central venous system above the SVC can lead to thrombosis and increased risk of infection.

Insertion Technique

Most catheters are placed using the Seldinger technique. A rolled towel is placed directly under the vertebral column at the shoulders to extend the clavicles. A peripheral line is established, and the patient is connected to EKG monitor and pulse oximeter. Intravenous sedation is typically established using small doses of benzodiazepines. The fluoroscopy operating table and patient are placed in the Trendelenburg position. The skin of the neck and entire upper anterior thorax is prepared, and sterile drapes are positioned. The skin and deep tissues are anesthetized with 1% lidocaine using a 25-gauge needle for the skin followed by a 22-gauge needle for the anticipated insertion tract (Fig. 52-4A).

For subclavian vein puncture, the site of skin puncture is usually 1 cm below the angle of the lateral third of the clavicle. The long insertion needle, as depicted in Figure 52-4A, is inserted slowly horizontal to the clavicle and below the clavicle, aiming for a point approximately one fingerbreadth above the sternal notch. While inserting slowly, a very small amount of negative pressure is maintained on the syringe. With experience, the physician develops a feel for the actual puncture of the vein, and when this occurs, the syringe fills easily with venous blood.

Maintaining careful position of the needle, the syringe is removed, and the catheter or guidewire is inserted (Fig. 52-4B). If the patient experiences discomfort in the neck, the catheter or guidewire is withdrawn somewhat. Turning the patient's head away from the site of insertion and exerting a downward pull on the ipsilateral arm could facilitate entrance of the catheter or guidewire into the SVC. Cardiac ectopy indicates that the guidewire has entered the right atrium, and the wire should be withdrawn slightly. Fluoroscopy may be used to pass the wire when difficulty is experienced. The correct position of the catheter is confirmed by fluoroscopy or chest x-ray before securing the catheter with a 3-0-nylon suture at the skin exit site. The tip of the catheter is positioned 1 cm above the SVC-atrial junction when the patient is in the Trendelenburg position. Chest radiograph is obtained in the recovery unit to document absence of pneumothorax.

When it is necessary to use the veins in the neck, the right internal jugular provides more direct access to the SVC and right atrium. In this case, the patient's head is turned to the opposite side. The insertion site is located just lateral to the carotid and approximately two fingerbreadths above the head of the clavicle. Another useful landmark for the insertion site is the angle formed by the

TABLE 52-1

General Guidelines for Catheter and Port Use

	ADVANTAGES	USES	DRESSINGS	FLUSHING	COMMENTS
Central Line	Placed at the bedside Easy removal One or multiple lumens Can change over wire	Recommended for hospital use only	Sterile gauze or sterile transparent dressing Change dressing twice weekly or if dressing becomes damp, loose or soiled	5 mL heparinized saline (10 units/mL) in each lumen daily or after each use	Antibiotic ointments may promote antibiotic resistance and fungal infections
PICC Catheter	Easy to insert and remove Infrequent insertion complications	Any patient needing one week to six months of IV access Patient must have accessible upper extremity vein	After insertion transparent dressing placed over site with gauze pad for 24 hours In-house transparent dressing over site with antimicrobial impregnated foam dressing (Biopath) Change every 6 days At home transparent dressing with Biopatch changed every week Change dressing when damp, loose, or soiled	In house: 3 mL heparinized saline (10 units/mL after each use or bid) At home: As in-house or may flush with 3 mL heparinized saline (100 units/mL) if only using once or twice daily	Flush and draw blood slowly as too much pressure can cause catheter tip to migrate
Hickman Catheter	Multiple sizes and numbers of lumens for variable patient populations Tunneled under skin	Continuous infusion therapy Long-term need for venous access	Newly placed line—Sterile gauze with Biopatch for 7–10 days. Remove sutures after 21 days In-house: Transparent dressing with Biopatch changed twice per week. At home: Gauze dressing preferred for active patients who perspire and should be changed twice per week Change any dressing when it is damp, loose, or soiled	5 mL heparinized saline (10 units/mL) daily or after each use	All sites should be cleaned with chlorhexidine prep during dressing changes Well healed sites might not require dressings after four weeks and may be cleaned with antimicrobial soap and water
Groshong Catheter	Slit valve requires no clamp or heparinized flushes Requires infrequent flushing Smaller, more flexible catheter	Single- or double-lumen catheter for long-term use			
Port	Positioned under skin Minimal care required	A patient needing one-lumen access and a low-maintenance catheter Intermittent infusion therapy	No dressing needed when not being accessed When being accessed with Huber needle, transparent dressing should be applied over needle and both are changed every 5 days	5 mL heparinized saline (10 units/mL) daily or after each use Flush with 20 mL normal saline after blood draws Monthly flush with 5 mL heparinized saline (100 units/mL)	Site should be cleaned with chlorhexidine prep before use Must access with noncoring needle Anything larger than 20-gauge needle can damage the port septum Always assess for blood return after accessing port May use EMLA cram before accessing port

sternal and clavicular heads of the sternocleidomastoid muscle (Fig. 52-5).

Placement of a permanent Silastic catheter, such as a Hickman, is depicted in Figure 52-6. Placement of the introducing needle and guidewire are as described in previous figures except that a 1-cm incision is made before inserting the introduction needle. A prophylactic antibiotic is given before the procedure. It is often beneficial to provide the patient with intravenous sedation.

A second 1-cm incision is placed lower on the anterior chest, usually at the level of the fourth or fifth interspace. The skin and subcutaneous tissues are first anesthetized with 1% lidocaine. The projected course of the tunneled catheter is also infiltrated with lidocaine. A tunneler is passed from the lower incision to the upper incision, where the guidewire is exiting. A heavy suture is tied to the end of the tunneler and brought down through the tract. The suture is tied to the end of the catheter and used

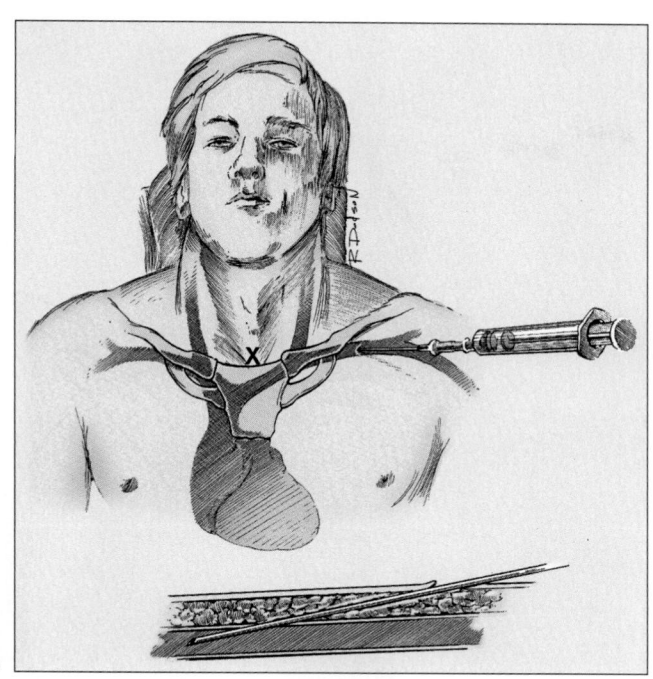

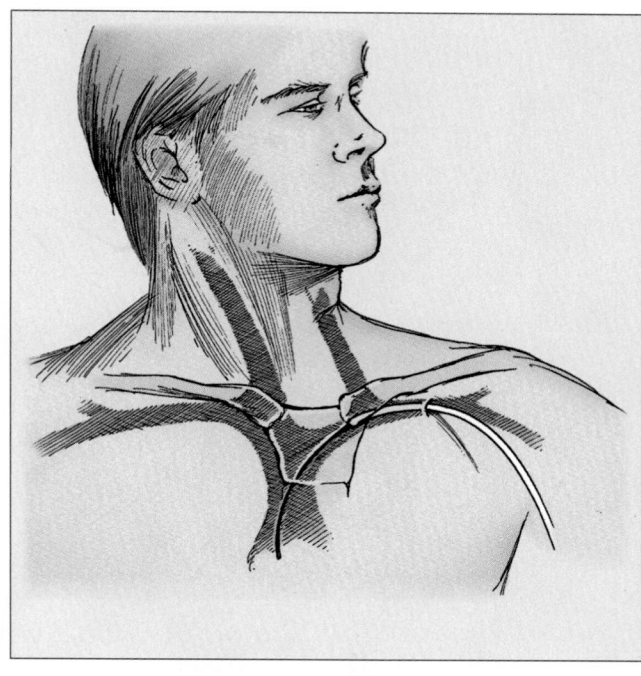

Figure 52-4. A, Placement of catheter using the Seldinger technique. Long insertion needle shown entering the vein through skin and subcutaneous tissues. **B,** Demonstration of catheter passing over guidewire.

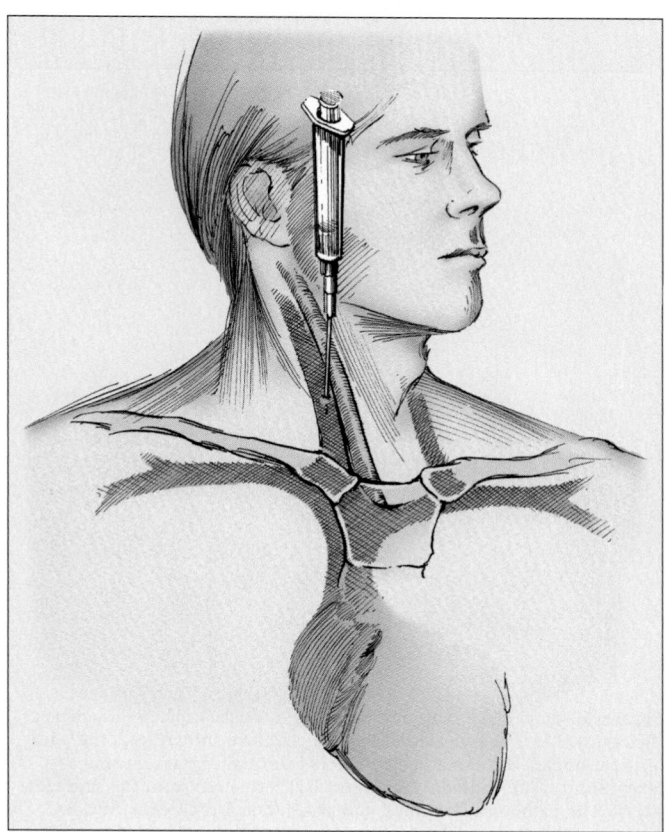

Figure 52-5. Demonstration of catheter insertion technique when utilizing a vein in the neck (right internal jugular).

to pull the catheter up through the tract, securing the cuff 3–4 cm from the skin exit site. The catheter is trimmed to the correct length that will position it about 1 cm above the SVC-RA junction with the patient in Trendelenburg position. This location is approximately four finger-breadths below the sternal notch. Care is taken to cut the catheter squarely and smoothly. An appropriate introducer and tear-sway sheath are passed over the guidewire into the vein (Fig. 52-7). A slight rotary motion facilitates the introduction of the sheath and avoids crimping. Care is taken to withdraw the guidewire occasionally as the introducer is inserted. This prevents the guidewire from being forced further into the right atrium and avoids the problem of developing a false passage rather than sliding along the wire. The guidewire is then removed, and a syringe is attached to the introducer to confirm that blood can be aspirated. The introducer is removed, and the thumb is used to control bleeding or air intake through the sheath. It is important to have the catheter tip poised to insert as the introducer is removed. The passage of the catheter could meet some resistance as it is passed between the clavicle and first rib.

Fluoroscopy or chest x-ray is obtained to confirm correct position, especially the tip location. The catheter is aspirated and flushed to confirm function. Care should be taken to avoid any angulations of the catheter through the subcutaneous tract, especially at the bend toward the subclavian vein. The incision below the clavicle is closed with a subcutaneous absorbable suture. The catheter is secured at the exit site with a 3-0 nylon suture, which is maintained for approximately three weeks to allow the fibrous tissue in growth into the subcutaneous cuff. The exit site is covered with a sterile gauze dressing.

Problems Common to Cancer and Its Therapy

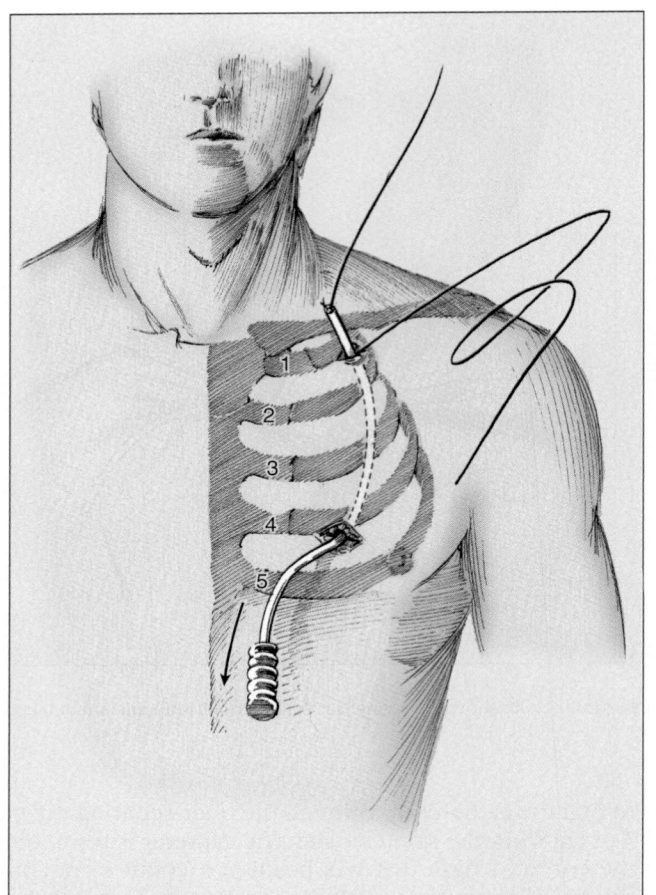

A

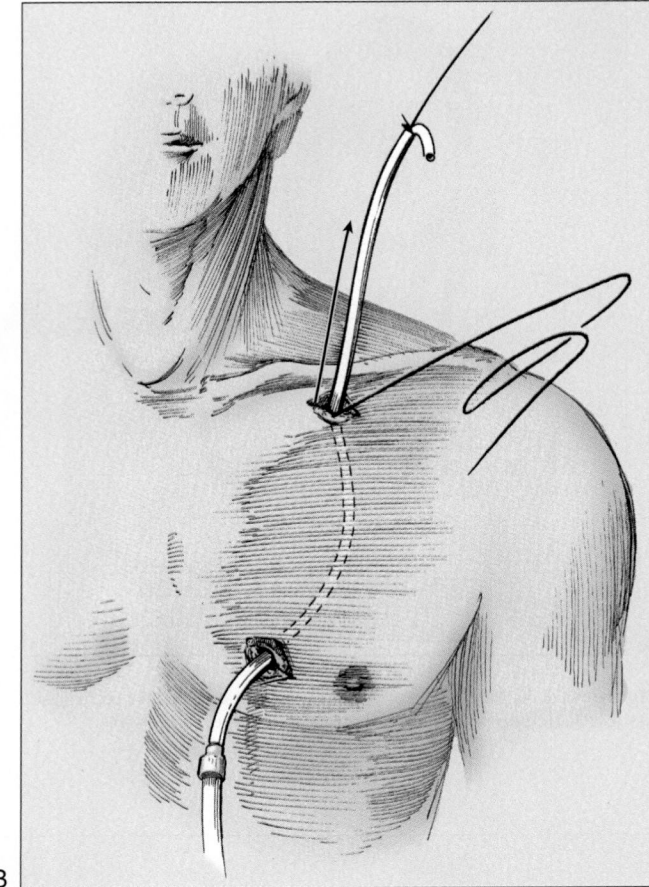

B

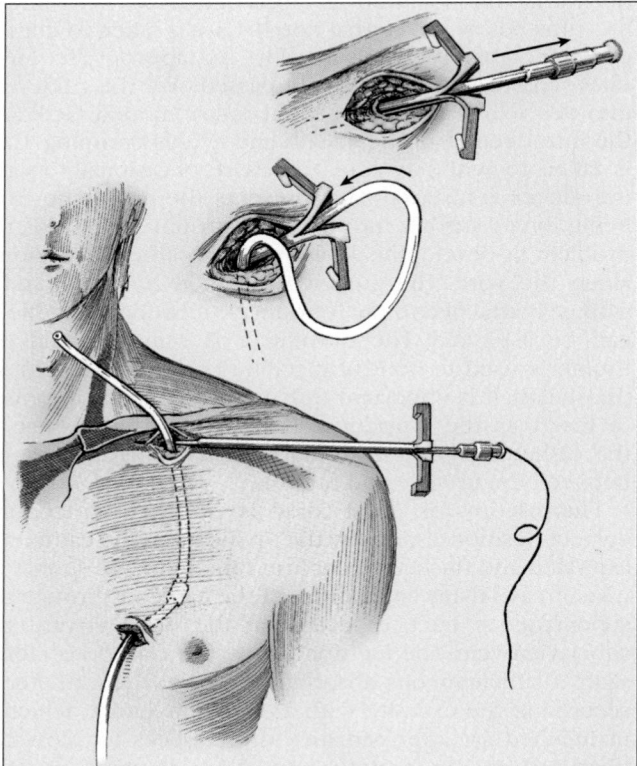

C

Figure 52-6. A, Placement of a permanent Silastic catheter (such as a Hickman). The first and second incision sites are shown, as is the path of the tunneler. **B,** The catheter is pulled through the tract using a heavy suture. The catheter cuff is secured 3 to 4 cm from the skin exit site. **C,** The catheter is trimmed and positioned 1 cm below SVC-RA junction. Introducer and tear-away sheath are shown passing over the guidewire. The catheter is inserted into the sheath and the sheath and introducer are removed.

Figure 52-7. Example of an introducer kit. The kit includes guidewire and introducer (dilator) with tear-away sheath (two different sizes shown). The upper, longer blunt object is a tunneler, which is included in some kits.

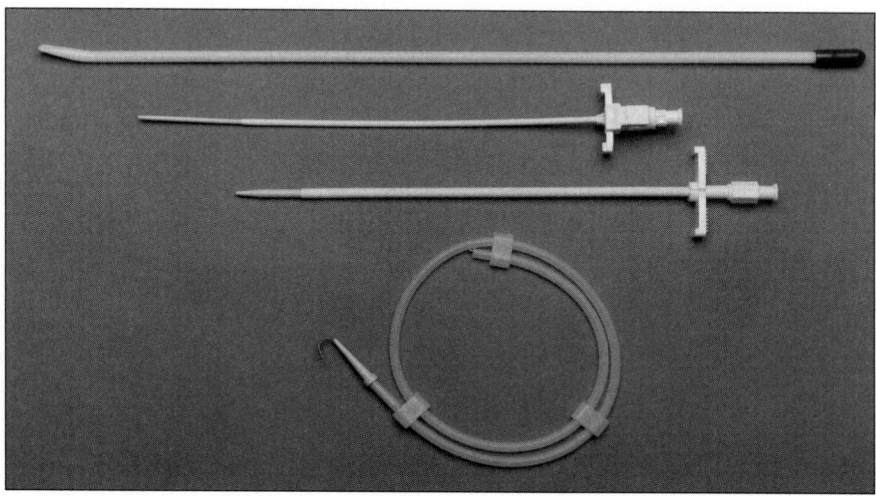

Similar techniques apply to the use of neck veins. The catheter is simply tunneled over the clavicle, the exit site being the same as for subclavian vein placement. When other sites are required (e.g., the femoral vein with the catheter tip in the inferior vena cava), direct cut-down exposure of the saphenous vein or other large femoral branch is preferred.

Figure 52-8 illustrates the placement of an implanted injection port. A 1-cm incision is placed below the clavicle at the site planned for subclavian venipuncture. A second, 3-cm incision is placed lower on the chest in a position that provides a relatively flat surface and stability for the port chamber. Local anesthesia is 1% lidocaine with

1:200,000 epinephrine. A subcutaneous pocket just large enough to accommodate the port is dissected inferior to the incision. Ideally, the level of this pocket is over the underlying pectoral fascia. The skin coverage needs to be thick, but the port must be easily accessible by percutaneous stick.

A tunneler is passed subcutaneously from the pocket through the intraclavicular incision. A suture is tied to the tunneler and brought down through the tract. The suture is tied to the end of the port catheter and used to pull the catheter through the tract to the intraclavicular incision. Care should be taken to position with gentle curve and to avoid catheter angulation. The port is secured in the

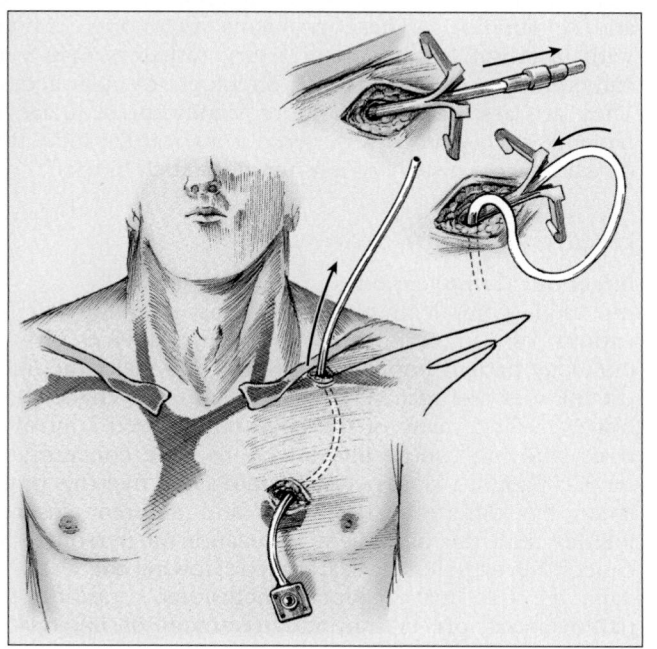

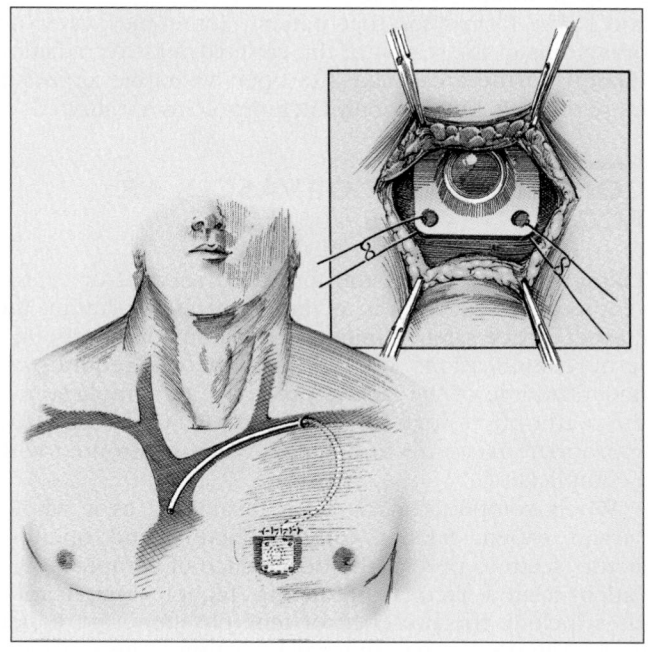

A

B

Figure 52-8. A, Placement of an implanted injection port. First and second inclusion sites are shown, as is dissected pocket to accommodate port. **B,** Demonstration of placement of port into subcutaneous pocket.

pocket with three sutures of 0-prolene. It is necessary to anchor the port adequately to prevent flipping or rotation of the device.

The guidewire is inserted as described, and the dilator and sheath are passed over it. The catheter is cut to the desired length. The dilator and guidewire are removed, and the catheter is inserted through the sheath as described. The incision for the port pocket is closed with interrupted 3-0 absorbable sutures placed in the subcutaneous layer. The skin is approximated with a running 4-0 absorbable suture. A transparent nonpermeable dressing is used at the port incision.

Open insertion methods are quite safe in a skilled surgeon's hands. The major complication of the open technique (due to the vein being directly opened) is the possibility of air embolus during the actual catheter insertion. This is most likely to occur in patients who are hypovolemic, cachectic, or unable to tolerate positioning in Trendelenburg position. Air embolus happens most frequently when the internal jugular vein is used, and extreme care with the use of the purse-string suture around the insertion site and venous occlusion with vascular clamps should limit the possibility of introduction of air into the vascular system. All who perform such open insertions should be well versed in the resuscitation measures for an air embolus. With open direct surgical placement, although it takes considerably longer than the closed Seldinger technique, complications should be much lower than 5%.[38-42] In the Hopkins series, the open method results in a complication rate of less than 1%. Although this is a safer technique, it requires more training, more experienced operative personnel, and larger incisions. Any patient who has had repeated problems with closed insertions should be approached in an open fashion, however, as this is the most controlled and safest format for that patient. Sometimes, previous operations in the region of the cardinal veins or radiation therapy to the area make the open operative approach more difficult, but generally such problems are limited.

COMPLICATIONS OF VASCULAR ACCESS DEVICES

Taking steps to ensure the long-term survival of central venous access devices is as important as implanting the correct device safely. Minimizing the immediate and long-term complications of central catheters requires an understanding of the factors predictive of complications, the pathophysiology of line complications, and the appropriate measures to be taken when confronted with a complication.

When complication rates are examined as a whole, certain patient factors, catheter factors, and operator factors seem to predict the occurrence of complications. Patient-related factors predicting higher complication rates include the presence of multiple comorbid conditions, atherosclerosis, abnormal anatomy, thrombocytopenia, immunocompromise, prior radiation therapy to insertion area, recent myocardial infarction, and patient restlessness.[43] In addition, multiple-lumen or stiffer catheters carry increased risks of complications.[44-47] Factors related to the person performing the insertion of the catheter also influence risk of complications. Risk increases if the operator has inserted fewer than 50 central venous catheters, if more than two tries at cannulating the vein are required, or if the insertion of the catheter is difficult.[15,48-50] Risk factors for specific complications are discussed in the sections that follow.

Immediate Complications

Pneumothorax
Published complication rates for pneumothorax after jugular vein central line placement are approximately 0.5% and up to four times higher for subclavian vein procedures.[15,51-53] The risk of this technical complication can be reduced dramatically among experienced operators or physicians who have experienced supervisors.[43]

Bleeding
Many patients with cancer are at increased risk of bleeding complications due to thrombocytopenia, uremia, other platelet dysfunction, or anticoagulant therapy. Bleeding complications are associated most frequently with thrombocytopenia.[54] For patients with platelet counts less than 50 or International Normalized Ratio (INR) greater than 2.0, we consider administration of platelets or fresh-frozen plasma. Experienced physicians should perform these procedures with access to ultrasound guidance if necessary.

Cardiac Arrhythmias
Disruptions in the normal cardiac conduction pathway can be caused by contact between the catheter and the right atrium. Most of these arrhythmias are short-lived and self-limiting.[15] These problems are more common with insertion of pulmonary artery catheters than with catheters typically inserted for oncologic vascular access. They are associated with more significant sequelae in patients having recently suffered a myocardial infarction or who have a history of left bundle branch block.[55,56]

Delayed Complications

Infectious Complications
Infectious complications are the most common complications of long-term vascular access devices in the oncology patient population. Two factors make the interpretation of this relatively well-studied topic challenging, however. First, many of the large randomized controlled trials studying central line infections have concentrated on ICU patients. Most people would agree that this population has different risk factors and different susceptibilities than the outpatient population of persons with cancer. Nevertheless, by carefully reviewing the available data, we can make some conclusions regarding the pathogenesis, prevention, and treatment of line-related infections among oncology patients. In studies of ICU patients with central lines, factors predisposing to line infection have included malignancy, neutropenia, extended duration of indwelling time, and coincident

parenteral nutrition. All of these factors obviously can contribute to the incidence of infection among patients with vascular access for oncologic treatment.[57-60]

Second, the confusing (but vastly important) terminology regarding line-related infections can make the literature on this topic difficult to interpret. Local infection is a positive culture at the catheter insertion site. Catheter colonization or infection is the positive culture of a segment of removed catheter. Catheter-associated bacteremia is bacteremia evidenced by a positive blood culture from a site other than the catheter and the positive culture of a segment of removed catheter with the same pathogen.

Understanding the pathophysiology of catheter-associated-bacteremia (CAB) can help us limit the incidence of this complication. At least 50% of CAB is caused by coagulase-negative staphylococcus. This common skin flora can colonize the catheter during insertion or later. Thrombus forming at the catheter tip or along the catheter tip can become a nidus for bacterial proliferation with resultant bacteremia. Central access catheter thrombosis significantly increases the risks of colonization and infection.[61] Bacteria can also be introduced into the bloodstream by hub contamination, by hematogenous seeding from another focus of infection, and, rarely, by the infusate itself.

Factors increasing the risk of catheter infection include prolonged duration of indwelling time, multiple-lumen catheters, femoral or internal jugular vein location, difficult catheter placement, and non–catheter-related bacteremia.[57-60,62] As mentioned previously, nontunneled catheters are at increased risk of catheter infection compared with tunneled catheters, and totally implantable devices are even less susceptible than tunneled catheters.[63-67]

Multiple-lumen catheters have demonstrated higher infection rates than single-lumen catheters. The addition of each lumen exponentially increases incidence of infection.[68-73] There are two possible explanations for this observation. First, the increased internal lumen diameter of the line is associated with a higher thrombosis rate and accumulation of loose thrombus tags at the catheter tip. Thrombosis causes more breaking of the line and more line manipulation when attempting to declot, leading to subsequent infection. Second, the multiple ports invite multiple interruptions of the line for access and result in a greater likelihood of introduction of bacteria. Despite their greater risk of iatrogenic infection, multiple-lumen catheters have great appeal for patients who need multiple simultaneous infusions of incompatible drugs. Very strict nursing guidelines must be followed in the management of multiple-lumen catheters to prevent iatrogenic infections and thrombosis.[74] Quality assurance activities must include close surveillance for potential preventable problems in maintaining vascular access in the patient with cancer.

Diagnosis and management of catheter-related infection differs between nontunneled and tunneled catheters. As mentioned previously, tunneled catheters are less susceptible to serious line infections and are typically more challenging to remove and replace.

Some diagnostic principles apply to both tunneled and nontunneled catheters. Routine surveillance blood cultures should not be performed. When a catheter-related infection is suspected due to fever, chills, purulence around the catheter site, paired percutaneous and catheter blood samples should be submitted for quantitative cultures.[75-80] Qualitative culture with continuously monitored differential time to positivity compares the time to positivity for catheter blood cultures to percutaneous peripheral-blood cultures. This technique has demonstrated excellent specificity and sensitivity for detecting catheter-related infection in tunneled catheters.[81,82]

In most patients with nontunneled central venous catheters, the line should be removed if the patient demonstrates signs of site infection or sepsis or if blood culture results from the catheter and percutaneous blood samples are positive.[81,82] Seven to ten days of narrow-spectrum antibiotic therapy is generally recommended. In certain cases of clinically stable patients with their first episode of coagulase-negative staphylococcus, a trial of antibiotic therapy might salvage the catheter.[70] For any patient with persistent bacteremia despite antibiotic therapy and removal of the infected catheter, a thorough investigation of possible septic sources such as endocarditis or septic thrombus is warranted.

Tunneled catheters or infusion ports should be removed in cases of sepsis, complicated infections, tunnel tract infections, or port abscesses.[83] A thorough evaluation confirming the surgically implanted catheter as the source of infection should precede the removal of any of these vascular access devices. In the absence of complicated infection, catheter salvage could be indicated. Antibiotic lock therapy is a reasonable approach for attempting to salvage lines with common coagulase-negative staphylococcus, *S. aureus*, or gram-negative bacilli intraluminal infections. This therapy consists of instilling the catheter lumen with high concentrations of antibiotics and leaving them there for several days.[84-87] If salvage therapy fails, a new tunneled catheter can be placed after removing the infected catheter, treating with an appropriate course of antimicrobial therapy, and repeating blood cultures with negative results.

As mentioned previously, catheter-related infection is associated with catheter-related thrombus. Flushing catheters with heparin solution can minimize infectious complications.[88] Several trials have demonstrated reduction in catheter infection by initiating oral anticoagulation, subcutaneous low-molecular weight heparin, or oral anticoagulation at the time of line placement.[89-92] Initiating delayed anticoagulant therapy after the line is placed could precipitate the embolization of a previously formed thrombus. The benefits of reduced infectious complications must be weighed against the risks of bleeding and heparin-induced thrombocytopenia before recommending these therapies to any patient.

Catheter Thrombus

Thrombus of central vein access devices predisposes to both line malfunction and line infection. The most common site of thrombus formation with prolonged indwelling central catheters is where the catheter enters the vein. At this point, a fibrin sleeve progresses distally towards the tip of the catheter. The precipitating event is likely local trauma from line insertion with subsequent endothelial damage and disruption of intraluminal laminar flow. The venous intima exposed to blood flow activates the coagulation cascade. Understanding this pathophysiology helps to explain why difficult line placements often lead to shorter catheter survival and increased rates of infection.

The incidence of central venous catheter-related thrombus as demonstrated by ultrasound is greater than 30% for catheters in place longer than seven days.[48,89] This problem typically presents as progressive difficulty in flushing the catheter. A change in posture or the Valsalva maneuver could allow aspiration of blood. Occasionally, thrombosis can present as extremity edema. This can be especially devastating after axillary nodal resection or axillary irradiation.

When a patient presents with symptoms suggesting the presence of a flow-obstructing clot, several steps should be taken before performing thrombolysis. A chest x-ray will demonstrate many of the line problems not amenable to lysis. Gravity flow and the ability to draw blood should be examined in multiple positions, including standing, sitting, and lying down. A fibrin sheath is suggested by excellent gravity flow and no blood return whatsoever. An occluded catheter is suggested by the inability to infuse solutions or draw blood in any position. The fibrin sheath and the occluded catheter are the only two conditions appropriate for lysis therapy. No lysis should be attempted within two weeks of line placement or if the chest x-ray is abnormal. See Tables 52-2 and 52-3 for our guidelines regarding the management of other potential catheter-related problems.

For many years, physicians used urokinase to clear clot from obstructed vascular access devices. Studies have demonstrated up to 95% success rates in opening thrombosed surgically implanted catheters using urokinase.[93] Recently, however, the FDA has raised concerns regarding potential infectious contamination of urokinase during manufacturing. Many centers now use alteplase or tissue plasminogen activator for lysing obstructive thrombus.[31,93,94]

Acute line obstruction can also be caused by precipitation of incompatible medications. Common offenders include total parenteral nutrition, etoposide salts, lipid emulsions, calcium salts, antibiotics, and sodium bicarbonate. Infusion of a solution specifically matched to the precipitated material might flush the line.[95]

Extravasation

Extravasation is defined here as the leaking of infusate into the subcutaneous tissue surrounding a central venous catheter. This complication can be caused by needle displacement from an implanted port, a defect in the catheter tubing within the subcutaneous tunnel, or withdrawal of the catheter from the vein due to inadequate fixation. Additionally, "backtracking" can occur when the catheter is partially occluded and infusate tracks up along the fibrin sleeve and into the subcutaneous tissue. Findings suggestive of extravasation include sudden swelling at line site, increased patient discomfort during infusion, and sudden loss of blood return.[96]

Clavicular–First Rib Compression

This infrequently discussed complication may occur up to 1% of the time in long-term indwelling catheters.[97] When the subclavian vein is cannulated more medially than usual in the narrow space between the clavicle and first rib, the line can be compressed between the first rib and the clavicle. Patients reporting difficulty infusing while in the sitting position or when the ipsilateral arm is elevated or abducted should be suspected of this compression. This malposition can be observed on chest x-ray as kinking of the line over the first rib. The catheter can break free and embolize if the line is not promptly removed. An interventional radiologist using a percutaneous retrograde femoral catherization approach can retrieve an embolized section of catheter.

MANAGEMENT OF NONFUNCTIONING CATHETERS

When a central venous catheter does not return blood or infuse solution, the malfunction should be assessed systematically to maximize catheter durability and to minimize the incidence of catheter-related complications. The first step in this assessment is reviewing the most recent chest radiograph to confirm appropriate place-

TABLE 52-2

Guidelines for Management of a Suspected Clot			
COMPLICATIONS	**CAUSE**	**GRAVITY FLOW OBSERVATION**	**CORRECTIVE ACTION**
Fibrin sheath	Fibrin collects on the tip or encases the catheter	Gravity flow is excellent in all positions, but no blood returns in any position	This catheter may be declotted following the declotting procedure*
Occluded catheter	Fibrin and platelets collect inside the catheter	Inability to infuse solutions and to draw blood	This catheter may be declotted following the declotting procedure* Note: Drug precipitant cannot be corrected with urokinase or heparin†

*These are the only two instances in which it is safe to declot after checking the chest radiograph for proper placement.
†Urokinase is very expensive ($50/vial) and should not be used indiscriminately.

TABLE 52-3

Guidelines for Management of an Unknown Clot

COMPLICATION	CAUSE	GRAVITY FLOW OBSERVATION	CORRECTIVE ACTION
Do not attempt to declot any of the following conditions:			
Malposition	Catheter cut too short and abuts against the vessel wall	Gravity flow is very positional and no blood returns in any position	This catheter must be removed—*do not* attempt to declot with urokinase, which may cause erosion of the vessel wall
Pinch-off syndrome	Insertion site is too close to the rib and first clavicle	Gravity flow is excellent when the patient is lying down, but stops when the patient sits up	This catheter must be removed or it will eventually develop a hole at the insertion site, causing extravasation of infusion or total catheter fragmentation and emboli into the heart
Transverse catheter	Catheter crosses over into the opposite subclavian	Gravity flow may be positional; slow blood return; position will be noted on chest radiograph	CVDL can go into the femoral vein and pull the catheter down to its proper position
Arrhythmias	Catheter tip too long—in the right atrium	Gravity flow may be positional; cardiac arrhythmias seen on electrocardiogram; poor blood return may be intermittent; positional will be noted on chest radiograph	Catheter must be pulled back into the SVC
Flipped up	Catheter tip in the jugular vein; can occur any time after placement due to extreme vomiting or coughing; most common with catheter tips cut too short and placed high in the SVC, or catheters that bulge at the entrance site due to catheter backing out of the vessel	Gravity flow and blood return may be positional; patient may complain of ringing in the ear or a "funny" sensation when flushing the catheter, position can be picked up on chest radiograph	CVDL may be able to reposition in the SVC if the catheter was not cut too short when it was initially placed
Major vessel thrombus	External thrombus in a blood vessel probably due to insertion trauma	No change in gravity flow or blood return; patient will develop swelling in the arm, hand, and neck, most commonly on the same side as the catheter	Documentation of major vessel thrombus by venogram or Doppler is required before treatment with high-dose thrombolytics can be instituted; consultation with hematology should follow thrombus diagnosis before treatment is started

CVDL, Cardiovascular and Diagnostic Laboratory; SVC, superior vena cava.

ment. The next step is checking for gravity flow. Connecting a bag of normal saline to gravity flow and asking the patient to change position, cough, and breathe deeply will demonstrate whether flow is positional. If the catheter is patent to gravity flow, lower the bag below the catheter and assess for blood return. With this information, one can make a decision as to whether to remove, reposition, or declot the catheter.

If the catheter has positional gravity flow and no blood return, the catheter is likely abutting the vessel wall. This situation has a high likelihood of causing erosion of the vessel wall with catastrophic results, so these catheters must be removed. When the catheter is pinched between the first rib and the clavicle, solution will flow to gravity when the patient is lying down and cease when the patient is sitting. These catheters also need to be removed, as they are at increased risk of line fracture and emboliz-ation. A malpositioned catheter tip can present with positional gravity flow and positional or slow blood return. Patients with this problem often complain of tinnitus or neck paresthesia with infusion of solution into the catheter. They also might have documented arrhythmias depending on the position of the misplaced

catheter tip. A chest radiograph could demonstrate that the catheter tip either has crossed into the contralateral subclavian vein or has flipped up into the internal jugular vein. These catheters should either be removed or repositioned by experienced interventional radiologists. Patients with arrhythmias may have catheters that have migrated into the right atrium and need to be removed or withdrawn.

There are two conditions appropriate for thrombolysis of the catheter with alteplase or tissue plasminogen activator (TPA): fibrin sheaths and intraluminal thrombus occlusions. Contraindications for declotting procedures include high bleeding risk and known recent or current episode of bleeding.

Catheter malfunction caused by fibrin sheaths usually demonstrates good gravity flow and no blood return because the sheath acts as a one-way valve, allowing outflow but not inflow through the catheter. When intraluminal fibrin and platelets occlude the catheter, the catheter will demonstrate neither gravity flow nor return regardless of any positional changes. If the caregiver is convinced that the catheter malfunction fits one of these categories and appropriate catheter position is confirmed

PROBLEM SOLVING IN CATHETER USE

TROUBLESHOOTING GUIDELINES

If a catheter does not have a blood return or will not infuse solution, before proceeding with the declotting procedure perform these troubleshooting techniques to diagnose the problem:

1. Connect a flush bag of NS or D_5W to the catheter and open the roller clamp to allow the fluid to flow to gravity.
2. Have the patient change position, take deep breaths, and cough while observing the drip rate.
3. When the fluid infuses at the fastest rate, lower the bag and observe for a blood return.
4. If a blood return is observed, use the catheter as indicated, making a note that it is positional.
5. If no blood return is observed in any position, if gravity flows freely in all positions, and if last chest radiograph verifies catheter tip in the SVC, proceed to declot the catheter with a known clot (catheter has a fibrin sheath).
6. If the radiograph shows that the catheter tip position is questionable, obtain a dye study. Dye study is contrast injected through the lumen of the catheter to verify exact location of the catheter tip, integrity of catheter, and flow of solution.

Before urokinase can be instilled, a dye study must be done if the radiograph shows the catheter tip position to be questionable.

DECLOTTING PROCEDURE

See the preceding guidelines before proceeding to declot, as follows:

1. Using a 1-mL syringe, create a vacuum by aspirating back on the plunger (at the hub) and clamp. Repeat once.
2. Instill 2 mL 1:1000 U heparin solution (in each lumen) and let dwell for 1 hour. Assess for a blood return.
3. If line remains clotted, instill the appropriate amount of urokinase and normal saline solution (listed following) using the same technique as with the heparin.
4. Let dwell for 30 minutes to 1 hour and then assess for a blood return. May repeat as long as the recommendation of 30,000 U/d is not exceeded. Complete aspiration of the solution may not be possible and systemic urokinase may be harmful.

CATHETER TYPE	UROKINASE (mL)	NORMAL SALINE (mL)
Central line, 14 gauge	0.7	0
Central line, 16 gauge	0.5	0
Hickman, 12 F	1	0.6
Hickman, 10 F	1	0.3
PIC	0.5	0
Groshong	1	0.6
Plasmapheresis	1	0.4

on chest radiograph, catheter thrombolysis is indicated. Contrast venography is not necessary before using TPA to open nonmechanical catheter occlusions.

Techniques for declotting catheters vary from institution to institution but follow the same general principles. We recommend instilling 500 mcg of TPA and allowing the infusate to dwell for one hour. If patency is not restored after one hour, instill an additional milligram of TPA and allow the infusate to dwell for another hour. Using a very similar technique, the authors of the Cardiovascular Thrombolytic to Open Occluded Lines Trial (COOL-2) studied nearly 1000 patients with occluded central venous catheters. These patients in a predominantly oncology population did not undergo prethrombolysis contrast studies. There were no deaths or major bleeding episodes directly attributable to the thrombolysis. More than 87% of the catheters were opened with the TPA. At three-month follow-up, nearly 75% of the catheters were still patent.[98]

VASCULAR ACCESS DEVICE MAINTENANCE

The risk of complications with a long-term vascular access device does not end with insertion of the device. Proper care and maintenance of each type of central catheter can reduce the incidence of catheter-related bacteremia, catheter thrombosis, and line failure dramatically. Maintenance is performed not only by qualified staff of oncology centers but also by patients and family members in the outpatient setting. In the nearby box we have detailed our recommendations for central catheter care after a thorough review of the best available literature.

SUMMARY

Patients and physicians have a large variety of vascular access devices from which to choose, and no individual catheter is the ideal solution for all clinical situations. By understanding the strengths and weaknesses of each catheter system, insertion site, and maintenance technique, we hope to minimize the morbidity associated with these commonly used devices. Clearly, having a great deal of experience with placing vascular access devices in the oncology population minimizes the number of problems. Line care is the joint responsibility of the health care team and can be a major source of patient morbidity if each and every member of the oncology team does not maintain the highest quality of care.

More than 500,000 vascular access devices are used in the United States each year. We must continue to conduct clinical studies to determine the safest, most cost-effective device for each cancer situation.

REFERENCES

1. Mayhall CG: Diagnosis and management of infections of implantable devices used for prolonged venous access [Review]. Curr Clin Top Infect Dis 1992;12:83–110.
2. Dryden MS, Samson A, Ludlam HA, Wing AJ, Phillips I: Infective complications associated with the use of the Quinton 'Permcath' for long-term central vascular access in haemodialysis. Journal of Hosp Infect 1991;19:257–262.
3. Pegues D, Axelrod P, McClarren C, et al: Comparison of infections in Hickman and implanted port catheters in adult solid tumor patients. J Surg Oncol 1992;49:156–162.
4. Elliott TS: Can antimicrobial central venous catheters prevent associated infection? [Review]. Br J Haematol 1999;107:235–241.
5. Muller H, Zierski J: The Huber needle as a special cannula for the puncture of implanted ports and pumps—a mistake in multiple variations [German]. Klin Woch 1988;66:963–969.
6. Niederhuber JE, Ensminger W, Gyres JW, Liepman M, Doan K and Cozzi E: Totally implanted venous and arterial access system to replace external catheters in cancer treatment. Surgery 1982;92:706–712.
7. Brothers TE, Von Moll LK, Niederhuber JE, Roberts JA, Walker-Andrews S, Ensminger WD: Experience with subcutaneous infusion ports in three hundred patients. Surg Gynecol Obstet 1988;166:295–301.
8. Brincker H, Saeter G: Fifty-five patient years' experience with a totally implanted system for intravenous chemotherapy. Cancer 1986;57:1124–1129.
9. Khoury MD, Lloyd LR, Burrows J, Berg R, Yap J: A totally implanted venous access system for the delivery of chemotherapy. Cancer 1985;56:1231–1234.
10. McGovern B, Solenberger R, Reed K: A totally implantable venous access system for long-term chemotherapy in children. J Pediat Surg 1985;20:725–727.
11. Bothe A Jr, Piccione W, Ambrosino JJ, Benotti PN, Lokich JJ: Implantable central venous access system. Am J Surg 1984;147:565–569.
12. Wobbes T, Slooff MJ, Sleijfer DT, Mulder NH, Postma A: Five years' experience in access surgery for polychemotherapy. An analysis of results in 100 consecutive patients. Cancer 1983;52:978–982.
13. Parkinson R, Gandhi M, Harper J, Archibald C: Establishing an ultrasound guided peripherally inserted central catheter (PICC) insertion service. Clin Radiol 1998;53:33–36.
14. Kearns PJ, Coleman S, Wehner JH: Complications of long arm-catheters: A randomized trial of central vs peripheral tip location. Jpen J Parent Ent Nutr 1996;20:20–24.
15. Rosen M, Latto I, Ng W: Handbook of Percutaneous Central Venous Catheterization. London, WB Saunders, 1992.
16. Patel NH: Percutaneous translumbar placement of a Hickman catheter into the azygous vein [comment]. AJR Am J Roentgenol 2000;175:1302–1304.
17. Collignon P, Soni N, Pearson I, Sorrell T, Woods P: Sepsis associated with central vein catheters in critically ill patients. Intensive Care Med 1988;14:227–231.
18. Pearson ML: Guideline for prevention of intravascular device-related infections. Part I. Intravascular device-related infections: an overview. The Hospital Infection Control Practices Advisory Committee [Review]. AJIC Am J Infect Control 1996;24:262–277.
19. Ruesch S, Walder B, Tramer MR: Complications of central venous catheters: Internal jugular versus subclavian access—a systematic review [comment] [Review]. Crit Care Med 2002;30:454–460.
20. Darouiche RO, Raad II, Heard SO, et al: A comparison of two antimicrobial-impregnated central venous catheters. Catheter Study Group [comment]. New Engl J Med 1999;340:1–8.
21. Raad I, Darouiche R, Dupuis J, et al: Central venous catheters coated with minocycline and rifampin for the prevention of catheter-related colonization and bloodstream infections. A randomized, double-blind trial. The Texas Medical Center Catheter Study Group [comment]. Ann Intern Med 1997;127:267–274.
22. Raad II, Hohn DC, Gilbreath BJ, et al: Prevention of central venous catheter-related infections by using maximal sterile barrier precautions during insertion [comment]. Infect Contr Hosp Epidemiol 1994;15:231–238.
23. Vassilomanolakis M, Plataniotis G, Koumakis G, et al: Central venous catheter-related infections after bone marrow transplantation in patients with malignancies: A prospective study with short-course vancomycin prophylaxis [comment]. Bone Marrow Transplant 1995;15:77–80.
24. Spafford PS, Sinkin RA, Cox C, Reubens L, Powell KR: Prevention of central venous catheter-related coagulase-negative staphylococcal sepsis in neonates. J Pediatr 1994;125:259–263.
25. Shaul DB, Scheer B, Rokhsar S, et al: Risk factors for early infection of central venous catheters in pediatric patients. J Am Coll Surg 1998;186:654–658.
26. Duggan J, O'Connell D, Heller R, Ghosh H: Causes of hospital-acquired septicaemia—a case control study. Quart J Med 1993;86:479–483.
27. Keenan SP: Use of ultrasound to place central lines [Review]. J Crit Care 2002;17:126–137.
28. Gualtieri E, Deppe SA, Sipperly ME, Thompson DR: Subclavian venous catheterization: Greater success rate for less experienced operators using ultrasound guidance [comment]. Crit Care Med 1995;23:692–697.
29. Shivnan JC, McGuire D, Freedman S, et al: A comparison of transparent adherent and dry sterile gauze dressings for long-term central catheters in patients undergoing bone marrow transplant. Oncol Nurs Forum 1991;18:1349–1356.
30. Bosserman G, McGuire DB, McGuire WP, Nicholls D: Multi-disciplinary management of vascular access devices. Oncol Nurs Forum 1990;17:879–886.
31. Cunningham RS, Bonam-Crawford D: The role of fibrinolytic agents in the management of thrombotic complications associated with vascular access devices [Review]. Nurs Clin North Am 1993;28:899–909.
32. Druy EM, Trout HH III, Giordano JM, Hix WR: Lytic therapy in the treatment of axillary and subclavian vein thrombosis. J Vasc Surg 1985;2:821–827.
33. Holcombe B: Restoring patency of long-term central venous access devices. J Intraven Nurs 1993;16:195.
34. Edwards RL, Klaus M, Matthews E, McCullen C, Bona RD, Rickles FR: Heparin abolishes the chemotherapy-induced increase in plasma fibrinopeptide A levels. Am J Med 1990;89:25–28.
35. Greenberg S, Kosinski R, Daniels J: Treatment of superior vena cava thrombosis with recombinant tissue type plasminogen activator. Chest 1991;99:1298–1301.
36. Rubin RN: Local installation of small doses of streptokinase for treatment of thrombotic occlusions of long-term access catheters. J Clin Oncol 1983;1:572–573.
37. Gilon D, Schechter D, Rein AJ, et al: Right atrial thrombi are related to indwelling central venous catheter position: Insights into time course and possible mechanism of formation. Am Heart J 1998;135:457–462.
38. Gauderer MW: Vascular access techniques and devices in the pediatric patient [Review]. Surg Clin North Am 1992;72:1267–1284.
39. Matsumoto T, Pavlides C, McDonald B, Brodsky I: Subcutaneous venous access for chemotherapy. Pennsylv Med 1984;87:56.
40. Lameris JS, Post PJ, Zonderland HM, Gerritsen PG, Kappers-Klunne MC, Schutte HE: Percutaneous placement of Hickman catheters: Comparison of sonographically guided and blind techniques. Am J Roentgenol 1990;155:1097–1099.
41. Fabri PJ: Permanent right atrial catheter insertion. Am J Surg 1982;143:394–396.
42. Stacey RG, Filshie J, Skewes D: Percutaneous insertion of Hickman-type catheters [comment]. Br J Hosp Med 1991;46:396–398.
43. Polderman KH, Girbes AJ: Central venous catheter use. Part 1: Mechanical complications [Review]. Intensive Care Med 2002;28:1–17.
44. Reed CR, Sessler CN, Glauser FL, Phelan BA: Central venous catheter infections: Concepts and controversies [comment] [Review]. Intensive Care Med 1995;21:177–183.
45. Lee RB, Buckner M, Sharp KW: Do multi-lumen catheters increase central venous catheter sepsis compared to single-lumen catheters? J Trauma Inj Infect Crit Care 1988;28:1472–1475.
46. Hilton E, Haslett TM, Borenstein MT, Tucci V, Isenberg HD, Singer C: Central catheter infections: Single- versus triple-lumen catheters. Influence of guide wires on infection rates when used for replacement of catheters [comment]. Am J Med 1988;84:667–672.

47. McCarthy MC, Shives JK, Robison RJ, Broadie TA: Prospective evaluation of single and triple lumen catheters in total parenteral nutrition. Jpen J Parent Ent Nutr 1987;11:259–262.

48. Bernard RW, Stahl WM: Subclavian vein catheterizations: A prospective study. I. Non-infectious complications. Ann Surg 1971;173:184–190.

49. Maki D: Nosocomial infections in the intensive care unit. In Parillo J, Bone R (eds): Critical Care Medicine: Principles of Diagnosis and Management. St. Louis, Mosby, 1995, pp 893–954.

50. Koksoy C, Kuzu A, Erden I, Akkaya A: The risk factors in central venous catheter-related thrombosis. Aust N Z J Surg 1995;65:796–798.

51. Kincaid EH, Davis PW, Chang MC, Fenstermaker JM, Pennell TC: "Blind" placement of long-term central venous access devices: Report of 589 consecutive procedures. Am Surg 1999;65:520–523.

52. Hagley MT, Martin B, Gast P, Traeger SM: Infectious and mechanical complications of central venous catheters placed by percutaneous venipuncture and over guidewires. Crit Care Med 1992;20:1426–1430.

53. Lucey B, Varghese JC, Haslam P, Lee MJ: Routine chest radiographs after central line insertion: Mandatory postprocedural evaluation or unnecessary waste of resources? Cardiovasc Intervent Radiol 1999;22:381–384.

54. Doerfler ME, Kaufman B, Goldenberg AS: Central venous catheter placement in patients with disorders of hemostasis. Chest 1996;110:185–188.

55. Thomson IR, Dalton BC, Lappas DG, Lowenstein E: Right bundle-branch block and complete heart block caused by the Swan-Ganz catheter. Anesthesiology 1979;51:359–362.

56. Morris D, Mulvihill D, Lew WY: Risk of developing complete heart block during bedside pulmonary artery catheterization in patients with left bundle-branch block. Arch Int Med 1987;147:2005–2010.

57. Press OW, Ramsey PG, Larson EB, Fefer A, Hickman RO: Hickman catheter infections in patients with malignancies. Medicine 1984;63:189–200.

58. Howell PB, Walters PE, Donowitz GR, Farr BM: Risk factors for infection of adult patients with cancer who have tunnelled central venous catheters. Cancer 1995;75:1367–1375.

59. Fuchs PC, Gustafson ME, King JT, Goodall PT: Assessment of catheter-associated infection risk with the Hickman right atrial catheter. Infect Contr 1984;5:226–230.

60. Thomas JH, MacArthur RI, Pierce GE, Hermreck AS: Hickman-Broviac catheters. Indications and results. Am J Surg 1980;140:791–796.

61. Barzaghi A, Dell'Orto M, Rovelli A, Rizzari C, Colombini A, Uderzo C: Central venous catheter clots: Incidence, clinical significance and catheter care in patients with hematologic malignancies. Pediatr Hematol Oncol 1995;12:243–250.

62. Band J: Pathogenesis of and risk factors for central venous catheter-related infections. UpToDate Online 11.1 . 2003. 5-28-2003. http://www.uptodate.com.

63. Pessa ME, Howard FM: Complications of Hickman-Broviac catheters. Surg Gynecol Obstet 1985;161:257–260.

64. Darbyshire PJ, Weightman NC, Speller DC: Problems associated with indwelling central venous catheters. Arch Dis Child 1985;60:129–134.

65. Groeger JS, Lucas AB, Thaler HT, et al: Infectious morbidity associated with long-term use of venous access devices in patients with cancer [comment]. Ann Int Med 1993;119:1168–1174.

66. Ross MN, Haase GM, Poole MA, Burrington JD, Odom LF: Comparison of totally implanted reservoirs with external catheters as venous access devices in pediatric oncologic patients. Surg Gynecol Obstet 1988;167:141–144.

67. Carde P, Cosset-Delaigue MF, Laplanche A, Chareau I: Classical external indwelling central venous catheter versus totally implanted venous access systems for chemotherapy administration: A randomized trial in 100 patients with solid tumors. Eur J Cancer Clin Oncol 1989;25:939–944.

68. Eastridge BJ, Lefor AT: Complications of indwelling venous access devices in cancer patients. J Clin Oncol 1995;13:233–238.

69. Franson TR, Zak O, van den Broek P: Evaluation of new anti-infective drugs for the treatment of vascular access device-associated bacteremia and fungemia. The European Working Party of the European Society of Clinical Microbiology and Infectious Diseases. Clin Infect Dis 1993;17:789–793.

70. La Quaglia MP, Lucas A, Thaler HT, Friedlander-Klar H, Exelby PR, Groeger JS: A prospective analysis of vascular access device-related infections in children. J Pediatr Surg 1992;27:840–842.

71. Larson EB, Wooding M, Hickman RO: Infectious complications of right atrial catheters used for venous access in patients receiving intensive chemotherapy. Surg Gynecol Obstet 1981;153:369–373.

72. Jacobs MB, Yeager M: Thrombotic and infectious complications of Hickman-Broviac catheters. Arch Intern Med 1984;144:1597–1599.

73. Benezra D, Kiehn TE, Gold JW, Brown AE, Turnbull AD, Armstrong D: Prospective study of infections in indwelling central venous catheters using quantitative blood cultures. Am J Med 1988;85:495–498.

74. Lobe TE, Schropp KP, Rogers DA, Rao BN: A "smart needle" to facilitate difficult vascular access in pediatric patients. J Pediatr Surg 1993;28:1401–1402.

75. Brun-Buisson C, Abrouk F, Legrand P, Huet Y, Larabi S, Rapin M: Diagnosis of central venous catheter-related sepsis. Critical level of quantitative tip cultures. Arch Intern Med 1987;147:873–877.

76. Schmitt SK, Knapp C, Hall GS, Longworth DL, McMahon JT, Washington JA: Impact of chlorhexidine-silver sulfadiazine-impregnated central venous catheters on in vitro quantitation of catheter-associated bacteria [comment]. J Clin Microbiol 1996;34:508–511.

77. Cleri DJ, Corrado ML, Seligman SJ: Quantitative culture of intravenous catheters and other intravascular inserts. J Infect Dis 1980;141:781–786.

78. Irwig L, Tosteson AN, Gatsonis C, et al: Guidelines for meta-analyses evaluating diagnostic tests [comment]. Ann Intern Med 1994;120:667–676.

79. Siegman-Igra Y, Anglim AM, Shapiro DE, Adal KA, Strain BA, Farr BM: Diagnosis of vascular catheter-related bloodstream infection: A meta-analysis. J Clin Microbiol 1997;35:928–936.

80. DesJardin JA, Falagas ME, Ruthazer R, et al: Clinical utility of blood cultures drawn from indwelling central venous catheters in hospitalized patients with cancer [comment]. Ann Intern Med 1999;131:641–647.

81. Blot F, Schmidt E, Nitenberg G, et al: Earlier positivity of central-venous- versus peripheral-blood cultures is highly predictive of catheter-related sepsis. J Clin Microbiol 1998;36:105–109.

82. Blot F, Nitenberg G, Chachaty E, et al: Diagnosis of catheter-related bacteraemia: A prospective comparison of the time to positivity of hub-blood versus peripheral-blood cultures. Lancet 1999;354:1071–1077.

83. Peacock SJ, Eddleston M, Emptage A, King A, Crook DW: Positive intravenous line tip cultures as predictors of bacteraemia. J Hosp Infect 1998;40:35–38.

84. Messing B, Peitra-Cohen S, Debure A, Beliah M, Bernier JJ: Antibiotic-lock technique: A new approach to optimal therapy for catheter-related sepsis in home-parenteral nutrition patients. Jpen J Parent Ent Nutr 1988;12:185–189.

85. Douard MC, Arlet G, Leverger G, et al: Quantitative blood cultures for diagnosis and management of catheter-related sepsis in pediatric hematology and oncology patients. Intensive Care Med 1991;17:30–35.

86. Krzywda EA, Andris DA, Edmiston CE Jr, Quebbeman EJ : Treatment of Hickman catheter sepsis using antibiotic lock technique. Infect Contr Hosp Epidemiol 1995;16:596–598.

87. Benoit JL, Carandang G, Sitrin M, Arnow PM: Intraluminal antibiotic treatment of central venous catheter infections in patients receiving parenteral nutrition at home [comment]. Clin Infect Dis 1995;21:1286–1288.

88. Rackoff WR, Weiman M, Jakobowski D, Hirschl R, Stallings V, Bilodeau J, et al: A randomized, controlled trial of the efficacy of a heparin and vancomycin solution in preventing central venous catheter infections in children [comment]. J Pediatr 1995;127:147–151.

89. Randolph AG, Cook DJ, Gonzales CA, Andrew M: Benefit of heparin in central venous and pulmonary artery catheters: A meta-analysis of randomized controlled trials [comment]. Chest 1998;113:165–171.

90. Monreal M, Alastrue A, Rull M, et al: Upper extremity deep venous thrombosis in cancer patients with venous access devices— prophylaxis with a low molecular weight heparin (Fragmin). Thromb Haemost 1996;75:251–253.

91. Bern MM, Lokich JJ, Wallach SR, et al: Very low doses of warfarin can prevent thrombosis in central venous catheters. A randomized prospective trial. Ann Intern Med 1990;112:423-428.

92. Boraks P, Seale J, Price J, et al: Prevention of central venous catheter associated thrombosis using minidose warfarin in patients with haematological malignancies. Br J Haematol 1998;101:483-486.

93. Seigel EL, Jew AC, Delcore R, Iliopoulos JI, Thomas JH: Thrombolytic therapy for catheter-related thrombosis. Am J Surg 1993;166: 716-718.

94. Bagnall-Reeb H, Ruccione K: Practical application of an algorithm for the thrombolytic treatment of occluded vascular access devices. J Pediatr Oncol Nurs 1993;10:79-82.

95. Ulz L, Petersen FB, Ford R, et al: A prospective study of complications in Hickman right-atrial catheters in marrow transplant patients. Jpen J Parent Ent Nutr 1990;14:27-30.

96. Wickham R, Purl S, Welker D: Long-term central venous catheters: Issues for care [Review]. Sem Oncol Nurs 1992;8:133-147.

97. Andris DA, Krzywda EA, Schulte W, Ausman R, Quebbeman EJ: Pinch-off syndrome: A rare etiology for central venous catheter occlusion. Jpen J Parent Ent Nutr 1994;18:531-533.

98. Deitcher SR, Fesen MR, Kiproff PM, et al: Cardiovascular thrombolytic to open occluded lines. Safety and efficacy of alteplase for restoring function in occluded central venous catheters: Results of the cardiovascular thrombolytic to open occluded lines trial. J Clin Oncol 2002;20:317-324.

Problems Common to Cancer and Its Therapy

II

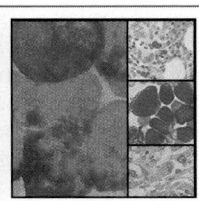

53

ACUTE ABDOMEN, BOWEL OBSTRUCTION, AND FISTULA

Kathleen M. Diehl
Alfred E. Chang

SUMMARY OF KEY POINTS

GASTROINTESTINAL BLEEDING
- Bleeding affects approximately 15% of patients with acute abdominal emergencies.
- It is more commonly seen in patients with leukemia or lymphoma who are undergoing intensive chemotherapy.
- Endoscopy is critical to identify the source of bleeding and could even be therapeutic.
- Nonoperative therapy is successful for most patients.

GASTROINTESTINAL PERFORATION
- Perforation affects approximately 20% of patients with acute abdominal emergencies.
- Bowel perforation can be due to spontaneous tumor rupture, tumor necrosis secondary to chemotherapy or radiation, drugs (e.g., steroids), and inflammatory conditions.
- Operative intervention is mandated unless the patient's overall prognosis is poor.

NEUTROPENIC ENTEROCOLITIS
- Also termed necrotizing enterocolitis, neutropenic enterocolitis typically affects the terminal ileum, cecum, and ascending colon in patients with chemotherapy-induced neutropenia.
- Most patients respond to conservative management with broad-spectrum antibiotics and bowel rest.
- Surgical intervention should be considered for perforation, uncontrolled sepsis, or persistence of symptoms despite correction of neutropenia.

BOWEL OBSTRUCTION
- Obstruction affects approximately 40% of patients with cancer who experience acute abdominal emergencies.
- One-fourth of patients requiring surgical intervention have a benign cause of their obstruction.
- Partial bowel obstruction can initially be treated nonoperatively by

tube decompression and is successful 25% of the time.
- Clinical suspicion of bowel ischemia or complete obstruction mandates urgent surgical intervention.

FISTULAE
- Presenting symptoms rarely match those of intra-abdominal malignancy and more commonly represent complications after surgery or radiation therapy, or both.
- Fistulae occur most often as a result of treatment of gynecologic malignancies.
- Medical management consisting of nutritional support and bowel rest allows spontaneous closure of most enterocutaneous fistulae.
- Causes for persistence of a fistula include undrained infection, luminal obstruction distal to the fistula, prior radiation, epithelialization of the fistulous tract, cancer within the tract, presence of a foreign body, and malnutrition.

INTRODUCTION

The management of patients with malignant disease has undergone significant changes. Multimodality therapy involving surgery, radiation therapy, chemotherapy, and immunotherapy is now commonplace. The clinician caring for the patient with cancer must be cognizant of the potential complications associated with these therapeutic modalities. Often, they can manifest as unique surgical problems. This chapter reviews the common abdominal complications and emergencies encountered in patients with a diagnosis of cancer. Topics include gastrointestinal bleeding and perforation, intra-abdominal inflammatory conditions, intestinal obstruction, and intestinal fistula. In addition, unique abdominal problems seen in patients undergoing bone marrow transplantation (BMT) are reviewed.

GENERAL CONSIDERATIONS

The term *acute abdomen* implies the presence of a life-threatening problem that needs to be evaluated for potential surgical intervention. A review of approximately 200 abdominal emergencies requiring surgical therapy at Memorial Sloan-Kettering Cancer Center during a five-year period showed that 39% were for obstruction, 22% for perforation, 15% for hemorrhage, 10% for inflammatory processes, and 14% for other miscellaneous problems (Table 53-1).[1,2] Because of the potential need for surgical intervention, it is critical to have a surgeon involved in the early evaluation of patients with significant abdominal complaints. In patients with cancer, the decision to intervene with surgical therapy can be difficult due to abnormal physiologic responses to injury, complications associated with previous cancer therapies, or ethical

TABLE 53-1

Acute Abdominal Emergencies in Cancer Patients Who Required Surgery: Memorial Sloan-Kettering Cancer Center*

CONDITION	TOTAL (%)
Obstruction	83 (39)
Hemorrhage	31 (15)
Intra-abdominal	
Ruptured tumor (7)	7 (23)
Unknown source (1)	1 (3)
Gastrointestinal	
Gastric (6)	6 (19)
Duodenum (5)	5 (16)
Small bowel (3)	3 (10)
Colon (9)	9 (29)
Perforation	47 (22)
Gastric (7)	7 (15)
Duodenum (9)	9 (19)
Small bowel (11)	11 (23)
Colon (20)	20 (43)
Inflammatory	22 (10)
Cholecystitis (7)	7 (32)
Appendicitis (5)	5 (23)
Bile peritonitis (4)	4 (18)
Cholangitis (3)	3 (14)
Septic ascites (1)	1 (4)
Neutropenic enterocolitis (1)	1 (4)
Crohn's disease (1)	1 (4)
Miscellaneous	30 (14)
Diagnostic error (15)	15 (50)
Incarcerated hernia (6)	6 (20)
Mesenteric vascular occlusion (6)	6 (20)
Rectal fistula (2)	2 (7)
Emergency splenectomy (1)	1 (3)
Total	213 (14)

*Excluding any case requiring surgery for postoperative complications.
From Turnbull ADM: Abdominal and upper gastrointestinal emergencies. In Turnbull ADM (ed): Surgical Emergencies in the Cancer Patient. Chicago, Year Book, 1987, p 152; and Starnes HF, Turnbull ADM, Daly JM: Colon and rectal emergencies. In Turnbull ADM (ed): Surgical Emergencies in the Cancer Patient. Chicago, Year Book, 1987, p 195.

considerations. In some instances, medical management is the mainstay of therapy when acute abdominal findings are evident.

Abdominal pain is the single most important symptom in the patient with an acute abdomen. In patients with a diagnosed intra-abdominal malignancy who are undergoing chemotherapy, radiation therapy, or both, abdominal pain must be evaluated and investigated carefully. Care must be taken not to attribute these complaints perfunctorily to the progression of the malignancy. An acute abdomen always cause pain unless the patient has an altered sensorium or spinal cord injury or is taking corticosteroids. The patient taking steroids might have diffuse peritonitis and yet remain pain-free and afebrile. Other abdominal complaints, such as vomiting, distention, lack of passage of flatus, and fever associated with pain should raise the examiner's index of suspicion that an acute abdomen is present.[3,4]

On physical examination, tenderness to palpation is one of the most important signs to elicit. Peritonitis almost invariably produces tenderness as a localized or diffuse finding. Even patients taking steroids usually (but not always) demonstrate tenderness. Percussion performed in a gentle manner can localize pain without alarming or hurting the patient and elicit involuntary guarding, another sign of peritonitis. Palpation of the abdomen might also demonstrate evidence of organomegaly or abdominal masses that could be contributing to the symptoms. An often forgotten examination technique is determination of loss of liver dullness to percussion over the right lower rib cage; this can be a hallmark of free air within the abdomen secondary to a bowel perforation. In the patient with a distended abdomen, percussion helps determine whether the distension is secondary to bowel gas or to the presence of ascites, which causes shifting dullness. Auscultation should be directed at identifying the presence and quality of bowel sounds or a succussion splash in a dilated stomach. In all patients with abdominal complaints, both pelvic and rectal examination must be part of the physical examination. These examinations are helpful to identify masses, evidence of peritoneal irritation, fistulous drainage, occult blood, or the presence of abscesses in the perirectal tissues.

Ultimately, the surgeon must make the determination as to whether the patient has an acute abdomen that requires surgical intervention. Although this decision is often made solely on the basis of the history and physical examination, laboratory and diagnostic imaging studies can help define the nature of the problem more accurately. Standard laboratory studies should include a complete blood count and electrolytes, including a serum bicarbonate level. Leukocytosis will normally be evident if an intra-abdominal infection is present. Unfortunately, chemotherapy-induced neutropenia might prevent the white cell count from adequately reflecting an inflammatory process. Similarly, patients on immunosuppressive doses of steroids will not mount a leukocytosis in response to an infection. In these situations, if an intra-abdominal inflammatory process is suspected, diagnostic imaging studies with ultrasonography or computed tomography (CT) could be helpful in identifying fluid collections or abscesses. In addition, CT is helpful in identifying free air, intestinal pneumatosis, and portal vein gas. Liver function studies and a serum amylase are helpful in patients with upper abdominal complaints when hepatobiliary or pancreatic organ pathology is suspected. Patients with evidence of gastrointestinal (GI) bleeding require serial hemoglobin or hematocrits, or both, to assess the severity and magnitude of the bleeding. Localization of the bleeding source by endoscopy or arteriography is important and could even be therapeutic. When abdominal distension is present, plain flat and upright films of the abdomen are important to determine whether evidence of obstruction or ileus exists and whether free air is present under the diaphragm. The specific roles of these studies are discussed as individual problems are reviewed.

Decisions to undertake surgical intervention in acutely ill patients with cancer should be directed at improving the patient's well-being. Whenever possible, the patient's definition of well-being should be respected.[5] If these principles are accepted, it is apparent that a number of situations might be encountered in the cancer patient with an acute abdomen in which surgical intervention is not appropriate. Unfortunately, few data are available to assist with the determination of the futility of surgery in patients with cancer.[6] Some evidence shows the efficacy of cardiopulmonary resuscitation (CPR) in patients with metastatic cancer.[7] If the CPR experience is applicable to surgical decisions, a preponderance of evidence demonstrates that survival to discharge is virtually never achieved in patients with metastatic cancer who require CPR. Emergency abdominal operations in patients with metastatic cancer receiving chemotherapy might be equally futile; one series reported that only one patient of 21 survived to return home after such surgery.[8]

GASTROINTESTINAL BLEEDING

The true incidence of significant gastrointestinal (GI) bleeding in patients with cancer is not accurately known. At one major cancer center, approximately 15% of patients with abdominal emergencies requiring surgery had abdominal hemorrhage, most of them secondary to GI tract bleeding (see Table 53-1). Patients with lymphoma or leukemia on intensive combination chemotherapy regimens are more likely to experience GI tract bleeding. Kemeny and Brennan[9] found that the most common cause of upper GI tract bleeding in patients with cancer was gastritis (36% of patients), followed by peptic or stress ulceration (26%) and tumor necrosis (23%)[10-14] (Table 53-2). Other, less common causes of bleeding include *Candida* esophagitis, Mallory-Weiss mucosal tears, hemorrhage from inflammatory conditions (i.e., neutropenic enterocolitis), or radiation-associated complications (i.e., arterial-enteric fistulae, radiation enteropathy). This multitude of potential causes of bleeding underscores the need to evaluate these patients thoroughly; the tumor cannot be presumed to be the source of bleeding.

The pathogenesis of upper GI bleeding can be multifactorial. Chemotherapeutic agents can damage or irritate the mucosa and depress platelet production. Gastritis or peptic ulcers can be induced by a variety of agents that patients might take, such as aspirin, alcohol, steroids, indomethacin, or phenylbutazone. The use of cortico-steroids increases the risk of hospitalization for upper GI bleeding more than fourfold.[15] Stress secondary to aggressive chemotherapy could also contribute to the development of upper GI bleeding. Hepatic arterial infusion of fluorodeoxyuridine (FUDR) utilizing an implanted pump for the treatment of liver tumors has been reported to result in a significant incidence of upper GI toxicity with gastritis and peptic ulcers.[16,17] Meticulous dissection is necessary to ensure ligation of small branches of the hepatic artery distal to the tip of the catheter; otherwise, FUDR infusion can result in gastritis and duodenitis with subsequent hemorrhage or perforation.

The development of rapid tumor necrosis with subsequent significant hemorrhage has been reported during chemotherapy. This problem is more commonly observed in patients with GI lymphomas. The incidence of significant GI bleeding in this patient population secondary to tumor lysis from therapy is approximately 5%[14,18-22] (Table 53-3). Surgical resection of GI lymphoma before systemic or radiation therapy (or both) has been advocated to avoid potential hemorrhage or perforation. This procedure could be beneficial for lesions that are amenable to resection with minimal morbidity.

Another etiology of upper GI bleeding is *Candida* infection of the GI tract. The esophagus can be affected in 10%–20% of patients being treated for hematologic malignancies. Esophageal candidiasis can be documented by endoscopy with esophageal washings. Treatment includes oral nystatin or ketoconazole; intravenous amphotericin B may be used in patients who cannot tolerate oral treatments.

Treatment of upper GI tract bleeding requires defining its source. Endoscopy should be performed early on for diagnosis. In most patients, nonoperative treatment is successful. Supportive measures with antacids, H_2-receptor blockers, and blood products will control the bleeding in 60% of patients with gastritis or ulceration. Endoscopic coagulative laser or bipolar cautery can sometimes control bleeding from isolated ulcerations or tumors. If medical management fails to stop bleeding from erosive gastritis or if more than 6 units of blood have been transfused (or both), surgery should be considered. Indications to proceed with surgery should also be

TABLE 53-2

Upper GI Tract Bleeding in Patients with Malignancy

| STUDY | DIAGNOSIS | NO. OF PATIENTS | TYPE OF HEMORRHAGE | | | |
			GASTRITIS	ULCER	TUMOR	OTHER
Padmanabhan et al.[10]	Malignancy	55	24	11	10	10
Klein et al.[11]	Malignancy	49	18	19	6	6
Hande et al.[12]	DHL-GI	3	0	0	3	0
Fleming et al.[13]	Gastric lymphoma	4	0	0	4	0
Kemeny et al.[14]	Burkitt's lymphoma	10	1	2	5	2
Total		121 (100%)	43 (36%)	32 (26%)	28 (23%)	18 (15%)

DHL, diffuse histiocytic lymphoma.
From Kemeny MM, Brennan M: The surgical complications of chemotherapy in the cancer patient. Curr Probl Surg 1987;24:613–675.

Problems Common to Cancer and Its Therapy

TABLE 53-3

Perforation or Bleeding of GI Tract Lymphomas Secondary to Tumor Lysis Induced by Chemotherapy, Radiation, or Both

STUDY	NO. OF PATIENTS	DIAGNOSIS	PERFORATION (NO. OF PATIENTS)	BLEEDING (NO. OF PATIENTS)
Kemeny et al.[14] (1982)	41	Burkitt's	0	5
Meyers et al.[18] (1985)	92	Non-Hodgkin's	4	NR
Talamonti et al.[19] (1990)	24	Non-Hodgkin's	2	3
Maor et al.[20] (1990)	34	Gastric non-Hodgkin's	0	0
Salles et al.[21] (1991)	77	Non-Hodgkin's	1	1
Rackner et al.[22] (1991)	15	Non-Hodgkin's	2	0
Total	283		9/283 (3%)	9/191 (5%)

NR, not reported.

predicated on the patient's potential quality of life and disease prognosis. For erosive gastritis, total or near-total gastrectomy is the most effective means of controlling hemorrhage but is associated with a high morbidity and mortality due to the underlying medical condition of these patients. Bleeding from duodenal ulcer disease in a patient with cancer is probably best treated by oversewing the ulcer and performing a truncal vagotomy with pyloroplasty. When extensive bleeding occurs from tumor, operative resection might be the only recourse.

For lower GI tract bleeding, colonoscopy, radionuclide imaging, or mesenteric angiography might be required to identify the source. Colonoscopy should be performed as the initial diagnostic study. Vigorous bleeding might limit the usefulness of colonoscopy. For GI bleeding at a rate greater than 1 mL/minute, selective mesenteric arteriography is the most accurate method for localization. Technetium-labeled red blood cell scans can be helpful in localizing the site of hemorrhage when bleeding is less in amount or intermittent. Surgical therapy is required for patients who fail medical management. Prior localization of the bleeding source is necessary to identify the segment of bowel to resect. When it is not possible to localize the source of colonic bleeding, subtotal colectomy should be performed. In poor-risk patients, therapy with selective infusion of vasopressin or embolization of the bleeding vessel can be performed, but the risk of bowel infarction exists.

PERFORATION

Perforation of the GI tract mandates operative intervention unless the patient's prognosis from the underlying malignancy is judged to be poor. Approximately 20% of patients with malignancy requiring emergent laparotomy have a bowel perforation (see Table 53-1). Excluding iatrogenic causes of bowel perforation (i.e., postoperative complications), the causes of perforation can be categorized into the following subgroups: spontaneous tumor rupture or erosion into bowel, or both; tumor necrosis secondary to therapy; drug-induced perforations; and inflammatory conditions. Spontaneous perforations of GI tract malignancies are unusual. Occasionally, gastric carcinomas might present with perforation as

the precipitating event.[23] Primary colon cancers might present as localized perforative lesions or can cause obstruction with subsequent perforation. Spontaneous perforation of GI tumors is probably more common in patients with lymphomas, although this still represents an unusual event. Large malignant retroperitoneal lymphomas, renal cell carcinomas, and testicular cancers metastatic to aortocaval nodes can invade adjacent duodenum and cause perforation.

Patients with GI lymphomas could have perforation or bleeding related to regression of their primary tumor during treatment with chemotherapy, radiation therapy, or both. The incidence of these problems in unresected patients with GI lymphomas is summarized in Table 53-3.[14,18-22] Perforation or bleeding from treatment-induced tumor lysis occurs in approximately 3% and 5% of patients, respectively. Some feel that low-grade, earlier-stage GI lymphomas are less likely to manifest these complications.[19] Although resection of larger, higher grade GI lymphomas can be associated with increased morbidity, the mortality rate is greater than 50% when surgical intervention is urgently required for perforation or bleeding in the setting of neutropenia and thrombocytopenia.[24,25] It is therefore reasonable to consider surgical resection of high-grade GI lymphomas in patients with acceptable risk before chemotherapy, radiation therapy, or both.

Drugs are the presumed cause of perforation when bowel wall injury cannot be associated with tumor necrosis or other specific factors in patients with cancer undergoing drug therapy. The drugs most commonly implicated are corticosteroids, which can give rise to ulcers and perforations in various portions of the GI tract. Nonsteroidal anti-inflammatory agents used for pain management can also predispose patients to peptic ulcer disease. Bowel necrosis with perforation has been described with the use of cytosine arabinoside. In 50 patients treated for leukemia, Jones and Abramson[26] reported on seven patients with bowel necrosis and peritonitis at autopsy. It was theorized that cytosine arabinoside was responsible as a result of a direct toxic effect on the GI mucosa. Taxol, which commonly is used to treat patients with ovarian and breast cancers, has also been reported as a chemotherapeutic agent that can cause bowel perforation unrelated to tumor lysis.[27] With the use of interleukin-2 (IL-2) for immunotherapy, occasional cases of colonic infarction and perforation have occurred.[28] The causes of these perforations are unknown, but it has been postulated that they arise from impaired perfusion due to hypotension, tissue edema, and vasoconstriction secondary to the use of pressor agents.

Treatment of bowel perforations from inflammatory processes varies with the site and cause. For gastric perforations secondary to benign ulcers, plication or subtotal resection is indicated. If ulceration is related to malignancy, then subtotal or total gastrectomy might be required. For perforated duodenal ulcers, various surgical options (from simple plication to antrectomy and vagotomy) can be employed depending on the circumstances. Small bowel perforations should be resected with re-anastomosis using healthy bowel. Colonic perforations, especially in the setting of the unprepped bowel and in the immunosuppressed patient, should be treated with resection and colostomy. Given the high mortality rate associated with perforation of the bowel in this immunosuppressed and potentially malnourished population, early diagnosis and treatment are of utmost importance.[29]

INFLAMMATORY CONDITIONS IN THE CANCER PATIENT

Increasingly, aggressive chemotherapeutic regimens are being employed in the treatment of patients with cancer. Unfortunately, these aggressive treatments can expose patients to life-threatening complications related to bone marrow suppression and neutropenia. The incidence of acute illnesses necessitating surgical intervention in the setting of the neutropenic patient with cancer is approximately 7% (Table 53-4).[30] Unique inflammatory abdominal problems in patients with cancer receiving aggressive therapies are reviewed in the following sections.

Neutropenic Enterocolitis

Neutropenic enterocolitis is a clinicopathologic syndrome involving the gastrointestinal tract of patients receiving chemotherapy for hematologic and solid malignancies.

TABLE 53-4

Conditions Found at Surgery in Neutropenic Patients with Cancer Undergoing Emergency Laparotomy	
CONDITION	**PERCENT**
Neutropenic enterocolitis	60
Bowel perforation	7
Hemorrhage (i.e., tumor site, gastritis, gastric ulcers)	9
Other (appendicitis, cholecystitis, incarcerated hernia, and so forth)	20
No disease	4

From Glenn J, Funkhouser WK, Schneider PS: Acute illnesses necessitating urgent abdominal surgery in neutropenic cancer patients: Description of 14 cases and review of the literature. Surgery 1989;105:778–789.

The clinical condition has been given a variety of names in the past, including typhlitis, ileocecal syndrome, and necrotizing enteropathy. Most commonly seen in patients undergoing treatment for leukemia, neutropenic enterocolitis is a rare occurrence, with an incidence of less than 5% in this patient population.[31-33] It is, however, the most common gastrointestinal complaint requiring surgical attention in neutropenic patients. In a literature review of 56 neutropenic patients with cancer requiring urgent laparotomy at the National Cancer Institute, neutropenic enterocolitis was diagnosed in 60%.[30]

The pathophysiologic basis of this clinical entity has not been established clearly and is undoubtedly multifactorial. Neutropenic enterocolitis characteristically affects the terminal ileum, cecum, and ascending colon in patients with chemotherapy-induced neutropenia. Although any part of the GI tract can be involved, the cecum appears to be the most severely affected, with mucosal ulceration, gangrene, and perforation. Some investigators have suggested that the cecum is more prone to this injury due to its greater distensibility, relatively lower blood flow, and increased stasis of luminal contents compared with the rest of the gastrointestinal tract.[34] The presence of microorganisms such as *Clostridium*, *Pseudomonas*, *Escherichia coli*, *Klebsiella*, and *Candida* in areas of necrotic bowel and in blood cultures from affected patients suggests that enterocolitis is primarily an infectious process in an immunocompromised host. The primary mucosal insult that allows bacterial invasion might result from a number of mechanisms, including chemotherapy-induced mucosal injury, shock leading to low flow and mucosal ischemia, abnormal intestinal flora secondary to aggressive, broad-spectrum antibiotics, or necrosis of tumor infiltrates. The invasion of bacteria itself can cause further necrosis of the bowel wall, leading to full-thickness infarction and perforation of the intestine.

The clinical presentation of neutropenic enterocolitis is extremely variable, and there are no strict criteria that must be fulfilled to make the diagnosis. Furthermore, the symptoms are nonspecific and can be similar to those of a number of gastrointestinal processes. Consequently, the true incidence of the disease might be different than reported in most clinical series. In 50 necropsies performed on children with leukemia, Moir and Bale[35] found evidence of enterocolitis in 23 children (46%). Most of these cases were not suspected clinically. Conversely, Wade and colleagues[36] reported on 15 patients with the clinical diagnosis of neutropenic enterocolitis who underwent either laparotomy or autopsy. The diagnosis was confirmed in only eight patients; no abnormalities of the bowel were found in four patients, appendicitis was found in two patients, and a small bowel volvulus was found in one patient. The common underlying characteristic of patients with neutropenic enterocolitis is the neutropenia, which is usually a result of chemotherapy but might also be a result of conditions such as aplastic anemia or cyclic neutropenia.[37,38] Affected patients typically present with fever, abdominal pain and distension, and diarrhea. Abdominal tenderness is frequently localized to the right lower quadrant but can also be diffused.

Problems Common to Cancer and Its Therapy

Peritonitis suggests intestinal perforation. Portal venous gas, low serum bicarbonate levels, and generalized peritonitis are ominous findings and suggest a poor outcome.[3,39] Stools are generally positive for occult blood, and sometimes significant gastrointestinal bleeding can be associated with the disease. A right lower quadrant mass might be palpable, indicating a dilated cecum or a focal inflammatory phlegmon or abscess. Advanced stages of the process can present with systemic sepsis and multiorgan failure.

No specific laboratory or radiologic findings are diagnostic for neutropenic enterocolitis. Plain abdominal radiographs can demonstrate dilated loops of bowel, thickening of the bowel wall, "thumbprinting" resulting from bowel wall edema, or indications of a right lower quadrant mass or phlegmon. Free intraperitoneal air indicates perforation of the bowel wall. Pneumatosis intestinalis is often seen and is not itself an indication for surgical intervention.[40,41] Ultrasound and CT might demonstrate concentric thickening of the bowel wall, pericolic fluid collections or abscesses, and pneumatosis intestinalis (Fig. 53-1). CT scans are superior in their ability to evaluate the entire abdomen for pathology, especially in patients with distended loops of bowel and ileus for whom ultrasound would not be possible.

The initial treatment for neutropenic colitis is supportive, with the administration of broad-spectrum antibiotics, nasogastric decompression, intravenous fluids,

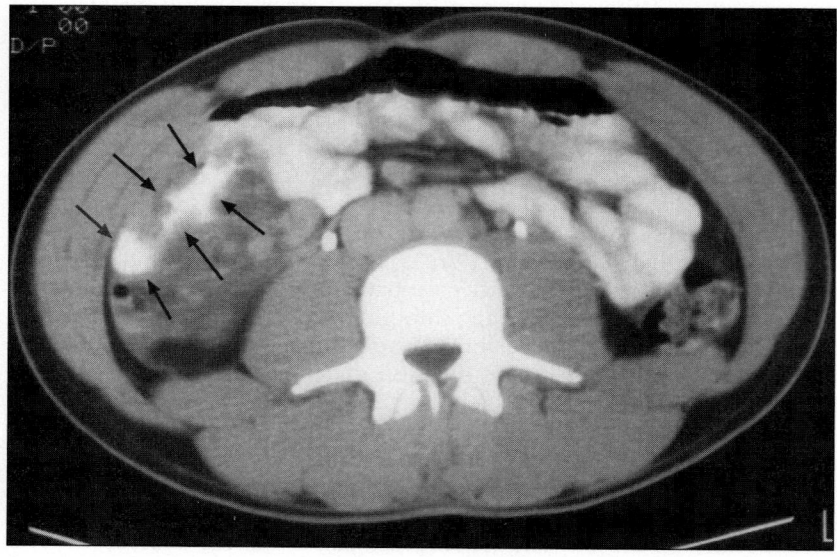

A

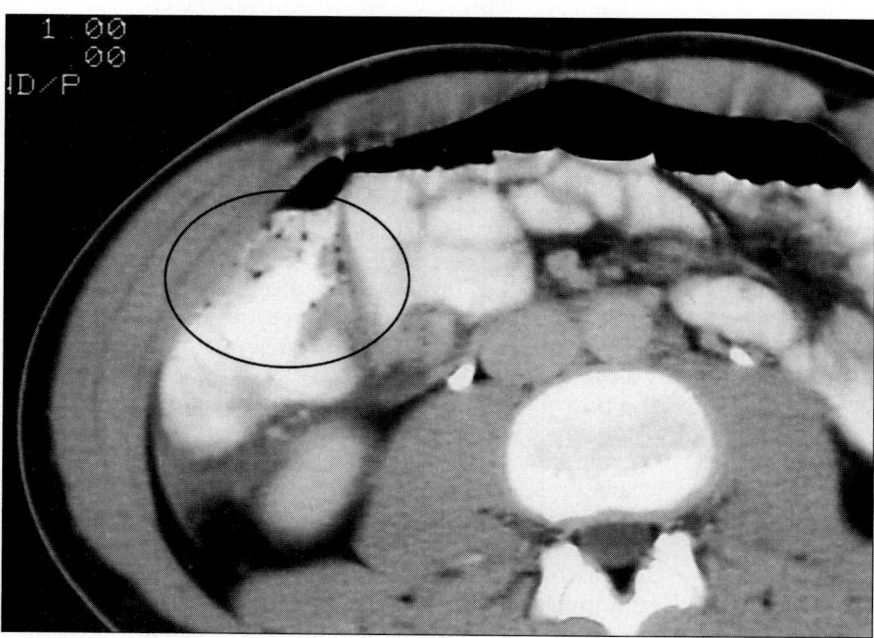

B

Figure 53-1. Neutropenic enterocolitis in a patient treated for acute myelogenous leukemia. **A,** CT scan of the abdomen showing concentric wall thickening (*arrows*) and adjacent inflammation of the cecum, ascending colon, and terminal ileum. **B,** Suggestion of pneumatosis intestinalis of colon wall (*circle*). (Courtesy of Charles Marn MD, University of Michigan Medical Center.)

bowel rest, and serial abdominal examinations.[42] In most patients, these measures are sufficient, and symptoms resolve after correction of the neutropenia. The indications for and timing of surgical intervention is controversial. Many authors believe that surgery is rarely helpful, citing high rates of operative morbidity and mortality in neutropenic patients with cancer.[43,44] Others have advocated an aggressive surgical approach to avoid further bowel necrosis, perforation, and sepsis.[31,32,45,46] Sound surgical judgment should be exercised in determining which patients require surgery, and the decision should not be clouded by the presence of neutropenia. Accepted indications for surgery in neutropenic enterocolitis include the following:

1. Persistent GI bleeding after correction of thrombocytopenia and coagulopathy;
2. Evidence of free intraperitoneal perforation;
3. Clinical deterioration despite aggressive supportive measures; and
4. Inability to rule out other intra-abdominal processes normally requiring surgery, such as bowel obstruction or acute appendicitis.[47,48]

The role of granulocyte macrophage colony-stimulating factor in neutropenic enterocolitis is yet unproved, although it has been used successfully in anecdotal cases.[43]

If exploratory surgery is performed, resection of grossly involved bowel is necessary. This typically involves a right hemicolectomy. The decision to perform a primary anastomosis or form an intestinal stoma must be based on the condition of the patient, the amount of intraperitoneal infection, and the appearance and viability of the remnant bowel. Primary anastomosis in the immunocompromised patient is associated with an increased incidence of anastomotic leak.[30,32] This complication is almost always fatal, thus formation of an anastomosis should be considered only for early, uncomplicated cases in patients with no systemic sepsis or organ failure.

In summary, very few neutropenic patients with cancer who have abdominal pain require surgery; most can be successfully treated medically. Aggressive supportive care, frequent clinical evaluations, and a high index of suspicion are necessary to determine which patients require surgical intervention. Specific situations that dictate surgery include uncontrollable GI bleeding, intestinal perforation, and deteriorating clinical course on medical management. Other intra-abdominal conditions, such as appendicitis, could be indistinguishable from neutropenic enterocolitis and should be considered in the differential diagnosis.

Appendicitis

Acute appendicitis can be extremely difficult to distinguish from neutropenic enterocolitis in patients receiving chemotherapy. In large series of children with leukemia or other malignancies, the incidence of appendicitis has been reported to be between 0.2% and 2%, which is equivalent to the incidence in the general pediatric population.[32,49-51] Typically, acute appendicitis presents with right lower quadrant pain and localized tenderness. The diagnosis of appendicitis can be made

based on "classic" symptoms and clinical findings in approximately half of affected patients. Angel and coworkers at St. Jude Children's Hospital[49] reported on 16 patients who developed appendicitis, of whom only nine presented with classic symptoms. Similarly, Silliman and colleagues[50] described seven children with cancer who were suspected to have acute appendicitis on preoperative evaluation. Only four of these patients proved to have appendicitis, while two had no abnormalities found and one had a small bowel perforation. There are no laboratory or radiologic tests that are diagnostic for appendicitis, and therefore, the diagnosis must be made on clinical grounds. CT scanning has been reported to be both sensitive and specific for acute appendicitis. Findings suggestive of appendicitis include a thickened, edematous appendix, periappendiceal inflammation or abscess, or a calcified appendicolith.[52] The odds that right lower quadrant pain is due to appendicitis or typhlitis are even. In 400 leukemic patients seen over a period of 15 years at the National Institutes of Health, acute appendicitis was identified at the time of emergency laparotomy in eight patients, and typhlitis was identified in seven.[53] The inability to differentiate between the two conditions has led to frequent delays in both diagnosis and treatment. In the report by Angel and colleagues,[49] the diagnosis of acute appendicitis was delayed in six out of 16 patients.

Whereas the treatment of neutropenic enterocolitis is primarily medical, the treatment of acute appendicitis is surgical. Conservative, nonoperative management of appendicitis is associated with a high mortality in patients with leukemia.[46] In the immunosuppressed patient with right lower quadrant pain, a trial of broad-spectrum antibiotics and bowel rest should be initiated, and frequent examinations should be made to ascertain any change in clinical status. The persistence of a septic course manifest by large fluid volume and vasopressor requirements mandates surgical exploration. With the resolution of neutropenia, continued signs of localized peritonitis should prompt surgical exploration. Delay in diagnosis results in a higher incidence of perforation, peritonitis, and death. Appendectomy is the treatment of choice for appendicitis. Cases complicated by perforation or abscess formation could necessitate the placement of drains, and the surgical incision should be left to close by secondary intention. Despite the poor medical condition and immunocompromised state of leukemic patients, prompt diagnosis and surgical treatment of acute appendicitis can be accomplished with low complications and mortality.

Pancreatitis

Pancreatitis in the oncology patient is likely to be caused by the same factors implicated in the normal population, such as gallstones or alcohol abuse. More specific to the oncology patient, however, pancreatitis can result from direct tumor infiltration into the gland or as complications of either medical or surgical therapy. Primary adenocarcinoma of the pancreas is seldom a cause of acute pancreatitis. Metastases to the pancreas have been reported from a variety of tumors, including renal cell carcinoma, melanoma, and cancers of the prostate, breast, and lung. In autopsy series, as many as 40% of patients with small cell cancer of the lung harbor metastatic disease in the pancreas. The vast majority of these metastases are asymptomatic, and fewer than 5% of patients develop acute pancreatitis.[54] Rare cases have been reported in which a bout of acute pancreatitis secondary to metastatic disease was the initial manifestation of cancer.[55,56] In general, prognosis of patients with metastasis-induced pancreatitis is poor.

Pancreatitis is a recognized complication of a number of antineoplastic chemotherapeutic agents, although the drug with which it is most commonly reported is L-asparaginase. The incidence of pancreatitis associated with this agent is as high as 16%.[57,58] Other antineoplastic drugs known to induce pancreatitis are corticosteroids, didanosine, and less commonly, cytarabine, cisplatin, interleukin-2, vincristine, methotrexate, mitomycin C, cyclophosphamide, doxorubicin, and ifosfamide.[59,60] The clinical course of patients with chemotherapy-induced pancreatitis is most often mild and self-limiting but can progress to necrotizing pancreatitis or pseudocyst formation. In patients treated with L-asparaginase-induced pancreatitis, there is an associated mortality rate as high as 12%.[58]

Pancreatitis is also a complication of other cancer treatments. Transarterial embolization (TAE) of the liver for primary or metastatic tumors is thought to cause pancreatitis by either misperfusion of chemotherapeutic agent and direct pancreatic toxicity or from disruption of pancreatic blood flow and resultant ischemia of the gland. Consistent with these hypotheses, when superselective TAE was used, no cases of pancreatitis were noted.[61,62] Manipulation of the ampulla of Vater or pancreas for malignant disease, such as with endoscopic retrograde cholangiopancreatography (ERCP), pancreatectomy, or splenectomy, can also result in pancreatic inflammation.

The clinical presentation of pancreatitis includes epigastric pain, nausea, vomiting, generalized ileus, tachycardia, and fever. The diagnosis is usually confirmed by elevations in the serum amylase and lipase levels. CT of the abdomen with intravenous contrast is useful to confirm the presence of pancreatic inflammation or phlegmon and to document necrosis or pseudocyst. Ultrasound scanning is often not feasible due to the associated ileus and bowel gas overlying the pancreas. Some investigators advocate the routine use of ultrasound as a screening study in patients being treated with L-asparaginase to monitor for pancreatic abnormalities that might indicate a need to stop therapy.[63] The treatment of pancreatitis is generally supportive and includes bowel rest, hydration, and intravenous hyperalimentation. If possible, the causative agent should be eliminated or discontinued, if it can be identified. Surgical intervention is reserved for patients with bleeding, infection, severe necrosis, or persistent pseudocyst.

Perianal and Perirectal Infections in Patients with Cancer

Perianal and perirectal infections develop most frequently in patients with acute leukemia under treatment with chemotherapy but can also be encountered in patients with other hematologic malignancies, solid tumors, or after bone marrow transplantation. In most series in the literature, the incidence of perianal infections in patients with leukemia is between 2% and 8%.[64-66] The vast majority of these patients have acute myelogenous leukemia. In a series of patients with small cell lung carcinomas being treated with intensive chemotherapy, 7% of patients developed perianal infections.[67] The exact pathogenesis of perianal infections in the oncology patient is not well defined. An underlying theme in most cases is either neutropenia, immunosuppression, or dysfunction of granulocytic cells. Many patients have a history of preexisting anorectal problems, including previous perianal or perirectal abscesses, fistula in ano, anal fissures, or hemorrhoids. Another common symptom associated with perianal infections is diarrhea, which can predispose a patient to perianal excoriation or ulceration with subsequent infection. Once established, the infection can spread into the ischiorectal fossa, supralevator space, retroperitoneum, or perineum. In the presence of a compromised immune function, this spread can be quite rapid, and systemic sepsis is present in approximately half of all patients. Ninety percent of the time, the perianal infections contain multiple aerobic and anaerobic organisms. The bacteria most frequently cultured from the abscess and blood are *E. coli*, *Ps. aeruginosa*, *Klebsiella*, *Enterococcus*, and *B. fragilis*.

The most common presenting symptoms are perianal pain and fever. On examination, the perianal region could be erythematous, indurated, and extremely tender to palpation. Spontaneous drainage of an abscess can result in ulceration, purulent discharge, or bleeding. Spread of the infection in the perineum can lead to a fulminant necrotizing fasciitis, termed Fournier's gangrene. In the profoundly neutropenic patient, however, suppuration and abscess formation might be absent. In the past, it was recommended that rectal examinations be deferred in neutropenic patients being evaluated for perianal infections for fear of causing mucosal trauma and providing a route of entry for bacteria into the perianal tissues or blood. There is little evidence to support this practice, as there is no higher rate of positive blood cultures in neutropenic patients with perianal infections who had rectal examinations compared with patients who did not.[68,69] In fact, thorough examination of the perianal region and rectum is imperative to diagnose the presence of a fluctuant mass indicating a drainable abscess. In rare instances, perianal sepsis could be the initial presenting symptom of a malignancy. Failure of an infection to resolve or heal after appropriate therapy should prompt biopsy of the area to exclude malignant infiltration.[70,71]

The optimal management of perianal infections is controversial. The initial course of therapy taken is the administration of broad-spectrum antibiotic and symptomatic relief using sitz baths, warm compresses, stool softeners, and analgesics. The antibiotic regimen must be active against enteric organisms, including anaerobes, *Enterococcus*, and *Ps. aeruginosa*. More than half of all neutropenic patients can be managed successfully using a nonoperative approach, prompting some investigators to advocate a medical approach.[65,66,72-74] It was felt that there was rarely a purulent collection to drain and that incision and drainage of purely indurated tissues would result in continued sepsis, poor wound healing, and hemorrhage. Many authors, however, feel that early surgical intervention is important in decreasing the morbidity and mortality in this disorder.[67,75] Dogmatic approaches to perianal infections should be avoided. It is generally agreed in the literature that the presence of a fluctuant mass in the perianal or perirectal region is an indication for surgery, as are continued deterioration and sepsis despite medical management. Several reports indicate that the timing of surgery in relation to the resolution of neutropenia is important. When incision and drainage is performed in the presence of neutropenia, there is no pus and no improvement in sepsis. Those patients without neutropenia and with fluctuant abscesses appear to benefit most from surgery.[76] There are currently no data regarding the use of colony-stimulating factors in the management of perianal infections. Surgery should include complete drainage of pus, debridement of necrotic tissue, and packing. Extensive perineal involvement or poorly controlled fecal soilage of the wound might necessitate a proximal diverting colostomy to promote healing.

INTESTINAL OBSTRUCTION

Obstruction of the GI tract is a common problem among patients with cancer. This was the most common indication for emergency laparotomy for acute abdomen

in one reported experience (see Table 53-1). Intestinal obstruction results in abdominal distension, pain, nausea, and vomiting. These symptoms are identical to those of adynamic ileus, a condition that needs to be distinguished from obstruction. Adynamic ileus in patients with cancer can be related to chemotherapeutic agents or can be secondary to other metabolic problems, such as sepsis. Vincristine sulfate and the vinca alkaloids are known to produce peripheral neuropathies and a paralytic ileus. Drug-induced ileus is estimated to occur in 10% of patients receiving these agents and could be due to their neurotoxic effects.[77] Flat and upright abdominal films are very helpful in differentiating adynamic ileus from an obstruction. With an adynamic ileus, generalized small bowel and colonic distension is apparent on x-ray without the multiple air-fluid levels and absence of colonic gas seen with mechanical obstruction. Patients with vincristine-induced adynamic ileus should be monitored for the need of possible surgical intervention. If distension of the colon becomes so marked that the cecum becomes greater than 14 cm in diameter, the risk of perforation is significant. Therapeutic options include colonoscopy for decompression, laparotomy with cecostomy tube placement, or colostomy.

Patients with a history of previous malignancy who present with bowel obstruction should be treated like any patient with intestinal obstruction (Fig. 53-2). One cannot assume that the obstructive problem is secondary to a recurrence of the previous cancer. Approximately 25% of patients who require laparotomy to treat their obstructions are found to have benign disease, and 4% have a new

Problems Common to Cancer and Its Therapy

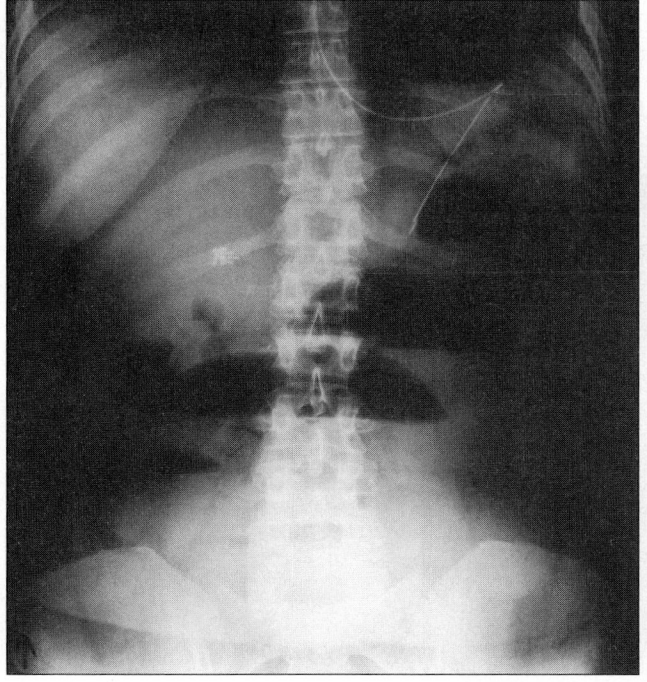
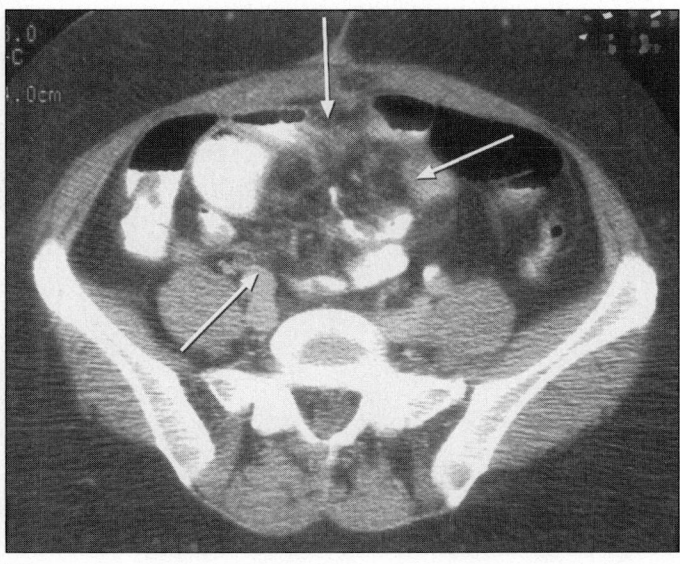

A   B

Figure 53-2. Small bowel obstruction in a patient with recurrent small bowel carcinoid tumor. **A,** Plain, upright radiograph of the abdomen demonstrating dilated loops of small bowel and multiple air-fluid levels. **B,** CT scan of the abdomen documenting recurrent tumor mass (*arrows*) involving small bowel and mesentery.

TABLE 53-5

Causes of Intestinal Obstruction in Patients with Cancer Identified at Laparotomy

STUDY	NO. OF PATIENTS	CAUSE OF OBSTRUCTION [NO. (%)]			OPERATIVE MORTALITY (%)*
		BENIGN	NEW PRIMARY	RECURRENT CANCER	
Ketcham et al.[78]	117	21 (18)	10 (9)	86 (73)	14[†]
Osteen et al.[79]	53	21 (32)	0 (9)	32 (60)	9[†]
Weiss et al.[80]	57	13 (23)	2 (4)	42 (73)	11[†]
Gallick et al.[81]					
Tang et al.[82]	43	10 (23)	0	33 (76)	12
Total	309	77 (25)	12 (4)	220 (71)	12

*30-day operative mortality rate.
[†]Mean.

primary malignancy (Table 53-5).[78-82] Operative mortality for patients with cancer undergoing laparotomy for intestinal obstruction is approximately 12% and is comparable to patients without a history of malignancy. The decision to proceed immediately with surgery vs. initial nonoperative management must be made based on the clinical presentation. A surgeon should be involved in the evaluation of the patient even if nonoperative therapy is chosen. Contrast studies may be employed to identify the site of obstruction, which could be multiple in location. In one series, the presence of both small bowel and large bowel obstructions was observed in 8% of patients.[82] Surgery is required if bowel strangulation is suspected because of fever, leukocytosis, and localized peritoneal tenderness. Radiographic evidence of complete bowel obstruction with loss of air in the distal large bowel and absence of flatus should likewise prompt urgent surgery. If a nonoperative approach is chosen, bowel decompression with a nasogastric tube (along with fluid and electrolyte resuscitation) is the mainstay of therapy. Nonoperative management succeeds in relieving the obstruction in up to 25% of these patients. In at least two reported series, nasogastric decompression relieved the obstruction within three days when it was effective.[79,80]

The reported results of surgical treatment for intestinal obstruction in this patient population vary significantly. Relief of obstruction has been reported in 35%–80% of patients.[83] Patients found to have benign causes for their obstruction (i.e., adhesions or radiation enteritis) obviously fare best (Fig. 53-3). Patients with a good performance status before intestinal obstruction, those with primary colorectal cancer, those without ascites, and those with a preoperative albumin greater than 3.0 mg/dL also appear to realize significant benefit from surgical therapy compared with patients who have advanced disease and a poor performance status.[84,85] In patients

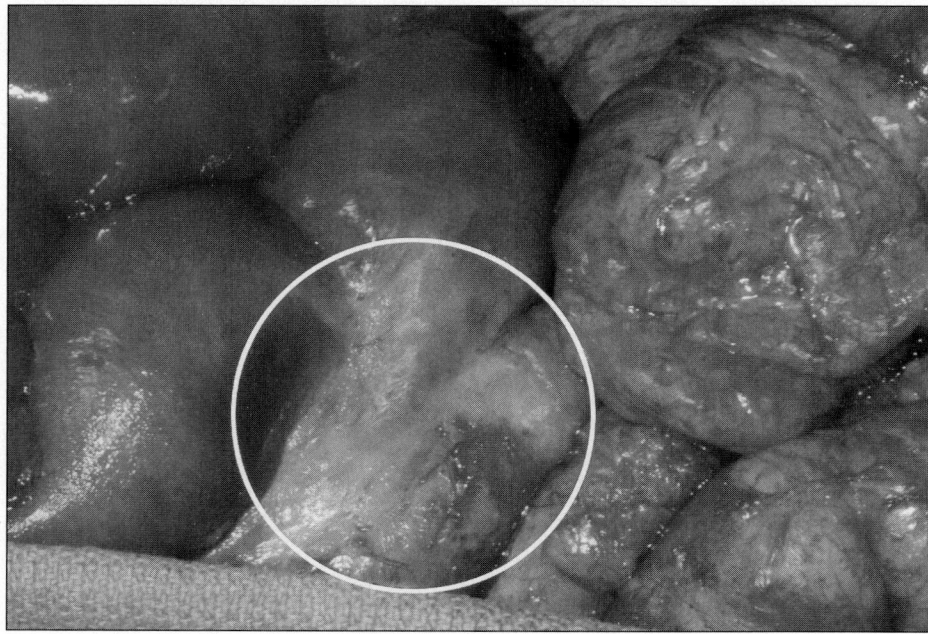

Figure 53-3. Radiated small bowel with stricture (*circle*). Dilated loops of small bowel proximal to this area demonstrate obstruction due to stricture.

with recurrent cancer as the cause for intestinal obstruction, approximately one-third develop another bowel obstruction from their disease after resolution of their first obstructive event.[86]

Stomach and Duodenum

The most common causes for upper GI obstruction involving the stomach or duodenum in patients with cancer are benign peptic ulcer disease, primary carcinoma of the gastric antrum, and gastric outlet obstruction secondary to a pancreatic or biliary tract carcinoma. Symptoms due to obstruction at this level include non-bilious vomiting, postprandial pain, and epigastric fullness. On physical examination, a succussion splash or palpable mass is present in approximately one-third of cases. Endoscopy is helpful for differentiating the site and cause of upper GI obstruction.

For benign, obstructive ulcer disease, operative therapy is generally required after initial stabilization with nasogastric decompression and fluid resuscitation. Pyloroplasty with vagotomy is the treatment of choice, particularly for patients with cancer who might be debilitated. For obstructing primary gastric carcinomas, a curative or palliative resection with reconstruction of GI continuity is recommended if technically feasible. When gastric outlet obstruction is due to an unresectable pancreatic or biliary tract neoplasm, treatment with creation of a gastrojejunostomy is the best approach for bypassing the obstruction.

Small Intestine

Most malignant obstructions of the small intestines are a result of metastatic deposits; primary tumors of the small bowel are rare. The most common malignancies giving rise to obstructive metastatic deposits are intra-abdominal tumors such as colorectal, ovarian, pancreatic, and gastric cancers. Symptoms of small bowel obstruction include crampy abdominal pain, distension, nausea, and vomiting. Physical examination usually reveals percussion tympany and high-pitched bowel sounds. Plain films of the abdomen reveal multiple air-fluid levels within the small intestine. A contrast study of the large bowel should be performed to determine whether distal obstruction is present, as carcinomatosis can involve multiple areas of the bowel. If a partial small bowel obstruction is diagnosed (i.e., presence of gas in the large bowel), then conservative management with tube decompression is appropriate. If resolution is not apparent after three days of conservative therapy, surgical exploration should be considered.

If a patient's small bowel obstruction has a benign cause such as adhesive bands, standard treatment should be performed. For carcinomatosis, aggressive attempts at freeing involved bowel loops or resection are not indicated. It is preferable to perform the simplest procedure with conservation of bowel length, which can be accomplished by a side-to-side bypass procedure. If malignant disease involves a significant portion of distal small bowel, the transverse colon can be used to establish the bypass anastomosis. At least one-third of patients successfully relieved of malignant small bowel obstruction experience recurrence of the obstruction. Survival after bypass surgery for malignant obstruction averages no longer than 11 months.

Colon and Rectum

Obstruction of the colon and rectum occurs approximately half as frequently as small bowel obstruction. Large bowel obstruction is more often a result of malignancy (i.e., primary or recurrent tumor) as opposed to benign causes such as volvulus or diverticulitis. Symptoms include vomiting, crampy abdominal pain, bleeding, lack of flatus or stool, or change in bowel habits. Flat and upright abdominal films are important in the initial assessment of these patients. A barium enema is key in localizing the site of obstruction.

Initial treatment should consist of nasogastric tube decompression and fluid resuscitation. If a total colonic obstruction is present, dilation of the proximal colon can lead to perforation of the cecum, especially if a competent ileocecal valve is present. Cecal dilation of 12–14 cm is associated with a high risk of perforation, and a decompressive procedure should be performed urgently to avoid this complication. A diverting colostomy relieves the obstruction and avoids perforation. This is also the surgical therapy of choice if there is evidence of peritoneal carcinomatosis. If the obstruction is related to a primary left colon cancer, resection followed by colostomy take-down several weeks later can be accomplished. For obstructing primary or metastatic tumors of the right colon, colectomy with primary anastomosis or a bypass procedure, respectively, should be performed. Obstructive tumors of the rectum are often a harbinger of locally advanced primary rectal tumors or recurrent carcinomas after a previous low anterior resection. These tumors are often associated with evidence of distant metastatic disease or a high local recurrence rate if resection is performed. Proximal diverting colostomy should be performed for unresectable tumors to palliate the obstruction. Another alternative for an unresectable tumor is to consider endoscopic ablative laser therapy to maintain intestinal continuity and avoid a colostomy.

Nonoperative Treatment of Bowel Obstruction

As noted previously, operative treatment of bowel obstruction in patients with cancer who fail a short, initial attempt at conservative management is almost always indicated. The cause of the obstruction is frequently not tumor related, and many patients with malignant bowel obstruction are able to undergo successful tumor resection or bypass for palliation. In some patients, however, recurrent malignant bowel obstruction soon (six to 12 months) after palliative bypass, deterioration of their general medical condition, or their wishes make an attempt at operative treatment of bowel obstruction inappropriate. In these patients, medical management might alleviate the abdominal pain, vomiting, and

WHEN OPERATIVE THERAPY IS NOT APPROPRIATE

The instances in which invasive treatments are not appropriate may be divided into two categories:

1. The patient's definition of well-being will not be achieved with operative intervention.
2. Operative treatment of the acute problem is "futile."

This critical point in the management of patients with cancer requires the recognition by the treating physician that specific disease-oriented treatments intended for cure or control of the cancer need to be redefined and explained to the patient and the family.

ISSUES RELATED TO THE PATIENT'S DEFINITION OF WELL-BEING

- It is important for the patient to determine what well-being means. The physician should inform the patient about the prognosis and quality of life with an operative intervention and about the odds for achieving them.
- Surgical treatment of some acute problems, although technically indicated (i.e., plication of a perforated ulcer in a patient with metastatic lung cancer), might be inappropriate if it is unlikely that such treatment will contribute to the overall well-being of the patient as measured by survival to discharge or even by elimination of the need for mechanical ventilation.
- Nonoperative, palliative management should be explained to the patient as a switch from a strategy of cure or control of the disease to one of symptom control and relief of distress.

ISSUES RELATED TO THE DETERMINATION OF THERAPEUTIC FUTILITY

- Futility must be defined in terms of the goals of therapy. The goals of the patient might differ significantly from those of the physician, in which case a consensus should be achieved.
- Futile treatments can be defined as the absolute inability to postpone death.
- It is not the obligation of the physician to offer futile treatments to the patient in an attempt to do "everything possible."

---

dehydration that result from inoperable malignant bowel obstruction. Aggressive use of narcotics, anticholinergics, antiemetics, phenothiazines, butyrophenones, tricyclic antidepressants, corticosteroids, and somatostatin analogs might palliate malignant bowel obstruction.[87,88] Baines and colleagues[89] described 38 patients who were treated in this fashion with a mean survival of almost 4 months; 7 patients survived for more than 7 months. The authors concluded that the distressing symptoms of inoperable malignant bowel obstruction could often be controlled pharmacologically.

An alternative approach that has been described for the therapy of these patients is the use of a venting gastrostomy in conjunction with either enteral or parenteral fluids. In one study in which venting gastrostomy was supplemented by intravenous hydration with a 10% dextrose-containing saline solution, mean duration of survival was approximately 64 days.[90] Malone and associates[84] used only enteral support; in the seven patients who had died at the time of reporting, mean survival was 35 days (range, 26–56 days). Three patients were alive at 77, 150, and 150 days, respectively. Neither of these reports commented on the adequacy of enteral nutrient intake in these patients nor the extent to which malnutrition could have contributed to mortality.

August and colleagues[91] have suggested the use of home parenteral nutrition in selected patients with inoperable malignant bowel obstruction, in whom pharmacologic palliation is not adequate and enteral intake is minimal. Home parenteral nutrition must often be combined with gastric drainage via gastrostomy (usually placed percutaneously) or nasogastric tube. These authors state that this approach should be considered only when other measures have failed and when survival beyond 40 days is probable. They reported that in the latter stages of their trial, 80% of these patients discharged on home parenteral nutrition after failing more conservative measures survived longer than 40 days. As judged by patients and families, 13 of 17 patients treated in this fashion experienced beneficial results. Recently, some authors have advocated nonoperative relief of malignant obstructions with the use of endoscopically placed endoluminal wall stents. This procedure is still experimental, but early reports show 70% relief of symptoms with low complication rates. Perforation (0%–15%) and stent migration (0%–40%) were the most common complications reported.[86,88]

ABDOMINAL PROBLEMS IN PATIENTS UNDERGOING BONE MARROW TRANSPLANTATION

Evaluation of acute abdominal complaints in patients who have had bone marrow transplants (BMT) is difficult and represents a major diagnostic challenge for the surgical oncologist. Virtually all patients who have undergone BMT will experience gastrointestinal problems at some point in the post-transplant period, and these can include nausea, vomiting, alterations in liver function tests, diarrhea, and abdominal pain. The surgeon is not infrequently faced with an acutely ill patient with abdominal pain and sepsis and the dilemma of whether an operation is necessary and will be of benefit. The spectrum of acute abdominal processes from which BMT patients can suffer is similar in most respects to that of any neutropenic or immunocompromised patient discussed in this chapter. There are, however, several disease entities that are unique to the BMT patient, and these will be discussed in this section.

There are three causes of abdominal complaints in the BMT patient that are unique:

1. High-dose induction chemotherapy or chemoradiation therapy given before transplantation.
2. Graft-vs.-host disease (GVHD) in recipients of allogeneic transplants.
3. Infections of the gut that occur before bone marrow recovery.[92]

The post-transplant period at which each of these potential complaints becomes problematic differs. Injury to the gastrointestinal tract and liver after high-dose chemotherapy and radiation is usually present by day 10, is transient, and resolves after several weeks. Acute GVHD appears between two and eight weeks after allogeneic BMT, while chronic GVHD is manifest from three to 15 months after BMT. In a large series of patients with leukemia transplanted with bone marrow from HLA-identical siblings, the median interval from transplant to the onset of acute and chronic GVHD was 17 and 111 days, respectively.[93] In patients receiving HLA-mismatched marrow, the onset of acute GVHD could be as early as seven days. Infections of the gut caused by bacteria and fungus are most often seen before day 30 after transplantation during the period of neutropenia, while infections by virus are usually seen after 30 days. Although there are reports of late (five months to one year) re-actuation of varicella zoster infection associated with acute abdominal pain, hepatitis and pancreatitis, or disseminated disease. Mortality rates are from 50% to 100%.[94,95]

The gastrointestinal complaints or symptoms are similar for the most part, no matter what the cause. For example, in a prospective study of patients who developed nausea and vomiting after BMT, Spencer and colleagues[96] found that 30% had gastrointestinal infections (predominantly herpesvirus), 26% had GVHD, 16% had both intestinal infection and GVHD, and 28% had either a nonintestinal etiology or no known cause for the nausea and vomiting. In another report by the same group, 13 cases of diffuse intestinal ulceration after BMT were described. The causes of this pathology were chemo-radiation toxicity in two patients, acute GVHD in five patients, opportunistic infection with either GVHD or chemotherapy toxicity in four patients, and Epstein-Barr virus-associated lymphoproliferative disorder in two patients.

GVHD is a process in which donor T-cells react to recipient cells; it develops in 30%–50% of patients receiving allogeneic grafts.[93,97] The main clinical manifestations of GVHD are skin rash, hepatic dysfunction, jaundice, diarrhea, bleeding from the gut mucosa, and abdominal pain. The diagnosis can usually be made based on these findings and can be confirmed with a rectal biopsy or upper gastrointestinal endoscopy with biopsy. The clinical severity of the GVHD is judged using the Seattle criteria, which take into account skin, liver, and gut findings (Table 53-6).[98] Despite the prominence of intra-abdominal organs and symptoms in the manifestations of GVHD, it is surprisingly rare that surgical intervention is necessary. The most common indications for abdominal surgery in patients with GVHD are gastrointestinal bleeding and obstruction.[97,99] Perforation of the bowel is uncommon. The finding of pneumatosis intestinalis on abdominal radiography has been reported to be present in as many as 18% of BMT patients with acute GVHD.[100] The majority of these cases do not require surgical exploration and can be managed medically with steroids and immuno-suppressive agents.[95,100-102] Pneumatosis intestinalis might also be associated with findings of retroperitoneal, mediastinal, or free intraperitoneal air. Although usually an indication for surgery, free air in the peritoneal cavity in this setting need not be associated with a frank bowel perforation, and there are reports of managing this problem without an operation.[101,103] Evidence of peritonitis and a persistent septic state despite adequate medical support should mandate surgical exploration, however.

Another frequent intra-abdominal complication of BMT is venoocclusive disease (VOD) of the liver. The etiology of VOD is thought to be damage to the hepatic venules and sinusoids induced by the high-dose cytoreductive therapy used to prepare patients for both allogeneic and autologous BMT. Cellular debris and consequent activation of the coagulation cascade result in obstruction of hepatic sinusoids and a clinical picture similar to that of portal hypertension. VOD occurs in more than half of BMT patients and is associated with significant mortality rates. In a study of 355 consecutive BMT patients, McDonald and colleagues[104] reported the overall incidence of VOD to be 54%, and the mortality rates for mild, moderate, and severe disease were 9%, 23%, and 98%, respectively. The incidence of VOD is thought to be increasing, probably due to the more aggressive conditioning regimens currently in use. The clinical signs of VOD include fluid retention, ascites, hyperbilirubinemia, hepatomegaly and right upper quadrant pain. Certain patients are at higher risk for developing VOD, including those with elevation

TABLE 53-6

Clinical Staging of Organ Involvement in Acute GVHD			
STAGE	SKIN	LIVER	GUT
+	Maculopapular rash <25% body surface	Bilirubin 2–3 mg/dL	Diarrhea 500–1000 mL/day
++	Maculopapular rash 25–50% body surface	Bilirubin 3–6 mg/dL	Diarrhea 1000–1500 mL/day
+++	Generalized erythroderma	Bilirubin 6–15 mg/dL	Diarrhea >1500 mL/day
++++	Desquamation and bullae	Bilirubin >15 mg/dL	Pain or ileus

of pretransplant transaminases, those receiving intensive conditioning regimens or mismatched marrow grafts, those treated with vancomycin or acyclovir at the beginning of the conditioning regimen, and those with a previous history of hepatitis or abdominal radiation.[104-106]

The differential diagnosis of VOD is lengthy and includes any disorder that could result in right upper quadrant pain, jaundice, or ascites. A partial list would include such disorders as hepatitis, drug- or parenteral nutrition-induced liver dysfunction, acute cholecystitis, cholangitis or liver abscess, and GVHD or tumor infiltration of the liver. In addition, the clinical picture of sudden onset of hepatomegaly and severe ascites is similar to that of Budd-Chiari syndrome. The diagnosis of VOD can usually be made on clinical signs, with liver biopsy being reserved for patients in whom the diagnosis is not certain. Doppler ultrasound has also been proposed as a means of diagnosing VOD. The ultrasonographic findings that have been described are decreased or reversed flow in the portal vein and elevations in the hepatic artery resistive index.[107,108] The ultrasound findings, however, might also serve as a source of confusion for the clinician, as it is common to find gallbladder distension, wall thickening, and sludge in patients after BMT, making the differentiation between VOD and acute cholecystitis difficult.[108] Most patients with hyperbilirubinemia after BMT do not require surgery. In a series of 180 patients treated with BMT for hematologic malignancies, Wasserheit and associates[109] found that 46 patients (26%) became jaundiced. The major causes of the hyperbilirubinemia was VOD in 22 patients; acute cholecystitis was diagnosed in only one of the 46 patients.

The treatment of VOD is supportive, with emphasis on maintaining intravascular volume and renal perfusion while limiting the amount of sodium and extravascular fluid accumulation. Promotion of diuresis is accomplished with loop diuretics, spironolactone, or renal dose dopamine.[105] The use of anticoagulants or thrombolytics (e.g., tissue plasminogen activator) to prevent hepatic venular and sinusoidal obstruction is controversial.[110,111] Symptomatic relief of ascites in VOD patients could require paracentesis. Successful surgical treatment of ascites with a portosystemic shunt has been reported, as has the use of transjugular intrahepatic portosystemic shunts (TIPS).[112,113] Although intriguing, the indications for and role of portosystemic shunting in VOD is unclear, as variceal bleeding is infrequently encountered in these patients, and the other manifestation, such as ascites, can be managed in a less invasive way.

In summary, BMT has become a proven and accepted treatment for a number of hematologic and solid malignancies. Transplant-related complications, such as GVHD and VOD, remain a major cause of mortality. The presentation and sequelae of both of these disease entities present difficult diagnostic and management challenges for the clinician. Although the management of GVHD and VOD are primarily medical, surgical consultation could be required for evaluation of abdominal pain and distension, nausea, vomiting, diarrhea, hyperbilirubinemia, or other gastrointestinal complaints. An understanding of the manifestations of these complications, together with vigilant clinical evaluation, are paramount to determine when surgical intervention is necessary in this complex patient population.

FISTULA

Fistula formation, although becoming somewhat less common, is still an important complication of cancer and its treatment. The anatomy of fistulous complications in patients with cancer cannot be categorized and is seemingly limited only by the imagination. Fistulae complicating cancers have been reported between the stomach and pericardium, the biliary and bronchial trees, the portal and systemic circulations, and the alimentary canal and vascular system, to name a few. This overview concentrates on the more routine fistulae connecting the skin, alimentary canal, and genitourinary tract in various combinations.

Fistulae are seen as complications in patients with cancer because multiple risk factors for fistula development are often present in these patients. Fistulae are rarely the presenting symptom of an intra-abdominal malignancy; they most often present as complications during or after treatment. Most agree that contributing factors include abdominal surgery, inflammatory bowel disease, radiation therapy, cancer, malnutrition, intra-abdominal sepsis, and exposure of GI serosa to the external environment. Many of these factors are prevalent in patients with cancer.

Despite the use of total parenteral nutrition (TPN), more sophisticated means of enteral nutrition, antibiotics, and wound care adjuvants, mortality rates from gastrointestinal fistulae remain high. Although mortality rates as low as 7% are reported, numbers in the range of 10%–30% are more representative.[114] The exact incidence of GI fistula formation in patients with cancer is not known but is likely quite low.

Etiology

According to one report, more than one-third of enterocutaneous fistulae occur in patients who have cancer or who have received radiation therapy, or both.[115] Cancers can cause fistulae through a number of mechanisms. Direct invasion with subsequent tumor necrosis can result in an abnormal connection between viscera and the skin. Ischemic necrosis secondary to neoplastic vascular invasion or secondary to small vessel occlusion from host reaction and sclerosis likewise can lead to fistula formation. Finally, tumor-induced perforation with abscess and subsequent erosion can cause a fistula to form. This latter mechanism is particularly troublesome, as it can lead to diagnostic confusion and can complicate management.

Ionizing radiation could have both acute and chronic effects on the gut. The acute effects—a result of the depletion of rapidly proliferating mucosal cells causing diarrhea, nausea, vomiting, abdominal pain, and GI tract bleeding—are generally self-limiting. Acute radiation injury to the GI tract can be predictive of subsequent long-term complications. Chronic radiation damage can become evident as early as one month after radiation therapy, or it might not be clinically apparent for as long as 30 years after treatment.[116] Although radiation injury to the bowel can arise as a complication in as many as 15% of patients receiving abdominal fields, fistulae occur rarely; the exact incidence is unknown but is likely less than 3%. Fistulae make up approximately 15% of the radiation-induced complications requiring surgical intervention. Factors related to the incidence of radiation-induced injury include the total radiation dose and fractionation, the sensitivity of exposed normal organs within the radiation port, anatomic considerations, the presence of comorbid conditions, and concomitant administration of other drugs. Rubin and Casarett[117] helped to define organ tolerance of radiation therapy. Small bowel, stomach, and colon are the least tolerant organs (maximum tolerable dose [MTD] = 45 Gy), followed by rectum (MTD = 55 Gy) and esophagus (MTD = 60 Gy). The more the dose is fractionated and the greater the number of ports used, the less likely it is that normal tissue injury will occur.[118] Thinner patients are thought to be at higher risk for developing radiation enteritis, colitis, and gastritis. Clearly, the greater the amount and extent of exposure to the radiation beam, the greater the risk of injury. For these reasons, many techniques have been developed to limit GI tract exposure to radiation, including the following:

- Filling the bladder and using the Trendelenburg position to displace bowel from the pelvis during pelvic irradiation
- The use of shielding and multiple ports
- Intra-operative radiation therapy, whereby normal visceral structures can be shielded from the radiation ports
- The operative creation of "slings" to exclude small bowel from the pelvis after an abdominoperineal resection for rectal cancer

Conversely, factors that tend to fix the bowel in a single location, such as postoperative adhesions, increase the likelihood of radiation enteritis. Preexistent large-vessel atherosclerosis and small-vessel diabetic vasculopathy can increase sensitivity to radiation injury. Finally, the effects of many chemotherapeutic agents—especially doxorubicin, 5-fluorouracil, gemcitabine, and mitomycin-C—can potentiate the effects of radiation therapy on normal tissues. In this regard, pyrimidine analogues such as bromodeoxyuridine and iododeoxyuridine are being studied as tumor-selective radiation sensitizers; normal tissue sensitization with these agents is not yet known.

Prevention

Fistulae complicating cancer generally occur during active treatment or subsequent follow-up. Fistulae can arise after emergency or complex primary cancer operations. There is little one can do when faced with an emergency cancer operation to reduce the risk of fistula formation other than adhere to good surgical principles and techniques. Systemic antibiotics might help to prevent complications (including fistulae) in these situations. Elective operations offer the opportunity to undertake preventive measures to avoid fistulae. Proper antimicrobial bowel prophylaxis, including a mechanical bowel preparation, nonabsorbable enteric antibiotics, and systemic antibiotics, clearly reduce the risk of perioperative complications. Perioperative hydration and cardiovascular support to prevent hypoperfusion and secondary end-organ injury are important. In patients undergoing elective pancreatic resections for cancer, such as pancreaticoduodenectomy (Whipple procedure), the perioperative administration of the somatostatin analogue, octreotide, could be beneficial in preventing subsequent pancreatic fistulae and in reducing postoperative complications and deaths.[119,120] During an operation, recognition of possible predisposing factors for fistula formation and use of prophylactic measures can be helpful. Intra-operative risk factors for fistula formation include active infection, extensive adhesions, creation of serosal injuries, prior radiation therapy, prior fistulization, and presence of ischemic tissue. In addition to careful dissection and anastomotic technique, thorough drainage of all intra-abdominal infection and debridement of all devitalized and ischemic tissue can reduce the incidence of fistulae. Protection of sites of anastomosis or extensive dissection could also be important, particularly in the previously irradiated abdomen. Vascularized flaps, including serosa, omentum, and muscle, have all been described to fill soft tissue defects and exclude small bowel from areas of dissection. In patients undergoing bowel resection for a nonmalignant complication (i.e., radiation enteritis), it could be helpful to undertake resection close to the bowel wall, leaving behind well vascularized mesentery. This mesentery can then be mobilized, keeping a vascular pedicle intact, to fill tissue defects or wrap anastomoses. Many investigators have demonstrated the relationship of nutritional status to operative morbidity and mortality, including fistulae. In a series of 40 patients with cancer who developed postoperative gastrointestinal fistulas, Spiliotis and colleagues[121] noted that an albumin level of less than 3.0 grams/dL was a poor prognostic factor for fistula closure. Although the role of delaying an operation to allow preoperative nutrition support and repletion is controversial, attention to postoperative protein, calorie, fluid, electrolyte, and micronutrient needs is basic to help avoid complications. No patient should need to become further malnourished postoperatively before a decision to initiate nutrition support is made.

Natural History

GI fistulae occur most often during the treatment of gynecologic malignancies. Although less common, they also occur in the settings of bladder and rectal cancer. Fistulae resulting from the treatment of other cancers are much less common (Table 53-7). Three factors contribute to this distribution:

1. Radiation therapy is most often used to treat cancer of the cervix, endometrium, and rectum. Postoperative irradiation after the extensive pelvic operations often

Problems Common to Cancer and Its Therapy

II

TABLE 53-7

Primary Cancer Site in Cancer Patients with Gastrointestinal Fistulae

SITE OF PRIMARY CANCER	NO. OF PATIENTS
Cervix	36
Endometrium	15
Ovary	13
Bladder	13
Colon/rectum	7
Other	4

From Jahnson S, Westerborn O, Gerdin B: Prognosis of surgically treated radiation-induced damage to the intestine. Eur J Surg Oncol 1992;18:487–493.

used to treat these diseases frequently exposes adhesed bowel to high doses of ionizing radiation.

2. The structures in the pelvis that are dose-limiting to radiation therapy are generally the colon and small intestine. To maximize antitumor effects, doses are often pushed to or beyond the limits of intestinal tolerance. In contrast, upper abdominal radiation is generally limited by hepatic, renal, and spinal cord toxicity before severe GI injury can occur.

3. Finally, structures fixed to the retroperitoneum (e.g., the duodenum, ligament of Treitz, terminal ileum, cecum, and distal sigmoid colon) are more likely to be injured by external beam radiation therapy. Other than the duodenum, these structures are the most likely to be irradiated during pelvic therapy for gynecologic and rectal cancers.

A number of factors decrease the likelihood of spontaneous closure of a fistula. The most common is undrained infection in proximity to the tract. Also common is luminal obstruction distal to the fistula. Other factors include prior radiation or chemotherapy, epithelialization of the fistula tract, cancer within the tract, granulomatous disease (i.e., inflammatory bowel disease or mycobacterial infection) within the fistula, presence of a foreign body, and malnutrition. Although predictive of morbidity due to fistulae, fistula output does not appear to be related to the probability of spontaneous fistula closure. Given proper nutritional support and attention to these factors, as many as 60% of GI fistulae might close spontaneously.[114]

Treatment

Complications routinely encountered with GI fistula include fluid and electrolyte disorders, sepsis, malnutrition, and impaired skin integrity. The frequency and severity of these complications relates to the daily volume of fistula output and to the composition of the output. High-output fistulae (>1 L/day) tend to originate more proximally in the GI tract. Because of the specialized composition of gastric juice, bile, and succus pancreaticus, these more proximal fistulae not only tend to lead to dehydration but are also more prone to cause electrolyte and acid-base imbalances. Low-output fistulae generally originate more distally in the alimentary canal, resulting in

EVALUATION AND TREATMENT OF GASTROINTESTINAL FISTULAE IN PATIENTS WITH CANCER

PHASE	OBJECTIVES
Resuscitation	Restoration of fluid and electrolyte homeostasis within first 12–48 hours. Treatment of organ dysfunction.
Stabilization	Definitive evaluation and treatment of sepsis. Restoration and maintenance of skin integrity. Control and minimization of fistula output (i.e., nasogastric suction, use of H_2 blockers and somatostatin analogs). Assessment of nutritional status.
Nutrition	Repletion and maintenance of nutrition status (enterally or parenterally). Correction of trace nutrient deficiencies.
Investigation	Determination of anatomy of fistula and associated abnormalities (i.e., CT scan and fistulogram).
Definitive treatment	Nonoperative management for a period of 3–6 weeks successful in the majority of patients in whom no factors preventing spontaneous closure are present. Surgical intervention indicated if there is persistent sepsis, high-output fistula precluding nutritional repletion, or other factors precluding spontaneous closure (i.e., epithelialized tract, distal luminal obstruction, radiated bowel, and so forth.

low-volume outputs that are generally isotonic. For these reasons, the classification of fistulae according to their daily output volume can help predict the likelihood and kinds of complications to be expected.

To treat GI tract fistulae appropriately, the goals that must be achieved include the following:

- Resuscitation
- Stabilization
- Nutrition
- Investigation
- Definitive treatment

Although many of these activities occur simultaneously, it is helpful to consider each objective sequentially.

Resuscitation

Resuscitation of patients with GI fistulae follows the principles of general fluid and electrolyte assessment and management. A urinary catheter and, if necessary, central venous pressure monitoring are quite helpful. Specific fluid, electrolyte, and acid-base disturbances, organ dysfunction, and nutritional status should be identified with the initial bloodwork and treated appropriately. Most patients require 2–6 L of crystalloid resuscitation over the initial 24-hour period. Signs of sepsis should be assessed to help guide subsequent evaluation. Antibiotics should be started only if a specific infection is identified. Blood products should be used only when specifically indicated, to restore red cell mass or to treat coagulation abnormalities. Subsequent diagnostic and therapeutic maneuvers must await completion of the resuscitation phase, so these issues must be dealt with promptly, over the initial 12–48 hours after presentation.

Stabilization

The stabilization phase is aimed at preventing further complications. The goals are to treat any sources of sepsis, maintain fluid and electrolyte balance, and protect skin integrity. Ongoing sepsis dooms any attempts at completing and maintaining fluid and nutritional resuscitation and ultimately leads to organ failure. Patients exhibiting signs of sepsis must be evaluated aggressively to identify the source. Intra-abdominal and perifistular abscesses are common and must be identified quickly. Thorough physical examination (including digital examination of the rectum, vagina, stomas, and wounds) is absolutely necessary. CT scan of the abdomen and pelvis using intravenous and enteric contrast and contrast in the rectum, fistula tract, and drainage tubes is often the most enlightening radiologic study (Fig. 53-4). Any undrained

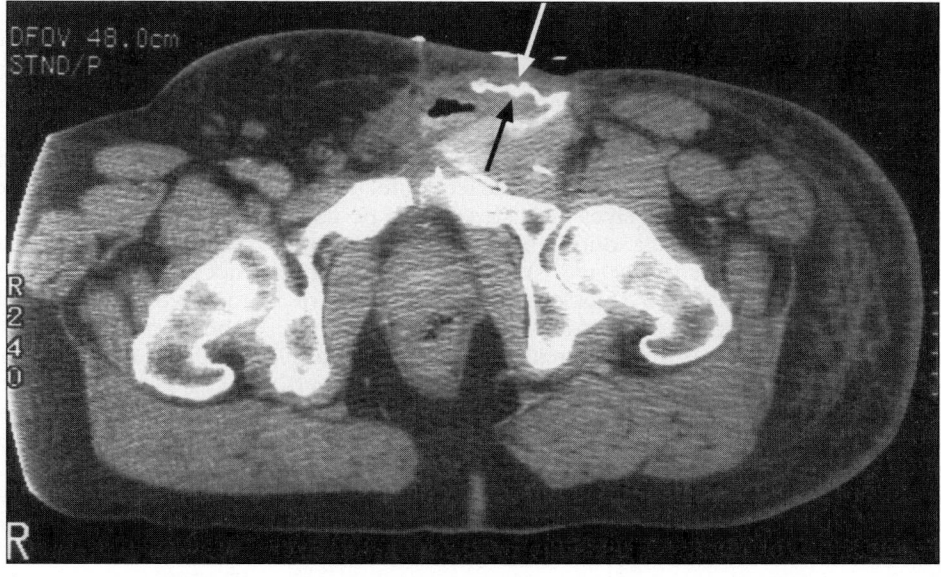

A

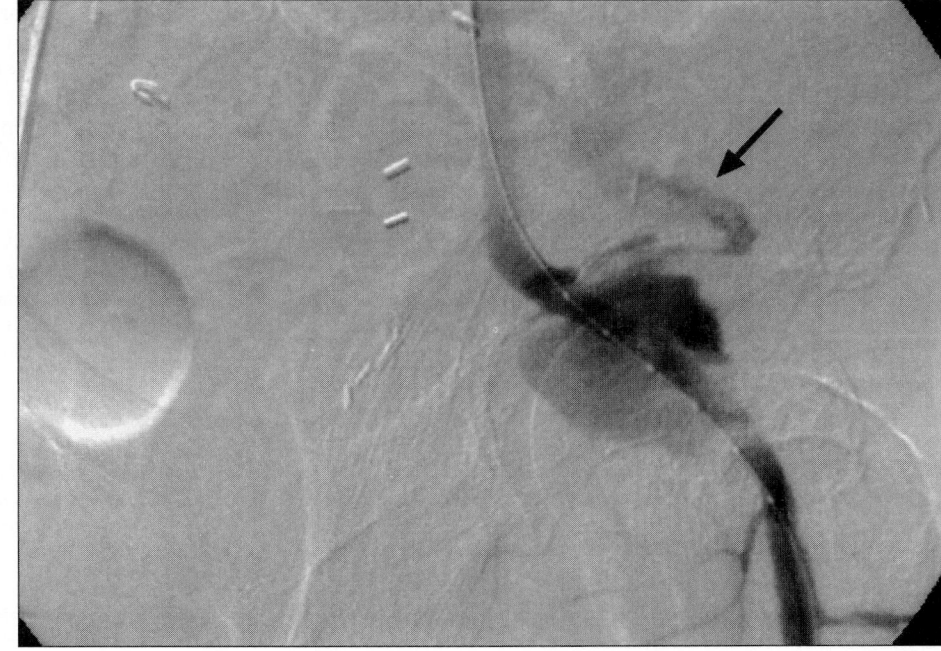

B

Figure 53-4. Arterioenterocutaneous fistula. Patient with a multiply recurrent high-grade liposarcoma of the spermatic cord treated with radical surgical resection and radiation therapy. After the most recent surgery, the patient developed an enterocutaneous fistula that was managed conservatively. He later presented with brisk bleeding from the fistula and per rectum. **A,** CT scan of the pelvis demonstrating recurrent tumor and tract (*arrows*) of enterocutaneous fistula. **B,** Arteriogram with contrast extravasation from the left external iliac artery and communication of the bowel (*arrow*).

foci of infection must be addressed aggressively and drained either percutaneously or operatively. Vascular access catheters and devices should be suspected of harboring infection and treated appropriately. Fluid and electrolyte homeostasis is best achieved by matching intake and output. This often requires collection, measurement, and laboratory analysis of nasogastric tube output, fistula drainage, and urine output. Significant fistula output should be replaced with an intravenous fluid of similar electrolyte composition. In general, for most small bowel, biliary, or pancreatic fistulae, the appropriate fluid would be lactated Ringer's solution. Once the acute electrolyte imbalances have been corrected and the fistula output has stabilized, intravenous fluid and nutritional infusions may be combined to simplify fluid management. Definitive treatment of fistulae ultimately requires the re-establishment of normal skin integrity; macerated skin and large open wounds complicate and delay spontaneous or operative closure. Thus, skin protection must be an early goal of fistula care. Enterostomal and wound care nursing specialists are invaluable. Techniques such as sump drainage, stoma bag application, and barrier protection of the skin using special adhesives or pastes should be used liberally. Minimizing fistula output simplifies both fluid and electrolyte homeostasis and skin care. Nasogastric suction and the use of H_2 blockers to decrease gastric secretory contribution to fistula output, although of theoretical benefit, only occasionally result in clinically significant benefits. The use of somatostatin or its longer-acting analog, octreotide, in the medical management of gastrointestinal fistulas is controversial. A number of small, nonrandomized series have demonstrated the ability of octreotide to reduce the volume of fistula drainage and shorten the time to fistula closure.[122-124] The results of prospective, randomized trials, however, have failed to demonstrate any advantage of octreotide over placebo.[125,126]

Nutrition

Malnutrition either preexists or will develop in nearly all patients with GI fistulae unless specific, aggressive nutrition support is initiated early in the treatment course. Either enteral or parenteral nutrition support can generally be started within 48 hours of presentation, as soon as the initial resuscitative and stabilization measures have been accomplished. With the advent of TPN in the early 1970s, many felt that mortality due to fistulae could be reduced substantially. Experience since then, however, suggests that TPN itself is of no special benefit; rather, maintenance of adequate nutrition by whatever means are feasible helps prevent fistula-related complications.[115] More recent paradigms regarding bacterial translocation and maintenance of gut barrier function, in fact, suggest that although TPN is better than no nutrition, enteral feeding is ideal. Wound and fistula losses of protein and calories are often difficult to measure. They must, however, be reckoned with in assessing nutritional requirements. Formal nitrogen balance studies and indirect calorimetric measurement of energy expenditure are the gold standards for adjusting protein and calorie intake to meet needs. Once requirements are determined, the route of administration chosen depends on overall patient status and the nature of the fistula. In general, early initiation of parenteral nutrition is helpful to ensure adequate support without delay. Subsequent aggressive attempts should be made to meet some or all of the patient's nutritional requirements enterally. Little evidence suggests that elemental enteral feedings or formulas containing specialized micronutrients (glutamine, short chain fatty acids, omega-3 oils, arginine, and so forth) offer incremental benefit. Generally, enteral formulas associated with the least volume of diarrhea and fistula output that meet the nutritional requirements of the patient should be used.

Investigation

Fistulae can be managed appropriately only when their anatomic features and associated potentiating factors are well defined. Reversible causes for fistulae failing to close spontaneously must be identified. Careful examination of the fistula with appropriate biopsies is necessary to rule out epithelialization or the presence of cancer, foreign bodies, or granulomatous processes within the tract. Generally, the entire GI tract should be investigated with radiographic contrast studies to rule out distal obstruction, to determine the origin of the fistula accurately, and to identify all involved organs and poorly drained associated abscesses. A fistulogram, obtained in the presence of an experienced surgeon, can provide valuable anatomic information and help the formulation of surgical plans. The utility of CT scans has already been discussed. In patients with cancer, a thorough search for recurrent and metastatic disease is also important. Discovery of incurable recurrences can temper the aggressiveness with which fistulae are treated and change the goals from definitive resection to palliation.

Definitive Treatment

In most patients who can be stabilized adequately and in whom no factors preventing spontaneous fistula closure are present, a trial period of three to six weeks of nonsurgical management is generally indicated. The availability of home parenteral and enteral nutrition support programs makes such a waiting period more palatable for patients who are otherwise doing well. Home care also can serve well those patients whose fistulae are gradually improving (spontaneous closure can be slow, particularly in patients with fistulae arising from the pancreas or a duodenal stump), those in whom general medical considerations or the presence of widespread metastatic disease make surgical exploration inappropriate, or those who have highly complex or recurrent fistulae. In some patients, adequate stabilization cannot be achieved. Ongoing fistula output or sepsis in these patients precludes nutritional repletion, adequate skin care, and protection of end-organ function. In this setting, early operation is mandatory.

The operative goals for treating intestinal fistulae are as follows:

1. Complete exploration of the peritoneal cavity to find undrained abscesses, unsuspected cancer, and associated complications

2. If possible, excision of the fistula tract and associated diseased tissue
3. If possible, restoration of continuity of the GI tract
4. Prevention of refistulization

Appropriate biopsies and cultures must be obtained. Use of vascularized omental, mesenteric, bowel, or muscular flaps to fill inflamed cavities and protect anastomoses is often helpful and should be planned for in conjunction with appropriate consultants preoperatively. The definitive operation is a good opportunity to simplify subsequent management of the patient through the insertion of enteric tubes for feeding and GI drainage. Bypass of fistulae can be a useful palliative technique when definitive resection is technically impossible or is felt to be associated with prohibitive morbidity.

REFERENCES

1. Turnbull ADM: Abdominal and upper gastrointestinal emergencies. In Turnbull ADM (ed): Surgical Emergencies in the Cancer Patient. Chicago, Year Book, 1987, p 152.
2. Starnes HF, Turnbull ADM, Daly JM: Colon and rectal emergencies. In Turnbull ADM (ed): Surgical Emergencies in the Cancer Patient. Chicago, Year Book, 1987, p 195.
3. Horowitz NS, Cohn DE, Herzog TJ, et al: The significance of pneumatosis intestinalis or bowel perforation in patients with gynecologic malignancies. Gynecol Oncol 2002;86:79–84.
4. Morita T, Tsunoda J, Inoue S, et al: Intestinal perforation in terminally ill cancer patients: Clinical characteristics. Am J Gastroenterol 1999;94:541–542.
5. Lynne J: Choices of curative and palliative care for cancer patients. Cancer 1986;36:100–104.
6. Haines I, Zalberg J, Buchanan J: Not-for-resuscitation orders in cancer patients—principles of decision-making. Med J Aust 1990;153:225–229.
7. Faber-Langendoen K: Resuscitation of patients with metastatic cancer: Is transient benefit still futile? Arch Intern Med 1991;151:235–239.
8. Ferrara J, Martin E, Carey L: Morbidity of emergency operations in patients with metastatic cancer receiving chemotherapy. Surgery 1982;92:605–609.
9. Kemeny MM, Brennan M: The surgical complications of chemotherapy in the cancer patient. Curr Probl Surg 1987;24: 613–675.
10. Padmanabhan A, Douglass HO Jr, Nava HR : Role of endoscopy in upper gastrointestinal bleeding in patients with malignancy. Endoscopy 1980;12:101–104.
11. Klein MS, Ennis F, Sherlock P et al: Stress erosions: A major cause of gastrointestinal hemorrhage in patients with malignant disease. Am J Dig Dis 1973;18:167–173.
12. Hande KR, Fisher R, DeVita V et al: Diffuse histiocytic lymphoma involving the gastrointestinal tract. Cancer 1978;41:1984–1989.
13. Fleming ID, Mitchell S, Dilawari RA: The role of surgery in the management of gastric lymphoma. Cancer 1982;49:1135–1141.
14. Kemeny MM, Magrath IT, Brennan M: The role of surgery in the management of American Burkitt's lymphoma and its treatment. Ann Surg 1982;196:82–86.
15. Nielsen GL, Sorensen HT, Mellemkjoer L, et al: Risk of hospitalization resulting from upper gastrointestinal bleeding among patients taking corticosteroids: a register-based cohort study. Am J Med 2001;111:541–545.
16. Kemeny N, Daly J, Oderman P et al: Hepatic artery pump infusion: Toxicity and results in patients with metastatic colorectal carcinoma. J Clin Oncol 1984;2:595–600.
17. Chang AE, Schneider P, Sugarbaker PH, et al: A prospective randomized trial of regional versus systemic continuous 5-fluorodeoxyuridine chemotherapy in the treatment of colorectal liver metastases. Ann Surg 1987;206:685–693.
18. Meyers PA, Potter V, Wollner N, Exelby P: Bowel perforation during initial treatment for childhood non-Hodgkin's lymphoma. Cancer 1985;56:259–261.
19. Talamonti MS, Dawes LG, Joehl RJ, Nahrwold DL: Gastrointestinal lymphoma. A case for primary surgical resection. Arch Surg 1990;125:972–977.
20. Maor MH, Velasques W, Fuller LM, Silvermintz KB J: Stomach conservation in stages IE and IIE gastric non-Hodgkin's lymphoma. Clin Oncol 1990;8:266–271.
21. Salles G, Herbrecht R, Tilly H et al: Aggressive primary gastrointestinal lymphomas: Review of 91 patients treated with the LNH-84 regimen. A study of the Groupe d'Etude des Lymphomes Agressifs. Am J Med 1991 Jan;90(1):77–84.
22. Rackner VL, Thirlby RC, Ryan JA Jr: Role of surgery in multimodality therapy for gastrointestinal lymphoma. Am J Surg 1991;161:570–575.
23. Gertsch P, Yip SKH, Chow LWC, Lauder IJ: Free perforation of gastric carcinoma. Arch Surg 1995;130:177–181.
24. List AF, Greer JP, Cousar JC, et al: Non-Hodgkin's lymphoma of the gastrointestinal tract: An analysis of clinical and pathologic features affecting outcome. J Clin Oncol 1988;6:1125–1133.
25. Yanchar NL, Bass J: Poor outcome of gastrointestinal perforations associated with childhood abdominal non-Hodgkin's lymphoma. J Pediatr Surg 1999;34:1169–1174.
26. Jones GT, Abramson N: Gastrointestinal necrosis in acute leukemia: A complication of induction therapy. Cancer Inv 1983;1:315–320.
27. Seewaldt V, Cain JM, Greer BE, Tamimi H, Figge DC: Correspondence, bowel complications with taxol therapy. J Clin Oncol 1993;11:1198.
28. Schwartzentruber D, Lotze MT, Rosenberg SA: Colonic perforation. An unusual complication of therapy with high-dose interleukin-2. Cancer 1988;62:2350–2353.
29. Yokota T, Yamada Y, Murakami Y, et al: Abdominal crisis caused by perforation of ileal lymphoma. Am J Emerg Med 2002;20:136–137.
30. Glenn J, Funkhouser WK, Schneider PS: Acute illnesses necessitating urgent abdominal surgery in neutropenic cancer patients: Description of 14 cases and review of the literature. Surgery 1989;105:778–789.
31. Mower WJ, Hawkins JA, Nelson EW: Neutropenic enterocolitis in adults with acute leukemia. Arch Surg 1986;121:571–574.
32. Villar HV, Warneke JA, Peck MD, Durie B, Bjelland JC, Hunter TB: Role of surgical treatment in the management of complications of the gastrointestinal tract in patients with leukemia. Surg Gynecol Obstet 1987;165:217–222.
33. Sloas MM, Flynn PM, Kaste SC, Patrick CC: Typhlitis in children with cancer: A 30-year experience. Clin Infect Dis 1993;17:484–490.
34. Williams N, Scott ADN: Neutropenic colitis: A continuing surgical challenge. Br J Surg 1997;84:1200–1205.
35. Moir DH, Bale PM: Necropsy findings in childhood leukemia, emphasizing neutropenic enterocolitis and cerebral calcification. Pathology 1976;8:247–258.
36. Wade DS, Nava HR, Douglass HO: Neutropenic enterocolitis: Clinical diagnosis and treatment. Cancer 1992;69:17–23.
37. Mulholland MW, Delaney JP: Neutropenic colitis and aplastic anemia. Ann Surg 1983;197:84–90.
38. Geelhoed GW, Kane MA, Dale DC, Wells SA: Colon ulceration and perforation in cyclic neutropenia. J Pediatr Surg 1973;8:379–382.
39. Kurbegov AC, Sondheimer JM: Pneumatosis intestinalis in non-neonatal pediatric patients. Pediatrics 2001;108:402–406.
40. de Magalhaes-Silverman M, Simpson J, Ball E: Pneumoperitoneum without peritonitis after allogeneic peripheral blood stem cell transplantation. Bone Marrow Transplant 1998;21(11):1153–1154.
41. Heng Y, Schuffler MD, Haggitt RC, et al: Pneumatosis intestinalis: A review. Am J Gastroenterol 1995;90:1747–1758.
42. Safdar A, Armstrong D: Infectious morbidity in critically ill patients with cancer. Crit Care Clin 2001;17:531–570, vii–viii.
43. Shaked A, Shinar E, Freund H: Neutropenic typhlitis: A plea for conservatism. Dis Colon Rectum 1983;26:351–352.
44. Schlatter M, Snyder K, Freyer D: Successful nonoperative management of typhlitis in pediatric oncology patients. J Pediatr Surg 2002;37:1151–1155.
45. Alt B, Glass NR, Sollinger H: Neutropenic enterocolitis in adults: Review of the literature and assessment of surgical intervention. Am J Surg 1985;149:405–408.

46. Schaller RT, Schaller JF: The acute abdomen in the immunologically compromised child. J Pediatr Surg 1983;6:937–944.

47. Shamberger RC, Weinstein HJ, Delorey MJ, Levey RH: The medical and surgical management of typhlitis in children with acute nonlymphocytic (myelogenous) leukemia. Cancer 1986;57:603–609.

48. Urbach DR, Rotstein OD: Typhlitis. Can J Surg 1999;42:415–419.

49. Angel CA, Rao BN, Wrenn E, Lobe TE, Kumar APM: Acute appendicitis in children with leukemia and other malignancies: Still a diagnostic dilemma. J Pediatr Surg 1992;27:476–479.

50. Silliman CC, Haase GM, Strain JD, et al: Indications for surgical intervention for gastrointestinal emergencies in children receiving chemotherapy. Cancer 1994;74:203–216.

51. Wallace J, Schwaitzberg S, Miller K: Sometimes it really is appendicitis: Case of a CML patient with acute appendicitis. Ann Hematol 1998;77:61–64.

52. Jacobs JE, Birnbaum BA: CT of inflammatory disease of the colon. Semin Ultrasound CT MRI 1995;16:91–101.

53. Skibber JM, Matter GJ, Pizzo PA, et al: Right lower quadrant pain in young patients with leukemia. A surgical perspective. Ann Surg 1987;206:711–716.

54. Chowhan NM, Madajewicz S: Management of metastases-induced acute pancreatitis in small cell carcinoma of the lung. Cancer 1990;65:1445–1448.

55. Gutman M, Inbar M, Klausner JM: Metastases-induced acute pancreatitis: A rare presentation of cancer. Eur J Surg Oncol 1992;19:302–304.

56. Stewart KC, Dickout WJ, Urschel JD: Metastasis-induced acute pancreatitis as the initial manifestation of bronchogenic carcinoma. Chest 1993;104:98–100.

57. Oettgen HF, Stephenson PA, Schwartz MK, et al: Toxicity of E. coli L-asparaginase in man. Cancer 1970;25(2):253–278.

58. Land VJ, Sutow WW, Fernbach DJ, Lane DM, Williams TE: Toxicity of L-asparaginase in children with advanced leukemia. Cancer 1972;30:339–347.

59. Izraeli S, Adamson PC, Blaney SM, Balis FM: Cancer: Acute pancreatitis after ifosfamide therapy. Cancer 1994;74:1627–1628.

60. Underwood TW, Frye CB: Drug-induced pancreatitis. Clin Pharm 1993;12:440–448.

61. Kishimoto W, Nakao A, Takagi H, Hayakawa T: Acute pancreatitis after transcatheter arterial embolization for hepatocellular carcinoma. Am J Gastroenterol 1989;84:1396–1399.

62. Khan KN, Nakata K, Shima M, et al: Pancreatic tissue damage by transcatheter arterial embolization for hepatoma. Dig Dis Sci 1993;38:65–70.

63. Samuels BI, Culbert SJ, Okamura J, Sullivan MP: Early detection of chemotherapy-related pancreatic enlargement in children using abdominal ultrasound. Cancer 1976;38:1515–1523.

64. North JH Jr, Weber TK, Rodriguez-Bigas MA, Meropol NJ, Petrelli NJ: The management of infectious and noninfectious anorectal complications in patients with leukemia. J Am Coll Surg 1996;183:322–328.

65. Grewal H, Guillem JG, Quan SHQ, Enker WE, Cohen AM: Anorectal disease in neutropenic leukemic patients. Dis Colon Rectum 1994;37:1095–1099.

66. Barnes SG, Sattler FR, Ballard JO: Perirectal infections in acute leukemia: Improved survival after incision and debridement. Ann Intern Med 1984;100:515–518.

67. Earle MF, Fossieck BE, Cohen MH, Ihde DC, Bunn PA, Minna JD: Perirectal infections in patients with small cell lung cancer. JAMA 1981;246:2464–2466.

68. Boddie AW, Bines SD: Management of acute rectal problems in leukemic patients. J Surg Oncol 1986;33:53–56.

69. Cohen JS, Paz IB, O'Donnell MR, Ellenhorn JDI: Treatment of perianal infection following bone marrow transplantation. Dis Colon Rectum 1996;39:981–985.

70. Porter AJ, Meagher AP, Sweeney JL: Anal lymphoma presenting as a perianal abscess. Austr N Z J Surg 1994;64:279–281.

71. Winslet MC, Allan A, Ambrose NS: Anorectal sepsis as a presentation of occult rectal and systemic disease. Dis Colon Rectum 1988;31:597–600.

72. Glenn J, Cotton D, Wesley R, Pizzo P: Anorectal infections in patients with malignant disease. Rev Infect Dis 1988;10:42–52.

73. Carlson GW, Ferguson CM, Amerson JR: Perianal infections in acute leukemia. Am Surgeon 1988;54:693–695.

74. Vanheuverzwyn R, Delannoy A, Michaux JL, Dive C: Anal lesions in hematologic diseases. Dis Colon Rectum 1980;23:310–312.

75. Buyukasik Y, Ozcebe OI, Sayinalp N, et al: Perianal infections in patients with leukemia: Importance of the course of neutrophil count. Dis Colon Rectum 1998;41:81–85.

76. Shaked AA, Shinar E, Freund H: Managing the granulocytopenic patient with acute perianal inflammatory disease. Am J Surg 1986;152:510–512.

77. Skibber JM, Matter GJ, Pizzo PA, Lotze MT: Right lower quadrant pain in young patients with leukemia. A surgical perspective. Ann Surg 1987;206:711–716.

78. Ketcham AS, Hoye RC, Pilch YH, Morton DL: Delayed intestinal obstruction following treatment for cancer. Cancer 1970;25:406–410.

79. Osteen RT, Guyton S, Steele G Jr, Wilson RE: Malignant intestinal obstruction. Surgery 1980;87:611–615.

80. Weiss SM, Skibber JM, Rosato FE: Bowel obstruction in cancer patients: Performance status as a predictor of survival. J Surg Oncol 1984;25:15–17.

81. Gallick HL, Weaver DW, Sachs RJ, Bouwman DL: Intestinal obstruction in cancer patients. An assessment of risk factors and outcome. Am Surg 1986;52:434–437.

82. Tang E, Davis J, Silberman H: Bowel obstruction in cancer patients. Arch Surg 1995;130:832–837.

83. Sise JG, Crichlow RW: Obstruction due to malignant tumors. Semin Oncol 1978;5:213–224.

84. Malone JM, Koonce T, Larson DM, et al: Palliation of small bowel obstruction by percutaneous gastrostomy in patients with progressive ovarian carcinoma. Obstet Gynecol 1986;68:431–433.

85. Blair SL, Chu DZ, Schwarz RE: Outcome of palliative operations for malignant bowel obstruction in patients with peritoneal carcinomatosis from nongynecological cancer. Ann Surg Oncol 2001;8:632–637.

86. Krouse RS, McCahill LE, Easson AM, et al: When the sun can set on an unoperated bowel obstruction: Management of malignant bowel obstruction. J Am Coll Surg 2002;195:117–128.

87. Muir JC, von Gunten CF: Antisecretory agents in gastrointestinal obstruction. Clin Geriatr Med 2000;16:327–334.

88. Ripamonti C, Twycross R, Baines M, et al: Clinical-practice recommendations for the management of bowel obstruction in patients with end-stage cancer. Support Care Cancer 2001;9:223–233.

89. Baines M, Oliver DJ, Carter RI: Medical management of intestinal obstruction in patients with advanced malignant disease: A clinical and pathological study. Lancet 1985;2:990–993.

90. Gemlo B, Rayner AA, Lewis B, et al: Home support of patients with end-stage malignant bowel obstruction using hydration and venting gastrostomy. Am J Surg 1986;152:100–104.

91. August DA, Thorn D, Fisher RL, Welchek CM: Home parenteral nutrition for patients with inoperable malignant bowel obstruction. J Parenter Enteral Nutr 1991;15:323–327.

92. Wolford JL, McDonald GB: A problem oriented approach to intestinal and liver disease after marrow transplantation. J Clin Gastroenterol 1988;10:419–433.

93. Bortin MM, Ringden O, Horowitz MM, Rozman C, Weiner RS, Rimm AA: Temporal relationships between the major complications of bone marrow transplantation for leukemia. Bone Marrow Transplant 1989;4:339–344.

94. Yagi T, Karasuno T, Hasegawa T, et al: Acute abdomen without cutaneous signs of varicella zoster virus infection as a late complication of allogeneic bone marrow transplantation: Importance of empiric therapy with acyclovir. Bone Marrow Transplant 2000;25:1003–1005.

95. Horak DA, Forman SJ: Critical care of the hematopoietic stem cell patient. Crit Care Clin 2001;17:671–695.

96. Spencer GD, Shulman HM, Myerson D, Thomas ED, McDonald GB: Diffuse intestinal ulceration after marrow transplantation: A clinicopathologic study of 13 patients. Hum Pathol 1986;17:621–633.

97. McGregor GI, Shepard J, Phillips GL: Acute graft-versus-host disease of the intestine: A surgical perspective. Am J Surg 1988;155:680–682.

98. Thomas ED, Storb R, Clift RA, et al: Bone marrow transplantation. N Engl J Med 1975;292:1-7.

99. Kaur S, Cooper G, Fakult S, Lazarus HM: Incidence and outcome of overt gastrointestinal bleeding in patients undergoing bone marrow transplantation. Dig Dis Sci 1996;41:598-603.

100. Maile CW, Frick MP, Crass JR, Snover DC, Weisdorf SA, Kersey JH: The plain abdominal radiograph in acute gastrointestinal graft -vs-host disease. Am J Roentgenol 1985;145:289-292.

101. Day DL, Ramsay NKC, Letourneau JG: Pneumatosis intestinalis after bone marrow transplantation. Am J Roentgenol 1988;151:85-87.

102. Chirletti P, Caronna R, Arcese W, et al: Gastrointestinal emergencies in patients with acute intestinal graft-versus-host disease. Leuk Lymph 1998;29:129-137.

103. Lipton J, Patterson B, Mustard R, et al: Pneumatosis intestinalis with free air mimicking intestinal perforation in a bone marrow transplant patient. Bone Marrow Transplant 1994;14:323-326.

104. McDonald GB, Hinds MS, Fisher LD, et al: Veno-occlusive disease of the liver and multiorgan failure after bone marrow transplantation: A cohort study of 355 patients. Ann Intern Med 1993;118:255-267.

105. Baron F, Deprez M, Beguin Y: The veno-occlusive disease of the liver. Haematologica 1997;82:718-725.

106. Jones RJ, Lee KSK, Beschorner WE, et al: Venoocclusive disease of the liver following bone marrow transplantation. Transplantation 1987;44:778-783.

107. Brown BP, Abu-Yousef M, Farner R, LaBrecque D, Gingrich R: Doppler sonography: A noninvasive method for evaluation of hepatic venocclusive disease. AJR Am J Roentgenol 1990;154:721-724.

108. Herbetko J, Grigg AP, Buckley AR, Phillips GL: Venoocclusive liver disease after bone marrow transplantation: Findings at duplex sonography. AJR Am J Roentgenol 1992;158:1001-1005.

109. Wasserheit C, Acaba L, Gulati S: Abnormal liver function in patients undergoing autologous bone marrow transplantation for hematologic malignancies. Cancer Inv 1995;13:347-354.

110. Korte W: Veno-occlusive disease of the liver after bone marrow transplantation: Is hypercoagulability really part of the problem? Blood Coag Fibrinol 1997;8:367-381.

111. Bearman SI, Lee JL, Baron AE, McDonald GB: Treatment of hepatic venocclusive disease with recombinant human tissue plasminogen activator and heparin in 42 marrow transpant patients. Blood 1997;89:1501-1506.

112. Smith FO, Johnson MS, Scherer LR: Transjugular intrahepatic portosystemic shunting (TIPS) for treatment of severe hepatic veno-occlusive disease. Bone Marrow Transplant 1996;18:643-646.

113. Fried MW, Connaghan DG, Sharma S, et al: Transjugular intrahepatic portosystemic shunt for the management of severe venoocclusive disease following bone marrow transplantation. Hepatology 1996;24:588-591.

114. Tarazi R, Steiger E: Enterocutaneous fistulas. In Kinney JM, John M, Hill GL, Owen OE (eds): Nutrition and Metabolism in Patient Care. Philadelphia, WB Saunders, 1988, p 243.

115. Reber H, Roberts C, Way LW, Dunphy JE: Management of external gastrointestinal fistulas. Ann Surg 1978;188:460-467.

116. Jahnson S, Westerborn O, Gerdin B: Prognosis of surgically treated radiation-induced damage to the intestine. Eur J Surg Oncol 1992;18:487-493.

117. Rubin P, Casarett GW: A direction for clinical radiation pathology. In Vaeth J (ed): Frontiers of Radiation Therapy and Oncology. Baltimore, University Park Press, 1972, p 1.

118. Novak J, Collins J, Donowitz M, et al: Effects of radiation on the human gastrointestinal tract. J Clin Gastroenterol 1979;3:9-39.

119. Montorsi M, Zago M, Mosca F, et al: Efficacy of octreotide in the prevention of pancreatic fistula after elective pancreatic resections: A prospective, controlled, randomized clinical trial. Surgery 1995;117:26-31.

120. Buchler M, Friess H, Klempa I, et al: Role of octreotide in the prevention of postoperative complications following pancreatic resection. Amer J Surg 1992;163:125-130.

121. Spiliotis J, Briand D, Gouttebel M-C, et al: Treatment of fistulas of the gastrointestinal tract with total parenteral nutrition and octreotide in patients with carcinoma. Surg Gynecol Obstet 1993;176:575-580.

122. Rosenberg L, Brown RA: Sandostatin in the management of nonendocrine gastrointestinal and pancreatic disorders: A preliminary study. Can J Surg 1991;34:223-229.

123. Borison DI, Bloom AD, Pritchard TJ: Treatment of enterocutaneous and colocutaneous fistulas with early surgery or somastatin analog. Dis Colon Rectum 1992;35:635-639.

124. Paran H, Neufeld D, Kaplan O, Klausner J, Freund U: Octreotide for treatment of postoperative alimentary tract fistulas. World J Surg 1995;19:430-434.

125. Sancho JJ, DiCostanzo J, Nubiola P, et al: Randomized double-blind placebo-controlled trial of early octreotide in patients with postoperative enterocutaneous fistula. Br J Surg 1995;82:638-641.

126. Scott NA, Finnegan S, Irving MH: Octreotide for treatment of postoperative alimentary tract fistulas. Acta Gastroenterol Belg 1993;56:266-270.

Problems Common to Cancer and Its Therapy

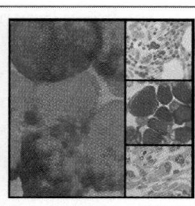

54 SUPERIOR VENA CAVA SYNDROME

Janessa Laskin

Anthony J. Cmelak

John Roberts

Steven G. Meranze

David H. Johnson

SUMMARY OF KEY POINTS

ETIOLOGY

- Superior vena cava (SVC) syndrome is usually due to neoplastic process—primary lung carcinoma is most prominent, with a disporportionate number of patients having small cell histology; non-Hodgkin's lymphoma and metastatic tumors are the next most common.
- SVC can be iatrogenic—sometimes seen as a complication of central venous line or cardiac surgery.

ANATOMY AND PHYSIOLOGY

- Junction of the braciocephalic veins forms the thin-walled, low-pressure SVC, which is subjected to obstruction from a variety of mediastinal components.
- External compression often precedes direct tumor invasion or thrombus formation.
- SVC has an extensive collateral network.

CLINICAL FEATURES

- Usual symptoms are head "fullness," dyspnea, cough, and chest pain, typically with insidious onset.
- More severe symptoms are infrequent and life-threatening, neurologic symptoms are rare.
- Diagnosis is based on clinical findings.

EVALUATION

- Chest radiograph typically shows mediastinal widening; a mass is often seen in the region of the SVC.
- Small-dose cavagrams can be safely accomplished to define exact location and routes of collateral flow.
- Computed tomography (CT) scanning demonstrates the mass and collateral flow and is the most helpful study to guide treatment.
- Treatment of an identified mass prior to histologic diagnosis rarely justified unless prior diagnosis is established.
- Methods used to define histology are sputum cytology, bronchoscopy, lymph node biopsy, thoracentesis, percutaneous biopsy, mediastinoscopy, and thoracotomy; previously reported high risks associated with these procedures are not justified in current data.

TREATMENT

- Radiation therapy fractionation schedule depends on tumor histology, stage, prognosis, patient's general condition, and whether obstruction is acute or subacute.
- Chemotherapy alone or with radiation therapy is the preferred treatment in small cell lung cancer; also used in non-Hodgkin's lymphoma.
- Surgery is usually reserved for selective patients with benign causes of obstruction and consists of a bypass procedure.
- Percutaneously placed, self-expanding intravascular wire stents provide an option or adjunct to other procedures in the pallative treatment of patients (usually with malignant disease).

INTRODUCTION

Obstruction of the superior vena cava (SVC) may occur as an acute or subacute process producing a syndrome with characteristic features including facial edema and plethora, dilation of chest wall and neck veins, mild to moderate respiratory difficulty, and, less commonly, conjunctival edema, central nervous system complaints such as headache, or, more rarely, visual disturbances and altered states of consciousness signs.[1-4] The first recorded description of superior vena cava obstruction (SVCO) occurred in 1757 when William Hunter described the entity in a patient with syphilitic aortic aneurysm.[5] For nearly two centuries thereafter, nonmalignant processes such as aortic aneurysms, syphilitic aortitis, or chronic mediastinitis due to tuberculosis were the predominant etiologic factors.[2,4,6,7] However, these diseases are now quite rare, and cancer has become the leading cause of SVCO primarily because of the rapid increase in the incidence of bronchogenic carcinoma after World War II.[2,4,6,8-10] Although SVCO was once considered a medical emergency, it is now well established that patients with SVCO rarely experience immediate, life-threatening complications.[6,11-13] Consequently, in cases in which a diagnosis is not known, it is appropriate to proceed with a biopsy to establish the underlying cause firmly, because optimal management is dependent on etiology.[14]

ANATOMY AND PATHOPHYSIOLOGY

The SVC is formed by the junction of the brachiocephalic veins, which in turn are formed by the joining of the internal jugular and subclavian veins. Thus the SVC represents the major drainage system of venous blood from the head, neck, arms, and upper thorax.[15] The right and left brachiocephalic veins join at about the level of the sternal angle to form the SVC. The SVC descends on the right side of the ascending aorta and empties into

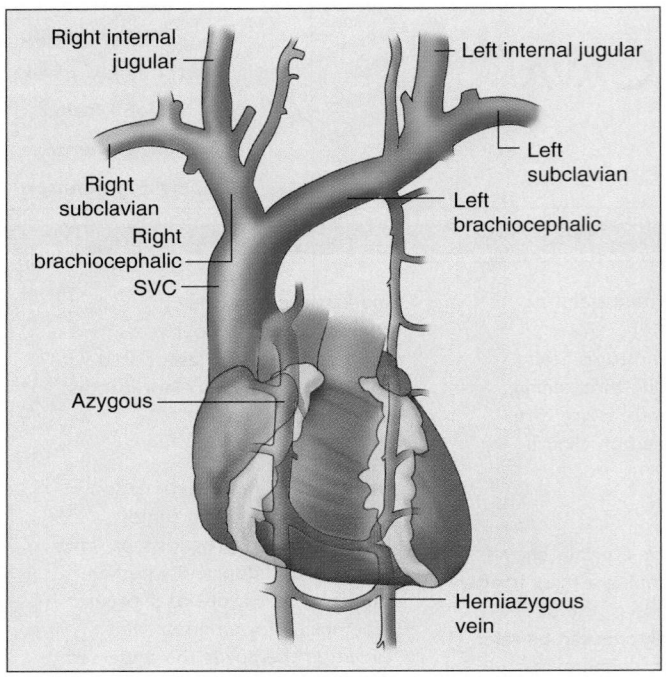

Figure 54-1. Normal anatomy and drainage pattern of the superior vena cava.

the right atrium, with its distal 2 cm lying within the pericardial sac (Fig. 54-1).

Because of its mediastinal location surrounded by several rigid structures including the sternum, trachea, pulmonary artery, right mainstem bronchus, and numerous lymph nodes, the SVC is particularly vulnerable to obstruction. Despite being a relatively large vessel, its thin vascular walls and low intravascular pressure contribute to the ease with which the SVC can be obstructed.[15] Obstruction of the SVC can be caused by external compression due to tumor or by lymph nodes enlarged by inflammation or metastases (Fig. 54-2). SVCO also can be caused by direct tumor invasion or by a thrombus. Secondary thrombus is reported to occur in up to 50% of cases[1] and may contribute to the lack of response to appropriate therapeutic maneuvers. In general, obstruction of the SVC above the orifice of azygos vein is better tolerated than is blockage below this level.[9,15,16] The azygos vein represents an important collateral system of the SVC and is formed by the junction of the right subcostal and right ascending lumbar veins. Additional routes of collateral flow include the mammary, vertebral, lateral thoracic, paraspinous, and esophageal vessels. The azygos vein ascends through the posterior and superior mediastinum, arches over the hilum of the right lung, and ends in the SVC. Fortunately, extensive anastomoses are formed between the SVC, azygos, and vertebral systems, providing multiple routes of collateral blood flow. Thus if an obstruction occurs above the

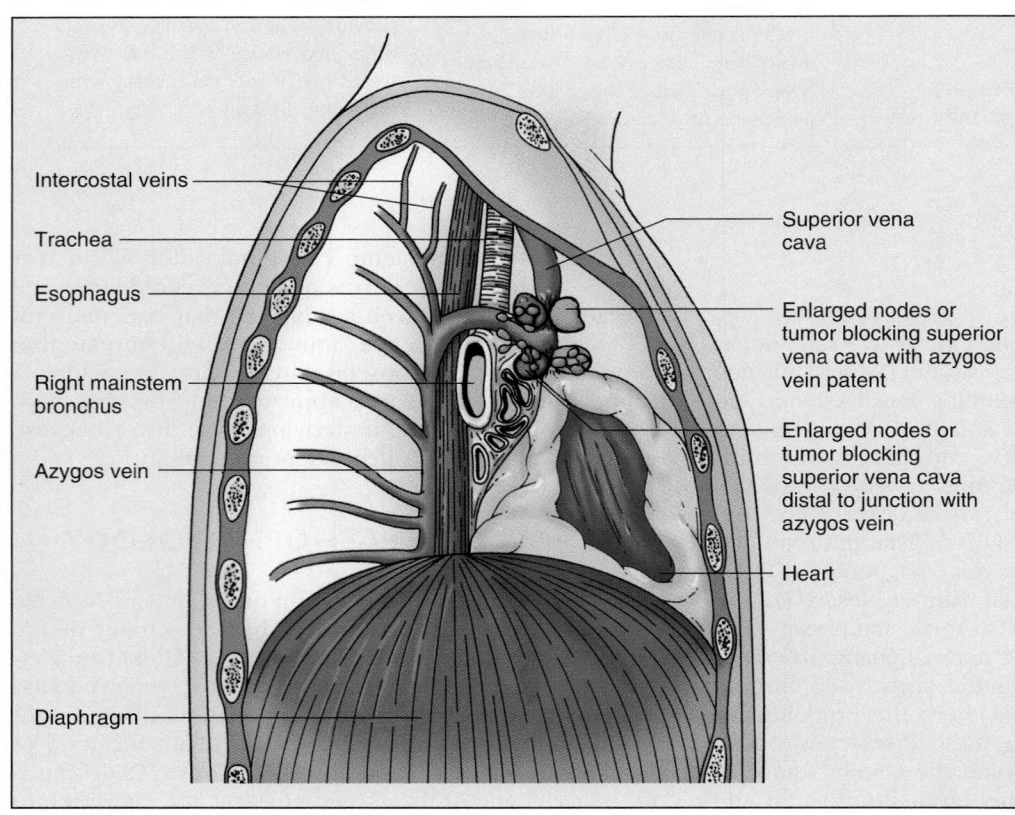

Figure 54-2. Lateral view of the thorax with superior vena cava obstruction.

azygos vein, blood can be diverted through chest-wall veins into the thoracic and iliac veins and enter the heart by way of the inferior vena cava (IVC) and azygos systems. Blood from the head and neck also can return to the heart via the vertebral plexus. If the SVC is obstructed between the azygos vein and the heart, the only route of blood return is via the IVC.

ETIOLOGY

Since the middle part of the 20th century, cancer has been the principal cause of SVCO, with bronchogenic carcinoma accounting for up to 85% of cases (Table 54-1).[1,2,4,10,11,17-20] The two most frequent lung cancer histologic types associated with SVCO are small cell and squamous cell carcinoma.[4,15,21-23] Although small cell lung cancer (SCLC) accounts for just 15% to 20% of newly diagnosed lung cancers, it is the underlying cause of up to 65% of all cases of SVCO.[4,6,9,24,25] The tendency of SCLC to occur centrally within the lung, as well as its high incidence of mediastinal lymph node metastases, most likely accounts for this consistent observation. Although lung cancer is the leading cause of SVCO, the incidence of this syndrome in patients with lung cancer ranges from 3% to 30%, with most series tending toward the lower figure.[3,12,26]

Non-Hodgkin's lymphoma is the second most common cause of SVCO.[2,6,27,28] Perez-Soler and colleagues[28] identified 36 cases among 915 lymphoma patients treated at the M.D. Anderson Cancer Center. SVCO was most commonly observed with diffuse large cell and lymphoblastic lymphomas.[28] The frequency of mediastinal presentations with the latter histologic types may account for this association, because up to 65% of patients with lymphoblastic lymphomas are first seen with a mediastinal mass. The incidence of SVCO in these categories of non-Hodgkin's lymphoma is reported to be 7% and 20%, respectively.[28] SVCO rarely is observed in small cleaved cell lymphomas or Hodgkin's disease, both of which are more common than lymphoblastic lymphoma.[28]

Metastatic cancers account for approximately 5% to 10% of SVCOs (see Table 54-1).[2,4,10,11,17,19,20,29-31] The most common primary tumor sites are, in approximate order of frequency, breast cancer, germ cell malignancies, and gastrointestinal cancers. Less common primary sites include sarcomas (including primary sarcomas of the great vessels),[32-34] transitional cell carcinoma, prostate cancer, and melanomas.[30] However, virtually any cancer capable of metastasizing to the mediastinum can result in SVCO.

Nonmalignant causes of SVCO account for up to 5% of cases. An increasingly common benign cause of SVCO is central venous catheter–induced thrombosis, which may occur with cardiac pacemakers, LaVeen shunts, hyperalimentation lines, and Swan-Ganz catheters, as well as those used for chemotherapy administration.[10,35-41] SVCO appears to be more common when the tip of the catheter is placed in the left subclavian vein in the upper part of the vena cava.[38] Contrast venography can help establish the diagnosis.[42,43] Treatment consists of thrombolytic agents and heparin.[39-41,44] The incidence of catheter-related thrombosis may be reduced with the application of very low dose warfarin (1 mg/day) before insertion of the catheter and continued afterward and possibly by ensuring fluoroscopically that the catheter tip is located below the third vertebra.[45,46] Additional rare benign causes of SVCO include chronic mediastinitis secondary to histoplasmosis, retrosternal goiters, *Nocardia*, and congestive heart failure.[2,47-51]

In children, SVCO is most frequently related to iatrogenic causes secondary to cardiovascular surgery for congenital heart disease or ventriculoatrial shunts for hydrocephalus.[52-54] The most common malignant causes of SVCO in children are non-Hodgkin's lymphoma, acute lymphoblastic leukemia, Hodgkin's disease, neuroblastomas, and yolk sac tumors.[53,54]

CLINICAL FEATURES

Typically, SVCO has a relatively insidious onset. Patients frequently complain of a sense of head "fullness," mild

TABLE 54-1

Causes of Superior Vena Cava Syndrome

	PARISH[2]	YELLIN[20]	LOCHRIDGE[17]	DAVENPORT[1]	BELL[4]	ARMSTRONG[11]	SCARANTINO[18]	LITTLE[19]
Total patients	86	63	66	35	159	125	60	42
Lung cancer	45	30	52	26	129	99	36	35
Non–small cell lung cancer	33	26	44	6	64	57	23	28
Small cell lung cancer	12	4	8	20	65	42	13	7
Lymphoma	8	13	8	1	3	18	8	3
Metastases	12	4	4	4	4	8	4	3
Thymoma/Thyroid	2	4	—	1	—	—	—	1
Benign	19	11	2		2	—	—	—
Biopsy not done	—	—	—	3	21	—	12	—

Data compiled from references 1, 2, 4, 11, and 17–20.

HISTOLOGIC CONFIRMATION OF UNDERLYING CAUSE OF SVCO

In most cases the distinction between carcinoma and lymphoma is readily accomplished with routine H&E stains. Special studies sometimes required to distinguish these entities include:

1. Immunoperoxidase stains
   a. Common leukocyte antigen; positive in lymphoma, negative in carcinomas
   b. Epithelial membrane antigen or keratin; positive in carcinomas, negative in lymphomas
   c. Surface immunoglobulins; positive in B-cell lymphomas, negative in carcinomas
2. Electron microscopy
   a. Desmosomes and intracellular junctions typical of carcinomas
   b. Microvilli typical of adenocarcinomas
   c. Dense-core granule (neurosecretory) present in neuroendocrine tumors (e.g., small cell lung cancer)
   d. Transformed lymphocytes, identified from a paucity of organelles, abundant free ribosomes, prominent nucleoli, and occasional presence of nuclear blebs

Immunoperoxidase studies can usually be obtained relatively quickly and are most helpful in distinguishing a lymphoma from a carcinoma. However, expensive pathology studies are avoided unless necessary to help guide therapeutic decisions.

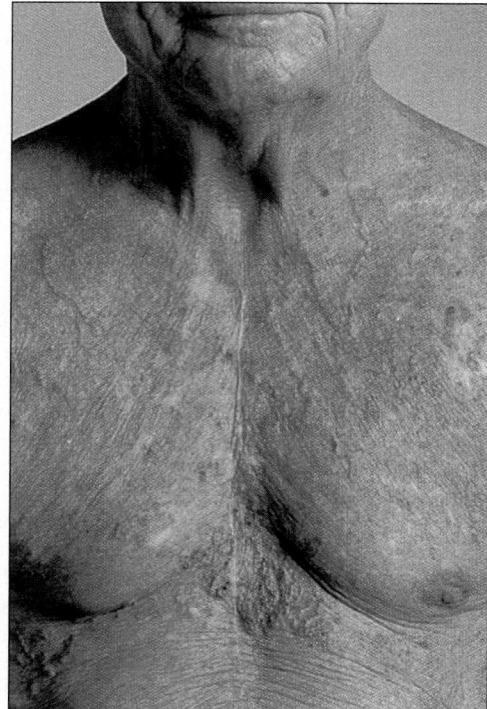

Figure 54-3. A patient with characteristic venous dilation and facial edema.

dyspnea, cough, chest pain, and occasionally dysphagia (Table 54-2).[2,4,13,20,25,54] Less frequently arm edema, stridor, upper body cyanosis, and neurologic symptoms (e.g., headaches or lethargy) may occur. All symptoms may be aggravated by positional changes, particularly those associated with lowering of the head. To some extent, the frequency of respiratory distress seems to be related to the underlying etiology, being less common with lymphomas.[28] The prospect of catastrophic neurologic events has led to the characterization of SVCO as an "oncologic emergency."[3,9,54] However, experimental studies in dogs as well as several recent reviews have conclusively demonstrated that life-threatening neurologic symptoms such as seizures, syncope, or coma rarely occur.[6,10,13,14,16]

The physical findings accompanying SVCO are diagnostic (Fig. 54-3). The overwhelming majority of patients exhibit dilated neck and/or chest-wall veins and facial edema, occasionally with cyanosis or plethora.[4,6,11,17-20,29] Arm edema occurs in 15% to 20% of patients. Only rarely is a patient seen without overt venous dilatation.[2] Although the duration of symptoms may range from a few days to several weeks, a majority of patients have symptoms of 4 weeks' duration or less.[4] Individuals with a longer duration of symptoms are more likely to have a benign cause of SVCO.[13,47] Another clinical feature suggesting a nonmalignant etiology of SVCO is the age of the patient, with those younger than 50 years being more likely to have a benign cause.[47]

TABLE 54-2

![] **Signs and Symptoms of Superior Vena Cava Obstruction**								
	PARISH	**YELLIN**	**LOCHRIDGE**	**MADDOX**	**BELL**	**ARMSTRONG**	**SCARANTINO**	**LITTLE**
Total patients	86	63	66	56	159	125	60	42
Suffusion	69	54	55	49	62	56	55	35
Dyspnea	54	19	55	—	112	69	47	22
Cough	47	13	46	—	11	29	11	26
Pain	17	4	—	—	20	19	—	—
Dysphagia	10	4	1	—	—	16	6	3
Syncope	6	—	2	—	6	—	—	—
Arm edema	3	20	—	19	13	49	—	—
Stridor	1	—	22	—	1	—	—	—
Neurologic	2	—	23	—	0	0	—	—
Hemoptysis	—	5	—	—	—	—	—	5

RADIOGRAPHIC FINDINGS AND DIAGNOSTIC STUDIES

Imaging Studies

A standard chest radiograph is the first radiographic procedure performed when SVCO is suspected, with the most common abnormality being mediastinal widening. Typically, a mass is found in the superior mediastinum, right hilum or perihilar region, or right upper lobe.[2,3] Less often the chest radiograph may reveal a pleural effusion, right upper lobe collapse, or rib notching. However, a normal chest radiograph is not inconsistent with the diagnosis of SVCO.[2]

A contrast-enhanced chest computed tomography (CT) scan provides visualization of extravascular and intravascular tumor, as well as thrombus formation within the SVC, and also demonstrates collateral flow.[55-61] A CT diagnosis depends on diminished or absent contrast opacification of central venous structures such as the innominate vein or the SVC inferior to the obstruction, and opacification of collateral venous routes,[59] especially anterior subcutaneous collaterals (Fig. 54-4).[60] Because dilution of the contrast medium by unopacified blood or the displacement of blood by laminar flow may simulate an intraluminal filling defect, both criteria must be present for the diagnosis of SVCO to be made.[59] The anatomy defined by CT scan may help to guide a fine-needle aspiration biopsy or another diagnostic procedure if a histologic diagnosis has not been previously established. The current-generation helical CT scans also have been used to diagnose SVCO with results that correlate well with regular contrast CTs.[62] Three-dimensional recon-

structions of the images may well replace venography in most cases. Helical scans can potentially reveal more information regarding the site and extent of disease and the collateral pathways involved, as well as define soft tissue abnormalities.

Contrast venacavograms may still play an occasional role in determining management strategy, particularly when surgical bypass is being considered.[63] In the past, contrast venacavography entailed the administration of large amounts of contrast material into peripheral veins, which sometimes resulted in complications such as phlebitis, thrombosis, and prolonged bleeding. The use of low-osmolarity contrast has eliminated most of these complications. Current techniques entail positioning a small catheter in the desired vascular location under fluoroscopic guidance with injection of only small amounts of contrast dye necessary to define the pattern of venous flow and degree of SVCO.[63] Collateral circulation is usually identified readily, and complications are uncommon. Cavography also is possible by using nuclear medicine techniques.[43,64-66] The more common collateral routes well seen in contrast cavography can be distinguished with radionuclide studies as well. Less common collateral pathways such as cerebral sinus route, venous shunts between systemic veins and the left heart, and shunting in the liver also have been demonstrated.[66]

In the majority of cases of SVCO, the CT scan will be the most useful radiographic study, although occasionally other studies provide helpful data.[55,56] For example, transesophageal echocardiography can be used to distinguish thrombus formation from extrinsic compression of the SVC.[67] Single-photon emission computed tomography (SPECT) has been used to identify obstruction of the SVC by an intravascular metastasis from an adenocarcinoma.[68]

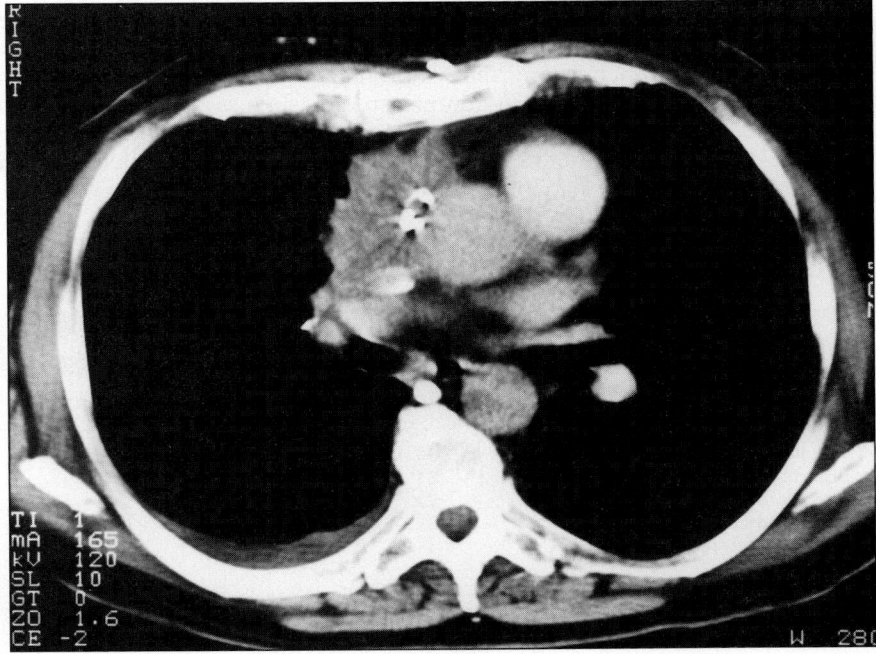

Figure 54-4. Chest computed tomography scan of a patient with superior vena cava obstruction. Note chest-wall vein contrast dye in anterior chest wall. Superior vena cava is severely compressed by metastatic malignancy.

Invasive Diagnostic Studies

Except in rare circumstances, a histologic diagnosis should be obtained before treating a patient with SVCO for two reasons.[6,10,13,14] First, a definitive diagnosis is necessary to plan therapy, and second, radiation therapy before establishing a diagnosis can make histologic diagnosis difficult or even impossible.[14,69,70] Until recently, a brief course of irradiation was often administered before obtaining a histologic diagnosis, largely because malignancy was known to be the most common cause and because it was generally assumed a short course of irradiation was relatively benign. Both of these suppositions have been criticized.[6,13]

Procedures commonly used to establish a tissue diagnosis include sputum cytology, bronchoscopy, lymph node biopsy, thoracotomy, and mediastinoscopy, although the diagnosis is sometimes obtained through other means such as thoracentesis and percutaneous lung biopsy with or without ultrasound guidance.[6,19,71-73] The complication rate of invasive procedures in the face of SVCO is fairly modest. Schraufnagel and associates[13] reviewed the outcome of 93 invasive procedures in 62 patients with diagnostic problems. None of the procedures was associated with a fatal outcome. Prolonged bleeding was observed in a few patients after venipuncture, but it was easily controlled with local pressure. "Excessive" bleeding was only observed in two cases: once during bronchoscopy and once during a mediastinoscopic procedure. Both procedures were abandoned without serious sequelae. In one case, the diagnosis was later established by thoracotomy. In a single patient with a mediastinal seminoma, respiratory distress followed a surgical biopsy. However, rapid reversal of the symptoms was possible with administration of oxygen, steroids, epinephrine, and furosemide. Yellin and colleagues[20] performed 27 invasive diagnostic procedures in 63 patients with SVCO. No mortality or major bleeding episodes were observed, and diagnostic material was obtained in 89% of patients. Ahmann[6] reported that complications of bronchoscopy and lymph node biopsies are virtually nonexistent and that contrast studies, such as nuclear medicine venography, are remarkably safe in the presence of SVCO. Of the various invasive procedures used to obtain tissue in patients with SVCO, mediastino-scopy appears to be the most risky. However, even this procedure has a relatively low complication rate. Mineo and colleagues[74] reviewed the outcome of 80 patients who underwent diagnostic mediastinoscopy for SVCO by a single surgeon over a 23-year period. Five patients had significant bleeding, but only one required an urgent sternotomy, and no perioperative mortality was recorded. A definitive diagnosis was made in all of the patients; therefore mediastinoscopy should be considered if less-invasive procedures are unsuccessful at determining a diagnosis (Table 54-3).[19,72,76]

The diagnostic yield from various noninvasive and invasive procedures ranges from approximately 20% for cytologic studies to virtually 100% with thoracotomy and mediastinoscopy (see Table 54-3).[73,74] Although these findings may reflect publication bias, the existing data argue against the need for immediate irradiation without a histologic diagnosis in most cases. Irradiation should be undertaken without tissue confirmation of the underlying etiology only in those cases with rapid progression of symptoms associated with severe respiratory distress. Conversely, prudence dictates that prolonged attempts to establish a histologic diagnosis should be discouraged in the presence of severe dyspnea due to tracheal compression or rapidly progressive neurologic symptoms. Furthermore, in circumstances in which SVCO occurs in an individual with an established diagnosis of cancer or other known cause, an attempt to reestablish the histology of the underlying cause clearly is not a productive exercise.[13]

DIAGNOSTIC APPROACH

In the absence of a known cause of SVCO, every effort should be made to obtain a histologic diagnosis before initiation of therapy. The least invasive diagnostic technique should be performed initially, followed by more invasive procedures as necessary. Induced sputum for cytologic examination may be all that is required. Cytologic examination of pleural fluid also may provide adequate information. If the patient has a palpable lymph node, a biopsy should be performed, or it should be subjected to fine-needle aspiration for cytologic material. However, fine-needle aspiration biopsies may fail to

TABLE 54-3

Diagnostic Procedures, Yield, and Complication Rate in Superior Vena Cava Obstruction

PROCEDURE	NO. PERFORMED	NO. DIAGNOSTIC	COMPLICATIONS
Sputum cytology	30	8	0
Bronchoscopy	84	39	1
Thoracotomy	22	21	0
Mediastinoscopy	132	124	13
Lymph node biopsy	44	30	0
Bone marrow	13	3	0

Data compiled from references 13, 20, 29, 55, 62, 74, and 75.

provide adequate material for distinction between sub-types of lymphoma. In the absence of nodal enlargement or pleural fluid, a bronchoscopic examination may be needed. If this procedure fails to provide a diagnosis, fine-needle aspiration of the intrathoracic mass by using CT guidance may yield adequate diagnostic material. Finally, if all other efforts fail, a more invasive procedure such as mediastinoscopy or thoracotomy may be required. Special pathological studies may be needed to establish a diagnosis when routine histologic assessment is unclear or available tissue is scant. Selected immunoperoxidase stains (e.g., common leukocyte antigen and epithelial membrane antigen) can be helpful in distinguishing a carcinoma from a lymphoma. Likewise, surface immuno-globulin determination can distinguish a lymphoma from a carcinoma. On rare occasions, electron microscopy may be needed to make a distinction between these two entities. Other laboratory studies such as serum tumor maker (e.g., β-human chorionic gonadotropin [HCG] and α-fetoprotein) determination may be useful in selected cases. For example, the presence of an elevated β-HCG and/or an abnormal α-fetoprotein in a young male patient with SVCO is virtually diagnostic of an underlying germ cell malignancy. In the latter situation, no further workup is needed before initiation of chemotherapy.

In rare circumstances, a definitive tissue diagnosis cannot be made in a timely manner. In such cases, it is appropriate to proceed with radiotherapy or placement of an endovascular stent because either therapy is effective for most underlying causes of SVCO. Subsequent treatment decisions may be made based on the clinical setting in which SVCO developed. For example, in an older adult smoker, lung cancer is the probable etiology, and further radiotherapy may be appropriate. Conversely, in a younger adult who does not smoke tobacco, lymph-oma is a more likely cause. In such cases, initiation of chemotherapy appropriate for non-Hodgkin's lymphoma can be justified after completion of initial radiotherapy.

TREATMENT

Radiotherapy

Radiotherapy is the most commonly used treatment modality for SVCO after a malignant etiology has been established. Three factors must be considered before radiation delivery: (1) dose fractionation (fraction size and timing), (2) total dose to be delivered, and (3) volume to be irradiated, or "field size."[9]

Dose Fractionation

Considerable controversy is found in the radiation oncology literature over the past 40 years regarding fractionation in patients with SVCO. Prior to 1960, treatment of SVCO generally consisted of low-dose (i.e., 50 to 100 cGy) fractions to avoid inducing "radiation edema," which was assumed to cause further compromise of SVC patency and worsen associated symptoms.[77] Experimental models using laboratory mice suggested this might be a concern. In reality, however, the fear of producing further SVC compromise by radiation-induced edema was largely unfounded, and symptoms previously ascribed to radiation edema were predominantly due to inadequately treated tumor, causing progressive obstruction.[22]

Rubin and associates[22] undertook a retrospective comparison of a high-fraction regimen (400 cGy/day) with historical controls treated with lower-fraction schedules (200 cGy/day). They noted more prompt relief of facial swelling after an initial high-dose-per-fraction schedule. The apparent superiority of high-dose-per-fraction regimens in providing faster symptom relief has been corroborated in several other retrospective nonrandomized studies.[1,4,13,14,16,18,21,78] In contrast, Perez and colleagues[3] found the high-dose-per-fraction regimen only slightly better than conventional fractions. It is our belief that for the management of potentially curable patients, 400-cGy fractions for the first 2 to 3 days is reasonable for those experiencing rapidly progressive and distressing SVCO. Thereafter, the daily fraction size can be safely reduced, and the total dose adjusted to compensate for

---

AN APPROACH TO PATIENTS WITH SUPERIOR VENA CAVA OBSTRUCTION

Diagnosis is established by physical examination and clinical presentation (see text).

Respiratory status should be assessed promptly. Only patients in extremis should be treated urgently with radiation without a histologic diagnosis. Emergency radiation therapy is necessary in fewer than 5% of all SVCO cases. Stent insertion can also be considered as first-line therapy for patients with malignant cases of SVCO.

Diagnostic evaluation should proceed with least invasive procedures performed initially followed by more invasive procedures as needed to obtain histologic diagnosis:

Chest radiograph
Sputum cytology
Thoracentesis with cytologic evaluation of fluid
Node biopsy if palpable node is present, avoid fine-needle aspiration if lymphoma suspected
Fiberoptic bronchoscopy
Mediastinoscopy
Thoracostomy

Evaluation may vary depending on the age and sex of the patient.

In older adults (i.e., ≥50), the most common cause of SVCO is lung cancer; lymphoma or metastatic cancer are less common and benign processes are uncommon.

In young adults (<50 years old), the most common cause of SVCO is lymphoma (usually large cell lymphoma or lymphoblastic lymphoma; rarely Hodgkin's disease); lung cancer or rare thoracic malignancy are less common, and germ cell cancer (almost never in females) and benign causes all uncommon. The above evaluation should be modified to include the following studies prior to more invasive procedures:

Serum tumor markers (i.e., β-HCG, α-fetoprotein, lactate dehydrogenase)
Bone marrow aspiration and biopsy

Problems Common to Cancer and Its Therapy

the number of initial high-dose fractions. Patients with subacute SVCO treated with curative intent should be managed with conventional (e.g., 200 to 300 cGy) fractions throughout their treatment course. Effects on surrounding normal tissues treated to tolerance doses are more predictable with standard fractions. Appropriate oblique fields with spinal cord shielding can later be used to boost the target volume.

In patients with extrathoracic disease who are treated with palliative intent, total radiotherapy doses will likely be lower, and the use of higher fraction sizes (e.g., ≥300 cGy) for the entire course of radiation is appropriate. With two hypofractionated regimens with 8-Gy fractions, Rodrigues and colleagues[79] concluded that 24 Gy given over a 3-week period produced better relief of symptoms, more durable responses, and better median survival than did 16 Gy given in 1 week. Consideration of spinal cord tolerance is still essential in all patients, however, to avoid injury to the small percentage who may have prolonged tumor responses and survivals.

Concern has been voiced regarding the tolerability of systemic therapy or radiation in patients who are elderly or who have a compromised performance status. Lonardi and associates[80] demonstrated that elderly patients with SVCO from solid tumors have been successfully palliated with short-course, large-fraction radiation. Twenty-three patients with a median age of 75 years and a median electrocorticography performance status of 2 were treated with a total dose of 12 Gy, given in two 6-Gy fractions 1 week apart. The overall clinical response rate was 87%, with minimal reported toxicity.

Total Dose

In the individual with SVCO, the planned total radiation therapy dose should take into account the specific type and extent of underlying malignancy and normal tissue tolerance. Other considerations include prognosis and performance status, the speed at which SVCO symptoms developed, and whether chemotherapy is to be included in the treatment program. The radiation oncologist must also decide if the goal of treatment is curative or palliative and treat accordingly. If radiation alone is to be used for the curative treatment of lymphoma in adults, 3600 to 4400 cGy is commonly recommended.[81,82] More commonly, however, combined-modality treatment is given, and total radiation dose can then be reduced.[83,84] In SCLC, typically 4500 cGy with concomitant chemotherapy is given,[85,86] and for non-SCLC, 6000 cGy or more is usually used sequentially or simultaneous with chemotherapy.[87-90]

Field Size

Radiation field size is determined by the extent of disease, baseline pulmonary reserve as determined by pulmonary function tests and split perfusion-ventilation scans, and the type of chemotherapy, if any, the patient will receive. Toxicity of treatment, in particular radiation pneumonitis (RP), pericarditis, and fibrosis, can carry significant morbidity and mortality if severe. Mortality from severe RP approaches 50% in some reports.[91] Others have shown that the degree of pneumonitis correlates strongly with overall survival after definitive treatment of lung cancer.[92]

Therefore efforts to minimize radiation field size carry considerable importance in the treatment of SVCO. Risk of pneumonitis is a function of many patient- and treatment-related factors: pretreatment performance status, gender (women more likely than men), forced expiratory volume in 1 second (FEV_1), low PaO_2 (<80 torr), mean lung dose (MLD), and volume of lung irradiated to 20 Gy (V_{20}).[92-94] To reduce the risk of pulmonary and cardiac toxicity, some groups have used induction chemotherapy followed by thoracic irradiation with a reduced treatment volume. With bronchogenic carcinoma, retrospective and prospective studies have shown that the postchemotherapy tumor volume can be treated without significantly compromising local control or survival.[95,96] In addition, CT scan–based treatment planning, particularly with intensity-modulated radiation therapy (IMRT), provides better assurance of the target volume and allows a reduction in the lung volumes irradiated.[97-100] Volumes should be constricted if high total doses are used (>4000 cGy) or if methotrexate, mitomycin C, doxorubicin, or bleomycin is used concomitantly.

Whenever possible, treatment recommendations should be determined by a multidisciplinary team to include the radiation oncologist, medical oncologist, and a surgeon or pulmonologist when appropriate. Patients with lymphoma or SCLC will need chemotherapy for control of systemic as well as local disease. The sequencing of treatment modalities will vary from one patient to the next and, as discussed earlier, may affect the overall dose and fractionation plan. Fraction size and total dose to the spinal cord should be carefully considered in patients with lymphoma who may subsequently undergo a bone marrow transplant requiring total body irradiation.

Response to Radiotherapy

Clinical response of SVCO signs and symptoms to various radiotherapeutic dose-fractionation schedules is high (Table 54-4).[1,11,18,20,29] Radiographic and postmortem pathologic studies, however, indicate that reestablishment of vena cava patency is rare, and therefore collateral flow rather than therapeutic intervention may be responsible for symptomatic improvement. Ahmann[6] reported the response to radiation therapy for SVCO based on a literature review of more than 90 publications since 1934. Overall, approximately 50% to 70% of treated patients achieve symptomatic improvement within 2 weeks of initiation of therapy. In circumstances in which serial venograms were obtained, normal venous flow through the SVC was rarely observed after completion of radiation therapy.[18,23,101] In some instances, complete obstruction remained despite clinical improvement in the patient's signs and symptoms.[18,23,101] Experimental studies conducted by Carlson[16] in dogs are consistent, showing that acute occlusion of the SVC above the azygous vein was never fatal. Improvement in symptoms usually occurred within 7 days and was accompanied by a rapid development of collateral flow. Furthermore, ligation of the azygous vein after SVCO resulted in a recrudescence of symptoms followed by recovery without sequelae.[16]

TABLE 54-4

Clinical Response of Superior Vena Cava Obstruction to Radiation Therapy			
AUTHOR	**NO. OF PATIENTS**	**RESPONSE RATE**	**RECOMMENDATION**
Yellin[20]	23	78%	SVCO not emergency; obtain biopsy before RT
Armstrong[11]	125	78%–83%	Use initial 4-Gy fractions
Maddox[29]	14	64%	Chemotherapy and RT are equally effective
Scarantino[18]	60	86%	Use initial high-dose RT fractions
Davenport[1]	35	91%	Use initial 4-Gy fractions
Howard[23]	253	86%	Use 30-Gy total dose

RT, radiation therapy; SVCO, superior vena cava obstruction.

SVC patency after radiation also has been assessed in autopsy studies.[6,12] After radiotherapy, the SVC usually is not sufficiently patent to allow adequate blood flow through the vessel. Ahmann's literature review[6] found that among 99 postmortem examinations of which most patients had achieved symptomatic relief after radiation therapy, only 14 patients had complete or partial SVC patency. Although autopsy studies may be less reliable than venography obtained in living patients, these results are entirely consistent with reported radiographic data. Although radiotherapy is associated with improvement or relief of clinical signs and symptoms in most patients, the majority of patients do not actually achieve any measurable increase in vena cava blood flow. The development of collateral blood flow probably contributes to the clinical improvement in some patients and is the sole reason for improvement in others. Thus the literature does not support the traditional dogma that emergency irradiation is needed in all patients with SVCO.

Chemotherapy

Small Cell and Non–Small Cell Lung Cancer

SVCO has been reported to occur in 7% to 12% of SCLC patients at diagnosis.[24,29,102-105] With rare exception,[29] the literature indicates that the presence of SVCO has little impact on the prognosis of SCLC patients, provided that therapy is appropriately instituted.[24,104-106] Even in the presence of SVCO, chemotherapy (with or without thoracic radiotherapy) is the preferred initial treatment of SCLC.[107] The choice of treatment is dictated by the patient's stage and performance status. Those with limited-stage disease, good performance status, and no contraindication to cisplatin are best treated with cisplatin plus etoposide and concurrent chest irradiation.[85] In extensive-stage disease, it is reasonable to proceed with chemotherapy alone—either cisplatin-based therapy or a cyclophosphamide-based regimen in those in whom excessive hydration is to be avoided.[24,102,104-106] Alternatively, carboplatin can be substituted for cisplatin if there is a need to avoid aggressive hydration.[108] A majority of patients will experience partial or complete resolution of signs and symptoms within 7 days of initiation of treatment, and in most series, complete resolution of symptoms has occurred within 2 weeks. Although the rapidity of symptom resolution suggests that a direct treatment effect on tumor regression is the principal cause of symptom improvement, the development of collateral drainage undoubtedly plays an equally significant role, as noted earlier. Thoracic radiotherapy does not caused transient worsening of symptoms. Although SVCO reoccurs in approximately 25% of patients, reinstitution of therapy with salvage chemotherapy alone, radiotherapy alone, or a combination of these modalities has effected prompt resolution of symptoms in most cases.[24] Unfortunately, sequential thoracic radiotherapy on completion of chemotherapy has not proved advantageous with regard to reducing the incidence of SVCO relapse.[109]

Chemotherapy alone also has been used for the treatment of SVCO in non-SCLC with positive results.[110] However, this approach is less effective with non–small cell tumors, and thus radiotherapy or combined modality therapy remains the preferred initial treatment.[89] Unlike SCLC, the presence of SVCO in non-SCLC seems to have a negative impact on the prognosis of patients with locally advanced disease.[111]

Non-Hodgkin's Lymphoma

Chemotherapy alone also can effectively palliate the symptoms of SVCO in non-Hodgkin's lymphoma,[28] although symptoms can be well controlled with radiotherapy. However, because lymphoma is usually a systemic process and death is rarely due to localized disease, radiotherapy should never be used in isolation except when dealing with recurrent disease. Local recurrences tend to occur primarily in patients with large mediastinal masses and large cell histologic types.[28] Therefore local consolidation with radiotherapy after a few cycles of chemotherapy can be justified in patients with large cell lymphoma and mediastinal masses larger than 10 cm.[28] Conversely, in lymphoblastic lymphoma, recurrences are uniformly systemic, obviating the need for radiotherapy in this histologic type of non-Hodgkin's lymphoma.[28] As in SCLC, the optimal chemotherapy regimen for treatment for lymphoma-associated SVCO has not been determined and is dictated to a much greater degree by the underlying histologic type, further underscoring the need to establish a tissue diagnosis before institution of therapy. Lymphoblastic lymphoma is more aggressive than large cell lymphomas and generally requires more aggressive chemotherapy.[112-114]

Surgery

Surgery generally plays a limited role in the management of the patient with SVCO, although reconstruction of the obstructed SVC may be indicated in highly selected patients.[63,115-118] Surgical intervention is reserved most often for patients with SVCO due to a benign cause such as granulomatous disease, aortic aneurysm, or retrosternal goiter.[119] When symptomatic malignant obstruction is refractory to radiotherapy, chemotherapy, or both, and when anticipated survival approaches 6 months, operation may be considered. Surgical intervention also may prove beneficial in the setting of recurrent SVCO after chemotherapy and radiation, and when caval thrombosis is the primary problem and fails to improve symptomatically with anticoagulants or thrombolytic therapy.[101,120-122]

Surgical bypass of the obstructed SVC may be accomplished with synthetic grafts (Dacron or Goretex), autologous pericardium, or autogenous vein graft, with preference for the later because of a better potential for long-term patency.[115-118,123,124] The spiral vein graft, initially described by Doty and associates,[116,125] is constructed by using saphenous vein, which is slit longitudinally and wrapped around a stent (usually a chest tube) of the desired diameter. The edges of the vein are joined by using continuous suture, resulting in a large-bore conduit. The bypass is constructed between the brachiocephalic or left internal jugular vein and the right atrial appendage. Long-term relief of symptoms may be achieved.[124-126] When SVCO is the result of a primary tumor of the SVC or right atrium, resection (with cardiopulmonary bypass) and reconstruction is recommended. These tumors may be relatively slow growing sarcomas (angiosarcomas or leiomyosarcomas), and long-term palliation is sometimes possible.[32-34]

Stents

Percutaneously placed, self-expanding intravascular wire stents can offer an attractive adjunct to other procedures in the palliative treatment of patients with SVCO in the presence or absence of an underlying malignant disease.[127] These devices have been placed before radiotherapy, during the course of radiotherapy or chemotherapy, and after maximum-tolerance radiation therapy.[128-146] This percutaneous treatment option offers the ability to increase the lumen diameter of the SVC and does not usually require general anesthesia. Complete symptom relief is often obtained within 24 to 48 hours in 75% to 95% of patients, depending on the underlying cause of SVCO and type of stent deployed (Table 54-5). Dyspnea appears to be the least likely symptom to improve, whereas facial and upper-body edema improve within 48 hours in virtually all patients.[137] Possible complications include acute thrombosis, retroperitoneal hemorrhage, and death due to cardiac arrhythmias, and reocclusion may occur (especially in the absence of anticoagulant therapy).[132,138,139] Because all currently available expandable stents have a metallic composition, their presence may preclude or limit serial follow-up with magnetic resonance imaging. This point should be taken into account before this course of treatment is chosen.

Venous access is accomplished through a femoral, jugular, or subclavian vein. It is necessary to traverse the obstruction with a guidewire to allow deployment of the stent, and in many cases, a preplacement venous angioplasty is indicated. The presence of acute thrombosis superimposed on the chronic SVCO may indicate the need for preprocedure thrombolytic therapy. Although thrombolytic therapy is associated with a known risk of hemorrhage, it may minimize the risk of thromboembolization and permit greater accuracy of stent placement.[127,144] Careful consideration should be given to a preprocedure cerebral CT scan to help rule out the presence of cerebral metastases before the use of thrombolytic therapy.[144]

Whereas a variety of metallic stents is currently available, most reports address one or more of three general device designs, the Gianturco-Rösch (sometimes referred to as the "Z-stent"; Cook, Bloomington, IN), Wallstent (Schneider, Plymouth, MN), and Palmaz stent (Johnson & Johnson Interventional Systems, Warren, NJ) (Figs. 54-5 and 54-6). No rigorous comparisons of outcomes have been made among the various stent designs. Each has particular qualities with respect to flexibility and radial strength, which may make one or another particularly well suited under certain clinical circumstances. Although the Wallstent and Z-stent are "self-expanding" devices, balloon dilatation may be required after stent deployment to provide a clinically adequate effect.[147]

TABLE 54-5

Evaluation of Intravascular Stents

AUTHOR	NO. OF PATIENTS	PRIMARY PATENCY RATE (%)	CLINICAL SUCCESS (%)	OVERALL COMPLICATION RATE (%)
Kee[127]	51	95	78	10
Smayra[140]	30	74	100	7
Chatziioannou[146]	18	100	89	0
Lanciego[141]	52	92	100	25
Gregorio[145]	82	93	95	0
Miller[142]	23	100	83	13
Thony[143]	26	83	90	4
Nicholson[144]	76	100	90	9

Figure 54-5. A, Gianturco-Rösch Z-stents–15-mm and 60-mm lengths. **B,** Palmaz stent, closed and expanded. **C,** Schneider Wallstent.

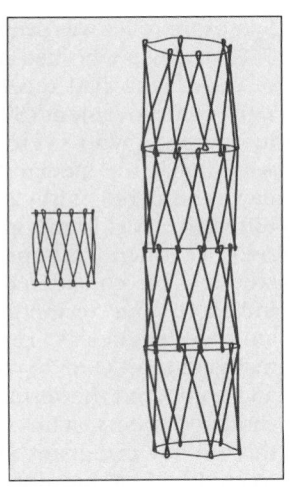
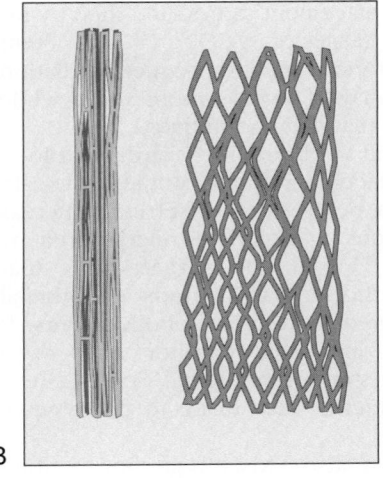
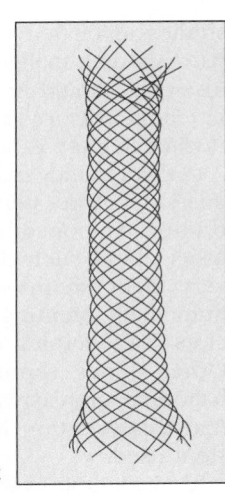

Technical and clinical success and long-term venous patency have been demonstrated by a number of trials summarized in Table 54-5.[127,140-146] The overall complication rate is relatively low, although considerable variation is found in the reporting of complications, as some studies include reocclusion as a complication.[146] The majority of the more serious complications involve graft migration. Many patients require more than one stent either to maintain SVC confluence with adjacent vessels or because the vascular lesion is too extensive to be covered by a single stent. Close follow-up is required to monitor venous patency, and stent occlusion can generally be alleviated by a second procedure. Many studies report that stented patients experience a rapid and almost complete resolution of the symptoms associated with SVCO.[137,138,140-143,145,148] For this reason, several recent

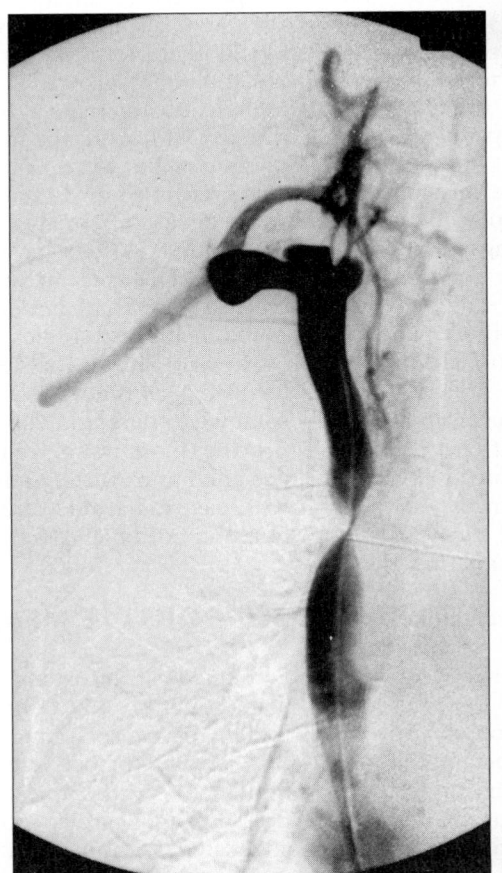
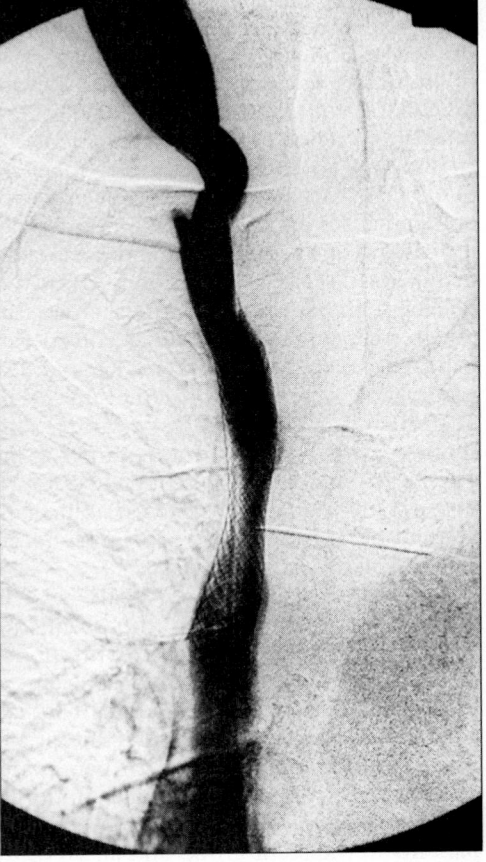

Figure 54-6. A, A 60-year-old man after radiotherapy for lung cancer with recurrent superior vena cava obstruction. **B,** Placement of a Wallstent resulted in immediate relief of symptoms. Radiograph at 6-month follow-up.

studies advocated stent placement as first-line therapy for patients with malignant causes of SVCO.[137,141-143,146] Stent insertion should not interfere with subsequent radiation or chemotherapy and may allow symptom relief while further therapy is being planned and initiated.

A discrepancy exists in the literature regarding balloon dilation before stent placement. Some studies advocate routine balloon dilation before stent insertion, whereas others limit such dilations to situations necessitated by very tight stenoses.[137,140,141,145] The suggestion is that immediate stenting without dilation traps endothelial clots, thus helping to prevent distant embolic events.[140] Other series reported improved patency rates with balloon angioplasty after stent placement.[143] Some believe that this variation in practice may relate to the type of stent used.

Considerable variation also exists regarding routine anticoagulation after stent placement. Chatziioannou and colleagues[146] recommend oral anticoagulation therapy with coumarin "for life." Kee and associates[127] recommend continuous oral anticoagulation for all of their patients with an underlying malignancy. In both the studies of Lanciego and co-workers[141] and Chacon Lopez-Muniz and associates,[137] patients were initially given anticoagulation with heparin and warfarin; however, over time, their standard of practice changed to recommend antiplatelet agents alone, with seemingly no adverse effects. Thony and colleagues[143] treated a few selected patients with heparin for up to 3 days after the procedure and otherwise recommend aspirin therapy for 3 months after stent placement. This shift in practice may reflect parallel studies of anticoagulation for coronary artery stents. As no standard recommendations exist now, the risks and benefits of full anticoagulation versus antiplatelet agents must be weighed for individual patients.[149]

Although a definite role exists for stents in malignant SVCO, the results of endothelial stent placement for benign causes are more mixed, and few long-term follow-up data are available.[147] Life expectancy for patients with malignant disease is often limited, but the same may not be true with benign SVCO, and therefore in these patients, long-term patency is a critical consideration. The underlying cause of the initial SVCO and the likelihood of recurrence may be more relevant in these situations. Technical success and symptom relief have been reported, primarily for venous catheter–induced SVCO.[145] The gold standard for benign SVCO remains surgical bypass, although, given the variability and rarity of this condition; no studies have been done comparing these two modalities.

Although no randomized trials have been done, two studies directly compared the results of endovascular stenting with radiation with or without chemotherapy for malignant SVCO. Tanigawa and colleagues[148] reported the results of 33 patients treated with radiation therapy or stents. These patients were selected for a specific therapy and not randomized. Of the 23 patients who underwent a stenting procedure, 11 had undergone ineffective radiation therapy for their obstructions. The majority of patients in the stent group and all 10 of the patients who received radiation therapy had a primary lung cancer.

Symptom relief was seen in 78% of the stent group overall; 75% of those who had not had previous therapy and 82% of those who had received prior radiation. Although the rate of improvement (80%) in clinical signs and symptoms in patients who were treated with radiation therapy was similar, the median time to respond was longer at 5.5 days compared with 24 to 48 hours after stenting. No difference was found in the overall survival between the two treatment groups. These authors suggested that stenting be considered first-line therapy and certainly indicated after an ineffective trial of radiation. Nicholson and colleagues[144] reported their experience with malignant SVCO of 76 patients treated with stent insertion and compared the results retrospectively with those of 25 similar patients who had been treated with radiation therapy for malignant SVCO. Of the 76 patients, 26 were treated with stents alone, and the remainder were treated with chemotherapy or radiation before or after stent placement. The report of Nicholson and coworkers confirms the more rapid resolution of clinical symptoms in the stent group versus the radiation-alone group; however, it should be noted that the radiation group was examined retrospectively. The mean asymptomatic time was significantly longer in the stent group at 21.8 weeks compared with 11.7 weeks in the radiation-only group. Although 83% of patients treated with a stenting procedure continued to have minor symptoms of swelling or venous distention, major symptoms were relieved in all 76 patients. In addition, more than 90% of patients in the stent group died without a recurrence of their SVCO symptoms compared with only 12% in the radiation-only group. The figures for the stent group include the patients who were treated with additional therapy, although the trends are the same for the 26 patients who were only stented. Poststent venography was preformed on 19 patients. Interestingly, although they were all asymptomatic, seven of these patients had a reoccluded SVC, suggesting that collateral vessels play a significant role in symptom relief. This finding is consistent with the reocclusion after radiation therapy noted in autopsy studies.[6,13]

No randomized trials are likely to compare treatments for SVCO, as the goals of each therapeutic modality are somewhat different. Although endovascular stents may provide more rapid relief of symptoms, they are not designed to treat the underlying cause of the obstruction, whereas radiation, chemotherapy, and surgery may function both palliatively and therapeutically.

SUPPORTIVE MEASURES

Few medical measures are of proven benefit in the management of SVCO, other than therapy directed at the underlying cause. General recommendations include bed rest, head-of-the-bed elevation, and oxygen administration.[9,20] These therapies are designed to reduce venous pressure and cardiac output. Diuretics also have been advocated without clear evidence of efficacy, although they are thought to lessen edema.[9] Steroids also are sometimes administered without good documentation as to their efficacy. These agents have been advocated for their putative benefit in lessening the likelihood of radiation-induced edema. However, in experimental systems, little inflammation or edema has been observed with irradiation.[77] Anticoagulation and thrombolytic therapy may be of benefit when the underlying cause is an indwelling catheter, but otherwise they have not been shown to alter the course of recovery.[30,40,41,115] Furthermore, because anticoagulation may impair diagnostic efforts, it should be avoided until a clear indication for its use is identified.

Survival in the face of SVCO is dependent on the underlying cause and proper treatment.[4,11,28,150] Overall, median survival is around 6 months and is clearly related to the underlying cause. One-year survival may range from as little as less than 1% in non-SCLC to more than 40% in patients with non-Hodgkin's lymphoma.[4,11]

SUMMARY

SVCO is usually not a true oncologic emergency, except in rare situations in which a patient experiences respiratory compromise secondary to tracheal obstruction. Administration of irradiation before histologic confirmation of the underlying cause can lead to inappropriate therapy and should be discouraged. Excessive concern about the risk of invasive procedures in the face of SVCO is likewise without foundation. Numerous reports have demonstrated the relative safety of bronchoscopy, thoracentesis, lymph node biopsy, and similar invasive procedures. In the past 5 years, numerous studies have demonstrated the palliative benefit of endovascular stent placement, particularly for malignant causes of SVCO. Stent placement does not preclude the use of additional therapy such as chemotherapy or radiation. In experienced hands, the procedure has a low rate of complications and often provides rapid and lasting relief of symptoms. Depending on availability, endovascular stenting should be considered early in the treatment of SVCO and certainly when a different primary therapy has failed. In many institutions, radiotherapy remains the treatment of choice, with exceptions made for those causes known to be relatively sensitive to chemotherapy (e.g., SCLC or non-Hodgkin's lymphoma).

REFERENCES

1. Davenport D, et al: Radiation therapy in the treatment of superior vena caval obstruction. Cancer 1978;42:2600-2603.
2. Parish JM, et al: Etiologic considerations in superior vena cava syndrome. Mayo Clin Proc 1981;56:407-413.
3. Perez CA, Presant CA, van Amburg AL: Management of superior vena cava syndrome. Semin Oncol 1978;5:23-134.
4. Bell DR, Woods RL, Levi JA: Superior vena caval obstruction: A 10 year experience. Med J Aust 1986;145:566-568.
5. Hunter W: History of aneurysm of the aorta with some remarks on aneurysms in general. Med Obs Inq 1957;1:323-357.
6. Ahmann FR: A reassessment of the clinical implications of the superior vena caval syndrome. J Clin Oncol 1984;8:961-969.
7. McIntire FT, Sykes EM: Obstruction of the superior vena cava. A review of the literature and report on two personal cases. Ann Intern Med 1949;30:925-960.
8. Parker SL, et al: Cancer statistics, 1997. Cancer J Clin 1997;4-7: 5-27.
9. Lokich JJ, Goodman R: Superior vena cava syndrome. Clinical management. JAMA 1975;231:58-61.
10. Escalante CP: Causes and management of superior vena cava syndrome. Oncology 1993;7:61-68; discussion 71-72, 75-77.
11. Armstrong BA, et al: Role of irradiation in the management of superior vena cava syndrome. Int J Radiat Oncol Biol Phys 1987;1-3:531-539.
12. Salsali M, Cliffton EE: Superior vena caval obstruction with lung cancer. Ann Thorac Surg 1968;6:437-442.
13. Schraufnagel DE, et al: Superior vena caval obstruction. Is it a medical emergency? Am J Med 1981;70:1169-1174.
14. Ostler PJ, et al: Superior vena cava obstruction: A modern management strategy [Review]. Clin Oncol (R Coll Radiol) 1997;9(2):83-89.
15. Roswit B, Kaplan G, Jacobson HG: The superior vena cava obstruction syndrome in bronchogenic carcinoma: Pathologic physiology and therapeutic management. Radiology 1953;61:722-737.
16. Carlson HA: Obstruction of the superior vena cava: An experimental study. Arch Surg 1934;29:669-677.
17. Lochridge SK, Knibbe WP, Doty DB: Obstruction of the superior vena cava. Surgery 1979;8-5:14-24.
18. Scarantino C, et al: The optimum radiation schedule in treatment of superior vena caval obstruction: Importance of 99mTc scintiangiograms. Int J Radiat Oncol Biol Phys 1979;5:1987-1995.
19. Little AG, et al: Malignant superior vena cava obstruction reconsidered: The role of diagnostic intervention. Ann Thorac Surg 1985;40:285-288.
20. Yellin A, et al: Superior vena cava syndrome: The myth—the facts. Am Rev Respir Dis 1990;141:1114-1118.
21. Davenport D, et al: Response of superior vena cava syndrome to radiation therapy. Cancer 1976;38:1577-1580.
22. Rubin P, et al: Superior vena cava syndrome: Slow low-dose versus rapid high-dose schedules. Radiology 1963;81:388-401.
23. Howard N: Mediastinal Obstruction. E & S Livingstone, 1967.
24. Sculier JP, et al: Superior vena caval obstruction syndrome in small cell lung cancer. Cancer 1986;57:847-851.
25. Hsu JW, et al: Superior vena cava syndrome in lung cancer: An analysis of 54 cases. Kao-Hsiung i Hsueh Ko Hsueh Tsa Chih [Kaohsiung J Med Sci] 1995;11:568-573.
26. Gauden SJ: Superior vena cava syndrome induced by bronchogenic carcinoma: Is this an oncological emergency? Australas Radiol 1993;37:363-366.
27. Enders GC, Sodums MT: Local thrombolytic therapy in superior vena cava syndrome secondary to malignant thymoma: A case report and literature review. Cathet Cardiovasc Diagn, 1994;31:215-218.
28. Perez-Soler R, et al: Clinical features and results of management of superior vena cava syndrome secondary to lymphoma. J Clin Oncol 1984;2:260-266.
29. Maddox A-M, et al: Superior vena cava obstruction in small cell bronchogenic carcinoma: Clinical parameters and survival. Cancer 1983;52:2165-2172.
30. Montalban C, et al: Metastatic carcinoma of the prostate presenting as a superior vena cava syndrome. Chest 1993;104:1278-1280.
31. Biswal BM, et al: Carcinoma of the uterine cervix presenting as superior vena cava syndrome: Report of three cases and a review of literature. J Obstet Gynaecol 1995;21:437-442.
32. Sumiyoshi Y, Kikuchi M: Leiomyosarcoma of the superior vena cava producing superior vena cava syndrome and heart tamponade. Pathol Int 1995;45:691-694.
33. Rytina ER, et al: Intimal sarcoma of the right brachiocephalic vein presenting as the superior vena caval syndrome. J Clin Pathol 1996;49:347-349.
34. Tovar-Martin E, et al: Intraluminal leiomyosarcoma of the superior vena cava: A cause of superior vena cava syndrome. J Cardiovasc Surg 1997;38:33-35.
35. Schwarz RE, Groeger JS, Coit DG: Subcutaneously implanted central venous access devices in cancer patients: A prospective analysis. Cancer 1997;79:1635-1640.
36. Bertrand M, et al: Iatrogenic superior vena cava syndrome. A new entity. Cancer 1984;54:376-378.

37. Woodyard TC, et al: Acute superior vena cava syndrome after central venous catheter placement. Cancer 1993;71:2621-2623.

38. Puel V, et al: Superior vena cava thrombosis related to catheter malposition in cancer chemotherapy given through implanted ports. Cancer 1993;72:2248-2252.

39. Morales M, Llanos M, Dorta J: Superior vena cava thrombosis secondary to Hickman catheter and complete resolution after fibrinolytic therapy. [Review]. Support Care Cancer 1997:5:67-69.

40. Presant CA: Tunneled central venous catheter complications and the iatrogenic superior vena cava syndrome. NY J Med 1992:92:43-44.

41. Kerr HD: Superior vena cava syndrome associated with a Hickman catheter. N Y J Med 1990;90:208-210.

42. Anderson AJ, et al: Thrombosis: the major Hickman catheter complication in patients with solid tumor. Chest 1989;95:71-75.

43. Mahmud AM, et al: Radionuclide venography and its functional analysis in superior vena cava syndrome. J Nucl Med 1996;37:1460-1464.

44. Matthews JA, Blake HA, Hall DJ: Iatrogenic superior vena cava syndrome treated with streptokinase. Gynecol Oncol 1987;26: 119-122.

45. Eastridge BJ, Lefor AT: Complications of indwelling venous access devices in cancer patients. J Clin Oncol 1995;13:233-238.

46. Bern MM, et al: Very low doses of warfarin can prevent thrombosis in central venous catheters: A randomized prospective trial. Ann Intern Med 1990;112:423-428.

47. Mahajan V, et al: Benign superior vena cava syndrome. Chest 1975;68:32-35.

48. Chen JC, Bongard F, Klein SR: A contemporary perspective on superior vena cava syndrome. Am J Surg 1990;160:207-211.

49. Urschel HC Jr, et al: Sclerosing mediastinitis: Improved management with histoplasmosis titer and ketoconazole. Ann Thorac Surg 1990;50:215-221.

50. Lee Y, Doering R, Jihayel A: Radiation-induced superior vena cava syndrome. Texas Heart Instit J 1995;22:103-104.

51. Abdelkafi S, et al: Superior vena cava syndrome associated with *Nocardia farcinica* infection. Thorax 1997;52:492-493.

52. Issa PY, et al: Superior vena cava syndrome in childhood: Report of ten cases and review of the literature. Pediatrics 1983;71:337-341.

53. Ingram L, Rivera GK, Shapiro DN: Superior vena cava syndrome associated with childhood malignancy: Analysis of 24 cases. Med Pediatr Oncol 1990;18:476-481.

54. Kelly KM, Lange B: Oncologic emergencies. [Review]. Pediatr Clin North Am 1997;44:809-830.

55. Moncada R, et al: Evaluation of superior vena cava syndrome by axial CT and CT phlebography. Am J Roentgenogr 1984;143:731-736.

56. Schwartz EE, Goodman LR, Haskin ME: Role of CT scanning in the superior vena cava syndrome. Am J Clin Oncol 1986;9:71-78.

57. Raptopoulos V: Computed tomography of the superior vena cava. Crit Rev Diagn Imaging 1986;25:373-429.

58. Yedlicka JW Jr, et al: Computed tomography of superior vena cava obstruction. J Thorac Imaging 1987;2:72-78.

59. Yedlicka JW, et al: CT findings in superior vena cava obstruction. Semin Roentgenol 1989;24:84-90.

60. Trigaux JP, Van Beers B: Thoracic collateral venous channels: Normal and pathologic CT findings. J Comput Assist Tomogr 1990;14:769-773.

61. Kim HJ, Kim HS, Chung SH: CT diagnosis of superior vena cava syndrome: Importance of collateral vessels. Am J Roentgenol 1993;161:539-542.

62. Qanadli SD, et al: Helical CT phlebography of the superior vena cava: Diagnosis and evaluation of venous obstruction. Am J Roentgenol 1999;172:1327-1333.

63. Stanford W, et al: Superior vena cava obstruction: A venographic classification. Am J Radiol 1987;148:259-262.

64. Son YH, Wetzel RA, Wilson WJ: ^{99m}Tc pertechnetate scintiphotography as diagnostic and follow-up aids in major vascular obstruction due to malignant neoplasm. Radiology 1968;91:349-357.

65. Rivera JV, Robert F, Ficek MA: Radionuclide angiography: Superior vena caval obstruction. Semin Nucl Med 1981;4:325-326.

66. Muramatsu T, et al: Hot spots on liver scans associated with superior or inferior vena caval obstruction. Clinl Nucl Med 1994;19:622-629.

67. Ayala K, et al: Diagnosis of superior vena caval obstruction by transesophageal echocardiography. Chest 1992;101:874-876.

68. Swayne LC, Kaplan IL: Gallium SPECT detection of neoplastic intravascular obstruction of the superior vena cava. Clin Nucl Med 1989;14:823-826.

69. Shimm DS, Logue GL, Rigsby LC: Evaluating the superior vena cava syndrome. JAMA 1981;245:951-953.

70. Loeffler JS, et al: Emergency prebiopsy radiation for mediastinal masses: Impact on subsequent pathologic diagnosis and outcome. J Clin Oncol 1986;4:716-721.

71. Ko, JC, et al: Superior vena cava syndrome: Rapid histologic diagnosis by ultrasound-guided transthoracic needle aspiration biopsy. Am J Respir Crit Care Med 1994;149:783-787.

72. Callejas MA, et al: Mediastinoscopy as an emergency diagnostic procedure in superior vena cava syndrome. Scand J Thor Cardiovasc Surg 1991;25:137-139.

73. Painter TD, Karpf M: Superior vena cava syndrome: Diagnostic procedures. Am J Med Sci 1983;285:2-6.

74. Mineo TC, et al: Mediastinoscopy in superior vena cava obstruction: Analysis of 80 consecutive patients. Ann Thorac Surg 1999;68:223-226.

75. Jahangiri M, Taggart DP, Goldstraw P: Role of mediastinoscopy in superior vena cava obstruction. Cancer 1993;71:3006-3008.

76. Bigsby R, Greengrass R, Unruh H: Diagnostic algorithm for acute superior vena caval obstruction (SVCO). J Cardiovasc Surg 1993;34:347-350.

77. Green J, Rubin P, Holzwasser G: The experimental production of superior vena cava obstruction. Radiology 1963;81:406-414.

78. Fisherman WH, Bradfield JS: Superior vena caval syndrome: response with initially high daily dose irradiation. South Med Assoc J 1973;66:677-680.

79. Rodrigues CI, Njo KH, Karim AB: Hypofractionated radiation therapy in the treatment of superior vena cava syndrome. Lung Cancer 1993;10:221-228.

80. Lonardi F, et al: Double-flash, large-fraction radiation therapy as palliative treatment of malignant superior vena cava syndrome in the elderly. Support Care Cancer 2002;10:156-160.

81. Kaplan HS, Evidence for a tumoricidal dose level in the radiotherapy of Hodgkin's disease. Cancer Res 1966;26:1221-1224.

82. Vijaykumar S, Myrianthropoulos LC: An updated dose-response analysis in Hodgkin's disease. Radiother Oncol 1992;24:1-13.

83. Connors JM, et al: Brief chemotherapy and involved field radiation therapy for limited-stage, histologically aggressive lymphoma. Ann Intern Med 1987;107:25-30.

84. Hoppe RT, et al: Progress in the treatment of Hodgkin's disease in the United States, 1973 versus 1983: The Patterns of Care Study. Cancer 1994;74:3198-3203.

85. Johnson DH, et al: Cisplatin and etoposide + thoracic radiotherapy administered once or twice daily in limited stage small cell lung cancer: Final report of Intergroup study 0096. Proc Am Soc Clin Oncol 1996;15:374.

86. Johnson DH, et al: Combination chemotherapy with or without thoracic radiotherapy in limited-stage small-cell lung cancer: A randomized trial of the Southeastern Cancer Study Group. J Clin Oncol 1993;11:1223-1229.

87. Choy H, et al: Phase I trial of outpatient weekly paclitaxel and concurrent radiation therapy for advanced non-small-cell lung cancer. J Clin Oncol 1994;12:2682-2686.

88. Dillman RO, et al: Improved survival in stage III non-small-cell lung cancer: Seven-year follow-up of Cancer and Leukemia Group B (CALGB) 8433 Trial. J Natl Cancer Instit 1996;88:1210-1215.

89. Roberts JR, Bueno R, Sugarbaker DJ: Multimodality treatment of malignant superior vena caval syndrome. Chest 1999;116: 835-837.

90. Sause WT, Turrisi AT: Principles and application of preoperative and standard radiotherapy for regionally advanced non-small cell lung cancer In Pass HI, et al (eds): Lung Cancer: Principles and Practice, Philadelphia, Lippincott-Raven, 1996, p 697-710.

91. Wang JC, Wang KY, Chen JT, et al: Outcome and prognostic factors for patients with non-small cell lung cancer and severe radiation pneumonitis. Int J Radiat Oncol Biol Phys 2002;54:735-741.

92. Inoue A, et al: Radiation pneumonitis in lung cancer patients: A retrospective study of risk factors and the long-term prognosis. International J Radiat Oncol Biol Phys 2001;49:649–655.

93. Robnett TJ, et al: Factors predicting severe radiation pneumonitis in patients receiving definitive chemoradiation for lung cancer. Int J Radiat Oncol Biol Phys 2000;48:89–94.

94. Seppenwoolde Y, Lebesque JV: Partial irradiation of the lung. Semin Radiat Oncol 2001;11:247–258.

95. Shank B, Scher HI: Controversies in treatment of small cell carcinoma of the lung. Cancer Invest 1985;3:367–387.

96. Kies MS, et al: Multimodal therapy for limited small-cell lung cancer: A randomized study of induction combination chemotherapy with or without thoracic radiation in complete responders; and with wide-field versus reduced-field radiation in partial responders: A Southwest Oncology Group Study. J Clin Oncol 1987;5:592–600.

97. Armstrong JG, et al: Three-dimensional conformal radiation therapy may improve the therapeutic ratio of high dose radiation therapy for lung cancer. Int J Radiat Oncol Biol Phys 1993;26:685–689.

98. Graham MV, et al: Three-dimensional radiation treatment planning study for patients with carcinoma of the lung. International J Radiat Oncol Biol Phys 1994;29:1105–1117.

99. Emami B, et al: Three-dimensional treatment planning for lung cancer. International J Radiat Oncol Biol Phys 1991;21:217–227.

100. Nutting CM, et al: A comparison of conformal and intensity-modulated techniques for oesophageal radiotherapy. Radiother Oncol 2001; 61:157–163.

101. Greenberg S, Kosinski R, Daniels L: Treatment of superior vena cava thrombosis with recombinant tissue type plasminogen activator. Chest 1991;99:1298–1301.

102. Kane RC, et al: Superior vena caval obstruction due to small-cell anaplastic lung carcinoma. JAMA 1976;235:1717–1718.

103. Dombernowsky P, Hansen HH: Combination chemotherapy in the management of superior vena caval obstruction in small-cell anaplastic carcinoma of the lung. Acta Med Scand 1978;204:513–516.

104. Urban T, et al: Superior vena cava syndrome in small-cell lung cancer. Arch Intern Med 1993;153:384–387.

105. Wurschmidt F, Bunemann H, Heilmann HP: Small cell lung cancer with and without superior vena cava syndrome: A multivariate analysis of prognostic factors in 408 cases. Int J Radiat Oncol Biol Phys 1995;33:77–82.

106. Chan RH, et al: Superior vena cava obstruction in small-cell lung cancer. Int J Radiat Oncol Biol Phys 1997;38:513–520.

107. Blanke CD, Johnson DH: Treatment of small cell lung cancer. Semin Thorac Cardiovasc Surg 1997;9:101–110.

108. Skarlos DV, et al: Randomized comparison of etoposide-cisplatin vs. etoposide-carboplatin and irradiation in small-cell lung cancer: A Hellenic Co-operative Oncology Group study. Ann Oncol 1994;5:601–607.

109. Spiro SG, et al: Treatment of obstruction of the superior vena cava by combination chemotherapy with and without irradiation in small cell carcinoma of the bronchus. Thorax 1983;38:501–505.

110. Citron MC, et al: Superior vena cava syndrome due to non-small cell lung cancer: Resolution with chemotherapy alone. JAMA 1983;250:71–72.

111. Martins SJ, Pereira JR: Clinical factors and prognosis in non-small cell lung cancer. Am J Clin Oncol 1999;22:453–457.

112. Coleman CN, et al: Treatment of lymphoblastic lymphoma in adults. J Clin Oncol 1986;4:1628–1637.

113. Kirn D, et al: Large-cell and immunoblastic lymphoma of the mediastinum: Prognostic features and treatment outcome in 57 patients. J Clin Oncol 1993;11:1336–1343.

114. Zinzani PL, et al: Adult lymphoblastic lymphoma: Clinical features and prognostic factors in 53 patients. Leukemia Lymphoma 1996;23:577–582.

115. Anderson RP, Li W: Segmental replacement of superior vena cava with spiral vein graft. Ann Thorac Surg 1983;36:85–88.

116. Doty DB: Bypass of superior vena cava: Six years experience with spiral vein graft for obstruction of superior vena cava due to benign and malignant disease. J Thorac Cardiovasc Surg 1982;83:326–338.

117. Nieto AF, Doty DB: Superior vena cava obstruction: Clinical syndrome, etiology and treatment. Curr Probl Cancer 1986;10:442–484.

118. Magnan PE, et al: Surgical reconstruction of the superior vena cava. Cardiovasc Surg 1994;2:598–604.

119. Lagerstrom CF, et al: Chronic fibrosing mediastinitis and superior vena caval obstruction from blastomycosis. Ann Thorac Surg 1992;54:764–765.

120. Patel V, et al: Superior vena cava syndrome: Current concepts of management. N J Med 1995;92:245–248.

121. Rantis PC Jr, Littooy FN: Successful treatment of prolonged superior vena cava syndrome with thrombolytic therapy: A case report. J Vasc Surg 1994;20:108–113.

122. Gray BH, et al: Safety and efficacy of thrombolytic therapy for superior vena cava syndrome. Chest 1991;99:54–59.

123. Piccione W Jr, Faber LP, Warren WH: Superior vena caval reconstruction using autologous pericardium. Ann Thorac Surg 1990;50:417–419.

124. Gloviczki P, et al: Reconstruction of large veins for nonmalignant venous occlusive disease. J Vasc Surg 1992;16:750–761.

125. Doty DB, Doty JR, Jones KW: Bypass of superior vena cava: Fifteen years' experience with spiral vein graft for obstruction of superior vena cava caused by benign disease. J Thorac Cardiovasc Surg 1990;99:889–895; discussion 895–896.

126. Gloviczki P, et al: Reconstruction of the vena cava and of its primary tributaries: A preliminary report. J Vasc Surg 1990;11:373–381.

127. Kee ST, et al: Superior vena cava syndrome: treatment with catheter-directed thrombolysis and endovascular stent placment. Radiology 1998;206:187–193.

128. Rosch J, et al: Gianturco expandable wire stents in the treatment of superior vena cava syndrome recurring after maximum-tolerance radiation. Cancer 1987;60:1243–1246.

129. Rosch J, et al: Gianturco-Rosch expandable Z-stents in the treatment of superior vena cava syndrome. Cardiovasc Intervent Radiol 1992;15:319–327.

130. Putnam JS, et al: Superior vena cava syndrome associated with massive thrombosis: Treatment with expandable wire stents. Radiology 1988;167:727–728.

131. Charnsangavej C, et al: Stenosis of the vena cava: Preliminary assessment of treatment with expandable metallic stents. Radiology 1986;161:295–298.

132. Hennequin LM, et al: Superior vena cava stent placement: Results with the Wallstent endoprosthesis. Radiology 1995;196:353–361.

133. Stock KW, et al: Treatment of malignant obstruction of the superior vena cava with the self-expanding Wallstent. Thorax 1995;50:1151–1156.

134. Chin DH, et al: Stent-graft in the management of superior vena cava syndrome. Cardiovasc Intervent Radiol 1996;19: 302–304.

135. Shah R, et al: Stenting in malignant obstruction of superior vena cava. J Thorac Cardiovasc Surg 1996;112:335–340.

136. Oudkerk M, et al: Self-expanding metal stents for palliative treatment of superior vena caval syndrome. Cardiovasc Intervent Radiology 1996;19:146–151.

137. Chacon Lopez-Muniz JI, et al: Treatment of superior and inferior vena cava syndromes of malignant cause with Wallstent catheter placed percutaneously. Am J Clin Oncol 1997;20:293–297.

138. Gross CM, et al: Stent implantation in patients with superior vena cava syndrome. Am J Roentgenol 1997;169:429–432.

139. Oudkerk M, Heystraten FM, Stoter G: Stenting in malignant vena caval obstruction. Cancer 1993;71:142–146.

140. Smayra T, et al: Long-term results of endovascular stent placement in the superior caval venous system. Cardiovasc Intervent Radiol 2001;24:388–394.

141. Lanciego C, et al: Stenting as first option for endovascular treatment of malignant superior vena cava syndrome. Am J Roentgenol 2001;177:585–593.

142. Miller JH, et al: Malignant superior vena cava obstruction: Stent placement via the subclavian route. Cardiovasc Intervent Radiol 2000;23:155–158.

143. Thony F, et al: Endovascular treatment of superior vena cava obstruction in patients with malignancies. Eur Radiol 1999;9:965–971.

144. Nicholson AA, et al: Treatment of malignant superior vena cava obstruction: Metal stents or radiation therapy. J Vasc Intervent Radiol 1997;8:781-788.

145. de Gregorio Ariza MA, Gamboa P, Gimeno MJ, et al: Percutaneous treatment of superior vena cava syndrome using metallic stents. Eur Radiol 2003;13:853-862.

146. Chatziioannou A, Alexopoulos T, Mourikis D, et al: Stent therapy for malignant superior vena cava syndrome: Should it be first line therapy or simple adjunct to radiotherapy. Eur J Radiol 2003;47:247-250.

147. Schindler N, Vogelzang RL: Superior vena cava syndrome: Experience with endovascular stents and surgical therapy. Surg Clin North Am 1999;79:683-694.

148. Tanigawa N, et al: Clinical outcome of stenting in superior vena cava syndrome associated with malignant tumors: Comparison with conventional treatment. Acta Radiol 1998;39:669-674.

149. Yim CD, Sane SS, Bjarnason H: Superior vena cava stenting. Radiol Clin North Am 2000;38:409-424.

150. Nogeire C, Mincer F, Botstein C: Long survival in patients with bronchogenic carcinoma complicated by superior vena caval obstruction. Chest 1979;75:325-329.

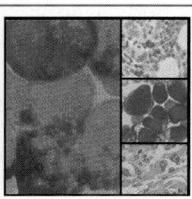

SPINAL CORD COMPRESSION

John C. Ruckdeschel

SUMMARY OF KEY POINTS

INCIDENCE

- Spinal cord compression is diagnosed in more than 30% of all patients with disseminated cancer, but only 5% experience cord dysfunction.
- Back pain almost always precedes neurologic injury.
- Spinal cord compression has a devastating effect on quality of life.
- Spinal cord compression is frequently, and unnecessarily, diagnosed late.

ETIOLOGY

- In 85% of cases destruction of the anterior portion of vertebral body occurs with subsequent.
- Demyelination.
- Arterial compromise.

- Venous occlusion.
- Vasogenic edema.

EVALUATION

- Any new or worsening back pain in a cancer patient mandates urgent radiographic evaluation.
- Limited-sagittal-views only magnetic resonance imaging (MRI) is the most rapid and cost-effective means of diagnosis and should be the first procedure performed.
- Computed tomographic myelography can be used when MRI is contraindicated.
- No characteristics of back pain safely differentiate cord compression from other benign or malignant spinal diseases.

GRADING OF THE COMPLICATION

- Any evidence of myelopathy signals impending catastrophic loss of cord function.
- Full paraplegia for more than 48 hours is rarely reversible.

TREATMENT

- Most patients can be treated with corticosteroids and radiation alone.
- Posterior laminectomy is almost never indicated unless the bulk of the tumor is posterior.
- Anterior spinal decompression is helpful in some patients.

INTRODUCTION

One of the most striking features found at rounds on a medical oncology service in the late 1960s was the disproportionate number of patients paralyzed by metastatic cancer to the spine and ensuing cord compression. In that era, before the advent of hospice and the availability of extensive home care options, the only chance these patients had to regain dignity was to be transferred to a rehabilitation service, which was unlikely given these patients' generally poor "rehabilitation potential." By the late 1970s the pathophysiologic mechanisms of spinal cord compression had been delineated,[1,2] and treatment options had been improved by the addition of corticosteroids to traditional surgical and radiotherapeutic options.[3,4] Outcome remained poor for most patients, however, because the diagnosis was only rarely made before the onset of neurologic damage. Gilbert and colleagues[5] and Greenberg and associates[6] outlined the diagnostic and therapeutic state of the art up to 1980. They found that a significant proportion of patients entering the hospital in an ambulatory state (and almost all patients entering nonambulatory) left with varying degrees of paresis and paralysis. The recurring theme in all of the reports from that era was the need for "earlier diagnosis."[7] Other than use of "an increased degree of

clinical suspicion" and seeking more precise signs of early cord dysfunction, no algorithms existed for early diagnosis of spinal cord compression.

All of the available results at the time of Gilbert and Greenberg's reports showed onset of back pain for periods ranging from weeks to months.[5-7] Rodichok and colleagues[8] proposed a diagnostic algorithm in which myelography (then the only available diagnostic tool) was used for evaluation of new back pain in cancer patients rather than being performed after development of early signs of spinal cord damage. Despite early opposition to this "overly aggressive" use of myelography, Rodichok and coworkers demonstrated that fully 60% of patients with new back pain, abnormal findings on a plain spinal radiograph, and normal findings at neurologic examination had epidural cord compression; that the extent of compression was less when epidural cord compression was diagnosed in this manner; and that 95% of these patients remained ambulatory when treated with radiation alone.[8,9] Even after recommendations from this trial were widely adopted in the United States, reports of series of patients treated in this manner were rare.[10-14] Subsequent reports from Denmark,[15] Australia,[16] Great Britain,[17] and Germany [18] described a staggering proportion of patients (48%-96%) with motor weakness, bladder dysfunction, and inability to walk.[15-18]

In the literature in this area, all reports before the mid-1980s are skewed by the change in diagnostic approach and the subsequent change in clinical manifestations of the syndrome. In almost all articles before 1985, most cases of spinal compression are described as manifesting as neurologic deficits.[5,6,19-28] In some reports, all cases are described as manifesting as myelopathy.[28] Therapeutic options are quite limited in this setting, and early reports of therapy based on these late manifestations are not fully relevant to cases diagnosed early. This chapter attempts to place the earlier data in context but focuses heavily on more recent data.

PATHOPHYSIOLOGY

Figure 55-1 shows the relevant anatomy of the spinal cord, spine, and associated structures and the location of metastatic lesions in these areas. Most malignant lesions causing spinal cord compression do so by invasion of the epidural space, most often as direct extension of metastatic lesions of the vertebral body. Tumor cells can get to the epidural space in several ways, hematogenous spread to the marrow being the most common.[29-31] This same pathway of dissemination also can lead to direct metastasis to the cord (intramedullary) or to the epidural space itself, both of which are highly unusual.[25] An alternative route of "hematogenous" spread to the spine is Batson's vertebral venous plexus, a low-pressure, valveless system that allows retrograde flow of tumor cells during any period of increased intra-abdominal or intrathoracic pressure.[32] Finally, tumor can reach the epidural space through the intervertebral foramina.[25] This mechanism is unusual unless the primary tumor preferentially forms paraspinal masses, a feature of lymphoma, neuroblastoma, and, on occasion, some types of carcinoma, such as small cell lung cancer.[25]

Once a malignant lesion has arrived at the epidural space, it begins what is usually a prolonged period of growth, eventually leading to compression of the spinal cord. It is not clear whether this compression manifests as direct pressure on the neural structures of the cord with subsequent demyelination, as arterial insufficiency with subsequent neural degeneration, or as venous blockage with secondary vasogenic edema due to disruption of the blood–spinal cord barrier. Animal models exist that demonstrate all three mechanisms.[33-35] At least one human pathologic study clearly demonstrated the presence of cord edema.[28] It is likely that all three mechanisms are operative to varying degrees. Investigators in Great Britain used magnetic resonance imaging (MRI) to confirm that soft-tissue epidural disease was the predominant (73% of cases) cause of cord compression as opposed to bony collapse (24%) or intrathecal disease (3%).[36] Results of various animal experiments have shown that the spinal cord can tolerate prolonged pressure if the onset of the pressure is slow and the neural degeneration is not irreversible.[37-39] Rades and colleagues[18] found that slower clinical progression of neurologic symptoms before diagnosis led to improved outcome. These data should give cause for hope in the management of spinal cord compression, because they mean there is leeway in treatment if the diagnosis can be made early. It is also in keeping with clinical experience that although the onset may be prolonged, once cord damage begins, the process can proceed exponentially.

EARLY DIAGNOSIS

A clear understanding of the pathophysiologic mechanism and clinical progression of spinal cord compression led to an algorithm used for early diagnosis with myelography and as a guide to therapy.[8] However, advances in MRI technology and availability have led to a new diagnostic algorithm.[40] It is necessary, however, to define the patient population for whom this algorithm is appropriate.

The Cancer Patient with Back Pain

The number of patients with back pain is enormous. Back pain is said to strike 80% of Americans at one time

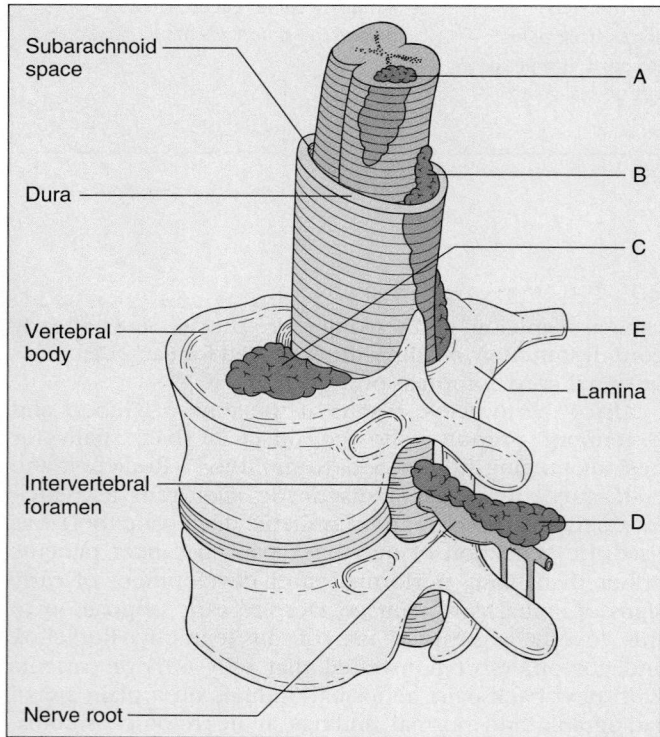

Figure 55-1. Locations of metastatic lesions of the spine. **A,** Intramedullary lesions are located within the spinal cord. **B,** Leptomeningeal lesions in the subarachnoid space are extramedullary and intradural. Epidural lesions arise from extension of metastatic lesions in the adjacent vertebral column **C,** in the paravertebral spaces through the intervertebral foramina **D,** or rarely, in the epidural space itself **E.** As they grow, these epidural metastatic lesions compress adjacent blood vessels, nerve roots, and spinal cord. The result is local and referred pain, radiculopathy, and myelopathy. (From Byrne TN: Spinal cord compression from epidural metastases. N Engl J Med 1992;327:614. Copyright 1992 Massachusetts Medical Society, 1992, with permission.)

Labels on figure: Subarachnoid space; Dura; Vertebral body; Intervertebral foramen; Nerve root; A; B; C; E; Lamina; D

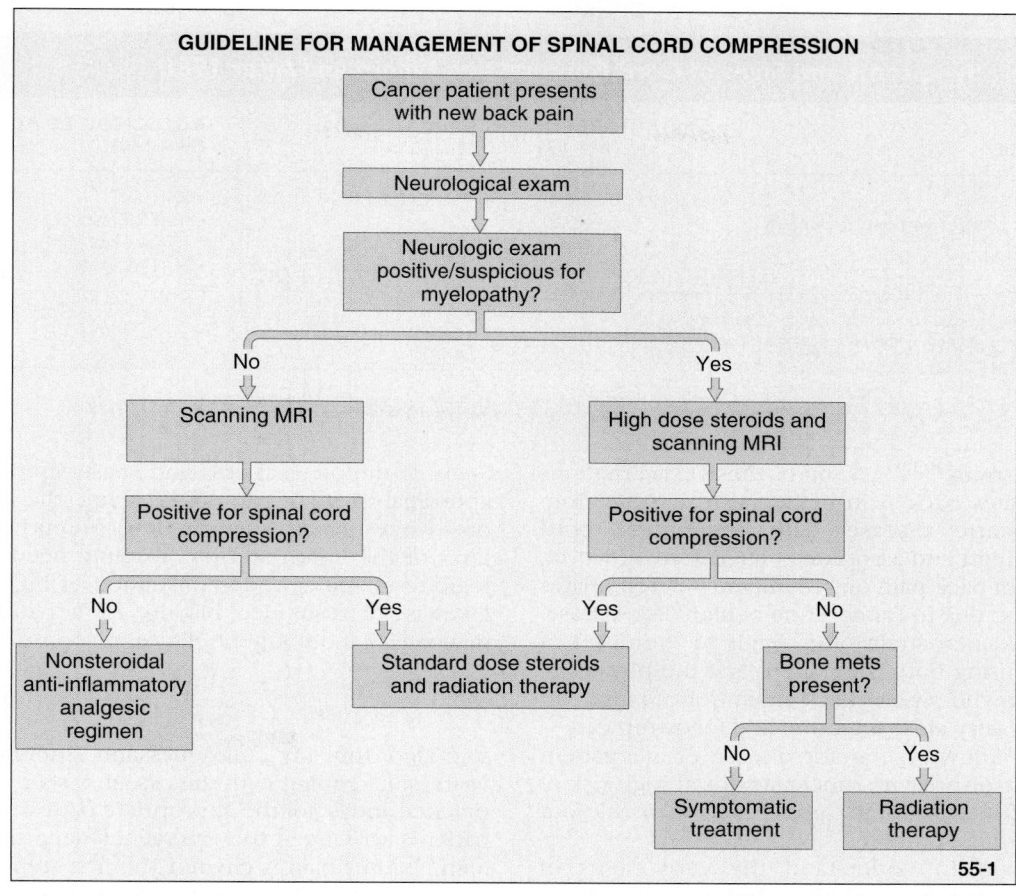

GUIDELINE FOR MANAGEMENT OF SPINAL CORD COMPRESSION

55-1

or another.[41] It also resolves with relatively minor interventions, such as rest and non-narcotic analgesics, most of the time. A cancer patient with impending cord compression is not well served, however, by a period of conservative therapy because of the propensity for the process to progress rapidly and the poorer outcome when any neurologic damage has occurred. How then does one decide to enter this algorithm? Care of any cancer patient who has new back pain or an exacerbation of previous symptoms should be started with at least the first phase of the algorithm. It is often stated that a patient has "no evidence of cord compression" (on the basis of careful neurologic examination) and therefore does not need radiographic evaluation. This miscalculation can be catastrophic for the patient.

The approach outlined in the algorithm is not the appropriate answer for patients *without* a known or suspected diagnosis of cancer. The number of patients with cancer that manifests solely as new back pain is quite small, but such a diagnosis should be suspected when an older patient does not respond to conservative therapy.

Signs and Symptoms

The first symptom of cord compression is back pain at the affected site.[5-14] This pain is often, but not always, accompanied by tenderness to percussion.[13] Perusing the

early literature gives one a false view of the presentation. Table 55-1 shows the symptoms and signs seen both initially and when the patient arrived for evaluation as described in a 1980 report by Greenberg and colleagues[6] and a 1981 report by Rodichok and associates[8] after introduction of the initial myelography-based algorithm. The initial symptom, invariably pain, did not differ between the two series, but the symptoms and signs at presentation clearly differed—far less loss of neurologic function occurred in the later study. It is important to note differences in these studies, however. The Greenberg study required an 80% or greater myelographic block, and no mention was made of how many patients were not considered because of a lesser degree of block. Nor did Greenberg and coworkers differentiate sensorimotor changes reflective of myelopathy from those reflecting only radiculopathy or plexopathy.[6] Table 55-1 presents only Greenberg's notation of "autonomic dysfunction" as clear evidence of myelopathy. Even so, the rate of myelopathy at evaluation was still nearly 2.5 times greater (44.5% versus 18.5%).[6,8,9] The main differences between the two trials were early use of myelography at the first sign of back pain and an abnormal plain radiograph in the Rodichok study[8,9] and untimed reliance on searching for subtle signs of early myelopathy in the Greenberg series.[6]

Back pain can be exacerbated by movement, change in position, cough, any act resulting in a Valsalva maneuver,

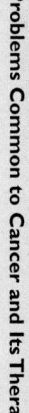

TABLE 55-1

Presenting Symptoms and Signs of Cord Compression Before and After 1981

SIGN/SYMPTOM	GREENBERG ET AL[6] (N = 83)	RODICHOK ET AL[8] (N = 140)
Pain	82 (98.8)	140 (100)*
Sensory or motor changes without myelopathy	58 (69.8) motor	46 (55.4) sensory
		37 (26.4) motor
Myelopathy	37 (44.5)	26 (18.5)

Data represent number of patients, with percentage in parentheses.
*Entry to the study was defined by the presence of back pain.

or any physical strain.[10,12-14] None of these exacerbations safely differentiates back pain of benign causation from that of metastatic disease with impending cord compression.[9] Grant and associates[12] suggested, however, that worsening of back pain on recumbency differentiates cord compression due to cancer from benign disk disease.

Totally coincidental strain often leads to the onset of symptoms, confusing both the patient and the physician. A cancer patient who reports back strain from a particular event still needs very close attention and follow-up care.[14] In the setting of known metastatic disease, or in a patient with lung, breast, or prostate cancer who is at high risk of development of metastasis, my preference is to rule out spinal cord compression first.

It is important to understand the early signs of myelopathy, however, because their presence dictates a far more urgent approach to diagnosis and therapy. Table 55-2 lists the signs of myelopathy. Understanding of the pathophysiologic mechanism suggests the order in which the signs most often occur.[10,12-14] The first sign after development of pain usually is weakness, closely followed by sensory loss in the affected distribution. Sensory loss occasionally precedes weakness. Weakness plus a proprioceptive deficit often manifests as ataxia; intramedullary metastasis occasionally causes ataxia as the first symptom. Autonomic dysfunction with urinary retention, constipation, and loss of control of bowel or bladder function is a later and particularly ominous finding, because full paraplegia can follow within hours.[14]

TABLE 55-2

Symptoms and Signs of Myelopathy

Weakness
Sensory loss
Hypoesthesia
Anesthesia
Diminished proprioception
Ataxia
Spasticity
Reflex hyperactivity
Autonomic dysfunction
Bladder incontinence
Bowel incontinence

Signs of motor weakness and spasticity often are found, abnormal plantar responses being the most common positive test result. A sensory level points both to the likely level of the lesion and the absolute need to stop neurologic tests and start administration of high-dose steroids. Likewise, a distended bladder or a patulous sphincter mandates a more urgent clinical response.

The Diagnostic Algorithm

The algorithm my colleagues and I developed over the years is in keeping with the case mix seen in an oncologic practice and is not the appropriate pathway for noncancer patients arriving in the emergency department with back pain.[8,9,] After pain is elicited, the first step is a neurologic examination. If the presence of an abnormal finding is in question, assistance should be sought from a neurologist. Any sign of myelopathy (see Table 55-2) should lead to prompt MRI of the entire spine with institution of high-dose dexamethasone therapy before the patient is sent to the MRI suite. Awaiting MRI confirmation of the diagnosis before instituting administration of steroids is almost never warranted. Even if the diagnosis is incorrect, the single bolus of steroid is extremely unlikely to cause any significant side effects. My colleagues and I have found MRI and myelography equivalent with respect to accuracy of diagnosis of cord compression. Although computed tomographic (CT) myelography gained favor for a brief period, most clinicians prefer to use MRI.[42-50] We order a myelogram only when the patient is unable to tolerate claustrophobia or cannot lie in the supine position. In addition, any suspicion of neoplastic meningitis is an indication for myelography. We prefer MRI because it gives information about the presence of early metastatic lesions elsewhere and is noninvasive. MRI depicts evidence of multiple epidural metastatic lesions.[48] Schiff and co-workers[48] showed that as many as 21% of silent thoracic or lumbar epidural metastatic lesions are missed when imaging studies are directed solely at the area of pain. When patients have myelopathy, MRI results are abnormal more than 80% of the time, but not 100%. In our original series (Table 55-3), three of the four patients with myelopathy in the presence of a normal myelogram had radiation myelopathy with Brown-Sequard syndrome. The fourth patient had conus medullaris involvement

TABLE 55-3

Myelographic Findings in Cancer Patients with Back Pain			
GROUP	**N**	**ABNORMAL MYELOGRAM* PERCENT**	
Patients with abnormalities at neurologic examination			
Myelopathy	18	14	78
Radiculopathy	28	17	61
Plexopathy	5	0/2	0
Patients with no abnormalities at neurologic examination			
Abnormal radiologic findings	25	15	60
Normal radiologic findings	17	0/7	0

*For purposes of this study, if the myelogram showed evidence of extramedullary metastatic tumor in the symptomatic area, it was considered abnormal.
From Rodichok LD, Harper GR, Ruckdeschel JC, et al: Early diagnosis of spinal epidural metastases. Am J Med 1981;70:1181.

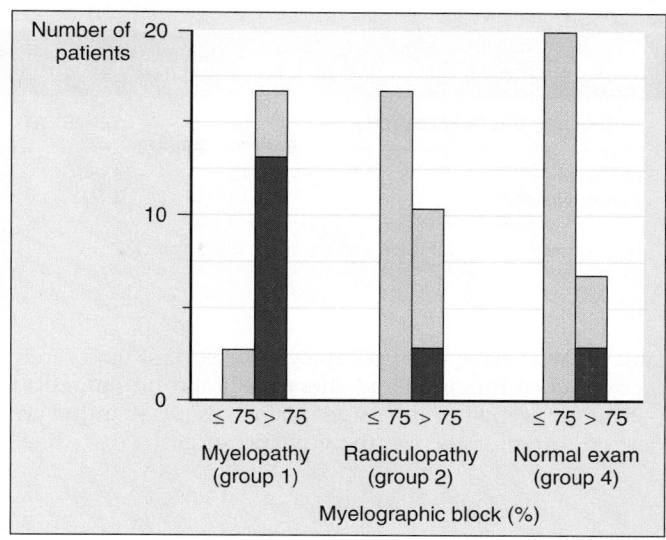

Figure 55-2. Extent of myelographic block as a function of clinical presentation. *Purple bar* represents complete obstruction. (From Rodichok LD, Ruckdeschel JC, Harper GR, et al: Early detection and treatment of spinal epidural metastases: The role of myelography. Ann Neurol 1986;20:696.)

with a normal-appearing myelogram.[8,9] When findings at the initial neurologic examination suggest plexus involvement, the patient is probably better served by a myelogram (preferably a CT myelogram), because spinal fluid can be assessed at the same time.[10] Only one of our plexopathy patients had an abnormal myelogram, but neoplastic meningitis and cord compression often are present in the same setting.[8,9]

When a patient has either local or radicular back pain with no evidence of myelopathy, the first step in the algorithm is what we have termed *scanning MRI.*[47] This study involves a series of T_1-weighted sagittal images extending from the cervical spine to the sacrum. If metastatic lesions of bone are found, in particular if there is a suggestion of epidural extension, the procedure is converted to a set of multiview images with and without gadolinium enhancement. This method is a faster and more cost-effective approach to early diagnosis of spinal cord compression[47] than the previous approach of plain radiography or bone scan followed by full MRI.[40] This approach has been supported by other investigators.[51-54]

Although the clinical realities of trying to perform diagnostic studies in the middle of the night often preclude performing MRI on an emergency basis, it should be remembered that nearly 10% of the neurologically intact patients in our original study had complete block at myelography.[8] In most settings the radiologic procedure is performed the following morning. my practice is to add steroids empirically until MRI can be performed. On occasion, it is difficult to ascertain the difference between an osteoporotic compression fracture and a compression fracture due to weakening of the vertebral body by metastatic disease. This is especially true because the age distributions of cancer and osteoporosis overlap. In both settings, MRI is extremely sensitive with respect to detection of metastatic disease within the marrow cavity.[49,50] If MRI findings are normal, I generally treat the patient conservatively with bed rest and non-narcotic analgesics. A very small group of patients have paraspinal

masses that do not cause bone erosion and yet can cause significant cord compression by advancement of tumor up the neural canal.[12-14] The intraspinal component of the disease is depicted at MRI, however, and further imaging with MRI or CT can be done to elucidate the extent of the paraspinal mass so it can be managed properly.

Figure 55-2 demonstrates extent of myelographic block according to clinical manifestations. Most patients with myelopathy have high-grade block and complete obstruction to flow of contrast medium in the epidural space.[8] In patients with radiculopathy, high- and low-grade blocks are equally distributed, and overall, only one third of lesions produce complete obstruction. Most patients encountered at the stage of back pain only, with no neurologic changes, have low-grade lesions; however, a small percentage have complete obstruction.[8]

It is less expensive to move directly from a report of back pain by a cancer patient with the appropriate findings to MRI than to proceed with the earlier algorithm.[40] Alternative clinical algorithms suggested by Choucair[10,11] are excessively complex and can be greatly enhanced by prompter use of MRI.[47-50]

TREATMENT

Bone metastatic lesions unresponsive to non-narcotic pain medications and anti-inflammatory agents are generally irradiated as the most effective means of relieving pain, although bisphosphonates are an increasingly used option.[55,56] In the presence of epidural metastatic lesions, therapy is indicated for all patients who have not had prolonged paraplegia. Treatment of patients who have paraplegia is successful in some instances, but only when the duration of paraplegia has been extremely brief.

Problems Common to Cancer and Its Therapy

TABLE 55-4

Primary Treatment of 48 Patients with Established Epidural Metastasis				
CLINICAL PRESENTATION	N	SURGERY	RADIATION THERAPY	OTHER
Myelopathy	12	6 (50)	6 (50)	0
Nonmyelopathy	36	2 (6)	29 (81)	5 (13)

Data represent number of patients with percentage in parentheses.
Adapted from Rodichok LD, Harper GR, Ruckdeschel JC, et al: Early diagnosis of spinal epidural metastases. Am J Med 1981;70:1181.

Patients who have been paraplegic for several days rarely recover cord function, and therapy should be limited to palliation of pain. The three mainstays of therapy are corticosteroids, radiation therapy, and surgery.

Corticosteroids

Solid experimental evidence has shown that steroids can relieve edema due to cord compression and that these drugs are clinically valuable.[57] What is less clear is the dosage required. Physicians at Memorial Sloan-Kettering Cancer Center in New York have popularized a high-dose regimen: a loading dose of 100 mg dexamethasone followed by 6 mg given four times a day (total dose 24 mg).[6,13] This regimen was based on results of laboratory studies demonstrating a dose-response benefit of dexamethasone.[58] Results of other comparative trials suggested no benefit of 100 mg dexamethasone over 10 mg dexamethasone given as a bolus, but controversy reigns in this area.[59] The controversy is less over the dose of dexamethasone than over for which patients high-dose therapy is appropriate. Almost no one questions starting high-dose dexamethasone in the care of patients with any degree of myelopathy, no matter how subtle. Without controlled trials, doses ranging from 10 to 100 mg of dexamethasone given as a bolus would appear appropriate. Clinical judgment usually leads to use of higher dosages as the severity of the myelopathy increases, particularly when the neurologic changes appear to be progressing at a rapid pace. Whether administration of steroids should be started in high doses for patients with radiculopathy or back pain and normal results of neurologic examination is another question. I usually start a lower dose of steroids, either 4 mg every 6 hours or a

bolus of 10 mg when MRI is delayed for unavoidable reasons. Whatever dose is initiated, tapering of the steroid should begin during the course of radiation therapy.[56] Long-term use of corticosteroids is fraught with serious clinical side effects.[50] Higher doses of steroids rarely are needed beyond the first 48 to 72 hours and in most situations are rarely needed after the initial bolus. The mainstay of treatment administered by our group has been 4–6 mg every 6 hours. If neurologic symptoms continue to progress with either this standard dose or the high-dose regimen, a highly unstable clinical situation exists that may be an indication for prompt surgical intervention.[14] During tapering, recrudescence of symptoms is an indication for increasing the steroid dose. If this step is not entirely and immediately effective, surgical decompression should be considered. Our usual practice is to reduce the dose of steroids by one third every 3 to 4 days so that near the end of the course of radiation therapy, the steroids have been almost completely tapered.[14]

Radiation Therapy

Reliance on treatment reports is most misleading in the area of radiation therapy. Several small studies were conducted to explore either posterior laminectomy or radiation therapy, or both, as therapy for spinal cord compression. These studies failed to demonstrate a difference in neurologic outcome between radiation therapy alone and laminectomy followed by radiation treatment.[5,60-63] A fair amount of leeway seemed left to proceed down either clinical pathway, depending on one's particular expertise. Tables 55-4 and 55-5 show the outcome among patients in our earlier study.[9] Of the

TABLE 55-5

Ambulatory Status After Treatment as a Function of Initial Ambulatory Status					
AMBULATORY STATUS AT DIAGNOSIS		NO. WALKING/NO. ALIVE (%)			
	N	1 MO	3 MO	6 MO	12 MO
0, 1, 2	56	51/56 (91.1)	34/40 (85)	22/25 (88)	15/16 (93.8)
3, 4	15	4/13 (30.8)	3/8 (37.5)	2/4 (50)	2/3 (66.7)

Ambulatory status: 0, walks normally; 1, walks without assistance; 2, walks with assistance (cane, walker); 3, stands only, cannot walk; 4, cannot stand or walk.
From Rodichok LD, Ruckdeschel JC, Harper GR, et al: Early detection and treatment of spinal epidural metastases: the role of myelography. Ann Neurol 1986;20:696.

TABLE 55-6

Sites of Disease Progression in Patients Treated for Epidural Cord Compression				
CLINICAL GROUP	N	SYSTEMIC CANCER	ESTABLISHED EPIDURAL METASTASIS	NEW EPIDURAL METASTASIS
Myelopathy	18	15 (83.3)	2 (11.1)	1 (5.5)
Nonmyelopathy	53	48 (90.6)	4 (7.5)	4 (7.5)
Overall	71	63 (88.7)	6 (8.4)	5 (7.0)

Data represent number of patients with percentage in parentheses.
Adapted from Rodichok LD, Harper GR, Ruckdeschel JC, et al: Early diagnosis of spinal epidural metastases. Am J Med 1981;70:1181.

patients who had myelopathy, fully one half needed surgical decompression because of rapidly progressive symptoms. Half were treated with radiation therapy alone. Among patients who had epidural cord compression without evidence of myelopathy, only two patients (6%) needed surgery for changes in clinical status. Fully 81% of patients were treated with radiation therapy alone; five patients (13%) were not treated either because death due to other causes was imminent or because the patient chose not to be treated. Only one or two patients were treated with systemic therapy as the primary treatment. Table 55-5 shows that patients treated in this manner maintain ambulatory status, if they were ambulatory at the beginning of treatment; some recover from varying stages of myelopathy.[8,9] When recovery occurs, it is stable, so these patients remain ambulatory until they die of systemic cancer. Table 55-6 shows the longer-term follow-up data on these patients. Only 8.7% of patients had progression of disease at the site of previously irradiated epidural metastatic lesions.[8,9] In 7% of patients, new epidural metastatic lesions developed at other sites during the follow-up period.

These data and data from several similar reports indicate that stabilization with corticosteroids followed by standard doses of radiation therapy (30–50 Gy over 2–4 weeks) is the treatment of choice.[61-66] Radiation usually is administered to two vertebral spaces above and below the site of the lesion to encompass the epidural disease, which frequently extends over several vertebral spaces.[62] Spinal cord tolerance is quite acceptable within this range. No results of controlled trials have suggested an advantage of one dose, or fractionation of radiation, over another.[14]

Surgery

The traditional surgical approach to epidural cord compression was posterior laminectomy.[15,60] Although this operation often resulted in prompt relief of pressure-related symptoms, the procedure is not used as often as it once was.[14] Structurally, posterior laminectomy further weakens the spine when the bulk of the destructive process is in the anterior vertebral body, which occurs in 85% of cases.[14] With increasing emphasis on quality of palliation, this further deterioration of the spine is not often in the patient's best interest. With a policy of early diagnosis, the need for emergency decompressive laminectomy should be almost eliminated. Except for

presence of the bulk of the tumor in the posterior elements, no indications for posterior laminectomy exist.

A procedure that has gained increasing acceptance is anterior decompression of the spine with subsequent reconstruction.[67-71] Several reports have described excellent palliation of pain for prolonged periods. This procedure has the advantage of stabilizing a spine that is structurally unstable and removing the bulk of the tumor causing compression. However, when judging the relative aspects of palliation, it is important to note that an anterior approach to the spine requires an intrathoracic or intra-abdominal approach, which greatly increases the complexity of the surgery involved. For a patient whose life expectancy is more than 6 months, this approach may make a great deal of sense, because the benefits of mobility and pain reduction far outweigh the short-term operative and postoperative complications. However, for a patient whose life expectancy is less than 3 months, it rarely makes sense to embark on a procedure that necessitates hospitalization for most of the remaining time. This is a highly individualized decision for most patients.

Questions have been raised about whether anterior decompression with radiation therapy is superior to radiation therapy alone. The 95% maintenance of ambulation rate with radiation alone attained in our study would be difficult to improve upon with additional surgery.[9] Only in the care of patients with evidence of myelopathy would this type of study be warranted. Patchell and colleagues[72] reported results of a study showing that surgery plus radiation was superior to radiation alone in treatment of patients who already had signs of myelopathy. It is important to note that the trial had a large number of patients who sought evaluation with myelopathy or diminished ambulation and that the role of surgery in earlier presentations has not been examined. The final indication for surgery is a spinal lesion as the presenting symptom when the spine is the sole site of clinical disease. This situation is associated most often with multiple myeloma with isolated plasmacytoma, but it can occur with other cancers.

CONCLUSIONS

Epidural cord compression due to cancer should progress to paralysis only when the patient delays seeking medical attention. A diagnosis can be readily made, as indicated in the management algorithm. The presence of new or worsening back pain in a patient with cancer should be a clarion call to action. It dictates performance of MRI. Nonsurgical therapy can maintain ambulation in most patients, but surgical intervention may be required for stabilization of the spine in a small number of patients.

REFERENCES

1. Ushio Y, Posner R, Posner JB, et al: Experimental spinal cord compression by epidural neoplasms. Neurology 1977;27:422.
2. Ikeda H, Ushio Y, Hayakawa T, et al: Edema and circulatory disturbances in the spinal cord compressed by epidural neoplasms in rabbits. J Neurosurg 1980;52:203.
3. Cantu RC: Corticosteroids for spinal metastases [letter]. Lancet 1968;2:912.
4. Posner JB, Howieson J, Cvitkovic E: "Disappearing" spinal cord compression: Oncolytic effect of glucocorticoids (and other chemotherapeutic agents) on epidural metastases. Ann Neurol 1977;2:409.
5. Gilbert RW, Kim J-H, Posner JB: Epidural spinal cord compression from metastatic tumor: Diagnosis and treatment. Ann Neurol 1978;3:40.
6. Greenberg HS, Kim J-H, Posner JB: Epidural spinal cord compression from metastatic tumor: Results with a new treatment protocol. Ann Neurol 1980;8:361.
7. Posner JB: Neurological complications of systemic cancer. Med Clin North Am 1979;63:783.
8. Rodichok LD, Harper GR, Ruckdeschel JC, et al: Early diagnosis of spinal epidural metastases. Am J Med 1981;70:1181.
9. Rodichok LD, Ruckdeschel JC, Harper GR, et al: Early detection and treatment of spinal epidural metastases: The role of myelography. Ann Neurol 1986;20:696.
10. Choucair AK: Myelopathies in the cancer patient: Incidence, presentation, diagnosis and management, I. Oncology 1991;5(6):71.
11. Choucair AK: Myelopathies in the cancer patient: Incidence, presentation, diagnosis and management, II. Oncology 1991;5(7):25.
12. Grant R, Papadopoulos SM, Greenberg HS: Metastatic epidural spinal cord compression. Neurol Clin 1991;9:825.
13. Posner JB: Back pain and epidural spinal cord compression. Med Clin North Am 1987;71:185.
14. Byrne TN: Spinal cord compression from epidural metastases. N Engl J Med 1992;327:614.
15. Helweg-Larsen S: Clinical outcome in metastatic spinal cord compression: A prospective study of 153 patients. Acta Neurol Scand 1996;94:269.
16. Milross CG, Davies MA, Fisher R, et al: The efficacy of treatment for malignant spinal cord compression. Australas Radiol 1997;41:137.
17. Hill ME, Richards MA, Gregory WM, et al: Spinal cord compression in breast cancer: A review of 70 cases. Br J Cancer 1993;68:969.
18. Rades D, Heidenreich F, Karstens JH: Final results of a prospective study of the prognostic value of the time to develop motor deficits before irradiation in metastatic spinal cord compression. Int J Radiat Oncol Biol Phys 2002;53:975.
19. Dunn RC, Kelly WA, Wohns RNW, et al: Spinal epidural neoplasia. J Neurosurg 1980;52:47.
20. Botterell EH, Fitzgerald CW: Spinal cord compression produced by extradural malignant tumors: Early recognition, treatment and results. Can Med Assoc J 1959;80:791.
21. Khan FR, Glicksman AS, Chu FCH, et al: Treatment by radiotherapy of spinal cord compression due to extradural metastases. Radiology 1967;89:495.
22. Rubin P: Extradural spinal cord compression by tumor, I: Experimental production and treatment trials. Radiology 1969;93:1243.
23. Longeval E, Hildebrand J, Vollont GH: Early diagnosis of metastases in the epidural space. Acta Neurochir 1975;31:177.
24. Stark RJ, Henson RA, Evans SJW: Spinal metastases: A retrospective survey from a general hospital. Brain 1982;105:189.
25. Posner JB: Spinal cord compression: A neurologic emergency. Clin Bull 1971;1:65.
26. Bruckman JE, Bloomer WD: Management of spinal cord compression. Semin Oncol 1978;5:135.
27. Raichle ME, Posner JB: The treatment of extradural spinal cord compression. Neurology 1970;20:391.
28. Barron KD, Hirano A, Araki S, et al: Experiences with metastatic neoplasms involving the spinal cord. Neurology 1959;9:91.
29. Arguello F, Baggs RB, Duerst RE, et al: Pathogenesis of vertebral metastasis and epidural spinal cord compression. Cancer 1990;65:98.
30. Batson OV: The function of the vertebral veins and their role in the spread of metastases. Ann Surg 1940;112:138.
31. Abrams HI, Spiro R, Goldstein N: Metastases in carcinoma. Cancer 1950;3:74.
32. Batson OV: The vertebral vein system, Caldwell lecture 1956. In Weiss L, Gilbert HA (eds): Bone Metastasis. Boston, GK Hall, 1981, p 21.
33. Gledhill RF, Harrison BM, McDonald WI: Demyelination and remyelination after acute spinal cord compression. Exp Neurol 1973;38:472.
34. Doppman JL: The mechanism of ischaemia in anteroposterior compression of the spinal cord. Invest Radiol 1975;10:543.
35. Kato A, Ushio Y, Hayakawa T, et al: Circulatory disturbances of the spinal cord with epidural neoplasm in rats. J Neurosurg 1985;63:260.
36. Pigott KH, Baddeley H, Maher EJ: Pattern of disease in spinal cord compression on MRI scan and implications for treatment. Clin Oncol (R Coll Radiol) 1994;6:7.
37. Tarlov IM, Klinger H, Vitale S: Spinal cord compression studies, I: Experimental techniques to produce acute and gradual compression. Arch Neurol Psychiatry 1957;70:813.
38. Tarlov IM, Klinger H: Spinal cord compression studies, II: Time limits for recovery after acute compression in dogs. Arch Neurol Psychiatry 1954;71:271.
39. Tarlov IM: Spinal cord compression studies, III: Time limits for recovery after gradual compression in dogs. Arch Neurol Psychiatry 1954;71:588.
40. Ruckdeschel JC: Spinal cord compression. In Abeloff M, Armitage J, Lichter A, et al (eds): Clinical Oncology. New York, Churchill Livingstone, 1995, p 619.
41. Bonica JJ: Historical, socioeconomic and diagnostic aspects of the problem, I: The nature of the problem. In Carron H, McLaughlin RE (eds): Management of Low Back Pain. Bristol, UK, Stonebridge Press, 1982, p 1.
42. Li KC, Poon PY: Sensitivity and specificity of MRI in detecting malignant spinal cord compression and in distinguishing malignant from benign compression fractures of vertebrae. Magn Reson Imaging 1988;6:547.
43. Carmody RF, Yang PJ, Seely GW, et al: Spinal cord compression due to metastatic disease: Diagnosis with MR imaging versus myelography. Radiology 1989;173:225.
44. Smoker WRK, Godersky JC, Knutzon RK, et al: The role of MR imaging in evaluating metastatic spinal disease. Am J Roentgenol 1987;149:1241.
45. Sze G, Abramson A, Krol G, et al: Gadolinium-DTPA in the evaluation of intradural extramedullary spinal disease. Am J Neuroradiol 1988;9:153.
46. Sze G, Krol G, Zimmerman RD, et al: Intramedullary disease of the spine: Diagnosis using gadolinium-DTPA–enhanced MR imaging. Am J Neuroradiol 1988;9:847.
47. Ruckdeschel JC: Rapid, cost-effective diagnosis of spinal cord compression due to cancer. Cancer Control 1995;2:320.
48. Schiff D, O'Neill BP, Wang C, et al: Neuroimaging and treatment implications of patients with multiple epidural spinal metastases. Cancer 1998;83:1593.
49. Jordan JE, Donaldson SS, Enzman DR: Cost effectiveness and outcome assessment of magnetic resonance imaging in diagnosing spinal cord compression. Cancer 1995;75:2579.
50. Godersky JC, Smoker WR, Knutson R: Use of magnetic resonance imaging in the evaluation of metastatic spinal disease. Neurosurgery 1987;21:676.
51. Jones KM, Schwartz RB, Mantello MT, et al: Fast spin-echo MR in the detection of vertebral metastases: Comparison of three sequences. Am J Neuroradiol 1994;15:401.
52. Mehta RC, Marks MP, Hinks RS, et al: MR evaluation of vertebral metastases: T1-weighted, short-inversion time inversion recovery,

fast spin-echo, and inversion-recovery fast spin-echo sequences. Am J Neuroradiol 1995;16:281.

53. Dwyer AJ, Frank JA, Sank VJ, et al: Short T1 inversion-recovery pulse sequence: Analysis and initial experience in cancer imaging. Radiology 1988;168:827.

54. Stimac GK, Porter BA, Olson DO, et al: Gadolinium-DTPA–enhanced MR imaging of spinal neoplasms: Preliminary investigation and comparison with unenhanced spin-echo and STIR sequences. Am J Roentgenol 1988;151:1185.

55. Hortobagyi GN, Theriault RL, Lipton A, et al: Long term prevention of skeletal complications of metastatic breast cancer with pamidronate: Protocol 19 Aredia breast cancer study group. J Clin Oncol 1998;16:2038.

56. Berenson JR, Lichtenstein A, Porter L, et al: Efficacy of pamidronate in reducing skeletal events in patients with advanced multiple myeloma. N Engl J Med 1996;334:488.

57. Weissman DE: Glucocorticoid treatment for brain metastases and epidural spinal cord compression: A review. J Clin Oncol 1988;6:543.

58. Delattre JY, Arbit E, Thaler HT, et al: A dose response study of dexamethasone in a model of spinal cord compression caused by epidural tumor. J Neurosurg 1989;70:920.

59. Vecht CJ, Haaxma-Reiche H, van Putten WLJ, et al: Initial bolus of conventional versus high dose dexamethasone in metastatic spinal cord compression. Neurology 1989;39:1255.

60. Black P: Spinal metastasis: Current status and recommended guidelines for management. Neurosurgery 1979;5:726.

61. Mones RJ, Dozier D, Berrett A: Analysis of medical treatment of malignant extradural spinal cord tumors. Cancer 1966;19:1842.

62. Young RF, Post EM, King GA: Treatment of spinal epidural metastases: Randomized prospective comparison of laminectomy and radiotherapy. J Neurosurg 1980;53:741.

63. Kornblith PL, Cassady JR: Central nervous system emergencies. In DeVita VT, Hellman S, Rosenberg SA (eds): Principles and Practice of Oncology, 2nd ed. Philadelphia, JB Lippincott, 1985, p 1960.

64. Friedman M, Kim TM, Panahon AM: Spinal cord compression in malignant lymphoma. Cancer 1976;37:1485.

65. Loeffler JS, Glicksman AS, Tefft M, et al: Treatment of spinal cord compression: A retrospective analysis. Med Pediatr Oncol 1983;11:347.

66. Maranzano E, Latini P, Beneventi S, et al: Radiotherapy without steroids in selected metastatic spinal cord compression patients: A phase II trial. Am J Clin Oncol 1996;19:179.

67. Sundaresan N, DiGiancinto GV, Krol G, et al: Spondylectomy for malignant tumors of the spine. J Clin Oncol 1989;7:1485.

68. Harrington KD: Anterior cord decompression and spinal stabilization for patients with metastatic lesions of the spine. J Neurosurg 1984;61:107.

69. Siegal T, Siegal T: Surgical decompression of anterior and posterior malignant epidural tumors compressing the spinal cord: A prospective study. Neurosurgery 1985;17:424.

70. Harrington KD: Anterior decompression and stabilization of the spine as a treatment for vertebral body collapse and spinal cord compression from metastatic malignancy. Clin Orthop 1988;233:177.

71. Perrin RG, McBroom RJ: Anterior versus posterior decompression for symptomatic spinal metastases. Can J Neurol Sci 1987;14:75.

72. Patchell R, Tibbs PA, Regine WF, et al: A randomized trial of direct decompressive surgical resection in the treatment of spinal cord compression caused by metastasis. In Program/Proceedings of the 39th Annual Meeting of the American Society of Clinical Oncology, Chicago, May 31–June 3, 2003. Alexandria, Va: ASCO, 2003. Available at www.asco.org/ac/1,1003,_12-002489-00_18-002003-00_19-00101474-00_29-00A,00.asp?.

Problems Common to Cancer and Its Therapy

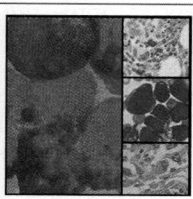

56

BRAIN METASTASES AND CARCINOMATOUS MENINGITIS

Penny K. Sneed

Kim Huang

James L. Rubenstein

SUMMARY OF KEY POINTS

- Central nervous system metastases are common, affecting up to 25% of cancer patients. Most central nervous metastases involve the brain; less often, the dura, leptomeninges, skull base, or cranial nerves may be affected. The term *carcinomatous meningitis* refers to the dissemination of cancer cells into the leptomeningeal space.
- The primary tumor types that most commonly give rise to brain metastases include lung cancer, melanoma, breast cancer, and renal cell carcinoma.
- Brain metastases are best detected with contrast-enhanced magnetic resonance imaging (MRI) and generally appear as enhancing, well-circumscribed lesions with surrounding vasogenic edema.
- Biopsy or resection may be indicated to confirm the diagnosis, particularly in a patient with a single lesion and no cancer diagnosis or no known metastatic disease.
- Carcinomatous meningitis often eludes early detection, because meningeal enhancement is visible on MRI in only about 50% of cases, and cerebrospinal fluid cytology may be negative in 40% to 50% of cases.
- The most important factors predicting longer survival of patients with brain metastases include age less than 60, good performance

status, control of the primary tumor, and lack of extracranial metastases.
- The most common treatment for brain metastases is whole-brain radiotherapy, although patients with a good prognosis who have a limited number of brain metastases may benefit from more aggressive therapy such as surgery (especially for a single brain metastasis) or radiosurgery, with or without adjuvant whole-brain radiation therapy.
- After whole-brain radiation therapy alone, at least 60% of symptomatic patients improve significantly. The median survival time is 3 to 6 months, with one third to one half of patients dying of brain metastases and the rest dying of systemic disease. About 24% of brain metastases have a complete response to whole-brain radiation therapy, and another 35% of lesions have a partial response, but the 1-year actuarial local control probability is on the order of 15% or less.
- Among patients with newly diagnosed brain metastases selected for surgery or radiosurgery with or without whole-brain radiation therapy, the median survival time is approximately 9 to 11 months. One-year actuarial local control is about 35% for surgery alone, 85% for

surgery and adjuvant whole-brain radiation therapy, and 75% to 90% for radiosurgery with or without adjuvant whole-brain radiotherapy. However, the increased local control achievable with surgery and radiation or with radiosurgery may be meaningful only in patients likely to live at least 6 or 12 months from the standpoint of their systemic disease.
- Chemotherapy is not generally used as a primary treatment for brain metastases, but it has some efficacy on its own, and there is increasing interest in combining drugs with whole-brain radiation therapy.
- Intrathecal chemotherapy plays a major role in the management of carcinomatous meningitis, alone or in combination with radiation therapy. Because craniospinal radiation therapy causes significant acute toxicity as well as long-lasting myelosuppression, carcinomatous meningitis may be managed using intrathecal chemotherapy combined with more limited radiation therapy, such as a lumbar field for gross disease in the cauda equina, skull base fields for cranial nerve involvement, or whole-brain radiation therapy in patients with hydrocephalus stemming from diffuse brain leptomeningeal involvement.

INTRODUCTION

Central nervous system (CNS) metastases result from the intracranial spread of tumor cells that originate outside of the CNS. Most CNS metastases involve the brain parenchyma, dura, or leptomeninges; less commonly, metastases involve the base of skull, cranial nerves, or dural sinuses. This chapter deals with both parenchymal brain metastases and leptomeningeal metastases, which is also known as carcinomatous meningitis.

BRAIN METASTASES

Epidemiology

Brain metastases appear to be more common than primary malignant brain tumors, although the exact incidence is unknown. In a Memorial Sloan-Kettering Cancer Center autopsy series, 24% of cancer patients had CNS metastases and 15% had brain metastases,[1] and in a Roswell Park Memorial Institute autopsy study of 216 melanoma patients, 55% had brain metastases.[2] A recent population-based study in the Netherlands found that 8.5% of 2724 patients with melanoma or lung, breast, colorectal, or renal cell carcinoma developed brain metastases; the 5-year cumulative incidence of brain metastases was 7.4% in patients with melanoma and 16.3%, 9.8%, 5.0%, and 1.2% for patients with lung, renal cell, breast, or colorectal carcinoma, respectively.[3] If these cumulative incidence estimates by tumor type are applied to the 2003 estimates of new cancer cases in the United States,[4] these tumor types alone could give rise to over 58,000 cases of brain metastases. If autopsy-based incidence figures are used instead, the estimated number of cases of brain metastases is much higher. It has been theorized that the incidence of brain metastases may be increasing as a result of improvements in cancer management leading to longer survival times and increased sensitivity of lesion detection made possible by contrast-enhanced, high-resolution MRI, although Schouten and colleagues found no evidence of an increasing incidence of brain metastases over the period from 1986 through 1995.[3]

The primary tumors most commonly responsible for brain metastases include lung cancer (40%–50% of cases), breast cancer (15%), melanoma (10%), and unknown primary (5%–10%), followed by renal cell carcinoma, colorectal cancer, gynecologic cancers, and other miscellaneous tumors.[5,6] Brain metastases may arise from any primary cancer, but certain tumors such as melanoma and carcinomas of the lung, kidney, and breast have a predilection for spread to the CNS. Some tumors, however, rarely metastasize to the brain, such as prostate, oropharyngeal, and skin carcinomas. In children, the solid malignancies most commonly responsible for brain metastases include sarcomas, neuroblastoma, and germ cell tumors.[7]

Cancer may spread to the brain at various points in the course of disease. Synchronous brain metastases, found within 1 month of the primary cancer diagnosis, occur in up to one third of patients,[3] including cases in which brain metastases are responsible for a patient's presenting signs or symptoms. More commonly, however, brain metastases are discovered after the diagnosis of cancer, often after other systemic metastases have developed. Among patients who develop brain metastases, metastases to the brain are diagnosed at a median of less than 1 year after diagnosis of lung cancer and at a median of 2 to 3 years after diagnosis of melanoma, breast cancer, gynecologic cancer, or renal cell carcinoma.[6] Overall, in cases where cancer metastases to the brain, the median time from primary diagnosis to diagnosis of brain metastases is 12 months.[6]

Pathophysiology

Brain metastases arise primarily from arterial hematogenous spread to the brain, with tumor cells tending to become trapped where blood vessels decrease in caliber at the gray/white matter junction and the most distal vasculature (the border zones or "watershed" zones between arterial territories).[8] Metastatic cells then adhere to the endothelial cells, penetrate into the brain parenchyma, and proliferate. Larger aggregates of tumor cells that gain access to the venous circulation are filtered out in lung capillaries before entering the systemic arterial circulation, but individual tumor cells may pass through the lung to lodge in the brain. Tumor emboli also may break off from lung metastases or primary lung cancers to travel to the brain via the arterial circulation. It has also been theorized that cells from pelvic or abdominal cancers may gain access to the posterior fossa or leptomeninges through Batson's vertebral venous plexus without passing through the lungs.[5] Intracranial spread also may occur via direct extension from bone or dural metastases or perineural involvement along cranial nerves. The distribution of metastases is roughly proportional to the relative blood flow to different regions; approximately 80% of brain metastases are located in the cerebral hemispheres, 10% to 15% in the cerebellum, and 1% to 5% in the brain stem.[5,6] A disproportionate number of posterior fossa metastases appear to arise from pelvic or abdominal primary tumors.[5]

Most brain metastases are very well circumscribed. Although there may be extensive associated edema, the tumor cells do not tend to infiltrate into surrounding brain tissue, in contrast to primary malignant brain tumors. Most brain metastases are solid, but they may appear cystic because of necrosis, keratin deposits in squamous cell carcinoma, or mucin secretion from adenocarcinoma. Brain metastases may be hemorrhagic, particularly from melanoma, renal cell carcinoma, choriocarcinoma, and, less frequently, bronchogenic carcinoma.[9] Well-differentiated metastases may be identified easily by the pathologist, but immunohistochemistry or electron microscopy may be needed to help make the diagnosis of metastatic disease (as opposed to a primary brain neoplasm) and to suggest the likely site of origin of poorly differentiated metastases.

Based on computed tomographic (CT) imaging, about 50% of patients are diagnosed as having a single brain metastasis.[5] Now that MRI is available, the actual percentage of patients diagnosed with a single metastasis is likely to be lower than this, because contrast-enhanced MRI is more sensitive than CT,[10] and, furthermore, triple-dose gadolinium is much more sensitive than single-dose gadolinium-enhanced MRI.[11] Single brain metastases are more common than multiple metastases in patients with renal cell, gastrointestinal, or unknown primaries.[6] Of note, the term *solitary brain metastasis* implies that a single brain metastasis is the only known site of metastatic disease, whereas the term *single brain metastasis* refers to a single cerebral lesion without implying whether or not there is other systemic disease.

Clinical Presentation

The possibility of brain metastases should be suspected in any cancer patient developing new neurologic signs or symptoms. Two thirds of cancer patients found to have brain metastases at autopsy had experienced neurologic symptoms from the metastases,[12] and only 10% of a series of 729 patients diagnosed by CT or MRI from 1973 through 1993 were asymptomatic.[6] The most common presenting symptoms are headache (24%–53%), focal weakness (16%–40%), altered mental status (24%–31%), seizures (15%–16%), and ataxia (9%–20%).[6,13] Symptoms may worsen gradually from a growing tumor and the associated edema. Less often, acute neurologic symptoms may occur from hemorrhage into a brain metastasis. The histologic types of tumor with the greatest propensity to produce hemorrhagic brain metastases include melanoma, renal cell carcinoma, and choriocarcinoma.

Diagnosis

Magnetic resonance imaging is the best diagnostic test to detect brain metastases. Standard imaging includes T2-weighted and pre- and post–gadolinium-enhanced T1-weighted sequences; a postcontrast fluid attenuated inversion recovery (FLAIR) sequence also is helpful in visualizing small metastases near cerebrospinal fluid (CSF) spaces (Fig. 56-1). Gadolinium-enhanced MRI is much more sensitive than either nonenhanced MRI or contrast-enhanced CT imaging.[10,14] In one study, 17 of 55 patients (31%) with a single metastasis based on contrast-enhanced CT imaging were found to have multiple metastases on contrast-enhanced MRI.[15] The sensitivity of MRI is improved by using "triple-dose" gadolinium (0.3 mmol/kg instead of 0.1 mmol/kg gadoteridol)[11] to increase contrast enhancement and by using contiguous axial 3-mm slices without skips and coronal 3-D spoiled gradient echo recovery (SPGR) volume imaging so that small lesions are not missed between slices. Functional imaging techniques such as positron emission tomography, magnetic resonance spectroscopy, and perfusion and diffusion MRI may aid in distinguishing metastatic lesions from necrosis, primary brain tumor, or nonmalignant processes.[16–18]

The differential diagnosis of an enhancing or hemorrhagic intracranial lesion includes brain metastasis, primary brain tumor, CNS lymphoma, abscess, encephalitis, cerebral infarct or hemorrhage, progressive multifocal leukoencephalopathy, tumefactive demyelinating disease, and radiation necrosis. Factors that aid in making a diagnosis based on imaging include characteristic appearance, a known cancer diagnosis, and multiplicity of lesions. However, a biopsy may be warranted if there is doubt about the diagnosis or if a single brain lesion is seen in a patient with a history of cancer but no other known metastatic disease, because management and prognosis may vary widely depending on the diagnosis. In a study by Patchell and coworkers in which patients received biopsy or surgery before whole-brain radiation therapy, 6 of 54 patients (11%) with a single brain lesion thought to be a metastasis were discovered to have, instead, glioblastoma, low-grade astrocytoma, abscess, or an inflammatory process.[19] A stereotactic biopsy series in 100 patients with multifocal brain lesions and no known primary cancer diagnosed malignant gliomas in 37% of patients, primary CNS lymphoma in 15%, brain metastases in 15%, low-grade gliomas in 12%, infectious processes in 10%, and ischemic lesions in 6% of patients.[20]

Prognostic Factors

In general, brain metastases are associated with a poor prognosis. In the pre-CT era, the median survival time of patients with symptomatic brain metastases was approximately 1 to 2 months without treatment,[21–23] 2 to 2.5 months with corticosteroid therapy,[24] and 3 to 6 months with whole-brain radiation therapy.[25–27] Despite some major advances in cancer diagnosis and treatment and imaging that allow earlier detection of brain metastases, the overall survival time of unselected patients with brain metastases treated with whole-brain radiation therapy has remained at 3 to 6 months since the 1950s.[6,28–30] Most patients with brain metastases have or soon will develop disseminated systemic disease, and overall survival is often determined by the extent and activity of the extracranial disease. In patients with a relatively short life expectancy, the treatment goal is to achieve rapid palliation and a remission free of neurologic symptoms commensurate with the patient's life expectancy. However, long-term survival or cure is possible in a small proportion of patients with brain metastases, and patients with a longer life expectancy from the standpoint of their systemic disease may benefit from more aggressive therapies that will yield more durable control of their brain metastases.

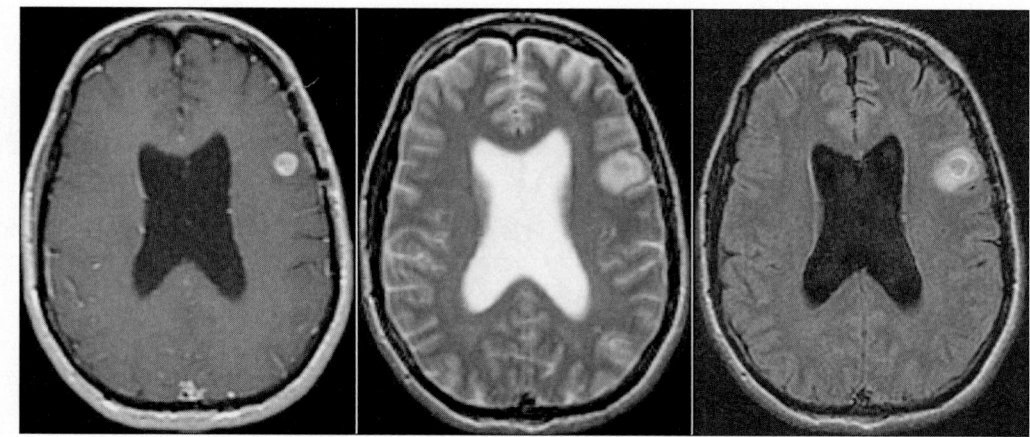

Figure 56-1. Typical appearance of a brain metastasis on magnetic resonance imaging. The lesion is well circumscribed and brightly enhancing on the postcontrast T1-weighted image *(left)*. Both edema and cerebrospinal fluid appear as increased signal on the T2-weighted image *(center)*. On the postcontrast fluid-attenuated inversion-recovery (FLAIR) image *(right)*, the brain edema surrounding the metastasis appears bright while the cerebrospinal fluid signal is suppressed.

Two large series that evaluated prognostic factors in patients with brain metastases were reported by Lagerwaard and coworkers and Gaspar and coworkers. Lagerwaard and coworkers studied 1292 patients with CT-diagnosed brain metastases treated at Daniel den Hoed Cancer Center in Rotterdam from 1981 through 1990.[31] The overall median survival time was 3.4 months, and the most important patient and tumor characteristics prognostic for improved survival included better performance status, no systemic tumor activity (limited vs. extensive activity), and normal serum lactate dehydrogenase level, followed by lesser factors, including breast cancer vs. other primary sites, age less than 70 years, and one or two versus three or more brain metastases.[31] Gaspar and coworkers identified three prognostic groups using a recursive partitioning analysis (RPA) of more than 1100 evaluable patients enrolled in three consecutive Radiation Therapy Oncology Group (RTOG) trials conducted from 1979 through 1993.[32] The median survival time was 7.1 months for the subgroup with the best prognosis, RPA class 1, consisting of patients less than 65 years old with a Karnofsky performance status (KPS) of at least 70, a controlled primary tumor, and no extracranial metastases (Table 56-1). The subgroup with the poorest prognosis, RPA class 3, including patients with KPS less than 70, had a median survival time of only 2.3 months; and the median survival time was 4.2 months for the remaining patients who made up RPA class 2 (see Table 56-1).[32] The prognostic value of these RPA classes has been validated in 569 patients with single or multiple brain metastases treated with radiosurgery with or without adjuvant whole-brain radiation therapy, with median survival times of 14.0 to 15.2 months for RPA class 1, 7.0 to 8.2 months for RPA class 2, and 5.3 to 5.5 months for RPA class 3 (see Table 56-1).[33] Similarly, median survival times were 14.8, 9.9, and 6.0 months for 125 RPA class 1, 2, and 3 patients, respectively, who underwent surgical resection and whole-brain radiotherapy (see Table 56-1).[34]

Treatment

The symptoms resulting from brain metastases may be ameliorated with corticosteroids or osmotic therapy for the peritumoral edema or with anticonvulsants for seizure control. Direct antitumor therapies include surgery, radiotherapy (external beam radiotherapy, radiosurgery, and brachytherapy), and chemotherapy.

Corticosteroids

Corticosteroid therapy generally is instituted in symptomatic patients as soon as brain metastases are diagnosed, to help alleviate symptoms until the brain metastases and edema improve from specific antitumor treatment. Corticosteroids reduce the permeability of leaky tumor blood vessels and thereby reduce the mass effect and edema caused by brain metastases.[35] Dexamethasone is the corticosteroid most commonly used because of its relatively low mineralocorticoid activity. It often is given as a loading dose of 10 mg followed by 4 mg every 6 hours. Higher doses are rarely needed, and lower doses (2–4 mg twice daily or 2–4 mg three times a day) may be adequate in many situations, with higher doses rarely needed. Patients commonly improve within hours after the first dose, attaining maximal benefit after approximately 3 to 7 days. After patients become asymptomatic or reach maximal benefit, the dose should be tapered gradually and either discontinued or else maintained at the lowest dose level needed to manage symptoms. If headaches recur or neurologic symptoms worsen during the course of the taper, the dose should be increased as needed and then the taper should proceed more gradually. Occasional patients develop steroid-withdrawal symptoms of depression, fatigue, nausea, or poor appetite, necessitating reinstitution of low-dose dexamethasone and a gradual taper schedule in the low-dose range. Corticosteroids have numerous adverse effects, particularly with long-term usage. Common short-term side effects include insomnia, increased appetite, fluid retention, mood changes, acne, and exacerbation of diabetes, and some of the serious long-term side effects include significant weight gain, steroid myopathy, immunosuppression, and aseptic necrosis of the femoral heads. It should be noted that steroid myopathy can cause fairly profound weakness in large proximal muscles, making it difficult for patients to get up and walk; this dysfunction may be mistaken for a sign of progression of CNS metastases and be seen as an indication to continue or increase corticosteroids when it is actually a complication of corticosteroid therapy.

TABLE 56-1

Median Survival Time by Radiation Therapy Oncology Group Recursive Partitioning Analysis Class					
	RPA CLASS 1		**RPA CLASS 2**		**RPA CLASS 3**
TREATMENT	**NO. OF PATIENTS**	**MST (MO)**	**NO. OF PATIENTS**	**MST (MO)**	**NO. OF PATIENTS**	**MST (MO)**
WBRT alone[32]	236	7.1	765	4.2	175	2.3
RS alone initially[33]	39	14.0	197	8.2	29	5.3
RS + upfront WBRT[33]	64	15.2	222	7.0	9	5.5
Surgery + WBRT[34]	26	14.8	63	9.9	36	6.0

MST, median survival time; RPA, recursive partitioning analysis; RS, radiosurgery; WBRT, whole-brain radiotherapy.

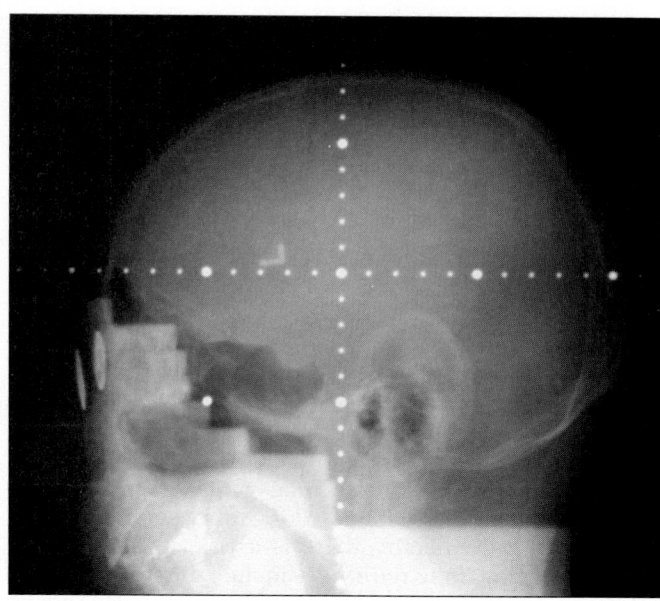

Figure 56-2. Double-exposed portal image of a typical whole-brain radiotherapy field, showing radiation covering the entire brain with blocking of the eyes and other extracranial structures.

Anticonvulsants

Seizures are very unlikely to occur from infratentorial metastases, but may be triggered by supratentorial metastases. About 15% of patients with brain metastases present with seizures, and 30% to 40% experience seizures at some point in the course of their disease.[36] Any patient with brain metastases who experiences a seizure should be started on an anticonvulsant such as phenytoin or carbamazepine, but prophylactic anticonvulsants are not generally recommended because prospective and retrospective studies have failed to demonstrate a benefit for prophylactic anticonvulsants in patients with brain metastases.[35-37] Furthermore, anticonvulsants may have

adverse side effects or cause allergic reactions, such as the Stevens-Johnson syndrome, that can be serious.

External Beam Radiotherapy

The most standard treatment for brain metastases consists of whole-brain radiotherapy covering the entire intracranial contents with shielding of the eyes (Fig. 56-2). The benefits of whole-brain radiotherapy were first described in the 1950s and 1960s. In these early studies, significant symptomatic improvement was noted in about 60% of patients, and the median survival time ranged from about 3 to 6 months with whole-brain radiotherapy[25-27] compared with an expected median survival time of 1 to 2 months without treatment.[21-23]

Whole-Brain Radiotherapy Randomized Trials. Multiple large phase III randomized trials of whole brain radiotherapy have been conducted by the RTOG since 1970 (Table 56-2). The first two trials compared various whole-brain radiotherapy fractionation schemes in over 1800 patients treated from 1971 through 1976 and gathered a wealth of data.[28,38] Complete or partial response of specific neurologic symptoms was observed in 60% to 90% of symptomatic patients; 47% to 52% of patients improved to a higher neurologic function class; the median duration of improvement was 10 to 12 weeks; and 75% to 80% of patients' remaining survival time was spent in an improved or stable neurologic state. The overall median survival times were 18 weeks (4.1 months) in the first study and 15 weeks (3.4 months) in the second study, and brain metastases were reported to be the cause of death in 49% and 31% of patients, respectively. There were no significant differences in symptomatic response rates, duration of response, or survival time according to the treatment regimen: 40 Gy in 20 fractions, 40 Gy in 15 fractions, 30 Gy in 15 fractions, 30 Gy in 10 fractions, or 20 Gy in 5 fractions. With the ultrarapid fractionation schemes tested by the RTOG (10 Gy in 1 fraction or 12 Gy

TABLE 56-2

Selected Randomized Trials of Whole-Brain Radiotherapy Alone for Brain Metastases

PROTOCOL	YEARS	NO. OF PATIENTS	FRACTIONATION SCHEME	MEDIAN SURVIVAL TIME (MO)
RTOG 6901[28,38]	1971–1973	233	30 Gy/10 fractions/2 wk	4.8
First study		217	30 Gy/15 fractions/3 wk	4.1
		233	40 Gy/15 fractions/3 wk	4.1
		227	40 Gy/20 fractions/4 wk	3.7
RTOG 7361[28,38]	1973–1976	447	20 Gy/5 fractions/1 wk	3.4
Second study		228	30 Gy/10 fractions/2 wk	3.4
		227	40 Gy/15 fractions/3 wk	4.1
RTOG 6901[39]	1971–1973	26	10 Gy/1 fraction/1 day	3.4
RTOG 7361[39]	1973–1976	33	12 Gy/2 fractions/2 days	3.0
Ultrarapid				
RTOG 7606[29]	1976–1979	130	30 Gy/10 fractions/2 wk	4.1
Favorable patients		125	50 Gy/20 fractions/4 wk	3.9
RTOG 9104[30]	1991–1995	213	30 Gy/10 fractions/2 wk	4.5
Accelerated hyperfractionation		216	54.4 Gy at 1.6 twice daily	4.5

RTOG, Radiation Therapy Oncology Group.

in 2 fractions; see Table 56-1), there was some concern that irradiation may have led to herniation and death within 48 hours of treatment in a small number of cases and time to neurologic progression was shorter than with more protracted regimens.[39,40] Both of these findings agreed with conclusions of a Memorial Sloan-Kettering Cancer Center evaluation of 15 Gy in 2 fractions over 3 days compared with 30 Gy in 15 fractions.[41] Two later RTOG trials failed to show any advantage of administering 50 Gy in 20 fractions or 54.4 Gy at 1.6 Gy twice daily over 30 Gy in 10 fractions (see Table 56-1),[29,30] further supporting the use of 30 Gy in 10 fractions over 2 weeks as the most common whole-brain radiotherapy treatment regimen. Other common treatment regimens include 35 to 37.5 Gy at 2.5 Gy per fraction, 40 to 50 Gy at 2.0 Gy per fraction, and 45 to 50.4 Gy at 1.8 Gy per fraction. Shorter regimens may be selected in patients with a shorter life expectancy or in cases when whole-brain radiotherapy is delaying chemotherapy needed to treat systemic disease. Longer regimens may be selected in patients with longer life expectancy, based on a suspicion that smaller fraction size may give less risk of late neurotoxicity.

Response and Local Control.   Nieder and coworkers studied CT response of brain metastases to whole-brain radiotherapy (30 Gy in 10 fractions).[42] Analyzed by lesion rather than by patient, the complete response rate was 24% and the partial response rate was 35%. The overall (complete plus partial) response rates were 81% for small cell carcinoma, 65% for breast cancer, 56% for squamous cell carcinoma, 50% for nonbreast adenocarcinoma, 46% for renal cell carcinoma, and 0% for melanoma. Absence of necrosis and smaller volume were associated with improved response rate. Complete response rates were as follows[42]:

Solid metastases, 39%
Lesions with less than 50% necrosis, 15%
Lesions with at least 50% necrosis, 11%
Lesions with a volume up to 0.5 cc, 52%
Lesions with a volume of 0.6 to 1.0 cc, 39%
Lesions with a volume of 1.1 to 3.0 cc, 17%
Lesions with a volume of 3.1 to 6.0 cc, 20%
Lesions with a volume of 6.1 to 10.0 cc, 5%
Lesions with a volume more than 10 cc, 0%

Another study by the same group suggested that a higher response rate was obtained with 40 Gy at 2 Gy per fraction with or without a partial brain boost to 50 or 60 Gy than with 30 Gy at 3 Gy per fraction.[43] Data on long-term local control of brain metastases are limited, but 1-year actuarial local control probabilities by patient after whole-brain radiotherapy alone ranged from 0% to 14% in the whole-brain radiotherapy-only arms of randomized trials reported by Kondziolka and coworkers[44] and Patchell and colleagues.[19]

Partial-Brain Radiotherapy.   Partial-brain radiotherapy can be considered for a single metastasis in lieu of whole-brain radiotherapy, but it is generally not advisable because it would complicate or preclude later whole-brain radiotherapy if needed (unlike radiosurgery, which delivers a much more focal radiation dose). Caution is advised when postoperative radiotherapy to the posterior fossa alone is contemplated, because cerebellar metastases appear to be associated with an increased risk of leptomeningeal dissemination postresection.[45,46] Partial-brain radiotherapy may be useful, however, for treating recurrent brain metastases that are not suitable for resection or radiosurgery.

Toxicity of Whole-Brain Radiotherapy.   Acute toxicity of whole-brain radiotherapy includes hair loss, fatigue, and modest skin reaction in essentially all patients as well as mild acute ototoxicity in some patients. The skin reaction resolves by several weeks, fatigue improves gradually over 1 to several months, and hair generally regrows by 6 months following whole-brain radiotherapy. In the minority of patients who are long-term survivors after whole-brain radiotherapy, there is a risk of late hearing loss, retinopathy if the retina was included in the radiation field, and permanent neurocognitive toxicity. DeAngelis and coworkers reported an 11% risk of severe radiation-induced dementia among 1-year survivors after resection of a single brain metastasis followed by postoperative whole-brain radiotherapy to 20 to 40 Gy using high-dose daily fractions.[45] A separate report from the same group described 12 patients cured of brain metastases who developed severe radiation-induced dementia with associated ataxia and urinary incontinence.[47] Imaging with CT showed atrophy, ventricular dilatation, and hypodense white matter. The whole-brain radiotherapy fractionation schemes included mostly mixtures of 3 or 4 Gy fractions with 5 or 6 Gy fractions, but two of the affected patients had received the standard regimen of 30 Gy in 10 fractions.[47] Nieder and coworkers reported a 42% 2-year actuarial probability of symptomatic mild, moderate, or severe late radiation toxicity in patients treated with resection of a single brain metastasis followed by whole-brain radiotherapy to 30 Gy in 10 fractions or 40 Gy in 20 fractions, but no details were provided regarding the nature of the toxicity.[48] Current trials for treatment of brain metastases are gathering needed prospective data on neurotoxicity.

Surgery
Surgery plays important roles in certain subsets of patients: confirming the diagnosis when needed; relieving mass effect from a large, symptomatic lesion (Fig. 56-3); improving the likelihood of durable local control for a single metastasis; and salvaging a progressing metastasis after previous therapy. Resection of brain metastases has become safer with advances in neuroimaging and neurosurgery such as image guidance, preoperative and intraoperative functional mapping, and intraoperative ultrasound and MRI.[49]

Randomized Trials of Whole-Brain Radiotherapy with or without Surgery.   Three prospective, randomized trials have been performed to evaluate the addition of surgery to whole-brain radiotherapy (Table 56-3). In the trial

Figure 56-3. Preoperative *(left),* immediate postoperative *(center),* and 2-month postoperative *(right)* contrast-enhanced T1-weighted magnetic resonance images of a single metastasis treated with surgical resection.

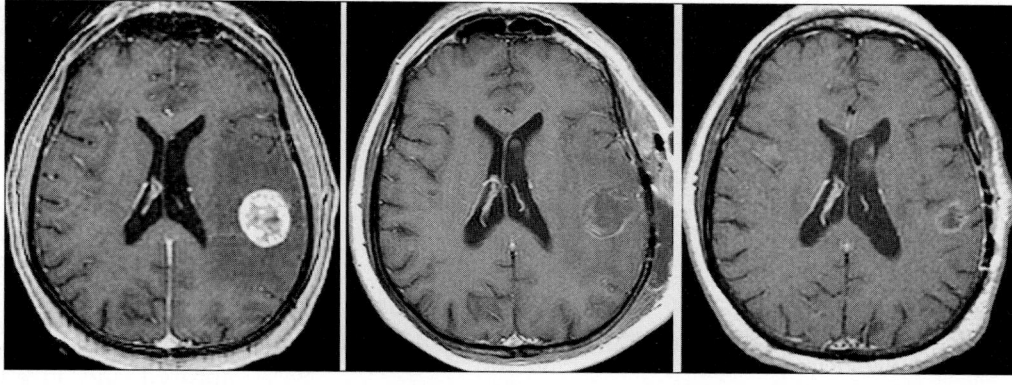

reported by Patchell and coworkers, 48 patients with single brain metastases were randomized to two groups: (1) biopsy and whole-brain radiotherapy vs. (2) resection and whole-brain radiotherapy to 36 Gy in 12 fractions.[19] Patients who underwent resection had significantly improved local control (80% vs. 48% for resection and whole-brain radiotherapy vs. biopsy and whole-brain radiotherapy; $P < 0.02$), duration of functional independence (median, 38 weeks vs. 8 weeks; $P < 0.005$), and survival (median, 40 weeks vs. 15 weeks; $P < 0.01$). Factors associated with longer survival included younger age, no extracranial disease, surgical resection, and a longer interval from primary diagnosis to brain metastasis diagnosis.[19]

A trial performed in the Netherlands randomized 63 evaluable patients with a single brain metastasis to surgery plus whole-brain radiotherapy vs. whole-brain radiotherapy alone (40 Gy at 2 Gy twice daily) (see Table 56-3).[50] Patients on the surgery arm of the trial had longer functionally independent survival (median, 7.5 months for

surgery and whole-brain radiotherapy vs. 3.5 months for whole-brain radiotherapy alone; $P = 0.06$) and longer survival time (median, 10 months vs. 6 months; $P = 0.04$). The survival benefit was seen only in patients without active extracranial disease, in whom the median survival time was 12 months for surgery and whole-brain radiotherapy versus 7 months for whole-brain radiotherapy alone ($P = 0.02$). The median survival time was 5 months for patients with active extracranial disease regardless of the treatment arm. Older age (over 60 vs. 60 years or younger) also was confirmed as an important, unfavorable prognostic factor ($P = 0.003$; hazard ratio = 2.74).[50]

A third trial failed to show a benefit for surgery in addition to whole-brain radiotherapy (30 Gy in 10 fractions over 2 weeks) (see Table 56-3).[51] The median survival times were 5.6 months among 41 patients randomized to surgery with whole-brain radiotherapy vs. 6.3 months among 43 patients randomized to whole-brain radiotherapy alone (of these 43 patients, 4 had surgery before whole-brain radiotherapy and 6 had surgery after

TABLE 56-3

Randomized Trials of Surgery or Radiosurgery and WBRT for Brain Metastases

STUDY (YEARS)	TREATMENT	NO. OF PATIENTS	PATIENTS WITH EXTRA CRANIAL DISEASE (%)	MEDIAN LOCAL FFP (MO)	MEDIAN FUNCTIONALLY INDEPENDENT SURVIVAL (MO)	MEDIAN SURVIVAL (MO)
Patchell et al. (1985–1988)[19]	Biopsy + WBRT	23	83	4.8	1.8	3.4
	Surgery + WBRT (36 Gy/12 fx)	25	76	>13.6 (P < 0.0001)	8.7 (P < 0.005)	9.2 (P < 0.01)
Noordijk et al. (1985–1990)[50]	WBRT	31	68	—	3.5	6
	Surgery + WBRT (40 Gy at 2 Gy BID)	32	69	—	7.5 (P = 0.06)	10 (P = 0.04)
Mintz et al. (1989–1993)[51]	WBRT	43	84	—	—	6.3
	Surgery + WBRT (30 Gy/10 fx)	41	73	—	— (P = NS)	5.6 (P = 0.24)
Kondziolka et al. (1985–1988)[44]	WBRT	14	71	6	—	7.5
	WBRT + RS (36 Gy/12 fx)	13	62	36 (P = 0.0005)	—	11.0 (P = 0.22)
Patchell et al. (1989–1997)[55]	Surgery	46	65	6.2	8.0	9.9
	Surgery + WBRT (50.4 Gy/28 fx)	49	63	>12.0 (P < 0.001)	8.5 (P = 0.61)	11.0 (P = 0.39)

FFP, freedom from progression; fx, fractions; NS, not significant; RS, radiosurgery; WBRT, whole-brain radiotherapy.

Problems Common to Cancer and Its Therapy

whole-brain radiotherapy). There was no difference in duration of functional independence between patients in the two treatment arms. The authors concluded that further trials or a meta-analysis was indicated,[51] but overall, these studies and previous nonrandomized experience[52-54] support the use of surgery in addition to whole-brain radiotherapy in patients with good performance status, controlled extracranial disease, and a single brain metastasis.

Randomized Trial of Surgery with or Without Whole-Brain Radiotherapy.
Postoperative whole-brain radiotherapy may help prevent recurrence at the resection cavity and prevent appearance of new brain metastases by treating any microscopic metastases elsewhere in the brain. Following up on multiple retrospective studies suggesting a benefit for postoperative whole-brain radiotherapy after resection of a brain metastasis, Patchell and associates[55] performed a randomized trial (see Table 56-3). Ninety-five adults were randomized to observation vs. postoperative whole-brain radiotherapy to 50.4 Gy in 28 fractions after complete resection of a single brain metastasis. The observation arm had a significantly increased risk of local failure (46% for observation vs. 10% for whole-brain radiotherapy), distant brain failure (37% vs. 14%), and any brain failure (70% vs. 18%); shorter time to local failure (median, 27 weeks vs. more than 52 weeks [6.2 months vs. more than 12 months]; $P < 0.001$; hazard ratio 6.03); and shorter time to any brain failure (median, 26 weeks vs. more than 70 weeks [6.0 months vs. more than 16.1 months]; $P < 0.001$; hazard ratio 4.94). Patients randomized to observation were more likely to die neurologic deaths ("brain death") (44% vs. 14%; $P = 0.003$), but, interestingly, had similar duration of functional independence (median, 35 weeks [8.0 months] for observation vs. 37 weeks [8.5 months] for whole-brain radiotherapy; $P = 0.61$) and similar survival time (median, 43 weeks vs. 48 weeks [9.9 months vs. 11.0 months]; $P = 0.39$).[55] Topics not addressed in the report included the use or success of salvage therapy and acute and late toxicity of whole-brain radiotherapy and salvage therapies.

Surgery for Multiple Metastases.
Surgical resection also may be used successfully to manage selected patients with more than one brain metastasis. Bindal and coworkers reported a median survival time of 14 months among 26 patients with multiple brain metastases who underwent resection of all of their brain lesions in a single operation, identical to the survival time of matched patients who had had resection of a single metastasis.[56] The complication rate was 9% per craniotomy, the 30-day mortality rate was 4%, and only 6% of symptomatic patients worsened while 83% improved and 11% remained stable.[56] A different group that described results of surgery and whole-brain radiotherapy had noted significantly poorer survival among 18 patients with multiple brain metastases compared with 28 patients with a single metastasis, but apparently only one patient with multiple metastases had undergone gross total resection of all (two) metastases, and this patient survived 46 months.[57]

Toxicity of Surgery for Brain Metastases.
The morbidity and mortality associated with surgical resection of brain metastases have decreased over the years as techniques have improved. In modern series, the 30-day mortality rate is about 4% to 5% (essentially identical to the 30-day mortality rate in patients managed with whole-brain radiotherapy alone).[49] The most common types of postoperative morbidity include wound infection, hemorrhage, meningitis, pneumonia, deep venous thrombosis, and pulmonary embolism, occurring in about 10% to 15% of patients on average.[49,58] Most patients are symptomatic preoperatively. One surgical series reported that 0 to 13% of patients worsened neurologically, 65% to 84% improved, and 11% to 22% remained stable after resection of single or multiple brain metastasis.[56]

Radiosurgery
Radiosurgery implies the delivery of carefully targeted, very focal radiation to one or more intracranial targets, usually using a specially adapted linear accelerator[59] or a Gamma Knife.[60] A stereotactic frame may be applied before to the procedure under local anesthesia to allow very precise targeting. Multiple beams or arcs provide for very steep fall-off of dose outside the target or targets, minimizing dose to surrounding normal brain tissue, but a thin shell of tissue around the target receives a potentially damaging dose of radiation (Fig. 56-4). Because the risk of radiation injury increases with increasing volume, lower doses usually are prescribed for larger target volumes, and radiosurgery targets tend to be limited to about 2.5 to 3 cm in diameter. An RTOG dose escalation trial concluded that the maximum tolerated doses of single fraction radiosurgery were 24 Gy for tumors 2 cm or smaller, 18 Gy for tumors measuring 2.1 to 3.0 cm, and 15 Gy for tumors 3.1 to 4.0 cm in maximum diameter.[61]

General Results of Radiosurgery.
Table 56-4 summarizes results of selected large series of radiosurgery for single or multiple, newly diagnosed or recurrent brain metastases treated with or without adjuvant whole-brain radiotherapy.[62-75] For median target volumes ranging from 1.7 to 7.5 cc and median prescribed doses ranging from 15.0 to 27.0 Gy in a single fraction, the crude local control rates were 85% to 96%; the 1-year actuarial local control probabilities were 82% to 88% by lesion, with a 0 to 17% risk of symptomatic radiation necrosis (average risk, 4%). In most of the series, the median survival times ranged from 7 to 11 months. Based on the data set of 518 lesions analyzed by Goodman and coworkers,[69] 1-year actuarial local freedom from progression probabilities were 88%, 75%, and 29% for doses of 18 Gy or greater, 15.0 to 17.9 Gy, and less than 15.0 Gy, respectively, and 92%, 83%, 69%, and 37% for maximum target diameters 1.0 cm or less, 1.1 to 2.0 cm, 2.1 to 3.0 cm, and greater than 3.0 cm, respectively.

Randomized Trials of Whole-Brain Radiotherapy with or Without Radiosurgery.
The first reported randomized trial of whole-brain radiotherapy with or without radiosurgery boost was performed in patients with a KPS of at

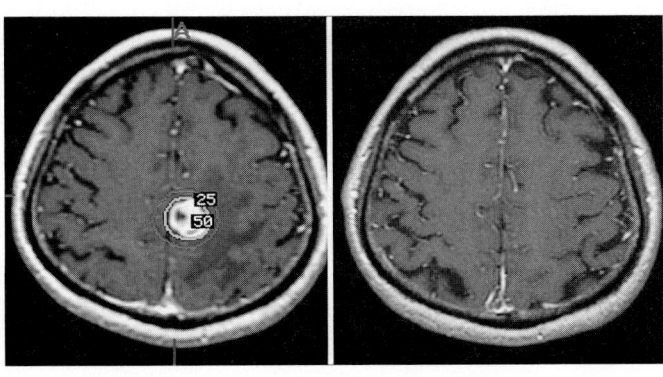

Figure 56-4. Postcontrast T1-weighted magnetic resonance imaging of a brain metastasis shown on the day of radiosurgery, with superimposed 50% and 25% isodose contours *(left)* and follow-up imaging 11 months later *(right)* showing near complete response. A dose of 17.5 Gy was prescribed to the 50% isodose contour.

62% of those randomized to whole-brain radiotherapy plus radiosurgery. Compared with whole-brain radiotherapy alone, radiosurgery plus whole-brain radiotherapy yielded significantly improved time to local failure (median, 36 months vs. 6 months; $P = 0.0005$) and time to any brain failure (median, 34 months vs. 5 months; $P = 0.002$); however, survival was not significantly different for the two arms (median, 7.5 months for whole-brain radiotherapy vs. 11 months for whole-brain radiotherapy plus radiosurgery; $P = 0.22$). Multiple patients who failed whole-brain radiotherapy alone underwent salvage radiosurgery.[44]

An RTOG trial from 1996 through June 2001 randomized 333 patients to whole-brain radiotherapy (37.5 Gy in 15 fractions) with or without radiosurgery boost.[76] The final publication should be an important contribution to the literature.

Radiosurgery Without Whole-Brain Radiotherapy for Newly Diagnosed Brain Metastases. Because of concern about possible late toxicity of whole-brain radiotherapy, several groups have tried managing patients using radiosurgery alone initially, followed by later salvage surgery, radiosurgery, whole-brain radiotherapy, or chemotherapy as needed.[33,73,77-79] Retrospective comparisons of initial radiosurgery only to radiosurgery with upfront whole-brain radiotherapy are summarized in Table 56-5. Survival was similar for radiosurgery alone initially vs. radiosurgery with upfront whole-brain radiotherapy for three of four studies. In those three studies, survival was about 5 months vs. about 6 months,[73] 11.3 months vs. 11.1 months,[77] and 8.2 vs. 8.6 months,[33] for radiosurgery alone or radiosurgery plus radiotherapy, respectively. In the fourth study, median survival time was thought to

least 70 and two to four brain metastases less than or equal to 2.5 cm in diameter, at least 5 mm from the optic chiasm (see Table 56-3).[44] The whole-brain radiotherapy regimen was 30 Gy in 12 fractions, and the radiosurgery dose was 16 Gy, given before, during, or after whole-brain radiotherapy, within 1 month of whole-brain radiotherapy. The study accrued only 27 patients because of early stopping rules based on a significant difference in brain control between the two arms. The median KPS was 100 in each arm of the study, and the median patient age was 58 years in the group receiving radiotherapy alone and 59 years in the group receiving radiosurgery as well. There was extracranial disease in 71% of the patients randomized to whole-brain radiotherapy alone but in only

TABLE 56-4

Results of Radiosurgery with or Without WBRT for Newly Diagnosed or Recurrent Brain Metastases						
FIRST AUTHOR	**NO. OF METASTASES/ PATIENTS**	**MEAN OR MEDIAN DOSE**	**MEDIAN TARGET VOLUME**	**LOCAL CONTROL BY LESION (%)**	**MEDIAN SURVIVAL (MO)**	**NECROSIS (%)**
Single metastases						
Auchter[62]	122/122	17.0 Gy	2.7 mL	86*/85†	12.9	0
Flickinger[63]	116/116	17.5 Gy	—	85*	11	4
Simonova[64]	237/237	21.5 Gy	7.5 mL	95*	9	2.5
Single or multiple metastases						
Chen[65]	431/190	20 Gy	2.8 mL	86†	7.8	3
Flickinger[66]	229/157	16.0 Gy	3.0 mL	89*	10	1
Fukuoka[67]	>215/130	>25 Gy	5.5 mL	≥96*	8	5
Gerosa[68]	343/225	21.1 Gy	5.7 mL	88†	9.2	—
Goodman[69]	682/258	18.5 Gy	1.7 mL	82†	9.1	—
Joseph[70]	189/120	26.6 Gy	5.3 mL	94*	7.4	17
Kihlstrom[71]	235/160	27.0 Gy	4.5 mL	94*	7	5
Moriarty[72]	643/353	15.0 Gy	2.5 mL	88†	10.5	3–6
Pirzkall[73]	311/236	20 Gy	—	92*	5.5	2
Sansur[74]	411/193	20 Gy	—	82 by pt.	7.5	2
Young[75]	669/250	—	—	91*	7	<4

pt, patient.
*Crude.
†1-yr actuarial.

TABLE 56-5

Nonrandomized Comparisons of Radiosurgery Alone Initially to Radiosurgery Plus Upfront WBRT for Single or Multiple Newly Diagnosed Brain Metastases

STUDY (YEARS)	TREATMENT	NO. OF PATIENTS	SINGLE BRAIN METASTASIS (%)	EXTRA CRANIAL DISEASE (%)	1-YEAR LOCAL FFP	MEDIAN BRAIN FFP (MO)	MEDIAN SURVIVAL (MO)
Pirzkall et al.	RS	158	76	68	89	—	~5
(1984–1997)[73]	RS + WBRT	78	71	67	92	—	~6
					(P = 0.13)	—	(P = NS)
Sneed et al.	RS	62	58	74	71	8.3 (19.8*)	11.3
(1991–1997)[77]	RS + WBRT	43	33	65	79	15.9 (18.1*)	11.1
					(P = 0.30)	(P = 0.008; 0.31*)	(P = 0.80)
Chidel et al.	RS	78	74	—	~62	9.2	10.5
(1989–1998)[78]	RS + WBRT	57	60	—	~75	35.1	6.4
					(P = 0.034)	(P = 0.027)	—
Sneed et al.	RS	268	63	70–71	—	—	8.2
(1989–1998)[33]	RS + WBRT	301	58	64–68	—	—	8.6
							(P = 0.93)

FFP, freedom from progression; NS, not significant; RS, radiosurgery; WBRT, whole-brain radiotherapy.
*Median brain FFP and P value allowing for successful salvage therapy.

be worse in the whole-brain radiotherapy group because of worse prognostic factors in this group.[78] Multivariate analyses adjusting for known prognostic factors confirmed that giving whole-brain radiotherapy up front had no influence on survival time.[33,73,77,78] Comparing initial radiosurgery only to radiosurgery with upfront whole-brain radiotherapy in the multi-institutional retrospective review, RPA class 1, 2, and 3 patients had 1-year survival probabilities of 56% vs. 56%, 38% vs. 29%, and 21% vs. 11%, respectively, with median survival times of 14.0 vs. 15.2 months (P = 0.98), 8.2 vs. 7.0 months (P = 0.38), and 5.3 vs. 5.5 months (P = 0.51), respectively (see Table 56-1).[33] In the other series, summarized in Table 56-5, local control was slightly worse for radiosurgery alone initially, with 1-year actuarial local freedom from progression probabilities of 89% vs. 92%,[73] 71% vs. 79%,[77] and approximately 62% vs. 75%.[78] Because of a much greater risk of developing new brain metastases when upfront whole-brain radiotherapy was not done, freedom from progression in the brain was significantly worse in the group receiving radiosurgery alone initially: median, 8.3 months vs. 15.9 months[77] and 9.2 months vs. 35.1 months.[78] In one series, the median time during which the brain was controlled (allowing for salvage therapy) was 19.8 months for radiosurgery alone initially vs. 18.1 mo. for radiosurgery with upfront whole-brain radiotherapy, and only 26% of radiosurgery-alone patients ultimately received whole-brain radiotherapy.[77] The authors concluded that selected patients may be appropriately managed with radiosurgery alone initially, given the success of salvaging new or recurrent brain metastases as needed. However, others have pointed out that a potential danger of this approach is that a significant proportion of brain metastases that develop or progress after radiosurgery alone may be symptomatic.[80] Furthermore, salvage therapy may not be successful, and radiosurgery plus later salvage therapy could be more costly than approaches including upfront whole-brain radiotherapy. Thus, although omission of upfront whole-brain radiotherapy does not appear to compromise length of survival, it could compromise ultimate intracranial control or neurologic outcome and add monetary cost. Prospective trials are underway to compare radiosurgery alone initially to radiosurgery with upfront whole-brain radiotherapy.

Radiosurgery Compared with Surgery. Radiosurgery has potential advantages over surgery in that it is less invasive and can more easily address inaccessible or multiple lesions. In addition, the border zone between the metastasis and normal brain tissue may receive a radiation dose sufficient to decrease the risk of local recurrence. The two major disadvantages of radiosurgery are that it generally is applicable only to lesions less than about 2.5 to 3.0 cm in diameter and that it results in slow tumor shrinkage over weeks or months rather than relieving mass effect immediately.

In the absence of data to date from prospective, randomized trials, several authors have compared their own results for radiosurgery patients with results cited in the literature for surgical patients Auchter and co-workers[62] reported a four-institution experience of radiosurgery and whole-brain radiotherapy in 122 adults who met selection criteria similar to those used in randomized trials of whole-brain radiotherapy with or without surgical resection:[19,50] KPS of at least 70 and newly diagnosed, surgically resectable single brain metastases with "nonsensitive" histology (excluding lymphoma, leukemia, multiple myeloma, small cell lung cancer, and germ cell tumors) and no urgent indication for resection. Local control was achieved in 86% of lesions with a 1-year actuarial local control probability of 85%, a median duration of functional independence of 10.1 months, and median survival time of 12.9 months (see Table 56-4),[62]

TABLE 56-6

Nonrandomized Comparisons of Radiosurgery with and Without WBRT to Surgery with and Without WBRT for Single Newly Diagnosed Brain Metastases

STUDY (YEARS)	TREATMENT	NO. OF PATIENTS	SINGLE BRAIN METASTASIS (%)	EXTRA CRANIAL DISEASE (%)	LOCAL FFP (%)	MEDIAN SURVIVAL
Bindal et al. (1991-1994)[81]	RS ± WBRT	31	77	42	61*	7.5 mo
	Surgery ± WBRT	62	74	52	87*	16.4 mo
					(P = 0.0001)	(P = 0.0018)
Muacevic et al. (1990–1997)[58]	RS alone	56	100	—	83†	8.0 mo
	Surgery ± WBRT	52	100	—	75†	15.6 mo
					(P = 0.49)	(P = 0.19)
O'Neill et al. (1991–1999)[82]	RS + WBRT	23	100	74	100	56% 1 yr
	Surgery ± WBRT	74	100	55	85	62% 1 yr
					(P = 0.020)	(P = 0.15)

FFP, freedom from progression; RS, radiosurgery; WBRT, whole-brain radiotherapy.
*Crude.
†1-yr actuarial.

comparable to the results of the "surgery plus whole-brain radiotherapy" arms of the randomized trials reported by Patchell and coworkers[19] and Noordijk and coworkers[50] (see Table 56-3).

Three other retrospective comparisons of radiosurgery and surgery are summarized in Table 56-6, with somewhat differing results.[58,81,82] Bindal and coworkers reported 61% crude local control rates for radiosurgery (with or without whole-brain radiotherapy) compared with a rate of 87% with conventional surgery (with or without whole-brain radiotherapy) and median survival times of 7.5 months and 16.4 months for radiosurgery and conventional surgery, respectively, with or without whole-brain radiotherapy.

In another retrospective study, Muacevic and coworkers compared outcome for patients with single metastases 3.5 cm or less in diameter treated with radiosurgery alone (56 patients) or surgery with whole-brain radiotherapy (52 patients). One-year local freedom from progression probabilities were 83% for radiosurgery compared with 75% for surgery with whole-brain radiotherapy (P = 0.49); new brain metastases developed in 11 (20%) of the radiosurgery patients and 6 (12%) of the surgery-plus-whole-brain-radiotherapy patients, but salvage radiosurgery was successful in all 6 radiosurgery patients who were offered salvage therapy. Median survival times were 8.0 months after radiosurgery compared with 15.6 months after surgery with whole-brain radiotherapy. Death rates from neurologic causes and complication rates were similar for the two treatment approaches, and corticosteroid requirements tended to be less among the radiosurgery patients.[58]

A third retrospective study compared patients with single metastases who were candidates for either surgery or radiosurgery. Most patients received adjuvant whole-brain radiotherapy in conjunction with radiosurgery (23 patients) or surgery (74 patients). Pretreatment performance status was worse in the radiosurgery group. Crude local control rates were 100% compared with 85%

(P = 0.02), and 1-year survival probabilities were 56% and 62% for radiosurgery and surgery, respectively (univariate P = 0.15; multivariate P = 0.62 with adjustment for age, performance status, and systemic disease status). Short-term complications occurred in 0% of patients undergoing radiosurgery compared with 13.5% of patients having conventional surgery; long-term complications occurred in 17.4% and 17.6% of radiosurgery and surgery patients, respectively.

Because of the difficulties in overcoming selection bias and other confounding factors in retrospective studies, a prospective, randomized trial is planned to better compare radiosurgery vs. surgery for single brain metastases.

Toxicity of Radiosurgery. Acute complications of radiosurgery occur in about 10% of patients, including seizures, headaches, exacerbation of preexisting neurologic deficits, nausea, and hemorrhage.[58,77,83] Early delayed and late complications may include transient perifocal edema responding to a short course of steroids in 7% to 18% of patients[58,73,83] or symptomatic radiation necrosis in an average of 4% of patients (see Table 56-4), causing headaches, seizures, or neurologic deficits. Symptoms usually respond to corticosteroids, but surgery may be needed if a patient requires a prolonged course of corticosteroids, tolerates them poorly, or remains symptomatic on corticosteroids, or if there is uncertainty as to whether a lesion represents progressive tumor or radiation necrosis.

Brachytherapy

Brachytherapy, the insertion of radioactive sources directly within a tumor or tumor bed, allows delivery of a high dose of radiation to the target volume with steep fall-off of dose outside of the intended region, because dose intensity decreases with the square of the distance from point sources and also decreases because of attenuation in tissue. Temporary brachytherapy has been applied to brain metastases using high-activity sources, often

TABLE 56-7

Results of Brachytherapy for Newly Diagnosed or Recurrent Brain Metastases

STUDY (YEARS)	TECHNIQUE/ ISOTOPE	PATIENTS (NO./TYPE)	ADJUVANT WBRT GIVEN?	CRUDE LOCAL FFP (%)	MEDIAN SURVIVAL (MO)	NECROSIS (%)
Bernstein et al. (?–1994)[84]	Temporary/ I-125	10 recurrent	no	60	10.5	30
Bogart et al. (1991–1996)[85]	Permanent/ I-125	15 new	no	80	14	0
McDermott et al. (1979–1994)[86]	Temporary/ I-125	5 new	yes (4/5)	—	68.2	10
		25 recurrent	no	—	13.9	
Ostertag and Kreth (1982–1992)[87]	Temporary/ I-125	38 new	yes	89	17	0
		34 new	no	91	15	
		21 recurrent	no	95	6	
Schulder et al. (1987–?)[88]	Permanent/ I-125	1 new	no	82	9	15
		12 recurrent	no			
Huang K. (1997–2001)*	Permanent/ I-125	16 new	no	94	12.1	21
		12 recurrent	no	83	8.9	

FFP, freedom from progression; I-125, iodine-125–labeled; WBRT, whole-brain radiotherapy.
*Unpublished data from the University of California San Francisco.

within afterloading catheters inserted under stereotactic guidance into gross tumor or a resection cavity. Permanent brachytherapy usually is accomplished by lining a tumor bed with low-activity radiation sources intraoperatively after gross total resection of a metastasis. Results of brachytherapy for brain metastases are summarized in Table 56-7.[84-88] In patients treated for recurrent brain metastases, crude local freedom from progression rates ranged from 60% to 95% and median survival times from 6 to 13.9 months. Among patients treated for newly diagnosed brain metastases, local freedom from progression rates ranged from 80% to 94% and median survival times from 12 to 17 months (except for an outlier median survival time of 68.2 months in 5 patients). The incidence of symptomatic radiation necrosis ranged from 0% to 30%, with an average of about 7%. These data support the use of brachytherapy as a treatment option in selected patients with brain metastases; in patients managed surgically, permanent radiation sources placed at the time of resection give an excellent probability of local control, eliminating one of the two roles for postoperative whole-brain radiotherapy. However, if upfront whole-brain radiotherapy is withheld, there is a significantly higher risk of later development of distant brain metastases. There is a risk that these metastases may be symptomatic, and they may or may not be salvageable with later radiosurgery, whole-brain radiotherapy, or other therapy. This strategy of surgery with brachytherapy needs to be investigated prospectively and compared with surgery with whole-brain radiotherapy.

Chemotherapy

Most clinicians have considered chemotherapy to be relatively ineffective for brain metastases, presumably because the blood-brain barrier prevents adequate access of chemotherapy to these tumors. However, some chemotherapeutic agents partially or even readily cross the blood-brain barrier, and the fact that brain metastases enhance with contrast on CT or MRI shows that the blood-brain barrier is broken down within metastases. Chemotherapy with cisplatin at 100 mg/m^2 on day 1 and etoposide at 100 mg/m^2 on days 4, 6, and 8 every 3 weeks was used as the primary treatment in a phase II study of 22 breast cancer patients with brain metastases, resulting in a 23% complete response rate and 32% partial response rate.[89] This regimen was then used as first-line therapy in a prospective study conducted from 1986 to 1993 by a group of nine institutions: 116 patients with recently diagnosed, previously untreated brain metastases from breast cancer, non–small cell lung cancer, or melanoma were enrolled, and 107 were evaluable.[90] None of the melanoma patients achieved an objective response, but the complete response rates were 13% and 7% and partial response rates 25% and 23% among the patients with breast and lung cancer, respectively. The median duration of response was 7 to 8 months, the median overall time to progression was 3.9 months for breast and lung cancer patients, and the median survival times were 7.1 months for breast cancer patients, 7.4 months for lung cancer patients, and 3.9 months for melanoma patients.[90] Data were not collected on further therapy given after chemotherapy. Other regimens that have been studied in patients with brain metastases from non–small cell lung cancer include vinorelbine, gemcitabine, and carboplatin (with 15% complete response and 30% partial response in 20 patients)[91] and paclitaxel and cisplatin combined with either vinorelbine or gemcitabine (resulting in a 38% complete and partial response rate among 25 patients).[92] There also has been interest in temozolomide, an oral alkylating agent that crosses the blood-brain barrier. At Memorial Sloan-Kettering Cancer Center, 41 patients with recurrent or progressive brain metastases were treated with temozolomide at 150 to 200 mg/m^2 daily for 5 days, repeated monthly. The partial response rate was 5%; 37% of patients had stable disease; and the median survival time was 6.6 months.[93]

Follow-up and Salvage Therapy

In patients who are doing reasonably well from the standpoint of their systemic disease, we recommend follow-up MRI every 3 months after treatment for brain metastases to detect new, progressive, or recurrent brain metastases that may need to be addressed with salvage therapy. It is important to note that a contrast-enhancing lesion seen after high-dose external beam radiation, radiosurgery, or brachytherapy could represent radiation necrosis rather than recurrent tumor, and additional analyses may be needed before considering retreatment.[94] The same therapeutic options available for newly diagnosed brain metastases may be considered for new, progressive, or recurrent metastases, although the type of previous therapy given may influence therapeutic options at recurrence. In general, retreatment options include whole-brain radiotherapy; radiosurgery (especially for lesions less than about 3 cm in diameter); surgery (especially for a single large or symptomatic progressive lesion), perhaps with permanent brachytherapy to help prevent local recurrence; and chemotherapy. If repeat whole-brain radiotherapy is given, lower doses and smaller fraction sizes generally are used, such as 20 to 25 Gy in 10 fractions or 30 Gy at 1.0 Gy twice daily. Results are similar to those reported for a first course of whole-brain radiotherapy, with symptomatic improvement in 42% to 75% of patients and median or mean survival time of 3.2 to 5 months after reirradiation.[95-97]

CARCINOMATOUS MENINGITIS

Dissemination of cancer cells into the leptomeningeal space is an extremely serious complication that affects approximately 5% of patients with cancer. With incremental improvements in outcomes in systemic cancer, the incidence of metastatic disease to the leptomeninges appears to be on the rise. Neoplastic meningitis presents significant diagnostic and therapeutic challenges; early diagnosis can be elusive, and effective control for leptomeningeal carcinoma usually is difficult to achieve. With current therapies, the median survival time is 3 to 6 months.

Epidemiology

Virtually any type of cancer can disseminate into the leptomeningeal space. Acute leukemias and intermediate or high-grade lymphomas are common causes of neoplastic meningitis. Among solid tumors, melanoma and small cell carcinoma exhibit the strongest propensity for leptomeningeal dissemination, with up to 25% of patients with metastatic disease from these diagnoses developing this complication. Ultimately, between 2% and 5% of breast cancer patients develop carcinomatous meningitis. Leptomeningeal dissemination also has been documented in less common neoplasms such as sarcomas, squamous cell carcinomas, and germ cell tumors. Primary tumors of the central nervous system such as medulloblastoma or ependymoma often seed the leptomeningeal space as well.[98-102]

Pathophysiology

The biological basis for dissemination and multifocal seeding of the leptomeninges by malignant cells is not well understood. At least three distinct pathways exist: (1) as a consequence of drop metastases, which may occur during resection of metastatic foci within the brain, especially after resection of posterior fossa tumors; (2) infiltration through arachnoid vessels or the choroid plexus following hematogenous dissemination of the tumor; or (3) direct extension along peripheral nerves to the subarachnoid space or perivenous spread from the bone marrow within the skull. Spread of tumor cells along the meningeal surface is facilitated by bulk CSF flow. In turn, meningeal deposits also may invade parenchyma as well as cranial or spinal nerve roots. The regions of the CNS most frequently affected are the basilar cisterns, the posterior fossa, and the cauda equina, where gravity promotes deposition of circulating cells.

Clinical Presentation

Leptomeningeal dissemination of cancer elicits several distinct neurologic presentations. Local tumor infiltration in the brain or spinal cord may cause headache, alterations in mental status, cranial nerve deficits causing diplopia, hearing loss, decreased taste, problems with swallowing and hoarseness, as well as incontinence, lower motor neuron weakness, and back or radicular pain. Metabolic dysfunction caused by disturbances in regional blood flow in the affected nervous tissue may cause seizures, isolated neurologic deficits including stroke-like symptoms, and even generalized encephalopathy. Obstruction of normal CSF flow pathways by focal tumor deposits may cause increased intracranial pressure and hydrocephalus.[98-103]

Diagnosis

CSF Evaluation

A high index of suspicion is required to make an early diagnosis of neoplastic meningitis; this ultimately requires a detailed examination of the CSF. Routine measurements include opening pressure, cell count, differential, protein, glucose, and direct cytologic evaluation of the CSF. The CSF is abnormal in terms of protein or glucose concentration in most patients with neoplastic meningitis, however, cytologic evaluation of the CSF, the gold standard, is an extremely insensitive test, and 40% to 50% of patients with neoplastic meningitis have negative CSF cytology.[98] Repeat CSF cytologic evaluations over time will increase diagnostic sensitivity, but the eventual conversion to positive cytology usually occurs in pace with neurologic deterioration secondary to overt tumor progression. Because of the importance of early diagnosis and intervention, there has been a significant effort to identify surrogate biomarkers for CNS and leptomeningeal metastases. For example, in the early 1980s, Posner's group demonstrated that the tumor antigen carcinoembryonic antigen (CEA) as well as the enzymatic activity of beta-glucuronidase could be detected in the CSF in patients with brain and leptomeningeal metastases.[104] The presence of these markers was shown to precede clinical detection of neoplastic meningitis and to rise and fall in parallel with the clinical course. Unfortunately, no biomarker with adequate sensitivity and specificity has emerged to date, and the diagnosis relies heavily on cytology and clinical impression.

Radiologic Features

The most common radiographic presentation is hydrocephalus without an identifiable mass lesion. Meningeal contrast enhancement is suggestive of neoplastic meningitis (Fig. 56-5) but also may be seen after lumbar puncture and with infection, inflammatory disease, trauma, subdural hematoma, or changes occurring postcraniotomy. Although gadolinium-enhanced MRI is more sensitive than CT in identifying leptomeningeal enhancement, only about 50% of patients with neoplastic meningitis and spinal symptoms have abnormal imaging studies.[98]

Treatment

Current therapeutic goals for most patients with neoplastic meningitis are to prevent further neurologic deterioration, to cytoreduce leptomeningeal tumor burden, and to prolong survival. Typically, untreated carcinomatous meningitis is associated with an advanced stage of systemic disease, often with concomitant parenchymal brain metastases and with an anticipated survival time of 4 to 6 weeks. Because of the inefficient regenerative capacity of the central nervous system, early aggressive intervention is critical to preserve neurologic function. Therapeutic intervention relies on traditional approaches with radiation, chemotherapy, or both, with the goal of treating the entire neuroaxis.

Radiotherapy

Radiotherapy is the most effective means of palliation, with the focus on symptomatic sites and regions where

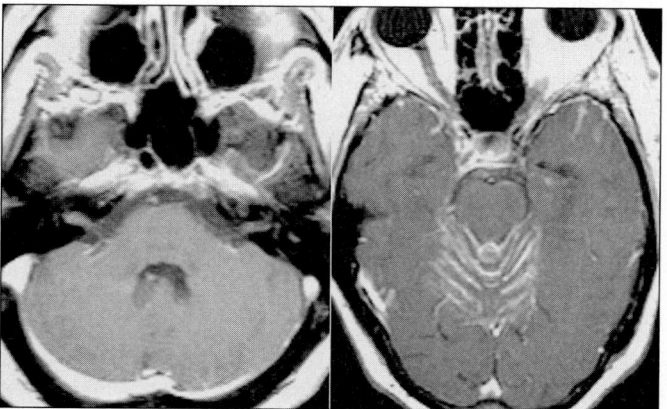

Figure 56-5. Postcontrast T1-weighted magnetic resonance imaging appearance of carcinomatous meningitis in two patients. Enhancement of both acoustic nerves is seen in the example on the *left*, and enhancement of the fissures of the cerebellar vermis is visible in the example on the *right*.

imaging studies have demonstrated bulk disease. There is substantial acute toxicity of craniospinal axis irradiation, with nausea, vomiting, marked fatigue, and myelosuppression. There is also a long-lasting negative impact on bone marrow function, compromising the safe administration of subsequent myelosuppressive chemotherapy. One strategy is to apply external beam irradiation selectively to symptomatic sites of disease and to rely on intrathecal chemotherapy to suppress the remainder of the disease in the neuroaxis. For example, in patients presenting with cranial nerve deficits, one approach is to treat only the base of the skull with radiation. In patients who present with cauda equina syndrome, external beam irradiation may be directed to the lumbosacral spine. Patients who present with seizure or hydrocephalus caused by extensive cranial leptomeningeal disease may best be palliated with whole-brain irradiation.[99-102]

Intrathecal Chemotherapy

The most reliable means of administering intrathecal chemotherapy is to use an implanted subcutaneous reservoir and ventricular catheter (Ommaya device). Although subarachnoid injections of chemotherapy result in high local CSF concentrations, studies of administration by lumbar administration suggest that 10% to 15% of lumbar punctures fail to deliver all of the drug to the subarachnoid space.[102] In addition, retrospective analysis suggests that intraventricular administration may result in prolonged remission in patients with leptomeningeal leukemia compared with administration by lumbar puncture.[105] Chemotherapeutic agents administered into the ventricle are carried through the neuroaxis by bulk CSF flow. Cerebrospinal fluid flow abnormalities are common in patients with leptomeningeal metastases, who often present with hydrocephalus and increased intracranial pressure as a result of disease that impedes CSF flow. Radionuclide ventriculography in patients with neoplastic meningitis has demonstrated that as many as 70% have ventricular outlet obstruction, abnormal flow in the spinal canal, or impaired flow over the CSF convexities.[106] These CSF flow abnormalities may be reversed with local irradiation. Because of the potential risk of irreversible neurotoxicity from high sustained concentrations of intrathecal chemotherapy, a CSF flow study is recommended for every patient beginning intrathecal chemotherapy via a ventricular catheter.[99,100]

Methotrexate and cytarabine are the agents most widely used for intrathecal chemotherapy. Intraventricular injection of methotrexate results in therapeutic concentrations (more than $1\ \mu M$) that persist for up to 48 hours; serum levels peak at approximately $0.1\ \mu M$ and fall more slowly. Treatment of active neoplastic meningitis typically consists of twice-weekly intrathecal therapy until CSF clears followed by weekly and then monthly maintenance therapy unless there is disease progression. The combination of twice-weekly methotrexate plus radiation results in an approximate 50% rate of disease stability or clinical improvement. Response should be assessed both in the ventricle and in the lumbar sac, where cytology is more likely to be positive. Intrathecal methotrexate can cause myelosuppression as well as mucositis, toxicities that can be attenuated by leucovorin. Leucovorin does not efficiently cross the blood-brain barrier in amounts sufficient to interfere with intra-CNS effects of methotrexate.

Cytosine arabinoside (Ara-C) also is commonly used but may have less efficacy in the treatment of neoplastic meningitis. Ara-C is inactivated by deamination by the enzyme cytidine deaminase. Low CNS levels of this enzyme result in relatively slow deamination of Ara-C within the brain and CSF, resulting in an extended half-life in the CNS compartment.[102]

Treatment-Related Toxicity

Placement of an intraventricular catheter is associated with less than 1% risk of perioperative hemorrhage. Extended use of the device is associated with at least a 5% risk of infection, usually with *Staphylococcus epidermidis* or *Staphylococcus aureus*. Impaired CSF flow of chemotherapy secondary to obstruction may result in seizures as well as acute arachnoiditis, characterized by nausea, vomiting, and mental status changes. For this reason, many practitioners obtain a radionuclide CSF flow study before initiation of intra-Ommaya chemotherapy. Ultimately the most significant toxicity associated with the treatment of leptomeningeal carcinomatosis is the development of a necrotizing leukoencephalopathy. This is most common in patients who have received intrathecal methotrexate following cranial irradiation. Initial findings are radiographic changes, usually symmetric abnormalities in white matter. Many of these patients subsequently develop progressive dementia that can progress to substantial debility and to death.[102]

Systemic Chemotherapy and New Approaches

A significant fraction of contrast-enhancing tumor visualized on neuroimaging studies theoretically is accessible by systemic chemotherapy, which is able to reach this fraction of tumor supplied by an abnormally permeable neovasculature. However, water-soluble chemotherapy drugs are limited by the intact blood-brain barrier, and systemic therapy fails to treat microscopic, nonenhancing disease both in brain parenchyma and in the subarachnoid space. One exception is high-dose systemic administration of methotrexate, which results in therapeutic levels in the CSF for a longer duration than the intrathecal route; this therapeutic strategy has been shown to be active in neoplastic meningitis in both lymphoma and in solid tumors. Moreover, systemic administration of methotrexate at high doses overcomes the problems associated with CSF flow obstruction, which may compromise subarachnoid administration. However, because high-dose methotrexate administration requires detailed inpatient monitoring of fluid status, urine alkalinization, and renal function, systemic administration of methotrexate at high doses is not appropriate or practical for all patients.[107]

Finally, in the current era of targeted therapeutics, there is increasing interest in the application of biologic

therapies in the leptomeningeal compartment, particularly small molecule inhibitors of signal-transducing molecules such as protein kinases or monoclonal antibodies against tumor-associated cell surface molecules. There is increasing evidence that when these agents are administered systemically they penetrate the leptomeningeal space inefficiently. For example, relatively low CSF levels of monoclonal antibodies that target CD20 in B-cell lymphomas or of small molecules that inhibit the bcr-abl tyrosine kinase have been documented recently after systemic administration.[108,109] Direct intra-CSF administration of monoclonal antibodies and immunotoxins is an area of current early phase investigation in the treatment or prophylaxis of neoplastic meningitis.[108,110]

REFERENCES

1. Posner JB, Chernik NL: Intracranial metastases from systemic cancer. Adv Neurol 1978;19:579-592.
2. Patel JK, Didolkar MS, Pickren JW, Moore, RH: Metastatic pattern of malignant melanoma. Am J Surg 1978;135:807-810.
3. Schouten LJ, Rutten J, Huveneers HAM, Twijnstra A: Incidence of brain metastases in a cohort of patients with carcinoma of the breast, colon, kidney, and lung and melanoma. Cancer 2002;94:2698-2705.
4. Jemal A, Murray T, Samuels A, Ghafoor A, Ward E, Thun MJ: Cancer statistics, 2003. CA Cancer J Clin 2003;53:5-26.
5. Delattre JY, Krol G, Thaler HT, Posner JB: Distribution of brain metastases. Arch Neurol 1988;45:741-744.
6. Nussbaum ES, Djalilian HR, Cho KH, Hall WA: Brain metastases histology, multiplicity, surgery, survival. Cancer 1996;78:1781-1788.
7. Graus F, Walker RW, Allen JC: Brain metastases in children. J Pediatr 1983;103:558-561.
8. Hwang TL, Close TP, Grego JM, Brannon WL, Gonzales F: Predilection of brain metastasis in gray and white matter junction and vascular border zones. Cancer 1996;77:1551-1555.
9. Hojo S, Hirano A: Pathology of metastases affecting the central nervous system. In Takakura K, Sano K, Hojo S, et al (eds): Metastatic Tumors of the Central Nervous System. Tokyo, Igaku-Shoin, 1982, pp 5-35.
10. Sze G, Milano E, Johnson C, Heier L: Detection of brain metastases: Comparison of contrast-enhanced MR with unenhanced MR and enhanced CT. Am J Neuroradiol 1990;11:785-791.
11. Yuh WTC, Fisher DJ, Runge VM, et al: Phase III multicenter trial of high-dose gadoteridol in MR evaluation of brain metastases. Am J Neuroradiol 1994;15:1037-1051.
12. Cairncross JG, Kim J-H, Posner JB: Radiation therapy for brain metastases. Ann Neurol 1980;7:529-541.
13. Posner JB: Management of central nervous system metastases. Semin Oncol 1977;4:81-91.
14. Davis PC, Hudgins PA, Peterman SB, Hoffman JC Jr: Diagnosis of cerebral metastases double-dose delayed CT vs contrast-enhanced MR imaging. Am J Neuroradiol 1991;12:293-300.
15. Schellinger PD, Meinck HM, Thron A: Diagnostic accuracy of MRI compared to CCT inpatients with brain metastases. J Neurooncol 1999;44:275-281.
16. Cha S, Knopp EA, Johnson G, Wetzel SG, Litt AW, Zagzag D: Intracranial mass lesions: dynamic contrast-enhanced susceptibility-weighted echo-planar perfusion MR imaging. Radiology 2002;223:11-29.
17. Law M, Cha S, Knopp EA, Johnson G, Arnett J, Litt AW: High-grade gliomas and solitary metastases: Differentiation by using perfusion and proton spectroscopic MR imaging. Radiology 2002;222:715-721.
18. Schaefer PW, Budzik RF Jr, Gonzalez RG: Imaging of cerebral metastases. Neurosurg Clin North Am 1996;7:393-423.
19. Patchell RA, Tibbs PA, Walsh JW, et al: A randomized trial of surgery in the treatment of single metastases to the brain. N Engl J Med 1990;322:494-500.

20. Franzini A, Leocata F, Giorgi C, Allegranza A, Servello D, Broggi G: Role of stereotactic biopsy in multifocal brain lesions: Considerations on 100 consecutive cases. J Neurol Neurosurg Psychiatry 1994;57:957–960.

21. Lang EF, Slater J: Metastatic brain tumors. Results of surgical and nonsurgical treatment. Surg Clin North Am 1964;44:865–872.

22. Markesbery WR, Brooks WH, Gupta GD, Young AB: Treatment for patients with cerebral metastases. Arch Neurol 1978;35:754–756.

23. Richards P, McKissock W: Intracranial metastases. BMJ 1963;1:15–18.

24. Horton J, Baxter DH, Olson KB: The management of metastases to the brain by irradiation and corticosteroids. Am J Roentgenol 1971;111:334–336.

25. Chao JH, Phillips R, Nickson JJ: Roentgen-ray therapy of cerebral metastases. Cancer 1954;7:682–689.

26. Chu FCH, Hilaris BB: Value of radiation therapy in the management of intracranial metastases. Cancer 1961;14:577–581.

27. Order SE, Hellman S, von Essen CF, Kligerman MM: Improvement in quality of survival following whole-brain irradiation for brain metastasis. Radiology 1968;91:149–153.

28. Borgelt B, Gelber R, Kramer S, et al: The palliation of brain metastases: Final results of the first two studies by the Radiation Therapy Oncology Group. Int J Radiat Oncol Biol Phys 1980;6:1–8.

29. Kurtz JM, Gelber R, Brady LW, Carella RJ, Cooper JS: The palliation of brain metastases in a favorable patient population: A randomized clinical trial by the Radiation Therapy Oncology Group. Int J Radiat Oncol Biol Phys 1981;7:891–895.

30. Murray KJ, Scott C, Greenberg HM, et al: A randomized phase III study of accelerated hyperfractionation versus standard in patients with unresected brain metastases: a report of the Radiation Therapy Oncology Group (RTOG) 9104. Int J Radiat Oncol Biol Phys 1997;39:571–574.

31. Lagerwaard FJ, Levendag PC, Nowak PJCM, Eijkenboom WMH, Hanssens PEJ, Schmitz PIM: Identification of prognostic factors in patients with brain metastases: A review of 1292 patients. Int J Radiat Oncol Biol Phys 1999;43:795–803.

32. Gaspar L, Scott C, Rotman M, et al: Recursive partitioning analysis (RPA) of prognostic factors in three Radiation Therapy Oncology Group (RTOG) brain metastases trials. Int J Radiat Oncol Biol Phys 1997;37:745–751.

33. Sneed PK, Suh JH, Goetsch SJ, et al: A multi-institutional review of radiosurgery alone vs. radiosurgery with whole brain radiotherapy as the initial management of brain metastases. Int J Radiat Oncol Biol Phys 2002;53:519–526.

34. Agboola O, Benoit B, Cross P, et al: Prognostic factors derived from recursive partitioning analysis (RPA) of Radiation Therapy Oncology Group (RTOG) brain metastases trials applied to surgically resected and irradiated brain metastatic cases. Int J Radiat Oncol Biol Phys 1998;42:155–159.

35. Batchelor T, DeAngelis LM: Medical management of cerebral metastases. Neurosurg Clin North Am 1996;7:435–446.

36. Cohen N, Strauss G, Lew R, Silver D, Recht L: Should prophylactic anticonvulsants be administered to patients with newly-diagnosed cerebral metastases? A retrospective analysis. J Clin Oncol 1988;6:1621–1624.

37. Glantz MJ, Cole BF, Friedberg MH, et al: A randomized, blinded, placebo-controlled trial of divalproex sodium prophylaxis in adults with newly-diagnosed brain tumors. Neurology 1996;46:985–991.

38. Coia LR: The role of radiation therapy in the treatment of brain metastases. Int J Radiat Oncol Biol Phys 1992;23:229–238.

39. Borgelt B, Gelber R, Larson M, Hendrickson F, Griffin T, Roth R: Ultra-rapid high dose irradiation schedules for the palliation of brain metastases: Final results of the first two studies by the Radiation Therapy Oncology Group. Int J Radiat Oncol Biol Phys 1981;7:1633–1638.

40. Hindo WA, DeTrana FAI, Lee M-S, Hendrickson FR: Large dose increment irradiation in treatment of cerebral metastases. Cancer 1970;26:138–141.

41. Young DF, Posner JB, Chu F, Nisce L: Rapid-course radiation therapy of cerebral metastases: Results and complications. Cancer 1974;34:1069–1076.

42. Nieder C, Berberich W, Schnabel K: Tumor-related prognostic factors for remission of brain metastases after radiotherapy. Int J Radiat Oncol Biol Phys 1997;39:25–30.

43. Nieder C, Berberich W, Niewald M, Walter K, Schnabel K: Relation between local result and total dose of radiotherapy for brain metastases. Int J Radiat Oncol Biol Phys 1995;33:349–355.

44. Kondziolka D, Patel A, Lunsford LD, Kassam A, Flickinger JC: Stereotactic radiosurgery plus whole brain radiotherapy versus radiotherapy alone for patients with multiple brain metastases. Int J Radiat Oncol Biol Phys 1999;45:427–434.

45. DeAngelis LM, Mandell LR, Thaler HT, et al: The role of postoperative radiotherapy after resection of single brain metastases. Neurosurgery 1989;24:798–805.

46. van der Ree RC, Dippel DW, Avezaat CJ, Sillevis Smitt PA, Vecht CJ, van den Brent MJ: Leptomeningeal metastasis after surgical resection of brain metastases. J Neurol Neurosurg Psychiatry 1999;66:225–227.

47. DeAngelis LM, Delattre JY, Posner JB: Radiation-induced dementia in patients cured of brain metastases. Neurology 1989;39:789–796.

48. Nieder C, Schwerdtfeger K, Steudel W-I, Schnabel K: Patterns of relapse and late toxicity after resection and whole-brain radiotherapy for solitary brain metastases. Strahlenther Onkol 1998;174:275–278.

49. Lang FF, Sawaya R: Surgical management of cerebral metastases. Neurosurg Clin North Am 1996;7:459–484.

50. Noordijk EM, Vecht CJ, Haaxma-Reiche H, et al: The choice of treatment of single brain metastasis should be based on extracranial tumor activity and age. Int J Radiat Oncol Biol Phys 1994;29:711–717.

51. Mintz AH, Kestle J, Rathbone MP, et al: A randomized trial to assess the efficacy of surgery in addition to radiotherapy in patients with a single cerebral metastasis. Cancer 1996;78:1470–1476.

52. Hendrickson FR, Lee M-S, Larson M, Gelber RD: The influence of surgery and radiation therapy on patients with brain metastases. Int J Radiat Oncol Biol Phys 1983;9:623–627.

53. Patchell RA, Cirrincione C, Thaler HT, Galicich JH, Kim J-H, Posner JB: Single brain metastases: Surgery plus radiation or radiation alone. Neurology 1986;36:447–453.

54. Sause WT, Crowley JJ, Morantz R, et al: Solitary brain metastasis: results of an RTOG/SWOG protocol evaluation surgery + RT versus RT alone. Am J Clin Oncol 1990;13:427–432.

55. Patchell RA, Tibbs PA, Regine WF, et al: Postoperative radiotherapy in the treatment of single metastases to the brain: A randomized trial. JAMA 1998;280:1485–1489.

56. Bindal RK, Sawaya R, Leavens ME, Lee, JJ: Surgical treatment of multiple brain metastases. J Neurosurg 1993;79:210–216.

57. Hazuka MB, Burleson WD, Stroud DN, Leonard CE, Lillehei KO, Kinzie JJ: Multiple brain metastases are associated with poor survival in patients treated with surgery and radiotherapy. J Clin Oncol 1993;11:369–373.

58. Muacevic A, Kreth FW, Horstmann GA, et al: Surgery and radiotherapy compared with gamma knife radiosurgery in the treatment of solitary cerebral metastases of small diameter. J Neurosurg 1999;91:35–43.

59. Kooy HM: Linear accelerators in stereotactic radiosurgery. In Alexander E 3rd, Loeffler JS, Lunsford LD (eds): Stereotactic Radiosurgery. New York, McGraw-Hill, 1993, pp 67–76.

60. Wu A, Lindner G, Maitz AH, et al: Physics of gamma knife approach on convergent beams in stereotactic radiosurgery. Int J Radiat Oncol Biol Phys 1990;18:941–949.

61. Shaw E, Scott C, Souhami L, et al: Single dose radiosurgical treatment of recurrent previously irradiated primary brain tumors and brain metastases: Final report of RTOG protocol 90-05. Int J Radiat Oncol Biol Phys 2000;47:291–298.

62. Auchter RM, Lamond JP, Alexander E 3rd, et al: A multiinstitutional outcome and prognostic factor analysis of radiosurgery for resectable single brain metastasis. Int J Radiat Oncol Biol Phys 1996;35:27–35.

63. Flickinger JC, Kondziolka D, Lunsford LD, et al: A multi-institutional experience with stereotactic radiosurgery for solitary brain metastasis. Int J Radiat Oncol Biol Phys 1994;28:797–802.

64. Simonova G, Liscak R, Novotny J Jr, Novotny J: Solitary brain metastases treated with the Leksell gamma knife: Prognostic factors for patients. Radiother Oncol 2000;57:207–213.

65. Chen JCT, Petrovich Z, O'Day S, et al: Stereotactic radiosurgery in the treatment of metastatic disease to the brain. Neurosurgery 2000;47:268–281.

66. Flickinger JC, Lunsford LD, Somaza S, Kondziolka D: Radiosurgery: Its role in brain metastasis management. Neurosurg Clin North Am 1996;7:497–504.

67. Fukuoka S, Seo Y, Takanashi M, Takahashi S, Suematsu K, Nakamura J: Radiosurgery of brain metastases with the Gamma Knife. Stereotact Funct Neurosurg 1996;66:193–200.

68. Gerosa M, Nicolato A, Severi F, et al: Gamma knife radiosurgery for intracranial metastases: From local tumor control to increased survival. Stereotact Funct Neurosurg 1996;66:184–192.

69. Goodman KA, Sneed PK, McDermott MW, et al: Relationship between pattern of enhancement and local control of brain metastases after radiosurgery. Int J Radiat Oncol Biol Phys 2001;50:139–146.

70. Joseph J, Adler JR, Cox RS, Hancock SL: Linear accelerator-based stereotaxic radiosurgery for brain metastases: The influence of number of lesions on survival. J Clin Oncol 1996;14:1085–1092.

71. Kihlstrom L, Karlsson B, Lindquist C: Gamma Knife surgery for cerebral metastases. Implications for survival based on 16 years experience. Stereotact Funct Neurosurg 1993;61:45–50.

72. Moriarty TM, Loeffler JS, Black PM, et al: Long-term follow-up of patients treated with stereotactic radiosurgery for single or multiple brain metastases. In Kondziolka D (ed): Radiosurgery 1995, vol 1. Basel, Karger, 1996, pp 83–91.

73. Pirzkall A, Debus J, Lohr F, et al: Radiosurgery alone or in combination with whole-brain radiotherapy for brain metastases. J Clin Oncol 1998;16:3563–3569.

74. Sansur CA, Chin LS, Ames JW, et al: Gamma knife radiosurgery for the treatment of brain metastases. Stereotact Funct Neurosurg 2000;74:37–51.

75. Young RF: Radiosurgery for the treatment of brain metastases. Semin Surg Oncol 1998;14:70–78.

76. Sperduto PW, Scott C, Andrews D, et al: Stereotactic radiosurgery with whole brain radiation therapy improves survival in patients with brain metastases: report of Radiation Therapy Oncology Group phase III study 95-08 (abstract). Int J Radiat Oncol Biol Phys 2002;54(Suppl 2):3.

77. Sneed PK, Lamborn KR, Forstner JM, et al: Radiosurgery for brain metastases: is whole brain radiotherapy necessary? Int J Radiat Oncol Biol Phys 1999;43:549–558.

78. Chidel MA, Suh JH, Reddy CA, Chao ST, Lundbeck MF, Barnett GH: Application of recursive partitioning analysis and evaluation of the use of whole brain radiation among patients treated with stereotactic radiosurgery for newly diagnosed brain metastases. Int J Radiat Oncol Biol Phys 2000;47:993–999.

79. Hasegawa T, Kondziolka D, Flickinger JC, Germanwala A, Lunsford DL: Brain metastases treated with radiosurgery alone: An alternative to whole brain radiotherapy? Neurosurgery 2003;52:1318–1326.

80. Regine WF, Huhn JL, Patchell RA, et al: Risk of symptomatic brain tumor recurrence and neurologic deficit after radiosurgery alone in patients with newly diagnosed brain metastases: results and implications. Int J Radiat Oncol Biol Phys 2002;52:333–338.

81. Bindal AK, Bindal RK, Hess KR, et al: Surgery versus radiosurgery in the treatment of brain metastasis. J Neurosurg 1996;84:748–754.

82. O'Neill BP, Iturria NJ, Link MJ, Pollock BE, Ballman KV, O'Fallon JR: A comparison of surgical resection and stereotactic radiosurgery in the treatment of solitary brain metastases. Int J Radiat Oncol Biol Phys 2003;55:1169–1176.

83. Shiau C-Y, Sneed PK, Shu H-KG, et al: Radiosurgery for brain metastases: relationship of dose and pattern of enhancement to local control. Int J Radiat Oncol Biol Phys 1997;37:375–383.

84. Bernstein M, Cabantog A, Laperriere N, Leung P, Thomason C: Brachytherapy for recurrent single brain metastasis. Canadian Journal of Neurological Science 1995;22:13–16.

85. Bogart JA, Ungureanu C, Shihadeh E, et al: Resection and permanent I-125 brachytherapy without whole brain irradiation for solitary brain metastasis from non-small cell lung carcinoma. J Neurooncol 1999;44:53–57.

86. McDermott MW, Cosgrove GR, Larson DA, Sneed PK, Gutin PH: Interstitial brachytherapy for intracranial metastases. Neurosurg Clin North Am 1996;7:485–495.

87. Ostertag CB, Kreth FW: Interstitial iodine-125 radiosurgery for cerebral metastases. Br J Neurosurg 1995;9:593–603.

88. Schulder M, Black PM, Shrieve DC, Alexander E 3rd, Loeffler JS: Permanent low-activity iodine-125 implants for cerebral metastases. J Neurooncol 1997;33:213–221.

89. Cocconi G, Lottici R, Bisagni G, et al: Combination therapy with platinum and etoposide of brain metastases from breast carcinoma. Cancer Invest 1990;8:327–334.

90. Franciosi V, Cocconi G, Michiara M, et al: Front-line chemotherapy with cisplatin and etoposide for patients with brain metastases from breast carcinoma, nonsmall cell lung carcinoma, or malignant melanoma. Cancer 1999;85:1599–1605.

91. Bernardo G, Cuzzoni Q, Strada MR, et al: First-line chemotherapy with vinorelbine, gemcitabine, and carboplatin in the treatment of brain metastases from non-small-cell lung cancer: A phase II study. Cancer Invest 2002;20:293–302.

92. Cortes J, Rodriguez J, Aramendia JM, et al: Front-line paclitaxel/cisplatin-based chemotherapy in brain metastases from non-small-cell lung cancer. Oncology 2003;64:28–35.

93. Abrey LE, Olson JD, Raizer JJ, et al: A phase II trial of temozolomide for patients with recurrent or progressive brain metastases. J Neurooncol 2001;53:259–265.

94. Sundaresan N, Galicich JH, Deck MDF, Tomita T: Radiation necrosis after treatment of solitary intracranial metastasis. Neurosurgery 1981;8:329–333.

95. Cooper JS, Steinfeld AD, Lerch IA: Cerebral metastases: Value of reirradiation in selected patients. Radiology 1990;174:883–885.

96. Kurup P, Reddy S, Hendrickson FR: Results of re-irradiation for cerebral metastases. Cancer 1980;46:2587–2589.

97. Wong WW, Schild SE, Sawyer TE, Shaw EG: Analysis of outcome in patients reirradiated for brain metastases. Int J Radiat Oncol Biol Phys 1996;34:585–590.

98. Chamberlain M: Neoplastic meningitis: A guide to diagnosis and treatment. Curr Opin Neurol 2000;13:641–648.

99. Grossman SA, Krabak MJ: Leptomeningeal carcinomatosis. Cancer Treat Rev 1999;25:103–119.

100. Grossman SA, Spence A: Cacinomatous/lymphomatous meningitis. The NCCN Clinical Practice Guidelines in Oncology 1999;13:144–160.

101. Jayson GC, Howell A: Carcinomatous meningitis in solid tumors. Ann Oncol 1996;7:773–786.

102. Posner JB: Neurologic complications of cancer. Philadelphia, FA Davis, 1995, pp 165–171.

103. DeAngelis LM: Current diagnosis and treatment of leptomeningeal metastasis. J Neurooncol 1998;38:245–252.

104. Schold SC, Wasserstrom WR, Fleisher M, Schwartz MK, Posner JB: Cerebrospinal fluid biochemical markers of central nervous system metastases. Ann Neurol 1980;8:597–604.

105. Bleyer WA, Poplack DG: Intraventricular versus intralumbar methotrexate for central-nervous-system leukemia: Prolonged remission with the Ommaya reservoir. Med Pediatr Oncol 1979;6:207–213.

106. Grossman SA, Trump DL, Chen DC, Thompson G, Camargo EE: Cerebrospinal fluid flow abnormalities in patients with neoplastic meningitis. An evaluation using [111]Indium-DTPA ventriculography. Am J Med 1982;73:641–647.

107. Glantz MJ, Cole BF, Recht L, et al: High-dose intravenous methotrexate for patients with nonleukemic leptomeningeal cancer: is intrathecal chemotherapy necessary? J Clin Oncol 1998;16:1561–1567.

108. Rubenstein JL, Combs D, Rosenberg J, et al: Rituximab therapy for CNS lymphomas: Targeting the leptomeningeal compartment. Blood 2003;101:466–468.

109. Petzer AL, Gunsilius E, Hayes M, et al: Low concentrations of STI571 in cerebrospinal fluid: A case report. Br J Haematol 2002;117:623–625.

110. Laske DW, Muraszko KM, Oldfield EH, et al: Intraventricular immunotoxin therapy for leptomeningeal neoplasia. Neurosurgery 1997;41:1039–1051.

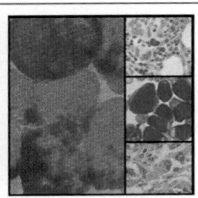

57

BONE METASTASES

Robert E. Coleman

Robert D. Rubens

SUMMARY OF KEY POINTS

INCIDENCE
- A major cause of (often prolonged) morbidity in cancer.
- Especially prevalent in breast and prostatic cancer.

CAUSES
- Osteolytic damage is mediated largely by stimulation of osteoclasts via tumor-derived cytokines; intermediary cells, including immune cells and osteoblasts, are involved.
- The vertebral-venous system of vessels is a significant anatomic pathway for metastatic spread to the skeleton.

DIAGNOSIS
- Differential diagnosis includes osteoporosis, degenerative disease, and Paget's disease.
- The isotope bone scan is a sensitive test to detect the presence of skeletal pathology but gives little information about its nature.
- Structural information on skeletal damage from metastatic bone

disease is best obtained by skeletal radiography supplemented by computerized tomography or magnetic resonance imaging.

EVALUATION OF THE PATIENT
- An assessment of patients' symptom and activity status is essential.
- Skeletal radiography assesses response to treatment, but the information is delayed and the method insensitive.
- Early indications of response of bone metastases to treatment can be obtained by monitoring biochemical markers, including the bone isoenzyme of alkaline phosphatase, osteocalcin, and pyridinium crosslinking amino acids.
- Isotopic bone scanning is not useful in monitoring response to treatment.

TREATMENT
- Antitumor treatments, such as radiation therapy, endocrine therapy, cytotoxic chemotherapy, and

targeted radio-isotope therapy, all have roles in palliating metastatic bone disease.
- The bisphosphonates are inhibitors of osteoclast activity and have become important agents for the treatment of metastatic bone disease, as they relieve symptoms, enable bone healing, and delay complications.

COMPLICATIONS
- Complications include pain, impaired mobility, pathologic fracture, spinal cord compression, cranial nerve palsies, nerve root lesions, hypercalcemia, and suppression of bone marrow function.
- Bisphosphonates together with intravenous rehydration are the treatments of choice for hypercalcemia.
- Orthopedic surgery has a role in the treatment and prophylaxis of pathologic fractures and spinal stabilization and in the relief of spinal cord compression.

INCIDENCE

Primary Tumors Leading to Bone Metastases

Primary bone cancer occurs predominantly among children and adolescents and is rare. By contrast, secondary bone cancer—particularly from carcinomas of the breast, lung, prostate, kidney, and thyroid—is common. The incidence of bone metastases from different primary sites recorded in postmortem studies is summarized in Table 57-1. Although the variability in these metastatic patterns is probably related to molecular and cellular biological characteristics of both the tumor cells and those of the tissues to which they metastasize, other factors, such as vascular pathways and blood flow, are also important.

Given the high prevalence of carcinomas of the breast, bronchus, and prostate, these cancers probably account for more than 80% of cases of metastatic bone disease. The

distribution of bone metastases is predominently to the axial skeleton—particularly the spine, pelvis, and ribs—rather than to the appendicular skeleton, although lesions in the humeri and femora are also common.[1]

Breast cancer, the most common malignancy in women of Western Europe and North America and which, in the areas of its highest incidence, accounts for some 10% of all cancers, is the tumor most often associated with metastatic bone disease. Because of the long clinical course this disease potentially can follow even after metastases have developed, morbidity from bone deposits presents a major problem for health care systems. There are no powerful predictors of which patients are at high risk of developing skeletal disease, but the incidence of bone metastases has been found to be significantly raised in association with steroid receptor-positive and well differentiated tumors.[2] A study of 587 patients dying from breast cancer showed that 69% had radiologic evidence of skeletal metastases before death, compared with 27% each for lung and liver metastases.[2] In this study, in which 2240 patients had presented with breast cancer over a ten-year

TABLE 57-1

Incidence of Skeletal Metastases from Autopsy Studies			
		INCIDENCE (%) OF BONE METASTASES	
PRIMARY TUMOR	**NO. OF STUDIES**	**MEDIAN**	**RANGE**
Breast	5	73	47–85
Prostate	6	68	33–85
Thyroid	4	42	28–60
Kidney	3	35	33–40
Bronchus	4	36	30–55
Esophagus	3	6	5–7
Gastrointestinal tract	4	5	3–11
Rectum	3	11	8–13

Modified from Galasko CSB: The anatomy and pathways of skeletal metastases. In Weiss L, Gilbert AH (eds): Bone Metastasis. Boston, GK Hall, 1981, p 49.

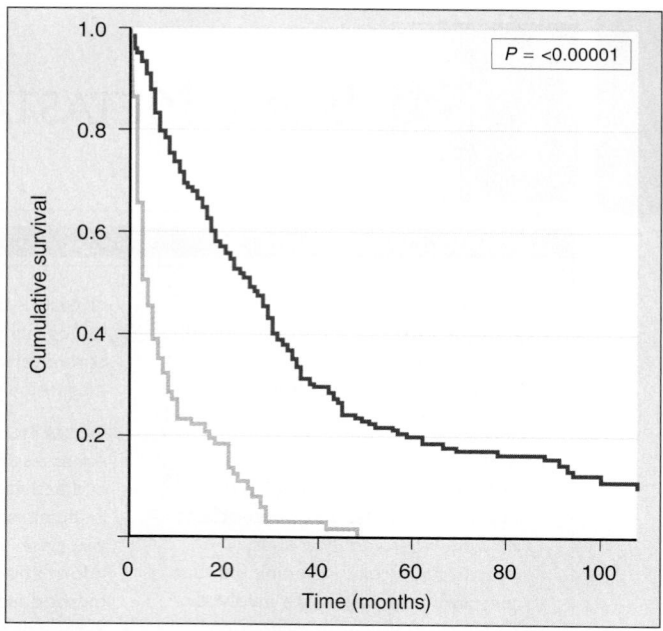

Figure 57-1. Survival of patients with breast cancer after first relapse in bone (*red curve*) compared with survival after first relapse in liver (*yellow curve*). (From Coleman RE, Rubens RD: The clinical course of bone metastases in breast cancer. Br J Cancer 1987;55:61–66.)

period, 681 patients (30%) had relapsed after a median follow-up of five years; 395 of these (58%) had distant metastases. One hundred eighty-four patients had their first relapse in bone, accounting for 47% of all those with first distant relapse, 24% of the total with any relapse (both local and distant), and 8% of the whole study population.

Although patients with first relapse in skeleton did not differ from those with first relapse in the liver either in terms of age, menstrual status, or median postoperative disease-free interval, the survival experience was markedly different for these two metastatic categories. Median survival after first relapse in bone was 20 months, compared to only three months after first relapse in liver (Fig. 57-1). For patients with metastatic bone disease apparently remaining confined to the skeleton, the median duration of survival was 24 months. These results show how protracted a problem bone metastases can be for many patients with breast cancer.

The prognosis after first relapse in bone is, however, influenced by other factors, as demonstrated in a further series of 367 patients.[3] Of this group, 139 women whose disease remained confined to the skeleton were significantly older and more likely to have lobular cancers and to have presented with little or no axillary lymph node involvement. The 228 women who subsequently developed extra-osseous metastases were more likely to have had poorly differentiated tumors and heavy nodal involvement at primary diagnosis. Favorable factors for a longer survival after first relapse in bone were low histologic grade, positive estrogen receptor status, long postoperative disease-free interval, and lack of development of extra-osseous disease.

The skeleton is by far the most common site of metastatic disease in prostatic cancer. Unlike breast cancer, in which radiologically the lesions frequently show a mix of osteoblastic and osteolytic appearances, osteosclerotic disease predominates in prostatic cancer. Nevertheless, computed tomography often identifies lytic areas within these ostensibly sclerotic lesions. Histologic studies also have demonstrated increased bone resorption in

metastatic prostatic cancer.[4] As in breast cancer, metastatic bone disease in prostatic cancer can follow a relatively long course. For example, patients of good performance status and bone-only disease affecting the axial skeleton have a median survival of about 53 months, compared with 30 months for those with additional visceral disease and only 12 months for poor-performance status patients with both bone and visceral disease.[5]

In lung cancer, the incidence of bone metastases identifiable at the time of primary diagnosis is highest in the small cell variety and lowest with squamous cell tumors, but at autopsy the incidence of bone metastases is similar for all four main histologic types of lung cancer (squamous cell, small cell, large cell anaplastic, and adenocarcinoma) at about 30%.[6] Survival from primary diagnosis of lung cancer is poor, and fewer than 10% of patients are alive after five years. Once metastatic disease is evident, most patients die within a few months. Bone metastases from lung cancer are usually of the osteolytic type, but because of the poor survival prospects, morbidity from them is much less of a long-term health care problem than for either breast or prostatic cancers.

CAUSES

Mechanisms of Metastases

The predominant distribution of bone metastases in the axial skeleton, in which most of the red bone marrow is situated, suggests that the slow blood flow at these sites could assist in the attachment of metastatic cells. Contrast

this, for example, with the circulation in the kidneys, which accounts for a high proportion of cardiac output and in which metastatic disease is extremely rare. This explanation alone does not account adequately for metastatic patterns, however. It seems likely that molecular properties of both the malignant cells and those of the tissue in which metastases develop must also be important. Furthermore, the high incidence of bone metastases, without corresponding lesions in the lungs, has raised questions about the precise route cancer cells take from primary tumors to the skeleton. The absence of lung deposits makes it unlikely that malignant cells pass through the pulmonary circulation. Even if lung tissue is not receptive as a site for the establishment of metastatic disease, tumor cells are unlikely to pass through its narrow capillaries, particularly when they are aggregated as tumor emboli.

The experiments of Batson[7] in animal and human cadavers, which demonstrated the vertebral-venous plexus, provide a good explanation for the predilection of metastatic spread from certain cancers to the skeleton. He demonstrated how venous blood from both the pelvis and the breast flowed not only into the venae cavae but also directly into the vertebral-venous plexus. Moreover, the flow into the vertebral veins predominated when intrathoracic or intra-abdominal pressure was elevated, as, for example, during Valsalva's maneuver and so, presumably, during its physiologic counterparts, such as coughing.

These experiments helped to explain the tendency of prostatic and breast cancers to produce metastases in the axial skeleton and limb girdles. Further studies demonstrated the extent of this network of valveless vessels, which involve the epidural veins, perivertebral veins, veins of the thoroco-abdominal wall, and veins of the head and neck, all carrying blood under low pressure. In this system, blood is continually subjected to arrest and reversal of the direction of flow. This vertebral-venous system parallels, connects with, and provides bypasses for the portal, pulmonary, and caval system of veins and so provides a pathway for the spread of disease between distant organs. Primary lung tumors invade the pulmonary venous system directly to gain access to the arterial circulation for dissemination.

Pathogenesis

Bone is a specialized connective tissue with a matrix consisting predominantly of type I collagen; it consists of an inner core of trabecular or spongiform bone covered by an outer shell of cortical bone. Although trabecular bone contains only 20%–25% of the total body calcium, its great surface area gives structural rigidity to the skeleton.

Shaping of the skeleton and the buildup of bone mass during childhood and adolescence result from bone growth and bone modelling processes. After reaching the so-called "peak bone mass" in early adult life, the bone remains an active tissue, and within focal sites scattered throughout the skeleton, microscopic quantities of old bone are continuously being replaced. In the normal adult skeleton, there are approximately two million of these remodeling units. Bone remodeling is an orderly process of resorption followed by new bone formation, which is essential for bone strength and occurs in response to mechanical stress. Bone resorption is mediated by the osteoclast, a multinucleated giant cell derived from granulocyte-macrophage precursors, whereas bone formation requires the presence and function of osteoblasts, derived from mesenchymal fibroblast-like cells. In a healthy individual, bone remodeling is regulated carefully by a mechanism known as coupling, which is mediated by a complex interaction of hormones, paracrine growth factors, and cytokines. Under normal circumstances and at any one time, 80%–95% of the adult bone surface is in a quiescent state, while the rest is involved in various stages of the remodeling cycle (Fig. 57-2).

The total duration of a remodeling cycle in young adults is estimated to be around 200 days. If the osteoblasts have deposited exactly the same amount of bone as has been removed previously by the osteoclasts, the remodeling cycle is in balance. In the situation of an imbalance of remodeling, a remodeling cycle will end with either a small gain in bone (positive balance) or, as is more frequently the case in malignancy, a small loss of bone (negative balance).

In metastatic bone disease, damage to the skeleton is usually much more extensive than could be expected simply from the number of malignant cells present. Much evidence has now accumulated showing that most of the tumor-induced skeletal destruction is mediated by osteoclasts (Fig. 57-3). Although tumor masses can damage the skeleton in other ways—possibly by compression of vasculature and consequent ischaemia in the late stages of cancer—these processes are believed to be of less importance than the destruction of bone by osteoclasts.

Malignant cells secrete factors that stimulate osteoclastic activity both directly and indirectly.[8] These factors include prostaglandin-E (PGE) and a variety of cytokines and growth factors, such as transforming growth factor (TGF) α and β, epidermal growth factor (EGF), tumor necrosis factor (TNF), and interleukin-1 (IL-1). For example, IL-1, the most powerful stimulator of bone resorption in vitro, is produced by squamous carcinoma cells.[9] Several human breast cancer lines have also been shown to produce osteoclast stimulating factors, including TGF-α, TGF-β, EGF, parathyroid hormone-related protein (PTH-rP), and prostaglandins.[10] Procathepsin D, another osteoclast stimulating factor, has also been shown to be a breast cancer cell product; this enzyme is under the regulatory control of estrogens in the MCF-7 cell line.[11,12] The active form of this enzyme stimulates bone resorption in vitro and is associated with proteolysis of collagen chains and the activation of TGF-β. Normal bone trabeculae are lined by a thin layer of uncalcified matrix, which protects the calcified bone from osteoclastic activity, and the action of these proteolytic enzymes might be a prerequisite for osteoclastic bone resorption.[13]

Malignant cells might also stimulate bone resorption by stimulating tumor-associated immune cells to release osteoclast-activating factors.[14] It has been shown that human melanoma cells produce a factor that stimulates macrophages to release TNF and IL-1 in vitro. Further-

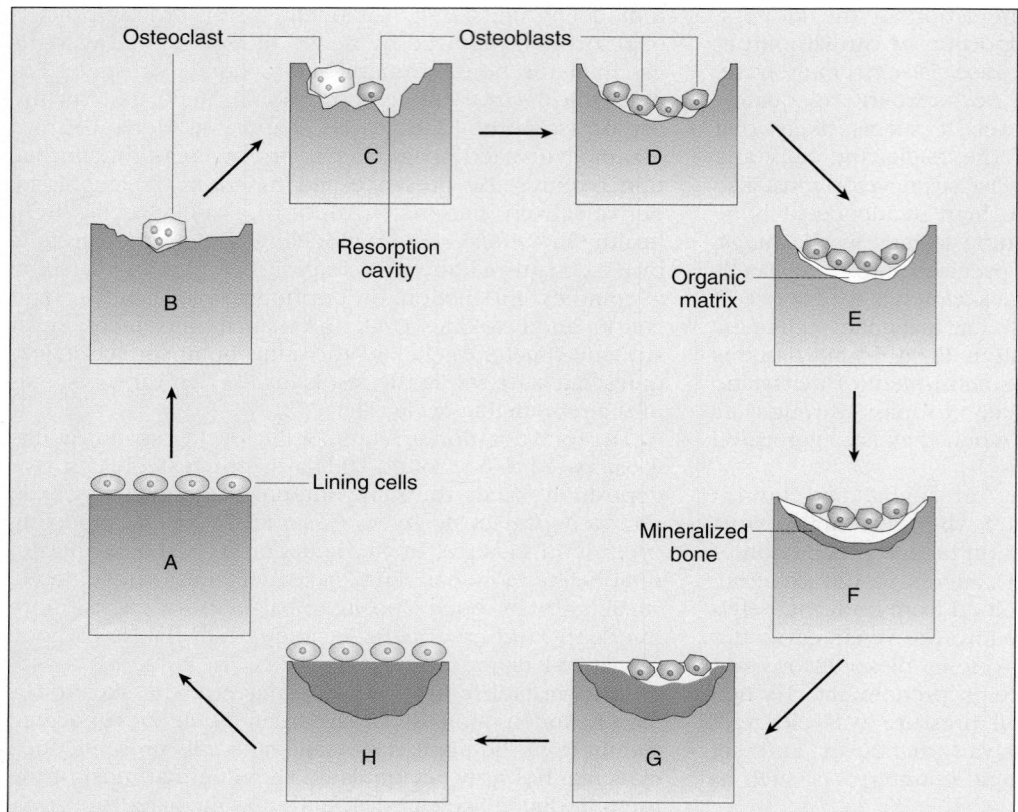

Figure 57-2. Schematic diagram illustrating the normal bone (A) remodeling cycle. Osteoclasts attracted to a site of fatigued bone create an erosion cavity (B and C). Osteoblasts are attracted and synthesize the organic matrix, which will fill the resorption cavity (D–F). The new bone is then remineralized to complete the remodeling process (G and H).

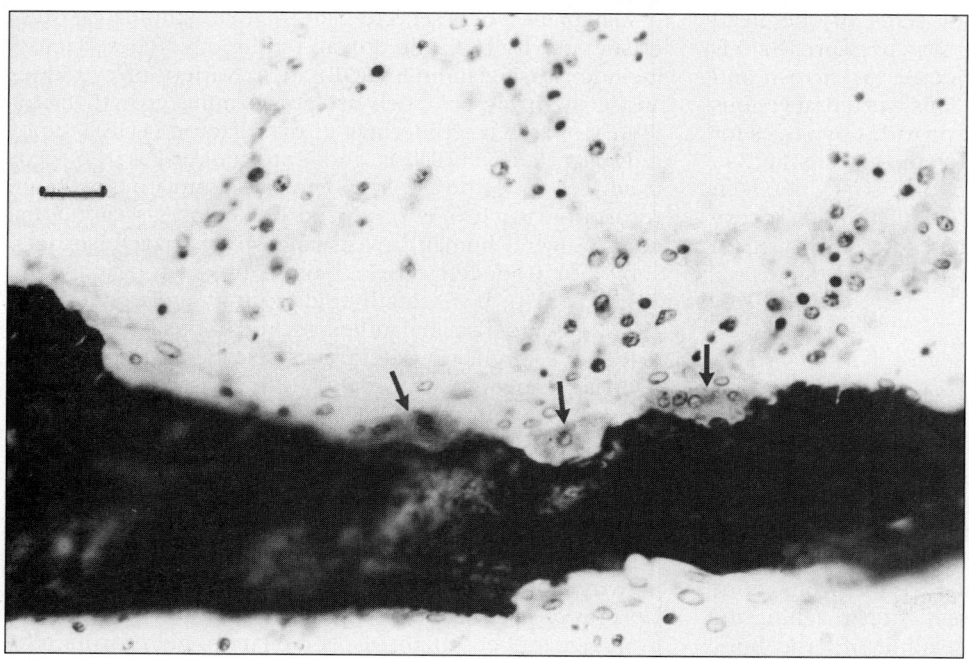

Figure 57-3. Histological section showing resorption lacunae on a bone trabeculum. Multinuclate osteoclasts (*arrows*) are resorbing bone in close association with mononuclear hemopoietic cells. The bar represents 20 μm. (From Boyce BF: Normal bone remodeling and its disruption in metastatic bone disease. In Rubens RD, Fogelman I [eds]: Bone Metastases—Diagnosis and Treatment. London, Springer Verlag, 1991, p 14, with permission).

more, purification of a cytokine-releasing factor from medium conditioned by melanoma cells has identified it as granulocyte-macrophage colony stimulating factor (GM-CSF) which activates osteoclastic bone resorption.[15] The complex interaction between tumor cells, osteoblasts, osteoclasts, and associated immune cells is summarized in Figure 57-4.

In addition to the local paracrine factors just described, osteoclastic activity can also be stimulated in malignant disease by systemic factors, particularly PTH-rP. This peptide is immunologically distinct from parathyroid hormone, but the two hormones have significant homology at the amino terminus of the molecule, which is necessary for osteoclast stimulation.[16] Ectopic production of this hormone, particularly in lung cancer, is a cause of osteoclastic bone resorption and hypercalcemia even in the absence of bone metastases.

It appears that these factors act only indirectly on osteoclasts, as these cells lack the required surface receptors. The receptors are expressed on osteoblasts, however, and these cells appear to control bone resorption by their influence on osteoclasts. In vitro studies of isolated osteoclasts show that they are not stimulated when exposed to any of the stimulating factors alone.[17] When exposed to these factors in the presence of osteoblasts, however, osteoclastic activity is increased; this does not depend upon direct cell-to-cell contact but rather is due to a diffusable factor. A further function of osteoblasts in controlling bone resorption is probably the production of collagenase, which can degrade the bone matrix.[18]

Although osteolytic disease is usually most evident at sites of bone metastases, osteosclerosis sometimes can predominate, particularly in prostatic cancer. In some instances, new bone formation is not necessarily preceded by bone resorption.[19] Osteoblast growth factors, such as TGF-β and platelet-derived growth factor, have been purified from prostatic tumor cells.[20]

Recently, the importance of PTHrP in the pathogenesis of osteolysis induced by metastatic breast cancer has been described.[21] In bone metastases, the secreted PTHrP acts in a paracrine manner to stimulate osteoclastic bone resorption. Not only does this lead to skeletal damage, but it also appears to confer a selective growth advantage on the tumor cells. This results from the release of factors for tumor growth from bone during the osteolytic process. Hence, a vicious circle is established in which the growth of metastatic cells is potentiated, leading to enhanced osteolysis and secretion of further growth factors to stimulate tumor cell proliferation.[22] This paracrine activity occurs even in the absence of hypercalcemia or increased circulating PTHrP levels. PTHrP stimulates osteoclastic resorption by increasing osteoblast and stromal cell production of receptor activator of nuclear factor κ B (RANK) ligand.[23] RANK ligand binds to its receptor, RANK, on osteoclast lineage cells, resulting in differentiation to mature osteoclasts and stimulation of osteoclast activity. In the normal bone environment, osteoblast secretion of osteoprotegerin (OPG) neutralises RANK ligand, so terminating its stimulatory effects on osteoclasts. In bone harboring cancer cells, however, there is a deregulation of the microenvironment. The MCF-7 estrogen-dependent breast cancer cell line has been found to decrease osteoblastic OPG mRNA levels, so enhancing osteoclast formation.[23] This imbalance is further compounded by release of transforming growth factor-beta (TGF-β) and insulin-like growth factor (IGF-1) resorbing bone, which further promotes tumor production of PTHrP, so promoting a perpetuating cycle of osteolytic bone destruction.[24]

Tumor cells might also have direct cell-to-cell interaction with bone marrow cells. One study recently found that prostate cancer cells are able to express a soluble form of RANKL (sRANKL) on the cell surface, a finding that implies a direct ability of prostate cancer cells to affect bone resorption.[25,26]

Prostate cancer, in contrast to breast cancer, tends to cause osteoblastic lesions in bone, leading to dense, sclerotic-looking metastases on plain radiographs. One of the factors that might be involved in prostatic bone lesions is the growth factor endothelin-1 (ET-1), which is produced by prostate cancer cells. Circulating levels have been found to be increased in patients with osteoblastic bone metastases from androgen-refractory prostate cancer, compared with patients whose cancer is confined to the prostate and normal controls.[27] Endothelin-1 has been found to stimulate osteoblast activity in animal models and to inhibit osteoclast activity, while antagonists of endothelin have been found to inhibit bone formation in vivo.[28,29] Furthermore, a recent study found that endothelin-1 production by prostate cancer cells is reduced by androgens but is stimulated in androgen-insensitive prostate cancer cells by factors (such as TGF-β).[30] This finding is clinically relevant, as metastatic prostate cancer typically develops androgen resistance. It

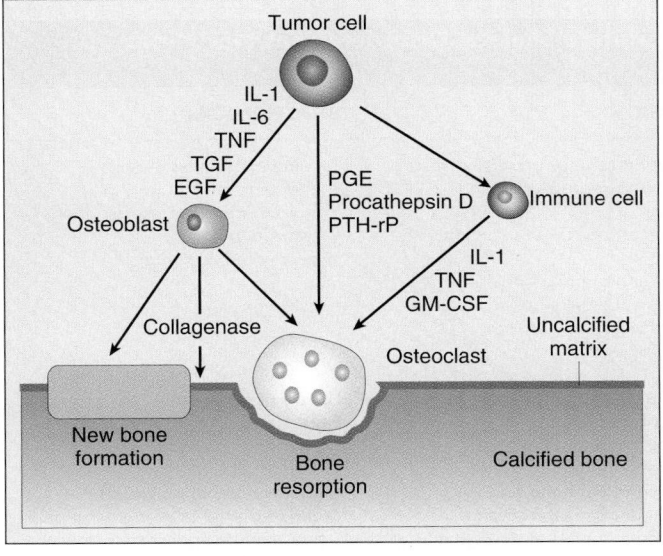

Figure 57-4. Diagrammatic summary of the cellular and molecular interactions involved in bone resorption and new bone formation in metastatic disease of the skeleton. EGF, epidermal growth factor; GM-CSF, granulocyte macrophage colony stimulating factor; IL-1, interleukin 1; IL-6, interleukin 6; PGE, prostaglandin-E; PTH-rP, parathyroid hormone-related protein; TGF, transforming growth factor (α and β); TNF, tumor necrosis factor.

is possible that PTHrP is also involved in the pathogenesis of prostate cancer bone metastases, as coexpression of PTHrP and its receptor has been found in both the primary tumor and in bone metastases of patients with prostate cancer.[31]

Evidence from morphometric studies and measurement of urinary markers of osteolytic bone resorption has led to the hypothesis that initially, osteoclastic bone resorption in prostate cancer is important, followed by intense osteoblastic activity.[32] This might not necessarily always be the case, however. A recent study found that the prostate cancer cell line PC-3 implanted into tibia of SCID mice caused osteolytic lesions, possibly through secretion of RANK ligand.[33] When another prostate cancer cell line (LAPC-9) was used, however, osteoblastic lesions developed even when no osteoclasts were present. Therefore, in this study the authors concluded that osteoclastic activity might not be a prerequisite for the formation of osteoblastic lesions.

In myeloma bone disease, bone marrow stromal cells are important for the pathogenesis of multiple myeloma.[34] Interleukin-6 appears to be an important growth and survival factor for myeloma cells and for conferring resistance to treatment with dexamethasone, a commonly used treatment for multiple myeloma. Barille and colleagues[35] also found that metalloproteinases (MMPs), known to be important in normal and malignant remodeling, contribute to the pathogenesis of myeloma. Bone marrow stromal cells secrete interstitial collagenases (MMP-1) and gelatinase A (MMP-2). MMP-1 initiates bone resorption, degrading type I collagen, which becomes a substrate for MMP-2.[35] Malignant plasma cells have been found to upregulate MMP-1 and activate MMP-2.[34]

DIAGNOSIS

Differential Diagnosis

Metastatic involvement of the skeleton typically affects multiple sites and causes pain, bony tenderness, and increasing disability. The diagnosis is often straightforward but occasionally can be difficult to make, and confusion with benign pathology is particularly a problem for elderly patients, in whom degenerative disease and osteoporosis are common. Particularly difficult clinical situations include elderly women with painful collapsed vertebrae who have a past history of breast cancer and in whom it can be difficult to distinguish osteoporotic collapse from metastatic destruction, and elderly men with prostatic cancer and pelvic pain with sclerotic radiologic changes in the pelvis attributable to either metastases or Paget's disease of bone.

In all cases, appropriate imaging tests are necessary and need to be interpreted in conjunction with the clinical picture, information from measurement of biochemical markers of bone metabolism and, when appropriate, serum tumor markers. Occasionally, bone biopsy under radiologic control or at open operation is necessary. Table 57-2 summarizes the typical clinical, radiologic, bone scan, and biochemical abnormalities of the more common skeletal pathologies.

TABLE 57-2

Clinical, Radiologic, and Biochemical Features of Common Skeletal Disorders That May Mimic Bone Metastases

DIAGNOSIS	CLINICAL FEATURES	RADIOLOGIC	BIOCHEMICAL
Bone metastases	Pain common Usually multiple sites Axial skeletal involvement typical	Bone scan very rarely completely normal Discrete lytic or sclerotic lesions on radiographs Fracture/vertebral pedicle destruction common Soft tissue extension on CT/MRI	Alkaline phosphatase usually elevated Increased urinary markers of bone resorption Hypercalcemia common
Degenerative disease	Elderly Limb involvement common Pain and stiffness Long history	Spinal involvement results in symmetric increased tracer uptake on scan Radiographs usually confirmatory	Usually normal
Osteoporosis	Elderly female Painless unless fracture or vertebral collapse	Normal scan unless recent fracture or vertebral collapse Diffuse osteopenia on radiographs Normal marrow on MRI	Usually normal serum parameters Slight elevation of urinary indices of bone resorption No hypercalcemia
Paget's disease of bone	Elderly Bone deformity common Involved site warm due to increased blood flow Skull often involved and enlarged	Diffuse involvement of bone on scan Sclerotic expanded appearance on radiographs	Alkaline phosphatase greatly elevated Increase in urinary hydroxyproline excretion Hypercalcemia very rare
Traumatic fractures	History of trauma usual Spontaneous rib fractures after chest wall irradiation common	Intense linear uptake on scan Rib lesions typically aligned, not randomly distributed No evidence of destruction around fracture site on radiographs (unless radiation induced)	Usually normal

Diagnostic Methods

Skeletal Radiograph

A skeletal radiograph indicates the net result of bone resorption and repair. For a destructive lesion in trabecular bone to be recognized on a plain radiograph, it must be greater than 1 cm in diameter, with loss of approximately 50% of the bone mineral content.[36] When radiographs are used as the primary investigation for bone metastases, such as in multiple myeloma, a skeletal survey is performed. Based on the usual distribution of metastases, this normally includes radiographs of the lateral skull and cervical spine, antero-posterior (AP) and lateral thoracic and lumbar spine, and AP pelvis and chest radiographs taken at low KVp to visualize the ribs optimally.

It is the predominance of lysis or sclerosis that gives rise to the characteristic radiographic appearances of bone metastases. When bone resorption predominates, focal bone destruction occurs, and bone metastases have a lytic appearance. Conversely, in bone metastases characterized by increased osteoblast activity and associated with a fibrous stroma (e.g., in prostate cancer), the lesions appear sclerotic. Even when one element predominates, both processes are greatly accelerated in the affected bone. Although probably a general phenomenon, this is most apparent in the appropriately termed "mixed" lesions, seen most commonly in breast cancer, in which both lytic and sclerotic components are clearly visible.

Lytic metastases are the most common type arising from breast, lung, thyroid, renal, melanoma, and gastrointestinal malignancies (Fig. 57-5). There is thinning of trabeculae, and the margins are usually ill defined, representing regions of partially destroyed trabeculae between the central destruction and the radiologically normal bone. The width of the margin reflects the aggressiveness of the lesion, with a narrow zone of transition in the less aggressive lesions. If the metastasis is in the medulla, there could be endosteal scalloping, while cortical lesions produce subperiosteal scalloping or a focal cortical defect.

Sclerotic metastases are usually from prostate cancer but also arise from breast, lung, and carcinoid tumors (Fig. 57-6). Excessive new bone formation gives rise to thickened, coarse trabeculae, which usually appear on radiographs as nodular, rounded, fairly well circumscribed sclerotic areas. Sometimes, less well defined, mottled, irregular areas of increased bone density occur, which can coalesce to produce a diffuse sclerotic appearance to the skeleton.

Radionucleotide Bone Scan

The radionuclide bone scan provides quite different information from the skeletal radiograph. The bone-seeking radiopharmaceutical is absorbed onto the calcium of hydroxyapatite in bone, a reaction which is influenced by osteoblastic activity and skeletal vascularity, with preferential uptake of tracer at sites of active bone formation. The bone scan, therefore, reflects the metabolic reaction of bone to the disease process, whether neoplastic, traumatic, or inflammatory. When bone metastases develop, there is usually sufficient increase in blood flow and reactive new bone formation to produce a focal increase in tracer uptake, often before bone destruction can be seen radiologically. Scintigraphic and radiographic appearances, therefore, do not necessarily correlate,

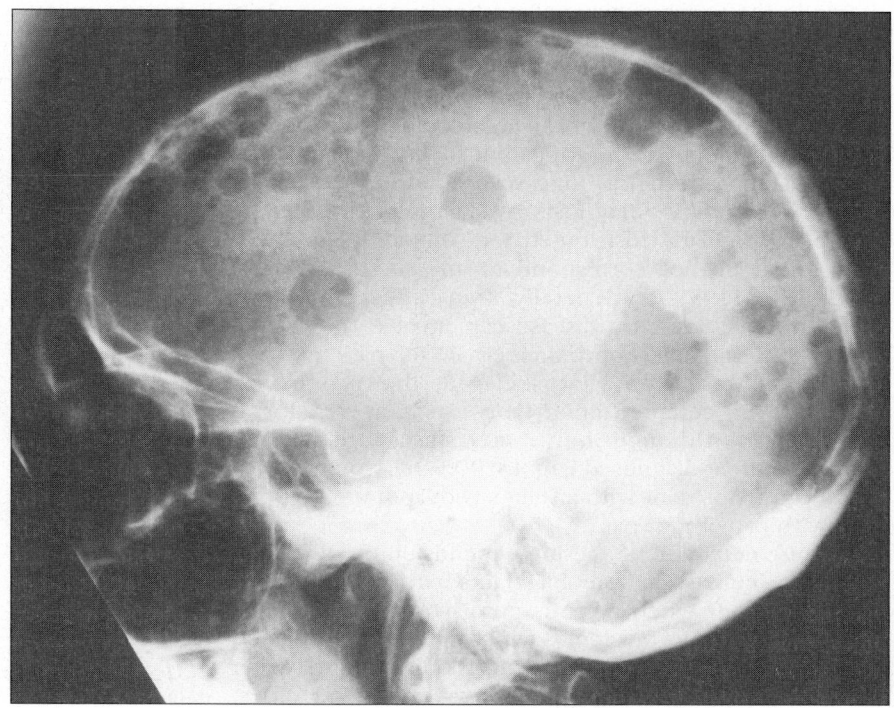

Figure 57-5. Lytic metastases in the skull.

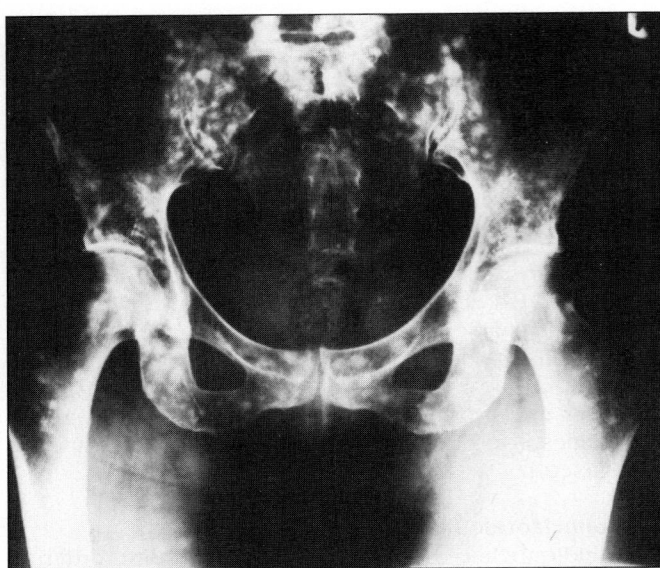

Figure 57-6. Sclerotic metastases in the pelvis.

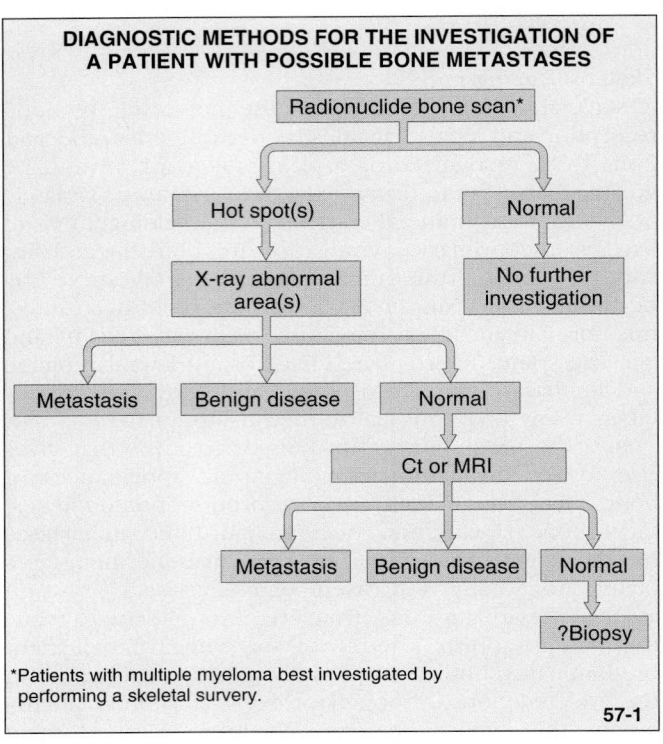

DIAGNOSTIC METHODS FOR THE INVESTIGATION OF A PATIENT WITH POSSIBLE BONE METASTASES

*Patients with multiple myeloma best investigated by performing a skeletal survey.

57-1

although the majority of comparative studies have found the bone scan to be the more sensitive of the two investigative techniques.[37] Lesions in the pubis, ischium, and sacrum can on occasion be obscured on the bone scan as a result of bladder activity, and not all established metastases are apparent on the scan.

A bone scan is generally performed by acquiring multiple images of the skeleton three to four hours after the intravenous injection of 550 MBq of [99m]technetium-labelled methylene-diphosphonate (MDP). If a lesion is identified, particularly when solitary, further investigation is necessary. A suggested protocol for investigation is shown in the accompanying algorithm. Appropriate plain radiographs of a focal lesion should be obtained in the first instance. If these are normal and clinically a metastasis is likely, then computed tomography (CT) or magnetic resonance imaging (MRI) of the area could be diagnostic.

Although bone scan appearances are nonspecific, recognizable patterns of bone scan abnormalities might suggest a specific diagnosis. Metastases are usually multiple, irregularly distributed foci of increased tracer uptake that do not correspond to any single anatomic structure (Fig. 57-7). Generally, they affect the axial skeleton, but metastatic disease can involve the appendicular skeleton, and approximately 7% of patients have involvement of the distal skeleton, the proportion increasing in certain tumor types such as renal cell carcinoma.[37] Although bone metastases are usually multiple when diagnosed, up to 20% of women with breast cancer present with a solitary hot spot on the bone scan with or without pain.[38]

Because detection of a lesion depends on the presence of a focal increase in osteoblast activity, a false negative scan will occur when there is pure lytic disease. This is typical of multiple myeloma, which is best investigated radiographically but also can occur in other tumors when there are rapidly growing lytic lesions. In extreme cases,

where there has been significant bony destruction, a photon-deficient area (cold spot) can develop (Fig. 57-8). Sclerotic metastases, on the other hand, are generally clearly visualized on the bone scan, the only exception being very slow-growing metastases, in which the alteration in metabolic activity is so subtle that it might not be distinguishable from normal background activity.

When there are extensive skeletal metastases, the focal lesions might coalesce to produce diffusely increased

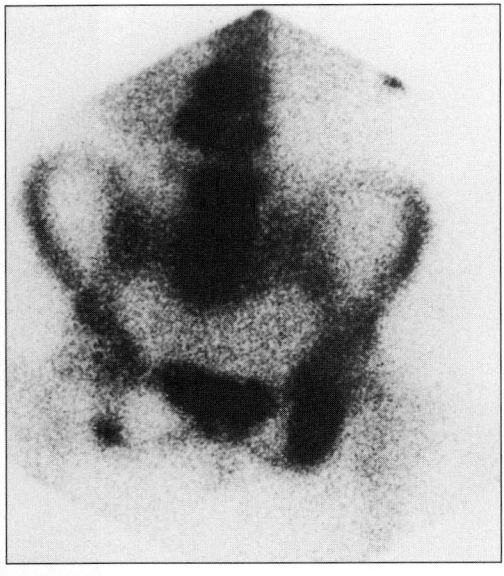

Figure 57-7. Radionuclide bone scan appearances of metastases in the lumbar spine and pelvis.

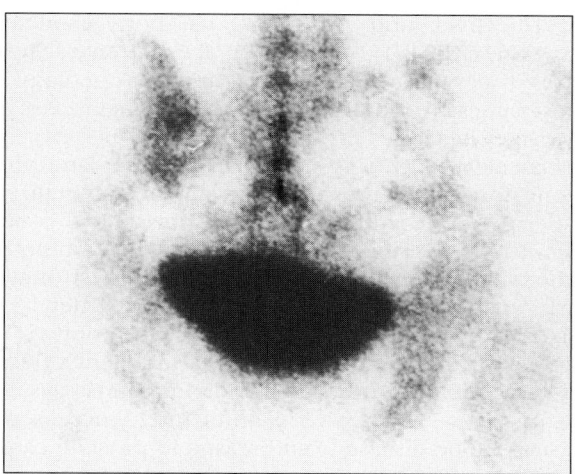

A

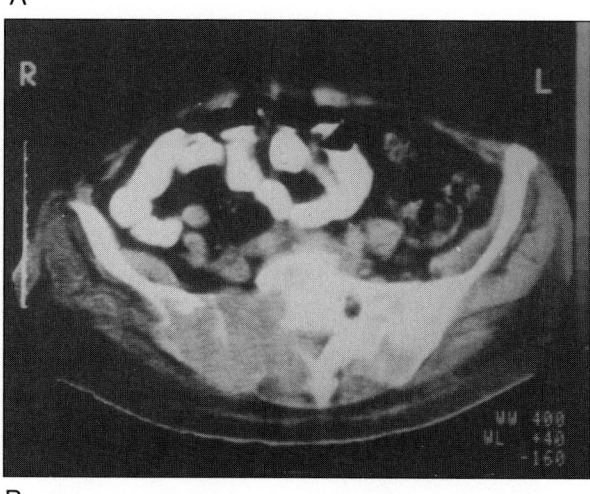

B

Figure 57-8. A, Photodeficient (cold lesion) in the sacrum resulting from a rapidly progressive destructive bone metastasis as demonstrated by CT scan slice taken through the lesion (**B**).

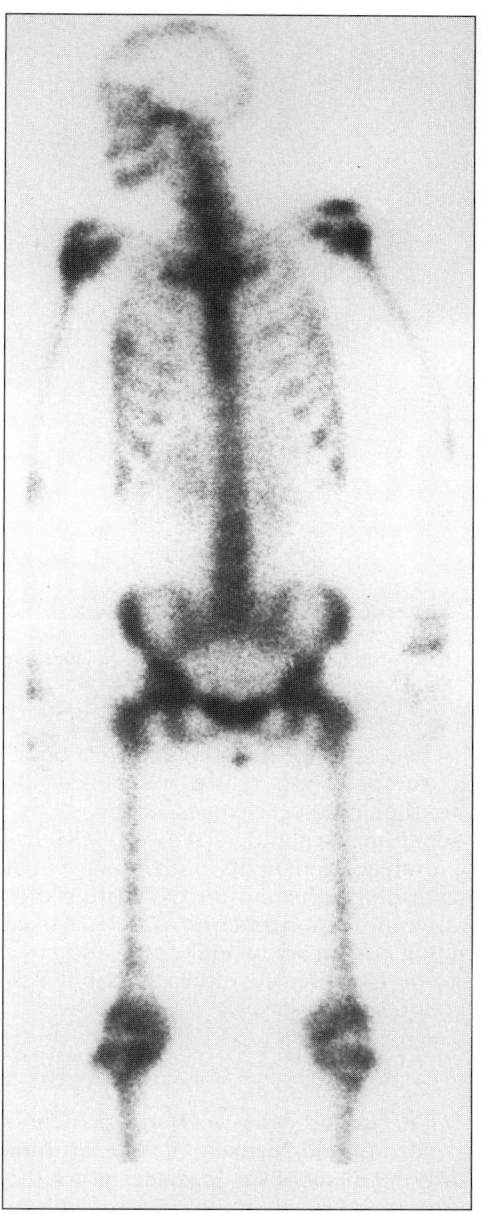

Figure 57-9. "Super scan" of malignancy. Note absent renal images and diffuse uptake of tracer throughout the skeleton.

uptake—the so-called "super scan" of malignancy (Fig. 57-9). This occurs most often in prostatic cancer but also is seen in other tumors, such as breast cancer. An increase in the contrast between bone and background soft tissue and faint or absent renal images are the typical appearances.

Computed Tomography

A computed tomography (CT) scan produces images with excellent soft tissue and contrast resolution. Bony destruction and sclerotic deposits are well shown (Fig. 57-10), and any soft-tissue extension of bone metastases is demonstrated clearly. CT is most appropriate for diagnosing spinal metastases, but as the whole spine cannot be scanned readily, CT is normally reserved for assessment of patients with positive bone scans and negative radiographs in an attempt to clarify the pathology. In one series of such patients with breast cancer, 50% had obvious metastases on CT, 25% had a benign cause, and no

abnormality could be demonstrated in 25%; none of these patients subsequently developed metastases.[39]

Magnetic Resonance Imaging

Magnetic resonance imaging (MRI) has the advantage over CT of providing multiplanar images that enable (as one example) imaging of the entire spine in the sagittal plane (Fig. 57-11).[37] The solid constituents of cortical bone give no signal on MRI and appear black, while the high water content of fat and bone marrow results in strong signals, making these tissues appear white. This signal is variable depending on the pulse sequence used. Detection of bone metastases by MRI depends on differences in MR signal

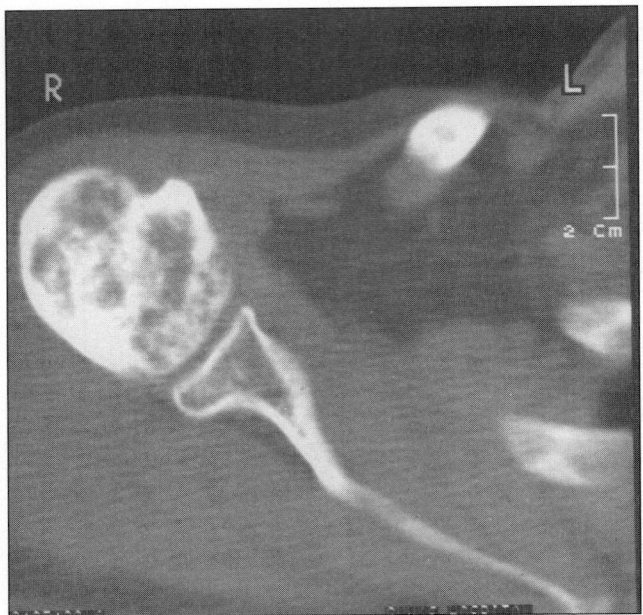

Figure 57-10. CT scan image through the right shoulder showing mixed lytic and sclerotic disease.

intensity between tumor tissue and normal bone marrow. Metastatic tumor is, therefore, visualized directly, in contrast to the indirect changes observed by x-ray or radionuclide bone scanning. Like CT, MRI has proved useful for evaluating patients with positive bone scans and normal radiographs and for elucidating the cause of a vertebral compression fracture.[40] MRI is excellent for demonstrating bone marrow infiltration and has also been reported to be more sensitive than the bone scan for the early detection of metastases.[41]

Biochemical Markers of Bone Metabolism

The effects of tumor cells on bone cell function can influence serum and urinary levels of biochemical markers of bone metabolism. In recent years, the number of available markers and the clinical relevance has increased rapidly; their value in the diagnosis of bone metastases has been studied in several tumor types.

Bone Formation Markers
Type 1 collagen is the major protein of bone and accounts for about 90% of the organic matrix. It is synthesized by osteoblasts to enable bone matrix deposition as a large precursor protein, Type 1 procollagen. Assay of the carboxy terminal propeptide of Type 1 procollagen (PICP) is now possible by radioimmunoassay and is believed to be a marker of early bone formation, appearing principally during the phase of osteoblast proliferation.[42,43]

Osteoblasts are naturally rich in alkaline phosphatase, and release of the enzyme into the circulation, predominantly in the middle stages of bone formation during the matrix maturation phase, gives some indication of osteoblast activity. Measurement of total alkaline phosphatase is routine, but to exclude the contribution

from the liver and other organs, bone isoenzyme estimation (ALP-BI) is required. Raised levels reflect increased new bone formation, and in oncology, the highest values are found with osteoblastic metastases or in response to healing.[44]

Osteocalcin (BGP) is a marker of the late phases of bone formation, appearing during the mineralization phase.[43] It is also synthesized in osteoblasts and contains three residues of the vitamin K-dependent amino acid γ-carboxy glutamic acid. Osteocalcin binds strongly to hydroxyapatite, but a small fraction of the newly synthesized protein appears in the circulation, from which it is rapidly cleared by the kidney. Measurement of serum levels is possible by a variety of radioimmunoassays.

Osteocalcin levels are significantly increased in metastatic bone disease from breast and prostate cancers

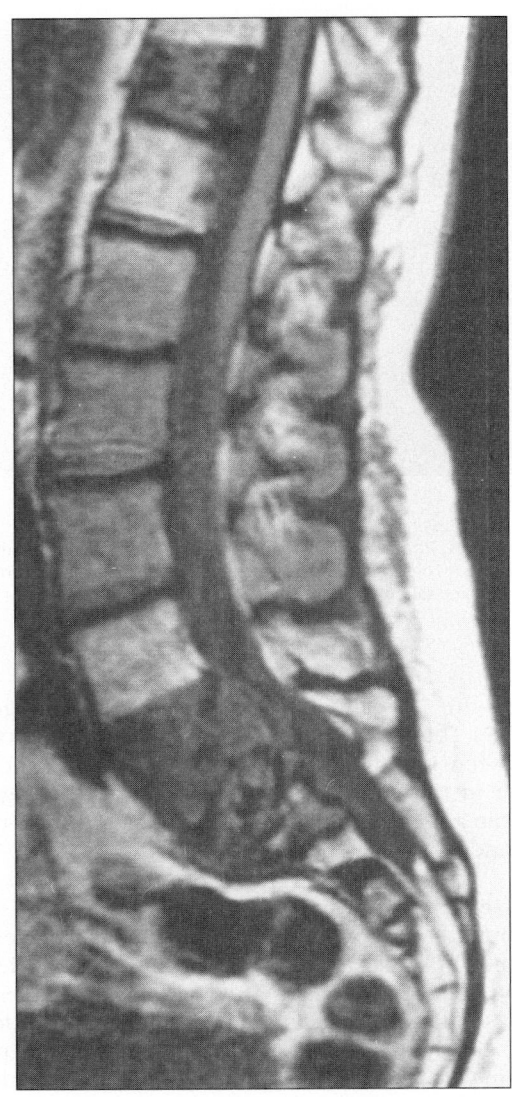

Figure 57-11. T1-weighted magnetic resonance image of spine with metastases in T11 and L5 appearing darker than normal marrow (From Richards MA: Magnetic resonance imaging. In Rubens RD, Fogelman I [eds]: Bone Metastases—Diagnosis and Treatment. London, Springer Verlag, 1991, p 91, with permission).

compared with levels in normal subjects, but not in multiple myeloma.[45,46] Levels are significantly higher in patients with blastic rather than lytic metastases and show some correlation with tumor bulk in prostate cancer.[47] Similar trends are reported with ALP-BI, with the highest levels occuring among patients with multiple blastic metastases.[44] Correlation between ALP-BI and osteocalcin is variable, reflecting their relationship to different phases of the bone formation process.[43] PICP levels typically correlate well with ALP-BI, especially for patients with blastic metastases. Increased levels are seen in over 50% of patients with prostatic metastases and in around 25% of patients with breast cancer but are usually normal in patients with multiple myeloma.[44,48,49] Neither ALP-BI, osteocalcin, or PICP is useful for early diagnosis of bone metastases.

Bone Resorption Markers

Resorption of bone releases calcium, hydroxyproline, and collagen fragments into the circulation. These are cleared by the kidney and excreted largely unchanged into the urine. Serum calcium measurements are performed routinely, but changes within the normal range give little guide to disease activity. Hypocalcemia is seen when osteoblastic metastases predominate; this is more typically associated with prostate cancer but does sometimes occur in advanced breast cancer.

Urinary calcium excretion is a more sensitive indicator of alterations in calcium homeostasis. The molar ratio of calcium to creatinine in an early morning urine sample collected after an overnight fast is a convenient, reproducible method of quantifying calcium excretion. The problem with urinary calcium is that it is not a specific resorption inhibitor, but only reflects the net effects of bone formation and resorption and is influenced by diet, the circulating levels of both parathyroid hormone (PTH) and parathyroid-related peptide (PTHrP), and the concomitant administration of drugs such as bisphosphonates (which influence bone resorption independently of any tumor related effects).[50] Urinary calcium excretion is not increased significantly in the majority of patients with metastatic bone disease, a finding that reflects the effects of bone formation and the renal handling of calcium.[50]

Urinary hydroxyproline excretion is a conventional parameter for measuring bone resorption in benign bone disease; it indicates matrix destruction more specifically but has been generally unreliable in the monitoring of metastatic bone disease due to contributions from both diet and soft tissue destruction by metastases.[50,51] Hydroxyproline excretion is typically increased in breast cancer and myeloma, but variable results have been found in prostate cancer.[51,52,53]

It is hoped that the recently introduced measurements of the intermolecular crosslinking compounds of collagen will overcome the poor specificity of the old markers. Pyridinoline (Pyr) and deoxypyridinoline (Dpd), also called hydroxy-lysylpyridinoline and lysyl-pyridinoline, respectively, are two crosslinking amino acids that hold together the extracellular telopeptide region at the ends of adjacent collagen chains. Pyr is found in bone, cartilage, and, to a lesser extent, in other connective tissues, while Dpd is almost exclusive to bone. They can be measured accurately in urine by reverse-phase high-peformance liquid chromatography (HPLC) and/or enzyme-linked immunosorbent assay (ELISA) and have been reported as specific measures of the rate of bone resorption.[54] Their excretion relative to creatinine is only minimally affected by renal function but does vary substantially throughout the day with a circadian rhythm, and from day to day. Therefore, samples must be taken at the same time each day.

Although both Pyr and Dpd have provided useful information in benign and malignant skeletal conditions, the HPLC assays are too complex and time-consuming to be suitable for routine laboratory practice. Crosslinks exist in both free (40%) and peptide-bound (60%) forms, and recently, new enzyme-linked immunoassays (ELISA) have been developed to measure the protein-bound cross-linking molecule at either the N-terminal part (NTx), the C-terminal part (Crosslaps) of type I collagen, and the free portions of both pyridinoline (F-Pyr) and deoxypyridinoline (F-Dpd), thereby providing a range of relatively simple assays for specific assessment of the rate of bone resorption.[55-57] A recent study in hypercalcemia of malignancy has shown that the simpler ELISA assays correlate closely with the HPLC-based Dpd and Pyr measurements and that they reflect the clear clinical differences observed between treatment with pamidronate or clodronate for hypercalcemia of malignancy.[58]

Bone resorption markers have been shown to be useful in the diagnosis of bone metastases in patients with cancer. Many studies have now shown a positive relationship between various bone markers and the presence of metastatic bone disease. Early work was focused on measurements of urinary calcium and hydroxyproline.[50,52,59] Both can be elevated in patients with metastatic bone disease, but the specificity and sensitivity of these measurements are too low to be clinically useful. More recently, attention has been focused on the various breakdown products of type I collagen, including pyridinoline (PYD), Dpd, N-terminal of type 1 collagen (Ntx), and C-terminal of type 1 collagen (Ctx).

Several studies have shown elevated PYD and Dpd in patients with bone metastases, and it is apparent that these are more reliable indicators of metastatic bone disease.[60-63] In the majority of patients with bone metastases, excretion of pyridinium crosslinks is typically increased by 2.5-fold compared with healthy controls and is also significantly elevated when compared with measurements in patients with cancer who have no bone metastases.[62] In a study that compared breast patients with cancer with bone metastases with healthy premenopausal women, the percentages of elevated values for the cancer group were 47% for urinary calcium, 74% for hydroxyproline, 83% for Ctx, and 100% for the collagen crosslinks PYD and Dpd. Alkaline phosphatase (but not urinary calcium) correlated significantly with the other four bone markers.[62] Patients with breast cancer but without bone metastases might also exhibit slightly increased PYD and Dpd excretion, possibly due to systemic stimulation of bone resorption by circulating tumor-derived parathyroid hormone-related protein.[63]

Problems Common to Cancer and Its Therapy

Other studies have confirmed these findings but also have highlighted the particular diagnostic value of Ntx. On the basis of radiographic and bone scan findings, 127 patients with cancer were divided into three groups, including 83 patients with no bone metastases, 22 patients with one or two bone metastases, and 22 patients with three or more metastases. PYD, Ntx, and Ctx were increased significantly in both groups with bone involvement, indicating the specificity and sensitivity of these markers.[63-65] Lipton and associates[64] attempted to determine which marker best correlates with skeletal metastases and concluded that Ntx was the most predictive for the presence of bone metastases. There are data, however, to show that some patients have indolent bone metastases or only an isolated one or two lesions that do not break down sufficient bone matrix to influence serum or urinary concentrations of bone resorption markers significantly. It should also be emphasized that bone markers are not specific for malignant disease and can be elevated in a number of benign bone diseases.[66,67] Therefore, there is still a need for skeletal imaging to diagnose bone metastases with certainty.

Although bone metastases in prostate cancer are primarily osteosclerotic, increased bone resorption is also evident, and elevated Ctx levels correlate with skeletal involvement.[68-70] In a study of 39 patients with prostate cancer with bone metastases, urinary serum Ctx was increased approximately twofold compared with values in 355 healthy, age-matched men.[46] Increases in bone resorption markers were not detected in prostate patients without bone metastases (n = 9) or in patients with benign prostatic hyperplasia (n = 9). Levels of bone resorption markers correlate with the extent of bone metastasis in prostate cancer and could be important in predicting clinical outcomes.[47,71] Biochemical markers of bone formation, including bone-specific alkaline phosphatase and the amino- and carboxy-terminal propeptides of type I procollagen, have also been shown to correlate with bone metastases in patients with prostate cancer.[71,72]

Bone formation markers can also be expected to be raised in metastatic bone disease because of increased turnover of bone remodeling. Compared with bone resorption markers, there are much fewer data available. Osteocalcin levels and bone-specific alkaline phosphatase levels have both been shown to be increased significantly in patients with metastatic bone disease from breast cancer compared with normal controls.[44,45] In such patients, levels of these two formation markers are significantly higher in those with blastic rather than lytic metastases; however, neither of these markers appears to be useful for early detection of bone metastases. It would be useful if markers, in addition to correlating with the presence of bone metastases, could give an indication of the extent of bone disease. There is evidence from several studies that a range of markers—including PYD, Dpd, and alkaline phosphatase—correlated with the number of skeletal areas involved.[64,73]

Bone Markers as Predictive/Prognostic Indicators

Because commonly used radiographic methods do not detect bone metastases in the very early stages of development, the question arises whether serial measurements of bone markers might identify the impending development of bone metastases. As yet, data relating to this question are sparse. Studies carried out on bone sialoprotein (BSP) have proved particularly interesting. Bone sialoprotein is a bone matrix integrin-binding protein synthesized by osteoblasts and osteoclasts; it is expressed ectopically by malignant breast, prostate, and other cancer cells.[74] The observations that serum BSP levels were significantly higher in patients with bone metastases than in those without (P < .05) and that levels were 142% greater in postmenopausal women than in premenopausal women suggested that BSP measurement might be useful for monitoring bone resorption.[54,75] The measurement of serum BSP levels is currently under evaluation as a prognostic factor for bone metastases, disease progression, and survival. In an analysis of 388 patients with primary breast cancer without metastasis, Diel and colleagues[76] showed that a BSP value in excess of 24 ng/mL was highly predictive of subsequent bone metastases. Of the 19 patients who subsequently developed skeletal metastases, only two had normal BSP levels.

Among patients diagnosed with bone metastases as the only site of metastatic involvement, the average survival time is two years. Is the degree of elevation of bone marker related to survival time? There is evidence that this is the case. In a study by Ali and colleagues,[64,77] serum Ntx levels were measured in 250 postmenopausal patients with breast cancer who had bone-only metastases. There was a highly significant correlation between a raised Ntx level and poor survival time. Furthermore, when the data were analysed according to quartiles of Ntx level, these differences became even more marked.

EVALUATION OF THE PATIENT

A variety of treatments, including radiotherapy, endocrine treatment, chemotherapy, and bisphosphonates, are used for the treatment of metastatic bone disease, and evaluation of their effects is important for both routine clinical practice and research. The current imaging methods used to assess response to these treatments are qualitative and routinely include plain radiographs, radionuclide bone scans and, in particular situations, CT scans. Assessing the response of bone metastases to therapy is notoriously difficult; the events in the healing process are slow to evolve and quite subtle, with sclerosis of lytic lesions only beginning to appear three to six months after the start of therapy.[74] Bone is the only site of metastatic disease that has separate criteria for evaluation of response to treatment, based on bone repair and destruction rather than on changes in tumor volume.[75] A complete review of the bone radiographs since the start of treatment is necessary to evaluate response—a slow and tedious process.

Assessing response to treatment in bone is more difficult than evaluation of disease in viscera and soft tissues, where tumor measurements can usually be taken. This results in reports of lower response frequencies to systemic treatments in the skeleton compared with other sites of disease. Complete response in nonosseus sites affected by breast cancer occurs in 10%–20% of patients, but a complete response (CR) in bone with return of normal trabecular pattern or resolution of sclerotic metastases is very rare. Although a low rate of CR might represent some biological phenomenon of site-specific resistance, this is unlikely, and the discrepancy in response frequency is almost certainly a reflection of the insensitivity of the assessment methods. Consequently, patients with metastatic disease confined to the bone are frequently excluded from many therapeutic trials, and patients with widespread metastatic disease (including bone) rely on the changes observed in soft tissue or visceral disease to judge response to treatment.

Although we recognize that the changes seen on serial radiographs remain the "gold standard" for evaluating response to therapy, new methods of assessing response are needed, both to improve patient management and to evaluate specific treatments. A number of alternatives or adjuncts to assessment based on plain radiographs have been suggested. None is ideal, each having advantages and disadvantages as outlined in the following sections. However, as will be shown later, developments in biochemic evaluation of bone metabolism offer the possibility of real progress in this area.

Assessment of Symptoms and Activity Status

The relief of symptoms is the principal aim of palliative therapy and rationally should be the most important marker of response to treatment. The use of pain as a marker of response in clinical trials has not found universal acceptance, however, and there is still no single internationally accepted pain questionnaire in oncology. Subjective response to treatment for bone disease requires information on pain intensity, analgesic consumption, and mobility, all of which need to be recorded. A simple questionnaire that amalgamates these three components has been adopted by us for use in a number of recent trials of bisphosphonate therapy for metastatic bone disease.[74] Validation of this questionnaire in terms of close correlations with objective response to treatment, quality of life measurement, and more complex pain assessment methods has been demonstrated.[76]

Quality-of-life assessment is now an important aspect of clinical trials methodology and, notwithstanding all the difficulties of analysis and interpretation, well validated tools such as the Functional Living Index in Cancer patients (FLIC) and the EORTC QOL-C30 questionnaire can provide useful information on subjective response to treatment in the routine clinical setting.[77,78]

Imaging of Bone Metastases

Radiologic assessment of response is based on radiographic evidence of bone healing. It is generally accepted that sclerosis of lytic metastases with no radiologic evidence of new lesions constitutes tumor regression (a partial response, or PR). Confounding factors include the appearance of sclerosis in an area that was previously normal on the radiograph. This could represent progression of a new metastasis but could also indicate a response, reflecting a radiographic example of the healing flare phenomenon within a lesion that was present at the start but was not destructive enough to be radiologically visible.[74,79] Interpretation is further complicated by variations in film exposure and by the effects of overlying bowel gas. The evaluation of response in osteosclerotic lesions is even more difficult, with most patients with sclerotic metastases eventually classified as either "no change" (NC) in response to therapy or unassessable. Here, decisions about the efficacy of treatment have to be based on symptomatic response or (when present) on change in extraskeletal disease.

Although the plain radiograph remains the assessment tool for judging response in clinical trials, it is clearly an inadequate technique. This lack of precision for radiographic assessment of response is exemplified by the observation that, in terms of survival, patients with radiographic evidence of sclerosis (PR) and those with no change in radiographic appearance for at least three months have a similar outcome.[80]

The use of bone scanning for assessment of response to therapy has always been contentious; when lytic metastases predominate, it is often unreliable. A reduction in the intensity and number of lesions (hot spots) on the bone scan was previously considered to represent response, and progressive disease was assumed if an increase in intensity or number of hot spots was seen. This interpretation is too simplistic, however.

After successful therapy for metastatic disease, the healing processes of new bone formation cause an initial increase in tracer uptake (akin to callus formation), and scans performed during this phase (less than six months) are likely to show increased intensity and number of hot spots. After treatment for six months, the bone scan appearances might improve, as the increased production of immature new bone—the cause of the hot spots—eventually ceases and isotope uptake gradually falls. This "deterioration" followed by subsequent "improvement" in the bone scan appearances after successful therapy has been termed the *flare response* and is now a well-recognized phenomenon in both breast and prostate cancers (Fig. 57-12).[79,81,82]

Conversely, a reduction in isotope uptake can occasionally be seen in rapidly progressive disease, when overwhelming bone destruction allows little chance for new bone formation, sometimes culminating in a photon-deficient (cold spot) lesion on the bone scan. Bone scanning in advanced disease should certainly be interpreted with great caution when performed within six months of a change in therapy; it is most useful for restaging at the time of relapse, to identify sites for radiologic assessment, and to bring to the attention of the clinician those sites at risk of pathologic fracture where prophylactic surgery could be indicated.

CT evaluation is effective for diagnosing metastases, particularly in the spine, but it is also occasionally valuable as a parameter of response to metastatic disease. Metastatic lesions are selected that are considered to be representative of the metastatic process (target lesions)

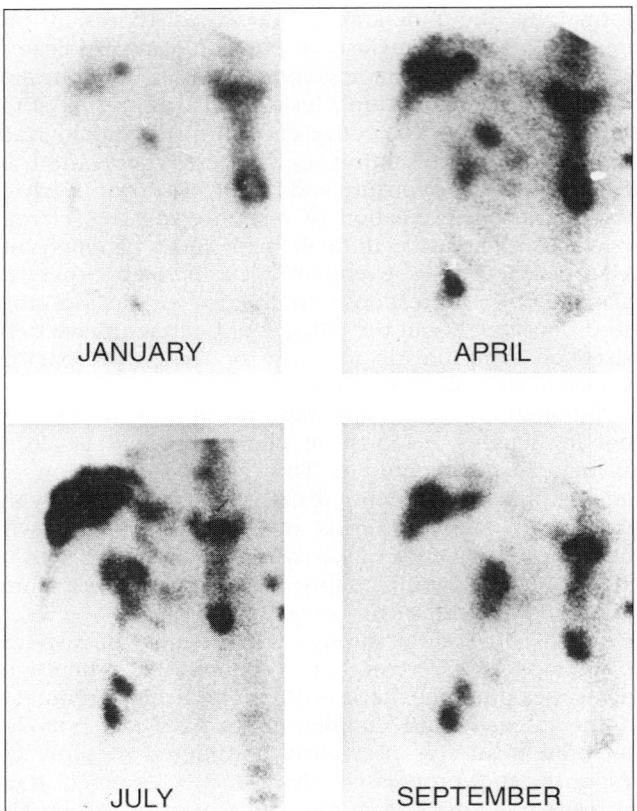

Figure 57-12. Flare response following effective palliative systemic therapy. Treatment was commenced in April after progression of previously asymptomatic disease. Follow-up scan three months later appears worse, but at six months the scan appearances are beginning to improve.

and suitable for serial examination. Because of the need for accurate repositioning of the patient, only target lesions in the spine and proximal ends of humerus or femur should be used. Transverse sections 3–4 mm thick with a standard window width and level appropriate for bone are optimum. If required, a region of interest (ROI) can be defined and the spectrum of Hounsfield values within it calculated by the computer. Changes in the spectrum with time can be determined, with a shift to the right (more positive) indicating replacement of lytic bone (which has a low Hounsfield value) by new sclerotic bone (which has a relatively high Hounsfield number). In one small prospective study, computed tomography correlated with clinical assessment in 13 patients (65%), whereas correlation between plain radiographs of the target lesion and clinical assessment of response was obtained in only 10 patients (50%).[83]

CT evaluation is particularly useful for assessing areas that are poorly visualized on plain radiographs (e.g., the sacrum) and might enable assessment of sclerotic bone disease. Within sclerotic metastases, areas of osteolysis are usually present and can be identified by CT. Sclerosis of this lytic component would suggest response to treatment, while new areas of lysis appearing within a sclerotic region probably represent progression of disease.[84]

The use of magnetic resonance imaging (MRI) for monitoring response to treatment is at present anecdotal, and in many parts of the world, limited equipment availability makes MRI unlikely to be suitable for routine use. As in primary bone tumors, however, MRI could have a role for detailed evaluation of a specific lesion, for example before surgery.

Tumor Markers

In breast cancer, unlike the germ cell malignancies, there is no highly specific tumor marker for either diagnosis or monitoring of disease. Some breast tumors, however, do produce tumor antigens that can be detected by radio-immunoassay. The most widely studied are carcino-embryonic antigen (CEA), which is elevated in 50%–80% of patients with metastatic breast cancer, and CA 15-3, which is elevated in 60%–90% of cases with advanced disease.

In a study by Kiang and associates,[85] the kinetics of CEA and CA 15-3 were assessed in 30 patients with advanced breast cancer immediately after chemotherapy. Although some patients showed the expected increase in markers with progression and decrease in markers with regression, others who responded showed an initial surge in tumor marker followed later by the expected decline.

Using an index derived from CEA and CA 15-3 in combination with erythrocyte sedimentation rate, an initial study of 65 patients with metastatic breast cancer found a significant correlation with clinical assessment of response using UICC criteria at two, four, and six months after systemic endocrine treatment.[86] More recently, this study was widened to include several European centers, using the same index to assess response to therapy in patients with breast cancer.[87] The authors concluded that changes in the markers were in line with and often predated therapeutic outcome criteria for both remission and progression.

It seems unlikely that any single tumor marker will be adequate for response assessment and that the most promising direction will be the establishment of combinations of markers together with an appropriate quantitative model.

Prostate specific antigen (PSA). is a marker of prostatic pathology and can be elevated in any prostate disease: benign prostatic hypertrophy (BPH), prostatitis, and cancer. The highest tissue production occurs in prostate cancer, and PSA has proved useful in the early diagnosis, staging, and follow-up of patients. The level of PSA is dependent on the volume of cancer, the volume of BPH in the prostate, and the differentiation of the tumor, with less production of PSA from poorly differentiated tumors. PSA levels usually decline after androgen deprivation and provide a reliable guide to response; elevations of PSA usually antedate other clinical evidence of progression by at least six months.[88]

Biochemical Assessment of Response

The stimulation of osteoclast function that results in osteolysis and disruption of the normal coupling between osteoblast and osteoclast function leads to changes in a variety of biochemical parameters. When treatment is prescribed for a patient with bone metastases, the effects of that treatment on the tumor cell population will influence bone cell activity. These changes can be appreciated within the first few weeks of starting effective therapy; for this reason, biochemical markers that reflect the rates of bone formation and resorption, respectively, might provide an early assessment of response to treatment (Table 57-3).

In the mid-1980s, several studies investigated the use of biochemical assessment of response to systemic therapy.[51,52,89] These generally showed that radiologic response correlated with a reduction in bone resorption. But, perhaps because at the time urinary calcium and hydroxyproline were the only available resorption markers, the reliability of biochemical monitoring was not established.

Hypercalcemia is usually indicative of progressive disease, and this is certainly the case if the hypercalcemia has developed more than a few weeks after the start of a new systemic treatment. Rarely, hypercalcemia can be a manifestation of the tumor flare, occuring within a week or so of starting tamoxifen, and in this case it might herald a response to treatment.[90]

Urinary calcium excretion was initially reported as a marker of response more than ten years ago; follow-up studies have confirmed that a rapid fall in urinary calcium excretion is typical of response.[59] In one prospective study of 70 unselected patients with advanced breast cancer receiving systemic treatment, 15 of 16 patients radiographically confirmed objective responders (94%) had a greater than 10% reduction in calcium excretion compared with 10 of 21 patients (48%) with progressive disease ($p < 0.01$).[52] Markers of osteoblast activity were also evaluated in this study. After one month, 15 of 16

responding patients (94%) showed a greater than 10% rise in both ALP-BI and osteocalcin, compared with 7 of 22 patients (31%) with radiologic evidence of progression ($p < 0.001$). The serum concentrations of ALP-BI and osteocalcin subsequently fell steadily after one to two and three to four months, respectively. Variable changes in bone formation have been reported by others researchers, depending on the timing of sample collection and the confounding changes induced by the healing flare.[90]

More recently, attention has turned to the possible use of collagen crosslink measurements for the assessment of response in bone. Walls and colleauges[91] studied the collagen crosslinks PYD and DPD in 36 patients with breast cancer with bone metastases. In 19 women who developed progressive disease, both markers increased, with significant changes becoming apparent by eight weeks. This evidence preceded radiologic evidence by a median of two months. By contrast, in 17 women who responded to hormone therapy, the markers did not change significantly.

In a study designed to evaluate bone resorption and tumor markers as possible alternatives to plain radiographs for the assessment of response to bisphosphonate therapy, Vinholes and associates[92] studied 37 patients with newly diagnosed bone metastases from breast cancer. Ntx levels were significantly lower than baseline values ($P \le .05$) at one and four months in responding patients, compared with values for patients with progressive disease. Similarly, Ntx levels at four months were significantly lower for patients with a time to progression (TTP) of less than seven months, compared with patients who progressed rapidly (TTP less than or equal to seven months). Furthermore, a greater than 50% increase in Ntx excretion correctly predicted disease progression in 78% of patients. In a larger, more recent study, 97 evaluable patients with metastatic bone disease from a variety of primary sites were followed during systemic therapy to correlate marker changes with response to treatment.[93] Good correlations of urinary Ntx, type 1 C terminal peptide (ICTP), and bone alkaline phosphatase changes with response were observed, with a rise in Ntx of greater than or equal to 52% having the highest positive predictive value (71%) for identifying progression of disease.

Although it is now well accepted that bone-targeted systemic therapy—particularly the use of the bisphosphonates—can reduce morbidity of skeletal metastases of breast cancer substantially, the optimization and timing of these therapies remains to be established. Bone markers potentially offer a powerful and relatively simple tool to assist the clinician in developing the most appropriate treatment strategies. Moreover, there is a prospect of using bone markers to tailor treatment to the individual patient.

Several comparative trials have examined bone resorption markers in patients with bone metastases who were treated with bisphosphonates.[74] First, in a study of 19 patients with breast cancer with extensive bone metastases, mean baseline levels of urinary calcium, hydroxyproline, Ctx, and collagen crosslinks (PYD and Dpd) were elevated in 47%, 74%, 83%, and 100% of

TABLE 57-3

Biochemical Markers of Bone Resorption and Formation

RESORPTION	FORMATION
Urine	**Serum**
Calcium	Alkaline phosphatase
Hydroxyproline	Osteocalcin
Pyridinoline	PICP
Deoxypyridinoline	PIIINP
Nx	
Crosslaps	
Free Dpd	
Free Pyr	
Galactosyl hydroxylysine	
Serum	
Calcium	
ICTP	
Galactosyl hydroxylysine	

Dpd, deoxypyridinoline; ICTP, type I collagen C telopeptide; NTx, N-telopeptide of type I collagen; PIIINP, procollagen type III propeptide; PICP, C-terminal propeptide or type I procollagen; Pyr, pyridinoline.

patients, respectively.[62] All of these markers decreased after pamidronate therapy, with the largest decrease observed in Ctx. In a second study of 29 patients with breast cancer with progressing bone metastases, the mean baseline values of Ntx, Ctx, and Dpd were elevated approximately twofold compared with age-matched controls, and after pamidronate therapy, levels of Ntx and Ctx again decreased significantly ($p = .001$).[94] In a third, double-blind study of 32 patients with hypercalcemia of malignancy, mean baseline levels of Ntx were sevenfold above normal, and mean Dpd and Ctx levels were each fivefold higher than normal.[58] Again, Ntx and Ctx showed the greatest decrease after pamidronate therapy, reaching 15% and 2% of the baseline values, respectively ($P < 0.01$).

There is also evidence that the individual pretreatment values of a bone marker, particularly Ntx, correlates with response to treatment. In patients with metastatic bone pain treated with pamidronate, the baseline values of Ntx in nonresponding patients were significantly higher ($p < 0.02$) than those of the clinical responders.[95] None of the patients with an initial Ntx value above twice the upper limit of normal responded, compared with more than 50% of those whose initial marker values were normal or below twice the upper level of normal. This study also showed that normalization of bone resorption markers correlated with response to treatment. Clinical benefit, as indicated by an improvement in a pain score, was seen only among those patients (17 of 32 [60%]) achieving a normal bone resorption rate after administration of pamidronate. No response was seen in the 11 patients (35%) with persistently elevated levels ($p = <0.01$). This suggested that the aim of bisphosphonate therapy should be to produce a fall in marker levels, preferably into the normal range.

A subsequent study has shown that this principle may be extended to the use of bone markers to distinguish between the benefits of different bisphosphonates.[96] In one study, 51 patients were allocated randomly to treatment with either oral clodronate, intravenous clodronate, or intravenous pamidronate. Symptomatic response was more frequent in the pamidronate group than in patients receiving clodronate, and this was reflected by a correspondingly greater decrease in the bone resorption markers Ctx and Ntx.

The ability of bisphosphonate therapy to reduce the frequency of skeletal complications also appears to be correlated with a reduction in bone resorption markers. Lipton and colleagues[97] investigated the fracture rate in 21 patients with cancer with bone metastases treated with intravenous pamidronate. In 12 patients, Ntx levels were normalized throughout a six-month period of follow-up, while in nine patients, urinary Ntx excretion remained above normal. In the former group, 42% developed fractures, whereas in the latter group (which failed to normalize), the corresponding figure was 89% ($p = 0.07$). Disease progression rates in bone were 25% and 78% for the two groups, respectively ($p = 0.03$). These data suggest, albeit in only a small number of patients, that normalization of bone resorption is necessary if the fracture rate in metastatic bone disease patients is to be reduced.

TREATMENT

In general, the treatment of bone metastases is aimed at palliating symptoms, with cure only rarely a realistic aim (e.g., in lymphoma); treatment varies depending on the underlying disease. External beam radiotherapy, endocrine treatments, chemotherapy, and radioisotopes are all important. In addition, orthopedic intervention might be necessary for the structural complications of bone destruction, and many patients with bone metastases develop hypercalcemia requiring specific treatment (see Chapter 48). Optimal management requires a multidisciplinary team that includes not only medical and radiation oncologists, orthopedic surgeons, general physicians, radiologists, and nuclear medicine physicians but also palliative medicine specialists and the symptom control team.

A schema for the management of bone metastases is shown in the accompanying algorithm. Treatment decisions depend on whether the bone disease is localized or widespread, the presence or absence of extraskeletal metastases, and the nature of the underlying malignancy. Radiotherapy is frequently relevant throughout the clinical course of the disease. Resistance to systemic treatments can be expected to develop, necessitating periodic changes of therapy in an effort to regain control of the disease.

External Beam Radiation Therapy

Shortly after the discovery of x-rays by Roentgen in 1895, radiation therapy was tried as an empiric treatment for bone metastases, and relief of bone pain was observed. Since these early reports, radiotherapy has become established as the treatment of choice for the palliation of painful single sites.[98]

Most treatments for bone pain use an external beam of ionizing radiation, either gamma rays or x-rays. Bones lying just below the skin surface, such as the ribs, skull, and clavicles, can be treated efficiently with an orthovoltage beam of 250–300 KeV. The beam is directed by an applicator to suit the required area of treatment and gives sufficient penetration to treat the affected area adequately. For the long bones—pelvis and spine—which are more deeply seated, a megavoltage beam is required to achieve sufficient penetration. Opposing anterior and posterior fields are often necessary to produce an even dose distribution across the volume to be treated. Although surface anatomy can be used to localize the treatment area, use of a treatment simulator is often preferable for accurate localization, particularly if treatment of adjacent areas is likely in the future.

Irradiation of bone can result in a number of pathologic changes that can include atrophy, osteitis, necrosis, and sarcomatous change. Postmortem studies have provided some insight into the structural effects of irradiation on bone-containing metastases. Initially, there is degeneration and necrosis of tumor cells, followed by a proliferation of collagen. Subsequently, a rich vascular fibrous stroma is produced, within which intense osteoblast activity lays

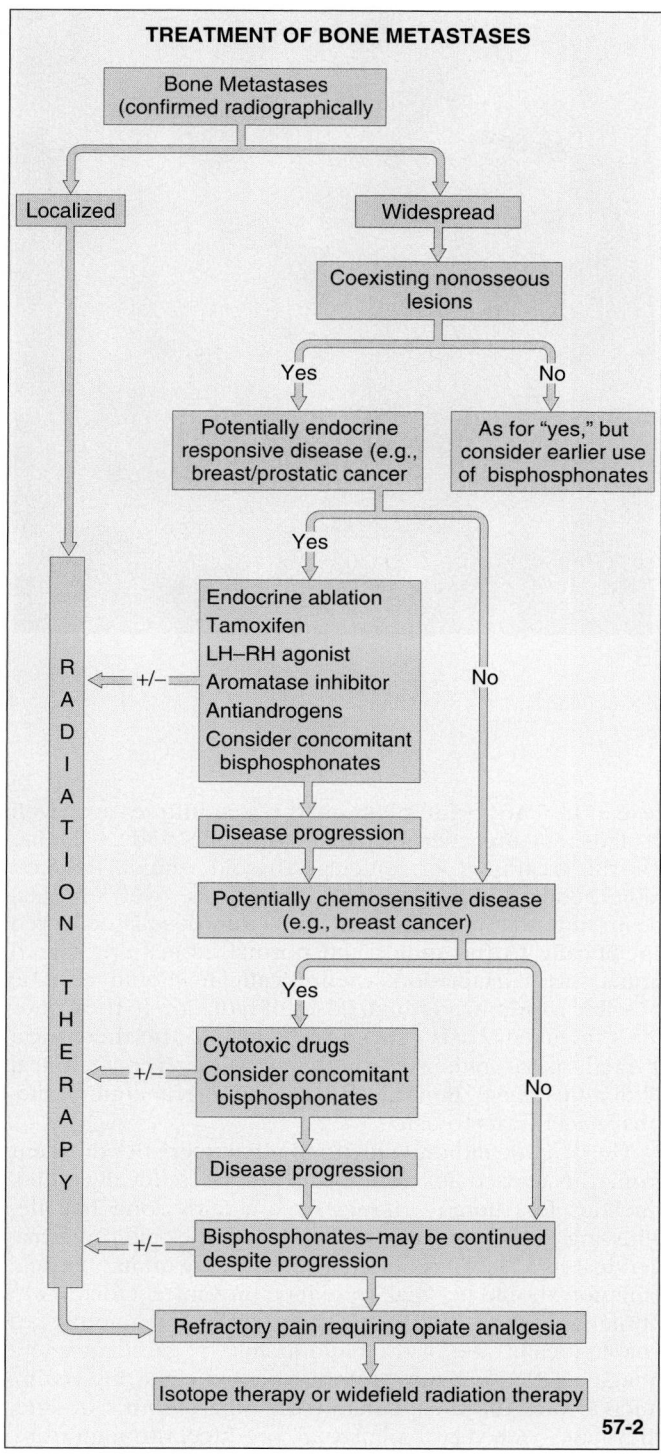

TREATMENT OF BONE METASTASES

Bone Metastases
(confirmed radiographically

Localized

Widespread

Coexisting nonosseous
lesions

Yes

No

Potentially endocrine
responsive disease (e.g.,
breast/prostatic cancer)

As for "yes," but
consider earlier use
of bisphosphonates

Yes

R A D I A T I O N   T H E R A P Y

Endocrine ablation
Tamoxifen
LH–RH agonist
Aromatase inhibitor
Antiandrogens
Consider concomitant
bisphosphonates

+/–

No

Disease progression

Potentially chemosensitive disease
(e.g., breast cancer)

Yes

Cytotoxic drugs
Consider concomitant
bisphosphonates

+/–

No

Disease progression

Bisphosphonates–may be continued
despite progression

+/–

Refractory pain requiring opiate analgesia

Isotope therapy or widefield radiation therapy

57-2

There is no doubt that local irradiation is effective for bone pain. Overall, response rates of around 85% are reported, with complete relief of pain achieved in one-half of patients.[101] Pain relief usually occurs rapidly, with more than 50% of responders showing benefit within one to two weeks. If improvement in pain has not occurred by six weeks or more after treatment, it is unlikely to be achieved.

Traditionally, treatment techniques and doses have varied considerably between different centers, with no particular approach appearing to be superior in terms of pain relief. In a large American study, the Radiation Therapy and Oncology Group (RTOG) reported the results of a prospective randomized study of more than 1000 treatments for metastatic bone pain. A variety of dose fractionation schedules were used, ranging from 15 Gy in five fractions to 40.5 Gy in 15 fractions. An overall response rate of 90% was observed, with approximately half of responders maintaining pain relief until death. Median duration of pain relief in the complete responders was 12–15 weeks. The complete response rate was 35% after 40.5 Gy in 15 fractions, compared with a response rate of only 28% after 25 Gy in five fractions (*p* = 0.0003).[102,103] On the other hand, two other prospective randomized studies have shown no difference in response rates between single or short-course radiotherapy and fractionated courses given over a period of two to three weeks.[104,105] In a more recent study, 30 Gy in 2-Gy fractions given over a three-week period was compared to 20 Gy given in 4-Gy fractions over five days. Although there was a trend toward improved pain relief and recalcification with the higher dose, no significant differences were observed.[106]

In a large Dutch trial, 1157 patients with painful bone metastases were randomized to receive either a single fraction of 8 Gy or a treatment schedule of six fractions of 4 Gy each.[107] No statistically significant differences in pain response, analgesic consumption, treatment side effects, or quality of life were identified. The only outcome measure that favored the multiple-fraction regimen over single-fraction treatment was the probability of retreatment (7% and 25%, respectively). Given that a single fraction is far less burdensome than multiple treatments for a patient with metastatic bone disease, it seems likely that the possibility of a retreatment is of limited importance. A cost-utility analysis of the study showed no difference in quality-adjusted life expectancy between the two regimens, while the financial cost was significantly lower for single fraction treatment.[108] Hence, accumulating evidence strongly favors single-fraction radiotherapy as the treatment of choice for many patients with painful bone metastases.

Retreatment of a painful site is usually possible, but a careful review of previous treatment fields, dose, and fractionation is needed to ensure that normal tissue tolerance, particularly of the spinal cord, is not exceeded. When higher radiation doses are administered, retreatment is precluded, and targeted radioisotope therapy is an alternative approach to palliation in those settings in which further external beam treatment is considered hazardous (see the discussion later in this chapter). After

down new woven bone. This is then gradually replaced by lamellar bone, and the intratrabecular stroma is repopulated by bone marrow tissue. Radiologically, it can be seen that recalcification of lytic areas begins three to six weeks after irradiation, with maximum recalcification occurring two to three months after the time of irradiation (Fig. 57-13).[99,100]

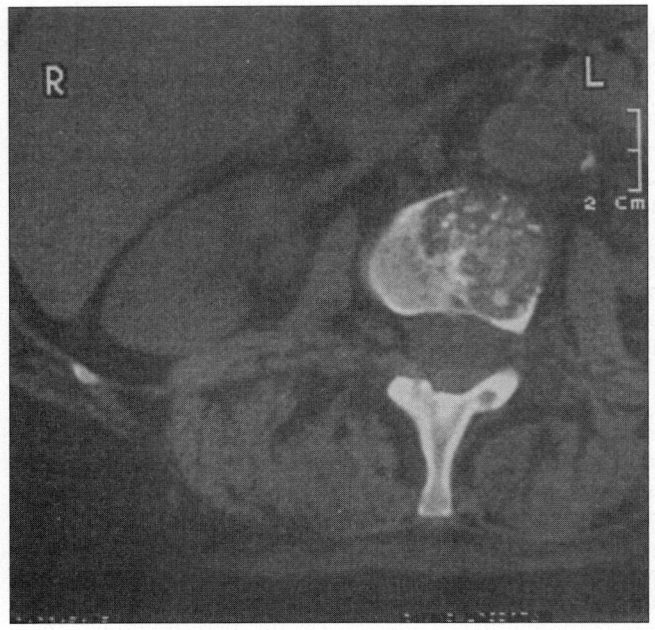

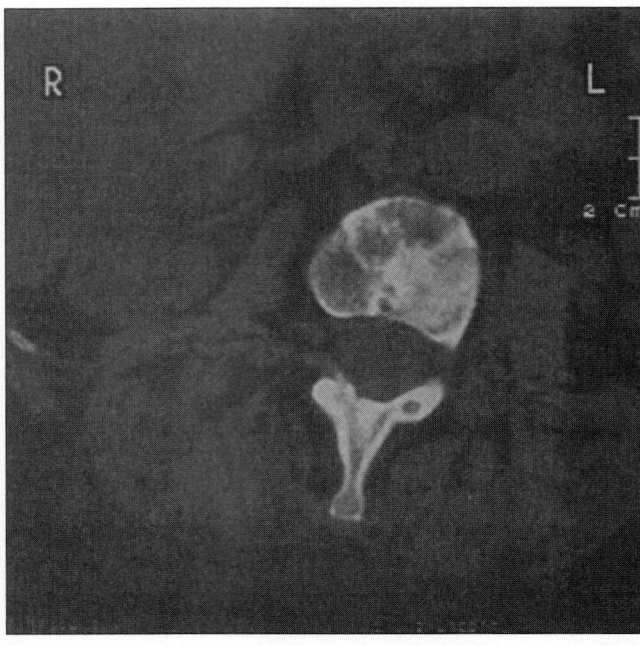

A

B

Figure 57-13. A, CT appearances of metastases in a lumbar vertebra. **B,** Evidence of bone healing two months after irradiation.

a single 8 Gy fraction, however, retreatment is possible, with more than 50% of patients with recurrence of bone pain responding to a second 8 Gy treatment—a finding that further supports the move occuring in many centers toward single-fraction treatments for routine palliation of metastatic bone pain.[109]

When there are multiple scattered sites of painful bone metastases, wide field/hemibody irradiation is often preferable to treating each site individually with local irradiation. Using single fractions of 6–7 Gy to the upper hemibody and 6–8 Gy to the lower hemibody, pain relief is reported in about 75% of patients, often occurring rapidly and sometimes within 24–48 hours of treatment.[110]

Hemibody irradiation is inevitably more toxic than localized external beam treatment. Virtually all patients who receive lower hemibody irradiation suffer gastrointestinal toxicity with nausea and diarrhoea. Premedication with intravenous hydration, steroids, and antiemetics is recommended to reduce these effects. The serious toxicities of hemibody irradiation are bone marrow suppression and radiation pneumonitis. Significant bone marrow suppression is seen in about 10% of patients receiving a single half-body treatment and in most patients who have sequential upper and lower hemibody treatment; these developments often compromise the use of subsequent chemotherapy. Radiation pneumonitis is both dose- and dose-rate-dependent; the occasional cases that do occur are difficult to treat and can be fatal.

Targeted Radioisotope Therapy

The therapeutic use of radioactive-labeled tracer molecules is currently an area of considerable interest and research. The principles of the technique are well established after decades of experience with ^{131}iodine for the treatment of follicular thyroid cancer. Targeted radiotherapy has theoretical advantages over external beam radiotherapy in that the radiation dose is delivered specifically to the tumor and normal tissues are spared unnecessary irradiation. Theoretically, it should also be possible to administer high doses of radiation to the tumor on a recurrent basis if necessary. Despite the theoretical attractions of radioisotope therapy, however, technical difficulties have limited the use of therapeutic radiopharmaceuticals to date.

Therapeutic radionuclides have characteristics different from those used for diagnostic purposes. Ideally, radionuclides for therapy should have a fairly long half-life, allowing adequate accumulation of the radiopharmaceutical within the target tissue. The gamma particle emission should be small to reduce unwanted radiation to nontarget tissues, but present in sufficient amounts to enable localization of the radionuclide by gamma camera imaging. Predominantly alpha- or beta-emitting radionuclides are the most suitable but, apart from ^{131}iodine, they have been very expensive to produce. Although many alpha- and beta-emitting radionuclides exist, relatively few have been evaluated clinically.

As follicular carcinoma of the thyroid commonly metastasize to bone, the treatment of bone metastases with ^{131}iodine is now well established, and excellent results can be obtained. In patients with a significant uptake of ^{131}iodine into the metastases, long-term palliation is usually possible, with 25% and 10% of patients still alive at 10 and 15 years, respectively. Conversely, those patients who do not concentrate ^{131}iodine in the metastases have a 10-year survival rate of only 8%, with no survivors reported at 15 years.[111] Treatment is generally well tolerated, although some patients develop a radiation reaction in the salivary glands. More important, however, is the 1%–2% incidence of radiation-induced leukemias.[112]

Neuroblastomas—and tumors of neuroectodermal origin in general—frequently metastasize to bone. Some 90% of these neoplasms incorporate the radiopharmaceutical ^{131}I-meta-iodo benzyl guanidine (I-MIBG), and this has now been used to treat many children with metastatic neuroblastoma. 5% of all patients have undergone CR, 40% have experienced PR, and 10% have progressed.[113] Bone marrow suppression is often severe, and ideally, bone marrow harvesting should be performed as a precautionary measure on patients with extensive bone metastases.

^{131}I-MIBG has also been used therapeutically to treat bone metastases from malignant phaeochromacytoma, medullary carcinoma of the thyroid, and carcinoid tumors, but with only limited success.[114] Between one-third and one-half of patients have had symptomatic benefit, but long-term remissions have not been recorded.

[89]Strontium is a beta emitter that imitates calcium and is taken up preferentially at sites of new bone formation. It has been shown to localize at the sites of prostatic bone metastases, with greater accumulation occurring in the metastatic lesions than is observed in normal bone.[115] The biologic half-life of strontium in metastases is long compared with that of normal bone, with whole-body retention of [89]strontium treatments ranging from 11% to 88% depending on the degree of skeletal involvement. The radiation dose to individual vertebral metastases from a single 150 MBq dose of [89]strontium has been shown to vary from 9 Gy to 92 Gy depending on the extent of metastatic spread. Of great clinical importance is the low dose of radiation to the bone marrow, which is only about one-tenth of that to the bone metastases.[116]

The selective beta-particle irradiation provides pain relief in up to 80% of patients, with 10%–20% becoming pain free.[117,118] On average, the response lasts for six months, with only mild hematologic toxicity. A number of randomized clinical trials have been performed. These have included a double-blind trial comparing the effects of [89]strontium with strontium chloride (placebo) as palliative therapy, with the radioactive [89]strontium clearly superior in terms of pain relief (p <.01).[119] In a more recent study, [89]strontium has been compared with conventional radiotherapy (hemibody or local) for the palliation of bone metastases from prostatic cancer.[120] [89]Strontium was at least as effective as external beam radiotherapy in achieving palliation and appeared also to delay or prevent the development of new sites of pain.

Widespread use of [89]strontium has been inhibited by the high price of this pharmaceutical. When the total cost of treatment is taken into account, however (including the use of hospital beds), the overall cost per patient is less than conventional field external beam therapy, although slightly more expensive than hemibody irradiation.[120]

[153]Samarium is both a beta- and a gamma-ray emitter, making it suitable for combined therapy and imaging. It has a short half-life (46 hours) and, linked to ethylene diamine tetramethylene phosphonate (EDTMP) for use as a radiopharmaceutical, concentrates preferentially in skeletal metastases.[121] Clinical reports indicate that [153]samarium-EDTMP can provide excellent palliation of pain. In one study, 22 of 34 patients (65%) with bone metastases who were unresponsive to conventional treatment experienced palliation within 14 days of a treatment with [153]samarium-EDTMP. The duration of response ranged from four to 35 weeks.[122] The short half-life also makes [153]samarium-EDTMP suitable for repeated treatments and in the same study, recurrence of pain was successfully controlled in four of nine patients. The safety and efficacy of this agent was confirmed in a larger, randomized, dose-controlled study.[123]

[186]Rhenium, an investigational radiopharmaceutical, which is also a beta- and a gamma-ray emitter, is complexed to hydroxyethylidene diphosphonate (HEDP) for therapeutic use. In a phase II trial of 28 patients with painful bone metastases, rhenium-HEDP led to significant pain reduction in eight of 12 men (67%) with prostatic cancer and in five of 16 women (36%) with breast cancer. The mean durations of response were 47 and 33 days for the prostate and breast patients, respectively.[124] Comparative studies of this agent with other therapeutic radionuclides are needed before its clinical role can be defined clearly.

Systemic Therapy

Systemic therapy for bone metastases can be directed against the tumor cell to reduce both cell proliferation and, in consequence, the production of cytokines and growth factors. Alternatively, systemic treatment is directed toward blocking the effect of these substances on host cells. Chemotherapy, endocrine treatments, and bone-seeking isotopes have direct antitumor effects, whereas agents such as the bisphosphonates and calcitonin are effective by preventing host cells (primarily osteoclasts) from reacting to tumor products. Systemic therapy, therefore, has either direct or indirect actions.

In general, the systemic treatment for metastatic bone disease is the same as that available for other metastatic manifestations of the malignancy. Treatment must therefore be discussed according to tumor type. Breast and prostate cancers are the most important, first because there are effective (albeit palliative) systemic treatments available and second because these two tumors represent the majority of patients with bone metastases. For a fuller discussion of systemic cancer management, the relevant site-specific chapters should be consulted.

Breast Cancer

For breast cancer, endocrine therapy is the treatment of choice for the initial treatment of metastatic disease. Exceptions to this are when visceral disease is so extensive and/or aggressive that it is inadvisable to wait six to eight weeks for a possible response—for example, when there are lymphangitic pulmonary metastases or liver metastases with compromised hepatic function.[125] In these two situations, cytotoxic chemotherapy is the initial treatment of choice.

Hormones act predominantly on cancer cells that express high affinity binding proteins (receptors) for estrogen (ER) and progesterone (PgR). These hormone-receptor complexes, in turn, act on the cell nucleus to mediate the specific cell response of the hormone. Significant (>50%) tumor shrinkage (a complete or partial objective response) after endocrine treatment occurs in one-third of unselected patients but is more likely among those with either steroid-receptor-positive tumors, a long disease-free interval from diagnosis to relapse, or bone or soft tissue metastases rather than visceral disease.[126]

Selection of specific endocrine treatment for patients is based on menopausal status. Premenopausal patients are now usually treated with a combination of tamoxifen and ovarian ablation, the latter of which is achieved by surgical bilateral oophorectomy, ovarian irradiation, or the use of LHRH agonists. For the past 30 years, tamoxifen has been the preferred treatment for postmenopausal patients, although recent trials of the aromatase inhibitors letrozole and anastrozole are challenging this dogma.[127] Although in general the median duration of response to endocrine therapy is around 15 months, prolonged responses to first-line hormone treatments lasting several years are not uncommon in patients with bone metastases.

Numerous recent developments in endocrine and cytotoxic treatments are of relevance to the patient with metastatic bone disease. In breast cancer, the highly specific aromatase inhibitors have displaced the older agents, megestrol acetate and aminoglutethimide.[128] Patients with disease progressing after endocrine therapy, and those with rapidly progressive life-threatening disease or those who are known to have ER- and PgR-negative tumors, should be considered for cytotoxic chemotherapy. Objectively responding patients usually gain relief of symptoms (including bone pain) and might become able to resume their previous activities.

Responses among women with bone metastases are nearly always only partial, with a median duration of response of nine to 12 months. The precise choice of drugs and schedule of administration to obtain the best results is not yet certain and vary from one patient or clinical problem to another. The anthracyclines (doxorubicin and epirubicin) and the taxoids (docetaxel and paclitaxel) are particularly active but also sometimes too toxic for elderly or frail patients. Chemotherapy can be especially hazardous for patients with extensive bone disease, due to both poor bone marrow tolerance after replacement of functioning marrow by tumor and the effects of previous irradiation. In view of this, regimens with relatively little myelotoxicity are usually preferable. Theoretically, the use of hematopoietic growth factors might allow patients with extensive bone metastases to receive more aggressive chemotherapy regimens but, for palliative treatment, the clinical benefit of this approach has not been demonstrated.

Prostate Cancer

In prostate cancer, bone is the dominant site for metastatic disease and in many patients is the only symptomatic problem. The appearances on plain radiography are predominantly osteoblastic and because of this, radiologic response is notoriously difficult to evaluate. Nevertheless, at least 80% of prostate tumors exhibit some degree of hormone responsiveness.[129]

Worldwide, the most commonly used form of endocrine therapy remains surgical castration. Stilbestrol is no longer appropriate therapy because of its feminizing effects and cardiovascular risks. Many new forms of endocrine treatment have been introduced recently, including the LHRH agonists and the anti-androgens. These pharmacologic alternatives are not necessarily any more effective than surgical orchidectomy, but for many patients they are aesthetically preferable to castration.[130] The role of combined endocrine therapy causing total androgen blockade (LHRH + antiandrogen) and the timing of endocrine intervention have, and continue to be, areas of intense clinical trial investigation.[131]

Patients with advanced prostate cancer tend to be elderly and often of poor performance status. Because of this and the presence of widespread bone involvement, their tolerance of toxic chemotherapy regimens is often poor, which has limited the use of this treatment modality significantly. To date, there is little evidence that cytotoxic drugs prolong survival for patients with advanced prostate cancer, although, in a randomized trial performed in 161 patients, mitoxantrone and prednisone have been shown to provide greater palliation of symptoms and improved quality of life than can be achieved with prednisone alone.[132] Treatment with chemotherapy should, however, still largely be restricted to use within the context of a clinical trial with careful evaluation of pain control, mobility, and quality of life in addition to tumor response.

Other Tumors

Skeletal morbidity is a major problem in multiple myeloma, and either widespread lytic metastases or diffuse osteopenia can occur. Around 50% of patients respond to chemotherapy, with a reduction in paraprotein levels and subjective improvement. Alkylating agents such as melphalan, anthracyclines, vinca alkaloids, and the corticosteroids are the most frequently prescribed agents. Despite the subjective improvement that is seen, bone healing is rare, with lytic lesions persisting despite control of the disease for months or years. Recently, survival in multiple myeloma has been shown to be improved by the selective use of high-dose chemotherapy with bone marrow or peripheral blood stem cell support.[133]

Bone involvement in curable malignancies is uncommon. In patients with germ cell tumors, bone involvement is an adverse prognostic feature, but despite this, cure with chemotherapy is usual. Bone involvement at diagnosis in lymphoma is relatively uncommon. When localized, it does not significantly affect the prognosis in Hodgkin's disease, but it does carry an adverse prognosis in non–Hodgkin's lymphoma. Curative therapy is still possible, however, and there is no evidence that bone represents a "sanctuary site."

Chemotherapy is of only limited and temporary benefit in relatively chemotherapy-resistant solid tumors such as non–small cell lung cancer or melanoma. Patients with skeletal metastases from these tumors derive most benefit from local palliative radiotherapy, and alternative (and more effective) systemic treatment approaches are needed.

Bisphosphonates

In the last ten years, the bisphosphonates have emerged as a valuable additional approach to the range of current treatments. All bisphosphonates are pyrophosphate analogues, characterized by a P-C-P containing central structure rather than the P-O-P of pyrophosphate, and a variable R′ chain that determines the relative potency, side effects, and (probably) the precise mechanism of action.[134] The P-C-P backbone renders bisphosphonates resistant to phosphatase activity and promotes their binding to the mineralized bone matrix. The structures of the commonly used bisphosphonates are illustrated in Figure 57-14.

After administration, bisphosphonates bind avidly to exposed bone mineral around resorbing osteoclasts, leading to very high local concentrations of bisphosphonate in the resorption lacunae (up to 1000 μM). On release from the bone surface, bisphosphonates are internalized by the osteoclast, where they cause disruption of the biochemical processes involved in bone resorption. These include destruction of the osteoclast cytoskeleton, disruption of the sealing zone at the bone surface, and loss of the ruffled border across which the hydrolytic enzymes and protons necessary for bone dissolution are normally secreted.[135]

Bisphosphonates also cause osteoclast apoptosis, with the appearance of distinctive changes in cell and nuclear morphology.[136] Although the precise molecular targets responsible for promoting this apoptosis are unknown, the bisphosphonates have recently been shown to inhibit enzymes of the mevalonate pathway, which are ultimately responsible for events that lead to the post-translational modification of GTP-binding proteins such as Ras and Rho.[137] Recent studies also suggest that bisphosphonates could have direct apoptotic effects on tumor cells.[138]

The different bisphosphonates vary in terms of the ratios of their inhibitory activity on bone mineralization to that on bone resorption. Etidronate, in particular, impairs the mineralization of normal calcified tissues such as bone, cartilage, and dentine.[139] On the other hand, clodronate and the aminobisphosphonates have relatively little effect on in vivo mineralization, a feature that makes them much more attractive for long-term administration in metabolic and metastatic bone diseases.[140]

After intravenous administration of a bisphosphonate, approximately 25%–40% of the injected dose is excreted by the kidney, and the remainder is taken up by bone.[141] All bisphosphonates suffer from poor bioavailability when given by mouth. They must be taken on an empty stomach, as they bind to calcium in the diet and can cause gastrointestinal toxicities such as nausea, vomiting, indigestion, and diarrhea.[142]

Irrespective of the mechanism(s) of action, bisphosphonates have been used successfully in the treatment of conditions characterized by increased osteoclast-mediated bone resorption, such as Paget's disease of bone or osteoporosis. In oncology, they have become the standard

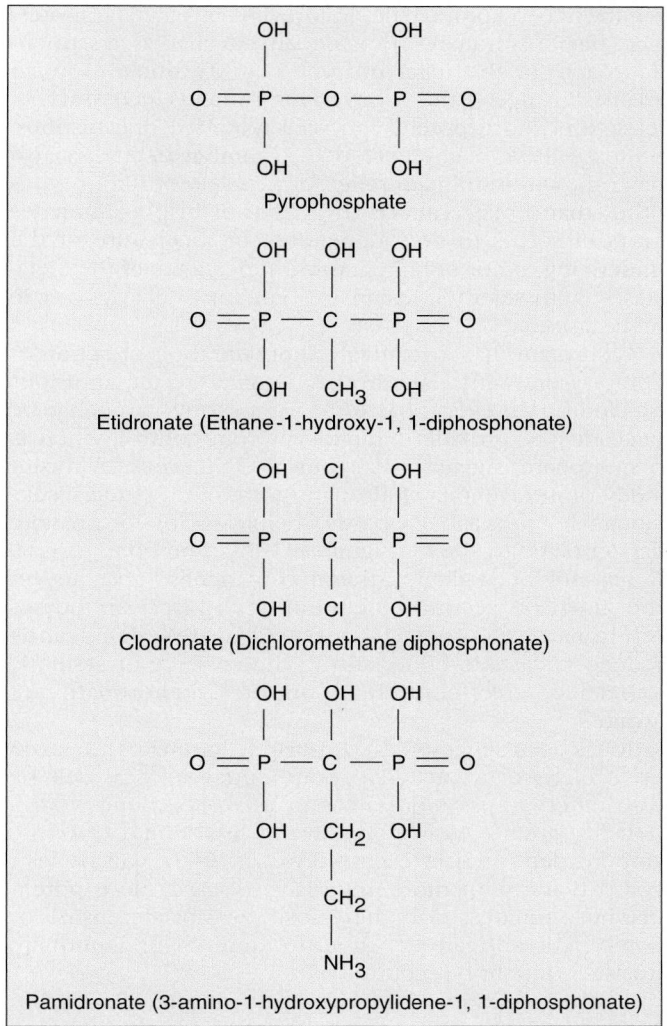

Figure 57-14. Structural formulae of commonly used bisphosphonates in relation to pyrophosphate.

treatment for tumor-induced hypercalcemia (TIH) and a valuable, new form of medical therapy for bone metastases.[143]

Rationale for the Wider Use of Bisphosphonates

As indicated previously, it is now generally accepted that osteoclast activation is the key step in the establishment and growth of all bone metastases. Biochemical data indicate that bone resorption is of importance not only in classic "lytic" diseases such as myeloma and breast cancer but also in prostate cancer, with values of resorption markers in the latter at least as high as those seen in breast cancer and other solid tumors.[144] As a result, the osteoclast is a key therapeutic target for skeletal metastases irrespective of the tissue of origin.

Bisphosphonates for Bone Pain

Although radiotherapy is the treatment of choice for localized bone pain, many patients have widespread, poorly localized bone pain, while others experience recurrence of bone pain in previously irradiated sites. The bisphosphonates provide an alternative treatment approach for the relief of bone pain. To obtain optimal analgesic effects, the intravenous route is necessary, at least until more potent and well tolerated oral bisphosphonates have been developed. A number of studies also have shown useful pain relief for a variety of tumor types other than breast cancer. The effect of bisphosphonates on pain seems to be independent of the nature of the underlying tumor or radiographic appearance of the metastases, with sclerotic lesions responding similarly to lytic metastases.

Clodronate has a relatively short duration of action in comparison with pamidronate.[58] As a result, infusions of clodronate every 10 to 14 days would probably be necessary to provide durable symptom control, whereas pamidronate is given every four to eight weeks. A recent study of intravenous clodronate given every three weeks alongside mitoxantrone-based chemotherapy for prostate cancer failed to show a significant effect on bone pain.[145] It has not been demonstrated convincingly that any of the first- or second-generation oral bisphosphonates (etidronate, clodronate, or pamidronate) significantly reduce metastatic bone pain in the absence of systemic anticancer treatment. Data on oral ibandronate are awaited.

It has been suggested that as bisphosphonates are taken up preferentially at active bone surfaces, they will be distributed across more areas of increased bone resorption in patients with more severe disease and thus, the amount deposited in each individual lesion will be less. For patients with more aggressive disease, more potent bisphosphonates, a higher dose or dose-intensity, or combined anticancer therapy and bisphosphonate treatment might be required.

The recognition of a possible symbiotic relationship between cancer cells and bone has raised the question as to whether bisphosphonate treatment, through suppression of the release of growth factors and cytokines from resorbing bone, has any effect on tumor burden. Anecdotal reports exist of falls in tumor markers in breast and prostate cancers treated in phase II studies with pamidronate, but these data are difficult to interpret, whereas in multiple myeloma there is laboratory evidence of apoptosis of human multiple myeloma cells in the presence of bisphosphonates.[146-148] Any anticancer activity of bisphosphonates is probably going to be discernable and of clinical relevance only in the adjuvant setting.

Bisphosphonates to Prevent Skeletal Morbidity

Breast Cancer. The absorption of bisphosphonates from the gut is poor, variable, and dramatically inhibited by food intake. To make matters worse, the absorbed fraction of oral bisphosphonates decreases even further when the absolute ingested amount is lower, thus the more potent bisphosphonates are even less well absorbed than etidronate and clodronate. Nevertheless, two randomized studies in advanced breast cancer have been performed: one placebo controlled study with clodronate and one open study with pamidronate (Table 57-4).[149,150]

Paterson and colleagues randomized 173 patients with bone metastases from breast cancer to receive either clodronate capsules, 1600 mg daily, or placebo capsules of identical appearance in addition to appropriate anticancer treatment(s).[149] The patients in each study group were comparable in their clinical, radiographic, and biochemical characteristics. In the patients who received clodronate, there was a significant reduction in skeletal morbidity. Overall, the combined rate of all skeletal events was 219 per 100 patient years for patients receiving clodronate compared with 305 for patients on placebo. Most of the benefit was accounted for by a reduction in hypercalcemic episodes (28 vs. 52, $p = <.01$) and the incidence of vertebral fractures (84 vs. 124 per 100 patient years, $p = <.025$). There was no significant effect on nonvertebral fractures, radiotherapy requirements, changes in antitumor therapy, or survival. There was a reduction in the absolute number of patients requiring spinal radiotherapy in the clodronate-treated group (32 vs. 42), but, disappointingly, no significant effect of clodronate treatment on the overall spinal radiotherapy requirements (75 vs. 89 courses per 100 patient-years, $p = $ NS). Oral clodronate was well tolerated, but difficulty swallowing the large capsules was encountered, to such an extent that 26% of patients receiving treatment for more than six months were noncompliant. These results indicate that oral clodronate can modify the course of skeletal disease in metastatic bone disease from breast cancer; however, the benefits seen were relatively small, and the overall clinical utility of clodronate remains poorly defined in advanced breast cancer.

There are currently no plans for oral pamidronate to be marketed. van Holten and colleagues,[150] however, reported an influential study of enteric-coated oral pamidronate. In their study, 161 women with bone metastases from breast cancer were randomized to standard anticancer treatment with or without oral pamidronate, initially at a dose of 600 mg/day but subsequently at a reduced dose of 300 mg/day because of poor gastrointestinal toleration of the drug. This was not a placebo-controlled study and required six years to recruit patients, suggesting possible selection bias. An initial analysis reported a significant reduction in skeletal morbidity with a reduction in pathologic fractures, episodes of severe bone pain, and hypercalcemia, leading to a reduction in radiotherapy requirements and the need to change the underlying systemic treatment. A subsequent analysis, however, revealed that most of this benefit accrued to the patients who received the initial planned dose of 600 mg pamidronate daily.[151]

In the first randomized study of intravenous pamidronate, Conte and coworkers[152] randomized 295 patients with breast cancer and bone metastases to one of two regimens:

1. Standard chemotherapy—generally cyclophosphamide and fluorouracil with one of the following: methotrexate (CMF), epirubicin (FEC), or doxorubicin (FAC)
2. Chemotherapy plus intravenous pamidronate, 45 mg every three weeks (a dose intensity of pamidronate which is now considered suboptimal)

TABLE 57-4

Effects of Bisphosphonates on Skeletal Morbidity: Results of Randomized Trials

BREAST CANCER

Agent and Route	N	Results	Investigator
Pamidronate 600 mg po vs. control	161	Reduced skeletal morbidity rate (SMR) – 94 vs. 52 events/100 women years (p = <0.01) 600 mg poorly tolerated No benefit with reduced dose (300 mg)	Van Holten[150,151]
Clodronate 1600 mg po vs. placebo	173	Reduced SMR – 305 vs. 219 events/100 woman years (p = <0.001)	Paterson[149]
Pamidronate 45 mg IV vs. control	295	Increased time to bone progression – 168 vs. 249 days (p = 0.02)	Conte[152]
Pamidronate 90 mg IV vs. placebo	382	Reduced proportion experiencing SRE – 65% vs. 46% (p = <0.001) Delay in first SRE 7.0 months vs. 13.1 (p = 0.0005)	Hortobagyi[154]
Pamidronate 60 mg IV vs. control	401	Median time to skeletal progression – 9 vs. 14 months (p = <0.01)	Hultborn[153]
Pamidronate 90 mg IV vs. placebo	374	Reduced proportion experiencing SRE – 67% vs. 56% (p = 0.027) Delay in first SRE 6.9 months vs. 10.4 (p = 0.049)	Theriault[155]
Ibandronate 2/6 mg IV vs. placebo	467	Reduced SMR with 6 mg dose, 2 mg ineffective SMR 2.18 vs. 1.61 (p = 0.03)	Body[162]

MULTIPLE MYELOMA

Agent and Route	N	Results	Investigator
Clodronate 1600 mg po vs. placebo	350	Improved two-year progression-free survival 24% vs. 12% (p < .05)	Lahtinen[165]
Pamidronate 90 mg IV vs. placebo	392	Reduced proportion experiencing SRE 24% vs. 41% (p < .001)	Berenson[167]
Clodronate 1600 mg po vs. placebo	614	Less skeletal morbidity and pain on progression	McCloskey[166]

MULTIPLE MYELOMA AND BREAST CANCER

Agent and Route	N	Results	Investigator
Zoledronic acid 4/8 mg IV vs. pamidronate 90 mg IV	1648	Zoledronic acid (4 mg) showed clinical activity equivalent to that of pamidronate (90 mg) In breast cancer patients, 43% had a SRE with 4 mg zoledronic acid, compared with 45% with pamidronate. In myeloma, 47% of patients had a SRE with zoledronic acid and 49% with pamidronate	Rosen[159]

PROSTATE CANCER

Agent and Route	N	Results	Investigator
Clodronate (4 x 520) mg oral vs. placebo	311	Reduction in number of SREs vs. placebo not significant (49% vs. 41%, p = NS)	Dearnaley[173]
Pamidronate 90 mg iv vs. placebo	378	Number of SREs equal in pamidronate and placebo arms, p = 1.0	Lipton[174]
Zoledronic acid 4/8 mg vs. placebo	643	Proportion of patients experiencing at least one SRE during the study was 25% lower in the zoledronate arm than in the placebo arm (p = .021)	Saad[175]

OTHER TUMOR TYPES

Agent and Route	N	Results (Bisphosphonate vs. Placebo/Control)	Investigator
Zoledronic acid 4/8 mg vs. placebo	773	Significant delay to time of first skeletal event in Zoledronic acid arm compared with placebo (p = 0.023) Significant reduction in proportion of patients having an event (47% vs. 38%, p = .039)	Rosen[176]

SRE, skeletal related event

A blinded, extramural review of the serial radiographs was performed. There were sufficient imaging studies available to assess response in bone in 224 patients. Of these, 141 (63%) had developed progressive disease in bone—72 patients receiving pamidronate and 69 control patients. A 48% increase in the median time to progression in bone in favor of the patient group who received pamidronate (249 vs. 168 days, $p = 0.02$) was identified. Sclerosis of lytic disease was noted in 53% and 44% of pamidronate and control patients, respectively. The other major endpoint of this trial was bone pain. A marked improvement in pain was seen more often in the pamidronate group (44% vs. 30%, $p = .025$), indicating that intravenous pamidronate adds to the symptom relief achieved by chemotherapy alone. There were also fewer complications in the pamidronate-treated group, including fewer long bone fractures (4 vs. 12) and a longer median time to requirement for radiotherapy (697 days vs. 571 days). Chemotherapy-related side effects and overall survival time were not influenced by pamidronate.

Similar results were reported in a Scandinavian trial, in which 401 patients receiving chemotherapy for advanced breast cancer were randomly allocated to receive either an intravenous pamidronate infusion (60 mg every four weeks) or a placebo infusion of the same dose intensity of pamidronate that was given in the Conte study.[136,153] The time to first skeletal complication and the number of events was significantly less with pamidronate. The median times to symptoms of skeletal progression were nine and 14 months for the pamidronate and placebo groups, respectively. No differences in pathologic fractures, radiotherapy requirements, or the need for a change in systemic therapy were seen.

The results of two double-blind, placebo-controlled trials of 90 mg pamidronate infusions every three to four weeks in addition to cytotoxic or endocrine treatments for patients with breast cancer and lytic bone metastases established bisphosphonate treatment as the standard of care in breast cancer.[154,155] These two studies were of similar design, with the exception of the systemic anticancer treatment at study entry, and the demographic and tumor characteristics were well balanced. The primary endpoint was the influence of pamidronate on skeletal-related events (SRE), namely:

- Pathologic long bone and vertebral fractures
- Spinal cord compression
- Radiation for pain relief or to treat or prevent pathologic fractures or spinal cord compression
- Surgery to bone
- Hypercalcemia of malignancy (HCM)

Treatment effects were expressed in terms of time to first SRE, the proportion of patients experiencing any SRE, the proportion of patients experiencing each individual type of SRE, and the skeletal morbidity rate (SMR), which was defined as the number of skeletal events per patient per year. In both studies, pamidronate was well tolerated, and no serious drug-related toxicity was identified.

In the chemotherapy study, 382 patients were randomized to chemotherapy and either monthly pamidronate (n = 185) or placebo infusions (n = 197).[154] The time to first SRE (excluding HCM) was seven months in the placebo group (i.e., those receiving chemotherapy alone) and 14 months in the pamidronate group ($p = <.01$). The SMR was significanctly lower throughout the study period and at 24 months was 2.5 compared with 3.6 ($p = <.001$). Benefits were maintained for at least two years. The proportion of pamidronate patients with an SRE(s) up to 24 months was 46% compared with 65% for the placebo patients ($p = <.001$). There were no differences in the types of chemotherapy or the dose intensity of treatments received during the study. The time to a change of treatment and the number of systemic treatments required during the study period were the same for both groups. Pain, analgesic use, and ECOG performance status were monitored throughout the study period. As there was inevitably a tendency for the underlying cancer to progress during the study period, there was an overall deterioration in mean performance status, pain, and analgesic consumption. The deterioration, however, was significantly less in the pamidronate group for all of these endpopoints. Quality of life was also better maintained in the pamidronate group. There was no difference in survival by treatment group, with the Kaplan-Meir estimate of median survival being 14.8 and 13.9 months for the pamidronate and placebo groups, respectively ($p = .82$).

In the endocrine study, 374 patients were randomized to receive hormone therapy with pamidronate (n = 182) or placebo (n = 192) infusions every month.[155] As in the chemotherapy study, pamidronate reduced the number and rate of SREs. The time to first SRE (excluding HCM) was six months for the placebo group and ten months for those receiving pamidronate ($p = <.049$). The benefits of pamidronate were slower to appear than in the chemotherapy study, but again the effect was maintained for at least two years. The SMR at 24 months was 2.4 for the pamidronate group compared with 3.8 for the control group ($p = .008$), and the proportion of pamidronate patients experiencing SRE(s) was 56% compared with 67% for the placebo patients ($p = .027$). The effects on pain and analgesic consumption were even more clearly evident in this study. Again, there was no difference in survival by treatment group; the Kaplan-Meier estimates of median survival were 23.1 and 23.5 months for the pamidronate and placebo groups, respectively ($p = .69$).

Zoledronic acid is the most potent bisphosphonate in clinical development and in in vitro systems has 100–1000 times the potency of pamidronate. A phase I study of thirty patients with hypercalcemia indicated that dose levels as low as 0.02 mg/kg (1-2 mg total dose) were effective in achieving normocalcemia.[156] In normocalcemic patients receiving zoledronic acid, a dose-dependent reduction in deoxypyridinoline, a specific marker of bone resorption, was identified.[157] These biochemical responses were at least as large as those previously reported after infusions of pamidronate (90 mg), and subsequently, a randomized, double-blind, dose finding, phase II study of zoledronic acid tested doses of 0.5 g, 2 g, and 4 mg zoledronic acid given on a four-weekly schedule. This study showed that 4 mg zoledronic acid was of similar efficacy to pamidronate and merited formal evaluation and development.[158]

Recently, a large international, multicenter, stratified, randomized, double-blind, phase III trial of zoledronic acid compared with pamidronate in the treatment of malignant bone disease for patients with breast cancer has been completed.[159] The trial was designed as a noninferiority trial, in which the primary efficacy variable was the proportion of patients experiencing at least one SRE. Secondary efficacy variables included the time to first SRE, skeletal morbidity rate (SMR), and an Andersen-Gill multiple events analysis.[160] The proportions of patients experiencing individual SREs, time to progression, response, performance status, analgesic and pain scores, and markers of bone resorption and formation were also assessed.

In the trial, 1130 patients with advanced breast cancer and at least one metastatic bone lesion were randomized to receive either 4 mg zoledronic acid or 8 mg zoledronic acid via a short intravenous infusion, or 90 mg pamidronate via a two-hour infusion. Treatments were administered every three to four weeks. Initially, zoledronic acid was administered as a five-minute infusion in 50 mL of 0.9% saline or 5% dextrose. This was amended to a 15-minute infusion in 100 mL of saline or dextrose due to concerns over renal toxicity. Similarly, the 8 mg dose of zoledronic acid was reduced to 4 mg due to continuing concerns over renal safety.

An initial analysis of the first 13 months of the study has been published.[159] Some 44%–46% of patients experienced at least one SRE, with this finding similar across all three treatment groups. Differences that were seen included a reduction in radiotherapy requirements between the zoledronic acid 4 mg and pamidronate groups (15% vs. 20%; $p = 0.031$). This difference was most marked among the patients with breast cancer who were receiving hormonal therapy (16% vs. 25%; $p = 0.022$). More recently, the final 25-month data have become available.[161] These show superiority for zoledronic acid 4 mg over pamidronate. Using the preplanned Andersen-Gill multiple-event analysis, a reduction of 20% in the risk of developing an SRE was observed (hazard ratio 0.799; $p = 0.025$).

There were no significant differences between the groups in terms of pain scores, analgesic use, or performance status. Pain was reduced in all groups, and analgesic use decreased or stabilized. There were no appreciable differences in the response of bone lesions to therapy or the time to progression between the study groups. All markers of bone resorption or formation decreased from baseline to the end of the study. At all time points, the urinary marker of bone resorption Ntx was significantly less in the zoledronic acid 4 mg group than in the pamidronate group (e.g., 64% vs. 57% below baseline at the end of one year; $p = 0.015$). Median overall survival was similar at approximately two years in the study groups. The most common adverse events were bone pain, nausea, fever, and fatigue, and as with the other adverse effects, they occurred generally with a similar frequency in each group. The incidence of renal dysfunction among the patients receiving 4 mg zoledronic acid (given on the 15-minute schedule) was indistinguishable from that for the pamidronate patients.

Ibandronate is another highly potent amino-bisphosphonate that is licensed in Europe for the treatment of hypercalcemia of malignancy; it is in clinical development for both the treatment of metastatic bone disease and the prevention and treatment of osteoporosis. Preliminary analysis of a phase III placebo-controlled trial of monthly infusions in breast cancer has shown a significant reduction in skeletal-related morbidity with ibandronate 4 mg.[162] Additionally, a film-coated tablet has been developed that has been shown to produce a dose-dependent reduction (at doses that are generally well tolerated) in both urinary calcium and collagen crosslink excretion.[163] Preliminary reports of phase III placebo-controlled trials of the oral formulation indicate that the oral formulation is active, with an impact on skeletal morbidity that is broadly similar to that observed in earlier placebo-controlled trials with other bisphosphonates.[164] The oral formulation has obvious attractions to both patients and health care providers, but the place of ibandronate cannot be defined until comparative data with zoledronic acid are available.

Multiple Myeloma. Multiple myeloma is typically characterized by a marked increase in osteoclast activity and proliferation. This excessive resorption of bone can be detected histomorphometrically at an early phase in the development of the disease and this itself could, through the release of interleukin-6 by the osteoclasts, play a contributory role to the growth of myeloma cells in bone. Bisphosphonates could thus be of great benefit in these patients, and recently performed trials support this view.

In a randomized, placebo-controlled trial of 350 patients with newly diagnosed myeloma, it was demonstrated that 2.4 g of clodronate daily for two years results in a significant reduction in the proportion of patients developing progression of osteolytic bone lesions (24% vs. 12% in an intention-to-treat analysis). There was only a mild, albeit significant, effect on the incidence of bone pain, however, and no effect on the occurrence of fractures or overall survival.[165] Another randomized, placebo-controlled trial of 614 patients evaluated the efficacy of 1600 mg daily of clodronate given from the time of diagnosis. Treatment with clodronate was associated with a 50% decrease in the proportion of patients with severe hypercalcemia (5.1% vs. 10.1%, $p = 0.06$) and a reduction in reported nonvertebral fractures (6.8% vs. 13.2%, $p = 0.04$). Additionally, a 30% reduction in the number of vertebral fractures (80 vs. 146, $p = 0.012$) was observed in a subset of patients with serial spine radiographs available for review.[166]

In the last five to ten years, monthly pamidronate infusions have become routine clinical management for myeloma, following the very clear results demonstrated in a large, double-blind, placebo-controlled trial. In that study, 392 patients with at least one osteolytic lesion received either 90 mg pamidronate or placebo infusions monthly for 21 months in addition to their antimyeloma chemotherapy regimens.[167] The proportion of patients developing SRE(s) was significantly lower in the group receiving pamidronate than the group receiving placebo (24% vs. 41%, $p = <.001$). The therapeutic benefit was independent of the line (first or subsequent) of antimyeloma therapy. The SMR was 2.1 in the placebo group vs. 1.1 with pamidronate ($p < 0.02$). Quality-of-life scores, performance status, pain scores, the incidence of pathologic fractures, and the need for radiotherapy treatments were all favorably influenced by pamidronate therapy.

Zoledronic acid has also been evaluated in multiple myeloma; 450 patients with advanced myeloma were included in a randomized trial comparing zoledronic acid with pamidronate.[159] No significant differences between the two agents were identified. Of the patients treated with zoledronic acid 4 mg, 47% experienced one or more SREs, compared with 49% in the group receiving pamidronate. The risk of an SRE was 7% lower with zoledronic acid, but this difference was not statistically significant (hazard rate 0.932, $p = 0.59$).[160] Intravenous ibandronate has been investigated in a randomized trial; however, the 2 mg dose chosen was unfortunately inactive and not statistically different from placebo.[168] It is now known that a dose of ibandronate 6 mg is required to reduce skeletal morbidity from metastatic bone disease.[162]

Prostate Cancer. Bisphosphonates have traditionally been evaluated in patients with osteolytic lesions, such as those associated with breast cancer and multiple myeloma. They have also been shown to reduce biochemical markers of bone resorption in patients with osteoblastic bone lesions that are associated with advanced prostate cancer.[4,169] Additionally, several phase II studies have assessed bone pain and analgesic use with some benefit in these acute end points.[147,170,171] These trials were statistically underpowered to detect significant effects on skeletal complications, and the results were not sufficiently convincing to lead to either regulatory approval for or widespread use of bisphosphonates for metastatic bone disease in prostate cancer. Furthermore, until recently, randomized, placebo-controlled trials of bisphosphonates had failed to demonstrate a significant reduction in skeletal complications from bone metastases in patients with advanced prostate cancer.

In a study of 57 patients with hormone-refractory prostate cancer and bone pain at study entry, Smith and colleagues[172] concluded that intravenous etidronate (5 mg/kg) followed by oral etidronate (400 mg/day) had no significant effects on pain levels or analgesic usage over and above placebo. A more recent clinical trial involving 208 patients investigated both pain and analgesic usage. In this study, intravenous clodronate was added to a background treatment of mitoxantrone and prednisolone. The study also included objectively measurable skeletal complications as clinical endpoints. No significant differences between clodronate and placebo were seen.[145]

The Medical Research Council in the United Kingdom has reported preliminary data from a phase III trial of oral clodronate in 311 men with metastatic bone disease from prostate cancer.[173] Quite a high dose of oral clodronate (Loron, 1040 mg twice daily) was administered for a median duration of 43 months. The early analysis reported a slight reduction in the proportion of patients receiving clodronate who were experiencing a skeletal event (41% vs. 49%), an improvement in time to progression (24 vs. 19 months), and increased median survival (37 vs.

28 months). None of these differences was statistically significant, however. Further follow-up could clarify the results of this trial, although, like the other studies mentioned previously, the study was probably underpowered to show the likely impact of a bisphosphonate on the course of disease.

Pamidronate has also been studied in patients with advanced prostate cancer.[174] In a multicenter, randomized, placebo-controlled trial, 236 patients with prostate cancer and bone metastases were treated with intravenous pamidronate (90 mg) or placebo every three weeks for nine months. This trial assessed bone pain as the primary endpoint and included an assessment of skeletal events as a secondary endpoint. Patients in this trial had very advanced disease (median baseline PSA = 97.8 ng/mL in the pamidronate group), very high levels of bone resorption, and substantial bone pain at study entry. As in the previous trials, pamidronate did not reduce the incidence of skeletal events and had only a slight effect on bone pain.

Despite the failure of all other bisphosphonates, zoledronic acid was investigated in patients with advanced prostate cancer to determine whether the increased potency of this compound would translate into improved clinical benefit. In this study, 643 patients with hormone-refractory prostate cancer and documented bone metastases were randomized to one of three different treatment groups:

1. 4 mg zoledronic acid ($n = 214$)
2. 8 mg zoledronic acid ($n = 221$)
3. Placebo ($n = 208$)[175]

In the 8-mg arm, the dose was reduced by a protocol amendment to 4 mg because of concerns over renal safety, and conclusions on the efficacy of this cohort are difficult to make. Zoledronic acid or placebo were administered every three weeks for 15 months, followed by an extension phase of a further 10 months. All patients received daily oral supplements of calcium and vitamin D. The disposition, demographics, and prognostic factors of patients in the zoledronic acid and placebo treatment groups were well balanced. The primary endpoint was the proportion of patients with a skeletal event, defined as before with the addition of changes in chemotherapy resulting from bone pain. Secondary endpoints included the time to first skeletal complication, an Andersen-Gill multiple-event analysis, levels of bone pain, and biochemical markers of bone resorption.

Zoledronic acid was significantly more effective than placebo across all primary and secondary endpoints. The zoledronic acid 4 mg treatment group experienced significantly fewer SRE(s) (33% vs. 44% with placebo; $p = .021$). Furthermore, there were consistent reductions in the proportion of patients with each type of skeletal complication, including nonvertebral fractures. Zoledronic acid also prolonged the time to first skeletal complication by more than four months ($p = .011$). Zoledronic acid 4 mg remained superior to placebo when fractures were excluded, indicating that the beneficial effect was not simply as a result of the prevention of osteoporotic fractures. Using the Andersen-Gill multiple-event analysis, it was calculated that zoledronic acid 4 mg reduced the overall risk of skeletal complications by 36%. Zoledronic acid reduced bone pain at all time points, and significant reductions in the markers of bone resorption were documented for the zoledronic acid group compared with the placebo group throughout the duration of the study. Despite the favorable effects on skeletal morbidity, however, there were no significant effects on disease-related endpoints such as time to progression and survival.

As a class, bisphosphonates are known to affect renal function; however, the risk of renal function deterioration in patients treated with zoledronic acid (4 mg via a 15-minute intravenous infusion) was found to be similar to that of placebo-treated patients. The only adverse events that occurred at increased frequency with zoledronic acid were fatigue, anemia, myalgia, and pyrexia. The majority of these events were manageable with simple supportive care measures and are as expected with any intravenous amino-bisphosphonate therapy.[174]

Other Tumors. Until recently, there had only been anecdotal reports of the use of bisphosphonates in other tumors associated with bone metastases. The pathophysiology of bone metastases is broadly similar in all tumor types, however, and bisphsophonates could thus be expected to be of value in preventing skeletal morbidity, especially if metastatic bone disease was a patient's dominant site of disease. As part of the development program for zoledronic acid, a phase III randomized, placebo-controlled trial has been performed in the management of bone metastases from solid tumors other than breast or prostate cancer.[176] The study included 773 patients with a wide variety of solid malignancies; 51% had lung cancer (mainly non–small cell), and the other most frequent tumor types were small cell lung cancer and renal cancer. As before, the patients were randomized in a double-blind fashion to one of three arms: zoledronic acid 4 mg, zoledronic acid 8 mg (reduced to 4 mg), or placebo every three weeks. The endpoints and changes to the infusion time and dose were similar to the two previously described phase III studies.

The study found that 4 mg of zoledronic acid significantly reduced the proportion of patients with at least one SRE (39% vs. 48%, $p = 0.039$) and significantly prolonged the time to the first SRE compared with placebo (314 days vs. 168 days, respectively, $p = 0.021$). This is a particularly important result in a population of patients with a very short median survival time (six months). Overall, zoledronic acid reduced the risk for SRE(s) by about 30% (hazard ratio 0.693 vs. placebo, $p = 0.003$). The adverse effects, excluding increases in serum creatinine associated with the 8/4 mg group, were very similar in all groups apart from the anticipated acute-phase response of fever and myalgia with the early infusions.

Optimum Use of Bisphosphonates in Metastatic Bone Disease

Criteria need to be determined regarding when in the course of metastatic bone disease bisphosphonates should be started and stopped.[177] Because of the logistics and cost of delivering monthly intravenous infusions for all patients with metastatic bone disease, certain empiric

recommendations on who should receive treatment are needed. These should take into account the underlying disease type and extent, the life expectancy of the patient, the probability of the patient experiencing a SRE, and the ease with which the patient can attend for treatment (or be treated by a domiciliary service).

In the authors' opinion, all patients with multiple myeloma should receive bisphosphonates from the time of diagnosis, and the highest priority should be given to patients with symptomatic bone metastases from breast cancer, particularly if they have already experienced a skeletal event. In the context of life-threatening visceral disease, bisphosphonate treatment for bone metastases from breast cancer is probably unececessary, particularly if the bone disease is asymptomatic. It is hoped that biochemical monitoring of bone resorption might prove to be relevant in identifying patients most likely to experience a reduction in skeletal morbidity from bisphosphonate treatment; if so, biochemical predictors could be incorporated into a "treatment priority" scoring system. Bisphosphonate treatment—specifically zoledronic acid—is also appropriate for patients with endocrine-resistant metastatic bone disease from prostate cancer. Patients with other tumors and symptomatic metastasis to bone should be considered for bisphosphonate treatment if bone is the dominant site of metastasis, especially if the prognosis is reasonable (> six months). Patients with renal cell cancer particularly appear to benefit from treatment.

Because bisphosphonates are providing supportive care, reducing the rate of skeletal morbidity but not necessarily abolishing it, the criteria for stopping their administration are different from those used for classical antineoplastic drugs. They should not necessarily be stopped when a skeletal event occurs or when there is progression in bone.

Despite the obvious clinical benefits of bisphosphonates, it is clear that only a proportion of events is prevented, and some patients do not experience a skeletal event despite the presence of metastatic bone disease. It is currently impossible to predict whether an individual patient needs or will benefit from a bisphosphonate. Overall, bisphosphonates reduce the frequency of skeletal events by 25%–40%; however, bisphosphonates are a relatively costly additional intervention in cancer care that is now potentially applicable to a very large proportion of patients with advanced malignancy. The cost effectiveness of routine long-term treatment has been questioned, and prioritization of bisphosphonate use is needed.[178]

A recent preliminary report on the use of the bone resorption marker Ntx suggests that biochemical monitoring could be useful to identify patients at high risk of skeletal complications. In this study of 121 patients with metastatic bone, monthly measurements of urinary Ntx were made during treatment with a range of bisphosphonates.[179] All SREs, hospital admissions for control of bone pain, and deaths during the period of observation were recorded. Ntx was strongly correlated with the number of SREs and/or deaths ($p < 0.001$). Patients with Ntx values above 100 nmol/mmol creatinine were many times more likely to experience an SRE or death than those with Ntx below this level ($p < 0.01$). Thus, a more cost-effective use of bisphosphonates might be to reserve them until patients have Ntx levels above either 50 or 100 nmol/mmol creatinine, and to adjust the dose and schedule to maintain a normal (<50nmol/mmol creatinine) rate of bone resorption. Randomized trials to assess this approach are planned.

Protecting the Skeleton

Prevention of Bone Metastases

Bone is the most frequent site of distant relapse, accounting for around 40% of all first recurrences.[2] In addition to the well-recognized release of bone cell activating factors from the tumor, it is now appreciated that release of bone-derived growth factors and cytokines from resorbing bone can both attract cancer cells to the bone surface and facilitate their growth and proliferation.[180] Inhibition of bone resorption could, therefore, have an effect on the development and progression of metastatic bone disease and is an adjuvant therapeutic strategy of potential importance.

Encouraging animal studies with a variety of animal tumor models and a range of bisphosphonates have shown inhibition of bone metastasis development and a reduction in tumor burden within bone.[181] More recently, several clinical trials have been reported using the relatively low-potency oral bisphosphonate, clodronate (Table 57-5). In the largest study, 1079 women with primary operable breast cancer were randomized to receive either clodronate 1600 mg daily or placebo for two years in addition to standard adjuvant systemic treatment. Recent data presented with a median follow-up time of five years revealed a nonsignificant reduction in the frequency of bone metastases in the patients treated with clodronate (63 [12%] vs. 80 [15%] patients).[182] During the two years on active treatment, however, there was a reduction in bone metastases, but this disappeared on discontinuation of the study drug, suggesting that

adjuvant bisphosphonate treatment trials in the future should test a longer duration of treatment. There was no effect on nonbone recurrence (112 [21%] vs. 128 [24%] patients), but, despite little effect on the primary endpoint (bone recurrence), patients randomized to the clodronate arm had a better survival (82% vs. 77%, $p = 0.047$).

In a second study, Diel and associates[183] studied 302 patients with breast cancer randomly allocated to either oral clodronate 1600 mg daily ($n = 157$) for three years or a control group ($n = 145$). These women had no overt evidence of metastatic disease but were selected for the trial on the basis of immunocytochemical detection of tumor cells in the bone marrow, a known risk factor for the subsequent development of distant metastases. Patients received appropriate adjuvant chemotherapy and endocrine treatment. There were no discernible prognostic or treatment imbalances between the two groups, and the follow-up schedules were similar. The median observation period was 36 months. The incidence of osseous metastases was significantly lower in the clodronate group (11 [7%] vs. 25 [17%] patients, $p < 0.002$). There was also a large, unexpected reduction in the incidence of visceral metastases in the clodronate group (19 [13%] vs. 42 [29%] patients, $p < 0.001$). These results have subsequently been updated and show similar results, although the striking effect on extraskeletal visceral relapse seen in the earlier report was less dramatic and no longer statistically significant.[184]

The exciting findings of the Diel study must be viewed in the light of a further trial that produced conflicting results. Saarto and colleagues[185] randomized 299 women with primary node-positive breast cancer to oral clodronate 1600 mg daily ($n = 149$) or a control group ($n = 150$). The median follow-up time was five years. Treatment with clodronate in this study did not lead to a reduction in the development of bone metastases (29 [19%] vs. 24 [16%] patients, $p = 0.27$ for the clodronate and control groups, respectively). Additionally, the development of nonskeletal recurrence was significantly higher in the clodronate

TABLE 57-5

The Use of Adjuvant Clodronate in Primary Operable Breast Cancer Trials

NO. OF PATIENTS	PERIOD OF CLODRONATE TREATMENT (YRS)	OCCURRENCE OF BONE METASTASES (CLODRONATE VS. PLACEBO)	OCCURRENCE OF NONBONE METASTASES (CLODRONATE VS. PLACEBO)	DEATHS (CLODRONATE VS. PLACEBO)	REFERENCE
1079	2	At two years, 2% vs. 5% p = .016 At >2 years 10% vs. 10% p = 0.73	At >2 years 21% vs. 24% p = 0.26	At 2 years 8% vs. 8% (approx) At 5 years 17% vs. 22% p = .047	Powles et al.[182]
299	3	21% vs. 17% p = .27	43% vs. 25% p = .009	At 5 years 30% vs. 17% p = .01	Saarto et al.[185]
302	2	14% vs. 24% p = .044	16% vs. 26% p = .091	At 5 years 10% vs. 22% p = .002	Diel et al.[183,184]

In all cases 1600 mg clodronate was given orally. Average follow-up time was 4.5–5.5 years.

group (60 [40%] vs. 36 [24%] patients, $p = .0007$) and, most important, the overall five-year survival was significantly lower in the clodronate group (70% vs. 83%, $p = .009$). It is possible that there were some prognostic imbalances favoring the control group, but the safest assumption is to consider that the Diel and Saarto studies cancel each other out and probably reflect the usual heterogeneity of results seen in relatively small studies of adjuvant treatment.

To identify a definite adjuvant role for bisphosphonates will require further large, randomized studies. The National Surgical Adjuvant Breast Project (NSABP) recently started a placebo-controlled trial of oral clodronate (n = >3000) in an attempt to resolve the value or otherwise of adjuvant clodronate. Adjuvant trials are just beginning with zoledronic acid. It is hoped that the added potency of zoledronic acid might have beneficial effects, not only through the inhibition of bone resorption, but also through direct effects on tumor cells in the bone marrow. There is increasing evidence, from a range of cell line experiments, that zoledronic acid can inhibit tumor cell adhesion and invasion.[186] Additionally, zoledronic acid promotes apoptosis both directly and in synergy with paclitaxel.[187] These effects are mediated through the mevalonate pathway, using the same molecular pathway that aminobisphosphonates exploit to inhibit osteoclast function. Finally, there are experimental data from animal models indicating that zoledronic acid can suppress angiogenesis.[188]

Effects of Cancer Treatments on Skeletal Health

There are now increasing numbers of long-term survivors from breast cancer who have received combination chemotherapy, radiotherapy, and hormonal cancer treatment. Many of these individuals are at increased risk of osteoporosis, largely because of the endocrine changes induced by treatment. There might also be clinically relevant, direct effects of cytotoxic drugs on bone. Treatment-induced bone loss is a particularly important long-term problem for women with breast cancer, for whom there are concerns about the safety of hormone replacement therapy.

Estrogen is known to be critical in the maintenance of normal bone mass in women. After menopause, a reduction in bone mineral density (BMD) occurs; the loss is most pronounced during the first three years, when the rate can be as high as 5% annually, but it then reduces to a rate of about 0.5% annually thereafter. The aromatase inhibitor anastrozole leads to nearly complete suppression of circulating estradiol and causes accelerated bone loss. In consequence, these women could be at greater risk of suffering a low-trauma fracture. Preliminary data from the large adjuvant trial of anastrozole vs. tamoxifen (ATAC) indicate that the rate of fractures is increased to 5.8% for patients taking anastrozole compared with 3.7% for women taking tamoxifen.[189] Part of this difference can be attributed to the bone-sparing effect of tamoxifen; however, a contribution from the direct effect of anastrozole on BMD and bone strength is also assumed.

The bisphosphonates, as potent inhibitors of bone resorption, have emerged as an important class of agents in the management of postmenopausal osteoporosis. The use of alendronate, an aminobisphosphonate, has demonstrated a significant reduction in osteoporotic fractures. A dose of 10 mg of alendronate in postmenopausal women resulted in an increase in BMD of 6% and 9% at the lumbar spine and femoral neck, respectively, with a concomitant decrease in fracture rates.[190] A meta-analysis of five studies with alendronate in this population has shown a 30% reduction in the incidence of non-vertebral fractures.[191] On the other hand, only a few studies address the effectiveness of these compounds in the management of cancer treatment-induced bone loss, especially among populations in which the use of hormone replacement therapy could be undesirable.

A few studies have evaluated women with breast cancer and a treatment-induced premature menopause. In the first, Saarto and colleagues[192] studied the effect of clodronate 1600 mg in 148 premenopausal women receiving adjuvant chemotherapy for breast cancer. They observed that rapid bone loss occurred in the women who became amenorhoeic after chemotherapy (6% and 2% losses at two years in the spine and hip, respectively). Among those receiving clodronate, however, the bone effects of chemotherapy-induced premature menopause were attenuated (2% loss and 1% gain at two years in the spine and hip, respectively). In a comparison of risedronate with placebo in a postmenopausal group of patients receiving tamoxifen, Delmas and associates[193] observed an approximately 2.5% increase in BMD at the lumbar spine and femoral neck in the risedronate group compared with the group receiving placebo.

Intravenous bisphosphonate administration is used widely in oncology in the treatment of metastatic disease and could be an attractive option for preventing bone loss in a cancer population. In a recent study, Reid and coworkers[194] investigated the use of three-monthly, six-monthly, and annual intravenous zoledronic acid administration in a general population of osteoporotic, postmenopausal women. It was found that a single 4 mg intravenous dose of zoledronic acid resulted in an increase in BMD of 4.6% at the spine and of 3.3% at the hip, both measured one year later. This was comparable to the increase in BMD achieved by giving the same total dose at three or six monthly intervals. Among patients with breast cancer, six-monthly zoledronic acid has also been shown to reverse the bone loss induced by a combination of the LHRH analog goserelin plus further estrogen suppression with anastrozole. In this study, a 10% loss of bone in the lumbar spine occurred with this combination without bisphosphonate, compared with a small 1% gain in BMD with six-monthly zoledronic acid.[195]

COMPLICATIONS OF BONE METASTASES

Bone metastases cause considerable morbidity: pain, impaired mobility, hypercalcemia, pathologic fracture, spinal cord or nerve root compression, and bone marrow

Problems Common to Cancer and Its Therapy

infiltration. In a study of 498 patients with first relapse in bone from breast cancer, 145 (29%) developed one or more major complications of metastatic bone destruction. Hypercalcemia occurred in 86 patients (17%), pathologic long bone fractures in 78 (16%), and spinal cord compression in 13 (3%).[2] Similar results were identified in a more recent report from the same institution.[3] In a study of multiple myeloma, the prevalence of skeletal complications at diagnosis was assessed in 254 patients.[196] Bone pain was reported in 75% of these patients—in the back in 50%, in the ribs in 20%, in the upper limbs in 7%, and in the lower limbs in 11%. Radiographic evaluation revealed the presence of vertebral fracture(s) in 54%, and 33% had hypercalcemia at diagnosis.

In two large randomized trials that included patients of breast cancer and multiple myeloma receiving chemotherapy, the mean skeletal morbidity rates (number of skeletal events per year) in the absence of bisphosphonates were 3.5 and 2.0, respectively, indicating that a skeletal event occurs in metastatic bone disease from breast cancer on the average of every three to four months and in multiple myeloma every 6 months.[154,167] Despite the clinical importance of metastatic bone disease and the huge expenditure on medical care for skeletal complications, however, there has, until recently, been relatively little academic interest in this condition or sufficient thought given as to how best to coordinate clinical management and deliver optimum care.[178,197,198]

Extensive infiltration of the bone marrow by metastatic disease causes leucoerythroblastic anaemia and pancytopaenia predisposing to infection and haemorrhage. Radiotherapy, often needed for the treatment of bone metastases, can exacerbate this problem, which in turn can compromise the ability to give chemotherapy effectively. Animal experiments have shown that cytotoxic drugs can interfere with osteoblastic function and new bone formation, but the clinical significance of these findings is unknown. Other iatrogenic factors might also aggravate morbidity from bone metastases. For example, endocrine ablation and corticosteroids might predispose a patient to osteoporotic fractures.

Bone Pain

Bone pain is the most common type of pain from cancer and a significant problem in both hospital and community practice. Pain is usually the presenting symptom and is caused by a variety of factors, including periosteal stretching, compression or infiltration of nerve roots, reflex muscle spasm, and the local effects of cytokines. Features of bone pain are that it is often poorly localized, has a deep, boring quality that aches or burns, and is accompanied by episodes of stabbing discomfort. It is often worse at night, being little helped by sleep and not necessarily relieved by lying down. There is often disturbance of the highly innervated periosteum—possibly giving this pain its neurogenic-like qualities and adding to its intractability.

Spinal instability is the cause of back pain in 10% of patients with cancer.[199] This can cause excruciating pain that is mechanical in origin. The patient is comfortable only when lying still, and any movement reproduces severe pain. Consequently, the patient might not be able to sit, stand, or walk. Becuse the pain is mechanical in origin, radiation therapy or systemic treatment cannot help; the only solution is stabilization of the spine. Stabilization requires major surgery, with risks of significant morbidity and mortality, but with careful selection of patients, excellent results can be obtained.

Hypercalcemia of Malignancy

Hypercalcemia (see also Chapter 48) is another emergency associated with metastatic bone disease. Its clinical features include nausea, vomiting, dehydration, and confusion. Although malignant hypercalcemia is usually associated with demonstrable bone metastases, this is not always the case. In a review of 147 patients with advanced breast cancer having hypercalcemia, 125 patients (85%) had definite radiographic evidence of bone metastases, but in 22 patients (15%) there was no such evidence of skeletal involvement.[200] In the latter group, there was a significantly higher incidence of liver metastases and inappropriately high renal tubular reabsorption of calcium, circumstances which suggested that liver involvement could be facilitating a humoral component in the pathogenesis of hypercalcemia in these patients.

Hypercalcemia causes a number of signs and symptoms, which vary considerably from patient to patient. These are often nonspecific, affecting many systems in the body, and can be mistaken for symptoms of the underlying cancer or associated treatment if there is not an astute awareness of the possibility of hypercalcemia. If untreated, a progressive rise in serum calcium leads to a deterioration in renal function and level of consciousmess. Death ultimately ensues as a result of cardiac arrhythmias and renal failure.

It is now clear that various mechanisms are involved in the pathogenesis of malignant hypercalcemia. These include increased bone resorption (osteolysis) and systemic release of humoral hypercalcemic factors. Bone metastases are common but not invariably present.[201] In some tumors, such as squamous cell cancers, humoral mechanisms are dominant, increasing both renal tubular calcium reabsorption and phosphate excretion. In others—multiple myeloma and lymphoma, for example—osteolysis predominates, while in breast cancer, both osteolysis and humoral mechanisms appear to be important.

Doubt about the aetiology of hypercalcemia in patients with cancer is unusual, but nonmalignant causes must be considered, particularly in the absence of metastases. In the community, hyperparathyroidism is the most common cause of hypercalcemia and may be encountered also in patients with cancer.[202] Measurement of parathyroid hormone (PTH) using a modern, specific radioimmunoassay is worthwhile if there is any doubt about the diagnosis; levels of PTH tend to be low or undetectable in malignancy and inappropriately high in hyperparathyroidism.

Intravenous bisphosphonates, in conjunction with rehydration, are now established as the treatment of choice for hypercalcemia. Approximately 70%–90% of patients will achieve normocalcemia, resulting in relief of symptoms and improved quality of life.[203] Zoledronic acid is the most effective bisphosphonate for the acute treatment of this metabolic emergency.[204]

Pathologic Fractures

Metastatic destruction of bone reduces its load-bearing capabilities, resulting initially in trabecular disruption and microfractures and, subsequently, in total loss of bony integrity. Rib fractures and vertebral collapse are the most common occurrences, resulting in loss of height, kyphoscoliosis, and a degree of restrictive lung disease. The most severe disability, however, is caused by fracture of a long bone or epidural extension of tumor into the spine.

The incidence of pathologic fracture in patients with bone metastases is somewhat uncertain and is dependent on whether rib and vertebral fractures are included. In one series, 150 (8%) of 1800 patients with metastatic bone disease developed a fracture of the femur or humerus; these were secondary to metastases from the breast in 53%, from the kidney in 11%, from the lung in 8%, from the thyroid in 5%, from lymphoma in 5%, and from the prostate in only 3% of patients.[205] In another smaller series of patients with breast cancer, the incidence of pathologic fractures was 57%, with rib fractures occuring first in 29%, vertebral collapse in 9%, long bone fractures in 9%, and pelvic fractures in 8% of patients.[206] Vertebral collapse is probably underreported in most series. Paterson and colleagues,[149] who systematically reviewed serial radiographs in patients participating in a clinical trial of oral clodronate, showed that a woman with bone metastases from breast cancer can expect to experience an average of 1.3 vertebral and 0.4 nonvertebral fractures a year.

The probability of developing a pathologic fracture increases with the duration of metastatic involvement and is therefore, somewhat paradoxically, more common in those patients with bone-only disease who have a relatively good prognosis. A retrospective analysis of 859 patients with bone metastases from breast cancer showed that those with bone-only disease had almost a fourfold increase in the incidence of subsequent pathologic long-bone fractures compared with patients who also had concomitant liver metastases. This finding was attributed to the different survival outcomes between the two groups; the median survival from diagnosis of bone metastases for patients with bone-only disease was 2.2 years, compared with 5.5 months for those with concomitant liver disease.[207] The study also showed that scintigraphic evidence of metastases in the femora and humeri at the time of diagnosis significantly predicted an increased risk of future fractures.

Because the development of a fracture is so devastating to a patient with cancer, increased emphasis is now being placed on attempts to predict metastatic sites at risk of fracture, the use of prophylactic surgery, and long-term administration of bisphosphonates.[208] Assessment of patients with symptomatic bone metastases by a specialist orthopedic and/or spinal surgeon should be a much more frequent component of multidisciplinary management than has been the case until now.

Fractures are common through lytic metastases and weight-bearing bones, the proximal femora being the most commonly affected sites. Damage to both trabecular and cortical bone are structurally important, but it is the relevance of cortical destruction that is most clearly appreciated. Several radiologic features that could predict imminent fracture have been identified.[208] Risk factors that have been taken into account include pain, the anatomic site of a lesion, its radiologic characteristics, and its size. Although intensity of pain, which is difficult to quantify, is not clearly associated with fracture risk, pain that is exacerbated by movement appears to be an important factor in predicting impending fracture. Presumably, such functional pain indicates diminution in the mechanical strength of a bone and in one series was followed invariably by fracture.

As far as radiologic appearances are concerned, there is a general consensus that lytic lesions carry a much higher risk of fracture than either mixed or osteosclerotic lesions. Accordingly, a particularly high fracture rate is found in association with metastases from lung cancer. Given the poor prognosis of this tumor, however, such fractures rarely lead to prolonged disability. By contrast, in breast cancer, which follows a much more protracted course, pathologic fracture is a major cause of prolonged disability. In prostatic cancer, with its predominantly sclerotic nature, pathologic fracture is less common but by no means rare.[175]

Radiologic assessment also yields information about the size of a lesion and the extent to which the bone is destroyed. When less than two-thirds of the diameter of a long bone is affected, pathologic fracture is relatively unusual, but above this limit the fracture rate increases markedly, with an incidence of approximately 80% for such lesions. A practical scoring system incorporating the foregoing factors has been described to give valuable guidance in the selection of patients for prophylactic fixation.[208]

Prophylactic internal fixation is the treatment of choice for such lesions, followed by radiotherapy to inhibit further tumor growth and avoid further bone destruction. It is easier to stabilize a bone while it is still intact and while rehabilitation and convalescence are shorter and easier. Depending on the primary lesion, endocrine treatment or chemotherapy could also be necessary. Providing the lesion is irradiated, there is no evidence to suggest that surgery increases the risk of disseminating tumor cells either locally or into the circulation. Indeed, there is some experimental evidence that pathologic fractures are associated with an increased incidence of pulmonary metastases and that prophylactic stabilization decreases this incidence.[209] If a given patient is not fit for surgery, radiotherapy and avoidance of weight-bearing activity are indicated.

Before surgery, a radionuclide bone scan and radiographs of the entire length of the affected bone should be obtained. These measures ensure that any other metastases that might subsequently develop into a pathologic fracture are also stabilized and included in the radiotherapy field. A pathologic fracture at the edge of a plate or of an intramedullary nail, particularly when fixed with methylmethacrylate, is more difficult to treat than if there were no implant in the bone.

Pathologic fractures are not necessarily a manifestation of terminal disease, and primary internal stabilization followed by radiotherapy are usually the treatments of choice, and certainly the only modalities likely to both restore mobility and relieve pain. Untreated pathologic fractures rarely heal, and although radiotherapy might achieve local tumor control, bony union remains unlikely. Radiotherapy inhibits chondrogenesis (a prerequisite for fracture healing), and with large areas of bone destruction there could be insufficient matrix remaining for adequate repair.

The type of internal stabilization chosen depends on the site of the lesion. When feasible, closed intramedullary nailing is preferred; however, at the end of the long bones, intramedullary nailing alone is inadequate, and alternative techniques are necessary. It is essential that the internal stabilization provide sufficient strength to allow un-supported use of the limb and for the legs to bear weight. Fulfilling this demand could require supplementation with methylmethacrylate (which is inserted into the tumor cavity with the implant fixed across the methyl-methacrylate while still soft) and bridging normal bone above and below the lesion.

Pathologic femoral neck fractures do not unite despite internal fixation, and in this situation, replacement arthroplasty is needed. Careful preoperative assessment of the pelvis and femur is necessary, and for this, CT scanning or MRI could be helpful. If there is no metastatic involvement of the acetabulum, a hemiarthroplasty could be all that is required. If the acetabulum is involved, however, total replacement arthroplasty is indicated, and sometimes pelvic reconstruction is necessary.[210] Many patients have metastases in the distal femur together with proximal involvement, and for these patients, a long-stemmed femoral prosthesis is recommended.

For humeral fractures, internal fixation is also useful, providing more rapid and greater pain relief compared with conservative treatment. Although patients with a very short life expectancy can be managed adequately with conservative treatment, those patients expected to survive longer than three months are best managed by internal fixation to ensure pain relief and restoration of function. Replacement arthroplasty could be necessary if the proximal humerus is involved, but most pathologic fractures of the humerus can be treated by intramedullary nailing.

Occasionally, patients present with an isolated metastasis in the distal skeleton. If on careful evaluation there is no other evidence of dissemination of the tumor, resection of the lesion should be considered. Local resection and prosthetic replacement are usually possible, but occasionally, amputation is indicated.

Spinal Instability

Spinal instability can cause excruciating pain that is mechanical in origin and not relieved by radiotherapy or systemic treatment. As with pathologic fractures of long bones, stabilization is required for pain relief and involves major surgery, which is associated with significant morbidity and mortality. There are several methods for spinal stabilization, but in general, the posterior approach is technically easier and allows stabilization of a larger area of the spine. With careful selection of patients, excellent results can be obtained. An associated neurologic deficit is not a contraindication to these procedures, and in one series, 20 of 29 patients with instability of the dorsal lumbar spine and an associated neurologic deficit obtained significant recovery of function.[211]

Percutaneous vertebroplasty, a new approach to treating spinal pain and instability, involves injecting an acrylic polymer into a diseased vertebral body. The technique was developed initially for the treatment of painful vertebral haemangiomas, and considerable experience with it has been obtained in the treatment of osteoporotic compression fractures. Its use has now been extended to the treatment of malignant spinal disease.[212] The technique provides effective pain relief, which is achieved more rapidly than with radiotherapy, and it confers the added benefit of providing structural support to the spinal column, thus reducing the risk of vertebral collapse and instability. Although generally a safe procedure, it can be complicated by leakage of the polymer, which predisposes to spinal cord or nerve root compression. The technique seems to have the potential for wider use, particularly among patients with limited vertebral disease and those for whom major surgical spinal stabilization procedures are unsuitable.

Compression of the Spinal Cord or Cauda Equina

Compression of the spinal cord or cauda equina in patients with metastatic disease of the spine is a medical emergency necessitating prompt diagnosis and treatment (see also Chapter 55). Its causes include pressure from an enlarging extradural mass, spinal angulation after vertebral collapse, vertebral dislocation after pathologic fracture or, rarely, pressure from intradural metastases. The most common primary tumors producing this complication, in decreasing order of frequency, are carcinoma of the breast, lung cancer, prostatic cancer, lymphoma, and renal carcinoma.

Back pain is the most common initial symptom of spinal cord compression; it affected 125 of 130 patients (96%) in one series.[213] Two types of pain can occur—local spinal or radicular. Radicular pain varies with the location of the tumor, being common in the cervical (79%) and lumbosacral (90%) regions and less common with thoracic lesions (55%). Both local spinal and radicular pain are experienced close to the site of the lesion identified at myelography. Motor weakness, sensory loss, and autonomic dysfunction are all common at presentation of spinal cord or cauda equina compression.

The development of back pain in a patient with cancer, coincident with an abnormality on a plain spinal radiograph, should serve as a warning for the possible development of spinal cord compression. In this situation, more than 60% of patients experience myelographic abnormalities or evidence of epidural disease on MRI.[214,215] Compression of the spinal cord or cauda equina can occur in association with spinal stability or in isolation. When there is a greater than 50% vertebral collapse, compression of the spinal cord becomes more likely. The keys to successful rehabilitation are early diagnosis, high-dose corticosteroids, rapid assessment, and urgent referral for either decompression and spinal stabilization or radiotherapy. Neurologic recovery is unlikely if the spinal compression is not relieved within 24-48 hours.

A detailed study of spinal cord compression complicating breast cancer in 70 patients has been reported.[215] Over the period of this review, 1684 patients had presented with metastatic disease, giving an incidence of cord compression of 4%. The median time to the development of spinal cord compression from diagnosis of breast cancer was 42 months. All patients had radiologic evidence of bone metastases, and only five of them were not known to have bone metastases previously. The most frequent symptom was motor weakness (96%), followed by pain (94%), sensory disturbance (79%), and sphincter disturbance (61%); 91% of patients had had at least one symptom for more than a week. Radiotherapy was given as primary treatment to 43 patients, while 21 had decompressive surgery (seven of whom had subsequent postoperative radiotherapy); six patients were too unwell for either treatment.

After treatment, 96% of those who were ambulatory before treatment maintained the ability to walk. In those unable to walk, 45% regained ambulation, radiotherapy and surgery being equally effective in achieving this result. Median survival after cord compression was four months, with no significant difference being seen between those treated by either radiotherapy or surgery. The most important predictor of survival was the ability to walk after treatment. The conclusion from the study was that the majority of patients had had prior warning symptoms of cord compression, and nearly all had previous evidence of spinal bone metastases before the complication occurred. These findings stress the importance of prompt presentation, diagnosis, and treatment and suggest that earlier diagnosis and intervention should improve outcome.

The choice between surgical decompression and radiotherapy depends on a variety of clinical features. Surgical decompression is indicated for patients with recent onset of symptoms and with progressive paraplegia and urinary retention of less than 30 hours duration. The site of compression should be localized to no more than two or three vertebral segments, and the patient should have a life expectancy of at least several weeks. For patients in whom the paraplegia has been established for several days or urinary retention has been present for more than 30 hours, surgical decompression rarely results in the recovery of bladder or motor function. Radiotherapy is indicated for those who are either unfit for surgery or do not meet the criteria for surgical decompression.

Several studies have suggested that surgical decompression has no advantage over radiotherapy.[216,217] It should be appreciated, however, that these studies compared dorsal laminectomy—an outdated and now inappropriate procedure—with irradiation; surgical decompression should be followed by spinal stabilization. The choice of management should be decided on an individual basis, and there are undoubtedly patients who have benefited greatly from appropriate and prompt surgical management.

SUMMARY

The management of bone metastases requires an experienced multidisciplinary team to ensure timely diagnosis and the appropriate integration of local and systemic treatments. The effects of tumor cells on bone cell function (especially on osteoclast activity) underpin the rationale for the use of bisphosphonate treatment to reduce skeletal morbidity. These bone-specific treatments are now an accepted part of routine clinical management.[218] Additionally, the disruption of bone remodeling results in release of collagen fragments, which appears to have value in predicting skeletal events, prognosis, and monitoring of response.

Further developments in our understanding of the pathophysiology of bone metastases can be expected to provide new therapeutic strategies. Already, improved knowledge of the signaling molecules involved in regulating osteoclast function—notably osteoprotogerin and RANK ligand—has led to the development of highly active targeted therapies for bone diseases, including cancer.[219,220]

REFERENCES

1. Galasko CSB: The anatomy and pathways of skeletal metastases. In Weiss L, Gilbert AH (eds): Bone Metastasis. Boston, GK Hall, 1981, pp 49–63.
2. Coleman RE, Rubens RD: The clinical course of bone metastases in breast cancer. Br J Cancer 1987;55:61–66.
3. Coleman RE, Smith P, Rubens RD: Clinical course and prognostic factors following recurrence from breast cancer. Br J Cancer 1998;77:336–340.
4. Urwin GH, Percival RC, Harris S, et al: Generalised increase in bone resorption in carcinoma of the prostate. Br J Urol 1985;57:721.
5. Robson M, Dawson N: How is androgen dependent metastatic prostate cancer best treated? Hematol Oncol Clin North Am 1996;10:727–747.
6. Muggia FM, Chervu LR: Lung cancer: Diagnosis in metastatic sites. Semin Oncol 1974;1:217.
7. Batson OV: The role of the vertebral veins in metastatic process. Ann Intern Med 1942;16:38.
8. Roodman GD: Role of stromal-derived cytokines and growth factors in bone metastasis. Cancer 2003;97:733–738.
9. Sato K, Fujii Y, Kasono K, Tsushima T, Shizume K: Production of Interleukin-1 alpha and a parathyroid hormone-like factor by a squamous cell carcinoma of oesophagus (EC-G1) derived from a patient with hypercalcaemia. J Clin Endocrinol Metab 1988;67:592.
10. Travers MT, Barrett-Lee PJ, Berger U, et al: Growth factor expression in normal, benign and malignant breast tissue. Br Med J 1988;296:1621.

11. Wo Z, Bonewald LF, Oreffo ROC, et al: The potential role of procathepsin D secreted by breast cancer cells in bone resorption. In Cohn DV, Glorieux FH, Martin TJ (eds): Calcium Regulation and Bone Metabolism. Amsterdam, Elsevier, 1990, p 304.

12. Cavailles V, Garcia M, Rochefort H: Regulation of cathepsin D and P52 gene expression by growth factors in MCF-7 human breast cancer cells. Mol Endocrinol 1989;3:552.

13. Chambers TJ, Fuller K: Bone cells predispose endosteal surface to resorption by exposure of bone mineral to osteoclastic contact. J Cell Sci 1985;76:155.

14. McBride WH: Phenotype and functions of intratumoral macrophages. Biochem Biophys Acta 1986;865:27.

15. Sabatini M, Chavez J, Mundy GR, Bonewald LF: Stimulation of tumor necrosis factor release from monocyte cells by the A375 human melanoma via granulocyte-macrophage colony stimulating factor. Cancer Res 1990;50:2673.

16. Suva LJ, Winslow GA, Moseley JM, et al: A parathyroid hormone-related protein implicated in malignant hypercalcaemia: Cloning and expression. Science 1987;237:893.

17. Chambers TJ, McSheehy PMJ, Thomson BM, Fuller K: The effect of calcium-regulating hormones and prostaglandins on bone resorption by osteoclasts disaggregated from neonatal rabbit bones. Endocrinology 1985;116:234.

18. Sakamoto S, Sakamoto M: Bone collagenase, osteoblasts and cell-mediated bone resorption. In Peck WA (ed): Bone and Mineral Research, vol 4. Amsterdam, Elsevier, 1986, p 49.

19. Valentin OA, Edouard C, Charhon S, Meunier PJ: Histomorphometic analysis of iliac bone metastases of prostatic origin. In Donath A, Huber H (eds): Bone and Tumors. Geneva, Switzerland, Medicine et Hygiene, 1980, p 24.

20. Koutsilieris M, Rabbini SA, Bennett HPJ, Goltzman D: Characteristics of prostate-derived growth factors for cells of the osteoblast phenotype. J Clin Invest 1987;80:941.

21. Guise TA, Yin JJ, Taylor SD, et al: Evidence for a causal role of parathyroid hormone-related protein in the pathogenesis of human breast cancer-mediated osteolysis. J Clin Invest 1996;98:1544-1549.

22. Thomas RJ, Guise TA, Yin JJ, et al: Breast cancer cells interact with osteoblasts to support osteoclast formation. Endocrinology 1999;140:4451-4458.

23. Guise TA: Molecular mechanisms of osteolytic bone metastases. Cancer 2000;88:2892-2898.

24. Hofbauer LC, Khosla S, Dunstan CR, Lacey DL, Boyle WJ, Riggs BL: The roles of osteoprotegerin and osteoprotegerin ligand in the paracrine regulation of bone resorption. J Bone Miner Res 2000;15:2-12.

25. Chikatsu N, Takeuchi Y, Tamusa Y, et al: Interactions between cancer and bone marrow cells induce osteoblast differentiation factor expression and osteoclast-like cell formation in vitro. Biochem Biophys Res Commun 2000;267:632-637.

26. Zhang J, Dai J, Qi Y, et al: Osteoprotegerin inhibits prostate cancer-induced osteoclastogenesis and prevents prostate tumor growth in the bone. J Clin Invest 2001;107:1235-1244.

27. Nelson JB, Hedican SP, George DJ, et al: Identification of endothelin-1 in the pathophysiology of metastatic adenocarcinoma of the prostate. Nature Med 1995;1:944-949.

28. Takuwa Y, Masaki T, Yamashita K: The effects of the endothelin family peptides on cultured osteoblastic cells from rat calvariae. Biochem Biophys Res Commun 1990;170:998-1005.

29. Chiao JW, Moonga BS, Yang YM, et al: Endothelin-1 from prostate cancer cells is enhanced by bone contact which blocks osteoclastic bone resorption. Br J Cancer 2000;83(3):360-365.

30. Granchi S, Bronechi S, Bonaccorsi L, et al: Endothelin-1 production by prostate cancer cell lines is up-regulated by factors involved in cancer progression and down-regulated by androgens. Prostate 2001;49:267-277.

31. Bryden AA, Hoyland JA, Freemont AJ, Clarke NW, George NJ: Parathyroid hormone related peptide and receptor expression in paired primary prostate cancer and bone metastases. Br J Cancer 2002;86(3):322-325.

32. Clarke NW, McClure J, George NJ: Morphometric evidence for bone resorption and replacement in prostate cancer. Br J Urol 1991;68:74-80.

33. Lee YP, Schwerz EM, Davies M, et al: Use of zoledronate to treat osteoblastic versus osteolytic lesions in a severe-combined-immunodeficient mouse model. Cancer Res 2002;62:5564-5570.

34. Derenne S, Amiot U, Barille S, et al: Zoledronate is a potent inhibitor of myeloma cell growth and secretion of IL-6 and MMP-1 by the tumoral environment. J Bone Miner Res 1999;14(12):2048-2056.

35. Barille S, Akhoundi C, Collette M, et al: Metalloproteinases in multiple myeloma: production of matrix metalloproteinase-9 (MMP-9), activation of pro-MMP-2, and induction of MMP-1 by myeloma cells. Blood 1997;90:1649-1655.

36. Edelstyn GA, Gillespie PJ, Grebbel FS: The radiological demonstration of osseous metastasis: Experimental observations. Clin Radiol 1967;18:158-162.

37. Fogelman I, Coleman RE: The bone scan and breast cancer. In Freeman L, Weissman H (eds): Nuclear medicine annual. New York, Raven Press, 1988, pp 1-38.

38. Boxer DI, Todd CEC, Coleman R, Fogelman I: Bone secondaries in breast cancer: The solitary metastasis. J Nucl Med 1989;30:1318-1320.

39. Muindi J, Coombes RC, Golding S, Powles TJ, Kahn O, Husband JE: The role of computed tomography in the detection of bone metastases in breast cancer patients. Br J Radiol 1983;56:233-236.

40. Yuh WT, Zachar CK, Barloon TJ, Sato Y, Sickels WJ, Hawes DR: Vertebral compression fractures: Distinction between benign and malignant causes with MR imaging. Radiology 1989;172:215-218.

41. Jones AL, Williams MP, Powles TJ, et al: Magnetic resonance imaging in the detection of skeletal metastases in patients with breast cancer. Br J Cancer 1990;62:296-298.

42. Melkko J, Niemi S, Risteli J, Risteli L: Radioimmunoassay for human procollagen. Clin Chem 1990;36:1328-1332.

43. Koizumi M, Maeda H, Yoshimura K, Yamauchi T, Kawai T, Ogata E: Dissociation of bone formation markes in bone metastasis of prostate cancer. Br J Cancer 1997;75:1601-1604.

44. Berruti A, Panero A, Angelli A, et al: Different mechanisms underlying bone collagen resorption in patients with bone metastases from prostate and breast cancer. Br J Cancer 1996;73:1581-1587.

45. Coleman RE, Mashiter G, Fogelman I, Rubens RD: Osteocalcin: A marker of metastatic bone disease. Eur J Cancer 1988;24:1211-1217.

46. Roux C, Ravaud P, Cohen-Solal M, et al: Biologic, histologic and densitometric effects of oral residronate in patients with multiple myeloma. Bone 1994;15:41-49.

47. Kymala T, Ristell J, Elomaa I: Type 1 collagen degradation product (ICTP) gives information about the nature of bone metastases and has prognostic value in prostate cancer. Br J Cancer 1995;71:1061-1064.

48. Kylmala T, Tammela T, Risteli L, Risteli J, Taube T, Elomaa I: Evaluation of the effect of oral clodronate on skeletal metastases with type I collagen metabolites. A controlled trial of the Finnish Prostate Cancer Group. Eur J Cancer 1993;29A:821-825.

49. Elomaa I, Virkkunrn P, Risteli L, Risteli J: Serum concentration of the cross-linked carboxyterminsl telopeptide of type I collagen (ICTP) is a useful prognostic indicator in multiple myeloma. Br J Cancer 1992;66:337-341.

50. Vinholes J, Coleman R, Eastell R: Effects of bone metastases on bone metabolism: Implications for diagnosis, imaging and assessment of response to cancer treatment. Cancer Treat Rev 1996;22:289-331.

51. Coombes RC, Dady P, Parsons C, McCready VR, Gazet J-C, Powles TJ: Assessment of response of bone metastases to systemic treatment in patients with breast cancer. Cancer 1983;52:610-614.

52. Coleman RE, Whitaker KD, Moss DW, Mashiter G, Fogelman I, Rubens RD: Biochemical monitoring predicts response in bone to systemic treatment. Br J Cancer 1988;58:205-210.

53. Myamato KK, McSherry SA, Robins SP, Besterman J, Mohler JL: Collagen crosslink metabolites in urine as markers of bone metastases in prostate cancer. J Urol 1994;151:909-913.

54. Siebel MJ, Robins SP, Bilezikian JP: Urinary pyridinium crosslinks of collagen. Specific marker of bone resorption in metabolic bone disease. Trends Endocrinol Metab 1992;3:263-270.

55. Hanson D, Weis MAE, Bollen AM, et al: A specific immunoassay for monitoring human bone resorption: Quantification of type 1 collagen cross-linked N-telopeptides in urine. J Bone Miner Res 1992;7:1251-1258.

56. Bonde M, Qvist P, Chriastensen C, et al: Applications of an enzyme immunoassay for a new marker of bone resorption (Crosslaps): Follow-up on hormone replacement therapy and osteoporosis risk assessment. J Clin Endocrinol Metab 1995;80:864-868.

57. Robins SP, Woitge H, Lindsay R, et al: Direct, enzyme-linked immunoassay for urinary deoxypyridinoline as a specific marker for measuring bone resorption. J Bone Miner Res 1994;9:1643-1649.

58. Vinholes JJ, Purohit OP, Abbey ME, Eastell R, Coleman RE: Evaluation of new bone resorption markers in a randomized comparison of pamidronate or clodronate for hypercalcaemia of malignancy. J Clin Oncol 1997;15:131-138.

59. Campbell FC, Blamey RW, Woolfson AM, Elston CW, Hosking DJ: Calcium excretion (CaE) in metastatic breast cancer. Br J Surg 1983;70:202-204.

60. Pecherstorfer M, Zimmer-Roth I, Schilling T, et al: The diagnostic value of urinary pyridinium crosslinks of collagen, serum, total alkaline phosphatase and urinary calcium excretion in neoplastic bone disease. J Clin Endocrinol Metabol 1995;80:97-103.

61. Massidda B, Ionta MT, Foddi MR, et al: Usefulness of pyridinium crosslinks and CA 15-3 as markers in metastatic bone breast carcinoma. Anticancer Res 1996;16:2221-2224.

62. Body JJ, Dumon JC, Gineyts E, Delmas PD: Comparative evaluation of markers of bone resorption in patients with breast cancer-induced osteolysis before and after bisphosphonate therapy. Br J Cancer 1997;75:408-412.

63. Demers LM, Costa L, Chinchilli VM, Gaydos L, Curley E, Lipton A: Biochemical markers of bone turnover in patients with metastatic bone disease. Clin Chem 1995;41:1489-1494.

64. Lipton A, Costa L, Ali SM, Demers LM: Bone markers in the management of metastatic bone disease. Cancer Treat Rev 2001;27:181-185.

65. Miura H, Yamamoto I, Takada M, et al: Diagnostic validity of bone metabolic markers for bone metastasis. Endocr J 1997;44:751-757.

66. Christianson RH: Biochemical markers of bone metabolism: An overview. Clin Biochem 1997;30:573-593.

67. Watts NB: Clinical utility of biochemical markers of bone remodeling. Clin Chem 1999;45:1359-1368.

68. Tamada T, Sone T, Tomomitsu T, Jo Y, Tanaka H, Fukunaga M: Biochemical markers for the detection of bone metastasis in patients with prostate cancer: Diagnostic efficacy and the effect of hormonal therapy. J Bone Miner Metab 2001;19:45-51.

69. Akimoto S, Furuya Y, Akakura K, Ito H: Comparison of markers of bone formation and resorption in prostate cancer patients to predict bone metastasis. Endocr J 1998;45:97-104.

70. Garnero P, Buchs N, Zekri J, Rizzoli R, Coleman RE, Delmas PD: Markers of bone turnover for the management of patients with bone metastases from prostate cancer. Br J Cancer 2000;82:858-864.

71. Garnero P: Markers of bone turnover in prostate cancer. Cancer Treat Rev 2001;27:187-192.

72. Koizumi M, Yonese J, Fukui I, Ogata E: The serum level of the amino-terminal propeptide of type I procollagen is a sensitive marker for prostate cancer metastasis to bone. BJU Int 2001;87:348-351.

73. Berruti A, Torta M, Piovesan A, et al: Biochemical picture of bone metabolism in patients with bone metastases. Anticancer Res 1995;2871-2876.

74. Brown JE, Coleman RE: Assessment of the effects of breast cancer on bone and the response to therapy. Breast 2002;11:1-11.

75. Hayward JL, Carbone PP, Heuson JC, Kumaoka S, Segaloff A, Rubens RD: Assessment of response to therapy in advanced breast cancer. Cancer 1977;3:1389-1394.

76. Purohit OP, Anthony C, Radstone CR, Owen J, Coleman RE: High-dose intravenous pamidronate for metastatic bone pain. Br J Cancer 1994;70:554-558.

77. Schipper H, Clinch J, McMurray A, Levitt M: Measuring the quality of life of cancer patients. The functional living index-cancer: Development and validation. J Clin Oncol 1984;2:472-483.

78. Aaronson NK, Ahmedzai S, Begman B, et al: The EORTC QLQ-C30. A quality of life instrument for use in International Clinical Trials in Oncology. J Natl Cancer Inst 1999;85:365-369.

79. Coleman RE, Rubens RD, Fogelman I: The bone scan flare following systemic treatment for bone metastases. J Nucl Med 1988;29:1354-1359.

80. Howell A, Mackintosh J, Jones M, Radford J, Wagstaff J, Selwood RA: The definition of the "no change" category in patients treated with endocrine therapy and chemotherapy for 6 advanced carcinoma of the breast. Eur J Cancer 1988;24:1567-1572.

81. Rossleigh MA, Lovegrove FTA, Reynolds PM, Byrne MJ, Whitney BP: The assessment of response to therapy of bone metastases in breast cancer. Aust NZ J Med 1984;14:19-22.

82. Pollen JJ, Witztun KF, Ashburn WL: The flare phenomenon on radionuclide bone scan in metastatic prostate cancer. Am J Radiol 1984;142:773-776.

83. Bellamy EA, Nicholas D, Ward M, Coombes RC, Powles TJ, Husband JE: Comparison of computed tomography and conventional radiology in the assessment of treatment response of lytic bony metastases in patients with carcinoma of the breast. Clin Radiol 1987;38:351-355.

84. Coleman RE: Assessment of response to treatment. In Rubens RD, Fogelman I (eds): Bone Metastases: Diagnosis and Treatment. London, Springer Verlag, 1991, pp 99-120.

85. Kiang DT, Greenberg LJ, Kennedy BJ: Tumour marker kinetics in the monitoring of breast cancer. Cancer 1990;65:193-199.

86. Robertson JFR, Pearson D, Price MR, Selby C, Blamey RW, Howell A: Objective measurement of therapeutic response in breast cancer using tumor markers. Cancer 1991;64:757-763.

87. Robertson JFR, Jaeger W, Syzmendera JJ, et al: The objective measurement of remission and progression in metastatic breast cancer by use of serum tumor markers. Eur J Cancer 1999;35:47-53.

88. Killian CS, Emrich LJ, Vargas FP, et al: Relative reliability of five serially measured markers for prognosis of progression in prostate cancer. J Natl Cancer Inst 1986;76:179.

89. Hortobagyi GN, Libshitz HI, Seabold JS: Osseus metastases of breast cancer. Clinical, biochemical, radiographic and scintigraphic evaluation of response to therapy. Cancer 1984;53:577-582.

90. Villalon AH, Tattersall MH, Fox RM, Woods RL: Hypercalcaemia after tamoxifen for breast cancer: A sign of tumor response. Br Med J 1979;20:1329-1330.

91. Walls J, Assiri A, Howell A, et al: Measurement of urinary collagen cross-links indicate response to therapy in patients with breast cancer and bone metastases. Br J Cancer 1999;80:1265-1270.

92. Vinholes J, Coleman R, Lacombe D, et al: Assessment of bone response to systemic therapy in an EORTC trial: Preliminary experience with the use of collagen cross-link excretion. European Organization for Research and Treatment of Cancer. Br J Cancer 1999;80:221-228.

93. Costa L, Demers LM, Gouveia-Oliveira A, et al: Prospective evaluation of the peptide-bound collagen type I cross-links N-telopeptide and C-telopeptide in predicting bone metastases status. J Clin Oncol 2002;20:850-856.

94. Vinholes JJ, Guo C-Y, Purohit OP, Eastell R, Coleman RE: Metabolic effects of pamidronate in patients with metastatic bone disease. Br J Cancer 1996;73:1089-1095.

95. Vinholes JJ, Purohit OP, Abbey ME, Eastell R, Coleman RE: Relationships between biochemical and symptomatic response in a double-blind trial of pamidronate for metastatic bone disease. Ann Oncol 1997;8:1243-1250.

96. Jagdev SP, Purohit OP, Heatley S, Herling C, Coleman RE: Comparison of the effects of intravenous pamidronate and oral clodronate on symptoms and bone resorption in patients with metastatic bone disease. Ann Oncol 2001;12:1433-1438.

97. Lipton A, Demers L, Curley E, et al: Markers of bone resorption in patients treated with pamidronate. Eur J Cancer 1998;34:2021-2026.

98. Leddy ET: Roentgen treatment of metastasis to the vertebrae and bones of the pelvis from carcinoma of the breast. Am J Roentgenol Radiat Ther 1930;24:657-672.

99. Matsubayashi T, Koga H, Nishiyama Y, Tominaga S, Sourada T: The reparative process of metastatic bone lesions after radiotherapy. Jpn J Clin Oncol 1981;11:253-259.

Problems Common to Cancer and Its Therapy

100. Hoskin, PJ: Radiotherapy in the management of bone metastases. In Rubens RD, Fogelman I (eds): Bone Metastases-Diagnosis and Treatment. London, Springer Verlag, 1991, pp 207–222.

101. Hoskin, PJ: Scientific and clinical aspects of radiotherapy in the relief of bone pain. Cancer Surv 1988;7:69–86.

102. Blitzer PH: Reanalysis of the RTOG study of the palliation of symptomatic osseous metastasis. Cancer 1985;55:1468–1472.

103. Tong D, Gillick L, Hendrickson F: The palliation of symptomatic osseous metastases: Final results of the study by the Radiation Therapy Oncology Group. Cancer 1982;50:893–899.

104. Price P, Hoskin PJ, Easton D, Austin D, Palmer SG, Yarnold JR: Prospective randomised trial of single and multifraction radiotherapy schedules in the treatment of painful bony metastases. Radiother Oncol 1986;6:247–255.

105. Madsen, EL: Painful bone metastasis: Efficacy of radiotherapy assessed by the patients: A randomised trial comparing 4 Gy x 6 versus 10 Gy x 2. Int J Radiat Oncol Biol Phys 1983;9:1775–1779.

106. Niewald M, Tkocz HJ, Abel U, et al: Rapid course radiation therapy vs more standard treatment: A randomised trial for bone metastases. Int J Radiat Oncol Biol Phys 1996;36:1085–1089.

107. Steenland E, Leer J, van Houwelingen H, et al: The effect of a single fraction compared to multiple fractions on painful bone metastases: A global analysis of the Dutch Bone Metastasis Study. Radiother Oncol 1999;52:101–109.

108. van den Hout W, van der Linden Y, Steenland E, et al: Single- versus multiple-fraction radiotherapy in patients with painful bone metastases: Cost-utility analysis based on a randomised trial. J Natl Cancer Inst 2003;95:222–229.

109. Janjan NA: Radiation for bone metastases: Conventional techniques and the role of systemic radiopharmaceuticals. Cancer 1997;80(Suppl 8):1628–1645.

110. Hoskin PJ, Ford HT, Harmer CL: Hemibody irradiation for metastatic bone pain. Clin Oncol 1989;1:41–42.

111. Charbord P, L'heritier C, Cukerstein W, Lumbros J, Tubiana M: Radio-iodine treatment in differentiated thyroid carcinomas. Treatment of first local recurrences and of bone and lung metastases. Ann Radiol 1977;20:783–786.

112. Pochin EE: Long term hazards of radio-iodine treatment of thyroid carcinoma. In Hedinger CE (ed): Thyroid Cancer. UICC Monograph Series, vol 12. Berlin, Springer Verlag, 1969, p 293.

113. Clarke SEM: Isotope therapy for bone metastases In Rubens RD, Fogelman I (eds): Bone Metastases—Diagnosis and Treatment. London, Springer Verlag, 1991, pp 187–206.

114. Hoefnagel CA, Voute PA, DeKraker J, Marcuse HR: Radionuclide diagnosis and therapy of neural crest tumors using 131I-MIBG. J Nucl Med 1987;28:308–314.

115. Blake GM, Zivanovic MA, McEwan AJ, Ackery DM: Strontium-89 therapy: Strontium kinetics in disseminated carcinoma of the prostate. Eur J Nucl Med 1986;12:447–454.

116. Blake GM, Zivanovich MA, Blaquiere RM, Fine DR, McEwan AJ, Ackery DM: Strontium-89 therapy: Measurement of absorbed dose to skeletal metastases. J Nucl Med 1988;29:549–557.

117. Robinson R, Spicer JA, Preston DF, Wegst AV, Martin NL: Treatment of metastatic bone pain with strontium-89. Nucl Med Biol 1987;14:219–222.

118. Laing AH, Ackery DM, Bayly RJ, et al: Strontium chloride for pain palliation in prostatic skeletal malignancy. Br J Radiol 1991;64:816–822.

119. Lewington VJ, McEwan AJ, Ackery DM, et al: A prospective, randomised double-blind crossover study to examine the efficacy of strontium-89 in pain palliation in patients with advanced prostate cancer metastatic to bone. Eur J Cancer 1991;27:954–958.

120. Quilty PM, Kirk D, Bolger JJ, et al: A comparison of the palliative effects of Strontium 89 external beam radiotherapy in metastatic prostatic cancer. Radiother Oncol 1994;31:33–40.

121. Ketring A: Sm-153-EHDP and rhenium-186 HEDP as bone therapeuticradiopharmaceuticals. Int J Rad Appl Instrum 1987;14:223–232.

122. Turner JH, Claringbold BG, Heatherington EL, Sorby P, Martindal AA: A phase I study of samarium-153 ethylenediamenetetramethylene phosphonate therapy for disseminated skeletal metastases. J Clin Oncol 1987;7:1926–1931.

123. Resche I, Chatal J-F, Pecking A, et al: A dose-controlled study of 153Sm-ethylenediaminetetramethylenephosphonate (EDTMP) in the treatment of patients with painful bone metastases. Eur J Cancer 1997;33:1583–1591.

124. Kolesnikov-Gauthier H, Carpentier P, Depreux P, Vennin P, Caty A, Sulman C: Evaluation of toxicity and efficacy of 186re-hydroxy-ethylidene diphosphonate in patients with painful bone metastases of prostate or breast cancer. J Nucl Med 2000;41: 1689–1694.

125. O'Reilly SM, Richards MA, Rubens RD: Liver metastases from breast cancer: The relationship between clinical, biochemical and pathological features and survival. Eur J Cancer 1990;26:574–577.

126. Clark GM, Sledge GW, Osborn CK, McGuire WL: Survival from first recurrence: Relative importance of prognostic factors in 1015 breast cancer patients. J Clin Oncol 1987;5:55–61.

127. Mouridsen H, Gershanovic M, Sun Y et al: Superior efficacy of letrozole versus tamoxifen as firstline therapy for postmenopausal women with advanced breast cancer: Results of a phase III study of the International Letrozole Breast Cancer Group. J Clin Oncol 2001;19:2596–2606.

128. Dowsett M: Aromatase inhibitors come of age. Ann Oncol 1997;8:631–632.

129. Solowat MS: Newer methods of hormonal therapy for prostate cancer. Urology 1984;24(Suppl 5):30–38.

130. Mauriac L, Coste P, Richaud P, Lamarche P, Mage P, Bonichon F: Clinical study of an LHRH agonist (ICI 118.630, Zoladex) in the treatment of prostatic cancer. Am J Clin Oncol 1988;11: 8117–8119.

131. Scher HI: Prostate carcinoma: Defining therapeutic objectives and improving overall outcomes. Cancer 2003;97(Suppl 3):758–771.

132. Tannock IF, Osaba D, Stockler MR, et al: Chemotherapy with mitoxantrone plus prednisone or prednisone alone for symptomatic hormone-resistant prostate cancer: A Canadian randomised trial with pallaitve endpoints. J Clin Oncol 1996;14:1756–1764.

133. Savarase DMF, Hsieh C-C, Stewart FM: Clinical impact of chemotherapy dose escalation in patients with haematologic malignancies and solid tumors. J Clin Oncol 1997;15:2981–2995.

134. Shinoda H, Adamek G, Felix R, et al: Structure-activity relationship of various bisphosphonates. Calcif Tissue Int 1983;35:87–99.

135. Rogers MJ, Xiong X, Ji X, et al: Inhibition of growth of Dictyostelium discoideum amoebo by bisphosphonates is dependent on cellular uptake. Pharmacol Res 1997;14:625–630.

136. Hughes DE, Wright KR, Uy HL, et al: Bisphosphonates promote apoptosis in murine osteoclasts in vitro and in vivo. J Bone Miner Res 1995;10:1478–1487.

137. Luckman SP, Hughes DE, Coxon FP, Graham R, Russell RGG, Rogers MJ: Nitrogen-containing bisphosphonates inhibit the mevalonate pathway and prevent post-translational prenylation of GTP-binding proteins, including Ras. J Bone Miner Res 1998;13: 581–589.

138. Neville-Webbe H, Holen I, Coleman RE: The anti-tumor effects and potential of bisphosphonates. Cancer Treat Rev 2002;28:305–320.

139. Schenk R, Merz WA, Muhlbauer R, et al: Effect of ethane-1-hydroxy-1,1- diphosphonate (EHDP) and dichloromethylene diphosphonate (Cl2MDP) on the calcification and resorption of cartilage and bone in the tibial epiphysis and metaphysis of rats. Calcif Tissue Res 1983;11:196–214.

140. Schenk R, Eggli P, Felix R, et al: Quantitative morphometric evaluation of the inhibitory activity of new aminobisphospho-nates on bone resorption in the rat. Calcif Tissue Int 1986;38:342–349.

141. Daley-Yates PT, Dodwell DJ, Pongchaidechma M, et al: The clearance and bioavailability of pamidronate in patients with breast cancer and bone metastases. Calcif Tissue Int 1991;49:433–435.

142. De Groen PC, Lubbe DF, Hirsch LJ, et al: Oesophagitis associated with the use of alendronate. New Engl J Med 1996;335:1016–1021.

143. Body JJ, Coleman RE, Piccart M: Use of bisphosphonates in cancer patients. Cancer Treat Rev 1996;22:265–287.

144. Lipton A, Costa L, Ali S, et al: Use of bone turnover for monitoring bone metastases and the response to therapy. Semin Oncol 2001;4(Suppl 11):54–59.

145. Ernst DS, Tannock IF, Venner PM, et al: Randomized placebo controlled trial of mitoxantrone/prednisone and clodronate versus mitoxantrone/prednisone alone in patients with hormone

refractory prostate cancer (HRPC) and pain: National Cancer Institute of Canada Clinical Trials Group study [abstract]. Proc Am Soc Clin Oncol 2002;21:177a.

146. Coleman RE: Skeletal complications of malignancy. Cancer 1997;80(Suppl):1588–1594.

147. Coleman RE, Purohit OP, Vinholes JJ, Zekri J: High dose pamidronate—Clinical and biochemical effects in metastatic bone disease. Cancer 1997;80:1686–1690.

148. Clarke NW, Holbrook IB, McClure J, et al: Osteoclast inhibition by pamidronate in metastatic prostate cancer: A preliminary study. Br J Cancer 1991;63:420–423.

149. Patterson AHG, Powles TJ, Kanis, JA, McCloskey EV, Hanson J, Ashley S: Double-blind controlled trial of oral clodronate in patients with bone metastases from breast cancer. J Clin Oncol 1993;11:59–65.

150. van Holten-Verzantvoort AT, Bijvoet OLM, Cleton FJ, et al: Reduced morbidity from skeletal metastases in breast cancer patients during long term bisphosphonate (APD) treatment. Lancet 1987;ii:983–985.

151. van Holten-Verzantvoort AT, Kroon HM, Bijvoet OLM, et al: Palliative bone treatment in patients with bone metastases from breast cancer. J Clin Oncol 1993;11:491–498.

152. Conte PF, Mauriac L, Calabresi F, et al: Delay in progression of bone metastases treated with intravenous pamidronate: Results from a multicentre randomised controlled trial. J Clin Oncol 1996;14:2552–2559.

153. Hultborn R, Ryden S, Gunderson S, Holmberg E, Wallgren U-B: Efficacy of pamidronate on skeletal complications from breast cancer metastases. A randomised prospective double blind placebo controlled trial. Acta Oncol 1996;35(Suppl 5):73–74.

154. Hortobagyi GN, Theriault RL, Porter L, et al: Efficacy of pamidronate in reducing skeletal complications in patients with breast cancer and lytic bone metastases. New Engl J Med 1996;335:1785–1791.

155. Theriault RL, Lipton A, Hortobagyi GN, et al: Pamidronate reduces skeletal morbidity in women with advanced breast cancer and lytic bone lesions: A randomised, placebo-controlled trial. J Clin Oncol 1999;17:846–854.

156. Body JJ, Lortholary A, Romieu G, Vigneron AM, Ford J: A dose-finding study of zoledronate in hypercalcaemic cancer patients. J Bone Miner Res 1999;14:1557–1661.

157. Berenson JR, Vescio R, Henick K, et al: A phase I, open label, dose ranging trial of intravenous bolus zoledronic acid, a novel bisphosphonate, in cancer patients with metastatic bone disease. Cancer 2001;91:144–154.

158. Berenson JR, Rosen LS, Howell A, et al: Zoledronic acid reduces skeletal-related events in patients with osteolytic metastases. Cancer 2001;91:1191–1200.

159. Rosen LS, Gordon D, Kaminski M, et al: Zoledronic acid versus pamidronate in the treatment of skeletal metastases in patients with breast cancer or osteolytic lesions of multiple myeloma: A phase III, double-blind, comparative trial. Cancer J 2001;7(5):377–387.

160. Andersen PK, Gill RD: Cox's regression model for counting processes: A large sample study. Ann Statistics 1982;10:1100–1120.

161. Rosen LS, Gordon D, Kaminski M, et al: Long-term efficacy and safety of zoledronic acid compared with pamidronate disodium in treatment of skeletal complications in patients with advanced multiple myeloma or breast cancer: A randomized, double-blind, multicenter, comparative trial. Cancer 2003;98:1735–1744.

162. Body JJ, Lichinitser MR, Diehl IE, et al: Double-blind placebo controlled trial of ibandronate in breast cancer metastatic to bone. Proc Amer Soc Clin Oncol 1999;18:575a.

163. Coleman RE, Purohit OP, Black C, et al: Double-blind, randomised, placebo-controlled study of oral ibandronate in patients with metastatic bone disease. Ann Oncol 1999;10:311–316.

164. Tripathy D, Lazarev A, Lichinitser MR, et al: Oral ibandronate lowers the incidence of skeletal complications in breast cancer patients with bone metastases. Proc Amer Soc Clin Oncol 2002;21:45a.

165. Lahtinen R, Laakso M, Palva I, Virkkunen P, Elomaa I, for the Finnish Leukaemia Group: Randomised, placebo-controlled multicentre trial of clodronate in multiple myeloma. Lancet 1992;340:1049–1052.

166. McCloskey EV, Maclennan ICM, Drayson M, Chapman C, Dunn J, Kanis JA: A randomised trial of the effect of clodronate on skeletal morbidity in multiple myeloma. Br J Haematol 1998;100:317–325.

167. Berenson JR, Lichtenstein A, Porter L, et al: Efficacy of pamidronate in reducing skeletal events in patients with advanced multiple myeloma. N Engl J Med 1996;334:488–493.

168. Menssen HD, Sakalova A, Fontana A, et al: Effects of long-term intravenous ibandronate therapy on skeletal-related events, survival, and bone resorption markers in patients with advanced multiple myeloma. J Clin Oncol 2002;20:2353–2359.

169. Garnero P, Buchs N, Zekri J, et al: Markers of bone turnover for the management of patients with bone metastases from prostate cancer. Br J Cancer 2000;82:858–864.

170. Purohit OP, Radstone SH, Anthony C, Kanis JA, Coleman RE: A randomized double-blind comparison of intravenous pamidronate and clodronate in the hypercalcaemia of malignancy. Br J Cancer 1995;72:1289–1293.

171. Adami S, Mian M: Clodronate therapy of metastatic bone disease in patients with prostatic carcinoma. Recent Results Cancer Res 1989;116:67–72.

172. Smith JR: Palliation of painful bone metastases from prostate cancer using sodium etidronate: Results of a randomized, prospective, double-blind, placebo-controlled study. J Urol 1989;141:85–87.

173. Dearnaley DP, Sydes MR on behalf of the MRC PR05 collaborators: Preliminary evidence that oral clodronate delays symptomatic progression of bone metastases from prostate cancer: First results of the MRC PR05 trial [abstract]. Proc Am Soc Clin Oncol 2001;20:174a.

174. Lipton A, Small E, Saad F, et al: The new bisphosphonate, Zometa (zoledronic acid), decreases skeletal complications in both osteolytic and osteoblastic lesions: A comparison to pamidronate. Cancer Invest 2002;20(Suppl 2):45–54.

175. Saad F, Gleason DM, Murray R, et al: A randomized, placebo-controlled trial of zoledronic acid in patients with hormone-refractory metastatic prostate carcinoma. J Natl Cancer Inst 2002;94:1458–1468.

176. Rosen L, Gordon D, Tchekmedyian S, et al: Zoledronic acid versus placebo in the treatment of skeletal metastases in patients with lung cancer and other solid tumours: a phase III double-blind, randomized trial. The Zoledronic Acid Lung Cancer and Other Solid Tumour Study Group. J Clin Oncol 2003;21:3150–3157.

177. Plunkett TA, Rubens RD: Bisphosphonate therapy for patients with breast carcinoma: Who to treat and when to stop. Cancer 2003;97(Suppl 3):854–858.

178. Body J-J: Effectiveness and cost of bisphosphonate therapy in tumor bone disease. Cancer 2003;97(Suppl 3):859–865.

179. Brown JE, Ellis S, Gutcher S, et al: The bone resorption marker Ntx is strongly correlated with skeletal events in metastatic bone disease and is influenced by dose escalation of clodronate [abstract]. Proc Am Soc Clin Oncol 2002;21:385a.

180. Boissier S, Ferreras M, Peyruchaud O, et al: Bisphosphonates inhibit breast and prostate carcinoma cell invasion, an early event in the formation of bone metastases. Cancer Res 2000;60:2949–2954.

181. Yoneda T, Michigami T, Yi B, et al: Use of bisphosphonates for the treatment of bone metastasis in experimental animal models. Cancer Treat Rev 1999;25:293–299.

182. Powles T, Paterson S, Kanis JA, et al: Randomised, placebo-controlled trial of clodronate in patients with primary operable breast cancer. J Clin Oncol 2002;20:3219–3224.

183. Diel IJ, Solomayer EF, Costa SD, et al: Reduction in new metastases in breast cancer with adjuvant clodronate treatment. N Engl J Med 1998;339:357–363.

184. Diel IJ, Solomayer E, Gollan C, Schutz F, Bastert G: Bisphosphonates in the reduction of metastases in breast cancer—Results of the extended follow-up of the first study population [abstract]. Proc Am Soc Clin Oncol 2000;20:82a.

185. Saarto T, Blomqvist C, Virkkunen P, Elomaa I: Adjuvant clodronate treatment does not reduce the frequency of skeletal metastases in node-positive breast cancer patients: 5 year results of randomised controlled trial. J Clin Oncol 2001;19:10–17.

186. Van der Pluijm G, Vloedgraven H, van Beek E, et al: Bisphosphonates inhibit adhesion of breast cancer cells to bone matrices in vitro. J Clin Invest 1996;98:698–701.

187. Jagdev S, Coleman RE, Shipman CM, Croucher P: The bisphosphonate zoledronic acid induces apoptosis of breast cancer cells: Evidence for synergy with paclitaxel. Br J Cancer 2001;84:1126–1134.

188. Wood J, Schnell C, Green J: Novel anti-angiogenic effects of the bisphosphonates compound zoledronic acid. JPET 2002;302:1055–1061.

189. ATAC Trialists' Group: Anastrozole alone or in combination with tamoxifen versus tamoxifen alone for adjuvant treatment of postmenopausal women with early breast cancer: First results of the ATAC randomised trial. Lancet 2002;359:2131–2139.

190. Black DM, Cummings SR, Karpf DB, et al: Randomised trial of the effect of alendronate on the risk of fracture in women with existing vertebral fractures. Lancet 1996;148:1535–1541.

191. Karpf DB, Shapiro DR, Seeman E, et al: Prevention of nonvertebral fractures by alendronate. JAMA 1997;277:1159–1164.

192. Saarto S, Blomqvist C, Valimaki M, Makela P, Sarna S, Elomaa I: Chemical castration induced by adjuvant cyclophosphamide, methotrexate, and fluorouracil chemotherapy causes rapid bone loss which is reduced by clodronate: A randomised study in premenopausal patients. J Clin Oncol 1997;15:1341–1347.

193. Delmas PD, Balena R, Confravreux E, et al: Bisphosphonate Risedronate prevents bone loss in women with artificial menopause due to chemotherapy of breast cancer: A double-blind, placebo-controlled study. J Clin Oncol 1997;15:955–962.

194. Reid IR, Brown JP, Burckhardt P, et al: Intravenous zoledronic acid in postmenopausal women with low bone mineral density. N Engl J Med 2002;346:653–661.

195. Gnant M, Hausmaninger H, Samonigg H, et al: Changes in bone mineral density caused by anastrozole or tamoxifen in combination with goserelin (+/- zoledronate) as adjuvant treatment for hormone receptor premenopausal breast cancer: Results of a randomised multicentre trial. Breast Cancer Res Treat 2002;76(Suppl 1):S31.

196. McCloskey EV, Spector T, Khan S, Sirtori P, Nagatsuka K, Kanis JA: Prevalence of vertebral deformity and concordance between definitions of fracture. In Christiansen C, Riis B (eds): Osteoporosis Proceedings. Copenhagen, Osteopress APS, 1993, pp 62–64.

197. Richards MA, Brayser S, Gregory WM, Rubens RD: Advanced breast cancer: Use of resources and cost implications. Br J Cancer 1993;67:856–860.

198. Biermann WA, Cantor RI, Fellin FM, Jakobowski J, Hopkins L, Newbold RC: An evaluation of the potential cost reductions resulting from the use of clodronate in the treatment of metastatic carcinoma of the breast. Bone 1997;12(Suppl 1):37–42.

199. Harrington KD: Orthopaedic surgical management of skeletal complications of malignancy. Cancer 1997;80(Suppl):1614–1627.

200. Coleman RE, Fogelman I, Rubens RD: Hypercalcaemia and breast cancer—An increased humoral component in patients with liver metastases. Eur J Surg Oncol 1988;14:423.

201. Ralston SH: Pathogenesis and management of cancer-associated hypercalcaemia. In Rubens RD, Fogelman I (eds): Bone Metastases—Diagnosis and Treatment. London, Springer Verlag, 191, pp 149–169.

202. Fisken RA, Heath DA, Bold AM: Hypercalcaemia—A hospital survey. Q J Med 1980;6:405–418.

203. Coleman RE: Pamidronate disodium in the treatment and management of hypercalcaemia. Rev Contemp Pharmacother 1998;9:147–164.

204. Major PP, Lortholary A, Hon J, et al: Zoledronic acid is superior to pamidronate in the treatment of hypercalcemia of malignancy—A pooled analysis of two randomized, controlled clinical trials. J Clin Oncol 2001;19:558–567.

205. Higinbotham NL, Marcove RC: The management of pathological fractures. J Trauma 1965;5:792.

206. Galasko CSB: The role of the orthopaedic surgeon in the treatment of skeletal metastases. In Rubens RD, Fogelman I (eds): Bone Metastases—Diagnosis and Treatment. London, Springer Verlag, 1991, pp 207–222.

207. Plunkett TA, Smith P, Rubens RD: Risk of complications from bone metastases in breast cancer: Implications for management. Eur J Cancer 2000;36:476–482.

208. Mirels H: Metastatic disease in long bones. A proposed scoring system for diagnosisng impending pathological fracture. Clin Orthop Rel Res 1989;249:256–264.

209. Bouma WH, Mulder JH, Hop WCJ: The influence of intramedullary nailing upon the development of metastases in the treatment of an impending pathological fracture: An experimental study. Clin Exp Metastasis 1983;1:205–212.

210. Harrington KD: The management of acetabular insufficiency secondary to metastatic malignant disease. J Bone Joint Surg [Am] 1981;63:653–684.

211. Siegal T, Siegal T: Vertebral body resection for epidural compression by malignant tumors. Results of forty-seven consecutive operative procedures. J Bone Joint Surg [Am] 1985;67:375–382.

212. Jensen ME, Kallmes DF: Percutaneous vertebroplasty in the treatment of malignant spine disease. Cancer J 2002;8:194–206.

213. Gilbert RW, Kim J-H, Posner JB: Epidural spinal cord compression from metastatic tumor diagnosis and treatment. Ann Neurol 1978;3:40.

214. Kamholtz R, Sze G: Current imaging in spinal metastatic disease. Semin Oncol 1991;18:158–169.

215. Hill ME, Richards MA, Gregory WM, Smith P, Rubens RD: Spinal cord compression in breast cancer: A review of 70 cases. Br J Cancer 1993;68:969–973.

216. Findlay GFG: Adverse effects of the management of malignant spinal cord compression. J Neurol Neurosurg Psychiatry 1984;47:761–768.

217. Cobb CA III, Leavens ME, Eckles N: Indications for nonoperative treatment of spinal cord compression due to breast cancer. J Neurosurg 1977;47:653–658.

218. Hillner BE, Ingle JN, Berenson JR, et al: American Society of Clinical Oncology guideline on the role of bisphosphonates in breast cancer. J Clin Oncol 2000;18:1378–1391.

219. Kong Y-Y, Yoshida H, Sarosi O, et al: OPGL is a key regulator of osteoclastogenesis, lymphocyte development and lymph-node organogenesis. Nature 1999;397:315–323.

220. Body J-J, Greipp P, Coleman RE, et al: A phase I study of AMGN-0007, a recombinant osteoprotogerin construct, in patients with multiple myeloma or breast carcinoma related bone metastases. Cancer 2003;97(Suppl 3):887–892.

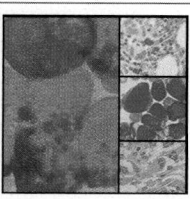

58

LUNG METASTASES

Michael J. Weyant

Valerie W. Rusch

SUMMARY OF KEY POINTS

INCIDENCE

- Lungs are the second most common site of metastases.
- Lungs are the sole site of metastasis in 80% of patients with sarcoma and in 2% to 10% of patients with carcinoma.

ETIOLOGY

- Hematogenous spread.
- Lymphangitic spread in carcinomas can occur early or late in the natural progression of all cancers.
- It is not well understood why lung metastases take several years to develop.

EVALUATION

- Few lung metastases are symptomatic—only 15% to 20% of patients complain of cough or pain. All patients with isolated pulmonary metastasis from extrathoracic malignancy should be evaluated for the possibility of resection.
- Initial imaging studies should consist of a plain chest x-ray followed by computed tomographic (CT) examination to predict resectability. Newer imaging modalities, such as 18F-fluorodeoxyglucose positron emission tomography (FDG-PET) and MRI, have not been shown to be as accurate or cost effective as CT.

- CT is unable to distinguish reliably between malignant and benign lesions.
- CT differs from the final pathology report in 42% of cases.
- CT underestimates the number of malignant lesions in 25% of cases.
- The accuracy of radiologic imaging is only 37%, underestimating the number of lesions by 39% and overestimating them by 25% for patients undergoing bilateral exploration.

PROGNOSTIC FACTORS

- Number of metastases.
- Disease-free interval (<36 months or >36 months).
- Histology/organ site of primary tumor.

SURGICAL TREATMENT

- First described case of pulmonary metastectomy was by Weinlechner in 1882.
- Alexander and Haight described the first series of patients—12 patients remained disease-free for 1 to 12 years.
- General guidelines that should be met before undertaking a resection include the following:
  - Control of the primary tumor, or ability to resect the primary tumor.

- Ability to resect metastatic disease completely.
- Ability of the patient to withstand the extent of pulmonary resection required to remove all gross tumor.
- Absence of extrathoracic metastasis.
- Absence of better alternative treatment.
- The location of metastases determines the extent and type of resection:
  - Peripheral metastasis— parenchymal sparing.
  - Central metastasis—lobectomy or pneumonectomy.
  - Solitary endobronchial metastasis—lobectomy, sleeve lobectomy, or pneumonectomy.
- Ensure that all grossly palpable tumors are resected with clear margins.
- More radical resection (lobectomy, pneumonectomy) does not increase survival.
- Bilateral metastases and recurrence of pulmonary metastases are not contraindications to resection and should not deter resection in lesion(s) that can be removed completely.

INTRODUCTION

The first described case of pulmonary metastectomy was reported in 1882 by a German surgeon named Weinlechner, who removed two incidental pulmonary nodules during a chest wall resection for sarcoma.[1] In 1938, Barry and Churchill[2] reported the first long-term survivor of pulmonary metastectomy, a patient with metastatic renal cell cancer. Their patient survived 23 years after surgery. Subsequently, Alexander and Haight described the first series of patients undergoing pulmonary metastectomy and its correlation to survival.[3] Twelve patients in their study remained free of disease for 1 to 12 years. Most important, from this early study came the first generally accepted criteria for pulmonary metastectomy:

1. The primary tumor should be removed completely.
2. There should be no evidence of extrapulmonary disease.
3. The patient should be able to tolerate the planned operation from the standpoint of overall medical condition.

Subsequently, these criteria were modified by other authors to reflect our improved understanding of the

TABLE 58-1

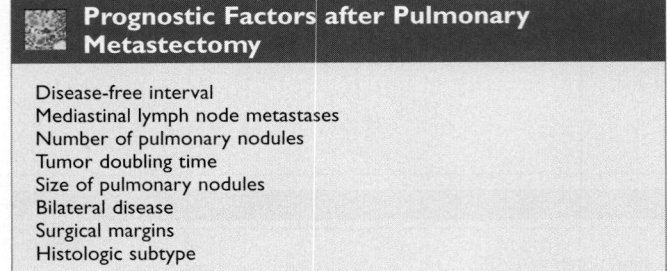

Prognostic Factors after Pulmonary Metastectomy

Disease-free interval
Mediastinal lymph node metastases
Number of pulmonary nodules
Tumor doubling time
Size of pulmonary nodules
Bilateral disease
Surgical margins
Histologic subtype

management of pulmonary metastases. Current additional criteria include the following:[4]

1. Control of the primary tumor, or ability to resect the primary tumor completely simultaneously with resection of metastasis.
2. Ability to resect metastatic disease completely.
3. Ability of the patient to tolerate the extent of pulmonary resection required to remove all gross tumor.
4. Absence of extrathoracic metastasis.
5. Absence of better alternative treatment.

Although these criteria are used widely, attempts continue to refine the selection of patients for pulmonary metastasectomy.

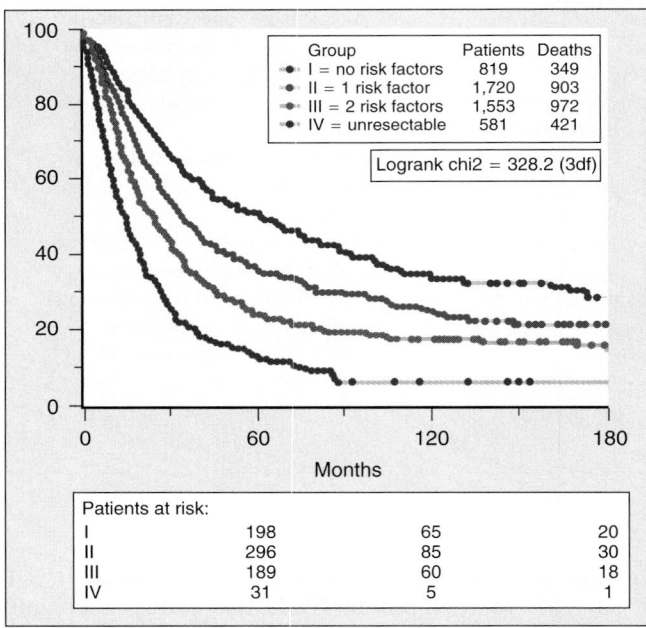

Group	Patients	Deaths
I = no risk factors	819	349
II = 1 risk factor	1,720	903
III = 2 risk factors	1,553	972
IV = unresectable	581	421

Logrank chi2 = 328.2 (3df)

Patients at risk:

I	198	65	20
II	296	85	30
III	189	60	18
IV	31	5	1

Figure 58-1. Survival of the four prognostic groups based on the analysis of 5206 patients entered into the International Registry of Lung Metastases. Group I includes patients who had completely resectable disease with a single metastasis and a disease-free interval after resection of the primary tumor (DFI) of 36 months or more; Group II, patients who had completely resectable disease with multiple metastases *or* a DFI of less than 36 months; Group III, patients who had completely resectable disease with multiple metastases *and* a DFI of less than 36 months; and Group IV, patients with unresectable disease. (From Pastorino U, Buyse M, Friedel G, et al: Long-term results of lung metastasectomy: Prognostic analyses based on 5206 cases. J Thorac Cardiovasc Surg 1997;113:37.)

Several prognostic factors that are not universal across all tumor histologies have been reported to affect outcome after pulmonary metastectomy (Table 58-1). The largest series of pulmonary metastectomy reported to date is from the International Registry of Lung Metastasis, which analyzed 5206 cases.[5] The overall 5-year survival after pulmonary metastectomy without stratifying for tumor type was 36%. Factors associated with better prognosis included a long disease-free interval, complete resection, and a small number of lung nodules. A staging system based on these prognostic factors was proposed (Fig. 58-1).

The role of surgery in the treatment of pulmonary metastases will continue to evolve as better systemic therapies become available. Currently, only a minority of patients with metastatic disease from any source are candidates for pulmonary metastectomy; however, improved imaging studies and the widespread use of computed tomography (CT) might detect more patients who have small-volume pulmonary metastases and are therefore candidates for metastasectomy. A current perspective of the evaluation and treatment of patients with isolated lung metastases is presented in this chapter.

DIAGNOSIS

Few patients with pulmonary metastasis are symptomatic. It is estimated that only 15% to 20% of patients present with cough or nonspecific chest pain and even fewer still with hemoptysis. Traditionally, chest x-ray has been the most commonly used and most cost-effective modality for screening patients for metastasis from extrathoracic malignancy. The most frequent radiographic appearance of a pulmonary metastasis is a peripherally located, well circumscribed nodule (Fig. 58-2).[6,7] Several less common radiographic characteristics have also been described. Cavitating lesions are associated with a differential diagnosis that includes benign, infectious, and malignant causes (Fig. 58-3). When malignant, cavitary lesions are usually squamous cell carcinomas. The frequency of cavitation in metastatic nodules is approximately 4%; however, squamous cell malignancy is responsible for 69% percent of these lesions. Spontaneous pneumothorax also can occur with metastatic lung lesions and is thought to be caused by cavitation and erosion into a bronchiole wall. Spontaneous pneumothorax is most frequently seen in patients with sarcoma. It is said that a spontaneous pneumothorax in a patient with history of a sarcoma should prompt an evaluation for possible occult metastatic lung lesions. Calcification of pulmonary nodules is usually related to a benign process such as a hamartoma; however, metastatic lesions of many types (especially osteogenic sarcoma) are known to produce calcification (Fig. 58-4).[6,7] Calcification in metastatic lesions are thought to be produced by several processes in different tumor types, including bone formation in osteogenic sarcoma, mucinous calcification of adenocarcinomas, or dystrophic calcification of lesions such as synovial sarcoma or giant cell tumors of the bone.[6] Hemorrhage

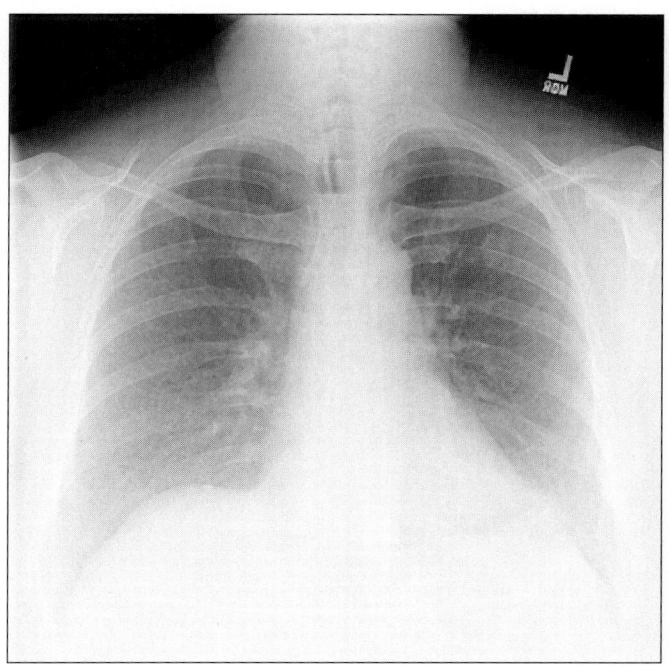
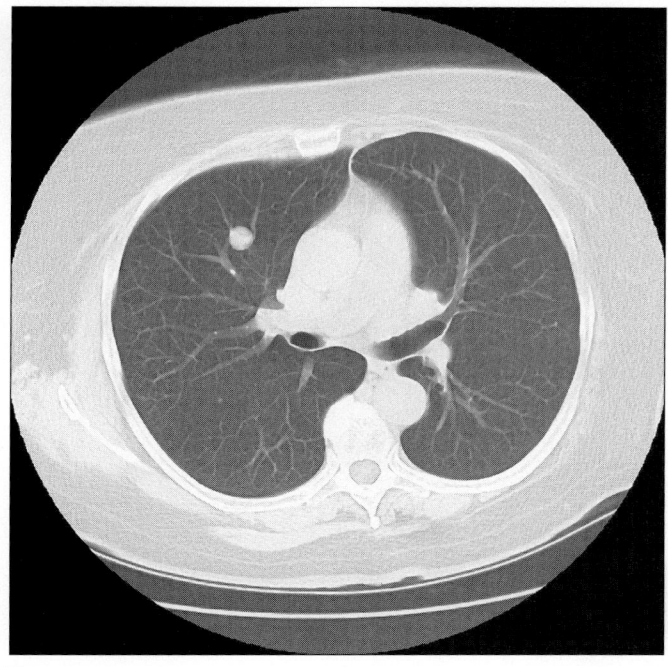

A   B

Figure 58-2. Two patients with metastatic sarcoma demonstrating typical findings of well circumscribed peripheral lesions. **A,** Plain chest radiograph. **B,** Computed tomographic image.

around lung nodules is also seen more frequently in benign lung lesions (e.g., fungal or mycobacterial infections) and is visualized as a halo around the lung nodule. This can be seen in metastatic lesions also and should raise the suspicion of metastasis among patients with a prior history of malignancy.

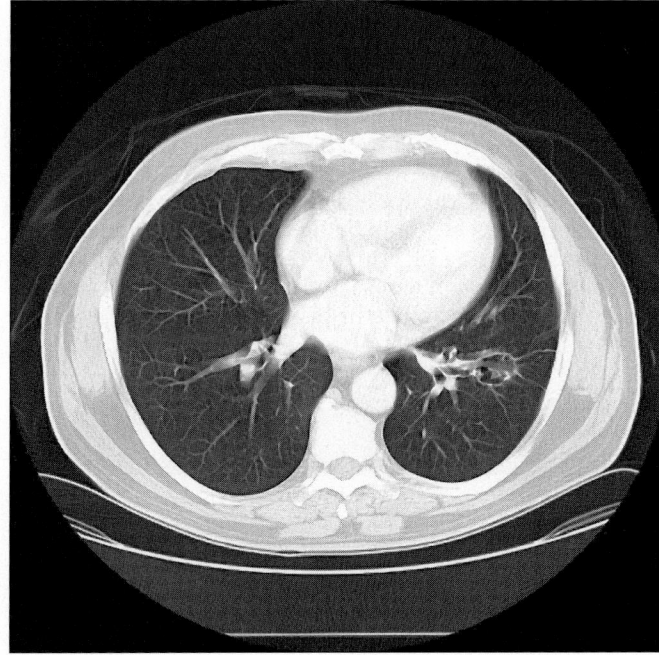

Figure 58-3. Chest CT demonstrating cavitary lesion in a patient with metastatic colorectal cancer.

Computed Tomography

The use of computed tomography (CT) as an adjunct to plain film radiography for the diagnosis of pulmonary metastases has increased dramatically during the last decade. This has been facilitated by the development of high-speed helical scanners. It is clear that CT is able to visualize more lesions than chest x-ray.[5,8-17] Chang and colleagues[11] reported that when compared to conventional radiography, CT was able to visualize nearly twice as many nodules.[18] CT is not able to distinguish reliably between malignant and benign lesions, however. McCormack and coworkers[8] retrospectively studied 144 patients who had had both a chest x-ray and a CT scan to identify metastatic lesions. The CT scan results differed from the final pathology reports in 42% of cases, with CT scan underestimating the number of malignant nodules in 25% of patients. Pastorino and associates[5] reported results of imaging for 2988 patients undergoing pulmonary metastectomy. The overall accuracy of radiologic assessment of the number of metastatic nodules was 61%, underestimating metastasis in 25% of patients. Interestingly, among those patients (1134) who had bilateral exploration, the accuracy of imaging was only 37%, with the number of lesions underestimated for 39% and overestimated for 25%. The accuracy and sensitivity of CT also depends on the size of the lesions (Table 58-2): the larger the lesion, the greater the sensitivity and accuracy. Munden and colleagues[14] reported on the clinical significance of pulmonary lesions less than 1 cm in diameter, finding malignant pulmonary lesions in 81% of patients with a history of prior malignancy. Multiple authors have described the ability of CT to detect a greater number of pulmonary nodules, while acknowledging a decreasing

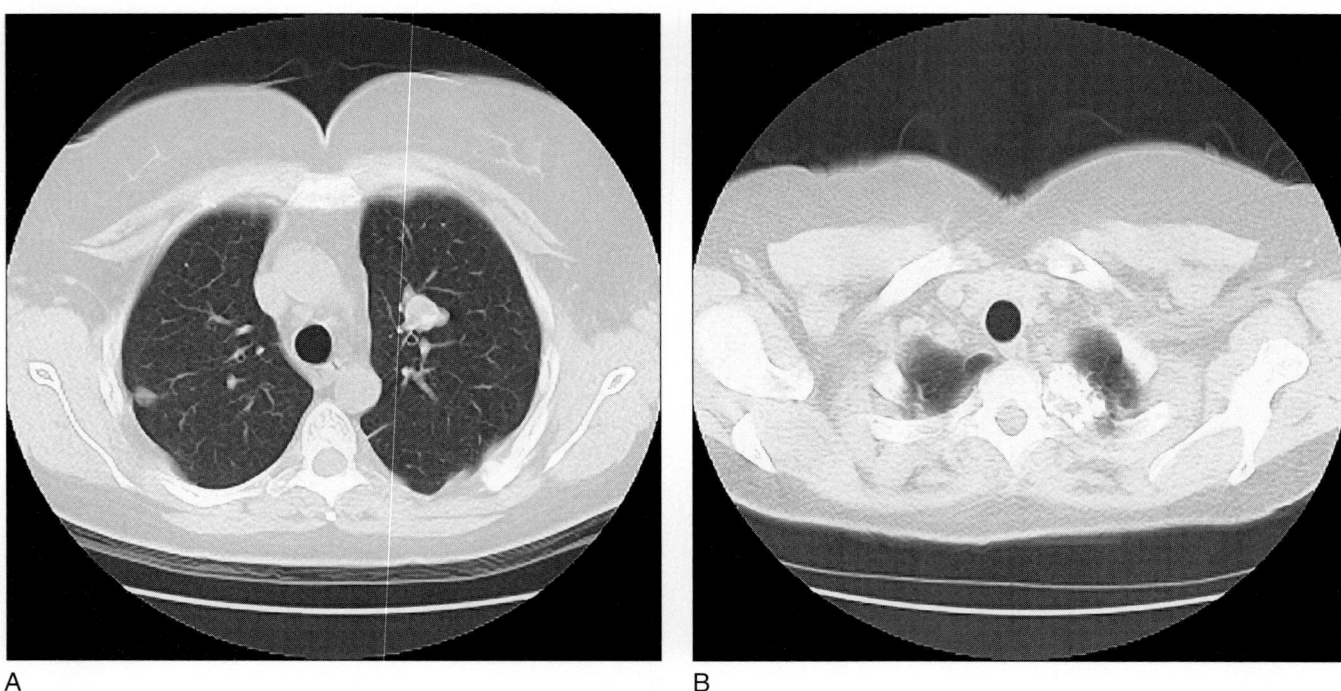

A   B

Figure 58-4. Metastatic osteosarcoma demonstrating the presence of calcifications in metastatic lesions. **A** and **B,** Chest CTs.

specificity of identifying malignant nodules with this diagnostic tool.[11,15] Therefore, not all small pulmonary nodules in patients with a past cancer history can be assumed to represent metastatic disease. Currently, there are no established guidelines for routine screening for pulmonary metastases. Many institutions still use periodic chest x-ray as the only imaging modality to rule out pulmonary metastasis. Other authors suggest that the use of CT for routine screening is indicated for groups of patients whose primary tumors have an unusually high propensity to spread to the lungs.[13,16] As the quality and speed of CT scanning progresses, it will likely become the sole screening tool for identifying pulmonary metastases.[11,15]

Magnetic Resonance Imaging

Magnetic resonance imaging (MRI) provides the benefits of reduced radiation exposure (of particular interest for cases involving younger patients) and the ability to detect

lesions at lung-mediastinal interfaces. MRI has not gained wide acceptance as a screening tool, however, mainly due to its increased time constraints and cost. Further technical considerations that are unfavorable include motion-related artifacts and an inability to detect calcified lesions. Kersjes and coworkers[19] performed a study comparing MRI with helical CT in the detection of pulmonary metastasis and showed MRI to have an overall accuracy of 84%. For lesions smaller than 5 mm, however, the sensitivity of MRI was only 36%. The routine use of MRI is currently not advocated as a screening tool for patients with pulmonary metastasis.

Nuclear Imaging

Imaging with ^{18}F-fluorodeoxyglucose positron emission tomography (FDG-PET) is being used more frequently to assist in the staging of primary tumors. Most often, this is used at the time of diagnosis to rule out distant metastasis, but it is used occasionally to assess response to therapy.

TABLE 58-2

Detection of Pulmonary Metastasis by Computed Tomography				
YEAR	**AUTHOR**	**NO. OF NODULES**	**SENSITIVITY FOR SMALL LESIONS**	**SENSITIVITY FOR LARGER LESIONS**
1998	Waters et al[*,18]	144	44% (≤5 mm)	91% (>5 mm)
1999	Diederich et al[9]	90	69% (≤6 mm)	95% (>6 mm)
2002	Margaritora et al[†,10]	188	48% (≤6 mm)	87% (>6 mm)

*Canine model.
†High-resolution CT group.

Currently, FDG-PET is not used as a screening tool to identify pulmonary metastasis, but multiple authors support the eventual use of this modality as a screening tool.[20,21] Dose and associates[21] studied 50 patients with breast cancer who had FDG-PET evaluations to determine the presence of metastatic disease. FDG-PET had a sensitivity of 78.6% in identifying pulmonary metastasis compared with conventional chest x-ray, which had a sensitivity of 41.6%.[21] Other authors report that FDG-PET might not be superior to conventional imaging techniques in identifying pulmonary metastasis from bone and soft tissue sarcomas.[22,23] Lucas and colleagues[22] studied 62 patients with soft tissue sarcoma who had FDG-PET during initial evaluation. The sensitivity of FDG-PET in detecting lung metastasis was 86.7% compared with 100% for CT, leading the authors to conclude that CT is a superior imaging tool for identifying these lesions. Further study is warranted to determine the true benefit, if any, of using FDG-PET as a routine screening tool for identifying patients with pulmonary metastasis. Because PET is currently unable to detect subcentimeter lung lesions reliably it is likely that CT will remain the most sensitive imaging modality.

SURGICAL APPROACHES TO LUNG METASTASIS

The goal of pulmonary metastectomy is to achieve complete resection of all visible and palpable tumor in the lung. The surgical approach is dictated by the extent and location of disease and by the patient's performance status. There are several approaches available depending on the size, number, and location of the lesions. The advantages and disadvantages of these approaches are outlined in Table 58-3.

The standard approach to the patient with disease localized to one hemithorax is a unilateral posterolateral thoracotomy. The thorax is usually entered through the fifth intercostal space. Several variations of this include muscle-sparing incisions, axillary incisions, or an anterior thoracotomy. All of these approaches allow full visual inspection and manual palpation of the entire lung.

During the past decade, the use of video-assisted thoracoscopy (VATS) has been described for pulmonary metastasectomy. This approach is controversial, however.[24-28] McCormack and coworkers[25] performed a prospective study evaluating the role of VATS to treat pulmonary metastasis. Eighteen patients had preoperative CT followed by VATS resection of all visible and CT detected lesions. All patients then immediately underwent thoracotomy with resection of any additional lung nodules. Additional malignant lesions were found in 56% of patients after attempted VATS resection of the nodules found on preoperative imaging. The authors concluded that this high failure rates of CT and VATS warranted closure of the study before the intended 50 patients could be enrolled. Recently, other authors have advocated the use of VATS for patients with a solitary pulmonary metastasis. Mutsaerts and associates[24,28] described their experiences with 20 patients who underwent either VATS or thoracotomy for resection for single pulmonary metastasis. The 5-year survival and recurrence rates for VATS appeared to be similar to those seen with thoracotomy.[28] Other authors have described localization methods using radiotracer injection to help identify small or deeply located lesions during VATS resections.[26] Currently, the practice in our institution is to use VATS primarily for the diagnosis of metastatic disease. Thoracotomy or other open procedures remain our preferred approach to pulmonary metastasectomy because of the prognostic importance of complete resection and the potential for missing small metastases with VATS.

The approach to bilateral disease is more variable, but the principles remain the same. The use of median sternotomy, "clamshell" thoracotomy (bilateral anterior thoracotomy with transverse sternotomy), sequential bilateral thoracotomies, and simultaneous bilateral posterolateral thoracotomies are employed as standard surgical approaches to the resection of bilateral metastases.[29-31] In general, resection of bilateral metastases is preferably done as a single operation. Sequential thoracotomies are performed only when the anatomical location of a lesion requires a complex or extensive operation, or when the patient's comorbidities dictate a more conservative approach to management.

In contrast to primary lung cancers, pulmonary metastases require only a local excision with a surrounding rim (1–2 cm) of benign lung tissue. This is accomplished most frequently by wedge resection performed by precision

TABLE 58-3

Surgical Approaches to Resection of Pulmonary Metastases		
SURGICAL APPROACH	**ADVANTAGES**	**DISADVANTAGES**
Unilateral Disease		
Posterolateral thoracotomy	Superior exposure and palpation of lung	Painful, large incision
Videothoracoscopy (VATS)	Less painful	Inability to palpate, poor ability to detect deep lesions
Bilateral Disease		
Clamshell thoracotomy	Excellent bilateral exposure	Painful; sacrifice of both internal mammary arteries
Simultaneous bilateral thoracotomies	One hospital stay/procedure	Painful
Staged (sequential) bilateral thoracotomy	Allows technically complex procedures	Two hospitalizations and procedures
Median sternotomy	Bilateral exposure, less painful	Poor exposure to posterior lung fields

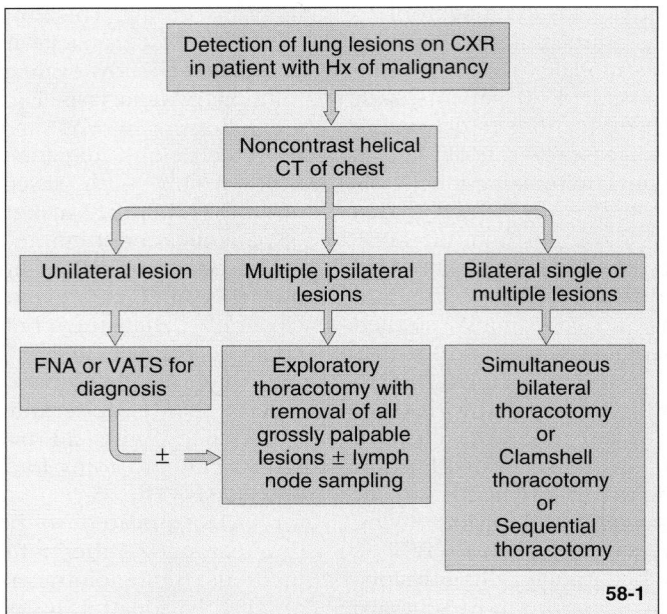

electrocautery or with a stapling instrument (Fig. 58-5). Segmentectomy, lobectomy, and pneumonectomy are used less commonly. It is important to note that survival after metastectomy is not increased by a more radical resection such as lobectomy or pneumonectomy. These procedures might be required technically to remove the lesion, however, and they should be applied to do so if needed. The most important principle of these techniques is a clear margin of resection.

The risks of resection of pulmonary metastasis using standard wedge resection is very low, with mortality generally 1% or less. Complications include bleeding, infection in the wound, pneumonia, or prolonged air leak. More extensive resections such as lobectomy or pneumonectomy carry only slightly higher morbidity rates, and these operations are well tolerated by most patients.

The preoperative evaluation for these patients is similar to that for patients undergoing lung resection for any other cause. Pulmonary function testing should be obtained for all patients to assure that the volume of lung resection will not compromise overall respiratory function. Thorough evaluation of underlying cardiovascular disease should also be undertaken, with preoperative stress testing as clinically indicated.

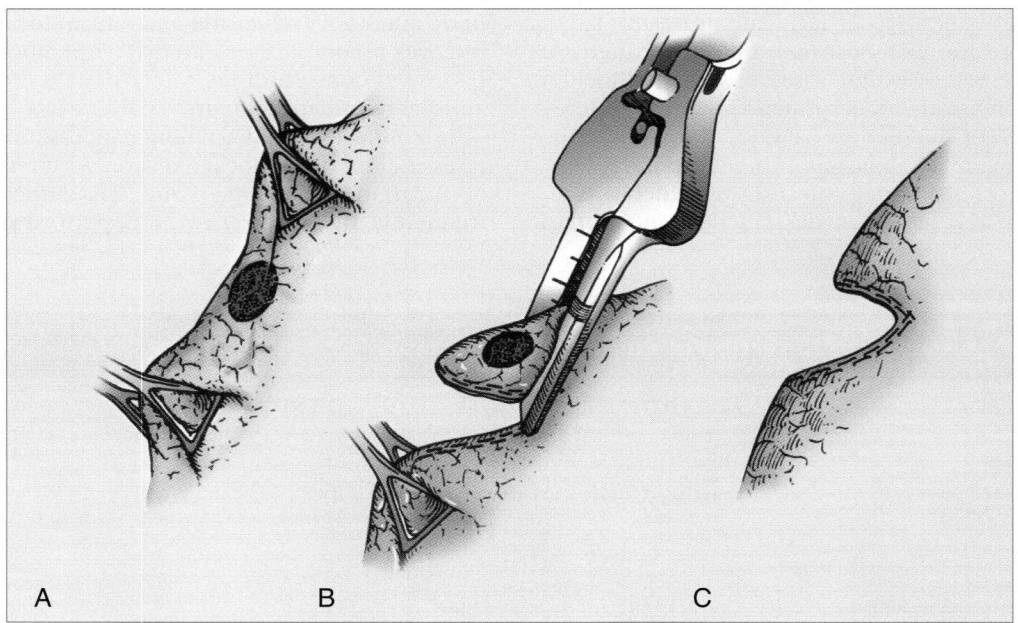

Figure 58-5. Method of wedge resection by using a stapling device. This technique is most suitable for peripherally located metastases adjacent to the fissures or edges of the lung. (From Rusch VW: Surgical techniques for pulmonary metastasectomy. Sem Thorac Cardiovasc Surg 2002;14:4.)

PULMONARY METASTASECTOMY FOR SPECIFIC TUMOR TYPES

Colorectal Cancers

It is estimated that 10% to 25% of patients with primary colorectal tumors have detectable metastases at the time of diagnosis.[32] Despite advances in adjuvant therapy and surgery, 50% of all patients with colorectal cancer will develop some form of metastasis during their lifetimes.[33] Approximately 15% of patients having curative resections of their primary colorectal tumors will develop distant metastasis, including metastasis to the lung.[34] Pulmonary metastasis can occur even with favorable primary tumor characteristics. Okumura and associates[35] reported that 26% of pulmonary metastectomies were performed in patients with Duke's A or B primary colorectal cancer. Since Blalock[36] reported the first pulmonary metastectomy for colorectal cancer in 1944, several authors have reported their experiences regarding overall survival and prognostic factors. The 5- and 10-year survival rates range from 30% to 40% and from 27% to 37%, respectively (Table 58-4).[37-40] It is clear from the literature that pulmonary metastectomy for colorectal cancer is associated with long-term survival, especially when a complete resection is performed. McCormack and colleagues[41] reviewed 144 patients who underwent pulmonary metastectomy for colorectal cancer and showed that survival for patients who underwent complete resection was approximately 40% at 5 years, whereas incomplete resection was associated with a poor prognosis.

As for other primary tumors, studies evaluating the disease free interval, the number of lesions (multiple vs. single), and the presence of lymph node involvement have shown these to be significant prognostic factors after pulmonary metastectomy for colorectal cancer.[35,37-46] Colorectal cancer is also unique in the fact that the serum tumor marker carcinoembryonic antigen (CEA), used as a marker for follow-up, has been shown to be a prognostic indicator for patients with pulmonary metastases.[37-46]

There is some disagreement as to whether single, ipsilateral metastases are associated with a better prognosis than either multiple ipsilateral or bilateral metastases. The presence of bilateral metastases was previously thought to be a contraindication to metastectomy. Recently, though, several authors have reported that the survival for patients with bilateral lesions is not significantly reduced compared with patients who have multiple ipsilateral lesions.[38,43] Although a solitary metastasis might be associated with a better prognosis than multiple metastases (either unilateral or bilateral), the main criteria used to select patients with multiple lesions is whether removal of these lesions is technically feasible and whether removal of the volume of lung parenchyma does not appear to compromise the patient's lung function to a significant extent.

CEA levels are elevated in 40% to 70% of patients prior to pulmonary metastectomy. Most authors report elevated CEA levels as an adverse prognostic factor.[39,40,44,45] The reason for this is unclear, although it has been postulated that the presence of CEA could promote adhesion or attachment of tumors cells or could be due to undetected extrathoracic metastasis.[47] Although an elevated CEA level is not used currently to exclude patients from resection, it could be useful to consider this in the context of other known prognostic factors. For instance, a patient who rapidly develops pulmonary metastases after resection of the primary tumor and has multiple lung nodules and an elevated CEA level might be treated initially with chemotherapy rather than going directly to pulmonary metastasectomy.

Hilar or mediastinal lymph node metastases are reported to occur in 1% to 28% of patients with colorectal pulmonary metastasis.[35,40-43,45] Saito and associates[40] reported that 20 of 138 patients (14.5%) who underwent lymph node sampling had positive nodes. The 5-year survival was 48.5% for the patients without hilar or mediastinal lymph node metastasis vs. 6.2% at 4 years for the patients with lymph node metastasis. Okumura and colleagues[35] performed systematic lymph node dissection on 100 patients with colorectal pulmonary metastasis. Fifteen of these patients had positive lymph nodes with a 5-year survival of 6.7%, compared with a 50% survival for those with negative lymph nodes, indicating that complete lymph node dissection does not increase survival. The routine use of mediastinal lymph node dissection in patients with pulmonary metastases appears to be the exception rather than the norm. The presence of malignant lymph nodes could indicate a group of patients otherwise thought to be disease-free who might benefit from additional adjuvant therapy. We favor doing media-

TABLE 58-4

	Survival of Patients Undergoing Pulmonary Metastectomy for Colorectal Cancer			
YEAR	AUTHOR	NUMBER	5-YEAR SURVIVAL (%)	10-YEAR SURVIVAL (%)
1992	McAfee et al[37]	139	30.5	N/A
1996	Okumura[35]	159	40.5	27.7
1998	McCormack et al[38]	287	40.0	32.0
2001	Zink et al[39]	110	32.6	N/A
2002	Saito et al.[40]	165	39.6	37.2

Studies represent analysis of 100 or more patients.

stinal lymph node sampling or dissection for these patients. Although these procedures might not have a therapeutic effect, they certainly provide important prognostic information.

Previously, the presence of both liver and lung metastases from colorectal cancer was thought to be a contraindication to metastectomy. Synchronous or metachronous lung and liver metastasis occurs in approximately 5% of patients with colorectal cancer. Headrick and coworkers[48] reported 5- and 10-year survivals of 30% and 16%, respectively, for 58 patients who underwent resection of both liver and lung metastases from colorectal cancer. Decreasing morbidity and mortality rates for liver resection now make resection of both lung and liver metastases a viable option for carefully selected patients.

Bone and Soft Tissue Sarcoma

Bone and soft tissue sarcomas comprise a histologically diverse group of tumors accounting for 1% of all adult malignancies, with approximately 6600 cases occurring in the United States annually.[49,50] Metastasis will occur in 25% to 70% of patients with localized disease, and 10% present with metastasis at the time of diagnosis.[50] Isolated pulmonary metastases occur in up to 20% of sarcoma patients during the course of their disease, with the lung being the site of failure after treatment in up to 90% of cases.[51,52] Factors associated with an increased risk of pulmonary metastasis include high tumor grade, primary tumor size greater than 5 cm, lower extremity site, and histological subtype.[51] The lack of effective systemic therapy for most soft tissue sarcomas makes surgical resection the best treatment for pulmonary metastases. Several studies have shown that the complete resection of pulmonary metastases is associated with long-term survival.[5,49,51,53] Billingsley and associates[49] reported that the 3-year actuarial survival was 46% for patients who had complete resection compared with 17% (p < 0.001) for those with incomplete resection of pulmonary metastasis. The cumulative 5-year survival for patients with bone and soft tissue sarcomas after pulmonary metastectomy ranges from 31% to 40% (Table 58-5).[5,49,53-55]

The histological subtype of sarcoma influences both the development of pulmonary metastasis and overall survival. High-grade, undifferentiated, and alveolar soft part sarcomas produce pulmonary metastasis in approx-

imately 60% of patients.[49] Tumors that are high grade and histologic variants such as liposarcoma, malignant fibrous histiocytoma, and malignant peripheral nerve tumor have all been reported as unfavorable prognostic factors.[49,51,56] Longer disease-free intervals, fewer lesions, and unilaterality have also been reported as favorable prognostic factors.

The incidence of hilar or mediastinal lymph node metastasis in patients with lung metastasis from sarcoma is 2%.[5] This low propensity for lymph node involvement is also a feature of primary sarcomas. Therefore, it seems that routine mediastinal lymph node sampling or dissection is unlikely to offer significant prognostic information or therapeutic benefit.

The rate of recurrence after pulmonary metastectomy for sarcoma ranges from 45% to 83%; however, the role of repeat resection of pulmonary metastases has been studied by few authors.[51,55-58] Weiser and colleagues[59] reported experience from Memorial Sloan Kettering concerning 86 patients who underwent re-resection of pulmonary metastases for soft tissue sarcoma. The 5-year survival after undergoing at least two operations for pulmonary metastectomy was 36%. Patients who had a complete re-resection had a median survival of 51 months, compared to 6 months for those who could not be completely re-resected. Poor prognostic indicators for re-resection included three or more nodules, lesions greater than 2 cm in size, and high-grade primary tumors. This study strongly suggested a benefit for repeat or multiple procedures for clearance of pulmonary disease in carefully selected patients.

Melanoma

Patients with metastatic melanoma have an especially poor prognosis. The most common sites of metastasis from melanoma are the lungs, distant subcutaneous tissue, and distant lymph nodes, with isolated lung metastasis occurring in 1.9% to 11% of patients.[60,61] Tafra and colleagues[62] reported their experience with 106 patients with metastatic melanoma who underwent pulmonary metastasectomy. Sixty-five of these patients underwent a complete resection. Although the benefit of a complete (vs. an incomplete) resection on survival could not be demonstrated in a univariate analysis, a multivariate analysis found that surgical resection (vs. no operation) was associated with a significantly better survival (p = 0.0001). Other authors have reported that complete resection is associated with prolonged survival.[63,64] Overall, the 5-year survival rates after resection of pulmonary metastasis from malignant melanoma vary from 4.5% to 27% (Table 58-6).[20,61-63,65-67] This wide range of values probably reflects the relatively small numbers of patients included in some studies. Prognostic factors that have been reported include operation, number of nodules, prior immune therapy, histologic type, disease-free interval, and tumor doubling time.[20,60,61-67] Harpole and coworkers[64] reported on a large series of patients who had pulmonary metastases from melanoma. Of the 945 patients, 112 (11.8%) underwent pulmonary metastasectomy. Histological type (nodular and acral lentiginous lesions), high Clark level, and thicker primary tumors were significantly

TABLE 58-5

Survival of Patients Undergoing Pulmonary Metastectomy for Bone and Soft Tissue Sarcomas

YEAR	AUTHOR	NUMBER	5-YEAR SURVIVAL (%)
1995	Choong et al[53]	214	40
1996	van Geel et al[54]	255	38
1997	Pastorino et al[5]	1917	31
1999	Billingsley et al[49]	138	37

Studies represent analysis of 100 patients or more.

TABLE 58-6

Survival of Patients Undergoing Pulmonary Metastectomy for Malignant Melanoma

YEAR	AUTHOR	NUMBER	5-YEAR SURVIVAL (%)
1985	Thayer et al[65]	18	11.1
1990	Karp et al[63]	22	4.5
1991	Gorenstein et al[61]	54	25.0
1995	Tafra et al[62]	106	27.0
1998	Ollila et al[67]	45	15.6
2002	Dalrymple-Hay et al[20]	121	22.1

TABLE 58-7

Survival of Patients Undergoing Pulmonary Metastectomy for Renal Cancer

YEAR	AUTHOR	NUMBER	5-YEAR SURVIVAL (%)
1994	Cerfolio et al[74]	96	36
1997	Fourquier et al[70]	50	44
1999	Friedel et al[72]	77	39
2002	Pfannschmidt et al[71]	149	42
2002	Piltz et al[73]	105	40

Studies represent analysis of 50 patients or more.

associated with pulmonary metastasis. The overall 5-year survival in this group was 4%. Patients who had a complete resection had a significantly higher median survival rate compared with those who had only partial resection, although all patients who underwent operations survived longer than those who had no operation. An analysis of the subset of patients who had a solitary metastasis found that patients who underwent resection had a significantly better median survival than patients managed nonsurgically. Important prognostic factors after surgery included complete resection, a long disease-free interval from treatment of the primary tumor to the diagnosis of the pulmonary metastasis, treatment with chemotherapy, and the total number of nodules. These data suggest that appropriately selected patients with metastatic melanoma confined to the lungs can benefit from pulmonary metastasectomy.

Renal Cell Carcinoma

Barry and Churchill[2] performed the first pulmonary metastectomy from renal adenocarcinoma in 1938. Approximately 30% of patients with renal cell carcinoma present with metastasis, and approximately 30%–50% of patients with initially localized tumors develop distant metastases.[68] One-half of patients who have a radical nephrouterectomy develop pulmonary metastases later, and only 16% of these patients will have disease confined to the lung.[69,70] The 5-year survival of patients with un-resected metastasis is approximately 2.7%.[71] The 5-year survival after resection of isolated pulmonary metastasis is reported to range from 36% to 44% (Table 58-7).[70-74] Several prognostic factors for survival have been identified, including complete resection, the disease-free interval between primary tumor treatment and metastasis, the number of metastases, and the presence or absence of lymph node metastases.[70,71,73]

Pfannschmidt and associates[71] reported on one of the largest series of pulmonary metastasectomy for renal cell cancer; they found that complete resection was possible in 78% of patients, and that these patients had a 5-year survival of 41.5% vs. 22.1% for those with incomplete resection This survival rate of 22.1% percent in incompletely resected patients was better than that for patients who had no resection at all.

Hilar and mediastinal lymph node metastases are seen in 22% to 30% of patients with metastatic renal cell cancer.[70,71] Fourquier and colleagues[70] and Pfannschmidt and associates[71] performed systematic mediastinal lymph node dissection on 50 and 191 patients, respectively. Both studies found that the presence of lymph node involvement was associated with a poorer survival. Although it is unknown whether lymph node dissection is therapeutic, it offers important prognostic information and should probably be performed on these patients.

Synchronous metastases are traditionally thought to be a relative contraindication to resection. The true incidence of synchronous vs. metachronous metastases in renal cell cancer is unclear, although in reported series of resected patients, synchronous lesions are less frequent and are thought to indicate a worse prognosis.[70,71] On the other hand, Fourquier and colleagues[70] examined survival among completely resected patients with synchronous lung metastases. Although the overall survival rate was lower for patients with synchronous lesions (48% vs. 20%), this was not statistically significant and again appeared to offer a survival benefit relative to no resection at all.

Head and Neck Cancer

Approximately 60,000 new cases of head and neck cancer occur each year in the United States.[75] The potential for metastatic spread is dependent on the stage of the primary tumor, with the rate of lung metastasis ranging from 4.3% to 25.1%.[76] Head and neck tumors and especially squamous cell cancers have a predilection for metastasizing to the lung, which is often the only site of metastasis.[77] The diagnosis of lung nodules in these patients is made even more challenging by the fact that 10% to 40% of lung nodules in these patients are actually second primary lung tumors.[78] There are few effective systemic therapy options for the treatment of lung metastasis from head and neck tumors, which leaves surgical resection as the most viable option. The estimated 5-year survival after pulmonary metastectomy in these patients ranges from 29% to 59% (Table 58-8).[75,76,78,79] The wide range of survival rates could be related to the heterogeneous histological groups reported in most series. Squamous cell tumors of head and neck origin have a worse prognosis than their glandular counterparts such as thyroid, adenoid cystic, and mucoepidermoid

TABLE 58-8

Survival of Patients Undergoing Pulmonary Metastectomy for Head and Neck Cancer			
YEAR	AUTHOR	NUMBER	5-YEAR SURVIVAL (%)
1992	Finley et al*,[78]	18	29
1996	Wedman et al[79]	21	59
1997	Nibu et al[76]	32	32
1999	Liu et al[75]	83	50

*Included only patients with squamous cell carcinoma metastasis.

tumors.[75,76,79] Liu and coworkers[75] reported on 83 patients undergoing pulmonary metastectomy from head and neck tumors. In their series, the 5-year overall survival for squamous cell tumors was 34%, compared with 64% for tumors of glandular origin (p = 0.14). Bilateral metastasis and recurrence of metastasis are not contraindications to resection and have not been shown to be adverse prognostic factors at this time.

Germ Cell Tumors

Germ cell tumors comprise only 1% of cancers but are the most common neoplasm in men aged 15 to 35 years. The vast majority of these tumors arise in the testis, with an annual incidence of five cases per 100,000.[80] The survival of patients with germ cell tumors has increased dramatically during the past 30 years because of cisplatin-based chemotherapy.[80] Monitoring of treatment and recurrence has been made possible by the use of sensitive tumor markers, including alpha fetoprotein (AFP) and human chorionic gonadotropin (BHCG).

Pulmonary metastasis at the time of presentation in these patients is common, approaching 50% for patients with retroperitoneal disease.[81] Residual masses after chemotherapy are present in approximately 50% of patients and could contain viable malignancy, mature teratoma, or only fibrosis and/or necrosis.[81] Surgical resection of these lesions is crucial to identify which of the above components is present, to predict outcome, and to determine whether any further therapy is warranted. The estimated 5-year survival rate after pulmonary metastectomy ranges from 59% to 77% (Table 58-9).[80–82] The most significant prognostic factor is the presence of viable tumor cells in the resected specimen. Liu and associates[80] reviewed the experience at Memorial Sloan-Kettering Cancer Center over a 28-year period of 157

TABLE 58-9

Survival after Pulmonary Metastectomy for Germ Cell Tumors			
YEAR	AUTHOR	NUMBER	5-YEAR SURVIVAL (%)
1998	Cagini et al[81]	141	77
1994	Anyanwu et al[82]	104	59
1998	Liu et al[80]	157	68

patients undergoing pulmonary metastectomy for germ cell tumors. After resection, viable tumor was found in 70 patients (44.5%), necrosis in 47 patients (29.9%), and mature teratoma in 40 patients (25.4%). Survival was significantly poorer in those patients with viable tumor cells (43% over 10-years) compared with those patients with necrosis/fibrosis (86% 10-year survival) or mature teratoma (84% 10-year survival).[80] The presence of mature teratoma in a specimen did not significantly worsen prognosis. The inability to make an accurate determination of the presence or absence of viable tumor cells in all residual lesions after treatment for germ cell tumors mandates that all of these lesions be resected to determine overall prognosis and potential for further therapy.

Breast Cancer

Breast cancer is the most prevalent cancer among women in the United States, with approximately 100,000 cases occurring annually.[83] Approximately 15% to 25% of patients with metastatic disease have their disease confined to the thorax. The data regarding pulmonary metastectomy is controversial, with most studies analyzing the outcome of encompassing small groups of patients treated over several decades. The largest series reported to date is by Friedel and colleagues[84] from the International Registry of Lung Metastases. They reported on 467 patients undergoing pulmonary metastectomy for breast cancer. Complete resection of all metastasis was possible in 84% of patients. The 5-year overall survival was 38% for patients who underwent complete resection, compared with 18% of patients with incomplete resection (p = 0.0009). A long disease-free interval and fewer lesions were associated with a longer survival in this group.[84] McDonald and associates[85] reported on 60 patients undergoing pulmonary metastectomy for breast cancer and failed to show a survival benefit for surgical management. Because breast cancer also frequently progresses to extrathoracic disease and is sensitive to current systemic therapies, pulmonary metastasectomy is rarely an appropriate treatment option. Indeed, breast cancer is an example of the evolution of the role of pulmonary metastasectomy. Before the advent of effective hormonal and chemotherapy, pulmonary metastasectomy was performed commonly for breast cancer with metastases confined to the lungs. Surgery is now considered infrequently for treatment.

ACKNOWLEDGMENT

The authors wish to thank Melody Owens for her expert assistance in manuscript preparation.

REFERENCES

1. Downey RJ: Surgical treatment of pulmonary metastases. Surg Oncol Clin N Am 1999;8:341.
2. Barry JD, Churchill BJ: Adenocarcinoma of the kidney with metastases to the lung. J Urol 1939;42:269.

3. Martini N, McCormack PM: Evolution of the surgical management of pulmonary metastases. Chest Surg Clin N Amer 1998;8:13.

4. Rusch VW: Pulmonary metastectomy: Current indications. Chest 1995;107:322S.

5. Pastorino U, Buyse M, Friedel G, et al: Long-term results of lung metastasectomy: Prognostic analyses based on 5206 cases. J Thorac Cardiovasc Surg 1997;113:37.

6. Libshitz HI, North LB: Pulmonary metastases. Radiol Clin N Am 1982;20:437.

7. Seo JB, Im J-G, Goo JM, et al: Atypical pulmonary metastases: Spectrum of radiologic findings. RadioGraphics 2001;21:403.

8. McCormack PM, Ginsberg KB, Bains MS, et al: Accuracy of lung imaging in metastases with implications for the role of thoracoscopy. Ann Thorac Surg 1993;56:863.

9. Diederich S, Semik M, Lentschig MG, et al: Helical CT of pulmonary nodules in patients with extrathoracic malignancy: CT-surgical correlation. Am J Roentgenol 1999;172:353.

10. Margaritora S, Porziella V, D'Andrilli A, et al: Pulmonary metastases: Can accurate radiological evaluation avoid thoracotomic approach? Eur J Cardiothorac Surg 2002;21:1111.

11. Chang AE, Schaner EG, Conkle DM, et al: Evaluation of computed tomography in the detection of pulmonary metastases. Cancer 1979;43:913.

12. Picci P, Vanel D, Briccoli A, et al: Computed tomography of pulmonary metastases from osteosarcoma: The less poor technique. A study of 51 patients with histological correlation. Ann Oncol 2001;12:1601.

13. Davis SD, Westcott J, Fleishon H, et al: Screening for pulmonary metastases. In American College of Radiology ACR Appropriateness Criteria, published online 2002, p. 655 (http://www.acr.org/dyna/?id=appcrit&pdf=0655-622_screening-pulmonary_mets_ac)

14. Munden RF, Pugatch RD, Liptay MJ, et al: Small pulmonary lesions detected at CT: Clinical importance. Radiology 1997;202:105.

15. Dinkel E, Mundinger A, Schopp D, et al: Diagnostic imaging in metastatic lung disease. Lung 1990;168(Suppl):1129.

16. Davis SD: CT evaluation for pulmonary metastases in patients with extrathoracic malignancy. Radiology 1991;180:1.

17. Woodard PK, Dehdashti F, Putman CE: Radiologic diagnosis of extrathoracic metastases to the lung. Oncology 1998;12:431.

18. Waters DJ, Coakley FV, Cohen MD, et al: The detection of pulmonary metastasis by helical CT: A clinicopathologic study in dogs. J Comput Assist Tomogr 1998;22:235.

19. Kersjes W, Mayer E, Buchenroth M, et al: Diagnosis of pulmonary metastases with turbo-SE MR imaging. Eur Radiol 1997;7:1190.

20. Dalrymple-Hay MJ, Rome PD, Kennedy C, et al: Pulmonary metastatic melanoma—the survival benefit associated with positron emission tomography scanning. Eur J Cardiothorac Surg 2002;21:611.

21. Dose J, Bleckmann C, Bachmann S, et al: Comparison of fluoro-deoxyglucose positron emission tomography and 'conventional diagnostic procedures' for the detection of distant metastases in breast cancer patients. Nucl Med Comm 2002;23:857.

22. Lucas JD, O'Doherty MJ, Wong JCH, et al: Evaluation of fluorodeoxyglucose positron emission tomography in the management of soft-tissue sarcomas. J Bone Joint Surg (Br) 1998;80:441.

23. Franzius C, Daldrup-Link HE, Sciuk J, et al: FDG-PET for detection of pulmonary metastases from malignant primary bone tumors: Comparison with spiral CT. Ann Oncol 2001;12:479.

24. Mutsaerts EL, Zoetmulder FA, Meijer S, et al: Outcome of thoracoscopic pulmonary metastasectomy evaluated by confirmatory thoracotomy. Ann Thorac Surg 2001;72:230.

25. McCormack PM, Bains MS, Begg CB, et al: Role of video-assisted thoracic surgery in the treatment of pulmonary metastases: Results of a prospective trial. Ann Thorac Surg 1996;62:213.

26. Burdine J, Joyce LD, Plunkett MB, et al: Feasibility and value of video-assisted thoracoscopic surgery wedge excision of small pulmonary nodules in patients with malignancy. Chest 2002;122:1467.

27. Davidson RS, Nwogu CE, Brentjens MJ, et al: The surgical management of pulmonary metastasis: Current concepts. Surg Oncol 2001;10:35.

28. Mutsaerts ELAR, Zoetmulder FAN, Meijer S, et al: Long term survival of thoracoscopic metastasectomy vs. metastasectomy by thoracotomy in patients with a solitary pulmonary lesion. Eur J Surg Oncol 2002;28:864.

29. van der Veen AH, van Geel AN, Hop WCJ, et al: Median sternotomy: The preferred incision for resection of lung metastases. Eur J Surg 1998;164:507.

30. Regal AM, Reese P, Antkowiak J, et al: Median sternotomy for metastatic lung lesions in 131 patients. Cancer 1985;55:1334.

31. Rusch VW: Surgical techniques for pulmonary metastasectomy. Sem Thorac Cardiovasc Surg 2002;14:4.

32. Niederhuber JE: Colon and rectum cancer. Patterns of spread and implications for workup. Cancer 1993;71(12 Suppl):4187.

33. Kindler HL, Shulman KL: Metastatic colorectal cancer. Curr Treat Options Oncol 2001;2:459.

34. Obrand DI, Gordon PH: Incidence and patterns of recurrence following curative resection for colorectal carcinoma. Dis Colon Rectum 1997;40:15.

35. Okumura S, Kondo H, Tsuboi M, et al: Pulmonary resection for metastatic colorectal cancer: Experiences with 159 patients. J Thorac Cardiovasc Surg 1996;112:867.

36. Blalock A: A recent advance in surgery. N Engl J Med 1944;231:261.

37. McAfee MK, Allen MS, Trastek VF, et al: Colorectal lung metastases: Results of surgical excision. Ann Thorac Surg 1992;53:780.

38. McCormack PM, Ginsberg RJ: Current management of colorectal metastases to lung. Chest Surg Clin N Am 1998;8:119.

39. Zink S, Kayser G, Gabius HJ, et al: Survival, disease-free interval, and associated tumor features in patients with colon/rectal carcinomas and their resected intrapulmonary metastases. Eur J Cardiothorac Surg 2001;19:908.

40. Saito Y, Omiya H, Kohno K, et al: Pulmonary metastasectomy for 165 patients with colorectal carcinoma. A prognostic assessment. J Thorac Cardiovasc Surg 2002;124:1007.

41. McCormack PM, Burt ME, Bains MS, et al: Lung resection for colorectal metastases. 10-year results. Arch Surg 1992;127:1403.

42. Ike H, Shimada H, Ohki S, et al: Results of aggressive resection of lung metastases from colorectal carcinoma detected by intensive follow-up. Dis Colon Rectum 2002;45:468.

43. Sakamoto T, Tsubota N, Iwanaga K, et al: Pulmonary resection for metastases from colorectal cancer. Chest 2001;119:1069.

44. Rena O, Casadio C, Viano F, et al: Pulmonary resection for metastases from colorectal cancer: Factors influencing prognosis. Twenty-year experience. Eur J Cardio-thorac Surg 2002;21:906.

45. Inoue M, Kotake Y, Nakagawa K, et al: Surgery for pulmonary metastases from colorectal carcinoma. Ann Thorac Surg 2000;70:380.

46. Wang CY, Hsie CC, Hsu HS, et al: Pulmonary resection for metastases from colorectal adenocarcinomas. Zhonghua Yi Xue Za Zhi (Taipei) 2002;65:15.

47. Gutman M, Fidler IJ: Biology of human colon cancer metastasis. World J Surg 1995;19:226.

48. Headrick JR, Miller DL, Nagorney DM, et al: Surgical treatment for hepatic and pulmonary metastases from colon cancer. Ann Thorac Surg 2001;71:975.

49. Billingsley KG, Burt ME, Jara E, et al: Pulmonary metastases from soft tissue sarcoma: Analysis of patterns of diseases and postmetastasis survival. Ann Surg 1999;229:602.

50. Komdeur R, Hoekstra HJ, van den Berg E, et al: Metastasis in soft tissue sarcomas: Prognostic critera and treatment perspectives. Cancer Metast Rev 2002;21:167.

51. Gadd MA, Casper ES, Woodruff JM, et al: Development and treatment of pulmonary metastases in adult patients with extremity soft tissue sarcoma. Ann Surg 1993;218:705.

52. Bacci G, Avella M, Picci P, et al: Metastatic patterns in osteosarcoma. Tumori 1988;74:421.

53. Choong PFM, Pritchard DJ, Rock MG, et al: Survival after pulmonary metastasectomy in soft tissue sarcoma. Prognostic factors in 214 patients. Acta Orthop Scan 1995;66:561.

54. van Geel AN, Pastorino U, Jauch KW, et al: Surgical treatment of lung metastases: The European Organization for Research and Treatment of Cancer—Soft Tissue and Bone Sarcoma Group study of 255 patients. Cancer 1996;77:675.

55. Casson AG, Putnam JB, Natarajan G, et al: Five-year survival after pulmonary metastasectomy for adult soft tissue sarcoma. Cancer 1992;69:662.

Problems Common to Cancer and Its Therapy

56. van Geel AN, van Coevorden F, Blankensteijn JD, et al: Surgical treament of pulmonary metastases from soft tissue sarcomas: A retrospective study in The Netherlands. J Surg Oncol 1994;56:172.

57. Rizzoni WE, Pass HJ, Wesley MN, et al: Resection of recurrent pulmonary metastases in patients with soft-tissue sarcomas. Arch Surg 1986;121:1248.

58. Pogrebniak HW, Roth JA, Steinberg SM, et al: Reoperative pulmonary resection in patients with metastatic soft tissue sarcoma. Ann Thorac Surg 1991;52:197.

59. Weiser MR, Downey RJ, Leung DH, et al: Repeat resection of pulmonary metastases in patients with soft-tissue sarcoma. J Am Coll Surg 2000;191:184.

60. Karakousis CP, Velez A, Driscoll DL, et al: Metastasectomy in malignant melanoma. Surgery 1994;115:295.

61. Gorenstein LA, Putnam JB Jr., Natarajan G, et al: Improved survival after resection of pulmonary metastases from malignant melanoma. Ann Thorac Surg 1991;52:204.

62. Tafra L, Dale PS, Wanek LA, et al: Resection and adjuvant immunotherapy for melanoma metastatic to the lung and thorax. J Thorac Cardiovasc Surg 1995;110:119.

63. Karp NS, Boyd A, Depan HJ, et al: Thoracotomy for metastatic malignant melanoma of the lung. Surgery 1990;107:256.

64. Harpole DH Jr., Johnson CM, Wolfe WG, et al: Analysis of 945 cases of pulmonary metastatic melanoma. J Thorac Cardiovasc Surg 1992;103:743.

65. Thayer JO Jr., Overholt RH: Metastatic melanoma to the lung: Long-term results of surgical excision. Am J Surg 1985;149:558.

66. Pogrebniak HW, Stovroff M, Roth JA, et al: Resection of pulmonary metastases from malignant melanoma: Results of a 16-year experience. Ann Thorac Surg 1988;46:20.

67. Ollila DW, Stern SL, Morton DL: Tumor doubling time: A selection factor for pulmonary resection of metastatic melanoma. J Surg Oncol 1998;69:206.

68. van der Poel HG, Roukema JA, Horenblas S, et al: Metastasectomy in renal cell carcinoma: A multicenter retrospective analysis. Eur Urol 1999;35:197.

69. Weiss L, Harlos JP, Torhorst J, et al: Metastatic patterns of renal carcinoma: An analysis of 687 necropsies. J Cancer Res Clin Oncol 1988;114:605.

70. Fourquier P, Regnard J-F, Rea S, et al: Lung metastases of renal cell carcinoma: Results of surgical resection. Eur J Cardiothorac Surg 1997;11:17.

71. Pfannschmidt J, Hoffmann H, Muley T, et al: Prognostic factors for survival after pulmonary resection of metastatic renal cell carcinoma. Ann Thorac Surg 2002;74:1653.

72. Friedel G, Hurtgen M, Penzenstadler M, et al: Resection of pulmonary metastases from renal cell carcinoma. Anticancer Res 1999;19:1593.

73. Piltz S, Meimarakis G, Wichmann MW, et al: Long-term results after pulmonary resection of renal cell carcinoma metastases. Ann Thorac Surg 2002;73:1082.

74. Cerfolio RJ, Allen MS, Deschamps C, et al: Pulmonary resection of metastatic renal cell carcinoma. Ann Thorac Surg 1994;57:339.

75. Liu D, Labow DM, Dang N, et al: Pulmonary metastasectomy for head and neck cancers. Ann Surg Oncol 1999;6:572.

76. Nibu K-I, Nakagawa K, Kamata S-E, et al: Surgical treatment for pulmonary metastases of squamous cell carcinoma of the head and neck. Am J Otolaryngol 1997;18:391.

77. Younes RN, Gross JL, Silva JF, et al: Surgical treatment of lung metastases of head and neck tumors. Am J Surg 1997;174:499.

78. Finley RK III, Verazin GT, Driscoll DL, et al: Results of surgical resection of pulmonary metastases of squamous cell carcinoma of the head and neck. Am J Surg 1992;164:594.

79. Wedman J, Balm AJ, Hart AA, et al: Value of resection of pulmonary metastases in head and neck cancer in patients. Head Neck 1996;18:311.

80. Liu D, Abolhoda A, Burt ME, et al: Pulmonary metastasectomy for testicular germ cell tumors: A 28-year experience. Ann Thorac Surg 1998;66:1709.

81. Cagini L, Nicholson AG, Horwich A, et al: Thoracic metastasectomy for germ cell tumours: Long-term survival and prognostic factors. Ann Oncol 1998;9:1185.

82. Anyanwu E, Krysa S, Buelzebruck H, et al: Pulmonary metastasectomy as secondary treatment for testicular tumors. Ann Thorac Surg 1994;57:1222.

83. Lanza LA, Natarajan G, Roth JA, et al: Long-term survival after resection of pulmonary metastases from carcinoma of the breast. Ann Thorac Surg 1992;54:244.

84. Friedel G, Pastorino U, Ginsberg RJ, et al: Results of lung metastasectomy from breast cancer: Prognostic criteria on the basis of 467 cases of the international registry of lung metastases. Eur J Cardiothorac Surg 2002;22:335.

85. McDonald ML, Deschamps C, Ilstrup DM, et al: Pulmonary resection for metastatic breast cancer. Ann Thorac Surg 1994;58:1599.

59

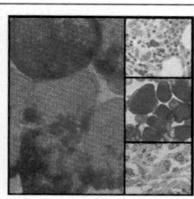

LIVER METASTASES

Nancy E. Kemeny

Margaret Kemeny

Theodore S. Lawrence

SUMMARY OF KEY POINTS

INCIDENCE

- Liver metastases are most frequently seen in patients with colorectal cancer (nearly 15% of patients presenting and an additional 60% developing subsequent spread); they are less common in patients with breast cancer (4% of initial failures), lung cancer (15%), and melanoma (24%).

ETIOLOGY

- The liver has a rich blood supply from both the hepatic artery and the portal vein; metastases can reach the liver from any organ, but the direct passage of blood from the gastrointestinal tract to the liver via the portal circulation plays a critical role in explaining the high rate of liver metastases from these sites.

DETECTION

- Contrast computed tomography (CT) and magnetic resonance imaging (MRI) can detect approximately two thirds of liver metastases.
- CT angiography, CT portography, and intraoperative ultrasound appear to have increased sensitivity compared with standard techniques.
- Positron emission tomography (PET) is more useful to detect extrahepatic disease.
- Of laboratory tests, carcinoembryonic antigen (CEA) can be useful for patients with metastatic colorectal cancer to the liver.

TREATMENT

Hepatic Resection

- There is general agreement that surgical resection is the treatment of choice for patients with one to three metastases from colorectal cancer, producing a 5-year survival of about 30%.

- Significant advances in surgical technique include the ability to perform metastasectomies (rather than formal lobectomies) and total vascular exclusion.
- The liver is the chief site of relapse after hepatic resection (50% of all patients).
- Prognostic variables that influence survival after hepatic resection include the presence of extrahepatic disease, the stage of the primary colon cancer, the time interval between primary and the development of hepatic metastases, and the number of metastases and positive margins.
- The use of adjuvant hepatic artery infusion (HAI) after liver resection has produced positive results in two American trials. There is a clear decrease in hepatic recurrence with adjuvant HAI.

Chemotherapy—Systemic

- The objective response rate with intravenous chemotherapy is improving, with response rates of 40% to 50% among patients with breast cancer, gastric cancer, and now even colon cancer.

Hepatic Artery Infusion

- Eight randomized trials demonstrate a higher response rate for HAI than for systemic infusion (42%–64% vs. 0%–38%, respectively). Survival advantage difficult to interpret: Two large U.S. studies allowed a crossover from systemic therapy to HAI after tumor failure. Other U.S. studies were too small (averaging 60 patients per study). The chief toxicity of HAI is biliary enzyme elevations in 40% and biliary sclerosis in 5% to 35% of patients.

Hepatic Artery Embolization

- Embolization could play a role in highly vascular tumors (neuroendocrine tumors and hepatocellular carcinoma).
- Embolization agents include gelfoam, lipiodol, and degradable starch microspheres.
- Embolization is rarely useful for patients with metastatic colorectal cancer.
- Chemoembolization involves the local entrapment of drug in the embolization agent in an attempt to provide a prolonged exposure of the tumor to drug locally, with less systemic exposure.

Ablative Techniques

- Cryosurgery involves destruction of tissue using a freezing probe.
- Limitations include the difficulty of controlling freezing and the typical requirement for laparotomy.
- Radiofrequency ablation destruction by frictional heat can be used percutaneously but is rarely good for lesions greater than 3 cm in size.

Absolute Ethanol Injection

- Ethanol is injected into the tumor under ultrasound guidance and could be of use for small hepatocellular carcinomas.

Radiation

- Whole-liver external-beam irradiation therapy (EBRT) alone is limited by the occurrence of radiation hepatitis to about 30 Gy.
- Parts of the liver can be treated to doses greater than 30 Gy using yttrium-90 (^{90}Y) microspheres, interstitial brachytherapy, and EBRT guided by three-dimensional treatment planning.

INTRODUCTION

Not that long ago, an oncology textbook would not have devoted an entire chapter to liver metastases. Oncologists were so pessimistic about the appearance of such metastases that "no treatment" was often the recommendation. Enormous changes have occurred, so that now, diagnosing liver metastases early can lead to effective treatment and even cure for a growing percentage of patients.

The liver is the primary site of metastases for many malignant neoplasms. Gastrointestinal malignancies are especially prone to spread to the liver because of its portal venous drainage. Extra-abdominal tumors such as bronchogenic carcinoma, breast cancer, and malignant melanoma often spread hematogenously to the liver.

For gastrointestinal tumors, differences are seen in the natural history of the hepatic metastases. In some circumstances, hepatic metastases are a sign of disseminated disease. When gastric and pancreatic cancers metastasize to the liver, the mean survival is short, and widespread metastases often exist, so that radical measures such as hepatic resection or hepatic artery infusion are rarely appropriate. In contrast, for colorectal cancer the liver might be the sole site of metastatic disease, and a significant fraction of these patients might have isolated liver metastasis. In this setting, progress has been significant in the areas of hepatic resection, regional chemotherapy, and radiation therapy as discussed in this chapter.

For nongastrointestinal tumors, metastases to the liver are less common as the initial site of relapse. Although breast, lung, and melanoma are the main extragastrointestinal cancers to metastasize to the liver, initial isolated metastases in the liver occur in 4%, 15%, and 24% of these patients, respectively.

Treatment of these types of metastases varies according to the sensitivity of the tumor type to chemotherapy. Those that are more sensitive to antineoplastic agents might benefit from systemic therapy or aggressive regional approaches (breast), while those that have limited response to chemotherapy (such as melanoma) may be approached regionally in the setting of a clinical trial. Special care must be exercised in choosing patients for regional therapy who do not have colorectal cancer, as diseases such as breast cancer and melanoma are rarely confined to the liver.

The last 20 years have witnessed new and more accurate methods of detecting and quantifying liver metastases, more advanced surgical techniques facilitating hepatic resection, and biologic advances that have increased the spectrum of available regional therapies. This chapter discusses advances in detection and treatment of liver metastases.

DETECTION

The need for early and accurate detection of liver metastases has become more critical as the guidelines for resectability of liver metastases have become more liberal.

Currently available modalities and their usefulness are listed in the sections that follow.

Imaging Techniques

Computed Tomography

CT images should be routinely evaluated by two different window levels in order to maximize detection of lesions (see Chapter 80). A soft tissue window (width of 300–500 Hounsfield units) is used for the initial examination of the liver; this allows for evaluation of adjacent abdominal architecture. A second setting with a narrow window and a lower width (100–150 H) is then used to evaluate the liver, as this setting increases contrast differences between the normal liver parenchyma and abnormalities.

Noncontrast CT. Noncontrast CT is usually used for patients with a history of contrast allergic reactions or renal impairment, but it also helps in identifying hypervascular metastases (especially carcinoid tumors, islet cell tumors, and renal cell carcinomas) or visualizing calcifications or hemorrhage. This form of CT often fails to distinguish hypovascular tumors from the liver parenchyma. One of the pitfalls of the procedure is that nonenhanced blood vessels can appear as low-attenuation masses and be confused with metastases.[1]

Contrast CT. Contrast is infused intravenously over the course of 2 minutes, with imaging done during the infusion. This method is better than noncontrast CT for detecting tumors that are hypovascular, such as colorectal carcinomas. One problem with this modality is that lesions might not be distinguishable from liver parenchyma during the equilibrium phase of the contrast injection (when the intravascular and interstitial concentrations equilibrate).[1]

CT Angiography. Currently the most accurate method for detecting metastases, CT angiography employs a bolus of contrast that is given into the hepatic artery (CT angiography) or via the superior mesenteric artery (CT portography). Liver imaging during arterial phase is critical for detection of hepatocellular carcinoma.

CT Portography (CTP). CTP dramatically enhances the liver parenchyma, as dye returned via the portal vein gives excellent contrast to the normal liver. Metastases appear as filling defects, surrounded by liver parenchyma that is contrast enhanced, as the majority of parenchymal blood supply is from the portal vein.[1]

Delayed CT. Sometimes CT is done 4 to 6 hours after 60 g of intravenous iodine has been given. It is most useful as an adjunct to increase the sensitivity and accuracy of CT portography. It has been shown to be a relatively sensitive technique for detection of liver tumors, as neoplastic lesions usually do not retain the iodine and appear as hypodense areas, while the iodine enhances the normal liver parenchyma.[1]

Magnetic Resonance Imaging

Magnetic resonance imaging (MRI) can be done in multiple planes, either axial (like the CT), sagittal, or coronal. Axial scanning is usually preferred for detecting liver metastases. The coronal or sagittal views, however, can be used to define better a tumor's proximity to adjacent structures, such as the portal veins and the vena cava. The most common pulse sequences are either a T1- or T2-weighted spin echo. The T1 images generally show metastases as low-intensity lesions, whereas in T2-weighted images, metastases are areas of high signal intensity (Fig. 59-1A). At all field strengths, T2-weighted sequences are generally superior for detection and characterization of liver masses. Benign cysts and hemangiomas are generally homogenous and have a bright appearance (termed a *light bulb sign*), whereas metastatic lesions are more heterogeneous and not as bright. Benign lesions tend to have sharply marginated borders, whereas malignant lesions tend to have irregular or indistinct margins.[1,2] Several new MRI contrast agents and pulse sequences are being evaluated to improve detection. The advantage to MRI is its lack of radiation and the low frequency of reaction to contrast agents.

Intraoperative Ultrasonography

Intraoperative ultrasonography (IOUS) is now being utilized to increase the ability to detect small and deep hepatic lesions that are not palpable, even by bimanual technique. In a study of 84 Japanese patients with colorectal cancer who were undergoing colon resection, IOUS detected 14 lesions that were missed on surgical palpation. Almost all of these lesions detected by IOUS were deep tumors less than 1.6 cm in size.[3] The authors believed that IOUS was a critical adjunct to surgical palpation to ascertain correctly the extent of metastatic liver disease. Another study confirmed this finding, stating that in a series of 70 patients, IOUS detected seven nonpalpable lesions.[4]

Positron Emission Tomography

5-18-Fluorodeoxglucose (18-FDG) is an imaging modality that allows direct evaluation of cellular glucose metabolism. Studies are now being performed to evaluate its usefulness to detect early disease, to find disease missed by other diagnostic tests, and to evaluate treatment.[5] There might be some argument on how useful PET is for diagnosing liver metastases, but clearly it is useful in diagnosing peritoneal recurrences. In 23 patients with elevated CEA, peritoneal recurrences were suspected in six patients who had PET scans. The sensitivity of PET was 88% and its diagnostic accuracy 78%, whereas the sensitivity and accuracy of CT were 38% and 44%, respectively.[6] Other studies have demonstrated that by the use of PET, some surgery can be avoided by the documentation of widespread disease.[7] Ruers and coworkers,[8] in a study of 51 patients analyzed for resection of colorectal liver metastases, found that 20% of patients had their management decisions changed because of PET scans demonstrating either unresectable liver disease or extrahepatic disease. In 27 patients undergoing liver resection, PET scans detected disease in 11 patients that was missed by conventional radiology.[9] Fong and associates[10] studied 40 patients who were being evaluated for resection and found that PET directly changed management in 23%. The number of lesions missed by PET, however—including 15 out of 52 pathologically proven metastases—demonstrates that there are still some problems in relying entirely on this modality to evaluate liver metastases.

PET can be used to help evaluate patients undergoing chemoembolization for liver metastases from adenocarcinoma. In one study, 6 of 34 lesions demonstrated persistent or increased 18-FDG, which led to further intervention.[11]

Comparison of Modalities

Several studies have compared imaging modalities for the detection of liver metastases. A German study prospectively compared CT (dynamic, noncontrast, or delayed contrast) with MRI and ultrasound.[12] In this study, 75 patients with known gastrointestinal tumors underwent imaging examinations prior to exploratory laparotomy, and 32 patients had 95 discrete hepatic lesions found at laparotomy.[13] Of the 95 lesions, 68% were detected by CT, 63% by MRI, and 53% by sonography, suggesting that CT was the best modality. Another prospective study involving 69 patients came to the same conclusion but also demonstrated the superiority of MRI T2-weighted images over T1.[14] Additional studies are needed to look at new MR pulse sequences and new contrast agents.

External ultrasonography has a lower rate of accuracy than CT or MRI. A unique study of ultrasonography prior to liver transplantation allowed the true accuracy to be determined pathologically.[15] Of 200 transplant patients, 34 patients had 80 tumors; only 36 of these were detected by ultrasonography, indicating a sensitivity of 45%. Of the 44 lesions not detected, 24 were smaller than 1 cm, 12 were 1 cm to 3 cm, and 8 were greater than 3 cm.

A French retrospective study of 28 consecutive patients compared CTP and dynamic CT prior to surgical resection.[16] Of the 69 metastases identified at surgery, dynamic CT had demonstrated only 52 (75%), whereas CTP identified 64 (93%). In a comparison of conventional CT with CT angiography in 60 patients, the sensitivity of CT angiography was higher (94% vs. 52%), but the false-positive rate was also higher. Because CTP is a relatively new procedure, technical causes of failure are still being recognized, including injection into the aorta or pancreaticoduodenal artery and reflux into a replaced right hepatic artery.[17] A comparison of PET imaging with CT and CTP in 52 patients with colorectal cancer revealed 92% accuracy for PET vs. 78% accuracy for CT and 80% accuracy for CTP.[18] Currently, the standard of care should be a spiral contrast CT scan. If the patient is about to undergo liver resection, CTP and intraoperative ultrasound should also be performed.

Lesions Confused with Liver Metastases

Several entities cannot always be reliably distinguished from metastases. Hemangiomas are common benign entities that often present a diagnostic dilemma. On MRI, hemangiomas can be confused with highly vascular

Problems Common to Cancer and Its Therapy

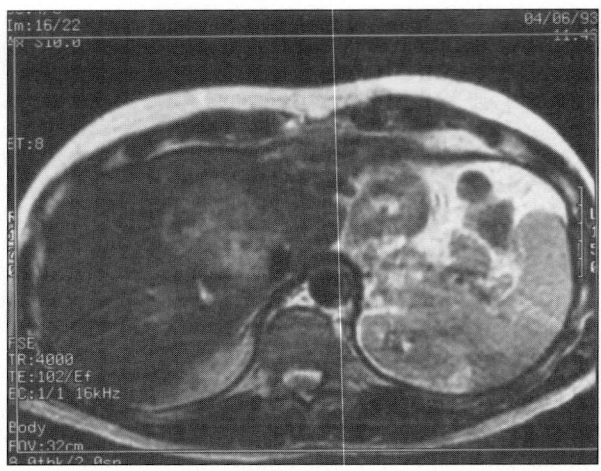
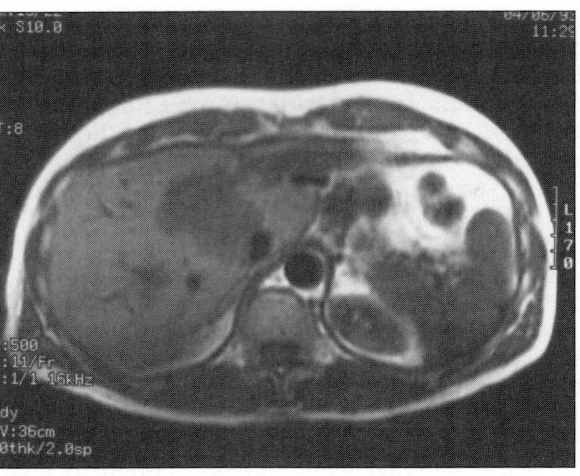

A

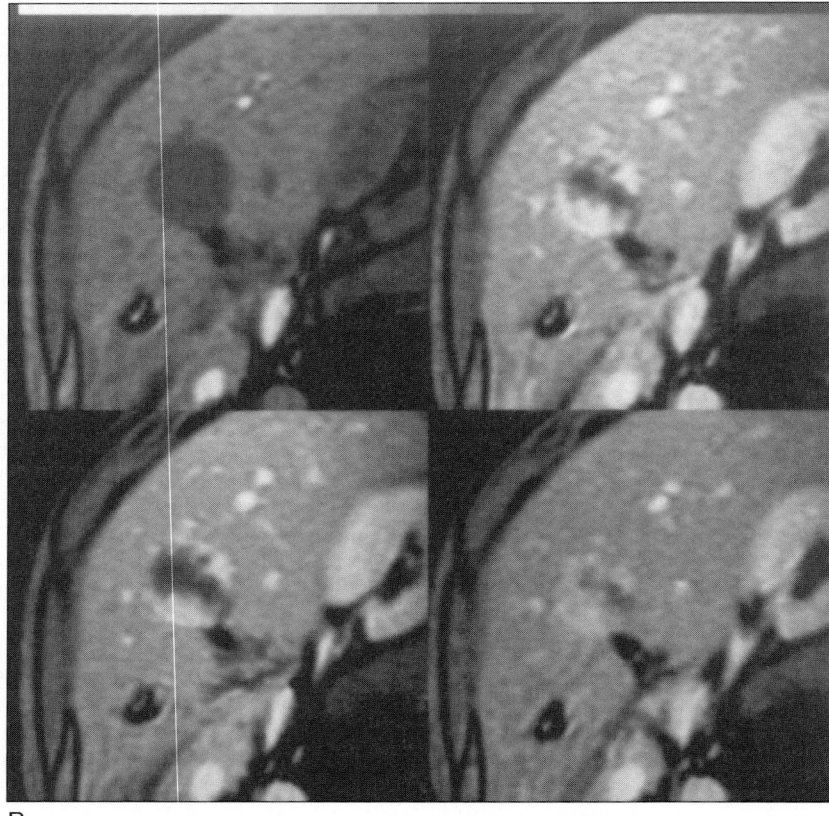

B

Figure 59-1. A, T2-weighted spin-echo image (*left*); T1-weighted spin echo image (*right*). In T2-weighted images, the metastases are areas of high signal intensity. In T1-wieghted images, metastases have a low intensity. **B,** Dynamic gadolinium-enhanced MRI demonstrating peripheral nodular enhancement in a hepatic hemangioma. Enhancement increases as the study advances over time from *upper left* to *lower left* and then to *upper* and *lower* right.

tumors and with cysts; however, if dynamic gadolinium injections are given, then hemangiomas can be more accurately diagnosed (Fig. 59-1B). Hemangiomas can also be mistaken for metastases in noncontrast CT scans and CTP. In fact, although CTP is highly sensitive in picking up small hepatic lesions, it has a high false-positive rate because benign lesions such as hemangiomas, cysts,

adenomas, or flow artifacts can be confused with metastases. Technetium-99 (^{99m}Tc) red blood cell scintigraphy is the most specific noninvasive test to diagnose hepatic hemangioma. One of the problems with the test is picking up small lesions; this problem has been improved by the use of single photon emission computed tomography (SPECT) (Fig. 59-2).[19] Table 59-1 lists some of the lesions

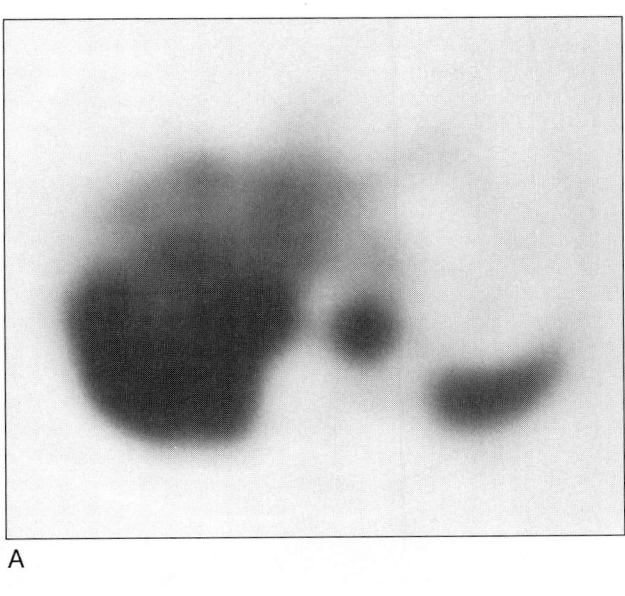

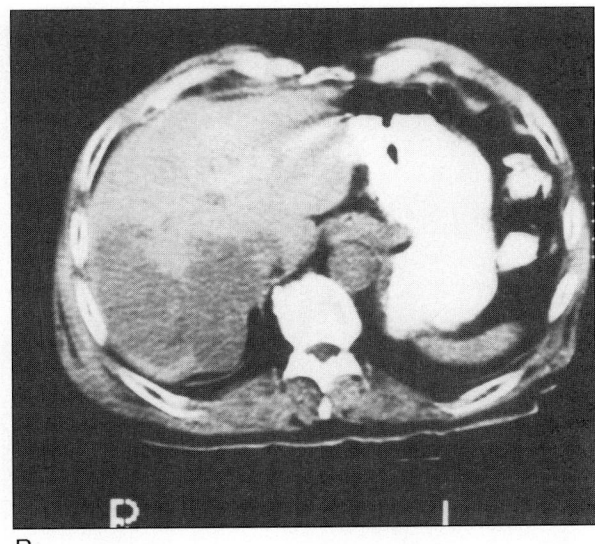

A   B

Figure 59-2. Hepatic hemangiomas. **A,** Transaxial SPECT image obtained 2 hours after injection of [99m]TC-labeled RBC. Normal blood activity is seen in the liver, and increased blood pooling activity is seen in the aorta and spleen (which is normal). There is a large area of increased blood pooling activity in the posterior section of the right lobe of the liver that corresponds to an area of reduced attenuation on the CT scan. **B,** The CT scan is obtained from the same plane as the SPECT scan. An increase in blood pooling activity with an increase in intensity from earlier images is specific for hemangioma.

confused with liver metastases and suggests the best test to differentiate among those entities. A rare but occasional entity that can on occasion be confused with metastases is focal fatty infiltration of the liver (Fig. 59-3). This could be especially prevalent in patients receiving hyperalimentation. MRI is helpful for distinguishing these lesions.

Biochemical Laboratory Tests

Unlike imaging techniques, the laboratory tests that are available for liver function assessment are not very sensitive. The basic liver function tests include the alkaline phosphatase (AP), prothrombin time (PT), lactate dehydrogenase (LDH), and serum transaminases. For patients who have metastatic colon cancer, CEA is also extremely useful. Several studies have looked at the usefulness of these tests to detect liver metastases, especially metastases from colorectal cancer.[14,20,21] CEA remains the most sensitive test for colorectal cancer, but even this test can be normal in the presence of liver metastases, especially with minimal hepatic disease. In a prospective study at the City of Hope Hospital (Durante, California) in patients with metastatic liver disease deemed resectable by CT, the average AP and LDH levels were within normal limits, while CEA was elevated in 73% of the patients.[22] LDH is useful as a prognostic indicator, with high LDH denoting a poorer survival.[23]

HEPATIC RESECTION

Because of recent advances in techniques for liver surgery, hepatic resection has become increasingly safe and used

more frequently in treatment over the last two decades. Hepatic resection of metastases was first attempted just before World War II. Experience gained from trauma centers during the war led to the emergence of techniques applicable to resection of metastatic hepatic lesions. In general, a major surgery such as a liver resection has been reserved for a situation in which the operation can be curative. Experience has shown that the resection

TABLE 59-1

Benign Liver Lesions That May Be Confused with Malignancy

TECHNIQUE	BENIGN LESIONS	MALIGNANCY
MRI T2	Vessels	Small metastatic lesions
	Hemangiomas	Highly vascular tumor (islet, cell, renal, carcinoid)
	Cysts	Cystic tumors
	Cysts	Highly vascular tumors (islet, cell, renal, carcinoid)
CT	Fatty infiltration	Metastases
	Fatty infiltration	Hepatocellular cancer
	Nonenhanced vessels	Metastases
	Adenoma	Abscess
CTP	Hemangioma	Metastases
	Cysts	
	Adenoma	
	Flow artifacts	
Angiography	Focal nodular hyperplasia	Metastases
	Hemangioma	

CT, computed tomography; CTP, CT portography; MRI, magnetic resonance imaging.

Problems Common to Cancer and Its Therapy

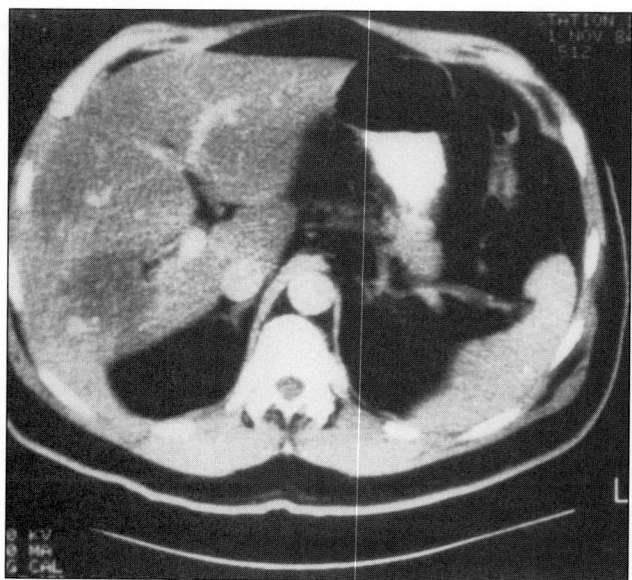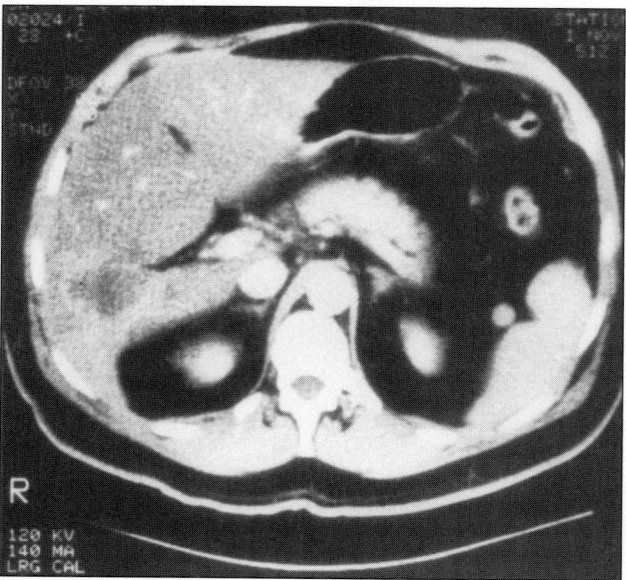

Figure 59-3. Fatty infiltration. This lesion was thought to represent metastatic disease; surgery revealed it was only fatty replacement.

of colorectal metastases to the liver can be curative in at least one quarter of patients with certain requirements. The curability by resection of liver metastases from other primary cancers is not quite as clear. The resection of metastases from other gastrointestinal malignancies, such as stomach and pancreas, has been disappointing because of the aggressive nature of these tumors by the time they become metastatic.[24,25]

Occasionally, a solitary hepatic metastasis from a breast carcinoma is found and resected with good results, but this is generally not advisable because breast cancer is a systemic disease. Liver metastases from gastrointestinal tumors can be considered regional spread, but for the metastases to go from the breast to the liver requires release of the tumor cells into the systemic circulation. Thus the concept that the liver could be the only site of spread is harder to prove, and as a result, curative intent is more difficult to achieve. A Parisian team reported their experience from 1988 to 1997 with 49 liver resections for metastatic breast cancer. They reported no mortality and a morbidity of 11.5%. The 1-, 2-, and 3-year survival was 86%, 79%, and 65%, respectively. Recurrence in the remaining liver was seen in 49% of the patients at 3 years after resection. Recurrent disease anywhere in the body was seen in 63.8% of patients at 3 years after the resection. The only factor that correlated with survival was the disease-free interval between diagnosis of the primary breast cancer and the appearance of the liver metastases, with a 3-year survival of 45% if the liver metastases appear in less than 4 years after the primary breast cancer vs. a 3-year survival of 82% if the breast cancer was more than 4 years from the appearance of the liver metastases.[26]

Another study from Paris reported on a smaller number of resections of solitary hepatic metastases from breast cancer.[27] Of the 32 patients with isolated liver metastases, 27 were found to have actual metastatic disease, while

5 had benign disease. Six of the 27 had diffuse disease that was not amenable to resection, while of the 21 who underwent hepatic resection, the average survival time was 26 months. For both of these studies, there is no way of judging the usefulness of hepatic resection vs. chemotherapy for these patients. It is interesting to note that the more recent study has a superior survival time. This could signify a number of factors, including better drugs and improved selection. The fact that the disease-free survival is still quite low, however, underscores the fact that even with strict patient selection, the chance of cure with a liver resection is quite limited, but real.

The role of hepatic resection for metastatic neuro-endocrine tumors has not been formally studied in a prospective manner because of the rarity of the disease. At the Mayo Clinic, over a 20-year period from 1970 to 1990, only 37 patients had a resection (17 curative resections and 20 palliative resections).[28] Eleven of the 17 patients with curative resections were alive 1 to 92 months after surgery (median 19 months) without evidence of disease. Of the 20 patients who underwent palliative resection, 1 died in the postoperative period, 8 died of disease 9 to 76 months after resection, and 19 patients had some relief of symptoms. The authors concluded that resection is reasonable in cases in which the bulk of tumor can be removed and the patients are symptomatic. A second report from the Mayo Clinic reviewed their hepatic resections for neuroendocrine tumors from 1984 to 1992, with a total of 74 cases.[29] Because this is a report from the same institution and there is some overlap of the time period, clearly many more resections were done in the later years (1990–1992) than in the two decades previous. The study included patients whose primary tumors were either completely resected or potentially completely resectable. Patients with carcinoid syndrome were injected with subcutaneous somatostatin pre-operatively. The tumor type breakdown can be seen in

TABLE 59-2

Types of Neuroendocrine Tumors in Mayo Clinic Series

TUMOR TYPE	NO. OF PATIENTS
Carcinoid	50
Glucagonoma	8
Multihormonal islet cell carcinoma	7
Nonfunctioning islet cell carcinoma	5
Gastrinoma	2
Insulinoma	1
Neuroendocrine	1

Table 59-2. Most patients (38) had nonanatomic resections, although 36 had a lobectomy or greater. The mortality rate was 2.7%, and the morbidity was 24.3%. Overall survival at 4 years was 73%, with a mean follow-up of 2.2 years. All of the 12 patients who died had tumor progression. There was no significant survival difference among those patients who had curative resections (that is, removal of all gross disease) vs. those who had palliative resections. Symptom relief was seen in 90% of patients. The authors concluded that resection should precede hepatic arterial occlusion and systemic chemotherapy because it provides an excellent response rate and good survival. Other studies with considerably fewer patients also support this conclusion.[30-32]

The other noncolorectal tumors metastatic to the liver that have been resected enough to have reported studies are the sarcomas. The group at Memorial Sloan-Kettering reviewed their experience with hepatic resections for sarcomas in the period from 1982 to 2000. There were 331 patients with liver metastases from a variety of primary sarcomas, 56 of whom had a hepatic resection. Thirty-four of the 56 patients had a gastrointestinal stromal tumor (GIST). Ten of the 56 patients have actually survived for 5 years, but only 2 are disease free. The disease-specific survival rate for 3 and 5 years was 50% and 30%, respectively. The patients with GIST had the same survival as those with other types of sarcoma. The time interval (less than or greater than 2 years) between the appearance of the primary sarcoma and that of the liver metastases had a significant influence on survival and was the only independent prognostic variable in a multivariate analysis.[33] All of the other reports in the literature are anecdotal, with far fewer patients in each study.[34-36]

Unlike these other primary tumors, the data on the resection of colorectal metastases to the liver has been advancing exponentially over the last 30 years. In the United States, there are more than 50,000 patients each year with liver metastases from colorectal cancer, and the resection of these metastases has been increasing because of expanding patient eligibility criteria. In the last decade, there have been a number of studies of resection of hepatic metastases from colorectal primaries—some with more than 1000 patients—that have added to the knowledge of which patients will benefit from resection.[10,37-41] In the two largest series, the 5-year survival for patients with one to three metastases who had a resection

DATA INTERPRETATION FOR HEPATIC RESECTION

Hepatic resection of one to three metastases from a colorectal primary is the only available treatment that will result in a 25 percent 5-year survival.

Hepatic resection of four or more metastases from a colorectal primary cannot be universally recommended at this time and should be confined to centers that are doing studies on these treatment modalities.

Patients with hepatic metastases synchronous with their primary colorectal lesions will have a poorer survival after hepatic resection than patients with hepatic metastases that developed 12 months after primary colon cancer resection. However, even patients with synchronous tumors have a 5-year survival of 20 percent and should have resection of one to three hepatic metastases if that is the only site of the disease.

Dukes' stage C of the primary colorectal resection is a poor prognostic indicator for patients undergoing resection of hepatic metastases, but should not exclude patients from hepatic resection.

Patients with extrahepatic abdominal metastases should not have an hepatic resection performed, unless the extrahepatic disease is part of a local recurrence in the colorectal area that can be completely removed.

Bilobar hepatic disease and previous response to chemotherapy are not factors that influence success with hepatic resection.

was 30% or greater.[10,37] In an earlier registry of more than 800 hepatic resections for colorectal metastases, which had been compiled from multiple institutions by Hughes and colleagues,[42-44] the 5-year survival for patients with one to three hepatic metastases who had complete resection was 37%. Because of the strong feeling over the last three decades that resection was the optimal treatment for a solitary metastasis, no randomized study of resection vs. any other treatment has been performed. Two studies compared the survival of matched historical control patients who underwent resection with those who had solitary hepatic lesions but did not undergo surgery.[45,46] In both studies, not 1 of the 120 patients without resection survived for more than 3 years, underscoring the rationale for resection of solitary lesions.

The retrospective series from Memorial Sloan-Kettering reviewed their experience with 1001 liver resections in patients with colorectal metastases from the years 1985 to 1998.[10] Because the study was reported in early 1999, there were many patients who did not have a 5-year follow-up; in fact, the median follow-up of survivors was 32 months, which might not be long enough to tell us which patients really would survive to 5 years. The median number of liver tumors was two, with 517 patients having solitary lesions and 330 having two or three lesions. The operative mortality was 2.8%. The 3-, 4-, and 5-year survival was 89%, 57%, and 37%, respectively; however, only 24.6% of patients resected before 1994 are 5-year survivors. The number of tumors removed (one or greater than one), the size of the tumors removed (greater or less than 5 cm), the preoperative CEA level (greater or less than 200 ng/mL), the extent of resection (less than or greater than a lobectomy), the resection margin in the hepatic specimen (negative or positive), and the presence of extrahepatic disease all were highly significant univariate and multivariate predictors of postsurgical survival. From this data, a Clinical Risk Score (CRS) was devised using five clinical criteria—the nodal status of the primary colorectal cancer, the disease-free interval from the primary colorectal cancer to the development of liver metastases, the number of hepatic tumors, the prehepatic resection CEA level, and the size of the hepatic tumors. Each criterion was given one point if the inferior condition existed, and then the points were added to give the score. The 5-year actuarial survival for a CRS of zero was 60% vs. a 14% survival for a score of 5. This gives surgeons a good handle on the prognostic expectations, but the score was not really intended for exclusion of patients from resection.

The other large series was a multi-institutional report from France reviewing 1568 patients who underwent resection of liver metastases from colorectal cancer.[37,47] Like the previous report, this study also looked at the effect of numerous prognostic indicators on overall survival after liver resection and then combined seven indicators into a prognostic scoring system. In this study, the 5-year survival among patients who had a resection of four or more lesions was 14% vs. 30% for three or fewer nodules ($P = 0.001$). Both large studies, together with others, underline the fact that the resection of more than four hepatic lesions results in significantly fewer cures, while for patients with one to three metastases, agreement exists that resection is worthwhile and can offer at least a 30% 5-year survival[10,37,39-48] (Table 59-3).

The French series found that one of the most significant prognostic variables was the stage of the primary lesion (Table 59-4). For patients with colorectal cancer and negative lymph nodes (Stage II), the 5-year survival after hepatic resection was 35% vs. 26% for patients with mesenteric lymph node involvement ($P < 0.001$). Other studies addressing the issue of stage are listed in Table 59-5.[42,48-52] In the French study, preoperative serum CEA was also significant; patients with a CEA value of less

than 5 had a 2-year survival of 70% vs. a 56% 2-year survival for patients whose CEA was greater than 30. For patients with tumor nodules less than 5 cm in size, survival was 30% vs. 26% for larger nodules ($P = 0.002$). The age of the patient was not found to be significant in this study or others.[53] The time between the primary tumor and the development of liver metastases in this and other studies was significant for prognosis if the time periods were divided to include at least the first year with the synchronous lesions (Table 59-6).[48-52]

There have been conflicting reports as to the importance of the margin of resection when removing

TABLE 59-4

Prognostic Variables in the Multi-Institutional Study from France

PROGNOSTIC VALUES	5-YEAR SURVIVAL (%)	P VALUE
Age		
<60 y	28	0.06
>60 y	27	
Tumor size		
<5 cm	30	0.002
>5 cm	26	
Stage of primary		
Dukes B	35	0.001
Dukes C	21	
Disease-Free interval		
<2 years	26	0.002
>2 years	32	
No. of nodules resected		
<4	30	0.0001
>3	14	
Resection margin		
>1 cm	32	0.0006
<1 cm	16	
CEA		
<5	70*	0.0001
>30	56*	

*2-year survival (%).
Data from Nordlinger B, Guiglet M, Vallant JC, et al: Surgical resection of colorectal carcinoma metastases to the liver. Cancer 1996;77:1254.

TABLE 59-3

Five-Year Survival After Hepatic Resection of Colorectal Cancer Metastases Based on Number of Lesions Resected

STUDY GROUP	NO. OF PATIENTS	5-YEAR SURVIVAL			
		1 METASTASIS	2–3 METASTASES	>1 METASTASIS	>3 METASTASES
Memorial Sloan Kettering[10]	441	44%			
	510			28%	23%
France[36]	1350	30%			
	183		30%		14%
Mayo Clinic[40]	187	31%			
	70				
	23		29%		9%
Italy[47]	134	20%			
	78			17%	
Hepatic Registry[42]	789	37%	37%		18%

TABLE 59-5

Survival after Hepatic Resection Based on Stage of Primary Colorectal Cancer

STUDY GROUP	NO. OF PATIENTS	DUKES STAGE	NO. OF PATIENTS	5-YEAR SURVIVAL	P VALUE
Milan[49]	95	B	29	47	0.02
		C	50	24	
United States[42]	789	B	226	47	0.001
		C	317	23	
Paris[50]	97	B	39	52	NS
		C	58	53	
Rotterdam[51]	117	B	53	26	NS
		C	54	11	
Erlangen[236]	173	B	49	53	0.01
		C	119	32	
Italy[48]	212	B	69	32	0.001
		C	116	11	

hepatic metastases. Although a different cutoff was used in the French study than in the Memorial study, the margin of normal hepatic tissue around the resected metastases was significant. For those patients with a margin greater than 1 cm, 32% of patients survived for 5 years, vs. a 16% survival for those with a margin less than 1 cm ($P = 0.006$). A report from Germany in 1991, however, showed no significant difference in survival among over 170 patients relative to their margins of resection.[52] This study broke down the margins into three groups: 1–4 mm, 5–9 mm, and greater than 10 mm. More recent studies support this study by showing that if there is no margin of clearance between the tumor and normal liver parenchyma, patients do worse, but whenever there is a margin, the difference between 1 mm, 10 mm, or greater is not significant (Table 59-7).[40,41,52,54] These data are understandable from a pathologic standpoint, as these tumors tend to be firm nodules with pushing borders and even a small margin would remove all of the tumor, whereas a positive margin would leave cells behind. This would not be true for primary hepatocellular carcinomas, as they can have more diffuse, infiltrative borders.

The French authors created a scoring system by using these seven variables, giving 1 point for each bad factor and 2 points for a CEA value greater than 30. Patients were calculated to have a 2-year survival of 79% if they had a score of 0 to 2 points, 60% if they had scores of 3 to 4 points, and 43% if they scored 5 to 7 points.[37] These prognostic scoring systems from the French study and the Memorial study are valuable tools to estimate patients' survival after a resection. For patients with poorer prognoses, other therapies might be added to surgery to try to improve their chances.

Several studies have addressed the issue of extrahepatic intra-abdominal metastases at the time of hepatic resection. In most instances, surgeons do not proceed with liver resection in the presence of extrahepatic metastases. In the series from New York, 88 patients with extrahepatic disease were included.[10] More than half of these patients had direct extension into other organs such as the diaphragm. Only 10 patients had positive portal nodal disease. Looking at all 88 patients with extrahepatic disease, the 5-year actuarial survival was 18%. The breakdown between those with discontinuous disease or

TABLE 59-6

Survival after Hepatic Resection Based on Synchronicity of the Hepatic Lesions and the Primary Colorectal Cancer

STUDY GROUP	NO. OF PATIENTS	SYNCHRONOUS	NO. OF PATIENTS (IN EACH GROUP)	5-YEAR SURVIVAL	P VALUE
Milan[49]	95	Yes	28	31	NS
		No	67	28	
Rotterdam[51]	117	Yes	38	15	NS
		No	79	22	
Erlangen[236]	173	Yes	85	32	0.05
		No	88	45	
Heidelberg[237]	122	Yes	48	2	0.01
		No	74	16	
United States[42]	789	Yes	259	27	
		1–12 mo	206	31	
		>12 mo	333	42	0.02
Paris[50]	97	Yes	35	52	NS
		No	62	52	
Italy[48]	212	Yes	85	18	NS
		No	113	22	

TABLE 59-7

Significance of Hepatic Resection Margin

INSTITUTION	MARGIN OF RESECTION	NO. OF PATIENTS	5-YEAR SURVIVAL	P VALUE
Erlangen[52]	0–4 mm	67	23	NS
	5–9 mm	40	29	
	>10 mm	65	39	
Mayo[41]	0–1 mm	17	29	NS
	1–10 mm	123	30	
	>10 mm	31	36	
	None	24	17	
Pittsburgh[40]	0–10 mm	92	25	
	>10 mm	95	29	
	None	17	0	0.006
Memorial[54]	1–10 mm	248	43	
	>10 mm	113	43	
	None	65	17	0.00003

direct extension was not made. In the Mayo Clinic report on hepatic resections in patients with extrahepatic disease, none of the 22 patients survived for 5 years, and only 1 survived for 3 years.[55] In the Hepatic Registry, of the 61 patients with extrahepatic involvement undergoing hepatic resection, none had a 5-year disease-free survival.[43] These data support the view that hepatic resection in the presence of noncontiguous extrahepatic intra-abdominal disease, with the exception of a local recurrence, is rarely curative and, in general, is inadvisable.

For extrahepatic disease not in the abdomen, the usefulness of resection could be different for disease in the lungs, especially solitary lesions in the lung. A recent study from the Mayo Clinic reviewed their experience with resection of both hepatic and pulmonary metastases from colorectal primaries. There were 58 patients, with no operative mortalities and a 5-year survival rate of 30%. These authors felt that the resection of both lung and liver of selected cases was justified.[56]

SURGICAL GUIDELINES FOR HEPATIC RESECTION

The existence of extrahepatic intra-abdominal metastases should be excluded before attempting a hepatic resection. Since the periportal lymph nodes are the most common site for intra-abdominal extrahepatic metastases, they should be biopsied and sent for frozen section. If extrahepatic disease is present the hepatic resection should not be carried out.

The extent of a hepatic resection can span from one small nodule to a trisegmentectomy by which 75 percent of the liver is removed. The assessment of patients for trisegmentectomy is very difficult, since no tests are currently available to delineate accurately which patients can survive with a 75 percent loss of liver mass. In general, however, if a patient has cirrhosis, an extensive resection is discouraged.

Debilitated (poor performance status) patients are not good candidates for major hepatic resection.

Age alone should not preclude a patient's eligibility for hepatic resection.

Does surgical technique affect survival? No one technique has been proven superior to others. For some surgeons who have experience with hepatic resections, the finger fracture technique works as well as the ultrasonic dissector (Cavitron), while for other surgeons who have learned the Cavitron technique, it is an invaluable tool. The laser dissector, another technique that is not universally available, has not proven superior to other surgical techniques. In one of the major advances of the last 15 years, more hepatic resections have been performed along nonanatomic lines. Metastasectomies, or removal of tumor plus a rim of hepatic tissue, can be done rather than a formal lobectomy. With the greater familiarity of the hepatic anatomic segments of Couinaud (Fig. 59-4),[35] current resections are more frequently being performed along these lines. This technique allows for both a reduction in the amount of normal liver removed and resection of disease from both lobes.

One relatively newer operative technique is the use of total vascular exclusion (TVE) for hepatic resections (i.e., the vena cava is cross-clamped in two areas—supra-

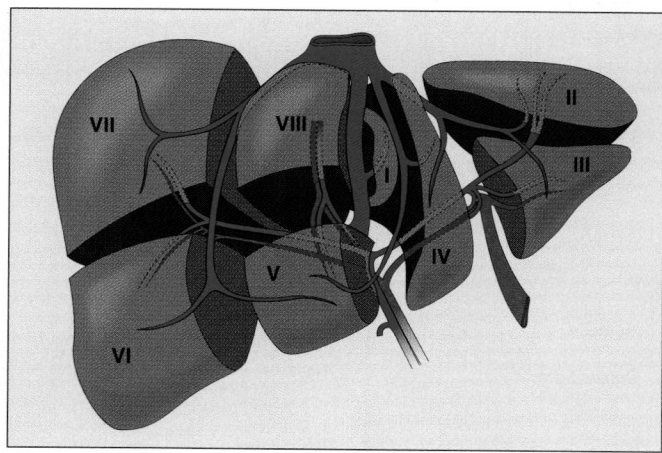

Figure 59-4. Couinaud's eight hepatic segments. (From Iwalsuki S, Sheahan DG, Starzl TE: The changing face of hepatic resection. Curr Probl Surg 1989;25:281.)

TABLE 59-8

Recurrence after Hepatic Resection

AUTHOR	NO. OF PATIENTS	NO. OF RECURRENCES	NO. OF LIVER ONLY	NO. OF LIVER AND EXTRAHEPATIC	NO. OF EXTRAHEPATIC ONLY
Van Ooijen et al.[51]	117	69	20 (29%)	14 (21%)	34 (50%)
Codi et al.[49]	93	69	28 (41%)	13 (19%)	28 (41%)
Hohenberger et al.[237]	122	80	17 (21%)	55 (69%)	8 (10%)
Hughes et al.[44]	607	424	148 (27%)	154 (27%)	106 (28%)
Rees et al.[238]	89	61	25 (41%)	9 (15%)	27 (44%)
Fong et al.[54]	465	235	96 (41%)	16 (7%)	123 (52%)

hepatic and subhepatic—and the porta hepatis is also occluded).[57,58] In Bismuth's[59] report on 54 patients using TVE, the average duration of cross-clamping was 46 minutes, and the average operating time was 6 hours. The transfusion requirements were low and no intraoperative deaths occurred. The application of vascular occlusion seemed to be useful for tumors close to the vena cava or for large central tumors.

The use of the autotransfuser, a technique pioneered in trauma patients, had been avoided initially for patients with malignancies because of fear that tumor cells might be disseminated into the bloodstream with this instrument. Prospective studies on patients undergoing hepatic resection for tumors have not shown this to be true.[60,61] Animal studies also support the concept that metastatic cells are organ specific and would not disseminate if introduced into the bloodstream. Because of these studies, many centers are using the autotransfusers during hepatic resection and reducing the need for multiple blood transfusions.

Another technical advance for hepatic surgery has been the use of fibrin glue, which can aid in sealing up the large, raw surfaces of the liver left after major resections.[62]

The question of drainage after hepatic resection has been addressed prospectively in a study that showed no difference in complications in the drained group vs. the undrained group. When the data are analyzed more carefully, however, it becomes clear that patients with lobectomies or greater did benefit from drains, whereas those patients with smaller resections did not need drains placed.[63,64]

Relapse rates after liver resections are described in Table 59-8. In the larger studies, it seems that approx-

imately 40% of patients who have hepatic resections will have recurrent disease in the liver as the first sign of the relapse. Of the 69 patients who had relapse in the Milan study, 28 (41%) had relapse in the liver only, 19 (28%) had only extra-abdominal relapse, 9 (13%) had intra-abdominal extrahepatic relapse, and 13 (19%) had relapse in both the liver and at an extrahepatic site.[49] Although extrahepatic failure is of concern, the liver remains the main site of relapse, appearing in more than 60% of patients.

Because of the increased use of hepatic resection for metastatic liver disease, the incidence of repeat hepatic resection has also increased. Approximately 10% of patients who have had a hepatic resection can have a repeat resection (Table 59-9). A study from Paris of 116 patients who underwent repeat hepatic resection reported a low operative mortality of 0.9% and a 3-year survival of 33%.[38] Of the patients who underwent repeat hepatic resection, 55% had recurrence in their liver after this operation. There were 170 patients in a registry report who had repeat hepatic resections with a 5-year survival of 26%, which was comparable to the 5-year survival for the original hepatic resection.[65] A recent study from Memorial Sloan-Kettering reviewed 126 second liver resections for recurrent colorectal metastases; the 5-year actuarial survival was 34%, with 19 actual 5-year survivors. The operative mortality was 1.6%, and morbidity was 28%.[66] A study of recurrence among these patients revealed a liver recurrence in 67% of the patients. Repeat hepatic resection, when feasible, can be done safely, and the outcome is comparable to that for the original hepatic resection.[67] Thus, if patients have isolated liver metastases (preferably solitary lesions) after hepatic resection, they should be candidates for repeat resection.

TABLE 59-9

Survival after Repeat Hepatic Resections for Colorectal Metastases

AUTHOR	NO. OF PATIENTS	OPERATIVE MORTALITY	SURVIVAL (%)		
			2-YEAR	3-YEAR	5-YEAR
Nordlinger et al.[38]	116	0.9%	57	33	
Petrowsky et al.[66]	126	1.6%		51	34
Fernandez-Trigo et al.[65]	170			37	26
Que et al.[239]	21			50	

Adjuvant Therapy after Liver Resection

Despite the high curative resection rate of hepatic resections, the recurrence of metastases is high, with 50% recurring in the liver. The use of hepatic artery infusion (HAI) of chemotherapy after liver resection was studied in a small prospective randomized fashion at the City of Hope Medical Center.[68,69] The patients with solitary metastases all had resection of their tumors, and half received postoperative continuous HAI of fluorodeoxy-uridine (FUDR). Patients with multiple but resectable metastases were randomized to either receive pump therapy alone with no resection or to undergo resection of all metastatic disease followed by HAI of FUDR. For the six patients who had resection only, their median time to failure was 8.7 months, and three of the six metastases recurred in the liver. For the five patients with resection plus pump, none had recurrence in the liver, and their median time to failure was 30.7 months. There was no difference in median survival between the two groups.

At Memorial Sloan-Kettering Cancer Center (MSKCC), 156 patients were randomized after liver resection to either HAI with systemic chemotherapy (HAI+SYS) or systemic chemotherapy alone (SYS). Chemotherapy was administered for 6 months. The endpoint of this study was 2-year survival. HAI therapy used was FUDR and dexa-methasone, and the systemic therapy was 5-Flourouracil (FU) and Leucovorin (LV). Patients were stratified by type of previous chemotherapy or no chemotherapy and the number of liver metastases (1, 2–4, >4). Survival was increased in the group receiving HAI+SYS (86%) vs. 72% for SYS ($P = 0.03$). Median survival is presently 67 months for the HAI+SYS group and 57 months for the group receiving SYS alone, with 5-year survivals of 56% and 45%, respectively. Hepatic disease-free survival is clearly better for the HAI group (Fig. 59-5). Overall, disease-free survival is also increased, but not as dramatically (Fig. 59-6). Toxicity was increased in the combined group with increased diarrhea and increased liver function test abnormalities. A total bilirubin greater than 3 mg/dL occurred in 18% of patients receiving HAI.[70]

The Eastern Cooperative Group (ECOG) and the Southwestern Oncology Group (SWOG) conducted a randomized study of hepatic resection alone vs. resection followed by four cycles of HAI–FUDR and 12 cycles of systemic infusion of FU. Only patients with three or fewer metastases were enrolled in the study. The study was powered to answer the question of whether HAI would increase PFS. Of the 110 patients randomized, only 75 are actually in the study, as a number of patients were excluded because of extrahepatic disease, unresectable disease, or no tumor. Four-year liver recurrence-free survival was 67% in the chemotherapy group and 43% in the control group ($P = 0.03$). Median survival was 63.7 months for the chemotherapy group and 49% for the control group.[71]

A German Cooperative group enrolled patients from 26 different centers and entered 226 patients into a study of resection followed by adjuvant hepatic arterial therapy with 5-FU and LV vs. a control group receiving no chemotherapy after resection. Although 113 were entered into the hepatic arterial group, only 87 were treated. Only

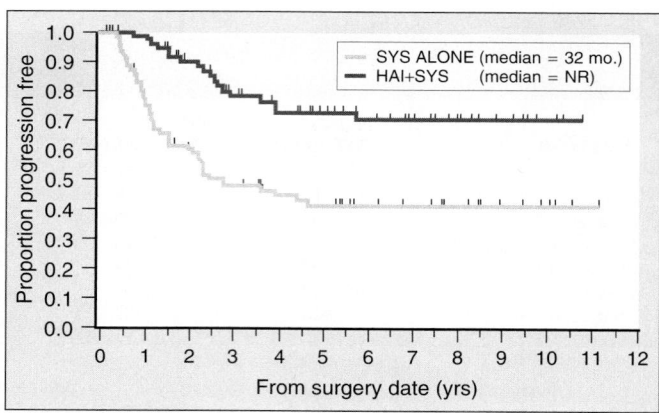

Figure 59-5. With FUDR plus LV, 60% of patients were alive at 2 years and 22% were alive at 4 years, while with FUDR alone, 40% were alive at 2 years and 19% were alive at 4 years.

64% had chemotherapy data available, and only 34 patients (30%) completed treatment. At an 18-month interim analysis, the relapse rate was 33% in the group receiving adjuvant therapy and 36% in the group treated with resection alone. If one looks only at those who were treated, the median survival was 44.8 months from the treated group vs. 39.7 months in the control group.[72]

In a nonrandomized study comparing two groups of patients in Nagoya,[73] the survival was increased with the use of adjuvant regional therapy after hepatectomy for colon cancer. The 3- and 5-year survivals were 53% and 23% using surgery alone, and 57% and 57%, respectively, when adjuvant chemotherapy with FU, doxorubicin, and mitomycin C were given after surgery.

Very few trials have evaluated systemic chemotherapy alone. Portier and colleagues[74] entered 173 patients in a randomized study of systemic therapy vs. control after liver resection. Two-year progression-free survival (PFS)

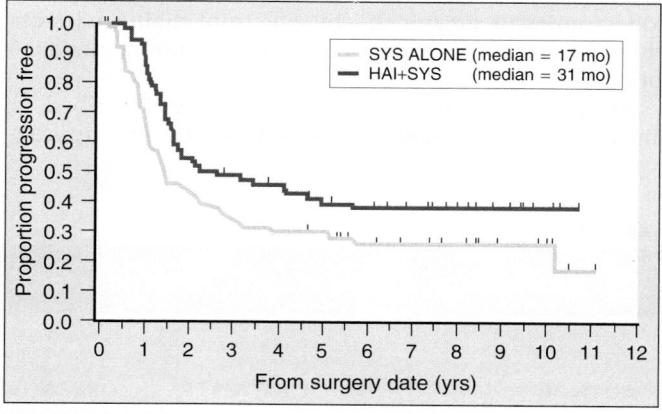

Figure 59-6. French study: survival curves for the HAI group (*magenta line*) and the systemic group (*yellow line*). (From Rougier P, Laplanche A, Huguier M, et al: Hepatic arterial infusion of floxuridine in patients with liver metastases from colorectal carcinoma: Long-term results of a prospective randomized trial. J Clin Oncol 1992;10(7):1112.)

was 40% and 36.6%, respectively. At 5 years, PFS was 32.2% vs. 25.5% ($P = 0.12$). Survival at 5 years was 50% vs. 40% ($P = 0.15$). In this group of patients, 69% had only one metastasis, vs. 38% in the MSKCC study.

In patients with hepatocellular carcinoma (HCC), a randomized study compared hepatic arterial injection of epirubicin and oral 1-hexycarbamoyl-5-fluorouracil (HCFU) to no further treatment in 57 patients after liver resection of HCC.[75] There was no significant difference between the two groups, and the authors felt that the chemotherapeutic agents chosen might not have been appropriate. Postoperative adjuvant therapy could compromise survival if the treatment is not effective, as it suppresses host immunity. In a small, randomized study of intravenous epirubicin with hepatic arterial iodized oil and cisplatin vs. no further treatment after liver resection for hepatocellular carcinoma, the disease-free survival was shorter in the treated group. There was an increase in extrahepatic metastases in the treated group.[76]

Factors that inhibit hepatic carcinogenesis might be more useful as adjuvant therapies for hepatocellular carcinoma. Retinoic acid inhibits chemically induced hepatocarcinogenesis in rats, spontaneous hepatocellular carcinoma in mice, and the production of α-fetoprotein in human hepatoma cell lines. In a study by the Hepatoma Prevention Study Group, 89 patients were randomized to polyphenolic acid (acyclic retinoid) or placebo for 12 months after liver resection. The polyphenolic group had a significant reduction in recurrent or new hepatomas ($P = 0.04$). The drug also improved overall survival, but not significantly.[77]

CHEMOTHERAPY

Systemic Chemotherapy

Responses of liver metastases to systemic chemotherapy are variable but usually reflect the response of the primary tumor. For patients with metastases from breast cancer, response rates can be as high as 60% with systemic chemotherapy, while for patients with metastatic colorectal carcinoma, the response rates are 30% or less.[78,79] Most studies of systemic therapy do not differentiate patients who have only liver metastases from those with generalized metastatic disease, making it difficult to draw conclusions about the usefulness of systemic chemotherapy to treat liver metastases. In some cases, however, the response rates of liver metastases are well documented.

In breast cancer, liver metastases represent a poor prognostic indicator, with median survival of 10 months in some series.[80] Visceral metastases, including liver metastases, have been reported to have fewer estrogen-positive receptors. Insulin-like growth factors are present in the liver and the lung and could be important to the growth and motility factors for breast cancer and lung cancer.[81] In looking at prognostic factors that predict response, patients with liver metastases were the ones who tended to respond the least.[82] Carter's[83] review of single agents (5- fluorouracil [5-FU] or cyclophosphamide [CTX]) demonstrated a 20% response in liver metastases vs. 32% and 27% in soft tissue and osseous metastases, respectively. The combination of halotestin, prednisone, and 5-FU produced objective responses in 26 of 52 patients (50%) with liver metastases from breast carcinoma.[84] Although combination chemotherapy has substantially improved the response rates obtained in treating breast cancer, liver metastases still have a lower response rate than soft tissue or pulmonary disease. Table 59-10 shows that the response rates for patients with liver metastases were similar to the overall responses but lower than the response rates found in soft-tissue metastases. In a Southwest Oncology Group study of 262 patients, 41 of 88 patients (47%) with liver metastases responded, vs. 110 of 154 patients (71%) without liver involvement ($P = 0.001$).[85] There is a suggestion that taxoids might be more effective against liver metastases.[86]

TABLE 59-10

Response of Different Metastatic Sites in Advanced Breast Carcinoma in Selected Series of Combination Chemotherapy

INVESTIGATORS	DRUGS	NO. OF PATIENTS	RESPONSE BY METASTASIS SITE (%)		
			TOTAL	LIVER	SOFT TISSUE
Mattsson et al.[240]	ADR, CTX, MTX, VCR, Pred	50	78	75	87
Muss et al.[241]	ADR, CTX, 5-FU, VCR, Pred	76	58	52	58
Gabra et al.[242]	ADR, 5-FU, infusion	56	56	76	76
Tranum et al.[243]	ADR, CTX, 5-FU, MTX	105	49	38	46
Jones et al.[244]	ADR, CTX	55	73	70	79
Chauvergne et al.[245]	ADR, MTX	209	43	40	46
Russell et al.[246]	ADR, VCR, Pred	50	67	67	70
Smalley et al.[247]	5-FU, CTX, MTX, VCR, Pred	75	37	30	42
Canellos et al.[248]	5-FU, CTX, MTX, Pred	40	68	38	91
Canellos et al.[248]	5-FU, CTX, MTX	93	53	48	47
Millward et al.[249]	ADR, IfoS	31	71	10	50
Airoldi et al.[250]	Docetaxel-epir	60	75	55	78
Wada et al.[251]	ADR, CTX, 5-FU	34	—	13	—
Dieras et al.[86]	Docetaxel	39	52	44	—

TABLE 59-11

Response of Liver Metastases in Gastric Carcinoma in a Selected Series of Combination Chemotherapy Treatments

| INVESTIGATORS | DRUGS | NO. OF PATIENTS | TOTAL RESPONSE (%) | LIVER METASTASES | |
				NO.	RESPONSE (%)
Franks[252]	ADR, MTX	14	71	6	50
Bitran et al.[253]	5-FU, ADR, Mit-C	11	53	8	25
GITSG[254]	5-FU, ADR, MeCCNU	15	47	8	25
Macdonald et al.[255]	5-FU, ADR, Mit-C	62	42	22	36
Seligman et al.[256]	5-FU, Strep	12	33	4	20
GISTG[254]	5-FU, ADR, MeCCNU	15	17	13	7
Bunn et al.[257]	5-FU, MeCCNU, ADR, Mit-C	18	11	6	17
Wagner et al.[258]	FU, ADR, cisplatin	20	50	2	50
Preusser et al.[259]	VP16, ADR, cisplatin	67	51	26	69
Levi et al.[260]	ADR	93	13	24	4
Levi et al.[260]	ADR, 5-FU, BCNU	94	40	25	28
Pazdur et al.[261]	FU + interferon	94	20	18	44
Wilke et al.[262]	Etoposide ADR, cisplatin	33	70	—	—
Lerner et al.[263]	Etoposide ADR, cisplatin	36	33	11	27
Webb et al.[264]	Epirubicin, cisplatin, FU	50	45	—	—

Metastases from gastric carcinoma are more responsive to chemotherapy than other gastrointestinal malignancies. One of the more commonly used regimens (5-FU, doxorubicin, and mitomycin C) produces a mean response of 35%, whereas for those with hepatic metastasis, the response rate was 28%.[87] The cumulative response for liver metastases (Table 59-11) was 34%, while the overall mean response rate was 36% for combination chemotherapy in the treatment of gastric carcinoma. Some newer regimens are included in the table, but they do not separate out response in liver metastases.

For patients with colorectal cancer, the liver is the most common site of dissemination, with up to 70% of patients with metastatic disease developing liver metastases.[88] Table 59-12 lists chemotherapy trials in patients with colorectal cancer in which the response of liver metastases is discussed separately. The 5-FU and leucovorin trials are included, but none of these studies describes the response of liver metastases separately. The overall response rate of 5-FU and leucovorin is generally around 20%. Sometimes with infusional methods, response rates are as high as 30%; however, the addition of new agents such as topoisomerase inhibitor, CPT-11, and a new platinum drug, oxaliplatinum, to 5-FU/leucovorin has increased both response rate and survival among patients with colorectal cancer.[89] In a randomized study using continuous-infusion 5-FU, the response rate was 31% with 5-FU and LV vs. 49% for those treated with CPT-11, 5-FU, and LV.[90] Survival was 14 months with the two drugs and 17 months with the three drugs. Using bolus 5-FU and +/- CPT-11/LV in a randomized study, the response rate was 21% with FU/LV vs. 39% with the three drugs, and the survival was 12.6 months vs. 14.8 months, respectively.[91] The addition of oxaliplatinum to the combination of 5-FU and LV also resulted in a significant improvement in response rates—50% vs. 22% with the three drugs vs. two drugs, respectively.[89] In a large U.S. study comparing the oxaliplatinum/5-FU/LV with CPT-11/5-FU/LV, the response

TABLE 59-12

Treatment of Metastatic Colorectal Carcinoma

	NO. OF PATIENTS	TOTAL RESPONSE (%)	NO. WITH LIVER METS	RESPONSE FOR LIVER METS (%)
FU[265]	42	10	11	0
FU[266]	31	23	31	23
MeCCNU + FU[265]	152	32	41	31
MeCCNU + FU[267]	133	16	93	18
MeCCNU + FU + Vin[268]	69	11	41	11
MOF-Strep[268]	75	32	60	37
FU + Interferon[269]	35	26	24	29
FU + Leucovorin[270]	63	33	46	—
FU + Leucovorin[23]	36	44	24	—
CPT-11[271]	41	33	35	28
CPT-11, FU, LV[91]	231	39	—	—
Oxal FU LV[92]	246	38		

rates and survival were increased with the oxaliplatinum combination—38% and 18.6 months vs. 29% and 14.1 months, respectively.[92]

When does one start systemic chemotherapy for patients with metastatic disease to the liver from breast, gastric, or colon cancer? For patients with colon or gastric cancer who are asymptomatic and have a small volume of disease (<20% of the liver involved with tumor and not resectable), three studies suggest that earlier treatment increases survival and increases the time with good performance status.[93-95] If the patient has rapidly progressive disease or is symptomatic, chemotherapy should be initiated immediately. One should have a baseline CT scan and laboratory values before starting treatment. To assess response, scans should be repeated at 2- to 3-month intervals to evaluate whether the tumor is responding, and therapy should be continued. Because hepatic metastases from a primary breast cancer usually progress rapidly and response rates to chemotherapy are high, patients are usually started on therapy early.

Neoadjuvant Chemotherapy

Neoadjuvant chemotherapy has been evaluated as a way to decrease hepatic tumor burden for the purpose of proceeding with hepatic resection. Although no randomized prospective trial has been completed regarding this as a treatment strategy, the results of a retrospective analysis have been presented, and the results appear promising.

Giachetti and colleagues[96] conducted a retrospective review of 151 patients with unresectable liver-only metastases from CRC who were treated with FU/LV and oxaliplatin followed by attempted liver resection. The criteria used to define unresectability were as follows: (1) more than four liver metastases (30%), (2) single tumor larger than 5 cm (34%), (3) tumor in both hepatic lobes, (4) invasion of the intrahepatic vascular structures, and (5) high percentage of liver involvement (>25% liver involvement) (48%).

Their analyses revealed that of this group, 77 patients (51%) became resectable after neoadjuvant therapy and 58 of 77 (75%) were able to undergo complete resections. The 5-year survival rate for the 77 patients who underwent hepatic resection was 50%, progression-free survival was 17 months, and 72% had relapsed within a median of 12 months.[96,97]

A prospective trial is under way at the Mayo clinic enrolling patients considered unresectable due to the following factors: (1) involvement of all three major hepatic veins, the portal vein bifurcation, or the retrohepatic vena cava; (2) involvement of the main right or main left portal vein and the main hepatic vein of the opposite lobe; (3) disease requiring more than a right or left trisegmentectomy; or (4) six or more metastatic lesions distributed diffusely in both lobes of the liver.

Additionally, the EORTC plans to enroll 300 patients with resectable liver metastases either in three to six cycles of FU/LV and oxaliplatin before undergoing resection (followed by additional cycles of treatment in the adjuvant setting) or to surgery alone.

TABLE 59-13

 Rationale for Hepatic Artery Infusion

Liver metastases are perfused by the hepatic artery. Normal liver is primarily supplied by the portal vein.
Certain drugs have high hepatic extraction.
The liver is often the first site of metastases—eliminating liver metastases would prevent extrahepatic disease.
Many drugs have a steep dose-response curve.
Drugs with a high total-body clearance are more effective.

Hepatic Arterial Chemotherapy

The rationale for hepatic arterial chemotherapy has an anatomic and pharmacologic basis (Table 59-13):

1. Liver metastases are perfused almost exclusively by the hepatic artery, while normal hepatocytes derive their blood supply both from the portal vein and minimally from the hepatic artery.[98]
2. Certain drugs are largely extracted by the liver during the first pass through the arterial circulation. This results in high local concentrations of drug with minimal systemic toxicity. Ensminger and coworkers[99] demonstrated that 94% to 99% of FUDR is extracted by the liver during the first pass, compared with 19% to 55% of 5-FU. This makes FUDR an optimal drug for hepatic arterial chemotherapy. The pharmacologic advantages of various chemotherapeutic agents for hepatic arterial infusion are summarized in Table 59-14.[100] Newer drugs, such as irinotecan and etoposide, do not as yet show an advantage when given by HAI.[101]
3. Drugs with a steep dose–response curve will be more useful when given by the intrahepatic route because a large dose can be given regionally.
4. Drugs with a high total body clearance are more useful for hepatic infusion. If a drug is not cleared rapidly, recirculation through the systemic circulation diminishes the advantage of hepatic arterial delivery.[102]
5. The liver is often the first and only site of metastatic disease. The theory of the stepwise pattern of metastatic progression states that hematogenous spread

TABLE 59-14

Drugs for Hepatic Arterial Infusion

DRUG	ESTIMATED HALF-LIFE	INCREASED (MIN) EXPOSURE BY HAI
Fluorouracil (FU)	10	5–10-fold
5-Fluoro-2-deoxyuridine (FUDR)	<10	100–400-fold
Bischlorethyl nitrosourea (BCNU)	<5	6–7-fold
Mitomycin C	<10	6–8-fold
Cisplatin	20–30	4–7-fold
Adriamycin (doxorubicin hydrochloride)	60	2-fold

HAI, hepatic arterial infusion.

TABLE 59-15

Hepatic Artery Infusion with External Pump

INVESTIGATORS	NO. OF PATIENTS	DRUG	RESPONSE (%)	CATHETER COMPLICATIONS OR BLEED (%)
Old Studies				
Tandon et al.[272]	122	5-FU 25 mg/kg × 9 d	65	42
Ansfield et al.[273]	419	5-FU 25 mg/kg × 4 d	55	21
Watkins et al.[274]	184	5-FU 25 mg/kg × 10 d	71	28
Cady and Oberfield[275]	55	FUDR 20 mg/kg	67	39
Smiley et al.[276]	166	5-FU 25 mg/kg × 4 d	25	30
New Studies				
Metzger et al.[127]	30	5-FU 2 g × 5 d	57	33
Denck[277]	50	5-FU 6 g × 3 d	58	5
Schlag et al.[128]	33	5-FU 1 g × 5 d	27	20
Rougier et al.[278]	43	5-FU 1 g weekly	56	65
Arai et al.[279]	32	FU 1000 × 5 h qw Mit-C 10-12 mg/m² q6w	78	25

occurs first via the portal vein to the liver, then from the liver to the lungs, and then to other organs.[103,104] Thus aggressive treatment of metastases confined to the liver (resection and/or hepatic infusion) could yield prolonged survival for some patients.

Regional hepatic arterial therapy can be done by using either a hepatic arterial port or a percutaneously placed catheter connected to an external pump or to a totally implantable pump. Early studies with percutaneously placed hepatic artery catheters produced high response rates, but clotting of the catheters and the hepatic artery, as well as bleeding, led physicians to abandon this method (Table 59-15). The development of a totally implantable pump allowed long-term hepatic artery infusion with good patency of the catheter and the hepatic artery and a low incidence of infection. One study compared three groups relative to placement of the hepatic artery catheter:

1. Surgical placement of a hepatic artery catheter
2. Percutaneous placement of the hepatic artery catheter
3. An operative implantable reservoir connected to the hepatic artery catheter

The reported ability of each technique to administer chemotherapy for the three groups of patients was 31, 25, and 115 days, respectively.[105] A number of trials using the implantable pump produced high response rates with good survivals (Table 59-16).

Toxicity of Hepatic Arterial FUDR Infusion

Most trials of hepatic arterial infusion given via an internal implantable pump use FUDR. A summary of the toxicities encountered are listed in Table 59-17. Myelosuppression, nausea, vomiting, and diarrhea do not occur with HAI of FUDR. If diarrhea does occur, shunting to the bowel should be suspected.[106] The most common problems with HAI are hepatic toxicity and ulcer disease.[107] Hepatobiliary toxicity is the most problematic toxicity seen with hepatic arterial chemotherapy. Most studies point to a combined ischemic and inflammatory effect on the bile ducts as the etiology of this complication. The bile ducts derive their blood supply almost exclusively from the hepatic artery and thus are undoubtedly perfused with high doses of chemotherapy.[108]

Clinically, biliary toxicity manifests as elevations of serum glutamic-oxaloacetic transaminase (SGOT), AP, and

TABLE 59-16

Hepatic Arterial FUDR Infusion with Internal Pump: Responses

INVESTIGATOR	NO. OF PATIENTS	PRIOR CHEMOTHERAPY (%)	PR (%)	DECREASE IN CEA (%)	MEDIAN SURVIVAL (MO)
Niederhuber et al.[280]	70	45	83	91	25
Balch and Urist[281]	50	40	—	83	26
Kemeny et al.[282]	41	43	42	51	12
Shepard et al.[283]	53	42	32	—	17
Cohen et al.[284]	50	36	51	—	—
Weiss et al.[285]	17	85	29	57	13
Schwartz et al.[286]	23	—	15	75	18
Johnson et al.[287]	40	—	47	—	12
Kemeny et al.[288]	31	50	52	—	22

TABLE 59-17

Hepatic Arterial FUDR Infusion with Internal Pump: Toxicities

INVESTIGATORS	NO. OF PATIENTS	GASTRITIS (%)	ULCER (%)	SGOT (%)	BILIRUBIN (%)	DIARRHEA (%)	BILIARY SCLEROSIS (%)
Niederhuber et al.[280]	70	56	8	32	24	—	—
Balch and Urist[281]	50	—	6	23	23	0	—
Kemeny et al.[282]	41	29	29	71	22	0	5
Shepard et al.[283]	53	—	20	49	24	—	—
Cohen et al.[284]	50	—	40	10	25	—	—
Weiss et al.[285]	17	50	11	80	23	23	—
Schwartz et al.[286]	23	53	—	77	20	10	—
Johnson et al.[287]	40	—	8	50	13	–0	5
Kemeny et al.[109]	31	17	6	47	—	–8	29
Hohn et al.[114]	61	35	2	0	78	11	29

bilirubin. Elevation of AST is an early manifestation of toxicity; elevation of AP or bilirubin is evidence of more severe damage. In the early stages of toxicity, hepatic enzyme elevation returns to normal when the drug is withdrawn and the patient is given a rest period, whereas in more advanced cases it does not resolve.

In patients who develop jaundice, endoscopic retrograde cholangiopancreatography (ERCP) might demonstrate lesions resembling idiopathic sclerosing cholangitis in 5% to 29%.[109] Because the ducts are sclerotic and nondilated, sonograms usually do not show dilation. In some patients, the strictures are more focal and usually worse at the hepatic duct bifurcation; drainage procedures either by ERCP or by transhepatic cholangiogram could be helpful.[110] Duct obstruction from metastases should first be excluded by CT of the liver.

Close monitoring of liver function tests is necessary to avoid the biliary complications. If serum bilirubin rises to 3 mg/dL or higher, no further treatment should be given until the bilirubin returns to normal and then only after a long rest period, to prevent the development of sclerosing cholangitis. With proper monitoring, this complication occurs in fewer than 10% of patients.

Severe ulcer disease results from inadvertent perfusion of the stomach and duodenum with drug via small collateral branches from the hepatic artery and can be prevented via careful dissection of these collaterals at the time of pump placement. Even without radiologically visible perfusion of the stomach, however, mild gastritis and duodenitis still can occur.

Complications of Hepatic Artery Infusion Pump Placement and Use

Incomplete or extrahepatic perfusion is usually a surgical problem. It is necessary to mobilize the entire gastroduodenal artery and ligate all branches supplying the stomach, duodenum, bile duct, or pancreas. The postoperative ^{99m}Tc macroaggregated albumin perfusion scan, when compared with the liver scan, can show incomplete perfusion of the liver from either an accessory or replaced hepatic artery not detected preoperatively or an incompletely isolated hepatic artery that is supplying vessels to the pancreas or gastrointestinal tract. These abnormalities can be assessed by performing a side port pump injection. (Most implantable pumps have a main chamber with a central port in which the drugs, such as FUDR, are placed for constant infusion. These pumps also have a side port that bypasses the main chamber and goes directly into the main catheter.) Often, an accessory left hepatic artery arising from the left gastric artery, or an accessory right hepatic artery arising from the superior mesenteric artery, has not been identified. In such instances, it might be possible to embolize the accessory vessel, which will allow collateral flow to develop from the main hepatic artery. A common technical error during catheter insertion is placing the catheter too far from the junction of

DOSE MODIFICATION FOR HEPATIC TOXICITY

SGOT	BILIRUBIN	AP	FUDR DOSE REDUCTION (%)
<2 × baseline	—	—	80
3 × baseline	or 1.5×	or 1.5×	50
>3 × baseline	or 2×	or 2×	Hold

Baseline, day 1 or previous FUDR dose. If elevations continue on reduced doses, decrease duration of FUDR to 1 week. If bilirubin >2 mg/dL, do not retreat for 2 months. If bilirubin levels return to and remain normal, use 25 percent of the previous FUDR dose for 1 week.

INTRAHEPATIC THERAPY MANAGEMENT OF TOXICITY

Ulcer	Denude vessels that supply stomach and duodenum
Hepatitis	Monitor SGOT, AP; decrease or hold hose for enzyme elevations
Biliary sclerosis	Monitor liver enzymes, document by ERCP; if present, do not retreat even if enzymes normalize
Cholecystitis	Remove gallbladder
Diarrhea	May be misperfusion or very extensive liver disease (repeat hepatic flow scan)

TECHNICAL ASPECTS OF PUMP INSERTION

1. Rule out extrahepatic disease by colonoscopy, chest radiograph, or CT scan of abdomen and pelvis.
2. Intraoperatively; portal lymph nodes should be biopsied to rule out extrahepatic disease.
3. Celiac and SMA arteriogram to identify arterial anatomy of liver and vessels to stomach and duodenum and pancreas.
4. Portal vein must be patent.
5. Portal lymph nodes should be biopsied intraoperatively to rule out extrahepatic disease.
6. Place catheter into gastroduodenal artery, not directly into hepatic artery, which could lead to thrombosis; secure catheter with nonabsorbable ties.
7. Identify and ligate branches to pancreas and duodenum.
8. Check whole-liver perfusion with 5 mL of fluorescein through side port.
9. Postsurgery macroaggregated albumin (MAA) scan should be performed through side port of pump to check perfusion of the liver and to ensure no extrahepatic perfusion.

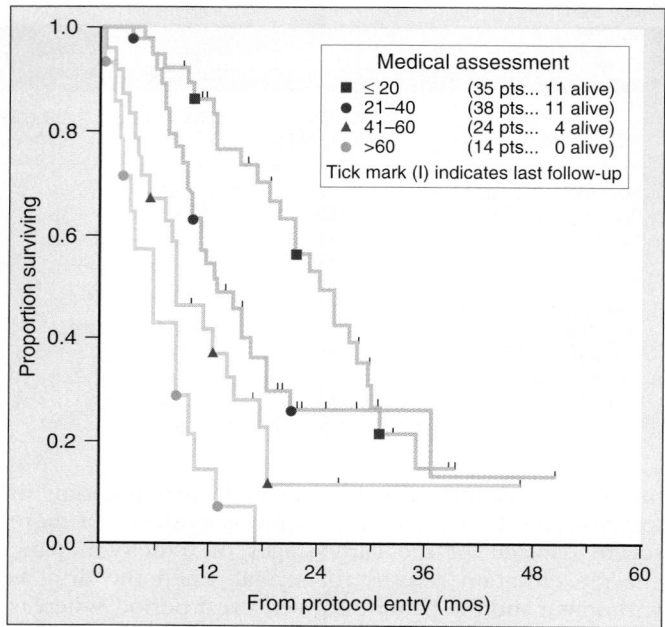

Figure 59-7. Survival distributions by percent of liver involvement (medical assessment). The median survival was 25 months for patients with less than 20% involvement vs. 6 months for patients with greater than 60% involvement. (From Kemeny N, Daly J, Oderman P, et al: Prognostic variables in patients with hepatic metastases from colorectal cancer: Importance of medical assessment of liver involvement. Cancer 1989;63:742.)

the gastroduodenal artery and hepatic artery. The segment of gastroduodenal artery continuously exposed to full-dose chemotherapy will eventually thrombose. There is a learning curve for both the surgeons and the medical oncologists. In one series, technical complications were seen in 37% of patients with inexperienced surgeons and in 6.6% of patients with experienced surgeons.[111]

Randomized Studies

It is difficult to assess the impact of hepatic infusional therapy on tumor response and patient survival without a prospective randomized study comparing it with systemic chemotherapy. In such studies, patients would have to be stratified for parameters known to influence tumor response rates and patient survivals, such as performance status, extent of liver involvement, and initial LDH level.

The influence of the extent of liver involvement on survival has been demonstrated by many investigators. The median survival for patients with less than 20% involvement was greater than 20 months, whereas survival was only 6 months for those with more than 60% involvement (Fig. 59-7).[112] The influence of certain laboratory parameters on tumor response and patient survival was evaluated at Memorial Sloan-Kettering Cancer Center, where the initial LDH level proved to be the most significant factor.[113] Patients whose initial LDH and CEA levels were normal had a median survival of 32 months vs. only 8 months for those with abnormal values (Fig. 59-8).

In a randomized study at Memorial Sloan-Kettering, patients were stratified by percent liver involvement and baseline LDH. All patients underwent exploratory laparotomy for pump placement; patients with extrahepatic disease were excluded from entry. Both groups received a 14-day continuous infusion of FUDR, but the dose was lower (0.125 mg/kg/day) in the systemic group than in the HAI group (0.3 mg/kg/day), as the higher dose

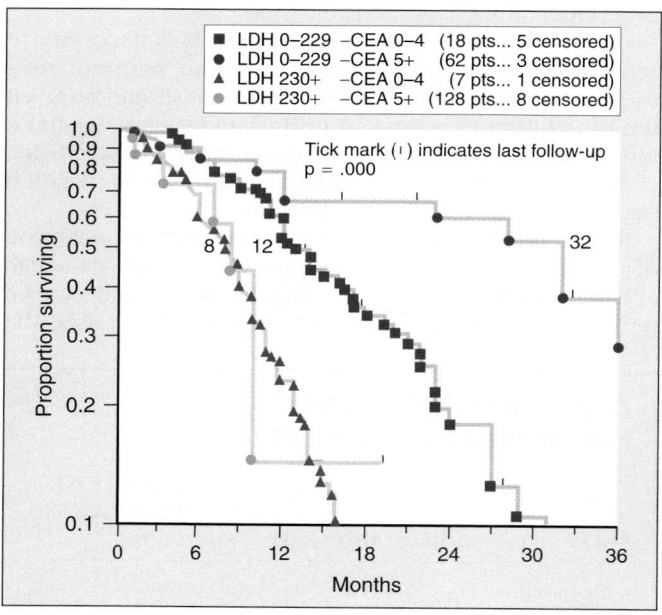

Figure 59-8. Metastatic colorectal carcinoma (survival). Survival curves based on initial LDH and CEA levels. The median survival of patients with normal LDH and CEA levels at initiation of chemotherapy was 32 months, whereas it was 8 months if both values were abnormal ($P < 0.001$). (From Kemeny N, Braun DW: Prognostic factors in advanced colorectal carcinoma: The importance of lactic dehydrogenase, performance status, and white blood cell count. Am J Med 1983;74:786.)

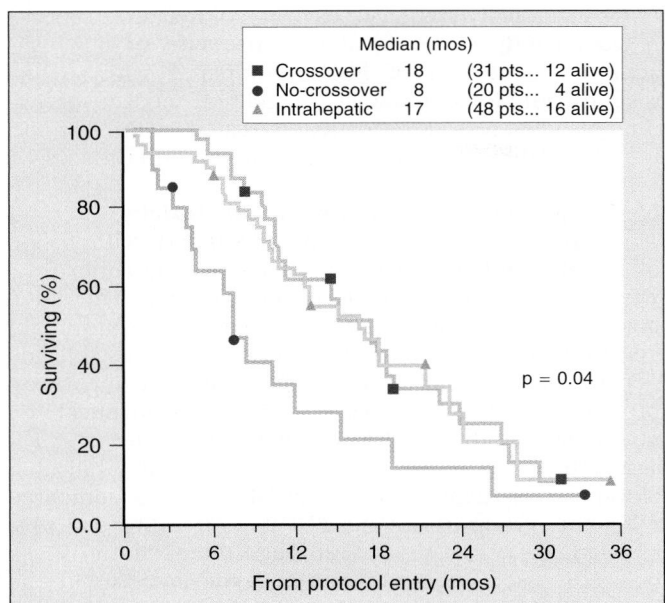

Figure 59-9. Memorial Sloan-Kettering study: Survival curves of HAI group (▲), crossover group (■), and noncrossover group (●). (From Kemeny N, Daly J, Reichman B, et al: Intrahepatic or systemic infusion of fluorodeoxyuridine in patients with liver metastases from colorectal carcinoma. Ann Intern Med 1987;107:459.)

could not be tolerated by systemic infusion. In this study, the doses actually delivered were lower than the doses quoted because no recalculation was done for residual volume. In patients randomized to systemic therapy, crossover from systemic therapy to HAI was permitted. Of the 99 evaluable patients, partial responses were seen in 53% and 21% of the HAI and systemic groups, respectively (P = 0.001). Of the patients who crossed over from systemic to HAI therapy, 25% had a partial response after the crossover and 60% had a decrease in CEA levels. The median survivals for the HAI and systemic groups were 17

and 12 months, respectively (P = 0.424). The interpretation of survival is difficult because 60% of the systemic patients crossed over. Those who did not cross over had a median survival of 8 months, compared with 18 months for those who crossed over to HAI (P = 0.04) (Fig. 59-9). An analysis of baseline characteristics in the crossover and noncrossover groups revealed no significant differences. Randomized studies are outlined in Table 59-18.

A similar randomized study conducted by the Northern California Oncology Group also used FUDR infusion in both the HAI and systemic groups.[114] Patients were stratified by extent of liver involvement, baseline bilirubin values, and performance status. The doses of FUDR were 0.2 and 0.075 mg/kg/day for 14 days in the HAI and systemic groups, respectively. The original HAI dose of 0.3 mg/kg/day was quickly reduced due to excessive toxicity. These were the actual doses administered, as recalculation was done taking into account the residual volume in the pump. Of the 117 eligible patients, 42% responded to HAI and 10% to systemic therapy (P = <0.001). The median time to progression was 401 and 201 days for the HAI and systemic groups, respectively (P = 0.009), while median survivals were 503 days and 484 days, respectively. Although a crossover design was not built into the study, 43% of the patients on systemic therapy eventually received HAI, which could have obscured survival differences between the two groups. Furthermore, this study, like most of the other randomized studies, included patients with metastases to hepatic lymph nodes, who not only have a poorer prognosis than patients with liver-only metastases but also might not respond to HAI as well, as the nodes are not being treated by direct liver perfusion.

A National Cancer Institute (NCI) study compared HAI with systemic infusion of FUDR.[115] In 64 patients, the response rates were 62% and 17% for the HAI and systemic groups, respectively (P = <0.003). Interpretation of survival data is difficult, as 34% of the HAI group never received chemotherapy, and 38% of the HAI group had positive portal lymph nodes. Despite these limitations, in the subset of patients without extrahepatic disease, the

TABLE 59-18

Randomized Studies of Intrahepatic versus Systemic Chemotherapy for Hepatic Metastases from Colorectal Cancer

GROUP	NO. OF PATIENTS	RESPONSE (%) HAI	SYS	P VALUE*	SURVIVAL (MO) HAI	SYS	P VALUE*
MSKCC[288]	162	52	20	.001	18*	12	
NCOG[114]	143	42	10	.0001	16.6	16	
NCI[115]	64	62	17	.003	20	11	
Consortium[289]	43	58	38	NS	—	NS	
City of Hope	41	56	0				
Mayo Clinic[116]	69	48	21	.02	12.6	10.5	
French[117]	163	49	14	NS	15	11	.02
English[95]	100	50	0	.001	13	6.3	.03
German[290]	168	43	20	.019	12.7	18	

NS, not stated.
*Only significant P values reported.

2-year survival was 47% in the HAI group vs. 13% in the systemic group ($P = 0.03$).

Another small study conducted by the Mayo Clinic (69 patients) compared HAI FUDR with systemic bolus 5-FU 500 mg/m^2 for 5 days.[116] The trial permitted entry of symptomatic patients only and did not allow a crossover. Objective tumor response was observed in 48% and 21% of patients in the HAI and systemic groups, respectively ($P = 0.02$), and time to hepatic progression was 15.7 and 6 months, respectively ($P = 0.001$). Despite the increase in response rate and time to hepatic progression, survival was similar in the two groups (12.6 and 10.5 months, respectively). This survival information is difficult to interpret, however, because 48% of the HAI groups were either not adequately treated or had extrahepatic disease.

In a French trial of 163 patients randomized to HAI of FUDR vs. systemic bolus 5-FU, the patients were stratified by extent of liver involvement and baseline LDH levels.[117] The response rates were 49% and 14% in the HAI and systemic groups, respectively. Median time to hepatic progression was 15 and 6 months, and median survival was 14 and 10 months for the HAI and systemic groups, respectively. The 2-year survival was 22% for HAI and 10% for the systemic group ($P < 0.02$). One of the criticisms of this trial is that some patients in the systemic group received chemotherapy only when they became symptomatic.

In a similar study done in England, 100 patients were randomized to HAI FUDR vs. systemic 5-FU (which was given to symptomatic patients only).[95] Quality of life and survival were improved significantly for the HAI group. Median survival was 405 days vs. 198 days for the HAI and systemic groups, respectively ($P = 0.03$).

The German Cooperative Group on Liver Metastases randomized 168 patients in a multicenter trial to one of three treatment groups:

1. HAI of FUDR
2. HAI FU/LV
3. Systemic FU/LV[118]

The median time to progression was 5.9, 9.2, and 6.6 months, and median survival was 12.7, 18.7, and 17.6 months, respectively. Tumor response rates were 43.2%, 45%, and 19.7%, and development of extrahepatic disease was 40.5%, 12.5%, and 18.3%, respectively. Toxicity data was more toxic with FU. The incidence of stomatitis was 8%, 75%, and 64.6%, while the incidence of diarrhea was 0%, 11%, and 11%, respectively. It should be pointed out that an intention-to-treat analysis was used, though 70% of patients randomized to HAI of FU/LV and 68.5% randomized to HAI of FUDR were treated.

The Medical Research Council/European Organization for the Research and Treatment of Cancer (MRC/EORTC) Colorectal Cancer Groups conducted a randomized trial of IV vs. HAI administration of FU/LV for 290 patients. Median and 2-year survival rates were 13.4 months and 23% in the intravenous (IV) arm vs. 14.7 months and 20% in the HAI arm; however, 37% of patients allocated to the HAI arm did not receive the assigned treatment.[119]

A meta-analysis combining the results of seven trials supports the use of HAI of FUDR in the treatment of nonresectable liver metastases from colorectal cancers.[120] A significantly better local response rate of 41% was achieved with HAI of FUDR compared with a 14% response rate for systemic FU. In addition, median survival time was increased in patients treated with HAI—16 months vs. 13 months for those treated with FU.

New Approaches to Decrease Hepatic Toxicity

The hepatic toxicity induced by hepatic arterial infusion of FUDR could be related to portal triad inflammation, which could lead to ischemia of the bile ducts. Therefore, hepatic arterial administration of dexamethasone might decrease biliary toxicity. In patients with established hepatobiliary toxicity from HAI, dexamethasone (Dex) promotes resolution of liver function abnormalities. In a randomized study of FUDR with dexamethasone vs. FUDR alone, there was a trend toward decreased bilirubin elevation in patients receiving FUDR plus Dex compared with the group receiving FUDR alone (9% vs. 30%, respectively [$P = 0.07$]).[121] Although the addition of Dex was not associated with a significant increase in the amount of FUDR that could be administered, the response rate was increased by 71% for the FUDR plus Dex group vs. by 40% for the group receiving FUDR alone ($P = 0.03$). Survival was also improved: 23 months for patients receiving FUDR plus Dex vs. 15 months for those receiving FUDR alone ($P = 0.06$)

The use of circadian modification of HAI with FUDR is another method to decrease hepatic toxicity. In a nonrandomized study at the University of Minnesota, a comparison of constant (flat) infusion vs. circadian-modified hepatic arterial FUDR infusion was conducted in 50 patients with metastatic colorectal carcinoma.[122] The initial dose was 0.25 to 0.3 mg/kg/day for a 14-day infusion. The group with circadian modification received 68% of each daily dose between 3:00 P.M. and 9:00 P.M. The patients with circadian modified infusion tolerated almost twice the daily dose of FUDR, with a decrease in hepatic toxicity compared with patients receiving flat infusions, but the study was not a prospective randomized study.

Another approach to decrease toxicity from HAI is to alternate drugs such as HAI FUDR with hepatic arterial 5-FU. A weekly hepatic arterial bolus of 5-FU does not cause hepatobiliary toxicity; however, it frequently produces treatment-limiting systemic toxicity or arteritis. Stagg and colleagues[123] used alternating HAI of FUDR (0.1 mg/kg/day for 7 days) followed by a hepatic arterial bolus of 5-FU (15 mg/kg on days 14, 21, and 28 via the pump side port every 35 days). The response rate was 51%, and median survival was 22.4 months. In contrast to the experience with single-agent HAI of FUDR, no patient on the alternating plan has had treatment terminated because of drug toxicity. Davidson and colleagues,[124] using a similar alternating regimen on 54 patients, produced a 54% response rate, with 3.5% of patients developing biliary sclerosis. Patt and associates,[125] using HAI of FU and interferon in FU- and LV-refractory patients, produced a 33% response rate with a median survival of 15 months and no hepatobiliary toxicity. Because 5-FU is less toxic to the biliary tract than FU, some investigators have returned to a strategy of using external pumps connected to a surgically placed hepatic artery catheter to infuse 5-FU. The dose of 5-FU needed for infusion is large, which would not fit into a small reservoir and therefore requires external pumps.

Warren and colleagues,[126] using weekly HAI FU infusion and systemic leucovorin, produced a 45% response rate in 31 patients without hepatic toxicity and mild systemic toxicity. Metzger and coworkers[127] treated 30 patients with an infusion of 5-FU at 2000 mg per day for 5 days plus mitomycin C 10 mg/m[2] on day 1; the courses were repeated every 6 weeks. The median survival was 18 months, with a 57% partial response rate. No patients developed sclerosing cholangitis, but mucositis and leukopenia were seen. Catheter complications occurred in 33%, which led to premature termination of treatment in one third of the patients. Schlag and associates,[128] using HAI of 5-FU (1000 mg/day for 5 days) via a surgically placed port connected to an external pump, reported a 27% partial response in 33 patients and a median survival of 14 months. Hepatobiliary toxicity was seen in only 5% of the patients. Table 59-19 lists some of the studies using FU and other agents by this technique.

Methods to Increase Response Rate

The potential benefit of multidrug hepatic arterial therapy has been evaluated. A randomized trial of a three-drug regimen (mitomycin C, BCNU, and FUDR) vs. FUDR alone was conducted in 67 patients with disease progression after previous treatment with systemic chemotherapy.[129] The overall response rate and survival were similar. The response rates in both groups were higher than would be expected with a second systemic regimen after failure of first-line treatment. For patients who had been treated previously for metastatic disease rather than receiving previous adjuvant therapy, the response rate was 48% for the three drugs vs. 24% for FUDR alone ($P = 0.03$). There was no difference in response rate among patients who had not received chemotherapy for metastatic disease and had received only prior adjuvant therapy. The use of high-dose mitomycin C (20 mg/m[2]) via the side port with FUDR and dexamethasone in the body of the pump increased the response rate, especially in previously treated patients, but it also increased toxicity.[130]

Based on success of systemic 5-FU/LV regimens and on laboratory studies suggesting that LV might actually be a better modifier of FUDR than of 5-FU, 64 patients were treated with FUDR and LV by HAI. The overall response rate was 62%, but 15% of patients developed biliary sclerosis. The toxicity of the combination was higher than of FUDR alone, but the survival was improved: 86% of the patients were alive at 1 year, 62% at 2 years, 33% at 3 years, and 10% at 5 years after treatment.[131,132]

To further increase response rate without an increase in toxicity, the combination of FUDR, Dex, and LV was tested.[132] The response rate was 78% in previously untreated patients, with only 3% of these developing sclerosing cholangitis. The median survival was 24.8 months, and the 1- and 2-year survivals were 91% and 57%, respectively. In patients who had received previous chemotherapy, the response rate was 52%.

Methods to Decrease Extrahepatic Disease

Extrahepatic disease develops in 40% to 70% of patients undergoing HAI. Such metastases can occur even when the patient's liver is still responding. The use of systemic therapy plus HAI might produce a decrease in extrahepatic disease. In Safi and associates,[133] study comparing FUDR (0.2 mg/kg/day for 14 of 28 days) with a combination of intra-arterial FUDR (0.21 mg/kg/day) and intravenous FUDR (0.09 mg/kg/day) given concurrently for 14 of 28 days (IA/IV), the response rates were 60% for both arms of the study. The incidence of extrahepatic disease, however, was 56% for the group receiving IA/IV treatment compared with 79% for those receiving HAI alone ($P < 0.01$). There was no difference in survival between the two groups ($P = 0.08$).[133] In Lorenz and colleagues,[134] study of 52 patients, combined HAI/IV did not increase survival or decrease the development of extrahepatic disease (60% and 62% for HAI/IV vs. HAI alone, respectively). Wanebo and coworkers[135] used continuous infusion FU and leucovorin for 14 days alternating with intrahepatic FUDR, dexamethasone, and leucovorin.

TABLE 59-19

Hepatic Arterial Therapy: FU Plus Other Agents				
INVESTIGATOR	**NO. OF PATIENTS**	**DOSE (MG/M²)**	**RESPONSE (%)**	**MEDIAN SURVIVAL**
Cortesi et al.[291]	109	FU 500 × 5 Cisplat 24 × 5	46	16
Warren et al.[126]	31	FU 1500 × 24 h LV 400 weekly × 6	48	17
Sugihara[292]	58	FU 360 × 7 then 100 × 7 d	50	11
Kerr et al.[293]	43	LV 200 FU 400 then FU 1800 22 h	36	—
Howell et al.[294]	40	LV 200 FU 400 then FU 1600 – 22 h q2w	46	19
Patt et al.[295]	48	Interf 5 mu FU 1000 × 5 h qw	33	15
Borner et al.[296]	28	5-FU 750/m² × 5 d	50	

Two other studies produced median survivals of 12 and 18 months administering HAI FUDR plus systemic FU.[136,137] Further studies of combined systemic and HAI regimens are necessary.

Attempts to decrease the development of extrahepatic disease in patients undergoing HAI also have focused on combining other agents that might be more effective than FUDR or FU. An important biochemical observation is that colorectal metastases in the lung—a common site of extrahepatic involvement—frequently have elevated levels of thymidylate synthase (TS) when compared with hepatic metastases.[138] This is important, as high TS levels in metastases have been reported to predict resistance to FU therapy.[139] Unlike FU, CPT-11 has been shown to retain activity in tumors with high TS levels.[140] Therefore, the drug could be more effective in controlling lung metastases. At Memorial Sloan-Kettering Cancer Center, 38 patients with unresectable hepatic metastases were treated with a combination of systemic CPT-11 with HAI of FUDR plus dexamethasone. The overall response rate was 74% (complete plus partial responses) in previously treated patients, but the development of extrahepatic disease remained a problem.[70] A similar study testing this combination in the adjunct setting after liver resection is almost completed.

Hepatic Arterial Infusion: Conclusions

HAI has several advantages. From a pharmacologic standpoint, HAI is more effective than systemic therapy, as higher drug levels are achieved at the sites of metastatic disease. Utilizing agents with high hepatic extraction virtually eliminates the systemic toxicity observed with "standard" chemotherapy.

Should every patient with unresectable liver metastases and no extrahepatic disease undergo HAI? Hepatic arterial therapy produces higher response rates compared with systemic therapy, but randomized studies have not definitely proved a survival advantage. More recent HAI trials demonstrate median survivals of 28 to 30 months, with 2-year survivals of 66%. Therefore, in a patient with extensive hepatic disease (30%–60% liver involvement) who can tolerate an operation, hepatic arterial therapy as the first treatment could be preferable. In patients with greater than 60% liver involvement, the response rate and duration of response are lower; therefore, some physicians might feel that this group should not undergo an operation. For patients with less than 20% involvement, one might have time to start with systemic chemotherapy, as survival is longer. If their tumor fails to respond, they can then undergo regional infusion. In institutions in which physicians are not familiar with placement of the hepatic arterial catheter and the pump or with the management of patients on regional infusion, systemic chemotherapy is a reasonable option. We have demonstrated that patients who fail systemic chemotherapy can still go on to respond to hepatic arterial therapy.

In eight randomized trials, the response rate was higher using HAI compared with systemic therapy (see Table 59-19). The time to hepatic progression was significantly longer in the HAI groups vs. the systemic groups (Table 59-20). The randomized pump studies do not

TABLE 59-20

Randomized Studies of HAI versus Systemic Chemotherapy: Time to Hepatic Progression

GROUP	NO. OF ELIGIBLE PATIENTS	TIME TO HEPATIC PROGRESSION (MO) HAI	TIME TO HEPATIC PROGRESSION (MO) SYS
Memorial Sloan-Kettering[288]	99	9	6
NCOG[114]	117	13	6.7
Mayo Clinic[116]	64	15.7	6
France[117]	163	15	6

HAI, hepatic arterial infusion; SYS, systemic.

evaluate the issue of survival clearly, for the following reasons:

1. In some studies, a crossover was allowed.
2. The number of patients was small.
3. Positive portal nodes were included in the HAI-treated groups.

Because the liver is often the initial site of metastatic disease in patients with colorectal carcinoma, early intensive therapy with surgical resection or intrahepatic infusion (or both) at a time when the tumor burden is small might prevent the progression of metastases to other sites. Although hepatic arterial therapy is applicable to only a minority of patients with metastatic colorectal carcinoma (those with only hepatic metastases), it might be the best available therapy for these patients (Fig. 59-10). Therefore, the CALGB recently completed a study comparing HAI with systemic therapy without a crossover. The trial randomized 143 patients and also addressed the differences in cost and quality of life obtained by the different treatments. HAI of FUDR, Dex, and LV was compared with systemic FU and LV; the response was 54% vs. 26%, respectively, and the survival was significantly increased, 29.8 months vs. 22.7 months, respectively (P = 0.027).[141]

In the future, molecular markers could help determine the optimal type of treatment. In one small study, patients with low thymidylate synthetase levels had a fourfold greater chance of responding after FU-based infusion.[142] In another study, patients with mutated p53 had a shorter survival.[143] These markers will be studied in the CALGB study of HAI therapy vs. systemic therapy mentioned previously.

The use of HAI for other tumor types has not been studied as extensively. Some of the breast studies using HAI are shown in Table 59-21. Most of these studies are on patients whose tumors are failing to respond to systemic therapy, and yet response rates of 50% or greater are seen in five of the eight studies.

HEPATIC ARTERIAL EMBOLIZATION

Because both hepatic metastases and primary liver tumors derive their blood supplies from the hepatic artery, hepatic arterial ligation (HAL) and embolization have

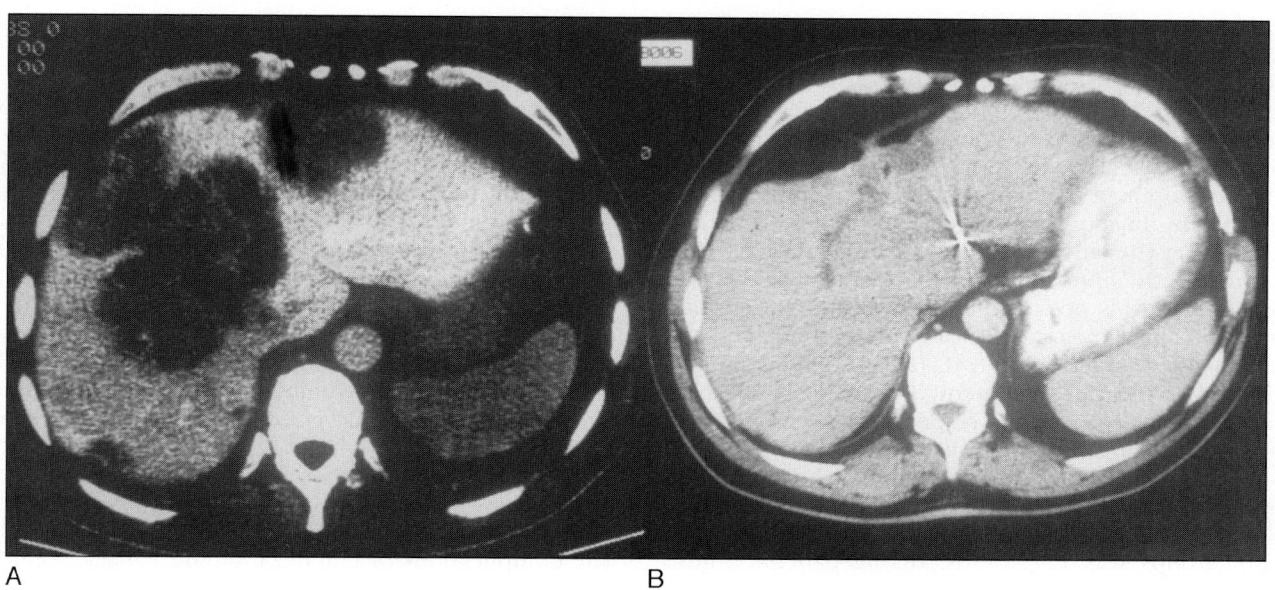

Figure 59-10. A, Patient's CT before treatment, demonstrating massive liver involvement. **B,** Patient's CT after hepatic arterial therapy, showing an excellent partial response after HAI FUDR and LV.

TABLE 59-21

HAI for Breast Cancer*

INVESTIGATORS	NO. OF PATIENTS	DRUGS	PARTIAL RESPONSE (%)	SURVIVAL (MO)
Fraschini et al.[297]	34	Cisplatin + vinblastine	33	11
Estape et al.[298]	16	VP-16-cytoxan	50	16
Fraschini et al.[299]	25	Vinblastine	52	11†
Fraschini et al.[300]	26	Cisplatin	19	11
Maral et al.[301]	15	Mitomycin-C + FUDR	53	18‡
Arai et al.[302]	56	FU + doxo + mitomycin	81	12.5
Tada et al.[303]	45	Doxorubicin + mitomycin-C	37	7.5

ADR, adriamycin; 5-FU, 5-fluorouracil; FUDR, fluorodeoxyuridine; HAI, hepatic arterial infusion; Mit-C, mitomycin C; MTX, methotrzate;
*Most studies consist of patients whose tumor progressed after previous systemic chemotherapy.
†Mean survival only for responders.
‡Some patients in study also had colon cancer.

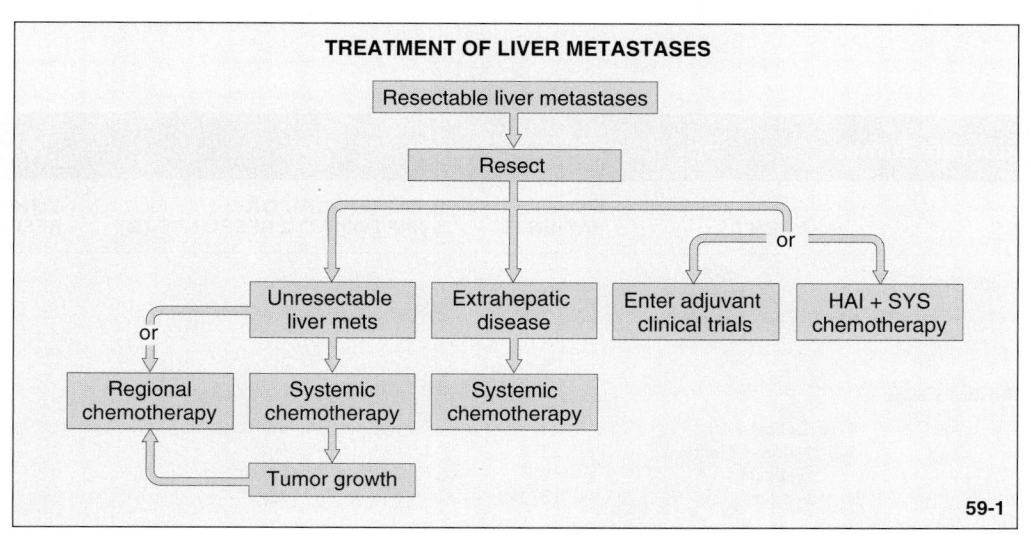

been used to reduce the tumor's blood supply.[144] In most hepatic tumors, HAL produces only a transient benefit because of the rapid development of collateral vessels. In vascular neuroendocrine tumors, HAL produces objective tumor reduction, while in colon metastases (which are typically less vascular), minimal regression occurs.

The development of a collateral blood supply might be minimized by injecting vaso-occlusive particles into the hepatic artery (hepatic artery embolization [HAE]), which also provides the opportunity for retreatment, as only the microvasculature is occluded.[103] In one study of 61 individuals with liver metastases from colorectal carcinoma, patients were randomized to HAE, HAL plus microspheres (HAE), or no further treatment. The median survivals were 8.7, 13, and 9.6 months, respectively, suggesting that embolization or ligation alone had no effect on survival for patients with colorectal carcinoma.[145] Gerard and associates[146] randomized 67 patients to HAL alone vs. HAL and portal vein infusion of 5-FU. The median survival in both groups was 12 months; among patients whose median extent of liver involvement was 30%, only one patient responded. Both studies suggest that this technique is not useful for colorectal cancer.

HAE has a definite role in highly vascular tumors, such as neuroendocrine tumors of the liver.[147] These tumors usually grow slowly, and a reduction in tumor bulk can result in significant palliation. Ajani and coworkers[148] treated 22 patients who had islet cell carcinoma with HAE using polyvinyl alcohol particles (Ivalon) and gelatin sponge particles (Gelfoam). The median survival in this study was 33 months from initiation of embolization (range, 1 month to 72 months); 12 patients had a partial response associated with subjective improvement and decrease in hormone levels. Other studies using HAE are listed in Table 59-22; all demonstrate an improvement in symptoms and a decrease in hormone levels. Gelfoam (size, 1–2 mm), one of the agents used for embolization, does not lead to peripheral vascular occlusion and has an inconsistent duration of occlusion (owing to absorption), while Ivalon (size, 150–500 μm), a smaller particle, allows for more peripheral occlusion and is not absorbable, allowing for a more persistent arterial occlusion.[148-150] A collagen particle (Angiostat; size, 20–250 μm) and a

biodegradable albumin microsphere (Spherex; size, 15–40 μm) are currently being tested, especially in combination with chemotherapy.

Interference with hepatic blood flow can exacerbate the underlying liver disease and can be dangerous in patients with portal venous thrombosis, which is present more often in patients with primary liver tumors vs. in those with metastatic disease. In a study by Carr and associates,[151] four patients with hepatocellular cancer had reversal of tumor-induced portal vein thrombus. The researchers obtained objective responses in 22 of 35 patients (63%) using Spherex (biodegradable) starch microspheres, doxorubicin, and cisplatin. There is clear evidence that arterial embolization causes antitumor effects, but some randomized studies have not shown increased survival.[152]

Complications of Embolization

The complications of embolization are nausea, vomiting, fever, pain, and changes in liver function tests (Table 59-23). Problems less commonly encountered include the following:

1. Injury of the gallbladder by retrograde flow through the cystic artery
2. Ischemic necrosis of the bowel by embolization of one of the vessels to the intestinal tract
3. Pancreatic infarction and pancreatitis by embolization of one of the pancreatic vessels
4. Dyspnea by embolization of the lungs[148-150,153-155]

In neuroendocrine tumors responding to HAE, rapid cell death can result in tumor lysis syndrome with symptomatic hyperuricemia, leading to uric acid nephropathy and oliguria. Vigorous hydration and prophylactic allopurinol might prevent this problem. In carcinoid tumors, HAE could cause a life-threatening carcinoid crisis from the rapid release of hormones from tumor cells. Somatostatin analogs may be given, either prior to the procedure or if a carcinoid crisis should occur.[156] To avoid some of the serious complications of HAE, patients with cirrhosis, portal vein occlusion, and biliary tract obstruction are usually excluded.

TABLE 59-22

Neuroendocrine Tumors				
INVESTIGATORS	**AGENT**	**NO. OF PATIENTS**	**BIOCHEMICAL OR SYMPTOMATIC RESPONSE (%)**	**TUMOR RESPONSE (%)**
Hepatic Artery Ligation				
Martin et al.[153]		8	76	
Moertel[154]		10	70	
Melia et al.[155]		6	50	17
Hepatic Artery Embolization				
Carrasco et al.[149]	Gelfoam	23	87	—
Ajani et al.[148]	Ivalon + Gelfoam	22	60	
Marlink et al.[150]	Gelfoam	10	100	90
Maton et al.[304]	Lyodura	13	76	—

TABLE 59-23

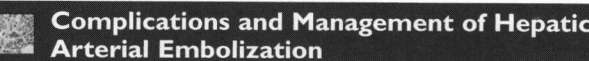

Complications and Management of Hepatic Arterial Embolization

Complication

Pain
Fever
Nausea and vomiting
↑WBC ↑LDH ↑SGOT
Cholecystitis
Hepatic gas formation and abscess
Renal insufficiency
Ileus

Pre-embolization

Hydration
Allopurinol
Somatostatin (only in neuroendocrine carcinomas)*
Analgesics just prior to procedure

Postembolization

Analgesics
Follow SBC, LDH, SGOT, Creatinine
Treat by appropriate measures nausea, fever, abscess, infection, ileus

*150–250 μg SC, q6–8 prior.

CHEMOEMBOLIZATION

An extension of the work with embolization is chemo-embolization. This process involves a local entrapment of drug in the embolization agent and provides a prolonged exposure of the tumor to the drug locally with less systemic drug circulation. A nonrandomized study by Daniels and colleagues[157] suggested that the addition of chemotherapy to the embolic agent (angiostat) produced an increase in response rate over the embolic agent alone. In a study by Venook and coworkers,[158] 51 patients with unresectable hepatocellular carcinoma were treated with Gelfoam and a mixture of three drugs—doxorubicin, mitomycin C, and cisplatin—given via a percutaneous hepatic artery catheter. Twelve (24%) had a partial response, and tumor liquefaction was noted in 70% of patients on CT, with a more than 50% reduction in α-fetoprotein in 68% of patients. Using this technique and the same drugs, these investigators also treated liver metastases from neuroendocrine tumors. In 12 patients with a median liver involvement of 60%, 33% had a partial response with a reduction in hormone levels.[159] Median survival from treatment initiation was 7 months (range, 3 months to 3 years). Lipiodol has been found to remain selectively in the primary and secondary liver cancers when injected into the hepatic artery, allowing visualization of tumors as small as 4 mm.[160] Thus Lipiodol can be used to deliver either chemotherapy or local radiation by combining with an agent such as iodine-131 (^{131}I).[160] Chemoembolization is rarely used for colorectal cancer, as median survivals are usually not increased; average survival is approximately 9 months.[161] Adding systemic therapy to hepatic chemoembolization could improve results. In one trial using regional cisplatin in a polyvinyl alcohol suspension with systemic FU, the partial response rate was 40%, and median survival was 19.3 months.[162]

Another form of chemoembolization is to enclose the chemotherapeutic agents in a microsphere.[163] Degradable starch microspheres injected intra-arterially are trapped in an extracapillary network formed in liver metastases.[163,164] Drug dissolved in the microsphere suspension is retained in the blood vessels of the target organ as long as the blood flow is blocked and then gradually releases the chemotherapeutic agents, resulting in a longer duration of tumor exposure to the drug. The most appropriate agents for microspheres would be those which, like mitomycin C, are preferentially toxic to cells under hypoxic conditions. Another useful drug to use with microspheres is doxorubicin. In a rabbit study, the mean tumor drug level was significantly higher when this drug was used with the microsphere compared with doxorubicin alone, whereas hepatic uptake of the drug by normal tissue was similar in the two groups.[165] Monoclonal antibodies can also be attached to the microspheres.[166]

Radioembolization attempts have been made using glass microspheres containing ^{90}Y, a β emitter with tissue penetrance of 2.5 mm. Andrews and coworkers[166] reported 5 of 23 responses with yttrium embolization. A study of ^{131}I- labeled lipiodol administered to 20 patients (15 HCC, 5 metastatic) produced an α-fetoprotein drop in 11 of 12 patients and a response in 9.[167] The response rates for radioembolization of metastatic tumors are far less than those reported for treatment of primary HCC, perhaps because most metastatic tumors except for neuroendocrine primaries are far less vascular than HCC.

CRYOSURGERY

Cryosurgery is an in situ destruction of tissue using subzero temperatures. The rapid freeze/thaw of tissues results in cellular damage and death. One advantage of cryosurgery is the ability to use local treatment without sacrificing normal tissue. Among the difficulties with this technique are defining the full extent of the tumor and the inability to monitor the amount of freezing, and thus the possibility of overtreatment of surrounding vulnerable normal tissue. Two technical developments have improved the use of cryosurgery:

1. Cryoprobes cooled by liquid nitrogen allowed more precise freezing, even within the liver.
2. Intraoperative ultrasound allowed precise placement of the cryoprobe and more accurate monitoring of the freezing process.

Cryosurgery has been used intraoperatively but also can be used percutaneously. In a series of 32 patients with liver tumors (24 with colorectal carcinoma), 28% percent remained free of disease for 5 to 60 months.[168] In another series using intraoperative cryosurgery on 18 patients who had metastatic colorectal carcinoma with 1 to 12 lesions, Onik and colleagues[169] reported that 4 patients had complete remission with a median survival of 28 months, while 14 patients were considered inadequately treated and had a 21-month median survival.

Weaver and coworkers[170] treated 47 patients with cryosurgery with occasional operative resection. The number of metastases ranged from 1 to 12. The 2-year survival was 62%. Morris and Ross,[171] reporting on 67 patients, noted that 75% of patients undergoing cryosurgery had an increase in CEA by 6 months later. Occasionally, the surgeon feels that all disease has been destroyed but, as seen by this study's positron emission tomography results after cryosurgery, tumor can still be present even though the surgeon feels that no disease has been left behind.

The 2-year survival after cryosurgery varies from 72% to 12%. The Boston series reported the highest survival, which might reflect the type of patient being selected for cryosurgery (i.e., lesser extent of disease and a smaller number of metastases).[172] Adam and associates[173] reported a 2-year survival rate of 50% for patients with colorectal metastases vs. 67% for patients with hepatocellular carcinoma. They reported a local recurrence rate of 44% for the colorectal patients. Because local recurrence is high, the use of HAI after cryosurgery could be useful. One small, nonrandomized study doubled survival with the use of HAI after cryosurgery.[174] Other trials are now evaluating the use of HAI plus or minus systemic therapy. In a series of 185 nonrandomized patients, 71 received adjuvant CPT-11 and/or HAI of FUDR after cryosurgery. Two-year survival was 75% for patients receiving postcryosurgery therapy vs. 35% if no adjuvant therapy was given.[175] Cryoablation can also be used after hepatic resection with close margins or to remove central lesions. Cryoprobes can be used as a handle to assist in segmental resections. An ice ball is produced with 1 cm margins around the tumor; then, the probe is used for traction so that a segmental resection can be performed.[176]

The addition of cryosurgery to conventional surgical procedures was evaluated by Korpan[177] in a randomized study. Those receiving surgical procedures plus cryosurgery had a slight increase in survival (49% vs. 36%), and there was a decrease in liver recurrence for both the cryo and noncryo groups (85% vs. 95%, respectively). The only statistical difference was a greater decrease in CEA in the group receiving cryosurgery.

Cryosurgery does involve some technical issues, including the following:

1. Adequate hydration before surgery, as myoglobinuria and tumor lysis can occur
2. Attention to bile ducts, as biliary fistula can occur
3. Two freeze/thaw cycles are preferred
4. The probe should not be pulled or twisted vigorously, as that could cause cracking[178]

Complications include hepatic cracking secondary to the thermal stresses that occur during rapid freezing; these are usually associated with hemorrhage, which could require packing. Other complications include biliary fistula requiring percutaneous drainage (which occurred in one patient) and myoglobinuria, resulting in acute tubular necrosis.

Published data do not support the use of cryosurgery in patients with resectable disease outside of a clinical trial.[179]

RADIOFREQUENCY ABLATION AND MICROWAVE COAGULATION

Just as tumors can be destroyed by cold, they can also be destroyed by heat. Techniques such as radiofrequency and microwave have been used to destroy tumors. Radiofrequency ablation involves placing a small electrode within the tumor and is used to deliver energy to the tissue. The radiofrequency current generates ionic agitation, which is converted into frictional heat and results in breakdown of proteins and cellular membranes. The larger tumors can be destroyed by cryoablation. For radiofrequency ablation, tumors need to be less than 4 cm or 5 cm in size. During the ablation, a hyperechoic area is formed around the tip of the needle, which corresponds to the area treated. It is sometimes difficult to evaluate whether all tumors have been treated. One of the advantages of radiofrequency ablation as opposed to cryoablation is that it can be performed percutaneously, as the probes are 10 mm in length. Solbiati and colleagues[180] treated 109 patients with colorectal metastases. He found a local control of 70%. Recurrence was significantly more frequent among patients with lesions greater than 3 cm. New metastases developed in 50% of patients, and survival rates were 67% and 33% at 2 and 3 years, respectively.[180] Bilchik and coworkers[181] proposed an algorithm for unresectable hepatic neoplasms, using cryosurgery for larger lesions and radiofrequency for tumors smaller than 3 cm, as local recurrences occurred in 38% of those receiving radiofrequency ablation and only in 17% of patients receiving cryosurgery. Among the most useful situations in which to use radiofrequency ablation are for patients with hepatocellular cancer who also have cirrhosis. Curley and associates[182] presented a series of 110 patients with cirrhosis who received radiofrquency ablation for hepatocellular cancer, with no recurrences occurring in 50%.

Cancer cells could be more sensitive than normal cells to heat due to the decreased vasodilation capacity of the neurovascular bed.[183] Microwave coagulation (MC) was initially developed for coagulation. When microwaves are applied to living tissue, they act mainly on the watery component. Using a probe to deliver 80-watt output for a 30-second duration creates a column of coagulated area of 10 mm. In 19 patients with hepatocellular carcinoma, 28 of 31 nodules underwent complete tumor ablation. Ten of the 19 patients are still free of disease (follow-up, 14–64 months). Advocates of this therapy suggest that microwave coagulation does not have inhomogeneous distribution within the tumor as seen with percutaneous ethanol injection therapy (PEIT).[184] MC is useful only in very small tumors (<3 cm). Both modalities (MC and PEIT) might be more useful if combined with embolization. Lesions near hilar structures are not good candidates for microwave coagulation, but lesions adjacent to hepatic veins can be treated.

PERCUTANEOUS ETHANOL INJECTION

PEIT was first performed in 1983 in Japan. Ultrasound guidance is used to place up to 30 mL of absolute ethanol into the lesion.[185] In patients with primary hepatoma, this treatment produced 5-year survivals of 43% for small lesions. Suzuki and colleagues[186] assigned 42 patients with HCC less than 3 cm to three groups—chemolipiodolization (C-LIP), C-LIP followed by gelatin sponge TAE (transcatheter embolization), or PEIT—and demonstrated a decrease in local recurrence with PEIT. Local recurrences at 1 year were 61%, 29%, and 20% for groups 1, 2, and 3, respectively. Shiina and coworkers[187] reported a 10-year survival of 66 percent using PEIT on single hepatocellular lesions smaller than 2 cm. In pooled data on 11,000 patients with hepatocelluar carcinoma from Japan, 3-year survival for surgical resection, PEIT, or embolization was 58%, 53%, and 20%, respectively. Other researchers, however, report a higher recurrence rate after PEIT vs. surgical resection. The size of the lesion also affects outcome. In an Italian study on 26 patients with metastatic disease, 13 of 15 patients with lesions smaller than 2 cm had responses, while among the six patients with lesions larger than 4 cm, no response was seen.[187] Yamamoto and associates[188] randomized 100 patients to TAE vs. TAE and PEIT. The 3-year survival was 20% for the TAE group and 50% for the TAE plus PEIT group, respectively ($P = 0.05$). This technique was also useful for treating small neuroendocrine tumors, possibly because they are highly hypervascular. At present, the technique needs further study to determine where it fits into the therapeutic armamentarium and whether it will increase survival for patients with metastatic liver tumors. Pending further study, it appears that percutaneous ethanol injection and cryosurgery could be applicable to patients with small metastatic lesions who cannot undergo surgical resection. Whether these techniques will be more beneficial than regional hepatic arterial therapy is not clear, as they only treat visible disease and do not deal with possible small metastases that are not visible.

ISOLATION PERFUSION

To administer high drug concentrations locally, the liver can be isolated by clamping the hepatic arteries, vena cava, and portal vein and then placing a catheter in the hepatic artery to perfuse the liver. A catheter in the retrohepatic vena cava drains the liver, and extracorporeal filters allow removal of chemotherapeutic agents and simplify the technique of isolated perfusion. With a double balloon inferior vena cava catheter, doses as high as 5000 mg/m^2 of FU and 120 mg/m^2 of doxorubicin have been administered. An initial trial using 30 mg/m^2 of mitomycin C produced veno-occlusive disease in four of the nine patients.[189] With the use of melphalan (L-PAM), toxicity was decreased, and with doses of 0.5 to 3.0 mg/kg, complete responses were seen in 2 of 17 patients.[190] Hyperthermic isolation perfusion of tumor necrosis factor

(TNF) and melphalan is being investigated. Melphalan (1.5 mg/kg) and TNF (1 mg) over 60 minutes of hyperthermic infusion produced a 75% response rate.[191]

GENE THERAPY

Tumors largely restricted to the liver (primary or metastatic) can potentially be treated by gene therapy. The gene transfer agents can be injected locally or via the hepatic artery. One trial involves the use of an adenovirus vector carrying the wild-type *p53* gene. Alteration in *p53* function is present in more than half of all malignancies, and re-expression of wild-type *p53* can result in apoptosis and in tumor shrinkage in rodents. A phase I study of recombinant adenovirus encoding wild-type *p53* administered via the hepatic artery produced no responses in 19 patients.[192] Transgene expression in tumor tissue was seen in patients receiving the highest dose levels. Other gene therapies involve the use of prodrug genes to convert innocuous drugs into active chemotherapeutic agents (cytosine deaminase converts 5-fluorocytosine to FU).[193]

To deliver directed immunotherapy, Rubin and associates[194] injected *HLA-B7* gene on a liposomal vector into liver tumors. No responses were seen in 15 patients in the phase I study, but plasmid DNA was detected in 14 of 15 patients. Another concept being evaluated is to have cells express a gene such as thymidine kinase and then kill the cells by use of a ganciclovir, which is converted by thymidine kinase to an active metabolite.[195]

RADIATION

In this section, the role of "traditional" whole liver irradiation (with or without systemic or regional chemotherapy) will be summarized. The recent development of conformal (three-dimensional [3-D] and intensity-modulated) radiation treatment planning has expanded the potential role for radiation therapy significantly in the treatment of localized intrahepatic cancers and will be emphasized.

Results of Whole-Liver Irradiation with or Without Chemotherapy

The traditional approach of using whole-liver irradiation has been limited by the low tolerance of the liver to whole-organ irradiation. It was discovered in the early 1960s that if doses greater than 30 to 35 Gy were given to the entire liver, patients often developed a condition that has become known as "radiation hepatitis," which is more appropriately called "radiation-induced liver disease" (RILD), as the pathologic evaluation reveals no evidence of hepatitis (see the discussion that follows).[196-198] Patients who suffer this complication present 3 weeks to 3 months after the completion of radiation therapy with anicteric ascites and painful hepatomegaly. Laboratory evaluation demonstrates a marked elevation of alkaline phosphatase out of proportion to the modest increases in ALT, AST, and bilirubin. Paracentesis and radiological

TABLE 59-24

Results of Treatment of Metastatic Cancer to the Liver Treated with Whole-Liver Irradiation Alone

REFERENCE	HISTOLOGY*	DOSE (GY/# FRACTIONS)	NO. OF PATIENTS	RESPONSE (% TOTAL)	MEDIAN SURVIVAL (MO)	HEPATITIS[†] TOXICITY
Borgelt et al.[305] RTOG 76-05	38% colorectal	21–30/7–19	103	55[‡]	3	0
Leibel et al.[306] RTOG 80-03	48% colorectal	21/7 (± misonidazole)	187	80[‡]/7[§]	4	0
Phillips et al.[307]	56% GI	≈20–37.5/8	36	72[‡]	ND	1
Prasad et al.[308]	33% colorectal	≈25/16	27	70[‡]	4	0
Russell et al.[201] RTOG 84-05	60% colorectal	27/15	53		4	0
		30/20	69	ND	4	0
		33/22	51		4	2

ND, not determined.
*Predominant histology.
[†]Number of patients with ≥ grade 3 radiation hepatitis.
[‡]Subjective decrease in pain.
[§]Objective (CT scan).

studies (CT and/or MRI) fail to show evidence of progressive disease. Liver biopsy reveals veno-occlusive disease pathologically identical to that resulting from a variety of insults. Although the majority of patients recover in 1 to 2 months, a small fraction develop overt liver failure (characterized by coagulopathies, thrombocytopenia, and changes in mental status) and death.[199,200]

Based on experience with other solid tumors, it is not surprising that whole-liver irradiation of approximately 30 Gy has had modest efficacy for patients with intrahepatic cancers. These doses can produce palliation of painful hepatic lesions in the majority of cases, but both the duration of the responses and patient survival tend to be short

(Table 59-24). Unfortunately, the use of hyperfractionation (1.5 Gy fractions given more than once daily), which has permitted increased dose delivery in the treatment of head and neck cancers, improves neither patient survival nor radiation tolerance.[201]

In an attempt to improve on the modest results of whole-liver irradiation alone, radiation has been combined with either systemic or regional chemotherapy. The most widely used drugs in this effort have been the fluoropyrimidines because in addition to their cytotoxicity against colorectal cancer, fluorouracil (5-FU) and floxuridine have been shown in laboratory studies to be radiation sensitizers.[202-204] The results of a number of

TABLE 59-25

Results of Treatment of Metastatic Cancer to the Liver Treated with Whole-Liver Irradiation with Chemotherapy

REFERENCE	DOSE (GY/ FRACTIONS)	CHEMO	ROUTE	NO. OF PATIENTS	RESPONSE (% TOTAL)	MEDIAN SURVIVAL (MO)	HEPATIC* TOXICITY
Ajlouni et al.[309]	21–30/14–20	FUDR	IAH	10	30[†]	9	0
Byfield et al.[310]	15–30/12[‡]	FUDR	IAH	28	ND	9	1
Friedman et al.[311]	13.5–21/5–7	5-FU, Dox	IAH	22	48[†]	>3	1
Herbsman et al.[312]	25–30/15	FUDR	IAH	13	70[§]	16	0
Lawrence et al.[313]	33/22	FUDR	IAH	19	39[†]	7	0
	36/24			13	ND	ND	3
Lokich et al.[314]	19.5–30/10–12	5-FU or FUDR	IAH	12	63[§]	ND	0
McCracken et al.[206]	19.5/13	5-FU, Mito C	IAH	13	(adjuvant)	ND	1
Raju et al.[315]	21/1.5	FUDR or FU	IAH or IV[¶]	12	83[§]	14	0
Rotman et al.[316]	≈22.5–32.3/15	5-FU	IV	27	83[§]	6	0
Sherman et al.[317]	15–30/7–10	5-FU or Pro ± HU ± Cy ± 5-FU	IV	50[9]	90[§]	4	0
Webber et al.[318]	25/10	FUDR	IAH	25	72[§]	12	0
Wiley et al.[319]	25.5/17	5-FU	IAH	19	37[†]	6	0
Volberding et al.[320]	21/7	5-FU, Dox, MTX	IAH	27	33[†]	7	0

Cy, cyclophosphamide; Dox, doxorubicin; 5-FU, 5-fluorouracil; FUDR, fluorodeoxyuridine; HU, hydroxyurea; IAH, intra-arterial hepatic infusion; IV, intravenous infusion; Mito, mitomycin C; MTX, methotrexate; ND, not determined; Pro, procarbazine.
*Number of patients with ≥grade 3 radiation hepatitis.
[†]Objective response (CT or radionuclide scan documenting 50% decrease in bidimensional product).
[‡]Split course therapy.
[§]Subjective response (e.g., decrease in pain).
[¶]FUDR (IAH) in four patients, 5-FU IV in eight patients.

such trials are summarized in Table 59-25. In general, the objective response rates and reported survival after combined modality therapy appear to be slightly superior to those obtained by radiation alone. A recent study, however, has demonstrated that whole-liver radiation (20 Gy in 10 fractions) does not improve the efficacy of 5-FU for patients who have widespread metastatic disease that includes liver metastases.[205] The tolerance of the liver to whole-organ irradiation does not appear to be affected markedly by the concomitant use of fluoropyrimidines, in contrast to the combination of whole-liver irradiation with other chemotherapeutic agents such as alkylating agents or mitomycin C, which do increase the risk of RILD[199,200,206-208]

Localized Radiation Therapy for Patients with Intrahepatic Cancers

The low tolerance of the liver to whole-organ irradiation has prompted investigators to treat parts of the liver with a high dose. One method of delivering high dose localized radiation is through the use of yttrium-90 (Y^{90}) microspheres. In Y^{90} therapy, Y^{89} oxide is incorporated into a stable glass matrix, which resists leaching. Under neutron bombardment, Y^{89} is converted to Y^{90}, a pure beta emitter with half-life of 64.5 hours and an average electron range of approximately 2.5 cm. The microspheres are then infused into the hepatic artery as a form of regional therapy for well-vascularized tumors.[209-211] Interest in this form of therapy has increased since the results of a randomized trial were published showing that the combination of microspheres and hepatic arterial floxuridine was superior to hepatic arterial floxuridine alone in the treatment of colorectal cancer confined to the liver. In this Australian study, 74 patients with unresectable colorectal metastases undergoing implantation of an hepatic arterial infusion pump were randomly assigned to receive a single dose of microspheres (2–3 GBq) through the hepatic artery within 4 weeks of surgery. Patients then went on to receive chronic floxuridine treatment in 12-day cycles at 4-week intervals. The overall response rate and median time to progression were increased in the group receiving microspheres (44% vs. 18% [$P < 0.01$] and 16 months vs. 10 months [$P < 0.001$], respectively), and there was a trend toward an improvement in overall survival.[212] It should be noted that the response rate for floxuridine alone in this study was substantially less than is typically reported (see earlier in this chapter).

Although the initial clinical results using microspheres are promising, their wider use has been hampered by a lack of understanding of dosimetry and by technical factors. Radiation dose is currently calculated by assuming that the microspheres are distributed uniformly throughout the liver and using MIRD calculations to determine the total dose delivered by the complete decay of the yttrium. The assumption of uniform deposition is clearly false, as brehmstrallen scans and biopsies show selective microsphere deposition in the tumor.[166] Significant strides have been made to better quantify the dosimetry of this technique by using techniques similar to those of standard brachytherapy (placement of radioactive sources inside the tumor).[213-215] A better understanding of both dosimetric and technical factors, such as the potential for pulmonary shunting (which can lead to radiation pneumonitis) is required before the safe use of microspheres can become routine.[216]

A second method of delivering high doses of radiation to parts of the liver is to use interstitial brachytherapy. One group of investigators has administered a single high dose of radiation to localized hepatic metastases by employing a high-dose-rate iridium-192 after-loader placed at the time of laparotomy.[217] ^{125}I seed implants, which delivers low-dose-rate irradiation (< about 0.15 Gy/hr) over several months also have been evaluated.[218] A relative disadvantage of this approach is that sources can be placed only at the time of a laparotomy. Furthermore, a homogeneous dose distribution is difficult to obtain with interstitial brachytherapy techniques when the tumor exceeds 3 to 5 cm in size.

More recently, efforts have been directed toward developing external beam irradiation techniques for delivering high doses of radiation to parts of the liver for patients with localized, unresectable intrahepatic cancers. These efforts have been based on the clinical observation that, just as the surgeon can resect substantial fractions of the liver if the remaining liver is functional, parts of the liver can be treated with high doses of radiation without causing toxicity if sufficient normal liver is spared. Conformal 3-D treatment planning, in which beams can enter the patient from almost any angle (Fig. 59-11), can reduce irradiation of normal liver substantially.[219,220] The incorporation of functional imaging modalities, such as PET scanning, into the planning process (Fig. 59-12) can increase the accuracy of treatment. 3-D treatment planning also can quantify the fraction of normal liver receiving irradiation. For instance, the liver is typically divided into approximately 2000 cubes (voxels), and the dose to each voxel is calculated. These dose calculations can be summarized in the form of a dose-volume histogram (DVH), which condenses the complex 3-D dose distribution into an easily interpreted format.

A series of Phase I/II trials for patients with unresectable intrahepatic cancer have used 3-D conformal external beam irradiation concurrently with hepatic arterial floxuridine. In one early study, 22 patients with localized unresectable colorectal cancer metastatic to the liver were treated with hepatic arterial floxuridine (0.2 mg/kg/day) combined with up to 72.6 Gy.[221] An objective response rate of 50% (2 CR, 9 PR) was reported, with the remaining patients showing stable disease. The overall median survival was 20 months, approaching that achieved by resection in a more favorable group of patients. Similar results were obtained in another series of 12 patients treated with high-dose partial-liver radiation without using 3-D conformal techniques.[222] A more recent trial using higher doses of radiation (up to 90 Gy) confirmed these results and demonstrated that escalated radiation dose was independently associated with improved progression-free and overall survival. The median survival of patients treated with 70 Gy or more was not reached (>16.4 months) compared with 11.6 months for patients treated with lower radiation doses ($P = 0.0003$).[223]

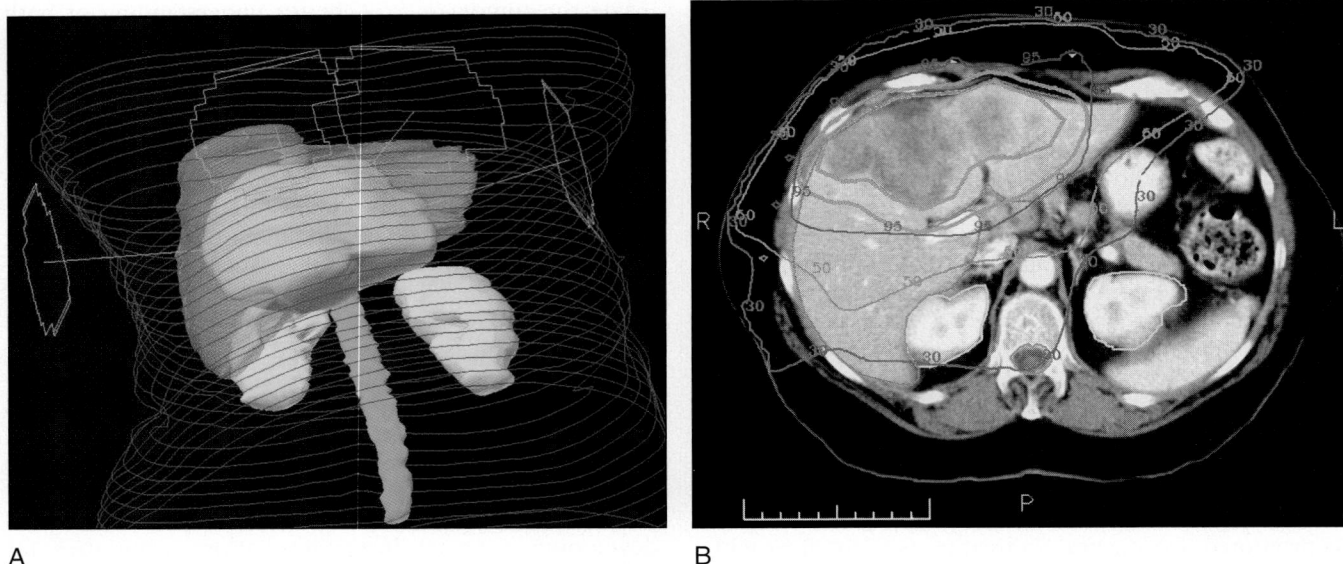

A   B

Figure 59-11. Treatment of intrahepatic cancer using conformation radiation. **A,** 3-D view of beam arrangement for treatment of an intrahepatic bile duct cancer. The (pink) planning target volume (PTV) is shown inside the liver. The external contour is shown in blue wireframe, the kidneys in yellow, and the spinal cord in green. Four multileaf collimator-shaped beams are shown in green. **B,** Dose distribution produced by field arrangement shown in **(A).** The gross tumor volume (GTV) and the expansion of the GTV (for potential tumor invasion, patient set-up uncertainty, and ventilatory motion) to form the PTV are shown in pink. Isodose lines indicate the doses delivered to various regions and demonstrate that all of the PTV receives at least 95% of the prescribed dose (70.5 Gy, delivered with concurrent hepatic arterial fluorodeoxyuridine). This patient is without evidence of toxicity or progression more than 3 years after treatment.

Another approach to delivering localized radiation to parts of the liver involves the use of a single large dose of radiation.[224,225] This has sometimes been referred to as "stereotactic" radiation, although current methods of liver treatment lack the precision in setup and tumor localization that are typical of stereotactic brain radiation. Doses of 8 to 30 Gy have been delivered in a single fraction to small tumors. In one study, small tumors (median size 10 cm³) showed an 81% rate of freedom from

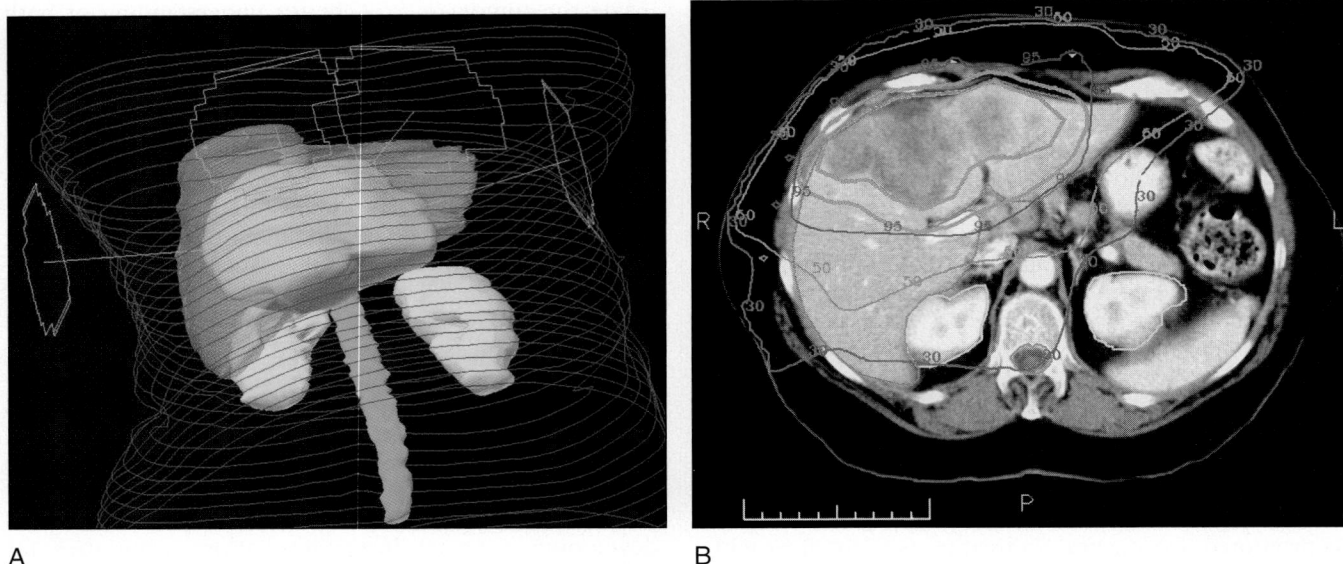

Figure 59-12. PET-CT registration for treatment planning. **A,** CT image obtained for radiation treatment planning of patient with recurrent colorectal cancer metastatic to the liver, who had undergone both resection and radiofrequency ablation. Brown and yellow lines show liver and kidney estimated on the CT image, whereas the red line represents tumor estimated from a PET scan. **B,** Images have been registered to each other using 3-D image registration techniques. Note that the abnormal appearing liver (produced by previous RFA) on CT image lateral to the actual tumor is not PET avid and, therefore, unlikely to contain tumor. (Courtesy of Marc Kessler, University of Michigan.)

progression at 18 months after this form of treatment.[225] The development of better methods for localization and targeting should permit improvement of this technique.[226]

Using 3-D Treatment Planning to Predict Hepatic Toxicity

Although 3-D techniques permit parts of the liver to be treated with doses of radiation far higher than what the entire liver can tolerate, it is possible that both higher doses and larger volumes than have been used in current studies could be employed safely. A first step in defining these limits is to develop a normal tissue complication probability (NTCP) model to describe the dependence of liver tolerance on the combination of dose and volume. A number of theoretical models (all of which require a knowledge of the 3-D dose distribution) have been proposed to estimate the volume dependence of normal tissue tolerance.[227-229] Initial investigations suggested that it would be possible to derive a quantitative model to predict RILD.[230] More recently, an NTCP model with parameters calculated from previous patient data has been used prospectively to prescribe a dose that would subject each patient to a 10% complication risk. Twenty-one patients have completed treatment on such a protocol. The mean dose delivered was 56.6 plus or minus 2.31 Gy (range, 40.5–81 Gy). This dose was significantly higher than the dose that would have been prescribed by the previous protocol (46.0 ± 1.65 Gy; range, 33–66 Gy; $P < 0.01$). One of 21 patients developed RILD. The complication rate of 4.8% (95% confidence interval 0%–23.8%) did not differ significantly from the predicted

8.8% NTCP (based on dose delivered). These results suggest that an NTCP model can be used prospectively to deliver safely far higher doses of radiation for patients with intrahepatic cancer than with previous approaches.[231] A recent analysis of 203 patients treated with conformal radiation (17 of whom developed RILD) refined the estimates of the parameters of the NTCP model and showed that mean dose is an excellent predictor of the risk of complication. It was also found that patients with primary hepatobiliary cancer were at significantly greater risk for complication than patients with colorectal cancer metastatic to the liver.[232]

Future Directions

There are at least four methods by which the outcome of treatment with conformal high-dose radiation combined with chemotherapy could be improved. One possibility would be to combine this form of acute therapy with repeated cycles of hepatic arterial and systemic chemotherapy as described previously. It also seems possible that further dose and volume escalation could be carried out by the development of true stereotactic radiation, which would minimize the volume of normal liver treated. A third potential plan would be to employ better radiation sensitizers, although one such sensitizer—bromodeoxyuridine, which appeared in laboratory studies to be more potent than floxuridine—produced only modest results in a clinical trial and increased toxicity significantly.[232-234] The converse approach could involve radiation protection of the normal liver. For instance, the free radical scavenger, amifostine, protects the normal liver (but not tumor) from radiation in preclinical studies.[235] It is hoped that these approaches will permit a greater fraction of patients to benefit from high-dose therapy and will increase local control in patients with localized unresectable intrahepatic cancers.

CONCLUSIONS

Liver metastases, especially from colorectal primaries, are treatable and potentially curable. Imaging techniques such as CT, MRI, and sonography have advanced in recent years and have led to increased sensitivity and specificity in the diagnosis of liver metastases. When properly applied, the techniques are nearly as sensitive as surgical exploration in the detection of hepatic lesions and in differentiating benign from malignant processes.

Liver surgery has been revolutionized in the past two decades. Dissections along nonanatomic lines have permitted the resection of multiple lesions that might previously have been considered unresectable. The new technique of vascular exclusion might improve the safety of major hepatic resections. Resection of solitary hepatic metastases or up to two to four metastases from colorectal carcinoma should be regarded as the best treatment for this condition. In older patients (>70 years), or in patients with medical conditions preventing surgery, expectant follow-up can be endorsed. As long as the tumor remains stable, withholding treatment is acceptable, but when the

tumor starts growing rapidly and local techniques cannot be used, systemic chemotherapy should be considered. In patients with progressive metastatic disease in the liver, systemic therapy or HAI may be initiated. In young patients with metastatic disease, even when disease is indolent or is symptomatic, it could be difficult not to treat. These patients may be considered for either local regional therapy (resection or regional infusion) or systemic chemotherapy followed by regional therapy.

External localized radiation or interstitial radiation can be used for patients who fail first-line treatment or in new protocols to delineate its value, perhaps in concert with chemotherapy. In patients with neuroendocrine tumors metastatic to the liver, the first approach is not to treat, as there could be a long period of stable disease. Symptoms may be treated with sandostatin. If the tumor progresses and the symptoms are not controlled, these vascular tumors can be treated by embolization or chemoembolization, with high expectations of response. Newer approaches to liver metastases such as cryosurgery, chemoembolization, interstitial radiation, or alcohol injections are available. The usefulness of these techniques compared with surgery or regional therapy is being investigated.

REFERENCES

1. Baron RL, Freeny PC, Moss AA: The liver. In Moss AA, Gamsu G, Genant HK (eds): Computed Tomography of the Body with Magnetic Resonance Imaging. Philadelphia, WB Saunders, 1992, pp 735-821.
2. Phillips V, Bernardino M: The liver and spleen. In Putman D, Ravin C (eds): Diagnostic Imaging, vol I. Philadelphia, WB Saunders, 1988, p 937.
3. Machi J, Isomoto H, Yamashita, Y, et al: Intraoperative ultrasonography in screening for liver metastases from colorectal cancer: Comparative accuracy with traditional procedures. Surgery 1987;101:678-684.
4. Russo A, Sparacino G, Plaja S, et al: Role of intraoperative ultrasound in the screening of liver metastases from colorectal carcinoma: Initial experiences. J Surg Oncol 1989;42:249-255.
5. Rydzewski B, Dehdashti F, Gordon BA, Teefey SA, Strasberg SM, Siegel BA: Usefulness of intraoperative sonography for revealing hepatic metastases from colorectal cancer in patients selected for surgery after undergoing FDG PET. Am J Roentgenol 2002;178:353-358.
6. Tanaka T, Kawai Y, Kanai M, et al: Usefulness of FDG-positron emission tomography in diagnosing peritoneal recurrence of colorectal cancer. Am J Surg 2002;184:433-436.
7. Kalff V, Hicks RJ, Ware RE, Greer B, Binns DS, Hogg A: Evaluation of high-risk melanoma: Comparison of [18F]FDG PET and high-dose 67Ga SPECT. Eur J Nucl Med Mol Imaging 2002;29:506-515.
8. Ruers TJ, Langenhoff BS, Neeleman N, et al: Value of positron emission tomography with [F-18]fluorodeoxyglucose in patients with colorectal liver metastases: A prospective study. J Clin Oncol 2002;20:388-395.
9. Lai D, Fulham M, Stephen M, et al: The role of whole-body positron emission tomography with [18F]fluorodeoxyglucose in identifying operable colorectal cancer metastases to the liver. Arch Surv 1996;131:703-707.
10. Fong Y, Fortner J, Sun RL, Brennan MF, Blumgart LH: Clinical score for predicting recurrence after hepatic resection for metastatic colorectal cancer: Analysis of 1001 consecutive cases. Ann Surg 1999;230:309-318; discussion 318-321.
11. Vitola J, Delbeke D, Meranze S, et al: Positron emission tomography with F-18-fluorodeoxyglucose to evaluate the results of hepatic chemoembolization. Cancer 1996;78:2039-2042.

12. Wernecke K, Rummeny E, Bongartz G, et al: Detection of hepatic masses in patients with carcinoma: Comparative sensitivities of sonography, CT and MR imaging. Am J Roentgenol 1991;157: 731–739.

13. Kemeny M, Subarbaker PH, Smith TJ, et al: A prospective analysis of laboratory tests and imaging studies to detect hepatic lesions. Ann Surg 1982;195:163–167.

14. Vassiliades VG, Foley WD, Alarcon J, et al: Hepatic metastases: CT versus MR imaging at 1.5T. Gastrointest Radiol 1991;16:159–163.

15. Dodd GD 3rd, Miller WJ, Baron RL, Skolnick ML, Campbell WL: Detection of malignant tumors in end-stage cirrhotic livers: Efficacy of sonography as a screening technique. Am J Roentgenol 1992;159:727–733.

16. Soyer P, Levesque M, Elias D, Zeitoun G, Roche A: Preoperative assessment of resectability of hepatic metastases from colonic carcinoma: CT portography vs sonography and dynamic CT. Am J Roentgenol 1992;159:741–744.

17. Paulson EK, Baker ME, Hilleren DJ, et al: CT arterial portography: Causes of technical failure and variable liver enhancement. Am J Roentgenol 1992;159:745–749.

18. Delbeke D, Vitola JV, Sandler M, et al: Staging recurrent metastatic colorectal carcinoma with PEG. J Nucl Med 1997;37:1196–1201.

19. Ziessman HA, Silverman PM, Patterson J, et al: Improved detection of small cavernous hemangiomas of the liver with high-resolution three-headed SPECT. J Nucl Med 1991;32:2086–2091.

20. Tartter P, Slater G, Gelernt I, Aufses A: Screening for liver metastases from colorectal cancer with carcinoembryonic antigen and alkaline phosphatase. Ann Surg 1981;193:357–360.

21. Ranson J, Adams P, Localio S: Preoperative assessment for hepatic metastases in carcinoma of the colon and rectum. Surg Gynecol Obstet 1973;137:435–438.

22. Kemeny M, Hogan J, Ganteaume B, et al: Preoperative staging with computerized axial tomography and biochemical laboratory tests in patients with hepatic metastases. Ann Surg 1986;203:169–172.

23. Doroshow J, Multhauf P, Leong L, et al: Prospective randomized comparison of fluorouracil versus fluorouracil and high-dose continuous infusion leucovorin calcium for the treatment of advanced measurable colorectal cancer in patients previously unexposed to chemotherapy. J Clin Oncol 1990;8:491–501.

24. Miyazaki M, Hiroshi I, Nakagawa K, et al: Hepatic resection of liver metastases from gastric cancer. AJG 1997;92:490.

25. Harrison L, Brennan M, Newman E, et al: Hepatic resection for noncolorectal, non-neuroendocrine metastases: A 15-year experience with 96 patients. Surgery 1997;121:625.

26. Pocard M, Pouillart P, Asselain B, Salmon R: Hepatic resection in metastatic breast cancer: Results and prognostic factors. Eur J Surg Oncol 2000;26:155–159.

27. Elias D, Lasser PH, Montrucolli D, Bonvallot S, Spielmann M: Hepatectomy for liver metastases from breast cancer. Eur J Surg Oncol 1995;21:510–513.

28. McEntee GP, Nagorney DM, Kvols LK, Moertel CG, Grant CS: Cytoreductive hepatic surgery for neuroendocrine tumors. Surgery 1990;108:1091–1096.

29. Que F, Nagorney D, Batts K, et al: Hepatic resection for metastatic neuroendocrine carcinomas. Am J Surg 1995;169:36–43.

30. Elias D, Rougier P, Lasser P, et al: Reductional major surgery and chemotherapy in multimetastatic apudomas. Ann Chir 1988;42:474–481.

31. Cobourn CS, Makowka L, Langer B, Taylor BR, Falk RE: Examination of patient selection and outcome for hepatic resection for metastatic disease. Surg Gynecol Obstet 1987;165:239–246.

32. Wolf R, Goodnight J, Krag D, Schneider P: Results of resection and proposed guidelines for patient selection in instances of noncolorectal hepatic metastases. Surg Gynecol Obstet 1991;173:454–460.

33. DeMatteo RP, Shah A, Fong Y, Jarnagin WR, Blumgart LH, Brennan MF: Results of hepatic resection for sarcoma metastatic to liver. Ann Surg 2001;234:540–547; discussion 547–548.

34. Sesto ME, Vogt DP, Hermann RE: Hepatic resection in 128 patients: A 24-year experience. Surgery 1987;102:846–851.

35. Iwalsuki S, Sheahan D, Starzl T: The changing face of hepatic resection. Curr Probl Surg 1989;26:281.

36. Lang H, Nussbaum KT, Kaudel P, Fruhauf N, Flemming P, Raab R: Hepatic metastases from leiomyosarcoma: A single-center experience with 34 liver resections during a 15-year period. Ann Surg 2000;231:500–505.

37. Nordlinger B, Guiget M, Vaillant JC, et al: Surgical resection of colorectal carcinoma metastases to the liver. Cancer 1996;77: 1254–1262.

38. Nordlinger B, Vaillant J, Guiguet M, et al: Survival benefit of repeat liver resections for recurrent colorectal metastases: 143 cases. J Clin Oncol 1994;12:1491.

39. Taylor M, Forster J, Langer B, et al: A study of prognostic factors for hepatic resection for colorectal metastases. Am J Surg 1997;173:467.

40. Gayowski T, Iwatsuki S, Madariaga J, et al: Experience in hepatic resection for metastatic colorectal cancer: Analysis of clinical and pathologic risk factors. Surg 1994;116:703–711.

41. Jamison R, Donohur J, Nagorney D, et al: Hepatic resection for metastatic colorectal cancer results in cure for some patients. Arch Surg 1997;132:505–511.

42. Registry of Hepatic Metastases: Resection of the liver for colorectal carcinoma metastases: A multi-institutional study of indications for resection. Surg 1988;103:278–288.

43. Hughes K, Scheele J, Sugarbaker P. Surgery for colorectal cancer metastatic to the liver. Surg Clin N Am 1989;69:340–359.

44. Hughes KS, Simon R, Songhorabodi S, et al: Resection of the liver for colorectal carcinoma metastases: A multi-institutional study of patterns of recurrence. Surgery 1986;100:278–284.

45. Scheele J, Stang R, Altendorf-Hofmann A: Hepatic metastases from colorectal carcinoma: Impact of surgical resection on the natural history. Br J Surg 1990;77:1241–1246.

46. Wilson S, Adson M: Surgical treatment of hepatic metastases from colorectal cancers. Arch Surg 1976;111:330–334.

47. Nordlinger B, Vaillant J, et al: A scoring system to select candidates for resection of colorectal liver metastases based on 1568 cases. SSO Abstract Book 1996;17:11.

48. Fegiz G, Ramacciato G, Gennari L, et al: Hepatic resection for colorectal metastases: The Italian multicenter experience. J Surg Onc 1991;2:144–154.

49. Codi R, Gennari L, Bignami P, et al: One hundred patients with hepatic metastases from colorectal cancer treated by resection: Analysis of prognostic determinants. Br J Surg 1991;78:797.

50. Elias D, Lasser P, Rougier P, et al: Another failure in the attempt of definition of the indications to the resection of liver metastases of colorectal origin. [French] J Chir (Paris) 1992;129:59–65.

51. Van Ooijen B, Wiggers T, Meijer S, et al: Hepatic resections for colorectal metastases in the Netherlands—a multi-institutional 10-year study. Cancer 1992;70:28–34.

52. Scheele J, Stangl R, Altendorf-Hofmann A, et al: Indicators of prognosis after hepatic resection for colorectal secondaries. Surgery 1991;110:13–29.

53. Fong Y, Blumgart L, Fortner J, et al: Pancreatic or liver resection for malignancy is safe and effective for the elderly. Ann Surg 1995;222:426.

54. Fong Y, Cohen AM, Fortner JG, et al: Liver resection for colorectal metastases. J Clin Oncol 1997;15:938–946.

55. Adson M, Van Heerden J, Adson M, et al: Resection of hepatic metastases from colorectal cancer. Arch Surg 1984;119:647–651.

56. Headrick JR, Miller DL, Nagorney DM, et al: Surgical treatment of hepatic and pulmonary metastases from colon cancer. Ann Thorac Surg 2001;71:975–979; discussion 979–980.

57. Stephen M, Ross Sheil A, Thompson J, et al: Aortic occlusion and vascular isolation allowing avascular hepatic resection. Arch Surg 1990;125:1482.

58. Delva E, Camus Y, Norlinger B, et al: Vascular occlusions for liver resections—operative management and tolerance to hepatic ischemia: 142 cases. Ann Surg 1989;2:209–211.

59. Bismuth H, Castaing D, Garden J: Major hepatic resection under total vascular exclusion. Ann Surg 1989;210:13–19.

60. Zulim RA, Rocco M, Goodnight JE, Jr., Smith GJ, Krag DN, Schneider PD: Intraoperative autotransfusion in hepatic resection for malignancy. Is it safe? Arch Surg 1993;128:206–211.

61. Fujimoto H, Okamoto E, Yamanaka N, et al: Efficacy of autotransfusion in hepatectomy for hepatocellular carcinoma. Arch Surg 1993;128:1065.

62. Giakoustidis E, Drosinopoulos P, Agouridakis K, Galanis N: Surgical treatment of liver injuries by application of Fibrinkleber. World J Surg 1985;9:144–148.

63. Fong Y, Brennan M, Brown K, et al: Drainage is unnecessary after elective liver resection: Results of a randomized trial. Am J Surg 1996;171:158.

64. Burt BM, Brown K, Jarnagin W, DeMatteo R, Blumgart LH, Fong Y: An audit of results of a no-drainage practice policy after hepatectomy. Am J Surg 2002;184:441-445.

65. Fernandez-Trigo V, Shamsa F, Aldrete J, et al: Repeat liver resections from colorectal metastasis. Repeat Hepatic Resection Registry. Cancer Treat Res 1994;69:185-196.

66. Petrowsky H, Gonen M, Jarnagin W, et al: Second liver resections are safe and effective treatment for recurrent hepatic metastases from colorectal cancer: A bi-institutional analysis. Ann Surg 2002;235:863-871.

67. Fong Y, Blumgart L, Cohen A, et al: Repeat hepatic resections for metastatic colorectal cancer. Ann Surg 1994;220:657.

68. Kemeny M, Goldberg D, Beatty J, et al: Results of a prospective randomized trial of continuous regional chemotherapy and hepatic resection as treatment of hepatic metastases from colorectal cancer. Cancer 1986;57:492-498.

69. Wagman L, Kemeny M, Leong L, et al: A prospective randomized evaluation of the treatment of colorectal cancer metastatic to the liver. J Clin Oncol 1990;8:1885-1893.

70. Kemeny N, Huang Y, Cohen AM, et al: Hepatic arterial infusion of chemotherapy after resection of hepatic metastases from colorectal cancer. N Engl J Med 1999;341:2039-2048.

71. Kemeny MM, Adak S, Gray B, et al: Combined-modality treatment for resectable metastatic colorectal carcinoma to the liver: surgical resection of hepatic metastases in combination with continuous infusion of chemotherapy—an intergroup study. J Clin Oncol 2002;20:1499-1505.

72. Lorenz M, Muller H-H, Schramm H, et al: Randomized trial of surgery versus surgery followed by adjuvant hepatic arterial infusion with 5-fluorouracil and folinic acid for liver metastases of colorectal cancer. Surg 1998;228:756-762.

73. Nonami T, Takeuchi Y, Yasui M, et al: Regional adjuvant chemotherapy after partial hepatectomy for metastatic colorectal carcinoma. Semin Oncol 1997;24:56-130.

74. Portier G, Rougier P, Milan C, et al: Adjuvant systemic chemotherapy using 5-fluorouracil and folinic acid after resection of liver metastases from colorectal origin. Proc Am Soc Clin Oncol 2002;21:133a.

75. Ono T, Nagasue N, Kohno H, et al: Adjuvant chemotherapy with epirubicin after radical resection of hepatocellular carcinoma: A prospective randomized study. Semin Oncol 1997;24:S6-18-S6-25.

76. Lai E, Lo C-M, Fan S-T, et al: Postoperative adjuvant chemotherapy after curative resection of hepatocellular carcinoma. Arch Surg 1998;133:183.

77. Muto Y, Moriwaki H, Ninomiya M, et al: Prevention of second primary tumors by an acyclic retinoid, polyprenoic acid, in patients with hepatocellular carcinoma. N Eng J Med 1996;334:1561-1567.

78. Carbone PP, Bauer M, Band P, Tormey D: Chemotherapy of disseminated breast cancer. Current status and prospects. Cancer 1977;39:2916-2922.

79. Kemeny N, Lokich JJ, Anderson N, Ahlgren JD: Recent advances in the treatment of advanced colorectal cancer. Cancer 1993;71:9-18.

80. Pritchard KI: Liver metastases: Can our understanding of their biology and prognostic value contribute to a strategy for optimum therapeutic management? Eur J Cancer 1997;33(Suppl 7):S11-S14.

81. Nicholson G: Differential organ tissue adhesion, invasion and growth properties of metastatic rat mammary adenocarcinoma cells. Breast Cancer Res Treat 1988;12:167.

82. Nash CI, Jones SE, Moon T, Davis S, Salmon S: Prediction of outcome in metastatic breast cancer treated with adriamycin combination chemotherapy. Cancer 1980;46:2380-2388.

83. Carter S: Single and combination nonhormonal chemotherapy in breast cancer. Cancer 1972;30:1543-1555.

84. Kaufman R, Rothschild E, Escher G, et al: Hypercalcemia in mammary carcinoma following the administration of a progestational agent. J Clin Endocrinol Metab 1964;24:1235.

85. George SL, Hoogstraten B: Prognostic factors in the initial response to therapy by patients with advanced breast cancer. J Natl Cancer Inst 1978;60:731-736.

86. Dieras V, Chevallier B, Kerbrat P, et al: A multicentre phase II study of docetaxel 75 mg m-2 as first-line chemotherapy for patients with advanced breast cancer: Report of the Clinical Screening Group of the EORTC. European Organization for Research and Treatment of Cancer. Br J Cancer 1996;74:650-656.

87. Kemeny N: The systemic chemotherapy of hepatic metastases. Semin Oncol 1983;10:148-158.

88. Kemeny N, Yagoda A, Braun D, et al: Therapy for metastatic colorectal carcinoma with combination of methyl-CCNU, 5-fluorouracil, vincristine and streptozotocin (MOF-Strep). Cancer 1980;45:876-881.

89. de-Gramont A, Bosset J-F, Milan C, et al: Randomized trial comparing monthly low-dose leucovorin and fluorouracil bolus with bimonthly high-dose leucovorin and fluorouracil bolus plus continuous infusion for advanced colorectal cancer: A French Intergroup study. J Clin Oncol 1997;15:808-815.

90. Douillard JY, Cunningham D, Roth AD, et al: Irinotecan combined with fluorouracil compared with fluorouracil alone as first-line treatment for metastatic colorectal cancer: A multicentre randomised trial. Lancet 2000;355:1041-1047.

91. Saltz LB, Cox JV, Blanke C, et al: Irinotecan plus fluorouracil and leucovorin for metastatic colorectal cancer. Irinotecan Study Group. N Engl J Med 2000;343:905-914.

92. Goldberg R, Morton R, Sargent D, et al: Oxaliplatin (Oxal) or CPT-11 + 5-fluorouracil (5FU)/leucovorin (LV) or oxal + CPT-11 in advanced colorectal cancer (CRC). Proc Am Soc Clin Oncol 2002;21:511.

93. Glimelius B, Hoffman K, Olafsdottir M, Pahlman L, Sjoden PO, Wennberg A: Quality of life during cytostatic therapy for advanced symptomatic colorectal carcinoma: A randomized comparison of two regimens. Eur J Cancer Clin Oncol 1989;25:829-835.

94. Scheithauer W, Rosen H, Kornek GV, Sebesta C, Depisch D: Randomised comparison of combination chemotherapy plus supportive care with supportive care alone in patients with metastatic colorectal cancer. BMJ 1993;306:752-755.

95. Allen-Mersh T, Earlam S, Fordy C, Abrams K, Houghton J: Quality of life and survival with continuous hepatic artery floxuridine infusion for colorectal liver metastases. Lancet 1994;344:1255-1260.

96. Giacchetti S, Zidani R, Perpoint B, et al: Phase III trial of 15-fluorouracil (5-FU), folinic acid (FA), with or without oxaliplatin (OXA) in previously untreated patients (pts) with metastatic colorectal cancer (MCC) [abstract]. Proc Am Soc Clin Oncol 1997;16:229a.

97. Bismuth H, Adam R, Levi F: Resection of nonresectable liver metastases from colorectal cancer after neoadjuvant chemotherapy. Farabos Annals Surg 1996;224:509-520.

98. Breedis C, Young C: The blood supply of neoplasms in the liver. Am J Pathol 1954;30:969.

99. Ensminger WD, Rosowsky A, Raso V: A clinical pharmacological evaluation of hepatic arterial infusions of 5-fluoro-2-deoxyuridine and 5-fluorouracil. Cancer Res 1978;38:3789-3792.

100. Ensminger WD, Gyves JW: Clinical pharmacology of hepatic arterial chemotherapy. Semin Oncol 1983;10:176-183.

101. Van Groeningen C, Vandervijgh W, Giaccone G, et al: Phase I clinical and pharmacokinetic study of 5 day CPT-11 hepatic arterial infusion (HAI) chemotherapy. Proc ASCO 1997;16:A768.

102. Collins JM: Pharmacologic rationale for regional drug delivery. J Clin Oncol 1984;2:498-504.

103. Weiss L, Grandmann E, Torhost J, et al: Hematogenous metastatic patterns in colonic carcinoma: An analysis of 1541 necropsies. J Pathol 1986;150:195-203.

104. Weiss L: Metastatic inefficiency and regional therapy for liver metastases from colorectal carcinoma. Regul Cancer Treat 1989;2:77-81.

105. Yasuda S, Noto T, Ikeda M, et al: Hepatic arterial infusion chemotherapy using implantable reservoir in colorectal liver metastasis. GanTo Kagaku Ryoho 1990;8:1815-1819.

106. Gluck W, Akwari O, Kelvin F, et al: A reversible enteropathy complicating continuous hepatic artery infusion chemotherapy with 5-fluoro 2-deoxyuridine. Cancer 1985;56:2424.

107. Hohn D, Stagg R, Price D, et al: Avoidance of gastroduodenal

toxicity in patients receiving hepatic arterial 5-fluoro-2-deoxyuridine. J Clin Oncol 1985;3:1257-1260.

108. Northover J, Terblance J: A new look at the arterial supply of the bile duct in man and its surgical implications. Br J Surg 1979;66:379-384.

109. Kemeny M, Battifora H, Flayney D, et al: Sclerosing cholangitis after continuous hepatic artery infusion of FUDR. Ann Surg 1985;202:176-181.

110. Brown K, Kemeny N, Berger M, et al: Obstructive jaundice in patients receiving hepatic artery infusional chemotherapy: Etiology, treatment implications, and complications after transhepatic biliary drainage. J Vasc Interv Radiol 1997;8:229-234.

111. Campbell KA, Burns RC, Sitzmann JV. Lipsett PA, Grochow LB, Niederhuber JE: Regional chemotherapy devices: Effect of experience and anatomy on complications. J Clin Oncol 1993;11:822-826.

112. Kemeny N, Daly J, Oderman P, et al: Prognostic variables in patients with hepatic metastases from colorectal cancer: Importance of medical assessment of liver involvement. Cancer 1989;63:742-747.

113. Kemeny N, Braun D: Prognostic factors in advanced colorectal carcinoma: The importance of lactic dehydrogenase, performance status, and white blood cell count. Am J Med 1983;74:786-794.

114. Hohn D, Stagg R, Friedman M, et al: A randomized trial of continuous intravenous versus hepatic intra-arterial floxuridine in patients with colorectal cancer metastatic to the liver: The Northern California Oncology Group Trial. J Clin Oncol 1989;7:1646-1654.

115. Chang AE, Schneider PD, Sugarbaker PH: A prospective randomized trial of regional versus systemic continuous 5-flouoroxyuridine chemotherapy in the treatment of colorectal liver metastases. Ann Surg 1987;206:685-693.

116. Martin JKJ, O'Connell MG, Wieland HS, et al: Intra-arterial floxuridine vs systemic fluorouracil for hepatic metastases from colorectal cancer. A randomized trial. Arch Surg 1990;125:1022.

117. Rougier P, Laplanche A, Huguier M, et al: Hepatic arterial infusion of floxuridine in patients with liver metastases from colorectal carcinoma: Long-term results of a prospective randomized trial. J Clin Oncol 1992;10:1112-1118.

118. Lorenz M, Muller HH: Randomized, multicenter trial of fluorouracil plus leucovorin administered either via hepatic arterial or intravenous infusion versus fluorodeoxyuridine administered via hepatic arterial infusion in patients with nonresectable liver metastases from colorectal carcinoma. J Clin Oncol 2000;18:243-254.

119. McArdle C, Kerr D, Ledermann J, et al: Intravenous (IV) vs intrahepatic arterial (IHA) 5FU/leucovorin for colorectal (CRC) liver metastases: Preliminary results of the MRC CR05/EORTC 40972 randomised trial. Am Soc Clin Oncol 2001;20:126a.

120. Meta-Analysis GiC: Reappraisal of HAI in the treatment of nonresectable liver metastases from colorectal carcinoma. J Natl Cancer Inst 1996;88:252-258.

121. Kemeny N, Steiter K, Diedzweiecki D, et al: A randomized trial of intrahepatic infusion of fluorouridine (FUDR) with dexamethasone versus FUDR alone in the treatment of metastatic colorectal cancer. Cancer 1992;69:327-334.

122. Hrushesky W, Von Roemelling R, Lanning R, Rabtini J: Circadian-shaped infusions of floxuridine for progressive metastatic renal cell carcinoma. J Clin Oncol 1990;8:1504-1513.

123. Stagg R, Venook A, Chase J, et al: Alternating hepatic intra-arterial floxuridine and fluorouracil: A less toxic regimen for treatment of liver metastases from colorectal cancer. J Natl Cancer Inst 1991;83:423-428.

124. Davidson B, Izzo F, Chase J, et al: Alternating floxuridine and 5-fluorouracil hepatic arterial chemotherapy for colorectal liver metastases minimizes biliary toxicity. Am J Surg 1996;172:244-247.

125. Patt Y, Charnsangavej C, Yoffe B, et al: Hepatic arterial infusion of floxuridine, leucovorin, doxorubicin, and cisplatin for hepatocellular carcinoma: Effects of hepatitis B and C viral infection on drug toxicity and patient survival. J Clin Oncol 1994;12:1204-1211.

126. Warren H, Anderson J, O'Gorman P, et al: A Phase II study of regional 5-fluorouracil infusion with intravenous folinic acid for colorectal liver metastases. Br J Cancer 1994;70:677-680.

127. Metzger U, Weder W, Rothlin M, Largiader F: Phase II study of intra-arterial fluorouracil and mitomycin-C for liver metastases of colorectal cancer. Recent Results Cancer Res 1991;121: 198-204.

128. Schlag P, Hohenberger P, Holting T, et al: Hepatic arterial infusion (HAI) chemotherapy for liver metastases of colorectal cancer using 5-FU. Eur J Surg Oncol 1990;16:99-104.

129. Kemeny N, Cohen A, Steiner K, et al: Randomized trial of hepatic arterial FUDR, Mitomycin and BCNU versus FUDR alone: Effective salvage therapy for liver metastases of colorectal cancer. J Clin Oncol 1993;11:330-335.

130. Kemeny N, Conti J, Blumgart L, et al: Hepatic arterial infusion of floxuridine (FUdR), dexamethasone (Dex) and high dose Mitomycin-C: Comparable response to FUdR/Leucovorin/Dex but with greater toxicity [abstract]. Proc ASCO 1995;14:201.

131. Kemeny N, Cohen A, Bertino J, et al: Continuous intrahepatic infusion of floxuridine and leucovorin through an implantable pump for the treatment of hepatic metastases from colorectal carcinoma. Cancer 1990;65:2446-2450.

132. Kemeny N, Conti JA, Cohen A, et al: Phase II study of hepatic arterial floxuridine, leucovorin, and dexamethasone for unresected liver metastases from colorectal carcinoma. J Clin Oncol 1994;12:2288-2295.

133. Safi F, Bittner R, Roscher R, Schuhmacher K, Graus W, Beger G: Regional chemotherapy for hepatic metastases of colorectal carcinoma (continous intra-arterial versus continuous intra-arterial/intravenous therapy). Cancer 1989;64:379-387.

134. Lorenz M, Hottenrott C, Inglis R, Kirkowa-Reimann M: Prevention of extrahepatic disease during intra-arterial floxuridine of colorectal liver metastases by simultaneous systemic 5-fluorouracil treatment? A prospective multicenter study. Gan To Kagaku Ryoho 1989;12:3662.

135. Wanebo H, Levy A, Vezeridis M, Cummings F. Hepatic artery infusion (HAI) of 5-fluorodeoxyuridine (FUdR) and dexamethasone (Dex) with low dose leucovorin (LV) (10 days) alternating with continuous intravenous infusion (CI) of 5-fluorouracil (5FU) with simultaneous low dose leucovorin (14 day) of unresectable metastases of colorectal cancer (CRC) [meeting abstract]. Proc Am Soc Clin Oncol 1996;15:224.

136. Allen-Mersh T, Kemeny N, Niedzwiecki D, Shurgot B, Daly J: Significance of a fall in serum CEA concentration in patients treated with cytotoxic chemotherapy for disseminated colorectal cancer. Gut 1987;28(12):1625-1629.

137. O'Connell M, Nagorney D, Bernath A, et al: Sequential intrahepatic fluorodeoxyuridine and systemic fluorouracil plus leucovorin for the treatment of metastatic colorectal cancer confined to the liver. J Clin Oncol 1998;16:2528-2533.

138. Leichman L, Lenz HJ, Leichman CG, et al: Quantitation of intratumoral thymidylate synthase expression predicts for resistance to protracted infusion of 5-fluorouracil and weekly leucovorin in disseminated colorectal cancers: Preliminary report from an ongoing trial. Eur J Cancer 1995;31A:1306-1310.

139. Gorlick R, Metzger R, Danenberg KD, et al: Higher levels of thymidylate synthase gene expression are observed in pulmonary as compared with hepatic metastases of colorectal adeno-carcinoma. J Clin Oncol 1998;16:1465-1469.

140. Saltz L, Danenberg P, Paty P, et al: High thymidylate synthase (TS) expression does not preclude activity of CPT-11 in colorectal cancer (CRC). Proc Am Soc Clin Oncol 1998;17:281a.

141. Kemeny N, Niedzweicki D, Hollis D, et al: Hepatic arterial (HAI) versus systemic therapy for hepatic metastases from colorectal cancer: A CALGB randomized trial of efficacy, quality of life (QOL), cost effectiveness, and molecular markers. Proc Am Soc Clin Oncol 2003;(abstract):22.

142. Kornmann M, Link K, Lenz H, et al: Thymidylate synthase is a predictor for response and resistance in hepatic artery infusion chemotherapy. Cancer Letters 1997;118:29-35.

143. Belluco C, Guillem J, Kemeny N, et al: p53 nuclear protein overexpression in colorectal cancer: A dominant predictor of survival in patients with advanced hepatic metastases. J Clin Oncol 1996;14:2696-2701.

144. Markowitz J: The hepatic artery. Surg Gynecol Obstet 1952;95:644-646.

145. Hunt TM, Flowerdew AD, Birch SJ, Williams JD, Mullee MA, Taylor I: Prospective randomized controlled trial of hepatic arterial

embolization or infusion chemotherapy with 5-fluorouracil and degradable starch microspheres for colorectal liver metastases. Br J Surg 1990;77:779-782.

146. Gerard A, Buyse M, Pector JC, et al: Hepatic artery ligation with and without portal infusion of 5-FU. A randomized study in patients with unresectable liver metastases from colorectal carcinoma. The E.O.R.T.C. Gastrointestinal Cancer Cooperative Group (G.I. Group). Eur J Surg Oncol 1991;17:289-294.

147. Martenson H, Nobin A, Bengmark S, et al: Embolization of the liver in the management of metastatic carcinoid tumors. J Surg Oncol 1984;27:152-158.

148. Ajani J, Carrasco CH, Charnsanpavej C, et al: Islet cell tumors metastatic to the liver: Effective palliation by sequential hepatic artery embolization. Ann Intern Med 1988;108:340-344.

149. Carrasco C, Charnsanparej C, Ajani J, et al: The carcinoid syndrome: Palliation by hepatic artery embolization. Am J Roentgenol 1986;147:149-154.

150. Marlink R, Lokich J, Robins J, Clouse M: Hepatic arterial embolization for metastatic hormone-secreting tumors. Cancer 1990;65:2227-2232.

151. Carr B, Zajko A, Bron K, et al: Phase II study of spherex (degradable starch microspheres) injected into the hepatic artery in conjunction with doxorubicin and cisplatin in the treatment of advanced-stage hepatocellular carcinoma: Interim analysis. Semin Oncol 1997;24:56.

152. Bruix J, Llovet J, Castells A, et al: Transarterial embolization versus symkptomatic treatment in patients with advanced hepatocellular carcinoma: Results of a randomized controlled trial in a single institution. Hepatology 1998;27:1578-1583.

153. Martin J, Moertel C, Adson M, et al: Surgical treatment of functioning metastatic carcinoid tumors. Arch Surg 1983;118:537-541.

154. Moertel C: Treatment of the carcinoid tumor and the malignant carcinoid syndrome. J Clin Oncol 1983;1:727-740.

155. Melia W, Nunnerly H, Johnson P, et al: Use of arterial devascularization and cytotoxic drugs in 30 patients with the carcinoid syndrome. Br J Cancer 1982:331-339.

156. Kvols L, Buck M, Moertel C, et al: Treatment of metastatic islet cell car inoma with a somatostatin analogue (SMS 201-995). Ann Intern Med 1987;107:162-168.

157. Daniels J, Daniels A, Quinn M, et al: Phase I trial with cisplatin or mitomycin hepatic chemoembolization (CE) with Angiostat collagen for embolization (CFE) in patients with colorectal cancer. Proc ASCO 1988;7:101.

158. Venook A, Stagg R, Lewis B, et al: Chemoembolization for hepatocellular carcinoma. J Clin Oncol 1990;8:1108-1114.

159. Venook A, Stagg R, Frye J, et al: Embolization of patients with liver metastases from carcinoid and islet cell tumors [abstract]. Proc Ann Meet ASCO 1991;10:A386.

160. Raoul J, Bourquet P, Bretagne J, et al: Hepatic artery injection of I-131 labeled Lipidol: Part I. Biodistribution study in patients with hepatocellular carcinoma and liver metastases. Radiology 1988;168:541-545.

161. Popov I, Lavrnic S, Jelic S, Jezdic S, Jasovic A: Chemoembolization for liver metastases from colorectal carcinoma: Risk or a benefit. Neoplasma 2002;49:43-48.

162. Bavisotto LM, Patel NH, Althaus SJ, et al: Hepatic transcatheter arterial chemoembolization alternating with systemic protracted continuous infusion 5-fluorouracil for gastrointestinal malignancies metastatic to liver: A phase II trial of the Puget Sound Oncology Consortium (PSOC 1104). Clin Cancer Res 1999;5:95-109.

163. McVie J, Hoefnagel C, Burger J: Tumor targeting of cytostatic compounds using intra-arterial biodegradable microspheres. Ann Rep Netherlands Cancer Inst 1985:83.

164. Sigurdson E, Ridge J, Daly J: Intra-arterial infusion of doxorubicin with degradable starch microspheres. Arch Surg 1986;121: 1277-1281.

165. Ball A: Regional chemotherapy for colorectal hepatic metastases using degradable starch microspheres. Acta Oncol 1991;30:309.

166. Andrews J, Walker S, Ackermann R, Cotton L, Ensminger W, Shapiro B: Hepatic radioembolization with Yttrium-90 containing glass microspheres: Preliminary results and clinical followup. J Nucl Med 1994;35:1637-1644.

167. Bretagne J, Raoul J, Bourguet P, et al: Hepatic artery injection of

I-131-labeled lipiodol. Part II. Prelimiinary results of therapeutic use in patients with hepatocellular carcinoma and liver metastases. Radiology 1988;168:547-550.

168. Ravikumar T, Kane R, Cady B, et al: A 5-year study of cryosurgery in the treatment of liver tumors. Arch Surg 1991;126:1520-1524.

169. Onik G, Rubinsky B, Zemel R, et al: Ultrasound-guided hepatic cryosurgery in the treatment of metastatic colon carcinoma. Cancer 1991;67:901-907.

170. Weaver ML, Atkinson D, Zemel R: Hepatic cryosurgery in treating colorectal metastases. Cancer 1995;76:210-214.

171. Morris D, Ross W: Australian experience of cryoablation of liver tumors: Metastases. Surg Oncol Clin NA 1996;5:391-397.

172. Steele G Jr, Ravikumar T, Benotti P: New surgical treatments for recurrent colorectal cancer [review]. Cancer 1990;65:723-730.

173. Adam R, Akpinar E, Johann M, Kunstlinger F, Majno P, Bismuth H: Place of cryosurgery in the treatment of malignant liver tumors. Ann Surg 1997;225:39-38.

174. Preketes A, Caplehorn J, King J, et al: Effect of hepatic artery chemotherapy on survival of patients with hepatic metastases from colorectal carcinoma treated with cryotherapy. World J Surg 1995;19:768-771.

175. Litvak DA, Wood TF, Tsioulias GJ, et al: Systemic irinotecan and regional floxuridine after hepatic cytoreduction in 185 patients with unresectable colorectal cancer metastases. Ann Surg Oncol 2002;9:148-155.

176. Welling R, Lamping K: Cryoprobe as a "handle" for resection of metastatic liver tumors. J Surg Oncol 1990;45:227-228.

177. Korpan N: Hepatic cryosurgery for liver metastases. Long-term followup. Ann Surg 1997;225:193.

178. Ravikumar TS, Steele GJ, Kane R, et al: Experimental and clinical observations on hepatic cryosurgery for colorectal metastases. Cancer Res 1991;51:6233-6237.

179. Tandan V, Harmantas A, Gallinger S: Long-term survival after hepatic cryosurgery versus surgical resection for metastatic colorectal carcinoma: A critical review of the literature. Can J Surg 1997;40:175-181.

180. Solbiati L, Ierace T, Tonolini M, Osti V, Cova L: Radiofrequency thermal ablation of hepatic metastases. Eur J Ultrasound 2001;13:149-158.

181. Bilchik AJ, Wood TF, Allegra D, et al: Cryosurgical ablation and radiofrequency ablation for unresectable hepatic malignant neoplasms: A proposed algorithm. Arch Surg 2000;135:657-662; discussion 662-664.

182. Curley SA, Izzo F, Ellis LM, Nicholas V, Vallone P: Radiofrequency ablation of hepatocellular cancer in 110 patients with cirrhosis. Ann Surg 2000;232:381-391.

183. Sugiyama A, Katayama M, Matsuda T, et al: Hepatic arterial infusion chemotherapy combined with hyperthermia for metastatic liver tumors of colorectal cancer. Semin Oncol 1997;24(Suppl 6): 135-138.

184. Sata M, Watanabe Y, Ueda S, et al: Microwave coagulation therapy for hepatocellular carcinoma. Gastroenterology 1996;110: 1507-1514.

185. Livraghi T, Baietta E, Matricardi L, et al: Fine needle percutaneous intratumoral chemotherapy under ultrasound guidance: A feasibility study. Tumori 1986;72:81-87.

186. Suzuki M, Suzuki H, Yamamoto T, et al: Indication of chemoembolization therapy withoutu gelatin sponge for hepatocellular carcinoma. Semin Oncol 1997;24(Suppl 6): 56-110.

187. Shiina S, Imamura M, Obi S, Teratani T, et al: Percutaneous ethanol injection therapy for small hepatocellular carcinoma. Gan to Kagaku Ryoho 1996;23:835-839.

188. Yamamoto K, Masuzawa M, Kato M, et al: Evaluation of combined therapy with chemoembolization and ethanol injection for advanced hepatocellular carcinoma. Semin Oncol 1997;24(Suppl 6):50-55.

189. Marinelli A, de Brauw LM, Beerman H, et al: Isolated liver perfusion with mitomycin C in the treatment of colorectal cancer metastases confined to the liver. Jpn J Clin Oncol 1996;26: 341-350.

190. Van Zuidewign D, de Brauw L, Marinelli A, et al: Isolated liver perfusioni with Mitomycin-C or melphalan in patients with hepatic metastases. Soc Surg Oncol 1993;46:198.

191. Alexander H, Bartlett D, Libutti S, Fraker D, Moser T, Rosenberg S: Isolated hepatic perfusion with tumor necrosis factor and melphalan for unresectable cancers confined to the liver. J Clin Oncol 1998;16:1479–1489.

192. Venook A, Bergsland E, Ring E, et al: Gene therapy of colorectal liver metastases using a recombinant adenovirus encoding wt p53 (SCH 58500) via hepatic artery infusion: A Phase I study [abstract]. Proc Am Soc Clin Oncol 1998;17:431a.

193. Trinh Q, Austin E, Murray D, et al: Enzyme/prodrug gene therapy: Comparison of cytosine deaminase/5-fluorocytosine versus thymidine kinase/ganciclovir enzyme/prodrug systems in a human colorectal carcinoma cell line. Cancer 1995;55:4808–4812.

194. Rubin J, Galanis E, Pitot H, et al: Phase I study of immunotherapy of hepatic metastases of colorectal carcinoma by direct gene transfer of an allogeneic histocompatability antigen, HLA-B7. Gene Therapy 1997;4:419–425.

195. Wills K, Huang W, Harris M, et al: Gene therapy for hepatocellular carcinoma: Chemosensitivity conferred by adenovirus-mediated transfer of the HSV-1 thymidine kinase gene. Cancer Gene Therapy 1995;2:191.

196. Ingold D, Reed G, Kaplan H, Bagshaw M: Radiation hepatitis. Am J Roentgenol 1965;93:200.

197. Ogata K, Hizawa K, Yoshida M, et al: Hepatic injury following irradiation—a morphologic study. Tukushima J Exp Med 1963;9:240.

198. Reed G, Cox A: The human liver after radiation injury. Am J Pathol 1966;48:597–612.

199. Lawrence T, Robertson J, Ensminger W, Anscher M, Jirtle R, Fajardo L: Hepatic toxicity resulting from cancer treatment. Int J Radiat Oncol Biol Phys 1995;31:1237–1248.

200. Jirtle R, Anscher M, Alati T: Radiation sensitivity of the liver. Adv Radiat Biol 1990;14:269–311.

201. Russell AH, Clyde C, Wasserman TH, Turner SS, Rotman M: Accelerated hyperfractionated hepatic irradiation in the management of patients with liver metastases: Results of the RTOG dose escalating protocol. Int J Radiat Oncol Biol Phys 1993;27:117–123.

202. Byfield J, Calabro-Jones P, Klisak I, Kulhanian F. Pharmacologic requirements for obtaining sensitization oif human tumor cells in vitro to combined 5-fluorouracil or ftorafur and x-rays. Int J Radiat Oncol Biol Phys 1982;8:1923–1933.

203. Bruso CE, Shewach DS, Lawrence TS: Fluorodeoxyuridine-induced radiosensitization and inhibition of DNA double strand break repair in human colon cancer cells. Int J Radiat Oncol Biol Phys 1990;19:1411–1417.

204. Heimburger DK, Shewach DS, Lawrence TS: The effect of fluorodeoxyuridine on sublethal damage repair in human colon cancer cells. Int J Radiat Oncol Biol Phys 1991;21:983–987.

205. Witte RS, Cnaan A, Mansour EG, Barylak E, Harris JE, Schutt AJ: Comparison of 5-fluorouracil alone, 5-fluorouracil with levamisole, and 5-fluorouracil with hepatic irradiation in the treatment of patients with residual, nonmeasurable, intra-abdominal metastasis after undergoing resection for colorectal carcinoma. Cancer 2001;91:1020–1028.

206. McCracken J, Weatherall T, Oishi N, Janaki L, Boyer C: Adjuvant intrahepatic chemotherapy with mitomycin and 5-FU combined with hepatic irradiation in high risk patients with carcinoma of the colon: A Southwest Oncology Group Phase II pilot study. Cancer Treat Rep 1985;69:129–131.

207. Haddad E, Le Bourgeois JP, Kuentz M, Lobo P: Liver complications in lymphomas treated with a combination of chemotherapy and radiotherapy: Preliminary results. Int J Radiat Oncol Biol Phys 1983;9:1313–1319.

208. Schacter L, Crum E, Spitzer T, Maksem J, Diwan V, Kolli S: Fatal radiation hepatitis: A case report and review of the literature. Gynecol Oncol 1986;24:373–380.

209. Gray B, Anderson JE, Burton MA, et al: Regression of liver metastases following treatment with yttrium-90 microspheres. Aust N Z J Surg 1992;62:105–110.

210. Tian J, BX X, Zhang J, Dong B, Liang P, Wang X: Ultrasound-guided internal radiotherapy using yttrium-90-glass microspheres for liver malignancies. J Nuclear Med 1996;37:958–963.

211. Stubbs R, Cannan R, Mitchell A: Selective internal radiation therapy (SIRT) with 90Yttrium microspheres for extensive colorectal liver metastases. Hepatogastroenterology 2001;48:333–337.

212. Gray B, Van Hazel G, Hope M, et al: Randomised trial of SIR-Spheres plus chemotherapy vs. chemotherapy alone for treating patients with liver metastases from primary large bowel cancer. Ann Oncol 2001;12:1711–1720.

213. Ho S, Lau W, Leung T, Chan M, Johnson P, Li A: Clinical evaluation of the partition model for estimating radiation doses from yttrium-90 microspheres in the treatment of hepatic cancer. Eur J Nuclear Med 1997;24:293–298.

214. Yorke ED, Jackson A, Fox RA, Wessels BW, Gray BN: Can current models explain the lack of liver complications in Y-90 microsphere therapy? Clin Cancer Res 1999;5:3024s–3030s.

215. Campbell A, Bailey I, Burton M: Tumour dosimetry in human liver following hepatic yttrium-90 microsphere therapy. Phys Med Biol 2001;46:487–498.

216. Leung T, Lau W, Ho S, et al: Radiation pneumonitis after selective internal radiation treatment with intraarterial 90-yttrium-microspheres for inoperable hepatic tumors. Int J Radiat Oncol Biol Phys 1995;33:919–924.

217. Thomas D, Nauta R, Rodgers J, et al: Intraoperative high dose rate interstitial irradiation of hepatic metastases from colorectal carcinoma. Results of a Phase I-II trial. Cancer 1993;71:1977–1981.

218. Donath D, Nori D, Turnbull A, Kaufman N, Fortner J: Brachytherapy in the treatment of solitary colorectal metastases to the liver. J Surg Oncol 1990;44:55–61.

219. Ten Haken R, Lawrence T, McShan D, Tesser R, Fraass B, Lichter A: Technical considerations in the use of 3-D beam arrangements in the abdomen. Radiother Oncol 1991;22:19–28.

220. Lawrence T, Tesser R, Ten Haken R: An application of dose volume histograms to the treatment of intrahepatic malignancies with radiation therapy. Int J Radiat Oncol Biol Phys 1990;19:1041–1047.

221. Robertson JM, Lawrence TS, Walker S, et al: The treatment of colorectal liver metastases with conformal radiation therapy and regional chemotherapy. Int J Radiat Oncol Biol Phys 1995;32:445–450.

222. Mohiuddin M, Chen E, Ahmad J: Combined liver radiation and chemotherapy for palliation of hepatic metastases from colorectal cancer. J Clin Oncol 1996;14:722–728.

223. Dawson LA, McGinn CJ, Normolle D, et al: Escalated focal liver radiation and concurrent hepatic artery fluorodeoxyuridine for unresectable intrahepatic malignancies. J Clin Oncol 2000;18:2210–2218.

224. Blomgren H, Lax I, Naslund I, et al: Stereotactic high dose fraction radiation therapy of extracranial tumors using an accelerator. Clinical experience of the first 31 patients. Acta Oncol 1995;34:861–870.

225. Herfarth KK, Debus J, Lohr F, et al: Stereotactic single-dose radiation therapy of liver tumors: Results of a phase I/II trial. J Clin Oncol 2001;19:164–170.

226. Balter J, Brock K, Litzenberd D, et al: Daily targeting of intrahepatic tumors for radiotherapy. Int J Radiat Oncol Biol Phys 2002;52:266–271.

227. Lyman J: Complication probability as assessed from dose volume histograms. Radiat Res 1985;8(Suppl):513.

228. Niemierko A, Goitein M: Calculation of normal tissue complication probability and dose-volume histogram reduction schemes for tissues with a critical element architecture. Radiother Oncol 1991;20:166.

229. Emami B, Lyman J, Brown A, et al: Tolerance of normal tissue to therapeutic irradiation. Int J Radiat Oncol Biol Phys 1991;21:109.

230. Lawrence TS, Ten Haken RK, Kessler ML, et al: The use of 3-D dose volume analysis to predict radiation hepatitis. Int J Radiat Oncol Biol Phys 1992;23:781–738.

231. McGinn C, Ten Haken R, Ensminger W, et al: The potential superiority of bromodeoxyuridine to iodeoxyuridine as a radiation sensitizer in the treatment of colorectal cancer. Cancer Res 1992;52:3698.

232. Dawson LA, Normolle D, Balter J, et al: Analysis of radiation-induced liver disease using the Lyman NTCP model. Int J Radiat Oncol Biol Phys 2002;53:810–821.

233. Lawrence T, Davis M, Maybaum J, et al: The treatment of intrahepatic cancers with radiation doses based on a normal

tissue complication probability model. J Clin Oncol 1998;16:2246.

234. Robertson J, McGinn C, Walker S, et al: A Phase I trial of hepatic arterial bromodeoxyuridine and conformal radiation therapy for patients with primary hepatobiliary cancers or colorectal liver metastases. Int J Radiat Oncol Biol Phys 1997;39:1087.

235. Symon Z, Levi M, Ensminger W, et al: Selective radioprotection of hepatocytes by systemic and portal vein infusions of amifostine in rat liver model. Int J Radiat Oncol Biol Phys 2001;50:473–478.

236. Scheele J, Stang R, Altendorf-Hofmann A, Paul M: Resection of colorectal liver metastases. World J Surg 1995;19:59–71.

237. Hohenberger P, Schlag P, Schwarz V, Herfarth C: Tumor recurrence and options for further treatment after resection of liver metastases in patients with colorectal cancer. J Surg Oncol 1990;44:245–251.

238. Rees M, Plant G, Bygrave S: Late results justify resection for multiple hepatic metastases from colorectal cancer. Br J Surg 1997;84:1136–1140.

239. Que FG, Nagorney DM: Resection of "recurrent" colorectal metastases to the liver. Br J Surg 1994;81:255–258.

240. Mattsson W, Arwidi A, von Eyben F, et al: Phase II study of combined vincristine, Adriamycin, cyclophosphamide, and methotrexate with citrovorum factor rescue in metastatic breast cancer. Cancer Treat Rep 1977;61:1527.

241. Muss HB, White DR, Richards F 2nd, et al: Adriamycin versus methotrexate in five-drug combination chemotherapy for advanced breast cancer: A randomized trial. Cancer 1978;42:2141–2148.

242. Gabra H, Cameron DA, Lee LE, Mackay J, Leonard RC: Weekly doxorubicin and continuous infusional 5-fluorouracil for advanced breast cancer. Br J Cancer 1996;74:2008–2012.

243. Tranum B, Hoogstraten B, Kennedy A, et al: Adriamycin in combination for the treatment of breast cancer: A Southwest Oncology Group study. Cancer 1978;41:2078–2083.

244. Jones SE, Durie BG, Salmon SE: Combination chemotherapy with adriamycin and cyclophosphamide for advanced breast cancer. Cancer 1975;36:90–97.

245. Chauvergne J, Gary-Bobo J, Klein T, et al: Polychemotherapy of advanced breast cancer. Triple combination with doxorubicin. Analysis of 209 observation. Bull Cancer 1977;64:667–680.

246. Russell JA, Baker JW, Dady PJ, et al: Combination chemotherapy of metastatic breast cancer with vincristine adriamycin and prednisolone. Cancer 1978;41:396–399.

247. Smalley RV, Carpenter J, Bartolucci A, Vogel C, Krauss S: A comparison of cyclophosphamide, adriamycin, 5-fluorouracil (CAF) and cyclophosphamide, methotrexate, 5-fluorouracil, vincristine, prednisone (CMFVP) in patients with metastatic breast cancer: A Southeastern Cancer Study Group project. Cancer 1977;40:625–632.

248. Canellos GP, Pocock SJ, Taylor SG 3rd, Sears ME, Klaasen DJ, Band PR: Combination chemotherapy for metastatic breast carcinoma. Prospective comparison of multiple drug therapy with L-phenylalanine mustard. Cancer 1976;38:1882–1886.

249. Millward M, Harris A, Cantwell B: Phase II study of doxorubicin plus ifosfamide/mesna in patients with advanced breast cancer. Cancer 1990;65:2421.

250. Airoldi M, Cattel L, Pedani F, et al: Clinical and pharmacokinetic data of a docetaxel-epirubicin combination in metastatic breast cancer. Breast Cancer Res Treat 2001;70:185–195.

251. Wada T, Nishiyama K, Nakatani Y, et al: CAF versus CAF plus Medroxyprogesterone Acetate for Treatment of Liver Metastases of Breast Cancer. Breast Cancer 1995;2:65–70.

252. Franks CR: Adriamycin and methotrexate in metastatic gastric cancer: A pilot study. Clin Oncol 1980;6:309–315.

253. Bitran JD, Desser RK, Kozloff MF, Billings AA, Shapiro CM: Treatment of metastatic pancreatic and gastric adenocarcinomas with 5- fluorouracil, adriamycin, and mitomycin C (FAM). Cancer Treat Rep 1979;63:2049–2051.

254. Gastrointestinal TSG: Phase II-III chemotherapy studies in advanced gastric cancer. Cancer Treat Rep 1979;63:1871.

255. Macdonald JS, Kisner DF, Smythe T, Woolley PV, Smith L Jr, Schein PS: 5-Fluorouracil (5-FU), methyl-CCNU, and vincristine in the treatment of advanced colorectal cancer: Phase II study utilizing weekly 5-FU. Cancer Treat Rep 1976;60:1597–1600.

256. Seligman M, Bukowski R, Groppe C, et al: Chemotherapy of metastatic gastrointestinal neoplasms with 5-fluorouracil and streptozotocin. Cancer Treat Rep 1977;61:1374.

257. Bunn PA Jr, Nugent JL, Ihde DC, Cohen MH, Eddy JL, Minna JD: 5-fluorouracil, methyl-CCNU, adriamycin, and mitomycin C in the treatment of advanced gastric cancer. Cancer Treat Rep 1978;62:1287–1293.

258. Wagner D, Yap S, Wobbes T, et al: Phase II trial of 5-flourouracil, Adriamycin and cisplatin (FAP) in advanced gastric cancer. Cancer Cheomother Pharmacol 1985;15:86.

259. Preusser P, Wilke H, Achterrath W, et al: Phase II study with the combination etoposide, doxorubicin, and cisplatin in advanced measurable gastric cancer. J Clin Oncol 1989;7:1310–1317.

260. Levi JA, Fox RM, Tattersall MH, Woods RL, Thomson D, Gill G: Analysis of a prospectively randomized comparison of doxorubicin versus 5-fluorouracil, doxorubicin, and BCNU in advanced gastric cancer: implications for future studies. J Clin Oncol 1986;4:1348–1355.

261. Pazdur R, Ajani JA, Winn R, et al: A phase II trial of 5-fluorouracil and recombinant alpha-2a-interferon in previously untreated metastatic gastric carcinoma. Cancer 1992;69:878–882.

262. Wilke H, Preusser P, Fink U, et al: Preoperative chemotherapy in locally advanced and nonresectable gastric cancer: A phase II study with etoposide, doxorubicin, and cisplatin. J Clin Oncol 1989;7:1318–1326.

263. Lerner A, Gonin R, Steele GD Jr, Mayer RJ: Etoposide, doxorubicin, and cisplatin chemotherapy for advanced gastric adenocarcinoma: Results of a phase II trial. J Clin Oncol 1992;10:536–540.

264. Webb A, Cunningham D, Scarffe JH, et al: Randomized trial comparing epirubicin, cisplatin, and fluorouracil versus fluorouracil, doxorubicin, and methotrexate in advanced esophagogastric cancer. J Clin Oncol 1997;15:261–267.

265. Baker L, Talley R, Maiter R, et al: Phase III comparison of the treatment of advanced gastrointestinal cancer with bolus weekly 5-FU vs methyl CCNU plus bolus weekly 5-FU. Cancer 1976;38:1.

266. Grage T, Vassilopoulos P, Shingleton W, et al: Results of a prospective randomized study of hepatic artery infusion with 5-fluorouracil vs intravenous 5-fluorouracil in patients with hepatic metastases from colorectal cancer: A Central Oncology Group study. Surgery 1979;86:550–555.

267. Buyroker T, Kim P, Groppe C, et al: 5FU infision with methyl-CCNU in the treatment of advanced colon cancer. Cancer 1978;42:1228.

268. Kemeny N, Yagoda A, Braun DJ, Golbey R: A randomized study of two different schedules of methyl CCNU, 5-FU and vincristine for metastatic colorectal carcinoma. Cancer 1979;43:78–81.

269. Kemeny N, Younes A, Seiter K, et al: Combination fluorouracil (FU) and recombinant alpha-interferon (Ifn) in advanced colorectal carcinoma: Activity but significant toxicity. Cancer 1990;66:2470–2475.

270. Ehrlichman C, Fine S, Wong A, Elhakim T: Randomized trial of fluorouracil and folinic acid in patients with metastatic colorectal carcinoma. J Clin Oncol 1988;6:469–475.

271. Conti J, Kemeny N, Saltz L, et al: Irinotecan is an active agent in untreated patients with metastatic colorectal cancer. J Clin Oncol 1996;14:709–715.

272. Tandon R, Bunnell I, Copper R: The treatment of metastatic carcinoma of the liver by percutaneous selective hepatic artery infusion of 5-fluorouracil. Surgery 1973;73:118.

273. Ansfield FJ, Ramirez G, Davis HLJ, et al: Further clinical studies with intrahepatic arterial infusion with 5-fluorouracil. Cancer 1975;36:2413–2417.

274. Watkins EJ, Khazei A, Nahra K: Surgical basis for arterial infusion chemotherapy of disseminated carcinoma of the liver. Surg Gynecol Obstet 1970;130:581.

275. Cady B, Oberfield R: Regional infusion chemotherapy of hepatic metastases from carcinoma of the colon. Am J Surg 1974;127:220.

276. Smiley S, Schouten J, Chang A, et al: Intrahepatic arterial infusion with 5-FU for liver metastases of colorectal carcinoma. Proc ASCO 1981;22:391.

277. Denck H: Ergebnisse einer intraarteriellen intermittierenden Chemotherapie mit 5-FUbei metastasenleber sowie inoperablen tumoren des gastrointestinal und urogenitaltrakts. Onkologie 1984;7:167–176.

278. Rougier P, Laser P, Elias D, et al: Intraarterial hepatic chemotherapy

(IAHC) for liver metastases (LM) from colorectal (CR) origin [abstract]. Proc ASCO 1987;6:369.

279. Arai Y, Inaba Y, Takeuchi Y, Ariyoshi Y: Intermittent hepatic arterial infusion of high-dose 5FU on a weekly schedule for liver metastases from colorectal cancer. Cancer Chemother Pharmacol 1997;40:526–530.

280. Niederhuber J, Ensminger W, Gyves J, et al: Regional chemotherapy of colorectal cancer metastatic to the liver. Cancer 1984;53:1336.

281. Balch CM, Urist MM: Intra-arterial chemotherapy for colorectal liver metastases and hepatomas using a totally implantable drug infusion pump. Recent Results Cancer Res 1986;100:123–147.

282. Kemeny N, Daly J, Oderman P, et al: Hepatic artery pump infusion toxicity and results in patients with metastatic colorectal carcinoma. J Clin Oncol 1984;2:595–600.

283. Shepard K, Levin B, Karl R, et al: Therapy for metastatic colorectal cancer with hepatic artery infusion chemotherapy using a subcutaneous implanted pump. J Clin Oncol 1985;3:161.

284. Cohen A, Kaufman S, Wood W, et al: Regional hepatic chemotherapy using an implantable drug infusion pump. Am J Surg 1983;145:529–533.

285. Weiss G, Garnick M, Osteen R, et al: Long-term arterial infusion of 5-fluorouracil for liver metastases using an implantable infusion pump. J Clin Oncol 1983;1:337–344.

286. Schwartz S, Jones L, McCune C: Assessment of treatment of intrahepatic malignancies using chemotherapy via an implantable pump. Ann Surg 1985;201:560–567.

287. Johnson L, Wasserman P, Rivkin S: FUDR hepatic arterial infusion via an implantable pump for treatment of hepatic tumors. Proc ASCO 1983;2:119.

288. Kemeny N, Daly J, Reichman B, et al: Intrahepatic or systemic infusion of fluorodeoxyuridine in patients with liver metastases from colorectal carcinoma—a randomized trial. Ann Intern Med 1987;107:459–467.

289. Niederhuber J: Arterial chemotherapy for metastatic colorectal cancer in the liver. Giessen, West Germany, Conference on Advances in Regional Cancer Therapy, 1985.

290. Lorenz M, Muller HH: Randomized, multicenter trial of fluorouracil plus leucovorin administered either via hepatic arterial or intravenous infusion versus fluorodeoxyuridine administered via hepatic arterial infusion in patients with nonresectable liver metastases from colorectal carcinoma. J Clin Oncol 2000;18:243–254.

291. Cortesi E, Capussotti L, DiTora P, et al: Bolus vs continuous hepatic arterial infusion of cisplatin plus intravenous 5-fluorouracil chemotherapy for unresectable colorectal metastases. Dis Colon Rectum 1994;37:S138–S143.

292. Sugihara K: Continuous hepatic arterial infusion of 5-fluorouracil for unresectable colorectal liver metastases: Phase II study. Surgery 1995;117:624–628.

293. Kerr D, Ledermann J, McArdle C, et al: Phase I clinical and pharmacokinetic study of leucovorin and infusional hepatic arterial fluorouracil. J Clin Oncol 1995;13:2968–2972.

294. Howell JD, McArdle CS, Kerr DJ, et al: A phase II study of regional 2-weekly 5-fluorouracil infusion with intravenous folinic acid in the treatment of colorectal liver metastases. Br J Cancer 1997;76:1390–1393.

295. Patt Y, Hoque A, Lozano R, et al: Phase II trial of hepatic arterial infusion of fluorouracil and recombinant human interferon alfa-2b for liver metastases of colorectal cancer refractory to systemic fluorouracil and leucovorin. J Clin Oncol 1997;15:1432–1438.

296. Borner M, Laffer U, Ludwig C, et al: Effectiveness and low toxicity of hepatic artery iinfusion with fluorouracil and mitomycin for metastatic colorectal cancer confined to the liver. From the Swiss Group for Clinical and Epidemiological Cancer Research (SAKK). Ann Oncol 1990;1:227–228.

297. Fraschini G, Charngangavej C, Carrasco C, et al: Percutaneous hepatic arterial infusion of cisplatin-vinblastine for refractory cancer metastatic to the liver. Am J Clin Oncol 1988;11:34–38.

298. Estape J, Daniels M, Vinolas N, et al: Combination chemotherapy with oral etoposide plus intravenous cyclophosphamide in liver metastases of breast cancer. Amer J Clin Oncol 1990;13:98–100.

299. Fraschini G, Flesihman G, Charnsangavej C, et al: Continuous 5-day infusion of vinblastine for percutaneous hepatic arterial chemotherapy for metastatic breast cancer. Cancer Treat Rep 1987;71:1001–1005.

300. Fraschini G, Fleishman G, Yap H-Y, et al: Percutaneous hepatic arterial infusion of cisplatin for metastatic breast cancer. Cancer Treat Rep 1987;71:313–315.

301. Maral J, Baumer R, Curet P, et al: Intra-arterial chemotherapy for liver metastases of colon and breast cancer [abstract]. Stockholm, Third European Conference on Clinical Oncology and Cancer Nursing, 1985.

302. Arai Y, Sone Y, Inaba Y, Ariyoshi Y, Kido C: Hepatic arterial infusion chemotherapy for liver metastases from breast cancer. Cancer Chemother Pharmacol 1994;33(Suppl):142–144.

303. Tada A, Ogawa M, Ingaki J, et al: Arterial infusion of combination chemotherapy consisting of adriamycin and mitomycin-C for liver metastases of breast cancer. Gan to Kagaku ryoho (Tokyo) 1986;13:70–74.

304. Maton P, Camilleri M, Griffin G, et al: Role of hepatic arterial embolization in the carcinoid syndrome. BMJ 1983;287:932–935.

305. Borgelt B, Belber R, Brady L, et al: The palliation of hepatic metastases: Results of the Radiation Therapy Oncology Group pilot study. Int J Radiat Oncol Biol Phys 1981;7:587.

306. Leibel S, Pajak T, Massullo V, et al: A comparison of misonidazole sensitized radiation therapy to radiation therapy alone for the palliation of hepatic metastases: Results of a Radiation Therapy Oncology Group randomized prospective trial. Int J Radiat Oncol Biol Phys 1987;7:1057.

307. Phillips R, Karnofsky D, Hamilton L, Nickson J: Roentgen therapy of hepatic metastases. Am J Roentgenol 1954;71:826.

308. Prasad B, Lee MS, Hendrickson FR: Irradiation of hepatic metastases. Int J Radiat Oncol Biol Phys 1977;2:129–132.

309. Ajlouni MI, Merrick HW, Skeel RT, Dobelbower RR Jr: Concomitant radiation therapy and constant infusion FUdR for unresectable hepatic metastases. Am J Clin Oncol 1990;13:532–535.

310. Byfield J, Barone R, Frankel S, Sharp T: Treatment with combined intraarterial 5-FUdR infusion and whole liver radiation for colon metastatic to the liver. Am J Clin Oncol 1984;7:319.

311. Friedman M, Cassidy M, Levine M, Phillips T, Spivack S, Resser KJ: Combined modality therapy of hepatic metastasis. Northern California Oncology Group Pilot Study. Cancer 1979;44:906–913.

312. Herbsman H, Hassan A, Gardner B, et al: Treatment of hepatic metastases with a combination of hepatic artery infusion chemotherapy and external radiotherapy. Surg Gynecol Obstet 1978;147:13–17.

313. Lawrence T, Dworzanin L, Walker-Andrews S, et al: Treatment of cancers involving the liver and porta hepatis with external beam irradiation and intraarterial hepatic fluorodeoxyuridine. Int J Radiat Oncol Biol Physiol 1990;20:555–561.

314. Lokich J, Kinsella T, Perri J, Malcolm A, Clouse M: Concomitant hepatic radiation and intraarterial fluorinated pyrimidine therapy: Correlation of liver scan, liver function tests, and plasma CEA with tumor response. Cancer 1981;48:2569–2574.

315. Raju PI, Maruyama Y, DeSimone P, MacDonald J: Treatment of liver metastases with a combination of chemotherapy and hyperfractionated external radiation therapy. Am J Clin Oncol 1987;10:41–43.

316. Rotman M, Kuruvilla AM, Choi K, et al: Response of colorectal hepatic metastases to concomitant radiotherapy and intravenous infusion 5 fluorouracil. Int J Radiat Oncol Biol Phys 1986;12:2179–2187.

317. Sherman DM, Weichselbaum R, Order SE, Cloud L, Trey C, Piro AJ: Palliation of hepatic metastasis. Cancer 1978;41:2013–2017.

318. Webber BM, Soderberg CH Jr, Leone LA, Rege VB, Glicksman AS: A combined treatment approach to management of hepatic metastasis. Cancer 1978;42:1087–1095.

319. Wiley AL Jr, Wirtanen GW, Stephenson JA, Ramirez G, Demets D, Lee JW: Combined hepatic artery 5-fluorouracil and irradiation of liver metastases. A randomized study. Cancer 1989;64:1783–1789.

320. Volberding PA, Friedman MA, Resser KJ, Phillips TL: Therapy of liver tumors metastatic from colorectal cancer with whole-liver radiation combined with 5-FU, adriamycin, and methotrexate. Cancer Chemother Pharmacol 1982;9:17–21.

60

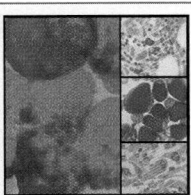

EFFUSIONS

Alexander I. Spira

Julie R. Brahmer

SUMMARY OF KEY POINTS

MALIGNANT PLEURAL EFFUSION

Background
- Common complication of cancer
- Frequently seen with breast and lung cancers and lymphoma
- Often asymptomatic

Incidence
- Presenting sign of malignancy in about one-half of patients who develop an effusion
- Approximately 40 cases of malignant pleural effusion are diagnosed for every 10,000 hospital admissions

Diagnosis
- Exudative effusions (high protein, LDH, or cholesterol) are very concerning for malignancy
- Cytology is the gold standard
- Pleural biopsy rarely adds information beyond that seen in other studies
- If an exudative effusion exists but is undiagnosed by other means, video-assisted thorascopic surgery (VATS) should be used for evaluation of the pleura

Evaluation
- Cytology should be evaluated by an experienced pathologist
- Low pH (<7.3) is associated with burden of disease, less likelihood of response to pleurodesis, and decreased survival
- Patient should be assessed for symptoms of dyspnea and survival probability (less than one to three months or not)

Treatment
- Asymptomatic effusions can be monitored
- Systemic chemotherapy can be effective in stable patients
- For patients symptomatic from their effusions, effective options include systemic therapy for patients with very responsive disease (e.g., hematologic malignancies, germ cell

tumors, breast cancer, small cell lung cancer) or repeated thoracentesis
- For patients requiring frequent thoracentesis or who rapidly redevelop effusions, options include:
  - Pleurodesis with talc (favored), doxycycline, or bleomycin
  - Pleurodesis with placement of a drainage catheter only
  - VATS with mechanical abrasion
  - Open surgical procedure in highly selected patients
- For patients refractory to pleurodesis, options include Denver-type drainage catheter or clinical trial

MALIGNANT PERICARDIAL EFFUSION

Background
- Less common complication of cancer than pleural effusion or ascites
- Frequently seen with breast and lung cancers and lymphoma
- Size of effusion does not correlate with symptoms; rather, acuity of collection and compliance of pericardium are most associated with tamponade physiology
- Often a preterminal event
- Tumors metastatic to pericardium often seen at autopsy in patients with advanced cancer

Incidence
- Found in 2%–30% of patients with cancer at autopsy
- Only about 10%–20% of patients with pericardial metastases develop tamponade

Diagnosis
- Cytology is the gold standard but not very sensitive
- Patients should be carefully evaluated for other causes, particularly those with other comorbidities or history of mediastinal or cardiac irradiation

Evaluation
- Cytology should be evaluated by an experienced pathologist
- Pericardial biopsy could be required if cytology is negative
- Patients should be evaluated for clinical signs of cardiac tamponade (hypotension, signs of low cardiac output, abnormal pulsus paradoxus)
- ECG should be evaluated for low voltages and electrical alternans
- Echocardiogram should be obtained for all patients

Treatment
- Asymptomatic effusions can be monitored
- Systemic chemotherapy might be effective for stable patients, even those with solid tumors
- Those with hypotension/clinical instability should proceed to emergent pericardiocentesis. Pericardial drainage catheters should be placed. There is a high likelihood of fluid recurrence with drainage only
- Stable patients requiring drainage should undergo subxiphoid pericardiostomy, which is a more definitive procedure
- Open procedures or pericardial sclerosis, usually with bleomycin, should be saved for refractory patients

MALIGNANT ASCITES

Background
- Common complication of cancer
- Frequently seen with ovarian cancer (most common cause), gastrointestinal malignancies, and carcinoma of unknown primary
- Survival is often poor but a distinct subset (i.e., those with ovarian cancer) might benefit with moderate long-term survival
- Rarely life-threatening

SUMMARY OF KEY POINTS—cont'd

Incidence
- Accounts for approximately 10% of all patients with ascites
- Often (about 50% of the time) can be a presenting feature of malignancy

Diagnosis
- Effusions with low serum-to-ascites-albumin gradient (SAAG) concerning for malignancy rather than portal hypertension
- Cytology is the gold standard
- Cross-sectional imaging (i.e., computed tomography scan) could demonstrate a primary malignancy
- Women with only ascites and no identifiable primary should undergo laparoscopy with biopsies for

evaluation of potential ovarian cancer

Evaluation
- Cytology should be evaluated by an experienced pathologist
- Patient should be assessed for symptoms and likely response to systemic chemotherapy

Treatment
- Asymptomatic effusions can be monitored
- Systemic chemotherapy is effective for many patients, particularly women with ovarian cancer. These patients should be treated with aggressive surgical debulking

- Intraperitoneal chemotherapy should be considered if easily available or on clinical trial
- For patients symptomatic from their effusions, effective options include:
  - Diuresis with spironolactone/furosemide; not very effective in most patients except for those with ascites due to portal hypertension from extensive hepatic metastases
  - Repeated paracentesis as needed
  - Patients with moderate long-term survival can be considered for either percutaneous tunneled drainage catheter or peritoneovenous shunt

MALIGNANT PLEURAL EFFUSIONS

A malignant pleural effusion is a common complication of cancer and is encountered frequently by oncologists and other physicians caring for such patients. Their effects can range from causing no symptoms whatsoever to being markedly symptomatic, and treatments must be tailored appropriately.

Collections of pleural fluid are likely to be directly related to tumor involvement of the pleura. For the patient with cancer, diagnostic accuracy in the assessment of pleural effusion is of the utmost importance. In many instances, the existence of a malignant pleural effusion drastically alters the treatment modalities that a patient will ultimately undergo; likewise, it drastically alters the likelihood of curing a patient with cancer. Nevertheless, many patients with cancer might have undergone surgery, have had radiation, or have other possible reasons for an effusion; there could, therefore, be alternative, benign reasons for an accumulation of pleural fluid. With this in mind, it is important to determine the appropriate cause of an effusion to provide optimal care.

Etiology and Pathogenesis

The Pleural Space

The pleural space is a real space completely surrounding the lung up to the hilar root; the visceral pleura covers the lung and interlobar fissures, and the parietal pleura covers the chest wall, diaphragm, and mediastinum. The small amount of normal physiologic pleural fluid allows transmission of the breathing effort from the lung to the chest wall, thereby allowing respiration to occur.[1] With the aid of a lavage technique in humans, each normal lung has been found to have approximately 0.13 mL pleural fluid/kg body mass (about 7 mL per lung).[2]

Pleural fluid appears to originate from systemic (i.e., not pulmonary) vessels in the pleural membranes and is reabsorbed by either pleural microvessels or lymphatics. Pleural fluid turnover is approximately 0.15 mL/kg/hr. Lymphatics tend to absorb the protein, while capillaries absorb fluid. Under normal conditions, the body is highly efficient in controlling the amount of pleural fluid present; a tenfold increase in the production rate of fluid results in only a 15% increase in pleural fluid volume.[3] With a turnover rate of greater than one pleural fluid volume per hour, a large amount of fluid flows through the pleural space daily.

Fluid Regulation

Fluid dynamics are governed mainly by the Starling equation, which is a measure of water flow out of the vessel balanced by resorption. This is shown in equation 1:

$$\text{Flow} = k \times [(P_{hyd} - P_{if}) - (O_{cap} - O_{if})] \qquad \text{(Eq. 1)}$$

where k = permeability constant; P_{hyd} = hydrostatic pressure of the capillary; P_{if} = hydrostatic pressure of the interstitial fluid; O_{cap} = oncotic pressure of the capillary; and O_{if} = oncotic pressure of the interstitial fluid.

The driving pressure (P_d) of fluid across a capillary is defined by the difference in pressures, Flow/k, as shown in equation 2:

$$P_d = [(P_{hyd} - P_{if}) - (O_{cap} - O_{if})] \qquad \text{(Eq. 2)}$$

Normally, there is equilibrium between flow into (entry) and out of (exit) the pleural space, leading to only a small, physiologic volume. Increased fluid entry into the pleural space can be a result of any of the following:

- Increase in permeability of the endothelial barriers (shown as k).
- Increase in microvascular pressure (P_{hyd} in the preceding equation), such as occurs with congestive heart

failure (CHF). Pulmonary capillary wedge pressure (PCWP) has the strongest correlation with the incidence of effusion in CHF.[4]

- Decrease in pleural pressure, which can happen with atelectasis or trapped lung. This indirectly affects P_{if}.
- Decrease in plasma oncotic pressure (affecting O_{cap}), such as occurs in conditions causing hypoproteinemia, usually due to hypoalbuminemia. Although this causation has a sound theoretical basis, it is rare that isolated hypoalbuminemia brings about a pleural effusion.[5]

Mechanisms of decreased fluid exit can include any of the following:

- Cytokine-mediated lymphatic constriction, which can result from conditions such as infection or tumor. This also can affect fluid entry by altering k, the permeability constant.
- Damage to lymphatics from drugs (e.g., chemotherapy), radiation, or surgery (e.g., ligation of the thoracic duct).[6]
- Involvement of the lymphatics by malignancy.
- Increase in systemic venous pressure, which is reflected as an elevated right atrial pressure. Although this is a reflection of overall volume status, it does not correlate as well with the incidence of pleural effusion as does the PCWP. Pulmonary emboli (PE), an example of an event that causes isolated elevations in right atrial pressure without affecting the volume of the left side of the heart and PCWP (it often decreases the PCWP), rarely cause pleural effusions that arise simply from increased venous pressure.[4] Effusions that arise from PE usually are cytokine mediated.

Malignant effusions are caused by both increased entry and decreased exit of fluid. Increased fluid entry appears to be the principal abnormality, however, as there are multiple pathways and channels of fluid resorption. Because of this, one can, in part, physiologically determine which mechanism is primarily responsible for the creation of an effusion. For example, among patients whose effusion reaccumulates rapidly after drainage, it is likely that the patient has mainly an increased production of fluid. Patients with mainly exit blocks do exist, however. It is important to keep such patients in mind, as they are more likely to have transudative effusions (see the discussions that follow). Exit blocks probably account for the small number of patients (5%–10%) with a malignant effusion that appears as a transudate upon analysis.[7] In evaluating the cause of an effusion, it is helpful to classify effusions according to their mechanism (Table 60-1).

The molecular biology of pleural effusions has begun to be understood, with vascular endothelial growth factor (VEGF) emerging as a major role player.[8] Because it induces endothelial vasodilation and enhances the permeability of the mesothelium 50,000 times more potently than histamine, VEGF is thought to be a major, if not the most important, cytokine in the etiology of effusions.[9-12] It might one day be part of the diagnostic evaluation of effusions. Novel approaches that use anti-VEGF mechanisms will likely be evaluated once this is better understood.[13,14]

TABLE 60-1

Differential Diagnosis of Pleural Effusion by Mechanism

Increased Permeability of Capillaries/Lymphatics

Malignancy
  Metastatic malignancy
  Intrathoracic malignancy (lung cancer)
  Malignant mesothelioma
Infection
  Bacterial, viral, fungal, mycobacterial, mycoplasmal, parasitic empyema
Pulmonary embolism
Connective tissue disorders
Drug induced (nitrofurantoin, procarbazine, amiodarone)
Esophageal rupture
Pancreatitis
Uremia
Postradiation
Collagen vascular disorders
  Rheumatoid arthritis, systemic lupus erythematosis, Wegener's granulomatosis, polyarteritis nodosa, Churg-Strauss syndrome
Dressler's syndrome (post myocardial infarction syndrome)
Subdiaphramatic abcess
Systemic capillary leak syndrome/adult respiratory distress syndrome
Vascular trauma
Postsurgical (including thoracic and abdominal surgeries)
Sarcoid
Yellow-nail syndrome
Myxedema

Increased Venous Hydrostatic Pressure

Congestive heart failure
Superior vena cava syndrome
Massive pulmonary embolism

Increased Lymphatic Pressure

Malignancy
Metastatic malignancy
Lymphoma
Sarcoidosis
Chylothorax
Post lymph node irradiation
Meig's syndrome
Peritoneal dialysis

Decreased Oncotic Pressure

Hypoalbuminemia (often from cancer cachexia)
Hypoproteinemia
Cirrhosis
Nephrotic syndrome
Glomerulonephritis

Altered Intrapleural Dynamics

Trapped lung (infection, malignancy)
Atelectasis

Incidence

More than a million pleural effusions occur each year, with about one-half arising from congestive heart failure. About one-fifth of effusions are malignant, but malignancy is the most common cause of symptomatic effusions. Underreporting in most series might also be a significant issue.[15] The causes of malignant pleural effusions are shown in Table 60-2 and reflect the incidence of cancers in general, with lung and breast cancers at the top of the list.[16-23]

TABLE 60-2

Malignant Neoplasms Associated with Pleural Effusion*

CAUSE	NO.	(%)
Total malignant effusions	1,283	(100)
Lung cancer	450	(35)
Breast cancer	256	(20)
Lymphomas and leukemia	256	(20)
Unknown primary (adenocarcinoma)	154	(12)
Unknown primary (all types)	95	(7)
Reproductive tract	70	(5)
Gastrointestinal tract	90	(7)
Genitourinary tract	66	(5)
All other	39	(3)

*Includes causes of malignant effusion each less than 1%: endocrine, head and neck cancer, mesothelioma, soft tissue sarcoma, bone cancer, and myeloma.

Diagnosis and Evaluation of a Pleural Effusion

Pleural effusions are apparent on a chest x-ray when a volume of 200 mL or greater of fluid is present.[24] In evaluating a patient with an pleural effusion of unknown etiology that is potentially malignant, Hausheer and Yarbro[25] have divided patients into four potential groups for purposes of establishing a diagnosis, based upon what is known about the patients' medical histories and initial clinical findings:

- Patients with a history of malignancy who develop an effusion
- Patients with no history of malignancy, condition, sign, or symptom that provides a clue to the etiology of their effusion
- Patients for whom diagnosis is not made by the usual approach and evaluation and for which more complicated and in-depth evaluations of their effusions are required
- Patients with clinical and historical reasons to suggest malignant pleural mesothelioma

Most patients in an oncologist's care fit into the first group. This first group can be subdivided into patients with clear advanced disease and very likely malignant pleural effusion and patients who have a history of malignancy but in whom the effusions might or might not be malignant. Among patients with advanced cancer, there is often no question as to whether the effusion is directly related to the malignancy, or the question is unimportant in terms of the patient's overall clinical management. In such a case, one can simply observe the patient unless he or she is symptomatic. For the patient in which an effusion *could* be malignant, however, accurate diagnosis becomes imperative for patient care and management, and one must consider all alternative causes in the etiology of the effusion. These include the possibility of other coexisting illnesses (e.g., CHF, infection), consequences of treating a prior malignancy (e.g., sequelae of prior surgery, radiation, or chemotherapy), and

the possibility that the effusion is indeed malignant. Most locally advanced solid-tumor malignancies will be downgraded to an incurable stage if the effusion is malignant, and thus treatments and goals of treatment will become dramatically different. In some cases, however, such as for childhood tumors (e.g., Ewing's sarcoma) or germ cell tumors, patients might remain curable but treatment plans can become radically different. Hematologic malignancies (e.g., lymphomas) might be upstaged, and this step might or might not affect the planned treatments. Lung cancer, the most common etiology of malignant effusions, can cause effusions both via direct involvement of pleura by tumor (e.g., increased fluid production according to the model previously discussed) and by decreased exit (lymphatic blockage). Patients with non–small cell lung cancer and transudative effusions on multiple evaluations of their pleural fluid are, in fact, considered early stage and are usually treated with curative intent, as if the effusion were caused by lymphatic blockage and not direct involvement of the pleura. Those with exudative effusions are considered to have advanced disease, even if malignant cells cannot be found, and are treated in a palliative manner. Patients with small cell lung cancer with exudative effusions are considered to be "extensive stage" because the field cannot be covered in a single, tolerable radiation port; and so they are also treated in a palliative manner with chemotherapy alone. Patients with other nonmalignant clinical reasons for effusions (e.g., large amount of ascites and cirrhosis, CHF, advanced malignancy) may be observed, but the physician should have a low threshold for reevaluation should clinical conditions change (e.g., a new fever or new shortness of breath) or if the effusion fails to resolve with appropriate measures.[26]

History and Physical Examination

Patients with pleural effusions usually present with dyspnea, chest pain, cough, orthopnea, or pleuritic chest pain. Other symptoms, such as hemoptysis, fever, and dysphagia, might also occur but are less common. Physical examination usually demonstrates dullness to percussion, decreased or absent breath sounds, and absence of fremitus. Due to atelectasis of adjacent lung, one can often hear crackles at the superior borders of the effusion. Both sides should be listened to equally to determine whether the effusion is unilateral or bilateral; bilateral, symmetric effusions might be more associated with volume overload states such as CHF, although this is a nonspecific finding. The exam should also pay attention to signs of systemic infection or other clues about the etiology of the effusion.

Radiologic Evaluation

The use of a chest x-ray to evaluate a suspected pleural effusion is the most valuable and easiest tool. Lateral views should be obtained along with posterioanterior (PA) views, as the latter miss up to 500 mL of fluid hidden behind the dome of the diaphragm. At least 75 mL of fluid is needed to obscure the posterior costophrenic angle; up to 175 mL of fluid is needed to obscure the lateral costophrenic angle. If the effusion reaches the fourth rib, 1000 mL is present; as little as 10 mL can be seen on a decubitus film. In terms of sampling for thoracentesis, a general rule of thumb is that an effusion that is thicker than 1 cm on a decubitus film is large enough for sampling by thoracentesis.[27-29] Computed tomography (CT) scanning is even more accurate in detecting small effusions, including as little as 2 mL of fluid. The volume of the fluid present can best be determined radiographically by using three-dimensional reconstruction and measuring the volume.[30] Neither magnetic resonance imaging (MRI) nor CT scan can distinguish transudates from exudates accurately, although both can be helpful in evaluating the pleural contents for masses, nodules, and pleural-based thickening once the fluid is removed.[31] Ultrasound is certainly useful for evaluating an effusion and as a guide during thoracentesis and might be able to distinguish an exudate (echogenic) from a tranduate (anechoic), although not in a definitive manner.[32]

Thoracentesis

Among patients with an effusion that requires evaluation, the x-ray should be evaluated to determine whether the effusion is loculated. If the effusion is not free-flowing on the decubitus film and is therefore loculated, or if the volume insufficient to attempt a safe, unguided thoracentesis, ultrasound guidance should be employed[33,34] When obtaining fluid, samples should be collected into tubes containing heparin to prevent clot formation; cloudy fluids should be centrifuged before the analysis described shortly.[35] Relative contraindications to thoracentesis include a skin infection at the site of needle insertion, an abnormal coagulation profile (PT or PTT >1.8 times normal, platelets <25,000/mm^3, or creatinine >6 mg/dL), or uneasiness of the operator in performing the procedure.[36] Mechanical ventilation does not appear to increase the risk of pneumothorax, but there could be a higher likelihood of developing a tension physiology if a pneumothorax does occur.[37-40] Complications of the procedure include pain, bleeding (hemothorax or hematoma), infection, splenic or hepatic laceration, seeding of the needle tract with tumor, or, most commonly, pneumothorax.[41] Studies show that in thoracenteses performed by trained physicians, pneumothoracies occur approximately 10% of the time, with a much higher rate when performed by trainees.[26,40,42] Small pneumothoracies can be observed in nonventilated patients, while larger ones might require chest-tube decompression. Although chest x-ray is often obtained after thoracentesis, it is not required for patients who are clinically asymptomatic after the procedure (absence of cough, chest pain, shortness of breath, and a normal lung exam), who do not experience aspiration of air, and for whom only one needle pass was used during the procedure.[43-45] The use of a therapeutic thoracentesis is discussed shortly.

Evaluation of Fluid: Transudates and Exudates

Fluids are classified as either transudates or exudates. Transudates arise from a disturbance in the hydrostatic or colloid forces (see Starling's equation, Eq. 1) across a barrier and have low protein and cellular contents. By definition, this is a noninflammatory process without pleural disease. A classic example of a transudative effusion is one due to CHF. Transudates may be thought of as volume overload states, and, in general, they are easily identified because of other medical conditions and are benign. Exudates, on the other hand, are formed by active secretion, inflammation, leakage, or permeability of a lymphovascular barrier and have a high cellular or protein content. They have a broader list of potential causes, can be more serious in their effects, and mandate a more thorough evaluation. In reality, most effusions that will be referred to an oncologist will be exudative in nature, as transudative effusions often present with a known systemic disease—for example, heart failure, cirrhosis, or nephrotic syndrome.[25]

Dividing effusions into one of these two categories is conceptually useful in classifying patients with unknown effusions. In 1972, Richard Light[46] published what has become the classic criteria for the biochemical classification of a pleural effusion and now is commonly known as Light's Criteria. According to this system, the values of lactate dehydrogenase (LDH) and protein are measured in both the pleural fluid and in serum, and the effusion is classified as an exudate if any one or more of the following three criteria are met:

1. Ratio of pleural/serum protein greater than 0.5
2. Pleural LDH greater than two-thirds of the upper limit of normal for the serum reference range
3. Ratio of pleural/serum LDH greater than 0.6

Criterion number 2 reflects a modification from the original published manuscript to account for the wide variation in the normal range of LDH in various reference labs.[35,47,48] The use of these criteria reported in the original work of Light and colleagues uses positive and negative predictive values, for a true exudative effusion, of 99% and 98% respectively.[46] Subsequent studies failed to confirm these high accuracies and led to further attempts to improve the accuracy of their classification.[35,49-52] A recent reevaluation of Light's criteria comes from Keller,[53] demonstrating that Light's criteria have an overall sensitivity for an exudate of near 100%, but a specificity of only approximately 80%.

Visual Evaluation

The first step in the evaluation of pleural fluid is visual observation as it is removed. Straw-like fluid is more likely to be benign and transudative in nature. Fluid containing pus-like fluid is more likely to be infective in nature. Bloody fluid is related to causes such as pulmonary infarction, malignancy, or a postoperative state. In general, these clues can be helpful, but no diagnosis can be made definitively. No studies have accurately assessed the visual appearances of fluid as an indication of malignancy.

Cholesterol

The level of cholesterol is higher in exudative than transudative effusions for unclear reasons. The higher level is likely to be a direct reflection of the permeability of the pleura. In one prospective study, using a cutoff value of 60 mg/dL, only 5% of patients had their known effusion misclassified.[54] Costa and colleagues[47] were able to demonstrate that a cholesterol greater than 45 mg/dL and an LDH greater than 200 IU/L in the pleural fluid alone identified exudates with a very high sensitivity (99%) and specificity (98%) without the requirement for a serum sample. A second study demonstrated slightly lower values for both sensitivity and specificity.[55] Using a pleural/serum cholesterol ratio threshold of 0.3, Valdes and associates[56] were able to provide fewer misclassifications than when applying Light's criteria. In short, the level of cholesterol in pleural fluid appears useful in distinguishing exudates from transudates.

Bilirubin

A ratio of pleural/serum bilirubin greater than 0.6 was initially found to correlate well with the presence of an exudate, even among patients with jaundice.[57] A subsequent study, however, found that the use of a pleural/serum bilirubin ratio was not very good in distinguishing an exudate from transudate when compared with traditional Light's criteria (75% accuracy in this study), and thus it should not be used routinely in this regard.[58]

Albumin Gradient

It has been pointed out by several investigators that diuresis can alter pleural fluid chemistry. In several studies, patients with an effusion because of CHF had their classification changed inappropriately from a transudate to an exudate after dieuresis, due to excess loss of free water compared with protein content in the fluid; these effusions have been described as a "pseudoexudate."[59] Because of this, Roth and colleagues,[60] in a manner extrapolated from Runyon's work on ascites (see later), used an albumin gradient (serum albumin minus pleural albumin) to distinguish transudates from exudates. This study compared the use of an albumin gradient cutoff of 1.2 g/dL (i.e., effusions with a gradient lower than 1.2 were classified as exudates) with standard Light's criteria; this criteria misclassified only 2 out of 59 patients with CHF as having an exudate, compared with 5 out of 59 misclassified when Light's criteria was used. A subsequent study, however, demonstrated that pleural fluid LDH (from Light's criteria) was in fact superior to methods using albumin gradients in both sensitivity and specificity.[61] Although it potentially offers some assistance in the appropriate classification of effusions among patients with CHF, the use of protein gradients has not been definitively shown to be superior to Light's criteria. In light of this information, the best approach is to use caution in evaluating patients having both pleural effusions and CHF. It is best to use more standard criteria and to defer classification of patients with CHF as having either an exudative or transudative effusion until a patient's fluid status has been stabilized and is in a reasonable equilibrium.

Optimal Testing

What can be stated conclusively is that Light's criteria has stood the test of time and is the most widely regarded.

A meta-analysis of eight studies including 1448 patients was unable to define an optimal diagnostic technique.[62] Based on these results, however, a 21st-century version of Light's criteria, modified only slightly from Light's original work by the addition of cholesterol as a marker, could be suggested as the best means of determining an exudate. According to these updated criteria, a patient can be said to have an exudate if any of the following criteria are met:[62]

1. Pleural fluid protein greater than 2.9 g/dL
2. Pleural fluid cholesterol greater than 45 mg/dL
3. Ratio of pleural fluid LDH to serum LDH greater than 0.6

The aforementioned meta-analysis demonstrated no superior combination (paired or triplet) to any one of these single tests. In most cases, particularly in the presence of obvious, known cancer, one should not have to delve beyond these criteria in the initial evaluation of a pleural effusion.

Other Testing

There are other situations in which a specific test might not differentiate between an exudate and a transudate but still might be helpful in narrowing down a diagnosis. In general, however, although these tests are useful, they are not 100% specific but merely point the clinician in a general direction that must be evaluated further.

Glucose. In general, the concentration of glucose in a pleural effusion is not very helpful. Usually, the appropriate preservative is not used, nor is concurrent plasma glucose measured.[35] Furthermore, glucose levels are extremely variable and not usually useful in defining the etiology of an effusion.[63] The only exception is that effusions due to rheumatoid arthritis frequently have a glucose level of less than 30 mg/dL and often less than 10 mg/dL.[64]

pH. In a diagnostic thoracentesis, pleural fluid pH should always be measured. For proper analysis, pleural fluid should be collected into a single syringe and a sample then transferred to a smaller, heparinized syringe for analysis.[65] Analysis should be via a blood gas machine, not on litmus paper, as the latter is unreliable and not an acceptable alternative.[66] Normal pleural fluid pH ranges from 7.60 to 7.64.[67] In one study, 46 patients with a pleural fluid pH less than 7.30 all had an exudate and one of the following six diagnoses: malignancy, empyema, collagen vascular disease, tuberculosis, esophageal rupture, or hemothorax.[68] Furthermore, patients with known malignant effusions and a pH less than 7.30 have a worse prognosis, shorter mean survival, poorer response to tetracycline pleurodesis, and a high rate of finding malignant cells on initial fluid cytology.[69] It should be remembered that patients with a parapneumonic effusion with either a pH less than 7.3 or gross pus should be considered for chest tube placement for drainage. The reader is referred to other texts for the management of empyemas.

Amylase. Pleural effusions with a high concentration of amylase (fluid amylase greater than the upper limit of normal for serum amylase or pleural/serum amylase ratio greater than 1.0) have been associated with pancreatitis, pancreatic pseudocyst rupture, or esophageal rupture.[26,70,71] Some patients with malignancy-induced effusion have an elevated pleural fluid amylase, including those with esophageal rupture due to tumor or those with metastatic lung or ovarian tumors.[72] If doubt is present, amylase isoenzyme subtyping may be performed. Patients with a pancreatic subtype profile are likely to have benign pancreatic disease, whereas those with a salivary isoamylase profile are likely to have carcinoma, often of the lung; either result should prompt an evaluation for malignancy.[73]

Cell Count. Cell counts are often obtained on pleural fluids but are rarely useful or diagnostic. Very high nucleated cell counts (>50,000/mL) are associated with complicated parapneumonic effusions and empyema but rarely are diagnostic.[26] As most cells are normally neutrophils or monocytes, a predominance of lymphocytes (>50%) should make one more seriously entertain the idea of a carcinomatous pleural effusion, and greater than 85% lymphocytes should make one entertain the diagnosis of lymphoma, sarcoidosis, chylothorax, rheumatoid pleurisy, or yellow nail syndrome.[26,74] An increase in pleural fluid eosinophilia (>10% of nucleated cells) might be associated with benign disease (hemo- or pneumothorax), but also can be associated with all types of malignancy.[75-77] The presence of mesothelial cells is not helpful in terms of diagnosis.[74,78,79]

Pleural fluid cytology is the simplest and most definitive method of diagnosing a malignant effusion. The sensitivity depends on the type of malignancy, extent of disease, and experience of the cytopathologist. Fluids should be concentrated first for optimal detection of malignancy.[80] In general, the sensitivity is on the order of 62%–90% and, as the gold standard, pleural fluid cytology is virtually 100% specific in the hands of an expert cytopathologist.[81,82] If an effusion demonstrates carcinoma and breast cancer is a diagnostic possibility, the cytologic specimen can be stained for estrogen and progesterone receptors as a means of both diagnosis and selection of potential treatment. In short, the presence of an abnormal cell population should prompt a further workup for the aforementioned causes, including malignancy.

Other tests have been evaluated in numerous studies as a means to refine the diagnosis of pleural effusions. For example, an elevated adenosine deaminasse has a high association with tuberculosis.[83] Elevated lipids (triglycerides) can be associated with a chylothorax and obstruction of the thoracic duct by any number of means, including malignancies.[84] In clinical experience, this and other tests (e.g., creatine kinase, LDH isoenzyme analysis, β2 microglobulin, albumin, ferritin, lysozyme, and others) are rarely used and/or specific, rarely associated with malignancy, and are therefore discussed elsewhere.[35]

Tumor Markers. Carcinoembryonic antigen (CEA) is probably the most widely used tumor marker and is indicative of an epithelial malignancy. Many series have evaluated pleural effusion CEA levels as a marker of malignancy.[85] Using a cutoff of 5 ng/mL, a Japanese group found that 50% of patients with cancer (and 68% of patients with lung cancer) had an elevated pleural fluid CEA; a more recent study found similar results.[86,87] Interestingly, in both of these studies, a large number of patients with negative fluid cytology (9 of 13 and 12 of 16, respectively) had elevated tumor markers. One study demonstrated that 9% of patients with abnormal pleural fluid CEA values (>10 ng/mL) had benign effusions (mainly empyemas and complicated parapneumonic effusions).[85] Using a cutoff of 7.2 ng/mL, CEA has a positive predictive value of 64% and a negative predictive value of 78%, although both this work and others have shown that very high levels of CEA are more likely to be associated with malignancy than with benign causes.[86,88] In short, an elevation of CEA in a pleural effusion is not very helpful unless it is extremely high, but as most patients have only modest elevations, their accuracy is insufficient to make a clear-cut diagnosis of an epithelial malignancy.

Other tumor markers have been studied to a lesser extent than CEA. Carbohydrate Antigen 19-9 (CA19-9), often elevated in pancreatic and gastrointestinal malignancies, and CYFRA 21-1 (for cytokeratin fragments) have demonstrated some correlation between levels in a pleural effusion and the presence of malignancy; the latter marker could be helpful in diagnosing a pleural effusion because of malignant mesothelioma.[87,89] CA125, although useful in following a patient with a known ovarian carcinoma, is not at all useful in the evaluation of effusions, as 77% of benign effusions have CA125 levels greater than three times the upper limit of normal.[90] As a marker of small cell lung cancer, neuron-specific enolase has been found to be useful by some investigators but not by others, and thus it has not been well evaluated so far.[88,91,92] Although many of these markers have some correlation with the presence of a tumor-involved effusion, the false positive and negative rates are high. Therefore, in circumstances in which they could be clinically useful (i.e., the effusion is cytologically negative, and there are no other radiographic or clinical sites of metastatic disease for evaluation), the use of tumor marker evaluation on the effusion is likely to add little, if any, helpful information. Further, a clinician would be hard-pressed to alter definitive treatment plans (e.g., add or withhold surgery or chemotherapy) on the basis of only a tumor marker, without cytologic evidence of disease. At best, tumor markers may be used for troubling circumstances in which a physician finds them useful in determining whether to pursue a potential malignant cause of an undiagnosed effusion or take a more watchful approach.

Evaluation of a Suspected Malignant Effusion

Although most malignant effusions occur among patients with known cancers, they can be the first indication of the presence of malignancy in up to 30% of patients.[93] In some patients, an effusion often can be the only site of a potential malignancy after a thorough evaluation. Once a patient is diagnosed with an exudative effusion, a malignant cause must be high on the list of differential diagnoses. A thorough history and complete physical examination must be performed, with careful attention to any potential causes or risk factors of malignancy. Once this evaluation takes place, the physician must gather some definitive evidence to institute appropriate evaluation. Frequently, such evidence involves consultation between the patient's primary physician and either a pulmonologist or an oncologist. Many clues as to the etiology of the effusion are obtained when further evaluations, such as chest x-rays, CT scans, or mammograms, are performed. Alternatively, cytologic evaluation of an exudative effusion can reveal the presence and type of malignancy directly.

It is important to keep in mind the most common malignancies that cause effusions. Not surprisingly, a majority of these are caused by lung cancer. Breast cancers and lymphomas also cause a significant number of these, with approximately one-third of all malignant pleural effusions being caused by other types of malignancies (see Table 60-2).[94] Appropriate evaluations should be performed as indicated (e.g., careful breast exam and mammogram in women with effusions; particular attention for lung cancer among patients with a history of smoking). It should be noted that there is a recently established entity, primary effusion lymphoma. This is found in HIV-positive patients; it is associated with human herpesvirus 8 (HHV-8) infection and has a pathogenesis similar to Kaposi's sarcoma.[95] This syndrome also can include pericardial effusions and ascites. Patients with mesothelioma often have a history of asbestos exposure and show evidence of both effusion and pleural thickening on CT scan. These patients can be considered for CT-guided biopsy of the appropriate areas, which is often effective in making a diagnosis.[96] A small percentage will be diagnosed with carcinoma of unknown primary, whose management, usually via chemotherapy, is also discussed in Chapter 97.[97] Even after an extensive evaluation, results can be nondiagnostic, and the patient must undergo further evaluation to determine the etiology of the effusion because no other cause has been identified although malignancy is still suspected. These further evaluations will now be discussed.

Closed Pleural Biopsy

These refer to blind, percutaneous biopsies of the parietal pleura using a special needle, such as a Cope's needle. Risks associated with this procedure are similar to those for a thoracentesis. Unfortunately, among patients with a cytology-negative malignant effusion, the yield of this procedure is only about 7%.[98] This yield is so low because the procedure is essentially a blind, random biopsy of the pleura that easily could miss a site of disease, particularly among patients without a significant disease burden. Novel approaches to this procedure, such as the use of brushings or a Tru-cut needle, might ultimately prove to be better diagnostically, but the procedure is currently rarely used in such situations because of its poor yield.[99,100]

Thoracoscopy

Several types of thoracoscopy are available. Medical thoracoscopy refers to the evaluation of the pleural space, usually under conscious sedation and local anesthesia, in nonintubated patients. This procedure is often performed by pulmonologists using a nondisposable, rigid thoracoscope. It is similar to chest tube placement by means of a trocar, but the pleural cavity can be directly imaged, biopsies and drainage can be performed, and talc poudrage pleurodesis can be done if necessary.[101] The procedure is generally safe and effective. Although it is highly accurate diagnostically, there are few pulmonologists able to perform the procedure well, particularly in the United States.[102,103]

Video-assisted thoracoscopic surgery (VATS) is more commonly used in the United States and is usually performed by thoracic surgeons. This is a more extensive procedure, using several ports and trochars, and it requires general anesthesia with single-lung ventilation and many single-use disposable instruments.[104,105] Although VATS is well tolerated, it does have some risks and carries with it a significant expense, due to general anesthesia and the requirement for expensive instruments. On occasion, it requires conversion to an open procedure if there are significant adhesions or if there are undue risks noted with the insertion of a thoracoscope.[94] Single-lung ventilation is also required and might be difficult for patients with significant lung disease.

With these techniques, fewer than 10% of malignant pleural effusions go undiagnosed, and thus thoracoscopy of some sort has become part of the evaluation algorithm when necessary if other methods fail.[106-108] Interestingly, a recent technique uses a semirigid pleuroscope, which is similar to bronchoscopes currently in use by pulmonologists but easier to employ. These can be used to drain and pleurodese effusions and might ultimately decrease the need for VATS in diagnosing potentially malignant effusions if comparison studies demonstrate its effectiveness.[109]

Treatment

For most malignancies, the existence of a malignant effusion places the patient into a noncurable, advanced staging category, but one that is often treatable nonetheless. In light of this, a palliative approach is often the mainstay of therapy, with several important exceptions that will be addressed in the discussion that follows. For patients with relatively small effusions that do not cause a high degree of dyspnea or impairment of functional status, consideration of systemic therapy of the malignancy, usually chemotherapy, is indicated. If, on the other hand, dyspnea is a primary concern, immediate management of the effusion is necessary. Unfortunately, for many patients with advanced disease, chemotherapy might not be able to provide rapid enough resolution of dyspnea or other symptoms, and thus one must employ mechanical means of reducing the effusion. First and foremost, the clinician should consider the individual patient's situation, with particular attention to overall prognosis, prior therapies (if any), age, and performance status. The physician must also weigh the likelihood of progression of other systemic disease during the time required for resolution of an effusion. For patients with large effusions who are in the terminal stage of their disease, supplemental oxygen with hospice referral might be the only appropriate intervention.

Systemic Therapy in Specific Malignancies

Hematologic Malignancies. Approximately 10% of malignant pleural effusions are due to lymphomas. Approximately 10% of patients with non-Hodgkin's Lymphoma (NHL), 5%–33% of patients with Hodgkin's disease, and about 2%–4% of patients with leukemia develop effusions.[110,111] Effusions are usually a manifestation of late disease but can be seen among patients at all stages. If a patient still has good chemotherapy treatment options, they should be considered as front-line therapy. These tumors are usually highly responsive to therapy, and there is a signficant possiblity of systemic dissemination in the time it takes to resolve an effusion by nonsystemic means. Initial treatment for NHL usually consists of CHOP (cyclophosphamide, doxorubicin, vincristine, prednisone), with or without rituximab, or a variant of this combination depending on the grade and nature of the lymphoma. Various related regimens are used for relapse, but ESHAP (etoposide, prednisolone, doxorubicin, cytarabine, and cisplatin), possibly combined with high-dose therapy with autologous stem cell rescue, is often considered. Therapy for Hodgkin's disease usually consists of doxorubicin, bleomycin, vincristine, and dacarbazine. The reader is guided to Chapters 111 and 112 in this text.

Effusions related to leukemia are rare but do occur. Because of their rapid proliferation time and rates of response when given chemotherapy, the patient is usually given chemotherapy consisting of an anthracycline (daunorubicin or idarubicin) with cytarabine, with various salvage regimens available, such as gemtuzumab. Multiple myeloma is an even rarer cause of an effusion but can be seen on occasion. These effusions typically have a high protein count (>8 g/L), and immunoelectropheresis of the effusions can be diagnostic.[112] The effusion might arise from marrow involvement of the adjacent ribs and chest wall. Unfortunately, multiple myeloma is more chemotherapy-resistant than other hematologic malignancies, making management more difficult with chemotherapy alone. Because steroids alone have a fairly good response rate, either alone or given in conjunction with a nonmyelosuppressive agent such as thalidomide, they are probably the best option when treatment is considered, as a nonresponding patient can proceed quickly to other alternatives without undue delay due to hematopoeitic toxicity from standard therapy.[113]

Solid Tumors. Many advanced solid tumors do not respond well to chemotherapy, so primary management of the effusion is often required. There are notable exceptions. Small cell lung cancer is unlikely to be curable, but effusions from this cause respond well to either cisplatin/etoposide or cisplatin/irinotecan therapy.[114,115] Testicular and other germ-cell neoplasms are not only responsive but also very curable, even at an advanced state, and thus early systemic treatment should be employed if at all possible.[116] Even patients with advanced germ cell tumors have good responses and should be considered for aggressive systemic therapy. Breast cancer might respond well to hormonal therapy or chemotherapy, particularly among patients who have not received prior systemic therapy. Mesothelioma is a unique tumor that arises directly from pleural or peritoneal surfaces. Effusions are often associated with the tumor and are not included in the staging system. Patients amenable for aggressive local therapy, even with an effusion, should be considered for such therapy, which can include surgery (extrapleural pneumonectomy) with concomitant resection of adjacent structures (diaphragm and/or pericardium) followed by chemotherapy and radiotherapy. Five-year survival (11%) is still quite limited for these patients, however.[117] Interestingly, a novel agent, pemetrexed (a multitargeted antifolate), has demonstrated remarkable benefit recently for patients with advanced disease when it is combined with standard cisplatin therapy. Future studies will undoubtedly examine this agent for patients with earlier-stage disease in an attempt to improve the cure rate. Because patients with solid organ tumors and advanced disease have relatively poor responses to chemotherapy overall, however, early direct management of the effusion among patients with dyspnea should be considered at the outset for patients who are unlikely to achieve rapid responses to chemotherapy.

Systemic Chemotherapy and Effusions. It should be remembered that the pharmacokinetics of drugs in the presence of effusions are poorly understood, as drug might accumulate in effusions and only slowly redistribute throughout the body. Methotrexate is a classic example of this phenomenon. Methotrexate is slowly released from all of the "third spaces," and those of large volumes (ascites, pleural effusions, or anasarca) might dramatically prolong the terminal half-life and lead to potential increased toxicity.[118] There are no direct guidelines for the use of methotrexate or other chemotherapies when large effusions exist, but the clinician should consider drainage of the effusion before the use of methotrexate, or the use of alternative therapies. Patients with pleural effusions receiving new chemotherapy agents should be monitored closely for treatment-induced toxicity.

Effusion-Targeted Therapy

Therapeutic Thoracentesis. Animal studies have demonstrated that effusions increase the volume of the hemithorax more than they compress lung parenchyma.[119] Because of this phenomenon, total lung capacity (TLC) increases by only one-third the volume of the fluid removed, and the forced vital capacity (FVC) after thoracentesis increases by only one-half the increase in TLC. Changes in TLC and FVC are variable, with the largest increases seen in those individuals with the healthiest lung tissue due to their high lung compliance.[120] Physiologically, patients with effusions have a large intrapulmonary shunt, and therefore effect of a given effusion on gas exchange and Pa_{O_2} can be highly variable; it is therefore difficult to predict the degree of resolution of dyspnea after fluid removal based solely on the size of the effusion.[121-123] Furthermore, lung expansion after fluid removal might be delayed, and thus its effects on the resolution of dyspnea might be delayed also.[124]

Therapeutic thoracentesis might serve as the main or sole therapy for management of an effusion in many patients. Thoracentesis, unlike other procedures, might permit rapid relief of symptoms without need of hospitalization. If systemic disease is a significant concern, thoracentesis might allow for a window of opportunity in which to gain control over a patient's symptoms before systemic chemotherapy is given. Similarly, it might also allow for palliation of symptoms for those patients with far advanced disease.

Therapeutic thoracenteses are performed similarly to diagnostic procedures. Although a pneumothorax usually occurs when air leaks into the pleural space through the needle, it can occur if the visceral pleura is lacerated with the needle. The latter complication may be avoided if a plastic catheter is threaded through the needle, directed inferiorly, and the needle is then removed; this procedure minimizes the chances that a pneumothorax will occur via perforation when the visceral and parietal surfaces become opposed after fluid removal. If a pneumothorax occurs, the leak usually seals itself quickly, but closure can be hastened by having the patient lie on the affected side, which decreases the pressure gradient between the alveoli and the pleural space.[125] The volume of pleural fluid that can be removed safely is unknown. One study by Light and colleagues[15] demonstrated that pleural fluid removal could be considered safe as long as pleural fluid pressure does not decrease below –20 cmH$_2$O. Because most clinicians do not measure pleural pressure, current recommendations are that no more than 1.0–1.5 L of fluid be removed at any one time, and that amount only if there are no signs of any adverse events such as dyspnea, pleural pain, or cough, which are indications of the rapid restoration of a strong negative pleural pressure. Patients with contralateral mediastinal shift can have larger amounts of fluid removed safely, as these adverse events are unlikely to occur. Rapid re-expansion might bring on the phenomenon of re-expansion pulmonary edema, which is due to the rapid resoration of capillary permeability through unknown mechanisms; this can occur when air or fluid is removed from the pleural space.[125] Patients with ipsilateral mediastinal shift are unlikely to obtain significant relief from thoracentesis, as this condition indicates a large amount of either trapped lung or mainstem bronchial occlusion.[95]

There have been no randomized or comparison trials examining the use of repeated thoracentesis compared with the use of other procedures. It is also difficult to predict the length of time within which an effusion might recur; some patients recur rapidly (within days), while others might benefit from slower recurrence. Most oncologists and pulmonologists often make an initial attempt at a therapeutic thoracentesis to allow immediate symptomatic relief and time for systemic therapy to take benefit, and to gauge the extent to which a pleural effusion causes dyspnea. For patients whose effusions recur rapidly, more invasive procedures might be required; those whose effusions recur more slowly might be managed solely with repeat thoracentesis.

Radiation Therapy. In general, radiation of the hemithorax, as a means of controlling an effusion, is contraindicated in most patients with malignant pleural effusions. This is because of the high incidence of radiation pneumonitis that is likely when a sufficient dose of radiation is given to large areas potentially involved with malignant effusions.[126] Certain situations, such as lymphatic obstruction from focal areas of lymphadenopathy (which may arise in lymphoma or in lung cancer), might benefit from radiation applied to these specific areas. Radiation doses are dependent on the nature of the malignancy.

Chemical Pleurodesis. Pleurodesis is intended to achieve a "symphysis between the parietal and visceral pleura, in order to prevent accumulation of either air (pneumothorax) or fluid (pleural effusion) in the pleural space," and malignant pleural effusions are the largest indications for pleurodesis.[127,128] The mechanism by which this symphysis occurs is poorly understood, but in general, it depends on pleural irritation to cause a cycle of inflammation, activation of the pleural coagulation cascade, fibrin placement and fibroblast recruitment, and, finally, collagen deposition that ultimately results in the fusion of both pleural surfaces.[127,129,130] Nevertheless, the exact mechanisms and factors that influence pleural sclerosis and effect pleurodesis are not well known and require further research. Many agents have been used in the past with various success rates reported; much of this information is based on personal and anecdotal experiences. These agents include, as a minimum list:

- Talc
- Tetracycline
- Minocycline
- Doxycycline
- Quinacrine
- Mepacrine
- Bleomycin
- Mitomycin
- Thiotepa
- Nitrogen mustard
- 50% glucose and water
- Interferon-α
- Interferon-γ
- Iodopovidone
- Radioactive colloidal gold
- Autologous blood
- Fibrin glue
- Bacille Calmette-Guérin
- Silver nitrate
- Killed *Corynebacterium parvum*[127]

The exact mechanism by which these agents effect pleurodesis probably differs slightly from one agent to another, but all lead to a final common pathway that activates the pleural coagulation cascade and the appearance of a fibrin network that yields a symphysis between the two surfaces.[128-130] The various agents have different properties and methods of administration.

Method of Pleurodesis. It should be recalled that patients must demonstrate that symptoms (usually dyspnea) respond to drainage of the pleural fluid, as patients with malignancy often have numerous reasons for dyspnea—pulmonary metastases, anemia, pulmonary embolus, trapped lung, or poor gas exchange—and might be unlikely to benefit from a resolution of the effusion. Thus it is important for patients to undergo a trial of therapeutic thoracentesis initially rather than proceed directly to chest-tube drainage. At the time that pleurodesis is performed, the effusion must be drained. For successful sclerosis, there should be evidence of complete lung re-expansion after initial drainage. Traditionally, one gauged the optimal time for sclerosis when there was minimal pleural fluid drainage (less than 150 mL per day), but this appears to be less relevant for success in sclerosis than does the confirmation of complete radiologic lung re-expansion.[131,132] This finding is the sole criterion by which the appropriate time for thoracentesis should be judged.

Traditionally, chest tube drainage has been performed with a standard size (24-32 Fr) chest tube. Tubes in this size range are associated with a great deal of pain and discomfort. More recent work has supported the use of smaller-bore (8-16 Fr) catheters. A prospective, randomized study of 18 patients found improved comfort and no difference in success or complication rates when small-bore catheters were used.[133] Several larger, non-randomized trials have shown good success rates with decreased complications when small-bore tubes were used compared with the historical experience with large-bore tubes.[134-137] One study demonstrated a good rate of sclerosis (79%) when a small-bore chest tube was used for outpatients in combination with either doxycycline or bleomycin.[136] In light of this finding, small-bore tube placement with consideration for outpatient management is an emerging standard of care.[138]

Ideally, the chest tube is placed posteriorly towards the diaphragm. After radiographic determination of lung re-expansion and drainage of fluid, sclerosis can be performed. Before installing sclerosing agents, intravenous narcotics or sedation is used frequently due to the pain associated with many agents. The agent of choice is added to the tube in 50-100 mL of sterile saline, and the tube is clamped for one hour. Classically, patients were rotated after intrapleural administration of the agent, but this is no longer believed to be necessary.[131] Recent evidence using radiolabelled tetracycline has shown fairly uniform dispersion throughout the pleural space within seconds of administration, and a subsequent randomized clinical trial showed no difference in the success of pleurodesis between rotated and nonrotated patients.[139,140] The issue of clamping is debated, with some clinicians recommending clamping of the chest tube for one hour and others recommending against it because of the rapid distribution of the sclerosing agent and the potential complications (e.g., tension pneumothorax) that might arise from a persistent air leak when the tube is clamped.[96,131] Suction is then restored for 24-72 hours, and, providing the lung remains fully expanded and the fluid output from the tube is low (generally less than 150 mL per 24-hour period), the chest tube may be removed.

Sclerosing Agents

Tetracycline/Doxycycline. Tetracycline was the most widely used sclerosing agent until it was discontinued by the manufacturer in 1992, although it might still be available in some countries.[141,142] Doxycycline has been recommended as a replacement, but there are no direct studies comparing the two agents. Historical comparisons demonstrate similar success rates with doxycycline compared with tetracycline, both on the order of 80%-85%.[143,144] Most studies and investigators have used 500 mg of doxycycline mixed in 50 to 100 mL of sterile saline, and the primary complication is pain related to the doxycycline, requiring either narcotics or conscious sedation.[94,136,143,144]

Talc. Talc, a pulverized, natural silicate, was first described as a pleurodesis agent by Bethune in 1935.[145] It is currently the most widely used, the best studied, and probably the most controversial such agent. Virtually every talc product is unique in chemistry and morphology, and many nontalc minerals are included. It is passed through a mesh during processing, and the size of the final preparation is dependent on the size of the mesh. In general, particles are smaller than 50 µ. There is a well-described association between talc and the development of cancer in individuals who mine talc. This is most likely due to the asbestos in the natural, unrefined product.[146] Several studies have demonstrated no increase in the incidence of either lung cancer or mesothelioma among patients who underwent talc pleurodesis who were followed for as long as 35 years.[147] Because talc for use in the United States is certified asbestos free, and because most patients with cancer undergoing pleurodesis have advanced, incurable disease, this association should not be of concern. Talc is provided by the manufacturer in a nonsterile form, but U.S. Pharmacopoeia standards limit the number of bacteria to 500 microorganisms per gram. One study demonstrated that bacillus species could be cultured from six different species of talc.[148] A major advantage of talc is the cost; the average wholesale price for the amount of talc typically used for pleurodesis procedures is less than $1.00. Sterilization of the talc raises the cost to between $5 and $20, dependent on the methods used, and it remains sterile for at least a year on pharmacy shelves.[148,149] The cost of talc is therefore significantly less than for any of the other agents used. Talc may be introduced via slurry (i.e., mixed with saline) in the chest tube used to drain the effusion, or insufflated (poudrage) with a bulb syringe or atomizer at the time of a thoracoscopic drainage procedure. (Thoracoscopy will be discussed shortly.) Mager and colleagues[150] randomized 20 patients who received talc slurry pleurodesis to either rotation or no rotation and found no difference in the success rates between the two

Problems Common to Cancer and Its Therapy

groups. These investigators used ^{99m}Tc-sestamibi-labelled talc and were able to demonstrate that 75% of the patients did not have uniform distribution of the talc, but most had successful procedures nonetheless. This finding reemphasizes the poor understanding we have of the biology and physics of pleurodesis.

In 1994, Kennedy and Sahn reviewed all the published series using talc as a pleurodesis agent and found a 91% success rate (659 of 723 patients) for pleurodesis, with success judged by various clinical and radiologic findings.[151] Doses of talc ranged widely, from 1 to 14 g per procedure. There was no difference between poudrage and slurry. Animal studies suggest that concomitant use of steroids can decrease the efficacy of talc pleurodesis, and a small study in humans demonstrated a small, not statistically significant decreased response to talc slurry when steroids were used.[152,153] Although these studies are not conclusive, steroids should be discontinued or the dose reduced as much as possible before pleurodesis procedures when talc or any pleurodesis agent is used.

Adverse effects from talc are variable. Pain ranging from nonexistent to severe is not uncommon; there is an overall reported incidence of 7%.[154] Fever, up to 102°F, occurs within the first 12 hours and can last up to 72 hours.[26,154] Empyema is an occasional complication, more often with talc slurry than with poudrage. Cardiovascular complications (e.g., arrhythmia, chest pain) have been noted, but it is difficult to assess whether these are a result of the talc pleurodesis procedure itself or the patients' comorbidities.[151,153]

Pulmonary complications constitute the largest and most significant group of complications associated with talc pleurodesis. Acute respiratory distress syndrome (ARDS), pneumonitis, and respiratory failure all have been reported after pleurodesis with talc.[155-160] The mechanisms by which talc might produce acute lung injury are unclear. One hypothesis is that the pneumonitis is related to the systemic absorption of talc; this is supported by the findings of Rinaldo[161] and others who were able to demonstrate talc particles both in broncho-alveolar lavage fluid after talc pleurodesis and in virtually every organ at autopsy of one patient.[160-163] Animal studies also have confirmed that talc can disseminate systemically after intrapleural administration.[147] One of the most concerning studies comes from Rehse and associates,[164] who found that in a series of 78 patients, 33% developed respiratory complications or death after talc pleurodesis, and 9% developed ARDS—rates that are significantly higher than those previously reported. Some investigators feel that the incidence of pulmonary complications is related to the dose of talc used for pleurodesis. Talc pleurodesis is still commonly used, however, and the relative merits of this vs. other methods are fiercely debated among experts and will be discussed later in this chapter.[162,165]

Bleomycin. Bleomycin has been studied since the 1970s for its use as a sclerosing agent.[166-171] The recommended dose for intrapleural administration is 60 U or 1 U/kg body weight, and is often reduced to 40 U/kg in the elderly.[136] Administration and its side effects are similar to those with talc pleurodesis, with pleuritic pain, rigors, fever, and mild nausea as the main concerns.[136] Although it also is used commonly as a chemotherapeutic agent, only 40% is systemically absorbed from the pleural cavity, and bleomycin is not myelosuppressive when used in pleurodesis.[170] Several studies report mixed results for bleomycin compared with other agents. A large meta-analysis (1168 patients) from Walker-Renard and colleagues[154] demonstrated a 54% success rate with bleomycin vs. a 67% success rate with tetracycline and its derivatives (doxycycline, minocycline), and a 93% success rate with talc. Zimmer and coworkers,[172] in a subsequent prospective randomized trial, did not demonstrate a statistically significant difference in efficacy between talc (90% successful) and bleomycin (79% successful, p = 0.388). Patz and colleagues[136] directly compared bleomycin and doxycycline with a small-bore catheter and likewise did not find any statistically significant difference between the two agents. It is important to note that there are large cost differences between the different agents. In the aforementioned study by Zimmer, the cost of the bleomycin was $955 per patient, compared with only $12 per patient for talc.[172]

Pleurodesis Without the Use of Agents. Interestingly, two studies demonstrated that one could obtain relatively effective pleurodesis with thoracoscopy and chest tube placement for several days without instillation of a pleurodesis agent; these studies demonstrate a combined 62% success rate among 61 total patients.[173,174] Talc insufflation at the time of thoracoscopy does indeed increase the success rate to more than 90% of patients, however.[151] The fact that one can achieve decent pleurodesis and modest success rates without the use of any pleurodesis agent highlights our relatively poor understanding of the mechanism of pleurodesis and suggests that irritation of any sort can in fact lead to sclerosis and symphysis of the two pleural membranes. One potentially superior alternative to simple chest tube placement is to perform mechanical abrasion of the pleura. There are, however, no large series evaluating mechanical abrasion at the time of thoracoscopy for effectiveness, nor any comparing mechanical abrasion with any other techniques.[162,163,175] Two studies in dogs, however, demonstrated that mechanical abrasion was either equivalent or superior to the use of talc (poudrage and slurry, respectively).[176,177] Mechanical abrasion can be performed with a thoracoscope (usually VATS) or via an open procedure. Pleural abrasion, in conjunction with bleb stapling, has been shown to be effective in preventing recurrent pneumothorax as a method of sclerosis in this nonmalignant entity.[178,179]

Predicting the Effectiveness of Pleurodesis. It has been stated that low pleural fluid pH can identify patients who might experience a low likelihood of success with pleurodesis.[128] Low pH is thought to be a marker of increased metabolic activity of intrapleural tumor, and as such it represents a larger tumor burden.[69] Large tumor burdens might prevent apposition of the pleural membranes. Some studies have supported an association of a low pleural fluid pH with a poorer pleurodesis outcome, while others have not.[69,180-185] Heffner and associates[186] re-analyzed individual patient data from both published and unpublished studies in 2000. Their analysis of 433 patients demonstrated that pleural fluid pH was the only independent predictor of pleurodesis failure, with an odds ratio of 4.46 when pleural fluid pH was lower than 7.28. A pH value of 7.15 or lower had a positive predictive value of 45.7% for pleurodesis failure. Although pH certainly helps predict pleurodesis failure, it is only of modest benefit in predicting outcome in individual patients, as even those patients with a low pH in the analyzed studies had a greater than 50% success rate with pleurodesis. Because of these limitations, fluid pH should only be considered as an additional piece of information, not as a means to totally rule out pleurodesis.

Surgical Options Including Shunts

There are several surgical procedures—parietal pleurectomy, decortication, and pleuropneumonectomy—that may be attempted for management of a malignant pleural effusion. These procedures carry with them major morbidities, and they have proven to be no better than pleurodesis alone.[187] Surgical palliation might, however, be an option for some patients, particularly those who fail chemical pleurodesis, patients with loculated effusions, or those with large tumor rinds on the pleural surface. VATS permits direct visualization of the entire pleural surface, the potential for mechanical abrasion of the pleural surface, and removal of some adhesions and loculations. Talc poudrage via insufflation may be performed, and a pleuroperitoneal shunt may be inserted as well.[188] Surgical intervention should also be considered if lung re-expansion does not occur promptly after removal of an effusion via chest tube drainage; failure to re-expand suggests a cortex of malignant tissue surrounding the lung, which may be further confirmed by a radiograph demonstrating a large effusion without mediastinal shift.[187] If such a cortex is seen at the time of VATS, it may be removed by conversion of the VATS to an open thoracotomy. This procedure might make pleurodesis and the restoration of a trapped lung possible. There is, however, a perioperative mortality of 12% associated with open procedures for decortication in these situations, therefore, this choice of procedure must be limited to an appropriate patient population.[187,189-191] Pleuroperitoneal shunts have a complication rate of approximately 12%, which is manifested mainly by shunt occlusion requiring replacement.[192] Peritoneal seeding of intrathoracic malignancy is a potential hazard but has not been definitively studied.[187]

Intrapleural Therapy

The rationale of intrapleural therapy is very appealing: Agents given directly into the pleural space can be directly toxic to tumor cells or to stimulants of the immune system that would ultimately be cytotoxic to tumor cells, thereby causing resolution of an associated malignant effusion. It should be noted that it is difficult to separate the cytotoxic effects of intrapleural therapy from pleural irritation to determine whether resolution of an effusion is due to cytotoxicity or pleurodesis. Bleomycin is a classic example of this phenomenon in that it is used as a sclerotic agent but also possesses antineoplastic activity. Intrapleural therapy, particularly chemotherapy, offers hope for patients who have a malignancy confined to the pleural space (e.g., mesothelioma) or for patients who have a higher disease burden in this location compared with other sites. A similar approach of locally directed chemotherapy has been used with particular success in the abdominal cavity, in cases of intraperitoneal chemotherapy for ovarian cancer.

Most agents that have been tried over the years have had limited success, and thus the idea of intrapleural therapy is still highly experimental. Several authors have proposed using cytostatic drugs in microspheres to allow for high intrapleural concentrations of drug with minimal systemic distribution.[193] Cytokines such as IL-2, interferon-β, and interferon-γ have been tried in the treatment of malignant mesothelioma, with moderate success in early trials.[194-199] Corynebacterium parvum has been tried with modest success (76%), but it is available only in Europe and is associated with a high rate of fever.[183,200-204] Methyl-prednisolone has demonstrated a small rate of efficacy in one study, with minimal toxicity. In terms of cytotoxic chemotherapy, many agents have been tried, including intrapleural 5-FU, mitomycin, cisplatin, cytarabine, doxorubicin, and etoposide.[154] Shoji and colleagues[205] recently reported their phase II results using repeated intrapleural chemotherapy with an implantable access system (an infuse-a-port, similar to that used for subcutaneous venous access), placed by a VATS procedure. Patients received biweekly 5-FU and cisplatin. Such a system was used previously for the administration of γ-interferon in the treatment of malignant mesothelioma by Driesen and colleagues[206] and allows for repeated, easy administration of intrapleural drugs with minimal catheter related toxicity. There was virtually no systemic toxicity, not even of the type that is usually associated with systemic therapy of these drugs, although the doses (5-FU, 250 mg; cisplatin, 10 mg) were far less than those typically used intravenously. Because of this observation, such a system warrants further testing as a method of both pleurodesis and treatment (neither of which was an endpoint in this dose-finding trial), particularly for tumors sensitive to agents that can be given intrapleurally. Silver nitrate was tried in the 1980s by Wied and associates[207] and was found to be inferior compared with tetracycline. This finding has since been readdressed in an animal model by Vargas and colleagues,[208] in which silver nitrate was combined with talc slurry; pleurodesis was superior when silver nitrate was used in conjunction with talc, although the rate of some complications were higher.

As described in virtually all of these reports, the success rates with these cytotoxic agents are less than those seen with talc, doxycycline, and even intrapleural bleomycin. There is the potential for systemic absorption, and consequently potential associated systemic toxicity from such agents. The costs of antineoplastic agents are much higher than those for doxycycline and talc. Because talc is well studied, inexpensive, effective, and readily available, it would be difficult to find a superior agent for use solely in the treatment of effusions; for these reasons, intrapleural therapy still remains experimental excepting the use of agents that cause pleurodesis.

Long-Term Drainage Catheters

For some patients, effective pleurodesis will not be attainable. In others, the life expectancy could be too short to justify such invasive procedures or minor surgeries (such as VATS), but control of the effusion is still important. Therefore, other effective means for the palliation of pleural effusions are necessary. In 1986, Leff and colleagues[209] reported on the use of an intrapleural catheter connected to a subcutaneously implanted access port that was accessed twice a week for drainage to relieve dyspnea from a pleural effusion. Others subsequently described the connection of a standard chest tube to a urinary drainage bag with an intervening Heimlich valve, which allows one-way flow.[210] Because of the potential risk of catheter dislodgement, two reports subsequently used tunneled catheters that could be drained by patients or visiting nurses.[211,212] Effective palliation was achieved for all patients, with minimal complications (e.g., infection). It is noteworthy that in one of these series, two of four patients achieved pleurodesis with only the long-term presence of the catheter itself.[212] These preliminary, makeshift systems ultimately led to the development of the Denver Pleurx system (Denver Biomaterials Inc., Golden, CO), the only tunneled catheter approved by the U.S. Food and Drug Administration (FDA) for pleural effusion management.[213]

The details of the Denver catheter are described in detail elsewhere, but it consists primarily of a 15.5 Fr silicone catheter with side holes and a polyester cuff that induces fibrosis along the tunnel; fibrosis decreases the risks of dislodgement, infection, and pericatheter leakage.[213] There is a proximal hub that prevents air entry or fluid egress, and it is capped when not in use. The catheter is usually placed into a free-flowing effusion or large locule under local anesthesia at the bedside. After initial drainage of no more than 1500 mL, drainage usually is performed every other day by the patient, family member, or a visiting nurse. The tube may be removed if three drainages in a row are scant and imaging shows no reaccumulation of fluid, suggesting spontaneous pleurodesis. The pivotal, approval trial for the FDA in 1999 compared the Denver catheter with doxycycline sclerotherapy.[214] Quality-of-life benefits were the same for the two groups, and there was a greater improvement in dyspnea with the Denver catheter; hospitalization was shorter in the catheter group (one day vs. six and a half days), and spontaneous pleurodesis developed in 46% of catheter placements, but effusions did recur 13% of the time. Sclerotherapy may be given through the catheter as well. Follow-up studies to the original data continue to demonstrate similarly good results.[215,216] Catheter complications occur about 15%–20% the time and include poor drainage requiring replacement, external catheter migration, tumor tracking along the catheter route, and infection (pleural fluid and skin). A recent report demonstrates symptomatic benefit (but not pleurodesis) for 91% of patients with trapped lung or multiloculated effusions.[213] The Denver Pleurx system is likely to offer significant benefit to all patients with pleural effusion and might allow many stable patients to undergo drainage and sclerosis on an outpatient basis.

Approach to Management

This subject is not without controversy, particularly with respect to the method of pleurodesis. Surgeons are likely to favor a surgical approach, such as VATS or thoracoscopy with pleurodesis attempts using talc or pleural abrasion, while pulmonologists and oncologists are likely to favor chest tubes and talc. Newer approaches with smaller chest tubes allow for outpatient management of pleural effusions in a more stable patient population. Cost considerations are important as well; surgical approaches can add significant expense because of operating room time and the involvement of anesthesiologists, although some of these expenses can easily be recovered by quicker hospital discharges and elimination of complications. Certain physicians have strong feelings one way or the other based on their interpretations of the literature and their personal experiences; well-performed clinical trials are difficult to perform for these situations and unlikely to occur. For example, because of the low, but very real incidence of ARDS (and mortality) associated with the use of talc that has not been seen with the use of any other agents, some clinicians feel that intrapleural talc should never be used; others recommend talc as long as lower doses (2–5 g) are used, although ARDS can be associated even at these doses.[160,162,163,165] When pleurodesis is indicated, our approach is to use talc in low doses (maximum 5 g). Because many patients achieve pleurodesis through the presence of a chest tube alone, that sole measure might be sufficient for a good percentage of patients, and certainly a trial of this can be considered in stable patients. Although our general approach is shown in the algorithm, the overall scheme needs to be individualized for the patient, with one physician (usually the medical oncologist) as the coordinator to ensure optimal outcomes.

PERICARDIAL EFFUSION

Malignant pericardial effusions are much less common than both ascites and pleural effusions. They are often an event that occurs with end-stage disease, and patients are often switched to a purely palliative mode on discovery of a pericardial effusion, particularly if tamponade or near-tamponade physiology is present. Because intracardiac tumors are exceedingly rare, the most common cause of pericardial effusions is tumor metastatic to the heart or pericardium. About one-third of patients with end-stage lung or breast cancer have evidence of pericardial metastases and/or effusion present at autopsy, although only a small number of these are symptomatic.

Etiology and Pathogenesis

The pericardial space normally contains a tiny amount of fluid that serves to reduce friction, maintain position

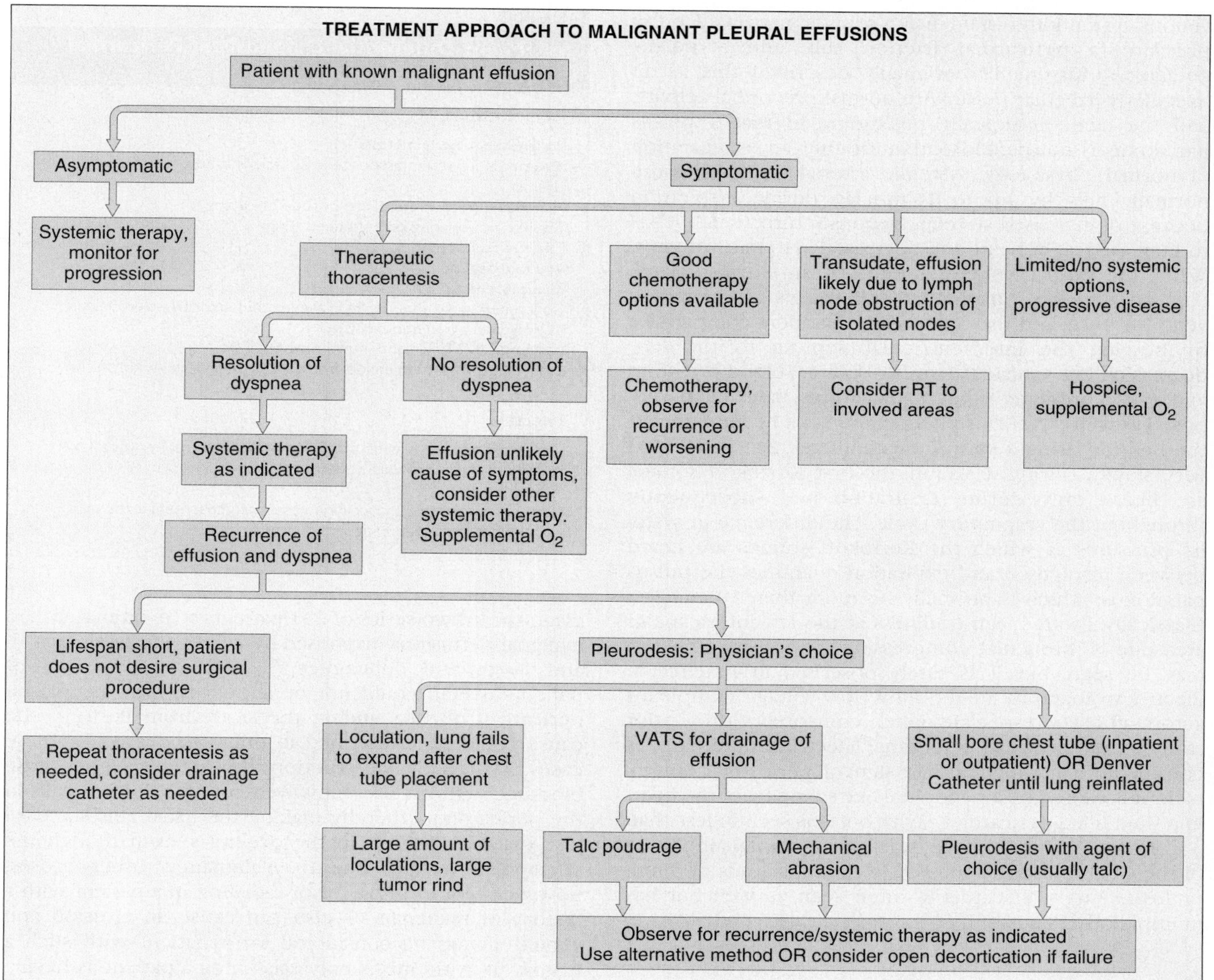

TREATMENT APPROACH TO MALIGNANT PLEURAL EFFUSIONS

Patient with known malignant effusion

Asymptomatic

Systemic therapy, monitor for progression

Symptomatic

Therapeutic thoracentesis

Good chemotherapy options available

Transudate, effusion likely due to lymph node obstruction of isolated nodes

Limited/no systemic options, progressive disease

Resolution of dyspnea

No resolution of dyspnea

Chemotherapy, observe for recurrence or worsening

Consider RT to involved areas

Hospice, supplemental O_2

Systemic therapy as indicated

Effusion unlikely cause of symptoms, consider other systemic therapy. Supplemental O_2

Recurrence of effusion and dyspnea

Lifespan short, patient does not desire surgical procedure

Pleurodesis: Physician's choice

Repeat thoracentesis as needed, consider drainage catheter as needed

Loculation, lung fails to expand after chest tube placement

VATS for drainage of effusion

Small bore chest tube (inpatient or outpatient) OR Denver Catheter until lung reinflated

Large amount of loculations, large tumor rind

Talc poudrage

Mechanical abrasion

Pleurodesis with agent of choice (usually talc)

Observe for recurrence/systemic therapy as indicated
Use alternative method OR consider open decortication if failure

60-1

---

of the heart in the pericardium and mediastinum, and provide a barrier against infection. It is essentially an ultrafiltrate of plasma enriched by pericardial and myocardial "substances."[217] Malignant cells obtain access to the space by either direct invasion from an adjacent tumor in the lung or mediastinum or by hematogenous or lymphatic spread. Retrograde progression of disease through the lymphatic channels draining the heart and pericardium results in a majority of effusions.[218,219] In terms of lymphatic drainage of the heart, the visceral pericardium is responsible for the majority of the pericardial drainage.[220] The subepicardial lymphatic drainage follows first along the coronary artery, then to other nodes that subsequently drain into either the thoracic duct or the mediastinal system.[221] Other drainage patterns occur as well, and systemic malignancy anywhere can progress to a malignant pericardial effusion. Fluid dynamics and physics in the pericardial cavity are iden-

tical to those in the pleural cavity, namely those governed by Starling's equation (Eq. 1). The potential space in the pericardial cavity is much less than in other potential areas of fluid accumulation (abdomen, lungs), and, depending on the compliance of the pericardium and the acuity of fluid collection, symptoms can develop rapidly. Further, because even a small amount of fluid that develops rapidly can compress the heart and thus impede diastolic filling, malignant pericardial effusions are often difficult to manage and tend to carry a grim prognosis.

Clinical Presentation

The most common clinical manifestations of pericardial effusion are dyspnea, cough, chest pain, orthopnea, palpitations, tachypnea, tachycardia, and edema. Physical examination might show signs of a low-output cardiac state (coolness of the extremities, diaphoresis), jugular

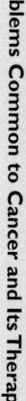

Problems Common to Cancer and Its Therapy

venous distention, distant heart sounds, narrowed pulse pressure, a pericardial friction rub, and a pulsus paradoxus. Kussmaul[222] originally described this as an irregularly irregular pulse with normal precordial activity, and the name is actually misleading in that a pulsus paradoxus is not paradoxical, but rather an exaggeration of normal physiology. Systemic arterial blood pressure normally falls by up to 10 mm Hg during inspiration because of increased systemic venous return, which leads to increased right heart and decreased systemic volumes. When the cardiac volume is fixed by an extrinsic force (i.e., an effusion), inspiration still causes an increased venous return, and the right heart chambers compensate by bowing the interventricular septum to the left, decreasing left ventricular stroke volume, blood pressure, and pulse pressure; other explanations have been proposed as well.[223-225] This phenomenon can be measured at the bedside using a sphygmomanometer that is deflated very slowly. During deflation, the first Kortokoff sounds are heard only during expiration and subsequently throughout the respiratory cycle. The difference in systolic pressures at which the Kortokoff sounds are heard between inspiration and expiration quantifies the pulsus paradoxus, which is normally no more than 10 mm Hg. Classically, Ewart's sign (dullness at the left infrascapular area due to bronchial compression by a large effusion) may be seen, but it is rarely observed in practice.[226] Electrocardiography might show low-voltage complexes across all leads (especially when compared with a prior study) and electrical alternans. Electrical alternans is considered a pathognemonic sign of pericardial tamponade; it is caused by a pendulum-like swinging of the heart in a fluid filled pericardial cavity, but it is seen in less than 3% of cases.[227] Low voltage is defined as a total amplitude of the QRS complexes in each of the limb leads of 5 mm or less. Sinus tachycardia is often seen as well but has multiple other causes.

Diagnosis and Evaluation

A patient with a pericardial effusion, like a patient with pleural effusion, should be classified according to the likelihood of the effusion being malignant. The causes of pericardial effusions are shown in Table 60-3 and should be considered for all patients, as benign effusions clearly portend much better diagnoses than malignant ones. Most effusions among patients with advanced cancer will, in fact, be due to that malignancy. In a series of 75 patients from Corey,[228] the most common causes of an unexplained pericardial effusion in a general population (with no known history of cancer) was malignancy in 25% and infection in 27%; among patients with known malignancy, one would expect a much higher rate. An autopsy series of 3314 patients found that cardiac metastases occur in 10% of patients dying of cancer.[229] Many patients with malignant effusions have known advanced cancer, and therefore, there is little diagnostic dilemma. In those patients in whom advanced cancer is unlikely, a more thorough evaluation should be done and is discussed in this portion of the chapter. Unfortunately, malignant pericardial effusion is often difficult to

TABLE 60-3

Major Differential Diagnosis of Pericardial Effusion by Etiology

Noninfectious

Malignancy (usually metastatic)
Myocardial infarction-associated (Dressler's syndrome)
Uremia
Myxedema (rare cause of tamponade physiology)
Trauma (penetrating or nonpenetrating)
Chylopericardium
Acute idiopathic
Rheumatic fever
Collagen vascular disease (SLE, rheumatoid arthritis, scleroderma, Wegener's granulomatosis)
Postsurgical (cardiac and intrathoracic)
Drug induced (procainamide, hydralazine, phenytoin, doxorubicin, isoniazide)

Infectious

Viral (coxsackievirus, echovirus, mumps, adenovirus, hepatitis, HIV)
Bacterial (pneumococcus, streptococcus, staphylococcus)
Tuberculous
Fungal (histoplasmosis, coccidiomycosis, candida, particularly in immunosuppressed patients)

diagnose. In two series of 241 patients who ultimately had malignant effusions diagnosed by Wilkes and associates[227] and Porte and colleagues,[230] approximately 50% of patients overall could not be shown to have neoplastic pericardial disease, and in the study from Porte,[227] the cause could be established in only one-quarter of these cases. Lymphatic obstruction by tumor might cause blockage without direct involvement of malignant cells in the pericardium, thereby making the usual gold-standard test, cytology, useless in the diagnosis, even though the effusion is in fact due to malignancy. Other causes, however—for example, prior radiation in a patient with a history of malignancy—also can cause an effusion and should always be considered for a patient with such a history to avoid mistakenly classifying a patient as having advanced cancer. Posner and coworkers[231] studied 31 patients with pericardial disease associated with various malignancies. Some 58% of patients had a malignant effusion, 32% had "idiopathic" pericarditis, and 10% had radiation-induced pericarditis. One study (using older radiotherapy equipment) from 1975 found that 30.9% of patients who underwent mantle radiotherapy for Hodgkin's disease were found to have "chest x-ray" evidence of pericardial effusion, and 13.6% required some intervention.[232]

Electrocardiogram and physical examination can be performed with particular attention to the foregoing findings. Chest radiograph can show a water bottle-shaped pericardium or an enlarged silhouette. Echocardiogram should be performed, emergently if there are clinical signs of tamponade, and to assess the hemodynamic impact of an effusion; this test can detect a volume of fluid as little as 15 mL. Echocardiographic findings have been reviewed elsewhere.[233] Fluid first appears as a lucent space between the pericardium and epicardium, visible only during systole and behind the left ventricle; once reaching 25–50 mL, it may be seen throughout the cardiac cycle. Once the effusion can separate the pericardium from the epicardium, the pericardial image becomes stationary; once it extends behind the atrium, atrial wall motion is markedly increased. When tamponade physiology is reached, the echo-Doppler shows compression of the right side of the heart, increased respiratory variation of mitral and tricuspid inflow velocity, and right atrial and ventricular collapse during diastole. Assessment of tamponade should be based on clinical and imaging evidence, not just on the volume of fluid present. CT scan is also sensitive for diagnosing an effusion. It can detect as little as 50 mL of pericardial fluid and, similar to an echocardiogram, can give an idea of intracardiac masses.[233] MRI also can provide direct imaging of the normal pericardium.[234] Both of these tests can give some clues as to the nature of the fluid (bloody, serous, chylous), but they rarely provide clinically useful information. If there is a small, questionable effusion present, MRI can differentiate between a small effusion and epicardial fat.[235] Because of the frequency with which oncology patients receive CT scans and MRIs, these studies often identify an effusion, prompting a further evaluation. Cardiac catheterization of the left and right sides of the heart can be used to confirm tamponade physiology (demonstrated by equivalence of pressures across all chambers) and improvement of these pressures after pericardiocentesis. This is usually not necessary, however.

Pericardiocentesis

Pericardiocentesis is usually performed with a 16- to 22-gauge needle (often a spinal needle) attached to a syringe inserted at roughly a 45-degree angle below the xiphoid process cephalad towards the tip of the left scapula. Advancement into the myocardium usually reveals an injury pattern on the ECG. Although this procedure is usually performed semi-electively, pericardiocentesis occasionally needs to be done in an emergent setting, where removal of as little as 50 mL of fluid can improve hemodynamic status.[236] Complications include ventricular perforation, arrythmias, and pneumothoracies and range from 5% to 20%. Complications are less likely (about 2%) when echocardiography is used to delineate the size and location of the fluid with respect to normal cardiac structures.[237] Among patients who are clinically unstable, with tamponade physiology and hypotension, vigorous volume resuscitation should be performed to increase cardiac filling pressures and cardiac output, even if signs of heart failure, such as edema or lung rales, are seen.[238]

Pericardial Fluid Evaluation

The evaluation of a patient with effusion depends on the category in which the physician places him or her. For those patients with small effusions and advanced malignancy found incidentally on imaging, nothing need be done except for a good physical examination and monitoring of the effusion. For patients with a suspicion of cancer, or those patients who are symptomatic due to tamponade physiology, attempts at diagnosis and therapy should be made. Pericardial effusion is rarely the initial manifestation of malignancy. Two studies both demonstrated that 7% of patients presenting with a pericardial effusion were ultimately given a new diagnosis of malignant pericardial disease.[239,240] Patients with no history of cancer who present with an effusion and absence of tamponade or significant clinical symptoms should be managed in a cautious, noninvasive manner. This approach usually includes treatment with anti-inflammatory therapy (such as NSAIDS) for potential idiopathic pericarditis for a period of one to two weeks.[239] Such management should be undertaken in cooperation with an experienced cardiologist. In terms of evaluating pericardial fluid, however, there are no specific guidelines for classifying an effusion as a transudate or exudate, or to further delineate the etiology of the effusion with criteria such as LDH, protein, glucose, pH, or cell count, as there are with pleural effusions. Interestingly, the best predictor for the behavior of a pericardial effusion of unknown etiology is from the clinical history of the patient. In a study of 322 patients from Sagrista-Sauleda and colleagues,[241] a large effusion with clinical signs of inflammation (two or more of the following: chest pain, fever, diffuse ST segment elevation, or friction rub) had a likelihood ratio of 20 for an idiopathic effusion, and those patients with tamponade without inflammation had a likelihood ratio of 2.9 for a malignant effusion.

It is worth repeating here that pericardial fluid, unlike pleural fluid, cannot be classified as a transudate or exudates. Nevertheless, aspirated fluid should be sent for cell count, cultures (if there is a possibility of infectious etiology), and cytology. The sensitivity of cytology for malignant pericardial disease varies widely, from 50% to 90%.[227,230,242-243] Reasons given for false-negative cytology include limited cellularlity in the specimen, shrouding by blood, or the absence of an expert cytopathologist. Interestingly, DNA diploidy obtained from flow cytometry has been found to correlate with benign cytology, and aneuploidy is associated with malignant cytology but is not sensitive enough to be definitive.[244] It is uncommon for pericardial fluid cytology to provide the first diagnosis of a malignancy. In one study of 47 pericardial fluid specimens, only 10 were positive for malignancy, and none of these represented the first diagnosis of a malignancy in a patient.[246] It is imperative, however, that the physician realize that a negative cytology does not exclude malignant pericardial disease. By the same token, patients with a history of cancer could have an effusion because of other reasons, particularly radiation.[247] One should be cautious, then, in providing the diagnosis of a malignant effusion (and usually advanced, incurable malignancy) unless definitive cytologic evidence is seen. For patients with a negative cytologic specimen but suspected malignancy, pericardial biopsy may be performed. Prospective studies have demonstrated a 5% to 20% positive yield for diagnostic pericardial biopsy specimens.[239,248] This is likely due to the blind nature of the biopsies and to the fact that biopsies are taken from the parietal pericardium, wheras the principal site of malignant involvement is the visceral pericardium, site of the epicardial lymphatics. The positive yield is much higher (54%) for biopsies performed during therapeutic (subxiphoid pericardiostomies) procedures; although there might be some selection bias, therapeutic procedures allow the pericardium to be visualized more directly and thus permit more accurate biopsy site selection.[239]

Pericardioscopy is a relatively new technique, available in specialized centers, that allows endoscopic inspection, aimed biopsies, and drainage of both pericardial surfaces and can even be used to obtain epicardial biopsies.[249,250] An expansion of this technique, using a perDUCER catheter, can be used for endocardial biopsies and thus far has been used for diagnosing and managing patients with nonmalignant pericarditis. This technique, however, also allows for guidewire and catheter placement, by which intrapericardial therapy may be administered. Ultimately, this technique might be expanded for use in evaluating and managing malignant pericardial etiologies.[251]

Treatment and Management

Asymptomatic malignant effusions do not require therapy. Volume depletion should be avoided, as adequate right ventricular preload is essential to allow sufficient cardiac output. For symptomatic patients, pericardiocentesis may be performed, either as initial therapy or to allow stabilization until a more definitive procedure can be performed. Unfortunately, up to three-quarters of patients recur and require treatment.[252,253]

Chemotherapy

A limited number of patients might benefit from systemic chemotherapy if such options are available (i.e., if they are expected to be chemotherapy responsive), or if a delay in treatment increases the risk of significant systemic progression. Such chemotherapy-sensitive tumors include leukemias, lymphomas, germ cell tumors, and even breast cancer. Although there might be reluctance on the physician's part to treat a malignant pericardial effusion with chemotherapy because of the feeling that even moderate effusions could become life threatening, there is ample evidence in the literature to support the use of chemotherapy in many circumstances. There are reports of successful resolution of effusions for patients with chronic myelomonocytic leukemia (CMML) with hydroyurea or chemotherapy.[254-257] Vaitkus and colleagues[252] reviewed the experience of treatment of 46 patients, mostly with breast cancer or lymphoma, who had malignant pericardial effusions treated with chemotherapy (38 of 46 patients initially having undergone therapeutic pericardiocentesis), and reported that systemic chemotherapy prevented recurrence in 67% of these patients. A special entity, primary cardiac lymphoma, although it responds to traditional chemotherapeutic regimens such as CHOP, is not responsive to radiotherapy and carries a poor prognosis, probably due to myocardial infiltration and tissue necrosis that might precede or result from chemotherapy.[258-260] Several researchers have reported pericardial effusions from leukemias with the presence of blast cells in the pericardial fluid, which were treated with emergent pericardiocentesis (because of tamponade) and immediate chemotherapy with good outcomes.[261,262] Other primary cardiac tumors, such as sarcoma and intrapericardial pheochromocytoma, tend not to be as responsive to chemotherapy, so control of the effusion should be the initial focus.[263] Vaitkus and associates[252] also reviewed the experience of 54 patients treated with radiotherapy and found that this procedure was successful two-thirds of the time, mainly in cases of hematologic malignancies and breast cancer (93% and 71% success rates, respectively) although 45% of patients with other solid tumors also had successful control. It should be noted, however, that radiotherapy might induce scarring or fibrosis that makes further interventions more difficult, so this procedure should be saved for end-stage patients declining other interventions. Those patients with physiology demanding immediate intervention should have some sort of drainage performed, while those that are stable and potentially chemotherapy-responsive should be considered for chemotherapy.

Percutaneous Tube Pericardiostomy

For patients not amenable to systemic therapy for whatever reasons, percutaneous drainage is performed. Because the rate of fluid reaccumulation is very high, prolonged catheter drainage is often employed in addition to pericardiocentesis. This is now common practice because it allows more a more complete drainage than that attainable by pericardiocentesis alone. After the pericardiocentesis, the needle is left in place, and a pigtail catheter is placed via the Seldinger catheter-over-a-guidewire technique. The catheter is left in place for several days and is not removed until the drainage is less than 20–30 mL per 24-hour period, at which point the catheter is removed. There is a small risk of infection with a catheter remaining in place for several days.[264] The catheter should be subject to intermittent rather than continuous drainage to maintain catheter patency. With this technique, however, there is still a relatively high likelihood that the fluid will reaccumulate unless other steps are taken. Unless the patient has a very short life expectancy (which still might require a repeat drainage) or, in the physician's mind, has a tumor from which one would expect a response from chemotherapy, other interventions will be required.

Surgical Approaches

Subxiphoid Pericardiostomy (Subxiphoid Pericardial Window). The subxipoid pericardial window, first reported by Napoleon's surgeon, Larrey, in 1829,[265] is now the most common surgical procedure for pericardial effusions. The procedure may be performed under local anesthesia with intravenous sedation; a small incision is made from the xiphoid process caudally for approximately 5 cm, and the xiphoid is either bisected or resected. After dissection to the pericardium, adhesions and masses are identified, a 2–4 cm^2 piece of pericardium is resected, and a chest tube is placed. The chest tube remains in place for postoperative drainage for several days, which could allow for sclerosis simply by acting as a pericardial irritant.[266] Allen and colleagues[267] retrospectively compared the experience of 117 patients who underwent either percutaneous catheter drainage with ultrasound or fluoroscopic guidance (n = 23) or subxiphoid pericardiostomy (n =

94). Complication rates were 17% in the percutaneous drainage group and 1% in the pericardiostomy group, with 4% mortality and a 30% recurrence rate in the percutaneous drainage group, compared with 0% mortality and 30% recurrence in the pericardiostomy group. In the percutaneous group, pigtail catheters remained in place for an average of 4.2 days, and mediastinal drainage was maintained for five days in the surgical group, so there was minimal difference in the number of days hospitalized. The advantages of the surgical group come with the caveat that the 23 patients who underwent percutaneous drainage did so because they were deemed to be too hemodynamically unstable to undergo a surgical procedure, and thus bias could account, at least in part, for the advantages of subxiphoid pericardiostomy. For all patients in this study, the median survival time of those patients having a malignant pericardial effusion was a paltry 2.2 months, with 13.8% of patients having a one-year survival. No patients who underwent pericardiostomy developed constrictive pericarditis. For patients who are hemodynamically stable, the subxiphoid pericardiostomy can and should be considered in lieu of percutaneous catheter drainage.

Alternative Surgical Techniques. Before the revival of the subxiphoid pericardial window, alternative surgical techniques had been used, including sternotomy and pericardiectomy or creation of a window via thoracotomy or VATS.[268-271] Initially, the experience of Piehler and associates[270] with 145 patients suggested that the extent of pericardial resection affected the recurrence rate, thus favoring open surgical drainage rather than the easier subxiphoid pericardiostomy. Several recent studies, however, have demonstrated no difference between the open or VATS procedures and subxiphoid pericardiostomies.[272,273] Vaitkus and coworkers[252] reported a decreased number of further pericardial complications when subxiphoid pericardiostomies, rather than open pericardiectomies, were performed. There is a much lower incidence of postoperative complications (including pneumonia, thrombosis, arrhythmia, respiratory failure) after subxiphoid pericardial drainage compared with transthoracic pericardial resection (10% vs. 50%, respectively).[272,273] VATS offers a minimally invasive technique for treatment of effusions but still requires general anesthesia and the ability to tolerate single-lung ventilation, so it offers little advantage over subxiphoid pericardiostomy. It should therefore be saved for situations in which the subxiphoid approach fails, in which a VATS approach would assist with evaluation or treatment of simultaneous lung pathology, or in which a larger specimen of pericardium is required for clearer observation and evaluation of an undiagnosed effusion.[273-275] A pericardial-peritoneal shunt with a Denver-type catheter and pump, similar to that used in pleural effusions, has been used for some patients with success, but its use should be limited to patients whose effusions are refractory to other management techniques.[275]

Percutaneous Balloon Pericardiotomy. Percutaneous balloon pericardiostomy is an extension of a percutaneous pigtail catheter, except that a balloon-dilating catheter (20 mm diameter and 3 cm length) introduced over a guidewire creates a nonsurgical pericardial window. Ziskind and colleagues[276] provided the results from the first 50 patients treated with this technique. The procedure was considered successful in 46 of the 50 patients, with two patients requiring early operation for a bleeding vessel and persistent drainage and two patients requiring late drainage for recurrent tamponade. Minor complications included fever, thoracentesis, requirement for chest tube placement, and pneumothorax. The most significant complications were the development of pleural effusions requiring drainage. Subsequent studies have reported up to 100% success rates.[277,278] Long-term outcome from these patients was still poor, with a mean survival time of 3.3 months. The procedure has been slow to gain acceptance because of the need for specialized training and equipment but could become a more popular option as interventional radiologists become adept in this technique.

Intrapericardial Sclerosing Agents and Chemotherapy. For pericardial effusions, as for pleural effusions, sclerosing agents may be used, and in general, do work.[279] Maher and colleagues[280] reported their experiences with 93 patients who underwent pericardial fluid drainage, followed by sclerosis with either doxycycline or tetracycline. A median of three instillations was required and was able to control the effusion 88% of the time. Shepherd and colleagues[281] reported similar results (75% success rate). The most common complaints with this procedure are pain (intrapericardial lidocaine should be injected before the sclerosing agent) and arrythmias. Bleomycin has been compared with doxycycline in a prospective, randomized study showing equal efficacy and less pain; therefore, it should probably be considered instead of doxycycline as the sclerosing agent of choice.[282]

The use of direct intrapericardial instillation of chemotherapy and biologic therapy has been examined in several settings with limited data. For pericardial as for pleural effusions, it is somewhat difficult to determine whether intrapericardial chemotherapy functions because of tumor cytotoxicity or pericardial irritation leading to sclerosis, as the physiology and mechanisms of sclerosis are poorly understood. Imamura[283] looked at the use of OK-432 (a heat-treated lyophilate of *Streptococcus Pyogenes A3*) instilled directly into the pericardium after fluid drainage. All ten patients in this study achieved complete control of the pericardial effusion, seven of the ten with only one treatment, for an average of 10.8 months. Complications were primarily fever and chest pain. Hypotension was also seen and was thought to be a result of rapid fluid reaccumulation in several patients. Moriya and associates[284] explored the use of intrapericardial carboplatin in ten patients with advanced non–small cell lung cancer; eight patients showed complete regression of the effusion with minimal toxicities and minimal systemic distribution of the carboplatin. Cisplatin is the best-studied therapy, with overall success rates of 67%–87%.[285] One of the earliest studies on the use of cisplatin comes from Fiorentino, who gave five patients intrapericardial cisplatin (50 mg over 5 minutes 5 days in a row, with courses repeated every 2 to 3 weeks if there was fluid recurrence).[285] There was a 60% complete response rate in the effusion. Side effects were limited to mild nausea with no hematologic or renal toxicities. Kawashima and colleagues[286] gave intrapericardial aclarubicin to five patients with pericardial tamponade secondary to malignant effusions; in four of the five, physicians were able to remove the pericardial catheter, and two of the five patients experienced a complete remission of the pericardial effusion. All patients demonstrated disappearance of the malignant cells from the pericardial space, with no cytopathologically demonstrable pericardial recurrence. Mitoxantrone and interferon have also been used, with similar results.[287,288] Used intrapericardially, however, there is a significant risk of pain, a requirement for multiple instillations, and a possibility of constrictive pericarditis for patients with a prolonged survival. Because of these factors, the use of pericardial sclerosis is declining, and intrapericardial chemotherapy remains highly experimental.

Summary

Malignant pericardial effusion is a dreaded complication of malignancy, indicative of advanced disease in most cases. The oncologist should take care to ensure that advanced disease is in fact present, and that the effusion has no other etiology in a patient who has a history of cancer. Management should be focused on immediate resuscitation and control of life-threatening symptoms. Asymptomatic patients with cancer and an effusion can be managed conservatively and observed with either repeat careful physical examination or serial echocardiograms. If there is a strong likelihood of tumor response to chemotherapy, or if chemotherapy is absolutely required (e.g., in cases of lymphoma or life-threatening systemic disease), it should be started as soon as possible. If emergent pericardiocentesis is required, it should be performed with placement of a percutaneous pigtail catheter. For patients who are clinically more stable but unable to be treated adequately with systemic chemotherapy, one could consider either percutaneous drainage

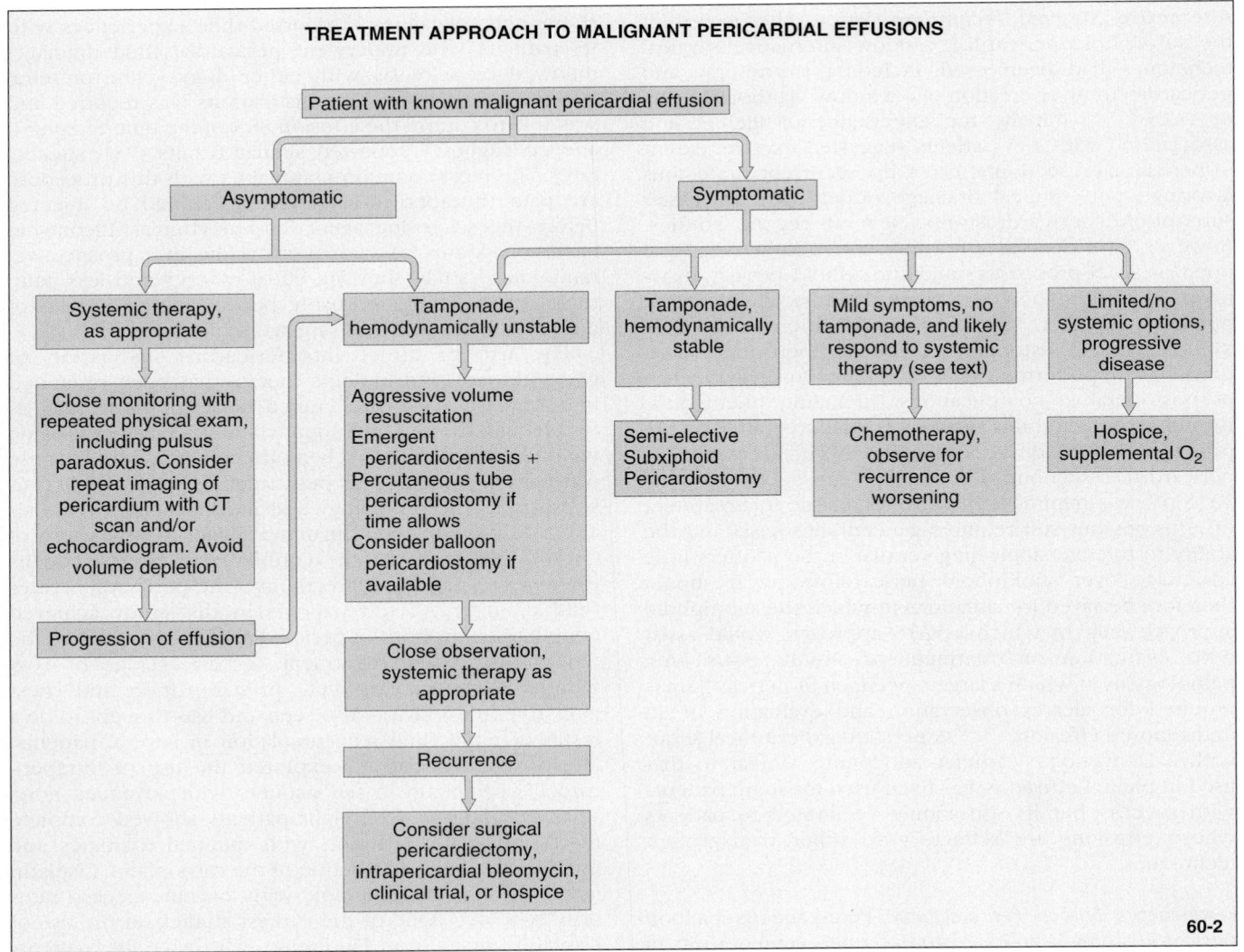

TREATMENT APPROACH TO MALIGNANT PERICARDIAL EFFUSIONS

60-2

or subxiphoid pericardiectomy under local anesthesia, with likely similar results; the latter demonstrates a lower rate of recurrence and is our procedure of choice. Such a management approach has been validated in several studies.[267,289] Use of other techniques, such as VATS, percutaneous balloon pericardiotomy, sclerosis, or intrapericardial chemotherapy offers new potential options for these patients should primary therapy fail.

ASCITES

Malignant ascites is a frequent occurrence in the patient with malignancy and is usually an indication of peritoneal carcinomatosis. Like malignant pericardial and pleural effusions, it is often a harbinger of advanced disease. It accounts for 10% of cases of ascites, and 1-year survival is less than 10%.[290]

Etiology and Pathogenesis

The peritoneal membrane contains lymphatics, which serve to collect fluid, proteins, cells, and other substances and return them to the systemic collection. There is a specialized anatomic feature, the stomata, which are relatively open connections that connect the abdominal cavity to submesothelial lymphatics, and which are the sites of most lymphatic drainage of the abdomen.[291,292] Fluid accumulations, as in the pleural and pericardial cavities, can occur if there is overproduction or decreased drainage of fluid. Again, fluid balance is mainly controlled by Starling's equation (Eq. 1).[293] Studies in adults have demonstrated that increased fluid production is a major cause of ascites among patients with peritoneal carcinomatosis.[294] Animal models in which mice were given intraperitoneal injections of tumor cells have demonstrated that obstruction to lymphatic flow can cause of ascites as well, and this has been confirmed using lymphoscintigraphy in humans.[295-298] Vascular endothelial growth factor (vEGF), an angiogenesis factor expressed by most tumors (including those that spread to the peritoneum), has been demonstrated, in vivo, to cause increased fluid production and to influence the development of ascites.[299-305] VEGF is probably the single biggest mediator of ascites production. IL-2, Tumor Necrosis Factor (TNF), interferon-α, and matrix metalloproteinases also have been implicated as factors contributing to the formation of ascites.[306-309] Intraperitoneal protein accumulation decreases the difference between plasma and peritoneal oncotic pressures and subsequently decreases filtration into the lymphatics.[310] Free fluid flow into the abdomen therefore increases according to Starling's equation. Fluid protein concentration can reach oncotic pressures similar to that reached in peritoneal dialysis, which is very effective in causing ultrafiltration.[311,312] One study in cats demonstrated that increased hepatic venous pressures alone could result in the production of ascites.[313] Unlike the case with cirrhotic patients, however, increased portal pressure probably contributes minimally to the development of ascites, except among patients with massive hepatic metastases.[294,312] The most common tumors that cause ascites are those of gastrointestinal and pelvic organs; the single most common type of tumor is ovarian cancer.

Diagnosis and Evaluation

Many patients with malignant ascites have small amounts of fluid first noticed on imaging studies, such as those done for staging or evaluation after therapy or for another complaint. Symptoms resulting from large amounts of fluid usually include abdominal distention, such that pants are no longer able to fit properly; early satiety; nausea; vomiting; an increase in weight; edema; and shortness of breath. Physical examination in the evaluation of ascites is notoriously difficult, especially among obese patients with lesser amounts of fluid. The physical examination has been shown to be from 50% to 94% sensitive and from 29% to 82% specific, with ultrasound as the gold standard of testing.[314] Physical examination can demonstrate a fluid wave, shifting, or flank dullness. The absence of flank dullness is the most accurate predictor against ascites, but one requires 1500 mL of fluid to be present to notice flank dullness. If there is suspicion of ascites in any patient, ultrasound is the easiest, fastest, and cheapest method of ascertaining a diagnosis of ascites; one series demonstrated that as little as 100 mL of fluid can be demonstrated on an ultrasound.[315,316] Radiologic studies such as CT or MRI can also give clear-cut evidence of ascites, but these are usually not necessary as part of the first-line evaluation. Plain film x-rays can show a ground glass appearance to the abdomen, loss of detail, haziness, or floating bowel on supine films but is nonspecific.

For many patients with known malignancy, the presence of ascites will not alter management, as advanced disease is already present. For some patients, particularly those without a known malignancy, the detection of ascites requires an appropriate evaluation to determine the etiology. For these patients, the differential diagnosis includes congestive heart failure, alcoholic cirrhosis, cirrhosis due to hepatitis B or C, previous abdominal surgeries, nonalcoholic steatohepatitis, and other causes of increased portal venous pressure. It should be remembered that patients with a history of cirrhosis have a predilection for hepatocellular carcinoma.

In most cases of ascites in which malignancy is a possibility, cross-sectional imaging, such as with a CT scan, should be performed to seek a primary tumor site, hepatic metastases, or other evidence of peritoneal seeding. Women in particular should have either an ultrasound or CT scan to evaluate the ovaries. After this, a diagnostic abdominal paracentesis is indicated. Ultrasound may be used during the procedure to localize ascites and minimize the risk of injury to abdominal organs (particularly the liver and intestine).[315] After local anesthesia, an 18-gauge needle attached to a 25- to 50-mL syringe is inserted into a site indicated by ultrasound or into the areas percussed as dull in the flanks, if sufficient fluid is present. If cytology is required, up to 1 L of fluid can be obtained using vacuum bottles. Even among patients with coagulopathies (such as cirrhosis), the risk of developing a hematoma is only 1% and that of causing

Problems Common to Cancer and Its Therapy

peritonitis or hemoperitoneum is 0.1%; therefore, one can usually proceed without the use of clotting factors or platelets.[317-319] Patients on therapeutic anticoagulation should have their anticoagulation withheld for several days before paracentesis.

Visualization of the fluid can provide some useful clues; clear fluid is usually associated with cirrhosis. Infected fluid is cloudy. Milky fluid can indicate chylous ascites, and should be sent for triglyceride evaluation. Such fluid often has triglyceride levels greater than 200 mg/dL and often as high as 1000 mg/dL. Some studies have demonstrated that the most common cause for chylous ascites is malignancy, although others have found cirrhosis as the primary cause.[320,321] Either way, if chylous fluid is found, it should heighten the physician's attention to the potential for malignancy. Heterogeneously bloody fluid is associated with a traumatic tap, while homogeneously bloody fluid indicates prior bleeding (i.e., a nontraumatic tap) and could indicate malignancy. Ascites is bloody in up to one-half of patients with hepatocellular carcinoma and in 22% of all patients with malignant ascites.[322-324] Spontaneous bacterial peritonitis (SBP) does not tend to develop to the extent that it does among patients with cirrhotic ascites, unless there has been previous surgery or a previous paracentesis. All patients should be evaluated for signs of SBP (including fever and abdominal pain) and a cell count on the ascitic fluid; a polymorphonuclear count greater than 250/mm^3 should prompt the use of empiric antibiotics in appropriate situations.[319,325]

The first and most important step in the evaluation of the patient with ascites of unknown etiology is to differentiate those causes arising from portal hypertension (usually cirrhosis) from other causes (including malignancy). The best test for this determination is the serum-to-ascites albumin gradient (SAAG), which is the difference between serum albumin and ascitic fluid albumin. Low-protein ascites, and thus an elevated gradient, can be thought of as arising mainly from pressure differentials brought upon by Starling's equation (Eq. 1); this is usually from portal venous hypertension. A gradient equal to or greater than 1.1 g/dL indicates portal hypertension with 97% accuracy, while a lower gradient indicates a lack of portal hypertension and possibly the presence of a malignancy.[321,326] The classical division of ascitic fluids into transudates and exudates using LDH, protein, and their serum/ascites ratios, akin to pleural effusions, has been shown to be not as useful. Total protein is not particularly useful for diagnosis of malignant ascites, although a a value of less than 1 g/dL is useful in predicting a patient's increased risk for SBP.[327,328] This range of values is usually seen in cirrhotic patients. A glucose value below 50 has been associated with malignancy but also can be indicative of infection.[9,43] An ascites/serum ratio of LDH greater than 1 indicates that the enzyme is actively being produced in the ascitic fluid and suggests malignancy, but not as specifically as with a pleural effusion.[327] Triglyceride levels should be obtained in milky ascites but might or might not be particularly helpful. Other chemistries and cultures should be obtained if diagnoses other than malignancy are entertained.[290,319,325,329] Siddiqui and colleagues[330] have

demonstrated that fibronectin is up to 100% sensitive and specific as a marker of malignant ascites in a small study of only 12 patients with malignant ascites; others feel that this test is not helpful, and it is not used routinely.[331]

The detection of tumor cells by cytology remains the gold standard for the detection of malignancy. For patients with peritoneal carcinomatosis due to cellular exfoliation into the ascitic fluid, malignant cells can be detected nearly 100% of the time.[323] On the other hand, patients with liver metastases and portal venous obstruction, chylous ascites from lymphomas and lymphatic obstruction, or hepatocellar carcinoma, might not have a positive ascitic fluid; the overall sensitivity for cytology is therefore on the order of 40%–75% when 500 mL of fluid is obtained.[330,332,333] To increase the detection of tumor cells and differentiate mesothelial cells from malignant cells, immunohistochemistry for cytokeratin, vimentin, leucocyte common antigen, S100, CEA, HMB45, and other markers may be performed on the cytologic specimen.[308] A small study by Loewenstein[334] has shown that an elevated CEA level in ascitic fluid is a good marker for malignancy, although this has not been well validated and requires further evaluation. Elevated serum or ascites CA-125 and CEA levels certainly should prompt a careful evaluation for malignancies, particularly for ovarian cancer in women with highly elevated CA-125, although neither marker is specific for any particular malignancy (or even malignancies in general) and might reflect only intra-abdominal pathology rather than malignant disease.[310] No known studies have correlated levels of CA-125 and CEA with the likelihood of a malignancy, but one would expect higher levels of tumor markers to have a greater association with malignancy.

Women with only ascites and no evidence of primary malignancy on cross-sectional imaging present an interesting situation. These patients should undergo laparoscopic evaluation, at which time both ovaries are biopsied, ascitic fluid is sampled, and random biopsies are performed throughout the abdomen. If ovarian carcinoma or adenocarcinoma consistent with ovarian carcinoma is seen, the procedure is converted to a laparotomy; it has been shown that aggressive surgical debulking to minimal residual disease improves response, survival time, and response to aggressive chemotherapy (usually taxane- and platinum-based) among patients with ovarian carcinoma. Such an approach can lead to a long disease-free interval and significant long-term survival. Even small, low-grade ovarian tumors, with the primary tumor not seen on imaging, can lead to diffuse peritoneal contamination, and hence, to the development of ascites.[335-337] Some patients might have papillary serous carcinoma of the peritoneum (PSCP), which arises from the peritoneal surface but shares a common histogenesis with ovarian tissue and also might be difficult to detect on cross-sectional imaging. It is important to remember that patients with ovarian cancer with ascites are classified as only stage III, and hence this rather large subgroup should be treated aggressively whenever possible. PSCP should be treated in a fashion similar to ovarian carcinoma.[338,339] Laparoscopy should be performed diligently. In a study from van Dam and associates[340] of 104 women with advanced ovarian cancer who underwent laparoscopy for diagnosis, 58% of patients had tumor implanted at the trocar site when only the skin was closed at the conclusion of the procedure, but in those in whom all abdominal wall layers were closed, only 2% had such implantation. For patients with ascites, there is a risk of prolonged fluid drainage at trocar placement sites. In one study, 2 of 92 patients developed peritonitis and died after undergoing laparascopic procedures in these circumstances.[341] For a more detailed discussion of the diagnosis and management of ovarian carcinoma, the reader is referred to Chapter 92.

Management

As with pleural and pericardial effusions, it is important to distinguish the appropriate situations in which to treat malignant ascites. Small amounts of ascites can be tolerated very well or not even noticed. On the other hand, when symptoms such as dyspnea, abdominal pain, fatigue, anorexia, or early satiety arise, treatment can be required. The most worrisome sign is dyspnea, which can arise both from an inordinate amount of weight being carried by the patient or by compression of the pleural cavity leading to a decrease in total lung capacity. Clearly, the overall clinical status of the patient should be taken into account when making these treatment decisions. In light of the fact that ascites does not usually pose a life-threatening situation, and that the disease might respond well to systemic therapy in instances such as ovarian cancer, systemic chemotherapy can be considered front-line therapy. For other situations, such as pancreatic cancer, because responses to therapy are much less frequent, one would consider an early direct approach to control of the fluid. Certainly, in either case, as most techniques to manage fluid (e.g., diuresis, paracentesis) are relatively easy and performed on an outpatient basis, one could combine systemic chemotherapy with these other options.

Fluid Balance Management

Third-spacing of fluid into nonvascular compartments results in decreased renal blood flow and consequently to sodium and water retention by the kidney, which ultimately leads to the propagation of third-spacing of fluids. The use of fluid management techniques to manage malignant ascites is controversial. Because tumors that arise from peritoneal seeding are not caused by pressure gradients shifts, some feel that management using diuretics and salt management techniques that effect renal handling of excess fluid and sodium are useless, while others believe they can be effective.[342,343] One can attempt dietary restriction of sodium to less than 2 g per day and also restrict free water intake to help decrease the amount of ascites. Unfortunately, to the patient with advanced malignancy, this strategy can prove overly burdensome, particularly when the patient is undergoing other treatments such as chemotherapy. At a minimum, however, the physician should restrict intravenous hydration as much as possible when chemotherapy is being administered.

The next step in this mode of management is the use of diuretics, which offers a noninvasive mechanism to help maintain fluid balance. The advantage of this approach is that it can be done easily on an outpatient basis with oral medications, and it is even possible for patients to perform minor self-adjustments in medication after instruction, which also restores to patients a degree control over their own health. A distal tubule diuretic, such as spironolactone, is usually used first. Such agents act on the distal nephron, thereby minimizing the chances for compensation by more distal renal elements. More important, it works at the site of the rennin-angtiotensin-aldosterone axis, which is upregulated due to decreased renal perfusion when significant third spacing occurs, as in ascites. Doses start at approximately 25–50 mg per day and can go as high as 200 mg per day. Painful gynecomastia can result, and if this proves bothersome, amiloride is an alternative. Spironolactone often is insufficient by itself and not immediate in its effects. In such cases, furosemide (usually starting at 20 mg per day and titrated to much higher doses) has been used for either a short period or, commonly, in combination. Razis and colleagues,[344] along with others, however, have pointed out that loop diuretics such as furosemide are minimally effective, if at all, in the management of ascites. The maximal ascitic reabsorption rate is 930 mL per day, and patients should therefore be instructed to weigh themselves daily and allow no more than a 0.5–1 kg per day loss in weight; in the presence of peripheral edema, slightly more weight can be lost per day.[292] Overdiuresis can result in hypotension, volume depletion, azotemia, and electrolyte abnormalities (particularly hyperkalemia with spironolactone, hypokalemia with furosemide), and thus patients should be monitored closely. Patients should be instructed to monitor their weights between physician visits and even to modify the doses of diuretics used when certain weight goals are met.

Unfortunately, although diuretics initially are used by many physicians for the control of ascites and certainly are easy to administer, they are not very effective.[345] Malignant ascites is usually not very responsive to diuresis because the pathogenesis is usually not related to increased portal pressure, as it is in cirrhosis, but rather is related to increased fluid production from the presence of tumor cells in the peritoneum.[346] In the rarer cases in which massive hepatic metastases are present and portal hypertension is the etiology of ascites, patients are much more likely to respond to diuretics.[347] Pockros and colleagues[346] confirmed this, finding that patients with a large amount of hepatic metastases (and hence elevated portal venous pressure) had a SAAG similar to cirrhotics and were more likely to respond to diuretics, while those patients with peritoneal carcinomatosis were less likely to respond to diuretic management of ascites. Although there are no direct comparative studies, it is because of these clinical experiences that diuresis is used much less frequently than paracentesis as a means of controlling ascites.[345]

Paracentesis

Paracentesis is the most frequently used and effective management approach to malignant ascites, but its effects are only temporary.[345] Large-volume paracentesis can improve shortness of breath and early satiety quickly. Because one removes the fluid and not the cause of the fluid, however, there is rapid redistribution to the peritoneal cavity. Because of this, large-volume paracentesis can result in intravascular volume depletion, hypotension, azotemia, and other consequences of dehydration.[292] Colloidal colume expansion has been tried as a means to prevent these sequelae. In a randomized trial in cirrhotics by Gines and colleagues,[348] 105 patients receiving large-volume paracentesis were randomly assigned to receive albumin or not. Patients not receiving albumin were more likely to show signs of hemodynamic deterioration, worsening renal function, and hyponatremia (20.8% vs. 3.8%). Most of these patients, however, simply had laboratory abnormalities, as no advantages in clinical morbidity or survival ever have been demonstrated in this or any other study.[319,349] Further, a 5L paracentesis would require approximately 50 g of albumin at a cost of of up to several thousand dollars and would change a quick procedure into either a day-long one or one requiring an overnight hospital stay, which is not easily justified for patients with advanced malignancies in the absence of proven benefit.[13] Because of this, the use of any colloidal expanders is difficult to justify.

Complications of repeated paracentesis include bleeding, pain, the induction of peritonitis, and bowel perforation. The presence of loculated ascites can make adequate removal of fluid to provide a symptomatic benefit nearly impossible, and it can increase the risk of the procedure. Ultrasound guidance should be employed to decrease the risk of complications.

Peritoneovenous Shunting

Peritoneovenous shunting, introduced by LeVeen for alcoholic liver disease, is effective in malignant ascites.[350] Because patients with intractable and debilitating ascites have a median survival of only 6 to 33 weeks and could probably be managed more easily with repeated paracentesis, patients selected for shunting should have an expected survival of several months requiring frequent paracentesis, as demonstrated by repeated recurrence of the ascites after drainage.[351-353] The device consists of a long, perforated tubing inserted in the peritoneal cavity, a tubing that inserts into the superior vena cava, and a one-way valve that connects the two. There are two types of shunts, the LeVeen shunt and the Denver shunt; the latter has a one-way pump that can be used by the patient or physician to clear debris in the shunt or valve. On inspiration, intrathoracic pressure is lowered and the one-way valve opens, allowing a baseline pressure difference between the thoracic cavity and abdominal cavity to increase by 3–5 cm H_2O from its baseline difference of 5–15 cm H_2O, causing fluid to flow across the pressure gradient and drain into the superior vena cava. Placement of the shunt can be done under local anesthesia, with two to three separate incisions made. Parsons and colleagues demonstrated no survival or quality-of-life advantage when peritoneovenous shunting was compared with repeated paracentesis.[354] Peritoneovenous shunting is effective in controlling ascites between 62% to 88% of the time.[355-359] Early studies demonstrated a large number of pump failures due to occlusion (up to nearly two-thirds), but more recent studies have demonstrated lesser rates of occlusion.[350,355,360-364] The manual pump present in the Denver device for clearing blockages has not demonstrated an advantage in the maintenance of shunt patency.[355,363] Flushing the pump and administration of thrombolytic agents might be able to restore patency and avoid pump removal and replacement in instances of pump failure.

Patients with ascites that is cytologically negative for tumor cells have a much longer shunt life than those patients with cytologic evidence of malignancy; this is probably due to sludging of the pump system with more viscous tumor cells or debris in the later case. Immediately after placement of the pump, congestive heart failure can occur due to a rapid increase in intravascular volume from infusion of a large amount of ascitic fluid; this risk can be minimized by performing a large-volume paracentesis just before the procedure.[351] Coagulopathy—specifically disseminated intravascular coagulation (DIC)—is common when the pumps are used in cirrhotic patients, but not in those with malignant ascites (rate of 4%).[356,365] DIC probably arises due to fibrinolytic activity of ascitic fluid, and fibrinolytic activity is decreased in patients with malignant ascites.[366] Those patients with malignant ascites and good preshunt hepatic function seem to be at an even particularly low or negligible risk for DIC.[367,368] Widespread dissemination of tumor cells from the peritoneum to the lungs has been demonstrated in several studies.[350,360,361,368] The clinical significance of additional tumor emboli among patients with advanced refractory malignancy, although it represents a major potential complication of shunt placement, is unclear. Infection also remains a concern, but the incidence of shunt-induced peritonitis is much lower among patients with malignant disease than among those with cirrhosis, probably due to the higher levels of protein and immunoglobulin in the ascites.[327,328]

With significant potential complications and alternatives available, Souter and colleagues[360,361] suggest the following criteria for patients who should be considered for shunt placement:

- The goal of care is palliative.
- Expected survival is longer than three months.
- The rate of fluid reaccumulation is rapid after large-volume paracentesis.
- There is no loculation.
- Accumulated fluid is not bloody or viscous, which could lead to early shunt dysfunction.

Patients with peritonitis or those not able to handle large, rapid fluid shifts (patients with significant cardiac or renal dysfunction) would also not be candidates for shunt placement.

Drainage Catheters

External drainage catheters offer a different method for palliation of ascites, namely a route available for repeated drainage that does not require repeated needle insertion. Patients are therefore offered the ability to perform repeated paracentesis without decreased morbidity and discomfort, possibly at home by themselves or with minimal assistance. Several different methods are available; most use vascular ports inserted into the peritoneum, tunneled catheters, or other similar devices to allow drainage after catheter access.[369-371] The best-described uses of this method are from Lomas and colleagues,[372] in which a patient with malignant ascites had 1 L of fluid removed per day for 3 months with a Tenckhoff catheter, and that from Belfort,[373] in which 17 patients were implanted with a 20 Fr silastic tube with a Dacron cuff at the peritoneal surface, all of whom did well with repeated removal of ascites.[374] A disadvantage of repeated drainage of ascites via any means is that, among patients who do survive and undergo a number of procedures, there is a large amount of protein loss, particularly when compared with peritoneovenous shunting, in which the fluid is rerouted to the vascular system and protein might be retained. The most impressive protein loss seen comes from Lomas' study,[375] in which the average albumin level fell from 2.8 g/dL to 1.8 g/dL. Other series, however, have demonstrated much smaller decreases in albumin level, especially when high-protein diets were used. If one considers that these patients have advanced, refractory malignancy, protein and albumin loss due to repeated drainage is probably not all that significant but should still be monitored.[370,373] There is a risk of infection with superficial catheters; in the aforementioned study by Belfort,[373] in which patients were given cuffed catheters, 47% of patients (8 of 17) developed postive ascitic fluid surveillance cultures, and 12% (2 of 17) required removal due to "significant infection." In a study using a tunneled catheter (the Denver Pleurx catheter), 0 of 10 patients developed infections requiring catheter removal.[370] Although no comparison studies have been done with peritoneal catheters, randomized studies involving other catheter systems clearly have demonstrated decreased infection rates when catheters had their cuffs placed subcutaneously in a tunnel rather than at the surface.[373] Percutaneous catheters therefore remain an option for some patients, although they are not used frequently.

Surgery

Sugarbaker[375] has been an advocate of peritonectomy, in which various parts of the peritoneum, omentum, and some intraabdominal organs are removed as a method of tumor cytoreduction (akin to debulking of ovarian cancer, which has now become a standard of care) in preparation for intraperitoneal chemotherapy. This approach has been used for patients with peritoneal carcinomatosis with the chemotherapy tailored towards the nature of the malignancy. Studies have shown modest success with this procedure in increasing survival time and in the prevention against the development of malignant ascites, but its use in the treatment of ascites has not been well evaluated.[376-378] It is likely to be of minimal use, as patients with advanced, malignant ascites often have chemotherapy-refractory disease and have too much systemic disease to benefit from cytoreduction; removal of ascites alone as palliation can usually be accomplished through much easier means. The role of intraperitoneal chemotherapy in the prevention of the development of ascites is intriguing, however, and is discussed next.

Intraperitoneal Therapy

Direct intraperitoneal therapy has been tried for quite some time in an attempt to deliver higher doses of chemotherapy locally with minimal systemic absorption and distribution.[379] Intraperitoneal therapy has been used to treat both ascites and intraabdominal malignancies, such as ovarian cancer. ^{32}P was used in the 1950s, with a reported response rate of 58% in the treatment of ascites.[380] More recently, colloidal suspensions of $^{32}CrPO_4$ have been used with modest success.[381] In 1955, Weisberger and colleagues[382] first reported the successful treatment of malignant ascites with intraperitoneal nitrogen mustard. Many different chemotherapies have been used in an attempt to help control ascites, including bleomycin, cisplatin, 5-FU, doxorubicin, and mitomycin.[169,383-387] Patients with disease responsive to chemotherapy are most likely to benefit from this procedure. In this manner, the intraperitoneal administration of cisplatin has been well studied, as ovarian cancer is one of the most common intraabdominal tumors with a predilection for causing ascites and is very responsive to systemic cisplatin chemotherapy. Simultaneous administration of intravenous thiosulfate might decrease systemic absorption of cisplatin.[388] Several investigators have found that intraperitoneal administration of cisplatin is indeed effective for control of intraabdominal ovarian cancer, with perhaps better efficacy than that given intravenously.[389] This conclusion remains quite controversial, however; the issue is discussed separately in Chapter 92, on ovarian malignancies. Gilly and colleagues[390] reported the resolution of ascites in 11 of 12 patients with either gastrointestinal or ovarian malignancy treated with surgical resection of bulk disease followed by intraperitoneal instillation of cisplatin and mitomycin-C in conjunction with hyperthermia. Loggie and colleagues[391] reported similar results with a similar protocol. It is interesting to note that in this study, 12 patients who did not present with ascites but had cytologically positive ascitic fluid at the time of surgery never developed malignant ascites and had a median survival of more than 32 months. Markman and associates[392] treated 19 patients with malignant peritoneal mesothelioma with a combination of intraperitoneal cisplatin and mitomycin. Of the 15 patients with malignant ascites, seven (47%) experienced control of fluid reaccumulation for a median of eight months (range 2 to 73 months), and some have achieved long-term survival.

Several intraperitoneal biological response modifiers have also been tried with modest success. Intraperitoneal administration of OK-432 plus IL-2 demonstrated a decrease in the amount of ascites in 18 of 22 patients with gastric cancer.[393] Correlative studies indicated that these biological factors might work to destroy tumor by activating complement and attracting neutrophils, lymphocytes, and activated macrophages.[394,395] Intraperitoneal administration of α-2β-interferon has demonstrated minimal toxicity but also minimal efficacy in the control of ascites.[396-398] A randomized study comparing interferon-α, interferon-β, and IL-2 demonstrated some minor responses, with intraperitoneal IL-2 showing ability to induce response in ascites for patients with intra-abdominal mesothelioma.[398] Complications include fever, leukopenia, and flulike malaise. Small pilot studies have demonstrated preliminary activity for radiolabelled monoclonal antibodies directed towards tumor markers, and for matrix metalloproteinase inhibitors.[399-401] The

complexity of these procedures, their limited availability, and the fact that many or most patients who present with intractable ascites have already undergone numerous treatments and are likely chemotherapy resistant, limits the role for intraperitoneal therapy in the management of ascites except in some special situations and, of course, in clinical trials. It is important for the role of intraperitoneal chemotherapy immediately after initial surgical explora-

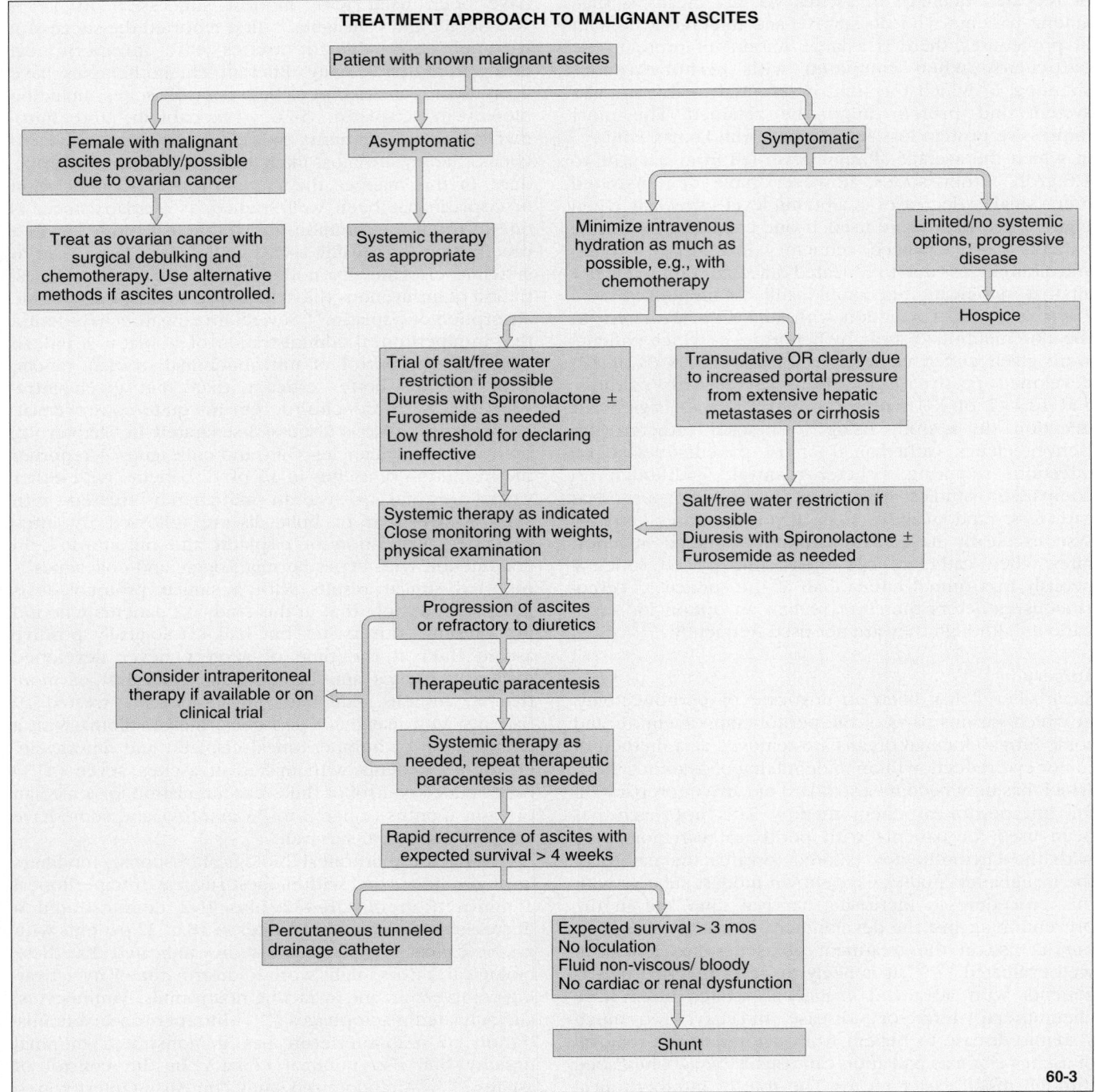

TREATMENT APPROACH TO MALIGNANT ASCITES

Patient with known malignant ascites

- Female with malignant ascites probably/possible due to ovarian cancer
  - Treat as ovarian cancer with surgical debulking and chemotherapy. Use alternative methods if ascites uncontrolled.

- Asymptomatic
  - Systemic therapy as appropriate

- Symptomatic
  - Minimize intravenous hydration as much as possible, e.g., with chemotherapy
    - Trial of salt/free water restriction if possible
      Diuresis with Spironolactone ± Furosemide as needed
      Low threshold for declaring ineffective
    - Transudative OR clearly due to increased portal pressure from extensive hepatic metastases or cirrhosis
      - Salt/free water restriction if possible
        Diuresis with Spironolactone ± Furosemide as needed
    - Systemic therapy as indicated
      Close monitoring with weights, physical examination
    - Progression of ascites or refractory to diuretics
      - Consider intraperitoneal therapy if available or on clinical trial
      - Therapeutic paracentesis
      - Systemic therapy as needed, repeat therapeutic paracentesis as needed
      - Rapid recurrence of ascites with expected survival > 4 weeks
        - Percutaneous tunneled drainage catheter
        - Expected survival > 3 mos
          No loculation
          Fluid non-viscous/ bloody
          No cardiac or renal dysfunction
          - Shunt
  - Limited/no systemic options, progressive disease
    - Hospice

60-3

tion for malignancy to be examined further to determine whether it produces a survival advantage or a reduction in the rate of development of malignant ascites.

Summary

The level of aggressiveness that one undertakes in the management of ascites is highly dependent on the overall clinical status of the patient. For those patients with chemotherapy-sensitive tumors who are not heavily pretreated, chemotherapy should be an early step in management, particularly in cases of ovarian and hematologic malignancies. Although diuretic therapy probably does not have much of an effect, we do recommend an early trial, as it is relatively easy to carry out and can be particularly helpful for patients with increased portal pressures due to massive hepatic metastases. For those patients with a limited life expectancy but a large amount of ascitic fluid causing symptoms, paracentesis on an as-needed basis should be used, with the caveat that recurrence of the effusion is virtually assured and repeat paracentesis required unless other steps are taken. Intraperitoneal therapy of many types can be considered where available, particularly for ascites due to ovarian cancer or in the setting of a clinical trial. Patients who are likely to live a long time without chemotherapy-responsive tumors should be considered for a shunt or catheter drainage device, or for any available clinical trial.

REFERENCES

1. Noppen M: Normal volume and cellular contents of pleural fluid. Curr Opin Pulm Med 2001;7:180.
2. Noppen M, De Waele MR, Li R, et al: Volume and cellular content of normal pleural fluid in humans examined by pleural lavage. Am J Respir Crit Care Med 2000;162:1023.
3. Miserocchi G: Physiology and pathophysiology of pleural fluid turnover. Eur Respir J 1997;10:219.
4. Wiener-Kronish JP, Matthay MA, Callen PW, Filly RA, Gamsu G, Staub NC: Relationship of pleural effusions to pulmonary hemodynamics in patients with congestive heart failure. Am Rev Respir Dis 1985;132:1253.
5. Eid AA, Keddissi JI, Kinasewitz GT: Hypoalbuminemia as a cause of pleural effusions. Chest 1999;115:1066.
6. Wemyss-Holden SA, Launois B, Maddern GJ: Management of thoracic duct injuries after oesophagectomy. Br J Surg 2001;88:1442.
7. Sahn SA: Malignant pleural effusions. Clin Chest Med 1985;6:113.
8. Grove CS, Lee YC: Vascular endothelial growth factor: The key mediator in pleural effusion formation. Curr Opin Pulm Med 2002;8:294.
9. Ku DD, Zaleski JK, Liu S, Brock TA: Vascular endothelial growth factor induces EDRF-dependent relaxation in coronary arteries. Am J Physiol 1993;265:H586.
10. Mohammed KA, Nasreen N, Hardwick J, Logie CS, Patterson CE, Antony VB: Bacterial induction of pleural mesothelial monolayer barrier dysfunction. Am J Physiol Lung Cell Mol Physiol 2001;281: L119.
11. Brown LF, Detmar M, Claffey K, et al: Vascular permeability factor/vascular endothelial growth factor: A multifunctional angiogenic cytokine. EXS 1997;79:233.
12. Cheng D, Lee YC, Rogers JT, et al: Vascular endothelial growth factor level correlates with transforming growth factor-beta isoform levels in pleural effusions. Chest 2000;118:1747.
13. Ishimoto O, Saijo Y, Narumi K, et al: High level of vascular endothelial growth factor in hemorrhagic pleural effusion of cancer. Oncology 2002;63:70.
14. Gary Lee YC, Melkerneker D, Thompson PJ, Light RW, Lane KB: Transforming growth factor beta induces vascular endothelial growth factor elaboration from pleural mesothelial cells in vivo and in vitro. Am J Respir Crit Care Med 2002;165:88.
15. Light RW: Pleural Diseases, 2nd ed. Philadelphia, Lea & Febiger, 1990.
16. Leuallen EC, Carr DT: Pleural effusion: Statistical study of 436 patients. N Engl J Med 1955;232:79.
17. Tinney WS, Olsen AM: The significance of fluid in the pleural space: A study of 274 cases. J Thorac Surg 1946;14:248.
18. Salyer WR, Eggleston JC, Erozan YS: Efficacy of pleural needle biopsy and pleural fluid cytopathology in the diagnosis of malignant neoplasm involving the pleura. Chest 1975;67:536.
19. Hirsch A, Ruffie P, Nebut M, Bignon J, Chretien J: Pleural effusion: Laboratory tests in 300 cases. Thorax 1979;34:106.
20. Chernow B, Sahn SA: Carcinomatous involvement of the pleura: An analysis of 96 patients. Am J Med 1977;63:695.
21. Johnston WW: The malignant pleural effusion. A review of cytopathologic diagnoses of 584 specimens from 472 consecutive patients. Cancer 1985;56:905.
22. Anderson CB, Philpott GW, Ferguson TB: The treatment of malignant pleural effusions. Cancer 1974;33:916.
23. Maghfoor I, Doll DC, Yarbro JW: Effusions. In Abeloff MA, Armitage JO, Lichter AS, Niederhuber JE (eds): Clinical Oncology. New York, Churchill-Livingstone, 2000, pp 922–949.
24. Colins JD, Burwell D, Furmanski S, Lorber P, Steckel RJ: Minimal detectable pleural effusions. A roentgen pathology model. Radiology 1972;105:51.
25. Hausheer FH, Yarbro JW: Diagnosis and treatment of malignant pleural effusion. SeminOncol 1985;12:54.
26. Sahn SA: State of the art. The pleura. Am Rev Respir Dis 1988;138:184.
27. Stark P: The Pleura. In Taveras A, Ferucci C, (eds): Radiology: Diagnosis, Imaging, Intervention. Philadelphia, Lippincott, 2003, pp 454–460.
28. Moskowitz H, Platt RT, Schachar R, Mellins H: Roentgen visualization of minute pleural effusion: An experimental study to determine the minimum amount of pleural fluid visible on a radiograph. Radiology 1973;109:33.
29. Woodring JH: Recognition of pleural effusion on supine radiographs: How much fluid is required? Am J Roentgenol 1984;142:59.
30. Mergo PJ, Helmberger T, Didovic J, Cernigliaro J, Ros PR, Staab EV: New formula for quantification of pleural effusions from computed tomography. J Thorac Imaging 1999;14:122.
31. Davis SD, Henschke CI, Yankelevitz DF, Cahill PT, Yi Y: MR imaging of pleural effusions. J Comput Assist Tomogr 1990;14:192.
32. Koh DM, Burke S, Davies N, Padley SP: Transthoracic US of the chest: Clinical uses and applications. Radiographics 2002;22:e1.
33. Lipscomb DJ, Flower CD, Hadfield JW: Ultrasound of the pleura: An assessment of its clinical value. Clin Radiol 1981;32:289.
34. Grogan DR, Irwin RS, Channick R, et al: Complications associated with thoracentesis. A prospective, randomized study comparing three different methods. Arch Intern Med 1990;150:873.
35. Tarn AC, Lapworth R: Biochemical analysis of pleural fluid: What should we measure? Ann Clin Biochem 2001;38:311.
36. McVay PA, Toy PT: Lack of increased bleeding after paracentesis and thoracentesis in patients with mild coagulation abnormalities. Transfusion 1991;31:164.
37. Godwin JE, Sahn SA: Thoracentesis: A safe procedure in mechanically ventilated patients. Ann Intern Med 1990;113:800.
38. McCartney JP, Adams JW, Hazard PB: Safety of thoracentesis in mechanically ventilated patients. Chest 1993;103:1920.
39. Zimmerman JE, Dunbar BS, Klingenmaier CH: Management of subcutaneous emphysema, pneumomediastinum, and pneumothorax during respirator therapy. Crit Care Med 1975;3:69.
40. Collins TR, Sahn SA: Thoracocentesis. Clinical value, complications, technical problems, and patient experience. Chest 1987;91:817.
41. Aguilar-Torres FG, Schlueter DP, Perlman L, Maskawa T: Subcutaneous implantation of an adenocarcinoma following thoracentesis. Wis Med J 1977;76:S19–21.
42. Sahn SA: Management of malignant pleural effusions. Monaldi ArchChest Dis 2001;56:394.

Problems Common to Cancer and Its Therapy

II

43. Capizzi SA, Prakash UB: Chest roentgenography after outpatient thoracentesis. Mayo Clin Proc 1998;73:948.

44. Doyle JJ, Hnatiuk OW, Torrington KG, Slade AR, Howard RS: Necessity of routine chest roentgenography after thoracentesis. Ann Intern Med 1996;124:816.

45. Aleman C, Alegre J, Armadans L, et al: The value of chest roentgenography in the diagnosis of pneumothorax after thoracentesis. Am J Med 1999;107:340.

46. Light RW, Macgregor MI, Luchsinger PC, Ball WC Jr : Pleural effusions: The diagnostic separation of transudates and exudates. Ann Intern Med 1972;77:507.

47. Costa M, Quiroga T, Cruz E: Measurement of pleural fluid cholesterol and lactate dehydrogenase. A simple and accurate set of indicators for separating exudates from transudates. Chest 1995;108:1260.

48. Light RW: Pleural effusions. Med Clin North Am 1977;61:1339.

49. Joseph J, Badrinath P, Basran GS, Sahn SA: Is the pleural fluid transudate or exudate? A revisit of the diagnostic criteria. Thorax 2001;56:867.

50. Vives M, Porcel JM, d'Vicente V, Ribelles E, Rubio M: A study of Light's criteria and possible modifications for distinguishing exudative from transudative pleural effusions. Chest 1996;109:1503.

51. Romero S, Candela A, Martin C, Hernandez L, Trigo C, Gil J: Evaluation of different criteria for the separation of pleural transudates from exudates. Chest 1993;104:399.

52. Antony VB, Holm KA: Testing the waters. Differentiating transudates from exudates. Chest 1995;108:1191.

53. Keller RR: Once more: Light's criteria revisited. Respiration 2000;67:11.

54. Hamm H, Brohan U, Bohmer R, Missmahl HP: Cholesterol in pleural effusions. A diagnostic aid. Chest 1987;92:296.

55. Gil SV, Martinez ME, Cases VE, Perpina TM, Leon FM, Sanchis AJ: Pleural cholesterol in differentiating transudates and exudates. A prospective study of 232 cases. Respiration 1995;62:57.

56. Valdes L, Pose A, Suarez J, et al: Cholesterol: A useful parameter for distinguishing between pleural exudates and transudates. Chest 1991;99:1097.

57. Meisel S, Shamiss A, Thaler M, Nussinovitch N, Rosenthal T: Pleural fluid to serum bilirubin concentration ratio for the separation of transudates from exudates. Chest 1990;98:141.

58. Burgess LJ, Maritz FJ, Taljaard JJ: Comparative analysis of the biochemical parameters used to distinguish between pleural transudates and exudates. Chest 1995;107:1604.

59. Pillay VKG: Total Proteins in serous fluids in cardiac failure. S Afr Med J 2002;39:142.

60. Roth BJ, O'Meara TF, Cragun WH: The serum-effusion albumin gradient in the evaluation of pleural effusions. Chest 1990;98:546.

61. Joseph J, Badrinath P, Basran GS, Sahn SA: Is albumin gradient or fluid to serum albumin ratio better than the pleural fluid lactate dehydroginase in the diagnostic of separation of pleural effusion? BMC Pulm Med 2002;2:1.

62. Heffner JE, Brown LK, Barbieri CA: Diagnostic value of tests that discriminate between exudative and transudative pleural effusions. Chest 1997;111:970.

63. Light RW, Ball WC Jr: Glucose and amylase in pleural effusions. JAMA 1973;225:257.

64. Sahn SA, Kaplan RL, Maulitz RM, Good JT Jr: Rheumatoid pleurisy. Observations on the development of low pleural fluid pH and glucose level. Arch Intern Med 1980;140:1237.

65. Goldstein LS, McCarthy K, Mehta AC, Arroliga AC: Is direct collection of pleural fluid into a heparinized syringe important for determination of pleural pH? A brief report. Chest 1997;112:707.

66. Lesho EP, Roth BJ: Is pH paper an acceptable, low-cost alternative to the blood gas analyzer for determining pleural fluid pH? Chest 1997;112:1291.

67. Sahn SA, Willcox ML, Good JT Jr, Potts DE, Filley GF: Characteristics of normal rabbit pleural fluid: Physiologic and biochemical implications. Lung 1979;156:63.

68. Good JT Jr, Taryle DA, Maulitz RM, Kaplan RL, Sahn SA: The diagnostic value of pleural fluid pH. Chest 1980;78:55.

69. Sahn SA, Good JT Jr: Pleural fluid pH in malignant effusions. Diagnostic, prognostic, and therapeutic implications. Ann Intern Med 1988;108:345.

70. Light RW: Exudative pleural effusions secondary to gastrointestinal diseases. Clin Chest Med 1985;6:103.

71. Kaye MD: Pleuropulmonary complications of pancreatitis. Thorax 1968;23:297.

72. Kramer MR, Saldana MJ, Cepero RJ, Pitchenik AE: High amylase levels in neoplasm-related pleural effusion. Ann Intern Med 1989;110:567.

73. Joseph J, Viney S, Beck P, Strange C, Sahn SA, Basran GS: A prospective study of amylase-rich pleural effusions with special reference to amylase isoenzyme analysis. Chest;102:1455.

74. Yam LT: Diagnostic significance of lymphocytes in pleural effusions. Ann Intern Med 1967;66:972.

75. Adelman M, Albelda SM, Gottlieb J, Haponik EF: Diagnostic utility of pleural fluid eosinophilia. Am J Med 1984;77:915.

76. Rubins JB, Rubins HB: Etiology and prognostic significance of eosinophilic pleural effusions. A prospective study. Chest 1996;110:1271.

77. Martinez-Garcia MA, Cases-Viedma E, Cordero-Rodriguez PJ, Hidalgo-Ramirez M, Perpina-Tordera M, Sanchis-Moret F, et al: Diagnostic utility of eosinophils in the pleural fluid. Eur Respir J 2000;15:166.

78. Light RW, Erozan YS, Ball WC Jr: Cells in pleural fluid. Their value in differential diagnosis. Arch Intern Med 1973;132:854.

79. Hurwitz S, Leiman G, Shapiro C: Mesothelial cells in pleural fluid: TB or not TB? S Afr Med J 1980;57:937.

80. Starr RL, Sherman ME: The value of multiple preparations in the diagnosis of malignant pleural effusions. A cost-benefit analysis. Acta Cytol 1991;35:533.

81. Hsu C: Cytologic detection of malignancy in pleural effusion: A review of 5,255 samples from 3,811 patients. Diagn Cytopathol 1987;3:8.

82. Johnston WW: The malignant pleural effusion. A review of cytopathologic diagnoses of 584 specimens from 472 consecutive patients. Cancer 1985;56:905.

83. Banales JL, Pineda PR, Fitzgerald JM, Rubio H, Selman M, Salazar-Lezama M: Adenosine deaminase in the diagnosis of tuberculous pleural effusions. A report of 218 patients and review of the literature. Chest 1991;99:355.

84. Sassoon CS, Light RW: Chylothorax and pseudochylothorax. Clin Chest Med 1985;6:163.

85. Garcia-Pachon E, Padilla-Navas I, Dosda MD, Miralles-Llopis A: Elevated level of carcinoembryonic antigen in nonmalignant pleural effusions. Chest 1997;111:643.

86. Tamura S, Nishigaki T, Moriwaki Y, et al: Tumor markers in pleural effusion diagnosis. Cancer 1988;61:298.

87. Salama G, Miedouge M, Rouzaud P, et al: Evaluation of pleural CYFRA 21-1 and carcinoembryonic antigen in the diagnosis of malignant pleural effusions. Br J Cancer 1998;77:472.

88. San Jose ME, Alvarez D, Valdes L, Sarandeses A, Valle JM, Penela P: Utility of tumour markers in the diagnosis of neoplastic pleural effusion. Clin Chim Acta 1997;265:193.

89. Niwa Y, Kishimoto H, Shimokata K: Carcinomatous and tuberculous pleural effusions. Comparison of tumor markers. Chest 1985;87:351.

90. Mezger J, Permanetter W, Gerbes AL, Wilmanns W, Lamerz R: Tumour associated antigens in diagnosis of serous effusions. J Clin Pathol 1988;41:633.

91. Shimokata K, Niwa Y, Yamamoto M, Sasou H, Morishita M: Pleural fluid neuron-specific enolase. A useful diagnostic marker for small cell lung cancer pleurisy. Chest 1989;95:602.

92. Pettersson T, Klockars M, Froseth B: Neuron-specific enolase in the diagnosis of small-cell lung cancer with pleural effusion: a negative report. Eur Respir J 1988;1:698.

93. van de Molengraft FJ, Vooijs GP: The interval between the diagnosis of malignancy and the development of effusions, with reference to the role of cytologic diagnosis. Acta Cytol 1988;32:183.

94. American Thoracic Society. Management of malignant pleural effusions. Am J Respir Crit Care Med 2000;162:1987.

95. Hengge UR, Ruzicka T, Tyring SK, et al: Update on Kaposi's sarcoma and other HHV8 associated diseases. Part 2: Pathogenesis, Castleman's disease, and pleural effusion lymphoma. Lancet Infect Dis 2002;2:344.

96. Beauchamp HD, Kundra NK, Aranson R, Chong F, MacDonnell KF:

The role of closed pleural needle biopsy in the diagnosis of malignant mesothelioma of the pleura. Chest 1992;102:1110.

97. Hainsworth JD, Greco FA: Treatment of patients with cancer of an unknown primary site. N Engl J Med 1993;329:257.

98. Prakash UB, Reiman HM: Comparison of needle biopsy with cytologic analysis for the evaluation of pleural effusion: Analysis of 414 cases. Mayo Clin Proc 1985;60:158.

99. Emad A, Rezaian GR: Closed percutaneous pleural brushing: A new method for diagnosis of malignant pleural effusions. Respir Med 1998;92:659.

100. Christopher DJ, Peter JV, Cherian AM: Blind pleural biopsy using a Tru-cut needle in moderate to large pleural effusion—An experience. Singapore Med J 1998;39:196.

101. Loddenkemper R: Thoracoscopy—State of the art. Eur Respir J 1998;11:213.

102. Tape TG, Blank LL, Wigton RS: Procedural skills of practicing pulmonologists. A national survey of 1,000 members of the American College of Physicians. Am J Respir Crit Care Med 1995;151:282.

103. Oldenburg FA Jr, Newhouse MT: Thoracoscopy. A safe, accurate diagnostic procedure using the rigid thoracoscope and local anesthesia. Chest 1979;75:45.

104. Weissberg D, Schachner A: Video-assisted thoracic surgery—State of the art. Ann Ital Chir 2000;71:539.

105. McKneally MF, Lewis RJ, Anderson RJ, et al: Statement of the AATS/STS Joint Committee on Thoracoscopy and Video Assisted Thoracic Surgery. J Thorac Cardiovasc Surg 1992;104:1.

106. Boutin C, Viallat JR, Cargnino P, Farisse P: Thoracoscopy in malignant pleural effusions. Am Rev Respir Dis 1981;124:588.

107. Martensson G, Pettersson K, Thiringer G: Differentiation between malignant and non-malignant pleural effusion. Eur J Respir Dis 1985;67:326.

108. Canto A, Blasco E, Casillas M, et al: Thoracoscopy in the diagnosis of pleural effusion. Thorax 1977;32:550.

109. Ernst A, Hersh CP, Herth F, et al: A novel instrument for the evaluation of the pleural space: an experience in 34 patients. Chest 2002;122:1530.

110. Weick JK, Kiely JM, Harrison EG Jr, Carr DT, Scanlon PW: Pleural effusion in lymphoma. Cancer 1973;31:848.

111. Hughes JC, Votaw ML: Pleural effusion in multiple myeloma. Cancer 1979;44:1150.

112. Rodriguez JN, Pereira A, Martinez JC, Conde J, Pujol E: Pleural effusion in multiple myeloma. Chest 1994;105:622.

113. Alexanian R, Barlogie B, Dixon D: High-dose glucocorticoid treatment of resistant myeloma. Ann Intern Med 1986;105:8.

114. Roth BJ, Johnson DH, Einhorn LH, et al: Randomized study of cyclophosphamide, doxorubicin, and vincristine versus etoposide and cisplatin versus alternation of these two regimens in extensive small-cell lung cancer: A phase III trial of the Southeastern Cancer Study Group. J Clin Oncol 1992;10:282.

115. Noda K, Nishiwaki Y, Kawahara M, et al: Irinotecan plus cisplatin compared with etoposide plus cisplatin for extensive small-cell lung cancer. N Engl J Med 2002;346:85.

116. Bosl GJ, Motzer RJ: Testicular germ-cell cancer. N Engl J Med 1997;337:242.

117. Antman KH, Corson JM: Benign and malignant pleural mesothelioma. Clin Chest Med 1985;6:127.

118. Chabner BA, Stoller RG, Hande K, Jacobs S, Young RC: Methotrexate disposition in humans: case studies in ovarian cancer and following high-dose infusion. Drug Metab Rev 1978;8:107.

119. Krell WS, Rodarte JR: Effects of acute pleural effusion on respiratory system mechanics in dogs. J Appl Physiol 1985;59:1458.

120. Light RW, Stansbury DW, Brown SE: The relationship between pleural pressures and changes in pulmonary function after therapeutic thoracentesis. Am Rev Respir Dis 1986;133:658.

121. Perpina M, Benlloch E, Marco V, Abad F, Nauffal D: Effect of thoracentesis on pulmonary gas exchange. Thorax 1983;38:747.

122. Karetzky MS, Kothari GA, Fourre JA, Khan AU: Effect of thoracentesis on arterial oxygen tension. Respiration 1978;36:96.

123. Brandstetter RD, Cohen RP: Hypoxemia after thoracentesis. A predictable and treatable condition. JAMA 1979;242:1060.

124. Brown NE, Zamel N, Aberman A: Changes in pulmonary mechanics and gas exchange following thoracocentesis. Chest 1978;74:540.

125. Kinasewitz G, Fishman N: Pleural Effusions. In Fishman N (ed): Pulmonary Diseases and Disorders. New York, McGraw-Hill, 1988, pp 750–801.

126. Gross NJ: Pulmonary effects of radiation therapy. Ann Intern Med 1977;86:81.

127. Bouros D, Froudarakis M, Siafakas NM: Pleurodesis: Everything flows. Chest 2000;118:577.

128. Rodriguez-Panadero F, Antony VB: Pleurodesis: State of the art. Eur Respir J 1997;10:1648.

129. Kroegel C, Antony VB: Immunobiology of pleural inflammation: Potential implications for pathogenesis, diagnosis and therapy. Eur Respir J 1997;10:2411.

130. Antony VB, Rothfuss KJ, Godbey SW, Sparks JA, Hott JW: Mechanism of tetracycline-hydrochloride-induced pleurodesis. Tetracycline-hydrochloride-stimulated mesothelial cells produce a growth-factor-like activity for fibroblasts. Am Rev Respir Dis 1992;146:1009.

131. Antunes G, Neville E: Management of malignant pleural effusions. Thorax 2000;55:981.

132. Villanueva AG, Gray AW Jr, Shahian DM, Williamson WA, Beamis JF Jr: Efficacy of short term versus long term tube thoracostomy drainage before tetracycline pleurodesis in the treatment of malignant pleural effusions. Thorax 1994;49:23.

133. Clementsen P, Evald T, Grode G, Hansen M, Krag JG, Faurschou P: Treatment of malignant pleural effusion: pleurodesis using a small percutaneous catheter. A prospective randomized study. Respir Med 1998;92:593.

134. Parker LA, Charnock GC, Delany DJ: Small bore catheter drainage and sclerotherapy for malignant pleural effusions. Cancer 1989;64:1218.

135. Seaton KG, Patz EF Jr, Goodman PC: Palliative treatment of malignant pleural effusions: Value of small-bore catheter thoracostomy and doxycycline sclerotherapy. Am J Roentgenol 1995;164:589.

136. Patz EF Jr, McAdams HP, Erasmus JJ, et al: Sclerotherapy for malignant pleural effusions: A prospective randomized trial of bleomycin vs doxycycline with small-bore catheter drainage. Chest 1998;113:1305.

137. Seaton KG, Patz EF Jr, Goodman PC: Palliative treatment of malignant pleural effusions: Value of small-bore catheter thoracostomy and doxycycline sclerotherapy. Am J Roentgenol 1995;164:589.

138. Saffran L, Ost DE, Fein AM, Schiff MJ: Outpatient pleurodesis of malignant pleural effusions using a small-bore pigtail catheter. Chest 2000;118:417.

139. Lorch DG, Gordon L, Wooten S, Cooper JF, Strange C, Sahn SA: Effect of patient positioning on distribution of tetracycline in the pleural space during pleurodesis. Chest 1988;93:527.

140. Dryzer SR, Allen ML, Strange C, Sahn SA: A comparison of rotation and nonrotation in tetracycline pleurodesis. Chest 1993;104:1763.

141. Heffner JE, Unruh LC: Tetracycline pleurodesis. Adios, farewell, adieu. Chest 1992;101:5.

142. Costabel U: Adieu, tetracycline pleurodesis (but not in Germany). Chest 1993;103:984.

143. Heffner JE, Standerfer RJ, Torstveit J, Unruh L: Clinical efficacy of doxycycline for pleurodesis. Chest 1994;105:1743.

144. Pulsiripunya C, Youngchaiyud P, Pushpakom R, Maranetra N, Nana A, Charoenratanakul S: The efficacy of doxycycline as a pleural sclerosing agent in malignant pleural effusion: A prospective study. Respirology 1996;1:69.

145. Bethune N: A new technique for the deliberate production of pleural adhesions as a preliminary to lobectomy. J Thorac Surg 1935;4:251.

146. Kleinfeld M, Messite J, Kooyman O, Zaki MH: Mortality among talc miners and millers in New York State. Arch Environ Health 1967;14:663.

147. Lange P, Mortensen J, Groth S: Lung function 22–35 years after treatment of idiopathic spontaneous pneumothorax with talc poudrage or simple drainage. Thorax 1988;43:559.

148. Kennedy L, Vaughan LM, Steed LL, Sahn SA: Sterilization of talc for pleurodesis. Available techniques, efficacy, and cost analysis. Chest 1995;107:1032.

149. Mattison LM, Steed LL, Sahn SA: More on talc sterilization. Chest 1996;109:1667.

150. Mager HJ, Maesen B, Verzijlbergen F, Schramel F: Distribution of talc suspension during treatment of malignant pleural effusion with talc pleurodesis. Lung Cancer 2002;36:77.

151. Kennedy L, Sahn SA: Talc pleurodesis for the treatment of pneumothorax and pleural effusion. Chest 1994;106:1215.

152. Xie C, Teixeira LR, McGovern JP, Light RW: Systemic corticosteroids decrease the effectiveness of talc pleurodesis. Am J Respir Crit Care Med 1998;157:1441.

153. Kennedy L, Rusch VW, Strange C, Ginsberg RJ, Sahn SA: Pleurodesis using talc slurry. Chest 1994;106:342.

154. Walker-Renard PB, Vaughan LM, Sahn SA: Chemical pleurodesis for malignant pleural effusions. Ann Intern Med 1994;120:56.

155. Rinaldo JE, Owens GR, Rogers RM: Adult respiratory distress syndrome following intrapleural instillation of talc. J Thorac Cardiovasc Surg 1983;85:523.

156. de Campos JR, Vargas FS, de Campos WE, et al: Thoracoscopy talc poudrage: A 15-year experience. Chest 2001;119:801.

157. Rehse DH, Aye RW, Florence MG: Respiratory failure following talc pleurodesis. Am J Surg 1999;177:437.

158. Bouchama A, Chastre J, Gaudichet A, Soler P, Gibert C: Acute pneumonitis with bilateral pleural effusion after talc pleurodesis. Chest 1984;86:795.

159. Nandi P: Recurrent spontaneous pneumothorax; an effective method of talc poudrage. Chest 1980;77:493.

160. Campos JR, Werebe EC, Vargas FS, Jatene FB, Light RW: Respiratory failure due to insufflated talc. Lancet 1997;349:251.

161. Rinaldo JE, Owens GR, Rogers RM: Adult respiratory distress syndrome following intrapleural instillation of talc. J Thorac Cardiovasc Surg 1983;85:523.

162. Light RW: Talc should not be used for pleurodesis. Am J Respir Crit Care Med 2000;162:2024.

163. Light RW: Diseases of the pleura: The use of talc for pleurodesis. Curr Opin Pulm Med 2000;6:255.

164. Rehse DH, Aye RW, Florence MG: Respiratory failure following talc pleurodesis. Am J Surg 1999;177:437.

165. Sahn SA: Talc should be used for pleurodesis. Am J Respir Crit Care Med 2000;162:2023.

166. Cunningham TJ, Olson KB, Horton J, et al: A clinical trial of intravenous and intracavitary bleomycin. Cancer 1972;29:1413.

167. Paladine W, Cunningham TJ, Sponzo R, Donavan M, Olson K, Horton J: Intracavitary bleomycin in the management of malignant effusions. Cancer 1976;38:1903.

168. Bitran JD, Brown C, Desser RK, Kozloff MF, Shapiro C, Billings AA: Intracavitary bleomycin for the control of malignant effusions. J Surg Oncol 1981;16:273.

169. Ostrowski MJ: An assessment of the long-term results of controlling the reaccumulation of malignant effusions using intracavity bleomycin. Cancer 1986;57:721.

170. Ostrowski MJ: Intracavitary therapy with bleomycin for the treatment of malignant pleural effusions. J Surg Oncol Suppl 1989;1:7.

171. Noppen M, Degreve J, Mignolet M, Vincken W: A prospective, randomised study comparing the efficacy of talc slurry and bleomycin in the treatment of malignant pleural effusions. Acta Clin Belg 1997;52:258.

172. Zimmer PW, Hill M, Casey K, Harvey E, Low DE: Prospective randomized trial of bleomycin vs talc slurry in pleurodesis for symptomatic malignant pleural effusions. Chest 1997;112:430.

173. Groth G, Gatzemeier U, Haussingen K, et al: Intrapleural palliative treatment of malignant pleural effusions with mitoxantrone versus placebo (pleural tube alone). Ann Oncol 1991;2:213.

174. Sorensen PG, Svendsen TL, Enk B: Treatment of malignant pleural effusion with drainage, with and without instillation of talc. Eur J Respir Dis 1984;65:131.

175. Light RW: Clinical practice. Pleural effusion. N Engl J Med 2002;346:1971.

176. Bresticker MA, Oba J, LoCicero J III, Greene R: Optimal pleurodesis: A comparison study. Ann Thorac Surg 1993;55:364.

177. Jerram RM, Fossum TW, Berridge BR, Steinheimer DN, Slater MR: The efficacy of mechanical abrasion and talc slurry as methods of pleurodesis in normal dogs. Vet Surg 1999;28:322.

178. Bertrand PC, Regnard JF, Spaggiari L, et al: Immediate and long-term results after surgical treatment of primary spontaneous pneumothorax by VATS. Ann Thorac Surg 1996;61:1641.

179. Mouroux J, Elkaim D, Padovani B, et al: Video-assisted thoracoscopic treatment of spontaneous pneumothorax: Technique and results of one hundred cases. J Thorac Cardiovasc Surg 1996;112:385.

180. Martinez-Moragon E, Aparicio J, Sanchis J, Menendez R, Cruz RM, Sanchis F: Malignant pleural effusion: prognostic factors for survival and response to chemical pleurodesis in a series of 120 cases. Respiration 1998;65:108.

181. Rodriguez-Panadero F, Segado A, Martin JJ, Ayerbe R, Torres GI, Castillo J: Failure of talc pleurodesis is associated with increased pleural fibrinolysis. Am J Respir Crit Care Med 1995;151:785.

182. Lan RS, Lo SK, Chuang ML, Yang CT, Tsao TC, Lee CH: Elastance of the pleural space: A predictor for the outcome of pleurodesis in patients with malignant pleural effusion. Ann Intern Med 1997;126:768.

183. Foresti V: Intrapleural Corynebacterium parvum for recurrent malignant pleural effusions. Respiration 1995;62:21.

184. Foresti V, Scolari N, Villa A, Parisio E, De Filippi G, Guareschi G: Malignant pleural effusions: Meaning of pleural-fluid pH determination. Oncology 1990;47:62.

185. Aelony Y, King RR, Boutin C: Thoracoscopic talc poudrage in malignant pleural effusions: Effective pleurodesis despite low pleural pH. Chest 1998;113:1007.

186. Heffner JE, Nietert PJ, Barbieri C: Pleural fluid pH as a predictor of pleurodesis failure: Analysis of primary data. Chest 2000;117:87.

187. American Thoracic Society. Management of malignant pleural effusions. Am J Respir Crit Care Med 2000;162:1987.

188. Petrou M, Kaplan D, Goldstraw P: Management of recurrent malignant pleural effusions. The complementary role talc pleurodesis and pleuroperitoneal shunting. Cancer 1995;75:801.

189. Fry WA, Khandekar JD: Parietal pleurectomy for malignant pleural effusion. Ann Surg Oncol 1995;2:160.

190. Khattab T, Smith S, Barbor P, Ghamdi SA, Abbas A, Fryer C: Extramedullary relapse in a child with mixed lineage acute lymphoblastic leukemia: chylous pleuropericardial effusion. Med Pediatr Oncol 2000;34:274.

191. Slichenmyer WJ, Fry DW: Anticancer therapy targeting the erbB family of receptor tyrosine kinases. Semin Oncol 2001;28:67.

192. al Kattan KM, Kaplan DK, Goldstraw P: The non-functioning pleuro-peritoneal shunt: Revise or replace? Thorac Cardiovasc Surg 1994;42:310.

193. Ike O, Shimizu Y, Hitomi S, Wada R, Ikada Y: Treatment of malignant pleural effusions with doxorubicin hydrochloride-containing poly(L-lactic acid) microspheres. Chest 1991;99:911.

194. Rosso R, Rimoldi R, Salvati F, et al: Intrapleural natural beta interferon in the treatment of malignant pleural effusions. Oncology 1988;45:253.

195. Astoul P, Viallat JR, Laurent JC, Brandely M, Boutin C: Intrapleural recombinant IL-2 in passive immunotherapy for malignant pleural effusion. Chest 1993;103:209.

196. Viallat JR, Boutin C, Rey F, Astoul P, Farisse P, Brandely M: Intrapleural immunotherapy with escalating doses of interleukin-2 in metastatic pleural effusions. Cancer 1993;71:4067.

197. Boutin C, Viallat JR, Van Zandwijk N, et al: Activity of intrapleural recombinant gamma-interferon in malignant mesothelioma. Cancer 1991;67:2033.

198. Boutin C, Nussbaum E, Monnet I, et al: Intrapleural treatment with recombinant gamma-interferon in early stage malignant pleural mesothelioma. Cancer 1994;74:2460.

199. Monti G, Jaurand MC, Monnet I, et al: Intrapleural production of interleukin 6 during mesothelioma and its modulation by gamma-interferon treatment. Cancer Res 1994;54:4419.

200. Foresti V: Corynebacterium parvum for malignant pleural effusions. Thorax 1995;50:104.

201. Salomaa ER, Pulkki K, Helenius H: Pleurodesis with doxycycline or Corynebacterium parvum in malignant pleural effusion. Acta Oncol 1995;34:117.

202. Leahy BC, Honeybourne D, Brear SG, Carroll KB, Thatcher N, Stretton TB: Treatment of malignant pleural effusions with intrapleural Corynebacterium parvum or tetracycline. Eur J Respir Dis 1985;66:50.

203. Millar JW, Hunter AM, Horne NW: Intrapleural immunotherapy with Corynebacterium parvum in recurrent malignant pleural effusions. Thorax 1980;35:856.

204. Bilaceroglu S, Cagirici U, Perim K, Ozacar R: Corynebacterium parvum pleurodesis and survival is not significantly influenced by pleural pH and glucose level. Monaldi Arch Chest Dis 1998;53:14.

205. Shoji T, Tanaka F, Yanagihara K, Inui K, Wada H: Phase II study of repeated intrapleural chemotherapy using implantable access system for management of malignant pleural effusion. Chest 2002;121:821.

206. Driesen P, Boutin C, Viallat JR, Astoul PH, Vialette JP, Pasquier J: Implantable access system for prolonged intrapleural immunotherapy. Eur Respir J 1994;7:1889.

207. Wied U, Halkier E, Hoeier-Madsen K, Plucnar B, Rasmussen E, Sparup J: Tetracycline versus silver nitrate pleurodesis in spontaneous pneumothorax. J Thorac Cardiovasc Surg 1983;86:591.

208. Vargas FS, Teixeira LR, Silva LM, Carmo AO, Light RW: Comparison of silver nitrate and tetracycline as pleural sclerosing agents in rabbits. Chest 1995;108:1080.

209. Leff RS, Eisenberg B, Baisden CE, Mosley KR, Messerschmidt GL: Drainage of recurrent pleural effusion via an implanted port and intrapleural catheter. Ann Intern Med 1986;104:208.

210. Hewitt JB, Janssen WR: A management strategy for malignancy-induced pleural effusion: Long-term thoracostomy drainage. Oncol Nurs Forum 1987;14:17.

211. Robinson RD, Fullerton DA, Albert JD, Sorensen J, Johnston MR: Use of pleural Tenckhoff catheter to palliate malignant pleural effusion. Ann Thorac Surg 1994;57:286.

212. Zeldin DC, Rodriguez RM, Glassford DM: Management of refractory MPEs with a chronic indwelling pleural catheter [Management of refractory malignant pleural effusions with a chronic indwelling pleural catheter {abstract}]. Chest 1991;100:87.

213. Pollak JS: Malignant pleural effusions: Treatment with tunneled long-term drainage catheters. Curr Opin Pulm Med 2002;8:302.

214. Putnam JB Jr, Light RW, Rodriguez RM, et al: A randomized comparison of indwelling pleural catheter and doxycycline pleurodesis in the management of malignant pleural effusions. Cancer 1999;86:1992.

215. Putnam JB Jr, Walsh GL, Swisher SG, et al: Outpatient management of malignant pleural effusion by a chronic indwelling pleural catheter. Ann Thorac Surg 2000;69:369.

216. Pollak JS, Burdge CM, Rosenblatt M, Houston JP, Hwu WJ, Murren J: Treatment of malignant pleural effusions with tunneled long-term drainage catheters. J Vasc Interv Radiol 2001;12:201.

217. Spodick DH: Intrapericardial therapeutics and diagnostics. Am J Cardiol 2000;85:1012.

218. Hancock EW: Neoplastic pericardial disease. Cardiol Clin 1990;8:673.

219. Fraser RS, Viloria JB, Wang NS: Cardiac tamponade as a presentation of extracardiac malignancy. Cancer 1980;45:1697.

220. Haagensen CD: The lymphatics in cancer. Philadelphia, WB Saunders, 2003, p 245.

221. Johnson RA: Lymphatics of blood vessels. Lymphology 1969;2:44.

222. Kussmaul A: Über schwielige Mediastino-Pericarditis und den paradoxen Puls. Berliner Klinische Wochenschrift 1878;461.

223. Shabetai RF: Pulsus paradoxus. J Clin Invest 1965;44:1882.

224. Reddy PS, Curtiss EI, Uretsky BF: Spectrum of hemodynamic changes in cardiac tamponade. Am J Cardiol 1990;66:1487.

225. McGregor M: Current concepts: Pulsus paradoxus. N Engl J Med 1979;301:480.

226. Ewart W: Practical aids in the diagnosis of pericardial effusion, in connection with the question as to surgical treatment. Br Med J 1896;1:717.

227. Wilkes JD, Fidias P, Vaickus L, Perez RP: Malignancy-related pericardial effusion. 127 cases from the Roswell Park Cancer Institute. Cancer 1995;76:1377.

228. Corey GR, Campbell PT, Van Trigt P, et al: Etiology of large pericardial effusions. Am J Med 1993;95:209.

229. Abraham KP, Reddy V, Gattuso P: Neoplasms metastatic to the heart: Review of 3314 consecutive autopsies. Am J Cardiovasc Pathol 1990;3:195.

230. Porte HL, Janecki-Delebecq TJ, Finzi L, Metois DG, Millaire A, Wurtz AJ: Pericardoscopy for primary management of pericardial effusion in cancer patients. Eur J Cardiothorac Surg 1999;16:287.

231. Posner MR, Cohen GI, Skarin AT: Pericardial disease in patients with cancer. The differentiation of malignant from idiopathic and radiation-induced pericarditis. Am J Med 1981;71:407.

232. Ruckdeschel JC, Chang P, Martin RG, et al: Radiation-related pericardial effusions in patients with Hodgkin's disease. Medicine (Baltimore) 1975;54:245–259.

233. Chong HH, GD Plotnick: Pericardial effusion and tamponade: Evaluation, imaging modalities, and management. Compr Ther 1995;21:378.

234. Sechtem U, Tscholakoff D, Higgins CB: MRI of the abnormal pericardium. Am J Roentgenol 1986;147:245.

235. Miller SW: Imaging pericardial disease. Radiol Clin North Am 1989;27:1113.

236. Kilpatrick ZM, Chapman CB: On pericardiocentesis. Am J Cardiol 1965;16:722.

237. Hall JB, Schmidt LD: Emergencies in critical care. In Hall JB, Schmidt GA, Wood LD, Crinc PF (eds): Principles of Crtical Care. New York, McGraw Hill, 1997, pp 1405–1410.

238. Gascho JA, Martins JB, Marcus ML, Kerber RE: Effects of volume expansion and vasodilators in acute pericardial tamponade. Am J Physiol 1981;240:H49.

239. Permanyer-Miralda, Sagrista-Sauleda J, Soler-Soler J: Primary acute pericardial disease: A prospective series of 231 consecutive patients. Am J Cardiol 1985;56:623.

240. Zayas R, Anguita M, Torres F, et al: Incidence of specific etiology and role of methods for specific etiologic diagnosis of primary acute pericarditis. Am J Cardiol 1995;75:378.

241. Sagrista-Sauleda J, Merce J, Permanyer-Miralda G, Soler-Soler J: Clinical clues to the causes of large pericardial effusions. Am J Med 2000;109:95.

242. Moores DW, Allen KB, Faber LP, et al: Subxiphoid pericardial drainage for pericardial tamponade. J Thorac Cardiovasc Surg 1995;109:546.

243. Hsu FI, Keefe D, Desiderio D, Downey RJ: Echocardiographic and surgical correlation of pericardial effusions in patients with malignant disease. J Thorac Cardiovasc Surg 1998;115:1215.

244. Bardales RH, Stanley MW, Schaefer RF, Liblit RL, Owens RB, Surhland MJ: Secondary pericardial malignancies: A critical appraisal of the role of cytology, pericardial biopsy, and DNA ploidy analysis. Am J Clin Pathol 1996;106:29.

245. Wiener HG, Kristensen IB, Haubek A, Kristensen B, Baandrup U: The diagnostic value of pericardial cytology. An analysis of 95 cases. Acta Cytol 1991;35:149.

246. Monte SA, Ehya H, Lang WR: Positive effusion cytology as the initial presentation of malignancy. Acta Cytol 1987;31:448.

247. Stewart JR, Fajardo LF, Gillette SM, Constine LS: Radiation injury to the heart. Int J Radiat Oncol Biol Phys 1995;31:1205.

248. Clarke DP, Cosgrove DO: Real-time ultrasound scanning in the planning and guidance of pericardiocentesis. Clin Radiol 1987;38:119.

249. Nugue O, Millaire A, Porte H, et al: Pericardioscopy in the etiologic diagnosis of pericardial effusion in 141 consecutive patients. Circulation 1996;94:1635.

250. Seferovic PM, Ristic AD, Maksimovic R, et al: Flexible percutaneous pericardioscopy: Inherent drawbacks and recent advances. Herz 2000;25:741.

251. Maisch B, Ristic AD, Rupp H, Spodick DH: Pericardial access using the PerDUCER and flexible percutaneous pericardioscopy. Am J Cardiol 2001;88:1323.

252. Vaitkus PT, Herrmann HC, LeWinter MM: Treatment of malignant pericardial effusion. JAMA 1994;272:59.

253. Celermajer DS, Boyer MJ, Bailey BP, Tattersall MH: Pericardio-centesis for symptomatic malignant pericardial effusion: A study of 36 patients. Med J Aust 1991;154:19.

254. Mani S, Duffy TP: Pericardial tamponade in chronic myelomonocytic leukemia. Chest 1994;106:967.

255. Strupp C, Germing U, Trommer I, Gattermann N, Aul C: Pericardial effusion in chronic myelomonocytic leukemia (CMML): A case report and review of the literature. Leuk Res 2000;24:1059.

256. Bradford CR, Smith SR, Wallis JP: Pericardial extramedullary haemopoiesis in chronic myelomonocytic leukaemia. J Clin Pathol 1993;46:674.

257. Yufu Y, Okada Y, Goto T, Nishimura J: Cardiac tamponade in chronic myelomonocytic leukemia: A case report. Jpn J Clin Oncol 1992;22:411.

258. Rolla G, Bertero MT, Pastena G, et al: Primary lymphoma of the heart. A case report and review of the literature. Leuk Res 2002;26:117.

259. Skalidis EI, Parthenakis FI, Zacharis EA, Datseris GE, Vardas PE: Pulmonary tumor embolism from primary cardiac B-cell lymphoma. Chest 1999;116:1489.

260. Ceresoli GL, Ferreri AJ, Bucci E, Ripa C, Ponzoni M, Villa E: Primary cardiac lymphoma in immunocompetent patients: Diagnostic and therapeutic management. Cancer 1997;80:1497.

261. Arya LS, Narain S, Thavaraj V, Saxena A, Bhargava M: Leukemic pericardial effusion causing cardiac tamponade. Med Pediatr Oncol 2002;38:282.

262. da Costa CM, de Camargo B, Lamelas R, et al: Cardiac tamponade complicating hyperleukocytosis in a child with leukemia. Med Pediatr Oncol 1999;33:120.

263. Saad MF, Frazier OH, Hickey RC, Samaan NA: Intrapericardial pheochromocytoma. Am J Med 1983;75:371.

264. Tsang TS, Seward JB, Barnes ME, et al: Outcomes of primary and secondary treatment of pericardial effusion in patients with malignancy. Mayo Clin Proc 2000;75:248.

265. Larrey EL: New surgical procedure to open the pericardium in the case of fluid in the cavity. Clin Chir 1829;36:303.

266. Okamoto H, Shinkai T, Yamakido M, Saijo N: Cardiac tamponade caused by primary lung cancer and the management of pericardial effusion. Cancer 1993;71:93.

267. Allen KB, Faber LP, Warren WH, Shaar CJ: Pericardial effusion: Subxiphoid pericardiostomy versus percutaneous catheter drainage. Ann Thorac Surg 1999;67:437.

268. Press OW, Livingston R: Management of malignant pericardial effusion and tamponade. JAMA 1987;257:1088.

269. Miller JI, Mansour KA, Hatcher CR Jr: Pericardiectomy: Current indications, concepts, and results in a university center. Ann Thorac Surg 1982;34:40.

270. Piehler JM, Pluth JR, Schaff HV, Danielson GK, Orszulak TA, Puga FJ: Surgical management of effusive pericardial disease. Influence of extent of pericardial resection on clinical course. J Thorac Cardiovasc Surg 1985;90:506.

271. Hazelrigg SR, Mack MJ, Landreneau RJ, Acuff TE, Seifert PE, Auer JE: Thoracoscopic pericardiectomy for effusive pericardial disease. Ann Thorac Surg 1993;56:792.

272. Naunheim KS, Kesler KA, Fiore AC, et al: Pericardial drainage: Subxiphoid vs. transthoracic approach. Eur J Cardiothorac Surg 1991;5:99.

273. Park JS, Rentschler R, Wilbur D: Surgical management of pericardial effusion in patients with malignancies. Comparison of subxiphoid window versus pericardiectomy. Cancer 1991;67:76.

274. Yim AP, Ho JK: Video-assisted subxiphoid pericardiectomy. J Laparoendosc Surg 1995;5:193.

275. Wang N, Feikes JR, Mogensen T, Vyhmeister EE, Bailey LL: Pericardioperitoneal shunt: An alternative treatment for malignant pericardial effusion. Ann Thorac Surg 1994;57:289.

276. Ziskind AA, Pearce AC, Lemmon CC, et al: Percutaneous balloon pericardiotomy for the treatment of cardiac tamponade and large pericardial effusions: Description of technique and report of the first 50 cases. J Am Coll Cardiol 1993;21:1.

277. Galli M, Politi A, Pedretti F, Castiglioni B, Zerboni S: Percutaneous balloon pericardiotomy for malignant pericardial tamponade. Chest 1995;108:1499.

278. Bertrand O, Legrand V, Kulbertus H: Percutaneous balloon pericardiotomy: A case report and analysis of mechanism of action. Cathet Cardiovasc Diagn 1996;38:180.

279. Fiocco M, Krasna MJ: The management of malignant pleural and pericardial effusions. Hematol Oncol Clin North Am 1997;11:253.

280. Maher EA, Shepherd FA, Todd TJ: Pericardial sclerosis as the primary management of malignant pericardial effusion and cardiac tamponade. J Thorac Cardiovasc Surg 1996;112:637.

281. Shepherd FA, Morgan C, Evans WK, Ginsberg JF, Watt D, Murphy K: Medical management of malignant pericardial effusion by tetracycline sclerosis. Am J Cardiol 1987;60:1161.

282. Liu G, Crump M, Goss PE, Dancey J, Shepherd FA: Prospective comparison of the sclerosing agents doxycycline and bleomycin for the primary management of malignant pericardial effusion and cardiac tamponade. J Clin Oncol 1996;14:3141.

283. Imamura T, Tamura K, Takenaga M, Nagatomo Y, Ishikawa T, Nakagawa S: Intrapericardial OK-432 instillation for the management of malignant pericardial effusion. Cancer 1991;68:259.

284. Moriya T, Takiguchi Y, Tabeta H, et al: Controlling malignant pericardial effusion by intrapericardial carboplatin administration in patients with primary non–small-cell lung cancer. Br J Cancer 2000;83:858.

285. Fiorentino MV, Daniele O, Morandi P, et al: Intrapericardial instillation of platin in malignant pericardial effusion. Cancer 1988;62:1904.

286. Kawashima O, Kurihara T, Kamiyoshihara M, Sakata S, Ishikawa S, Morishita Y: Management of malignant pericardial effusion resulting from recurrent cancer with local instillation of aclarubicin hydrochloride. Am J Clin Oncol 1999;22:396.

287. Kuhn K, Purea H, Selbach J, Westerhausen M: Treatment with locally applied mitoxantrone. Acta Med Austriaca 1989;16:87.

288. Wilkins HE III, Cacioppo J, Connolly MM, Marquez G, Grays P: Intrapericardial interferon in the management of malignant pericardial effusion. Chest 1998;114:330.

289. Laham RJ, Cohen DJ, Kuntz RE, Baim DS, Lorell BH, Simons M: Pericardial effusion in patients with cancer: Outcome with contemporary management strategies. Heart 1996;75:67.

290. Runyon BA: Care of patients with ascites. N Engl J Med 1994;330:337.

291. Gotloib L, Shostak A: The functional anatomy of the peritoneum as a dialyzing membrane. In Twardowski ZJ, Nolph KD, Khanna R (eds): Contemporary Issues in Nephrology Peritoneal Dialysis: New Concepts and Applications. New York, Churchill Livingstone, 2003, pp 1–50.

292. Lifshitz S: Ascites, pathophysiology and control measures. Int J Radiat Oncol Biol Phys 1982;8:1423.

293. Levendoglu-Tugal O, Weiss R, Ozkaynak MF, Sandoval C, Lentzner B, Jayabose S: T-cell acute lymphoblastic leukemia after renal transplantation in childhood. J Pediatr Hematol Oncol 1998;20:548.

294. Hirabayashi K, Graham J: Genesis of ascites in ovarian cancer. Am J Obstet Gynecol 1970;106:492.

295. Fastaia J, Dumont AE: Pathogenesis of ascites in mice with peritoneal carcinomatosis. J Natl Cancer Inst 1976;56:547.

296. Feldman GB, Knapp RC, Order SE, Hellman S: The role of lymphatic obstruction in the formation of ascites in a murine ovarian carcinoma. Cancer Res 1972;32:1663.

297. Coates G, Bush RS, Aspin N: A study of ascites using lymphoscintigraphy with 99m Tc-sulfur colloid. Radiology 1973;107:577.

298. Bronskill MJ, Bush RS, Ege GN: A quantitative measurement of peritoneal drainage in malignant ascites. Cancer 1977;40:2375.

299. Neufeld G, Cohen T, Gengrinovitch S, Poltorak Z: Vascular endothelial growth factor (VEGF) and its receptors. FASEB J 1999;13:9.

300. Senger DR, Perruzzi CA, Feder J, Dvorak HF: A highly conserved vascular permeability factor secreted by a variety of human and rodent tumor cell lines. Cancer Res 1986;46:5629.

301. Yamamoto S, Konishi I, Mandai M, et al: Expression of vascular endothelial growth factor (VEGF) in epithelial ovarian neoplasms: Correlation with clinicopathology and patient survival, and analysis of serum VEGF levels. Br J Cancer 1997;76:1221.

302. Zebrowski BK, Liu, Ramirez K, Akagi Y, Mills GB, Ellis LM: Markedly elevated levels of vascular endothelial growth factor in malignant ascites. Ann Surg Oncol 1999;6:373.

303. Mesiano S, Ferrara N, Jaffe RB: Role of vascular endothelial growth factor in ovarian cancer: Inhibition of ascites formation by immunoneutralization. Am J Pathol 1998;153:1249.

304. Luo JC, Toyoda M, Shibuya M: Differential inhibition of fluid accumulation and tumor growth in two mouse ascites tumors by an antivascular endothelial growth factor/permeability factor neutralizing antibody. Cancer Res 1998;58:2594.

305. Schlaeppi JM, Wood JM: Targeting vascular endothelial growth factor (VEGF) for anti-tumor therapy, by anti-VEGF neutralizing monoclonal antibodies or by VEGF receptor tyrosine-kinase inhibitors. Cancer Metastasis Rev 1999;18:473.

306. Bertoglio S, Melioli G, Baldini E, et al: Intraperitoneal infusion of recombinant interleukin-2 in malignant ascites in patients with gastrointestinal and ovarian cancer. Acta Med Austriaca 1989;16:81.

307. Ott MG, Mannel DN, Gallati H, Goerig M, Raeth U: Peripheral natural killer cell activity and intraperitoneal soluble p55 tumor necrosis factor receptor in patients with malignant ascites: Two possible indicators for response to intraperitoneal combined tumor necrosis factor alpha and interferon gamma treatment. Cancer Immunol Immunother 1996;42:31.

308. Aslam N, Marino CR: Malignant ascites: New concepts in pathophysiology, diagnosis, and management. Arch Intern Med 2001;161:2733.

309. Parsons SL, Watson SA, Steele RJ: Phase I/II trial of batimastat, a matrix metalloproteinase inhibitor, in patients with malignant ascites. Eur J Surg Oncol 1997;23:526.

310. Beatty JD, Romero C, Brown PW, Lawrence W Jr, Terz JJ: Clinical value of carcinoembryonic antigen: Diagnosis, prognosis, and follow-up of patients with cancer. Arch Surg 1979;114:563.

311. Mactier RA: Peritoneal lymphatics. In Twardowski ZJ, Nolph KD, Khanna R (eds): Kinetics of Ultrafiltration with Glucose and Alternative Osmotic Agents. New York, Churchill-Livingstone, 1990, pp 24–30.

312. Tamsma JT, Keizer HJ, Meinders AE: Pathogenesis of malignant ascites: Starling's law of capillary hemodynamics revisited. Ann Oncol 2001;12:1353.

313. Zink J, Greenway CV: Intraperitoneal pressure in formation and reabsorption of ascites in cats. Am J Physiol 1977;233:H185.

314. Cattau EL Jr, Benjamin SB, Knuff TE, Castell DO: The accuracy of the physical examination in the diagnosis of suspected ascites. JAMA 1982;247:1164.

315. Inadomi J, Cello JP, Koch J: Ultrasonographic determination of ascitic volume. Hepatology 1996;24:549.

316. Goldberg BB, Goodman GA, Clearfield HR: Evaluation of ascites by ultrasound. Radiology 1970;96:15.

317. Runyon BA: Paracentesis of ascitic fluid. A safe procedure. Arch Intern Med 1986;146:2259.

318. McVay PA, Toy PT: Lack of increased bleeding after paracentesis and thoracentesis in patients with mild coagulation abnormalities. Transfusion 1991;31:164.

319. Runyon BA: Management of adult patients with ascites caused by cirrhosis. Hepatology 1998;27:264.

320. Press OW, Press NO, Kaufman SD: Evaluation and management of chylous ascites. Ann Intern Med 1982;96:358.

321. Runyon BA, Montano AA, Akriviadis EA, Antillon MR, Irving MA, McHutchison JG: The serum-ascites albumin gradient is superior to the exudate-transudate concept in the differential diagnosis of ascites. Ann Intern Med 1992;117:215.

322. DeSitter L, Rector WG Jr: The significance of bloody ascites in patients with cirrhosis. Am J Gastroenterol 1984;79:136.

323. Akriviadis EA: Hemoperitoneum in patients with ascites. Am J Gastroenterol 1997;92:567.

324. Runyon BA, Hoefs JC, Morgan TR: Ascitic fluid analysis in malignancy-related ascites. Hepatology 1988;8:1104.

325. Such J, Runyon BA: Spontaneous bacterial peritonitis. Clin Infect Dis 1998;27:669.

326. Hoefs JC: Serum protein concentration and portal pressure determine the ascitic fluid protein concentration in patients with chronic liver disease. J Lab Clin Med 1983;102:260.

327. Runyon BA, Hoefs JC: Ascitic fluid chemical analysis before, during and after spontaneous bacterial peritonitis. Hepatology 1985;5:257.

328. Runyon BA: Low-protein-concentration ascitic fluid is predisposed to spontaneous bacterial peritonitis. Gastroenterology 1986;91:1343.

329. Runyon BA, Antillon MR: Ascitic fluid pH and lactate: Insensitive and nonspecific tests in detecting ascitic fluid infection. Hepatology 1991;13:929.

330. Siddiqui RA, Kochhar R, Singh V, Rajwanshi A, Goenka MK, Mehta SK: Evaluation of fibronectin as a marker of malignant ascites. J Gastroenterol Hepatol 1992;7:161.

331. Runyon BA: Malignancy-related ascites and ascitic fluid "humoral tests of malignancy". J Clin Gastroenterol 1994;18:94.

332. Cardozo PL: A critical evaluation of 3000 cytologic cases of

333. DiBonito L, Falconieri G, Colautti I, Bonifacio D, Dudine S: The positive peritoneal effusion. A retrospective study of cytopathologic diagnoses with autopsy confirmation. Acta Cytol 1993;37:483.

334. Loewenstein MS, Rittgers RA, Feinerman AE, et al: Carcinoembryonic antigen assay of ascites and detection of malignancy. Ann Intern Med 1978;88:635.

335. Gershenson DM, Silva EG, Tortolero-Luna G, Levenback C, Morris M, Tornos C: Serous borderline tumors of the ovary with noninvasive peritoneal implants. Cancer 1998;83:2157.

336. Gershenson DM, Silva EG, Levy L, Burke TW, Wolf JK, Tornos C: Ovarian serous borderline tumors with invasive peritoneal implants. Cancer 1998;82:1096.

337. Silva EG, Tornos C, Zhuang Z, Merino MJ, Gershenson DM: Tumor recurrence in stage I ovarian serous neoplasms of low malignant potential. Int J Gynecol Pathol 1998;17:1.

338. Strnad CM, Grosh WW, Baxter J, et al: Peritoneal carcinomatosis of unknown primary site in women. A distinctive subset of adenocarcinoma. Ann Intern Med 1989;111:213.

339. Ransom DT, Patel SR, Keeney GL, Malkasian GD, Edmonson JH: Papillary serous carcinoma of the peritoneum. A review of 33 cases treated with platin-based chemotherapy. Cancer 1990;66:1091.

340. van Dam PA, DeCloedt J, Tjalma WA, Buytaert P, Becquart D, Vergote IB: Trocar implantation metastasis after laparoscopy in patients with advanced ovarian cancer: Can the risk be reduced? Am J Obstet Gynecol 1999;181:536.

341. Menzies RI, Fitzgerald JM, Mulpeter K: Laparoscopic diagnosis of ascites in Lesotho. Br Med J 1985;291:473.

342. Osterlee J: Peritoneovenous shunting for ascites in cancer patients. Br J Surg 1980;67:145–160.

343. Greenway B, Johnson PJ, Williams R: Control of malignant ascites with spironolactone. Br J Surg 1982;69:441.

344. Razis DV, Athanasiou A, Dadiotis L: Diuretics in malignant effusions and edemas of generalized cancer. J Med 1976;7:449.

345. Lee CW, Bociek G, Faught W: A survey of practice in management of malignant ascites. J Pain Symptom Manage 1998;16:96.

346. Pockros PJ, Esrason KT, Nguyen C, Duque J, Woods S: Mobilization of malignant ascites with diuretics is dependent on ascitic fluid characteristics. Gastroenterology 1992;103:1302.

347. Parsons SL, Lang MW, Steele RJ: Malignant ascites: A 2-year review from a teaching hospital. Eur J Surg Oncol 1996;22:237.

348. Gines P, Tito L, Arroyo V, et al: Randomized comparative study of therapeutic paracentesis with and without intravenous albumin in cirrhosis. Gastroenterology 1988;94:1493.

349. Runyon BA: Patient selection is important in studying the impact of large-volume paracentesis on intravascular volume. Am J Gastroenterol 1997;92:371.

350. Straus AK, Roseman DL, Shapiro TM: Peritoneovenous shunting in the management of malignant ascites. Arch Surg 1979;114:489.

351. Reinhold RB, Lokich JJ, Tomashefski J, Costello P: Management of malignant ascites with peritoneovenous shunting. Am J Surg 1983;145:455.

352. Roussel JG, Kroon BB, Hart GA: The Denver type for peritoneovenous shunting of malignant ascites. Surg Gynecol Obstet 1986;162:235.

353. Edney JA, Hill A, Armstrong D: Peritoneovenous shunts palliate malignant ascites. Am J Surg 1989;158:598.

354. Parsons SL, Lang MW, Steele RJ: Malignant ascites: A 2-year review from a teaching hospital. Eur J Surg Oncol 1996;22:237.

355. Gough IR, GA Balderson: Malignant ascites. A comparison of peritoneovenous shunting and nonoperative management. Cancer 1993;71:2377.

356. Faught W, Kirkpatrick JR, Krepart GV, Heywood MS, Lotocki RJ: Peritoneovenous shunt for palliation of gynecologic malignant ascites. J Am Coll Surg 1995;180:472.

357. Qazi R, Savlov ED: Peritoneovenous shunt for palliation of malignant ascites. Cancer 1982;49:600.

358. Helzberg JH, Greenberger NJ: Peritoneovenous shunts in malignant ascites. Dig Dis Sci 1985;30:1104.

359. Schumacher DL, Saclarides TJ, Staren ED: Peritoneovenous shunts for palliation of the patient with malignant ascites. Ann Surg Oncol 1994;1:378.

360. Souter RG, Wells C, Tarin D, Kettlewell MG: Surgical and pathologic complications associated with peritoneovenous shunts in management of malignant ascites. Cancer 1985;55:1973.

361. Souter RG, Tarin D, Kettlewell MG: Peritoneovenous shunts in the management of malignant ascites. Br J Surg 1983;70:478.

362. Lacy JH, Wieman TJ, Shively EH: Management of malignant ascites. Surg Gynecol Obstet 1984;159:397.

363. Hyde GL, Dillon M, Bivins BA: Peritoneal venous shunting for ascites: A 15-year perspective. Am Surg 1982;48:123.

364. McLoud TC, Bourgouin PM, Greenberg RW, et al: Bronchogenic carcinoma: Analysis of staging in the mediastinum with CT by correlative lymph node mapping and sampling. Radiology 1992;182:319.

365. Ragni MV, Lewis JH, Spero JA: Ascites-induced LeVeen shunt coagulopathy. Ann Surg 1983;198:91.

366. Scott-Coombes DM, Whawell SA, Vipond MN, Crnojevic L, Thompson JA: Fibrinolytic activity of ascites caused by alcoholic cirrhosis and peritoneal malignancy. Gut 1993;34:1120.

367. Gleysteen JJ, Hussey CV, Heckman MG: The cause of coagulopathy after peritoneovenous shunt for malignant ascites. Arch Surg 1990;125:474.

368. Smith RR, Sternberg SS, Paglia MA, Golbey RB: Fatal pulmonary tumor embolization following peritoneovenous shunting for malignant ascites. J Surg Oncol 1981;16:27.

369. Borger JA, Pitel P, Crump G: Management of malignant ascites with a vascular port. J Pediatr Surg 1993;28:1605.

370. Richard HM III, Coldwell DM, Boyd-Kranis RL, Murthy R, Van Echo DA: Pleurx tunneled catheter in the management of malignant ascites. J Vasc Interv Radiol 2001;12:373.

371. Sabatelli FW, Glassman ML, Kerns SR, Hawkins IF Jr: Permanent indwelling peritoneal access device for the management of malignant ascites. Cardiovasc Intervent Radiol 1994;17:292.

372. Lomas DA, Wallis PJ, Stockley RA: Palliation of malignant ascites with a Tenckhoff catheter. Thorax 1989;44:828.

373. Belfort MA, Stevens PJ, DeHaek K, Soeters R, Krige JE: A new approach to the management of malignant ascites; a permanently implanted abdominal drain. Eur J Surg Oncol 1990;16:47.

374. Flowers RH III, Schwenzer KJ, Kopel RF, Fisch MJ, Tucker SI, Farr BM: Efficacy of an attachable subcutaneous cuff for the prevention of intravascular catheter-related infection. A randomized, controlled trial. JAMA 1989;261:878.

375. Sugarbaker PH: Peritonectomy procedures. Ann Surg 1995;221:29.

376. McClay EF, Braly PD, Kirmani S, et al: A phase II trial of intraperitoneal high-dose carboplatin and etoposide with granulocyte macrophage-colony stimulating factor support in patients with ovarian carcinoma. Am J Clin Oncol 1995;18:23.

377. Sugarbaker PH, Jablonski KA: Prognostic features of 51 colorectal and 130 appendiceal cancer patients with peritoneal carcinomatosis treated by cytoreductive surgery and intraperitoneal chemotherapy. Ann Surg 1995;221:124.

378. Sugarbaker PH: Intraperitoneal chemotherapy for treatment and prevention of peritoneal carcinomatosis and sarcomatosis. Dis Colon Rectum 1994;37:S115.

379. Dedrick RL, Myers CE, Bungay PM, DeVita VT Jr: Pharmacokinetic rationale for peritoneal drug administration in the treatment of ovarian cancer. Cancer Treat Rep 1978;62:1.

380. Jacobs ML, Duarte MD: Radioactive colloidal chromic phosphate to control pleural effusions and ascites. JAMA 1955;166:597.

381. Jackson GL, Blosser NM: Intracavitary chromic phosphate (32P) colloidal suspension therapy. Cancer 1981;48:2596.

382. Weisberger AS, Levine B, Sorasli JP: Use of nitrogen mustard in the treatment of serous effusions of neoplastic origin. JAMA 1955;159:1704.

383. Casper ES, Kelsen DP, Alcock NW, Lewis JL Jr: Ip cisplatin in patients with malignant ascites: Pharmacokinetic evaluation and comparison with the IV route. Cancer Treat Rep 1983;67:235.

384. Markman M: Intraperitoneal chemotherapy as treatment of ovarian carcinoma: Why, how, and when? Obstet Gynecol Surv 1987;42:533.

385. Markman M: Intraperitoneal chemotherapy for malignant diseases of the gastrointestinal tract. Surg Gynecol Obstet 1987;164:89.

386. Markman M: Intraperitoneal chemotherapy for ovarian carcinoma. Biomed Pharmacother 1987;41:420.

387. Ozols RF, Young RC, Speyer JL, et al: Phase I and pharmacological studies of adriamycin administered intraperitoneally to patients with ovarian cancer. Cancer Res 1982;42:4265.

388. Howell SB, Pfeifle CL, Wung WE, et al: Intraperitoneal cisplatin with systemic thiosulfate protection. Ann Intern Med 1982;97:845.

389. Alberts DS, Liu PY, Hannigan EV, et al: Intraperitoneal cisplatin plus intravenous cyclophosphamide versus intravenous cisplatin plus intravenous cyclophosphamide for stage III ovarian cancer. N Engl J Med 1996;335:1950.

390. Gilly FN, Carry PY, Brachet A, et al: Treatment of malignant peritoneal effusion in digestive and ovarian cancer. Med Oncol Tumor Pharmacother 1992;9:177.

391. Loggie BW, Perini M, Fleming RA, Russell GB, Geisinger K: Treatment and prevention of malignant ascites associated with disseminated intraperitoneal malignancies by aggressive combined-modality therapy. Am Surg 1997;63:137.

392. Markman M, Kelsen D: Efficacy of cisplatin-based intraperitoneal chemotherapy as treatment of malignant peritoneal mesothelioma. J Cancer Res Clin Oncol 1992;118:547.

393. Yamaguchi Y, Satoh Y, Miyahara E, et al: Locoregional immunotherapy of malignant ascites by intraperitoneal administration of OK-432 plus IL-2 in gastric cancer patients. Anticancer Res 1995;15:2201.

394. Kondo M, Kato H, Yoshikawa T, Sugino S: Treatment of cancer ascites by intraperitoneal administration of a streptococcal preparation OK-432 with fresh human complement—Eole of complement-derived chemotactic factor to neutrophils. Int J Immunopharmacol 1986;8:715.

395. Katano M, Torisu M: New approach to management of malignant ascites with a streptococcal preparation, OK-432. II. Intraperitoneal inflammatory cell-mediated tumor cell destruction. Surgery 1983;93:365.

396. Stuart GC, Nation JG, Snider DD, Thunberg P: Intraperitoneal interferon in the management of malignant ascites. Cancer 1993;71:2027.

397. Bezwoda WR, Seymour L, Dansey R: Intraperitoneal recombinant interferon-alpha 2b for recurrent malignant ascites due to ovarian cancer. Cancer 1989;64:1029.

398. Lissoni P, Barni S, Tancini G, et al: Intracavitary therapy of neoplastic effusions with cytokines: Comparison among interferon alpha, beta and interleukin-2. Support Care Cancer 1995;3:78.

399. Buckman R, De Angelis C, Shaw P, et al: Intraperitoneal therapy of malignant ascites associated with carcinoma of ovary and breast using radioiodinated monoclonal antibody 2G3. Gynecol Oncol 1992;47:102.

400. DeClerck YA, Perez N, Shimada H, Boone TC, Langley KE, Taylor SM: Inhibition of invasion and metastasis in cells transfected with an inhibitor of metalloproteinases. Cancer Res 1992;52:701.

401. Wojtowicz-Praga S, Low J, Marshall J, et al: Phase I trial of a novel matrix metalloproteinase inhibitor batimastat (BB-94) in patients with advanced cancer. Invest New Drugs 1996;14:193.

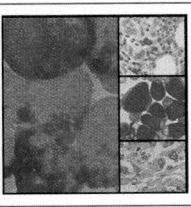
NEUROLOGIC COMPLICATIONS

Mark R. Gilbert

SUMMARY OF KEY POINTS

INCIDENCE OF CHEMOTHERAPY- AND RADIATION THERAPY–INDUCED NEUROTOXICITY

- The actual incidence is unknown but is increasing.
- Improvements in supportive care have allowed dose escalations of many drugs, resulting in neurotoxicity.
- Increased survival from cancer has resulted in neurotoxicity with a long latency.
- New treatments directed at tumors in the central nervous system often result in neurotoxicity, particularly with therapies administered directly into the brain.

ETIOLOGY OF NEUROTOXICITY

- Direct effects on neurons, myelin, and supporting glial cells have been implicated.

- Effects on neuronal cytoskeleton and axonal transport, neuronal metabolism, and neurotransmitter function are the most commonly hypothesized mechanisms of toxicity.

EVALUATION OF THE PATIENT

- Chemotherapy or radiation toxicity should be considered a diagnosis of exclusion in most cases.
- Specific diagnostic tests do not exist for most situations.
- The diagnosis often is made by recognition of a neurotoxic syndrome temporally related to treatment.

GRADING OF THE COMPLICATION

- Grading scales are of limited value for monitoring individual patients and are used only for study populations.

- More refined grading for management is a component of neurologic and neuropsychologic testing.

TREATMENT

- Most neurotoxic syndromes do not have specific treatment.
- Prevention or reduction of risk often is possible with proper monitoring or treatment planning.
- New agents are under development as management or prevention of neurotoxicity, but careful testing is required to ensure that the antineoplastic effect is not compromised.

INTRODUCTION

The neurotoxic effects of cancer chemotherapeutic agents and radiation therapy are of increasing importance in the treatment of cancer patients. Although the exact incidence of treatment-related neurotoxicity is unknown, the frequency is certainly increasing. Several factors are known to be responsible for this increase in incidence of treatment-related neurotoxicity.

First, recent advances in supportive care allow the use of much higher doses of chemotherapy. For example, granulocyte- and granulocyte-macrophage colony-stimulating factors allow use of drug doses that would previously have caused severe bone marrow suppression. Unfortunately, similar factors for prevention of development of neurotoxicity do not exist. In initial studies of paclitaxel, a novel antitubulin agent, myelosuppression was dose limiting. Use of colony-stimulating factors has allowed dose escalation, but severe peripheral neuropathy has developed in many patients treated at these higher doses.[1,2] Similarly, nephrotoxicity and myelosuppression had limited dose escalation of cisplatin in the past.

Innovative hydration schemes and colony-stimulating factors have reduced the risk of these toxicities. Dose escalation has resulted in severe neurotoxicity and ototoxicity, now considered the dose-limiting toxicities.[3]

Second, improvements in cancer treatment have increased the duration of survival from many malignant diseases. As a consequence, treatment-related neurotoxicity with a long latency between treatment and onset of symptoms is being recognized with increasing frequency. Childhood acute lymphoid leukemia often was fatal until recognition of the central nervous system (CNS) as a sanctuary for leukemia cells. Treatment of cerebrospinal fluid (CSF) with direct administration of methotrexate and use of cranial irradiation resulted in a marked increase in long-term remission and cure. This treatment of the CNS, however, also caused delayed neurotoxicity. Severe dementia developed in some patients, and many others experienced a decline in cognitive function years after completion of treatment.[4-8]

Third, new agents, including biologic response modifiers, or novel routes of administration designed specifically to target the nervous system for management of brain metastases or primary brain tumors will most likely result in an increase in neurotoxicity. Spiromustine, an experimental agent specifically designed to cross the blood-brain barrier, showed promising results in pre-clinical animal testing for the management of brain metastases. Unfortunately, administration to patients in phase I testing resulted in a high incidence of acute encephalopathy.[9] Likewise, use of disruption of the blood-brain barrier to improve drug delivery to brain tumors has led to a marked increase in neurotoxicity compared with standard systemic administration. Results of animal studies have demonstrated that chemical opening of the blood-brain barrier results in a marked increase in exposure of normal brain parenchyma to chemotherapy with a much smaller increase in delivery to the tumor.[10] Implantation of carmustine (BCNU)-impregnated polymer wafers into the resection cavity has shown a survival benefit for glioblastoma but with an increase in the incidence of brain necrosis and infection.[11]

Continued improvement in cancer treatment will result in prolonged survival and an increased rate of cure. Therefore long-term morbidity, particularly development of irreversible neurotoxicity, is a critical concern. This chapter discusses the agents most commonly responsible for neurotoxicity, describes differential diagnosis and evaluation of patients with neurologic dysfunction, and addresses management and prevention of chemotherapy- and radiation therapy–induced neurotoxicity.

SPECIFIC AGENTS

Cytosine Arabinoside

Cytosine arabinoside (ara-C) can cause a wide range of neurotoxicity. The toxicity that develops depends on the route of administration and the dose used.

Cerebellar Toxicity

Systemic administration of high-dose (>1 g/m^2) intravenous ara-C leads to acute cerebellar toxicity.[12-15] Onset of neurologic symptoms is generally acute and often is noticed during administration of a multiday regimen.[12,13,16] Patients have evidence of global cerebellar dysfunction, which manifests as truncal, limb, and gait ataxia, dysarthria, and nystagmus. In some cases, permanent cerebellar dysfunction develops; in others, a mild cerebellar syndrome develops that resolves promptly after completion of the chemotherapy.[12,13]

Patients with irreversible cerebellar damage have a characteristic and selective loss of Purkinje cells in the cerebellum.[15] The pathogenesis of the specific cellular damage is unknown, nor have the pathologic findings in the cerebella of patients who have recovered from transient cerebellar dysfunction been reported.

The incidence of irreversible cerebellar toxicity with high-dose ara-C regimens has been reported to be 8% to 20%. Reported risk factors for development of cerebellar toxicity include size of current dose, cumulative dose, age (persons older than 50 years are at higher risk), and renal dysfunction with impaired drug clearance.[13,14,17,18] Whether patients in whom reversible cerebellar dys-

function develops with previous treatment are at higher risk of development of permanent dysfunction is unknown.

Encephalopathy

Acute encephalopathy, often accompanied by seizures, occurs less frequently than cerebellar dysfunction in patients treated with high-dose intravenous ara-C.[13] In most cases, somnolence and lethargy completely resolve soon after completion of chemotherapy. Patients with persistent encephalopathy usually have had additional medical problems, such as severe infection.[18] In addition, leukoencephalopathy, clinically and pathologically indistinguishable from the leukoencephalopathy associated with methotrexate, has been reported as a late complication of high-dose intravenous ara-C administration and with administration of ara-C directly in the CSF.[13]

Spinal Cord Toxicity

Direct administration of ara-C into the lumbar thecal space has been reported to cause myeloradiculopathy.[19-23] Patients have evidence of both spinal cord and nerve root dysfunction. This complication is uncommon, usually being found only after an extensive course of intrathecal chemotherapy. In many instances, patients have received both intrathecal ara-C and methotrexate.[24,25] Neurologic signs are noticed days to weeks after treatment, although there have been reports of myelopathy developing within minutes. In most cases, loss of neurologic function progresses slowly over days, and only one half of patients have improvement or full recovery. Several hypotheses have been proposed for the mechanism of chemotherapy-induced myelopathy. Focal damage from injection of hyperosmolar solution,[26] barbotage from injection,[27] and direct toxic effects of chemotherapy on the spinal cord parenchyma[20] are the most common proposed mechanisms of subacute myelopathy. Histologic examination of the spinal cord shows focal areas of necrosis, most marked along the periphery of the spinal cord.[20,21,24] Microscopic examination shows axonal swelling with accompanying demyelination.[20,21,24]

Myelin basic protein levels in the CSF may be elevated before marked neurologic damage occurs.[24,25] For patients with early symptoms, such as paresthesia, back pain, or Lhermitte's sign, the level of myelin basic protein in the CSF should be measured. If the level is elevated, further lumbar administration of chemotherapy should be avoided.[25]

Other Neurotoxicity Associated with Cytosine Arabinoside

Peripheral neuropathy has been reported after administration of high-dose ara-C.[28] Symmetric sensorimotor polyneuropathy developed 2 weeks after completion of treatment. Nerve biopsy demonstrated axonal damage with patchy regions of demyelination. In addition, a case of reversible parkinsonism has been reported after administration of high-dose ara-C.[13] Onset of tremor, bradykinesia, and masked facies were found 3 weeks after completion of treatment. Treatment with carbidopa/levodopa provided only transient improvement. All parkinsonian features, however, resolved over 12 weeks.

L-Asparaginase

Cerebrovascular Events

Cerebrovascular events caused by L-asparaginase–induced coagulopathy constitute the most common neurotoxicity associated with L-asparaginase treatment. Both thrombotic and hemorrhagic strokes have been reported in patients receiving L-asparaginase.[29-31] Thrombosis of cerebral sinuses also has occurred in patients receiving this agent. The clinical manifestations of sinus thrombosis usually are acute, severe headache, nausea, and vomiting caused by the rapid increase in intracranial pressure. Changes in level of consciousness occur most frequently with sagittal sinus thrombosis because of bilateral cerebral hemisphere involvement. Although most patients with sinus thrombosis have acute and rapidly progressive changes in neurologic function, some patients experience only headache and mild neurologic dysfunction.[29]

Development of neurologic symptoms during L-asparaginase therapy should be evaluated with either head computed tomography (CT) or magnetic resonance imaging (MRI). MRI usually is preferred because it often depicts sinus thrombosis by absence of a flow void in the sinus. MRI also depicts early signs of ischemic brain injury and punctate hemorrhage.

Neuropsychiatric Effects

Less frequently, L-asparaginase treatment has been associated with development of neuropsychiatric symptoms,[32] most notably depression, delusions, hallucinations, disorientation, and altered levels of consciousness. In the series described by Holland and colleagues,[32] 5 of 19 patients with acute leukemia experienced psychiatric symptoms. The onset of symptoms occurred 2 to 19 days after treatment, and the symptoms reversed in three patients who lived longer than 6 weeks. Pathologic analysis in two cases revealed leukemic infiltration. The combination of leukemic involvement of the CNS and treatment-induced depletion of L-asparagine and L-glutamine in the brain has been proposed as a possible factor contributing to development of psychiatric symptoms.

Busulfan

Busulfan administration has been reported to cause generalized tonic-clonic seizures.[33] This reaction has been reported with high-dose treatment as a preparative regimen for bone marrow transplantation. Prophylactic treatment with anticonvulsants, particularly phenytoin, has been shown to reduce the risk of seizures.[34]

Methotrexate

Methotrexate can cause acute, subacute, and chronic neurotoxicity.

Acute Neurotoxicity

Administration of high-dose intravenous methotrexate (> 3 g/m^2) has been associated with development of acute encephalopathy characterized primarily by somnolence, confusion, and seizures.[5,35] Although the pathogenesis of this syndrome is unknown, laboratory studies with rats have shown profound metabolic alteration in the brain after intravenous administration of high-dose methotrexate.[36] In these experiments, a widespread decrease in glucose utilization and protein synthesis was found. In similar studies, folinic acid (leucovorin) markedly diminished these metabolic effects,[37] a finding that suggested a possible role for leucovorin in decreasing the severity of methotrexate-induced somnolence syndrome. Although the somnolence and confusion that occur with acute methotrexate toxicity resolve completely, evidence shows that patients in whom this syndrome develops are at greater risk of chronic methotrexate-induced neurotoxicity.[38] Cases have been reported in which, despite resolution of the clinical symptoms, white-matter changes persist on MR images.[39]

Subacute Toxicity

Subacute methotrexate-induced neurotoxicity generally develops weeks after methotrexate administration and occurs most frequently in patients who have also received cranial radiation therapy.[5] Transient inhibition of myelin formation is thought to be the mechanism of toxicity. The syndrome is completely reversible over weeks, and corticosteroid treatment may accelerate recovery.

Chronic Neurotoxicity

Chronic methotrexate neurotoxicity is known as *leukoencephalopathy*. This syndrome develops months to years after methotrexate administration and has been seen after both intravenous and intrathecal administration of methotrexate.[4-8,40-50] Cranial radiation therapy, particularly when it precedes methotrexate administration, greatly increases the risk of leukoencephalopathy.[5,51] In addition, elevated CSF methotrexate concentration has been associated with an increased risk of neurotoxicity.[42] Younger patients are at higher risk of leukoencephalopathy.[52] Clinically, patients show progressive loss of cognitive function and focal neurologic signs, which may progress to profound dementia, coma, or death.[4-6,8,43] Some patients have seizures as a consequence of widespread neuronal injury. There is no known treatment, and the neurologic deficits are generally irreversible. Brain imaging with MRI or CT often shows large areas of abnormalities in cerebral white matter (Fig. 61-1). Elevated levels of myelin basic protein in CSF have been reported in patients with progressive neurologic dysfunction from methotrexate-induced leukoencephalopathy.[44]

Pathologic examination shows wide areas of coagulative necrosis with swollen axonal cylinders and demyelination.[4,40,53,54] There are regions with vascular changes, particularly microangiopathic calcifications.[45,48,55] The pathogenesis of leukoencephalopathy is unknown, but results of laboratory studies with brain explant cultures suggest that the primary injury may be neuronal (axonal), and the characteristic demyelination may be a secondary phenomenon.[56]

Spinal Cord Toxicity

Chemotherapy-induced myelopathy is an uncommon toxicity of intrathecal treatment with methotrexate.[57-61]

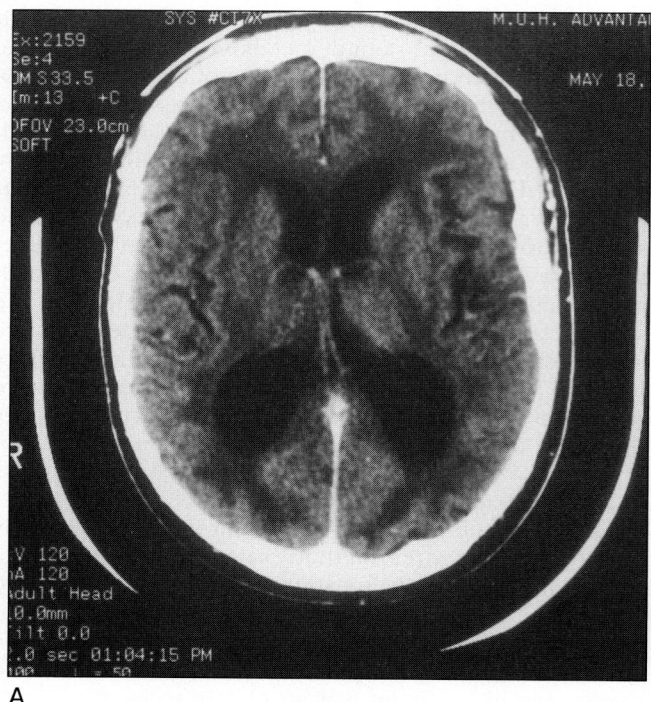
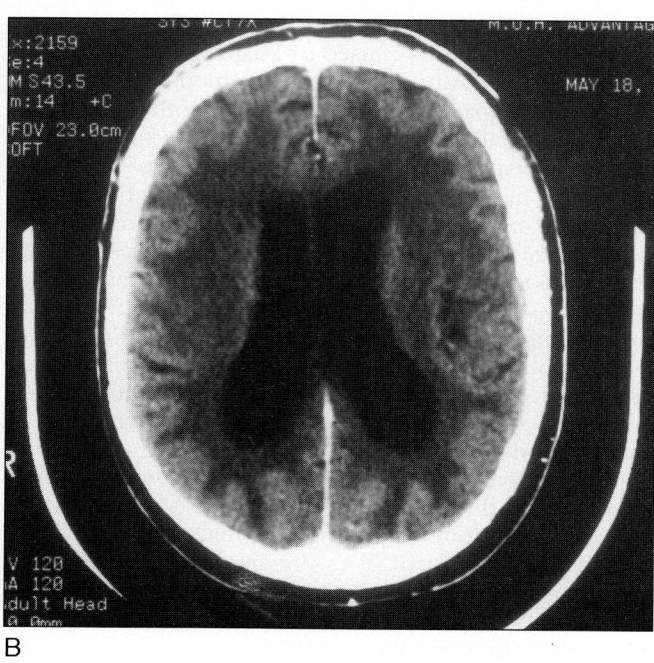

Figure 61-1. A and **B,** Methotrexate-induced leukoencephalopathy. CT scans obtained 6 months after completion of intrathecal chemotherapy. A 63-year-old man with meningeal lymphoma underwent whole-brain radiation therapy. Several months later, he had recurrent meningeal lymphoma and was treated with intrathecal methotrexate. Progressive dementia developed. Widespread destruction of white matter and diffuse atrophy are evident.

Myelopathy generally develops only after extensive intrathecal treatment. Both methotrexate and ara-C have been associated with myelopathy. The clinical syndrome of methotrexate-induced myelopathy is identical to that with ara-C (see earlier, Cytosine Arabinoside). Loss of neurologic function may be progressive; only approximately one half of patients have either complete or partial recovery. The onset of symptoms is generally subacute. Symptoms develop over days to weeks, usually beginning days to weeks after administration of chemotherapy. The histologic findings are identical to those of ara-C–induced myelopathy.

Vinca Alkaloids

Treatment with vinca alkaloids, particularly vincristine, is commonly associated with neurotoxicity.

Peripheral Neuropathy

Peripheral neuropathy is the toxicity associated most frequently with vincristine and correlates with the cumulative dose of the drug.[62-66] Loss of deep tendon reflexes occurs in nearly all patients who receive several vincristine treatments. Distal sensorimotor polyneuropathy develops with continued treatment.[62,64,66] The predominant neurologic finding is loss of pain and temperature sensation in a stocking-and-glove distribution. Motor and vibration/proprioceptive loss usually is milder and occurs later with continued treatment.

The mechanism of toxicity is unknown, but it is probably related to the effects of the vinca alkaloids on microtubules. Vinca-induced disruption of axonal microtubules causes marked disarray of the axonal cytoskeleton and formation of neurofilamentous masses[67-72] and reversible neurofilament-containing crystalloid inclusions.[73] These effects most likely influence axonal transport, which depends on microtubules as the transport mechanism.[74] Patients with underlying neuropathy, such as diabetic neuropathy or Charcot-Marie-Tooth disease, may have severe neuropathy even with low cumulative doses.[75,76] Severe, even life-threatening neuropathy has been reported after administration of as little as 2 mg to patients with Charcot-Marie-Tooth disease (hereditary motor sensory neuropathy type 1), and evidence suggests that patients should be screened before administration of vincristine.[77-79] Previous radiation treatment of peripheral nerves also increases the neurotoxic effects of vincristine.[80]

In addition to peripheral neuropathy, autonomic neuropathy and cranial nerve palsy have been reported. Autonomic neuropathy most commonly manifests as gastrointestinal dysmotility (obstipation or constipation). In severe cases, paralytic ileus and intestinal perforation have resulted.[62,81] Less frequently, orthostatic hypotension develops from autonomic involvement. Vincristine-induced mononeuropathy involving the femoral nerve has been reported. Vincristine can cause cranial nerve palsies, including the optic (II), oculomotor (III), trigeminal, abducens, facial, acoustic, and vagus nerves.[62,64,82,83] In addition, patients occasionally report facial pain with vincristine treatment, possibly a transient effect on the trigeminal nerve or ganglion.[62]

Central Nervous System Effects

Vincristine has been reported to cause encephalopathy, coma, and seizures.[84-88] These effects are rare and reversible. The underlying mechanism is unknown in most cases, although in some cases these neurologic effects have been attributed to vincristine-induced syndrome of inappropriate antidiuretic hormone secretion (SIADH) and hyponatremia.[87,89-92] The mechanism of SIADH is unknown, but serum antidiuretic hormone levels are elevated.

Other Toxicity Associated with Vinca Alkaloids

Quadriplegia with vincristine treatment has been reported, in one case in association with Guillain-Barré syndrome.[93-95] The time of onset of has been variable. In some patients quadriparesis develops soon after vincristine treatment, whereas in others it occurs several weeks after treatment. In most cases, the weakness is partially reversible.[93]

Myopathy has occurred with vincristine therapy.[63,96] There is no known clinical correlate with these results in which pathologic examination of muscle tissue has revealed spheromembranous degeneration.

Cisplatin

Peripheral Neuropathy

The most common neurotoxicity associated with cisplatin is peripheral neuropathy. The neuropathy predominantly involves the large sensory fibers, which mediate vibration and proprioceptive function. Deep tendon reflexes are lost because of toxic effects on the large myelinated sensory fibers, which provide the afferent arm of the reflex arc. Involvement of motor function is generally mild and is seen only in patients with severe sensory neuropathy. Development of neuropathy is dose related. The earliest signs are detected when the cumulative dose exceeds 300 mg/m^2.[97] Schedule of administration may be a significant factor, because patients receiving treatment on five consecutive days have been reported to have a higher incidence of neuropathy than patients treated with a shorter dose schedule but the same cumulative dose.[98-100] Continued treatment with cisplatin in patients with neuropathy can result in severe sensory ataxia, which often impairs ambulation. The neuropathy is partially reversible, and patients with mild impairment are generally more likely to have full recovery.[99] A longitudinal study confirmed there is often a delay in the onset of neuropathy. Eleven percent of patients had neuropathy at the end of treatment, but the incidence had increased to 65% 3 months later. One year later, most of the patients had recovered, only 17% having persistent symptoms.[101]

The pathogenesis of cisplatin-induced neuropathy is unknown. Neuropathologic studies have shown involvement of the large sensory fibers with regions of axonal swelling and myelin breakdown and, in more severe cases, axonal loss.[102] The spinal cord shows almost exclusive involvement of myelinated axons in the dorsal columns, consistent with the clinical features of vibratory and proprioceptive loss.[103] Platinum concentration in peripheral nerve and spinal ganglia was 20 times greater than in brain from patients at autopsy.[101] This finding may explain the predilection of cisplatin for sensory fibers and sparing of the CNS.

Spinal Cord Toxicity

Cisplatin treatment has been associated with the development of Lhermitte's sign, which is an electric shock sensation down the spine or into the extremities with neck flexion.[104,105] The phenomenon is most commonly associated with spinal cord demyelinating lesions in multiple sclerosis. A similar mechanism, cisplatin-induced demyelination, may be the cause in patients with this syndrome. Most patients achieve full recovery, although, like recovery from the cisplatin-induced neuropathy, improvement may take several months.

Other Neurotoxicity Associated with Cisplatin

Other neurotoxicities reported with cisplatin include optic neuropathy, seizures, encephalopathy, and cortical blindness. These complications of treatment are rare. Patients with optic neuropathy may have prolonged vision loss and pallor of the optic disk.[106,107] The reported cases of seizures and cortical blindness have been self-limited, all patients recovering fully.[108-110] The cause of the seizures and cortical blindness from cisplatin treatment is unknown but may be similar to toxicity that occurs with other heavy metals (lead, thallium), although endovascular injury has been proposed as a possible mechanism.[109,111] Many of these patients have white-matter abnormalities on brain MRI consistent with posterior reversible encephalopathy syndrome (see later, Encephalopathy). A syndrome has also been described in which patients experience focal neurologic deficits and seizures after intravenous administration of cisplatin. In these patients, findings at brain MRI were normal. One patient had reoccurrence of encephalopathy with cisplatin rechallenge, and a second patient died of status epilepticus. At autopsy, the brain showed only focal gliosis.[112]

Cisplatin Toxicity Associated with Intra-arterial Administration

Intra-arterial administration of cisplatin causes focal toxicity. Administration into the internal carotid artery can cause severe retinal toxicity.[113,114] Supraophthalmic administration can cause focal areas of brain parenchymal necrosis with resulting seizures and neurologic impairment.[114]

Ototoxicity

Ototoxicity is a dose-related effect of cisplatin. Patients receiving more than 200 mg/m^2 are at high risk of hearing loss.[115] Hearing loss, particularly when it is moderate to severe, often is permanent.[115,116] Results of most studies suggest that patients with underlying hearing loss are at greater risk of functional hearing loss, although a small series found no relation to previous hearing loss.[115,117,118] Additional risk factors include age older than 46 years and previous cranial radiation therapy involving the ears or temporal lobes.[116,117] Patients with normal hearing lose high-frequency hearing first but, with continued treatment, may lose hearing in all frequency ranges.[115] A rapid screening audiogram technique has been developed to monitor patients undergoing cisplatin treatment.[118] Pathologic examination of cochleae from patients with cisplatin-induced ototoxicity reveals extensive loss of the outer hair cells and less effect on the inner hair cells.[115]

Cyclophosphamide

Cyclophosphamide can indirectly cause metabolic encephalopathy and seizures. High-dose cyclophosphamide can lead to SIADH.[119-122] Unrecognized, this syndrome can lead to severe hyponatremia, coma, and seizures. Although not reported in the literature in association with cyclophosphamide-induced SIADH, rapid correction of hyponatremia can result in central pontine myelinolysis, which is irreversible loss of the central pontine pathways.[123] A locked-in syndrome may develop, or a chronic vegetative state can result from central pontine myelinolysis.

Ifosfamide

The most common neurotoxicity associated with ifosfamide is encephalopathy. Severe ifosfamide-induced encephalopathy has been reported in children and adults.[124-128] Neurologic deterioration usually begins within hours of administration of ifosfamide.[124,126,128] Confusion, hallucinations, and aphasia are the most common initial signs. Progression to coma is generally rapid. Some patients also exhibit clinical evidence of seizure activity or myoclonus with intermittent twitching of the extremities.[124,127] Electroencephalography (EEG) shows severe slowing with D activity and can display evidence of seizure activity.[124,127] In most cases, encephalopathy completely resolves over several days after cessation of therapy, although in one study, investigators found persistent mental status changes in some patients 10 weeks after treatment.[129] The incidence of ifosfamide neurotoxicity has been reported to be 5% to 20%. Several risk factors predispose patients to development of neurotoxicity from ifosfamide. These factors include low serum albumin concentration,[128] high serum creatinine concentration, pelvic cancer,[130] and previous treatment with cisplatin.[131] Ifosfamide treatment has been associated with an extrapyramidal syndrome characterized by choreoathetosis, blepharospasm, and opisthotonic posturing.[132] These symptoms resolved over several days.

5-Fluorouracil

Cerebellar Toxicity
5-Fluorouracil (5-FU) causes acute cerebellar dysfunction. Patients experience moderate to severe gait ataxia, scanning speech, appendicular ataxia marked by severe dysmetria, and often nystagmus.[133-136] These neurologic findings resolve completely within several days after completion of therapy. The incidence of cerebellar toxicity has been reported to be 3% to 7% and correlates with dose and the interval between treatments.[137]

Neuropsychiatric Symptoms
Organic brain syndrome has been reported with 5-FU treatment.[138] Confusion and disorientation develop without evidence of cerebellar dysfunction. Retreatment of a patient with 5-FU resulted in a similar episode of mental deterioration. Oculomotor disturbances, specifically vergence disturbances characterized by diplopia when viewing distant objects, were reported in two patients.[139] There also has been a report of a possible association of 5-FU treatment with recurrent acute toxic neuropathy.[140]

Other Neurotoxicity Associated with 5-Fluorouracil Treatment
Several cases have been reported of multifocal inflammatory leukoencephalopathy associated with use of 5-FU and levamisole in adjuvant therapy for colon carcinoma.[141] These patients have a subacute neurologic syndrome characterized by focal neurologic findings and cognitive dysfunction. MRI shows widespread patchy white-matter lesions that enhance with administration of gadolinium (Fig. 61-2). Pathologically these lesions are characterized by an intense inflammatory infiltrate with extensive loss of myelin, but the axons are generally spared. Complete recovery occurs over weeks after cessation of 5-FU and levamisole. The benefit of corticosteroid treatment is uncertain in accelerating recovery. The pathogenesis of this idiosyncratic reaction is unknown, although levamisole can affect blood-brain barrier function, and this effect may be potentiated by 5-FU. Recognition of this treatment-induced leukoencephalopathy can be important, because the clinical presentation and MRI findings can be misinterpreted as brain metastasis.

Fludarabine

Fludarabine can cause somnolence and a mild peripheral neuropathy at low doses.[142] At high doses, white-matter changes, particularly in the occipital lobes and brainstem, have been reported.[143] Encephalopathy and cerebellar signs are common with this leukoencephalopathy. Progressive symptoms, including coma, and death have been reported. Pathologic evaluation has shown necrotic changes in the involved white matter.[143] The risk of development of progressive multifocal leukoencephalopathy, an infection with the JC virus, may be increased with fludarabine treatment. Diagnosis requires biopsy of involved brain or polymerase chain reaction testing of CSF.[144]

Nitrosoureas

Central Nervous System Toxicity
Nitrosoureas, most commonly carmustine (BCNU), can cause encephalopathy characterized by a progressive

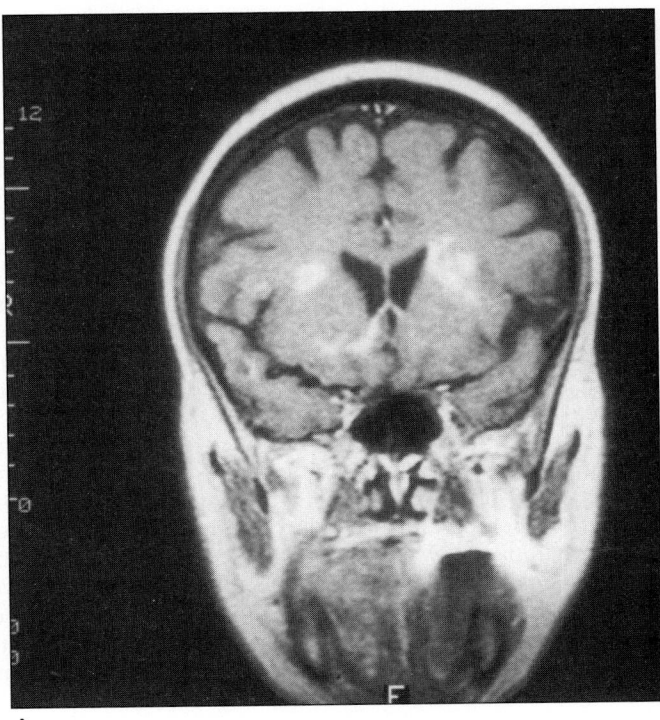

A

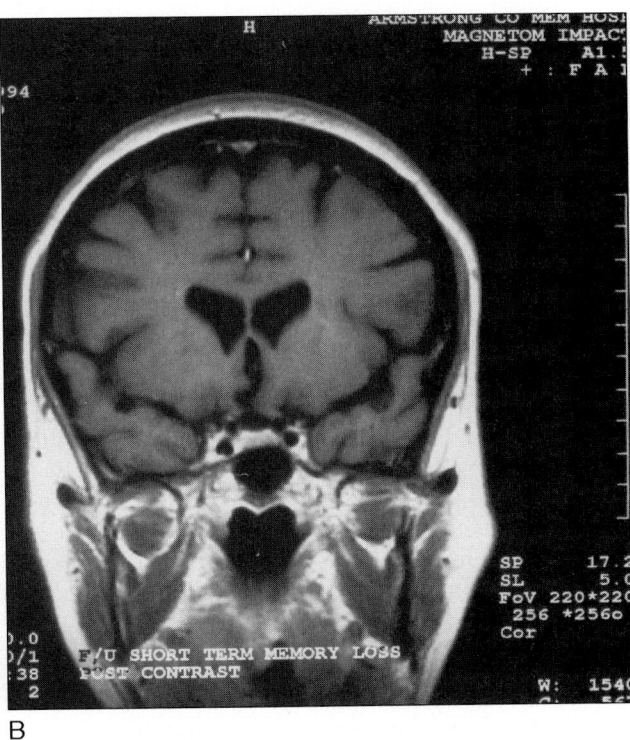

B

Figure 61-2. Levamisole–5-fluorouracil (5-FU) multifocal inflammatory leukoencephalopathy. **A,** A 54-year-old woman had progressive encephalopathy and focal neurologic signs 4 months after beginning adjuvant therapy with levamisole and 5-FU for colon carcinoma. Several white-matter lesions are present, many of which became enhanced with administration of gadolinium-EDTA. **B,** Six months later, the patient had fully recovered. Resolution of the enhanced lesions is evident.

decline in cognitive function, development of seizures and coma, and death.[145-147] This complication is most commonly observed with intracarotid or supraophthalmic arterial delivery of nitrosourea, although a similar syndrome has been reported in patients who receive very high-dose intravenous carmustine treatment.[148] Pathologically the toxicity associated with intra-arterial therapy is characterized by necrosis, regions of demyelination, edema, and axonal loss limited to the region perfused by the intra-arterial therapy. Because the predominant changes have been seen in the white matter, the condition is called leukoencephalopathy, indistinguishable from the changes seen with methotrexate and ara-C treatment. Similar pathologic changes are seen with high-dose intravenous carmustine, but both cerebral hemispheres are involved.[148] In addition, focal brain necrosis has been reported with intra-arterial nitrosourea treatment. This toxicity is thought to be a consequence of drug streaming along the vessel wall, without mixing with arterial blood.[149] This stream of concentrated drug may flow into a small branch of the artery. A small region of brain (or tumor) receives an enormous dose of drug, and focal necrosis results.

A biodegradable polymer containing BCNU has been shown effective in the management of recurrent malignant glioma. The BCNU-impregnated polymer also has been approved for treatment of patients with newly diagnosed glioblastoma. This treatment usually is followed by conventional external beam radiation therapy.[150] This combination may increase the incidence of treatment-associated necrosis. The wafers are placed into the tumor cavity after resection. Results of clinical trials indicate that the local therapy is well tolerated, although an increase in peritumoral edema necessitates a temporary increase in corticosteroid dose, and there are reports of treatment-associated necrosis.[151]

Retinal Toxicity

Retinal toxicity has been reported with intracarotid administration of nitrosoureas, particularly carmustine.[114,152] This retinopathy is painful and often results in permanent vision loss. Infusion above the ophthalmic artery eliminates this toxicity but may increase the likelihood of streaming (see earlier, Central Nervous System Toxicity).

Oxaliplatin

Oxaliplatin is a novel platinum compound that has demonstrated activity in several malignant tumors. Neurotoxicity, particularly peripheral neuropathy, has been dose limiting. Two types of neuropathy have been described. The first is typical, distal sensory neuropathy involving predominantly large fibers, similar to that seen with cisplatin therapy. The second type of neuropathy has been acute toxicity occurring within hours of drug infusion. Patients experience paresthesia and dysesthesia of the hands and feet, jaw tightness, and a sensation of loss of breathing without respiratory distress. The last syndrome has been called *pharyngolaryngodysesthesiea.* The acute neurotoxic syndrome caused by oxaliplatin is reversible. Administration of glutathione has been reported to hasten recovery.[153,154]

Lhermitte's sign and urinary retention have been reported with oxaliplatin therapy. All of the patients who had this syndrome received a cumulative dose of more than 1000 mg, and symptoms resolved within weeks.[155]

Procarbazine

Early reports of procarbazine use describe neurotoxicity, both peripheral and CNS toxicity, as common side effects of treatment.

Peripheral Neuropathy

The peripheral neuropathy described with procarbazine use is most commonly described as paresthesia, often subjective and generally transient. The incidence of paresthesia ranges from 2% to 20%; this variability may be related to dose or treatment schedule.[156-158]

Central Nervous System Toxicity

Signs of CNS depression, ranging from mild drowsiness to profound stupor, have been reported.[156,158] This toxicity worsens with use of phenothiazine to control emesis and may be related to the monoamine oxidase inhibitor qualities of procarbazine. No report has discussed the use of dietary restrictions in patients receiving procarbazine. CNS depression was reported to occur in 14% to 33% of patients in these series.[156-158]

Paclitaxel and Docetaxel

Paclitaxel and docetaxel are novel antineoplastic agents that bind to tubulin and promote formation and stabilization of microtubules.[140,159,160] In phase I and II testing of paclitaxel, myelosuppression was the dose-limiting toxicity. However, since colony-stimulating factors (e.g., granulocyte-macrophage and granulocyte colony-stimulating factors) have become widely available, peripheral neuropathy has become the dose-limiting toxicity.[1,2] The neuropathy is predominantly sensory, particularly affecting small-caliber (pain and temperature) sensory fibers.[161] The effect on motor fibers and large-caliber sensory fibers (vibration and proprioception) is less severe. Nerve conduction studies of large myelinated nerve fibers show evidence of both axonal injury and demyelination.[161] Neuropathy generally occurs at doses greater than 200 mg/m^2, and symptoms develop 1 to 3 days after treatment. Although much of the neurologic dysfunction reverses over several weeks, continued treatment causes progressive neurologic toxicity. The peripheral neuropathy associated with docetaxel appears to be similar to that of paclitaxel in preliminary reports, although in a randomized trial, the incidence and severity were less with docetaxel.[162,163]

Laboratory models used in evaluation of paclitaxel neuropathy have demonstrated that local administration of paclitaxel causes large regional accumulation of microtubules and inhibition of anterograde slow transport of microtubules.[164-167] Furthermore, paclitaxel administration inhibits nerve regeneration after experimental crush injury.[168] Studies with dorsal root ganglia explants have shown similar microtubule accumulations in the axons.[169,170] Toxic effects on Schwann cells have been found in both animal and tissue culture models.[141,171,172] Although it has not been elucidated, the precise mechanism of paclitaxel neurotoxicity is likely to be directly related to microtubule aggregation that disrupts the normal axonal cytoskeleton.[165-167,170,171] Treatment with nerve growth factor in both an animal model and tissue culture significantly decreased the neurotoxic effects of paclitaxel.[173,174]

Transient encephalopathy has been reported to occur within hours of administration of standard doses of paclitaxel. All patients had undergone previous brain radiation therapy, and all recovered within hours.[175] Acute encephalopathy was been reported to occur in six patients receiving a very high intravenous dose of paclitaxel (>600 mg/m^2). Encephalopathy developed between 7 and 23 days after treatment. Three patients recovered; the other 3 patients died of progressive coma. Autopsy revealed generalized white-matter atrophy.[176]

Tamoxifen

Tamoxifen can cause reversible retinal dysfunction at the conventional antiestrogen doses used for breast cancer therapy.[177-179] At higher doses, reversible encephalopathy with delusions, somnolence, and cerebellar dysfunction has been reported.[180-182]

BIOLOGIC RESPONSE MODIFIERS

Interleukin-2

Central Nervous System Toxicity

The vascular leak associated with intravenous interleukin-2 (IL-2) administration can result in encephalopathy and coma.[183] A high percentage of patients receiving both systemic IL-2 and lymphocyte-activated killer cells experience encephalopathy or a neuropsychiatric syndrome.[183] In most cases, severe but reversible cognitive impairment occurs. In the presence of an intracranial mass lesion, the increase in brain edema leads to an asymmetric shift in the brain, resulting in herniation. There also has been a single case report of development of multifocal white-matter lesions associated with intravenous administration of IL-2. The lesions resolved completely over several months.[184] Another case report described fatal leuko-encephalopathy associated with IL-2 treatment.[185]

Other Toxicity Associated with Interleukin-2 Treatment

The cases of five patients have been reported in which neuro-ophthalmic complications developed that were temporally associated with intravenous IL-2 treatment.[186,187] Transient scotomata, diplopia, amaurosis fugax, and visual-field cuts developed.

Interferons

Systemic administration of interferon affects both the central and peripheral nervous systems.

Central Nervous System Toxicity

Confusion, lethargy, mood changes, and loss of cognitive function are the most common CNS effects associated with use of interferons.[188-190] Encephalopathy, with perseveration and aphasia, also has been reported,[189] as has a parkinsonian syndrome with bradykinesia, masked facies, and micrographia.[191] In addition, major depression has occurred with use of interferon α (IFN-α).[192] The neurologic effects of interferon are dose related, but they are more severe in patients with underlying neurologic abnormalities.[193] Although the neurotoxic effects of interferon therapy usually resolve completely within a few weeks, some patients may have persistent behavioral changes.[188] Intraventricular administration of IFN-α caused severe neurologic toxicity in one study. Effects ranged from headache and confusion to coma. Additional side effects of intraventricular administration included parkinsonism, hearing loss, and seizures.[194]

Peripheral Nervous System Toxicity

Mild peripheral neuropathy manifesting as paresthesia has been reported with interferon use,[189] as has a case of brachial neuritis in a patient with underlying neuropathy.[195]

Metronidazole

Metronidazole is a nitroimidazole compound often used as an antimicrobial agent. Its chemical derivatives (e.g., misonidazole, etanidazole) are used in cancer treatment as radiosensitizers. The neurologic side effects associated with these agents include neuropathy, encephalopathy, cerebellar dysfunction, and seizures.[196-199] These neurotoxic effects are dose related, and the peripheral neuropathy can be the dose-limiting toxicity.[200] The neurologic side effects of metronidazole have been reversible, although the neuropathy may take several months to resolve.

Suramin

Suramin is an experimental agent that has been tested in therapy for a variety of cancers, including prostate cancer and glioma. The dose-limiting toxicity of suramin is peripheral neuropathy, which has been found to be concentration dependent. In one study investigators found a high incidence of neuropathy in patients with peak plasma levels greater than 350 µg/mL. Neuropathy can be severe, mimicking the acute flaccid paralysis that occurs with Guillain-Barré syndrome.[201,202]

Thalidomide

Thalidomide has both immunomodulatory and anti-angiogenic properties, has shown significant activity in multiple myeloma, and is being evaluated in the management of several other cancers.[203] Somnolence, the predominant side effect, is dose related, and the drug can be titrated in most patients to a level of tolerance. Peripheral neuropathy is treatment limiting. The neuropathy has been characterized as sensory-motor axonal polyneuropathy manifesting as painful paresthesia or numbness.[204] Severity of symptoms correlates with cumulative dose. Nerve biopsies reveal distal axonal degeneration and demyelination. A longitudinal study in patients with dermatologic disease confirmed the high incidence of neuropathy (25% in this study) and the association with daily dosing.[205]

RADIATION NEUROTOXICITY

Radiation neurotoxicity is becoming an increasingly important and recognized complication of cancer therapy. New therapeutic strategies for systemic cancer and for CNS metastasis have improved survival, uncovering a greater incidence of late, chronic toxicity from radiation and combined chemoradiotherapy treatments. Advances in technology, such as radiosurgery and brachytherapy, allow local dose intensification of radiation treatment. Furthermore, advances in development of radiosensitizers will increase the effects of radiation therapy on tumor and surrounding normal tissue.

Central Nervous System Effects

Cranial radiation therapy can cause acute, subacute, and chronic neurotoxicity. Volume of brain treated, total dose, and dose fraction are the most important determinants of toxicity, although there appears to be some variation in patient susceptibility.

Acute Toxicity

Acute toxicity manifests as rapid onset of alteration in level of consciousness. This disorder generally occurs within weeks of initiation of cranial radiation therapy.[206] Acute toxicity is most common in patients receiving whole-brain radiation therapy. The pathogenesis is unknown, and most patients have complete recovery of neurologic function.

Early-Delayed Toxicity

Early-delayed toxicity is noticed weeks to 3 months after completion of radiation treatment.[207] Most commonly, patients have drowsiness, nausea, headaches, ataxia, and worsening of underlying neurologic dysfunction. Complete resolution is expected, although rare patients have an idiosyncratic reaction with widespread brain necrosis.[208] The pathogenesis of early-delayed toxicity is unknown, but the reaction has been speculated to be related to reversible demyelination. CT reveals decreased attenuation in the cerebral white matter; MRI reveals increased signal intensity in white matter on T_2-weighted images.

Chronic, Late Radiation Injury

Chronic, late radiation injury usually appears 9 months to 2 years after completion of radiation treatment, although some patients have experienced symptoms 10 years after treatment.[208,209] Patients have focal areas of radiation necrosis or evidence of diffuse radiation injury. The incidence of each depends on the dose of treatment, fractionation schedule, and area of treatment.[210,211] Focal necrosis often manifests as focal neurologic deficits, such as hemiparesis or aphasia. Global signs such as obtundation can occur when the necrotic area causes increased intracranial pressure and herniation. Similarly, focal necrotic regions can cause seizures. Pathologic examination of the necrotic region reveals vascular injury to the small arteries and arterioles and evidence of coagulative necrosis with destruction of all elements of the nervous tissue.[212] Treatment is directed at decreasing edema and mass effect. Patients generally respond to corticosteroids.[213] Surgical resection, if feasible, can be curative.

Diffuse Injury

Diffuse injury manifests as global neurologic dysfunction, with personality change, confusion, and lethargy, and can progress to dementia, obtundation, or coma.[207,211] Diffuse white-matter changes are found on CT or MRI, manifesting as low attenuation on CT scans and high signal intensity in the periventricular and subcortical white matter on T_2-weighted and proton density MR images.[214-216] Mass effect and focal neurologic signs are not common, although late in the course, seizures and motor dysfunction can occur. The main risk factors for diffuse injury include the volume of brain treated, concurrent or adjuvant chemotherapy treatment of the CNS, and short-course, high-dose-fraction treatment. The incidence is difficult to determine, but reports have shown neurologic and imaging changes in 32% to 50% of patients treated.[214-216]

The pathogenesis of diffuse radiation injury is not known, although distinctive neuropathologic changes have been described. The most prominent pathologic finding is vascular changes in the small arteries and arterioles. Hyalinization of the vessel walls with occlusion is common.[211,217] In addition, areas of necrosis, gliosis, and demyelination are found. There is no established treatment. Corticosteroids may provide transient relief of associated edema but do not alter the course of the syndrome.

Necrotizing Leukoencephalopathy

Necrotizing leukoencephalopathy is the most severe neurologic toxicity associated with radiation therapy. It is most common when CNS-directed chemotherapy is combined with radiation therapy. This syndrome is described earlier, in the discussion of methotrexate-associated toxicity. The incidence of leukoencephalopathy is much greater in patients who receive chemotherapy after cranial radiation therapy than in patients receiving either treatment alone or those receiving chemotherapy before the initiation of radiation.[218,219]

Mineralizing angiopathy has occurred in pediatric patients treated with both intrathecal methotrexate and radiation therapy.[218] The changes are frequently diagnosed as dystrophic calcifications during neuroradiologic examinations. Pathologic analysis reveals deposits of calcium in small blood vessels, often with surrounding regions of necrotic brain. The clinical significance of these changes is uncertain.

Cranial radiation therapy has been associated with a wide spectrum of endocrinologic effects.[220] Most are attributed to damage to the hypothalamic-pituitary axis. These effects are generally dose dependent and may manifest several years after completion of the radiation treatment. Results of several studies have suggested there is differing vulnerability of the various endocrine loops.[221] Growth hormone deficiency and stimulation of precocious puberty have occurred at doses as low as 18 Gy.[222] Deficiency of gonadotropins, thyroid-stimulating hormone, and corticotropin usually are found only when the hypothalamic-pituitary axis receives more than 40 Gy.[223] Similarly, hyperprolactinemia occurs most often in young women receiving more than 40 Gy of radiation therapy. Careful long-term monitoring of these patients is critical.[224] Appropriate replacement therapy or prolactin suppression treatment should prevent sequelae.

Radiation Myelopathy

Several distinct syndromes have resulted from the effects of radiation injury to the spinal cord: an acute syndrome manifesting as paraplegia or quadriplegia; early transient myelopathy; delayed progressive myelopathy; and an anterior horn, lower motor neuron syndrome.

The acute syndrome is rare with current dosing schedules. Reports state that weakness evolves over a few hours or days.[225] The syndrome is most likely caused by acute necrotizing radiation injury due to rapidity of onset and failure of neurologic recovery.

The early transient form appears 6 to 12 weeks after treatment.[226] Most patients have Lhermitte's sign—electrical shock sensation down the spine with neck flexion. No neurologic deficits are found, and the symptoms resolve spontaneously over several weeks. Transient demyelination is hypothesized to be the cause of the symptoms.

Delayed progressive radiation myelopathy is the most common radiation-induced spinal cord disorder, although it is relatively rare. Symptoms generally develop 6 months to 1 year after completion of radiation therapy, although some data suggest that the latent period may be as long as 18 months to 2 years.[227] The signs may vary from patient to patient. Some patients have monoplegia, others paraplegia or quadriplegia. Sensory symptoms are generally more severe than motor symptoms. Some patients have Brown-Sequard syndrome. Progression may take several years.[225] The pathogenesis is thought to be similar to that of delayed neurotoxicity after cranial radiation therapy (see earlier).[225,226] Pathologic examination reveals rarefaction of spinal cord white matter with small areas of necrosis. Degeneration of myelin sheaths and loss of oligodendrocytes have been noted. Other causes of spinal cord dysfunction need to be excluded, including intramedullary tumor or infection, multiple sclerosis, vitamin B_{12} deficiency, sarcoidosis, and Lyme disease. There is no treatment, and most patients experience progressive neurologic dysfunction over months to years.

Lower motor neuron syndrome occurs after spinal cord radiation therapy. Patients have pure motor signs of weakness, atrophy, and fasciculations.[225] The syndrome manifests itself 3 months to 2 years after radiation treatment and is similar to polio. The pathogenesis is unknown. Hypotheses include loss of anterior horn cell neurons or radiation-induced injury to motor nerve roots. No treatment except supportive care exists.

Peripheral Nerve Toxicity

Peripheral nerves are relatively resistant to the effects of radiation therapy. Early effects, developing within 2 days of a single large-fraction treatment in an experimental animal system, include changes in vascular permeability of the nerve, changes in bioelectrical activity, and abnormal microtubule assembly in the axon.[228] Late changes include fibrosis in the nerve sheath and angiopathic changes in the small arterioles providing the vascular supply to the nerve.[229] Large (>25 Gy) single doses or extended fractionated treatment to a very high total dose (>80 Gy) are thought to be necessary for injury to the peripheral nerve. Similar changes have been found for some cranial nerves.

Brachial and lumbar plexopathy warrant a separate discussion. These syndromes result from radiation injury to the nerve fibers in the plexus. Brachial plexopathy is most common, caused by axillary radiation therapy for breast cancer.[230] Lumbar plexopathy is more commonly associated with pelvic external-beam radiation therapy, although local radioactive seed implantation (brachytherapy) may result in local nerve damage.[228]

The diagnosis of radiation plexopathy can be difficult and requires excluding tumor infiltration as the cause of the symptoms. This process is most difficult with brachial plexus dysfunction and in patients with apical lung cancer or metastatic breast cancer. The distinguishing features in comparing radiation with tumor brachial plexopathy have been described extensively.[230] None of the criteria are absolute, although tumor infiltration is more likely to be painful and involve the lower nerve roots (C7–T1) than is radiation injury, which is less likely to cause severe pain and generally involves higher roots (C5–C6). Acute reversible radiation injury to the brachial plexus has been described. This condition is often painful, although the pain is generally mild. Patients experience weakness and atrophy in a C6–T1 distribution. Spontaneous recovery is typical.

Radiation has been reported to accelerate vascular injury, causing segmental obstruction of the subclavian artery.[231] This condition usually is painless. The motor and sensory loss evolve quickly without subsequent progression or improvement.

Lumbosacral plexopathy is less common than radiation-related brachial plexopathy.[232] Symptoms usually occur at least 1 year after radiation treatment. Pain is usual and mild. The pathogenesis is uncertain, although fibrosis causing nerve compression and ischemia is a likely cause. The diagnosis of radiation-related lumbosacral plexopathy is made by excluding tumor infiltration. Imaging (MRI or CT) often is useful, although in select cases, surgical exploration is indicated.

Muscle Injury from Radiation Treatment

Muscle is thought to be relatively resistant to the effects of radiation therapy, although results of several studies have suggested that at higher doses (>50 Gy) significant late toxicity may occur.[229] Early effects are uncommon, symptoms are generally found after 1 year, and the onset of changes has been reported as late as 10 years after radiation therapy. Symptoms include muscle contractures, loss of function, pain, extremity edema, and pathologic fractures. The synergy of the toxic effects with chemotherapy is uncertain, although most patients have received both modalities of treatment.[229] No treatment other than conservative measures including physical therapy exists.

DIFFERENTIAL DIAGNOSIS

Dementia and Encephalopathy

Acute Encephalopathy

A common neurologic problem in patients with cancer is acute encephalopathy.[233] The differential diagnosis is extensive. Most commonly, however, acute encephalopathy is caused by toxic or metabolic derangement. Frequent causes include narcotic effects, electrolyte abnormalities, hypoxia, and renal or hepatic dysfunction. Meningeal carcinomatosis frequently manifests as mental status changes due to increased intracranial pressure, seizures, or infiltration of the cortex through the Virchow-Robin spaces surrounding surface blood vessels. Likewise, brain metastasis can cause an acute change in mental status when a sudden increase in tumor size (often hemorrhage) results in a rapid change in intracranial pressure or when tumor-induced seizures occur. A paraneoplastic syn-drome, limbic encephalitis, can manifest as a progressive dementia, which often is subacute. This paraneoplastic syndrome is most frequently associated with small cell lung cancer, but it has been described in association with other tumors. Patients often have serum anti-Hu antibodies, also found in paraneoplastic sensory neuropathy.[234-236]

Cancer treatment can directly or indirectly cause acute encephalopathy. High doses of intravenous methotrexate or ara-C can cause reversible encephalopathy, often accompanied by lethargy.[5,13,35] Results of studies with animals and with patients in which positron emission tomography was used after high-dose methotrexate showed temporary reduction in brain metabolic activity in both glucose utilization and protein synthesis.[36,237] Folinic acid (leucovorin) administration improved metabolic activity in laboratory studies.[37] Other agents known to cause encephalopathy include vincristine, ifosfamide, procarbazine, fludarabine, paclitaxel, and L-asparaginase. The immunostimulant levamisole causes reversible encephalopathy and has been associated with a demyelinating condition known as *multifocal inflammatory leukoencephalopathy*.[141] The radiation sensitizers metronidazole and misonidazole also can produce encephalopathy.[196-199] The hormonal agent tamoxifen has been reported to cause encephalopathy at high doses.

Biologic response modifiers such as the interferons and interleukins commonly cause reversible encephalopathy, although permanent neurologic sequelae may result from prolonged use of interferon.[188,189] Radiation therapy can cause an acute syndrome that manifests as lethargy that is generally reversible.

Posterior reversible encephalopathy syndrome (PRES) has been seen most frequently with use of the immuno-modulators cyclosporine and tacrolimus, but cisplatin, gemcitabine, and combination chemotherapy regimens also have been associated with the syndrome. The clinical manifestations are encephalopathy, cortical blindness, and variable loss of other higher cortical functions, such as aphasia and apraxia. Brain CT and MRI findings are patchy white-matter changes and are characteristic (Fig. 61-3). The pathogenesis of the syndrome is unknown, although hypertension and hypomagnesemia have been associated. Full recovery has occurred with cessation of treatment or adjustment of the dose of the immunosuppressant.[238-242]

Many chemotherapeutic agents provoke a change in mental status by causing secondary metabolic derangement. Cyclophosphamide and vincristine can stimulate SIADH.[89,90,120,121] The resulting hyponatremia can lead to seizures and encephalopathy. Hyponatremia secondary to cisplatin-induced salt wasting nephropathy can cause the same neurologic problems. Treatment with L-asparaginase, corticosteroids, and streptozocin can lead to glucose intolerance. Left untreated, this condition can result in nonketotic hyperosmolar coma. Many chemotherapeutic agents can cause hepatic and renal dysfunction with consequent development of secondary neurologic symptoms.

Chronic Encephalopathy and Dementia

Dementia, or chronic progressive loss of cognitive function, is most commonly associated with treatment directed at the CNS. Leukoencephalopathy, characterized histologically by white-matter changes consisting of axonal swelling and loss with regions of demyelination, is the classic chronic or late neurotoxic syndrome.[4,6] Cognitive changes are first noticed 6 months to 2 years after completion of treatment and are often progressive, leading to profound dementia, coma, or death.[4-6,8,43] Intrathecal chemotherapy with methotrexate, ara-C, or

thiotepa is most closely associated with leukoencephalopathy, although a similar syndrome occurs with high-dose intravenous methotrexate and ara-C and with intra-arterial chemotherapy (BCNU, cisplatin).[243,244] Previous treatment with cranial radiation therapy significantly increases the risk of leukoencephalopathy.[5,51] Cranial radiation therapy alone can cause leukoencephalopathy, although the incidence increases markedly when radiation is combined with chemotherapy. Other agents, such as ifosfamide, can cause prolonged encephalopathy and are associated with acute toxicity.[129]

Diagnostic Evaluation

A thorough search for a treatable underlying cause of encephalopathy should be undertaken in all cases. The diagnosis of chemotherapy-induced encephalopathy is made by excluding other causes. The order of diagnostic tests is based on findings on physical and neurologic evaluation. Patients with focal neurologic findings need early imaging studies (CT or MRI), although certain metabolic disorders (e.g., hypoglycemia) can manifest as focal neurologic deficits. A metabolic evaluation, including measurement of electrolytes, renal and liver function tests, measurement of oxygenation, serum calcium, serum magnesium, and serum ammonia, and possibly thyroid and adrenal function testing, should be performed for most patients. Careful review of prescribed and over-the-counter medications may provide critical information. In some cases, blood and urine toxicology screening may be necessary. EEG often is helpful in directing the evaluation by indicating the presence of structural abnormalities (periodic localizing epileptiform discharges or focal slowing) or may indicate a global metabolic process (e.g., diffuse slowing with D waves or triphasic waves in hepatic encephalopathy). Patients in subclinical status epilepticus may have encephalopathy; in these cases, the EEG findings are diagnostic. Lumbar puncture often is needed to exclude infectious or neoplastic meningitis. In most cases, head MRI or CT should be performed before lumbar puncture to look for a mass lesion in the brain that would make lumbar puncture unsafe. The search for the underlying cause often is revealing. One group of investigators reported uncovering the cause of encephalopathy in 31 of 37 patients.[233]

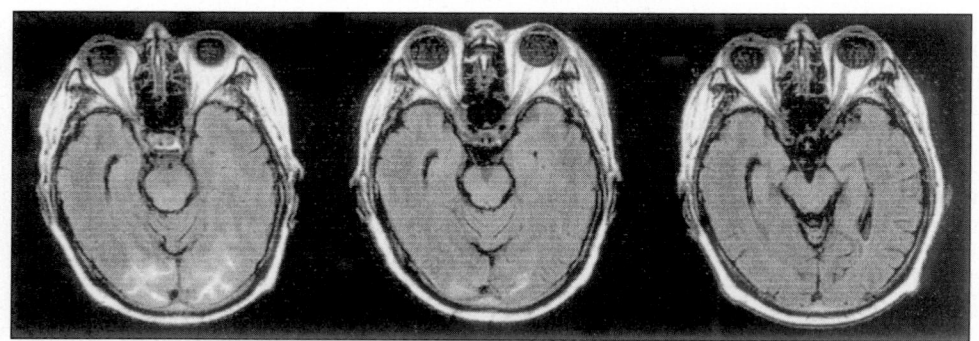

June 4, 2002   July 5, 2002   October 10, 2002

Figure 61-3. Posterior reversible encephalopathy syndrome. A 47-year-old man with acute monocytic leukemia who had undergone allogeneic bone marrow transplantation, had headache, nausea, and vomiting. **A,** Magnetic resonance fast fluid attenuated inversion recovery (FLAIR) images show changes consistent with the syndrome. **B** and **C,** Symptoms resolved within days of cessation of tacrolimus treatment. Repeated magnetic resonance images show resolution of the posterior abnormalities.

Seizures

Clinical Manifestations and Differential Diagnosis

The differential diagnosis of the causal factors of seizures in cancer patients is extensive. It can be broadly classified into toxic/metabolic and structural causes. Metabolic factors include hepatic and renal failure resulting from tumor growth or treatment toxicity, electrolyte abnormalities such as hypercalcemia from bone destruction or parathyroid hormone effect, hypomagnesemia from chemotherapy (cisplatin) or excessive vomiting, hyponatremia from SIADH or salt-wasting nephropathy (cisplatin), hypoxia, hyperglycemia from pancreatic failure (streptozocin), or glucose intolerance (corticosteroids). Several chemotherapeutic agents are known to be a direct cause of seizures (Table 61-1).

Structural causes of seizures include brain metastasis, dural metastasis, and meningeal carcinoma. Ischemic and hemorrhagic vascular events also provoke seizures. A tumor-induced hypercoagulable state may greatly increase risk of stroke or venous sinus thrombosis.[245] A similar hypercoagulable state can be seen with L-asparaginase treatment. The paraneoplastic syndrome marantic endocarditis often results in cerebrovascular events, as can infectious endocarditis, a potential complication of treatment-induced neutropenia.[191] Cisplatin can cause vasospasm of the intracranial vessels, producing a stroke.[246] Furthermore, immunocompromised patients are at greater risk of CNS infection (including bacterial and fungal meningitis), brain abscess, and viral encephalitis (including progressive multifocal leukoencephalopathy).

Diagnostic Evaluation

The type of seizure dictates the initial evaluation. Focal seizures are more commonly associated with structural brain lesions, although metabolic disorders can precipitate focal seizures if there is an underlying structural problem. Generalized seizures may be the consequence of structural or metabolic processes or both.

The diagnostic evaluation generally involves a metabolic evaluation similar to that described for encephalopathy. Electrolyte imbalances, such as hyponatremia, hypomagnesemia, hypocalcemia or hypercalcemia, hyperglycemia, and hyperphosphatemia, are possible metabolic causes. Similarly, hepatic and renal dysfunction increase the likelihood of seizures, particularly in a patient with an underlying structural brain lesion. Most cancer patients who experience a seizure need an imaging study of the brain (CT or MRI). These studies should be performed both with and without contrast material. EEG may be helpful in determining whether there is ongoing seizure activity, in confirming the diagnosis of seizure if the event was not witnessed or not accompanied by tonic-clonic activity, or possibly localizing a focal lesion or process. For example, herpes encephalitis often has bitemporal periodic localizing epileptiform discharges, even before abnormalities are seen on MR images. Lumbar puncture may be needed to evaluate for infectious and neoplastic meningitis. Lumbar puncture should be performed after brain imaging, except when there is concern regarding bacterial meningitis and obtaining the scan will delay lumbar puncture and administration of antibiotic therapy.

The diagnosis of chemotherapy-induced seizures is made after other causes are excluded. For most chemotherapeutic agents, seizures develop acutely, either during or immediately after treatment. Seizures often are accompanied by encephalopathy. In most instances, the prognosis for recovery from the acute development is good. Unfortunately, when seizures develop as a component of chronic or delayed neurotoxicity (leukoencephalopathy), the prognosis is poor, and neurologic dysfunction often progresses. The seizures are a manifestation of widespread brain destruction.

Cerebellar Dysfunction

Clinical Manifestations and Differential Diagnosis

Cerebellar dysfunction in cancer patients occurs most commonly with metastatic spread to the cerebellum or brainstem. Meningeal carcinoma occasionally causes cerebellar signs by infiltrating cerebellar pathways. Structural cerebellar lesions often show asymmetric dysfunction, which can be useful in differentiating this condition from drug-induced cerebellar toxicity. Paraneoplastic cerebellar degeneration is being recognized with increasing frequency. This syndrome is characterized by subacute progressive loss of cerebellar function.[235,247,248] Patients usually have symmetric loss of all cerebellar function and exhibit appendicular and truncal ataxia, nystagmus, and scanning speech. This paraneoplastic syndrome occurs most commonly with lung cancer but also has been associated with gynecologic cancers and Hodgkin's disease. Many patients have antibodies in the serum, designated anti-Yo, that bind to cerebellar tissue, specifically Purkinje cells, and cross-react with tumor tissue.[247]

TABLE 61-1

Chemotherapeutic Agents That Cause Seizures

AGENT	ROUTE OF ADMINISTRATION	COMMENT
L-Asparaginase	Intravenous	Associated with cerebrovascular events
Busulfan	Oral	Bone marrow transplant preparative regimen
Cisplatin	Intravenous	Rare; may be associated with cortical blindness, posterior reversible encephalopathy syndrome
Cytosine arabinoside	High-dose intravenous (acute)	Late with leukoencephalopathy
Ifosfamide	Intravenous	Associated with encephalopathy
Methotrexate	High-dose intravenous (acute)	Late with leukoencephalopathy
Metronidazole	Intravenous, oral	
Nitrosoureas	Intracarotid or supraophthalmic	Often associated with focal brain necrosis
Vincristine	Intravenous	

5-FU and ara-C can cause cerebellar toxicity from specific irreversible damage to the cerebellar Purkinje cells. The result is truncal ataxia, unsteady gait, dysarthria, and nystagmus.[12-15,133-136] The dysfunction usually is symmetrical. MRI findings immediately after chemotherapy are normal, but cerebellar atrophy often is detected at MRI months later.

Diagnostic Evaluation

Patients with cerebellar dysfunction need MRI with and without gadolinium enhancement in an evaluation for metastatic lesions. In addition, the MRI findings may suggest the presence of meningeal carcinoma if there is enhancement in the subarachnoid space. Patients with no evidence of brain metastasis need lumbar puncture in an evaluation for meningeal carcinoma. Examination for the presence of serum anti-Yo antibodies should be performed, particularly for patients who have malignant lesions associated with this paraneoplastic syndrome.

In patients with only appendicular ataxia, the possibility that sensory ataxia is present must be examined. The presence of sensory ataxia suggests the presence of severe sensory neuropathy, such as paraneoplastic sensory neuronopathy, dorsal column dysfunction from a structural lesion (e.g., epidural cord compression), or metabolic abnormality (e.g., vitamin B_{12} deficiency).

Cranial Neuropathy

Clinical Manifestations and Differential Diagnosis

The presence of cranial neuropathy in cancer patients most commonly indicates the presence of meningeal carcinoma, tumor involvement of the bones of the cranial base with encroachment of neural foramina, or rarely, brainstem metastasis.[249] Chemotherapy-induced cranial neuropathy is rare. Vincristine can cause cranial nerve palsy; extraocular eye movement abnormalities are most common.[62,64,82,83] Intraventricular administration of drugs and of biologic response–modifying agents can cause transient cranial nerve palsy, often due to abnormalities in CSF circulation.[250]

Clinical Manifestations and Differential Diagnosis

In both meningeal carcinoma and drug-induced cranial nerve palsy, the seventh (facial) cranial nerve is most commonly affected. Unfortunately, there is little to differentiate the clinical manifestations of drug-induced nerve palsy from those of meningeal carcinoma. Both conditions can involve several cranial nerves, be indolent in onset, and demonstrate spontaneous resolution. Therefore examination of the CSF is critical in the care of these patients. In addition to meningeal carcinoma, tumor encroachment on neural foramina at the skull base from bone metastasis can cause cranial nerve palsy, as can small intraparenchymal lesions (tumor, infarct, or hemorrhage), although such lesions are rare.

Diagnostic Evaluation

In the care of patients with cranial nerve palsy, several examinations of the CSF often are needed to determine whether tumor cells are present. Evaluation of the bones of the skull base with thin-section CT helps determine the presence of metastatic bone lesions. MRI of the brainstem is performed to evaluate for intraparenchymal lesions, although in most cases, other brainstem signs are present, in which case, this test should be part of the initial evaluation.

Optic Neuropathy and Ocular Toxicity

Clinical Manifestations and Differential Diagnosis

Optic neuropathy can be seen in patients with meningeal carcinoma, lymphoma, or leukemia with infiltration of the optic nerve.[251,252] In addition, compression from cranial base tumors can cause similar loss of vision. Optic neuritis, characterized by unilateral or bilateral loss of vision, has been reported as a rare paraneoplastic syndrome associated with small cell lung cancer.[253] Loss of vision often is accompanied by photosensitivity and papilledema. Antiretinal antibodies have been found in the serum of these patients. Retinopathy is most commonly associated with intracarotid administration of nitrosoureas and cisplatin.[113,114,151,152] High concentrations of drug flow into the ophthalmic artery, which supplies the retina, causing severe pain and often complete loss of vision. Newer techniques, allowing administration above the ophthalmic artery, have eliminated this local toxicity.

Intravenous cisplatin administration has been associated with optic disk swelling and optic neuropathy.[106,107] This reaction is idiosyncratic, and the mechanism is unknown.

Diagnostic Evaluation

Chemotherapy-induced retinopathy from intra-arterial administration occurs soon after treatment and is rarely difficult to diagnose. Optic neuropathy from cisplatin is more indolent, and other causes must be considered, particularly meningeal carcinoma. Other toxins, such as isoniazid, chlorpropamide, and ethambutol, also must be considered, as must paraneoplastic optic neuropathy. Optic nerve tumors and frontal lobe mass lesions can cause optic atrophy, although they are uncommon causes of isolated optic atrophy. MRI or CT may be helpful.

Spinal Cord Toxicity

Clinical Manifestations and Differential Diagnosis

The most common cause of spinal cord dysfunction in patients is epidural cord compression, either from direct extension of bone metastasis or from paravertebral spread through the intervertebral foramina. Intramedullary tumor and extramedullary intradural tumors can have myelopathic manifestations.[254] Similarly, epidural abscess and hematoma can be clinically indistinguishable from epidural tumor. Encephalomyelitis is a frequently described paraneoplastic syndrome associated with several types of tumors, particularly small cell lung cancer.[255] A rare paraneoplastic myelopathy has been described with lung cancer, renal cell carcinoma, and Hodgkin's disease. This syndrome is characterized by subacute progression of spinal cord dysfunction, usually in the thoracic region, although damage occasionally occurs at several levels. Pathologic examination reveals segmental necrosis.

Lumbar intrathecal administration of methotrexate and ara-C can causes focal myelopathy.[19-25] Symptoms appear hours to days after treatment. Symptoms associated with this myelopathy include sensory loss, upper and lower motor neuron dysfunction, radiating pain (similar to Lhermitte's syndrome), and bowel and bladder incontinence. The myelopathy may be transient or progressive; complete irreversible paraplegia is usually seen with progressive dysfunction. Myelopathy also has been reported with spinal radiation therapy. A rare, acute syndrome develops over days. The more common chronic myelopathy with radiation therapy develops months after completion of treatment.

Diagnostic Evaluation

The diagnostic evaluation of patients with spinal cord dysfunction is directed by findings at physical examination and history acquisition. Rapid progression of symptoms suggests the presence of a rapidly growing tumor causing cord compression, epidural hematoma, or abscess. This finding warrants emergency evaluation with either MRI or myelography. Most studies support the use of high-dose steroids at presentation, with a tapering schedule dependent on the radiographic findings. Early loss of bowel and bladder function or a suspended sensory level suggests the presence of an intramedullary lesion. Gadolinium-enhanced MRI is the study of choice.

Chemotherapy myelopathy may show edema on MRI and elevated myelin basic protein levels in CSF. The diagnosis of chemotherapy myelopathy is often made on the basis of temporal association with intrathecal treatment and absence of other causes. Carcinomatous meningitis can mimic spinal cord compression and requires CSF examination for diagnosis.

Peripheral Neuropathy

Clinical Manifestations and Differential Diagnosis

Peripheral neuropathy is a common paraneoplastic syndrome. Mild sensorimotor neuropathy is the most common neuropathy in patients with cancer.[256] The cause is unknown, but the condition is a distinct entity, separate from the diffuse weakness associated with cachexia. Rare pure motor and pure sensory paraneoplastic neuropathies have also been described. Sensory neuronopathy, most common with small cell lung cancer, causes severe sensory loss.[257,258] The intense inflammatory reaction and neuronal destruction in the dorsal root ganglia have led to the term *dorsal root ganglionitis*. Some patients have anti-Hu antibodies in serum.[235,258] Motor neuronopathy manifests as isolated lower motor neuron loss.[259] This syndrome has been found in both Hodgkin's and non-Hodgkin's lymphoma patients. The pathogenesis of this pure motor syndrome is unknown. Other causes of neuropathy that should be considered are diabetes, thyroid dysfunction, vitamin B_{12} deficiency, and alcoholic neuropathy.

TABLE 61-2

Agents That Cause Peripheral Neuropathy

AGENT	COMMENT
Cisplatin	Large sensory fiber (vibration, proprioception); dose and cumulative dose-related; dose-limiting
Cytosine arabinoside	Rare, symmetric sensorimotor polyneuropathy
Interferons	Transient paresthesia
Misonidazole, metronidazole	Sensorimotor polyneuropathy; dose-limiting
Oxaliplatin	Large sensory fiber (vibration, proprioception); dose and cumulative dose-related; dose-limiting; acute hyperexcitability syndrome
Paclitaxel, docetaxel	Dose-related sensorimotor; dose-limiting
Procarbazine	Transient paresthesia
Suramin	Incidence and severity of neuropathy related to peak plasma levels of suramin (>350 µg/mL highest risk)
Thalidomide	Sensory-motor axonal polyneuropathy; incidence related to duration and dose of treatment
Vincristine	Frequent; dose-related, autonomic, and sensorimotor; exacerbated in patients with underlying neuropathy; dose-limiting

Several cancer chemotherapeutic agents cause peripheral neuropathy. These are listed in Table 61-2. The peripheral neuropathy secondary to chemotherapy is temporally related to administration for most agents. Cisplatin is an exception, and delayed neuropathy occurs in some patients.

Carcinomatous meningitis can manifest as multilevel radiculopathy, initially mimicking peripheral neuropathy. Likewise, brachial and lumbar plexopathy from tumor infiltration or radiation therapy can mimic neuropathy, but careful neurologic examination determines the localized nature of the process.

Diagnostic Evaluation

The evaluation of a patient with neuropathy depends on the results of the neurologic examination. Determination of the components of the peripheral nervous system involved is critical in guiding evaluation. Pure motor loss in a patient with lymphoma strongly suggests the presence of a paraneoplastic process, although CSF analysis should be performed to exclude Guillain-Barré syndrome. Likewise, the presence of pure sensory neuropathy involving both small and large sensory fibers suggests dorsal root ganglionitis. Pure large-fiber sensory neuropathy is most common with cisplatin treatment. Nerve conduction testing and electromyelography (EMG) may be helpful in determining whether the process is axonal or demyelinating. Some patients should undergo lumbar puncture to exclude carcinomatous meningitis or evaluation for Guillain-Barré syndrome.

Problems Common to Cancer and Its Therapy

Myopathy

Clinical Manifestations and Differential Diagnosis

Myopathy is a rare symptom in cancer, usually the consequence of treatment. Dermatomyositis and poly-myositis are paraneoplastic syndromes characterized by inflammatory myopathy and the presence or absence of a rash, respectively.[260,261] Dermatomyositis and polymyositis have been associated with many tumors, most commonly lung and gastrointestinal tumors. Patients have an elevated serum creatine phosphokinase (CPK) level. Although myopathy is a rare complication of chemotherapy, it has been described with use of paclitaxel and vincristine.[63,86,262]

Interferon and other biologic response–modifying agents can cause myalgia but show no evidence of muscle dysfunction or breakdown. Cisplatin and other agents that cause electrolyte abnormalities (e.g., hypomagnesemia) can cause muscle cramping.

Diagnostic Evaluation

For patients with clinical evidence of myopathy, serum CPK level should be measured before EMG. An elevated CPK level suggests active muscle destruction, as with polymyositis/dermatomyositis and use of paclitaxel or vincristine. Measurement of electrolytes (e.g., magnesium and potassium) may be useful. In patients with loss of strength or muscle pain, EMG and muscle biopsy may be necessary.

GRADING OF NEUROTOXICITY

None of the uniform grading systems of neurotoxicity is suitable for serial evaluation of patients. The most commonly used neurotoxicity measures have been developed by the cooperative oncology groups (Eastern Cooperative Oncology Group [ECOG] and the Southwest Oncology Group [SWOG]) for monitoring the neuro-toxicity of protocol treatments. The ECOG neurotoxicity guide is shown in Table 61-3. Although they are useful in the evaluation of groups of patients, these toxicity tables are not sufficient for monitoring individual patients. Standard neurologic testing with careful recording is best suited for individual patient care. Textbooks review the techniques required for performing an in-depth neuro-logic evaluation.[263,264] Quantitative measures of mental status function, motor examination results, and sensory function have been published.[265-267]

TREATMENT

No specific treatment exists to prevent or reverse most chemotherapy-related neurotoxicity. Therefore the focus should be on monitoring for development of toxicity so that treatment can be modified before the development of severe dysfunction. Rational treatment guidelines for minimizing neurotoxicity are needed.

TABLE 61-3

ECOG Toxicity Table for Scoring Treatment-Related Neurotoxicity

		0	STAGE 1	STAGE 2	STAGE 3	STAGE 4
Sensory	Neurosensory	None or no change	Mild paresthesias; loss of deep tendon reflexes	Mild or moderate objective sensory loss; moderate paresthesias	Severe objective sensory loss or paresthesias that interfere with function	—
	Neurovision	None or no change	—	—	Symptomatic subtotal loss of vision	Blindness
	Neurohearing	None or no change	Asymptomatic, hearing loss on audiometry only	Tinnitus	Hearing loss interfering with function but correctable with hearing aid	Deafness, not correctable
Motor	Neuromotor	None or no change	Subjective weakness; no objective findings	Mild objective weakness without marked impairment of function	Objective weakness with impairment of function	Paralysis
	Neuroconstipation	None or no change	Mild	Moderate	Severe	Ileus >96 h
Psychological	Neuromood	No change	Mild anxiety or depression	Moderate anxiety or depression	Severe anxiety or depression	Suicidal ideation
Clinical	Neurocortical	None	Mild somnolence or agitation	Moderate somnolence or agitation	Severe somnolence or agitation, confusion, disorientation, or hallucinations	Coma, seizures, toxic psychosis
	Neurocerebellar	None	Slight incoordination, dysdiadokinesis	Intention tremor, dysmetria, slurred speech, nystagmus	Locomotor ataxia	Cerebellar necrosis
	Neuroheadache	None	Mild	Moderate or severe but transient	Unrelenting and severe	—

Prevention

The key to prevention of permanent neurologic damage is to initiate a system for monitoring for toxicity. For example, patients receiving intrathecal chemotherapy are at risk of chemotherapy-induced myelopathy, an often irreversible toxicity. These patients may report vague neurologic symptoms or radicular back pain during the course of treatment that may be an early sign of neurologic damage. Findings at neurologic examination may not indicate loss of function, but the finding of an elevated CSF myelin basic protein level indicates that with subsequent treatment, the risk of myelopathy is high.[24,25]

Vincristine treatment can cause peripheral neuropathy. Some patients have autonomic neuropathy out of proportion to the sensorimotor neuropathy. The autonomic dysfunction can lead to intestinal dysmotility, ileus, and viscous perforation. Therefore all patients receiving vincristine chemotherapy should be carefully evaluated if abdominal symptoms develop. Obstipation from vincristine would mandate avoiding further vincristine treatment.

Modification of Drug Dosing or Order

In certain treatment regimens, altering the order of drug administration can result in a marked decrease in the risk of a neurotoxic complications. The risk of methotrexate-induced leukoencephalopathy after therapy for meningeal leukemia or carcinoma is reduced if the chemotherapy treatments, particularly intrathecal chemotherapy, precede cranial radiation therapy.[5] The reason for this schedule-dependent toxicity is unknown. It has been suggested that radiation opens the blood-brain barrier, increasing exposure of the brain to subsequent chemotherapy treatment. Other regimens in which dose order seems important include combination chemotherapy with cisplatin and ifosfamide. Patients receiving cisplatin before ifosfamide are at greater risk of ifosfamide-induced encephalopathy.[131]

Despite concern for synergistic neurotoxicity, certain regimens have been shown not to cause excessive neurotoxic effects. For example, a phase I study of paclitaxel and cisplatin included frequent neurologic examinations as a critical component.[268] Despite the well-recognized effects of both drugs on the peripheral nervous system, minimal overlapping toxicity occurred. Cisplatin treatment caused dose-related loss of vibratory sensation, whereas paclitaxel treatment correlated with loss of peripheral motor function. These findings underscored the importance of including careful neurologic testing as a component of phase I and II trials of new drugs and combination therapies.

Protective Agents

Several promising reports have appeared of agents that either block development of certain chemotherapy-induced neuropathies or help reverse toxicity. In the former category, the agent ORG 2766 has been reported to protect against cisplatin neuropathy. This drug, a synthetic analog of corticotropin, was tested in a double-blind, placebo-controlled trial in which patients with ovarian cancer underwent intensive cisplatin therapy. A dose-related protective effect was found.[30] Although the mechanism of action is unknown, results of laboratory studies suggest that ORG 2766 works synergistically with trophic factors (e.g., nerve growth factors) to promote nerve regeneration.[269,270] Results of a study conducted with a tissue culture model suggested that corticotropin fragments may have a direct cellular protective role.[271] Amifostine, an organic thiophosphate, protects normal cells from the effects of radiation. Amifostine has been tested as a neuroprotectant for paclitaxel in 2 phase III studies. In a study of non–small cell lung cancer, there was a reduction in incidence of radiation esophagitis, but not in paclitaxel-induced neuropathy.[272] In the study of ovarian cancer, the incidence of grade 3 and 4 peripheral neuropathy was significantly reduced.[273] Glutamine has been evaluated as a neuroprotectant for the peripheral nervous system. In a study with a small group of patients, the incidence of peripheral neuropathy among patients treated with paclitaxel with glutamine (10 g orally, 3 times a day for 4 days after paclitaxel) was compared with the incidence when paclitaxel was given alone.[274] A statistically significant reduction in severe neuropathy was found in the glutamine-treated group with significant decreases in the incidence and severity of dysesthesia, motor weakness, worsening of gait, and impairment of activities of daily living. Other possible protective agents include WR 2721 (cisplatin) and nerve growth factor (paclitaxel).[99,173,275] Leucovorin may be helpful in reversing acute methotrexate-induced encephalopathy and somnolence.[37] There is no known therapy for chemotherapy-induced leukoencephalopathy.

Recognition of Groups at High-Risk of Development of Neurotoxicity

Certain patients are at high risk of neurotoxicity from treatment. Patients with underlying peripheral neuropathy (e.g., Charcot-Marie-Tooth disease, diabetic neuropathy) have been reported to be much more susceptible to development of severe neuropathy, including potentially fatal autonomic neuropathy.[75,76] These patients need careful monitoring and immediate cessation of treatment if autonomic dysfunction develops. Similarly, among patients with underlying neuropathy, the condition is more likely to become severe with paclitaxel therapy.[1,2]

Patients with meningeal tumors (carcinoma, leukemia, lymphoma) often need extensive intrathecal chemotherapy. An intraventricular reservoir often is placed for this purpose. Before the reservoir system is used to administer chemotherapy, it is essential that placement and normal CSF flow be confirmed. This procedure is most readily performed by injecting indium-111–labeled albumin into the lateral ventricle through the reservoir system.[276,277] Not only does this test help determine catheter placement, but also monitoring the flow of tracer at 6, 24, and 48 hours helps determine the presence of abnormalities of clearance from the ventricular system or drug resorption at the arachnoid granulations. Figure 61-4

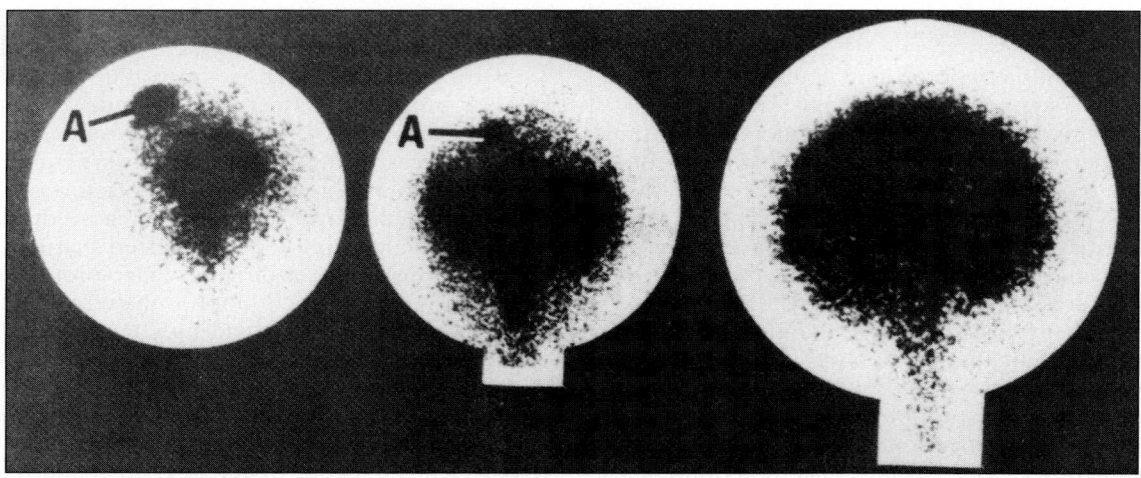

Figure 61-4. Normal cerebrospinal fluid indium-111–DTPA flow scan. Anterior cortical views immediately after injection (*left*), at 4 hours (*middle*), and at 24 hours (*right*). A, reservoir.

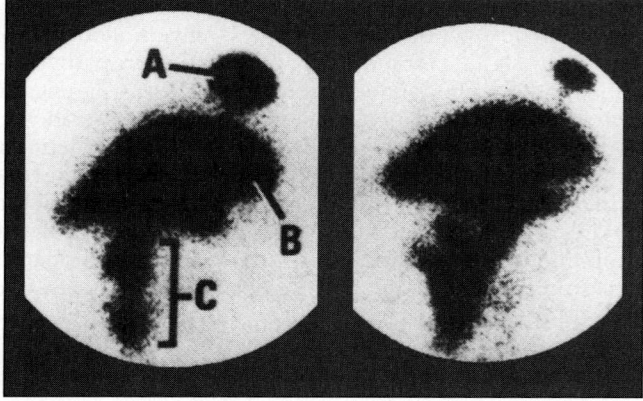

Figure 61-5. Ventricular outlet obstruction, lateral cortical view. Scans immediately after injection (*left*) and hours later (*right*). The reservoir (A), lateral ventricles (B), and fourth ventricle (C) are visible.

shows normal CSF flow and resorption of tracer through the arachnoid granulations. By contrast, Figures 61-5 and 61-6 show poor outflow from the lateral ventricles persisting 24 hours after contrast injection. Poor clearance of drug markedly increases the neurotoxicity of intraventricular treatment. These patients may need local radiation therapy for restoration of normal flow before instillation of chemotherapy.

Irreversible ototoxicity from cisplatin administration is more severe in patients with underlying hearing loss. Hearing loss with cisplatin also may be accelerated when the inner ear region and temporal lobe are treated with radiation.[116] Radiation treatment before or after cisplatin administration can cause this synergistic ototoxicity.

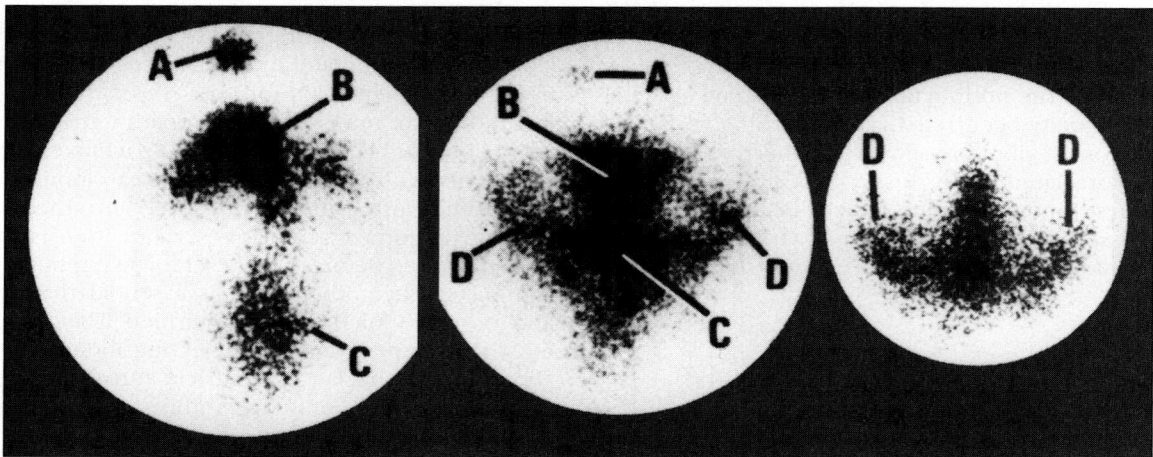

Figure 61-6. Obstruction of flow over cortical convexities. Scans immediately after injection (*left*), at 4 hours (*middle*), and at 24 hours (*right*). Visible are the reservoir (A), lateral ventricles (B), fourth ventricle (C), and tracer rising over the low portion of the cortical convexities (D).

CONCLUSIONS

The incidence of chemotherapy-induced neurotoxicity is increasing as a consequence of advances in supportive care, use of higher doses of drugs, new treatments targeted at the CNS, and prolonged patient survival, which allows toxicities with long latencies to become evident. The diagnosis of treatment-associated neurotoxicity is made after other diagnostic possibilities are excluded and when the pattern of toxicity is consistent with recognized neurotoxic effects. Management of most treatment-associated neurotoxicities is limited. The optimal strategy is early recognition of neurotoxicity, careful monitoring of patients at increased risk of toxicity, and modification of regimens to avoid synergistic toxicity when possible. Future directions should include investigation of the mechanisms of toxicity and development of techniques for protecting the nervous system without altering the antineoplastic effect of treatment.

REFERENCES

1. Rowinsky EK, Chaudhry V, Forastiere AA, et al: Phase I and pharmacologic study of paclitaxel and cisplatin with granulocyte colony-stimulating factor: Neuromuscular toxicity is dose-limiting. J Clin Oncol 1993;11:2010.
2. Chaudhry V, Rowinsky EK, Sartorius SE, et al: Peripheral neuropathy from Taxol and cisplatin combination chemotherapy: Clinical and electrophysiological studies. Ann Neurol 1994;5:304.
3. Neijstrom E, Gabriel DA, Capizzi RL: High-dose methotrexate-induced neurotoxicity associated with elevation of CSF myelin basic protein [letter]. J Clin Oncol 1985;3:593.
4. Price RA, Jamieson PA: The central nervous system in childhood leukemia. II. Subacute leukoencephalopathy. Cancer 1975;35:306.
5. Bleyer WA: Neurologic sequelae of methotrexate and ionizing radiation: A new classification. Cancer Treat Rep 1981;65 (suppl 1):89.
6. Ch'ien LT, Aur RJA, Verzosa MS, et al: Progression of methotrexate-induced leukoencephalopathy in children with leukemia. Med Pediatr Oncol 1981;9:133.
7. Hara T, Kishikawa T, Miyazaki S, et al: Central nervous system complications in childhood leukemia. Am J Pediatr Hematol Oncol 1984;6:129.
8. Meadows AT, Evans AE: Effects of chemotherapy on the central nervous system. Cancer 1976;37:1079.
9. Pazdur R, Redman BG, Corbett T, et al: Phase I trial of spiromustine (NSC 172112) and evaluation of toxicity and schedule in a murine model. Cancer Res 1987;47:4213.
10. Hiesiger EM, Voorhies RM, Basler GA, et al: Opening the blood-brain barrier and blood-tumor barriers in experimental rat brain tumors: The effect of intracarotid hyperosmolar mannitol on capillary permeability and blood flow. Ann Neurol 1986;19:50.
11. McGovern PC, Lautenbach E, Brennan PJ, Lustig RA, Fishman NO. Risk factors for postcraniotomy surgical site infection after 1,3-bis (2-chloroethyl)-1-nitrosourea (Gliadel) wafer placement. Clin Infect Dis 2003;36:759–765.
12. Grossman L, Baker MA, Sutten DMC: Central nervous system toxicity of high-dose cytosine arabinoside. Med Pediatr Oncol 1983;11:246.
13. Hwang T, Yung WKA, Estey EH, Fields WS: Central nervous system toxicity with high-dose ara-C. Neurology 1985;35:1475.
14. Benger A, Browman GP, Walker IR, Preisler HD: Clinical evidence of a cumulative effect of high-dose cytarabine on the cerebellum in patients with acute leukemia: A leukemia intergroup report. Cancer Treat Rep 1985;69:240.
15. Winkelman MD, Hines JD: Cerebellar degeneration caused by high-dose cytosine arabinoside: A clinicopathological study. Ann Neurol 1983;14:520.
16. McGuire WP, Rowinsky EK, Rosenshein NB, et al: Taxol: A unique antineoplastic agent with significant activity in advanced ovarian epithelial neoplasms. Ann Intern Med 1989;111:273.
17. Gottlieb D, Bradstock K, Koutts J, et al: The neurotoxicity of high-dose cytosine arabinoside is age-related. Cancer 1987;60:1439.
18. Damon LE, Mass R, Linker CA: The association between high-dose cytarabine neurotoxicity and renal insufficiency. J Clin Oncol 1989;7:1563.
19. Wolff L, Zighelboim J, Gale RP: Paraplegia following intrathecal cytosine arabinoside. Cancer 1979;43:83.
20. Breuer AC, Pitman SW, Dawson DM, Schoene WC: Paraparesis following intrathecal cytosine arabinoside: A case report with neuropathologic findings. Cancer 1977;40:2817.
21. Mena H, Garcia JH, Velandia F: Central and peripheral myelinopathy associated with systemic neoplasia and chemotherapy. Cancer 1981;48:1724.
22. Dunton SF, Nitschke R, Spruce WE, et al: Progressive ascending paralysis following administration of intrathecal and intravenous cytosine arabinoside. A Pediatric Oncology Group study. Cancer 1986;57:1083.
23. Hahn AF, Feasby TE, Gilbert JJ: Paraparesis following intrathecal chemotherapy. Neurology 1983;33:1032.
24. Clark AW, Cohen SR, Nissenblatt MJ, Wilson SK: Paraplegia following intrathecal chemotherapy. Neuropathologic findings and elevation of myelin basic protein. Cancer 1982;50:42.
25. Bates SE, Raphaelson MI, Price RA, et al: Ascending myelopathy after chemotherapy for central nervous system acute lymphoblastic leukemia: Correlation with cerebrospinal fluid myelin basic protein. Med Pediatr Oncol 1985;13:4.
26. Gagliano RG, Costanzi JJ: Paraplegia following intrathecal methotrexate: Report of a case and review of the literature. Cancer 1976;37:1663.
27. Bunge RP, Settlage PH: Neurological lesions in cats following cerebrospinal fluid manipulation. J Neuropathol Exp Neurol 1957;16:471.
28. Borgeat A, De Muralt B, Stadler M: Peripheral neuropathy associated with high-dose ara-C therapy. Cancer 1986;58:852.
29. Feinberg WM, Swenson MR: Cerebrovascular complications of l-asparaginase therapy. Neurology 1988;38:127.
30. van der Hoop RG, Vecht CJ, van der Burg ME, et al: Prevention of cisplatin neurotoxicity with an ACTH(4-9) analogue in patients with ovarian cancer. N Engl J Med 1990;322:89.
31. Priest JR, Ramsay NKC, Steinherz PG, et al: A syndrome of thrombosis and hemorrhage complicating l-asparaginase therapy for childhood acute lymphoblastic leukemia. J Pediatr 1982;100:984.
32. Holland J, Fasanello S, Ohnuma T: Psychiatric symptoms associated with l-asparaginase administration. J Psychiatr Res 1974;10:105.
33. Pichini S, Altieri I, Bacosi A, et al: High performance liquid chromatographic-mass spectrometric assay of busulfan in serum and cerebrospinal fluid. J Chromatogr 1992;581:143.
34. Gregg AP, Shepherd JD, Phillips GL: Busulphan and phenytoin [letter]. Ann Intern Med 1989;111:1049.
35. Walker RW, Allen JC, Rosen G, Caparros B: Transient cerebral dysfunction secondary to high-dose methotrexate. J Clin Oncol 1986;4:1845.
36. Phillips PC, Thaler HT, Berger CA, et al: Acute high-dose methotrexate neurotoxicity in the rat. Ann Neurol 1986;20:583.
37. Phillips PC, Thaler HT, Allen JC, Rottenberg DA: High-dose leucovorin reverses acute high-dose methotrexate neurotoxicity in the rat. Ann Neurol 1989;25:365.
38. Ch'ien LT, Aur RJA, Stagner S, et al: Long-term neurological implications of somnolence syndrome in children with acute lymphocytic leukemia. Ann Neurol 1990;8:273.
39. Cohen Y, Lossos A, Polliack A: Neurotoxicity with leukoencephalopathy after a single intravenous high dose of methotrexate in a patient with lymphoma. Acta Haematol 2002;107:185–186.
40. Norrell H, Wilson CB, Slagel DE, Clark DB: Leukoencephalopathy following the administration of methotrexate into the

cerebrospinal fluid in the treatment of primary brain tumors. Cancer 1974;33:923.

41. Nelson RW, Frank JT: Intrathecal methotrexate-induced neurotoxicities. Am J Hosp Pharm 1981;38:65.

42. Bleyer WA, Drake JC, Chabner BA: Neurotoxicity and elevated cerebrospinal-fluid methotrexate concentration in meningeal leukemia. N Engl J Med 1973;289:770.

43. Bleyer WA, Griffin TW: White matter necrosis, mineralizing microangiopathy, and intellectual abilities in survivors of childhood leukemia: Associations with central nervous system irradiation and methotrexate therapy. In Gilbert HA, Kagan AR (eds): Radiation Damage to the Nervous System. New York, Raven Press, 1980, p 155.

44. Gangji D, Reaman GH, Cohen SR, et al: Leukoencephalopathy and elevated levels of myelin basic protein in the cerebrospinal fluid of patients with acute lymphoblastic leukemia. N Engl J Med 1990;303:19.

45. Allen JC, Rosen G, Mehta BM, Horten B: Leukoencephalopathy following high-dose iv methotrexate chemotherapy with leucovorin rescue. Cancer Treat Rep 1980;64:1261.

46. Shalen PR, Ostrow PT, Glass PJ: Enhancement of the white matter following prophylactic therapy of the central nervous system for leukemia. Radiology 1981;140:409.

47. Geiser CF, Bishop Y, Jaffe N, et al: Adverse effects of intrathecal methotrexate in children with acute leukemia in remission. Blood 1975;45:189.

48. Kay HEM, Knapton PJ, O'Sullivan JP, et al: Encephalopathy in acute leukemia associated with methotrexate therapy. Arch Dis Child 1972;47:344.

49. Duttera MJ, Bleyer WA, Pomeroy TC, et al: Irradiation, methotrexate toxicity, and the treatment of meningeal leukemia. Lancet 1973;1:703.

50. Rosen G, Marcove RC, Caparros B, et al: Primary osteogenic sarcoma: Rationale for preoperative chemotherapy and delayed surgery. Cancer 1979;43:2163.

51. Ochs J, Mulhern R, Fairclough D, et al: Comparison of neuropsychologic functioning and clinical indicators of neurotoxicity in long-term survivors of childhood leukemia given cranial radiation or parenteral methotrexate: A prospective study. J Clin Oncol 1991;9:145.

52. Chessels JM, Cox TC, Kendall B, et al: Neurotoxicity in lymphoblastic leukaemia: Comparison of oral and intramuscular methotrexate and two doses of radiation. Arch Dis Child 1990;65:416.

53. Liu HM, Maurer HS, Vongsvivut S, Conway JJ: Methotrexate encephalopathy. A neuropathologic study. Hum Pathol 1978;9:635.

54. Nakazato Y, Ishida Y, Morimatsu M: Disseminated necrotizing leukoencephalopathy. Acta Pathol Jpn 1990;30:659.

55. Suzuki K, Takemura T, Okeda R, Hatakeyama S: Vascular changes of methotrexate-related disseminated necrotizing leukoencephalopathy. Acta Neuropathol 1984;65:145.

56. Gilbert MR, Harding BL, Grossman SA: Methotrexate neurotoxicity: In vitro studies using cerebellar explants from rats. Cancer Res 1989;49:2502.

57. Cohen ME, Duffner PK, Terplan KL: Myelopathy with severe structural derangement associated with combined modality therapy. Cancer 1983;52:1590.

58. Skullerud K, Halvorsen K: Encephalomyelopathy following intrathecal methotrexate treatment in a child with acute leukemia. Cancer 1978;42:1211.

59. Back EH: Death after intrathecal methotrexate. Lancet 1969;2:1005.

60. Bagshawe KD, Magrath IT, Golding PR: Intrathecal methotrexate. Lancet 1969;2:1258.

61. Luddy RE, Gilman PA: Paraplegia following intrathecal methotrexate. J Pediatr 1973;83:988.

62. Rosenthal S, Kaufman S: Vincristine neurotoxicity. Ann Intern Med 1974;80:733.

63. Bradley VG, Lassman LP, Pearce GW, Walton JN: The neuromyopathy of vincristine in man. Clinical, electrophysiological and pathological studies. J Neurol Sci 1907;10:107.

64. Sandler SG, Tobin W, Henderson ES: Vincristine-induced neuropathy: A clinical study of fifty leukemic patients. Neurology 1969;19:367.

65. Casey EB, Jellife AM, Le Quesne PM, Millett YL: Vincristine neuropathy: Clinical and electrophysiological observations. Brain 1973;96:69.

66. Guiheneuc P, Ginet J, Groleau JY, Rojouan J: Early phase of vincristine neuropathy in man. J Neurol Sci 1990;45:355.

67. Burdman JA: A note on the selective toxicity of vincristine sulfate on chick-embryo sensory ganglia in tissue culture. J Natl Cancer Inst 1966;37:331.

68. Mena MA, Pardo B, Casarejos MJ, et al: Neurotoxicity of levodopa on catecholamine-rich neurons. Mov Disord 1992;7:23.

69. Shelanski ML, Wisniewski H: Neurofibrillary degeneration induced by vincristine therapy. Arch Neurol 1969;20:199.

70. Seil FJ: Neurofibrillary tangles induced by vincristine and vinblastine sulfate in central and peripheral neurons in vitro. Exp Neurol 1968;21:219.

71. Journey LJ, Burdman J, Whaley A: Electron microscopic study of spinal ganglia from vincristine-treated mice. J Natl Cancer Inst 1969;43:603.

72. Donoso JA, Green LS, Heller-Bettinger IE, Samson FE: Action of the vinca alkaloids vincristine, vinblastine, and desacetyl vinblastine amide on axonal fibrillar organelles in vitro. Cancer Res 1977;37:1401.

73. Sato M, Miyoshi K: Ultrastructural observations on the vincristine-induced neuronal crystalloid inclusion in young rats. Acta Neuropathol (Berl) 1984;63:150.

74. Green LS, Donoso JA, Heller-Bettinger IE, Samson FE: Axonal transport disturbances in vincristine-induced peripheral neuropathy. Ann Neurol 1977;1:255.

75. Griffiths JD, Stark RJ, Ding JC, Cooper IA: Vincristine neurotoxicity in Charcot-Marie-Tooth syndrome. Med J Aust 1985;143:305.

76. Hogan-Dunne CM, Fellmeth WG, McGuire SA, Kiley VA: Polyneuropathy following vincristine therapy in two patients with Charcot-Marie-Tooth syndrome. JAMA 1984;252:2862.

77. Chauvenet AR, Shashi V, Selsky C, Morgan E, Kurtzberg J, Bell B: Vincristine-induced neuropathy as the initial presentation of Charcot-Marie-Tooth disease in acute lymphoblastic leukemia: A Pediatric Oncology Group study. J Pediatr Hematol Oncol 2003;25:316–320.

78. Trobaugh-Lotrario AD, Smith AA, Odom LF: Vincristine neurotoxicity in the presence of hereditary neuropathy. Med Pediatr Oncol 2003;40:39–43.

79. Naumann R, Mohm J, Reuner U, Kroschinsky F, Rautenstrauss B, Ehninger G: Early recognition of hereditary motor and sensory neuropathy type 1 can avoid life-threatening vincristine neurotoxicity. Br J Haematol 2001;115:323–325.

80. Cassady JR, Tonnesen GL, Wolfe LC, Sallan SE: Augmentation of vincristine neurotoxicity by irradiation of peripheral nerves. Cancer Treat Rep 1980;64:963.

81. Wheeler JS, Siroky MB, Bell R, Babayan RK: Vincristine-induced bladder neuropathy. J Urol 1983;30:342.

82. Sanderson PA, Kuwabara T, Cogan DG: Optic neuropathy presumably caused by vincristine therapy. Am J Ophthalmol 1976;81:146.

83. Vecchi V, Maccolini E, Bravetti GO, et al: Transient optic neuropathy secondary to MOPP chemotherapy in Hodgkin's disease: Report of a case. Tumori 1984;70:571.

84. Johnson FL, Bernstein ID, Hartmann JR, Chard RL: Seizures associated with vincristine sulfate therapy. J Pediatr 1973;82:699.

85. Martin J, Mainwaring D: Coma and convulsions associated with vincristine therapy. Br Med J 1973;4:782.

86. Whittaker JA, Parry DH, Bunch C, Weatherall DJ: Coma associated with vincristine therapy. Br Med J 1973;4:335.

87. Slater LM, Wainer RA, Serpick AA: Vincristine neurotoxicity with hyponatremia. Cancer 1969;23:122.

88. Scheithauer W, Ludwig H, Maida E: Acute encephalopathy associated with continuous vincristine sulfate combination therapy: Case report. Invest New Drugs 1985;3:315.

89. Suskind RM, Brusilow SW, Zehr J: Syndrome of inappropriate secretion of antidiuretic hormone produced by vincristine toxicity (with bioassay of ADH level). J Pediatr 1972;81:90.

90. Fine RS, Clarke RR, Shore NA: Hyponatremia and vincristine therapy. Am J Dis Child 1966;112:256.

91. Stuart MJ, Cuaso C, Miller M, Oski FA: Syndrome of recurrent

increased secretion of antidiuretic hormone following multiple doses of vincristine. Blood 1975;45:315.

92. Robertson GL, Bhoopalam N, Zelkowitz LJ: Vincristine neurotoxicity and abnormal secretion of antidiuretic hormone. Arch Intern Med 1973;132:717.

93. Mueller JM, Flaherty MJ: Vincristine-induced quadriparesis. South Med J 1978;71:1310.

94. Wheeler RH, Votaw M: Vincristine and quadriparesis. Ann Intern Med 1974;81:709.

95. Norman M, Elinder G, Finkel Y: Vincristine neuropathy and Guillain-Barré syndrome: A case with acute lymphatic leukemia and quadriparesis. Eur J Haematol 1987;39:75.

96. Slotwiner P, Song SK, Anderson PJ: Spheromembranous degeneration of muscle induced by vincristine. Arch Neurol 1966;15:172.

97. Roelofs RI, Hrushesky W, Rogin J, Rosenberg L: Peripheral sensory neuropathy and cisplatin chemotherapy. Neurology 1984;34:934.

98. Pollera CF, Pietrangeli A, Giannarelli D: Cisplatin-induced peripheral neurotoxicity: Relationship to dose intensity [letter]. Ann Oncol 1991;2:212.

99. Mollman JE, Glover DJ, Hogan WM, Furman RE: Cisplatin neuropathy: Risk factors, prognosis, and protection by WR-2721. Cancer 1988;61:2192.

100. Cavaletti G, Marzorati L, Bogliun G, et al: Cisplatin-induced peripheral neurotoxicity is dependent on total-dose intensity and single-dose intensity. Cancer 1992;69:203.

101. von Schlippe M, Fowler CJ, Harland SJ: Cisplatin neurotoxicity in the treatment of metastatic germ cell tumour: Time course and prognosis. Br J Cancer 2001;85:823–826.

102. Thompson SW, Davis LE, Kornfeld M, Hilgers RD, Standefer JC: Cisplatin neuropathy: Clinical, electrophysiologic, morphologic, and toxicologic studies. Cancer 1984;54:1269–1275.

103. Walsh TJ, Clark AW, Parhad IM, Green WR: Neurotoxic effects of cisplatin therapy. Arch Neurol 1982;39:719.

104. Eeles R, Tait DM, Peckham MJ: Lhermitte's sign as a complication of cisplatin-containing chemotherapy for testicular cancer. Cancer Treat Rep 1986;70:905.

105. Walther PJ, Rossitch E, Bullard DE: The development of Lhermitte's sign during cisplatin chemotherapy. Cancer 1987;60:2170.

106. Wilding G, Caruso R, Lawrence TS, et al: Retinal toxicity after high-dose cisplatin therapy. J Clin Oncol 1985;3:1683.

107. Becher R, Schutt P, Osieka R, Schmidt CG: Peripheral neuropathy and ophthalmologic toxicity after treatment with cis-dichlorodiaminoplatinum II. J Cancer Res Clin Oncol 1980;96:219.

108. Berman IJ, Mann MP: Seizures and transient cortical blindness associated with cis-platinum (II) diamminedichloride (PDD) therapy in a thirty-year-old man. Cancer 1990;45:764.

109. Cattaneo MT, Filipazzi V, Piazza E, et al: Transient blindness and seizure associated with cisplatin therapy. J Cancer Res Clin Oncol 1988;114:528.

110. Mead GM, Arnold AM, Green JA, et al: Epileptic seizures associated with cisplatin administration. Cancer Treat Rep 1982;66:1719.

111. Lyass O, Lossos A, Hubert A, Gips M, Peretz T: Cisplatin-induced non-convulsive encephalopathy. Anticancer Drugs, 1998;9:100–104.

112. Steeghs N, De Jongh FE, Smitt PA, Bent MJ: Cisplatin-induced encephalopathy and seizures. Anticancer Drugs 2003;14:443–446.

113. Maiese K, Walker RW, Gargan R, Victor JD: Intra-arterial cisplatin-associated optic and otic toxicity. Arch Neurol 1992;49:83.

114. Kupersmith MJ, Frohman LP, Choi IS, et al: Visual system toxicity following intra-arterial chemotherapy. Neurology 1988;38:284.

115. Schaefer SD, Post JD, Close LG, Wright CG: Ototoxicity of low- and moderate-dose cisplatin. Cancer 1985;56:1934.

116. Aguilar-Markulis NV, Beckley S, Priore R, Mettlin C: Auditory toxicity effects of long-term cis-dichlorodiammineplatinum II therapy in genitourinary cancer patients. J Surg Oncol 1981;16:111.

117. Helson L, Okonkwo E, Anton L, Cvitkovic E: Cis-platinum ototoxicity. Clin Toxicol 1978;13:469.

118. Durrant JD, Rodgers G, Myers EN, Johnson JT: Hearing loss: risk factor for cisplatin ototoxicity? Observations. Am J Otol 1990;11:375.

119. Fausti SA, Henry JA, Schaffer HI, et al: High-frequency monitoring for early detection of cisplatin toxicity. Arch Otolaryngol Head Neck Surg 1993;119:661.

120. DeFronzo RA, Braine H, Colvin OM, Davis PJ: Water intoxication in man after cyclophosphamide therapy. Ann Intern Med 1973;78:861.

121. Webberley MJ, Murray JA: Life-threatening acute hyponatremia induced by low dose cyclophosphamide and indomethacin. Postgrad Med J 1989;65:950.

122. DeFronzo RA, Colvin OM, Braine H, et al: Cyclophosphamide and the kidney. Cancer 1974;33:483.

123. Sterns RH, Riggs JE, Schochet SS Jr: Osmotic demyelination syndrome following correction of hyponatremia. N Engl J Med 1986;314:1535.

124. Gieron MA, Barak LS, Estrada J: Severe encephalopathy associated with ifosfamide administration in two children with metastatic tumors. J Neurooncol 1988;6:29.

125. Meanwell CA, Blake AE, Kelly KA, et al: Prediction of ifosfamide/mesna associated encephalopathy. Eur J Clin Oncol 1986;22:815.

126. Miller LJ, Eaton VE: Ifosfamide-induced neurotoxicity: A case report and review of the literature. Ann Pharmacother 1992;26:183.

127. Pratt CB, Green AA, Horowitz ME, et al: Central nervous system toxicity following the treatment of pediatric patients with ifosfamide/mesna. J Clin Oncol 1986;4:1253.

128. Curtin JP, Koonings PP, Gutierrez M, et al: Ifosfamide-induced neurotoxicity. Gynecol Oncol 1991;42:193.

129. Cabral FR: Isolation of Chinese hamster ovary cell mutants requiring the continuous presence of Taxol for cell division. J Cell Biol 1983;97:22.

130. Cabral F, Wible L, Brenner S, Brinkley BR: Taxol-requiring mutant of Chinese hamster ovary cells with impaired mitotic spindle assembly. J Cell Biol 1983;97:30.

131. Pratt CB, Goren MP, Meyer WH, et al: Ifosfamide neurotoxicity is related to previous cisplatin treatment for pediatric solid tumors. J Clin Oncol 1990;8:1399.

132. Anderson NR, Tandon DS: Ifosfamide extrapyramidal neurotoxicity. Cancer 1991;68:72.

133. Riehl JB, Brown WB: Acute cerebellar syndrome secondary to 5-fluorouracil therapy. Neurology 1964;14:961–967.

134. Bixenman WW, Nicholls JVV, Warwick OH: Oculomotor disturbances associated with 5-fluorouracil chemotherapy. Am J Ophthalmol 1977;83:789.

135. Moertel CG, Reitemeier RJ, Bolton CF, Shorter RG: Cerebellar ataxia associated with fluorinated pyrimidine therapy. Cancer Chemother Rep 1964;41:15.

136. Moore DH, Fowler WC Jr, Crumpler LS: 5-Fluorouracil neurotoxicity. Gynecol Oncol 1990;36:152.

137. Antin PB, Forry-Schaudies S, Friedman TM, et al: Taxol induces postmitotic myoblasts to assemble interdigitating microtubule-myosin arrays that exclude actin filaments. J Cell Biol 1981;90:300.

138. Mole-Bajer J, Bajer AS: Action of Taxol on mitosis: Modification of microtubule arrangements and function of the mitotic spindle in Haemanthus endosperm. J Cell Biol 1983;96:527.

139. Vallee RB: A Taxol-dependent procedure for the isolation of microtubules and microtubule-associated proteins (MAPs). J Cell Biol 1982;92:435.

140. Manfredi JJ, Parness J, Horwitz SB: Taxol binds to cellular microtubules. J Cell Biol 1982;94:688.

141. Hook CC, Kimmel DW, Kvols LK, et al: Multifocal inflammatory leukoencephalopathy with 5-fluorouracil and levamisole. Ann Neurol 1992;31:262.

142. Grever MR, Kopecky KJ, Cottman CA, et al: Fludarabine monophosphate: A potentially useful agent in chronic lymphocytic leukemia. Nouv Rev Fr Hematol 1988;30:457.

143. Chun HG, Leyland-Jones B, Caryk SM, et al: Central nervous system toxicity of fludarabine phosphate. Cancer Treat Rep 1986;70:1225.

144. Vidarsson B, Mosher DF, Salamat MS, Isaksson HJ, Onundarson PT: Progressive multifocal leukoencephalopathy after fludarabine therapy for low-grade lymphoproliferative disease. Am J Hematol 2002;70:51–54.

Problems Common to Cancer and Its Therapy

145. Mahaley MS Jr, Whaley RA, Blue M, Bertsch L: Central neurotoxicity following intracarotid BCNU chemotherapy for malignant gliomas. J Neurooncol 1986;3:297.

146. Kleinschmidt-DeMasters BK: Intracarotid BCNU leukoencephalopathy. Cancer 1986;57:1276.

147. Rosenblum MK, Delattre JY, Walker RW, Shapiro WR: Fatal necrotizing encephalopathy complicating treatment of malignant gliomas with intra-arterial BCNU and irradiation: A pathological study. J Neurooncol 1989;7:269.

148. Burger PC, Kamenar E, Schold SC, et al: Encephalomyelopathy following high-dose BCNU therapy. Cancer 1981;48:1318.

149. Blacklock JB, Wright DC, Dedrick RL, et al: Drug streaming during intra-arterial chemotherapy. J Neurosurg 1986;64:284.

150. Westphal M, Hilt D, Bortey, et al: A phase 3 trial of local chemotherapy with biodegradable carmustine (BCNU) wafers (Gliadel wafers) in patients with primary malignant glioma. Neurooncology 2003;5:79–88.

151. Brem H, Mahaley MSJ, Vick NA, et al: Interstitial chemotherapy with drug polymer implants for the treatment of malignant gliomas. J Neurosurg 1991;74:441.

152. Grimson BS, Mahaley MS Jr, Dubey HD, Dudka L: Ophthalmic and central nervous system complications following intracarotid BCNU (carmustine). J Clin Neuroophthalmol 1981;1:261.

153. Wilson RH, Lehky T, Thomas RR, Quinn MG, Floeter MK, Grem JL: Acute oxaliplatin-induced peripheral nerve hyperexcitability. J Clin Oncol 2002;20:1767–1774.

154. Cascinu, S, Catalano, V, Cordella, L, et al: Neuroprotective effect of reduced glutathione on oxaliplatin-based chemotherapy in advanced colorectal cancer: A randomized, double-blind, placebo-controlled trial. J Clin Oncol 2002;20:3478–3483.

155. Taieb S, Trillet-Lenoir V, Rambaud L, Descos L, Freyer G: Lhermitte sign and urinary retention: Atypical presentation of oxaliplatin neurotoxicity in four patients. Cancer 2002;94:2434–2440.

156. Stolinsky DC, Solomon J, Pugh RP, et al: Clinical experience with procarbazine in Hodgkin's disease, reticulum cell sarcoma, and lymphosarcoma. Cancer 1970;26:984.

157. Brunner KW, Young CW: A methylhydrazine derivative in Hodgkin's disease and other malignant neoplasms. Ann Intern Med 1965;63:69.

158. Samuels ML, Leary WV, Alexanian R, et al: Clinical trials with N-isopropyl-a-(2-methylhydrazino)-p-toluamide hydrochloride in malignant lymphoma and other disseminated neoplasia. Cancer 1967;20:1187.

159. Horwitz SB, Lothstein L, Manfredi JJ, et al: Taxol: Mechanisms of action and resistance. Ann N Y Acad Sci 1986;466:733.

160. Black MM: Taxol interferes with the interaction of microtubule-associated proteins with microtubules in cultured neurons. J Neurosci 1987;7:3695.

161. Lipton RB, Apfel SC, Dutcher JP, et al: Taxol produces a predominantly sensory neuropathy. Neurology 1989;39:368.

162. Bissett D, Setanoians A, Cassidy J, et al: Phase I and pharmaco-kinetic study of taxotere (RP56976) administered as a 24-hour infusion. Cancer Res 1993;53:532.

163. Vasey PA, Atkinson, R, Coleman, R, et al: Docetaxel-carboplatin as first line chemotherapy for epithelial ovarian cancer. Br J Cancer 2001;84:170–178.

164. Roytta M, Horwitz SB, Raine CS: Taxol-induced neuropathy: Short-term effects of local injection. J Neurocytol 1984;13:685.

165. Vuorinen V, Roytta M, Raine CS: The long-term cellular response to Taxol in peripheral nerve: Schwann cell and endoneurial cell changes. J Neurocytol 1989;18:785.

166. Vuorinen V, Roytta M, Raine CS: The long-term effects of a single injection of Taxol upon peripheral nerve axons. J Neurocytol 1989;18:775.

167. Komiya Y, Tashiro T: Effects of Taxol on slow and fast axonal transport. Cell Motil Cytoskeleton 1988;11:151.

168. Vuorinen V, Roytta M, Raine CS: The acute effects of Taxol upon regenerating axons after nerve crush. Acta Neuropathol (Berl) 1988;76:26.

169. Masurovsky EB, Peterson ER, Crain SM, Horwitz SB: Morphological alterations in dorsal root ganglion neurons and supporting cells of organotypic mouse spinal cord-ganglion cultures exposed to Taxol. Neuroscience 1983;10:491.

170. Masurovsky EB, Peterson ER, Crain SM, Horwitz SB: Microtubule arrays in Taxol-treated mouse dorsal root ganglion–spinal cord cultures. Brain Res 1981;217:392.

171. Vuorinen V, Roytta M, Raine CS: The acute response of Schwann cells to Taxol after nerve crush. Acta Neuropathol (Berl) 1988;76:17.

172. Roytta M, Peltonen J, Vuorinen V: Schwann cells and collagen synthesis in Taxol-treated nerve crush: An electron microscopic study. Coll Relat Res 1988;8:123.

173. Apfel SC, Lipton RB, Arezzo JC, Kessler JA: Nerve growth factor prevents toxic neuropathy in mice. Ann Neurol 1991;29:87.

174. Peterson ER, Crain SM: Nerve growth factor attenuates neurotoxic effects of Taxol on spinal cord-ganglion explants from fetal mice. Science 1982;217:377.

175. Ziske CG, Schottker B, Gorschluter M, et al: Acute transient encephalopathy after paclitaxel infusion: Report of three cases. Ann Oncol 2002;13:629–631.

176. Nieto Y, Cagnoni PJ, Bearman SI, et al: Acute encephalopathy: A new toxicity associated with high-dose paclitaxel. Clin Cancer Res 1999;5:501–506.

177. Gorin MB, Day R, Costantino JP, et al: Long-term tamoxifen citrate use and potential ocular toxicity. Am J Ophthalmol 1998;125:493–501.

178. Noureddin BN, Seoud M, Bashshur Z, Salem Z, Shamseddin A, Khalil A. Ocular toxicity in low-dose tamoxifen: A prospective study. Eye 1999;13:729–733.

179. Ashford AR, Doney I, Tiwari RP, et al: Reversible ocular toxicity related to tamoxifen therapy. Cancer 1988;61:33.

180. Pluss JL, DiBella NJ: Reversible central nervous system dysfunction due to tamoxifen in a patient with breast cancer. Ann Intern Med 1984;10:652.

181. Love RR: Tamoxifen therapy in primary breast cancer: Biology, efficacy, and side effects. J Clin Oncol 1989;7:803.

182. Ron IG, Inbar MJ, Barak Y, et al: Organic delusional syndrome associated with tamoxifen treatment. Cancer 1992;69:1415.

183. Denicoff KD, Rubinow DR, Papa MZ, et al: The neuropsychiatric effects of treatment with interleukin-2 and lymphokine-activated killer cells. Ann Intern Med 1987;107:293.

184. Somers SS, Reynolds JV, Guillou PJ: Multifocal neurotoxicity during interleukin-2 therapy for malignant melanoma. Clin Oncol (R Coll Radiol) 1992;4:135.

185. Vecht C, Keohane C, Menon RS, et al: Acute fatal leukoencephalopathy after interleukin-2 therapy. N Engl J Med 1990;323:1146.

186. Bernard JT, Ameriso S, Kempf RA, et al: Transient focal neurologic deficits complicating interleukin-2 therapy. Neurology 1990;40:154.

187. Friedman DI, Hu EH, Sadun AA: Neuro-ophthalmic complications of interleukin-2 therapy. Am J Ophthalmol 1991;109:1679.

188. Collins CA, Vallee RB: Temperature-dependent reversible assembly of Taxol-treated microtubules. J Cell Biol 1987;105:2847.

189. Mattson K, Niiranen A, Iivanainen M, et al: Neurotoxicity of interferon [letter]. Cancer Treat Rep 1983;67:958.

190. Mattson K, Niiranen A, Laaksonen R, Cantell K: Psychometric monitoring of interferon neurotoxicity [letter]. Lancet 1984;1:275.

191. Rosen P, Armstrong D: Nonbacterial thrombotic endocarditis in patients with malignant neoplastic disease. Am J Med 1973;54:23.

192. Capuron L, Gumnick JF, Musselman DL, et al: Neurobehavioral effects of interferon-alpha in cancer patients: Phenomenology and paroxetine responsiveness of symptom dimensions. Neuropsychopharmacology 2002;26:643–652.

193. Schibler MJ, Cabral F: Taxol-dependent mutants of Chinese hamster ovary cells with alterations in alpha- and beta-tubulin. J Cell Biol 1986;102:1522.

194. Meyers CA, Obbens EA, Scheibel RS, Moser RP: Neurotoxicity of intraventricularly administered alpha-interferon for leptomeningeal disease. Cancer 1991;68:88.

195. Bernsen PLJA, Chung REW, Vingerhoets HM, Janssen JTP: Bilateral neuralgic amyotrophy induced by interferon treatment. Arch Neurol 1988;45:449.

196. Bailes J, Willis J, Priebe C, Strub R: Encephalopathy with metronidazole in a child. Am J Dis Child 1983;137:290.

197. Frytak S, Moertel CH, Childs DS: Neurologic toxicity associated with high-dose metronidazole therapy. Ann Intern Med 1978;88:361.

198. Kusumi R, Plouffe JF, Wyatt RH, Fass RJ: Central nervous system toxicity associated with metronidazole therapy. Ann Intern Med 1990;93:59.

199. Rose GP, Dewar AJ, Stratford IJ: A biochemical neurotoxicity study relating the neurotoxic potential of metronidazole and nitrofurantoin with misonidazole. Int J Radiat Oncol Biol Phys 1982;8:781.

200. Coleman CN, Buswell L, Noll L, et al: The efficacy of pharmacokinetic monitoring and dose modification of etanidazole on the incidence of neurotoxicity: Results from a phase II trial of etanidazole and radiation therapy in locally advanced prostate cancer. Int J Radiat Oncol Biol Phys 1992;22:565.

201. Chaudhry V, Eisenberger MA, Sinibaldi VJ, Sheikh K, Griffin JW, Cornblath DR: A prospective study of suramin-induced peripheral neuropathy. Brain 1996;119:2039–2052.

202. Soliven B, Dhand UK, Kobayashi K, et al: Evaluation of neuropathy in patients on suramin treatment. Muscle Nerve 1997;20:83–91.

203. Singhal S, Mehta J: Thalidomide in cancer. Biomed Pharmacother 2002;56:4–12.

204. Chaudhry V, Cornblath DR, Corse A, Freimer M, Simmons-O'Brien E, Vogelsang G: Thalidomide-induced neuropathy. Neurology 2002;59:1872–1875.

205. Bastuji-Garin S, Ochonisky S, Bouche P, et al: Incidence and risk factors for thalidomide neuropathy: A prospective study of 135 dermatologic patients. J Invest Dermatol 2002;119:1020–1026.

206. McLean AS: Early adverse effects of radiation. Br Med Bull 1973;29:69.

207. Valk PE, Dillon WP: Radiation injury of the brain. AJNR Am J Neuroradiol 1991;12:45.

208. Watne K, Hager B, Heier M, et al: Reversible oedema and necrosis after irradiation of the brain: Diagnosis procedures and clinical manifestations. Acta Oncol 1990;29:891.

209. Late complications of radiotherapy. Drug Ther Bull 1997;35:13.

210. Morris JG, Gratton-Smith P, Panegyres PK, et al: Delayed cerebral radiation necrosis. Q J Med 1994;87:119.

211. Marks JE, Wong J: The risk of cerebral radionecrosis in relation to dose, time and fractionation: A follow-up study. Prog Exp Tumor Res 1985;29:210.

212. Rottenberg DA, Chernik NL, Deck MD, et al: Cerebral necrosis following radiotherapy of extracranial neoplasms. Ann Neurol 1977;1:339.

213. Shaw PJ, Bates D: Conservative treatment of delayed cerebral radiation necrosis. J Neurol Neurosurg Psychiatry 1984;47:1338.

214. Curnes JT, Laster DW, Ball MR, et al: MRI of radiation injury to the brain. AJNR Am J Neuroradiol 1986;147:119.

215. Packer RJ, Zimmerman RA, Bilaniuk CT: Magnetic resonance imaging in the evaluation of treatment related central nervous system damage. Cancer 1986;58:635.

216. Constine LS, Konski A, Ekholm S, et al: Adverse effects of irradiation correlated with MR and CT imaging. Int J Radiat Oncol Biol Phys 1988;15:319.

217. Marshall VG, Bradley WGJ, Marshall CE, et al: Deep white matter infarction: Correlation of MR imaging with histopathologic findings. Radiology 1988;167:517.

218. Price RA: Histopathology of CNS leukemia and complications of therapy. Am J Pediatr Hematol Oncol 1979;1:21.

219. Pizzo PA, Poplack DG, Bleyer WA: Neurotoxicities of current leukemia therapy. Am J Pediatr Hematol Oncol 1979;1:127.

220. Sklar CA, Constine LS: Chronic neuroendocrinological sequelae of radiation therapy. Int J Radiat Oncol Biol Phys 1995;31:1113.

221. Littley MD, Shalet SM, Bearwell CG: Radiation and the hypothalamic-pituitary axis. In Gutin PH, Leibel SA, Sheline GE (eds): Radiation Injury of the Nervous System. New York, Raven Press, 1991, p 303.

222. Leventhal BG, Shearer PD: Recognizing and managing the late effects of cancer treatment. Oncology (Huntingt) 1989;3:73.

223. Lam KS, Tse VK, Wang C, et al: Effects of cranial irradiation on hypothalamic-pituitary function: A 5-year longitudinal study in patients with nasopharyngeal carcinoma. Q J Med 1991;286:165.

224. Byrd RL: Late effects of treatment of cancer in children. Pediatr Ann 1983;12:450.

225. Goldwein JW: Radiation myelopathy: A review. Med Pediatr Oncol 1987;15:89.

226. Schultheiss TE, Stephens LC: Invited review: Permanent radiation myelopathy. Br J Radiol 1992;65:737.

227. Schultheiss TE, Higgins EM, El-Mahdi AM: The latent period in clinical radiation myelopathy. Int J Radiat Oncol Biol Phys 1984;10:1109.

228. Kinsella TJ, Weichgelbaum RR, Sheline GE: Radiation injury of cranial and peripheral nerves. In Gilbert HA, Kagan AR (eds): Radiation Damage to the Nervous System: A Delayed Therapeutic Hazard. New York, Raven Press, 1980, p 145.

229. Gillette EL, Mahler PA, Powers BE, et al: Late radiation injury to muscle and peripheral nerves. Int J Radiat Oncol Biol Phys 1995;31:1309.

230. Olsen NK, Pfeiffer P, Mondrup K, et al: Radiation-induced brachial plexus neuropathy in breast cancer patients. Acta Oncol 1990;29:885.

231. Gerard JM, Franck N, Moussa Z, et al: Acute ischemic brachial plexus neuropathy following radiation therapy. Neuropathy 1989;39:450.

232. Kinsella TJ, Sindelar WF, DeLuca AM, et al: Tolerance of peripheral nerve to intraoperative radiotherapy (IORT): Clinical and experimental studies. Int J Radiat Oncol Biol Phys 1985;11:1579.

233. Gilbert MR, Grossman SA: The incidence and nature of neurologic problems in patients with solid tumors. Am J Med 1986;81:951.

234. Henson RA, Hoffman HL, Ulrich H: Encephalomyelitis with carcinoma. Brain 1965;88:449.

235. Posner JB, Furneaux HM: Paraneoplastic syndromes. In Waksman BH (ed): Immunologic Mechanisms in Neurologic and Psychiatric Disease. New York, Raven Press, 1990, p 187.

236. Jaekle KA: Autoimmune paraneoplastic limbic encephalitis. Neurology 1988;38(suppl 1):390.

237. Phillips PC, Dhawan V, Strother SC, et al: Reduced cerebral glucose metabolism and increased brain capillary permeability following high-dose methotrexate chemotherapy: A positron emission tomographic study. Ann Neurol 1987;21:59.

238. Sanchez-Carpintero R, Narbona J, Lopez de Mesa R, Arbizu J, Sierrasesumaga L: Transient posterior encephalopathy induced by chemotherapy in children. Pediatr Neurol 2001;24:145–148.

239. Honkaniemi J, Kahara V, Dastidar P, et al: Reversible posterior leukoencephalopathy after combination chemotherapy. Neuroradiology 2000;42:895–899.

240. Russell MT, Nassif AS, Cacayorin ED, Awwad E, Perman W, Dunphy F: Gemcitabine-associated posterior reversible encephalopathy syndrome: MR imaging and MR spectroscopy findings. Magn Reson Imaging 2001;19:129–132.

241. Wong R, Beguelin GZ, De Lima M, et al: Tacrolimus-associated posterior reversible encephalopathy syndrome after allogeneic haematopoietic stem cell transplantation. Br J Haematol 2003;122:128–134.

242. Cosottini M, Lazzarotti G, Ceravolo R, Michelassi MC, Canapicchi R, Murri L: Cyclosporine-related posterior reversible encephalopathy syndrome (PRES) in non-transplant patient: A case report and literature review. Eur J Neurol 2003;10:461–462.

243. Gutin PH, Weiss HD, Wiernik PH, Walker MD: Intrathecal N, N', N''-triethylenethiophosphoramide [thio-TEPA (NSC 6396)] in the treatment of malignant meningeal disease: Phase I-II study. Cancer 1976;38:1471.

244. Gutin PH, Levi JA, Wiernik PH, Walker MD: Treatment of malignant meningeal disease with intrathecal thioTEPA: A phase II study. Cancer Treat Rep 1977;61:885.

245. Collins RC, Al-mondhiry H, Chernik NL, Posner JB: Neurologic manifestations of intravascular coagulation in patients with cancer: A clinical-pathological analysis of 12 cases. Neurology 1975;25:795.

246. Stefenelli T, Kuzmits R, Ulrich W, Glogar D: Acute vascular toxicity after combination chemotherapy with cisplatin, vinblastine, and bleomycin for testicular cancer. Eur Heart J 1988;9:552.

247. Anderson NE, Rosenblum MK, Posner JB: Paraneoplastic cerebellar degeneration: Clinico-immunological correlations. Ann Neurol 1988;24:559.

248. Furneaux HM, Rosenblum MK, Dalmau J, et al: Selective expression of Purkinje-cell antigens in tumor tissue from patients with paraneoplastic cerebellar degeneration. N Engl J Med 1990;322:1844.

249. Greenberg HS, Deck MD, Vikram B, et al: Metastasis to the base of the skull: Clinical findings in 43 patients. Neurology 1981;31:530.

250. Brown T, Havlin K, Weiss G, et al: A phase I trial of Taxol given by a 6-hour intravenous infusion. J Clin Oncol 1991;9:1261.

251. Moore RY, Oda Y: Malignant lymphoma with diffuse involvement of peripheral nerves. Neurology 1962;12:186.

252. Teoh R, Barnard RO, Gautier-Smith PC: Polyneuritis cranialis as a presentation of malignant lymphoma. J Neurol Sci 1990;48:399.

253. Grunwald GB, Kornguth SE, Towfighi J, et al: Autoimmune basis of visual paraneoplastic syndrome in patients with small cell lung carcinoma. Cancer 1987;60:780.

254. Byrne TN: Spinal cord compression from epidural metastases. N Engl J Med 1992;327:614.

255. Henson RA, Ulrich H: Encephalomyelitis. In Cancer and the Nervous System. Oxford, UK, Blackwell Scientific, 1980, p 314.

256. Croft PB, Wilkinson M: The incidence of carcinomatous neuromyopathy in patients with various types of carcinoma. Brain 1965;88:427.

257. Horwich MS, Cho L, Porro RS, Posner JB: Subacute sensory neuropathy: A remote effect of carcinoma. Ann Neurol 1977;19:2.

258. Grisold W, Drlicek M, Popp W, Jellinger K: Paraneoplastic sensory neuropathy, revisited. Neurology 1988;38:508.

259. Schold SC, Cho ES, Somasundaram M, Posner JB: Subacute motor neuropathy: A remote effect of lymphoma. Ann Neurol 1979;5:271.

260. DeVere R, Bradley WG: Polymyositis: Its presentation, morbidity and mortality. Brain 1976;98:637.

261. Barnes BE: Dermatomyositis and malignancy: A review of the literature. Ann Intern Med 1976;84:68.

262. Hildebrand J, Joffroy A, Vauthier J, Flament-Durand J: [Neuro-toxicity of formyl leurosine: An experimental and clinical study (author's transl)]. Acta Neurol Belg 1979;79:322.

263. Mayo Clinic and Mayo Foundation: Clinical Examinations in Neurology, 6th ed. St. Louis, Mosby–Year Book, 1991.

264. Haerer AF: DeJong's The Neurologic Examination, 5th ed. Philadelphia, JB Lippincott, 1992.

265. Strub RA, Black FW: The Mental Status Examination in Neurology, 2nd ed. Philadelphia, FA Davis, 1992.

266. O'Brien MD (ed): Aids to the Examination of the Peripheral Nervous System. London, Bailliere-Tindall, 1986.

267. Elderson A, Gerritsen van der Hoop R, Haanstra W, et al: Vibration perception and thermoperception as quantitative measurements in the monitoring of cisplatin induced neurotoxicity. J Neurol Sci 1989;93:167.

268. Rowinsky EK, Gilbert MR, McGuire WP, et al: Sequences of Taxol and cisplatin: A phase I and pharmacologic study. J Clin Oncol 1991;9:1692.

269. Gerritsen van der Hoop R, de Koning P, Boven E, et al: Efficacy of the neuropeptide ORG.2766 in the prevention and treatment of cisplatin-indued neurotoxicity in rats. Eur J Cancer Clin Oncol 1988;24:637.

270. Muller LJ, Gerritsen van der Hoop R, Moorer-van Delft CM, et al: Morphological and electrophysiological study of the effects of cisplatin and ORG-2766 on rat spinal ganglion neurons. Cancer Res 1990;50:2437.

271. Windebank AJ, Smith AG, Russell JW: The effect of nerve growth factor, ciliary neurotrophic factor, and ACTH analogs on cisplatin neurotoxicity in vitro. Neurology 1994;44:488.

272. Leong SS, Tan EH, Fong KW, et al: Randomized double-blind trial of combined modality treatment with or without amifostine in unresectable stage III non-small-cell lung cancer. J Clin Oncol 2003;21:1767–1774.

273. Lorusso D, Ferrandina G, Greggi S, et al: Phase III multicenter randomized trial of amifostine as cytoprotectant in first-line chemotherapy in ovarian cancer patients. Ann Oncol 2003;14:1086–1093.

274. Vahdat L, Papadopoulos K, Lange D, et al: Reduction of paclitaxel-induced peripheral neuropathy with glutamine. Clin Cancer Res 2001;7:1192–1197.

275. Gandara DR, Wiebe VJ, Perez EA, et al: Cisplatin rescue therapy: Experience with sodium thiosulfate, WR2721, and diethyldithiocarbamate. Crit Rev Oncol Hematol 1990;10:353.

276. Grossman SA, Trump DL, Chen DC, et al: Cerebrospinal fluid flow abnormalities in patients with neoplastic meningitis: An evaluation using 111indium-DTPA ventriculography. Am J Med 1982;73:641.

277. Chamberlain MC, Corey-Bloom J: Leptomeningeal metastases: 111indium-DTPA CSF flow studies. Neurology 1991;41:1765.

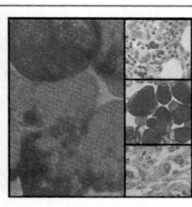

62

PULMONARY COMPLICATIONS OF ANTICANCER TREATMENT

Mitchell Machtay

SUMMARY OF KEY POINTS

RADIATION PNEUMONITIS: RISK FACTORS

- Older age
- Lower performance status
- Lower baseline pulmonary function
- Large radiation volume treated with more than 20 Gy
- ?Cumulative radiation dose
- ?Lower lobe primary tumor
- ?Transforming growth factor β serum levels

RADIATION PNEUMONITIS: DIAGNOSIS

- The most predominant symptoms are dyspnea and hypoxia, especially on exertion.
- Fever (usually low grade) is common.
- Diffusing capacity of the lung for carbon dioxide is the most sensitive value during pulmonary function testing.
- Interstitial or ground-glass infiltrate usually, but not always, corresponds well to the irradiated volume.
- Findings at bronchoscopy are relatively unremarkable (bronchial lavage may reveal lymphocytosis).
- Pulmonary embolism, infection, and progressive tumor must be ruled out. These conditions can coexist with radiation pneumonitis.
- Response to corticosteroids is rapid.

RADIATION PNEUMONITIS: TREATMENT

- The best treatment is prevention. Patients must be selected carefully for thoracic radiation, and irradiated volumes must be limited.

- Corticosteroids have no prophylactic or therapeutic value in the management of long-term radiation fibrosis but are very useful in the management of acute and subacute pneumonitis.
- Consultation with a pulmonologist is necessary.
- Oxygen is administered as indicated to prevent hypoxia.
- High doses of corticosteroids (60 mg/day of prednisone) with slow tapering are needed for severe grade 2 or any grade 3 radiation pneumonitis.
- If prolonged corticosteroid treatment is anticipated, prophylaxis against corticosteroid complications is needed. These measures include gastrointestinal prophylaxis, diet and pharmacologic management of hyperglycemia, infection prophylaxis, and osteoporosis prophylaxis.
- Antibiotics, bronchodilators, diuretics, and anticoagulation are administered as indicated for coexisting cardiopulmonary illnesses.

DRUG-INDUCED LUNG INJURY: RISK FACTORS

- Usually bleomycin, nitrosoureas, and mitomycin
- Bone marrow transplantation
- Concurrent or recent thoracic radiation therapy
- Lower baseline pulmonary function

DRUG-INDUCED LUNG INJURY: DIAGNOSIS

- Dyspnea and hypoxia are predominant, but a wide range of possible symptoms exist.

- Interstitial or ground-glass infiltrate usually is diffuse throughout both lungs and may be worse in the lower lobes.
- Findings at bronchoscopy are relatively unremarkable (bronchial lavage may reveal lymphocytosis).
- Pulmonary embolism, infection, and progressive tumor must be ruled out and may coexist with drug-induced lung injury.
- Injury is usually (but not universally) corticosteroid responsive.

DRUG-INDUCED LUNG INJURY: TREATMENT

- When the diagnosis is suspected, the suspected causative agent should be discontinued.
- Consultation with a pulmonologist is necessary.
- Oxygen is administered as indicated to prevent hypoxia.
- High doses of corticosteroids (≥ 60 mg/day of prednisone) with slow taper may be needed for severe grade 2 or any grade 3 pneumonitis.
- If prolonged corticosteroid treatment is anticipated, prophylaxis against corticosteroid complications entails gastrointestinal prophylaxis, diet or pharmacologic management of hyperglycemia, infection prophylaxis, and osteoporosis prophylaxis.
- Antibiotics, bronchodilators, diuretics, and anticoagulation are administered as indicated to manage coexisting cardiopulmonary illnesses.

INTRODUCTION

Although relatively uncommon, pulmonary disorders are among the most feared complications of anticancer therapy. Many cancer patients have some degree of underlying respiratory dysfunction; thus a relatively minor challenge to the lungs can result in respiratory failure and death.

The two major categories of pulmonary complications are radiation pneumonopathy and drug-induced pneumonopathy. These conditions do not include other major categories of pulmonary disease in cancer patients, such as pulmonary embolism, infection (community acquired, atypical, and aspiration pneumonia), and anatomic complications of tumor or surgery, such as pulmonary hemorrhage and fistula. Radiation therapy or chemotherapy can contribute to these multifactorial problems of the respiratory system.

Radiation pneumonopathy and drug-induced pneumonopathy share several important features, most notably that they are usually processes of the interstitium of the lung and thus can cause marked impairment of gas exchange and dyspnea. Corticosteroids are the mainstay of management of both types of pneumonopathy but may provide at best a Pyrrhic victory and at worst can cause life-threatening infections or other complications. Better techniques for avoiding treatment-related pneumonop-

athy—and better therapy for established pneumonopathy—will come only from improved understanding of and intervention against the complex molecular processes that cause and maintain these pathologic states.

PULMONARY TOXICITY OF THORACIC RADIATION THERAPY

Thoracic radiation is probably the most important cause of pulmonary toxicity in oncology. Lung toxicity from radiation is a clinically relevant issue for lymphoma, breast cancer, bone marrow transplantation (BMT), esophageal cancer, and lung cancer. Figure 62-1 illustrates a typical case of radiation pneumonitis and its sequelae.

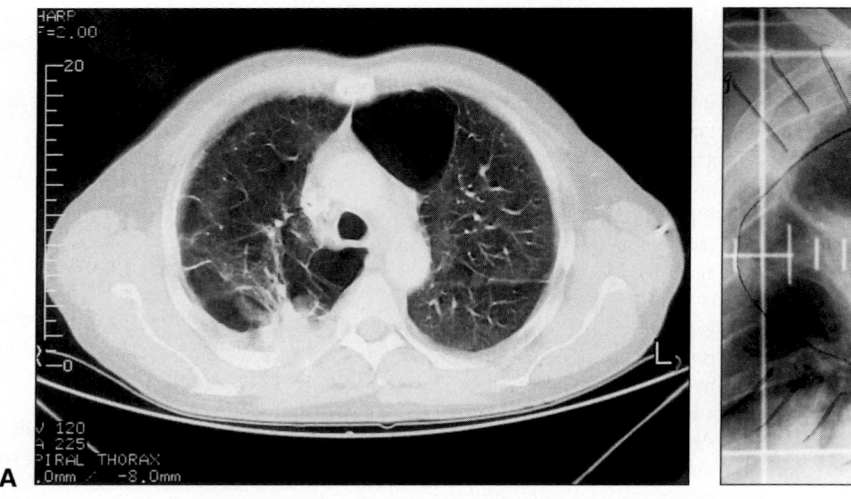
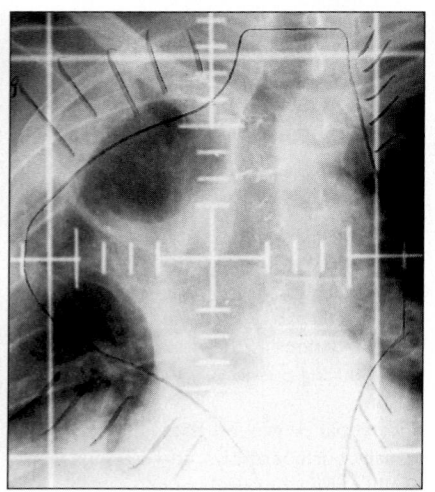
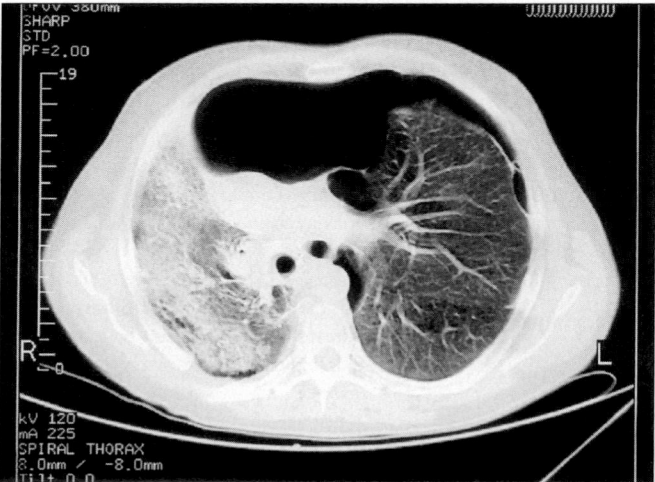
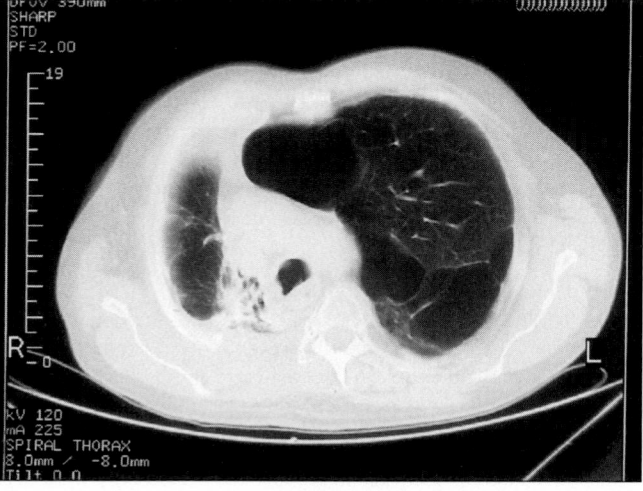

Figure 62-1. Case example of radiation pneumonopathy. **A,** Diagnostic computed tomographic (CT) scan shows signs of advanced chronic obstructive pulmonary disease with bullous disease in an elderly man who had dyspnea and chest pain. Posteriorly located adenocarcinoma of the lung was found and clinically staged $T_3N_0M_0$. **B,** Radiation simulation image. The patient underwent gross total surgical resection but was found to have positive tumor margins and received radical radiation therapy to the chest. **C,** CT scan. Approximately 6 weeks after radiation therapy progressively severe dyspnea developed, culminating in profound dyspnea necessitating hospitalization. Grade 3 acute radiation pneumonitis in the right lung was found with left-sided pneumothorax. The patient was treated with steroids, antibiotics, and a Pleurx catheter. **D,** CT scan. Approximately 1 year later the patient's condition was stable with no evidence of recurrent cancer. The patient had discontinued steroid therapy but needed intermittent oxygen therapy for radiation fibrosis of the right lung.

The mechanisms behind radiation-induced lung injury remain poorly understood despite decades of study. A detailed review of the histopathologic and molecular events occurring in radiation pneumonopathy is beyond the scope of this chapter, and several excellent reviews have been published.[1-3] Irradiation damages endothelial cells, epithelial cells (particularly surfactant-producing type II pneumocytes), and reticuloendothelial cells within the lung through several mechanisms, including apoptosis and induction of stress response genes. It is now generally agreed that cytokines, such as transforming growth factor β (TGF-β), play a major role in promoting radiation pneumonopathy, including development of long-term fibrosis.[4] It can be difficult histopathologically (or molecularly) to differentiate established radiation lung injury from other forms of end-stage lung disease, such as idiopathic pulmonary fibrosis, drug-induced injury, or even very advanced chronic obstructive pulmonary disease (COPD). Traditional clinical understanding of radiation lung injury recognizes two distinct syndromes: (1) radiation pneumonitis and (2) radiation fibrosis of the lung. Radiation pneumonitis is characterized by intense interstitial inflammation and alveolar exudate. It develops over several weeks to months after irradiation and (if the host/patient survives) resolves within 6 to 12 months. Radiation pulmonary fibrosis, in contrast, generally does not begin until several months after radiation therapy but progresses relentlessly over years. Radiation pneumonitis usually responds well to corticosteroids. Many oncologists confirm the diagnosis on the basis of an empirical trial of steroids. In contrast, corticosteroids do not influence progression of radiation pulmonary fibrosis.

In most cases, radiation lung injury is confined to the regions of lung within the radiation field or portal. This conventional wisdom has been challenged by several researchers who have found evidence of "out-of-field" radiation injury, which may manifest in a syndrome similar to bronchiolitis obliterans with organizing pneumonia (BOOP).[5] In the most severe cases, diffuse acute respiratory distress syndrome may result from partial lung irradiation.[6] Autoimmunity has been hypothesized as a mechanism of out-of-field radiation lung injury, with the possibility that localized lung damage triggers diffuse lymphocyte-mediated hypersensitivity against pulmonary self antigens.[7]

Radiation lung injury may have any of a variety of clinical and radiographic presentations, but the hallmark is generally dyspnea out of proportion to other findings. The most common imaging finding is an interstitial infiltrate corresponding to the radiation portals, but it is not unusual to find consolidation, nodularity, or even pleural effusions. This problem can make the differential diagnosis among recurrent/progressive cancer, infection, and radiation lung injury extremely difficult, particularly in patients with lung cancer. Positron emission tomography with fluorodeoxyglucose (FDG) may be helpful for differentiating recurrence from radiation toxicity, although intense radiation pneumonitis and even actively developing fibrosis can cause elevated FDG uptake.[8,9]

Incidence of Radiation Lung Injury and Predictive Factors

The most important factor influencing development of clinically relevant radiation lung injury is the volume of lung irradiated.[10-14] In radiation oncology, the lung is considered a parallel-architecture organ, meaning that destruction of very small portions of it should not cause overall organ dysfunction. In contrast, other organs, such as the spinal cord, are considered series-architecture organs, in which destruction of one region will lead to irreversible dysfunction downstream from that injury.[15]

Irradiation of the entire lung volume (bilateral lungs) is uncommon today, except as part of total body irradiation for selected BMT conditioning regimens. The therapeutic index for whole lung irradiation is extraordinarily narrow. For example, upper hemibody irradiation (for diffuse bone metastasis) has relatively little toxicity at a single dose of 6 Gy,[16] but an increase to 8 Gy results in high risk of life-threatening pulmonary toxicity.[17] A single-fraction dose of 10 Gy to the entire lungs is nearly universally lethal. The safety of total body irradiation for BMT has been enhanced by use of fractionation, partial lung transmission shielding,[18] and decreased radiation dose rate.[19]

At the other extreme, irradiation of small lung volumes rarely results in radiation pneumonitis. For example, in tangential irradiation of the breast (after lumpectomy) or chest wall (after mastectomy), the risk of clinically significant radiation pneumonitis is approximately 1%, increasing to approximately 5% with addition of irradiation of the regional (axillary/supraclavicular) nodes.[20] Radiation pneumonitis after small-volume thoracic radiation therapy such as this may be relatively mild and usually resolves completely.

Understanding the true incidence of radiation pneumonopathy is complicated by limitations of the historical and current standards for defining and grading this illness. Grade 1 radiation lung injury (Table 62-1) is almost certainly underreported, and the distinction between grade 2 and grade 3 toxicity is highly subjective.[21] Furthermore, the Radiation Therapy Oncology Group (RTOG) and others have arbitrarily divided toxicity scales into early versus late, on the basis of a 90-day cutoff point from the start of radiation therapy. This distinction is useful for some radiation therapy effects but extremely inappropriate for lung toxicity, in which the "early" or acute toxicity (pneumonitis) might not begin for several months after completion of radiation therapy. Finally, the current toxicity scales do not account for intercurrent organ dysfunction from tumor, infection, or chronic illnesses such as COPD, all of which are particularly common in patients with malignant thoracic tumors. It is important to remember that COPD by itself (in the absence of lung cancer) has an extremely high rate of morbidity and mortality.[22]

The National Cancer Institute and its cooperative groups, including RTOG, have finalized CTC version 3.0, renamed *Common Terminology Criteria for Adverse Events*, an extensive update and reorganization of the common toxicity scales.[23] The CTCv3.0 preliminary definitions and grading for selected pulmonary events are

TABLE 62-1

Traditional Scoring System for Radiation Lung Injury[21]

EVENT	GRADE 1	GRADE 2	GRADE 3	GRADE 4
Radiation pneumonitis (RTOG criteria)	Mild symptoms of dry cough or dyspnea on exertion	Persistent cough requiring narcotic antitussive agents/dyspnea with minimal effort but not at rest	Severe cough, unresponsive to narcotic antitussive agents, dyspnea at rest, clinical or radiographic evidence of acute pneumonitis, intermittent oxygen requirements, or requirements for steroids	Severe respiratory insufficiency with requirements for continuous oxygen
Radiation lung fibrosis (RTOG/EORTC criteria)	Asymptomatic or mild symptoms—dry cough, slight radiographic changes	Moderate symptomatic fibrosis	Severe symptomatic fibrosis, dense radiographic changes	Severe respiratory insufficiency, oxygen required, or assisted ventilation

Grade 0 (not shown), absence of the adverse event; Grade 5 (not shown) death related to the adverse event; EORTC, European Organization for Research and Treatment of Cancer; RTOG, Radiation Therapy Oncology Group.

shown in Table 62-2. There have been numerous changes to the scoring criteria in the pulmonology section, and separate scales are no longer used for early and late radiation therapy–related events.

Despite limitations of the scoring systems for radiation lung injury, some clinical studies provide insight into the complex relations among volume of lung irradiated, regions of lung irradiated, radiation dose, and host factors.[14] Table 62-3 summarizes the literature on this topic. Most clinical radiation oncology studies have focused on the concept of the dose-volume histogram (DVH), in which percentage of total lung irradiated is plotted against radiation dose.[10,11,24] With modern radiation planning software integrating findings at computed tomography (CT), DVHs are easy to generate. However, there is no consensus on how to interpret these plots. Some researchers suggest the most relevant information obtained from DVHs is the V20 (percentage of total lung volume irradiated to >20 Gy (conventionally fractionated radiation therapy).[11] The concept of DVH and V20 is shown in Figure 62-2.

Some experts have recommended using V30 (percentage of total lung volume irradiated to >30 Gy),[25] mean lung dose,[26] or a variety of other values. Retrospective studies conducted with moderate to large samples of patients with analyzable DVHs and clinical courses have clearly shown that lung toxicity is associated with lung DVH characteristics that reflect large volumes of irradiated lung. However, studies have not clearly defined a safe lung DVH in therapy for lung cancer.

A major problem with the tool of DVH analysis that may explain its limited reliability is that it is based purely on anatomic data with no consideration of lung physiology or other patient-related factors. In a DVH every cubic centimeter of lung tissue is considered to have the same physiologic utility to the patient. To minimize this problem, radiation oncologists may exclude grossly nonfunctional lung (e.g., consolidation, tumor, bleb) from analysis, but subtle differences in gas-exchange ability in different areas of the lung almost certainly still exist. In an

effort to address this issue, some investigators have integrated nuclear medicine lung ventilation/perfusion scanning into radiation planning.[27,28] This technique has not become readily available, partly because of difficulties in fusing nuclear medicine images (which often have poor anatomic delineation) with CT scans.

Studies of DVHs have been conducted almost entirely with patients treated with conventionally fractionated radiation therapy (1.8–2.15 Gy once daily) without use of concurrent chemotherapy. It is clear that large daily fractions of radiation therapy are more toxic than conventional fraction sizes. In a literature review of the cases of 1911 lung cancer patients treated with chemoradiotherapy, Roach and colleagues[29] found that the most important predictor of radiation pneumonitis was radiation fraction size, specifically fraction size ≥2.67 Gy.

Although neoadjuvant (before radiation therapy) chemotherapy probably does not greatly affect the risk of radiation pneumonitis, concurrent chemotherapy appears to increase the risk of pulmonary toxicity. Certain chemotherapy agents given during radiation therapy, in particular the anthracyclines (such as doxorubicin or dactinomycin),[30-32] bleomycin,[33,34] and gemcitabine,[35] appear to carry a higher risk of sensitizing the lung to radiation injury. The data regarding paclitaxel, which has become one of the most popular agents to give during thoracic radiation therapy, are less certain and controversial.[36-39] Some experts have suggested that taxane-containing concurrent chemoradiotherapy regimens are more likely to induce radiation lung injury than is a traditional platin/vinca or platin/etoposide regimen.

Nontreatment factors that appear to be predictive of radiation lung injury have been studied. Not surprisingly, pretreatment performance status has been shown to correlate with development of clinical radiation pneumonopathy.[40] Pretreatment pulmonary function is probably an important factor,[41] although its utility is confounded by the fact that medium to large thoracic tumors typically adversely affect results of pulmonary function tests, which may improve after successful radiation therapy. Advanced

TABLE 62-2

CTC v3 (as of May 2003)[23] Selected Common Terminology Criteria for Adverse Events

EVENT	GRADE 1	GRADE 2	GRADE 3	GRADE 4
ARDS	N/A	N/A	Present; intubation not required	Present; intubation required
Aspiration	Asymptomatic "silent" aspiration	Symptomatic (e.g., altered eating habits, coughing/choking); medical intervention indicated (e.g., antibiotics, suction or oxygen)	Clinical or radiographic signs of pneumonia or pneumonitis; unable to aliment orally	Life-threatening (e.g., aspiration pneumonia or pneumonitis)
Atelectasis	Asymptomatic	Symptomatic; medical intervention indicated (e.g., bronchoscopic suctioning)	Operative (e.g., stent, laser) intervention indicated	Life-threatening respiratory compromise
Carbon monoxide diffusion capacity abnormality	90%–75% of predicted	<75%–50% of predicted	<50%–25% of predicted	<25% of predicted
Cough	Symptomatic, nonnarcotic medication only indicated	Symptomatic and narcotic medication indicated	Symptomatic and significantly interfering with sleep or ADL	N/A
Dyspnea	Dyspnea on exertion but can walk 1 flight of stairs without stopping	Dyspnea on exertion; unable to walk 1 flight of stairs or 1 city block (0.1 km) without stopping	Dyspnea with ADL (dressing, undressing, talking, eating)	Dyspnea at rest; intubation/ventilator indicated
FEV_1	90%–75% of predicted	<75%–50% of predicted	<50%–25% of predicted	<25% of predicted
Fistula	Asymptomatic Radiographic findings only	Symptomatic, tube thoracostomy or medical management indicated; associated with altered respiratory function but not interfering with ADL	Symptomatic and associated with altered respiratory function interfering with ADL; endoscopic (e.g., stent) or primary closure by operative intervention indicated	Life-threatening consequences; operative intervention with thoracoplasty, long-term open drainage or multiple thoracotomies indicated
Hypoxia	N/A	Decreased O_2 saturation with exercise (e.g., pulse oximeter <88%); intermittent supplemental oxygen	Decreased O_2 saturation at rest; continuous oxygen indicated	Life-threatening; intubation/ventilation indicated
Pleural effusion (nonmalignant)	Asymptomatic	Symptomatic; intervention such as diuretics or up to two therapeutic thoracenteses indicated	Symptomatic and supplemental oxygen, more than two therapeutic thoracenteses, tube drainage or pleurodesis indicated	Life-threatening (e.g., causing hemodynamic instability or ventilatory support indicated)
Pneumonitis, infiltrates	Asymptomatic; radiographic fiindings	Symptomatic, not interfering with ADL	Symptomatic, interfering with ADL; O_2 indicated	Life-threatening or ventilatory support indicated
Pneumothorax	Asymptomatic; radiographic findings	Symptomatic; intervention indicated (e.g., hospitalization for observation, tube placement without sclerosis)	Sclerosis and/or operative intervention indicated	Life-threatening, causing hemodynamic instability (e.g., tension pneumothorax) or ventilatory support indicated
Prolonged chest tube drainage or air leak after lung operation	N/A	Sclerosis or additional tube thoracostomy indicated	Operative intervention indicated (e.g., thoracotomy with stapling or sealant)	Life-threatening or debilitating or organ resection indicated
Prolonged intubation after pulmonary resection	N/A	Extubated within 24–72 hr postoperatively	Extubated >72 hr postoperatively but before tracheostomy indicated	Tracheostomy indicated
Pulmonary fibrosis (radiographic changes)	Minimal findings (or patchy or bibasilar changes); estimated radiographic portion of total lung volume that is fibrotic of <25%	Patchy or bibasilar changes with estimated total lung volume that is fibrotic or 25%–50%	Dense or widespread infiltrates/consolidation with estimated radiographic proportion of total lung that is fibrotic of 50%–74%	Estimated radiographic proporton or total lung volume that is fibrotic is > 75%; honeycombing

Grade 0 (not shown), absence of the adverse event; Grade 5 (not shown), death related to the adverse event; ADL, activities of daily living (e.g., feeding self, toileting; ARDS, acute respiratory distress syndrome; FEV_1, forced expiratory volume in 1 second; N/A, not applicable.

Problems Common to Cancer and its Therapy

II

TABLE 62-3

Selected Clinical Studies of the Incidence and Severity of Radiation Pneumonopathy

STUDY	NO. OF PATIENTS CHARACTERISTICS	GRADE 2+ PNEUMONOPATHY	GRADE 3+ PNEUMONOPATHY	FATAL	COMMENTS
Studies in Lung Cancer					
Byhardt/RTOG[119] 1998	388 pts with lung CA treated with chemo and RT	NS	17%	1.5%	
	136 pts with sequential chemo followed by RT	NS	10%	1%	
	252 pts with concurrent chemo RT	NS	20%	2%	
Keller/Intergroup[120] 2000	488 pts with lung CA treated with RT +/– chemo after surgery	NS	3.5%	1%	No difference with or without chemo
Turrisi/Intergroup[121] 1999	417 pts limited stage small cell lung CA treated with concurrent RT/chemo	12%	5%	1%	No difference for once-daily vs twice-daily RT
Hernando/Duke[25] 2001	201 pts with lung CA	18%	4%	NS	RP correlated with V30 above/below 18% (24 vs 6%)
Sim/MSKCC[122] 2002	152 pts with lung CA	33%	14%	2%	Grade 3+ RP correlated with mean lung dose in a substudy[13]
Robnett[40] 2000	148 pts with lung CA	NS	8%	1%	Grade 3+ RP was 16% for PS1 vs 2% for PS0
Graham/Washington Univ.[11] 1999	99 pts with lung CA	22%	8%	4%	
	54 pts wih V20 <32%	6%	0%	0%	
	45 pts with V20 >32%	27%	18%	9%	
Studies of Other Thoracic Malignant Tumors					
Lind (breast CA)[20] 2002	613 pts with breast CA	2.4%	NS	NS	RP was 1% for tangent RT vs 5% for regional RT
Hughes-Davies/JCRT (Hodgkin's)[123] 1998	172 pts with bulky intrathoracic Hodgkin's disease	14%	NS	1%	
Cooper/RTOG (esophagus)[124] 1999	117 pts with esophagus CA treated with chemo RT	NS	3%	1%	

CA, cancer; JCRT, Joint Center for Radiation Therapy; MSKCC, Memorial Sloan-Kettering Cancer Center; NS, not significant; PS, performance status; RP, radiation pneumonopathy; RT, radiation therapy; RTOG, Radiation Therapy Oncology Group; V20, V30, percentage of total lung volume irradiated to ≥20 Gy, >30 Gy.

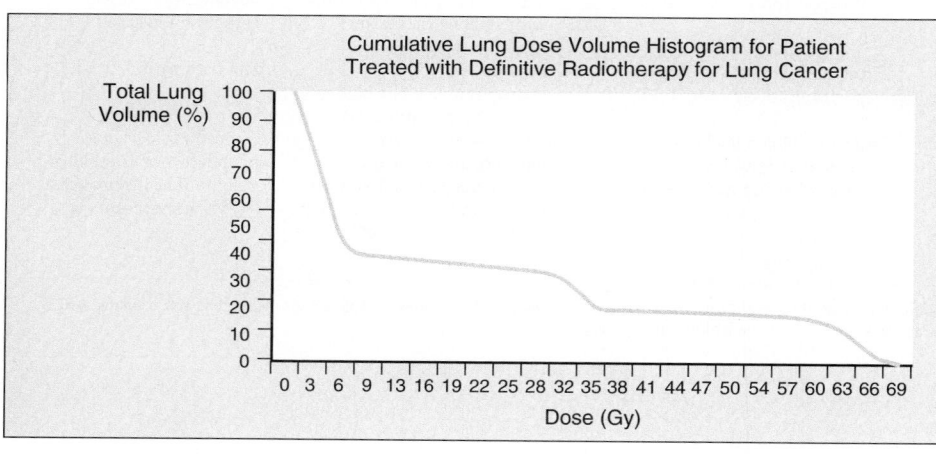

Figure 62-2. Graphic representation (*yellow curve*) of dose-volume histogram for total lung volume irradiated to a nominal dose of 63 Gy in a patient with lung cancer. In this case the V20 (the percentage of total lung volume receiving >20 Gy) is approximately 36%, which is considered a moderate-risk dose level for clinical radiation pneumonopathy.

age, perhaps as a surrogate marker for pulmonary reserve, seems to be associated with a higher risk of radiation pneumonopathy and its severity.[42]

Diagnosis and Management of Radiation Pneumonitis

With modern, conformal, multifield radiation therapy, it is no longer possible to simply look for pathognomonic rectangular infiltrates on a chest radiograph. A patient who has recently undergone radiation treatment and has dyspnea or other pulmonary symptoms of greater than grade 1 intensity needs a thorough evaluation that includes CT of the thorax.[43] In selected circumstances the evaluation should include high-resolution thin-section scanning to rule out pulmonary embolism. Pulse oximetry or arterial blood gas testing should be performed to assess the need for supplemental oxygen. The tests and procedures to be considered in evaluation of cancer patients with suspected pneumonopathy are summarized in Table 62-4.

If the clinical manifestations and test results are consistent with grade 2 or greater radiation pneumonitis, administration of corticosteroids should be instituted in most cases. Controlled randomized trials of corticosteroids for radiation pneumonitis have not been conducted with human subjects. However, the efficacy of corticosteroids has been well established in nonrandomized clinical studies[44] and in preclinical models.[45,46] A large variety of initial and tapering steroid regimens exist, and the exact schedule must be tailored to the individual patient. In general, for severe (grade 3) radiation pneumonitis, prednisone approximately 1 mg/kg/day is indicated for 2 weeks. Brief hospitalization for intravenous administration of steroids may be indicated. After several weeks, the dose should be tapered gently, by approximately 10 mg every 2 weeks. It is not unusual for patients to have a symptomatic relapse in the setting of steroid taper.[47] If relapse occurs, it is important to rule out concomitant infection. If the diagnosis of recurrent radiation pneumonitis is confirmed, the steroid dose should be increased and titrated accordingly.

With these guidelines, the typical patient with grade 3 or intense grade 2 radiation lung injury must take steroids for approximately 3 months. Some patients need steroids for considerably longer, although the benefit after 6 months is dubious (when radiation pneumonitis has generally resolved and may be superseded by fibrosis). At the outset, the physician should explain to the patient the potential need and implications of longer-term steroid use. A proton-pump inhibitor or histamine$_2$-blocker should be prescribed to counteract gastritis. Consideration should be given to evaluation for and medical prophylaxis against osteoporosis. Patients should be counseled about exercise (as tolerated by their pulmonary symptoms) and diet to minimize problems with steroid-induced hyperglycemia and muscle wasting. Blood chemistry values, including fasting glucose, liver function tests, and albumin, should be checked periodically. If a diuretic is being used with steroids, it is important to check serum electrolyte levels frequently.

It is uncertain whether a low-dose "prophylactic" antibiotic should be prescribed. In light of the profound lymphopenia that most patients have after chemoradiation therapy and steroid treatment (as with typical concurrent paclitaxel–radiation therapy regimens), it may be appropriate to prescribe an every-other-day dose of trimethoprim-sulfamethoxazole (Bactrim) when starting high-dose steroids.[48] If findings at chest CT suggest the presence of coexistent active infection, broader and more intense antibiotics are indicated. The patient should undergo bronchoscopy if there is no improvement after several days of steroid and antibiotic therapy.

TABLE 62-4

Evaluation of Patient with Dyspnea or Suspected Radiation or Chemotherapy Pneumonopathy

STUDY	RATIONALE
CT of chest with and without contrast material	Assess extent and appearance of infiltrates and other findings, correlate with radiation therapy data. Rule out recurrent progressive cancer.
High-resolution pulmonary embolism protocol CT	Rule out pulmonary embolism.
Pulse oximetry (at rest and after ambulation)	Assess need for supplemental oxygen.
Pulmonary function tests (spirometry, D$_{LCO}$)	Assess extent of impairment of pulmonary function; especially useful if baseline measurements exist.
Complete blood count	Assess white blood cell count (signs of infection) and hemoglobin concentration (anemia contributes to dyspnea).
Blood culture	Rule out sepsis and infectious endocarditis.
Electrocardiogram	Assess for dysrhythmia, signs of cardiac ischemia or inflammation.
Echocardiogram	Assess for pericarditis and percardial effusion, heart failure.
Ventilation/perfusion lung scan, pulmonary angiogram, or both	Rule out pulmonary embolism.
Bronchoscopy	Assess for infection (particularly atypical infection) and recurrent or progressive cancer.
Open lung biopsy (e.g., thoracoscopic biopsy)	Avoid because of risks of general anesthesia; may be necessary if diagnosis remains uncertain and there is no response to steroids.

D$_{LCO}$, diffusing capacity of the lung for carbon dioxide.

The prognosis of grade 1–2 radiation pneumonitis is relatively good with meticulous supportive care and the use of steroids as needed. Grade 3 radiation pneumonitis, however, at least in lung cancer patients, has a poor prognosis.[49] It is uncertain whether this is the direct result of radiation pneumonitis or coexisting problems, including tumor recurrence and infection.

Management of Radiation Pulmonary Fibrosis

Although radiation pneumonitis usually is relieved with steroids, radiation pulmonary fibrosis does not. Some patients undergoing steroid therapy for radiation pneumonitis eventually start to experience worsening pulmonary function. This decline may be caused by pulmonary fibrosis but also may be caused at least in part by disorders such as infection, cardiac problems, and pulmonary embolism, and reevaluation is indicated. If it has been more than 6 months since the patient has undergone radiation therapy (or chemotherapy, because some chemotherapy drugs can induce radiation recall reactions in the lung), increasing the steroid dose is unlikely to yield benefit.

Management of radiation pulmonary fibrosis is supportive. Emphasis is on administration of oxygen, management of acute infection, bronchodilator therapy, and maximization of the other components of oxygen delivery (e.g., cardiac and blood pressure medications and correction of anemia). It is unknown whether pulmonary rehabilitation programs involving exercise and weight maintenance are helpful for radiation pulmonary fibrosis. Tobacco should be strictly avoided.

Trials of Prevention or Management of Radiation Pulmonary Fibrosis

As shown in Table 62-5, results of studies have suggested that prophylactic administration of amifostine during thoracic radiation therapy ameliorates radiation pneumonitis.[50,51] These studies were relatively immature and conducted in a patient population with a short life expectancy (locally advanced lung cancer), so it is unclear at this time whether this drug will have long-term antifibrotic protection. Preclinical data support the role of amifostine as a protective agent against radiation pulmonary fibrosis.[52]

Other nonspecific antioxidants have been studied as means of decreasing radiation fibrosis, although they are not necessarily specific for the lung.[53] Gene therapy to deliver antioxidants to the lung is under study. Researchers from the University of Pittsburgh have developed a system in which the gene for the potent antioxidant enzyme manganese superoxide dismutase (MnSOD) can be transfected into a plasmid and administered by inhalation.[54-56] This approach, still highly experimental, may offer a treatment without the systemic effects induced by amifostine and steroids.

The use of angiotensin-converting enzyme (ACE) inhibitors, particularly captopril, has shown promise in preclinical rodent studies.[57] The mechanism of efficacy is unclear and may be related to the beneficial vasodilatory effects of these drugs on small blood vessels or may be due to antioxidant activity. The laboratory data can be criticized for being based on use of relative doses of captopril far in excess of the usual human dose. The only clinical (retrospective) study of ACE inhibitors did not show a protective effect.[58] However, clinical data have shown efficacy of captopril for radiation-induced renal dysfunction. The RTOG is developing an open-label randomized clinical trial of captopril (standard dose similar to that used for hypertension or heart disease) versus usual supportive care of patients receiving radiation therapy to the lung. The projected sample size is 178 patients, the primary end point being "long-term" (12-month) pulmonary damage attributable to radiation by CTC criteria.

Increased understanding of the cytokine-based mechanisms of radiation lung injury may offer opportunities for intervention.[3,59] Because TGF-β is thought to be the dominant profibrotic cytokine and perhaps even a cause of radiation pneumonitis, attempts are underway to develop molecules with anti–TGF-β activity.

TABLE 62-5

			GRADE 2+ RADIATION PNEUMONITIS CONTROL (WITHOUT AMIFOSTINE)	**GRADE 2+ RADIATION PNEUMONITIS WITH AMIFOSTINE**	
STUDY	**NO. OF PATIENTS/ CHARACTERISTICS**	**AMIFOSTINE DOSE**			**P VALUE**
Antonadou[50] 2001	97 stage III NSCLC treated to 55–60 Gy (no chemo)	340 mg/m²/day	43%	9%	.001
Antonadou[125] 2002	45 stage III NSCLC treated to 55–60 Gy + chemo	340 mg/m²/day	65%	32%	.038
Komaki[51] 2002	53 stage III NSCLC treated 69.6 Gy	500 mg twice weekly	23%	4%	.037

Randomized Trials of Effect of Amifostine on Radiation Pneumonitis After Thoracic Radiation Therapy with or Without Chemotherapy for Lung Cancer

NSCLC, non–small cell lung cancer.

Other Forms of Radiation Lung Injury

There is increasing recognition that high-dose radiation can contribute to other serious problems within the lung. One of the most feared complications is bronchopleural fistula, a postoperative complication that is significantly increased by the use of preoperative radiation therapy or chemoradiotherapy and is very difficult to manage.[60,61] Patients who receive neoadjuvant chemoradiation for stage III lung cancer should be considered for additional bronchial stump reinforcement (e.g., intercostal muscle flap) at the time of surgery in an effort to minimize this risk.

Endobronchial brachytherapy for palliation of obstructive endobronchial malignant tumors is associated with approximately 10% risk of severe pulmonary complications, including massive hemoptysis and bronchial stenosis.[62-64] It often is difficult to differentiate the contribution of irradiation to these serious events from the contribution of the tumor itself. Many of these patients have undergone brachytherapy as salvage treatment after previous full-dose external beam radiation therapy. Thus lifetime irradiation doses to the walls of the bronchi and adjacent blood vessels may be extremely high. Careful brachytherapy technique and smaller brachytherapy fraction size appear to reduce the risk of severe hemoptysis.[63,65]

External beam radiation therapy or chemoradiation may be associated with severe bronchial stenosis when radiation therapy doses are exceptionally high.[66] With increasing interest in intensified-dose radiation therapy with high-technology conformal techniques, this problem may become an increasing concern in the management of lung cancer. Prospective studies are in progress.[67]

As shown in the case example in Figure 62-1, radiation lung injury can be associated with pneumothorax, perhaps as a result of radiation fibrosis causing increased traction on the lung as well as direct radiation injury to the pleura.[68]

PULMONARY TOXICITY OF SYSTEMIC ANTICANCER THERAPIES

Many chemotherapy drugs can cause pulmonary toxicity, the incidence ranging from <1% to >30%. The drugs most associated with pulmonary toxicity are bleomycin, methotrexate, cytosine arabinoside, mitomycin, and the nitrosoureas (especially carmustine [BCNU]). Table 62-6 is a broad categorization of anticancer therapies into high, moderate, and low risks of pneumotoxicity, although any individual patient may experience severe lung problems from any agent.

Unlike thoracic radiation therapy, which usually affects only the portion of lung within the radiation field, systemic agents often cause diffuse pneumonopathy. Although it is relatively rare compared with radiation pneumonopathy, chemotherapy-induced lung injury can be extremely intense and even have a higher fatality rate than radiation pneumonitis. As with radiation pneumonitis, corticosteroids are commonly used and may be effective, particularly in early stages of injury. It is particularly important to rule out alternative and concurrent diagnoses (see Table 62-4). Unlike radiation injury, drug-induced lung toxicity can occur in a timeframe during which it is possible to discontinue the offending agent. A review of some of the agents associated with pulmonary toxicity follows.

Bleomycin

Bleomycin is the chemotherapy drug most commonly associated with lung damage. The reported incidence ranges from 3% to 40%.[69-71] This drug is predominantly used in the management of Hodgkin's disease and germ cell tumors, cancers that occur mainly in younger patients with less underlying pulmonary comorbidity than lung cancer patients. There are a number of similarities between bleomycin pneumonopathy and radiation

TABLE 62-6

 Anticancer Therapies Categorized by Risk of Pneumotoxicity

Highly pneumotoxic agents (risk of pulmonary SAE probably >5%)	Bleomycin; BCNU; mitomycin; interleukins. Bone marrow transplantation (with or without TBI). Large-volume thoracic radiation therapy (e.g., T$_4$N3 lung cancer). Surgical resection for lung cancer.
Moderately pneumotoxic agents (risk of pulmonary SAE probably 1%–5%)	Methotrexate; busulfan; melphalan; CCNU/MeCCNU; cyclophosphamide; ifosfamide; fludarabine; gemcitabine; paclitaxel/docetaxel. Small-volume thoracic radiation therapy (e.g., breast cancer). Non–lung cancer oncologic surgery.
Uncommonly pneumotoxic agents (risk of pulmonary SAE probably <1%)	5-FU; capecitabine; cisplatin/carboplatin; doxorubicin; actinomycin-D; etoposide; topotecan/irinotecan; vincristine/vinblastine; vinorelbine; temozolomide; tamoxifen; aromatase inhibitors for breast cancer. Hormonal therapies for prostate cancer; steroids.
Pneumotoxicity risks present but of uncertain frequency	Anti-EGFR agents (e.g., ZD-1839); monoclonal antibodies (e.g., anti-VEGF MoAb); imatinib (Gleevac).

BCNU, carmustine; CCNU, lomustine; EGFR, epidermal growth factor receptor; 5-FU, 5-fluorouracil; MeCCNU, semustine; MoAb, monoclonal antibody; SAE, serious adverse event; TBI, total body irradiation; VEGF, vascular endothelial growth factor.

pneumonopathy, including two patterns of disease (pneumonitis and fibrosis). As with radiation, the clinical manifestations of bleomycin lung toxicity usually occur weeks to months after the initiation of treatment. The infiltrates can be diffuse or limited to basilar and subpleural aspects of the lungs.[72] A nodular pattern occasionally occurs, mimicking cancer progression.

As in radiation pneumonopathy, dyspnea is the primary symptom of bleomycin lung toxicity. Pulmonary function testing shows a restrictive pattern. Diffusing capacity of the lung for carbon dioxide (DLCO), or carbon monoxide transfer (TLCO), appears to be a sensitive indicator of bleomycin pneumonopathy and should be measured before bleomycin is started and periodically between cycles.[73,74] A significant decrease in DLCO should prompt consideration of discontinuation of this drug.[75] There appears to be an association between cumulative bleomycin dose and risk of pneumonopathy. The general recommendation is to limit the cumulative bleomycin dose to <400 mg.[70]

Other factors that may predispose to bleomycin lung toxicity include smoking,[76] cisplatin-related renal dysfunction,[77] and mediastinal irradiation.[34,78,79] The potential for high doses of oxygen to worsen bleomycin lung toxicity is a concern, as shown by animal data,[80] although controversy exists in clinical practice.[81,82]

Bleomycin pneumonitis is rarely fatal. Most patients achieve complete or near-complete recovery.[83-85] Corticosteroids may have some benefit,[86] although the data are not as clear as those for radiation pneumonitis. Some cases of steroid-responsive bleomycin pneumonitis/fibrosis may represent early hypersensitivity, BOOP-like events. After bleomycin chemotherapy, cancer survivors may have significant declines in pulmonary function for approximately 6 months, but by 2 years after chemotherapy few have significant respiratory dysfunction.[83]

Antimetabolites

Methotrexate, which is commonly used in therapy for rheumatoid arthritis as well as for cancer, is the antimetabolite drug most commonly linked to pulmonary injury. It can cause interstitial pneumonitis similar to that caused by bleomycin and other drugs.[87,88] Steroid therapy may be indicated for severe cases.

Gemcitabine has become one of the most commonly used chemotherapy drugs for solid tumors, including lung cancer. It has been associated with a small (<10%) risk of very severe respiratory insufficiency that may be related to capillary leak syndrome[89-93] similar to that seen with cytosine arabinoside.[94] Steroid therapy can be a useful adjunct to supportive treatment and may improve radiologic findings.[91,95] Extreme caution is advised in the use of gemcitabine with thoracic radiation therapy. An early report that combined full doses of both modalities resulted in unacceptable life-threatening pneumonitis.[35] Gemcitabine may also be associated with radiation recall pneumonitis, even a year or more after thoracic radiation therapy.[92]

Fludarabine is now commonly used to manage hematologic malignant disease, including chronic lymphocytic

leukemia, and as are other antimetabolite drugs is relatively well tolerated. in approximately 8% of cases, fludarabine causes pulmonary toxicity characterized by fever and interstitial pneumonitis.[96,97] Although this syndrome is probably steroid responsive, it is critical to rule out opportunistic infection given the patient population usually treated with this drug.

Alkylators and Nitrosoureas

Alkylators and nitrosoureas are frequent components of conditioning regimens for BMT, a procedure associated with a high rate of pulmonary toxicity. It is difficult to isolate the effect of these drugs in this setting, in which many other insults to the lung often occur, but it is likely that they contribute, particularly at BMT dose intensity.[98,99] Results suggest that pulmonary toxicity from BMT with total body irradiation–containing regimens is similar to that from regimens without total body irradiation.[100,101]

In the non-BMT setting, classic alkylators, such as cyclophosphamide, ifosfamide, and melphalan, have occasionally been associated with interstitial pneumonitis and acute or subacute dyspnea that may be steroid responsive.[102-105] However, these drugs have caused long-term pulmonary fibrosis, even several decades after treatment.[102]

For nitrosoureas such as BCNU, pulmonary injury is considered a dose-limiting toxicity. The predominant problem with these agents is pulmonary fibrosis, which appears to be chronic and dose dependent.[106-108] In one study, BCNU pulmonary fibrosis in patients treated for glioma was rare at cumulative doses less than 960 mg/m².[108] The association between other nitrosoureas and pulmonary toxicity is not commonly reported but does occur.[109] The pulmonary fibrosis caused by nitrosoureas does not appear to be steroid responsive.

Anthracyclines and Other Antitumor Antibiotics

Anthracyclines, including doxorubicin, are rarely associated with direct pulmonary injury on their own (although dyspnea from cardiac injury can clinically mimic lung toxicity). However, these drugs are extremely potent radiosensitizers and appear to sensitize normal lung to radiation pneumonopathy. For example, a randomized trial of concurrent versus sequential chemoradiotherapy (including doxorubicin) for small cell lung carcinoma was closed early because of development of 6 fatal cases of pneumonopathy among 82 patients treated concurrently. There may be a risk of radiation recall–like reactions in patients receiving doxorubicin after high-dose thoracic radiation therapy, at least in the vulnerable lung cancer population.[110]

Unlike the anthracyclines, which have a modest lung toxicity profile, mitomycin is well known as a potentially pneumotoxic agent that can cause noncardiogenic pulmonary edema, pneumonitis, and pleural effusion. Toxicity is difficult to predict and not clearly dose related[111] but is estimated to occur in 5% of patients or more.[112-114] In a prospective study of patients treated with mitomycin, 28% of patients tested had significant (>20%) declines in D_{LCO}, and 5% had grade 3+ lung toxicity.[112] A favorable response to steroids has been reported.[115]

Biologic Agents

Immunomodulatory anticancer agents, particularly interleukin-2, can cause pulmonary toxicity such as noncardiogenic pulmonary edema, pneumonitis, and pleural effusion. In one study, high-dose interleukin-2 was associated with the presence of diffuse radiographic infiltrates in 41% of patients. A study of interferon γ added to chemotherapy for small cell lung cancer showed a 5% incidence of severe pneumonitis, including one death.[116] Excessive increase in radiation pneumonitis also has been seen with concurrent interferon therapy.[117]

The most recently heralded class of anticancer agents are targeted therapies against malignant signal transduction pathways. One such agent is trastuzumab (Herceptin). There is insufficient information about the pulmonary effects of these new agents. However, interstitial pneumonitis, some cases fatal, has occurred in postmarketing studies of gefitinib (also known as ZD-1839 or Iressa), a small-molecule inhibitor of the tyrosine kinase activity of endothelial growth factor receptor 1.[118]

REFERENCES

1. Morgan GW, Pharm B, Breit SN: Radiation and the lung: A reevaluation of the mechanisms mediating pulmonary injury. Int J Radiat Oncol Biol Phys 1995;31:361-369.
2. Vujaskovic Z, Marks LB, Anscher MS: The physical parameters and molecular events associated with radiation-induced lung toxicity. Semin Radiat Oncol 2000;10:296-307.
3. Vujaskovic Z, Groen HJM: TGF-beta, radiation induced pulmonary injury and lung cancer. Int J Radiat Oncol Biol Phys 2000;76:511-516.
4. Rubin P, Johnston CJ, Williams JP, et al: A perpetual cascade of cytokines postirradiation leads to pulmonary fibrosis. Int J Radiat Oncol Biol Phys 1995;33:99-109.
5. Arbetter KR, Prakash VB, Tazelaar HD, et al: Radiation-induced pneumonitis in the non-irradiated lung. Mayo Clin Proc 1999;74:27-36.
6. Byhardt R, Abrams R, Almagro U: The association of adult respiratory distress syndrome (ARDS) with thoracic irradiation (RT). Int J Radiat Oncol Biol Phys 1988;15:1441-1444.
7. Roberts CM, Foulcher E, Zaunders JJ, et al: Radiation pneumonitis: A possible lymphocyte-mediated hypersensitivity reaction. Ann Intern Med 1993;118:696-700.
8. Zhuang H, Pourdehnad M, Lambright ES, et al: Dual time point 18F-FDG PET imaging for differentiating malignant from inflammatory processes. J Nucl Med 2001;42:1412-1417.
9. Strauss LG: Fluorine-18 deoxyglucose and false positive results: A major problem in the diagnostics of oncological patients. Eur J Nucl Med 1996;23:1409-1415.
10. Martel MK, Ten Haken R, Hazuka MB, et al: Dose-volume histogram and 3-D treatment planning evaluation of patients with pneumonitis. Int J Radiat Oncol Biol Phys 1994;28:575-581.
11. Graham MV, Purdy JA, Emami B, et al: Clinical dose-volume histogram analysis for pneumonitis after 3D treatment for non-small cell lung cancer (NSCLC). Int J Radiat Oncol Biol Phys 1999;45:323-329.
12. Poulson JM, Vujaskovic Z, Gillette SM, et al: Volume and dose-response effects for severe symptomatic pneumonitis after fractionated irradiation. Int J Radiat Biol 2000;76:463-468.
13. Yorke ED, Jackson A, Rosenzweig KE, et al: Dose-volume factors contributing to the incidence of radiation pneumonitis in non-small-cell lung cancer patients treated with three-dimensional conformal radiation therapy. Int J Radiat Oncol Biol Phys 2002;54:329-339.
14. Byhardt RW, Martin L, Pajak TF, et al: The influence of field size and other treatment factors on pulmonary toxicity following hyperfractionated irradiation for inoperable non-small cell lung cancer (NSCLC): Analysis of a Radiation Therapy Oncology Group (RTOG) protocol. Int J Radiat Oncol Biol Phys 1993;27:537-544.
15. Emami B, Lyman J, Brown A, et al: Tolerance of normal tissue to therapeutic irradiation. Int J Radiat Oncol Biol Phys 1991;21:109-122.
16. Poulter CA, Cosmatos D, Rubin P, et al: A report of RTOG 8206: A phase III study of whether the addition of single dose hemibody irradiation to standard fractionated local field irradiation is more effective than local field irradiation alone in the treatment of symptomatic osseous metastases. Int J Radiat Oncol Biol Phys 1992;23:207-214.
17. Fryer C, Fitzpatrick P, Rider W, et al: Radiation pneumonitis: Experience following a large single dose of radiation. Int J Radiat Oncol Biol Phys 1978;4:931-936.
18. Weshler Z, Breuer R, Or R, et al: Interstitial pneumonitis after total body irradiation: Effect of partial lung shielding. Br J Haematol 1990;74:61-64.
19. Travis EL, Peters LJ, McNeill J, et al: Effect of dose-rate on total body irradiation: Lethality and pathologic findings. Radiother Oncol 1985;4:341-351.
20. Lind PARM, Marks LB, Hardenbergh PH, et al: Technical factors associated with radiation pneumonitis after local +/- regional radiation therapy for breast cancer. Int J Radiat Oncol Biol Phys 2002;52:137-143.
21. Trotti A, Byhardt R, Stetz J, et al: Common toxicity criteria: Version 2.0. an improved reference for grading the acute effects of cancer treatment—impact on radiotherapy. Int J Radiat Oncol Biol Phys 2000;47:13-47.
22. Anthonisen NR: Prognosis in chronic obstructive pulmonary disease: Results from multicenter clinical trials. Am Rev Respir Dis 1989;140:S95-S99.
23. Common Terminology Criteria for Adverse Events. Available at http://ctep.cancer.gov/forms/CTCAEv3.pdf.
24. Armstrong JG, Berman C, Leibel S, et al: 3-Dimensional conformal therapy may improve the therapeutic ratio of high dose radiation therapy for lung cancer. Int J Radiat Oncol Biol Phys 1993;26:685-689.
25. Hernando ML, Marks LB, Bentel GC, et al: Radiation-induced pulmonary toxicity: A dose-volume histogram analysis in 201 patients with lung cancer. Int J Radiat Oncol Biol Phys 2001;51:655-659.
26. Kwa SL, Lebesque JV, Theuws JC, et al: Radiation pneumonitis as a function of mean lung dose: An analysis of pooled data of 540 patients. Int J Radiat Oncol Biol Phys 1998;42:1-9.
27. Marks LB, Spencer DP, Bentel GC, et al: The utility of SPECT lung perfusion scans in minimizing and assessing the physiologic consequences of thoracic irradiation. Int J Radiat Oncol Biol Phys 1993;26:659-668.
28. Marks LB, Spencer DP, Sherhouse DW, et al: The role of three dimensional functional lung imaging in radiation treatment planning: The functional dose volume histogram. Int J Radiat Oncol Biol Phys 1995;33:65-75.
29. Roach MR, Gandara DR, Yuo HS, et al: Radiation pneumonitis following combined modality therapy for lung cancer: Analysis of prognostic factors. J Clin Oncol 1995;13:2606-2612.
30. Cassady JR, Richter MP, Piro AJ, et al: Radiation-adriamycin interactions: Preliminary clinical observations. Cancer 1975;36:946-949.
31. Verschoore J, Lagrange JL, Boublil JL, et al: Pulmonary toxicity of a combination of low-dose doxorubicin and irradiation for inoperable lung cancer. Radiother Oncol 1987;9:281-288.
32. Phillips TL, Fu KK: Quantification of combined radiation therapy and chemotherapy effects on critical normal tissues. Cancer 1976;37:1186-1200.
33. Catane R, Schwade J, Turrisi A, et al: Pulmonary toxicity after radiation and bleomycin: A review. Int J Radiat Oncol Biol Phys 1979;5:1513-1518.

34. Mah K, Keane TJ, VanDyk J, et al: Quantitative effect of combined chemotherapy and fractionated radiotherapy on the incidence of radiation-induced lung damage: A prospective clinical study. Int J Radiat Oncol Biol Phys 1994;28:563–574.

35. Scalliet P, Goor C, Galdermans D, et al: Gemzar (Gemcitabine) with thoracic radiotherapy: A phase II pilot study in chemonaive patients with advanced non-small cell lung cancer (NSCLC) [abstract 1923]. Proc Am Soc Clin Oncol 1998;17:499.

36. Willner J, Schmidt M, Kirschner J, et al: Sequential chemo- and radiochemotherapy with weekly paclitaxel (Taxol) and 3D-conformal radiotherapy of stage III inoperable non-small cell lung cancer: Results of a dose escalation study. Lung Cancer 2001;32:163–171.

37. Taghian AG, Assaad SI, Niemierko A, et al: Risk of pneumonitis in breast cancer patients treated with radiation therapy and combination chemotherapy with paclitaxel. J Natl Cancer Inst 2001;93:1806–1811.

38. Hanna YM, Baglan KL, Stromberg JS, et al: Acute and subacute toxicity associated with concurrent adjuvant radiation therapy and paclitaxel in primary breast cancer therapy. Breast J 2002;8:149–153.

39. Socinski MA, Rosenman JG, Halle J, et al: Dose-escalating conformal thoracic radiation therapy with induction and concurrent carboplatin/paclitaxel in unresectable stage IIIA/B NSCLC: A modified phase I/II trial. Cancer 2001;92:1213–1223.

40. Robnett TJ, Machtay M, Vines EF, et al: Factors predicting severe radiation pneumonitis in patients receiving definitive chemoradiation for lung cancer. Int J Radiat Oncol Biol Phys 2000;48:89–94.

41. Rubenstein JH, Richter MP, Moldofsky PJ, et al: Prospective prediction of post-radiation therapy lung function using quantitative lung scans and pulmonary function testing. Int J Radiat Oncol Biol Phys 1988;15:83–87.

42. Koga K, Kusumoto S, Watanabe K, et al: Age factor relevant to the development of radiation pneumonitis in radiotherapy of lung cancer. Int J Radiat Oncol Biol Phys 1988;14:367.

43. Mah K, Poon PY, Van Dyk J, et al: Assessment of acute radiation-induced pulmonary changes using computed tomography. J Comput Assist Tomogr 1986;10:736–743.

44. Moss WT, Haddy FJ, Sweany SK: Some factors altering the severity of acute radiation pneumonitis: Variation with cortisone, heparin and antibiotics. Radiology 1960;75:50–54.

45. Gross NJ, Narine KR, Wade R: Protective effect of corticosteroids on radiation pneumonitis in mice. Radiat Res 1988;113:112–119.

46. Ward HE, Kemsley L, Davies L, et al: The effect of steroids on radiation-induced lung disease in the rat. Radiat Res 1993;136:22–28.

47. Castellino R, Glatstein E, Turbow M, et al: Latent radiation injury of lungs or heart activated by steroid withdrawal. Ann Intern Med 1974;80:593–599.

48. Reckzeh B, Merte H, Pfluger KH, et al: Severe lymphocytopenia and interstitial pneumonia in patients treated with paclitaxel and simultaneous radiotherapy for non-small-cell lung cancer. J Clin Oncol 1997;14:1071–1076.

49. Wang JY, Chen KY, Wang JT, et al: Outcome and prognostic factors for patients with non-small-cell lung cancer and severe radiation pneumonitis. Int J Radiat Oncol Biol Phys 2002;54:735–741.

50. Antonadou D, Coliarakis N, Synodinou M, et al: Randomized phase III trial of radiation treatment +/– amifostine in patients with advanced-stage lung cancer. Int J Radiat Oncol Biol Phys 2001;51:915–922.

51. Komaki R, Lee JS, Kaplan B, et al: Randomized phase III study of chemoradiation with or without amifostine for patients with favorable performance status inoperable stage II-III non-small cell lung cancer: Preliminary results. Semin Radiat Oncol 2002;12:46–49.

52. Vujaskovic Z, Feng QF, Rabbani ZN, et al: Assessment of the protective effect of amifostine on radiation-induced pulmonary toxicity. Exp Lung Res 2002;28:577–590.

53. Delanian S, Balla-Mekias S, Lefaix J: Striking regression of chronic radiotherapy damage in a clinical trial of combined pentoxifylline and tocopherol. J Clin Oncol 1999;17:3283–3290.

54. Epperly M, Bray J, Kraeger S, et al: Prevention of late effects of irradiation lung damage by manganese superoxide dismutase gene therapy. Gene Therapy 1998;5:196–208.

55. Epperly MW, Bray JA, Krager S, et al: Intratracheal injection of adenovirus containing the human MnSOD transgene protects athymic nude mice from irradiation-induced organizing alveolitis. Int J Radiat Oncol Biol Phys 1999;43:169–181.

56. Epperly MW, Epstein CJ, Travis EL, et al: Decreased pulmonary radiation resistance of manganese superoxide dismutase (MnSOD)-deficient mice is corrected by human manganese superoxide dismutase–plasmid/liposome (SOD2-PL) intratracheal gene therapy. Radiat Res 2000;154:365–374.

57. Ward WF, Lin PJ, Wong PS, et al: Radiation pneumonitis in rats and its modification by the angiotensin-converting enzyme inhibitor captopril evaluated by high-resolution computed tomography. Radiat Res 1993;135:81–87.

58. Wang LW, Fu XL, Clough R, et al: Can angiotensin-converting enzyme inhibitors protect against symptomatic radiation pneumonitis? Radiat Res 2000;153:405–410.

59. Anscher MS, Kong FM, Marks LB, et al: Changes in plasma transforming growth factor beta during radiotherapy and the risk of symptomatic radiation-induced pneumonitis. Int J Radiat Oncol Biol Phys 1997;37:253–258.

60. Vester SR, Faber LP, Kittle CF, et al: Bronchopleural fistula after stapled closure of bronchus. Ann Thorac Surg 1991;52:1253–1257.

61. Sonobe M, Nakagawa M, Ichinose M, et al: Analysis of risk factors in bronchopleural fistula after pulmonary resection for primary. Eur J Cardiothorac Surg 2000;18:519–523.

62. Taulelle M, Chauvet B, Vincent P, et al: High dose rate endobronchial brachytherapy: Results and complications in 189 patients. Eur Respir J 1998;11:162–168.

63. Yao MS, Koh WJ: Endobronchial brachytherapy. Chest Surg Clin N Am 2001;11:813–827.

64. Huber RM, Fischer R, Hautmann H, et al: Palliative endobronchial brachytherapy for central lung tumors: A prospective randomized comparison of two fractionation schedules. Chest 1995;107:463–470.

65. Hara R, Itami J, Aruga T, et al: Risk factors for massive hemoptysis after endobronchial brachytherapy in patients with tracheobronchial malignancies. Cancer 2001;92:2623–2627.

66. Hayakawa K, Mitsuhashi N, Furuta M, et al: High-dose radiation therapy for inoperable non-small cell lung cancer without mediastinal involvement. Strahlenther Onkol 1996;172:489–495.

67. Rosenman JG, Halle JS, Socinski MA, et al: High-dose conformal radiotherapy for treatment of stage IIIA/IIIB non-small-cell lung cancer: Technical issues and results of a phase I/II trial. Int J Radiat Oncol Biol Phys 2002;54:348–356.

68. Pezner RD, Horak DA, Sayegh HO, et al: Spontaneous pneumothorax in patients irradiated for Hodgkin's disease. Int J Radiat Oncol Biol Phys 1990;18:193–198.

69. Dearnaley DP, Horwich A, A'Hern R, et al: Combination chemotherapy with bleomycin, etoposide and cisplatin (BEP) for metastatic testicular teratoma: Long-term follow-up. Eur J Cancer 1991;27:684–691.

70. Sleijfer S: Bleomycin-induced pneumonitis. Chest 2001;120:617–624.

71. Saxman SB, Nichols CR, Einhorn LH: Pulmonary toxicity in patients with advanced stage germ cell tumors receiving bleomycin with and without granulocyte colony stimulating factor. Chest 1997;111:657–660.

72. Rimmer MJ, Dixon AK, Flower CDR, et al: Bleomycin-lung: CT observations. Br J Radiol 1985;58:1041–1045.

73. Comis RL, Kuppinger MS, Ginsberg SJ, et al: Role of single-breath carbon monoxide diffusing capacity in monitoring the pulmonary effects of bleomycin in germ cell tumor patients. Cancer Res 1979;39:5076–5080.

74. Wolkowicz J, Sturgeon J, Ravji M, et al: . Bleomycin-induced pulmonary function abnormalities. Chest 1992;101:97–101.

75. Comis RL: Bleomycin pulmonary toxicity: Current status and future directions. Semin Oncol 1992;19:64–70.

76. Parvinen LM, Kilkku P, Makinen E, et al: Factors affecting the pulmonary toxicity of bleomycin. Acta Radiol 1983;22:417–422.

77. Sleijfer S, Van der Mark TW, Schraffordt Koops H, et al: Enhanced effects of bleomycin on pulmonary function assessments in patients with decreased renal function due to cisplatin. Eur J Cancer 1996;32A:550–552.

78. Hirsch A, Vander Els N, Straus DJ, et al: Effect of ABVD chemotherapy with and without mantle or mediastinal irradiation on pulmonary function and symptoms in early-stage Hodgkin's disease. J Clin Oncol 1996;14:1297–1305.

79. Horning SJ, Adhikari A, Rizk N, et al: Effect of treatment for Hodgkin's disease on pulmonary function: Results of a prospective study. J Clin Oncol 1994;12:297–305.

80. Blom-Muilwijk MC, Vriesendorp R, Veninga TS, et al: Pulmonary toxicity after treatment with bleomycin alone or in combination with hyperoxia. Br J Anaesth 1988;60:91–97.

81. Ingrassia TS 3rd, Ryu JH, Trastek VF, et al: Oxygen-exacerbated bleomycin pulmonary toxicity. Mayo Clin Proc 1991;66:173–178.

82. Donat SM, Levy DA: Bleomycin associated pulmonary toxicity: Is perioperative oxygen restriction necessary? J Urol 1998;160: 1347–1352.

83. Marina NM, Greenwald CA, Fairclough DL, et al: Serial pulmonary function studies in children treated for newly diagnosed Hodgkin's disease with mantle radiotherapy plus cycles of cyclophosphamide, vincristine, and procarbazine alternating with cycles of doxorubicin, bleomycin, vinblastine, and dacarbazine. Cancer 1995;75:1706–1711.

84. Jensen JL, Goel R, Venner PM: The effect of corticosteroid administration on bleomycin lung toxicity. Cancer 1990;65:1291–1297.

85. Simpson AB, Paul J, Graham J, et al: Fatal bleomycin pulmonary toxicity in the west of Scotland 1991–95: A review of patients with germ cell tumours. Br J Cancer 1998;78:1061–1066.

86. White DA, Stover DE: Severe bleomycin-induced pneumonitis: Clinical features and response to corticosteroids. Chest 1984;86:723–728.

87. Imokawa S, Colby TV, Leslie KO, et al: Methotrexate pneumonitis: Review of the literature and histopathological findings in nine patients. Eur Respir J 2000;15:373–381.

88. Cannon GW: Methotrexate pulmonary toxicity. Rheum Dis Clin North Am 1997;23:917–937.

89. Vansteenkiste JF, Vandebroek JE, Nackaerts KL, et al: Clinical-benefit response in advanced non-small-cell lung cancer: A multicentre prospective randomised phase III study of single agent gemcitabine versus cisplatin-vindesine. Ann Oncol 2001;12:1221–1230.

90. DePas T, Curigliano G, Franceschelli L, et al: Gemcitabine-induced systemic capillary leak syndrome. Ann Oncol 2001;12:1651–1652.

91. Briasoulis E, Pavlidis N: Noncardiogenic pulmonary edema: An unusual and serious complication of anticancer therapy. Oncologist 2001;6:153–161.

92. Sauer-Heilborn A, Kath R, Schneider CP, et al: Severe non-hematological toxicity after treatment with gemcitabine. J Cancer Res Clin Oncol 1999;125:637–640.

93. Pavlakis N, Bell DR, Millward MJ, et al: Fatal pulmonary toxicity resulting from treatment with gemcitabine. Cancer 1998;80: 286–291.

94. Andersson BS, Cogan BM, Keating MJ, et al: Subacute pulmonary failure complicating therapy with high-dose ara-C in acute leukemia. Cancer 1985;56:2181–2184.

95. Boiselle PM, Morrin MM, Huberman MS: Gemcitabine pulmonary toxicity: CT features. J Comp Assist Tomogr 2000;24:977–980.

96. Helman DL, Byrd JC, Ales NC, et al: Fludarabine-related pulmonary toxicity: A distinct clinical entity in chronic lymphoproliferative syndromes. Chest 2002;122:785–790.

97. Stoica GS, Greenberg HE, Rossoff LJ: Corticosteroid fludarabine pulmonary toxicity. Am J Clin Oncol 2002;25:340–341.

98. Chap L, Shpiner R, Levine M, Norton L, Lill M, Glaspy J: Pulmonary toxicity of high dose chemotherapy for breast cancer: A non-invasive approach. Bone Marrow Transplant 1997;20:1063–1067.

99. Wilcyzynski SW, Erasmus JJ, Petros WP, et al: Delayed pulmonary toxicity syndrome following high-dose chemotherapy and bone marrow transplantation for breast cancer. Am J Respir Crit Care Med 1998;157:565–573.

100. Hartsell WF, Czyzewski EA, Ghalie R, et al: Pulmonary complications of bone marrow transplantation: A comparison of total body irradiation and cyclophosphamide to busulfan and cyclophosphamide. Int J Radiat Oncol Biol Phys 1995;32:69–73.

101. Hartman AR, Williams SF, Dillon JJ: Survival, disease-free survival and adverse effects of conditioning for allogeneic bone marrow transplantation with busulfan/cyclophosphamide vs total body irradiation: A meta-analysis. Bone Marrow Transplant 1998;22:439–443.

102. Malik SW, Myers JL, DeRemee RA, et al: Lung toxicity associated with cyclophosphamide use. Two distinct patterns. Am J Respir Crit Care Med 1996;154:1851–1856.

103. Baker W, Fistel SJ, Jones RV, et al: Interstitial pneumonitis associated with ifosfamide therapy. Cancer 1990;65:2217–2221.

104. Spector I, Zimbler H, Ross S: Early-onset cyclophosphamide induced interstitial pneumonitis. JAMA 1979;242:2852–2854.

105. Akasheh MS, Freytes CO, Vesole DH: Melphalan-associated pulmonary toxicity following high-dose therapy with autologous hematopoietic stem cell transplantation. Bone Marrow Transplant 2000;26:1107–1109.

106. O'Driscoll BR, Hasleton PS, Taylor PM, et al: Active lung fibrosis up to 17 years after chemotherapy with carmustine (BCNU) in childhood. N Engl J Med 1990;323:378–382.

107. O'Driscoll BR, Kalra S, Gattamaneni HR, et al: Late carmustine lung fibrosis: Age at treatment may influence severity and survival. Chest 1995;107:1355–1357.

108. Nelson DF, Diener-West M, Weinstein AS, et al: A randomized comparison of misonidazole sensitized radiotherapy plus BCNU and radiotherapy plus BCNU for treatment of malignant glioma after surgery: Final report of an RTOG study. Int J Radiat Oncol Biol Phys 1986;12:1793–1800.

109. Block M, Lachowiez RM, Rios C, et al: Pulmonary fibrosis associated with low-dose adjuvant methyl-CCNU. Med Pediatr Oncol 1990;18:256–260.

110. Maurer LH, Herndon JE 2nd, Hollis DR, et al: Randomized trial of chemotherapy and radiation therapy with or without warfarin for limited-stage small-cell lung cancer: A Cancer and Leukemia Group B study. J Clin Oncol 1997;15:3378–3387.

111. Okuno SH, Frytak S: Mitomycin lung toxicity: Acute and chronic phases. Am J Clin Oncol 1997;20:282–284.

112. Castro M, Veeder MH, Mailliard JA, et al: A prospective study of pulmonary function in patients receiving mitomycin. Chest 1996;109:939–944.

113. deReijke TM, Keuppens FI, Whelan P, et al: Orchiectomy and orchiectomy plus mitomycin C for metastatic prostate cancer in patients with poor prognosis: The final results of a European Organization for Research in Cancer Therapy Genitourinary Group Trial. J Urol 1999;162:1658–1664.

114. Twohig KJ, Matthay RA: Pulmonary effects of cytotoxic agents other than bleomycin. Clin Chest Med 1990;11:31–54.

115. Chang AY, Kuebler JP, Pandya KJ, et al: Pulmonary toxicity induced by mitomycin C is highly responsive to glucocorticoids. Cancer 1986;57:2285–2290.

116. vanZandwijk N, Groen HJ, Postmus PE, et al: Role of recombinant interferon-gamma maintenance in responding patients with small cell lung cancer: A randomised phase III study of the EORTC Lung Cancer Cooperative Group. Eur J Cancer 1997;33:1759–1766.

117. Shaw EG, Deming RL, Creagan ET, et al: Pilot study of human recombinant interferon gamma and accelerated hyperfractionated thoracic radiation therapy in patients with unresectable stage IIIA/B nonsmall cell lung cancer. Int J Radiat Oncol Biol Phys 1995;31:827–831.

118. Reuters Health News: At least 173 deaths linked to Iressa use in Japan. Reuters, February 6, 2003.

119. Byhardt RW, Scott C, Sause WT, et al: Response, toxicity, failure patterns, and survival in five Radiation Therapy Oncology Group (RTOG) trials of sequential and/or concurrent chemotherapy and radiotherapy for locally advanced non-small cell carcinoma of the lung. Int J Radiat Oncol Biol Phys 1998;42:469–478.

120. Keller SM, Adak S, Wagner H, et al: A randomized trial of postoperative adjuvant therapy in patients with completely resected stage II or IIIA non-small cell lung cancer. N Engl J Med 2000;343:1217–1222.

121. Turrisi AT 3rd, Kim K, Blum R, et al: Twice-daily compared with once-daily thoracic radiotherapy in limited small cell lung cancer treated concurrently with cisplatin and etoposide. N Engl J Med 1999;340:265–271.

122. Sim S, Rosenzweig KE, Schindelheim R, et al: Induction chemotherapy plus three-dimensional conformal radiation

therapy in the definitive treatment of locally advanced non-small cell lung cancer. Int J Radiat Oncol Biol Phys 2002;51:665–665.

123. Hughes-Davies L, Tarbell NJ, Coleman CN, et al: Stage IA-IIB Hodgkin's disease: Management and outcome of extensive thoracic involvement. Int J Radiat Oncol Biol Phys 1998;39:361–369.

124. Cooper JS, Guo M, Herskovic A, et al: Chemoradiotherapy of locally advanced esophageal cancer: Long-term followup of a prospective randomized trial (RTOG 85-01). JAMA 1999;281:1623–1627.

125. Antonadou D: Radiotherapy or chemotherapy followed by radiotherapy with or without amifostine in locally advanced lung cancer. Semin Radiat Oncol 2002;12:50–58.

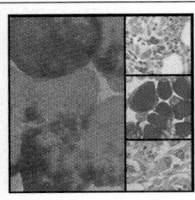

63

CARDIAC EFFECTS OF CANCER THERAPY

James L. Speyer

Michael S. Ewer

Robin S. Freedberg

SUMMARY OF KEY POINTS

INCIDENCE

Cardiomyopathy/Congestive Heart Failure
- Anthracyclines: 5% to 20% of patients receiving cumulative doxorubicin more than 450 mg/m², higher in children
- Other antineoplastics (mitoxantrone, cyclophosphamide): less than 2%
- HER2/neu antibody
- Radiation therapy: Common 5 to 20 years after single anteroposterior port

Arrhythmias
- Paclitaxel: less than 1%
- Amsacrine: less than 1%
- Dihydroazacytidine*
- Interleukin-2, interleukin-6*
- Interleukin-11*
- Rituxan*

Myocardial Ischemia
- Radiation therapy
- 5-Fluorouracil (5-FU): 1% to 4.5% with infusion schedules

Pericardial Disease
- Radiation therapy: Effusions in 6% to 30% of patients receiving radiation

therapy to the chest: constriction in 2% of patients receiving radiation therapy to the chest with current techniques
- Acute pericarditis and hypotension also occur

Fluid Retention
- Docetaxel, interleukins, interferons, tumor necrosis factor (TNF), cytokines, granulocyte-macrophage colony stimulating factor (GM-CSF), monoclonal antibody (CD20)

ETIOLOGY OF COMPLICATION
- Anthracycline-induced cardiomyopathy
- Radiation-induced cardiomyopathy
- Radiation-induced myocardial ischemia
- Decreased systemic vascular resistance

DIAGNOSIS
- Clinical cardiac symptoms—New York Heart Association Classification
- Hemodynamics—Bristow Staging Score
- Radionuclide scans—serial scans including baseline

- Endomyocardial biopsy— Billingham Histopathologic Scoring System
- Doppler echocardiography— Pericardial effusion/constriction; LV systolic/diastolic dysfunction

TREATMENT
- Discontinue offending agent

Risk Reduction with Anthracyclines
- Anthracyclines: limit dose (e.g., doxorubicin <450 mg/m²). Use less toxic analogs.
- Alteration of dose schedule
- Unique delivery systems (e.g., liposomes)
- Blocking agents (dexrazoxane: ICRF-187, ADR 529) (Zinecard)

Cardiomyopathy/Congestive Heart Failure
- Sodium and fluid restriction, diuretics, afterload reduction (ACE inhibitors)

Radiation-Induced Pericardial Disease
- Acute pericarditis: nonsteroidal anti-inflammatory drugs, steroids
- Constriction: pericardiectomy

*Database too small to adequately estimate.

INTRODUCTION

The cardiac side effects of cancer therapies include the entire breadth of cardiac pathology. They provide a considerable challenge to the clinician, because they produce signs and symptoms of disease not specific to treatment, and their differential diagnosis therefore includes a broad spectrum of other etiologies. The sequelae of the tumors being treated, underlying cardiac disease, and effects of nononcologic interventions may affect the heart in ways that often cannot be distinguished clinically from the cardiac effects of cancer treatment. These factors make the diagnosis, assessment, and clinical course of the cardiac effects of cancer therapy especially challenging. Despite these considerations, it is clear that dysrhythmias, ischemia, congestive heart failure, peripheral vascular disease, and pericardial disease can be

caused by a variety of cancer therapies and the various combinations of agents and modalities used in the treatment of malignancy.

A variety of approaches can be used to evaluate patients with these side effects effectively. The patient with cancer who presents with cardiac problems can be approached by considering all known side effects associated with the therapy or therapies that he or she is receiving or has received in the past. Alternatively, the entire spectrum of treatment-related, as well as non-treatment-related, causes of his or her cardiac presentation can be considered.

Because the latter approach is closer to the usual clinical process of differential diagnosis, this chapter is organized in that manner. However, in order to consider side effects by therapeutic agent and modality, a summary is organized according to the effects of specific agents (Table 63-1).

TABLE 63-1

Cardiovascular Complications of Cancer Therapies

THERAPY	COMPLICATIONS
Chemotherapy Drugs	
Anthracyclines (e.g., doxorubicin [adriamycin])	Cardiomyopathy, CHF*
	Dysrhythmias
Epirubicin	Pericardial effusion
Anthrapyrazoles	Cardiomyopathy, CHF
Piroxantrone	Cardiomyopathy
Mitoxantrone	Cardiomyopathy, CHF*
Amsacrine	Dysrhythmias
Cyclophosphamide	CHF
	Hemorrhagic myocarditis*
	Pericardial effusion
Ifosfamide	CHF
5-Fluorouracil	Myocardial ischemia*
	Cerebrovascular ischemia
Vinca alkaloids	Angina
	Raynaud phenomenon
Dihydro-5-azacytidine	Dysrhythmias, pericardial effusion
Paclitaxel (Taxol)	Dysrhythmias, ECG changes, ischemia
Docetaxel (Taxotere)	Fluid retention
Cisplatin	Raynaud phenomenon*
Bleomycin	Raynaud phenomenon*
Taxol + doxorubicin	Cardiomyopathy
Thalidomide in combination	Thromboembolic events
Biologic Response Modifiers	
IFN-α	Hypotension
	Tachycardia
IFN-β	Hypotension
TFN-γ	Hypotension
Interleukin-1α	Hypotension
Interleukin-2	CHF
	Hypotension
	Dysrhythmias
	Ischemia
Interleukin-4	Myocarditis
Interleukin-6	Dysrhythmias
Interleukin-11	Atrial dysrhythmias
TNF	Hypotension*
GM-CSF	Hypotension
	Pericardial effusion
Monoclonal Ab to CD20	Hypotension, angina, dysrhythmias
Monoclonal Ab to Her2/neu	CHF
Radiation Therapy	CHF
	Coronary artery disease*
	Pericarditis*
	Pericardial effusion
	Constriction*

Ab, antibody; CHF, congestive heart failure; ECG, electrocardiographic; IFN, interferon; GM-CSF, granulocyte macrophage colony-stimulating factor; TNF, tumor necrosis factor.
*Significant effect.

CONGESTIVE HEART FAILURE

Anthracyclines

Chemotherapy that incorporates an anthracycline antibiotic is a significant cause of congestive heart failure in cancer patients treated with these agents (Table 63-2).

The anthracyclines are of special interest, in part because congestive heart failure (CHF) resulting from these agents can progress to death from iatrogenic causes. We now are able, in large part, to prevent the potentially deadly aspects of CHF from anthracylcine use. Most information relating to anthracycline-induced cardiomyopathy is derived from studies with doxorubicin and, to a lesser extent, with daunorubicin. However, other clinically available drugs of this class also have been associated with clinically indistinguishable cardiotoxic effects.

Cardiac biopsy specimens have demonstrated that the dose-related cardiomyopathy associated with anthracyclines is biventricular. Retrospective studies indicate that the incidence of clinically recognizable congestive failure with doxorubicin is 7% to 15% in patients who have received a cumulative dose greater than 450 mg/m^2 to 500 mg/m^2 without cardioprotection (Fig. 63-1).[1,2] Above this dose the incidence of clinical congestive heart failure (CHF) rises more steeply. (Cumulative cardiotoxic doses associated with the use of other anthracyclines vary, but the shape of the curve plotting cumulative dose against the likelihood of congestive heart failure is similar for all anthracyclines that have been studied.) Caution must be exercised when evaluating patients receiving anthracyclines, because this cardiomyopathy is not an all-or-none phenomenon, and isolated instances of CHF have been observed at lower cumulative doses.[3]

The actual incidence of clinical CHF may be higher than was reported previously in retrospective trials.[4-8] Prospective clinical trials suggest that, when patients are observed closely, the number developing early signs of CHF at cumulative doses of 450 mg/m^2 may exceed 25%. The cardiotoxic effects of anthracyclines probably start with the first dose. Each subsequent administration constitutes a sequential stress superimposed on existing cardiac injury that may have resulted from prior doses of anthracyclines or from other causes. In addition, non–anthracycline-related stress or damage occurring months or years later finds the heart with preexisting damage and adds a cumulative burden or sequential stress.[9]

Factors associated with an increased risk of anthracycline-induced chronic cardiomyopathy are derived from retrospective studies in adults.[1] They include age greater than 70 years, exposure to ionizing radiation to the chest wall, and preexisting cardiac disease or risk factors. Prior cardiac risks include active CHF, history of myocardial infarction (MI) within the preceding year, hypertension, aortic stenosis, diabetes mellitus, and prior exposure to anthracyclines. The relative contributions of each of these factors are not well-defined, and when an individual patient has more than one risk factor the damage may be increased considerably. One possible common denominator among these entities is increased wall stress; any condition resulting in increased wall stress warrants heightened scrutiny and efforts to mitigate the cardiotoxic effects of anthracyclines. Children also are at increased risk for developing anthracycline cardiac toxicity.

The natural history of the cardiomyopathy from anthracylcine use varies. In some patients it worsens despite maximal medical therapy and can lead inexorably to

TABLE 63-2

Anthracyclines and Cardiotoxicity

ASSOCIATED WITH CARDIOMYOPATHY IN CLINICAL USE	ASSOCIATED WITH CARDIOTOXICITY IN CLINICAL TRIALS
Doxorubicin (Adriamycin)	Aclarnomycin A
Daunorubicin (Daunomycin)	Anthrapyrazoles
4′Epidoxorubicin (Epiadriamycin/Epirubicin)	Marcellomycin
4′-Deoxydoxorubicin (Esorubicin)	Carminomycin
Demethoxydaunorubicin (Idarubicin)	Detorubicin
Pegylated doxorubicin (Doxil)	Pirarubicin (4′-O-tetrahydropyromyl Adriamycin)
Liposomal daunorubicin (Daunosome)	Cyanomorpholinodoxorubicin
Mitoxantrone (anthracycline analog)	Menogaril
	TLC D99 (Myocet)

death. Other patients are left with permanent reduction in left ventricular ejection fraction (LVEF) and persistent symptoms of CHF. Still others can experience gradual improvement in symptoms and LVEF,[10] perhaps due, in part, to compensation and myocardial remodeling.[11]

Pathophysiology

Anthracycline-induced cardiomyopathy is the result of a series of repeated chemical injuries to the myocardium (possibly with some recovery) that gradually impair cellular defenses, resulting in cell damage with decreased contractility and, eventually, cell death. This is consistent with the gradual onset, variability of course, risk factors for increased susceptibility, and laboratory and pathologic findings of the cardiomyopathy that results from use of these drugs.

The common mechanism for anthracycline cardiomyopathy appears to be via free radical damage. Reduction of the quinone groups on the *B* ring of the anthracene structure (Fig. 63-2) results in a semiquinone radical before further reduction to the alcohol (e.g., doxorubicinol). Interaction with oxygen yields free radical oxygen

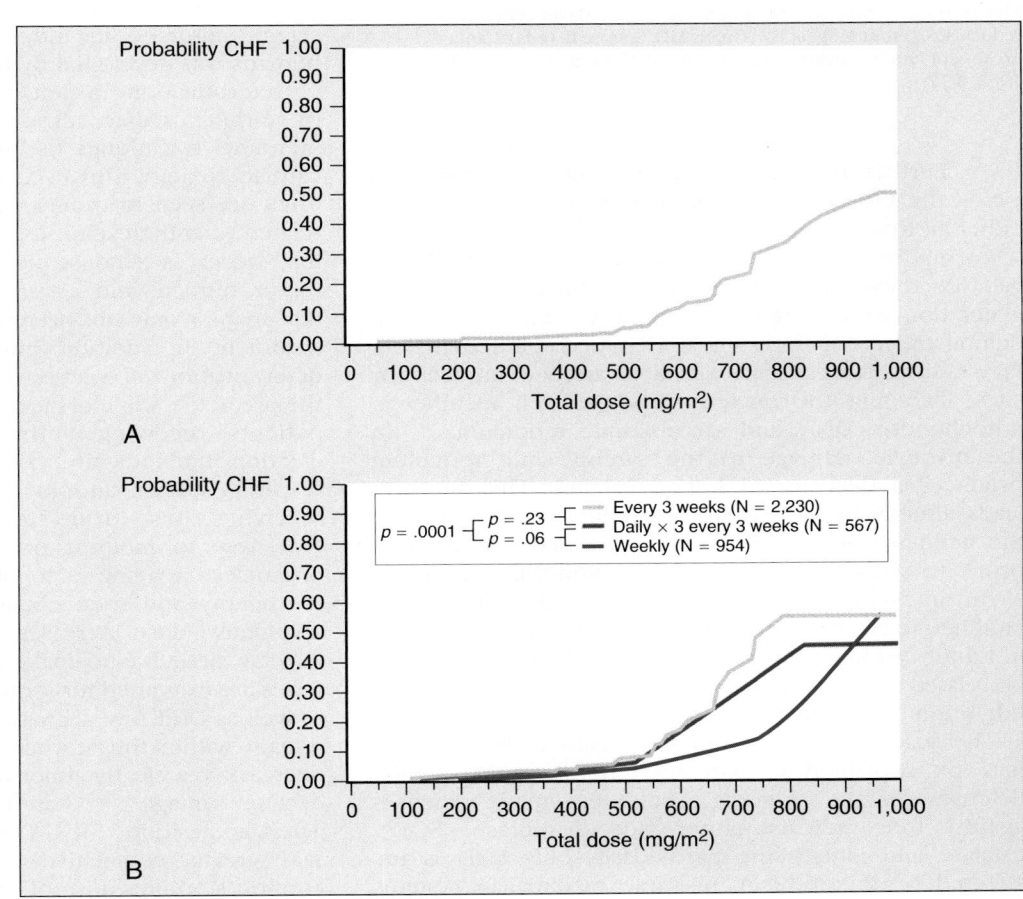

Figure 63-1. Incidence of clinical congestive heart failure according to cumulative dose of doxorubicin. **A,** All patients. **B,** By schedule. (From Von Hoff DD, Layard MW, Basa P, Davis HL, Von Hoff AL, Rozencweig M, Muggia FM: Risk factors for doxorubicin-induced congestive heart failure. Ann Intern Med 1979;91:710-717.)

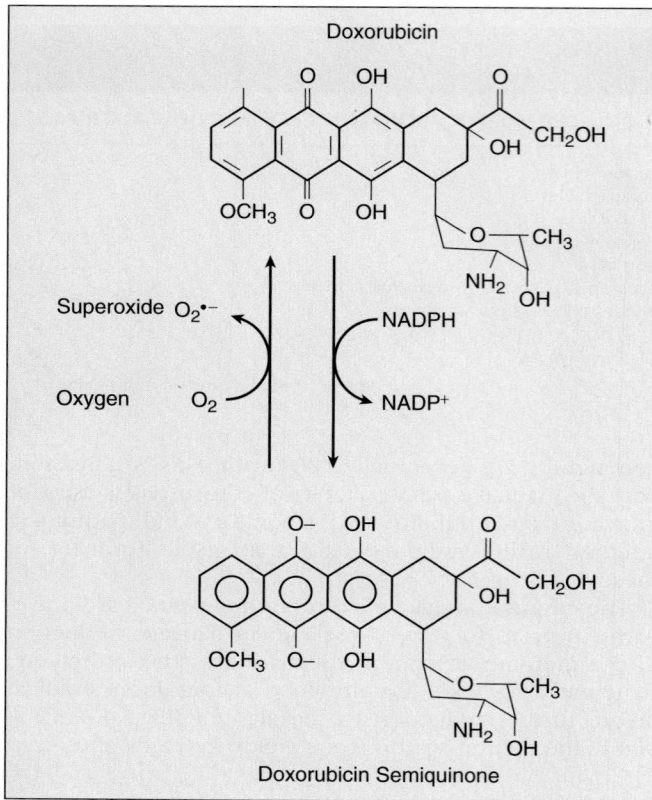

Doxorubicin

Superoxide $O_2^{\bullet-}$ ← NADPH

Oxygen O_2 → NADP$^+$

Doxorubicin Semiquinone

Figure 63-2. Redox cycling of doxorubicin by flavin-centered reductases. (From Muggia FM, Green MD, Speyer JL (eds): Cancer Treatment and the Heart. Baltimore, Johns Hopkins University Press, 1992, p 12.)

(O_2^*). Further reaction of the semiquinone with H_2O_2 yields the OH$^-$ radical. These reactions can proceed in either an iron-independent or iron-dependent fashion.[12,13]

Formation of an Fe^{3+}–doxorubicin complex can catalyze these reactions, greatly enhancing free radical generation. An Fe^{3+}–doxorubicin DNA complex has been demonstrated which results in increased cell destruction. Free radicals can cause damage at a variety of intracellular sites, including the nuclear envelope, cell membrane, mitochondria, DNA, and sarcoplasmic reticulum.[13,14] In the myocyte, damage to the sarcoplasmic reticulum produces a decrease in bound calcium. This, in turn, leads directly to decreased contractility by its action on the actin-myosin complex. Free Ca^{++} also may activate proteases within the heart, causing myofibrillar damage.

Anthracycline-induced free radical damage is not confined to the myocardium. It may indeed play some role in tumor cell killing, although this is primarily thought to be related to other mechanisms (e.g., DNA intercalation, inhibition of topoisomerase II).

The susceptibility of myocardial cells to free radicals may be explained in part by differences in cellular defenses. Of the primary cellular enzymatic defenses against free radicals—superoxide dismutase (SOD), catalase and glutathione peroxidase—only SOD is unaffected by doxorubicin. In some mammalian systems

myocytes contain very low catalase compared to other cells, e.g. liver cells.[15] Furthermore, doxorubicin can decrease cellular glutathione peroxidase. The complete translation of the observations from the rodent system to humans is not clear.[16]

In clinical practice, the anthracyclines appear to have a mechanism of activity similar to that just described. The mechanisms do not, however, fully explain the cardiac effects of the related anthracene compounds (e.g., mitoxantrone). In isolated myocyte models, specific inhibitory agents (dexrazoxane) inhibit anthracycline-induced cardiac damage, but not that of mitoxantrone, suggesting that some other mechanism for cardiac toxicity also may exist.[17] In a spontaneously hypertensive rat model, though, dexrazoxane inhibits both doxorubicin and mitoxantrone-induced cardiac toxicity.[18] Some investigators have suggested that in addition to the preceding mechanism, cardiac damage in children is due at least in part to interference with cell growth.[19]

Diagnosis

Patients may present with any or all symptoms of CHF, including decreased exercise tolerance, dyspnea, or signs of pulmonary and circulatory congestion. In our experience, sinus tachycardia and an inability to return promptly to basal cardiac rate after exertion in an otherwise oncologically stable patient are the earliest sign of myocardial toxicity, and usually predate more classic symptoms of heart failure. These can be graded by the well-established system for grading CHF.[20] A system of staging anthracycline-induced hemodynamic changes in humans was developed by Bristow (Table 63-3).[21]

Determination of left ventricular ejection fraction, by either cardiac ultrasound or gated radionuclide scanning techniques, is used to assess anthracycline cardiac toxicity. However, changes in systolic function often are seen in cancer patients, and they may not be related to anthracycline-associated damage. Such changes may occur as a consequence of anemia, the extent of tumor burden, and a variety of metabolic aberrations that may or may not be related to the malignancy or its treatment. In addition, interobserver variability in the determination of ejection fraction may further diminish the predictive value of ejection fraction alone in following patients receiving anthracyclines. Nevertheless, LV ejection fractions are used most commonly in both research studies and in clinical follow-up of patients receiving these drugs to assess their cardiotoxicity. One way to monitor patients with echocardiography or nuclear imaging is to obtain a baseline study prior to therapy and then obtain values at intervals as the cumulative dose increases. At high cumulative doses, it may be desirable to make more frequent observations. Scans are examined for sequential changes in wall motion as well as LVEF. Any decrease in LVEF, including those that remain within the "normal" range as well as those that decrease to a clearly abnormal value, may indicate anthracycline damage.[4,6,22] Careful monitoring with multiple gated acquisition (MUGA) scans may permit treatment with greater cumulative doses of doxorubicin than an empiric stopping dose of 450 to 500 mg/m^2.[4,5,6,23] Serial

TABLE 63-3

Clinical Staging of Doxorubicin Cardiac Toxicity

GRADE	ABNORMALITY
0	Within normal limits
1	Mild abnormality, any of the following:
	Resting hemodynamics:
	RVEDP >8 to <12 mm Hg or mean RAP ≥7 to <10 mm Hg
	LVEDP ≥12 to <15 mm Hg or mean PCW >10 to <15 mm Hg
	CI ≥2.2 and <2.5 L/min/m² with AVDO₂ >5 vol%
	Exercise hemodynamics:
	RVEDP >5 to <9 mm Hg above resting pressure
	PCCW >5 to <11 mm Hg above resting pressure, exercise factor (change in cardiac output/change in oxygen consumption) ≥4 to 6
2	Moderate abnormality, any of the following:
	2 or more of the above factors
	Pressure at rest:
	PCW or LVEDP ≥15 to <20 mm Hg
	RVEDP ≥12 to <17 mm Hg or RA >10 to ≤15
	CI <2.2 to ≥1.8 with AVDO₂ difference >5 vol%
	Exercise hemodynamics:
	RVEDP ≥9 mm Hg above resting pressure
	PCW ≥10 mm Hg above resting pressure at rest, exercise factor <4
3	Severe abnormality, any of the following:
	2 or more moderate abnormalities
	Hemodynamics at rest:
	PCW to LVEDP ≥20 mm Hg
	RVEDP ≥18 or ≥16 mm Hg
	CI <1.8 L/min/m² with AVDO₂ difference >5 vol%

AVDO₂, ateriovenous oxygen difference; CI, cardiac index; LVEDP, left ventricular end-diastolic pressure; PCW, pulmonary capillary wedge; RAP, right arterial pressure; RVEDP, right ventricular end-diastolic pressure.
Adapted from Bristow MR, Mason JW, Billingham ME, Daniels JR: Dose-effect and structure-function relationships in doxorubicin cardiomyopathy. Am Heart J 1981;102:709.

determinations may, however, result in premature abandonment of an important therapy because of false-positive results on an ultrasound or MUGA scan. It is important to bear in mind that the likelihood of congestive heart failure follows an exponential curve, that early toxicity may be difficult to quantify, and that an additional two or three cycles of chemotherapy may expose patients to life-threatening cumulative dosages. Decreases in the absolute value of LVEF by 10% to 20% or to less than the lower limit of normal for the laboratory warrants discontinuation of therapy. The key is that a decrease in LVEF usually precedes the development of clinical CHF and that termination of drug therapy may stop the progression of the biochemical process before clinical symptoms became apparent. Algorithmic validation of this approach has been published and supports this approach, but it is not fail-safe. When exceeding recommended cumulative dosages can be anticipated, cardioprotective strategies are clearly appropriate.

Although MUGA scans have been used in most investigational studies and for clinical follow-up, Doppler echocardiography is a useful tool for both preanthracycline evaluation of the heart (allowing assessment of underlying valvular and pericardial pathology, as well as myocardial systolic and diastolic function) and clinical follow-up during treatment. Newer computer-assisted echocardiographic technologies, including automated border detection-derived quantification of cardiac volumes and left ventricular ejection fraction, may make nuclear quantification modalities (which require radioisotopes) obsolete in patients whose hearts can be imaged ultrasonically.[24] Doppler evaluation of diastolic parameters, including rates of isovolemic relaxation and rapid filling, may be useful in the early detection of anthracycline-induced myocardial dysfunction.[25-27] Echocardiography has been used extensively in children, in whom the shorter periods of time needed to acquire data are helpful. In patients with cardiac dysrhythmias, the rhythm disturbance may interfere with cardiac gating, and echocardiography offers advantages. Patients who have received radiation to the left side of the chest may be difficult to study with cardiac ultrasound and often are better candidates for nuclear imaging.[28]

Myoscint scans are a newer investigational technique that may compliment MUGA scans. In trials using Myoscint scans, a monoclonal antibody to cardiac myosin is tagged with iodine 131–labeled, which may provide more direct evidence of myocardial damage and overcome some of the lack of specificity of MUGA scans.[29] These scans have been used as an adjunct to MUGA scans in a randomized trial of epirubicin and dexrazoxane. To date, neither the parameters of diastolic dysfunction nor any of the newer nuclear imaging techniques are sufficiently sensitive to replace MUGA scans.[30,31]

Recent evidence indicates that quantification of the cardiac contractile proteins known as troponins is a highly sensitive method of detecting myocardial cell injury in acute coronary syndromes, and has led investigators to study the applicability of such measurements to assessing anthracycline-induced myocardial cell damage. Elevated serum troponin T levels in children receiving doxorubicin for acute lymphoblastic leukemia (ALL) have been demonstrated to predict the echocardiographic findings of LV dilatation and LV wall thinning months later.[32] In an experimental model of hypertensive rats receiving doxorubicin, rises in troponin T correlated with, but preceded, the histopathologic changes associated with anthracycline-induced myocardial toxicity.[33] Troponin T levels also were used in this model to monitor cardio-protection by dexrazoxane.[18] In at least one series,[34] troponin I levels rose in anthracycline-treated patients before deterioration in LVEF was visible by MUGA scanning. Troponin I levels were elevated and correlated with a fall in LVEF in breast cancer patients receiving high-dose chemotherapy with and without anthracyclines.[35] Markers of cardiac damage have not yet been demonstrated to help in making clinical decisions to continue or stop the administration of anthracyclines. A number of additional markers currently are being investigated.[36]

The pathology of anthracycline-induced myocardial cell damage can be observed by histologic examination obtained by endomyocardial biopsy (Table 63-4). A continuum of change is well described, from dilation of vacuoles, to mitochondrial swelling, myofibrillar dropout, and, ultimately, cell death.[37] The changes seen on endomyocardial biopsy appear to parallel the clinical findings, and there is a good correlation with the clinical examination and results of MUGA scans.[38,39] The consistency of these findings among nonmammalian species has provided the basis for a number of animal models of anthracycline cardiomyopathy.[40,41]

The principal advantage of endomyocardial biopsy is the relative specificity of the test. The procedure usually is done by performing a right heart catheterization (more commonly the left heart in Europe) and using a specialized instrument to obtain a number of small tissue fragments from the interventricular septum. These are fixed for routine histologic examination using hematoxylin & eosin or fixed in glutaraldehyde for examination

under the electron microscopic. The procedure usually is performed on an outpatient basis, and in experienced hands the incidence of serious complication is less than 1%.[42]

The disadvantages of endomyocardial biopsy (EMB) include the necessity for special expertise in obtaining and interpreting the biopsies, the cost, and the possible, although low, risk of complications. In addition, many investigators, but not all, do not find serial EMB a practical option, limiting its potential clinical utility.

Decreasing Anthracycline Cardiotoxicity

Risk Reduction. Prevention is vitally important in reducing chronic anthracycline cardiac toxicity. Current approaches to risk reduction include changes in dose and schedule, and use of analogs, new delivery systems, and specific blocking agents. Dose adjustment may be achieved by limiting anthracycline doses in patients at increased risk for toxicity or by empiric limitation of cumulative doses of doxorubicin to 400 mg/m^2 to 450 mg/m^2. Both of these approaches have merit, but neither prevents toxicity in all patients. Moreover, limiting therapy or discontinuing therapy prematurely may deprive those patients who are not experiencing toxicity of therapy from which they are continuing to benefit. As noted, a combination of dose restriction with careful cardiac monitoring may offer the safest practical approach to patients receiving doxorubicin.[4,5,41] However, such strategies do have some risk of both suboptimal tumor management and cardiotoxicity.

Dose Schedule Changes. Alterations in the dose schedule of anthracyclines are based on the hypothesis that chronic cardiac toxicity is related primarily to peak drug concentration, whereas the antitumor effect is more related to total drug exposure (concentration × time, or area under the curve [AUC]). Clinical trials of weekly schedules versus those in which the drug is given every 21 days support this hypothesis: weekly schedules resulted in decreased clinical toxicity[1,43,44] and improved endomyocardial biopsy scores.[45] Extending this approach

TABLE 63-4

Histopathologic Scale of Doxorubicin Cardiomyopathy*	
Grade 0	Within normal limits
Grade 1	Minimal numbers of cells (<5% of total number of cells per blocks) with early change (early myofibrillar loss or distended sarcoplasmic reticulum)
Grade 1.5	Small group of cells involved (5% to 15% of total number), some of which have definite change (marked myofibrillar loss or cytoplasmic vacuolization)
Grade 2	Groups of cells (16%–25% of total number), some of which have definite change (marked myofibrillar loss or cytoplasmic vacuolization)
Grade 2.5	Groups of cells involved (26%–35%), some of which have definite change (marked myofibrillar loss or cytoplasmic vacuolization)
Grade 3	Diffuse cell damage (>35% of total number of cells) with marked change (total loss of contractile elements, loss of organelles, mitochondrial, and nuclear degeneration)

*Other grading scales that may incorporate an intermediate grade of 0.5 are sometimes encountered. The individual defined grades are uniform between these various scales.[202]

Adapted from Billingham ME, Mason JW, Bristow MR, Daniels JR: Anthracycline cardiomyopathy monitored by morphologic changes. Cancer Treat Rep 1978;62:865.

to continuous infusion maximizes the reduction in plasma drug concentration while still maintaining oncologic effect. Several studies have demonstrated decreased cardiac toxicity with prolonged continuous infusions (e.g., 24 to 96 hours) compared with standard rapid infusion schedules.[46,47] The cardiac toxicity is less when measured by clinical exam, MUGA scan, or cardiac biopsy, without apparent loss of antitumor efficacy. While all of the studies demonstrate that continuous infusion schedules clearly reduce cardiac toxicity, they do not totally prevent it. They do, however, allow significantly higher cumulative dosages to be administered with acceptable cardiotoxicity. In the case of doxorubicin, for example, approximately 900 mg/m^2, or twice the usual cumulative dosage, can be given when the drug is administered by 96-hour continuous infusion. Mucositis is the factor that limits the duration of infusional regimens to a maximum of 96 hours. Continuous infusion schedules have not been universally accepted, in part, because of the increased cost and the necessity for long-term or implantable access lines and infusion pumps.

New Delivery Systems.

Liposomal drugs are a new class of agents that may permit more specific organ targeting of anthracyclines, thereby producing less systemic and cardiac toxicity. Drug can be incorporated into a variety of liposomal drug preparations.[48-51] Initial activity was reported in Kaposi sarcoma for daunorubicin[48,49] and doxorubicin.[51] More recently, activity also has been reported in ovarian cancer[52] and breast cancer,[50] and clinical trials are in progress. In animal models, the pegylated liposomal preparation of doxorubicin Doxil is less cardiotoxic than is the free drug. In one trial, patients treated with Doxil had lower cardiac biopsy scores (0.5 vs. 2.25) than did controls treated with the standard doxorubicin protocol.[53,54] Similar reductions in cardiac toxicity, as measured by biopsy score, were reported in a group of 29 women with breast cancer being treated with TLC D-99 liposomal doxorubicin.[55] Other unique delivery systems include starch microspheres,[56] albumic microspheres,[57] and lipiodol.[58]

Analogs.

Analog development holds the promise of good antitumor activity with decreased cardiac toxicity. Many anthracyclines in clinical use (e.g., epirubicin and esorubicin) have been shown to produce less cardiac toxicity in preclinical animal models and were developed as potentially less cardiotoxic compounds than doxorubicin.[59] Although this is still an important avenue of research, it has not yet resulted in a major reduction in clinical cardiac toxicity when the drugs are administered at equimyelotoxic doses.[60,61] Twenty-five of 261 patients who received more than 600 mg/m^2 of epirubicin (with single doses of epirubicin 45–90 mg/m^2 day 1 and day 8 q 28 days) developed CHF (10%), including seven who died of cardiac toxicity.[60,61] In a later analysis, the same group reported that 59% of patients who had received 850 to 1000 mg/m^2 of epirubicin exhibited a 25% fall in ejection fraction 3 years after the completion of epirubicin, and 20% developed symptoms of congestive heart failure. Therapy with ACE inhibitors reversed the clinical symptoms in most, but not all, cases.[62] Biopsy studies have been limited, but suggest some cardiac protection over the native compound.[63] Some degree of cardiac toxicity indicated by a change in LVEF or development of clinical CHF was observed in patients receiving adjuvant therapy[63] with high doses (epirubicin 200 mg/m^2 and cyclophosphamide 4 g/m^2)[64] or in combination with paclitaxel,[65] although in all of these the incidence of clinical CHF was low. In the Canadian trial that compared FEC (5-fluorouracil, epirubicin, and cyclophosphamide) to CMF (cyclophosfomide, methotrexate, and 5-fluorouracil) there was no clinical cardiac toxicity in the 351 patients in the FEC arm; one of the 359 patients in the CMF arm did show cardiac toxicity, however.[61]

Blocking Agents.

Differences in the biochemical mechanisms of antitumor activity and cardiac toxicity provide a potential avenue of selectively inhibiting or preventing the adverse effect. Targets for this approach include agents that prevent free radical generation or salvage free radicals. Several free radical scavengers, including alpha tocopherol (vitamin E),[66] N-acetyl cysteine,[67] coenzyme Q-10,[68] and prenylamine,[69,70] have been tested as selective cardiac protectors with negative or inconclusive results. Dexrazoxane has been approved for use in the United States and is clearly cardioprotective. The compound is a bisdioxopiperazine that is hydrolyzed intracellularly to form a bidentate chelator, similar in structure to EDTA; it effectively binds intracellular iron. The putative mechanism of cardioprotection is that dexrazoxane strips Fe^{2+} from the iron–doxorubicin complex, thereby preventing free radical generation (Fig. 63-3). Randomized trials in patients with breast cancer[23,71-74] and small cell lung cancer[75] indicate that dexrazoxane can reduce doxorubicin-induced cardiac damage as measured by clinical examination, MUGA scan or endomyocardial biopsy. Dexrazoxane's limiting toxicity of myelosuppression did not add significantly to the toxicity of the regimens. Conflicting results for its effect on antitumor activity have been reported, but most trials indicate no negative effects.[5,71,72,74] However, a possible increase in early disease progression in one large study has led to some concern.[76] Additional trials have suggested that the drug affords cardioprotection in breast cancer without interfering with antitumor efficacy.[77-79] Furthermore, analysis of randomized trials in breast cancer suggests that even when dexrazoxane is added after the sixth course of chemotherapy (300 mg/m^2), there is significant cardioprotection while maintaining the antitumor activity of the regimen. While these analyses argue for the use of this agent in the management of breast cancer, it is now clear that anthracyclines cause cardiac damage considerably earlier than had been previously appreciated, and protection after multiple cycles of chemotherapy may not represent the optimal approach to cardioprotection.[80]

Further evaluation of dexrazoxane as a means of cardiac protection from other anthracyclines is currently underway. Coadministration of dexrazoxane with a less cardiotoxic doxorubicin analog may offer the best future

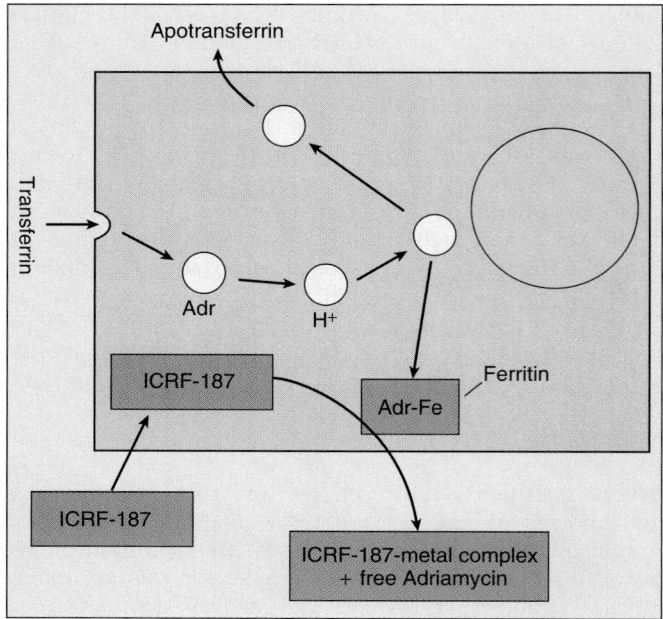

Figure 63-3. Proposed mechanism for ICRF-187 inhibition of doxorubicin Fe complex formation. (From Muggia FM, Green MD, Speyer JL (eds): Cancer Treatment and the Heart. Baltimore, Johns Hopkins University Press, 1992, p 27.)

means of reducing anthracycline-related cardiac toxicity. Of interest, dexrazoxane has been shown in animal systems to protect against the cardiotoxic effects of epidoxorubicin but may have less effect with mitoxantrone.[17,81] Clinical testing of dexrazoxane in combination with epidoxorubicin has been shown in randomized trials in women with breast cancer to protect against cardiac toxicity without inhibiting antitumor activity,[82] and these results have been extended to sarcoma treated with high-dose epirubicin.[30]

Pediatrics

Children appear to be more sensitive to the cardiotoxicity of anthracycline than are adults, and younger children are at the greatest risk.[27,83] Retrospective studies suggest that anthracycline toxicity occurs in children at lower cumulative doses.[27,84,85] Improved survival in childhood cancers has permitted the study of long-term effects of treatment. In contrast to adult patients, who rarely develop late CHF without having manifested early-onset cardiotoxicity, delayed-onset cardiac decompensation has been described in children 6 to 10 years after treatment.[86,87] Anthracyclines may cause reduction in cardiac growth, or latent functional or structural damage that may not manifest itself until the children outgrow their limited cardiac capacity. Children treated with doxorubicin have been found to have a progressive increase in left ventricular afterload,[88] possibly resulting from inappropriately thin left ventricular walls, which produces increased wall stress. In addition, a variety of factors that increase cardiac stress (e.g., drug use, weight lifting, pregnancy) increase the risk of late cardiac dysfunction in patients who received anthracycline treatment in childhood.[89,90] Viral

infection may represent a sequential stress that may account for some of the cases of late cardiotoxicity in children.[9]

In contrast to adults, echocardiograms measuring fractional shortening and LVEF are used more commonly in children.[27] Possible limitations of radionuclide scans in children include the infusion of radioactive isotopes, the requirement for lying still, and the variable quality of studies, because increased variability of cardiac cycle time in children can affect cardiac gating.

As in adults, factors not related to cancer treatment may contribute to cardiac toxicity in children. In one study, 12 of 103 children with ALL (12%) demonstrated elevated cardiac troponin T levels at the time of diagnosis. In this randomized Children's Oncology Group trial, dexrazoxane also significantly decreased the amount of doxorubicin-induced troponin T level elevation without interfering with the rate of complete clinical remission.[91]

Other Causes of Congestive Heart Failure

Chemotherapy

Mitoxantrone. Mitoxantrone was developed primarily as a non-cardiotoxic analog of the anthracyclines. It is an anthracendione that lacks the amino sugar common to anthracyclines. Data from collected single-agent studies and two randomized studies indicate that mitoxantrone may result in a congestive cardiomyopathy, but at a lower incidence than doxorubicin when equimyelotoxic doses are compared.[92-94] The incidence of cardiotoxicity at cumulative doses of greater than 160 mg/m^2 is about 5%, although the incidence of clinical congestive heart failure is less than 2%.

The clinical presentation is similar to that seen with doxorubicin. The diagnostic evaluation and endomyocardial biopsy changes are similar to those seen with doxorubicin.[95]

The biochemical mechanism of damage is not clear. Prior therapy with doxorubicin increases the risk of mitoxantrone cardiac toxicity; changing from one anthracycline to another, or to an analog, may not protect from cardiotoxicity. As stated previously, the mechanism of cardiac toxicity may not be the same as for doxorubicin.

Phosphoramide Mustards. High-dose intravenous cyclophosphamide infusion (120–240 mg/kg over 1 to 4 days) has been associated with congestive heart failure and death from hemorrhagic myocarditis.[96-98] In contrast to that from anthracyclines, cardiac toxicity from cyclophosphamide is acute and is not related to the cumulative dose. Mortality is high in the face of fulminant hemorrhagic myocarditis, the majority of patients treated with high-dose cyclophosphamide will demonstrate a decrease in QRS voltage and a decrease in systolic function, which often are asymptomatic and reversible. Postmortem studies and an experimental animal model suggest that the loss of systolic function is due to direct endothelial injury resulting in capillary microthrombosis and interstitial fibrin deposition.

Ifosfamide. Iphosphamide also has been associated with the development of CHF in a dose-dependent fashion. In one series of 52 patients receiving a high dose ($10-18$ g/m^2) as part of high-dose chemotherapy with ABMT, 9 patients (17%) developed CHF (8 severe enough to require admission to the intensive care unit) at a mean of 12 days (range, 6–23 days) after therapy.[99] Most of these patients received prior doxorubicin, raising the possibility of sequential stress. Of interest, autopsy data (endomyocardial biopsies were not performed) did not reveal hemorrhagic myocarditis.

Interleukin-2. The major cardiovascular effects of interleukin-2 (IL-2) include hypotension (secondary to decreased peripheral vascular resistance), dysrhythmias, and ischemia. Primary myocardial suppression is also suggested by a decrease in LVEF and an increased end-diastolic volume. This results from inadequate cardiac compensation in the face of changes in peripheral resistance.[100]

Piroxantrone. Piroxantrone is an anthrapyrazole developed in part to avoid the cardiac toxicity of anthracyclines. In a Phase II trial of women with breast cancer,[101] piroxantrone was associated with a decrease in LVEF in 2 of 30 patients.

Monoclonal Antibody to Her2/neu. The monoclonal antibody to Her2/neu receptor, trastuzumab (Herceptin), is now available for the treatment of breast cancers that overexpress Her2/neu. Cardiac toxicity was reported in the single-agent Phase II trial reported by Cobleigh and coworkers.[102] In the pivotal Stage III trial, an unexpectedly high incidence of cardiac toxicity was observed—27% when an anthracycline and cyclophosphamide were combined with trastuzumab compared with 8% with the chemotherapy alone. A similar though smaller effect (13% versus 1%) was observed when paclitaxel was combined with trastuzumab. It should be noted that all of the patients treated with paclitaxel had received prior anthracyclines.[103] Seidman and colleagues[104] reviewed the records of 1219 patients in seven trastuzumab trials. They report an incidence of cardiac dysfunction of 3% to 7% with trastuzumab alone, 27% with anthracycline and cyclophosphamide, and 13% with paclitaxel. Further data from prospective trials are necessary to better quantify the contribution of trastuzumab to chemotherapy-induced toxicity.[105] The mechanism for trastuzumab toxicity has not been elucidated, but there is in vitro evidence that Her2 may be involved in myocyte resistance to stress and repair.[106,107] Decreased repair mechanisms combined with the known cardiotoxic effects of other agents could explain the clinical observations. Recent studies have demonstrated that the biopsy changes seen with doxorubicin are not present with trastuzumab toxicity.[108] Anecdotal case reports have suggested that the cardiac toxicity associated with trastuzumab is reversible and may not recur with retreatment.[109] Additional questions being addressed in several large trials include the relative effects of the duration and sequence of trastuzumab therapy combined with chemotherapy. The addition of carboplatin to paclitaxel and trastuzumab does not appear to increase cardiac toxicity[110] nor does the combination of vinorelbine and trastuzumab.[111,112] Cardiac observations with combinations of trastuzumab and gemcitabine, capecitabine, and other drugs are underway.

Other Combinations. Combinations of chemotherapeutic agents have been reported to cause varying degrees of CHF. When doxorubicin was first combined with paclitaxel, an 18% incidence of CHF was reported with cumulative doxorubicin doses of 400 mg/m^2.[113] Not all investigators reported this high rate, however.[114] When the paclitaxel initially was administered as a 24-hour infusion, increased plasma and tissue concentrations of doxorubicin and the doxorubicinol metabolite were observed. Limiting the doxorubicin dose and allowing for an interval between doxorubicin and paclitaxel administration reduced the incidence of CHF to 4.7% of 657 patients, with a higher incidence of 25% in patients who received greater than 440 mg/m^2.[115] Combinations of doxorubicin with docetaxel have not been associated with increased cardiac toxicity.[116] In a randomized trial comparing doxorubicin and docetaxel with doxorubicin and cyclophosphamide in 429 women with breast cancer, CHF was not increased (3% vs. 4%), and the decline in LVEF—30 points from baseline—was less (1% compared with 6%).[117,118] The incidence of CHF has been reported to be 6% for the combination of epidoxorubicin with paclitaxel.[119] Several trials have raised the possibility of increased cardiac toxicity when doxorubicin is combined with high-dose cyclophosphamide[120] in the transplant setting.

Radiation

Radiation to the myocardium can cause interstitial myocardial fibrosis. This occurs through capillary damage, organization of fibrinous exudates with microcirculatory damage, and fibrosis.[121] Echocardiography and MUGA scans can help to differentiate primary myocardial damage from the pericardial damage that often occurs in the same patients.[122] Repeated doses or very high radiation doses (>6000 cGy) are associated with a greater risk of radiation damage. Biventricular dysfunction is a common, although usually asymptomatic finding, occurring 5 to 20 years after radiation therapy. This is especially likely in patients who have been treated through a single anteroposterior port.[123] As a result of advances in radiotherapy techniques, clinically significant radiation-induced myocarditis is rare, and presumably the rates of late dysfunction will become rare as well.

Increased caution must be exercised, however, when radiation therapy is combined with doxorubicin therapy, because there appears to be a synergistic toxic effect on the myocardium. This may occur even if the two therapies are temporally separated by long time periods. Prior radiation is a well recognized risk factor for developing doxorubicin toxicity.[124] Conversely, radiation can cause a

Problems Common to Cancer and Its Therapy

DOXORUBICIN-INDUCED CARDIOMYOPATHY

MONITORING

- Physical examination is the best way to monitor patients for doxorubicin-induced cardiomyopathy (e.g., sinus tachycardia is a nonspecific early sign), with radionuclide scans or echocardiograms at baseline, 300 mg/m^2, 450 mg/m^2, and each 100 mg/m^2 thereafter.
- Patients at increased risk—for instance, those who have had prior treatment with anthracyclines, are older than 70 years of age, have had prior chest radiation therapy, or have preexisting cardiac disease—may need to be observed more closely. Therapy should be withheld if the left ventricular ejection fraction falls to less than 0.45 or to 0.2 below baseline (other investigators have used a fall of 0.15 as the cutoff for discontinuing therapy).
- Most centers still use endomyocardial biopsy as the confirmatory tool. Biopsy should be considered in patients with a cumulative dose of 450 mg/m^2 or more, and therapy should be withheld in any case if the Billingham biopsy score is 2 or greater.
- Cardiac troponin C and I are under investigation for monitoring purposes.

CUMULATIVE DOSE LIMITATION

If monitoring strategies are in place, most patients who are thought to be benefiting from therapy can be safely treated to doses exceeding 450 mg/m^2.

DOSAGE SCHEDULE MODIFICATION

The incidence of cardiomyopathy may be decreased by modifying the dose schedule. For example, intravenous bolus schedules may be adjusted by dividing the 21-day dose into three weekly doses, or a continuous infusion schedule in which the full dose is given over 72 to 96 hours through central catheters with portable infusion pumps.

CARDIOPROTECTION

Dexrazoxane (ICRF-187: ADR 529), a chelating agent that binds intracellular iron and prevents free radical production, has been shown in clinical trials to markedly reduce the incidence and severity of cardiomyopathy.

TREATMENT

- The first step in treatment is to stop the doxorubicin, and then not to use it again in the future. As with other cardiomyopathies, fluid intake is limited.
- Sodium, diuretics, afterload, and cautious use of afterload reduction, especially with angiotensin-converting enzyme inhibitors, may result in clinical improvement.
- The course is variable and can vary, ranging from improvement to steady worsening with biventricular failure and death as the outcome.

sudden decrease in ventricular function in a patient who either is receiving or has received doxorubicin.

Therapy

Treatment of all cardiomyopathies is similar, regardless of their etiology. Ceasing treatment with the offending agent is of prime importance, and changing from one agent to another will not protect from further cardiotoxicity. Fluid and sodium restriction and the use of diuretics may provide some relief in acute situations. Afterload reduction with agents such as ACE inhibitors is clearly beneficial, and in stable patients, beta-adrenergic blockers such as carvedilol appear to be of significant benefit.[125] Clinical improvement in anthracycline-induced CHF has been demonstrated, as has improvement in LVEF as measured by serial MUGA scans.[6,126] Currently no therapy is available that can reverse the damage done to the injured myocardium, and dexrazoxane, despite its mechanism of protection in the acute stage of cardiac damage, would not be expected to repair existing damage.

CONGESTIVE STATES ASSOCIATED WITH OTHER CANCER TREATMENT

General considerations of fluid and electrolyte management should be carefully considered when administering anticancer treatment. Possible fluid overload states may result from intensive hydration regimens (e.g., for cisplatin), or with transfusion. Patients with anemia and low serum albumin are more susceptible to high output

states. Malignant pleural and pericardial effusions, as well as ascites or intrathoracic malignancies, can cause external compression of the heart with resulting symptoms of congestive heart failure. Thyroid dysfunction sometimes is identified in cancer patients and responds to the usual therapeutic interventions.

DYSRHYTHMIAS

Dysrhythmias are commonly seen in the course of treatment of malignancies. The entire spectrum of supraventricular and ventricular brady- and tachydysrhythmias may be seen in cancer patients for a variety of reasons that may or may not be related to the cancer or its treatment. These include intra- or paracardiac tumor, electrolyte imbalances, fever, or hyperadrenergic states. Dysrhythmias related to therapy may, in turn, be related to coronary or myocardial disease resulting from anticancer therapy, or to the direct dysrhythmogenic effects of the anticancer therapy itself.

Radiation injury has been implicated in the development of sinus node dysfunction, atrioventricular block, and conduction disturbances below the bundle of His.[127,128]

Occasional dysrhythmias have been reported with the anthracyclines. While these usually occur in the setting of the drug-induced cardiomyopathy, the dysrhythmias are not a prominent part of the clinical picture. Sinus tachycardia, however, is exceeding common in patients with an anthracycline-induced cardiomyopathy and may be the earliest sign of the cardiomyopathic effect of anthracyclines. Supraventricular dysrhythmias also may occur with the development of pulmonary venous hypertension. Ventricular dysrhythmias occur in the setting of left ventricular failure. Sudden death, however, remains rare.

In contrast to the anthracyclines, the primary cardiac toxicity of amsacrine is its deleterious electrophysiologic effects. The incidence of life-threatening dysrhythmias in patients receiving amsacrine has been reported to be 1%.[129] Amsacrine infusion also has been associated with QT prolongation. This effect appears to be the basis of ventricular dysrhythmias that have been observed in clinical practice. However, malignant ventricular dysrhythmias in patients treated with amsacrine have been seen most frequently in association with hypokalemia. It has been suggested, therefore, that patients receive prophylactic administration of potassium chloride in anticipation of amsacrine infusion.[130] Arsenic trioxide, an agent that is being used increasingly in the treatment of promyelocytic leukemia, also is associated with prolongation of the QT interval, and some deaths have been reported following the use of this agent.[131,132]

Taxol has been implicated in the development of dysrhythmias. A 30% incidence of asymptomatic bradycardia has been observed with this agent; however, the bradycardia seldom requires termination of the agent. In addition, atrioventricular block of varying degrees, bundle branch block, and ventricular tachycardia have been described[133,134] and may require specific therapy.

Supraventricular tachycardias were reported in 8 of 41 (20%) patients receiving therapy with dihydro-5-azacytidine, an investigational pyrimidine, for mesothelioma.[135]

Interleukin-11 (Neumega) recently has been introduced for the reduction of chemotherapy-induced thrombocytopenia. In one trial, 6 of 58 patients (10%) developed symptomatic dysrhythmias[136]—5 patients had atrial fibrillation and 1 patient had atrial flutter. The authors speculated that these effects might have been secondary to fluid retention. Dysrhythmias also have been reported with the monoclonal antibody to CD20 (Rituxan).[137,138] Nonspecific dysrhythmia is common in cancer patients, and may be due to fluid and electrolyte shifts associated with vomiting, as well as hyperadrenergic states that may accompany anemia and a variety of other factors. Most of these rhythm disturbances may be managed with correction of the underlying abnormality and do not require specific antidysrhythmic therapy.

MYOCARDIAL ISCHEMIA

A variety of ischemic syndromes have been ascribed to oncologic therapy. Much of the data, however, is anecdotal, as there is a high incidence of coronary artery disease in the population in which cancer is also common. Chemotherapy may shift a previously stable oxygen supply and demand balance in favor of an increased demand in the face of a fixed supply that results in the ischemic syndrome. The clinical picture is further confused by the high incidence of intercurrent intrathoracic malignant disease, anemia, fever, and infections, and concomitant treatment with other drugs, all of which

may affect the balance. Furthermore, the malignancy itself may cause chest pain in a patient with noncritical ischemic disease.

There is, however, convincing evidence that thoracic radiation therapy is associated with the development of coronary artery disease.[139] In addition to the very substantial body of evidence that radiation causes small vessel damage, which ultimately leads to myocardial fibrosis and cardiomyopathy, there also are data that implicate radiation therapy in the development of epicardial (particularly ostial) coronary artery disease.[139,140] The original data came largely from case reports of myocardial ischemia and infarction in young adults (without other risk factors for coronary atherosclerosis) following mediastinal radiation therapy.[141-143] Two basic pathologic mechanisms have been implicated. The first relates to the direct effects of radiation on the endothelial cells of epicardial coronary arteries leading to accelerated atherogenesis. The second—and more typical—pathology is that of severe medial and adventitial fibrosis, perhaps mediated through radiation damage to the vasa vasorum. Typically, this vessel fibrosis is associated with a paucity of the intimal lipid deposition that characterizes atherosclerotic lesions.[143-146] With newer cardiac-sparing radiation therapy techniques, the likelihood of cardiac damage has been reduced.

Much less is known about the ischemia-producing effects of oncologic drug therapies. The largest number of cases of ischemia ascribed to anticancer therapy is associated with treatment with 5-fluorouracil.[147-153] Several case reports called attention to this possible association. There have been isolated reports of patients with normal coronary angiography who developed typical symptoms and electrocardiographic (ECG) evidence of ischemia after 5FU infusion,[148] but a review of over 1000 patients receiving 5FU revealed an incidence of cardiac toxicity of 4.5% in patients in whom coronary disease was known to predate treatment versus an incidence of 1.1% in those not known to have coronary artery disease (CAD) prior to therapy.[149] Thus it was not surprising that an early prospective analysis[146] was not convincing for a causative role of this drug in the development of angina or myocardial infarction. In a prospective series of 910 patients,[150] however, 5 patients (0.55%) developed signs and symptoms consistent with coronary artery spasm. All five patients had ST segment elevation and ventricular dysrhythmias. Four had documented infarction, and two had cardiac arrests, leading to the hypothesis that there may be 5FU- or metabolite-mediated increases in coronary vasomotor tone. Coronary artery spasm as a mechanism for 5FU-associated ischemia could explain the increased incidence of ischemia in patients with underlying coronary disease as well as in those with angiographically normal coronary vessels. Interestingly, however, nitrates and calcium blockers do not appear to render a protective effect.[153] Multiple studies have suggested that the association of 5FU with myocardial ischemic events is more striking in patients treated with continuous infusion therapy.[147,150-153] The association is more common in patients receiving concomitant radiation therapy[153] or treatment with cisplatin.[152]

Although the vinca alkaloids also have been reported to precipitate angina and myocardial infarction,[154,155] this observation is strictly anecdotal.

PERIPHERAL VASCULAR DISEASE

Raynaud phenomenon has been described in patients receiving cisplatin-based therapy.[156] It also has been described after therapy with vinblastine, vincristine, and bleomycin. These may be similar in mechanism to other ischemic syndromes (e.g., coronary ischemia or cerebral vascular ischemia), which have been described with these agents as well as 5FU.

Increased thromboembolism has been observed when thalidomide is combined with doxorubicin,[157] and with gemcitabine and infusional 5-fluorouracil.[158] A similarly high incidence of thromboembolic events was reported with the combination of gemcitabine, cisplatin, and SU5416.[159] As is the case for radiation-induced coronary artery disease, clinically significant occlusive lesions in other arteries, such as the carotids,[160] have been reported following irradiation.

PERICARDIAL DISEASE

Most pericardial disease presenting in cancer patients may be attributed to the underlying malignancy. Patients may have metastatic disease to the pericardium or obstruction of lymphatic or venous flow, producing a pericardial effusion. Even in patients without clinically manifest disease, asymptomatic pericardial effusions are common. Pericardial effusions have been ascribed to the anthracyclines[161] as well as cyclophosphamide[162] and dihydro-5 azacytidine.[135] With the exception of irradiation, pericardial manifestations of cancer treatment are seldom troublesome. Interestingly, in series in which pericardial effusions were reported with doxorubicin or cyclophosphamide, most patients ultimately went on to demonstrate evidence of myocardial toxicity from the drugs. Isolated pericarditis was rare.

Docetaxel (Taxotere), an active taxane analog of paclitaxel (Taxol), has broad antitumor activity, but is associated with fluid retention in some patients. Severe fluid retention and congestive heart failure is rare. This syndrome is progressive with more treatment cycles. It does not appear to be of cardiac or renal origin.[163] Premedication with steroids substantially reduces this problem.[163,164]

Radiation-Induced Pericardial Disease

Pericardial disease is a well-known side effect of thoracic radiation therapy. Effusions have been reported in 6% to 30% of patients receiving radiation therapy to the chest.[165] Since the 1960s there have been numerous reports of patients who had received high-dose mediastinal radiation for the treatment of lymphoma and ultimately developed pericardial disease.[166-168] Similar reports ascribing pericardial disease to radiation therapy for breast cancer also appeared in the late 1960s.[169]

The clinical spectrum of radiation-induced pericardial disease is wide. Acute pericarditis occurs in 10% to 15% of patients with Hodgkin disease who receive more than 4000 rads to the mediastinum.[170] The clinical onset of symptoms related to the pericarditis is anywhere from 0 to 85 months after therapy, with a peak occurring between 5 and 9 months. The acute pericarditis may be symptomatic, with the patient experiencing chest pain and fever and the physician noting a pericardial friction rub. However, acute pericardial inflammation probably is often asymptomatic. In any event, the acute pericarditis usually resolves spontaneously. In symptomatic patients, treatment with nonsteroidal anti-inflammatory drugs (including aspirin) or corticosteroids probably is warranted.[171]

The acute effects of radiation on the pericardium appear to be due to an increase in capillary permeability in the pericardium resulting in a fibrinous exudate. Ultimately, fibrosis and calcification may occur. Less than half of symptomatic and asymptomatic patients with acute pericarditis will go on to develop chronic pericardial disease or tamponade.[172] Constrictive pericarditis has been described anywhere from 2 to 20 years after radiation.[173] Signs of constriction may include a pericardial knock, Kussmaul's sign, peripheral edema, and evidence of bowel edema or hepatic congestion. The pericardium may appear thickened on a thoracic CAT scan or an echocardiogram. The diagnosis of constrictive physiology almost always can be confirmed by Doppler echocardiography. In such patients pericardiectomy may be warranted; however. the surgery is often difficult and carries significant morbidity and mortality.

Radiation-induced pericardial disease appears to depend on the extent to which the heart has received radiation and the dose of radiation delivered to the heart. With current techniques in mediastinal radiation, including the use of modern megavoltage equipment and the delivery of divided radiation to the anterior and posterior thorax with a subcorinal shell, it is likely that the incidence of pericardial disease has been significantly decreased, perhaps to the range of 2% to 2.5%.[173,174]

CARDIOCIRCULATORY EFFECTS OF BIOLOGIC RESPONSE MODIFIERS

Recombinant technology has made a number of new agents available for clinical trial. As expected, they have a variety of side effects. In some cases they may actively be the molecular indicator of a variety of cellular interactions. Hypotension and tachycardia are observed with a number of agents. With interferon alpha, these have been reported in 6% to 14% of patients.[175,176] It is difficult in these studies to separate changes in blood pressure from dysrhythmias or ischemic events. Hypotension is a more consistent feature of interferon and,[177-181] although fewer patients have received other biologic therapies.

Hypotension (along with dysrhythmias, ischemia, and decreased contractility) is a major side effect of interleukin-2, and was observed to occur in more than 70% of patients in the early IL2/LAK trials.[182,183] The primary mechanism appears to be decreased vascular resistance.[100,182-184] In the early days of therapy, patients develop increased heart rate, increased cardiac index, and decreased left ventricular stroke volume work index, peripheral vascular resistance, and mean arterial blood pressure. The clinical presentation is similar to that of septic shock, with a vascular leak syndrome, fluid retention, and noncardiogenic pulmonary edema. The mechanism may be similar to septic shock, with induction of cytokines and effector cells and the release of vaso-active agents.[185,186] Reductions in dose and continuous infusion schedules have lessened these toxicities[187-190] but also may decrease the antitumor effects.[191,192] In one study,[193] oral L-carnitine appeared to decrease these complications. IL-2 toxicity often requires ICU management, support with pressors, and, at times, ventilatory support.

Hypotension also has been described with tumor necrosis factor (TNF),[194] granulocyte macrophage colony-stimulating factor (GM-CSF),[195] interleukin-11,[136] and monoclonal antibodies.[137,138] With TNF the hypotension often is dose-limiting.[194] With GM-CSF it is observed at high doses and is associated with a capillary leak syndrome and decreased peripheral resistance.[195] The mechanism with these two agents is not as well defined nor is the clinical problem as acute as it is with IL-2. Hypotension also has been reported with interleukin-1 in Phase I trials.[196]

The possibility of cardiac toxicity was raised in early trials of interleukin-4, especially when one patient was found to have biopsy-proven myocarditis.[197,198] Interleukin-6 has been associated with cardiac dysrhythmias.[199] Syncope or near-syncope was reported in 6 of 58 patients in a trial of IL-11 (5 patients at the 50 mg/kg level and 1 patient in the in placebo group). Six patients also had documented dysrhythmias.[136]

Changes in peripheral vascular resistance and hypotension may be generalized effects of biologic therapies. Further elucidation of their mechanisms and management is required.

The complexities of bone marrow transplantation have led to cardiac toxicity in a number of patients. In a series of 170 patients monitored prospectively, life-threatening pericardial effusions or cardiac arrest were observed in less than 2% of cases.[200] Decreased ejection fraction was observed in 17 patients. In a retrospective study of 138 patients treated with high-dose therapy and stem cell rescue, cardiotoxicity occurred in 17 patients. It occurred more frequently in patients with lymphoma and breast cancer.[201] It is difficult, however, to determine which of the many drugs used in the regimen, particularly the chemotherapy induction, is responsible for these changes.

LONG-TERM EFFECTS OF CHEMOTHERAPY

One additional caution must be raised. As an increasing number of patients are long-term survivors—survivors of childhood cancers, adult patients who received adjuvant therapy without disease recurrence, or long-term survivors of more advanced adult malignancies—

unanticipated cardiovascular effects may be observed. Long-term observation and study of these patients is necessary. Identification of such effects may bring into question the overall risk/benefit ratio of the original treatment. In a long-term (median, 10.2 years) follow-up study of 992 males in the United Kingdom who had been treated with chemotherapy or radiation for testicular cancer, the incidence of cardiac events (angina, chest pain, or MI) was increased when compared to controls treated with orchiectomy alone: chemotherapy alone RR 2.59; radiation therapy RR 2.40; and chemotherapy plus radiation RR 2.78. Neither the radiation fields nor the specific chemotherapeutic agent (bleomycin, vinblastine, cisplatin or carboplatin) fully explained these findings.[202]

REFERENCES

1. Von Hoff DD, Layard MW, Basa P, Davis HL, Von Hoff AL, Rozencweig M, Muggia FM: Risk factors for doxorubicin-induced congestive heart failure. Ann Intern Med 1979;91:710–717.
2. Von Hoff DD, Rozencweig M, Layard M, Slavik M, Muggia FM: Daunomycin-induced cardiotoxicity in children and adults. A review of 110 cases. Am J Med 1977;62:200–208.
3. Bristow M, Thompson P, Martin R, Mason J, Billingham M, Harrison D: Early anthracycline cardiotoxicity. Am J Med 1978; 65:823–832.
4. Schwartz RG, McKenzie WB, Alexander J, et al: Congestive heart failure and left ventricular dysfunction complicating doxorubicin therapy: A seven year experience using serial radionuclide angiocardiography. Am J Med 1987;82:1109–1118.
5. Speyer JL, Green MD, Zeleniuch-Jacquotte A, et al: ICRF-187 permits longer treatment with doxorubicin in women with breast cancer. J Clin Oncol 1992;10:117–127.
6. Schwartz RG, Zaret BL: The diagnosis and treatment of drug-induced myocardial disease. In Muggia FM, Green MD, Speyer JL (eds): Cancer Treatment and the Heart. Baltimore, Johns Hopkins University Press, 1992, pp 173–197.
7. Swain S, Whaley F, Gerber M, et al: Congestive heart failure after doxorubicin containing therapy in advanced breast cancer patients treated with or without dexrazoxane. Proc Am Soc Clin Oncol 1996;15:A536.
8. Swain SM, Whaley FS, Ewer MS: Congestive heart failure in patients treated with doxorubicin: A retrospective analysis of three trials. Cancer 2003;97:2869–2879.
9. Ali M, Ewer M, Gibbs H, Swafford J, Graff K: Late doxorubicin-associated cardiotoxicity in children: The possible role of intercurrent viral infection. Cancer 1994;74:182.
10. Saini J, Rich MW, Lyss AP: Reversibility of severe left ventricular dysfunction due to doxorubicin cardiotoxicity: Report of three cases. Ann Intern Med 1987;106:814–816.
11. Dries DL, Strong MH, Cooper RS, et al: Efficacy of angiotensin-converting enzyme inhibition in reducing progression from asymptomatic left ventricular dysfunction to symptomatic heart failure in black and white patients. JACC 2002;40:311–317.
12. Gianni L, Corden BJ, Myers CE: The biochemical basis of anthracycline toxicity and antitumor activity. In Hodgson E, Bend JR, Philport RM (eds): Reviews in Biochemical Toxicology. Amsterdam, Elsevier, 1983, pp 1–82.
13. Gianni L, Myers CE: The role of free radical formation in the cardiotoxicity of anthracycline. In Muggia FM, Green MD, Speyer JL (eds): Cancer Treatment and the Heart. Baltimore, Johns Hopkins University Press, 1992, pp 9–46.
14. Doroshow JH: Effect of anthracycline antibiotics on oxygen radical formation in rat heart. Cancer Res 1983;43:460–472.
15. Doroshow JH, Locker GY, Myers CE: The enzymatic defenses of the mouse heart against reactive metabolites. J Clin Invest 1980;65:128–135.
16. Green MD, Alderton P, Sobol MM, Gross J, Muggia FM, Speyer JL. ICRF-187 (ADR-529) cardioprotection against anthracycline-

induced cardiotoxicity: Clinical and preclinical studies. Cancer Treat Res 1991;58:101–117.

17. Alderton PM, Gross J, Green MD: Comparative study of doxorubicin, mitoxantrone, and epirubicin in combination with ICRF-187 (ADR-529) in a chronic cardiotoxicity animal model. Cancer Res 1992;52:194–201.

18. Herman EH, Zhang J, Rifai N, et al: The use of serum levels of cardiac troponin T to compare the protective activity of dexrazoxane against doxorubicin- and mitoxantrone-induced cardiotoxicity. Cancer Chemother Pharmacol 2001;48:297–304.

19. Lipshultz S, Giantris A, Lipsitz S, et al: Doxorubicin administration by continuous infusion is not cardioprotective: the Dana-Farber 91-01 Acute Lymphoblastic protocol. J Clin Oncol 2002;20:1677–1682.

20. The Criteria Committee of the New York Heart Association: Nomenclature and Criteria for Diagnosis of Diseases of the Heart and Great Vessels. 8th ed. Boston, Little, Brown, 1979.

21. Bristow MR, Mason JW, Billingham ME, Daniels JR: Dose-effect and structure-function relationships in doxorubicin cardiomyopathy. Am Heart J 1981;102:709–718.

22. Speyer JL, Green MD, Dubin N, et al: Prospective evaluation of cardiotoxicity during a 6 hour doxorubicin infusion regimen in women with adenocarcinoma of breast. Am J Med 1985;78:555–563.

23. Speyer JL, Green MD, Kramer E, et al: Protective effect of the bispiperazinedione ICRF-187 against doxorubicin-induced cardiac toxicity in women with advanced breast cancer. N Engl J Med 1988;319:745–752.

24. Gorcsan J III, Schulman DS, Koch L, Thornton J, Follansbee W: Echocardiographic automated border detection-derived left ventricular ejection fraction: Comparison with radionuclide angiography. Abstract. Circulation 1991;84(Suppl II):585.

25. Marchandise B, Schroeder E, Bosly A, et al: Early detection of doxorubicin cardiotoxicity: Interest of Doppler echocardiographic analysis of left ventricular filling dynamics. Am Heart J 1989;118:92–98.

26. Stoddard M, Seeger J, Liddell N, et al: Prolongation of isovolumetric relaxation time as assessed by Doppler echocardiography predicts doxorubicin-induced systolic dysfunction in humans. J Am Coll Cardiol 1992;20:62–69.

27. Grenier MA, Lipshultz SE: Epidemiology of anthracycline cardiotoxicity in children and adults. Semin Oncol 1985;25(Suppl 10):72–85.

28. Ali M, Ewer M: Cancer and the Cardiopulmonary System. New York, Raven Press, 1984.

29. Carrio I, Estorch M, Berna L, et al: Assessment of anthracycline-induced myocardial damage by quantitative indium 111 myosin-specific monoclonal antibody studies. Eur J Nucl Med 18:806–812, 1991.

30. Lopez M, Vici P, Lauro LD, et al: Randomized prospective clinical trial of high-dose epirubicin and dexrazoxane in patients with advanced breast cancer and soft tissue sarcomas. J Clin Oncol 1998;16:1–7.

31. Ewer M, Ali M, Gibbs H, et al: Cardiac diastolic function in pediatric patients receiving doxorubicin. Acta Oncol 1994;33:645–649.

32. Lipshultz SE, Ottlinger M, Lipsitz SR, et al: Predictive value of serum cardiac troponin T (cTnT) in pediatric patients at risk for myocardial injury. J Am Coll Cardiol 1977;29:A431.

33. Herman EH, Lipshultz SE, Rifai N, et al: Use of cardiac troponin T levels as an indicator of doxorubicin-induced cardiotoxicity. Cancer Res 1998;58:195–197.

34. Missov E, Pau F, Calzolari C: Increased circulating levels of cardiac troponin in anthracycline-treated patients. Circulation 1996;94(8, Supplement 1):1–732.

35. Cardinale A, Sandri MT, Martinoni A, et al: Myocardial injury revealed by plasma troponin I in breast cancer treated with high-dose chemotherapy. Ann Oncol 2002;13:710–715.

36. Okumura H, Iuchi K, Yoshida T, et al: Brain natriuretic peptide is a predictor of anthracycline-induced cardiotoxicity. Acta Haematol 2000;104:158–163.

37. Billingham ME, Mason JW, Bristow MR, Daniels JR: Anthracycline cardiomyopathy monitored by morphologic changes. Cancer Treat Rep 1978;62:865–872.

38. Ewer MS, Ali MK, Mackay B, et al: A comparison of cardiac biopsy grades and ejection fraction estimations in patients receiving Adriamycin. J Clin Oncol 1984;2:112–117.

39. Benjamin RS, Chawla SP, Ewer MS: Adriamycin cardiac toxicity—An assessment of approaches to cardiac monitoring and cardioprotection. In Hacker MP, Lazo JS, Tritton TR (eds): Organ-directed Toxicities of Anticancer Therapy. Boston, Martinus Nijhoff, 1987.

40. Ferrans VJ, Sanchez JA, Herman EH: Pathologic anatomy of animal models of the cardiotoxicity of anthracyclines. In Muggia FM, Green MD, Speyer JL (eds): Cancer Treatment and the Heart. Baltimore, Johns Hopkins University Press, 1992, pp 89–113.

41. Herman EH, Ferrans VJ, Sanchez JA: Methods of reducing the cardiotoxicity of anthracyclines. In Muggia FM, Green MD, Speyer JL (eds): Cancer Treatment and the Heart. Baltimore, Johns Hopkins University Press, 1992, pp 114–169.

42. Ewer M, Carrasco C, MacKay B, Ali M, Benjamin R: Cardiac biopsy procedures at a cancer center. Proc Am Soc Clin Oncol 1991;10:336.

43. Carlson RW: Reducing the cardiotoxicity of the anthracyclines. Oncology 1992;6:95–100.

44. Weiss AJ, Metter GE, Fletcher WS, Wilson WL, Grage TB, Ramirez G: Studies on Adriamycin using a weekly regimen demonstrating its clinical effectiveness and lack of cardiac toxicity. Cancer Treat Rep 1976;60:813–822.

45. Torti FM, Bristow MR, Howes AE, et al: Reduced cardiotoxicity of doxorubicin delivered on a weekly schedule: Assessment by endomyocardial biopsy. Ann Intern Med 1983;99:745–749.

46. Benjamin RS: The schedule dependency of the cardiotoxicity of Adriamycin: Its relevance to pharmacokinetic parameters. In Muggia FM, Green MD, Speyer JL (eds): Cancer Treatment and the Heart. Baltimore, Johns Hopkins University Press, 1992, pp 278–285.

47. Legha SS, Benjamin RS, Mackay B, et al: Reduction of doxorubicin cardiotoxicity by prolonged continuous intravenous infusion. Ann Intern Med 1982;96:133–139.

48. Treat J, Roh JK, Woolley PV, Neefe J, Schein PS, Rahman A: A Phase I study: Liposome encapsulated doxorubicin (LED) [abstract 117]. Proc Am Soc Clin Oncol 1987;6:117.

49. Sharma D, Muggia F, Lucci L, et al: Liposomal Daunorubicin (VS-103): Tolerance and clinical effects in AIDS-related Kaposi's sarcoma (KS) during a Phase I study [abstract]. Proc Am Soc Clin Oncol 1990;9:4:9.

50. Treat J, Greenspan A, Forst D, Rahman A: A Phase II study in recurrent breast cancer patients (pts) with liposomal encapsulated doxorubicin (LED) [abstract 166]. Breast Cancer Res Treat 1988;12:148.

51. Berry G, Billingham M, Alderman E, Torti F, Lum B, DuMond C, Martin F: Reduced cardiotoxicity of Doxil (pegylated liposomal doxorubicin) in AIDS Kaposi's sarcoma patients compared to a matched control group of cancer patients given doxorubicin. Proc Am Soc Clin Oncol 1996;15:A843.

52. Muggia FM, Hainsworth J, Jeffers S, et al: Phase II study of Doxil in refractory ovarian cancer: Antitumor activity and toxicity modification by liposomal encapsulation. J Clin Oncol 1997;15:987–993.

53. Sparano JA, Winer EP: Liposomal anthracyclines for breast cancer. Semin Oncol 2001;28(4 suppl 12):32–40.

54. Safra T, Muggia F, Jeffers S, et al: Pegylated liposomal doxorubicin (Doxil): Reduced clinical cardiotoxicity in patients reaching or exceeding cumulative doses of 500 mg/m². Ann Oncol 2000;11:1029–1033.

55. Harris L, Batist G, Belt R, et al: The TLC D-99 study group. Liposome-encapsulated doxorubicin compared with conventional doxorubicin in a randomized multicenter trial as first-line therapy of metastatic breast carcinoma. Cancer 2002;94:25–36

56. Teder H, Nilsson B, Aronsen KF, Jonsson K, Hellekant C, Aspergren K: Hepatic arterial infusion of Adriamycin and degradable starch microspheres; pharmacokinetic studies in man [abstract 82]. Proc Am Soc Clin Oncol 1983;2:21.

57. Noteborn HPJM, McVie JG: Chemoembolisation in regional chemotherapy. In Domelof L (ed): Drug Delivery in Cancer Treatment (ESO monographs). Berlin, Springer-Verlag, 1989, p 55.

58. Nakamura H, Hashimoto T, Taguchi T, et al: Chemoembolization. Gan To Kagaku Ryoho 1987;14:1656–1663.

59. McVie JG: Anthracycline analogues and carriers. In Muggia FM, Green MD, Speyer JL (eds): Cancer Treatment and the Heart. Baltimore, Johns Hopkins University Press, 1992, pp 217–245.

60. Nielsen D, Hansen OP, Dombernowsky P: Epirubicin cardiac toxicity in patients with advanced breast cancer. Ann Oncol 1992;3(Suppl 5):114.

61. Levine M, Bramwell VH, Pritchard KI, et al: Randomized trial of intensive cyclophosphamide, epirubicin, and fluorouracil chemotherapy compared with cyclophosphamide, methotrexate and fluorouracil in premenopausal women with node-positive breast cancer. J Clin Oncol 1998;16:2651–2658.

62. Jensen BV, Skovsgaard T, Nielsen SL: Functional monitoring of anthracycline cardiotoxicity: a prospective, blinded, long-term observational study of outcome in 120 patients. Ann Oncol 2002;13:699–709.

63. Meinardi MT, van der Graaf WTA, Gietema JA, et al: Evaluation of long term cardiotoxicity after epirubicin containing adjuvant chemotherapy for breast cancer using various detection techniques. Heart 2002;88:81–82.

64. Basser RL, Abraham R, Bik To L, Fox RM, Green MD: Cardiac effects of high-dose epirubicin and cyclophosphamide in women with poor prognosis breast cancer. Ann Oncol 1999;10:53–58.

65. Gennari A, Salvadori B, Donati S, et al: Cardiotoxicity of epirubicin/paclitaxel-containing regimens: Role of cardiac risk factors. J Clin Oncol 1999;17:3596–3602.

66. Legha SS, Wang Y-M, Mackay B, Ewer M, Hortobagyi GN, Benjamin RS, Ali MK: Clinical and pharmacologic investigation of the effects of alpha-tocopherol on Adriamycin cardiotoxicity. Ann NY Acad Sci 1982;393:411–418.

67. Myers C, Bonow R, Palmeri S, et al: A randomized controlled trial assessing the prevention of doxorubicin cardiomyopathy by N-acetylcysteine. Semin Oncol 1983;10:53–55.

68. Judy MV, Hall JH, Dugan W, Toth PD, Folkers K: Coenzyme Q$_{10}$ reduction of Adriamycin cardiotoxicity. In Folkers K, Yamamura Y (eds): Biomedical and Clinical Aspects of Coenzyme Q$_{10}$. New York, Elsevier, 1984, pp 241–245.

69. Milei J, Marantz A, Ale J, Vazquez A, Buceta JE: Prevention of Adriamycin-induced cardiotoxicity by prenylamine: A pilot double blind study. Cancer Drug Del 1987;4:129–136.

70. Milei J, Vazquez A, Boveris A, Llesuy S, Molina HA, Storino R, Marantz A: The role of prenylamine in the prevention of Adriamycin-induced cardiotoxicity. A review of experimental and clinical findings. J Intern Med Res 1988;16:19–30.

71. Koning J, Palmer P, Franks CR, Mulder DE, Speyer JL, Green MD, Hellmann K: Cardioxane-ICRF-187. Towards anticancer drug specificity through selective toxicity reduction. Cancer Treatment Rev 1991;18:1–19.

72. Rosenfeld CS, Weisberg SR, York RM, et al: Prevention of adriamycin cardiomyopathy with dexrazoxane (ADR-529, ICRF-187). Proc Am Soc Clin Oncol 1992;11;62.

73. Weisberg SR, Rosenfeld CS, York RM, et al: Dexrazoxane (ADR-529, ICRF-187, Zinecard) protects against doxorubicin induced chronic cardiotoxicity. Proc Am Soc Clin Oncol 1992; 11:91.

74. Maillaird JA, Speyer JL, Hanson K, et al: Prevention of chronic adriamycin cardiotoxicity with the bisdioxopiperazine dexrazoxane (ICRF-187, ADR-529, Zinecard) in patients with advanced or metastatic breast cancer. Proc Am Soc Clin Oncol 1992;11:91.

75. Feldmann JF, Jones SE, Weisberg SR, et al: Advanced small cell lung cancer treated with CAV (cyclophosphamide + Adriamycin + vincristine) chemotherapy and the cardioprotective agent dexrazoxane (ADR-529, ICRF-187, Zinecard"). Proc Am Soc Clin Oncol 1992;11:296.

76. Swain SM, Whaley FS, Gerber MC, et al: Cardioprotection with dexrazoxane for doxorubicin-containing therapy in advanced breast cancer. J Clin Oncol 1997;15:1318–1332.

77. Kolaric K, Bradamante V, Cervek J, et al: A Phase II trial of cardioprotection with cardioxane (ICRF-187) in patients with advanced breast cancer receiving 5-fluorouracil, doxorubicin and cyclophosphamide. Oncology 1995;52:251–255.

78. Ten Bokkel Huinink W, Schreuder J, Dubbelman R, et al: ICRF 187 protects against doxorubicin induced cardiomyopathy. Ann Oncol 1992;3:114A, 1992.

79. Maral J. Personal communication. Chiron Therapeutics, Amsterdam, The Netherlands, 1998.

80. Swain SM, Whaley FS, Gerber MC, Ewer MS, Bianchine JR, Gams RA: Delayed administration of dexrazoxane provides cardioprotection for patients with advanced breast cancer treated with doxorubicin-containing therapy. J Clin Oncol 15:1333–1340, 1997.

81. Filppi JA, Imondi AR, Wolgemuth RL: Characterization of the cardioprotective effect of (S)(+)-4,4'-propylene-2,6-piperazinedione (ICRF-187) on anthracycline cardiotoxicity. In Hacker MP, Lazo JS, Tritton TR (eds): Organ-directed toxicities of anticancer drugs. Boston, Martinus Nijhoff, 1988, p 225.

82. Venturini M, Michelotti A, Mastro L, et al: Multicenter randomized controlled clinical trial to evaluate cardioprotection in women receiving epirubicin chemotherapy for advanced breast cancer. J Clin Oncol 1996;3112–3120.

83. Ali MK, Ewer MS: The natural history of anthracycline cardiotoxicity in children. In Muggia FM, Green MD, Speyer JL (eds): Cancer Treatment and the Heart. Baltimore, Johns Hopkins University Press, 1992, pp 246–255.

84. Gottdiener JS, Mathisen DJ, Borer JS, et al: Doxorubicin cardiotoxicity. Chest 1980;78:880–882.

85. Dresdale A, Bonow RO, Wesley R: Prospective evaluation of doxorubicin-induced cardiomyopathy resulting from postsurgical adjuvant treatment of patients with soft tissue sarcomas. Cancer 1983;52:51–60.

86. Goorin AM, Borow KM, Goldman A: Congestive heart failure due to Adriamycin cardiotoxicity: Its natural history in children. Cancer 1981;47:2810–2816.

87. Goorin AM, Chauvenet AR, Perez-Atayde AR, Cruz J, McCone R, Lipshultz SE: Initial congestive heart failure, six to ten years after doxorubicin chemotherapy for childhood cancer. J Pediatr 1990;116:144–147.

88. Lipshultz SE, Colan SD, Gelber RD: Late cardiac effects of doxorubicin therapy for acute lymphoblastic leukemia in childhood. N Engl J Med 1991;324:808–815.

89. Steinherz LJ, Graham T, Hurwitz R, et al: Guidelines for cardiac monitoring of children during and after anthracycline therapy: Report of the Cardiology Committee of the Children's Cancer Study Group. Pediatrics 1992;89:942–949.

90. Steinherz L, Steinherz P: Delayed cardiac toxicity from anthracycline therapy. Pediatrician 1991;18:49–52.

91. Lipshultz SE, Colan SD, Silverman LB, et al: Dexrazoxane reduces incidence of doxorubicin-associated acute myocardiocyte injury in children with acute lymphoblastic leukemia (ALL) [abstract 1557]. Proc Am Soc Clin Oncol 2002;21:390a.

92. Posner LE, Kukart G, Goldberg J, Bernstein T, Cartwright K: Mitoxantrone: An overview of safety and toxicity. Invest New Drugs 1985;3:123–132.

93. Cowan JD, Osborne CK, Neidhart JA, von Hoff DD, Constanzi JJ, Vaughn CB: A randomized trial of doxorubicin, mitoxantrone, and bisantrene in advanced breast cancer (a Southwest Oncology Group study). Invest New Drugs 1985;3:147–152.

94. Henderson IG, Allegra JC, Woodcock T, et al: Randomized clinical trial comparing mitoxantrone with doxorubicin in previously treated patients with metastatic breast cancer. J Clin Oncol 1989;7:560–571.

95. Benjamin RS, Chawla SP, Ewer MS, Carrasco CH, Mackay B, Holmes F: Evaluation of mitoxantrone cardiac toxicity by nuclear angiography and endomyocardial biopsy: An update. Invest New Drugs 1985;3:117–121.

96. Gottdiener JS, Appelbaum FR, Ferrans VJ, Deisseroth A, Ziegler J: Cardiotoxicity associated with high-dose cyclophosphamide therapy. Arch Intern Med 1981;141:758–763.

97. Appelbaum FR, Strauchen JA, Graw RG Jr: Acute lethal carditis caused by high dose combination chemotherapy. A unique clinical and pathological entity. Lancet 1976;1:58–62.

98. Cazin B, Gorin NC, Laporte JP, et al: Cardiac complications after bone marrow transplantation. A report on a series of 63 consecutive transplantations. Cancer 1986;57:2061–2069.

99. Quezado ZMN, Wilson WH, Cunnion RE, Parker MM, Reda D, Bryant G, Ognibene FP: High-dose ifosfamide is associated with severe, reversible cardiac dysfunction. Ann Intern Med 1993;118:31–36.

100. Ognibene FP, Rosenberg SA, Lotze M, Skibber J, Parker MM, Shelhamer JH, Parrillo JE: Interleukin-2 administration causes reversible hemodynamic changes and left ventricular dysfunction similar to those seen in septic shock. Chest 1988;94:750–754.

101. Ingle JN, Kuross JA, Mailliard JA, Loprinzi CL, Jung SH: Evaluation of piroxantrone in women with metastatic breast cancer and failure on non-anthracycline chemotherapy. A North Central Cancer Treatment Group Trial. Proc Am Soc Clin Oncol 1993;12:A140.

102. Cobleigh MA, Vogel CL, Tripathy D, et al: Multinational study of the efficacy and safety of humanized anti-HER2 monoclonal antibody in women who have HER2-overexpressing metastatic breast cancer that has progressed after chemotherapy for metastatic disease. J Clin Oncol 1999;17:2639–2648.

103. Slamon DJ, Leyland-Jones B, Shak S, et al: Use of chemotherapy plus a monoclonal antibody against HER2 for metastatic breast cancer that overexpresses HER2. N Engl J Med 2001;344: 783–792.

104. Seidman A, Hudis C, Pierri MK, et al: Cardiac dysfunction in the trastuzumab clinical trials experience. J Clin Oncol 2002;20:1215–1221.

105. Speyer J: Cardiac dysfunction in the trastuzumab clinical trials experience. J Clin Oncol 2002;20:1156–1157.

106. Chien KR: Myocyte survival pathways and cardiomyopathy implications for trastuzumab cardiac toxicity. Semin Oncol 2000;27(suppl 11):9–14.

107. Feldman A, Lorell B, Reis S: Trastuzumab in the treatment of metastatic breast cancer: American therapy versus cardiotoxicity. Circulation 2000;102:272–274.

108. Ewer MS, Vooletich M, Valero V, Higano CS, Benjaminj RS: Trastuzumab (Herceptin) cardiotoxicity: clinical course and cardiac biopsy correlations [abstract 489]. Proc Am Soc Clin Oncol 2002;21:123a.

109. Ewer MS, Vooletich M, Valero V, Benjamin RS: Reversibility of trastuzumab-associated cardiotoxicity [abstract]. Proceedings of the annual meeting of the European Society of Medical Oncology (ESMO), October 2002, Nice, France.

110. Robert N, Leyland-Jones B, Asmar L, et al: Phase III comparative study of trastuzumab and paclitaxel with and without carboplatin win patients with HER-2/*neu* positive advanced breast cancer [abstract 35]. Breast Cancer Res Treat 2002;76(suppl 1): S37.

111. Burstein HJ, Kuter I, Campos SM, et al: Clinical activity of trastuzumab and vinorelbine in women with her2-overexpressing metastatic breast cancer. J Clin Oncol 2002;20:1800–1808.

112. Jahanzeb M, Mortimer JE, Furhan Y, et al: Phase II trial of weekly vinorelbine and trastuzumab as first-line therapy in patients with Her2+ metastatic breast cancer. Oncologist 2002;7:410–417.

113. Gianni L, Munzone E, Giuseppe C, et al: Paclitaxel by 3-hour infusion in combination with bolus doxorubicin in women with untreated metastatic breast cancer: high antitumor efficacy and cardiac effects in a dose-finding and sequence-finding study. J Clin Oncol 1995;13:2688–2699.

114. Sparano JA: Use of dexrazoxane and other strategies to prevent cardiac toxicity associated with doxorubicin–Taxane combinations. Semin Oncol, 1998;25(4 suppl 10): 61–65.

115. Gianni L, Dombernowsky P, Sledge G, et al: Cardiac function following combination therapy with paclitaxel and doxorubicin: An analysis of 657 women with advanced breast cancer. Ann Oncol 2001;12:1067–1073.

116. Valero V, Perez E, Dieras V: Doxorubicin and taxane combination regimens for metastatic breast cancer: Focus on cardiac effects. Semin Oncol 2001;28(suppl 12):15–23.

117. Nabholtz JM, Falkson C, Campos D, et al: Tax 306 study group. Docetaxel and doxorubicin compared with doxorubicin and cyclophosphamide as first-line chemotherapy for metastatic breast cancer: results of a randomized, multicenter, phase III trial. J Clin Oncol 2003;21:968–975.

118. Nabholtz JM, Reese DM, Lindsay MA, Riva A: Docetaxel in the treatment of breast cancer: an update on recent studies. Semin Oncol 2002;29(3 suppl 12):28–34.

119. Conte PF, Michelotti A, Baldini E, et al: A dose-finding study of epirubicin in combination with paclitaxel in the treatment of advanced breast cancer. Semin Oncol 1996;23(5 suppl 11):28–31.

120. Somlo G, Doroshow JH, Forman SJ, et al: High-dose chemotherapy and stem-cell rescue in the treatment of high-risk breast cancer: prognostic indicators of progression-free and overall survival. J Clin Oncol 1997;15:2882–2893.

121. Stewart JR, Fajardo LF: Radiation-induced heart disease: An update. Prog Cardiovasc Dis 1984;27:173.

122. Renzi RH, Straus KL, Glatstein E: Radiation-induced myocardial disease. In Muggia FM, Green MD, Speyer JL (eds): Cancer Treatment and the Heart. Baltimore, Johns Hopkins University Press, 1992, pp 289–295.

123. Gottdiener JS, Katin MJ, Borer JS, et al: Late cardiac effects of therapeutic mediastinal irradiation. Assessment by echocardiography and radionuclide angiography. N Engl J Med 1983;308:569.

124. Kinsella TJ, Ahmann DL, Giuliani ER, Lie JT: Adriamycin cardiotoxicity in stage IV breast cancer: Possible enhancement with prior left chest radiation therapy. Int J Radiat Oncol Biol Phys 1979;5:1997.

125. Lenihan D, Tong A, Woods M, et al: Withdrawal of ACE inhibitors and beta blockers in chemotherapy-induced heart failure leads to severe adverse cardiovascular events. J Cardiac Failure 2003; 9:S77.

126. Jensen BV, Nielsen SL, Skovsgaard T: Treatment with angiotensin-converting-enzyme inhibitor for epirubicin-induced dilated cardiomyopathy. Lancet 1996;347:297–299.

127. Cohen IS, Bharati S, Glass J, Lev M: Radiotherapy as a cause of complete atrio-venticular block in Hodgkin's disease. Arch Int Med 1981;141:676.

128. Pohjola-Sintonen S, Totterman KJ, Salmo M, Sitanen P: Late cardiac effects of mediastinal radiotherapy in patients with Hodgkin's disease. Cancer 1987;60:31.

129. Weiss RB, Moquin D, Adams JD, Griffin JD, Zimbler H: Electrocardiogram abnormalities induced by Amsacrine. Cancer Chemother Pharmacol 1983;10:133–134.

130. Feldman EJ, Arlin ZA, Sullivan P, Engelking C: Preventing Amsacrine induced cardiac arrhythmias. J Clin Oncol 1987;5:2041.

131. Kazunori O, Hitoshi Y, Kazuyuki S, et al: Prolongation of the QT interval and ventricular tachycardia in patients treated with arsenic trioxide for acute promyelocytic leukemia. Ann Intern Med 2001;133:881–885.

132. Unnikrishnan D, Dutcher J, Varshneya N, et al: Torsades de pointes in 3 patients with leukemia treated with arsenic trioxide. Blood 2001;97:1514–1516.

133. Rowinsky EK, McGuire WP, Guarnieri T, Fisherman JS, Christian MC, Donehower RC: Cardiac disturbances during the administration of Taxol. J Clin Oncol 1991;9:1704–1712.

134. Arbuck SG, Strauss H, Rowinsky E, et al: A reassessment of cardiac toxicity associated with Taxol. Monogr Natl Cancer Inst 1993;15:117–130.

135. Vogelzang NJ, Herndon JE 2nd, Cirrincione C, et al: Dihydro-5-azacytidine in malignant mesothelioma. A phase II trial demonstrating activity accompanied by cardiac toxicity. Cancer and Leukemia Group B. Cancer 1997;79:2237–2242.

136. Tepler I, Elias L, Smith JW II, et al: A randomized placebo-controlled trial of recombinant human Interleukin-11 in cancer patients with severe thrombocytopenia due to chemotherapy. Blood 1996;87:3607–3614.

137. Genetech Corporation. San Francisco, CA. Rituxan, 1997. Data on file.

138. Maloney DG, Grillo-Lopez AJ, Bodkin D, et al: IDEC-C2B8: Results of a phase I multiple-dose trial in patients with relapsed non-Hodgkin's lymphoma. J Clin Oncol 1997;15:3266–3274.

139. McEniery PT, Dorosti K, Schiavone WA, et al: Clinical and angiographic features of coronary artery disease after chest irradiation. Am J Cardiol 1987;60:1020.

140. Tracy GP, Brown DE, Johnson LW, Gottlieb AJ: Radiation-induced coronary artery disease. JAMA 1974;228:1660.

141. Pearson HES: Incidental dangers of x-ray therapy. Lancet 1958;2:223.

142. Prentice RTW: Myocardial infarction following radiation. Lancet 1965;1:338.

143. Dollinger MR: Myocardial infarction due to postirradiation fibrosis of the coronary arteries. JAMA 1966;195:316.

144. Simon EB, Ling J, Mendizabal RC, Midawell J: Radiation-induced coronary artery disease. Am Heart J 1984;108:1032.

145. Kopelsen G, Herwig KJ: The etiologies of coronary artery

disease in cancer patients. Int J Radiat Oncol Biol Phys 1978;4:895.

146. Brosius FC, Walker BF, Roberts WC: Radiation heart disease: Analysis of 16 young (aged 15 to 33 years) necropsy patients who received over 3500 rads to the heart. Am J Med 1981;7:519.

147. de Forni M, Malet-Martino MC, Jaillais P, et al: Cardiotoxicity of high-dose continuous infusion fluorouracil: A prospective clinical study. J Clin Oncol 1992;10:1795–1801.

148. Freeman NJ, Costanza ME: 5-fluorouracil associated cardiotoxicity. Cancer 1988;61:36–45.

149. Labianca R, Beretta G, Clerici M, Fraschini P, Luporini G: Cardiac toxicity of 5-FU: A study of 1083 patients. Tumori 1982;68: 505–510.

150. Keefe DL, Roistacher N, Pierri MK: Clinical cardiotoxicity of 5-fluorouracil. J Clin Pharmacol 1993;33:1060–1070.

151. Ensley J, Kish J, Tapazoglou E, Patel B, Kloner R, Wynne J, Al-Sarraf M: 5-fluorouracil infusions associated with an ischemic cardiotoxicity syndrome. Proc Am Soc Clin Oncol 1986;5:142 (Abs. 554).

152. Jakubowski AA, Kemeny N: Hypotension as a manifestation of cardiotoxicity in 3 patients receiving cisplatin and 5-fluorouracil. Cancer 1988;62:266–269.

153. Anand AJ: Fluorouracil cardiotoxicity. Ann Pharmacother 1994;28:374–378.

154. Lejonc JL, Vernant JP, MacQuin J, Castaigne A: Myocardial infarction following vinblastine treatment (Letter). Lancet 1980;2:692.

155. Mandel EM, Lewinski V, Djaldetti M: Vincristine-induced myocardial infarction. Cancer 1975;36:1979–1982.

156. Doll DC, List AF, Greco FA, Hainsworth JD, Hande KR, Johnson DH: Acute vascular ischemic events after cisplatin-based combination chemotherapy for germ-cell tumors of the testis. Ann Intern Med 1986;105:48–51.

157. Zangari M, Siegel E, Barlogie B, et al: Thrombogenic activity of doxorubicin in myeloma patients receiving thalidomide: implications for therapy. Blood 2002;100:1168–1171.

158. Desai AA, Vogelzang NJ, Rini BI, Ansari R, Krauss S, Stadler WM: A high rate of venous thromboembolism in a multi-institutional phase II trial of weekly intravenous gemcitabine with continuous infusion fluorouracil and daily thalidomide in patients with metastatic renal cell carcinoma. Cancer 2002;95:1629–1636.

159. Kuenen BC, Rosen L, Smit EF, et al: Dose-finding and pharmacokinetic study of cisplatin, gemcitabine, and SU5416 in patients with solid tumors. J Clin Oncol 2002;20:1657–1667.

160. Silverberg GO, Britt RH, Goffinet DR: Radiation induced carotid artery disease. Cancer 1978;41:130.

161. Bristow MR, Thompson PD, Martin RP, Mason JW, Billingham ME: Early anthracycline cardiotoxicity. Am J Med 1978;65:823–832.

162. Cazin B, Gorin NC, Laporte JP, et al: Cardiac complications after bone marrow transplantation. A report on a series of 63 consecutive transplantations. Cancer 1986;57:2061–2069.

163. Ravdin PM, Valero V: Review of docetaxel (Taxotere), a highly active new agent for the treatment of metastatic breast cancer. Semin Oncol 1995;22(2 Suppl 4):17–21.

164. Rittenberg CN, Gralla RJ, Cole JT, Marques CB, Robertson CL: Preventing docetaxel-induced fluid retention: the efficacy of corticosteroids. Proc Am Soc Clin Oncol 1996;15:A1719.

165. Martin RG, Ruckdeschel JC, Chang P, Byhardt R, Bouchard RJ, Wiernik PH: Radiation-related pericarditis. Am J Cardiol 1975;35:216.

166. Stewart JR, Cohn KE, Fajardo LF, Hancock EW, Kaplan HS: Radiation-induced heart disease: A study of twenty-five patients. Radiology 1967;89:302–310.

167. Pierce RH, Hafermann MD, Kagan AR: Changes in the transverse cardiac diameter following mediastinal irradiation for Hodgkin's disease. Radiology 1969;93:619–624.

168. Glicksman AS, Nickson JJ: Acute and late reactions to irradiation in the treatment of Hodgkin's disease. Arch Intern Med 1973;131:369.

169. Masland DS, Rotz CT, Harris JH: Postradiation pericarditis with chronic pericardial effusion. Ann Intern Med 1968;69:97–102.

170. Taymore-Luria H, Kohn K, Pasternak RC: Radiation heart disease. J Cardiovasc Med 1993;8:113.

171. Stewart JR, Fajardo LF: Radiation-induced heart disease: An update. Prog Cardiovasc Dis 1984;27:173–194.

172. Applefeld MM, Slawson RG, Hall-Craigs M, Green DC, Singleton RT, Wiernik PH: Delayed pericardial disease after radiotherapy. Am J Cardiol 1981;47:210–213.

173. Carmel RJ, Kaplan HS: Mantle irradiation in Hodgkin's disease. Cancer 1976;37:2813.

174. Tarbell NJ, Thompson L, Mauch P: Thoracic irradiation in Hodgkin's disease: Disease control and long-term complications. Int J Radiat Oncol Biol. Phys 1990;18:275.

175. Spiegel RJ: The alpha interferons: Clinical overview. Semin Oncol 1987;14:1–12.

176. Jones GJ, Itri LM: Safety and tolerance of recombinant interferon alfa-2A (Roferon-A) in cancer patients. Cancer 1986;57: 1709–1715.

177. Hawkins M, Horning S, Konrad M, et al: Phase I evaluation of a synthetic mutant of B-interferon. Cancer Res 1985;45:5914–5920.

178. Rinehart JJ, Malspeis L, Young D, Neidhart J: Phase I/II trial of human recombinant interferon gamma in renal cell carcinoma. J Biol Response Mod 1986;5:300–308.

179. Rinehart J, Malspeis L, Young D, Neidhart J: Phase I/II trial of human recombinant beta-interferon serene in patients with renal cell carcinoma. Cancer Res 1986;46:5364–5367.

180. Goldstein D, Gockerman J, Krishnan R: Effects of gamma-interferon on the endocrine system: Results from a Phase I study. Cancer Res 1987;47:6397–6401.

181. Brown TD, Koeller J, Beougher K, Golando J, Bonnem EM, Spiegel RJ, Von Hoff DD: A Phase I clinical trial of recombinant DNA gamma interferon. J Clin Oncol 1987;5:790–798.

182. Lee RE, Lotze MT, Skibber JM, et al: Cardiorespiratory effects of immunotherapy with interleukin-2. J Clin Oncol 1989;7:7–20.

183. Margolin KA, Rayner AA, Hawkins MJ, et al: Interleukin-2 and lymphokine-activated killer cell therapy of solid tumors: Analysis of toxicity and management guidelines. J Clin Oncol 1989;7: 485–498.

184. Gaynor ER, Vitek L, Sticklin L, et al: The hemodynamic effects of treatment with interleukin-2 and lymphokine-activated killer cells. Ann Intern Med 1988;109:953–958.

185. Parker MM, Parrillo JE: Septic shock. Hemodynamics and pathogenesis. JAMA 1983;250:3324–3327.

186. Parker MM, Shelhamer JH, Bacharach SL, et al: Profound but reversible myocardial depression in patients with septic shock. Ann Intern Med 1984;100:483–490.

187. West WH, Tauer KW, Yannelli JR, Marshall GO, Orr DW, Thurman GB, Oldham RK: Constant-infusion recombinant interleukin-2 in adoptive immunotherapy of advanced cancer. N Engl J Med 1987;316:898–905.

188. Mitchell MS, Kempf RA, Harel W, Shau H, Boswell WD, Lind S, Bradley EC: Effectiveness and tolerability of low dose cyclophosphamide and low dose IL-2 in disseminated melanoma. J Clin Oncol 1988;6:409–424.

189. Whitehead RP, Kopecky KJ, Samson MK, Costanzi JJ, Natale R, Feun L, Hersh EM: A Phase II study of iv bolus recombinant interleukin 2 (IL-2) in metastatic malignant melanoma: A Southwest Oncology Group Study [abstract 1108]. Proc Am Soc Clin Oncol 1989;8:286.

190. Weiss GR, Margolin K, Aronson FR, Sznol M, Atkins MB, Gucalp R, Fisher RI: A randomized Phase II trial of continuous infusion (CI) interleukin-2 (IL-2) or bolus injection (BI) IL-2 plus lymphokine-activated killer cells (LAK) for advanced renal cell carcinoma (Abs. 509). Proc Am Soc Clin Oncol 1989;8:132.

191. Dutcher JP, Gaynor E, Boldt DH: Phase II study of high dose intravenous continuous infusion (IVCI) interleukin-2 (IL2) and lymphokine activated killer (LAK) cells in patients (PTS) with metastatic melanoma (MM). Proc Am Soc Clin Oncol 1989; 8:282.

192. Bradley EC, Louie AC, Paradise CM, Carlin PA, Bleyl KL, Groves ES, Rudolph AR: Antitumor response in patients with metastatic renal cell carcinoma is dependent upon regimen intensity. (Abs. 519). Proc Am Soc Clin Oncol 1989;8:134.

193. Lissoni P, Galli MA, Tancini G, Barni S: Prevention by L-carnitine of interleukin-2 related cardiac toxicity during cancer immuno-therapy. Tumori 1993;79:202–204.

194. Hawkins MJ, Sznol M: The cardiovascular effects of human recombinant cytokines. In Muggia FM, Green MD, Speyer JL (eds): Cancer Treatment and the Heart. Baltimore, Johns Hopkins University Press, 1992, pp 296–328.

195. Shogan JE, Brandt SJ, Jones RB, et al: Toxicity from recombinant human granulocyte-macrophage colony stimulating factor (rHuGM-CSF) after high dose chemotherapy and autologous bone marrow transplant (ABMT). Proc Am Assoc Cancer Res 1988;29:A209.

196. Dennis D, Chachoua A, Caron D, et al: Biologic activity of interleukin 1 (IL-1) alpha in patients with refractory malignancies. Proc ASCO 1992;11:255.

197. Trehu EG, Isner JM, Mier JW, Karp DD, Atkins MB: Possible myocardial toxicity associated with interleukin-4 therapy. J Immunother 1993;14:348–351.

198. Leach MW, Snyder EA, Sinha DP, Rosenblum IY: Safety evaluation of recombinant human interleukin-4. I. Preclinical studies. Clin Immunol Immunopathol 1997;83:8–11.

199. Weber J, Yang JC, Topalian SL, et al: Phase I trial of subcutaneous interleukin-6 in patients with advanced malignancies. J Clin Oncol 1993;11:499–506.

200. Hertenstein B, Stefanic M, Schmeiser T, et al: Cardiac toxicity of bone marrow transplantation: predictive value of cardiologic evaluation before transplant. J Clin Oncol 1994;12:998–1004.

201. Brockstein B, Mick R, Smiley C, Zimmerman T, Grinblatt D, Williams SF: Risk factors for pulmonary and cardiac toxicity after high dose chemotherapy and stem cell rescue in breast cancer and lymphoma. Proc Am Soc Clin Oncol 1996;15:A1749.

202. Huddart RA, Norman A, Shahidi M, Horwich A, Coward D, Nicholls J, Dearnaley DP: Cardiovascular disease as a long-term complication of treatment for testicular cancer. J Clin Oncol 2003;21:1513–1523.

64

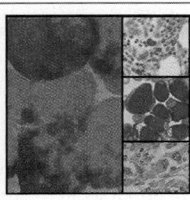

REPRODUCTIVE COMPLICATIONS

Marwan Fakih

Annette Sunga

Donald L. Trump

SUMMARY OF KEY POINTS

- Reproductive complications associated with cancer or its treatment are expected to increase as the number of cancer survivors increases.

CANCER-RELATED

- Oligospermia is present in more than 50% of patients with Hodgkin's disease and testicular cancer.
- Patients with baseline oligospermia are more likely to become infertile after treatment.
- Central nervous system involvement and hormonal disturbance are infrequent causes of reproductive complications.

TREATMENT-RELATED COMPLICATIONS

- Surgery
- Radiation therapy
- Hormonal therapy
- Chemotherapy and bone marrow transplantation (BMT)

SURGERY

- Prostatectomy and other pelvic surgeries are associated with erectile dysfunction; retroperitoneal dissection is associated with retrograde ejaculation.
- Nerve-sparing surgery improves potency and decreases retrograde ejaculation rates in patients with prostate, testicular, and rectal cancers.
- Gynecologic surgery may have a direct impact on sexual function by altering the normal female genital anatomy.
- Altered body image (mastectomy or colostomy) may have a profound impact on sexual function.

RADIATION THERAPY

- Prepubertal testicles and ovaries are more resistant to the effects of radiation.
- Testicular spermatogenesis is affected by doses as low as 15 cGy,

and complete aspermia may occur with a dose of 600 cGy.
- Leydig's cell dysfunction occurs at doses exceeding 2000 cGy.
- Ovarian function is more resistant to the effects of radiation. The effects are age-related with a significantly increased risk of permanent menopause in patients older than 40 years at dosages exceeding 150 to 400 cGy.
- Erectile dysfunction occurs within 2 years of treatment in 60% to 80% of patients with prostate cancer receiving external beam radiation. Most cases are attributed to vascular insufficiency.

HORMONAL THERAPY

- Gonadotropin-releasing hormone (GnRH) agonists and antagonists result in medical castration with resultant loss of libido and impotence.
- Antiandrogen therapy results in a lesser degree of impotence compared with GnRH analogs in the treatment of prostate cancer.

CHEMOTHERAPY AND BONE MARROW TRANSPLANTATION

- Alkylating agents are associated with the highest rates of infertility.
- Doses and duration of treatment are directly associated with risk of infertility.
- Risks for infertility and amenorrhea are related to age, dose, and duration of therapy.
- Prepubertal males and females have the highest tolerance to chemotherapy. Normal puberty has been reported in both genders after chemotherapy.
- Premature ovarian failure is age-related, with the highest risk in patients older than 40 years. The younger the female, the lower is the risk of amenorrhea and the higher

are the chances that menstruation will resume on completion of chemotherapy.
- High doses of alkylating agents such as cyclophosphamide doses of greater than 7.5 g/m^2 are likely to be associated with abnormal sperm counts in adolescent boys. Doses of greater than 9 g/m^2 are associated with prolonged infertility. The mechlorethamine, vincristine, procarbazine, and prednisone (MOPP) regimen used in Hodgkin's disease is particularly associated with male infertility. In some males, fertility is recovered several years after completion of therapy.
- Females who resume menstruation after treatment are at higher risk for early menopause.
- Radiation therapy during BMT conditioning results in male infertility and a high rate of premature ovarian failure. BMT without radiation has been associated with a high rate of fertility preservation in females treated before puberty or at a very young age.

CANCER AND PREGNANCY

- Cancer complicates 1 in every 1000 pregnancies.
- Chemotherapy
  - Highest risk of congenital abnormalities is during first trimester of pregnancy and is especially common with antimetabolites such as methotrexate.
  - Data available from patients with leukemia and breast cancer suggest that chemotherapy during the second and third trimesters of pregnancy results in normal offspring. No long-term complications have been identified so far.
- Radiation therapy

SUMMARY OF KEY POINTS, continued

- Risks are highest during the organogenesis period (first trimester).
- Mental retardation and microcephaly may occur with second-trimester and early third-trimester exposure.

PREVENTION AND TREATMENT
- Sperm cryopreservation should be discussed with all males

undergoing treatments that may cause sterility.
- Use of GnRH analogues may have a protective effect on ovarian function, but no protective effects on spermatogenesis have been established. Their use is considered experimental.
- Gonadal shielding and ovarian transposition ameliorate effects of radiation on gonadal function.

- Assistive reproductive technologies and alternative methods of sperm collection have resulted in successful pregnancies for couples with severe male infertility caused by cancer or its treatment.
- The use of sildenafil has reestablished potency in a large number of patients with surgery- or radiation-induced erectile dysfunction.

INTRODUCTION

Advances in the treatment of cancer have resulted in marked improvements in survival and cure rates. Hence, the number of cancer survivors continues to rise.

Patients with cancer often have immediate and long-term complications related to cancer and its treatment. Insults to reproductive health constitute an often overlooked dimension. Sexual dysfunction and infertility can have a major impact on patient well-being, interpersonal relationships, and family building.

Attention to reproductive health issues and patient involvement in treatment planning early in the course of the disease and its treatment are key. This review focuses on the reproductive complications of cancer and its treatment.

REPRODUCTIVE PHYSIOLOGY

Gonadal Form and Function

The ovaries produce mature fertilizable ova, as well as sex steroids and reproductive/gonadal peptides (inhibin and activin). These activities are carried out in an integrated manner by the different compartments of the ovarian functional unit, the follicle. The granulosa cells are the source of the sex steroids estradiol and progesterone, as well as the peptides, inhibin, activin, and follistatin. De novo synthesis of progesterone by the theca cells is dependent on an abundant supply of cholesterol. Granulosa cells also produce progesterone independently.[1] Estrogen biosynthesis, on the other hand, requires cooperation of both the granulosa and the theca-interstitial cells. Precursor steroids (mainly androstenedione), synthesized in the theca cells, are transferred across the basement membrane of the follicle to the granulosa cells where they are aromatized to estrogens. The peptides inhibin, activin, and follistatin are expressed in various tissues including the ovaries and anterior pituitary.

There are approximately one million follicles at birth. During the reproductive years, typical cyclic follicular recruitment, selection, and dominance eventually deplete the ovaries of follicles, leading to cessation of ovarian function and menopause.

In males, the testes secrete androgenic hormones and produce mature spermatozoa. These two processes are highly interrelated and regulated by multiple factors. Compartments of the testes, much like those of the ovaries, serve different functions. The seminiferous tubules consist of Sertoli's cells that support the developing sperm and germ cells and are the sites of spermatogenesis. The interstitial cells, or Leydig's cells, are essential for testosterone synthesis. Testosterone is transported from the Leydig's cells to the seminiferous tubules, where it acts to enhance spermatogenesis. Testicular hormones are also responsible for the induction of male development during embryogenesis.

Hypothalamic-Pituitary-Gonadal Axis

The main regulators of testicular and ovarian function are the gonadotropins, follicle-stimulating hormone (FSH) and luteinizing hormone (LH). Both the biosynthesis and secretion of gonadotropins are modulated by an interplay of (1) hypothalamic factors (gonadotropin releasing hormone [GnRH]), (2) intrapituitary factors (the pituitary peptides activin and follistatin), and (3) gonadal feedback (steroids and peptides).[1] Gonadotropin expression is controlled by the hypothalamus primarily through the action of GnRH. GnRH is produced in the medial basal hypothalamus and is released in a pulsatile fashion to the anterior pituitary where it binds to plasma membrane receptors on the gonadotropes and stimulates release of FSH and LH (Fig. 64-1). Depending on the reproductive stage, estrogens can either increase or decrease gonadotropin production. Increased levels of estrogen in females or increased levels of testosterone in males down-regulate gonadotropin secretion. However, increased levels of estrogens at the time of a surge in LH exert a positive feedback effect. In addition to steroid hormones, the gonadal proteins activin, inhibin, and follistatin modulate release of FSH.[2] Inhibin decreases and activin stimulates gonadotropin function. Follistatin also inhibits FSH but is less potent than inhibin.

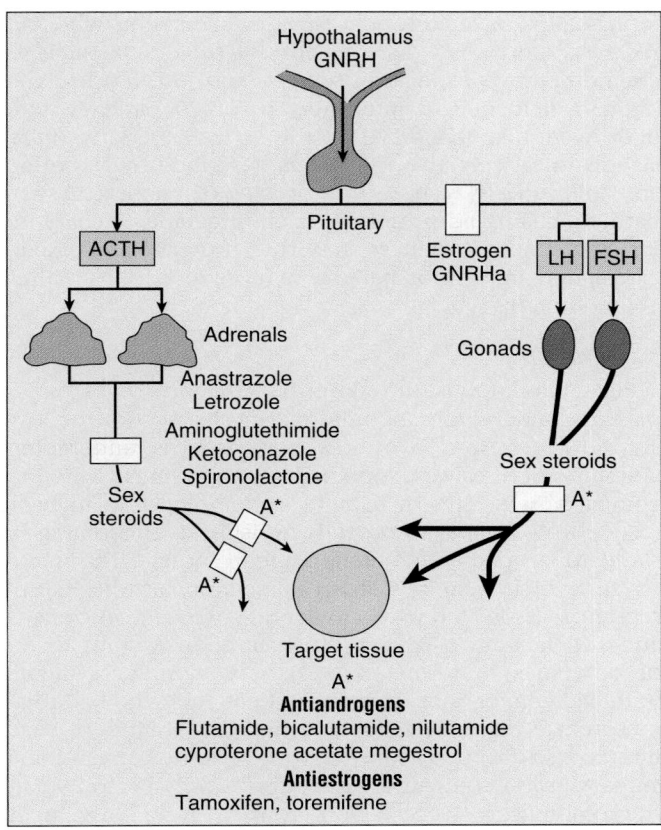

Figure 64-1. Diagram illustrating trophic factors controlling adrenal and gonadal sex steroid secretion and approaches available to inhibit the secretion (□) and action (A*) of sex steroid hormones.

Regulatory control of gonadotropins in the ovaries and testes is similar. In the testes, LH interacts with high-affinity cell surface receptors on the plasma membranes of Leydig's cells, and through a cyclic adenosine monophosphate–activated series of steps, stimulates the synthesis of the enzymes of testosterone production. The epithelium of the seminiferous tubules is the primary site of action of FSH. FSH binds to cell surface receptors of Sertoli's cells, stimulating the synthesis of androgen-binding proteins and an aromatase enzyme complex that convert testosterone to estradiol. LH and FSH effects on the ovaries strongly resemble those on the testes. Activation of gonadotropin receptors on the plasma membranes of the granulosa and theca cells stimulates the adenylate cyclase system, thereby inducing the regulation of female steroid hormone production and follicular maturation.[3]

DIRECT EFFECTS OF CANCER ON REPRODUCTIVE FUNCTION

Although this chapter concentrates on the impact of cancer therapy on reproductive function, it is important to note that cancer itself can have important direct effects on sexual and reproductive function.

Gonadal tumors may result in reproductive dysfunction caused by gonadal germinal tissue destruction, as well as aberrations in hormonal balance. Ovarian sex cord–stromal tumors are often associated with hormonal effects such as precocious puberty, amenorrhea, virilizing symptoms, and postmenopausal bleeding. Male sex cord–stromal tumors may be associated with precocious puberty, feminization syndrome, and gynecomastia. Reproductive organ cancers and other cancers involving the pelvis may interfere with coitus directly as a result of anatomic changes or indirectly as a result of pain. Females with invasive vulvar and vaginal cancers and advanced cervical cancers often experience postcoital bleeding or dyspareunia. Males with testicular cancer often have diffuse testicular pain, swelling, and tenderness that interfere with intercourse. Penile cancer usually presents as a penile sore or mass, which when neglected, may result in ulceration, bleeding, or secondary infection, which may interfere with coitus.

Central nervous system involvement, directly with primary cancer or by metastatic disease and indirectly through paraneoplastic involvement, can have a considerable impact on reproductive function. Pituitary prolactin-secreting adenomas are commonly associated with impotence in men and amenorrhea and galactorrhea in women. Other pituitary adenomas can affect reproductive function by destroying gonadotropes that produce LH and FSH. Craniopharyngiomas and other metastatic cancers can directly invade the pituitary gland and produce hypothalamic-pituitary dysfunction. Similarly, metastatic disease that affects the hypothalamic-pituitary axis will also lead to reproductive dysfunction.

Paraneoplastic syndromes are an infrequent but well-documented cause of reproductive dysfunction. Ectopic corticotropin secretion (e.g., as in small cell lung cancer) can result in Cushing-like disease including amenorrhea. Other neurologic paraneoplastic syndromes can have a direct impact on reproductive function through the involvement of the autonomic nervous system, as in Lambert-Eaton syndrome, or an indirect impact by resulting in personality changes, as in limbic encephalitis.[4]

Cancer, especially Hodgkin's disease and testicular cancer, is associated with an increased rate of infertility. Men with Hodgkin's disease may have abnormal spermatogenesis. Whitehead and colleagues[5] noted that 4 of 19 untreated males had suboptimal sperm counts and motility. Hendry and colleagues[6] reported that only 27% of 49 men with Hodgkin's disease had normal semen analysis findings before initiation of treatment. Chapman and colleagues[7] performed testicular biopsies before treatment in patients with Hodgkin's disease; they performed semen analysis and examined tissue specimens. Sixteen of 37 patients had abnormal semen analysis findings. Histologic abnormalities were noted in 8 of 9 pretreatment biopsy specimens from men with abnormal semen analysis findings. Tubular hyalinization and basement membrane thickening were the most common findings.

Infertility data are even more compelling in patients with testicular cancer. The degree of spermatogenic abnormalities in these patients is greater than what would be accounted for by local tumor effect or degree of

Problems Common to Cancer and Its Therapy

systemic involvement. Studies show that as many as 93% of patients may have substandard sperm quality before chemotherapy or radiation.[6,8,9] Histologic investigations have revealed a high prevalence of dysfunctional spermatogenesis even in the contralateral testicle uninvolved with cancer.[10] It is also interesting to note that an increased risk of testicular cancer has been suggested among patients with abnormal semen analysis findings. An analysis of association between testicular cancer and subfertility was conducted in a group of 3530 Danish men. This analysis showed that men with testicular cancer had reduced fertility before the diagnosis of cancer was made. Men with nonseminomatous testicular cancer were more likely to have been found to have preexisting reduced fertility than men with seminomas.[11] The specific links between the pathologic events that cause infertility and testicular cancer remain unclear.

Cancer can also indirectly alter sexual function in patients with cancer as a result of depression, anxiety, fatigue, pain, alteration in body image, and strained interpersonal relationships.

EFFECTS OF CANCER THERAPY ON SEXUAL AND REPRODUCTIVE FUNCTION

Surgery

Surgical treatments with the most significant impact on reproductive function are those involving the pelvis. These include radical prostatectomy, radical cystectomy, rectal cancer surgery, orchiectomy, retroperitoneal dissection, and radical hysterectomy.

Prostate Cancer

Erectile dysfunction in patients undergoing radical prostatectomy is commonly seen after surgery.[12-15] In a study in which 376 patients were randomly assigned to undergo radical prostatectomy versus watchful waiting, the incidence of erectile dysfunction was significantly higher in the surgical group (80%) than in the observation group (45%).[16] Identification and sparing of the neurovascular bundles that carry cavernous nerves is associated with a significant improvement in potency rate after radical prostatectomy.[17] Bilateral nerve-sparing surgeries are considerably more effective in maintaining erectile function compared with unilateral nerve-sparing surgeries. Potency rates after bilateral nerve-sparing surgery at 3 years were 76% compared with 30% after unilateral nerve-sparing surgery in previously potent patients younger than 60 years. The rates of potency are lower in older patients and in patients with known erectile dysfunction before surgery.[18]

Testicular Cancer

Retroperitoneal lymph node dissection (RPLND) frequently damages the sympathetic nerves innervating the seminal vesicles and the bladder neck. This leads to loss of seminal vesicle emission or emission without bladder neck closure (retrograde ejaculation).[19,20] In the series reported by Hartmann and colleagues,[21] patients who had received more than one modality of treatment (such as chemotherapy or radiation therapy and RPLND) had the highest incidence of infertility. Six of 29 patients who underwent bilateral RPLND in this series experienced dry ejaculation. A selective RPLND, as described by Donohue and colleagues,[22] results in the sparing of a unilateral sympathetic chain and preservation of antegrade ejaculation. Jacobsen and colleagues[23] reported preserved antegrade ejaculation in 89% of patients undergoing RPLND after chemotherapy.

Rectal Cancer

Williams and Johnston[24] described the outcomes of 78 patients undergoing abdominoperineal resection or low anterior resection. Two thirds of patients undergoing abdominoperineal resection had impaired sexual function compared with 30% of patients undergoing low anterior resection.[24] Total mesorectal excision is becoming a standard procedure in rectal cancer surgery. This technique, which requires sharp dissection of the mesorectum, is associated with a lower rate of local recurrences and a higher rate of potency preservation. A comparison of outcomes in terms of sexual function for patients who had conventional surgery and patients who had total mesorectal resection showed that the ability to have intercourse dropped from 75% to 13% in the conventional surgery group compared with a drop from 67% to 29% in the total mesorectal resection group.[25] The improvement in sexual function with total mesorectal resection is a result of the identification and sparing of the preaortic superior hypogastric plexus (responsible for ejaculation) and the bilateral hypogastric nerves that form the inferior hypogastric plexus (responsible for erection). Nerve-sparing techniques have resulted in a potency preservation rate of 88% to 90%, although 19% to 59% of patients with preserved erectile function were unable to ejaculate.[26-28] There is less information available on sexual dysfunction in women with rectal cancer. However, physical factors such as vaginal stenosis, urinary and fecal incontinence, and dyspareunia may have a significant impact on female sexual function.

Other Surgeries

Gynecologic surgeries can alter sexual function directly by affecting the anatomy of the female genital tract. Changes in genital sensation such as pain or numbness or inability to reach orgasm can occur after gynecologic surgery. Mastectomies may have a profound impact on a woman's self-image, overall sexual satisfaction, and frequency of sexual activity. Women who undergo breast conservation surgery or reconstruction are more likely to enjoy breast caressing but do not differ significantly from patients undergoing mastectomy regarding frequency of sex, reaching orgasm, or overall sexual satisfaction.[29,30]

Radiation Therapy

Radiation therapy affects reproductive function through direct effects on the pituitary, hypothalamus, gonads, uterus, and penile arterial and nerve supply.

Central Nervous System Effects

The endocrinologic and fertility effects of central nervous system irradiation have not been adequately evaluated in survivors of childhood cancer. However, mounting evidence suggests that cranial irradiation reduces fertility and sexual function. External irradiation to the brain can cause damage to the hypothalamus and impair its function; pituitary cells are more resistant to irradiation. Pituitary dysfunction caused by irradiation is attributed to disturbance in the hypothalamic-pituitary axis. Hypopituitarism develops slowly after brain irradiation and can be associated with an increase in prolactin levels.[31] Hypothalamic-pituitary function was studied in 31 patients with nasopharyngeal tumors treated with primary radiation therapy (4000–6000 cGy).[32] All patients had a normal baseline pituitary function. At 1 year after treatment, elevations in thyroid-stimulating hormone levels and blunted responses in LH to luteinizing hormone–releasing hormone (LHRH), suggesting an abnormality in the pulsatile release of LHRH, were noted in males. Three females had amenorrhea in association with elevated prolactin levels.[32] A dose-dependent response has been suggested, with thyroid-stimulating hormone (TSH) and gonadotropin abnormalities more commonly seen with brain irradiation doses exceeding 3000 cGy.[33] A recent multicenter study of 593 long-term survivors of acute lymphoblastic leukemia disclosed an increased rate of infertility among children treated with whole-brain radiation.[34] The study suggests that cranial irradiation affects fertility by disturbing gonadotropins necessary for the normal function and maturation of the testis and ovaries. The fertility of female survivors who were treated around the time of menarche was significantly lower than that of sibling control subjects (rate ratio = 0:59). Fertility in male patients who received cranial radiation doses of 2400 cGy before the age of 9 years was only one third that of control subjects (rate ratio = 0:35). Survivors treated at other ages did not have fertility deficits when compared with control subjects; this suggests a window period in which normal gonadotropin function is most essential for gonadal maturation.[34] This study also shows that reproductive dysfunction may occur as a result of brain irradiation (1200–2400 cGy) at doses lower than previously suggested. In another study in which the effects of acute lymphoblastic leukemia treatment on onset of menarche were evaluated, survivors receiving 1800 cGy of cranial radiation before the age of 8 years had early onset of menarche, whereas survivors treated with 2400 cGy craniospinal radiation had delayed onset of menarche.[35] Ninety percent of survivors of acute lymphoblastic leukemia in this study had normal onset of menarche compared with control subjects.

Testicular Function

Radiation therapy that includes the testes in the field of treatment can result in gonadal failure. Permanent Leydig's cell dysfunction occurs with a dose of 2000 to 3000 cGy. Therapeutic radiation doses (2400 cGy) to the testes given to patients with acute leukemia cause Leydig's cell dysfunction manifested by low testosterone levels or a poor testosterone response to gonadotropins.[34,36] Spermato-genic elements are much more sensitive to radiation than Leydig's cells. Radiation doses as low as 15 cGy transiently suppress spermatogenesis, and doses higher than 600 cGy permanently destroy the germinal elements.[37] Berthelsen[38] evaluated the effects of adjuvant irradiation for seminoma on gonadal function; retroperitoneal and ipsilateral iliac irradiation resulted in an estimated scatter of 200 to 1300 cGy to the unaffected contralateral testicle. Two thirds of patients had azoospermia, and it took a median of 540 days from the end of treatment before spermatozoa were again found in semen samples. A median of 1250 days passed before the pretreatment sperm count was reached. One to five years after treatment, sperm counts were still low (median, 6×10^6 per ejaculate) and serum FSH levels were elevated (median, 61 IU/L).[38] The time to recovery has been shown to be dose dependent, at least in the range of 19 to 148 cGy.[39] There was no increase in post-treatment congenital abnormalities, and the conception rate after treatment was 60% to 70%.[38]

Ovarian Function

Information on the effects of radiation therapy on the ovaries is more limited. Irradiation that does not involve the pelvis usually does not result in ovarian failure. Madsen and colleagues[40] described menstrual function and fertility in 36 women, ages 10 to 40 years, with supradiaphragmatic Hodgkin's lymphoma. The average radiation dose to mantle and paraaortic fields was 4000 to 4400 cGy; the calculated scatter radiation dose to the pelvis at the ovaries was 3200 Gy. There were 38 pregnancies in 18 women; all offspring were healthy. One of 36 women (2.7%) experienced premature menopause.[40] This report confirms the relative resistance of ovarian function to radiation therapy compared with testicular spermatogenesis. The effect of radiation on the ovaries is dose dependent. Single doses of 500 cGy produce menstrual irregularities in women of all ages. For women older than 40 years, a single 600-cGy dose usually induces menopause. Dose fractionation results in higher dose tolerability; women between the ages of 20 and 30 years can tolerate up to 3000 cGy when the dose is fractionated over 6 weeks.[41] Goldman and Johnson[42] reviewed the effects of radiation on the ovaries and confirmed a dose-dependent and age-dependent response to radiation. Although a dose of 150 cGy had no deleterious effects on fertility in women younger than 40 years, those older than 40 had a moderate risk of infertility. At doses of 250 to 400 cGy, women younger than 40 had a 60% risk of infertility, and the risk approached 100% in women older than 40.[42]

Pelvic Radiation

Radiation therapy is commonly used as definitive treatment for patients with localized or locally advanced prostate cancer. Although the etiology of erectile dysfunction after definitive radiation therapy for prostate cancer is likely a multifactorial phenomenon, mounting evidence suggests that the arteriogenic mechanism is more important in this setting than the cavernosal mechanism. Maintenance of normal erection requires both vasodilatation of penile arteries (arteriogenic element) and concomitant relaxation of the corporal smooth muscles (cavernosal element). Duplex ultrasonography can be used to assess arteriogenic function by measuring peak penile blood flow and cavernosal function by measuring distension of the corpora cavernosa in the setting of normal penile flow.[43] Duplex ultrasonography in patients with prostate cancer who have radiation therapy–induced erectile dysfunction confirmed a 63% rate of arteriogenic dysfunction.[43] This contrasts with prostatectomy-induced erectile dysfunction: only 32% of patients who underwent prostatectomy had arteriogenic dysfunction, whereas 52% had cavernosal dysfunction.[43] Erectile dysfunction is frequently seen after treatment of prostate cancer with external beam radiation and increases in frequency with time. Potency and age before treatment are risk factors for erectile dysfunction after completion of therapy. Data from one institution on 802 patients before and after treatment for prostate cancer show that only 15% of patients (24.5% of previously potent) who elected radiation therapy had normal erectile function at a median of 53 months of follow-up.[44] Others have shown higher rates of potency, especially when preradiation baseline erectile dysfunction is taken into account. In 290 patients with prostate cancer treated with radiation, 62% and 42% of those who were potent before treatment maintained potency at 12 and 24 months, respectively.[45] These potency rates drop further with time. Conformal radiation therapy limits the radiation field while delivering a high dose of radiation to the prostate and may be associated with a lower degree of impotence.[46,47] Mantz and colleagues[47] described a 5-year potency rate of 53% among 287 patients with prostate cancer treated with 6000 to 7200 cGy conformal radiation therapy. The use of brachytherapy in the treatment of prostate cancer has also been associated with a lower incidence of impotence. Prostate brachytherapy as monotherapy was associated with 5-year and 6-year potency rates of 76% and 52%, respectively, among previously potent patients.[48,49] The addition of external beam radiation or antiandrogen therapy to brachytherapy decreases the rates of potency substantially.[48,49]

Prior radiation therapy below the diaphragm has also been associated with an increased rate of preterm delivery, low-birth-weight infants, and increased perinatal morbidity. Among 114 pregnancies in women who had received abdominal radiotherapy for Wilms' tumor, an adverse pregnancy outcome occurred in 34 (30%). Women who received radiotherapy had an eightfold increase in the perinatal mortality rate and a fourfold increase in low-birth-weight infants. Women with Wilms' tumor who did not receive radiotherapy did not exhibit any increased risks.[50] Other data suggest a particularly high risk of preterm delivery and low birth weight but no congenital malformations in women who conceive within 1 year after completion of radiotherapy, suggesting uterine or hormonal defects as the cause of these abnormalities.[51]

Hormonal Therapy

Ablative hormonal therapy is often applied in patients with androgen- or estrogen-sensitive tumors. The most common applications are prostate cancer and breast cancer.

Gonadotropin-Releasing Hormone Agonists and Antagonists

Leuprolide and goserelin are two potent GnRH analogues that are commercially available in the United States. These two analogues are much more potent in stimulating gonadotropin release than GnRH. Initial treatment with GnRH agonists will result in LH and FSH surges with resultant gonadal steroid synthesis stimulation. However, after 10 to 14 days of continuous exposure to GnRH analogues, GnRH receptors on gonadotropin cells in the pituitary are down-regulated, resulting in inhibition of LH and FSH release and gonadal suppression. After prolonged GnRH analogue therapy, testosterone and estrogen levels are suppressed to castration levels. In males, this is usually associated with complete loss of sexual desire and marked changes in frequency, magnitude, duration, and rigidity of nocturnal erections.[52] Treatment exceeding 2 years results in atrophic testes, which may not recover even if administration of GnRH is discontinued.[53] In females, the use of GnRH in the adjuvant treatment of breast cancer is associated with an increased rate of sexual dysfunction, but the symptoms are usually reversible on discontinuation of therapy.[54]

Abarelix, a GnRH antagonist, has recently been approved for use in the treatment of hormone-sensitive prostate cancer. Abarelix was not associated with an initial testosterone surge, whereas LHRH agonists were associated with a transient testosterone surge of more than 80% in the first week of therapy.[55] Medical castration occurred in 75% of patients receiving abarelix in the first week of therapy compared with 0% of those receiving LHRH analogues.[55] When compared with a combination of LHRH agonist (leuprolide) and antiandrogen (bicalutamide), abarelix was associated with a more rapid decrease in testosterone to castrate levels and avoidance of a testosterone surge with the initiation of treatment.[56] The effects on reproductive function are similar to those of LHRH agonists and are a direct consequence of castrate testosterone levels.

Antiandrogens

Antiandrogens exert their activity by directly binding to and blocking the activity of androgen receptors. Androgen blockage is associated with a rise in FSH and LH levels and a resultant rise in the serum testosterone level.[57] Antiandrogens (such as flutamide, bicalutamide, or nilutamide) are commonly used in the management of prostate cancer either as an adjunct therapy to LHRH analogues or when treatment with LHRH agonists or antagonists fails. When combined with LHRH analogues, antiandrogens do not add to the incidence of gynecomastia (12%–13%) or hot flashes (60%–64%) and do not affect the incidence of impotence, which is universal in these patients.[58] High-dose bicalutamide has been compared with maximum androgen blockade as monotherapy in patients with advanced prostate cancer. There was comparable clinical activity but significantly less impotence and loss of libido.[59] Recent reports, however, suggest that the ability to maintain potency during antiandrogen monotherapy is limited. A study in which flutamide was evaluated as monotherapy for 147 patients with previously untreated prostate cancer demonstrated preservation of sexual activity in 22% of patients and preservation of morning erection in 20% at 2 to 6 years from the start of therapy.[60] The median time to loss of morning erections and sexual activity was 12.9 and 13.7 months, respectively.[60]

Selective Estrogen Receptor Modulators and Aromatase Inhibitors

Tamoxifen is the most commonly prescribed adjuvant hormonal therapy. This selective estrogen receptor modulator has estrogenic effects in bone and endometrium and antiestrogenic effects in breast tissue. This results in an effective antitumor effect and maintenance of bone density. In premenopausal women, the antiestrogen effect is perceived by the hypothalamus as a state of estrogen deficiency, resulting in increases in LH and FSH levels and hyperestrogenemia. In postmenopausal women, in whom FSH and LH levels are elevated and estrogen levels are depressed, tamoxifen reduces gonadotropin secretion.

Treatment with tamoxifen after primary therapy for breast cancer is associated with a high incidence of hot flashes (20%–50%); little information is available on the incidence of sexual function.[61] A small study evaluated the incidence of sexual dysfunction in 57 women receiving adjuvant tamoxifen.[62] Pain, burning, or discomfort with intercourse were reported by 54% of patients and did not correlate with age, surgical treatment of the primary cancer, or chemotherapy.[62] Berglund and colleagues[54] have reported no significant effects on sexuality after treatment with adjuvant tamoxifen in premenopausal females. Aromatase inhibitors such as anastrozole and letrozole have been associated with a lower incidence of hot flashes and have been generally better tolerated than tamoxifen. No clear sexual dysfunction has been associated with these agents. This may be because their use has been largely limited to postmenopausal patients.

Estrogens/Progesterone

GnRH analogues have largely replaced estrogens in the management of prostate cancer, and aromatase inhibitors have replaced progestational agents in the management of estrogen receptor–positive breast cancer.

The use of the estrogen diethylstilbestrol in the treatment of prostate cancer induces effective suppression of FSH and LH production and castrate levels of testosterone.[63] However, estrogen use is associated with higher rates of gynecomastia and unacceptable cardiovascular toxicity. High-dose treatment with the progestational agent megestrol results in LH, FSH, estrogen, testosterone, and adrenal steroid suppression.[64–66] The use of high-dose megestrol acetate as an appetite stimulant is associated with an 18% rate of impotence in males, and its use has been associated with testosterone suppression.[66,67] The extent and permanency of effects of estrogenic and progestational agents on reproductive function depend on the dose and duration of their use.

Chemotherapy

Effects in Men

Among chemotherapeutic agents, alkylating agents have the most profound effects on male fertility. Chlorambucil and cyclophosphamide deplete the testicular germinal epithelium in a dose-dependent fashion. Cumulative dosages of chlorambucil in excess of 400 mg and cyclophosphamide in excess of 6 g are associated with prolonged azoospermia.[68,69] Both sperm counts and sperm motility are markedly reduced after cyclophosphamide-containing regimens in the treatment of soft-tissue sarcomas. Antimetabolites have little effect on spermatogenesis when used in standard dosages. The use of high-dose methotrexate in the adjuvant treatment of patients with osteosarcoma has been associated with transient oligospermia.[70] Similarly, doxorubicin has been associated with reversible testicular injury in patients with osteosarcoma.[71] Cisplatin seems to affect spermatogenesis in a dose-dependent fashion.[72]

Combination chemotherapies containing alkylating agents are far more fertility-impairing than nonalkylating combinations. The majority of men treated with mechlorethamine, vincristine, procarbazine, and prednisone (MOPP) have severe oligospermia or azoospermia, and findings from testicular biopsies confirm germinal aplasia.[5,73] Procarbazine seems to have significant effects on testicular spermatogenesis and its effects are often irreversible. Regimens that do not include procarbazine such as cyclophosphamide, vincristine, and prednisone (CVP) are usually associated only with transient FSH level elevations and oligospermia.[74] Chapman and colleagues[75] followed up 64 patients with Hodgkin's lymphoma treated with mechlorethamine, vinblastine, procarbazine, and prednisone (MVPP). Only 4 of 64 patients treated with the procarbazine-based regimen recovered spermatogenesis after a median follow-up of 51 months.[75] Comparison of the procarbazine-containing regimen MOPP with Adriamycin, bleomycin, vinblastine, dacarbazine (ABVD) in patients with Hodgkin's disease revealed a considerably higher rate of azoospermia with MOPP (100%) than with ABVD (35%). Reversal of azoospermia rarely occurred with MOPP but did occur in the majority of patients receiving ABVD.[76] Dose dependency of infertility is also clearly evident in patients with Hodgkin's disease receiving combination chemotherapy. Azoospermia occurred considerably less often in patients receiving two cycles of MOPP compared with those receiving six cycles.[77]

Combination chemotherapy for testicular cancers has also been associated with FSH level elevation and oligospermia. These results are complicated further by the fact that the majority of patients with testicular cancer have abnormal spermatogenesis before initiation of therapy. Cisplatin-based regimens are associated with suppression of spermatogenesis at 1 year after completion of therapy. However, by 1.5 to 3 years after treatment, spermatogenesis usually returns to pretreatment baseline.[78,79] Patients with testicular cancer with pretreatment oligospermia or with persistent FSH level elevation at 2 years after treatment are unlikely to recover normal spermatogenesis after treatment.

Effects in Women

Follicular growth and maturation are affected by chemotherapy. Histologic evaluation of ovaries of females treated with cytotoxic chemotherapy shows fibrosis and follicular destruction.[80,81] Premature ovarian failure is a common result of chemotherapy and is dependent on patient age, dose, duration, and type of chemotherapy administered. Alkylating agents have been strongly associated with ovarian dysfunction. Daily cyclophosphamide treatment for periods exceeding 1 year has been associated with amenorrhea in females younger than 40 years.[82,83] In most series, an incidence of amenorrhea of 50% or higher is reported within 1 month of initiation of cyclophosphamide therapy.[84] Younger females are more tolerant of the effects of chemotherapy and have a better chance of resuming menstruation after completion of chemotherapy. In an assessment of the effects of adjuvant cyclophosphamide, fluorouracil, and methotrexate (CMF) on reproductive function in patients with breast cancer, Mehta and colleagues[85] reported medians of 5.5, 2.3, and 1.1 months to onset of amenorrhea in patients younger than 35 years, between the ages of 35 and 45 years, and older than 45 years, respectively. In another study, patients 30 to 40 years of age required a median dose of 9.3 g of cyclophosphamide before amenorrhea developed, whereas patients older than 40 required a median dose of 5.2 g.[86] A median of 20.4 g was required before the onset of amenorrhea in patients younger than 30 years.[86] Menses resumed in 50% of those younger than 40, but it rarely resumed in females older than 40 years.[86] Treatment with the alkylating agent melphalan resulted in amenorrhea in 73% of patients between the ages of 40 and 49 years compared with 22% in patients younger than 40 years.[87] Similar results have been described with other alkylating agents such as busulfan and chlorambucil. Younger women have a larger number of oocytes in reserve and thus a lesser likelihood of experiencing permanent ovarian damage after alkylating agent chemotherapy in comparison with older women.

Other nonalkylating chemotherapies such as antimetabolites, bleomycin, vinca alkaloids, and daunorubicin are not a frequent cause of amenorrhea.

Combination chemotherapies have been evaluated more extensively as a cause of premature ovarian failure. Doxorubicin-based regimens in the adjuvant treatment of breast cancer resulted in a 96% frequency of amenorrhea in women 40 to 49 years of age compared with 0% among women 30 years of age or younger.[88] These regimens frequently incorporated other alkylating agents. Data collected from patients treated with MOPP for Hodgkin's disease similarly confirm the importance of age at the time of treatment.[89] Treatment of women with lymphoma with regimens that do not include procarbazine (e.g., ABVD) results in a lower incidence of premature menopause.[74,90] The importance of age and chemotherapy intensity has been stressed by a survey of 96 female patients treated with combinations of ifosfamide, methotrexate, cisplatin, etoposide, and doxorubicin for localized osteosarcoma. The study evaluated the incidence of treatment-related amenorrhea and post-treatment fertility.[91] All 24 patients treated at a prepubertal age

experienced menarche at a median age of 13 years. After menarche, 16 had normal menses and 8 had permanently irregular cycles.[91] Sixty-eight patients (11 to 43 years) had entered puberty on initiation of chemotherapy. Sixty-nine percent of these had amenorrhea, typically after one cycle of therapy. A four-drug regimen was associated with 89% amenorrhea, whereas a three-drug regimen was associated with only 53%. Amenorrhea was also related to age: 19 of 51 patients younger than 20 years continued to menstruate during chemotherapy compared with only 2 of 17 patients older than 20 at the time of treatment. The majority resumed menstruation on completion of chemotherapy. Among 22 patients who married after treatment, 20 became pregnant at a median age of 27 years. None of the pregnancies resulted in congenital anomalies.[91]

The duration of combination chemotherapy is also of paramount importance in induction of amenorrhea. Treatment of premenopausal women with a combination of cyclophosphamide, methotrexate, fluorouracil, vincristine, and prednisone resulted in amenorrhea in 55% of patients treated for 12 weeks and in 83% of patients treated for 36 weeks.[92]

Chemotherapy Effects in Children

Testicular Function in Boys

The prepubertal testes are more resistant to the effects of chemotherapy than the adult testes. This relative resistance may be due to the nonproliferative status of the prepubertal germinal layer. Although it may take years, a certain degree of spermatogenesis recovery usually occurs in most boys who have received a total dose of cyclophosphamide of less then 10 g.[93] Gonadal function was assessed in 17 male survivors of childhood sarcomas treated with vincristine, actinomycin, and cyclophosphamide with or without doxorubicin.[94] Only two patients who received less than 7.5 g/m^2 had normal findings on semen analysis. All patients who received more than 7.5 g/m^2 had abnormal findings on semen analysis and all 5 who received more than 25 g/m^2 had azoospermia more than 5 years after therapy.[94] Most patients (15 of 16) maintained a normal testosterone level.[94] MOPP therapy leads to a considerably higher rate of testicular damage, presumably because of the added effect of procarbazine. Nine of 19 prepubertal patients receiving MOPP or cyclophosphamide-based therapy (exceeding 9 g of cyclophosphamide) were sterile at a median follow-up period of 9 years.[95] Alkylating therapy during puberty may have more detrimental effects on sexual function than therapy before the onset of puberty. In a cohort of 12 prepubertal and pubertal patients receiving MOPP therapy, all pubertal patients had irreversible azoospermia but two prepubertal patients were able to recover spermatogenesis. Pubertal treatment with MOPP was also associated with a high incidence of gynecomastia in association with low-normal testosterone levels and elevated LH and FSH levels.[96]

Ovarian Function in Girls

Prepubertal ovaries are relatively resistant to the effects of chemotherapy in comparison with postpubertal ovaries. Most prepubertal females receiving MOPP therapy for Hodgkin's disease achieved normal puberty and were subsequently able to have normal pregnancies.[97,98] Treatment of females with acute leukemia with a multidrug regimen of prednisone, vincristine, methotrexate, and 6-mercaptopurine with or without cyclophosphamide resulted in ovarian failure in only one of 17 prepubertal females.[99] Byrne and colleagues[100] retrospectively evaluated fertility rates in survivors of childhood and adolescent cancer. Two thousand two hundred eighty-three survivors were compared with 3270 siblings included as control subjects. There was no apparent effect of alkylating-agent therapy administered alone (relative fertility, 1.02), and only a moderate fertility deficit was evident when alkylating-agent therapy was combined with radiation below the diaphragm (relative fertility, 0.81) among women. The overall relative fertility in women was 0.93 and compared favorably with men's relative fertility of 0.76.[100] Childhood cancer therapy has also been associated with an increased risk of early menopause. In a large cohort of childhood cancer survivors, the principal risks for early menopause were found to be treatment after onset of puberty, treatment with radiotherapy below the diaphragm, and treatment with alkylating agents.[101] Survivors who received the diagnosis after puberty and treated with radiation therapy below the diaphragm were 8.5 times more likely to reach menopause in their twenties. The average age for menopause in survivors treated with both an alkylating agent and radiation therapy below the diaphragm was 31 years.[101]

High-Dose Chemotherapy (Bone Marrow Transplantation)

High-Dose Chemotherapy in Females
Gonadal dysfunction after high-dose chemotherapy is dependent on age, sex, type of conditioning regimen, and previous therapy. In women, increased age and treatment with an alkylating conditioning regimen including total body irradiation (TBI) are associated with a high rate of ovarian failure. In 144 women with leukemia who underwent bone marrow transplantation (BMT) after TBI and treatment with cyclophosphamide, amenorrhea was present for 3 years after transplantation. Only nine patients eventually recovered their ovarian function.[102] The likelihood of recovering ovarian function decreased by a factor of 0.8 per year of age.[102] TBI enhances the risk of ovarian failure. Ovarian failure usually occurs within 3 months of TBI. A single nonfractionated dose of 10 Gy is more likely to result in damage to the ovaries and decrease the chance of ovarian recovery than a fractionated 12-Gy total dose.[102] Recovery of ovarian function is more likely with chemotherapy-only conditioning regimens but is usually limited to females younger than 30 years of age. In a study of a conditioning regimen of cyclophosphamide of 200 mg/kg, all females 26 years of age or younger recovered their ovarian function, whereas only 5 of 16 females older than 26 did so.[102] In another report on patients with non-Hodgkin's lymphoma treated with consolidation high-dose chemotherapy (cyclophosphamide, carmustine, and etoposide), 9 of 56 patients were able conceive despite receiving a total dose of 10,800 mg/m²

cyclophosphamide.[103] Pregnancies were limited to females younger then 29 years of age; no birth defects were reported.[103] The addition of busulfan to cyclophosphamide is rarely associated with ovarian recovery, even in younger patients.[104]

BMT may also be complicated by graft-versus-host disease. When severe, graft-versus-host disease can cause vaginal strictures and adhesions that interfere with intercourse.[105]

High-Dose Chemotherapy in Males
The majority of males who undergo BMT with or without TBI have marked elevations in their LH and FSH levels. Testosterone levels may be depressed but are usually maintained in the normal range, reflecting an adequate compensatory reaction by Leydig's cells to the rise in the LH level. Infertility is the rule in adult and young males receiving high-dose chemotherapy with or without TBI, reflecting the relative sensitivity of the germinal component to chemotherapy and radiation therapy relative to Leydig's cells. Decreased libido has been reported in patients who have undergone BMT. This is probably multifactorial and results from psychologic stress, mild suppression of testosterone levels, and vascular and neurologic damage. Testosterone levels were found to be in the low to normal range in a study of 24 males with features of hypogonadism and erectile dysfunction after BMT.[106] Although supplementation with testosterone resulted in an improvement in libido, there were no clear beneficial effects on erectile dysfunction.[106] Doppler studies in these patients confirmed evidence of cavernosal arterial insufficiency and strongly correlated with prior TBI therapy.[106,107]

High-Dose Chemotherapy in Children
Permanent ovarian failure is less commonly seen in prepubertal females than in adults. A combination of high-dose chemotherapy and TBI is associated with a higher incidence of ovarian failure than chemotherapy alone. Sarafoglou and colleagues[108] reported a median age of 8.6 years for prepubertal females with acute leukemia treated with BMT (TBI-based regimen) in whom ovarian failure developed. The median age for prepubertal females who went on to enter puberty was 6.1 years.[108] Even in those who enter puberty, normal uterine maturation is impaired and the endometrium is atrophic as a result of radiation therapy. Supplementation with hormone replacement improves mucosal thickness, but the total volume of the uterus remains contracted.[109] Long-term follow-up of survivors of childhood acute leukemia reveals that TBI is indeed the most important factor in development of gonadal failure. Among 77 survivors of leukemia, three groups of treatment were identified: chemotherapy, chemotherapy and cranial irradiation, and chemotherapy and TBI.[110] Forty-four of 44 patients treated with chemotherapy entered and progressed through puberty without sex hormone supplementation. Only 1 of 18 of patients treated with chemotherapy and cranial irradiation experienced early amenorrhea accompanied by elevated gonadotropin levels. Eight of 15 patients treated with chemotherapy and

Problems Common to Cancer and Its Therapy

TBI had gonadal failure (3 men and 5 women) requiring long-term sex hormone supplementation.[110]

CHEMOTHERAPY AND RADIATION DURING PREGNANCY

Cancer complicates 1 in 1000 pregnancies.[111] The most frequent cancers detected during pregnancy are cervical cancer, breast cancer, melanoma, ovarian cancer, thyroid cancer, and leukemia.[112] With an increasing median age at which pregnancy is occurring, more cancers are expected to be diagnosed during pregnancy. Chemotherapy has an essential role in the management of many of these tumors. The timing and selection of chemotherapeutic agents should be optimized to maximize the clinical benefit to the patient while minimizing the risk to the fetus.

Fetal Stage of Development and Pregnancy Outcome

The most important factor influencing fetal outcome in patients with cancer treated during pregnancy is the stage of fetal development on treatment initiation. The first trimester is the most susceptible period. The blastocyst is relatively resistant to teratogens for the first 2 weeks because it lacks an established circulation. After implantation but prior to organogenesis, the blastocyst may exhibit damage secondary to chemotherapy resulting in abortion or may survive without manifesting any abnormalities. Organogenesis begins during the fifth gestational week and continues until the eighth week. During organogenesis, the stem cell population is limited, and damage from chemotherapy may result in major defects. Exposure to chemotherapy during the first trimester may result in a malformation rate of 10% to 20% compared with an estimated rate of 3% in the general population.[113] By the thirteenth week of gestation, all organs have developed with the exception of the brain and gonads.[114] Exposure to chemotherapy on completion of organogenesis (second and third trimesters) is thus unlikely to result in major birth defects but may result in fetal growth retardation. Treatment of patients with hematologic malignancies and breast cancer during the second and third trimesters has not been associated with any increase in the rate of congenital anomalies.[115-117]

Effects of Different Classes of Chemotherapeutic Agents on Pregnancy Outcome

Different classes of chemotherapeutic agents have varying teratogenic potential. Alkylating agents and antimetabolites appear to have a greater potential for causing detrimental effects than antitumor antibiotics, platinum analogues, and vinca alkaloids.[118]

Alkylating Agents

Fetal abnormalities have been reported as a result of first-trimester exposure to cyclophosphamide, chlorambucil, and busulfan.[119-123] No definite causal relationship has been established for other agents such as thiotepa, melphalan, and dacarbazine; but first-trimester exposure data for these compounds are limited.

Antibiotic Agents

No definite causal relationship between congenital malformations and treatment with dactinomycin or bleomycin has been documented. Births of healthy children to patients exposed during the first, second, and third trimesters have been reported.

Antimetabolites

Methotrexate is known for its teratogenic effects and has been used as an abortifacient. Congenital anomalies associated with first-trimester use have been described. Malformations include severe skull abnormalities, heart defects such as dextroposition, and digital anomalies.[124,125] Exposure starting as late as 11 weeks has been associated with anomalies.[125] 5-Fluorouracil may be similarly associated with congenital anomalies when administered in the first trimester. One case of multiple congenital anomalies including radial dysplasia, absent digits, and hypoplasia of multiple organs has been reported as a result of first-trimester exposure.[126] Cytarabine has been commonly used to treat hematologic malignancies in the second and third trimesters of pregnancy without a reported increase in congenital defects. First-trimester exposure has been associated with congenital abnormalities including microtus and auditory canal atresia, lobster claw hand and other digital anomalies, and lower limb defects.[127,128] Caligiuri and Mayer[129] have reported normal pregnancy outcome after first-trimester exposures. There is currently no information on pregnancy outcomes in patients treated with the newer antimetabolite gemcitabine.

Anthracyclines

First-trimester exposures to anthracyclines have been associated with normal and abnormal fetal outcomes. Imperforate anus, rectovaginal fistula, and microcephaly have been described after first-trimester exposure to doxorubicin.[130]

Vinca Alkaloids

Definite fetal anomalies associated with vinca alkaloids have not been reported. Sporadic anomalies have been reported in patients receiving combination therapy. Several women who were treated with vinca alkaloids during the first trimester of pregnancy have given birth to healthy neonates.[113,131]

Platinum Compounds

Ten pregnant women with cancer have been reported to receive cisplatin during the second or third trimester of pregnancy.[132] None of the neonates demonstrated any congenital anomalies, but fetal growth was restricted in 50% of pregnancies.

Taxanes

Limited clinical information is available on the clinical effects of taxanes on pregnancy. Review of the literature reveals one report of a patient with ovarian cancer treated during the third trimester of pregnancy with carboplatin and paclitaxel without any adverse events on the newborn.[133] A woman with metastatic breast cancer treated with docetaxel during the second and third trimesters of pregnancy gave birth to a normal healthy infant.[134]

Topoisomerase II Inhibitors

Etoposide has not been reported to cause congenital malformations. However, fetal marrow suppression manifesting as severe neonatal anemia and leukopenia has been reported in a pregnant woman treated for leukemia.[135]

In general, chemotherapy has not been associated with an increased risk of congenital malformations if administered in the second or third trimester, but an increased incidence of growth restriction and premature birth has been noted. An increased risk of congenital anomalies has been associated with treatment in the first trimester. Doll and colleagues[136] reported an incidence of fetal malformations of 15% in association with first-trimester chemotherapy exposure versus 1.3% for second- and third-trimester exposure. This risk is apparently highest when antimetabolites, especially methotrexate, are used. If cancer occurs in the first trimester and systemic cytotoxic therapy is clearly indicated, termination of the pregnancy should be considered. Delay of chemotherapy until it can be given more safely in the second or third trimester should be considered if the risk for a poor outcome in the mother is not increased. The long-term effects of different chemotherapeutic agents on progeny have not been adequately evaluated. Anecdotal data suggest that most offspring exposed in utero exhibit normal physical and mental development. Eighty-four children born to patients with hematologic malignancies and exposed to chemotherapeutic agents in utero were followed up for a median of 18.7 years.[137] In all the children studied, learning and educational performance were normal and no congenital, neurologic, or psychologic abnormalities were observed. There was no apparent increase in malignancies. Some of these individuals became parents during the period of follow-up. Twelve second-generation offspring were evaluated and all of them were healthy.[137]

Targeted Therapy

Several newer agents have been developed to target specific growth receptors, antigens, or kinases that are essential for cell growth and development. Two commercially available agents are the anti-Her-2/neu antibody trastuzumab and the anti-CD-20 antibody rituximab. Reproductive data for monkeys given 25 times the human equivalent of trastuzumab did not show any evidence of teratogenicity. However, trastuzumab diffuses through the placental circulation and immediate and long-term effects on human progeny have not been evaluated. Rituximab has not been evaluated extensively in reproductive animal models. A 29-year-old patient with diffuse large cell lymphoma was treated during her second and third weeks of pregnancy with a combination of rituximab and cyclophosphamide, hydroxydaunomycin, Oncovin, and prednisone (CHOP) therapy.[138] She delivered a healthy female infant at 36 weeks. Other targeted agents such as the anti-epidermal growth factor receptor (EGFR) antibody C225 or EGFR-tyrosine kinase inhibitors are still in clinical trials, and no data are available regarding potential teratogenicity; therefore these agents should be avoided during pregnancy.

Immunomodulators

Limited data are available on the effects of interferons and interleukins on pregnancy. In animals, interferon-α and interleukin-2 have abortifacient and embryolethal effects. More than 20 case reports of pregnancy during interferon-α treatment in all three trimesters have been published.[139-141] None of the cases were associated with congenital anomalies, but growth retardation and premature births were more frequent than expected.[141]

Effects of Radiation Therapy on Pregnancy Outcome

Human data regarding the effects of radiation on fetal outcome are limited to accidental exposure and findings in victims of nuclear disaster. Similar to chemotherapy, the effects of radiation seem to be most pronounced during the period of organogenesis. During the first 8 to 25 weeks of pregnancy, the central nervous system is particularly sensitive to the effects of radiation. The most comprehensive review of clinical effects of pelvic radiation therapy was reported by Dekaban.[142] Pelvic irradiation up to 3 weeks after conception did not result in severe congenital anomalies, although a considerable number of embryos may have been resorbed or aborted.[142] Irradiation between weeks 4 and 11 led to the development of severe congenital anomalies in many organs. Exposure between weeks 11 and 16 led to anomalies of the eye, skeleton, and genital organs; stunted growth; microcephaly; and mental retardation.[142] Exposure during weeks 16 to 20 was associated with mild microcephaly, mental retardation, and stunted growth; whereas later exposures were unlikely to cause structural abnormalities.[142]

Data from Hiroshima and Nagasaki atomic bomb survivors suggest a dose-dependent effect of radiation on congenital anomalies, with a dose of 50 cGy resulting in a 40% risk of microcephaly. Doses in excess of 10 cGy may result in cognitive impairment, and higher exposures may result in further exacerbation of mental retardation. In utero radiation exposure also results in an increased risk of carcinogenesis with an estimated 6% risk of cancer by the age of 15 years per Gy of exposure.[143]

Radiation therapy should be avoided during pregnancy because of the significant physical, functional, and mental dysfunction that can result from exposure in the first and second trimesters. Even in cases of breast cancer when breast irradiation is given with abdominal shielding, the estimated fetal dose with 5000 cGy to the primary tumor is 14 to 18 cGy. This is well above the proposed threshold for microcephaly and mental retardation.[144]

CHEMOTHERAPY AND RADIATION DURING PREGNANCY

The risk of congenital anomalies is highest for first-trimester exposure and is most commonly associated with antimetabolites such as methotrexate. Decision making should be individualized, and decisions regarding termination or continuation of pregnancy should take into consideration the risks to the mother and the fetus. For women in the first trimester of pregnancy who require initiation of chemotherapy, termination of pregnancy should be considered. For patients who elect to proceed with pregnancy, the choice of chemotherapy should take into account the risks of congenital malformations. Chemotherapy choice is also important for women in the second trimester of pregnancy. Reports of congenital malformations and myocardial toxicity have been described with second-trimester exposure to methotrexate and doxorubicin. A delay in chemotherapy for a few weeks or until delivery for women in the third trimester can be considered if the mother's outcome is unlikely to be compromised. Delivery induction for gestations of more then 32 weeks is also another acceptable option for women in the third trimester of pregnancy.

Radiation therapy should be avoided during all stages of pregnancy. First- and second-trimester exposures are associated with congenital abnormalities, and third-trimester exposure can result in cognitive dysfunction.

PREVENTION

Modifying the treatment and its timing as discussed earlier may reduce reproductive complications, but care must be taken to avoid compromising treatment efficacy, and detailed discussions with patients are mandatory.

Retroperitoneal nerve-sparing dissections result in significant improvements in potency rates after radical prostatectomy. Similar results are reported in rectal surgeries with nerve-sparing dissection. Alternative chemotherapeutic regimens with low gonadal toxicity potential should be considered when possible. The substitution of ABVD therapy has resulted in similar or better efficacy in the treatment of Hodgkin's lymphoma and a lower rate of ovarian and testicular failure.

Unfortunately, most cancer diagnoses have limited treatment options, and the choice of a regimen with a low potential for gonadal toxicity is often not feasible. Spermatogenesis and follicular growth and maturation are particularly sensitive to the effects of chemotherapy because of their high mitotic rate. Thus treatment interventions that suppress germinal function during administration of cytotoxic therapy may limit the gonadal toxicity. GnRH analogs have been shown to inhibit spermatogenesis in various animals and in humans. The use of GnRH analogues has been reported to protect rat testes from chemotherapy and radiation.[145,146] However, treatment of testicular cancer and patients with Hodgkin's disease with LHRH analogues has failed to show any protective effects against the development of azoospermia.[147-149] Effective inhibition of spermatogenesis may require several weeks of hormonal manipulation with GnRH analogues. Treatment with GnRH analogues for several weeks before initiation of chemotherapy is often not feasible clinically and may account for the failure of previous studies to show a protective effect on gonadal function.

Similar attempts to protect the ovaries from cytotoxic chemotherapy by suppressing cycling through GnRH analogues and oral contraceptives have been made. A small study of patients with Hodgkin's disease receiving alkylating agent–based chemotherapy and oral contraceptives showed that five of six patients resumed normal menstrual function at 26 months.[150] Other studies of oral contraceptives and GnRH analogues failed to show any protective effects in patients with Hodgkin's disease in comparison with control subjects.[148,151] However, one prospective study in patients with lymphoma showed significant protection against ovarian failure with co-treatment with GnRH analogues.[152] Eighteen patients with lymphoma were treated with a monthly depot injection of GnRH agonist, starting before chemotherapy and continuing for a maximum of 6 months. Most of these patients (15 of 18) were treated with the MOPP/ABV(D) combination chemotherapy, followed by mantle field irradiation in 10 patients. This group of patients with prospectively treated lymphoma was compared with a matched control group of 18 women. Only 39% of the patients receiving chemotherapy alone resumed spontaneous ovulation in comparison with 94% of those receiving GnRH analogues along with chemotherapy.[152,153]

Other means of protection from radiation effects include gonadal shielding. In females receiving pelvic radiation, transposition of the ovaries may be one means of preventing radiation damage. Transposition of one or two ovaries can be done at time of laparotomy or laparoscopically. Spontaneous pregnancy rates after ovarian transposition are low, presumably because of the distorted tubo-ovarian anatomy caused by the procedure itself or the local therapy (radiation) to the pelvic area.[154]

TREATMENT

Treatment of reproductive complications is aimed at relieving the symptoms related to gonadal failure and providing assistance in achieving reproduction. This section focuses on hormone replacement, treatment measures for impotence, and reproductive assistance technologies.

Hormone Replacement

Premature ovarian failure results in sudden onset of menopausal symptoms caused by an abrupt decrease in estrogen levels. Sexual symptoms related to ovarian failure include vaginal atrophy, thinning of vulvar tissues and the vagina, decreased vaginal lubrication and elasticity, mood swings and irritability, and hot flashes. Estrogen replacement therapy (in combination with progesterone in patients without hysterectomy) can reverse most of these symptoms and should be discussed with all patients with iatrogenic ovarian failure. Risks including increased rate of cardiovascular and cerebral accidents and benefits such as osteoporosis prevention should be addressed before initiation of therapy. Hormone replacement in patients with breast cancer continues to be an area of concern because of the theoretical potential of promoting tumor growth. However, no reports have yet shown a detrimental effect of estrogen replacement in this population. Patients who are not candidates for or who refuse systemic estrogen replacement can be treated symptomatically with vaginal moisturizers and water-based lubricants. Vaginal estrogen therapy has also resulted in improvements in symptoms of vaginal dryness, dyspareunia, and a decrease in the incidence of urinary tract infections.

Male hypogonadism caused by chemotherapy and radiation therapy is associated with loss of libido, hot flashes, and impotence. Testosterone replacement as a depot injection or in a transdermal formulation may restore sexual function in such cases.[155,156]

Management of Erectile Dysfunction

The advent of sildenafil citrate (Viagra) marks an important milestone in the treatment of male impotence. The physiologic mechanism of penile erection involves release of nitrous oxide in the corpus cavernosum during sexual stimulation. Nitrous oxide results in an increase in cyclic guanosine monophosphate, which in turn results in corpus cavernosum smooth muscle relaxation, allowing an increase in blood flow. Sildenafil improves the ability to achieve and maintain an erection by blocking the degradation of cyclic guanosine monophosphate.

Sildenafil leads to successful intercourse in patients with prostate cancer who experience erectile dysfunction after prostatectomy, external beam radiation, or brachy-therapy. Response rates typically range between 70% and 80%.[157-160] The ease of oral administration and efficacy of this agent have made it the most commonly prescribed agent for erectile dysfunction.[161] Because sildenafil potentiates the hypotensive effects of nitrates, prescribers should ensure that patients taking sildenafil do not have any significant cardiac history and are not receiving any concomitant nitrate medications. Other alternative therapies include penile injections, vacuum devices, and intraurethral suppositories. These are more cumbersome to the patient and are associated with high dropout rates.[162] In refractory situations, surgical intervention with penile implants may be considered.

Assisted Reproductive Technologies

Once germinal testicular aplasia or premature ovarian failure occurs as a result of cancer therapy, the damage may be irreversible. Unless sperm banking or storage of embryos is done before treatment, these patients will not be able to parent their own biologic children. This issue has not been given adequate attention, and its importance to patients has been long overlooked. A survey of 904 men who were given a diagnosis of cancer revealed that 51% wanted children in the future.[163] Only 60% of men recalled being informed about infertility and only 51% were offered sperm banking.[163] Lack of prior discussion about sperm banking with patients was the most common reason for failing to bank sperm.[163]

Several advances in reproductive technologies allow for fertility preservation in patients undergoing gonadal toxic therapies. Intrauterine insemination is accomplished by selecting washed sperm with high motility and injecting them directly into the uterus at the time of ovulation. This procedure requires cryopreservation of 5 to 10 million normal sperm. In vitro fertilization with embryo transfer (IVF-ET) involves culturing the aspirated oocytes and spermatozoa in vitro, followed by the transcervical replacement of the embryo into the uterine cavity. With IVF-ET, the number of sperm required is 0.5 to 1 million.[164] Intracytoplasmic sperm injection (ICSI) involves the injection of a single sperm into the cytoplasm of the oocyte with transcervical placement of the embryo into the uterine cavity. ICSI reduces the criteria for sperm cryopreservation, theoretically, to the presence of one motile sperm. This makes almost any male patient with cancer who is not completely azoospermic a candidate for sperm cryopreservation. Even in patients with complete ejaculatory azoospermia, testicular sperm extraction, followed by ICSI and embryo cryopreservation, may represent an option for fertility preservation.[165,166] Testicular sperm extraction is typically achieved by performing open biopsy of testicular tissues with or without microdissection.[167] ICSI is now performed in 60% to 80% of assisted reproductive procedures in some metropolitan U.S. areas and is the procedure of choice for couples with a male infertility factor. In cases in which sperm has been stored or extracted successfully, success-ful pregnancy rates in the range of 30% are expected.[166,168] Transrectal electroejaculation is yet another viable method for sperm collection for the purpose of cryo-preservation or in vitro fertilization (IVF) in patients with retrograde ejaculation.[169] Other options for sperm collec-tion in patients with retrograde ejaculation are insemina-tion with sperm-rich urine (after masturbation) or bladder washings. Successful reports of insemination with these collection methods in conjunction with techniques ranging from intrauterine insemination to ICSI have been reported.[170]

Oocyte cryopreservation has been associated with few pregnancies. Low pregnancy yield and the need to delay chemotherapy to achieve appropriate follicular stimula-tion limit the use of this technique for female fertility preservation. Ovarian tissue cryopreservation is a novel technique under investigation. The procedure involves oophorectomy and cryopreservation before initiation of cancer treatments. On completion of cancer-directed therapy and when conception is planned, the frozen banked ovarian tissue is thawed and autotransplanted in the patient. Successful ovulation after autotransplantation has been reported, and the procedure continues to be under investigation.[171] Another option for fertility preservation involves IVF and embryo cryopreservation before initiation of treatment. The technique is cumber-some and expensive, may delay the initiation of effective chemotherapy, and constitutes an ethical dilemma.

PREVENTION AND TREATMENT OF SEXUAL AND REPRODUCTIVE DYSFUNCTION OF CANCER THERAPY

PREVENTION

The best prevention is selection of equally effective treatments with lesser toxic effects. Treatment of Hodgkin's disease with ABVD rather than MOPP will often result in fertility preservation. Selection of bone marrow conditioning regimens that do not incorporate total-body radiation should be considered for patients receiving bone marrow transplants. Ovarian and testicular suppression with GnRH analogues has not been shown conclusively to protect gonadal function and should be limited to clinical studies.

All males who are still contemplating future fatherhood and for whom chemotherapy that has been associated with infertility (such as alkylating agents) or pelvic radiation is planned should be offered sperm banking. Oocyte banking and ovarian cryopreservation continue to be investigated in females and have not yet been standardized. In vitro fertilization with embryo cryopreservation may represent another alternative in females undergoing gonadal toxic treatments.

TREATMENT

Treatment involves hormone replacement for patients with premature ovarian failure and low testosterone levels.

Estrogen replacement ameliorates menopausal symptoms including hot flashes, vaginal dryness, and dyspareunia. Vaginal estrogen therapy ameliorates the local vaginal symptoms in patients with relative contraindications to systemic estrogen replacement.

Testosterone replacement in men improves libido and reduces hot flashes and may improve potency in cases of severe androgen deficiency. Impotence caused by surgery or radiation therapy may be successfully treated with sildenafil. This agent should be avoided in patients with significant cardiovascular illness and is contraindicated in patients receiving nitrates. Sildenafil therapy should be considered as a first-line pharmacologic therapy in impotent patients with normal testosterone levels and in whom psychosocial causes are not suspected.

Assisted reproductive technologies such as intrauterine insemination, in vitro fertilization, and intracytoplasmic sperm injection should be considered as options for restoring fertility in couples who have difficulty conceiving after cancer therapy.

For patients who are unable to conceive because of uterine or cervical abnormalities attributed to the cancer or its treatment, IVF with implantation in a surrogate has been described.[172]

REFERENCES

1. Yen R, Barbieri, Jaffe R: Reproductive endocrinology: Physiology, pathophysiology, and clinical management, 4th ed. Philadelphia, WB Saunders, 1999, p 153.
2. Welt CK: The physiology and pathophysiology of inhibin, activin and follistatin in female reproduction. Curr Opin Obstet Gynecol 2002;14:317.
3. Wilson J, et al: Williams textbook of endocrinology, 9th ed. Philadelphia, WB Saunders, 1998, p 212.
4. O'Suilleabhain P, Low PA, Lennon VA: Autonomic dysfunction in the Lambert-Eaton myasthenic syndrome: Serologic and clinical correlates. Neurology 1998;50:88.
5. Whitehead E, et al: The effects of Hodgkin's disease and combination chemotherapy on gonadal function in the adult male. Cancer 1982;49:418.
6. Hendry WF, et al: Semen analysis in testicular cancer and Hodgkin's disease: Pre- and post-treatment findings and implications for cryopreservation. Br J Urol 1983;55:769.
7. Chapmam RM, Sutcliffe SB, Malpas JS: Male gonadal dysfunction in Hodgkin's disease. A prospective study. JAMA 1983;245:1323.
8. Berthelsen JG, Skakkebaek NE: Gonadal function in men with testis cancer. Fertil Steril 1983;39:68.
9. Fossa SD, Abyholm T, Aakvaag A: Spermatogenesis and hormonal status after orchiectomy for cancer and before supplementary treatment. Eur Urol 1984;10:173.
10. Petersen PM, Skakkebaek NE, Giwercman A: Gonadal function in men with testicular cancer: Biological and clinical aspects. APMIS 1998;106:24, discussion 34.
11. Jacobsen R, et al: Risk of testicular cancer in men with abnormal semen characteristics: Cohort study. BMJ 2000;321:7789.
12. Walsh PC, Epstein L, Lowe F: Potency following radical prostatectomy with wide unilateral excision of the neurovascular bundle. J Urol 1987;138:823.
13. Talcott JP, Rieker P, Clark J: Patient-reported symptoms after primary therapy for early prostate cancer: Results of a prospective cohort study. J Clin Oncol 1998;16:275.
14. Seigel T, Moul J, Spevak M: The development of erectile dysfunction in men treated for prostate cancer. J Urol 2001;165:430.
15. Kao T, Cruess TD, Garner D: Multicenter patient self-reporting questionnaire on impotence, incontinence and stricture after radical prostatectomy. J Urol 2000;163:858.
16. Steineck G, et al: Quality of life after radical prostatectomy or watchful waiting. N Engl J Med 2002;347:790.
17. Walsh PC, Lepor H, Eggleston JC: Radical prostatectomy with preservation of sexual function: Anatomical and pathological considerations. Prostate 1983;4:473.
18. Rabbani F, et al: Factors predicting recovery of erections after radical prostatectomy. J Urol 2000;164:1929.
19. Kom C, Mulholland SG, Edson M: Etiology of infertility after retroperitoneal lymphadenectomy. J Urol 1971;105:528.
20. Leiter E, Brendler H: Loss of ejaculation following bilateral retroperitoneal lymphadenectomy. J Urol 1967;98:375.
21. Hartmann JT, et al: Long-term effects on sexual function and fertility after treatment of testicular cancer. Br J Cancer 1999;80:801.
22. Donohue JP, et al: Nerve-sparing retroperitoneal lymphadenectomy with preservation of ejaculation. J Urol 1990;144:287, discussion 291.
23. Jacobsen KD, et al: Ejaculation in testicular cancer patients after post-chemotherapy retroperitoneal lymph node dissection. Br J Cancer 1999;80:249.
24. Williams NS, Johnston D: The quality of life after rectal excision for low rectal cancer. Br J Surg 1983;70:460.
25. Maurer CA, et al: Total mesorectal excision preserves male genital function compared with conventional rectal cancer surgery. Br J Surg 2001;88:1501.
26. Maas CP, et al: Radical and nerve-preserving surgery for rectal cancer in The Netherlands: A prospective study on morbidity and functional outcome. Br J Surg 1998;85:92.

27. Leveckis J, et al: Bladder and erectile dysfunction before and after rectal surgery for cancer. Br J Urol 1995;76:752.
28. Masui H, et al: Male sexual function after autonomic nerve-preserving operation for rectal cancer. Dis Colon Rectum 1996;39:1140.
29. Schover LR: Sexuality and body image in younger women with breast cancer. J Natl Cancer Inst Monogr 1994;16:177.
30. Schover LR: Partial mastectomy and breast reconstruction. A comparison of their effects on psychosocial adjustment, body image, and sexuality. Cancer 1995;75:54.
31. Samaan NA, et al: Hypopituitarism after external irradiation. Evidence for both hypothalamic and pituitary origin. Ann Intern Med 1975;83:771.
32. Lam KS, et al: Early effects of cranial irradiation on hypothalamic-pituitary function. J Clin Endocrinol Metab 1987;64:418.
33. Littley MD, et al: Radiation-induced hypopituitarism is dose-dependent. Clin Endocrinol (Oxf) 1989;31:363.
34. Boughton B: Childhood cranial radiotherapy reduces fertility in adulthood. Lancet Oncol 2002;3:330.
35. Mills JL, et al: Menarche in a cohort of 188 long-term survivors of acute lymphoblastic leukemia. J Pediatr 1997;131:598.
36. Brauner R, et al: Leydig-cell function in children after direct testicular irradiation for acute lymphoblastic leukemia. N Engl J Med 1983;309:25.
37. Ash P: The influence of radiation on fertility in man. Br J Radiol 1980;53:271.
38. Berthelsen JG: Sperm counts and serum follicle-stimulating hormone levels before and after radiotherapy and chemotherapy in men with testicular germ cell cancer. Fertil Steril 1984;41:281.
39. Hahn EW, et al: Recovery from aspermia induced by low-dose radiation in seminoma patients. Cancer 1982;50:337.
40. Madsen BL, Giudice L, Donaldson SS: Radiation-induced premature menopause: A misconception. Int J Radiat Oncol Biol Phys 1995;32:1461.
41. Lushbaugh CC, Casarett GW: The effects of gonadal irradiation in clinical radiation therapy: A review. Cancer 1976;37:1111.
42. Goldman S, Johnson FL: Effects of chemotherapy and irradiation on the gonads. Endocrinol Metab Clin North Am 1993;22:617.
43. Zelefsky MJ, Eid JF: Elucidating the etiology of erectile dysfunction after definitive therapy for prostatic cancer. Int J Radiat Oncol Biol Phys 1998;40:129.
44. Siegel T, et al: The development of erectile dysfunction in men treated for prostate cancer. J Urol 2001;165:430.
45. Turner SL, et al: Sexual dysfunction after radical radiation therapy for prostate cancer: A prospective evaluation. Urology 1999;54:124.
46. al-Abany M, et al: Improving the preservation of erectile function after external beam radiation therapy for prostate cancer. Radiother Oncol 2000;57:201.
47. Mantz CA, et al: Potency preservation following conformal radiotherapy for localized prostate cancer: Impact of neoadjuvant androgen blockade, treatment technique, and patient-related factors. Cancer J Sci Am 1999;5:230.
48. Potters L, et al: Potency after permanent prostate brachytherapy for localized prostate cancer. Int J Radiat Oncol Biol Phys 2001;50:1235.
49. Merrick GS, et al: Erectile function after permanent prostate brachytherapy. Int J Radiat Oncol Biol Phys 2002;52:893.
50. Li FP, et al: Outcome of pregnancy in survivors of Wilms' tumor. JAMA 1987;257:216.
51. Mulvihill JJ, et al: Pregnancy outcome in cancer patients. Experience in a large cooperative group. Cancer 1987;60:1143.
52. Marumo K, Baba S: Erectile function and nocturnal penile tumescence in patients with prostate cancer undergoing luteinizing hormone-releasing hormone agonist therapy. Int J Urol 1999;6:19.
53. Smith JA Jr, Urry RL: Testicular histology after prolonged treatment with a gonadotropin-releasing hormone analogue. J Urol 1985;133:612.
54. Berglund G, et al: Effect of endocrine treatment on sexuality in premenopausal breast cancer patients: A prospective randomized study. J Clin Oncol 2001;19:2788.
55. Tomera K, et al: The gonadotropin-releasing hormone antagonist abarelix depot versus luteinizing hormone releasing hormone agonists leuprolide or goserelin: Initial results of endocrinological and biochemical efficacies in patients with prostate cancer. J Urol 2001;165:1585.
56. Trachtenberg J, et al: A phase 3, multicenter, open label, randomized study of abarelix versus leuprolide plus daily antiandrogen in men with prostate cancer. J Urol 2002;167:1670.
57. Migliari R, et al: Short-term effects of flutamide administration on hypothalamic-pituitary-testicular axis in man. J Urol 1988;139:637.
58. Crawford ED, et al: A controlled trial of leuprolide with and without flutamide in prostatic carcinoma. N Engl J Med 1989;321:419.
59. Boccardo F, et al: Bicalutamide monotherapy versus flutamide plus goserelin in prostate cancer patients: Results of an Italian Prostate Cancer Project study. J Clin Oncol 1999;17:2027.
60. Schroder FH, et al: Prostate cancer treated by anti-androgens: Is sexual function preserved? EORTC Genitourinary Group. European Organization for Research and Treatment of Cancer. Br J Cancer 2000;82:283.
61. Osborne CK: Tamoxifen in the treatment of breast cancer. N Engl J Med 1998;339:1609.
62. Mortimer JE, et al: Effect of tamoxifen on sexual functioning in patients with breast cancer. J Clin Oncol 1999;17:1488.
63. Kitahara S, et al: Stronger suppression of serum testosterone and FSH levels by a synthetic estrogen than by castration or an LH-RH agonist. Endocr J 1997;44:527.
64. Pommier RF, Woltering EA, Fletcher WS: Changes in serum sex steroid levels during megestrol acetate therapy. Surg Oncol 1994;3:351.
65. Lundgren S, Helle SI, Lonning PE: Profound suppression of plasma estrogens by megestrol acetate in postmenopausal breast cancer patients. Clin Cancer Res 1996;2:1515.
66. Weisberg J, et al: Megestrol acetate stimulates weight gain and ventilation in underweight COPD patients. Chest 2002;121:1070.
67. Jatoi A, et al: Dronabinol versus megestrol acetate versus combination therapy for cancer-associated anorexia: A North Central Cancer Treatment Group study. J Clin Oncol 2002;20:567.
68. Richter P, et al: Effect of chlorambucil on spermatogenesis in the human with malignant lymphoma. Cancer 1970;25:1026.
69. Fairley KF, Barrie JU, Johnson W: Sterility and testicular atrophy related to cyclophosphamide therapy. Lancet 1972;1:568.
70. Shamberger RC, et al: Effects of high-dose methotrexate and vincristine on ovarian and testicular functions in patients undergoing postoperative adjuvant treatment of osteosarcoma. Cancer Treat Rep 1981;65:739.
71. Meistrich ML, et al: Recovery of sperm production after chemotherapy for osteosarcoma. Cancer 1989;63:2115.
72. Stuart NS, et al: Long-term toxicity of chemotherapy for testicular cancer—the cost of cure. Br J Cancer 1990;61:479.
73. Sherins RJ, DeVita V: Effects of drug treatment for lymphoma on male reproductive capacity. Ann Intern Med 1973;79:216.
74. Bokemeyer C, et al: Long-term gonadal toxicity after therapy for Hodgkin's and non-Hodgkin's lymphoma. Ann Hematol 1994;68:105.
75. Chapman RM, et al: Cyclical combination chemotherapy and gonadal function. Retrospective study in males. Lancet 1979;1:285.
76. Santoro A, et al: Long-term results of combined chemotherapy-radiotherapy approach in Hodgkin's disease: Superiority of ABVD plus radiotherapy versus MOPP plus radiotherapy. J Clin Oncol 1987;5:27.
77. da Cunha MF, et al: Recovery of spermatogenesis after treatment for Hodgkin's disease: Limiting dose of MOPP chemotherapy. J Clin Oncol 1984;2:571.
78. Fossa SD, et al: Semen quality after treatment for testicular cancer. Eur Urol 1993;23:172.
79. Hansen PV, et al: Testicular function in patients with testicular cancer treated with orchiectomy alone or orchiectomy plus cisplatin-based chemotherapy. J Natl Cancer Inst 1989;81:1246.
80. Sobrinho LG, Levine RA, DeConti RC: Amenorrhea in patients with Hodgkin's disease treated with antineoplastic agents. Am J Obstet Gynecol 1971;109:135.
81. Miller JJ III, Williams GF, Leissring JC: Multiple late complications of therapy with cyclophosphamide, including ovarian destruction. Am J Med 1971;50:530.

82. Uldall PR, Kerr DN, Tacchi D: Sterility and cyclophosphamide. Lancet 1972;1:693.

83. Warne GL, et al: Cyclophosphamide-induced ovarian failure. N Engl J Med 1973;288:1159.

84. Schilsky RL, et al: Gonadal dysfunction in patients receiving chemotherapy for cancer. Ann Intern Med 1980;93:109.

85. Mehta RR, Beattie CW, Das Gupta TK: Endocrine profile in breast cancer patients receiving chemotherapy. Breast Cancer Res Treat 1992;20:125.

86. Koyama H, et al: Cyclophosphamide-induced ovarian failure and its therapeutic significance in patients with breast cancer. Cancer 1977;39:1403.

87. Fisher B, et al: 1-Phenylalanine mustard (L-PAM) in the management of premenopausal patients with primary breast cancer: Lack of association of disease-free survival with depression of ovarian function. National Surgical Adjuvant Project for Breast and Bowel Cancers. Cancer 1979;44:847.

88. Hortobagyi GN, et al: Immediate and long-term toxicity of adjuvant chemotherapy regimens containing doxorubicin in trials at M.D. Anderson Hospital and Tumor Institute. NCI Monogr 1986;1:105.

89. Schilsky RL, et al: Long-term follow up of ovarian function in women treated with MOPP chemotherapy for Hodgkin's disease. Am J Med 1981;7:552.

90. Muller U, Stahel RA: Gonadal function after MACOP-B or VACOP-B with or without dose intensification and ABMT in young patients with aggressive non-Hodgkin's lymphoma. Ann Oncol 1993;4:399.

91. Longhi A, et al: Reproductive functions in female patients treated with adjuvant and neoadjuvant chemotherapy for localized osteosarcoma of the extremity. Cancer 2000;89:1961.

92. Reyno L, Levine M, Skingley P: Chemotherapy induced amenorrhea in a randomized trial of adjuvant chemotherapy duration in breast cancer (abstract). Eur J Cancer 1993;21:29A.

93. Etteldorf JN, et al: Gonadal function, testicular histology, and meiosis following cyclophosphamide therapy in patients with nephrotic syndrome. J Pediatr 1976;88:206.

94. Kenney LB, et al: High risk of infertility and long term gonadal damage in males treated with high dose cyclophosphamide for sarcoma during childhood. Cancer 2001;9:613.

95. Aubier F, et al: Male gonadal function after chemotherapy for solid tumors in childhood. J Clin Oncol 1989;7:304.

96. Sherins RJ, Olweny CL, Ziegler JL: Gynecomastia and gonadal dysfunction in adolescent boys treated with combination chemotherapy for Hodgkin's disease. N Engl J Med 1978;1299:12.

97. Ortin T, Shostak C, Donaldson S: Gonadal status and reproductive function following treatment for Hodgkin's disease in childhood: The Stanford experience. Int J Radiat Oncol Biol Phys 1990;19:873.

98. Green D, Brecher M, Lindsay A: Gonadal function in pediatric patients following treatment for Hodgkin's disease. Med Pediatr Oncol 1981;9:235.

99. Siris ES, Leventhal BG, Vaitukaitis JL: Effects of childhood leukemia and chemotherapy on puberty and reproductive function in girls. N Engl J Med 1976;294:1143.

100. Byrne J, et al: Effects of treatment on fertility in long-term survivors of childhood or adolescent cancer. N Engl J Med 1987;317:1315.

101. Byrne J, et al: Early menopause in long-term survivors of cancer during adolescence. Am J Obstet Gynecol 1992;166:788.

102. Sanders J, Buckner C, Amos D: Ovarian function following marrow transplantation for aplastic anemia or leukemia. J Clin Oncol 1988;6:813.

103. Brice P, et al: Pregnancies after high-dose chemotherapy and autologous stem cell transplantation in aggressive lymphomas. Blood 2002;100:736.

104. Grigg A, McLachlan R, Zajac J: Reproductive status in long-term bone marrow transplant survivors receiving busulfan-cyclophosphamide (120mg/kg). Bone Marrow Transplant 2000;26:1089.

105. Schubert MA, et al: Gynecological abnormalities following allogeneic bone marrow transplantation. Bone Marrow Transplant 1990;5:425.

106. Chatterjee R, et al: Cavernosal arterial insufficiency is a major component of erectile dysfunction in some recipients of high-dose chemotherapy/chemo-radiotherapy for hematological malignancies. Bone Marrow Transplant 2000;25:1185.

107. Chatterjee R, et al: Management of erectile dysfunction by combination therapy with testosterone and sildenafil in recipients of high-dose therapy for hematological malignancies. Bone Marrow Transplant 2002;29:607.

108. Sarafoglou K, Boulad F, Gillio A: Gonadal function after bone marrow transplantation for acute leukemia during childhood. J Pediatr 1997;130:210.

109. Bath LE, et al: Ovarian and uterine characteristics after total body irradiation in childhood and adolescence: Response to sex steroid replacement. Br J Obstet Gynaecol 1999;106:1265.

110. Leung W, et al: Late effects of treatment in survivors of childhood acute myeloid leukemia. J Clin Oncol 2000;18:3273.

111. Potter JF, Schoeneman M: Metastasis of maternal cancer to the placenta and fetus. Cancer 1970;25:380.

112. Buekers TE, Lallas TA: Chemotherapy in pregnancy. Obstet Gynecol Clin North Am 1998;25:323.

113. Gilliland J, Weinstein L: The effects of cancer chemotherapeutic agents on the developing fetus. Obstet Gynecol Surv 1983;38:6.

114. Sorosky JI, Sood AK, Buekers TE: The use of chemotherapeutic agents during pregnancy. Obstet Gynecol Clin North Am 1997;24:591.

115. Aviles A, et al: Growth and development of children of mothers treated with chemotherapy during pregnancy: Current status of 43 children. Am J Hematol 1991;36:243.

116. Berry DL, et al: Management of breast cancer during pregnancy using a standardized protocol. J Clin Oncol 1999;17:855.

117. Greenlund LJ, Letendre L, Tefferi A: Acute leukemia during pregnancy: A single institutional experience with 17 cases. Leuk Lymphoma 2001;41:571.

118. Wiebe VJ, Sipila PE: Pharmacology of antineoplastic agents in pregnancy. Crit Rev Oncol Hematol 1994;16:75.

119. Enns G, Roeder E, Chan R: Apparent cyclophosphamide (Cytoxan) embryopathy: A distinct phenotype? Am J Med Genet 1999;86:237.

120. Shotton D, Monie I: Possible teratogenic effect of chlorambucil in a human fetus. JAMA 1963;186:745.

121. Steege J, Caldwell D: Renal agenesis after first trimester exposure to chlorambucil. South Med J 1980;73:1414.

122. Lee R, Johnson C, Hanlon D: Leukemia during pregnancy. Am J Obstet Gynecol 1962;84:455.

123. Diamond I, Anderson M, McCreadie S: Transplacental transmission of busulfan in a mother with leukemia: Production of fetal malformation and cytomegaly. Pediatrics 1960;25:85.

124. Milunsky A, Graef JW, Gaynor MF Jr: Methotrexate-induced congenital malformations. J Pediatr 1968;72:790.

125. Bawle EV, Conard JV, Weiss L: Adult and two children with fetal methotrexate syndrome. Teratology 1998;57:51.

126. Stephens JD, et al: Multiple congenital anomalies in a fetus exposed to 5-fluorouracil during the first trimester. Am J Obstet Gynecol 1980;137:747.

127. Wagner VM, et al: Congenital abnormalities in baby born to cytarabine treated mother. Lancet 1980;2:98.

128. Schafer AI: Teratogenic effects of antileukemic chemotherapy. Arch Intern Med 1981;141:514.

129. Caligiuri MA, Mayer RJ: Pregnancy and leukemia. Semin Oncol 1989;16:388.

130. Murray CL, et al: Multimodal cancer therapy for breast cancer in the first trimester of pregnancy. A case report. JAMA 1984;252:2607.

131. Schapira DV, Chudley AE: Successful pregnancy following continuous treatment with combination chemotherapy before conception and throughout pregnancy. Cancer 1984;54:800.

132. Tomlinson MW, Treadwell MC, Deppe G: Platinum based chemotherapy to treat recurrent Sertoli-Leydig cell ovarian carcinoma during pregnancy. Eur J Gynaecol Oncol 1997;18:44.

133. Sood AK, Shahin MS, Sorosky JI: Paclitaxel and platinum chemotherapy for ovarian carcinoma during pregnancy. Gynecol Oncol 2001;83:599.

134. De Santis M, et al: Metastatic breast cancer in pregnancy: First case of chemotherapy with docetaxel. Eur J Cancer Care (Engl) 2000;9:235.

135. Murray NA, et al: Fetal marrow suppression after maternal chemotherapy for leukemia. Arch Dis Child Fetal Neonatal Ed 1994;7:F209.

136. Doll DC, Ringenberg QS, Yarbro JW: Antineoplastic agents and pregnancy. Semin Oncol 1989;16:337.

137. Aviles A, Neri N: Hematological malignancies and pregnancy: A final report of 84 children who received chemotherapy in utero. Clin Lymphoma 2001;2:173.

138. Herold M, Sabine S, Bittrich H: Efficacy and safety of combined rituximab chemotherapy during pregnancy. J Clin Oncol 2001;19:3439.

139. Mubarak A, Kalil R, Awidi A: Normal outcome of pregnancy in chronic myeloid leukemia treated with interferon-alpha in 1st trimester: Report of 3 cases and review of the literature. Am J Hematol 2002;69:115.

140. Trotter J, Zygmunt A: Conception and pregnancy during interferon-alpha therapy for chronic hepatitis C. J Clin Gastroenterol 2001;32:76.

141. Hiratsuka M, Minakami H, Koshizuka S: Administration of interferon-alpha during pregnancy: Effects on fetus. J Perinatal Med 2000;28:372.

142. Dekaban AS: Abnormalities in children exposed to x-radiation during various stages of gestation: Tentative timetable of radiation injury to the human fetus. I. J Nucl Med 1968;9:471.

143. Greskovich JF Jr, Macklis RM: Radiation therapy in pregnancy: Risk calculation and risk minimization. Semin Oncol 2000;27:633.

144. Otake M, Schull WJ: Radiation-related small head sizes among prenatally exposed A-bomb survivors. Int J Radiat Biol 1993;63:255.

145. Schally AV, et al: Protective effects of analogs of luteinizing hormone-releasing hormone against x-radiation-induced testicular damage in rats. Proc Natl Acad Sci USA 1987;84:851.

146. Ward JA, et al: Protection of spermatogenesis in rats from the cytotoxic procarbazine by the depot formulation of Zoladex, a gonadotropin-releasing hormone agonist. Cancer Res 1990;50:568.

147. Kreuser ED, et al: Reproductive toxicity with and without LHRHA administration during adjuvant chemotherapy in patients with germ cell tumors. Horm Metab Res 1990;22:494.

148. Waxman JR, Ahmed R, Smith D: Failure to preserve fertility in patients with Hodgkin's disease. Cancer Chemother Pharmacol 1987;19:159.

149. Krause W, Pfluger K: Treatment with the gonadotropin-releasing hormone agonist buserelin to protect spermatogenesis against cytotoxic treatment in young men. Andrologia 1989;21:265.

150. Chapman RN, Sutcliffe SB: Protection of ovarian function by oral contraceptives in women receiving chemotherapy for Hodgkin's disease. Blood 1981;58:849.

151. Whitehead E, Shalet S, Blackledge G: The effect of combination chemotherapy on ovarian function in women treated for Hodgkin's disease. Cancer 1993;52:988.

152. Blumenfeld Z, et al: Prevention of irreversible chemotherapy-induced ovarian damage in young women with lymphoma by a gonadotrophin-releasing hormone agonist in parallel to chemotherapy. Hum Reprod 1996;1:1620.

153. Blumenfeld Z, Haim N: Prevention of gonadal damage during cytotoxic therapy. Ann Med 1997;29:199.

154. Gabriel D, Bernard S, Croom R: Oopheropexy and the management of Hodgkin's disease. Arch Surg 1986;121:183.

155. Burris AS, et al: A long-term, prospective study of the physiologic and behavioral effects of hormone replacement in untreated hypogonadal men. J Androl 1992;13:297.

156. Harlap S: The benefits and risks of hormone replacement therapy: An epidemiologic overview. Am J Obstet Gynecol 1992;166:1986.

157. Merrick G, Butler W, Lief J: Efficacy of sildenafil citrate in prostate brachytherapy patients with erectile dysfunction. Urology 1999;53:1112.

158. Kedia S, Zippe C, Agarwal A: Treatment of erectile dysfunction with sildenafil citrate (Viagra) after radiation therapy for prostate cancer. Urology 1999;54:308.

159. Valicenti R, Choi E, Chen C: Sildenafil citrate effectively reverses sexual dysfunction induced by three-dimensional conformal radiation therapy. Urology 2001;57:769.

160. Incrocci L, Koper P, Hop W: Sildenafil citrate (Viagra) and erectile dysfunction following external beam radiotherapy for prostate cancer: A randomized, double blind, placebo-controlled, cross-over study. Int J Radiat Oncol Biol Phys 2001;51:1190.

161. Hatzichristou DG: Sildenafil citrate: Lessons learned from 3 years of clinical experience. Int J Impot Res 2002;14(suppl 1):S43.

162. Dewire DM, Todd E, Meyers P: Patient satisfaction with current impotence therapy. Wis Med J 1995;94:542.

163. Schover LR, et al: Knowledge and experience regarding cancer, infertility, and sperm banking in younger male survivors. J Clin Oncol 2002;20:1880.

164. Ohl DA, Sonksen J: What are the chances of infertility and should sperm be banked? Semin Urol Oncol 1996;14:36.

165. Schrader M, et al: Testicular sperm extraction in azoospermic patients with gonadal germ cell tumors prior to chemotherapy—a new therapy option. Asian J Androl 2002;4:9.

166. Chan PT, et al: Testicular sperm extraction combined with intracytoplasmic sperm injection in the treatment of men with persistent azoospermia postchemotherapy. Cancer 2001;92:1632.

167. Okada H, Dobashi M, Yamazaki T: Conventional versus microdissection testicular sperm extraction for nonobstructive azoospermia. J Urol 2002;168:1063.

168. Blackhall FH, et al: Semen cryopreservation, utilisation and reproductive outcome in men treated for Hodgkin's disease. Br J Cancer 2002;87:381.

169. Ohl DA, et al: Electroejaculation following retroperitoneal lymphadenectomy. J Urol 1991;145:980.

170. Silva PD, et al: Successful treatment of retrograde ejaculation with sperm recovered from bladder washings. A report of two cases. J Reprod Med 2000;45:957.

171. Oktay K: Ovarian tissue cryopreservation and transplantation: Preliminary findings and implications for cancer patients. Hum Reprod Update 2001;7:526.

172. Giacalone PL, et al: Successful in vitro fertilization-surrogate pregnancy in a patient with ovarian transposition who had undergone chemotherapy and pelvic irradiation. Fertil Steril 2001;76:388.

Problems Common to Cancer and Its Therapy

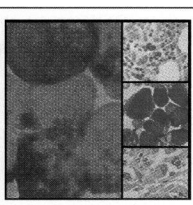

65

ENDOCRINE COMPLICATIONS

Tracey O'Connor
Donald L. Trump

SUMMARY OF KEY POINTS

- Endocrine dysfunction results from cancer therapy and is sometimes the goal of therapy.
  - Surgery, irradiation, and medical or hormonal therapy may be used to treat tumors arising in endocrine organs or to reduce hormone secretion for palliation of hormone-sensitive tumors.
- Endocrine dysfunction may occur as an unintended consequence of antineoplastic therapy.
  - Hypopituitarism may result from surgery or irradiation and is associated with clinically significant deficiencies of growth hormone, thyrotropin, gonadotropin, and corticotropin.
  - Thyroid dysfunction is related to neck irradiation, total body irradiation, and immune therapy.
  - Gonadal dysfunction from surgery, radiotherapy, or chemotherapy results in disruption of puberty, infertility, and premature menopause.
  - Adrenal dysfunction from medical therapy or chemotherapy (ketoconazole, aminoglutethimide)

may result in glucocorticoid or mineralocorticoid deficiency.
- Chemotherapy can cause pancreatitis (L-asparaginase) and occasionally pancreatic exocrine or endocrine deficiencies.

DIAGNOSTIC CONSIDERATIONS
- Many symptoms associated with cancer or cancer therapy may be confused with those associated with pituitary, adrenal, thyroid, or gonadal dysfunction.
- The occurrence of growth deficiency, delayed or precocious puberty, fatigue, weight loss or gain, hair loss, amenorrhea, orthostatic hypotension, hyperpigmentation, or electrolyte abnormalities must raise consideration of an endocrine deficiency resulting from a primary tumor or therapy.

EVALUATION
Pituitary
- Hypopituitarism is related to hypothalamic or pituitary dysfunction, and patients often have more than one deficiency.
- Basal serum hormone

measurements can confirm pituitary insufficiency; dynamic tests may be required if results are equivocal or in the case of partial deficiency.
Thyroid
- Evaluation of thyroid function includes serum assays of the free thyroxine level and thyroid-stimulating hormone (TSH).
- Primary hypothyroidism is characterized by low thyroxine and elevated TSH levels.
- Central hypothyroidism is characterized by low thyroxine levels and inappropriately normal or low TSH levels.
Adrenals
- Adrenal function may be assessed by early morning cortisol concentration.
- The corticotropin stimulation test (250 mg intravenously of cosyntropin, with serum cortisol measured at 30 and 60 minutes) is the most commonly used test for the diagnosis of primary adrenal insufficiency.

INTRODUCTION

Cancer therapy may disrupt the usual function of endocrine organs intentionally or as an unavoidable side effect of therapy. This disruption will affect the patient whether the dysfunction is therapeutic (suppressing gonadal function as a means of treating breast[1] or prostate cancers[2]) or an unintended effect (osteoporosis as a result of premature menopause).[3] This chapter discusses the disruption of endocrine function by surgery, chemotherapy, and radiotherapy. The proper evaluation of endocrine function also is reviewed.

DIRECT EFFECTS OF CANCER THERAPY ON THE ENDOCRINE SYSTEM

Surgical Therapy

The anterior pituitary gland secretes a number of vital hormones that control multiple metabolic functions [growth hormone (GH), thyroid-stimulating hormone (TSH), follicle-stimulating hormone (FSH), luteinizing hormone (LH), adrenocorticotropin, prolactin]. Secretion of these substances from the anterior pituitary is controlled through hypothalamic factors that reach the anterior pituitary through the hypothalamic-hypophyseal portal vessels. Secretion of the two posterior pituitary hormones [antidiuretic hormone (ADH) and oxytocin] is controlled by nerve fibers that originate in the hypothalamus and terminate in the posterior pituitary. The two hormones associated with the posterior pituitary are synthesized by neurons within the hypothalamus and transported to the posterior pituitary for storage and later release into the peripheral circulation.

Normal pituitary function may be altered by surgical resection of pituitary tumors, or from disruption of the hypothalamic-pituitary axis (HPA). Surgical resection of pituitary tumors may result in deficiencies in anterior pituitary hormones. Posterior pituitary hormone deficiency does not generally result from surgery if the hypothalamus remains intact.

Deficiencies also may result from resection of primary tumors involving the thyroid (hypothyroidism), pancreas (diabetes mellitus), ovaries (estrogen deficiency), or testes (testosterone). Rarely, bilateral adrenalectomy, which results in glucocorticoid and mineralocorticoid deficiencies, may be indicated for the treatment of bilateral primary adrenal tumors.

Permanent disruption of parathyroid function as a result of surgery is rarely a goal of surgical intervention. Hypoparathyroidism may result from attempted subtotal removal of parathyroid glands as a therapy for parathyroid hyperplasia, but is rarely permanent. More commonly, removal of all parathyroid glands occurs at the time of extensive neck surgery for advanced head and neck tumors, or as part of a total thyroidectomy. It is often possible to transplant parathyroid tissue to other parts of the body to maintain parathyroid hormone secretion. However, permanent hypoparathyroidism can follow thyroidectomy; the reported incidence is up to 40%,[4] and such an occurrence will require life-long calcium and vitamin D supplementation.

Historically, surgery has been used as a means of disrupting normal endocrine function with therapeutic intent.[5] Response rates of 15% to 30% were reported after hypophysectomy or adrenalectomy in advanced breast cancer.[6,7] However, these procedures resulted in significant morbidity, including hypoadrenalism and hypopituitarism, requiring life-long replacement therapy. These procedures have been replaced by pharmacologic means of suppressing pituitary secretion of gonadotropins [luteinizing hormone–releasing hormone (LHRH) agonists or antagonists] and adrenal steroidogenesis (aromatase inhibitors).[8] For premenopausal patients, ovarian ablation by surgical oophorectomy remains a therapeutic option in the metastatic and adjuvant settings. Currently, however, most trials investigating the role of ovarian ablation in breast cancer therapy use LHRH agonists to achieve functional castration.[9] Orchiectomy reduces the level of circulating androgens in men by approximately 95%, and this procedure remains a therapy option alone or in conjunction with antiandrogens (so-called combined androgen blockade or total androgen deprivation) for men with metastatic prostate cancer.[10] It is important to note, however, that a large randomized trial comparing bilateral orchiectomy with or without flutamide for metastatic prostate cancer was unable to demonstrate a survival benefit in the combined androgen-blockade group.[11] Androgen suppression is increasingly being used as part of multimodality therapy (with irradiation) for localized prostate cancer and as an adjuvant after potentially curative irradiation or prostatectomy.

Radiation Therapy

Endocrine organs may be intentionally, or unavoidably, exposed to ionizing radiation during treatment for malignancy, with resulting dysfunction. Endocrine abnormalities also may result from hypothalamic-pituitary dysfunction after radiation therapy for central nervous system tumors. A consideration of the complications of gonadal radiation may be found in Chapter 64, which discusses reproductive complications. Other specific sites are discussed subsequently.

Hypothalamic-Pituitary Axis

Anterior pituitary dysfunction may result when external radiation is directed at the HPA during the course of treatment for hormone-secreting or nonfunctioning pituitary adenomas and craniopharyngiomas. Hypopituitarism also is possible in patients who receive radiation therapy for nasopharyngeal, extracranial, or primary brain tumors.[12] Two years after cranial radiation for nasopharyngeal carcinoma, 19% of patients demonstrated a deficiency in one or more anterior pituitary hormones.[13] Total-body irradiation (TBI) delivered as part of a bone marrow transplant preparative regimen[14] and prophylactic cranial radiation also may cause hypopituitarism.[15]

A number of observations indicate that the hypothalamus is more radiosensitive than the anterior pituitary and that growth hormone (GH) deficiency is an early feature of radiation-induced damage to the HPA. Pulsatile GH secretion is controlled by growth hormone–releasing hormone (GHRH) and somatostatin,[16] which are produced by the hypothalamus. It appears that the hypothalamic damage related to radiation is a result of direct injury to hypothalamic neurons rather than to vascular structures.[17]

The incidence of anterior pituitary hormone deficiency is related to total radiation dose and the number of fractions with which the dose is delivered. The total dose of radiation delivered to the hypothalamic-pituitary region is the major determinant of the speed of onset as well as the incidence and severity of anterior pituitary deficiencies. The greater the dose, the more likely the patient is to have panhypopituitarism, and the earlier the deficiencies will occur.[12] Prospective studies of pituitary function after radiotherapy indicate that the onset and frequency of pituitary hormone deficiency are variable. In a study of 22 patients treated for pituitary adenoma, conventional pituitary radiation given as a dose of 50 Gy over a 4-week period caused deficiencies in thyrotropin, corticotropin, and gonadotropin in more than 50% of patients at a mean of 4.2 years after treatment.[18] In a larger series of 66 patients treated with external radiation for pituitary tumors, high percentages of deficiencies were reported. GH deficiency (GHD) was reported in

100% of patients at 5 years; 91% demonstrated deficient gonadotropin, and 77%, deficient corticotropin.[19]

As these data suggest, the most common hormonal abnormality after radiation to the HPA is GHD, which may occur as an isolated finding. The clinical ramifications of GHD are most evident in the growing child, with a reduction in growth velocity that may lead to short stature. Although poor linear growth is very common in children with GHD, it is not universal or immediately apparent. Several studies suggest that the slowing of growth may not occur for the first year or two after onset of GHD.[20] Although it is less likely to produce clinical symptoms, GHD in the postpubertal individual may be associated with a relative decrease in muscle mass and increase in adiposity.[21] In a higher proportion of children treated with TBI or cranial radiation, GHD develops, as compared with adults, and they are more likely to require replacement, suggesting that the GH status of children is more vulnerable to irradiation effects.[22] In contrast to the pediatric series, GH secretion does not appear to be affected by TBI administered to adults. Littley and colleagues[23] studied 18 adults 17 to 55 months after treatment with TBI and bone marrow transplantation (BMT) between 17 and 55 months earlier. They reported that all the patients had a normal peak GH response to a GH provocation test.

In addition to GHD, abnormalities in the secretion of gonadotropin, corticotropin, and thyrotropin are reported in patients when the HPA is included in the treatment field. In children treated for acute lymphoblastic leukemia (ALL) with prophylactic cranial irradiation, doses of 18 to 24 Gy have been associated with early puberty in girls. Together with a reduction in GH secretion, the early puberty has been suggested to contribute to the reduced final height in survivors of childhood ALL.[24] Central precocious puberty has been described in 6 of 15 girls and 3 of 14 boys treated with 30 to 55 Gy of external irradiation for brain tumor.[25] Hypogonadotrophic hypogonadism also may develop later.[26] Although GHD and premature sexual development can occur after doses as low as 18 Gy fractionated radiation, deficiencies in thyroid-stimulating hormone (TSH) and adrenocorticotropin are seen primarily in individuals treated with more than 40 Gy HPA radiation. Five years after treatment, a study of 251 patients treated for pituitary disease with external radiotherapy described an incidence of TSH deficiency of 9% at 20 Gy, increasing to 52% at 42 to 45 Gy. A similar relation was described for adrenocorticotropic hormone (ACTH) and gonadotropin deficiency when the 20-Gy group was compared with the 35- to 45-Gy dose range.[27] Hyperprolactinemia can be seen after high-dose radiotherapy (>40 Gy) and has been described in both sexes and all age groups, but is most common in young women.[20] Constine and associates[28] described a 50% frequency of hyperprolactinemia in 32 patients treated with radiation for brain tumor with doses ranging from 39.6 to 70.2 Gy. Other investigators reported rates of 20% after treatment for nasopharyngeal carcinoma.

Hyperprolactinemia can cause pubertal delay or arrest in children, galactorrhea and/or amenorrhea in women, and decreased libido and impotence in adult males.[13] Most neuroendocrine disturbances that result as a consequence of HPA radiation are treatable, and patients at risk require long-term endocrine follow-up.[20]

Thyroid

The thyroid gland is the largest pure endocrine gland in the body and one of the organs most susceptible to clinically significant damage after therapeutic external radiation. Irradiation of the thyroid may produce hypothyroidism, Graves' disease, silent thyroiditis, benign nodules, and thyroid cancers.[29] Thyroid neoplasms, both benign and malignant, are known to occur with increased frequency after neck irradiation, and the incidence is related to the radiation dose and length of follow-up.[30] The association of thyroid cancer and irradiation is discussed in detail in Chapter 74.

Hancock and colleagues[31] described their experience with thyroid disease (hypothyroidism, hyperthyroidism, and thyroid cancer) among patients treated with irradiation and with or without chemotherapy for Hodgkin's disease at the Stanford University Center. Of 1787 patients, 1677 received irradiation to the thyroid. At 26 years of follow-up, the actuarial risk of thyroid disease was 67%. In the majority of patients (47%), hypothyroidism developed. Approximately half of this risk was manifested within 5 years of radiation; however, hypothyroidism developed more than 20 years after exposure in some individuals. The risk of thyroid cancer was 15.6 times the expected risk, and the risk of Graves' disease was 7.2 to 20.4 times that for normal subjects. These data should remind clinicians to observe thyroid function closely in patients who have previously been treated with upper mantle or cervical radiation.

The most frequent complication of neck irradiation is hypothyroidism. In one series of children treated for Hodgkin's disease, the actuarial risk of developing overt or subclinical hypothyroidism was 60% by 11 years, with the median time to development of hypothyroidism, 6 years. Of the 51 patients, 39 had undergone mantle radiation only (median dose, 45 Gy), 11 had received mantle irradiation and chemotherapy (median dose, 31 Gy), and one patient had not received radiation to the mantle region.[32] Many risk factors have been associated with the suppression of thyroid function, the most consistent association being with higher radiation dose.[33] Controversy continues regarding the effect of age at time of irradiation, gender, and association with the prior use of lymphangiograms.[30]

TBI is associated with thyroid dysfunction in adults and children, and the effects may be transient.[34] The incidence appears to be significantly less after fractionated TBI (15% to 16%) than after single-dose TBI (46% to 48%).[22] Whereas TSH elevation is frequent and occurs at a mean of 3.2 years after TBI, clinical hypothyroidism is uncommon.[35]

The development of hyperthyroidism after neck irradiation for Hodgkin's disease has been described by several groups,[29,36] primarily in adult subjects treated with neck irradiation. The clinical picture resembles Graves' disease and is characterized by diffuse thyroid enlargement, suppressed TSH, high levels of thyroid hormone, and development of autoantibodies to the thyroid.[22] The incidence of hyperthyroidism after cervical irradiation is unclear due to the small number of cases reported. Eye changes (exophthalmos) have occasionally been reported after external-beam radiation to the neck, and by inference appear to be related to immune reactions in which antithyroid antibodies crossreact with ocular structures.[37]

Acute radiation thyroiditis has been described rarely after external neck irradiation[38] and is more commonly associated with therapeutic doses of radioiodine for thyroid diseases. Radiation thyroiditis may be associated with fever, pain in the anterior cervical region, and transient exacerbation of hyperthyroidism.

Parathyroid

Several studies suggest that individuals with a history of head and neck irradiation are at risk for developing hyperparathyroidism related to parathyroid adenoma or carcinoma.[39,40] Cohen and coworkers[41] identified a cohort of 4297 patients previously treated with radiation to the tonsils before the age of 16 years. Among the 2923 patients able to be identified, 32 patients reported clinical hyperparathyroidism. This represents a 2.5- to 2.9-fold increase compared with the general population in the same age group. Additionally, 31% of patients in whom hyperparathyroidism developed also had a thyroid cancer, compared with 11% prevalence of thyroid cancer in the treated group that did not exhibit parathyroid dysfunction. Generally, a long latency period between exposure and onset of hyperparathyroidism is observed (> 25 years). These findings support an association between radiation exposure and parathyroid abnormalities. Although some cases of hyperparathyroidism are asymptomatic and do not require surgery, others cause significant morbidity, including nephrolithiasis and metabolic bone disease, and can be disabling. Therefore individuals with a history of head and neck radiation should be monitored with calcium levels periodically (every 1 to 2 years) and indefinitely.[42]

Chemotherapy

Historically, exogenous hormones have been administered to suppress the growth of cancer. The effects of the administration of androgens, estrogens, and high-dose glucocorticoids for the treatment of breast cancer, prostate cancer, and lymphomas are well recognized and are discussed in the chapters specifically designated for the discussion of these diseases. The following discussion is limited to those situations in which systemic use of nonhormonal agents for the therapy of cancer results in disruption of endocrine function. A discussion of the effects of systemic chemotherapy on ovarian and testicular function is found in Chapter 64.

Hypothalamic-Pituitary Axis

The administration of chemotherapeutic agents has been reported to disrupt GH secretion in children in the absence of cranial radiotherapy. Roman and colleagues[43] studied growth and GH secretion in 60 children in complete remission after treatment with chemotherapy and surgery for solid tumors. None received cranial radiotherapy. They observed GHD in 45% of those studied,

and found that these children were more likely to have received high doses of actinomycin D, but could find no correlation with duration of treatment, length of follow-up, tumor type, sex, or age.

Growth retardation during treatment for acute leukemia is partially counteracted by a "catch-up" phase after cessation of maintenance chemotherapy. However, depending on the intensity of chemotherapy, significant height loss can be detected in 40% to 70% of patients at a 6-year follow-up.[44] Chemotherapy can also aggravate the growth failure of children with brain tumors receiving craniospinal radiation.[45]

Pharmacologic induction of the syndrome of inappropriate secretion of antidiuretic hormone (SIADH) either by potentiation of ADH effect or by increased ADH secretion has been attributed to multiple antineoplastic agents. Cyclophosphamide and the vinca alkaloids are most frequently associated. The vinca alkaloids are reported to stimulate the central release of ADH from the neurohypophyseal system,[46] whereas the alkylating agents enhance ADH activity.[47] Regardless of the mechanism, the result is an increase in water reabsorption by the kidney, leading to expansion and dilution of body compartments. Recent case reports also implicate platinum agents,[48] vinorelbine,[49] taxanes,[50] and methotrexate.[51] Clinically significant hyponatremia may occur with the administration of these agents.

Thyroid

Clinically evident thyroid dysfunction is rarely associated with the use of standard systemic chemotherapy agents. However, a growing body of literature is investigating the prevalence of endocrine function after BMT. Although most patients with clinically evident dysfunction are treated with TBI and chemotherapy, there are reports of thyroid dysfunction in nearly 50% of allogeneic BMT recipients treated with chemotherapy (busulfan and cyclophosphamide) alone. This is manifest as low T_3 syndrome [free thyroxine (FT_4) and TSH within, and free triiodothyronine (FT_3) below the respective ranges of normality], chronic thyroiditis, and transient subclinical hyperthyroidism and hypothyroidism.[52] Chemotherapy may potentiate the degree of hypothyroidism seen with radiotherapy. One study of 32 patients treated for medulloblastoma in childhood found that in 18 (56%), hypothyroidism developed at a median time after radiotherapy of 41 months. Hypothyroidism was documented in 10 of 12 (83%) who had 2340 cGy + chemotherapy [vincristine, N-(2-chloroethyl)-N'-cyclohexyl-N-nitrosourea (CCNU), cisplatin, or cyclophosphamide], 6 of 10 (60%) who had 3600 cGy + chemotherapy (vincristine, CCNU, prednisone), and 2 of 10 (20%) treated with 3600 cGy without chemotherapy.[53]

Aminoglutethimide, an inhibitor of cholesterol conversion to pregnenolone, has been reported to cause thyroid dysfunction with long-term use. This effect is due to blockade of the iodination of tyrosine.[54] Figg and associates[55] reported 9 of 29 men treated with aminoglutethimide for metastatic prostate cancer with clinical and biochemical evidence of hypothyroidism, which reversed with levothyroxine.

Immune therapies are well-recognized causes of thyroid dysfunction. Atkins and colleagues[56] were the first to describe an association between therapy with recombinant interleukin-2 (IL-2) and thyroid abnormalities. Thyroid dysfunction, particularly hypothyroidism, has been commonly described in patients receiving IL-2 therapy. Among initially euthyroid patients, 32% had hypothyroidism during and 14% after IL-2 therapy.[57] The proposed mechanism is autoimmune, because elevated levels of antithyroglobulin and antithyroid microsomal antibodies have been identified.[58] The incidence of thyroid dysfunction has been related to the length of therapy with IL-2, increasing with longer treatment duration. The frequency of thyroid dysfunction also has been linked to response rate; however, this observation is biased because patients who respond are more likely to receive IL-2 for a longer duration.[59] The thyroid function of individuals receiving IL-2 therapy should be monitored, and those that manifest biochemical evidence of hypothyroidism should receive thyroid replacement.

5-Fluorouracil and L-asparaginase have been shown to modify circulating thyroid hormone levels. 5-Fluorouracil increases total thyroxine and triiodothyronine levels. The free thyroxine index and TSH levels remain normal as a result either of increased levels of thyroxine-binding globulin or of binding capacity.[60] L-Asparaginase causes transient thyroxine-binding globulin deficiency by diminishing hepatic synthesis and also inhibits TSH secretion by the pituitary gland, resulting in decreased total thyroxine levels and decreased free thyroxine concentrations.[61] Transient hyperthyroidism after L-asparaginase therapy for ALL also has been observed.[62] These thyroid-function abnormalities are not severe, are short-lived, and generally do not require specific therapy.

Thyroid-function test changes have been examined with the use of adjuvant tamoxifen, and the results are conflicting.[63] Some authors have concluded that tamoxifen therapy in the postmenopausal woman causes an increase in thyroid-binding globulin and associated increases in measured thyroxine uptake and T_4; TSH levels remained unchanged.[63] Others report a significant increase in TSH initially, a decrease by 6 months, and no change in T_3 or T_4 concentrations.[64] All women remain eumetabolic and did not require treatment. Although tamoxifen administration can change thyroid hormone concentrations, free thyroid hormone levels remain unchanged, and patients remain euthyroid after long-term tamoxifen therapy.[65]

Adrenal

A method of medically ablating or reducing adrenal function was sought for a number of years as an alternative to surgical resection of the adrenal glands, a procedure used primarily for the treatment of advanced breast cancer. Aminoglutethimide and ketoconazole both suppress adrenal function. These drugs appear to have their effect through their ability to inhibit important cytochrome P-450 isozymes, which are necessary for adrenal steroidogenesis.[66,67] Aminoglutethimide, at doses of 1000 to1500 mg/day, and ketoconazole, at doses of 800 to 1200 mg/day, will produce adrenal insufficiency in 30% to 40% of patients. The antiadrenal effects of ketoconazole

and aminoglutethimide are reversible with treatment discontinuation. Although standard glucocorticoid treatment is generally required in these patients during treatment, mineralocorticoid replacement is usually not required. If aminoglutethimide or ketoconazole is discontinued and steroid compounds are replaced, the adrenal gland generally recovers promptly. Full recovery within 1 to 2 weeks is usual.

Mitotane (o,p′-DDD) is an oral chemotherapy agent most often used to treat adrenal carcinoma. It possesses potent antiadrenal effects.[68] It is used primarily to treat adrenal hyperfunction associated with adrenal carcinomas or ectopic production of corticotropin. It has been reported to result in sustained remission for some patients with metastatic adrenal carcinoma with long-term administration.[69] Although the mechanism of action is incompletely understood, adrenal necrosis and permanent adrenal insufficiency can result, necessitating life-long glucocorticoid administration.

Pancreas

Pancreatic exocrine or endocrine insufficiency attributable to chemotherapy is uncommon. Acute pancreatitis has been described as a complication of L-asparaginase therapy, particularly in children, and can be fulminant and fatal.[70] Although unusual, several cases of diabetes mellitus have been induced during asparaginase therapy.[71] Hyperglycemia is usually transient and responds to intravenous fluids, drug discontinuation, and insulin therapy. The exact mechanism of asparaginase-induced diabetes mellitus is unclear; however, insulin-production interference caused by protein-synthesis inhibition has been proposed.[72]

Streptozotocin is a nitrosurea, used primarily for the treatment of pancreatic endocrine tumors. Preclinical models demonstrate beta-cell necrosis destruction and insulin-dependent diabetes in many species.[73] Mild glucose intolerance has been described in patients receiving this agent; however, specific treatment is rarely required.[74] Because this drug is used infrequently, streptozotocin-associated islet cell dysfunction is an uncommon issue in the practice of oncology.

EVALUATION OF ENDOCRINE DEFICIENCY

As previously discussed, endocrine dysfunction may arise in cancer patients for a number of reasons. These include growth of the primary tumor; the desired effects of curative or palliative treatment with surgery, irradiation, or chemotherapy; or the unavoidable consequence of treatment. Evaluation of specific endocrine deficiencies or abnormalities should be directed by the patient's clinical history and physical examination, as well as knowledge regarding the location of the primary tumor and past and current therapies.

Hypopituitarism may be caused by either hypothalamic or pituitary dysfunction, and patients may have single or multiple hormone deficiencies. When one hormonal deficiency is identified, others must be sought. Although basal serum hormone measurements may be all that is needed to confirm pituitary insufficiency, dynamic tests are used if the results of serum hormone tests are equivocal or to diagnose partial deficiencies. Both the target hormone concentration and the pituitary hormone concentrations should be measured to assess the appropriateness of both values.[75] Assessment of appropriate pituitary hormone secretion may be performed by dynamic testing (GH), by direct measurement of serum concentration (FSH, LH, TSH, prolactin), or by evaluating the hormone production of the target organ (testosterone, estradiol, thyroxine, cortisol).

The diagnosis of GHD is difficult because of the nature of GH release and individual variability. A single measurement of serum GH is rarely useful, because the serum concentration is low most of the day, and growth hormone is secreted in a pulsatile fashion. A stimulatory test is therefore required to assess the somatotrophin reserve.[75] GHD frequently accompanies other pituitary hormone deficiencies. According to the Consensus Guidelines for the Diagnosis and Treatment of Adults with GH deficiency,[76] the insulin hypoglycemia test is the diagnostic test of choice, and the criterion for diagnosing GHD that warrants therapy is peak GH of less than 3 mg/L. The Food and Drug Administration (FDA) has approved GH therapy for adults only if there is evidence of hypothalamic or pituitary disease and a subnormal serum GH response to a stimulation test. The FDA considers that the peak serum GH concentration in response to hypoglycemia or other stimulus should be less than 5 mg/L, if measured by radioimmunoassay, or less than 2.5 mg/L, if measured by immunoradiometric assay.[77] Insulin-induced hypoglycemia is the preferred provocative test. Patients with disease of the pituitary are more likely to have an abnormal response to this test than to levodopa, arginine, glucagons, and clonidine. The insulin hypoglycemia test is contraindicated in the debilitated, in patients with cardiovascular or cerebrovascular disease, and in patients with a history of seizure, abnormal electroencephalogram (EEG), or history of brain surgery.[78] In patients with a contraindication, the combined arginine/ GHRH stimulation test may be used. GHD is diagnosed if the maximum stimulated serum GH concentration is less than 5 µg/mL (polyclonal radioimmunoassay) or less than 2.5 µg/mL (immunochemiluminescent assay).

The diagnosis of GHD in childhood is a complex process requiring clinical and growth assessment, combined with biochemical tests and radiologic evaluation. GHD may be an isolated finding or a component of multiple pituitary hormone deficiency. In a child with clinical criteria for GHD, a peak GH concentration less than 10 mg/L has traditionally been used to support the diagnosis after a provocative GH test. However, the diagnosis must also be based on very short height (more than 2.5 standard deviations below the mean height for normal children of the same age), delayed bone age, poor growth velocity (less than the 25th percentile), and a predicted adult height substantially below the mean parental height. In the absence of a gold standard, it is important that the clinician integrate all available data when making a diagnosis.[77] Great care should be taken in using insulin or

glucagon in a young child, and testing requires close monitoring by an experienced team.[79]

Controversy remains about the optimal biochemical diagnosis of corticotropin deficiency. In moderate to severe corticotropin deficiency, the early morning serum cortisol concentrations are consistently less than 250 nM.[80] Of the several dynamic tests developed to assess HPA function, the most common is the corticotropin stimulation test (250 mg intravenously of corticotropin, with serum cortisol concentration measured at baseline and 30 and 60 minutes). If corticotropin and adrenal secretion are normal, the serum cortisol concentration should increase to 20 mg/dL or higher.[81] In patients with severe corticotropin deficiency, the serum cortisol response will be lower, or absent, as a result of adrenal atrophy. However, some patients with pituitary failure of recent onset in whom there has been insufficient time for adrenal atrophy to occur or some patients with partial deficiency may have a normal serum cortisol level.[75] Additional testing may be required in these individuals.

Thyroid dysfunction is readily evaluated by serum immunoassays for TSH and FT$_4$, which is not affected by variations in protein binding. In central hypothyroidism, low thyroxine levels are accompanied by normal or low TSH levels. In primary hypothyroidism, thyroxine levels are low, and TSH is elevated. In hyperthyroidism, thyroxine levels are elevated, and TSH levels are suppressed.[82]

The best test of gonadotrophin deficiency in a premenopausal woman is the menstrual history, as hypogonadotrophic hypogonadism leads to menstrual disturbances. Low serum estradiol levels in the presence of low or normal concentrations of FSH are the main indications for the diagnosis of hypogonadotrophic hypogonadism.[83] In the male patient, low serum testosterone in combination with low or normal concentrations of FSH are demonstrated. Low testosterone or estradiol levels in association with low or normal gonadotropin levels suggest pituitary or hypothalamic dysfunction; elevated gonadotropin levels suggest primary gonadal failure.

After high-dose radiotherapy to the HPA axis, hyperprolactinemia can occur, primarily in young women. It may be assessed with a random serum measurement. Dynamic testing of the lactotrophin reserve with thyrotropin-releasing hormone is not useful, because it does not differentiate between the different causes of hyperprolactinemia.[75] Presenting symptoms of clinically significant hyperprolactinemia can include amenorrhea, galactorrhea, and infertility.[84]

HORMONE REPLACEMENT THERAPY

Children with proven GHD should be treated with recombinant GH as soon as possible after diagnosis, with the goal being to maximize height attainment before the onset of puberty. Although growth velocity improves significantly after the initiation of GH therapy, children with GHD as a consequence of cranial radiotherapy or TBI/BMT respond less well than children with idiopathic GHD.[85] This suboptimal response may also reflect factors such as radiation-induced skeletal dysplasia and early onset of puberty.[86] The routine follow-up of pediatric patients with GHD is best performed by a pediatric endocrinologist with a pediatrician or other primary care provider on a 3- to 6-month basis. GH is routinely used in the range of 25 to 50 µg/kg/day and should be administered subcutaneously in the evening on a daily basis.[79]

GH also is administered to adults with documented GHD, and reverses many of the associated findings, such as reduced muscle mass and increased fat mass, lower bone density, and higher serum lipid concentrations, as well as decreased vitality, sexual disturbance, and fatigue.[77] However, not all adults with GHD have these symptoms, and the ultimate clinical efficacy of GH replacement in adults remains controversial.

Hyperprolactinemia may result in amenorrhea or infertility in women and infertility and impotence in men. Care must be taken to rule out hypothyroidism as a possible contributing cause, as well as stopping medications that may contribute, if possible. Dopamine agonists such as cabergoline or bromocriptine are frequently prescribed.[87]

Hypothyroidism is treated with thyroid hormone replacement with the goal of normalization of thyroxine levels (5 to 12 mg/dL) and also TSH levels (0.5 to 5.0 mU/L). Treatment with thyroxine replacement is generally recommended for those patients found to have a normal thyroxine level but elevated TSH levels.

Adrenal insufficiency requires glucocorticoid, and at times, mineralocorticoid supplementation. Pituitary or isolated ACTH deficiency is generally not characterized by mineralocorticoid deficiency. No universal agreement exists on appropriate doses, timing, and monitoring of hydrocortisone-replacement therapy. Patients with symptomatic adrenal insufficiency should be treated with hydrocortisone or cortisone in the early morning and afternoon. The usual initial oral dose is 25 mg of hydrocortisone (15 mg in the morning, 10 mg in the evening). This may be decreased over time, with the goal of using the minimal effective dose to prevent weight gain and osteoporosis.[88] Patients with primary adrenal insufficiency require mineralocorticoid replacement with fludrocortisone (0.05 to 2.0 mg orally each day). During periods of minor febrile illness or stress, patients with adrenal insufficiency require double to triple the usual dose of hydrocortisone. Severe illness or surgery warrants treatment with high-dose intravenous hydrocortisone (100 to 150 mg hydrocortisone per day for 2 to 3 days), dependent on the severity of the illness or surgery.[89]

Hormone-replacement therapy (HRT) is indicated in hypogonadotrophic hypogonadism and primary gonadal failure in prepubertal children and in many adult men and women with hypogonadism. Pubertal development in children who have been treated for malignancy should be carefully monitored. As mentioned earlier, precocious puberty may be induced by cranial irradiation, and this may be followed by hypogonadotrophic hypogonadism. Precocious puberty may require treatment with gonadotropin-releasing hormone (GnRH) analogue therapy.[90] At the time of expected puberty, children with hypothalamic or pituitary dysfunction, or isolated ovarian

HORMONE REPLACEMENT THERAPY

Children with proven GHD should receive recombinant growth hormone as soon as possible after diagnosis, with the goal being to maximize height attainment before puberty. GH is routinely used in the range of 25 to 50 µg/kg/day subcutaneously in the evening.

GH therapy in adults is given as replacement for documented GHD. The goal of therapy is to improve muscle and cardiac function, restore normal body composition, improve serum lipids, and positively affect quality of life.

Thyroxine therapy (levothyroxine; usual maintenance dose, 100 to 200 µg/day) is indicated for the treatment of hypothyroidism.

Adrenal insufficiency requires glucocorticoid supplementation. Hydrocortisone may be used with the usual initial oral dose of 15 mg in the morning and 10 mg in the evening. Patients with primary adrenal insufficiency also require mineralocorticoid replacement with oral fludrocortisone, 0.05 to 0.2 µg daily.

Testosterone may be given intramuscularly (200 mg of testosterone enanthate or propionate administered every 2 weeks) or by a transdermal system to maintain secondary sexual characteristics and behavior in androgen-deficient men.

Women with hypogonadotropic hypogonadism require sex-hormone replacement for relief of symptoms and long-term prevention of osteoporosis and premature atherosclerosis. Ovulation can be induced if desired.

HRT in women with a history of breast cancer remains controversial. Nonhormonal treatments to alleviate the symptoms of menopause are indicated. Consideration of estrogen replacement therapy in these patients must include a thorough discussion of the potential risks and benefits, and emphasize the uncertainty of the impact on breast cancer recurrence.

or testicular deficiency as a result of cancer treatment, require the administration of either testosterone or cyclic estrogens and progestins for the normal progression of puberty to occur.

Chemotherapy is well documented to play a role in the induction of premature menopause. The use of HRT in these women to alleviate symptoms and prevent chronic disease remains controversial. The large Women's Health Initiative trial recently stopped the combined estrogen-progestin arm after reporting more harmful than beneficial outcomes in this arm versus placebo, with the therapy group demonstrating increases in the numbers of invasive breast cancers, congestive heart disease (CHD), stroke, and pulmonary embolism that were not offset by the smaller reductions in the numbers of hip fractures and colorectal cancers.[91] A parallel trial of estrogen alone in women who have had hysterectomy is continuing, and the planned end of this trial is March 2005.

Androgen-deprivation therapy with a GnRH agonist is the mainstay of treatment for metastatic prostate cancer. Evidence that early androgen-deprivation therapy improves outcomes has led to the increased use of GnRH agonists in men without distant metastasis.[92] Toxicities of these therapies are now noted to include fatigue, weight gain, osteopenia, gynecomastia, loss of libido, decreased muscle mass, and hot flashes.[93] Once therapy is initiated, many men continue treatment with androgen deprivation for years, and debilitating osteoporosis can result. Bisphosphonates such as pamidronate have demonstrated protection of bone mineral density in the lumbar spine, greater trochanter, and total hip in men receiving leuprolide.[92] In a randomized, placebo-controlled study of men with androgen-independent prostate cancer, zoledronic acid reduced skeletal-related events and pathologic fractures.[94]

HRT has traditionally been withheld from women with a history of breast cancer, although its effect on the risk of breast cancer recurrence in breast cancer survivors remains uncertain.[95] Data on the effect of HRT among breast cancer survivors are limited to nonrandomized studies and qualitative reviews of these studies. A recent meta-analysis of this literature performed by Col and associates[95] failed to demonstrate a significant effect of HRT on breast cancer recurrence, but these findings are based on observational data with a variety of biases. A randomized, prospective trial evaluating this issue has yet to be completed.

A number of nonhormonal interventions may be helpful in addressing the symptoms of menopause and androgen deprivation. Vasomotor symptoms have been demonstrated to have a significant impact on the quality of life of breast cancer patients,[96] and if mild, may respond to behavioral changes in conjunction with vitamin E (800 IU/day).[97] More significant symptoms may respond to therapy with venlafaxine, which decreases hot flashes by about 60%.[98] Low-dose megestrol acetate is frequently prescribed.[99] Gabapentin appears promising in preliminary studies, and further trials of this agent are under way. Vaginal symptoms may be treated with nonhormonal vaginal lubricants. The risks of osteoporosis may be decreased with calcium and vitamin D supplementation and weight-bearing exercise as well as bisphosphonates. The risk of cardiovascular disease may be modified by lifestyle changes including proper diet, exercise, avoidance of smoking, and hypertension and lipid control.

In those patients with a history of breast cancer who have unacceptable menopausal symptoms despite the interventions listed, HRT may be considered, but only after a detailed discussion regarding potential benefits and risks. Until more data are available, women with a history of breast cancer who contemplate taking HRT should understand the uncertain impact of this therapy on recurrence risk.

REFERENCES

1. Conte CC, Menoto T, Rosner D, et al: Therapeutic oophorectomy in metastatic breast cancer. Cancer 1989;64:150.
2. Jackson IM, Matthews MJ, Diver JM, et al: LHRH analogues in the treatment of cancer. Cancer Treat Rev 1989;16:161.
3. Pouilles JM, Tremollieres F, Bonneu M, et al: Influence of early age at menopause on vertebral bone mass. J Bone Miner Res 1994;9:311.
4. Lo CY: Parathyroid autotransplantation during thyroidectomy. ANZ J Surg 2002;72:902.
5. Beatson GT: On the treatment of inoperable cases of carcinoma of the mamma: Suggestions for a new method of treatment. Lancet 1896;2:104, 162.
6. Schwarz M, Tindall GT, Nixon DW: Transsphenoidal hypophysectomy in disseminated breast cancer. South Med J 1981;74:315.
7. Silverstein MJ, Byron RL, Yonemoto RH: Bilateral adrenalectomy for advanced breast cancer. Surgery 1975;77:825.
8. Buzdar A: Endocrine therapy in the treatment of metastatic breast cancer. Semin Oncol 2001;28:291.
9. Dees EC, Davidson NE: Ovarian ablation as adjuvant therapy for breast cancer. Semin Oncol 2001;28:322.
10. Samson DJ, Seidenfeld J, Schmitt B, et al: Systematic review and meta-analysis of monotherapy compared with combined androgen blockade for patients with advanced prostate carcinoma. Cancer 2002;95:361.
11. Eisenberger M, Blumenstein B, Crawford E, et al: Bilateral orchiectomy with or without flutamide for metastatic prostate cancer. N Engl J Med 1998;339:1036.
12. Shalet S: Radiation and pituitary dysfunction. N Engl J Med 1993;328:131.
13. Lam KS, Tse VK, Wang C, et al: 1987;64:418.
14. Mills W, Chatterjee R, McGarrigle HH, et al: Partial hypopituitarism following total body irradiation in adult patients with hematological malignancy. Bone Marrow Transplant 1994;14:471.
15. Hata M, Ogino I, Aida N, et al: Prophylactic cranial irradiation of acute lymphoblastic leukemia in childhood: Outcomes of late effects on pituitary function and growth in long-term survivors. Int J Cancer 2001;96:117.
16. Toogood A, Nass R, Pezzoli S, et al: Preservation of growth hormone pulsatility despite pituitary pathology, surgery, and irradiation. J Clin Endocrinol Metab 1997;82:2215.
17. Chieng PU, Huang TS, Chang CC, et al: Reduced hypothalamic blood flow after radiation treatment of nasopharyngeal cancer: SPECT studies in 34 patients. Am J Neuroradiol 1991;12:1661.
18. Snyder FJ, Fowble BF, Schatz NJ, et al: Hypopituitarism following radiation therapy of pituitary adenomas. Am J Med 1986;81:457–462.
19. Littley MD, Shalet SM, Beardwell CG, et al: Hypopituitarism following external radiotherapy for pituitary tumors in adults. Q J Med 1989;70:145.
20. Sklar CA, Constine LS: Chronic neuroendocrinological sequelae of radiation therapy. Int J Radiat Oncol Biol Phys 1995;31:1113.
21. Salamon F, Cuneo R, Hesp R, et al: The effects of treatment with recombinant human growth hormone on body composition and metabolism in adults with growth hormone deficiency. N Engl J Med 1989;321:1797.
22. Brennan B, Shalet S: Endocrine late effects after bone marrow transplant. Br J Haematol 2002;118:58.
23. Littley M, Shalet S, Morganstern G, et al: Endocrine and reproductive dysfunction following total body irradiation in adults. Q J Med 1991;287:265.
24. Didcock E, Davies HA, Didi M, et al: Pubertal growth in young adult survivors of childhood leukemia. J Clin Oncol 1995;13:2503.
25. Oberfield SE, Chin D, Uli N, et al: Endocrine late effects of childhood cancers. J Pediatr 1997;131:S37.
26. Muller J: Disturbance of pubertal development after cancer treatment. Best Pract Res Clin Endocrinol Metab 2002;16:91.
27. Littley MD, Shalet SM, Beardwell CG, et al: Radiation–induced hypopituitarism is dose-dependent. Clin Endocrinol (Oxf) 1989;31:363.
28. Constine LS, Woolf PD, Cann D, et al: Hypothalamic-pituitary dysfunction after radiation for brain tumors. N Engl J Med 1993;328:87.
29. Hancock SL, McDougall IR: Thyroid abnormalities after therapeutic external radiation. Int J Radiat Oncol Biol Phys 1995;31:1165.
30. Sklar C, Whitton J, Mertens A, et al: Abnormalities of the thyroid in survivors of Hodgkin's disease: Data from the childhood cancer survivor study. J Clin Endocrinol Metab 2000;85:3227.
31. Hancock SL, Cox RS, McDougall IR: Thyroid diseases after treatment of Hodgkin's disease. N Engl J Med 1991;325:599.
32. Bhatia S, Ramsay N, Bantle J: Thyroid abnormalities after therapy for Hodgkin's disease in childhood. Oncologist 1996;1:62.
33. Hancock SL, Cox RS, McDougall IR: Thyroid diseases after treatment of Hodgkin's disease. N Engl J Med 1991;325:599.

34. Katsanis E, Shapiro R, Robison L, et al: Thyroid dysfunction following bone marrow transplantation: Long term follow-up of 80 pediatric patients. Bone Marrow Transplant 1990;5:335.

35. Thomas O, Mahe MA, Campion L, et al: Long-term complications of total body irradiation in adults. Int J Radiat Oncol Biol Phys 2001;49:125.

36. Loeffler JS, Tarbell NJ, Garber JR, et al: The development of Graves' disease following radiation therapy in Hodgkin's disease. Int J Radiat Oncol Biol Phys 1988;14:175.

37. Jacobson DR, Fleming BJ: Graves' disease with ophthalmopathy following radiotherapy for Hodgkin disease. Am J Med Sci 1984;288:217.

38. Nishiyama K, Kozuka T, Higashihara T: Acute radiation thyroiditis. Int J Radiat Oncol Biol Phys 1996;36:1221.

39. Christmas TJ, Chapple CR, Noble JG, et al: Hyperparathyroidism after neck irradiation. Br J Surg 1988;75:873.

40. Ron E, Saftlas AF: Head and neck radiation carcinogenesis: epidemiologic evidence. Otolaryngol Head Neck Surg 1996;115:403.

41. Cohen J, Gierlowski, TC, Schneider AB: A prospective study of hyperparathyroidism in individuals exposed to radiation in childhood. JAMA 1990;264:581.

42. Schneider AB, Gierlowski TC, Shore-Freedman E, et al: Dose-response relationships for radiation-induced hyperparathyroidism. J Clin Endocrinol Metab 1995;80:254.

43. Roman J, Villaizan, CJ, Garcia-Foncillas J, et al: Growth and growth hormone secretion in children with cancer treated with chemotherapy. J Pediatr 1997;131:105.

44. Spoudeas H: Growth and endocrine function after chemotherapy and radiotherapy in childhood. Eur J Cancer 2002;38:1748.

45. Olshan JS, Gubernick J, Packer J, et al: The effects of adjuvant chemotherapy on growth in children with medulloblastoma. Cancer 1992;70:2013.

46. Antony A, Robinson WA, Roy C, et al: Inappropriate antidiuretic hormone secretion after high dose vinblastine. J Urol 1980;123:783.

47. DeFronzo RA, Braine H Clovin M, et al: Water intoxication in man after cyclophosphamide therapy: Time course and relation to drug activation. Ann Intern Med 1973;78:861.

48. Ishii K, Aoki Y, Sasaki M, et al: Syndrome of inappropriate secretion of antidiuretic hormone induced by intraarterial cisplatin chemotherapy. Gynecol Oncol 2002;87:150.

49. Garrett CA, Simpson TA Jr: Syndrome of inappropriate antidiuretic hormone associated with vinorelbine therapy. Ann Pharmacother 1998;32:1306.

50. Langer-Nitsche C, Luck HJ, Heilmann M: Severe syndrome of inappropriate antidiuretic hormone secretion with docetaxel treatment in metastatic breast cancer. Acta Oncol 2000;39:1001.

51. Frahm H, von Hulst, M: Increased secretion of vasopressin and edema formation in high dosage methotrexate therapy. Z Gesamte Int Med 1988;43:411.

52. Tauchmanova L, Selleri C, Rosa GD: High prevalence of endocrine dysfunction in long-term survivors after allogeneic bone marrow transplantation for hematologic diseases. Cancer 2002;95:1076.

53. Paulino AC: Hypothyroidism in children with medulloblastoma: A comparison of 3600 and 2340 cGy craniospinal radiotherapy. Int J Radiat Oncol Biol Phys 2002;53:543.

54. Product Information Cytadren, aminoglutethimide. East Hanover, NJ, Novartis Pharmaceuticals Corporation, 2000.

55. Figg WD, Thibault A, Sartor AO, et al: Hypothyroidism associated with aminoglutethimide in patients with prostate cancer. Arch Intern Med 1994;154:1023.

56. Atkins MG, Mier JW, Parkinson DR: Hypothyroidism after treatment with interleukin-2 and lymphokineactivated killer cells. N Engl J Med 1988;318:1557.

57. Schwartzentruber DJ, White DE, Zweig, MH, et al: Thyroid dysfunction associated with immunotherapy for patients with cancer: Cancer 1991;68:2384.

58. Kruit WJ, Bolhuis RL, Goey SH, et al: Interleukin-2-induced thyroid dysfunction is correlated with treatment duration but not with tumor response. J Clin Oncol 1993;11:921.

59. Phan G, Attia P, Steinberg S: Factors associated with response to high-dose interleukin-2 in patients with metastatic melanoma. J Clin Oncol 2001;19:3477.

60. Shalet SM: Endocrine sequelae of cancer therapy. Eur J Endocrinol 1996;135:135.

61. Garnick MB, Larsen PR: Acute deficiency of thyroxine-binding globulin during L-asparaginase therapy. N Engl J Med 1979;301:252.

62. Fadilah SA, Faridah I, Cheong SK: Transient hypothyroidism following L-asparaginase therapy for acute lymphoblastic leukemia: Med J Malaysia 2000;55:513.

63. Mamby CC, Love RR, Lee KE: Thyroid function test changes with adjuvant tamoxifen therapy in postmenopausal women with breast cancer. J Clin Oncol 1995;13:854.

64. Zidan J, Rubenstein W: Effect of adjuvant tamoxifen therapy on thyroid function in postmenopausal women with breast cancer. Oncology 1999;56:43.

65. Kostoglou-Athanassiou I, Ntalles K, Markopoulous G, et al: Thyroid function in postmenopausal women with breast cancer on tamoxifen. Eur J Gynaecol Oncol 1998;19:150.

66. Santen RJ, Samojlik E, Lipton A: Kinetic, hormonal and clinical studies with aminoglutethimide in breast cancer. Cancer 1977;39:2948.

67. Trump DL, Havlin KH, Messing EM: High dose ketoconazole in advanced hormone-refractory prostate cancer: Endocrinologic and clinical effects. J Clin Oncol 1989;7:1093.

68. Lubitz JA, Freeman L, Ikun R: Mitotane in inoperable adrenal cortical carcinoma. JAMA 1973;223:1109.

69. Ilias I, Alevizaki M, Philippou G, et al: Sustained remission of metastatic adrenal carcinoma during long-term administration of low-dose mitotane. J Endocrinol Invest 2001;24:532.

70. Lamelas RG, Chapchap P, Magalhaes AC, et al: Successful management of a child with asparaginase-induced hemorrhagic pancreatitis. Med Pediatr Oncol 1999;32:316.

71. Jaffe N: Diabetes mellitus secondary to L-asparaginase therapy. J Pediatr 1972;81:1270.

72. Ettinger IJ, Ettinger AG, Avaramis VI, et al: Acute lymphoblastic leukemia: A guide to asparaginase and pegaspargase therapy. BioDrugs 1997;7:30.

73. Yang H, Wright J: Human (beta) cells are exceedingly resistant to streptozocin in vivo. Endocrinology 2002;143:2491.

74. Broder LE, Carter SK: Pancreatic islet cell carcinoma: Results of treatment with streptozocin in 52 patients. Ann Intern Med 1973;79:108.

75. Vance ML: Hypopituitarism. N Engl J Med 1994;330:1651.

76. Anonymous: Consensus guidelines for the diagnosis and treatment of adults with growth hormone deficiency: Summary statement of the Growth Hormone Research Society workshop on adult growth hormone deficiency. J Clin Endocrinol Metab 1998;83:379.

77. Vance ML, Mauras N: Growth hormone therapy in adults and children. N Engl J Med 1999;341:1206.

78. Fitzgerald PA: Endocrinology. In Tierney LN Jr., McPhee SJ, Papadakis, M (eds): Current Medical Diagnoses and Treatment, 42nd ed. New York, McGraw-Hill, 2003, p 1067-1151.

79. GH Research Society: Consensus guidelines for the diagnosis and treatment of growth hormone deficiency in childhood and adolescence: Summary statement of the GH research society. J Clin Endocrinol Metab 2000;85:3990.

80. Lamberts SW, deHerder WW, van der Lely AJ: Pituitary insufficiency. Lancet 1998;352:127.

81. May ME, Carey RM: Rapid adrenocorticotropic hormone test in practice: Retrospective review. Am J Med 1985;79:679.

82. Dayan CM: Interpretation of thyroid function tests. Lancet 2001;357:619.

83. Wood DF, Franks S: Hypogonadism in women. In Grossman A, ed. Clinical Endocrinology. Oxford, Blackwell Scientific, 1998, p 702.

84. Suliman AM, al-Saber F, Hayes F: Hyperprolactinemia: Analysis of presentation, diagnosis, and treatment in the endocrine service of a general hospital. Ir Med J 2000;93:74.

85. Papadimitriou A, Uruena M, Hamill G, et al: Growth hormone treatment of growth failure secondary to total body irradiation and bone marrow transplantation. Arch Dis Child 1991;66:689.

86. Holm K, Nysom K, Rasmussen MH, et al: Growth, growth hormone, and final height after BMT: Possible recovery of irradiation-induced growth hormone insufficiency. Bone Marrow Transplant 1996;18:163.

87. Sabuncu T, Arikan E, Tasan E, et al: Comparison of the effects of cabergoline and bromocriptine on prolactin levels in hyperprolactinemic patients. Intern Med 2001;40:857.

Problems Common to Cancer and Its Therapy

88. Oelkers W: Adrenal insufficiency. N Engl J Med 1996;335:1206.

89. Lamberts SW, Bruining HA, deJong FA: Corticosteroid therapy in severe illness. N Engl J Med 1997;337:1285.

90. Muller J: Disturbance of pubertal development after cancer treatment. Best Pract Res Clin Endocrinol Metab 2002;16:91.

91. Writing Group for the Women's Health Initiative Investigators: Risks and benefits of estrogen plus progestin in health postmenopausal women. JAMA 2002;288:321.

92. Smith M, McGovern F, Zietman A, et al: Pamidronate to prevent bone loss during androgen-deprivation therapy for prostate cancer. N Engl J Med 2001;345:948.

93. Hellerstedt BA, Pienta KJ: The current state of hormonal therapy for prostate cancer. CA Cancer J Clin 2002;52:154.

94. Saad F, Murray R, Venner P, et al: A randomized, placebo-controlled trial of zoledronic acid in patients with hormone-refractory metastatic prostate carcinoma. J Natl Cancer Inst 2002;94:1458.

95. Col N, Hirota LK, Orr RK, et al: Hormone replacement therapy after breast cancer: A systematic review and quantitative assessment of risk. J Clin Oncol 2001;19:2357.

96. Couzi RJ, Helzlsouer KJ, Fetting JH: Prevalence of menopausal symptoms among women with a history of breast cancer and attitudes toward estrogen replacement therapy. J Clin Oncol 1995;13:2737.

97. Shanafelt TD, Bsrton DL, Adjei AA, et al: Pathophysiology and treatment of hot flashes. Mayo Clin Proc 2002;77:1155.

98. Loprinzi CL, Kugler JW, Sloan JA, et al: Venlafaxine in management of hot flashes in survivors of breast cancer: A randomized controlled trial. Lancet 2000;356:2059.

99. Quella SK, Loprinzi CL, Sloan JA, et al: Long term use of megestrol acetate by cancer survivors for the treatment of hot flashes. Cancer 1998;82:1784.

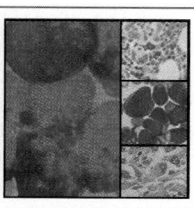

66

SECOND MALIGNANT NEOPLASMS

Daniel M. Green

Giulio J. D'Angio

SUMMARY OF KEY POINTS

EPIDEMIOLOGY

- Pediatric patients who survive their primary cancer are at increased risk of developing a new malignancy.
- Magnitude of this risk is modulated by several factors, including the genetic susceptibility of the patient, the type of surgical procedure employed for removal of the tumor, the use of radiation therapy as part of the treatment plan, the chemotherapeutic agents employed, the severity of immune suppression present at the completion of all treatment, and environmental exposures.
- The potential risk of a second malignant process following treatment of adults should not lead to therapeutic compromises when treatment, often aggressive, is of known benefit.

GENERAL RECOMMENDATIONS

- All former patients should remain under a physician's care indefinitely.
- All former patients should undergo an annual physical examination (preferably by a physician who is familiar with the problem of therapy-induced malignancy).
- Physicians should counsel cancer survivors regarding the potential for the adverse effects of tobacco use, including the potential to interact with the adverse effects of their prior therapy, such as irradiation or oropharynx, esophagus, and/or lungs.

EXPOSURE SPECIFIC RECOMMENDATIONS

- Patients who have been irradiated should have plain radiographs obtained whenever local pain occurs in previously irradiated bone.

- Patients who have received irradiation to volumes that include the breast, uterine cervix, or intestine should undergo routine evaluation with available screening tests, such as mammography, Pap smear, and stool examination for the presence of occult blood.
- Annual mammography should be initiated no later than ten years after breast irradiation.
- Careful physical examination will facilitate the early identification of thyroid nodules and skin cancer.
- All patients treated with an alkylating agent, procarbazine, or a topoisomerase II inhibitor, should have a complete blood count every 6 to 12 months for a minimum of 12 years after diagnosis.
- Presence of macrocytosis and/or cytopenia should prompt evaluation of the bone marrow.

INTRODUCTION

Second malignant neoplasms (SMNs) develop in patients as a result of genetic and iatrogenic factors and their interplay. The therapies employed are different for children and adults because of the differences in the primary cancers encountered. Primary cancers in adults are usually of epithelial origin, unlike the embryonal and sarcomatous neoplasms encountered at earlier ages. In addition, some of the SMNs encountered in adults are the result of therapies they received for nonmalignant conditions treated when they were children. This discussion therefore has been divided into two parts according to the age group being considered (i.e., children and adolescents and adults).

CHILDREN AND ADOLESCENTS

SMNs are a recognized complication of successful treatment of children and adolescents for cancer. The frequency of these had been reported to be 1.9% at 10 years after diagnosis, 5.0% to 12.0% at 25 years after diagnosis,

3.3% to 4.9% at 25 years after diagnosis among 3-year survivors, 3.2% to 12.0% at 20 years after diagnosis among 5-year survivors, and 7.8% at 25 years after diagnosis among five-year survivors.[1-10] These series differed with respect to the time period during which the patients were treated, the completeness of follow-up, and the treatment exposures experienced by the patients. Increasingly, the data suggest that although specific exposures (whether to a particular chemotherapeutic agent or to ionizing radiation) might be linked to the occurrence of a new malignancy, the most important factor in the pathogenesis of many SMNs could well be the genetic susceptibility of the patient. We will review those genetic and treatment factors that have been associated with the occurrence of SMNs and discuss the follow-up and evaluation of the successfully treated pediatric patient with cancer.

Genetic Factors

The importance of genetic predisposition to the occurrence of a SMN has been demonstrated most clearly in patients with hereditary retinoblastoma. Among 1604 children treated for retinoblastoma at several medical centers in Boston, Massachusetts between 1937 and 1984 and several medical centers in New York City between 1914 and 1984 and who survived for one year after diagnosis, 961 had the hereditary form of the disease. The cumulative percentage of those who developed a SMN was 51.0% (± 6.2%) 50 years after retinoblastoma diagnosis, compared with 5.0% (± 3.0%) among those with nonhereditary retinoblastoma (Fig. 66-1A). Among those patients with hereditary retinoblastoma, the cumulative percentage who developed SMNs was 58.3% (± 8.9%) among those whose treatment included radiation therapy (RT), compared with 26.5% (± 10.7%) among those whose treatment did not include RT (Fig. 66-1B).[11-13]

Other researchers, although confirming the susceptibility of patients with hereditary retinoblastoma to the development of new cancers, did not identify an effect of the same magnitude as that reported by Eng and colleagues.[11] Draper and coworkers,[14] in a report based on the experience of the Oxford Childhood Cancer Research Group, estimated the risk of a SMN after treatment for retinoblastoma at 4.2% 18 years after diagnosis among all patients with retinoblastoma, and at 8.4% 18 years after diagnosis among those with genetic retinoblastoma. The rate reported among patients with genetic retinoblastoma was approximately one-fifth the rate reported by Eng and colleagues. The explanation for this difference in the rates of SMNs is not clear, but it could be related to differences in the frequency of administration of chemotherapy (especially alkylating agents) to these patients; to biased follow-up of patients who developed a second malignant tumor; or to differences in the median duration of follow-up of the two series. Chemotherapy was administered to 6.7% (26 of 384) of the British patients with genetic retinoblastoma and to an unreported fraction of the American patients.[12,14]

The Li-Fraumeni syndrome consists of sarcoma diagnosed in the proband before age 45 years, with additional cancers (frequently soft tissue sarcoma or breast cancer) diagnosed in other children and young adults within the family.[15] The genetic defect in some families with the Li-Fraumeni syndrome was demonstrated to be a mutation within the p53 gene.[16-19] Because the pattern of first and second malignant tumors in some patients with SMNs resembles the distribution observed within some families with the Li-Fraumeni syndrome, a series of patients with SMNs was evaluated for the occurrence of mutations at this locus. Mutations were identified in 5.1% of 59 patients examined.[20,21] Mutations within the p53 gene have been demonstrated in neurofibrosarcomas (but not in the germline) of some patients with neurofibromatosis type 1 (NF1).[22] Pediatric patients with cancer who have neurofibromatosis have a relative risk of 8.1 of developing a SMN compared with pediatric patients with cancer without neurofibromatosis.[23] Future research could demonstrate that those NF1 patients who develop SMNs have coexistent germline p53 mutations.

Genetic loci associated with the occurrence of Wilms' tumor have been identified at 11p13 (WT1), 11p15, 17q 12-q21, and 19q13.[24-26] Some patients have germline mutations in WT1, the only Wilms' tumor-associated gene that has been sequenced.[27,28] Li and associates[29] reported that the frequency of SMNs in a cohort of successfully treated Wilms' tumor patients was 6% 20 years after diagnosis. SMNs were diagnosed only in irradiated patients. Patients who had received dactinomycin were not protected from the occurrence of SMNs, in contrast to the results of a prior case-control study.[29,30] Breslow and colleagues[31] reviewed the occurrence of SMNs among patients entered on the National Wilms Tumor Studies. The cumulative risk of SMN was 1.6% 15 years after diagnosis (Fig. 66-2). The relative risk of developing SMN was increased in patients who had received RT, with the relative risk increasing with increasing radiation dose. Administration of doxorubicin increased the relative risk at each level of radiation exposure.[31] Other researchers have reported a cumulative frequency of SMN after treatment for Wilms' tumor at 3.9% at 20 years, with a relative risk of 11.0.[32]

One group of investigators reported SMNs in 33.3% of patients (two of six) with bilateral Wilms' tumor.[33] In

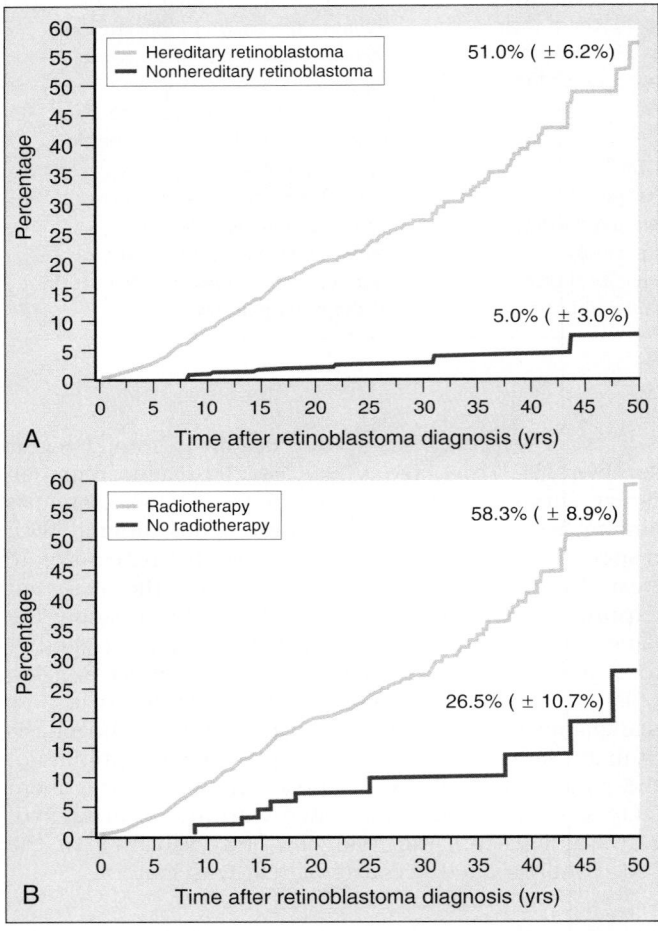

Figure 66-1. A, The cumulative incidence of second malignant tumors is increased in children with familial retinoblastoma. **B,** The cumulative risk of second malignant tumors is increased in children with familial retinoblastoma who are treated with radiation therapy. (Reprinted from Wong FL, Boice JD Jr, Abramson DH, et al: Cancer incidence after retinoblastoma: Radiation dose and sarcoma risk. JAMA 1997;1262:278, with permission.)

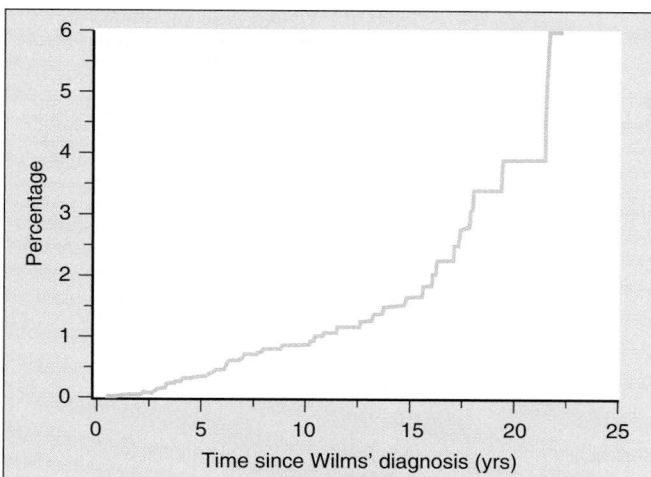

Figure 66-2. Children successfully treated for Wilms' tumor have a significant risk of developing a second malignant tumor. (Reprinted from Bresolow NE, Takashima JR, Whitton JA, et al: Second malignant neoplasms following treatment for Wilms' tumor: A report from the National Wilms Tumor Study Group. J Clin Oncol 1995;13:1851, with permission.)

this group of patients, many would be expected to have germline abnormalities in a Wilms' tumor-associated gene, but patients with bilateral Wilms' tumor were not at increased risk for SMNs according to the National Wilms Tumor Study Group analysis.[31]

Treatment Factors

Surgery

Surgical procedures can increase the risk of subsequent malignancy. Adenocarcinoma of the colon has been reported in several patients after ureterosigmoidostomy. The incidence of adenocarcinoma in these patients was approximately 9.9 per 1000, compared with an incidence rate of 9.9 per 100,000 in the general population.[34] The majority of reported patients have undergone this procedure for treatment of exstrophy of the bladder. The median interval between ureterosigmoidostomy and the diagnosis of colon carcinoma was 22 years.[35] Carcinoma might develop at the ureterocolonic suture line after temporary ureterosigmoidostomy despite rediversion of urine away from the colonic mucosa and has been reported in one patient with ileal loop urinary diversion, suggesting that the complication cannot be avoided by the use of a different surgical procedure.[36,37]

Radiation Therapy

Thyroid carcinoma is a known complication of neck irradiation for benign conditions during infancy.[38] Patients who receive neck irradiation for malignant diseases are at risk for the subsequent occurrence of thyroid malignancies. These have been reported after treatment of patients with medulloblastoma, rhabdomyosarcoma, acute lymphoblastic leukemia, and Hodgkin's disease (HD).[39-50] The incidence of thyroid cancer in survivors of HD was 0.8% (1 in 119) among children treated at Stanford University.[59] Malignant thyroid tumors can develop from

3 to 30.1 years after completion of RT.[51,52] Malignant thyroid tumors occurred at lower RT doses than did benign lesions.[52] Ron and colleagues[53] reported that a linear-exponential model fit the dose-response data for thyroid cancer after treatment for childhood cancer better than a linear model. This finding is consistent with the data of Upton,[54] who demonstrated that the dose-response relationship for some radiation-induced experimental tumors was quadratic rather than linear. These data led Gray[55] to hypothesize that the shape of the dose-response curve was the sum of two radiation-induced processes—mutation induction and cell death.

Central nervous system tumors, including meningiomas and gliomas, have been reported with increasing frequency after direct or incidental irradiation of the brain, a finding that was anticipated based on the occurrence of brain tumors in children treated with low doses of RT for tinea capitis.[56-62] Neglia and colleagues[63] reported that the relative risk of a secondary central nervous system malignancy among children treated for acute lymphoblastic leukemia was 21.7. The most significant factors for the occurrence of these tumors were previous prophylactic cranial irradiation and age less than six years at diagnosis (Fig. 66-3).[63] Other researchers have confirmed the increased risk of central nervous system tumors in children whose treatment for acute lymphoblastic leukemia included cranial irradiation.[64,65]

Sarcomas of bone have been reported both in patients with hereditary retinoblastoma and in those surviving other types of childhood cancer. The cumulative risk of SMN in bone was estimated to be 2.8% among 9170 patients evaluated but was 14.1% among those with retinoblastoma and 22.1% among those treated for Ewing sarcoma at 20 years after diagnosis (Fig. 66-4).[66] The relative risk was 2.7 among patients whose treatment

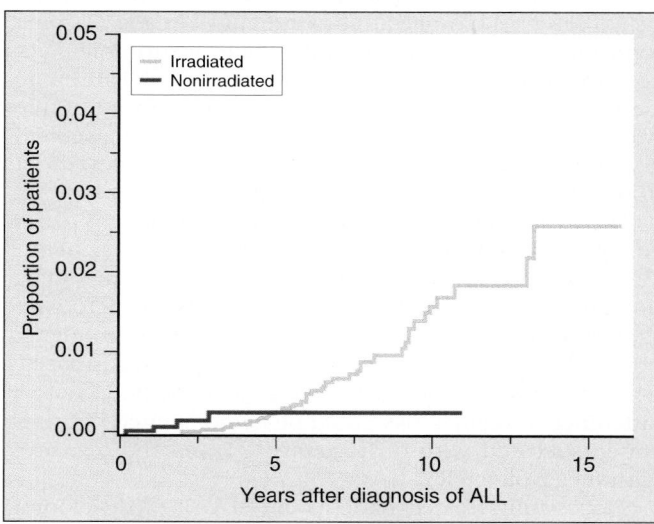

Figure 66-3. The cumulative incidence of second malignant tumors is increased in children whose treatment for acute lymphoblastic leukemia included radiation therapy. (Reprinted from Neglia JP, Meadows AT, Robinson LL, et al: Second neoplasms after acute lymphoblastic leukemia in childhood. N Engl J Med 1991;325:1330, with permission. Copyright 1991 Massachusetts Medical Society.)

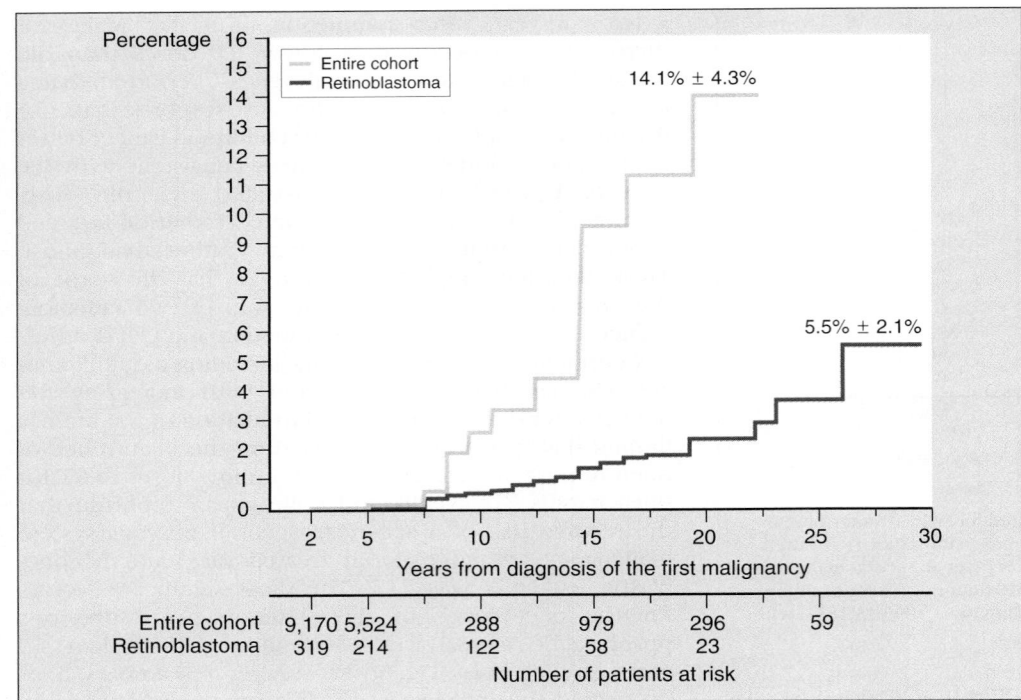

Figure 66-4. The cumulative incidence of bone sarcoma as a second malignant tumor is increased in children treated for retinoblastoma compared with those treated for other forms of childhood cancer. (Reprinted from Tucker MA, D'Angio GJ, Boice JD Jr, et al: Bone sarcomas linked to radiography and chemotherapy in children. N Engl J Med 1987;317:588, with permission. Copyright 1987 Massachusetts Medical Society.)

had included RT, with the relative risk increasing with increasing RT dose and more intensive use of alkylating agents.[66] Other researchers reported a relative risk for osteosarcoma of 87.9–1515 in patients treated for retinoblastoma; the relative risk rises to 800 after treatment for Ewing sarcoma.[67,68] Hawkins and colleagues[69] calculated the cumulative frequency of bone cancer in previously irradiated childhood cancer survivors as 0.5% among those not treated for retinoblastoma and as 7.2% among those treated for heritable retinoblastoma. The dramatic risk of sarcoma of bone after treatment of Ewing sarcoma, reported earlier from several single institutions, was confirmed in a multi-institutional review.[70,71] The cumulative frequency of a SMN in patients treated successfully was 9.2% at 20 years after diagnosis, and that of a secondary sarcoma was 6.5%. No secondary sarcomas developed in patients who had received less than 4800 cGy.[72]

The evolution of RT technique from the use of orthovoltage radiation apparatuses (which produce a higher absorbed dose in bone) to the use of megavoltage radiation apparatuses (which does not have this characteristic) should result in a lower frequency of SMNs in irradiated bones.[73–75] When this expectation was addressed in a case-control study of bone sarcoma as a SMN, however, no difference in relative risk could be demonstrated between patients treated with orthovoltage RT and those treated with megavoltage RT.[66]

Successfully treated patients are at risk of developing carcinomas (e.g., of the skin) within prior RT treatment volumes given at a very early age.[76] Breast cancer, first reported in three young women (22, 34, and 38 years of age, respectively) after irradiation for Wilms' tumor to a volume that included part or all of the breast,[77,78] occurs with a relative risk of 17–136 among irradiated survivors

of pediatric HD.[79–82] The finding of an increased risk for breast cancer after breast irradiation is consistent with several studies of women who received incidental breast irradiation from diagnostic radiographs to evaluate pulmonary tuberculosis or scoliosis; who received therapeutic low-dose irradiation for mastitis, benign breast disease, thymic enlargement, or tinea capitis; or who received incidental whole-body irradiation as the result of atomic bomb detonations in Hiroshima and Nagasaki.[83–90]

Adenocarcinoma of the colon occurred within the volume of irradiation in three patients at the ages of 12, 27, and 27 years, respectively.[91–93] It is possible that these patients had germline mutations in a cancer predisposition gene that contributed to their susceptibility to radiation carcinogenesis.

Total body irradiation, a component of most preparative regimens for allogeneic bone marrow transplantation for malignant diseases, is associated with a cumulative risk for the occurrence of a second solid neoplasm of 8.3% at 13 years after treatment, although the RR for a second solid cancer was not significantly increased among those who received pretransplant RT or total body irradiation[94–96]

Chemotherapy

The significance of prior treatment with chemotherapy in the pathogenesis of SMNs was first evaluated in detail in cohorts of adults treated successfully for HD. The risk factors for the occurrence of SMNs in pediatric patients after treatment for HD have been evaluated less thoroughly.

Bhatia and coworkers[80] reported that the cumulative risk of developing any SMN after treatment for HD in childhood was 7% at 15 years after diagnosis. The risk of developing non-Hodgkin's lymphoma was 1.1%, and the risk of developing any type of leukemia was 2.8% at 15 years after diagnosis. The investigators calculated the cumulative dose per square meter of each alkylating agent received, divided the cumulative dose distributions for each agent into thirds, and assigned a numerical value (0,1,2,3) for each agent received, depending on whether the patient had received none of the drug or had a cumulative drug dose in the lower, middle, or upper third of the dose distribution. A summary score (alkylating agent dose [AAD] score) was derived by adding the results for each agent received. The relative risk of leukemia increased by 1.5 for each unit increase in the AAD score.[80,97] The actuarial risk of developing acute myelogenous leukemia 10 years after diagnosis was 11% among pediatric patients treated at Stanford University with low-dose (2500 cGy) RT and MOPP (nitrogen mustard [M], vincristine [O], procarbazine [P], and prednisone [P]) chemotherapy, which has an AAD score of 2.[98] The risk was 1.1% 15 years after diagnosis among pediatric patients treated with involved or extended field RT and various chemotherapy regimens that did not contain nitrogen mustard (vincristine, prednisone, doxorubicin, with or without procarbazine; cyclophosphamide, vincristine, prednisone, procarbazine, or methotrexate).[99]

Other investigators have studied the risk of developing SMNs after various chemotherapeutic agent exposures. Tucker and colleagues[100] reported that prior treatment with an alkylating agent increased the risk of developing bone cancer or leukemia (Fig. 66-5) as SMN.[66] De Vathaire and coworkers[101] demonstrated that actinomycin D increased the risk of a bone or soft tissue SMN (RR = 8.7). Garwicz and associates[23] reported that treatment with classical alkylating agents (nitrogen mustard, cyclophosphamide, CCNU), nonclassical alkylating agents (procarbazine), vinca alkaloids (vinblastine, vincristine), or prednisone each increased the relative risk of SMN. Only

procarbazine increased the relative risk of SMN when it was included in a two-factor multivariate model.[23] Klein and colleagues[102] reported an increased relative risk for SMN with higher doses of several agents, including cyclophosphamide (RR –6.3 for doses >8000 mg/m², cisplatinum (RR –2.8 for doses >435 mg/m²), and 6-mercaptpuurine (RR –4.5 for doses >5000 mg/m²). Neglia and associates[9] reported that treatment with anthracycline (RR –1.51 for doses of 101–300 mg/m²; RR –1.44 for doses >300 mg/m²) or epipodophyllotoxin (RR –2.78 for doses >4001 mg/M²) but did not demonstrate an increased relative risk with increasing AAD score or cisplatinum exposure.

The epipodophyllotoxins have been identified as important leukemogens. Pui and coworkers[103] reported the risk of secondary acute myelogenous leukemia (AML) as 4.7% at six years after diagnosis among patients treated for acute lymphoblastic leukemia. The risk was substantially higher (19.1%) among patients with T-cell leukemia. These investigators subsequently demonstrated that the risk of secondary AML in this population was related to the administration of epipodophyllotoxins, with the cumulative frequency of AML being 12.3% among those treated twice weekly and 12.4% among those treated weekly, compared with a frequency of 1.6% among those treated with the drug less frequently or not at all (Fig. 66-6).[104]

The risk of secondary AML depends on the cumulative dose of drug administered and the schedule of administration, with the frequency reported to be 0% among germ cell tumor patients treated with less than 2000 mg/m², 5.9% among childhood acute lymphoblastic leukemia patients treated with 1800–9900 mg/m², 11.3% among germ cell tumor patients who received more than 2000 mg/m², and 18.4% among pediatric NHL patients who received 4200–5600 mg/m².[105-107] Hawkins and asso-

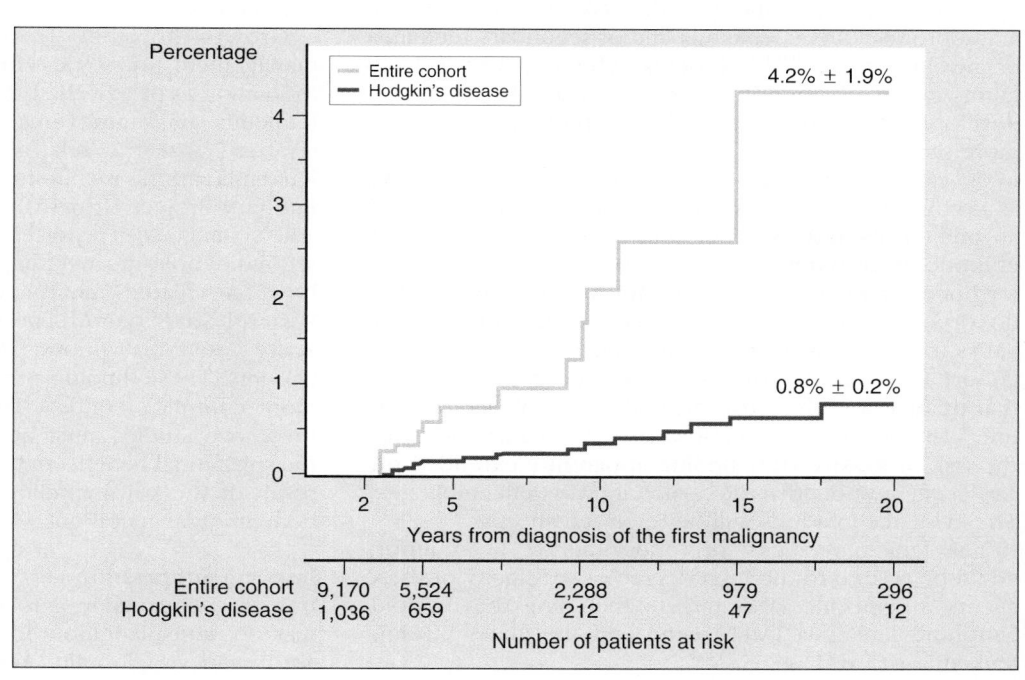

Figure 66-5. The cumulative incidence of leukemia as a second malignant tumor is increased in children treated for Hodgkin's disease compared with those treated for other forms of childhood cancer. (Reprinted from Tucker MA, Meadows AT, Boice JD Jr, et al: Leukemia after therapy with alkylating agents for childhood cancer. J Natl Cancer Inst 1987;78:459, with permission.)

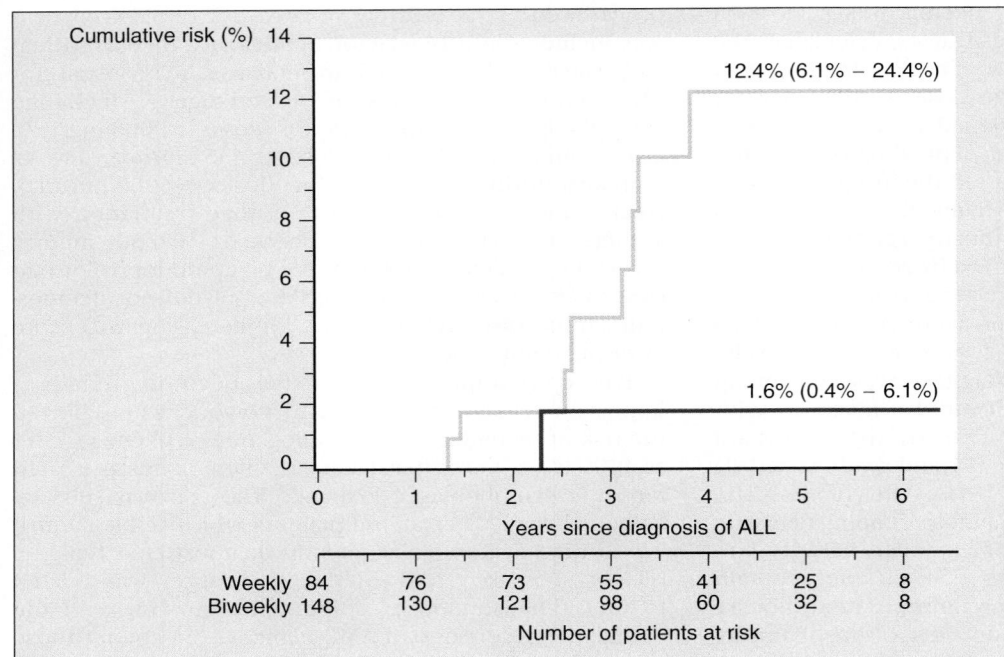

Figure 66-6. The cumulative incidence of acute myelogenous leukemia after treatment for acute lymphoblastic leukemia is increased among children whose therapy includes weekly epipodophyllotoxin. (Reprinted from Pui C-H, Behm FG, Raimondi SC, et al: Secondary acute myeloid leukemia. N Engl J Med 1989;321:136, with permission. Copyright 1989 Massachusetts Medical Society.)

ciates[108] reported an increased risk of secondary leukemia with increasing cumulative dose of epipodophyllotoxin but did not find that the risk of secondary leukemia was zero for cumulative doses below 2000 mg/m^2.[108]

The carcinogenic potential of the anthracycline, doxorubicin, was suggested by the results of a previous case-control study of risk factors for leukemia as a SMN, in which increasing doxorubicin dose was associated with an increasing relative risk of leukemia as a SMN after adjustment for the AAD score.[100] More recently, prior treatment with anthracyclines or epipodophyllotoxins have been shown to increase the risk of therapy-related acute promyelocytic leukemia and of secondary leukemia or myelodysplasia.[109,110] Patients who received 1.2–6.0 grams/m^2 of epipodophyllotoxin had a relative risk of developing leukemia of 3.9, whereas those who received more than 170 mg/m^2 of anthracycline had a relative risk of developing leukemia of 3.0.[110] This finding is of interest, as doxorubicin is now known to have topoisomerase II as one of its targets—the same target as that of the epipodophyllotoxins. A case-control study of risk factors for bone sarcoma as a SMN did not identify any effect of doxorubicin therapy on the risk of developing such SMNs.[66] An analysis of risk factors for any SMN in a large cohort of pediatric patients with cancer demonstrated that treatment with doxorubicin was the only factor identified (other than treatment with BCNU) that increased the risk of a SMN; (this finding apparently extended the earlier suggestion that doxorubicin was leukemogenic.[3] The evidence in adults will be reviewed shortly.

The leukemogenicity of topoisomerase II inhibitors could be related to the high degree of specificity of these agents for specific DNA targets, including the myeloid-lymphoid leukemia (MLL) gene and the acute myeloid leukemia 1 (AML1) gene.[111-113]

Although most studies of carcinogenicity of chemotherapeutic agents have focused on the development of leukemia after treatment, it is clear that solid tumor induction is also possible after exposure to one or more chemotherapeutic agents. The best example of this is the occurrence of solid SMNs in genetically predisposed retinoblastoma patients who were treated with cyclophosphamide only after enucleation.[14] As our ability to identify genetically predisposed patients improves, our understanding of the apparent anomaly of solid tumor induction after systemic exposure to a carcinogenic agent will increase.

Growth hormone treatment is necessary for the management of some children who received cranial irradiation as part of their therapy for acute lymphoblastic leukemia or brain tumors. Fradkin and associates[114] reported that the relative risk for the occurrence of leukemia among members of the National Hormone and Pituitary Project Growth Hormone cohort was 2.6. Sklar and colleagues[115] reported a relative risk of 3.21 for a second neoplasm (including meningioma) among growth hormone-treated members of the Childhood Cancer Survivor Study cohort. There were no cases of secondary acute leukemia among the growth hormone-treated patients. These findings require confirmation in larger, more complete cohorts. The possible risk identified by these two studies must be considered in the context of the substantial benefits that accrue to these patients as the result of therapy, including improved linear growth and bone mineral accretion.

Immune Suppression

Immune suppression is a component of allogeneic bone marrow transplantation. To prevent graft-vs.-host disease, antithymocyte globulin (ATG) can be administered to the

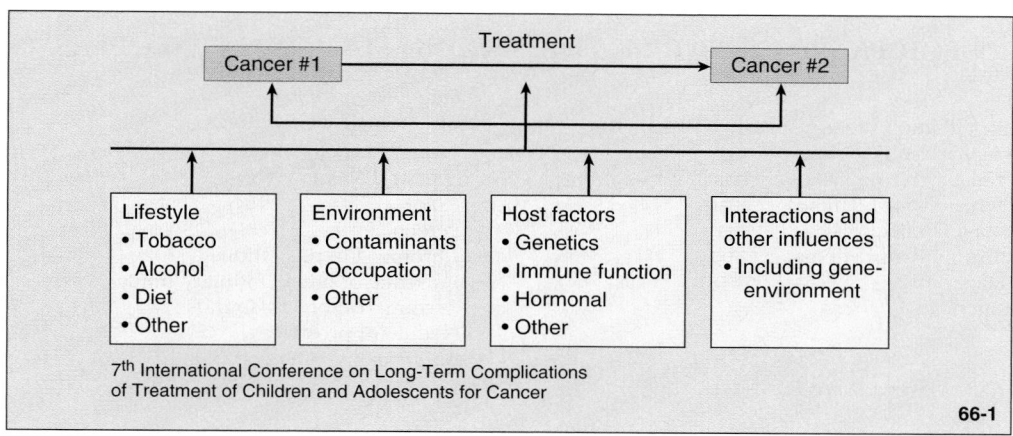

Treatment

Cancer #1 ────────────────→ Cancer #2

Lifestyle	Environment	Host factors	Interactions and other influences
• Tobacco	• Contaminants	• Genetics	• Including gene-environment
• Alcohol	• Occupation	• Immune function	
• Diet	• Other	• Hormonal	
• Other		• Other	

7th International Conference on Long-Term Complications
of Treatment of Children and Adolescents for Cancer

66-1

recipient, or the bone marrow can be manipulated to remove T cells. These manipulations and bone marrow transplantation from an unrelated bone marrow donor increase the risk of Epstein-Barr virus–associated B-cell lymphoproliferative disorder. The cumulative incidence rates at 10 years after bone marrow transplantation were 11.3% among those treated with ATG, 11.4% among those who received T-cell–depleted bone marrow, and 2.3% among those who received bone marrow from unrelated donors.[94]

Recommendations

Pediatric patients who survive their primary cancer are at increased risk of developing a new malignancy. The magnitude of this risk is modulated by several factors, including the genetic susceptibility of the patient,[116] the type of surgical procedure employed for removal of the tumor, the use of RT as part of the treatment plan, the chemotherapeutic agents employed, the severity of immune suppression present at the completion of all treatment, and environmental exposures.

All former patients should remain under a physician's care indefinitely and should undergo an annual physical examination, preferably by a physician who is familiar with the problem of therapy-induced malignancy.

Patients who have been irradiated should have plain radiographs obtained whenever local pain occurs in a previously irradiated bone. Patients who have received irradiation to volumes that include the breast, uterine cervix, or intestine should undergo routine evaluation with available screening tests, such as mammography, pap smear, and stool examination for the presence of occult blood. Annual mammography should be initiated no later than ten years after breast irradiation. Careful physical examination will facilitate the early identification of thyroid nodules and skin cancer.

All patients who have been treated with an alkylating agent, procarbazine, or a topoisomerase II inhibitor should have a complete blood count every 6 to 12 months for a minimum of 12 years after diagnosis. The presence of macrocytosis and/or cytopenia should prompt evaluation of the bone marrow.

The adverse health consequences of tobacco use, including carcinogenesis, are well documented. One-third of childhood cancer survivors use tobacco.[117-122] Physicians should counsel childhood cancer survivors regarding the potential for the adverse effects of tobacco use to interact with the adverse effects of their prior therapy, such as irradiation of the oropharynx, esophagus, and/or lung.

ADULTS

Genetic Factors

Travis[123] provides an excellent, comprehensive overview and update of research concerning SMNs focusing on solid tumors in the adult age group. She stresses that several factors besides chemotherapy, radiotherapy, and their interplays need to be considered; these are shown in Figure 66-7. For example, the complex potential interactions of alkylating agents, RT, and tobacco smoking are developed extensively in her discussion of lung cancers as SMNs, especially in HD patients. She points out the additional variable in HD patients (i.e., impaired immunologic responses), so that data derived from long-term survivors of HD cannot be extrapolated with confidence to patients with other SMNs.

The potential importance of immunodeficiency in the appearance of SMNs was the hypothesis explored by Hemminki and coworkers[124] in an imaginative epidemiologic investigation. They noted that skin cancers and non–Hodgkin's lymphomas (NHLs) were the most frequent malignant lesions to appear in immune deficient patients (e.g., in renal transplant patients given needed post-transplant immune-suppressing agents). Using the Swedish nation-wide database, they found 4301 secondary skin cancers and 1672 NHLs in a period of about 40 years among 10.2 million survivors of a primary cancer. The researchers found increased risks—up to 12-fold depending on patient sex and primary tumor site—for these two neoplastic entities. These results suggest that immunodeficiency could play a role in the appearance of SMNs.

EVALUATION FOR PATIENTS AT RISK FOR SECOND MALIGNANT NEOPLASMS

RISK FACTORS
- Treatment with radiation therapy, an alkylating agent, and/or a topoisomerase II inhibitor
- History of hereditary retinoblastoma (unilateral with a positive family history or bilateral)
- Carrier of ataxia-telangiectasia
- Postsurgical chronic lymphedema
- Ureterosigmoidostomy
- Estrogen treatment

HISTORY
- Pain in any previously irradiated area
- Bruising
- Gum bleeding
- Pallor
- Easy fatigability
- Breast lump
- Cough
- Chest pain
- Hemoptysis
- Blood in stool
- Constipation
- Tenesmus
- Hematuria
- Increased urinary frequency/incontinence

- Difficulty voiding
- Intermenstrual bleeding

PHYSICAL EXAMINATION
- Pallor
- Petechiae
- Chronic skin ulceration
- Presence of lump (mobility, tenderness, consistency)
- Asymmetric breath sounds
- Nodule in prostate
- Abnormal uterine cervix

EVALUATION
- Plain radiographs of any painful area or mass in a previously irradiated area
- Stool examination for occult blood (any patient who received any abdominal irradiation)
- Pap smear
- Urine cytology (any patient with hematuria and a history of bladder irradiation and/or treatment with an oxazophosphorine alkylating agent)
- Mammogram
- Additional tests as indicated by the history and physical examination

---

Several sites of primary tumors in both males and females were encompassed in their study, making therapy-induced immunosuppression unlikely. This points to possible underlying genetic factors as contributory influences.

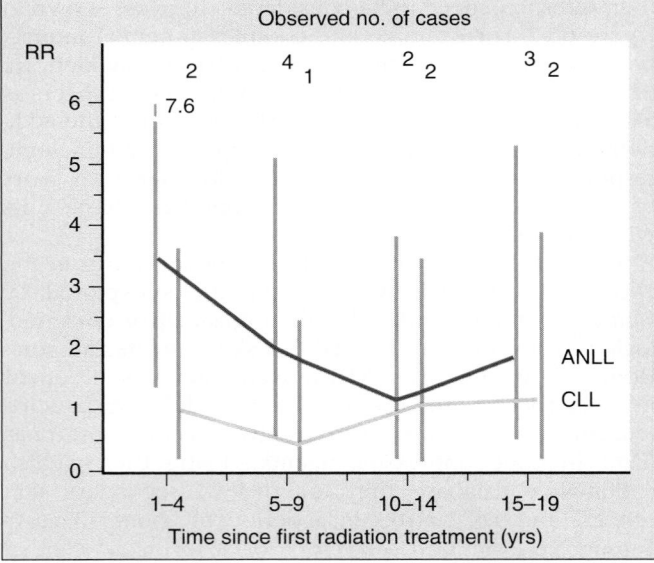

Figure 66-7. Schematic illustration of risk factors for second primary cancers. (Adapted from Storm HH: Second primary cancer after treatment for cervical cancer. Later effects after radiotherapy. Cancer 1998;61:679, with permission. Copyright 1998 American Cancer Society.)

The importance of the Li-Fraumeni syndrome as a risk factor for cancer in young adults has been discussed previously.[116] Lalle and associates[125] screened seven older SMN patients and did not find p53 mutations in exons 4–8 among these individuals. They concluded that there is genetic heterogeneity for SMN development in patients who are older at the time of the first diagnosis.

Cancer families provide evidence supporting laboratory studies of the genetic bases of adult cancers. Cancer predisposition genes for breast cancer (BRCA1, BRCA2), colon cancer (MSH1, MSH2, APC, DCC), malignant melanoma (CDK2), and renal cell carcinoma (RCC) have all been identified.[124]

Genetic factors related to irradiation carcinogenesis were discussed in a workshop dealing largely with laboratory studies.[126] At the clinical level, carriers of the ataxia-telangiectasia gene (ATM) are more likely to develop cancer; Swift and colleagues[127] estimate a 3 to 4 excess relative risk of cancer in male and female carriers. Female breast cancer was the most frequent cancer reported (excess risk of about 5) and was more likely to occur in those exposed to ionizing radiation. Little and coworkers[128] compared the relative risks of developing post-therapeutic irradiation SMNs to those among Japanese survivors of the atomic bomb blasts. They found the relative risks of developing leukemia or lung, bone, or ovarian cancer to be higher among the Japanese survivors than for treated patients. Neither chemotherapy nor underlying genetic factors seemed to play a role in their results.

The cytogenetics of SMNs have been the subject of intensive investigation. Le Beau and associates[129] described characteristic abnormalities of chromosome 5 [del (5q)] and 7[del (7q)] in patients with treatment-associated acute myeloid leukemia.[129] (The terms "acute myeloid leukemia" [AML] and "acute non-lymphoblastic leukemia" [ANLL] will be used interchangeably in this discussion. In most cases, the term used will be that employed by the authorities being cited.)

Detourmignies and colleagues[130] found t(15;17) in treatment-associated acute promyelocytic leukemia (t-APL) and the other forms of acute myeloid leukemia (t-AML), the same translocation as found in those diseases de novo. In addition, t(8;21), t(9;11) and inv(16) were found in t-APL and other t-AMLs. They tend to arise in patients with solid tumors, have short latent periods, and are associated with prior therapy with drugs that inhibit topoisomerase II. Cytogenetic evaluations of solid SMNs have demonstrated chromosome 22 deletions in meningiomas and deletions in chromosomes 10 and 17 in malignant astrocytomas.[131,132] These cytogenetic findings could have important implications regarding early identification and early treatment of SMNs.

Treatment Factors

Surgery

The appearance of epithelial tumors at the suture line of ureterosigmoidostomies has been cited previously.[34-37] In adults, perhaps the most common SMN ascribed to surgery is angiosarcoma in a lymphedematous structure (the Stewart-Treves syndrome), a complication that has been described most often after radical mastectomy.[133] The tumors tend to arise in the edematous arm rather than in irradiated areas.[134] Angiosarcoma developing in RT fields have been reported after tylectomy (lumpectomy) and breast irradiation.[135] Marchal and coworkers[136] conducted a survey of breast angiosarcomas developing in women treated with breast-conserving techniques. They found nine cases among almost 20,000 women but found no conclusive evidence linking therapy as a causative factor.

Radiation Therapy

The factors involved in radiation carcinogenesis have been reviewed recently by Cosset[137] and by Lindsay and colleagues.[138] Breast, thyroid, bone and soft tissues, and organs and tissues that are prone to develop SMNs after RT given in childhood are also vulnerable to radiation oncogenesis when treatment is given during the adult years.

Bone and Soft Tissue. Lagrange and coworkers[139] reported 80 radiation-associated sarcoma cases collected by a consortium of French cancer centers. The median dose of RT was 50 Gy (range: 9–110Gy) delivered to adults (median age 44 years) for a variety of primary diagnoses. Of the histologically proven secondary sarcomas, 70% were bone and 30% were soft tissue sarcomas, with osteosarcomas and malignant fibrous histiocytomas predominating among them. Unlike the earlier study by Tountas and colleagues,[140] these authors could not demonstrate a correlation with increasing dose. The outcomes were

poor despite aggressive treatment based largely on surgical maneuvers.

RT-associated soft-tissue sarcomas such as those found by Lagrange and coworkers[139] are of particular interest. Kim and associates[141] reported the detailed histopathology of the soft-tissue sarcomas developing in irradiated tissues in their 20 patients, some of whom were children and/or were irradiated for nonmalignant disorders. Sarcomas in 14 patients (70%) were of the spindle cell variety, which includes fibrosarcoma. (An angiosarcoma developed in one child among the 20.) The latent period measured from the time of irradiation ranged from 3 to 40 years (median = 12 years), compared with 4 to 27 years (median = 11 years) for 27 cases of bone sarcoma identified by the researchers during the same study period. The median doses were lower for the soft-tissue sarcomas than for the bone sarcomas, and no sarcomas developed in patients receiving less than the equivalent of 30 Gy over 3 weeks in this early series.

Chest irradiation preceded the appearance of the rare mesothelioma as a SMN in four men and four women who served as the basis for an epidemiologic study conducted by Cavazza and colleagues.[142] The evolution of the mesotheliomas in the study patients followed the same temporal and other patterns as in those contracting asbestos-related tumors. The authors conclude that therapy might have been a factor for some patients.

Storm[143] reviewed the frequency of SMNs in a cohort of 24,970 Danish women with invasive cervical cancer and 19,470 who had carcinoma in situ followed for 30 or more years. Taken together, there was an increased relative risk of 1.9 in irradiated patients surviving 30 or more years, representing an excess of 64 cases per 10,000 women annually.

Werner-Wasik and coworkers[144] analyzed the frequency and patterns of SMNs they found in women with cervical cancer and came to a different conclusion. They found 11 SMNs among 10 of the 125 women with FIGO stages I and II cervical carcinoma who received radiotherapy in a recent ten-year period (1980–1990). Two of the SMNs were synchronous (bladder and thyroid), and four of the nine metachronous cancers appeared in the breast. Lung (two cases) and myeloma, NHL, and vulva (one case each) accounted for the other five SMNs. All of the SMNs were outside the fields of irradiation, and none of the women had received chemotherapy. The researchers concluded that the increased relative risk of a SMN might be genetically based, as treatments did not appear to be factors. This again emphasizes the need to consider the multiple possible contributing factors (see Fig. 66-7).

Sturgeon and associates[145] found an excess of SMNs among women with vulvar or vaginal cancers. Most of the SMNs were smoking related (lung, upper airways) or in patients infected with the human papillomavirus (HPV), which is known to be associated with cancers of the genital tract. A related observation by Hemminki and Dong[146] is of interest. They found an increase in anal cancers in both women with cervical cancer and their husbands, implicating HPV in the etiology of anal cancer.

An increased risk of ovarian cancer as a SMN was found by Hall and colleagues[147] in certain sets of women. These were those younger than 50 years of age with melanoma or cancer of the colon, breast, cervix, uterine corpus, or ovary. The relative risks for women in these groups ranged from about 5 to almost 20.

A reputed increase in breast cancers among women with ovarian cancer could not be substantiated by Bergfeldt and coworkers.[148] Their case-control study from a pool of 5060 Swedish women led them to conclude that increased surveillance (mammography) of surviving patients with ovarian cancer was not warranted. Travis and associates[149] likewise attribute secondary breast cancers to factors other than therapy, although they attribute soft-tissue, bladder, and rectal malignancies to RT and leukemia to chemotherapy.

A population-based study of second primary cancers was reported by Buiatti and colleagues.[150] They considered only the 463 metachronous SMNs that developed among the 19,252 adults with primary cancers of the colon, rectum, lung, stomach, and female breast who constituted the study population. Significantly higher risks of developing another cancer were found in patients under 65 years of age. Associations of three types were found:

1. Between primary rectal and secondary kidney cancers.
2. Between colon and later ovarian malignancies.
3. Between female breast and subsequent rectal cancers, although cancer in the opposite breast constituted the highest risk in this group.

No correlations were made between the treatments used for the primary tumor and the secondary cancer. This report, together with that of Werner-Wasik and associates,[144] highlights the fact that not all SMNs should be assumed to have an iatrogenic basis.

In their review, Mark and colleagues[151] focused on 13 women with radiation-associated uterine sarcomas among the total pool of 114 patients with sarcoma of the uterus seen by them. The estimated absolute risk for such a second malignant neoplasm was less than 1%. The investigators concluded that RT should not be avoided in the management of gynecologic malignancies for fear of post-RT SMNs. This point is underlined by the results of a study by Koyama and coworkers,[152] who found multiple primary malignant neoplasms—chiefly in the gastrointestinal tract, prostate, and bladder—among 104 patients with urologic cancers of various types.

Long-term follow up is not available for large numbers of men receiving RT for prostatic carcinoma. Movsas and associates[153] found no increase in the risk of SMN among 543 of their patients when compared with a matched set of 18,135 men derived from the Connecticut Tumor Registry. Most of the SMNs developed outside the RT fields and were associated with lifestyles predisposing to cancer (e.g., smoking and alcohol abuse). No definite increase was found by Johnstone and colleagues[154] either, but Brenner and coworkers differed.[155] The latter group reported analyses based on tens of thousands of men who did or did not receive prostate RT. They found a small but statistically significant increase in the solid tumor rate that included sarcomas in the treated field and bladder and rectal carcinomas.

SMNs occurring in men with testicular cancers have been studied by several investigators. Wanderas and associates[156] found an increased risk of second germ cell cancer, usually of the same histology, among 2201 patients, the risk being highest among men younger than 30 years of age at first diagnosis. More SMNs than expected were found by Ruther and colleagues[157] in their multicenter collection of men with pure seminomas. These included both nontesticular and testicular SMNs. A variety of SMNs was reported by Travis and coworkers[158] in a large cohort study of 29,000 survivors. SMNs of the gastrointestinal and genitourinary tracts and thyroid were represented, along with connective tissue malignancies, NHL, leukemia, and melanoma. The authors point out that multiple factors could be contributing to the apparent increase in risk. Nichols and Loehrer,[159] commenting on the Travis paper, stress that these SMNs were the result of treatments given years before and no longer in use. Historically, RT was used routinely for even relatively low-stage disease, and extended fields were often employed, albeit at comparatively low total doses. More recently, RT was combined with chemotherapeutic agents, thus increasing the exposure to potential carcinogens. Current therapy minimizes exposure to both these oncogens. (See the "Epithelium" section next for relevant examples of SMNs in such patients.)

Epithelium. Both basal cell and squamous cell carcinomas (SCC) have long been known to be consequences of skin irradiation, as are other sites of squamous epithelium, including the vagina and the esophagus.[143,160,161]

Sherrill and coworkers[161] reported two cases of SCC in men who received mediastinal RT for testicular teratocarcinomas. The authors provide no estimation of risk but do record eight additional SCCs of the esophagus (some as SMNs) after thoracic irradiation for various reasons. Glanzmann and associates[162] reported 16 SMNs in 289 men surviving infradiaphragmatic RT for testicular neoplasm. One of eight within an RT field was diagnosed as cancer of the esophagus, not otherwise specified. Cancers of the colon and rectum, bladder, lung, and penis were also documented. Other researchers, who have studied larger numbers of patients, have documented increased relative risks for carcinomas of some of these and for other organs ranging from 1.2 to 2.3, and higher risks for leukemia [RR = 2.4] and soft-tissue sarcomas [RR – 3.0±].[163] The SMNs tended to develop in irradiated fields.

Breast Cancer. Obedian and colleagues[164] reviewed the frequency of second breast cancers in women treated with and without RT after lumpectomy. The rate was about 10% in both groups, each encompassing about 1000 patients. Rubino and coworkers,[165] however, found a 1.6-fold increase in the risk of a SMN when second breast cancers and nonmelanomatous skin cancers were excluded from the analyses. A more comprehensive review by Fowble and associates[166] evaluated several risk factors in women who had been treated uniformly with wide local excision, axillary dissection, and postoperative

TABLE 66-1

Relative Risk of Contralateral Breast Cancer after Radiation Therapy

AGE AT TREATMENT	NO. EXPOSED	TOTAL NO.	RR
(10-yr survivors)			(95% CI)
<45 yrs old	45	143	1.85 (1.15–2.97)
>45 yrs old	55	298	1.08 (0.74–1.57)

CI, confidence interval; RR, relative risk.
Adapted from Boice JD, Harvey EB, Blettren M, et al: Cancer in the contralateral breast after radiotherapy for breast cancer. N Engl J Med 1992;326:781.

irradiation. Their cumulative 10-year SMN rate was 16% in the 1253 women reviewed. These neoplasms included cancers occurring anywhere, including skin and the opposite breast. The rate was halved when only nonbreast malignant tumors (e.g., skin most commonly, gynecological or gastrointestinal tumors) were in the sample.

The accumulating interest and concern regarding the risk of cancer in the contralateral breast after the use of RT for the management of breast cancer is due to the fact that the RT doses received by the opposite breast are in the range known to be carcinogenic, especially in young women.[167] Boice and colleagues,[168] in a review of their case-control study of 41,109 women with breast cancer, reported a 2.7% risk of developing breast cancer on the opposite side attributable to prior irradiation. Some of the more important variables they considered in their analyses are shown in Table 66-1. An increase in relative risk was observed in irradiated women surviving 10 or more years, but only in those treated when under 45 years of age (RR = 1.85). The risk among this sample increased with increasing RT dose, the analyzed range extending from 1.99 Gy to 4 Gy, and the RRs from 1.54 to 2.35, respectively (p = 0.003). Levitt and Mandel[169] have pointed out the difficulties inherent in studies of radiation oncogenesis in the opposite breast and emphasize weighing the risk-benefit factors entailed. Although the issue remains highly controversial, it would seem prudent to conclude from these data that the dose to the contralateral breast in patients with breast cancer under 45 years of age should be reduced to a minimum.[170]

Lungs. The lungs are included incidentally in many RT treatment volumes, including those for the treatment of mediastinal HD and those for treatment of the remaining ipsilateral breast tissue after lumpectomy for breast cancer. The relative risk of cancer in the ipsilateral lung was 8.1 ten years after irradiation and was 2.8 for cancer in either lung 15 years after irradiation.[171,172] The relative risk for cancer in the ipsilateral lung is 76.6 in irradiated patients with breast cancer who also smoke, compared with 6.7 among irradiated patients with breast cancer who do not smoke.[173] The relative risk of lung cancer in patients treated with RT only for HD was 3.09, although two other studies did not demonstrate such an increased risk.[174-176]

Nervous System. Jones[177] conducted an extensive retrospective analysis of brain tumors occurring in patients after RT for pituitary lesions, a unique group that receives relatively high doses of RT for nonmalignant lesions. He concluded that the risk of RT oncogenesis in adults is low after small-field RT in the doses usually used for the control of pituitary disorders. The tumors most often ascribed to RT are meningiomas and high-grade astrocytomas.[178,179] Other factors, including younger age, higher dose, and larger fields, might increase the risk and shorten the latency period, as suggested by Soffer and colleagues[179] and Cavin and coworkers.[178] Jones' thorough discussion of both irradiated and unirradiated adults with pituitary tumors who developed regional fibrosarcomas, gliomas, and meningiomas raises questions regarding the role of therapeutic RT in the genesis of such SMNs. His paper and that of Erfurth and associates[180] provide important perspectives for evaluating the reports of RT-associated brain tumors. Erfurth and associates not only find no clear evidence implicating RT but also again raise the possibility of underlying genetic factors being responsible.

Leukemia. High doses of irradiation lead to bone marrow inactivation.[181] Marrow beyond the high-dose region receives less than inactivating doses, which could be mutagenic. Storm[143] described a significantly increased relative risk of acute nonlymphoblastic leukemia (ANLL) (RR = 3.5), manifest in the early postirradiation years, but not chronic lymphoblastic leukemia (CLL). The decrease in relative risk by the 10th year after diagnosis, which approximated that of the general population by the 15th year after diagnosis, was unlike the experience with solid tumors. The relative risks for the latter continued to increase with time. Other investigators reported a relative risk of 2.4 for the occurrence of ANLL or myelodysplastic syndrome after only RT for breast cancer.[182] These results differ from earlier data reported by Hutchinson[181] alone and Boice and Hutchinson,[183] who found no increase in the leukemia rate of a cohort of women with 60,000 person-years of follow-up who were evaluated at five and ten years after irradiation for cancer of the cervix.

Chemotherapy

Leukemia–Lymphoma. Most of the SMNs reported after chemotherapy have been AML or NHL. The alkylating agents were the first to be implicated in the etiology of these SMNs and remain the most frequently implicated agents.[184,185] By the early 1970s, AML had been recorded in patients treated with alkylating agents for multiple myeloma and for breast, lung, colon, and ovarian cancers.[184-188] Subsequently, the leukemogenicity of the nitrosoureas was recognized.[189,190] The increased relative risk of AML in patients with brain tumors who had been given carmustine was estimated to be about 25 by Greene and colleagues.[191] More recently, other agents have been associated with AML. These include the epipodophyllotoxins, the platinum compounds, and their combinations.[192,193]

AML that developed in women with ovarian cancer who had been given alkylating agents was one of the first iatrogenic chemotherapy-related SMNs reported in convincing numbers.[185] The relative risk reported by Reimer and associates[185] was more than 170 for women receiving alkylating agents compared with those who did not. That estimate was updated by Greene and colleagues,[194] who found a relative risk of 110 and the excess risk of ANLL to be 5.8 cases per 1000 women per year. Melphalan and chlorambucil were the two agents most strongly implicated (relative risks of 122 and 159, respectively), with the risk of leukemia being dose-related.

Kaldor and coworkers,[195] in an international case-control study of women with ovarian cancer, found increased risks of leukemia in those who had received cyclophosphamide, chlorambucil, melphalan, thiotepa, or dihydroxybusulfan (Treosulfan) as single agents. The relative risks, which increased with larger administered doses, ranged from 2.2 for low-dose cyclophosphamide to 23.0 for chlorambucil and melphalan and 33.0 for Treosulfan in high doses as defined by the researchers. The risk estimates were relative to women receiving only RT or surgery, there being no increased leukemia risk identified in patients who had radiotherapy alone. The risk of leukemia was also increased in patients treated with the combination of doxorubicin and cisplatin, agents not generally considered carcinogenic by themselves in humans. Kaldor and coworkers[195] concluded that at least one of the two drugs was leukemogenic. The controversies engendered by large-scale studies of this kind are reflected in the editorial that accompanied the article and the brisk correspondence that followed.[196,197]

Travis and associates[198] underscore these issues by their findings regarding the 4402 10-year survivors among the 32,251 women with ovarian cancer on whom they collected data. They found 1296 SMNs rather than the expected 1014 in such a cohort, the cumulative risk at 20 years of follow-up being 18.2% vs. the 11.5% expected in the general population. Although leukemias appeared to be related to chemotherapy and cancers in infradiaphragmatic sites appeared to be related to radiotherapy, there were also increased risks of tumors in other sites—for example, breast cancer and ocular melanoma—that are not obviously related to the treatments used. Travis and associates[198] therefore postulated genetic or other factors that predispose to ovarian cancer as being responsible. In this way, they echo the surmises of Werner-Wasik and colleagues[144] concerning the SMNs that develop in women with cervical cancer.

Fisher and coworkers[199] reviewed the extensive experience accumulated in women treated for breast cancer following the protocols of the National Surgical Adjuvant Breast and Bowel Project (NSABP). Using data from the Surveillance, Epidemiology and End Results (SEER) Registry for comparison, they reported a relative risk of 24.0 for AML among all patients treated with surgery and chemotherapy. The risk was found to be 39.3 among patients under 50 years of age, compared with a relative risk of 19.9 among those age 50 or older. The relative risks of AML were 2.6 among all women treated with surgery only and 10.3 among those treated

with surgery and RT. These data confirm the leukemogenicity of l-phenylalanine mustard, the alkylating agent employed in the chemotherapy trials conducted by the NSABP.[195] Curtis and associates[182] reported relative risks for ANLL or myelodysplastic syndrome of 10.0 and 17.4 among unirradiated and irradiated patients with breast cancer, respectively, who were treated with an alkylating agent.

Greene[193] reviewed the evidence concerning the carcinogenicity of cisplatin in animals and humans and provided a concise survey of the oncogenic potential of other chemotherapeutic agents in common use in adults with cancer. He pointed out that cisplatin has many of the properties of an oncogen and is carcinogenic in animal systems, where its effects can be reversed by MESNA (2-mercaptoethane-sulfonate). The evidence implicating cisplatin as a leukemogen in humans is found in situations where it has been used together with etoposide or doxorubicin. It is not clear whether cisplatin is a cofactor in leukemogenesis when used with other drugs, or whether these other drugs, rather than cisplatin, are responsible.

AML, usually of French-American-British M5 morphology, having a characteristic translocation that involves 11q23, is being detected in patients given topoisomerase II inhibitors.[200-202] The anthracyclines, epipodophyllotoxins, and dactinomycin are such inhibitors.[202] Detourmignies and colleagues[130] implicated inhibitors of topoisomerase II in their report of therapy-associated acute promyelocytic leukemia (t-APL). They pointed out that the same translocation, t(15;17), can be identified in both de novo and treatment-related acute promyelocytic leukemias that develop after therapy with drugs of this class.

van Leeuwen[203] provided an extensive analysis of AML and myelodysplasia developing after cancer treatments of various kinds and at different ages. In general, the findings authoritatively confirm the observations of others in that chemotherapy was found to be more leukemogenic than irradiation, and the latent periods for the appearance of nonlymphatic leukemias after therapy with topoisomerase II inhibitors and alkylating agents tended to be short (<5 years) and long (5–10 years), respectively. There has been a recent report of a 23-year interval between treatment of HD and the appearance of secondary erythroleukemia. This was attributed to the alkylating agents used as part of the HD therapy.[204] van Leeuwen's detailed analyses by original tumor type, treatments employed, and age factors are worthy of careful reading by students of this problem.

Solid Tumors. Solid tumors are not often associated with anticancer drugs. Four breast carcinomas were listed by Greene[193] among the few solid tumors that appeared in cisplatin-treated women without there being a convincing causative relationship. A dose-effect relationship between alkylating agent treatment and the occurrence of secondary bone sarcomas was identified in children, and there have been several reports of urothelial carcinomas and other tumors in adults treated with cyclophosphamide.[66,204-208] That alkylating agents can be responsible for bladder cancer was established by the experience with

TABLE 66-2

Estimated Risk of Acute Nonlymphoblastic Leukemia in Adults Treated for Hodgkin Disease at the Istituto Nazionale Tumori, Milan, Italy

TREATMENT	NO. OF PATIENTS	MEDIAN FOLLOW-UP (YEARS)	ANLL OBSERVED	ANLL EXPECTED	ACTUARIAL RISK (%)
RT alone	307	11	0	5.1	0
CT alone	96	8	1	0.9	1.4±2.3
RT ± ABVD	180	8.5	0	2.4	0
RT ± MOPP	335	9	9	4.8	10.2±5.2
RT ± ALK	411	11	9	5.8	4.8±1.6

ALK, various regimens containing alkylating agents and/or procarbazine; ANLL, acute nonlymphoblastic leukemia; CT, chemotherapy; RT, radiotherapy.
Adapted from Valagussa P, Santoro A, Fossati-Bellani F, et al: Second acute leukemia and other malignancies following treatment for Hodgkin's disease. J Clin Oncol 1986;4:830–837.

chlornaphazine, an agent no longer marketed for this reason.[209] Although the data of Fairchild and coworkers[210] and others[211] suggested that cyclophosphamide was not a significant etiologic factor for bladder cancer, Travis and associates[212] reported a relative risk of 4.5 of bladder cancer among patients with NHL treated with cyclophosphamide. The relative risk increased with increasing cumulative dose, being 6.3 for cumulative doses of 20–49 g and 14.5 for cumulative doses of 50 g or more. Topical nitrogen mustard has been held responsible for the appearance of skin cancers in patients with mycosis fungoides treated in that way.[213]

Hodgkin's Disease. There is a voluminous literature concerning the leukemias, NHLs, and solid tumors that are encountered in adults with HD, with often conflicting reports. Major focus here will be placed on two recent analyses of large series that studied the solid tumor and leukemia risks. Results of past reviews are shown in Tables 66-2 and 66-3.[214-219]

The relative and absolute excess risks of site-specific SMNs in long-term HD survivors was assessed by Dores and colleagues.[220] They analyzed data from 32,591 HD patients that included 1111 25-year survivors and found 1726 solid tumors among those patients. Cancers of the lung, GI tract, and female breast were the most frequently observed. The actuarial SMN rate among 25-year survivors was about 20%, with the risk being about the same in all age groups. Of interest was an apparent decrease in SMN risk after the 25th year of survival. The leukemia risk in HD survivors was reviewed by Brusamolino and coworkers.[221] Their 1659-patient sample was analyzed according to age, splenectomy, combined modality therapy, and cumulative drug doses, especially of alkylating agents, including nitrosourea derivatives. The overall actuarial risk of leukemia at 15 years was 4.2%, with two peaks. These occurred at three and eight years after initiation of therapy, and the curve flattened at 12 years. The risks after RT alone, chemotherapy alone, and combined modality treatments were 0.3%, 2.8%, and 5.4%, respectively. Risks were higher among patients receiving extended field RT, lomustine, or mechlorethamine. Neither age nor splenectomy proved to be significant independent variables. No leukemias were found in patients treated with ABVD (Adriamycin, bleomycin, vinblastine, dacarbazine).

The difficulties in reaching conclusions regarding cause and effect are brought out sharply by a historic paper by Rosner,[222] who 20 years ago reviewed 82 HD patients with AML. His analyses necessarily reflected the treatments in use before that time—RT in various doses and field

TABLE 66-3

Second Malignant Solid Tumors Following Treatment of Adults for Hodgkin's Disease*

AUTHOR	XRT ONLY	XRT ± CHEMO (ADJUVANT)	XRT ± CHEMO (SALVAGE)	CHEMO ONLY
Coltman et al[215]	1.5%	3.0%	2.6%	2.9%
Glicksman et al[216]			9.5% (IF) 7.5%, 7.1% (EF) 6.6% (TNI)	
Tester et al[217]	7.0%	7.0%	9.0%	7.0%
Tucker et al[218]	7.0%	11.7%	16.5%	5.5%
Valagussa et al[214†]	8.9%		9.9% (MOPP) 5.8% (ABVD)	0.0%

EF, extended field radiation therapy; IF, involved field radiation therapy; TNI, total nodal radiation therapy.
*Excludes non-Hodgkin's lymphomas.
†See also the 1997 report of Swerdlow et al.[219] that gives standardized incidence ratios for various treatments employed.

arrangements. He found three patients in whom the two diseases appeared to coexist, but he nonetheless implicated RT as the major oncogenic factor, despite the fact that 3 of the 82 patients with AML had not been irradiated. He concluded that "It is...possible that acute leukemia is part of the natural history of HD..."[222] Indeed, it is difficult to escape the implication that therapy could play a role in disengaging the two conditions rather than being a causative factor. The appeal by Aisenberg and Finkelstein[223] for great care in the collection of data and their analyses resonates today.

Secondary non–Hodgkin's Lymphoma. The cumulative incidence rate of secondary NHL among HD patients, which increased during the first five years after treatment before reaching a plateau, was not correlated with any specific treatment or combinations of therapies. Swerdlow and colleagues[219] suggest that immunosuppression could be a contributing factor to the occurrence of secondary NHL in HD patients, most if not all of whom have long been known to be immunologically impaired at diagnosis.[224,225]

Other Primary Sites. An extensive review of SMNs among more than 600,000 Swedish patients was conducted by Dong and Hemminki,[226] who found standardized cumulative incidence rates of 8.4% and 8.7% for males and females, respectively. The risks were very high (more than tenfold) for certain concordant sites such as the nose, skin squamous cell cancers, bone, and connective tissue for both males and females. In males, this held true for breast cancer and cancers of the upper aerodigestive tract; and in females, it held true for leukemia. Boysen and Loven[227] studied the SMN problem in 714 survivors of head and neck cancers. They found 84 SMNs in 81 patients, 10 of the 84 SMNs being synchronous with the index squamous cell carcinoma. The annual incidence of SMNs was 3.5%, and the relative risk was 2.4. Ancillary features (sex, age, stage) were not governing factors, but Boysen and Loven[227] point out that SMNs become a greater concern than local tumor recurrence after three years of follow-up. Reynolds and coworkers,[228] in a similar study, implicated lifestyle and environmental factors. They seem to be important cofactors in the genesis of SMNs in patients with head and neck cancers.

Shingaki and associates[229] also found SMNs in 20 of 61 patients with stage I and II squamous cell carcinomas of the oral cavity who had been treated with surgery alone, thus absolving ancillary therapies as contributing factors.

The importance of possible genetic factors in the etiology of SMNs has been mentioned by several authors (e.g., Travis[123]). Jefferies and colleagues[230] investigated whether the suppressor gene CDKN2A (p16) on chromosome 9 might have played a role in the SMNs that developed in 40 patients with squamous cell cancer of the head and neck region. This was done because of the frequent loss of heterozygosity in that region in patients with such primary tumors. No mutations were found, however, leading the authors to conclude that p16 loss was not a factor.

Evidence for possible underlying genetic influences (or at least, common etiologic factors) comes forward when cancers develop in nonconcordant structures. Osteosarcoma and hereditary retinoblastoma, discussed earlier in this chapter, is a prime example. Malmer and coworkers[231] found a similar disconnect in their very large cohort study of patients with colorectal cancer, representing more than 570,000 person-years at risk. They found an increased risk of meningioma (especially in women) among these survivors, a relationship that has yet to be explained.

Immunosuppression

Drugs and drug combinations that produce profound immunosuppression could be responsible for the appearance of lymphomas and other tumors.[232] Such neoplasms have long been known to be associated with deliberate immunosuppression in transplant patients and in those with acquired immunodeficiency syndrome.[233,234]

Kinlen and associates[232] were among the first to conduct a systematic study of cancers appearing in patients who had been given immunosuppressive drugs. In 1979, they reported an increase in the risk of NHL (especially in the brain) in renal transplant recipients (RR = 58.6).

Curtis and colleagues[96] have revisited this issue recently and reported that bone marrow transplant (BMT) survivors are at risk of developing solid tumors with the passage of time. Their analyses were based on 20,000 BMT recipients; many different types of SMNs were encountered, including brain and thyroid tumors. These developed only in patients who were given brain and total body irradiation (TBI). The highest risk was in young children (<10 years of age). Although Lai and coworkers[235] criticized the choice of controls, the Curtis[96] results are generally in keeping with those reported by others.[236,237]

The risks of myelodysplastic syndrome (MDS) and acute myelogenous leukemia (AML) after therapy were discussed by Hosing and associates.[238] They studied almost 500 patients with NHL who received high-dose chemotherapy and autologous stem cell transplantation and found 22 patients with MDS or AML. The risk was highest among patients receiving total body irradiation together with cyclophosphamide and etoposide.

Prolonged immunosuppression is associated with the appearance of skin cancers.[188,232] Kinlen and colleagues[232] estimated increased risks of basal cell, squamous cell, and melanotic malignancies to be 1.2, 23, and 8, respectively, in renal transplant patients. Liddington and coworkers[239] reported cutaneous carcinomas (mostly of the squamous cell type) in renal transplant patients and estimated the increase in risk to be approximately 100-fold. Penn[188] found four instances of de novo, unrelated malignant tumors, one of them a skin cancer, in a review of 101 patients with cancer undergoing organ transplantation. Other investigators have described similar cases.[240]

Hormones

Hormones and hormonal manipulations have been held responsible in oncogenesis. Various second tumors have been reported in men with prostatic cancer treated with estrogens. These include breast cancers, hepatomas, and desmoids.[241-243] In women, the use of oral contraceptives that emphasize the estrogenic component has been held responsible for the subsequent appearance of endometrial cancer. This is a potential source of SMNs in female patients with cancer managed by hormonal manipulations or in women who use hormone-based contraceptives.[244]

Recommendations and Conclusions

The recommendations made previously for children apply equally to adults, suitably modified for the age group. In adults particularly, for whom the prognosis often is worse than in children, the potential risk of a second malignant process should not lead to therapeutic compromises when treatment, often aggressive, is of known benefit. As shown in Figure 66-7, further SMN research must take into fuller account possible contributory genetic, immunologic, environmental, and other factors beyond which drugs and what RT doses were used.

ACKNOWLEDGMENTS

The authors thank Mrs. Diane Piacente and Mrs. Lee Sucher for preparation of the manuscript.

REFERENCES

1. Westermeier T, Kaatsch P, Schoetzau A, Michaelis J: Multiple primary neoplasms in childhood: Data from the German Children's Cancer Registry. Eur J Cancer 1998;34:687.
2. Tucker MA, Meadows AT, Boice JD, et al: Cancer risk following treatment of childhood cancer. In Boice JD Jr, Fraumeni JF Jr.(ed): Radiation Carcinogenesis, Epidemiology and Biological Significance. New York, Raven Press, 1984, p 211.
3. Green DM, Zevon MA, Reese PA, et al: Second malignant tumors following treatment during childhood and adolescence for cancer. Med Pediatr Oncol 1994;22:1-10.
4. Olsen JH, Garwicz S, Hertz H, et al: Second malignant neoplasms after cancer in childhood or adolescence. Br Med J 1993;307:1030-1036.
5. Hawkins MM, Draper GJ, Kingston JE: Incidence of second primary tumors among childhood cancer survivors. Br J Cancer 1987;56:339-347.
6. De Vathaire F, Hawkins M, Campbell S, et al: Second malignant neoplasms after a first cancer in childhood: Temporal pattern of risk according to type of treatment. Br J Cancer 1999;79:1884-1893.
7. Li FP: Second malignant tumors after cancer in childhood. Cancer 1977;40:1899-1902.
8. Li FP, Cassady JR, Jaffe N: Risk of second tumors in survivors of childhood cancer. Cancer 1975;35:1230-1235.
9. Neglia JP, Friedman DL, Yasui Y, et al: Second malignant neoplasms in five-year survivors of childhood cancer: Childhood Cancer Survivor Study. J Natl Cancer Inst 2001;93:618-629.
10. de Vathaire F, Schweisguth O, Rodary C, et al: Long-term risk of a second malignant neoplasm after a cancer in childhood. Br J Cancer 1989;59:448-452.
11. Eng C, Li FP, Abramson DH, et al: Mortality from second tumors among long-term survivors of retinoblastoma. J Natl Cancer Inst 1993;85:1121-1128.
12. Wong FL, Boice JD Jr, Abramson DH, et al: Cancer incidence after retinoblastoma: Radiation dose and sarcoma risk. JAMA 1997;278:1262-1267.
13. Kitchin FD, Ellsworth RM: Pleiotropic effects of the gene for retinoblastoma. J Med Genet 1974;11:244-246.
14. Draper GJ, Sanders BM, Kingston JE: Second primary neoplasms in patients with retinoblastoma. Br J Cancer 1986;53:661-671.
15. Li FP, Fraumeni JF Jr, Mulvihill JJ, et al: A cancer family syndrome in twenty-four kindreds. Cancer Res 1988;48:5358-5362.
16. Law JC, Strong LC, Chidambaram A, Ferrell RE: A germ line mutation in exon 5 of the p53 gene in an extended cancer family. Cancer Res 1992;51:6385-6387.
17. Santibanez MF, Birth JM, Hartley AL, et al: p53 germline mutations in Li-Fraumeni syndrome. Lancet 1991;338:1490.
18. Malkin D, Li FP, Strong LC, et al: Germ line p53 mutations in a familial syndrome of breast cancer, sarcomas and other neoplasms. Science 1990;250:1233-1238.
19. Srivastava S, Zou Z, Pirollo K, Blattner W, Chang EH: Germ-line transmission of a mutated p53 gene in a cancer-prone family with Li-Fraumeni syndrome. Nature 1990;348:747-749.
20. Malkin D, Jolly KW, Barbier N, et al: Germ line mutations of the p53 tumor-suppressor gene in children and young adults with second malignant neoplasms. N Engl J Med 1992;326:1309-1315.
21. Malkin D, Friend SH, Li FP, Strong LC. Germ-line mutations of the p53 tumor-suppressor gene in children and young adults with second malignant neoplasms [letter]. N Engl J Med 1997;336:734.
22. Menon AG, Anderson KM, Riccardi VM, et al: Chromosome 17p deletions and p53 gene mutations associated with the formation of malignant neurofibrosarcomas in von Recklinghausen neurofibromatosis. Proc Natl Acad Sci USA 1990;87:5435-5439.
23. Garwicz S, Anderson H, Olsen JH, et al: Second malignant neoplasms after cancer in childhood and adolescence: A population-based case-control study in the 5 Nordic countries. Int J Cancer 2000;88:672-678.
24. Rapley EA, Barfoot R, Bonaiti-Pellie C, et al: Evidence for susceptibility genes to familial Wilms tumor in addition to WT1, FWT1 and FWT2. Br J Cancer 2000;83:177-183.
25. McDonald JM, Douglass EC, Fisher R, et al: Linkage of familial Wilms' tumor predisposition to chromosome 19 and a two-locus model for the etiology of familial tumors. Cancer Res 1998;58:1387-1390.
26. Rahman N, Arbour L, Tonin P, et al: Evidence for a familial Wilms tumor (FWT1) on chromosome 17q12-q21. Nat Genet 1996;13:461-463.
27. Pelletier J, Bruening W, Kashtan CE, et al: Germline mutations in the Wilms' tumor suppressor gene are associated with abnormal urogenital development in Denys-Drash syndrome. Cell 1991;67:437-447.
28. Bruening W, Bardeesy N, Silverman BL, et al: Germline intronic and exonic mutations in the Wilms' tumour gene (WT1) affecting urogenital development. Nature Genet 1992;1:144-148.
29. Li FP, Yan JC, Sallan S, et al: Second neoplasms after Wilms' tumor in childhood. J Natl Cancer Inst 1983;71:1205-1209.
30. D'Angio GJ, Meadows A, Mike V, et al: Decreased risk of radiation associated second malignant neoplasms in actinomycin D treated patients. Cancer 1976;37:1177-1185.
31. Breslow NE, Takashima JR, Whitton JA, et al: Second malignant neoplasms following treatment for Wilms tumor: A report from the National Wilms Tumor Study Group. J Clin Oncol 1995;13:1851-1859.
32. Hartley AL, Birch JM, Blair V, Morris-Jones P, Gattamaneni HR, Kelsey AM: Second primary neoplasms in a population-based series of patients diagnoses with renal tumours in childhood. Med Pediatr Oncol 1994;22:318-324.
33. Wikstrom S, Parkkulainen KV, Louhimo I: Bilateral Wilms' tumor and secondary malignancy. J Pediatr Surg 1982;17:269-272.
34. Sooriyaarachchi GS, Johnson RO, Carbone PP: Neoplasms of the large bowel following ureterosigmoidostomy. Arch Surg 1977;112:1174-1177.
35. Recht KA, Belis JA, Kandzari SJ, Milam DF: Ureterosigmoidostomy followed by carcinoma of the colon. Cancer 1979;44:1538-1542.
36. Gittes RF: Carcinogenesis in ureterosigmoidostomy. Urol Clin North Am 1986;13:201-205.
37. Shousa S, Scott S, Polak J: Ileal loop carcinoma after cystectomy for bladder exstrophy. Br Med J 1978;2:397-398.
38. Refetoff S, Harrison J, Karanfilski BT, Kaplan EL, DeGroot LJ, Beckerman C: Continuing occurrence of thyroid carcinoma after irradiation to the neck in infancy and childhood. N Engl J Med 1975;292:171-175.

39. Andrew DS, Kerr IF: Carcinoma of thyroid following irradiation for medulloblastoma. Clin Radiol 1965;16:282.

40. Raventos A, Duszynski DO: Thyroid cancer following irradiation for medulloblastoma. Am J Roentgenol 1965;89:175.

41. Roggli VL, Estrada R, Fechner RE: Thyroid neoplasia following irradiation for medulloblastoma. Cancer 1979;43:2232-2238.

42. Vane D, King DR, Boles ET Jr: Secondary thyroid neoplasms in pediatric cancer patients: Increased risk with improved survival. J Pediatr Surg 1984;9:855-860.

43. Tang TT, Holcenberg JS, Duck SC, Hodach AE, Oechler HW, Camitta BM: Thyroid carcinoma following treatment for acute lymphoblastic leukemia. Cancer 1980;46:1572-1576.

44. Bakri K, Shimaoka K, Rao U, Tsukada Y: Adenosquamous carcinoma of the thyroid after radiotherapy for Hodgkin's disease. Cancer 1983;52:465-470.

45. Cryer PE, Kissane JM: A functioning thyroid nodule in a patient previously treated with irradiation for Hodgkin's disease. Am J Med 1980;68:429.

46. Getaz EP, Shimaoka K, Rao U: Anaplastic carcinoma of the thyroid following external irradiation. Cancer 1979;43:2248-2253.

47. McDougall IR, Coleman CN, Burke JS, Saunders W, Kaplan HS: Thyroid carcinoma after high-dose external radiotherapy for Hodgkin's disease. Cancer 1980;45:2056-2060.

48. Moroff SV, Fuks JV: Thyroid cancer following radiotherapy for Hodgkin's disease: A case report and review of the literature. Med Pediatr Oncol 1986;14:216-220.

49. Weshler Z, Krasnokuki D, Peshin Y, Biran S: Thyroid carcinoma induced by irradiation for Hodgkin's disease. Acta Radiol (Oncol) 1978;17:383-386.

50. Constine LS, Donaldson SS, McDougall IR, Cox RS, Link MP, Kaplan HS: Thyroid dysfunction after radiotherapy in children with Hodgkin's disease. Cancer 1984;53:878-883.

51. De Vathaire F, Hardiman C, Shamsaldin A, et al: Thyroid carcinomas after irradiation for a first cancer during childhood. Arch Int Med 1999;159:2713-2719.

52. Acharya S, Sarafoglou K, LaQuaglia M, et al: Thyroid neoplasms after therapeutic radiation for malignancies during childhood or adolescence. Cancer 2003;97:2397-2403.

53. Ron E, Lubin JH, Shore RE, et al: Thyroid cancer after exposure to external radiation: A pooled analysis of seven studies. Radiat Res 1995;141:259-277.

54. Upton AC: The dose-response relation in radiation-induced cancer. Cancer Res 1961;21:717.

55. Gray LH: Cellular Radiation Biology. Baltimore, Williams and Wilkins Company. 1965.

56. Takaue Y, Sullivan MP, Ramirez I, Cleary KR, van Eys J: Second malignant neoplasm in treated Hodgkin's disease. JAMA 1986;140:49-51.

57. Chung CK, Stryker JA, Cruse R, Vannuci R, Towfighi J: Glioblastoma multiforme following prophylactic cranial irradiation and intrathecal methotrexate in a child with acute lymphocytic leukemia. Cancer 1981;47:2563-2566.

58. Rimm IJ, Li FP, Tarbell NJ, Winston KR, Sallan SE: Brain tumors after cranial irradiation for childhood acute lymphoblastic leukemia. Cancer 1987;59:1506-1508.

59. Marus G, Levin CV, Rutherford GS: Malignant glioma following radiotherapy for unrelated primary tumors. Cancer 1986;58:886-894.

60. Kumar PP, Good RR, Skultety FM, Leibrock LG, Severson GS: Radiation-induced neoplasms of the brain. Cancer 1987;59:1274-1282.

61. Nygaard R, Garwicz S, Haldorsen T, et al: Second malignant neoplasms in patients treated for childhood leukemia. Acta Paediatr Scand 1991;80:1220-1228.

62. Ron E, Modan B, Boice JD Jr, et al: Tumors of the brain and nervous system after radiotherapy in childhood. N Engl J Med 1988;319:1033-1039.

63. Neglia JP, Meadows AT, Robison LL, et al: Second neoplasms after acute lymphoblastic leukemia in childhood. N Engl J Med 1991;325:1330-1336.

64. Loning L, Zimmerman M, Reiter A, et al: Secondary neoplasms subsequent to Berlin-Frankfurt-Munster therapy of acute lymphoblastic leukemia in childhood: Significantly lower risk without cranial radiotherapy. Blood 2000;95:2770-2775.

65. Kimball Dalton VM, Gelber RD, Li F, Donnelly MJ, Tarbell NJ, Sallan SE: Second malignancies in patients treated for childhood acute lymphoblastic leukemia. J Clin Oncol 1998;16:2848-2853.

66. Tucker MA, D'Angio GJ, Boice JD Jr, et al: Bone sarcomas linked to radiotherapy and chemotherapy in children. N Engl J Med 1987;317:588-593.

67. Olsen JH, Garwicz S, Hertz H, et al: Second malignant neoplasms after cancer in childhood or adolescence. Br Med J 1993;307:1030-1036.

68. Le Vu B, De Vathaire F, Shamsaldin A, et al: Radiation dose, chemotherapy and risk of osteosarcoma after solid tumours during childhood. Int J Cancer 1998;77:370-377.

69. Hawkins MM, Wilson LM, Burton HS, et al: Radiotherapy, alkylating agents, and risk of bone cancer after childhood cancer. J Natl Cancer Inst 1996;88:270-278.

70. Strong LC, Herson J, Osborne BM, Sutow WW: Risk of radiation-related subsequent malignant tumors in survivors of Ewing's sarcoma. J Natl Cancer Inst 1979;62:1401-1406.

71. Greene MH, Glaubiger DL, Mead GD, Fraumeni JF Jr: Subsequent cancer in patients with Ewing's sarcoma. Cancer Treat Rep 1979;63:2043-2046.

72. Kuttesch JF Jr, Wexler LH, Marcus RB, et al: Second malignancies after Ewing's sarcoma: Radiation dose-dependency of secondary sarcomas. J Clin Oncol 1996;14:2818-2825.

73. Haselow RE, Nesbit M, Dehner LP, Khan FM, McHugh R, Levitt SH: Second neoplasms following megavoltage radiation in a pediatric population. Cancer 1978;42:1185-1191.

74. Potish RA, Dehner LP, Haselow RE, Kim TH, Levitt SH, Nesbit M: The incidence of second neoplasms following megavoltage radiation for pediatric tumors. Cancer 1985;56:1534-1537.

75. Gold DG, Neglia JP, Dusenberry KE. Second neoplasms after megavoltage radiation for pediatric tumors. Cancer 2003;97:2588-2596.

76. O'Malley B, D'Angio GJ, Vawter GF: Late effects of roentgen therapy given in infancy. Am J Roentgenol 1963;89:1067.

77. Li FP, Corkery J, Vawter G, Fine W, Sallan SE: Breast carcinoma after cancer therapy in childhood. Cancer 1983;51:521-523.

78. Reimer RR, Fraumeni JF Jr, Reddick F, Moorhead EL II: Breast carcinoma following radiotherapy of metastatic Wilms' tumor. Cancer 1977;40:1450-1452.

79. Hancock SL, Tucker MA, Hoppe RT: Breast cancer after treatment of Hodgkin's disease. J Natl Cancer Inst 1993;85:25-31.

80. Bhatia S, Robison LL, Oberlin O, et al: Breast cancer and other second neoplasms after childhood Hodgkin's disease. N Engl J Med 1996;334:745-751.

81. Aisenberg AC, Finklestein DM, Doppke KP, Koerner FC, Boivin JF, Willet CG: High risk of breast carcinoma after irradiation of young women with Hodgkin's disease. Cancer 1997;79:1203-1210.

82. Sankila R, Garwicz S, Olsen JH, et al: Risk of subsequent malignant neoplasms among 1,641 Hodgkin's disease patients diagnosed in childhood and adolescence: A population based cohort study in the five Nordic countries. J Clin Oncol 1996;14:1442-1446.

83. Miller AB, Howe GR, Sherman GJ, et al: Mortality from breast cancer after irradiation during fluoroscopic examinations in patients being treated for tuberculosis. N Engl J Med 1989;321:1285-1289.

84. Boice JD Jr, Preston D, Davis FG, Monson RR: Frequent chest x-ray fluoroscopy and breast cancer incidence among tuberculosis patients in Massachusetts. Radiat Res 1991;125:214-222.

85. Hoffman DA, Lonstein JE, Morin MM, Visscher W, Harris BS 3rd, Boice JD Jr: Breast cancer in women with scoliosis exposed to multiple diagnostic X rays. J Natl Cancer Inst 1989;81:1307-1312.

86. Shore RE, Hildreth N, Woodard E, Dvoretsky P, Hempelmann L, Pasternack B: Breast cancer among women given X-ray therapy for acute post partum mastitis. J Natl Cancer Inst 1986;77:689-696.

87. Mattson A, Ruden B-I, Hall P, Wilking N, Rutqvist LE: Radiation-induced breast cancer: Long-term follow-up of radiation therapy for benign breast disease. J Natl Cancer Inst 1993;85:1679-1685.

88. Hildreth NG, Shore RE, Dvoretsky PM: The risk of breast cancer after irradiation of the thymus in infancy. N Engl J Med 1989;321:1281-1284.

89. Modan B, Chetrit A, Alfandary E, Katz L: Increased risk of breast cancer after low-dose irradiation. Lancet 1989;i:629-631.

90. Tokunaga M, Land CE, Yamamoto T, et al: Incidence of female breast cancer among atomic bomb survivors, Hiroshima and Nagasaki, 1950-1980. Radiat Res 1987;112:243-272.

91. Li FP: Colon cancer after Wilms' tumor [letter]. J Pediatr 1980;96:954-955.

92. Opitz JM: Adenocarcinoma of the colon following Wilms' tumor [letter]. J Pediatr 1980;96:774-775.

93. Sabio H, Teja K, Elkon D, Shaw A: Adenocarcinoma of the colon following the treatment of Wilms' tumor. J Pediatr 1979;95:424-426.

94. Bhatia S, Ramsay NKC, Steinbuch M, et al: Malignant neoplasms following bone marrow transplantation. Blood 1996;87:3633-3639.

95. Bhatia S, Louie AD, Bhatia R, et al: Solid cancers after bone marrow transplantation. J Clin Oncol 2001;19:464-471.

96. Curtis RE, Rowlings PA, Deeg HJ, et al: Solid cancers after bone marrow transplantation N Engl J Med 1997;336:897-904.

97. Meadows AT, Obringer AC, Marrero O, et al: Second malignant neoplasms following childhood Hodgkin's disease: Treatment and splenectomy as risk factors. Med Pediatr Oncol 1989;17:477-484.

98. Donaldson SS, Link MP: Combined modality treatment with low-dose radiation and MOPP chemotherapy for children with Hodgkin's disease. J Clin Oncol 1987;5:742-749.

99. Schellong G, Riepenhausen M, Creutzig U, et al: Low risk of secondary leukemias after chemotherapy without mechlorethamine in childhood Hodgkin's disease. J Clin Oncol 1997;15:2247-2253.

100. Tucker MA, Meadows AT, Boice JD Jr, et al: Leukemia after therapy with alkylating agents for childhood cancer. J Natl Cancer Inst 1987;78:459-464.

101. De Vathaire F, Francois P, Hill C, et al: Role of radiotherapy and chemotherapy in the risk of second malignant neoplasms after cancer in childhood: Temporal pattern of risk according to type of treatment. Br J Cancer 1989;59:792-796.

102. Klein G, Michaelis J, Spix C, et al: Second malignant neoplasms after treatment of childhood cancer. Eur J Cancer 2003;39:808-817.

103. Pui C-H, Behm FG, Raimondi SC, et al: Secondary acute myeloid leukemia in children treated for acute lymphoid leukemia. N Engl J Med 1989;321:136-142.

104. Pui C-H, Ribaeiro RC, Hancock ML, et al: Acute myeloid leukemia in children treated with epipodophyllotoxins for acute lymphoblastic leukemia. N Engl J Med 1991;325:1682-1687.

105. Pedersen-Bjergaard J, Daugaard G, Hansen SW, Philip P, Larsen SO, Rorth M: Increased risk of myelodysplasia and leukaemia after etoposide, cisplatin, and bleomycin for germ cell tumours. Lancet 1991;338:359-363.

106. Winick NJ, McKenna RW, Shuster JJ, et al: Secondary acute myeloid leukemia in children with acute lymphoblastic leukemia treated with etoposide. J Clin Oncol 1993;11:209-217.

107. Sugita K, Furukawa T, Tsuchida M, et al: High frequency of etoposide (VP-16)-related secondary leukemia in children with non-Hodgkin's lymphoma. Am J Pediatr Hematol/Oncol 1993;15:99-104.

108. Hawkins MM, Kinnier Wilson LM, Stovall MA, et al: Epipodophyllotoxins, alkylating agents and radiation and risk of secondary leukaemia after childhood cancer. Br Med J 1992;304:951-958.

109. Beaumont M, Sanz M, Carli PM, et al: Therapy-related acute promyelocytic leukemia. J Clin Oncol 2003;21:2123-2137.

110. LeDeley MC, Leblanc T, Shamsaldin A, et al: Risk of secondary leukemia after a solid tumor in childhood according to the dose of epipodophyllotoxins and anthracyclines: A case-control study by the Societe Francaise d'Oncologie Pediatrique. J Clin Oncol 2003;21:1074-1081.

111. Aplan PD, Chervinsky DS, Stanulla M, Burhans WC: Site-specific DNA cleavage within the MLL breakpoint cluster region induced by topoisomerase II inhibitors. Blood 1996;87:2649-2658.

112. Stanulla M, Wang J, Chervinsky DS, Thandala S, Aplan PD: DNA cleavage within the MLL breakpoint cluster region is a specific event which occurs as part of higher-order chromatin fragmentation during the initial stages of apoptosis. Mol Cell Biol 1997;17:4070-4079.

113. Stanulla M, Wang J, Chervinsky DS, Aplan PD: Topoisomerase II inhibitors induce DNA double-strand breaks at a specific site within the AML1 locus. Leukemia 1997;11:490-496.

114. Fradkin JE, Mills JL, Schonberger LB, et al: Risk of leukemia after treatment with pituitary growth hormone. JAMA 1993;270:2829-2832.

115. Sklar CA, Mertens AC, Mitby P, et al: Risk of disease recurrence and second neoplasms in survivors of childhood cancer treated with growth hormone: A report from the Childhood Cancer Survivor Study. J Clin Endocrinol Metabol 2002;87:3136-3141.

116. Mulhern RK, Tyc VL, Phipps S, et al: Health-related behaviors of survivors of childhood cancer. Med Pediatr Oncol 1995;25:159-165.

117. Troyer H, Holmes GE: Cigarette smoking among childhood cancer survivors [letter]. Am J Dis Child 1988;142:123.

118. Corkery JC, Li FP, McDonald JA, Hanley JA, Holmes GE, Holmes FF: Kids who really shouldn't smoke [letter]. N Engl J Med 1979;300:1279.

119. Haupt R, Byrne J, Connelly RR, et al: Smoking habits in survivors of childhood and adolescent cancer. Med Pediatr Oncol 1992;20:301-306.

120. Green DM, Zevon MA, Hall B: Cigarette smoking among survivors of cancer diagnosed during childhood or adolescence [abstract]. Proc Am Soc Clin Oncol 1997;16:519a.

121. Tao ML, Guo MD, Weiss R, et al: Smoking in adult survivors of childhood acute lymphoblastic leukemia. J Natl Cancer Inst 1998;90:219-225.

122. Li FP: Cancer families: Human models of susceptibility to neoplasia—the Richard and Linda Rosenthal Foundation Award Lecture. Cancer Res 1998;48:5381-5386.

123. Travis LB: Therapy-associated solid tumors. Acta Oncol 2002;41:323-333.

124. Hemminki K, Jiang Y, Steineck G: Skin cancer and non-Hodgkin's lymphoma as second malignancies: Markers of impaired immune function? Eur J Cancer 2003;39:223-229.

125. Lalle P, Moyret C, Bignon YJ: Lack of germ-line mutations in the p53 gene exons 4 to 8 in patients with late-onset second malignant neoplasms. Cancer Genet Cytogenet 1994;76:148-150.

126. Elkind MM, Bedford JS, Benjamin SA, et al: Oncogenic mechanisms in radiation-induced cancer. Cancer Res 1991;51:2740-2747.

127. Swift M, Morrell D, Massey RB, Chase CL: Incidence of cancer in 161 families affected by ataxia-telangiectasia. N Engl J Med 1991;325:1831-1836.

128. Little MP, Muirhead CR, Haylock RG, Thomas M: Relative risks of radiation-associated cancer: Comparison of second cancer in therapeutically irradiated populations with the Japanese atomic bomb survivors. Radiat Environ Biophy 1999;38:267-283.

129. Le Beau MM, Albain KS, Larson RA, et al: Clinical and cytogenetic correlations in 63 patients with therapy-related myelodysplastic syndromes and acute non-lymphocytic leukemia: Further evidence for characteristic abnormalities of chromosomes no. 5 and 7. J Clin Oncol 1986;4:325-345.

130. Detourmignies L, Castaigne S, Stoppa AM, et al: Therapy-related acute promyelocytic leukemia: A report on 16 cases. J Clin Oncol 1992;10:1430-1435.

131. Collins VP, Nordenskjold M, Dumanski JB: Molecular aspects of meningiomas. Brain Pathol 1970;1:19.

132. el Azouzi M, Chung RY, Farmer GE, et al: Loss of distinct regions on the short arm of chromosome 17 associated with tumorigenesis of human astrocytomas. Proc Natl Acad Sci USA 1989;86:7186-7190.

133. Stewart FW, Treves N: Lymphangiosarcoma in postmastectomy lymphedema. A report of three cases. Cancer 1948;1:64.

134. Edeiken S, Russo DP, Knecht J, Parry LA, Thompson RM: Angiosarcoma after tylectomy and radiation therapy for carcinoma of the breast. Cancer 1992;70:644-647.

135. Benda JA, Al-Jurf AS, Benson AB 3rd: Angiosarcoma of the breast following segmental mastectomy complicated by lymphedema. Am J Clin Pathol 1987;87:651-655.

136. Marchal C, Weber B, de Lafontan B, et al: Nine breast angiosarcomas after conservative treatment for breast carcinoma: A survey from French comprehensive cancer centers. Int J Radiat Oncol 1999;44:113-119.

137. Cosset JM: Radiation-induced cancers: State of the art in 1997. Cancer Radiother 1997;1:823-835.

138. Lindsay KA, Wheldon EG, Deehan C, et al: Radiation carcinogenesis modeling for risk of treatment-related second tumours following radiotherapy. Br J Radiol 2001;74:529–536.

139. Lagrange J-L, Ramaioli A, Chateau M-C, et al: Sarcoma after radiation therapy: Retrospective multi-institutional study of 80 histologically confirmed cases. Radiol 2000;216:197.

140. Tountas AA, Fornasier VL, Harwood AR, Leung PM: Postirradiation sarcoma of bone: A perspective. Cancer 1979;43:182–187.

141. Kim JH, Chu FCH, Woodard HQ, Huvos AG: Radiation induced sarcomas of bone following therapeutic radiation. Int J Radiat Oncol Biol Phys 1983;9:107–110.

142. Cavazza A, Travis LB, Travis WD, et al: Post-irradiation malignant mesothelioma. Cancer 1997;79:192.

143. Storm HH: Second primary cancer after treatment for cervical cancer. Late effects after radiotherapy. Cancer 1988;61:679–688.

144. Werner-Wasik M, Schmid CH, Bornstein L, Madoc-Jones H: Increased risk of second malignant neoplasms outside radiation fields in patients with cervical carcinoma. Cancer 1995;75: 2281–2285.

145. Sturgeon SR, Curtis RE, Johnson K, Ries L, Brinton LA: Second primary cancers after vulvar and vaginal cancers. Am J Obstet Gynecol 1996;174:929–933.

146. Hemminki K, Dong C: Cancer in husbands of cervical cancer patients. Epidemiology 2000;11:347–349.

147. Hall HI, Jamison P, Weir HK: Second primary ovarian cancer among women diagnosed previously with cancer. Cancer Epidemiol Biom Preven 2001;10:995–999.

148. Bergfeldt K, Nilsson B, Einhorn S, Hall P: Breast cancer risk in women with a primary ovarian cancer: A case-control study. Eur J Cancer 2001;37:2229–2234.

149. Travis LB, Curtis RE, Boice JD Jr, Platz CE, Hankey BF, Fraumeni JF Jr: Second malignant neoplasms among long-term survivors of ovarian cancer. Cancer Res 1996;56:1564–1570.

150. Buiatti E, Crocetti E, Acciai S et al: Incidence of second primary cancers in three Italian population-based cancer registries. Eur J Cancer 1997;33:1829–1834.

151. Mark RJ, Poen J, Tran LM, Fu YS, Heaps J, Parker RG: Postirradiation sarcoma of the gynecologic tract. A report of 13 cases and a discussion of the risk of radiation-induced gynecologic malignancies. Am J Clin Oncol 1996;19:59–64.

152. Koyama K, Furukawa Y, Tanaka H: Multiple primary malignant neoplasms in urologic patients. Scand J Urol Nephrol 1995;29: 483–490.

153. Movsas B, Hanlon AL, Pinover W, Hanks GE: Is there an increased risk of second primaries following prostate irradiation? Internat J Radiat Oncol Biol Phys 1998;41:251–255.

154. Johnstone PA, Powell CR, Riffenburgh R, Rohde DC, Kane CJ: Second primary malignancies in T1-3N0 prostate cancer patients treated with radiation therapy with 10-year follow-up. J Urol 1998;159:946–949.

155. Brenner DJ, Curtis RE, Hall EJ, Ron E: Second malignancies in prostate carcinoma patients after radiotherapy compared with surgery. Cancer 2000;88:398–406.

156. Wanderas EH, Fossa SD, Tretli S: Risk of a second germ cell cancer after treatment of a primary germ cell cancer in 2201 Norwegian male patients. Eur J Cancer 1997;33:244–252.

157. Ruther U, Dieckmann K, Bussar-Maatz R, Eisenberger F: Second malignancies following pure seminoma. Oncol 2000;58:75–82.

158. Travis LB, Curtis RE, Storm H, et al: Risk of second malignant neoplasms among long-term survivors of testicular cancer. J Natl Cancer Inst 1997;89:1429–1439.

159. Nichols CR, Loehrer PJ Sr: The story of second cancers in patients cured of testicular cancer: Tarnishing success or burnishing irrelevance? J Natl Cancer Inst 1997;89:1394–1395.

160. MacKee GM, Cipollaro AC: X-Rays and Radium in the Treatment of Diseases of the Skin, 4th ed. Philadelphia, Lea and Febiger, 1946.

161. Sherrill DJ, Grishkin BA, Galal FS, Zajtchuk R, Graeber GM: Radiation associated malignancies of the esophagus. Cancer 1984;54:726–728.

162. Glanzmann CH, Schultz G, Lutolf UM: Long-term morbidity of adjuvant infradiaphragmatic irradiation in patients with testicular cancer and implications for the treatment of stage I seminoma. Radiother Oncol 1991;22:12–18.

163. Moller H, Mellemgaard A, Jacobsen GK, Pedersen D, Storm HH: Incidence of second primary cancer following testicular cancer. Eur J Cancer 1993;29A:672–676.

164. Obedian E, Fischer DB, Haffty BG: Second malignancies after treatment of early-stage breast cancer: lumpectomy and radiation therapy versus mastectomy. J Clin Oncol 2000;18:2406–2412.

165. Rubino C, de Vathaire F, Diallo I, Shamsaldin A, Le MG: Increased risk of second cancers following breast cancer: role of the initial treatment. Breast Cancer Res Treat 2000;61:183–195.

166. Fowble B, Hanlon A, Freedman G, Nicolaou N, Anderson P: Second cancers after conservative surgery and radiation for stages I-II breast cancer: identifying a subset of women at increased risk. Int J Radiat Oncol Biol Phys 2001;51:679–690.

167. Frass BA, Roberson PL, Lichter AS: Dose to the contralateral breast due to primary breast irradiation. Int J Radiat Oncol Biol Phys 1985;11:485–497.

168. Boice JD, Harvey EB, Blettner M, et al: Cancer in the contralateral breast after radiotherapy for breast cancer. N Engl J Med 1992;326:781–785.

169. Levitt SH, Mandel JS: Breast carcinogenesis: risk of radiation [editorial]. Int J Radiat Oncol Biol Phys 1985;11:1421–1423.

170. Correspondence. Cancer in the contralateral breast after radiotherapy for breast cancer. N Engl J Med 1992;327:430-ff.

171. Neugut AI, Robinson E, Lee WC, Murray T, Karowski K, Kutcher GJ: Lung cancer after radiation therapy for breast cancer. Cancer 1993;71:3054–3057.

172. Inskip PD, Stovall M, Flannery JT: Lung cancer risk and radiation dose among women treated for breast cancer. J Natl Cancer Inst 1994;86:983–988.

173. Neugut AI, Murray T, Santos J, Amols H, Hayes MK, Flannery JT: Increased risk of lung cancer after breast cancer radiation therapy in cigarette smokers. Cancer 1994;73:1615–1620.

174. Travis LB, Curtis RE, Bennett WP, Hankey BF, Travis WD, Boice JD: Lung cancer after Hodgkin's disease. J Natl Cancer Inst 1995;87:1324–1327.

175. Kaldor JM, Day NE, Bell J, Clark EA, Langmark F, Karjalainen S: Lung cancer following Hodgkin's disease: A case-control study. Int J Cancer 1992;52:677–681.

176. Van Leeuwen FE, Klokman WJ, Stovall M, Hagenbeek A, van den Belt-Dusebout AW, Noyon R: Roles of radiotherapy and smoking in lung cancer following Hodgkin's disease. J Natl Cancer Inst 1995;87:1530–1537.

177. Jones A: Radiation oncogenesis in relation to the treatment of pituitary tumours. Clin Endocrinol 1991;35:379–397.

178. Cavin LW, Dalrymple GV, McGuire EL, Maners AW, Broadwater JR: CNS tumor induction by radiotherapy: A report of four new cases and estimate of dose required. Int J Radiat Oncol Biol Phys 1990;18:399–406.

179. Soffer D, Gomori JM, Siegl T, Shalit MN: Intracranial meningiomas after high-dose irradiation. Cancer 1989;63:1514–1519.

180. Erfurth EM, Bulow B, Mikoczy Z, Svahn-Tapper G, Hagmar L: Is there an increase in second brain tumours after surgery and irradiation for a pituitary tumour? Clin Endocrinol 2001;55: 613–616.

181. Hutchinson GB: Leukemia in patients with cancer of the cervix uteri treated with radiation: A report covering the first 5 years of an international study. J Natl Cancer Inst 1968;40:951.

182. Curtis RE, Boice JD Jr, Stovall M, Bernstein L, Greenberg RS, Flannery JT: Risk of leukemia after chemotherapy and radiation treatment for breast cancer. N Engl J Med 1992;326:1745–1751.

183. Boice JD, Hutchison GB: Leukemia in women following radiotherapy for cervical cancer. Ten-year follow-up of an international study. J Natl Cancer Inst 1980;65:115–129.

184. Kyle RA, Pierre RV, Bayrd ED: Multiple myeloma and acute myelomonocytic leukemia: Report of four cases possibly related to melphalan. N Engl J Med 1970;283:1121–1125.

185. Reimer RR, Hoover R, Fraumeni JF Jr, Young RC: Acute leukemia after alkylating-agent therapy of ovarian cancer. N Engl J Med 1977;297:177–181.

186. Rosner F, Grunwald H: Multiple myeloma terminating in acute leukemia: report of 12 cases and review of the literature. Am J Med 1974;57:927–939.

187. Kaslow RA, Wisch N, Glass JL: Acute leukemia following cytotoxic chemotherapy. JAMA 1972;219:75–76.

188. Penn I: Second malignant neoplasms associated with immunosuppressive medications. Cancer 1976;37:1024-1032.
189. Cohen RJ, Wiernik PH, Walker MD: Acute non-lymphocytic leukemia associated with nitrosourea chemotherapy: Report of two cases. Cancer Treat Rep 1976;60:1257-1261.
190. Boice JD Jr, Greene MH, Killen JY Jr, et al: Leukemia and preleukemia after adjuvant treatment of gastrointestinal cancer with semustine (methyl CCNU). N Engl J Med 1983;309:1079-1084.
191. Greene MH, Boice JD Jr, Strike TA: Carmustine as a cause of acute non-lymphocytic leukemia. N Engl J Med 1985;313:579.
192. Brenez D, Devriendt J, Lenclud C, Schmerber J: Acute non-lymphocytic leukemia following chemotherapy with cisplatin and etoposide for non-small-cell carcinoma of the lung: A case report. Cancer Chemother Pharmacol 1990;26:235-236.
193. Greene MH: Is cisplatin a human carcinogen? J Natl Cancer Inst 1992;84:306-312.
194. Greene MH, Boice JD, Greer BE, Blessing JA, Dembo AJ: Acute non-lymphocytic leukemia after therapy with alkylating agents for ovarian cancer. N Engl J Med 1982;307:1416-1421.
195. Kaldor JM, Day NE, Pettersson F, Clarke EA, Pedersen D, Mehnert W: Leukemia following chemotherapy for ovarian cancer. N Engl J Med 1990;322:1-6.
196. Coltman CA Jr, Dahlberg S: Treatment-related leukemia. N Eng J Med 1990;322:52-53.
197. Correspondence. N Engl J Med 1990;322:1818-ff.
198. Travis LB, Curtis RE, Boice JD Jr, Platz CE, Hankey BF, Fraumeni JF Jr: Second malignant neoplasms among long-term survivors of ovarian cancer. Cancer Res 1996;56:1564-1570.
199. Fisher B, Rockette H, Fisher ER, Wickerham DL, Redmond C, Brown A: Leukemia in breast cancer patients following adjuvant chemotherapy or postoperative radiation: The NSABP experience. J Clin Oncol 1985;3:1640-1658.
200. Albain KS, LeBeau MM, Ullirsch R, Schumacher H: Implication of prior treatment with drug combinations including inhibitors of topoisomerase II in therapy-related monocytic leukemia with a 9;11 translocation. Genes Chromosom Cancer 1990;2:53-58.
201. Pedersen-Bjergaard J, Sigsgaard TC, Nielsen D, Gjedde SB, Philip P, Hansen M: Acute monocytic or myelomonocytic leukemia with balanced chromosome translocations to band 11q23 after therapy with 4-epi-doxorubicin and cisplatin or cyclophosphamide for breast cancer. J Clin Oncol 1992;10:1444-1451.
202. Smith MA, Rubinstein L, Ungerleider RS: Therapy-related acute myeloid leukemia following treatment with epipodophyllotoxins: Estimating the risks. Med Pediatr Oncol 1994;23:86-98.
203. van Leeuwen FE: Risk of acute myelogenous leukemia and myelodysplasia following cancer treatment. Baillieres Clin Haematol 1996;9:57-85.
204. Scully RE, Mark EJ, McNeely WF, Ebeling SH, Phillips LD: Case records of the Massachusetts General Hospital—Case 38-1997. N Engl J Med 1997;337:1895-1903.
205. Carney CN, Stevens PS, Fried FA, Mandell J: Fibroblastic tumor of the urinary bladder after cyclophosphamide therapy. Arch Pathol Lab Med 1982;106:247-249.
206. Fuchs EF, Kay R, Poole R, Barry JM, Pearse HD: Uroepithelial carcinoma in association with cyclophosphamide ingestion. J Urol 1981;126:544.
207. Durkee C, Benson R: Bladder cancer following administration of cyclophosphamide. Urology 1980;16:145-148.
208. Chasko SB, Keuhnelian JG, Gutowski WT, Gray GF: Spindle cell cancer of bladder during cyclophosphamide therapy for Wegener's granulomatosis. Am J Surg Path 1980;4:191-196.
209. Videbaek A: Chlornaphazine (Erysan) may induce cancer of the urinary bladder. Acta Med Scand 1964;176:45.
210. Fairchild WV, Spence CR, Solomon HD, Gangai MP: The incidence of bladder cancer after cyclophosphamide therapy. J Urol 1979;122:163-164.
211. Pearson RM, Soloway MS: Does cyclophosphamide induce bladder cancer? Urology 1978;XI:437-447.
212. Travis LB, Curtis RE, Glimelius B, Holowaty EJ, Van Leeuwen FE, Lynch CF: Bladder and kidney cancer following cyclophosphamide therapy for non-Hodgkin's lymphoma. J Natl Cancer Inst 1995;87:524-530.
213. Lee LA, Fritz KA, Golitz L, Fritz TJ, Weston WL: Second cutaneous malignancies in patients with mycosis fungoides treated with topical nitrogen mustard. J Am Acad Dermatol 1982;7:590-598.
214. Valagussa P, Santoro A, Fossati-Bellani F, Bonfi A. Bonadonna G: Second acute leukemia and other malignancies following treatment for Hodgkin's disease. J Clin Oncol 1986;4:830-837.
215. Coltman CA Jr, Dixon DO: Second malignancies complicating Hodgkin's disease: A Southwest Oncology Group 10-years follow-up. Cancer Treat Rep 1982;66:1023-1033.
216. Glicksman AS, Pajak TF, Gottlieb A, Nissen N, Stutzman L, Cooper MR: Second malignant neoplasms in patients successfully treated for Hodgkin's disease: A Cancer and Leukemia Group B study. Cancer Treat Rep 1982;66:1035-1044.
217. Tester WJ, Kinsella TJ, Waller B, Makuch RW, Kelley PA, Glatstein E: Second malignant neoplasms complicating Hodgkin's disease: The National Cancer Institute experience. J Clin Oncol 1984;2:762-769.
218. Tucker MA, Coleman CN, Cox RS, Varghese A, Rosenberg SA: Risk of second cancers after treatment for Hodgkin's disease. N Engl J Med 1988;318:76-81.
219. Swerdlow AJ, Barber JA, Horwich A, et al: Second malignancy in patients with Hodgkin's disease treated at the Royal Marsden Hospital. Br J Cancer 1997;75:116-123.
220. Dores GM, Metayer C, Curtis RE, Lynch CF, Clarke EA, Glimelius B: Second malignant neoplasms among long-term survivors of Hodgkin's disease: a population-based evaluation over 25 years. J Clin Oncol 2002;20:3484-3494.
221. Brusamolino E, Anselmo AP, Klersy C, Santoro M, Orlandi E. Pagnucco G: The risk of acute leukemia in patients treated for Hodgkin's disease is significantly higher after combined modality programs than after chemotherapy alone and is correlated with the extent of radiotherapy and type and duration of chemotherapy: A case-control study. Haematol 1998;83:812-823.
222. Rosner F: Acute leukemia as a delayed consequence of cancer chemotherapy. Cancer 1976;37:1033-1036.
223. Aisenberg AC, Finkelstein DM: Second malignancies in Hodgkin's disease. J Clin Oncol 2000;18:2186-2187.
224. Parker F Jr, Jackson H Jr, Fitzhugh G, Spies TD: Studies of diseases of the lymphoid and myeloid tissues. IV. Skin reactions to human and avian tuberculin. J Immunol 1932;22:277.
225. Van Rijswijk REN, Sybesma JPHB, Kater L: A prospective study of changes in immune status following radiotherapy for Hodgkin's disease. Cancer 1984;53:62-69.
226. Dong C, Hemminki K: Second primary neoplasms in 633,964 cancer patients in Sweden, 1958-1996. Int J Cancer 2001;93:155-161.
227. Boysen M, Loven JO: Second malignant neoplasms in patients with head and neck squamous cell carcinomas. Acta Oncol 1993;32:283-288.
228. Reynolds W, Firkins R, Aguiar S: Primary cancer of the head and neck. Iowa Med 1993;83:63-65.
229. Shingaki S, Kobayashi T, Suzuki I, Kohno M, Nakajima T: Surgical treatment of stage I and II oral squamous cell carcinomas: analysis of causes of failure. Br J Oral Maxillofacial Surg 1995; 33:304-308.
230. Jefferies S, Edwards SM, Hamoudi RA, A'Hern R, Foulkes W, Goldgar D: No germline mutations in CDKN2A (p16) in patients with squamous cell cancer of the head and neck and second primary tumours. Br J Cancer 2001;85:1383-1386.
231. Malmer B, Tavelin B, Henriksson R, Gronberg H: Primary brain tumours as second primary: a novel association between meningioma and colorectal cancer. Int J Cancer 2000;85:78-81.
232. Kinlen LJ, Sheil AGR, Peto J, Doll R: Collaborative United Kingdom–Australasian study of cancer in patients treated with immunosuppressive drugs. Br Med J 1979;2:1461-1466.
233. Penn I, Hammond W, Brettschneider L, Starzl TE: Malignant lymphomas in transplantation patients. Transplant Proc 1969;1:106-112.
234. Snider WD, Simpson DM, Aronyk K: Primary lymphoma of the nervous system associated with acquired immune-deficiency syndrome [letter]. N Engl J Med 1983;308:45.
235. Lai S, Page JB, Lai H: Solid cancers after bone marrow transplantation. N Engl J Med 1997;337:345-346.
236. Riddler SA, Breinig MC, McKnight JL: Increased levels of circulating Epstein-Barr virus (EBV)-infected lymphocytes and decreased EBV nuclear antigen antibody responses are associated with the development of post-transplant lymphoproliferative

disease in solid-organ transplant recipients. Blood 1994;84: 972–984.

237. Hanto DW, Gajl-Peczalska KJ, Frizzera G, Arthur DC, Balfour HH Jr, McClain K: Epstein-Barr virus (EBV) induced polyclonal and monoclonal B-cell lymphoproliferative diseases occurring after renal transplantation: Clinical, pathologic, and virologic findings and implications for therapy. Ann Surg 1983;198:356–369.

238. Hosing C, Munsell M, Yazji S, Anderson B, Couriel D, deLima M: Risk of therapy-related myelodysplastic syndrome/acute leukemia following high-dose therapy and autologous bone marrow transplantation for non-Hodgkin's lymphoma. Ann Oncol 2002;13:450–459.

239. Liddington M, Richardson AJ, Higgins RM, Endre ZH, Venning VA, Murie JA: Skin cancer in renal transplant recipients. Br J Surg 1989;76:1002–1005.

240. Morland BJ, Radford M: Cutaneous squamous cell carcinoma following treatment for acute lymphoblastic leukaemia. Med Pediatr Oncol 1993;21:150–152.

241. Dore B, Dombriz M, Denis P, Darracq-Paries JC: Cancer of the breast in patients having prostatic cancer treated with estrogens. Report of three cases. J Urol 1982;88:247–252.

242. Brooks JJ: Hepatoma associated with diethylstilbestrol therapy for prostatic carcinoma. J Urol 1982;128:1044–1045.

243. Svanvik J, Knutsson F, Jansson R, Ekman H: Desmoid tumor in the abdominal wall after treatment with high dose Estradiol for prostatic cancer. Acta Chir Scand 1982;148:301–303.

244. Weiss NS, Sayvetz TA: Incidence of endometrial cancer in relation to the use of oral contraceptives. N Engl J Med 1980;302: 551–554.

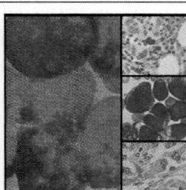

CANCER IN THE ELDERLY: BIOLOGY, PREVENTION, AND TREATMENT

Lodovico Balducci

Claudia Beghé

SUMMARY OF KEY POINTS

INCIDENCE

- Cancer in the older person is increasingly common.
- Data about the prevention and the management of cancer in the older person are limited.

EPIDEMIOLOGY OF AGING AND CANCER

- The older population continues to expand due to reduced mortality and birth rates. Currently 60% of all malignancies occur in persons aged 65 and older, and this proportion is expected to rise to 70% by the year 2030. Although cancer-related mortality is declining among younger persons, it is increasing among the oldest ones.
- Of special interest, cancer appears to affect mainly older individuals who are otherwise healthy and would have lived longer were it not for the cancer.

AGING AND CARCINOGENESIS

The association of cancer and age may be explained by three mechanisms that are not mutually exclusive:

1. Carcinogenesis is a time-consuming process, the end-product of which, cancer, is more likely to develop at an advanced age.
2. Aging is associated with molecular changes that mimic carcinogenesis; older cells are primed to the effects of environmental carcinogens.
3. Aging is associated with environmental phenomena such as immune senescence or proliferative senescence that favor the development of cancer.

AGING AND CANCER BIOLOGY

The biology of common malignancies such as breast cancer, ovarian cancer, non-Hodgkin's lymphoma, and acute myeloid leukemia (AML) may change with age. In some cases the tumor may become more indolent, whereas in others it becomes more aggressive.

Two mechanisms underlie these changes:

1. The biology of the tumor cells (e.g., the prevalence of MDR1 in AML increases after age 60, causing a worse prognosis).
2. The aging of the patient: an age-related increase in circulating concentrations of interleukin 6 (IL-6) may favor the growth of lymphomas, whereas hormonal senescence may inhibit the growth of breast cancer.

ASSESSMENT OF THE OLDER PERSON

- Aging involves a progressive shortening of life expectancy and reduction in the functional reserve of multiple organ systems.
- Personal and social resources to cope with stress may become more limited.
- Reduced life expectancy and reduced stress tolerance lessen the benefits and enhance the risks of medical intervention.
- A comprehensive geriatric assessment (CGA), evaluating the patient's function, comorbidity, cognition, nutrition, medications, and living resources, is a currently available, reliable instrument for predicting life expectancy and the risk of treatment-related complications.
- The CGA may unveil preexisting situations such as undiagnosed disease, poor nutrition, depression, or lack of adequate social support that are remediable and may influence the outcome of treatment.
- A number of laboratory tests, including the circulating levels of IL-6 and D-dimer, and tests of physical performance may complement the CGA.

CANCER PREVENTION

- Older individuals may be primary candidates for chemoprevention of

cancer, but none of the current chemopreventative agents have demonstrated efficacy definitively.
- Screening asymptomatic patients for cancer of the breast and of the large bowel appears reasonable when the life expectancy is 5 years or longer.

CANCER TREATMENT

- *Surgery:* Age by itself, up to age 100, does not appear to increase the risk of surgical mortality, although the risk of surgical complications and length of postoperative hospitalization increase with age. Age is a definitive risk factor for mortality related to emergency surgery.
- *Radiation therapy:* Tolerance for radiation therapy seems to remain high, even for individuals aged 80 and older.
- *Cytotoxic chemotherapy:* The main pharmacologic changes of age include decreased excretion of drugs and of their active metabolites from the kidneys; decreased volume of distribution of water-soluble drugs, which may in part be accounted for by anemia; increased susceptibility to myelodepression, mucositis, and peripheral and central neuropathy; and cardiomyopathy. The National Cancer Center Network (NCCN) has issued the following guidelines for the management of older cancer patients:
  1. Dose adjustment according to individual glomerular filtration rate (GFR), for patients aged 65 and older.
  2. Prophylactic use of filgrastim or pegfilgrastim for patients aged 65 and older treated with combination chemotherapy of dose-intensity comparable to that of cyclophosphamide, doxorubicin, vincristine, and prednisone (CHOP).
  3. Maintenance of hemoglobin levels of 12 g/dL or greater.

INTRODUCTION

The progressive aging of the population is an epidemiologic hallmark of our times. People aged 65 and older represented 12% of the population in 1990; the percentage in this age group is expected to grow to 20% by 2030.[1] The segment of the older population undergoing the most rapid growth is that older than 85, the so-called "oldest old."

Aging is the most important risk factor for cancer. The incidence of common malignancies increases with age—in fact, currently more than 50% of all neoplasms occur in persons aged 65 and older[2] (Fig. 67-1), and this proportion is expected to increase to 70% by 2030. Cancer-related mortality has decreased for persons younger than 65 since 1950, but has remained stable or even increased for older persons.[2] Clearly, improved cancer control involves effective management of cancer in older individuals.

This chapter explores the association between cancer and aging, the influence of aging on cancer biology, and prevention and treatment of cancer in older persons, after reviewing the biologic and the clinical aspects of aging. The main goal is to provide a frame of reference allowing the practitioner to estimate risks and benefits of preventive and therapeutic interventions in each individual.

BIOLOGY OF AGING

Molecular and Cellular Biology

Cellular aging "in vitro" (cells aging in the plate or test tube) is associated with a number of molecular events, some of which may favor and others inhibit the development of cancer. Formation of DNA adducts, DNA hypomethylation, and point mutation[3] mimic the early stages of carcinogenesis, are associated with activation of oncogenes and inhibition of antiproliferative genes, and may prime the aging cell to the effects of environmental carcinogens, which explains, in part, the association between cancer and age. Other changes, including a progressive reduction in telomere length and telomerase activity[4] and activation of the P14 antiproliferative gene, encoding the CDK16 inhibitor, are contrary to those

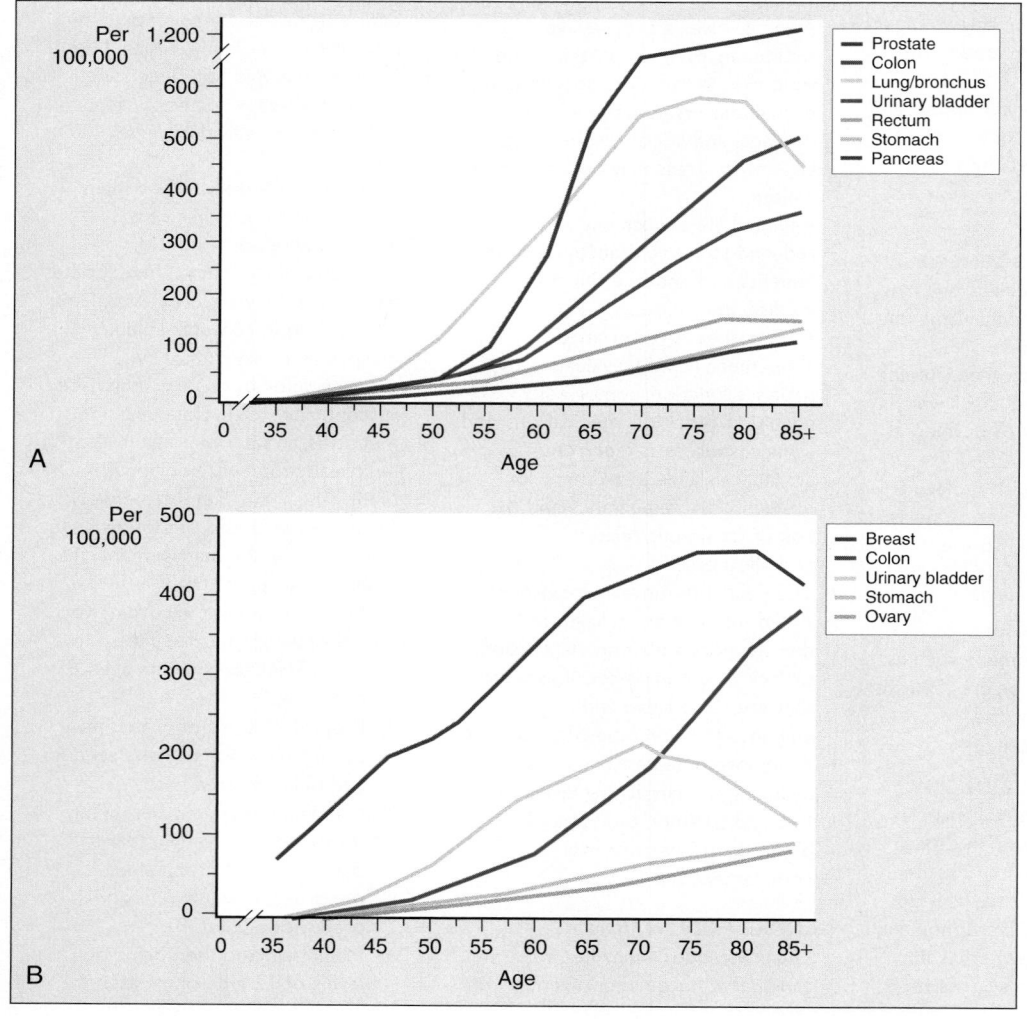

Figure 67-1. Incidence of different neoplasms with age. **A,** Men. **B,** Women.

observed in neoplastic cells.[5] Of special interest are age-related abnormalities in protein synthesis, with reduced activity of DNA-repairing and drug-metabolizing enzymes, which may both accelerate carcinogenesis and enhance the complications of cytotoxic chemotherapy in normal tissues.[6]

Paradoxically, proliferative senescence may enhance the risk of cancer, because together with the ability to replicate themselves the senescent cells lose the ability to undergo apoptosis and do acquire immortality.[7,8] Proliferative senescence also is associated with the production of tumor growth factors and of proteolytic enzymes that may favor metastatic spread.[7,8]

Physiology of Aging

Aging involves a progressive reduction in the functional reserve of multiple organ systems, with reduced tolerance of stress, including cancer and cancer treatment. The mechanisms may include increased prevalence of chronic diseases;[9] progressive accumulation of catabolic cytokines, including interleukins 6 and 10 and tumor necrosis factor in the circulation;[10] and reduction in the stem cell reserve of different tissues.[11] Catabolic cytokines appear pivotal in physiologic aging: their accumulation is associated with increased prevalence of geriatric syndromes,[12] increased risk of mortality and functional decline,[11] and a generalized catabolic status.[13]

From the standpoint of cancer treatment the most significant changes include gastrointestinal, renal, hepatic, hematopoietic, and mucosal changes, which may alter the pharmacokinetics of antineoplastic agents and may increase the risk of complications from cancer treatment.

BIOLOGICAL INTERACTIONS OF CANCER AND AGING

Aging may affect tumor biology at two levels: carcinogenesis and tumor growth.

Aging and Carcinogenesis

The association of aging with carcinogenesis may be explained by at least three mechanisms: duration of carcinogenesis, increased susceptibility of aging tissues to environmental carcinogens,[3] and changes in body environment, including proliferative senescence[7] and immune senescence.[14] Both experimental and epidemiologic findings support the theory that aging tissues are more susceptible to environmental carcinogens. Several murine tissues, including cutaneous, hepatic, lymphatic, and nervous tissues, have been found to be more likely to develop cancer after exposure to carcinogens if they are obtained from older animals.[3] In humans, the incidence of some cancers, such as nonmelanomatous skin cancer and prostate cancer, increases geometrically with age, suggesting enhanced carcinogenesis.[2] In addition, the incidence of some neoplasms, including non-Hodgkin's lymphomas,[15] anaplastic astrocytomas, and glioblastoma multiforme,[16] has increased several-fold among older

individuals during the past 30 years, suggesting that older individuals may be more susceptible than the younger ones to new environmental carcinogens. In the Italian city of Trieste, Barbone and coworkers found that the incidence of lung cancer after exposure to environmental pollutants increased in relation to the patient's age at the time of exposure.[17] The increased susceptibility of older individuals to environmental carcinogens indicates that primary cancer prevention, including elimination of environmental carcinogens and chemoprevention, may be particularly effective in older individuals. This is a new concept, directly opposed to common wisdom, which has held that preventative interventions are less efficacious for older individuals.

Aging and Tumor Growth

Aging may influence tumor growth at two levels, the neoplastic cell itself and the host environment in which the tumor grows. It is reasonable to expect a concentration of more indolent tumors among older individuals (Fig. 67-2), by a process of natural selection. This is certainly the case with breast cancer, as the prevalence of well-differentiated, hormone receptor–rich tumors increases with age.[18]

The influence of the tumor host on cancer growth was demonstrated in a now-classic experiment by Ershler and coworkers, who demonstrated that the same load of Lewis lung carcinoma and B16 melanoma were associated with shorter survival and higher incidence of metastasis in younger animals.[19] In successive studies, these authors demonstrated that the tumor growth rate seemed to decrease for poorly immunogenic and increase for highly immunogenic tumors as the host age increased, highlighting the influence of immune senescence on tumor growth. In humans, Kurtz and coworkers demonstrated a reduction in the growth rate of primary breast cancer among older women, related directly to the degree of mononuclear cell reactions.[20] This observation suggested that immune senescence may mitigate tumor growth in poorly immunogenic tumors.

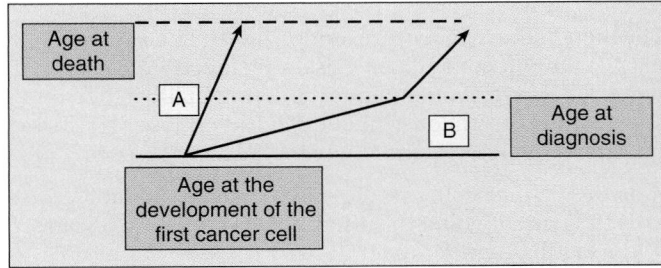

Figure 67-2. The prevalence of more indolent tumors may increase with age for a process of natural selection. In this figure, two persons start developing cancer, both at the age of 35 years. One cancer (A) is very aggressive, and will become manifest at age 37 and cause death at age 39. The other (B) is very indolent, will not become manifest until age 65, and will not cause the patient's death until age 75. By a process of natural selection, due to the earlier deaths of the bearers of more aggressive tumors, one can expect to find a higher prevalence of indolent tumors among older individuals.

TABLE 67-1

Age and Changes in Cancer Prognosis		
NEOPLASM	**AGE-RELATED CHANGES IN PROGNOSIS**	**MECHANISM (S)**

Acute myelogenous leukemia[73]	Worse with age:
	    Increased resistance to chemotherapy
	    Increased mortality during induction
		Neoplastic cell
		    Increased prevalence of MDR1-expressing cells
		    Increased prevalence of stem cell leukemia

Non-Hodgkin's lymphoma[21]	Worse with age:
	    Decreased duration of complete remission
		Tumor host
		    Increased circulating concentration of interleukin-6

Breast cancer[20]	More indolent disease	Neoplastic cell
		    Increased prevalence of hormone receptor-rich,
		    well-differentiated tumors
		Tumor host
		    Decreased production of sex hormones
		    Immune senescence

Celomic ovarian cancer[21]	Worse with age:
	    Decreased remission duration
	    Decreased survival
		Unknown

Non–small cell lung cancer[21]	Better prognosis with age Presentation at an earlier stage	Unknown

The clinical behavior of several human malignancies may change with the age of the patient.[21] Table 67-1 reveals that the biology of both the tumor cell and the tumor host may influence the change in prognosis. Another important observation is that in some cases the prognosis becomes worse with age, contrary to the generally held view. In any case, age by itself should not be considered a prognostic factor. If it is true that approximately 80% of breast cancers in women aged 70 and older are rich in hormone receptors, the converse is also true: 20% of cancers of women in this age group are *not* rich in hormone receptors and may require cytotoxic chemotherapy. If MDR1 is present in 67% of patients over age 60 with AML, it also is true that 33% of these patients have a disease responsive to chemotherapy and potentially curable. Each case should be treated on its own merits based on an estimate of risks and benefits.

CLINICAL EVALUATION OF THE OLDER PATIENT

The benefit of cancer prevention and cancer treatment may be reduced and the risk enhanced in the older person, due to a simultaneous reduction in life expectancy and in the tolerance of medical interventions. The basic questions of geriatric oncology include the following:

- Is the patient going to die with cancer or of cancer?
- Is the patient going to suffer the consequence of cancer during his/her lifetime?
- Is the patient able to tolerate cancer treatment?

The answer to these questions may be provided by a comprehensive geriatric assessment (CGA) (Table 67-2) involving the patient's level of functioning and his or her coexisting medical conditions (e.g., comorbidity, geriatric syndromes, polypharmacy, malnutrition) and the social resources available to ensure compliance with and safety of cancer treatment.

General Principles of Geriatric Assessment

In general geriatrics, the CGA has succeeded in reducing the rate of functional dependence and of admission to the hospital and to adult living facilities.[22-24] In geriatric oncology, the CGA may unearth conditions that may compromise cancer treatment. In a pilot study involving 15 women aged 70 and older with early breast cancer, the performance of the CGA resulted in, on average, an additional 17.2 interventions per patient.[25] Three studies exploring the effects of CGA in older cancer patients demonstrated some degree of functional dependence in approximately 70% of those patients; some degree of comorbidity in more than 70% of them; and dementia, malnutrition, and depression in approximately 20%.[26-28]

The CGA also helps to make a gross estimate of the patient's life expectancy and expected tolerance of treatment. Life expectancy declines with the degree of functional dependence and also with the seriousness of comorbidity and of geriatric syndromes.[29-31] Two recent studies demonstrated that the risk of chemotherapy-induced myelosuppression increased for patients who were dependent in some instrumental activities of daily living.[32,33]

The CGA also provides a common language for use in the classification of older individuals undergoing cancer treatment or enrolled in clinical trials. For this purpose, the subdivision of age into four different functional states as proposed by Hamerman is particularly helpful[34] (Table 67-3). The two definitions of frailty are not mutually exclusive.[35,36] The alternative definition is more comprehensive and makes it possible to classify as frail some of the individuals who do not fit the original definition. The group of highest interest in geriatric oncology is the intermediate group, because the majority of cancer patients probably fall in this group. Unfortunately the scope of this group is poorly defined, with one side bordering on full independence and the other bordering on frailty. This group of patients may be referred to as

TABLE 67-2

Comprehensive Geriatric Assessment and Clinical Implications

ASSESSMENT	CLINICAL IMPLICATIONS
Functional Status	
Activities of daily living (ADL) and instrumental activities of daily living (IADL)	Relation to life expectancy, functional dependence, and tolerance of stress
Comorbidity	
Number of comorbid conditions and comorbidity indices	Relation to life expectancy and tolerance of stress
Mental Status	
Folstein Mini Mental Status	Relation to life expectancy and dependence
Emotional Conditions	
Geriatric Depression Scale (GDS)	Relation to life expectancy; may indicate motivation to receive treatment
Nutritional Status	
Mini Nutritional Assessment (MNA)	Reversible condition; possible relationship to survival
Polypharmacy	Risk of drug interactions
Geriatric Syndromes	
Delirium, dementia, depression, falls, incontinence, spontaneous bone fractures, neglect and abuse, failure to thrive, vertigo	Relationship to survival Functional dependence

vulnerable. A user-friendly questionnaire, the Vulnerable Elderly Survey 13 (VES 13), scores vulnerability on the basis of functional impairment.[37] A number of issues related to the VES 13 still need clarification, including its relationship with comorbidity and cognitive, social, and emotional conditions.

Clinical Aspects of Geriatric Assessment

Function

Function is assessed based on performance status, activities of daily living (ADLs), and instrumental activities of daily living (IADLs). The ADLs include transferring,

TABLE 67-3

Taxonomy of Age

GROUP	CHARACTERISTICS	TREATMENT IMPLICATIONS
Primary	No functional dependence Negligible comorbidity	Standard treatment
Intermediate (functional reserve substantially reduced; some degree of reversibility)	Dependence in one or more IADLs Stable comorbidity (e.g., stable angina, chronic renal insufficiency)	Attempts at rehabilitation and correction of reversible conditions Special precautions such as provision of caregiver and reduction of initial chemotherapy dose.
Secondary, or frailty (negligible functional reserve, no reversibility; rehabilitation directed only to prevent further deterioration)	One of the following criteria: Dependence in one or more ADLs Three or more comorbid conditions or one poorly controlled comorbid conditions One or more geriatric syndromes Alternative definition: at least three of the following: Involuntary weight loss (≥ 10% original weight over 1 year) Steady fatigue Difficulty in initiating movements Slow movements Reduced grip strength	Symptom management, which may include chemotherapy at low doses, is the main goal of treatment.
Near death (irreversible decline toward death)		Terminal care

ADLs, activities of daily living; IADLs, instrumental activities of daily living.
Modified from Hamerman DL: Toward an understanding of frailty. Ann Intern Med 1999;130:945–950.

CLINICAL EVALUATION OF THE FRAIL PERSON

The diagnosis of frailty indicates an almost complete exhaustion of the functional reserve and negligible ability to tolerate even minimal stress. Because the implications of this diagnosis for cancer treatment are critical, it is important to highlight a few points:

- Frailty is a chronic condition, which in general predates the diagnosis of cancer. A delirious older person with a neoplasm of the stomach who was completely independent before the start of vomiting and becoming dehydrated clearly is not frail. That person is experiencing an acute complication of her or his malignancy that should be treated with all determinate speed and aggressiveness.
- Even frail patients may benefit from palliative chemotherapy for symptom management. Although frailty is associated with reduced life expectancy, that does not necessarily mean that death is imminent: about 60% of frail individuals are alive 2 years after the diagnosis of frailty. Some of these patients include older women with breast cancer metastatic to the bones or older men with prostate cancer metastatic to the bones, who require palliation for their pain. Opioids are not always desirable in these patients because of unpleasant side effects, which may include nausea, constipation, and delirium. Under such circumstances, the use of chemotherpay in low doses (e.g., capecitabine, navelbine, gemcitabine, doxil, weekly taxanes) may represent the most effective form of symptom management.

The definition of frailty is evolving as more effective rehabilitation approaches become available and a number of biological markers of aging emerge (e.g., IL-6, D-dimer). The clinician should stay in touch with developments in this field.

bathing, dressing, eating, toileting, and continence; dependence in one or more of these activities, with the exception of continence, is considered a sign of frailty and is associated with a 2-year mortality rate around 40%.[26,27,35] The IADLs are those activities necessary to maintain an independent life, including use of transportation shopping ability to take medications, to provide one's own meals, to use the telephone, to manage one's own finances, and to take care of laundry and housecleaning. Dependence in one or more IADLs (with the exceptions of laundry and housecleaning) is associated with a 2-year mortality rate of 16% and a 50% risk of developing dementia over 2 years.[26,27,38,39] In addition, dependence in IADLs is associated with increased risk of neutropenia from cytotoxic chemotherapy.[32,33] In two prospective studies, functional dependence and performance status (PS) appeared poorly correlated; consequently, it is recommended that they be evaluated independently.[26,27]

Comorbidity

Comorbidity is an independent cause of mortality for older cancer patients[9] and may be associated with reduced tolerance of cancer treatment. The best way to assess comorbidity is still being investigated. Satariano and Ragland identified seven conditions associated with reduced life expectancy and demonstrated that the risk of mortality increased with the number of comorbid conditions.[40] Other authors have devised comorbidity scales that take into account the degree of severity of each condition. Of these, the Cumulative Index of Related Symptoms-Geriatrics (CIRS-G) proved in some studies to be the most sensitive.[41] Another advantage of the CIRS-G is that its final score may be translated into the score of another scale of common use in epidemiologic studies, the Charlson's scale.

Anemia is of special interest among the comorbid conditions,[42] because its incidence and prevalence increase with age. Anemia is an independent risk factor for death and for myelosuppression from cytotoxic chemotherapy,[43] is a main cause of fatigue and functional dependence,[42] and may be associated with congestive heart failure and dementia.[42] An unsolved question is what level of hemoglobin defines anemia. Of special interest is the Women's Health Study, showing that hemoglobin levels lower than 13.4 g/dL were an independent risk factor for death among 556 home-dwelling women aged 65 and over, followed prospectively for a period of 8 years.[44] In cancer patients anemia was associated with

ASSESSMENT OF OLDER INDIVIDUALS: SCREENING TESTS

The comprehensive geriatric assessment (CGA) is time-consuming. A number of provisions that save office time may render its use more cost-effective. Proposed strategies include the following:

- Home assessment, in which questionnaires are mailed to the patient at home and completed there before the office visit. The advantage is reduction of the visit time. Disadvantages include dependence on self-reported function and comorbidity, patient's inability to assess his or her own cognition, and inability of a significant proportion of patients to complete the questionnaire.
- Administration of screening tests before the visit, with a more complete CGA then performed for patients who screen positive. The Vulnerable Elderly Survey 13 (VES 13), one of the best-validated screeing tests, can be completed in less than 1 minute. This is our favorite approach, because it saves time and has been validated with functional and survival outcomes. Potential disadvantages include disagreement among clinicians on the score above which the test is considered positive and lack of a way to provide information about comorbidy, nutrition, cognition, and emotional disorders.
- Use of laboratory tests or physical performance tests to screen patients at risk of death and disability. This approach is promising but needs validation, and shoud be considered at present to be in clinical trials.
- An additional issue is the age at which screening should begin. We have selected an age of 70 and older, because previous studies have shown that the steepest increase in prevalence of age-related changes is seen between age 70 and 75.

reduced survival, whereas correction of anemia with erythropoietin was shown possibly to improve survival.[45]

Geriatric Syndromes

Geriatric syndromes include a number of conditions typical, if not specific, of aging, such as dementia, depression, delirium, incontinence, vertigo, falls, spontaneous bone fractures, failure to thrive, and neglect and abuse. Geriatric syndromes are associated with reduced life expectancy and are considered a hallmark of frailty.[35] To be considered a geriatric syndrome, these conditions must interfere with a person's daily life. Dementia must be moderate to severe; delirium must occur as a result of medications or organic diseases that do not commonly affect the central nervous system (e.g., urinary or upper respiratory infections); incontinence must be complete and irreversible; and falls must occur at least three times a month or the fear of falling must prevent regular activities such as walking. Depression is of special interest, because it is associated with decreased life expectancy, even when it is subclinical.[46] Depression also interferes with treatment compliance and in many cases may be fully reversible by medication. A simple 15-item questionnaire, the Geriatric Depression Scale 15 (GDS 15) speedily and reliably detects individuals with subclinical depression and is part of the CGA.[46]

Social Resources

Pivotal among the social resources is the home caregiver. The ideal caregiver should be able to recognize and manage emergencies, to support the patient physically and emotionally, to mediate conflicts among family members, and to act as spokesperson for the family with the health care provider.[47] Under the best circumstances, the caregiver is the practitioner's best ally in ensuring compliance with treatment and smooth interactions with the patient. For this reason, it behooves the practitioner to participate in the selection, training, and support of the caregiver. In reality, the caregiver of an older person often is an older spouse with health problems of his or her own or a married daughter who needs to balance her caregiving duties with other family and work responsibilities.

Nutrition

The prevalence of protein/calorie malnutrition increases with age. Isolation, depression, economic restriction, and reduced appreciation of hunger may all contribute to insufficient food intake, while chronic diseases and inflammatory cytokines may impede the synthesis of new proteins.[48] The Mini Nutritional Assessment (MNA) is a simple nutritional screening test used worldwide that identifies patients who are malnourished and those at risk of becoming malnourished, thereby permitting the prevention and early reversal of malnutrition.[49]

Polypharmacy

The prevalence of polypharmacy increases with age and among cancer patients aged 70 and older has been found to be as high as 41%.[26,27] The problem of polypharmacy exemplifies a common problem of elderly patients in developed countries: the absence of a primary care provider.[50] According to a recent study, more than 50% of individuals aged 70 and older in the United States, Canada, and Israel, although attending multiple specialty clinics, lacked a primary care physician.

Other Forms of Geriatric Assessment

The CGA is the standard form of geriatric assessment, but it may be complemented by laboratory data and by so-called "proofs" of physical performances.

Laboratory Markers of Aging

The recognition that the concentration of catabolic cytokines in the circulation increases with age and usually is correlated with the presence of geriatric syndromes prompted a number of studies aimed at establishing whether these substances may predict functional dependence and decreased survival. In a recent study, Cohen and coworkers demonstrated that increased concentrations of either interleukin-6 (IL-6) or D-dimer were associated with a 50% increase in the risk of functional dependence and death.[10] When the concentration of both substances was elevated (in the upper quartile), however, the risk increased more than threefold.

Tests of Physical Performance

Difficulty in performing some activities is considered a predictor of functional dependence and disability. Of particular interest, a recent study has shown that the risk of mortality and functional dependence can be predicted by the "get up and go" test.[51] In this test, an older individual is asked to get up from an armchair and walk 10 feet forward and back. Both inability to get up without using the chair arms and requiring more than 10 seconds to walk the distance are highly predictive of functional decline.

Issues Related to the Geriatric Assessment

A number of issues related to the application of the CGA in clinical practice need further study. Among these are the questions of which patients should undergo a CGA, who should perform the test, and whether the complete test is always necessary.

Who should undergo a CGA? In three prospective studies of cancer patients aged 70 and older, the CGA unearthed a number of conditions that were reversible and might interfere with cancer treatment.[26-28] Based on these findings. The National Cancer Center Network (NCCN) recommended some form of CGA for all cancer patients aged 70 and older.[52]

Who should perform the CGA? Ideally, the CGA should be performed by a primary care provider at periodic intervals, and the results should be part of the patient's permanent record. Any physician involved in the management of older patients should be familiar with the principles of CGA and its interpretation.

Is a full CGA necessary in all patients? Because the CGA is time-consuming, more cost-effective alternatives have been explored. Their value has not yet been determined. These include the use of a screening instrument to identify patients at high risk of functional dependence. For this purpose, the VES 13 questionnaire[37] and the "get up and go" test appear promising.[51] The problem with both of these, however, is that they do not provide any direct assessment of comorbidity, depression, cognition, and social resources. Another interesting approach was proposed by Ingram and coworkers, which involved sending to the patient's home a package including questionnaires about function, comorbidity, depression, and social resources.[28] In a population of veterans with cancer, more than 70% of the patients returned the questionnaires fully completed. Currently, a task force of the International Society of Geriatric Oncology is studying the most cost- and time-effective form of assessment for older cancer patients.

CANCER PREVENTION IN OLDER INDIVIDUALS

Some aspects of aging favor and others interfere with cancer prevention. Based on the fact that the incidence of cancer increases with age, older individuals might appear to be the population most likely to benefit from cancer prevention. At the same time, reduced life expectancy and decreased tolerance of chemopreventive therapy may lessen the benefits of some types of prevention. The study of cancer prevention in older persons is complicated by a lack of general agreement on what represents a meaningful endpoint. Should it be reduction in cancer-related mortality, as commonly accepted in prevention trials, or should it, instead, be an improvement in quality of life, given the limited life expectancy of these individuals?[53]

In this section we provide a brief review of the evidence supporting chemoprevention and early detection of cancer among older individuals.

Chemoprevention

At least three groups of substances, the selective estrogen receptor modulators (SERMs), the retinoids, and the nonsteroidal anti-inflammatory drugs (NSAIDs), have demonstrated cancer preventive activity in randomized clinical trials,[54] but these substances are used only to a limited degree in current clinical practice for cancer prevention. The SERM tamoxifen has a number of potential side effects, including endometrial cancer, deep vein thrombosis, strokes, and vasomotor and genito-urinary manifestations of menopause, the incidence of which increases with age.[53] In a decision analysis, Gail and coworkers calculated that tamoxifen may be beneficial for women aged 70 if their risk of developing breast cancer over 5 years is as high as 7% and if they do not present other contraindications to the drug; the threshold of risk at which this agent may be beneficial increases with the age of the patient.[55]

Older individuals may represent ideal candidates for future studies of chemoprevention in virtue of their increased risk of cancer, but none of the current options for chemoprevention appears optimal.

Screening and Early Detection

Because the prevalence of common cancers increases with age, one might expect that the positive predictive value of screening tests also would increase.[53] At the same time, older individuals have in general undergone screening for common cancers earlier in life. Previous examinations may have eliminated all prevalence cases and minimized the diagnostic yield of subsequent examinations.

Breast Cancer

Most of the randomized controlled studies have established that serial mammograms reduce by 20% to 30% the cancer-related mortality among women aged 50 to 70.[56] The benefits of mammography after age 70 have been suggested by three reports. A historically controlled cohort study, the Nijmegen study, showed a reduction in cancer-related mortality up to age 75[57]; a retrospective study of the Survey Epidemiology and End Results (SEER) data showed a more than twofold decrement of breast cancer–related mortality for women aged 70 to 79 who had undergone at least two mammograms after age 70[58]; and another retrospective analysis of the same data showed that women over 70 who had not undergone screening mammography presented with breast cancer at a more advanced stage than did those who had been screened.[59] An important question is the role of clinical examination of the breast (CBE). The Canadian study suggested that CBE may be as effective as screening mammography in women aged 50 to 60,[60] and the Breast Cancer Detection Demonstration Project (BCCDP) showed that mammography was superior to CBE only in the diagnosis of ductal carcinoma in situ (DCIS).[61] The CBE appears particularly attractive for older women who undergo multiple clinic visit in the course of the year, as it may be performed with no additional cost and inconvenience. A decision analysis by Kerlikowske offered a frame of reference for making screening mammography more cost-effective: this study demonstrated that limiting screening mammography to women aged 70 to 79 in the upper quintile of bone density, who are those at higher risk for breast cancer, would still detect 92% of all cancer at half the cost of screening the entire population.[62] Additional questions concern the role of new techniques such as digital mammography and MRI in older women.

Colorectal Cancer

Early detection of cancer of the large bowel reduces the cancer-related mortality for persons aged 50 to 80, but controversy lingers concerning the most appropriate screening strategy.[53] According to a recent decision analysis, full colonoscopy every 10 years is more cost-effective than yearly examination of the stool for fecal occult blood or more frequent flexible rectosigmoidoscopy.[63] Virtual colonoscopy, which appears to be as sensitive as endoscopy, may be a more comfortable alternative for older individuals.

Prostate Cancer

The value of screening asymptomatic men for prostate cancer with serial PSA determinations, and the most cost-effective screening strategies, are controversial.[53] If screening is instituted, it should be continued up to age 75, as a recent Swedish study demonstrated that radical prostatectomy reduces prostate cancer-related mortality in men up to age 75.[64]

Other Cancers

No benefits of screening women over 60 for cervical cancer have been recognized, if these women have undergone regular Papanicolaou examinations of the cervix earlier in life[53] and have had normal results. Interest in screening ex-smokers for lung cancer has been renewed by the demonstration that spiral computed tomography is able to detect small and curable cancer.[53] This approach remains controversial but may have particular interest for older individuals, because the incidence of lung cancer is increasing after age 80, probably because smoking cessation has resulted in a decrease in early coronary deaths and an increase in indolent lung cancers.[65]

Clearly, early detection of breast and colorectal cancer may reduce the mortality of older individual and may improve their quality of life. It appears reasonable to institute some form of screening for persons whose life expectancy is 5 years or longer, as the initial benefits of screening are seen after 5 years.

CANCER TREATMENT

Surgery

Although the risk of surgical mortality and other surgical complications increases with the age of the patient, elective surgery appears safe in general, even in patients over 80.[66] Individuals who are 70 years of age and older are substantially more vulnerable to the complications of emergency surgery, especially surgery related to the digestive tract. Regular screening of these individuals for colorectal cancer may minimize the incidence of emergency surgery. A number of recent advances in surgery and anesthesia have rendered cancer surgery even safer for older individuals. These include more limited surgical excisions (e.g., transanal resection of rectal cancer) and the use of anesthetic agents with a shorter half-life and minimal respiratory suppression.[67]

Radiation Therapy

Two large patient series from Europe and one from the United States attest to the feasibility and safety of radiation therapy in individuals of all ages.[68-70] Combined chemotherapy and radiation therapy in the management of cancer of the head and neck, the esophagus, the bladder, and the lung also appear well tolerated up to age 80 at least. Among the newer radiation techniques, brachyherapy and high-dose intraoperative radiation are of special interest for treatment of older patients: brachytherapy minimizes the risk of complications to normal tissues, and intraoperative radiation eliminates the inconvenience of serial visits. Data on hyperfractionated radiation in older individuals are wanted. Among the

complications of radiation therapy, mucositis is of special concern to older individuals, because age is associated with a more limited reserve of mucosal stem cells and increased proliferation of epithelial superficial cells,[71] two conditions that predispose to more prolonged and severe mucositis in older individuals. In the case of cancer of the upper airways or upper digestive tract, where the risk of mucositis is highest, nutritional management is essential and may involve prophylactic position of a percutaneous endoscopic gastrostomy tube.[70]

Cytotoxic Chemotherapy

Age is associated with changes in the pharmacokinetics and pharmacodynamics of cytotoxic drugs and increased susceptibility of certain organ systems to therapeutic complications.[71] The pharmacokinetic changes of major interest involve absorption, renal excretion, and volume of distribution of drugs.

The intestinal absorption of nutrients decreases with age, secondary to a reduction in the absorbing surface area, in the splanchnic circulation, and in gastric motility and secretions,[72] but the bioavailability of oral agents (e.g., capecitabine) does not appear to be compromised. Oral drugs are particularly appropriate for older individuals because of the convenience of administration and adjustability of doses.

A progressive reduction in glomerular filtration rate (GFR) is an almost universal consequence of aging, and it may lead to a more prolonged half-life of medications that are excreted from the kidneys (e.g., methotrexate, bleomycin, carboplatin) and of active and toxic metabolites of drugs excreted through other avenues.[71] These metabolites include daunorubicinol and idarubicinol, responsible for approximately 80% of the activity of the parent compounds,[71] and arauridine, responsible for the cerebellar toxicity of high-dose cytarabine.[71] Dose adjustment of these agents to the individual's GFR may improve tolerability.

The volume of distribution (Vd) of a drug is determined by the body composition and the concentration of serum albumin and of hemoglobin.[71] Hemoglobin is important because most antineoplastic agents are bound to red blood cells. In the presence of anemia, the free concentration in plasma and toxicity of these substances in the circulation increase.[43] Correction of anemia may then ameliorate the toxicity of chemotherapy. Among the pharmacodynamic changes associated with age, the most significant are the increased prevalence of multidrug resistance, abnormal intracellular metabolisms of drugs, and abnormal repair of DNA damage. Multidrug resistance may be caused by increased expression of the MDR1 gene, as is the case in acute myelogenous leukemia,[73] increased prevalence of anoxic tumor cells, and resistance to apoptosis.[71] Abnormal drug metabolism and delay in DNA repair may enhance the toxicity of these agents.[6]

Myelosuppression and mucositis are particularly common and severe complications of cytotoxic chemotherapy.

The risk of neutropenia and neutropenic infections with moderately toxic chemotherapy (such as cyclophosphamide, doxorubicin, vincristine, and prednisone [CHOP]) increases with age and appears particularly marked after age 70; fortunately, hemopoietic growth factors in pharmacologic doses prevent this complication in 50% to 75% of individuals over 70 years of age.[74] Neutropenic infection may be lethal and may occur after the first course of treatment, a fact that prompted the recommendations to use growth factors prophylactically in patients aged 65 and older.[75]

The risk of mucositis also increases with age, and this complication may be lethal if not treated promptly.[76] A keratinocyte growth factor, undergoing clinical trials, appears promising for the prevention of mucositis.[77] Other interventions to ameliorate this complication include substitution for intravenous fluorinated pyrimidines by capecitabine, which is associated with a lower risk of mucositis, and hydration for older individuals who develop diarrhea or severe dysphagia.

PRACTICAL DECISIONS RELATED TO THE MANAGEMENT OF OLDER INDIVIDUALS

Informed decision making is the key to effective and safe treatment of older individuals. Any oncologic decision for these patients has two components: the person and the neoplasm. For example, cytotoxic chemotherapy is rarely indicated in a woman aged 90 or older with stage 1 or 2 breast cancer, given the negligible benefit and the substantial risk of treatment. Extermann and coworkers demonstrated that adjuvant chemotherapy is beneficial to an 80-year-old woman when her chances of dying of breast cancer are only about 30%, if a 1% reduction in breast cancer–related mortality is desirable; in a 90-year-old woman, however, the risk of dying of breast cancer must be close to 70% to justify the use of chemotherapy.[78] Chemotherapy seems definitively indicated if the same patient has a chemotherapy-responsive disease that may shorten her survival, such as large cell non-Hodgkin's lymphoma. The nearby algorithm depicts a useful frame of reference for the use of chemotherapy in older individuals. The two points that deserve emphasis are (1) the rapidly evolving classification of older individuals; and (2) in some circumstances chemotherapy may represent the best palliation of frail individuals. Several agents with minimal toxicity, including capecitabine at low doses, weekly taxanes, gemcitabine, and vinorelbine, may be used safely in these patients.[35]

NATIONAL AND INTERNATIONAL INITIATIVES RELATED TO CANCER AND AGE

The issues of cancer in the older person have been well recognized throughout the Western world, and have prompted a number of important responses.

Governmental Responses

The National Cancer Institute in cooperation with the National Institute of Aging has held a number of conferences related to cancer and aging. As a consequence of these conferences 6 to 8 program grants (P20), for the development of geriatric programs within comprehensive cancer centers have been offered. In addition, a number of requests for proposals for the study of management of cancer in the older person have been offered.

All major cooperative groups in the United States and Europe now have a committee or subcommittee whose aim is promotion of enrollment of older individuals into existing clinical trials and promotion of clinical trials devoted to older individuals.

Professional Associations and Private Foundations

The American Association for Cancer Research (AACR), the American Society of Clinical Oncology (ASCO), and

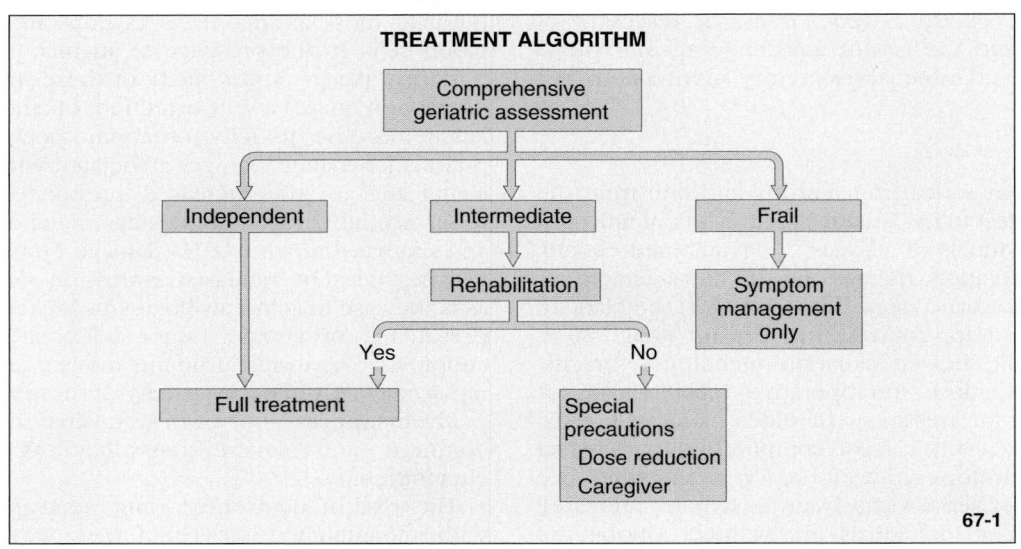

TREATMENT ALGORITHM

Comprehensive geriatric assessment → Independent / Intermediate / Frail

Intermediate → Rehabilitation → Yes → Full treatment; No → Special precautions / Dose reduction / Caregiver

Independent → Full treatment

Frail → Symptom management only

67-1

TABLE 67-4

 Guidelines for the Management of the Older Person with Cancer Established by the National Cancer Center Network

1. All patients aged 65 and older should undergo some form of geriatric assessment prior to institution of treatment.
2. The dose of compounds that are excreted through the kidneys or that give origin to active and toxic metabolites excreted through the kidneys should be adjusted to individual GFRs in persons aged 65 and older. The doses should be escalated if no toxicity is encountered.
3. Patients aged 65 and older treated with moderately toxic chemotherapy (of dose intensity comparable to CHOP) should receive prophylactic growth factors (G-CSF or pegylated G-CSF).
4. Hemoglobin levels should be maintained at ≥12 g/dL with epoietin.
5. Patients aged 65 and older experiencing grade 3–4 mucositis should be admitted to the hospital and receive aggressive fluid resuscitation.

CHOP, cyclophosphamide, doxorubicin, vincristine, and prednisone; G-CSF, granulocyte colony-stimulating factor; GFR, glomerular filtration rate.

the European Society of Medical Oncology (ESMO) have dedicated special scientific and educational sessions to the issues of cancer and aging. ASCO also has developed a special curriculum on cancer and age. Of the private foundations, special mention is deserved by the Hartford Foundation, which has founded, through ASCO, 12 3-year fellowships for special training in geriatric oncology.

A number of industry-funded cooperative efforts for studying the management of cancer in the elderly also have been developed, including the Geriatric Oncology Consortium in the United States, the Geriatric Radiation Oncology Group (GROG) in Italy, and the Italian Group of Geriatric Oncology (GioGER), which, although it originated in Italy, incorporates the effort of several European countries.

Practice Guidelines

In 1999 the National Cancer Center Network (NCCN) established a panel for the issuance of guidelines for the management of older individuals. The first set of guidelines (Table 67-4) was published in 2000.[52] These guidelines are based on the clinical evidence reviewed in this chapter and are meant as a frame of reference for clinical practice and as a building block to accommodate emerging data. Other associations, including the EORTC and the Canadian Cancer Institute, are preparing their own guidelines.

CONCLUSIONS

This chapter describes the scope of geriatric oncology, which includes changes in tumor and patient biology as well as a comprehensive evaluation of the older person, aimed to establish life expectancy, treatment tolerance, risk of cancer-related complication, and need for rehabilitative intervention. Biological changes and CGA are the two poles of preventative and therapeutic interventions. Treatment-related guidelines may help establish a uniform approach to older cancer patients and thus facilitate the

interpretation of clinical data. A number of initiatives developed during the past 5 years promote clinical research in older cancer patient and promise to fill the current gaps in clinical evidence. In any case, no circumstances should age alone represent a contraindication to effective cancer treatment.

REFERENCES

1. Yancik R, Ries LAG: Aging and cancer in America: Demographic and epidemiologic perspectives. Hematol Oncol Clin North Am 2000;14:17–24.
2. Yancik RM, Ries L: Cancer and age: Magnitude of the problem. In Balducci L, Lyman GH, Ershler WB (eds): Comprehensive Geriatric Oncology. London, Harwood Academic Publishers, 1998, pp 95–104.
3. Anisimov VN: Age as a risk factor in multistage carcinogenesis. In Balducci L, Lyman GH, Ershler WB (eds): Comprehensive Geriatric Oncology, 2nd ed. London, Taylor & Francis, 2004.
4. Collins K: Mammalian telomeres and telomerase. Curr Opin Cell Biol 2000;12:378–383.
5. Liggett WH, Sidransky D: Role of the P16 tumor suppressor gene in cancer. J Clin Oncol 1998;16:1197–1206.
6. Rudd GN, Hartley GA, Souhani RL: Persistence of cisplatin-induced interstrand crosslinking in peripheral blood mononuclear cells from elderly and younger individuals. Cancer Chemother Pharmacol 1995;35:323–326.
7. Campisi J: Cancer and age: The double-edged sword of proliferative senescence. J Am Geriatr Soc 1997;45:482–488.
8. Warner HR: Aging and regulation of apoptosis. Curr Top Cell Regul 1997;35:107–121.
9. Yancik R, Ganz PA, Varriccio CG, et al: Perspectives on comorbidity and cancer in the older patient: Approach to expand the knowledge base. J Clin Oncol 2001;19:1147–1151.
10. Cohen HJ, Harris T, Pieper CF: Coagulation and activation of inflammatory pathways in the development of functional decline and mortality in the elderly. Am J Med 2003;114:180–187.
11. Van Zant G: Stem cells and genetics in the study of development, aging and longevity. In Hekimi S (ed): Results and problems in cell differentiation, Vol. 29. Berlin/Heidelberg, Springer-Verlag, 2000, pp 203–235.
12. Ershler WB, Keller ETR: Age-associated increased interleukin-6 gene expression, late life disease and frailty. Ann Rev Med 2000;51: 245–270.
13. Hamerman D, Berman JV, Albers W, et al: Emerging evidence of inflammation in conditions frequently affecting older adults: Reports of a symposium. J Am Geriatr Soc 1999;47:1016–1102.
14. Burns EA, Goodwin JS: Immunological changes of aging. In Balducci L, Lyman GH, Ershler WB (eds): Comprehensive Geriatric Oncology, 2nd ed. London, Taylor & Francis, 2004.
15. Monfardini S, Carbone A: Non-Hodgkin's lymphomas. In Balducci L, Lyman GH, Ershler WB (eds): Comprehensive Geriatric Oncology. London, Harwood Academic Publishers, 1998, pp 577–595.
16. Flowers A: Brain tumors. In Balducci L, Lyman GH, Ershler WB (eds): Comprehensive Geriatric Oncology. London, Harwood Academic Publishers, 1998, pp 703–720.
17. Barbone F, Bovenzi M, Cavallieri F, et al: Air pollution and lung cancer in Trieste, Italy. Am J Epidemiol 1995;141:1161–1169.
18. Martoni F, Cucinotta A, Piana E, et al: Breast cancer in the older woman. Crit Rev Oncol Hematol 2003;46:207–209.
19. Ershler WB: Influence of tumor host on the tumor growth in older patients. In Balducci L, Lyman GH, Ershler WB (eds). Comprehensive Geriatric Oncology, 2nd ed. London, Taylor & Francis, 2004.
20. Kurtz JM, Jacquemier J, Amalric R, et al: Why are local recurrences after breast-conserving therapy more frequent in younger patients? J Clin Oncol 1990;10:141–152.
21. Repetto L, Balducci L: A case for geriatric oncology. Lancet Oncology 2002;3:289–297.
22. Cohen HJ, Feussner JR, Weinberger M, et al: A controlled trial of inpatient and outpatient geriatric assessment. N Engl J Med 2002;346,905–912.

23. Reuben DB, Franck J, Hirsch S, et al: A randomized clinical trial of outpatient geriatric assessment (CGA), coupled with an intervention, to increase adherence to recommendations. J Am Ger Soc 1999;47:269-276.

24. Bula CJ, Berod AC, Stuck AE, et al: Effectiveness of preventive in-home geriatric assessment in well functioning, community dwelling older people: Secondary analysis of a randomized trial. J Am Ger Soc 1999;47:389-395.

25. Balducci L, Extermann M, Meyer J, et al: Comprehensive geriatric intervention in older breast cancer patients. A pilot [abstract 3008]. Proc Am Soc Clin Oncol 2001;20:314b.

26. Extermann M, Overcash J, Lyman GH, et al: Comorbidity and functional status are independent in older cancer patients. J Clin Oncol 1998;16;1582-1587.

27. Repetto L, Fratino L, Audisio RA, et al: Comprehensive geriatric assessment adds information to the Eastern Cooperative Group performance status in elderly cancer patients. An Italian Group for Geriatric Oncology Study. J Clin Oncol 2002;20;494-502.

28. Ingram SS, Seo PH, Martell RE, et al: Comprehensive assessment of the elderly cancer patient: The feasibility of self-report methodology. J Clin Oncol 2002;20:770-775.

29. Inouye SK, Peduzzi PN, Robison JT, et al: Importance of functional measures in predicting mortality among older hospitalized patients. JAMA 1998;279:1187-1193.

30. Stump TE, Callahan CM, Hendrie HC: Cognitive impairment and mortality in older primary care patients. J Am Geriatr Soc 2001;49:934-940.

31. Blazer DG, Hybels CF, Pieper CF: The association of depression and mortality in elderly persons: a case for multiple independent pathways. J Gerontol Med Sci 2001;56A:M505-509.

32. Extermann M, Chen A, Cantor AB, et al: Predictors of toxicity from chemotherapy in older patients. Eur J Cancer 2002;38:1466-1473.

33. Zagonel V, Fratino L, Piselli P, et al: The comprehensive geriatric assessment predicts mortality among elderly cancer patients [abstract 1458]. Proc Am Soc Clin Oncol 2002;21:365a.

34. Hamerman D: Toward an understanding of frailty. Ann Intern Med 1999;130:945-950.

35. Balducci L, Stanta G: Cancer in the frail patient: A coming epidemic. Hematol Oncol Clin North Am 2000;14:235-250.

36. Fried LP, Tangen CM, Walston J, et al: Frailty in older adults: Evidence for a phenotype. J Gerontol Med Sci 2001;56A: M146-M156.

37. Saliba D, Elliott M, Rubenstein LZ, et al: The Vulnerable Elders Survey: A tool for identifying vulnerable older people in the community. J Am Geriatr Soc 2001;49:1691-1699.

38. Reuben DB, Rubenstein LV, Hirsch SH, et al: Value of functional status as predictor of mortality. Am J Med 1992;93:663-669.

39. Barberger-Gateau P, Fabrigoule C, Helmer C, et al: Functional impairment in instrumental activities of daily living: An early clinical sign of dementia? J Am Geriatr Soc 1999;47:456-462.

40. Satariano WA, Ragland DR: The effect of comorbidity on 3-year survival of women with primary breast cancer. Ann Intern Med 1994;120:104-110.

41. Extermann M: Measuring comorbidity in older cancer patients. Eur J Cancer 2000;36:453-471.

42. Balducci L: Epidemiology of anemia in the elderly: Information on diagnostic evaluation. J Am Geriatr Soc 2003;51(3 Suppl):S2-S9.

43. Schrijvers D, Highley M, DeBruyn E, et al: Role of red blood cell in pharmacokinetics of chemotherapeutic agents. Anticancer Drugs 1999;10:147-153.

44. Chaves PH, Volpato S, Fried L: Challenging the World Health Organization criteria for anemia in the older woman [abstract]. J Am Geriatr Soc 2001;49:S3,A10.

45. Littlewood TJ, Bajetta E, Nortier JW, et al: Effects of epoetin alfa on hematologic parameters and quality of life in cancer patients receiving nonplatinum chemotherapy: results of a randomized, double-blind, placebo-controlled trial. J Clin Oncol 2001;19: 2865-2874.

46. Lyness JM, Ling DA, Cox C, et al: The importance of subsyndromal depression in older primary care patients. Prevalence and associated functional disability. J Am Geriatr Soc 1999;47:647-652.

47. Weitzner MA, Haley WE, Chen H: The family caregiver of the older cancer patient. Hematol Oncol Clin North Am 2000:14: 269-282.

48. Melton LJ, Khosla S, Crowson CS, et al: Epidemiology of sarcopenia. J Am Geriatr Soc 2000;48:625-630.

49. Guigoz Y, Vellas B, Garry PJ: Mininutritional assessment: A practical assessment tool for grading the nutritional state of elderly patients. In Guigoz Y, Vellas B, Garry PJ (eds): Facts, Research, Interventions in Geriatrics. New York, Serdi Publishing, 1997, pp 15-60.

50. Clarfield AM, Bergman H, Kane R: Fragmentation of care for frail older people—an international problem. Experience from three countries: Israel, Canada, and the United States. J Am Geriatr Soc 2001;49:1714-1721.

51. Gill TM, Baker DI, Gottschalk M, et al: A program to prevent functional decline in physically frail elderly persons who live at home. N Engl J Med 2002;347:1068-1074.

52. Balducci L, Yates G: General guidelines for the management of older patients with cancer. NCCN Proceedings. Oncology (Huntingt.) 2000;14:221-227.

53. Balducci L, Beghé C: Cancer prevention in the older person. Clin Geriatr Med 2002;18:505-528.

54. Hong WK, Spitz MR, Lippman SM: Chemoprevention in the 21st century: Genetics, risk modeling, and molecular targets. J Clin Oncol 2000;18(Suppl):9s-18s.

55. Gail MH, Costantino JP, Bryant J, et al: Weighing the risks and benefits of tamoxifen treatment for preventing breast cancer. J Natl Cancer Inst 1999;91:1829-1846.

56. Kerlikowske K, Grady D, Rubin SM, et al: Efficacy of screening mammography. A meta-analysis. JAMA 1995;273:149-154.

57. Van Dijck JAAM, Holland R, Verbeeck ALM, et al: Efficacy of mammographic screening in the elderly: A case-referent study in the Nijmegen program in the Netherlands. J Natl Cancer Inst 1994;86:934-938.

58. McCarthy EP, Burns RB, Freund KM, et al: Mammography use, breast cancer stage at diagnosis, and survival among older women. J Am Geriatr Soc 2000;48:1226-1233.

59. Randolph WM, Goodwin JS, Mahnken JD, et al: Regular mammography use is associated with elimination of age-related disparities in size and stage of breast cancer at diagnosis. Ann Int Med 2002;137:783-790.

60. Miller AB, Baines CJ, To T, et al: Canadian National Breast Screening Study 2: Breast cancer detection and death rates among women aged 50-59 years. Can Med Assoc J 1992;147:1477-1488.

61. Mitra I: Breast screening: the case for physical examination without mammography. Lancet 1994;343:342-344.

62. Kerlikowske K, Salzman P, Phillips KA, et al: Continuing screening mammography in women aged 70 to 79 years. JAMA 1999;282: 2156-2163.

63. Frazier AL, Colditz GA, Fuchs CS: Cost-effectiveness of screening for colorectal cancer in the general population. JAMA 2000;284:1954-1961.

64. Holmberg L, Bill-Axelson A, Hegelsen F, et al: A randomized trial comparing radical prostatectomy with watchful waiting in early prostate cancer. N Engl J Med 2002;347:781-789.

65. Halpern MT, Gillespie BW, Warner KE: Patterns of absolute risk of lung cancer mortality in former smokers. J Natl Cancer Inst 1993;17:457-464.

66. Kemeny MM, Bush-Devereaux E, Merriam LT, et al: Cancer surgery in the elderly. Hematol Oncol Clin North Am 2000;14:169-192.

67. Davila H, Miguel R: Anesthesia in older cancer patients. In Balducci L, Lyman GH, Ershler WB (eds): Comprehensive Geriatric Oncology, 2nd edition. London, Taylor & Francis, 2004.

68. Olmi P, Ausili Cefaro GP, Balzi M, et al: Radiotherapy in the aged. Clin Geriatr Med 1997;13:143-168.

69. Scalliet P, Pignon T: Radiotherapy in the elderly. In Balducci L, Lyman GH, Ershler WB (eds): Comprehensive Geriatric Oncology. London, Harwood Academic Publishers, 1998, pp 421-428.

70. Zachariah B, Balducci L: Radiation therapy of the older patient. Hematol Oncol Clin North Am 2000;14:131-167.

71. Cova D, Balducci L: Cytotoxic chemotherapy in the older patient. In Balducci L, Lyman GH, Ershler WB (eds): Comprehensive Geriatric Oncology, 2nd ed. London, Taylor & Francis, 2004.

72. Balducci L, Carreca I: Oral chemotherapy of cancer in the elderly. Am J Cancer 2002;1:101-108.

73. Lancet JE, Willman CL, Bennett JM: Acute myelogenous leukemia and aging: Clinical interactions. Hematol Oncol Clin North Am 2000;16:251-268.

74. Balducci L, Hardy CL, Lyman GH: Hemopoietic growth factors in the older cancer patient. Current Opin Hematol 2001;8:170-187.

75. Gomez H, Mas L, Casanova L, et al: Elderly patients with aggressive non-Hodgkin's lymphoma treated with CHOP chemotherapy plus granulocyte-macrophage colony-stimulating factor: Identification of two age subgroups with differing hematologic toxicity. J Clin Oncol 1998;16:2352-2358.

76. Jacobson SD, Cha S, Sargent DJ, et al: Tolerability, dose intensity and benefit of 5FU based chemotherapy for advanced colorectal cancer (CRC) in the elderly. A North Central Cancer Treatment Group Study [abstract 1534]. Proc Am Soc Clin Oncol 2001;20:384.

77. Spielberger RT, Stiff P, Emmanouilides C, et al: Efficacy of recombinant human keratinocyte growth factor (rhukgf) in reducing mucositis in patients with hematologic malignancies undergoing autologous peripheral blood progenitor cell transplantation after radiation-based conditioning. Results of a phase 2 trial [abstract 25]. Proc Am Soc Clin Oncol 2001;20:7a.

78. Extermann M, Balducci L, Lyman GH: What threshold for adjuvant therapy in older breast cancer patients? J Clin Oncol 2000;18:1709-1717.

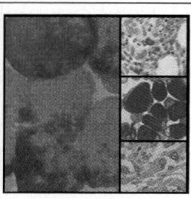

68

SPECIAL ISSUES IN PREGNANCY

James E. Wooldridge
Donald C. Doll

SUMMARY OF KEY POINTS

INCIDENCE
- Cancer is the second leading cause of death in women between the ages of 20 and 39 years.
- Cancer complicates 1 in 1000 pregnancies.
- The most common cancers during pregnancy are breast, cervical, and thyroid cancer; lymphoma; melanoma; and leukemia.
- Seventeen percent of fetuses exposed to single-agent chemotherapy and 23% exposed to combination chemotherapy during the first trimester have been reported to have malformations.

ETIOLOGY OF COMPLICATIONS
- Altered maternal physiology
- Rapid fetal development

- Chemotherapy during the first trimester
- Therapeutic radiation during gestation

EVALUATION OF THE PATIENT
- Careful determination of gestational age of the fetus
- Careful maternal staging, with limited exposure to ionizing radiation
- Determination of maternal prognosis based on malignancy and best staging efforts

TREATMENT
- Important factors in treatment planning include gestational age, maternal symptoms, maternal and fetal prognosis, and potential therapeutic benefit.

- Chemotherapy during the first trimester is generally associated with a high risk of fetal malformations; however, chemotherapy during the second and third trimesters may enhance maternal outcome without significant fetal risk.
- Therapeutic radiation jeopardizes fetal outcome and should be reserved for the postpartum period when possible.
- Pregnancy after cancer diagnosis and therapy is possible but deserves prepregnancy risk counseling and close follow-up.

INTRODUCTION

Few situations in life can span the emotions of joy and fear as that experienced by a pregnant patient diagnosed with cancer. Cancer is the second leading cause of death in women between the ages of 20 and 39, and it complicates 1 in 1000 pregnancies. The most common cancers diagnosed in pregnant patients are those seen in nonpregnant women of similar age: breast, cervix, thyroid, lymphoma, melanoma, and leukemia. There are essentially no clinical trials and there are few integrated or prospective data available to make clear recommendations based on science; however, a significant clinical experience is available in the published literature from which reasonable recommendations can be made. Pregnancy-associated cancer typically includes cancer during gestation and in the immediate postpartum period. This chapter focuses primarily on the issues related to cancer care during the gestational period.

A number of factors must be considered in diagnosis, staging, treatment, and follow-up of the pregnant patient and child. Physiologic changes affect the pharmacology of drugs and present specific challenges in surgical and radiation treatment. Medications, radiation, and surgery comprise a short list of potentially harmful situations for the fetus. Between 10% and 15% of all pregnancies result in miscarriage or spontaneous abortion, and 2% to 3%

of all newborns may have congenital abnormalities.[1] Approximately 1% of congenital abnormalities are due to drugs but most have no clear etiology.[2] Clearly, the physician, patient, and family must work together to develop a treatment plan based not only on medical information but also on ethical, moral, religious, and legal grounds.

MATERNAL-FETAL PHYSIOLOGY

Pregnancy induces a number of important physiologic changes, and these changes may, in total or in part, cause significant alterations in the metabolism and efficacy of commonly used medications. Many of these adaptations are also relevant to the surgical treatment of patients with cancer. Because of the risk involved, use of chemotherapeutic and supportive care drugs is largely anecdotal, and clinical trials do not exist. Understanding these changes is important in anticipating efficacy and toxicity of these agents in pregnant patients with cancer.

Plasma volume in pregnancy is increased by as much as 50%, resulting in an increased volume of distribution and decreased peak plasma concentration. A dilutional anemia results from the increased plasma volume. The serum creatinine level is decreased, whereas glomerular filtration is increased, resulting in enhanced clearance of drugs. Gastric emptying and gastrointestinal motility are delayed, and drug absorption may be altered. Enterohepatic circulation is increased, which may lead to increased drug bioavailability, and enhanced hepatic oxidation may enhance drug clearance. Although albumin levels are decreased because of the expanded plasma volume, levels of plasma proteins, including coagulation factors, are increased as a result of estrogen stimulation, which may alter the pharmacokinetics of drugs with significant protein binding. Thus drug-specific characteristics such as route of administration, lipophilicity, protein binding, and mechanisms of metabolism and clearance become important considerations in anticipating effects in pregnant patients, although few data exist to guide physicians in adjustment of drug dosing.

The importance of physiologic changes in pregnancy is not limited to pharmacology; such changes also affect surgical treatment planning. In addition to the increased plasma volume and dilutional anemia, pregnancy is accompanied by reduced mean arterial pressure, increased oxygen consumption, and a narrow respiratory reserve. Cardiac output in the pregnant patient is increased by 30% to 50% as early as the second trimester and can be affected by patient positioning. In the supine position, the gravid uterus can compress the inferior vena cava, resulting in decreased venous return and reduction in cardiac output. Compression of the aorta can result in decreased uterine blood flow, and either mechanism can result in insufficient blood flow to the placenta. Fetal development or viability may be jeopardized by hypotension and hypoxemia, which can result from a lack of understanding of these circulatory and respiratory changes.

FETAL DEVELOPMENT

Fetal development is divided into three phases: implantation, organogenesis, and growth. It is important to recognize the stage of fetal development in determining the potential harm that may occur with a given intervention in pregnant patients with cancer. The implantation phase lasts from conception to 2 weeks and often ends in spontaneous abortion in the face of a noxious stimulus. Organogenesis begins after the second week and ends between 7 and 12 weeks. During this time the major organs are formed, and noxious stimuli may lead to organ dysgenesis, which may result in congenital malformation or fetal death. The growth phase begins in the second trimester and lasts until term. During this time, noxious stimuli may affect somatic growth, as well as development of the nervous system. Fetal growth retardation results in low birth weight, which is associated with abnormal brain development and subsequent learning disabilities. It is therefore important to consider the effects of cancer therapy on the future of the child as well as the development of the fetus.

MATERNAL-FETAL PHARMACOKINETICS

The placenta is the connection between the maternal and fetal circulation, making it the gateway for drugs to reach the fetus. It is easier for uncharged, lipophilic, low molecular weight drugs with minimal protein binding to cross the placenta than for drugs with the opposite characteristics to do so.[3,4] With the exception of large proteins such as L-asparaginase and interferon alfa, most antineoplastic agents possess these properties and thus cross the placenta and enter the fetal circulation. It is interesting that p-glycoprotein has been described in the gravid endometrium, which may provide a natural barrier for some antineoplastic agents, such as vinca alkaloids and the anthracycline antibiotics.[5] This may be particularly relevant in treatment of acute leukemia in pregnancy, for which many drugs affected by the multidrug-resistant phenotype have been used throughout gestation, often without unfavorable fetal outcome.

The fetal liver can metabolize drugs through oxidation, dehydrogenation, reduction, glucuronidation, methylation, and acetylation as early as 7 to 8 weeks of pregnancy.[6] The fetal kidneys may also be involved in drug elimination, but the extent to which both fetal organs participate in drug elimination is minimal. Drug excretion into the amniotic fluid may actually increase exposure and risk of adverse effects, particularly with antimetabolites that are excreted in active form. In contrast, some agents such as nitrogen mustard are utilized and bound to tissue with essentially no active drug or metabolites excreted. Because the movement of drug molecules is bidirectional, the placenta is also a route of drug elimination, and in fact, the placenta is the primary portal of exit of waste products and toxins from the fetus. Transplacental passage of antineoplastic agents has been reported in association with doxorubicin[7] and cisplatin.[8] In general, the metabolites are more polar than the parent compound and may not cross the placenta as easily. As a result, metabolites may accumulate in fetal tissues or amniotic fluid.[9]

Teratogenicity

More than 2500 elements have been catalogued as being potentially teratogenic in animal experiments; however, clear evidence of toxicity to the human fetus is available only for a few of these.[10,11] Extrapolation of teratogenic and mutagenic effects of chemotherapeutic agents from animals to human organogenesis is dangerous because of differences in species susceptibility.[12] The vinca alkaloids cause malformations in a hamster model,[13] yet based on clinical experience, vinblastine is recommended by lymphoma experts for the treatment of Hodgkin's lymphoma during the first trimester when therapy is necessary and therapeutic abortion is refused.[14] The U.S. Food and Drug Administration defined risk categories for all drugs based on the evidence available for fetal harm (Table 68-1). The majority of chemotherapeutic agents are considered to have undefined or definite evidence of fetal risk, but the benefits from use in pregnant women may be acceptable despite the risk, if the drug is needed in a life-threatening situation for which safer drugs are not available. Multiple factors likely influence the probability of teratogenesis including phase of embryo organogenesis,[15-22] frequency of administration, duration of exposure, synergistic effects of drugs,[21,22] radiation,[23-25]

TABLE 68-1

Food and Drug Administration Risk Categories for Drugs Administered During Pregnancy

Category A	Controlled studies in women do not show risk to the fetus during first trimester, there is no evidence of risk in later trimesters, and possibility of fetal harm is remote.
Category B	Animal-reproduction studies have not shown a fetal risk, but there are not controlled studies in pregnant women; or animal-reproduction studies have shown an adverse effect (other than a decrease in fertility) but this has not been confirmed in controlled studies in women in first trimester (no evidence of a risk in later trimesters).
Category C	Studies in animals have revealed adverse effects on the fetus (teratogenic, embryocidal, or both) and there are no controlled studies in women, or studies in animals and women are unavailable. Drug should only be given if potential benefit justifies the risk to the fetus.
Category D	There is positive evidence of human fetal risk, but the benefits from use in pregnant women may be acceptable despite the risk (if the drug is needed in life-threatening situation for which other safer drugs are not available).
Category X	Studies in humans and animals have shown fetal malformations, there is evidence of fetal risk based on human experience, or both. The risk of use in a pregnant woman clearly outweighs any potential benefit. This drug is contraindicated in women who are or may become pregnant.

Reprinted from Federal Register 1980;44:37434-37467.

and individual genetic susceptibility.[26] Nonetheless, the use of systemic antineoplastic therapy alone appears to be accompanied by significantly lower risk than is commonly appreciated.

SYSTEMIC ANTINEOPLASTIC THERAPY DURING PREGNANCY

The timing of fetal drug exposure is critical and may be associated with immediate and delayed deleterious effects.[1] Drugs administered within 1 week of conception may produce an "all or nothing" phenomenon, that is, a spontaneous abortion or a healthy fetus. During the first trimester, when organogenesis occurs, drugs can produce congenital malformations and/or result in spontaneous abortion. Doll and colleagues[27] reviewed the literature on patients treated with chemotherapy during pregnancy and reported that 17% of pregnancies exposed to a single chemotherapeutic and 23% exposed to combination chemotherapy during the first trimester resulted in fetal malformations and 1.5% exposed during the latter two trimesters resulted in fetal malformation. This review was recently updated by Maghfoor and Doll[28] without significant change (Tables 68-2 and 68-3). In the second and third trimesters, drugs are less likely to cause significant malformations; however, they may impair fetal growth and development, which affects childhood development. Specifically, neuronal growth in the brain continues and damage beyond the first trimester can produce microcephaly, mental retardation, and impaired learning. A variety of antineoplastic drugs are known to be secreted in breast milk, and breastfeeding during chemotherapy should be avoided (Table 68-4).

Antimetabolites

Aminopterin is the chemotherapeutic most clearly linked to congenital malformations. Although no longer used in modern chemotherapy regimens, another folate antagonist, methotrexate, is commonly used. Both drugs

are highly associated with fetal abnormalities when given during the first trimester.[27,29-32] The "aminopterin syndrome" is characterized by cranial dysostosis, hypertelorism, micrognathia, limb deformities, and mental retardation.[33]

TABLE 68-2

Chemotherapy During First Trimester of Pregnancy

CLASS	NO. OF EXPOSED PATIENTS	NO. OF FETAL MALFORMATIONS
Alkylating Agents		
Busulfan	24	2
Chlorambucil	6	1
Cyclophosphamide	7	3
Nitrogen mustard	6	0
Triethylenemelamine	4	0
Antimetabolites		
Aminopterin	52	10
Methotrexate	9	3
6-Mercaptopurine	20	0
Cytarabine	1	1
5-Fluorouracil	1	1
Hydroxyurea	3	0
Plant Alkaloids		
Vinblastine	14	1
Antibiotics		
Daunorubicin	1	0
Miscellaneous		
Procarbazine	1	1
Amsacrine	1	1
Cisplatin	1	0
Total	151	24 (15%)
Combination Chemotherapy	54	9 (16%)

From Maghfoor I, Doll DC: Chemotherapy in pregnancy. In Perry MC (ed): The Chemotherapy Source Book, 3rd ed. Philadelphia, Lippincott Williams & Wilkins, 2001, p 537.

TABLE 68-3

Chemotherapy During Second and Third Trimesters of Pregnancy

CLASS	NO. OF EXPOSED PATIENTS	NO. OF FETAL MALFORMATIONS
Alkylating agents	26	1
Antimetabolites	38	0
Antibiotics	1	0
Plant alkaloids	6	0
Combinations	142	2
Total	213	3 (1.4%)

From Maghfoor I, Doll DC: Chemotherapy in pregnancy. In Perry MC (ed): The Chemotherapy Source Book, 3rd ed. Philadelphia, Lippincott Williams & Wilkins, 2001, p 537.

Although it is not recommended for use during the first trimester, methotrexate does not uniformly cause malformations. Eight women experiencing 10 pregnancies after low-dose exposure to methotrexate during first trimester for treatment of rheumatic disease had five healthy term babies, three spontaneous abortions, and two elective abortions.[34] Such findings suggest that methotrexate is not always teratogenic when given in the first trimester and that there may be a critical dose above which fetal malformations occur. Exposure to methotrexate in the latter trimesters has not been associated with significant malformations.[16,27,35,36]

5-Fluorouracil (5-FU) was associated with multiple congenital malformations in the fetus of a patient who was found to be pregnant at week 14, after she began receiving chemotherapy for colon cancer at week 12.[37] Vaginal administration of 5-FU to five patients during the first trimester was associated with delivery of five healthy infants, although amniocentesis performed on one mother showed the fetus to have a 47, XXX genotype.[38] Use of 5-FU in the latter trimesters has not been associated with adverse events, and 5-FU is an integral component of the multidisciplinary care of patients with breast cancer in one center.[39] Among 20 patients exposed to single-agent 6-mercaptopurine during the first trimester, no fetal anomalies were documented[27]; however, first trimester use of single agent 6-mercaptopurine for the treatment of malignant lymphoma has resulted in spontaneous abortion.[40] Cytosine arabinoside, alone and in combination with other drugs, during the first trimester has also been associated with congenital anomalies.[36,41–43]

TABLE 68-4

Common Chemotherapy Drugs Found in Breast Milk

Cisplatin
Cyclophosphamide
Doxorubicin
Etoposide
Hydroxyurea
Interferon alfa
Methotrexate
Mitoxantrone

Alkylating Agents

Alkylating agents are commonly used in the treatment of lymphoma, acute lymphocytic leukemia, and breast cancer. Specifically, cyclophosphamide is commonly used in the adjuvant therapy of breast cancer and curative treatment of non-Hodgkin's lymphoma. Among 47 at-risk pregnancies, 6 malformations were reported when alkylating agents were used in the first trimester.[28] Four of these six mothers had also received radiation therapy. In the same review, three of seven pregnancies in which cyclophosphamide was used in the first trimester resulted in fetal malformations. Daily administration of cyclophosphamide with intermittent administration of prednisone throughout a twin pregnancy resulted in a delivery of healthy female infant and a male infant with multiple congenital anomalies.[44] The male child ultimately had papillary thyroid cancer at age 11 and a neuroblastoma at age 14. Exposure to chlorambucil during the first trimester has been reported to cause renal aplasia, cleft palate, and skeletal abnormalities.[16] Administration of busulfan during the first trimester leads to malformation in 8% to 12% of pregnancies, although this may be confounded by radiation.[28,45]

Platinum

A number of case reports documenting platinum use during pregnancy have surfaced over the past decade. At least 12 patients have received cisplatin during pregnancy,[46–57] and one patient also received carboplatin.[53] No congenital malformations were noted, although all patients received treatment after the first trimester.

Microtubule Targeting Drugs

Although vinblastine is highly teratogenic in animal models,[13] a literature review identified one malformation in 14 women treated with vinblastine in the first trimester.[27] The use of vinblastine in the first trimester may be relatively safe, and it is recommended as an approach to defer definitive chemotherapy for the treatment of lymphoma until the second trimester when therapeutic abortion is declined.[14] Fewer reports on the use of vincristine during the first trimester are available. No congenital malformations were reported in 11 pregnancies exposed to vincristine, with three being in the first trimester.[20] The vinca alkaloids, like the alkylating agents, are frequently included in curative regimens. In another review, three anomalies were reported in 13 patients treated with either agent in combination with other drugs in the first trimester, and 24 more pregnancies were exposed in latter trimesters without malformation.[45] Vinorelbine has been used to treat four patients during the latter trimesters without fetal harm.[49,58]

Limited information on taxane use during pregnancy is available. A patient with stage IIIC ovarian cancer was treated with paclitaxel after cytoreductive surgery at 27 weeks' gestation. She received three cycles of chemotherapy with paclitaxel and cisplatin during pregnancy, and the infant experienced normal physical and mental development at 30 months.[46] A second patient received docetaxel for rapidly progressive metastatic breast cancer immediately after the first trimester. She received three cycles through 30 weeks' gestation, and a healthy infant was delivered at 32 weeks. The child's development was normal at 2 years.[59]

Anthracyclines

Doxorubicin, daunorubicin, and idarubicin are integral agents for the treatment of leukemia, lymphoma, and breast cancer. Each of these agents has been used during pregnancy with no reports of fetal malformations.[28,45,60] Reversible cardiomyopathy in an infant exposed to idarubicin and all-trans-retinoic acid has been reported.[61]

Bleomycin

Bleomycin can induce chromosomal changes in vitro[62]; however, no reports suggest a similar effect during pregnancy in humans. In a recent series of 84 women with lymphoma, 16 women received bleomycin for treatment of Hodgkin's lymphoma, and an undisclosed number received it for treatment of for non-Hodgkin's lymphoma.[63] No malformations were reported. Bleomycin has been used in all trimesters without report of malformation.[56,63-67]

Topoisomerase Inhibitors

Etoposide is one of the most commonly used topoisomerase inhibitors and has been shown to be teratogenic in rodents, with the potential for cranial and skeletal abnormalities.[68] Topoisomerase II inhibitors (i.e., etoposide and teniposide) have been used during pregnancy, and teniposide was given to two patients without fetal compromise.[69,70] Etoposide has been used in all trimesters of pregnancy for the treatment of lymphoma,[66] leukemia,[71,72] and neuroblastoma,[73] and no fetal malformations have been reported in any of the infants. There are no data on use of topoisomerase I inhibitors (i.e., topotecan, irinotecan) during pregnancy.

Immunotherapy

Interferon-alpha has been used in 21 patients (including 10 in the first trimester) during pregnancy for a variety of disorders, and there were no abnormal fetal outcomes.[74] A patient with a refractory T-cell lymphoma responded to interferon alfa during the third trimester.[75] Rituximab has been used in one patient during the second trimester of pregnancy with a normal outcome.[76] Use of interleukin-2 during pregnancy has not been reported.

Miscellaneous

Corticosteroids are commonly used in curative therapy for non-Hodgkin's lymphoma. Although animal models have suggested an increase in fetal malformations, only recently did a case-control study show a significant association between first trimester exposure to corticosteroids and cleft palate in newborns.[77]

No information is available on use of capecitabine and other new agents; therefore, clear recommendations cannot be made concerning these drugs. It is important to bear in mind that combinations of agents may have synergistic teratogenic activity, and as newer, targeted antineoplastic drugs are developed, it will be important to monitor and report such findings. The potential risks and benefits of newer drugs must be carefully weighed against the same evidence-based information on older drugs.

RADIATION EXPOSURE DURING PREGNANCY

Radiation can be divided into ionizing and nonionizing radiation. Ionizing radiation has the ability to penetrate tissue and damage cellular DNA, resulting in mutation and ultimately affecting the development and viability of the fetus. Ionizing radiation clearly causes fetal abnormalities or death. Limited exposure to ionizing sources, such as the amount required for some medically necessary radiographic studies, may have little or no effect on development. Numerous studies of radiation exposure after atomic bomb detonations in Japan confirmed that this effect is dependent on dose and stage of fetal development at the time of exposure. Common fetal abnormalities after exposure to ionizing radiation include microcephaly, eye malformations, and growth retardation.[78] Fetal irradiation may result in an increased risk for acute leukemia during childhood. For these reasons, it is recommended that cumulative radiation exposure during gestation not exceed 500 mrem (5 mGy) and that exposure from 8 to 15 weeks after conception should be kept below 100 mrem (1 mGy) because of the increased incidence of mental retardation.[79]

Imaging

Routine cancer care requires staging of the malignancy. The benefits of precise staging must be carefully weighed against the risk of fetal malformation, mental retardation, and death caused by radiation. Fetal radiation during computed tomography in the latter trimesters ranges from 2910 to 4260 mrem (29.1 to 42.6 mGy),[80] and thus computed tomography is contraindicated during pregnancy. In contrast, a two-view chest x-ray examination delivers a dose of 60 mrem (0.6 mGy) to the fetus, which may be less with shielding.[81] Nonetheless, reasonable staging assessment can be performed during pregnancy with chest x-ray examination, sonography, and magnetic resonance imaging (MRI).[79,81] Sonography may be particularly useful in assessing the breasts and liver. MRI can be used sparingly when precise lymph node staging in the chest or abdomen is required. Unfortunately, MRI is subject to motion artifact, which may hamper image quality.

Therapeutic Radiation

Radiation therapy is commonly USED in the treatment of patients with breast cancer, cervical cancer, and lymphoma, all of which are common cancers in women of childbearing age. Systemic Iodine 131 is often used for treatment of thyroid cancer. The importance of radiation therapy in achieving cure or significant survival enhancement must be carefully considered, and when appropriate, delayed until after delivery. In breast cancer treatment, radiation therapy to the breast and/or axillary lymph nodes commonly follows adjuvant chemotherapy, and therefore radiation is not initiated until 14 to 18 weeks after surgery. Radiation in the treatment of lymphoma, likewise, typically follows chemotherapy, which can "buy time" until fetal maturity. Several studies indicate good outcomes when treatment with radioiodine is delayed for pregnant patients with thyroid cancer. In contrast, the curative treatment of cervical and anus cancers depends on therapeutic radiation to the pelvic region, and immediate delivery, followed by definitive treatment, is typically recommended. Radiation is extremely important for palliation of cancer-related symptoms and has been carefully used during pregnancy without fetal harm.[82,83] The fetal radiation dose during treatment of brain metastases has been estimated at 100 mGy without shielding.[84]

SPECIFIC CANCERS AND PREGNANCY

The optimal approach to caring for pregnant patients with cancer is not clearly defined; however, it is important to weigh the ability to provide the optimal cancer care to the mother with potential fetal risk. The desired outcome is the preservation of life and future livelihood of two individuals, although this is clearly not possible in all situations. Surgery can be performed during pregnancy, although there is a small but increased risk of low birth weight and infant death within 7 days[85] or spontaneous abortion.[86] An increase in malformations was not seen. Chemotherapy can likewise be used in carefully controlled circumstances.[87] Although therapeutic abortion is rarely recommended or accepted without significant deliberation, it remains an important consideration for certain situations.

Breast Cancer

Breast cancer is the most common malignancy in women and is not uncommon in women of childbearing age.[88]

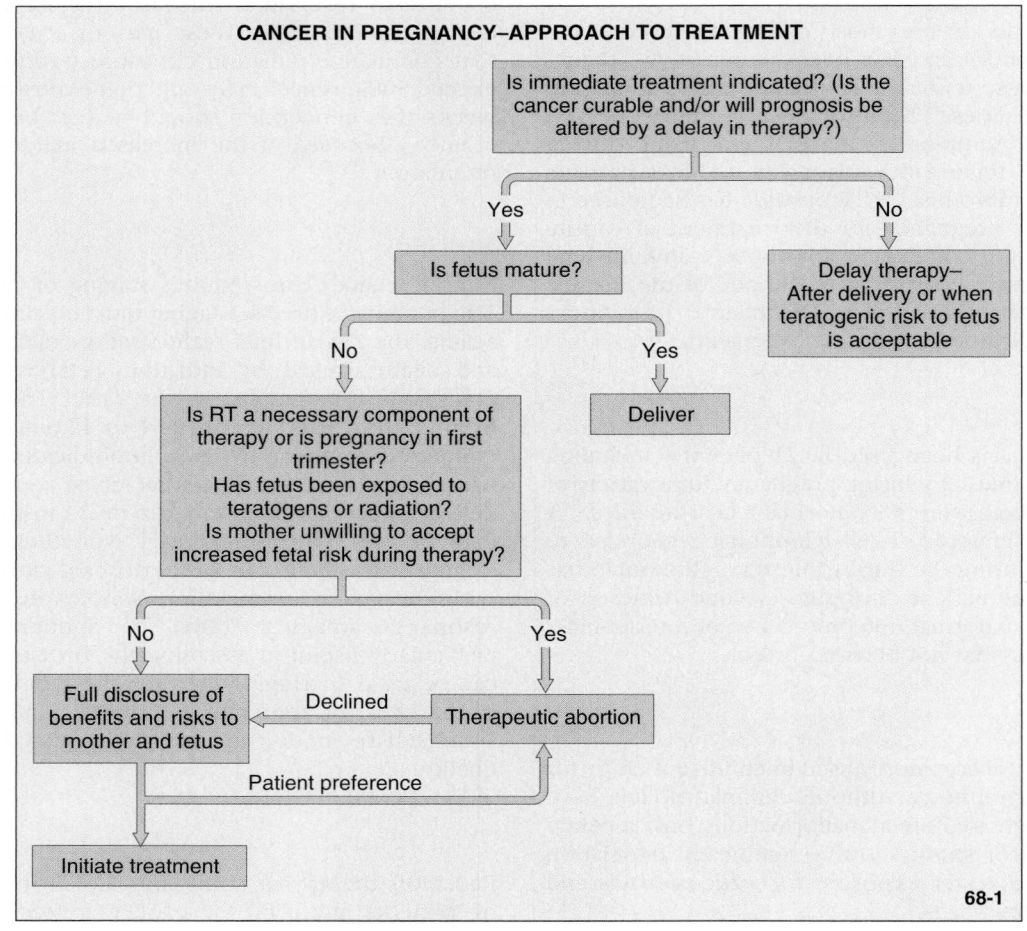

CANCER IN PREGNANCY–APPROACH TO TREATMENT

68-1

Therefore it is not surprising that breast cancer is the most commonly diagnosed malignancy in the pregnant patient in modern reports, and this is unlikely to change as women delay pregnancy until later in life.[89,90] Breast cancer during pregnancy appears to be more advanced and more likely to involve axillary lymph nodes[91], and it has been associated with a higher incidence of Her-2/neu positivity.[92] The more advanced stage appears to be due to diagnostic delay rather than direct effects of pregnancy on the cancer, and stage-specific survival is similar to that for nonpregnant patients.[93,94]

The most important factor in the diagnosis of breast cancer during pregnancy is suspicion. Imaging can be accomplished with mammography (with abdominal shielding) or sonography, although the false-positive rate with mammography is higher in pregnant patients.[88] Biopsy specimens should be obtained from mass lesions that suggest malignancy, even if results of imaging studies are negative. Biopsy can be accomplished with fine-needle aspiration, core needle biopsy, or surgical excision. Milk fistulas have been associated with core needle biopsy,[95] and fine-needle aspiration is preferred.[96] Surgical excision is often done when results of needle biopsy are nondiagnostic, as well as for surgical treatment.

The treatment of breast cancer during pregnancy is difficult. It is generally accepted that therapeutic abortion does not alter survival of the mother,[88,96,97] although treatment decisions may be somewhat easier. Termination of pregnancy is clearly an issue to be resolved through discussion and counseling with the patient and her significant others. Treatment options include surgery and systemic chemotherapy, the latter of which should be reserved for the second or third trimesters when indicated. Therapeutic radiation is contraindicated during pregnancy; however, it can be incorporated into the plan when the timing of initial treatment results in delivery before radiation. Treatment of the breast cancer should not be delayed, and timing should be similar to that for the nonpregnant patient with breast cancer.

A standardized protocol has been reported by a multidisciplinary breast cancer group at M.D. Anderson Cancer Center, where patients underwent extensive assessment by a number of specialists, followed by diagnostic biopsy and treatment.[98] This represents one of the few (if not the only) prospective reports on the care of pregnant women with breast cancer in the literature. Surgical treatment often includes modified radical mastectomy, especially in early gestation when radiation therapy would be significantly delayed. It is clear, however, that breast-conserving procedures can also be successfully employed,[39,99] and adjuvant or neoadjuvant chemotherapy may facilitate this approach. In the updated, prospective M.D. Anderson experience, 39 women received FAC (5-FU, Adriamycin [doxorubicin], cyclophosphamide) chemotherapy for a median of four cycles during the second and third trimesters with no reported spontaneous abortions, stillbirths, or fetal anomalies.

Recommendations regarding pregnancy after treatment for breast cancer are based on limited data. Recent studies indicate cancer-related prognosis is not affected by subsequent pregnancy[100,101] and subsequent pregnancy may even be protective,[101] although this remains controversial.[102,103] Nonetheless, most experts currently recommend an interval of 2 years between diagnosis of breast cancer and subsequent pregnancy,[104] although continued research is needed to refine such recommendations.[105]

Cervical Cancer

Cervical cancer appears to be the most common malignancy diagnosed during pregnancy, although it is still relatively uncommon in pregnant women. Fortunately, cervical cancer is curable in the early stages, and stage-specific survival for pregnant patients is similar to that for nonpregnant patients.[106-109] Papanicolaou smears are a standard component of the prenatal examination, but despite this fact, some cancers go undetected and do not manifest until after delivery.[110] An abnormal Papanicolaou test result should prompt immediate investigation, including colposcopy and biopsy if indicated.[111] Cone biopsy has been performed in pregnancy but should be only be done if necessary for diagnosis of invasive malignancy. Nearly 5% of cone biopsies performed during pregnancy resulted in fetal death.[112-115]

Management of early- and late-stage cervical cancer during pregnancy differs. Evidence suggests that deferred therapy for early-stage disease does not alter prognosis.[116,117] Therefore some experts recommend conization before 24 weeks' gestation for diagnosis, and deferred treatment after 24 weeks when the likelihood of advanced disease is small.[111] Appropriate definitive therapy should be instituted as soon as it is feasible after delivery. If late-stage disease is confirmed, immediate treatment is typically recommended; however, this raises many difficult issues. Standard therapy for late-stage cervical cancer involves radiotherapy, often with chemotherapy.[118-120] Sood and colleagues[117] reported on a series of 26 patients treated with radiotherapy, and when the diagnosis was made in the third trimester, immediate delivery was followed by radiation therapy 2 weeks later. Two of 15 infants died as a result of complications of prematurity at 27 and 29 weeks; however, all remaining infants did well with gestatations of 34 weeks. Six patients in the second trimester had hysterotomies, followed by radiation, and all fetuses died. Three patients in the first trimester had radiation with the fetus in place, all of which resulted in spontaneous abortion. Cesarean section is the preferred method of delivery because vaginal delivery appears to increase the risk of relapse.[110] Smith and colleagues[89] reported an increased risk of neonatal death for patients with cervical cancer associated with pregnancy.

Ovarian Cancer

Because of the frequent use of sonography during pregnancy, the discovery of an adnexal mass during pregnancy is not uncommon. Fortunately, invasive epithelial ovarian cancer is uncommon during pregnancy, with the majority of ovarian neoplasms in pregnancy having germ cell or low malignant potential histology.[121] Surgical staging and treatment of ovarian neoplasms include debulking surgery, including omentectomy, lymph node and peritoneal biopsy, and assessment of peritoneal washings. Germ cell tumors are typically treated with bleomycin, etoposide, and cisplatin; and experience with these agents in the latter trimesters of pregnancy is limited.[56,122] Low malignant potential neoplasms are treated with surgery alone. Invasive epithelial ovarian cancer is treated with postoperative chemotherapy consisting of cisplatin and paclitaxel. Only one case report of this combination in a pregnant patient is presently available, and the combination was safely used for three cycles in a pregnant woman with stage IIIC papillary serous ovarian adenocarcinoma.[46] The child had normal growth and development at 30 months of age.

Choriocarcinoma

Choriocarcinoma concurrent with pregnancy is exceedingly rare. In a series reviewed by Steigrad and colleagues,[123] only 35 cases were available in the medical literature, which revealed mortality rates of 62% for mothers and 65% for fetuses. This is in stark contrast to the generally favorable outcome of women who have gestational trophoblastic tumors after pregnancy. Patients may present with vaginal bleeding, abdominal pain, cough, breathlessness, or neurologic symptoms. Choriocarcinoma can metastasize to the fetus. Choriocarcinoma metastatic to the fetus was previously known as the *infantile choriocarcinoma syndrome*,[124] and a few case reports suggest that it is treatable with chemotherapy.[125,126]

Acute Leukemia

Acute leukemia during pregnancy presents a particularly challenging clinical situation. A number of case series exist,[63,127-129] and it is clear that the prognosis of the pregnant patient with acute leukemia has improved as the treatment for leukemia has evolved.[128] Commonly used drugs for induction and consolidation chemotherapy of acute leukemia include cytarabine, anthracyclines, cyclophosphamide, methotrexate, mercaptopurine, corticosteroids, and vinca alkaloids. Each of these drugs has been used in all phases of pregnancy; however, fetal malformations are more common when the drugs are administered in the first trimester,[27] and fetal prognosis is better when therapy is delivered in the second or third trimesters.[45] ATRA (all-trans-retinoic acid) has been used in patients with acute promyelocytic leukemia (APL) in the latter trimesters safely and effectively.[130-133] Transient cardiomyopathy was reported in an infant whose mother was treated for APL with ATRA and idarubicin beginning at 13 weeks' gestation.[61] There is limited experience with hydroxyurea in pregnancy, and it may be reasonable to consider leukapheresis in place of hydroxyurea when immediate leukoreduction is necessary.[134]

Despite initial reports of certain mortality,[129] pregnancy no longer appears to adversely affect the outcome of the pregnant patient with acute leukemia.[134] Because maternal prognosis may be jeopardized by treatment delay, most experts recommend treatment of the leukemia concordant with standard treatment of the disease. Aviles

and colleagues reported on their relatively modern experience of pregnant women with acute lymphocytic leukemia (n = 10) who received induction and consolidation chemotherapy with cyclophosphamide, vincristine, prednisone, and doxorubicin and acute myeloid leukemia (n = 19) who received induction and consolidation chemotherapy with cytarabine with an anthracycline.[63] At the time of the report, 20 of 29 mothers were alive and leukemia-free after therapy, and seven had died of disease. It is interesting to note that 29 children were born without congenital anomalies, 11 of whom were reportedly exposed to chemotherapy during the first trimester.

Lymphoma

Lymphoma is the fourth most common malignancy diagnosed during pregnancy,[89,90] and despite the fact that the non-Hodgkin lymphomas (NHLs) are more common than Hodgkin's lymphomas in the general population, Hodgkin's lymphoma is more prevalent in the childbearing years.[14] Thus Hodgkin's lymphoma is the most common lymphoma diagnosed during pregnancy, and nodular sclerosis is the most common histologic finding. When NHL is seen concurrent with pregnancy, it is more likely to be an aggressive form of the disease, which is consistent with the fact that indolent lymphomas are uncommon in young adults. A lymph node biopsy specimen must be obtained and reviewed by an experienced pathologist is necessary to confirm the diagnosis, and staging typically involves CT scans and a bone marrow biopsy. Computed tomography is contraindicated during pregnancy; however, abdominal sonography and a chest x-ray examination with shielding can be performed to complete staging.[14] Magnetic resonance imaging may be an alternative when it is used sparingly for situations requiring precise staging. Available evidence suggests that pregnancy does not alter the prognosis of lymphoma.

Aggressive NHL is typically treated with chemotherapy, and commonly used drugs include cyclophosphamide, doxorubicin, vincristine, and prednisone (CHOP). Cyclophosphamide is associated with fetal malformations when given in the first trimester[27]; however, all drugs have been given safely and effectively in the second and third trimesters. Rituximab, an anti-CD20 monoclonal antibody, is commonly used with CHOP chemotherapy; however, only one report of its use in pregnancy is available,[76] and it was used with doxorubicin, vincristine, and prednisone safely, beginning in the twenty-first week of pregnancy. Indolent NHLs often do not require immediate therapy, and when possible, observation is the treatment of choice.

The standard therapy for Hodgkin's lymphoma has evolved over the past decade. Previously, definitive radiation therapy was the treatment of choice for limited-stage disease; however, many experts now recommend chemotherapy with doxorubicin, bleomycin, vinblastine, and dacarbazine (ABVD) with or without involved-field radiation. Advanced-stage disease is typically treated with chemotherapy. During pregnancy, ABVD without dacarbazine has been recommended by some experts.[14,135] The older literature reflects the use of MOPP (mechlorethamine, vincristine, procarbazine, prednisone) chemotherapy for Hodgkin's lymphoma, and MOPP has also been used during pregnancy.[63] Procarbazine and mechlorethamine have been associated with fetal malformations,[27,45] and this regimen has fallen out of favor with most oncologists. Although radiation has been used with a favorable outcome during pregnancy for the treatment of lymphoma, there are few, if any, circumstances in the current era in which radiation would be the treatment of choice in this setting.

Timing of therapy is a difficult issue with lymphoma and pregnancy. Prognosis is related to stage in both Hodgkin's and non-Hodgkin's lymphoma, and therefore, curative therapy should not be delayed any longer than is necessary to optimize the outcome for both mother and infant. Single-agent vinblastine has been used safely during all trimesters of pregnancy, and many experts recommend it as an alternative to therapeutic abortion when immediate treatment is required.[14] When pregnancy adversely affects the mother's prognosis, most experts recommend consideration of therapeutic abortion.

Chronic Leukemia

Chronic lymphocytic leukemia has been reported in pregnancy[136] but is very rare.[137] most likely because it is uncommon in adults younger than 40 years. There are a number of case reports of chronic myeloid leukemia (CML) during pregnancy, although all of them represent a limited experience. Recent advances in the treatment of this disease have resulted in a shift from interferon alfa to imatinib mesylate as standard initial therapy. There are currently no reports on the use of imatinib during pregnancy; however, in a review of 21 patients (including 10 in the first trimester) treated with interferon alfa during pregnancy for a variety of disorders including CML and hairy cell leukemia, there were no abnormal fetal outcomes.[74] Leukopheresis[138-140] and hydroxyurea[141-143] have also been used to control an elevated leukocyte count in pregnant patients with CML.

Colorectal Cancer

Colorectal cancer is uncommon in pregnancy, and fewer than 100 cases are reported in the literature.[144-148] The majority of cases present in the rectum (64% to 86%) and with advanced disease (60% stage III or greater).[144] Colonoscopy has been performed during pregnancy.[149] Barium enema is contraindicated during pregnancy. Abdominal sonography may be useful to identify a mass lesion.[146] Common symptoms include rectal bleeding, abdominal pain and distension, and nausea and vomiting. The rarity of colon cancer in the setting of pregnancy, coupled with attribution of these symptoms to pregnancy, may lead to a delay in diagnosis.[145] Many reports detail cesarean delivery at the time of fetal maturity, followed by definitive colorectal surgery; however, cancer resection has been performed during pregnancy before fetal maturity.[148] The administration of adjuvant 5-FU has typically followed delivery,[149,150] and in most reports of 5-FU use during pregnancy, lower doses are given to patients with breast cancer.[39,151,152]

Gastric Cancer

Gastric symptoms are common in pregnancy, but fortunately, gastric cancer is not. The prevalence of gastric symptoms may delay diagnosis in the uncommon situation of concurrent gastric malignancy in the pregnant woman. From a review of 131 cases,[153] maternal outcome appears to be poor, with a 20% survival at 1 year. Fetal outcome is generally good, with 72% alive at birth, and no reports of disease metastatic to the fetus or infant.

Hepatocellular Carcinoma

Hepatocellular carcinoma is more commonly detected in men and tends to occur in patients beyond childbearing age. Nonetheless, this disease has been reported during pregnancy, and in a review of 28 cases, maternal outcome was typically poor. Stage-specific survival does not appear to differ from that for age-matched, nonpregnant women.[154] Pain in the right upper quadrant in patients at high risk should prompt consideration of the diagnosis of hepatocellular carcinoma, as well as spontaneous rupture.[155] A marked elevation in alpha-fetoprotein can be diagnostic.

Lung Cancer

Lung cancer is the most common malignancy in the United States and the most common cause of cancer death in women; however, lung cancer diagnosed during pregnancy is exceedingly rare. In a recent review of 16 cases, both non–small cell (n = 11) and small cell (n = 5) types were found, primarily in advanced stages.[49] Only one patient was reported to be alive more than 12 months from diagnosis. One patient was treated with chemotherapy consisting of cisplatin and vinorelbine at 27 weeks' gestation in an attempt to palliate the mother's severe dyspnea. Delivery by cesarean section ensued 4 days later, and the infant was healthy at the time of the report. Metastasis of small cell carcinoma from mother to fetus has been reported.[156] The child received aggressive chemotherapy and autologous transplantation and was reported to be well at 1 year of age.

Genitourinary Malignancies

Renal cell carcinoma has been reported in pregnancy. Presenting symptoms and signs included recurrent urine infection, flank pain, flank mass, and hemolytic anemia.[157,158] Sonography can be used for diagnosis, and surgery is the treatment of choice when feasible.[159] Bladder cancer has been reported during pregnancy, but the paucity of reports precludes discussion.[160]

Melanoma

Melanoma is not uncommon in women of childbearing age and therefore is an important consideration for the obstetrical team. Changing nevi or nevi suggestive of melanoma should be evaluated by a dermatologist, because pregnancy does not affect these lesions.[161]

Reviews of the literature suggest that stage-specific melanoma prognosis, primary tumor location, and treatment are similar to those for the nonpregnant patient.[162] Decisions regarding pregnancy after melanoma are difficult and should be based on risk of relapse. Some experts suggest pregnancy 3 years or more after diagnosis may be reasonable. Melanoma has one of the highest propensities for metastasis to the placenta of any malignancy, and melanoma can metastasize to the fetus.[163] The use of adjuvant interferon for melanoma during pregnancy has not been reported.

Thyroid Cancer

Some studies suggest thyroid cancer may be one of the most prevalent malignancies during pregnancy.[89] The most common presentation is that of an asymptomatic thyroid nodule. In a retrospective study, the outcomes of 61 women with thyroid cancer during pregnancy were compared with the outcomes of 528 age-matched nonpregnant women.[164] There were no significant differences in age, treatment choice (total or subtotal thyroidectomy with or without subsequent ^{131}I), or outcomes; however, there was a significant difference in treatment delay among pregnant women, with 77% choosing to have surgery after delivery. Radioiodine treatment was always administered after pregnancy. These and other data have led experts to recommend surgery during the second trimester when the diagnosis is made in early pregnancy; otherwise, most women can defer therapy until after delivery without altering prognosis.[165,166]

Sarcoma

Sarcomas are rarely diagnosed during pregnancy, and they represent a heterogenous group of diseases with varying natural histories. Ewing's sarcoma has been reported during pregnancy on a number of occasions, with successful delivery of chemotherapy to the mother during gestation.[167,168] A series of 18 pregnant patients with osteogenic sarcoma was compared with a group of nonpregnant control subjects matched for age, tumor location, and histologic findings.[169] There appeared to be no reciprocal effects on outcome between pregnancy and sarcoma.

PREGNANCY AFTER CANCER THERAPY

Completion of cancer therapy is accompanied by new anxieties and questions for the patient and her family. In addition to concerns about relapse, issues of family frequently arise. Is pregnancy possible? What is the risk for fetal anomaly? What happens in the event of relapse? A number of studies have indicated that the risk of fetal anomaly after cancer therapy is low and is likely similar to that of the general population.[170,171] Fertility issues must be considered in the treatment planning for any patient of childbearing age, male or female. Sperm cryopreservation is commonly available and effective; however, ova preservation is difficult, expensive, and not routinely available at present.[172] Nonetheless, it can be successful and has even been performed after bone marrow transplantation.[173]

Optimal timing of pregnancy after cancer in women is difficult, controversial, and based on opinion rather than data. Most experts recommend deferring pregnancy for 2 to 3 years, according to relapse risk for the specific malignancy.[104] Special concerns arise in patients with breast cancer desiring pregnancy, given hormonal issues and potential for stimulation of hormone-responsive malignant cells. Fortunately, several reports suggest that risk of breast cancer relapse in the face of pregnancy is not increased.[101,103] Patients with Wilms' tumor who have been treated with radiation to the flank have an increased risk for fetal malposition, premature labor, and infants with low birth weight and congenital malformations.[174,175] Oncologists must be sensitive to the needs of the young patient with cancer who desires a family, and recommendations should be individualized based on experience reflected in the literature and patient preference.

REFERENCES

1. Beeley L: Adverse effects of drugs in the first trimester of pregnancy. Clin Obstet Gynecol 1986;13:177.
2. Brent RL: The complexities of solving the problem of human malformations. Clin Perinatol 1986;13:491.
3. Wan SH, Huffman DH, Azarnoff DL, et al: Effect of route of administration and effusions on methotrexate pharmacokinetics. Cancer Res 1974;34:3487.
4. Powis G: Anticancer drug pharmacodynamics. Cancer Chemother Pharmacol 1985;14:177.
5. Arceci RJ, Croop JM, Horwitz SB, Housman D: The gene encoding multidrug resistance is induced and expressed at high levels during pregnancy in the secretory epithelium of the uterus. Proc Natl Acad Sci USA 1988;85:4350.
6. Juchau M, Chao S, Omiecinski C: Drug metabolism by the human fetus. In Gibaldi M, Prescott LF (eds): Handbook of Clinical Pharmacokinetics. New York, ADIS Health Science Press, 1983, p 58.
7. Karp GI, von Oeyen P, Valone F, et al: Doxorubicin in pregnancy: Possible transplacental passage. Cancer Treat Rep 1983;67:773.
8. Shamkhani H, Anderson LM, Henderson CE, et al: DNA adducts in human and patas monkey maternal and fetal tissues induced by platinum drug chemotherapy. Reprod Toxicol 1994;8:207.
9. Koren G: Changes in drug disposition during pregnancy and their clinical implications. In Koren G, Lishner M, Farine D (eds): Cancer in Pregnancy: Maternal and Fetal Risks. Cambridge, England, Cambridge University Press, 1996, p 27.
10. Brent RL: Evaluating the alleged teratogenicity of environmental agents. Clin Perinatol 1986;13:609.
11. Shepard TH: Catalog of Teratogenic Agents, 10th ed. Baltimore, MD, Johns Hopkins University Press, 2001.
12. Koren G, Pastuszak A, Ito S: Drugs in pregnancy. N Engl J Med 1998;338:1128.
13. Ferm V: Congenital malformation in hamster embryos after treatment with vinblastine and vincristine. Science 1963;141:426.
14. Pohlman B, Macklis RM: Lymphoma and pregnancy. Semin Oncol 2000;27:657.
15. Sokal J, Lessman E: Effects of cancer chemotherapeutic agents on the human fetus. JAMA 1960;172:1765.
16. Nicholson HO: Cytotoxic drugs in pregnancy. Review of reported cases. J Obstet Gynaecol Br Commonwealth 1968;75:307.
17. Blatt J, Mulvihill JJ, Ziegler JL, et al: Pregnancy outcome following cancer chemotherapy. Am J Med 1980;69:828.
18. Sweet DL Jr, Kinzie J: Consequences of radiotherapy and antineoplastic therapy for the fetus. J Reprod Med 1976;17:241.

19. Barber HR: Fetal and neonatal effects of cytotoxic agents. Obstet Gynecol 1981;58:41S.

20. Gililland J, Weinstein L: The effects of cancer chemotherapeutic agents on the developing fetus. Obstet Gynecol Surv 1983;38:6.

21. Antman K, Mayer R, Frei E: Vascular, hormonal, teratogenic and miscellaneous toxicities of chemotherapeutic agents. In Perry MC, Yarbro JW (eds): Toxicity of Chemotherapy. Orlando, FL, Grune & Stratton, 1984, p 521.

22. Mulvihill JJ, McKeen EA, Rosner F, Zarrabi MH: Pregnancy outcome in cancer patients. Experience in a large cooperative group. Cancer 1987;60:1143.

23. Diamond I, Anderson M, McCreadie S: Transplacental transmission of busulfan (myleran) in a mother with leukemia. Production of fetal malformations and cytomegaly. Pediatrics 1960;25:85.

24. Toledo TM, Harper RC, Moser RH: Fetal effects during cyclophosphamide and irradiation therapy. Ann Intern Med 1971;74:87.

25. Abramovici A, Shaklai M, Pinkhas J: Myeloschisis in a six weeks embryo of a leukemic woman treated by busulfan. Teratology 1978;18:241.

26. Cahen RL: Experimental and clinical chemoteratogenesis. Adv Pharmacol 1966;4:263.

27. Doll DC, Ringenberg QS, Yarbro JW: Management of cancer during pregnancy. Arch Intern Med 1988;148:2058.

28. Maghfoor I, Doll DC: Chemotherapy in pregnancy. In Perry MC (ed): The Chemotherapy Source Book, 3rd ed. Philadelphia, Lippincott Williams & Wilkins, 2001, p 537.

29. Bawle EV, Conard JV, Weiss L: Adult and two children with fetal methotrexate syndrome. Teratology 1998;57:51.

30. Doll DC, Ringenberg QS, Yarbro JW: Antineoplastic agents and pregnancy. Semin Oncol 1989;16:337.

31. Ebert U, Loffler H, Kirch W: Cytotoxic therapy and pregnancy. Pharmacol Ther 1997;74:207.

32. Buckley LM, Bullaboy CA, Leichtman L, Marquez M: Multiple congenital anomalies associated with weekly low-dose methotrexate treatment of the mother. Arthritis Rheum 1997;40:971.

33. Warkany J: Aminopterin and methotrexate: Folic acid deficiency. Teratology 1978;17:353.

34. Kozlowski RD, Steinbrunner JV, MacKenzie AH, et al: Outcome of first-trimester exposure to low-dose methotrexate in eight patients with rheumatic disease. Am J Med 1990;88:589.

35. Pizzuto J, Aviles A, Noriega L, et al: Treatment of acute leukemia during pregnancy: Presentation of nine cases. Cancer Treat Rep 1980;64:679.

36. Schleuning M, Clemm C: Chromosomal aberrations in a newborn whose mother received cytotoxic treatment during pregnancy. N Engl J Med 1987;317:1666.

37. Stephens JD, Golbus MS, Miller TR, et al: Multiple congenital anomalies in a fetus exposed to 5-fluorouracil during the first trimester. Am J Obstet Gynecol 1980;137:747.

38. Van Le L, Pizzuti DJ, Greenberg M, Reid R: Accidental use of low-dose 5-fluorouracil in pregnancy. J Reprod Med 1991;36:872.

39. Gwyn K, Theriault R, Sahin A, et al: Treatment of breast cancer (br ca) during pregnancy (pg) using a standard protocol: Update of the M.D. Anderson experience. In Grunberg S (ed): American Society of Clinical Oncology Proceedings. San Francisco, CA. American Society of Clinical Oncology, 2001, A1821.

40. Zemlickis D, Lishner M, Degendorfer P, et al: Fetal outcome after in utero exposure to cancer chemotherapy. Arch Intern Med 1992;152:573.

41. Maurer LH, Forcier RJ, McIntyre OR, Benirschke K: Fetal group C trisomy after cytosine arabinoside and thioguanine. Ann Intern Med 1971;75:809.

42. Schafer AI: Teratogenic effects of antileukemic chemotherapy. Arch Intern Med 1981;141:514.

43. Wagner VM, Hill JS, Weaver D, Baehner RL: Congenital abnormalities in baby born to cytarabine treated mother. Lancet 1980; 2:98.

44. Zemlickis D, Lishner M, Erlich R, Koren G: Teratogenicity and carcinogenicity in a twin exposed in utero to cyclophosphamide. Teratog Carcinog Mutagen 1993;13:139.

45. Wiebe VJ, Sipila PE: Pharmacology of antineoplastic agents in pregnancy. Crit Rev Oncol Hematol 1994;16:75.

46. Sood AK, Shahin MS, Sorosky JI: Paclitaxel and platinum chemotherapy for ovarian carcinoma during pregnancy. Gynecol Oncol 2001;83:599.

47. Otton G, Higgins S, Phillips KA, Quinn M: A case of early-stage epithelial ovarian cancer in pregnancy. Int J Gynecol Cancer 2001;11:413.

48. Marana HR, de Andrade JM, da Silva Mathes AC, et al: Chemotherapy in the treatment of locally advanced cervical cancer and pregnancy. Gynecol Oncol 2001;80:272.

49. Janne PA, Rodriguez-Thompson D, Metcalf DR, et al: Chemotherapy for a patient with advanced non-small-cell lung cancer during pregnancy: A case report and a review of chemotherapy treatment during pregnancy. Oncology 2001;61:175.

50. Ohara N, Teramoto K: Successful treatment of an advanced ovarian serous cystadenocarcinoma in pregnancy with cisplatin, Adriamycin and cyclophosphamide (CAP) regimen. Case report. Clin Exp Obstet Gynecol 2000;27:123.

51. Bayhan G, Aban M, Yayla M, et al: Cis-platinum combination chemotherapy during pregnancy for mucinous cystadeno-carcinoma of the ovary. Case report. Eur J Gynaecol Oncol 1999; 20:231.

52. Tomlinson MW, Treadwell MC, Deppe G: Platinum based chemotherapy to treat recurrent Sertoli Leydig cell ovarian carcinoma during pregnancy. Eur J Gynaecol Oncol 1997;18:44.

53. Henderson CE, Elia G, Garfinkel D, et al: Platinum chemotherapy during pregnancy for serous cystadenocarcinoma of the ovary. Gynecol Oncol 1993;49:92.

54. King LA, Nevin PC, Williams PP, Carson LF: Treatment of advanced epithelial ovarian carcinoma in pregnancy with cisplatin-based chemotherapy. Gynecol Oncol 1991;41:78.

55. Malfetano JH, Goldkrand JW: Cis-platinum combination chemotherapy during pregnancy for advanced epithelial ovarian carcinoma. Obstet Gynecol 1990;75:545.

56. Christman JE, Teng NN, Lebovic GS, Sikic BI: Delivery of a normal infant following cisplatin, vinblastine, and bleomycin (PVB) chemotherapy for malignant teratoma of the ovary during pregnancy. Gynecol Oncol 1990;37:292.

57. Kim DS, Park MI: Maternal and fetal survival following surgery and chemotherapy of endodermal sinus tumor of the ovary during pregnancy: A case report. Obstet Gynecol 1989;73:503.

58. Cuvier C, Espie M, Extra JM, Marty M: Vinorelbine in pregnancy. Eur J Cancer 1997;33:168.

59. De Santis M, Lucchese A, De Carolis S, et al: Metastatic breast cancer in pregnancy: First case of chemotherapy with docetaxel. Eur J Cancer Care (Engl) 2000;9:235.

60. Claahsen HL, Semmekrot BA, van Dongen PW, Mattijssen V: Successful fetal outcome after exposure to idarubicin and cytosine-arabinoside during the second trimester of pregnancy—a case report. Am J Perinatol 1998;15:295.

61. Siu BL, Alonzo MR, Vargo TA, Fenrich AL: Transient dilated cardiomyopathy in a newborn exposed to idarubicin and all-trans-retinoic acid (ATRA) early in the second trimester of pregnancy. Int J Gynecol Cancer 2002;12:399.

62. Bornstein RS, Hungerford DA, Haller G, et al: Cytogenetic effects of bleomycin therapy in man. Cancer Res 1971;31:2004.

63. Aviles A, Neri N: Hematological malignancies and pregnancy: A final report of 84 children who received chemotherapy in utero. Clin Lymphoma 2001;2:173.

64. Falkson HC, Simson IW, Falkson G: Non-Hodgkin's lymphoma in pregnancy. Cancer 1980;45:1679.

65. Rawlinson KF, Zubrow AB, Harris MA, et al: Disseminated Kaposi's sarcoma in pregnancy: A manifestation of acquired immune deficiency syndrome. Obstet Gynecol 1984;63:2S.

66. Rodriguez JM, Haggag M: Vacop-b chemotherapy for high grade non-Hodgkin's lymphoma in pregnancy. Clin Oncol 1995;7:319.

67. Nantel S, Parboosingh J, Poon MC: Treatment of an aggressive non-Hodgkin's lymphoma during pregnancy with macop-b chemotherapy. Med Pediatr Oncol 1990;18:143.

68. Sieber SM, Adamson RH: Toxicity of antineoplastic agents in man, chromosomal aberrations antifertility effects, congenital malformations, and carcinogenic potential. Adv Cancer Res 1975;22:57.

69. Lambert J, Wijermans PW, Dekker GA, Ossenkoppele GJ: Chemotherapy in non-Hodgkin's lymphoma during pregnancy. Neth J Med 1991;38:80.

70. Lowenthal RM, Funnell CF, Hope DM, et al: Normal infant after combination chemotherapy including teniposide for Burkett's lymphoma in pregnancy. Med Pediatr Oncol 1982;10:165.

71. Brunet S, Sureda A, Mateu R, Domingo-Albos A: Full-term pregnancy in a patient diagnosed with acute leukemia treated with a protocol including VP-16. Med Clin (Barc) 1993;100:757.

72. Aviles A, Niz J: Long-term follow-up of children born to mothers with acute leukemia during pregnancy. Med Pediatr Oncol 1988;16:3.

73. Arango HA, Kalter CS, Decesare SL, et al: Management of chemotherapy in a pregnancy complicated by a large neuroblastoma. Obstet Gynecol 1994;84:665.

74. Mubarak AA, Kakil IR, Awidi A, et al: Normal outcome of pregnancy in chronic myeloid leukemia treated with interferon-alpha in 1st trimester: Report of 3 cases and review of the literature. Am J Hematol 2002;69:115.

75. Echols KT, Gilles JM, Diro M: Mycosis fungoides in pregnancy: Remission after treatment with alpha-interferon in a case refractory to conventional therapy: A case report. J Matern Fetal Med 2001;10:68.

76. Herold M, Schnohr S, Bittrich H: Efficacy and safety of a combined rituximab chemotherapy during pregnancy. J Clin Oncol 2001;19: 3439.

77. Rodriguez-Pinilla E, Martinez-Frias ML: Corticosteroids during pregnancy and oral clefts: A case-control study. Teratology 1998;58:2.

78. Miller RW: Delayed radiation effects in atomic-bomb survivors. Major observations by the Atomic Bomb Casualty Commission are evaluated. Science 1969;166:569.

79. Pelsang RE: Diagnostic imaging modalities during pregnancy. Obstet Gynecol Clin North Am 1998;25:287.

80. Damilakis J, Perisinakis K, Voloudaki A, Gourtsoyiannis N: Estimation of fetal radiation dose from computed tomography scanning in late pregnancy: Depth-dose data from routine examinations. [erratum appears in Invest Radiol 2000 35:706]. Invest Radiol 2000;35:527.

81. Nicklas AH, Baker ME: Imaging strategies in the pregnant cancer patient. Semin Oncol 2000;27:623.

82. Willemse PH, van der Sijde R, Sleijfer DT: Combination chemotherapy and radiation for stage IV breast cancer during pregnancy. Gynecol Oncol 1990;36:281.

83. Magne N, Marcie S, Pignol JP, et al: Radiotherapy for a solitary brain metastasis during pregnancy: A method for reducing fetal dose. Br J Radiol 2001;74:638.

84. Mazonakis M, Damilakis J, Theoharopoulos N, et al: Brain radiotherapy during pregnancy: An analysis of conceptus dose using anthropomorphic phantoms. Br J Radiol 1999;72:274.

85. Mazze RI, Kallen B: Reproductive outcome after anesthesia and operation during pregnancy: A registry study of 5405 cases. Am J Obstet Gynecol 1989;161:1178.

86. Duncan PG, Pope WD, Cohen MM, Greer N: Fetal risk of anesthesia and surgery during pregnancy. Anesthesiology 1986;64:790.

87. Williams SF, Schilsky RL: Antineoplastic drugs administered during pregnancy. Semin Oncol 2000;27:618.

88. Keleher AJ, Theriault RL, Gwyn KM, et al: Multidisciplinary management of breast cancer concurrent with pregnancy. J Am Coll Surg 2002;194:54.

89. Smith LH, Dalrymple JL, Leiserowitz GS, et al: Obstetrical deliveries associated with maternal malignancy in California, 1992 through 1997. Am J Obstet Gynecol 2001;184:1504.

90. Pavlidis NA: Coexistence of pregnancy and malignancy. Oncologist 2002;7:279.

91. Petrek J: Breast cancer and pregnancy. In Harris JR (ed): Diseases of the Breast. Philadelphia, Lippincott-Raven Publishers, 1996, p 883.

92. Elledge RM, Ciocca DR, Langone G, McGuire WL: Estrogen receptor, progesterone receptor, and her-2/neu protein in breast cancers from pregnant patients. Cancer 1993;71:2499.

93. Zemlickis D, Lishner M, Degendorfer P, et al: Maternal and fetal outcome after breast cancer in pregnancy. Am J Obstet Gynecol 1992;166:781.

94. Petrek JA, Dukoff R, Rogatko A: Prognosis of pregnancy-associated breast cancer. Cancer 1991;67:869.

95. Schackmuth EM, Harlow CL, Norton LW: Milk fistula: A complication after core breast biopsy. Am J Roentgenol 1993;161:961.

96. Sorosky JI, Scott-Conner CE: Breast disease complicating pregnancy. Obstet Gynecol Clin North Am 1998;25:353.

97. Gwyn K, Theriault R: Breast cancer during pregnancy. Oncology (Huntingt) 2001;15:39.

98. Berry DL, Theriault RL, Holmes FA, et al: Management of breast cancer during pregnancy using a standardized protocol. J Clin Oncol 1999;17:855.

99. Kuerer HM, Gwyn K, Ames FC, Theriault RL: Conservative surgery and chemotherapy for breast carcinoma during pregnancy. Surgery 2002;131:108.

100. von Schoultz E, Johansson H, Wilking N, Rutqvist LE: Influence of prior and subsequent pregnancy on breast cancer prognosis. J Clin Oncol 1995;13:430.

101. Gelber S, Coates AS, Goldhirsch A, et al: Effect of pregnancy on overall survival after the diagnosis of early-stage breast cancer. J Clin Oncol 2001;19:1671.

102. Guinee VF, Olsson H, Moller T, et al: Effect of pregnancy on prognosis for young women with breast cancer. Lancet 1994;343:1587.

103. Surbone A: Too early to say that pregnancy has an antitumor effect on breast cancer. J Clin Oncol 2001;19:3707.

104. Petrek JA: Pregnancy safety after breast cancer. Cancer 1994;74:528.

105. Surbone A, Petrek JA: Childbearing issues in breast carcinoma survivors. Cancer 1997;79:1271.

106. Manuel-Limson GA, Ladines-Llave CA, Sotto LS, Manalo AM: Cancer of the cervix in pregnancy: A 31-year experience at the Philippine General Hospital. J Obstet Gynaecol Res 1997;23:503.

107. van der Vange N, Weverling GJ, Ketting BW, et al: The prognosis of cervical cancer associated with pregnancy: A matched cohort study. Obstet Gynecol 1995;85:1022.

108. Hopkins MP, Morley GW: The prognosis and management of cervical cancer associated with pregnancy. Obstet Gynecol 1992;80:9.

109. Zemlickis D, Lishner M, Degendorfer P, et al: Maternal and fetal outcome after invasive cervical cancer in pregnancy. J Clin Oncol 1991;9:1956.

110. Sood AK, Sorosky JI, Mayr N, et al: Cervical cancer diagnosed shortly after pregnancy: Prognostic variables and delivery routes. Obstet Gynecol 2000;95:832.

111. Method MW, Brost BC: Management of cervical cancer in pregnancy. Semin Surg Oncol 1999;16:251.

112. Kuoppala T, Saarikoski S: Pregnancy and delivery after cone biopsy of the cervix. Arch Gynecol 1986;237:149.

113. Ludviksson K, Sandstrom B: Outcome of pregnancy after cone biopsy—a case-control study. Eur J Obstet Gynecol Reprod Biol 1982;14:135.

114. Hannigan EV, Whitehouse HH III, Atkinson WD, Becker SN: Cone biopsy during pregnancy. Obstet Gynecol 1982;60:450.

115. Averette HE, Nasser N, Yankow SL, Little WA: Cervical conization in pregnancy. Analysis of 180 operations. Am J Obstet Gynecol 1970;106:543.

116. Sood AK, Sorosky JI, Krogman S, et al: Surgical management of cervical cancer complicating pregnancy: A case-control study. Gynecol Oncol 1996;63:294.

117. Sood AK, Sorosky JI, Mayr N, et al: Radiotherapeutic management of cervical carcinoma that complicates pregnancy. Cancer 1997;80:1073.

118. Keys HM, Bundy BN, Stehman FB, et al: Cisplatin, radiation, and adjuvant hysterectomy compared with radiation and adjuvant hysterectomy for bulky stage IB cervical carcinoma. N Engl J Med 1999;340:1154.

119. Rose PG, Bundy BN, Watkins EB, et al: Concurrent cisplatin-based radiotherapy and chemotherapy for locally advanced cervical cancer. N Engl J Med 1999;340:1144.

120. Morris M, Eifel PJ, Lu J, et al: Pelvic radiation with concurrent chemotherapy compared with pelvic and para-aortic radiation for high-risk cervical cancer. N Engl J Med 1999;340:1137.

121. Zanotti KM, Belinson JL, Kennedy AW: Treatment of gynecologic cancers in pregnancy. Semin Oncol 2000;27:686.

122. Buller RE, Darrow V, Manetta A, et al: Conservative surgical management of dysgerminoma concomitant with pregnancy. Obstet Gynecol 1992;79:887.

123. Steigrad SJ, Cheung AP, Osborn RA: Choriocarcinoma co-existent with an intact pregnancy: Case report and review of the literature. J Obstet Gynaecol Res 1999;25:197.

124. Witzleben CL, Bruninga G: Infantile choriocarcinoma: A characteristic syndrome. J Pediatr 1968;73:374.

125. Belchis DA, Mowry J, Davis JH: Infantile choriocarcinoma. Re-examination of a potentially curable entity. Cancer 1993;72:2028.

126. McNally OM, Tran M, Fortune D, Quinn MA: Successful treatment of mother and baby with metastatic choriocarcinoma. Int J Gynecol Cancer 2002;12:394.

127. Caligiuri MA, Mayer RJ: Pregnancy and leukemia. Semin Oncol 1989;16:388.

128. Catanzarite VA, Ferguson JE II: Acute leukemia and pregnancy: A review of management and outcome, 1972–1982. Obstet Gynecol Surv 1984;39:663.

129. McLain CR Jr: Leukemia in pregnancy. Clin Obstet Gynecol 1974;17:185.

130. Stentoft J, Nielsen JL, Hvidman LE: All-trans retinoic acid in acute promyelocytic leukemia in late pregnancy. Leukemia 1994;8(Suppl 2): S77.

131. Hoffman MA, Wiernik PH, Kleiner GJ: Acute promyelocytic leukemia and pregnancy. A case report. Cancer 1995;76:2237.

132. Delgado-Lamas JL, Garces-Ruiz OM: Malignancy: Case report: Acute promyelocytic leukemia in late pregnancy. Successful treatment with all-trans-retinoic acid (ATRA) and chemotherapy. Hematol Oncol 2000;4:415.

133. Giagounidis AA, Beckmann MW, Giagounidis AS, et al: Acute promyelocytic leukemia and pregnancy. Eur J Haematol 2000;64:267.

134. Brell J, Kalaycio M: Leukemia in pregnancy. Semin Oncol 2000; 27:667.

135. Dhedin N, Coiffier B: Lymphoma and pregnancy. In Canellos GP, Lister TA, Sklar JL (eds): The lymphomas, 1st ed. Philadelphia, WB Saunders, 1998, p 549.

136. Chrisomalis L, Baxi LV, Heller D: Chronic lymphocytic leukemia in pregnancy. Am J Obstet Gynecol 1996;175:1381.

137. Adami HO, Tsaih S, Lambe M, et al: Pregnancy and risk of non-Hodgkin's lymphoma: A prospective study. Int J Cancer 1997;70:155.

138. Strobl FJ, Voelkerding KV, Smith EP: Management of chronic myeloid leukemia during pregnancy with leukapheresis. J Clin Apheresis 1999;14:42.

139. Fitzgerald D, Rowe JM, Heal J: Leukapheresis for control of chronic myelogenous leukemia during pregnancy. Am J Hematol 1986;22:213.

140. Bazarbashi MS, Smith MR, Karanes C, et al: Successful management of ph chromosome chronic myelogenous leukemia with leukapheresis during pregnancy. Am J Hematol 1991;38:235.

141. Celiloglu M, Altunyurt S, Undar B: Hydroxyurea treatment for chronic myeloid leukemia during pregnancy. Acta Obstet Gynecol Scand 2000;79:803.

142. Baykal C, Zengin N, Coskun F, et al: Use of hydroxyurea and alpha-interferon in chronic myeloid leukemia during pregnancy: A case report. Eur J Gynaecol Oncol 2000;21:89.

143. Patel M, Dukes IA, Hull JC: Use of hydroxyurea in chronic myeloid leukemia during pregnancy: A case report. Am J Obstet Gynecol 1991;165:565.

144. Bernstein MA, Madoff RD, Caushaj PF: Colon and rectal cancer in pregnancy. Dis Colon Rectum 1993;36:172.

145. Balloni L, Pugliese P, Ferrari S, et al: Colon cancer in pregnancy: Report of a case and review of the literature. Tumori 2000;86:95.

146. Komurcu S, Ozet A, Ozturk B, et al: Colon cancer during pregnancy. A case report. J Reprod Med 2001;46:75.

147. Vitoratos N, Salamalekis E, Makrakis E, Creatsas G: Sigmoid colon cancer during pregnancy. Eur J Obstet Gynecol Reprod Biol 2002;104:70.

148. Caforio L, Draisci G, Ciampelli M, et al: Rectal cancer in pregnancy: A new management based on blended anesthesia and monitoring of fetal well being. Eur J Obstet Gynecol Reprod Biol 2000;88:71.

149. Chan YM, Ngai SW, Lao TT: Colon cancer in pregnancy. A case report. J Reprod Med 1999;44:733.

150. Heise RH, Van Winter JT, Wilson TO, Ogburn PL Jr: Colonic cancer during pregnancy: Case report and review of the literature. Mayo Clin Proc 192;67:1180.

151. Dreicer R, Love RR: High total dose 5-fluorouracil treatment during pregnancy. Wis Med J 1991;90:582.

152. Gwyn KM, Theriault RL: Breast cancer during pregnancy. Curr Treat Options Oncol 2000;1:239.

153. Jaspers VK, Gillessen A, Quakernack K: Gastric cancer in pregnancy: Do pregnancy, age or female sex alter the prognosis? Case reports and review. Eur J Obstet Gynecol Reprod Biol 1999;87:13.

154. Lau WY, Leung WT, Ho S, et al: Hepatocellular carcinoma during pregnancy and its comparison with other pregnancy-associated malignancies. Cancer 1995;75:2669.

155. Hsu KL, Ko SF, Cheng YF, Huang CC: Spontaneous rupture of hepatocellular carcinoma during pregnancy. Obstet Gynecol 2001;98:913.

156. Tolar J, Coad JE, Neglia JP: Transplacental transfer of small-cell carcinoma of the lung. N Engl J Med 2002;346:1501.

157. Smith DP, Goldman SM, Beggs DS, Lanigan PJ: Renal cell carcinoma in pregnancy: Report of three cases and review of the literature. Obstet Gynecol 1994;83:818.

158. Monga M, Benson GS, Parisi VM: Renal cell carcinoma presenting as hemolytic anemia in pregnancy. Am J Perinatol 1995;12:84.

159. Walker JL, Knight EL: Renal cell carcinoma in pregnancy. Cancer 1986;58:2343.

160. Loughlin KR, Ng B: Bladder cancer during pregnancy. Br J Urol 1995;75:421.

161. Katz VL, Farmer RM, Dotters D: Focus on primary care: From nevus to neoplasm: Myths of melanoma in pregnancy. Obstet Gynecol Surv 2002;57:112.

162. Borden EC: Melanoma and pregnancy. Semin Oncol 2000;27:654.

163. Baergen RN, Johnson D, Moore T, Benirschke K: Maternal melanoma metastatic to the placenta: A case report and review of the literature. Arch Pathol Lab Med 1997;121:508.

164. Moosa M, Mazzaferri EL: Outcome of differentiated thyroid cancer diagnosed in pregnant women. J Clin Endocrinol Metab 1997;82:2862.

165. Morris PC: Thyroid cancer complicating pregnancy. Obstet Gynecol Clin North Am 1998;25:401.

166. Vini L, Hyer S, Pratt B, Harmer C: Management of differentiated thyroid cancer diagnosed during pregnancy. Eur J Endocrinol 1999;140:404.

167. Haerr RW, Pratt AT: Multiagent chemotherapy for sarcoma diagnosed during pregnancy. Cancer 1985;56:1028.

168. Merimsky O, Le Chevalier T, Missenard G, et al: Management of cancer in pregnancy: A case of Ewing's sarcoma of the pelvis in the third trimester. Ann Oncol 1999;10:345.

169. Huvos AG, Butler A, Bretsky SS: Osteogenic sarcoma in pregnant women. Prognosis, therapeutic implications, and literature review. Cancer 1985;56:2326.

170. Mulvihill JJ, Myers MH, Connelly RR, et al: Cancer in offspring of long-term survivors of childhood and adolescent cancer. Lancet 1987;2:813.

171. Byrne J: Long-term genetic and reproductive effects of ionizing radiation and chemotherapeutic agents on cancer patients and their offspring. Teratology 1999;59:210.

172. Shahin MS, Puscheck E: Reproductive sequelae of cancer treatment. Obstet Gynecol Clin North Am 1998;25:423.

173. Lipton JH, Virro M, Solow H: Successful pregnancy after allogeneic bone marrow transplant with embryos isolated before transplant. J Clin Oncol 1997;15:3347.

174. Li FP, Gimbrere K, Gelber RD, et al: Outcome of pregnancy in survivors of Wilms' tumor. JAMA 1987;257:216.

175. Green DM, Peabody EM, Nan B, et al: Pregnancy outcome after treatment for Wilms tumor: A report from the national Wilms Tumor Study Group. J Clin Oncol 2002;20:2506.

Problems Common to Cancer and Its Therapy

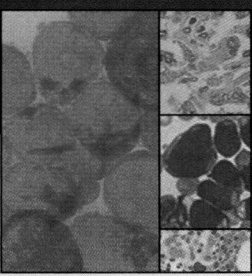

PART III

SPECIFIC MALIGNANCIES

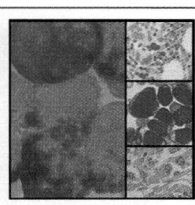

69

CANCER OF THE CENTRAL NERVOUS SYSTEM

Amit Maity

Amy A. Pruitt

Kevin D. Judy

Peter C. Phillips

SUMMARY OF KEY POINTS

INCIDENCE

- In 2002, 39,500 new cases of primary central nervous system (CNS) tumors were diagnosed in the United States; 17,000 of these tumors were malignant.
- Of all primary CNS tumors, 85% are intracranial; the remaining 15% occur in the spinal axis. An estimated 3110 new cases of primary benign and malignant brain tumors were diagnosed in children (ages 0 to 19 years) in 2002.
- Primary CNS malignancies account for 1% of all adult cancers and 2% of all adult cancer deaths. Among children 14 years old or younger, primary CNS malignancies account for approximately 23% of all cancers and 26% of all deaths due to cancer.

PATHOLOGY AND CLASSIFICATION

- Among intracranial tumors, the histologic types include meningiomas (27%), glioblastomas (21%), other astrocytomas (11%), neuromas (8%), pituitary adenomas (7%), oligodendrogliomas (4%), ependymomas (2%), and embryonal tumors including medulloblastomas (2%).
- Among children aged 14 years or younger, the histologic types of tumors include pilocytic astrocytomas (20%), glioblastomas (4%), other astrocytomas (13%), ependymomas (7%), oligodendrogliomas (2%), embryonal tumors including medulloblastomas (19%), craniopharyngiomas (3%), and germ cell tumors (4%).
- Most brain tumors are supratentorial; notable exceptions include brainstem gliomas, cerebellar pilocytic astrocytomas, medulloblastomas, and ependymomas, which involve the posterior fossa.
- Glioblastoma multiforme (WHO grade IV astrocytoma) and brainstem gliomas in children have the poorest prognosis. Pilocytic astrocytomas have the most favorable prognosis.

CLINICAL MANIFESTATIONS

- General symptoms, deriving from the mass effect, include increased intracranial pressure, edema, and shift and destruction of surrounding brain tissue, producing changes in personality and cognitive function, headaches, nausea, vomiting, seizures, and papilledema.
- Focal symptoms include focal seizures, visual changes, speech abnormalities, gait abnormalities, and cranial nerve deficits.
- Posterior fossa tumors often compress the fourth ventricle, causing hydrocephalus, and frequently present with ataxia and intractable nausea and vomiting.
- Brainstem gliomas often present with combination of cranial nerve palsies and "long-tract" signs such as hemianesthesia or hemiparesis coupled with ataxia if there is cerebellar involvement.
- Pineal region tumors (germ cell tumors, pineocytoma, and pineoblastoma as well as gliomas of this region) may compress the aqueduct of Sylvius, causing hydrocephalus. Compression of pretectal area produces Parinaud's syndrome with paralysis of upgaze, ptosis, and loss of pupillary light reflexes along with retraction-convergence nystagmus.

DIAGNOSTIC STUDIES

- Magnetic resonance imaging (MRI) with gadolinium contrast medium is the most sensitive technique.
- Computed tomographic (CT) scan is good for visualizing intratumoral calcifications and bone erosion but poor at visualizing the posterior fossa.
- Positron emission tomography (PET) may help discriminate between tumor recurrence and radiation necrosis.
- MR spectroscopy may help distinguish high-grade tumor from low-grade tumor or radiation necrosis.

THERAPY

- For most brain tumors, tissue diagnosis is required (the exception may be selected brainstem gliomas).
- Treatment for brain tumors is highly dependent on histologic characteristics. For many tumors (for example, gliomas, meningiomas, primitive neuroectodermal tumors, ependymomas), maximal surgical resection that is safely feasible is the primary treatment.
- For some tumors (for example, glioblastomas, primitive neuroectodermal tumors, germ cell tumors), radiation therapy is an essential adjunct treatment after surgery.
- For some tumors (for example, acoustic neuromas and glomus tumors), either radiation or surgery can offer successful control; decision between the two is based on assessment of side effects.
- Chemotherapy is assuming an increasingly important role in the management of many brain tumors (for example, germ cell tumors, anaplastic oligodendrogliomas, primitive neuroectodermal tumors, and CNS lymphomas).

INTRODUCTION

An estimated 39,500 new cases of primary CNS tumors were diagnosed in the United States in 2002.[1] Approximately 17,000 of those tumors were malignant, representing 1.3% of all cancers diagnosed that year.[2] Malignant CNS tumors caused approximately 13,000 deaths in 2002.[2] According to SEER (Surveillance, Epidemiology, and End Results) data, between 1991 and 1995, malignant tumors of the brain and spinal cord accounted for 1% of newly diagnosed adult cancers and 2% of deaths due to cancer.[3]

For most patients with primary CNS tumors, the initial therapy is usually operative. Radiation therapy is often an important component of therapy following surgery, but for those with malignant disease, chemotherapy has had an expanding role. A great deal of knowledge has been amassed over the past 15 years regarding the biology of brain tumors, and it is hoped that this information will lead to improved treatments in the future.

EPIDEMIOLOGY

The different histologic types of CNS tumors are shown in Table 69-1. Meningiomas, glioblastomas, and astrocytomas constitute over half of all CNS tumors. The incidence of different histologic types varies with age, as shown in

TABLE 69-2

Distribution of All Primary CNS Tumors in Childhood by Histologic Type		
TUMOR	**AGE 0–14 (N = 2302)**	**AGE 15–19 (N = 731)**
	FREQUENCY (%)	**FREQUENCY (%)**
Pilocytic astrocytoma	19.6	12.2
Glioblastoma	3.8	3.8
All other astrocytomas	13.0	13.0
Ependymoma	6.9	5.2
Oligodendroglioma	2.3	4.5
Embryonal, including PNET/medulloblastomas	18.7	7.3
Pituitary	0.7	10.4
Craniopharyngioma	3.4	3.3
Germ cell tumor	3.5	6.8
All others	27.9	33.5

Gliomas account for 57% of all tumors in the age group 0–14 years and 46% of all tumors in the age group 15–19 years.
Data from Central Brain Tumor Registry of the United States, Statistical Report 2002–2003, analysis of data collected from 1995 to 1999.

Figure 69-1. For gliomas and meningiomas, the incidence increases with age, reaching a peak in late adulthood. The range of histologic types that affect children differ from those that affect adults (Table 69-2). For example, glioblastomas and meningiomas, which together account for half of all adult CNS tumors, are rare in the pediatric population. Conversely, pilocytic astrocytomas and embryonal tumors including primitive neuroectodermal tumors (PNETs) are very common in children aged 0 to 14 years, accounting for 20% and 19%, respectively, of all CNS tumors.

Overall survival rates for patients with different histologic types are shown in Table 69-3. Among subtypes of astrocytomas, the prognosis from best to poorest is seen with pilocytic astrocytomas, diffuse astrocytomas, anaplastic astrocytomas, and glioblastomas. Oligodendrogliomas do significantly better than diffuse astrocytomas. One striking observation is that the outcome is worse in older patients than younger ones for every histologic type of tumor listed, with the exception of ependymoma. This finding is true for the most curable tumor listed, pilocytic astrocytoma, as well as for the least curable, glioblastoma. Based on 1973–1999 Surveillance, Epidemiology, and End Results (SEER) data, the 5-year survival rates following the diagnosis of a primary malignant brain tumor were 63% for patients 0 to 19 years old at diagnosis, 50% for those 20 to 44 years old, 14% for those 45 to 64 years old, and 5% for those 65 years and older.

In comparing SEER data from 1975 to 1979 versus 1991 to 1995, it is evident that there was a significant increase in the incidence of primary CNS malignancies from the earlier period to the later period in two age groups: children below the age of 14 and adults older than 70.[3] In particular, adults over the age of 85 have shown a particularly dramatic increase in the incidence of primary CNS malignancies from 1975 to 1995. It has been postulated that the increased use of MRI is a factor;

TABLE 69-1

Cell of Origin and Distribution of Primary CNS Tumors by Histologic Type		
TUMOR	**CELL OF ORIGIN**	**FREQUENCY (%)**
Meningioma	Arachnoidal fibroblast	27.4
Glioblastoma	Astrocyte	23.0
Astrocytoma	Astrocyte	11.3
Ependymoma	Ependymal cell	2.2
Oligodendroglioma	Oligodendrocyte	4.0
Embryonal, including primary neuroectodermal tumor (PNET)/ medulloblastoma	Unknown*	1.9
Pituitary adenoma	Pituitary	6.6
Craniopharyngioma	Cells from Rathke's pouch	0.8
Nerve sheath	Schwann cell	7.5
Lymphoma	Lymphocyte	2.7
All others		12.6
Choroid plexus papilloma or carcinoma	Choroid epithelial cell	
Hemangioblastoma	Endothelial cell	
Germ cell tumor	Primitive germ cell	
Pineocytoma	Pineal parenchymal cell	
Chordoma	Notochordal remnant	

Gliomas (glioblastomas, astrocytomas, oligodendrogliomas, and ependymomas) and neuroepithelial tumors account for 44.4% of all tumors.
*The cell of origin for CNS PNET is of great debate among neuropathologists.
Data from Central Brain Tumor Registry of the United States, Statistical Report 2002–2003, analysis of data collected from 1995 to 1999 (n = 37,788).

Figure 69-1. Age-specific incidence of primary CNS tumors by histology. The category "All brain tumors" includes some specific types not individually shown (tumors of the cranial and spinal nerves, hemangioblastomas, CNS lymphomas, germ cell tumors, tumors of the sellar region). The "Astrocytoma" category includes diffuse astrocytomas, anaplastic astrocytomas, unique astrocytoma variants, and astrocytomas not otherwise specified. (From Central Brain Tumor Registry of the United States: Statistical Report: Primary Brain Tumors in the United States 1992–1997.)

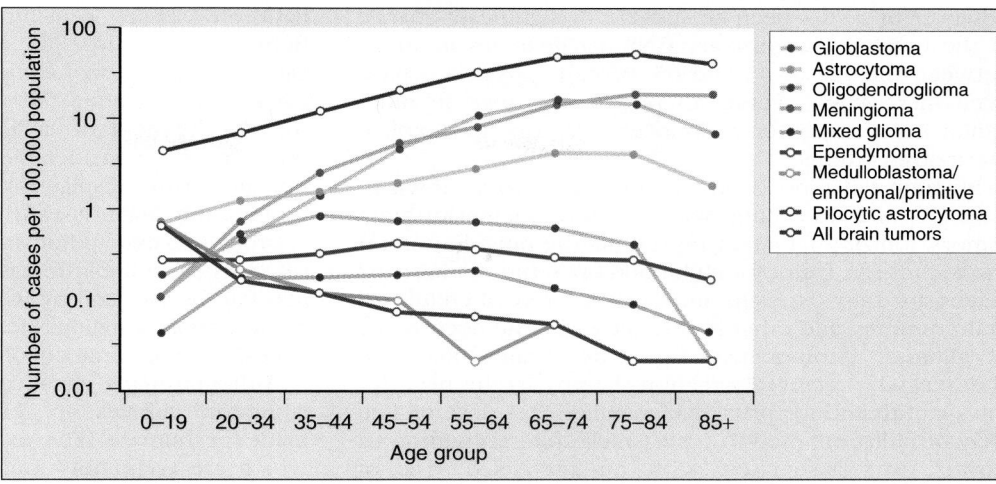

TABLE 69-3

Survival Rates for Selected CNS Tumors by Age Groups

TUMOR	AGE GROUP	NO. OF CASES	SURVIVAL RATES (%)			
			1-YR	2-YR	5-YR	10-YR
Pilocytic astrocytoma	0–19	634	97	96	93	91
	20–44	201	93	90	87	82
	45–64	42	88	86	72	58
	65+	18	*	*	*	*
Diffuse astrocytoma	0–19	124	93	87	82	80
	20–44	268	90	82	57	38
	45–64	163	59	36	24	14
	65+	104	29	16	6	6
Anaplastic astrocytomas	0–19	158	78	61	52	48
	20–44	771	86	73	50	33
	45–64	598	54	32	16	12
	65+	471	20	6	2	2
Glioblastoma	0–19	244	51	29	19	16
	20–44	1643	59	30	13	8
	45–64	5872	35	8	2	1
	65+	5974	13	2	0.3	0.2
Oligodendroglioma	0–19	152	92	86	82	76
	20–44	773	95	91	81	62
	45–64	453	86	74	54	32
	65+	146	57	46	29	10
Anaplastic oligodendroglioma	0–19	8	*	*	*	*
	20–44	109	91	74	50	31
	45–64	93	72	57	39	29
	65+	46	44	24	18	*
Ependymoma	0–19	380	85	71	52	44
	20–44	364	91	89	84	76
	45–64	219	85	81	69	58
	65+	75	74	74	71	50
Mixed gliomas	0–19	101	87	80	71	65
	20–44	318	92	85	69	49
	45–64	188	80	59	35	22
	65+	57	49	35	16	8
Embryonal/PNET	0–19	926	79	69	53	46
	20–44	287	86	75	57	45
	45–64	47	74	69	55	38
	65+	9	*	*	*	*

*Too few cases to estimate.
Data from SEER (Surveillance, Epidemiology, and End Results), 1973–1999.

however, there has been no statistically significant change in the incidence of primary CNS malignancies in adults between the age of 45 and 65. Perhaps physicians have been increasingly willing to pursue diagnosis in older adults. However, other undiscovered factors may explain these observations.

Ionizing radiation is one of the few factors shown to have a strong association with the development of brain tumors. Ionizing radiation represents the most important exogenous risk factor for childhood brain tumors. Prenatal diagnostic x-ray exposure increases the risk of childhood brain tumors,[4] and other reports describe the occurrence of gliomas, meningiomas, and other brain tumors in children who received radiation therapy to the head for tinea capitis and for prior malignancies.[5-8] A dose of 1 to 2 Gy of radiation, used to treat Israeli children with tinea capitis, was associated with an increased risk of developing brain tumors, specifically meningiomas, gliomas, and nerve sheath tumors.[9] A dose response in the induction of brain tumors was seen with a relative risk of 3.0 at 1 Gy. Tumors developed at least 6 years following irradiation, with a mean interval greater than 15 years. Even lower doses of radiation delivered with ^{226}Ra used to treat hemangiomas in Swedish infants (mean dose to brain of 7 cGy) were found to be associated with an excess risk of intracranial tumors, including pituitary adenomas, gliomas, meningiomas, and nerve sheath tumors.[10]

A large amount of data exists on the incidence of brain tumors in patients who received cranial irradiation for the treatment of acute lymphoblastic leukemia (ALL). The estimated cumulative risk of secondary malignant brain tumors after childhood ALL therapy is 0.5% by 10 years after completion of therapy.[11] In a study from St. Jude Children's Research Hospital the actuarial 20-year probability of developing a brain tumor in these patients was 1.4%.[12] The probability of developing a high-grade glioma was greater in children who were younger than 5 years of age when diagnosed than in those 6 years or older (1.08% versus 0.45%; $P = .045$). A dose response appears likely, with a 20-year risk of developing a brain tumor of 3.2% in patients who received more than 30 Gy versus 1.03% in those who received 21 Gy or less ($P = .015$). No CNS malignancies were seen in patients who did not receive cranial irradiation. The latency period between radiation and the diagnosis of a brain tumor ranged from 5.9 to 29 years (median 12.6 years), but this time was longer for meningiomas (median 19 years) than for high-grade gliomas (median 9.1 years). Very similar results regarding the frequency of brain tumors, latency period, and dependence on prior cranial radiation were seen in studies from the German BFM group[13] and the Children's Cancer Study Group (CCSG).[14] The types of brain tumors that have been reported in these series include gliomas, meningiomas, and medulloblastomas. Patients who received cranial irradiation for ALL also often received intrathecal chemotherapy. It has been suggested that cranial radiation and intrathecal chemotherapy may work synergistically to increase the incidence of glial tumors.[15,16]

Viruses can induce brain tumors in animals in the experimental setting.[17] However, there are no conclusive data on viruses causing brain tumors in humans.[18] Between 1955 and 1963, a limited number of poliovirus vaccine lots were contaminated with live simian virus 40 (SV40). The potential involvement of polyomaviruses in the development of childhood brain tumors has been the subject of considerable debate.[19] Monkey and human polyomaviruses display a strong oncogenic potential after inoculation into rodent brain.[20] Ependymomas and choroid plexus papillomas can be induced by SV40 and BK virus; medulloblastomas, ependymomas, and astrocytomas can be induced by JC virus. However, recent studies argue against a major role of these viruses in the pathogenesis of human medulloblastomas and ependymomas.[21]

Although many chemicals can induce brain tumors in laboratory animals, no definitive associations have been made in humans. For example, N-nitroso compounds, which are commonly found in foods, are known to be neurocarcinogenic in animals. Oxidants in the environment can cause DNA damage, so it has been hypothesized that antioxidants such as vitamin E found in certain foods may protect against the development of cancers. However, epidemiologic studies have provided mixed support for the idea that the intake of N-nitroso compounds, antioxidants, or specific nutrients in foods can influence the risk of developing brain tumors (reviewed by Berleur and Cordier[18]).

Also, no conclusive evidence indicates that occupational exposure to industrial chemicals leads to the development of brain tumors, although a number of studies suggest a link.[22] Some of the chemicals that can induce brain tumors in laboratory animals, such as polycyclic aromatic hydrocarbons, can do so only when administered by direct contact or transplacentally but not by inhalation or dermal contact, which are more relevant in the cases of occupational exposure. Specific chemicals that have been examined include cosmetics containing N-nitroso compounds, organic solvents, chemicals used in the manufacture of synthetic rubber, formaldehyde, phenols, polycyclic aromatic compounds, polyvinyl chloride, and pesticides. Vinyl chloride can induce brain tumors in rats; however, a recent review found that the association in humans in inconclusive.[23] Bohnen and Kurland reviewed studies examining the incidence of brain tumors in agricultural workers exposed to pesticides and found that the results were inconclusive.[24] A large meta-analysis of studies examining workers in the petrochemical industry found no increased risk of brain tumors in this population.[25]

Recently, a great deal of interest in the media and the lay public has centered on the use of cellular telephones and the risk of brain tumors. However, several epidemiologic studies have failed to show any statistically significant association between the two. In a case-control study, Inskip and coworkers were unable to show a correlation between the duration of cell phone use and the development of gliomas, meningiomas, and acoustic neuromas.[26] Another large case-control study also found no association between cell phone use and the risk of developing a brain tumor.[27] In spite of these negative findings, because of the increasing use of cellular phones and the use of digital phones, which operate at a higher frequency (1600

TABLE 69-4

Hereditary Syndromes Associated with Brain Tumors

HEREDITARY SYNDROME	ASSOCIATED CNS TUMORS	GENE	CHROMOSOMAL LOCUS	DEFECTIVE PROTEIN AND NORMAL FUNCTION
Neurofibromatosis 1	Optic pathway gliomas, meningiomas, neuromas	NF1	17q11-12	Neurofibromin; GTPase-activating protein (GAP) negatively regulates Ras
Neurofibromatosis 2	Bilateral acoustic neuromas, meningiomas, gliomas	NF2	22q12	Merlin; related to membrane cytoskeleton linker protein 4.1 superfamily
Tuberous sclerosis	Cerebral hamartomas	TSC1	9q34	Hamartin
	Subependymal giant cell astrocytoma (SEGA)	TSC2	16p13	Tuberin; associates with hamartin; both are involved in signaling downstream of AKT
von Hippel–Lindau syndrome	Hemangioblastomas	VHL	3p25-29	VHL protein; degrades HIF-1a under normoxia
Li-Fraumeni syndrome	Malignant gliomas	p53	17p13	p53; maintains genomic stability
Cowden's syndrome	Meningiomas	PTEN	10q23	PTEN; lipid phosphatase, counters PI(3) kinase activation
Gorlin's syndrome (nevoid basal cell carcinoma syndrome)	Medulloblastomas	PTCH	9q22	Cell surface receptor; regulates normal brain development
Turcot's syndrome	Medulloblastomas	APC	5q21	APC; part of β-catenin/Wnt signaling pathway
	Malignant gliomas	hMLH1	3p21	Involved in mismatch repair
	Malignant gliomas	PMS2	7p22	Involved in mismatch repair
Familial retinoblastoma	Pineoblastomas	Rb	13q14	Rb protein; regulates entry into S phase
Ataxia-telangiectasia	CNS lymphoma	ATM	11q22-23	ATM protein; involved in DNA damage sensing
Multiple endocrine neoplasia syndrome 1 (MEN-1)	Pituitary adenomas	MEN-1	11q13	Menin; function unknown

to 2000 MHz) than the older analog phones (800 to 900 MHz), undoubtedly interest in this issue will continue.

Other factors that have been analyzed for their possible relationship to the development of brain tumors include a history of head trauma and injury, drugs and medications, allergies, seizures, smoking and alcohol consumption, and exposure to power frequency electromagnetic fields (EMFs). However, none of these factors have been shown to be conclusively important.[22]

Most brain tumors represent sporadic cases; however, familial clustering has been noted. It is estimated that hereditary syndromes account for 2% of childhood brain tumors, although this may be an underestimate because some hereditary syndromes may not be diagnosed.[28] Some hereditary syndromes known to be associated with brain tumors are listed in Table 69-4.[29] Some of these associations are extremely strong. Nearly 70% of all optic pathway gliomas occur in patients with neurofibromatosis type 1 (NF1),[30] and acoustic neuromas commonly occur in patients with NF2.[31] Hereditary immunosuppression disorders such as the Wiskott-Aldrich syndrome as well as treatment-associated immunosuppression seen in organ-transplant recipients or exogenous immunosuppression in HIV infection are all associated with an increased risk of primary CNS lymphoma.

BIOLOGY

In the past decade, the field of oncology has seen explosive growth in the understanding of basic biologic processes. Normal cells have constraints in their ability to grow; for example, their growth is generally inhibited when they contact other cells. However, tumor cells have sustained genetic mutations that allow them to overcome these constraints. Some of these changes allow them to proliferate in the absence of external cues. Other genetic changes allow them to induce angiogenesis and develop their own blood supply. Still other changes make it possible for tumor cells to invade adjacent normal tissues.

Cell Proliferation

Normal cells rely on growth factors secreted in their local environment to stimulate their growth. However, many CNS tumors have developed the ability to express their own growth factors along with the respective receptors, resulting in an autocrine loop that allows for self-stimulation.[32] Platelet-derived growth factor (PDGF)-related genes including both the ligands and the receptors are expressed in gliomas and meningiomas.[33] The receptor PDGFR-α is overexpressed in all grades of astrocytomas, but only higher grade tumors overexpress the ligands PDGF-A and PDGF-B.[34] Insulin-like growth factors and their receptors are both expressed in brain tumors, including gliomas and meningiomas.[35] The epidermal growth factor receptor (EGFR) is amplified in 40% to 60% of glioblastomas, and expression of transforming growth factor-α (TGF-α), a ligand that binds to this receptor, is increased in gliomas and meningiomas.[36] Both scatter factor (also known as hepatocyte growth factor, or HGF) and its receptor c-met are expressed in gliomas with the highest level of expression seen in the most malignant tumors.[37,38] Antisense and dominant negative strategies directed against insulin-like growth factors, PDGF, EGFR, and TGF-α have been used to inhibit the growth of many glioma cell lines, indicating the importance of these growth factors in their proliferation.[39]

Specific Malignancies

As a result of increasing expression of receptors and ligands, increased signaling occurs in many brain tumors, resulting in activation of many different pathways that are important in proliferation. The best studied of these pathways is the MAP kinase pathway, which involves Ras and Raf. Another pathway that has attracted much attention recently is the PI(3) kinase pathway which leads to activation of Akt. Both of these pathways can be activated in brain tumors through stimulation of receptor tyrosine kinases.[40] Mutation of PTEN, which occurs in 30% to 40% of glioblastomas, can also lead to increased Akt activation in GBMs.[41] Another signaling molecule that may be activated by tyrosine kinase receptor signaling in brain tumors is phospholipase C-γ, which in turn increases protein kinase C (PKC) expression.[32] Couldwell and associates showed that PKC activity is induced by exposure of glioma cells to epidermal growth factor and that PKC is expressed at higher levels in human malignant glioma specimens than in normal brain tissue.[42]

Ras activation is commonly seen in human astrocytomas and neurifibromas in spite of the fact that these tumors rarely contain *ras* mutations.[43,44] In astrocytomas, Ras activation likely occurs through activation of growth factor receptors such as EGFR and PDGFR.[45] Farnesyl transferase inhibitors (FTIs), which block Ras function, can prevent the growth of glioblastomas both in vitro and in vivo.[46] Furthermore, the ability of FTIs to inhibit glioblastoma growth correlates well with the presence of activated Ras.[47] However, other mechanisms of activation of aberrant G proteins occur in other CNS tumors.[48] In neurofibromatosis type I, there is loss of expression of neurofibromin, an inactivator of Ras (see Table 69-4). This loss of neurofibromin leads to the increased Ras activation seen in NF1-associated astrocytomas. Pituitary adenomas often show activation of the G-α subunit of the large heterotrimeric G_s protein, resulting in mitogenic signaling.

Cell proliferation is intimately tied to cell cycle regulation. For many tumors, mutations in two different pathways are important for deregulating the cell cycle. The first of these is the p16/cdk4 or cdk6/cyclin D/Rb pathway. The second is the p21/p53/mdm2/p19ARF pathway. Mutations in both of these pathways are common in many brain tumors and are thought to play a causal role in the genesis of these tumors. Mutations in these pathways are common in gliomas and will be discussed in greater detail in the section devoted to these tumors in this chapter. However, other brain tumors may also have mutations in some of these genes, for example, homozygous deletions at the *CDKN2A* locus in anaplastic meningiomas.[49]

Angiogenesis

In order for a tumor to grow beyond a certain size, it must develop a blood supply. The process of angiogenesis is described in detail in Chapter 9 in this text. A number of growth factors are known to be important in angiogenesis. The most prominent of these is vascular endothelial growth factor (VEGF), which is overexpressed in many brain tumors including high-grade gliomas,[37,50] meningiomas,[51] and ependymomas.[50] In one study,

increasing VEGF expression correlated with increasing malignant grade in astrocytomas, oligodendrogliomas, and ependymomas.[50] Likewise, increased expression of the VEGF receptors Flt-1 and KDR in tumor vasculature was found to correlate with increasing VEGF expression and malignant grade. Growth factors other than VEGF that may play a role in angiogenesis in gliomas include members of the TGF-β family, PDGF, basic fibroblast growth factor, and scatter factor/HSF.[52] As discussed in the previous section, many of these factors and their receptors are overexpressed in brain tumors.

Angiogenesis can also be negatively regulated by factors such as thrombospondin 1 (TSP1) and 2. TSP1 is positively regulated by p53, so loss of p53, which commonly occurs in gliomas, can lead to decreased TSP1 expression and increased angiogenesis. Introduction of chromosome 10 into glioma cells resulted in increased expression of TSP1 and in human glioblastoma cell lines and inhibition of angiogenesis, suggesting that TSP1 may also be negatively regulated by a gene on this chromosome.[53]

Invasion

Many brain tumors, particularly gliomas, display an invasive phenotype with infiltration of tumor cells into surrounding tissues. For this reason, it is difficult to cure these tumors. Numerous proteins have been identified that may be important in this invasive phenotype. The matrix metalloproteases (MMPs) are a family of proteins that can degrade components of the extracellular matrix (ECM). In one study, MMPs were found to be expressed at higher levels in high-grade astrocytomas than in low-grade tumors.[54] Antisense MMP-9 can decrease glioblastoma invasion, indicating the importance of this protease in the invasive phenotype.[55]

The urokinase system also plays a role in glioma invasion.[56] Urokinase plasminogen activator (uPA) binds to its receptor uPAR and converts plasminogen to plasmin, which can degrade the ECM. uPAR may also be involved in other processes such as cell adhesion and transmission of extracellular signals across the plasma membrane. uPA and uPAR are both expressed at higher levels in high-grade astrocytomas than in low-grade astrocytomas and are absent in non-neoplastic brain tissue.[57] Suppression of uPAR function using an antisense strategy or a uPA fragment resulted in decreased tumor invasion in human glioblastoma cells both in vitro and in vivo.[58,59] In order for tumor cells to invade, they must first be able to adhere to the ECM and migrate. Integrins, which are transmembrane proteins expressed as heterodimers, are required to allow cells to adhere to various matrix substrates such as laminin, fibronectin, and vitronectin. A myriad of different integrins are expressed in gliomas.[60] Many of these integrins such as a_vb_3 have increased expression in gliomas compared to normal brain and may contribute to their invasive phenotype.[61] The ECM in brain tissue is limited to the perivascular space, which is often infiltrated by glioma cells. However, evidence shows that glioma cells can also induce normal brain tissue to make ECM components such as laminin and fibronectin.[62] Glioblastoma cells injected intracerebrally were found to secrete the matrix protein vitronectin into the ECM at the invading tumor margin.[57] If this behavior is a general phenomenon, it may be another means by which gliomas can modulate adhesion and invasion.

CLINICAL PRESENTATION

Pathophysiology of Signs and Symptoms

Parenchymal brain tumors produce symptoms by three main mechanisms, each of which has important implications for therapy: (1) Infiltration along nerve fiber tracts is typical of low-grade astrocytomas and oligodendrogliomas. The first symptom may be a single seizure. Normal brain tissue may be present within areas appearing abnormal on MRI, and functional mapping may be necessary for safe resection of these slowly growing tumors.[63-66] (2) Displacement of brain tissue and production of vasogenic edema is typical of cerebral metastases. Such tumors sometimes can be resected or irradiated focally with less risk to adjacent normal brain tissue than is the case with infiltrating tumors. (3) Rapidly growing aggressive tumors such as high-grade astrocytomas may grow as a mass *and also destroy* surrounding neuropil to such an extent that surgical resection, though helpful for the reduction of mass effect and intracranial pressure, may not alleviate local symptoms.

Intracranial neoplasms tend to produce progressive symptoms. Location and rate of growth determine both general and specific localizing symptoms and signs. Thus a patient with a low-grade glial tumor may have seizures for many years or behavioral alteration for many months before developing focal signs. A patient with a more aggressive glial neoplasm may develop headache and focal signs over a few weeks. Acute apoplectic onset is associated with hemorrhage or the development of hydrocephalus.

Brain tumor symptoms may be general, localizing, or falsely localizing. *General symptoms* include headache, lethargy, nausea, vomiting, and vague balance difficulties. These symptoms tend to be manifestations of increased intracranial pressure from a combination of expanding tumor volume and the production of associated vasogenic cerebral edema. Tumors may also cause raised intracranial pressure by obstruction of the ventricular system or blockage of the venous sinuses. Abrupt headache and exacerbation of neurologic signs may accompany the plateau waves of sudden increased intracranial pressure.

Sustained intracranial pressure in excess of 200 mm H_2O causes brain shifts that can displace brain tissue through fixed intracranial openings, producing life-threatening herniation syndromes (Fig. 69-2 and Table 69-5).[67] The *uncal herniation syndrome* is caused by tumors arising in the lateral aspect of the brain, most commonly the temporal lobe. The earliest, most consistent sign of uncal herniation is a unilaterally dilated pupil due to compression of the ipsilateral third cranial nerve. This first sign is followed by extraocular movement abnormalities consistent with an oculomotor palsy.

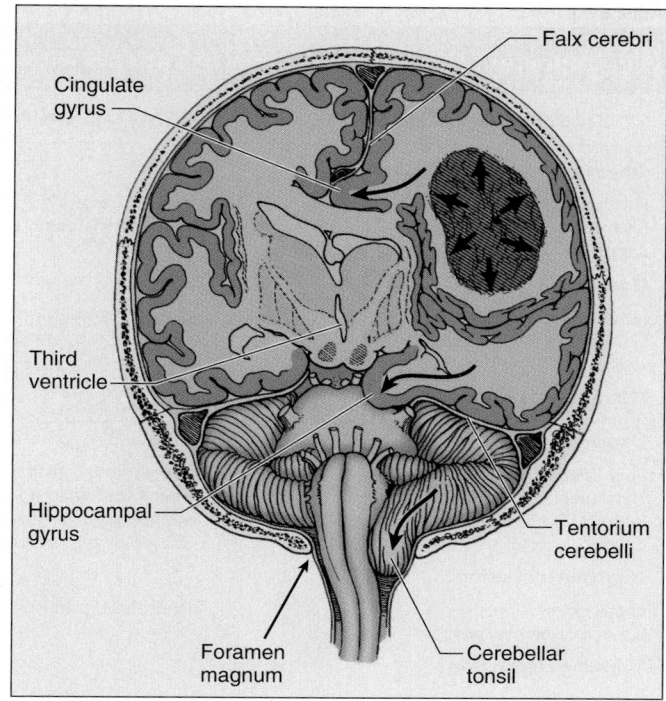

Figure 69-2. Intracranial herniation syndromes evoked by supratentorial masses. The tumor and its edema (*arrows*) have produced the following (*curved arrows*): cingulate gyrus herniation under the falx cerebri; diencephalic herniation across the midline compressing the ipsilateral ventricle and producing the hydrocephalus in the contralateral ventricle; hippocampal gyrus herniation through the tentorial notch compressing the posterior cerebral artery and brainstem; and herniation of the cerebellar tonsils through the foramen magnum. (Adapted from Plum F, Posner JB: The Diagnosis of Stupor and Coma, 3rd ed. Philadelphia, FA Davis, 1980.)

Also, the posterior cerebral artery may be compressed against the tentorium, leading to homonymous hemianopia. Brainstem compression can cause contralateral hemiparesis or on occasion ipsilateral hemiparesis, which is a result of the contralateral cerebral peduncle compressing against the edge of the tentorium, causing what is known as Kernohan's notch.[68] Patients with uncal herniation may be initially awake, but progression to obtundation, coma, and death may occur rapidly, within hours.

The *central herniation syndrome* results from tumors that arise along the midline axis of the brain, especially those deep in the basal ganglia and thalamus regions. The initial signs and symptoms are due to diencephalic compression. The first evidence for this is often an alteration in the level of alertness and behavior. Some patients become agitated; others become very drowsy. They may develop hemisensory or hemiparetic deficits and periodic Cheyne-Stokes respirations. Initially with diencephalic compression, pupils are small (1 to 3 mm), but as the syndrome progresses and the midbrain and upper pons are compressed, the pupils dilate moderately and fix at midposition (3 to 5 mm). As the syndrome progresses, patients become progressively lethargic and apathetic and may develop Cushing's signs of hyper-

TABLE 69-5

Important Clinical Syndromes in Patients with Brain Tumors

SYNDROME/SIGNS AND SYMPTOMS	LOCALIZATION/PATHOGENESIS	COMMON TUMOR TYPES
Obstructive Hydrocephalus		
Headache, papilledema Nausea, vomiting Ataxia, stiff neck	Posterior fossa Third ventricle compressed due to tumor growth/cyst	Medulloblastoma, ependymoma, astrocytomas
Communicating Hydrocephalus		
Headache/pressure waves Gait apraxia	Arachnoid granulation Scarring from treatment, hemorrhage or infection	Meningeal gliomatosis, any primary or metastatic tumor type
Venous Sinus Thrombosis	Sinus	Meningioma
Uncal Herniation		
Pupil dilation, oculomotor palsy Hemianopia Ipsilateral hemiparesis Coma	Temporal lobe herniates through tentorial notch leading to posterior cerebral artery compression, contralateral peduncle compression, midbrain compression	Any tumor type
Central Herniation		
Lethargy, small pupils Cheyne-Stokes respiration	Diencephalic compression	Any tumor type
Tonsillar Herniation		
Posterior headache Stiff neck Opisthotonos	Cerebellar tonsil herniates into foramen magnum	Posterior fossa tumor (astrocytoma ependymoma, medulloblastoma)
Pituitary Apoplexy		
Headache, diplopia Third cranial nerve palsy Hypotension	Hemorrhage into pituitary	Pituitary adenoma, meningioma, craniopharyngioma

tension and bradycardia due to direct compression of the hemodynamic control nuclei within the brainstem.[69,70]

Tonsillar herniation may be caused by an expanding mass in the posterior fossa, the region of the brain between the tentorium and the foramen magnum. This expansion results in the cerebellar tonsils being pushed through the foramen magnum. The syndrome is characterized by posterior headache, vomiting, stiff neck, and sometimes opisthotonic posturing. Dysconjugate eye movements and syncope may occur with cough or sudden postural change. Frequently, these patients complain of visual dysfunction due to progressive papilledema affecting visual acuity. As a result of direct compression of the medulla and its respiratory center, these patients may develop irregular breathing and acute apnea. Further compression of the brainstem can lead to Cushing's signs of hypertension and bradycardia. Tumors in the posterior fossa may also completely obstruct the fourth ventricle, leading to an obstructive hydrocephalus, which, if left untreated, will present as a central herniation syndrome. From a clinical standpoint, patients with tonsillar herniation can be very difficult to diagnose. Patients are often agitated at the onset of the syndrome and are frequently sedated with narcotics only to develop further respiratory compromise and death.

These herniation syndromes can rapidly progress from the onset of symptoms to death. They can be precipitated by medical procedures. Lumbar puncture may lead to tonsillar herniation, and ventriculostomy may result in upward herniation in which the brainstem is forced upward through the tentorial notch. A high index of suspicion is required in order to successfully diagnose and treat these patients by emergent intubation and administration of appropriate therapy (see the later section on acute raised intracranial pressure).

General Signs and Symptoms

Headache results from traction on pain-sensitive structures of the intracranial contents, including the large cerebral vessels, the dura and meninges, the venous sinuses, and cranial nerves V and IX. Headache is the most common symptom of a brain tumor and occurs in approximately 50% of these patients at some time during the course of the illness.[71] Headache more frequently accompanies rapidly growing than slowly growing tumors. However, tumors located in neurologically noneloquent areas such as the nondominant frontal and temporal lobes may present with headache as the sole manifestation of tumor. The "classic" brain tumor–associated headache is often worse in the morning and lateralized to the side of the mass. Brain tumor–associated headache may be worsened by coughing or straining. However, the majority of brain tumor patients do not have these classic symptoms but instead have headaches that are deep, aching, and difficult to distinguish from tension headache. As a general rule, headaches from posterior fossa tumors are localized to the back of the head or neck, whereas those of the anterior and middle cranial fossas may be referred to the forehead or eye, at times being misconstrued as "sinus" headache.

Brain tumor–associated cognitive changes may be initially subtle and are frequently misdiagnosed as depression or, in the older patient, age-associated forgetfulness or early Alzheimer's disease. The patient may complain of additional nonspecific symptoms such as fatigue, concentration problems, irritability, and loss of interest in usual activities. Frontal lobe tumor location is the most common site for tumors producing these symptoms as the initial manifestation of neoplasm. Hypomania and psychosis are less common cognitive symptoms and when occurring as the presenting symptoms are usually associated with temporal lobe tumors.

Roughly paralleling cognitive decline and of poor localizing value by themselves, several other symptoms may emerge. Dysphagia is a common complaint, and the patient's caregivers may note that the cognitively impaired patient seems to take a long time to chew and swallow. Oral candidiasis is a potential complicating issue in patients on long-term corticosteroid therapy, and appropriate treatment should be instituted. Similarly, incontinence tends to parallel the degree of cognitive impairment. Urinary retention may occur in patients with bifrontal brain disease or with spinal cord problems. Opiate medications may exacerbate the urologic symptoms.

Seizures occurring for the first time in adults are more likely to be due to focal brain pathology, particularly neoplasms, than are seizures occurring in childhood. Intracranial tumors produce both generalized tonic-clonic seizures, secondarily generalized tonic-clonic seizures, and partial, localization-related seizures. The tumors most likely to present with seizures are slowly growing astrocytomas and oligodendrogliomas or oligoastrocytomas. Seizures occur at some time in 25% to 50% of patients with brain tumors.[72-74] Tumors in the cortical and subcortical cerebral hemispheres, particularly the insula, are the tumors most likely to produce seizures. Such seizures may be more difficult to control than those of idiopathic epilepsy, and many patients require more than one anti-epileptic drug (AED) (see later section on "Treatment"). Seizure frequency may increase during radiation treatment and continue at an increased frequency for several months thereafter because of localized swelling.

Papilledema, swelling of the optic nerve head with engorgement of retinal veins, usually indicates raised intracranial pressure. Before CT and MRI came into use, papilledema was a more frequent finding in brain tumors than it is today because diagnosis now occurs earlier in the patient's course. Currently, fewer than 20% of patients have papilledema at presentation, down from 59% in the 1971 report by Huber.[75]

The development of papilledema is dependent on the location of the tumor and the rate of growth. Papilledema is more common in patients with infra-tentorial tumors than in those with supratentorial tumors.

Other papilledema-producing tumor areas include the third ventricle, cerebral aqueduct, and fourth ventricle. Thus, in adults, medulloblastomas, glial tumors of the cerebellum, hemangioblastomas, and tumors of the cerebellopontine angle are most commonly associated with papilledema.

Vomiting, with or without nausea, may occur as a result of direct simulation of emetic centers in the floor of the fourth ventricle. This mechanism explains the nausea and vomiting seen with raised intracranial pressure, particularly when the rise in pressure has been rapid and associated with hemorrhage or herniation. Patients with posterior fossa tumors frequently experience nausea and vomiting. More commonly, however, nausea is a nonlocalizing symptom and the differential diagnosis of this symptom must include adverse drug reactions from AEDs, analgesics, or other concurrent medications and gastritis from high-dose corticosteroid treatment.

Localizing Signs of Intracranial Tumor

Focal clinical signs of intracranial reflect the location of the mass and its associated vasogenic edema, which is often of much greater volume. This chapter will not provide a detailed discussion of every possible localizing sign, but rather will focus on the general principle of neurologic localization and the specific emergent syndromes that should be recognized because of their localizing and management importance (see Table 69-5).

Disorders associated with *frontal lobe lesions* include early impairment of intellectual function and language function if the dominant frontal lobe is involved. Patients with bilateral frontal tumors appear to lack initiative and spontaneity, a state called abulia. Such patients may have an impaired gait with difficulty initiating walking. Personality changes include inattentiveness, apathy, and depression as well as the less common disinhibition and inappropriate affect leading to socially inappropriate behaviors. As tumors enlarge to involve the motor cortex, patients may develop contralateral motor problems such as hemiparesis or monoparesis.

Receptive language, auditory discrimination, and memory are all important functions of the dominant temporal lobe. Patients with *nondominant temporal lobe tumors* may have seizures involving visual, olfactory, or gustatory hallucinations. Deep temporal tumors may cause a contralateral visual field cut (superior quadrantanopia).

The parietal lobe is demarcated form the frontal lobe by the central sulcus. Parietal lobe functions include tactile perceptions; integration of sensory, visual, and auditory information; and visual discrimination in the inferior contralateral quadrant. When tumor involves the nondominant *parietal lobe*, inattention to the deficit (anosognosia) may be a prominent feature of the presentation.

Tumors in the occipital lobes cause a contralateral quadrantic or hemianopic defect, sometimes with sparing of central macular vision.

Tumors of the brainstem cause a great many focal deficits early in their course. Typically, a combination of cranial nerve palsies and "long-tract" signs such as hemianesthesia or hemiparesis coupled with ataxia reflecting cerebellar involvement give a clue to the localization. Patients with brainstem tumors experience difficulty with swallowing and speech articulation. They are at risk for aspiration.

Cerebellopontine angle tumors such as acoustic neuromas impair function of the eighth cranial nerve and produce unilateral hearing loss tinnitus, and later vertigo. Involvement of adjacent cranial nerves VII and V leads to facial palsy and facial anesthesia. Later cerebellar dysfunction reflects tumor growth in this area.

Tumors of the pituitary and suprasellar region produce endocrinologic abnormalities either by hormonal production by secretory adenomas or by impingement on hypothalamic-pituitary connections. Visual defects reflect chiasmatic involvement. The most common pituitary region field defect is a bitemporal hemianopia.

Pineal region tumors (germ cell tumors, pineocytoma, and pineoblastoma as well as gliomas of this region) may compress the aqueduct of Sylvius, causing hydrocephalus. The pretectal area produces a characteristic syndrome (Parinaud's syndrome) with paralysis of upgaze, ptosis, and loss of pupillary light reflexes along with retraction-convergence nystagmus.

Many primary tumors are capable of *diffuse infiltration of the meninges.* Gliomas, lymphomas, and oligodendrogliomas all may invade the subarachnoid space, producing a meningeal reaction that may mimic chronic infection. They produce variable cranial nerve and spinal root dysfunction and diffuse headache, sometimes with a picture of communicating hydrocephalus. Elevated cerebrospinal fluid (CSF) protein, low CSF glucose, and positive cytologic findings are the diagnostic hallmarks.

On occasion the clinician will be faced with symptoms that appear to give a clue to the patient's tumor site but are *false localizing symptoms.* Abducens (cranial nerve VI) palsies may reflect brainstem involvement but commonly are a nonlocalizing symptom of raised (or, much less commonly, low) intracranial pressure. Ocular pain is of little localizing value as it may reflect any of the structures innervated by the first division of cranial nerve V. Thus eye pain may reflect any process in the anterior or middle cranial fossas. Diplopia may result from cranial nerve invasion by brainstem or leptomeningeal tumor, but can also be caused by excess levels of antiepileptic drugs.

Posterior head pain may reflect posterior fossa disease, but also may come from the upper cervical segments, and spinal cord tumor or caudal extension of a primary brainstem tumor should be considered if the patient presents with pain in the occiput. Another sign of cervical cord disease is bilateral upper limb weakness or numbness.

Gait disorders pose another potential hazard for falsely localizing symptoms. A frontal lobe gait ataxia may mimic basal ganglia or even cerebellar disease. The patient walks slowly with a wide-based gait and seems to have difficulty initiating movements. Proximal leg weakness could reflect spinal metastases from intracranial or systemic tumor, but probably the most common cause of proximal leg weakness is corticosteroid-induced myopathy.

Treatment of Brain Tumor Symptoms

Acute Raised Intracranial Pressure

The most immediate life-threatening syndromes are the herniation syndromes, but rapid increase in vasogenic edema also mandates aggressive treatment of evolving neurologic symptoms. If the patient is rapidly deteriorating, intubation and hyperventilation aiming for a PCO_2 of 25 to 30 mm Hg is required. Mannitol is administered intravenously with a loading dose of 1 to 2 g/kg followed by 0.5 to 1 g/kg every 6 hours as needed to control intracranial pressure. Mannitol may be transiently effective, but rebound sometimes develops after 24 to 48 hours. Dexamethasone in a loading dose of 20 mg followed by 6 to 10 mg IV every 4 to 6 hours is appropriate to start as initial treatment as well. Electrolytes and glucose levels must be followed, and gastritis prophylaxis is required. Acute neurosurgical interventions include intracranial pressure (ICP) monitoring devices and ventricular drainage or tumor decompression in cases of obstruction. Fluid management requires avoidance of hyponatremia.

Chronic Increased Intracranial Pressure

Dexamethasone in doses of 8 to 40 mg/day repairs the "leaky" blood-brain barrier of tumor vasculature. Controlling the edema helps to control headache, nausea, and seizures as well. Chronic raised ICP can cause visual loss, and careful ophthalmologic follow-up with visual fields is essential. Acetazolamide therapy for symptomatic plateau waves has been useful for some patients with raised ICP from intracerebral or leptomeningeal tumor.[76]

In the doses required to treat cerebral edema, corticosteroids produce many adverse effects, ranging from the easily managed gastritis symptoms and glucose intolerance to insomnia, steroid psychosis, intractable hiccoughs, and disabling myopathy. The psychosis may respond easily to reduction of steroid dose and addition of neuroleptics. However, the steroid myopathy requires weeks of physical therapy with attempts at steroid reduction. Anecdotal reports suggest that substitution of a nonfluorinated steroid such as methylprednisolone for fluorinated steroids such as dexamethasone may help reverse the weakness.[77]

Many brain tumor patients remain on corticosteroids for prolonged periods. They are thus susceptible to infection particularly with *Pneumocystis carinii*, which carries a 50% mortality rate. Among solid tumors, primary and metastatic brain tumors have the highest rate of *Pneumocystis* infection, which occurs in 2% of these patients and proves fatal to 40% of them.[78] The mean duration of steroid therapy before infection was 7 months with a mean dexamethasone equivalent dose of 1 to 2 mg/day.[79] In view of these statistics chemoprophylaxis with 1 tablet twice a day of trimethoprim/sulfamethoxazole twice weekly should be given to brain tumor patients on corticosteroids longer than 4 weeks.

Brain tumor patients who require long-term use of corticosteroids may develop an adrenal insufficiency state manifested by lethargy, hypotension, electrolyte imbalance, and diffuse weakness upon steroid withdrawal. Intercurrent systemic stressors such as surgery or systemic infection may lead to serious hypotension. Chronic glucocorticoid supplementation with hydrocortisone 10 to 20 mg per day is essential for these patients.[80,81]

Seizures

Neuro-oncologists often find themselves working closely with epileptologists as they seek to control seizures with minimal side effects. Because brain tumor patients frequently require corticosteroids, analgesics, anxiolytics, and antiemetics, drug-drug interactions make epilepsy management complex.

The potential interaction of AEDs with other medications required for brain tumor patients has led to reconsideration of prophylactic use of antiseizure drugs. Cytochrome P-450 enzyme-inducing drugs such as phenytoin and carbamazepine may interact with numerous chemotherapeutic agents (see the section, "Radiation Therapy: General Considerations"), reducing levels achieved and diminishing efficacy. AEDs may also increase the corticosteroid dose required for effective vasogenic edema treatment. For those patients with low-grade gliomas who may be on AEDs for many years, teratogenesis and osteoporosis are also a risk.

Approximately 20% of patients with gliomas treated with phenytoin or carbamazepine and cranial irradiation develop a rash, and a few develop the most serious and sometimes life-threatening reaction, the Stevens-Johnson syndrome. This reaction is seen in the setting of hypersensitivity to AEDs unmasked during the taper of high-dose corticosteroids. The mechanism may be depletion of suppressor T cells by radiation, allowing emergence of the hypersensitivity syndrome.[82,83] Treatment is controversial, but often the corticosteroid dose is doubled as AEDs are withdrawn abruptly.

Given all the potential hazards of AEDs, it is worthwhile to consider whether their prophylactic use is justified in the brain tumor patient population. A controlled prospective study of brain tumor patients addressing the question of prophylaxis for epilepsy showed an overall incidence of 26% with no difference in the seizure rate between patients taking AEDs and those without prophlyaxis.[84] A second study involving 100 patients confirmed the lack of efficacy of AEDs in preventing seizures or altering survival outcome in brain tumor patients.[85] These findings are consistent with those of Foy and colleagues who conducted a prospective trial involving 276 craniotomy patients (not all of whom had tumors) who were randomized postoperatively to receive phenytoin, carbamazepine, or no treatment. There was no difference in the incidence of seizures (37%) or postoperative complications among the groups.[86] For all these reasons, a recent practice parameter by the Quality Standards Subcommittee of the American Academy of Neurology concluded that there was no benefit to routine prophylactic use of AEDs in patients with brain tumors.[87]

Even after the acute phases of successful tumor treatment, epilepsy management may continue to be a major issue in quality of life for long-term survivors of low-grade brain neoplasms. A particularly dangerous late consequence of chronic AED therapy with phenytoin, carbamazepine, and phenobarbital is osteoporosis; therefore, long-term survivors should be screened regularly with DEXA scans.

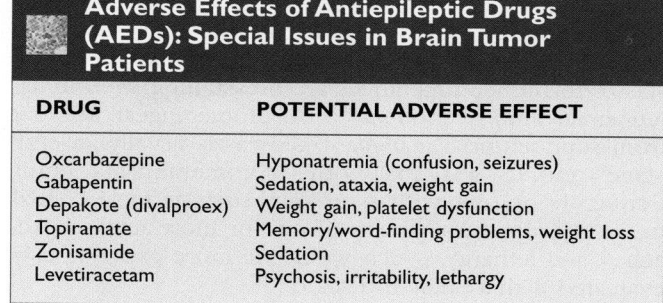

TABLE 69-6

Adverse Effects of Antiepileptic Drugs (AEDs): Special Issues in Brain Tumor Patients	
DRUG	**POTENTIAL ADVERSE EFFECT**
Oxcarbazepine	Hyponatremia (confusion, seizures)
Gabapentin	Sedation, ataxia, weight gain
Depakote (divalproex)	Weight gain, platelet dysfunction
Topiramate	Memory/word-finding problems, weight loss
Zonisamide	Sedation
Levetiracetam	Psychosis, irritability, lethargy

In the last 15 years several new AEDs have been introduced that offer new choices for brain tumor patients and the possibility of limiting side effects while achieving excellent seizure control. However, the clinician must be familiar with some side effects specific to these drugs (Table 69-6) in order to diagnose symptoms accurately, eliminate the offending drug, and avoid unnecessary diagnostic and therapeutic interventions.

Deep Venous Thrombosis

Deep venous thrombosis is extremely common in brain tumor patients and has a reported incidence of 28% to 45%.[88,89] Among brain tumor patients, those with gliomas and meningiomas are at the highest risk for thromboembolism, which is a common cause of fever of unknown origin in this population. Alterations in fibrinolysis, immobility, paresis, tumor necrosis factor, steroids, and neurosurgical procedures all combine to make brain tumor patients a high-risk group. Many of these patients receive vena caval filters because of the perceived risk of hemorrhage into their intracranial tumors. However, retrospective studies have suggested a very low risk of hemorrhage and in addition have demonstrated an incidence of complications of vena caval filters of greater than 60% in this patient group. Complications included pulmonary embolism, filter thrombosis, and postphlebitic syndrome.[90] Low-molecular-weight heparins have been found to have a good safety profile in the neurosurgical population.[91] Prophylaxis with enoxaparin 40 mg subcutaneously daily plus external compression stockings has been found to be superior to compression stockings alone in the prevention of venous thromboembolism after neurosurgery.[92,93] Although no absolute guidelines are available, most neurosurgeons would be reluctant to fully anticoagulate patients within 3 weeks of surgery. Also, a subset of patients with late white matter changes due to radiation therapy may be at special risk of brain hemorrhage on heparin.

DIAGNOSTIC IMAGING

Lumbar Puncture

Lumbar punctures are not commonly employed for the diagnosis of brain tumors. With primary gliomas the yield from CSF cytologic examination at initial diagnosis is extremely low. Carcinomatous meningitis is usually found in the late stages of solid tumors but can be the initial presentation in 5% to 10% of patients with systemic cancer.[94,95] The most common systemic tumors to metastasize to the leptomeninges are breast, lung, melanoma, leukemia, and lymphoma.[96,97] Leptomeningeal seeding from supratentorial malignant gliomas is usually an end-stage finding. Patients with leptomeningeal tumor frequently present with symptoms such as focal cranial nerve neuropathies, paresis of one or more limbs, headaches, and lethargy, which would be more expeditiously evaluated with a brain MRI scan.

Skull X-rays

Plain films of the skull have been used in the past to determine evidence of mass effect due to shift of the calcified pineal gland. This modality has been largely replaced with the modern use of CT scans and MRI. Plain x-rays of the skull are still useful for evaluating skull lesions such as dermoids and epidermoids as well as eosinophilic granulomas. These primary lesions of the skull frequently can be best seen with plain skull x-rays. Epidermoid and dermoid tumors of the bone are congenital tumors derived from ectopic epithelium. These painless benign lesions can grow to be quite large, causing deformity of the skull. Eosinophilic granulomas may be associated with Hand-Schüller-Christian disease, a triad of diabetes insipidus, exophthalmos, and bone lesions usually found in the skull. Other primary bone lesions that can be found on plain skull x-rays include multiple myeloma and plasmacytoma. Bone foramen abnormalities occurring in the skull include fibrous dysplasia and Paget's disease. Fibrous dysplasia can be cystic or sclerotic, usually occurs in the anterior middle fossa, and can cause proptosis of the eye and compression of the cranial nerves exiting the middle fossa, causing pain and entrapment syndromes. Paget's disease is benign but thought to be a premalignant condition causing symptoms similar to those of fibrous dysplasia because of thickening of the bone at the skull base, constricting neural foramen. Occasionally, meningiomas can grow selectively into the bone rather than into the intracranial compartment. This invasion causes thickening of the bone with compression syndromes as previously described causing proptosis of the eye, constriction of neural foramen causing cranial nerve deficits, and more commonly, complaints of headache syndromes. Owing to the thickening and sclerotic changes seen in the latter three disease states, these lesions are frequently evaluated with plain skull x-rays as part of the workup.

Computed Tomography

CT scans are usually the first study obtained when a patient presents with a neurologic complaint. CT scans can be obtained quickly in most hospitals as a screening tool. Hemorrhagic lesions can be seen owing to the increased density of blood. Infarcts will acutely present as edematous tissue and can be confused with tumors, especially low-grade gliomas, which may not enhance

with contrast agents. Iodinated contrast agents are useful to differentiate the tumor from the surrounding edematous brain tissue, as the contrast agent is able to leak out of the vascular space into the tumor owing to breakdown of the blood-brain barrier. The pattern of ring enhancement of tumors may be difficult to distinguish from the ring enhancement of a cerebral abscess, though brain tumors are far more common than brain abscesses in the United States. CT images have limitations at the skull base due to volume-averaging artifact as the x-ray beam slides over uneven bone ridges. This artifact makes it difficult to interpret findings in the skull base and in the posterior fossa (the region between the tentorium and foramen magnum). CT scans are still the study of choice in patients who cannot undergo MRI scans such as patients with implanted pacemakers, defibrillators, or other implanted metal that prevents imaging with an MRI scan.

Magnetic Resonance Imaging

MRI has become the study of choice for evaluating brain tumors. The high degree of definition of the anatomy of the brain as well as the absence of bony artifacts seen in CT scans has enabled MRI to provide exceptional images of the tumor. Localization of the lesion is precise as an MRI is done in three planes. The study of choice for evaluating brain tumors is an MRI with and without contrast material. Much like CT scan contrast, MRI contrast, gadolinium, is able to penetrate into the tumor because of breakdown in the blood-brain barrier and leak. This enables the tumor site to become white on the T1-weighted images. Gadolinium enhancement can be crucial in identifying leptomeningeal disease as thickened areas of the dura as well as "sugar-coating" of the brain itself.

Multiple sequences may be obtained from the MRI scans that highlight different properties of both the brain and the tumor. Of particular interest are the T2-weighted and FLAIR (fluid attenuated inversion-recovery) images showing the vasogenic edema created by the tumor. Evaluating this edema pattern is very important in assessing the degree of mass effect. The volume of edematous brain may represent the true limits of a glioma tumor, as tumor cells are present in the nonenhancing tissue surrounding the enhancing tumor.[98] This pattern provides the rationale for standard external beam radiation therapy to include the edematous volume of brain plus a margin of 1 to 2 cm. The edema pattern extending into the corpus callosum implies direct tumor invasion into the corpus callosum. The fiber tracks passing through the corpus callosum are so compact as to prevent edema from passing through along these fiber tracks so that any edema seen is created by local tumor infiltration. This feature is very important in assessing extent of tumor in a patient.

Endothelial proliferation with neovascularity is a hallmark of malignancy in brain neoplasms. MRI perfusion imaging can be performed in combination with conventional MRI examinations to determine the extent of neovascularity. There appears to be very good correlation between regional cerebral blood volume and grade of malignant glioma. In particular, this is especially helpful in distinguishing grade III from grade IV malignant gliomas.[99,100] It has been noted that anaplastic astrocytomas with gadolinium enhancement show a higher vascularity index than those without gadolinium enhancement. Perfusion imaging may enable us to follow the anti-angiogenic effects of treatment in brain tumors. Perfusion imaging appears to be useful in assessing benign tumors such as meningiomas to determine the vascularity of these tumors, which may be associated with progression.[101]

MRI techniques have been utilized to identify areas of brain activity in real time. This functional MRI technique has become quite useful in identifying regions of eloquent brain adjacent to tumors.[102,103] By identifying language and motor areas adjacent to tumors one can determine the degree of aggressive surgical resection that can be carried out and also the best way to preserve this functional activity.[104] Functional MRI scans are being imported into frameless stereotaxy units that are used for intra-operative surgical planning.[105] By using discrete motor, sensory, language, or visual paradigms one can activate the relevant part of the cortical brain for identification of functional activity. The one limitation to functional MRI scans is that it does not identify subcortical white matter tracks that are activated by the investigated activity.

There has been a great deal of interest in the ability of routine clinical MRI scanners to perform MR spectroscopy (MRS) as a technique to evaluate molecular components of a defined voxel within the brain tissue. The ability to obtain a smaller voxel size has provided the ability to be much more selective in evaluating components of a tumor. MRS has been applied quite extensively to malignant gliomas where the most important molecular components are N-acetylaspartate (NAA), creatine, choline, and a combined peak of lipids and lactate.[106] MRS can be used from the diagnostic perspective as malignant gliomas exhibit a higher choline peak relative to creatine and a lower NAA peak with increasing grade of malignancy (Fig. 69-3). An additional peak beyond the NAA peak identifies lipids and lactate, which are also a marker of malignancy and can be seen both in primary gliomas as well as metastatic tumors. MRS can be utilized to determine whether a region of enhancement in a previously treated tumor represents active tumor or radiation necrosis. MRS has been used to follow treatment effects over an extended period of time. Most useful has been the development of the multivoxel technique in which large areas of the brain can be mapped with individually small voxels so that one can determine small areas of active tumor within a large region of brain.

MRI has the ability to specifically identify vascular structures such as major arteries and veins. MR angiography (MRA) and MR venography (MRV) can be useful in evaluating major vessels at the base of the skull for skull base tumors. The quality of MRA and MRV has been steadily improving and provides a noninvasive means of evaluating these vascular structures without the need for angiography.

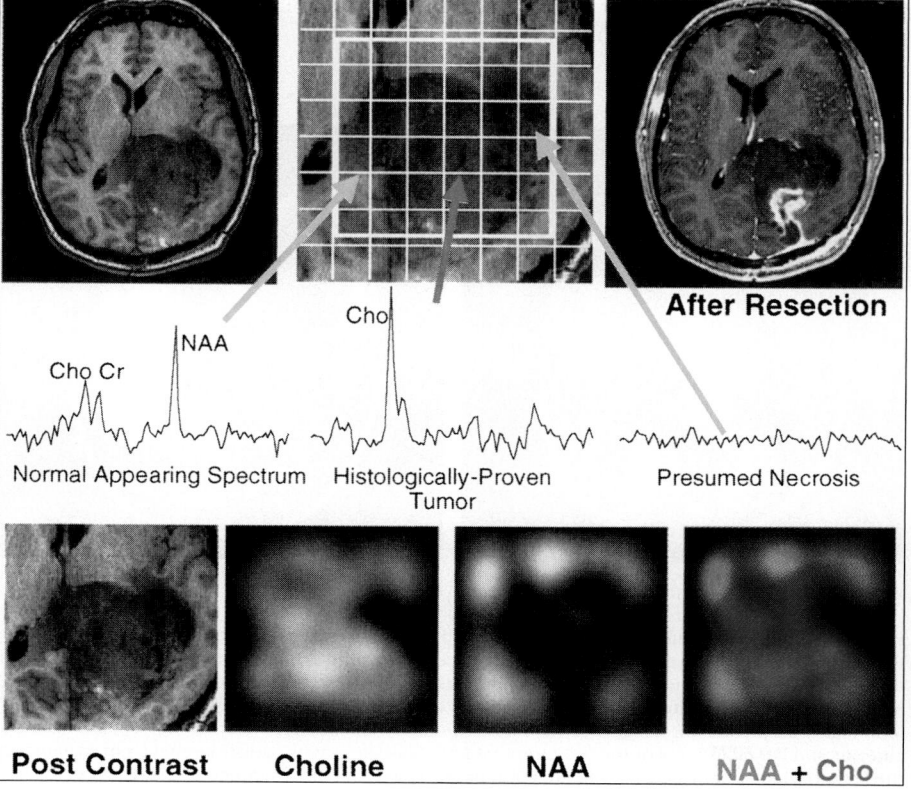

Figure 69-3. Magnetic resonance imaging (MRI) and magnetic resonance spectroscopic (MRS) studies of WHO grade II oligoastrocytoma. Axial T1-weighted postgadolinium MRI on day prior to surgery (*top left panel*) shows area of hypodensity that does not enhance (*bottom left panel*). MRS (*top middle panel*) showed area of high choline (1.8 times greater than adjacent brain) and low N-acetylaspartate (NAA) levels, as well as a smaller region of no significant metabolite levels, which is presumed necrosis. The resection was limited to a region of elevated choline with no significant NAA. (From Vigneron A, Bollen A, McDermott M, et al: Three-dimensional magnetic resonance spectroscopic imaging of histologically confirmed brain tumors. Magn Reson Imaging 2001;19:93.)

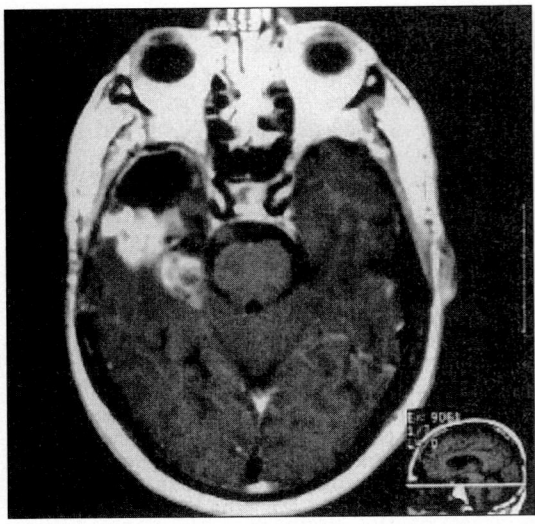 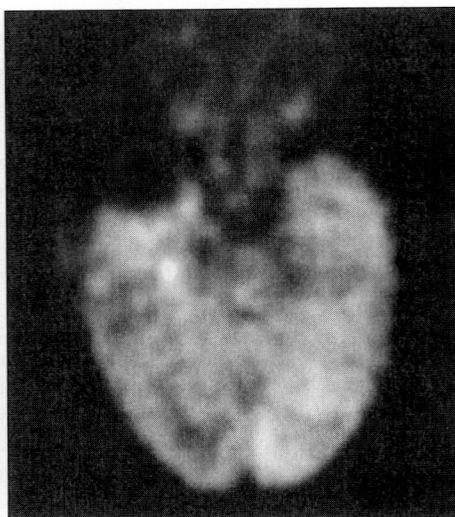

Figure 69-4. Positron emission tomographic (PET) scan of recurrent glioma. Patient had anaplastic oligodendroglioma surgically resected 15 months prior to date of studies. Areas of contrast enhancement on T1-weighted MRI scan (*left panel*) have high FDG accumulation consistent with recurrent high-grade tumor on coregistered FDG-PET image (*right panel*). (From Hagge RJ, Wong TZ, Coleman RE: Positron emission tomography. Brain tumors and lung cancer. Radiol Clin North Am 2001;39:874.)

Positron Emission Tomography

Positron emission tomography (PET) imaging utilizes a radioactive isotope, ^{18}F-fluorodeoxyglucose (FDG), to image metabolism of glucose in the brain. Because glucose is the sole fuel for brain tissue, this metabolic imaging allows visualization of brain physiology. PET scans will be positive in glioblastoma multiforme, primary CNS lymphoma, oligodendroglioma, and malignant meningioma due to the high uptake of FDG.[107] Anaplastic astrocytomas and oligodendrogliomas, meningiomas, and metastatic tumors show variable FDG uptake, but low-grade gliomas and radiation necrosis show little to no FDG uptake (Figs. 69-4 and 69-5).

Intraoperative Ultrasound

In general, brain tumors are echogenic so that real-time ultrasound can be used for localization. Ultrasound can be used to identify normal intracranial structures such as the ventricles, the falx, and the tentorium. Exact tumor localization is necessary owing to small operative exposures to the brain. The ultrasound can be used on the dura surrounding the brain or directly on the brain tissue. Ultrasound can be quite useful in finding large brain tumor cysts that cause herniation of the brain during surgery. By accurately localizing the cyst, ultrasound allows a needle to be inserted to drain the cyst and rapidly decompress the brain.

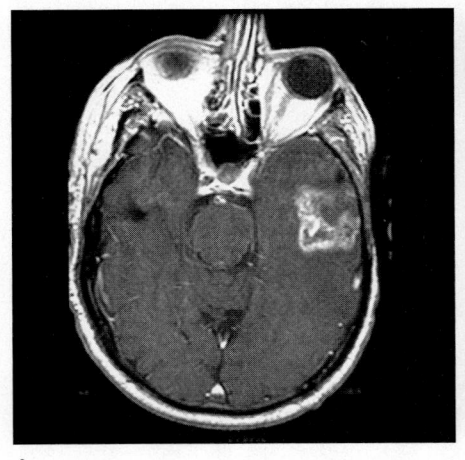 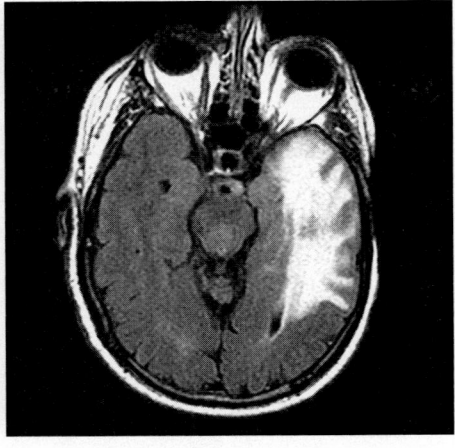 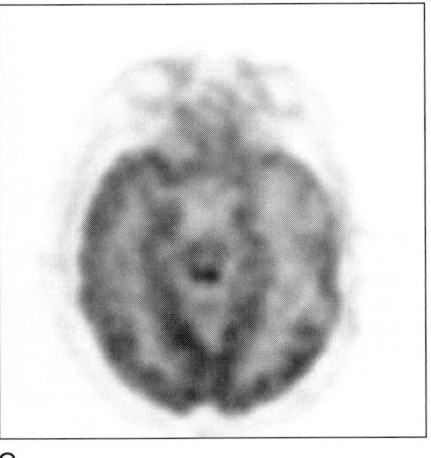

A   B   C

Figure 69-5. Positron emission tomographic (PET) and magnetic resonance imaging (MRI) scan of patient with radiation necrosis of the brain. Patient had a recurrence of a basal cell carcinoma involving the skin overlying the zygoma and the left periauricular region with extension into the temporalis muscle. He underwent surgical resection, but because of perineural invasion, he received 6400 cGy postoperatively to the tumor bed. Approximately 2 years later, he developed aphasia and confusion. **A,** T1-weighted postgadolinium MRI showed a ring-enhancing mass in left temporal lobe highly suspicious for malignancy. **B,** FLAIR MRI showed extensive edema. **C,** [18F]-FDG scan showed patchy areas of hypometabolism within the anterior and lateral aspects of the left temporal lobe consistent with radiation effect, not malignancy. Patient underwent surgery with resection of the lesion, which confirmed it to be radiation necrosis without any evidence of malignancy.

SURGERY: GENERAL CONSIDERATIONS

The successful resection of a brain tumor requires removing the tumor only without injuring the surrounding normal brain. The approach to removal of brain tumors follows the mantra of real estate agents, "location, location, location." Deep tumors that are in noneloquent brain can be easily accessed and removed, whereas superficial tumors may not be easily resectable because of their location within extremely eloquent brain tissue.

The goals of surgery are threefold. First, surgery is needed to establish the histologic type of the lesion; this procedure is frequently better performed through a craniotomy with a more aggressive debulking of the tumor, rather than a simple stereotactic biopsy so that there is no question of sampling error. Second, surgery is used to debulk the mass effect of the tumor to improve a neurologic deficit and to prevent imminent death in patients with large tumors and early herniation syndromes. Third, it also allows debulking the tumor to increase efficacy of radiation therapy and chemotherapy, which have the best response rate when they are used with minimal tumor burden.

Establishing a tissue diagnosis is extremely important for therapeutic and prognostic considerations. Frequently the histologic diagnosis may be straightforward; however, in a category of tumors that present as mixed gliomas, tissue sampling can induce errors in diagnosis.[108] A limited biopsy may show a solitary cell type; however, further examination of a more extensive biopsy may reveal that the tumor has other components. This information is particularly important when the other components identified might change the pathologic interpretation from a grade II glioma to an anaplastic grade III glioma. Noninvasive means of establishing tissue diagnosis have been pursued, primarily through the use of MRS.[109,110] Significant progress has been made to determine histologic diagnosis of tumors with MRS; however, MRS is still not specific enough to make major therapeutic decisions. Histopathologic determination remains the gold standard.

The most common presenting symptoms in glioma patients are headache and seizures.[111] Debulking large tumors will reduce the dural stretch, decreasing headaches. The incidence of seizures in patients with malignant gliomas can be decreased by at least 75% with attempts at gross total resection.[112] Improvement in other presenting symptoms such as hemiparesis, visual field loss, and aphasia depends on whether the impaired neurologic tissue is simply compressed by the tumor mass or whether the tumor itself has directly destroyed these neural tracts. In the former case, but not the latter, debulking the tumor will improve the patient's symptoms.

Owing to liberal use of CT and MRI scans, herniation syndromes with brain tumors, discussed in the earlier section on pathophysiology of signs and symptoms, are uncommon presentations. However, patients do occasionally present central or uncal herniation syndromes from late-stage brain tumors. These patients need to have an emergent CT or MRI scan and have rapid evaluation for possible surgery for reduction of mass effect as a life-saving measure.

Another rationale for maximal debulking is to reduce the tumor burden by one or two log orders of cells. By such cytoreduction, one can hopefully increase efficacy of both radiation and chemotherapy in the treatment of these tumors.

RADIATION THERAPY

Radiation is commonly used to treat many different types of brain tumors. The radiation oncologist must decide on many factors in the treatment of an individual patient, including treatment volume, dose, and fractionation. Although newer treatment techniques including stereotactic radiation, intensity modulated radiation therapy (IMRT), and proton beam therapy are being used for specific cases, the majority of patients treated for brain tumors still receive conventional external beam radiation therapy.

Technical Details

Before a patient can start receiving radiation, therapy must be carefully planned. Traditionally, this has involved using a simulator, a kilovoltage x-ray machine with fluoroscopic capabilities. The purpose of simulation is to take films of the region to be treated using appropriate field sizes and beam orientations in order to simulate the fields that will be used during actual treatment. Prior to the simulation, the patient often had a treatment planning CT scan performed in which the tumor volume was outlined and treatment fields were determined with the aid of computer-assisted dosimetry. In the treatment of brain tumors it has been particularly important to design fields that conform to the tumor volume, excluding as much of normal brain as possible in order to minimize side effects. The latest advances in computer hardware and software have allowed visualization of the target volume and normal structures in three dimensions; therefore, this approach has been termed *3D-conformal therapy*. More recently, departments have started using CT simulators in which CT scanning and simulation can be performed on the same machine. After a simulation has been performed and a treatment plan developed, films are taken on the treatment machine to verify that the correct fields are being treated.

The appropriate volume to be treated depends on the tumor type. Most brain tumors including gliomas and meningiomas are treated with focal radiation to the lesion with a margin. The actual abnormality seen on imaging studies is termed *gross tumor volume* (GTV). Additional tissue surrounding the GTV that is felt to potentially contain tumor cells is included in the clinical target volume (CTV). For some tumors such as glioblastomas, which can be highly infiltrative, the CTV might include a 1.5-cm margin surrounding the GTV as determined by T1-weighted MRI scans. However, for other tumors that do not infiltrate, such as meningiomas, pituitary adenomas, acoustic neuromas, and craniopharyngiomas, the CTV would typically be much tighter than that used for glioblastomas. An additional volume is included around the CTV to take into account day-to-day setup error and to allow for buildup of dose, resulting in patient treatment volume (PTV).

Most brain tumors are treated with focal radiation therapy; however, for some tumors such as PNETs and germ cell tumors of the CNS, it may be necessary to treat the entire craniospinal axis. In this case, a special technique must be used. Most brain tumors are treated optimally with the patient in a supine position. The patient is placed in a mask made of thermoelastic plastic during the simulation and during all treatments in order to ensure that the patient's head is immobilized. However, when craniospinal radiation is used, the optimal patient position is prone. This facilitates daily setup and treatment with the spinal canal treated with one or two fields entering from the patient's back and the entire cranial contents treated with opposed lateral fields. Because abutting fields are used to encompass the entire craniospinal axis, the possibility exists for overlap between fields, resulting in a potential overdosage to part of the spinal cord. Therefore, great care must be taken during the setup of these fields. In many institutions, a technique termed *feathering* is used in which the matchlines between fields are changed periodically to ensure that a hot or cold spot does not persist in the same region of the spinal cord throughout the entire treatment.

Stereotactic Radiotherapy

Stereotactic radiotherapy is a technique for delivering high-dose radiation to a target volume with very tight margins, thereby sparing surrounding normal tissues. This procedure can be done by using (1) a gamma knife machine, which contains 201 fixed cobalt sources that converge to a single point, (2) a conventional linear accelerator outfitted with additional hardware so that it can deliver focused radiation generally using between 3 and 5 arcs, or (3) charged particles such as protons which, because of their physical properties, deposit energy in a narrower region than do x-rays.

Stereotactic radiation can be delivered in a single large fraction. This approach is termed *stereotactic radiosurgery* (SRS). In spite of its name, however, no surgery is performed. A sterotactic head frame must be screwed to the skull. In adults this step can be done using local anesthesia, but in children conscious sedation or general anesthesia must be used. The headframe allows localization of the tumor in a 3D coordinate system and also immobilizes the head during treatment, thereby allowing for delivery of radiation with precision to a very tightly defined volume. The patient has a CT scan performed with the headframe in place. At our institution an MRI with gadolinium contrast material is performed prior to placement of the headframe. The MRI representations are then fused to the CT images, and a treatment plan is devised that targets the lesion while minimizing dose to normal structures. The doses of radiation that are used in stereotactic radiosurgery generally range from 10 to 20 Gy and are based on the volume of tissue irradiated, with higher doses used for smaller volumes. The doses generally used are based on the likelihood of developing radiation necrosis extrapolated from data originally generated using single doses of proton therapy.[113] The choice between a gamma knife and a linear accelerator is based on availability. The same linear accelerator used for conventional radiotherapy can be outfitted for use in stereotactic radiotherapy. In contrast, gamma knife machines must be dedicated to doing stereotactic radiotherapy only and are quite expensive with sources that need to be replaced every few years, so there are fewer of these machines around.

Stereotactic radiotherapy can also be delivered in a fractionated regimen over several days or weeks. Of course, in this case a headframe that is screwed into the skull cannot be used. Therefore, relocatable headframes have been developed. These headframes use custom-made moldings conforming to the patient's occiput and a bite block to maintain a precise and reproducible fit day to day.

A large experience supports using stereotactic radiotherapy, either in a single fraction or a fractionated regimen, for the treatment of intracranial metastases, arteriovenous malformations (AVMs), and primary brain tumors. Stereotactic radiotherapy for AVMs is beyond the scope of this chapter, and its use in treating intracranial metastases is covered in Chapter 56. Its use in the treatment of meningiomas, pituitary adenomas, and acoustic neuromas will be discussed in greater detail in the corresponding sections in this chapter.

Charged particles including protons have been used to treat brain tumors. Because of their physical properties, protons result in more limited dose to normal tissues than conventional x-rays. However, the availability of protons or other charged particles is extremely limited owing to the requirement of a high-energy cyclotron to produce these particles. Only a handful of centers in the United States have protons or other charged particles available for medical treatment.

Adverse Effects Following Irradiation of the Brain or Spine

Acute and Early Delayed Effects Following Cranial Irradiation

A variety of side effects can occur following radiation to the CNS.[114] These side effects can be divided into acute effects, which occur during the treatment, delayed early effects, which occur within a few months of radiation, and late effects, which occur months to years later.

Acute effects following cranial irradiation include fatigue, nausea, headaches, anorexia, and alopecia. Patients often complain of fatigue, not just with cranial radiation, but with radiation to other regions of the body, and as a result they often need to sleep longer than usual or take naps during the day. Patients may experience nausea within hours following the administration of the radiation and headaches during the course of treatment. Nausea is usually well controlled with antiemetics such as ondansetron or granisetron. Nausea and headaches are thought to be caused by radiation-induced edema and can be ameliorated with corticosteroids. Patients who are placed on steroids prior to radiation often continue them when radiotherapy is started. In patients receiving craniospinal radiation, the nausea and anorexia may be compounded by the radiation that the upper gastrointestinal tract receives as a result of exit dose from the spinal field. Hair loss generally starts after the scalp has received 20 to 30 Gy. It is not generally permanent, but regrowth of hair may take months, and often in the regrown hair is thinner or even a different color than the original. In areas that receive a high dose of radiation, especially with tangentially directed fields, alopecia may be permanent. Other acute side effects from cranial irradiation may include accumulation of cerumen in the ear canals and serous otitis media.

The most common delayed early effect from radiation is the somnolence syndrome, which is characterized by excessive drowsiness, nausea, and irritability.[115] If it occurs, it generally does so 1 to 3 months after radiation has been completed. This syndrome is thought to be due to transient, diffuse demyelination. It is usually seen following whole-brain irradiation for ALL but can also be seen after radiation for brain tumors. The syndrome resolves spontaneously, but steroids can shorten its duration. Delayed early effects following cranial irradiation can also take the form of focal neurologic signs due to intralesional reactions related to tumor response or perilesional reactions related to edema or demyelination.

Brain Necrosis and Neurocognitive Deficits Following Cranial Irradiation

The pathophysiology of late effects from CNS irradiation is poorly understood. Some of the effects may be caused by degenerative changes in the supporting glial cells, whereas others may be caused by vascular changes due to endothelial cell loss and capillary occlusion.

One of the most serious late effects from cranial irradiation is brain necrosis, which may cause significant and persistent neurologic injury.[116,117] It may also produce progressive cerebral edema and mass effect, requiring prolonged corticosteroid use or surgery. Third, it may be confused with tumor growth, resulting in the inappropriate use of antitumor therapies. The onset of radiation necrosis includes behavioral changes—lethargy and dementia, headache and papilledema, and seizure. Clinical signs and symptoms are usually identified from 2 to 3 years after radiation, though confirmed cases have been detected as early as 9 months and as late as 16 years after radiation. The signs and symptoms are strongly related to the site of radiation necrosis; however, the most common symptoms are focal motor deficits. Radionecrosis is often difficult to distinguish from recurrent tumor by CT or MRI, which may show increased signal intensity on T1-weighted images and contrast enhancement on T1-weighted images.[118] However, as discussed earlier in "Diagnostic Imaging," and as shown in Figure 69-5, PET scanning with FDG may help distinguish viable tumor from necrotic tissue.[119-121] Often surgical exploration is necessary, not only to establish a diagnosis, but also as a therapeutic intervention by removing the region of necrosis. Histopathologically, the changes seen in

radiation-induced necrosis are generally limited to the white matter and include focal coagulative necrosis and demyelination (Fig. 69-6).[122] Accurate data regarding the incidence of brain necrosis based on CT/MRI imaging comes from a randomized trial of radiation for low-grade gliomas.[123] In this study, the 2-year actuarial incidence of brain necrosis was 2.5% for patients receiving 50.4 Gy and 5% for those receiving 64.8 Gy.

Neurocognitive deficits are often observed following cranial radiation, especially in young children. Many of the sequelae manifest several years after treatment of children with brain tumors, which mandates long-term follow-up. Sequential assessments of neurocognitive function demonstrated progressive deterioration during 6 years after whole-brain radiotherapy in children with ALL treated with 18 Gy of whole-brain irradiation.[124] Numerous studies of neurocognitive function in children following whole-brain irradiation for ALL have been performed.[125-130] In summary, these studies show that whole-brain irradiation can lead to decline in neurocognitive function, an effect which appears to be greater with younger children and higher doses of radiation (24 Gy) but which can be seen with 18 Gy.[124] An interaction between methotrexate (intrathecal or high-dose systemic) and whole-brain irradiation may also be causing these late effects.[130]

Studies of patients treated for PNET/medulloblastoma have uniformly shown poor outcomes in terms of intelligence, memory, language, attention, academic skills, psychosocial function, and quality of life, even in patients

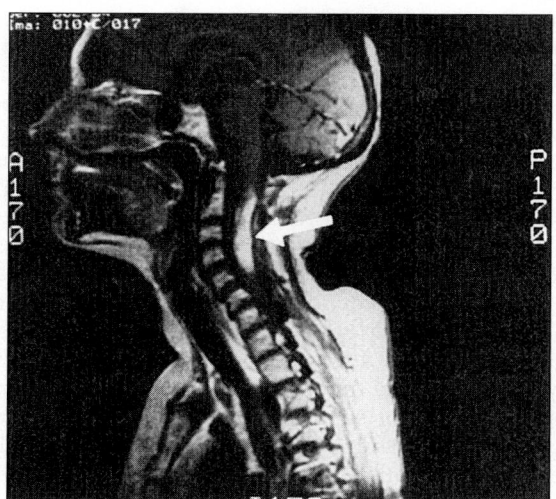

Figure 69-6. Magnetic resonance imaging (MRI) scan of patient with radiation necrosis of spinal cord. Patient received 45 Gy of radiation to the cervical cord (C1–C6) for grade II astrocytoma of the cord. Four years later she developed weakness of the upper extremities. T1-weighted postgadolinium MRI scan showed enlargement of the cervical cord and enhancement felt to be consistent with recurrence. Patient received chemotherapy without improvement and eventually died owing to respiratory failure. Autopsy of spinal cord showed chromic radiation changes and necrosis of the cervical cord but no evidence of recurrent tumor. (From Phuphanich S, Jacobs M, Murtagh FR, Gonzalvo A: MRI of spinal cord radiation necrosis simulating recurrent cervical cord astrocytoma and syringomyelia. Surg Neurol 1996;45:363.)

treated as adults.[131,132] Many of these patients received 36 Gy to the whole brain followed by a boost to a total dose of 54 to 55.8 Gy to the posterior fossa. Data suggest that these patients have a decline in their IQ values because of an inability to acquire new skills and information at a rate comparable to their healthy same-age peers, rather than to a loss of previously acquired information and skills.[133] These neurocognitive deficits have been correlated with loss of white matter in the brain, and the younger the patient when given radiation, the more severe the deficits.[134,135]

Mulhern and associates performed an analysis of neurocognitive function after treatment for brain tumors, pooling data from 22 studies with a total of 544 patients.[136] They showed that the most critical factors influencing intellectual outcome are the dose of radiation and young age at the time of radiation. Younger children (<4 years old) who received whole-brain radiation showed a 14-point decrease in IQ compared with older children. Accordingly, current therapeutic strategies do not use whole-brain radiation in children younger than 3 years and try to reduce radiation doses.

Accurate assessment of the effects of changes in cranial radiation on neurocognitive development in young children is complicated by important methodologic and study design problems. A common concern is that measurement of IQ, per se, is neither a sensitive nor specific method of assessing the cognitive impairments of these patients.[137] Accordingly, efforts have been made to establish and validate reliable and easy-to-use instruments for assessing IQ as well as other neuropsychological aspects.[138]

Another treatment complication associated with cranial radiotherapy is leukoencephalopathy, which is most often associated with intravenous or IT methotrexate (MTX) and cranial radiation.[116,117,139] Young age is also an important risk factor; however, leukoencephalopathy can affect all age groups. Histologically multifocal white matter destruction with loss of myelin occurs, especially in the periventricular regions. MRI scans show these periventricular abnormalities. CT scans may also show intracerebral microcalcifications due to mineralizing microangiopathy. The clinical expression of leukoencephalopathy ranges from mild evidence of white matter injury on neuroimaging studies to severe necrotizing leukoencephalopathy with profound neurologic impairment and, in some cases, death. Mild or subclinical cases are more common than severe necrotizing leukoencephalopathy. The bulk of the experience comes from children who received 24 Gy whole-brain radiation along with high doses of intravenous (IV) and intrathecal (IT) MTX. The incidence of leukoencephalopathy is low in patients who receive cranial radiation therapy (RT) and IT MTX or cranial radiation and IV MTX but may be as high as 45% in patients who receive all three treatments.[140] In general MTX is most toxic when given during or following radiation.

Although the majority of the literature on neurocognitive function following cranial irradiation concerns children, some data are available for adults. Taphoorn and associates found no significant differences in neurocognitive function in patients with low-grade gliomas who received radiation (45 to 63 Gy) versus those who did not.[141] In another retrospective study, young adults with low-grade brain tumors treated with 54 to 56 Gy of radiation to limited fields often showed a transient early delayed drop in neuropsychological performance at 6 months; however, the risk of long-term cognitive dysfunction was low, at least out to 4 years.[142]

In a North Central Cancer Treatment Group (NCCTG) randomized study of 64.8 versus 50.4 Gy for low-grade gliomas,[123] data regarding cognitive performance were collected prospectively. Analysis of this data with a median follow-up of 7.4 years in the patients still alive showed that the vast majority of patients with normal baseline MMSE (mini-mental status examinations) maintained these after radiotherapy.[143] Patients with abnormal MMSE prior to RT were more likely to have an improvement in cognitive abilities than deterioration after receiving RT. Armstrong and coworkers conducted prospective, comprehensive, longitudinal neuropsychological testing on 26 adult patients with low-grade supratentorial brain tumors, mostly gliomas, who had received radiotherapy.[144] Nine patients underwent testing 6 years following radiotherapy. No declines were noted in most neurocognitive tests. Seven of the 37 neuropsychological tests showed improvement over 6 years. However, declines in selected tests of cognitive function, such as visual memory, emerged only at 5 years.

Based on these and other studies, one recent review on the neurocognitive effects of radiotherapy on patients with low-grade gliomas came to the conclusion that the weight of evidence suggests only sporadic, limited neurocognitive damage from focal radiotherapy at the doses usually prescribed.[145] These patients do not appear to suffer from widespread cognitive impairment or dementia.

Less data are available on the cognitive functioning of survivors of high-grade gliomas. One study found that most long-term survivors of high-grade glioma experienced significant cognitive difficulties.[146] However, all the patients on this study had received whole-brain irradiation as part of their treatment, which is no longer standard treatment for high-grade gliomas.

Cranial irradiation can result in arterial vascular problems such as vessel obliteration or narrowing resulting in a stroke-like syndrome.[147] These complications are rare, but when they occur they are more likely to happen following radiation of the parasellar region.

Endocrine Deficits Following Cranial or Spinal Irradiation

Endocrine problems are common following cranial irradiation,[77] particularly in children.[148-150] They include growth hormone deficiency, thyroid dysfunction, and gonadal dysfunction.

The hypothalamus is more radiosensitive than the pituitary gland and is responsible for endocrine dysfunction at lower doses. However, at higher doses (>40 Gy), both the anterior pituitary gland and the hypothalamus contribute to endocrine dysfunction. Of all the hormones, growth hormone is the most likely to show deficiency following irradiation. Growth hormone deficiency is seen in the majority of children who have received whole-brain irradiation. One study found that in children with ALL given 24 Gy to the whole brain, 56% developed growth hormone deficiency, whereas no such problems were seen in children given 18 Gy, at least at 4 years.[151] The latency of onset is dose-dependent, being shorter with higher doses.[152] Growth may be further impaired by spinal irradiation, which directly affects vertebral body growth center.[153]

Precocious puberty may also occur following relatively low doses, on the order of 18 Gy.[154] However, deficiencies in the other hormones such as gonadotropins, thyroid-stimulating hormone (TSH), and adrenocorticotropic hormone (ACTH) are rare below 40 Gy.[149] Thyroid dysfunction is common in patients treated with high-dose radiotherapy for brain tumors.[155] Constine and coworkers studied endocrine function in 32 patients with brain tumors not involving the hypothalamic-pituitary region who received 39.6 to 70.2 Gy to this region.[156] Sixty-five percent of patients developed hypothalamic or pituitary hypothyroidism. Fourteen of 23 (61%) postpubertal patients had evidence of hypogonadism as manifested by oligomenorrhea or low estradiol levels or low testosterone levels. Fifty percent had mild hyperprolactinemia. Subtle abnormalities in adrenal function were seen in 35% of patients.

In patients receiving craniospinal radiation, hypothyroidism may also occur secondary to exit dose to the thyroid gland. In a study of patients treated for brain tumors not involving the hypothalamic-pituitary axis from the Christie Hospital in Manchester, the incidence of hypothyroidism was 15% versus 33% ($P = .013$), respectively, for patients receiving cranial or craniospinal irradiation.[157] The mean spinal dose was 29 Gy, and the exit dose to the thyroid gland ranged from 10 to 15 Gy.

Optic Neuropathy Following Cranial Irradiation

Irradiation of tumors that are close to the optic nerves or optic chiasm may result in sufficient dose to these structures so that optic neuropathy is a concern. Two major classes of optic neuropathy are recognized, anterior optic neuropathy and retrobulbar optic neuropathy.[158] The former is thought to be due to vascular injury affecting the nerve head inside the globe anterior or adjacent to the lamina cribrosa. This type is associated with swelling of the optic head, in contrast to retrobulbar optic neuropathy, which is due to more proximal injury to the optic nerve. Diagnostic criteria for retrobulbar optic neuropathy include (1) visual loss (monocular or binocular) accompanied by corresponding visual field defects, (2) funduscopic examination often showing a pale optic disk but without edema, (3) onset 6 months to several years following radiation therapy that delivered a significant dose to the optic nerve/chiasm, and (4) no radiologic evidence of visual pathway compression.[159] MRI scans may show pathologic contrast enhancement of the region of the optic nerve/chiasm that received a high dose of radiation.[160]

Parsons and coworkers examined radiation-induced optic neuropathy in patients treated for primary extracranial head and neck tumors at the University of Florida.[158] Out of 215 optic nerves at risk, they found

anterior optic neuropathy in five nerves and retrobulbar optic neuropathy in 12 nerves. No injuries were observed in 106 optic nerves that received less than 59 Gy. The 15-year actuarial risk of optic nerve neuropathy after 60 Gy or more was 11% when daily fractions less than 1.9 Gy were used versus 47% when 1.9 Gy or more were used.

The data cited here suggest that the optic nerve/chiasm tolerance is at least 59 Gy; however, the University of Florida population did not include patients with intracranial tumors compressing the optic nerve/chiasm. Possibly, in the latter situation the tolerance of the optic nerve/chiasm is lower because of ischemic injury. Patients with pituitary adenomas or craniopharyngiomas have been reported to develop optic neuropathy after doses as low as 45 to 50 Gy, although in many of these cases the daily fraction size was greater than 2 Gy.[159,161,162] Based on these results, most investigators currently recommend limiting the optic chiasm/nerve dose to 50 Gy in 1.8- to 2-Gy fractions in the treatment of pituitary adenomas or craniopharyngiomas. For other brain tumors requiring higher doses, most radiation oncologists would try to restrict the optic nerve/chiasm dose to 55 Gy or lower. Adherence to these guidelines should keep the risk of radiation-induced optic neuropathy extremely low (1% or less) but unfortunately will not completely eliminate it.

Second Neoplasms Following Cranial Irradiation

Second neoplasms including malignant gliomas and meningiomas remain relatively uncommon consequences of radiation therapy for brain tumors.[6,163] Recent reports raise concerns that the addition of adjuvant chemotherapy may increase the risk of second malignancies in long-term survivors of childhood brain tumors.[15,16] This finding may be especially true after prolonged use of alkylating agents and etoposide with or without radiation.

Myelopathy Following Spinal Irradiation

A delayed early effect that can be seen after irradiation of the cervical spine is Lhermitte's sign, which is characterized by an electric shock-like sensation precipitated by forward neck flexion.[164] The symptoms typically start weeks to a few months after radiation. They are maximal at first but abate with time without the development of any objective signs. The paresthesias most commonly occur in the lumbosacral region but can also involve the upper and lower extremities and the upper back. This transient form of Lhermitte's sign can occur after doses of radiation well within accepted spinal cord tolerance and is not associated with any permanent late sequelae. The pathogenesis is thought to due to an inhibitory effect on oligodendrocytes that results in transient reversible demyelination. However, a more ominous form of Lhermitte's sign can present after a longer latency period following radiation (at least a year), which then progresses to chronic radiation myelopathy.

Chronic myelopathy is the most catastrophic late effect that can occur following spinal cord irradiation. Nearly half of patients who develop chronic myelopathy will die from complications.[165] A biphasic distribution occurs in the latency period from radiation to the onset of

Specific Malignancies

III

myelopathy. The early peak is from 12 to 14 months and the second peak from 24 to 28 months. The pathologic insults that lead to myelopathy include damage to oligo-dendroglial cells, causing demyelination and white matter necrosis, and death of endothelial cells, resulting in vascular injury. Some patients develop partial neurologic dysfunction, and others progress to complete paraplegia or quadriplegia. No clinical or radiologic findings are pathognomonic for radiation-induced myelopathy. Therefore, the diagnosis is usually made by a combination of (1) neurologic findings corresponding to a level just below the irradiated region, (2) a history of spinal cord irradiation to a high dose (>45 Gy) at least 6 months prior to the onset of symptoms, (3) MRI findings of increased intensity on T2-weighted images in the irradiated region,[166] and (4) exclusion of other etiologies. The MRI findings in spinal cord myelopathy can mimic tumor recurrence with gadolinium enhancement on MRI (see Fig. 69-6).[6]

The probability of developing chronic radiation myelopathy is dependent not only on the total dose delivered to the spinal cord but also on the fraction size. It is now well recognized that larger fraction sizes are associated with more severe later effects. However, this relationship was not always appreciated, and many of the cases of chronic myelopathy described in the literature occurred in patients who received 40 to 60 Gy to the cord in large daily fractions (2.45 to 5 Gy).[114] Using standard fraction sizes (1.8 to 2 Gy/day), a commonly observed limit for dose to the spinal cord is 45 Gy. In a study of the incidence of myelitis after irradiation of the cervical cord, Marcus and Million found that out of 1112 patients, only 2 (0.18%) developed chronic radiation myelopathy.[167] Two of 471 patients (0.42%) receiving between 45 and 50 Gy developed this complication. No patient out of 442 who received between 40 and 45 Gy and no patient out of 75 who received greater than 50 Gy developed myelitis. The authors' conclusion was that even when going to 50 to 55 Gy to the cervical cord, the likelihood of developing chronic myelopathy was extremely low. However, it is possible to see myelitis even if the spinal cord dose is limited to 45 Gy. This paper mentioned reports in the literature of myelitis developing at doses less than 45 Gy or even less than 40 Gy, using 1.8 to 2 Gy daily fractions. However, this development would be extremely rare. It is estimated that the risk of developing chronic myelopathy at this dose is 0.2% or less.[114]

GENERAL PRINCIPLES OF CHEMOTHERAPY

Chemotherapy of brain tumors involves many of the same problems as chemotherapy for systemic cancer, including lack of specificity, intrinsic or developing cellular resistance, intolerance of normal tissue to drug toxicity, synergistic toxicity between chemotherapy and radiation therapy, and systemic toxicity. Brain tumor therapy also has specific problems of drug delivery across the blood-brain or blood-tumor barrier. Cerebral edema may impede drug delivery, and corticosteroids that effectively treat the edema may "repair" tumor vessels and impede the delivery

of chemotherapy to the tumor. Thus, a recurring disappointment in clinical chemotherapy trials has been the failure to translate promising preclinical chemotherapy findings into meaningful improvement in patient survival.

Further complicating assessment of chemotherapy in brain tumor patients is the observation that corticosteroids also often reduce MRI contrast enhancement and improve symptoms, making it difficult to distinguish chemotherapy effect from corticosteroid effect.[168] Further confusion may arise when neuroimaging documents enlargement of mass after stereotactic radiosurgery that may progress over many months. Because PET scanning may not reliably distinguish radiation necrosis from tumor progression, the results of concurrent chemotherapy may be ambiguous.[168] Conventional MRI response criteria of 25% to 50% reduction in contrast-enhancing tumor therefore may not always be a true measurement of chemotherapeutic efficacy. Radiation therapy also may result in endovascular changes making access to the brain more difficult for chemotherapeutic agents. Attempts to circumvent this problem by administering chemotherapy before radiation remain an area of active investigation.

Clinical criteria for chemotherapeutic success are similarly confusing. Performance status, measured in many clinical trials by the Karnofsky Performance Scale, is affected by tumor size, presence of seizures, and adverse effects of AEDs and steroids. Thus, appropriate measurement of chemotherapeutic efficacy should not be median survival alone. Median progression-free survival or 6-month progression-free survival and reduction in seizure frequency, corticosteroid requirement, and focal deficits are all parameters that must be measured. For long-term survivors cognitive impairment and other serious acute and chronic neurologic toxicities of cytotoxic chemotherapy and newer molecular strategies factor into the assessment of chemotherapeutic program efficacy.

Finally, chemotherapy of primary brain tumors for the past 20 years has been designed on the assumption that the problem is one of local control with few recurrences outside the original tumor site.[169] However, with longer survival times and local tumor control patients with high-grade glial tumors appear to be developing a higher rate of multicentric cerebral and even leptomeningeal disseminated disease, and oncologists may need to design future systemic regimens with these considerations in mind.

An important consideration in the chemotherapy of brain tumors is the ability of the drugs to cross the blood-brain barrier (BBB). The BBB defines the restricted transport between blood and the CNS of water-soluble, ionized molecules larger than about 200 daltons. The BBB is formed by the endothelial cells of brain capillaries with some contribution from astrocytes. Brain capillaries differ from capillaries elsewhere in the body by the presence of tight intercellular junctions. The brain's extracellular or interstitial fluid is an ultrafiltrate essentially identical to CSF. Capillaries of the choroid plexuses are fenestrated, allowing access of large protein molecules into the plexus stroma. However, the epithelial cells separating stroma from CSF have apical tight junctions. The brain lacks a lymphatic system.

These features of the BBB and blood-CSF barriers exclude entry of large molecules like proteins and limit entry of smaller molecules to their ability to cross the lipid bilayer of cells. Lipid-soluble molecules like nicotine, ethanol, heroin, and the alkylating agent BCNU (carmustine) pass readily across the BBB. Another function of the BBB may be that of pumping out chemicals potentially harmful to the brain. P-glycoprotein, a BBB protein, is present in the membrane of some brain tumor cells and serves to reduce the intracellular concentration of several chemotherapeutic agents.[170] The P-glycoprotein is encoded by a gene responsible for a form of resistance to chemotherapy: the *MDR1* gene (multidrug resistance).[171] Numerous studies have linked the expression of P-glycoprotein with resistance to topoisomerase inhibitors including VP-16 (etoposide), VM-26 (teniposide), campto-thecin, and other drugs such as paclitaxel and their derivatives. In preclinical studies in nude mice bearing human glioblastoma-implanted tumors, coadministration of P-glycoprotein inhibitors such as valspodar (SDZ PSC-833) resulted in marked improvement in access of paclitaxel and 90% reduction in tumor volume.[172] Not all malignant gliomas contain tumor cells that express P-glycoprotein, and the expression in such cells does not correlate with tumor grade. Little evidence links the expression of *MDDR1* gene to patient response to specific chemotherapeutic drugs.[173,174]

Other mechanisms involved in glioma cell BCNU resistance are O-6-methylguanine-DNA methyltransferase (MGMT) and glutathione-S-transferase π. MGMT repairs nitrosourea-induced DNA damage by catalyzing the transfer of a methyl group from the O-6 position of guanine to its own molecule through a cysteine acceptor site. Not all BCNU-resistant glioma cell lines have an overexpression of this enzyme, but the presence of MGMT recently has been shown to correlate with survival in GBM patients treated with nitrosoureas. Patients who had high levels of MGMT had a median survival of 9 months versus 15 months for those with low levels of MGMT. No such correlation was found for the level of activity of glutathione-S-transferase π.[175] MGMT inhibitors resulted in increasing the cytotoxic effects of BCNU.[176]

Quantitative examination of the blood-brain barrier (BBB) and the blood-tumor barrier (BTB) has resulted in new avenues of investigation for brain tumor chemotherapy. Methotrexate entry into brain tumors can be enhanced by intra-arterial delivery, but the use of hyperosmolar mannitol for this purpose results in a far greater increase of drug entry into normal brain tissue rather than tumor. Human and rat studies of BCNU, cisplatin, and other agents after BBB disruption in both primary glial tumors and primary CNS lymphoma have demonstrated significant toxicity.[177,178] Attempts to deliver BCNU and other drugs intra-arterially have been largely abandoned because of unfavorable survival compared to patients treated intravenously, the poor outcomes in large part due to marked cerebral and ocular toxicity.[179-181]

In brain tumors the BBB is impaired in many pathologic states including traumatic injuries, infections, ischemia, and neoplasms. In brain tumors, the degree to which BBB tight endothelial cell junctions are disrupted and vascular permeability thereby increased varies within even a single tumor. The persistence of a relatively intact barrier impedes entry of some water-soluble chemotherapeutic agents into areas of tumor, leading investigators to look for methods of opening the BBB that are less toxic than intra-arterial mannitol. Another method of opening the BBB has involved using the agent RMP-7, a bradykinin analog. Based on earlier promising studies in rat tumors in which intravenous RMP-7 selectively increased uptake of carboplatin into tumors, a randomized controlled trial of intravenous carboplatin and RMP-7 versus carboplatin and placebo was conducted in patients with recurrent malignant glioma. No significant differences were found in median survival times, median time to progression, or in neuropsychological assessments, functional independence, or quality of life assessments. The use of RMP-7 had no effect on the pharmacokinetics or toxicity of carboplatin.[182] Additional trials using larger doses of RMP-7 are under way.

SUPRATENTORIAL GLIOMAS

Clinical Considerations

Patients with supratentorial gliomas may present with general signs and symptoms such as changes in mental status, seizures, headaches, papilledema, and nausea and vomiting as discussed in the earlier section on general signs and symptoms. They may also have focal signs and symptoms dependent on tumor location (see the section on localizing signs of intracranial tumor).

Over the decades there has been a change in the presentation of patients with supratentorial low-grade astrocytomas. In the pre-CT era, these patients often presented with headaches, papilledema, and motor weakness.[183] However, in more recent series in which CT scans or MRI scans were performed routinely, 68% to 95% of patients presented with seizures and very few had other signs or symptoms.[183-185] A possible explanation for this is that in the pre-CT era, many of these patients would have been placed on antiseizure medication and would not have been diagnosed with a brain tumor until their tumor grew large enough to cause signs and symptoms of increased intracranial pressure.

A history of seizures is also extremely common in patients with oligodendrogliomas, occurring in 70% to 90% of cases. The duration of symptoms can be very long. In a study by Ludwig and coworkers, 55% of patients had symptoms for longer than 1 year prior to diagnosis, and 37% had symptoms for longer than 3 years.[186] A few patients had symptoms for 10 to 15 years prior to diagnosis.

Low-grade astrocytomas decrease in frequency with increasing age. Their incidence is highest between the ages of 20 and 40 and decreases in patients older than 50. Oligodendrogliomas display a similar age-related frequency. However, high-grade astrocytomas, including glioblastomas, increase in frequency with increasing age (>60 years) (see Fig. 69-1).

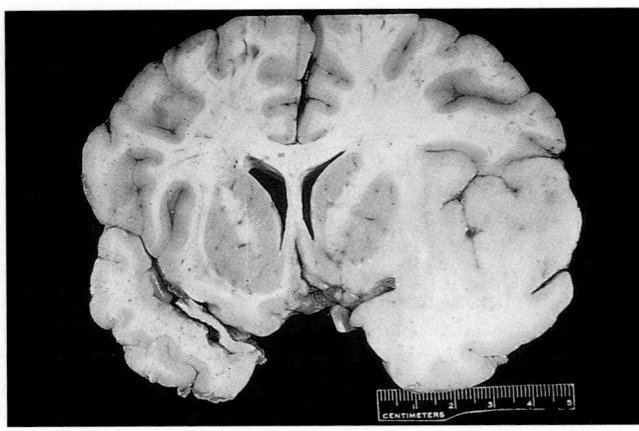

Figure 69-7. Diffuse low-grade astrocytoma: gross specimen. WHO grade II astrocytoma arises diffusely and infiltrates the right temporal lobe. Normal boundaries between the gray and white matter are obscured. Because borders are poorly defined, complete surgical resection is very difficult. (From Burns DK, Kumar V: The nervous system. In Collins T [ed]: Robbins Basic Pathology, 7th. ed. Philadelphia, WB Saunders, 2003, p 832.)

Pathology of Supratentorial Gliomas

Astrocytomas arise from astrocytes, the supporting cells of the central nervous system. GFAP (glial fibriallary acidic protein) is expressed in the cytoplasmic processes that extend from the astrocytes; therefore, antibodies against this protein can be used in immunohistochemical studies. Over the years, many different pathologic staging systems have been used. Kernohan devised a four-tiered system that classified tumors into grade 1, the slowest growing tumors, through grade 4, the most malignant tumors.[187] A three-tiered system including astrocytoma, anaplastic astrocytoma, and glioblastoma multiforme developed by Ringertz was used in many cooperative trials.[188]

More recently, Daumas-Duport and Scheithauer, reviewing cases from the Mayo Clinic and Sainte-Anne's Hospital in Paris, devised a system utilizing the presence of nuclear atypia, mitoses, endothelial proliferation, and necrosis to grade tumor from 1 through 4.[189] This system led to a better discrimination of outcome for patients treated at the Mayo Clinic than did the Kernohan system.

The most widely used system today for astrocytomas is the WHO system.[190] Grade I is reserved for pilocytic tumors, which are the most benign histologically, generally cured with surgery alone. Because they are more common in children than adults, they are discussed in greater detail in a later section, "Childhood Brain Tumors." The remaining categories are grade II (diffuse astrocytomas), grade III (anaplastic astrocytomas), and grade IV (glioblastomas).

Diffuse astrocytomas (grade II) are poorly defined, gray tumors that expand the parenchyma and obliterate normal gray/white matter boundaries (Fig. 69-7).[7,191] Microscopically increased numbers of irregularly distriuted astrocytes with mildly atypical nuclei are seen (Fig. 69-8A). Tumor cells can be seen infiltrating into normal brain tissue at some distance from normal tissue. Diffuse astrocytomas are often classifed into one of three subtypes: fibrillary (the most common subtype), protoplasmic, and gemistocytic.[192] Fibrillary astrocytomas are composed of tightly interlacing bundles of small, spindle-shaped cells amid a predominantly fibrillar matrix. Gemistocytic astrocytomas contain plump cells with distinct, round, pink cytoplasm arranged on a more delicately interlacing fibrillar matrix, whereas protoplasmic astrocytomas are composed of small, round, regular cells with indistinct cytoplasmic boundaries arranged on a loosely fibrillar stroma.

Microscopically, anaplastic astrocytomas (WHO grade III) are distinguished from grade II tumors by their greater cellularity, increased nuclear pleomorphism, and most important, mitotic activity (Fig. 69-8B). In both these and grade IV glioblastomas, tumor cells infiltrate into surrounding normal brain tissue, often at a great distance from the primary tumor mass. Histologically, glioblastomas are distinguished from anaplastic astrocytomas by the presence of endothelial proliferation or necrosis (Fig. 69-9). The necrosis can form a serpentine pattern referred to as "pseudopalisading" in which tumor cells crowd around the edges of the necrotic region. The presence of necrosis is of particular importance in grading gliomas and has been associated with shorter survival time.[193] Grade IV glioblastomas show areas of hemorrhage, necrosis, and cystic change on gross examination

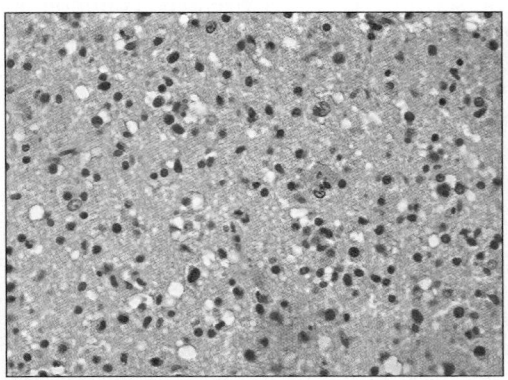

A

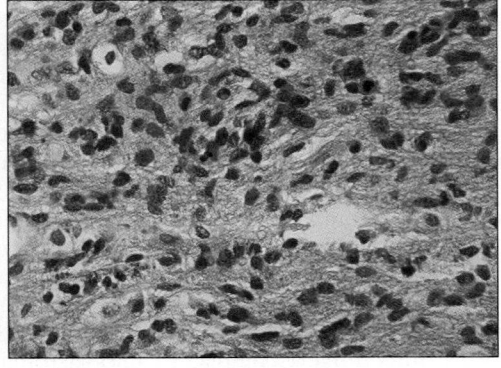

B

Figure 69-8. Histology of low-grade astrocytoma versus anaplastic astrocytoma. **A,** Low-grade astrocytoma (WHO grade II) shows low cellularity, slight nuclear pleomorphism, no endothelial proliferation, no necrosis. **B,** Anaplastic astrocytoma (WHO grade III) shows increased cellularity, pleomorphism, and mitotic activity compared to grade II astrocytoma in (**A**). Anaplastic astrocytoma also lacks endothelial proliferation and necrosis. (Courtesy of Dr. Daniel Skovronsky, Department of Pathology, University of Pennsylvania School of Medicine.)

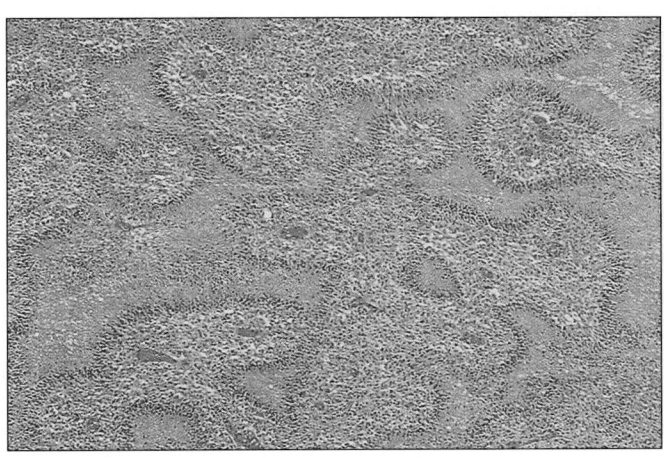
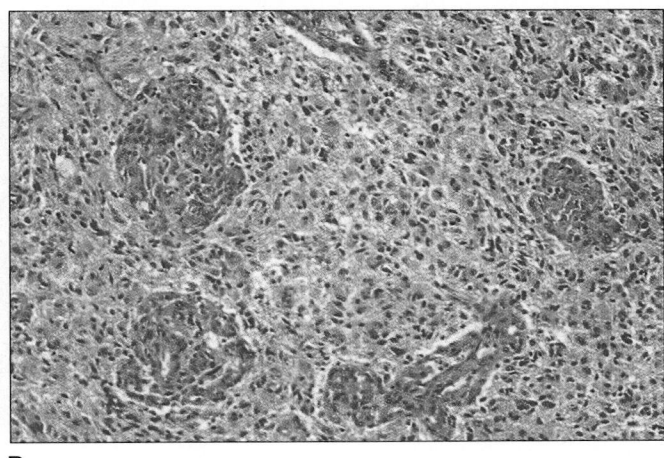

A   B

Figure 69-9. Glioblastoma multiforme (grade IV astrocytoma); histology. **A,** Pseudopalisading cells surrounding regions of necrosis. **B,** Endothelial proliferation, which in this case has reached dramatic proportions with the formation of tangled clusters of neovascular channels, often referred to as "glomeruloid" blood vessels because of their resemblence to renal glomeruli. (Maher EA, McKee AC: Neoplasms of the central nervous system. In Skarin AT [ed]: Dana-Farber Cancer Institute Atlas of Diagnostic Oncology, 3rd ed. St. Louis, Mosby, 2003, p 406.)

(Fig. 69-10).[191] Glioblastomas can present with multicentric disease, but occurs in less than 5% of cases as determined by autopsy of untreated patients.[169]

In addition to pathologic grading by morphology, techniques have been developed to measure cell kinetics based on the idea that faster growing tumors are more malignant. These techniques include immunohistochemical (ISHC) staining using antibodies directed against Ki-67 (MIB-1) or PNCA (proliferating cell nuclear antigen). Another technique involves calculation of an S phase fraction by measuring the incorporation of BUdR (bromodeoxyuridine) or IUdR (iododeoxyuridine) into tumor cells after intravenous injection of the agent. The predictive power of all three of these techniques has been compared to clinical parameters.[194] These methods still

have problems and are not routinely used, but there is some promise that they may offer prognostic information independent of histology. Likewise, ISHC stains for genetic changes found in glial tumors may also be used in the future to assess prognosis.

The different grades of astrocytoma carry very different prognoses. WHO grade I (pilocytic) astrocytomas generally have a greater than 90% cure following surgical resection alone. In contrast WHO grade IV tumors have a median survival of 1 to 2 years, even after aggressive combined modality therapy. WHO grade III tumors can have long-term survivors on the order of 20%, but the median survival time is approximately 2 years. WHO grade II tumors have a better prognosis than grade III tumors, but even in these, many patients will recur with a higher grade tumor, although this recurrence may take 6 to 8 years.

Most oligodendrogliomas occur in the cerebral hemispheres (80%), but they can occur in the lateral and third ventricles. Oligodendrogliomas arise from oligodendrocytes, which produce myelin. They often involve the subcortical white matter with extension into the cerebral cortex. On gross examination, oligodendrogliomas are often soft and gelatinous and are better circumscribed than astrocytomas.[191] They frequently have calcifications. In spite of their gross appearance, they can infiltrate surrounding tissues, including the subarachnoid space and leptomeninges.

Because of fixation artifact, microscopically, oligodendrogliomas appear as sheets of cells with nuclei surrounded by a clear halo of cytoplasm, giving them the appearance of a "fried egg" (Fig. 69-11A). Unlike astrocytomas, oligodendroglioma lack fibrillary cytoplasmic processes. Calcifications are present in 90% of these tumors. Often a network of capillaries gives them a "chicken wire" appearance. The current WHO classification for oligodendrogliomas is a two-tiered system with grade II (oligodendroglioma) and grade III (anaplastic oligodendroglioma).[190] Features suggestive of anaplasia

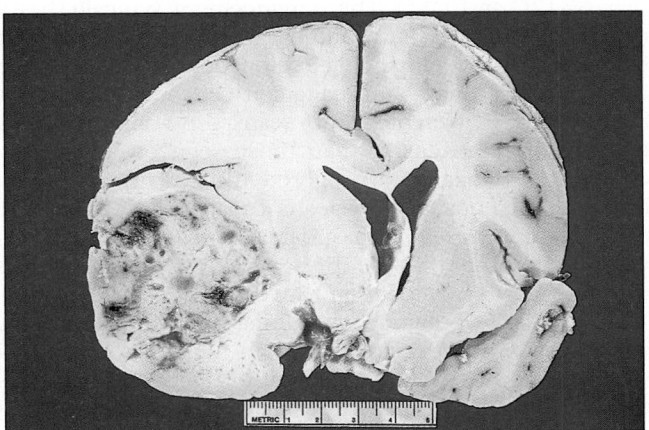

Figure 69-10. Glioblastoma multiforme: gross specimen. In contrast to the grade II astrocytoma shown in Figure 69-7, this WHO grade IV glioblastoma contains irregular areas of discoloration and cystic change, reflecting presence of hemorrhage and necrosis. These lesions are highly infiltrative and cause significant mass effect. Note shift of midline structures in this specimen to the right. (From Burns DK, Kumar V: The nervous system. In Collins T [ed]: Robbins Basic Pathology, 7th ed. Philadelphia, WB Saunders, 2003, p 832.)

Specific Malignancies

III

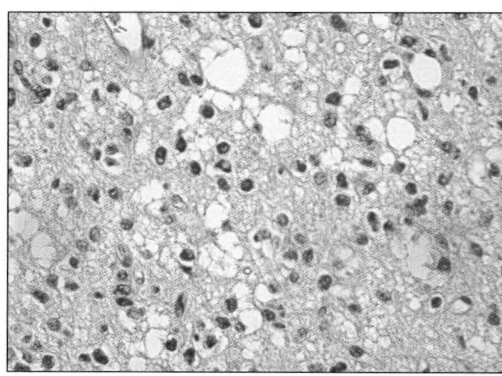 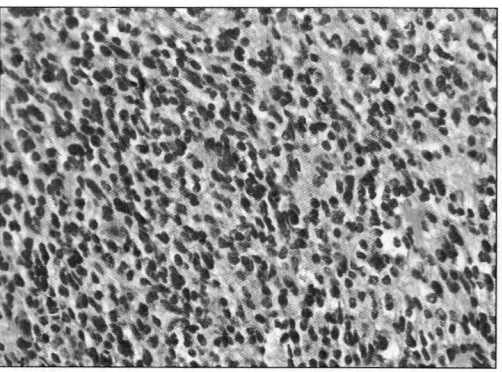

A   B

Figure 69-11. Histology of oligodendroglioma versus anaplastic oligodendroglioma. **A,** In WHO grade II oligodendroglioma, oliogodendrocytes are uniform cells with small, round nuclei and a characteristic perinuclear halo ("fried egg" cells). **B,** Grade III oligodendroglioma shows cytologic atypia and increased mitotic activity compared to **(A).** (Courtesy of Dr. Daniel Skovronsky, Department of Pathology, University of Pennsylvania School of Medicine.)

include cytologic atypia and increased mitotic activity (Fig. 69-11B). Two other features, microvascular proliferation and pseudopalisading necrosis, when present in an oligodendroglial tumor, would classify it as a grade III tumor, in contrast to an astrocytic tumor in which these features would make it a glioblastoma (grade IV). Anaplastic oligodendrogliomas have a poorer prognosis than low-grade tumors, but they are much more sensitive to chemotherapy than their astrocytoma counterparts (for more detail, see the section on chemotherapy for oligodendroglioma and mixed oligoastroctyomas). In the Mayo Clinic series, the 5- and 10-year survival rates and median survival rates for low-grade oligodendrogliomas were 75%, 46%, and 9.8 years, respectively, versus 41%, 20%, and 3.9 years for high-grade tumors.[195]

Distinct from oligodendrogliomas are mixed gliomas or oligoastrocytomas. According to the WHO classification, this latter category includes tumors that show "a conspicuous mixture of two distinct neoplastic cell types resembling the tumor cells in oligodendroglioma and diffuse astrocytoma."[195] The two components may be in different regions or diffusely mixed together. This definition is vague in that an oligodendroglioma with a very small astrocytic component might be classified by some pathologists as a pure oligodendroglioma but by others as a mixed oligoastrocytoma. In the WHO classification, these tumors are subdivided into oligoastrocytomas (grade II) and anaplastic oligoastrocytomas (grade III). Grading of these tumors is very difficult because the two components often differ in grade. In particular it is problematic how to classify a tumor that has oligodendroglioma-like regions in a background that otherwise appears like a glioblastoma. Some have referred to these tumors as glioblastomas with oligodendroglioma component, which may have a better prognosis than ordinary glioblastomas.[196]

Overall, patients with oligodendrogliomas have a better prognosis than patients with astrocytomas.[123] One might expect oligoastrocytomas to have an intermediate prognosis, and in some series this is the case. For example, in the Mayo Clinic experience, the 5- and 10-year survival rates and median survival times were 46%, 17%, and 4.7 years for low-grade diffuse astrocytomas compared to 73%, 49%, and 9.8 years for low-grade oligodendrogliomas.[197] The respective figures for patients with

oligoastrocytomas were in between these figures at 63%, 33%, and 7.1 years. However, in the UCSF series, 5- and 10-year survival rates for patients with pure oligodendrogliomas and oligoastrocytomas were identical.[198] The discrepancy between these series may be due to the difficulty in categorizing these tumors and interinstitutional differences in pathologic interpretation.

Imaging of Supratentorial Gliomas

WHO grade I (pilocytic) astrocytomas show enhancement on CT and MRI scans. In contrast, WHO grade II astrocytomas are typically poorly defined, hypodense, or isodense lesions on CT scans that do not enhance. However, either localized or homogenous enhancement can be seen in up to 30% to 40% of cases with calcification in 5% to 10% of cases.[184,199] MRI shows low signal intensity on T1-weighted images and high signal on T2-weighted images (Fig. 69-12A and B). Grade III anaplastic astrocytomas and grade IV glioblastomas generally enhance with contrast material, although in one study, enhancement was not seen in 40% of the former or in 4% of the latter (Fig. 69-12C and D).[200] The enhancement typically has a ringlike appearance surrounding an area of necrosis. The perimeter of the enhancing region does not define the border of the tumor, and malignant cells may be present beyond this. T2-weighted MRI scans show abnormalities that are more extensive than those seen on a contrast-enhanced CT scan or T1-weighted MRI scan. In one study in which stereotactic biopsies correlated with radiologic findings in patients with gliomas, isolated tumor cells were often found to be present as far as the region showing increased signal on T2-weighted images.[98]

At least 50% of oligodendrogliomas show calcifications, which can be appreciated on plain films of the skull as well as CT scans.[201] Enhancement of oligodendrogliomas can be seen on CT and MRI scans, but is often mild and poorly defined.

Biology of Supratentorial Gliomas

Genetics of Low-Grade Astrocytomas

A common genetic alteration in both low-grade and high-grade astrocytomas is the loss of one allele of the long arm of chromosome 17 (17p).[202,203] This change is determined

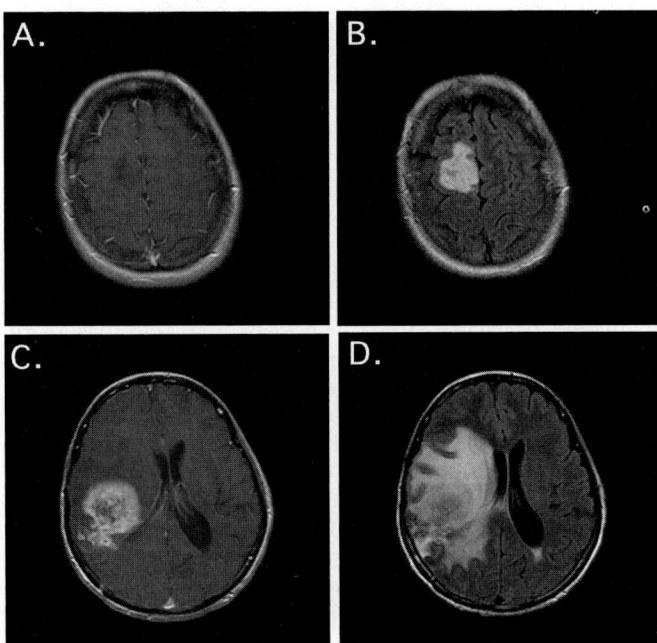

Figure 69-12. Low-grade astrocytoma versus glioblastoma multiforme. **A,** WHO grade II astrocytoma: Axial T1-weighted postgadolinium MRI shows no enhancing mass; however, region of hypodensity is seen. **B,** Corresponding FLAIR image of tumor in **(A)** shows abnormality consistent with edema. **C,** WHO grade IV glioblastoma multiforme: axial T1-weighted postgadolinium MRI shows presence of large mass compressing the right lateral ventricle (*left*). Rim of enhancement with central necrosis is typical of these tumors. **D,** Corresponding FLAIR image of tumor in **(C)** shows extensive peritumoral edema.

by loss of heterozygosity (LOH) studies, which use restriction fragment length polymorphisms (RFLPs) to distinguish the maternal and paternal chromosomes. In a given patient, if normal tissue showed the presence of two distinct alleles at a locus, the patient is heterozygous at that locus and "informative." If, in the tumor taken from that patient, only one of these alleles remains, this indicates that LOH or chromosomal loss of one allele has occurred. The consistent loss of a region of a chromosome in a specific tumor type suggests the presence of a tumor suppressor located in this region. If the remaining allele contains an inactivating mutation, this finding strongly suggests that the gene is in fact the target of the deletion. The *p53* tumor suppressor gene is located on 17p, raising the possibility that this may be the target for the chromosomal loss. Supporting this idea, approximately 50% of grade II and grade III astrocytomas have allelic loss of chromosome 17p, and mutations in the remaining p53 allele are seen exclusively in these tumors.[204]

p53 mutations are seen in 30% to 40% of all grades of astrocytomas, suggesting that it is an early event in glioma progression.[205] The majority of the mutations described in gliomas have been missense mutations. p53 is a transcription factor that has important functions in regulating apoptosis, cell cycle progression following DNA damage, and genomic instability. Mutation of p53 in grade II astrocytomas may possibly lead to genomic instability that

sets the stage for additional mutations that lead to the formation of higher grade tumors. In astrocytomas lacking p53 mutations, the p53 pathway may be deregulated by other means such as amplification of *MDM2* or loss of p14ARF. MDM2 is a protein that binds to p53 and abolishes its transcriptional activity. Therefore, overexpression of MDM2 effectively decreases p53 function. p14ARF binds to the p53/MDM2 complex and inhibits MDM2-mediated degradation of p53; therefore, loss of p14ARF effectively increases p53 degradation. In one study, disruption of the p53 pathway through mutation of p53, MDM2 amplification, or mutation/deletion of *p14ARF* was found to occur in 47% of astrocytomas, 72% of anaplastic astrocytomas, and 76% of glioblastomas.[206]

Another gene whose expression is altered in low-grade astrocytomas is *PDGFR-α*. The PDGF family consists of A and B subunits which can dimerize to form AA, BB, or AB units. Two PDGF receptors exist, the α receptor, which can bind PDGF AA and AB, and the β receptor, which can bind PDGF BB. By in situ hybridization, PDGFR-α mRNA was found to be overexpressed in 60% to 90% of grade II, III, and IV tumors, suggesting that it might be an early event in gliomagenesis.[207] The same study showed an excellent correlation between PDGFR-α overexpression and LOH on chromosome 17p, suggesting that there might be some relationship between the PDGF pathway and loss of p53. Overexpression of the PDGFR-α mRNA was confirmed to correlate with overexpression of the protein by immunohistochemical staining.[208] As will be discussed later, overexpression of the ligand (PDGF A or B) is not very common in low-grade gliomas but is seen in higher-grade tumor.

Loss of heterozygosity at chromosome 22q occurs in 20% to 30% of gliomas of all grades, suggesting that there is a tumor suppressor gene in this region.[209,210] Even though the neurofibromatosis 2 (*NF2*) gene is located in this region, it does not appear to be the one.

Genetics of Anaplastic Astrocytomas

In comparison to grade II astrocytomas, grade III anaplastic astrocytomas have a dramatic increase in mitotic rate. LOH of 13q and 9p has been identified in high-grade astrocytomas, and these deletions may be associated with changes in cell cycle regulation. In particular, the Rb (retinoblastoma) pathway is deregulated in these tumors. This pathway is described in detail in Chapter 5. Rb is a protein that binds to the transcription factor E2F, inhibiting its transcription of target genes and thereby transition from G1 into S phase. When Rb is phosphorylated by a cyclin-dependent kinase (CDK4 or 6), Rb dissociates from E2F, allowing the latter to promote cell cycle progression. An added level of regulation is the existence of cdk inhibitors such as p16 which inhibit cell cycle progression by binding to cdks and preventing them from phosphorylating Rb. Therefore, p16 opposes the effects of Rb and cdk4.

LOH of chromosome 13 occurs in 30% to 40% of higher grade astrocytomas, suggesting the presence of a tumor suppressor gene at this region.[209,210] The Rb gene maps to 13q14, and could be the target of this deletion. In one study, LOH specifically at the Rb locus was not found in any low-grade astrocytoma but was found in 20% of grade III and 32% of grade IV astrocytomas.[211] Mutations in the Rb gene were seen in 4 of 16 (25%) of grade III/IV tumors, further supporting the idea that Rb is the target of the deletion in chromosome 13q14. Other studies have found similar rates of Rb mutation or loss of expression in anaplastic astrocytomas and glioblastomas (10% to 33%).[212,213] A second component of the Rb pathway that is often altered in high-grade astrocytomas is the cdk inhibitor p16, whose gene *CDKN2A* is located on chromosome 9p, a common site of deletion in these tumors. In one study, homozygous deletion of the region encompassing the *CDKN2A* gene was seen in 19% of anaplastic astrocytomas and 41% of glioblastomas.[214] *CDK4* amplification was seen respectively in 19% of anaplastic astrocytomas and 20% of glioblastomas. Other studies have shown homozygous deletion of *CDKN2A* in the range of 30% to 60% and *CDK4* amplification in the range of 11% to 15% in glioblastomas.[213,215]

Ichimura and coworkers found complete loss of wild-type *CDKN2A* or *RB* gene or amplification of the *CDK4* gene in 38% of anaplastic astrocytomas and 64% of glioblastomas, but in none of 25 low-grade astrocytomas.[212] In this study, out of 120 glioblastomas, 111 (94%) had an abnormality in one of these genes. But only two had an abnormality in more than one. Therefore, these three genetic alterations, loss of *RB* expression, *CDKN2A* deletion, and *CDK4* amplification, appear to be mutually exclusive changes. This has been seen in other studies and strongly suggests that abnormalities in these three genes target the same pathway.[213,215] In some high-grade gliomas, *CDK6*, another cyclin-dependent kinase involved in the G1/S transition, has been found to be amplified; therefore, it may be another potential component of this pathway that can be deregulated during gliomagenesis.[216]

The CDKN2A locus encodes two different proteins through alternate splicing, p16 and p14[ARF]. Therefore, deletion at this locus results in loss of both proteins. p14[ARF] binds to the p53/MDM2 complex and inhibits MDM2-mediated degradation of p53; therefore, loss of p14[ARF] disrupts the p53 pathway. In one study, 40% of glioblastomas, 13% of anaplastic astrocytomas, but no low-grade astrocytomas were found to have deleted or mutated p14[ARF].[212]

There may be a tumor suppressor gene located on chromosome 19q that is important in the transition from low-grade astrocytoma to anaplastic astrocytoma. LOH of chromosome 19q was found to occur in 24% of glioblastomas and 44% of anaplastic astrocytomas but in zero of six grade II astrocytomas.[217]

Genetics of Glioblastomas

Glioblastomas can be distinguished from anaplastic astrocytomas by the presence of necrosis, endothelial cell proliferation, and neovascularization. As discussed earlier, many of the changes seen in anaplastic astrocytomas such as *RB* mutation and *CDK4* amplification are also seen in glioblastomas, although generally at a somewhat higher frequency. However, some genetic changes are fairly specific for glioblastomas and are rarely seen in anaplastic astrocytomas.

One genetic change that is restricted to glioblastomas is EGFR overexpression through amplification. EGFR amplification in seen in 40% to 50% of malignant human glioblastoma specimens[218-220] but rarely in anaplastic astrocytomas.[218-220] Approximately 40% of globastomas that have EGFR amplification contain a mutant form of the EGFR. The most common mutant is known as α-EGFR or EGFRvIII, which is missing exons 2 to 7, resulting in an in-frame deletion of 801bp of the coding sequence of the extracellular domain.[221-223] This particular mutant form of EGFR is constitutively activated and cannot be down-regulated. Its expression in glioblastoma cells has been associated with increased proliferation and decreased apoptosis and increased tumorigenicity and invasion in vivo.[223,224] Other mutant forms of the EGFR have been described in glioblastomas but are less common.[225]

Because glioblastomas often express EGF and TGF-α, which are both ligands for EGFR, overexpression of the receptor leads to the creation of an autocrine loop that may allow for self-stimulation.[226] Ras mutations are rarely seen in glioblastomas[44]; however, high levels of Ras-GTP are found in these tumors, suggesting that the Ras pathway is activated in these cells, perhaps by upstream events such as EGFR overexpression.[43] Another tyrosine kinase receptor family member that is often over-expressed in glioblastomas is PDGF. One study found mRNA and protein overexpression of PDGF-A and -B as well the PDGF-α receptor in glioblastomas and anaplastic astrocytomas, suggesting that this growth factor also participated in an autocrine loop in these tumors.[34]

A second genetic change that is common in glioblastomas but rarely seen in anaplastic astrocytomas is a structural alteration in chromosome 10, occurring in 53% to 90% of cases.[209,210,227,228] The entire chromosome 10 is often deleted in glioblastomas, and was deleted in 93% of cases in one study.[229] However, partial deletions at 10p, 10q23, and 10q25-26 can also occur, suggesting the existence of more than one tumor suppressor gene on this chromosome.[229-231] The tumor suppressor gene *PTEN* appears to be one of the targets of chromosome 10q deletion. Located on 10q23, *PTEN* (phosphatase and <u>ten</u>sin homolog deleted on chromosome <u>ten</u>) was cloned by two groups independently.[232,233] It encodes a phosphatase that dephosphorylates the D-3 position of phosphoinositide phosphates such as $PI(3,4,5) P_3$ to convert them to $PI(4,5) P_2$ (which is reviewed in more detail in Chapter 2). Inactivation of PTEN leads to unopposed PI(3) kinase activity and constitutive activation of downstream effectors such as Akt.[41] Mutation of *PTEN* is seen in 27% to 44% of glioblastomas.[234-237] A smaller number of glioblastomas can have homozygous deletion of both copies of the *PTEN* gene, leading to complete loss of expression.[237] The findings of one study suggested a potential association between lower *PTEN* levels and shorter survival times in patients with glioblastomas, although this figure did not reach statistical significance.[238] *PTEN* mutations have been found in anaplastic astrocytomas, although at a much lower frequency than in glioblastomas.[239] One study found the presence of *PTEN* mutations in anaplastic astrocytoma to be a powerful prognostic factor portending a poorer outcome.[239]

There may be some association between EGFR amplification and LOH of chromosome 10. In one study, von Deimling and associates found LOH of chromosome 10 in 100% of glioblastomas with EGFR amplification but in only 33% of glioblastomas without this amplification.[240] No consistent correlation has been found between EGFR amplification and PTEN mutation; therefore, most likely, some other tumor suppressor gene on chromosome 10 is associated with EGFR amplification.[234,237]

Primary versus Secondary Glioblastomas

Although the previous discussion suggests an orderly progression from low-grade astrocytomas to anaplastic astrocytoma to glioblastoma, this pattern may not always be true. In fact, evidence has revealed at least two different pathways for developing glioblastomas (Fig. 69-13).[241] One pathway, leading to the secondary glioblastoma, includes a history of a prior lower grade (grade II or III) astrocytoma, generally 5 to 10 years previously. This type of glioblastoma tends to arise in younger patients, with a median age of 40. However, in a primary glioblastoma, the pathway includes no antecedent history of a lower grade astrocytoma. The clinical history is usually short, on the order of months, and the patients tend to be older, with a median age of 55 when diagnosed. Primary glioblastomas are far more common than the secondary glioblastomas, accounting for more than 80% of all glioblastomas.[242]

Lang and coworkers analyzed genetic alterations in 34 astrocytomas and categorized them into three different groups.[227] One group consisted of 43 tumors with p53 mutations, which contained all grades of tumors. Of the 23 glioblastomas in this group, only one had EGFR amplification. A second group consisted of six tumors without p53 mutations but with other changes. Only high-grade tumors were in this group including five glioblastomas, and all five had EGFR amplification. The last group consisted of 16 tumors without any of these genetic changes.

p53 mutations rarely occur in primary glioblastomas (10% or less) but are common in secondary glioblastomas (>50%).[243,244] Conversely, EGFR amplification almost never occurs in secondary GBMs (<5%) but is common in primary glioblastomas (>40%).[234,243] Hence, these two genetic changes are mutually exclusive.[244] Also, a significant reciprocal correlation apparently exists between p53 mutation and PTEN mutation in glioblastomas, with not a single tumor out of 53 exhibiting both mutations in one study.[234] Consistent with this, the same study found that PTEN mutations are more common in primary glioblastomas (32%) than in secondary glioblastomas (4%). Another study also found that that PTEN mutations were rarely seen in glioblastomas containing p53 mutations.[236]

An alternate mechanism of p53 inactivation in some tumors may be MDM2 overexpression. In one study, MDM2 overexpression was found to occur in over 52% of primary glioblastomas as assessed by immunohistochemical staining but in only 11% of secondary glioblastomas (P = .0015).[245] One study found that the Rb/p16/cdk4 pathway is disrupted in primary and secondary glioblastomas to a similar extent (50% versus 39%).[215] However, in this study CDKN2A mutations were significantly more frequent in primary than secondary glioblastomas (36% versus 4%). The rate of CDK4 amplification or loss of Rb expression was not statistically significantly different between the two types of glioblastomas.

Angiogenesis and Hypoxia in Glioblastomas

One of the characteristic features of glioblastomas is endothelial proliferation and neovascularization. A variety of growth factors that can increase angiogenesis are expressed by glioblastomas. Foremost among these factors is VEGF (vascular endothelial growth factor). PDGF-A and -B are also overexpressed in these tumors. Endothelial cells in the vicinity of glioblastomas overexpress VEGF receptors and PDGF receptors, allowing for them to respond to their ligands. Therefore, the tumor cells may interact with the neighboring endothelial cells in a paracrine fashion to stimulate angiogenesis. VEGF, also known as vascular permeability factor (VPF), is a potent inducer of capillary permeability. The high levels of VEGF expression in glioblastoma may be responsible for the edema seen in these tumors. Some evidence shows that genetic changes common to glioblastomas such as EGFR

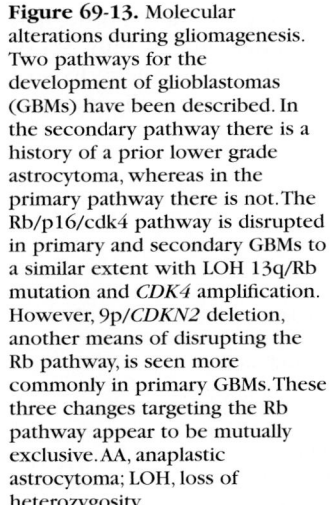

Figure 69-13. Molecular alterations during gliomagenesis. Two pathways for the development of glioblastomas (GBMs) have been described. In the secondary pathway there is a history of a prior lower grade astrocytoma, whereas in the primary pathway there is not. The Rb/p16/cdk4 pathway is disrupted in primary and secondary GBMs to a similar extent with LOH 13q/Rb mutation and CDK4 amplification. However, 9p/CDKN2 deletion, another means of disrupting the Rb pathway, is seen more commonly in primary GBMs. These three changes targeting the Rb pathway appear to be mutually exclusive. AA, anaplastic astrocytoma; LOH, loss of heterozygosity.

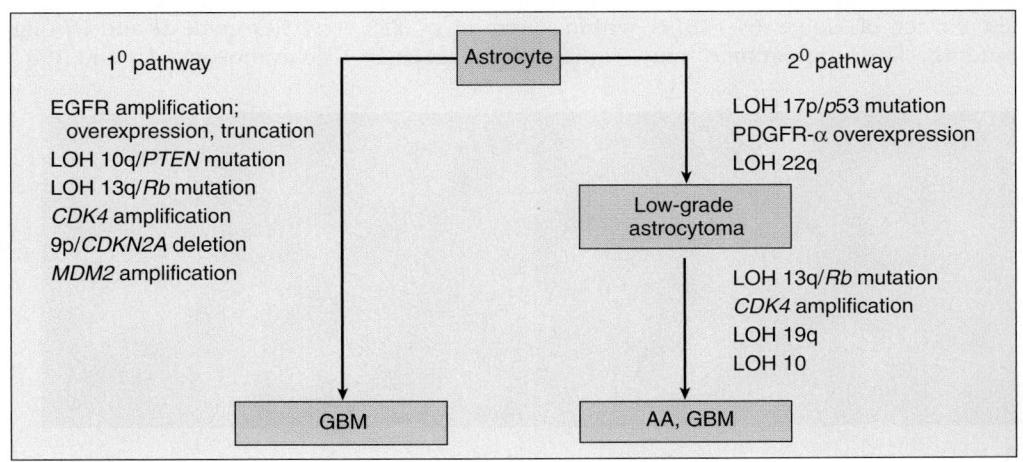

1⁰ pathway

EGFR amplification;
  overexpression, truncation
LOH 10q/PTEN mutation
LOH 13q/Rb mutation
CDK4 amplification
9p/CDKN2A deletion
MDM2 amplification

Astrocyte

2⁰ pathway

LOH 17p/p53 mutation
PDGFR-α overexpression
LOH 22q

Low-grade astrocytoma

LOH 13q/Rb mutation
CDK4 amplification
LOH 19q
LOH 10

GBM

AA, GBM

activation and PTEN mutation may contribute to high levels of VEGF expression, perhaps through activation of the PI(3) kinase pathway.[246-248]

In addition to expressing high levels of VEGF, glioblastomas are also thought to have significant regions of hypoxia, which may be a cause of treatment resistance. The presence of hypoxia is consistent with the histologic features commonly seen in glioblastoma including the presence of pseudopalisading necrosis and proliferative blood vessels. Hypoxia has been shown to be a characteristic of brain tumors using polarographic needle electrodes.[249-251] In other tumor sites such as cervix cancer, extremity sarcomas, and head and neck cancer, studies have demonstrated that hypoxia is associated with a poor prognosis.[252-256] Thus, further evaluation of the presence and level of hypoxia in brain tumors may lead to a better understanding and the development of additional therapeutic strategies.

The use of the electrode system is significantly limited by the difficulty of accessing tumors, the need for anesthesia, cost, dependence on a technically skilled user, interobserver variability,[243,257] failure to distinguish necrosis from hypoxia,[258] and inability to provide information regarding patterns of hypoxia. The use of 2-nitroimidazole binding agents as hypoxia detectors overcomes a number of these limitations. The reductive metabolism of these agents leads to their activation and subsequent formation of intracellular covalent bonds with macromolecules.[259] This process is greatly inhibited as a function of increasing oxygen concentration. EF5 is such an agent and its intracellular adducts can be detected using monoclonal antibodies and fluorescence immunohistochemical techniques. Investigators at our institution have previously described the clinical use of this agent in treating squamous cell tumors, brain tumors, and sarcomas.[260-263]

Figure 69-14A demonstrates the relationship between EF5 binding and Ki67 proliferation in gliobastoma sample. The highest EF5 binding in this tumor section corresponds to moderate to severe hypoxia (0.5% to 0.1% oxygen). In general, there is an inverse localization between these hypoxic regions and the location of the proliferating (Ki67+) cells. Figure 69-14B demonstrates that blood vessels are generally distant from hypoxic regions, suggesting diffusion-limited hypoxia. However, this is not always the case. One vessel, seen in the lower left corner of Figure 69-14B, is within a region of EF5 binding. This appearance may represent a recently infarcted vessel, acute (perfusion-limited) hypoxia, or a vessel with a longitudinal oxygen gradient.

Genetics of Oligodendrogliomas and Oligoastrocytomas

Two chromosomal abnormalities are frequently seen in oligodendrogliomas, deletion of chromosomes 1p and 19q. Oligodendrogliomas exhibit LOH at chromosome 19q in 63% to 81% of cases and LOH at 1p in 41% to 92% of cases.[264-267] LOH of 1p and 19q commonly occurs in both grade II and III oligodendrogliomas, so these changes probably occur early during tumorigenesis.[264,267] Neither gene on 1p or 19q has yet been identified. 19q loss can also be seen in astrocytomas; however, these tumors infrequently have accompanying 1p loss.[266,267]

Anaplastic oligodendrogliomas with 1p/19q deletions respond much more favorably to chemotherapy than tumors without these losses.[268] This finding is discussed in greater detail later in the section on chemotherapy for oligodendroglioma and mixed oligoastroctyomas. A correlation has been found between oligodendroglioma location and the presence of genetic alterations. Anaplastic oligodendrogliomas arising from the frontal, parietal, or occipital lobes were more likely to contain 1p/19q deletions than those arising in the temporal lobes, insula, or diencephalon.[269]

Other mutations have been described in oligodendrogliomas. LOH at chromosome 10 and 17p, both common abnormalities in astrocytomas, can be seen in oligodendrogliomas, but the incidence is lower, and generally these cases do not have 1p/19q deletions.[264] p53 mutations are much less common in oligodendrogliomas than in astrocytomas, occurring in only 5% to 10% of cases, and have an inverse correlation with loss of 1p/19q.[266,267] In one study, deletion of CDKN2A was seen in 21% of anaplastic oligodendrogliomas and was associated with a significantly poorer response to chemotherapy and worse prognosis.[268]

Oligoastrocytomas can have genetic changes characteristic of either oligodendrogliomas or astrocytomas. LOH of 1p and 19q have been seen, respectively, in as high as 63% and 72% of oligoastrocytomas.[266] Maintz and coworkers compared the genetic changes in oligoastrocytomas to pure astrocytomas and oligodendrogliomas.[267] p53 mutations were present in approximately one half of WHO grade II and III astrocytomas but in only 5% of WHO grade II and III oligodendrogliomas. Allelic loss of chromosome 1p and 19q were common in oligodendro-

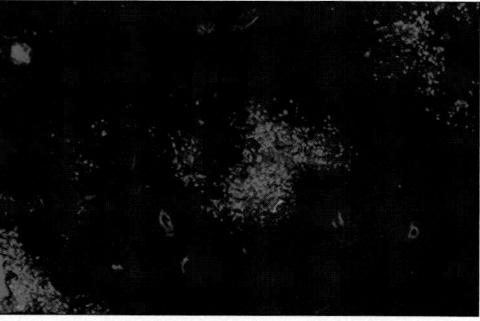

A   B

Figure 69-14. Staining for regions of hypoxia in glioblastoma multiforme with EF5. **A,** EF5 binding patterns (red) and proliferating cells (Ki67; green) are demonstrated in this image. **B,** Tissue from the same patient. EF5 binding is shown in red, and blood vessels, stained with PECAM, are shown in green. Each image is 2.0 × 1.4 mm.

gliomas (41% and 63%, respectively) but uncommon in astrocytomas (12% and 35%, respectively). Oligoastrocytomas contained p53 mutations in 32% of cases and allelic loss of 1p and 19q in 52% and 70% of cases, respectively. LOH of chromosomes 1p/19q and mutation in p53 were found to be inversely correlated, rarely occurring in the same tumor. Molecular findings were correlated with morphologic appearance in that tumors with 1p/19q deletions generally had a predominant oligodendroglial component whereas tumors with p53 mutations had an astrocytic component. These data suggest two subsets of oligoastrocytomas, one being genetically similar to astrocytomas and the other similar to oligodendrogliomas.

Surgery for Supratentorial Gliomas

Extent of Surgical Resection

The role of extent of surgical resection in the treatment of gliomas has been controversial for many years.[270-273] Virtually all the reviews in this area have been retrospective; therefore, they are subject to significant selection bias. Most likely, patients with the most favorable, easily resectable lesions within noneloquent brain have tended to undergo aggressive resections, whereas those with deeper lesions in more eloquent brain have been selected for stereotactic biopsy to minimize surgical morbidity. Some have advocated maximal resection for gliomas, reasoning that this approach is associated with improved survival.[274,275] A possible explanation for this view may be that fewer cells are left behind that need to be eradicated with radiation and chemotherapy.

Others have advocated stereotactic biopsy alone as the preferred mode of histologic diagnosis in the treatment of patients with gliomas.[270,272] Stereotactic biopsy affords a histologic diagnosis with a low complication rate (2% to 5%). However, stereotactic biopsy may lead to an inaccurate pathologic diagnosis. In a review of 81 consecutive patients initially diagnosed with stereotactic biopsy who subsequently underwent a craniotomy, Jackson and associates showed that the pathologic diagnosis based on the stereotactic biopsy was incorrect in 38% of the patients.[271] This figure represented sampling error in these patients, 96% of whom were biopsied at outside institutions. Despite the fact that these tumors were located in eloquent brain and previously treated by neurosurgeons, gross total resection could be achieved in 57% of these patients once they reached a major tertiary care hospital (M.D. Anderson Cancer Center, Houston, Texas). Major complications were seen in only 12.3% of these patients undergoing aggressive craniotomy for resection of the malignant glioma located in eloquent brain.

To specifically address the role of aggressive resection of gliomas in prolonging survival Lacroix and associates performed a retrospective multivariate analysis of 416 patients using prospectively collected data.[273] Postoperative volumetric MRI scans were obtained on all patients so that a blinded neuroradiologist was able to determine extent of resection given as a percentage of the original tumor. Patients with a resection of 98% or more of the tumor volume had a median survival time of 13 months versus patients with a less than 98% resection with a median survival time of 8.8 months. Also found to be significant were age, Karnofsky Performance Score, and extent of tumor necrosis. Even when statistical analysis controlled for these other three factors, extent of resection remained a significant variable.

Navigation During Surgery

Intraoperative MRI scanners have allowed for real-time evaluation of the extent of tumor resection. Patients can be imaged during surgery with MRI in order to provide real-time feedback of the surgical resection.[276,277] Schulder and associates reviewed 93 patients who underwent neurosurgery aided by a low-field intraoperative MRI scanner.[278] They found that surgery was directly affected by imaging in 51% of the operations. Second lesions not otherwise evident on the initial preoperative scan were seen in 21 patients, and in another 14 patients unnecessary dissection was avoided as a result of real-time imaging. Intraoperative MRI scanners with field strengths of 1.5 tesla are being utilized not only for anatomic

---

MANAGEMENT APPROACH

SUPRATENTORIAL ASTROCYTOMAS

- Grade I (pilocytic astrocytomas). Surgery is curative. If residual tumor is seen on postoperative imaging, the patient should have a second craniotomy to resect the entire tumor. Radiation therapy and chemotherapy have limited utility for these tumors.
- Grade II (low-grade astrocytoma). Surgery is the mainstay of therapy in noneloquent brain. In patients under the age of 40 who undergo gross total resection, no additional therapy is given. Patients under the age of 40 with incomplete resections and patients over the age of 40 with or without complete resections are treated with radiation therapy (54 to 60 Gy).
- Grade III astrocytoma (anaplastic astrocytoma). Surgery is required to establish a tissue diagnosis and debulk the mass. Patients should be treated with radiation therapy (60 Gy) and chemotherapy.
- Grade IV gliomas (glioblastoma multiforme). Surgery is required to establish tissue diagnosis and debulk the lesion. Surgery is followed by radiation therapy to a dose of 60 Gy. Chemotherapy consisting of carmustine, combination PCV (procarbazine, lomustine, and vincristine), or temozolomide can be used for tumor control.

imaging, but also perfusion imaging and MR angiographic imaging. Frameless stereotactic units have been available for many years allowing for downloading preoperative MRI scans to an intraoperative computer workstation creating a three-dimensional reconstruction of the images. The patient's head can be directly referenced to the images for precise intraoperative localization to less than 2 mm. Investigators have been able to import both PET and functional MRI data into the frameless stereotaxy units to map out functional brain during surgery.[105,279]

Intraoperative cortical and subcortical mapping has been used to define eloquent brain when resecting gliomas.[280,281] Intraoperative cortical mapping has enabled neurosurgeons to become more aggressive with tumors located within eloquent brain. This approach especially applies to resecting low-grade gliomas that occur immediately adjacent to motor and speech areas. Cortical mapping may be done with the patient lightly anesthetized but awake enough to respond to questions so that speech areas can be mapped.

Photodynamic Therapy During Surgery

Photodynamic therapy (PDT) utilizes fluorescing dyes activated by specific wavelengths of light to intraoperatively identify residual tumor and to destroy glioma cells.[282] Photodynamic dyes exhibit high selectivity for tumor versus normal surrounding glial cells. This increased selectivity can be as low as 10-fold to as high as 100-fold, depending on the specific agent. A unique aspect of photodynamic dyes is that at a lower wavelength of light the dye will fluoresce to identify residual tumor, whereas higher wavelengths of light activate the PDT dye, causing cytotoxicity to the depth of penetration of the lightwave. The PDT dye is given prior to surgery, then the tumor bed is illuminated using a laser or light diode of the optimum wavelength of light to activate the dye.[283,284] One of the drawbacks of this therapy is the long half-life of these agents, on the order of weeks to months, making it mandatory that patients must avoid direct sunlight for this time period.

Complications of Surgery

A recent analysis by the Glioma Outcome (GO) Project reviewed perioperative complications and neurologic outcomes of patients subjected to craniotomy for the diagnosis and treatment of gliomas.[285] The Glioma Outcome Project was a prospectively compiled database capturing information on 788 patients. Of these, 499 underwent either a first or second craniotomy for treatment of their malignant glioma, and the remaining 289 patients underwent stereotactic biopsy only. There was no difference in the characteristics of the patients who underwent first or second craniotomies. However, the analysis of the perioperative symptoms revealed that patients undergoing a second craniotomy had a higher incidence of altered level of consciousness and papilledema, whereas those undergoing a first craniotomy had a higher incidence of headache. The incidence of depression was higher in patients undergoing a second craniotomy, 11% in the group undergoing the first craniotomy versus 20% in the patients undergoing a second

craniotomy. This change may be a reflection of patients with a chronic disease state. Systemic infections were also higher in patients undergoing a second craniotomy at 4.4% versus 0% for patients undergoing a first craniotomy. This finding is not unexpected because these patients frequently have been heavily pretreated with radiation and chemotherapy as well as long-term steroid use, causing significant immunosuppression. When evaluating postoperative neurologic status, patients undergoing their first craniotomy had the same or better neurologic status in 92% of the patients, whereas this number dropped to 82% in patients undergoing their second craniotomy. Nevertheless, the overwhelming majority of patients are benefited by a debulking procedure to reduce neurologic deficits. As has been shown in multiple other studies, the most important preoperative factor associated with good neurologic outcome has been Karnofsky Performance Score (KPS). Those patients with higher KPS fared better with surgery than patients with lower KPS. This relationship is a reflection of degree of neurologic injury. The Glioma Outcome Project is perhaps the only prospectively collected database for evaluating outcomes of surgery in the treatment of malignant gliomas. The analysis of this data reveals that the incidence of further neurologic deficit with craniotomy is only 8% in patients undergoing their first operation versus 18% in patients undergoing a second craniotomy for resection of a malignant glioma. Given the severity of the disease this risk is certainly acceptable. More important, the objective prospectively obtained data show improvement in neurologic outcome with aggressive debulking surgery. One must realize that these data were compiled from participating institutions, and the decision for surgery was left to the discretion of the surgeon; therefore, certainly there was selection bias in terms of who underwent radical surgery versus stereotactic biopsy. The authors do not discuss the incidence of tumors in eloquent versus noneloquent brain. Nevertheless, this study would be representative of the general practice of surgical neurooncology throughout the country.

Radiation Therapy for Supratentorial Gliomas

Radiation Therapy for Olidodendrogliomas

Numerous retrospective reports have been published on the use of radiation therapy for low-grade oligodendrogliomas.[286] The results from these reports are mixed and inconclusive. Furthermore, these retrospective studies are plagued with a myriad of problems. In order to contain sufficient patient numbers, most of these reports span decades, sometimes going back as far as the 1940s. Obviously, prior to the advent of CT scans, accurate treatment planning would have been difficult, as well as good radiologic follow-up to document relapses. Prior to the 1960s, radiation was given using orthovoltage machines, which inadequately treat deep tissues. Many of the studies included high-grade tumors, thereby confounding the issue. The doses given to some of the patients would be considered inadequate by today's standards. An even larger problem is that these studies do not use chemotherapy. As discussed later in the section on genetics of oligodendrogliomas and oligoastrocytomas, at least a subset of these tumors are highly responsive to chemotherapy, which is rapidly becoming the standard frontline therapy for oligodendrogliomas following surgery.

Radiation Therapy for Low-Grade Astrocytomas

Numerous retrospective studies have been published on the outcome in low-grade astrocytomas. These suffer from the same deficits just noted with studies on oligo-dendrogliomas. However, in the case of low-grade astrocytomas, more studies are restricted to patients treated in the CT scan era (Table 69-7). Outcomes vary widely, with 5-year survival rates ranging from 55% to 90% and 10-year survival rates ranging from 36% to 77%. This underscores the tremendous heterogeneity among these patients, making it difficult to make comparisons across studies. One study from Philipon and associates with a large number of patients treated with surgery alone or surgery and radiation failed to find a significant difference in survival between the two.[199] However, analysis of patients over 40 years old with grade II tumors showed a significant difference with and without radiation (3-year survival rate: 50% versus 25%).

One often-cited large retrospective study that is not listed in Table 69-7 is from the Mayo Clinic.[287] This study included 126 patients with supratentorial astrocytomas (91 pure astrocytoma; 35 mixed oligoastrocytoma) diagnosed between 1960 and 1982: 35 received high-dose radiation (53 Gy or more), 67 received low-dose radiation (less than 53 Gy), and 19 underwent surgery alone. The 5-year survival rates were 68%, 47%, and 32% and the 10-year survival rates 39%, 21%, and 11%, respectively, for the three groups (P = .39). Patients older than 35 years of age had a significant improvement in survival when they received high-dose radiation compared with those who received low-dose radiation or no radiation, with a 5-year survival rate of 67% versus 37% (P = .008). This difference was not seen in patients younger than 35 years of age.

The results of these retrospective studies have largely been superseded by the results of the randomized trials discussed in the next section.

Randomized Trials of Radiation Therapy for Low-Grade Gliomas

To date, the results of three randomized trials for low-grade gliomas specifically addressing radiation therapy questions have been published, two from the European Organization for Research and Treatment of Cancer (EORTC) and one from the North Central Cancer Treatment Group (NCCTG) (Table 69-8). The EORTC 22844 trial randomized adults with supratentorial low-grade astrocytomas, oligodendrogliomas, or mixed oligoastrocytomas to receive either 45 Gy or 59.4 Gy of radiation after surgery.[288] The NCCTG study was similar except that patients were randomized to receive either 50.4 or 68.4 Gy following surgery.[123] Patients underwent a range of surgeries including biopsy, subtotal resection, or gross total resection. Neither study showed any benefit to the higher dose in terms of overall survival or progression-free survival. If anything, the NCCTG study showed a lower survival rate in patients receiving the higher dose of radiation (64.8 Gy). The 5-year survival rates in both studies ranged from 58% to 72%.

The EORTC also performed study 22845 in which patients with astrocytomas, oligodendrogliomas, or mixed oligoastrocytomas were randomized to 54 Gy versus no upfront radiation following surgery.[289] The latter arm had the option of receiving radiation if there was progression of disease. No difference was seen in overall survival (63% versus 66%). However, a statistically significant advantage was found in the group that received radiation in terms of progression-free survival, 42% versus 37% at 5 years and median time to progression 4.8 years versus 3.4 years (P = .02). The fact that there is no difference in survival has supported the position of those who advocate delaying radiation. Conversely, those favoring upfront radiation in the treatment of low-grade gliomas have cited the improved progression-free survival rate in the irradiated group.

TABLE 69-7

Treatment of Supratentorial Low-Grade Astrocytomas in the CT/MRI Era: Results of Selected Retrospective Series

| AUTHOR (INSTITUTION) | YEARS OF STUDY | TREATMENT GROUP | NO. OF PATIENTS | SURVIVAL RATES | | | |
				5-YEAR SURVIVAL (%)	10-YEAR SURVIVAL (%)	MEDIAN SURVIVAL (YRS)	P VALUE
Philippon[199] (Paris)	1978–1987	S	61	65	50	9 (all pts)	0.43
		S + RT	118	55	40		
Piepmeier[185] (Yale)	1982–1990	S or S + RT	55	90	77	12	—
McCormack[184] (NYU)	1977–1988	S or S + RT	53	64	47	7.3	—
Vertosick[183] (U. Pitt)	1978–1988	S or S + RT	79	66	36	8.2	—

RT, radiation therapy (immediate postoperative); S, surgery.

TABLE 69-8

Results of Randomized Trials for Low-Grade Gliomas

AUTHOR (STUDY)	YEARS OF STUDY	HISTOLOGIC TYPE	TREATMENT GROUP	NO. OF PATIENTS	5-YEAR SURVIVAL RATE	5-YEAR PFS
Karim,[288] EORTC 22844	1985–1991	9% astrocytoma (A), gr. I 60% astrocytoma, gr. II 22% oligodendroglioma (O) 9% mixed	45 Gy 59.4 Gy	171 172	58% P = .94 59%	47% P = .73 50%
Karim,[289] EORTC 22845	1986–1997	2% astrocytoma, gr. I 60% astrocytoma, gr. II 25% oligodendroglioma 10% mixed	Observation 54 Gy	140 150	66% P = .49 63%	37% P = .02 44%
Shaw,[123] NCCTG	1986–1994	32% astrocytoma or mixed (A>O) 68% oligodendroglioma or mixed (O>A)	50.4 Gy 64.8 Gy	101 102	72% P = .48 65%	55% P = .65 52%

These randomized trials confirmed the importance of certain prognostic factors in low-grade gliomas. In the NCCTG trial, three prognostic factors—histologic subtype, age, and tumor size—were consistently associated with overall survival in multivariate analysis.[123] The 5-year survival rates for patients with oligodendroglioma predominant tumors versus astrocytomas were 74% and 56%, respectively (P = .0001), for patients under age 40 years versus 77% and 60%, respectively (P = .025), for those aged 40 years and older, and 81% and 61%, respectively (P = .008), when preoperative tumor size was less than 5 cm versus 5 cm or more. In the EORTC 22844 study, the extent of resection had a great impact on overall survival, with patients who had more than 90% of their tumor removed doing much better than those who underwent a biopsy. Multivariate analysis of data from the two EORTC trials confirmed that astrocytoma histology, age over 40 years, and preoperative size greater than 6 cm were all unfavorable prognostic factors and also uncovered a few others, such as tumor crossing the midline and the presence of neurologic deficits prior to surgery.[290]

Based on these randomized trials, adults with low-grade gliomas show no difference in survival whether radiation therapy (RT) is given postoperatively or delayed until recurrence. Therefore, it would be reasonable to observe a patient with a completely resected low-grade glioma.

However, many investigators still advocate radiation after complete resections in older patients (>40 years) or after incomplete resection. Doses between 54 and 60 Gy are typically given in 1.8- to 2-Gy daily fractions over 5 to 6 weeks. It is common to treat the MRI-defined gross tumor volume (GTV) with a 2-cm margin.

The Radiation Therapy Oncology Group (RTOG) recently completed trial 9802 for histologically confirmed low-grade gliomas (Fig. 69-15); however, it is too early to analyze the data. Patients who had undergone total resection and were less than 40 years of age (low-risk group) were observed. The remaining patients were randomized to either radiation alone (54 Gy) or radiation followed by six cycles of procarbazine CCNU (lomustine) vincristine (PCV) chemotherapy. The RTOG will soon open a randomized phase II study of RT (54 Gy) followed by temozolomide or temozolomide both during and following RT.[291] The EORTC will soon open a phase III study randomizing between either RT (50 Gy) or temozolomide.[291]

Randomized Trials of Radiation Therapy for High-Grade Astrocytomas

The earliest randomized trial to demonstrate that radiation therapy was beneficial in the treatment of high-grade gliomas was conducted by the Brain Tumor Study Group

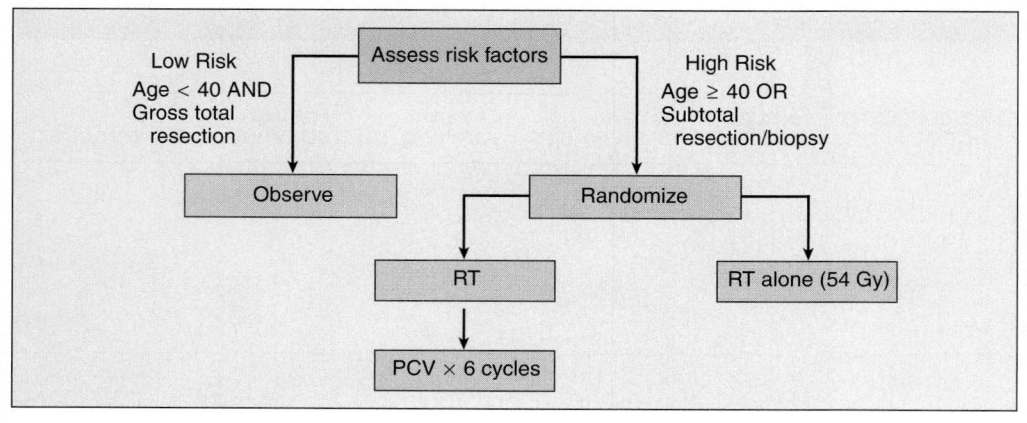

Figure 69-15. Schema for RTOG/Intergroup 9802 protocol for low-grade gliomas. Protocol was open to patients with histologically verified WHO grade II astrocytoma, oligodendroglioma, or oligoastrocytoma. Study was closed to accrual June 2002. CCNU, vincristine; PC, procarbazine.

(BTSG 69-01) (Table 69-9).[292] Patients were randomized to supportive care, whole-brain radiation therapy (WBRT), BCNU, or WBRT and BCNU. The role of BCNU is discussed later in the chemotherapy section ("Upfront Chemotherapy for High-Grade Astrocytomas"). This BTGS trial clearly showed a benefit to radiation alone versus supportive care with a median survival for 9 months versus 3.5 months and a 1-year survival rate of 24% versus 3% ($P = .001$). Based on this trial, radiation therapy has remained an essential component in the treatment of high-grade gliomas. A second randomized trial from the Scandinavian Glioblastoma Study Group confirmed the efficacy of radiation using a lower dose of WBRT (45 Gy) compared to supportive care (see Table 69-9).[293]

The results from BTSG 69-01 and two successive BTSG studies were pooled together to examine dose response.[294] The original studies were all randomized; however, patients were not randomly assigned to different radiation doses; therefore, the analysis of dose was a retrospective one. With this caveat in mind, the study showed a benefit to using 60 Gy versus 50 Gy (median survival 10.5 months versus 7 months; $P = .004$). The Medical Research Council in Great Britain performed a randomized study examining dose in high-grade astrocytomas.[295] After surgery, patients were randomly assigned to receive either 45 Gy or 60 Gy of radiation. The treatment volumes used in this study were very generous but less than whole brain. Patients receiving 45 Gy were treated mostly to the

TABLE 69-9

Results of Selected Randomized Trials for High-Grade Astrocytomas Focusing on Radiation and Radiation Modifiers

AUTHOR STUDY	YEARS OF STUDY	GBM (%)	TREATMENT GROUP	NO. OF PATIENTS	MEDIAN SURVIVAL (MOS)	18-MONTH SURVIVAL RATE (%)	COMMENTS
Walker,[292] BTSG 69-01	1969–1972	90	Supportive care	31	3.5	0	RT superior to supportive care ($P = .001$)
			BCNU	51	4.6	4	
			RT (60 Gy WBRT)	68	9	4	RT + BCNU superior to supportive care ($P = .001$)
			RT (60 Gy WBRT) + BCNU	72	8.6	18	
Kristiansen,[293] SGSG	1974–1978	—	Supportive care	38	5.2	0	RT superior to supportive care
			RT (45 Gy WB)	35	10.8	13	
			RT (45 Gy WB) + BLEO	45	10.8	13	
Bleehen[295]	1983–1988	—	RT (45 Gy)	144	—	11	60 Gy superior to 45 Gy ($P = .04$)
			RT (60 Gy)	299	—	18	
Chang,[300] RTOG 74-01	1974–1979	80	RT (60 Gy WB)	148	9.9	19	No difference between any group
			RT (60 Gy WB + 10 Gy boost	105	8.4	22	No improvement with 70 Gy
			RT (60 Gy WB) + BCNU	165	10.0	29	
			RT (60 Gy WB) + DTIC+ MeCCNU	136	9.8	26	
Selker,[297] BTCG 87-01	1987–1994 (10% AA)	85	[125]I implant (60 Gy) + BCNU + RT* (60.2 GY)	137	17	56	No improvement with implant
			RT* (60.2 Gy) + BCNU	133	14.8	44	
Laperriere,[304] PMH	1986–1996	92	RT (50 Gy) + BCNU	69	13.2		No improvement with implant
			RT (50 Gy) + BCNU + [125]I implant (60 Gy)	71	13.8		
Nelson,[308] RTOG 79-18	1979–1983	83	RT + BCNU	146	12.4	34	No improvement with misonidazole
			RT + MISO + BCNU	147	10.7	27	
Prados,[307] RTOG 94-04	1994–1997	0†	RT (60 Gy) + PCV	134	—	74	Preliminary analysis: no improvement with BUdR
			RT (60 Gy) + BUdR + PCV	134	—	62	
Souhami,[306] RTOG 93-05	1994–2000	100	RT (60 Gy) + BCNU	186	14.1	22 (2 years)	Preliminary analysis; no improvement with radiosurgery boost
			Radiosurgery boost + RT (60 Gy) + BCNU	(total in both arms)	13.7	18 (2 years)	

BLEO, bleomycin; BUdR, Bromodeoxyuridine; DTIC, Dacarbazine; MISO, misonidazole; PCV, procarbazine, cisplatin, vincristine; RT, radiation therapy; WB, whole-brain.
*During the early part of the study, external beam radiation was given to whole brain to a dose of 43 Gy followed by a boost to the tumor volume for an additional 17.2 Gy. From 5/89, WBRT was dropped, and entire dose was restricted to tumor volume.
†All patients on this trial had anaplastic astrocytomas.

entire supratentorial region. Those who received the higher dose were treated to 40 Gy to volumes similar to the first group, followed by an additional 20 Gy to the tumor volume with a 1-cm margin.

The early studies for high-grade gliomas including the preceding BTSG studies used WBRT. This choice was based on the assumption that it was impossible to accurately localize the true extent of these tumors because of inadequate imaging and the tendency of high-grade gliomas to infiltrate into surrounding brain tissue. This idea was challenged in a study that used CT imaging and autopsy data in patients who had died of glioblastomas to show that CT scans generally localized the tumor to within 2 cm of the pathologically determined margins.[169] In patients who had received radiation and subsequently failed, the relapse occurred within the site of the primary tumor in 90% of cases. Based on this study, the standard radiotherapy for high-grade gliomas started to change from WBRT to limited fields. Their results were validated by another study that showed that 78% of unifocal high-grade gliomas were found to recur within 2 cm of the initial tumor margin, defined as the enhancing edge of the tumor seen on CT scan.[296]

Cooperative group trials no longer use WBRT for the treatment of high-grade gliomas. In one study, BTCG 87-01, which was actually testing the value of brachytherapy, the radiation protocol changed during the course of the study.[297] At the beginning of the study, the external beam radiation consisted of WBRT to 43 Gy followed by a boost of 17.2 Gy to the enhancing tumor with a 3-cm margin. However, as the standard of care for radiation treatment began to change, the trial was amended in 5/89, so that the entire course of external beam radiotherapy was given to partial fields. Comparison of the outcome of patients who had received WBRT to those that received partial brain irradiation for the entire treatment showed no difference in survival. In numerous other studies, the elimination of WBRT and the use of partial brain irradiation for high-grade gliomas have led to outcomes no worse than those seen when WBRT was routinely administered. The current standard of care on RTOG studies is to define the initial volume as the preoperative lesion with edema as seen on T2-weighted MRI images with a 2-cm margin. This volume is treated to 46 Gy followed by a boost to the gadolinium-enhancing lesion seen on T1-weighted images with a 2.5-cm margin to 60 Gy.

By pooling the results of three RTOG studies and using a nonparametric recursive partitioning technique, Curran and associates identified several significant prognostic factors for survival in patients with high-grade gliomas: histology, Karnofsky performance status, age, neurologic function, and duration of symptoms.[298] Patients could be placed into groups I through IV with different outcomes on the basis of these factors.

Data are available regarding the radiologic response of high-grade astrocytomas to radiation therapy. In one multicenter trial patients had CT scans done preoperatively, at the end of radiation therapy, 6 to 8 weeks after the end of radiation coinciding with the start of chemotherapy, 8 weeks after the first course of chemotherapy, and then every 3 to 4 months.[299] The radiation dose consisted of 44 Gy to the whole brain followed by 14 Gy to the tumor volume. Twenty-two of 63 evaluable tumors (35%) responded to radiation, defined as showing a decrease in the enhancing tumor volume by 25% or greater. The vast majority of responding tumors, 20, showed a response by the end of radiation therapy. In two tumors the response occurred between the end of radiation and the start of chemotherapy (8 weeks later). Three tumors (5%) progressed by the end of radiation. Complete disappearance of the enhancing mass was extremely rare, occurring in only three tumors (5%). Response was more common in anaplastic astrocytomas (11 of 21 or 52%) than glioblastomas (11 of 42 or 26%), although this figure did not reach statistical significance.

Because of the poor survival of patients with high-grade astrocytomas, numerous strategies have been tried to improve the results with radiation. These efforts fall into two main classes: increasing radiation dose and modulating the radiation response. Doses higher than 60 Gy have been used to no avail. The RTOG 74-01/ECOG 1374 trial randomized between 60 Gy WBRT and a total dose of 70 Gy (60 Gy WBRT followed by a 10-Gy boost) but showed no improved survival with the additional dose.[300] Hyperfractionation has also been used to try to increase the total dose. In BTCG 77-02, patients who were randomly assigned hyperfractionated WBRT (66 Gy in 1.1-Gy twice daily fractions) with BCNU showed no difference in survival compared with those who received conventional WBRT (60 Gy).[301] In the RTOG 90-06 trial patients were randomized to receive either 60 Gy in conventional fractionation or 72 Gy in a hyperfractionated regimen (1.2 Gy twice a day). No differences were found in survival between the two groups.[302]

Radioactive implants have also been used to increase dose locally to the tumor bed. Single institution data suggested improved outcome with this approach over conventional radiotherapy.[303] In the BTCG 87-01 trial, patients were randomized to receive either an ^{125}I implant (60 Gy) or no implant at surgery. Following this, patients received 60 Gy via external beam radiation. Remarkably, no survival benefit was achieved with 120 Gy delivered with brachytherapy and external beam radiation.[297] In a trial conducted at the Princess Margaret Hospital, patients underwent surgery followed by 50 Gy of external beam radiation, then were randomized to either receive an ^{125}I implant (60 Gy) or not.[304] This study, too, showed no improvement with an implant.

Another means of increasing dose to the tumor region following conventional radiation has been stereotactic radiotherapy. Single institution studies have shown improved results with this approach, for example, from the Joint Center for Radiation Therapy at Harvard.[305] This approach was tested in the RTOG study 93-05, in which the control arm received standard fractionated radiotherapy (60 Gy in 30 fractions) with BCNU chemotherapy, whereas the experimental arm received a radiosurgery boost (15 to 24 Gy) prior to external beam radiation. Preliminary results abstracted from this trial indicate no benefit to the radiosurgery boost.[306]

Numerous agents have been tried in combination with radiation to try to improve survival. Conventional chemotherapy is discussed later in the section on upfront chemotherapy for high-grade astrocytomas. Halogenated pyrimidine analogs are incorporated preferentially into dividing cells and substitutes for the thymidine in DNA, sensitizing cells to double strand breaks. In vitro this can lead to radiosensitization by preventing the repair of double strand breaks. One halogenated pyrimidine, BUdR, has been tried in a randomized trial. Prados and associates randomized patients with anaplastic astrocytomas to receive radiation and PCV chemotherapy with or without the radiosensitizer which was given as a 96-hour infusion concurrently with the radiation.[307] However, no difference in survival was found.

Glioblastomas are thought to have regions of hypoxia that can lead to radioresistance. Therefore, agents that are hypoxic cell sensitizers have been used in conjunction with radiation (see Table 69-9). The hypoxic cell sensitizer misonidazole was tested in RTOG trial 79-18 but was not found to lead to an improvement in survival.[308] Misonidazole also showed no benefit in another randomized trial, BTSG 77-02.[300]

Therefore, in spite of numerous attempts to improve the radiation response in randomized trials, the prognosis of patients with high-grade astrocytomas remains bleak. As is apparent with the trials using a brachytherapy boost, even extraordinarily high doses do not control glioblastomas locally. In one study in which 90 Gy was given to these tumors using a 3-D conformal boost, 21 out of 23 patients failed in the high-dose volume. Only 2 of 23 failed marginally, and no patients failed distantly.[309]

Chemotherapy for Gliomas

General Considerations

Heterogeneity of glioma cell chemosensitivity has been demonstrated for nearly 30 years.[310] More recently, attempts have been made to correlate tumor sensitivity or resistance to BCNU with chromosomal anomalies underlying the progression from differentiated astrocytic cells to malignant gliomas.[311]

As discussed earlier in the section on primary versus secondary glioblastomas, glioblastomas may develop de novo (primary GBM) or via progression from low-grade or anaplastic astrocytoma (secondary GBM), the two types displaying distinct genetic evolutionary pathways.[241] Secondary GBMs contain a mutation or allelic loss of chromosome 17p, the target of which is the *p53* gene.[202-204] These genetic differences are reflected in different demographic characteristics of patients harboring these neoplasms. Almost 65% of patients ages 18 to 45 have secondary GBM characteristics, such as mutant *p53*, whereas only 8% of patients over 60 years old have this finding. Some patients whose secondary GBMs exhibit chromosome 7 amplification may be more responsive to BCNU. Furthermore, radiation and chemotherapy may alter the expression of molecular markers. Significant reductions in p53, EGFR, and MDM2 expression in paired initial and recurrent glioblastomas have been reported and suggest an eventual strategy for tailoring chemotherapy regimens to specific molecular tumor recurrence characteristics.[312]

Despite the foregoing developments, substitution of standard histologic classification and standard grading of astrocytic tumors by genotyping is not yet appropriate either for prognostic or for chemotherapeutic decision-making purposes. A recent study from Johns Hopkins examined the prognostic value of tumor markers in 32 GBM patients. Tumor cell ploidy, p53, and Ki-67 labeling as well as gender, age, race, location of tumor, and primary versus recurrent tumor yielded only the known association of increased age along with female gender and increasing Ki-67 index with decreased survival. Race, ploidy, and p53 had no prognostic value.[313]

Chemotherapy for Low-Grade Astrocytomas

Chemotherapy for low-grade astrocytomas is usually reserved for those patients whose unresectable tumors are progressively symptomatic. Radiation therapy has traditionally been used as a first-line treatment at progression. Potential toxicity of proposed therapy for

---

MANAGEMENT APPROACH

OLIGODENDROGLIOMAS AND MIXED OLIGOASTROCYTOMAS

- Optimal therapy and uniform grading systems (pure versus mixed; anaplastic) are not well established. Therefore, clinical trials may include patients with mixed histologic types, so outcome data must be interpreted cautiously.
- All tumors should be sent for genetic analysis. Advances in molecular genetic analysis have led to improvements in predicting response to chemotherapy. Pure oligodendrogliomas are more chemosensitive than mixed tumors (related to different proportions of loss of heterozygosity of chromosomes 1p and 19q).
- Primary treatment is maximal feasible resection.

Anaplastic tumors are treated with radiation therapy and 1 year of PCV chemotherapy. The role of preradiation chemotherapy is the subject of several ongoing clinical trials. At recurrence temozolomide is effective for anaplastic tumors; well-tolerated and probably equally effective is PCV used as adjuvant therapy.

- Low-grade oligodendrogliomas that are progressive by MRI can be treated with PCV or temozolomide. PCV is the best-studied regimen for recurrence but is associated with cumulative myelosuppression, nausea, vomiting, and peripheral neuropathy. Temozolomide is well tolerated and is emerging as a feasible first-line choice. Radiation therapy maybe useful for tumors that progress on chemotherapy.

low-grade gliomas must be balanced against the long natural history. Particularly in younger patients and in those who have an oligodendroglial component in their tumors, median survival times may exceed 10 years with 5-year survival rates as high as 89%.[314] Indeed, some authors have argued that quality of life considerations with particular attention to cognitive status dictate a prolonged "wait and see" policy in patients with suspected low-grade glioma.[315] Some variants of low-grade glial tumors have a more ominous prognosis and for the rare situation of multicentric gliomatosis cerebri, chemotherapy may be a reasonable first-line approach. A recent case report documents both MRI and MR spectroscopic improvement in this usually untreatable condition.[316] Potential considerations in the use of alkylating agents for patients with low-grade astrocytomas should include the risk of hematologic malignancies (5% at 5 years) or sterility. When the astrocytoma contains a portion of oligodendroglial cells an increasingly common practice is to recommend chemotherapy, but the percentage of oligodendroglial cells required to convey chemosensitivity to the entire mass is unknown. Molecular genetic analysis of oligoastrocytomas has suggested an inverse correlation between 1p/19q deletions and p53 mutations, rarely occurring in the same tumor (see the earlier section on genetics of oligodendrogliomas and oligoastrocytomas).[267] Tumors with 1p/19q deletions tend to have a predominant oligodendroglial component. It remains to be seen if patients with low-grade tumors can be reliably selected for chemotherapy based on these criteria.

Upfront Chemotherapy for High-Grade Astrocytomas

The infiltrating nature of high-grade astrocytomas precludes complete resection in most patients. Therefore, following maximal feasible surgical debulking, external beam radiation therapy is required. The role of chemotherapy has been investigated for more than 30 years but results have been inconclusive. Interpretation of clinical trials is hampered by the inclusion of variable mixtures of GBM, anaplastic astrocytoma (AA), and anaplastic oligodendroglioma (AO) patients in most studies, but some very general conclusions can be drawn from meta-analyses. One meta-analysis of 16 published phase II randomized prospective studies involving over 3000 patients showed primarily a higher proportion of 2-year survivors for patients primarily with AA but to a lesser extent with GBM who receive adjuvant chemotherapy.[317] Recently, Stewart performed a systematic review and meta-analysis from all available randomized studies to compare radiotherapy alone with radiotherapy plus chemotherapy.[318] The main results from 121 randomized trials including more than 3000 patients or 81% of patients from all known randomized trials showed a 15% relative decrease in the risk of death. This percentage was equivalent to an absolute increase of 1-year survival of 6% and a 2-month increase in median survival time irrespective of age, sex, histology, performance status, or extent of resection.[318] Although most studies have excluded patients over age 65, recent rethinking of this issue based on some small prospective studies of elderly patients with good postoperative performance status suggest that

radiation therapy plus adjuvant chemotherapy with temozolomide is well tolerated and doubles time to tumor progression (TTP).[319]

The earliest prospective brain tumor chemotherapy clinical trials were performed by the Brain Tumor Study/Cooperative Group (BTCG/BTSG). In Trial 69-01 Walker and colleagues found that median survival time was not significantly prolonged in patients receiving carmustine (BCNU), but at 18 months 19% of patients reciving chemotherapy, radiation, and surgery were alive compared with 4% of those treated with radiation and surgery alone.[320] In BTSG Trial 75-01 Green and coworkers showed that the addition of chemotherapy to surgery and radiation therapy significantly increased mean survival time from 40 weeks to 50 weeks and increased the percentage of patients surviving 18 months to 24%.[321] In these and most studies of chemotherapy as adjuvant therapy for high-grade astrocytoma the benefit was greater in patients with AA than in those with GBM.

Another well-studied and frequently used chemotherapy regimen is combination therapy with PCV: procarbazine, CCNU (lomustine), and vincristine (Table 69-10). Although initial reports suggested a survival advantage for patients with AA receiving PCV over those treated with BCNU, subsequent meta-analysis of four studies failed to confirm this finding.[322] The PCV regimen clearly is more toxic due to myelosuppression and peripheral neuropathy. Many additional trials of single-agent and combination chemotherapy have been conducted, but median time to tumor progression for patients with GBM remains about 6 to 8 months with median survival times consistently around 12 to 15 months.

This dismal situation has led to many attempts to design more effective single and combination drug regimens. The major agents studied in recent trials are carboplatin, paclitaxel, topotecan, irinotecan, and temozolomide. Of these drugs, temozolomide, an oral imidazotetrazine alkylating agent with excellent oral bioavailability and satisfactory brain tissue concentration, has been the most successful (see Table 69-10). A recent multicenter phase II trial with temozolomide enrolled 51 adult patients who received a maximum of four cycles of treatment before external beam radiotherapy.[323] There was an 11% complete response (CR) rate and a 16% partial response (PR) rate. However, overall survival rates of 23.5 months for AA and 13.2 months for GBM did not represent a significant prolongation of survival compared with PCV or BCNU.

There are several alternatives to the standard adjuvant regimens. A phase 3 trial of local chemotherapy with intracavitary biodegradable carmustine (BCNU) wafers has been reported. Two hundred forty patients received either BNCU or placebo wafers at the time or primary surgical resection and were then treated with external beam irradiation. Median survival time in the BCNU wafer group was 13.9 months versus 11.6 months. This modest survival advantage may have been partly outweighed by a higher incidence of adverse effects in the BCNU group including CSF leak and significant vasogenic edema.[324] Several institutions have reported a high rate of perioperative craniotomy infection after wafer placement.

TABLE 69-10

Chemotherapeutic Agents for the Treatment of Malignant Gliomas

SINGLE DRUG THERAPY

Drug	Dosage	Route	Toxicity
BCNU (carmustine)	80 mg/m^2/day for 3 consecutive days; or 200 mg/m^2 in 1 day; repeat q 6–8 wk	Intravenous	Delayed (3 weeks) thrombocytopenia, leukopenia, abnormal liver function tests
CCNU (lomustine)	130 mg/m^2 q 6–8 wk	Oral	Same as BCNU
Procarbazine	150 mg/m^2 daily for 28 days; repeat after 28-day rest	Oral	Leukopenia beginning 3–4 weeks; rarely, rash
Temozolomide	150–200 mg/m^2 daily for 5 days; repeat q 28 days	Oral	Leukopenia; thrombocytopenia

COMBINATION CHEMOTHERAPY (PCV)*

Drug	Dosage	Route	Toxicity
CCNU	110 mg/m^2 on day 1	Oral	See above
Procarbazine	60 mg/m^2 daily, days 8–21	Oral	See above
Vincristine	1.4 mg/m^2 on days 8 and 29	Intravenous	Peripheral neuropathy

*Procarbazine (Matulane), CCNU (lomustine), and vincristine (Oncovin) repeated in 6 to 8 weeks.

Another strategy to circumvent the problems of drug access and tumor resistance is high-dose chemotherapy followed by autologous hematopoietic stem cell transplantation. Durando and colleagues recently reported results in 114 patients with newly diagnosed AA, GBM, or AO. Five deaths associated with treatment occurred largely in patients with KPS 60 or less. Overall results were not significantly better than the standard regimens.[325]

In order to circumvent the problems of decreased drug delivery across the BBB, tissue hypoxia, and cell growth arrest due to radiation some groups have studied preirradiation chemotherapy. A phase III study comparing three cycles of BCNU and cisplatin followed by radiation therapy (ECOG Trial 2394) reported outcomes in 223 patients randomized to preirradiation chemotherapy versus standard BCNU. The groups showed no difference in median survival time or 1-year survival rate. Notably, only 56% of patients received all three planned chemotherapy courses underscoring the difficulty of delaying radiation therapy in this population.[326]

Chemotherapy for Recurrent High-Grade Astrocytomas

Chemotherapy has a meaningful palliative role in some patients with recurrent malignant astrocytic tumors. Although long-term disease-free survival occurs in fewer than 10% of patients, most such patients have been treated for multiple recurrences, often with more than one surgical resection and several different chemotherapy regimens.[327] Any benefit from chemotherapy for recurrent disease must be measured against the roughly 4- to 5-month median survival rate after repeat surgical removal of recurrent high-grade astrocytic tumors. Most published chemotherapy trials for recurrent tumor are small phase II studies, and very few studies directly compare one regimen with another.

Because benefits of available cytotoxic chemotherapy for AA and GBM are small, participation in clinical trials is appropriate for many patients. If the patient previously has received PCV or BCNU therapy, temozolomide can be used. It is currently Food and Drug Administration (FDA) approved only for recurrent GBM. On the basis of three open label multicentric controlled studies totaling more than 525 patients temozolomide appear to be a safe choice for such patients with 6-month progression-free survival rate of 46% and 12-month progression-free survival rate of 24%.[328] In another study that included both anaplastic oligodendrogliomas and anaplastic astrocytomas, median overall survival after recurrence was 13.6 months with objective MRI changes seen in 35% of patients.[329] Even heavily pretreated patients may respond to temozolomide.[330] However, although temozolomide may increase length of progression-free survival time, it has minimal impact on overall length of survival.[331] In direct comparison with procarbazine as a single agent therapy at relapse temozolomide appears superior both in progression-free survival and in quality of life.[332]

For patients whose tumors recur after initial treatment with the standard regimens, potentially useful strategies include targeted interstitial drug delivery using biodegradable microspheres and wafers. A placebo-controlled multicenter study in 22 patients reported a median survival of 31 weeks in patients receiving BCNU polymers compared to 23 weeks in the patients receiving placebo polymers.[333] The BCNU wafer system (Gliadel) is approved for recurrent high-grade astrocytoma. As is any direct tumor injection treatment method, the utility of Gliadel is limited to those patients who can have meaningful re-resection of tumors that are relatively well circumscribed, unilateral, and in noneloquent brain locations, a situation not typical of the majority of anaplastic astrocytic tumors.

Irinotecan, a topoisomerase I inhibitor, has been the subject of several studies in patients with recurrent malignant astrocytoma. A respectable 10% to 15% objective imaging response rate has been achieved after infusions every three weeks.[334] In two other studies seeking maximal tolerated dose a marked effect of concomitant enzyme-inducing antiepileptic drugs was found. Patients taking cytochrome P-450–inducing AEDs achieved lower levels of the active metabolite SN-38 (7-ethyl-10-hydroxy-camptothecin) than those not receiving AEDs.[335] Subsequent and ongoing irinotecan studies have stratified patients according to AED use.

Chemotherapy for Anaplastic Oligodendrogliomas

Increasing evidence has accumulated to confirm that anaplastic oligodendrogliomas and possibly anaplastic oligoastrocytomas are special types of malignant gliomas that are sensitive to chemotherapy.[329,336–342] Although the molecular markers of chemosensitivity, allelic loss of chromosomes 1p and 19q, have been shown to have prognostic significance in multiple studies, the reason for oligodendroglial chemosensitivity remains unknown. Zlatescu and colleagues have made the clinically interesting observation that allelic loss of 1p and 19q is related to tumor location and extent of tumor spread in the brain.[269] Anaplastic oligodendrogliomas located in the frontal, parietal, and occipital lobes were significantly more likely to harbor 1p/19q loss than histologically identical tumors arising in the temporal lobe, insula, or diencephalon. Frontal tumors tend to have greater bilateral diffuse spread, and investigation of the biologic significance of these growth and invasion differences eventually may have implications for management strategies. However, it is already feasible to begin to predict appropriate chemotherapy for patients based on their tumor genotype. It should be emphasized that many studies are hampered by inclusion of patients with mixed gliomas and variable components of anaplasia. However, a consensus about chemotherapy and radiation for oligodendroglial tumors is beginning to emerge based on correlation of molecular parameters and clinical outcomes.

In the first large study of chemotherapy for anaplastic oligodendrogliomas, Cairncross and the National Cancer Institute of Canada conducted a multicenter phase II trial of intensive PCV (iPCV), which differs from the regimen in Table 69-10 because of an increase dose of CCNU from 110 mg/m^2 to 130 mg/m^2 and an increased dose of procarbazine from 60 mg/m^2 to 75 mg/m^2.[336] This study included new or recurrent anaplastic oligodendrogliomas and reported a 75% overall response rate with 38% complete responses. Time to tumor progression was at least 16.3 months for the entire eligible group and at least 25.2 months for complete responders. Cairncross and colleagues have returned to their original cohort of patients in the Radiation Therapy Oncology Group Trial 94-02 (that had been designed to compare the effectiveness of radiation therapy alone versus radiation therapy plus PCV in AO and OA).[343] Blood specimens, slides, and paraffin blocks were obtained and the authors did a retrospective analysis of 1p/19q deletions in 26 tumors determining correlation of chemosensitivity with allelic loss on these chromosomes. These data are in agreement with a series of 162 tumors from the Mayo Clinic in which combined loss of 1p and 19q was a significant predictor of prolonged survival time in patients with pure oligodendroglioma independent of tumor grade. This favorable association was not demonstrated in patients with astrocytoma or mixed oligoastrocytoma.[344] Patients can be further subdivided for prognostic purposes. Those who have both 1p and 19q deletions have the longest survival with a response duration of greater than 31 months in the Cairncross study. Those with allelic loss of 1p only have a high initial response to chemotherapy but a response duration of only 11 months.[345] Patients with intact 1p and p53 mutations had only a 33% response to chemotherapy and a 7-month duration of response.

Similar retrospective chemosensitivity correlation with univariable 1p status has been found with temozolomide. In this retrospective study 90% of patients who had 1p allelic loss responded to temozolomide, but only 33% of patients with intact 1p benefited from treatment.[346] These correlations were independent of gender, age, and tumor grade.

Clinical trials reported thus far have not prospectively stratified patients by genetic status. However, overall chemotherapy response rates are impressive in newly diagnosed anaplastic oligodendroglial tumors.[336,337,339,340,342] Approximately two thirds of patients with anaplastic oligodendrogliomas have shown substantial response to first-line PCV therapy (see Table 69-11 for summary of clinical trials). Even patients with recurrent anaplastic oligodendrogliomas may respond to PCV chemotherapy (Table 69-12).[338,347] However, most patients with recurrent anaplastic oligodendrogliomas who received PCV at initial presentation are currently being treated with temozolomide at relapse. Several small trials have shown the safety and efficacy of temozolomide regardless of prior PCV therapy.[329,341,348] An open label phase II trial of temozolomide in 47 patients with oligodendrogliomas who relapsed after radiation and PCV chemotherapy demonstrated an objective response rate of 43%, median PFS of 7.5 months, and 34% rate of disease-free survival at 12 months.[341] In another phase II multicenter trial that included anaplastic oligodendroglioma and some cases of mixed oligoastrocytoma, a response rate was seen in 26% of patients who had previously received PCV therapy and in two out of three chemotherapy-naive patients.[348] A short time to tumor progression appears to be a bad prognostic factor for response to both first-line PCV chemotherapy and temozolomide

Chemotherapy for Oligodendroglioma and Mixed Oligoastroctyomas

The prognostic significance of alterations in chromosomes 1p and 19q have been studied in other diffuse gliomas of variable anaplastic morphology. Combined loss of 1p and 19q has been identified as a univariate predictor of prolonged survival among patients with pure oligodendroglioma and remains a significant predictor after adjusting for age and tumor grade. There has been increasing interest in identification of a subset of patients with well-differentiated oligodendroglioma or mixed glioma with poor prognosis in order to offer early appropriate therapy. In a recent small study, association of chromosome 10q LOH predicted a short survival time in oligoastrocytomas, and LOH on 1p again was associated with significantly longer survival time.[349]

TABLE 69-11

Chemotherapy Trials for Newly Diagnosed Low-Grade and Anaplastic Oligodendroglioma and Oligoastrocytoma

AUTHOR	THERAPY	TUMOR	N	CR/PR/SD	MTP (MOS)	6/12 MONTH PFS	MEDIAN SURVIVAL (MOS)
Cairncross[336]	iPCV before RT	AO, AOA*	24	38%/37%/17%	>16.3	NR/NR	NR
Boiardi[342]	BCNU + cisplatin Before and after RT	AOA	32	NR	54.6	NR/NR	70.1
Buckner[350]	PCV before RT	O, OA	28	52% (CR+PR)	NR	NR/100%	NR
Kim[337]	PCV before or after RT	AO, AOA	32	31%/59%/3%	15.4	NR	61.4
Jeremic[339]	PCV + RT	AO, AOA	23	NR	NR	100%/100%	>60
Paleologos[340]	PCV or I-PCV before RT	AO or AOA	30	40%/30%/27%	36	89%/NR	NR

AO, anaplastic oligodendroglioma; AOA, anaplastic oligoastrocytoma; CR, complete response; MTP, median time to progression; PFS, progression-free survival; NR, no response; O, oligodendroglioma; OA, olgioastrocytoma; PR, partial response; RT, radiation therapy; SD, stable disease.
*In this series, 14 patients had newly diagnosed anaplastic oligodendrogliomas; 10 had recurrent disease.

Because of the great range of survival times in patients with lower grade oligodendroglioma and mixed oligo-astroctyoma, objective evidence of substantial alteration of natural history is difficult to document. The most clear-cut way to demonstrate chemotherapy efficacy in these patients therefore would be to give chemotherapy before radiation therapy and document objective regression on MRI. Buckner and colleagues have done this for a small group of low-grade oligodendrogliomas (see Table 69-11).[350] They studied response rate and toxicity of PCV administered before radiation therapy in newly diagnosed patients. Fifty-two percent of patients demonstrated tumor regression on MRI after 4 cycles of PCV and prior to radiation therapy. Though the sample size was small in this study and responses did not correlate with loss of 1p and 19q, LOH of 1p and 19q were not seen in low-grade oligoastrocytoma and were inversely correlated with the presence of p53 mutation.

The EORTC conducted two studies using temozolomide for patients with low-grade oligodendrogliomas or oligoastroctyomas, one for patients who had received PCV chemotherapy and radiation for their initial disease,[351] and another for patients who had received surgery and radiation without chemotherapy initially.[352] These studies showed a 25% to 53% response rate to temozolomide (see Table 69-12).

Molecular information should be used in conjunction with radiographic characteristics, conventional histologic analysis of mitoses, and MIB-1 staining along with the demographic prognostic variables of age, duration of symptoms, and functional status (including seizure control). Translating these variables into chemotherapy guidelines for the lower grade oligodendrogliomas and oligoastrocytomas has led some clinicians to recommend initial chemotherapy without radiation therapy for patients whose tumors have both the 1p and 19q

TABLE 69-12

Chemotherapy Regimens for Recurrent Low-Grade and Anaplastic Oligodendroglioma and Oligoastrocytoma

AUTHOR	THERAPY	TUMOR	N	CR/PR/SD	MTP (MOS)	6/12 MONTH PFS	MEDIAN SURVIVAL (MOS)
Yung[329]	Temozolomide	AA* AOA, AO	111	8%/27%/26%	5.4	46%/24%	13.6
van den Bent[338]	iPCV or PCV	O, OA AO, AOA	52	17%/46%/19%	10	NR/NR	20
Cairncross[347]	iPCV, then high-dose thiotepa and transplant	AO, AOA	20†	20%/80%/0%	20	NR/NR	49
Chinot[341]	Temozolamide	AO, AOA	47	15%/28%/40%	7.5	NR/34%	8.8
van den Bent[348]	Temozolamide	AO, AOA	30	10%/21%/28%	NR	44%/27%	7
van den Bent[352]	Temozolamide‡	O, OA	38	53% (CR+PR)	10.4	71%/40%	NR
van den Bent[351]	Temozolamide	O, OA	28	25% (CR+PR)	8.0 (in responders)	29%/11%	NR

AA, anaplastic astrocytoma; AO, anaplastic oligodendroglioma; AOA, anaplastic oligoastrocytoma; MTP, median time to progression; MST, median survival time; CR, complete response; PFS, progression-free survival; PR, partial response; O, oligodendroglioma; OA, oligoastrocytoma.
*This study included AA and is included here for comparison. AOA and AO had better survival than AA.
†In this report, 38 patients with recurrent disease started induction chemotherapy with iPCV. However, only 20 patients made it to the high-dose thiotepa portion. Numbers are based on these 20 patients.
‡In this report, none of the patients had received any prior chemotherapy before being placed on temozolomide at relapse.

deletions. Patients with the 1p deletion only also may be candidates for initial therapy with either PCV or temozolomide. At recurrence patients with a favorable genetic profile who have previously been treated with PCV can be offered temozolomide. Progression through the chemotherapy regimen would dictate radiation therapy. Further larger trials should help to substantiate the safety and efficacy of chemotherapy as a sole modality for low-grade oligodendroglial tumors.

Patients with recurrent or progressive oligodendroglioma or oligoastrocytoma who carry neither of these deletions or who have p53 mutation and possibly 10q deletions should receive radiation therapy after maximal surgical resection.

Therapy of Elderly Patients with Malignant Gliomas

Elderly patients with malignant gliomas have a poorer outcome than younger patients (see Table 69-3). Brandes and associates evaluated the role of surgery, radiation therapy, and chemotherapy for the treatment of patients older than 65 years of age with newly diagnosed glioblastoma multiforme.[319] They found that the main predictive factor in evaluating this treatment was perioperative KPS. The higher the KPS, the better the patient fared, regardless the treatment. Patients were stratified into group A (surgery with radiation therapy to 59.4 Gy), group B (surgery, radiation therapy, and chemotherapy with procarbazine, lomustine, and vincristine [PCV]), and group C (surgery, radiation therapy, and temozolomide). The median time to disease progression was significantly better in group C patients. Overall survival was better in group C but did not reach statistical significance. Hematologic toxicity was higher in patients with a PCV regimen compared with temozolomide.

Another study evaluated the role of debulking craniotomy versus stereotactic biopsy in the treatment of patients over the age of 65 with malignant gliomas.[353] Patients in this study were randomized to either stereotactic biopsy or craniotomy for debulking of the tumor. Patients were evaluated with an intention to treat analysis. Median survival time was 171 days following craniotomy versus 85 days following biopsy. This difference was not statistically significant; however, it did suggest that patients undergoing a more aggressive craniotomy survived longer. Time to deterioration was 105 days in the craniotomy group and 72 days in the biopsy group. This increased time to deterioration corresponds to maintenance of quality of life during this period. Both groups of patients tolerated the radiation therapy well.

Based on these results, it appears that patients with malignant gliomas over the age of 65 may still benefit from aggressive therapy, if they have a reasonable performance status. Therefore, old age alone should not be a criteria for minimizing therapy.

Quality of Life Following Therapy for Gliomas

Quality of life (QOL) issues are paramount to treating patients with gliomas. Taphoorn and associates found that patients with low-grade gliomas complained of more drowsiness, fatigue, memory deficits, and concentration problems than control patients with hematologic malignancies. An analysis of QOL was performed on patients participating on an EORTC trial randomizing between 59.4 and 45 Gy for low-grade gliomas.[288] This analysis found that patients receiving the higher dose complained of more fatigue and insomnia immediately after radiotherapy and poorer emotional functioning 7 to 15 months after randomization.[354]

Data on QOL of patients with malignant gliomas are more limited than for those with low-grade tumors, probably because there are fewer survivors. Patients with malignant gliomas face the same burdens of dealing with a terminal disease as patients with breast cancer, lung cancer, and other malignancies, but they have unique perspectives in that they are uniformly concerned about the potential damage to their brain and cognitive function. These patients not only have to deal with concepts of dying and leaving behind their families and friends but also have a constant worry about being in a persistent vegetative state and being a burden to their family. Measurement of QOL is important for the understanding of the impacts of our treatments on the disease because the goal is to improve survival but not at the sacrifice of QOL issues.[355]

New Approaches to Therapy of Gliomas

The disappointing results of conventional cytotoxic chemotherapy have led to efforts to find more effective and better tolerated therapies. The challenge of neuro-oncology is to develop new compounds or procedures of gene transfer that specifically target the molecular alterations of glioma tumor cells and restore normal gene expression, cell cycle regulation, and apoptosis.[356] Significant progress is likely to come from some combination of cytotoxic chemotherapy with biologic agents directed at genetic alterations specific to brain tumors, such as growth factor receptors. Receptors are tempting targets because they are extracellular and easily accessible to drugs or antibodies.

As discussed in the section on genetics of glioblastomas, a major genetic alteration in GBM is overexpression of epidermal growth factor located on chromosome 7p13-p11.[218-220] Therefore the EGF receptor could be a good target in these tumors. To date the only example of such a strategy extensively evaluated in human gliomas is radioiodinated (^{125}I) monoclonal antibody 425, directed against the EGFR. Ten years of experience were recently summarized by Emrich and colleagues.[357] Median survival time and median survival time after recurrence were 51 months and 25 months in AA patients and 17 months and 9 months in GBM patients when the antibody was given intravenously or intrarterially. When given as adjuvant therapy in a phase II study of 180 patients, median survival times for GBM and AA were 13.4 and 50.9 months, respectively.

In a different EGFR-directed strategy of potential relevance to brain tumor therapy, the synthetic anilinoquinazoline molecule called *Iressa* targets EGFR by competition with ATP and both inhibits EGF-stimulated phosphorylation and downregulates VEGF, implying an additional antiangiogenic action.[358] Iressa is metabolized through cytochrome P-450 CYP3A4, and dose modifications likely will be necessary in upcoming trials in brain tumor patients on AEDs.

Many growth factor receptors possess tyrosine kinase activity, and a number of compounds that inhibit this activity have been identified. Combination therapy with irinotecan and the protein kinase C inhibitor tamoxifen has been reported to prolong survival in recurrent high-grade glioma in a phase I/II study.[359] Tamoxifen has also been combined in high dosage with carboplatin in a phase II study.[360]

Because gliomas produce specific angiogenic peptides such as VEGF (see molecular genetics section in this chapter) to stimulate new blood vessel formation, angiogenesis inhibitors are a logical drug development target. Hypoxic areas within gliomas may stimulate angiogenesis and promote invasiveness of glial cells.[361] Many of these changes in gene expression are mediated by hypoxia-inducible factor-1 (HIF-1). Further preclinical studies are necessary to assess the potential consequences of blocking HIF-1 target genes such as VEGF since these genes play regulatory roles in normal cellular differentiation and physiology.[362]

Additional targets for brain tumor therapy are matrix metalloproteinases (MMPs), a family of proteases that are secreted by inflammatory and tumor cells and digest the basement membrane and extracellular matrix, allowing infiltration of tumor cells into normal brain tissue and promoting the formation of new vessels. Marimastat, an MMP inhibitor, has been administered to recurrent GBM patients alone or in combination with temozolomide. Its major toxicity is diffuse muscle and joint pain.[363] In particular the EGFRvIII mutant, which lacks a part of the extracellular domain leading to constitutively activation,[221-223] is associated with increased MMP activity, consistent with an aggressive tumor with extensive brain invasion.[364,365] MMP inhibitors might be preferentially effective in this group.[365]

The transfer of genetic material to tumor cells to make them more susceptible to chemotherapy or to reverse the alterations that sustain the neoplastic phenotype has been studied in several centers. Gene therapy strategies include transfecting antioncogenes or drug-activating enzymes to glioma cells. The most extensively studied system is the "suicide gene therapy" with herpes simplex virus thymidine kinase (*HSV-tk*) gene inserted into a replication-defective murine retrovirus. Murine fibroblasts are engineered to produce these recombinant retroviruses and are injected into gliomas, infecting the proliferating tumor cells and making them produce thymidine kinase. The tumor cells then are susceptible to the antiherpes drug ganciclovir while nondividing brain cells are not infected. Clinical studies using this promising approach have been disappointing because of poor tumor cell transfection efficiency, although some long times to tumor progression have been reported.[366-368] A prospective controlled trial of patients with newly diagnosed GBM showed no improvement in survival or time to tumor progression when intraoperative HSV-tk therapy and standard radiation were compared to surgery and radiation alone.[369] Adenoviral and adeno-associated viral vector genes are being studied as well. A phase I study of stereotactic injection of an adenovirus vector to transfer wild-type p53 gene is among the early clinical trials now under way among those involving viral vectors to replace tumor suppressor genes.[370]

Other translational strategies that have moved to small preliminary human trials include glutamine depletion with phenylacetate and 13-cis-retinoic acid (CRA), a metabolite of beta-carotene that acts to promote differentiation.[371] Yung and colleagues administered CRA orally, but although toxicity was acceptable, the results were not better than temozolomide as a single agent.[372] Another strategy is based on the observation that cyclooxygenase-2 (COX-2), the inducible isoform of prostaglandin H synthase, is overexpressed in human gliomas. Investigators have tried to correlate the prognostic clinical relevance of such enzyme expression. Shono and colleagues analyzed immunohistochemistry of 66 tumor specimens and correlated the percentage of COX-2 expression with patient survival.[373] For gliomas, high COX-2 expression correlated with increasing histologic grade and poorer survival, independent of all other conventional variables. It did not correlate with positive p53 immunostaining or MIB-1 labeling index. These findings suggest that high COX-2 expression in tumor cells is associated with clinically more aggressive gliomas and poorer prognosis.[373] In another study, Prayson and colleagues studied the immunohistochemical profile of 47 GBM specimens and found that high COX-2 expresssion did correlate with MIB-1 (marker of cell proliferation) immunostaining.[374] As a group, tumors with a higher rate of cell proliferation tended to have increased expression of COX-2. These findings are potentially important as COX-2 inhibitors are currently available and may play a role in the management of high-grade glioma, offering a relatively easy and well-tolerated adjunct to cytotoxic therapies.

Despite effective neuroimaging and earlier diagnosis, advances in the understanding of cellular events that underlie progression of brain tumors, a steady stream of novel agents, and suggestive preclinical animal studies, clinical trials have proved disappointing. Because of the heterogeneity of malignant glial tumors, treatment strategies likely will require synergistic combinations of cytotoxic agents and noncytotoxic-specific molecular methods with the hope that genetic profiling eventually will help pinpoint appropriate choices for individual patients.

PRIMARY CENTRAL NERVOUS SYSTEM LYMPHOMA

Pathology

Primary central nervous system lymphoma (PCNSL) has been known previously by many other names, including reticulum cell sarcoma, diffuse histiocytic lymphoma, and microglioma. The cell of origin is the B lymphocyte

MANAGEMENT APPROACH

PRIMARY CENTRAL NERVOUS SYSTEM LYMPHOMA AT THE UNIVERSITY OF PENNSYLVANIA

1. Primary central nervous system lymphoma (PCNSL) is a non-Hodgkin's B-cell lymphoma arising in the brain, leptomeninges, spinal cord, or eyes. It should be considered a whole-brain disease and rarely spreads outside the nervous system.

2. Optimal treatment of PCNSL is not yet fully established, but experience with various combinations of radiation and chemotherapy suggests that initial induction treatment should be attempted with a methotrexate-based intravenous chemotherapy regimen and that concurrent intrathecal chemotherapy is not necessary. Median survival times of over 40 months have been reported with methotrexate monotherapy with significantly less cerebral white matter toxicity and its clinical correlate of cognitive decline than seen in earlier protocols that included cranial irradiation.

3. Methotrexate 8 g/m² given intravenously every 14 days for up to 8 cycles is induction therapy followed in complete response (CR) cases by 11 monthly cycles of the same dose of methotrexate. Leucovorin rescue is given and concurrent corticosteroids and antiepileptic drugs are prescribed as indicated.

4. Adequate delivery of chemotherapy to microscopically infiltrated areas of brain protected by the blood-brain barrier remains a significant problem and recurrence at multiple cerebral sites remains a problem for which effective therapy remains to be developed.

5. Retreatment of a prior complete responder at relapse with the preceding intensive methotrexate regimen is feasible. Alternatives include whole-brain radiation therapy, cytarabine, or investigational studies with temozolomide or rituximab.

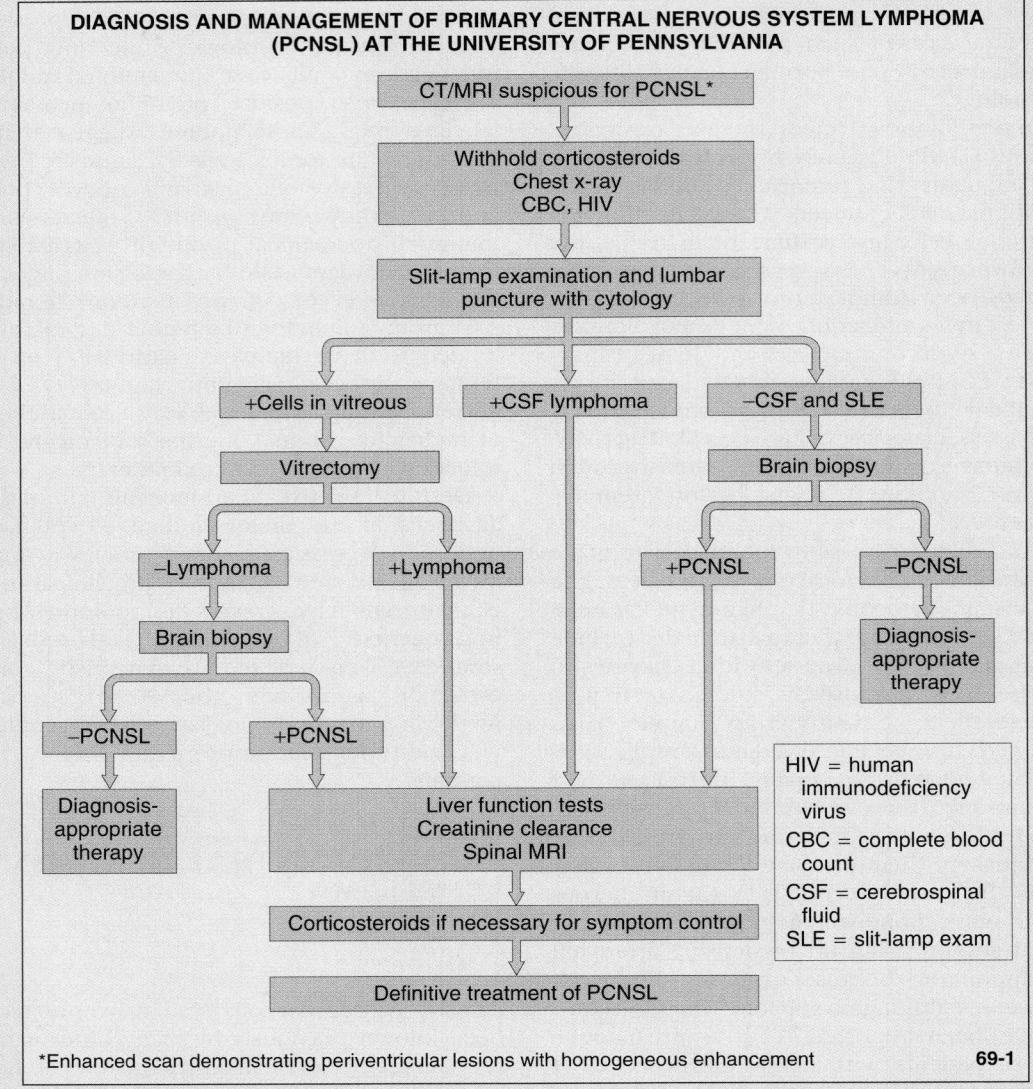

DIAGNOSIS AND MANAGEMENT OF PRIMARY CENTRAL NERVOUS SYSTEM LYMPHOMA (PCNSL) AT THE UNIVERSITY OF PENNSYLVANIA

CT/MRI suspicious for PCNSL*

Withhold corticosteroids
Chest x-ray
CBC, HIV

Slit-lamp examination and lumbar puncture with cytology

+Cells in vitreous → +CSF lymphoma → −CSF and SLE

Vitrectomy → Brain biopsy

−Lymphoma / +Lymphoma → +PCNSL / −PCNSL

Brain biopsy → Diagnosis-appropriate therapy

−PCNSL / +PCNSL

Diagnosis-appropriate therapy

Liver function tests
Creatinine clearance
Spinal MRI

Corticosteroids if necessary for symptom control

Definitive treatment of PCNSL

HIV = human immunodeficiency virus
CBC = complete blood count
CSF = cerebrospinal fluid
SLE = slit-lamp exam

*Enhanced scan demonstrating periventricular lesions with homogeneous enhancement

69-1

MANAGEMENT APPROACH—cont'd

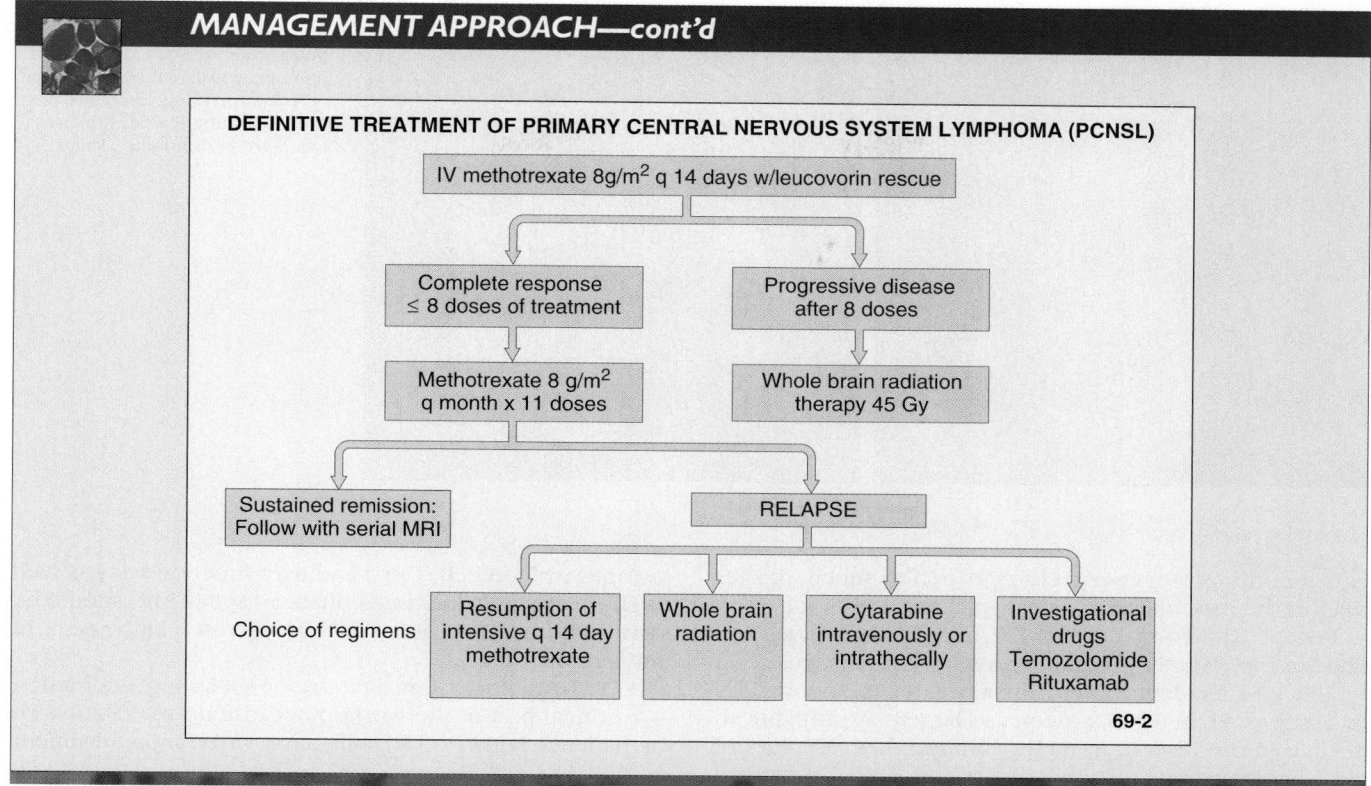

DEFINITIVE TREATMENT OF PRIMARY CENTRAL NERVOUS SYSTEM LYMPHOMA (PCNSL)

IV methotrexate 8g/m^2 q 14 days w/leucovorin rescue

Complete response ≤ 8 doses of treatment

Progressive disease after 8 doses

Methotrexate 8 g/m^2 q month x 11 doses

Whole brain radiation therapy 45 Gy

Sustained remission: Follow with serial MRI

RELAPSE

Choice of regimens

Resumption of intensive q 14 day methotrexate

Whole brain radiation

Cytarabine intravenously or intrathecally

Investigational drugs Temozolomide Rituxamab

69-2

and PCNSL is therefore a high-grade non-Hodgkin's B-cell neoplasm, usually diffuse large cell or large cell immuno-blastic type. Frequently, perivascular clusters of lympho-cytes and T-lymphocyte infiltrates are common in immunocompetent patients.[375] The Epstein-Barr virus genome has been found in HIV patients with PCNSL, but no consistent confirmation of viral etiology of PCNSL among immunocompetent patients has been made. Human herpesvirus 8 (Kaposi's sarcoma–associated herpesvirus) was reported in over 50% of both normal and immunocompromised patients with PCNS.[376] HTLV-1 and hepatitis C virus have not been associated with PCNSL.

Only 1% to 3% of PCNSLs are of T-cell origin. The incidence of T-cell PCNSL appears to be higher in Japan than in the United States.[377] Primary T-cell lymphoma has been diagnosed in both immunocompromised and immunocompetent patients. A younger age at diagnosis for T-cell lymphomas has been suggested, and it appears to present more frequently as an infratentorial lesion, with one third to one half of reported cases in the cerebellum or brainstem.[378] T-cell lymphoma may appear as a large cystic mass on MRI. The prognosis of T-cell PCNSL may be worse than that for comparably staged B-cell tumors. Authors of case reports available suggest that this tumor should be treated aggressively with regimens used for the more common B-cell lymphomas.[379]

Biology

PCNSL arises in the brain leptomeninges, spinal cord, or eyes and rarely spreads outside the central nervous

system. Its predilection for the periventricular white matter gives rise to the characteristic neuroimaging appearance of a hyperdense mass on unenhanced com-puted tomography or hypointense appearance on T2-weighted MRI. Three quarters of immunocompetent patients have a solitary enhancing mass lesion at presen-tation. Following contrast medium administration, most bulky masses of PCNSL enhance, most often homogen-eously but occasionally in a ring-like pattern (Fig. 69-16). PCNSLs, however, appear to be diffusely infiltrative at the time of presentation. These areas of disease are not visible on neuroimaging studies because they are behind a relatively intact blood-brain barrier. Postmortem correlates with MRI obtained shortly before death show that there are widespread areas of microscopic infiltration in areas that appear normal on MRI.[380] Therefore, PCNSL can be classified as stage 1E disease and should be considered for treatment purposes a *whole brain disease*.

Until the 1980s PCNSL was considered a rare tumor, accounting for about 2% of CNS malignancies in immuno-competent patients and 1% to 2% of all lymphomas.[381] However, the demographics of the disease have changed both among immunocompetent patients and among those with HIV and organ transplant recipients. The incidence of PCNSL among immunocompetent individuals has increased 25-fold to 51 cases per 10 million by 2000. Among immunocompetent patients with PCNSL, median age of diagnosis is 55 years and males outnumber females by 2:1. Among AIDS patients the median age is 35 years and 95% of HIV patients with PCNSL are male.[382] Among organ transplant recipients the peak incidence of PCNSL

Specific Malignancies

III

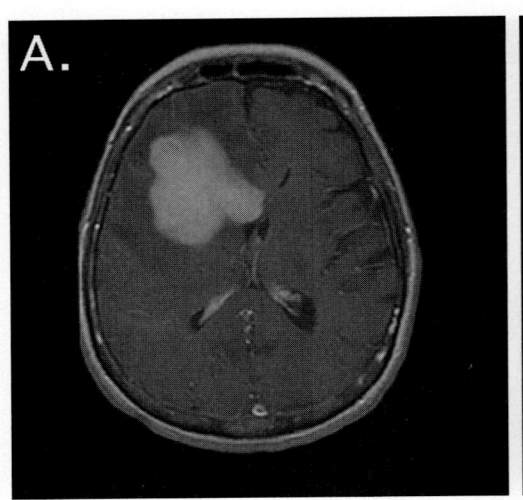
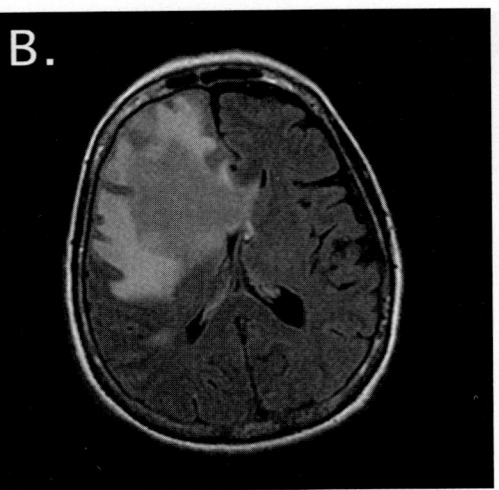

Figure 69-16. CNS lymphoma. **A,** Axial T1-weighted postgadolinium MRI shows homogeneously enhancing frontal mass compressing ventricles. **B,** Corresponding FLAIR MRI shows extensive peritumoral edema.

is 6 months post-transplantation, a period much shorter than in the precyclosporine transplant era.

Recent data from the Surveillance, Epidemiology, and End Results (SEER) program show an overall decline in total PCNSL incidence rates from a peak of 102 per million in 1995 to 51 in 1998, a decrease largely attributable to decline in the disease in males younger than 59 years of age. The annual rate among patients over 60 has remained unchanged since 1994.[383] The decline in the younger male population with PCNSL reflects the advent of effective antiretroviral therapy and a declining incidence of PCNSL in the HIV-infected population.[384] This chapter will discuss PCNSL and its treatment in the immunocompetent population. See Chapter 98 for discussion of PCNSL in HIV and organ transplant recipients.

Clinical Diagnosis and Staging

The most common clinical presentation consists of progressive focal symptoms. Seizures may occur. Less commonly, progressive cognitive decline without focal symptoms leads to the diagnosis. The several variant clinical presentations in the immunocompetent population include primary ocular, meningeal, relapsing-remitting disease; intravascular malignant lymphomatosis with stroke-like onset; and neurolymphomatosis with both peripheral and CNS involvement. The differential diagnosis of PCNSL includes high-grade glial tumor, CNS metastases, neurosarcoidosis, and tumefactive multiple sclerosis. Spinal cord PCNSL is very rare. Ocular lymphoma may be the first manifestation of the disease or its relapse. Patients with ocular lymphoma have a 50% to 80% chance of developing cerebral lymphoma.

Initial evaluation of patients with suspected PCNSL should include a thorough physical examination to exclude possible extraneural sources of lymphoma. Neurologic evaluation is directed at clarification of the extent of CNS disease. Extraneural sites are uncommon in patients without prior known lymphoma, and extensive abdominal and pelvic studies are not usually warranted. Chest x-ray should be performed and blood tests should include

complete blood cell (CBC) and liver function tests as well as HIV testing. Gadolinium-enhanced spinal MRI should be performed because bulky nodular disease can be seen in the leptomeninges.

Ophthalmologic consultation for slit-lamp examination is a critical part of the workup because up to 10% or 15% of patients with PCNSL will have vitreous involvement at the time of diagnosis and half of these patients will have no visual symptoms. Lumbar puncture should be performed if not contraindicated because of the intracranial mass location(s). Glucose, protein, blood cell count, and flow cytometry should be obtained. Recent reports of molecular diagnosis of PCNSL by the demonstration of monoclonality by amplification of the rearranged IgH genes by polymerase chain reaction (PCR) to the CDR-III region raises the possibility of definitive diagnosis, even with few cells present in the cerebrospinal fluid (CSF).[385] However, in several cases the PCR was negative even when conventional cytologic appearance was suspicious for malignancy. In another study, monoclonal patterns in the CSF were found in 77% of biopsy-proven cases with no false positives among control subjects.[386] At present, however, it is premature to make therapeutic decisions based on these promising early clinical findings.

When the preceding procedures fail to confirm the diagnosis, the surgical procedure of choice is a stereotactic brain biopsy. Aggressive surgical resection does not improve survival and may cause deterioration due to the deep location of many PCNSLs. It is most important to try to *withhold corticosteroids* from patients during initial evaluation and surgical confirmation. Corticosteroids repair the blood-brain barrier and also have a direct cytolytic effect on B-cell lymphomas. Although the patient's clinical symptoms may improve with early institution of corticosteroids, with frequent nearly complete resolution of MRI-enhancing abnormalities, diagnosis will be compromised, and corticosteroids will have to be withdrawn in order to proceed with definitive biopsy confirmation. Some interest has centered on immunohistochemical definition of morphologic markers of prognostic significance on the biopsy material (Fig. 69-17). Braaten and

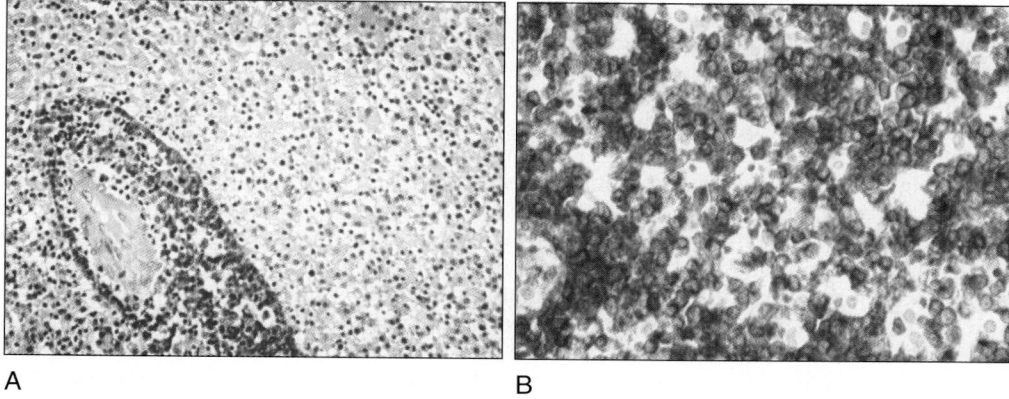

Figure 69-17. CNS lymphoma: histology. **A,** High-grade B cell lymphoma with dense perivascular lymphocytic cuffing (H&E stain). **B,** CD20 staining. Dense staining for CD20 (a B-cell marker) in same specimen.

A

B

colleagues studied the expression of BCL-6 antigen in PCNSL and found that the presence of this antigen predicted a median survival of 101 months compared to 14.7 months in patients without this marker.[387] Other groups, however, have found that the marker correlates with a negative prognosis, and thus, clinical decisions cannot be made on the basis of these early immunohistochemistry studies.[388]

Treatment

PCNSL is an aggressive disease for which the median survival time in untreated immunocompetent patients is only 3 months. Increasing age and poor performance status are important negative prognostic variables. The goal of treatment is to eradicate both contrast-enhancing mass lesions and microscopic infiltration of brain, spine, leptomeninges, and vitreous. Treatment must be designed to maximize efficacy but also to minimize toxicity to the brain. Optimal treatment has not been established. The reason for the lack of standardized treatment protocols is the relatively low number of patients and the absence of a phase III randomized trial.[389] However, in the past 10 years steady increases in median survival times have been achieved in patients with PCSNL. Five-year survival rates on the order of 40% are now being reported by many groups with median survival times of 3 to 4 years.[390-392]

Radiation treatment alone led to median survival times of 18 months in early clinical trials with only 3% to 4% 5-year survival rates.[393,394] Chemotherapy was first used as an adjunct to radiation therapy more than 20 years ago after methotrexate was found to be effective in the treatment of systemic lymphoma. Twelve studies totaling more than 450 patients have established the efficacy of multiple chemotherapeutic regimens. Initially, most were used along with or following a course of whole-brain radiation. The most commonly used drugs have been methotrexate, cytarabine, and cyclophosphamide. The first two agents have been used intravenously and intrathecally. Extension of median survivals for up to 4 years with combined regimens was achieved in the mid-1990s. The most frequently used combined regimen involved administration of intravenous methotrexate at doses ranging from 3.5 g/m^2 to 8 g/m^2 every 10 to 14 days for three cycles followed by whole-brain radiation therapy to 40 to 50 Gy with subsequent administration of cytarabine 3 g/m^2 for three cycles. DeAngelis and colleagues reported 58% complete response rates with additional 36% partial responses and progression-free median survival of 24 months.[395] A worse prognosis was associated with age greater than 60 years (50.4 months versus 21.8 months). With improved survival, however, increasing numbers of patients developed severe delayed neural toxicity. At 18 months 15% to 50% of patients treated with combined radiation and chemotherapy had extensive white matter abnormalities with severe cognitive decline.[396-398] Age and preexisting white matter disease due to hypertension may be relative risk factors.[394,399] This complication typically begins from 4 months to several years after treatment.[396]

Recognition of the serious sequelae of combined radiation and chemotherapy led to attempts to provide chemotherapy as the sole modality to newly diagnosed PCNSL patients. Initial response rates to chemotherapy vary from 50% to 100% with duration of response between 12 and 44 months. Typical of the successes of many clinical trials are the results of Cher and colleagues who reported complete responses in 17 of 19 patients receiving methotrexate alone with an event-free median survival time of 32 months and overall survival period of 53 months.[400] Therapeutic levels of methotrexate can be achieved in the CSF following intravenous drug administration, making it possible to achieve clearance of malignant cells from the CSF without intrathecal administration.[401]

Attempts to improve on the results of methotrexate have included a variety of other multidrug chemotherapy regimens. Standard regimens effective in the treatment of comparable systemic non-Hodgkin's lymphomas (CHOP, CHOD, or MACOP-B) are not effective for PCNSL.[402-405] Attempts to disrupt the blood-brain barrier with hyperosmolar intra-arterial mannitol do not provide additional survival benefit beyond intravenous methotrexate-based regimens.[406]

Many neuro-oncologists therefore have concluded that high-dose methotrexate should be offered to all patients as the first-line agent for PCNSL.[407] However, there are dissenting opinions. Herrlinger and colleagues reported only a 29.7% complete response rate with intravenous methotrexate while 37.8% of their patients progressed, and they revisit the question of whole-brain radiation therapy as a first-line treatment for PCNSL.[408] However, most centers have based their therapy on methotrexate regimens. Long-term follow-up of patients who achieved durable remissions for more than 1 year suggests that chemotherapy alone is associated with a low risk of neurotoxicty even in the elderly, although MRIs may show significant areas of clinically asymptomatic leukoencephalopathy.[409-411]

The following recommendations apply to immunocompetent patients only. The goal of treatment is to achieve a complete response and to avoid cranial irradiation. Patients with AIDS-related PCNSL must have individualized treatment based on their immune status and concurrent infections.[412] Transplant recipients similarly must have an initial attempt at reduction of immunosuppression, and their treatment also must be tailored to the extent of organ dysfunction due to the primary disease process and concurrent therapy.

No firmly established dose for methotrexate has been confirmed; doses in excess of 3.5 g/m^2 have been shown to achieve satisfactory CSF levels. PCNSL patients receive methotrexate 8 g/m^2 every 14 days for up to 8 cycles. The calculated dose is diluted in 500 mL D$_5$W and given intravenously over a 4-hour period. Patients with a complete response will receive two additional doses of methotrexate at 14-day intervals followed by 11 monthly doses of methotrexate 8 g/m^2 as long as a complete response is maintained. Monthly MRI scans are obtained during induction therapy and continued at 3-month intervals during maintenance therapy. The methotrexate protocol involves close clinical monitoring, adjustment of intravenous fluid, and calcium leucovorin rescue in addition to the frequent monitoring of urine pH, renal function, and methotrexate levels.

Contraindications to methotrexate therapy include allergy to methotrexate, inability to achieve adequate hydration because of cerebral edema, cardiac, or pulmonary problems and concurrent immunosuppressive treatment. Patients should not have received prior cranial irradiation. Patients with renal dysfunction resulting in a creatinine clearance of less than 50 mL/minute or serum creatinine levels greater than 2 mg/dL should not receive methotrexate. Patients with significant ascites or pleural effusions may experience delayed methotrexate clearance because of third space accumulation.

Calcium leucovorin "rescue" should begin 24 hours after the *start* of methotrexate infusion. The dose is adjusted based on methotrexate levels. Any dose of leucovorin greater than 50 mg should be given intravenously. If the level of methotrexate at 24 hours is greater than 10^{-5} M, 100 mg/m^2 is given intravenously every 6 hours until rescue is achieved and continued at 25 mg intravenously or orally every 6 hours until the methotrexate plasma concentration is less than 10^{-7}. Most patients clear to this level by 72 hours after the infusion.

Patients with an established PCNSL diagnosis may receive concurrent corticosteroid therapy to alleviate symptoms. Patients receiving methotrexate therapy should not receive concurrent salicylates, or nonsteroidal anti-inflammatory drugs or sulfonamide medications for at least 1 week prior to the initiation of methotrexate

therapy. Many patients with PCNSL will remain on corticosteroids for extended periods of time. The combination of corticosteroids and methotrexate may lead to a low CD4 count, and these patients will be at risk for *Pneumocystis carinii* pneumonia. Like other brain tumor patients, patients with PCNSL should receive prophylaxis with trimethoprim/sulfamethoxazole two to three times per week, this drug being discontinued 1 week prior to methotrexate therapy.[413] Concurrent antiepileptic drug therapy is acceptable and management of nausea associated with chemotherapy does not differ in this population from other patients receiving comparable regimens.

The management of progressive or recurrent PCNSL is not yet well established. Age and performance status of the patient must be taken into account. In general, greater than 25% enlargement of previous areas of gadolinium contrast enhancement, the appearance of new lesions, or the appearance of malignant cells in the CSF, vitreous, or, rarely, elsewhere in the body constitutes treatment failure. Cher and colleagues have reported that for patients who have completed their maintenance therapy, return to a more intensive methotrexate dosage regimen may lead to a second complete response.[400] For patients who have progressed through therapy, other chemotherapeutic agents such as cytarabine intravenously or intrathecally may be considered. At relapse or in the case of failure to achieve complete response after 8 cycles of methotrexate, many treating physicians would consider palliative radiation therapy. The immediate palliation of progressive symptoms is a realistic goal but must be weighed against the possibility that survival will be extended enough to allow emergence of late cognitive neurotoxicity. Most centers treat whole brain to 40 to 45 Gy in 20 doses over 4 to 5 weeks.

After initial diagnosis, surgical intervention usually has little role. However, the need for intrathecal chemotherapy may mandate placement of an Ommaya reservoir. Development of communicating hydocephalus with or after treatment of meningeal lymphoma may require shunting.

Parenchymal treatment failure is the most common pattern of relapse. Ocular, meningeal, and late rare extra-CNS relapses (breast, abdominal wall, bone, lymph nodes) have been described and may be seen with increasing frequency as patients survive longer. Temozolomide is under investigation as a treatment for progressive PCNSL. Rituximab, a monoclonal antibody against the B-cell–specific CD 20 antigen, has been demonstrated to be effective against various non-Hodgkin's lymphomas, but CSF levels following intravenous therapy are not high.[414] Attempts to circumvent this problem have involved intraventricular administration through an Ommaya reservoir with some early reports indicating total clearing of cells in leptomeningeal lymphoma.[415] Whether rituximab will clear parenchymal masses is not clear. Intensive chemotherapy followed by hematopoietic stem cell rescue using a regimen of cytarabine and etoposide has been reported to give a complete response rate of 70% with median progression-free survival of 3 years.[416] However, several of these patients had intraocular lymphoma only. The question of using a more intensive chemo-

MANAGEMENT APPROACH

MENINGIOMAS

- Extra-axial tumors arise from dura; common locations are cerebral convexity, parasagittal falx, sphenoid ridge.
- Tumors have a long natural history, mandating long follow-up.
- Over 90% are benign; remainder have atypical histologic features or frankly invade brain parenchyma.
- Primary treatment is surgical, if feasible.
- Radiation therapy is reserved for tumors that are incompletely resected, recur after surgery, are

- inaccessible to surgical resection, or have atypical/invasive features.
- Standard dose has been approximately 54 Gy for benign meningiomas; up to 60 Gy for those with atypical/invasive features.
- Stereotactic radiation therapy techniques have been used; however, follow-up is still short in these studies.
- Anecdotal reports exist of responses to medical therapy (hydroxyurea, antiestrogen, and antiprogesterone agents).

therapy protocol earlier in the course of the disease has led to an ongoing prospective multicenter trial.

MENINGIOMA

Clinical and Pathologic Considerations

Meningiomas comprise approximately 20% to 25% of all intracranial tumors (see Table 69-1). The male-to-female ratio is 1:2 with the incidence increasing with age, reaching a peak in the seventh decade.[417] They arise from arachnoidal cells in the meninges, not the brain parenchyma; therefore, they are extra-axial. They produce signs and symptoms by compressing normal tissues. The locations of meningiomas in two large series are shown in Table 69-13.[417,418] The specific signs and symptoms depend on the anatomic location of the meningioma. For example, meningiomas arising from the cerebral

convexity can cause altered mentation and seizures, whereas those arising from the suprasellar region are likely to cause loss of vision, bitemporal hemianopia, and optic atrophy.

Numerous potential etiologic agents for meningiomas have been investigated, including radiation, trauma, viruses, occupational exposure, diet, and exposure to sex hormones.[419] However, only ionizing radiation has been strongly implicated in the pathogenesis of these tumors, for example, following scalp irradiation for tinea capitis as discussed previously in the section on epidemiology.[9] This tumor appears to have some relationship with breast cancer because the likelihood of developing a meningioma after developing a breast cancer or breast cancer after meningioma is higher than in the general population.[420]

Meningiomas frequently contain deletions of chromosome 22. One study found complete loss of one copy of the chromosome in 52% of tumors and partial deletion of 22q in another 11% of meningiomas.[421] The target of this chromosomal deletion is likely the *NF2* gene, which is mutated in patients with neurofibromatosis 2. One of the tumor types commonly seen in these patients is meningioma.[31] The *NF2* gene also appears to have an important role in the pathogenesis of sporadic meningiomas. One study found *NF2* mutations in 60% of sporadic meningiomas, all of which had lost one copy of chromosome 22.[422] However, 40% of meningiomas have neither allelic loss of chromosome 22 nor *NF2* gene mutation; therefore, a second tumor suppressor gene is likely linked to the development of meningiomas.

Grossly, meningiomas appear as rounded masses, well circumscribed in contour, with a well-defined dural base that can be easily separated from the underlying brain tissue (Fig. 69-18). Often these tumors extend into the adjacent bone. Histologically the different subtypes of benign meningiomas include syncytial, fibroblastic (fibrous), transitional (mixed), psammomatous, microcystic, and papillary; however, these distinctions carry little prognostic significance.[192] Of more importance prognostically is whether the meningioma is benign, which is the case 90% of the time.[417] Features of atypical meningiomas are focal isolated necrosis, prominence of nucleoli, and mitotic figures with high cell density.[192] Malignant meningiomas are characterized by invasion into adjacent

TABLE 69-13

Anatomic Location of Meningiomas

TUMOR LOCATION	FREQUENCY (%)*	FREQUENCY (%)†
Convexity	34	21
Parasagittal	22	17
Sphenoid ridge	17	16
Lateral ventricle	5	—
Tentorium	4	—
Cerebellar convexity/ posterior fossa	5	14
Parasellar	3	12
Intraorbital	2	2
Cerebellopontine angle	2	—
Olfactory groove	3	10
Foramen magnum	1	—
Clivus	1	—
Spine	—	8
Other	1	—

*Out of 179 cases reported in Rohringer and associates[417]; this series included only cases of intracranial meningiomas, none of the spine.
†Out of 225 cases reported in Mirimanoff and associates.[418]

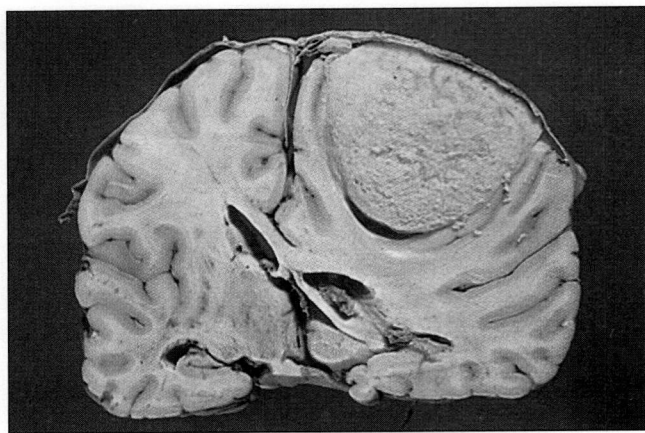

Figure 69-18. Meningioma: gross specimen. A large convexity meningioma severely displaces the underlying tissue downward and laterally, creating a midline shift and marked ventricular compression. (From Maher EA, McKee AC: Neoplasms of the central nervous system In Skarin AT [ed]: Dana-Farber Cancer Institute Atlas of Diagnostic Oncology, 3rd ed. St. Louis, Mosby, 2003, p 420.)

normal brain tissue. In one large study based on data from the National Cancer Data Base (NCDB), the overall 5-year survival rates in patients with benign, atypical, and malignant meningiomas were 70%, 75%, and 55%, respectively.[423]

Meningiomas have a distinctive appearance radiologically. On MRI scans, most meningiomas are isointense with gray matter on T1-weighted scans and enhance intensely with gadolinium (Fig. 69-19).[424] About 60% of meningiomas have peritumoral edema and 20% have associated bony changes, either destruction or hyperostosis.

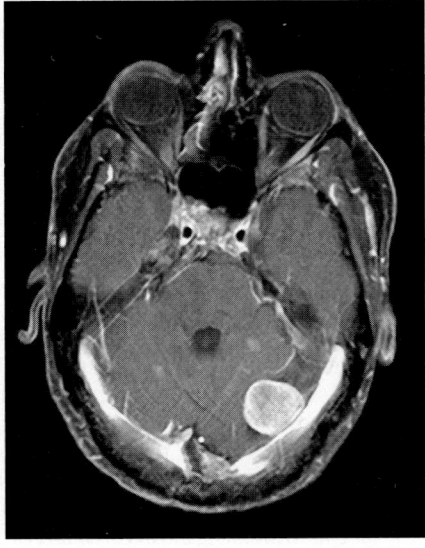

Figure 69-19. Meningioma. Axial T1-weighted postgadolinium MRI shows extra-axial enhancing mass that compresses the underlying brain tissue.

The bony changes are better visualized with CT scans than MRI scans.[424] Calcifications, central necrosis, or pseudocysts may be seen within the tumor.

Surgery and Conventional Radiation Therapy for Meningiomas

In a classic paper describing the outcome in 225 patients with meningiomas treated with surgery as the sole modality at Massachusetts General Hospital (MGH), Mirimanoff and associates found progression-free survival (PFS) rates of 93%, 80%, and 68% at 5, 10, and 15 years, respectively, for those who underwent a total resection versus 63%, 45%, and 9% for those who underwent a subtotal resection ($P < .0001$).[418] In general, sites associated with higher resectability rates had lower rates of progression. For example, meningiomas in the convexity, 96% of which underwent total resection, had a 5-year recurrence/progression rate of 3% versus 34% for lesions in the sphenoid ridge, which had only a 28% rate of total resection. These results suggested that surgery alone was inadequate therapy for meningiomas if total resection could not be achieved. In a subsequent study from MGH, Miralbell and associates reported on 17 patients who underwent subtotal resection of a meningioma followed by radiation therapy.[425] Their 8-year PFS was 88%, which was much better than the 48% rate calculated for the cohort of patients with subtotal resections who did not receive postoperative radiation.

Other retrospective studies from the University of Florida and UCSF have reached similar conclusions regarding the improvement in local control with postoperative radiation therapy in patients who have undergone a subtotal resection.[426-429] These series include mostly patients with benign meningiomas. Studies that have compared outcomes of patients with benign versus malignant meningiomas have found that the latter have a much worse outcome than the former.[429,430] For example, the UCSF series also found a much poorer outcome for patients with malignant versus benign meningiomas (5-year PFS rate of 89% versus 48%; $P = .001$).[429]

The foregoing studies have all used conventional fractionated radiation therapy, usually to doses ranging from 50 to 60 Gy of radiation via conventional fractionation and delivery techniques. Currently, most investigators would recommend approximately 54 Gy for benign meningiomas following incomplete resection and up to 60 Gy for meningiomas that have atypical or malignant features.

Stereotactic Radiation Techniques for Meningiomas

There is substantial experience in using stereotactic radiation techniques in the treatment of meningiomas. One of the centers that has extensive experience with this technique is the University of Pittsburgh. In their long-term follow-up of 99 patients with meningiomas treated with gamma-knife stereotactic radiosurgery (SRS) from 1987 to 1992 with 9 to 25 Gy (median marginal dose 16 Gy), the total rate of failure was 11% at 63 to 120 months following SRS.[431] The majority of meningiomas showed a decrease in size by MRI with time. At years 4 to 6, 69% of cases showed a decrease in size by MRI scan; by years 8 to 10 this number had increased to 88%. The Mayo Clinic and the Brigham and Women's Hospital have also reported rates of local control on the order of 89% in benign meningiomas using gamma-knife and linear accelerator–based SRS.[432,433] However, the follow-up period remains short, with the median ranging from 31 to 40 months. Furthermore, in both these series, patients with atypical or malignant features did poorly. In the Mayo Clinc series the 5-year local control rates were 93%, 68%, and 0% for benign, atypical, and malignant meningiomas, respectively ($P < .0001$). In spite of the goal to deliver an extremely conformal dose, SRS can still cause significant complications. Rates of complication, often involving cranial nerves, have been reported in the 5% to 13% range.[431-433]

A large experience supports using SRS for treating cavernous sinus meningiomas. Owing to their location, surgical resection can cause significant complications, particularly cranial nerve morbidity and resulting extra-ocular muscle paralysis.[434] A number of institutions have reported high local control rates in the 91% to 98% range using marginal doses that typically range from 12 to 18 Gy, but with very short follow-up (median 2 to 3 years).[435-437] Furthermore, cranial nerve V appears to be sensitive to single high-dose fractions because the incidence of trigeminal nerve dysfunction has ranged from 45% to 11% in these series.

In an effort to decrease late effects, fractionated stereotactic radiotherapy (FSRT) has also been used to treat meningiomas. At the University of Heidelberg they have used 56.8 Gy in 1.8-Gy daily fractions with a relocatable headframe for large base of skull meningiomas.[438] With a median follow-up period of 35 months, the 5-year progression-free survival rate was 94% for 180 patients with benign meningiomas but 78% for those with atypical features. Another instance when FSRS has been used instead of SRS is for optic nerve sheath meningiomas because of the potential risk of optic nerve injury with a single large dose of radiation. One group reported using FSRT with 50 to 54 Gy in 1.8-Gy fractions to treat these tumors.[439] Of 22 optic nerves that were treated, 42% showed improvement.

In summary, there are numerous reports using stereotactic techniques for delivering radiation to meningiomas as an alternative to surgery or following subtotal resection. However, considering the long natural history of these tumors, much longer follow-up will be needed to adequately evaluate these results. Furthermore, there are concerns regarding cranial neuropathies associated with single large fractions of radiation, especially to the cavernous sinus and optic nerve.

Medical Therapy for Meningiomas

The medical management of meningiomas has no proven role. On the basis of a report of dramatic shrinkage of tumors in three patients treated with hydroxyurea,[440] this drug has been used by other investigators in patients with recurrent or unresectable meningiomas who had already received or refused radiation. However, subsequent reports have not shown a dramatic reduction in the size of the meningiomas, although some patients treated with hydroxyurea appear to show a halt in the growth of the tumors or improvement in symptoms.[441,442]

Objective responses have been reported in patients treated with antiestrogen or antiprogesterone agents such as mifepristone (RU-486) or mepitiostane.[443,444] A large, multicenter phase IIII trial (SWOG 9005) was set up to test the efficacy of RU-486 in treating patients with meningiomas, but the results from this study have not been reported. Tamoxifen has also been reported to have modest activity against meningiomas.[445]

PITUITARY ADENOMA

Clinical and Pathologic Considerations

Pituitary adenomas account for 10% to 15% of all intracranial tumors. They arise from the anterior lobe of the pituitary gland. The pituitary gland and stalk are normally

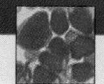

MANAGEMENT APPROACH

PITUITARY ADENOMAS

- Pituitary adenomas are extremely common as incidental findings (up to 10% of normal volunteers by MRI screening).
- Symptomatic adenomas come to medical attention as a result of hormone secretion, compression of nearby structures causing neurologic symptoms, or compression of pituitary stalk causing hypopituitarism.
- Classified by size as microadenomas (≤1 cm) or macroadenomas.
- Initial therapy for most prolactinomas is with dopamine agonist (e.g., bromocriptine, lisuride, pergolide), which usually decreases prolactin levels and shrinks tumor.

- Initial therapy for most other pituitary adenomas is transsphenoidal surgical resection, which is safe and rapidly reverses neurologic symptoms. Surgery normalizes hormone levels in most patients with microadenomas.
- Radiation therapy is currently reserved for residual disease or recurrence after surgery, or for patients who are medically inoperable. In patients with elevated hormones, normalization of levels after radiation may take years. A dose of 45 Gy in 180-cGy daily fractions should offer good control with extremely low risk of optic neuropathy.

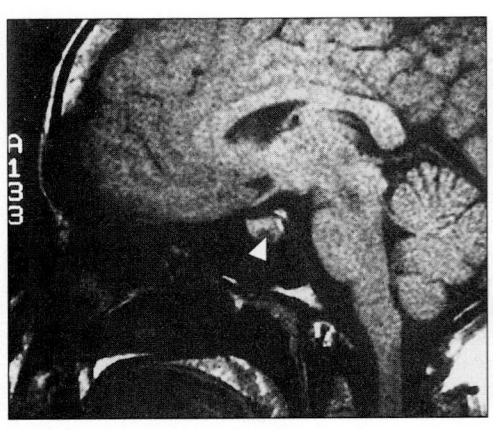

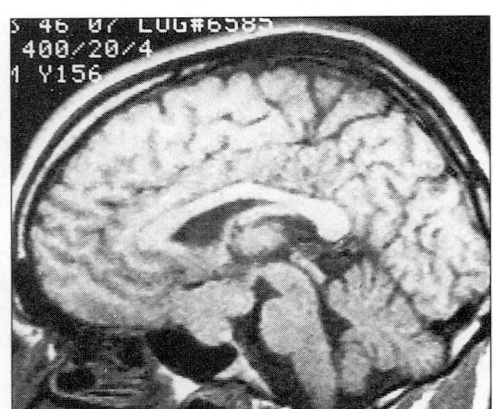

A   B

Figure 69-20. Pituitary adenomas. **A,** T1-weighted midline sagittal MRI demonstrates a local hypointensity within the pituitary gland, representing a microadenoma (*arrow*). **B,** Similar scan in another patient shows a large intrasellar mass (macroadenoma) with suprasellar extension. (From Moore FD, Socinski MA, Joste NE: Endocrine tumors and malignancies. In Skarin AT [ed]: Dana-Farber Cancer Institute Atlas of Diagnostic Oncology, 3rd ed. St. Louis, Mosby, 2003, p 306.)

isointense with brain on T1-weighted MRI scans. However, the gland and stalk intensely enhance following contrast medium administration because of the absence of a blood-brain barrier. Pituitary adenomas are generally seen as hypointense foci on T1-weighted MRI images and do not enhance with gadolinium (Fig. 69-20).[446] Other abnormalities that can appear as a hypointense, nonenhancing lesion in the pituitary include pars intermedia cysts, metastases, infarctions, epidermoid cysts, and abscesses.

Asymptomatic pituitary adenomas were found in 1.5% to 27% of autopsy cases and in 10% of normal adult volunteers by MRI scanning.[446] However, symptomatic pituitary adenomas are much less common. They can give rise to symptoms by secretion of hormones or by compression of nearby structures, causing neurologic disturbances such as headaches, bilateral bitemporal hemianopia from compression of the optic chiasm, and cranial nerve palsies from invasion into the cavernous sinus. Adenomas can also cause hypopituitarism from compression of the pituitary stalk.

Many investigators have studied the genetics of pituitary adenomas. Patients with MEN-1 (multiple endocrine neoplasia type 1) are predisposed to developing pituitary adenomas as well as parathyroid and pancreatic islet tumors.[447] Anterior pituitary tumors occur in 30% of patients with MEN-1, most commonly prolactinomas but also nonfunctional and growth hormone (GH) and ACTH-secreting tumors. These patients have a germline mutation in the *MEN-1* gene, and if they develop a pituitary tumor, there is deletion in the remaining wild-type allele in the tumor.[448] *MEN-1* mutations are not commonly found in sporadic pituitary adenomas[449]; however, one gene that is mutated in a substantial proportion of pituitary adenomas is that encoding the α-subunit of the GTP-binding protein G_s. Mutation of this gene leads to constitutive activation of the cyclic AMP (cAMP) pathway. The mutated form of this gene is called *gsp* and is found in 40% of GH-secreting adenomas, 10% of nonfunctioning adenomas, and 6% of ACTH-secreting adenomas.[449]

At one time pituitary adenomas were classified according to their staining characteristics (basophilic, eosinophilic, chromophobe). However, they are now classified according to secretion of hormones. In one series of 684 patients with pituitary adenomas who underwent surgery, prolactinomas were the most common (43%) followed by nonsecreting tumors (30%) (Table 69-14).[450] TSH-secreting tumors were rare in this series (2/684) as they are in others.

TABLE 69-14

Pituitary Adenomas and Clinical Presentation by Endocrine Secretion			
TYPE OF SECRETION	**FREQUENCY (%)***	**SYMPTOMS**	**TYPICAL SIZE AT DIAGNOSIS**
Prolactinoma	43	Women: amenorrhea, galactorrhea Men: impotence, hypopituitarism	Females: micoadenoma Males: macroadenoma
Nonsecreting Gonadotropin	30	Hypopituitarism	Macroadenoma
Growth hormone (GH)	17	Gigantism in children	Macroadenoma Acromegaly in adults
Adrenocorticotropic hormone (ACTH)	7	Cushing's disease Nelson's disease	Microadenoma
Thyroid-stimulating hormone (TSH)	<1	Hyperthyroidism	Can be microadenoma; often macroadenoma due to delayed diagnosis

*Frequency in 684 cases reported in Oruckaptan and associates.[450]

Adenomas are also classified on the basis of size as macroadenomas (>1 cm in diameter) or microadenomas. Nonsecreting adenomas are generally macroadenomas at the time of diagnosis because they usually come to medical attention fairly late when they are causing neurologic symptoms due to mass effect. The same is true for gonadotropin-secreting adenomas, which are inefficient producers and secretors of hormones. Growth-hormone secreting adenomas and prolactinomas in men are often macroadenomas at the time of diagnosis, probably because their clinical effects occur gradually and are often ignored early in their course. Because the same pituitary stem cell can produce both growth hormone and prolactin, many patients have adenomas that secrete both hormones. Prolactinomas in women and ACTH-secreting adenomas are usually microadenomas at diagnosis. Prolactinomas in women commonly cause amenorrhea and galactorrhea. ACTH-secreting adenomas often cause dramatic clinical signs and symptoms associated with hypercortisolism that rapidly bring patients to medical attention. ACTH-secreting pituitary adenomas can also be seen in approximately 25% of patients who have undergone bilateral adrenalectomies for Cushing's syndrome secondary to loss of negative feedback control by cortisol on the hypothalamus. The majority of these patients also develop hyperpigmentation due to ACTH hypersecretion. This condition is termed *Nelson's syndrome*, and in this setting the pituitary tumors are usually very large and often difficult to completely resect.[451]

Surgery for Pituitary Adenomas

The current therapy for most pituitary adenomas, excluding prolactinomas, involves surgery. For nonsecreting tumors, which tend to be large and present with neurologic symptoms, surgery offers rapid decompression of the visual pathways. For hormonally active tumors, surgery leads to a rapid drop in hormone secretion. The current preferred technique is the transsphenoidal approach, which was popularized by Harvey Cushing in the early 1900s. It then fell out of favor but regained popularity in the 1960s.[452] Transsphenoidal resection is fairly safe with a mortality rate less than 1%.[453] The most common complications arising from this surgery are nasal septum perforation, anterior pituitary insufficiency, postoperative diabetes insipidus, which is usually transient, and CSF leak, sometimes leading to meningitis.[453] Much rarer complications include carotid artery injury and loss of vision. A recent variation of this approach has been to use an endoscope through the nostril to gain access to the pituitary transsphenoidally, thus eliminating the need for conventional skin incisions and further improving postoperative recovery.[454] The transsphenoidal approach is used in more than 90% of pituitary operations. It is appropriate for microadenomas, enclosed macroadenomas with symmetrical suprasellar extension, and even some invasive adenomas. However, if the pituitary adenoma is very fibrous or shows significant extension into the middle cranial fossa, a transsphenoidal resection may be impossible, and an intracranial operation may be necessary.

The success of surgery alone in curing adenomas depends on the size of the tumor. In a review of transsphenoidal resection for GH-secreting adenomas, in most series hormonal normalization was seen in 67% to 91% of microadenomas but in only 48% to 65% of macroadenomas.[455] ACTH-secreting adenomas, which are generally less than 1 cm at diagnosis, show a normalization of hormones following resection in 75% to 96% of cases in most surgical series.[456] TSH-secreting adenomas are rare compared to other pituitary adenomas, and when diagnosed, they are often large. Normalization of TSH following resection of these tumors has varied widely in different series, ranging from 33% to 86%.[457]

The results of surgery for hormone-inactive adenomas are harder to document because the criteria for surgical success are less well defined. Clinical improvement can be seen even without total removal of the tumor. Series in which CT or MRI scans were performed a few months after surgery show a wide range of gross complete resection rates for these tumors, ranging from 28% to 84%.[458–460] A review of several surgical series showed that the likelihood of normalization of visual fields following surgery ranged from 16% to 53% and that visual field improvement occurred in 26% to 70% of cases.[461]

Medical Therapy for Pituitary Adenomas

Although surgical resection and radiation therapy are effective therapies for prolactinomas, the primary treatment for these tumors currently is medical. This choice is based on the availability of drugs that can suppress prolactin secretion and shrink these tumors. Surgical resection and radiotherapy are still used for prolactinomas in the minority of patients who fail to respond to drugs or who cannot tolerate them.

Clinical manifestations of prolactinomas differ between the sexes.[462] In premenopausal women, oligomennorhea/ amennorhea and galactorrhea are extremely common. Infertility may also be the presenting symptom, and women often have decreased libido. Estrogens have a marked stimulatory effect on prolactin synthesis and secretion; therefore, pregnancy can stimulate the growth of these tumors. In men and postmenopausal women, these tumors are generally asymptomatic until they are large enough to compress nearby structures, causing symptoms such as visual deficits, headaches, and panhypopituitarism. Chronic hyperprolactinemia leads to decreased libido and impotence in 90% of men. Galactorrhea is uncommon in men but can occur in 10% to 20% of these patients. The problems with reproductive/sexual function are due to inhibition of pulsatile gonadotropin secretion.

Secretion of prolactin by the lactotroph cells in the anterior pituitary gland is negatively regulated by dopamine produced by the hypothalamus. Therefore, dopamine agonists such as bromocriptine stimulate dopamine secretion by the hypothalamus and inhibit prolactin secretion by the lactotrophs. Bromocriptine has been the standard therapy for prolactinomas for decades. It has been shown to decrease tumor size and normalize prolactin levels in 70% to 90% of patients.[462] Bromocriptine also restores ovulation and menses and improves visual fields in a similar percentage of cases. Tumor shrinkage and decrease in prolactin levels can take anywhere from days to weeks to months to occur. Unfortunately, the action of bromocriptine is reversible; therefore, when the drug is discontinued, usually the tumor regrows and the prolactin level increases. Therefore, lifelong administration is the rule, and many patients can tolerate prolonged treatment for years. Bromocriptine has been used prophylactically during pregnancy to reduce symptomatic tumor enlargement. However, 10% to 20% of patients experience side effects such as nausea, vomiting, dizziness, postural hypotension, and headaches. In patients who have limiting toxicity with bromocriptine or whose tumors fail to respond to this drug, newer dopamine agonists such as lisuride, pergolide mesylate, and cabergoline have been used with some success.[463]

A few drugs are now available for the treatment of endocrine hypersecretion in pituitary tumors other than prolactinomas. For GH-secreting adenomas, somatostatin analogs such as octreotide and lanreotide have been shown to reduce GH levels in over 90% of patients with almost complete suppression in half.[464] Synthetic agents that block GH binding to its receptor or GH-releasing hormone to its receptors in the pituitary are being used experimentally. In general these drugs are not being used as first-line therapy in patients with GH-secreting adenomas but rather in patients in whom surgery has been unsuccessful.

TSH-secreting adenomas are often very large at diagnosis, making complete surgical resection difficult. Because these tumors express somatostatin receptors, octreotide and lanreotide can decrease tumor size and decrease TSH secretion.[464]

Radiation Therapy for Pituitary Adenomas

Radiation therapy is also highly effective in controlling pituitary adenomas. However, it is rarely given as sole treatment for newly diagnosed pituitary adenomas. In contrast to surgery, radiation will not result in as rapid a reversal of neurologic symptoms or drop in hormonal secretion. Radiation therapy is usually reserved for patients who either have residual disease after surgery or have a recurrence following surgery. Radiation therapy is occasionally used as sole primary therapy in patients who are inoperable.

The overall 10-year control rates using radiation therapy are on the order of 85% to 95% based on a number of large retrospective series.[465–469] In a study from the University of Heidelberg, in 138 patients with pituitary adenomas who received radiation as initial therapy or following recurrence, the overall local control rate was 95% with a mean follow-up of 6 years.[468] Likewise, in a study from the University of Florida with a median follow-up of 9.2 years, the overall local control rate at 10 years was 93%.[469] Ninety-eight patients in this series had surgery and radiotherapy as initial therapy, and their 10-year local control rate was 95%. This was comparable to the 10-year local control rate of 90% for the 23 patients who had radiotherapy alone for newly diagnosed adenomas, but

better than the 80% control rate seen in 20 patients who received radiation for a recurrence after their initial surgery ($P = .03$). Similar findings regarding improved local control in patients receiving surgery and radiation up front compared to those receiving radiation at recurrence were obtained from the Princess Margaret Hospital based on examining 160 patients with hormonally inactive pituitary adenomas.[466] Pituitary adenomas can occur in the pediatric population, although they are much less common than in adults. In one study, 11 patients with pituitary adenomas aged 19 or less were treated with surgery and radiation or radiation only.[470] With a median follow-up of 15.6 years, only two had failed.

In the previous studies, local control refers to lack of disease progression clinically and radiologically. However, many patients who have hormone elevations at the outset may not have complete normalization following radiation. In the University of Heidelberg series, out of 68 patients with hormonally active pituitary adenomas, 52% had some reduction in their hormonal overproduction, but only 38% had a complete normalization.[468] Furthermore, in patients who had a response, it often took years, in some cases up to 9 years. A study from the Princess Margaret Hospital specifically analyzed 145 patients who received radiation for hormonally active pituitary adenomas.[465] The progression-free rate was 96% at 10 years; however, the actuarial long-term biochemical remission rate was only 40%. Therefore, radiation is highly effective in preventing pituitary adenomas from growing; however, it is far less effective in normalizing hormone levels in patients with hormonally active tumors.

Late Effects Following Pituitary Irradiation

In the preceding series, the median doses ranged from 45 to 50 Gy.[465,466,468,469] In the University of Heidelberg study, a statistically significant dose-response relationship was found in favor of a dose of $\geq$45 Gy.[468] One of the worrisome potential late effects of using higher total doses is the possibility of radiation-induced optic neuropathy. In some series, a few patients develop visual problems following radiation, presumably due to optic nerve damage, but this incidence is low, ranging from 0.7% to 2%.[465,468,469] As discussed in the section on optic neuropathy following cranial irradiation, the risk of optic nerve/chiasm injury is dependent on both total dose and dose per fraction. At the doses commonly used to treat pituitary adenomas (45 to 50 Gy), the risk of radiation-induced optic neuropathy with standard fractionation (1.8 to 2 Gy/day) is very low but not zero.

Doses from 45 to 50 Gy to the pituitary gland carry a substantial risk of causing hypopituitarism. In patients who did not have hormonal deficiencies at the start, the risk of developing insufficiency of a given hormone ranged from 10% to 30% in the preceding series.[465,466,468,469] It is likely that half of all patients treated with 45 to 50 Gy will develop deficiency of at least one pituitary hormone 5 years after radiotherapy. However, this is an ongoing risk following radiation and can occur many years afterward; therefore, patients must be followed indefinitely for this complication.

Second malignant neoplasms are always a concern in patients who receive radiation and who are expected to be long-term survivors. In an analysis of 334 patients with pituitary adenomas treated at the Royal Marsden Hospital with surgery and radiation therapy (median dose 45 Gy) five patients developed a secondary brain tumor (two astrocytomas, two meningiomas, one meningeal sarcoma) for an actuarial risk of 1.3% at 10 years and 1.9% at 20 years.[471] The relative risk for developing a second tumor compared with the incidence in the normal population was 9.3. A report from the Princess Margaret Hospital came to similar conclusions. Out of 306 patients treated for pituitary adenomas, 4 developed gliomas of the brain with a latency of 8 to 15 years. The relative risk compared to the normal population was 16 with an actuarial risk of 1.7% at 10 years and 2.7% at 15 years.[472]

Stereotactic Radiation Techniques for Pituitary Adenomas

A number of institutions have reported using stereotactic means of delivering radiation therapy to pituitary adenomas, both in fractionated and single-dose regimens. Investigators have used fractionated stereotactic radiotherapy (FSRT) with 45 to 50 Gy in 1.8-Gy daily fractions using relocatable stereotactic head frames.[473,474] Stereotactic radiosurgery (SRS) has also been used with single fractions ranging from 10 to 27 Gy.[473-475] The local control rates using these techniques has been reported to be greater than 90%; however, the length of follow-up in these studies is too short to make definite conclusions. The rationale for using single large doses is the contention that the interval to normalization of hormonal levels is shorter with this approach than with conventionally fractionated radiation therapy. Yoon and associates reported that 11 of 13 patients with prolactinomas had normalization of their hormone level within 1 year.[475] Mitsumori and associates found that the average time to normalization with SRS was 8.5 months versus 18 months with FSRT (45 Gy in 1.8-Gy daily fractions).[474] In spite of this finding, this group did not advocate SRS for pituitary adenomas because the 3-year actuarial rate of adverse CNS effects was 28% with SRS but 0% with FSRT. This sentiment is shared by many radiation oncologists who would feel much safer using a fractionated regimen than a single large dose given the critical normal structures that are adjacent to the pituitary gland and the likelihood that these patients will survive for a long time with the potential of manifesting late complications.

ACOUSTIC NEUROMA

Clinical and Pathologic Considerations

This entity has many other names; in addition to neuromas, these tumors are also referred to as neurilemmomas, neurinomas, neurofibromas, schwannomas, and nerve sheath tumors. They are benign tumors that most commonly originate from cranial nerve VIII, usually in the vestibular region of the internal auditory foramen where the nerve acquires a Schwann sheath. For this reason, these tumors are also sometimes called vestibular schwannomas. Neuromas can affect other cranial nerves, for example, the trigeminal nerve and nerves in the jugular foramen region; however, these types are much less common than acoustic neuromas.[476,477]

Acoustic neuromas make up 8% to 10% of all primary intracranial tumors, generally affecting people in the fifth decade of life. These tumors characteristically grow very slowly. Early on they are asymptomatic, but as they enlarge, they lead to progressive hearing loss and tinnitus.[478] The hearing loss is typically in the conversational range. As the tumor expands and compresses cranial nerve VIII, it may cause vertigo and unsteadiness of gait. With growth into the cerebellopontine angle, cranial nerves V and VII may be compressed, resulting in otalgia, facial numbness, facial palsy, and change in taste. With continued growth, there may be brainstem compression and obstruction of the fourth ventricle causing hydrocephalus. Because these symptoms can arise insidiously, some patients have a progressive hearing loss and gait unsteadiness over years before they are diagnosed.

Patients with neurofibromatosis type 2 often have bilateral acoustic neuromas; in fact, the occurrence of the latter is diagnostic for NF2.[31] Therefore, acoustic neuromas in patients with NF2 contain mutations in the *NF2* gene and chromosome 22 deletions. Sporadic unilateral acoustic neuromas arising in patients without NF2 are also associated with chromosome 22 deletion and *NF2* mutation.[479,480]

Surgery for Acoustic Neuromas

Traditionally, acoustic neuromas have been treated by surgical resection. A number of different approaches can be taken, including the suboccipital approach, the translabyrinthine approach, and the middle fossa approach.[481] Some centers strongly favor one approach over the others, but many make a decision on a case-by-case basis. The translabyrinthine approach is the only procedure that inherently sacrifices hearing in the course of the procedure; therefore, it is generally not used in patients who have some residual useful hearing.[482] Hearing preservation is possible but not guaranteed with either the suboccipital or middle fossa approach. In one series of patients who underwent a resection using the suboccipital approach with an attempt to preserve hearing, 18 of 46 (39%) patients who had good preoperative hearing maintained good hearing after surgery.[483] The middle fossa approach is indicated in patients who have useful hearing and have tumors entirely contained within the internal auditory canal. In one series using this approach, total tumor removal was achieved in 98% of cases with hearing preservation in 59% of cases.[484] Eighty-nine percent of patients maintained normal or near normal facial nerve function.

Catastrophic complications such as brainstem stroke, postoperative cerebellar hemorrhage, or death are rare following surgery for acoustic neuromas.[485] Two other serious complications that are more common are CSF leak, which can lead to meningitis, and cranial nerve VII palsy. Some surgical teams feel that CSF leak and damage to the facial nerve are more likely with the suboccipital approach than the translabyrinthine approach; however, both complications have been described with both approaches.[482,486] In an effort to decrease damage to the facial nerve, many surgeons routinely perform intraoperative electromyographic monitoring.[485] Persistent headaches that last for months to a year are more common following surgery with the suboccipital approach, presumably as a result of aseptic meningitis from contamination of the subarachnoid space with bone dust when the internal acoustic canal is drilled intradurally.[481]

Radiotherapy for Acoustic Neuromas

Radiation therapy is often effective in cases in which total resection cannot be performed. In a series from UCSF, postoperative radiation therapy (>45 Gy) decreased the recurrence rate after subtotal resection from 46% (6 of 13 patients) to 6% (1 of 11; $P = .01$).[487] Radiation therapy is also effective in controlling acoustic neuromas that are not surgically resected. Proton beam therapy has been used to deliver single large fractions to acoustic neuromas. In the Massachusetts General Hospital series, 68 patients received a dose of 12 Gy to the tumor margin. With a median follow-up of 44 months, the 5-year actuarial control rate was 84%.[488]

Single large doses of radiation with stereotactic radiosurgery (SRS) have also been used (Fig. 69-21). The University of Pittsburgh has one of the largest experiences with this approach. An analysis of their first 5 years of using gamma knife radiosurgery with 12 to 20 Gy marginal dose showed a 98% local control rate.[489] However, of patients who had normal function of cranial nerves VII and V prior to radiosurgery, 15% and 16%, respectively, developed some dysfunction afterward. Furthermore, of patients with useful hearing prior to radiosurgery, only 47% maintained the same level of hearing. Other institutions also found high local control rates along with high rates of cranial nerve V and VII dysfunction following single large stereotactic doses using either a gamma knife[490] or a linear accelerator.[491] Based on their initial results, the investigators at the University of Pittsburgh changed their policy by decreasing the marginal dose and using MRI scans for treatment planning purposes.[492] One hundred ninety patients were treated with gamma knife radiosurgery from 1992 to 1997 delivering 11 to 18 Gy to the margin of the tumor (median dose 13 Gy). With a median follow-up of 30 months, the 5-year actuarial tumor control rate was 97%, and 71% of patients retained useful hearing. The 5-year rates for developing facial weakness and facial numbness were 1% and 2.7%, respectively.[492]

In order to potentially reduce late effects, a number of institutions have started using fractionated stereotactic radiation (FSRT). Both hypofractionation (25 Gy in 5-Gy fractions, 30 Gy in 3-Gy fractions, 21 Gy in 7-Gy fractions)[493,494] and conventional fractionation with 54 to 58 Gy in 1.8- to 2-Gy fractions[495,496] or 36 to 44 Gy in 1.8-Gy fractions[497] have been used. Although the follow-up is very short in some of these series, the control rates have ranged from 97% to 100% with a useful hearing rate ranging from 72% to 85% and low rates of cranial nerve V and VII dysfunction. Although the jury is still out on using single-dose SRS versus FSRT for acoustic neuromas, the experience at Jefferson University Hospital strongly favors the latter. Patients have been treated with either gamma

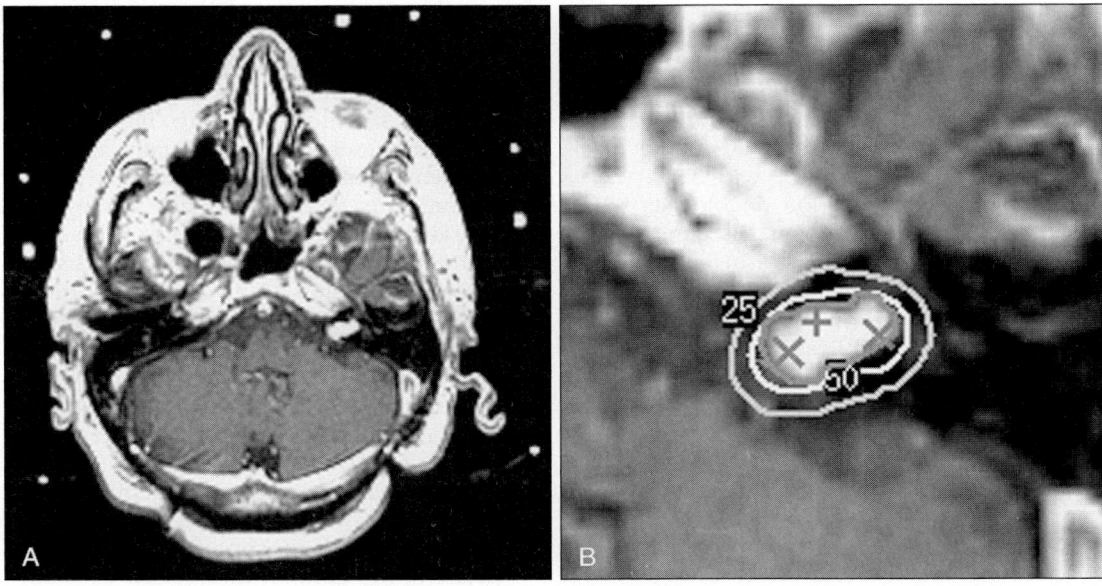

Figure 69-21. Acoustic neuroma targeted by gamma knife radiosurgery. **A,** Axial T1-weighted postgadolinium magnetic resonance imaging (MRI) scan shows enhancing mass in the left auditory canal. **B,** Enlarged view shows superimposed gamma knife isodose distribution using three isocenters. Target volume was 0.4 cm². Fifty percent and 25% isodose lines are shown in white around target volume. (From Larson DA, Shrieve D, Loeffler JS: Radiosurgery. In Leibel SA, Phillips TL [eds]: Textbook of Radiation Oncology. Philadelphia, WB Saunders, 1998, p 389.)

knife SRS (12 Gy marginal dose) or FSRT (50 Gy in 2-Gy fractions) in a nonrandomized fashion. The rates of cranial nerve V and VII preservation were equally high in both groups (93% to 98%) as were the local control rates (97% or better). However, there was a significant difference in the serviceable hearing (33% for gamma knife SRS versus 81% for FSRT).

Therefore, evidence suggests that radiation therapy can be an alternative to surgery to control the growth of acoustic neuromas. However, there will undoubtedly continue to be debate as to the merits of one treatment over the other as well as the optimal radiotherapy technique. Although the previous discussion has centered around the treatment of acoustic neuromas, there is evidence that SRS is effective in controlling the growth of trigeminal neuromas and alleviating trigeminal neuralgia, as either an alternative or adjunct to surgery.[498]

CEREBELLAR HEMANGIOBLASTOMAS

Clinical and Pathologic Considerations

Hemangioblastomas are low-grade vascular tumors that constitute 1% to 2% of intracranial tumors. They usually occur in the cerebellar hemispheres and vermis, although they can involve the pons, medulla, and spinal cord. Most cases occur sporadically, but 20% occur as part of the familial von Hippel–Lindau (VHL) syndrome.[499] Patients with VHL syndrome have a germline mutation in the *VHL* gene. Tumors that these patients develop have sustained a mutation in the second VHL allele, leading to loss of VHL protein function resulting in stabilization of the HIF-1α protein under normoxic conditions. Stabilization of HIF-1α leads to constitutive high levels of expression of target genes including VEGF (vascular endothelial growth factor).[500] For this reason, the tumors seen in patients with the VHL syndrome are highly vascular. Other abnormalities seen in these patients include retinal angiomas, renal cell carcinomas, and cysts involving many organs such as the pancreas, kidney, lungs, and liver. These patients may also develop pheochromocytomas, and they often display erythrocytosis as a result of increased erythropoietin production. Sporadic hemangioblastomas, which occur in patients not suffering from the VHL syndrome, also contain mutations in the VHL gene in at least 20% of cases.[501]

Patients with cerebellar hemangioblastomas often present in the third decade of life. Their presenting symptoms stem from cerebellar dysfunction, increased intracranial pressure, and involvement of nearby cranial nerves. These signs and symptoms include headaches, nausea, vertigo, diplopia, tinnitus, ataxia, and poor co-ordination.[502] The lesion is well visualized by CT scan or MRI scan. Angiography, which is generally performed prior to surgery, shows the highly vascular nature of these tumors.

Histologically hemangioblastomas show numerous capillary and sinusoidal channels lined with endothelial cells. Often there is a cystic component filled with xantho-chromic, proteinaceous fluid with a vascular nodule in the cyst wall. In one series, 6 of 19 cases (32%) had a solid lesion without a cystic component.[503] Lesions of this type are more likely to originate in the brainstem.

Therapy for Cerebellar Hemangioblastomas

The primary therapy for most patients with these tumors is surgical resection, if this can be done safely. If there is a cyst, it is drained, and then the solid component is dissected and removed. However, if the tumor involves the brainstem, surgery may be extremely risky with the potential for massive hemorrhage or extensive post-operative edema leading to death.[503] Surgical resection historically has been associated with high local control rates. In one series, only 13 patients of 112 (12%) had recurrences after surgery.[502] Six of these patients had the recurrence in the original tumor bed following incomplete removal, and 10 failed in a different site or in the same site following gross total resection.

For patients with unresectable or incompletely resected hemangioblastomas or for those who are medically inoperable, radiation therapy is usually given. In a series from the Mayo Clinic, 27 patients were treated with radiation, 6 because of microscopic positive margins following surgery and 20 for gross residual disease.[504] In patients with gross residual disease, the local control rate was 57% for those who received 50 Gy or more but only 33% for those receiving less than this dose. Four of the six patients with microscopic residual disease were controlled. For all 27 patients, the overall 15-year survival rate was 58%, and the relapse-free survival rate was 42%. Sung and associates also found that patients who received a higher dose (40 to 55 Gy) had a superior survival compared to these who received 20 to 36 Gy.[505] Therefore, based on these results it would be reasonable to use approximately 50 Gy in patients requiring radiation.

Radiosurgery has been used for cerebellar hemangio-blastomas. In a study from three institutions, 38 hemangioblastoma lesions in 22 patients were treated stereo-tactically with single fractions ranging from 12 to 20 Gy (median 15.5 Gy).[506] The vast majority of these tumors had not undergone gross total resection. With a median follow-up of 24.5 months, the 2-year actuarial overall survival rate was 88% and the 2-year progression-free survival rate was 86%.

CHORDOMAS AND CHONDROSARCOMAS INVOLVING THE BASE OF SKULL

Clinical and Pathologic Considerations

Chordomas constitute less than 0.1% to 0.2% of all intracranial tumors. They arise along the path of the primitive notochord, which stretches from the tip of the dorsum sellum to the coccyx. Half of all chordomas arise from the sacrococcygeal region, but a third arise from the base of skull, most commonly the clivus but occasionally the petrous bone. Chordomas rarely metastasize. Grossly, they are extradural, often multilobulated, and pseudo-encapsulated. Their consistency can range from extremely soft to woody or cartilaginous. Histologically, one sees nests and cords of large vacuolated epithelioid cells within a myxoid stroma. A chondroid subtype contains areas with a hyaline-appearing stroma. Previously it was thought that the chondroid subtype might have a more favorable outcome than the typical chordoma; however, this has not been substantiated in recent studies.

In a report from the Mayo Clinic, diplopia was the most common symptom followed by headaches, ptosis, retro-orbital pain, and neck pain. Cranial nerve deficits were very common, especially for cranial nerve VI, although deficits of cranial nerves III, IV, V, IX, X, and XII were also seen.[507] In the same study, MRI was demonstrated to be the best modality for demonstrating the entire extent of cranial chordomas and the involvement of adjacent structures. Typically these tumors appear hypointense (black) on T1-weighted images and hyperintense (white) on T2-weighted images (Fig. 69-22). Other possibilities in the differential diagnosis of a clival lesion that need to be considered include metastasis, myeloma, osteochondroma, meningioma, or chondrosarcoma.

Low-grade chondrosarcomas are often lumped together with chordomas. The former arise from primary mesenchymal cells or embryonal rests of cartilaginous matrix. Chondrosarcomas are composed of hyaline cartilage, myxoid cartilage, or a mixture of the two. The myxoid variant may be confused with chordoma.

In one large series of chondrosarcomas of the base of the skull, 6% arose from the sphenoethmoid complex, 28% from the clivus, and 66% from the temporo-occipital region.[508] Chordomas and low-grade chondrosarcomas show a similar radiologic appearance. Together they account for almost all primary malignant bone tumors arising from the base of skull. Both rarely metastasize; however, they can cause death and significant morbidity from local invasion. Even though they are treated similarly, low-grade chondrosarcomas appear to have a better prognosis than chordomas, as discussed subsequently.

Therapy for Chordomas and Chondrosarcomas Involving the Base of Skull

Surgery is almost always performed when a chordoma or chondrosarcoma in the base of skull is suspected in order to both establish a diagnosis and to alleviate symptoms. The surgery is often performed jointly by a neurosurgeon and a head and neck surgeon. Complete resection can be curative but may not be possible owing to extent of disease. In a series from the University of Pittsburgh, 60 patients (46 with chordomas; 14 with chondrosarcomas) were treated primarily with surgery.[509] Sixty-seven percent underwent total or near-total resection; 20% received postoperative radiation because of radiologic evidence of residual tumor. The 5-year recurrence-free survival rate for patients with chordomas was 65% and for chondrosarcomas 90% (P = .09). Two common problems following surgery were the development of CSF leakage and new cranial nerve deficits, which occurred in 30% and 80% of cases, respectively.

In a series from the Mayo Clinic, 51 patients with intracranial chordomas were treated with subtotal resection (78%) or biopsy (22%). Seventy-six percent received postoperative radiation (median dose 50 Gy).[510] However, in spite of this, the 5-year actuarial disease-free survival rate was only 33%. The most important factor for survival on multivariate analysis was young age. Those less than 40 years of age had a 10-year actuarial survival of 63% versus 11% for those over 40. The use of postoperative radiation did not improve overall survival but did show a trend toward improved disease-free survival, especially in patients less than 40 years old.

Because tumors in the base of skull are near critical structures within the brain, there has been a growing use of radiation techniques that can deliver doses to a tightly conformal treatment volume, such as stereotactic radiation and proton beam therapy. There have been reports using both stereotactic radiosurgery (SRS) to deliver single large fractions[511] and fractionated sterotactic radiotherapy (FSRT).[512] In one series, 45 patients (37 with chordoma and 8 with chondrosarcoma) received fractionated radiation using a stereotactic headframe but with conventional fractionation (1.8 Gy/day) to a total median dose of approximately 65 Gy.[512] Among the patients with chondrosarcomas, the local control rate was 100% at 5 years. However, patients with chordomas had local control rates of only 50% at 5 years and 40% at 8 years.

Some consider fractionated proton beam therapy to be the treatment of choice for incompletely resected skull base chondrosarcomas and chordomas, although the availability of facilities that can deliver such treatment is very limited. The advantage of proton beam therapy is that, unlike conventional x-rays, protons have a very sharp fall-off in dose. Proton beam therapy has been used since

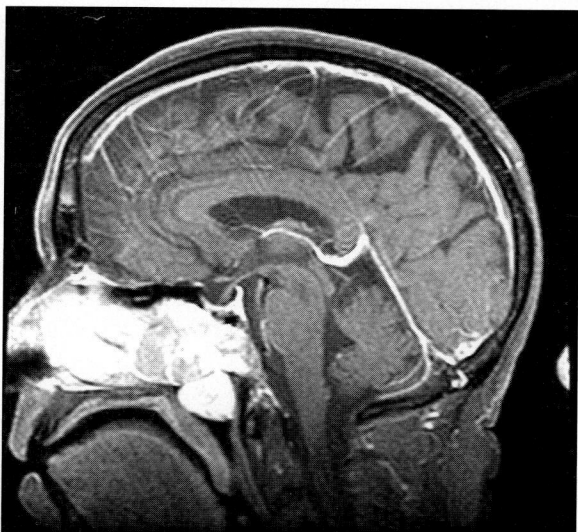

Figure 69-22. Clival chordoma. Sagittal T1-weighted postgadolinium MRI shows enhancing mass replacing the clival marrow that extends into the sphenoid sinus, the nasopharynx, and the posterior nasal cavity.

the 1970s at Massachusetts General Hospital. In a report from that institution, 200 patients with chondrosarcomas of the skull base were treated with surgery followed by radiation.[508] A gross total resection was achieved in only 5% of patients. Radiation was delivered using a combination of x-rays and proton beam therapy to a dose of 64.2 to 79.6 cobalt gray equivalents (median dose 72.1 CGEs in 38 fractions). The 10-year local control rate and progression-free survival rate were 98% and 99%, respectively. In contrast, the experience with almost 300 patients with skull base chordomas treated in a similar manner was not nearly as good with 5- and 10-year progression-free survival rates of 70% and 45%, respectively.

GLOMUS TUMORS OF THE BASE OF SKULL

Clinical and Pathologic Considerations

Glomus tumors are low-grade tumors of neural crest origin arising from the paraganglionic (glomus body) cells; therefore, they are also referred to as nonchromaffin paragangliomas. Becase they are thought to be associated with chemoreceptor tissue, they are also known as chemodectomas. Glomus tissue is found along the vagus nerve, the glossopharyngeal nerve, and the jugular ganglion. Glomus tumors are often divided into those arising in the soft tissue of the neck (glomus vagale and carotid body) and those involving the temporal bone/base of skull (glomus jugulare and glomus tympanicum). Only the latter group will be discussed in this chapter as they often have intracranial extension and are managed by neurosurgeons.

Glomus jugulare tumors originate from the jugular bulb in the base of skull, whereas glomus tympanicum tumors arise from the middle ear cavity along the nerve of Jacobsen (cranial nerve X) or Arnold (cranial nerve IX). In one series, 57 of 75 (76%) patients with glomus tumors of the head and neck region had glomus jugulare tumors, whereas 11 of 75 (15%) had glomus tympanicum tumors.[513] In this series, otologic signs and symptoms were common in patients with both of these tumors. Conductive hearing loss or tinnitus occurred in the majority of these patients. Over a third had bleeding from the ear, ear pain, a polyp visible in the ear canal, or a mass behind the tympanic membrane. Cranial nerve impairments were also very common, specifically cranial nerve VII in patients with glomus tympanicum tumors and cranial nerves V, VI, VII, VIII, IX, X, XI, and/or XII in patient with glomus jugulare tumors.

CT and MRI are often diagnostic for these tumors (Fig. 69-23). Cerebral angiography will demonstrate the extremely vascular nature of these tumors and is generally performed immediately prior to surgery.

Therapy for Glomus Tumors of the Base of Skull

The therapy for glomus tumors is very controversial with some experts strongly advocating surgery and others

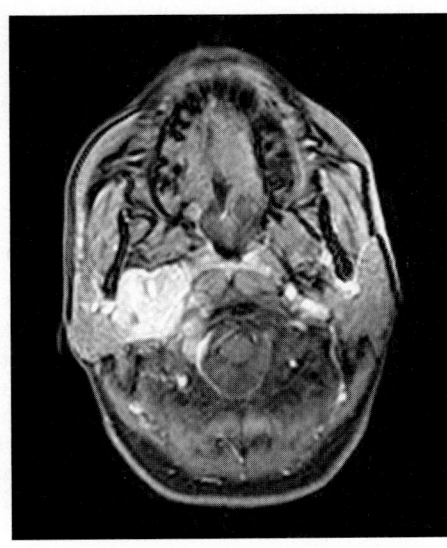

Figure 69-23. Glomus jugulare tumor. Axial T1-weighted postgadolinium MRI shows enhancing mass in the right base of skull.

strongly advocating radiation. When surgery is performed, it is generally preceded by embolization to reduce the subsequent operative time and blood loss. Surgery for glomus tumors involving the base of skull is usually performed jointly with a neurosurgeon and a head and neck surgeon, often using a combined suboccipital and transtemporal approach. The results following surgery in the modern era have been excellent with local control rates ranging from 83% to 95%.[514] The main complications following surgery have been cranial nerve palsies, especially of the facial nerve, and CSF leak.

The literature regarding radiation for glomus tumors is extensive. In a series of 46 patients treated with doses of radiation ranging from 35 to 66 Gy at the Royal Marsden Hospital, the 10-year local control rate was 90% with a median follow-up of 9 years.[515] There were some late relapses so that the 25-year local control rate dropped to 73%. Two patients, both of whom had received 64 Gy or higher, developed a facial nerve palsy as a late complication. In the University of Florida series, 53 patients with temporal bone glomus tumors (46 with jugulare and 9 with tympanicum tumors), most of whom had no prior therapy, received radiation ranging from 37.7 to 60 Gy (median dose 45 Gy).[514] The 10-year local control rate was 92% with a median follow-up of 15 years. Based on their experience, the authors recommended 45 Gy in 1.8-Gy fractions when radiation was used. Their review of the literature showed local control rates ranging from 83% to 100% in series using radiation therapy for temporal bone glomus tumors. A few reports exist on studies using single large fractions of stereotactic radiosurgery (20 to 25 Gy)[516,517]; however, the follow-up is short, and this approach cannot be considered to be a standard treatment for this disease.

Therefore, both surgery and radiation can offer excellent local control for glomus tumors. The decision between the two is often based on consideration of treatment complications. It may be reasonable to use primary resection for early-stage base of skull glomus tumors in which the risk of surgical complication should be low and to reserve radiation therapy for patients with large tumors or with incomplete surgical resections.

PINEAL REGION TUMORS

The pineal gland is located adjacent to the cerebral aqueduct and brainstem. Therefore, tumors in this location frequently obstruct the posterior aspect of the third ventricle and aqueduct of Sylvius, causing acute hydrocephalus with headaches, papilledema, nausea, vomiting, diplopia, and lethargy. As tumors grow anteriorly, the midbrain tegmentum and quadrigeminal plate are compressed, resulting in Parinaud's syndrome: paralysis of upward gaze, diminished pupillary response to light, and retractory or convergence nystagmus.

In the United States and Europe, tumors of the pineal region account for less than 0.5% to 1% of all intracranial tumors.[518] However, in Japan, they account for 3% of all intracranial tumors. Tumors in this location are much more common in childhood and account for 3% to 11% of intracranial tumors in this age group.[519]

In series from the United States and Europe, roughly a third of all pineal region tumors are germ cell tumors (GCTs), the majority of which are germinomas (Table 69-15).[518,520] In Japan, GCTs make up a larger percentage of all pineal region tumors because germinomas are much more common than in the West. Because GCTs occur most commonly in the second decade of life, these tumors are discussed in the section, "Childhood Brain Tumors." Approximately a third of pineal region tumors are of glial origin, mostly astrocytomas, but also glioblastomas, oligodendrogliomas, and ependymomas. These tumors are managed in a similar manner as their counterparts in other parts of the brain, as discussed in other sections in this chapter.

Pineal parenchymal tumors (PPTs) account for slightly less than a third of all pineal region tumors (see Table 69-15). A little less than half of PPTs are pineocytomas and the other half are pineoblastomas. Pineocytomas are histologically benign neoplasms composed of well-differentiated pineal parenchymal cells. These tumors generally affect young adults and rarely disseminate. In one study, the 5-year actuarial survival rate for nine patients with pineocytomas was 86%.[521] Following resection all these patients received local field radiotherapy to a dose of greater than 50 Gy without craniospinal irradiation.

In contrast, pineoblastomas consist of embryonal cells indistinguishable from primitive neuroectoermal tumors (PNETs) in other CNS sites, tend to disseminate through the CSF, and have a much poorer prognosis than pineocytomas. Pineoblastomas are rare in adults,[522] generally occurring in the first two decades of life. Management of these pineoblastomas is similar to that of other supratentorial PNETs as discussed in the section, "Childhood Brain Tumors." A small percentage of PPTs (<10%) do not fit either of the two categories discussed here.[523] These PPTs are either mixed pineocytoma/pineoblastoma tumors or PPTs of intermediate differentiation. These tumors, like pineoblastomas, have the capacity to seed the CSF; therefore, some have recommended craniospinal radiation therapy for them.[523] In one study, the 5-year survival rate of patients with PPTs excluding pineocytomas (15 pineoblastomas, 2 mixed PPTs, 4 PPTs with intermediate differentiation) was 49%.[521] A multicenter retrospective study examining adults with PPTs found that those with PPTs of intermediate differentiation had a better outcome than those with pineoblastomas (10-year survival rate of 72% versus 23%, $P = .001$; 10-year spinal control rate of 81% versus 50%; $P = .04$).[522]

TUMORS OF THE SPINAL AXIS

Clinical and Pathologic Considerations

Tumors of the spinal cord are far less common than intracranial tumors, accounting for only 15% of all CNS tumors. The distribution of histologic types involving the spinal axis is different from that affecting the brain (Table 69-16).[524] For example, neuromas (schwannomas) account for almost a quarter of all spinal axis lesions but are very uncommon in the brain. Most spinal axis tumors are intradural, although chordomas are extradural (see Table 69-16). Clinically, these tumors present in one of three ways: (1) radicular pain secondary to compression or infiltration of spinal cord roots, causing a kinfe-like sensation along the nerve distribution, (2) sensorimotor deficits dependent on the level of the tumor, characterized by muscle weakness, paresthesias (pain and temperature abnormalities contralateral to the side of muscle weakness), and (3) central syringomelia with destruction of the central gray matter causing motor neuron destruction, muscle wasting, and loss of pain and temperature sensation with preservation of touch.

TABLE 69-15

Distribution of Pineal Region Tumors by Histologic Type		
TUMOR	**FREQUENCY (%)***	**FREQUENCY (%)†**
Germ cell tumor (GCT)	34	31
Germinoma	(27)	(18)
Teratoma	(4)	(7)
Other GCT	(3)	(6)
Glial	33	27
Astrocytoma	(27)	(17)
Ependymoma	(4)	(11)
Other glial	(2)	(0)
Pineal parenchymal	24	27
Pineocytoma	(12)	(15)
Pineoblastoma	(12)	(12)
Miscellaneous (pineal cyst, meningioma, etc.)	11	15

*Frequency in 370 cases reported by Regis and associates.[520]
†Frequency in 282 cases reported by Konovalov and associates.[518]

TABLE 69-16

Distribution of Primary Spinal Axis Tumors by Histologic Type

TUMOR	LOCATION	FREQUENCY (%)
Meningioma	Intradural; extramedullary	42
Schwannoma	Intradural; extramedullary	22
Ependymoma*	Intradural; intramedullary	15
Astrocytoma	Intradural; intramedullary	11
Other		6

*Ependymomas of the spinal cord are intramedullary, but myxopapillary ependymomas of the cauda and filum terminale are intradural but extramedullary.
Data from Los Angeles County 1972–1985 (Preston-Martin[524])

The imaging modality of choice for spinal tumors is MRI.[525] Both meningiomas and schwannomas are intradural but extramedullary. The signal intensity of meningiomas on T1- and T2-weighted images is similar to that of the normal cord, whereas for neuromas the signal is increased on T2-weighted images. Meningiomas typically enhance with gadolinium. Spinal cord ependymomas and astrocytomas are generally intramedullary tumors. The exception is ependymoma involving the conus medullaris, which is not actually an intrinsic tumor of the spinal cord. Ependymomas and astrocytomas of the spinal cord have a similar appearance on MRI (Fig. 69-24). T1-weighted images show an enlarged spinal cord extending for several vertebral body segments. Both astrocytomas and ependymomas may have cysts that are visible on MRI. T2-weighted images show increased signal intensity in the region of the tumor with accompanying adjacent edema. Both tumor types typically enhance with gadolinium, although there are rare exceptions. The gadolinium enhancement in ependymomas tends to be very homogeneous with clear demarcation of the upper and lower extent, unlike astrocytomas, in which the true extent is often underestimated by MRI. Because they arise from cells in the central canal, ependymomas are centrally located and expand circumferentially. In contrast, astrocytomas can originate from anywhere in the spinal cord. The differential diagnosis of these tumors includes various nonmalignant conditions such as multiple sclerosis, transverse myelitis, and infarction of the cord. Hemangioblastomas are much less common than astrocytomas or ependymomas. They show enlargement of the spinal cord with multiple cysts. There may be one or more intensely enhancing nodules which may be in the cyst wall.

Chordomas Involving the Spinal Axis

Chordomas involving the base of skull were discussed in the section on chordomas and chondrosarcomas involving the base of skull; however, these tumors can also involve the sacrum or the mobile spine. Unlike the other histologic types listed in Table 69-16, chordomas are extradural tumors. Radiation therapy has been used but with poor results. In a series from the Princess Margaret Hospital, 48 patients with chordoma (23 of the sacrum, 5 of the mobile spine, and 20 of the base of skull) received radiation therapy, most immediately after initial diagnosis but some after local failure following surgery.[526] Survival rate was 54% at 5 years and 20% at 10 years, and patients with nonclival disease did just as poorly as patients with clival disease.

In patients with chordomas of the sacrum or spine who are able to undergo a radical resection, there is a reasonable chance for long-term local control and cure. In a series from the Sahlgrenska University Hospital in Sweden, 39 patients (30 tumors involving the sacrum; 9 involving the mobile spine) underwent surgery as the primary treatment.[527] Most presented with pain but many also had neurologic symptoms. En bloc surgical resection was performed in 35 cases. The final surgical margins were wide in 23 patients but marginal or positive in 16. With a mean follow-up of 8.1 years, 23 patients (59%) were disease-free at the time of last follow-up. Seventeen patients (44%) developed local recurrence, and 11 patients (28%) developed distant metastases. The estimated 10- and 15-year survival rates were 64% and 52%, respectively.

Spinal Meningiomas

Meningiomas are the most common spinal axis tumor (see Table 69-16). They are associated with neurofibromatosis 2 as are their intracranial counterparts.[31] They have an excellent prognosis with surgery. In a large series of meningiomas from MGH treated with surgery alone, 18

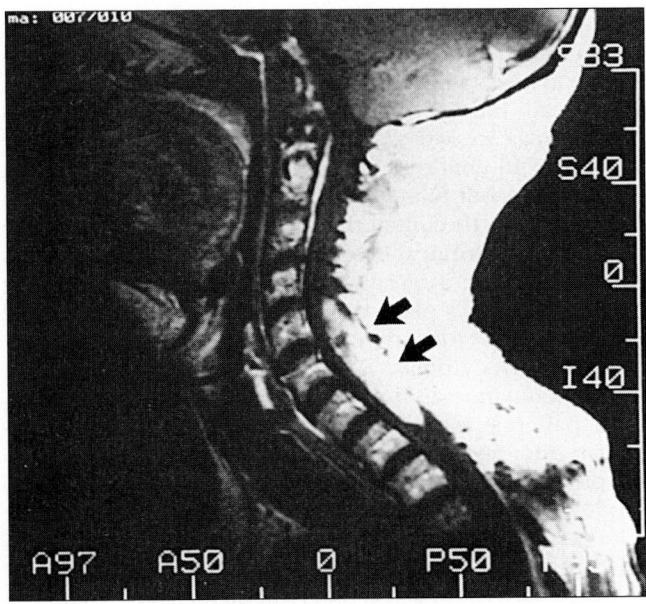

Figure 69-24. Spinal cord ependymoma. Patient had prior history of spinal ependymoma treated with surgery and 50 Gy of radiation. Eight years later he developed new neurologic symptoms. This sagittal T1-weighted postgadolinium MRI shows well-circumscribed, enhancing intramedullary mass extending from C4 through T1. He subsequently underwent complete resection of this tumor, which was histologically confirmed to be an ependymoma. (From Baldwin H, Hadlet MN, Pittman H, Spetzler RF, Drayer BP: Gadolinium DTPA enhancement of a recurrent intermedullary ependymoma: A case report. Surg Neurol 1989;31:222.)

(8%) involved the spine (see Table 69-13).[418] There were no failures at 5 years and a 13% recurrence rate at 10 years. In a report from the Milan Neurologic Insitute, the crude recurrence rate was 6% in 150 patients with spinal meningiomas who had a complete tumor resection versus 17% in the 6 patients who underwent subtotal resection.[528] Out of 80 patients who had undergone a total resection at the Cleveland Clinic, only one relapsed, at 8 years.[529] Even the seven patients who had a subtotal resection did well, with only two relapsing, one at 13 and one at 16 years. Therefore, these tumors do very well with total resection. In the event of subtotal resection, radiation therapy should be considered, as in the case of intracranial meningioma.

Spinal Schwannomas

Schwannomas (neuromas) arise from the Schwann sheath, which covers the extramedullary axons of the nerve roots. They are evenly distributed throughout the cervical, thoracic, and lumbar regions but uncommon in the sacral region. The lesions are benign and well encapsulated; therefore, total surgical resection is usually possible and is curative.

Spinal Cord Ependymomas

Although spinal cord ependymomas are less common that meningiomas and schwannomas involving the spinal axis (see Table 69-16), they account for 60% of all intramedullary tumors. They occur more frequently in the middle adult years and are rare in children. Because of their central location within the spinal cord, ependymomas often present with dysesthesias followed by progressive motor dysfunction but without objective evidence of sensory dysfunction.[530] A variety of histologic subtypes have been described, including cellular (the most common), epithelial, fibrillar, malignant, and myxopapillary. The last subtype is seen only in the filum terminale or the conus medullaris, and is therefore technically not an intramedullary tumor.

Spinal cord ependymomas have a more favorable outcome than intracranial ependymomas. The primary treatment of these tumors is surgery. Although not usually encapsulated, benign spinal cord ependymomas do not generally infiltrate adjacent normal tissue. Therefore, the surgeon can usually find a plane between tumor and normal tissue, allowing for gross total resection, which is associated with a very low rate of recurrence. In one series of 38 patients with spinal cord ependymomas who underwent a gross total resection, none had recurred after a mean follow-up of 24 months.[530] In another series, of 11 patients with spinal ependymomas who underwent gross total resection, only one patient required a second operation for recurrent tumor.[531] In contrast, of 13 patients who underwent a subtotal resection, continued tumor growth led to a second operation in 5 patients and death in 1 patient.

It is hard to assess the role of postoperative radiation for this tumor because of the limited number of retrospective studies with small numbers of patients. Generally, post-operative radiation has been given to patients who had a subtotal resection. In a review of 11 series using surgery followed by postoperative radiation for spinal ependymomas, both the 5- and 10-year survival rates ranged from 60% to 100% with most of the series showing 5-year survival rates in the 80% to 90% range and local relapse rates from 13% to 33%.[532] In two of the largest series from the Princess Margaret Hospital[533] and the Royal Marsden Hospital/Atkinson Morley's Hospital,[534] patients with high-grade tumors had a much higher relapse rate than those with low-grade tumors. In both these series, when failures occurred, they were usually local.

Based on the limited data available, it is difficult to make strong recommendations. However, for benign ependymomas that are totally resected, there does not appear to be a need for postoperative radiation. For incompletely resected benign ependymomas, it would be reasonable to give 45 to 50 Gy to the tumor bed. For high-grade ependymomas, some would advocate giving all patients postoperative radiation, regardless of the extent of surgical resection. The actual volume that should be irradiated is unclear. High-grade spinal ependymomas have been reported to fail intracranially. This has led some to advocate craniospinal radiation,[533] although there is little evidence that the addition of cranial irradiation adds any benefit.[534] If one considered craniospinal irradiation for a high-grade spinal ependymoma, a reasonable dose would be 36 Gy followed by a boost to the primary tumor bed to a dose of 50 to 54 Gy.

Spinal Cord Astrocytomas

Astrocytomas are slightly less common than ependymomas in the spinal cord, accounting for approximately 40% of all intramedullary spinal tumors. Most spinal astrocytomas are low grade; in adults only 10% to 15% are high grade. In children, high-grade astrocytomas are even less common, but pilocytic astrocytomas are seen. As with ependymomas, the initial therapy for astrocytomas of the spinal cord is surgical resection. However, astrocytomas tend to be more infiltrative than ependymomas, making it difficult to find a plane of resection between tumor and normal cord in order to perform a total resection.

Spinal astrocytomas have a poorer prognosis than spinal ependymomas. In a study from Hokkaido University, of 13 patients with astrocytomas and 22 with ependymomas, the 5-year actuarial survival rate for the two groups were 50% and 96%, respectively ($P = .007$). The histologic grade of the astrocytoma has as significant influence on prognosis. In a series from the Mayo Clinic, of 43 pilocytic astrocytomas and 25 diffuse fibrillary astrocytomas, the 10-year survival rates were 81% and 15%, respectively.[535] In a series from UCSF, 12 patients with low-grade spinal astrocytomas had a relapse-free survival rate of 53%, whereas the 3 patients with high-grade tumors all died within 8 months.[536] The 5-year survival rate for patients with low-grade astrocytomas has been in the 55% to 79% range in other series[537,538]; however, for high-grade astrocytomas, it is rare to have survivors at 5 years, with the median survival time being a year or less.[538,539]

As with spinal astrocytomas, it is hard to conclusively demonstrate that postsurgical radiation improves outcome; however, generally it has been given to patients who have had a subtotal resection. Most investigators have used 45 to 50 Gy to local fields for low-grade astrocytomas. High-grade astrocytomas have been known to recur with CNS dissemination, leading some to recommend craniospinal irradiation. However, in spite of such aggressive therapy, these tumors still recur.

No strong data support the use of chemotherapy for spinal cord astrocytomas. However, nitrosoureas and other agents used in intracranial astrocytomas have been used with anecdotal reports of efficacy.[540]

Miscellaneous Intramedullary Tumors

Of the 10% of intramedullary spinal cord tumors that are not ependymomas or astrocytomas, there is a mixture of uncommon tumors including hemangioblastomas, ependymomas, and gangliogliomas.[541] Although exceedingly rare, primary intramedullary germ cell tumors and PNETs have been reported.[540,542]

Hemangioblastomas are benign vascular lesions associated with von Hippel-Lindau disease in 10% to 30% of cases, as is the case for their cerebellar counterpart (see the section "Cerebellar Hemangioblastomas"). Typically they occur in males in their fourth decade of life. Most of these tumors appear as enhancing tumor nodule within a cyst or syrinx. Because they have well-defined margins, surgical resection usually provides a cure, although care must be taken to avoid excessive bleeding of these vascular tumors.[543]

Subependymomas are benign well-circumscribed lesions that affect men between 30 and 60 years of age. Subependymomas are generally avascular and well demarcated from the normal cord, making complete surgical resection likely. Gangliogliomas are generally benign tumors that have neuronal differentiation. Usually seen intracranially, they have been reported in the spinal cord. The primary treatment for these tumors is complete surgical resection; however, resection is associated with a significant risk of recurrence. In one series of 30 cases of spinal gangliogliomas, the 5-year actuarial survival rate was 84%, but the 5-year event-free survival rate was only 36%.[544]

CHILDHOOD BRAIN TUMORS

Primary CNS tumors are the most common solid tumors and the leading cause of cancer-related morbidity and death in children.[545] CNS neoplasms constitute 24% of all malignancies in children younger than 14 years of age in the United States. An estimated 3110 new cases of childhood (age 0–19) primary benign and malignant brain tumors were diagnosed in 2002.[1] Of these, 2330 were estimated to be in children under the age of 15. The annual age-adjusted incidence rate is currently approximately 3.9 per 100,000 children.[546,547] During the period from 1973 through 1994, the reported incidence of primary malignant brain tumors among children in the United States increased by 35%.[547] This increase may be due to improved detection and reporting facilitated by the availability of high-resolution neuroimaging.[548]

These observations also raise serious concerns that environmental factors may play a substantial causative or contributory role. Despite these concerns, epidemiologic studies investigating maternal nutritional intake, childhood diet, childhood exposure to electromagnetic fields, and parental occupational exposure have not established direct links between these factors and the development of childhood brain tumors.[549-552] However, as discussed in the section on epidemiology, strong data support a connection between cranial irradiation in childhood and the subsequent development of brain tumors.

Hereditary factors are estimated to be primarily responsible for approximately 2% of childhood brain tumors.[28] Nearly 70% of all optic pathway gliomas occur in patients with neurofibromatosis type 1 (NF1),[30] and almost all childhood vestibular schwannomas occur in patients with NF2. Hereditary immunosuppression disorders as seen in Wiskott-Aldrich syndrome and ataxia-

---

MANAGEMENT APPROACH

MEDULLOBLASTOMA/PRIMITIVE NEUROECTODERMAL TUMORS

- Medulloblastoma and related PNETs are the most common malignant childhood brain tumor.
- Surgical objectives include gross total resection to establish diagnosis, restore CSF flow, and improve survival.
- Postoperative staging should be undertaken in all patients and should include an MRI of the brain within 24 hours of surgery, an MRI of the entire spine 10 to 14 days after surgery, and CSF cytologic examination 10 to 14 days after surgery. These studies determine subsequent risk-based treatments.

- Standard risk patients must meet *all* the following criteria: older than 3 years of age, cerebellar location, little or no residual tumor (<1.5 cm³), *and* no evidence of metastatic tumor spread. All other patients are high-risk.
- Standard risk patients are treated with lower dose craniospinal radiation therapy to doses in the range of 24 Gy, tumor doses in the range of 56 cGy, and less intensive chemotherapy.
- High-risk MB/PNET patients are treated with craniospinal radiation to doses in the range of 36 Gy, tumor radiation doses in the range of 56 Gy, and intensive chemotherapy.

telangiectasia, as well as treatment-associate immuno-suppression as in organ-transplant recipients or exogenous immunosuppression as in HIV infection are all associated with an increased risk of primary CNS lymphomas.[553-555]

Primitive Neuroectodermal Tumors

Primitive neuroectodermal tumors (PNETs) constitute 23% of pediatric CNS tumors and are the most common malignant brain tumor in childhood.[550] When located in the cerebellar vermis, the site of approximately 85% of all CNS PNETs, these tumors are usually called medullo-blastomas. Other common locations include the pineal region (pineoblastoma, 10%) and supratentorial regions (5%).[326,556,557] The nosology of these tumors is the subject of longstanding controversy among neuropathologists. Rorke has suggested that they be grouped together as CNS PNETs based on the assumption that they each arise from neoplastic transformation of pluripotent uncommitted neuroectodermal precursors.[558,559] For cerebellar medullo-blastoma (MB/PNET), recent evidence supports the hypothesis that that these tumors arise from disordered cerebellar granular cell development.[560] The cells of origin for pineal and supratentorial PNETs have not been identified; however, microarray studies demonstrate different patterns of gene expression for medullo-blastoma, pineal, and supratentorial PNETs.[561]

A variety of cytogenetic and molecular genetic abnormalities have been observed in childhood PNETs. The most common, observed in 40% to 50% of cases, is a deletion of the short arm of chromosome 17, typically resulting in the formation of an isochromosome I (17q).[558] Putative tumor suppressor locations have been identified on chromosome 17p and 9q. Multivariate analysis has not clearly identified a clinical prognostic significance for 17p deletion either altering clinical outcome or associated with higher metastatic stage.[562] A putative tumor suppressor locus located on the long arm of chromosome 9 has been identified in 10% to 18% of PNETs.[563,564] The locus for nevoid basal cell carcinoma syndrome (Gorlin's syndrome) has been mapped to this region of chromosome 9. The gene responsible for nevoid basal

cell carcinoma syndrome is the human homolog of the *Drosophila* patched gene (*PTCH*).[565] It encodes a cell surface receptor which, among other functions, regulates normal brain development by repressing transcription of genes encoding members of the transforming growth factor-beta and Wnt families of signaling proteins.[566] Sonic hedgehog is a PTCH ligand that has many functions as an oncogene in mammalian tumors.[567] The incidence of MB/PNET among patients with nevoid basal cell carcinoma syndrome is reported to be approximately 4%.[568] Mutations in PTCH have been identified in nearly 12% of sporadic PNET/MB,[569] and one PNET/MB was shown to contain a mutation in the sonic hedgehog gene. These observations indicate that multiple genes in the sonic hedgehog PTCH signaling pathway contribute to PNET tumorigenesis.

The clinical presentation of PNET/MB is dominated by signs and symptoms of obstructive hydrocephalus and increased intracranial pressure: headache; nausea and vomiting; drowsiness and other behavior changes; and ataxia. These characteristics are often indistinguishable from other posterior fossa tumors, including ependymoma and cerebellar astrocytoma. To differentiate posterior fossa tumors, computer-based neural networks combining data from neuroimaging studies and patient characteristics have been successfully used (Fig. 69-25). In a series of 33 children with posterior fossa tumors, an experienced neuroradiologist was able to correctly predict the tumor type in 73% of cases, whereas the neural networks using different data sets had 95% accuracy.[570]

Preoperative management includes the assessment and treatment of increased intracranial pressure. Patients with papilledema and significant visual impairment require emergency placement of an external third ventricular drain followed immediately by tumor resection. Prolonged delay between ventricular drainage and tumor resection significantly increases the risk of transtentorial upward herniation. For patients with less severe signs and symptoms of increased intracranial pressure, cortico-steroids and acetazolamide may be used to relieve symptoms, reduce tumor swelling, and permit further surgical planning.

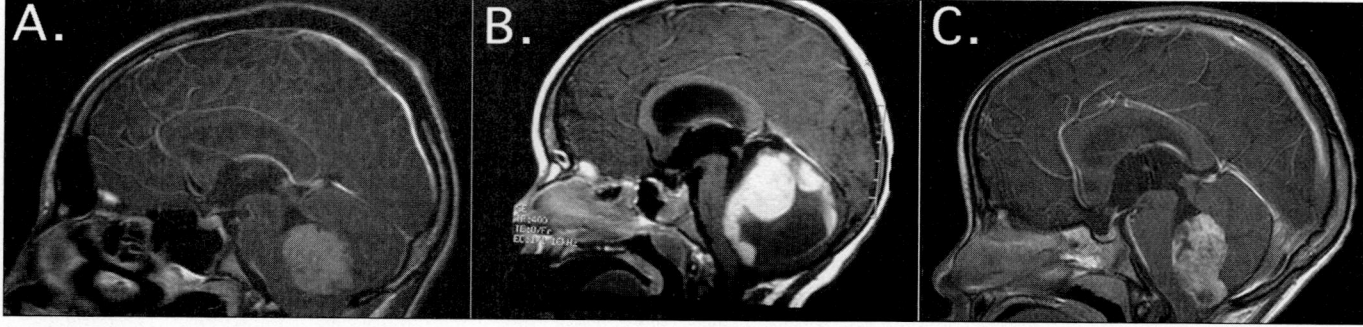

Figure 69-25. Posterior fossa tumors. Sagittal T₁-weighted postgadolinium MR images of three different posterior fossa tumors. **A,** Medulloblastoma shows homogeneous contrast enhancement without evidence of cyst formation. **B,** Cerebellar pilocytic astrocytoma shows prominent cyst or multicyst formation with one or more contrast enhancing mural nodules. **C,** Ependymoma arising from floor of fourth ventricle shows heterogeneous contrast enhancement pattern and extends inferiorly to the upper cervical spinal cord. Note that pilocytic astrocytoma shows intense enhancement, in spite of being a low-grade glioma (WHO grade I).

There are three surgical objectives in PNET/MB treatment. First, sufficient tissue must be obtained to permit accurate histopathologic diagnosis. Second, tumor removal should be complete or near complete because complete tumor removal favorably influences prognosis.[571] Third, every effort should be made to reestablish normal CSF flow. The majority of children with PNET/MB will not need a permanent ventriculoperitoneal (VP) shunt. The incidence of tumor dissemination to the abdomen by VP shunt is extremely low.[572]

Two postoperative syndromes may complicate the clinical course of patients with PNET/MB and other posterior fossa tumors. Aseptic meningitis may occur in up to 5% of patients undergoing posterior fossa surgery and is not limited to those with PNET/MB. Fever and meningismus, ranging from mild to severe in intensity, develop 5 to 10 days after surgery. Although this complication may occur more frequently in patients with large postoperative pseudomeningoceles under tension, there are no clinical features that reliably distinguish this presumed chemical meningitis from bacterial meningitis. Therefore, analysis and culture of CSF is essential. If no infectious etiology is identified, this complication is effectively treated with corticosteroids. A second syndrome, that of cerebellar mutism after resection of posterior fossa tumors, was noted in the early 1980s.[573,574] This condition is far more common than originally reported and occurs in up to 15% of children with large midline cerebellar tumors.[575] Complete or near-complete loss of speech is often accompanied by severe lower cranial nerve, cerebellar, and motor abnormalities as well as visual disturbances.[576] Cerebellar mutism typically presents 1 to 4 days after surgery and may be found more frequently in cases of aggressive surgical pursuit of PNET/MB adherent to or invading the brainstem. Most patients with this syndrome recover functional speech during a period of several weeks to months from symptom onset, although significant residual speech, lower cranial nerve, and motor coordination dysfunction are common.

Adjuvant therapy in PNET/MB is determined by postoperative staging for prognostic risk factor assessment. The most important clinical prognostic factor is metastatic stage followed by postoperative residual tumor volume, tumor location, and patient's age at diagnosis.[571,577,578] PNET/MB is commonly associated with seeding of the spinal cord (Fig. 69-26). Accordingly, three tumor staging studies are important for PNET/MB: (1) neuraxis staging evaluation by spinal MRI (preoperatively or 10 to 14 days after surgery) to identify metastatic tumor aggregates; (2) CSF cytologic examination (intraoperatively or 10 to 14 days after surgery) to identify leptomeningeal tumor spread; and (3) postoperative neuroimaging to assess residual tumor. Based on these studies, PNET/MB patients are classified into two risk-for-recurrence groups. Standard-risk patients must have no evidence of metastatic disease, 1.5 cm or less residual tumor, be older than 3 years at diagnosis, and have primary tumor located in the posterior fossa only.[579] High-risk patients have one or more of the following conditions: evidence of leptomeningeal tumor spread; more than 1.5 cm residual tumor; age less than 3 years at diagnosis; or primary tumor location outside the posterior fossa.

Clinical prognostic factors alone are not sufficient to distinguish a low-risk from a standard-risk group. Furthermore, a potentially very high risk group of patients may benefit from significantly different therapy regimens than standard- or high-risk PNET/MB. It is unlikely that additional clinical prognostic factors will be identified, and the identification of biologic prognostic factors will facilitate a more sensitive and specific stratification of patients to risk-adopted therapies. Accordingly, biologic studies of large, representative, and relatively homogeneously treated PNET/MB patients are of great interest. Independent retrospective studies of childhood PNET

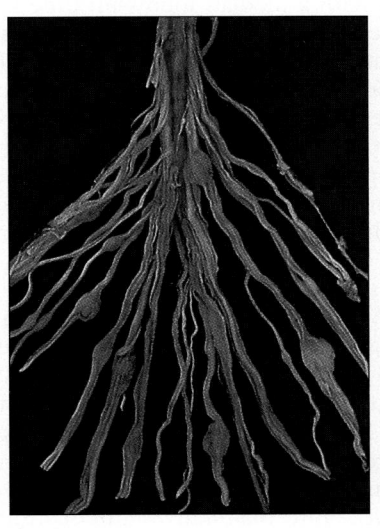

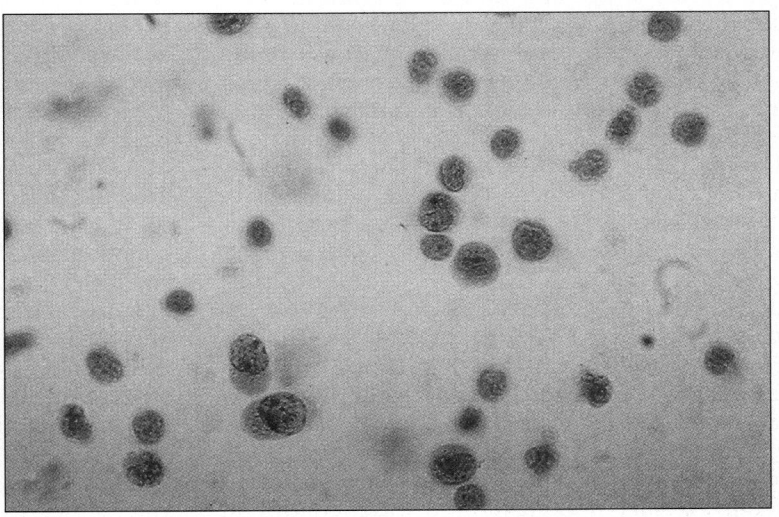

A   B

Figure 69-26. Disseminated medulloblastoma. **A,** Studding of caudal nerve roots from spinal arachnoid spread of tumor. **B,** Malignant cells identified by cytologic examination of CSF. (From Maher EA, McKee AC: Neoplasms of the central nervous system In Skarin AT [ed]: Dana-Farber Cancer Institute Atlas of Diagnostic Oncology, 3rd ed. St. Louis, Mosby, 2003, p 415.)

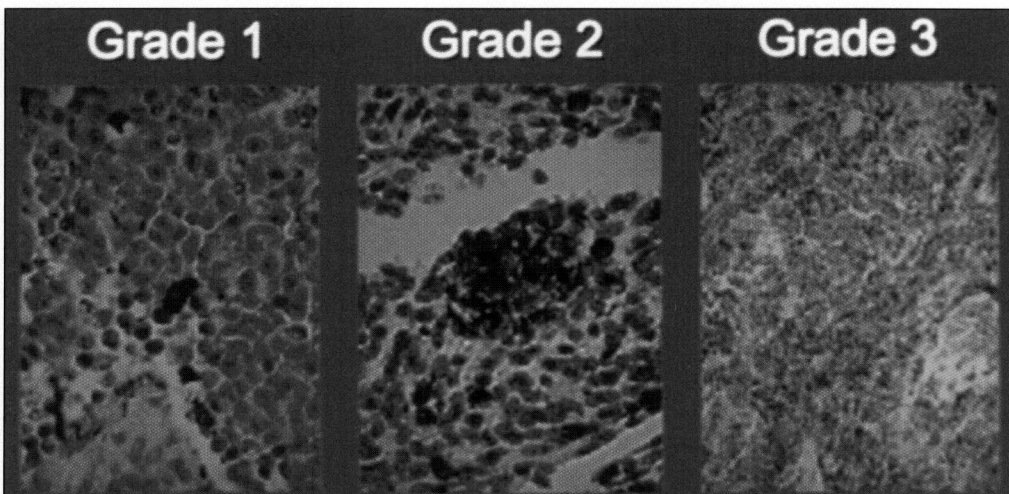

Figure 69-27. GFAP immunostaining of medulloblastoma. The expression of GFAP is an identified prognostic factor in the prognosis of patients with medulloblastomas. GFAP expression may include scattered or isolated cells (grade 1), clusters of GFAP positive cells (grade 2), or widespread staining (grade 3). Staining was performed as discussed in Janss and associates.[583]

patients demonstrates that tumor expression of the neurotrophin receptor TrkC is a potent biologic prognostic factor.[580,581] Other candidates include HER2/HER4 coexpression,[582] GFAP expression (Fig. 69-27),[583] *MYC* amplification,[564] and platelet-derived growth factor receptor expression.[584] Larger prospective studies are planned to determine if these new biologic factors will supplement, or supplant, the significance of clinical factors.

Treatment approaches for PNET/MB are determined by assignment to either a standard- or high-risk category. Four general trends have emerged. High-risk patients are treated with 36 Gy radiation to the craniospinal axis and chemotherapy. Standard-risk patients may be treated with less intensive approaches including reduced craniospinal radiation (e.g., 2400 cGy) to decrease the risk of significant treatment-associated toxicities. Infants and children under 3 or 4 years of age may be treated with intensive chemotherapy alone to postpone or avoid the neurotoxic effects of radiation on the developing brain. Newer protocols combine systemic and intrathecal chemotherapy with conformal XRT to the tumor bed. For recurrent tumors, the introduction of high-dose chemotherapy followed by peripheral blood stem cell (PBSC) rescue may offer some hope for retrieval, especially for patients with minimal residual disease before high-dose chemotherapy. However, the prognosis for recurrent PNET/MB remains very poor.

Radiation therapy is the mainstay of PNET/MB treatment. Cumulative local tumor doses should be approximately 56 Gy. Doses less than 50 Gy have been shown to be less effective.[585] Radiation should be delivered to the entire craniospinal axis, regardless of the tumor metastatic stage.[586] Treatment with craniospinal (36 Gy) and local boost radiotherapy (total dose 54 Gy) without adjuvant chemotherapy results in long-term disease control in approximately 60% of children with PNET/MB.[587] However, after whole-brain radiotherapy, many children will have significant long-term neurocognitive sequelae, including demonstrable drops in overall intelligence. This decline in intelligence is influenced by age at irradiation and dose. Silber and associates reported that patients who received a dose of 36 Gy to the whole brain scored 8.2 points less on IQ testing than those with 24 Gy, and 12.3 points less than those who received 18 Gy.[588] Older age at the time of irradiation was associated with less decline in subsequent IQ score.

Serious long-term side effects of radiotherapy on the developing nervous system prompted efforts to reduce the dose of craniospinal radiation therapy (CSRT) in nonmetastatic PNET/MB. The lowest craniospinal radiotherapy doses reported, 18 Gy in 10 fractions, with 50.4 to 55.8 Gy to the posterior fossa tumor bed, has been used in combination with vincristine during irradiation and subsequent vincristine, CCNU, and cisplatin.[589] Ten patients between 18 and 60 months of age, and without evidence of tumor dissemination, were treated according to this approach. With a median follow-up time for living patients of 6.3 years, survival rate at 6 years was 70% ± 20%. The three patients who relapsed all developed spinal metastases, in association with brain or posterior fossa recurrence. These data suggest that a subset of PNET/MB patients can be cured with chemotherapy and reduced doses of craniospinal irradiation. However, the optimal dose of CSRT remains uncertain. A prospective single-arm study reported the use of 23.4 Gy CSRT, standard local radiotherapy (55.8 Gy), and adjuvant vincristine, CCNU, and cisplatin chemotherapy given during and after radiotherapy.[590] After 3 years, the progression-free survival rate for 68 children aged 3 to 10 years with nondisseminated PNET/MB treated with this approach was 86% ± 4%.

Prospective studies demonstrate that chemotherapy has an important role in the treatment of high-risk PNET/MB. PNET/MBs are responsive to a variety of chemotherapeutic agents, including cisplatin, cyclophosphamide, vincristine, CCNU, and busulfan.[591] Incorporation of cisplatin, CCNU, and vincristine into a postradiation chemotherapy regimen for high-risk patients resulted in 5-year survival rates in excess of 80%.[592] Of note, this survival rate was significantly higher than survival rates for standard-risk patients treated with radiation therapy alone (i.e., historical controls). This and other single-institution studies have provided strong support for the use of effective adjuvant chemotherapy for all PNET/MB patients.

High-dose chemotherapy (HDCT) with peripheral blood stem cell (PBSC) rescue is a therapeutic strategy that has shown encouraging results in the treatment of relapsed PNET/MB.[593] In children with recurrent PNET/MB, Kalifa and associates used a high-dose busulfan-thiotepa regimen.[594] Of 28 patients evaluable for tumor response, complete tumor resolution was obtained in 36%, a partial response in 39%, and no response in 25%. Finlay and colleagues reported a series of 23 patients with recurrent PNET/MB.[595] The chemotherapy consisted of carboplatin, thiotepa, and etoposide followed by PBSC rescue. Three patients died of treatment-related toxicities. Overall, 7 of the 23 patients (30%) remained free from tumor recurrence at a median follow-up of 54 months after HDCT. These results are better than previously reported phase II trial results. Prospective collaborative national and international studies will determine different HDCT regimens not only in terms of survival but also in terms of toxicity and quality of life.

Low-Grade Astrocytomas of Childhood

Low-grade glioma/astrocytomas occur throughout the brain and spinal cord. The predominant histologic appearance of cerebellar astrocytomas is pilocytic, whereas optic pathway/hypothalamic low-grade gliomas are more commonly fibrillary in appearance. Optic pathway/hypothalamic gliomas may be classified by location into those anterior to but not involving the chiasm, chiasmal tumors with extension posteriorly along the optic radiations, and chiasmal/hypothalamic tumors for which the initial site of tumor growth cannot be determined.

Optic Nerve Gliomas

Optic nerve gliomas anterior to the chiasm present with symptomatic and progressive visual loss and proptosis. Their appearance on CT and MRI studies is usually sufficiently diagnostic so that routine biopsy is not necessary. Meningiomas of the optic nerve sheath can often be distinguished from optic nerve gliomas based on neuroimaging characteristics. Optic nerve gliomas should be treated conservatively. Progressive tumor growth together with severe visual dysfunction justifies surgical resection of the nerve. Surgical resection is curative and no further therapy is required. As a rule, optic nerve gliomas anterior to the chiasm do not invade the chiasm itself. For patients with progressive tumor growth and functional vision, radiation therapy is rarely indicated, and current chemotherapy is similar to that for chiasmal gliomas (see following section).

Chiasmal and Chiasmal/Hypothalamic Gliomas

Chiasmal and chiasmal/hypothalamic gliomas constitute 60% to 85% of all optic pathway/hypothalamic tumors. These tumors, especially very large chiasmal/hypothalamic glioma, often come to medical attention before patients are 5 years of age, with symptoms of visual loss and hydrocephalus. Older children are more likely to present with symptoms, which include endocrinopathies and behavioral symptoms. Children younger than 2 years of age may present with a diencephalic syndrome characterized by frequent vomiting, anorexia, and failure to thrive.[596] In children with chiasmal tumors involving the optic nerve, the diagnosis is frequently made by radiographic criteria alone. Especially in children with NF1, diffuse enlargement of the optic chiasm, with extension posteriorly along the optic radiations to the geniculate bodies and beyond, may be sufficiently characteristic to permit reliable diagnosis. Surgical biopsy and histologic confirmation is advisable for large globular tumors with hypothalamic involvement. Though diagnostic confusion is not common, these tumors may have a clinical and neuroimaging appearance similar to solid craniopharyngiomas or germ cell tumors.

Most chiasmal and chiasmal/hypothalamic gliomas are not "cured" by currently available surgical, radiation therapy, or chemotherapy. The slow and often erratic growth of these tumors has led some to conclude that most of these "benign" tumors will eventually be fatal.[597] In the past decade, the development of more effective chemotherapy strategies makes this conclusion far less certain, and the majority of patients remain alive without progressive tumor growth in excess of 10 years. In most cases, the decision to initiate treatment is based on clinical or radiographic evidence of tumor growth from serial observations rather than automatically initiating treatment at the time of tumor diagnosis. Patients with severe visual loss or clear historical evidence of rapid clinical worsening represent exceptions to this approach. Whereas some patients show significant changes in visual acuity or neuroimaging scans within weeks or months of initial diagnosis, many other remain stable for months or years without interval treatment.

For patients who retain a degree of useful vision, chiasmal and chiasmal/hypothalamic gliomas cannot be completely resected. However, there is growing recognition that surgical debulking of large chiasmal/hypothalamic gliomas may provide rapid relief of symptoms caused by mass effect and hydrocephalus, delay the need for radiation therapy in young children, result in years of clinical stability without tumor growth, and improve the effectiveness of subsequent radiation therapy.[598,599]

Local involved-field radiation therapy has been shown to be effective in arresting tumor growth and causing tumor shrinkage.[600,601] However, complete tumor regression is rare after radiation. Because more than 90% of patients with optic pathway/hypothalamic gliomas survive longer than 10 years,[600,602] the late effects of radiation therapy, including neurocognitive problems, endocrinopathy, optic nerve injury, and radiation-induced second neoplasms are important considerations. These issues have stimulated the investigation of alternative treatment approaches, including chemotherapy

Chemotherapy has a defined role in the treatment of optic pathway/hypothalamic gliomas. In a large multi-institutional trial of carboplatin and vincristine, 60% of progressive low-grade glioma patients had a significant reduction in tumor volume, and another 30% of patients had tumor stabilization.[603] A different regimen developed at University of California at San Francisco included procarbazine, 6-thioguanine, dibromodulcitol, CCNU, and vincristine. This treatment protocol resulted in prolonged periods of disease stabilization with a median time to tumor progression of 132 weeks in children with low-grade gliomas.[604] For younger children, particularly those less than 5 years of age, the use of chemotherapy delays or obviates the need for radiation therapy, thereby reducing or eliminating the neurologic morbidity associated with radiation therapy in young children. Currently used chemotherapy regimens for optic pathway tumors are generally well tolerated, can be administered in the outpatient setting, and do not have a high incidence of serious late effects. Because of the successful use of chemotherapy in younger children, attempts have been made to use chemotherapy in older patients. However, it remains to be proved whether the duration of progression-free survival for patients treated with chemotherapy is comparable to that for radiotherapy.

The incidence of optic pathway tumors in patients with neurofibromatosis type 1 (NF1) is markedly higher than in the general population. Up to 15% of children in whom the diagnosis of NF1 is confirmed have optic pathway tumors when they undergo screening neuroimaging.[605] Most optic nerve gliomas in NF1 patients are anterior to the optic chiasm. However, slightly more than half of all children with radiographically identifiable optic pathway tumors ultimately developed signs or symptoms directly related to their tumors. When studied systematically, these tumors appear to behave in a more indolent fashion than their counterparts in children who do not have NF1. However, low-grade gliomas in children with NF1 are notoriously erratic in their natural history. At times, these tumors appear to undergo rapid growth and then spontaneously arrest. Treatment of anterior optic nerve glioma is only necessary when there is significant symptomatic tumor progression. Consequently, routine screening neuroimaging of asymptomatic patients is unwarranted.[30] Because optic pathway tumors nearly always arise in children younger than 10 years of age, all such children should undergo yearly ophthalmologic evaluation and annual assessments of growth to monitor for signs of precocious puberty.

Similar to their non-NF1 counterparts, management of children with NF1 and optic pathway gliomas is dependent on the location of the tumor. Anterior optic pathway gliomas do not invade the chiasm in NF1 patients and are managed according to the clinical symptoms. Chiasmatic optic pathway gliomas are watched closely for neuroimaging or clinical evidence of tumor progression. Progressive chiasmal tumors are treated with chemotherapy strategies that have a relatively low incidence of second malignancies (e.g., carboplatin and vincristine). Use of nitrosoureas in children with NF1 is associated with an increased risk of myeloid leukemia. In addition, there is a pervasive concern that use of radiation therapy in this patient population with an increased incidence of glial brain tumors will result in an unacceptably high incidence of treatment-induced secondary brain tumors.

The challenge for the future is to determine the most appropriate treatment for each patient, based on rate of tumor progression, age, prior therapy, and visual/endocrine status.

Cerebellar Astrocytomas

Histologically, cerebellar astrocytomas of childhood are typically pilocytic or low-grade fibrillary. Malignant gliomas of the cerebellum in childhood are extremely rare. The survival rate is determined by the extent of resection, not by histologic features. Use of radiation therapy is limited to those cases of recurrent astrocytoma that cannot be resected because of extensive invasion into the cerebellar peduncles or brainstem. Cerebellar astrocytomas have, arguably, the best prognosis of any brain tumor, with 10-year survival rates approaching 100%.[606] If a postoperative MRI shows resectable tumor (see Fig. 69-25B), reexploration may be indicated to achieve complete resection.

Ependymoma

Childhood intracranial ependymomas represent approximately 5% to 10% of all childhood brain tumors (see Table 69-2) and behave primarily as localized, relatively noninvasive neoplasms that originate from the ventricular ependymal linings. Nearly 70% of childhood ependymomas are located in the posterior fossa arising from the floor of the fourth ventricle (see Fig. 69-25C). The remaining 30% are located in supratentorial periventricular regions. The classic histologic feature of ependymomas is the perivascular pseudorosette. Two general histologic classifications have been described. Well-differentiated ependymomas are moderately to highly vascular with low mitotic indices, little cellular pleomorphism, or evidence of necrosis. Malignant ependymomas exhibit higher mitotic rates, substantial cellular atypia, and prominent necrosis. The rare "ependymoblastoma" is best classified as a PNET with histologic evidence of ependymal differentiation and treated in a fashion identical to the PNETs. The role of standard histologic classification in prognosis is controversial; however, growing evidence suggests that biologic prognostic factors identified in tumors specimens, such as Erb receptor expression, may provide greater prognostic accuracy.[607]

The primary challenge in ependymoma treatment is local control because metastatic disease at initial diagnosis or first relapse is uncommon.[608,609] Surgical resection of these tumors is often difficult, and complete removal is achieved in less than 50% of the patients. Ependymomas are often located close to brainstem structures, which increases the risk of high morbidity when complete resection is attempted. Several studies confirmed the critical role of a radical surgical resection in patients with newly diagnosed ependymomas.[610,611] Five-year progression-free survival rates range from 50% to 70% after complete surgical resection and 0% to 30% after incomplete resection.[612-614] Better survival is noted in children who have undergone complete resection. The frequency of gross total resections has been increased by sophisticated technologies, including ultrasonic tissue dissociators, argon lasers, and robotic localizing devices; by experience of the surgeon with children; and by the intent and preoperative plan to perform a radical surgical resection.[615] The availability of an intraoperative neuroimaging may provide immediate confirmation of the degree of resection and allow the surgeon to reoperate, immediately, if necessary.[616] For patients with residual tumor after initial surgery, re-resection immediately after the postoperative MRI reveals residual tumor remains an option. Alternatively, deferral of second surgery until the patient child recovers and receives chemotherapy or radiotherapy may be considered.

Involved-field radiotherapy represents standard therapy for children older than 3 years who have intracranial ependymomas. Conventional radition therapy doses range from 54 to 56 Gy. Controversial aspects of radiation therapy for ependymomas include treatment volume and the necessity for craniospinal irradiation. Based on published reports that indicated a significant risk of CSF seeding, craniospinal radiation was recommended.[617] Subsequent studies indicate that the likelihood of a neuraxis relapse in ependymoma occurs in less than 5%.[608] Routine staging for these patients includes a postoperative MRI scan of the brain to characterize the extent of resection. MRI of the spine as well as lumbar puncture for CSF cytologic evaluation is critically important to therapeutic planning. For patients without disseminated disease at diagnosis, the pattern of relapse is local in the vast majority of cases and is not influenced by the delivery of craniospinal irradiation. Therefore, prophylactic craniospinal irradiation is no longer recommended. Currently evaluated strategies to enhance local tumor control in patients with residual or progressive disease include radiosurgery.[618]

The role of chemotherapy in the treatment of ependymoma is controversial as these tumors are considered to be relatively chemotherapy-resistant. In a study of 19 children with newly diagnosed ependymoma, a 74% 5-year progression-free survival rate was reported in children with postoperative residual tumor treated with radiation therapy and platinum-based chemotherapy.[619] This was higher than published results for radiotherapy alone for this group. Based on this finding, current clinical trials use chemotherapy for patients whose postoperative imaging studies are positive for residual tumor. For patients with recurrent ependymoma, options for further therapy other than re-resection are few; usually, maximal irradiation has already been administered, and high-dose chemotherapy is of modest benefit to only a minority of patients.[620,621] Therefore, management consists largely of symptom control and palliation.

Brainstem Glioma

Gliomas of the brainstem, distinctly uncommon in adults, represent a major tumor group in childhood. In past years, brainstem tumors were considered as a single entity; uniformly fatal despite the most intensive therapies. Despite this, some children had continuous progression-free survival rates in excess of 5 years,[622] whereas a larger number of children died from progres-

sive tumor within 18 months. To distinguish good- from poor-risk groups, investigators evaluated neuroimaging characteristics and biopsied these tumors.[622] Results from these studies identified two major classes of brainstem gliomas: (1) diffuse intrinsic brainstem gliomas, typically centered in the pons and upper medulla, which have a uniformly poor prognosis; (2) focal brainstem gliomas, typically located in the upper midbrain or lower medulla, which have a substantially better prognosis.

Factors responsible for the initiation and progression of brainstem and supratentorial gliomas in children are poorly understood. Although a model of tumor progression has been proposed for gliomas in adults, it is unlikely that this model is applicable to gliomas in younger children. Malignant transformation from low-grade astrocytoma to malignant glioma is distinctly uncommon in children. The genetic pathways leading to primary (de novo) glioblastoma of pediatric patients appear to be different from those of adult patients, as reflected by the comparatively low frequency of *EGFR* amplification (6%), *CDKN2A* deletion (19%), and the absence of *MDM2* amplification in childhood glial tumors.[623]

Diffuse Intrinsic Brainstem Gliomas

Diffuse intrinsic brainstem gliomas constitute more than 70% of all brainstem neoplasms. Their MRI characteristics include diffuse infiltrative enlargement of the pons or rostral medulla (Fig. 69-28).[624] T1-weighted MRI sequences usually show mass effect and reduced signal compared with normal brain. T2-weighted MRI sequences often reveal high-signal regions of tumor infiltration with rostral extension into the midbrain and brachium pontis and lateral extension into the cerebellar peduncles. Brainstem enlargement may be unilateral and is often asymmetrical at initial diagnosis. The fourth ventricle is usually distorted; however, obstructive hydrocephalus is distinctly uncommon at initial presentation. The clinical presentation of diffuse pontomedullary brainstem gliomas classically involves one or more of the following abnormalities: (1)

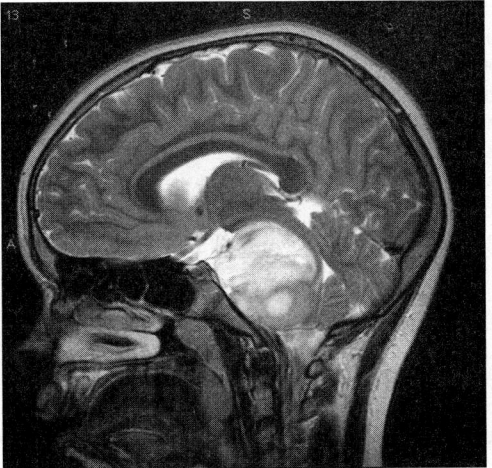

Figure 69-28. Diffuse pontine glioma. FLAIR image of sagittal magnetic resonance imaging (MRI) scans shows image of glioma diffusely infiltrating the pons.

cranial nerve palsies, typically of VI and VII; (2) ataxia; and (3) long tract signs, including hyper-reflexia and extensor plantar responses. The prediagnostic symptomatic interval is often less than 3 months.

The impetus for biopsy and autopsy studies of these tumors arose from efforts to correlate histologic features with clinical outcome. The brainstem is among the most eloquent brain structures, thereby reducing surgical accessibility. These studies showed that a limited surgical procedure, either stereotactic or via open biopsy, can be accomplished safely with acceptable risk of morbidity.[625] They did not, however, show that biopsy information was a uniformly accurate predictor of clinical outcome, possibly due to the difficulty of obtaining a sufficiently large, representative sample.[626] In many centers, current management for these tumors avoids routine diagnostic biopsy when the clinical and neuroimaging features typical of diffuse pontomedullary brainstem gliomas are identified. Diagnostic biopsy is clearly indicated for brainstem mass lesions with an unusual MRI appearance or a highly atypical clinical course. Examples of these circumstances include the young child with a several-year history of slowly progressive clumsiness and facial asymmetry who may have a ganglioglioma of the brainstem or the child with the acute onset of facial weakness, ataxia, fever, and CSF pleocytosis who may have a focal brainstem encephalitis.

In general, there is no established role for the routine resection of diffuse intrinsic brainstem gliomas. Early in the clinical course, tumor cells infiltrate widely throughout brainstem structures but still permit neurologic function to remain at normal or near-normal levels. Consequently, removal of tumor is likely to result in severe neurologic deficits. However, some diffuse pontomedullary brainstem gliomas may have a cystic projection dorsally or laterally. These surface projections may provide a limited opportunity for tumor resection. However, it is uncommon that more than 50% of the tumor can be removed, and it is unlikely that limited debulking affects progression-free or total survival.

Diffuse pontomedullary brainstem gliomas are among the least responsive and most treatment-resistant childhood solid tumors. Conventional therapy consists of 54 to 60 Gy involved-field radiation therapy administered in single daily fractions of approximately 1.8 to 2 Gy. This approach results in median survival times of 9 to 13 months from diagnosis.[626] Despite encouraging single institution reports suggesting prolonged progression-free survival for children treated with hyperfractionated radiation therapy in which total radiation doses reached 78 Gy, larger cooperative trials failed to demonstrate a therapeutic advantage for this approach.[627-629] Radiation implants (i.e., brachytherapy) are not appropriate for these tumors, and the role of stereotactic radiosurgery has not been evaluated.

Chemotherapy trials for diffuse pontomedullary brainstem gliomas have yielded similarly disappointing results. Preradiation single-agent or combination chemotherapy infrequently produces objective (i.e., radiographic) response rates that exceed 25%.[626] Furthermore, it is unlikely that even these limited response rates

translate into significantly longer total survival. A phase III trials using CCNU, vincristine, and prednisone after radiation therapy failed to show a survival advantage when compared with radiation therapy alone.[630] The use of more aggressive chemotherapy strategies including high-dose chemotherapy followed by PBSC reinfusion results in relatively brief duration responses and few instances of significant tumor reduction lasting 12 months or longer.[631] Accordingly, it is difficult to support the routine use of chemotherapy in brainstem gliomas outside the setting of well-structured clinical trials.

Dorsally Exophytic Tumors

Dorsally exophytic tumors arise from the floor of the fourth ventricle, often completely fill the ventricle, and may have few if any neurologic signs for years before developing symptoms of obstructive hydrocephalus. MRI demonstrates a well-demarcated lesion, hyperintense on T2-weighted images and hypointense on T1-weighted images but enhancing with gadolinium (Fig. 69-29). Usually these lesions are low-grade fibrillary or pilocytic astrocytomas that are amenable to surgical resection. If substantial surgical tumor removal is achieved, often no adjuvant treatment is necessary and the patient is closely observed with serial MRI scans. Use of local radiation therapy or chemotherapy is limited to the uncommon cases of malignant dorsally exophytic gliomas or the occurrence of significant tumor growth after surgery.[632]

Cervicomedullary Tumors

Cervicomedullary tumors occupy the inferior two thirds of the medulla and the upper portion of the cervical spinal cord. These histologically low-grade gliomas tend

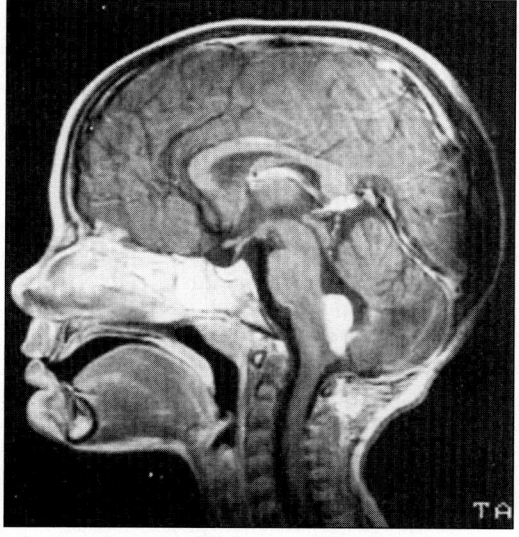

Figure 69-29. Dorsally exophytic brainstem glioma. Sagittal T1-weighted postgadolinium magnetic resonance imaging (MRI) scan shows intensely enhancing lesion filling fourth ventricle attached only at floor at level of pontomedullary junction. Enhancement is characteristic of juvenile pilocytic astrocytoma. (From Halperin EC, Constine LS, Tarbell NJ, Kun LE: Pediatric Radiation Oncology, 3rd ed. Lippincott, Williams & Wilkins, 1999, p 99.)

to extend from their cervicomedullary center in conformance with anatomic boundaries.[633] In contrast to midbrain tumors, intratumoral cysts are uncommon. The prediagnostic symptomatic interval may extend for several years. Surgical resection of these tumors is indicated upon clinical or radiographic evidence of tumor growth. Although near-total resection is possible, the poorly defined interface between tumor and normal brainstem often precludes complete surgical removal of these tumors. Long-term follow-up indicates that many patients will not have evidence of growth for more than 5 years. When tumor growth is observed, its rate is often extremely slow, and malignant transformation has not been observed. Similar to the dorsally exophytic tumors, radiation or chemotherapy is limited to those few cases in which progressive symptomatic tumor growth is observed and cannot be controlled by surgical approaches alone.

Cystic Nodular Brainstem Tumors

Cystic nodular brainstem tumors may be located in any region of the brainstem but are most often noted in the midbrain.[622] These tumors have a radiographic appearance identical to their cerebellar counterparts and histologically they typically resemble a juvenile pilocytic astrocytoma. Surgery is appropriate for those symptomatic patients with unequivocal evidence of tumor growth on neuroimaging studies. Where possible, resection of the mural nodule is usually curative. In cases in which the majority of the tumor is in the ventral midbrain, surgical options are limited to a diagnostic biopsy and treatment consists of radiation therapy or chemotherapy. Long-term survival for patients with these tumors is often in excess of 5 to 10 years and a conservative management approach is often advisable.

Adult Brainstem Gliomas

As discussed previously, brainstem gliomas in adults are much rarer than in children. They account for less than 2% of all adult brain tumors.[634] In one study of 48 adults with brainstem gliomas, the overall median survival was 5.4 years and the 3-year survival rate was 66%.[635] The authors categorized them into three different groups. The most frequent type (48% of cases) occurred in young adults and resembled the diffuse pontine glioma of childhood in terms of clinical and radiologic presentation. However, the overall outcome (median survival of 7.3 years) was much better than that of pediatric diffuse pontine gliomas. This may be because in adults many of these tumors were low-grade gliomas (9 of 11 patients who underwent biopsy had a benign histologic appearance). The other common tumor type (31%), which occurred in elderly patients, showed ringlike contrast enhancement and was associated with a median survival time of only 11 months. Tumors in this category that were biopsied were found to be high-grade gliomas. The third group (8%) consisted of focal tectal gliomas, which affected young adults and had a favorable outcome.

The conclusion that adults with this disease have a better prognosis than children was also reached in a study from Memorial Sloan-Kettering of 19 adult patients with brainstem gliomas. The authors found the median survival time to be 54 months and the 5-year survival rate to be 45%.[636]

Intracranial Germ Cell Tumors

Germ cell tumors (GCTs) constitute 12.5% to 16% of all childhood tumors in Japan but only 3% to 11% in the United States and Western European countries.[637] The majority are located in the pineal region, about a third in the suprasellar region. The clinical presentation of tumors involving the pineal region and their differential diagnosis is discussed ealier in the section, under "Tumors of the Spinal Axis." The clinical presentation of suprasellar GCTs includes panhypopituitarism, diabetes insipidus, and visual disturbances with usually long prediagnostic symptomatic intervals, often exceeding 1 year.

The neuroimaging characteristics of GCTs, suprasellar or pineal, do not provide sufficient differentiation between GCT histologic features to render biopsy unnecessary.[637,638] The diversity of tumor histologic types in the suprasellar/pineal region underscore the importance of adequate biopsy samples for accurate diagnosis. Small samples obtained from stereotactic biopsy may not identify mixed tumor types. Therefore, an open surgical biopsy approach, when possible, is preferred. Knowledge of histology influences surgical management. Complete resection is curative for well-differentiated teratomas. By contrast, chemotherapy and radiation therapies are ineffective for this tumor. The extent of surgical resection may be less important for germinomas, which are exquisitely sensitive to chemotherapy and radiation therapy or for the malignant nongerminomatous GCTs, which frequently spread throughout the CSF and are less responsive to radiation and chemotherapy.

Histologic findings also influence radiation treatment planning. Germinomas are very radiation sensitive. Of purely historical interest, 10 to 30 Gy "diagnostic" doses of radiation have been administered to unbiopsied suprasellar or pineal region tumors. If significant tumor reduction was observed, it was assumed to be a germinoma, and radiation therapy was continued to doses ranging from 40 to 56 Gy. This strategy is unacceptable in modern clinical practice for several reasons. Patients with mature teratoma and other radioresistant tumors are likely to be treated unnecessarily. Furthermore, nongerminomatous or mixed GCTs may respond briskly to radiotherapy, but may require craniospinal radiotherapy with then insufficient treatment volume. Finally, growing evidence shows that nongerminomatous or mixed GCTs benefit from chemotherapy and radiotherapy.

Identification of nongerminomatous or mixed GCTs may be facilitated by evaluation of specific markers in blood or CSF. α-Fetoprotein (AFP) is produced initially by the fetal yolk sac and later by hepatocytes. Detection of elevated levels of AFP in a CNS tumor patient implies the presence of primitive yolk sac elements (Table 69-17).[637] Beta human chorionic gonadotropin (β-HCG) is a marker for GCTs with syncytiotrophoblast activity. Although pure germinomas may express relatively low levels of β-HCG, choriocarcinomas produce the highest levels of this hormone (see Table 69-16). β-HCG expression is not a

TABLE 69-17

CSF and Serum Tumor Markers for Germ Cell Tumors

TUMOR	AFP	β-HCG
Germinoma	–	±
Nongerminomatous germ cell tumors		
Embryonal carcinoma	±	±
Yolk sac tumor	++	–
Choriocarcinoma	–	++
Teratoma, mature	–	–
Teratoma, immature-malignant	±	±
Mixed germ cell tumor	±	±

AFP, alpha-fetoprotein; β-HCG, beta-human chorionic gonadotropin.
Adapted from Kretschmar CS: Germ cell tumors of the brain in children; A review of current literature and new advances in therapy. Cancer Invest 1997;15:187.

marker of metastasis or tumor size. Placental alkaline phosphatase (PLAP) is another marker that has been found elevated in patients with GCTs.[639] Its diagnostic use lies more in immunohistochemistry. PLAP immunostaining is positive and diagnostically definitive for germinomas.[637]

Craniospinal radiation therapy is clearly indicated in cases of documented leptomeningeal metastasis from germinoma; however, its use in patients with normal CSF cytology and spinal MRI is controversial. In a series from the University of Pennsylvania in which 39 patients with biopsy-proved germinomas all received craniospinal irradiation, regardless of extent of disease, there have been no relapses with a median length of follow-up of 7.1 years and a 10-year survival rate of 97%.[640] However, other institutions using more limited radiation fields with or without chemotherapy for biopsy-proved germinomas have also reported 5-year survival rates exceeding 90%.[641,642]

In contrast to germinomas, nongerminomatous GCTs (choriocarcinoma, embryonal carcinoma, yolk sac tumors, and malignant teratomas) have a high incidence of leptomeningeal metastasis,[643] and craniospinal radiation therapy is an important component of their overall treatment plan. Well-differentiated teratomas are generally unresponsive to radiation, and use of radiation therapy is limited to unresectable recurrent or progressive teratomas in many centers. For these cases, stereotactic radiosurgery may prove to be of greater therapeutic benefit.

Chemotherapy has an important role in the treatment of many GCTs. Germinomas appear to be as sensitive to chemotherapy as they are to radiation.[644,645] Chemotherapy has been used effectively for germinomas in three settings: (1) chemotherapy without radiation therapy; (2) chemotherapy followed by reduced-dose radiation therapy for tumors with incomplete tumor response; (3) chemotherapy after radiation therapy for tumors with incomplete tumor response. Malignant nongerminomatous GCTs have a considerably worse prognosis than pure germinomas.[642] Accordingly, there have been attempts to improve survival in patients with nongerminomatous GCTs using intensified chemotherapy and multimodality therapeutic strategies.[646] A study of postoperative pre- and postradiation chemotherapy for patients with non-

germinomatous GCT, but no metastases, reported a 4-year progression-free survival rate of 74%.[647]

Craniopharyngioma

Craniopharyngiomas constitute 6% to 10% of all childhood brain tumors and represent one of the three major tumor groups frequently found in the suprasellar region. These tumors most likely arise from embryonic epithelial cell rests in the region of Rathke's cleft. Radiographically, their appearance typically includes a cystic or multicystic component as well as a solid component (Fig. 69-30). Calcifications are present in the majority of cases. Craniopharyngioma cyst fluid, similar to that of a Rathke's cleft cyst, is viscous and contains a high cholesterol content. Rupture of the cyst contents during surgical removal is well known to produce an intense chemical meningitis.

The clinical presentation of craniopharyngiomas is similar to other suprasellar tumors. The primary age of onset is in the first decade of life; however, presentation before 2 years of age is uncommon. Approximately 25% of craniopharyngiomas are detected in the third decade or later. The primary signs and symptoms include visual dysfunction, headache, optic pallor, endocrinopathies including growth failure and diabetes insipidus, and behavioral or learning dysfunction. Based on these findings, preoperative assessment of patients with suspected craniopharyngioma should include a thorough visual examination and endocrine evaluation.

Surgical removal of craniopharyngiomas is the primary therapeutic modality.[648] Complete surgical resection obviates the need for further therapy in the majority of cases. When postoperative MRI and intraoperative visual assessment show no evidence of tumor, the rate of recurrence is less than 20% and the majority of recurrences occur within the first 2 years after surgery.[649] However, the overall surgical approach to craniopharyngiomas remains

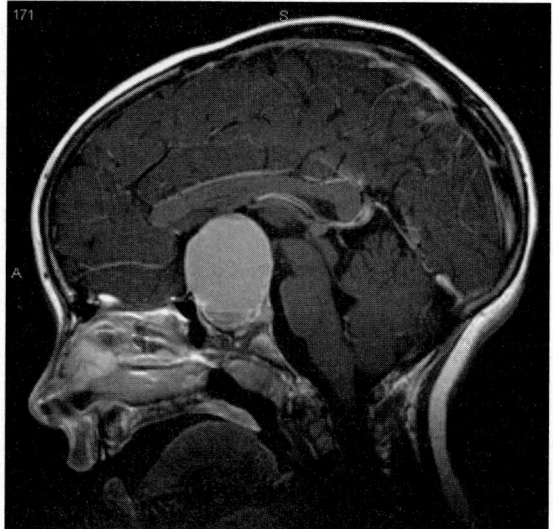

Figure 69-30. Magnetic resonance imaging (MRI) scan: Craniopharyngioma. Sagittal T1-weighted postgadolinium MRI shows enhancing cystic suprasellar mass.

the subject of considerable disagreement. Gross total resection is often achieved at the expense of panhypopituitarism and behavioral and neuropsychological dysfunction, which often severely affects the patient's quality of life.[650-652]

An alternative surgical strategy involves planned incomplete resection followed by radiation therapy. Radiation therapy represents standard treatment for patients with residual craniopharyngioma.[652-657] Less than 50% of patients with known postoperative residual disease who are not treated with radiation therapy will survive for 10 years. By contrast, those treated with local field radiation, typically using doses of 50 to 56 Gy, have disease-free survival rates of approximately 80% at 10 years. Recent studies suggest that quality of life may be better for these patients than for children treated with aggressive surgical resection alone.[654]

There is no established role for chemotherapy in the treatment of craniopharyngioma. However, in patients who recur following external beam radiation with primarily a cystic component, a technique that may be useful is the instillation of colloidal β-emitting radionuclides, such as ^{32}P or ^{90}Yt.[658-660] This technique has also been used in some patients as first-line therapy.

Brain Tumors in Infants

Approximately 20% of childhood brain tumors occur in infants and young children less than 3 years of age. Unfortunately, the survival outcomes in this age group have been significantly less favorable compared with older children, both overall and for specific tumor types.[661] These infants are also at increased risk for substantial radiation-related neurotoxicity, including mental retardation, growth failure, and leukoencephalopathy.[662,663] Therefore, primary postoperative chemotherapy approaches have been adopted with the aim to postpone or even to avoid radiation therapy. Between 1976 and 1988, 17 children younger than 3 years with PNET/MB or ependymoma were treated with a multiagent chemotherapy including mechlorethamine, vincristine, procarbazine, and prednisone (MOPP).[664] Radiotherapy was reserved for recurrent disease. Eight of 12 children with PNET/MB and 2 of 5 children with ependymoma survived, and those children who did not require radiation showed normal height and intellectual ability. Although a subset of infant PNET/MB can be cured by chemotherapy alone,[662,665] expectations that more of these children do well by using intensive multiagent chemotherapy have not been realized. Current cooperative group studies are testing chemotherapy dose intensification, addition of intrathecal chemotherapy, and earlier introduction of more limited radiation therapy, restricting treatment volume and further limiting normal tissue irradiation by using conformal techniques.

REFERENCES

1. CBTRUS (Central Brain Tumor Registry of the United States): 2002-2003 Report on Primary Brain Tumors in the United States. Chicago, Central Brain Tumor Registry of the United States, 2003.
2. Cancer Facts & Figures 2002. American Cancer Society, Surveillance Research, Atlanta, 2002.
3. Legler JM, Ries LA, Smith MA, et al: Cancer surveillance series [corrected]: Brain and other central nervous system cancers: Recent trends in incidence and mortality. J Natl Cancer Inst 1999;91:1382.
4. Shu XO, Jin F, Linet MS, et al: Diagnostic x-ray and ultrasound exposure and risk of childhood cancer. Br J Cancer 1994;70:531.
5. Shore RE, Albert RE, Pasternack BS: Follow-up study of patients treated by x-ray epilation for tinea capitis; resurvey of post-treatment illness and mortality experience. Arch Environ Health 1976;31:21.
6. Shapiro S, Mealey JJ, Sartorius C: Radiation-induced intracranial malignant gliomas. J Neurosurg 1989;71:77.
7. Relling MV, Rubnitz JE, Rivera GK, et al: High incidence of secondary brain tumours after radiotherapy and antimetabolities. Lancet 1999;354:34.
8. Liwnicz BH, Berger TS, Liwnicz RG, et al: Radiation-associated gliomas: A report of four cases and analysis of postradiation tumors of the central nervous system. Neurosurgery 1985;17:436.
9. Ron E, Modan B, Boice JD Jr, et al: Tumors of the brain and nervous system after radiotherapy in childhood. N Engl J Med 1988;319:1033.
10. Karlsson P, Holmberg E, Lundell M, et al: Intracranial tumors after exposure to ionizing radiation during infancy: A pooled analysis of two Swedish cohorts of 28,008 infants with skin hemangioma. Radiat Res 1998;150:357.
11. Jenkinson H, Hawkins M: Secondary brain tumours in children with ALL. Lancet 1999;354:1126.
12. Walter AW, Hancock ML, Pui CH, et al: Secondary brain tumors in children treated for acute lymphoblastic leukemia at St. Jude Children's Research Hospital. J Clin Oncol 1998;16:3761.
13. Loning L, Zimmermann M, Reiter A, et al: Secondary neoplasms subsequent to Berlin-Frankfurt-Munster therapy of acute lymphoblastic leukemia in childhood: Significantly lower risk without cranial radiotherapy. Blood 2000;95:2770.
14. Neglia JP, Meadows AT, Robison LL, et al: Second neoplasms after acute lymphoblastic leukemia in childhood. N Engl J Med 1991;325:1330.
15. Duffner PK, Krischer JP, Horowitz ME, et al: Second malignancies in young children with primary brain tumors following treatment with prolonged postoperative chemotherapy and delayed irradiation: A Pediatric Oncology Group Study. Ann Neurol 1998;44:313.
16. Shapiro S, Mealy JJ: Late anaplastic gliomas in children previously treated for acute lmphoblastic leukemia. Pediatr Neurosci 1989;15:176.
17. Barth RF: Rat brain tumor models in experimental neuro-oncology: The 9L, C6, T9, F98, RG2 (D74), RT-2 and CNS-1 gliomas. J Neurooncol 1998;36:91.
18. Berleur MP, Cordier S: The role of chemical, physical, or viral exposures and health factors in neurocarcinogenesis: Implications for epidemiologic studies of brain tumors. Cancer Causes Control 1995;6:240.
19. Butel JS, Lednicky JA: Cell and molecular bilogy of simian virus 40: Implications for human infections and disease. J Natl Cancer Inst 1999;91:119.
20. Walsh JW, Zimmer SG, Perdue ML: Role of viruses in the induction of primary intracranial tumors. Neurosurgery 1982;10:643.
21. Weggen S, Bayer TA, von Deimling A: Low frequency of SV40, JC and BK polyomavirus sequences in human medulloblastomas, meningiomas and ependymomas. Brain Pathol 2000;10:85.
22. Wrensch M, Minn Y, Chew T, et al: Epidemiology of primary brain tumors: Current concepts and review of the literature. Neurooncol 2002;4:278.
23. McLaughlin JK, Lipworth L: A critical review of the epidemiologic literature on health effects of occupational exposure to vinyl chloride. J Epidemiol Biostat 1999;4:253.
24. Bohnen NI, Kurland LT: Brain tumor and exposure to pesticides in humans: A review of the epidemiologic data. J Neurol Sci 1995;132:110.
25. Wong O, Raabe GK: A critical review of cancer epidemiology in the petroleum industry, with a meta-analysis of a combined

database of more than 350,000 workers. Regul Toxicol Pharmacol 2000;32:78.

26. Inskip PD, Tarone RE, Hatch EE, et al: Cellular-telephone use and brain tumors. N Engl J Med 2001;344:79.

27. Muscat JE, Malkin MG, Thompson S, et al: Handheld cellular telephone use and risk of brain cancer. JAMA 2000;284:3001.

28. Narod SA, Stiller C, Lenoir GM: An estimate of the heritable fraction of childhood cancer. Br J Cancer 1991;63:993.

29. Kimmelman A, Liang BC: Familial neurogenic tumor syndromes. Hematol Oncol Clin North Am 2001;15:1073.

30. Listerncik R, Louis DN, Packer RJ, et al: Optic pathway gliomas in children with neurofibromatosis 1: Consensus statement from the NF1 Optic Pathway Glioma Task Force. Ann Neurol 1997;41:143.

31. Evans DG, Huson SM, Donnai D, et al: A genetic study of type 2 neurofibromatosis in the United Kingdom. II. Guidelines for genetic counselling. J Med Genet 1992;29:847.

32. Feldkamp MM, Lau N, Guha A: Signal transduction pathways and their relevance in human astrocytomas. J Neurooncol 1997;35:223.

33. Kirsch M, Wilson JC, Black P: Platelet-derived growth factor in human brain tumors. J Neurooncol 1997;35:289.

34. Guha A, Dashner K, Black PM, et al: Expression of PDGF and PDGF receptors in human astrocytoma operation supports the existence of an autocrine loop. Int J Cancer 1995;60:168.

35. Glick RP, Lichtor T, Unterman TG: Insulin-like growth factors in central nervous system tumors. J Neurooncol 1997;35:315.

36. Tang P, Steck PA, Yung WK: The autocrine loop of TGF-alpha/EGFR and brain tumors. J Neurooncol 1997;35:303.

37. Schmidt NO, Westphal M, Hagel C, et al: Levels of vascular endothelial growth factor, hepatocyte growth factor/scatter factor and basic fibroblast growth factor in human gliomas and their relation to angiogenesis. Int J Cancer 1999;84:10.

38. Rosen EM, Laterra J, Joseph A, et al: Scatter factor expression and regulation in human glial tumors. Int J Cancer 1996;67:248.

39. Campbell JW, Pollack IF: Growth factors in gliomas: Antisense and dominant negative mutant strategies. J Neurooncol 1997;35:275.

40. Rempel SA: Molecular biology of nervous system tumors. Hematol Oncol Clin North Am 2001;15:979.

41. Haas-Kogan D, Shalev N, Wong M, et al: Protein kinase B (PKB/Akt) activity is elevated in glioblastoma cells due to mutation of the tumor suppressor PTEN/MMAC. Curr Biol 1998;8:1195.

42. Couldwell WT, Antel JP, Yong VW: Protein kinase C activity correlates with the growth rate of malignant gliomas: Part II. Effects of glioma mitogens and modulators of protein kinase C. Neurosurgery 1992;31:717.

43. Feldkamp MM, Lala D, Lau N, et al: Expression of activated epidermal growth factor receptors, Ras-guanosine triphosphate, and mitogen-activated protein kinase in human glioblastoma multiforme specimens. Neurosurgery 1999;45:1442.

44. Bos JL: ras oncogenes in human cancer: A review [published erratum appears in Cancer Res 1990;50(4):1352]. Cancer Res 1989;49:4682.

45. Guha A: Ras activation in astrocytomas and neurofibromas. Can J Neurol Sci 1998;25:267.

46. Feldkamp MM, Lau N, Guha A: Growth inhibition of astrocytoma cells by farnesyl transferase inhibitors is mediated by a combination of anti-proliferative, pro-apoptotic and anti-angiogenic effects. Oncogene 1999;18:7514.

47. Feldkamp MM, Lau N, Roncari L, et al: Isotype-specific Ras. GTP-levels predict the efficacy of farnesyl transferase inhibitors against human astrocytomas regardless of Ras mutational status. Cancer Res 2001;61:4425.

48. Woods SA, Marmor E, Feldkamp M, et al: Aberrant G protein signaling in nervous system tumors. J Neurosurg 2002;97:627.

49. Weber RG, Bostrom J, Wolter M, et al: Analysis of genomic alterations in benign, atypical, and anaplastic meningiomas: Toward a genetic model of meningioma progression. Proc Natl Acad Sci USA 1997;94:14719.

50. Chan AS, Leung SY, Wong MP, et al: Expression of vascular endothelial growth factor and its receptors in the anaplastic progression of astrocytoma, oligodendroglioma, and ependymoma. Am J Surg Pathol 1998;22:816.

51. Lamszus K, Lengler U, Schmidt NO, et al: Vascular endothelial growth factor, hepatocyte growth factor/scatter factor, basic fibroblast growth factor, and placenta growth factor in human meningiomas and their relation to angiogenesis and malignancy. Neurosurgery 2000;46:938.

52. Jensen RL: Growth factor-mediated angiogenesis in the malignant progression of glial tumors: A review. Surg Neurol 1998;49:189.

53. Hsu SC, Volpert OV, Steck PA, et al: Inhibition of angiogenesis in human glioblastomas by chromosome 10 induction of thrombospondin-1. Cancer Res 1996;56:5684.

54. Nakagawa T, Kubota T, Kabuto M, et al: Production of matrix metalloproteinases and tissue inhibitor of metalloproteinases-1 by human brain tumors. J Neurosurg 1994;81:69.

55. Lakka SS, Rajan M, Gondi C, et al: Adenovirus-mediated expression of antisense MMP-9 in glioma cells inhibits tumor growth and invasion. Oncogene 2002;21:8011.

56. Mohanam S, Gladson CL, Rao CN, et al: Biological significance of the expression of urokinase-type plasminogen activator receptors (uPARs) in brain tumors. Frontiers Biosci 1999;4:D178.

57. Gladson CL, Wilcox JN, Sanders L, et al: Cerebral microenvironment influences expression of the vitronectin gene in astrocytic tumors. J Cell Sci 1995;108(Pt 3):947.

58. Mohanam S, Jasti SL, Kondraganti SR, et al: Stable transfection of urokinase-type plasminogen activator antisense construct modulates invasion of human glioblastoma cells. Clin Cancer Res 2001;7:2519.

59. Mohanam S, Chandrasekar N, Yanamandra N, et al: Modulation of invasive properties of human glioblastoma cells stably expressing amino-terminal fragment of urokinase-type plasminogen activator. Oncogene 2002;21:7824.

60. Gladson CL: The extracellular matrix of gliomas: Modulation of cell function. J Neuropathol Exp Neurol 1999;58:1029.

61. Uhm JH, Gladson CL, Rao JS: The role of integrins in the malignant phenotype of gliomas. Frontiers Biosci 1999;4:D188.

62. Knott JC, Mahesparan R, Garcia-Cabrera I, et al: Stimulation of extracellular matrix components in the normal brain by invading glioma cells. Int J Cancer 1998;75:864.

63. Witwer BP, Moftakhar R, Hasan KM, et al: Diffusion-tensor imaging of white matter tracts in patients with cerebral neoplasm. J Neurosurg 2002;97:568.

64. Holodny AI, Ollenschlager M: Diffusion imaging in brain tumors. Neuroimaging Clin North Am 2002;12:107.

65. Sinha S, Bastin ME, Whittle IR, et al: Diffusion tensor MR imaging of high-grade cerebral gliomas. Am J Neuroradiol 2002;23:520.

66. Mori S, Frederiksen K, van Zijl PC, et al: Brain white matter anatomy of tumor patients evaluated with diffusion tensor imaging. Ann Neurol 2002;51:377.

67. Plum F, Posner JB: The Diagnosis of Stupor and Coma, 3rd ed. Philadelphia, Davis, 1980, pp 87–116.

68. Kernohan JW, Woltman HW: Incisura of the crus due to contralateral brain tumor. Arch Neurol Psychiatry 1929;21:274.

69. Cushing H: Concerning a definite regulatory mechanism of the vasomotor centre which controls blood pressure during cerebral compression. Bull Johns Hopkins Hosp 1901;12:290.

70. Cushing H: Some experimental and clinical observations concerning states of increased intracranial tension. 1902;124:375.

71. Forsyth PA, Posner JB: Headaches in patients with brain tumors: A study of 111 patients. Neurology 1993;43:1678.

72. Hughes JR, Zak SM: EEG and clinical changes in patients with chronic seizures associated with slowly growing brain tumors. Arch Neurol 1987;44:540.

73. Moots PL, Maciunas RJ, Eisert DR, et al: The course of seizure disorders in patients with malignant gliomas. Arch Neurol 1995;52:717.

74. Bartolomei JC, Christopher S, Vives K, et al: Low-grade gliomas of chronic epilepsy: A distinct clinical and pathological entity. J Neurooncol 1997;34:79.

75. Huber A: Eye Symptoms in Brain Tumors, 2nd ed. St. Louis, Mosby, 1971.

76. Watling CJ, Cairncross JG: Acetazolamide therapy for symptomatic plateau waves in patients with brain tumors. Report of three cases. J Neurosurg 2002;97:224.

77. Dropcho EJ, Soong SJ: Steroid-induced weakness in patients with primary brain tumors. Neurology 1991;41:1235.

78. Schiff D: Pneumocystis pneumonia in brain tumor patients: Risk factors and clinical features. J Neurooncol 1996;27:235.

79. Gluck T, Geerdes-Fenge HF, Straub RH, et al: Pneumocystis carinii pneumonia as a complication of immunosuppressive therapy. Infection 2000;28:227.

80. Krasner AS: Glucocorticoid-induced adrenal insufficiency. JAMA 1999;282:671.

81. Coursin DB, Wood KE: Corticosteroid supplementation for adrenal insufficiency. JAMA 2002;287:236.

82. Delattre JY, Safai B, Posner JB: Erythema multiforme and Stevens-Johnson syndrome in patients receiving cranial irradiation and phenytoin. Neurology 1988;38:194.

83. Mamon HJ, Wen PY, Burns AC, et al: Allergic skin reactions to anticonvulsant medications in patients receiving cranial radiation therapy. Epilepsia 1999;40:341.

84. Weaver S, DeAngelis LM, Fulton D, et al: A prospective radnomized study of prophylactic anticonvulsants in patients with primary or metastatic brain tumors or metastatic brain tumors with or without prior seizures. Ann Neurol 1997;42:430.

85. Forsyth PA, Weaver S, Fulton D, et al: Prophylactic anticonvulsants in patients with brain tumour. Can J Neurol Sci 2003;30:106.

86. Foy PM, Chadwick DW, Rajgopalan N, et al: Do prophylactic anticonvulsant drugs alter the pattern of seizures after craniotomy? J Neurol Neurosurg Psychiatry 1992;55:753.

87. Glantz MJ, Cole BF, Forsyth PA, et al: Practice parameter: anticonvulsant prophylaxis in patients with newly diagnosed brain tumors. Report of the Quality Standards Subcommittee of the American Academy of Neurology. Neurology 2000;54:1886.

88. Brandes AA, Scelzi E, Salmistraro G, et al: Incidence of risk of thromboembolism during treatment of high-grade gliomas: A prospective study. Eur J Cancer 1997;33:1592.

89. Chan AT, Atiemo A, Diran LK, et al: Venous thromboembolism occurs frequently in patients undergoing brain tumor surgery despite prophylaxis. J Thromb Thrombolysis 1999;8:139.

90. Levin JM, Schiff D, Loeffler JS, et al: Complications of therapy for venous thromboembolic disease in patients with brain tumors. Neurology 1993;43:1111.

91. Iorio A, Agnelli G: Low-molecular-weight and unfractionated heparin for prevention of venous thromboembolism in neurosurgery: A meta-analysis. Arch Intern Med 2000;160:2327.

92. Agnelli G, Piovella F, Buoncristiani P, et al: Enoxaparin plus compression stockings compared with compression stockings alone in the prevention of venous thromboembolism after elective neurosurgery. N Engl J Med 1998;339:80.

93. Goldhaber SZ, Dunn K, Gerhard-Herman M, et al: Low rate of venous thromboembolism after craniotomy for brain tumor using multimodality prophylaxis. Chest 2002;122:1933.

94. Chamberlain MC: Current concepts in leptomeningeal metastasis. Curr Opin Oncol 1992;4:533.

95. Grossman SA, Moynihan TJ: Neoplastic meningitis. Neurol Clin 1991;9:843.

96. Kaplan JG, DeSouza TG, Farkash A, et al: Leptomeningeal metastases: Comparison of clinical features and laboratory data of solid tumors, lymphomas and leukemias. J Neurooncol 1990; 9:225.

97. Wasserstrom WR, Glass JP, Posner JB: Diagnosis and treatment of leptomeningeal metastases from solid tumors: Experience with 90 patients. Cancer 1982;49:759.

98. Kelly PJ, Daumas-Duport C, Kispert DB, et al: Imaging-based stereotaxic serial biopsies in untreated intracranial glial neoplasms. J Neurosurg 1987;66:865.

99. Pruel C, Kuhn B, Lang E, et al: Differentiation of cerebral tumors using multi-section echoplanar MR perfusion imaging. Eur J Radiol 2003;48:244–251.

100. Uematsu H, Maeda M, Sadato N, et al: Blood volume of gliomas determined by double-echo dynamic perfusion-weighted MR imaging: A preliminary study. Am J Neuroradiol 2001; 22:1915.

101. Maeda M, Itoh S, Kimura H, et al: Vascularity of meningiomas and neuromas: Assessment with dynamic susceptibility-contrast MR imaging. Am J Roentgenol 1994;163:181.

102. Alsop DC, Detre JA, D'Esposito M, et al: Functional activation during an auditory comprehension task in patients with temporal lobe lesions. Neuroimage 1996;4:55.

103. Atlas SW, Howard RS 2nd, Maldjian J, et al: Functional magnetic resonance imaging of regional brain activity in patients with intracerebral gliomas: Findings and implications for clinical management. Neurosurgery 1996;38:329.

104. Roux FE, Boulanouar K, Ranjeva JP, et al: Usefulness of motor functional MRI correlated to cortical mapping in Rolandic low-grade astrocytomas. Acta Neurochir (Wien) 1999;141:71.

105. Maldjian JA, Schulder M, Liu WC, et al: Intraoperative functional MRI using a real-time neurosurgical navigation system. J Comput Assist Tomogr 1997;21:910.

106. Nelson SJ, Vigneron DB, Dillon WP: Serial evaluation of patients with brain tumors using volume MRI and 3D 1H MRSI. NMR Biomed 1999;12:123.

107. Wong F, Kim E: Nuclear medicine studies. In Levin V (ed): Cancer in the Nervous System. New York, Churchill Livingstone, 1996, p 50.

108. Hart MN, Petito CK, Earle KM: Mixed gliomas. Cancer 1974;33:134.

109. Bruhn H, Frahm J, Gyngell ML, et al: Noninvasive differentiation of tumors with use of localized H-1 MR spectroscopy in vivo: Initial experience in patients with cerebral tumors. Radiology 1989;172:541.

110. Sutton LN, Lenkinski RE, Cohen BH, et al: Localized 31P magnetic resonance spectroscopy of large pediatric brain tumors. J Neurosurg 1990;72:65.

111. McKeran RO, Thomas DGT: Clinical study of gliomas. In Graham DI (ed): Brain Tumors: Scientific Basis, Clinical Investigation, and Current Therapy. Boston, Butterswoth, 1980, p 194.

112. Telfeian AE, Philips MF, Crino PB, et al: Postoperative epilepsy in patients undergoing craniotomy for glioblastoma multiforme. J Exp Clin Cancer Res 2001;20:5.

113. Kjellberg RN, Hanamura T, Davis KR, et al: Bragg-peak proton-beam therapy for arteriovenous malformations of the brain. N Engl J Med 1983;309:269.

114. Schultheiss TE, Kun LE, Ang KK, et al: Radiation response of the central nervous system. Int J Radiat Oncol Biol Phys 1995;31:1093.

115. Freeman JE, Johnston PG, Voke JM: Somnolence after prophylactic cranial irradiation in children with acute lymphoblastic leukaemia. BMJ 1973;4:523.

116. Cohen ME, Duffner PK: Long-term consequences of CNS treatment for childhood cancer, Part I: Pathologic consequences and potential for oncogenesis. Pediatr Neurol 1991;7:157.

117. Duffner PK, Cohen ME: Long-term consequences of CNS treatment for childhood cancer, Part II: Clinical consequences. Pediatr Neurol 1991;7:237.

118. Constine LS, Konski A, Ekholm S, et al: Adverse effects of brain irradiation correlated with MR and CT imaging. Int J Radiat Oncol Biol Phys 1988;15:319.

119. Buchpiguel CA, Alavi JB, Alavi A, et al: PET versus SPECT in distinguishing radiation necrosis from tumor recurrence in the brain. J Nucl Med 1995;36:159.

120. Phillips PC: Positron emission tomography studies of transport and metabolism in brain tumors. In Packer R, Bleyer WA, Pochedly C (eds): Pediatric Neuro-Oncology. Philadelphia, Harwood Academic Publishers, 1992, pp 91–110.

121. Di Chiro G, Oldfield E, Wright DC, et al: Cerebral necrosis after radiotherapy and/or intraarterial chemotherapy for brain tumors: PET and neuropathologic studies. Am J Roentgenol 1988;150:189.

122. Burger PC, Mahley MS Jr, Dudka L, et al: The morphologic effects of radiation administered therapeutically for intracranial gliomas: A postmortem study of 25 cases. Cancer 1979;44:1256.

123. Shaw E, Arusell R, Scheithauer B, et al: Prospective randomized trial of low- versus high-dose radiation therapy in adults with supratentorial low-grade glioma: Initial report of a North Central Cancer Treatment Group/Radiation Therapy Oncology Group/ Eastern Cooperative Oncology Group study. J Clin Oncol 2002;20:2267.

124. Jankovic M, Brouwers P, Valsecchi MG, et al: Association of 1800 cGy cranial irradiation with intellectual function in children with acute lymphoblastic leukaemia. ISPACC. International Study Group on Psychosocial Aspects of Childhood Cancer. Lancet 1994;344:224.

125. Meadows AT, Gordon J, Massari DJ, et al: Declines in IQ scores and cognitive dysfunctions in children with acute lymphocytic leukaemia treated with cranial irradiation. Lancet 1981;2:1015.

Specific Malignancies

III

126. Ochs J, Mulhern R, Fairclough D, et al: Comparison of neuropsychologic functioning and clinical indicators of neurotoxicity in long-term survivors of childhood leukemia given cranial radiation or parenteral methotrexate: A prospective study. J Clin Oncol 1991;9:145.

127. Mulhern RK, Fairclough D, Ochs J: A prospective comparison of neuropsychologic performance of children surviving leukemia who received 18-Gy, 24-Gy, or no cranial irradiation. J Clin Oncol 1991;9:1348.

128. Mulhern RK, Wasserman AL, Fairclough D, et al: Memory function in disease-free survivors of childhood acute lymphocytic leukemia given CNS prophylaxis with or without 1,800 cGy cranial irradiation. J Clin Oncol 1988;6:315.

129. Halberg FE, Kramer JH, Moore IM, et al: Prophylactic cranial irradiation dose effects on late cognitive function in children treated for acute lymphoblastic leukemia. Int J Radiat Oncol Biol Phys 1992;22:13.

130. Waber DP, Tarbell NJ, Fairclough D, et al: Cognitive sequelae of treatment in childhood acute lymphoblastic leukemia: Cranial radiation requires an accomplice. J Clin Oncol 1995;13:2490.

131. Dennis M, Spiegler BJ, Hetherington CR, et al: Neuropsychological sequelae of the treatment of children with medulloblastoma. J Neurooncol 1996;29:91.

132. Kramer JH, Crowe AB, Larson DA, et al: Neuropsychological sequelae of medulloblastoma in adults. Int J Radiat Oncol Biol Phys 1997;38:21.

133. Palmer SL, Goloubeva O, Reddick WE, et al: Patterns of intellectual development among survivors of pediatric medulloblastoma: A longitudinal analysis. J Clin Oncol 2001;19:2302.

134. Mulhern RK, Palmer SL, Reddick WE, et al: Risks of young age for selected neurocognitive deficits in medulloblastoma are associated with white matter loss. J Clin Oncol 2001;19:472.

135. Mulhern RK, Reddick WE, Palmer SL, et al: Neurocognitive deficits in medulloblastoma survivors and white matter loss. Ann Neurol 1999;46:834.

136. Mulhern RK, Hancock J, Fairclough D, et al: Neuropsychological status of children treated for brain tumors: A critical review and integrative analysis. Med Pediatr Oncol 1992;20:181.

137. Jenney MEM: Theoretical issues pertinent to measurement of quality of life. Med Pediatr Oncol Suppl 1998;I:41.

138. Bradlyn AS, Ritchey AK, Harris CV, et al: Quality of life research in pediatric oncology. Research methods and barriers. Cancer 1996;78:1333.

139. Bleyer WA: Neurologic sequelae of methotrexate and ionizing radiation: A new classification. Cancer Treat Rep 1981;65(Suppl 1):89.

140. Griffin T: White matter necrosis, micoangiopathy and intellectual abilities in survivors of childhood leukemia. Association with central nervous system irradiation and methotrexate toxicity. In Gilbert HA, Kagan AR (eds): Radiation Damage to the Central Nervous System. New York, Raven, 1980, p 155.

141. Taphoorn MJ, Schiphorst AK, Snoek FJ, et al: Cognitive functions and quality of life in patients with low-grade gliomas: The impact of radiotherapy. Ann Neurol 1994;36:48.

142. Vigliani MC, Sichez N, Poisson M, et al: A prospective study of cognitive functions following conventional radiotherapy for supratentorial gliomas in young adults: 4-year results. Int J Radiat Oncol Biol Phys 1996;35:527.

143. Brown PD, Buckner JC, Brown CA, et al: The effects of radiation on cognitive function in patients with low-grade glioma. Int J Radiat Oncol Biol Phys 2001;51(Suppl 1):135.

144. Armstrong CL, Hunter JV, Ledakis GE, et al: Late cognitive and radiographic changes related to radiotherapy: Initial prospective findings. Neurology 2002;59:40.

145. Brown PD, Buckner JC, Uhm JH, et al: The neurocognitive effects of radiation in adult low-grade glioma patients. Neuro-oncology 2003;5:161.

146. Archibald YM, Lunn D, Ruttan LA, et al: Cognitive functioning in long-term survivors of high-grade glioma. J Neurosurg 1994;80:247.

147. Mitchell WG, Fishman LS, Miller JH, et al: Stroke as a late sequela of cranial irradiation for childhood brain tumors. J Child Neurol 1991;6:128.

148. Livesey EA, Hindmarsh PC, Brook CG, et al: Endocrine disorders following treatment of childhood brain tumors. Br J Cancer 1990;61:622.

149. Sklar CA, Constine LS: Chronic neuroendocrinological sequelae of radiation therapy. Int J Radiat Oncol Biol Phys 1995;31:1113.

150. Oberfield SE, Chin D, Uli N, et al: Endocrine late efects of childhood cancers. J Pediatr 1997;131:S37.

151. Rappaport R, Brauner R: Growth and endocrine disorders secondary to cranial irradiation. Pediatr Res 1989;25:561.

152. Clayton PE, Shalet SM: Dose dependency of time of onset of radiation-induced growth hormone deficiency. J Pediatr 1991;118:226.

153. Sklar CA: Growth and neuroendocrine dysfunction following therapy for childhood cancer. Pediatr Clin North Am 1997;44:489.

154. Leiper AD, Stanhope R, Kitching P, et al: Precocious and premature puberty associated with treatment of acute lymphoblastic leukaemia. Arch Dis Child 1987;62:1107.

155. Oberfield SE, Allen JC, Pollack J: Long-term endocrine sequeale after treatment of medulloblastoma: Prospective study of growth and thyroid function. J Pediatr 1986;108:219.

156. Constine LS, Woolf PD, Cann D, et al: Hypothalamic-pituitary dysfunction after radiation for brain tumors. N Engl J Med 1993;328:87.

157. Ogilvy-Stuart AL, Shalet SM, Gattamaneni HR: Thyroid function after treatment of brain tumors in children. J Pediatr 1991;119:733.

158. Parsons JT, Bova FJ, Fitzgerald CR, et al: Radiation optic neuropathy after megavoltage external-beam irradiation: Analysis of time-dose factors. Int J Radiat Oncol Biol Phys 1994;30:755.

159. Kline LB, Kim JY, Ceballos R: Radiation optic neuropathy. Ophthalmology 1985;92:1118.

160. Young WC, Thornton AF, Gebarski SS, et al: Radiation-induced optic neuropathy: correlation of MR imaging and radiation dosimetry. Radiology 1992;185:904.

161. Aristizabal S, Caldwell WL, Avila J: The relationship of time-dose fractionation factors to complications in the treatment of pituitary tumors by irradiation. Int J Radiat Oncol Biol Phys 1977;2:667.

162. Harris JR, Levene MB: Visual complications following irradiation for pituitary adenomas and craniopharyngiomas. Radiology 1976;120:167.

163. Hawkins MM, Draper GJ, Kingston JE: Incidence of second primary tumours among childhood cancer survivors. Br J Cancer 1987;56:339.

164. Jones A: Transient radiation myelopathy. Br J Radiol 1964;37:727.

165. Schultheiss TE, Stephens LC, Peters LJ: Survival in radiation myelopathy. Int J Radiat Oncol Biol Phys 1986;12:1765.

166. Wang PY, Shen WC, Jan JS: MR imaging in radiation myelopathy. Am J Neuroradiol 1992;13:1049.

167. Marcus RB Jr, Million RR: The incidence of myelitis after irradiation of the cervical spinal cord. Int J Radiat Oncol Biol Phys 1990;19:3.

168. Watling CJ, Lee DH, Macdonald DR, et al: Corticosteroid-induced magnetic resonance imaging changes in patients with recurrent malignant glioma. J Clin Oncol 1994;12:1886.

169. Hochberg FH, Pruitt A: Assumptions in the radiotherapy of glioblastoma. Neurology 1980;30:907.

170. Schinkel AH: The roles of P-glycoprotein and MRP1 in the blood-brain and blood-cerebrospinal fluid barriers. Adv Exp Med Biol 2001;500:365.

171. Toth K, Vaughan MM, Peress NS, et al: MDR1 P-glycoprotein is expressed by endothelial cells of newly formed capillaries in human gliomas but is not expressed in the neovasculature of other primary tumors. Am J Pathol 1996;149:853.

172. Fellner S, Bauer B, Miller DS, et al: Transport of paclitaxel (Taxol) across the blood-brain barrier in vitro and in vivo. J Clin Invest 2001;110:1309.

173. Scheck A: Molecular biology of chemotherapy and resistance. Barrow Neurol Inst Q 1998;14:43.

174. Becker I, Becker KF, Meyermann R, et al: The multidrug-resistance gene MDR1 is expressed in human glial tumors. Acta Neuropathol 1991;82:516.

175. Anda T, Shabani HK, Tsunoda K, et al: Relationship between expression of O6-methylguanine-DNA methyltransferase, glutathione-S-transferase pi in glioblastoma and the survival of the

patients treated with nimustine hydrochloride: An immunohisto-chemical analysis. Neurol Res 2003;25:241.

176. Ali-Osman F, Antoun G, Wang H, et al: Buthionine sulfoximine induction of gamma-L-glutamyl-L-cysteine synthetase gene expression, kinetics of glutathione depletion and resynthesis, and modulation of carmustine-induced DNA-DNA cross-linking and cytotoxicity in human glioma cells. Mol Pharmacol 1996;49:1012.

177. Mass M, Remsen L, McCormick C, et al: Neurotoxicity of chemotherapeutic agents and immunoconjugates delivered after blood-brain barrier modification neuropathoilogical studies (abstract). Ann Neurol 1995;38:342.

178. Shapiro WR, Green SB, Burger PC, et al: A randomized comparison of intra-arterial versus intravenous BCNU, with or without intravenous 5-fluorouracil, for newly diagnosed patients with malignant glioma. J Neurosurg 1992;76:772.

179. Kapp J, Vance R, Parker JL, et al: Limitations of high dose intra-arterial 1,3-bis(2-chloroethyl)-1-nitrosourea (BCNU) chemotherapy for malignant gliomas. Neurosurgery 1982;10:715.

180. Silvani A, Eoli M, Salmaggi A, et al: Intra-arterial ACNU and carboplatin versus intravenous chemotherapy with cisplatin and BCNU in newly diagnosed patients with glioblastoma. Neurol Sci 2002;23:219.

181. Watanabe W, Kuwubara R, Nakahaa T: Severe ocular and orbital toxicity after intracarotid injection of carboplatin for recurrent glioblastomas. Ophthalmology 2002;240:1033.

182. Prados MD, Schold SJS, Fine HA, et al: A randomized, double-blind, placebo-controlled, phase 2 study of RMP-7 in combination with carboplatin administered intravenously for the treatment of recurrent malignant glioma. Neuro-oncol 2003;5:96.

183. Vertosick FT Jr, Selker RG, Arena VC: Survival of patients with well-differentiated astrocytomas diagnosed in the era of computed tomography. Neurosurgery 1991;28:496.

184. McCormack BM, Miller DC, Budzilovich GN, et al: Treatment and survival of low-grade astrocytoma in adults—1977–1988. Neurosurgery 1992;31:636.

185. Piepmeier J, Christopher S, Spencer D, et al: Variations in the natural history and survival of patients with supratentorial low-grade astrocytomas. Neurosurgery 1996;38:872.

186. Ludwig CL, Smith MT, Godfrey AD, et al: A clinicopathological study of 323 patients with oligodendrogliomas. Ann Neurol 1986;19:15.

187. Kernohan J, Mabon R, Svien H: Symposium on new and simplified concept of gliomas. Proc Staff Meet Mayo Clin 1949;24:71.

188. Ringertz N: Grading of gliomas. Acta Pathol Microbiol Scand 1950;27:51.

189. Daumas-Duport C, Scheithauer B, O'Fallon J, et al: Grading of astrocytomas. A simple and reproducible method. Cancer 1988;62:2152.

190. Kleihues P, Louis DN, Scheithauer BW, et al: The WHO classification of tumors of the nervous system. J Neuropathol Exp Neurol 2002;61:215.

191. Burns DK, Kumar V: The Nervous System. In Collins T (ed): Robbins Basic Pathology, 7th ed. Philadelphia, WB Saunders, 2003, p 832.

192. Maher E, McKee A: Neoplasms of the central nervous system. In Skarin A (ed): Dana-Farber Cancer Institute Atlas of Diagnostic Oncology. St. Louis, Mosby, 2003, p 395.

193. Nelson JS, Tsukada Y, Schoenfeld D, et al: Necrosis as a prognostic criterion in malignant supratentorial, astrocytic gliomas. Cancer 1983;52:550.

194. McKeever PE, Ross DA, Strawderman MS, et al: A comparison of the predictive power for survival in gliomas provided by MIB-1, bromodeoxyuridine and proliferating cell nuclear antigen with histopathologic and clinical parameters. J Neuropathol Exp Neurol 1997;56:798.

195. Shaw EG, Scheithauer BW, O'Fallon JR, et al: Oligodendrogliomas: The Mayo Clinic experience. J Neurosurg 1992;76:428.

196. Kraus JA, Lamszus K, Glesmann N, et al: Molecular genetic alterations in glioblastomas with oligodendroglial component. Acta Neuropathol (Berl) 2001;101:311.

197. Shaw EG, Scheithauer BW, O'Fallon JR: Supratentorial gliomas: A comparative study by grade and histologic type. J Neurooncol 1997;31:273.

198. Wallner KE, Gonzales M, Sheline GE: Treatment of oligodendrogliomas with or without postoperative irradiation. J Neurosurg 1988;68:684.

199. Philippon JH, Clemenceau SH, Fauchon FH, et al: Supratentorial low-grade astrocytomas in adults. Neurosurgery 1993;32:554.

200. Chamberlain MC, Murovic JA, Levin VA: Absence of contrast enhancement on CT brain scans of patients with supratentorial malignant gliomas. Neurology 1988;38:1371.

201. Celli P, Nofrone I, Palma L, et al: Cerebral oligodendroglioma: prognostic factors and life history. Neurosurgery 1994;35:1018.

202. Fults D, Tippets RH, Thomas GA, et al: Loss of heterozygosity for loci on chromosome 17p in human malignant astrocytoma. Cancer Res 1989;49:6572.

203. el-Azouzi M, Chung RY, Farmer GE, et al: Loss of distinct regions on the short arm of chromosome 17 associated with tumorigenesis of human astrocytomas. Proc Natl Acad Sci USA 1989;86:7186.

204. von Deimling A, Eibl RH, Ohgaki H, et al: p53 mutations are associated with 17p allelic loss in grade II and grade III astrocytoma. Cancer Res 1992;52:2987.

205. Louis DN: The p53 gene and protein in human brain tumors. J Neuropathol Exp Neurol 1994;53:11.

206. Ichimura K, Bolin MB, Goike HM, et al: Deregulation of the p14ARF/MDM2/p53 pathway is a prerequisite for human astrocytic gliomas with G1-S transition control gene abnormalities. Cancer Res 2000;60:417.

207. Hermanson M, Funa K, Koopmann J, et al: Association of loss of heterozygosity on chromosome 17p with high platelet-derived growth factor alpha receptor expression in human malignant gliomas. Cancer Res 1996;56:164.

208. Hermanson M, Funa K, Hartman M, et al: Platelet-derived growth factor and its receptors in human glioma tissue: Expression of messenger RNA and protein suggests the presence of autocrine and paracrine loops. Cancer Res 1992;52:3213.

209. Fults D, Pedone CA, Thomas GA, et al: Allelotype of human malignant astrocytoma. Cancer Res 1990;50:5784.

210. James CD, Carlbom E, Dumanski JP, et al: Clonal genomic alterations in glioma malignancy stages. Cancer Res 1988;48:5546.

211. Henson JW, Schnitker BL, Correa KM, et al: The retinoblastoma gene is involved in malignant progression of astrocytomas. Ann Neurol 1994;36:714.

212. Ichimura K, Schmidt EE, Goike HM, et al: Human glioblastomas with no alterations of the CDKN2A (p16INK4A, MTS1) and CDK4 genes have frequent mutations of the retinoblastoma gene. Oncogene 1996;13:1065.

213. Ueki K, Ono Y, Henson JW, et al: CDKN2/p16 or RB alterations occur in the majority of glioblastomas and are inversely correlated. Cancer Res 1996;56:150.

214. Schmidt EE, Ichimura K, Reifenberger G, et al: CDKN2 (p16/MTS1) gene deletion or CDK4 amplification occurs in the majority of glioblastomas. Cancer Res 1994;54:6321.

215. Biernat W, Tohma Y, Yonekawa Y, et al: Alterations of cell cycle regulatory genes in primary (de novo) and secondary glioblastomas. Acta Neuropathol (Berl) 1997;94:303.

216. Costello JF, Plass C, Arap W, et al: Cyclin-dependent kinase 6 (CDK6) amplification in human gliomas identified using two-dimensional separation of genomic DNA. Cancer Res 1997;57:1250.

217. von Deimling A, Louis DN, von Ammon K, et al: Evidence for a tumor suppressor gene on chromosome 19q associated with human astrocytomas, oligodendrogliomas, and mixed gliomas. Cancer Res 1992;52:4277.

218. Wong AJ, Bigner SH, Bigner DD, et al: Increased expression of the epidermal growth factor receptor gene in malignant gliomas is invariably associated with gene amplification. Proc Natl Acad Sci USA 1987;84:6899.

219. Tuzi NL, Venter DJ, Kumar S, et al: Expression of growth factor receptors in human brain tumours. Br J Cancer 1991;63:227.

220. Libermann TA, Nusbaum HR, Razon N, et al: Amplification, enhanced expression and possible rearrangement of EGF receptor gene in primary human brain tumours of glial origin. Nature 1985;313:144.

221. Ekstrand AJ, Sugawa N, James CD, et al: Amplified and rearranged epidermal growth factor receptor genes in human glioblastomas reveal deletions of sequences encoding portions of the N-and/or C-terminal tails. Proc Natl Acad Sci USA 1992;89:4309.

Specific Malignancies

III

222. Ekstrand AJ, Longo N, Hamid ML, et al: Functional characterization of an EGF receptor with a truncated extracellular domain expressed in glioblastomas with EGFR gene amplification. Oncogene 1994;9:2313.

223. Nishikawa R, Ji XD, Harmon RC, et al: A mutant epidermal growth factor receptor common in human glioma confers enhanced tumorigenicity. Proc Natl Acad Sci USA 1994;91:7727.

224. Nagane M, Coufal F, Lin H, et al: A common mutant epidermal growth factor receptor confers enhanced tumorigenicity on human glioblastoma cells by increasing proliferation and reducing apoptosis. Cancer Res 1996;56:5079.

225. Frederick L, Wang XY, Eley G, et al: Diversity and frequency of epidermal growth factor receptor mutations in human glioblastomas. Cancer Res 2000;60:1383.

226. Ekstrand AJ, James CD, Cavenee WK, et al: Genes for epidermal growth factor receptor, transforming growth factor alpha, and epidermal growth factor and their expression in human gliomas in vivo. Cancer Res 1991;51:2164.

227. Lang FF, Miller DC, Koslow M, et al: Pathways leading to glioblastoma multiforme: A molecular analysis of genetic alterations in 65 astrocytic tumors. J Neurosurg 1994;81:427.

228. Rasheed BK, Fuller GN, Friedman AH, et al: Loss of heterozygosity for 10q loci in human gliomas. Genes Chromosomes Cancer 1992;5:75.

229. Ichimura K, Schmidt EE, Miyakawa A, et al: Distinct patterns of deletion on 10p and 10q suggest involvement of multiple tumor suppressor genes in the development of astrocytic gliomas of different malignancy grades. Genes Chromosomes Cancer 1988;22:9.

230. Fults D, Pedone C: Deletion mapping of the long arm of chromosome 10 in glioblastoma multiforme. Genes Chromosomes Cancer 1993;7:173.

231. Rasheed BK, McLendon RE, Friedman HS, et al: Chromosome 10 deletion mapping in human gliomas: A common deletion region in 10q25. Oncogene 1995;10:2243.

232. Li J, Yen C, Liaw D, et al: PTEN, a putative protein tyrosine phosphatase gene mutated in human brain, breast, and prostate cancer [see comments]. Science 1997;275:1943.

233. Steck PA, Pershouse MA, Jasser SA, et al: Identification of a candidate tumour suppressor gene, MMAC1, at chromosome 10q23.3 that is mutated in multiple advanced cancers. Nat Genet 1997;15:356.

234. Tohma Y, Gratas C, Biernat W, et al: PTEN (MMAC1) mutations are frequent in primary glioblastomas (de novo) but not in secondary glioblastomas. J Neuropathol Exp Neurol 1989;57:684.

235. Wang SI, Puc J, Li J, et al: Somatic mutations of PTEN in glioblastoma multiforme. Cancer Res 1997;57:4183.

236. Rasheed BK, Stenzel TT, McLendon RE, et al: PTEN gene mutations are seen in high-grade but not in low-grade gliomas. Cancer Res 1997;57:4187.

237. Liu W, James CD, Frederick L, et al: PTEN/MMAC1 mutations and EGFR amplification in glioblastomas. Cancer Res 1997;57:5254.

238. Ermoian RP, Furniss CS, Lamborn KR, et al: Dysregulation of PTEN and protein kinase B is associated with glioma histology and patient survival. Clin Cancer Res 2002;8:1100.

239. Smith JS, Tachibana I, Passe SM, et al: PTEN mutation, EGFR amplification, and outcome in patients with anaplastic astrocytoma and glioblastoma multiforme. J Natl Cancer Inst 2001;93:1246.

240. von Deimling A, Louis DN, von Ammon K, et al: Association of epidermal growth factor receptor gene amplification with loss of chromosome 10 in human glioblastoma multiforme. J Neurosurg 1992;77:295.

241. Kleihues P, Ohgaki H: Primary and secondary glioblastomas: From concept to clinical diagnosis. Neuro-oncol 1999;1:44.

242. Dropcho EJ, Soong SJ: The prognostic impact of prior low grade histology in patients with anaplastic gliomas: A case-control study. Neurology 1996;47:684.

243. Reifenberger J, Ring GU, Gies U, et al: Analysis of p53 mutation and epidermal growth factor receptor amplification in recurrent gliomas with malignant progression. J Neuropathol Exp Neurol 1996;55:822.

244. Watanabe K, Tachibana O, Sata K, et al: Overexpression of the EGF receptor and p53 mutations are mutually exclusive in the evolution of primary and secondary glioblastomas. Brain Pathol 1996;6:217.

245. Biernat W, Kleihues P, Yonekawa Y, et al: Amplification and overexpression of MDM2 in primary (de novo) glioblastomas. J Neuropathol Exp Neurol 1997;56:180.

246. Zundel W, Schindler C, Haas-Kogan D, et al: Loss of PTEN facilitates HIF-1-mediated gene expression. Genes Develop 2000;14:391.

247. Maity A, Pore N, Lee J, et al: Epidermal growth factor receptor (EGFR) transcriptionally upregulates VEGF expression in human glioblastoma cells via a pathway involving PI(3) kinase and distinct from that induced by hypoxia. Cancer Res 2000;60:5879.

248. Pore N, Liu S, Haas-Kogan DA, et al: PTEN mutation and epidermal growth factor receptor activation regulate vascular endothelial growth factor (VEGF) mRNA expression in human glioblastoma cells by transactivating the proximal VEGF promoter. Cancer Res 2003;63:236.

249. Cruickshank GS, Rampling RP, Cowans W: Direct measurement of the PO_2 distribution in human malignant brain tumours. Adv Exp Med Biol 1994;345:465.

250. Collingridge DR, Piepmeier JM, Rockwell S, et al: Polarographic measurements of oxygen tension in human glioma and surrounding peritumoural brain tissue. Radiother Oncol 1999;53:127.

251. Rampling R, Cruickshank G, Lewis AD, et al: Direct measurement of pO_2 distribution and bioreductive enzymes in human malignant brain tumors. Int J Radiat Oncol Biol Phys 1994;29:427.

252. Nordsmark M, Alsner J, Keller J, et al: Hypoxia in human soft tissue sarcomas: Adverse impact on survival and no association with p53 mutations. Br J Cancer 2001;84:1070.

253. Kaanders JH, Wijffels KI, Marres HA, et al: Pimonidazole binding and tumor vascularity predict for treatment outcome in head and neck cancer. Cancer Res 2002;62:7066.

254. Brizel DM, Sibley GS, Prosnitz LR, et al: Tumor hypoxia adversely affects the prognosis of carcinoma of the head and neck. Int J Radiat Oncol Biol Phys 1997;38:285.

255. Brizel DM, Scully SP, Harrelson JM, et al: Tumor oxygenation predicts for the likelihood of distant metastases in human soft tissue sarcoma. Cancer Res 1996;56:941.

256. Hockel M, Schlenger K, Aral B, et al: Association between tumor hypoxia and malignant progression in advanced cancer of the uterine cervix. Cancer Res 1996;56:4509.

257. Nozue M, Lee I, Yuan F, et al: Interlaboratory variation in oxygen tension measurement by Eppendorf "Histograph" and comparison with hypoxic marker. J Surg Oncol 1997;66:30.

258. Jenkins WT, Evans SM, Koch CJ: Hypoxia and necrosis in rat 9L glioma and Morris 7777 hepatoma tumors: Comparative measurements using EF5 binding and the Eppendorf needle electrode. Int J Radiat Oncol Biol Phys 2000;46:1005.

259. Koch CJ: Measurement of absolute oxygen levels in cells and tissues using oxygen sensors and the 2-nitroimidazole EF5. In Sen C, Packer SA (eds): Antioxidants and Redox Signaling. San Diego, Raven Press, 2001, pp 3–31.

260. Evans SM, Hahn S, Pook DR, et al: Detection of hypoxia in human squamous cell carcinoma by EF5 binding. Cancer Res 2000;60:2018.

261. Evans S, Hahn S, Magarelli D, et al: Hypoxia in human intraperitoneal and extremity sarcomas. Int J Radiat Oncol Biol Phys 2001;49:587.

262. Evans S, Hahn S, Magarelli D, et al: Hypoxic heterogeneity in human tumors: EF5 binding, vasculature, necrosis and proliferation. Am J Clin Oncol 2001;24:467.

263. Evans SM, Koch CJ: Prognostic significance of hypoxia in human tumors. Cancer Lett 2003;195:1.

264. Reifenberger J, Reifenberger G, Liu L, et al: Molecular genetic analysis of oligodendroglial tumors shows preferential allelic deletions on 19q and 1p. Am J Pathol 1995;145:1175.

265. Bello MJ, Vaquero J, de Campos JM, et al: Molecular analysis of chromosome 1 abnormalities in human gliomas reveals frequent loss of 1p in oligodendroglial tumors. Int J Cancer 1994;57:172.

266. Mueller W, Hartmann C, Hoffmann A, et al: Genetic signature of oligoastrocytomas correlates with tumor location and denotes distinct molecular subsets. Am J Pathol 2002;161:313.

267. Maintz D, Fiedler K, Koopmann J, et al: Molecular genetic evidence for subtypes of oligoastrocytomas. J Neuropathol Exp Neurol 1997;56:1098.

268. Cairncross JG, Ueki K, Zlatescu MC, et al: Specific genetic predictors of chemotherapeutic response and survival in patients with anaplastic oligodendrogliomas. J Natl Cancer Inst 1998;90:1473.

269. Zlatescu MC, TehraniYazdi A, Sasaki H, et al: Tumor location and growth pattern correlate with genetic signature in oligodendroglial neoplasms. Cancer Res 2001;61:6713.

270. Coffey RJ, Lunsford LD, Taylor FH: Survival after stereotactic biopsy of malignant gliomas. Neurosurgery 1988;22:465.

271. Jackson RJ, Fuller GN, Abi-Said D, et al: Limitations of stereotactic biopsy in the initial management of gliomas. Neuro-oncol 2001;3:193.

272. Kondziolka D, Lunsford LD: The role of stereotactic biopsy in the management of gliomas. J Neurooncol 1999;42:205.

273. Lacroix M, Abi-Said D, Fourney DR, et al: A multivariate analysis of 416 patients with glioblastoma multiforme: Prognosis, extent of resection, and survival. J Neurosurg 2001;95:190.

274. Wood JR, Green SB, Shapiro WR: The prognostic importance of tumor size in malignant gliomas: A computed tomographic scan study by the Brain Tumor Cooperative Group. J Clin Oncol 1988;6:338.

275. Laws ER Jr: Radical resection for the treatment of glioma. Clin Neurosurg 1995;42:480.

276. Trantakis C, Winkler D, Lindner D, et al: Clinical results in MR-guided therapy for malignant gliomas. Acta Neurochir Suppl 2003;85:65.

277. Nimsky C, Ganslandt O, Buchfelder M, et al: Glioma surgery evaluated by intraoperative low-field magnetic resonance imaging. Acta Neurochir Suppl 2003;85:55.

278. Schulder M, Sernas TJ, Carmel PW: Cranial surgery and navigation with a compact intraoperative MRI system. Acta Neurochir Suppl 2003;85:79.

279. Sobottka SB, Bredow J, Beuthien-Baumann B, et al: Comparison of functional brain PET images and intraoperative brain-mapping data using image-guided surgery. Comput Aided Surg 2002;7:317.

280. Matz PG, Cobbs C, Berger MS: Intraoperative cortical mapping as a guide to the surgical resection of gliomas. J Neurooncol 1999;42:233.

281. Duffau H, Capelle L, Denvil D, et al: Usefulness of intraoperative electrical subcortical mapping during surgery for low-grade gliomas located within eloquent brain regions: Functional results in a consecutive series of 103 patients. J Neurosurg 2003;98:764.

282. Muller PJ, Wilson BC, Lilge L, et al: Clinical trials in photodynamic therapy of malignant brain tumors. Proc Soc Photo-Opt Instr Eng 2000;3903:14.

283. Croce AC, Fiorani S, Locatelli D, et al: Diagnostic potential of autofluorescence for an assisted intraoperative delineation of glioblastoma resection margins. Photochem Photobiol 2003;77:309.

284. Yang VX, Muller PJ, Herman P, et al: A multispectral fluorescence imaging system: design and initial clinical tests in intra-operative Photofrin-photodynamic therapy of brain tumors. Lasers Surg Med 2003;32:224.

285. Chang SM, Parney IF, McDermott M, et al: Perioperative complications and neurological outcomes of first and second craniotomies among patients enrolled in the Glioma Outcome Project. J Neurosurg 2003;98:1175.

286. Shaw EG: Low-grade gliomas. In Tepper JE (ed): Clinical Radiation Oncology. Philadelphia, Churchill Livingstone, 2000, p 345.

287. Shaw EG, Daumas-Duport C, Scheithauer BW, et al: Radiation therapy in the management of low-grade supratentorial astrocytomas. J Neurosurg 1989;70:853.

288. Karim AB, Maat B, Hatlevoll R, et al: A randomized trial on dose-response in radiation therapy of low-grade cerebral glioma: European Organization for Research and Treatment of Cancer (EORTC) Study 22844. Int J Radiat Oncol Biol Phys 1996;36:549.

289. Karim AB, Afra D, Cornu P, et al: Randomized trial on the efficacy of radiotherapy for cerebral low-grade glioma in the adult: European Organization for Research and Treatment of Cancer Study 22845 with the Medical Research Council study BRO4: An interim analysis. Int J Radiat Oncol Biol Phys 2002;52:316.

290. Pignatti F, van den Bent M, Curran D, et al: Prognostic factors for survival in adult patients with cerebral low-grade glioma. J Clin Oncol 2002;20:2076.

291. Shaw EG, Wisoff JH: Prospective clinical trials of intracranial low-grade glioma in adults and children. Neuro-oncol 2003;5:153.

292. Walker MD, Alexander E Jr, Hunt WE, et al: Evaluation of BCNU and/or radiotherapy in the treatment of anaplastic gliomas. A cooperative clinical trial. J Neurosurg 1978;49:333.

293. Kristiansen K, Hagen S, Kollevold T, et al: Combined modality therapy of operated astrocytomas grade III and IV. Confirmation of the value of postoperative irradiation and lack of potentiation of bleomycin on survival time: A prospective multicenter trial of the Scandinavian Glioblastoma Study Group. Cancer 1981;47:649.

294. Walker MD, Strike TA, Sheline GE: An analysis of dose-effect relationship in the radiotherapy of malignant gliomas. Int J Radiat Oncol Biol Phys 1979;5:1725.

295. Bleehen NM, Stenning SP: A Medical Research Council trial of two radiotherapy doses in the treatment of grades 3 and 4 astrocytoma. The Medical Research Council Brain Tumour Working Party. Br J Cancer 1991;64:769.

296. Wallner KE, Galicich JH, Krol G, et al: Patterns of failure following treatment for glioblastoma multiforme and anaplastic astrocytoma. Int J Radiat Oncol Biol Phys 1989;16:1405.

297. Selker RG, Shapiro WR, Burger P, et al: The Brain Tumor Cooperative Group NIH Trial 87-01: A randomized comparison of surgery, external radiotherapy, and carmustine versus surgery, interstitial radiotherapy boost, external radiation therapy, and carmustine. Neurosurgery 2002;51:343.

298. Curran WJ Jr, Scott CB, Horton J, et al: Recursive partitioning analysis of prognostic factors in three Radiation Therapy Oncology Group malignant glioma trials. J Natl Cancer Inst 1993;85:704.

299. Gaspar LE, Fisher BJ, MacDonald DR, et al: Malignant glioma–timing of response to radiation therapy. Int J Radiat Oncol Biol Phys 1993;25:877.

300. Chang CH, Horton J, Schoenfeld D, et al: Comparison of postoperative radiotherapy and combined postoperative radiotherapy and chemotherapy in the multidisciplinary management of malignant gliomas. A joint Radiation Therapy Oncology Group and Eastern Cooperative Oncology Group study. Cancer 1983;52:997.

301. Deutsch M, Green SB, Strike TA, et al: Results of a randomized trial comparing BCNU plus radiotherapy, streptozotocin plus radiotherapy, BCNU plus hyperfractionated radiotherapy, and BCNU following misonidazole plus radiotherapy in the postoperative treatment of malignant glioma. Int J Radiat Oncol Biol Phys 1989;16:1389.

302. Scott CB, Scarantino C, Urtasun R, et al: Validation and predictive power of Radiation Therapy Oncology Group (RTOG) recursive partitioning analysis classes for malignant glioma patients: A report using RTOG 90-06. Int J Radiat Oncol Biol Phys 1998;40:51.

303. Prados MD, Gutin PH, Phillips TL, et al: Interstitial brachytherapy for newly diagnosed patients with malignant gliomas: The UCSF experience. Int J Radiat Oncol Biol Phys 1992;24:593.

304. Laperriere NJ, Leung PM, McKenzie S, et al: Randomized study of brachytherapy in the initial management of patients with malignant astrocytoma. Int J Radiat Oncol Biol Phys 1998;41:1005.

305. Loeffler JS, Alexander E 3rd, Wen PY, et al: Results of stereotactic brachytherapy used in the initial management of patients with glioblastoma. J Natl Cancer Inst 1990;82:1918.

306. Souhami L, Scott C, Brachman D, et al: Randomized prospective comparison of stereotactic radiosurgery (SRS) followed by conventional radiotherapy (RT) with BCNU to RT with BCNU alone for selected patients with supratentorial glioblastoma multiforme (GBM): Report of RTOG 93-05 protocol. Int J Radiat Oncol Biol Phys 2002;54:94.

307. Prados MD, Scott C, Sandler H, et al: A phase 3 randomized study of radiotherapy plus procarbazine, CCNU, and vincristine (PCV) with or without BUdR for the treatment of anaplastic astrocytoma: A preliminary report of RTOG 9404. Int J Radiat Oncol Biol Phys 1999;45:1109.

Specific Malignancies

308. Nelson DF, Diener-West M, Weinstein AS, et al: A randomized comparison of misonidazole sensitized radiotherapy plus BCNU and radiotherapy plus BCNU for treatment of malignant glioma after surgery: Final report of an RTOG study. Int J Radiat Oncol Biol Phys 1986;12:1793.

309. Chan JL, Lee SW, Fraass BA, et al: Survival and failure patterns of high-grade gliomas after three-dimensional conformal radiotherapy. J Clin Oncol 2002;20:1635.

310. Shapiro JR, Yung WK, Shapiro WR: Isolation, karyotype, and clonal growth of heterogeneous subpopulations of human malignant gliomas. Cancer Res 1981;41:2349.

311. Shapiro JR, Pu PY, Mohamed AN, et al: Chromosome number and carmustine sensitivity in human gliomas. Cancer 1993;71:4007.

312. Stark AM, Witzel P, Strege RJ, et al: p53, mdm2, EGFR, and msh2 expression in paired initial and recurrent glioblastoma multiforme. J Neurol Neurosurg Psychiatry 2003;74:779.

313. Reavey-Cantwell JF, Haroun RI, Zahurak M, et al: The prognostic value of tumor markers in patients with glioblastoma multiforme: Analysis of 32 patients and review of the literature. J Neurooncol 2001;55:195.

314. Allison RR, Schulsinger A, Vongtama V, et al: Radiation and chemotherapy improve outcome in oligodendroglioma. Int J Radiat Oncol Biol Phys 1997;37:399.

315. Reijneveld JC, Sitskoorn MM, Klein M, et al: Cognitive status and quality of life in patients with suspected versus proven low-grade gliomas. Neurology 2001;56:618.

316. Benjelloun A, Delavelle J, Lazeyras F, et al: Possible efficacy of temozolomide in a patient with gliomatosis cerebri. Neurology 2001;57:1932.

317. Fine HA, Dear KB, Loeffler JS, et al: Meta-analysis of radiation therapy with and without adjuvant chemotherapy for malignant gliomas in adults. Cancer 1993;71:2585.

318. Stewart LA: Chemotherapy in adult high-grade glioma: A systematic review and meta-analysis of individual patient data from 12 randomised trials. Lancet 2002;359:1011.

319. Brandes AA, Vastola F, Basso U, et al: A prospective study on glioblastoma in the elderly. Cancer 2003;97:657.

320. Walker MD, Green SB, Byar DP, et al: Randomized comparisons of radiotherapy and nitrosoureas for the treatment of malignant glioma after surgery. N Engl J Med 1980;303:1323.

321. Green SB, Byar DP, Walker MD, et al: Comparisons of carmustine, procarbazine, and high-dose methylprednisolone as additions to surgery and radiotherapy for the treatment of malignant glioma. Cancer Treat Rep 1983;67:121.

322. Dropcho EJ: Novel chemotherapeutic approaches to brain tumors. Hematol Oncol Clin North Am 2001;15:1027.

323. Gilbert MR, Friedman HS, Kuttesch JF, et al: A phase II study of temozolomide in patients with newly diagnosed supratentorial malignant glioma before radiation therapy. Neuro-oncol 2002;4:261.

324. Westphal M, Hilt DC, Bortey E, et al: A phase 3 trial of local chemotherapy with biodegradable carmustine (BCNU) wafers (Gliadel wafers) in patients with primary malignant glioma. Neuro-oncol 2003;5:79.

325. Durando X, Lemaire JJ, Tortochaux J, et al: High-dose BCNU followed by autologous hematopoietic stem cell transplantation in supratentorial high-grade malignant gliomas: A retrospective analysis of 114 patients. Bone Marrow Transplant 2003;31:559.

326. Grossman SA, O'Neill A, Grunnet M, et al: Phase III study comparing three cycles of infusional carmustine and cisplatin followed by radiation therapy with radiation therapy and concurrent carmustine in patients with newly diagnosed supratentorial glioblastoma multiforme: Eastern Cooperative Oncology Group Trial 2394. J Clin Oncol 2003;21:1485.

327. Tatter SB: Recurrent malignant glioma in adults. Curr Treat Options Oncol 2002;3:509.

328. Brada M, Hoang-Xuan K, Rampling R, et al: Multicenter phase II trial of temozolomide in patients with glioblastoma multiforme at first relapse. Ann Oncol 2001;12:259.

329. Yung WK, Prados MD, Yaya-Tur R, et al: Multicenter phase II trial of temozolomide in patients with anaplastic astrocytoma or anaplastic oligoastrocytoma at first relapse. Temodal Brain Tumor Group. J Clin Oncol 1999;17:2762.

330. Brandes AA, Ermani M, Basso U, et al: Temozolomide in patients with glioblastoma at second relapse after first line nitrosourea-procarbazine failure: A phase II study. Oncology 2002;63:38.

331. Dinnes J, Cave C, Huang S, et al: A rapid and systematic review of the effectiveness of temozolomide for the treatment of recurrent malignant glioma. Br J Cancer 2002;86:501.

332. Yung WK, Albright RE, Olson J, et al: A phase II study of temozolomide vs. procarbazine in patients with glioblastoma multiforme at first relapse. Br J Cancer 2000;83:588.

333. Brem H, Piantadosi S, Burger PC, et al: Placebo-controlled trial of safety and efficacy of intraoperative controlled delivery by biodegradable polymers of chemotherapy for recurrent gliomas. The Polymer-brain Tumor Treatment Group. Lancet 1995;345:1008.

334. Buckner JC, Reid JM, Wright K, et al: Irinotecan in the treatment of glioma patients: Current and future studies of the North Central Cancer Treatment Group. Cancer 2003;97:2352.

335. Cloughesy TF, Filka E, Kuhn J, et al: Two studies evaluating irinotecan treatment for recurrent malignant glioma using an every-3-week regimen. Cancer 2003;97:2381.

336. Cairncross G, Macdonald D, Ludwin S, et al: Chemotherapy for anaplastic oligodendroglioma. National Cancer Institute of Canada Clinical Trials Group. J Clin Oncol 1994;12:2013.

337. Kim L, Hochberg FH, Thornton AF, et al: Procarbazine, lomustine, and vincristine (PCV) chemotherapy for grade III and grade IV oligoastrocytomas. J Neurosurg 1996;85:602.

338. van den Bent MJ, Kros JM, Heimans JJ, et al: Response rate and prognostic factors of recurrent oligodendroglioma treated with procarbazine, CCNU, and vincristine chemotherapy. Dutch Neuro-oncology Group. Neurology 1998;51:1140.

339. Jeremic B, Shibamoto Y, Gruijicic D, et al: Combined treatment modality for anaplastic oligodendroglioma: A phase II study. J Neurooncol 1999;43:179.

340. Paleologos NA, Macdonald DR, Vick NA, et al: Neoadjuvant procarbazine, CCNU, and vincristine for anaplastic and aggressive oligodendroglioma. Neurology 1999;53:1141.

341. Chinot O: Chemotherapy for the treatment of oligodendroglial tumors. Semin Oncol 2001;28:13.

342. Boiardi A, Eoli M, Salmaggi A, et al: Cisplatin and BCNU chemotherapy for anaplastic oligoastrocytomas. J Neurooncol 2000;49:71.

343. Jenkins RB, Curran W, Scott CB, et al: Pilot evaluation of 1p and 19q deletions in anaplastic oligodendrogliomas collected by a national cooperative cancer treatment group. Am J Clin Oncol 2001;24:506.

344. Smith JS, Perry A, Borell TJ, et al: Alterations of chromosome arms 1p and 19q as predictors of survival in oligodendrogliomas, astrocytomas, and mixed oligoastrocytomas. J Clin Oncol 2000;18:636.

345. Ino Y, Zlatescu MC, Sasaki H, et al: Long survival and therapeutic responses in patients with histologically disparate high-grade gliomas demonstrating chromosome 1p loss. J Neurosurg 2000;92:983.

346. Chahlavi A, Kanner A, Peereboom D, et al: Impact of chromosome 1p status in response of oligodendroglioma to temozolomide: preliminary results. J Neurooncol 2003;61:267.

347. Cairncross G, Swinnen L, Bayer R, et al: Myeloablative chemotherapy for recurrent aggressive oligodendroglioma. Neuro-oncol 2000;2:114.

348. van den Bent MJ, Keime-Guibert F, Brandes AA, et al: Temozolomide chemotherapy in recurrent oligodendroglioma. Neurology 2001;57:340.

349. Bissola L, Eoli M, Pollo B, et al: Association of chromosome 10 losses and negative prognosis in oligoastrocytomas. Ann Neurol 2002;52:842.

350. Buckner JC, Gesme D Jr, O'Fallon JR, et al: Phase II trial of procarbazine, lomustine, and vincristine as initial therapy for patients with low-grade oligodendroglioma or oligoastrocytoma: Efficacy and associations with chromosomal abnormalities. J Clin Oncol 2003;21:251.

351. van den Bent MJ, Chinot O, Boogerd W, et al: Second-line chemotherapy with temozolomide in recurrent oligodendroglioma after PCV (procarbazine, lomustine and vincristine) chemotherapy: EORTC Brain Tumor Group phase II study 26972. Ann Oncol 2003;14:599.

352. van den Bent MJ, Taphoorn MJ, Brandes AA, et al: Phase II study of first-line chemotherapy with temozolomide in recurrent oligodendroglial tumors: The European Organization for Research and Treatment of Cancer Brain Tumor Group Study 26971. J Clin Oncol 2003;21:2525.

353. Vuorinen V, Hinkka S, Farkkila M, et al: Debulking or biopsy of malignant glioma in elderly people—a randomised study. Acta Neurochir (Wien) 2003;145:5.

354. Kiebert GM, Curran D, Aaronson NK, et al: Quality of life after radiation therapy of cerebral low-grade gliomas of the adult: Results of a randomised phase III trial on dose response (EORTC trial 22844). EORTC Radiotherapy Co-operative Group. Eur J Cancer 1998;34:1902.

355. Heimans JJ, Taphoorn MJ: Impact of brain tumour treatment on quality of life. J Neurol 2002;249:955.

356. Basso U, Ermani M, Vastola F, et al: Non-cytotoxic therapies for malignant gliomas. J Neurooncol 2002;58:57.

357. Emrich JG, Brady LW, Quang TS, et al: Radioiodinated (I-125) monoclonal antibody 425 in the treatment of high grade glioma patients: Ten-year synopsis of a novel treatment. Am J Clin Oncol 2002;25:541.

358. Ciardiello F, Caputo R, Bianco R, et al: Inhibition of growth factor production and angiogenesis in human cancer cells by ZD1839 (Iressa), a selective epidermal growth factor receptor tyrosine kinase inhibitor. Clin Cancer Res 2001;7:1459.

359. Chen TC, Su S, Fry D, et al: Combination therapy with irinotecan and protein kinase C inhibitors in malignant glioma. Cancer 2003;97:2363.

360. Mastronardi L, Puzzilli F, Couldwell WT, et al: Tamoxifen and carboplatin combinational treatment of high-grade gliomas. Results of a clinical trial on newly diagnosed patients. J Neurooncol 1998;38:59.

361. Brat DJ, Mapstone TB: Malignant glioma physiology: Cellular response to hypoxia and its role in tumor progression. Ann Intern Med 2003;138:659.

362. Oosthuyse B, Moons L, Storkebaum E, et al: Deletion of the hypoxia-response element in the vascular endothelial growth factor promoter causes motor neuron degeneration. Nat Genet 2001;28:131.

363. Groves MD, Puduvalli VK, Hess KR, et al: Phase II trial of temozolomide plus the matrix metalloproteinase inhibitor, marimastat, in recurrent and progressive glioblastoma multiforme. J Clin Oncol 2002;20:1383.

364. Lal A, Glazer CA, Martinson HM, et al: Mutant epidermal growth factor receptor up-regulates molecular effectors of tumor invasion. Cancer Res 2002;62:3335.

365. Choe G, Park JK, Jouben-Steele L, et al: Active matrix metalloproteinase 9 expression is associated with primary glioblastoma subtype. Clin Cancer Res 2002;8:2894.

366. Ram Z, Culver KW, Oshiro EM, et al: Therapy of malignant brain tumors by intratumoral implantation of retroviral vector-producing cells. Nat Med 1997;3:1354.

367. Palu G, Cavaggioni A, Calvi P, et al: Gene therapy of glioblastoma multiforme via combined expression of suicide and cytokine genes: A pilot study in humans. Gene Ther 1999;6:330.

368. Shand N, Weber F, Mariani L, et al: A phase 1-2 clinical trial of gene therapy for recurrent glioblastoma multiforme by tumor transduction with the herpes simplex thymidine kinase gene followed by ganciclovir. GLI328 European-Canadian Study Group. Hum Gene Ther 1999;10:2325.

369. Rainov NG: A phase III clinical evaluation of herpes simplex virus type 1 thymidine kinase and ganciclovir gene therapy as an adjuvant to surgical resection and radiation in adults with previously untreated glioblastoma multiforme. Hum Gene Ther 2000;11:2389.

370. Lang F, Fullger G, Prados M: Preliminary results of a phase I clinical trial of adenovirus-mediated p53 gene therapy for recurrent glioma. Neuro-oncol 2000;2:227.

371. Chang SM, Kuhn JG, Robins HI, et al: Phase II study of phenylacetate in patients with recurrent malignant glioma: A North American Brain Tumor Consortium report. J Clin Oncol 1999;17:984.

372. Yung WK, Kyritsis AP, Gleason MJ, et al: Treatment of recurrent malignant gliomas with high-dose 13-cis-retinoic acid. Clin Cancer Res 1996;2:1931.

373. Shono T, Tofilon PJ, Bruner JM, et al: Cyclooxygenase-2 expression in human gliomas: Prognostic significance and molecular correlations. Cancer Res 2001;61:4375.

374. Prayson RA, Castilla EA, Vogelbaum MA, et al: Cyclooxygenase-2 (COX-2) expression by immunohistochemistry in glioblastoma multiforme. Ann Diagn Pathol 2002;6:148.

375. Bashir R, Chamberlain M, Ruby E, et al: T-cell infiltration of primary CNS lymphoma. Neurology 1996;46:440.

376. Corboy JR, Garl PJ, Kleinschmidt-DeMasters BK: Human herpesvirus 8 DNA in CNS lymphomas from patients with and without AIDS. Neurology 1998;50:335.

377. Mineura K, Sawataishi J, Sasajima T, et al: Primary central nervous system involvement of the so called 'peripheral T-cell lymphoma'. Report of a case and review of the literature. J Neurooncol 1993;16:235.

378. Villegas E, Villa S, Lopez-Guillermo A, et al: Primary central nervous system lymphoma of T-cell origin: Description of two cases and review of the literature. J Neurooncol 1997;34:157.

379. Gijtenbeek JM, Rosenblum MK, DeAngelis LM: Primary central nervous system T-cell lymphoma. Neurology 2001;57:716.

380. Lai R, Rosenblum MK, DeAngelis LM: Primary CNS lymphoma: A whole-brain disease? Neurology 2002;59:1557.

381. Maher EA, Fine HA: Primary CNS lymphoma. Semin Oncol 1999;26:346.

382. Ciacci JD, Tellez C, VonRoenn J, et al: Lymphoma of the central nervous system in AIDS. Semin Neurol 1999;19:213.

383. Kadan-Lottick NS, Skluzacek MC, Gurney JG: Decreasing incidence rates of primary central nervous system lymphoma. Cancer 2002;95:193.

384. Chamberlain MC, Kormanik PA: AIDS-related central nervous system lymphomas. J Neurooncol 1999;43:269.

385. Gleissner B, Siehl J, Korfel A, et al: CSF evaluation in primary CNS lymphoma patients by PCR of the CDR III IgH genes. Neurology 2002;58:390.

386. Kros JM, Bagdi EK, Zheng P, et al: Analysis of immunoglobulin H gene rearrangement by polymerase chain reaction in primary central nervous system lymphoma. J Neurosurg 2002;97:1390.

387. Braaten KM, Betensky RA, de Leval L, et al: BCL-6 expression predicts improved survival in patients with primary central nervous system lymphoma. Clin Cancer Res 2003;9:1063.

388. Chang CC, Kampalath B, Schultz C, et al: Expression of p53, c-Myc, or Bcl-6 suggests a poor prognosis in primary central nervous system diffuse large B-cell lymphoma among immunocompetent individuals. Arch Pathol Lab Med 2003;127: 208.

389. Damek DM: Primary central nervous system lymphoma. Curr Treat Options Neurol 2003;5:213.

390. Abrey LE, DeAngelis LM, Yahalom J: Long-term survival in primary CNS lymphoma. J Clin Oncol 1998;16:859.

391. Herrlinger U, Schabet M, Brugger W, et al: Primary central nervous system lymphoma 1991–1997: Outcome and late adverse effects after combined modality treatment. Cancer 2001;91:130.

392. DeAngelis LM: Primary CNS lymphoma: treatment with combined chemotherapy and radiotherapy. J Neurooncol 1999;43:249.

393. Ling SM, Roach M 3rd, Larson DA, et al: Radiotherapy of primary central nervous system lymphoma in patients with and without human immunodeficiency virus. Ten years of treatment experience at the University of California San Francisco. Cancer 1994;73:2570.

394. Nelson DF, Martz KL, Bonner H, et al: Non-Hodgkin's lymphoma of the brain: Can high dose, large volume radiation therapy improve survival? Report on a prospective trial by the Radiation Therapy Oncology Group (RTOG): RTOG 8315. Int J Radiat Oncol Biol Phys 1992;23:9.

395. DeAngelis LM, Seiferheld W, Schold SC, et al: Combination chemotherapy and radiotherapy for primary central nervous system lymphoma: Radiation Therapy Oncology Group Study 93-10. J Clin Oncol 2002;20:4643.

396. Glass J, Gruber ML, Cher L, et al: Preirradiation methotrexate chemotherapy of primary central nervous system lymphoma: Long-term outcome. J Neurosurg 1994;81:188.

397. Keime-Guibert F, Napolitano M, Delattre JY: Neurological complications of radiotherapy and chemotherapy. J Neurol 1998;245:695.

Specific Malignancies

III

398. Sarazin M, Ameri A, Monjour A, et al: Primary central nervous system lymphoma: Treatment with chemotherapy and radiotherapy. Eur J Cancer 1995;31A:2003.

399. Abrey LE, Yahalom J, DeAngelis LM: Treatment for primary CNS lymphoma: The next step. J Clin Oncol 2000;18:3144.

400. Cher L, Glass J, Harsh GR, et al: Therapy of primary CNS lymphoma with methotrexate-based chemotherapy and deferred radiotherapy: Preliminary results. Neurology 1996;46:1757.

401. Glantz MJ, Cole BF, Recht L, et al: High-dose intravenous methotrexate for patients with nonleukemic leptomeningeal cancer: is intrathecal chemotherapy necessary? J Clin Oncol 1998;16:1561.

402. Schultz C, Scott C, Sherman W, et al: Preirradiation chemotherapy with cyclophosphamide, doxorubicin, vincristine, and dexamethasone for primary CNS lymphomas: Initial report of radiation therapy oncology group protocol 88-06. J Clin Oncol 1996;14:556.

403. Lachance DH, Brizel DM, Gockerman JP, et al: Cyclophosphamide, doxorubicin, vincristine, and prednisone for primary central nervous system lymphoma: Short-duration response and multifocal intracerebral recurrence preceding radiotherapy. Neurology 1994;44:1721.

404. Brada M, Dearnaley D, Horwich A, et al: Management of primary cerebral lymphoma with initial chemotherapy: Preliminary results and comparison with patients treated with radiotherapy alone. Int J Radiat Oncol Biol Phys 1990;18:787.

405. Bessell EM, Graus F, Lopez-Guillermo A, et al: CHOD/BVAM regimen plus radiotherapy in patients with primary CNS non-Hodgkin's lymphoma. Int J Radiat Oncol Biol Phys 2001;50:457.

406. Dahlborg SA, Henner WD, Crossen JR, et al: Non-AIDS primary CNS lymphoma: First example of a durable response in a primary brain tumor using enhanced chemotherapy delivery without cognitive loss and without radiotherapy. Cancer J Sci Am 1996;2:166.

407. Nasir S, DeAngelis LM: Update on the management of primary CNS lymphoma. Oncology 2000;14:228.

408. Herrlinger U, Schabet M, Brugger W, et al: German Cancer Society Neuro-Oncology Working Group NOA-03 multicenter trial of single-agent high-dose methotrexate for primary central nervous system lymphoma. Ann Neurol 2002;51:247.

409. Freilich RJ, Delattre JY, Monjour A, et al: Chemotherapy without radiation therapy as initial treatment for primary CNS lymphoma in older patients. Neurology 1996;46:435.

410. Kim L, Hochberg FH, Shaeffer P: White-matter abnormalities in unirradiated patients cured of primary central nervous system lymphoma. Neuroradiology 2000;42:406.

411. Fliessbach K, Urbach H, Helmstaedter C, et al: Cognitive performance and magnetic resonance imaging findings after high-dose systemic and intraventricular chemotherapy for primary central nervous system lymphoma. Arch Neurol 2003;60:563.

412. Slobod KS, Taylor GH, Sandlund JT, et al: Epstein-Barr virus-targeted therapy for AIDS-related primary lymphoma of the central nervous system. Lancet 2000;356:1493.

413. Mathew BS, Grossman SA: *Pneumocystis carinii* pneumonia prophylaxis in HIV negative patients with primary CNS lymphoma. Cancer Treat Rev 2003;29:105.

414. Harjunpaa A, Wiklund T, Collan J, et al: Complement activation in circulation and central nervous system after rituximab (anti-CD20) treatment of B-cell lymphoma. Leuk Lymphoma 2001;42:731.

415. Pels H, Schulz H, Manzke O, et al: Intraventricular and intravenous treatment of a patient with refractory primary CNS lymphoma using rituximab. J Neurooncol 2002;59:213.

416. Soussain C, Suzan F, Hoang-Xuan K, et al: Results of intensive chemotherapy followed by hematopoietic stem-cell rescue in 22 patients with refractory or recurrent primary CNS lymphoma or intraocular lymphoma. J Clin Oncol 2001;19:742.

417. Rohringer M, Sutherland GR, Louw DF, et al: Incidence and clinicopathological features of meningioma. J Neurosurg 1989;71:665.

418. Mirimanoff RO, Dosoretz DE, Linggood RM, et al: Meningioma: analysis of recurrence and progression following neurosurgical resection. J Neurosurg 1985;62:18.

419. Longstreth WT Jr, Dennis LK, McGuire VM, et al: Epidemiology of intracranial meningioma. Cancer 1993;72:639.

420. Helseth A, Mork S, Glattre E: Neoplasms of the central nervous system in Norway: V. Meningioma and cancer of other sites. APMIS 1989;97:738.

421. Dumanski JP, Rouleau GA, Nordenskjold M, et al: Molecular genetic analysis of chromosome 22 in 81 cases of meningioma. Cancer Res 1990;50:5863.

422. Ruttledge MH, Sarrazin J, Rangaratnam S, et al: Evidence for the complete inactivation of the NF2 gene in the majority of sporadic meningiomas. Nat Genet 1994;6:180.

423. McCarthy BJ, Davis FG, Freels S, et al: Factors associated with survival in patients with meningioma. J Neurosurg 1998;88:831.

424. Sheporatis L, Osborn A, Smirniotopoulous J, et al: Radiologic-pathologic correlation: Intracranial meningioma. Am J Neuroradiol 1992;13:29.

425. Miralbell R, Linggood RM, de la Monte S, et al: The role of radiotherapy in the treatment of subtotally resected benign meningiomas. J Neurooncol 1992;13:157.

426. Taylor BW Jr, Marcus RB Jr, Friedman WA, et al: The meningioma controversy: Postoperative radiation therapy. Int J Radiat Oncol Biol Phys 1988;15:299.

427. Condra KS, Buatti JM, Mendenhall WM, et al: Benign meningiomas: Primary treatment selection affects survival. Int J Radiat Oncol Biol Phys 1997;39:427.

428. Barbaro NM, Gutin PH, Wilson CB, et al: Radiation therapy in the treatment of partially resected meningiomas. Neurosurgery 1987;20:525.

429. Goldsmith BJ, Wara WM, Wilson CB, et al: Postoperative irradiation for subtotally resected meningiomas. A retrospective analysis of 140 patients treated from 1967 to 1990. J Neurosurg 1994;80:195.

430. Glaholm J, Bloom HJ, Crow JH: The role of radiotherapy in the management of intracranial meningiomas: The Royal Marsden Hospital experience with 186 patients. Int J Radiat Oncol Biol Phys 1990;18:755.

431. Kondziolka D, Levy EI, Niranjan A, et al: Long-term outcomes after meningioma radiosurgery: Physician and patient perspectives. J Neurosurg 1999;91:44.

432. Hakim R, Alexander E 3rd, Loeffler JS, et al: Results of linear accelerator-based radiosurgery for intracranial meningiomas. Neurosurgery 1998;42:446.

433. Stafford SL, Pollock BE, Foote RL, et al: Meningioma radiosurgery: tumor control, outcomes, and complications among 190 consecutive patients. Neurosurgery 2001;49:1029.

434. O'Sullivan MG, van Loveren HR, Tew JM Jr: The surgical resectability of meningiomas of the cavernous sinus. Neurosurgery 1997;40:238.

435. Spiegelmann R, Nissim O, Menhel J, et al: Linear accelerator radiosurgery for meningiomas in and around the cavernous sinus. Neurosurgery 2002;51:1373.

436. Morita A, Coffey RJ, Foote RL, et al: Risk of injury to cranial nerves after gamma knife radiosurgery for skull base meningiomas: Experience in 88 patients. J Neurosurg 1999;90:42.

437. Lee JY, Niranjan A, McInerney J, et al: Stereotactic radiosurgery providing long-term tumor control of cavernous sinus meningiomas. J Neurosurg 2002;97:65.

438. Debus J, Wuendrich M, Pirzkall A, et al: High efficacy of fractionated stereotactic radiotherapy of large base-of-skull meningiomas: long-term results. J Clin Oncol 2001;19:3547.

439. Andrews DW, Faroozan R, Yang BP, et al: Fractionated stereotactic radiotherapy for the treatment of optic nerve sheath meningiomas: Preliminary observations of 33 optic nerves in 30 patients with historical comparison to observation with or without prior surgery. Neurosurgery 2002;51:890.

440. Schrell UM, Rittig MG, Anders M, et al: Hydroxyurea for treatment of unresectable and recurrent meningiomas. II. Decrease in the size of meningiomas in patients treated with hydroxyurea. J Neurosurg 1997;86:840.

441. Newton HB, Slivka MA, Stevens C: Hydroxyurea chemotherapy for unresectable or residual meningioma. J Neurooncol 2000;49:165.

442. Mason WP, Gentili F, Macdonald DR, et al: Stabilization of disease progression by hydroxyurea in patients with recurrent or unresectable meningioma. J Neurosurg 2002;97:341.

443. Grunberg SM, Weiss MH, Spitz IM, et al: Treatment of unresectable

meningiomas with the antiprogesterone agent mifepristone. J Neurosurg 1991;74:861.

444. Oura S, Sakurai T, Yoshimura G, et al: Regression of a presumed meningioma with the antiestrogen agent mepitiostane. Case report. J Neurosurg 2000;93:132.

445. Chamberlain MC: Meningiomas. Curr Treat Options Neurol 2001;3:67.

446. Hall WA, Luciano MG, Doppman JL, et al: Pituitary magnetic resonance imaging in normal human volunteers: Occult adenomas in the general population. Ann Intern Med 1994;120:817.

447. Thakker RV: Multiple endocrine neoplasia. Horm Res 2001; 56(Suppl 1):67.

448. Weil RJ, Vortmeyer AO, Huang S, et al: 11q13 allelic loss in pituitary tumors in patients with multiple endocrine neoplasia syndrome type 1. Clin Cancer Res 1998;4:1673.

449. Suhardja AS, Kovacs KT, Rutka JT: Molecular pathogenesis of pituitary adenomas: A review. Acta Neurochir (Wien) 1999;141: 729.

450. Oruckaptan HH, Senmevsim O, Ozcan OE, et al: Pituitary adenomas: results of 684 surgically treated patients and review of the literature. Surg Neurol 2000;53:211.

451. Howlett TA, Plowman PN, Wass JA, et al: Megavoltage pituitary irradiation in the management of Cushing's disease and Nelson's syndrome: Long-term follow-up. Clin Endocrinol (Oxford) 1989;31:309.

452. Hardy J: Transphenoidal microsurgery of the normal and pathological pituitary. Clin Neurosurg 1969;16:185.

453. Ciric I, Ragin A, Baumgartner C, et al: Complications of transsphenoidal surgery: Results of a national survey, review of the literature, and personal experience. Neurosurgery 1997;40:225.

454. Jho HD: Endoscopic transsphenoidal surgery. J Neurooncol 2001;54:187.

455. Laws ER, Vance ML, Thapar K: Pituitary surgery for the management of acromegaly. Horm Res 2000;53(Suppl 3):71.

456. Ludecke DK, Flitsch J, Knappe UJ, et al: Cushing's disease: A surgical view. J Neurooncol 2001;54:151.

457. Sanno N, Teramoto A, Osamura RY: Thyrotropin-secreting pituitary adenomas. Clinical and biological heterogeneity and current treatment. J Neurooncol 2001;54:179.

458. Losa M, Franzin A, Mangili F, et al: Proliferation index of nonfunctioning pituitary adenomas: Correlations with clinical characteristics and long-term follow-up results. Neurosurgery 2000;47:1313.

459. Lillehei KO, Kirschman DL, Kleinschmidt-DeMasters BK, et al: Reassessment of the role of radiation therapy in the treatment of endocrine-inactive pituitary macroadenomas. Neurosurgery 1998;43:432.

460. Woollons AC, Hunn MK, Rajapakse YR, et al: Non-functioning pituitary adenomas: indications for postoperative radiotherapy. Clin Endocrinol (Oxford) 2000;53:713.

461. Losa M, Mortini P, Barzaghi R, et al: Endocrine inactive and gonadotroph adenomas: Diagnosis and management. J Neuro-oncol 2001;54:167.

462. Molitch ME: Diagnosis and treatment of prolactinomas. Adv Intern Med 1999;44:117.

463. Nomikos P, Buchfelder M, Fahlbusch R: Current management of prolactinomas. J Neurooncol 2001;54:139.

464. Colao A, Di Sarno A, Marzullo P, et al: New medical approaches in pituitary adenomas. Horm Res 2000;53(Suppl 3):76.

465. Tsang RW, Brierley JD, Panzarella T, et al: Role of radiation therapy in clinical hormonally active pituitary adenomas. Radiother Oncol 1996;41:45.

466. Tsang RW, Brierley JD, Panzarella T, et al: Radiation therapy for pituitary adenoma: Treatment outcome and prognostic factors. Int J Radiat Oncol Biol Phys 1994;30:557.

467. Breen P, Flickinger JC, Kondziolka D, et al: Radiotherapy for nonfunctional pituitary adenoma: Analysis of long-term tumor control. J Neurosurg 1998;89:933.

468. Zierhut D, Flentje M, Adolph J, et al: External radiotherapy of pituitary adenomas. Int J Radiat Oncol Biol Phys 1995;33:307.

469. McCord MW, Buatti JM, Fennell EM, et al: Radiotherapy for pituitary adenoma: Long-term outcome and sequelae. Int J Radiat Oncol Biol Phys 1997;39:437.

470. Grigsby PW, Thomas PR, Simpson JR, et al: Long-term results of radiotherapy in the treatment of pituitary adenomas in children and adolescents. Am J Clin Oncol 1988;11:607.

471. Brada M, Ford D, Ashley S, et al: Risk of second brain tumour after conservative surgery and radiotherapy for pituitary adenoma. BMJ 1992;304:1343.

472. Tsang RW, Laperriere NJ, Simpson WJ, et al: Glioma arising after radiation therapy for pituitary adenoma. A report of four patients and estimation of risk. Cancer 1993;72:2227.

473. Milker-Zabel S, Debus J, Thilmann C, et al: Fractionated stereotactically guided radiotherapy and radiosurgery in the treatment of functional and nonfunctional adenomas of the pituitary gland. Int J Radiat Oncol Biol Phys 2001;50:1279.

474. Mitsumori M, Shrieve DC, Alexander E 3rd, et al: Initial clinical results of LINAC-based stereotactic radiosurgery and stereotactic radiotherapy for pituitary adenomas. Int J Radiat Oncol Biol Phys 1998;42:573.

475. Yoon SC, Suh TS, Jang HS, et al: Clinical results of 24 pituitary macroadenomas with linac-based stereotactic radiosurgery. Int J Radiat Oncol Biol Phys 1998;41:849.

476. McCormick PC, Bello JA, Post KD: Trigeminal schwannoma. Surgical series of 14 cases with review of the literature. J Neurosurg 1988;69:850.

477. Goel A, Muzumdar D, Raman C: Trigeminal neuroma: analysis of surgical experience with 73 cases. Neurosurgery 2003;52:783.

478. Harner SG, Laws ER Jr: Clinical findings in patients with acoustic neurinoma. Mayo Clin Proc 1983;58:721.

479. Bijlsma EK, Brouwer-Mladin R, Bosch DA, et al: Molecular characterization of chromosome 22 deletions in schwannomas. Genes Chromosomes Cancer 1992;5:201.

480. Lekanne Deprez RH, Bianchi AB, Groen NA, et al: Frequent NF2 gene transcript mutations in sporadic meningiomas and vestibular schwannomas. Am J Hum Genet 1994;54:1022.

481. Jackler RK, Pitts LH: Selection of surgical approach to acoustic neuroma. Otolaryngol Clin North Am 1992;25:361.

482. Briggs RJ, Luxford WM, Atkins JS Jr, et al: Translabyrinthine removal of large acoustic neuromas. Neurosurgery 1994;34:785.

483. Post KD, Eisenberg MB, Catalano PJ: Hearing preservation in vestibular schwannoma surgery: What factors influence outcome? J Neurosurg 1995;83:191.

484. Shelton C, Brackmann DE, House WF, et al: Middle fossa acoustic tumor surgery: Results in 106 cases. Laryngoscope 1989;99:405.

485. Wiet RJ, Teixido M, Liang JG: Complications in acoustic neuroma surgery. Otolaryngol Clin North Am 1992;25:389.

486. Samii M, Matthies C: Management of 1000 vestibular schwannomas (acoustic neuromas): Hearing function in 1000 tumor resections. Neurosurgery 1997;40:248.

487. Wallner KE, Sheline GE, Pitts LH, et al: Efficacy of irradiation for incompletely excised acoustic neurilemomas. J Neurosurg 1987;67:858.

488. Harsh GR, Thornton AF, Chapman PH, et al: Proton beam stereotactic radiosurgery of vestibular schwannomas. Int J Radiat Oncol Biol Phys 2002;54:35.

489. Kondziolka D, Lunsford LD, McLaughlin MR, et al: Long-term outcomes after radiosurgery for acoustic neuromas. N Engl J Med 1998;339:1426.

490. Foote RL, Coffey RJ, Swanson JW, et al: Stereotactic radiosurgery using the gamma knife for acoustic neuromas. Int J Radiat Oncol Biol Phys 1995;32:1153.

491. Mendenhall WM, Friedman WA, Bova FJ: Linear accelerator-based stereotactic radiosurgery for acoustic schwannomas. Int J Radiat Oncol Biol Phys 1994;28:803.

492. Flickinger JC, Kondziolka D, Niranjan A, et al: Results of acoustic neuroma radiosurgery: An analysis of 5 years' experience using current methods. J Neurosurg 2001;94:1.

493. Williams JA: Fractionated stereotactic radiotherapy for acoustic neuromas. Int J Radiat Oncol Biol Phys 2002;54:500.

494. Poen JC, Golby AJ, Forster KM, et al: Fractionated stereotactic radiosurgery and preservation of hearing in patients with vestibular schwannoma: A preliminary report. Neurosurgery 1999;45:1299.

495. Varlotto JM, Shrieve DC, Alexander E 3rd, et al: Fractionated stereotactic radiotherapy for the treatment of acoustic neuromas: Preliminary results. Int J Radiat Oncol Biol Phys 1996;36:141.

Specific Malignancies

III

496. Fuss M, Debus J, Lohr F, et al: Conventionally fractionated stereotactic radiotherapy (FSRT) for acoustic neuromas. Int J Radiat Oncol Biol Phys 2000;48:1381.

497. Shirato H, Sakamoto T, Sawamura Y, et al: Comparison between observation policy and fractionated stereotactic radiotherapy (SRT) as an initial management for vestibular schwannoma. Int J Radiat Oncol Biol Phys 1999;44:545.

498. Huang CF, Kondziolka D, Flickinger JC, et al: Stereotactic radiosurgery for trigeminal schwannomas. Neurosurgery 1999;45:11.

499. Clifford SC, Maher ER: Von Hippel–Lindau disease: clinical and molecular perspectives. Adv Cancer Res 2001;82:85.

500. Kaelin WG Jr: Molecular basis of the VHL hereditary cancer syndrome. Nat Rev Cancer 2002;2:673.

501. Kanno H, Kondo K, Ito S, et al: Somatic mutations of the von Hippel–Lindau tumor suppressor gene in sporadic central nervous system hemangioblastomas. Cancer Res 1994;54:4845.

502. Mondkar VP, McKissock W, Russell RW: Cerebellar haemangioblastomas. Br J Surg 1967;54:45.

503. Okawara SH: Solid cerebellar hemangioblastoma. J Neurosurg 1973;39:514.

504. Smalley SR, Schomberg PJ, Earle JD, et al: Radiotherapeutic considerations in the treatment of hemangioblastomas of the central nervous system. Int J Radiat Oncol Biol Phys 1990;18:1165.

505. Sung DI, Chang CH, Harisiadis L: Cerebellar hemangioblastomas. Cancer 1982;49:553.

506. Patrice SJ, Sneed PK, Flickinger JC, et al: Radiosurgery for hemangioblastoma: Results of a multiinstitutional experience. Int J Radiat Oncol Biol Phys 1996;35:493.

507. Larson TC 3rd, Houser OW, Laws ER Jr: Imaging of cranial chordomas. Mayo Clin Proc 1987;62:886.

508. Rosenberg AE, Nielsen GP, Keel SB, et al: Chondrosarcoma of the base of the skull: A clinicopathologic study of 200 cases with emphasis on its distinction from chordoma. Am J Surg Pathol 1999;23:1370.

509. Gay E, Sekhar LN, Rubinstein E, et al: Chordomas and chondrosarcomas of the cranial base: Results and follow-up of 60 patients. Neurosurgery 1995;36:887.

510. Forsyth PA, Cascino TL, Shaw EG, et al: Intracranial chordomas: A clinicopathological and prognostic study of 51 cases. J Neurosurg 1993;78:741.

511. Muthukumar N, Kondziolka D, Lunsford LD, et al: Stereotactic radiosurgery for chordoma and chondrosarcoma: Further experiences. Int J Radiat Oncol Biol Phys 1998;41:387.

512. Debus J, Schulz-Ertner D, Schad L, et al: Stereotactic fractionated radiotherapy for chordomas and chondrosarcomas of the skull base. Int J Radiat Oncol Biol Phys 2000;47:591.

513. Spector GJ, Druck NS, Gado M: Neurologic manifestations of glomus tumors in the head and neck. Arch Neurol 1976;33:270.

514. Hinerman RW, Mendenhall WM, Amdur RJ, et al: Definitive radiotherapy in the management of chemodectomas arising in the temporal bone, carotid body, and glomus vagale. Head Neck 2001;23:363.

515. Powell S, Peters N, Harmer C: Chemodectoma of the head and neck: Results of treatment in 84 patients. Int J Radiat Oncol Biol Phys 1992;22:919.

516. Foote RL, Pollock BE, Gorman DA, et al: Glomus jugulare tumor: Tumor control and complications after stereotactic radiosurgery. Head Neck 2002;24:332.

517. Jordan JA, Roland PS, McManus C, et al: Stereotastic radiosurgery for glomus jugulare tumors. Laryngoscope 2000;110:35.

518. Konovalov AN, Pitskhelauri DI: Principles of treatment of the pineal region tumors. Surg Neurol 2003;59:250.

519. Abay EO 2d, Laws ER Jr, Grado GL, et al: Pineal tumors in children and adolescents. Treatment by CSF shunting and radiotherapy. J Neurosurg 1981;55:889.

520. Regis J, Bouillot P, Rouby-Volot F, et al: Pineal region tumors and the role of stereotactic biopsy: Review of the mortality, morbidity, and diagnostic rates in 370 cases. Neurosurgery 1996;39:907.

521. Schild SE, Scheithauer BW, Haddock MG, et al: Histologically confirmed pineal tumors and other germ cell tumors of the brain. Cancer 1996;78:2564.

522. Lutterbach J, Fauchon F, Schild SE, et al: Malignant pineal parenchymal tumors in adult patients: Patterns of care and prognostic factors. Neurosurgery 2002;51:44.

523. Schild SE, Scheithauer BW, Schomberg PJ, et al: Pineal parenchymal tumors. Clinical, pathologic, and therapeutic aspects. Cancer 1993;72:870.

524. Preston-Martin S: Descriptive epidemiology of primary tumors of the spinal cord and spinal meninges in Los Angeles County, 1972–1985. Neuroepidemiology 1990;9:106.

525. Lowe GM: Magnetic resonance imaging of intramedullary spinal cord tumors. J Neurooncol 2000;47:195.

526. Catton C, O'Sullivan B, Bell R, et al: Chordoma: Long-term follow-up after radical photon irradiation. Radiother Oncol 1996;41:67.

527. Bergh P, Kindblom LG, Gunterberg B, et al: Prognostic factors in chordoma of the sacrum and mobile spine: A study of 39 patients. Cancer 2000;88:2122.

528. Solero CL, Fornari M, Giombini S, et al: Spinal meningiomas: Review of 174 operated cases. Neurosurgery 1989;25:153.

529. Levy WJ Jr, Bay J, Dohn D: Spinal cord meningioma. J Neurosurg 1982;57:804.

530. Epstein FJ, Farmer JP, Freed D: Adult intramedullary spinal cord ependymomas: The result of surgery in 38 patients. J Neurosurg 1993;79:204.

531. Cooper PR: Outcome after operative treatment of intramedullary spinal cord tumors in adults: Intermediate and long-term results in 51 patients. Neurosurgery 1989;25:855.

532. Isaacson SR: Radiation therapy and the management of intramedullary spinal cord tumors. J Neurooncol 2000;47:231.

533. Waldron JN, Laperriere NJ, Jaakkimainen L, et al: Spinal cord ependymomas: A retrospective analysis of 59 cases. Int J Radiat Oncol Biol Phys 1993;27:223.

534. Whitaker SJ, Bessell EM, Ashley SE, et al: Postoperative radiotherapy in the management of spinal cord ependymoma. J Neurosurg 1991;74:720.

535. Minehan KJ, Shaw EG, Scheithauer BW, et al: Spinal cord astrocytoma: Pathological and treatment considerations. J Neurosurg 1995;83:590.

536. Linstadt DE, Wara WM, Leibel SA, et al: Postoperative radiotherapy of primary spinal cord tumors. Int J Radiat Oncol Biol Phys 1989;16:1397.

537. Sandler HM, Papadopoulos SM, Thornton AF Jr, et al: Spinal cord astrocytomas: Results of therapy. Neurosurgery 1992;30:490.

538. Jyothirmayi R, Madhavan J, Nair MK, et al: Conservative surgery and radiotherapy in the treatment of spinal cord astrocytoma. J Neurooncol 1997;33:205.

539. Cohen AR, Wisoff JH, Allen JC, et al: Malignant astrocytomas of the spinal cord. J Neurosurg 1989;70:50.

540. Balmaceda C: Chemotherapy for intramedullary spinal cord tumors. J Neurooncol 2000;47:293.

541. Miller DJ, McCutcheon IE: Hemangioblastomas and other uncommon intramedullary tumors. J Neurooncol 2000;47:253.

542. Matsuoka S, Itoh M, Shinonome T, et al: Intramedullary spinal cord germinoma: Case report. Surg Neurol 1991;35:122.

543. Spetzger U, Bertalanffy H, Huffmann B, et al: Hemangioblastomas of the spinal cord and the brainstem: Diagnostic and therapeutic features. Neurosurg Rev 1996;19:147.

544. Lang FF, Epstein FJ, Ransohoff J, et al: Central nervous system gangliogliomas. Part 2: Clinical outcome. J Neurosurg 1993;79:867.

545. Gurney JG, Severson RK, Davis S, et al: Incidence of cancer in children in the United States. Cancer J 1995;75:2186.

546. Grovas A, Fremgen A, Rauck A, et al: The national cancer data base report on patterns of childhood cancers in the United States. Cancer 1997;80:2321.

547. Ries LAG, Kosary CL, Hankey BF, et al: SEER cancer statistics review. DHHS. Publ. No. NIH 97-2789, 1998.

548. Smith MA, Freidlin B, Simon R: Trends in reported incidence of primary malignant brain tumors in children in the United States. J Natl Cancer Inst 1998;90:1269.

549. Lubin F, Farbstein H, Chetrit A, et al: The role of nutritional habits during gestation and child life in pediatric brain tumor etiology. Int J Cancer 2000;86:139.

550. Gurney JG, Smith MA, Bunin GR: CNS and miscellaneous intracranial and intraspinal neoplasms. SEER Pediatric Monograph, National Cancer Institute, 2000.

551. Feychting M, Floderus B, Ahlbom A: Parental occupational exposure to magnetic fields and childhood cancer. Cancer Causes Control 2999;11:151.

552. Bunin GR, Kuijten RR, Buckley LB, et al: Relation between maternal diet and subsequent primitive neuroectodermal brain tumors in young children. N Engl J Med 1993;329:536.

553. Penn I, Porat G: Central nervous system lymphomas in organ allograft recipients. Transplantation 1995;59:240.

554. Granovsky MO, Mueller BU, Nicholson HS, et al: Cancer in human immunodeficiency virus-infected children: A case series from the Children's Cancer Group and the National Cancer Institute. J Clin Oncol 1998;16:1729.

555. Spitzer A, Weis RA, Rapin I: Complications of immunosuppression. J Pediatr 1992;121:145.

556. Rorke LB: Pathology of brain and spinal cord tumors. Pediatr Neurosurg 1999;395.

557. Jakacki RI: Pineal and nonpineal supratentorial primitive neuroectodermal tumors. Childs Nerv Syst 1999;15:586.

558. Rorke LB, Trojanowski JQ, Lee VM, et al: Primitive neuroectodermal tumors of the central nervous system. Brain Pathol 1997;7:765.

559. Bruner JM, Inouye L, Fuller GN, et al: Diagnostic discrepancies and their clinical impact in neuropathology referral practice. Cancer 1998;79:796.

560. Pomeroy SL, Sutton ME, Goumnerova LC, et al: Neurotrophins in cerebellar granule cell development and medulloblastoma. J Neurooncol 1997;35:347.

561. Pomeroy SL, Tamayo P, Gaasenbeek M, et al: Prediction of central nervous system embryonal tumour outcome based on gene expression. Nature 2002;415:436.

562. Biegel JA, Janss AJ, Raffel C, et al: Prognostic significance of chromosome 17p deletions in childhood primitive neuroectodermal tumors (medulloblastoma) of the central nervous system. Clin Cancer Res 1997;3:473.

563. Schofield D, West DC, Anthony DC, et al: Correlation of loss of heterozygosity at chromosome 9q with histological subtype in medulloblastoma. Am J Pathol 1995;146:472.

564. Scheurlen EG, Schwabe GC, Joos S, et al: Molecular analysis of childhood primitive neuroectodermal tumors defines markers associated with poor outcome. J Clin Oncol 1998;16:2479.

565. Hahn H, Wicking C, Zaphiropoulous PG, et al: Mutations of the human homolog of *Drosophila* patched in the nevoid basal cell carcinoma syndrome. Cell 1996;85:841.

566. Hunter T: Oncoprotein networks. Cell 1997;88:333.

567. Oro AE, Higgis KM, Hu Z, et al: Basal cell carcinomas in mice overexpressing sonic hedgehog. Science 1997;276:817.

568. Evans DG, Farndon PA, Burnell LD, et al: The incidence of Gorlin syndrome in 173 consecutive case of medulloblastoma. Br J Cancer 1991;64:959.

569. Raffel C, Jenkins RB, Frederick L, et al: Sporadic medulloblastoma contain PTCH mutatuions. Cancer Res 1997;57:842.

570. Arle JE, Morris C, Wang ZJ, et al: Prediction of posterior fossa tumor type in children by means of magnetic resonance image properties spectroscopy. J Neurosurg 1997;86:755.

571. Zeltzer PM, Boyett JM, Finlay JL, et al: Metastasis stage, adjuvant treatment, and residual tumor are prognostic factors for medulloblastoma in children: Conclusion from the Children's Cancer Group 921 randomized phase III study. J Clin Oncol 1999;17:832.

572. Berger MS, Baumeister B, Geyer JR, et al: The risks of metastases from shunting in children with primary central nervous system tumors. J Neurosurg 1991;74:872.

573. Hirsch JF, Renier D, Czernichow P, et al: Medulloblasoma in childhood. Survival and functional results. Acta Neurochir 1979;48:1.

574. Wisoff JH, Epstein FJ: Pseudobulbar palsy after posterior fossa operation in children. Neurosurgery 1984;15:707.

575. Pollack IF: Posterior fossa syndrome. Int Rev Neurobiol 1997;41:411.

576. Liu GT, Phillips PC, Molloy P, et al: Visual Impairment associated with mutism after posterior fossa surgery in children. Neurosurgery 1998;42:253.

577. Garton GR, Schomberg PJ, Scheithauer BW, et al: Medulloblastoma —Prognostic factors and outcome of treatment: review of the Mayo Clinic experience. Mayo Clinic Proc 1990;65:1077.

578. Tait DM, Thorton-Jones H, Bloom HJG, et al: Adjuvant chemotherapy for medulloblastoma: The first multi-centre control trial of the International Society of Pediatric Oncology (SIOP). Eur J Cancer 1990;26:464.

579. Packer RJ, Cogen P, Vezina G, et al: Medulloblastoma: Clinical and biologic aspects. Neuro-oncol 1999;1:232.

580. Kim JYH, Sutton ME, Lu DJ: Activation of neurotrophin-3 receptor TrkC induces apoptosis in medulloblastoma. Cancer Res 1999;59:711.

581. Grotzer MA, Janns AJ, Fung KM: TrkC expression predicts good clinical outcome in primitive neuroectoderam brain tumors. J Clin Oncol 2000;18:1027.

582. Gilbertson RJ, Perry RH, Kelly PJ, et al: Prognostic significance of HER2 and HER4 coexpression in childhood medulloblastoma. Cancer Res 1997;57:3272.

583. Janss AJ, AT Y, JH S, et al: Glial differentiation predicts poor clinical outcome in primitive neuroectodermal brain tumors. Ann Neurol 1996;39:481.

584. MacDonald TJ, Brown KM, LaFleur B, et al: Expression profiling of medulloblastoma: PDGFRA and the RAS/MAPK pathway as therapeutic targets for metastatic disease. Nat Genet 2001;29:143.

585. Silverman CL, Simpson JR: Cerebellar medulloblastoma: The importance of posterior fossa dose to survival and patterns of failure. Int J Radiat Oncol 1982;8:1869.

586. Jenkin D: The radiation treatment of medulloblastoma. J Neurooncol 1996;29:45.

587. Evans AE, Jenkin DT, Sposto R, et al: The treatment of medulloblastoma. Results of a prospective randomized trial of radiation therapy with and without CCNU, vincristine, and prednisone. J Neurosurg 1990;72:572.

588. Silber JH, Radcliffe J, Peckham V, et al: Whole-brain irradiation and decline in intelligence: The influence of dose and age on IQ score. J Clin Oncol 1992;10:1390.

589. Goldwein JW, Radcliffe J, Johnson J, et al: Updated results of a pilot study of low dose craniospinal irradiation plus chemotherapy for children under five with cerebellar primitive neuroectodermal tumors (medulloblastoma). Int J Radiat Oncol Biol Phys 1996;34:899.

590. Packer RJ: Brain tumors in children. Arch Neurol 1999;56:421.

591. Friedman HS, Oakes WJ, Bigner SH, et al: Medulloblastoma tumor biological and clinical perspectives. J Neurooncol 1991;11:1.

592. Packer RJ: Chemotherapy for medulloblastoma/primitive neuro-ectodermal tumors of the posterior fossa. Ann Neurol 1990;28:823.

593. Kalifa C, Valteau D, Pizer B, et al: High-dose chemotherapy in childhood brain tumours. Child Nerv Syst 1999;15:498.

594. Kalifa C, Hartmann O, Demeocq F, et al: High-dose busulfan and thiotepa with autologous bone marrow transplantation in childhood malignant brain tumors: a phase II study. Bone Marrow Transplant 1992;9:227.

595. Dunkel IJ, Boyett JM, Yates A, et al: High-dose carboplatin thiotepa, and etoposide with autologous stem-cell rescue for patients with recurrent medulloblastoma. J Clin Oncol 1998;16:222.

596. Gropman AL, Packer RJ, Nicholson HS, et al: Treatment of diencephalic syndrome with chemotherapy: Growth, tumor response, and long term control. Cancer 1998;83:166.

597. Alvord ECJ, Lofton S: Gliomas of the optic nerve or chiasm. Outcome by patient's age tumor site, and treatment. J Neurosurg 1988;68:85.

598. Wisoff JH: Management of optic pathway tumors of childhood. Neurosurg Clin North Am 1992;3:791.

599. Sutton LN, Molloy P, Sernyak H, et al: Long-term outcome of hypothalamic/chiasmatic astrocytomas in children treated with conservative surgery. J Neurosurg 1995;83:583.

600. Pierce SM, Barnes PD, Loeffler JS, et al: Definitive radiation therapy in the management of symptomatic patients with optic glioma. Survival and long term effects. Cancer 1990;65:45.

601. Erkal HS, Serin M, Cakmak A: Management of optic pathway and chiasmatic-hypothalamic gliomas in children with radiation therapy. Radiother Oncol 1997;45:11.

602. Horwich A, Bloom HJ: Optic gliomas: Radiation therapy and prognosis. Int J Radiat Oncol Biol Phys 1985;11:1067.

603. Packer RJ, Ater JL, Allen J, et al: Carboplatin and vincristine chemotherpy for children with newly diagnosed progressive in low grade gliomas. J Neurosurg 1997;86:747.

604. Prados MD, Edwards MS, Rabbitt J, et al: Treatment of pediatric low-grade gliomas with a nitrosourea-based multiagent chemotherapy regimen. J Neurooncol 1997;32:235.

605. Listerncik R, Charrow J, Greenwald MJ, et al: Natural history of optic pathway tumors in children with neurofibromatosis type 1. J Pediatr 1994;125:63.

606. Sutton LN, Cnaan A, Klatt L, et al: Postoperative surveillance imaging in children with cerebellar astrocytomas. J. Neurosurg 1996;84:721.

607. Gilbertson RJ, Bentley L, Hernan R, et al: ERBB receptor signaling promotes ependymoma cell proliferation and represents a potential novel therapeutic target for this disease. Clin Cancer Res 2002;8:3054.

608. Goldwein JW, Corn BW, Finlay JL, et al: Is craniospinal irradiation required to cure children with malignant (anaplastic) intracranial epenymomas. Cancer 1991;67:2766.

609. Vanuystel L, Brada M: The role of prophylactic spinal irradiation in localized intracranial ependymoma. Int J Radiat Oncol 1991;21:825.

610. Nazar GB, Hoffman HJ, Becker LE, et al: Infratentorial ependymomas in childhood: Prognostic factors and treatment. J Neurosurg 1990;72:408.

611. Evans AE, Anderson JR, Lefkowitz-Boudreaux IB, et al: Adjuvant chemotherapy of childhood posterior fossa ependymoma: Cranio-spinal irradiation with or without adjuvant CCNU, vincristine, and prednisone; a Childrens Cancer Group study. Med Pediatr Oncol 1996;27:8.

612. Pollack IF, Gerszten PC, Martinez AJ, et al: Intracranial ependymomas of childhood: Long term outcome and prognostic factors. Neurosurgery 1995;37:655.

613. Sutton LN, Goldwein JW, Perilongo G, et al: Prognostic factors in childhood ependymomas. Pediatr Neurosurg 1991;16:57.

614. Robertson PL, Zeltzer PM, Boyett J, et al: Survival and prognostic factors following rediation therapy and chemotherapy for ependymomas in children: A report of the Children's Cancer Group. J Neurosurg 1998;88:695.

615. Allen J, Siffert J, Hukin J: Clinical manifestations of childhood ependymoma: A multitude of syndromes. Pediatr Neurosurg 1998;28:49.

616. Wirtz CR, Knauth M, Staubert A, et al: Clinical evaluation and follow-up results for intraoperative magnetic resonance imaging in neurosurgery. Neurosurgery 2000;46:1112.

617. Kim YH, Fayos JW: Intracranial ependymomas. Radiology 1977;124:805.

618. Grabb PA, Lunsford LD, Albright AL, et al: Stereotactic radiosurgery for glial neoplasms of childhood. Neurosurgery 1996;38:696.

619. Needle MN, Goldwein JW, Grass JW: Adjuvant chemotherapy for the treatment of intracranial ependymoma of childhood. Cancer 1997;80:341.

620. Goldwein JW, Glauser TA, Packer RJ, et al: Recurrent intracranial ependymomas in children. Cancer 1990;66:557.

621. Mason WP, Goldman S, Yates A, et al: Survival following intensive chemotherapy with bone marrow reconstitution for children with recurrent intracranial ependymoma. J Neurooncol 1998;37:135.

622. Greenberger JS, Cassady JR, Levene MB: Radiation therapy of thalamic gliomas. Radiology 1977;122:463.

623. Sung T, Miller DC, Hayes RL, et al: Preferential inactivation of th p53 tumor suppressor pathway and lack of EGFR receptor amplification distinguish de novo high grade pediatric astrocytomas from de novo adult astrocytomas. Brain Pathol 2000;10:249.

624. Albright AL, Packer RJ, Zimmerman RA, et al: Magnetic resonance scans should replace biopsies for the diagnosis of diffuse brain stem gliomas: A report from the Children's Cancer Group. Neurosurgery 1993;33:1026.

625. Epstein F, McCleary EL: Intrinsic brain-stem tumors of childhood: Surgical indications. J Neurosurg 1986;64:11.

626. Jennings MT, Freeman ML, Murray MJ: Strategies in the treatment of diffuse pontine gliomas: The therapeutic role of hyperfractionated radiotherapy and chemotherapy. J Neurooncol 1996;28:207.

627. Packer RJ, Boyett JM, Zimmerman RA, et al: Outcome of children with brain stem gliomas after treatment with 7800 cGy of hyperfrationated radiotherapy. A Children's Cancer Group Phase I/II Trial. Cancer 1994;74:1827.

628. Mandell LR, Kadota R, Freeman CR, et al: There is no role for hyperfractioneded radiotherapy in management fo children with newly diagnosed diffuse intrinsic brainstem tumors: Results of Pediatric Oncology Group phase III trial comparing conventional vs. hyperfractionaed radiotherapy. Int J Radiat Oncol Biol Phys 1999;43:959.

629. Kaplan AM, Albright AL, Zimmerman RA, et al: Brainstem gliomas in children. A Children's Cancer Group review of 119 cases. Pediatr Neurosurg 1996;24:185.

630. Jenkin RD, Boesel C, Ertel I, et al: Brain-stem tuors in childhood: A prospective randomized trial of irradiation with and without adjuvant CCNU, VCR, and prednisone. A report of the Children's Cancer Study Group. J Neurosurg 1987;66:227.

631. Bouffet E, Raquin M, Doz F, et al: Radiotherapy followed by high does busulfan and thiotepa: A prospective assesment of high dose chemotherapy in children with diffuse pontine gliomas. Cancer 2000;88:685.

632. Pollack IF, Hoffman HJ, Humphreys RP, et al: The long-term outcome after surgical treatment of dorsally exophytic brain stem gliomas. J Neurosurg 1993;78:859.

633. Robertson PL, Allen JC, Abbott IR, et al: Cervicomedullary tumors in children: A distinct subset of brainstem gliomas. Neurology 1994;44:1798.

634. Shrieve DC, Wara WM, Edwards MS, et al: Hyperfractionated radiation therapy for gliomas of the brainstem in children and in adults. Int J Radiat Oncol Biol Phys 1992;24:599.

635. Guillamo JS, Monjour A, Taillandier L, et al: Brainstem gliomas in adults: Prognostic factors and classification. Brain 2001;124:2528.

636. Landolfi JC, Thaler HT, DeAngelis LM: Adult brainstem gliomas. Neurology 1998;51:1136.

637. Kretschmar CS: Germ cell tumors of the brain in children: A review of current literature and new advances in therapy. Cancer Invest 1997;15:187.

638. Kang JK, Jeun SS, Hong YK, et al: Experience with pineal region tumors. Childs Nerv Syst 1998;14:63.

639. Shinoda J, Ymada H, Sakai N, et al: Placental alkaline phosphatase as a tumor marker for primary intracranial germinoma. J Neurosurg 1988;68:710.

640. Maity A, Shu H-KG, Janss A, et al: Craniospinal radiation in the treatment of biopsy proven intracranial germinomas: Twenty-five years experience in a single center. Int J Radiat Oncol Biol Phys (in press).

641. Wolden SL, Wara WM, Larson DA, et al: Radiation therapy for primary intracranial germ-cell tumors. Int J Radiat Oncol Biol Phys 1995;32:943.

642. Matsutani M, Sano K, Takakura K, et al: Primary intracranial germ cell tumors: A clinical analysis of 153 histologically verified cases. J Neurosurg 1997;86:446.

643. Jennings MT, Gelman R, Hochberg F: Intracranial germ-cell tumors: Natural history and pathogenesis. J Neurosurg 1985;63:155.

644. Bouffet E, Baranzelli MC, Patte C, et al: Combined treatment modality for intracranial germinomas: Results of a multicentre SFOP experience. Societe Francaise d'Oncologie Pediatrique. Br J Cancer 1999;79:1199.

645. Buckner JC, Peethambaram PP, Smithson WA, et al: Phase II trial of primary chemotherapy followed by reduced-dose radiation for CNS germ cell tumors. J Clin Oncol 1999;17:933.

646. Balmaceda C, Heller G, Rosenblum M, et al: Chemotherapy without irradiation—A novel approach for newly diagnosed CNS germ cell tumors: Results of an international cooperative trial. The First International Central Nervous System Germ Cell Tumor Study. J Clin Oncol 1996;14:2908.

647. Robertson PL, DaRosso RC, Allen JC: Improved prognosis of intracranial non-germinoma germ cell tumors with multimodality therapy. J Neuro-oncol 1997;32:71.

648. Sanford RA: Craniopharyngioma: Results of survey of the American Society of Pediatric Neurosurgery. Pediatr Neurosurg 1994;21(Suppl 1):39.

649. Hoffman HJ, De Silva M, Humphreys RP, et al: Aggressive surgical management of craniopharyngiomas in children. J Neurosurg 1992;76:47.

650. Duff JM, Meyer FB, Ilstrup DM, et al: Long-term outcomes for surgically resected craniopharyngiomas. Neurosurgery 2000;46:291.

651. Carpentieri SC, Waber DP, Scott RM, et al: Memory deficits among children with craniopharyngiomas. Neurosurgery 2001;49:1053.

652. Habrand JL, Ganry O, Couanet D, et al: The role of radiation therapy in the management of craniopharyngioma: A 25-year experience and review of the literature. Int J Radiat Oncol Biol Phys 1999;44:255.

653. Isaac MA, Hahn SS, Kim JA, et al: Management of craniopharyngioma. Cancer J 2001;7:516.

654. Merchant TE, Kiehna EN, Sanford RA, et al: Craniopharyngioma: The St. Jude Children's Research Hospital experience 1984–2001. Int J Radiat Oncol Biol Phys 2002;53:533.

655. Kalapurakal JA, Goldman S, Hsieh YC, et al: Clinical outcome in children with craniopharyngioma treated with primary surgery and radiotherapy deferred until relapse. Med Pediatr Oncol 2003;40:214.

656. Stripp D, Maity A, Janss A, et al: Surgery with or without radiation therapy in the management of craniopharyngiomas in children and young adults. Int J Radiat Oncol Biol Phys (in press).

657. Varlotto JM, Flickinger JC, Kondziolka D, et al: External beam irradiation of craniopharyngiomas: Long-term analysis of tumor control and morbidity. Int J Radiat Oncol Biol Phys 2002;54:492.

658. Blackburn TP, Doughty D, Plowman PN: Stereotactic intracavitary therapy of recurrent cystic craniopharyngioma by instillation of 90yttrium. Br J Neurosurg 1999;13:359.

659. Pollock BE, Lunsford LD, Kondziolka D, et al: Phosphorus-32 intracavitary irradiation of cystic craniopharyngiomas: Current technique and long-term results. Int J Radiat Oncol Biol Phys 1995;33:437.

660. Voges J, Sturm V, Lehrke R, et al: Cystic craniopharyngioma: Long-term results after intracavitary irradiation with stereotactically applied colloidal beta-emitting radioactive sources. Neurosurgery 1997;40:263.

661. Kun LE: Challenges and directions. Pediatr Clin North Am 1997;4:907.

662. Duffner PK, Horowitz ME, Krischer JP, et al: Postoperative chemotherapy and delayed radiation in children less than three years of age with malignant brain tumors. N Engl J Med 1993;328:1725.

663. Suc E, Kalifa C, Brauner R, et al: The price of survival. A retrospective study of 20 long term survivors. Acta Neurochir 1990;106:93.

664. Ater JL, van Eys J, Woo SY, et al: MOPP chemotherapy without irradiation as primary postsurgical therapy for brain tumors in infants and young children. J Clin Oncol 1997;32:243.

665. Geyer JR, Zeltzer PM, Boyett J, et al: Survival of infants with primitive neuroectodermal tumors or malignant ependymomas of the CNS treated with eight drugs in 1 day: A report from the Children's Cancer Group. J Clin Oncol 1994;12:1607.

Specific Malignancies

III

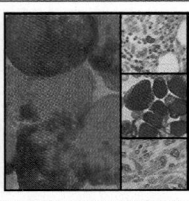

Leslie R. Holmes

John E. Munzenrider

Victor M. Elner

David S. Bardenstein

Allen S. Lichter

SUMMARY OF KEY POINTS

INCIDENCE
- Primary eye tumors are relatively uncommon (approximately 2000 per year) and cause 250 to 300 deaths annually.
- Many systemic lesions can involve the eye/orbit, especially breast and lung cancer, as well as lymphoma.
- The most common ophthalmic tumors are choroidal melanoma, retinoblastoma, rhabdomyosarcoma, optic nerve glioma, and squamous and melanocytic malignancies of the eyelid and conjunctiva.

ETIOLOGY
- The etiology of most tumors is unknown.
- Retinoblastoma is the prototypical model of a genetically transmissible tumor via loss of a tumor suppressor gene.
- Squamous tumors of the lids and conjunctiva are associated with sun exposure.
- Choroidal metastases are surprisingly frequent, due to the rich blood supply to this structure.

DIAGNOSIS
- Ocular tumors can be directly visualized, greatly facilitating diagnosis, but biopsy is difficult.
- For ocular tumors, a combination of funduscopic examination, ultrasonography, and CT/MRI can yield diagnostic accuracies of 98% to 99%.
- Orbital and adnexal tumors are diagnosed by CT findings and biopsy.

TREATMENT
- Intraocular tumors are treated with local modalities such as external radiation, episcleral plaque irradiation, and photocoagulation, with or without chemotherapy, if useful vision can be preserved; otherwise, the eye is enucleated.
- Orbital malignancies are frequently treated by radiation/chemotherapy, but exenteration may be necessary in far-advanced solid tumors.
- Eyelid and conjunctival malignancies are successfully managed by local excision or by irradiation.
- Metastatic disease is commonly palliated by irradiation.

INTRODUCTION

Ocular oncology is a discipline that presents unique clinical challenges. While it is often considered to focus on uveal melanoma, retinoblastoma, and metastases within the eye as well as lymphoma and rhabdomyosarcoma in the orbit and adnexal tissues, ocular oncology also includes tumors of dermal, osseous, neural, vascular, hematologic, soft tissue, mucous membrane, and glandular derivations. Neoplasms of ocular tissues, however, frequently differ in their clinical behaviors from their counterparts in other tissues. Moreover, each ocular tissue (conjunctiva, eyelid, orbit, optic nerve, and nasolacrimal apparatus) is distinct with respect to its oncologic behavior. Even the various tissue layers within the eye show remarkable differences with respect to the types of neoplasms affecting them and their tissue responses. Thus, for example, malignant melanomas of the conjunctiva, iris, and choroid display remarkably different patterns of clinical behavior and prognosis. Similar site-related behavior occurs with lymphoma of the conjunctiva, orbit, and eyelid so that a thorough understanding of the intricate anatomy of the eye and periocular tissues is needed in order to provide effective oncologic diagnosis and treatment. Thus generalizations about tumor types cannot be made. These patients should be managed in a multidisciplinary fashion by medical and radiation oncologists, and ophthalmologists with oncologic training.

Other important features of ocular oncology are that most intraocular tumors can be visualized directly with resolutions measured in fractions of millimeters so that neoplasms can be monitored noninvasively. Using only the clinical examination and noninvasive tests, many tumors can be diagnosed by ocular oncologists with accuracies approaching 98% to 99%. Because of the delicate functional equilibrium of the eye, invasive techniques or their sequelae can render an eye dysfunctional and so their use is limited. On the other hand, tumors affecting the eyelids, orbit, optic nerve, and nasolacrimal apparatus frequently require additional diagnostic studies to detect or characterize them.

Whereas a broad variety of ocular and adnexal neoplasms exists, such tumors are much less common than neoplasms of other systems. This has a number of implications. Extensive data concerning the natural history of ocular neoplasms are limited. This disadvantage is compounded in the eye, where loss of function can be induced by small lesions. Similarly, experience in treating many of these tumors is limited and so management is highly variable even among specialists.

Given these premises, this chapter seeks to provide a broad view of the spectrum of ocular oncology in combination with detailed discussions of management approaches. It is organized by discrete anatomic compartments: (1) the eye (see Table 70-1), (2) the orbit (see Table 70-6), (3) the eyelids (see Table 70-7), and (4) the conjunctiva (see Table 70-8). Ocular tumors and distinctive syndromes related to systemic neoplasia are also discussed (see Table 70-9). Some historical data are included to illuminate the rationale underlying certain currently preferred management regimens. General guidelines regarding the management of these tumors reflect the published literature and the authors' experience. Extensive discussion is reserved for regimens that provide proven effectiveness and safety of patients. When multiple methods of equal value exist, they are all presented; the authors' preferences are not used to exclude any of the various methods. Algorithmic guidelines cannot be provided, and the reader should consult an ophthalmologist trained in ocular oncology for assistance.

INTRAOCULAR NEOPLASIA

The intraocular neoplasms are listed in Table 70-1.

TABLE 70-1

Intraocular Neoplasms

Benign

Melanocytic nevus*
Melanocytoma*
Hemangioma*
Medulloepithelioma[†]
Neurofibroma
Osteoma
Neurilemmoma
Leiomyoma
  Fibrous histiocytoma
Glioneuroma
  Neuroepithelial adenoma[†]

Uncertain Behavior

Reactive lymphoid hyperplasia*[†]

Malignant

Malignant melanoma*[†]
Retinoblastoma*[†]
Primary lymphoma (reticulum cell sarcoma)*[†]
Leukemia/lymphoma*[†]
Medulloepithelioma[†]
Rhabdomyosarcoma
Leiomyosarcoma
Neuroepithelial adenocarcinoma[†]
Extension of local tumour
  Conjunctival carcinoma[†]
  Orbital sarcoma[†]
  Lacrimal gland carcinoma[†]
Metastatic tumor
  Carcinoma*[†]
  Neuroblastoma[†]
  Malignant melanoma[†]

*Common tumor.
[†]Discussed in text.

Primary Malignant Intraocular Tumors of Adults

Primary Malignant Intraocular Tumors of Adults

Malignant Melanoma of Choroid and Ciliary Body (Posterior Uveal Melanoma)

Uveal melanoma is the most common primary intraocular malignancy of adults; it is estimated to account for 12% of all melanomas and between 30% and 80% of noncutaneous melanomas.[1,2] This entity may be subclassified anatomically into iris, ciliary body, and choroidal melanoma (5% to 10%, 10% to 15%, and 80% of uveal melanomas, respectively).[3] Incidence estimates range from 5 to 7.2/million in a variety of countries.[4-6] The incidence of uveal melanoma in the United States over a 25-year period, between 1973 and 1997, has recently been described, based on the Surveillance, Epidemiology, and End Results (SEER) program database. The mean age-adjusted incidence in the U.S. is 4.3 per million, similar to that reported by European countries. The age-adjusted incidence rate has remained stable for the past 25 years. Males are significantly more likely to be diagnosed with melanoma than females (males 4.9 per million [4.6 to 5.2] 95% CI interval; females 3.7 [3.5 to 3.9] 95% CI interval. Eye melanomas represent 2.9% of all recorded cases of melanoma. Almost all (97.8%) uveal melanomas in the U.S. occur in the white population. There was no significant variation of incidence by geographic location.[7]

The lesions arise from uveal melanocytes and may occur de novo or in the setting of a nevus. Difficulties in understanding the nature of this tumor derive from its unpredictable clinical behavior and the absence of clinical signs that predict malignant potential.[8-13] The most commonly used clinical criteria for diagnosing malignancy in uveal melanocytic tumors are tumor size and thickness. Based on probabilistic data, a continuum exists between small pigmented lesions with little or no metastatic potential and large aggressive lesions with high malignant potential. The clinical term *nevoma* is used to describe the transition state between a benign nevus and an obvious malignant melanoma. While choroidal melanomas are sometimes classified separately from those arising in the ciliary body, they have common prognostic features and thus will be considered together in this chapter.

Choroidal melanomas are uncommon in heavily pigmented patients. White individuals have three times the risk that Asians have and eight times the risk that blacks have of developing uveal melanoma.[14,15] Melanomas are observed with increased frequency in patients with ocular or oculodermal melanocytosis (nevus of Ota).[16] They are uncommon in children and young adults and increase in incidence with age.[17]

Choroidal melanomas typically present as asymptomatic masses or cause painless visual loss or retinal detachment. The tumor may be suspected by the presence of enlarged sentinel vessels in the sclera overlying ciliary body or iris melanomas. Unilateral glaucoma or intraocular hemorrhage may also bring attention to these lesions. Rarely, patients will present with metastatic melanoma and an unknown primary tumor. In such cases, in addition to uveal melanoma, the differential diagnosis for primary melanoma includes skin, respiratory sinuses, viscera, and brain tumors. Melanomas can be found anywhere melanocytes exist and are rarely bilateral or multiple within the eye. Ten percent to 20% of choroidal melanomas are unsuspected.[18,19] This situation usually occurs in eyes with opaque media or those that are blind and painful. Patients with blind, painful eyes and opaque media require ophthalmic evaluation.

Diagnosis is primarily based on the ophthalmoscopic and ultrasonographic findings. Diagnostic rates by experienced observers approach 98% to 99%.[20,21] The clinical history may mislead the clinician to diagnose a uveal melanoma as a metastasis based on the history of a systemic malignancy and inadequate or atypical ultrasonographic examination. Ophthalmoscopically, uveal melanomas are usually pigmented (Fig. 70-1A), but they may be amelanotic or variegated (Fig. 70-1B). Uveal melanomas are usually dome-shaped, but 5% show a diffuse placoid growth pattern.[22] The so-called collar-button or mushroom growth pattern (Fig. 70-1C), indicative of tumor rupture through Bruch's membrane, the thin, innermost layer of the choroid proper, is almost pathognomonic for melanoma. Retinal detachment, when present, is small in comparison with the size of the tumor. This contrasts with the large exudative detachments associated with uveal metastases.

Ultrasonography remains the imaging modality of choice for intraocular tumors, which are currently evaluated by standardized echography consisting of B-mode (Fig. 70-1D) and quantitative A-mode ultrasonography. Melanomas are usually densely cellular tumors; the typical ultrasonographic picture shows homogeneous low attenuation of the echoes, sharp delineation between the tumor and the retina and sclera, choroidal excavation, and

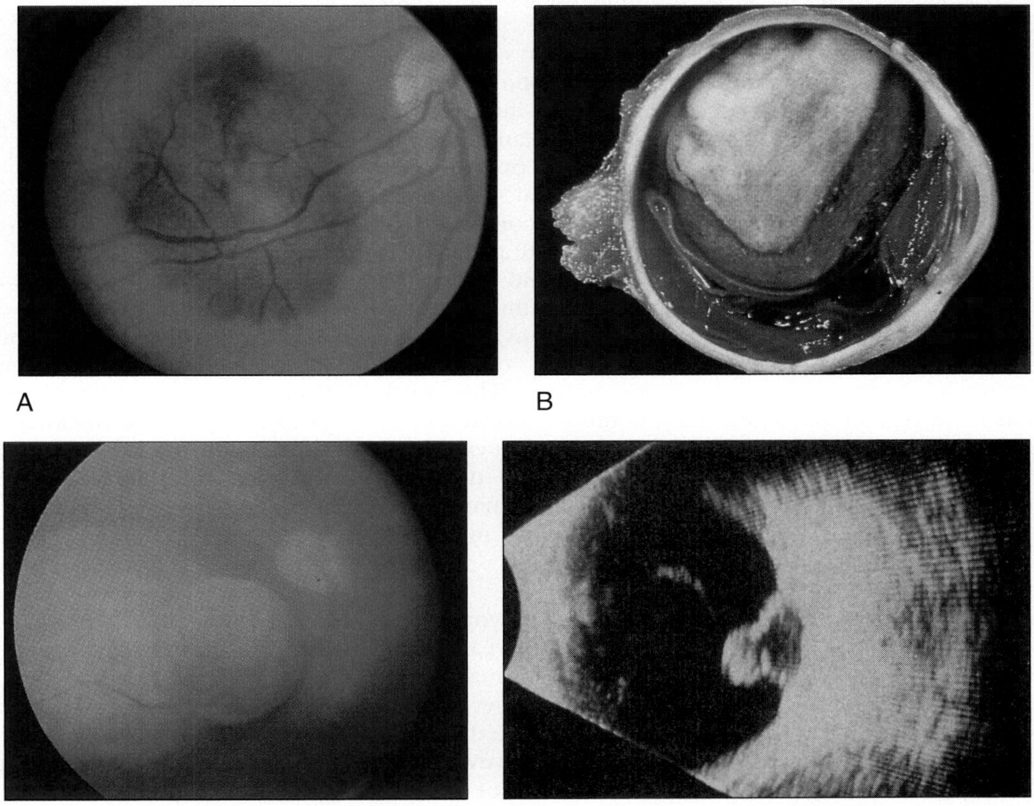

Figure 70-1. A, Pigmented choroidal melanoma with overlying orange pigment. **B,** Cut section of enucleated eye containing large choroidal melanoma with amelanotic and overlying darkly pigmented regions. **C,** Amelanotic choroidal melanoma with characteristic collar-button configuration corresponding to tumor growth through Bruch's membrane. **D,** Ultrasonogram of tumor in **(C)** showing collar-button and larger tumor base. Typical highly reflective surface overlies dark acoustic quiet zone. **E,** Spindle-shaped cohesive spindle B melanoma cells. **F,** Polygonal, poorly cohesive epithelioid melanoma cells with eosinophilic cytoplasm and prominent nucleoli. Tumor cells are surrounded by reactive lymphocytes.

A

B

C

D

E

F

Specific Malignancies

the presence of an intrinsic tumor vasculature.[23-25] Ultrasonography is diagnostic in 82% of cases.[26] Fluorescein angiography is of limited value and serves primarily to exclude other conditions such as hemorrhagic lesions and hemangiomas.[21,26] Fine-needle aspiration (FNA) biopsy can be of great assistance in atypical cases.[27-29] Extraocular extension can be detected with ultrasonography, computed tomography (CT), or magnetic resonance imaging (MRI).[30,31] MRI is primarily of value when hemorrhage obscures the lesion or for the assessment of extraocular extension.

Using a large number of enucleated eyes with available follow-up data, a histologic classification, the Callender system, has been used for grading uveal melanomas and assessing prognosis.[32] Tumor cell types were categorized as spindle A cells with slender nuclei, inconspicuous nucleoli, and fibrillar cytoplasm; spindle B cells with plump nuclei, distinct nucleoli, and fibrillar cytoplasm (Fig. 70-1E); and epithelioid cells, which were large polygonal cells with larger eosinophilic nucleoli and poor intercellular cohesion (Fig. 70-1F).

Careful studies of patient survival after enucleation have established that tumors composed of spindle A cells are mainly benign nevi. The Callender classification was modified by dividing uveal malignant melanomas into categories based on cell types that carry progressively higher risks of mortality. Currently, choroidal melanomas are classified as spindle cell melanomas comprised of spindle A and spindle B cells, mixed cell melanomas comprised of spindle cells and epithelioid cells, and epithelioid cell melanomas.[33-35] Meticulous multifactorial analysis of data shows that the most important pathologic factors predicting prognosis are cell type, tumor size, extrascleral extension, and mitotic activity. This work has been further advanced using computer-assisted cytomorphometry of the inverse of the standard deviation of the nucleolar area within tumor nuclei; this measures cellular atypia and correlates well with malignancy and mortality.[36-38] Discrete melanomas less than 3 mm thick have a less than 5% chance of metastasis.[39-41]

Management. Improvements in ophthalmoscopic and echographic techniques over the past 20 years have allowed better differentiation of melanomas from simulating lesions, thereby reducing the number of eyes enucleated for suspected melanoma. Clinical diagnosis accuracy can approach 99%. Even today, however, eyes with pigmented tumors of appreciable size or growth are often enucleated without knowledge of their true malignant potential. Ethical considerations have limited scientific study of untreated large or growing pigmented uveal tumors to determine their actual risk of metastasis and death.

Since tissue is not routinely obtained for histologic analysis, management is based solely on clinical criteria. Intervention is offered for lesions showing signs of active growth or whose size is felt to be significant for risk of metastasis. Such signs include increase in thickness or diameter, accumulation of subretinal fluid or orange deposits representing clusters of pigment-laden macrophages, and a collar-button tumor configuration. When

---

MANAGEMENT ALTERNATIVES FOR CHOROIDAL MELANOMA

OBSERVATION
Entire tumor visualized
Asymptomatic, without signs of growth
Diameter <10 mm, height <2 mm
Patient refuses intervention

LOCAL RESECTION (EXTERNAL)
Tumors not involving the posterior pole
Diameter <15 mm
Much higher rate of early complications
Good initial vision may be retained

RADIATION
Plaque or charged particle treatment successful
  Diameter <15 mm, height <10 mm
  Used when preservation of vision is possible
  Patient's only seeing eye
  Ocular retention in 90% of cases, vision preserved in
    more than 50% of eyes

ENUCLEATION
Used for eyes with no vision potential
Used for eyes when radiation will unequivocally lead to
  vision loss
Used for eyes with regrowth after radiation therapy
Used for eyes with complications (e.g., neovascularization,
  pain)

---

doubt regarding progression exists, serial examination, ultrasonography, and photography are indicated. Classification of melanomas by size is presented in Table 70-2.[42,43] Both diameter and thickness are classified and the tumor is placed in the lowest category (i.e., a tumor of medium thickness and large diameter would be considered medium sized). A staging system for uveal melanoma based on the tumor-node-metastasis (TNM) system has also been developed but is not widely used.[44]

Current management options include observation, thermal destruction, plaque irradiation, external-beam radiation, local resection of tumor, and enucleation of the eye.

Observation. Observation is applicable when the entire tumor is easily visualized, asymptomatic, less than 10 mm in diameter, less than 2 mm thick, and shows no signs of growth. The patient must understand that a potentially malignant condition is being observed and also be reliably available for serial clinical evaluations. In various series, 10% to 45% of observed lesions have shown growth.[41] When growth occurs, treatment is indicated.

TABLE 70-2

Classification of Uveal Melanoma by Size (mm)			
	SMALL	**MEDIUM**	**LARGE**
Diameter	<10	10–15	>15
Height	<2	2–5	>5

Thermal Therapies. Traditional thermal destruction (cryotherapy or photocoagulation) is applicable only for selected pigmented tumors of less than 10 mm diameter, less than 4 mm thickness, of specific locations. Data on the efficacy of these modalities are limited, since different indications for treatment have been used in various studies and many patients require multiple treatments for tumors, rendering the concepts of cure and tumor-free interval difficult to apply. Even though these are relatively small tumors at the initiation of therapy, less than 50% are controlled with these modalities, which are being used less frequently (generally when other modalities are refused by the patient).[45] Thermal destruction using photosensitizers such as hematoporphyrins is being evaluated for use in melanoma treatment.

Hyperthermia employing microwave ultrasonography and ferromagnetic techniques has been used to treat melanomas.[46-49] This was attempted both to explore hyperthermia as a primary modality and to use it in combination with plaque radiation therapy to lower the required radiation dose and thus the radiation-associated complications. Greater experience has shown early efficacy of combined episcleral plaque thermoradiotherapy in tumor shrinkage, but longer follow-up is required to assess ultimate efficacy and complication rates. These techniques show promise, and further evaluation is awaited, but the technical support required for these modalities is extensive.

Surgical. Enucleation (of the eye) has been the traditional method of treating choroidal melanomas, because it removed the tumor and because alternative techniques had not yet been developed. Only 1% to 2% of patients present with metastases from their uveal melanoma and the annual rate of metastasis is 1% to 2%.[50,51] After enucleation, mortality from metastasis rises eightfold in the first 2 years and tapers back to a rate of 1% to 2% over the next 6 years.[51] This increase in tumor-related mortality, which was not compensated for by later adjustments in the mortality curve, suggests that enucleation might predispose to metastasis (the Zimmerman-McLean hypothesis). Others suggested that tumor cells might be dispersed by particularly traumatic enucleations.[51-53] The validity of enucleation, the chief modality of the time, was questioned, and a variety of so-called no-touch techniques were introduced to reduce surgically induced spread of tumor cells.[53,54] Numerous observations and data suggest that tumor cells do not spread directly during enucleation, but that micrometastases already present grow after enucleation, perhaps abetted by alterations in immunologic homeostasis after enucleation.[55-57]

Mortality after enucleation is said to be up to 50% in some series, but this figure is difficult to interpret because the prognosis is also multifactorially dependent on cell type, tumor size, location, and extrascleral extension. Moreover, selection of patients for enucleation may be biased toward tumors with worse prognoses. Current indications for enucleation include: large tumors in eyes with useful vision in which vision and perhaps the eye itself would be lost after irradiation; tumors that cannot be treated with radiation since the tumor margins

cannot be visualized; tumors with optic nerve involvement; absence of useful vision in the eye; failure of previous alternative treatment; patient request; and a painful eye even in the presence of metastatic uveal melanoma. Complications of enucleation include hemorrhage, wound dehiscence, implant extrusion, implant migration, and altered cosmesis. Follow-up after enucleation includes physical examination, liver function tests, chest radiographs, and examination of the remaining eye at 3- to 4-month intervals. The role of modalities such as positron emission tomography (PET) scanning in melanoma is not yet known. Enucleated patients are advised to wear protective eyewear at all times.

Local resection of choroidal melanoma is a modality that has been used by only a few individuals. This technique has evolved from a full-thickness eye wall resection technique requiring a patch graft to tumor resection through a partial-thickness scleral flap in which the tumor and 10% of the overlying scleral thickness are excised.[58-61] Theoretically, this technique allows maximal retention of ocular function without the complications of radiation. It can be appropriate for equatorial melanomas less than 15 mm in diameter or less than one fourth of the ocular circumference, but it is extremely difficult technically. Hypotensive anesthesia is used to reduce intraoperative choroidal bleeding. The results of this technique are difficult to evaluate, since it is practiced with so many variations. The classical technique using an external approach and resection alone results in one fourth of patients with vision of 20/30 or better and rates of metastasis comparable to enucleation. Local resection using a transvitreal approach is also performed in a few centers.

Radiation Therapy. Charged particle radiotherapy with protons and plaque brachytherapy are the most commonly employed radiation modalities. Both are advantageous for treating ocular tumors because of the highly conformal dose that each can deliver. Choice of which radiation modality to employ is determined by the size and location of the tumor, the physical dose distribution characteristics of each modality, the local availability of the treatment, and the expertise and interests of the clinicians involved.

The proton beam delivers a homogeneous dose to the tumor, a potentially advantageous property for tumors abutting or involving the optic disc or the macula. Those structures would usually receive a greater dose than that prescribed if treated with a plaque, because of the dose gradient from the tumor base to its apex seen with that technique; dose to the tumor base may be significantly greater than dose to the tumor apex, especially for taller tumors. In some cases, the dose distribution with the proton beam can conform more closely to an irregularly shaped tumor than can the dose distribution from a standard plaque. Normal tissues in the entrance path of the beam may receive almost the prescribed dose with the proton beam, whereas the radiation dose from the plaque to normal structures in the forward direction from the tumor decreases relatively rapidly with increasing distance from the plaque. With most currently employed plaques, there is little or no dose to tissues behind the

TABLE 70-3

Radionuclides Commonly Used in Episcleral Plaque Therapy		
RADIONUCLIDE	**ENERGY (PARTICLE TYPE)**	**HALF-LIFE**
^{60}Co	1.2 MeV (X)	5 years
^{125}I	28 KeV (X)	60 days
^{106}Ru	3.5 MeV (B)	366 days
^{103}Pd	21 KeV (X)	17 days

plaque; the dose to tissues in the distal path of the beam falls off quite rapidly with the proton beam as well. Large tumors may not be adequately treated with the plaque techniques, and adequate plaque placement may be difficult with posterior tumors, due to both limited sclera access because of the narrowing of the orbit posteriorly, and the anatomic difficulty presented by the optic nerve exiting the eye in patients with peripapillary tumors. In contrast, proton-beam therapy can be given to a melanoma of any size located at any site within the eye. The dose conformality of both modalities offers specific advantages for treating eye tumors, by providing relative sparing of uninvolved ocular and orbital structures.

Historically, radiation therapy for choroidal melanomas developed after irradiation was used to treat other tumors, because of the radiosensitivity of ocular structures and because the high dose of radiation required for successful treatment prevented the use of external-beam photon

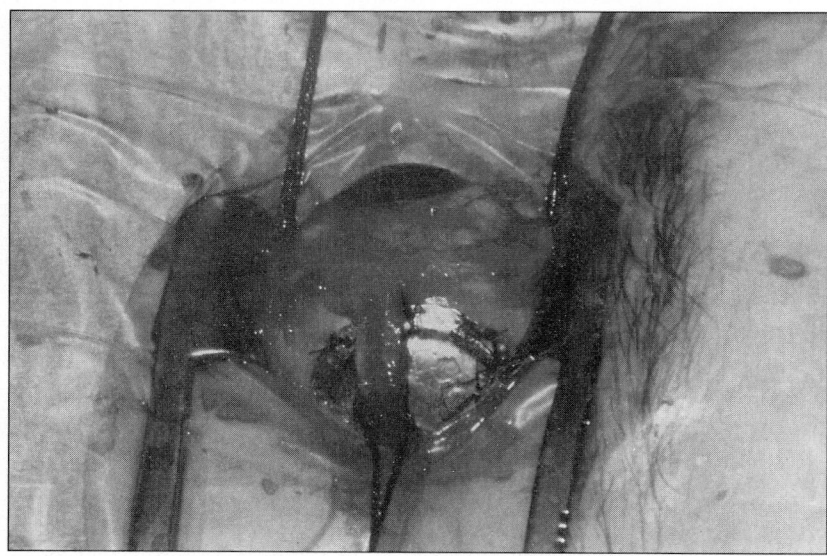

A

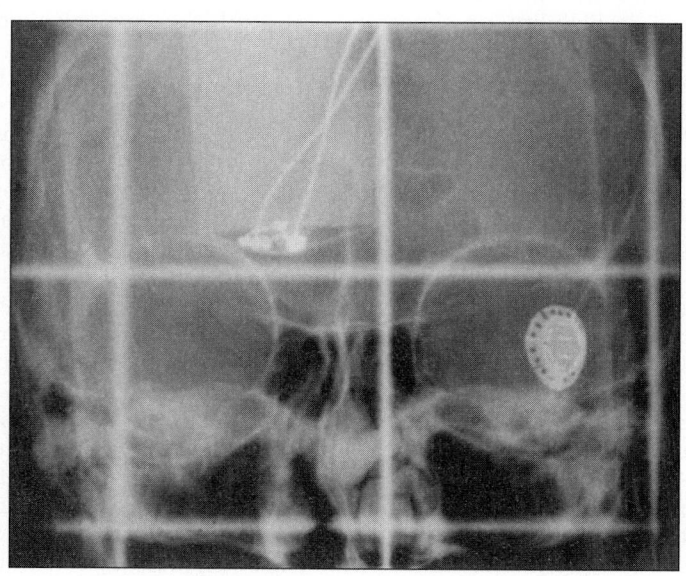

B

Figure 70-2. A, Eye plaque in place over a melanoma of the lateral side of the left eye. The metal plaque is placed beneath the ocular musculature and is fixed in place with small sutures. **B,** Anterior radiograph of the plaque in place. The small perforations around the exterior of the plaque accommodate the sutures that hold the plaque in place. The small, dense rods inside the plaque are the iodine seeds that provide the radiation.

therapy. Nonetheless, local radiation for uveal melanoma has been performed since 1929.[62,63] Initially, radon seeds were implanted directly into the tumor, but episcleral irradiation plaques (brachytherapy) soon became and continues to be the most widely used modality. Charged particle external-beam modalities (teletherapy) are relatively recent and extremely successful, but require far greater technical support than radiation plaques. Interest in irradiation of melanomas increased after the controversy raised by the Zimmerman-McLean hypothesis. Cobalt-60 (^{60}Co) was the first isotope to be used extensively in episcleral plaques.[63,64] In the 1980s, a shift to less energetic isotopes, such as iodine-125 (^{125}I), occurred in the United States,[65-67] making brachytherapy in this country similar to the low-energy ruthenium-106 (^{106}Ru) and palladium-103 (^{103}Pd) isotope treatment used in Europe[68] (Table 70-3). ^{125}I is currently the most frequently used isotope in the United States. Advantages of less energetic isotopes include the ability to shield adjacent structures, the surgeon, and the hospital staff from the radiation, in contrast to ^{60}Co, which cannot be completely shielded. Lower energy isotopes such as ^{125}I also allow more customized configuration of radiation dosing using rimmed plaques. However, ^{125}I is more expensive and it requires more complex dosimetry. The steeper dose gradient between the sclera and tumor apex with lower energy isotopes requires a higher scleral dose for adequate tumor treatment and increases the risk of complications in the surrounding retina and sclera.

Early large experiences with episcleral irradiation plaques came from a few centers.[69,70] Indications for brachytherapy of choroidal melanoma include small melanomas showing growth, medium and large tumors in eyes with vision potential, and melanomas in the patient's only seeing eye. In eyes without vision potential, plaques may also be used, since eyes treated with plaques allow preservation of the eye without a proven increased risk of metastatic disease. The published guidelines for the size range of melanomas that can be treated using brachytherapy vary slightly among centers. However, tumors more than 10 mm thick or 15 mm in diameter allow little chance of preserving useful vision in the eye, while tumors greater than 15 mm thick or 20 mm in diameter allow little chance of preserving the eye. Other considerations are that the entire tumor must be visualized to allow adequate plaque placement and post-tumor examination.

The technique of plaque application (Fig. 70-2A and B) is usually straightforward, but it may be extremely difficult in some cases. Both standard and customized plaques can be used.[71] Because of the life-threatening nature of the tumor being treated, the difficulty of episcleral plaque application should not be underestimated. Current dose recommendations vary, and range from 70 to 100 Gy at the tumor apex in most cases. The duration of treatment is guided by the total dose prescribed and the strength of the radiation source, but is typically in the range of 100 hours.

The results of brachytherapy at different centers are difficult to compare. Different isotopes, criteria for treatment, and dose regimens have been used. In addition, the histologic cell types and rate of growth of the tumors

TABLE 70-4

Results of Episcleral Plaque Therapy for Choroidal Melanoma

SERIES	NO. OF PATIENTS	RADIO-NUCLIDE	ENUCLEATION RATE (%)
Mameghan et al.*	53	^{125}I	8
Quivey et al.[73]	239	^{125}I	8
Fontanesi et al.†	144	^{125}I	10
Lean et al.‡	56	^{125}I	20
Kleineidam et al.§	184	^{106}Ru	11

*Mameghan H, Karolis C, Fisher R, et al: Iodine-125 irradiation of choroidal melanoma: Clinical experience from the Prince of Wales and Sydney Eye Hospital. Aust Radiol 1992;16:249.
†Fontanesi J, Meyer D, Xu S, et al: Treatment of choroidal melanoma with I-125 plaque. Int J Radiat Oncol Biol Phys 1993;26:619.
‡Lean EK, cohen DM, Liggett PE, et al: Episcleral radioactive plaque therapy: Initial clinical experience with 56 patients. Am J Clin Oncol 1990;13:185.
§Kleineidam M, Guthoff R, Bentzen SM: Rates of local control, metastasis, and overall survival in patients with posterior uveal melanomas treated with ruthenium-106 plaques. Radiother Oncol 1993;28:148.

in different series are not known. The effect of radiation from episcleral plaques is to damage the nucleic acid of tumor cells and render them incapable of reproducing. Since melanomas tend to grow slowly, massive shrinkage is rare. About 70% of irradiated melanomas will shrink, but only 10% will disappear entirely.[72,73] In experienced centers, retention of plaque-treated eyes is 90% (Table 70-4) and about half of all patients retain useful vision, but this is dependent on tumor size and location.[74] While highly successful and felt to be equal to enucleation at most centers of ocular oncology worldwide, the equivalence of plaque therapy to enucleation has not yet been prospectively established. As part of the Collaborative Ocular Melanoma Study (COMS), patients with medium-sized melanomas were randomized to receive either plaque or enucleation treatment.

Charged particle teletherapy of choroidal melanoma has been performed with helium ions or protons for 20 years.[75,76] This modality was initially thought to have a number of theoretical advantages over plaque radiation therapy. These included the physics of dose deposition, with sharp lateral drop-off of radiation to 10% of peak dose within 3 mm, allowing protection of radiosensitive structures in the eye, as well as the Bragg peak phenomenon, the ability of the beam to deposit most of its energy in a narrow range of depth. In addition, the particle energy was felt to be more tumoricidal at doses equivalent to those delivered using brachytherapy. The technique is available at only a few facilities, it is expensive, and it is technically very demanding.

More precise focusing of the radiation dose in the target can be achieved with charged particle beams than with x-ray beams. This ability to better spare noninvolved ocular and orbital structures makes charged particle beams ideal for treating ocular tumors. Charged particle beams were first used to treat uveal melanomas over a quarter of a century ago, in what continues to be a most fruitful collaborative effort between the Radiation Oncology Department of Massachusetts General Hospital (MGH), the Retina Service of the Massachusetts Eye and

Ear Infirmary (MEEI), and the Harvard Cyclotron Laboratory (HCL).[77-82] Well in excess of 10,000 patients have been treated with charged particle radiation throughout the world,[82] using techniques and doses similar to those developed by the MGH-MEEI-HCL group.

Surgical tumor localization is performed in most uveal melanoma patients.[77,78,83] The base of the tumor is defined by transillumination and/or indirect ophthalmoscopy and scleral depression, and outlined by suturing 2-mm-diameter radiopaque tantalum rings (T-rings) directly to the sclera. Three pairs of orthogonal radiographs of the eye, each with the eye to be treated looking at a different fixation point, are taken on the second or third day after surgery. T-ring positions from these radiographs are digitized into the planning program. Other input data for the planning program includes axial eye length and tumor height as determined from A- and B-mode ultrasound, tumor drawings by the ophthalmologist, and fundus photographs of the tumor. The tumor base is drawn manually on the computer screen with respect to the position of the T-rings, incorporating information from the ophthalmologist's sketches, the fundus photographs, and measurements of clip position relative to the tumor base taken at the time of surgical localization. A fixation point for the treatment is chosen, which minimizes the dose given to the lens, the optic nerve, and the macula. The treatment plan is reviewed with the ophthalmologist and the radiation oncologist before implementation.

A transparency generated by the planning program shows the desired clip positions for both anteroposterior (AP) and lateral radiographs when the eye is positioned at the angle chosen for treatment. The transparency can be overlaid on a radiograph taken through the treatment aperture with the eye in the treatment position at treatment setup. A transparency of the light field projection of the proton beam through the treatment aperture onto the front of the eye is used as a final check on patient alignment.

A light field setup only has been used for treatment of anterior ciliary body or iris tumors, and for other ocular lesions such as angiomas, hemangiomas, and choroidal metastases. In those cases, tumor location is determined by transillumination of anterior melanomas, or from fundus photographs and the ophthalmologist's tumor sketch in patients with other lesions. Dose volume histograms for the globe, lens, ciliary body, retina, macula, and disc are also routinely generated. The planning program also specifies an individualized brass aperture for each patient, which is fabricated by a computer-controlled milling machine. Treatment portals are relatively small, ranging from 10 to 35 mm in diameter. Tissue compensators have not been used for the ocular treatments in the MGH-MEEI program.

Patients are treated in the seated position, their head immobilized with an individually molded face mask and bite block. Eye position for treatment is established and maintained by voluntary patient fixation on a light positioned to define the prescribed fixation angle. The proton beam enters the eye to the extent possible through the sclera, reducing or eliminating direct irradiation of the cornea, anterior chamber, and lens. Eye position for treatment in patients who have had clips placed for tumor localization is determined radiographically, and verified before treatment by comparing the projection of the light field through the treatment aperture onto the front of the eye with the computer prediction of the light field position relative to the limbus. Patients who did not undergo surgical localization are treated with a light field setup only, with eye position determined as described. Irradiation of the eyelid is reduced or eliminated by lid retraction. Treatment setup is routinely accomplished in 5 to 10 minutes, with irradiation times being 1 to 2 minutes. During treatment, eye position is monitored by a video camera. Mean movement during treatment was 0.5 mm ± 0.3 mm, as determined during 41 treatments in 11 patients; maximum movement was 1.2 mm.[84] Using the MGH-MEEI techniques, 94% of patients received the standard dose of 70 CGE (cobalt Gy equivalents, CGE = proton Gy times relative biologic effectiveness [RBE] 1.1).[85-88] Ninety-nine percent received 5 fractions, and 94% completed treatment in 7 to 9 days.

The tumor margins are localized with four tantalum rings sewn to the sclera during an operative procedure. Treatment planning involves selecting a beam orientation and eye position to avoid radiosensitive structures, since the beam enters anteriorly. A method of fixing the patient's face and gaze must be used. Four to five treatments are given over 7 to 11 days to a total dose ranging from 50 to 80 Gy equivalents.

After either form of irradiation, the patient is examined at 3-month intervals, although some will observe the patient less frequently. Complete ophthalmologic examination is important to detect tumor recurrence, progression, complications of treatment, and any treatable disease in the contralateral eye. Ultrasonography and photographic documentation are also performed serially. Metastatic evaluations consisting of a general physical examination (with special attention to the skin), chest radiographs, and serum liver enzyme tests are also performed at periodic intervals. While abdominal ultrasonography, CT, and MRI are probably more sensitive in detecting early metastases than serum studies and chest radiographs, the inability to treat metastatic disease effectively and its low incidence make the cost-benefit ratio of the more extensive testing very high.

In the published MGH data,[79,89-95] local tumor control, defined as absence of increase in tumor height on serial ultrasound, or in lateral growth seen on ophthalmoscopy or fundus photography, was achieved in 96.3 ± 1.5% and 95.4 ± 3.3% at 60 and 84 months: 236 and 82 patients were available for follow-up at those intervals. Tumors recurred at the margin of the irradiated volume in 10 of 12 patients; regrowth in the other two patients recurred in the full dose (70 CGE) volume. Two failures were noted after 48 months.[90] Recurrences were observed between 2 months and 11.3 years after irradiation in 1922 patients with median ocular follow-up of 5.2 years after irradiation. Rates of tumor regrowth at 5 and 10 years, including both 45 patients with growth documented by ultrasound and/or sequential fundus photographs and 17 patients enucleated for suspected but unconfirmed tumor growth, were 3.2% (95% confidence interval [CI], 2.5% to 4.2%), and 4.3% (95% CI, 3.3% to 5.6%). Tumor recurrence was independently related to tumor-related death.[91]

Survival at 5 years after proton beam treatment has been approximately 80%.[79,92,93] Survival rates after proton beam treatment are at least as good as those observed in patients treated primarily with enucleation, based on survival comparisons made between 556 proton-treated patients and two groups treated with enucleation. During the same 10-year period that the proton treatments were being given (July 1975 to December 1984), 238 patients were enucleated, and 275 patients had been enucleated during the preceding decade (January 1965 to June 1975). Kaplan-Meier estimated survival rates at 5 years were 81 ± 2%, 68 ± 3%, and 74 ± 3% for irradiated patients, patients enucleated in the later period, and those enucleated in the earlier period, respectively. At 10 years, estimated survival rates were 63 ± 5%, 53 ± 4%, and 50 ± 3%, respectively. Median follow-up time for the three patient groups was 5.3, 8.8, and 17.0 years, respectively.[89]

Significant prognostic factors defined for both irradiated[93] and enucleated[94] patients were used to classify patients in each treatment group according to risk of distant failure. Younger patients with relatively small posterior tumors were at lower risk, older patients with larger tumors involving the ciliary body were at higher risk, and intermediate risk patients were of intermediate age and had tumors of intermediate size that extended anterior to the equator but did not involve the ciliary body. Estimated survival probabilities were better for proton treated patients in each risk category than for either enucleated group. This study also demonstrated that patients receiving conservation therapy with protons did not have a worse survival outcome than those undergoing enucleation.[95]

Probability of eye retention at 5 years is related to tumor size: 97%, 93%, and 78% of patients with small, intermediate, and large tumors, respectively. Multivariate analysis identified independent risk factors associated with greater likelihood of eye loss as ciliary body involvement, tumor height >8 mm, and distance between the posterior tumor edge and the fovea. Risk of eye loss was greatest in patients with two or more risk factors (238 patients). Eye loss risk was least for patients with no risk factors (213 patients), and intermediate for those with one risk factor (569 patients). Eye retention rates at 5 years were 99 ± 1% and 92 ± 2% for the low and intermediate risk groups, respectively. Only 76 ± 7% of patients in the highest risk group retained the eye at 5 years.[96] In a more recent analysis, the estimated eye retention rate was 84% at 15 years in 2069 patients treated through December 31, 1997, with median follow-up of 9.4 years.[97] Similar eye retention rates were observed after proton beam treatment of 2648 eyes in 2645 patients treated in Switzerland. With median time to follow-up of 44 months, eye retention rates were 89.8%, 86.2%, and 83.7% at 5, 10, and 15 years, respectively.[98]

In over 50% of treated eyes, visual acuity is unchanged or improved after proton treatment. In patients with useful vision (visual acuity 20/200 or better) before treatment, visual loss after treatment can be attributed to cataract progression, retinal detachment, and radiation retinopathy. Both initial tumor characteristics and radiation dose significantly influence visual prognosis after proton treatment. Initial tumor characteristics significantly related to post-treatment visual acuity include initial visual acuity, tumor height, distance between the posterior tumor margin and the optic disc and/or fovea, and presence of a pretreatment retinal detachment involving the macula. Radiation dose to the optic disc, fovea, and lens is also related to post-treatment visual acuity.[80] Useful vision was preserved in only 39% of 363 patients with tumor edge ≤3 mm from the optic disc and/or fovea; 83% of that group received >35 CGE to either or both of those structures. In contrast, useful vision was preserved in 67% of 199 patients with posterior tumor edge >3 mm from both the optic disc and the fovea; 91% of that group received <35 CGE to those structures.[81] Depending on risk group, the probability for visual loss (visual acuity worse than 20/200) ranged from 100% to 20% in 2069 patients treated through December 31, 1997, with median follow-up of 9.4 years.[97]

Acutely, the only morbidity frequently noted is moist eyelid desquamation, which occurs in patients whose lids could not be completely retracted from the irradiation field. The lid segment involved is relatively small, typically ranging in size from 2 to 5 mm by 8 to 15 mm. The desquamation heals in 4 to 6 weeks. Late lid sequelae include permanent eyelash loss, eyelid atrophy, and scarring within the desquamated area.

Late radiation injury to anterior ocular structures includes rubeosis iridis with neovascular glaucoma and cataract formation. Some degree of visual preservation or restoration can be achieved in some patients developing these complications. Posterior subcapsular opacities (PSCs) developed within three years of treatment in 42% of 388 patients with clear lenses initially. The probability of PSC formation was related to lens dose, tumor height, and older age.[99] Of the 1171 patients treated through December 1987, 42% (494) had lens opacities. Cataract extraction was performed on 84 such patients between 2 months and 11 years after treatment. Approximately one half of those patients had visual acuity 20/100 or better 1 year after surgery; in one third of patients, it was 20/40 or better. Larger tumor size was highly correlated with poorer visual outcome after cataract extraction. Six patients eventually underwent enucleation, five because of painful blind eyes after surgery and one in whom a "ring melanoma" was diagnosed after surgery.[100]

Late radiation injury to posterior ocular structures includes macular edema, maculopathy, papillopathy, and optic atrophy. Few if any treatment options exist for patients with these complications, all of which can result in significant visual loss. Generally similar posterior complication patterns are seen in radionuclide plaque–treated patients.[101,102] Focal laser therapy may be beneficial in the short term for some patients.[103]

A relationship has been suggested between the reason for enucleation and death from metastatic disease. In 1541 patients, with median follow-up of 8 years, the probability of eye retention at 10 years was 89% ± 2%. Thirty-four patients who lost the eye because of tumor growth after proton treatment were almost four times as likely to die from metastasis as were 103 patients whose eye was removed because of treatment complications (rate ratios 3.8 versus 0.9, 95% CI 2.3% to 6.3% and 0.6% to 1.4%, respectively).[104]

The results of ocular teletherapy are clearly difficult to compare with enucleation and brachytherapy. With both radiation methods, retention of the eye occurs in 90% of patients, and useful vision is preserved in the majority of cases.[105] Only one center has conducted randomized studies comparing plaque and particle irradiation.[106] Enucleation rates in this study were 17% in ^{125}I-treated patients compared with 9% in patients treated with charged particles. However, the dose of ^{125}I was 70 Gy, which is lower than the 80 to 100 Gy used by others, and the lateral brachytherapy treatment margin was only 1 mm, less than the 2 mm used for the helium teletherapy and brachytherapy at other centers. At the same time, complications from helium ion treatment were more common than with ^{125}I plaque therapy. Complications were related to the localization of the radiation dose within the eye. More posterior complications such as vitreous hemorrhage occurred with irradiation plaques, while anterior complications such as neovascular glaucoma occurred more often with particle beam therapy.[107] It should also be recognized that particle beam therapy is available in only a handful of centers in the United States. Brachytherapy complications include cataract, radiation retinopathy and optic neuropathy, neovascular glaucoma, vitreous hemorrhage, scleral necrosis, dry eye, lacrimal punctal stenosis, eyelash loss, and tumor progression.[101,102]

A retrospective study compared survival in 103 enucleated patients with that of 345 patients receiving conservation therapy with isotope plaque brachytherapy. At 15 years, metastasis-free survivals were 57.1% (SE 6.4%) and 61.8% (SE 3.3%) for the enucleated and the plaque-treated patients, respectively. There was no survival disadvantage for the irradiated patients.[108]

Because of questions concerning enucleation-induced tumor cell metastasis, interest developed in preoperative external-beam irradiation (20 Gy) to "sterilize" dispersed cells. While such irradiation has been shown to reduce mitotic activity, two small studies at major ocular oncology centers showed no apparent effect on clinical outcome.[109,110] This conclusion was confirmed by an arm of the COMS study that prospectively randomized large tumors with respect to irradiation.[111]

Recent series employing the immediate postoperative placement of a radioactive episcleral plaque showed highly variable recurrence rates. However, some patients will undergo expulsive choroidal hemorrhage intra-operatively, resulting in the need to enucleate the eye. Unpublished data suggest that visual function appears to decline with time in these patients. From its original description with significant complications, it has evolved to require placement of silicone oil in the eye and immediate postoperative brachytherapy and cryotherapy, raising the operative time with hypotensive anesthesia and cost. Complication rates are high for retinal detachment and cataract. Long-term follow-up is needed to assess the oncologic efficacy of this technique.

Stereo radiosurgery (gamma knife) techniques have been applied to intraocular tumors. While tumors have undergone regression, complications occur in a majority of patients. The role of this modality in intraocular melanoma is still unclear.

Melanomas extend directly from the eye by growth along emissary vessels passing through the sclera or, more rarely, by invasion through the sclera and by hematogenous spread to distant sites. Limited extrascleral extension of choroidal melanoma can be managed with enucleation and excision of the adjacent tumor or with brachytherapy in selected cases, although most data are anecdotal and lack long-term follow-up.[112] Orbital exenteration may be used when more extensive diffuse orbital involvement is present, but the data regarding survival after this disfiguring procedure are limited and controversial and have been obtained in poorly controlled series.[113]

Prognosis in choroidal melanoma is related to cell type, tumor size, and degree of extrascleral extension. A recent characterization of the intrinsic vascular pattern of choroidal melanoma has been found to be a good prognostic indicator. The presence of closed vascular loops indicates a poor prognosis. The strength of its prognostic predictions varies in different studies based on technical considerations, but it is thought that this should be included in histopathologic reports. Metastasis is a grim sign, with mean patient survival of less than 1 year after its discovery. Metastases can occur up to 30 years after initial diagnosis.[114,115] The tumor demonstrates a remarkable hepatotropism. Over 90% of patients dying of choroidal melanoma had liver involvement in both an early study and recent studies.[116] The liver is the initial site of metastasis in 56% of patients.[117] Skin, lung, bone, and brain are other common sites. Systemic chemotherapy remains the main form of therapy but is effective in very few cases.[118,119] Rarely, it may be combined with local infusion of chemotherapeutic agents through the hepatic artery.[119] Combined therapy with interleukin-2 (IL-2) or immunotherapy with sensitized lymphocytes may prove to be more effective, but the data are limited and the risks of immune suppression fostering tumor growth are unknown.[120] Rare cases have undergone partial hepatectomy, but most cases have progressed in spite of this surgery.[121]

Malignant Melanoma of Iris

Melanoma of the iris is about one twentieth as common as ciliary body and choroidal melanomas.[122] In early series, iris melanomas were thought to account for 3% to 10% of uveal melanomas, but other studies have since shown that most of the iris tumors reported in these series were in fact benign nevi and not malignant melanomas.[123,124] A similar review of a large series of iris tumors originally designated melanomas led to reclassification as benign nevi in 87%.

Iris melanomas may be pigmented or nonpigmented, and they occur in the inferior half of the iris in 80% of cases (Fig. 70-3A).[125,126] Iris melanomas arise from melanocytes in the iris stroma. Melanomas are most common in lightly pigmented individuals, particularly

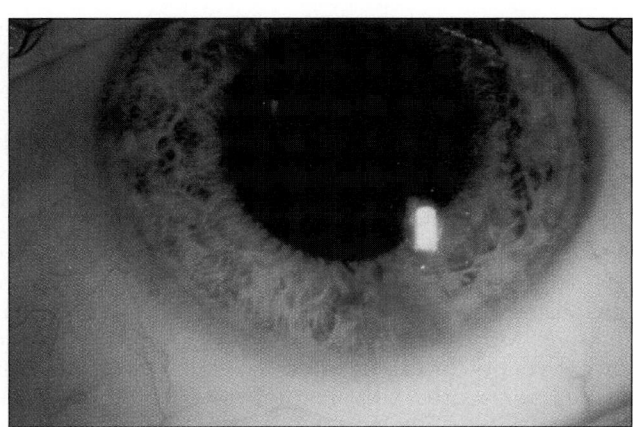

A

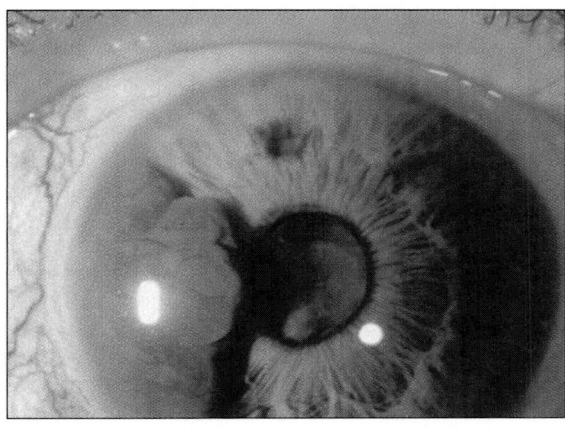

B

Figure 70-3. A, Small pigmented tumor, histologically confirmed to be iris melanoma. **B,** Larger iris melanoma growing into anterior chamber and touching cornea.

patients with blue irides. They exist in a continuum with iris nevi and share many common features. Both may be flat or elevated, circumscribed or diffuse, show prominent vascularity, or present with hemorrhage. Clinically, iris freckles are pigmented lesions that allow recognition of the delicate structure of the anterior iris stroma while melanomas and nevi obscure the superficial stromal architecture. Because of the overlap between iris nevi and melanoma, clinical diagnosis frequently cannot be made on the basis of a single examination. Signs suggestive of malignancy include growth, hemorrhage, distortion of the pupil, glaucoma, involvement of the anterior chamber angle, intractable glaucoma, and extension through the sclera (Fig. 70-3B). Nonetheless, only 5% of suspicious iris lesions managed by observation alone show growth within 5 years, and no finding other than extraocular spread indicates clinically malignant behavior.[127]

Management. The diagnosis is primarily made on the basis of the clinical examination. Ancillary tests such as ultrasonography are less helpful than for choroidal melanomas. High-frequency B-scan ultrasonography of the anterior segment can reveal the extent of the lesion but does not quantitatively evaluate the internal structure, and most lesions are too thin for internal structure analysis with quantitative A-scan ultrasonography. Fine-needle aspiration cytology may be helpful in selected cases, but sampling error may result in a false-negative diagnosis of malignancy.[128]

Management of iris melanocytic lesions has changed over recent years. Historically, many eyes underwent early enucleation for presumed melanoma. Current management is more conservative, since the biologic behavior of histologically malignant lesions is often indolent.[123,124] Circumscribed tumors are reevaluated every 6 months for evidence of progression. When indicated, tumors are excised using iridectomy or iridocyclectomy with preservation of the eye.[129] Infrequently, iris melanomas are treated with alternative techniques such as plaque brachytherapy. Diffuse iris melanomas pose management challenges. Vision is usually good and treatment often adversely affects vision. If refractory glaucoma exists, enucleation is the treatment of choice, since it treats all of the problems. If the diagnosis is questionable, iris biopsy may be performed. If the lesion is not growing and glaucoma develops, conventional treatment of the glaucoma using the usual indications for medication and surgery has been advocated. However, the authors have seen several cases in which melanomas grew posteriorly into the ciliary body while glaucoma was being treated medically and even surgically, exposing the patient to the risk of tumor dissemination. Occasionally, even diffuse, thin lesions may show histopathologic features of malignancy including discohesive tumor cells, nuclear pleomorphism, and mitoses. Even so, most iris melanomas follow a benign biologic course, and reported long-term mortality remains 1% to 4% with a combined figure from multiple series of 1%, further supporting conservative treatment for these tumors.[130]

Primary Intraocular Large Cell Lymphoma
Primary intraocular large cell lymphoma (PILCL), previously known as reticulum cell sarcoma, is probably better designated as primary central nervous system lymphoma (PCNSL) with ocular involvement (PCNSL-O), since it is most likely a subset of PCNSL.[131] This uncommon tumor typically presents as uveitis refractory to treatment. Elderly patients are most commonly affected, but all adults with new bilateral uveitis or refractory uveitis require evaluation for PCNSL-O.[132] PCNSL-O may also occur in patients with acquired immunodeficiency syndrome (AIDS).[133] It is associated with central nervous system (CNS) lymphoma. One third of patients have known CNS disease before ocular manifestations develop.[134] Conversely, 85% of patients with PILCL will eventually develop CNS disease.[135] Patients present with bilateral disease in two thirds of cases, and 85% will eventually manifest bilateral disease.[135] Clinical history can elicit symptoms of CNS involvement in 10% of patients, and clinical or laboratory findings increase the detection of CNS involvement to more than 30% at the time of ocular presentation.

PILCL patients present with painless decreased vision and frequently have been managed for putative refractory

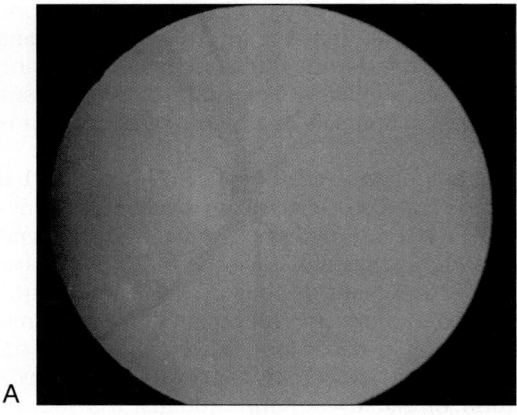

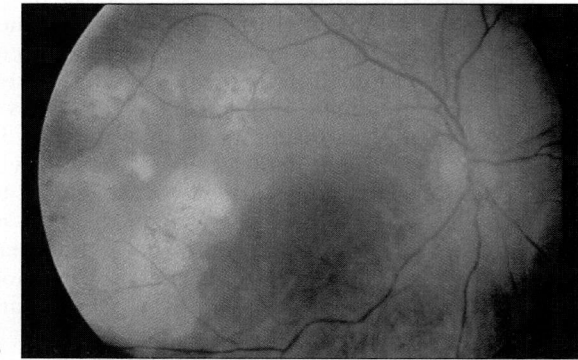

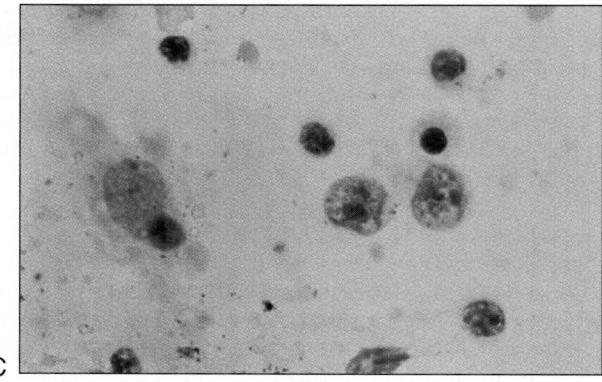

Figure 70-4. A, Primary intraocular large cell lymphoma with neoplastic cells in vitreous obscuring clear view of retina and optic nerve. **B,** Primary intraocular large cell lymphoma with yellow subretinal tumor infiltrates. **C,** Vitreous aspirate from eye in **(A)** showing malignant B lymphocytes with hyperchromatic nuclei containing large nuceoli. Small reactive lymphocytes are also seen.

uveitis. Cells are seen in the vitreous (Fig. 70-4A) and less often in the anterior chamber. Yellow to white subretinal infiltrates of tumor cells (Fig. 70-4B) are highly suggestive of PILCL, but retinal hemorrhage may occur, simulating cytomegalovirus retinitis. Lymphoid tumors with primary choroidal rather than retinal or vitreal involvement represent a different disease process. Rather than PILCL, such patients have ocular involvement as a manifestation of systemic lymphoma or a localized lymphoma that may extend into the orbit through emissary channels in the sclera.

Management. PILCL is most commonly diagnosed by vitreous biopsy, using either FNA or closed vitrectomy techniques. Multiple vitreous biopsies may be required to establish the diagnosis.[136] Chorioretinal biopsy and, rarely, enucleation may be required for diagnosis.[137] Diagnosis depends on the quality of the cytologic preparation and is based on the finding of neoplastic lymphocytes with coarse chromatin, prominent nucleoli, and convoluted nuclear membranes (Fig. 70-4C). Reactive inflammatory cells may present concurrently, complicating the pathologic diagnosis. If PILCL is strongly suspected, lumbar puncture for cerebrospinal fluid cytology and bone marrow biopsy may be performed while the patient is anesthetized for the vitreous biopsy. It should be noted that in only 25% of patients will large cell lymphoma have spread beyond the eye and CNS. Evaluation of this tumor must include brain imaging. MRI using gadolinium is more sensitive than CT in detecting early lesions of CNS lymphoma. Treatment of PILCL with brain and orbital irradiation produces good initial response, but these patients frequently relapse and recurrent CNS tumor causes death. Patients treated with radiation combined with intrathecal methotrexate have increased survival.[138,139] Treatment involves whole-brain irradiation that includes both eyes to a dose of 40 Gy. A 10-Gy boost is often given to the bulk of the intracranial disease.[140]

Patients with isolated ocular disease at presentation present a special challenge. The morbidity of radiation therapy and intrathecal chemotherapy is significant, resulting in a 10% incidence of decreased intellectual function.[139] Some authorities treat these patients conservatively with ocular irradiation and serial examinations of the CNS, while others irradiate the eyes and brain and may use intrathecal chemotherapy. Recent studies have shown that B-scan echography was abnormal in patients tested with eye findings.[141,142] Some investigators advocate using supplemental systemic chemotherapy.[142] Primary multiagent chemotherapy without radiation has shown some efficacy, while markedly reducing radiation-related cognitive deficits.[143] Patients treated for PILCL require thorough serial clinical evaluations. General physical and ophthalmologic examinations are performed every 3 months. MRI of the CNS and cerebrospinal fluid cytologic examinations are performed biannually for the first 5 years after treatment. Prognosis is related to the extent of the disease at the time of diagnosis.

Choroidal lymphoma is usually a manifestation of systemic lymphoma and not PILCL of the eye and CNS. After biopsy to establish the diagnosis, the lymphoma undergoes traditional staging. Systemic lymphoma is treated with standard lymphoma chemotherapeutic protocols that may be supplemented with orbital irradiation if vision is threatened while localized lymphoma is being treated by local irradiation.

Secondary Malignant Intraocular Tumors of Adults

Choroidal Metastases
Choroidal metastases are the most common intraocular malignancies in adults. The choroid is the most frequent

MANAGEMENT OF CHOROIDAL METASTASES

DIAGNOSIS

Choroidal metastasis should be considered in any cancer patient with new visual complaints, especially those with breast or lung primaries.

Ophthalmoscopy shows characteristic yellowish, low-lying lesion with poorly delineated margins.

Occasionally, this metastasis is the patient's presenting complaint and precedes the diagnosis of symptomatic disease.

TREATMENT

Radiation should be given to the eye through a lateral field—30 to 40 Gy in 2 to 4 weeks.

Contralateral eye should be carefully examined.

If negative, treatment fields should avoid this eye as much as possible. If metastases develop later, the fellow eye can then be treated.

Simultaneous brain metastases should be ruled out.

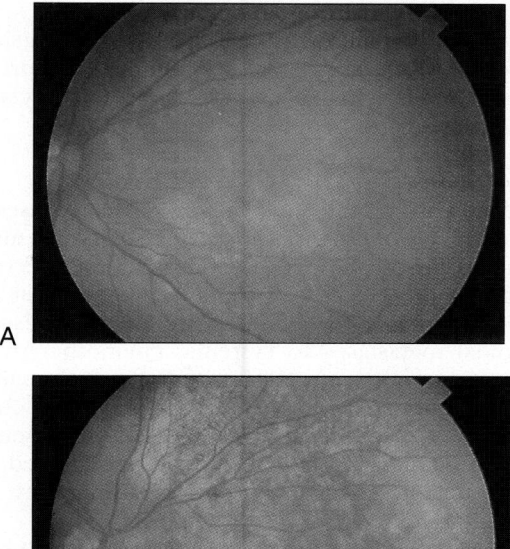

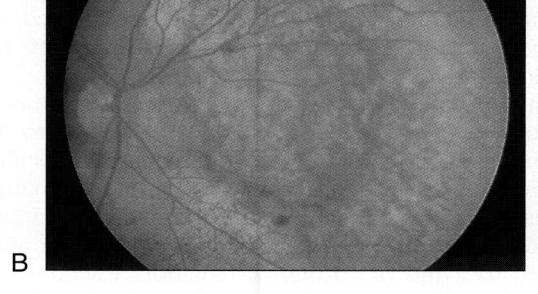

Figure 70-5. A, Metastatic breast carcinoma of choroid prior to radiation therapy. **B,** Involution of same tumor following external-beam irradiation. Reactive pigmentary choroidal atrophy is present.

site of ocular and orbital metastasis, being involved in 57% to 90% of cases.[144,145] Autopsy studies showed that up to 12% of eyes from patients with carcinoma were found to have choroidal metastases.[144,146] Clinical series have demonstrated rates of metastasis of up to 4.7%,[147] and the most recent series of breast carcinoma showed an overall metastasis rate of 27%.[148] Clinical series may underestimate the incidence of metastases, since ocular evaluations are deferred in terminally ill patients and many metastases are asymptomatic. For its overall size, the choroid is estimated to be the body tissue most prone to metastasis, presumably due to its very high blood circulation.[149]

Almost any type of tumor can metastasize to the eye. Choroidal metastases may be the first sign of malignancy in 25% to 50% of clinical cases in which they occur.[150-152] The most common primary tumors causing choroidal metastases are breast carcinoma (Fig. 70-5A) and lung carcinoma, comprising up to 64% and 30% of metastases, respectively.[145,150-152] Most patients are middle-aged or elderly. Two common clinical scenarios occur. In patients with breast carcinoma, 80% to 90% of metastases are discovered after the primary lesion and are associated with extensive systemic disease. With lung carcinoma, 70% to 90% of ocular metastases are discovered before the primary tumor.[145,150-152] Metastatic lesions are bilateral in up to 40% of cases and show multiple lesions in a single eye in 13% to 20% of cases.[144,145]

Although most clinically detected choroidal metastases produce symptoms, usually of vision loss or retinal detachment,[153] metastases are generally painless and may be discovered incidentally on routine eye examination. On ophthalmoscopy, metastases tend to be posteriorly located, amelanotic, yellowish, low-lying lesions with poorly defined margins (see Fig. 70-5A). Secondary changes in the overlying retinal pigment epithelium can occur, but these are easily distinguished from the pigmentation of choroidal melanoma by experienced observers.

The one exception is metastatic melanoma to the choroid in which the metastasis may be brown. However, unlike dome-shaped primary melanomas, metastatic lesions are placoid in configuration. Frequently, metastases induce a significant serous retinal detachment, presumably by inducing retinal pigment epithelial dysfunction. In contrast to choroidal melanomas, the amount of retinal detachment is great compared with the size of the tumor. Ultrasonography can frequently differentiate metastases from melanomas. Metastases are moderately to highly reflective and show internal heterogeneity but lack significant intrinsic vasculature. They are usually placoid and have a less steep spike of intersection with the sclera than choroidal melanomas. On fluorescein angiography, the tumors show late hyperfluorescence. Diagnosis of choroidal metastasis is usually made on the basis of clinical history, ophthalmoscopic examination, ultrasonography, and angiography. Diagnostic accuracy should exceed 95% with trained examiners. The presence of a known primary cancer, together with clinical and ultrasonographic features typical of a choroidal metastasis, allows the diagnosis to be made with confidence. If the clinical appearance or ultrasonography (or both) are atypical for metastasis, it should be recalled that 6% of patients with choroidal melanomas have a history of systemic malignancy.[154]

Serum studies for tumor-associated antigens such as carcinoembryonic antigen (CEA) and prostate-specific antigen (PSA) may be of assistance in arriving at the clinical diagnosis of choroidal metastasis.[155] When choroidal tumors occur in the absence of a known primary tumor, full systemic diagnostic evaluation should be performed in an attempt to identify the primary malignancy. In rare instances, FNA biopsy or incisional choroidal biopsy may be indicated.

Management. Management of choroidal metastases can include observation, chemotherapy, irradiation, enucleation, and (rarely) photocoagulation.[156-165] Observation is appropriate for inactive lesions or lesions that have responded to previously administered therapy. Response of choroidal metastases to systemic chemotherapy and hormonal therapy occurs in breast carcinoma, small cell carcinoma of the lung, thyroid carcinoma, and choriocarcinoma.[158,161,163,164] These modalities may represent the first choice of therapy, since they may be repeated, they have widespread effects on metastases, and they have fewer local side effects.[158]

Treatment usually consists of external-beam photon irradiation to a total dose of 30 to 40 Gy in 2- to 3-Gy fractions (see Fig. 70-5B).[165,166] If the prognosis for life is poor, but treatment is necessary, larger fractions can be administered over a shorter period. Before initiating choroidal radiation therapy, a brain CT or MRI should be obtained to avoid performing irradiation a second time for a brain metastasis, which could double the dose of radiation to the orbits and could increase treatment morbidity.[167] Treatment is given through lateral fields so that damage to the anterior structures of the eye, such as the cornea and lacrimal gland, can be avoided. Radiation retinopathy or optic neuropathy are dose related and rarely occur at the doses used for metastases. They are also long-term side effects that occur beyond the life expectancy of the patient in most cases.

Enucleation for suspected ocular metastasis is indicated for an eye with uncontrollable pain and with full patient understanding that the procedure will not affect the course of the cancer. In some cases, enucleations or local resection of eyes with solitary low-grade metastases, such as carcinoid tumors, have been performed in an attempt to eradicate the sole site of residual cancer, but often other metastatic lesions will appear.[168,169] Patient preference may be for enucleation of this metastasis, but this should be discouraged in most cases. Rarely, a tumor will be indistinguishable from a choroidal melanoma or no primary lesion will be found and enucleation will be appropriate. Because of the diffuse character and multiple or bilateral occurrence of choroidal metastases, radiation modalities requiring surgery (such as episcleral plaques and charged particle therapy) are rarely used.[170]

Choroidal metastases are successfully treated in 75% to 90% of cases (see Fig. 70-5B). Lesions usually flatten within 2 months and associated retinal detachments resolve within 6 months.[148] The visual outcome appears to be related to the pretreatment vision, the number and location of tumors, and the extent of retinal detachment. Historically, choroidal metastases have been felt to represent end-stage disease and survival was short. A mean survival of 8 to 9 months for metastatic breast carcinoma was reported several years ago.[148-151] However, one series

shows improved mean survival time of 18 months for patients with this cancer.[171,172]

Iris Metastases

Iris metastases are less common than choroidal metastases, comprising one tenth of uveal metastases.[173] They are typically white to pink tumors that may be solid masses or discohesive. Discohesive cells may cause a pseudohypopyon, a buildup of puslike fluid in the anterior of the eye. Iris metastases occur more commonly in the upper half of the iris and grow more rapidly than iris melanomas. Almost all cases are unilateral. They may cause vision loss, glaucoma (38% to 50%), or hemorrhage. Metastases must be differentiated from amelanotic melanomas, leiomyomas, lymphoid lesions, iritis, and infection. In two thirds of cases the iris metastasis is not the presenting manifestation of the primary tumor. The primary tumor in cases of iris metastasis is: breast (40%), lung (27%), various other carcinomas (24%), melanomas (7.5%), and no primary (2.5%).[174]

Diagnosis is made on the basis of the history and clinical examination. Systemic evaluation for a primary tumor is important. This should include physical examination, serum studies, and imaging studies. Diagnosis can often be made on the basis of FNA biopsy or incisional biopsy of the iris tumor.

Management. The treatment of iris metastases is guided by the same principles as that of posterior uveal metastases. However, specific limitations must be considered. The use of chemotherapy, if indicated for other metastases or residual tumor, is less damaging to the eye than radiation therapy. External-beam radiation with doses of 30 Gy can be effective. Brachytherapy has been used but has potential for more anterior segment complications and loss of the eye because of the high dose of radiation at the surface of the plaque. Local control of tumor has been excellent, but prognosis remains poor, with mean survival of 20 months in one large series.[175]

Intraocular Leukemia

A prospective study found intraocular tumor cell infiltrates in 3% of patients with leukemia, while 39% of leukemic patients had intraocular manifestations related to the leukemia.[176] Thirteen percent of patients have characteristic retinal hemorrhages with white centers that may contain either platelets or tumor cells. Ocular involvement can be found in 80% of leukemia patients on careful histologic evaluation of postmortem tissue.[177,178] Ocular involvement is most common in the acute or chronic myeloid leukemias.

Any intraocular structure may be involved. Iris masses, diffuse infiltration simulating uveitis, secondary glaucoma, solid tumor infiltrates, hemorrhages, and optic nerve infiltration (Fig. 70-6) may all occur. Tumor infiltrates are white-yellow, but optic nerve involvement, which has been reported in 0% to 30% of patients,[176,179] is usually pink-gray. Infiltration of the optic nerve by tumor must be differentiated from papilledema secondary to intracranial involvement.

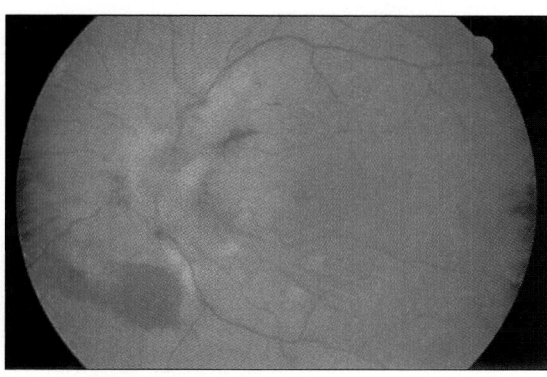

Figure 70-6. Leukemic involvement of the optic nerve head with yellow-white tumor infiltrate, retinal hemorrhages, and retinal folds.

Diagnosis in these patients is challenging, since hematologic abnormalities and opportunistic infections related to the leukemia or its treatment may simulate actual leukemic involvement. Consideration of all these entities in the diagnostic evaluation is critical for accurate diagnosis. Firm diagnosis may be established by aspiration biopsy, but incisional biopsy of a mass, choroid, or retina may be required. Presumptive clinical diagnosis is made based on the history, clinical findings, and response to treatment in patients too ill to undergo biopsy. Careful imaging studies, preferably MRI, are used to delineate CNS involvement.

Management. Ocular leukemia is managed with radiation and chemotherapy either alone or in combination. Optic nerve involvement is not responsive to intrathecal chemotherapy but responds to low-dose irradiation of 8 to 10 Gy in 90% of cases. Involvement of the iris or other anterior segment structures is managed with 5 to 10 Gy of radiation in addition to chemotherapy. Response to low-dose radiation can also be used to differentiate optic nerve involvement from papilledema.

Uncommon Intraocular Tumors

Neuroepithelial Tumors

The nonpigmented epithelium of the ciliary body and the pigmented epithelium of the ciliary body and retina are rarely the site of benign or malignant tumors. The nonpigmented ciliary epithelial tumors present as solid masses that can disrupt anterior segment anatomy.[180,181] Clinical and histologic differentiation of these tumors from amelanotic malignant melanoma or metastasis can be extremely difficult. The usual diagnostic modalities for intraocular tumors are used, but few data exist for differentiating these from other tumors.

In contrast to melanoma, tumors of the pigment epithelium are not infrequent in black patients.[182] These jet black tumors usually occur in the periphery or near the optic disk. The tumors are prechoroidal and tend to show an abrupt rise from adjacent tissue, presumably because they are not tenting up overlying tissue. These clinical features help to differentiate them from choroidal melanomas.

Few data exist on management of these rare tumors. If small or minimally progressive, they may be observed. When accessible and not excessive in size, they can be excised with retention of the eye. Eyes containing large or posterior tumors usually undergo enucleation.

Retinal Metastases

Tumors metastatic to the retina are conspicuously uncommon. Isolated cases have been reported and include carcinoma and melanoma.[183-188] While among choroidal metastases carcinomas greatly outnumber melanoma, this is not true with retinal metastases.

Primary Malignant Intraocular Tumors of Children

Retinoblastoma

Retinoblastoma is the most common primary malignant intraocular tumor of children. It is estimated to occur at a rate of 1 per 18,000 live births.[189-191] It represents the prototypic example of a genetically related tumor.[192] It occurs in sporadic nonheritable (60%) and familial heritable (40%) forms.[193] Knudson's two-hit hypothesis to explain retinoblastoma genesis has been substantiated by elegant genetic studies.[194-196] In this model, mutations of both copies of a gene are required for tumorigenesis. The affected gene is the *Rb1* gene, which is located on the short arm of chromosome 13 and codes for a tumor suppressor protein. In sporadic nonheritable cases, both mutations occur in a somatic retinal cell. In heritable cases the first mutation occurs in a germline cell and is found throughout the body, while the second occurs in a somatic retinal cell. The heritable mutation in the germline cell appears to be inherited as an autosomal dominant mutation with high penetrance, but is, in fact, a recessive mutation of a tumor suppressor protein.[195] Bilateral tumors imply a germinal mutation, and up to 10% of unilateral cases may involve germinal mutations.[193,196] Multiple separate tumors in one eye also suggest a germinal mutation, but the existence of separate tumors in an eye may be difficult to differentiate from the seeding of a single primary intraocular tumor in some cases. Multiple separate tumors in one eye have been said to suggest a germinal mutation, but the distinction between separate primary tumors and seeding can be difficult. In addition, one study demonstrated over 50% of unilateral sporadic tumors appeared multifocal on histologic evaluation.[197] Familial retinoblastoma, in which the mutation is transmitted to the patient from an affected parent, occurs in up to 25% of cases with germinal mutations, while the remaining heritable cases represent new germinal mutations.[198]

Clinically, retinoblastoma presents most often with leukokoria in 60% (Fig. 70-7A) and strabismus in 20% of cases. Less common presentations include decreased vision, family history, ocular or orbital inflammation, or glaucoma. Patients with bilateral tumors are diagnosed at a mean age of 12 months, while unilateral disease is

Specific Malignancies

III

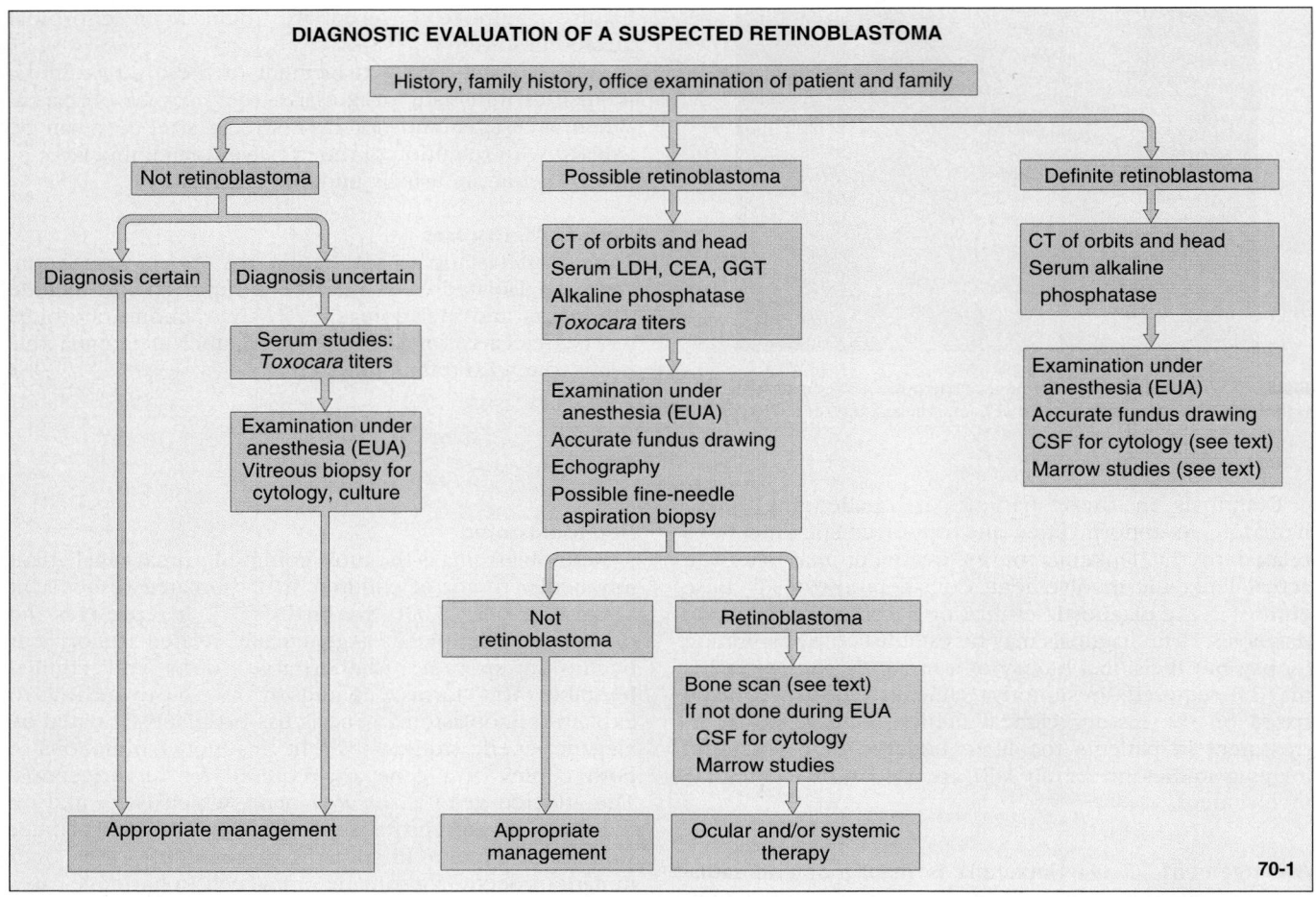

DIAGNOSTIC EVALUATION OF A SUSPECTED RETINOBLASTOMA

History, family history, office examination of patient and family

Not retinoblastoma — Possible retinoblastoma — Definite retinoblastoma

Not retinoblastoma
- Diagnosis certain
- Diagnosis uncertain
  - Serum studies: *Toxocara* titers
  - Examination under anesthesia (EUA) Vitreous biopsy for cytology, culture

Possible retinoblastoma
- CT of orbits and head Serum LDH, CEA, GGT Alkaline phosphatase *Toxocara* titers
- Examination under anesthesia (EUA) Accurate fundus drawing Echography Possible fine-needle aspiration biopsy
- Not retinoblastoma / Retinoblastoma
  - Bone scan (see text) If not done during EUA CSF for cytology Marrow studies

Definite retinoblastoma
- CT of orbits and head Serum alkaline phosphatase
- Examination under anesthesia (EUA) Accurate fundus drawing CSF for cytology (see text) Marrow studies (see text)

Appropriate management — Appropriate management — Ocular and/or systemic therapy

70-1

diagnosed at a mean age of 24 months.[199] Diagnosis of new tumors after the age of 6 years is very rare, but new tumors have been reported in patients through the sixth decade.[200-203] Leukokoria is notoriously difficult to detect during routine pediatric examination, especially in its early to moderate stages. Failure to identify leukokoria in the face of parental report of an abnormal pupil should not preclude urgent ophthalmologic referral.

Ophthalmoscopy is the most important modality in the diagnosis of retinoblastoma. Patients should undergo a dilated fundus examination in the ophthalmologist's office, but complete evaluation of the entire fundus to allow accurate staging and treatment planning once a tumor is detected requires examination under anesthesia. Parents and siblings should also undergo dilated fundus examination, since siblings may have unsuspected tumors and parents may have dormant or regressed tumors.

On examination, the tumors range from a translucent white to yellow-white (Fig. 70-7B). Calcium flecks may be seen and are characteristic. Overlying extensive retinal detachment may obscure the appearance of the tumor. Tumor may be seen in the vitreous and the anterior chamber and may layer out, simulating hypopyon from endophthalmitis. Infrequently, acute inflammation produced by tissue necrosis is seen.[204-206] If the intraocular

pressure rises, the cornea may become cloudy and even limit the view of the intraocular tumor. CT is valuable in detecting characteristic tumor calcifications (Fig. 70-7C), while MRI is superior in detecting extraocular extension.

Variants include diffuse and trilateral retinoblastoma. Diffuse retinoblastoma forms no discrete mass.[207,208] These may present as chronic inflammation, and the diagnosis is frequently delayed. Usually these are sporadic and unilateral cases. Children with suspected endophthalmitis must have this diagnosis excluded. Trilateral retinoblastoma is an infrequent variant in which ocular tumors are accompanied by a midline brain tumor.[209-212] The first cases were pineal tumors, but the definition has been broadened to include primitive neuroectodermal tumors in midline locations. The brain tumor usually presents after the eye tumors with symptoms and signs of increased intracranial pressure. The tumor is well imaged by CT or MRI. Treatment has been unsuccessful in almost all cases. The cases with longer survival may reflect very early diagnosis of a small tumor. Management, if elected by the family, involves surgery, chemotherapy, and radiation.

Retinoblastomas are pink to chalky-white tumors that contain calcium deposits (Fig. 70-7D). They derive from neuroblastic photoreceptor progenitor cells. Undifferentiated tumors may consist almost entirely of undifferen-

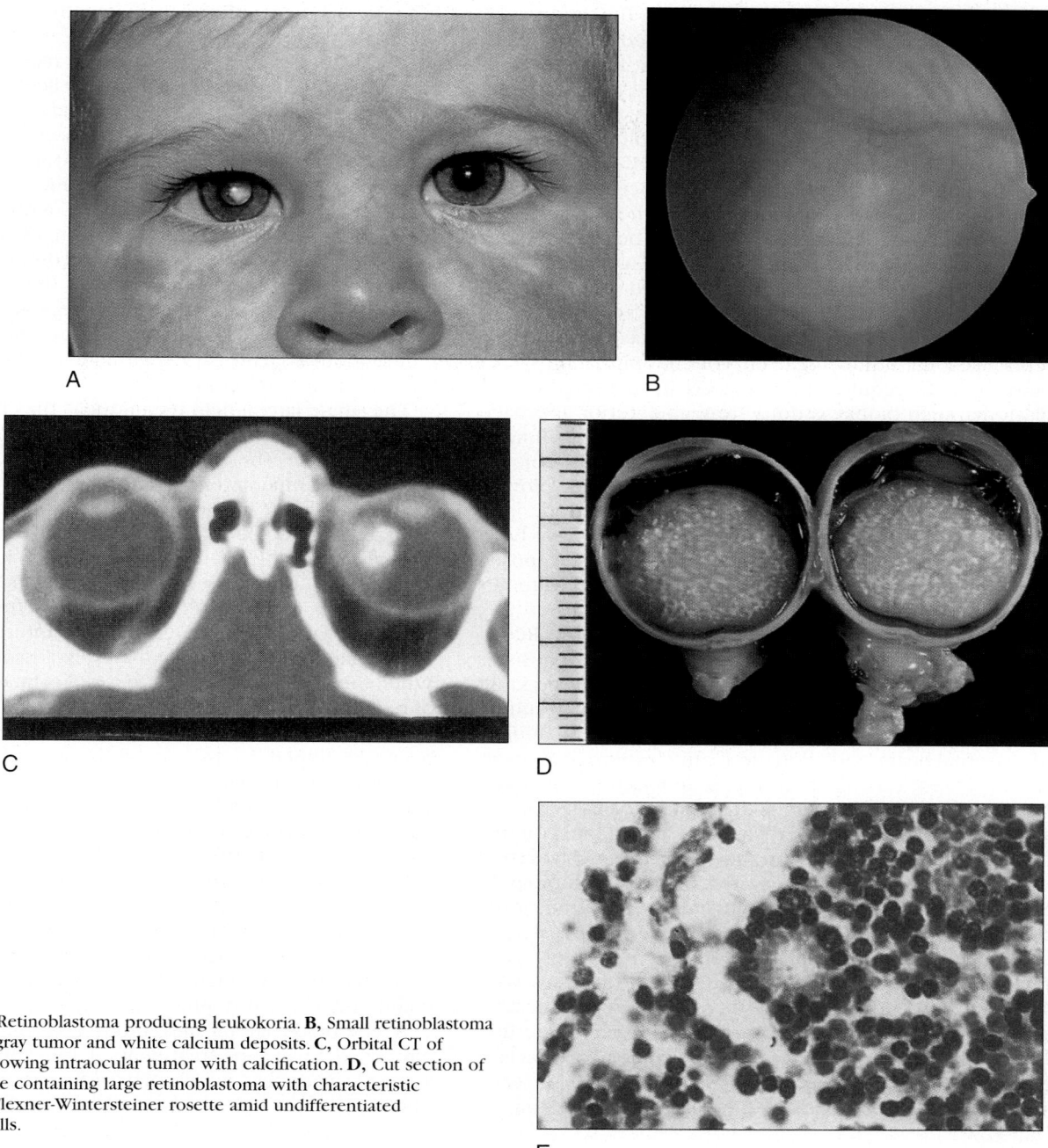

Figure 70-7. A, Retinoblastoma producing leukokoria. **B,** Small retinoblastoma with translucent gray tumor and white calcium deposits. **C,** Orbital CT of retinoblastoma showing intraocular tumor with calcification. **D,** Cut section of the enucleated eye containing large retinoblastoma with characteristic calcifications. **E,** Flexner-Wintersteiner rosette amid undifferentiated retinoblastoma cells.

tiated cells with high nuclear/cytoplasmic ratios, pleomorphism, and numerous mitoses. Zones of necrosis with dystrophic calcification are distinctive, with viable cells forming perivascular cuffs. Differentiated tumors exhibit photoreceptor differentiation with cells exhibiting polarity and forming Flexner-Wintersteiner rosettes (Fig. 70-7E) or fleurettes. Homer-Wright rosettes, also found in other neuroepithelial tumors, may be seen.

Retinocytoma is an infrequent benign counterpart of retinoblastoma.[213,214] These are small, translucent, fleshy tumors. Whereas some authors differentiate these from retinoblastoma on the basis of vascularity, their features

overlap with retinoblastoma, and failure to grow is the sole clinical criterion. Transformation to malignant retinoblastoma has occurred, so serial clinical observation is needed.[215] Pathologic studies have found these tumors to contain more differentiated cell types.

Management. The differential diagnosis of retinoblastoma is extensive and includes neoplastic, inflammatory, developmental, hereditary, and traumatic conditions.[216] In most cases, the diagnosis can be made on the basis of clinical history and the ocular and general physical

Specific Malignancies

examinations. When the appearance of the intraocular mass is atypical or obscured, CT is the study of choice to detect calcification, which is seen in most discrete tumors.[217,218] Spiral CT decreases the need for anesthesia, monitoring, and contrast without loss of diagnostic accuracy.[219] Diffuse retinoblastoma, tumors arising in adults, and very small tumors may not show calcification. The finding of calcification in an intraocular mass in a child is almost pathognomonic for retinoblastoma, but rare cases of intraocular calcification can be seen in other conditions. Involvement of the optic nerve in cases of tumor overlying the optic disc can be visualized with contrast-enhanced MRI or CT, but MRI is probably superior.

Infrequently, in atypical cases or cases of diffuse retinoblastoma simulating uveitis or endophthalmitis, FNA biopsy may be required for diagnosis. In suspected retinoblastoma, such biopsy is done from an anterior approach to avoid seeding other soft tissues. Fear of this technique has resulted from confusion between planned FNA biopsy with appropriate technique and vitrectomies, employing relatively large-caliber instruments, irrigation, and exposure of subconjunctival soft tissue, which have been performed on unsuspected retinoblastomas misdiagnosed as intraocular inflammation and which have led to tumor spread into the orbit.[220]

Retinoblastomas have long been staged by the Reese-Ellsworth system,[221] which relates to visual prognosis as opposed to survival and which is based on clinical extent of disease, not histopathologic features or extent of tumor. Also, this system is based only on the treatment options of external-beam radiation and enucleation. The more recent Essen classification for retinoblastoma management still does not address histopathologic factors or survival.[222] Efforts are under way to design a more comprehensive classification system, but even the most current working classification does not include pathology.[223] Staging evaluation historically included evaluation of the bone marrow and cerebrospinal fluid (CSF). Recent data suggest that bone marrow studies are of low yield in unselected cases and are positive only in cases with advanced disease. However, a recent case report demonstrated negative CSF cytology on lumbar puncture, but positive CSF cytology when the tumor was excised using a neurosurgical approach, suggesting that in early stages, CNS spread may be undetectable with lumbar puncture.[224,225]

Treatment of retinoblastoma represents one of the major successes in oncology. Before this century the mortality was 100%; 30 years ago it declined to 20%, and it is now less than 5% using enucleation. If the tumors involve only the eyes, local treatment is appropriate. If extraocular disease exists, other modalities are necessary. Enucleation gives the highest local control and cure rate but results in total loss of vision, altered cosmesis, and orbital hypoplasia. It has been shown repeatedly that if the tumor is confined to the globe, survival is greater than 90%.[226,227] As the tumor extends posteriorly into the optic nerve, survival may decrease to 30% when the surgical margin of the optic nerve is involved. Advances in treatment have been directed at tumor control with preservation of vision and have included external-beam

radiation therapy, thermal destructive modalities, and chemotherapy.

The introduction of external-beam radiation therapy in the middle of this century led to excellent tumor control, but ocular complications from irradiation were common and severe because of the high doses employed.[228-231] Advances for retinoblastoma treatment have since centered on modification of technique to maximize efficacy and decrease complications. With the advent of megavoltage techniques, preservation of life and vision was possible. Previously, it was recommended that in bilateral retinoblastoma, the eye with the larger tumor be enucleated while the smaller tumor receive external-beam radiation therapy. This dictum is no longer used, and enucleation as a primary treatment is reserved for eyes with no useful visual potential.

The single lateral field technique is the classic external-beam radiation therapy technique for retinoblastoma. In this technique, the anterior edge of a lateral beam is placed a few millimeters behind the limbus and either the beam is angled 2 to 5 degrees posteriorly to avoid beam divergence into the lens of the contralateral eye or the central axis of the beam is half-beam blocked.[232] Current total dosing using this straightforward and reproducible technique is 45 to 50 Gy in 1.5- to 2-Gy fractions. Its disadvantage is that it does not treat the anterior portions of the retina, and recurrence may develop in this region. While theoretically designed to avoid cataract, 20% to 30% of patients develop ipsilateral cataract.[233,234]

Precision lateral external-beam radiation therapy has been developed to treat retinoblastoma.[235-237] Using a vacuum contact lens and magnet to immobilize the eye and generate a highly reproducible position, a sharply collimated beam is used to treat the entire retina and vitreous, while attempting to minimize the lens exposure. If the tumor affects the posterior portions of the retina, the entire beam is placed posterior to the lens. Local control of 61% is obtained with this technique alone. One third of eyes developed cataracts, and one third of these cataracts were extracted. The main drawback of this technique is that it requires special equipment.

A combined lateral and anterior technique has been employed to ensure treatment of the entire retina. The anterior field may be treated with either electrons or photons.[238,239] A shield is sometimes used to protect the lens, but it shadows and thereby decreases the dose to the posterior portions of the retina. Results using this technique have been variable. Some investigators report worse tumor control with the use of a lens shield, but others do not use a shield and claim superior tumor control over single lateral field delivery with similar rates of cataract formation. Overall recurrence rates for unilateral tumors can approach 40% in referral centers. Recurrence is associated with larger tumor size and more extensive disease.[239,240] Complications of all forms of external-beam radiation therapy include cataract, orbital and midfacial maldevelopment, radiation retinopathy, optic neuropathy, hypopituitarism, and increased incidence of secondary tumors in the irradiation field.[231,237,241] The results are presented in Table 70-5. New techniques continue to be developed.[248]

TABLE 70-5

■ Results of External-Beam Radiation Treatment of Retinoblastoma

SERIES	NO. OF EYES	INITIAL LOCAL CONTROL (%)	ENUCLEATION (%)
Foote et al.[233]	25	44	20
Schipper et al.[235]	54	41	19
Cassady et al.[246]	223	49	31
Bedford et al.[245]	58	52	16
Thompson et al.[247]	34	56	29
Abramson et al.[242]	57	49	26
Howarth et al.[243]	12	33	0
Amendola et al.[244]	67	64	1

Plaque radiation therapy has been used infrequently for decades but has recently come into broader use.[249-251] The frequent presence of multiple lesions with diffuse edges as well as technical difficulties with the smaller pediatric eye and orbit limits the applicability of this technique. As with other ocular plaque radiation therapy, isotope use has shifted from ^{60}Co to ^{125}I. Treatment doses are 35 to 50 Gy. In appropriate cases this technique is successful, with 86% of eyes showing no tumor recurrence and 60% having good vision.[251] For primary lesions that can be covered by a single plaque, this treatment has potential. The inverse-square dosimetry of this modality results in higher relative radiation dosing to the retinal tumor with lower radiation doses to surrounding tissues than those that cause long-term complications after external-beam radiation therapy. Tumor response to plaques that are sequentially moved on the surface of the eye to treat an entire tumor are good, but the increased incidence and severity of radiation retinopathy and the difficulty of calculating overlapping fields suggest that this is not an appropriate technique. Plaque radiation therapy is also useful in treating solitary recurrences after external-beam radiation therapy.[251] However, the total radiation dose to treat the retina is at least 80 Gy. Further studies evaluating the long-term outcome of this method are needed.

Dose delivered to growth centers in the bony orbit, the brain, and the pituitary and hypothalamus can be significantly reduced with proton-beam therapy in treating children with retinoblastomas. Such patients are planned with the 3D planning program developed at MGH,[252,253] and treated under general anesthesia with fractionated 3D conformal proton-beam therapy, to doses in the 42 to 46 CGE range, at 2 CGE per fraction. Limitation of dose to normal tissues in general, and to orbital and skull bone in particular, is particularly important in treating patients with the hereditary form of the disease, who are at high risk for developing late second malignant neoplasms (SMNs).[254] The risk of SMN development appears to be greater in infants treated within the first year of life.[255] In an effort to avoid external-beam irradiation and its increased risk of second malignancies in these children, investigators have been experimenting with chemotherapy as initial treatment of retinoblastoma, to avoid external radiation and instead use local treatments such as laser or cryotherapy or focal radiation with plaque.[256-260] Typically the chemotherapy regimen includes carboplatin plus vincristine and etoposide. Objective response rates as high as 100% have been reported, but the authors have seen failures from these series.[251] Thus far, these early reports are encouraging and may lead to a reduction in the number of patients needing external-beam radiation, but longer follow-up in these series is required.[261]

Histopathologic features of prognostic significance for mortality due to retinoblastoma have been identified based on the examination of eyes from patients who have undergone enucleation. The most important histologic parameter is the extent of optic nerve involvement by tumor posterior to the lamina cribrosa, with progressively higher mortality occurring as tumor extends toward the surgical margin of resection.[226,227] Extraocular extension is ominous, while choroidal invasion is significant only if it is extensive.[227,262,263]

After enucleation, adjunctive irradiation is used when tumor is found at the surgical margin of the optic nerve in the enucleated specimen. Data on the role of chemotherapy in this scenario are limited and the criteria are subjective and controversial. Also, the long-term consequences of using chemotherapeutic agents in patients with a genetic predisposition to neoplasia remain to be seen. Chemotherapy is used when metastatic disease is present, when the optic nerve margin is involved, when CSF cytology is positive for tumor, and in trilateral cases. More controversial indications for chemotherapy are large tumors with vitreous seeding as an adjunct to external-beam radiation therapy and when poor prognostic parameters of optic nerve or orbital invasion are found at enucleation.

Patients with retinoblastoma require ophthalmologic evaluation every 3 months initially, and this interval is extended until age 6, after which the child may be examined yearly. Yearly systemic evaluation is also necessary. CT or MRI of bilateral cases to detect the few trilateral cases has a high cost-benefit ratio. Patients with metastases usually undergo a rapid demise.[264] Response to chemotherapy has been reported in a few cases.[265,266]

Second Primary Tumor. While primary treatment of retinoblastoma has become very successful, the challenge of treating second primary tumors (SPTs) remains, since these are more likely to be fatal than the primary tumor. In patients with systemic alteration of the *Rb1* gene, a significant risk of secondary tumors exists. The risk of a secondary tumor arising in a patient with hereditary retinoblastoma is substantial. Further study of a large series of retinoblastoma patients treated with radiation for SPTs showed a relative risk of 30 for heriditary retinoblastoma patients, with a cumulative SPT incidence of 50% at 50 years, 10 times greater than for nonheriditary cases.[267] Second primary tumors can occur within the field of irradiation (about 70% of the time) and outside the field of irradiation (approximately 30% of the time).[268,269]

The most common tumors are bone sarcomas, but soft tissue sarcomas are seen as well as melanoma, CNS malignancies, carcinoma, and lymphoma.[267,270-273] Some data suggest that most of the second cancer risk occurs in patients who are irradiated before the age of 1 year. Radiation before that age is felt to be associated with increased incidence of SPTs in the field of radiation and decreased survival.[274] Clearly, second tumors pose a major threat to patients who are cured of retinoblastoma, especially those who have hereditary disease, have been irradiated for cure, and were younger than 1 year old at time of treatment. These data provide an incentive to try to find alternative methods to treat these children that avoid external-beam radiation and yet preserve the high cure rate and maintain the patient's vision. Whether chemotherapy to shrink the tumor combined with aggressive local therapy can fill that role is the subject of active research.

Medulloepithelioma

Ocular medulloepithelioma, like retinoblastoma, is a tumor of the neuroepithelium. It usually occurs in the ciliary epithelium, although it can arise in other sites with neuroepithelium, including the optic disc. These tumors usually present in children between 2 and 4 years old; the mean age at diagnosis, which is frequently delayed for over a year, is 5 years.[275] They also occur in adults.[276] These tumors are almost always unilateral and they present insidiously with poor vision, glaucoma, pain, an ocular mass, or leukokoria.

Medulloepitheliomas may have teratoid or nonteratoid differentiation patterns and may be benign or malignant.[275] Nonteratoid tumors show neuroepithelial cells forming cords, tubules, or sheets. Teratoid elements include glial tissue, rhabdomyoblasts, cartilage, and both mesenchymal and ependymal tissue. Malignancy is based on the presence of undifferentiated neuroepithelial elements, high mitotic activity, sarcomatous areas, and invasion of the outer layers of the eye. Homer-Wright rosettes are common and Flexner-Wintersteiner rosettes may be seen, which makes the distinction between this tumor and retinoblastoma difficult.

Management. Because of the rarity and variability of these tumors, no typical set of findings is seen on ancillary examination, and the diagnosis is most often made at enucleation. Rarely, cells may be aspirated from the anterior chamber to provide the diagnosis while maintaining the integrity of the eye. No established treatment exists for this tumor. In the absence of a preoperative diagnosis, alternative measures such as radiation therapy or thermal destruction play a small role. Historically, some small tumors were excised, but in most cases, vision has been lost and enucleation is appropriate. Although evidence of malignancy can be found in about two thirds of cases, death has occurred in only 12 of the reported malignant cases, all after orbital recurrence.[275] When orbital extension by a malignant medulloepithelioma exists, exenteration, chemotherapy, and radiation therapy may be offered empirically.

ORBITAL NEOPLASIA

The benign, malignant, and diagnostically uncertain orbital neoplasms are listed in Table 70-6.

Primary Orbital Tumors of Adults

Lymphoproliferative Tumors (Lymphoma and "Reactive Lymphoid Hyperplasia")

Lymphoproliferative tumors of the orbit and periocular tissues are common and have a peak incidence in the seventh decade of life; women are affected more than men.[277-279] Approximately 15% of patients with orbital lymphoid tumors have a history of prior nonophthalmic lymphoma, but this is rare for conjunctival proliferations.[277,278,280,281] Lymphoma is characterized by an insidious, painless onset and a predilection for the superior portions of the orbit, particularly the levator and superior rectus muscles and lacrimal gland.[282] It may be bilateral. The tumor is of uniform, firm consistency and may project into the conjunctival fornices as a salmon-colored mass (Fig. 70-8). When involving the lacrimal gland, it usually affects both the orbital and palpebral lobes and may be palpable as a rubbery mass that may be fixed to the orbital rim.[279,283-285] In contrast to the benign propensity of lymphoproliferative lesions involving the lacrimal gland, most of those involving the eyelid and lacrimal sac are lymphomatous.[286,287] Chief clinical signs include proptosis, mass effect, ptosis, and a restriction of ocular motility that is less than that seen in thyroid ophthalmopathy and idiopathic inflammatory pseudotumor (IIP), since lymphoma induces much less fibrovascular tissue response. Although lymphomas are usually indolent, 10% to 25% of patients may display signs of conjunctival redness, pain, or acute orbital inflammation.[288] CT reveals a homogeneous mass with indistinct borders due to infiltration of surrounding orbital fibrofatty tissues that also molds to the contour of the eye and other orbital structures without bony alterations.[283,289] CT is preferred to MRI, since it is useful to rule out bone involvement. Benign reactive lymphoid hyperplasia also may be bilateral, may present insidiously with painless and gradual proptosis or globe displacement, and may show CT features similar to those of lymphoma. Thus clinical features and imaging studies of reactive lymphoid hyperplasias do not distinguish them from lymphoma, necessitating biopsy.

Orbital and periocular lymphomas are virtually all non-Hodgkin's B-cell lymphomas.[277-279,290] Grossly, the lesions appear salmon-pink or fish-flesh colored. Histologically, they are highly cellular proliferations, most of which are generally composed of neoplastic small lymphocytes with minimal cytologic atypia.[291] Lesions of IIP and thyroid ophthalmopathy, by contrast, are hypocellular when compared with orbital lymphoid tumors, including reactive lymphoid hyperplasia. The current prognostic classification of lymphoma upon which treatment is based is the working formulation for clinical usage first published in 1982.[292] In this classification, the most

TABLE 70-6

Orbital Neoplasms

Benign

Idiopathic inflammatory pseudotumor*[†]
Capillary hemangioma*
Cavernous hemangioma*
Neurilemmoma*
Lymphangioma*
Neurofibroma*
Osteoma*
Osteoblastoma
Lipoma
Fibroma
Ossifying fibroma
Leiomyoma
Granular cell myoblastoma
Rhabdomyoma
Chondroma
Glomus tumor
Paraganglioma
Juvenile xanthogranuloma
Sinus histiocytosis
Teratoma
Lacrimal gland tumors
   Pleomorphic adenoma (benign mixed tumor)*[†]

Uncertain Behavior

Reactive lymphoid hyperplasia*[†]
Optic nerve glioma*[†]
Meningioma*[†]
Fibrous histiocytoma*[†]
Hemangiopericytoma*[†]
Langerhans' cell histiocytosis[†]
Plasmacytoma[†]
Lacrimal gland tumor
   Benign lymphoepithelial lesion*[†]

Malignant

Lymphoma*[†]
Rhabdomyosarcoma*[†]
Granulocytic sarcoma[†]
Multiple myeloma[†]
Malignant peripheral nerve sheath tumor[†]
Alveolar soft part sarcoma[†]
Malignant melanoma[†]
Osteosarcoma[†]
Fibrosarcoma[†]
Leiomyosarcoma[†]
Chondrosarcoma[†]
Liposarcoma[†]
Malignant glioma of optic nerve[†]
Endodermal sinus tumor[†]
Extension of local tumor
   Paranasal sinus and nasal carcinoma*[†]
   Angiosarcoma[†]
   Esthesioneuroblastoma[†]
   Uveal melanoma[†]
   Retinoblastoma[†]
   Eyelid and conjunctival carcinoma[†]
   Retinal anlage tumor[†]
   Ameloblastoma[†]
Metastatic tumor
   Carcinoma*[†]
   Neuroblastoma[†]
   Nephroblastoma (Wilms' tumor)[†]
   Malignant melanoma[†]
   Sarcoma[†]
Lacrimal gland tumor
   Adenoid cystic carcinoma*[†]
   Carcinoma ex pleomorphic adenoma[†]
   Mucoepidermoid carcinoma[†]
   Poorly differentiated adenocarcinoma[†]

*Common tumor.
[†]Discussed in text.

common lymphomas occurring in the orbit and periocular tissues include small cell lymphocytic, small cell lymphocytic-plasmacytoid, and follicular small cleaved cell low-grade lymphomas as well as diffuse small cell intermediate-grade lymphoma. A substantial number of the small B-cell lymphomas are now classified as extra-

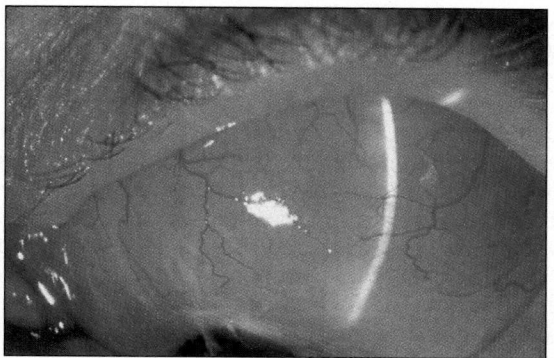

Figure 70-8. Salmon-colored conjuctival lymphoma in a patient with combined conjunctival and orbital lymphoma.

nodal marginal zone B-cell lymphomas, also known as low-grade B-cell lymphomas of mucosa-associated lymphoid tissue (MALT) type.[281,293,294] Involving orbital, adnexal, and conjunctival tissues, MALT-type lymphoma generally follows an indolent course with excellent response to therapy and long periods between relapses. If dissemination occurs, it is generally extranodal. Atypical CD5+ marginal zone lymphomas may occur, involve bone marrow, and relapse.[295,296]

The histologic classification of ocular lymphomas has important clinical and prognostic implications. Systemic lymphoma occurs in about 50% of patients with intermediate- and high-grade ocular lymphomas and 25% of patients with low-grade ocular lymphoma within 5 years of initial presentation.[278] Furthermore, up to 50% of patients with tumors exhibiting atypical cytologic features suggestive of but not diagnostic for lymphoma will develop systemic lymphoma within 5 years.[297] The site of tumor involvement is also important, since eyelid, orbital, and conjunctival involvement are associated with systemic lymphoma in two thirds, one third, and one fifth of patients, respectively.[278] Thus orbital lymphomas tend to be more aggressive than their conjunctival counterparts and intermediate-grade diffuse orbital lymphomas are associated with systemic disease in more than 75% of cases. Bilateral orbital lymphoid lesions are associated with a 35% incidence of systemic disease, which is not significantly higher than that seen in unilateral disease.[278,298]

Immunophenotyping may be important to determine clonality of lymphoid tumors. Monoclonal immunotyping of cytologically abnormal B lymphocytes in biopsies, even when reactive T lymphocytes are present, is strongly indicative of lymphoma and may allow for the diagnosis of lymphoma in otherwise indeterminate cases.[277,278,299,300] Histologically and immunophenotypically polyclonal infiltrates containing germinal centers, admixtures of mature B and predominantly T lymphocytes, plasma cells, mononuclear phagocytes, and occasional eosinophils and neutrophils characterize reactive lymphoid hyperplasia. Nevertheless, polyclonal staining of a lymphoid lesion does not rule out the possibility of supervening systemic lymphoma, since approximately two thirds of all ocular lymphoid tumors harbor subpopulations of monoclonal B lymphocytes, and systemic lymphomas arise in up to 25% of patients with immunophenotypically polyclonal reactive lymphoid proliferations of the conjunctiva and orbit.[297,301-303] Thus even the entity of reactive lymphoid hyperplasia is best classified as a lymphoid neoplasm with a potential for developing localized and systemic lymphoma.[297,298,304-306]

These findings indicate that patients with ocular lymphoid lesions, regardless of immunophenotype, should be evaluated and followed medically for the possibility of systemic lymphoma.[290] Recent advances that permit highly sensitive assessment of monoclonal B-lymphocyte populations by detecting heavy- and light-chain immunoglobulin genes have been applied to ocular adnexal and orbital lymphoproliferative lesions.[300,307,308] Immunoglobulin gene rearrangement studies have shown B-lymphocyte monoclonality in three quarters of lymphomas and in some lesions that appear polyclonal by immunophenotyping, the latter suggesting why lymphoma develops in patients with apparently reactive lymphoid proliferations. However, the lack of clonal detection in one quarter of proven lymphomas renders current polymerase chain reaction (PCR) techniques as research tools only.

Treatment of presumed lymphomas includes adequate biopsy to establish the diagnosis. Trials of systemic corticosteroids frequently reduce the lymphomas, which usually regrow after cessation of corticosteroid treatment and therefore should not generally be substituted for biopsy. Biopsy is usually done through an anterior approach but may require lateral orbitotomy with bone removal for posteriorly located lesions. In cases with bilateral involvement, only one side is sampled, since identical histopathologic and immunophenotypic patterns have been found in all cases biopsied bilaterally.[309] Subsequent careful systemic evaluation for disseminated disease is the best way to determine treatment and prognosis for patients with ostensibly reactive as well as atypical and frankly lymphomatous proliferations.[279] This evaluation should include a complete blood count, immunoelectrophoresis, bone marrow biopsy, and chest and abdominal/

LYMPHOMA OF THE EYE AND ORBIT

OCULAR LYMPHOMA
Diagnosis
Vitreous biopsy
Cerebrospinal fluid cytology
MRI of CNS
Systemic workup for lymphoma

Treatment
Brain and eye radiation to 40 Gy
Intrathecal methotrexate frequently used for cerebrospinal fluid prophylaxis
Systemic chemotherapy usually reserved for patients with known systemic tumor

ORBITAL LYMPHOMA
Diagnosis
Biopsy
    Distinction between benign lymphoid dysplasia and malignant lymphoma sometimes difficult, even with immunohistologic staining and immunoglobulin gene rearrangement studies
Systemic workup needed

Treatment
Low-grade lymphoma: localized radiation therapy to 15 to 30 Gy
High-grade lymphoma: CHOP × 3 plus radiation therapy (30 to 40 Gy)
Manifestation of systemic lymphoma: chemotherapy with or without radiation therapy

---

pelvic CT.[310-312] Treatment of orbital lymphomas is heavily dependent on the grade and location of the tumor. Low-grade lesions in the conjunctiva are typically controlled with low doses of radiation in the range of 15 to 20 Gy. Low-grade lesions involving the orbit are managed with doses in the range of 30 to 35 Gy. Intermediate and high-grade lymphomas are treated with three cycles of CHOP (cyclophosphamide, doxorubicin, vincristine, and prednisone) chemotherapy followed by orbital irradiation to 40 Gy.[313] Complications of radiation therapy including dry eye, cataract, and optic nerve and retinal vasculopathy are reduced by fractionating treatment and carefully planning the delivery of radiation using three-dimensional conformal techniques, and are increased when chemotherapy and irradiation are given concomitantly.[314] If systemic disease is found, chemotherapy is usually given as a first modality. Response in the eye can then be evaluated and a decision made as to whether to administer additional radiation therapy to this local site.[310] Clinical follow-up every 6 months for 2 years and then yearly is performed to rule out supervening systemic disease, since some patients who are cured of their local orbital tumor may develop systemic lymphoma and die.[302] However, patients without signs of systemic lymphoma at presentation or within 1 year after ophthalmic presentation have a 90% likelihood of remaining free of systemic disease.[278] In patients who develop orbital and adnexal involvement in the course of systemic lymphoma, chemotherapy and/or radiotherapy frequently result in prolonged remission.[280]

High-grade large B-cell lymphomas of the orbit may rarely occur in nonimmunocompromised patients and in patients with AIDS.[293,316-318] Combination chemotherapy and radiation therapy, or chemotherapy alone, or palliative treatment for AIDS patients is instituted to treat these tumors, which frequently cause massive proptosis and threaten vision by progressive tumor enlargement. Although rare in the United States,[319] Burkitt's lymphoma is a high-grade lymphoma that is common in Africa and may occur in the setting of AIDS.[316,320] It usually involves the maxilla and may extend into the orbit, resulting in rapidly progressive proptosis, superior globe dystopia, marked conjunctival chemosis, and visual loss.[321,322] Due to extremely rapid tumor growth, proptosis may be massive; CNS infiltration occurs in 30% of cases, resulting in cranial nerve palsies and epidural tumor masses. These tumors are associated with cytogenetic translocation of the c-*myc* oncogene at chromosomal locations corresponding to immunoglobulin heavy- and light-chain genes.[323] Pathologically, the tumor is formed by a redundant population of large B lymphocytes with numerous mitoses and interspersed mononuclear phagocytes that have abundant clear cytoplasm imparting a characteristic "starry-sky" histopathologic appearance. Management involves biopsy followed by chemotherapy and adjunctive local radiation therapy.[324]

Primary orbital T-cell lymphoma is rare.[325-328] Neoplastic T-cell involvement of the orbit and periocular tissues is usually found in established systemic mycosis fungoides.[329] This tumor displays prominent skin findings of scaling, redness, thickening, and ulceration as well as peripheral lymphadenopathy. Biopsy reveals characteristic neoplastic T lymphocytes containing convoluted nuclear profiles.

Orbital involvement by Hodgkin's lymphoma is rare and is usually associated with widespread disease or clinical relapse.[330,331] The tumor may affect the anterior orbit or orbital bones or may result from intraorbital extension of cranial involvement.[332] Histopathologic diagnosis, as elsewhere, relies on demonstration of Reed-Sternberg cells or their variants in known cases.

Plasma Cell Tumors

Plasma cell tumors may be either polyclonal reactive lesions or monoclonal malignant tumors formed by proliferations of highly differentiated B lymphocytes that produce immunoglobulin restricted to a single heavy chain and a single light chain.[333-335] Benign orbital plasmacytomas occur as solitary bone tumors (that may extend into adjacent soft tissue), extramedullary plasmacytomas of orbital soft tissues or conjunctiva, or plasmacytomas extending into the orbit from adjacent sinuses or the nasopharynx.[336-339] Benign plasmacytomas, like orbital involvement with multiple myeloma and Waldenström's macroglobulinemia, may exhibit manifestations of progressive proptosis, pain, diplopia, ptosis, and inferior or medial ocular dystopia, but they lack signs and symptoms of systemic involvement, including absent or only low levels of monoclonal immunoglobulins on serum immuno-

electrophoresis.[334] CT may reveal lytic bone lesions whose differential diagnosis includes benign plasmacytoma and multiple myeloma, Waldenström's macroglobulinemia, or metastatic carcinoma.[340] When a plasma cell tumor is found in the orbit, bone marrow biopsy, serum protein electrophoresis, and immunoglobulin electrophoresis of the serum and urine should be undertaken to rule out the systemic diseases of multiple myeloma or Waldenström's macroglobulinemia, both of which may result in bilateral orbital involvement.[333,341-344]

Multiple myeloma, which has a peak incidence in the seventh decade of life, results in clinically manifest bone pain, fatigue, and anemia.[333,334,336] Orbital involvement may occur any time during the disease course and may be its presenting manifestation. Hyperviscosity due to high concentrations of monoclonal immunoglobulins secreted by tumor cells into the blood may result in retinal vein occlusion. When they involve bone, plasma cell tumors frequently affect the orbital roof or lateral wall. Immunohistochemical staining of biopsied tissue to identify heavy and light immunoglobulin chain monoclonality of the plasma cell proliferation is extremely helpful for diagnosis. Even so, up to 50% of apparently benign solitary plasmacytomas will evolve into systemic multiple myeloma, so these lesions are also often treated with approximately 40 Gy to the site of involvement or by complete excision with radiation therapy. Multiple myeloma and Waldenström's macroglobulinemia are both treated with systemic chemotherapy and adjunctive radiation therapy to localized lesions.[334,336]

Benign Lymphoepithelial Lesion

The benign lymphoepithelial lesion involves the lacrimal and salivary glands of postmenopausal women and causes the severe xerophthalmia and xerostomia of Sjögren's syndrome.[345,346] Rheumatoid arthritis or other autoimmune diseases also occur in this syndrome. Clinically, brown eyelid discoloration accompanies lacrimal gland swelling. Histologically, diffuse and severe lymphocyte and plasma cell infiltration, progressive destruction of lacrimal glandular acini, reactive proliferation of terminal ductules forming "epimyoepithelial islands," and fibrosis of lacrimal gland lobules characterize the benign lymphoepithelial lesion.[346,347] These patients are at increased risk of developing nodal and extranodal lymphomas, including lesions that arise in affected lacrimal glands.[347-349] Mucosa-associated lymphoid tissue (MALT) lymphoma, a low-grade, indolent, localized small cell lymphoma that is effectively treated with local irradiation, is especially prone to develop in these lesions.[348]

Idiopathic Inflammatory Pseudotumor

IIP is a common orbital inflammation of adults that may be acute, subacute, or chronic depending on the degree of inflammatory symptoms and signs (Fig. 70-9A). It is discussed here to distinguish its features from the lymphoproliferative disorders with which it may be confused. Acute IIP is characterized by abrupt onset of pain, swelling, and redness, whereas chronic IIP may be insidious, progressing over weeks to months, often with only subtle manifestations of inflammation.[351,352] Symptoms in

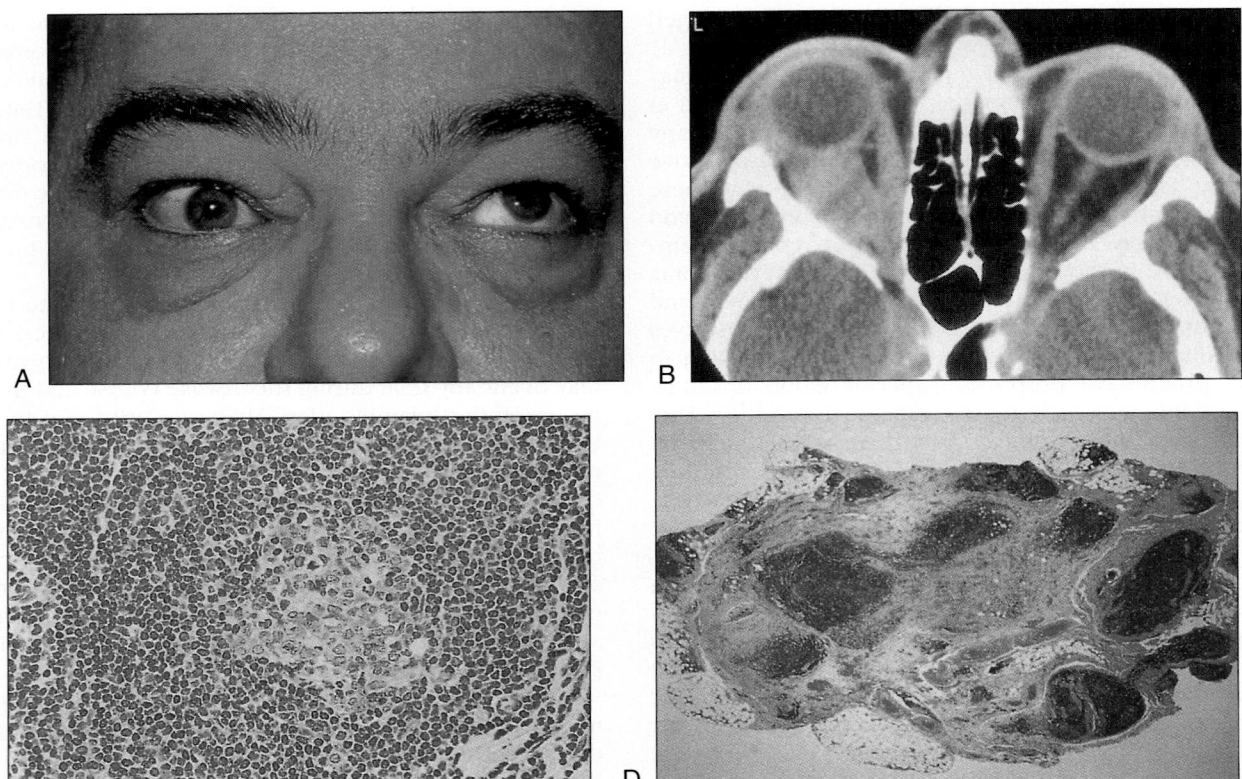

Figure 70-9. A, Right proptosis, redness, and decreased extraocular motility in a patient with idiopathic orbital inflammatory pseudotumor. **B,** Orbital CT of same patient showing enlarged rectus muscles and infiltration of orbital fat extending to surround optic nerve. **C,** Germinal center in reactive lymphoid infiltrate of orbital pseudotumor. **D,** Orbital biopsy of sclerosing form of orbital pseudotumor with fibrotic tissue supervening on chronic inflammation.

chronic IIP are generally due to secondary effects of proptosis and entrapment of structures by fibrosis. Inflammation and dense sclerosis of extraocular muscles and motor nerves results in diplopia, and similar involvement of the optic nerve causes visual loss.[352,353] IIP of motor and sensory nerves at the orbital apex may result in the painful ophthalmoplegia syndrome of Tolosa-Hunt. Orbital congestion may also occur due to impaired venous drainage through the superior orbital fissure. Intracranial extension may be associated with bony erosion and increased morbidity and mortality.[354,355] In some cases sclerosing IIP has been associated with chronic progressive fibrosis of the retroperitoneum, mediastinum, bile ducts, thyroid, or meninges.[356]

Approximately 10% of cases of IIP occur during the first two decades of life.[357] It is usually more fulminant and frequently bilateral, and it may be associated with anterior uveitis and papillitis. Cases with bilateral involvement and uveitis may be more recalcitrant and may recur. Systemic eosinophilia and increased numbers of eosinophils within tissue infiltrates may be present.[358]

IIP may affect specific tissues such as the lacrimal gland, extraocular muscle, episclera, optic nerve, or uvea, resulting in characteristic clinical patterns.[304,359] IIP has a particular propensity to involve the lacrimal gland and superotemporal orbit, causing acute pain, swelling, redness, and tenderness of the lateral upper eyelid that

may be associated with conjunctival chemosis, lateral rectus paresis, and pain on eye movement. Myositis results in painful paresis and muscle restriction.[360,361] Episcleritis and periscleritis result in pain and redness associated with eyelid and conjunctival swelling and secondary ptosis.[362] Uveal involvement may include choroidal effusion that results in exudative retinal detachment.[363] Optic nerve involvement causes visual loss, pain on eye movement, and papillitis visible on ophthalmoscopic examination.[359]

CT scanning reveals an ill-defined mass with shaggy margins that involves orbital structures and permeates orbital fat (Fig. 70-9B).[359,364] The infiltrates may extend along muscles and tendons, particularly the medial and superior rectus-levator muscles and may cause radiographic enhancement of the lacrimal gland, optic nerve sheath, apical fat, or sclera.[304,359,364] CT evidence of inflammation rarely extends into the paranasal sinuses.[365] Pathologically, the findings in IIP depend on the degree of inflammation and fibrovascular tissue response. Acute IIP shows a polymorphic infiltrate of lymphocytes, plasma cells, mononuclear phagocytes, neutrophils, and eosinophils.[351,358] The subacute and chronic forms of IIP demonstrate lymphoid follicles (Fig. 70-9C) as well as reactive fibrovascular stroma (Fig. 70-9D) that progressively replaces normal fat, muscle, and glandular tissue, entrapping and restricting the function of the orbital structures.[297]

Orbital pseudotumor usually occurs as a single episode but may recur in adults up to 10 years after the initial presentation.[366] Biopsy is not required for typical acute and subacute IIP, in which prompt response to high-dose corticosteroids, tapered over the course of weeks to months, is therapeutic and diagnostic.[304,359,367] Recurrent cases may be treated with additional courses of corticosteroids, but long-term treatment is avoided due to common and severe systemic complications.[368,369] IIP unresponsive to corticosteroids, chronic IIP, and IIP with osseous, extraorbital, or lacrimal gland involvement should be biopsied, in the latter circumstance because many systemic inflammatory and neoplastic processes may involve the lacrimal gland. In these cases, incisional biopsy is preferred over fine-needle biopsy, which is often inconclusive. Low-dose irradiation of 15 to 20 Gy in divided doses over 10 to 14 days often adequately treats cases that are not steroid responsive.[304,359,367] Cytotoxic agents including azathioprine, methotrexate, cyclophosphamide, and cyclosporine have been used in patients refractory to corticosteroids and radiation therapy.[367,370,371] Orbital decompression has been used to relieve optic nerve compression. In rare cases, locally progressive lesions may require excision or orbital exenteration to control the disease, since these tumors may extend intracranially and result in CNS morbidity and even death.[354,355,367] Overlaps occur between benign reactive hyperplasia and IIP both clinically and pathologically, but true IIP seldom, if ever, evolves into lymphoma.[305,351] Nonetheless, late development of lymphoma has occurred in treated or untreated ostensible IIP.

Fibrous Histocytic Tumors/Hemangiopericytoma
Orbital tumors composed of oval to spindle-shaped mesenchymal cells exhibit variable degrees of fibroplastic differentiation and are classified based on distinctive histopathologic growth patterns, vascularity, and immunoreactivity under several rubrics: fibrous histiocytoma,[372] hemangiopericytoma,[373] and solitary fibrous[374,375] and giant cell angiofibroma.[376] The precise interrelationship of these putative tumor types has yet to be determined, since there is histopathologic and immunohistochemical overlap and the follow-up required to assess the clinical significance of these subclassifications has not yet been possible because these tumors are uncommon and may recur many years after initial resection.

Fibrous histiocytoma is a common primary mesenchymal orbital tumor of adults with a mean age of onset of 43 years.[372] It may also occur in children and subsequent to radiotherapy for retinoblastoma.[377-380] Fibrous histiocytomas involving the orbit may be benign, locally aggressive, or frankly malignant.[372] Malignant tumors may follow previous orbital irradiation. Fibrous histiocytomas are unilateral tumors that produce proptosis, globe displacement, reduced vision, chemosis, muscle palsies, and pain. CT reveals a rounded, well-circumscribed mass that rarely erodes bone. The tumor arises from cells that show variable degrees of fibroblastic and histiocytic differentiation. Pathologically, benign lesions appear circumscribed and display a distinctive storiform pattern. Locally aggressive tumors, which comprise about 25%

of cases, show increased cellularity, significant atypia, mitoses, and hemangiopericytoma-like areas. In approximately 10% of cases, the tumors are poorly circumscribed with infiltrating margins. About 10% of tumors are frankly malignant and show considerable pleomorphism, numerous mitotic figures, atypical mitoses, and necrosis.[379,381,382] Rarely, malignant fibrous histiocytomas of the orbit are metastatic.[383] Fibrous histiocytomas are best treated by complete, wide, local excision, since incompletely removed benign lesions may recur and become locally aggressive.[372] Recurrent locally aggressive and malignant lesions require exenteration. Adjunctive radiation therapy does not appear to provide therapeutic benefit if exenteration is performed with clean surgical margins. Mortality occurs from malignant and locally aggressive tumors that become malignant upon recurrence. In these cases the average survival is 10 years after initial diagnosis, and death occurs from local extension or metastatic spread.[372]

Almost exclusively a tumor of adults, hemangiopericytoma affects men more often than women by a 2:1 ratio.[373] Clinical signs include subacute, progressive unilateral proptosis with reduced vision, diplopia, and mild pain accompanied by eyelid edema and engorgement of eyelid and episcleral vessels resulting in blue or red discoloration (Fig. 70-10A).[373] Most of these tumors occur superiorly in the orbit, producing inferior dystopia of the eye, but they may invade the orbit secondarily from nasal or ethmoidal sinus origin. They may also arise in the conjunctiva, episclera, or lacrimal gland.[384] CT and MRI reveal an enhancing, circumscribed mass with arterial feeders that may extend through bone into the cranial cavity (Fig. 70-10B).[385] Whereas they deceptively appear to be encapsulated, hemangiopericytomas are solid, purplish, friable tumors that bleed readily. Histopathologically, neoplastic pericytes form a dense proliferation of oval to spindle-shaped cells, among which are prominent ecstatic vessels.[373] A distinctive, rich capillary network ramifies to surround individual or groups of pericytes. The surgical margins frequently contain tumor on microscopic examination. Histologically benign hemangiopericytomas are distinguished from frankly malignant tumors by mitotic rate, cellularity, and nuclear pleomorphism.[373] Frankly malignant and borderline lesions have greater tendencies to recur locally and result in distant metastases. Although technically difficult to remove, complete excision with tumor-free margins should be attempted, since incompletely resected tumors recur, become locally aggressive or malignant, and spawn distant metastases. An alternative approach employing conservative excision and radiation therapy has also been advocated.[386] Clinical and histopathologic findings should be considered jointly in clinical management since histopathologic features are insufficient to predict biologic behavior.[387] All hemangiopericytomas, regardless of category, have the capacity to recur and metastasize, sometimes decades after initial resection.[388,389] Metastases to lung, bone, and liver may result in death.[373,387]

Solitary fibrous tumor, first described in the orbit in 1994, was initially described in the thoracic cavity, where it is distinguished from mesothelial tumors based on

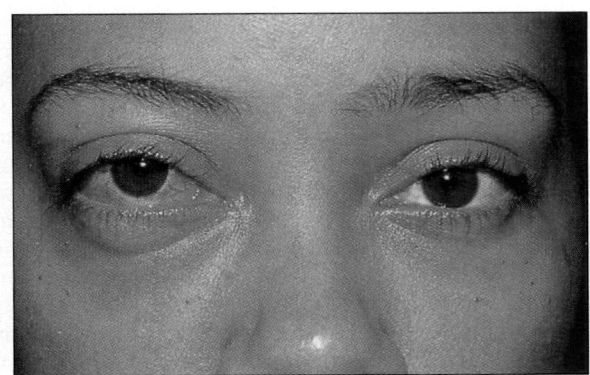

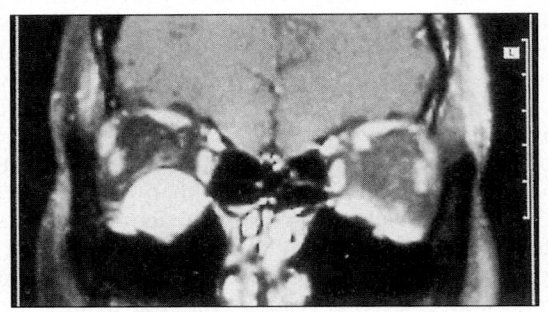

Figure 70-10. A, Right proptosis and inferior blue-red dislocation of eye and eyelid due to highly vascular hemangiopericytoma. **B,** Orbital MRI of same patient showing large enhancing mass inferiorly within the oribit.

its fibroblastic phenotype and immunoreactivity for CD34 and vimentin.[374,375] Giant cell angiofibroma, first described in the orbit in 1995, was described as distinct from solitary fibrous tumors by its vascularized spindle cell proliferation, hypocellular areas containing giant cells, and immunohistochemical positivity for CD34 and vimentin.[376,390] Both of these tumors, however, may be locally infiltrative, leading to recurrence, and display fibrous histocytoma- and hemangiopericytoma-like areas. Thus the precise relationship of these recently described histologically classified entities to fibrous histiocytoma and hemangiopericytoma has yet to be determined.[391,392]

Epithelioid sarcoma, a rare mesenchymal malignancy usually found in tendon sheaths in extremities, has also been reported in the orbit.[393] This entity requires aggressive surgical resection, since it may be fatal.

Optic Nerve Meningioma

Meningiomas may arise as primary tumors from the meninges of the orbital optic nerve, from the orbital surface of the sphenoid bone, or, more commonly, as secondary extensions from the cranium.[394,395] Rarely, ectopic meningiomas may arise in orbital soft tissues.[396,397] Optic nerve meningiomas are unilateral, unless associated with neurofibromatosis; they have a peak incidence in middle age and a female/male predilection of 3:1.[396-399] Optic nerve meningiomas may also occur in children and may be aggressive. Optic nerve meningiomas present as painless, slowly progressive proptosis (Fig. 70-11A) associated with progressive reduction in visual acuity

and visual field loss, afferent pupillary defect, optic disc edema, venous congestion, and optociliary shunt vessels on the surface of the optic disc.[400-403] In advanced cases, the optic disc shows atrophy or reactive proliferative glial tissue, or both. These meningiomas cause progressive central visual field scotomas by directly invading optic nerve tissue or circumferentially enveloping it, resulting in nerve compression and ischemia.[402] Meningiomas arising from the orbital surface of the sphenoid bone or (rarely) from rests of meningothelial cells extrinsic to the optic nerve grow into the orbital apex and compress the optic nerve, a process that may be aggravated by reactive hyperostosis. Optic nerve meningiomas that occur intracranially or within the optic canal do not produce proptosis. Chiasmal involvement is associated with bitemporal hemianopia.[404]

CT of primary optic nerve meningioma shows the nerve to be surrounded by an irregularly shaped mass that has extended through the dura into surrounding orbital tissue[394,395,405] (Fig. 70-11B). Optic canal erosion, hyperostosis at the orbital apex, or calcification within the tumor may be present. The optic nerve passing through the mass results in a radiolucent linear "railroad track" sign corresponding to the position of the nerve on axial CT and a double-ring sign on coronal sections.[394] Hyperostosis may occur adjacent to intracanalicular meningiomas that are best detected by MRI.[406,407] MRI has the advantage of demonstrating the proximal extent of optic nerve meningioma involvement. Rarely, optic nerve meningiomas may require biopsy to establish a definitive

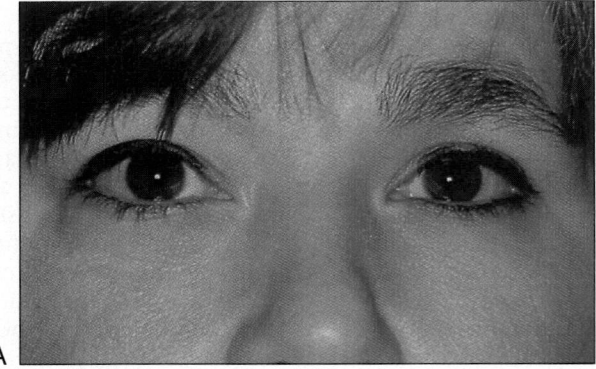

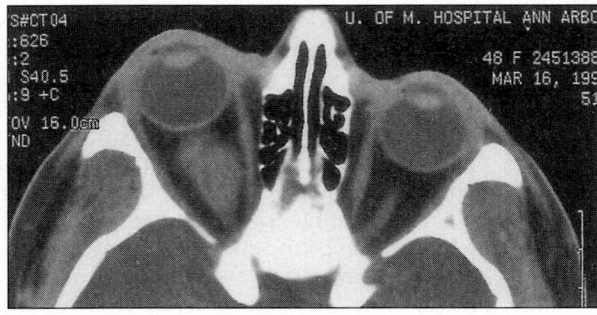

Figure 70-11. A, Right proptosis due to optic nerve meningioma. **B,** Orbital CT of same patient showing tumor around optic nerve that is seen as a linear radiolucent shadow within the center of the tumor (railroad track sign).

diagnosis.[408] Lateral orbitotomy is used for anterior tumors, and transcranial orbitotomy is necessary to approach orbital apical lesions or those arising intracranially. All meningiomas derive from rests of meningothelial cells, but they may assume different histopathologic patterns. The most common pattern is meningotheliomatous with whorls of plump cells containing vacuolated nuclei. These meningiomas sometimes exhibit concentrically laminated calcific (psammoma) bodies. All subtypes of meningioma affecting the orbit (whether meningotheliomatous, fibroblastic, syncytial, or transitional) have a similar prognosis. Immunohistochemical detection of vimentin and epithelial membrane antigens may aid in the histopathologic diagnosis.[409]

The natural history of meningioma is slowly progressive growth and blindness. Meningiomas arising in the orbit or optic canal may extend intracranially after a protracted clinical course.[401] Those within the cranium often may involve the chiasm and other adjacent structures. Treatment of intraorbital meningiomas is controversial and depends on vision, tumor size and location, and the age and overall health of the patient.[410] If the tumor is confined to the orbit in a patient with good vision, it may be followed clinically. If progressive tumor growth and visual loss is noted, carefully planned radiation treatment consisting of 55 Gy delivered over 6 weeks may stunt tumor growth and improve vision in some cases.[410,411] Untreated tumors and tumors unresponsive to radiation therapy may be treated surgically by optic nerve sheath decompression, sheath stripping, en bloc removal, or debulking, but these techniques frequently result in visual loss by interrupting the vascular supply to the optic nerve.[402,403,412] The degree of postoperative visual loss correlates with preoperative visual impairment and tumor size.[403,413] Stripping or incomplete resection of the meningioma from the optic nerve may also lead to recurrence.[400,402,403,412] Intracranial involvement frequently causes optic nerve compression and may be more amenable to surgery, which results in improvement in 40% to 60% of cases.[414,415] The effectiveness of radiation therapy is controversial for the treatment of intracranial meningiomas, but clinical improvement has been reported in some series of patients undergoing radiation therapy.[416,417] The observed progression of meningiomas during pregnancy and breast-feeding correlates with the presence of estrogen and progesterone receptors on meningiomas.[418-420] This has prompted attempts at hormonal treatment using the antiprogesterone drug mifepristone (RU-486), with tumor response in approximately one third of patients.[421]

Patients with optic nerve meningiomas have protracted clinical courses. Metastases are rare, but they may occur to liver, lung, thyroid, or subarachnoid space.[421] Ectopic orbital meningiomas are successfully treated with complete excision.[422]

Malignant Glioma of Optic Nerve and Chiasm

Malignant gliomas of the optic nerve and chiasm are rare tumors of middle-aged adults with no apparent sex predilection.[423-425] Clinical findings include rapidly progressive unilateral or bilateral visual loss, ocular pain, and headaches. Unilateral visual loss is frequently followed by bilateral blindness that occurs within weeks or months of clinical onset. Ophthalmoscopically, the optic disc may appear normal or may show edema or atrophy. Involvement of the intraorbital optic nerve results in proptosis, ophthalmoplegia, conjunctival chemosis, venous stasis retinopathy, and ocular ischemia.[423] Histopathologically, the tumor is a high-grade astrocytoma with high cellularity and pleomorphism, mitoses, and necrosis. In spite of aggressive surgical and radiation therapy, the tumor spreads rapidly to involve the intracranial contents, and death usually occurs within months.[423,424]

Malignant Peripheral Nerve Sheath Tumor (Malignant Schwannoma)

Malignant peripheral nerve sheath tumor is a rare orbital tumor that arises from peripheral nerves, predominantly branches of the trigeminal nerve.[426,427] It is a disease of older adults but may occur in young adults with preexisting orbital neurofibromas of von Recklinghausen's disease.[426,427] De novo tumors usually arise as nodular growths in the anterior, superomedial orbital quadrant in relation to the supraorbital nerve as circumscribed masses that displace the eye inferiorly. Pain and hypesthesia due to sensory nerve dysfunction may be localized or referred within the distribution of the sensory nerve. Best visualized by MRI, progressive perineural growth along the nerve through the superior orbital fissure may involve the midbrain, leading to death. Pathologically, the tumor consists of atypical, pleomorphic spindle and epithelioid cells involving the peripheral nerve of origin that stain for S100 and epithelial membrane antigens.[428] Treatment is by radical surgery to prevent invariably fatal brain involvement and metastases to lymph nodes, lungs, and bone. Successful radiotherapeutic tumor control has been reported,[429] but the use of primary or adjuvant radiotherapy is controversial, since it may increase tumor aggressiveness.[430] Radiation therapy and chemotherapy are palliative in most patients, since the 5-year mortality exceeds 50%.[426,427] Nevertheless, long-term survival and late recurrence after incomplete tumor excision has been reported.[430]

Malignant Melanoma of Orbit

Primary orbital melanomas are rare and usually arise in the setting of oculodermal melanocytosis (nevus of Ota) and from cellular blue nevi.[431-433] Seventy-five percent of cases occur in adults with a mean age of 42 years; the vast majority occurs in Caucasians.[433] The tumor causes proptosis, globe displacement, and chemosis, which may evolve rapidly or slowly, but always progressively. CT reveals an enhancing, circumscribed, round mass, but perineural intracranial spread (best detected by MRI) may occur. Pathologically, these tumors are characterized by a proliferation of atypical spindle melanoma cells arising from increased numbers of nonatypical spindle melanocytes of nevus of Ota or blue nevi. Tumors exhibiting mixed cell types are high mitotic count and portend poor prognosis.[433] Treatment includes wide surgical excision, exenteration, or extended exenteration for lesions with intracranial spread.[432,434] Overall, 5-year mortality exceeds 40%.

Leiomyosarcoma

Leiomyosarcomas are uncommon orbital tumors that may occur de novo[435,436] or after irradiation for retinoblastoma.[437,438] Unilateral proptosis and mass effect are the principal clinical manifestations. They are unencapsulated vascular tumors composed of a hypercellular population of spindle-shaped cells arranged in intertwining bundles and exhibiting pleomorphism and mitoses. Treatment is complete excision with tumor-free margins or orbital exenteration. Death may occur from metastatic spread.[435,436]

Liposarcoma

Liposarcoma principally affects adults, but occurs in children as young as 5 years.[439-442] Rare metastatic orbital liposarcomas have been described.[443] They result in insidious proptosis and globe displacement due to mass effect, but may cause pain.[442] These tumors are yellow to yellow-white, gelantinous to firm, lobular, poorly circumscribed, or invasive. CT or MRI reveals a mass of variably increased density over surrounding fat (Fig. 70-12). Two histopathologic variants usually occur in the orbit, both of which have a better prognosis than other types not found in the orbit. Myxoid liposarcomas have a rich vascular plexus separating malignant lipoblasts, whereas well-differentiated liposarcomas contain atypical lipoblasts and spindle-shaped cells separated by fibrous septae.[440,443] Treatment is by excision with possible adjunctive radiation for the myxoid and well-differentiated tumors; orbital exenteration is reserved for treatment recurrences. Exenteration of tumors is performed initially if the more anaplastic and aggressive pleomorphic liposarcoma is diagnosed on biopsy.

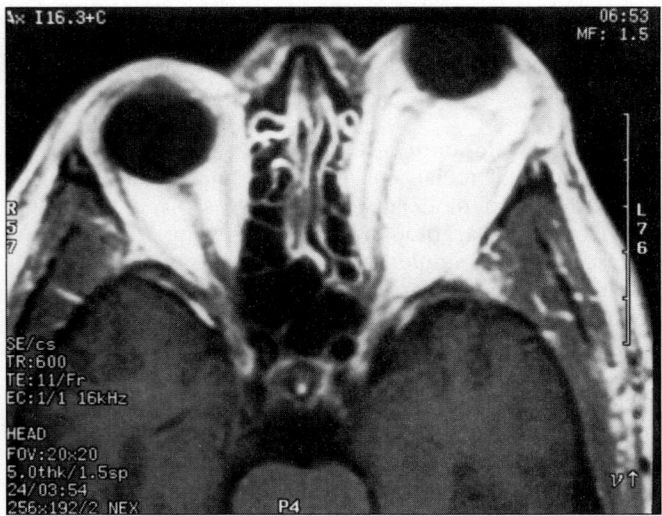

Figure 70-12. MRI of a low-grade orbital liposarcoma. A large mass of fat signal intensity fills the orbit, causing marked proptosis and deviation of the optic nerve.

Alveolar Soft Part Sarcoma

Alveolar soft part sarcomas are rare primary orbital tumors of young adults and adolescents that affect females more often than males by a ratio of 4:1.[444] These nodular, vascular tumors cause proptosis, edema, and dilation of conjunctival vessels and may simulate cavernous hemangioma on CT. Histopathologically, the tumor consists of polygonal cells arranged in a characteristic alveolar-like pattern; the cells contain distinctive periodic acid-Schiff (PAS)–positive crystal-like structures that are readily apparent on electron microscopy. Treatment consists of wide surgical excision and adjunctive radiation therapy.[445,446] Metastatic disease and death may occur many years after initial resection.[446]

Chondrosarcoma

An uncommon orbital tumor, chondrosarcoma usually develops as an extension from the paranasal sinuses and nose and usually presents with nasal drainage, epistaxis, and nasal obstruction.[447] Orbital invasion results in proptosis, globe displacement, diplopia, or epiphora. Posterior orbital involvement may result in optic nerve dysfunction or third nerve palsy. Mesenchymal or myxoid variants of primary orbital chondrosarcoma may begin along the orbital wall or within soft tissue.[448] Histopathologically, chondrosarcomas consist of malignant chondroblasts with increased cellularity and pleomorphism forming a cartilaginous matrix, often in a chicken-wire distribution. Variants occurring primarily in the orbit are mesenchymal or myxoid chondrosarcomas that may arise either in the bone or soft tissue of young adults.[449,450] CT of typical chondrosarcoma reveals an irregular mass with bony destruction, but a well-defined boundary or a heterogeneous, irregular mass in the mesenchymal or myxoid variants.[451] Mesenchymal or myxoid variants show well-differentiated hyaline cartilage admixed with malignant spindle-shaped cells, histopathologically. Treatment of typical chondrosarcoma consists of complete surgical excision, since the tumor may recur and metastasize over the course of years.[452] Since they are more aggressive, mesenchymal variants have been treated with exenteration and adjunctive radiotherapy. However, surgical excision with adjuvant chemotherapy and radiotherapy appears to provide adequate tumor control without exenteration.[453] Palliative radiation therapy has also been used in these advanced cases.

Primary Lacrimal Gland Neoplasms

About two thirds of lacrimal gland tumors are inflammatory or lymphoproliferative and the remaining one third are primary epithelial neoplasms. Lacrimal gland neoplasms may be categorized clinically by history, physical examination, and imaging studies.[284,285,289,454,455] Located in the lacrimal fossa, these lesions cause lateral upper eyelid fullness and deform the palpebral fissure. They may cause inferomedial globe displacement or proptosis if growth extends posteriorly in the orbit. Inflammatory and lymphoproliferative tumors include sarcoidosis, IIP, benign lymphoepithelial lesion, reactive lymphoid hyperplasia, atypical lymphoid hyperplasia, and frank lymphoma. They usually have short clinical histories, CT findings of ill-defined oblong tumors without bony changes, and a tendency to affect both lobes of the lacrimal gland.[289] Primary epithelial tumors result in proptosis, globe displacement, and blepharoptosis. They predominantly affect the orbital lobe of the lacrimal gland, but have been reported to arise from the palpebral lobe.[456] Tumors involving the orbital lobe typically exhibit bony alterations on CT. Of the epithelial tumors, 50% are benign pleomorphic adenomas and 50% are malignant tumors, of which 60% are adenoid cystic carcinoma, 20% are carcinoma ex pleomorphic adenoma, and 20% are other carcinomas.[454]

Pleomorphic Adenoma (Benign Mixed Tumor)

Pleomorphic adenoma is the most common epithelial neoplasm of the lacrimal gland. It occurs in early middle age (average, 40 years) and has no sex predominance.[454] This firm, nontender, nonpainful tumor develops insidiously and progresses slowly, often over the course of years, resulting in fullness of the lateral upper eyelid, inferomedial displacement of the eye, and mechanical restriction of motility on upgaze. CT shows a rounded, well-circumscribed mass in the lacrimal gland fossa, the bone of which frequently shows pressure-induced remodeling due to nodular tumor growth that occurs predominantly in the deep portions of the orbital lobe.[289] In rare cases, tumors may arise in the palpebral lobe or accessory lacrimal gland.[456-458] The tumor is derived from epithelial and myoepithelial cells, resulting in a biphasic picture of epithelial and stromal elements, the latter composed of proliferating metaplastic myoepithelial cells that secrete a chondroid matrix in which frank bone or cartilage may form.[455] The combination of epithelioid and mesenchymal structures gives rise to the term *benign mixed tumor* or *chondroid syringoma*. Treatment must consist of complete en bloc excision based on the clinical and radiologic features, since incomplete excision or incisional biopsy causes tumor cell spillage that frequently results in tumor recurrence and malignant transformation to an aggressive carcinoma.[434-463] Curative en bloc removal of the tumor with surrounding normal tissue may be difficult because the tumor frequently invades its pseudocapsule to involve the periosteum of the lacrimal fossa.[464] Malignancy may arise in 10% of untreated pleomorphic adenomas followed for 20 years and in 20% of tumors by 30 years.[454,455,461,462] En bloc resection with surrounding normal tissue should be performed to avoid these adverse sequelae.

Adenoid Cystic Carcinoma

Adenoid cystic carcinoma comprises 60% of malignant epithelial lacrimal gland tumors.[454,461] Occurring in middle age at an average onset of 45 years and without sex predilection, it usually causes a relatively abrupt onset of progressive pain, proptosis, globe displacement, and diplopia (Fig. 70-13A). This tumor may arise in a pre-existing pleomorphic adenoma that shows new progressive growth. Rarely, this tumor may arise in the palpebral lobe of the main gland or from an ectopic focus.[457,465] Pain is associated with the tumor's early and great propensity

for perineural infiltration,[438,439] but pain may be absent in a significant minority of cases.[468-470] The tumor frequently spreads medially to involve motor nerves to the extraocular muscles, causing diplopia. CT studies show a nonencapsulated soft tissue mass that may be associated with irregular erosion of the bony lacrimal fossa[289] (Fig. 70-13B). Bony changes may not be present, however.[454] MRI may be helpful in detecting perineural spread. Histopathologically, the tumor cells may exhibit the classic cribriform (Swiss-cheese) pattern sharply outlined by a characteristic surrounding hyaline-like stroma or other patterns[466] (Fig. 70-13C).

Of the five histopathologic patterns (cribriform, tubular, comedocarcinoma, sclerosing, and basaloid), the basaloid pattern is associated with the worst prognosis

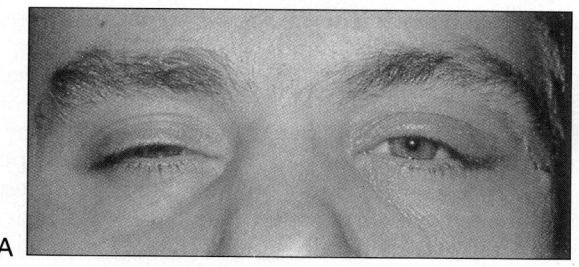

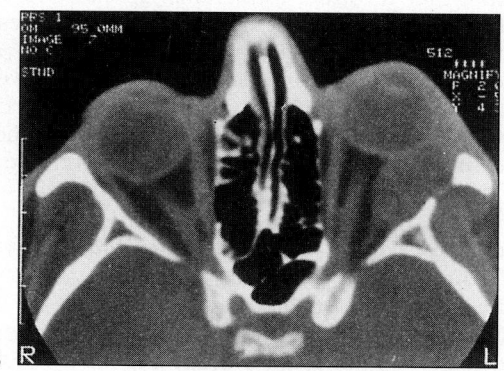

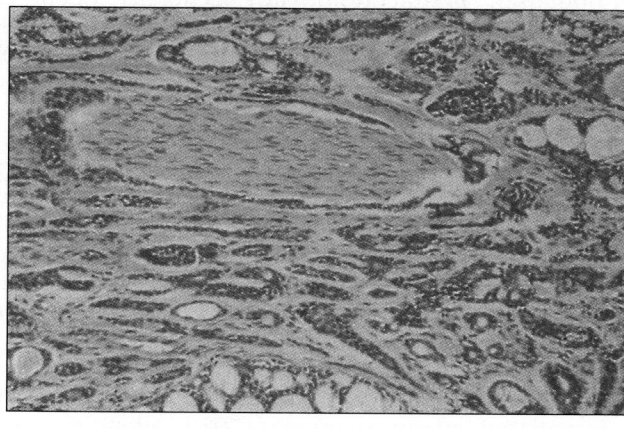

Figure 70-13. A, Left proptosis and eyelid swelling in a patient with adenoid cystic carcinoma of the lacrimal gland. **B,** Orbital CT of same patient showing circumscribed lacrimal gland mass and bone destruction. **C,** Photomicrograph of same tumor showing characteristic Swiss-cheese and histopathologic pattern, cylindroma histologic patterns, and perineural invasion.

Specific Malignancies

III

(5-year survival of only 20%).[471] By contrast, patients whose tumors lack the basaloid pattern have a 5-year survival of 70%. Nevertheless, the overall 15-year survival for all patients is only 20%, whereas the cribriform pattern may connote longer survival.[469,471] Adenoid cystic carcinoma invades anteriorly into the lid, posteriorly into the orbital tissues, and eventually into the brain. Invasion of perineural lymphatics is present in one fourth of cases and may be found beyond the grossly visible border of the tumor.[469] It may occur early in the course of the disease and may lead to preauricular and cervical lymph node metastases followed by hematogenous dissemination to lung, bone, and skin. Bone invasion, present in 80% of cases, also results in poor prognosis by portending death due to direct intracranial spread. Treatment includes incisional biopsy to establish the diagnosis followed by an interdisciplinary cranial base surgical approach including tumor excision and removal of adjacent orbital bone whose involvement by tumor may only be visible on microscopic examination.[472-475] Exenteration is avoided in the absence of intraconal or extensive orbital involvement. Surgery may be followed by radiation therapy of 50 to 60 Gy to the tumor bed.[466] The prognosis is poor, and local recurrences are common. Recurrent tumor may be treated with irradiation if not previously given. Chemotherapy is generally ineffective. Most patients succumb either to direct intracranial spread due to perineural involvement or to hematogenous metastases, most frequently to the lung. Many patients die within 3 years of clinical diagnosis, with a median survival of 5 years.[471] Long-term survival is uncommon and usually occurs in cases without apparent invasion of bone by tumor and with treatment by exenteration early in the course of the disease.

Carcinoma Ex Pleomorphic Adenoma (Malignant Mixed Tumor)

Carcinoma ex pleomorphic adenoma comprises 20% of malignant epithelial lacrimal gland tumors.[454] They arise in middle-aged adults at an average age of 57 years and without sex predilection. They generally occur as malignant transformations of long-standing pleomorphic adenomas or recurrent mixed tumors that have been incompletely removed.[455] Since the vast majority of these tumors do not contain malignant epithelium and stroma, they are more accurately referred to as carcinoma ex pleomorphic adenoma. True malignant mixed tumors, with sarcomatous change of the stromal component, are rare. Clinically, rapid acceleration of existing proptosis due to a preexisting pleomorphic adenoma occurs over the course of several months, or else a partially removed pleomorphic adenoma recurs multiple times with rapidly progressive tumor eventually developing. CT shows a heterogeneous enhancing mass with adjacent lytic bone destruction. Pathologically, superimposition of poorly differentiated adenocarcinoma (70%), adenoid cystic carcinoma (25%), or squamous cell carcinoma (rare) on a previously existing pleomorphic adenoma or its remnant is necessary for the diagnosis.[476] Treatment involves en bloc excision including involved bone or biopsy followed by exenteration with removal of adjacent involved orbital

bone. Adjunctive radiation therapy or palliative radiation may be used in selective cases. Prognosis is poor, with a mortality of 30% at 5 years and 50% by 12 years.[476]

Other Lacrimal Gland Carcinomas

Poorly differentiated carcinoma, adenocarcinoma, mucinous carcinoma, mucoepidermoid carcinoma, and squamous cell carcinoma may arise de novo in the lacrimal gland.[476] These tumors may be aggressive and show pleomorphism and high mitotic rates. They are treated as adenoid cystic carcinomas and malignant mixed tumors insofar as biopsy and exenteration are concerned.

Secondary Malignant Orbital Tumors of Adults

Extensions of Eyelid and Conjunctival Neoplasms

Eyelid and conjunctival neoplasms frequently invade the orbit by direct extension of tumor or by perineural invasion to reach sites distant from the main tumor mass.[477,478] Treatment in the case of eyelid and conjunctival carcinomas, for example, consists of combinations of extensive surgery,[477,479-482] radiation therapy,[482,483] or chemotherapy.[484,485] Eyelid and conjunctival neoplasms are discussed in detail later.

Extensions of Paranasal Sinus and Nasopharyngeal Neoplasms

Extensions of paranasal sinus and nasopharyngeal neoplasms are most often poorly differentiated squamous cell carcinomas, but they include transitional cell carcinoma, adenocarcinoma, and mucoepidermoid carcinoma. These malignant neoplasms may all be misdiagnosed as sinusitis, causing delay in treatment with resultant extensive tumor growth.[486,487]

Squamous carcinoma arising in the nasopharynx or paranasal sinuses accounts for 15% of all secondary orbital tumors.[486-488] Occurring in middle age, this neoplasm is two to three times more common in men and involves the orbit in more than half of cases with advanced disease.[489-491] Orbital invasion by nasopharyngeal and paranasal sinus carcinomas frequently results in ocular displacement, proptosis, palpable mass, swelling of the lower eyelid and/or cheek, chronic pain and/or paresis, multiple cranial nerve dysfunction, and visual loss due to optic nerve infiltration or compression.[486] Involvement of the posterior orbit, cavernous sinus, and base of the skull may result in massive congestion and conjunctival chemosis due to obstruction of venous outflow. Thus secondary tumors arising from the sinuses and nasopharynx are important in the differential diagnosis of cavernous sinus syndrome and painful ophthalmoplegia. CT is mandatory to image the soft tissue neoplasm and associated destruction so that treatment can be planned.[492] Paranasal squamous cell carcinoma is managed by biopsy followed by wide surgical excision that may be supplemented with radiation therapy of 50 to 60 Gy in 5 to 6 weeks. Overall 5-year survival using this combination therapy is as high as 75% but is reduced to 30% when orbital involvement occurs.[489-491] Tumor resection with preservation of the eye is possible in most cases, but exenteration may be required for tumor control.[492-496] Palliative chemotherapy with cisplatin may reduce tumor growth and control pain in advanced cases.[497] Nasopharyngeal carcinoma is best managed by biopsy followed by concurrent radiation and chemotherapy. The prognosis for this tumor is poor, with a 5-year survival of 0% to 10%, since widespread tumor extension occurs early, diagnosis is delayed, and regional lymph node metastases are common in early stages of the disease.[498] Death results from distant metastases or direct invasion into the brain, which is common and is due to the inability to excise or otherwise completely control these tumors, in most cases. With combined-modality therapy, however, local control and survival appear to be improving.

A subtype of poorly differentiated nasopharyngeal squamous cell carcinoma, the so-called lymphoepithelioma, shows severe chronic inflammation.[499] Lymphoepithelioma presentation in the orbit is accompanied by lymph node metastases in up to 70% of cases as well as destruction of bone at the base of the skull with associated cranial nerve palsies.[499] Radiation therapy is effective, with 5-year survival as high as 35%.

Inverted papillomas that invade the orbit from the nose, paranasal sinuses, and lacrimal sac are locally aggressive tumors that frequently contain areas of malignant transformation to squamous cell or transitional cell carcinoma. Recurrence after initial tumor excision is the rule, and intracranial extension may occur. Early wide surgical excision provides the best chance for cure.[500]

Adenoid cystic carcinoma, mucoepidermoid carcinoma, and carcinoma ex pleomorphic adenoma arising in accessory salivary glands may also invade the orbit.[486] Secondary adenoid cystic carcinomas of the orbit are as frequent as primary lacrimal gland tumors. They occur in middle age and affect men and women in equal numbers. Signs and symptoms are similar to those of secondary squamous cell carcinoma. These tumors are highly lethal and kill by brain extension or metastatic spread, principally to the lung. Average survival is 7.5 years.

Malignant melanomas may arise in the nose, mouth, and sinuses and are more common in Asians.[501] They are highly lethal tumors that are difficult to treat because the primary site is difficult to identify. They require wide local excision and exenteration, if necessary. Fibrosarcoma, chondrosarcoma, and glioblastoma multiforme may also arise primarily in the sinuses or nasopharynx and affect the orbit.[486,487]

Extensions of Odontogenic Neoplasms

Ameloblastoma is an odontogenic tumor that rarely involves the orbit of adults; it has a male predilection of nearly 5:1.[502] The tumor originates in the maxilla and grows gradually, insidiously, and painlessly. Initial symptoms generally are upper gingival swelling or tooth displacement. Progressive tumors, including recurrent tumors that have undergone incomplete resection, involve the maxillary antrum, orbital floor, nasal cavity, and ethmoid sinus.[503,504] Orbital signs include proptosis and displacement of the eye, while CT reveals progressive bone destruction.[502-504] Histopathologically, the tumor

consists of epithelial islands with pallisaded cells in fibrous stroma that arise from primitive tooth precursors. Treatment consists of wide, en bloc surgical excision. When incompletely resected, advanced tumors may invade the base of the skull and result in death.[505-507]

Extensions of Intracranial Neoplasms

Orbital extension of intracranial meningioma is common and may occur at initial presentation or may follow numerous resections.[508] Females are affected more than males by a ratio of 3:1. These meningiomas arise predominantly in the region of the sphenoid ridge, basofrontal region, or around the sella; they expand into the orbit, resulting in the otherwise unexplained edema of the upper eyelid (Fig. 70-14A), conjunctival chemosis, proptosis, transmission of intracranial pressure, and disturbances of ocular motility. Ophthalmoplegia and visual loss with only minimal proptosis may occur if the tumor grows medially along the lesser wing of the sphenoid bone in the region of the superior orbital fissure and optic canal. CT shows osteolytic and osteoblastic bony lesions due to tumor infiltration that may occur en plaque with only a minor soft tissue component evident on CT or MRI (Fig. 70-14B). Gadolinium-enhanced MRI may be the only

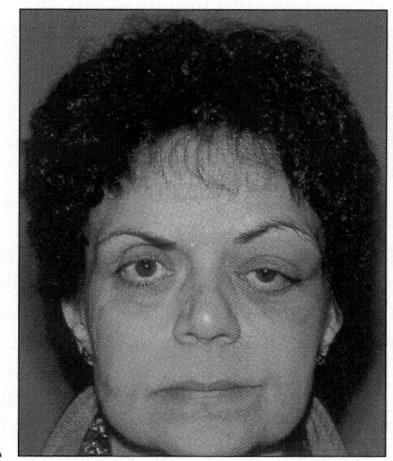

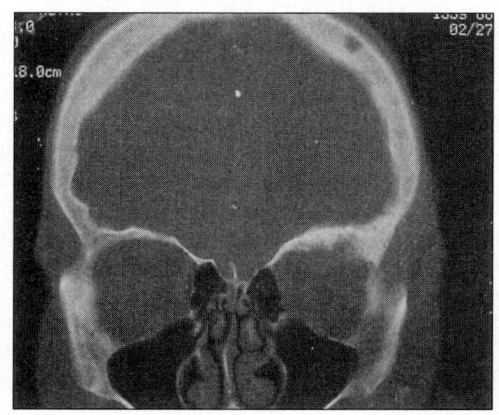

Figure 70-14. **A,** Upper eyelid edema, mild proptosis, and downward displacement of the eye due to en plaque sphenoid wing meningioma. **B,** CT of same patient demonstrating lytic bone lesions and diffuse reactive hyperostosis due to bone infiltration by meningioma.

means to detect soft tissue tumor involving the intracranial dura or compressing the optic nerve.[509] Intracranial extension may be associated with anosmia, ophthalmoplegia, pituitary dysfunction, and seizures. Sphenoidal wing meningiomas may result in direct compression of prechiasmal optic nerve and may result in the Foster-Kennedy syndrome, which consists of optic atrophy, ipsilateral visual field loss, and contralateral papilledema. These meningiomas are frequently associated with independent meningiomas within the cranium, particularly in neurofibromatosis. Treatment of initial or recurrent tumors includes surgical excision and radiation therapy of 50 to 55 Gy either alone or in combination.[508-510] Radiation treatment is particularly useful to treat patients with superior orbital fissure, cavernous sinus, or optic canal involvement.[509]

Aggressive astrocytoma may invade the orbit from its intracranial origin. Glioblastoma multiforme extension into the orbit is associated with proptosis and severe neurologic deficits. Treatment is palliative and consists of radiotherapy and chemotherapy.[511-513] Chordoma may occur at any age and most often presents with severe headache or pain and abducens palsy due to its growth along the clivus.[514,515] CT demonstrates sphenoid bone and sellar destruction as well as the expansile soft tissue neoplasm. Debulking and radiation therapy slow tumor growth, but a protracted clinical course with pain, blindness, and dysphagia usually ends in death.[515] Lymphoma, leukemia, and meningeal carcinomatosis may affect the optic nerve and extend into the orbit as a result of tumor spread along the subarachnoid space of the optic nerve sheath, causing blindness.[516-518]

Extensions of Intraocular Neoplasms

Malignant tumors of the eye that may invade the orbit include uveal melanoma, large cell lymphoma retinoblastoma, medulloepithelioma, and rarely pigmented and nonpigmented adenocarcinoma of the neuroepithelium of the eye. Invasion of the optic nerve and orbit by intraocular tumors is enhanced in eyes with glaucoma. Choroidal melanomas typically extend along the emissary nerves and vessels except for the diffuse type, which can grow directly through the sclera.[519,520] MRI is more sensitive than ultrasonography or CT in the detection of extraocular growth by uveal melanoma and retinoblastoma.[521,522] Extrascleral orbital extension of uveal melanoma to the surgical margin of an enucleated eye results in a poor prognosis, with two thirds of patients dying of metastatic disease.[523] Almost all patients with orbital recurrence after enucleation have metastatic disease and extremely poor prognosis. The management of extraorbital extension is controversial, since exenteration after prior enucleation does not appear to improve long-term survival of patients compared with enucleation alone.[524-527] When discovered primarily by MRI or other means, and localized, however, brachytherapy, en bloc resection of the eye and extrascleral tumor at the time of enucleation (with surrounding uninvolved orbital tissue), or primary exenteration may improve survival.[528] The use of preoperative radiation therapy before enucleation in these instances has also been advocated.

Orbital Metastases of Adults

Metastatic tumors and secondary extensions of malignant tumors are the most common malignancies involving the eye and orbit. Orbital involvement is less common than uveal involvement, but metastases nonetheless comprise approximately 10% to 15% of orbital tumors, with a peak incidence during the sixth and seventh decades of life.[529-531] The orbits are equally affected. Metastases are bilateral in 10% of cases.[529]

Abrupt clinical onset is followed by progressive symptoms and signs of pain, periorbital swelling, proptosis (Fig. 70-15A), extraocular motility dysfunction (Fig. 70-15B), ptosis, and decreased vision that are disproportionately severe for the amount of tumor involvement.[529-531] Metastatic lesions are frequently misdiagnosed as cellulitis, IIP, or thyroid ophthalmopathy.[529,532] CT is preferred to MRI for evaluation of these lesions, since metastatic tumors produce osteolytic or osteoblastic bone lesions in more than 50% of cases.[533] CT findings also include unencapsulated diffuse tumor with irregular margins (Fig. 70-15C).[533-536] Most patients have known primary malignancies at the time of orbital involvement, and 50% have widespread metastatic disease.[532] However, approximately 25% of metastatic tumors present in the orbit as the initial manifestation of the tumor.[532-537]

The most common orbital metastatic tumors are breast carcinoma (42%), lung carcinoma (11%), prostate carcinoma (8%), and cutaneous malignant melanoma (5%), while 10% arise from an unknown primary tumor.[529] Metastatic breast carcinoma has a predilection for fat, usually occurs late in the course of the disease, and may cause enophthalmos due to scirrhous reaction of infiltrated orbital tissue, a finding that may also occur in pulmonary and gastric carcinoma.[538] Orbital metastasis is frequently the first overt sign of lung carcinoma, which has the worst prognosis.[529,539] Prostate carcinoma has a strong tendency to metastasize to orbital bone.[529,540] Renal cell carcinoma may metastasize to the orbit many years after excision of the primary tumor or as the initial manifestation of a silent primary tumor and is a highly vascular lesion that tends to involve bone. Other metastatic lesions include gastrointestinal, hepatic, and thyroid carcinomas, and gastrointestinal and pulmonary carcinoid tumors.[541-544] Sarcomas rarely metastisize to the orbit, but include angiosarcoma, chondrosarcoma, and mesothelioma.[545-547] Uveal melanomas also may metastasize to the contralateral orbit.[548]

Solitary extraocular muscle metastasis causing muscle enlargement may occur, chiefly from breast carcinoma and cutaneous melanoma.[534,535,549] Metastatic tumors to extraocular muscle must be differentiated from various inflammatory and infiltrative lesions including thyroid ophthalmopathy and myositis. Secondary optic nerve involvement is common in leukemia. Optic nerve metastases may also occur from pulmonary, breast, or gastric carcinoma in adults and, chiefly in children, from acute leukemias.[517,518,550] This may occur as a result of direct extension of intraocular metastases into the nerve, as a discrete metastasis, or as a component of meningeal carcinomatosis that spreads along the meningeal sheaths

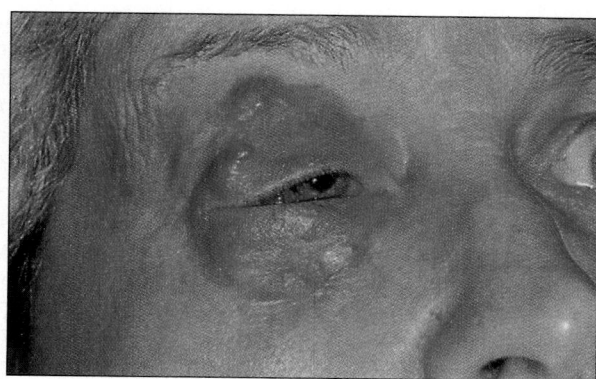

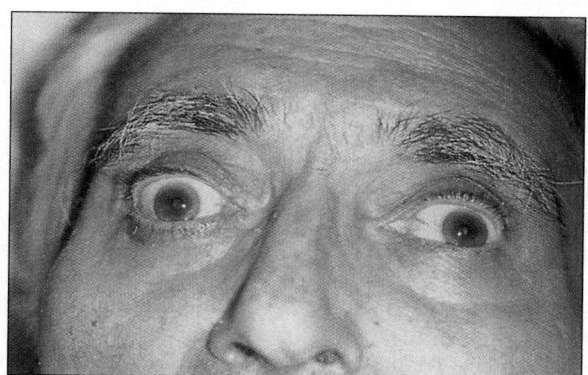

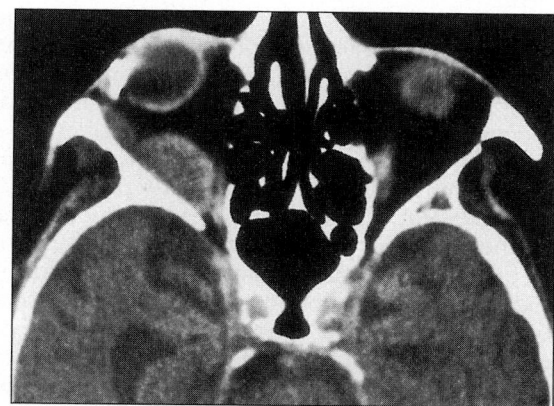

Figure 70-15. **A,** Eyelid and orbital involvement by metastatic breast carcinoma. **B,** Metastatic prostate carcinoma causing proptosis and ophthalmoplegia. **C,** CT-guided needle biopsy of orbital tumor of patient in **(B).**

of the optic nerve. The latter may cause unilateral or bilateral visual loss with ophthalmoscopically visible optic disc swelling and splinter hemorrhages. Tumor infiltration of the nerve results in ophthalmoscopically visible gray-pink tumor, swelling, and distortion of the nerve head. Leukemic infiltration of the disc usually responds to radiation, whereas secondary changes from meningeal carcinomatosis do not.[550]

Although 50% or more of patients with orbital lesions have signs of other systemic metastases,[529,530] open biopsy or (in selected cases) needle aspiration biopsy[551,552] of orbital and periocular lesions is often indicated to establish the orbital diagnosis.[537] Treatment consists of

local radiation therapy and systemic chemotherapy, but the prognosis is poor, with an average survival of about 1 year.[532-537] Patients who have pulmonary, renal, or gastrointestinal carcinoma or malignant melanoma have the poorest prognosis (<6 months average survival). By contrast, some patients with breast, prostate, or thyroid carcinomas or carcinoid tumors may have prolonged survival.[529,531,550] Nonetheless, accurate diagnosis of an orbital metastasis may allow detection of an unknown primary and permit curative or at least palliative treatment that may salvage vision and prolong patient survival. Radiation therapy to the orbit consisting of 30 to 50 Gy relieves symptoms and improves function in up to 90% of cases.[553]

Primary Orbital Tumors of Children

Rhabdomyosarcoma

Rhabdomyosarcoma is the most common primary orbital malignancy in children. These tumors collectively account for 15% to 20% of all rhabdomyosarcomas and less than 10% of orbital tumors in children.[554,555] The mean age of onset of primary orbital rhabdomyosarcomas is 7 years and that of secondary tumors is 12 years, with both groups showing a predilection for boys.[554,556,557] The typical clinical course is of rapid and progressive proptosis or displacement of the eye by a tumor that tends to occur superiorly, particularly superonasally, in the orbit (Fig. 70-16A). Ptosis or a lid mass (50%), proptosis (25%), and conjunctival mass (5%) are common presenting features. Alternatively, and even more commonly, the tumor may also secondarily invade the orbit from the paranasal sinuses or nasopharynx.[558] It may (rarely) arise from the conjunctiva.[559] CT or MRI of primary orbital tumors reveals a large circumscribed tumor or infiltrate that appears to be contiguous with an extraocular muscle (Fig. 70-16B). CT is preferred to MRI for evaluation of the rhabdomyosarcoma because its demonstration of bony invasion is important to treatment and survival. MRI may provide evidence of actual brain involvement, however. Bone destruction is always seen in secondary orbital rhabdomyosarcomas of parameningeal origin and in one third to one half of primary tumors; the superior medial orbital wall is the most commonly affected, followed by the lateral wall.

Biopsy must be obtained as rapidly as possible to establish a pathologic diagnosis upon which prompt systemic evaluation and initiation of therapy proceeds.[554,560,562] Arising from mesenchymal cells that exhibit variable degrees of striated muscle differentiation, the grossly white, fibrous orbital or periocular tumors may show three histologic subtypes: embryonal, alveolar, and botryoid.[562,564] The embryonal pattern is most common in the orbit and contains pleomorphic rounded and elongated spindle cells with scant eosinophilic cytoplasm and mitotic activity. Alveolar rhabdosarcoma, which is common in the inferior portion of the orbit in older children or adolescents and which has a poorer prognosis, is composed of polygonal cells arranged in sheets divided by fibrovascular septae. The central cells frequently

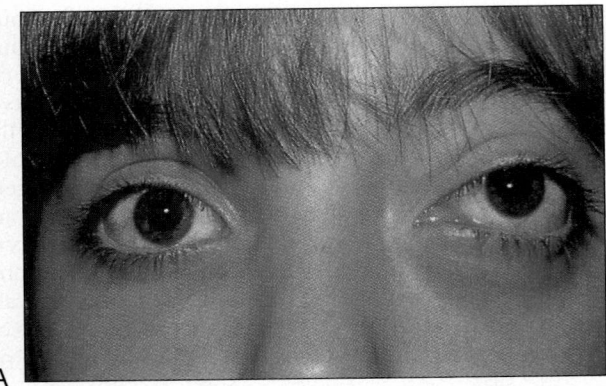

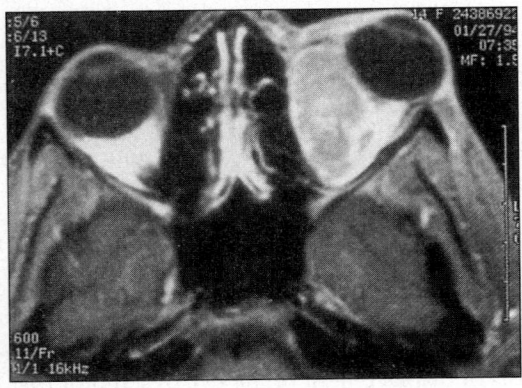

Figure 70-16. A, Left proptosis and lateral displacement of eye in a child with rhabdomyosarcoma. **B,** MRI showing large medial orbital mass. Bone destruction was present on CT.

undergo degeneration, leaving the so-called alveolar pattern with single tumor cells lining the fibrovascular septae.[563,564] The botryoid variant arises in the conjunctiva and resembles a grapelike mass that histologically contains embryonal cells in an edematous matrix. Immunostaining for desmin, actin, or myoglobin greatly assists in the histopathologic diagnosis of the tumor.[565,566]

Untreated rhabdomyosarcoma can lead to complete destruction of eye, orbit, and orbital bone with progressive intracranial spread and lymphatic and hematogenous metastases. Involvement of the orbital bone is considered a poor prognostic sign, since it is associated with the most common tumor-related cause of death, contiguous intracranial spread. Metastasis can also occur, however, typically to the lung. Diagnostic biopsy with or without limited surgical debulking is followed by staging. Treatment consists of combination external-beam irradiation and chemotherapy.[554,567,568] This combination treatment, although reducing 5-year mortality to less than 10%, is still associated with significant ocular morbidity including radiation keratitis, dry eye, cataract, lacrimal canalicular stenosis, radiation retinopathy, optic neuropathy, and orbital bone hypoplasia.[558,569] The cumulative outcome of these radiation-associated ocular effects results in complete blindness in two thirds of patients.[570] Recent reports indicate that the sole use of chemotherapy may not compromise survival rates while it reduces radiation-induced morbidity.[571,572] However, there appears to be a

higher incidence of cases with local treatment failure and/or recurrence that require retreatment with combined chemotherapy and radiotherapy.[572] Sole use of radiotherapy has also been reported to provide comparable survival to that of combined chemotherapy/radiotherapy protocols.[573] Since radiation therapy with conformal three-dimensional techniques can treat orbital tumors with considerably less damage to normal, uninvolved ocular structures, three-dimensional techniques are beginning to be evaluated in the treatment of this tumor. Recurrence indicates a poor prognosis and requires retreatment with chemotherapy and/or radiotherapy; in some cases exenteration is necessary, since large doses of radiation have already been given.[554,558,561,562] If the patient remains tumor-free for more than 3 years after diagnosis and treatment, recurrence is extremely unlikely but has been reported as late as 6 years after initial treatment.[574]

Granulocytic Sarcoma

Solid infiltrates of orbital and periocular tissue by leukemic cells may antedate peripheral blood and bone marrow involvement.[575-577] The greenish tumor, formed by neoplastic granulocytes of acute myelogenous leukemia, is the most common orbital leukemic involvement of children during the first decade of life.[516,578] In the Mediterranean basin and Africa, granulocytic sarcoma ranks second only to Burkitt's lymphoma as a cause of proptosis in children.[320] In contrast to adults, in whom chronic leukemia affects the orbit, orbital involvement by acute leukemia is much more common in children.[579] Based on postmortem series, orbital and eyelid involvement occurs in approximately 10% of cases.[516] The two typical presentations are only periocular disease, often of the eyelids, and leukemic relapse with periocular soft tissue involvement. Clinical manifestations include rapid onset of hemorrhage, proptosis, and visual loss that may mimic orbital cellulitis. CT shows an irregular or circumscribed homogeneous mass that may be associated with bony involvement. Diagnosis and treatment of cases before development of full-blown systemic disease may substantially improve prognosis. The diagnosis is made by biopsy demonstration of neoplastic granulocytes that show positivity with naphthyl-ASD-chloroacetate esterase (Leder stain), contain lyosomes when examined by electron microscopy, and stain immunohistochemically for common leukocyte antigen (CD45), lysozyme, and particularly MAC387.[577] Periocular tissue infiltration may also result from acute lymphoid leukemia, chronic myeloid leukemia, and chronic lymphoid leukemia.[516,580,581] Treatment includes systemic chemotherapy and local radiation therapy.

Fibrosarcoma

Fibrosarcoma is a rare primary orbital tumor of children occurring at a mean age of 4 years,[582] but case reports exist of this tumor in adults.[583,584] Primary orbital fibrosarcomas occur twice as often in females as in males. This tumor can also be secondary, with spread to the orbit from adjacent paranasal sinuses or nasal cavity always associated with bone destruction.[583] These tumors are also well known to occur after radiation therapy for familial retinoblastoma. Clinical findings include proptosis, eyelid swelling, restriction of ocular motility, and ptosis. CT usually reveals an irregular but well-circumscribed mass with adjacent bone destruction in cases due to secondary orbital involvement. Histologically, the highly cellular tumor contains spindle cells exhibiting nuclear pleomorphism in a fibrous stroma. Treatment involves wide surgical excision, usually exenteration; this is frequently effective in eradicating the tumor, which may be less aggressive in children. Death occurs due to local or metastatic spread. Adjunctive radiation therapy and chemotherapy may also be used, but they appear to be of little added benefit.

Osteosarcoma

Osteosarcoma is a highly malignant and destructive tumor of older children and young to middle-aged adults (overall average age, 40 years).[585] The *Rb1* gene responsible for hereditary retinoblastoma may also be involved in the genesis of heritable and nonheritable osteosarcoma.[586-588] This tumor may occur in patients with hereditary retinoblastoma, particularly after irradiation.[589] It has also arisen in the setting of Paget's disease of bone.[590] Osteosarcoma arises from orbital or sinus bone to produce rapid onset and progression of unilateral proptosis, globe displacement, pain, numbness, and periorbital edema.[591,592] Pathologically, this neoplasm consists of malignant osteoblasts and exhibits high cellularity, marked pleomorphism, and numerous mitoses.[591] Tumor cells form irregular trabeculae of osteoid, and malignant cartilaginous areas may also be present. Treatment consists of radical excision with adjunctive radiation and chemotherapy, but the prognosis is poor.[585]

Endodermal Sinus Tumor

Endodermal sinus tumor, also known as yolk sac tumor, is a malignant germ cell tumor that is a rare primary orbital neoplasm of children who average 13 months old at presentation.[593,594] All orbital tumors have resulted in rapid unilateral proptosis. Extraorbital extension may also occur. Histopathologically, the tumor exhibits a papillary-like pattern of anaplastic, embryonal epithelium arranged around vascular cores and numerous hyaline globules.[529] All tumors show immunopositivity for α-fetoprotein, levels of which are rarely detected in the sera of patients with orbital neoplasms.[595] Treatment consists of exenteration, radiation therapy, or chemotherapy either alone or in combination.[596] Orbital tumors appear to have a better prognosis than similar neoplasms arising at other sites, presumably due to their smaller size at the time of diagnosis.[528,529]

Optic Nerve Glioma

Optic nerve gliomas represent approximately 15% of orbital tumors in children and are unilateral unless associated with neurofibromatosis.[597,598] They are low-grade pilocytic astrocytomas, 70% of which occur in children during the first decade, with a female preponderance. Optic gliomas present with painless, progressive proptosis (Fig. 70-17A) and loss of vision, strabismus, nystagmus,

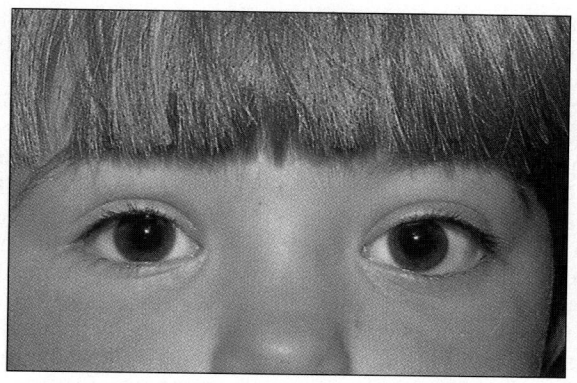

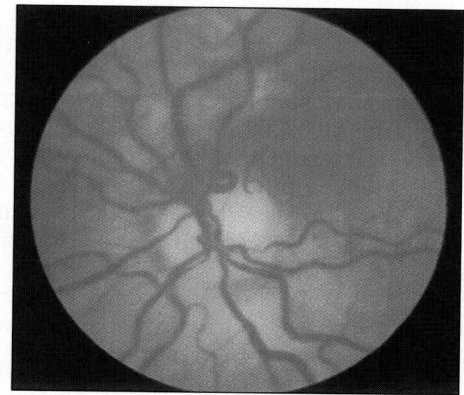

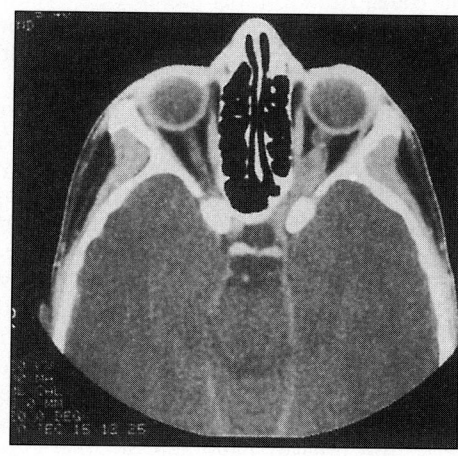

Figure 70-17. A, Left proptosis in child with optic nerve glioma. **B,** Optic atrophy due to optic nerve glioma. **C,** CT of fusiform optic nerve glioma extending intracranially to involve chiasm.

afferent pupillary defect, optic atrophy (Fig. 70-17B), reduced color vision, and central scotomas. Ocular involvement may include optic disc edema, venous stasis retinopathy, shunt vessels, and neovascular glaucoma.[594-596,599,600] The tumor may spread to involve the optic foramen, chiasm, and even the opposite optic nerve. Gliomas affect only the intraorbital optic nerve in 15% of cases, while 60% involve the chiasm and 25% involve other intracranial structures. Proptosis may be subtle and even absent in chiasmal gliomas. Intracranial extension may be associated with headache, papilledema, temporal or bitemporal visual field loss, and hypothalamic signs of precocious puberty, somnolence, or diabetes insipidus. Optic nerve glioma may be sporadic or may occur in the setting of neurofibromatosis (15% to 35% of cases).[601] Conversely, optic nerve glioma occurs in approximately 15% of patients with neurofibromatosis.[601]

CT or MRI reveals optic nerve thickening or fusiform nerve enlargement resulting in a kinked, S-shaped profile due to tumor proliferation confined to the nerve sheath[594-595] (Fig. 70-17C). Intracranial extension results in optic canal enlargement without hyperostosis and erosion of the sella turcica anteriorly into a J-shaped configuration best seen by CT. Chiasmal, optic tract, optic radiation, or suprasellar hypothalamic involvement are features best demonstrated by MRI.[598,602,604] Grossly, the tumor causes a smooth, fusiform enlargement of the optic nerve with intact dura. The glioma consists of a proliferation of bland, elongated spindle-shaped pilocytic astrocytes that may infiltrate the optic nerve substance or may grow primarily in the subarachnoid space, inciting meningothelial cell proliferation that may simulate a meningioma.[605,606] The fibrillar cytoplasm of the tumor cells contains collections of neurofilaments that may form characteristic Rosenthal's fibers containing β-B-crystalline.[607] Secretion of mucopolysaccharide results in pools of extracellular mucin that may imbibe water and result in abrupt exacerbation of proptosis.[599,608] These tumors show self-limited growth and do not undergo malignant transformation or metastases. Neurofibromatosis in children may be associated with optic nerve sheath meningioma as well as optic glioma with diffuse arachnoidal hyperplasia.[598,606]

Most gliomas have self-limited or very slow growth, but some may be more aggressive with progressive proptosis and visual loss.[609-611] Tumor growth is most likely to occur in patients with significant proptosis and optic disc swelling, and without neurofibromatosis. Progression to involve the chiasm and even the contralateral optic nerve may occur. Intracranial extension is associated with poor prognosis,[612] particularly in patients with hydrocephalus and exophytic growth into the hypothalamic region, in whom the 10-year mortality reaches 60%,[611,613] compared with the 20-year mortality of 20% in patients with only chiasmal tumor involvement.[612] Generally, gliomas posterior to the chiasm have the greatest potential for death, which usually occurs due to increased intracranial pressure or interference with pituitary-hypothalamic function.

Treatment of optic nerve glioma is controversial due to the variability in its natural history.[388,611,614] Careful monitoring without treatment may be prudent in patients with clinically stationary disease or only slowly progressive visual loss without evidence of optic foramen or intracranial involvement.[609,615,616] These patients should be evaluated clinically every 6 months and CT or MRI performed every 1 to 2 years. In patients demonstrating intracranial progression documented radiologically, radiation therapy may be used and may result in clinical and radiologic improvement.[611] Nonetheless, surgical excision via a transcranial superior orbitotomy, sparing the eye, may be preferable to prevent radiation damage

to immature brain tissue and radiotherapy-induced endocrine disturbances in these young patients.[598,617,618] In patients with an obviously blind, proptotic eye, surgical excision with retention of the eye is preferable, since it has the added benefit of improving cosmetic and functional results. Radiation or chemotherapy treatment for chiasmal gliomas is controversial, and many reserve this treatment only for patients with progressive visual loss, hydrocephalus, or other complications associated with hypothalamic dysfunction.[619-621] Radiation treatment is often the treatment of choice for hypothalamic involvement, but it is unclear if survival can actually be improved.[399,609,621,622] Intracranial surgery with adjunctive radiation therapy may be employed for large tumors with marked visual or CNS signs and symptoms, including aqueductal stenosis and hydrocephalus.[598,616] Chemotherapy consisting of combination actinomycin D and vinblastine has also been used, with success reported in more than 60% of patients with progressive chiasm and hypothalamic involvement.[623]

Langerhans' Cell Histiocytosis

Langerhans' cell histiocytosis, formally designated histiocytosis X, comprises three clinical presentations: eosinophilic granuloma of bone, Hand-Schüller-Christian disease, and Letterer-Siwe disease.[624,625] Affecting children and young adults, Langerhans' cell histiocytosis often presents with orbital manifestations and has an overall incidence of orbital involvement of 6% to 24% that is greater in young children.[626,633] Eosinophilic granuloma of bone may be either unifocal or multifocal. Unifocal disease occurs in older children and younger adults with a distinct predilection for superotemporal orbital bone.[628-630] These patients have unilateral proptosis, swelling of the lateral portions of the upper and lower eyelids, and superolateral inflammation that may simulate dacryoadenitis. CT reveals an irregular, lytic, expanding lesion of frontal or zygomatic bone that thins the cortex. Tumor extending into the orbital soft tissue shows contrast enhancement. Involvement of the orbit by multifocal eosinophilic granuloma, formerly designated Hand-Schüller-Christian disease, has classically been described as a triad of exophthalmos, lytic lesions of the skull, and diabetes insipidus.[630] This disease is a chronic form of Langerhans' cell histiocytosis with episodic progression that usually occurs in children.[625] It may also involve other soft tissue sites including viscera, lymph nodes, and skin. These patients show proptosis, papilledema, optic atrophy, ptosis, ophthalmoplegia, trigeminal hypoesthesia, and facial nerve palsy.[626,627] CT in these cases reveals lytic defects of the sella turcica and sphenoid bone as well as retro-orbital and orbital soft tissue involvement that account for the clinical manifestations. Acute and progressive Langerhans' cell histiocytosis with diffuse bone and soft tissue involvement was formerly designated Letterer-Siwe disease. This widespread disorder involves viscera, bone marrow, skin, mucous membranes, and soft tissues.[627]

Histopathologically, all these disorders result from proliferations of Langerhans' cells of the mononuclear phagocyte system. These cells are distinctive mononuclear and binucleated histiocytes that contain T-6 and S100 antigens and exhibit diagnostic Birbeck granules when viewed ultrastructurally.[631,632] The lesions of Langerhans' cell histiocytosis show these cells admixed with variable numbers of eosinophils, lymphocytes, plasma cells, and multinucleated mononuclear phagocytes.

Treatment options include surgical excision, local radiation therapy, or intralesional corticosteroid injection. In most cases biopsy is followed by either local radiation therapy of 5 to 10 Gy in divided doses to the orbital lesions[633] or by intralesional corticosteroid injection.[634,635] Either therapy resolves the neoplasm in most cases of localized disease. However, spontaneous remissions of isolated orbital tumors have also been reported.[636,637] In patients with severe multifocal osseous disease or diffuse soft tissue and bone involvement, corticosteroid and chemotherapy alone or in combination with localized radiation therapy has been used with mixed success.[627,630,632,633] The prognosis is much poorer for patients younger than 2 years of age with disseminated Langerhans' cell histiocytosis (of whom only 46% survive) than for older patients (87% survival).[624,625,630] Unfavorable prognostic signs include extensive bone marrow or pulmonary involvement.[630]

Secondary Malignant Orbital Tumors of Children

Extensions of Paranasal Sinus and Nasopharyngeal Neoplasms

Rhabdomyosarcoma may primarily arise in the paranasal sinuses or nasopharynx and secondarily invade the orbit.

Angiosarcomas (hemangiosarcoma) are rare orbital tumors that occur principally within the first two decades of life and cause acute proptosis, dystopia of the eye, ptosis, and ophthalmoplegia.[638-640] Angiosarcomas, also known as hemangioendotheliomas, derive as extensions from surrounding paranasal sinuses and bone or, less commonly, within the orbit. CT reveals either an apparently circumscribed or infiltrative tumor that enhances substantially with contrast and may be associated with lytic bone defects. Histopathologically, the infiltrative tumor contains vascular spaces lined by malignant endothelial cells that line intraluminal papillary projections and form highly cellular areas containing slitlike vascular spaces. Treatment of localized tumors consists of wide surgical excision, including exenteration, and adjunctive radiation therapy, since angiosarcomas are locally aggressive, recur after incomplete excision, and have a high potential for metastases, especially if the primary tumor is located in the posterior orbit.[639,640] Palliative radiation therapy may be used in patients with metastases.

Esthesioneuroblastoma, also known as olfactory neuroblastoma, usually arises near the olfactory plate in the superior portion of the nasal cavity, from where it may invade the orbit.[641,642] It occurs in a slightly older pediatric or adult population. Esthesioneuroblastoma may produce nasal blockage or bloody nasal discharge as its most common presenting symptom, but ophthalmic symptoms of proptosis and ophthalmoplegia are the initial manifestation in 10% of cases.[643,644] CT reveals a homogeneous mass with bone destruction.[645] Histopathologically, the tumor is composed of small undifferentiated cells with mitotic activity but may show differentiation with the formation of rosettes and the apices of cells showing hairlike processes and background neuropil. Immunohistochemical positivity of tumor cells for neural filamentary proteins, S100 antigen, or HNK-1 antigen may be indispensable for arriving at a diagnosis.[646] Esthesioneuroblastoma is locally aggressive and may metastasize. Combination treatment with surgical resection, chemotherapy, and radiation therapy may be curative in a substantial number of patients.[647]

Melanotic neuroectodermal tumor (retinal anlage tumor) is an uncommon secondary orbital tumor that usually originates in the maxilla or zygoma.[648-650] It generally occurs in infancy as a hard, painless mass displacing the globe medially and impairing fullness to the involved side of the face. CT reveals a lytic lesion of the lateral orbital wall with sclerosis of adjacent bone. The tumor is composed of cuboidal neuroepithelial cells containing pigment and lining fibrovascular septae. Treatment is wide surgical excision or biopsy followed by chemotherapy and radiotherapy.[650]

Extensions of Intraocular Neoplasms

Retinoblastoma may invade the orbit by direct trans-scleral extension of large retinal tumors. More often, however, it invades the orbit due to optic nerve extension or recurs in the orbit after seeding from the cut surgical margin of the optic nerve at the time of enucleation. Orbital recurrence may mimic orbital cellulitis[651,652] and usually occurs within 2 years of enucleation. Neglected cases may present with proptosis, lid swelling, and ecchymoses. Orbital involvement may be obscured in the anophthalmic socket by an orbital implant. Orbital extension worsens the prognosis, with a 5-year survival of only 10% in this group of patients.[653,654] Retinoblastoma invading the orbit grows rapidly to form masses of undifferentiated neuroblastic cells. The tumor gains access to the CNS via the optic nerve or along vessels that enter the orbit through the superior orbital fissure, resulting in death, typically within 1 year. Before enucleation, contrast-enhanced T_1-weighted MRI with fat suppression improves the detection of optic nerve invasion by retinoblastoma, whose extent may require that a long segment of optic nerve be delivered with the eye at enucleation.[522] After enucleation, treatment for localized extension at the cut margin of the optic nerve, orbital recurrence, or massive choroidal invasion includes radiation therapy and possibly chemotherapy also. However, no current basis exists for using chemotherapy for choroidal invasion alone. When orbital involvement is found, prompt chemotherapy and radiation therapy in conjunction with surgical debulking is used to limit the chance of CNS spread and distant metastases, which cause death, but surgical debulking and exenteration alone appear to be of little benefit.[655-657] Chemotherapy with adjunctive radiation therapy is used for systemic spread, and intrathecal chemotherapy and CNS radiotherapy are used for CNS spread.[656,658] Medulloepithelioma may also invade the orbit from its primary origin in the eye. Surgical excision, chemotherapy, and radiation therapy may be used in these rare cases.

Orbital Metastases of Children

Neuroblastoma is the most common metastatic tumor to the orbit in young children, occurring as the initial manifestation of disease in up to 20% of cases; most cases affect children between 1 and 4 years old.[659] It rarely represents a primary orbital neoplasm.[660] The tumor presents abruptly, with proptosis, globe displacement, and eyelid ecchymosis that may mimic trauma, including child abuse (Fig. 70-18A).[659,661,662] Bilateral metastases are present in approximately 50% of cases. Opsoclonus and Horner's syndrome secondary to mediastinal or cervical primary neuroblastoma may also occur. Systemic signs include malaise, pallor, weakness, and fever. CT and MRI reveal a large, irregular, poorly circumscribed orbital mass (Fig. 70-18B) with adjacent bone destruction and, frequently, brain metastases.[663] Children with metastatic orbital neuroblastoma often have a palpable abdominal mass, increased urinary vanillylmandelic acid in more than 80% of cases, and positive bone scan in 15% of cases in spite of negative initial skeletal surveys.[664] Histopathologically, the tumor is characterized by small undifferentiated neuroblasts demonstrating Homer-Wright rosettes and background fibrillar neuropil.[664] Treatment consists of systemic chemotherapy with adjunctive radiation therapy. No evidence suggests that debulking of orbital metastases improves prognosis. In general, survival is best in children under 11 months of age (72%).[661,665] Children older than 2 years, however, have only a 12% survival. Disseminated disease, including orbital involvement, is highly lethal in children older than 2 years.

Ewing's sarcoma occurs in older children and young adults.[666] Primary Ewing's sarcoma may involve any bone of the orbit but is rare. Orbital involvement by Ewing's sarcoma is more frequently seen in the setting of disseminated disease.[667-670] Clinically, the unilateral tumor presents with rapidly progressive proptosis and subconjunctival hemorrhage. CT reveals a soft tissue mass with bony involvement, usually in the lateral orbit. Biopsy reveals the tumor to be composed of featureless, small cells that may be of parasympathetic neural lineage[671] and contain cytoplasm that is PAS-positive. Patients with orbital involvement usually have unresectable tumor. Radiation therapy and adjunctive chemotherapy may prolong survival, but the prognosis is poor.[666] Nephroblastoma (Wilms' tumor) can rarely metastasize to the orbit in patients before the age of 5 and presents as a rapidly progressive unilateral proptosis with displacement of the globe and eyelid ecchymosis.[672] CT reveals a large irregular mass with bony invasion. Histopathologic evaluation reveals a biphasic tumor of embryonic renal cells forming epithelial tubules admixed with a malignant spindle cell stroma. Treatment consisting of surgical excision, radiation therapy, and chemotherapy results in an overall survival of nearly 90%.[673]

Rhabdomyosarcoma metastasis to the orbit is rare, resulting in proptosis, loss of vision, orbital pain, and motility dysfunction.[674,675] CT demonstrated the tumor in all reported cases. Prognosis is poor, with death occurring within 6 months of orbital involvement in spite of combination chemotherapy and radiotherapy.[674] Palliative radiotherapy, however, may be helpful.

NEOPLASIA OF THE EYELID AND CONJUNCTIVA

Tables 70-7 and 70-8 outline the types of neoplasms found in the eyelid and conjunctiva.

Primary Malignant Tumors of the Eyelid and Conjunctiva

Basal Cell Carcinoma

Basal cell carcinoma accounts for about 90% of all malignant eyelid tumors.[677] It is seen predominantly in light-skinned persons with chronic sun exposure and in individuals with genetic abnormalities, including xeroderma pigmentosa, nevus sebaceous, and basal cell nevus syndrome. Basal cell carcinoma is most frequent in the lower eyelid and medial canthus.[678-680] Basal cell carcinoma does not occur on non-hair-bearing surfaces, such as conjunctiva, since it arises from the basal cells of the hair shaft that then populate the surface epithelium and subsequently form thickened tumors.

Clinically, basal cell carcinoma has widely variable appearances.[677,680,681] In situ lesions exhibit scaling,

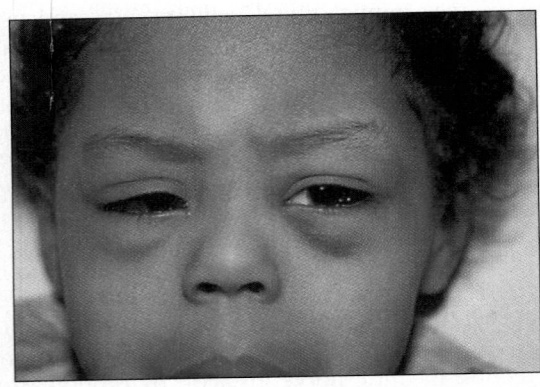

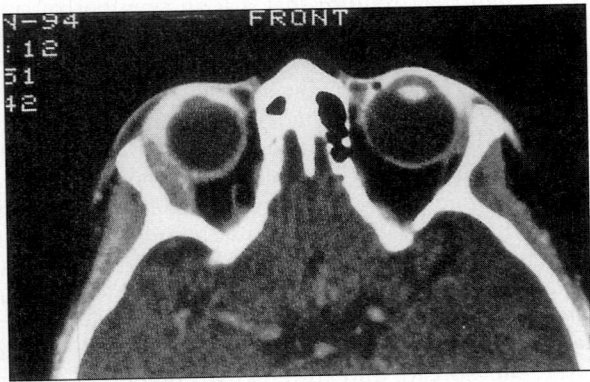

Figure 70-18. **A,** Left proptosis and lower eyelid ecchymosis in a child with metastatic neuroblastoma. **B,** CT of same patient showing orbital metastasis.

TABLE 70-7

 Eyelid Neoplasms

Benign

Benign keratosis*
Seborrheic keratosis*
Squamous papilloma*
Lentigo
Melanocytic nevus*
Keratoacanthoma*
Neurofibroma*
Benign apocrine tumors*
Benign eccrine tumors*
Benign pilar tumors*
Sebaceous adenoma†
Verruca vulgaris
Inverted follicular keratosis
Nevus verrucosus (Jadassohn)
Juvenile xanthogranuloma

Premalignant

Actinic keratosis*†
Lentigo maligna*†

Malignant

Basal cell carcinoma*†
Bowen's disease*†
Squamous cell carcinoma*†
Malignant melanoma*†
Sebaceous cell carcinoma*†
Trabecular (Merkel) cell carcinoma†
Lymphoma/leukemia*†
Kaposi's sarcoma†
Metastatic carcinoma†
Malignant eccrine tumors†
Malignant pilar tumors

*Common tumor.
†Discussed in text.

telangiectasia, inflammation, and superficial ulceration, but no thickening corresponding to invasion of dermis. Nodular basal cell carcinoma (Fig. 70-19A) presents as a pearly nodule with superficial telangiectatic vessels surrounded by compressed dermal structures. It may simulate a squamous papilloma, seborrheic keratosis, cutaneous horn, or inclusion cyst when central cystic degeneration occurs. Ulcerative basal cell carcinoma (rodent ulcer) shows a characteristic central ulcer surrounded by raised, vascularized, pearly epithelial tumor and chronic inflammation. Morphea or sclerosing basal cell carcinoma exhibits a pale, indurated plaque with ill-defined borders that corresponds to deeply invasive, thin, elongated strands of tumor cells eliciting dense scarring. Multicentric basal cell carcinoma may show an irregular, multinodular surface with telangiectatic vessels or diffuse involvement by basal cell carcinoma in situ.

The tumor growth pattern is the most important prognostic factor. Basal cell carcinoma may be either well circumscribed as in the nodular variants, aggressive with infiltrating margins as in the morphea variant, or multicentric with multiple tumors arising over a large sun-damaged or genetically susceptible area. The aggressive and multicentric types are biologically dangerous because tumor may extend beyond the margins seen on clinical

examination. The extent of tumor invasion is also prognostically important, since basal cell carcinoma rarely metastasizes but causes morbidity by local infiltration and destruction.[681] Neglected, incompletely resected, and aggressive basal cell carcinomas may invade the orbit and occasionally result in death by intracranial invasion.[679,680] The orbit is usually invaded anteriorly and pain is uncommon unless perineural invasion occurs. Diplopia may also result from extraocular muscle involvement.

The principal treatment is surgical excision, best performed with perioperative microscopic examination of the surgical margins.[682-684] Recurrence rates are less than 5% when microscopic monitoring is used, but they range from 12% to 34% without it.[682] Recurrence is greatest for medial canthal tumors because of the proximity of the skin to the bone and orbital tissues and the tendency to be less aggressive in resecting in this area.[678,685,686] Radical surgery including en bloc exenteration with removal of periorbital and orbital bone that may be involved yields the best chance for survival in advanced cases.

TABLE 70-8

Conjunctival Neoplasms

Benign

Squamous papilloma*†
Melanocytic nevus*
Lymphangioma*
Hemangioma*
Oncocytoma*
Neurofibroma
Fibroma
Myxoma*
Inverted follicular keratosis
Lacrimal sac tumors

Uncertain Behavior

Reactive lymphoid hyperplasia*†

Premalignant

Actinic keratosis*†
Carcinomatous intraepithelial neoplasia*†
Primary acquired melanosis*†

Malignant

Squamous cell carcinoma*†
Malignant melanoma*†
Sebaceous carcinoma*†
Lymphoma/leukemia*†
Kaposi's sarcoma*†
Rhabdomyosarcoma†
Mucoepidermoid carcinoma†
Spindle cell carcinoma†
Lacrimal sac tumor†
Extension of local tumor
    Uveal melanoma†
      Retinoblastoma†
      Orbital sarcoma†
      Eyelid carcinoma†
Metastatic tumor
    Carcinoma†

*Common tumor.
†Discussed in text.

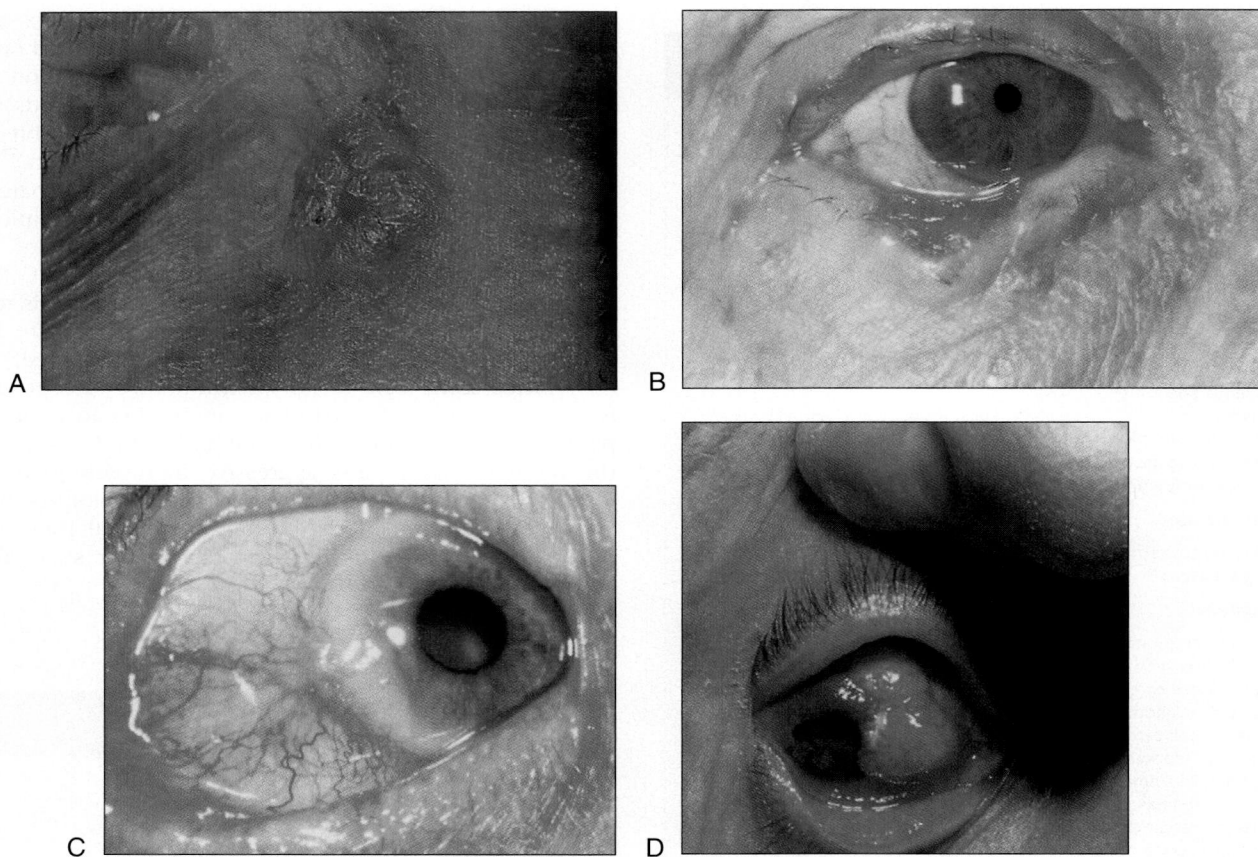

Figure 70-19. A, Basal cell carcinoma of medial canthus, nodular-ulcerative type. **B,** Squamous cell carcinoma of the eyelid with ulceration of eyelid margin and loss of lashes. **C,** Squamous cell carcinoma of conjunctiva showing vascularization. Thickened translucent tumor extends onto the corneal surface. **D,** Large exophytic squamous cell carcinoma of conjunctiva with corneal involvement.

Radiation therapy achieves 5-year tumor-free survival of up to 97%.[687] The use of low-energy electrons to deliver 35 to 50 Gy in 2.5- to 3.5-Gy fractions decreases radiation side effects of corneal damage, dry eye, conjunctival keratinization, eyelid atrophy, loss of eyelashes, obliteration of canaliculi, ectropion, cataract, and retinal and optic nerve vasculopathy.[688] These complications of radiation may result in a nonfunctional, painful eye when the eye cannot be adequately shielded. Radiation therapy is less effective for aggressive morphea basal cell carcinoma and may render detection of recurrent tumor difficult. Cryotherapy may achieve 5-year tumor control of up to 97% with circumscribed tumors less than 10 mm in diameter, while poorer results are obtained for larger or aggressive growth pattern tumors.[689,690]

Squamous Cell Carcinoma of the Eyelid and Its Precursors

Actinic keratosis is the most common precancerous lesion of the eyelids.[691] Occurring in adults after chronic sun exposure, actinic keratoses are well demarcated, roughened, scaling, often slightly erythematous patches that may evolve to squamous cell carcinoma in 10% to 15% of lesions.[692] Histopathologically, intraepithelial dysplasia, parakeratosis, and hyperkeratosis are associated

with solar elastosis of the underlying dermis. Slow progression to severe dysplasia is characterized by a progressive replacement of epidermis with disorganized, dysplastic tumor cells, but no violation of the epithelial basement membrane, which signifies the development of squamous cell carcinoma. Squamous cell carcinomas arising from actinic keratosis are less aggressive than other types of squamous cell carcinoma.[691-693] Conservative excision, with or without adjunctive cryotherapy, even of squamous cell carcinoma developing in actinic keratosis, is curative.

Bowen's disease (intraepithelial squamous cell carcinoma) may occur de novo and in immunosuppressed individuals. Clinically appearing as a reddened, well-demarcated, pigmented, and scaling patch on the periocular skin of the face, neck, or hands, de novo lesions are most common in middle-aged and elderly light-skinned patients.[691,694] Its variants may occur in the oral mucosa and conjunctiva.[694] Histopathologically, malignant cells invade throughout the full thickness of the surface epithelium and along skin appendages, frequently associated with underlying inflammation.[681,691] Progression to invasive squamous cell carcinoma occurs over a protracted course. Treatment is by surgical excision with microscopic examination of the resection margins to ensure complete excision.[694,695] Alternatively, radiation therapy or cryotherapy may be used in unresectable cases.[694,695]

Squamous cell carcinoma is responsible for approximately 5% of malignant eyelid tumors.[692,696] This tumor occurs in elderly light-skinned individuals, in whom it is related to sun exposure or irradiation.[697-699] It also occurs in the setting of Bowen's disease, in individuals exposed to hydrocarbons[700] or arsenic,[701] in immunosuppressed patients,[702] and in those with genetic abnormalities such as xeroderma pigmentosa.[703] Squamous cell carcinoma is more common in the lower eyelid than the upper eyelid, frequently arises at or near the lid margin, and is common in the medial canthus.[691,692,696] It may arise de novo, in Bowen's disease, or, most commonly, from actinic keratosis. Tumors arising de novo frequently are ill-defined, elevated, indurated plaques or nodules with irregular rolled edges and telangiectasia that may undergo ulceration (Fig. 70-19B). Squamous cell carcinoma developing in Bowen's disease exhibits thickening of the preexisting erythematous, scaling lesion. Carcinoma supervening in actinic keratosis is generally circumscribed in its growth. Squamous cell carcinomas often exhibit irregular surfaces due to underlying reactive inflammation. Histopathologically, squamous cell carcinomas range from well-differentiated lesions difficult to separate from keratoacanthoma to aggressive, poorly differentiated anaplastic tumors. They are frequently accompanied by chronic inflammation.

Squamous cell carcinomas are often aggressive and locally invasive tumors that cause extensive local tissue damage as tumor spreads along fascial planes, blood vessels, and nerves.[692,696,704] The likelihood of metastasis is related to the degree of differentiation, size, and depth of invasion.[692,705] Metastases occur by lymphatic spread to preauricular, submandibular, and cervical lymph nodes in advanced cases.[696] Treatment of squamous cell carcinoma is by local excision with microscopic examination of all surgical margins, preferably using a micrographic technique.[686,696,704,706] Orbital invasion usually occurs in tumors recurrent after irradiation, after multiple excisions and recurrences, and from neglected tumors.[696,707] These cases should be evaluated by CT or MRI, or both, to assess the extent of disease, including perineural and bony involvement.[706] Early perineural invasion results in ophthalmoplegia and pain and is more common than in basal cell carcinoma. Radiation therapy or cryotherapy has been used in patients who are unwilling or unable to undergo radical surgery, including extended exenteration.[686,687,695,709,710] Chemotherapy with cisplatin and doxorubicin has also been used in advanced cases.[711]

Squamous Cell Carcinoma of the Conjunctiva and Its Precursors

Squamous cell carcinoma and its precursor lesions are the most common conjunctival neoplasms. They typically occur in elderly patients, 75% of whom are men; however, when seen in young patients these tumors are frequently associated with human immunodeficiency virus (HIV) infection and may be more aggressive.[712-715] Preinvasive, dysplastic lesions are usually either discrete actinic keratoses when superimposed on pterygia or ill-defined lesions when arising de novo. Currently, the preferred term for partial-thickness dysplasia of the epithelium is conjunctival intraepithelial neoplasia (CIN) grade I or II, and for full-thickness dysplasia, the term is CIN grade III or carcinoma in situ. Patients with squamous cell carcinoma are a mean of 8 years older than patients with CIN at the time of diagnosis.[712,713]

CIN arising in actinic keratoses remains as an interpalpebral, thickened, leukoplakic lesion that may be pigmented due to reactive melanosis. It shows limited capacity for invasion. CIN arising de novo is usually a minimally thickened, gelatinous gray-pink, interpalpebral lesion that begins at the corneoscleral limbus. Extension onto the cornea results in a tumor veil and irregular vascularization that does not reach the edge of the CIN.[713] De novo CIN lesions may also thicken and keratinize, giving a leukoplakic appearance. The extent of CIN may be impossible to delineate by clinical inspection alone and may require numerous map biopsies of the conjunctiva and cornea. Most CIN lesions show a limited capacity to invade surrounding tissues if left undisturbed, but they may become aggressive after disruption of anatomic boundaries by biopsy or incomplete excision leading to ocular or orbital invasion. However, squamous cell carcinoma may also develop from dysplasia that evolves slowly over the course of years.

Squamous cell carcinoma developing from preinvasive lesions may appear as a sessile (Fig. 70-19C) or papillomatous growth of the conjunctiva and cornea that contains an intrinsic tumor vasculature; it may be leukoplakic if keratinization is present.[712] Alternatively, the tumor may remain chiefly thin and hazy if it consists primarily of intraepithelial tumor cell growth. Squamous cell carcinoma arising in actinic keratosis is usually delimited as opposed to derivation from CIN de novo. Squamous cell carcinoma may simulate a pterygium, but the tumor will often show location, extent of involvement, and tumor-associated vascular pattern that are atypical for pterygia. Histopathology of the tumor may show different areas with various grades of CIN as well as frankly invasive, usually well-differentiated, squamous cell carcinoma. Fully developed frankly carcinomatous tumors become elevated, fleshy, red, exophytic growths (Fig. 70-19D). Reactive pigmentation by activated melanocytes can occur, confusing the diagnosis with melanoma.

Primary treatment consists of complete excision of the squamous cell carcinoma and CIN components of these tumors with microscopic examination of surgical margins to monitor completeness of removal.[716] Adjunctive cryotherapy may be used to the margins of resection and to microscopic areas of unresectable tumor on the ocular surface. Tissue defects may be allowed to heal by secondary intention, closed primarily by mobilizing adjacent conjunctiva, or repaired with mucous membrane grafts. Limbal autografts from the contralateral eye may be used if the corneal and limbal defect is extensive.[717] Cases with diffuse involvement can be treated with irradiation. A small number of patients have been treated with cryoablation.[718] Other advanced cases have been treated with 50 Gy of photon radiation, but destruction of glands of the ocular surface usually results in severe dry eye that causes loss of vision and sometimes loss of the eye.[719] Squamous cell carcinomas with widespread conjunctival spread and those invading the eye or orbit may require exenteration to control the tumor, which is locally invasive.

Incompletely excised CIN and squamous cell carcinoma are 10 times as likely to recur (50% versus 5%) compared with completely excised neoplasms.[712] Recurrences usually appear within 2 years of removal, but may occur over a decade later.[720] In one series, one third of lesions treated with either resection or cryoablation alone recurred, while combined excision and cryotherapy resulted in a recurrence rate of less than 9%.[721] Recurrence rates of less than 5% have been seen in other series.[719]

New topical treatments whose long-term efficacy is yet unknown include short-term applications of 5-fluorouracil, mitomycin C, and interferon.[722-725] Orbital invasion and regional lymph node metastases may occur in up to 10% of patients, but prognosis for life is excellent.[726-728] Two variants of squamous cell carcinoma, spindle cell carcinoma and mucoepidermoid carcinoma, are much more aggressive than typical squamous cell carcinoma.[729-731]

Malignant Melanoma of the Eyelid and Its Precursors

Malignant melanomas constitute only 1% of malignant eyelid neoplasms, but they may be lethal.[691] Many are associated with ultraviolet light exposure. These tumors may originate from preexisting nevi, in premalignant melanosis, or de novo and are classified by distinctive clinical and histopathologic features.[681,732] In melanomas originating in nevi, the neoplastic melanocytes usually arise in areas of junctional activity resulting in clinically evident growth, variations in pigmentation, ulceration, or thickening. Lentigo maligna melanoma, the most common eyelid melanoma, arises in the sun-exposed areas of elderly light-skinned individuals from lentigo maligna, a flat, irregularly pigmented tan-brown patch of melanosis that may reach several centimeters in size due to a prolonged intraepithelial radial growth of atypical spindle-shaped melanocytes along the epidermal-dermal junction.[733,734] In 30% of cases, malignant melanoma develops and is heralded by thickening of the lesion corresponding to superficial invasion into the papillary dermis, frequently accompanied by inflammation. Melanomas arising de novo begin as intraepithelial neoplastic transformations of melanocytes that exhibit varying degrees of radial and vertical growth resulting in different morphologic patterns and mortality. Superficial spreading melanoma appears as a raised plaque of irregular outline and color ranging from white to brown-black. Neoplastic spindle-shaped and epithelioid melanocytes invade the overlying epithelium and infiltrate the dermis more rapidly and deeply than lentigo maligna melanoma, resulting in higher metastatic potential. Nodular melanoma, which may be deeply pigmented or amelanotic, has the shortest radial growth phase and an early, deep vertical component resulting in a rapidly growing, clinically detectable tumor with high metastatic potential. The tumor invades the dermis and is charac-terized by variable numbers of malignant epithelioid and spindle cells.

Mortality correlates with the type of melanoma and depth of invasion.[681,735] The best prognostic indicator for metastases and death is tumor thickness from the epidermal granular layer to the deepest tumor infiltration (Breslow's level), especially in the eyelid skin, in which rete ridges, upon which Clark's levels are based, are lacking.[735] Skin tumors invading less than 0.76 mm have an excellent prognosis (<1% mortality), whereas those more than 1.5 mm thick have a much poorer prognosis (37% mortality). Treatment consists of total surgical excision, but wide surgical margins[736] and regional lymph node dissection[737] do not appear to increase survival. Upon invasion of the dermis, the tumor frequently metastasizes to regional lymph nodes and distant sites including liver, lung, bone, and brain.

Malignant Melanoma of the Conjunctiva and Its Precursors

Conjunctival malignant melanomas are uncommon, unilateral tumors with probably one tenth to one twentieth the incidence of uveal melanomas.[738,739] Primarily arising in light-skinned individuals, these neoplasms are rare in blacks.[740-742] Most patients are middle aged or elderly. In the conjunctiva, junctional or compound nevi give rise to 25% of melanomas, whereas about 75% develop from primary acquired melanosis (PAM). Rarely, tumors arise de novo as intraepithelial proliferations of neoplastic melanocytes.[743]

Conjunctival nevi are usually pigmented and without prominent vascularity. They are usually flat or of minimal thickness. The presence of cysts within a pigmented lesion is most consistent with a nevus. Growth at puberty, presumably in response to hormonal stimuli, should not be confused with neoplastic transformation, but biopsy may be necessary to make this distinction. Melanomas arising in nevi show clinical growth, variation in color, thickening, increased vascularity, and loss of epithelial mobility over underlying tissue. They originate near the epithelial-stromal junction, infiltrate stroma, and are composed in variable proportions of spindled and epithelioid melanoma cells similar to those seen in the skin.

PAM is a unilateral, idiopathic premalignant melanosis of the conjunctival epithelium that begins in middle age or later as an insidious, subtle, golden-brown stippling of the epithelium (Fig. 70-20A). Any part of the conjunctiva may be involved. However, since reactive pigmentation is rare in the palpebral and forniceal conjunctiva, any pigmented lesion in these regions is highly suggestive of malignancy. PAM tends to be slowly progressive and may regress at its original site only to manifest in another location. Progression of intraepithelial neoplasia may be associated with underlying hyperemia and inflammatory infiltrates that may thicken the lesion, raising clinical concern of an incipient malignant melanoma. Biopsy is indicated for any lesion that develops in an area of thickening, fixation to deeper tissues, or a frank tumor.

The progression of PAM to malignant melanoma is established. The initial lesion of PAM consists of increased melanotic pigmentation of the otherwise normal conjunc-

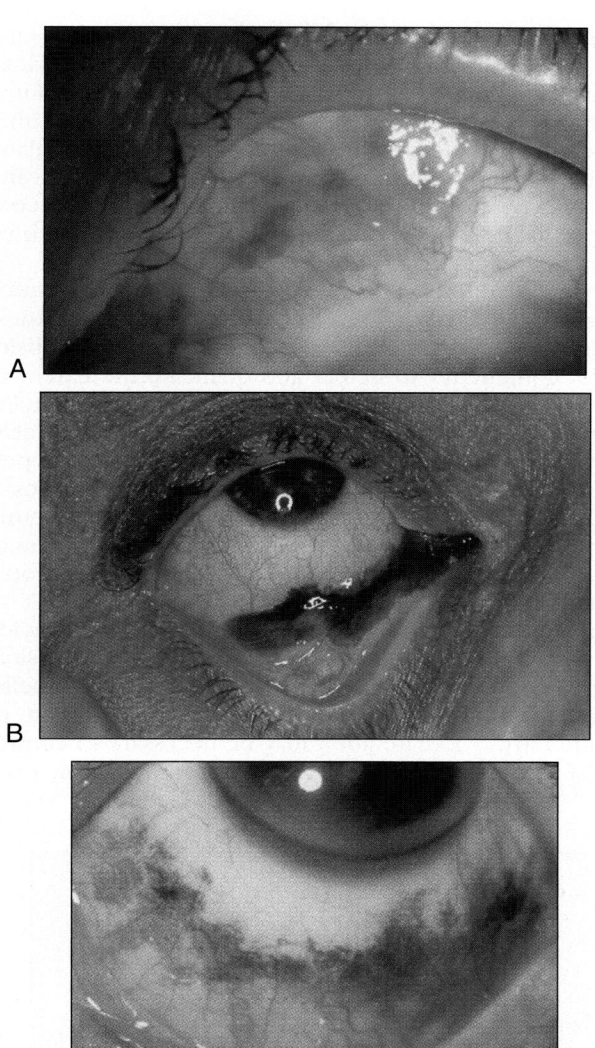

Figure 70-20. A, Primary acquired melanosis of conjunctiva. **B,** Conjunctival malignant melanoma arising in primary acquired melanosis. **C,** Ocular melanocytosis with slate-blue episcleral and scleral pigmentation. Overlying conjunctiva is normal.

tiva (stage Ia). This may progress to mild and then marked atypical melanocytic hyperplasia with pagetoid invasion of the conjunctival epithelium (malignant melanoma in situ) (stage Ib).[743,745] Invasive malignant melanoma may then ensue (stage II) (Fig. 70-20B), resulting in tumors less than 1.5 mm thick (stage IIa) and greater than 1.5 mm thick (stage IIb). Patients with intraepithelial PAM, characterized by atypical, discohesive melanocytes invading the epithelium (pagetoid spread), have a 90% chance of developing invasive melanoma within 10 years. Overall, 20% of patients with PAM will develop melanoma.[743-745]

The clinical differential diagnosis includes benign melanosis, which is frequently bilateral, ocular and oculodermal melanocytosis (nevus of Ota) (Fig. 70-20C), and secondary reactive pigmentation. Minimally suspicious lesions may be serially examined. Lesions showing

growth outside of puberty, thickening, or abnormal vascularity should be biopsied. A unilateral pigmented lesion in palpebral or forniceal conjunctiva in a light-skinned person should be biopsied. Patients suspected of having PAM require multiple map biopsies in areas of thickening because of this tumor's multicentric nature. Conjunctival melanoma arising de novo in apparently normal conjunctiva may rapidly increase in size to form an invasive tumor plaque or nodule.

Definitive treatment of malignant melanocytic lesions of the conjunctiva involves excision and cryotherapy. Corneal epithelial involvement requires scraping or chemical debridement.[746-748] Extensive involvement by PAM or melanoma in situ can be treated with extensive cryotherapy, irradiation, and extensive resection with mucous membrane grafting. Radiation treatment has included external-beam x-ray and strontium-90 (^{90}Sr) irradiation, as well as ^{125}I customized plaques, but complications of radiation therapy frequently result in poor vision or loss of the eye.[749-752] Radiation is not applicable in cases with palpebral or forniceal involvement or for recurrences after previous irradiation. If intraocular or intraorbital extension, recurrence after irradiation, or tumor whose resection is incompatible with a seeing eye are present, orbital exenteration may be necessary.[753] An evaluation for systemic metastasis is needed before performing this disfiguring procedure. Conjunctival melanoma, in contrast to uveal melanoma, spreads to the regional lymph nodes. Thus local excision with or without radical neck dissection may be offered to a patient, but the latter procedure probably does not improve prognosis.[754]

Survival of patients with conjunctival melanoma appears to be related primarily to the thickness, extent, and location of tumor. Diffuse disease and involvement of nonbulbar conjunctiva are prognostically unfavorable, while tumors less than 1.5 mm thick rarely metastasize and cause death.[743,746,755-757] The abundance of lymphatic channels in the conjunctiva makes early lymphatic spread common. This may lead to the development of local subconjunctival satellite lesions, regional lymph node metastases, and eventual hematogenous dissemination to the liver, bone, skin, and CNS. Overall, 5-year mortality for conjunctival melanomas is about 25%.[743,756] Nonetheless, mortality for invasive conjunctival melanoma is variable. Small, minimally invasive melanomas may be lethal, whereas large, even locally metastatic tumors, may not be. Other patients with conjunctival melanoma, especially from PAM, have had multiple tumor recurrences over one or two decades. Even regional lymph node metastasis may be surgically excised and may not be followed by death due to metastatic tumor.[743,758]

Rare cases of acquired melanosis show no pigment (acquired melanosis sine pigmento), and their diagnosis is usually delayed.[745] In these rare cases, early orbital exenteration may be required to prevent tumor metastasis progression and death.[759,760]

Sebaceous Carcinoma of the Eyelid

Sebaceous carcinoma accounts for approximately 1% to 5% of malignant eyelid tumors.[761,762] Peak incidence is in the seventh decade of life, with a female/male predominance of 2:1 and an increased incidence in Asians.[763] The tumor may arise in previously irradiated areas,[764] including in patients with hereditary retinoblastoma.[765] Sebaceous carcinoma may present as a discrete or multicentric tumor, or it may mimic a unilateral chronic blepharitis.[766,767]

Discrete tumors are painless, nontender nodules that arise in meibomian or Zeis' glands of the eyelid or in sebaceous glands of the caruncle to form invasive tumors. These tumors have a predilection for the upper eyelid and caruncle, but may occur on the eyebrow and lower eyelid.[761,765,767] Sebaceous carcinomas mimicking recurrent chalazia are enlarging yellow tumors that extend into the eyelid and only ulcerate superficially when they are advanced.[761] Diffuse intraepithelial spread by tumor cells may often spawn multicentric tumors of the upper and lower eyelids by populating multiple meibomian or Zeis' glands.[762,768] Diffuse intraepithelial spread is universally associated with underlying reactive chronic inflammation and may involve the lid margins, conjunctiva, conjunctival fornices, cornea, and skin, resulting in a clinical picture of chronic blepharoconjunctivitis with lid thickening, redness, and scaling (Fig. 70-21A).[761,762,768] Cancerization of the corneal epithelium leads to a veil. Delineation of extent of spread is difficult, if not impossible, on clinical examination. Intraepithelial spread to involve adnexal structures often results in diffuse loss of eyelashes (madarosis) and may lead to invasion of the lacrimal gland and lacrimal drainage system.[769,770] It has been proposed that intraepithelial sebaceous carcinoma may arise de novo within the epithelium, not requiring a meibomian or Zeis' gland origin.[771] The destruction of meibomian gland orifices and lash follicles may be helpful in distinguishing sebaceous carcinoma from recurrent chalazia or chronic blepharoconjunctivitis.

Early recognition and diagnosis result in much improved survival. Diagnosis may require full-thickness wedge biopsy of the eyelid or numerous random biopsies of the conjunctiva to detect and delineate the extent of tumor spread.[772,773] Histopathologically, intraepithelial or invasive tumor is composed of large basophilic cells containing foamy cytoplasm; pleomorphic, hyperchromatic nuclei; and numerous, often bizarre mitoses[762] (Fig. 70-21B). Invasion of the epithelium, or pagetoid spread, may lead to replacement of the entire thickness of the epithelium by tumor cells with underlying chronic inflammation.

Treatment of invasive nodular tumors is early wide excision, with margins of 5 mm or more, with possible lymph node dissection.[773-775] Delimited intraepithelial conjunctival disease may be treated with excision or cryotherapy.[776] Exenteration may be necessary to control diffuse intraepithelial tumor with extensive pagetoid inva-

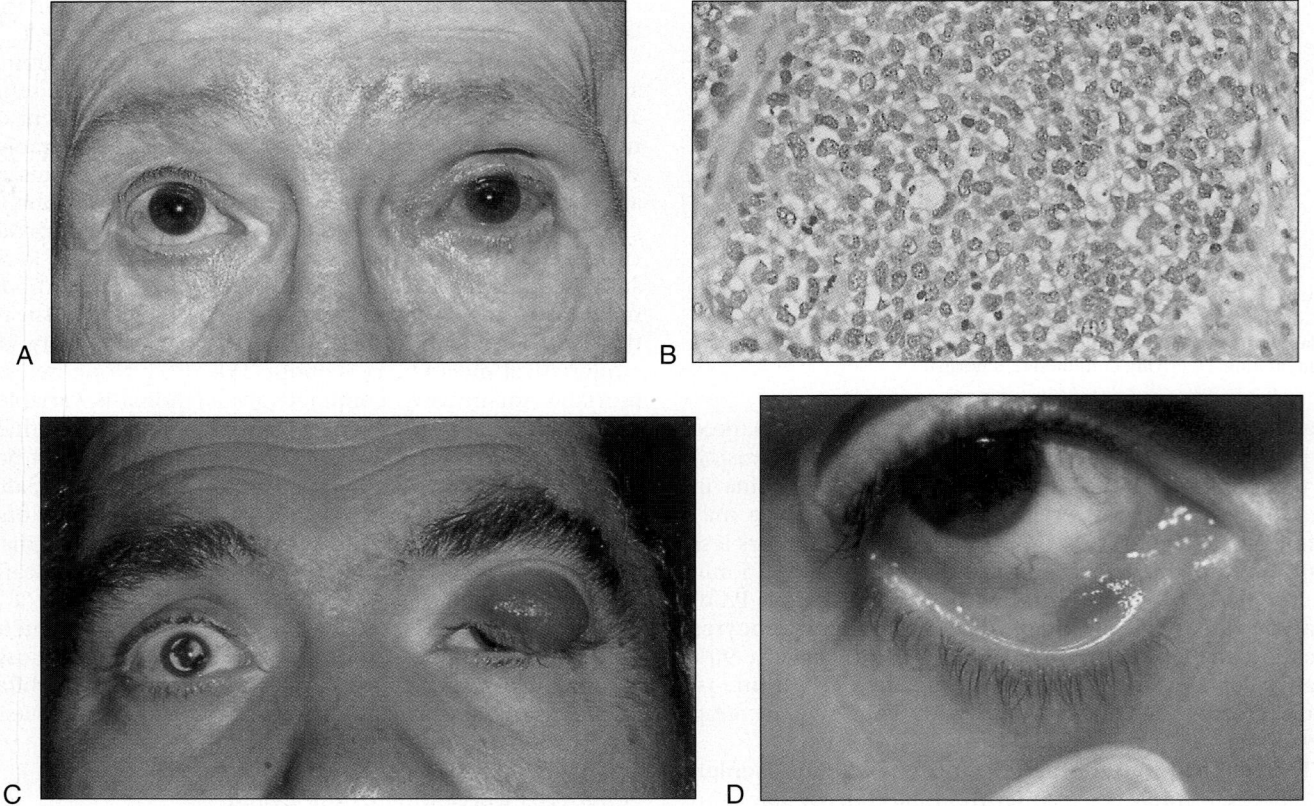

Figure 70-21. **A,** Sebaceous carcinoma with reactive conjunctival and eyelid inflammation simulating chronic blepharoconjunctivitis. **B,** Invasive nodule of sebaceous carcinoma showing tumor cells with foamy cytoplasm and numerous mitoses. **C,** Large violaceous Merkel cell tumor of eyelid. **D,** Kaposi's sarcoma of conjunctiva in patient with AIDS.

sion, since recurrence is common after lesser excisions.[777] The tumor is generally aggressive and eventually invades lymphatics and blood vessels. Metastases may occur to preauricular or cervical lymph nodes followed by tumor spread to lung, liver, and brain.[761,762] Intraepithelial or superficially invasive tumors result in a 5-year mortality of 20% to 25%, and mortality for invasive lesions approaches 40%. Orbital invasion is present in up to 35% of cases with regional lymph node metastases, and the 5-year mortality reaches 75% in patients with orbital extension who require exenteration for any hope of cure. Other risk factors for death include duration of symptoms for more than 6 months, tumor diameter greater than 10 mm, multicentricity, poor differentiation on histopathology, and highly infiltrative pagetoid invasion of overlying epithelium.[762] Overexpression of nuclear p53 protein has been correlated with recurrence, invasion, and metastasis.[778] Radiation therapy is only palliative, but control has been reported with doses of 50 to 60 Gy.[779]

Lymphoma of the Eyelid and Conjunctiva

Lymphoproliferative disorders are common in the conjunctiva. Reactive lymphoid hyperplasia with and without atypia, lymphoma, and leukemia can all affect the conjunctiva and have been discussed at length earlier in this chapter, so only a few specific comments are made here. These lesions present as soft, subepithelial, discrete or poorly demarcated growths with a fleshy or salmon color (see Fig. 70-8), but increased vascularity may render them reddish. The appearances of benign and malignant lesions overlap greatly except that epithelial scarring over a lesion suggests chronicity and thus a benign growth.[780] Eyelid lesions present as nontender, noninflamed masses that may be deep within the eyelid and even extend into the orbit. MRI with gadolinium and fat suppression may be superior to CT for detecting subtle lymphomas in the eyelid and conjunctiva. A large, carefully followed population showed that the site of ophthalmic involvement has prognostic value. Patients with conjunctival involvement were least likely to develop systemic disease, followed by patients with orbital involvement, while patients with eyelid involvement were most likely to have progression to systemic disease.[781]

Conjunctival and eyelid lymphoid lesions should be biopsied with as little damage as possible to adjacent structures. The surgeon must ensure that sufficient diagnostic material is obtained and promptly delivered to the pathology laboratory in an unfixed state for appropriate histologic and immunophenotypic studies. The pathologist should also be advised that a lymphoid lesion is being considered in the differential diagnosis to ensure proper handling and study selection.

Patients with malignant lymphoma should undergo a staging evaluation. Lymphomas limited to the eyelid or conjunctiva are generally treated with radiation therapy alone, shielding radiosensitive ocular structures. Patients who also have systemic disease are initially treated with chemotherapy alone, to avoid unnecessary ophthalmic complications of radiation. In those cases with systemic involvement, adjunctive irradiation is used only for large, vision-threatening tumors or as palliative therapy.

Merkel Cell Tumor of the Eyelid

Merkel cell tumor, also known as primary neuroendocrine carcinoma of the skin and trabecular carcinoma, is a highly aggressive tumor with a predilection for the head and neck region and a peak incidence in the seventh and eighth decades of life.[782,783] Rapid, progressive formation of a firm, raised, purple to red nontender nodule without overlying skin ulceration is the usual clinical presentation (Fig. 70-21C).[783] Histopathologically, the tumor consists of uniform hyperchromatic cells with scant cytoplasm and numerous mitoses. The tumor cells form trabecular patterns or sheets of cells that permeate the surrounding soft tissues. Immunohistochemical studies show distinctive staining for low-molecular-weight cytokeratin and positivity for other neuroendocrine markers. Electron microscopic demonstration of neurosecretory granules may also aid in the pathologic diagnosis.

Some local recurrence and extensive spread occur in more than one third and one fourth of cases, respectively,[784] and wide resection followed by adjunctive radiotherapy has been advocated to prevent recurrent disease. Lymph node dissection in conjunction with radiotherapy has also been proposed, either prophylactically or in the treatment of clinically evident lymph node metastases.[784] Nevertheless, mortality is as high as 50% within 2 years of diagnosis.[783,784]

Kaposi's Sarcoma of the Eyelid and Conjunctiva

Kaposi's sarcoma occurs most frequently in patients with AIDS, but may be seen in immunosuppressed patients undergoing allograft transplantation. The development of this tumor is related to the severity of immunosuppression, and its incidence has been reduced by high-activity antiretroviral therapy (HAART). This eyelid and conjunctival tumor appears as an ill-defined, flat, purple or red-brown plaque with indistinct margins. Progressive thickening forms a nodular lesion that may undergo late ulceration (Fig. 70-21D). Multiple tumors at different stages may be present. Dugel and colleagues[784] have classified them histologically into three stages. Histologically, the tumor is composed of a proliferation of spindle tumor cells with vascular or lymphatic differentiation and numerous mitoses. Located among the spindle cell proliferation are numerous vascular slits containing blood and hemosiderin deposits.

The diagnosis of Kaposi's sarcoma is made by history and clinical findings, and biopsy is rarely required for diagnosis. Treatment consists of systemic chemotherapy or local measures for isolated ophthalmic involvement.[785,786] Local treatment includes excision, cryotherapy, or irradiation. Radiation therapy is preferred for tumor response,[787] but bulbar lesions can be excised to avoid complications of conjunctival irradiation. Cryotherapy used alone is associated with increased recurrence compared with excision with or without adjunctive cryotherapy.

Malignant Dermal Adnexal Neoplasms of the Eyelids

Malignant sweat gland tumors include infiltrating signet-ring cell carcinoma, which may appear as a nodule with infiltrating margins in middle-aged or elderly men.[788]

Diffuse lid thickening results from soft tissue infiltration by vacuolated, mucin-containing tumor cells that may be difficult to differentiate from metastatic adenocarcinoma. These tumors frequently metastasize and may recur locally and invade the orbit.[788,789] Primary mucinous adenocarcinomas may occur predominantly in the eyelids of middle-aged and elderly men, where they appear as indurated nodules or cystic lesions that tend to recur and invade the orbit.[790] The tumor cells, frequently arranged in lobules and cords, lie in large pools of mucin. Adenocarcinoma of Moll's gland is rare[791-793] and is composed of lobules of malignant cells with apocrine differentiation, pleomorphism, and numerous mitotic figures.[792] Sclerosing sweat duct carcinoma has a predilection for the face and may involve the eyelid and eyebrow.[794] These tumors arise in young to middle-aged adults and may form indurations, plaques, or nodules. Although they frequently recur, they do not metastasize. Histopathologically, the tumors demonstrate strands of epithelial cells within sclerotic stroma and may demonstrate perineural invasion and calcification. Treatment of all of these lesions consists of wide local excision and possible lymph node dissection of involved nodes.

Secondary Malignant Eyelid and Conjunctival Tumors

Metastases of the Eyelid and Conjunctiva
Metastases represent less than 1% of eyelid and conjunctival tumors. Occurring most commonly in elderly patients, these tumors may present as a solitary painless nodule, a diffuse nontender fullness or induration, or as an ulcerating lesion of the skin.[795] The most common primary sites include carcinomas of the breast, gastrointestinal tract, lung, or genitourinary tract as well as cutaneous melanoma.[796,797] Due to the high incidence of breast metastases, females outnumber males. Eyelid metastases may be the initial presenting lesion or may occur in patients with histories of prior carcinoma, even though the primary tumor may antedate the eyelid metastasis by several years.

Diagnosis is made by open or fine-needle biopsy. When indicated, treatment consists of local excision or radiation therapy together with evaluation and systemic treatment of the primary and other metastatic tumors.

Lacrimal Sac Tumors
The most common lacrimal sac tumors derive from epithelium.[798] Clinical symptoms and signs include intermittent epiphora and dacryocystitis, a palpable mass, or spontaneous hemorrhage from the punctum.[799-801] Carcinomas outnumber benign tumors 3:1. The most common benign epithelial tumor is exophytic or sessile squamous papilloma, which may recur repeatedly after excision. Inverted papillomas may arise in the lacrimal sac or may extend into the sac from the nose or maxillary sinus; they frequently recur after incomplete excision and cause local destruction including bony erosion.[801,802] Squamous cell carcinoma or transitional cell carcinoma may supervene in up to 20% of inverted papillomas.

Squamous cell carcinoma is the most common tumor of the lacrimal sac and occurs at an average age of 55 years.[800-801] Adenocarcinoma and mucoepidermoid carcinoma are rare, the latter resulting in death in most cases.[803] The lacrimal sac may be invaded by medial canthal basal cell carcinoma or squamous cell carcinoma, presenting as lacrimal duct obstruction. Nonepithelial tumors are predominantly benign and include capillary hemangioma, cavernous hemangioma, and neurilemmoma, but fibrous histiocytoma hemangiopericytoma, and malignant melanoma have been reported.[804-806] Treatment for all these tumors is primarily surgical with resection of surrounding bone and orbital tissue including exenteration, if necessary, for malignant tumors. Radiation therapy may be used adjunctively for aggressive or inoperable lesions, and there is limited experience in treating with radiation as a sole modality.[807] Lymphoma is more common than inflammatory pseudo-tumor and is treated like other orbital and periocular lymphomas.[808]

NEOPLASIA-ASSOCIATED DISORDERS

The neoplasia-associated disorders are listed in Table 70-9.

Disorders Associated with Remote Neoplasia

Muir-Torre Syndrome
Patients with Muir-Torre syndrome, an autosomal dominant condition, have single or multiple eyelid sebaceous adenomas or keratoacanthomas.[810,811] Men are affected twice as often as women. Sebaceous adenomas of the eyelids are rare and strongly suggest the possibility of internal carcinoma, since 50% of patients with Muir-Torre syndrome have but a single sebaceous adenoma of the skin.[812,813] Colonic and gastric carcinomas are common in this syndrome and may arise multicentrically from adenomatous polyps, but other visceral carcinomas have been described. In fact, 75% of these patients have a familial history of visceral carcinoma. These patients may also have other benign adenomas, adenomatous hyperplasias, and fibrous proliferations. The eyelid lesions may precede or follow the visceral tumors.

Cowden's Disease
Cowden's disease (multiple hamartoma syndrome) is an autosomal dominant disorder characterized by a variety of cutaneous lesions associated with carcinomas of the breast and thyroid.[814] The affected patients have facial papules that are frequently seen to be trichilemmomas on histopathologic examination.[815] The eyelid is involved in approximately 40% of cases.[814] The finding of multiple trichilemmomas is virtually pathognomonic for Cowden's disease.[816] A recent association of Cowden's disease with Lhermitte-Duclos disease has been described.[817]

Basal Cell Nevus Syndrome
Basal cell nevus syndrome is an autosomal dominant trait with greater than 90% penetrance that affects men more

TABLE 70-9

Ocular Conditions Related to Malignancy

CONDITION	INHERITANCE	OCULAR FINDINGS	SYSTEMIC MALIGNANCY
Muir-Torre syndrome	AD	Sebaceous adenoma	Gastrointestinal carcinoma
Cowden's disease	AD	Trichilemmoma	Thyroid, breast carcinoma
Basal cell nevus syndrome	AD	Multiple cell carcinomas	Basal cell carcinoma, fibrosarcoma, medulloblastoma
Gardner's syndrome	AD	Congenital retinal pigment epithelial hypertrophy	Colonic carcinoma
Neurofibromatosis I	AD	Lisch nodules, eyelid neurofibroma, choroidal hamartoma, café au lait spots, optic nerve glioma, meningioma	Gliomas, meningioma, malignant astrocytoma, pheochromocytoma, malignant peripheral nerve sheath tumor
Neurofibromatosis 2	AD	Cataract, retinal hamartoma, optic nerve glioma, and meningioma	Meningioma, glioma
von Hippel-Lindau disease	AD	Retinal hemangioblastoma carcinoma, hemangioblastoma	Pheochromocytoma, renal cell
Tuberous sclerosis	AD	Retinal astrocytic hamartoma	Malignant astrocytoma
Retinoblastoma	AD	Retinoblastoma	Osteosarcoma, sebaceous carcinoma, fibrosarcoma
Bilateral uveal melanocytic tumors		Diffuse bilateral melanocytic tumor	Various cutaneous and visceral malignancies
Multiple endocrine neoplasia III/IIB	AD	Thickened corneal nerves	Pheochromocytoma, parathyroid carcinoma, medullary carcinoma of thyroid
Cancer-associated retinopathy	–	Retinal degeneration, blindness	Carcinomas of lung, breast, and cervix
Radiation dermatitis	–	Erythema, telangiectasia, pigmentation, atrophy, ulceration	Squamous cell carcinoma, basal cell carcinoma
Xeroderma pigmentation	AR	Erythema, telangiectasia, scaling, pigmentation, atrophy	Squamous cell carcinoma, melanoma, basal cell carcinoma, sarcoma
Ocular/oculodermal melanocytosis	–	Melanocytosis	Melanoma

than women.[818] Multiple basal cell carcinomas exhibiting a multicentric pattern of growth develop in the second decade of life with eyelid involvement in 20% to 25% of cases.[819] These develop as nodules that enlarge and increase in number in adulthood. Periocular basal cell carcinomas are more likely to develop after irradiation. Patients with this disorder may also develop other malignant tumors such as ovarian and mandibular fibrosarcomas and medulloblastoma. These patients also have a higher incidence of mandibular cysts, dyskeratosis and pitting of the skin of the palms and soles, and a variety of skeletal defects, as well as ocular findings of congenital blindness, cataract, glaucoma, and choroidal colobomas.[820,821]

Gardner's Syndrome

Gardner's syndrome is an autosomal dominant syndrome consisting of adenomatous polyposis of the colon, benign tumors of soft tissue and bone, dental abnormalities, extracolonic cancer, and desmoid tumors. All untreated patients will develop adenocarcinoma of the colon.[822] Congenital retinal pigment epithelial hypertrophy has been linked to Gardner's syndrome. This finding is present in two thirds of families with the syndrome.[823] Ophthalmoscopically, dark brown, flat, round to kidney bean–shaped lesions range from 0.2 to 1.5 mm in diameter and represent increased pigment in retinal pigment epithelial

cells.[824-827] Affected individuals may have from 1 to 30 lesions in each eye.

Neurofibromatosis

Neurofibromatosis (NF) is a phakomatosis with protean manifestations. It occurs in two main forms: NF-1 with café au lait spots, neurofibromas, iris melanocytic hamartomas, and optic nerve gliomas; and NF-2 with bilateral acoustic neuromas, optic nerve gliomas, and meningiomas. Less common varieties of neurofibromatosis also exist. Both common forms are autosomal dominant; the locus of NF-1 is on chromosome 17 and that of NF-2 is on chromosome 22.[828-831]

Patients with NF-1 may have neurofibromas in a variety of ocular tissues, including the eyelid, orbit, and uvea. Iris melanocytic hamartomas (Lisch nodules) are present in 90% of patients older than 5 years and 100% of patients older than 20 years.[832,833] Unaffected relatives do not show Lisch nodules. Other ocular hamartomas, including retinal astrocytic hamartomas, may be seen. Fifteen percent of NF-1 patients will have optic nerve gliomas on CT.[834,835] The plexiform neurofibromas of NF-1 may undergo malignant transformation.[836]

von Hippel-Lindau Disease

von Hippel-Lindau disease is an autosomally dominant phakomatosis manifested by multiple angiomas. Retinal

Specific Malignancies

III

disease alone is termed von Hippel disease, while retinal and cerebellar tumor involvement is designated von Hippel-Lindau disease. The locus for the gene is on chromosome 3.[837] The benign hemangioblastomas of the retina may frequently impair vision due to exudative retinal detachment and may lead to loss of the eye. The cerebellar hemangioblastomas can be fatal. Affected individuals may also have pheochromocytoma (3% to 10%) or renal cell carcinomas (25%) that also may be fatal.[838-840]

Tuberous Sclerosis (Bourneville's Disease)

Tuberous sclerosis is a phakomatosis characterized by facial or ungual fibromas, cortical tubers, subependymal hamartomas, and multiple retinal hamartomas.[841] The retinal lesions are translucent astrocytic hamartomas that may show calcification and mulberry configurations. They can be confused with retinoblastomas. Malignant astrocytomas may occur in this condition.[842]

Hereditary Retinoblastoma

Patients with treated heritable retinoblastoma may develop sarcomas, carcinomas, and melanomas in or out of the radiation field,[843,845] particularly after radiation therapy for residual retinoblastoma. The cumulative 30-year incidence of second malignant tumors ranges from 18% to 35%,[844,846-850] and the estimated cumulative probability of death from second primary tumors is 26% at 40 years. Radiation before age 12 months is associated with increased incidence and earlier development of second primary tumors in the field of irradiation.[845] Any orbital swelling, pain, or loss of vision should be promptly evaluated with CT and biopsy as needed. These patients are also at up to 10% risk (by age 5 years) of developing midline neuroectodermal brain tumors, most notably pineoblastoma, the so-called trilateral retinoblastoma.[844]

Bilateral Uveal Melanocytic Tumor

Bilateral uveal melanoma is exceedingly rare. Thus uncommon cases of bilateral or multiple uveal melanocytic lesions, reported in association with a wide variety of visceral and cutaneous malignancies, have received special attention.[851-853] Lesions can be flat or elevated and may be diffuse throughout the uvea. Many demonstrate atypical or frankly malignant histopathologic features. The cause of these tumors is unknown.

Multiple Endocrine Neoplasia Syndrome III/IIB

The multiple endocrine neoplasia syndrome III/IIB consists of the associated occurrence of medullary carcinoma of the thyroid, pheochromocytoma, and parathyroid adenocarcinomas.[854] The first manifestations of this autosomal dominant condition are often mucosal neuromas that appear in early childhood. They appear as multiple small nodules of the lips, tongue, and mouth. Conjunctival scleral and corneal neuromas may also occur, as may neuromas of the nasal skin and eyelids. These lesions lead to thickening of involved structures. Enlarged corneal nerves may be noted on routine eye examination and may lead to early detection of the syndrome.[855,856]

Cancer-Associated Retinopathy

A relatively uncommon but increasingly recognized condition is cancer-associated retinopathy. These patients develop retinal degeneration resulting in progressive painless visual loss that can progress to blindness over months to years. Most cases have been associated with small cell carcinomas of the lung, but carcinomas of the breast, uterus, and cervix and melanomas have also been implicated.[857-859]

Symptomatically, blurred vision, visual field defects, and distorted color vision are reported. Ophthalmoscopically, patients show alterations of the retinal pigment epithelium and retinal arteriolar attenuation. The electroretinogram is abnormal in all cases.[857] Histologically, a generalized loss of retinal ganglion cells and pigmentary retinopathy are seen. Decreases of other retinal cell types have also been noted.[860,861] The pathogenesis is thought to be autoimmune, since circulating antibodies reacting with retinal protein are found in sera of affected patients.[861]

Disorders Predisposing to Local Neoplasia

Radiation Dermatitis

Radiation changes within the skin include atrophy, fibrosis, and frequently chronic inflammation. These areas are also prone to develop neoplasms including squamous cell carcinoma, basal cell carcinoma, sebaceous carcinoma, or sarcoma including fibrosarcoma and osteogenic sarcoma.[862,863]

Xeroderma Pigmentosum

The underlying defect in xeroderma pigmentosum is an inherited autosomal recessive inability to repair ultraviolet-induced damage to cellular DNA.[864,865] This renders the skin and conjunctiva extremely sensitive to neoplasia induced by solar irradiation manifested by the development of crops of malignant tumors, especially in the head and neck regions. Up to 70% of patients develop cutaneous malignancies by a median age of 8 years.[866] Tumors of the skin and conjunctiva include squamous cell carcinomas, basal cell carcinomas, malignant melanoma, and sebaceous carcinoma in areas exposed to sunlight.[865,867]

Oculodermal Melanocytosis (Nevus of Ota)

Nevus of Ota is a unilateral blue-gray discoloration of the periorbital skin and sclera (see Fig. 70-20C) that may be associated with deeper hyperpigmentation of the choroid, orbit, and meninges.[868,869] Occurring in the first 2 decades of life, with an increased incidence in Asians and blacks, this lesion consists of a proliferation of fusiform and dendritic, heavily pigmented melanocytes. Malignant melanoma, although uncommon, may occur in any of the regions of involvement.[869-871] In white patients, nevus of Oto increases the predisposition to uveal melanoma.[872]

Dysplastic Nevus (Atypical Mole) Syndrome

Patients with dysplastic nevus (atypical mole) syndrome are prone to cutaneous melanoma. The incidence of this syndrome is increased in patients with uveal melanoma and may predispose to the development of ocular melanocytic tumors.[873]

REFERENCES

Intraocular Neoplasia

1. Albert DM, Earle JD, Sahel JA: Intraocular Melanoma. In DeVita VT Jr, Hellman S, Rosenberg SA (eds): Cancer: Principles & Practice of Oncology, 3rd ed. Philadelphia, JB Lippincott, 1985, p 1543.
2. Cutler SJ, Young JL (eds): Third national cancer survey: Incidence data. Natl Cancer Inst Monogr 1975;41:1.
3. Hogan MJ, Zimmerman LE: Ophthalmic Pathology: An Atlas and Textbook, 2nd ed. Philadelphia, WB Saunders, 1962.
4. Young JL, Percy CL, Asire AJ, et al: Cancer incidence and mortality in the United States: 1973–1977. Natl Cancer Inst Monogr 1981;57:1.
5. Egan EM, Seddon JM, Gragoudas ES, et al: Uveal melanoma in New England: Profile of cases diagnosed in 1984. Presented at the Massachusetts Eye and Ear Infirmary Alumni Association Award Meeting, April 9, 1987, Cambridge, Mass.
6. Abrahamson M: Malignant melanoma of the choroid and the ciliary body 1956–1975. Acta Ophthalmol (Copenh) 1982;61:600.
7. Singh AD, Topham A: Incidence of uveal melanoma in the United States: 1973–1997. Ophthalmology 2003;110:956–961.
8. Char DH, Heilbron DL, Juster RR, et al: Choroidal melanoma growth patterns. Br J Ophthalmol 1983;67:575.
9. Gass JDM: Comparison of uveal melanoma growth rates with mitotic index mortality. Arch Ophthalmol 1985;103:924.
10. Fribert TR, Finchberg E, McQuaig S: Extremely rapid growth of a primary choroidal melanoma. Arch Ophthalmol 1983;101:1375.
11. Sahel JA, Pesavento R, Frederick A Jr, et al: Uveal melanoma arising de novo over a 16-month period. Arch Ophthalmol 1988;106:381.
12. Augsburger JJ, Gonder JR, Amsel J, et al: Growth rates and doubling time of posterior uveal melanomas. Ophthalmology 1984;91:1709.
13. Lambert JR, Char DM, Howes E Jr, et al: Spontaneous regression of a choroidal melanoma. Arch Ophthalmol 1986;104:732.
14. Graham BJ, Duane TD: Meetings, conferences, symposia: Report of ocular melanoma task force. Am J Ophthalmol 1981;90:72.
15. Scotto J, Fraumeni JF, Lee JAH: Melanomas of the eye and other noncutaneous sites. J Natl Cancer Inst 1976;56:489.
16. Yanoff M, Zimmerman LE: Histogenesis of malignant melanoma of the uvea: III. The relationship of congenital ocular melanocytosis and neurofibromatosis to uveal melanomas. Arch Ophthalmol 1967;77:4331.
17. Barr CC, McLean IW, Zimmerman LE: Uveal melanoma in children and adolescents. Arch Ophthalmol 1981;99:2133.
18. Shields JA, Zimmerman LE: Lesions simulating malignant melanoma of the posterior uvea. Arch Ophthalmol 1973;86:466.
19. Zimmerman LE: Problems in the diagnosis of malignant melanoma of the choroid and ciliary body. Am J Ophthalmol 1973;75:917.
20. Char DH: The management of small choroidal melanomas. Surv Ophthalmol 1978;22:377.
21. Shields JA, McDonald PR: Improvements in the diagnosis of posterior uveal melanoma. Arch Ophthalmol 1974;91:259.
22. Font RL, Spaulding AG, Zimmerman LE: Diffuse malignant melanoma of the uveal tract: A clinicopathologic report of 54 cases. Trans Am Acad Ophthalmol Otolaryngol 1968;72:877.
23. Coleman DJ, Abramson DH, Jack RL, et al: Ultrasonic diagnosis of tumors of the choroid. Arch Ophthalmol 1974;91:344.
24. Ossoinig C, Bigar F, Kaefring SL: Malignant melanoma of the choroid and ciliary body: A differential diagnosis in clinical echography. Curr Concepts Ophthalmol 1975;83:141.
25. Coleman DJ, Lizzi FL, Jack RL: Ultrasonography of the Eye and Orbit. Philadelphia, Lea & Febiger, 1977.
26. Char DH, Stone RD, Irvine AR, et al: Diagnostic modalities in choroidal melanoma. Am J Ophthalmol 1980;89:223.
27. Kauffman ML: Aspiration biopsy of malignant melanoma of choroid. Arch Ophthalmol 1952;47:541.
28. Gonzalez Vanrell F, Pateyro P, Grosso O: Cytological contribution to the diagnosis of melanoma of the choroid. Arch Soc Oftal Hisp Am 1950;10:579.
29. Augsburger JJ, Shields JA, Folberg R, et al: Fine needle aspiration biopsy in the diagnosis of intraocular cancer: Cytologic-histologic correlations. Ophthalmology 1985;92:39.
30. Mafee MF, Peyman GA, McKusick MA: Malignant uveal melanoma and similar lesions studied by computed tomography. Radiology 1985;156:403.
31. Mafee MF, Peyman GA, Grisolan JE, et al: Malignant uveal melanomas and simulating lesions: MRI imaging evaluation. Radiology 1986;160:773.
32. Callender GR: Malignant melanotic tumors of the eye: A study of histologic types in 111 cases. Trans Am Acad Ophthalmol Otolaryngol 1931;36:131.
33. McLean IW, Foster WD, Zimmerman LE, Gamel JW: Modifications of Callender's classification of uveal melanoma at the Armed Forces Institute of Pathology. Am J Ophthalmol 1983;95:502.
34. McLean IW, Zimmerman LE, Evans RM: Reappraisal of Callender's spindle A type of malignant melanoma of choroid and ciliary body. Am J Ophthalmol 1978;86:557.
35. McLean IW, Foster WD, Zimmerman LE: Uveal melanoma: Location size, cell type and enucleation as risk factors in metastasis. Hum Pathol 1981;13:123.
36. Gamel JW, McLean IW: Quantitative analysis of the Callender classification of uveal melanoma cells. Arch Ophthalmol 1977;95:686.
37. Gamel JW, McLean IW: Modern developments in histopathologic assessment of uveal melanomas. Ophthalmology 1984;91:679.
38. Gamel JW, McLean IW, Grecky RA, et al: Objective assessment of the malignant potential of intraocular melanomas with standard microslides stained with hematoxylin-eosin. Hum Pathol 1985;16:689.
39. Thomas JV, Green WR, Maumenee AE: Small choroidal melanomas: A long-term follow-up study. Arch Ophthalmol 1979;97:861.
40. Char DH, Hogan MJ: Management of small elevated pigmented choroidal lesions. Br J Ophthalmol 1977;61:54.
41. Gass JD: Observation of suspected choroidal and ciliary body melanomas for evidence of growth prior to enucleation. Ophthalmology 1980;87:523.
42. Nauman GOH, Yanaff M, Zimmerman LE: Histogenesis of malignant melanoma of the uvea. I. Histopathologic characteristics of nevi of the choroid and ciliary body. Arch Ophthalmol 1966;76:784.
43. Zimmerman LE: Malignant melanoma of the uveal tract. In Spencer WH (ed): Ophthalmic Pathology: An Atlas and Textbook, 3rd ed. Philadelphia, WB Saunders, 1986, p 2075.
44. Beahrs OH, Myers MH: Manual for Staging of Cancer, 2nd ed. Philadelphia, JB Lippincott, 1983, p 197.
45. Shields JA, Shields CL: Intraocular Tumors: A Text and Atlas. Philadelphia, WB Saunders, 1992, p 178.
46. Finger PT, Packer S, Svitra P, et al: Hyperthermic treatment of intraocular tumors. Arch Ophthalmol 1986;102:1477.
47. Coleman DJ, Lizzi FL, Burgess SE, et al: Ultrasonic hyperthermia and radiation in the management of intraocular malignant melanoma. Am J Ophthalmol 1986;101:635.
48. Petrovich Z, Astrahan MA, Luxon G, et al: Episcleral plaque thermoradiotherapy in patients with choroidal melanoma. Int J Radiat Oncol Biol Phys 1992;23:599.
49. Burgess JE, Chang S, Svitra PP, et al: Effects of hyperthermia on experimental choroidal melanoma. Br J Ophthalmol 1985;69:584.
50. Zimmerman LE, McLean IW: Metastatic disease from untreated uveal melanomas. Am J Ophthalmol 1979;88:524.
51. Zimmerman LE, McLean IW, Foster WD: Does enucleation of the eye containing a malignant melanoma prevent or accelerate the dissemination of tumor cells? Br J Ophthalmol 1978;62:420.
52. Zimmerman LE, McLean IW: An evaluation of enucleation in the management of uveal melanomas. Am J Ophthalmol 1979;87:741.
53. Fraunfelder FT, Boozman FW, Wilson RS, et al: No-touch technique for intraocular malignant melanomas. Arch Ophthalmol 1977;95:1616.
54. Wilson RS, Fraunfelder FT: "No-touch" cryosurgical enucleation: A minimal trauma technique for eyes harboring intraocular malignancy. Ophthalmology 1978;85:1170.
55. Niederkorn JY, Streilen JW: Intracamerally induced concomitant immunity: Mice harboring progressively growing intraocular tumors are immune to spontaneous metastases and secondary tumor challenge. J Immunol 1983;131:2587.

Specific Malignancies

III

56. Niederkorn JY: Enucleation-induced metastasis of intraocular melanoma in mice. Ophthalmology 1984;91:692.

57. Seigel D, Myers M, Ferris F III, et al: Survival rates after enucleation of eyes with malignant melanomas. Am J Ophthalmol 1979;87:761.

58. Peyman GA, Juarez CT, Diamond IG, et al: Ten years' experience with eye wall resection for uveal malignant melanomas. Ophthalmology 1984;91:1720.

59. Naumann GOH: Block excision of tumors of the ciliary body and choroid. In Lommatzsch PK, Blodi FC (eds): Intraocular Tumors. Berlin, Akademie Verlag, 1983, p 386.

60. Foulds WS: Results of local excision of uveal tumors. In Lommatzsch PK, Blodi FC (eds): Intraocular Tumors. Berlin, Akademie Verlag, 1983, p 374.

61. Char DH: Clinical Ocular Oncology. New York, Churchill Livingstone, 1989, p 145.

62. Moore RF: Choroidal sarcoma treated by the intraocular insertion of radon seeds. Br J Ophthalmol 1930;14:14.

63. Stallard HB: Radiotherapy for malignant melanoma of the choroid. Br J Ophthalmol 1966;50:147.

64. Markoe AM, Brady LW, Shields JA, et al: Malignant melanoma of the eye: Treatment of posterior uveal lesions by Co-60 plaque radiotherapy versus enucleation. Radiology 1985;156:801.

65. Sealy R, Le Roux PLM, Rapley F, et al: The treatment of ophthalmic tumors with low energy sources. Br J Urol 1976;49:551.

66. Packer S, Rotman M: Radiotherapy of choroidal melanoma with iodine-125. Ophthalmology 1980;87:582.

67. Garretson BR, Robertson DM, Earl JD: Choroidal melanoma treatment with iodine-125 brachytherapy. Arch Ophthalmol 1987;105:1394.

68. Lommatsch PK: B-irradiation of choroidal melanoma within 106R/106Rh applicators: 16 years' experience. Arch Ophthalmol 1983;101:713.

69. Char DH: Clinical Ocular Oncology. New York, Churchill Livingstone, 1989, p 118.

70. Shields JA, Augsburger JJ, Brady LW, et al: Cobalt plaque therapy for posterior uveal melanomas. Ophthalmology 1982;89:1201.

71. Vine AK, Ten Haken RK, Diaz RF, et al: A new inexpensive customized plaque for choroidal melanoma iodine-125 plaque therapy. Ophthalmology 1989;94:543.

72. Abramson DH, Servodidio CA, McCormick B, et al: Changes in height of choroidal melanomas after plaque therapy. Br J Ophthalmol 1986;74:356.

73. Quivey JM, Char DH, Phillips TL, et al: High intensity of 125 iodine (125-I) plaque treatment of uveal melanomas. Int J Radiat Oncol Biol Phys 1993;26:613.

74. Shields CL, Shields JA, Karlsson U, et al: Reasons for enucleation after plaque radiotherapy for posterior uveal melanoma. Ophthalmology 1989;96:919.

75. Char DH, Saunders W, Castro JR, et al: Helium ion therapy for choroidal melanoma. Ophthalmology 1983;90:1219.

76. Gragoudas ES, Seddon J, Goitein M, et al: Current results of proton beam irradiation of uveal melanomas. Ophthalmology 1985;92:284.

77. Gragoudas ES, Goitein M, Koehler AM, et al: Proton irradiation of small choroidal malignant melanomas. Am J Ophthalmol 1977;83:655-673.

78. Gragoudas ES, Goitein M, Verhey LJ, et al: Proton beam irradiation: An alternative to enucleation for intraocular melanoma. Ophthalmology 1980;87:571-581.

79. Gragoudas ES, Seddon JM, Egan K, et al: Long-term results of proton beam irradiated uveal melanomas. Arch Ophthalmol 1987;94:349-353.

80. Seddon JM, Gragoudas ES, Polivogianis L, et al: Visual outcome after proton beam irradiation of uveal melanoma. Ophthalmology 1986;93:666-674.

81. Seddon JM, Gragoudas ES, Egan KM, et al: Uveal melanomas near the optic disc or fovea: Visual results after proton beam irradiation. Ophthalmology 1987;94:354-361.

82. Sisterson J: Ion beam therapy: Overview of the world experience. Application of Accelerators in Research and Industry. Proceedings of the Seventeenth International Conference, November 2002, Denton, Texas.

83. Goitein M, Miller T: Planning proton therapy of the eye. Med Phys 1983;10:275-283.

84. Verhey LJ, Goitein M, Munzenrider JE, et al: Precise positioning of patients for radiation therapy. Int J Radiat Oncol Biol 1982;8:289-294.

85. Urano M, Goitein M, Verhey LJ, et al: Relative biological effectiveness of modulated proton beams in various murine tissues. Int J Radiat Oncol Biol Phys 1984;10:509-514.

86. Miller DW: A review of proton beam radiotherapy. Med Phys 1995;22:1943-1954.

87. Yashkin PN, Silin DI, Zolotov VA, et al: Relative biologic effectiveness of proton medical beam at Moscow Synchotron determined by the Chinese hamster cells assay. Int J Radiat Oncol Biol Phys 1995;31:535-540.

88. Paganetti H, Niemierko A, Ancukiewicz M, et al: Relative biological effectiveness values for proton beam therapy. Int J Radiat Oncol Biol Phys 2002;53:407-421.

89. Seddon JM, Gragoudas ES, Albert DM, et al: Comparison of survival rates for patients with uveal melanoma after treatment with proton beam irradiation or enucleation. Am J Ophthalmol 1985;99:282-290.

90. Munzenrider JE, Verhey L, Gragoudas ES, et al: Conservative treatment of uveal melanoma: Dose distribution to tumors with local recurrence after proton beam therapy. Int J Radiat Oncol Biol Phys 1989;17:493-498.

91. Gragoudas ES, Lane AM, Munzenrider JE, et al: Long-term risk of local failure after proton therapy for choroidal/ciliary body melanoma. Trans Am Ophthalmol Soc 2002;100:43-48.

92. Gragoudas ES, Seddon JM, Egan KM, et al: Metastasis from uveal melanoma after proton beam irradiation. Ophthalmology 1988;95:992-999.

93. Gragoudas ES, Seddon JM, Polivogianis LL, et al: Prognostic factors for metastasis following proton beam irradiation of uveal melanomas. Ophthalmology 1986;93:675-680.

94. Seddon JM, Albert DM, Lavin P, et al: A prognostic factor study of disease-free interval and survival following enucleation for uveal melanoma. Arch Ophthalmol 101:1894-1899, 1983.

95. Seddon JM, Gragoudas ES, Egan KM, et al: Relative survival rates after alternative therapies for uveal melanoma. Ophthalmology 1990;97:769-777.

96. Egan K, Gragoudas ES, Seddon JM, et al: The risk of enucleation after proton beam irradiation of uveal melanoma. Ophthalmology 1989;96:1377-1383.

97. Gragoudas ES, Goitein M, Lane AM, et al: Evidence-based estimates of outcomes in patients irradiated for intraocular melanoma. Arch Ophthalmol 2002;120:665-671.

98. Egger E, Zografos L, Schalenbourg A, et al: Eye retention after proton beam radiotherapy for uveal melanoma. Int J Radiat Oncol Biol Phys 2003;55:867-880.

99. Gragoudas ES, Egan KM, Arrigg PG, et al: Cataract extraction after proton beam irradiation for malignant melanoma of the eye. Arch Ophthalmol 1992;110:475-479.

100. Gragoudas ES, Egan KM, Walsh SM, et al: Lens changes after proton beam irradiation for uveal melanoma. Am J Ophthalmol 1995;119:157-164.

101. Gunduz K, Shields CL, Shields JA, et al: Radiation complications and tumor control after plaque radiotherapy of choroidal melanoma with macular involvement. Am J Ophthalmol 1999;127:579-589.

102. Gunduz K, Shields CL, Shields JA, et al: Radiation retinopathy following plaque radiotherapy for posterior uveal melanoma. Arch Ophthalmol 1999;117:609-614.

103. Hykin PG, Shields CL, Shields JA, et al: The efficacy of focal laser therapy in radiation-induced macular edema. Ophthalmology 1998;105:1425-1429.

104. Egan KM, Ryan LM, Gragoudas ES: Survival implications of enucleation after definitive radiotherapy for choroidal melanoma: An example of regression on time-dependent covariates. Arch Ophthalmol 1998;116:366-370.

105. Castro JR, Char DH, Petti PL, et al: 15 years' experience with helium ion radiotherapy for uveal melanoma. Int J Radiat Oncol Biol Phys 1997;39:989.

106. Char DH, Quivey JM, Castro JR, et al: Helium ions versus iodine 125 brachytherapy in the management of uveal melanoma. Ophthalmology 1993;100:1547.

107. Daftari IK, Char DH, Verhey LJ, et al: Anterior segment spacing to

reduce charged particle radiotherapy complications in uveal melanoma. Int J Radiat Oncol Biol Phys 1997;39:997.

108. Augsburger JJ, Schneider S, Freire J, et al: Survival following enucleation versus plaque radiotherapy in statistically matched subgroups of patients with choroidal melanomas: Results in patients treated between 1980 and 1987. Graefes Arch Clin Exp Ophthalmol 1999;237:558–567.

109. Augsburger JJ, Lauritzen K, Gamel JW, et al: Matched group study of preenucleation radiotherapy alone for primary malignant melanoma of the choroid and ciliary body. Am J Clin Oncol 1990;13:382.

110. Char DH, Phillips TL: Pre-enucleation irradiation of uveal melanoma. Br J Ophthalmol 1985;69:177.

111. The Collaborative Ocular Melanoma Study (COMS) randomized trial of pre-enucleation radiation of large coroidal melanoma II: Initial mortality findings. COMS report no. 10. Am J Ophthalmol 1998;125:779.

112. Shields JA, Shields CL: Current management of posterior uveal melanoma. Mayo Clin Proc 1993;68:1196.

113. Kersten RC, Tse D, Anderson RL, et al: Role of orbital exenteration in malignant melanoma with melanoma with extrascleral extension. Ophthalmology 1985;92:436.

114. Hall WEB: Malignant melanoma of the uveal tract: Report of a case with death 30 years after enucleation. Arch Ophthalmol 1950;44:381.

115. Kirk HQ: Delayed metastasis from choroidal melanoma. Surv Ophthalmol 1966;11:651.

116. Jensen OA: Malignant melanomas of the uvea in Denmark, 1943–1952. Acta Ophthalmol 1963;(Suppl)75:221.

117. Char DH: Metastatic choroidal melanoma. Am J Ophthalmol 1978;86:76.

118. Young DW, Lever RS, English JS, MacKie RM: The use of BELD combination chemotherapy (bleomycin, vindesine, CCNU, and DTIC) in advanced malignant melanoma. Cancer 1985;55:1879.

119. Carrasco CH, Wallace S, Charnsangavej C, et al: Treatment of hepatic metastasis in ocular melanoma: Embolization of the hepatic artery with polyvinyl sponge and cisplatin. JAMA 1986;255:3152.

120. Rosenberg SA, Lotze MT, Muul LM, et al: A progress report on the treatment of 157 patients with advanced cancer using lymphokine activated killer cells and interleukin-2 or high dose interleukin-2 alone. N Engl J Med 1987;316:889.

121. Fornier GA, Albert DM, Arrigg CA, et al: Resection of solitary metastasis: Approach to palliative treatment of hepatic involvement with choroidal melanoma. Arch Ophthalmol 1984;102:80.

122. Howard G, Forrest AW: Incidence and location of melanocytomas. Arch Ophthalmol 1967;77:61.

123. Arentsen JJ, Green WR: Melanoma of the iris: Report of 72 cases treated surgically. Ophthalmic Surg 1975;6:23.

124. Jakobiec FA, Silbert G: Are most iris "melanomas" really nevi? A clinicopathological study of 189 lesions. Arch Ophthalmol 1981;99:2117.

125. Shields JA, Shields CL: Intraocular Tumors: A Text and Atlas. Philadelphia, WB Saunders, 1992, p 69.

126. Rones B, Zimmerman LE: The prognosis of primary tumors of the iris treated by iridectomy. Arch Ophthalmol 1958;60:193.

127. Territo C, Shields CL, Shields JA, et al: Natural course of melanocytic tumors of the iris. Ophthalmology 1988;95:1251.

128. Char DH, Crawford JB, Gonzales J, et al: Iris melanoma with increased intraocular pressure: Differentiation of focal solitary tumors from diffuse or multiple tumors. Arch Ophthalmol 1989;107:548.

129. Reese AB, Jones IS, Cooper WC: Surgery for tumors of the iris and ciliary body. Am J Ophthalmol 1968;66:173.

130. Geisse LJ, Robertson DM: Iris melanoma. Am J Ophthalmol 1985;99:638.

131. Bardenstein DS: Intraocular lymphoma. Cancer Control 1998;5:317.

132. Freeman LN, Schachat AP, Knox DL, et al: Clinical features, laboratory investigation, and survival in ocular reticulum cell sarcoma. Ophthalmology 1987;94:1631.

133. Matzkin DC, Slamovits TL, Rosenbaum PS: Simultaneous intraocular and orbital non-Hodgkin lymphoma in the acquired immune deficiency syndrome. Ophthalmology 1994;101:850.

134. Char DH, Ljung B-M, Miller TR, et al: Primary intraocular lymphoma (ocular reticulum cell sarcoma): Diagnosis and management. Ophthalmology 1988;95:625.

135. Char DH, Margolis L, Newman AB: Ocular reticulum cell sarcoma. Am J Ophthalmol 1981;91:480.

136. Char DH, Ljung B-M, Deschenes J, et al: Intraocular lymphoma: Immunological and cytological analysis. Br J Ophthalmol 1988;72:905.

137. Kirmani MH, Thomas EL, Rao NA, et al: Intraocular reticulum cell sarcoma: Diagnosis by choroidal biopsy. Br J Ophthalmol 1987;71:748.

138. Margolis L, Fraser R, Lichter A, Char DH: The role of radiation therapy in the management of ocular reticulum cell sarcoma. Cancer 1980;45:688.

139. Rosen ST, Makuch RW, Lichter AS, et al: Role of prophylactic cranial irradiation in prevention of central nervous system metastases in small cell lung cancer. Potential benefit restricted to patients with complete response. Am J Med 1983;74:615.

140. Merchant A, Foster CS: Primary intraocular lymphoma. Int Ophthalmol Clin 1997;37:101.

141. Ursea R, Heinemann MH, Silverman RH, et al: Ophthalmic ultrasonographic findings in primary central nervous system lymphoma with retinal involvement. Retina 1997;117:118.

142. Valluri S, Moorthy RS, Khan A, et al: Combination treatment of intraocular lymphoma. Retina 1995;15:125.

143. Plowman PN, Montefiore DS, Lightman S: Multiagent chemotherapy in the salvage cure of ocular lymphoma relapsing after radiotherapy. Clin Oncol (R Coll Radiol) 1993;5:315.

144. Bloch RS, Gartner S: The incidence of ocular metastatic carcinoma. Arch Ophthalmol 1971;85:673.

145. Stephens RF, Shields JA: Diagnosis and management of cancer metastatic to the uvea: A study of 70 cases. Ophthalmology 1979;86:1336.

146. Nelson CC, Hertzberg BS, Klintworth GK: A histopathologic study of 716 unselected eyes in patients with cancer at the time of death. Am J Ophthalmol 1983;95:788.

147. Albert DM, Rubenstein RA, Scheie HG: Tumor metastasis to the eye. Part I: Incidence in 213 adult patients with generalized malignancy. Am J Ophthalmol 1967;63:723.

148. Mewis L, Young SE: Breast carcinoma metastatic to the choroid: Analysis of 67 patients. Ophthalmology 1982;89:147.

149. Weiss L: Analysis of the incidence of intraocular metastasis. Br J Ophthalmol 1993;77:149.

150. Shields JA, Shields CL: Intraocular Tumors: A Text and Atlas. Philadelphia, WB Saunders, 1992, p 208.

151. Ferry AP, Font RL: Carcinoma metastatic to the eye and orbit. I: a clinicopathologic study of 227 cases. Arch Ophthalmol 92: 276, 1974.

152. Ferry AP, Font RL: Carcinoma metastatic to the eye and orbit. II: A clinicopathologic study of 26 patients with carcinoma metastatic to the anterior segment of the eye. Arch Ophthalmol 1975;29:472.

153. Freedman MI, Folk JC: Metastatic tumors to the eye and orbit: Patient survival and clinical characteristics. Arch Ophthalmol 1987;105:1215.

154. Kindy-Degnan N, Char DH: Coincident systemic malignancy in uveal melanoma patients. Can J Ophthalmol 1989;24:204.

155. Michelson JB, Felberg NT, Shields JA: Evaluation of metastatic cancer to the eye: Carcinoembryonic antigen and gamma glutamyl transpeptidase. Arch Ophthalmol 1977;95:692.

156. Maor M, Chan RC, Young SE: Radiotherapy of choroidal metastases: Breast cancer as primary site. Cancer 1977;40:2081.

157. Reddy S, Saxena VS, Hendrickson F, Deutsch W: Malignant metastatic disease of the eye: Management of an uncommon complication. Cancer 1981;47:810.

158. Letson AD, Davidorf FH, Bruce RA Jr: Chemotherapy for treatment of choroidal metastases from breast carcinoma. Am J Ophthalmol 1982;93:102.

159. Chu FC, Huh SH, Nisce LZ, Simpson LD: Radiation therapy of choroid metastasis from breast cancer. Int J Radiat Oncol Biol Phys 1977;2:273.

160. Brinkley JR Jr: Response of a choroidal metastasis to multiple-drug chemotherapy. Cancer 1980;45:1538.

161. Cogan DG, Kuwabara T: Metastatic carcinoma to eye from the breast: Effects of endocrine therapy. Arch Ophthalmol 1954;52:240.

162. Barondes MJ, Hamilton AM, Hungerford J, et al: Treatment of choroidal metastasis from choriocarcinoma [letter]. Arch Ophthalmol 1989;107:796.

163. Sierocki JS, Schafrank M, et al: Carcinoma metastatic to the anterior ocular segment: Response to chemotherapy. Cancer 1980;45:2521.

164. Weisenthal R, Brucker A, Lanciano R: Follicular thyroid cancer metastatic to the iris [letter]. Arch Ophthalmol 1989;107:494.

165. Jaeger EA, Frayer WC, Southard ME, et al: Effect of radiation therapy on metastatic choroidal tumors. Trans Am Acad Ophthalmol Otolaryngol 1971;75:94.

166. Rudoler SB, Shields CL, Corn BW, et al: Vision is improved in the majority of patients treated with extended-beam radiotherapy for choroidal metastases: A multivariate analysis of 188 patients. J Clin Oncol 1997;15:1244.

167. Char DH: Clinical Ocular Oncology. New York, Churchill Livingstone, 1989, p 143.

168. Bell RM, Bullock JD, Albert DM: Solitary choroidal metastasis from bronchial carcinoid. Br J Ophthalmol 1975;59:155.

169. Rodrigues M, Shields JA: Iris metastasis from a bronchial carcinoid tumor. Arch Ophthalmol 1978;96:77.

170. Gragoudas ES, Carroll JM: Multiple choroidal metastases from bronchial carcinoid treated with photocoagulation and proton beam irradiation. Am J Ophthalmol 1979;87:299.

171. Merrill CF, Kaufman DI, Dimitrov NV: Breast cancer metastatic to the eye is a common entity. Cancer 1991;68:623.

172. Shields JA, Shields CL: Intraocular Tumors: A Text and Atlas. Philadelphia, WB Saunders, 1992, p 235.

173. Char DH, Schwartz A, Miller TR, et al: Ocular metastases from systemic melanoma. Am J Ophthalmol 1980;90:702.

174. Shields JA, Shields CL, Kiratli H, de Potter P: Metastatic tumors to the iris in 40 patients. Am J Ophthalmol 1995;119:422.

175. Rudoler SB, Shields CL, Corn BW, et al: Vision is improved in the majority of patients treated with extended-beam radiotherapy for choroidal metastases. J Clin Oncol 1997;15:1244.

176. Schachat AP, Markowitz JA, Guyer DR, et al: Ophthalmic manifestations of leukemia. Arch Ophthalmol 1989;107:697.

177. Allen RA, Straatsma BR: Ocular involvement in leukemia and allied disorders. Arch Ophthalmol 1961;66:490.

178. Kincaid MC, Green WR: Ocular and orbital involvement in leukemia. Surv Ophthalmol 1983;27:211.

179. Ridge EW, Jaffe N, Walton DS: Leukemic ophthalmopathy in children. Cancer 1976;38:1744.

180. Rodrigues M, Hidayat A, Karesh J: Pleomorphic adenocarcinoma of ciliary epithelium simulating an epibulbar tumor. Am J Ophthalmol 1988;106:595.

181. Dryja TP, Albert DM, Horns D: Adenocarcinoma arising from the epithelium of the ciliary body. Ophthalmology 1981;88:1290.

182. Font RL, Rao NA, Zimmerman LE, et al: Pigmented tumors of the ciliary and retinal pigment epithelium: An analysis of 40 cases. Invest Ophthalmol Vis Sci 1983;24:50.

183. Cherington FJ: Metastatic adenocarcinoma of the optic nerve, head, and adjacent retina. Br J Ophthalmol 1961;45:227.

184. Duke JR, Walsh FB: Metastatic carcinoma to the retina. Am J Ophthalmol 1959;47:44.

185. Kennedy RJ, Rummel WD, McCarthy JL, et al: Metastatic carcinoma of the retina: Report of a case and the pathologic findings. Arch Ophthalmol 1958;60:12.

186. Kinderman WR, Shields JA, Eiferman RA, et al: Metastatic renal cell carcinoma to the eye and adnexae: A report of 3 cases and review of the literature. Ophthalmology 1981;88:1347.

187. Letson AD, Davidorf FH: Bilateral retinal metastases from cutaneous melanoma. Arch Ophthalmol 1982;100:605.

188. Riffenburgh RS: Metastatic malignant melanoma to the retina. Arch Ophthalmol 1961;66:487.

189. Barry G, Mullaney J: Retinoblastoma in the Republic of Ireland. Trans Ophthalmol Soc U K 1971;91:839.

190. Schappert-Kimmijser J, Hemmes GD, Niijland R: The heredity of retinoblastoma. Ophthalmologica 1966;151:197.

191. Tarkkanen A, Tuovinen E: Retinoblastoma in Finland 1912–1964. Acta Ophthalmol 1971;49:293.

192. Kundson AG Jr: Retinoblastoma: A prototypic hereditary neoplasm. Semin Oncol 1978;5:57.

193. Vogel F: Genetics of retinoblastoma. Hum Genet 1979;52:1.

194. Knudson AG Jr: Mutation and cancer: Statistical study of retinoblastoma. Proc Natl Acad Sci USA 1971;68:820.

195. Friend SH, Bernards R, Rogelj S, et al: A human DNA segment with properties of the gene that predisposes to retinoblastoma and osteosarcoma. Nature 1986;323:643.

196. Sparkes RS, Sparkes MC, Wilson MG, et al: Regional assignment of genes for human esterase D and retinoblastoma to chromosome band 13q14. Science 1980;208:1042.

197. Moll AC, Koten JW, Lindenmayer JA, et al: Three histopathological types of retinoblastoma and their relation to heredity and age of enucleation. J Med Genet 1996;33:923.

198. Sanders TE: Pseudoglioma: Clinicopathologic study of 15 cases. Trans Am Ophthalmol Soc 1950;48:575.

199. Ellsworth RM: The practical management of retinoblastoma. Trans Am Ophthalmol Soc 1969;67:462.

200. Sparkes RS, Murphree AL, Lingua RW, et al: Gene for hereditary retinoblastoma assigned to human chromosome 13 by linkage to esterase D. Science 1983;219:971.

201. Makley TA Jr: Retinoblastoma in a 52-year-old man. Arch Ophthalmol 1963;69:325.

202. Takahashi TT, Tamura S, Inoue M, et al: Retinoblastoma in a 26 year old adult. Ophthalmology 1983;90:179.

203. Verhoeff FH: Retinoblastoma: Report of case in man aged forty-eight. Arch Ophthalmol 1929;2:643.

204. Stafford WR, Yanoff M, Parnell BL: Retinoblastoma initially misdiagnosed as primary ocular inflammations. Arch Ophthalmol 1969;82:771.

205. Shields JA, Shield CL, Suvarnamani C, et al: Retinoblastoma manifesting as orbital cellulilitis. Am J Ophthalmol 1991;112:442.

206. Bardenstein DS, Katz NNR, Peiffer R: Retinoblastoma presenting with orbital cellulitis: A mechanistic hypothesis (submitted).

207. Schofield PB: Diffuse infiltrating retinoblastoma. Br J Ophthalmol 1960;44:35.

208. Nicholson DH, Norton EW: Diffuse infiltrating retinoblastoma. Trans Am Ophthalmol Soc 1980;78:265.

209. Jakobiec FA, Tso MO, Zimmerman LE, et al: Retinoblastoma and intracranial malignancy. Cancer 1977;39:2048.

210. Bader JL, Miller RW, Meadows AT, et al: Trilateral retinoblastoma [letter]. Lancet 1980;2:582.

211. Zimmerman LE: Trilateral retinoblastoma. In Blodi FC (ed): Retinoblastoma. New York, Churchill Livingstone, 1985, p 185.

212. Pesin SR, Shields JA: Seven cases of trilateral retinoblastoma. Am J Ophthalmol 1989;107:121.

213. Margo C, Hidayat A, Kopelman J, Zimmerman LE: Retinocytoma: A benign variant of retinoblastoma. Arch Ophthalmol 1983;101:1519.

214. Abramson DH: Retinoma, retinocytoma, and the retinoblastoma gene [editorial]. Arch Ophthalmol 1983;101:1517.

215. Eagle RC, Shields JA, Donoso LA, et al: Malignant transformation of spontaneously regressed retinoblastoma, retinoma/retinocytoma variant. Ophthalmology 1989;96:1389.

216. Shields JA, Shields CL: Intraocular Tumors: A Text and Atlas. Philadelphia, WB Saunders, 1992, p 341.

217. Bullock JD, Campbell RJ, Waller RR: Calcificiation in retinoblastoma. Invest Ophthalmol Vis Sci 1977;16:252.

218. Char DH, Hedges TR III, Norman D: Retinoblastoma, CT diagnosis. Ophthalmology 1984;91:1347.

219. O'Brien JM, Char DH, Tucker N, et al: Efficacy of unanesthetized spiral computed tomography scanning in initial evaluation of childhood leukocoria. Ophthalmology 1995;102:1345.

220. Stevenson KE, Hungerford J, Garner A: Local extraocular extension of retinoblastoma following intraocular surgery. Br J Ophthalmol 1989;73:739.

221. Ellsworth RM: The practical management of retinoblastoma. Trans Am Ophthalmol Soc 1969;67:462.

222. Hopping W: The new Essen prognosis classification for conservative sight saving treatment of retinoblastoma. In Lommatzsch PK, Blodi FC (eds): Intraocular Tumors. Berlin, Akademie Verlag, 1983, p 497.

223. De Sutter E, Hoepping W, Zeller G: Comparison between different retinoblastoma classifications. Bull Soc Belge Ophthalmol 1993;248:19.

224. Gimblett ML, Wellings PC, Lewis M, et al: Retinoblastoma with micrometastasis to CSF. Pathology 1995;27:27.

225. Pratt CB, Meyer D, Chenaille P, Crom DB: The use of bone marrow aspirations and lumbar punctures at the time of diagnosis of retinoblastoma. J Clin Oncol 1989;7:10.

226. Shidnia H, Hornback NB, Helveston EM, et al: Treatment results of retinoblastoma at Indiana University Hospitals. Cancer 1977;40: 2917.

227. Stannard C, Lipper S, Sealy R, et al: Retinoblastoma: Correlation of invasion of the optic nerve and choroid with prognosis and metastases. Br J Ophthalmol 1979;63:560.

228. Hilgartner HL: Report of a case of double glioma treated with x-ray. Texas J Med 1902–1903;18:322.

229. Martin HE, Reese AB: Treatment of retinal gliomas by fractionated or divided dose principle of Roentgen radiation: Preliminary report. Arch Ophthalmol 1936;16:733.

230. Reese AB, Merriam GR, Martin HE: Treatment of bilateral retinoblastoma by radiation and surgery: Report on 15 year follow-up. Am J Ophthalmol 1949;32:175.

231. Egbert PR, Donaldson SS, Moazed K, et al: Visual results and ocular complications following radiotherapy for retinoblastoma. Arch Ophthalmol 1978;96:1826.

232. Donaldson SS, Egbert PR, Lee W-H: Retinoblastoma. In Pizzo PA, Poplack DG (eds): Principles and Practice of Pediatric Oncology, 2nd ed. Philadelphia, JB Lippincott, 1993, p 683.

233. Foote RL, Garretson BR, Schomberg PJ, et al: External beam irradiation for retinoblastoma: Patterns of failure and dose-response analysis. Int J Radiat Oncol Biol Phys 1989;16:823.

234. Blach LE, McCormick B, Abramson DH: Int J Radiat Oncol Biol Phys 1996;35:45.

235. Schipper J, Tan KE, van Peperzeel HA: Treatment of retinoblastoma by precision megavoltage radiation therapy. Radiother Oncol 1985;3:117.

236. Harnett AN, Hungerford JL, Lambert GD, et al: Improved external beam radiotherapy for the treatment of retinoblastoma. Br J Radiol 1987;60:753.

237. Messmer EP, Fritze H, Mohr C, et al: Long-term treatment effects in patients with bilateral retinoblastoma: ocular and mid-facial findings. Graefes Arch Clin Exp Ophthalmol 1991;229:309.

238. Weiss DR, Cassady JR, Petersen R: Retinoblastoma: A modification in radiation therapy technique. Radiology 1975;114:705.

239. McCormick B, Ellsworth R, Abramson D, et al: Radiation therapy for retinoblastoma: Comparison of results with lens-sparing versus lateral beam techniques. Int J Radiat Oncol Biol Phys 1988;15:567.

240. Abramson DH, Servodidio CA, De Lillo AR, et al: Recurrence of unilateral retinoblastoma following radiation therapy. Ophthalmol Genet 1994;15:107.

241. McCormick B: Retinoblastoma. In Leibel SA, Phillips TL (eds): Textbook of Radiation Oncology. Philadelphia, WB Saunders, 1998, p 1149.

242. Abramson DH, Gerardi CM, Ellsworth RM, et al: Radiation regression patterns in treated retinoblastoma: 7 to 21 years later. J Pediatr Ophthalmol Strabismus 1991;28:102.

243. Howarth C, Meyer D, Hustu HO, et al: Stage-related combined modality treatment of retinoblastoma: Results of a prospective study. Cancer 1980;45:851.

244. Amendola BE, Lamm FR, Markoe AM, et al: Radiotherapy of retinoblastoma: A review of 63 children treated with different irradiation techniques. Cancer 1990;66:21.

245. Bedford MA, Bedotto C, Macfaul PA: Retinoblastoma: A study of 139 cases. Br J Ophthalmol 1971;55:19.

246. Cassady JR, Sagerman RH, Tretter P, et al: Radiation therapy in retinoblastoma: An analysis of 230 cases. Radiology 1969;93:405.

247. Thompson RW, Small RC, Stein JJ: Treatment of retinoblastoma. AJR Radium Ther Nucl Med 1972;114:16.

248. Steenbakkers RJ, Altschuler MD, D'Angio GJ, et al: Optimized lens-sparing treatment of retinoblastoma with electron beams. Int J Radiat Oncol Biol Phys 1997;39:589.

249. Stallard HB: The treatment of retinoblastoma. Ophthalmologica 1966;151:214.

250. Fass D, McCormick B, Abramson D, Ellsworth R: Cobalt 60 plaques in recurrent retinoblastoma. Int J Radiat Oncol Biol Phys 1991;21:625.

251. Shields CL: External beam radiation therapy and retinoblastoma: Long-term results in the comparison of two techniques. Am J Ophthalmol 1993;115:842.

252. Goitein M, Abrams M: Multi-dimensional treatment planning: I. Delineation of anatomy. Int J Radiat Oncol Biol Phys 1983; 9:777–787.

253. Goitein M, Abrams M, Rowell D, et al: Multi-dimensional treatment planning: II. Beam's-eye view, back projection, and projection through CT slices. Int J Radiat Oncol Biol Phys 1983;9-789-97.

254. Wong FL, Boice JD, Abramson DH, et al: Cancer incidence after retinoblastoma. JAMA 1997;278:1262–1267.

255. Abramson DH, Frank CM: Second nonocular tumors in survivors of bilateral retinoblastoma: A possible age effect on radiation relaed risk. Ophthalmology 1998;105:573–580.

256. Murphree AL, Villablanca JG, Deegan WF III, et al: Chemotherapy plus local treatment in the management of intraocular retinoblastoma. Arch Ophthalmol 1996;114:1348.

257. Gallie BL, Budning A, DeBoer G, et al: Chemotherapy with focal therapy can cure intraocular retinoblastoma without radiotherapy. Arch Ophthalmol 1996;114:1321.

258. Bornfeld N, Schuler A, Bechrakis N, et al: Preliminary results of primary chemotherapy in retinoblastoma. Klin Paediatr 1997;209:216.

259. Kingston JE, Hungerford JL, Madreperia SA, Plowman PN: Results of combined chemotherapy and radiotherapy for advanced intraocular retinoblastoma. Arch Ophthalmol 1996;114:1339.

260. Greenwald MJ, Strauss LC: Treatment of intraocular retinoblastoma with carboplatin and etoposide chemotherapy. Ophthalmology 1996;103:1989.

261. Carlos Hernandez MD: What is the evidence supporting chemotherapy for intraocular retinoblastoma? [letter]. Arch Ophthalmol 1997;115:1604.

262. Redler LD, Ellsworth RM: Prognostic importance of choroidal invasion in retinoblastoma. Arch Ophthalmol 1973;90:294.

263. Kopelman JE, McLean IW, Rosenberg SH: Multivariate analysis of risk factors for metastasis in retinoblastoma treated by enucleation. Ophthalmology 1987;94:371.

264. MacKay CJ, Abramson DH, Ellsworth RM: Metastatic patterns of retinoblastoma. Arch Ophthalmol 1984;102:391.

265. Judisch GF, Apple DJ, Fratkin JD: Retinoblastoma: A survivor 12 years after treatment for metastatic disease. Arch Ophthalmol 1980;98:711.

266. Petersen RA, Friend SH, Albert DM: Prolonged survival of a child with metastatic retinoblastoma. J Pediatr Ophthalmol Strabismus 1987;24:247.

267. Wong FL, Boice JD Jr, Abramson DH, et al: Cancer incidence after retinoblastoma. Radiation dose and sarcoma risk [see comments]. JAMA 1997;278:1262.

268. Abramson DH, Ellsworth RM, Kitchin FD, Tung G: Second nonocular tumors in retinoblastoma survivors. Are they radiation induced? Ophthalmology 1984;91:1351.

269. Abramson DH, Ronner HJ, Ellsworth RM: Second tumors in nonirradiated bilateral retinoblastomoa. Am J Ophthalmol 1979;87:624.

270. Meadows AR, D'Angio GJ, Mike V, et al: Patterns of second malignant neoplasms in children. Cancer 1977;40:1903.

271. Nuutinen J, Karja J, Sainio P: Epithelial second malignant tumours in retinoblastoma survivors. A review and report of a case. Acta Ophthalmol (Copenh) 1982;60:133.

272. Ferlito A, Recher G, Tomazzoli L: Radiation-induced fibrosarcoma of the mandible following treatment for bilateral retinoblastoma. J Laryngol Otol 1979;93:1015.

273. Roarty JD, McLean IW, Zimmerman LE: Incidence of second neoplasms in patients with bilateral retinoblastoma. Ophthalmology 1988;95:1583.

274. Abramson DH, Frank CM: Second nonocular tumors in survivors of bilateral retinoblastoma: A possible age effect on radiation-related risk. Ophthalmology 1998;105:573.

275. Broughton WI, Zimmerman LE: A clinicopathologic study of 56 cases of intraocular medulloepitheliomas. Am J Ophthalmol 1978;85:407.

276. Carrillo R, Streeten BW: Malignant teratoid medulloepithelioma in an adult. Arch Ophthalmol 1979;97:695.

Specific Malignancies

III

Orbital Neoplasia

277. Mederios LJ, Harris NL: Lymphoid infiltrates of the orbit and conjunctiva: Z monoclonal antibody study. Ophthalmology 1986;93:1276.

278. Knowles DM, Jakobiec FA, McNally L, Burke JS: Lymphoid hyperplasia and malignant lymphoma occurring in the ocular adnexa (orbit, conjunctiva, and eyelids): A prospective multiparametric analysis of 108 cases during 1977 to 1987. Hum Pathol 1990;21:959.

279. Henderson JW, Campbell RJ, Farrow GM, et al: Orbital Tumors, 3rd ed. New York, Raven Press, 1993, p 279.

280. Bairey O, Kremer I, Rakowsky E, et al: Orbital and adnexal involvement in systemic non-Hodgkin's lymphoma. Cancer 1994;73: 2395.

281. White WL, Ferry JA, Harris NL, Grove AS Jr: Ocular adnexal lymphoma: A clinicopathologic study with identification of lymphomas of mucosa-associated lymphoid tissue type. Ophthalmology 1995;102:1994.

282. Hornblass A, Jakobiec FA, Riefler DM, et al: Orbital lymphoid tumors located predominantly within extraocular muscles. Ophthalmology 1987;94:688.

283. Yeo JH, Jakobiec FA, Abbott GF, Trokel SL: Combined clinical and computed tomographic diagnosis of orbital lymphoid tumors. Am J Ophthalmol 1982;94:235.

284. Stewart WB, Krohel GB, Wright JE: Lacrimal gland and fossa lesions: An approach to diagnosis and management. Ophthalmology 1979;86:886.

285. Wright JE, Stewart WB, Krohel GB: Clinical presentation and management of lacrimal gland tumors. Br J Ophthalmol 1979;63:600.

286. Benger RS, Frueh BR: Lacrimal drainage obstruction from lacrimal sac infiltration by lymphocytic neoplasia. Am J Ophthalmol 1986;101:242.

287. Knowles DM, Jakobiec FA: Orbital lymphoid neoplasms: A clinicopathologic study of 60 patients. Cancer 1980;46:576.

288. Polito E, Galieni P, Leccisotti A: Clinical and radiological presentation of 95 orbital lymphoid tumors. Graefes Arch Clin Exp Ophthalmol 1996;234:504.

289. Jakobiec FA, Yeo JH, Trokel SL, et al: Combined clinical and computed tomographic diagnosis of primary lacrimal fossa lesions. Am J Ophthalmol 1982;94:785.

290. Cockerham GC, Jacobiec FA: Lymphoproliferative disorders of the ocular adnexa. Int Ophthalmol Clin 1997;37:39.

291. Jakobiec FA, Iwamoto T, Patell M, et al: Ocular adnexal monoclonal lymphoid tumors with a favorable prognosis. Ophthalmology 1986;93:1547.

292. National Cancer Institute: National Cancer Institute sponsored study of classifications of non-Hodgkin's lymphomas: Summary and description of a working formulation for clinical usage. Cancer 1982;49:2112.

293. Reifler DM, Warzynski MJ, Blount WR, et al: Orbital lymphoma associated with acquired immunodeficiency syndrome (AIDS). Surv Ophthalmol 1994;38:371.

294. Hardman-Lea S, Kerr-Muir M, Wotherspoon AC, et al: Mucosal-associated lymphoid tissue lymphoma of the conjunctiva. Arch Ophthalmol 1994;112:1207.

295. Ferry JA, Yang WI, Zukerberg LR, et al: CD5+ extranodal marginal zone B-cell (MALT) lymphoma: A low grade neoplasm with a propensity for bone marrow involvement and relapse. Am J Clin Pathol 1996;105:31.

296. Ballesteros E, Osborne BM, Matsushima AY: CD5+ low-grade marginal zone B-cell lymphomas with localized presentation. Am J Surg Pathol 1998;22:201.

297. Jakobiec FA, Font RL: Lymphoid tumors. In Spencer WH (ed): Ophthalmic Pathology: An Atlas and Textbook, Vol 3. Philadelphia, WB Saunders, 1986, p 2663.

298. White V, Rootman J, Quenville N, et al: Orbital lymphoproliferative and inflammatory lesions. Can J Ophthalmol 1987;22:362.

299. Jakobiec FA, Iwamoto T, Knowles DM: Ocular adnexal lymphoid tumors: Correlative ultrastructural and immunologic marker studies. Arch Ophthalmol 1982;100:84.

300. Jakobiec FA, Neri A, Knowles DM: Genotypic monclonality in immunophenotypically polyclonal orbital lymphoid tumors: A new model of tumor progression in the lymphoid system. Ophthalmology 1987;94:980.

301. Rootman J, Patel S, Jewell L: Polyclonal orbital and systemic infiltrates. Ophthalmology 1984;91:1112.

302. Barthold HJ, Harvey A, Markee AM, et al: Treatment of orbital pseudotumors and lymphoma. Am J Clin Oncol 1986;9:527.

303. Mittal BB, Deutsch M, Kennerdell J, et al: Paraocular lymphoid tumors. Radiology 1986;159:793.

304. Kennerdell JS, Dresner SC: The nonspecific orbital inflammatory syndromes. Surv Ophthalmol 1984;29:93.

305. Maureillo JA, Flanagan JC: Pseudotumor and lymphoid tumor: Distinct clinicopathologic entities. Surv Ophthalmol 1989;34:142.

306. Polito E, Leccisotti A: Prognosis of orbital lymphoid hyperplasia. Graefes Arch Clin Exp Ophthalmol 1996;234:150.

307. Mederios LJ, Andrade RE, Harris NL, Cossman J: Lymphoid infiltrates of the orbit and conjunctiva: Comparison of immunologic and gene rearrangement data. Lab Invest 1989;60:624.

308. White VA, Gascoyne RD, McNeil BK, et al: Histopathologic findings and frequency of clonality detected by the polymerase chain reaction in ocular adnexal lymphoproliferative lesions. Mod Pathol 1996;9:1052.

309. McNally L, Jakobiec FA, Knowles DM: Clinical, morphologic, immunophenotypic, and molecular genetic analysis of bilateral ocular adnexal lymphoid neoplasma in 17 patients. Am J Ophthalmol 1987;103:555.

310. Smitt MC, Donaldson SS: Radiotherapy is successful treatment for orbital lymphoma. Int J Radiat Oncol Biol Phys 1993;26:59.

311. Chao CK, Lin HS, Devineni VR, Smith M: Radiation therapy for primary orbital lymphoma. Int J Radiat Oncol Biol Phys 1995;31:929.

312. Esik O, Ikeda H, Mukai K, Kaneko A: A retrospective analysis of different modalities for treatment of primary orbital non-Hodgkin's lymphomas. Radiother Oncol 1996;38:13.

313. Miller TP, Dahlbert S, Cassady JR, et al: Chemotherapy alone compared with chemotherapy plus radiotherapy for localized intermediate and high-grade non-Hodgkin's lymphoma. N Engl J Med 1998;339:21.

314. Bessell EM, Henk JM, Whitelocke RAF, et al: Ocular morbidity after radiotherapy of orbital and conjunctival lymphoma. Eye 1987;1:90.

315. Reddy EK, Bhatia P, Evans RG: Primary orbital lymphomas. Int J Radiat Oncol Biol Phys 1988;15:1239.

316. Antle CM, White VA, Horsman DE, Rootman J: Large cell orbital lymphoma in a patient with acquired immunodeficiency syndrome: Case report and review. Ophthalmology 1990;97:1494.

317. Brooks HL Jr, Downing J, McClure JA, et al: Orbital Burkitt's lymphoma in a homosexual man with acquired immune deficiency. Arch Ophthalmol 1984;102:1533.

318. Nadal D, Caduff R, Frey E, et al: Non-Hodgkin's lymphoma in four children infected with the human immunodeficiency virus. Cancer 1994;8:73:224.

319. Blakemore WS, Ehrenberg M, Fritz KJ, et al: Rapidly progressive proptosis secondary to Burkitt's lymphoma: Origin in the ethmoidal sinuses. Arch Ophthalmol 1983;101:1741.

320. Templeton AC: Orbital tumours in African children. Br J Ophthalmol 1971;55:254.

321. Jakobiec FA, Nelson D: Lymphomatous plasmacytic, histiocytic, and hematopoietic tumors of the orbit. In Tasman LI, Jaeger EA (eds): Duane's Clinical Ophthalmology, revised ed, Vol 2. Philadelphia, JB Lippincott, 1993, p 161.

322. Edelstein C, Shields JA, Shields CL, et al: Non-African Burkitt lymphoma presenting with oral thrush and an orbital mass in a child. Am J Ophthalmol 1997;124:859.

323. Lombardi L, Newcomb E, Dalla-Favera R: Pathogenesis of Burkitt lymphoma: Expression of an activated c-myc oncogene causes the tumorigenic conversion of EBV-infected human B lymphoblasts. Cell 1987;49:161.

324. Ziegler JL: Treatment results of 54 American patients with Burkitt's lymphoma are similar to the African experience. N Engl J Med 1977;297:75.

325. Meekins B, Proia AD, Klintworth GK: Cutaneous T-cell lymphoma presenting as a rapidly enlarging ocular adnexal tumor. Ophthalmology 1985;92:1288.

326. Lauer SA, Fischer J, Jones J, et al: Orbital T-cell lymphoma in human T-cell leukemia virus I infection. Ophthalmology 1988;95:110.

327. Henderson JW, Banks PM, Yeatts RP: T-cell lymphoma of the orbit. Mayo Clin Proc 1989;64:940.

328. Leidenix MJ, Mamalis N, Olson RJ, et al: Primary T-cell immuno-blastic lymphoma in a pediatric patient with a 2-week history of painless periorbital swelling. Ophthalmology 1993;100:998.

329. Stenson S, Ramsay DL: Ocular findings in mycosis fungoides. Arch Ophthalmol 1981;99:272.

330. Kremer I, Loven D, Mor C, Lurie H: A solitary conjunctival relapse of Hodgkin's disease treated by radiotherapy. Ophthalmol Surg 1989;20:494.

331. Fratkin JD, Shammas HF, Miller SD: Disseminated Hodgkin's disease with orbital involvement. Arch Ophthalmol 1978;96:102.

332. Sapozink MD, Kaplan HS: Intracranial Hodgkin's disease: A report of 12 cases and review of the literature. Cancer 1983;52:1301.

333. deSmet MD, Rootman J: Orbital manifestations of plasmacytic lymphoproliferations. Ophthalmology 1987;94:995.

334. Knapp AJ, Gartner S, Henkind P: Multiple myeloma and its ocular manifestations. Surv Ophthalmol 1987;31:343.

335. Jonasson F: Orbital plasma cell tumors. Ophthalmologica 1978;177:152.

336. Rootman J, Robertson W, Lapointe JS, et al: Plasma cell tumors. In Rootman J (ed): Diseases of the Orbit: A Multidisciplinary Approach. Philadelphia, JB Lippincott, 1988, p 216.

337. Gonnering RS: Bilateral primary extramedullary orbital plasmacytomas. Ophthalmology 1987;94:267.

338. Tung G, Finger PT, Klein I, Chess Q: Plasmacytoma of the orbit. Arch Ophthalmol 1988;106:1622.

339. Adkins JW, Shields JA, Shields CL, et al: Plasmacytoma of the eye and orbit. Int Ophthalmol 1996;20:339.

340. Howling SJ, Tighe J, Patterson K, Shaw P: Case report: The CT features of orbital multiple myeloma. Clin Radiol 1998;53:304.

341. Jampol LM, Marsh JC, Albert DM, et al: IgA associated lympho-plasmacytic tumor involving the conjunctiva, eyelid, and orbit. Am J Ophthalmol 1975;79:279.

342. Terasaki H, Kikuchi S, Hoshi S: Ophthalmic tumor formation in Waldenström's macroglobulinemia. Jpn J Ophthalmol 1996;40:385.

343. Jackson A, Kwartz J, Noble JL, Reagan GE: Inadequately irradiated solitary extramedullary plasmacytoma of the orbit requiring exenteration. Am J Ophthalmol 1995;120:803.

344. Krishnan K, Adams PT: Bilateral orbital tumors and lacrimal gland involvement on Waldenström's macroglobulinemia [letter]. Eur J Haematol 1995;55:205.

345. Pokorny G, Nemeth J, Marczinovits I, et al: Primary Sjögren's syndrome from the viewpoint of an internal physician. Int Ophthalmol 1991;15:401.

346. Font RL, Yanoff M, Zimmerman LE: Benign lymphoepithelial lesions of the lacrimal gland and its relationship to Sjögren's syndrome. Am J Clin Pathol 1967;48:365.

347. McCurley TL, Collins RD, Ball E, et al: Nodal and extranodal lymphoproliferative disorders in Sjögren's syndrome. Hum Pathol 1990;21:482.

348. Pepose JS, Akata RF, Pflugfelder SC, et al: Mononuclear cell phenotypes and immunoglobulin gene rearrangement in lacrimal gland biopsies from patients with Sjögren's syndrome. Ophthalmology 1990;97:1599.

349. Fishleder A, Tubbs R, Hesse B, et al: Uniform detection of immunoglobulin-gene rearrangement in benign lymphoepithelial lesions. N Engl J Med 1987;316:1118.

350. Wotherspoon AC, Diss TC, Pan LX, et al: Primary low-grade B-cell lymphoma of the conjunctiva: A mucosa-associated lymphoid tissue type lymphoma. Histopathology 1993;23:417.

351. Jakobiec FA, Font RL: Non-infectious orbital inflammation. In Spencer WH (ed): Ophthalmic Pathology: An Atlas and Textbook, Vol 3. Philadelphia, WB Saunders Co, 1986, p 2777.

352. Weissler MC, Miller E, Fortune MA: Sclerosing orbital pseudo-tumor: A unique clinicopathologic entity. Ann Otol Rhinol Laryngol 1989;98:496.

353. Cervellini P, Volpin L, Curri D, et al: Sclerosing orbital pseudotumor. Ophthalmologica 1986;193:39.

354. Abramovitz JN, Kasdon DL, Sutula F, et al: Sclerosing orbital pseudotumor CT demonstrating of extension beyond orbit. Neurosurgery 1983;12:463.

355. Frohman LP, Kupersmith MJ, Lang J, et al: Intracranial extension and bone destruction in orbital pseudotumor. Arch Ophthalmol 1986;104:380.

356. Comings DE, Skubi KB, van Eyes J, et al: Familial multifocal fibrosclerosis: Findings suggesting that retroperitoneal fibrosis, mediastinal fibrosis, sclerosing cholangitis, Riedel's thyroiditis, and pseudotumor may be different manifestations of a single disease. Ann Intern Med 1967;66:884.

357. Mottow LS, Jakobiec FA: Idiopathic inflammatory orbital pseudo-tumor in childhood. I: Clinical characteristics. Arch Ophthalmol 1978;96:1410.

358. Noguchi H, Kephart GM, Campbell J, et al: Tissue eosinophilia and eosinophil degranulation in orbital pseudotumor. Ophthalmology 1991;98:928.

359. Rootman J, Nugent R: The classification and management of acute orbital pseudotumors. Ophthalmology 1982;89:1040.

360. Weinstein GS, Dresner SC, Slamovits TL, et al: Acute and subacute orbital myositis. Am J Ophthalmol 1983;96:209.

361. Bullen CL, Younge BR: Chronic orbital myositis. Arch Ophthalmol 1982;100:1749.

362. Rush JA, Kennerdell JS, Donin JF: Acute periscleritis: A variant of idiopathic orbital inflammation. Orbit 1982;1:221.

363. Benson WE: Posterior scleritis. Surv Ophthalmol 1988;32:297.

364. Curtin HD: Pseudotumor. Radiol Clin North Am 1987;25:583.

365. Pillai P, Saini JS: Bilateral sino-orbital pseudotumor. Can J Ophthalmol 1988;23:177.

366. Braig RF, Romanchuk KG: Recurrence of orbital pseudotumor after 10 years. Can J Ophthalmol 1988;23:187.

367. Kennerdell JS: Management of nonspecific inflammatory and lymphoid orbital lesions. Int Ophthalmol Clin 1991;31:7.

368. Leone CR Jr, Lloyd WC III: Treatment protocol for orbital inflammatory disease. Ophthalmology 1985;92:1325.

369. Jakobiec FA, Jones IS: Idiopathic inflammatory pseudotumor. In Jones IS, Jakobiec FA (eds): Diseases of the Orbit. Hagerstown, Maryland, Harper & Row, 1979, p 187.

370. Diaz-Llopis M, Menezo JL: Idiopathic inflammatory orbital pseudotumor and low-dose cyclosporine. Am J Ophthalmol 1989;107:547.

371. Paris GL, Waltuch GF, Egbert PR: Treatment of refractory orbital pseudotumors with pulsed chemotherapy. Ophthal Plast Reconstr Surg 1990;6:96.

372. Font RL, Hidayat AA: Fibrous histiocytoma of the orbit. Hum Pathol 1982;13:199.

373. Croxatto JO, Font RL: Hemangiopericytoma of the orbit: A clinicopathologic study of 30 cases. Hum Pathol 1982;13:210.

374. Dorfman DM, To K, Dickersin GR, et al: Solitary fibrous tumor of the orbit. Am J Surg Pathol 1994;18:281.

375. Westra WH, Gerald WL, Rosai J: Solitary fibrous tumor: Consistent CD34 immunoreactivity and occurrence in the orbit. Am J Surg Pathol 1994;18:992.

376. Dei Tos AP, Seregard S, Calonje E, et al: Giant cell angiofibroma: A distincitive orbital tumor in adults. Am J Surg Pathol 1995;19:1286.

377. Jakobiec FA, Klapper D, Maher E, et al: Infantile subconjunctival and anterior orbital fibrous histiocytoma. Ophthalmology 1988;95:516.

378. Liu D, McCann P, Kini RK, et al: Malignant fibrous histiocytoma of the orbit in a 3-year-old girl. Arch Ophthalmol 1987;105:895.

379. Larkin DFP, O'Donoghue HN, Mullaney J, et al: Orbital fibrous histiocytoma in an infant. Acta Ophthalmol (Copenh) 1988;66:585.

380. Cole CH, Magee JF, Gianoulis M, Rogers PC: Malignant fibrous histiocytoma in childhood. Cancer 1993;71:4077.

381. Caballero LR, Rodriguez AC, Sopelana AB: Angiomatoid malignant fibrous histiocytoma of the orbit. Am J Ophthalmol 1981;92:13.

382. Ros PR, Kursunoglu S, Batlle JF, et al: Malignant fibrous histiocytoma of the orbit. J Clin Neuroophthalmol 1985;5:116.

383. Stewart WB, Newman NM, Cavender JC, et al: Fibrous histiocytoma metastatic to the orbit. Arch Ophthalmol 1978;96:871.

384. Lee JT, Pettit TH, Glasgow BJ: Epibulbar hemangiopericytoma. Am J Ophthalmol 1997;124:547.

385. Jakobiec FA, Howard G, Jones IS, Wolff M: Hemangiopericytoma of the orbit. Am J Ophthalmol 1974;78:816.

Specific Malignancies

III

386. Setzkorn RK, Lee DJ, Iliff NT, et al: Hemangiopericytoma of the orbit treated with conservative surgery and radiotherapy. Arch Ophthalmol 1987;105:1103.

387. Karcioglu ZA, Nasr AM, Haik BG: Orbital hemangiopericytoma: Clinical and morphologic features. Am J Ophthalmol 1997;123:661.

388. Panda A, Dayal Y, Singhal V, et al: Haemangiopericytoma. Br J Ophthalmol 1984;68:124.

389. Rice CD, Kersten RC, Mrak RE: An orbital hemangiopericytoma recurrent after 33 years. Arch Ophthalmol 1989;107:552.

390. Ganesan R, Hammond CJ, van der Walt JD: Giant cell angiofibroma of the orbit. Histopathology 1997;30:93.

391. Heathcote JG: Pathology update: Solitary fibrous tumour of the orbit. Can J Ophthalmol 1997;32:432.

392. Burnstine MA, Morton AD, Font RL, et al: Lacrimal gland hemangiopericytoma. Orbit 1998;17:179.

393. White VA, Heathcote JG, Hurwitz JJ, et al: Epithelioid sarcoma of the orbit. Ophthalmology 1994;101:1680.

394. Jakobiec FA, Depot MJ, Kennerdell JS, et al: Combined clinical and computed tomographic diagnosis of orbital glioma and meningioma. Ophthalmology 1984;91:137.

395. Levin LA, Jakobiec FA: Optic nerve tumors of childhood: A decision-analytical approach to their diagnosis. Int Ophthalmol Clin 1992;32:223.

396. Karp LA, Zimmerman LE, Borit A, et al: Primary intraorbital meningiomas. Arch Ophthalmol 1974;91:24.

397. Rose GE: Orbital meningiomas: Surgery, radiotherapy, or hormones? Br J Ophthalmol 1993;77:313.

398. Eggers H, Jakobiec FA, Jones IS: Tumors of the optic nerve. Doc Ophthalmol 1976;41:43.

399. Bynke H, Kagstrom E, Tjernstrom K: Aspects of the treatment of gliomas of the anterior visual pathway. Acta Ophthalmol 1977;55:269.

400. Wright JE: Primary optic nerve meningiomas: Clinical presentation and management. Trans Am Acad Ophthalmol Otolaryngol 1977;83:617.

401. Sibony PA, Krauss HR, Kennerdell JS, et al: Optic nerve sheath meningiomas: Clinical manifestations. Ophthalmology 1984;91:1313.

402. Wilson BW: Meningiomas of the anterior visual system. Surv Ophthalmol 1981;26:109.

403. Crisante L: Surgical treatment of meningiomas of the orbit and optic canal: A retrospective study. Acta Neurochir (Wien) 1994;126:27.

404. Grant FC, Hedges TR Jr: Ocular findings in meningiomas of the tuberculum sellae. Arch Ophthalmol 1956;56:163.

405. Barnes PR, Robson CD, Robertson RL, Poussaint TY: Pediatric orbital and visual pathway lesions. Neuroimag Clin North Am 1996;6:179.

406. Zimmerman CF, Schatz NJ, Glaser JS: Magnetic-resonance imaging of optic nerve meningiomas: Enhancement with gadolinium-DTPA. Ophthalmology 1990;97:585.

407. Alper MG: Management of primary optic nerve meningiomas: Current status therapy in controversy. J Clin Neuroophthalmol 1981;1:101.

408. Hansen-Knarhoi M, Poole MD: Preoperative difficulties in differentiating intraosseous meningiomas and fibrous dysplasia around the orbital apex. J Craniomaxillofac Surg 1994;22:226.

409. Artlich A, Schmidt D: Immunohistochemical profile of meningiomas and their histological subtypes. Hum Pathol 1990;21:843.

410. Kennerdell JS, Maroon JC, Malton M, et al: The management of optic nerve sheath meningiomas. Am J Ophthalmol 1988;106:450.

411. Lee AG, Woo SY, Miller NR, et al: Improvement in visual function in an eye with a presumed optic nerve sheath meningioma after treatment with three-dimensional conformal radiation therapy. J Neuroophthalmol 1996;16:247.

412. Stern EW: Meningiomas in the cranio-orbital junction. J Neurosurg 1973;38:428.

413. Verheggen R, Markakis E, Muhlendyck H, Finkenstaedt M: Symptomatology, surgical therapy and postoperative results of sphenoorbital, intraorbital-intracanalicular and optic nerve sheaths. Acta Neurochirurg 1996(Suppl);65:95.

414. Andrews BT, Wilson CB: Suprasellar meningiomas: The effect of tumor location on postoperative visual outcome. J Neurosurg 1988;69:523.

415. Rosenstein J, Symon L: Surgical management of suprasellar meningioma. Part 2: Prognosis for visual function following craniotomy. J Neurosurg 1984;61:642.

416. Wara WM, Sheline GE, Newman H, et al: Radiation therapy of meningiomas. AJR Radium Ther Nucl Med 1975;123:453.

417. Kupersmith MJ, Warren FA, Newall J, et al: Irradiation of meningiomas of the intracranial anterior visual pathway. Ann Neurol 1987;21:131.

418. Wan WL, Geller JL, Felden SE, et al: Visual loss caused by rapidly progressive intracranial meningiomas during pregnancy. Ophthalmology 1990;97:18.

419. Cahill DW, Bashirelahi N, Solomon LW, et al: Estrogen and progesterone receptors in meningiomas. J Neurosurg 1984;60:985.

420. Lesch KP, Fahlbusch R: Simultaneous estradiol and progesterone receptor analysis in meningiomas. Surg Neurol 1986;26:257.

421. Grunberg SM, Weiss MH, Spitz IM, et al: Treatment of unresectable meningiomas with the antiprogesterone agent mifepristone. J Neurosurg 1991;74:861.

422. Johnson TE, Weatherhead RG, Nasr AM, Siqueira EB: Ectopic (extradural) meningioma of the orbit: A report of two cases in children. J Pediatr Ophthalmol Strabismus 1993;30:43.

423. Spoor TC, Kennerdell JS, Martinez AJ, et al: Malignant gliomas of the optic nerve pathways. Am J Ophthalmol 1980;89:284.

424. Rudd A, Rees JE, Kennedy P, et al: Malignant optic nerve gliomas in adults. J Clin Neuroophthalmol 1985;5:238.

425. Manor RS, Israeli J, Sandbank U: Malignant optic glioma in a 70-year-old patient. Arch Ophthalmol 1976;94:1142.

426. Jakobiec FA, Font RL, Zimmerman LE: Malignant peripheral nerve sheath tumors of the orbit: A clinicopathologic study of eight cases. Trans Am Ophthalmol Soc 1985;83:332.

427. Lyons CJ, McNab AA, Garner A, et al: Orbital malignant peripheral nerve sheath tumours. Br J Ophthalmol 1989;73:731.

428. Ariza A, Bilbao JM, Rosai J: Immunohistochemical detection of epithelial membrane antigen in normal perineural cells and perineurioma. Am J Surg Pathol 1988;12:678.

429. Ezurum SA, Melen O, Lissner G, et al: Orbital malignant peripheral nerve sheath tumors. Treatment with surgical resection and radiation therapy. J Clin Neuroophthalmol 1993;12:1.

430. Morton AD, Elner VM, Frueh B: Recurrent orbital malignant peripheral nerve sheath tumor 18 years after initial resection. Ophthal Plast Reconstr Surg 1997;13:239.

431. Dutton JJ, Anderson RL, Schelper RL, et al: Orbital malignant melanoma and oculodermal melanocytosis: Report of two cases and review of the literature. Ophthalmology 1984;91:497.

432. Rice CD, Brown HH: Primary orbital melanoma associated with orbital melanocytosis. Arch Ophthalmol 1990;108:1130.

433. Tellada M, Specht CS, McLean IW, et al: Primary orbital tumors. Ophthalmology 1996;103:929.

434. Polito E, Leccisotti A: Primary and secondary orbital melanomas: A clinical and prognostic study. Ophthal Plast Reconstr Surg 1995;11:169.

435. Meekins BB, Dutton JJ, Proia AD: Primary orbital leiomyosarcoma: A case report and review of the literature. Arch Ophthalmol 1988;106:82.

436. Jakobiec FA, Howard GM, Rosen M, et al: Leiomyoma and leiomyosarcoma of the orbit. Am J Ophthalmol 1975;80:1028.

437. Font RL, Jurco S III, Brechner RJ: Postradiation leiomyosarcoma of the orbit complicating bilateral retinoblastoma. Arch Ophthalmol 1983;101:1557.

438. Folberg R, Cleasby G, Flanagan JA, et al: Orbital leiomyosarcoma after radiation therapy for bilateral retinoblastoma. Arch Ophthalmol 1983;101:1562.

439. Lane CM, Wright JE, Garner A: Primary myxoid liposarcoma of the orbit. Br J Ophthalmol 1988;72:912.

440. Jakobiec FA, Rini F, Char D, et al: Primary liposarcoma of the orbit: Problems in the diagnosis and management of five cases. Ophthalmology 1989;96:180.

441. McNab AA, Moseley I: Primary orbital liposarcoma: Clinical and computed tomographic features. Br J Ophthalmol 1990;74:437.

442. Sabb PC, Syed NA, Sires BS, et al: Primary orbital myxoid liposarcoma presenting as orbital pain. Arch Ophthalmol 1996;114:353.

443. Nasr AM, Ossoinig KC, Kersten RF, et al: Standardized echographic-histopathologic correlations in liposarcoma. Am J Ophthalmol 1985;99:193.

444. Font RL, Jurco S, Zimmerman LE: Alveolar soft part sarcoma of the orbit: A clinicopathologic analysis of seventeen cases and a review of the literature. Hum Pathol 1982;13:569.

445. Simmons WB, Haggerty HS, Ngan B, et al: Alveolar soft part sarcoma of the head and neck. A disease of children and young adults. Int J Pediatr Otorhinolaryngol 1989;17:139.

446. Henderson JW, Campbell RJ, Farrow GM, et al: Miscellaneous tumors. In Orbital Tumors, 3rd ed. New York, Raven Press, 1993, p 413.

447. Henderson JW, Campbell RJ, Farrow GM, et al: Orbital Tumors, 3rd ed. New York, Raven Press, 1993, p 171.

448. Bras J, Gillissen JPA, Koornneff L, et al: Extraskeletal myxoid chondrosarcoma of the orbit. Orbit 1985;4:189.

449. Shimo-Oku M, Okamoto N, Ogita Y, et al: A case of mesenchymal chondrosarcoma of the orbit. Acta Ophthalmol (Copenh) 1980;58:831.

450. Rohrbach JM, Steuhl KP, Pressler H, et al: Primary extraskeletal mesenchymal chondrosarcoma of the lid. Graefes Arch Clin Exp Ophthalmol 1991;229:172.

451. Rosenthal DL, Schiller AL, Mankin HJ: Chondrosarcoma: Correlation of radiological and histological grade. Radiology 1984;150:21.

452. Finn DG, Goepfer H, Batsakis JG: Chondrosarcoma of the head and neck. Laryngoscope 1984;94:1534.

453. Lauer SA, Friedland S, Goodrich JT, Dorfman H: Mesenchymal chondrosarcoma with secondary orbital invasion. Ophthal Plast Reconstr Surg 1995;1:182.

454. Henderson JW, Campbell RJ, Farrow GM, et al: Primary epithelial neoplasms. In Orbital Tumors, 3rd ed. New York, Raven Press, 1993, p 323.

455. Jakobiec FA, Font RL: Lacrimal gland tumors. In Spencer WG (ed): Ophthalmic Pathology: An Atlas and Textbook, Vol 3. Philadelphia, WB Saunders, 1986, p 2496.

456. Tong JT, Flanagan JC, Eagle RC Jr, Mazzoli RA: Benign mixed tumor arising from an accessory lacrimal gland of Wolfring. Ophthal Plast Reconstr Surg 1995;11:136.

457. Vangveeravong S, Katz SE, Rootman J, White V: Tumors arising in the palpebral lobe of the lacrimal gland. Ophthalmology 1996;103:1606.

458. Vangveeravong S, Katz SE, Rootman J, White V: Tumors arising in the palpebral lobe of the lacrimal gland. Ophthalmology 1996;103:1606.

459. Auran J, Jakobiec FA, Krebs W: Benign mixed tumor of the palpebral lobe of the lacrimal gland: Clinical diagnosis and appropriate surgical management. Ophthalmology 1988;95:90.

460. Parks SL, Glover AT: Benign mixed tumors arising in the palpebral lobe of the lacrimal gland. Ophthalmology 1990;97:526.

461. Shields JA, Shields CL: Malignant transformation of presumed pleomorphic adenoma of lacrimal gland after 60 years. Arch Ophthalmol 1987;105:1403.

462. Perzin KH, Jakobiec FA, Livolsi VA, et al: Lacrimal gland malignant mixed tumors (carcinomas arising in benign mixed tumors): A clinicopathologic study. Cancer 1980;45:2593.

463. Wright JE: Factors affecting the survival of patients with lacrimal gland tumours. Can J Ophthalmol 1982;17:3.

464. Jones IS: Surgical consideration in the management of lacrimal gland tumors. Clin Plast Surg 1978;5:561.

465. Shields JA, Shields CL, Eagle RC Jr, et al: Adenoid cystic carcinoma developing in the nasal orbit. Am J Ophthalmol 1997;123:398.

466. Font RL, Gamel JW: Adenoid cystic carcinoma of the lacrimal gland: A clinicopathologic study of 72 cases. In Nicholson DH (ed): Ocular Pathology Update. New York, Masson, 1980, p 277.

467. Zimmerman LE, Sanders TE, Ackerman LV: Epithelial tumors of the lacrimal gland: Prognostic and therapeutic significance of histologic types. Int Ophthalmol Clin 1962;2:337.

468. Janecka I, Housepian E, Trokel S, et al: Surgical management of malignant tumors of the lacrimal gland. Am J Surg 1984;148:539.

469. Lee JA, Wolter JR: A clinicopathologic study of primary adenoid cystic carcinomas of the lacrimal gland. Ophthalmology 1985;92:128.

470. Stewart WB, Krohel GB, Wright JE: Lacrimal gland and fossa lesions: An approach to diagnosis and management. Ophthalmology 1979;86:886.

471. Gamel JW, Font RL: Adenoid cystic carcinoma of the lacrimal gland: The clinical significance of basaloid histologic pattern. Hum Pathol 1982;13:219.

472. Lee DA, Campbell RJ, Waller RR, et al: A clinicopathologic study of primary adenoid cystic carcinoma of the lacrimal gland. Ophthalmology 1985;92:128.

473. Byers RM, Berkeley RG, Luna M, et al: Combined therapeutic approach to malignant lacrimal gland tumors. Am J Ophthalmol 1975;79:53.

474. Marsh JL, Wise MD, Smith M, et al: Lacrimal gland adenoid cystic carcinoma: Intracranial and extracranial en bloc resection. Plast Reconstr Surg 1981;68:577.

475. Gormley WB, Sekhar LN, Wright DC, et al: Management and long-term outcome of adenoid cystic carcinoma with intracranial extension: a neurological perspective. Neurosurgery 1996;38:1105.

476. Font RL, Gamel JW: Epithelial tumors of the lacrimal gland: An analysis of 265 cases. In Jakobiec FA (ed): Ocular and Adnexal Tumors. Birmingham, Alabama, Aesculapius, 1978, p 787.

477. Glover TA, Grove AS Jr: Orbital invasion by malignant eyelid tumors. Ophthal Plast Reconstr Surg 1989;5:1.

478. Csaky KG, Custer P: Perineural invasion of the orbit by squamous cell carcinoma. Ophthalmic Surg 1990;21:218.

479. Grove AS Jr: Staged excision and reconstruction of extensive facial-orbital tumors. Ophthalmic Surg 1977;8:91.

480. Rosen HM: Periorbital basal cell carcinoma requiring ablative craniofacial surgery. Arch Dermatol 1987;123:376.

481. Hornblass A, Roen JL: A combined facial, orbital and intracranial resection of extensive basal cell carcinoma arising in the eyelid. Ophthalmic Surg 1985;16:769.

482. Johnson TE, Tabbara KF, Weatherhead RG, et al: Secondary squamous cell carcinoma of the orbit. Arch Ophthalmol 1997;115:7508.

483. Fitzpatrick PJ, Thompson GA, Easterbrook WM, et al: Basal and squamous cell carcinoma of the eyelids and their treatment by radiotherapy. Int J Radiat Oncol Biol Phys 1984;10:449.

484. Luxenberg MN, Guthrie TH Jr: Chemotherapy of eyelid and periorbital tumors. Trans Am Ophthalmol Soc 1985;83:162.

485. Luxenberg MN, Guthrie TH Jr: Chemotherapy of basal cell and squamous cell carcinoma of the eyelids and periorbital tissues. Ophthalmology 1986;93:504.

486. Henderson JW, Campbell RJ, Farrow GM, et al: Secondary epithial neoplasms. In Orbital Tumors, 3rd ed. New York, Raven Press, 1993, p 343.

487. Johnson LN, Krohel GB, Yeon EB, et al: Sinus tumors invading the orbit. Ophthalmology 1984;91:209.

488. Weber AL, Stanton AC: Malignant tumors of the paranasal sinuses: Radiologic, clinical, and histopathologic evaluation of 200 cases. Otolaryngol Head Neck Surg 1984;6:761.

489. Gullane PJ, Conley J: Carcinoma of the maxillary sinus: A correlation of the clinical course with orbital involvement, pterygoid erosion of pterygopalatine invasion and cervical metastases. J Otolaryngol 1983;12:141.

490. Flores AD, Anderson DW, Doyle PJ, et al: Paranasal sinus malignancy: A retrospective analysis of treatment methods. J Otolaryngol 1987;13:141.

491. Conley J: The risk to the orbit in head and neck cancer. Laryngoscope 1985;95:515.

492. Graamans K, Slootweg PJ: Orbital exenteration in surgery of malignant neoplasms of the paranasal sinuses: The value of preoperative computed tomography. Arch Otolaryngol Head Neck Surg 1989;115:977.

493. Larson DL, Christ JE, Jesse RH: Preservation of the orbital contents in cancer of the maxillary sinus. Arch Otolaryngol 1982;108:370.

494. Perry C, Levine PA, Williamson BR, et al: Preservation of the eye in paranasal sinus cancer surgery. Arch Otolaryngol Head Neck Surg 1988;114:632.

495. McCary WS, Levine PA, Cantrell RW: Preservation of the eye in the treatment of sinonasal malignant neoplasms with orbital involvement: A confirmation of original use. Arch Otolaryngol Head Neck Surg 1996;122:657.

Specific Malignancies

496. Ascaso FJ, Adiego MI, Garcia J, et al: Sinonasal undifferentiated carcinoma involving the orbit. Eur J Ophthalmol 1994;4:234.

497. Al-Sarraf M, LeBlanc M, Giri PG, et al: Chemoradiotherapy versus radiotherapy in patients with advanced nasopharyngeal cancer: Phase III randomized Intergroup study 0099. J Clin Oncol 1998;16:1310.

498. Jakobiec FA, Rootman J, Jones IS: Secondary and metastatic tumors of the orbit. In Tasman W, Jaeger EA (eds): Duane's Clinical Ophthalmology, revised ed, Vol 2. Philadelphia, JB Lippincott, 1993.

499. Batsakis J: Tumors of the Head and Neck. Baltimore, Williams & Wilkins, 1974.

500. Elner VM, Burstine MA, Goodman ML, Dortzbach RK: Inverted papillomas that invade the orbit. Arch Ophthalmol 1995;113:1178.

501. Takagi M, Ishikawa G, More W: Primary malignant melanoma of the oral cavity in Japan: With special reference to mucosal melanosis. Cancer 1974;34:358.

502. Henderson JW, Campbell RJ, Farrow GM, et al: Orbital Tumors, 3rd ed. New York, Raven Press, 1993, p 193.

503. Weiss JS, Bressler SB, Jacobs EF, et al: Maxillary ameloblastoma with orbital invasion. Ophthalmology 1985;92:710.

504. Daramola JO, Abioye AA, Ajagbe AH, et al: Maxillary malignant ameloblastoma with intraorbital extension: Report of a case. J Oral Surg 1980;38:203.

505. Bredenkamp JK, Zimmerman MC, Mickel RA: Maxillary ameloblastoma: A potentially lethal neoplasm. Arch Otolaryngol Head Neck Surg 1989;115:99.

506. Komisar A: Plexiform ameloblastomas of the maxilla with extension to the skull base. Head Neck Surg 1984;7:172.

507. Kyriazis AP, Karkazis GC, Kriazis AA: Maxillary ameloblastoma with intracerebral extension. Oral Surg 1971;32:582.

508. Henderson JW, Campbell RJ, Farrow GM, et al: Orbital Tumors, 3rd ed. New York, Raven Press, 1993, p 377.

509. Maroon JC, Kennerdell JS, Vidovich DV, et al: Recurrent spheno-orbital meningioma. J Neurosurg 1994;80:202.

510. Kupersmith MJ, Warren FA, Newell J, et al: Irradiation of meningiomas of the intracranial anterior visual pathway. Ann Neurol 1987;21:131.

511. Pompili A, Calvosa F, Caroli F, et al: The transdural extension of gliomas. J Neurooncol 1993;15:67.

512. Rainov NG, Holzhausen HJ, Meyer H, Burkert W: Local invasivity of glioblastoma multiforme with destruction of skull bone: Case report and review of literature. Neurosurg Rev 1996;19:183.

513. Brandes A, Carollo C, Gardiman M, et al: Unusual nasal and orbital involvement of glioblastoma multiforme: A case report and review of the literature. J Neurooncol 1998;36:179.

514. Henderson JW, Campbell RJ, Farrow GM, et al: Orbital Tumors, 3rd ed. New York, Raven Press, 1993, p 182.

515. Ferry AP, Haddad HM, Goldman JL: Orbital invasion by an intracranial chordoma. Am J Ophthalmol 1991;92:7.

516. Kincaid MC, Green WR: Ocular and orbital involvement in leukemia. Surv Ophthalmol 1983;27:211.

517. Ginsberg J, Freemond AS, Calhoun JB: Optic nerve involvement in metastatic tumors. Ann Ophthalmol 1970;2:604.

518. Christmas NJ, Mead M, Richardson EP, Albert DM: Secondary optic nerve tumors. Surv Ophthalmol 1988;36:96.

519. Starr HJ, Zimmerman LE: Extrascleral extension and orbital recurrence of malignant melanomas of the choroid and ciliary body. Int Ophthalmol Clin 1962;2:369.

520. Shamms HF, Blodi FC: Orbital extension of choroidal and ciliary body melanomas. Arch Ophthalmol 1977;95:2002.

521. Hosten N, Bornfeld N, Wassmuth R, et al: Uveal melanoma: Detection of extraocular growth with MR imaging and US. Radiology 1997;202:61.

522. Ainbinder DJ, Haik BG, Frei DF, et al: Gadolinium enhancement: Improved MRI detection of retinoblastoma extension into the optic nerve. Neuroradiology 1996;38:778.

523. Affeldt JC, Minckler DS, Azen SP, Yeh L: Prognosis in uveal melanoma with extraocular extension. Arch Ophthalmol 1980; 98:1975.

524. Shields JA, Augsburger JJ, Corwin S, et al: The management of uveal melanomas with extrascleral extension. Orbit 1986;5:31.

525. Shields JA, Shields CT: Massive orbital extension of posterior uveal melanomas. Ophthal Plast Reconstr Surg 1991;7:238.

526. Rini FJ, Jakobiec FA, Hornblass A, et al: The treatment of advanced choroidal melanoma with massive orbital extension. Am J Ophthalmol 1987;104:634.

527. Kersten RC, Tse DT, Anderson RL, et al: The role of orbital exenteration in choroidal melanoma with extrascleral extension. Ophthalmology 1985;92:436.

528. Shields JA, Shields CL, Augsburger JJ, et al: Solitary metastasis of choroidal melanoma to contralateral eyelid. Ophthal Plast Reconstr Surg 1987;3:9.

529. Goldberg RA, Rootman J, Cline RA: Tumors metastatic to the orbit: A changing picture. Surv Ophthalmol 1990;35:1.

530. Henderson JW, Farrow GM: Metastatic carcinomas. In Henderson JW: Orbital Tumors, 2nd ed. New York, BC Decker, 1980, p 361.

531. Shields CL, Shields JA: Metastatic tumors to the orbit. Int Ophthalmol Clin 1993;33:189.

532. Goldberg RA, Rootman J: Clinical characteristics of metastatic orbital tumors. Ophthalmology 1990;97:620.

533. Healy JF: Computed tomographic evaluation of metastases to the orbit. Ann Ophthalmol 1983;15:1025.

534. Capone A Jr, Slamovits TL: Discrete metastasis of solid tumors to extraocular muscles. Arch Ophthalmol 1990;108:237.

535. Slamovits TL, Burde RM: Bumpy muscles. Surv Ophthalmol 1988;33:189.

536. Peyster RG, Shapiro MD, Haik BG: Orbital metastasis: Role of magnetic resonance imaging and computed tomography. Radiol Clin North Am 1987;25:647.

537. Shields CL, Shields JA, Peggs M: Tumors metastatic to the orbit. Ophthal Plast Reconstr Surg 1988;4:73.

538. Cline RA, Rootman J: Enophthalmos: A clinic review. Ophthalmology 1984;91:229.

539. Freedman MI, Folk JC: Metastatic tumors to the eye and orbit: Patient survival and clinical characteristics. Arch Ophthalmol 1987;105:1215.

540. Boldt HC, Nerad JA: Orbital metastases from prostate carcinoma. Arch Ophthalmol 1988;106:1403.

541. Riddle PJ, Font RL, Zimmerman LE: Carcinoid tumors of the eye and orbit: A clinicopathologic study of 15 cases with histochemical and electron microscopic observations. Hum Pathol 1982;13:459.

542. Loo KT, Tsui WM, Chung KH, et al: Hepatocellular carcinoma metastasizing to the brain and orbit: Report of three cases. Pathology 1994;26:119.

543. Tranfa F, Cennamo G, Rosa N, et al: An unusual orbital lesion: Hepatoma metastatic to orbit. Ophthalmologica 1994;208:329.

544. Fan JT, Buettner H, Bartley GB, Bolling JP: Clinical features and treatment of seven patients with carcinoid tumor metastatic to the eye and orbit. Am J Ophthalmol 1995;119:211.

545. Burnstine MA, Frueh BR, Elner VM: Angiosarcoma metastatic to the orbit. Arch Ophthalmol 1996;114:9306.

546. George DP, Zamber RW: Chondrosarcoma metastatic to the eye. Arch Ophthalmol 1996;114:349.

547. Kubota K, Furuse K, Kawahara M, et al: A case of malignant pleural mesothelioma with metastasis to the orbit. Jpn J Clin Oncol 1996;26:469.

548. Coupland SE, Sidiki S, Clark BJ, et al: Metastatic choroidal melanoma to the contralateral orbit 40 years after enucleation. Arch Ophthalmol 1996;114:751.

549. Rothfus WE, Curtin HD: Extraocular muscle enlargement: A CT review. Radiology 1984;151:677.

550. Mack HG, Jacobiec FA: Isolated metastases to the retina or optic nerve. Int Ophthalmol Clin 1997;37:251.

551. Kennerdell JS, Slamovits TL, Dekker A, et al: Orbital fine needle aspiration biopsy. Am J Ophthalmol 1985;99:547.

552. Krohel GB, Tobin DR, Chavis RM: Inaccuracy of fine needle aspiration biopsy. Ophthalmology 1985;92:666.

553. Glasburn JR, Klionsky M, Brady LW: Radiation therapy for metastatic diseases involving the orbit. Am J Clin Oncol 1984;7:145.

554. Wharam M, Beltangady M, Hays D, et al: Localized orbital rhabdomyosarcoma: An interim report of the Intergroup Rhabdomyosarcoma Study Committee. Ophthalmology 1987;94:251.

555. Kodsi SR, Shetlar DJ, Campbell RJ, et al: A review of 340 orbital tumors in children during a 60-year period. Am J Ophthalmol 1994;117:177.

556. Henderson JW, Campbell RJ, Farrow GM, et al: Tumors of primitive mesoderm, smooth muscle, and adipose tissue. In Orbital Tumors, 3rd ed. New York, Raven Press, 1993, p 201.

557. Knowles DM II, Jakobiec FA, Potter GE, et al: The diagnosis and treatment of rhabdomyosarcoma of the orbit. In Jakobiec FA (ed): Ocular and Adnexal Tumors. Birmingham, Alabama, Aesculapius, 1978.

558. Haik BG, Jereb B, Smith ME, et al: Radiation and chemotherapy of parameningeal rhabdomyosarcoma involving the orbit. Ophthalmology 1986;93:1001.

559. Cameron D, Wick MR: Embryonal rhabdomyosarcoma of the conjunctiva. Arch Ophthalmol 1986;104:1203.

560. Ellsworth RM: Discussion. Ophthalmology 1987;94:254.

561. Maurer HM, Moon T, Donaldson M, et al: The intergroup rhabdomyosarcoma study: A preliminary report. Cancer 1977;40:2015.

562. Maurer HM: The Intergroup Rhabdomyosarcoma Study: Update, November 1978. Natl Cancer Inst Monogr 1981;56:61.

563. Tsokos M, Webber BL, Parham DM, et al: Rhabdomyosarcoma: A new classification scheme related to prognosis. Arch Pathol Lab Med 1992;116:847.

564. Dehner LP: Favorable versus unfavorable histologic appearance: The lexicon of pathologic grading of solid malignant neoplasms in children. Arch Pathol Lab Med 1992;116:817.

565. Azumi N, Ben-Ezra J, Battifora H: Immunophenotypic diagnosis of leiomyosarcomas and rhabdomyosarcomas with monoclonal antibodies to muscle-specific actin and desmin in formalin-fixed tissue: A clinicopathologic and immunohistochemical study. Mod Pathol 1988;1:469.

566. Altmannsberger M, Weber K, Droste R, et al: Desmin is a specific marker for rhabdomyosarcomas of human and rat origin. Am J Pathol 1985;118:85.

567. Newton WA, Soule EH, Hamoudi AB, et al: Histopathology of childhood sarcomas, Intergroup Rhabdomyosarcoma Studies I and II: Clinicopathologic correlation. J Clin Oncol 1988;6:67.

568. Abramson DH, Ellsworth RM, Tretter P, et al: The treatment of orbital rhabdomyosarcoma with irradiation and chemotherapy. Ophthalmology 1979;86:1330.

569. Heyn R, Raagab A, Raney RBJ, et al: Late effects of therapy in orbital rhabdomyosarcoma in children: A report from the intergroup rhabdomyosarcoma study. Cancer 1986;57:1738.

570. Abramson DH, Notis CM: Visual acuity after radiation for orbital rhabdomyosarcoma. Am J Ophthalmol 1994;118:808.

571. Alvarez Silvan AM, Garcia Canton JA, Pineda Cuevas G, Alfuro Gutierrez J: Successful treatment of orbital rhabdomyosarcoma in two infants using chemotherapy alone. Med Pediatr Oncol 1996;26:186.

572. Rousseau P, Flamant F, Quintana E, et al: Primary chemotherapy in rhabdomyosarcomas and other malignant mesenchymal tumors of the orbit: Results of the International Society of Pediatric Oncology MMT 84 Study. J Clin Oncol 1994;12:516.

573. Notis CM, Abramson DH, Sagerman RH, Ellsworth RM: Orbital rhabdomyosarcoma: Treatment or overtreatment. Ophthalmic Genet 1995;16:159.

574. Chestler FJ, Dorthzbach RK, Kronish JW: Late recurrence in primary orbital rhabdomyosarcoma [letter]. Am J Ophthalmol 1988;106:92.

575. Zimmerman LE, Font RL: Ophthalmic manifestations of granulocytic sarcoma (myeloid sarcoma or chloroma). Am J Ophthalmol 1975;9:975.

576. Davis JL, Parke DW, Font RL: Granulocytic sarcoma of the orbit. Ophthalmology 1985;92:1758.

577. Stockl FA, Dolmetsch AM, Saornil MA, et al: Orbital granulocytic sarcoma. Br J Ophthalmol 1997;81:1084.

578. Jordan DR, Neel LP, Carpenter BF: Chloroma. Arch Ophthalmol 1991;109:734.

579. Watkins LM, Remulla HD, Rubin PA: Orbital granulocytic sarcoma in an elderly patient. Am J Ophthalmol 1997;123:854.

580. Rubinfeld RS, Gootenberg JE, Chavis RM, et al: Early onset acute orbital involvement in childhood acute lymphoblastic leukemia. Ophthalmology 1988;95:116.

581. Skinnider LF, Romanchuk KG: Orbital involvement in chronic lymphocytic leukemia. Can J Ophthalmol 1984;19:142.

582. Weiner JM, Hidayat AA: Juvenile fibrosarcoma of the orbit and eyelid: A study of five cases. Arch Ophthalmol 1983;101:253.

583. Henderson JW, Campbell RJ, Farrow GM, et al: Fibrous connective tissue tumors. In Orbital Tumors, 3rd ed. New York, Raven Press, 1993, p 138.

584. Yanoff M, Scheie HG: Fibrosarcoma of the orbit: Report of two patients. Cancer 1966;19:1711.

585. Henderson JW, Campbell RJ, Farrow GM, et al: Orbital Tumors, 3rd ed. New York, Raven Press, 1993, p 165.

586. Benedict WF, Fung YK, Murphree AL: The gene responsible for the development of retinoblastoma and osteosarcoma. Cancer 1988;8(Suppl 62):1691.

587. Dryja TP, Rapaport JM, Epstein J, et al: Chromosome 13 homozygosity in osteosarcoma without retinoblastoma. Am J Hum Genet 1986;38:59.

588. Hansen MF, Koufos A, Gallie BL, et al: Osteosarcoma and retinoblastoma: A shared chromosomal mechanism revealing recessive predisposition. Proc Natl Acad Sci USA 1985;82:6216.

589. Lueder GT, Judisch GF, O'Gorman TW: Second nonocular tumors in survivors of heritable retinoblastoma. Arch Ophthalmol 1986;104:372.

590. Epley KD, Lasky JB, Karesh JW: Osteosarcoma of the orbit associated with Paget disease. Ophthal Plast Reconstr Surg 1998;14:62.

591. Fu YS, Perzin KH: Non-epithelial tumors of the nasal cavity, paranasal sinuses, and nasopharynx: A clinicopathologic study. II. Osseous and fibro-osseous lesions, including osteoma, fibrous dysplasia, ossifying fibroma, osteoblastoma, giant cell tumors, and osteosarcoma. Cancer 1974;3:1289.

592. Blodi FC: Pathology of orbital bones. Am J Ophthalmol 1976;81:1.

593. Katz NNK, Ruymann FB, Margo CE, et al: Endodermal sinus tumor (yolk sac carcinoma) of the orbit. J Pediatr Ophthalmol Strabismus 1983;19:270.

594. Margo CE, Folberg R, Zimmerman L, et al: Endodermal sinus tumor (yolk sac carcinoma) of the orbit. Ophthalmology 1983; 90:1426.

595. Roth A, Iris L: Tumeur du sac vitellin, de localisation primitive orbitaire. Ann Pediatr (Paris) 1984;31:693.

596. Kivela T, Tarkkanen A: Orbital germ cell tumors revisited: A clinicopathological approach to classification. Surv Ophthalmol 1994;38:541.

597. Porterfield JF: Orbital tumors in children: A report on 214 cases. Int Ophthalmol Clin 1962;2:319.

598. Pascual-Castroviejo I, Martinez Bermejo A, Lopez Martin V, et al: Optic gliomas in neurofibromatosis type 1 (NF-1): Presentation of 31 cases. Neurologica 1994;9:173.

599. Charles NC, Nelson L, Brookner AR, et al: Pilocytic astrocytoma of the optic nerve with hemorrhage and extreme cystic degeneration. Am J Ophthalmol 1981;92:691.

600. Buchanan TAS, Hoyt WF: Optic nerve glioma and neovascular glaucoma: Report of a case. Br J Ophthalmol 1982;66:96.

601. Lewis RA, Gerson LP, Axelson KA, et al: Von Recklinghausen neurofibromatosis. II. Incidence of optic gliomata. Ophthalmology 1984;91:929.

602. Holman RE, Grimson BS, Drayer BP, et al: Magnetic resonance imaging of optic nerve gliomas. Am J Ophthalmol 1985;100:596.

603. Haik BG, Saint Louis L, Bierly J, et al: Magnetic resonance imaging in the evaluation of optic nerve gliomas. Ophthalmology 1987;94:709.

604. Imes RK, Hoyt WF: Magnetic resonance imaging signs of optic nerve gliomas in neurofibromatosis 1. Am J Ophthalmol 1991;111:729.

605. Cooling RJ, Wright JE: Arachnoid hyperplasia in optic nerve glioma: Confusion with orbital meningioma. Br J Ophthalmol 1979;63:596.

606. Zimmerman L: Arachnoid hyperplasia in optic nerve glioma. Br J Ophthalmol 1980;64:638.

607. Goldman JE, Corbin E: Rosenthal fibers contain ubiquitinated alpha B-crystallin. Am J Pathol 1991;139:933.

608. Anderson DR, Spencer WH: Ultrastructural and histochemical observations of optic nerve gliomas. Arch Ophthalmol 1970;83:324.

609. Hoyt WF, Baghdassarian SA: Optic glioma of childhood: Natural history and rationale for conservative management. Br J Ophthalmol 1969;53:793.

610. Stern J, Jakobiec FA, Housepian EM: The architecture of optic nerve gliomas with and without neurofibromatosis. Arch Ophthalmol 1980;98:505.

611. Alvord EC Jr, Lofton S: Gliomas of the optic nerve or chiasm: Outcome by patients' age, tumor site, and treatment. J Neurosurg 1988;68:85.

612. Imes RK, Hoyt WF: Childhood chiasmal gliomas: Update on the fate of patients in the 1969 San Francisco Study. Br J Ophthalmol 1986;70:179.

613. Fletcher WA, Imes RK, Hoyt WF: Chiasmal gliomas: Appearance and long-term changes demonstrated by computerized tomography. J Neurosurg 1986;65:154.

614. Rush JA, Younge BR, Campbell RJ, et al: Optic glioma. Long-term follow-up of 85 histopathologically verified cases. Ophthalmology 1982;89:1213.

615. Miller NR, Iliff WJ, Green WR: Evaluation and management of gliomas of the anterior visual pathways. Brain 1974;97:743.

616. Thompson CR, Lessell S: Anterior visual pathway gliomas. Int Ophthalmol Clin 1997;37:261.

617. Henderson JW, Campbell RJ, Farrow GM, et al: Miscellaneous tumors of presumed neuroepithelial origin. In Orbital Tumors, 3rd ed. New York, Raven Press, 1993, p 244.

618. Kun LE, Mulhern RK, Crisco JJ: Quality of life in children treated for brain tumors: intellectual, emotional, and academic function. J Neurosurg 1983;58:1.

619. Giuffre R, Bardelli AM, Taverniti L, et al: Anterior optic pathways gliomas: The dilemma of treatment. J Neurosurg Sci 1982;26:61.

620. McFadzean RM, Brewin TB, Doyle D, et al: Glioma of the optic chiasm and its management. Trans Ophthalmol Soc U K 1983;103:199.

621. Glaser JS, Hoyt WF, Corbett J: Visual morbidity with chiasmal glioma: Long-term studies of visual fields in untreated and irradiated cases. Arch Ophthalmol 1971;85:3.

622. Packer RJ, Savino PJ, Bilaniuk LT, et al: Chiasmatic gliomas of childhood: A reappraisal of natural history and effectiveness of cranial irradiation. Childs Brain 1983;10:393.

623. Packer RJ, Sutton LN, Bilaniuk LT, et al: Treatment of chiasmatic-hypothalamic gliomas of childhood with chemotherapy: An update. Ann Neurol 1988;23:79.

624. Char DH, Ablin A, Beckstead J: Histiocytic disorders of the orbit. Ann Ophthalmol 1984;16:867.

625. MacCumber MW, Hoffman PN, Wand GS, et al: Ophthalmic involvement in aggressive histiocytosis X. Ophthalmology 1990;97:22.

626. Henderson JW, Campbell RJ, Farrow GM, et al: Histiocytic disorders. In Orbital Tumors, 3rd ed. New York, Raven Press, 1993, p 309.

627. Moore AT, Pritchard J, Taylor DSI: Histiocytosis X: An ophthalmological review. Br J Ophthalmol 1985;69:7.

628. Feldman RB, Moore DM, Hood CI, et al: Solitary eosinophilic granuloma of the lateral orbital wall. Am J Ophthalmol 1985;100:318.

629. Jakobiec FA, Trokel SL, Aron-Rosa D, et al: Localized eosinophilic granuloma (Langerhans' cell histiocytosis) of the orbital frontal bone. Arch Ophthalmol 1980;98:1814.

630. Nolph MB, Luikin GA: Histiocytosis X. Otolaryngol Clin North Am 1982;15:635.

631. Favara BE, McCarthy RC, Mierau GW: Histiocytosis X. Hum Pathol 1983;14:663.

632. Fartasch M, Vigneswaran N, Diepgen TL, et al: Immunohisto-chemical and ultrastructural study of histiocytosis X and non-X histiocytosis. J Am Acad Dermatol 1990;23:885.

633. Harnett AN, Doughty D, Hirst A, et al: Radiotherapy in benign orbital disease. II: ophthalmic Graves' disease and orbital histiocytosis X. Br J Ophthalmol 1988;72:289.

634. Cohen M, Zornoza J, Cangir A, et al: Direct injection of methylprednisolone sodium succinate in the treatment of solitary eosinophilic granuloma of the bone: A report of 9 cases. Radiology 1980;136:289.

635. Wirtschafer JD, Nesbit M, Anderson P, et al: Intralesional methylprednisolone for Langerhans' cell histiocytosis of the orbit and cranium. J Pediatr Ophthalmol Strabismus 1987;24:194.

636. Glover AT, Grove AS Jr: Eosinophilic granuloma of the orbit with spontaneous healing. Ophthalmology 1987;94:1008.

637. Sommer JE, Marre E: Spontanecheilung beim Eosinophen Granulom der orbita. Folia Ophthalmol 1979;4:116.

638. Tsuda N, Takaku I: A case report of malignant vascular tumor of the orbit in a newborn infant. Folia Ophthalmol Jpn 1970;21:728.

639. Hufnagel T, Ma L, Kuo TT: Orbital angiosarcoma with subconjunctival presentation: Report of a case and literature review. Ophthalmology 1987;94:72.

640. Shields JA: Vasculogenic tumors and malformations. In Shields JA (ed): Diagnosis and Management of Orbital Tumors. Philadelphia, WB Saunders, 1989, p 132.

641. Rakes SM, Yeatts RP, Campbell RJ: Ophthalmic manifestations of esthesioneuroblastoma. Ophthalmology 1985;92:1749.

642. Mills SE, Frierson HF Jr: Olfactory neuroblastoma: A clinicopathologic study of 21 cases. Am J Surg Pathol 1985;9:317.

643. Valles San Leandro L, Arcas Martinez-Slaas I, Villegas Perez MP, et al: Esthesioneuroblastoma: An atypical form of manifestation. Eur J Ophthalmol 1994;4:118.

644. Bobele GB, Sexauer C, Barnes PA, et al: Esthesioneuroblastoma presenting as an orbital mass in a young child. Med Pediatr Oncol 1994;22:269.

645. Regenbogen VS, Zinreich SJ, Kim KS, et al: Hyperostotic esthesioneuroblastoma: CT and MR findings. J Comput Assist Tomogr 1988;12:52.

646. Axe S, Kuhajda FP: Esthesioneuroblastoma: Intermediate filaments, neuroendocrine, and tissue-specific antigens. Am J Clin Pathol 1987;88:139.

647. McCaffrey TV, Olsen KD, Yohanan JM, et al: Factors affecting survival of patients with tumors of the anterior skull base. Laryngoscope 1994;104:940.

648. Lamping KA, Albert DM, Lack E, et al: Melanotic neuroectodermal tumor of infancy (retinal anlage tumor). Ophthalmology 1985;92:143.

649. Hall WC, O'Day DM, Glick AD: Melanotic neuroectodermal tumor of infancy: An ophthalmic appearance. Arch Ophthalmol 1979;97:922.

650. Singh AD, Husson M, Shields CL, et al: Primitive neuroectodermal tumor of the orbit. Arch Ophthalmol 1994;112:217.

651. Kovanlikaya A, Nelson MD Jr, Murphree AL: Radiological case of the month: Retinoblastoma presenting with orbital cellulitis. Arch Pediatr Adolesc Med 1996;150:873.

652. Foster BS, Mukai S: Intraocular retinoblastoma presenting as ocular and orbital inflammation. Int Ophthalmol Clin 1996;36:153.

653. Ellsworth RM: Orbital retinoblastoma. Trans Am Ophthalmol Soc 1974;72:79.

654. Rootman J, Ellsworth RM, Hofbauer J, et al: Orbital extension of retinoblastoma: A clinicopathological study. Can J Ophthalmol 1978;13:72.

655. Kopelman JE, McLean IW, Rosenberg PH: Multivariate analysis of risk factors for metastasis in retinoblastoma. Ophthalmology 1987;94:371.

656. Doz F, Khelfaoui F, Mosseri V, et al: The role of chemotherapy in orbital involvement of retinoblastoma: The experience of a single institution with 33 patients. Cancer 1994;74:722.

657. Kiratli H, Bilgic S, Ozerdem U: Management of massive orbital involvement of intraocular retinoblastoma. Ophthalmology 1998;105:322.

658. Redler LD, Ellsworth RM: Prognostic importance of choroidal invasion in retinoblastoma. Arch Ophthalmol 1973;90:294.

659. Henderson JW, Campbell RJ, Farrow GM, et al: Miscellaneous tumors of presumed neuroepithelial origin. In Orbital Tumors, 3rd ed. New York, Raven Press, 1993, p 252.

660. Rootman J: Secondary tumors of the orbit. In Rootman J (ed): Diseases of the Orbit: A Multidisciplinary Approach. Philadelphia, JB Lippincott, 1988, p 427.

661. Musarella MA, Chan HSL, DeBoer G, et al: Ocular involvement in neuroblastoma: Prognostic implications. Ophthalmology 1984;91:936.

662. Bohdiewicz PJ, Gallegos E, Fink-Bennett D: Raccoon eyes and the MIBG super scan: Scintigraphic signs of neuroblastoma in a case of child abuse. Pediatr Radiol 1995;25(Suppl 1):S90-92.

663. Gallet BL, Egelhoff JC: Unusual CNS and orbital metastases of neuroblastoma. Pediatr Radiol 1989;19:287.

664. Enzinger FM, Weiss SW: Soft Tissue Tumors, 2nd ed. St. Louis, Mosby, 1988, p 816.

665. Finklestein JZ: Neuroblastoma: The challenge and frustration. Hematol Oncol Clin North Am 1987;1:675.

666. Wilkins RM, Pritchard DJ, Burgert EO Jr, et al: Ewing's sarcoma of bone: Experience with 140 patients. Cancer 1986;58:2551.

667. Albert DM, Rubenstein RA, Scheie HG: Tumor metastases to the eye. Am J Ophthalmol 1967;63:727.

668. Alvarez-Berdecia A, Schut L, Bruce DA: Localized primary intracranial Ewing's sarcoma of the orbital roof: Case report. J Neurosurg 1979;50:811.

669. Woodruff G, Thorner P, Skarf B: Primary Ewing's sarcoma of the orbit presenting with visual loss. Br J Ophthalmol 1988;72:786.

670. Lim TC, Tan WT, Lee YS: Congenital extraskeletal Ewing's sarcoma of the face: A case report. Head Heck 1994;16:75.

671. Horowitz ME, Tsokos MG, DeLaney TF: Ewing's sarcoma. Cancer J Clin 1992;42:300.

672. Fratkin JD, Purcell JJ, Krachmer JH, et al: Wilms' tumor metastatic to the orbit. JAMA 1977;238:1841.

673. D'Angio GJ: Oncology seen through the prism of Wilms' tumor. Med Pediatr Oncol 1985;13:53.

674. Barnes PD, Robson CD, Robertson RL, Poussaint TY: Pediatric orbital and visual pathway lesions. Neuroimaging Clin North Am 1996;6:179.

675. Fekrat S, Miller NR, Loury MC: Alveolar rhabdomyosarcoma that metastasized to the orbit. Arch Ophthalmol 1993;111:1662.

Neoplasia of the Eyelid and Conjunctiva

676. Loeffler M, Hornblass A: Characteristics and behavior of eyelid carcinoma (basal cell, squamous cell, sebaceous gland and malignant melanoma). Ophthalmic Surg 1990;21:513.

677. Doxanas MT, Green WR, Iliff CE: Factors in the successful surgical management of basal cell carcinoma in the eyelid. Am J Ophthalmol 1981;91:726.

678. Payne JW, Duke JR, Butner R, et al: Basal cell carcinoma of the eyelids: A long-term follow-up study. Arch Ophthalmol 1969;81:553.

679. Beard C: Observations on the treatment of basal cell carcinoma of the eyelids. Trans Am Acad Ophthalmol Otolaryngol 1975;79:664.

680. Lever WF, Schaumburg-Lever G: Histopathology of the Skin, 7th ed. Philadelphia, JB Lippincott, 1990.

681. Robins P, Rodriguez-Sains R, Rabinovitz H, et al: Mohs' surgery for periocular basal cell carcinomas. J Dermatol Surg Oncol 1985;11:1203.

682. Baylis HI, Cies WA: Complications of Mohs' chemosurgical excision of eyelid and canthal tumors. Am J Ophthalmol 1975;80:116.

683. Mohs FE: Micrographic surgery for the microscopically controlled excision of eyelid cancers. Arch Ophthalmol 1986;104:901.

684. Wiggs EO: Morpheaform basal cell carcinomas of the canthi. Trans Am Acad Ophthalmol Otolaryngol 1975;79:649.

685. Beard C: Management of malignancy of the eyelids. Am J Ophthalmol 1981;92:1.

686. Schlienger P, Brunin F, Desjardins L, et al: External radiotherapy for carcinoma of the eyelid: Report of 850 cases treated. Int J Radiat Oncol Biol Phys 1996;34:277.

687. Gladstein AH: Efficacy, simplicity, and safety of x-ray therapy of basal cell carcinomas on periocular skin. J Dermatol Surg Oncol 1978;4:586.

688. Margo CE, Waltz K: Basal cell carcinoma of the eyelid and periocular skin. Surv Ophthalmol 1993;38:169.

689. Tuppurainen K: Cryotherapy for eyelid and periocular basal cell carcinomas: Outcome in 166 cases over an 8-year period. Graefes Arch Clin Exp Ophthalmol 1995;233:205.

690. Font RL: Eyelids and lacrimal drainage system. In Spencer WH (ed): Ophthalmic Pathology: An Atlas and Textbook, Vol 3. Philadelphia, WB Saunders, 1986, p 2141.

691. Doxanas MT, Iliff WJ, Iliff NT, et al: Squamous cell carcinoma of the eyelids. Ophthalmology 1987;94:538.

692. Moller R, Reymann F, Hou-Jensen K: Metastases in dermatological patients with squamous cell carcinoma. Arch Dermatol 1979;115:703.

693. Lee MM, Wick MM: Bowen's disease. Cancer 1990;40:237.

694. Fraunfelder FT, Zacarian SA, Limmer BL, Wingfield D: Cryosurgery for malignancies of the eyelid. Ophthalmology 1980;87:461.

695. Reifler DM, Hornblass A: Squamous cell carcinoma of the eyelid. Surv Ophthalmol 1986;30:349.

696. Aubry F, MacGibbon B: Risk factors of squamous cell carcinoma of the skin: A case-control study in the Montreal region. Cancer 1985;55:907.

697. Glass AG, Hoover RN: The emerging epidemic of melanoma and squamous cell skin cancer. JAMA 1989;262:2097.

698. Stern RS, Lange R: Non-melanoma skin cancer occurring in patients treated with PUVA five to ten years after treatment. J Invest Dermatol 1988;91:120.

699. Hueper WC: Chemically induced skin cancers in man. Natl Cancer Inst Monogr 1963;10:377.

700. Neubauer O: Arsenical cancer: A review. Br J Cancer 1947;1:192.

701. Rao NA, Dunn SA, Romero JL, et al: Bilateral carcinomas of the eyelid. Am J Ophthalmol 1986;101:480.

702. Kraemer KH, Lee MM, Scotto J: Xeroderma pigmentosum: Cutaneous, ocular, and neurologic abnormalities in 830 published cases. Arch Dermatol 1987;123:241.

703. Trobe JD, Hood I, Parsons JT, et al: Intracranial spread of squamous carcinoma along the trigeminal nerve. Arch Ophthalmol 1982; 100:608.

704. Friedman HI, Cooper PH, Wanebo HJ: Prognostic and therapeutic use of microstaging of cutaneous squamous cell carcinoma of the trunk and extremities. Cancer 1985;56:1099.

705. Mohs FE: Chemosurgical treatment of cancer of the eyelid: A microscopically controlled method of excision. Arch Ophthalmol 1948;39:43.

706. Shields JA: Diagnosis and Management of Orbital Tumors. Philadelphia, WB Saunders, 1989, p 340.

707. Glover AT, Grove AS Jr: Orbital invasion by malignant eyelid tumors. Ophthal Plast Reconstr Surg 1989;5:1.

708. Fraunfelder FT, Zacarian SA, Wingfield DL, Limmer BL: Results of cryotherapy for eyelid malignancies. Am J Ophthalmol 1984;97:184.

709. Lederman M: Radiation treatment of cancer of the eyelids. Br J Ophthalmol 1976;60:794.

710. Guthrie TH Jr, McElveen LJ, Porubsky ES, Harmon JD: Cisplatin and doxorubicin: An effective chemotherapy combination in the treatment of advanced basal cell and squamous carcinoma of the skin. Cancer 1985;55:1629.

711. Erie JC, Campbell RJ, Liesegang TJ: Conjunctival and corneal intraepithelial and invasive neoplasia. Ophthalmology 1986;93:176.

712. Waring GO III, Roth AM, Ekins MB, et al: Clinical and pathologic description of 17 cases of corneal intraepithelial neoplasia. Am J Ophthalmol 1984;97:547.

713. Muccioli C, Belfort R Jr, Burnier M, Rao N: Squamous cell carcinoma of the conjunctiva in a patient with the acquired immunodeficiency syndrome. Am J Ophthalmol 1996;121:94.

714. Karp CL, Scott IU, Chang TS, Pflugfeldder SC: Conjunctival intraepithelial neoplasia: A possible marker for human immunodeficiency virus infection? Arch Ophthalmol 1996; 114:257.

715. Buus DR, Tse DT, Folberg R: Microscopically controlled excision of conjunctival squamous cell carcinoma. Am J Ophthalmol 1994;117:551.

716. Copeland RA Jr, Char DH: Limbal autograft reconstruction after conjunctival squamous cell carcinoma. Am J Ophthalmol 1990;110:412.

717. Lommatzsch P: Beta-ray treatment of malignant epithelial tumors of the conjunctiva. Am J Ophthalmol 1976;81:198.

718. Fraunfelder FT, Wingfield D: Management of intraepithelial conjunctival tumors and squamous cell carcinomas. Am J Ophthalmol 1983;95:359.

719. Tabin G, Levin S, Snibson G, et al: Late recurrences and the necessity for long-term follow-up in corneal and conjunctival intraepithelial neoplasia. Ophthalmology 1997;104:485.

720. Devron HC: Clinical Ocular Oncology. New York, Churchill Livingstone, 1989, p 70.

721. Yeatts RP, Ford JG, Stanton CA, Reed JW: Topical 5-fluorouracil in treating epithelial neoplasia of the conjunctiva and cornea. Ophthalmology 1995;102:1338.

722. Frucht-Pery J, Rozenman Y: Mitomycin C therapy for corneal intraepithelial neoplasia. Am J Ophthalmol 1994;117:164.

723. Frucht-Pery J, Sugar J, Baum J, et al: Mitomycin C treatment for conjunctival-corneal intraepithelial neoplasia: A multicenter experience. Ophthalmology 1997;104:2085.

724. Hu FR, Wu MJ, Kuo SH: Interferon treatment for corneolimbal squamous dysplasia. Am J Ophthalmol 1998;125:118.

725. Devron HC: Clinical Ocular Oncology. New York, Churchill Livingstone, 1989, p 69.

726. Stokes JJ: Intraocular extension of epibulbar squamous cell carcinoma of the limbus. Trans Am Acad Ophthalmol Otolaryngol 1955;59:143.

727. Iliff WJ, Marback R, Green WR: Invasive squamous cell carcinoma of the conjunctiva. Arch Ophthalmol 1975;93:119.

728. Carroll JM, Kuwabara T: A classification of limbal epitheliomas. Arch Ophthalmol 1965;73:545.

729. Cohen BH, Green WR, Iliff NT, et al: Spindle cell carcinoma of the conjunctiva. Arch Ophthalmol 1980;98:1809.

730. Rao NA, Font RL: Mucoepidermoid carcinoma of the conjunctiva: A clinicopathologic study of five cases. Cancer 1976;38:1699.

731. Mihm MC Jr, Clark WH Jr, From L: The clinical diagnosis, classification and histogenetic concepts of the early stages of cutaneous malignant melanomas. N Engl J Med 1971;284:1078.

732. Wayte DM, Helwig EB: Melanotic freckle of Hutchinson. Cancer 1968;21:893.

733. Cramer SF, Kiehn CL: Sequential histologic study of evolving lentigo maligna melanoma. Arch Pathol Lab Med 1982;106:121.

734. Breslow A: Thickness, cross-sectional areas, and depth of invasion in the prognosis of cutaneous melanoma. Ann Surg 1970;172:902.

735. Day CL Jr, Mihm MC Jr, Sober AJ, et al: Narrower margins for clinical stage I malignant melanoma. N Engl J Med 1982;306:479.

736. Turkula LD, Woods JE: Limited or selective nodal dissection for malignant melanoma of the head and neck. Am J Surg 1984;148:446.

737. Keller AZ: Histology, survivorship and related factors in the epidemiology of eye cancers. Am J Epidemiol 1973;97:386.

738. Scotto J, Fraumeni JF Jr, Lee JA: Melanomas of the eye and other non-cutaneous sites: epidemiologic aspects. J Natl Cancer Inst 1976;56:489.

739. Charles NC, Stenson S, Taterka HB: Epibulbar malignant melanoma in a black patient. Arch Ophthalmol 1979;97:316.

740. Welsh NH, Jhavery Y: Malignant melanoma of the cornea in an African patient. Am J Ophthalmol 1971;72:796.

741. Kalski R, Lomeo M, Kirhgrader P, et al: Caruncular malignant melanoma in a black patient. Ophthalmic Surg 1995;26:139.

742. Folberg R, McLean IW, Zimmerman LE: Malignant melanoma of the conjunctiva. Hum Pathol 1985;16:136.

743. Reese AB: Precancerous and cancerous melanosis of conjunctiva. Am J Ophthalmol 1955;39:96.

744. Jakobiec FA, Folberg R, Iwamoto T: Clinicopathologic characteristics of premalignant and malignant melanocytic lesions of the conjunctiva. Ophthalmology 1989;96:147.

745. Jakobiec FA, Brownstein S, Wilkinson RD, et al: Combined surgery and cryotherapy for diffuse malignant melanoma of the conjunctiva. Arch Ophthalmol 1980;98:1390.

746. Jakobiec FA, Brownstein S, Albert D, et al: The role of cryotherapy in the management of conjunctival melanoma. Ophthalmology 1982;89:502.

747. Brownstein S, Jakobiec FA, Wilkinson RD, et al: Cryotherapy for precancerous melanosis (atypical melanocytic hyperplasia) of the conjunctiva. Arch Ophthalmol 1981;99:1224.

748. Lommatzsch PK: Beta-ray treatment of malignant epibulbar melanoma. Graefes Arch Clin Exp Ophthalmol 1978;209:111.

749. Lederman M, Wybar K, Busby E: Malignant epibulbar melanoma: Natural history and treatment by radiotherapy. Br J Ophthalmol 1984;68:605.

750. Discussion of pigmented tumors of the conjunctiva. In Boniuk M (ed): Ocular and Adnexal Tumors: New and Controversial Aspects. St. Louis, Mosby, 1964, p 24.

751. Lederman M: Radiotherapy of malignant melanomata of the eye. Br J Radiol 1961;34:21.

752. Paridaens AD, Minassian DC, McCartney AC, Hungerford JL: Prognostic factors in primary malignant melanoma of the conjunctiva: A clinicopathological study of 256 cases. Br J Ophthalmol 1994;78:252.

753. Travis LW, Rice DH, McClatchey KD, et al: Malignant melanoma of conjunctiva metastatic to parotid gland: Reports of cases and discussion of surgical management. Laryngoscope 1977;87:2000.

754. Silvers DN, Jakobiec FA, Freeman TR, et al: Melanoma of the conjunctiva: A clinicopathologic study. In Jakobiec FA (ed): Ocular and Adnexal Tumors. Birmingham, Alabama, Aesculapius, 1978, p 583.

755. Jeffrey IJM, Lucas DR, McEwan C, et al: Malignant melanoma of the conjunctiva. Histopathology 1986;10:363.

756. Paridaens AD, Minassian DC, McCarthy AC, Hungerford JL: Prognostic factors in primary malignant melanoma of the conjunctiva: A clinicopathological study of 256 cases. Br J Ophthalmol 1994;78:252.

757. Zimmerman LE: Melanocytic tumors of interest to the ophthalmologist. Ophthalmology 1980;87:497.

758. Jakobiec FA, Rini FJ, Fraunfelder FT, Brownstein S: Cryotherapy for conjunctival primary acquired melanosis and malignant melanoma. Ophthalmology 1988;95:1058.

759. Paridaens ADA, McCartney ACE, Hungerford JL: Multifocal amelanotic conjunctival melanoma and acquired melanosis sine pigmento. Br J Ophthalmol 1992;76:163.

760. Kass LG, Hornblass A: Sebaceous carcinoma of the ocular adnexa. Surv Ophthalmol 1989;33:477.

761. Rao NA, Hidayat AA, McLean JW, et al: Sebaceous carcinomas of the ocular adnexa: A clinicopathologic study of 104 cases with five-year follow-up data. Hum Pathol 1982;13:113.

762. Ni C, Searl SS, Kuo PK, et al: Sebaceous cell carcinomas of the ocular adnexa. Int Ophthalmol Clin 1982;22:23.

763. Lemos LB, Santa Cruz DJ, Baba N: Sebaceous carcinoma of the eyelid following radiation therapy. Am J Surg Pathol 1978; 2:305.

764. Boniuk M, Zimmerman LE: Sebaceous carcinoma of the eyelid, eyebrow, caruncle, and orbit. Trans Am Acad Ophthalmol Otolaryngol 1968;72:619.

765. Yeatts RP, Waller RR: Sebaceous carcinoma of the eyelid: Pitfalls in diagnosis. Ophthal Plast Reconstr Surg 1985;1:35.

766. Doxanas MT, Green WR: Sebaceous gland carcinoma: Review of 40 cases. Arch Ophthalmol 1984;102:245.

767. Wolfe JT III, Yeatts RP, Wick MR, et al: Sebaceous carcinoma of the eyelid: Errors in clinical and pathologic diagnosis. Am J Surg Pathol 1984;8:597.

768. Shields JA, Font RL: Meibomian gland carcinoma presenting as a lacrimal gland tumor. Arch Ophthalmol 1974;92:304.

769. Khan JA, Grove AS Jr, Joseph MP, Goodman M: Sebaceous carcinoma: Diuretic use, lacrimal system spread, and surgical margins. Ophthal Plast Reconstr Surg 1989;5:227.

770. Margo CE, Lessner A, Stern GA: Intraepithelial sebaceous carcinoma of the conjunctiva and skin of the eyelid. Ophthalmology 1992;99:227.

771. Leibsohn J, Bullock J, Waller R: Full-thickness eyelid biopsy for presumed carcinoma in situ of the palpebral conjunctiva. Ophthalmic Surg 1982;13:840.

772. Putterman AM: Conjunctival map biopsy to determine pagetoid spread. Am J Ophthalmol 1986;102:87.

773. Tenzel RR, Stewart WB, Boynton JR, Zbar M: Sebaceous adeno-carcinoma of the eyelid: Definition of surgical margins. Arch Ophthalmol 1977;95:2203.

774. Dogru M, Matsuo H, Inoue M, et al: Management of eyelid sebaceous carcinomas. Ophthalmologica 1997;211:40.

775. Lisman RD, Jakobiec FA, Small P: Sebaceous carcinoma of the eyelids: The role of adjunctive cryotherapy in the management of conjunctival pagetoid spread. Ophthalmology 1989;96:1021.

776. Folberg R, Whitaker DC, Tse DT, et al: Recurrent and residual sebaceous carcinoma after Mohs' excision of the primary lesion. Am J Ophthalmol 1987;103:817.

777. Gonzalez-Fernandez F, Kaltreider SA, Patnaik BD, et al: Sebaceous carcinoma: Tumor progression through mutational inactivation of p53. Ophthalmology 1998;105:4987.

778. Nunery WR, Welsh MG, McCord CD Jr: Recurrence of sebaceous carcinoma of the eyelid after radiation therapy. Am J Ophthalmol 1983;96:10.

779. Morgan G, Harry J: Lymphocytic tumours of indeterminate nature: A 5-year follow-up of 98 conjunctival and orbital lesions. Br J Ophthalmol 1978;62:381.

780. Jakobiec FA, Knowles DM: An overview of ocular adnexal lymphoid tumors. Trans Am Ophthalmol Soc 1989;87:420.

781. Searl SS, Boynton JR, Markowitch W, et al: Malignant Merkel cell neoplasm of the eyelid. Arch Ophthalmol 1984;102:907.

782. Kivela T, Tarkkanen A: The Merkel cell and associated neoplasma in the eyelid and periocular region. Surv Ophthalmol 1990;35:171.

783. Shaw JH, Rumball E: Merkel cell tumor: Clinical behavior and treatment. Br J Surg 1991;78:138.

784. Dugel PU, Gill PS, Frangieh GT, Rao NA: Treatment of ocular adnexal Kaposi's sarcoma in acquired immune deficiency syndrome. Ophthalmology 1992;99:1127.

785. Shuler JD, Holland GN, Miles SA, et al: Kaposi sarcoma of the conjunctiva and eyelids associated with the acquired immunodeficiency syndrome. Arch Ophthalmol 1989;107:858.

786. Le Bourgeois JP, Frikha H, Piedbois P, et al: Radiotherapy in the management of epidemic Kaposi's sarcoma of the oral cavity, the eyelid, and the genitals. Radiother Oncol 1994;30:263.

787. Jakobiec FA, Austin P, Iwamoto T, et al: Primary infiltrating signet ring carcinoma of the eyelids. Ophthalmology 1983;90:291.

788. Grizzard WS, Torczynski E, Edwards WC: Adenocarcinoma of eccrine sweat glands. Arch Ophthalmol 1976;94:2119.

789. Wright JD, Font RL: Mucinous sweat gland adenocarcinoma of eyelid: A clinicopathologic study of 21 cases with histochemical and electron microscopic observations. Cancer 1979;44:1757

790. Aurora AL, Luxenberg MN: Case report of adenocarcinoma of glands of Moll. Am J Ophthalmol 1970;70:984.

791. Ni C, Wagoner M, Kieval S, et al: Tumors of the Moll's glands. Br J Ophthalmol 1988;68:502.

792. Thomson SJ, Tanner NSB: Carcinoma of the apocrine glands at the base of eyelashes: A case report and discussion of histological diagnostic criteria. Br J Plast Surg 1989;42:598.

793. Cooper PH, Mills SE, Leonard DD, et al: Sclerosing sweat duct (syringomatous) carcinoma. Am J Surg Pathol 1985;9:422.

794. Arnold AC, Bullock JD, Foos RY: Metastatic eyelid carcinoma. Ophthalmology 1985;92:114.

795. Mansour AM, Hidayat AA: Metastatic eyelid disease. Ophthalmology 1987;94:667.

796. Kiratli H, Shields CL, Shields JA, DePotter P: Metastatic tumors to the conjunctiva: Report of 10 cases. Br J Ophthalmol 1996;80:5.

797. Pe'er J, Hidayat AA, Ilsar M, et al: Glandular tumors of the lacrimal sac: Their histopathologic patterns and possible origins. Ophthalmology 1996;103:10.

798. Flanagan JC, Stokes DP: Lacrimal sac tumors. Trans Am Acad Ophthalmol Otolaryngol 1978;85:1282.

799. Ryan SJ, Font RL: Primary epithelial neoplasms of the lacrimal sac. Am J Ophthalmol 1973;76:73.

800. Hornblass A, Jakobiec FA, Bosniak S, et al: The diagnosis and management of epithelial tumors of the lacrimal sac. Ophthalmology 1980;87:476.

801. Verner FL, Maguda TA, Young JM: Epithelial papillomas of the nasal cavity and sinuses. Arch Otolaryngol 1959;70:574.

802. Ni C, Wagoner MD, Wang WJ, et al: Mucoepidermoid carcinomas of the lacrimal sac. Arch Ophthalmol 1983;101:1572.

803. Gurney N, Chalkley T, O'Grady R: Lacrimal sac hemangiopericytoma. Am J Ophthalmol 1971;71:757.

804. Farkas TG, Lamberson RE: Malignant melanoma of the lacrimal sac. Am J Ophthalmol 1968;66:45.

805. Pe'er JJ, Stefanyszyn M, Hidayat AA: Nonepithelial tumors of the lacrimal sac. Am J Ophthalmol 1994;118:650.

806. Sagerman RH, Fariss AK, Chung CT, King GA, Yuo HS, Fries PD: Radiotherapy for nasolacrimal tract epithelial cancer. Int J Radiat Oncol Biol Phys 1994;29:177–181.

807. Saccogna P, Strauss ML, Bardenstein DS: Lymphoma of the nasolacrimal system. Otolaryngol Head Neck Surg 1994; 111:647.

Neoplasia-Associated Disorders

808. Graham R, McKee P, McGibbon D, et al: Torre-Muir syndrome: An association with isolated sebaceous carcinoma. Cancer 1985;55:2868.

809. Jakobiec FA, Zimmerman LE, LaPiana F, et al: Unusual eyelid tumors with sebaceous differentiation in the Muir-Torre syndrome. Ophthalmology 1988;95:1543.

810. Jakobiec FA: Sebaceous adenoma of the eyelid and visceral malignancy. Am J Ophthalmol 1974;78:952.

811. Tillawi I, Katz R, Pellettiere EV: Solitary tumors of meibomian gland origin and Torre's syndrome. Am J Ophthalmol 1987;104:179.

812. Bardenstein DS, McLean IW, Nerney J, et al: Cowden's disease. Ophthalmology 1988;95:1038.

813. Brownstein MH, Mehregan AH, Bikowski JB, et al: The dermatopathology of Cowden's syndrome. Br J Dermatol 1979;100:667.

814. Brownstein MH, Mehregan AH, Bikowski JB: Trichilemmomas in Cowden's disease [letter]. JAMA 1977;238:26.

815. Wells GB, Lasner TM, Yousem DM, Zager EL: Lhermitte-Duclos disease and Cowden's syndrome in an adolescent patient: Case report. J Neurosurg 1994;81:133.

816. Feman SS, Apt L, Roth AM: The basal cell nevus syndrome. Am J Ophthalmol 1974;78:222.

817. Zackheim HS, Loud AV, Howell JB: Nevoid basal cell carcinoma syndrome: Some histologic observations on the cutaneous lesions. Arch Dermatol 1966;93:317.

818. Howell JB, Freeman RG: Structure and significance of the pits with their tumors in the nevoid basal cell carcinoma syndrome. J Am Acad Dermatol 1980;2:224.

819. Gorlin RJ: Nevoid basal cell carcinoma syndrome. Medicine 1987;66:98.

820. Wennstrom J, Pierce ER, McKusick VA: Hereditary benign and malignant lesions of the large bowel. Cancer 1974;34(Suppl):850.

821. Lewis RA, Crowder WE, Eierman LA, et al: The Gardner syndrome: Significance of ocular features. Ophthalmology 1984;91:916.

822. Traboulsi EI, Maumenee IH, Krush AJ, et al: Pigmented ocular fundus lesions in the inherited gastrointestinal polyposis syndromes and in hereditary nonpolyposis colorectal cancer. Ophthalmology 1988;95:964.

823. Stein EA, Brady KD: Ophthalmologic and electro-oculographic findings in Gardner's syndrome. Am J Ophthalmol 1988;106:326.

824. Blair NP, Trempe CL: Hypertrophy of the retinal pigment epithelium associated with Gardner's syndrome. Am J Ophthalmol 1980;90:661.

825. Shields JA, Tso MOM: Congenital grouped pigmentation of the retina: Histopathologic description and report of a case. Arch Ophthalmol 1975;93:1153.

826. Barker D, Wright E, Nguyen K, et al: Gene for von Recklinghausen neurofibromatosis is in the pericentromeric region of chromosome 17. Science 1987;236:1100.

827. Seizinger BR, Rouleau GA, Ozelius LJ, et al: Genetic linkage of von Recklinghausen neurofibromatosis to the nerve growth factor receptor gene. Cell 1987;49:589.

828. Rouleau GA, Wertelecki W, Haines JL, et al: Genetic linkage of bilateral acoustic neurofibromatosis to a DNA marker on chromosome 22. Nature 1987;329:246.

829. Wertelecki W, Rouleau GA, Superneau DW, et al: Neurofibromatosis 2: Clinical and DNA linkage studies of a large kindred. N Engl J Med 1988;319:278.

830. DeAngelis LM, Kelleher MB, Post KD, et al: Multiple paragangliomas in neurofibromatosis: A new neuroendocrine neoplasia. Neurology 1987;37:129.

831. Lubs M-Le, Bauer M, Formas ME, et al: Iris hamartomas in the diagnosis of neurofibromatosis-1. Int Pediatr 1990;5:261.

832. Lewis RA, Gerson LP, Axelson KA, et al: Von Recklinghausen neurofibromatosis. II. Incidence of optic gliomata. Ophthalmology 1984;91:929.

833. Listernick R, Charrow J, Greenwald MJ, et al: Optic gliomas in children with neurofibromatosis type 1. J Pediatr 1989;114:788.

834. Ariel IM: Tumors of the peripheral nervous system. CA Cancer J Clin 1983;33:282.

835. Seizinger BR, Rouleau GA, Ozelius LJ, et al: Von Hippel-Lindau disease maps to the region of chromosome 3 associated with renal cell carcinoma. Nature 1988;332:268.

836. Maher ER, Yates JRW, Harries R, et al: Clinical features and natural history of von Hippel-Lindau disease. Q J Med 1990;77:1151.

837. Hardwig P, Robertson DM: Von Hippel-Lindau disease: A familial, often lethal, multisystem phakomatosis. Ophthalmology 1984;91:263.

838. Horton JC, Harsh GR IV, Fisher JW, et al: Von Hippel-Lindau disease and erythrocytosis: Radioimmunoassay of erythropoietin in cyst fluid from a brainstem hemangioblastoma. Neurology 1991; 41:753.

839. Williams R, Taylor D: Tuberous sclerosis. Surv Ophthalmol 1985;30:143.

840. Monaghan HP, Krafchik BR, MacGregor DL, et al: Tuberous sclerosis complex in children. Am J Dis Child 1981; 135:912.

841. Eng C, Li FP, Abramson DH, et al: Leiomyosarcoma of the bladder eighteen years after cyclophosphamide therapy for retino-blastoma. Urol Int 1993;51:49.

842. Moll AC, Imhof SM, Bouter LM, et al: Second primary tumors in patients with hereditary retinoblastoma: A register-based follow-up study, 1945–1954. Int J Cancer 1996;67:515.

843. Abramson DH, Frank CM: Second nonocular tumors in survivors of bilateral retinoblastoma: A possible age effect on radiation-related risk. Ophthalmology 1998;105:573.

844. Abramson DH, Ronner HJ, Ellsworth RM: Second tumors in nonirradiated bilateral retinoblastoma. Am J Ophthalmol 1979;87:624.

845. Draper GJ, Sanders BM, Kingston JE: Second primary neoplasms in patients with retinoblastoma. Br J Cancer 1986;53:661.

846. Roarty JD, McLean IW, Zimmerman LE: Incidence of second neoplasms in patients with bilateral retinoblastoma. Ophthalmology 1988;95:1583.

847. Traboulsi EI, Zimmerman LE, Manz HJ: Cutaneous malignant melanoma in survivors of heritable retinoblastoma. Arch Ophthalmol 1988;106:1059.

848. Margo CE, Pavan PR, Gendelman D, et al: Bilateral melanocytic uveal tumors associated with systemic non-ocular malignancy: Malignant melanomas or benign paraneoplastic syndrome? Retina 1987;7:137.

849. Tucker MA, D'Angio GJ, Boice JD Jr, et al: Bone sarcomas linked to radiotherapy and chemotherapy in children. N Engl J Med 1987;317:588.

850. Mullaney J, Mooney D, O'Connor M, McDonald GSA: Bilateral ovarian carcinoma with bilateral uveal melanoma. Br J Ophthalmol 1984;68:261.

851. Barr CC, Zimmerman LE, Curtin VT, et al: Bilateral diffuse melanocytic uveal tumors associated with systemic malignant neoplasms: A recently recognized syndrome. Arch Ophthalmol 1982;100:249.

852. Block MB, Roberts JP, Kadair RB, et al: Multiple endocrine adenomatosis, type IIB. JAMA 1975;234:710.

853. White MP, Goel KM, Connor JM, et al: Mucosal neuroma syndromea phenotype for malignancy. Arch Dis Child 1985;60:876.

854. Khairi MRA, Dexter RN, Surzynski NJ, et al: Mucosal neuroma, pheochromocytoma and medullary thyroid carcinoma, multiple endocrine neoplasia, type 3. Medicine 1975;54:89.

855. Thirkill CE, Roth AM, Keltner JL: Cancer-associated retinopathy. Arch Ophthalmol 1987;105:372.

856. Crofts JW, Bachynski BN, Odel JG: Visual paraneoplastic syndrome associated with undifferentiated endometrial carcinoma. Can J Ophthalmol 1988;23:128.

857. Wolf JE, Arden GB: Selective magnocellular damage in melanoma-associated retinopathy: comparison with congenital stationary nightblindness. Vision Res 1996;36:2369.

858. Buchanan TAS, Gardiner TA, Archer DB: An ultrastructural study of retinal photoreceptor degeneration associated with bronchial carcinoma. Am J Ophthalmol 1984;97:277.

859. Grunwald GB, Kornguth SE, Towfighi J, et al: Autoimmune basis for visual paraneoplastic syndrome in patients with small cell lung carcinoma. Retinal immune deposits and ablation of retinal ganglion cells. Cancer 1987;60:780.

860. Martin H, Strong E, Spiro RH: Radiation-induced skin cancer of the head and neck. Cancer 1970;25:61.

861. Lazar P, Cullen SI: Basal cell epithelioma and chronic radio-dermatitis. Arch Dermatol 1963;88:172.

862. Kraemer KH, Lee MM, Scotto J: Xeroderma pigmentosum: Cutaneous, ocular, and neurologic abnormalities in 830 published cases. Arch Dermatol 1987;123:241.

863. Robbins JH, Moshell AN: DNA repair processes protect human beings from premature solar skin damage: evidence from studies on xeroderma pigmentosum. J Invest Dermatol 1979;73:102.

864. Kraemer KH, Lee MM, Andrews AD, Lambert WC: The role of sunlight and DNA repair in melanoma and nonmelanoma skin cancer. The xeroderma pigmentosum paradigm. Arch Dermatol 1994;130:1018.

865. Gaasterland DE, Rodrigues MM, Moshell AN: Ocular involvement in xeroderma pigmentosum. Ophthalmology 1982;89:980.

866. Kopf AW, Weidman AI: Nevus of Ota. Arch Dermatol 1962;85:195.

867. Hidano A, Kajima H, Ikeda S, et al: Natural history of nevus of Ota. Arch Dermatol 1967;95:187.

868. Gonder JR, Shields JA, Albert DM, et al: Uveal malignant melanoma associated with ocular and oculodermal melanocytosis. Ophthalmology 1982;89:953.

869. Dutton JJ, Anderson RL, Schelper RL, et al: Orbital malignant melanoma and oculodermal melanocytosis: Report of two cases and review of the literature. Ophthalmology 1984;91:497.

870. Singh AD, DePotter P, Fijal BA, et al: Lifetime prevalence of uveal melanoma in white patients with oculo(dermal) melanocytosis. Ophthalmology 1998;105:195.

871. Bataille V, Pinney E, Hungerford JL, et al: Five cases of coexistent primary ocular and cutaneous melanoma. Arch Dermatol 1993;129:198.

872. van Hees CL, de Boer A, Jager MJ, et al: Are atypical nevi a risk factor for uveal melanoma? A case-control study. J Invest Dermatol 1994;103:202.

873. Hammer H, Olah J, Toth-Molnar E: Dysplastic nevi are a risk factor for melanoma. Eur J Ophthalmol 1996;6:472.

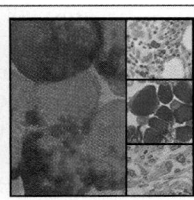

71

CANCER OF THE HEAD AND NECK

Harry Quon

Diane Hershock

Michael Feldman

Duane Sewell

Randal S. Weber

SUMMARY OF KEY POINTS

INCIDENCE
- Over 37,000 estimated new cases per year in the United States.
- Over 11,000 estimated deaths per year in the United States.

EPIDEMIOLOGY AND RISK FACTORS
- The dominant risk factors are tobacco and alcohol use.
- Other risk factors may include immunosuppression and viral infection (human papillomaviruses and Epstein-Barr virus).

PATHOLOGY/BIOLOGY
Majority are squamous cell carcinomas (HNSCC) with well-delineated local-regional spread pattern.

CLINICAL FINDINGS
- Depends on the anatomic site of involvement.
- Common symptoms may include hoarseness of voice, dysphagia, odynophagia, and referred otalgia.

DIFFERENTIAL DIAGNOSIS
Lymphoma, sarcoma, other solid malignancies.

STAGING
- Clinical evaluation including endoscopic evaluation of the upper aerodigestive tract.
- Local-regional anatomic imaging to include computed tomography (CT) or magnetic resonance imaging (MRI).
- Chest radiograph.
- Ultrasound of the neck in select cases.
- Chest CT, bone scan, positron emission tomography (PET) in select cases.
- Complete blood count (CBC).

PRIMARY THERAPY, SALVAGE THERAPY
- Early Stage Definitive Therapy: subsite specific with either definitive surgery or radiotherapy. Involvement of sites important for speech or swallowing function or sites where surgical risks are prohibitive may favor therapy that provides functional organ preservation. This often favors primary radiotherapy.
- Advanced Stage Definitive Therapy: subsite specific with either definitive surgery with postoperative radiotherapy as indicated or chemoradiotherapy with concurrent chemoradiotherapy often favored. Involvement of sites important for speech or swallowing function may favor therapy that provides functional organ preservation. This often favors chemoradiotherapy. Altered fractionated radiotherapy may be used in patients not able to receive chemotherapy or as a alternative therapeutic option for nonbulky primary but advanced stage disease.
- Advanced Stage Palliative Therapy: treatment options may include radiotherapy. Systemic chemotherapy or treatment on protocol with systemic chemotherapy often favored due to more favorable toxicity profile.
- Local-Regional Recurrent Salvage Therapy: for resectable disease with no prior irradiation, surgery with postoperative radiotherapy favored; for resectable disease with prior irradiation, surgery with considerations for reirradiation +/– brachytherapy implant favored. For unresectable disease without prior irradiation, chemoradiotherapy favored; for unresectable disease with prior irradiation, reirradiation on protocol or systemic chemotherapy.

COMPLICATIONS
- Surgery: Nerve injury, hematoma formation, organ dysfunction.
- Radiotherapy: *Acute*: skin desquamation, mucositis, dysphagia, odynophagia, xerostomia, taste alterations; *late*: xerostomia, skin/soft tissue/mucosal atrophy, soft tissue fibrosis, permanent swallowing dysfunction, hypothyroidism, transverse myelitis, blindness.
- Chemotherapy: bone marrow suppression.

PROGNOSIS
Subsite specific and histology specific. For locally advanced HNSCC, the long-term disease control rate is less than 40%.

FUTURE DIRECTIONS
- Further improvements in local-regional management with the integration of novel targeted agents in combination with current chemotherapy and radiotherapy regimens.
- Continued development of novel radiotherapy techniques including intensity-modulated radiotherapy and proton radiotherapy.

INTRODUCTION

In the United States for the year 2003, cancer of the head and neck represented 2.8% of all new cancer cases and 2% of all cancer deaths.[1] Being a relatively uncommon disease, misdiagnosis along with patient neglect not uncommonly contributes to an advanced stage at presentation and limited survival.[2] Despite being relatively uncommon, research and management of head and neck cancers continue to receive significant emphasis due to the rich anatomic and functional complexity of this body site, which is critical to issues of self-esteem, communication, and social integration. Though squamous cell carcinomas constitute the majority of adult histopathologies (95%)[3] that may arise in the head and neck site, the various histopathologies and anatomic subsites of involvement result in tremendous discordant variability in the natural course of the diseases for this small anatomic site.

The site begins at the base of the skull and extends only to the clavicles, and includes the base of the skull, temporal bone (external auditory canal, middle and inner ear), paranasal sinuses, nasopharynx, oropharynx (soft palate, tonsil structures, base of tongue, oropharyngeal wall), larynx, hypopharynx (pyriform sinuses, postcricoid, posterior pharyngeal wall), oral cavity (lips, buccal mucosa, alveolar ridges, floor of mouth, oral tongue, retromolar trigone), major and minor salivary glands, skin, and the neck.

As such, management of head and neck cancers has evolved to require a multidisciplinary approach with effective integration of various skills and treatment modalities to achieve the desired goals of cure and functional organ preservation. Despite improvements in the diagnosis and local-regional management of head and neck cancer, little significant increases in long-term survival rates over the past 30 years have been realized. The desire for more effective yet organ-preserving therapies with acceptable toxicity is currently being addressed with recent technological advancements in surgical and radiotherapy techniques and the development of novel biologic agents. These agents are particularly attractive, as they have been demonstrated in cell model systems to target various aberrant molecular proteins that appear to have dominant roles in mediating biologic aggressiveness or therapeutic resistance. These advances coupled with tremendous clinical research activity have resulted in a number of therapeutic options for patients with head and neck cancer.

EPIDEMIOLOGY

Approximately 37,000 new cases of head and neck squamous cell carcinoma (HNSCC) will be seen in the United States in 2003 with 68% being diagnosed in males, accounting for approximately 11,000 cancer deaths with 71% in males.[1] Additionally, cancers of the oral cavity and oropharynx represent 3% of all malignancies in men and 2% in women in the United States.[4] Worldwide, 15% of male cancers, 600,000 cases annually, are HNSCC. Head and neck cancers do affect both sexes and all races, but there continues to be a preponderance in males, African Americans, and Asians.[4] Oral and pharyngeal cancers have decreased significantly in white males over the past 20 years and in white females younger than age 65.[5] Conversely, the incidence and mortality rates have significantly increased in African American males, but decreased in black women. The incidence of laryngeal cancer appears to mimic that of lung cancer; there appears to be a small decline in the incidence in white men younger than age 65, but the incidence continues to increase in white and black males older than 65 and in women of all age categories.[6]

There is limited knowledge concerning the epidemiology of in situ head and neck cancers (lip, oral cavity, larynx, and pharynx). Data extrapolated from population-based cancer registries in the National Cancer Institute's Surveillance, Epidemiology, and End Results (SEER) program revealed annual age-adjusted incidence rates for in situ HNSCC rose from 6.33/1,000,000 person-years in 1976 to 8.04/1,000,000 in 1995 (35% change).[7] The predominant anatomic sites of change were the larynx and lip, with this significant rise felt to be attributable to improved surveillance.

Of significant concern are the rising trends of head and neck malignancies in the pediatric population and younger adults. Again using data from SEER, the average annual rate in children younger than 15 years rose 35% from 1.10 to 1.49 between 1973 to 1975 and 1994 to 1996, respectively.[8] This incidence reflects a greater increase than childhood cancer in general, which increased 25% during that same period. In a selected population at the MD Anderson Cancer Center, the percentage of adults younger than age 40 with oral tongue squamous cell carcinomas rose from 4% to 18% between 1971 and 1993.[9] This finding has been substantiated by SEER data where the incidence of tongue cancer (oral cavity and oropharynx) increased by 60% in adults younger than 40.[10] The prognosis tended to be worse in black males compared to white in the same age category. Trends in laryngeal cancers, documented most accurately in the VA system increased as well between 1983 and 1993 but more notably amongst those older than 65 years.[11]

Successful therapy for HNSCC may be limited by the recognized risk of second primary malignancies in the aerodigestive tract. Using data from a population-based cancer registry, investigators from the United Kingdom observed 5.5% of males and 3.6% of females to have developed a second primary cancer after an initial diagnosis of head and neck cancer.[12] There was a significantly increased risk for a second cancer in most of the upper aerodigestive tract sites commonly associated with tobacco exposure, with a standardized incidence ratio for subsequent oral cancer of 5.56 in men and 15.31 in women. Excluding these tobacco-associated sites resulted in a nonsignificant risk for a second malignancy. Those with a first detected pharyngeal cancer experienced the highest incidence of a second malignancy. The relative risk for multiple primary cancers was higher in younger patients and among patients who received radiotherapy for their first primary. These investigators estimated that within 20 years of the first primary HNSCC, 30% of males and 20% of females would develop subsequent primary malignancies.

ETIOLOGY AND PATHOGENESIS

Tobacco and alcohol continue to remain the two major risk factors for HNSCC in developed countries, with their carcinogenic risks summarized in several working group reports by the International Agency for Research on Cancer (IARC).[13,14] It is estimated that 75% to 90% of all head and neck carcinomas are attributable to tobacco consumption, particularly cigarette smoking.[15,16] The cumulative evidence easily fulfills the criteria for causality between cigarette smoking and the development of HNSCC.[17,18] Supporting a causal relationship has been the demonstration that the risk of developing HNSCC rises with increasing numbers of cigarettes smoked per day and increasing years' duration of the habit.[3,19] Current smokers have an approximate 20-fold higher risk of oropharyngeal and laryngeal cancers than lifelong nonsmokers.[19,20] The increased relative risk of developing head and neck cancer in the heaviest smokers is quoted as 20 to 40 times that of nonsmokers.[19,20,21] Even light or occasional use of cigarettes leads to an increased risk of cancer.[3,19,21] In addition to the duration of smoking and number of cigarettes, the type of cigarettes and the age, sex, and race of the smoker also influence the relative risk. In contrast, it has been estimated that the relative risk of developing head and neck cancer for heavy consumers of alcohol is two to sixfold.[22]

There are 300 carcinogens present in tobacco, with tobacco-specific N-nitrosamines (TSNAs) being the most harmful.[23] These substances are metabolites of nicotine, the major alkaloid responsible for addiction to tobacco.[17] TSNAs are known to bind to DNA and to cause mutations that can activate proto-oncogenes or inactivate tumor suppressor genes.[24] Other harmful mutagenic compounds found in tobacco include polycyclic aromatic hydrocarbons (PAHs), carbon monoxide, and hydrogen cyanide.[23]

Despite limited data, there appears to be an association between cigar and pipe smoking and an increased risk for HNSCC. Cigar consumption in the United States has increased substantially since 1993. Cigars are known to contain even higher concentrations of TSNAs than cigarettes.[25] With regard to environmental smoke, cigars emit 20 times the carbon monoxide and twice the PAHs as cigarettes, due in large part to their greater size.[25] The increased risk of HNSCC associated with cigar smoking is between 1.9 and 10.3 times that of nonsmokers.[15,25-28] Smoking more than 4 cigars per day increases the risk more than 20-fold.[29] A recent study analyzed prospectively the rates of cancer deaths amongst cigar-smoking men. Men who ever smoked cigarettes or pipes were excluded. Risk of death from oral cavity/pharynx and larynx cancers was 4.0 (95% CI 1.5 to 10.3) and 10.3 (95% CI 2.6 to 41.0), respectively.[26] Although fewer dedicated studies have been performed, pipe smoking has been similarly implicated.[15,30,31]

Active cigarette smoking is not the only form of tobacco exposure that poses a risk. Exposure to second-hand, or environmental, smoke has also been implicated in several publications as a risk factor for the development of head and neck cancer.[32-34] A recent study of over 300 patients and controls found that secondhand smoke increased the risk of HNSCC with a dose-response pattern. Individuals who were exposed to the highest levels of environmental cigarette smoke were up to four times more likely to develop HNSCC.[34]

Tobacco is consumed in a smokeless form in many cultures around the world. In the West the most common form of smokeless tobacco is termed snuff, while in parts of Asia it often takes the form of betel quid. Betal quids consist of a betel pepper leaf wrapped around a mixture of areca nut, slaked lime, and tobacco; the slaked lime releases an alkaloid that causes a sense of euphoria in the user. Approximately 200 million persons throughout the western Pacific basin and south Asia regularly chew betel quid.[35] Betel quid can lead to a progressive scarlike formation known as oral submucous fibrosis. The data regarding an increased risk of oral cancer in those who chew betel are incontrovertible, with an estimated odds ratio of 17 for the development of HNSCC.[35-38]

In Europe and the Americas, there is a large variation in the amounts of TSNA among the various brands and forms of smokeless tobacco available.[39] Therefore a discrepancy is found for the estimated cancer risk associated with smokeless tobacco consumption in Europe and the Americas.[18,39] Recent studies of Swedish moist snuff users showed no increase in cancer incidence over control individuals,[18,40] which could be due to the lower concentrations of TSNA in Swedish snuff.[39] However, the link between other forms of smokeless tobacco and oral cancer is well established.[41-43] A recent review of the known literature found relative risks ranging from 0.6 to 13, depending on the type of smokeless tobacco studied.[42]

Alcohol consumption is also a known independent risk factor for HNSCC.[19,44-47] For those individuals that drink heavily but do not smoke, the increased relative risk reportedly ranges from 5.0 to 11.6, increasing in significance with higher numbers of drinks consumed.[45,46] When alcohol and tobacco are consumed together, the risk increases multiplicatively rather than additively.[15,19,48] Extremely high odds ratios have recently been quoted for heavy consumers of both tobacco and alcohol.[19,44] Franceschi and colleagues reported an odds ratio of 228 for oral cancer in consumers of more than 25 cigarettes per day and more than 11 drinks per day.[44] One other report noted an odds ratio of 177 for laryngeal cancer in heavy tobacco and alcohol users.[19]

The mechanism for alcohol-induced carcinogenesis is not fully understood. Pure ethanol has been shown not to be carcinogenic.[49] However, alcohol is often regarded more as a co-carcinogen, facilitating carcinogenesis rather than initiating it.[50] Several mechanisms for this have been proposed. It has been suggested that alcohol may increase the penetration of carcinogens across the oral mucosa,[51] as well as cause mucosal atrophy, which may result in an enhanced susceptibility to chemical carcinogens.[52] It has also been suggested that alcohol may have an effect on

DNA repair mechanisms.[53] Other suggested mechanisms include nutritional deficiencies associated with heavy drinking, the effects of contaminants and congeners in alcoholic beverages, and the induction of microsomal enzymes that enhance the metabolic activation of tobacco or other carcinogens.[3] These mechanisms may also explain the observation of an increased risk of cancer with heavy alcohol consumption in nonsmokers. Several reports suggest that women may be more susceptible than men to alcohol-induced carcinogenesis in the head and neck.[46,54,55]

Several studies have implicated the lack of vitamin and fresh fruit intake as a risk factor for head and neck cancer.[56-61] However, it is often difficult to separate malnutrition from other confounding variables, including alcohol and cigarette consumption. Related to malnutrition is the problem of poor oral hygiene, which has also been found to be associated with HNSCC.[62-64]

It has been proposed that HNSCC patients have increased chromosomal sensitivity to carcinogen exposure that predisposes them to developing cancer.[65-68] In vitro laboratory studies have shown that cells from HNSCC patients suffer more chromosome breaks upon exposure to a mutagen than do normal control cells.[67,69] In addition, young HNSCC patients who were nonsmokers demonstrated mucosa that was particularly mutagen sensitive.[70]

Immunosuppression may predispose individuals to an increased risk of HNSCC. The risk of carcinomas of the lip is particularly increased in renal transplant patients.[71-73] Cutaneous malignancies including lip appear to be increased in cardiothoracic transplant patients.[74] Other sites of malignancies may include the oral cavity though the risk does not appear to be as significantly increased as it is with cutaneous malignancies including the lip in transplant patients. An increased risk of oral cavity carcinomas has been reported in HIV patients.[75] These tumors are generally more aggressive, with decreased patient survival[74,76] and a demonstrated association between the degree of medical immunosuppression, most notably involving prednisone, and advanced stage presentation and an adverse survival.[76]

A potential causal relationship is believed to exist between viral infections and carcinomas of the head and neck. Human papillomaviruses (HPVs) have been associated with a risk for oral cavity[77,78] and oropharyngeal carcinomas.[78,79] Interestingly, these carcinomas may have a better prognosis[80,81] and response to therapy such as radiotherapy.[79] A nested case control study suggested that the risk may be with the HPV-16 serotype, with 50% and 14% of oropharyngeal and oral tongue carcinomas containing HPV-16 DNA, respectively. In a large retrospective study, 90% of HPV positive tumors were of the HPV-16 subtype. Two oncoproteins encoded by HPVs, E6 and E7, are known to inactivate p53 and the tumor suppressor protein retinoblastoma, presenting potential mechanisms of action.[82,83] The Epstein-Barr virus (EBV) is a human herpes virus that has been implicated in a number of human malignancies, including nasopharyngeal carcinoma. A consistent association between EBV and less differentiated types of nasopharyngeal carcinoma

(NPC) has been reported.[84-86] While the extent to which EBV infection may contribute to NPC carcinogenesis has not been completely elucidated, an early role is supported by evidence of clonal EBV infection in preinvasive lesions (carcinoma in situ).[87] The expression of various viral gene products, EBV nuclear antigen (EBNA), and latent membrane proteins (LMP1, LMP2) has been demonstrated to have the capacity to induce transformation in vitro consistent with a carcinogenic role for EBV infection.

PATHOLOGY

Squamous Cell Carcinoma

Oral Cavity

Squamous cell carcinoma accounts for 95% of all malignant tumors in the oral cavity. Other malignancies involving the oral cavity include malignant salivary gland lesions, mucosal melanoma, lymphoma, and sarcoma. While squamous cell carcinoma can occur anywhere in the oral cavity, the most common locations include the floor of the mouth, tongue, and hard palate. In the earliest recognizable stage, squamous cell carcinoma appears as firm, pearly plaques or as irregular, roughened, or verrucous areas of mucosal thickening, which can be mistaken for leukoplakia, a premalignant lesion. Larger lesions are seldom mistaken for leukoplakia and form either exophytic masses (Fig. 71-1A) or endophytic lesions often with associated ulceration and heaped-up edges (Fig. 71-1B).

Histologic examination frequently reveals an association with in situ lesions, sometimes with surrounding areas of epithelial dysplasia of varying degrees (Fig. 71-1C). Histologically, these tumors range from well-differentiated keratinizing neoplasms to poorly differentiated squamous cell carcinoma without keratinization to anaplastic and sometimes sarcomatoid growth patterns (Fig. 71-1D). Less common patterns include verrucous carcinoma.

Larynx

Epithelial changes in the larynx include a spectrum of pathologic changes beginning with hyperplasia and progressing through dysplasia, carcinoma in situ, and invasive carcinoma.[88] Similar to the oral cavity, these early pathologic lesions appear as white (leukoplakia) or reddened (erythroplakia) thickenings and cannot be reliably distinguished from early invasive carcinoma. The earliest lesions (hyperplasia) have little or no malignant transformation potential, whereas mild dysplasia progresses to carcinoma in 1% to 2% of cases over a 10-year period and rises to 5% to 10% with high-grade dysplasia over a similar time span. In general, the more severe the dysplasia the greater the risk of progression to carcinoma.

About 95% of laryngeal carcinomas are the typical squamous cell carcinoma. Squamous cell carcinoma may develop on the vocal cords, but it may also develop in a supraglottic or subglottic location. Similar to oral squamous cell carcinomas, these lesions begin as in situ carcinoma and, left untreated, grow into infiltrating,

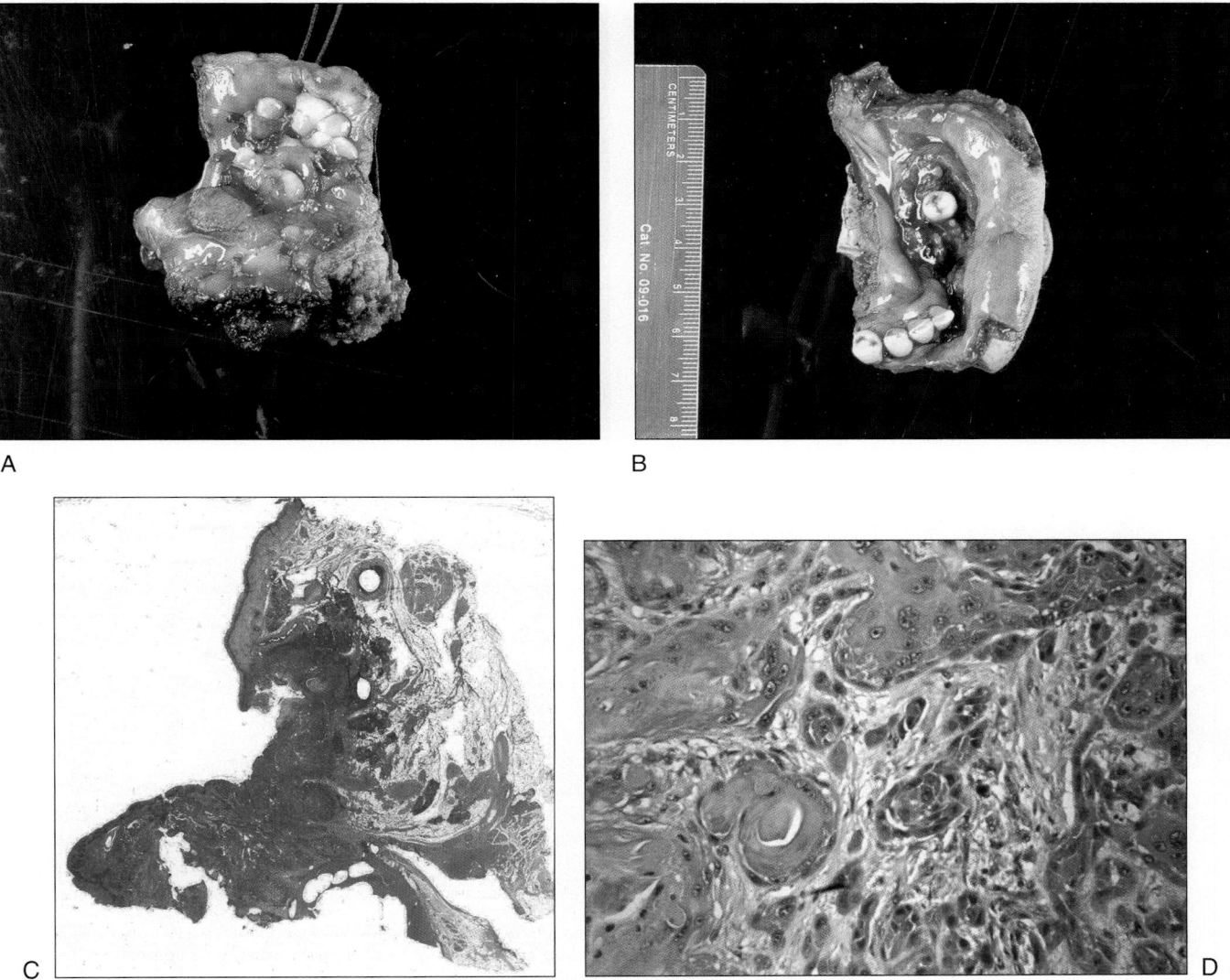

Figure 71-1. A, Squamous cell carcinoma growing as an exophytic lesion in the floor of the mouth. **B,** Squamous cell carcinoma growing as an ulcerated endophytic lesion along the alveolar ridge of the mandible. **C,** Invasive squamous cell carcinoma and adjacent precursor lesion of the tongue. **D,** Squamous cell carcinoma, moderately differentiated, of the tongue.

ulcerated, and fungating lesions (Fig. 71-2A to C). The degree of differentiation of squamous carcinoma is highly variable and similar to the oral cavity. Rare cases show sarcomatoid differentiation.

Nasal Sinus and Nasopharynx

Epithelial carcinomas in the nasal sinus are clustered under the term *nasopharyngeal carcinoma.* Within this clustered entity are three distinct histopathologically recognizable tumor patterns: (a) keratinizing squamous cell carcinoma; (b) nonkeratinizing squamous cell carcinoma; and (c) undifferentiated carcinoma, also referred to as lymphoepithelial type of nasopharyngeal carcinoma. The nonkeratinizing and undifferentiated carcinoma is most closely associated with EBV infection.

Keratinizing and nonkeratinizing squamous cell carcinoma in the nasopharynx is morphologically similar to lesions found in the larynx and oral cavity. The non-keratinizing forms may also take the appearance of transitional epithelium, hence the designation of some nasal carcinomas as transitional type. In contrast, the undifferentiated form of nasopharyngeal carcinoma shows a unique morphology characterized by the growth of large tumor cells with round to oval nuclei, prominent nucleoli, fine vesicular chromatin, and indistinct cell borders (which produces a syncytial appearance). There is an abundant lymphoid response within this tumor, sometimes obscuring the malignant epithelial cells. EBV genome is frequently found within the epithelial tumor cells (Fig. 71-3A to C).

A rare and highly aggressive variant of squamous cell carcinoma, the so-called basaloid squamous cell carcinoma, can be found in the upper aerodigestive and nasopharynx and less commonly in other sites within the

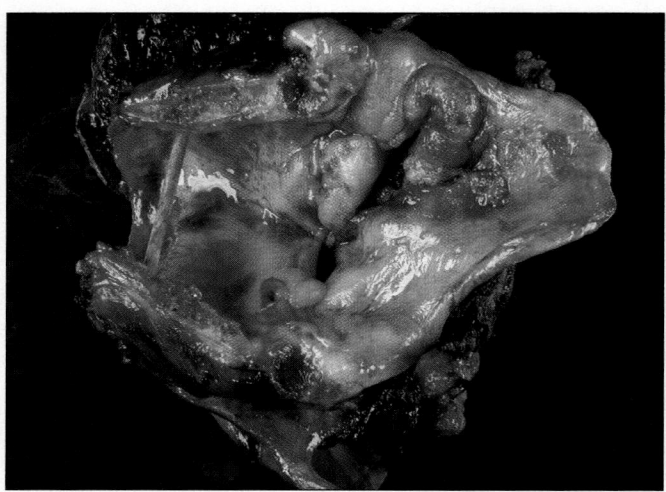
A

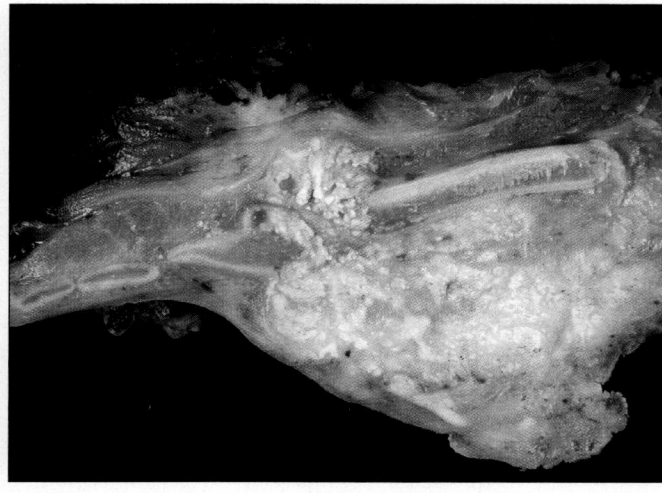
B

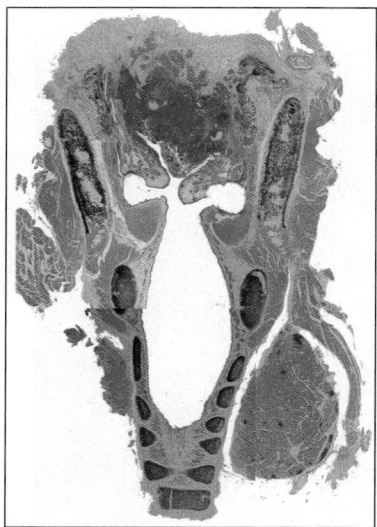
C

Figure 71-2. A, Squamous cell carcinoma of the larynx, supraglottic opened posteriorly. **B,** Squamous cell carcinoma of the larynx invading between thyroid and cricoid cartilages. **C,** Coronal section of larynx showing a supraglottic squamous cell carcinoma.

head and neck.[89,90] This tumor is characterized by cells infiltrating in small to large nests with prominent central comedo-type necrosis. At the edges of the nests, the tumor cells form an organized palisade. In addition, variable areas of the tumor show malignant squamous cell morphology with keratinization. Cytologically, the tumor cells show marked nuclear pleomorphism with single cell necrosis and high mitotic rates (Fig. 71-3D).

A rare and highly aggressive carcinoma found within the nasal sinus is the sinonasal undifferentiated carcinoma (SNUC) believed to originate from the schneiderian mucosa.[91] These lesions may present with or without neuroendocrine differentiation but without evidence of squamous or glandular differentiation. SNUCs are distinguished from undifferentiated nasopharyngeal carcinoma by the absence of a surrounding lymphoid reaction. SNUC cells are medium in size and grow in nests. Cytologically, the tumor cells show fine chromatin pattern, hyperchromasia, and variably sized nucleoli. Mitotic rates are high and necrosis is common.

Malignant Salivary Gland Neoplasms

Salivary gland tumors are a rare and interesting heterogenous group of tumors. The vast majority of salivary gland tumors are benign and develop in the parotid gland. However, a subset of salivary gland tumors is malignant. Malignant salivary gland tumors are more common in the minor salivary glands (50% to 60%) and sublingual salivary glands (80% to 90%) in contrast to the parotid (20% to 30%) and submandibular (30% to 40%). A brief discussion of the major types of malignant salivary gland tumors follows.

Mucoepidermoid Carcinoma

Mucoepidermoid carcinomas are the most frequent type of malignant salivary gland tumor. While occurring most often in the parotid gland, they can also be seen with high frequency in the minor salivary glands. These tumors, as the name implies, are composed of a mixture of squamous cells (epidermoid component) and mucous secreting cells

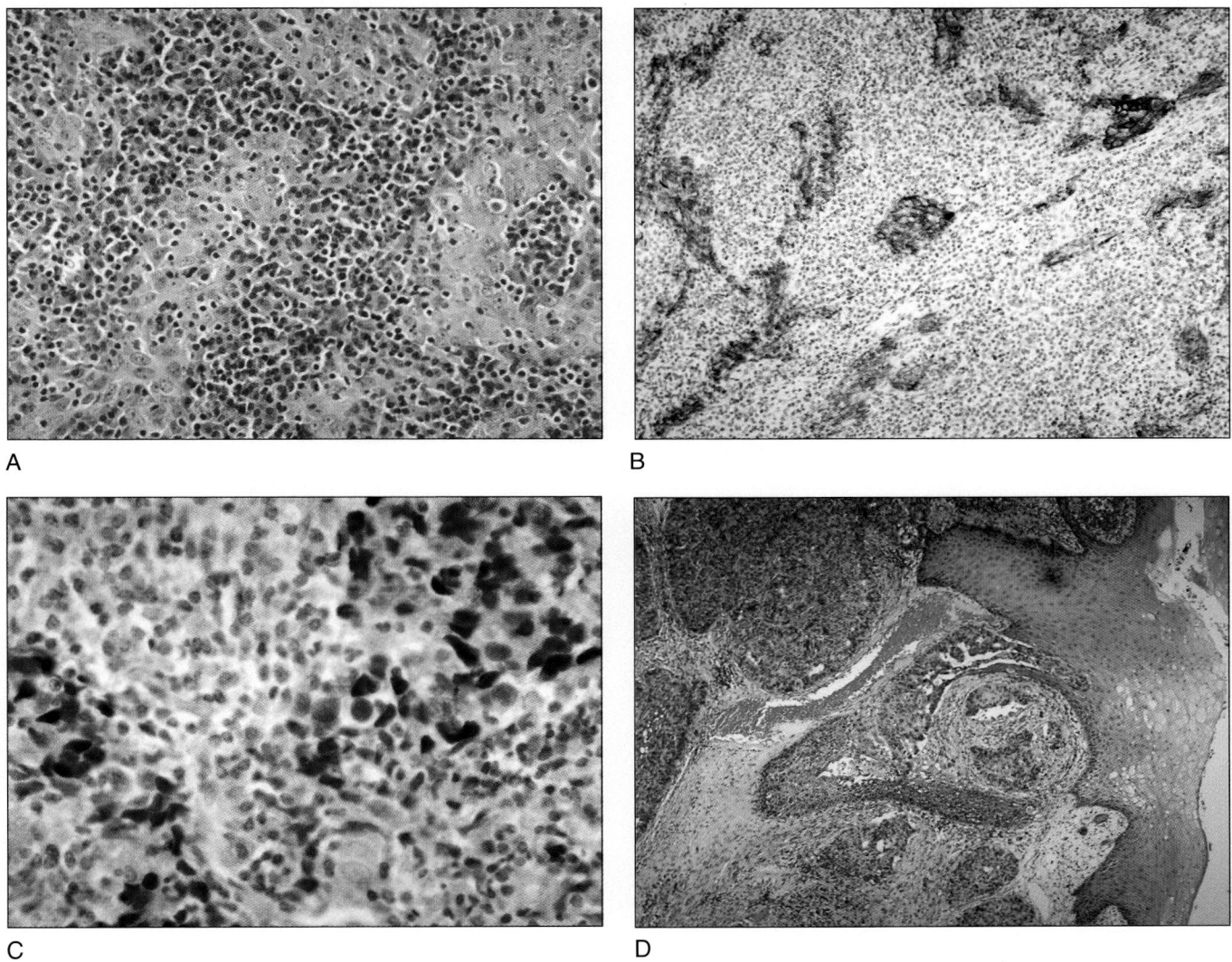

Figure 71-3. A, Nasopharyngeal carcinoma, undifferentiated type, lymphoepithelial type (H&E). **B,** Nasopharyngeal carcinoma, undifferentiated type, lymphoepithelial type (Cytokeratin). **C,** Nasopharyngeal carcinoma, undifferentiated type, lymphoepithelial type EBV in situ hybridization. **D,** Basaloid squamous cell carcinoma of nasopharynx showing in situ squamous cell carcinoma.

(mucoid component). A third cell type found within these lesions is the intermediate cell.

Mucoepidermoid carcinomas vary in size and lack a well-defined capsule. Microscopically, the tumor shows a pushing or infiltrative border. They vary in appearance from white to grey and frequently have small to microscopic mucinous cysts (Fig. 71-4A). Microscopically, the tumor is composed of cells arranged in cords, nests, and sheets with varying amounts of squamous, mucous, and intermediate cells. These tumors can vary from being well differentiated to highly aggressive, poorly differentiated histopathology. Various grading schemes to account for these differences cluster tumors into low-, intermediate-, and high-grade categories based on the amount of mucinous cells, solid squamous nests, mitotic rate, necrosis, and pleomorphism.[92,93] These tumor grades also correlate with patient outcome. Low-grade tumors (Fig. 71-4B) rarely metastasize, are often locally infiltrative,

and recur in 10% to 15% of cases, and therefore have an excellent 5-year survival rate of greater than 90%. In contrast, high-grade tumors (Fig. 71-4C) are highly infiltrative, recur in 30% to 40% of cases, and metastasize in 30% to 40% of cases at presentation, producing 5-year survival rate of only 50%.[94-96] Grading appears to have less prognostic importance when the submandibular glands are involved. Involvement of this site appears to be associated with an increased risk of distant relapse regardless of grade.[96,97]

Adenocarcinoma, NOS

These tumors are now restricted to lesions which do not show histopathologic patterns of the other salivary gland tumor types. These tumors can occur in the parotid gland as well as minor salivary glands and typically present in the sixth to eighth decade of life. At presentation, varying histologic patterns including tubular, papillary (with

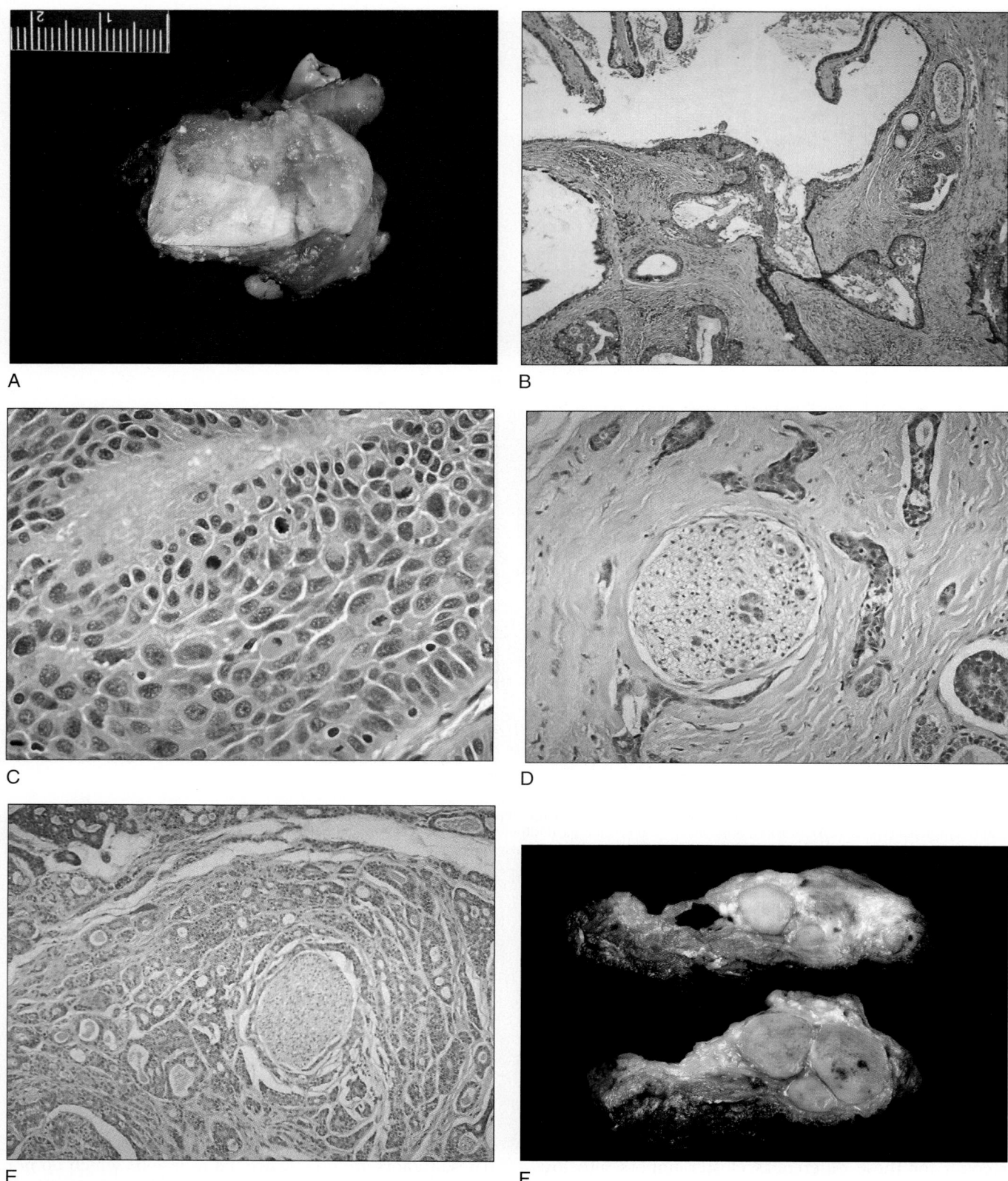

Figure 71-4. A, Mucoepidermoid carcinoma of the minor salivary gland eroding mandibular bone. **B,** Mucoepidermoid carcinoma, low grade of the palate showing microcystic architecture. **C,** Mucoepidermoid carcinoma, high grade showing solid growth and high mitotic rate (other areas of the tumor showed focal mucinous pattern). **D,** Minor salivary gland with adenoid cystic carcinoma growing in a typical cribriform pattern with many lumens showing eosinophilic basement membrane material. **E,** Parotid gland with adenoid cystic carcinoma growing in cribriform plates and cords with perineural invasion. **F,** Parotid gland with carcinoma ex pleomorphic adenoma.

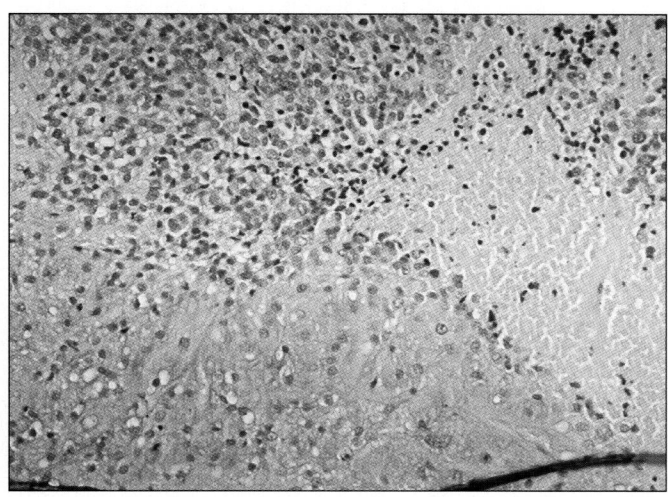

G

Figure 71-4, *cont'd.* **G,** Parotid gland with Carcinoma ex pleomorphic adenoma showing adenocarcinoma NOS with comedo type necrosis.

varying degrees of differentiation from well to poorly differentiated) adenocarcinoma may be observed. Important in the work-up of these patients is to exclude an adenocarcinoma from another body site as salivary gland adenocarcinomas can mimic adenocarcinomas from other organ sites.

Adenoid Cystic Carcinoma

Adenoid cystic carcinomas account for some 20% of malignant salivary gland tumors. They are frequently located in the minor salivary glands (40% to 50% of cases) and less often in the parotid gland (20% to 30%). The most common histologic pattern is the classic cribriform type or "Swiss cheese" pattern, characterized by neoplastic cells forming oval or circular spaces or nests. Within these nests is dark, eosinophilic, hyaline-like basement membrane material. The amount of the hyaline material can distort the cell nests and produce a small acinar- or cord-like appearance to the tumor nests (Fig. 71-4D). Perineural invasion is almost invariably observed in these tumors (Fig. 71-4E) and a diagnosis of adenoid cystic carcinoma without finding perineural invasion should be carefully reconsidered. Adenoid cystic carcinomas are graded into low-, intermediate- and high-grade tumors based upon the amount of solid growth, mitoses, necrosis, and pleomorphism[98]; like mucoepidermoid carcinoma, the degree of differentiation is correlated with long-term survival.

Acinic Cell Carcinoma

More than 90% of acinic cell carcinomas arise in the parotid gland. These tumors occur between the ages of 50 to 70, with men affected more than women (2:1 M:F ratio). The gross appearance of these tumors varies but is often white-tan in color and shows a well-circumscribed but unencapsulated mass. Microscopically, the most common histologic pattern consists of solid sheets of cells with low-grade cytology and granular basophilic cytoplasm similar to the serous acinar cells of a normal salivary gland. Less common variants include a cystic and microcystic pattern in which the tumor cells are arranged at the edges of the cyst, and cells with granular basophilic cytoplasm are arranged among cells with a tombstone appearance and capitation-type secretion as well as cells with a bubbly vacuolated appearance. Rare cases of acinic cell carcinoma have been reported to undergo de-differentiation into a high-grade aggressive malignancy[99] while most acinic cell carcinomas behave in a more indolent fashion.[100,101]

Malignant Mixed Tumor (Carcinoma Ex Pleomorphic Adenoma)

Malignant mixed tumors of the salivary gland are predominantly tumors that started as pleomorphic adenomas and the epithelial component of the adenoma underwent malignant transformation. This transformation may be confined to the adenoma, resulting in the noninvasive carcinoma ex pleomorphic adenoma.[102] However, the majority of carcinomas that arise out of pleomorphic adenomas are infiltrative and aggressive lesions (Fig. 71-4F and G). The transformation to a malignant phenotype is heralded by a change in the behavior of the patient's underlying pleomorphic adenoma characterized by a sudden enlargement of an otherwise stable adenoma or the onset of pain in a previously asymptomatic adenoma. Morphologically, the malignant transformation can take on any malignant epithelial salivary tumor phenotype, with the most common being adenocarcinoma NOS.[103] Occasionally, multiple recognizable histologic patterns may be present. These tumors are highly aggressive with 5-year survival rates as low as 25%. Another form of the malignant mixed tumor is the true carcinosarcoma, which again often arises from a pleomorphic adenoma background. These tumors have both malignant epithelial and malignant stromal elements.

Polymorphous Low-grade Carcinoma

Polymorphous low-grade adenocarcinoma (PLGA) is a rare low-grade carcinoma of minor salivary glands. These tumors grow as infiltrative masses and are composed of uniformly low-grade tumor cells arranged in a variety of histologic patterns including tubular, solid, papillary, microcystic, cribriform (with true lumens), pseudo-adenoid cystic (without true lumens), fascicular, single file, and cordlike.[104] Perineural invasion is common. In contrast to adenoid cystic carcinoma, PLGA stains positively for EMA and may be relied upon to distinguish these two pathologies. Rare cases of PLGA have metastasized and these cases have been associated with more than focal areas of papillary growth. Rare cases have dedifferentiated into high-grade aggressive carcinomas.[105]

Salivary Duct Carcinoma

Salivary duct carcinomas are rare tumors with a male predilection. These are rapidly growing tumors that can produce pain and nerve palsies. Morphologically, these tumors resemble comedo-type duct carcinoma of the breast and may also grow in a cribriform or papillary pattern. Cytologically, these tumors tend to be high grade with nuclear pleomorphism, single cell necrosis and high mitotic rate. Clinically, these tumors behave in an aggressive fashion with poor long-term survival.[106,107]

Lymphoid Tumors of Head and Neck

Extranodal Lymphoma

Extranodal lymphomas of the head and neck can take on the same morphologic spectrum as that seen anywhere in the body. While large cell lymphoma predominates, any morphologic pattern can be seen. While many of these lymphomas arise in association with lymphoid tissue within Waldeyer's ring, they are not limited to this location.

Angiocentric Lymphoma

Formerly called by a variety of terms (polymorphic reticulosis, lethal midline granulomatosis), this lymphoid malignancy presents as an aggressive destructive lesion characterized by ulceration and tissue necrosis. The tumor cells are visible, growing in an angiocentric location. Immunophenotypically, these tumors are often either NK or T cells with rare B cell phenotype reported.[108-110] It is important to distinguish this entity from nonmalignant sinonasal lesions, such as Wegener's granulomatosis, that can also produce an ulcerating and necrotizing lesion.

Plasmacytoma

Extramedullary plasmacytomas occur in the area of Waldeyer's ring of lymphoid tissue. These tumors represent clonal plasma cell tumors. Some 30% of patients with plasmacytomas will eventually develop multiple myeloma if followed for 20 years. Cytologically, the plasma cells can vary from well-differentiated plasma cells to very atypical-appearing plasmablasts. Occasionally, plasmacytomas with increased plasmablasts are misdiagnosed as poorly differentiated carcinoma unless the pathologist considers plasmacytoma in the differential diagnosis and orders the appropriate immunohistochemical studies.

Olfactory Neuroblastoma

Olfactory neuroblastomas or esthesioneuroblastomas are rare tumors that arise from the olfactory neuroepithelium. This epithelium can be found along the roof of the nasal cavity to the midportion of the nasal septum and onto the superior turbinate. These tumors appear morphologically similar to neuroblastomas that arise in the adrenal gland. They are characterized by proliferation of small round blue cells arranged in nests and surrounded by a vascular network in a loose connective tissue stroma. Rosette formations can be seen as well as neurofibrillary material in the center of the rosette and within the connective tissue matrix. These tumors stain for neuroendocrine markers including S100, NSE, chromogranin, and Leu-7, which aids in distinguishing them from poorly differentiated carcinoma.[111,112]

Melanoma

In addition to cutaneous melanomas that can occur anywhere on the head and neck, melanomas may also involve the mucosal surface of the oral cavity or nasal sinus. These tumors often present in the fifth or sixth decade of life. Mucosal melanomas often appear histologically similar to their cutaneous counterparts and may display a similar range of architectural and cytologic variability as exhibited by cutaneous melanomas. One interesting exception is that some mucosal melanomas display a small cell phenotype that on biopsy can easily be mistaken for a nonkeratinizing squamous cell carcinoma (Fig. 71-5A and B).

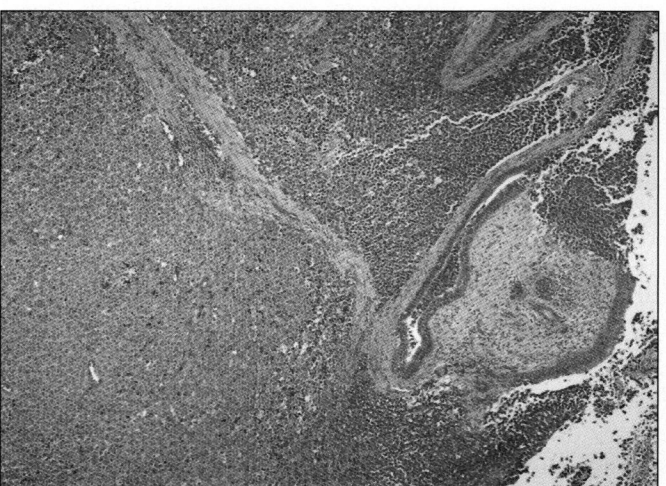

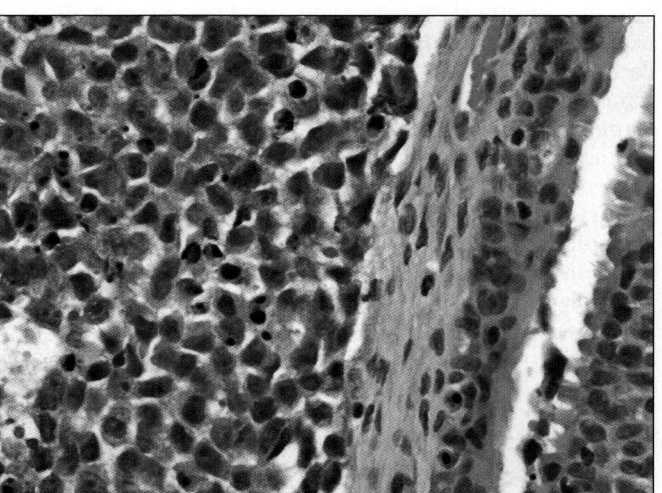

A   B

Figure 71-5. A, Sinus with primary mucosal melanoma showing infiltrative destructive growth by large epithelioid cells beneath respiratory mucosa. **B,** Sinus with primary mucosal melanoma showing infiltrative destructive growth by large epithelioid cells beneath respiratory mucosa. Cells exhibit a blastic appearance with prominent single cell necrosis and high mitotic rate.

Sarcomas

Angiosarcoma

Angiosarcomas may occur in the head and neck and most commonly present in the face and scalp usually in the sixth or seventh decade of life. Angiosarcomas of the oral or nasal cavity are exceedingly rare. Morphologically, these tumors show anastomosing vascular channels with varying degrees of nuclear atypia in the malignant endothelial cells. Those with better differentiation have a better prognosis.

Chondrosarcoma

Chondrosarcomas may arise in any bone within the head and neck as well as within the larynx. They are typically seen in the sixth or later decade of life. Similar to chondrosarcomas occurring in other areas, malignancy is defined by infiltrative, permeative growth as nuclear crowing and atypia within cartilage lacunae.

Osteosarcoma

Osteosarcomas may occur in any bone of the head and neck. This lesion is often seen in younger patients with a peak in the third decade. In addition, osteosarcomas have been seen after radiation therapy or in association with Paget's disease.[113,114] Morphologically, these tumors are characterized by infiltrative and destructive growth of surrounding bone and soft tissue.

Chordoma

Chordomas are low-grade tumors derived from notochord remnants. The two most common locations for the tumors are at the base of the skull (spheno-occiput) and sacrum. In the head and neck area, these tumors may involve the clivus, sphenoid, upper nasopharynx, occipital bone, maxilla, ethmoid, pterygoids, or cervical vertebrae.[115] These tumors grow as lobulated, infiltrative lesions that destroy adjacent normal structure. Microscopically, a myxoid matrix predominates with epithelioid cells growing singly or in small nests. These epithelioid cells are granular or vacuolated (physalipherous cells) and show staining for both keratin and S100 by immunohisto-chemistry, helping differentiate them from low-grade chondrosarcomas, which are keratin negative.

BIOLOGY

In the simplest of terms, cancer formation can be regarded as the escape of cells from the normal regulatory mechanisms of the cell cycle. Consequently, the cells proliferate without regard to their surroundings. Their progeny often become less differentiated, and they become able to invade surrounding tissues and spread to distant sites.

The genetic alterations associated with these changes are myriad. With regard to head and neck squamous cell carcinoma, much of the seminal work has elucidated the potential role of the tumor suppressor gene in the pathogenesis of cancer. These genes are expressed at appropriate levels in normal tissue and have a negative effect on cellular growth. If one or more of these genes is inactivated via mutation, chromosomal deletion, or DNA methylation, however, the loss of negative regulatory control may lead to unregulated growth and subsequently to cancer. The tumor suppressor genes p53, p16, and p19^{ARF} are the major tumor suppressor genes involved in HNSCC pathogenesis. p53 lies on chromosome 17p and is a negative regulator of the cell cycle via the cyclin/cyclin-dependent kinase complex. It is frequently mutated in HNSCC, with 40% to 70% of tumors harboring muta-tions.[116,117] p16 and p19ARF are also cell cycle inhibitors, and they are also frequently inactivated in HNSCC.[118] The method of inactivation, however, is not only gene mutation but also chromosomal deletion and promoter methylation.[119] Approximately 70% to 80% of cancers have allelic loss of the chromosomal region 9p, where p16 resides.[120,121] The loss of these cell cycle inhibitors is thought to contribute to progression from normal mucosa to preneoplastic lesions to invasive cancer.[122]

There are genes that are overexpressed in HNSCC as well. These oncogenes include cyclin D1, c-myc, and epidermal growth factor, and their increased expression can also contribute to the pathogenesis of HNSCC.[123-125] More recently, attention has turned to cell adhesion receptors such as integrins and E-cadherin with regard to tumor invasion and recurrence.[126,127] E-cadherin has been shown to be highly underexpressed in oral tongue carcinomas, and weak expression of the molecule was significantly correlated with a higher recurrence rate and worse 5-year survival.[127] Integrin expression is closely tied to the invasiveness of HNSCC cell lines.[126]

Theoretically, many of these genetic alterations should result in the expression of altered proteins that the host immune system would recognize as foreign. The cells would then be identified and targeted for immune-mediated destruction. It is clear, however, that tumor cells are able to escape from the host immune system through a variety of mechanisms.[128] A significant propor-tion of tumor cells have decreased expression of human leukocyte antigen (HLA), Class I, a molecule necessary for the presentation of foreign peptides to the immune system.[129] Furthermore, T lymphocytes that infiltrate the tumor are not as competent at killing tumor cells, presum-ably due to factors within the tumor microenvironment.[128]

New technologies will soon enable researchers to analyze further the genetic and immunological changes that occur in HNSCC. Complementary DNA microarrays allow for large-scale analysis of gene expression. Researchers have already identified hundreds of genes that are either overexpressed or underexpressed in HNSCC.[130,131] Future studies will elucidate the relation-ship of these genes to the pathogenesis of cancer, and novel tumor markers will be identified against which new chemotherapeutic and immunotherapeutic modalities can be targeted.

CLINICAL PRESENTATION/PATIENT EVALUATION

Patients who develop head and neck cancer present with certain symptoms according to the location of the tumor.

Some symptoms and patient characteristics are common to many head and neck patients regardless of the site of origin, however. Head and neck cancer patients are mostly male and in their sixth decade of life or older. Most have a history of tobacco and alcohol use. They often present with cachexia due to either dysphagia, tumor burden, or malnutrition. Rapid weight loss is sometimes seen. Hemoptysis is also frequently found. Pain, either primary or referred to the ipsilateral ear, is also often encountered. Many tumors present with cervical metastasis as the first sign of disease, and a thorough examination must be performed to identify the primary site.

More specifically, symptoms associated with oral cavity tumors include bleeding, dysphagia, dysarthria, and halitosis. Ill-fitting dentures are sometimes encountered. Oropharyngeal tumors cause similar symptoms. In addition, pain is often experienced at the site within the oropharynx or referred to the ear. A neck mass is often the presenting sign of an oropharyngeal tumor. Supraglottic tumors can present with dyspnea, dysphagia, and voice change. Glottic and subglottic tumors are likely to cause hoarseness and dyspnea. Dysphagia and ear pain is often experienced by patients with hypopharyngeal cancer.

The Initial Head and Neck Examination

An initial examination of the head and neck should be performed with the patient sitting upright in a chair. A standard and complete head and neck examination should then be performed. All 12 cranial nerves are examined. Otoscopy and anterior rhinoscopy are conducted. Examination of the oral cavity is preferably done with a head light to allow bimanual examination of the lips, buccal mucosa, gingiva, floor of mouth, and oral tongue. Palpation of the tongue and base of tongue is often forgotten, but is crucial for a thorough evaluation. The tongue base can be further examined with a mirror and with a flexible fiberoptic laryngoscope. The larynx is also visualized with these instruments. While viewing the larynx fiberoptically, the physician should ask the patient to perform several maneuvers: vocalization to allow assessment of vocal cord motion; tongue protrusion to aid in viewing the vallecula; and filling the cheeks with air to help visualize the pyriform sinuses. After the subglottis is evaluated, the laryngoscope can be removed and the examination completed with palpation of the neck for masses. Finally, the neck is palpated for masses. The size, mobility, and consistency of any mass should be carefully noted.

Staging Investigations

Radiography is a necessary component of the evaluation. It is now standard to order a CT scan of the head and neck for any patient with suspected cancer. Not only does this exam help to evaluate the size and location of the primary, but also any possible metastasis. An MRI scan can provide useful additional information in certain cases, such as in previously treated patients or in those lesions in which skull base involvement must be ruled out. Routine preoperative laboratory values should be obtained, as well as appropriate medical consults as indicated.

If accessible in the clinic, a biopsy of any suspicious mucosal lesion should be taken after local administration of anesthetic. Generally, oral cavity lesions and selected oropharyngeal lesions are easily biopsied in the clinic. For most lesions of the base of tongue, larynx, and hypopharynx, direct laryngoscopy with biopsy under anesthesia is required. During this procedure, flexible esophagoscopy should be undertaken to rule out tumor spread into the cervical esophagus. In addition, a tracheostomy and/or gastrostomy tube should be placed at this time if indicated. If no primary is identified, but a firm node 1 cm or greater is present, the node should be sampled via fine-needle aspiration (FNA). An open biopsy of a neck node in an adult suspected of head and neck cancer should be undertaken only after FNA diagnosis is inconclusive and a primary site cannot be identified.

Based on this extensive clinical and radiologic evaluation, the cancer is assigned a stage. Generally, T1, T2, and T3 represent an increasing tumor size, whereas T4 is defined by invasion of a surrounding structure (skin, nerve, vessel, cartilage). The node, or N, stage is identical for all head and neck cancer sites and is defined in Table 71-1. The absence or presence of distant metastases is defined as M0 or M1. The T, N, and M stages are combined into overall groupings that are presented in Table 71-1. Since the natural history of head and neck cancer varies somewhat according to specific anatomic location of the primary disease and since stages III and IV include a large number of different T and N stages, it is customary to refer to specific head and neck cancers by their individual T, N, and M stage and the primary site.

Follow-up

After completion of initial treatment, patients are seen every 4 to 6 weeks for 2 years in the office; during this period a complete set of laboratory data and chest

TABLE 71-1

Overall Group Staging of Head and Neck Cancer			
STAGE	**GROUPING**		
0	Tis	N0	M0
I	T1	N0	M0
II	T2	N0	M0
III	T3	N0	M0
	T1	N1	M0
	T2	N1	M0
	T3	N1	M0
IVA	T4a	N0	M0
	T4a	N1	M0
	T1	N2	M0
	T2	N2	M0
	T3	N2	M0
	T4a	N2	M0
IVB	T4b	Any N	M0
	Any T	N3	M0
IVC	Any T	Any N	M1

From American Joint Committee on Cancer: American Joint Committee on Cancer Staging Manual, 6th ed., 2002, p 65.

radiographs are checked every 6 months to look for metastatic disease or second malignancies. It is important to follow the level of thyroid-stimulating hormone, since many patients who have received therapeutic radiation to the neck will become hypothyroid and will require thyroid hormone supplementation. A baseline post-treatment CT scan (or MRI after skull-base procedures) is obtained about 2 months after the end of postoperative radiation as a reference point for comparison in the event that disease recurs.

During the third year, the patient is seen every 3 months, and every 4 months during the fourth year. After five years, the patient should be examined once per month.

PROGNOSIS

Prognostic and treatment predictive factors play a central role in the treatment decision-making process as the current therapeutic approach utilizes a risk-stratification paradigm. This recognizes that current accepted treatment modalities are associated with significant risk and a spectrum of toxicities. These factors facilitate this risk assessment and guide decisions on whether to initiate therapy and may also influence what type of therapy to administer. An ideal prognostic factor would provide information about the biological behavior of a tumor, permitting the prediction of the outcome and response to therapy. The use of such factors has become confusing, however, due to the spectrum of factors reported, often with conflicting results. This has led to efforts to systematically classify head and neck prognostic factors based on the level of significance and reliability including a recent meta-analysis.[132]

This heterogeneity results from several sources, including statistical underpowered studies, absence of statistical modeling for independent prognostic effects, variability in the nature of the therapy applied, the composition of prognostic factors as represented in the study group, and the inherent biologic heterogeneity of cancer. The heterogeneity is compounded further by the heterogeneity associated with the tests and instruments that are often utilized to measure aspects of the tumor biology. While it may be said that clinical prognostication is often imprecise, several clinical factors have an established role. In the head and neck, tumor site is a strong prognostic factor for survival, regardless of the treatment modality, and reflects the precision in which it can be identified by the clinician, though exceptions may exist, particularly for large tumors that overlap anatomic subsites.[133-135] Within each subsite, the current AJCC (American Joint Committee on Cancer) TNM staging criteria have been demonstrated to have prognostic significance and continue to evolve through efforts to stratify further the staging classification based on prognosis.[136] Most problematic are patients that constitute the heterogeneous locally advanced AJCC stage IV group.

The recent sixth edition of the TNM classification introduces a distinction of the heterogeneous T4 disease group based upon the probability of disease control, with T4a disease representing a reasonable probability and T4b disease representing such extensive disease that an adverse outcome is certain. In essence, the watershed between T4a and T4b reflects for most subsites the transition to unresectable disease that has been a recognized prognostic factor. Criteria for T4 subclassification by each anatomic subsite have been developed.[137] When considered with the N and M staging, this facilitates three distinct prognostic groups: advanced lower-risk stage IVA (potentially curable); advanced high-risk stage IVB (of dubious curability); and stage IVC with distant metastatic disease (undoubtedly incurable).[137] The critical distinction is the definition of IVB as N3 disease or T4b with any N category (excluding the nasopharynx subsite), for which aggressive local-regional therapy may be undertaken but with a potentially low expectation of success, a philosophical view that has been termed aggressive palliation. In this subgroup of patients, other patient-based prognostic factors, such as performance status, comorbidities, and a patient's ability to tolerate and comply with local-regional aggressive therapy, may have significant effect and influence on the anticipated outcome and hence treatment decisions. While the committee acknowledges that comparative outcome data do not exist for these new stage IV groupings, these groupings are likely to be surrogate groupings for tumor volume and resectability that have established prognostic effects and form the basis for the current therapeutic paradigm.

Within each subsite, various tumor features, noteworthy for their prognostic impact and not necessarily reflected in the new TNM staging criteria, warrant additional comments. In the oral cavity, tumor thickness/depth of invasion has been well recognized to influence the risk of nodal metastases[138,139] and reflect biologic aggressive disease with an adverse survival.[138,139] Po and colleagues recently demonstrated that tumor thickness in oral tongue carcinomas was the only significant factor that had significant predictive value for subclinical nodal metastasis, local recurrence, and survival in multivariate analysis. With the use of 3-mm and 9-mm division, tumor of up to 3-mm thickness has 8% risk of subclinical nodal metastasis, 0% local recurrence, and 100% 5-year actuarial disease-free survival; tumor thickness of more than 3 mm and up to 9 mm had a risk of 44% subclinical nodal metastasis, 7% local recurrence, and 76% 5-year actuarial disease-free survival; tumor of more than 9 mm had 53% risk of subclinical nodal metastasis, 24% local recurrence, and 66% 5-year actuarial disease-free survival.[139] For the nasopharynx, the staging classification reflects the prognostic importance of soft tissue extension beyond the nasopharynx, particularly the presence and the degree of extension into the parapharyngeal space.[140] In this regard, MRI is superior to CT imaging for providing this prognostication. For well-differentiated thyroid carcinomas, young age (younger than 45 years old) is an important favorable prognostic factor such that patients with other favorable prognostic factors including small tumors (1 to 1.5 cm) that are well encapsulated and confined to the thyroid may be observed with no adjuvant therapy recommended.[141] Anaplastic thyroid carcinomas carry an adverse prognosis irrespective of the local disease extension at the time of presentation.

For patients treated with radiotherapy, CT-based tumor volume assessment[142-146] and the presence of anemia[144,147-151] appear to be prognostic for local-regional control and survival. Interestingly, in a series of 258 patients with T1-4 glottic carcinoma treated with surgery only, anemia and positive surgical margins were independently associated with an adverse 5-year local-regional control rate.[151] Protracted overall treatment duration for a course of radiotherapy is well established as an adverse prognostic factor for local-regional control.[152-156] Limited data suggest that this adverse prognostic factor may also be important in patients receiving concurrent chemoradiotherapy where the risk of toxicity and treatment interruptions is increased.[157] For early-stage glottic larynx carcinomas treated with radiotherapy, a dose per fraction less than 2 Gy appears to be associated with poor local control rates in various univariate analyses, but this has not been conclusively demonstrated to be independent of other time-dose parameters.[156,158,159] Despite this, current consensus recommendations are for dose per fraction of 2 to 2.25 Gy.[160] Tumor response to radiotherapy has been demonstrated in a large prospective series of 228 patients with HNSCC treated uniformly with conventionally fractionated radiotherapy to be associated with local control. Multivariate analysis showed that the probability of local relapse was significantly and independently increased for minor regression at 5 weeks (<75%) (relative risk (RR): 2.3), for nonlaryngeal tumors (RR: 2.4) and for T3-T4 disease (RR:2.4).[134]

In patients requiring postoperative radiotherapy who demonstrate high-risk adverse prognostic features, the time interval between surgery and radiotherapy and the overall treatment time from the time of surgery to completion of the radiotherapy appear to be important.[161] Investigators from the MD Anderson have previously demonstrated that the most adverse prognostic postoperative risk factor is the presence of extracapsular extension (ECE).[162] These investigators have proposed and prospectively validated a risk stratification criterion that identifies patients as high-risk if ECE is present or two or more pathologic risk factors are present. These include oral cavity primary, mucosal margins close or positive, nerve invasion, more than one positive lymph node, more than one positive nodal group, the largest node greater than 3 cm, and treatment delay longer than 6 weeks.[161,162] Cooper and colleagues noted similar risk factors in a review of the Radiation Therapy Oncology Group (RTOG) database.[163] In the high-risk group of patients, progressively protracted treatment time was associated with progressively adverse local-regional control rates ($p = 0.005$) and overall survival ($p = 0.027$) with the most favorable outcome occurring when the overall treatment time was less than 11 weeks.[161] Other retrospective series have noted similar observations.[164,165]

The heterogeneity and imprecision of clinical prognostic factors have encouraged recent efforts to evaluate the potential prognostic significance of various molecular factors[166] and various quantitative measures describing functional tumor imaging such as magnetic resonance spectroscopy.[167,168] Grandis and colleagues reported a strong independent prognostic value for the epidermal growth factor receptor (EGFR) and its ligand, transforming growth factor–alpha (TGF-α), in a mature but heterogeneous group of 91 patients with a mixture of stages and sites treated with surgery and adjuvant therapy. Of the 91 patients, 56 (62%) received postoperative external-beam radiation therapy and 16 (18%) received adjuvant chemotherapy. Protein expression was quantitated by computer immunohistochemistry image analysis on paraffin-embedded specimens. Increasing levels of overexpression of either EGFR or TGF-α were associated with an increasing adverse disease-free and cause-specific survival. Other investigators using various quantitative assays of this surface receptor have also demonstrated an independent prognostic effect of EGFR overexpression.[169-172] These series are noteworthy for the strong prognostic significance observed in multivariate analysis, possibly due to the reduced test heterogeneity with such quantitative assays and the biologic significance of EGFR overexpression.

PRIMARY TREATMENT AND TREATMENT COMPLICATIONS

General Principles

Effective management of head and neck cancers requires comprehensive consideration of several often-competing treatment goals. This routinely requires the efficient integration of various treatment modalities and supportive services for appropriate patient care. As such, representation from disciplines including head and neck surgery, reconstructive surgery, radiation oncology, medical oncology, pathology, neuroradiology, dentistry, oral and maxillofacial surgery, nutrition, nursing, rehabilitation medicine, social services, and psycho-oncology is routinely required.

Before the start of any therapy, it is not only important to evaluate issues of histologic diagnosis and the anatomical extent of disease, but also to review issues that may impact on treatment compliance. This should include a review of the level of social support a patient has, with appropriate referrals to support services as indicated. Similarly, effective attention to nutritional support and pain management can significantly improve patient compliance to any subsequent therapeutic plan. Depending upon the treatment modalities that are required, pretreatment evaluation by oral and maxillofacial services may be indicated. If radiotherapy is indicated, prophylactic enteral tube placement for nutritional support may be appropriate, especially if concurrent chemoradiotherapy is used. Wherever possible, review of a patient's case within the context of a multidisciplinary tumor conference is strongly advocated.

On establishment of a histologic diagnosis of cancer in the head and neck, subsequent treatment decisions follow from a hierarchy of considerations. As treatment for head and neck cancer is associated with significant risk and spectrum of toxicities, it becomes important to identify patients with a poor prognosis, for whom treatment may be appropriately tailored. Determining a poor prognosis can be complex and imprecise, influenced not only by the anticipated clinical outcome, but also by various patient factors including treatment tolerance and toxicity. In large part, the imprecision of prognostication results from the clinical heterogeneity of established prognostic and treatment predictive factors, as already discussed. Where a poor prognosis is uncertain, it may be appropriate to adopt a curative intent, but with discussions held with the patient regarding the potentially low expectations of treatment success.

In tailoring treatment to the prognosis, it is the hope that patients with a poor prognosis will only be subjected to treatment toxicities that are appropriate for the goals of any palliative treatment. Hence palliative (or curative) intent should be clearly distinguished from palliative (or curative) treatment goals. Unfortunately, palliative treatment goals for advanced head and neck carcinomas (HNSCC) often require achieving some degree of local-regional disease control but with constraints to minimize toxicities. While various palliative radiotherapy schedules have been reported, in general, it may be more appropriate to consider the role of systemic chemotherapy to minimize the adverse quality of life that results from radiotherapy-induced xerostomia and taste alteration. In appropriate circumstances, surgical intervention including the use of high-dose rate brachytherapy implants may achieve treatment goals with the most favorable therapeutic ratio. When and how best to achieve such palliative treatment goals become issues of judgment that follow from engaging a thoughtful dialogue between various members of the multidisciplinary team and the patient and family members.

In treating patients felt to be appropriate for potentially curative therapy, a higher threshold for unacceptable toxicity on the part of the treating physician and patient is implicitly accepted. As a result, an evidence-based approach in deciding between various treatment options is preferred to justify the increased tolerance of toxicity. This has favored a systematic categorization of the quality of clinical reports reflecting the study methodology employed and the confidence that the results reported are free of biases and random variability. In general, randomized trials with sufficient statistical power provide the greatest unbiased level of evidence and confidence that the results are reproducible. Not uncommonly, treatment effects are often smaller than anticipated, leading to variable results among similar randomized trials, which limit consensus treatment recommendations. For head and neck carcinomas, competing comorbidities and the risk of second malignancies contribute to underpowered trials in demonstrating improvements in patient survival. As a result, prospective and retrospective comparative analyses of different treatment options are often relied upon to provide significant treatment guidance. These studies are, however, subject to potential biases from patient selection and the generalizability of the reported results may be limited by the nature of the patients selected. Attempts to match groups by stage are often performed to ensure their comparability, leaving only the treatment to vary. However, this strategy may be limited by the effects of stage migration and should be carefully reviewed for this potential influence. For HNSCC, this is particularly important in light of the significance anatomic tumor extent can influence treatment prognosis[137] and the recent evolution of various sensitive imaging modalities. Lastly, institutional series, case series, and reports may also be limited by the size of the sample study population and the absence of comparative analysis of different therapeutic strategies. They often provide insight into the management of rare histologic diagnoses, however. Where insufficient evidence-based literature exists, consensus treatment principles have evolved to further guide treatment recommendations. Alternative systematic quantitative tools such as decision-tree analysis techniques and cost-effectiveness analysis have not been well studied and remain limited in their impact in the management of head and neck cancers.

For HNSCC, therapeutic principles have traditionally considered competing treatment goals of local-regional control and the level of risk and spectrum of toxicity in defining the concept of a therapeutic ratio. For toxicity, both quantitative and qualitative issues are important to consider, as a severe but low probability toxicity may be important in defining what is an acceptable therapeutic ratio for the patient. This concept of a therapeutic ratio is important, as a dose-response relationship exists for both disease control and toxicity in several treatment modalities, including chemotherapy and radiotherapy and may even be extended conceptually to surgery. While treatment toxicities are an important consideration in evaluating treatment options, there continues to be an emphasis on local-regional control as a principal measure of treatment success. This underscores the natural history of the disease and the cosmetic and functional impact of cancer in this body site. As such, definitive therapeutic decisions often involve evaluation of surgery- or radiotherapy-based strategies. While there is a paucity of rigorous randomized comparisons of these two treatment approaches, several generalizations may be noted.

Where local-regional control rates appear comparable between competing treatment modalities, such as surgery and radiotherapy, the use of a single modality associated with the most favorable therapeutic ratio is preferred. This principle is most applicable to the use of surgery or radiotherapy for early-stage disease (typically T1-2 N0-1). For early-stage disease, local-regional control rates reported from surgical and radiotherapy institutional series appear to be comparable, with the possible notable exception of the oral tongue subsite where anecdotal experience suggests that local control rates with external-beam radiotherapy are inferior. (Rather, the incorporation of a brachytherapy implant appears to provide comparable results to surgery.) Surgery is often preferred for disease involving sites that are readily accessible, such as the oral cavity site, whereby the risk of complications are low. In contrast, early stage nasopharyngeal carcinoma is typically treated with radiotherapy due to the risks associated with surgery in this location.

Radiotherapy has traditionally been considered to be more attractive for early stage tumors involving sites where surgical resection may compromise organ function, such as involvement of the oropharynx, larynx, and hypopharynx. Again, this consideration is appropriate where local control rates appear comparable. However, evolving experience and sophistication with various organ-preserving surgical techniques offer the potential for good function preservation with no apparent compromise in oncologic results. Examples include various innovative larynx-preservation techniques that have been described including the supracricoid laryngectomy.[173,174] These techniques are influenced by patient and tumor selection, with some techniques being very operator-dependent and thus not necessarily generalizable. Where available, these techniques provide a patient in the early stage of disease that involves critical sites of organ function such as the larynx a potential single treatment modality without the issues of radiotherapy-induced late complications. It also provides the patient and the treating physician the ability to reserve radiotherapy for the management of relapses and second head and neck malignancies. Currently, the relative efficacy with regard to oncologic results and organ function between these surgical options and radiotherapy remains unexplored.

This single modality principle for early-stage disease attempts to minimize toxicity and emphasizes the importance of patient and tumor selection. Where postoperative radiotherapy appears likely, definitive radiotherapy may be more appropriate, particularly for small volume disease, as it is unclear that combined modality therapy is superior to radiotherapy alone. This consideration is particularly relevant where initial definitive en bloc resection may in combination with postoperative radiotherapy further complicate treatment toxicity and organ function. Not uncommonly, these issues are encountered with more extensive early-stage HNSCC or where the anatomic location limits achieving adequate surgical margins. For these and more advanced lesions, the role of debulking surgery has also been proposed.[175] This has been favored as a strategy for efficient reduction of the number of tumor clonogens without the surgical morbidity of more extensive tissue resection. Though attractive, the value of this approach remains controversial as it has not been subjected to critical scientific scrutiny and remains ill defined in the scientific literature.

For more advanced primary lesions (typically defined as T3-4 disease), increased treatment-related toxicities have generally been accepted due to more inferior local control rates. As such, a combined modality approach has typically been employed. Traditionally, this has included surgery and radiotherapy with either preoperative or postoperative conventionally fractionated radiotherapy. The latter approach has typically been favored due to the ability to delineate more accurately the tumor extent of disease and to permit pathologic stratification of patients requiring postoperative radiotherapy (PORT).[176] When evaluated in a randomized trial of 277 patients with supraglottic larynx and hypopharynx carcinomas (RTOG 73-03), PORT demonstrated superior mature local-regional control rates though the results were confounded by a higher dose delivered in the postoperative setting.[177] Recent randomized trials have permitted optimization of not only selection of patients requiring PORT,[161] but the dose required[162] and the identification of prognostic factors adversely influencing the outcome particularly in high-risk patients.[161] More significantly, it is now clear that the time from surgery to the start of PORT and the overall treatment time of PORT are important determinants of local-regional control in patients with high-risk features. As the issue of patients with more extensive disease undergoing higher risk surgical resection may confound these observations, the magnitude of benefit from manipulating these time variables remains to be determined. Nevertheless, it remains prudent to regard these observations, emphasizing the importance for effective coordinated management, which is best achieved in the context of a multidisciplinary team of health-care providers. Strategies to improve upon the results of surgery and PORT have included adjuvant chemotherapy, concurrent postoperative chemoradiotherapy, and altered fractionated radiotherapy schedules such as various accelerated radiotherapy schedules. These strategies remain subjects of ongoing study to further define their role and efficacy in patients with resectable locally advanced HNSCC.

For unresectable advanced disease, conventionally fractionated radiotherapy alone has been traditionally recommended. Results of suboptimal local-regional disease control in the absence of surgical options, however, have favored an acceptance of intensifying treatment with increased treatment toxicities. Despite this acceptance, it is important to recognize that the increased toxicity associated with this strategy warrants careful patient selection as the therapeutic ratio is clearly reduced. This has included the use of concurrent chemotherapy with daily-fractionated radiotherapy,[178] altered fractionated radiotherapy alone,[179] and recent combinations of concurrent chemotherapy with altered fractionated radiotherapy schedules.[180] In general, modest success has been realized with both daily-fractionated chemoradiotherapy and altered fractionated radiotherapy and they are regarded as acceptable therapeutic options. For concurrent chemoradiotherapy, determining the optimal agents and schedule remains largely undefined and the subject of ongoing evaluation. While a recent updated patient-based meta-analysis has demonstrated a modest survival benefit with concurrent chemoradiotherapy,[181] the generalizability of these results to current popular taxane-based chemoradiotherapy regimens is unclear.[157,182] Randomized data currently also support the use of either a dose-escalated hyperfractionated schedule or an accelerated schedule reducing the overall treatment time by 1 week with twice daily treatments in the final 2.4 weeks for this group of patients.[179] Determining the relative efficacy and indications for these two treatment strategies also remains largely undefined. Despite the improvements in local-regional control rates observed with the various altered fractionated schedules, the predominant relapse patent continued to be local-regional (approaching 50%) with distant relapses being less than 20%, leading current opinion to favor the use of concurrent chemoradiotherapy for large volume disease presenting at the primary site and/or in the neck.[183] The integration of chemotherapy has been particularly favored for bulky neck disease, as the risk of distant relapses is increased with some chemoradiotherapy regimens, demonstrating activity in impacting on this risk.[135]

In recent years, treatment decisions have been progressively influenced by obligations to achieve functional organ preservation for advanced but resectable HNSCC. This treatment goal has been buoyed by the fact that the superiority of altered fractionated radiotherapy schedules[179] and concurrent chemoradiotherapy[178] demonstrated in randomized trials have, in general, been in study populations that have been unselected based on the resectability of the disease.[184] This treatment goal has been particularly paramount for the larynx[185,186] and oropharynx subsites[187] and continues to evolve, as the optimal definitions, methodology, and instruments for studying functional organ preservation remain to be defined. As surgical resection for more advanced disease often results in greater normal tissue extirpation and loss of function, radiotherapy-based management strategies have typically been favored. It is noteworthy, however, that the relative oncologic efficacy of surgical resection often followed by PORT to these radiotherapy-based strategies has not been rigorously evaluated. In fact, studies have demonstrated that patients will prioritize length of life if compromises in speech or swallowing function are required.[188] As such, surgical resection remains an appropriate treatment consideration, particularly where organ function has already been compromised by tumor. Invasion of bony or cartilaginous structures by advanced HNSCC has also been considered an indication for surgery on the basis of historic experience of poor responsiveness to radiation therapy, though this is debated.[189] Recent results with treatment intensive intra-arterial chemoradiotherapy strategies have challenged this indication.[190]

In general, two therapeutic paradigms involving radiotherapy have been adopted for organ preservation. A nonselective strategy may be adopted whereby the tumor response serves as an in vivo test for radiosensitivity reserving surgery for salvage.[191] This poses increased risks of difficulties and complications with salvage surgery, but increases the number of patients achieving organ preservation. It is also limited by the recognition that not all patients who fail at the primary site after radiotherapy are amenable to surgical salvage. Alternatively, selecting tumors and patients who may have a more favorable probability of local control with radiotherapy minimizes the proportion of patients subjected to increased surgical complication rates, but may subject patients with radiosensitive lesions to unnecessary surgery. A hybrid strategy that continues to have proponents utilizes treatment response to either chemotherapy[187,192,193] or an intermediate radiotherapy dose typically between 50 and 55 Gy.[134,135] Responses to chemotherapy have been argued to predict for biologically favorable and responsive disease to subsequent radiotherapy. It has also been argued that significant radiotherapy responses possess sufficient predictive power, allowing for the selection of patients who are destined to require salvage surgery, in turn limiting the subsequent toxicity from cumulative therapy with higher radiotherapy doses. A large prospective radiotherapy series has demonstrated this to have independent prognostic value for local control.[134]

Early experiences of organ preservation with conventionally fractionated radiotherapy were limited to the larynx, and the results were disappointing.[143,194-197] Salvage surgery was possible in 50% to 80% of early stage disease treated with radiotherapy.[194-196] Inferior local-regional control rates reported for bulky disease such that the majority of patients required salvage surgery, with 50% being successful, and were also associated with increased surgical complication rates.[191,197] This gave rise to the use of various neoadjuvant chemoradiotherapy regimens in attempts to achieve organ preservation. However, the value of the neoadjuvant chemotherapy in contributing to local disease control was questioned. In a recently completed randomized trial, it was subsequently demonstrated to have minimal value and the trial indicated that intensive local-regional therapy was a more appropriate strategy.[198] Recent studies have now demonstrated that the use of an altered fractionation schedule (hyperfractionated and accelerated schedules)[179] or the use of concurrent chemotherapy[135,198] in combination with daily-fractionated radiotherapy offers superior local-regional control rates. However, this gain in local-regional control rate may still come at the increased risk of surgical complications with salvage surgery. The risk of pharyngocutaneous fistula increased from 15% to 30% in patients treated randomized to radiotherapy alone or concurrent chemoradiotherapy with cisplatin for larynx preservation, respectively.[185] It remains to be demonstrated whether this risk is observed with other treatment-intensive regimens (and for other head and neck disease sites) that aim to improve upon local-regional disease control.

As such, patients deciding between initial surgical therapy and organ-preservation therapy must balance the issues of immediate organ loss with lower complication rates and a reduced probability of delayed organ extirpation but at an increased risk of surgical complications. To guide these decisions, attention has focused on the probability of organ preservation with radiotherapy-based strategies and the degree of function that will be achieved. To date, radiotherapy predictive factors remain limited to considerations of clinical tumor features such as tumor volume.[142,143,146] While predictive factors of organ function remain in evolution, it is clear that where nonexisting pretreatment function is observed, successful radiotherapy is unlikely to restore function.

In the evolution of organ preservation as a curative treatment goal, several additional concerns have been raised. Initial concerns focused on the potential risk of an adverse outcome due to the potential risk of ongoing tumor metastasis. Early randomized trials comparing surgery and PORT with neoadjuvant chemoradiotherapy have demonstrated that organ preservation could be achieved without immediate surgical extirpation and with no compromise in overall survival.[192,193] The second trial has centered on treatment toxicity, especially with recent evidence favoring the concurrent integration of chemoradiotherapy for organ preservation.[185,186,198]

With concurrent chemoradiotherapy, increased swallowing dysfunction and secondary risks of aspiration, events contrary to the goal of functional organ preservation have been observed.[187,199] The mechanisms contributing to these events remain to be fully understood, but in general may relate to the severity and location of the treatment-induced mucosal edema and subsequent fibrosis and/or damage to peripheral nerves, all compounded by significant radiotherapy-induced xerostomia. Despite these concerns, preliminary data suggest that patient quality of life may still be improved due to organ preservation.[200]

Traditionally, the management of the primary tumor site dictated the treatment modality for the neck as a strategy to facilitate efficient management of HNSCC. Treatment decision-making for the neck has adopted a similar therapeutic paradigm of risk stratification to optimize the therapeutic ratio, but with the decision-making further complicated by the primary treatment considerations. Conceptually, the issue of functional organ preservation may also be extended to the neck as neck dissection may result in cosmetic changes and compromised neck and shoulder function. Similarly, radiotherapy-induced edema and fibrosis may compromise the goal of functional neck preservation and may be exacerbated by a neck dissection.

Typically, single modality treatment is favored for early stage neck disease and combined modality for advanced neck disease. In the clinically negative neck, where surgical resection has been elected for the primary site management, elective neck dissection may be omitted if preoperative evaluation determines a high risk of requiring PORT and the risk of occult nodal metastasis is sufficiently high to warrant elective management. Where radiotherapy has been selected for management of the primary site, neck dissection in the clinically negative neck is not indicated. In fact, preradiotherapy neck dissection may alter the lymphatic flow of the neck, necessitating larger volumes of the neck to be irradiated and requiring surgical wounds to be irradiated to higher doses. It may also contribute to delays in the delivery of radiotherapy that have been reported to contribute to an adverse overall survival when compared in a retrospective comparative analysis to postradiotherapy neck dissection.[201]

In the clinically positive neck with adverse risk features, combined modality (surgery and radiotherapy) has also been favored due to the increased risk and morbidity associated with regional relapses and the limited salvage options. Postoperative radiotherapy after a neck dissection is indicated based on the presence of adverse pathologic nodal risk factors such as extracapsular extension. Again, delays in the start of PORT may be detrimental, particularly when high-risk nodal factors are present.

Where conventionally fractionated radiotherapy alone has been employed for locally advanced HNSCC, suboptimal regional control rates coupled with the morbidity and the limited success of subsequent salvage neck dissection have prompted the incorporation and general acceptance of a planned neck dissection. This approach is generally accepted in the presence of residual adenopathy after radiotherapy. This approach has also been selectively applied to patients with adverse risk factors such as large nodal size (typically 3 cm or greater). This risk stratifica-

tion follows from radiotherapy series demonstrating an inverse relationship between nodal size and control rate.[202,203] Dubray and colleagues reported on the neck control rate in 1251 patients treated with radiotherapy alone and noted 3-year neck control rates by maximum nodal size of: 0.5 cm, 77%; 2 cm, 67%; 4 cm, 60%; 6 cm, 52%; 8 cm, 37%; and 10 cm, 7%. Multivariate analysis noted that regional relapses independently increased with increased nodal size ($p = 0.0001$), decreasing radiation dose ($p = 0.0001$), T4 primary disease ($p = 0.0001$), node fixation ($p = 0.02$), bilateral neck disease ($p = 0.03$), and geographic miss ($p = 0.0001$).[203]

However, there continues to be controversy regarding the benefit of a planned neck dissection in the setting of a complete clinical response in the neck, particularly in large pretreatment lymph nodes, after completion of radiotherapy.[204] Treatment with conventionally fractionated radiotherapy has demonstrated that the prognosis of large neck nodes with a complete response is associated with a prognosis comparable to that of smaller nodal metastases, and that the risk of relapse is low.[202,205] This suggests that perhaps the subgroup of patients with a complete response in the neck may have more favorable radiosensitive disease and may not require a neck dissection. However, a neck dissection continues to be favored, particularly for advanced neck disease, as the likelihood of achieving a complete response with radiotherapy alone is limited. The efficacy of this approach is further supported by several retrospective series demonstrating improved regional control rates[205-207] with a possible improvement in survival[208] despite the absence of a randomized trial. Attempts to definitively treat advanced neck disease also increase the risk of subsequent wound complications with any subsequent salvage neck dissection,[209] if that is even possible given that salvage options are almost always limited due to disease encasing critical structures such as the carotid artery.[210,211]

This issue has been further compounded by the use of concurrent chemoradiotherapy strategies that have reported improved local-regional control rates. One trial of concurrent hyperfractionated chemoradiotherapy versus hyperfractionated radiotherapy suggested a lower frequency of residual disease in the dissected neck specimen in favor of the concurrent chemoradiotherapy arm (21% vs. 37.5%).[212] No neck relapses occurred in either arm in cases where a planned neck dissection was performed. McHam and colleagues retrospectively reported on 109 patients treated with concurrent chemoradiotherapy with or without a neck dissection for indications of residual neck disease or as a planned procedure.[211] Residual neck disease was observed in 33% of the neck specimens (25% and 39% of neck specimens with complete clinical responses or partial clinical responses, respectively). Neck relapses were observed in 5 out of 76 (6.6%) and 4 out of 33 (12%) patients receiving and not receiving a neck dissection, respectively. The only factor significantly correlating with neck relapses was the presence of residual disease (5 out of 25 vs. 0 out of 51). These findings would suggest that both chemoradiotherapy and neck dissection are contributing to high neck control rates, with clinical evaluation of the neck

not possessing sufficient predictive power to select for a subgroup of patients where a planned neck dissection may be held. The role of positron emission tomography (PET) imaging, including a risk of false negative results, remains to be defined.[213,214] While there appears to be no appreciable increased risk of surgical complications with the addition of concurrent chemotherapy,[215-217] increased neck and mucosal edema, particularly with bilateral neck dissections, may significantly contribute to the treatment morbidity.

Management of patients with HNSCC is further complicated by the risk of developing second primary carcinomas and relapses within an aerodigestive tract that may have been extensively exposed to prior treatment. This further emphasizes the single modality treatment principle where appropriate and favors surgery alone where possible. An irradiated aerodigestive tract limits not only reirradiation, but can also limit an effective surgical salvage, as concerns of residual microscopic disease in cases that would otherwise warrant considerations of postoperative radiotherapy often exist. In general, repeat surgery is associated with fewer normal tissue toxicity constraints but greater immediate functional consequences than reirradiation. As such, where a second primary or relapse occurs within a previously irradiated field, surgical resection should be the primary treatment option.[218] Experiences with various repeat external-beam radiotherapy strategies, including the integration of chemotherapy, have unfortunately demonstrated limited success, often at the risk of significant toxicities.[218] The exception appears to be nasopharyngeal carcinomas that are more radiosensitive. Even then, significant late complications may arise, but may be more accepted given the limited surgical options.

As institutional series have demonstrated that higher repeat radiation doses are more likely to be successful, this has favored the incorporation of conformal radiotherapy techniques where possible. These may include stereotactic radiosurgery/radiotherapy, 3-D conformal radiotherapy, intensity-modulated radiotherapy, and brachytherapy techniques. The first option has been used as a preferred strategy for the nasopharynx where infiltrative disease extends beyond the limits of an intracavitary brachytherapy implant. The last has been particularly favored where the disease is well defined and for its ability to deliver a biologically effective dose to a limited volume. In fact, limited institutional series have reported on the efficacy of a brachytherapy implant for the base of tongue, tonsil for selected well-defined lesions as an alternative to surgery for lesions that are also suitable for surgical resection. In general, a coordinated brachytherapy implant at the time of complete gross surgical resection of either the second primary relapse or in the neck dissected neck may facilitate successful reirradiation. Where surgical reconstruction and wound closure incorporate the introduction of unirradiated tissue, the risk of complications from brachytherapy reirradiation may be reduced. This approach is limited by the ability to define the extent of microscopic disease in the head and neck where normal anatomic barriers and lymphatic drainage patterns have been altered from prior therapies. It thus becomes important to apply a brachytherapy implant appropriately, as these results are not necessarily generalizable.

Treatment Modality Considerations

Surgery

General. The decision to treat HNSCC with surgical therapy must be undertaken carefully. In order to assess whether a patient is a surgical candidate, the input of a multidisciplinary team is invaluable. Of the many issues to be considered, among the most important is the medical condition of the patient. Severe cardiac or pulmonary disease, profound malnutrition, and generalized debilitation are relative contraindications to immediate surgical intervention. Therefore a detailed assessment by a trusted internist or cardiologist is mandatory when a major resection is planned.

The next important consideration is whether the lesion can be removed safely with adequate margins. The "resectability" of a tumor is assessed via physical examination and radiographic studies. In general, tumor involvement with certain anatomic landmarks, including the base of skull and the prevertebral fascia, renders the lesion unresectable. This is due to the inability to achieve an adequate normal tissue margin in these areas. In addition to tumor location, massive tumor size can also preclude total extirpation. In these cases, negative margins may be impossible to obtain. In addition, adequate reconstruction may be exceedingly difficult, and other forms of therapy should be considered.

Postoperative function is also a primary concern when considering surgical therapy. The ability to speak clearly and swallow effectively is greatly affected by surgery in the head and neck. While complete resection of the malignancy is our paramount importance, reconstruction of the surgical defect must be designed so that the patient has an opportunity to regain as much speech and swallowing function as possible. Site-specific considerations will be discussed in the following sections.

The cognitive ability of the patient to undergo postoperative rehabilitation should be reviewed as well. Patients who are neurologically or emotionally unable to participate should be identified early in the decision-making process. They may be better served with different forms of therapy. The social situation of the patient should also be considered. Patients who live alone may require admission to a nursing home or skilled nursing facility in order to ensure adequate postoperative care.

In general, primary surgical therapy is reserved for patients with tumors of the oral cavity, selected early staged larynx cancer, skin cancer, salivary gland tumors, paranasal sinus tumors, and thyroid neoplasms. Patients with very advanced tumors invading bone, destroying cartilage, or extending into the soft tissues of the neck are considered for primary surgical therapy. When patients have severe organ dysfunction due to cancer infiltration, surgery should also be considered since functional restoration with nonsurgical therapy is unlikely.

Neck Dissection. It is important to understand the different types of neck dissections that can be performed

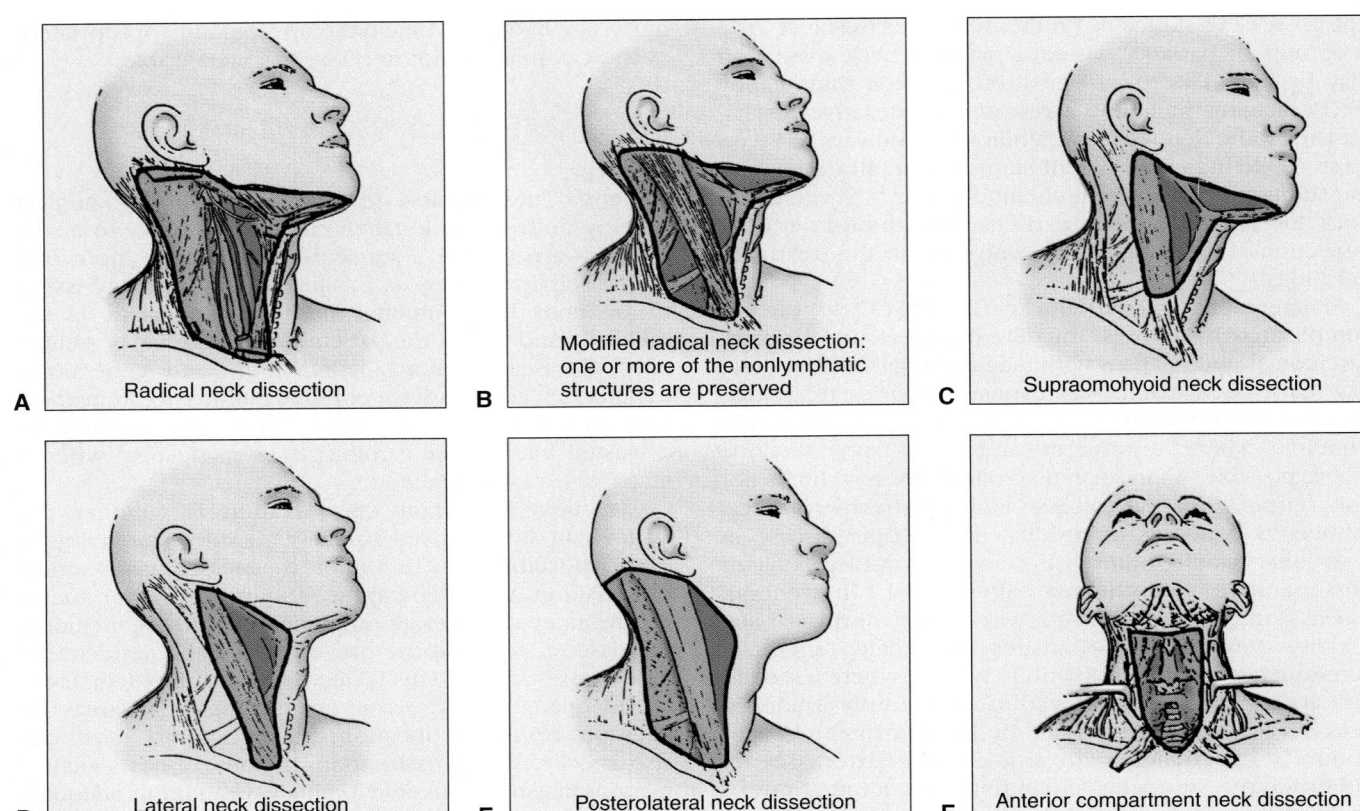

Figure 71-6. Types of neck dissection. **A,** Radical. **B,** Modified radical: One or more of the nonlymphatic structures are preserved. **C,** Supraomohyoid. **D,** Lateral. **E,** Posterolateral. **F,** Anterior compartment.

(Fig. 71-6). The radical neck dissection is a procedure wherein the lymph nodes from all five levels of the neck, the sternocleidomastoid muscle, the internal jugular vein, and the spinal accessory nerve are all removed. The specimen is removed en bloc, theoretically so that there is no spillage of tumor and so that there is a complete resection of any metastases. This procedure is indicated only in the setting of massive neck metasases involving most of the levels of the neck as well as the nonlymphatic structures.

A modified radical neck dissection removes all of the lymph nodes in the neck but spares one or more of the nonlymphatic structures. There are three types of modified radical neck dissection. Type I spares the spinal accessory nerve, type II spares the nerve and the internal jugular, and type III spares the nerve, vein, and sternocleidomastoid muscle. A type III dissection is also termed a functional or Bocca neck dissection, named after the Italian surgeon who pioneered the surgery.[219]

Selective neck dissections do not involve the resection of all five levels of lymph nodes, but usually three or more according to the site of the primary cancer. These neck dissections are usually perfomed in the setting of the N0 neck. There is some controversy regarding the use of a selective neck dissection versus a modified radical or radical neck dissection when known metastases are present, although a consensus is forming that a selective

neck dissection is appropriate for patients with N1 and selected N2 disease.[220-222]

Radiotherapy
General. Historical experiences with external-beam radiotherapy (EBRT) have demonstrated that acute treatment-limiting radiotherapy-induced dermatitis may be limited by fractionation and the use of higher energy radiotherapy. which results in less surface dose. As such, current standard radiotherapy practices have evolved to utilize a fractionated radiotherapy prescription using modern linear accelerated (LINAC) radiotherapy machines that can produce a spectrum of beam energies. With fractionation, issues of patient immobilization and treatment setup reproducibility become important considerations. For the head and neck, several critical normal tissue structures such as the spinal cord and optic chiasm are often in close proximity to the irradiated target. For these reasons, a prerequisite treatment simulation whereby patients are immobilized with various devices including a custom-made face mask and frame with the setup referenced to a laser light coordinate system in the treatment rooms is required before treatment may be initiated (Figs. 71-7 and 71-8).

Various immobilization devices exist, achieving differential degrees of immobilization. Immobilization addresses the issue of the precision of the treatment

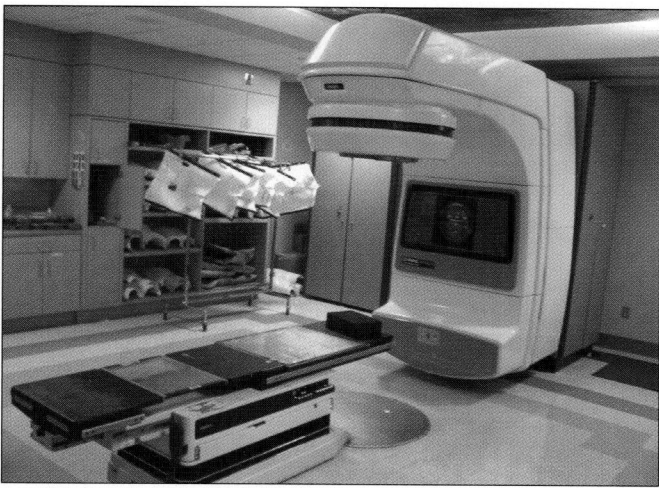

Figure 71-7. Linear accelerator with reference laser lights shown for reproducible patient setup.

delivery as a strategy to optimize the therapeutic ratio. The most examples of this are recently described stereotactic radiotherapy and radiosurgery techniques that involve immobilization of the patient in a rigid head frame system that may be removed daily for fractionated treatments in the former case or bolted to the cranium for a single large dose of radiation in the latter case.

More sophisticated treatment planning may involve obtaining axial images, typically with a dedicated CT scanner, of the immobilized referenced patient to facilitate non-coplanar three-dimensional beam arrangements or the use of intensity-modulated radiotherapy (IMRT) techniques. The former utilizes geometric shielding to effect shaping of the radiotherapy beam; the latter utilizes various approaches that result in modulation of the radiotherapy beam fluence to achieve additional degrees of radiotherapy beam conformality. Increasing the conformality provides an additional strategy to optimize the therapeutic ratio separate from the issue of radiotherapy beam precision. Radiotherapy beam conformality, however, is often dependent on achieving beam precision for it to be successful. This again places emphasis on achieving sufficient reproducible patient immobilization.

While these new conformal techniques are often advantageous in the sparing of dose to critical head and

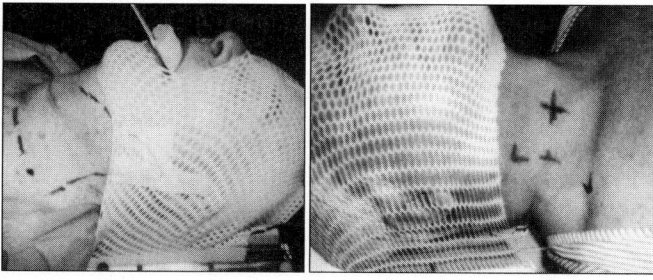

Figure 71-8. Patient in mask in the treatment position. **A,** Supraglottic carcinoma. **B,** Glottic cancer. (From Liebel and Phillips: Clinical Radiation Oncology, p 503.)

neck normal structures, it is important to recognize that this benefit comes at the expense of increasing the volume of normal tissue that is exposed to low doses of the entry and exit radiotherapy beams. This issue is particularly emphasized with the IMRT technique that may often dose many small segments of a radiotherapy beam or exploit the automated delivery process to deliver many more radiotherapy beams to achieve the degree of conformality sought. Concerns have been raised with regard to the potential long-term consequences of exposing larger volumes of normal tissue to low doses of irradiation. In particular, a genotoxic and possibly carcinogenic effect has been speculated. These concerns remain to be fully evaluated, but they emphasize the importance of judiciously and appropriately applying these techniques when counseling young patients, particularly those with an anticipated good prognosis.

The success of these techniques is also dependent on the ability to accurately identify anatomic sites that may harbor subclinical disease. Currently, the basis for this determination is derived from surgical and clinical documentation of disease extension that is often unique to each head and neck subsite. Recent functional imaging techniques, such as positron emission tomography–based studies, remain promising active areas of investigation. As a result, the transition to the use of axial images for radiation treatment planning places a significant emphasis on the knowledge and experience of the radiation oncologist with regard to the natural history of the disease as it pertains in axial anatomy. In particular, the identification of nodal groups that are typically at risk for harboring subclinical nodal metastases may more problematic. To aid in this regard, several reports have been published delineating axial anatomic structures that may be used to delineate the various nodal groups (Table 71-2).[223] The incidence of nodal metastases has also been summarized and can significantly aid the radiation oncologist. (Table 71-3) It is important to remember, however, that where prior treatment to the neck has occurred, altered flow of lymphatics is a significant concern. As with the head and neck surgeon, skill and judgment must be exercised with these precise treatment techniques. The alternative may be particularly detrimental.

External-Beam Radiotherapy Time-Dose-Fractionation Considerations. Conventional or daily radiotherapy fractionation (typically daily 1.8 to 2 Gy fractions to a total dose of 70 Gy) has permitted the delivery of higher radiotherapy doses that are currently limited by normal tissue tolerances such as the mandible. Conceptually, radiotherapy failures may result from insufficient doses of radiotherapy relative to the number of tumor clonogens or may be due to cellular mechanisms of radioresistance. The former has proven to be more amenable to therapeutic manipulation with the study of various altered fractionation schedules that may be generalized into two groups: hyperfractionation or accelerated fractionation (Fig. 71-9). Various randomized trials have been conducted and have been recently summarized.[183]

A hyperfractionated schedule or the use of lower doses per treatment fraction has been hypothesized to reduce

TABLE 71-2

Recommendation for the Radiologic Boundaries of the Neck Node Levels

LEVEL	ANATOMIC BOUNDARY					
	CRANIAL	CAUDAL	ANTERIOR	POSTERIOR	LATERAL	MEDIAL
Ia	Geniohyoid m.	Platysma m.	Symphysis menti; platysma m.	Body of hyoid bone	Medial edge of anterior belly of digastric m.	n.a.*
Ib	Mylohyoid m., cranial edge of submandibular gland or caudal edge of medial pterygoid m.	Platysma m.	Symphysis menti	Body of hyoid bone; posterior edge of submandibular gland	Basilar edge of mandible; platysma m.	Lateral edge of anterior belly of digastric m.
II	Bottom edge of the body of CI	Bottom edge of the body of hyoid bone	Posterior edge of submandibular gland; posterior edge of posterior belly of digastric m.	Posterior border of sternocleido-mastoid m.	Medial edge of sternocleido-mastoid m.	Internal edge of internal carotid artery, paraspinal (levator scapulae) m.
III	Bottom edge of the body of hyoid bone	Bottom edge of cricoid cartilage	Posterolateral edge of sternohyoid m.	Posterior edge of sternocleido-mastoid m.	Medial edge of sternocleido-mastoid m.	Internal edge of carotid artery, paraspinal (scalenius) m.
IV	Bottom edge of cricoid cartilage	Cranial border of clavicle	Posterolateral edge of sternohyoid m.	Posterior edge of sternocleido-mastoid m.	Medial edge of sternocleido-mastoid m.	Internal edge of internal carotid artery, paraspinal (scalenius) m.
V	Skull base	Cranial border of clavicle	Posterior edge of sternocleido-mastoid m.	Anterior border of trapezius m.; scalenius m.	Platysma m: skin	Paraspinal (levator scapulae, splenius capitalis) m.
VI	Bottom edge of the body of hyoid bone	Sternal manutrium	Skin; platysma m.	Posterolateral edge of sternohyoid m.	Medial edge of common carotid artery, skin and anterior-medial edge of sterno-cleidomastoid m.	n.a.
Retro-pharyngeal	Base of skull	Cranial edge of the body of hyoid bone	Levator veli palatini m.	Prevertebral m. (longus colli, longus capitals)	Medial edge of internal carotid artery	Midline

*Midline structure lying between the medial borders of the anterior belly of the digastric muscle.
From Gregoire, et al: Radiother and Oncol 2000;56:144.

TABLE 71-3

Distribution of Clinical Metastatic Neck Nodes from Head and Neck Squamous Cell Carcinomas[3,28,49]

TUMOR SIZE	PATIENTS WITH N+ (%)	DISTRIBUTION OF METASTATIC LYMPH NODES PER LEVEL (PERCENTAGE OF THE NODE-POSITIVE PATIENTS)					
		I	II	III	IV	V	OTHER*
Oral cavity (n = 787)	36	42/3.5†	79/8	18/3	5/1	1/0	1.4/0.3
Oropharynx (n = 1479)	64	13/2	81/24	23/5	9/2.5	13/3	2/1
Hypopharynx (n = 847)	70	2/0	80/13	51/4	20/3	24/2	3/1
Supraglostic larynx (n = 428)	55	2/0	71/21	48/10	18/7	15/4	2/0
Nasopharynx (n = 440)	80	9/5	71/56	36/32	22/15	32/26	15/10

*Parotid buccal nodes.
†Ipslateral/contralateral nodes.
From Gregoire, et al. Radiother and Oncol 2000; 56:137.

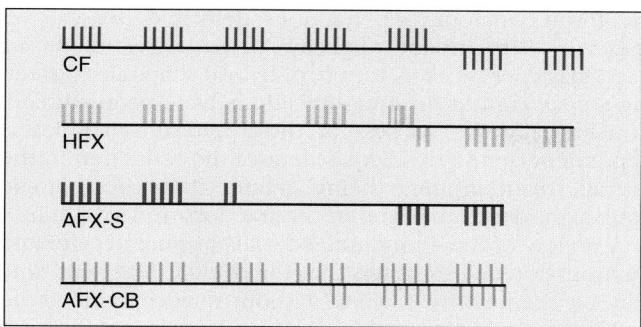

Figure 71-9. Schematic illustration of the fractionation regimens investigated by the Radiation Therapy Oncology Group. Each bar represents one radiation fraction. Bars above the lines represent large-field irradiation and those below the lines stand for coned-down boost irradiation. CF, conventional fractionation; 70 Gy in 35 fractions over 7 weeks. HFX, hyperfractionation; 81.6 Gy in 68 fractions over 6.8 weeks. AF-S, accelerated split-course fractionation; 67.2 Gy in 42 fractions over 6 weeks. AFX-CB, accelerated fractionation with concomitant boost strategy; 72 Gy in 42 fractions over 6 weeks. (From Nguyen LN, Ang KK: Radiotherapy for cancer of the head and neck: Altered fractionation regimens. Lancet Oncol 2002;3:693–701.)

the risk of late radiotherapy-induced complications associated with an increase in the total radiotherapy dose. Typically, the dose per fraction is reduced to 1.15 to 1.2 Gy and exploits a differential radiosensitivity between normal late-responding tissues and most cancers, including HNSCC. To ensure that the overall treatment time is not adversely protracted, fractions are often delivered twice a day with an interfraction time period of 6 hours.

Several randomized trials reported support the concept of hyperfractionation as a strategy to increase the biologically effective dose delivered without a significant

increase in the risk of late radiotherapy-induced complications (Table 71-4).[179,224–226] In general, improved local-regional control rates were observed with improved survival rates observed in two trials.[225,226] The largest trial (RTOG 90-03) of radiotherapy fractionation schedules randomized over 1000 patients with locally advanced AJCC stage III and IV HNSCC (>60% stage IV) for all subsites except nasopharynx (stage II disease permitted for base of tongue and hypopharynx) to one of four fractionation schedules including hyperfractionation to a dose of 81.6 Gy in 1.2 Gy per fraction twice daily in 68 fractions over 7 weeks treated every Monday to Friday.[179] The standard control arm consisted of 70 Gy in 2 Gy per day in 35 fractions over 7 weeks. With a median follow-up of 23 months, the 2-year local-regional control rate, 2-year disease-free survival rate, and 2-year overall survival rate was 54.4% (vs. standard arm of 46%, $p = 0.045$; see Fig. 71-10), 37.6% (vs. 31.7%, $p = 0.067$) and 54.5% (vs. 46.1%, NS), respectively. The modest but superior local-regional control rates in the hyperfractionated schedule reflected a 2-year local relapse rate and 2-year regional relapse rate of 37.8% (vs. 43.7% in the control arm) and 26.6% (vs. 32.1%), respectively. A planned neck dissection was permitted for residual neck abnormalities and for N2 and N3 neck disease regardless of the response. The 2-year distant relapse rate was 16.8% (vs. 17.8%).

Increased acute mucositis was the predominant acute toxicity with the hyperfractionated arm in the RTOG 90-03 trial. No increased risks of late toxicities were observed through the follow-up at the time of report, although this report would be regarded as immature for this endpoint. However, a prior prospective dose-escalation hyperfractionation study (also using 1.2 Gy per

TABLE 71-4

	Phase III Trials Addressing Hyperfractionation in Patients with Head and Neck Cancer							
REF	**TUMOR SITE AND STAGE**	**N**	**DOSE PER FRACTION (GY)**	**FRACTIONS PER DAY**	**TOTAL DOSE (GY)**	**OVERALL TREATMENT TIME (WEEKS)**	**TUMOR RESPONSE**	**COMPLICATIONS**
179	Various sites stage III–IV, stage II of tongue base, hypopharynx	1073	1.2 1.8* 1.6 2.0	2 1–2 2 1	81.6 72.0 67.2 70.0	6.0 7.0 6.0 7.0	LRC, higher with HF and CB (p=0.045 and 0.05); DFS, trend in favour of HF and CB (p=0.067 and 0.054); no difference in OS	More acute mucositis with all altered fractionations; no difference in late complication rate
224	Oropharynx T2-3 N0-1	356	1.15 2.0	2 1	80.5 70.0	7.0 7.0	5-year LRC, 59% vs 40% (p=0.02); improved local control of T3 tumors	More acute mucositis with HF: no difference in late complication rate
225	Oropharynx stage III–IV	98	1.1 2.0	2 1	70.4 66.0	6.5 6.5	Tumor response, 84% vs 64% (p=0.02) 3-5 year OS, 27% vs 8% (p=0.03)	Earlier onset of acute reactions with HF, late complications, no details
226	Various sites, T3–4, N0 or any TN	331	1.45 2.55	2 1	58.0 51.0	4.0 4.0	5-year LRC, 45% vs 37% (p=0.01); 5-year OS, 40% vs 30% (p=0.01)	More acute mucositis with HF; 5-year grade 3-4 late toxic effects, 8% vs 14% (p=0.31).

*Boost dose given in 1.5 Gy fractions.
CB, constant boost; DFS, disease-free survival; HF, hyperfractionation; LRC, locoregional control; OS, overall survival.
From Nguyen LN, Ang KK: Radiotherapy for cancer of the head and neck: Altered fractionation regimens. Lancet Oncol 2002;3:693–701.

fraction BID) conducted by the RTOG (83-13) demonstrated that the risk of late toxicities was significantly increased with an interfraction time of less than 4.5 hours.[227] A large retrospective review also observed the importance of interfraction time.[228] As this strategy can be logistically demanding for the patient, it becomes important to recognize that the current recommended interfraction time of 6 hours should be maintained.

Alternatively, an accelerated radiotherapy schedule attempts to deliver the prescribed total dose over a shorter treatment duration. This strategy is founded on observations of adverse local-regional control rates with protracted treatment durations (with conventional fractionated schedules) such that higher total doses are required to maintain the same probability of tumor control. These results have been interpreted to be consistent with a model whereby tumor clonogens surviving each daily radiotherapy fraction undergo an accelerated rate of repopulation. As a consequence, a larger tumor burden would be expected with increasing duration of treatment interruptions. It has been rationalized that by reducing the overall treatment time, the opportunity and impact of accelerated tumor repopulation would be minimized. As the severity of acute toxicities is increased, some accelerated schedules studied have attempted to modify the risk of unacceptable acute toxicities by modifying either the dose per fraction or the total dose as a strategy to achieve an acceptable therapeutic ratio. Accelerated radiotherapy schedules may therefore be categorized into two groups: schedules that do not modify the dose per fraction or the total dose (pure accelerated schedules)[229-232] (Table 71-5); and those that do (hybrid accelerated schedules)[179,233-236] (Table 71-6). Examples of

the former include two fractions delivered per day on some or all treatment weekdays or daily treatments for 6 to 7 days per week. A variety of hybrid schedules reflecting a spectrum of dose modifications have been studied. Conceptually, the success of these hybrid schedules is dependent on the dose equivalent of the reduction in the overall treatment time being greater than the biologic equivalent dose reduction in the fractionation schedule.

A review of the 4 randomized trials of pure accelerated fractionation demonstrates that the overall treatment time may be reduced by 1 week without unacceptable acute and late toxicities, achieving modest improvements in local-regional control with no evidence of consistent survival gains.[229-231,237] The most aggressive of these schedules was conducted at the BC Cancer Agency where the experimental arm consisted of 66 Gy in 33 fractions with twice-daily fractions of 2 Gy with an interfraction time of 6 hours resulting in an overall treatment time of 3.4 weeks (vs. 6.6 weeks). Patients receiving the accelerated schedule were more likely to experience RTOG Grade 3-4 acute toxicities (27/41 versus 8/41, $p = 0.00005$). Increased grade 4 late toxicities (8/41 versus 2/41) resulted in premature termination of the study, which precluded definitive conclusions regarding the therapeutic efficacy of this schedule. Of the eight cases of late toxicities, four occurred after salvage surgery, two were soft tissue necroses, and two followed from persistent acute toxicities. Investigators at the Sklodowska-Curie Institute observed similar observations of consequential late effects involving the mucosa in their experimental arm of 70 Gy in 35 fractions with daily fractions of 2 Gy 7 days per week with an overall treatment time of 5 weeks. These investigators observed no

TABLE 71-5

Phase III Trials of Pure Accelerated Fractionation in Patients with Head and Neck Cancer

REF	TUMOUR SITE AND STAGE	N	DOSE PER FRACTION (GY)	FRACTIONS PER DAY	TOTAL DOSE (GY)	OVERALL TREATMENT TIME (WEEKS)	TUMOR RESPONSE	COMPLICATIONS
229	Various sites, stage III-IV	82	2.0	2 (at least 6h apart)	66.0	3.4	CR, 35% vs 29% (p=0.18)	Grade 3-4 reactions, 27 vs 8 (p=0.00005); grade 4 late toxicity, 8 vs 2 (p=0.10)
			2.0	1	66.0	6.8	No difference in 3-year relapse-free survival	
230	Various sites, T2-4, N0-1	100	1.8-2.0	1	–70.0	5.0	3-year LC, 82% vs 37% (p<0.0001);	Severe mucositis, 62% vs 26%; late complications, 10% vs 0%
			1.8-2.0	1	–70.0	7.0	3-year OS, 78% vs 32% (p<0.0001)	
232	Various sites, all stages	1485	2.0	1	–66.0	6.0	5-year LRC, 66% vs 57% (p-0.01);	More acute mucositis with AF; no difference in late complication rate
			2.0	1	–66.0	7.0	5-year DFS, 72% vs 66% (p=0.04); no difference in OS	
231	Laryngeal carcinomas, T1-3, N0	396	2.0	1-2 (at least 6 h apart)	66.0	5.5		
			2.0	1	66.0	6.5	LRC, higher with AF (p=0.03)	More acute reactions with AF; no difference in late complications except for telangiectasia

AF, accelerated fractionation; CR, complete response; DFS, disease-free survival; LC, local control; LRC, locoregional contract; OS, overall survival.
From Nguyen LN, Ang KK: Radiotherapy for cancer of the head and neck: Altered fractionation regimens. Lancet Oncol 2002;3:693–701.

TABLE 71-6

Phase III Trials of Hybrid Accelerated Fractionation in Patients with Head and Neck Cancer

REF	TUMOR SITE AND STAGE	N	DOSE PER FRACTION (GY)	FRACTIONS PER DAY	TOTAL DOSE (GY)	OVERALL TREATMENT TIME (WEEKS)	TUMOR RESPONSE	COMPLICATIONS
Accelerated Fractionation with Total Dose Reduction								
233	Various sites, mainly stage II–IV	918	1.5	3 (every 6 h)	54.0	2.0	No difference in LRC, disease-free interval, or 08 ulceration,	More acute mucositis, less epidermal telangiectasia, mucosal ulceration, and edema with AF
			2.0	1	66.0	6.5		
234	Various sites, stage III–IV	350	1.8	2 (at least 6 hrs apart)	59.4	3.5	5-year LRC, 52% vs 47% (p=0.30); 5-year DFS, 41% vs 35% (p=0.32); 5-year DSS, 46% vs 40% (p=0.40)	More severe acute mucositis (p=0.00008) but lower frequency of grade ≥2 late soft-tissue effects (p<0.05) with AF (except for mucosal late effect)
			2		70.0	7.0		
235	All sites, oropharynx, 75%; T4.70%	269	2.0	2	−63.0	3.3	2-year LRC, 68% vs 34% (p<0.01) No difference in OS	Grade 3-4 mucositis, 83% vs 28% (p<0.01); similar late toxic effects
			2.0	1	70.0	7.0		
Accelerated Fractionation with Split-Course (Type B) or Concomitant Boost (Type C)								
236	Various sites, T2–4 N0–1	500	1.6	3	72.0	5.0	5-year LRC, 59% vs 46% (p=0.02); trend for higher 5-year DFS (p=0.08); no difference in OS (p=0.95)	More severe acute mucositis and higher frequency of severe late morbidity (p<0.001) with AF
			2.0	1	70.0	7.0		
179	Various sites, stage III–IV stage II of tongue base, hypopharynx	1073	1.8*	1–2	72.0	6.0	LRC, higher with CB and HF (p=0.06 and 0.045); DFS, strong trend in favour of CB and HF (p=0.054 and 0.067); no difference in OS	More acute mucositis with all altered fractionations: no difference in late complication rate
			1.2	2	81.6	7.0		
			1.6	2	67.2	6.0		
			2.0	1	70.0	7.0		

*Boost dose given in 1.5 Gy fractions.
AF, accelerated fractionation; CB, conconstant boost; DFS, disease-free survival DSS, disease-specific survival; HF, hyperfractionation; LRC, locoregional control; OS, overall survival.
From Nguyen LN, Ang KK: Radiotherapy for cancer of the head and neck: Altered fractionation regimens. Lancet Oncol 2002;3:695.

additional late toxicities when the dose per fraction was reduced to 1.8 Gy per day. While a significant gain in local-regional control and overall survival was observed, concerns regarding the validity of these observations have been raised due to the unexpected poor outcome of the control arm, especially where the study did not include patients with N2 or N3 disease.

In contrast, investigators from both the Danish[232] and Polish[238] Cooperative Groups conducted randomized trials accelerating treatment with six treatments per week, either as an additional treatment on the weekend[232,238] or as a single second daily fraction, with no evidence of any increased late toxicities[232] Acute toxicities were increased as would be expected. Significant improvements in local-regional control rates were observed with no survival gains. Hence the evidence to date would suggest that late toxicities possibly resulting from severe acute toxicities that exceed normal tissue repair capacities limit the increased biologic effect to only approximately a 1-week reduction in the overall treatment time. It may be possible to realize additional therapeutic gains with a modest reduction in the dose per fraction to 1.8 Gy, but this needs to be further validated.

Various hybrid accelerated radiotherapy schedules have been studied as strategies to further achieve increased biologic effects with greater reductions in the overall treatment time (see Table 71-6).[179,233-236] These schedules may be further differentiated depending on whether (type A) or not the total dose was reduced (type B and C). Typically, the total dose has been reduced where more than a 2-week treatment time reduction (from a conventional 7-week course) has been attempted. The most aggressive schedule was the CHART schedule that reduced the treatment time by 4.5 weeks by delivering 1.5 Gy TID with an interfraction time of 6 hours over a total duration of 2 weeks to a total dose of 54 Gy (representing a 18% dose reduction).[233] In a randomized trial of 918 patients with stage II-IV HNSCC involving various sites (majority laryngeal carcinomas), no improvement in local-regional control or overall survival was observed. While this trial did demonstrate increased acute toxicities that occurred earlier, it is noteworthy that fewer late radiotherapy toxicities were observed in the accelerated arm. Poulsen and colleagues performed a randomized trial of 350 patients with stage III-IV HNSCC through the Trans-Tasman Radiation Oncology Group

(TROG) studying a schedule with a 3.5-week reduction in the treatment time and a 10.6 Gy (15%) total dose reduction.[234] The experimental arm consisted of 1.8 Gy BID (6-hour interfraction time) to a total dose of 59.4 Gy. No improvement in local-regional control rates, disease-free survival, or survival was noted. Again, acute toxicities were more severe and occurred earlier, but no increased late toxicities were observed. Lastly, a French Cooperative Group Study (GORTEC 94-02) reported the preliminary results of a randomized trial of 268 patients with the majority having advanced T4 oropharyngeal carcinomas with the experimental arm receiving a 4-week reduction in treatment time and a modest 10% (7Gy) reduction in the total dose.[235] The schedule employed consisted of 2 Gy BID over 3 weeks to 62-62 Gy versus 70 Gy in 2 Gy per day. With only a median follow-up of 28 months, a significant improvement in 2-year actuarial local-regional control rate was observed (58% vs. 34%, $p < 0.01$) with no difference in overall survival. Increased acute mucosal toxicities were reported with no increased late toxicities noted with the limited follow-up. Hence the data to date would suggest that with only a modest total dose reduction of 10%, reducing the overall treatment time by more than 3 weeks could achieve improvements in local-regional control. With only a modest total dose reduction, however, it remains to be seen if late toxicities are increased.

Two other randomized trials have attempted to accelerate the overall treatment but without reductions in the total dose. The European Organization for Treatment of Cancer (EORTC) Radiotherapy Cooperative Group randomized 512 patients with T2-4 HNSCC of all sites excluding the hypopharynx to conventional arm of 70 Gy in 35 fractions daily over 7 weeks or 72 Gy in 45 fractions over 5 weeks (EORTC 22851).[236] The experimental arm introduced a split in the treatment duration with the first half delivering 28.8 Gy in 18 fractions over 8 days with 1.6 Gy per fraction TID. This was followed by a 12 to 14 day treatment interruption followed by a second course of 43.2 Gy in 27 fractions over 17 days again with 1.6 Gy per fraction TID. While the 5-year local-regional control rate improved 13% (59% vs. 46%, 95% CI 3%–23% with a 24% reduction in local failure rate, this treatment regimen was associated with unacceptable toxicities including twice as many grade 3–4 acute morbidities with grade 5 toxicity reported. Significantly more grade 3 fibrosis ($p < 0.001$) and severe neurological complications, including permanent peripheral neuropathy, occurred in the accelerated arm. In contrast, the RTOG conducted a 4-arm randomized trial of 1073 patients with stage III-IV HNSCC (stage II base of tongue and hypopharynx permitted) with one of two accelerated schedules also employing a treatment interruption and a 4% total dose reduction (RTOG 90-03).[179] This arm consisted of 1.6 Gy BID (6-hour interfraction time) to a dose of 67.2 Gy in 42 fractions over 6 weeks. No improvement in local-regional control or overall survival was noted, suggesting that the treatment interruption employed also contributed to the absence of treatment benefit that was not sufficiently compensated in the dose-intensity of fractionation schedule.

In the RTOG 90-03, a second accelerated schedule employing twice-daily fractions in the final 2.4 weeks with the second fraction delivered with a 6-hour interfraction interval and limited to only the boost volume.[179] A total dose of 72 Gy was delivered with the morning fraction 1.8 Gy and the afternoon boost fraction 1.6 Gy in the final 2.4 weeks of a 6-week treatment schedule. This limitation in volume was developed as a strategy to minimize the toxicity with the twice-daily fractionation. The timing of the concomitant followed from prior work by Ang and colleagues who demonstrated slightly better local control rates than if the concomitant boost was delivered at the beginning of the radiotherapy schedule.[239] The results of the RTOG 90-03 demonstrated that the local-regional control rate was significantly improved (2-year: 54.2% vs. 46.1%) with a trend to improved disease-free survival (Fig. 71-10). The modest but superior local-regional control rates with this delayed concomitant boost accelerated schedule reflected a 2-year local relapse rate and 2-year regional relapse rate of 36.9% (vs. 43.7% in the control arm) and 33.3% (vs. 32.1%), respectively. A planned neck dissection was permitted for residual neck abnormalities and for N2 and N3 neck disease regardless of the response. The 2-year distant relapse rate was 16.6% (vs. 17.8%). No improvement in overall survival was observed. Comparable increased acute toxicities were observed as with the other altered fractionation schedules including the hyperfractionated arm. No significantly increased late toxicities were observed though the incidence of late toxicities was higher in the accelerated schedule. As the

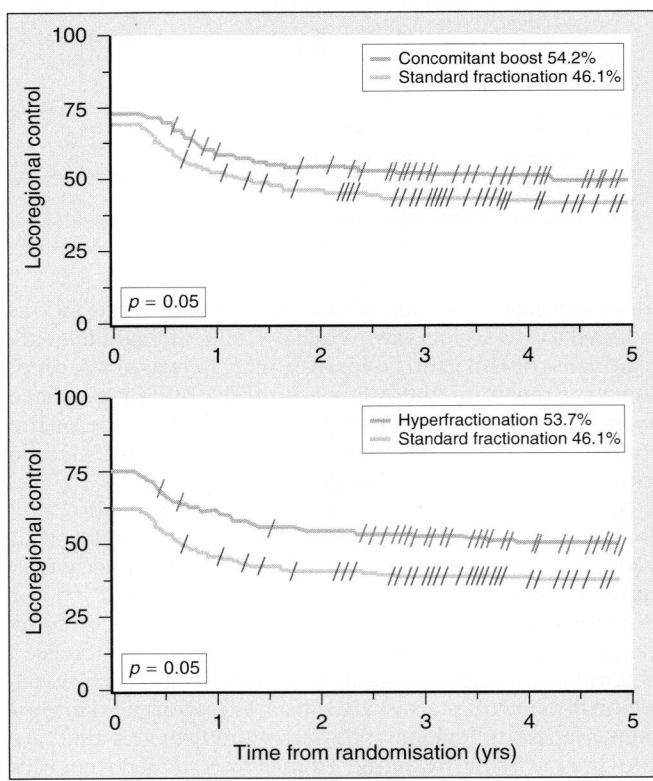

Figure 71-10. Local-regional control rates of concomitant boost accelerated and hyperfractionation regimens relative to that of conventional fractionation. (From Nguyen LN, Ang KK: Radiotherapy for cancer of the head and neck: Altered fractionation regimens. Lancet Oncol 2002;3:695.)

benefits from this fractionation schedule appear to be comparable to the hyperfractionated schedule reported in RTOG 90-03, investigators have concluded that an accelerated schedule with a delayed concomitant boost may be preferred due to the more favorable logistical treatment delivery issues.[183]

While the use of an altered fractionated radiotherapy schedule offers an improved local-regional control rate of approximately 15%, this comes at the price of increased acute toxicities. Most notable is the increased mucositis, which can occur earlier and be more severe depending on how the various dose and time parameters are manipulated. The results from the Conventional Accelerated Irradiation (CAIR) trial highlight the potential for excessive mucosal toxicities to exceed their normal repair capacity, leading to consequential late effects.[238,240] A similar potential for increased mucosal toxicities with consequential late effects also appears to have emerged with various concurrent chemoradiotherapy schedules including both conventionally fractionated[187,199] and altered fractionated schedules.[241] These results highlight that a limit to local-regional intensive therapy does in fact exist and have led to interest in the development of normal tissue protectants.

Treatment Toxicities and Normal Tissue Protectants. The most developed of these normal tissue protectants is amifostine. This thiol-containing compound and its metabolite, WR-2721, are believed to function as a free-radical scavenger and appear to have preferential normal tissue uptake with the highest concentration found in salivary glands and kidneys.[242,243] Amifostine has been shown to reduce cisplatin-induced nephrotoxicity.[244] It has received tremendous clinical interest initially for the protection of salivary glands from radiotherapy-induced xerostomia and most recently, as a mucosal normal tissue protectant. To date, clinical trials have reported improvements in radiation-induced xerostomia,[245-248] reduced hematologic effects particularly with concurrent chemoradiotherapy,[245] and reduced radiotherapy-induced mucositis with altered fractionated radiotherapy and from concurrent chemoradiotherapy.[246,249] No compromise in treatment outcome has been reported, including by a small randomized trial using definitive chemoradiotherapy[246] and a larger randomized trial containing a mixture of patients receiving postoperative radiotherapy and definitive therapy.[247] The latter trial led to the current approved indication for amifostine limited to the postoperative setting, due to concerns of potential tumor protection that may not be adequately detected.

This trial randomized 315 patients receiving conventionally fractionated radiotherapy to receive an intravenous 3-minute infusion of amifostine (200 mg/m^2) 15 to 30 minutes before each daily fraction.[247] The main toxicities were nausea (any grade 44% vs. 16%, $p < 0.001$), vomiting (any grade 37% vs. 7%, $p < 0.001$), hypotension (any grade 15% vs. 2%, $p < 0.001$), and a hypersensitivity reaction (any grade 5% vs. 0%, $p = 0.003$) with 21% discontinuing the amifostine before completing the scheduled treatment. The mean quantity of unstimulated

saliva 1 year after treatment was significantly higher, correlating with a lower frequency of late grade ≥ 2 xerostomia in the group receiving amifostine. In this trial, mucositis was not reduced (grade ≥ 3: 35% with amifostine vs. 39% no amifostine, $p = 0.48$), contrary to the results of other randomized trials.[246,249] It has been postulated that this discrepancy may relate to dose, as Buntzel administered 500 mg as a flat dose and only on the days during which daily concurrent carboplatin was administered (days 1 to 5 and days 21 to 26).[246] Ongoing trials are under way to verify these results. It is clear, however, that the toxicities related to amifostine are dose-related, particularly the emetogenic side effects. These concerns along with logistical issues with coordinated daily administration have prompted studies with a subcutaneous schedule of administration. Promising early results from a French Cooperative Group study (GORTEC) compared intravenous amifostine as 3-minute infusion of amifostine (200 mg/m^2) 15 to 30 minutes before each daily fraction to a subcutaneous schedule delivering 500 mg 20 to 60 minutes before each daily fraction.[248] Early reporting describes reduced incidence of hypotension (6% vs. 0% in favor of the subcutaneous route), with nausea and vomiting remaining dominant side effects in both treatment arms. The rate of acute xerostomia appeared to be similar, offering a potential alternative schedule for administration.

Intensity-Modulated Radiotherapy. In recent years, significant technological advances have enabled the ability to vary the fluence of the radiotherapy beam, permitting an additional degree of dose conformality and some exciting potential therapeutic applications. These may include an improved therapeutic ratio when irradiating near the base of skull, parotid sparing to minimize the risk of xerostomia, and manipulation of the effective radiotherapy dose per fraction that is delivered to the tumor or surgical bed. Coupled with promising advances in functional imaging, there exists the potential to manipulate the dose to critical areas within the tumor that may harbor radioresistant cells. In particular, interest has focused on identifying areas of tumor hypoxia that may be amenable to in vivo hypoxia imaging with various promising compounds including Cu-ATSM[250] and EF-5.[251] While this technique remains promising, it is important to recognize its evolving nature and the potential for geographic tumor "misses," particularly areas of subclinical tumor extension that may also be complicated by a lower dose per fraction delivered. In addition, successful sparing of normal tissues requires knowledge of the dose and volume constraints that are associated with acceptable risks for toxicities. This knowledge base remains in evolution. The generalizability of not only the technique but also target delineation is the subject of several ongoing trials through the RTOG. Nevertheless, early reports are promising.

Several prospective reports demonstrated that with intensity-modulated radiotherapy (IMRT), dose and volume constraints to the parotid glands may be successful in reducing the xerostomia associated with radiotherapy to the head and neck.[252-255] Quality of life instruments have been used and suggest that there may be additional benefits resulting from reduced xerostomia.[256] These investigators noted that the probability of a geographic tumor miss was low,[255,257] with the majority of relapses within field, emphasizing the importance to identify potential radioresistant subvolumes.[254,257] Lee and colleagues reported a promising 4-year local-regional progression free rate of 98% without any increased acute toxicities for 67 patients with stage I-IV nasopharyngeal carcinoma with 70% having stage III or IV disease.[255] While toxicities to important critical structures may be manipulated, this may come at the expense of increased skin toxicities[258] as a result of increased irradiation dose resulting from multiple complex beam arrangements that expose more normal tissues that would otherwise have been excluded with conventional techniques. It is this observation that has lead to concerns regarding potential long-term adverse effects and a call for prudence in the application of IMRT.[259]

Postoperative Radiotherapy. The indications for postoperative radiotherapy (PORT) may follow a risk-stratification paradigm that identifies patients as low, intermediate, or high risk for local-regional relapse, based upon the absence, presence of one, or presence of two or more risk factors, respectively (Fig. 71-11). These risk factors include: oral cavity primary, mucosal margins close or positive, nerve invasion, more than one positive lymph node, more than one positive nodal group, largest node greater than 3 cm, and treatment delay longer than 6 weeks.[161,162] In addition, the presence of nodal extracapsular extension by itself placed patients in the high-risk group.[162,163] While no randomized trial exists to demonstrate the efficacy of postoperative radiotherapy, Ang and colleagues demonstrated in a prospective trial of patients with an intermediate risk of relapse a comparable local-regional control rate (> 90%) as that of patients with no adverse risk factors, deemed to be low risk, and not treated with PORT (see Fig. 71-11).[161] While the overall survival for the intermediate group appeared to be inferior to the low-risk group, PORT continues to be recommended due to the importance of local-regional control.

Peters and colleagues previously reported on a dose-finding randomized trial demonstrating that a minimum tumor dose of 57.6 Gy to the whole operative bed should be delivered with a boost of 63 Gy being given to sites of increased risk, especially regions of the neck where extracapsular nodal disease is present.[162] These investigators did not find any benefit with dose escalation above 63 Gy at 1.8 Gy per day and postulated that this might be offset by tumor repopulation. As such, Ang and colleagues recently reported the results of a multi-institution prospectively registered trial of 288 patients with HNSCC deemed to require PORT.[161] Of these 288 patients, 151 patients were stratified as high-risk and subsequently randomized between a conventionally fractionated schedule versus an accelerated schedule utilizing the delayed concomitant boost technique with a

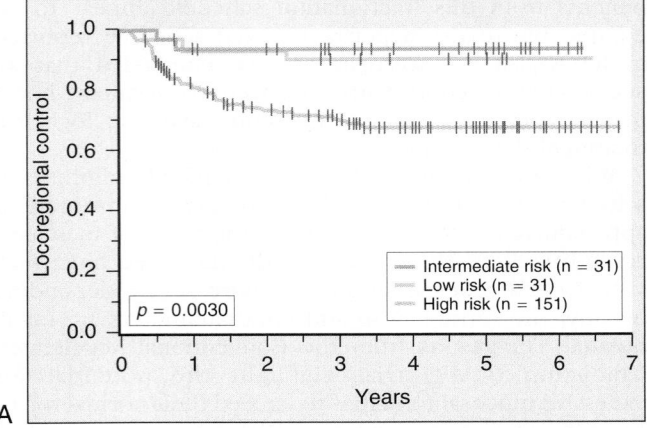

A

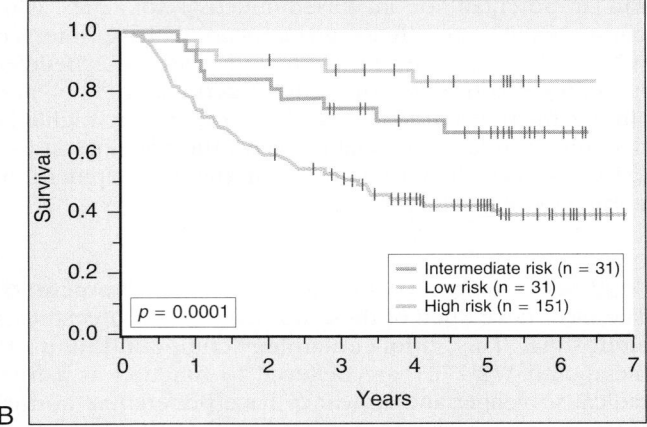

B

Figure 71-11. Actuarial local-regional control rates and overall survival by postoperative risk stratification. (From Ang, et al: Int J Radiat Oncol Biol Phys 2002;51:574.)

total dose of 63 Gy delivered in each arm. The authors report in this mature trial a nonsignificant trend for higher local-regional control ($p = 0.11$) and survival ($p = 0.08$) in favor of the accelerated schedule that appeared to result from an underpowered sample size (Fig. 71-12). Acute confluent mucositis (62% vs. 36%) was significantly greater in the experimental arm as would be expected. The actuarial probability of a patient sustaining one or more late complications between the two fractionation schedules ($p = 0.94$) did not significantly differ between the two arms. As such, these investigators concluded that the benefits of an accelerated PORT schedule had not been definitively established, but comment that, in practice, an accelerated PORT schedule may be used to keep the overall treatment time to less than 11 weeks in unavoidable situations where there has been protracted time before PORT. The latter follows from the demonstration of a significant adverse impact on both local-regional control and survival rates when analyzed by the overall treatment time (Fig. 71-13). These results must be interpreted with caution, however, as the study design did not stratify by the time interval before starting PORT. Care should be exercised in the use of an accelerated schedule as concern has also been raised of a possible

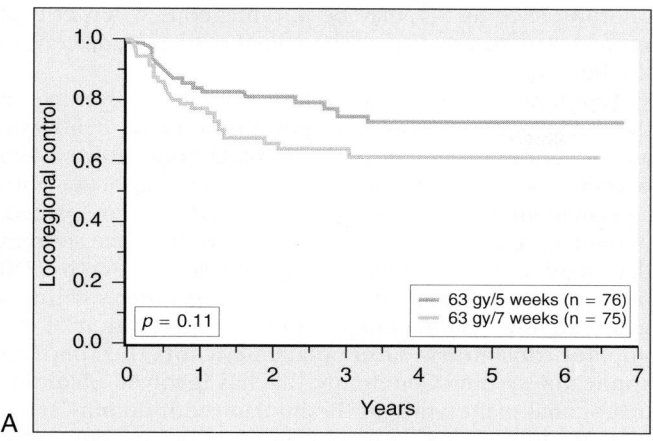

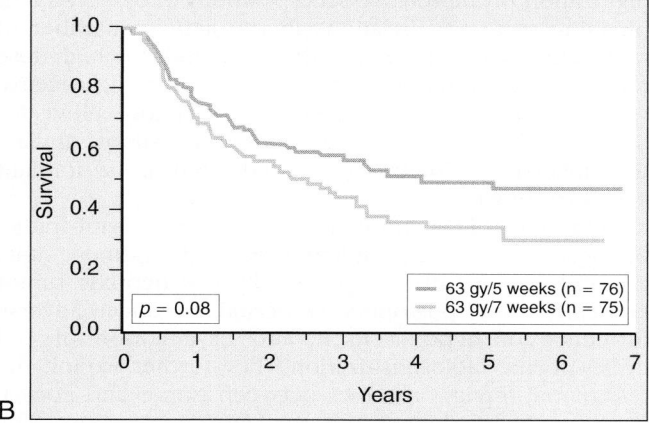

Figure 71-12. Actuarial local-regional control rates and overall survival for high-risk patients according to the postoperative radiotherapy fractionation schedule. (From Ang, et al: Int J Radiat Oncol 2002;51:574.)

increased risk of late toxicities in the postoperative setting.[260] Rather, patients anticipated to require postoperative radiotherapy should be appropriately identified with the appropriate arrangements made for the patient so as to prevent unnecessary interruptions to starting PORT. Trotti and colleagues demonstrated in a prospective comparative trial with a median follow-up of 6 years that patients initiating PORT within 4 weeks had a significantly lower rate of crude in-field relapses (0/10 vs. 10/32).[260]

It has also been proposed that the integration of chemotherapy with postoperative radiotherapy be favored in light of the increased risk of distant relapses also observed in the high-risk group. Ang and colleagues noted a 5-year actuarial distant relapse rate of 33% (vs. 3% in the low-risk group). While attractive, this remains an active area of investigation with no established chemoradiotherapy regimen. Two randomized trials of postoperative chemoradiotherapy with concurrent cisplatin and daily fractionated radiotherapy have been reported.[261,262] Bachaud and colleagues reported the results of a prematurely closed randomized trial due to poor patient accrual, demonstrating improved local-regional control rate, disease-free survival, and overall survival with weekly

concurrent cisplatin. Only 88 patients with stage III or IV disease with the presence of extracapsular extension (ECE) were randomized, however, with the authors concluding that these results require validation in a larger study. Recently, the RTOG presented the preliminary results of a randomized trial of 459 patients with high-risk postoperative features including ECE receiving radiotherapy or radiotherapy and bolus cisplatin on weeks 1, 4, and 7 (RTOG 9501).[262] Modest improvement in local-regional disease control and disease-free survival (54% vs. 43%, p = 0.049) in favor of the chemoradiotherapy arm with no difference in overall survival was reported.

Several institutional retrospective reports have suggested that the addition of a brachytherapy implant to postoperative radiotherapy where surgical margins are positive or close may improve upon the local control rates for a mixture of tumor sites.[263-267] This strategy may be particularly attractive for early oral cavity lesions where the risk of nodal metastasis is low, avoiding the morbidity with external-beam radiotherapy. Site-specific indications for the floor of mouth[263] and the oral tongue[264] have been reported. Pernot and colleagues reported on a 5-year local control rate of 89% for 97 patients treat with either

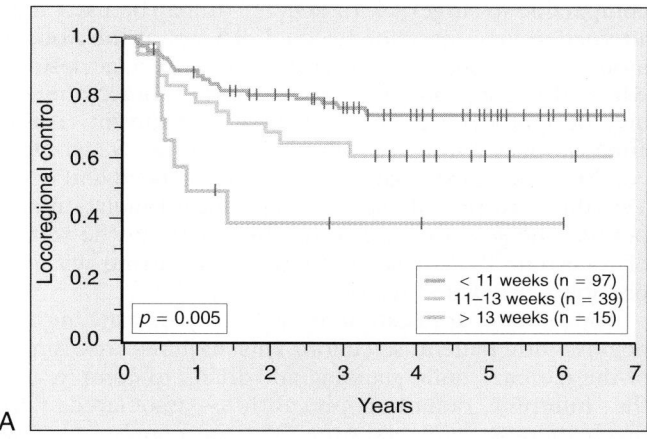

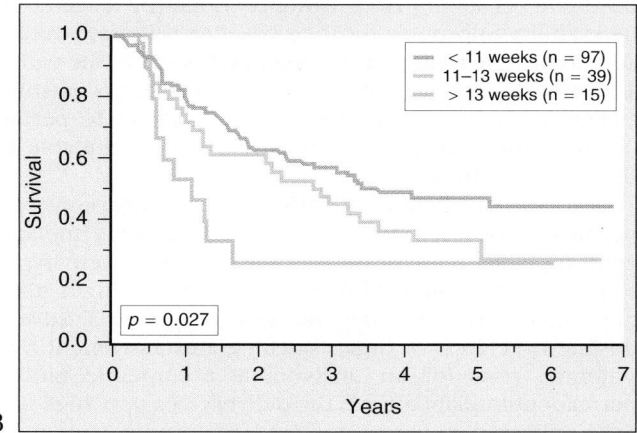

Figure 71-13. Actuarial local-regional control rates and overall survival for high-risk patients according to the overall treatment time (from the time of surgery to the completion of radiotherapy). (From Ang, et al: Int J Radiat Oncol 2002;51:574.)

postoperative EBRT followed by an implant or an implant alone for oral cavity tumors.[265] Self-resolving grade 1 and 2 complications occurred in 19% and 12% respectively with only 6% of complications requiring surgical intervention (grade 3). These results are particularly promising in light of the fact that one third of the patients treated included T3 and T4 lesions. As such, this therapeutic may be considered where the surgical margin of concern can be located and where experience exists for the safe administration of the implant.

Brachytherapy. Brachytherapy has a significant role in the management of head and neck squamous cell carcinomas[268,269] with various techniques described.[270] Due to the unique physical properties, treatment morbidity is minimized as a result of reduced irradiation in the surrounding normal tissues. An implant may be used in the definitive setting for several tumor sites including the tonsil and soft palate,[271-276] oral tongue,[277-280] base of tongue,[281-288] and lip.[289,290] The use of an implant in the base of tongue has the advantage of being a functional organ-preserving treatment strategy validated with quality of life instruments,[291,292] with the results suggested to be superior to external-beam radiotherapy alone and comparable to surgery with PORT.[284] It may be used as an alternative to surgery for selected cancers of the floor of mouth in specific circumstances. In early stage lesions, where the risk of nodal metastases is low, brachytherapy may be employed definitively or in an adjuvant fashion after surgery. In more advanced lesions, it is often combined with external irradiation of the head and neck. The ability to provide specific high local irradiation also permits the selective use of brachytherapy in the setting of recurrent[293,294] or second HNSCC occurring within a previously irradiated region.[295]

Appropriate application of a brachytherapy implant begins with patient selection. This requires assessment of the patient's understanding and ability to comply with the inherent radiation precautions associated with brachytherapy implants, especially for continuous low-dose rate (LDR) implants. Patients should be selected for their ability to provide for their baseline self-care needs in addition to the treatment-related needs such as the care of a tracheostomy, nasogastric feeds, and a patient-controlled analgesic pump as indicated. Patients subject to periods of confusion and disorientation may not be suitable for this mode of therapy.

Several considerations influence the decision of a permanent or a temporary implant. Permanent implants, emitting radiation over the lifetime of its radioactivity, use sources that provide LDR irradiation. Suboptimal placement of a permanent implant and the potential adverse dosimetric effects of organ swelling and movement pose potential risks for an unfavorable therapeutic ratio. A permanent implant affords the delivery of a very high total dose delivered, however, and may be advantageous when implanting complex and irregular surfaces not amenable to placement of temporary catheter-based implants where chinking of the catheters is a significant risk. The judicious use of permanent sources with low energy photons, such as ^{125}I, may be advantageous when critical normal structures, such as the spinal cord, are adjacent to the implant.

Temporary implants are more commonly applied in the head and neck as that permits a more deliberate and accurate placement of the implant applicator system without the radiation exposure concerns that occur with a permanent implant. Typically, nylon catheters are placed, mimicking the desired position of the radioactive sources that may then be subsequently afterloaded with LDR radioactive seeds embedded at defined positions within a nylon strand. This technique affords optimization of the implant dosimetry after placement of the implant applicator system. Commonly, this has involved obtaining orthogonal plain x-rays of the implant with dummy seeds placed within the selected applicator system, with digitization of the relative seed positions into a treatment planning software. Variations in the activity, number of radioactive sources, loading duration, and, for high-dose rate (HDR) computer-guided remote afterloading systems, variations in the dwell time and position allow for dosimetric optimization. Optimization cannot obviate the adverse dosimetry associated with poor implant geometry, however.

Temporary LDR implants also offer several radiobiologic advantages, including a reduced treatment time, the ability to irradiate a potentially less hypoxic tumor bed early in the postoperative period, a reduced adverse influence of hypoxia itself, and exploitation of cell cycle-specific radiosensitization. They further exploit the differential repair capacities between tumor and normal tissues, reducing the risk of normal late complications. The risk of radiation exposure to staff, however, necessitates good source handling skills and strict radiation precautions. Alternatively, HDR sources with computer-guided remote afterloading significantly reduce the exposure risks and required precautions. Fractionated radiotherapy is delivered with a single ^{192}Ir source fixed to the end of a cable wire that may be variably stepped along the length of each catheter. HDR implants have greater flexibility in conforming the implant dosimetry to the target volume, yield a relatively more homogeneous dose distribution to those of LDR implants, and, as the delivery of the radiation occurs over a shorter time period, are less subject to the effects of organ movement. This may yield a lower complication rate as a result of this precise geometric sparing. Concerns remain, however, with regard to the risk of increased late complications from the higher dose rate of radiation.[296] This has prompted ongoing studies to define the optimal fractionation schedules to reduce this risk. Several other promising but investigational techniques include the use of pulsed dose rate (PDR) radiation, which has been studied as a technique to exploit the logistical advantages and reduced radiation exposure of remote afterloading and the LDR biologic advantages that may be mimicked by this technique.[268,297,298] High-dose rate intraoperative radiation therapy (HDR-IORT) remains a promising investigational technique that has the advantage of accurately delivering radiation to the areas at risk of tumor recurrence potentially at a time when the tumor burden is the lowest.[299]

Chemotherapy

General. The role of chemotherapy in the primary treatment of locally advanced disease became more prominent in the 1970s due to the poor outcome of stage III and IV disease treated with surgery and/or radiation. Definitive treatments with chemotherapy emerged in nasopharyngeal cancer, organ-preservation protocols for the larynx[193] and the hypopharynx,[192] and, most recently, the oropharynx.[300] Systemic chemotherapy continues to have a role for palliation in patients with locally advanced stage disease, locally recurrent disease beyond salvage techniques such as surgery, and for metastatic disease.

Prognostic Factors. The decision to treat with chemotherapy remains dependent on various factors that can contribute to response. Those factors include the patient's performance status, nutritional status, the tumor burden and extent, disease stage, degree of tumor differentiation, and primary cancer site.[192,301-303]

Neoadjuvant/Induction Chemotherapy. Over the last 10 to 15 years, approaches to the treatment of patients with stage III and IV disease began to include the use of chemotherapy as induction therapy before planned surgical resection and, more recently, before radiotherapy. The concept of induction chemotherapy arose from several principles. It has been postulated that chemotherapy might promote regression of tumor, enhancing local-regional therapy through sensitization, and also may identify patients who might be candidates for a more conservative surgical approach as the need for improved quality of life through functional preservation has arisen. Thus organ preservation, rather than extensive, morbid surgical procedures came into vogue as a philosophical consideration in the management of advanced stage disease. An additional attractive feature with this approach was the conceptual ability to treat micrometastatic disease in hopes of reducing distant failure rates, which can be 40% or greater with conventional local-regional surgical/radiation approaches. Lastly, it was felt that the use of chemotherapy before the tumor and vascular bed are altered by surgery or radiation might improve the ability to identify responding tumorus that might benefit from adjuvant chemotherapy.

Nonrandomized phase II trials in the 1970s utilized single-agent chemotherapy based on strategies used in the recurrent and metastatic setting. These single-agent trials reported 30% to 40% responses.[304] Induction strategies subsequently involved multiple chemotherapy regimens. The first reported trials by Wittes and colleagues[304] showed a 71% response rate with complete responses (CR) noted in 21% of patients using cisplatin and continuous infusion bleomycin in 21 patients. Other studies followed, using cisplatin/bleomycin with other drugs such as hydrea and revealing increased toxicity with no improvement in response rates or survival.[305] Investigators from Wayne State reported the first trial using neoadjuvant cisplatin with infusional 5-fluorouracil (5-FU) with an overall response rate of 88% and a complete response rate of 54%.[306] The investigators reported that 120-hour infusional 5-fluorouracil showed improvement

over 96-hour infusions and that complete responses were two times higher after three total cycles compared to two.[305-307] More recent studies appear to confirm that complete response rates will increase after three to five cycles; other studies have confirmed the activity of this combination but at varied response rates (38% to 100%) and complete response rates (13% to 54%).[308,309] A 38% complete response rate was also achieved by the RTOG.[310] Numerous other combinations reported have included: high-dose cisplatin with fixed-dose 5-fluorouracil, high-dose 5-fluorouracil with fixed-dose cisplatin, intra-arterial cisplatin, and additional drugs with cisplatin/5-FU such as bleomycin, cyclophosphamide, mitoguazone, taxanes, and methotrexate have been given with significant toxicity and no overall differences in response or survival.[307,310-312] Trials using carboplatin with 5-FU have shown similar response rates of 70% to 80% and complete response rates of 30% to 40%, which are similar to those of cisplatin/5-FU.[313]

Although these experiences with chemotherapy plus radiation included several randomized trials with neoadjuvant chemotherapy, many were characterized by methodological problems. In 1985, the increasing interest in laryngeal preservation coupled with disappointing experiences with upfront radiotherapy for advanced disease, laid the foundation for the Veterans Affairs Cooperative Studies Program (VACSP) to initiate a multi-institutional randomized trial of neoadjuvant chemotherapy as an organ-preservation strategy.[193] Previously untreated patients with locally advanced but potentially resectable stage III (T2-3/N1, T3/N0) or stage IV (T1-3/N2-3, T4/N0-1) disease of the supraglottic or glottic larynx were randomized to either neoadjuvant chemotherapy or to surgical resection (Fig. 71-14). The chemotherapy regimen was cisplatin (CDDP) with continuous infusion 5-FU for 5 days with response after 2 cycles used to stratify patients to either continue with an additional cycle of chemotherapy followed by radiotherapy or, for non-responders, salvage surgery followed by postoperative radiotherapy. In total, 332 patients were enrolled, 216 patients with T3, 85 with T4, and 240 patients with N0-1 disease. Laryngeal preservation was noted in 64% of patients enrolled in the chemotherapy arm. Local failure was significantly higher in the chemotherapy/radiation arm, but distant failure was significantly lower in this arm. Long-term overall survival was approximately 30% in each arm. On subset analysis, sequential chemotherapy/radiation was less effective in the T4 tumors or those with N2 or greater disease; 50% of these patients required salvage laryngectomies. While this trial demonstrated that laryngeal conservation was achievable in 64% of patients with advanced laryngeal carcinoma, the incremental role neoadjuvant chemotherapy contributed to this is unclear. This laryngeal preservation rate appears to be comparable to the results achieved with radiotherapy alone followed by salvage surgery, which ranged from 50% to 73%.[191,197] The value of neoadjuvant chemotherapy has also been questioned as only a subset of patients with advanced laryngeal cancers had chemoresponsive tumors.

These results were subsequently mimicked in a similar randomized trial conducted by the EORTC.[192] The

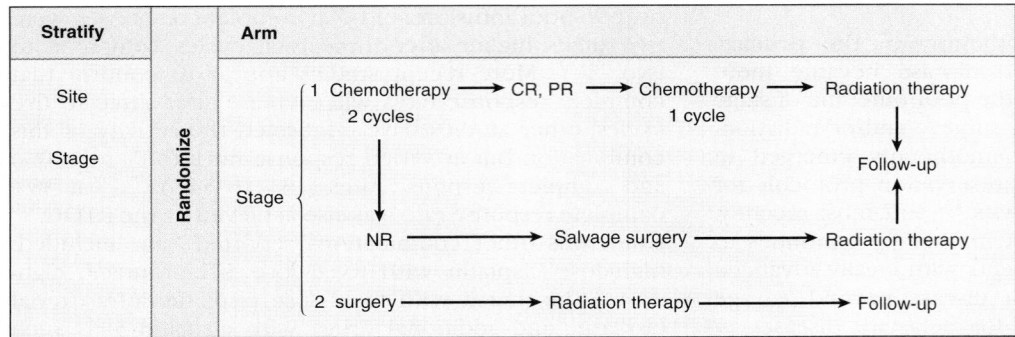

Stratify	Arm
Site	
Stage	

Randomize

Stage
{
1 Chemotherapy → CR, PR → Chemotherapy → Radiation therapy
   2 cycles   1 cycle

                                              Follow-up

NR → Salvage surgery → Radiation therapy

2 surgery → Radiation therapy → Follow-up
}

Figure 71-14. Study schema of VA larynx preservation trial. (From Department of Veterans Affairs Laryngeal Cancer Study Group: N Engl J Med 1991;324:1685–1690.)

EORTC randomized a smaller population of 194 patients with locally advanced hypopharyngeal cancer (6% with stage II, 57% with stage III, and 37% with stage IV) to either cisplatin/5-FU versus total laryngectomy/partial pharyngectomy/radical neck dissection with adjuvant radiation therapy. Only patients who achieved a complete response received radiation alone; 54% had a complete response at the primary site, 51% at the nodal site, and 43% achieving a CR both at the primary and nodal site. Treatment failures at the local, regional, and second primary sites occurred at approximately the same frequencies in the immediate-surgery arm (12%, 19%, and 16%, respectively) and in the induction-chemotherapy arm (17%, 23%, and 13%, respectively). In contrast, there were fewer failures at distant sites in the induction-chemotherapy arm than in the immediate-surgery arm (25% versus 36%, respectively; $p = .041$). The median duration of survival was 25 months in the immediate-surgery arm and 44 months in the induction-chemotherapy arm that the investigators concluded was equivalent. The 3- and 5-year estimates of retaining a functional larynx in patients treated in the induction-chemotherapy arm were 42% (95% confidence interval = 31% to 53%) and 35% (95% confidence interval = 22% to 48%), respectively. It would appear that with a more stringent response to chemotherapy, fewer local relapses might be anticipated in contrast to the results of the VA study.[193]

Recently, a French Cooperative trial (GETTEC) reported the randomized results using a neoadjuvant chemotherapy approach for organ preservation for the oropharynx site.[300] Patients with a squamous cell carcinoma of the oropharynx for whom curative radiotherapy or surgery was considered feasible were randomized to either three cycles of neoadjuvant chemotherapy followed by local-regional treatment determined by the treating physician or the same local-regional treatment without chemotherapy. The local-regional treatment consisted either of surgery plus radiotherapy or of radiotherapy alone. The chemotherapy consisted of cisplatin (100 mg/m^2) on day 1 followed by a 24-hour intravenous infusion of fluorouracil (1000 mg/m^2/day) for 5 days delivered every 21 days. A total of 318 patients were enrolled in the study between 1986 and 1992; the study was prematurely closed due to a loss of clinical equipoise as the treating physicians believed that neoadjuvant chemotherapy was efficacious. The authors note, however, that this decision was inde-

pendent of any knowledge of the trial results, minimizing the impact of any bias. Overall survival was significantly better ($p = 0.03$) in the neoadjuvant chemotherapy group than in the control group, with a median survival of 5.1 years versus 3.3 years in the no-chemotherapy group. The effect of neoadjuvant chemotherapy on event-free survival was less and of borderline significance ($p = 0.11$). In summary, it is clear that systemic chemotherapy can impact on the risk of distant relapses, with possible improvements in overall survival.

The preceding studies led to the more recent intergroup trial, RTOG 9111, conducted in patients with stage III/IV resectable disease of the larynx.[198] Patients were randomized to three arms: chemotherapy (cisplatin/5-FU) followed by radiation therapy; concurrent chemoradiation with high-dose cisplatin as the radiosensitizer; or standard fractionated external-beam radiation daily. Patients with T4 lesions were not included in this trial. If a patient initially had N2 or N3 neck disease, a modified neck dissection was performed independent of response. Two-year laryngectomy-free survival was superior in the group of patients receiving concurrent chemoradiotherapy ($p = 0.018$), reducing the number of laryngectomies performed by approximately 50%, with the number of larygectomies performed identical in the other two treatment arms (43 vs. 21 vs. 49, respectively). Two-year local-regional control rates were also superior in the concurrent chemoradiotherapy arm (61%, 78%, 56%, respectively), with the overall survival (~75%) not differing among the treatment arms.

Efforts continue to improve on the clinical efficacy of neoadjuvant chemotherapy in hopes of achieving significant activity to yield consistent survival benefits.[314] Recent strategies have focused on the use of neoadjuvant chemotherapy followed by concurrent chemoradiotherapy. Various phase II studies[187,301,315-318] have been reported. These also include variations of the "gold standard" chemotherapy regimen, cisplatin and 5-FU, incorporating leucovorin (PFL regimen) with or without interferon-α, efforts pioneered by Vokes and colleagues in Chicago.[301,317] A recently completed Eastern Cooperative Oncology Group (ECOG) phase II trial of neoadjuvant carboplatin and paclitaxel followed by concurrent weekly paclitaxel and daily-fractionated radiotherapy for oropharynx carcinomas included functional swallowing assessments as a measure of functional preservation. This trial follows from promising preliminary data reported by Machtay and colleagues who noted a major clinical response rate of 89% after induction chemotherapy, with a 90% complete response rate after concomitant chemotherapy.[187] The 3-year survival rate and 3-year progression-free survival was 68% and 60%, respectively. Local-regional control was 82% and the 3-year distant failure rate was reported at 18%. Organ preservation was achieved in 77% of all patients. In general, increased toxicities have been observed in these trials with promising activity that will require study in the context of a randomized trial. These strategies offer the promise of not only improved local-regional control rates with organ preservation, but also with a reduced risk of late distant relapses and more consistent improvements in overall survival. Recent results from a large patient-based meta-analysis, however, have drawn attention to the potential negative effects of neoadjuvant chemotherapy when used as a larynx preservation strategy, as a nonsignificant hazard ratio of death (1.19, 0.97-1.46) was noted.[181]

Concurrent/Concomitant Chemoradiotherapy.

A significant body of literature exists including numerous randomized trials of concurrent chemotherapy that have been systematically summarized by several investigators.[181,319-321] These independent reviews have consistently favored the concurrent integration of chemotherapy. Pignon and colleagues reported the largest and recently updated of these meta-analyses.[181] This patient-based meta-analysis of over 10,000 patients derived from 63 randomized trials confirmed an absolute survival benefit of 4% at 2 and 5 years with the greatest benefit of 8% observed in the group receiving concurrent chemotherapy. The group that contributed to this survival benefit was found to be the group of studies that utilized radiotherapy as the local-regional treatment. The survival benefit was found to be significantly greater with multi-agent versus single-agent concurrent chemotherapy. A

nonsignificant increase in the risk of death was noted with multi-agent chemotherapy regimens containing a platinum agent (Fig. 71-15). When analyzed with co-variants, a significant decreasing benefit on survival for concurrent chemotherapy was noted with increasing age, which might be partly explained by lower compliance and higher toxicities (Fig. 71-16). These results are consistent with anecdotal clinical experiences and high-light the importance of patient selection for concurrent chemoradiotherapy in light of the small incremental benefit. No survival benefit was observed with either neo-adjuvant or adjuvant chemotherapy, leading the authors to recommend its use only within the context of a clinical trial.

While concomitant chemoradiotherapy is probably the most promising and feasible approach in locally advanced patients, there remains several issues including the generalizability of these survival benefits to specific subsites, specific chemoradiotherapy regimens, including recent popular taxane-based regimens, and whether or not, differences exist between resectable and unresectable disease. The latter distinction becomes important, as concurrent chemoradiotherapy has emerged as a popular strategy to achieve functional organ preservation.[198] Because the addition of concurrent chemotherapy increases mucosal toxicity and poses the potential of adversely affecting swallowing function,[187,199] if the survival benefits, particularly with multi-agent regimens, are generalizable to those patients with resectable disease, compromises in organ function may result. Even if survival benefits are not observed, multi-agent regimens may still be preferred, as recently noted by Adelstein and associates[135] In their mature report of 100 patients with resectable HNSCC of various tumor sites, improved local-regional control rates without surgical salvage (77% vs. 45%, $p < 0.001$) with no survival benefits was observed with concurrent chemotherapy (both 5-FU [1000 mg/m^2/day] and cisplatin [20 mg/m^2/day] given as a conti-

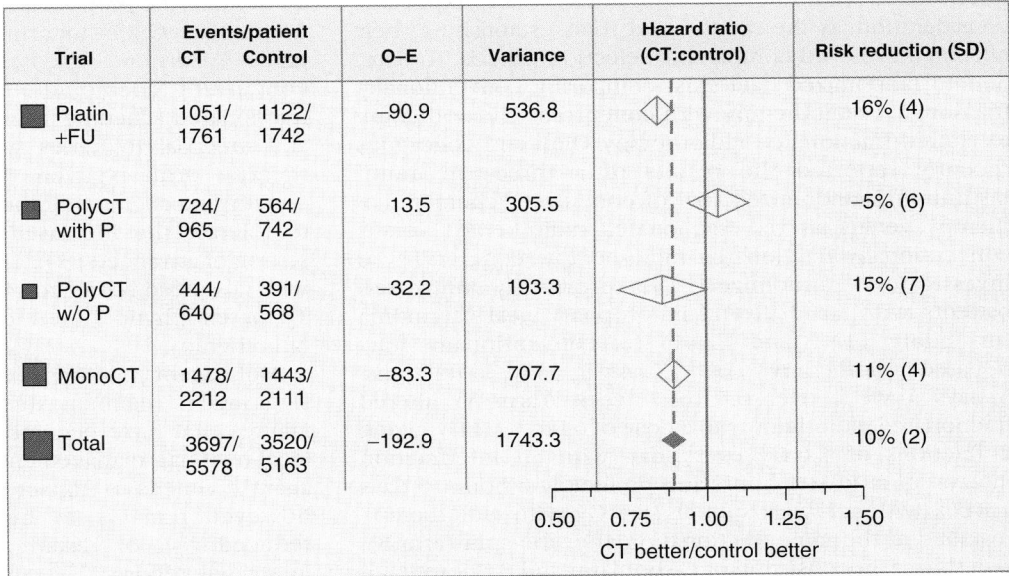

Trial	Events/patient CT	Events/patient Control	O–E	Variance	Hazard ratio (CT:control)	Risk reduction (SD)
▪ Platin +FU	1051/ 1761	1122/ 1742	−90.9	536.8		16% (4)
▪ PolyCT with P	724/ 965	564/ 742	13.5	305.5		−5% (6)
▪ PolyCT w/o P	444/ 640	391/ 568	−32.2	193.3		15% (7)
▪ MonoCT	1478/ 2212	1443/ 2111	−83.3	707.7		11% (4)
▪ Total	3697/ 5578	3520/ 5163	−192.9	1743.3		10% (2)

0.50   0.75   1.00   1.25   1.50
CT better/control better

Figure 71-15. Hazard ratio of death with local-regional treatment plus chemotherapy with local-regional treatment by types of chemotherapy. Platin (cisplatin or carboplatin) + fluorouracil (FU), combination CT with platin (poly CT + P), combination CT without platin (poly CT w/o P), single-agent CT (mono CT) including platin. Test for heterogeneity between types of chemotherapy, $p = 0.02$. (From Pignon, et al: Lancet 2000;355:949-955.)

| Covariate/ | Events/patient | | O–E | Variance | Hazard ratio |
category	CT	Control			(CT:control)
Age					
50 or less	784/1206	879/1379	−60.9	383.5	
51–60	1303/1871	1284/1914	−77.5	617.8	
61+	1306/1811	1433/2017	−25.4	642.3	
Sex					
Male	2928/4165	3117/4530	−137.9	1452.8	
Female	486/779	428/818	−31	222.5	
Performance status					
0	754/1264	744/1380	−49.8	360.7	
1	994/1299	1071/1457	−71.8	486.4	
2+	245/292	272/303	−12.6	115	
Stage					
I–II	228/534	213/519	−7.1	104	
III	1013/1672	1088/1835	−33.9	499.1	
IV	2148/2746	2252/3003	−154	1044.1	
Site					
Oral cavity	1041/1553	1105/1678	−75.6	500.2	
Oropharynx	1097/1539	1101/1629	−49.8	522	
Larynx	510/793	553/892	−31	250.8	
Hypopharynx	664/911	668/947	−38.6	310.5	
Others	165/281	222/344	10.4	88.2	

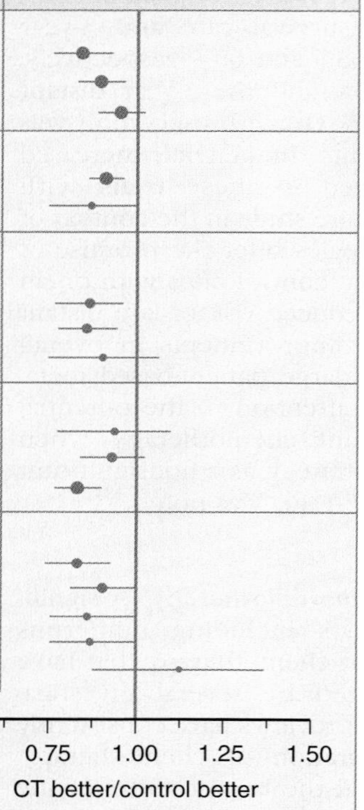

0.50   0.75   1.00   1.25   1.50
CT better/control better

Figure 71-16. Hazard ratio of death with local-regional treatment with or without chemotherapy by age, sex, performance status, stage, or tumor site. Test for trend for age was significant ($p = 0.05$). (From Pignon, et al: Lancet 2000;355:949–955.)

nuous intravenous infusion over 4 days beginning on days 1 and 22). Successful primary salvage surgery was possible in 73% of cases, which contributed to the absence of any demonstrable survival benefit.

While concurrent chemoradiotherapy has been studied in patients with stage III and IV HNSCC, often without selection for resectability, it becomes important to recognize in its application the narrowed therapeutic ratio.[184] In this regard, the relative efficacy of altered fractionated radiotherapy schedules is an important consideration, as the randomized trials establishing their efficacy have used comparable selection criteria. To date, limited randomized data exist comparing conventionally fractionated radiotherapy with concurrent chemotherapy to altered fractionated radiotherapy. Olmi and colleagues recently reported the results of a three-arm multi-institutional randomized trial of concurrent chemoradiotherapy versus altered fractionated radiotherapy versus conventionally fractionated radiotherapy alone.[322] These investigators randomized 192 previously untreated patients with stage III and IV oropharyngeal carcinoma (excluding T1N1 and T2N1) to: conventionally fractionated radiotherapy to 66 to 70 Gy in 33 to 35 fractions, 5 days a week over 6.5 to 7 weeks (arm A); altered fractionated radiotherapy to a dose of 64 to 67.2 Gy, giving 2 fractions of 1.6 Gy every day with an interfraction interval of at least 4 hours and preferably 6 hours, 5 days a week with a 2-week split at 38.4 Gy, with radiotherapy resumed at the same fractionation after the split (arm B); or a third arm consisting of carboplatin and 5-fluorouracil

(CBDCA 75 mg/m(2), days 1 to 4; 5FU 1,000 mg/m(2) I.V. over 96 hours, days 1 to 4, every 28 days (at 1st, 5th, and 9th week) (arm C), using the same daily fractionation schedule as the standard arm (arm A). No significant differences were detected in overall survival ($p = 0.129$): 40% of arm A, 37% of arm B, and 51% of arm C were alive at 24 months. The 2-year disease-free survival, however, was significantly different among the three arms ($p = 0.022$), in favor of the chemoradiotherapy arm. At 24 months, the proportion of patients without relapse was 42% for arm C, 23% for arm A, and 20% for arm B. Increased grade 3 skin and mucosal toxicities were noted in the concurrent chemoradiotherapy arm and the altered fractionated schedule. A suggestion of increased late skin and mucosal toxicities was noted in the chemoradiotherapy arm. Nguyen and Ang have also favored concurrent chemoradiotherapy in patients who are able to tolerate the increased toxicities, particularly in the setting of advanced T3 or T4 primary disease or in patients with advanced N2-3 neck disease, stratifying patients with T2 or exophytic T3 N1 disease to altered fractionated radiotherapy.[183]

Multi-agent regimens continue to be favored over single-agent regimens due to concerns of late distant failures that have become more evident with improved local-regional management. The ability of many multi-agent regimens to impact on the risk of distant relapses, however, remains to be clearly established.[178,323] A reduced risk of distant relapse has been suggested in several reports[135,324] and may suggest that the local-regional therapy is effective in addressing micrometastases, but one has to control the local-regional disease for this benefit to manifest. As such, significant interest has been focused on the incorporation of altered fractionated radiotherapy schedules with concurrent chemotherapy (Table 71-7). In total, six randomized trials have been reported and may be characterized by the type of altered fractionation used.[212,241,323-326] Of the trials combining an accelerated schedule, acute mucosal toxicities were significantly increased with two trials demonstrating unacceptable toxicity,[241,326] with one trial noting a high rate of chronic swallowing dysfunction.[326] Jeremic and colleagues reported an improved 5-year local-regional control rate (50% vs. 36% at 5 years; p = .041), 5-year overall survival (46% vs. 25% at 5 years; p = .0075), and distant metastasis-free survival (86% vs. 57% at 5 years; p =.0013) with the concurrent administration of daily cisplatin (6 mg/m^2) with a hyperfractionated schedule delivering 77 Gy in 1.1 Gy twice daily in 70 fractions over

7 weeks compared to this same hyperfractionated schedule alone.[324] No significantly increased acute or late toxicities were reported. This remains a promising aggressive regimen that requires further validation of the concept of daily radiosensitization with an altered fractionation schedule. Lastly, both 5-fluorouracil and cisplatin with or without leucovorin have been administered concurrently with a split-course schedule. Wendt and colleagues demonstrated improved local-regional control rates with an accelerated split-course schedule with concurrent bolus schedule of cisplatin, 5-fluorouracil, and leucovorin, but the results were overall disappointing (36% vs. 17%, p = 0.004).[323] A significant reduction in the total dose was used. Brizel and colleagues administered concurrent cisplatin and 5-fluorouracil with a split-course hyperfractionated schedule of 1.25 Gy twice daily over 47 days with a 7- to 10-day treatment interruption after 40 Gy.[212] Improved local-regional control rates with no difference in overall survival were noted, with increased

TABLE 71-7

Phase III Trials of Concurrent Chemotherapy and Altered Fractionation in Patients with Head and Neck Cancer

REF	TUMOR SITE AND STAGE	N	THERAPY REGIMENS	TUMOR RESPONSE	COMPLICATIONS
Accelerated fractionation plus chemotherapy					
325	Various sites T1–4 N0–3	188	55.3 Gy over 17 days (2.5 Gy on day 1, then 1.65 Gy, twice a day) plus/minus mitomycin c; conventional fractionation, 60 Gy over 7 weeks	Combination treatment yielded higher LRC (p<0.05) and survival (p<0.03)	More mucositis than in the combination group but not intensified by mitomycin c; late toxic effects not reported
241	Various sites, stage III–IV	240	69.9 Gy over 5.5 weeks plus carboplatin (70 mg/m^2 per day) and fluorouracil (600 mg/m^2 per day) for 2 cycles of 5 days; 69.9 Gy over 5.5 weeks (1.8 Gy once daily for 3.5 weeks, then, individual fractions of 1.8 Gy and 1.5 Gy, daily for 2 weeks)	2-year OS, 48% vs 39% (p=0.11); 2-year LC, 51% vs 45% (p=0.14); patients receiving radiochemotherapy had worse LRC (p=0.007)	Grade 3-4 mucositis, 68% vs 52% (p=0.01); grade 3–4 vomiting, 8.2% vs 1.6% (p=0.02); late swallowing problems and feeding tube dependency, 51% vs 25% (p=0.02)
326	Various sites, advanced-inoperable	109	62.64 Gy over 5 weeks plus cisplatin (100 mg/m^2 on day 1, 16, and 32) and fluorouracil (1 g/m^2 on days 1–5, and 31–35); 62–64 Gy over 3 weeks	Not yet reported	Early stopping due to higher treatment-related deaths in the combined-treatment group
Hyperfractionation plus chemotherapy					
324	Various sites, stage III–IV	130	77 Gy over 7 weeks plus cisplatin (6 mg/m^2 per day); 77 Gy over 7 weeks (1.1 Gy, twice daily)	5-year LRPFS, 50% vs 35% (p=0.04); 5-year PFS, 46% vs 25% (p=0.007); 5-year DMFS, 86% vs 57% (p=0.001); 5-year OS, 46% vs 25% (p=0.008)	No significant difference in acute morbidity (except for leucopenia, p=0.006) or late toxic effects
Split-course altered-fractionation plus chemotherapy					
323	Various sites, stage III–IV	270	70.2 Gy over 51 days plus cisplatin, fluorouracil, and leucovorin; 70.2 Gy over 51 days (23.4 Gy in 1.8-Gy fractions, twice daily × 3 cycles with a 10-day break)	3-year LRC, 36% vs 17% (p<0.004); 3-year OS, 48% vs 24% (p<0.0003)	Grade 3-4 acute mucositis, 38% vs 16% (p<0.001); serious late side-effects, 10% vs 6.4% (NS)
212	Various sites, T2-4 N0–3	122	70 Gy over 47 days as 1.25 Gy twice daily (7–10 day break after 40 Gy) plus cisplatin and fluorouracil in weeks 1 and 6 75 Gy over 42 days as 1.25 Gy, twice daily	3-year LRC, 70% vs 44% (p=0.01); 3-year RFS, 61% vs 41% (p=0.07); 3-year OS, 55% vs 34% (p=0.07)	Similar mucositis; increased enteral feeding and sepsis with combination therapy; similar late complications

DMFS, distant-metastasis-free survival; LC, local control; LRC, locoregional control; LRPFS, locoregional progression-free survival; NS, not significant; OS, overall survival; PFS, progression-free survival.
From Nguyen LN, Ang KK: Radiotherapy for cancer of the head and neck: Altered fractionation regimens. Lancet Oncol 2002;3:698.

risk of sepsis and enteral feeding noted in the experimental arm. To date, the generalizability of any of these regimens is limited not only by the increased toxicity, but also by the intensive resources required on the part of the treating team and the patients.

Postoperative/Adjuvant Chemotherapy. The use of postoperative adjuvant chemotherapy in patients at high risk for local and regional recurrence from HNSCC remains under evaluation.[181] Patients with two or more positive regional nodes, extracapsular extension of disease, positive resected margin, or perineural/perivascular invasion are considered to be in a high-risk category. Ang and colleagues noted a 5-year actuarial distant relapse rate of 33% (vs. 3% in the low-risk group).[161] A comparable level of risk for distant relapses in various chemoradiotherapy series with patients treated nonsurgically has been described ranging from 15% to 30%.[135,178,212] Laramore and colleagues reported the results of a randomized trial conducted through the Intergroup (0034), randomizing patients after surgical resection to either three cycles of cisplatin and 5-fluorouracil chemotherapy followed by postoperative radiotherapy (CT/RT) or postoperative radiotherapy alone (RT). Patients were stratified as having either low-risk or high-risk treatment volumes depending on whether the surgical margin was greater than or equal to 5 mm, there was extracapsular nodal extension, and/or there was carcinoma in situ at the surgical margins. Radiation doses of 50 to 54 Gy were given to low-risk volumes and 60 Gy were given to high-risk volumes. A total of 442 patients were analyzable with no difference noted in the overall survival (4-year actuarial survival rate was 44% on the RT arm and 48% on the CT/RT arm [*p* = n.s.]), 4-year disease-free survival (38% vs. 46%, respectively), and 4-year local-regional control rates (29% vs. 26%, respectively). However, the overall incidence of distant metastases was 23% on the RT arm compared to 15% on the CT/RT arm (*p* = 0.03), again confirming activity as noted in trials employing neoadjuvant chemotherapy, but with no improvement in overall survival as noted in the recently updated meta-analysis reported by Pignon and colleagues.[181] There have been a limited number of other randomized trials reported. These include a small randomized trial of adjuvant chemotherapy for oral cavity lesions reported in abstract only that favored the control arm,[327] and a second also limited to the oral cavity that did not demonstrate any improvement in disease-free survival or overall survival.[328]

Chemoprevention. Retinoids have been increasingly used in the treatment of oral leukoplakia and dysplasia of the head and neck since the 1960s. Studies have been published using retinoids in the treatment of head and neck cancers in conjunction with interferon. 13 cis-retinoic acid (13c-RA) has also been looked at in the adjuvant setting. More recently, retinoids have been evaluated in the "preventive" setting after definitive therapy.

A phase I/II study looked at cis-retinoic acid, cisplatin, and ifosfamide in patients with advanced or recurrent HNSCC.[329] Patients were given cisplatin at 20 mg/m²/day

for 5 days every 3 weeks with cis-retinoic acid at 0.5 mg/kg orally for 5 days/week and dose-escalating ifosfamide at 1000 to 1500 mg/m². A response rate of 72% was reported with median time to progression of 10.4 months and overall survival of 13 months.

The combination of retinoids and interferons has synergistic effects in modulating proliferation, differentiation, and apoptosis. A German study evaluated 30 patients after treatment for stage IV HNSCC in which adjuvant "chemopreventive" cis-retinoic and interferon were administered for 6 months.[330] The dose of cis-retinoic acid was 0.5 mg/kg/day orally and the dose of interferon was 3 million IU per week subcutaneously. Sixteen patients remained disease free 1 year after definitive treatment. Associated side effects were weight loss, flushing, cachexia, worsening xerostomia, and dysphagia from cis-retinoic acid. Interferon side effects were reported as pyrexia and hematological changes.

Based on the preceding data, a phase II study was conducted in this country using cis-retinoic acid, alpha-tocopherol, and interferon as adjuvant therapy in patients definitively treated for locally advanced HNSCC.[331] Three million units of interferon were given subcutaneously three times weekly with alpha-tocopherol at 1200 IU/day orally and cis-retinoic acid at 50 mg/m²/day orally for 12 months. Forty-five patients were enrolled; 38 completed the year trial. At a median of 24 months follow-up, the local and regional failure rate was 9% with 5% failing distantly. Median survival at 2 years was reported as 84%. This adjuvant regimen is being tested at the phase III level.

Celecoxib is a novel compound that specifically inhibits the inducible form of the enzyme cyclooxygenase (COX-2) (prostaglandin G/H synthase). Celecoxib is an oral anti-inflammatory agent indicated for the treatment of rheumatoid arthritis and osteoarthritis. Nonsteroidal anti-inflammatory drugs (NSAIDs) and related drugs such as COX-2 inhibitors are attractive candidates for prevention based on recent epidemiologic and case-control studies suggesting that the risk of several malignancies such as colon, esophagus, gastric, and bladder is reduced in chronic NSAID users.[332-336] Many tumors, both human and animal, express elevated levels of COX-2 compared to normal tissue.[337,338] This elevation is also noted in premalignant lesions.[339] In the head and neck area, COX-2 overexpression is seen in oral leukoplakia as well as squamous cell carcinomas. Increased levels of COX-2 can contribute to carcinogenesis by modulating xenobiotic metabolism, apoptosis, immune surveillance, and angiogenesis. In animal models, selective COX-2 inhibitors suppress the formation of tumors, including tongue cancer. Selective COX-2 inhibitors can also suppress the growth and metastasis of established tumors and enhance the anticancer activity of both radiation and chemotherapy. Celecoxib is now being evaluated for efficacy and safety as an adjunct in the prevention of cancer and the prevention of recurrence and metastasis after therapy. Thus COX-2 inhibitors may be a promising strategy to prevent and treat HNSCC.

Targeted Therapy/Novel Approaches. Novel biologic agents have been developed to target multiple specific regions of cancer cells. Protein tyrosine kinases are major components of cell signaling pathways. Various subfamilies of these kinases include receptors for the epidermal growth factor (EGFRs), platelet-derived growth factor (PDGF), vascular endothelial growth factor (VEGF), fibroblast growth factor and hepatocyte growth factor. EGFR is one of four receptors involved in cellular proliferation, differentiation, and survival and is widely expressed in many malignant tissues. EGFR inhibitors such as anti-EGRF monoclonal antibodies, tyrosine kinase inhibitors, ligand conjugates, and antisense oligonucleotides have received significant attention in patients with HNSCC as the EGFR is commonly overexpressed in 80% to 90% of patients.

Epidermal Growth Factor Receptor. Epidermal growth factor receptor (EGFR–erb-B1) is part of the erb-B family of receptor tyrosine kinases, which includes erb-B2/Her2/neu, erb-B3/Her3, and erb-B4/Her4.[340,341] EGFR is composed of three domains: an extracellular ligand-binding domain; a transmembrane lipophilic region; and an intracellular protein tyrosine kinase domain.[342,343] Endogenous ligands to EGFR include EGF, TGF-alpha, and heparin-binding EGF. When activated, phosphorylation of the intracellular tyrosine residues results in a cascade of protein phosporylations, resulting in turn in the activation of various downstream signal transduction pathways, including ras/MAP kinase, phosphatidylinositol-3 kinase, and STAT-3. The signal transduction pathway can lead to cell proliferation, tumor growth, and progression of invasion and metastasis signals.[344,345] Based on its overexpression in many cell types (particularly HNSCC cell lines) and the fact that EGFR-based signals can mediate resistance to chemotherapy and radiotherapy, it has been hypothesized that inhibition of EGFR may result in a synergistic antitumor effect.

Numerous EGFR inhibitors have been evaluated, including anti-EGFR monoclonal antibodies, tyrosine kinase inhibitors, ligand conjugates, immunoconjugates, and antisense oligonucleotides. Small molecules such as the tyrosine kinase inhibitors target intracellular tyrosine kinase signaling and inhibit EGFR; antibodies are more directed at the extracellular domain.

IMC-C225 (ImClone Systems, Somerville, New Jersey) is a monoclonal antibody targeting the EGFR and has been studied in several tumor types. In vitro, this antibody appears to enhance the antitumor activity of chemotherapy such as cisplatin (CDDP) and doxorubicin as well as the radiosensitivity of HNSCC cell lines.[346] Similar in vitro data have shown C225 to enhance radiosensitivity.[347,348]

Recent evidence now supports a role for EGFR to mediate a cytoprotective stress response to ionizing radiation. Therapeutically relevant doses of ionizing radiation have been demonstrated to increase expression of EGFR[349] and cytosolic release of TGF-μ from its membrane-bound form,[350] modulate an activated EGFR autophosphorylation profile[350-353] with increased mitogenic signals involving the MAPK pathway with cellular proliferation,[352,354] and protect from radiation-induced cell death.[350] In a series of experiments with the radioresistant vulva squamous carcinoma cell line A431, inhibition of EGFR with the tyrosine kinase inhibitor tyrphostin AG1478 was associated with reduced MAPK activation and reduced EGFR-mediated tumor cell proliferation.[352] Taken collectively, it is intriguing to postulate that such a response may serve to mediate the clinical phenomenon of accelerated tumor repopulation during radiotherapy for HNSCC.[152] This hypothesis may be particularly relevant in HNSCC in light of the significant body of clinical data supporting the notion of tumor clonogen repopulation contributing to radiation failure.[179,238]

Early phase I trials of C225 alone and in combination with CDDP were reported. Fifty-two patients were initially treated with dose-escalation of C225 as well as CDDP weekly.[355] C225 was dose escalated to 200 to 400 mg/m², but CDDP dosing was found to be optimal only at 60 mg/m² due to toxicity at higher doses. One patient developed a humoral response. Toxicities included acneiform rashes, gastrointestinal distress, seborrheic dermatitis, flushing, asthenia, and transaminitis. This led to subsequent studies in the metastatic setting.

A phase I trial with 12 patients with metastatic HNSCC with high levels of EGFR expression were given 3 doses of C225 with 100 mg/m² of CDDP every 3 weeks.[356] Weekly maintenance of C225 was given at 250 mg/m². Responses were seen in 67% of the 12 patients enrolled with minimum toxicity. A follow-up study with C225/CDDP in patients with recurrent HNSCC was presented at the American Association for Cancer Research (AACR) in 2001. Sixty-three patients were evaluated and given a loading dose of 400 mg/m² of C225 followed by weekly maintenance of 250 mg/m² and CDDP at 75 or 100 mg/m². The overall response was 24%. C225 by itself has reported response rates of 10% and thus this was encouraging. ECOG recently compared single-dose CDDP to CDDP/C225 in a double blind randomized trial in patients with previously untreated recurrent or metastatic HNSCC with 35% to 40% stable disease in both arms.[357]

Anti-EGFR antibodies have radiosensitization properties in cell cultures and preclinical animal studies. A phase I study with C225 and radiation in 16 patients with locally advanced disease (13 with stage IV) was recently reported with an overall clinical response rate of 100% and CR of 87%.[358] The impressive complete response rate has been interpreted to be consistent with radiosensitization. A multi-institutional phase III trial comparing radiation therapy alone versus radiation therapy plus C225 in locally advanced HNSCC has recently closed to accrual with results currently being analyzed.

Tyrosine Kinase Inhibitors. ZD1839 (Iressa, AstraZeneca Pharmaceuticals LP, Wilmington, Delaware) is a selective EGFR tyrosine kinase inhibitor, recently approved by the FDA as palliative therapy in non–small cell lung cancer. Preclinically, ZD1839 potentiates the antitumor and apoptotic effects of several cytotoxic agents including CDDP and taxanes.[359,360] In combination with radiation, ZD1839 shows dose-dependent inhibition of cellular proliferation in human SCC cell lines. ZD1839 can also inhibit tumor angiogenesis in tumor zenograft models in vivo.[348]

Four phase I trials using ZD1839 as monotherapy mostly on patients with prostate, lung, colorectal, ovarian, and head and neck cancer have reported modest toxicity such as diarrhea, nausea and vomiting, transient transaminitis, and rash. Most patients had been heavily pretreated and most were lung cancer patients. The results of the non–small cell lung cancer (NSCLC) monotherapy trial were presented. The overall response rate in 208 patients was 53% and the median progression-free survival rate was 84 days.[361] This study as well as several other trials led to recent FDA approval.

The role of ZD1839 as a radiosensitizer is the subject of an ongoing NCI-sponsored multi-institutional trial in combination with a delayed concomitant boost accelerated radiotherapy schedule and with concurrent chemoradiotherapy. The chemoradiotherapy employs a weekly cisplatin schedule. The use of oral tyrosine kinase inhibitors may be particularly attractive for its flexible daily dosing schedules. It is hypothesized that this may permit continued arrest of tumor repopulation during any unplanned radiotherapy treatment interruptions. As such, this clinical trial seeks to continue daily dosing of ZD1839 during these unplanned interruptions and during the weekends in light of the provocative positive results of an accelerated schedule that delivered radiotherapy through the weekends.[238]

A phase II trial in recurrent/metastatic squamous cell carcinoma of the head and neck was also recently published.[362] Fifty-two patients previously treated with only one other strategy were allowed to enroll. Patients were given the higher dose of 500 mg/day orally; 250 mg/day is the approved dose based on phase I data in NSCLC. Patients were able to tolerate this drug through feeding tubes. The observed response rate was 10.6%. Median time to progression and overall survival was 3.4 and 8.1 months, respectively.

OSI-774 (Genetech, San Francisco, California) is also an orally active quinazoline and potent selective inhibitor of EGFR tyrosine kinase. This results in cell cycle arrest at G1. Phase I studies with OSI-774 were well tolerated, again with toxicities including diarrhea, skin rash, and gastrointestinal upset. OSI-774 has been tested in HNSCC patients refractory to chemotherapy at 150mg/day dosing. In a phase II trial with 114 patients, 13% of patients had a partial response and 29% had stable disease.[363] Toxicities were as previously noted and included acneiform rash, diarrhea, nausea, vomiting, headache, and fatigue.

Ras Inhibitors. It has been suggested that oral cavity cancers have a 27% mutation rate in h-ras.[364] Farnesyl transferase inhibitors (FTIs) inhibit a critical enzymatic step in the post-translational modification of ras, allowing the constitutive expression of mutated ras genes. Several FTIs are available in the study setting: R115777 (Janssen Pharmaceutica, Titusville, New Jersey); BMS214662 (Bristol-Meyers Squibb); and SCH66336 (Schering Plough, Kenilworth, New Jersey).

R115777 is a nonpeptidomimetric orally available FTI. It can be used alone in patients or in combination with chemotherapy. Toxicity has been minimal. Reversible myelosuppression is the most common dose-limiting toxicity, as well as fatigue, nausea, renal dysfunction, and peripheral neuropathy. A phase I trial using R115777 with irinotecan was reported.[365] Another with docetaxel is being conducted, as is a third with gemcitibine.[366,367]

BMS214662 has preferential cytotoxicity against nonproliferating cells. Combination chemotherapy from preclinical human colon cancer cell lines has exhibited synergy with paclitaxel, irinotecan, gemcitabine, and an epothilone analog, BMS247550.[368] Phase I studies are ongoing in advanced solid tumors, including using this drug with CDDP at 75 mg/m^2 every 3 weeks.

p53 Targets. As discussed elsewhere in this chapter, p53 mutations occur in 45% to 70% of HNSCC patients and are associated with continual tobacco and alcohol use.[29,30] p53 is a multifunctional protein that can be induced by DNA damage and plays a significant role in the detection and repair of damaged DNA. P53 can induce apoptosis in severely damaged cells and has been associated with both carcinogenesis and poor prognosis in many cancers, including HNSCC.

ONYX-015 is an E1B-55kD gene-deleted replication-selective adenovirus that replicates and causes cytopathogenicity in certain cancer cell lines.[369,370] Selective intratumoral replication and tumor-selective tissue destruction of ONYX-015 have been demonstrated in phase I and II trials in refractory/recurrent HNSCC patients.[371,372] Clinical benefit was seen in 15% of patients. A phase II multicenter trial of intratumoral ONYX-015 in combination with CDDP and 5-FU in patients with recurrent HNSCC was reported.[373] Forty patients received injections, 30 for 5 consecutive days and 10 twice daily for 2 weeks. Responses and stable disease were noted in both groups. Pain was noteworthy in the twice-daily injected, but otherwise this was well-tolerated.

Thus novel modalities involving molecular targets are actively being investigated. Cytotoxic agents have limited efficacy as demonstrated throughout many sections of this chapter, and thus targeted therapies may improve treatment in the recurrent, metastatic, and, eventually, the definitive setting.

Site-Specific Treatment Considerations

Nasopharynx

The nasopharynx is a cuboidal structure bounded by the sphenoid bone superiorly, the posterior choanae anteriorly, the clivus and the first two cervical vertebrae posteriorly, and the soft palate inferiorly. The eustachian tube enters through the lateral wall with the posterior portion of the tube being cartilaginous and forming the portion of the lateral nasopharyngeal wall known as the torus tubarus. Just posterior to this is the fossa of Rosenmuller.

The vast majority of malignancies in the nasopharynx are epithelial neoplasms and arise from the lateral wall, particularly from the fossa of Rosenmuller. Local spread may include extension anteriorly through the submucosa including the nasal cavity, laterally and superiorly through the foramen lacerum with cranial nerve involvement, and inferiorly into the oropharynx. Extension into the cavernous sinus commonly results in a sixth cranial nerve palsy. Two cranial nerve syndromes have been characterized. The petrosphenoidal syndrome describes involvement of the third, fourth, fifth, and sixth cranial nerves. The retroparotidian syndrome describes involvement of the 9th, 10th, 11th, and 12th cranial nerves. Metastatic spread to the adjacent upper cervical lymph nodes and to the retropharyngeal lymph nodes that are located in the retropharyngeal space that lies between the lateral border of the posterior nasopharyngeal wall and medial to the carotid artery may extend inferiorly to the level of the hyoid bone.

Both the tumor stage and the histologic grade of epithelial malignancies are prognostic. The WHO identifies three histopathologic types: type 1, differentiated; type 2, nondifferentiated and type 3, undifferentiated or lymphoepithelial, which highlights the presence of numerous infiltrating lymphocytes. The presence of keratin is an adverse prognostic feature for local control and overall survival. Other malignancies may include lymphoma, plasmacytomas, melanomas, and, in the pediatric population, juvenile angiofibromas and rhabdomyosarcomas. Approximately 60% to 90% of patients with nasopharyngeal cancer present with palpable adenopathy and up to 50% of patients with involved nodes have bilateral disease.[374-376] Patients with adenopathy at the mastoid tip require exclusion of a malignancy in the nasopharynx due to the characteristic lymphatic drainage pattern from the retropharyngeal space. Staging follows the recently revised sixth edition of the AJCC TNM criteria. No modifications have been recommended, including subdivision of the T4 stage that is new to this sixth edition.[137] Both MRI and CT scans are complementary in this tumor site, with the former favored in most cases and the latter beneficial where there is bone invasion or destruction.

Due to the anatomic location of the nasopharynx, surgical resection has not typically been recommended due to the inherent surgical complication rates with surgery in this area including the inability to achieve margins. As such, radiation therapy is the treatment of choice. Fortunately, nasopharyngeal carcinomas (NPCs) are both sensitive and responsive to radiotherapy and chemotherapy, the two principle treatment modalities that are used. For early stage disease, radiotherapy alone may be used with excellent results reported, with 3-year overall survival rates ranging from 70% to 100%[374,377-379] and 65% to 100%[374,377-379] for stage I and II disease, respectively, based on the AJCC 1997 staging system. Typical local control rates to current treatments have been summarized by Lee[380]: approximately 80% (72% to 90%) for T1 and approximately 70% (5% to 100%) for T2. Even with locally confined disease (T1), generous initial radiotherapy margins are advised.

Unfortunately, the majority of patients present with locally advanced disease. Local control for T3-4 disease may be expected to be about 50% (39% to 72%).[380] For locally advanced stage III and IV disease, concurrent chemoradiotherapy has emerged as the standard treatment option following from the results of the Intergroup 0099 (IG0099) study reported by al-Sarraf and coworkers.[381] These investigators reported the results of 147 evaluable patients of 193 registered randomized to radiotherapy alone or radiotherapy with concomitant cisplatin (100 mg/m^2 IV on days 1, 22, and 43) followed by adjuvant chemotherapy with cisplatin 80 mg/m^2 on day 1 and fluorouracil 1000 mg/m^2/day on days 1 to 4 administered every 4 weeks for 3 courses. An improvement in the 3-year progression-free survival rate (69% vs. 24%, $p < 0.001$) and overall survival (76% vs. 46%, $p = 0.001$) was observed on interim analysis, prompting premature study closure. These results are not without debate, however.[380]

Several investigators have questioned whether this positive study may have resulted from inferior outcomes in the control arm rather than a therapeutic effect. Chow and investigators from the Princess Margaret Hospital recently published the results of a large institutional series using radiotherapy alone administered in a homogenous manner to 172 patients with advanced stage disease, demonstrating a 5-year disease-free survival and overall survival rate of 48% and 62%, respectively.[382] Though these authors acknowledge that direct comparisons with the control arm of IG0099 have limited validity, these observations made during a similar time period as the IG0099 provide a context within which the positive results of the IG0099 should be interpreted. In a similar report by Cooper and colleagues, 86 patients with locally advanced disease treated with radiotherapy alone had a 3-year actuarial disease-free survival and overall survival rate of 43% and 61%, respectively.[383] These investigators also observed that in 35 patients treated with the IG0099 protocol, the projected 3-year disease-free survival and overall survival rates were 63% and 93%, respectively, suggesting benefit. Recently, Cheng and colleagues reported the results of 107 patients treated with concurrent 5-fluorouracil and cisplatin (weeks 1 and 6) and radiotherapy followed by 2 cycles of adjuvant 5-fluorouracil and cisplatin. The 5-year overall survival rate, disease-free survival rate, and local-regional control rate were 84.1%, 74.4%, and 89.8%, respectively. The 3-year overall survival rates for stage II, III, and IV were 100%, 92.8%, and 69.4% ($p = 0.0002$), and the 3-year disease-free survival rates were 96.9%, 87.7%, and 51.9% ($p = 0.0001$). While a confirmatory randomized trial is noted to be under way,[384] the current consensus opinion continues to recommend the concurrent chemoradiotherapy. These results further suggest that Asian patients may also benefit from concurrent chemoradiotherapy, which has been questioned due to geographic differences in the histologic subtype between North America and Asia. A pilot trial of a modified schedule of the IG0099 regimen (reduced cisplatin dose) has been demonstrated to be safe and has given rise to a phase III trial to confirm the generalizability of these results to the Asian population.[384]

With concurrent chemoradiotherapy, toxicities are clearly increased. In addition, the late toxicities with concurrent chemoradiotherapy have not been well reported upon. Increased acute toxicites include not only mucosal toxicities that are further compounded by the large volume of normal mucosa that is irradiated, but also the asthenia and emetogenic side effects of concurrent high-dose cisplatin. As Cooper describes,[383] the observations by Cheng and colleagues[382] may suggest that other alternative regimens may be equally if not more effective. The impact of these toxicities is important to consider in patient management, as treatment interruptions during radiotherapy have also been demonstrated to result in inferior local-regional control rates and disease-free survival.[385] These investigators estimated that local-regional relapses increased 3.3% per day of treatment interruption. The timing of the interruption, including interruptions early in the course of treatment, appeared to be equally detrimental. While it is unclear if NPC tumor kinetics may be different with concurrent administration of chemotherapy, close attention to the toxicities of treatment and causes for interruption during a course of radiotherapy may be prudent.

One attractive strategy to minimize toxicities associated with concurrent chemoradiotherapy has been to employ lower but more frequent doses of chemotherapy. Chan and colleagues recently reported the results of a randomized trial of 350 patients to concurrent weekly cisplatin (40 mg/m^2) with daily fractionated radiotherapy.[386] Though no improvement was observed overall for the primary endpoint of progression-free survival, subgroup analysis demonstrated benefit in Ho's T3 stage due to an improved time to first distant failure. The treatment was well tolerated. The results of a second randomized trial of concurrent 5-fluorouracil and cisplatin, however, showed a significant improvement in progression-free survival.[387]

Despite the improved outcome that appears to have been realized with concurrent chemoradiotherapy for locally advanced NPC, a proportion of patients may continue to have persistent disease that is slow to respond. The therapeutic options recommended have been further irradiation or observation. A limited number of studies have reported on the role of an implant in patients with persistent disease after standard therapy.[388-393] These studies have suggested that further irradiation in early stage disease that is amenable to intracavitary and interstitial techniques may result in comparable local control rates as achieved in patients demonstrating a prompt complete response.[389] Hence dose escalation may be adequate in compensating for tumors demonstrating a low radioresponsiveness. The optimal dose schedule remains to be determined with both 60 Gy LDR and 22.5 to 25 Gy HDR schedules reported. Stereotactic radiosurgery has been used with preliminary data, suggesting that up to 70% of patients with organ-confined recurrences may achieve local control out to 2 years.[394] Late toxicities do not appear to be increased. In light of the poorer local control rates and survival rates in patients managed for local recurrences, a brachytherapy implant or stereotactic radiosurgery may be considered in the management of patients demonstrating persistent disease.

Neck control for NPC is unique for its increased sensitivity to radiotherapy compared to the typical HNSCC.[395] In the clinically negative neck, elective irradiation is recommended due to the high probability of subclinical nodal metastases with a risk of 40% neck relapse if untreated, which is associated with a significantly higher incidence of distant failure (21% versus 6%) despite successful nodal salvage.[396,397] With appropriate doses of irradiation (50 Gy), the probability of relapse is less than 5%.[398] In the clinical positive neck, doses of 60 Gy or greater are typically recommended; average regional control rates of 90% (range = 86% to 96%) and 75% (range = 71% to 87%) might be expected for neck nodes 3 cm or less and greater than 6 cm, respectively.[380] As such, the role of a planned neck dissection is typically not recommended but may be appropriate. Where a residual abnormality remains, a neck dissection is typically recommended. This may be complicated, however, by the recognition that in some NPC lesions, gross disease response can be slow at both the primary site and in the neck. As well, the integration of a neck dissection can create conflicts with regard to the prompt initiation of adjuvant chemotherapy. In light of the association between local-regional relapses and the subsequent risk of distant metastases,[397] a neck dissection continues to be a prudent recommendation at this time.

Various strategies have been used in attempts to improve upon the survival rates, particularly for locally advanced disease. The first is to optimize local-regional control not only as this is a major pattern of relapse in this group of patients, but also for the potential impact on the risk of distant metastases. The second is the integration of various chemotherapy agents with definitive radiotherapy. As a dose-response relationship appears to exist for local control[399] and the overall treatment time[385] also appears to impact adversely on treatment outcome, several institutions have reported their results using altered fractionation for locally advanced NPC with[400] or without concurrent chemotherapy.[401] Jian and colleagues employed the same chemotherapy regimen as Cheng and colleagues with cisplatin and 5-fluorouracil on weeks 1 and 6, with concurrent hyperfractionated radiotherapy to 74.4 Gy in 48 patients. With a median follow-up of 57 months, 3-year local-regional control rate was 93%, the disease-free survival rate was 71%, and the overall survival rate was 72%. In particular, T4 patients had a 3-year local-regional control rate of 91%, disease-free survival of 62%, and an overall survival of 63%. The major acute toxicity was grade 3 mucositis in 73% and grade 2 weight loss in 31% of patients. The authors concluded that the treatment was well tolerated with 88% of patients completing their radiation treatment within 8 weeks.[400] These promising results require further validation of the results and definition of the increased toxicity risks, particularly in light of the unacceptable toxicities observed in other non-nasopharyngeal concurrent chemoradiotherapy series employing altered fractionation.[326]

Various randomized trials incorporating various sequences of chemotherapy and radiotherapy have been reported. To date, a number of randomized trials have failed to demonstrate a benefit with either neoadjuvant[402-406] or adjuvant chemotherapy.[404,407,408] These results are consistent with a recent large patient-based meta-analysis.[181] As such, the use of adjuvant chemotherapy particularly with definitive chemoradiotherapy should be judiciously applied.

As nasopharyngeal carcinomas are radiosensitive, locally recurrent carcinomas may be amenable to reirradiation. As the risk of late complications, including soft tissue and brain necrosis and neuropathies, are very much dose and volume dependent with reirradiation, the general strategy has been to incorporate conformal radiotherapy techniques for the boost component of the reirradiation. As with treatment for persistent disease, this may take the form of either a brachytherapy or stereotactic radiosurgery boost.[409] In a series of over 891 patients reirradiated, the extent of the recurrence was prognostic. Overall, about 30 % achieved local disease control with local control best seen when a repeat radiation dose of 60 Gy or greater was delivered.[410] The selection of small EBRT fraction size and the use of a brachytherapy implant was associated with a reduced risk of late complications. Several other institutional series have reported sustained local control rates of 20% to 60%, with the variability due to the extent of initial disease presentation and at recurrence and the dose of reirradiation.[388,390-392] In selected series treating only disease confined to the nasopharynx mucosa amenable to either an intracavitary or interstitial implant, sustained local control rates of 50 to 60% may be realized. These series have also demonstrated, however, a significant risk of developing late radiation-related complications including soft tissue and bone necrosis, trismus, fistula formation, and neurologic complications such as radiation myelitis and temporal lobe necrosis.

Salvage surgery is now being performed in Taiwan for NPC in selected patients. Large prospective studies are needed to determine efficacy, but small retrospective studies have demonstrated feasibility and success in local control.[411,412] Hsu and colleagues studied 60 patients who underwent salvage surgery, and showed that the results of surgical resection in terms of local control and overall survival were slightly better than those patients undergoing high-dose reirradiation for local relapse, with fewer late complications.[412] These authors favored salvage surgery for rT1-2 and limited rT3 disease, due to the fewer complications. This therapeutic option may be considered for selected lesions and in appropriate centers with expertise in this technique, as its relative efficacy to high-dose reirradiation remains to be defined.

Locally recurrent and metastatic nasopharyngeal cancers generally remain chemosensitive. Many patients have been previously treated with combined modality strategies involving a platinum agent and 5-FU. Several phase II trials have evaluated carboplatin and paclitaxel in this setting. Carboplatin at an AUC 7 with 3-hour infusional paclitaxel at 200 mg/m^2 revealed an overall response rate of 57% in the metastatic setting.[413] Another phase II study investigated carboplatin at AUC 6 with 135 mg/m^2 paclitaxel over three hours with an overall response rate of 59%.[414] Two other phase II studies again using similar dosing schedules of Carboplatin AUC 6 or 5.5 with 175 mg/m^2 paclitaxel demonstrated 75% and 25% responses with median overall survival rates of 12 and 9.5 months, respectively.[415,416]

Paranasal Sinus and Nose

Malignant tumors of the sinonasal tract are relatively rare, constituting approximately 3% of upper respiratory tract cancers. As such, the scientific literature is limited to multiple small retrospective reports describing the treatment and outcome of these patients. This has limited progress in defining the optimal management for these malignancies. While squamous cell carcinoma is the most common, several other types of epithelial tumors are less commonly found, including melanoma, adenocarcinoma, adenoid cystic carcinoma, and esthesioneuroblastoma.[417] Nonepithelial malignancies arising in the sinonasal tract include sarcomas and lymphoma.

Among the different subsites within the paranasal sinuses, squamous cell carcinomas occur most commonly in the maxillary sinus.[418] The second most common location is the nasal cavity. The ethmoid sinus is more frequently the site of adenocarcinoma or esthesioneuroblastoma. Cancer arises rarely in the frontal and sphenoid sinuses.[418] The prognosis of these lesions is based upon staging classification, as well as upon their relationship to Ohngren's line. This theoretical plane extends from the medial canthus of the eye to the angle of the mandible. Tumors anteromedial to this plane are thought to have a considerably better prognosis. Staging follows the sixth edition AJCC staging criteria. The nasoethmoid complex was added as a tumor site with subdivision of the T4 stage made for both maxillary sinus and nasal cavity and ethmoid sinus.[137]

Most malignancies are advanced at presentation and commonly involve one or more adjacent structures (Fig. 71-17). Orbital invasion often occurs early with cancers of the maxilla and of the ethmoid sinuses, while it

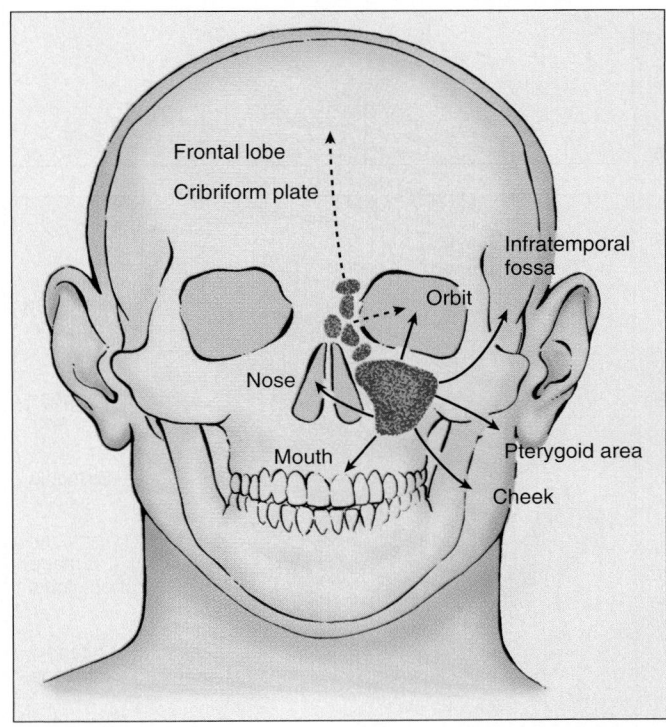

Figure 71-17. Routes of spread of cancer of the paranasal sinuses. *Solid arrows*, maxillary sinus cancer; *dashed arrows*, ethmoid sinus cancer.

is often a late event for nasal cavity tumors. Malignancies beginning in the anterolateral infrastructure of the maxilla often erode through the inferolateral wall and extend into the oral cavity with involvement of the maxillary gingival or the adjacent gingivobuccal sulcus. In general, the risk of cervical nodal metastases is low unless the tumor has involved mucosal surfaces with abundant lymphatics such as the oral cavity.

Management of paranasal sinus malignancies is primarily surgical, with adjunctive radiation and possibly chemotherapy for advanced lesions.[419,420] For maxillary sinus tumors, a partial or total maxillectomy is required to excise the tumor with negative margins, depending upon its location. The maxilla can be accessed via a variety of approaches. For smaller, medially based tumors, a medial maxillectomy can be performed via a mid-face degloving approach, in which incisions are made under the lip. For larger lesions, well-placed skin incisions in the nasal crease and upper lip are often required for access. Reconstruction in these cases usually involves a skin graft or acellular dermal graft to reline the mucosal surface, as well as a dental appliance to recreate the hard palate.

Tumors that involve the ethmoid sinuses frequently require a craniofacial resection for surgical access because of the proximity to the skull base. This procedure not only requires an anterior approach to the sphenoethmoid area, but also a craniotomy by a skilled neruosurgeon to address the skull base and dura. Orbital exenteration must be

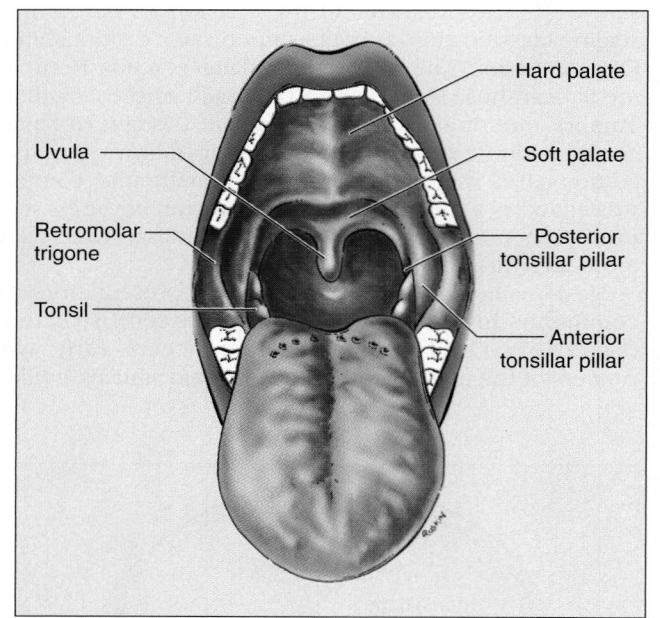

A

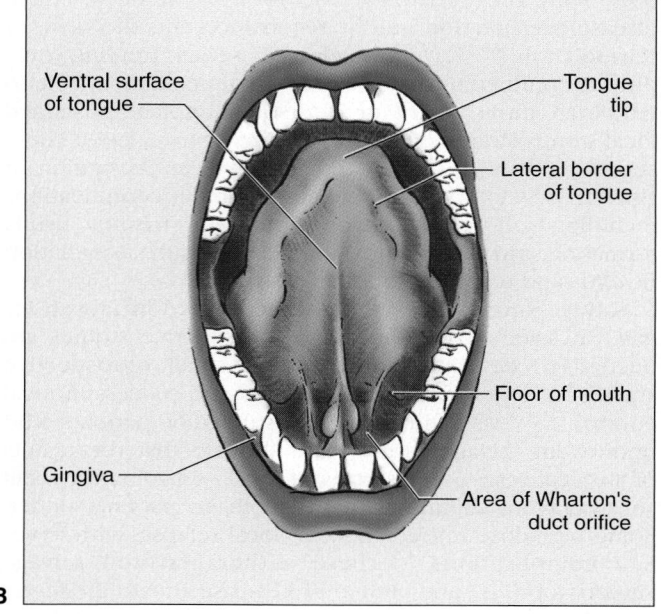

B

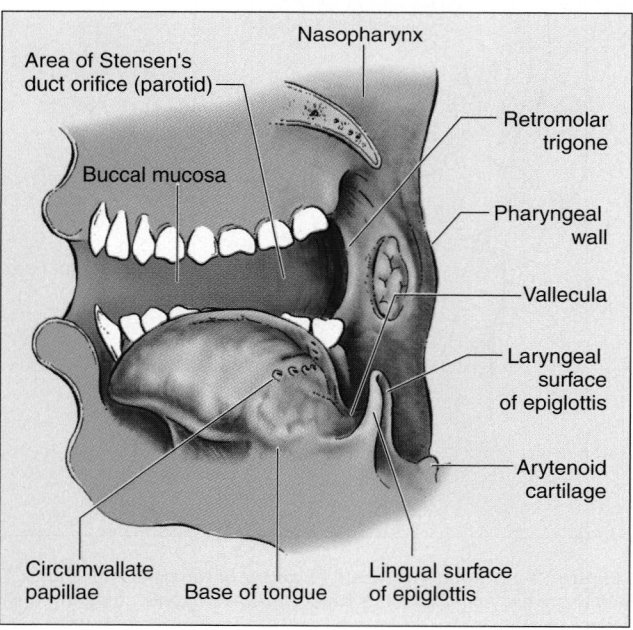

C

Figure 71-18. Oral cavity and oropharynx anatomy. **A,** Open mouth view. **B,** Tongue elevated showing floor of mouth. **C,** Sagittal view.

considered if the tumor involves the periorbital fat and/or extraocular muscles. The surgical indications for this vary, however, with an inclination toward eye conservation and an evolving consensus that bone erosion is not an absolute indication. The decision is an intraoperative decision.

Where surgical resection is not feasible, either medically or surgically, definitive radiotherapy may be used. It has also been favored as an organ-preservation strategy to avoid an orbital exenteration. In this capacity, it may be used definitively, reserving surgery for salvage,[421] or as preoperative radiation as a strategy to downstage the tumor. Given the proximity to many critical normal structures, new radiotherapy techniques including intensity-modulated radiotherapy, stereotactic radiosurgery, or fractionated stereotactic radiotherapy are recommended as they are likely to improve the therapeutic ratio. These techniques are an important consideration in light of evidence suggesting a potential dose-response relationship with dose greater than 65 Gy recommended.[422] Other technical considerations include the use of computer image fusion software that can permit the use of MRI images and the superiority of delineating soft tissue disease during the radiotherapy treatment planning process. While the current literature does not necessarily support the potential incremental therapeutic efficacy, this is due to the relative rarity of this disease and not due to the absence of any effect. As well, the value of concurrent chemotherapy as a radiosensitizer, including early interests in the use of intra-arterial chemotherapy, remains to be established.[423] The value of elective management of the neck remains unclear. As this often increases the treatment morbidity, it may be omitted. Where considered, most nodal metastases occur in the level I and II regions.

The overall 5-year survival rate for patients with maxillary sinus cancer is 30% to 50%.[422,424,425] Cervical metastases occur in less than 10% of maxillary sinus cancers.[426] Therefore a prophylactic neck dissection is not indicated in the N0 neck. Cervical metastases are associated with a very poor prognosis, with 5-year survival rates less than 10%.

Oral Cavity

The oral cavity (Fig. 71-18) is composed of the lip, anterior two thirds of the tongue (oral tongue), floor of mouth, buccal mucosa, gingiva, hard palate, and retromolar trigone. The floor of the mouth is bounded by the lower alveolar ridge anteriorly and laterally and the ventral tongue surface and anterior tonsillar pillar posteriorly. The oral tongue lies anterior to the circumvallate papillae. The buccal mucosa overlies the buccinator muscle, is bounded superiorly and inferiorly by the gingiva, and extends posteriorly to the retromolar trigone. The gingiva is the soft tissue overlying the alveolar ridges of the mandible and maxilla. The hard and soft palates form the roof of the mouth. The retromolar trigone mucosa overlies the mandibular ramus and is bounded anteriorly by the buccal mucosa and posteriorly by the anterior tonsillar pillar. As elsewhere in the head and neck, squamous cell cancer is the most common type except in

TABLE 71-8

AJCC Tumor Classification System for Staging Cancer of the Oral Cavity

STAGE	CHARACTERISTICS
Tis	Carcinoma in situ
T1	Tumor 2 cm or less in greatest dimension
T2	Tumor more than 2 cm but not more than 4 cm in greatest dimension
	Tumor more than 4 cm in greatest dimension
T3	Tumor invades adjacent structures (e.g., through cortical bone, into deep [extrinsic] muscle of tongue, maxillary sinus, skin)

From the American Joint Committee on Cancer: Manual on Staging of Cancer, 4th ed. Philadelphia, JB Lippincott, 1992, with permission.

the hard palate, where most tumors originate in the minor salivary glands. For staging of cancers of the oral cavity, the American Joint Committee on Cancer (AJCC) classification system is used (Table 71-8). The principle management approach is surgical resection followed by postoperative radiotherapy. Carcinomas of the oral cavity have an adverse prognosis and often require postoperative radiotherapy.[162]

Lip. Surgical management of squamous cell carcinoma of the lip is complex, due to the challenges in reconstruction of this unique part of the body. Although secondary to the complete resection of the lesion, the preservation of speech, oral competence, and cosmesis must be considered. Surgical therapy is considered to be equally effective to radiation in treating early, T1, or T2 lesions.[427-430] Small lesions of the lip can be managed surgically via wide local excision and primary closure. The morbidity associated with this often is less than would be experienced with radiation. Larger lesions that require resection of more than one half of the lip require local flap reconstruction. These flaps involve the mobilization of remaining lip tissue, or even the use of tissue from the opposite lip.

Metastases from lip carcinoma is relatively rare, with the incidence reported at 12% or less.[431,432] In the N0 neck, occult metastases are estimated to occur in 5% to 10% of cases. Therefore elective neck dissection is not routinely performed in the N0 neck. Neck dissections are generally performed when cervical metastases are clinically or radiographically apparent.

Predictably, the results of these procedures depend upon the extent of disease. Five-year survival for T1 and T2 cancers of the lip is greater than 90%, whether treated with surgery or radiation.[428] For larger cancers, especially those that have metastasized, the cure rates are in the range of 40% to 50%.[428,433] Thus for stage III and IV cancers, a combined approach with surgery and postoperative radiation is indicated. For smaller lesions, surgery and radiation are equally effective, however, surgery is often recommended because of shorter treatment time and excellent rehabilitation with minimal morbidity.

Buccal Mucosa. Malignant tumors arising from the buccal mucosa are rare, and early lesions are treated primarily with surgery. While surgical management of T1 buccal mucosa lesions can be managed with transoral wide local excision, larger tumors may require more complex resections. Extension to the mandible or maxilla may lead to a partial mandibulectomy or maxillectomy. Reconstructive options for smaller lesions include primary closure, fat grafting, or a split-thickness skin graft. Larger defects would require local mucosal flaps, myocutaneous rotational flaps, or free flaps, depending on the size and extent of the lesion. Neck dissections are indicated only for clinically positive cervical metastases. The treatment algorithm for carcinoma is similar to other sites in the oral cavity, with surgery indicated for early lesions, and combined therapy with surgery and radiation for advanced lesions

Oral Tongue. Oral tongue carcinomas represent approximately 25% of oral cavity carcinomas. These lesions are characterized by early infiltration into the underlying tongue musculature with an early and high risk for regional metastases. Surgical resection has been favored as external radiotherapy results alone have been disappointing.[434,435] While it has been shown that radiation and surgery are equally effective in treating early lesions,[436] a recent review of 332 patients revealed that disease-free survival was better with surgery alone than radiation alone.[435] In general, surgery is often the treatment of choice for early lesions because of the ease of surgical access, excellent reconstruction options, and quick treatment time. For stage III and IV lesions, a combined treatment approach is favored. For select lesions, various series describe comparable results with the use of external beam and a brachytherapy implant as definitive therapy.

Surgical management for squamous cell carcinoma of the oral tongue can take a variety of forms depending on the size and location of the lesion. Small T1 or T2 tumors are treated with a partial glossectomy with a transoral approach. Larger lesions may require a total or near-total glossectomy, often requiring a mandibulotomy or a cervical pull-through procedure. T4 lesions that involve the mandible require composite resection including either a marginal or segmental mandibular resection.

Reconstruction of the surgical defects also depends upon their size and location. After resection of smaller lesions, allowing healing through secondary intention may best preserve function. For larger defects resulting from resection of T2 or T3 defects, healing is facilitated by primary closure, or split-thickness skin graft. For near-total or total glossectomy defects, a pedicled myocutaneous flap or free-tissue transfer is needed for reconstruction. For those patients with mandibular involvement, reconstruction options vary with the location of the defect. Mandibular defects that are large and are located near the mandibular symphysis often require vascularized composite free-flaps to restore mandibular continuity with acceptable function and cosmesis.

Surgical or radiation treatment of the neck is indicated in most cases of oral tongue squamous cell carcinoma.

The rates of occult cervical metastases exceed 30% for lesions T2 and greater.[277,278,433,437,438] Therefore for the N0 neck a selective neck dissection is indicated in T2-T4 lesions, or T1 lesions with depth of invasion greater than 3 to 4 mm.[139,438-440] Patients with clinical or radiographic evidence of cervical metastasis may require more radical procedures depending upon the number and size of nodal involvement.

A significant body of literature exists supporting a role for brachytherapy in the management of selected oral tongue carcinomas that tend to be well defined and, hence, likely less infiltrative. Brachytherapy has been used alone or in combination with EBRT, demonstrating local control efficacy. The largest experience of over 600 patients from the Curie Institute reported local control rates of 86%, 78%, and 71% for T1, T2, and T3 lesions, respectively.[277] Early T1 and T2 lesions were treated with temporary interstitial LDR iridium-192 implants alone, delivering 70 Gy in 6 to 9 days. Larger T2 and T3 lesions were treated with EBRT (50 to 55 Gy) followed by an implant (20 to 30 Gy). Other investigators have demonstrated comparable results demonstrating a high rate of local control.[280,296,441-445] Several series reported local control rates of 90% or greater for very selected lesions often amenable to a single plane implant alone with a lesion thickness of less than 1 cm.[296,441] Mazeron and colleagues reported their series of 121 patients with T1 or T2 N0 tumors treated with 60 to 70 Gy by the Paris system.[442] The crude local control rates for T1, T2a (2.1-3 cm), and T2b (3.1-4 cm) reported were 86%, 89%, and 74%, respectively. The dose prescribed was found to be significantly associated with the risk of local control, with doses less than 65 Gy associated with a fivefold risk of relapse. Selection by the growth pattern has been shown to influence the 5-year local control rates with 85%, 79%, and 45% reported for superficial, exophytic, and infiltrative lesions, respectively.[445] Implant of the oral tongue has been associated with a 10% to 20% risk of mild-moderate self-limiting soft tissue ulceration and a low risk (< 10%) of mandibular osteoradionecrosis in experienced hands. Custom lead-embedded mandibular prostheses and spacers are recommended and have been demonstrated to reduce the risk of bone complications.[441] A predicted 5-year probability of osteoradionecrosis of 38% was reduced to 4% with the use of a spacer. When used in combination with external beam, the overall treatment time and the proportion of dose delivered with the implant may be important.[446]

Several studies suggest treating selected early stage T1 and T2 node negative lesions with HDR brachytherapy alone may facilitate treatment delivery.[296,444,447] One promising schedule comes from a small randomized trial of 29 patients comparing LDR brachytherapy (70 Gy over 4 to 9 days) to an HDR schedule (60 Gy in 10 fractions of 6 Gy/fraction delivered twice daily over 6 days) for a selected group of patients with T1 or T2 N0 squamous cell carcinoma of the lateral oral tongue (OT).[444] The lesions had a thickness of 10 mm or less such that they were treated with a single plane HDR implant with the dose prescribed at 0.5 cm from the reference plane. The 1-year local control (LC) rates were 86% and 100% ($p = 0.157$)

in the LDR (n = 15) and HDR (n = 14) groups, respectively. The 2-year LC was identical, though the median follow-up of 24 months (10 to 32 months) limits this observation. One soft tissue ulceration and one bone exposure complication arose in the HDR arm, though a prosthetic spacer was not used in the latter case. Leung and colleagues have reported preliminary results treating 8 patients with the same HDR schedule showing 100% local control rate with a median follow-up of 26 months.[447] Though promising, the short follow-up and the significant risk of a false negative error limits any definitive conclusions regarding the generalized application of HDR brachytherapy in place of standard LDR implants for the oral tongue.

A subset of patients with a close or positive surgical excision margin and no indication for neck irradiation have been treated with a brachytherapy implant alone (iridium-192 LDR to 60 Gy). This obviates the risk of further major surgery or EBRT-related toxicities, including xerostomia. A promising mature local control rate of 89% has been observed in a small retrospective series.[263] Similar results have been reported.[448,449]

Floor of Mouth. Most floor of mouth (FOM) cancers are amenable to surgical treatment. T1 and T2 cancers that do not involve the mandible are often treated with wide local excision with 1 cm margins. In contrast to lip cancers, postoperative loss of speech and swallowing function is not as prevalent with small FOM tumors. Therefore reconstruction can be performed simply with via primary closure, secondary intention, skin graft, or an acellular dermis graft. Although not always necessary, it is recommended that the patient undergo preoperatively extraction of any decaying teeth close to the lesion.

For those tumors that approach the mandible, a more complex procedure is indicated. Tumors that involve in periosteum of the mandible require a marginal mandibulectomy, where the top half of the involved bone is removed. The overall continuity of the mandible remains intact. T4 tumors that have invaded the cortex of the mandible require a segmental resection of the involved bone. Reconstruction mandates either composite free-flap reconstruction or no reconstruction if the defect is laterally based.

Surgical management of the neck must take into consideration that occult metastases occur frequently in floor of mouth cancers. The incidence is between 23% and 35% of lesions.[277,278,450,451] Therefore most authors recommend treatment of the N0 neck in all T2 lesions or greater.[450–452] For T1 lesions, tumors greater than 2 to 4mm in thickness have been found to have a high rate of metastasis, and treatment is also recommended.[453,454] If surgical rather than radiation treatment is pursued, a selective neck dissection that includes the first echelon nodes (level I and upper level II regions of the neck) should be performed. Unless the lesion is clearly unilateral, a bilateral neck dissection is recommended. Floor of mouth primaries generally call for a supraomohyoid neck dissection with resection of levels I, II, and III. Level IV should be included when performing a dissection for cancers of the oral tongue and oropharynx.[455] Levels I and

V are rarely involved with laryngeal cancer, therefore a lateral neck dissection of levels II, III, and IV is the procedure of choice for these lesions.[222]

The cure rates of surgical therapy for floor of mouth have been quoted as 95% for stage I cancers and 86% for stage II cancers.[456] Another study where the vast majority of patients were treated surgically also demonstrated cure rates of 80% or greater for early lesions.[457] The cure rates for similarly staged cancers treated with radiation are reported by one study as 88% and 47% for T1 and T2 lesions, respectively.[265] Another study showed, however, that surgery and radiation are equally effective in treating early lesions, and that stage III and IV lesions should be treated with combined therapy.[458] In general, the early lesions of the floor of mouth are best managed surgically unless there is contraindication. Combined therapy is necessary for larger lesions.

Hard Palate. The type of surgical management indicated for lesions originating in the hard palate depends largely on the presence of bone involvement. With those lesions that do not involve the periosteum, the tumor can be excised without the underlying bone with an adequate mucosal margin. Tumors invading the periosteum, however, require full-thickness resection of the involved bone. Larger tumors may require partial or total maxillectomy. Reconstruction usually involves a skin graft and a dental prosthesis for large palatal defects. Neck metastases are rare, and should be managed surgically with a neck dissection. The role of primary radiation is limited in this disease, but postoperative radiation is indicated for advanced lesions.

Oropharynx

Although radiation therapy plays a large role in the treatment of squamous cell carcinoma of the oropharynx, surgery is often indicated in combination with radiation for larger T3 and T4 lesions.[459] Although there are site-specific considerations, certain principles apply to surgery in the oropharynx whether the lesion is in the tonsil, base of tongue, or the soft palate. Selected T1 tumors can be approached transorally. A transoral approach, however, may not provide the access necessary to excise larger lesions completely and safely. In these cases, an anterior or lateral mandibulotomy is often utilized in order to gain access. Mandibular involvement by oropharyngeal lesions necessitates marginal or segmental mandibular resection. A neck dissection can be performed in continuity with or separately from the primary tumor.

The goal of reconstruction in this region is to minimize the severe disfigurement and functional compromise that may result from oropharyngeal procedures. Reconstruction options for surgical defects of the oropharynx depend on the size and location of the lesion. Defects from small T1 lesions can be repaired via secondary intention, primary closure, or a split-thickness skin graft. Reconstruction options for larger lesions include a skin graft, a tongue flap, a myocutaneous flap, or free-tissue transfer. Reconstruction after segmental mandibular resection preferably includes osseous free-tissue transfer to replace the excised bone. If a marginal or small segmental resection is performed, however, the bone does not need to be replaced. The complications involved with surgical treatment of oropharyngeal tumors are similar to those encountered with the treatment of oral cavity tumors. Because the tongue base is critical to swallowing function, dysphagia and aspiration are frequently seen after tongue base resection. This can be treated with aggressive swallowing rehabilitation. There are site-specific surgical and nonsurgical considerations within the oropharynx.

Tonsil. Though T1 and T2 tonsil lesions are generally best treated with radiation, large T2, T3 and T4 lesions are often treated with combined therapy. If the mandible is not involved, the procedure of choice is a radical tonsillectomy that includes the tonsil, the tonsillar pillars, and a portion of the underlying muscle. If the mandible is involved, a composite resection including a segmental mandibulectomy is required.

Some authors argue that early tonsil lesions are best treated with surgery. One small study of 18 patients was recently published. It cited a 5-year survival rate of 92% for surgically treated patients with T1 or T2 cancers of the tonsil.[460] Similar results are found in patients treated with irradiation alone with less functional morbidity, however.[461,462] In addition, the use of radiotherapy alone for early tonsil lesions allows the retropharyngeal lymph nodes to be addressed, particularly for progressively more posterior lesions and those involving the posterior pillar. While early lesions are best treated with radiation, advanced stage III and IV cancers required combined surgical therapy with radiotherapy for best results.[459,463] The relative efficacy of this approach to an increasing role for concurrent chemoradiotherapy in advanced oropharyngeal carcinomas including tonsil carcinomas is unknown. With increasing involvement of the soft palate and of the pharyngeal wall, however, surgical resection becomes less favored (though often preferred due to concomitant bulky tumor) due to the functional consequences and increased risk of complications, respectively. For more advanced lesions, with increasing posterior disease extension, the risk of parapharyngeal involvement and retropharyngeal lymph node metastases increases, necessitating radiotherapy as either definitive therapy or in the postoperative setting. Where surgical resection is not indicated, concurrent chemoradiotherapy is emerging as a favored definitive strategy on the basis of recent randomized trials and meta-analyses.[181] This treatment approach is limited by the uncertainty with regard to the optimal chemoradiotherapy schedule and the potential for these results not to be generalizable to the tonsil site specifically. It is also recognized that salvage surgery, when chemoradiotherapy is used for potential organ preservation indications, is limited by the proportion of recurrences able to undergo salvage surgery and then the proportion of salvage surgery that is successful.

Despite these concerns, several prospective studies have demonstrated high local-regional control rates (80% to 90%) where oropharyngeal and tonsil sites were the predominant tumor sites. It is not clear if these results are superior to local-regional control rates that have been reported for treatment with radiotherapy alone. Several institutional series have outlined the results that may be expected from fractionated radiotherapy alone. It is recognized, however, that the fractionation schedule may in turn influence the results.

To address these concerns, Withers and colleagues reported the results of a remarkable collaborative retrospective multi-institutional study of carcinoma of the tonsil fossa treated with radiotherapy alone as part of the Patterns of Fractionation Study.[153] In total, 676 patients from 9 participating institutions provided sufficient treatment variability in fractionation schedules resulting from institutional treatment policies to permit study. Several noteworthy observations were made. With the exception of T1 disease, decreased local control rates were observed with the presence of clinically evident nodal disease across each T-stage. Cox regression modeling demonstrated that T-stage, N-stage, total dose, and the overall treatment time were independent significant factors. Though the optimal fractionation schedule could not be identified, a nonsignificant reduction in local relapse was observed with altered fractionated schedules consistent with the observations of RTOG 90-03.[179] Modeling of the relationship between local tumor control and the overall treatment time suggested that an accelerated growth rate may occur at about day 30, but did not significantly improve upon the basic model of a constant tumor growth rate throughout the treatment duration. Whether or not these tumor kinetics differ with perturbations from the use of concurrent chemotherapy is unclear but should remain respected.

Hence where radiotherapy is used as definitive therapy alone, an altered fractionation schedule is preferred with particular attention paid to minimize any treatment interruptions at any time in the treatment duration. Several reports provide a basis for selection of lesions appropriate for homolateral irradiation.[464-466] The advantages of homolateral irradiation include reduced acute toxicities, less risk of treatment interruptions, reduced dose to the contralateral parotid, and less risk of complete xerostomia. O'Sullivan and colleagues reported the results of a large retrospective analysis of 228 patients treated with daily fractionated radiotherapy alone with mature follow-up.[464] Based upon an institutional policy of homo-lateral irradiation for lesions that did not cross midline structures, these investigators were able to demonstrate a spectrum of risk of contralateral neck relapses to guide treatment selection. Patients at low risk (less than 5%) of contralateral neck relapse include those with T1-2 lateralized lesions with involvement of even then lateral two thirds of the soft palate or lateral one third of the base of the tongue. However, the involvement of these structures requires judicious use of ipsilateral irradiation.

Soft Palate. Soft palate lesions that are large may require a partial maxillectomy for complete excision. In general, soft palate tumors are amenable to definitive radiotherapy for cure. The fields should cover the draining lymphatics and the retropharyngeal lymph nodes. With this modality palatal function can usually be preserved. Reconstruction of this defect may include a skin graft along with a prefabricated prosthesis to maintain swallowing function. Radiation has been shown to be effective in controlling early lesions, while combined therapy is needed for stage III and IV lesions.[467-469]

Cervical metastases should be treated with surgery, radiation, or both. Neck dissections can be performed before or after radiation therapy. The decision to perform surgery or radiation first depends upon how the primary is to be treated, and upon the size and extent of the neck metastasis. If the metastasis is of sufficient size to require a radical neck dissection or if it encases the carotid artery, primary treatment with radiation is preferred so that the neck mass might become smaller and more resectable. Bilateral treatment should be considered in large oropharyngeal tumors or those that cross the midline.

The clinically negative neck should also be treated by surgery or radiation when the primary originates from the oropharynx. The risk of occult disease is 30% or greater, and these nodes can be found anywhere in levels I to IV of the neck.[470-472] Therefore if an elective neck dissection is performed rather than radiation therapy, a selective neck dissection is performed addressing these levels. For midline lesions, bilateral treatment of the neck must be performed.

Base of Tongue. Treatment options for carcinomas of the base of tongue may include surgery or radiotherapy-based strategies. Limited comparative studies have been published to guide the treatment decision-making process. Given the functional impact of therapy to this site, considerations of functional organ preservation have received increasing consideration as comparable local-regional control and survival rates have been suggested. In this regard, while radiotherapy has typically been preferred, several surgical issues are important to consider.

With regard to the tongue base, there are additional considerations depending on the size and location of the lesion. If a small tumor lies posteriorly and inferiorly in the base of tongue, a transhyoid approach through the neck can be considered rather than a mandible splitting approach. For small tumors that lie laterally in the tongue base or on the pharyngeal walls, a lateral pharyngotomy can be considered. For larger tumors, resection of a significant portion may result in chronic aspiration because the tongue base is critical to swallowing function. Recurrent pulmonary infections in the elderly or immunocompromised can be life threatening. Thus a laryngectomy is often considered when more than half of the tongue base is to be removed, especially in high-risk patients. If the larynx is preserved, postoperative functional results can be optimized with swallowing therapy or laryngeal suspension.[473]

For base of tongue tumors, the data show that early tumors are best treated by radiotherapy or surgery while patients with advanced lesions should receive combined treatment. In one study of 173 patients, early primary tumors treated with surgery or radiotherapy had a control rate of 83% (5 of 6 tumors) and 89% (40 of 45 tumors),

respectively. For advanced primary tumors, definitive radiotherapy produced a local control rate of 55% (42 of 76 tumors), compared with 79% (23 of 29 tumors) for surgery and postoperative radiotherapy.[474] Radiotherapy is preferred for early lesions because of the decreased treatment morbidity compared with base of tongue surgery.

In this regard, data exist to demonstrate that the local control rates for external beam followed by a brachytherapy implant are superior to those achieved with external-beam radiotherapy alone.[284] One retrospective review demonstrated comparable local control rates between external-beam radiotherapy with an implant and surgery, both of which were superior to external-beam radiotherapy alone.[287] Several independent investigators have consistently demonstrated that a brachytherapy implant boost (20 to 30 Gy) after EBRT (45 to 55 Gy) is associated with effective local control rates. No significant functional deficits with this organ-preserving strategy have been reported when several quality of life domains were studied, even for advanced lesions.[291,292] The greatest experience has been with temporary interstitial LDR iridium-192 implants. Mature local control rates of 85% or greater may be expected for T1 and T2 lesions and 80% to 85% with T3 lesions.[281] Similar results have been reported.[282-288,475,476] In general, the more advanced lesions treated have been selected based upon favorable exophytic growth patterns. The experience of a brachytherapy implant in T4 lesions remains limited.[281,283,284,288,475] Concurrent chemoradiotherapy techniques are favored, particularly for the more advanced T3-4 lesions. Puthawala and colleagues reported a mature crude local control rate of 67% with more relapses observed in patients with more advanced neck disease[288] and used a higher brachytherapy boost dose of 30 to 40 Gy compared to 20 to 25 Gy for T1-2 lesions. The value of an implant for T4 lesions appears promising but requires further evaluation, particularly when combined with combination chemoradiotherapy, as late swallowing complications may compromise the benefits of an organ-preserving treatment strategy.

Larynx

From the standpoint of staging and treatment, the larynx is divided into supraglottic, glottic, and subglottic regions (Table 71-9 and Fig. 71-19). The supraglottic region is composed of the epiglottis, arytenoid cartilages, aryepiglottic folds, false cords, and laryngeal ventricles. The glottic larynx includes the true vocal cords as well as the anterior and posterior commissures. The subglottic region extends to the inferior edge of the cricoid cartilage. Transglottic tumors involve the glottic level as well as another site within the larynx.

Supraglottic Larynx. With regard to early lesions, surgical management of supraglottic tumors varies depending upon the exact location of the lesion. T1 tumors of the suprahyoid epiglottis are readily managed endoscopically via CO_2 laser excision. Tumors of the infrahyoid epiglottis are not amenable to this type of resection because of the

Specific Malignancies

TABLE 71-9

AJCC Classification for Staging Primary Laryngeal Cancer

STAGE	CHARACTERISTICS
Supraglottis	
T1	Tumor limited to once subsite of supraglottis, with normal vocal cord mobility
T2	Tumor invades more than one subsite of supraglottis or glottis, with normal vocal cord mobility
T3	Tumor limited to larynx with vocal cord fixation and/or invades postcricoid area, medial wall of pyriform sinus, or pre-epiglottic tissues
T4	Tumor invades thyroid cartilage and/or extends to other tissue beyond the larynx (e.g., to oropharynx, soft tissue of neck)
Glottis	
T1	Tumor limited to vocal cord(s) (may involve anterior or posterior commissures) with normal mobility
T1a	Tumor limited to one vocal cord
T1b	Tumor involves both vocal cords
T2	Tumor extends to supraglottis or subglottis, or both, with or without impaired vocal cord mobility
T3	Tumor limited to the larynx with vocal cord fixation
T4	Tumor invades through thyroid cartilage and/or extends to other tissue beyond the larynx (e.g., oropharynx, soft tissue of neck)
Subglottis	
T1	Tumor limited to the subglottis
T2	Tumor extends to vocal cord(s) with normal or impaired mobility
T3	Tumor limited to larynx with vocal cord fixation
T4	Tumor invades through cricoid or thyroid cartilage and/or extends to other tissues beyond the larynx (e.g., oropharynx, soft tissues of neck)

From the American Joint Committee on Cancer: Manual on Staging of Cancer, 4th ed Philadelphia, JB Lippincott, 1992, with permission.

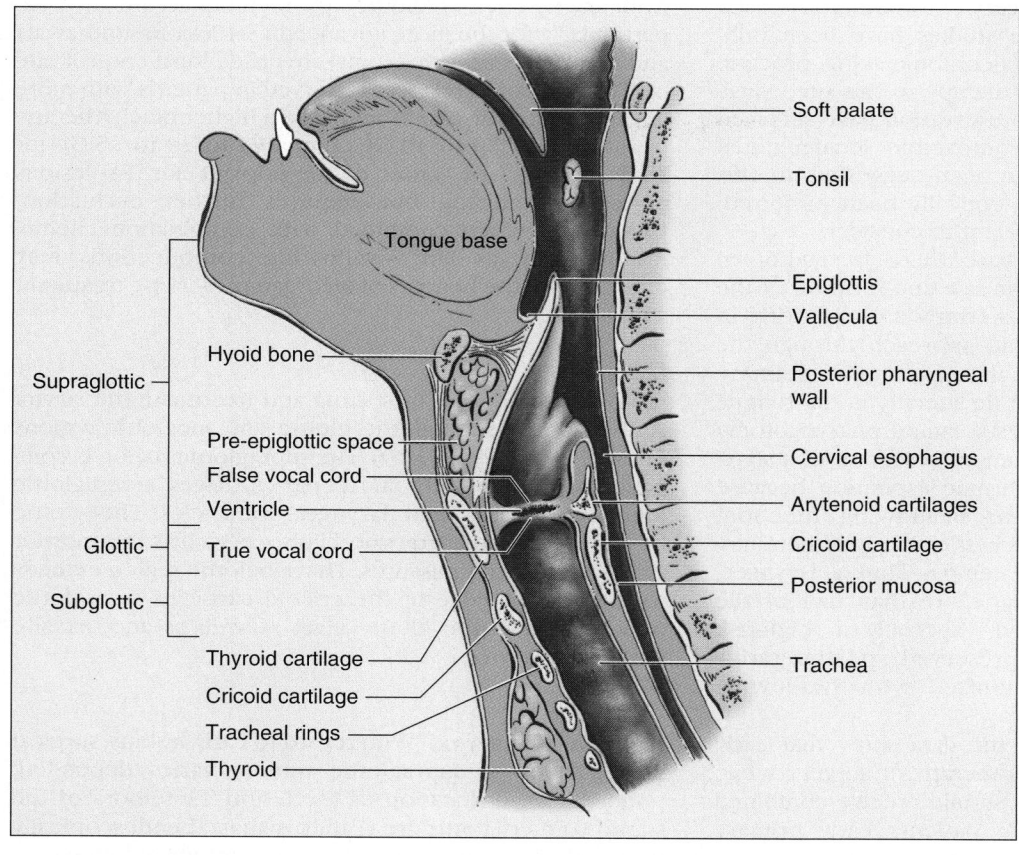

Figure 71-19. Anatomy of larynx and hypopharynx: Sagittal view. (From Gregoire, et al: Radiotherapy and Oncology 2000;56:135–150.

possibility of pre-epiglottic space invasion.[477] An open procedure is more oncologically sound in these cases.

Surgical treatment of early lesions of the false vocal folds often requires a supraglottic laryngectomy, which spares the true vocal folds. If a supraglottic tumor extends to the true cords, the patient may be a candidate for a supracricoid laryngectomy, which spares at least one arytenoid cartilage but not the true cords. Patients who undergo this procedure generally have excellent functional results with regard to speech and swallowing.[478,479]

Surgical treatment of T4 lesions requires a total laryngectomy in most cases. This procedure involves the resection of the entire larynx, including the epiglottis, the true and false vocal cords, the thyroid cartilage, one lobe of the thyroid gland, and the involved mucosa of the hypopharynx or base of tongue. The remaining pharyngeal mucosa is then closed, either primarily or with additional tissue from a free or rotational flap. The long-term functional swallowing results from this procedure are generally excellent, especially if the pharynx was closed primarily.[480-482] Speech rehabilitation is performed with a number of devices and techniques, including esophageal speech, an electrolarynx, or a tracheoesophageal puncture device.

Due to the high rate of occult metastasis, bilateral treatment of the neck is recommended in most cases of squamous cell carcinoma of the supraglottis. In the clinically N0 neck, surgical treatment includes a selective neck dissection including levels II, III, and IV, as these are the most likely locations for occult metastases.[221,483]

The decision to treat T1, T2, and T3 lesions with radiation or surgery can be difficult. Recent studies in the surgical literature show good 5-year survival rates with either modality.[484-487] Radiation with surgical salvage may be the best option for patients that have pulmonary disease who are at a high risk for severe complications from aspiration.

Salvage surgery often entails a total laryngectomy. Patients who are surgical candidates for a partial laryngectomy retain glottic function without compromising oncologic outcome.[488] The status of the cervical nodes also must be taken into consideration when deciding on treatment modality. Surgery is certainly indicated when large metastatic nodes are present, as this allows for combined therapy. Surgery or radiation is sufficient to treat the N0 neck.

Glottic Larynx. Early lesions of the true vocal cords that are not treated with radiation can be treated surgically in a number of ways. Carcinomas in situ may be managed endoscopically with vocal cord stripping or with the CO_2 laser. T1 lesions of the true vocal cords may be treated surgically with via cordectomy or CO_2 laser excision. T2 lesions often require open procedures for adequate surgical resection, although radiotherapy is an equally effective option. Operations geared toward organ-preservation surgery such as a vertical hemilaryngectomy or a supracricoid laryngectomy should be considered before total laryngectomy for T2 lesions. T3 and T4 lesions of the glottis almost always require a total laryngectomy

if surgical management is chosen, although selected patients with T3 cancers are candidates for a supracricoid hemilaryngectomy.[489]

Management of the neck in glottic carcinoma differs from supraglottic carcinoma because the risk of occult metastasis is less, ranging from 3% to 21%.[490-493] Observation is the treatment of choice for the neck in T1 and T2 primary glottic cancers, but some authors recommend treatment of the N0 neck in T3 and T4 cancers.[494] If surgical management is chosen, a selective neck dissection of levels II to IV is the procedure of choice. In the N+ neck, a selective or modified radical neck dissection may be indicated depending upon the size and location of the metastasis.

The oncologic results for T1 lesions of the glottis are good. Endoscopic cordectomy is equal to radiotherapy for most lesions, with cure rates above 90%.[495,496] Several factors should determine which modality to use. Patient concerns and health are of paramount importance. It must be made clear that while radiation can often be used for salvage after surgery, the salvage procedure indicated after failed radiation may be a total laryngectomy. Lesions of the anterior commissure, though classified as T1, are not as effectively treated with radiation and are difficult to excise endoscopically.[497,498] An open partial laryngeal procedure such as a hemilaryngectomy or supracricoid laryngectomy can be considered depending on the extent of the lesion.

T2 lesions can be managed with radiation or surgery equally well. The 5-year local control rate has been estimated to be greater than 80% after either primary surgical therapy or radiation therapy.[489,496,499-502] It is more likely, however, that an open partial laryngectomy approach rather than a simpler endoscopic approach is needed for adequate surgical treatment.[489,496,501] Therefore it becomes very important to choose surgical candidates carefully with regard to pulmonary function, intelligence, motivation, and home situation.

For advanced stage tumors, it has been shown that survival is similar between patients treated with an organ-preservation protocol and those treated with surgery.[503,504] It should be noted that in the landmark Veterans Affairs study, although 66% of patients in the organ-preservation arm preserved their larynges, 39% were tracheostomy dependent. Patients should be offered chemotherapy and radiation therapy as an alternative to total laryngectomy, however. It has been recently shown that salvage laryngectomy after organ-preservation therapy is associated with acceptable morbidity, and that survival after the surgery was not affected by the initial organ-preservation treatment.[185]

Subglottic Larynx. Primary cancers originating in the subglottis are relatively rare.[505] Because conservative endoscopic procedures would fail to clear the tumor, management of these tumors most often requires total laryngectomy. A paratracheal lymph node dissection and ipsilateral thyroidectomy should also be considered. Subglottic extension of T3 or T4 subglottic cancers should be managed similarly. Postoperative radiation therapy should be added to decrease the risk of a stomal recurrence.

Hypopharynx. Surgical management of hypopharyngeal cancers is particularly challenging because the mucosa of the hypopharynx is vital to swallowing function. Thus surgical extirpation of large tumors often requires complex reconstructions to minimize postoperative dysphagia.

The surgical options vary with the size and precise location of the tumor within the hypopharynx. Selected small tumors of the pyriform sinuses can be managed using conservation procedures that maintain laryngeal function. These procedures include the partial laryngopharyngectomy and supracricoid hemilaryngopharyngectomy.[506,507] To be a candidate for these procedures, a patient must have a small lesion that does not involve surrounding structures or impair vocal cord motion. In addition, the patient must have good pulmonary function and motivation to undergo rigorous swallowing rehabilitation.

For most tumors of the pyriform sinus T2 and larger, a total laryngectomy with partial pharyngectomy is indicated. This procedure can carry significant morbidity, especially when performed as salvage after failed radiation therapy. To reconstruct the pharynx, surgical options include myocutaneous flaps such as the pectoralis flap, fasciocutaneous flaps such as the deltopectoral flap, and free-tissue transfer from the forearm or jejunum. A gastric transposition procedure, facilitated by a general surgeon in the operating room, is also used in cases where there is a circumferential pharyngeal defect.

Tumors of the posterior pharyngeal wall are more accessible anatomically, making surgical management less complex than for pyriform sinus cancers. Most pharyngeal wall cancers can be resected directly, without laryngectomy, via a suprahyoid or lateral pharyngotomy approach. Reconstruction is often performed with a split-thickness skin graft or acellular dermal graft. Larger tumors may require myocutaneous or free-flap reconstruction.

Cancers that involve the postcricoid region of the hypopharynx require an extensive procedure if they are to be managed surgically. A total laryngectomy, partial pharyngectomy, and cervical esophagectomy are usually required. A total esophagectomy may be indicated depending upon the inferior extent of the lesion.

Occult metastases from hypopharyngeal cancers are present in greater than 30% of N0 necks.[490,508] Therefore selective neck dissection of levels II, III, and IV are indicated, even in patients staged N0. In addition, if the tumor approaches the midline, bilateral neck dissections should be performed.[508,509]

The outcome for patients with hypopharyngeal cancer is poor, especially if the tumor originates in the pyriform sinus. Marks and colleagues estimated 5-year survival to be 14% for advanced pyriform sinus cancers.[510] In the same retrospective study, it was demonstrated that surgery alone was significantly superior to radiotherapy, with or without chemotherapy, in the treatment of the disease. Another retrospective study showed that surgery is superior to combined chemotherapy and radiation therapy, although the difference was not statistically significant.[511] A prospective study showed that organ preservation is superior in terms of survival, but again the difference was not statistically significant.[192] The treatment of advanced hypopharyngeal cancer must be individualized for each patient.

Major and Minor Salivary Glands. Surgical treatment is the mainstay of salivary gland cancer management, whether arising from the parotid, submandibular, sublingual, or minor salivary glands. Surgery for parotid gland malignancy is perhaps the most challenging because of the location of the facial nerve coursing between the superficial and deep lobes. Most parotid tumors are located in the superficial lobe of the gland, and therefore are treated with a superficial parotidectomy via a transcervical approach, sparing the facial nerve. Those tumors within the deep lobe of the gland require a total parotidectomy. The facial nerve is spared in these cases if it is not involved with the malignancy. For deep lobe malignancies, additional access via a submandibular or, rarely for massive tumors, a mandible splitting approach.

Submandibular gland tumors are usually contained within the gland, and therefore resection is limited to the submandibular triangle. The marginal mandibular, lingual, and hypoglossal nerves should be spared. If there is spread to the surrounding tissues, these structures, as well as surrounding bone, floor of mouth, and skin may need to be removed surgically. The extent of surgery for malignancies of the sublingual glands and minor salivary glands depend upon the size and location of the tumor within the oral cavity.

Combined therapy is usually recommended for high-grade malignancies of the salivary gland such as high-grade mucoepidermoid carcinoma. Postoperative radiation has been shown to improve local-regional control in several studies.[512,513] Neck dissections are indicated in the event of known cervical metastasis.

Unknown Primary. The treatment for unknown primary squamous carcinoma may include neck dissection followed by postoperative radiotherapy alone or radiotherapy followed by a neck dissection. The relative efficacy of these two strategies has not been evaluated. There is no role established at this time for the addition of concurrent chemotherapy, though this remains an attractive therapeutic strategy. However, the increased mucosal toxicities including the potential long-term swallowing dysfunction must be balanced against unclear benefits including regional control and survival. Currently, irradiation may include the neck alone or elective mucosal irradiation of potential primary sites. Weir and colleagues noted no survival benefits with elective mucosal irradiation,[514] though Reddy and colleagues continued to recommend elective mucosal irradiation due to reduced risk of contralateral nodal and primary relapses.[515] The latter depends on the location of the nodal metastases. For level II nodal metastases, this may require elective irradiation of the oropharynx and laryngeal structures.

Recurrent HNSCC and Second HNSCC. The optimal management for recurrent non-nasopharyngeal HNSCC and second primary HNSCC remains to be defined and is complicated by retrospective series reporting on heterogeneous groups of patients treated. Reirradiation of the head and neck is possible, however, with increased but potentially acceptable toxicities. Various investigators have studied combinations of chemotherapy and radiotherapy in hopes of realizing significant radiosensitization such that the total required for reirradiation is reduced. The results have been summarized by Kao and associates[218] Unfortunately, only a select few demonstrate benefit with survival prolongation. Higher total doses appear to be important, with a reirradiation dose of 60 Gy typically recommended.[516] As such, one must balance the limited potential gains with an increased risk of complications including soft tissue necrosis and neurologic damage. Currently, reirradiation with external-beam radiotherapy and chemotherapy remains limited to clinical trials at centers with ongoing systematic experience with particular protocols. Various conformal radiotherapy techniques may facilitate safer reirradiation. These include recent techniques such as IMRT. However, the use of brachytherapy implant for reirradiation can play an important role in improving the therapeutic ratio, as full-dose irradiation is required for any potential for cure.

Surgery is preferred and offered for resectable lesions in the absence of unacceptable functional and cosmetic sequelae. In this setting, there is often a need for management of microscopic residual disease with radiotherapy. A planned introduction of nonirradiated tissue flaps with coordination of the implant placement and of the wound reconstruction can reduce the risk of wound complications. Both pedicled myocutaneous flaps[517] and microvascular free flaps have been described.[518] Despite this, complication rates of 20% to 50%, including a risk of carotid rupture when the neck is implanted, have been reported. Factors other than the radiation may be contributing to this increased risk of complications. This is tempered by local control rates of 44% to 80%, suggesting a limited therapeutic ratio.[519-522] Hence patient selection is particularly important for this indication.

A brachytherapy implant alone may be used for selected second primary HNSCC. Peiffert and colleagues reported the results of a ^{192}Ir implant alone for 73 patients with tonsil carcinoma treated at the Centre Alexis Vautrin.[295] The majority presented with early node negative disease with a median dose of 60 Gy prescribed according to the Paris dosimetry system. The 5-year actuarial local control rate for T1 N0 and T2 N0 lesions was 80% and 67%, respectively. Acceptable grade 2 self-resolving complications were observed in 10 cases (13%) with the majority being soft tissue necrosis due to a dose greater than 60 Gy. This appeared to be increased when compared to the same institution's series when tonsil implants were prescribed in unirradiated tissues.[272] The 5-year actuarial disease-specific survival and overall survival was 64% and 30%, respectively. No long-term survivors were observed, reflecting the increased risk of other malignancies and other alcohol and smoking related comorbidities in this patient population.

Other retrospective series have reported the results of reirradiation with an implant, but include both patients with a second primary HNSCC and recurrent HNSCC,

confounding the overall analyses. Treatment of recurrent HNSCC may be expected to have lower local control rates due to the treatment of more radioresistant clonogens, an observation consistent with clinical data.[293,294,523] Langlois and colleagues reported the reirradiation results of a larger and heterogeneous group treated at the Centre Alexis Vautrin for 123 patients with T1-3 disease treated with a ^{192}Ir implant with a mean dose of 62 Gy.[294] A 5-year actuarial local control rate of 59% was observed. Local control correlated with size less than 3 cm, second primary (vs. recurrent lesions), dose greater than 60 Gy, and tumor site (oral cavity favorable compared to oropharynx). Only a 5-year actuarial survival rate of 24% was realized, with local control achieved, and a time interval between reirradiation of more than 2 years associated with a better prognosis. Mucosal necrosis was observed in 28 cases (23%). Stevens and colleagues also noted favorable local control rates with second primary HNSCC, a reirradiation dose of 60 Gy or greater for second primary HNSCC, a treatment interval longer than 1 year for recurrent lesions, and the use of an implant in addition to EBRT.[523] Mazeron and colleagues reported a 5-year actuarial local control rate of 69% for 70 patients with oropharyngeal carcinomas reirradiated with a ^{192}Ir implant alone delivering a mean dose of 60 Gy with the Paris system.[524] Similarly, tumor site (glossotonsillar sulcus and base of tongue being unfavorable) and tumor size (> 2 cm) adversely influenced the local control rate, though larger lesions occurred more frequently in the base of tongue. Regional nodal irradiation was not intentionally treated, with only 7 of 69 (10%) developing nodal relapses. Soft tissue necrosis was the main complication (27%), was self-resolving in 13 of 14 patients, and appeared to be increased when a large lesion was implanted.

Levandag reported the results of 73 patients with either second primary HNSCC or recurrent HNSCC comparing EBRT reirradiation with implant with or without EBRT reirradiation (18 patients), though significant heterogeneity existed in the treatment applied in each of the patient cohorts, precluding definitive conclusions.[525] Selection bias was minimized as the two cohorts represented sequential treatment periods resulting from an institutional policy change. A crude local control rate of 29% and 50% were reported, respectively, suggesting improved control rates with an implant though this was confounded by the higher mean dose delivered in the implant cohort compared to the EBRT cohort. The high rate of temporary mucosa ulcerations (13/18 vs. 9/55) was likely related to the implant technique used. To reduce the increased risk of mucosal ulceration associated with an implant, Housset and colleagues employed a planned treatment interruption, delivering the intended dose in two separate implants with a source shift.[293] In total, 55 patients with both recurrent and second primary base of tongue (BOT) SCC was implanted, with 31 patients receiving a single course implant of 60 Gy and 24 patients receiving a split course implant delivering 35 Gy and 30 Gy with a 1-month interruption. A significant reduction in the risk of mucosal necrosis was observed with the introduction of a treatment interruption (16% vs. 43%), though a trend toward a lower crude local control rate (37.5% vs.

52%) suggests that such a strategy warrants further investigation.

In summary, a brachytherapy implant may be selectively applied for reirradiation in view of the poor prognosis associated with this patient population. Favorable local control rates may be expected in patients with second primary HNSCC, small tumor sizes, tumor sites other than the base of tongue, and the delivery of 60 Gy or greater. For recurrent HNSCC, treatment intervals of longer than 1 year appear to select for lesions that are less radioresistant. Soft tissue complications appear to be increased and range from 20% to 30% with the majority being self-resolving.

SUMMARY AND FUTURE DIRECTIONS

A paradigm shift has occurred in the management of squamous cell carcinoma of the upper aerodigestive tract over the past 25 years. In the 1970s and 1980s, Fletcher and others demonstrated the ability to preserve function through the use of definitive radiation for patients with cancers of the larynx and oropharynx. In the mid-1980s, Wolf and Hong introduced the concept of laryngeal preservation by combining induction chemotherapy and definitive radiation for patients who obtained a significant response to the induction phase of treatment. For the first time, organ preservation was achieved without a deleterious effect on survival. After this favorable report by the Veterans Affairs Cooperative Group, treatment intensification trials were designed to increase the rate of organ preservation and to improve survival rates. Concomitant chemotherapy and radiation therapy were demonstrated to provide a survival benefit over neoadjuvant chemotherapy and radiation, albeit with increased toxicity. The Radiation Therapy Oncology Group implemented a three-arm trial for laryngeal preservation in 1992 to test this concept. Preliminary results from this trial demonstrated a higher rate of organ preservation among patients receiving concomitant chemotherapy compared to induction chemotherapy and radiation therapy or radiation alone. Despite an increased rate of laryngeal preservation, however, treatment intensification did not translate into improved survival.

Current therapeutic approaches have been designed to improve local-regional cancer control and survival through further treatment intensification. Phase III trials are evaluating different chemotherapeutic agents combined with altered fractionated radiation schemes and take advantage of the radiosensitizing effects of chemotherapy when administered concurrently with radiation. While the outcome from these trials will not be reported for some time, the toxicity associated with aggressive combination therapy is of increasing concern. Anatomic organ preservation through nonsurgical means has been convincingly demonstrated; nevertheless outcome data that demonstrate effective functional preservation of the organ are lacking. Assessment of organ function and quality of life are now integrated into these trials and will provide longitudinal data on pre- and post-treatment organ function and how these relate to the patient's perceived quality of life. In the future, the success of anatomic as well as functional organ preservation will be clarified.

Further treatment intensification will likely be associated with unacceptable toxicity and will require new approaches to ameliorate the side effects of cytotoxic therapy. Toxicity scoring schemes are being developed and implemented to provide a more quantitative assessment of early and late treatment side effects. Mucosal injury, an early treatment effect, and fibrosis, a late effect, will constrain further attempts to intensify treatment. Mucositis contributes to nutritional deficits and may lead to circumferential scarring and stenosis of the pharynx. Fibrosis contributes to laryngeal and pharyngeal dysfunction through loss of neuromuscular coordination and muscle function. Intensity-modulated radiotherapy to limit exposure of normal tissues and agents to mitigate these side effects are being studied in clinical trials. To date, none of the systemic agents to lessen toxic side effects has convincingly demonstrated effectiveness.

While current therapeutic approaches destroy neoplastic cells, collateral damage to normal tissues is responsible for the toxic side effects and long-term functional impairment. Future directions may come from continued technological advancements including organ-preserving surgical techniques and the use of more precise radiotherapy techniques such as IMRT. The greatest potential for gain, however, comes from capitalizing on the molecular mechanisms specific to cancer cells that are responsible for tumor progression. The hope is for more cancer-specific therapy without the increased toxicity. The results from clinical trials conducted with several of these agents alone support the notion that there may be more specific tumor targeting, as the toxicity profiles have to date been very modest. Activity has also been modest, however, and this has lead to the use of surrogate measures to determine if, in fact, these agents are inhibiting the molecular targets in vivo. While the head and neck site lends itself to tissue biopsies for these assays, the hope is for the continued development of functional imaging to provide us with these answers. Given the modest activity with these agents alone, the challenge that exists at this moment is to develop novel strategies of combining these targeted biologic agents with cytotoxic drugs and radiation in a rational manner. This will depend on successful translation of knowledge gained from laboratory investigations, particularly about the molecular mechanisms of treatment resistance. We are at the threshold of realizing our long-sought goal of effective cancer control through the use of targeted therapy that will optimize local-regional control and enhance survival within the context of acceptable toxicity.

REFERENCES

1. Jemal A, et al: Cancer statistics, 2003. CA Cancer J Clin 2003;53(1): 5-26.
2. Collins SL: Avoiding delay and misdiagnosis of head and neck cancer: Rare tumors with common symptoms. Compr Ther 1995;21(2):59-67.
3. Franceschi S, et al: Smoking and drinking in relation to cancers of the oral cavity, pharynx, larynx, and esophagus in northern Italy. Cancer Res 1990;50(20):6502-6507.

4. Society AC: Cancer facts and figures 2002. Atlanta, Georgia, American Cancer Society, 2002.

5. Silverman S, Jr: Demographics and occurrence of oral and pharyngeal cancers: The outcomes, the trends, the challenge. J Am Dent Assoc 2001;132 Suppl:7S-11S.

6. Shiboski CH, Shiboski SC, Silverman S, Jr: Trends in oral cancer rates in the United States, 1973-1996. Community Dent Oral Epidemiol 2000;28(4):249-256.

7. Reid BC, et al: Head and neck in situ carcinoma: Incidence, trends, and survival. Oral Oncol 2000;36(5):414-420.

8. Albright JT, Topham AK, Reilly JS: Pediatric head and neck malignancies: US incidence and trends over 2 decades. Arch Otolaryngol Head Neck Surg 2002;128(6):655-659.

9. Myers JN, et al: Squamous cell carcinoma of the tongue in young adults: Increasing incidence and factors that predict treatment outcomes. Otolaryngol Head Neck Surg 2000;122(1):44-51.

10. Schantz SP, Yu GP, Head and neck cancer incidence trends in young Americans, 1973-1997, with a special analysis for tongue cancer. Arch Otolaryngol Head Neck Surg 2002;128(3):268-274.

11. Fedele DJ et al: Oral/pharyngeal, laryngeal, and lung cancer discharge trends in Department of Veterans Affairs hospitals. J Public Health Dent 1998;58(4):309-312.

12. Warnakulasuriya KA, Robinson D, Evans H. Multiple primary tumors following head and neck cancer in southern England during 1961-98. J Oral Pathol Med 2003;32(8):443-449.

13. IARC Working Group, Lyon, 23-30 October 1986: Tobacco smoking. IARC Monogr Eval Carcinog Risk Chem Hum 1986;38:1-421.

14. IARC Working Group, Lyon, 13-20 October 1987: Alcohol drinking. IARC Monogr Eval Carcinog Risks Hum 1988;44:1-378.

15. Blot WJ, et al: Smoking and drinking in relation to oral and pharyngeal cancer. Cancer Res 1988;48(11):3282-3287.

16. Johnson N: Tobacco use and oral cancer: A global perspective. J Dent Educ 2001;65(4):328-339.

17. Gupta PC, Murti PR, Bhonsle RB: Epidemiology of cancer by tobacco products and the significance of TSNA. Crit Rev Toxicol 1996;26(2):183-198.

18. Lewin F, et al: Smoking tobacco, oral snuff, and alcohol in the etiology of squamous cell carcinoma of the head and neck: A population-based case-referent study in Sweden. Cancer 1998;82(7):1367-1375.

19. Talamini R, et al: Combined effect of tobacco and alcohol on laryngeal cancer risk: A case-control study. Cancer Causes Control 2002;13(10):957-964.

20. Dietz A, Heller WD, Maier H: [Epidemiologic aspects of cancers of the head-neck area]. Offentl Gesundheitswes 1991;53(10):674-680.

21. Tuyns AJ, et al: Cancer of the larynx/hypopharynx, tobacco and alcohol: IARC international case-control study in Turin and Varese (Italy), Zaragoza and Navarra (Spain), Geneva (Switzerland) and Calvados (France). Int J Cancer 1988;41(4):483-491.

22. Jacobs CD: Etiologic considerations for head and neck squamous cancers. Cancer Treat Res 1990;52:265-282.

23. Das BR., Nagpal JK: Understanding the biology of oral cancer. Med Sci Monit 2002;8(11):RA258-267.

24. Hoffmann D, et al: Nicotine-derived N-nitrosamines (TSNAs) and their relevance in tobacco carcinogenesis. Crit Rev Toxicol 1991;21(4):305-311.

25. Baker F, et al: Health risks associated with cigar smoking. JAMA 2000;284(6):735-740.

26. Shapiro JA, Jacobs EJ, Thun MJ: Cigar smoking in men and risk of death from tobacco-related cancers. J Natl Cancer Inst 2000;92(4):333-337.

27. Iribarren C, et al: Effect of cigar smoking on the risk of cardiovascular disease, chronic obstructive pulmonary disease, and cancer in men. N Engl J Med 1999;340(23):1773-1780.

28. Schlecht NF, et al: Effect of smoking cessation and tobacco type on the risk of cancers of the upper aerodigestive tract in Brazil. Epidemiology 1999;10(4):412-418.

29. Garrote LF, et al: Risk factors for cancer of the oral cavity and oropharynx in Cuba. Br J Cancer 2001;85(1):46-54.

30. Franceschi S, et al: Risk factors for cancer of the tongue and the mouth: A case-control study from northern Italy. Cancer 1992;70(9):2227-2233.

31. De Stefani E, Barrios E, Fierro L: Black (air-cured) and blond (flue-cured) tobacco and cancer risk. III: Oesophageal cancer. Eur J Cancer 1993;29A(5):763-766.

32. Strome M, et al: Carcinoma of the tonsil. Head Neck 1993;15(5):465-468.

33. Tan EH, et al: Squamous cell head and neck cancer in nonsmokers. Am J Clin Oncol 1997;20(2):146-150.

34. Zhang ZF, et al: Environmental tobacco smoking, mutagen sensitivity, and head and neck squamous cell carcinoma. Cancer Epidemiol Biomarkers Prev 2000;9(10):1043-1049.

35. Norton SA: Betel: Consumption and consequences. J Am Acad Dermatol 1998;38(1):81-88.

36. Reichart PA: Oral cancer and precancer related to betel and miang chewing in Thailand: A review. J Oral Pathol Med 1995;24(6):241-243.

37. Chen PC, et al: Risk of oral cancer associated with human papillomavirus infection, betel quid chewing, and cigarette smoking in Taiwan: An integrated molecular and epidemiological study of 58 cases. J Oral Pathol Med 2002;31(6):317-322.

38. Thomas S, Wilson A: A quantitative evaluation of the aetiological role of betel quid in oral carcinogenesis. Eur J Cancer B Oral Oncol 1993;29B(4):265-271.

39. Nilsson R: A qualitative and quantitative risk assessment of snuff dipping. Regul Toxicol Pharmacol 1998;28(1):1-16.

40. Schildt EB, et al: Oral snuff, smoking habits and alcohol consumption in relation to oral cancer in a Swedish case-control study. Int J Cancer 1998;77(3):341-346.

41. Winn DM, et al: Snuff dipping and oral cancer among women in the southern United States. N Engl J Med 1981;304(13):745-749.

42. Rodu B, Cole P: Smokeless tobacco use and cancer of the upper respiratory tract. Oral Surg Oral Med Oral Pathol Oral Radiol Endod 2002;93(5):511-515.

43. IARC Working Group, Lyon, 23-30 October 1984: Tobacco habits other than smoking; betel-quid and areca-nut chewing; and some related nitrosamines. IARC Monogr Eval Carcinog Risk Chem Hum 1985;37:1-268.

44. Franceschi S, et al: Comparison of the effect of smoking and alcohol drinking between oral and pharyngeal cancer. Int J Cancer 1999;83(1):1-4.

45. Franceschi S, et al: Cessation of alcohol drinking and risk of cancer of the oral cavity and pharynx. Int J Cancer 2000;85(6):787-790.

46. Talamini R, et al: Cancer of the oral cavity and pharynx in nonsmokers who drink alcohol and in nondrinkers who smoke tobacco. J Natl Cancer Inst 1998;90(24):1901-1903.

47. Schlecht NF, et al: Interaction between tobacco and alcohol consumption and the risk of cancers of the upper aerodigestive tract in Brazil. Am J Epidemiol 1999;150(11):1129-1137.

48. Maier H, et al: Tobacco and alcohol and the risk of head and neck cancer. Clin Investig 1992;70(3-4):320-327.

49. Obe G, Ristow H: Mutagenic, cancerogenic and teratogenic effects of alcohol. Mutat Res 1979;65(4):229-259.

50. Wight AJ, Ogden GR: Possible mechanisms by which alcohol may influence the development of oral cancer: A review. Oral Oncol 1998;34(6):441-4417.

51. Squier CA: The permeability of oral mucosa. Crit Rev Oral Biol Med 1991;2(1):13-32.

52. Maier H, et al: Effect of chronic alcohol consumption on the morphology of the oral mucosa. Alcohol Clin Exp Res 1994;18(2):387-391.

53. Hsu TC, Furlong C, Spitz MR: Ethyl alcohol as a cocarcinogen with special reference to the aerodigestive tract: A cytogenetic study. Anticancer Res 1991;11(3):1097-1101.

54. Blume SB: Women and alcohol: A review. JAMA 1986;256(11):1467-1470.

55. Franceschi S, et al: Alcohol and cancers of the upper aerodigestive tract in men and women. Cancer Epidemiol Biomarkers Prev 1994;3(4):299-304.

56. La Vecchia C, et al: Dietary indicators of laryngeal cancer risk. Cancer Res 1990;50(15):4497-4500.

57. Pelucchi C, et al: Fibre intake and laryngeal cancer risk. Ann Oncol 2003;14(1):162-167.

58. Esteve J, et al: Diet and cancers of the larynx and hypopharynx: The IARC multicenter study in southwestern Europe. Cancer Causes Control 1996;7(2):240-252.

Specific Malignancies

III

59. Kjaerheim K, Gaard M, Andersen A: The role of alcohol, tobacco, and dietary factors in upper aerogastric tract cancers: A prospective study of 10,900 Norwegian men. Cancer Causes Control 1998;9(1):99-108.

60. Negri E, et al: Selected micronutrients and oral and pharyngeal cancer. Int J Cancer 2000;86(1):122-127.

61. Petridou E, et al: The role of diet and specific micronutrients in the etiology of oral carcinoma. Cancer 2002;94(11):2981-2988.

62. Graham S, et al: Dentition, diet, tobacco, and alcohol in the epidemiology of oral cancer. J Natl Cancer Inst 1977;59(6): 1611-1618.

63. Balaram P, et al: Oral cancer in southern India: The influence of smoking, drinking, paan-chewing and oral hygiene. Int J Cancer 2002;98(3):440-445.

64. Homann N, et al: Poor dental status increases acetaldehyde production from ethanol in saliva: A possible link to increased oral cancer risk among heavy drinkers. Oral Oncol 2001;37(2):153-158.

65. Schantz SP, et al: Genetic susceptibility to head and neck cancer: Interaction between nutrition and mutagen sensitivity. Laryngoscope 1997;107(6):765-781.

66. Sturgis EM, Wei Q: Genetic susceptibility: Molecular epidemiology of head and neck cancer. Curr Opin Oncol 2002;14(3):310-317.

67. Cloos J, et al: Genetic susceptibility to head and neck squamous cell carcinoma. J Natl Cancer Inst 1996;88(8):530-535.

68. Forastiere A, et al: Head and neck cancer. N Engl J Med 2001; 345(26):1890-1900.

69. Spitz MR et al: Chromosome sensitivity to bleomycin-induced mutagenesis, an independent risk factor for upper aerodigestive tract cancers. Cancer Res 1989;49(16):4626-4628.

70. Schantz SP, et al: Young adults with head and neck cancer express increased susceptibility to mutagen-induced chromosome damage. JAMA 1989;262(23):3313-3315.

71. van Zuuren EJ, de Visscher JG, Bouwes Bavinck JN: Carcinoma of the lip in kidney transplant recipients. c 1998;38(3):497-499.

72. Harris JP, Penn I: Immunosuppression and the development of malignancies of the upper airway and related structures. Laryngoscope 1981;91(4):520-528.

73. King GN, et al: Increased prevalence of dysplastic and malignant lip lesions in renal-transplant recipients. N Engl J Med 1995; 332(16):1052-1057.

74. Pollard JD, et al: Head and neck cancer in cardiothoracic transplant recipients. Laryngoscope 2000;110(8):1257-1261.

75. Flaitz CM, et al: Intraoral squamous cell carcinoma in human immunodeficiency virus infection: A clinicopathologic study. Oral Surg Oral Med Oral Pathol Oral Radiol Endod 1995;80(1):55-62.

76. Preciado DA, Matas A, Adams GL: Squamous cell carcinoma of the head and neck in solid organ transplant recipients. Head Neck 2002;24(4):319-325.

77. Sugerman PB, Shillitoe EJ: The high risk human papillomaviruses and oral cancer: Evidence for and against a causal relationship. Oral Dis 1997;3(3):130-147.

78. Mork J, et al: Human papillomavirus infection as a risk factor for squamous-cell carcinoma of the head and neck. N Engl J Med 2001;344(15):1125-1131.

79. Lindel K, et al: Human papillomavirus positive squamous cell carcinoma of the oropharynx: A radiosensitive subgroup of head and neck carcinoma. Cancer 2001;92(4):805-813.

80. Sisk EA, et al: Human papillomavirus and p53 mutational status as prognostic factors in head and neck carcinoma. Head Neck 2002;24(9):841-849.

81. Gillison ML, et al: Evidence for a causal association between human papillomavirus and a subset of head and neck cancers. J Natl Cancer Inst 2000;92(9):709-720.

82. Werness BA, Levine AJ, Howley PM: Association of human papillomavirus types 16 and 18 E6 proteins with p53. Science 1990;248(4951):76-79.

83. Munger K, et al: The E6 and E7 genes of the human papillomavirus type 16 together are necessary and sufficient for transformation of primary human keratinocytes. J Virol 1989; 63(10):4417-4421.

84. Neel HB, III, et al: Application of Epstein-Barr virus serology to the diagnosis and staging of North American patients with nasopharyngeal carcinoma. Otolaryngol Head Neck Surg 1983;91(3):255-262.

85. Andersson-Anvret M, et al: Relationship between the Epstein-Barr virus and undifferentiated nasopharyngeal carcinoma: Correlated nucleic acid hybridization and histopathological examination. Int J Cancer 1977;20(4):486-494.

86. Hawkins EP, et al: Nasopharyngeal carcinoma in children—a retrospective review and demonstration of Epstein-Barr viral genomes in tumor cell cytoplasm: A report of the Pediatric Oncology Group. Hum Pathol 1990;21(8):805-810.

87. Pathmanathan R, et al: Clonal proliferations of cells infected with Epstein-Barr virus in preinvasive lesions related to nasopharyngeal carcinoma. N Engl J Med 1995;333(11):693-698.

88. Crissman JD, Zarbo RJ: Dysplasia, in situ carcinoma, and progression to invasive squamous cell carcinoma of the upper aerodigestive tract. Am J Surg Pathol 1989;13(Suppl 1):5-16.

89. Muller E, Beleites E: The basaloid squamous cell carcinoma of the nasopharynx. Rhinology 2000;38(4):208-211.

90. Paulino AF, et al: Basaloid squamous cell carcinoma of the head and neck. Laryngoscope 2000;110(9):1479-1482.

91. Frierson HF, Jr, et al: Sinonasal undifferentiated carcinoma: An aggressive neoplasm derived from schneiderian epithelium and distinct from olfactory neuroblastoma. Am J Surg Pathol 1986;10(11):771-779.

92. Auclair PL, Goode RK, Ellis GL: Mucoepidermoid carcinoma of intraoral salivary glands: Evaluation and application of grading criteria in 143 cases. Cancer 1992;69(8):2021-2030.

93. Batsakis JG, Luna MA: Histopathologic grading of salivary gland neoplasms: I. Mucoepidermoid carcinomas. Ann Otol Rhinol Laryngol 1990;99(10 Pt 1):835-838.

94. Clode AL, et al: Mucoepidermoid carcinoma of the salivary glands: A reappraisal of the influence of tumor differentiation on prognosis. J Surg Oncol 1991;46(2):100-106.

95. Evans HL: Mucoepidermoid carcinoma of salivary glands: A study of 69 cases with special attention to histologic grading. Am J Clin Pathol 1984;81(6):696-701.

96. Moz U, et al: [Mucoepidermoid carcinoma of salivary glands: Histologic grading as prognostic factors.] Acta Otorhinolaryngol Ital 1993;13(6):559-564.

97. Spiro RH, et al: Mucoepidermoid carcinoma of salivary gland origin: A clinicopathologic study of 367 cases. Am J Surg 1978;136(4):461-468.

98. Szanto PA, et al: Histologic grading of adenoid cystic carcinoma of the salivary glands. Cancer 1984;54(6):1062-1069.

99. Henley JD, et al: Dedifferentiated acinic cell carcinoma of the parotid gland: A distinct rarely described entity. Hum Pathol 1997;28(7):869-873.

100. Lewis JE, Olsen KD, Weiland LH: Acinic cell carcinoma: Clinico-pathologic review. Cancer 1991;67(1):172-179.

101. Oliveira P, Fonseca I, Soares J: Acinic cell carcinoma of the salivary glands: A long term follow-up study of 15 cases. Eur J Surg Oncol 1992;18(1):7-15.

102. Ohtake S, et al: Precancerous foci in pleomorphic adenoma of the salivary gland: Recognition of focal carcinoma and atypical tumor cells by P53 immunohistochemistry. J Oral Pathol Med 2002; 31(10):590-597.

103. Lewis JE, Olsen KD, Sebo TJ: Carcinoma ex pleomorphic adenoma: Pathologic analysis of 73 cases. Hum Pathol 2001;32(6): 596-604.

104. Evans HL, Luna MA: Polymorphous low-grade adenocarcinoma: A study of 40 cases with long-term follow-up and an evaluation of the importance of papillary areas. Am J Surg Pathol 2000;24(10): 1319-1328.

105. Simpson RH, et al: Polymorphous low-grade adenocarcinoma of the salivary glands with transformation to high-grade carcinoma. Histopathology 2002;41(3):250-259.

106. Delgado R, Vuitch F, Albores-Saavedra J: Salivary duct carcinoma. Cancer 1993;72(5):1503-1512.

107. Hellquist HB, Karlsson MG, Nilsson C: Salivary duct carcinoma—a highly aggressive salivary gland tumor with overexpression of c-erbB-2. J Pathol 1994;172(1):35-44.

108. Aviles A, et al: Angiocentric T-cell lymphoma of the nose, paranasal sinuses and hard palate. Hematol Oncol 1992;10(3-4):141-147.

109. Aviles A, et al: Angiocentric nasal T/natural killer cell lymphoma: A single centre study of prognostic factors in 108 patients. Clin Lab Haematol 2000;22(4):215-220.

110. Koch M, et al: [Angiocentric T/NK cell lymphoma: A special clinical-pathological entity of lethal midline granuloma. A case report]. Laryngorhinootologie 2001;80(7):410–415.

111. Harrison D: Surgical pathology of olfactory neuroblastoma. Head Neck Surg 1984;7(1):60–64.

112. Argani P, et al: Olfactory neuroblastoma is not related to the Ewing family of tumors: Absence of EWS/FLI1 gene fusion and MIC2 expression. Am J Surg Pathol 1998;22(4):391–398.

113. Unni KK, Dahlin DC: Premalignant tumors and conditions of bone. Am J Surg Pathol 1979;3(1):47–60.

114. Unni KK, Dahlin DC: Osteosarcoma: Pathology and classification. Semin Roentgenol 1989;24(3):143–152.

115. Campbell WM, et al: Nasal and paranasal presentations of chordomas. Laryngoscope 1980;90(4):612–618.

116. Somers KD, et al: Frequent p53 mutations in head and neck cancer. Cancer Res 1992;52(21):5997–6000.

117. Boyle JO, et al: The incidence of p53 mutations increases with progression of head and neck cancer. Cancer Res 1993;53(19):4477–4480.

118. Liggett WH, Jr, et al: p16 and p16 beta are potent growth suppressors of head and neck squamous carcinoma cells in vitro. Cancer Res 1996;56(18):4119–4123.

119. Reed AL, et al: High frequency of p16 (CDKN2/MTS-1/INK4A) inactivation in head and neck squamous cell carcinoma. Cancer Res 1996;56(16):3630–3633.

120. van der Riet P, et al: Frequent loss of chromosome 9p21-22 early in head and neck cancer progression. Cancer Res 1994;54(5):1156–1158.

121. Nawroz H, et al: Allelotype of head and neck squamous cell carcinoma. Cancer Res 1994;54(5):1152–1155.

122. Califano J, et al: Genetic progression model for head and neck cancer: Implications for field cancerization. Cancer Res 1996;56(11):2488–2492.

123. Grandis JR, Tweardy DJ: Elevated levels of transforming growth factor alpha and epidermal growth factor receptor messenger RNA are early markers of carcinogenesis in head and neck cancer. Cancer Res 1993;53(15):3579–3584.

124. Saranath D, et al: Oncogene amplification in squamous cell carcinoma of the oral cavity. Jpn J Cancer Res 1989;80(5):430–437.

125. Jares P, et al: PRAD-1/cyclin D1 gene amplification correlates with messenger RNA overexpression and tumor progression in human laryngeal carcinomas. Cancer Res 1994;54(17):4813–4817.

126. Dyce OH, et al: Integrins in head and neck squamous cell carcinoma invasion. Laryngoscope 2002;112(11):2025–2032.

127. Chow V, et al: A comparative study of the clinicopathological significance of E-cadherin and catenins (alpha, beta, gamma) expression in the surgical management of oral tongue carcinoma. J Cancer Res Clin Oncol 2001;127(1):59–63.

128. Whiteside TL: Immunobiology and immunotherapy of head and neck cancer. Curr Oncol Rep 2001;3(1):46–55.

129. Grandis JR, et al: Human leukocyte antigen class I allelic and haplotype loss in squamous cell carcinoma of the head and neck: Clinical and immunogenetic consequences. Clin Cancer Res 2000;6(7):2794–2802.

130. Sok JC, et al: Tissue-specific gene expression of head and neck squamous cell carcinoma in vivo by complementary DNA microarray analysis. Arch Otolaryngol Head Neck Surg 2003;129(7):760–770.

131. Ha PK, et al: A transcriptional progression model for head and neck cancer. Clin Cancer Res 2003;9(8):3058–3064.

132. Chiesa F, et al: Prognostic factors in head and neck oncology: A critical appraisal for use in clinical practice. Anticancer Res 1998;18(6B):4769–4776.

133. Grandis JR, et al: Levels of TGF-alpha and EGFR protein in head and neck squamous cell carcinoma and patient survival [see comments]. J Natl Cancer Inst 1998;90(11):824–832.

134. Jaulerry C, et al: Prognostic value of tumor regression during radiotherapy for head and neck cancer: A prospective study. Int J Radiat Oncol Biol Phys 1995;33(2):271–279.

135. Adelstein DJ, et al: Mature results of a phase III randomized trial comparing concurrent chemoradiotherapy with radiation therapy alone in patients with stage III and IV squamous cell carcinoma of the head and neck. Cancer 2000;88(4):876–883.

136. Cooper JS, et al: Recursive partitioning analysis of 2105 patients treated in Radiation Therapy Oncology Group studies of head and neck cancer. Cancer 1996;77(9):1905–1911.

137. O'Sullivan B, Shah J: New TNM staging criteria for head and neck tumors. Semin Surg Oncol 2003;21(1):30–42.

138. O-charoenrat P, et al: Tumour thickness predicts cervical nodal metastases and survival in early oral tongue cancer. Oral Oncol 2003;39(4):386–390.

139. Po Wing Yuen A, et al: Prognostic factors of clinically stage I and II oral tongue carcinoma: A comparative study of stage, thickness, shape, growth pattern, invasive front malignancy grading, Martinez-Gimeno score, and pathologic features. Head Neck 2002;24(6):513–520.

140. Xiao GL, Gao L, Xu GZ: Prognostic influence of parapharyngeal space involvement in nasopharyngeal carcinoma. Int J Radiat Oncol Biol Phys 2002;52(4):957–963.

141. Cady B, Rossi R: An expanded view of risk-group definition in differentiated thyroid carcinoma. Surgery 1988;104(6):947–953.

142. Pameijer FA, et al: Can pretreatment computed tomography predict local control in T3 squamous cell carcinoma of the glottic larynx treated with definitive radiotherapy? Int J Radiat Oncol Biol Phys 1997;37(5):1011–1021.

143. Pameijer FA, et al: Evaluation of pretreatment computed tomography as a predictor of local control in T1/T2 pyriform sinus carcinoma treated with definitive radiotherapy. Head Neck 1998;20(2):159–168.

144. Rudat V, et al: Prognostic impact of total tumor volume and hemoglobin concentration on the outcome of patients with advanced head and neck cancer after concomitant boost radiochemotherapy. Radiother Oncol 1999;53(2):119–125.

145. Kawashima M, et al: Local-regional control by conventional radiotherapy according to tumor volume in patients with squamous cell carcinoma of the pharyngolarynx. Jpn J Clin Oncol 1999;29(10):467–473.

146. Doweck I, Denys D, Robbins KT: Tumor volume predicts outcome for advanced head and neck cancer treated with targeted chemoradiotherapy. Laryngoscope 2002;112(10):1742–1749.

147. Canaday DJ, et al: Significance of pretreatment hemoglobin level in patients with T1 glottic cancer. Radiat Oncol Investig 1999;7(1):42–48.

148. Fein DA, et al: Pretreatment hemoglobin level influences local control and survival of T1-T2 squamous cell carcinomas of the glottic larynx. J Clin Oncol 1995;13(8):2077–2083.

149. Grant DG, Hussain A, Hurman D: Pretreatment anaemia alters outcome in early squamous cell carcinoma of the larynx treated by radical radiotherapy. J Laryngol Otol 1999;113(9):829–833.

150. Henke M, et al: Erythropoietin for patients undergoing radiotherapy: A pilot study. Radiother Oncol 1999;50(2):185–190.

151. Lutterbach J, Guttenberger R: Anemia is associated with decreased local control of surgically treated squamous cell carcinomas of the glottic larynx. Int J Radiat Oncol Biol Phys 2000;48(5):1345–1350.

152. Withers HR, Taylor JM, Maciejewski B: The hazard of accelerated tumor clonogen repopulation during radiotherapy. Acta Oncol 1988;27(2):131–146.

153. Withers HR, et al: Local control of carcinoma of the tonsil by radiation therapy: An analysis of patterns of fractionation in nine institutions. Int J Radiat Oncol Biol Phys 1995;33(3):549–562.

154. Nishimura Y, et al: Radiation therapy for T1,2 glottic carcinoma: Impact of overall treatment time on local control. Radiother Oncol 1996;40(3):225–232.

155. Fein DA, et al: Do overall treatment time, field size, and treatment energy influence local control of T1-T2 squamous cell carcinomas of the glottic larynx? Int J Radiat Oncol Biol Phys 1996;34(4):823–831.

156. Le QT, et al: Influence of fraction size, total dose, and overall time on local control of T1-T2 glottic carcinoma. Int J Radiat Oncol Biol Phys 1997;39(1):115–126.

157. Suntharalingam M, et al: Predictors of response and survival after concurrent chemotherapy and radiation for locally advanced squamous cell carcinomas of the head and neck. Cancer 2001;91(3):548–554.

158. Mendenhall WM, et al: T1-T2 squamous cell carcinoma of the glottic larynx treated with radiation therapy: relationship of

dose-fractionation factors to local control and complications. Int J Radiat Oncol Biol Phys 1988;15(6):1267-1273.

159. Kim RY, Marks ME, Salter MM: Early-stage glottic cancer: Importance of dose fractionation in radiation therapy. Radiology 1992;182(1):273-275.

160. Kaanders JHAM, Hordijk GJ: Carcinoma of the larynx: The Dutch national guideline for diagnostics, treatment, supportive care and rehabilitation. Radiother Oncol 2002;63(3):299-307.

161. Ang KK, et al: Randomized trial addressing risk features and time factors of surgery plus radiotherapy in advanced head-and-neck cancer. Int J Radiat Oncol Biol Phys 2001;51(3):571-578.

162. Peters LJ, et al: Evaluation of the dose for postoperative radiation therapy of head and neck cancer: First report of a prospective randomized trial. Int J Radiat Oncol Biol Phys 1993;26(1):3-11.

163. Cooper JS, et al: Precisely defining high-risk operable head and neck tumors based on RTOG #85-03 and #88-24: Targets for postoperative radiochemotherapy? Head Neck 1998;20(7): 588-594.

164. Rosenthal DI, et al: Importance of the treatment package time in surgery and postoperative radiation therapy for squamous carcinoma of the head and neck. Head Neck 2002;24(2):115-126.

165. Muriel VP, Tejada MRG, de Dios Luna del Castillo J: Time-dose-response relationships in postoperatively irradiated patients with head and neck squamous cell carcinomas. Radiother Oncol 2001;60(2):137-145.

166. Quon H, Liu FF, Cummings BJ: Potential molecular prognostic markers in head and neck squamous cell carcinomas. Head Neck 2001;23(2):147-159.

167. Hendrix RA: 31P localized magnetic resonance spectroscopy of head and neck tumors—preliminary findings. Otolaryngol Head Neck Surg 1990;103(5 Pt 1):775-783.

168. Mukherji SK, et al: Proton MR spectroscopy of squamous cell carcinoma of the extracranial head and neck: in vitro and in vivo studies. AJNR Am J Neuroradiol 1997;18(6):1057-1072.

169. Maurizi M, et al: EGF receptor expression in primary laryngeal cancer: Correlation with clinico-pathological features and prognostic significance. Int J Cancer 1992;52(6):862-866.

170. Maurizi M, et al: Prognostic significance of epidermal growth factor receptor in laryngeal squamous cell carcinoma. Br J Cancer 1996;74(8):1253-1257.

171. Dassonville O, et al: Expression of epidermal growth factor receptor and survival in upper aerodigestive tract cancer. J Clin Oncol 1993;11(10):1873-1878.

172. Magne N, et al: The relationship of epidermal growth factor receptor levels to the prognosis of unresectable pharyngeal cancer patients treated by chemo-radiotherapy. Eur J Cancer 2001;37(17):2169-2177.

173. Tufano RP: Organ preservation surgery for laryngeal cancer. Otolaryngol Clin North Am 2002;35(5):1067-1080.

174. Teknos TN, Hogikyan ND, Wolf GT: Conservation laryngeal surgery for malignant tumors of the larynx and pyriform sinus. Hematol Oncol Clin North Am 2001;15(2):261-276.

175. Gourin CG, Johnson JT: Surgical treatment of squamous cell carcinoma of the base of tongue. Head Neck 2001;23(8):653-660.

176. Bartelink H, et al: The value of postoperative radiotherapy as an adjuvant to radical neck dissection. Cancer 1983;52(6):1008-1013.

177. Tupchong L, et al: Randomized study of preoperative versus postoperative radiation therapy in advanced head and neck carcinoma: Long-term follow-up of RTOG study 73-03. Int J Radiat Oncol Biol Phys 1991;20(1):21-28.

178. Calais G, et al: Randomized trial of radiation therapy versus concomitant chemotherapy and radiation therapy for advanced-stage oropharynx carcinoma. J Natl Cancer Inst 1999; 91(24):2081-2086.

179. Fu KK, et al: A radiation therapy oncology group (RTOG) phase III randomized study to compare hyperfractionation and two variants of accelerated fractionation to standard fractionation radiotherapy for head and neck squamous cell carcinomas: First report of RTOG 9003. Int J Radiat Oncol Biol Phys 2000;48(1): 7-16.

180. Harrison LB, et al: Concomitant chemotherapy-radiation therapy followed by hyperfractionated radiation therapy for advanced unresectable head and neck cancer. Int J Radiat Oncol Biol Phys 1991;21(3):703-708.

181. Pignon JP, et al: Chemotherapy added to locoregional treatment for head and neck squamous-cell carcinoma: Three meta-analyses of updated individual data. Lancet 2000;355(9208):949-955.

182. Wanebo H, et al: Surgical resection is necessary to maximize tumor control in function-preserving, aggressive chemoradiation protocols for advanced squamous cancer of the head and neck (stage III and IV). Ann Surg Oncol 2001;8(8):644-650.

183. Nguyen LN, Ang KK: Radiotherapy for cancer of the head and neck: Altered fractionation regimens. Lancet Oncol 2002;3(11): 693-701.

184. Forastiere AA, Trotti A: Radiotherapy and concurrent chemotherapy: A strategy that improves locoregional control and survival in oropharyngeal cancer. J Natl Cancer Inst 1999;91(24): 2065-2066.

185. Weber RS, et al: Outcome of salvage total laryngectomy following organ preservation therapy: The Radiation Therapy Oncology Group trial 91-11. Arch Otolaryngol Head Neck Surg 2003;129(1):44-49.

186. Wolf GT: Commentary: Phase III trial to preserve the larynx: Induction chemotherapy and radiotherapy versus concurrent chemotherapy and radiotherapy versus radiotherapy—Intergroup trial R91-11. J Clin Oncol 2001;19(18 Suppl):28s-31s.

187. Machtay M, et al: Organ preservation therapy using induction plus concurrent chemoradiation for advanced resectable oropharyngeal carcinoma: A University of Pennsylvania phase II trial. J Clin Oncol 2002;20(19):3964-3971.

188. List MA, et al: How do head and neck cancer patients prioritize treatment outcomes before initiating treatment? J Clin Oncol 2000;18(4):877-884.

189. Million RR: The myth regarding bone or cartilage involvement by cancer and the likelihood of cure by radiotherapy. Head Neck 1989;11(1):30-40.

190. Samant S, et al: Bone or cartilage invasion by advanced head and neck cancer: Intra-arterial supradose cisplatin chemotherapy and concomitant radiotherapy for organ preservation. Arch Otolaryngol Head Neck Surg 2001;127(12):1451-1456.

191. Parsons JT, et al: T4 laryngeal carcinoma: Radiotherapy alone with surgery reserved for salvage. Int J Radiat Oncol Biol Phys 1998;40(3):549-552.

192. Lefebvre JL, et al: Larynx preservation in pyriform sinus cancer: Preliminary results of a European Organization for Research and Treatment of Cancer phase III trial. EORTC Head and Neck Cancer Cooperative Group. Natl Cancer Inst 1996;88(13): 890-899.

193. Department of Veterans Affairs Laryngeal Cancer Study Group: Induction chemotherapy plus radiation compared with surgery plus radiation in patients with advanced laryngeal cancer. N Engl J Med 1991;324(24):1685-1690.

194. McLaughlin MP, et al: Salvage surgery after radiotherapy failure in T1-T2 squamous cell carcinoma of the glottic larynx. Head Neck 1996;18(3):229-235.

195. Rodriguez-Cuevas S, et al: Partial laryngectomy as salvage surgery for radiation failures in T1-T2 laryngeal cancer. Head Neck 1998;20(7):630-633.

196. Harwood AR, et al: Management of early supraglottic laryngeal carcinoma by irradiation with surgery in reserve. Arch Otolaryngol 1983;109(9):583-585.

197. Croll GA, et al: Primary radiotherapy with surgery in reserve for advanced laryngeal carcinoma: Results and complications. Eur J Surg Oncol 1989;15(4):350-356.

198. Maor MH, et al: Larynx preservation and tumor control in stage III and IV laryngeal cancer: a three-arm randomized intergroup trial; RTOG 91-11. Int J Radiat Oncol Biol Phys 2002;54(1):2-3.

199. Eisbruch A, et al: Objective assessment of swallowing dysfunction and aspiration after radiation concurrent with chemotherapy for head-and-neck cancer. Int J Radiat Oncol Biol Phys 2002;53(1): 23-28.

200. Nguyen NP, et al: Combined chemotherapy and radiation therapy for head and neck malignancies: Quality of life issues. Cancer 2002;94(4):1131-1141.

201. Byers RM, et al: Resection of advanced cervical metastasis prior to definitive radiotherapy for primary squamous carcinomas of the upper aerodigestive tract. Head Neck 1992; 14(2):133-138.

202. Bataini JP, et al: Impact of neck node radioresponsiveness on the regional control probability in patients with oropharynx and pharyngolarynx cancers managed by definitive radiotherapy. Int J Radiat Oncol Biol Phys 1987;13(6):817–824.

203. Dubray BM, et al: Is reseeding from the primary a plausible cause of node failure? Int J Radiat Oncol Biol Phys 1993;25(1):9–15.

204. Corry J, Smith JG, Peters LJ: The concept of a planned neck dissection is obsolete. Cancer J 2001;7(6):472–474.

205. Mendenhall WM, et al: Planned neck dissection after definitive radiotherapy for squamous cell carcinoma of the head and neck. Head Neck 2002;24(11):1012–1018.

206. Lee HJ, et al: Long-term regional control after radiation therapy and neck dissection for base of tongue carcinoma. Int J Radiat Oncol Biol Phys 1997;38(5):995–1000.

207. Barkley HT, Jr, et al: Management of cervical lymph node metastases in squamous cell carcinoma of the tonsillar fossa, base of tongue, supraglottic larynx, and hypopharynx. Am J Surg 1972;124(4):462–467.

208. Mendenhall WM, et al: Radiation therapy for squamous cell carcinoma of the tonsillar region: A preferred alternative to surgery? J Clin Oncol 2000;18(11):2219–2225.

209. Taylor JM, et al: The influence of dose and time on wound complications following postradiation neck dissection. Int J Radiat Oncol Biol Phys 1992;23(1):41–46.

210. Mabanta SR, et al: Salvage treatment for neck recurrence after irradiation alone for head and neck squamous cell carcinoma with clinically positive neck nodes. Head Neck 1999;21(7):591–594.

211. McHam SA, et al: Who merits a neck dissection after definitive chemoradiotherapy for N2-N3 squamous cell head and neck cancer? Head Neck 2003;25(10):791–798.

212. Brizel DM, et al: Hyperfractionated irradiation with or without concurrent chemotherapy for locally advanced head and neck cancer. N Engl J Med 1998;338(25):1798–1804.

213. Schechter NR, et al: Can positron emission tomography improve the quality of care for head-and-neck cancer patients? Int J Radiat Oncol Biol Phys 2001;51(1):4–9.

214. Greven KM, et al: Serial positron emission tomography scans following radiation therapy of patients with head and neck cancer. Head Neck 2001;23(11):942–946.

215. Stenson KM, et al: The role of cervical lymphadenectomy after aggressive concomitant chemoradiotherapy: The feasibility of selective neck dissection. Arch Otolaryngol Head Neck Surg 2000;126(8):950–956.

216. Lavertu P, et al: Comparison of surgical complications after organ-preservation therapy in patients with stage III or IV squamous cell head and neck cancer. Arch Otolaryngol Head Neck Surg 1998;124(4):401–406.

217. Newman JP, et al: Surgical morbidity of neck dissection after chemoradiotherapy in advanced head and neck cancer. Ann Otol Rhinol Laryngol 1997;106(2):117–122.

218. Kao J, et al: Reirradiation of recurrent and second primary head and neck malignancies: A comprehensive review. Cancer Treat Rev 2003;29(1):21–30.

219. Bocca E, et al: Functional neck dissection: An evaluation and review of 843 cases. Laryngoscope 1984;94(7):942–945.

220. Muzaffar K: Therapeutic selective neck dissection: A 25-year review. Laryngoscope 2003;113(9):1460–1465.

221. Shah JP: Patterns of cervical lymph node metastasis from squamous carcinomas of the upper aerodigestive tract. Am J Surg 1990;160(4):405–409.

222. Ferlito A, Rinaldo A: Selective lateral neck dissection for laryngeal cancer with limited metastatic disease: Is it indicated? J Laryngol Otol 1998;112(11):1031–1033.

223. Gregoire V, et al: Selection and delineation of lymph node target volumes in head and neck conformal radiotherapy. Proposal for standardizing terminology and procedure based on the surgical experience. Radiother Oncol 2000;56(2):135–150.

224. Horiot JC, et al: Hyperfractionation versus conventional fractionation in oropharyngeal carcinoma: Final analysis of a randomized trial of the EORTC cooperative group of radiotherapy. Radiother Oncol 1992;25(4):231–241.

225. Pinto LH, et al: Prospective randomized trial comparing hyperfractionated versus conventional radiotherapy in stages III

226. Cummings B, O'Sullivan B, Keane T: 5-year results of a 4 week/ twice daily radiation schedule. Radiother Oncol 2000;56:S8.

227. Fu KK, et al: Late effects of hyperfractionated radiotherapy for advanced head and neck cancer: Long-term follow-up results of RTOG 83-13. Int J Radiat Oncol Biol Phys 1995;32(3):577–588.

228. Garden AS, et al: Hyperfractionated radiation in the treatment of squamous cell carcinomas of the head and neck: A comparison of two fractionation schedules. Int J Radiat Oncol Biol Phys 1995;31(3):493–502.

229. Jackson SM, et al: A randomised trial of accelerated versus conventional radiotherapy in head and neck cancer. Radiother Oncol 1997;43(1):39–46.

230. Skladowski K, et al: Randomized clinical trial on 7-day-continuous accelerated irradiation (CAIR) of head and neck cancer: Report on 3-year tumor control and normal tissue toxicity. Radiother Oncol 2000;55(2):101–110.

231. Hliniak A, et al: A multicentre randomized/controlled trial of a conventional versus modestly accelerated radiotherapy in the laryngeal cancer: Influence of a 1 week shortening overall time. Radiother Oncol 2002;62(1):1–10.

232. Overgaard J, et al: Five compared with six fractions per week of conventional radiotherapy of squamous-cell carcinoma of head and neck: DAHANCA 6 and 7 randomised controlled trial. Lancet 2003;362(9388):933–940.

233. Dische S, et al: A randomised multicentre trial of CHART versus conventional radiotherapy in head and neck cancer. Radiother Oncol 1997;44(2):123–136.

234. Poulsen MG, et al: A randomised trial of accelerated and conventional radiotherapy for stage III and IV squamous carcinoma of the head and neck: A Trans-Tasman Radiation Oncology Group Study. Radiother Oncol 2001;60(2):113–122.

235. Bourhis J, et al: Very accelerated versus conventional radiotherapy in HNSCC: Results of the GORTEC 94-02 randomized trial. Int J Radiat Oncol Biol Phys 2000;48(1):111.

236. Horiot JC, et al: Accelerated fractionation (AF) compared to conventional fractionation (CF) improves loco-regional control in the radiotherapy of advanced head and neck cancers: Results of the EORTC 22851 randomized trial. Radiother Oncol 1997;44(2):111–121.

237. Overgaard J, Hansen HS, Garau C: The DAHANCA 6 & 7 trial: A randomized multicenter study of 5 versus 6 fractions per week of conventional radiotherapy of squamous cell carcinoma (SCC) of the head and neck. Radiother Oncol 2000;56(Suppl):S4.

238. Skladowski K, et al: Randomized clinical trial on 7-day-continuous accelerated irradiation (CAIR) of head and neck cancer: Report on 3-year tumor control and normal tissue toxicity. Radiother Oncol 2000;55(2):101–110.

239. Ang KK, et al: Concomitant boost radiotherapy schedules in the treatment of carcinoma of the oropharynx and nasopharynx. Int J Radiat Oncol Biol Phys 1990;19(6):1339–1345.

240. Maciejewski B, et al: Randomized clinical trial on accelerated 7 days per week fractionation in radiotherapy for head and neck cancer: Preliminary report on acute toxicity. Radiother Oncol 1996;40(2):137–145.

241. Staar S, et al: Intensified hyperfractionated accelerated radiotherapy limits the additional benefit of simultaneous chemotherapy—results of a multicentric randomized German trial in advanced head-and-neck cancer. Int J Radiat Oncol Biol Phys 2001;50(5):1161–1171.

242. Utley JF, Marlowe C, Waddell WJ: Distribution of 35S-labeled WR-2721 in normal and malignant tissues of the mouse 1,2. Radiat Res, 1976;68(2):284–291.

243. Rasey JS, et al: Biodistribution of the radioprotective drug 35S-labeled 3-amino-2-hydroxypropyl phosphorothioate (WR77913). Radiat Res 1985;102(1):130–137.

244. Kemp G, et al: Amifostine pretreatment for protection against cyclophosphamide-induced and cisplatin-induced toxicities: Results of a randomized control trial in patients with advanced ovarian cancer. J Clin Oncol 1996;14(7):2101–2112.

245. McDonald S, et al: Preliminary results of a pilot study using WR-2721 before fractionated irradiation of the head and neck to

reduce salivary gland dysfunction. Int J Radiat Oncol Biol Phys 1994;29(4):747–754.

246. Buntzel J, et al: Selective cytoprotection with amifostine in concurrent radiochemotherapy for head and neck cancer. Ann Oncol 1998;9(5):505–509.

247. Brizel DM, et al: Phase III randomized trial of amifostine as a radioprotector in head and neck cancer. J Clin Oncol 2000;18(19): 3339–3345.

248. Bardet E, et al: Preliminary data of the GORTEC 2000-02 phase III trial comparing intravenous and subcutaneous administration of amifostine for head and neck tumors treated by external radiotherapy. Semin Oncol 2002;29(6 Suppl 19):57–60.

249. Bourhis J, Rosine D: Radioprotective effect of amifostine in patients with head and neck squamous cell carcinoma. Semin Oncol 2002;29(6 Suppl 19):61–62.

250. Chao KSC, et al: A novel approach to overcome hypoxic tumor resistance: Cu-ATSM-guided intensity-modulated radiation therapy. Int J Radiat Oncol Biol Phys 2001;49(4):1171–1182.

251. Koch CJ, Evans SM: Noninvasive PET and SPECT imaging of tissue hypoxia using isotopically labeled 2-nitroimidazoles. Adv Exp Med Biol 2003;510:285–292.

252. Chao KSC, et al: Intensity-modulated radiation therapy reduces late salivary toxicity without compromising tumor control in patients with oropharyngeal carcinoma: A comparison with conventional techniques. Radiother Oncol 2001;61(3):275–280.

253. Chao KSC, et al: A prospective study of salivary function sparing in patients with head-and-neck cancers receiving intensity-modulated or three-dimensional radiation therapy: Initial results. Int J Radiat Oncol Biol Phys 2001;49(4):907–916.

254. Dawson LA, et al: Patterns of local-regional recurrence following parotid-sparing conformal and segmental intensity-modulated radiotherapy for head and neck cancer. Int J Radiat Oncol Biol Phys 2000;46(5):1117–1126.

255. Lee N, et al: Intensity-modulated radiotherapy in the treatment of nasopharyngeal carcinoma: An update of the UCSF experience. Int J Radiat Oncol Biol Phys 2002;53(1):12–22.

256. Lin A, et al: Quality of life after parotid-sparing IMRT for head-and-neck cancer: A prospective longitudinal study. Int J Radiat Oncol Biol Phys 2003;57(1):61–70.

257. Chao KSC, et al: Patterns of failure in patients receiving definitive and postoperative IMRT for head-and-neck cancer. Int J Radiat Oncol Biol Phys 2003;55(2):312–321.

258. Lee N, et al: Skin toxicity due to intensity-modulated radiotherapy for head-and-neck carcinoma. Int J Radiat Oncol Biol Phys 2002;53(3):630–637.

259. Glatstein E: Intensity-modulated radiation therapy: The inverse, the converse, and the perverse. Semin Radiat Oncol 2002;12(3): 272–281.

260. Trotti A, et al: Postoperative accelerated radiotherapy in high-risk squamous cell carcinoma of the head and neck: Long-term results of a prospective trial. Head Neck 1998;20(2):119–123.

261. Bachaud JM, et al: Combined postoperative radiotherapy and weekly cisplatin infusion for locally advanced head and neck carcinoma: Final report of a randomized trial. Int J Radiat Oncol Biol Phys 1996;36(5):999–1004.

262. Cooper JS, et al: Patterns of failure for resected advanced head and neck cancer treated by concurrent chemotherapy and radiation therapy: an analysis of RTOG 9501/intergroup phase III trial. Int J Radiat Oncol Biol Phys 2002;54(1):2.

263. Lapeyre M, et al: Postoperative brachytherapy: A prognostic factor for local control in epidermoid carcinomas of the mouth floor. Eur J Surg Oncol 1997;23(3):243–246.

264. Chao KS, et al: The impact of surgical margin status and use of an interstitial implant on T1, T2 oral tongue cancers after surgery. Int J Radiat Oncol Biol Phys 1996;36(5):1039–1043.

265. Pernot M, et al: Indications, techniques and results of post-operative brachytherapy in cancer of the oral cavity. Radiother Oncol 1995;35(3):186–192.

266. Beitler JJ, et al: Close or positive margins after surgical resection for the head and neck cancer patient: The addition of brachytherapy improves local control. Int J Radiat Oncol Biol Phys 1998;40(2):313–317.

267. Vikram B, Mishra S: Permanent iodine-125 implants in postoperative radiotherapy for head and neck cancer with positive surgical margins. Head Neck 1994;16(2):155–157.

268. Mazeron JJ, et al: How to optimize therapeutic ratio in brachytherapy of head and neck squamous cell carcinoma? Acta Oncol 1998;37(6):583–591.

269. Quon H, Harrison LB: Brachytherapy in the treatment of head and neck cancer. Oncology (Huntingt) 2002;16(10):1379–1393; discussion 1393, 1395–1396.

270. Pierquin B, Marinello G: A Practical Manual of Brachytherapy. Madison, Wisconsin, Medical Physics, 1997.

271. Mazeron JJ, et al: Place of Iridium 192 implantation in definitive irradiation of faucial arch squamous cell carcinomas. Int J Radiat Oncol Biol Phys 1993;27(2):251–257.

272. Pernot M, et al: Velotonsillar squamous cell carcinoma: 277 cases treated by combined external irradiation and brachytherapy—results according to extension, localization, and dose rate. Int J Radiat Oncol Biol Phys 1992;23(4):715–723.

273. Hoffstetter S, et al: Treatment duration as a prognostic factor for local control and survival in epidermoid carcinomas of the tonsillar region treated by combined external beam irradiation and brachytherapy. Radiother Oncol 1997;45(2):141–148.

274. Esche BA, et al: Interstitial and external radiotherapy in carcinoma of the soft palate and uvula. Int J Radiat Oncol Biol Phys 1988;15(3):619–625.

275. Leborgne JH, et al: The place of brachytherapy in the treatment of carcinoma of the tonsil with lingual extension. Int J Radiat Oncol Biol Phys 1986;12(10):1787–1792.

276. Puthawala AA, Syed AM, Gates TC: Iridium-192 implants in the treatment of tonsillar region malignancies. Arch Otolaryngol 1985;111(12):812–815.

277. Decroix Y, Ghossein NA: Experience of the Curie Institute in treatment of cancer of the mobile tongue: II. Management of the neck nodes. Cancer 1981;47(3):503–508.

278. Decroix Y, Ghossein NA: Experience of the Curie Institute in treatment of cancer of the mobile tongue: I. Treatment policies and result. Cancer 1981;47(3):496–502.

279. Mazeron JJ, et al: Prognostic factors of local outcome for T1, T2 carcinomas of oral tongue treated by iridium 192 implantation. Int J Radiat Oncol Biol Phys 1990;19(2):281–285.

280. Pernot M, et al: The study of tumoral, radiobiological, and general health factors that influence results and complications in a series of 448 oral tongue carcinomas treated exclusively by irradiation. Int J Radiat Oncol Biol Phys 1994;29(4):673–679.

281. Harrison LB, et al: Long term results of primary radiotherapy with/without neck dissection for squamous cell cancer of the base of tongue. Head Neck 1998;20(8):668–673.

282. Lusinchi A, et al: External irradiation plus curietherapy boost in 108 base of tongue carcinomas. Int J Radiat Oncol Biol Phys 1989;17(6):1191–1197.

283. Horwitz EM, et al: The impact of temporary iodine-125 interstitial implant boost in the primary management of squamous cell carcinoma of the oropharynx. Head Neck 1997;19(3):219–226.

284. Regueiro CA, et al: Influence of boost technique (external beam radiotherapy or brachytherapy) on the outcome of patients with carcinoma of the base of the tongue. Acta Oncol 1995;34(2): 225–233.

285. Crook J, et al: Combined external irradiation and interstitial implantation for T1 and T2 epidermoid carcinomas of base of tongue: The Creteil experience (1971–1981). Int J Radiat Oncol Biol Phys 1988;15(1):105–114.

286. Goffinet DR, et al: 192-Ir pharyngoepiglottic fold interstitial implants: The key to successful treatment of base tongue carcinoma by radiation therapy. Cancer 1985;55(5):941–948.

287. Housset M, et al: A retrospective study of three treatment techniques for T1-T2 base of tongue lesions: Surgery plus postoperative radiation, external radiation plus interstitial implantation and external radiation alone. Int J Radiat Oncol Biol Phys 1987;13(4):511–516.

288. Puthawala AA, et al: Limited external beam and interstitial 192-iridium irradiation in the treatment of carcinoma of the base of the tongue: A ten year experience. Int J Radiat Oncol Biol Phys 1988;14(5):839–848.

289. Jorgensen K, Elbrond O, Andersen AP: Carcinoma of the lip: A series of 869 cases. Acta Radiol Ther Phys Biol 1973;12(3): 177–190.

290. Beauvois S, et al: Brachytherapy for lower lip epidermoid cancer: Tumoral and treatment factors influencing recurrences and complications. Radiother Oncol 1994;33(3):195-203.

291. Harrison LB, et al: Detailed quality of life assessment in patients treated with primary radiotherapy for squamous cell cancer of the base of the tongue. Head Neck 1997;19(3):169-175.

292. Horwitz EM, et al: Excellent functional outcome in patients with squamous cell carcinoma of the base of tongue treated with external irradiation and interstitial iodine 125 boost. Cancer 1996;78(5):948-957.

293. Housset M, et al: Split course interstitial brachytherapy with a source shift: The results of a new iridium implant technique versus single course implants for salvage irradiation of base of tongue cancers in 55 patients. Int J Radiat Oncol Biol Phys 1991;20(5):965-971.

294. Langlois D, Hoffstetter S, Pernot M: Selection of patients for reirradiation with local implants in carcinomas of oropharynx and tongue. Acta Oncol 1988;27(5):571-573.

295. Peiffert D, et al: Salvage irradiation by brachytherapy of velotonsillar squamous cell carcinoma in a previously irradiated field: Results in 73 cases. Int J Radiat Oncol Biol Phys 1994;29(4):681-686.

296. Lau HY, et al: Seven fractions of twice daily high-dose-rate brachytherapy for node-negative carcinoma of the mobile tongue results in loss of therapeutic ratio. Radiother Oncol 1996;39(1):15-18.

297. Levendag PC, et al: Fractionated high-dose-rate and pulsed-dose-rate brachytherapy: First clinical experience in squamous cell carcinoma of the tonsillar fossa and soft palate. Int J Radiat Oncol Biol Phys 1997;38(3):497-506.

298. Peiffert D, et al: Pulsed dose rate brachytherapy in head and neck cancers: Feasibility study of a French cooperative group. Radiother Oncol 2001;58(1):71-75.

299. Nag S, et al: Pilot study of intraoperative high dose rate brachytherapy for head and neck cancer. Radiother Oncol 1996;41(2):125-130.

300. Domenge C, et al: Randomized trial of neoadjuvant chemotherapy in oropharyngeal carcinoma. French Groupe d'Etude des Tumeurs de la Tete et du Cou (GETTEC). Br J Cancer 2000;83(12):1594-1598.

301. Kies MS, et al: Induction chemotherapy followed by concurrent chemoradiation for advanced head and neck cancer: Improved disease control and survival. J Clin Oncol, 1998;16(8):2715-2721.

302. Cognetti F, et al: Prognostic factors for chemotherapy response and survival using combination chemotherapy as initial treatment of advanced head and neck squamous cell cancer. J Clin Oncol 1989;7(7):829-837.

303. Wolf GT, Makuch RW, Baker SR: Predictive factors for tumor response to preoperative chemotherapy in patients with head and neck squamous carcinoma. The Head and Neck Contracts Program. Cancer 1984;54(12):2869-2877.

304. Wittes R, et al: cis-Dichlorodiammineplatinum(II)-based chemotherapy as initial treatment of advanced head and neck cancer. Cancer Treat Rep 1979;63(9-10):1533-1538.

305. Shapshay SM, et al: Prognostic indicators in induction cis-platinum bleomycin chemotherapy for advanced head and neck cancer. Am J Surg 1980;140(4):543-548.

306. Rooney M, et al: Improved complete response rate and survival in advanced head and neck cancer after three-course induction therapy with 120-hour 5FU infusion and cisplatin. Cancer 1985;55(5):1123-1128.

307. Weaver A, et al: Superior clinical response and survival rates with initial bolus of cisplatin and 120 hour infusion of 5-fluorouracil before definitive therapy for locally advanced head and neck cancer. Am J Surg 1984;148(4):525-529.

308. Crissman JD, et al: Improved response and survival to combined cisplatin and radiation in non-keratinizing squamous cell carcinomas of the head and neck: An RTOG study of 114 advanced stage tumors. Cancer 1987;59(8):1391-1397.

309. Tapazoglou E, et al: The activity of a single-agent 5-fluorouracil infusion in advanced and recurrent head and neck cancer. Cancer 1986;57(6):1105-1109.

310. Al-Sarraf M: Clinical trials with fluorinated pyrimidines in patients with head and neck cancer. Invest New Drugs 1989;7(1):71-81.

311. Ensley JF, et al: Correlation between response to cisplatinum-combination chemotherapy and subsequent radiotherapy in previously untreated patients with advanced squamous cell cancers of the head and neck. Cancer 1984;54(5):811-814.

312. Kish JA, et al: Evaluation of high-dose cisplatin and 5FU infusion as initial therapy in advanced head and neck cancer. Am J Clin Oncol 1988;11(5):553-557.

313. Eisenberger M, et al: Carboplatin (NSC-241-240): An active platinum analog for the treatment of squamous-cell carcinoma of the head and neck. J Clin Oncol 1986;4(10):1506-1509.

314. Urba SG, et al: Intensive induction chemotherapy and radiation for organ preservation in patients with advanced resectable head and neck carcinoma. J Clin Oncol 1994;12(5):946-953.

315. Giralt JL, et al: Preoperative induction chemotherapy followed by concurrent chemoradiotherapy in advanced carcinoma of the oral cavity and oropharynx. Cancer 2000;89(5):939-945.

316. Mantovani G, et al: Induction chemotherapy followed by concomitant chemoradiation therapy in advanced head and neck cancer: A phase II study for organ-sparing purposes evaluating feasibility, effectiveness and toxicity. Int J Oncol 2002;20(2):419-427.

317. Mantz CA, et al: Induction chemotherapy followed by concomitant chemoradiotherapy in the treatment of locoregionally advanced oropharyngeal cancer. Cancer J 2001;7(2):140-148.

318. Papadimitrakopoulou VA, et al: Cisplatin, fluorouracil, and L-leucovorin induction chemotherapy for locally advanced head and neck cancer: The MD Anderson Cancer Center experience. Cancer J Sci Am 1997;3(2):92-99.

319. Browman GP, et al: Choosing a concomitant chemotherapy and radiotherapy regimen for squamous cell head and neck cancer: A systematic review of the published literature with subgroup analysis. Head Neck 2001;23(7):579-589.

320. El-Sayed S, Nelson N: Adjuvant and adjunctive chemotherapy in the management of squamous cell carcinoma of the head and neck region. A meta-analysis of prospective and randomized trials. J Clin Oncol 1996;14(3):838-847.

321. Munro AJ: An overview of randomised controlled trials of adjuvant chemotherapy in head and neck cancer. Br J Cancer 1995;71(1):83-91.

322. Olmi P, et al: Locoregionally advanced carcinoma of the oropharynx: Conventional radiotherapy vs. accelerated hyperfractionated radiotherapy vs. concomitant radiotherapy and chemotherapy—a multicenter randomized trial. Int J Radiat Oncol Biol Phys 2003;55(1):78-92.

323. Wendt TG, et al: Simultaneous radiochemotherapy versus radiotherapy alone in advanced head and neck cancer: A randomized multicenter study. J Clin Oncol 1998;16(4):1318-1324.

324. Jeremic B, et al: Hyperfractionated radiation therapy with or without concurrent low-dose daily cisplatin in locally advanced squamous cell carcinoma of the head and neck: A prospective randomized trial. J Clin Oncol 2000;18(7):1458-1464.

325. Dobrowsky W, Naude J: Continuous hyperfractionated accelerated radiotherapy with/without mitomycin C in head and neck cancers. Radiother Oncol 2000;57(2):119-124.

326. Bourhis J, et al: Preliminary results of the GORTEC 96-01 randomized trial, comparing very accelerated radiotherapy versus concomitant radio-chemotherapy for locally inoperable HNSCC. Int J Radiat Oncol Biol Phys 2001;51(1):39.

327. Bitter K: Postoperative chemotherapy versus postoperative cobalt 60 radiation in patients with advanced oral carcinoma: Report on a randomized study. Head Neck Surg 1981;3(abstract):264.

328. Szpirglas H, Chastang C, Bertrand JC: Adjuvant treatment of tongue and floor of the mouth cancers. Recent Results Cancer Res 1978;68:309-317.

329. Recchia F, et al: Ifosfamide, cisplatin, and 13-Cis retinoic acid for patients with advanced or recurrent squamous cell carcinoma of the head and neck: A phase I-II study. Cancer 2001;92(4):814-21.

330. Buntzel J, Kuttner K: Chemoprevention with interferon alfa and 13-cis retinoic acid in the adjunctive treatment of head and neck cancer. Auris Nasus Larynx 1998;25(4):413-418.

331. Shin DM, et al: Combined interferon-alfa, 13-cis-retinoic acid, and alpha-tocopherol in locally advanced head and neck squamous

cell carcinoma: Novel bioadjuvant phase II trial. J Clin Oncol 2001;19(12):3010-3017.

332. Giovannucci E, et al: Aspirin and the risk of colorectal cancer in women. N Engl J Med 1995;333(10):609-614.

333. Giovannucci E, et al: Relationship of diet to risk of colorectal adenoma in men. J Natl Cancer Inst 1992;84(2):91-98.

334. Thun MJ, Namboodiri MM, Heath CW, Jr: Aspirin use and reduced risk of fatal colon cancer. N Engl J Med 1991;325(23):1593-1596.

335. Thun MJ, et al: Aspirin use and risk of fatal cancer. Cancer Res 1993;53(6):1322-1327.

336. Paganini-Hill A, et al: Aspirin use and chronic diseases: A cohort study of the elderly. BMJ 1989;299(6710):1247-1250.

337. Kargman SL, et al: Expression of prostaglandin G/H synthase-1 and -2 protein in human colon cancer. Cancer Res 1995;55(12):2556-2559.

338. DuBois RN, et al: Increased cyclooxygenase-2 levels in carcinogen-induced rat colonic tumors. Gastroenterology 1996;110(4):1259-1262.

339. Lin DT, et al: Cyclooxygenase-2: A novel molecular target for the prevention and treatment of head and neck cancer. Head Neck 2002;24(8):792-799.

340. Carpenter G: Receptors for epidermal growth factor and other polypeptide mitogens. Annu Rev Biochem 1987;56:881-914.

341. Carpenter G, Cohen S: Epidermal growth factor. J Biol Chem 1990;265(14):7709-7712.

342. Harari PM, Huang SM: Modulation of molecular targets to enhance radiation. Clin Cancer Res 2000;6(2):323-325.

343. Schlessinger J: The epidermal growth factor receptor as a multifunctional allosteric protein. Biochemistry 1988;27(9):3119-3123.

344. Thompson DM, Gill GN: The EGF receptor: Structure, regulation and potential role in malignancy. Cancer Surv 1985;4(4):767-788.

345. Shin DM, et al: Dysregulation of epidermal growth factor receptor expression in premalignant lesions during head and neck tumorigenesis. Cancer Res 1994;54(12):3153-3159.

346. Baselga J, et al: Antitumor effects of doxorubicin in combination with anti-epidermal growth factor receptor monoclonal antibodies. J Natl Cancer Inst 1993;85(16):1327-1333.

347. Huang SM, Bock JM, Harari PM: Epidermal growth factor receptor blockade with C225 modulates proliferation, apoptosis, and radiosensitivity in squamous cell carcinomas of the head and neck. Cancer Res 1999;59(8):1935-1940.

348. Huang SM, Harari PM: Modulation of radiation response after epidermal growth factor receptor blockade in squamous cell carcinomas: Inhibition of damage repair, cell cycle kinetics, and tumor angiogenesis. Clin Cancer Res 2000;6(6):2166-2174.

349. Peter RU, et al: Increased expression of the epidermal growth factor receptor in human epidermal keratinocytes after exposure to ionizing radiation. Radiat Res 1993;136(1):65-70.

350. Dent P, et al: Radiation-induced release of transforming growth factor alpha activates the epidermal growth factor receptor and mitogen-activated protein kinase pathway in carcinoma cells, leading to increased proliferation and protection from radiation-induced cell death. Mol Biol Cell 1999;10(8):2493-2506.

351. Schmidt-Ullrich RK, et al: Radiation-induced autophosphorylation of epidermal growth factor receptor in human malignant mammary and squamous epithelial cells. Radiat Res 1996;145(1):81-85.

352. Schmidt-Ullrich RK, et al: Radiation-induced proliferation of the human A431 squamous carcinoma cells is dependent on EGFR tyrosine phosphorylation. Oncogene 1997;15(10):1191-1197.

353. Todd DG, et al: Ionizing radiation stimulates existing signal transduction pathways involving the activation of epidermal growth factor receptor and ERBB-3, and changes of intracellular calcium in A431 human squamous carcinoma cells. J Recept Signal Transduct Res 1999;19(6):885-908.

354. Balaban N, et al: The effect of ionizing radiation on signal transduction:antibodies to EGF receptor sensitize A431 cells to radiation. Biochim Biophys Acta 1996;1314(1-2):147-156.

355. Baselga J, et al: Phase I studies of anti-epidermal growth factor receptor chimeric antibody C225 alone and in combination with cisplatin. J Clin Oncol 2000;18(4):904-914.

356. Shin DM, et al: Epidermal growth factor receptor-targeted therapy with C225 and cisplatin in patients with head and neck cancer. Clin Cancer Res 2001;7(5):1204-1213.

357. Burtness B, et al: Phase III trial comparing cisplatin (C) + placebo (P) to C + anti-epidermal growth factor antibody (EGFR) C225 in patients with metastatic/recurrent head and neck cancer (HNC). Proc Am Soc Clin Oncol 2002;21:901.

358. Robert F, et al: Phase I study of anti-epidermal growth factor receptor antibody cetuximab in combination with radiation therapy in patients with advanced head and neck cancer. J Clin Oncol 2001;19(13):3234-3243.

359. Sirotnak FM, et al: Efficacy of cytotoxic agents against human tumor xenografts is markedly enhanced by coadministration of ZD1839 (Iressa), an inhibitor of EGFR tyrosine kinase. Clin Cancer Res 2000;6(12):4885-4892.

360. Baselga J, Averbuch SD: ZD1839 (Iressa) as an anticancer agent. Drugs 2000;60 Suppl 1:33-40; discussion 41-42.

361. Baselga J, et al: Initial results from a phase II trial of ZD1839 (Iressa) as second-and third-line monotherapy for patients with advanced non-small cell lung cancer (IDEAL-1). Proc AACR-NCI-EORTC Int Conf, 2001;630:abstract.

362. Cohen EE, et al: Phase II trial of ZD1839 in recurrent or metastatic squamous cell carcinoma of the head and neck. J Clin Oncol 2003;21(10):1980-1987.

363. Senzer N, Soulieres D, et al: Phase II evaluation of OSI-774, a potent oral antagonist of the EGRF-TK in patients with advanced squamous cell carcinoma of the head and neck. Proc Am Soc Clin Oncol 2001;6:abstract.

364. Glisson S, et al: Smokeless tobacco induced oral cavity tumors in Kentucky have a high incidence of h-ras mutations. Proc Am Soc Clin Oncol 1998;17:abstract.

365. Kehrer D, et al: Clinical pharmacokinetics of irinotecan given in combination with farnesyl transferase inhibitor Zanestra. Proc AACR-NCI-EORTC Int Conf, 2001;449:abstract.

366. Awada A, et al: A phase I clinical and pharmacokinetic trial of Zanestra (farnesyl transferase inhibitor, R115777) and docetaxel: A promising combination in patients with solid tumors. Proc AACR-NCI-EORTC Int Conf 2001;602:abstract.

367. Adjei A, et al: A phase I trial of the farnesyl transferase inhibitor R115777, in combination with gemcitabine and cisplatin in patients with advanced cancer. Proc Am Soc Clin Oncol 2001;320:abstract.

368. Lee F, et al: The pro-apoptotic FT inhibitor BMS-213662 produced synergistic antitumor activity in combination chemotherapy with antiproliferative cytotoxic agents. Proc AACR-NCI-EORTC Int Conf 2001;401:abstract.

369. Bischoff JR, et al: An adenovirus mutant that replicates selectively in p53-deficient human tumor cells. Science 1996;274(5286): 373-376.

370. Heise C, et al: ONYX-015, an E1B gene-attenuated adenovirus, causes tumor-specific cytolysis and antitumoral efficacy that can be augmented by standard chemotherapeutic agents. Nat Med 1997;3(6):639-645.

371. Kirn D, Hermiston T, McCormick F: ONYX-015: Clinical data are encouraging. Nat Med 1998;4(12):1341-1342.

372. Ganly I, et al: A phase I study of Onyx-015, an E1B attenuated adenovirus, administered intratumorally to patients with recurrent head and neck cancer. Clin Cancer Res 2000;6(3):798-806.

373. Khuri FR, et al: A controlled trial of intratumoral ONYX-015, a selectively-replicating adenovirus, in combination with cisplatin and 5-fluorouracil in patients with recurrent head and neck cancer. Nat Med 2000;6(8):879-885.

374. Qin DX, et al: Analysis of 1379 patients with nasopharyngeal carcinoma treated by radiation. Cancer 1988;61(6):1117-1124.

375. Mesic JB, Fletcher GH, Goepfert H: Megavoltage irradiation of epithelial tumors of the nasopharynx. Int J Radiat Oncol Biol Phys 1981;7(4):447-453.

376. Hoppe RT, Goffinet DR, Bagshaw MA: Carcinoma of the nasopharynx: Eighteen years' experience with megavoltage radiation therapy. Cancer 1976;37(6):2605-2612.

377. Lee AW, et al: Staging of nasopharyngeal carcinoma: From Ho's to the new UICC system. Int J Cancer 1999;84(2):179-187.

378. Cooper JS, Cohen R, Stevens RE: A comparison of staging systems for nasopharyngeal carcinoma. Cancer 1998;83(2):213-219.

379. Ozyar E, et al: Comparison of AJCC 1988 and 1997 classifications for nasopharyngeal carcinoma. American Joint Committee on Cancer. Int J Radiat Oncol Biol Phys 1999;44(5):1079-1087.

380. Lee AW: Contribution of radiotherapy to function preservation and cancer outcome in primary treatment of nasopharyngeal carcinoma. World J Surg 2003;27(7):838-843.

381. al-Sarraf M, et al: Chemoradiotherapy versus radiotherapy in patients with advanced nasopharyngeal cancer: Phase III randomized Intergroup study 0099. J Clin Oncol 1998;16(4):1310-1317.

382. Chow E, et al: Radiotherapy alone in patients with advanced nasopharyngeal cancer: Comparison with an intergroup study. Is combined modality treatment really necessary? Radiother Oncol 2002;63(3):269-274.

383. Cooper JS: Concurrent chemotherapy and radiation therapy for advanced stage carcinoma of the nasopharynx. Int J Radiat Oncol Biol Phys 2000;48(5):1277-1279.

384. Tan EH, et al: Concurrent chemoradiotherapy followed by adjuvant chemotherapy in Asian patients with nasopharyngeal carcinoma: Toxicities and preliminary results. Int J Radiat Oncol Biol Phys 1999;45(3):597-601.

385. Kwong DL, et al: The effect of interruptions and prolonged treatment time in radiotherapy for nasopharyngeal carcinoma. Int J Radiat Oncol Biol Phys 1997;39(3):703-710.

386. Chan ATC, et al: Concurrent chemotherapy-radiotherapy compared with radiotherapy alone in locoregionally advanced nasopharyngeal carcinoma: Progression-free survival analysis of a phase III randomized trial. J Clin Oncol 2002;20(8):2038-2044.

387. Lin JC, et al: Phase III study of concurrent chemoradiotherapy versus radiotherapy alone for advanced nasopharyngeal carcinoma:positive effect on overall and progression-free survival. J Clin Oncol 2003;21(4):631-637.

388. Leung TW, et al: High dose rate intracavitary brachytherapy in the treatment of nasopharyngeal carcinoma. Acta Oncol 1996;35(1):43-47.

389. Leung TW, et al: Salvage brachytherapy for patients with locally persistent nasopharyngeal carcinoma. Int J Radiat Oncol Biol Phys 2000;47(2):405-412.

390. Syed AM, et al: Brachytherapy for primary and recurrent nasopharyngeal carcinoma: 20 years' experience at Long Beach Memorial. Int J Radiat Oncol Biol Phys 2000;47(5):1311-1321.

391. Pryzant RM, et al: Retreatment of nasopharyngeal carcinoma in 53 patients. Int J Radiat Oncol Biol Phys 1992;22(5):941-947.

392. Kwong DL, et al: Long term results of radioactive gold grain implantation for the treatment of persistent and recurrent nasopharyngeal carcinoma. Cancer 2001;91(6):1105-1113.

393. Teo PM, et al: A retrospective study of the role of intracavitary brachytherapy and prognostic factors determining local tumor control after primary radical radiotherapy in 903 nondisseminated nasopharyngeal carcinoma patients. Clin Oncol (R Coll Radiol) 1996;8(3):160-166.

394. Chua DT, et al: Linear accelerator-based stereotactic radiosurgery for limited, locally persistent, and recurrent nasopharyngeal carcinoma: Efficacy and complications. Int J Radiat Oncol Biol Phys 2003;56(1):177-183.

395. Chow E, et al: Enhanced control by radiotherapy of cervical lymph node metastases arising from nasopharyngeal carcinoma compared with nodal metastases from other head and neck squamous cell carcinomas. Int J Radiat Oncol Biol Phys 1997;39(1):149-154.

396. Lee AW, et al: Retrospective analysis of 5037 patients with nasopharyngeal carcinoma treated during 1976-1985: Overall survival and patterns of failure. Int J Radiat Oncol Biol Phys 1992;23(2):261-270.

397. Kwong D, Sham J, Choy D: The effect of loco-regional control on distant metastatic dissemination in carcinoma of the nasopharynx:an analysis of 1301 patients. Int J Radiat Oncol Biol Phys 1994;30(5):1029-1036.

398. Wang C: Carcinoma of the nasopharynx. In Wang CC (ed): Radiation Therapy for Head and Neck Neoplasm, 3rd ed. New York, Wiley-Liss, 1997, pp 257-280.

399. Lee AW, et al: Effect of time, dose and fractionation on local control of nasopharyngeal carcinoma. Radiother Oncol 1995;36(1):24-31.

400. Jian JJ, et al: Improvement of local control of T3 and T4 nasopharyngeal carcinoma by hyperfractionated radiotherapy and concomitant chemotherapy. Int J Radiat Oncol Biol Phys 2002; 53(2):344-352.

401. Jen YM, et al: Dose escalation using twice-daily radiotherapy for nasopharyngeal carcinoma: Does heavier dosing result in a happier ending? Int J Radiat Oncol Biol Phys 2002;54(1):14-22.

402. Chua DT, et al: Preliminary report of the Asian-Oceanic Clinical Oncology Association randomized trial comparing cisplatin and epirubicin followed by radiotherapy versus radiotherapy alone in the treatment of patients with locoregionally advanced nasopharyngeal carcinoma. Asian-Oceanic Clinical Oncology Association Nasopharynx Cancer Study Group. Cancer 1998;83(11):2270-2283.

403. Cvitkovic E, et al: Neoadjuvant chemotherapy (NACT) with epirubicin (EPD), cisplatin (CDDP), bleomycin (BLEO) (BEC) in undifferentiated nasopharyngeal cancer (UCNT): Preliminary results of an international phase III trial. Proc Am Soc Clin Oncol, 1994;13:283.

404. Chan ATC, et al: A prospective randomized study of chemotherapy adjunctive to definitive radiotherapy in advanced nasopharyngeal carcinoma Int J Radiat Oncol Biol Phys 1995;33(3):569-577.

405. Ma J, et al: Results of a prospective randomized trial comparing neoadjuvant chemotherapy plus radiotherapy with radiotherapy alone in patients with locoregionally advanced nasopharyngeal carcinoma. J Clin Oncol 2001;19(5):1350-1357.

406. Hareyama M, et al: A prospective, randomized trial comparing neoadjuvant chemotherapy with radiotherapy alone in patients with advanced nasopharyngeal carcinoma. Cancer 2002;94(8):2217-2223.

407. Chi K-H, et al: A phase III study of adjuvant chemotherapy in advanced nasopharyngeal carcinoma patients. Int J Radiat Oncol Biol Phys 2002;52(5):1238-1244.

408. Rossi A, et al: Adjuvant chemotherapy with vincristine, cyclophosphamide, and doxorubicin after radiotherapy in local-regional nasopharyngeal cancer: Results of a 4-year multicenter randomized study. J Clin Oncol 1988;6(9):1401-1410.

409. Pai PC, et al: Stereotactic radiosurgery for locally recurrent nasopharyngeal carcinoma. Head Neck 2002;24(8):748-753.

410. Lee AW, et al: Retrospective analysis of patients with nasopharyngeal carcinoma treated during 1976-1985: Survival after local recurrence [see comments]. Int J Radiat Oncol Biol Phys 1993;26(5):773-782.

411. Hao SP, Tsang NM, Chang CN: Salvage surgery for recurrent nasopharyngeal carcinoma. Arch Otolaryngol Head Neck Surg 2002;128(1):63-67.

412. Hsu MM, et al: Factors affecting the overall survival after salvage surgery in patients with recurrent nasopharyngeal carcinoma at the primary site: Experience with 60 cases. Arch Otolaryngol Head Neck Surg 2001;127(7):798-802.

413. Fountzilas G, et al: Paclitaxel by three-hour infusion and carboplatin in advanced carcinoma of nasopharynx and other sites of the head and neck: A phase II study conducted by the Hellenic Cooperative Oncology Group. Ann Oncol 1997; 8(5):451-455.

414. Yeo W, et al: A phase II study of combination paclitaxel and carboplatin in advanced nasopharyngeal carcinoma. Eur J Cancer 1998;34(13):2027-2031.

415. Tan EH, et al: Phase II trial of a paclitaxel and carboplatin combination in Asian patients with metastatic nasopharyngeal carcinoma. Ann Oncol 1999;10(2):235-237.

416. Airoldi M, et al: Carboplatin plus taxol is an effective third-line regimen in recurrent undifferentiated nasopharyngeal carcinoma. Tumori 2002;88(4):273-276.

417. Sisson GA, Sr, Toriumi DM, Atiyah RA: Paranasal sinus malignancy: A comprehensive update. Laryngoscope 1989;99(2):143-150.

418. Lewis JS, Castro EB: Cancer of the nasal cavity and paranasal sinuses. J Laryngol Otol 1972;86(3):255-262.

419. Sakai S, et al: Multidisciplinary treatment of maxillary sinus carcinoma. Cancer 1983;52(8):1360-1364.

420. Shidnia H, et al: The role of radiation therapy in the treatment of malignant tumors of the paranasal sinuses. Laryngoscope 1984;94(1):102-106.

421. Waldron J, Witterick I: Paranasal sinus cancer: Caveats and controversies. World J Surg 2003;27(7):849-855.

422. Le QT, et al: Treatment of maxillary sinus carcinoma: A comparison of the 1997 and 1977 American Joint Committee on Cancer staging systems. Cancer 1999;86(9):1700-1711.

423. Tsujii H, et al: The role of radiotherapy in the management of maxillary sinus carcinoma. Cancer 1986;57(12):2261-2266.

424. Stern SJ, et al: Squamous cell carcinoma of the maxillary sinus. Arch Otolaryngol Head Neck Surg 1993;119(9):964-969.

425. Giri SP, et al: Management of advanced squamous cell carcinomas of the maxillary sinus. Cancer 1992;69(3):657-661.

426. Lee F, Ogura JH: Maxillary sinus carcinoma. Laryngoscope 1981;91(1):133-139.

427. Ashley FL, et al: Carcinoma of the lip: A comparison of 5-year results after irradiation and surgical therapy. Am J Surg 1965. 110(4):549-551.

428. Baker SR, Krause CJ: Carcinoma of the lip. Laryngoscope 1980;90(1):19-27.

429. Cerezo L, et al: Squamous cell carcinoma of the lip: Analysis of the Princess Margaret Hospital experience. Radiother Oncol 1993;28(2):142-147.

430. de Visscher JG, et al: Surgical treatment of squamous cell carcinoma of the lower lip: Evaluation of long-term results and prognostic factors—a retrospective analysis of 184 patients. J Oral Maxillofac Surg 1998;56(7):814-820; discussion 820-821.

431. Hosal IN, et al: Squamous cell carcinoma of the lower lip: Am J Otolaryngol 1992;13(6):363-365.

432. McGregor GI, Davis NL, Hay JH: Impact of cervical lymph node metastases from squamous cell cancer of the lip. Am J Surg 1992;163(5):469-471.

433. Zitsch RP, III, et al: Outcome analysis for lip carcinoma. Otolaryngol Head Neck Surg 1995;113(5):589-596.

434. Bamberg M, Schulz U, Scherer E: Postoperative split course radiotherapy of squamous cell carcinoma of the oral tongue. Int J Radiat Oncol Biol Phys 1979;5(4):515-519.

435. Sessions DG, et al: Analysis of treatment results for oral tongue cancer. Laryngoscope 2002;112(4):616-625.

436. Fein DA, et al: Carcinoma of the oral tongue: A comparison of results and complications of treatment with radiotherapy and/or surgery. Head Neck 1994;16(4):358-365.

437. Ho CM, et al: Occult lymph node metastasis in small oral tongue cancers. Head Neck 1992;14(5):359-363.

438. Asakage T, et al: Tumor thickness predicts cervical metastasis in patients with stage I/II carcinoma of the tongue. Cancer 1998;82(8):1443-1448.

439. Byers RM, et al: Can we detect or predict the presence of occult nodal metastases in patients with squamous carcinoma of the oral tongue? Head Neck 1998;20(2):138-144.

440. Kurokawa H, et al: Risk factors for late cervical lymph node metastases in patients with stage I or II carcinoma of the tongue. Head Neck 2002;24(8):731-736.

441. Miura M, et al: Factors affecting mandibular complications in low dose rate brachytherapy for oral tongue carcinoma with special reference to spacer. Int J Radiat Oncol Biol Phys 1998;41(4):763-770.

442. Mazeron JJ, et al: Iridium 192 implantation of T1 and T2 carcinomas of the mobile tongue. Int J Radiat Oncol Biol Phys 1990;19(6):1369-1376.

443. Pernot M, et al: Iridium-192 brachytherapy in the management of 147 T2N0 oral tongue carcinomas treated with irradiation alone: Comparison of two treatment techniques. Radiother Oncol 1992;23(4):223-228.

444. Inoue T, et al: Phase III trial of high and low dose rate interstitial radiotherapy for early oral tongue cancer. Int J Radiat Oncol Biol Phys 1996;36(5):1201-1204.

445. Shibuya H, et al: Brachytherapy for stage I and II oral tongue cancer: An analysis of past cases focusing on control and complications. Int J Radiat Oncol Biol Phys 1993;26(1):51-58.

446. Mendenhall WM, et al: T2 oral tongue carcinoma treated with radiotherapy: Analysis of local control and complications. Radiother Oncol 1989;16(4):275-281.

447. Leung TW, et al: Technical hints for high dose rate interstitial tongue brachytherapy. Clin Oncol (R Coll Radiol) 1998;10(4):231-236.

448. Ange DW, Lindberg RD, Guillamondegui OM: Mangement of squamous cell carcinoma of the oral tongue and floor of mouth after excisional biopsy. Radiology 1975;116(1):143-146.

449. Brown M, Hu K, Harrison L: Adjuvant interstitial brachytherapy for resected T1 and T2 cancer of the oral cavity with close or positive margins. In American Brachytherapy Society Proceedings, 2001, Vancouver, British Columbia.

450. McGuirt WF, Jr, et al: Floor of mouth carcinoma: The management of the clinically negative neck. Arch Otolaryngol Head Neck Surg 1995;121(3):278-282.

451. Teichgraeber JF, Clairmont AA: The incidence of occult metastases for cancer of the oral tongue and floor of the mouth: treatment rationale. Head Neck Surg 1984;7(1):15-21.

452. Dias FL, et al: Elective neck dissection versus observation in stage I squamous cell carcinomas of the tongue and floor of the mouth. Otolaryngol Head Neck Surg 2001;125(1):23-29.

453. Kligerman J, et al: Supraomohyoid neck dissection in the treatment of T1/T2 squamous cell carcinoma of oral cavity. Am J Surg 1994;168(5):391-394.

454. Spiro RH, et al: Predictive value of tumor thickness in squamous carcinoma confined to the tongue and floor of the mouth. Am J Surg 1986;152(4):345-350.

455. Byers RM, et al: Frequency and therapeutic implications of "skip metastases" in the neck from squamous carcinoma of the oral tongue. Head Neck 1997;19(1):14-19.

456. Hicks WL, Jr, et al: Squamous cell carcinoma of the floor of mouth: A 20-year review. Head Neck 1997;19(5):400-405.

457. Shaha AR, et al: Squamous carcinoma of the floor of the mouth. Am J Surg 1984;148(4):455-459.

458. Panje WR, Smith B, McCabe BF: Epidermoid carcinoma of the floor of the mouth: surgical therapy vs. combined therapy vs. radiation therapy. Otolaryngol Head Neck Surg 1980;88(6):714-720.

459. Denittis AS, et al: Advanced oropharyngeal carcinoma treated with surgery and radiotherapy: Oncologic outcome and functional assessment. Am J Otolaryngol 2001;22(5):329-335.

460. Watkinson JC, et al: Conservation surgery in the management of T1 and T2 oropharyngeal squamous cell carcinoma: The Birmingham UK experience. Clin Otolaryngol 2002;27(6):541-548.

461. Wang CC, Montgomery W, Efird J: Local control of oropharyngeal carcinoma by irradiation alone. Laryngoscope 1995;105(5 Pt 1):529-533.

462. Remmler D, et al: Treatment of choice for squamous carcinoma of the tonsillar fossa. Head Neck Surg 1985;7(3):206-211.

463. Wang MB, et al: Tonsillar carcinoma: analysis of treatment results. J Otolaryngol 1998;27(5):263-269.

464. O'Sullivan B, et al: The benefits and pitfalls of ipsilateral radiotherapy in carcinoma of the tonsillar region. Int J Radiat Oncol Biol Phys 2001;51(2):332-343.

465. Kagei K, et al: Ipsilateral irradiation for carcinomas of tonsillar region and soft palate based on computed tomographic simulation. Radiother Oncol 2000;54(2):117-121.

466. Jackson SM, et al: Cancer of the tonsil: the results of ipsilateral radiation treatment. Radiother Oncol 1999;51(2):123-128.

467. Weber RS, et al: Squamous cell carcinoma of the soft palate, uvula, and anterior faucial pillar. Otolaryngol Head Neck Surg 1988; 99(1):16-23.

468. Keus RB, et al: Results of irradiation in squamous cell carcinoma of the soft palate and uvula. Radiother Oncol 1988;11(4):311-317.

469. Erkal HS, et al: Squamous cell carcinomas of the soft palate treated with radiation therapy alone or followed by planned neck dissection. Int J Radiat Oncol Biol Phys 2001;50(2):359-366.

470. Candela FC, Kothari K, Shah JP: Patterns of cervical node metastases from squamous carcinoma of the oropharynx and hypopharynx. Head Neck 1990;12(3):197-203.

471. O'Brien CJ, et al: The use of clinical criteria alone in the management of the clinically negative neck among patients with squamous cell carcinoma of the oral cavity and oropharynx. Arch Otolaryngol Head Neck Surg 2000;126(3):360-365.

472. Stoeckli SJ, et al: Histopathological features of occult metastasis detected by sentinel lymph node biopsy in oral and oropharyngeal squamous cell carcinoma. Laryngoscope 2002;112(1):111-115.

473. Weber RS, et al: Functional results after total or near total glossectomy with laryngeal preservation. Arch Otolaryngol Head Neck Surg 1991;117(5):512–515.

474. Weber RS, et al: Treatment selection for carcinoma of the base of the tongue. Am J Surg 1990;160(4):415–419.

475. Kaylie DM, et al: External beam radiation followed by planned neck dissection and brachytherapy for base of tongue squamous cell carcinoma. Laryngoscope 2000;110(10 Pt 1):1633–1636.

476. Vikram B, et al: A non-looping afterloading technique for base of tongue implants: Results in the first 20 patients. Int J Radiat Oncol Biol Phys 1985;11(10):1853–1855.

477. McDonald TJ, DeSanto LW, Weiland LH: Supraglottic larynx and its pathology as studied by whole laryngeal sections. Laryngoscope 1976;86(5):635–648.

478. Naudo P, et al: Functional outcome and prognosis factors after supracricoid partial laryngectomy with cricohyoidopexy. Ann Otol Rhinol Laryngol 1997;106(4):291–296.

479. Naudo P, et al: Complications and functional outcome after supracricoid partial laryngectomy with cricohyoidoepiglottopexy. Otolaryngol Head Neck Surg 1998;118(1):124–129.

480. Davis RK, et al: The anatomy and complications of "T" versus vertical closure of the hypopharynx after laryngectomy. Laryngoscope 1982;92(1):16–22.

481. Hillman RE, et al: Functional outcomes following treatment for advanced laryngeal cancer. Part I—Voice preservation in advanced laryngeal cancer. Part II— Laryngectomy rehabilitation: The state of the art in the VA System. Research Speech-Language Pathologists. Department of Veterans Affairs Laryngeal Cancer Study Group. Ann Otol Rhinol Laryngol 1998;172 (Suppl):1–27.

482. Ward EC, et al: Swallowing outcomes following laryngectomy and pharyngolaryngectomy. Arch Otolaryngol Head Neck Surg 2002;128(2):181–186.

483. Wenig BL, Applebaum EL: The submandibular triangle in squamous cell carcinoma of the larynx and hypopharynx. Laryngoscope 1991;101(5):516–518.

484. Spaulding CA, et al: Partial laryngectomy and radiotherapy for supraglottic cancer:a conservative approach. Ann Otol Rhinol Laryngol 1989;98(2):125–129.

485. Scola B, et al: Management of cancer of the supraglottis. Otolaryngol Head Neck Surg 2001;124(2):195–198.

486. Mendenhall WM, et al: Radiotherapy for squamous cell carcinoma of the supraglottic larynx:an alternative to surgery. Head Neck 1996;18(1):24–35.

487. Hinerman RW, et al: Carcinoma of the supraglottic larynx: Treatment results with radiotherapy alone or with planned neck dissection. Head Neck 2002;24(5):456–467.

488. DeSanto LW: Early supraglottic cancer. Ann Otol Rhinol Laryngol 1990;99(8):593–597.

489. Laccourreye H, et al: Supracricoid laryngectomy with cricohyoidoepiglottopexy: A partial laryngeal procedure for glottic carcinoma. Ann Otol Rhinol Laryngol 1990;99(6 Pt 1):421–426.

490. Ogura JH, Biller HF, Wette R: Elective neck dissection for pharyngeal and laryngeal cancers: An evaluation. Ann Otol Rhinol Laryngol 1971;80(5):646–650.

491. Hao SP, Myers EN, Johnson JT: T3 glottic carcinoma revisited: Transglottic vs. pure glottic carcinoma. Arch Otolaryngol Head Neck Surg 1995;121(2):166–170.

492. Yang CY, et al: Nodal disease in purely glottic carcinoma: Is elective neck treatment worthwhile? Laryngoscope 1998;108(7):1006–1008.

493. Greene RM, Dewitt AI, Otto RA, Management of T3 N0 and T4 N0 glottic carcinomas: Results of a national survey. Otolaryngol Head Neck Surg 2003;128(2):191–195.

494. Johnson JT: Carcinoma of the larynx: Selective approach to the management of cervical lymphatics. Ear Nose Throat J 1994;73(5):303–305.

495. Cragle SP, Brandenburg JH: Laser cordectomy or radiotherapy: Cure rates, communication, and cost. Otolaryngol Head Neck Surg 1993;108(6):648–654.

496. Bron LP, et al: Treatment of early stage squamous-cell carcinoma of the glottic larynx:endoscopic surgery or cricohyoidoepiglotto-pexy versus radiotherapy. Head Neck 2001;23(10):823–829.

497. Dickens WJ, et al: Treatment of early vocal cord carcinoma: A comparison of apples and apples. Laryngoscope 1983;93(2):216–219.

498. Maheshwar AA, Gaffney CC: Radiotherapy for T1 glottic carcinoma:impact of anterior commissure involvement. J Laryngol Otol 2001;115(4):298–301.

499. Howell-Burke D, et al: T2 glottic cancer: Recurrence, salvage, and survival after definitive radiotherapy. Arch Otolaryngol Head Neck Surg 1990;116(7):830–835.

500. Bergqvist M, et al: Radiation treatment of T1-T4 squamous cell carcinoma of the larynx: A retrospective analysis and long-term follow-up of 135 patients. Anticancer Res 2002;22(2B):1239–1242.

501. de Campora E, Radici M, de Campora L: External versus endoscopic approach in the surgical treatment of glottic cancer. Eur Arch Otorhinolaryngol 2001;258(10):533–536.

502. Garden AS, et al: Results of radiotherapy for T2N0 glottic carcinoma: does the "2" stand for twice-daily treatment? Int J Radiat Oncol Biol Phys 2003;55(2):322–328.

503. Editorial. Radiother Oncol 1997;44(2):97–99.

504. Clayman GL, et al: Laryngeal preservation for advanced laryngeal and hypopharyngeal cancers. Arch Otolaryngol Head Neck Surg 1995;121(2):219–223.

505. Shaha AR, Shah JP: Carcinoma of the subglottic larynx. Am J Surg 1982;144(4):456–458.

506. Ogura JH, Marks JE, Freeman RB: Results of conservation surgery for cancers of the supraglottis and pyriform sinus. Laryngoscope 1980;90(4):591–600.

507. Laccourreye H, et al: Supracricoid hemilaryngopharyngectomy: Analysis of 240 cases. Ann Otol Rhinol Laryngol 1987;96(2 Pt 1):217–221.

508. Buckley JG, MacLennan K: Cervical node metastases in laryngeal and hypopharyngeal cancer: A prospective analysis of prevalence and distribution. Head Neck 2000;22(4):380–385.

509. Marks JE, et al: The risk of contralateral lymphatic metastases for cancers of the larynx and pharynx. Am J Otolaryngol 1992;13(1):34–39.

510. Marks SC, et al: Outcome of pyriform sinus cancer: A retrospective institutional review. Laryngoscope 1996;106(1 Pt 1):27–31.

511. Zelefsky MJ, et al: Combined chemotherapy and radiotherapy versus surgery and postoperative radiotherapy for advanced hypopharyngeal cancer. Head Neck 1996;18(5):405–411.

512. North CA, et al: Carcinoma of the major salivary glands treated by surgery or surgery plus postoperative radiotherapy. Int J Radiat Oncol Biol Phys 1990;18(6):1319–1326.

513. Harrison LB, et al: Postoperative radiation therapy for major salivary gland malignancies. J Surg Oncol 1990;45(1):52–55.

514. Weir L, et al: Radiation treatment of cervical lymph node metastases from an unknown primary: An analysis of outcome by treatment volume and other prognostic factors. Radiother Oncol 1995;35(3):206–211.

515. Reddy SP, Marks JE: Metastatic carcinoma in the cervical lymph nodes from an unknown primary site:results of bilateral neck plus mucosal irradiation vs. ipsilateral neck irradiation. Int J Radiat Oncol Biol Phys 1997;37(4):797–802.

516. Eisbruch A, Dawson L: Reirradiation of head and neck tumors: Benefits and toxicities. Hematol Oncol Clin North Am 1999;13(4):825–836.

517. Stafford N, Dearnaley D: Treatment of 'inoperable' neck nodes using surgical clearance and postoperative interstitial irradiation. Br J Surg 1988;75(1):62–64.

518. Moscoso JF, et al: Simultaneous interstitial radiotherapy with regional or free-flap reconstruction, following salvage surgery of recurrent head and neck carcinoma: Analysis of complications. Arch Otolaryngol Head Neck Surg 1994;120(9):965–972.

519. Chen KY, Mohr RM, Silverman CL: Interstitial iodine 125 in advanced recurrent squamous cell carcinoma of the head and neck with follow-up evaluation of carotid artery by ultrasound. Ann Otol Rhinol Laryngol 1996;105(12):955–961.

520. Lee DJ, et al: Intraoperative I-125 seed implantation for extensive recurrent head and neck carcinomas. Radiology 1991;178(3):879–882.

Specific Malignancies

III

521. Park RI, et al: Iodine-125 seed implantation as an adjunct to surgery in advanced recurrent squamous cell cancer of the head and neck. Laryngoscope 1991;101(4 Pt 1):405–410.

522. Vikram B, et al: Intraoperative radiotherapy in patients with recurrent head and neck cancer. Am J Surg 1985;150(4):485–487.

523. Stevens KR, Jr, Britsch A, Moss WT: High-dose reirradiation of head and neck cancer with curative intent. Int J Radiat Oncol Biol Phys 1994;29(4):687–698.

524. Mazeron JJ, et al: Salvage irradiation of oropharyngeal cancers using iridium 192 wire implants: 5-year results of 70 cases. Int J Radiat Oncol Biol Phys 1987;13(7):957–962.

525. Levendag PC, Meeuwis CA, Visser AG: Reirradiation of recurrent head and neck cancers: External and/or interstitial radiation therapy. Radiother Oncol 1992;23(1):6–15.

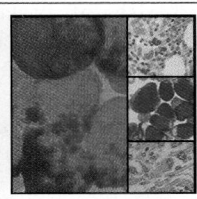

72

MELANOMA

Julie R. Lange

William H. Sharfman

Rhoda M. Alani

Charles M. Balch

SUMMARY OF KEY POINTS

INCIDENCE

- The incidence of melanoma has risen dramatically over the past century.
- Approximately 55,100 new cases of invasive melanoma are diagnosed each year in the United States, and it is estimated that 1 in 75 persons in the U.S. will be diagnosed with melanoma in their lifetime.

ETIOLOGY/EPIDEMIOLOGY

- Risk of melanoma is strongly related to exposure to UV irradiation, and to a susceptible host phenotype, namely, fair hair and skin, a tendency to burn, and numerous benign or atypical nevi.
- Family and personal history of skin cancers are also important risk factors.

PATHOLOGY/BIOLOGY

- The single most important pathologic feature of the primary lesion is the thickness in mm.
- Histologic ulceration is also a strong prognostic feature.

CLINICAL FINDINGS

- Many primary melanomas display typical features of border irregularity and variegated pigmentation.
- Others may be recognized by a patient report of a change in the size or color of a pigmented lesion or by a report of itching or bleeding from a skin lesion.
- Other primary melanomas may lack these features and therefore may be more difficult to recognize.

DIFFERENTIAL DIAGNOSIS/ STAGING

- Any suspicious lesion or questionable new or changing lesion should have a full-thickness biopsy.
- Microstaging of the primary lesion relies on accurate determination of the depth of the lesion, and determination of whether histologic ulceration is present.
- The current AJCC staging system includes the thickness and presence or absence of ulceration of the primary tumor, the number of positive nodes, and whether the nodes are microscopically or macroscopically positive.

PRIMARY THERAPY/SALVAGE THERAPY: SURGICAL

- All primary melanomas need a wide local excision for local control.
- Margins of excision are determined by the thickness of the primary lesion.
- For patients presenting with a new primary melanoma ≥1 mm and a clinically negative regional node basin, sentinel node biopsy can be used to determine the node status.
- For patients with known metastatic nodes, regional node dissection is performed.

PRIMARY THERAPY/SALVAGE THERAPY: SYSTEMIC

- Adjuvant therapy should be offered to patients with high-risk, resected disease (e.g., nodal metastases or a primary ≥4 mm), either with

interferon alpha or as part of a clinical trial.
- Although approved by the FDA in 1996 for high-risk patients, subsequent clinical trials of interferon have failed to show a clear overall survival benefit, although they consistently show a DFS benefit, and its routine use remains controversial.
- For advanced melanoma, DTIC and high-dose IL-2 are the only FDA approved agents.
- Durable responses can occur but are rare, and systemic therapy for advanced metastatic disease is usually palliative.

COMPLICATIONS

- Primary surgical therapy can usually be accomplished with preservation of full function and reasonable cosmesis. Node dissection is accompanied by a risk of lymphedema.

PROGNOSIS

- Prognosis is strongly related to the thickness of the tumor at its original presentation and the nodal status.
- Today, patients are diagnosed early and will have an excellent prognosis.
- Once systemic metastatic disease is recognized, median survival is approximately 6 to 9 months.
- With current therapies, the outcome for patients with advanced disease is poor, and further research is needed to improve systemic therapies for melanoma patients.

INTRODUCTION

In the early part of the 20th century, melanoma was considered a rare disease, and was frequently only recognized at an advanced stage. Today, melanoma is one of the most common malignancies, but is usually recognized at an early stage, when survival rates are high, often with surgery as the only necessary treatment. Melanoma occurs throughout the adult years, and therefore is associated with potential loss of many years of productive life. When diagnosed early, it is one of the most treatable malignancies. A better understanding of the natural history of melanoma and a number of well-run studies of surgical treatment of melanoma have resulted in surgical procedures that are much less radical than those commonly performed just a few decades ago. Advanced melanoma is one of the most difficult diseases to treat and presents opportunities for further research and improvement in treatment strategies. Interest in the biology of this disease continues to increase; ongoing research in molecular biology and its potential application to the medical treatment of melanoma may lead to improved management strategies. This chapter reviews the current treatment of melanoma.

EPIDEMIOLOGY

According to the American Cancer Society, there were expected to be approximately 55,100 new cases of melanoma and 7910 deaths attributable to melanoma in the United States in 2004. It is the fifth most frequently diagnosed malignancy in men and the seventh most frequently diagnosed malignancy in women. It is slightly more common in men than in women. Additionally, approximately 37,700 new cases of in situ melanoma are diagnosed each year. The incidence of melanoma has risen dramatically over the last few decades, and it is now estimated that the lifetime risk of melanoma in the United States is approximately 1 in 57 for men and 1 in 81 for women.[1] Mortality from melanoma is significant. The overall mortality attributable to melanoma has increased because of the great increase in the incidence of the disease; however, because case mortality rates have improved, today 89% of patients are alive 5 years after their diagnosis.[1] However, because melanoma often affects young and middle-aged adults, the potential for years of life lost is great. For most of the 20th century, the incidence of melanoma in populations of European origin rose faster than any other cancer except lung cancer.[2] There are now reports that the incidence of melanoma is stabilizing or slightly decreasing, particularly among younger adults.[3]

Most known risk factors for melanoma fall into one of two categories: susceptibility of the host and exposure to ultraviolet irradiation. Persons who are most susceptible to melanoma are fair-skinned, with a tendency to sunburn. They may have more than 20 benign moles, atypical moles, or congenital moles. A family history of melanoma is also associated with increased risk.

Skin Type

Fair-skinned persons with a tendency to burn are at higher risk than darker-skinned persons. Red or blond hair and blue or green eyes are associated with increased risk. Freckling is common.[4,5]

Common and Atypical Nevi

Common benign nevi, if numerous, are associated with increased risk.[6-8] Atypical nevi are flat macules greater than 5 mm, with variable pigmentation, asymmetrical outlines, and indistinct borders. Atypical nevi are found in 2% to 7% of the white population, but in approximately 40% of patients with melanoma. The presence of atypical nevi implies a greatly increased risk of melanoma, particularly if there is also a family history of melanoma. There is a rare, autosomal dominant syndrome of atypical nevi with variable penetrance. These nevi may occur on non–sun-exposed areas. The lifetime risk of melanoma in some affected families is nearly 100%, with many melanomas occurring de novo and apparently not in preexisting atypical nevi.[9,10]

Giant Congenital Nevi

Patients with large nevi present at birth or in early childhood are at increased risk for melanoma. Giant congenital melanocytic nevi are often elevated, and are usually large, prominent, irregular pigmented lesions. They may follow a dermatome distribution and cover large areas. They occur in fewer than 1 in 20,000 births. Malignant changes may occur in the deeper areas of the dermis and may therefore be difficult to detect.[11] Excision early in life when possible is advised.

Personal History of Melanoma

In patients with a personal history of melanoma, there is an approximately 5% lifetime risk of a second melanoma. Persons who have had melanoma need lifelong skin screening.

Exposure

Ultraviolet (UV) radiation exposure to both UVA and UVB is strongly associated with subsequent development of melanoma. The exposure history that is most strongly associated with subsequent melanoma development is intermittent intense exposure, particularly a history of blistering sunburns in childhood. Exposure to UV radiation is of great interest because it is a modifiable risk factor. However, UV radiation is not necessary for the development of melanoma; areas without sun exposure, such as the soles of the feet and the anal area, can be sites of primary melanoma. The development of melanoma is, like many cancers, a result of a complex interaction between patient susceptibility and carcinogen exposure.

ETIOLOGY AND PATHOGENESIS

Melanoma arises from transformation of melanocytes, which are of neural crest origin. Most melanocytes reside in the basal layer of the epidermis or within benign common nevi. Melanocytes synthesize melanin using the enzyme tyrosinase, and thus under normal conditions, help to protect against UV damage. Melanoma induction by UV radiation is a multistep process, involving both UVB and UVA. The initial event is DNA injury by UVB, followed by promotion of malignancy by both UVB and UVA damage. Melanoma has been conceptualized as growing first in a radial growth phase with little risk of metastatic behavior. This phase is followed by the vertical growth phase with the capacity for metastasis.[12] Different clinical and histologic features are associated with the different phases. Tumor progression likely is the consequence of multiple genetic events.

Melanoma can arise in a preexisting nevus or de novo. Most melanomas probably do not arise from preexisting benign nevi. Only approximately 20% to 30% of melanomas are pathologically associated with melanocytic nevi, and epidemiologic studies strongly suggest that the risk of an individual nevus undergoing malignant transformation is low.[13-15] Thus, although having large numbers of nevi is associated with increased risk of melanoma, the actual precursor lesion is still in question. It is likely that the stepwise evolution of melanocytic nevi to melanoma and the de novo onset of melanoma from malignant conversion of epidermal melanocytes are both mechanisms of tumorigenesis.

PATHOLOGY

Most melanomas can be diagnosed accurately on routine histologic examination. Common melanomas arise from melanocytes in the basal layer of the epidermis, and can be classified based on the growth pattern observed. Melanoma in situ clinically is usually a flat or slightly elevated pigmented lesion and must be distinguished from atypical nevus and from invasive melanoma.

Histologically, in situ melanoma shows atypical melanocytes in a "pagetoid" growth pattern confined to the epidermis. The atypical cells are usually seen throughout the epidermis and usually include mitotic figures. There are no atypical melanocytes in the dermis. Melanoma in situ presumably has no ability to metastasize. It is unknown how often melanoma in situ progresses to invasive melanoma. Conservative excision with a 5-mm margin is essentially curative.

Early invasive melanoma has a radial growth phase. There are small aggregates of melanoma cells in the papillary dermis that are smaller than the aggregates in the epidermis, lack mitotic activity, and are less than 15 cells wide. A vertical growth phase is seen in invasive melanomas that have progressed beyond the radial growth phase. Clinically, these are raised lesions that sometimes occur within a preexisting lesion. In the dermis, atypical melanocytes are found in expanded aggregates that are larger than those in the epidermis. Mitotic figures are present.

Primary melanoma can almost always be diagnosed by routine histologic examination. On recognition of invasive melanoma, proper microstaging is of great importance, because the thickness of the lesion is the most important prognostic factor at the time of diagnosis, and essentially all decisions about the extent of evaluation and appropriate clinical management are based on the report of microstaging. The importance of the depth of invasion into the dermis was recognized by Wallace Clark, who described an association between increasing depth of penetration into the dermis and worsening prognosis.[16] Clark designated melanoma as invading to a maximum of one of five "levels." In level I, melanoma is confined to the epidermis and is in situ melanoma; in level II, it is found in the papillary dermis; in level III, melanoma cells are found throughout the papillary dermis; in level IV, melanoma invades the reticular dermis; and in level V, it invades the subcutaneous fat. Alexander Breslow showed that the thickness of a melanoma measured in millimeters also correlates with prognosis.[17] The thickness is readily reproducible and is measured through an ocular micrometer, from the top of the epidermis to the deepest melanoma cells. Thickness is more strongly correlated with survival than is the level of invasion. Based on a review of outcomes from a large database, we now know that for lesions greater than 1 mm, using the Clark's level does not add any prognostic information beyond the thickness. For lesions thinner than 1 mm, Clark's level adds prognostic information and should therefore always be reported in thin melanoma.[18]

Histologic ulceration is a poor prognostic feature. Ulceration is included in the current staging system and is such a poor prognostic feature that its presence increases the patient's implied risk of recurrence to that of the next higher T stage grouping.[19] Ulceration is recognized by absence of the epidermis overlying the melanoma; presumably, the tumor has eroded through the epidermis rather than pushing it upward. A histologically ulcerated melanoma does not necessarily have a grossly recognizable ulcer crater.

A minimally acceptable pathology report includes the thickness measured in millimeters and the presence of ulceration; in thin (≤1 mm) melanoma, the level should also be reported. Many other features are associated with prognosis and are frequently reported as well. High mitotic rate is associated with poorer survival; further study may determine whether it should be reported routinely.[20] Regression is recognized by the absence of melanoma with fibroplasia, inflammatory cells, and melanophages with edema and telangiectasia. Regression has sometimes been associated with an unfavorable prognosis.[21] Although an uncommon finding, angiolymphatic invasion can be associated with a poorer prognosis and should be reported whenever seen.[22]

Recognized Variants

Desmoplastic Melanoma

The cellular morphology is spindled, and there is a marked desmoplastic response of the surrounding stroma. The tumor may be poorly defined and may extend deeply into the reticular dermis, and perineural infiltration is often seen. The lesion may resemble a schwannoma or neurofibroma, and can also resemble sclerosing blue nevi or a desmoplastic Spitz variant. Desmoplastic tumor cells almost always express S-100, and many express neuronspecific enolase. Desmoplastic melanoma clinically is sometimes nonpigmented, and may resemble a fibroma, basal cell carcinoma, or scar. These lesions are most often found on the head and neck and the upper body, and are somewhat more common in older men.[23] Desmoplastic melanoma is associated with a somewhat lower risk of metastasis, but a higher risk of local recurrence, compared with common melanoma.[24]

Malignant Blue Nevus

Malignant blue nevus is an unusual variant of melanoma that arises in a preexisting blue nevus and shows highly infiltrative, pleomorphic spindle cells, often with areas of bizarre giant cells and necrosis. The mitotic rate is usually high, and often there is blood vessel invasion as well as irregular invasion of the subcutaneous fat. These melanomas clinically are most commonly found on the scalp, and the risk of metastasis is high.[25,26]

Minimal Deviation Melanoma

Minimal deviation melanoma appears as an expanding nodule of moderately atypical melanocytes with a uniform appearance. Nuclei are enlarged, chromatin is irregular, and the nuclear-to-cytoplasmic ratio is increased compared with ordinary nevus cells. There is no necrosis, and mitotic figures are rare. Clinically, these lesions usually arise on the trunk of young adults and are of low metastatic potential.[27,28]

Melanoma of Soft Parts

Also known as clear cell sarcoma, neoplasm of soft tissue usually presents as a soft tissue nodule in the extremities of young adults.[29] Cells are uniform and cohesive and show melanocytic differentiation and prominent nucleoli, with abundant cytoplasm with a clear or granular appearance. Multinucleated giant cells are usually present, and mitoses are few. Cells are almost always positive for S-100, are usually positive for HBM-45 and Melan-A, and ultrastructurally show melanosomes. Most show a t(12;22)(q13;q13) translocation that is not seen in common melanoma.[30,31] Long-term survival is poor.

BIOLOGY

Over the last decade, much progress has been made in defining the genetic events that influence melanoma development; however, few of these discoveries have translated to improved therapies or the development of useful diagnostic or prognostic markers. Most recently, a systematic approach to identifying cancer-associated genetic defects has been attempted because most of the human genome has been sequenced. Such studies have brought new molecular pathways to light in the area of melanoma investigation. Greater knowledge of the molecular events that govern melanoma development is expected to result in the design of targeted therapeutic strategies that may soon significantly improve patient outcomes.

Cell-Cycle Regulatory Proteins in the Development of Melanoma

p16/INK4A and the Retinoblastoma Pathway

Cell-cycle regulatory proteins are necessary to regulate the capacity for cell growth and division and are therefore critical targets in all tumors. Virtually every factor involved in cell-cycle regulation is altered in particular tumor types. Frequent deletions in the 9p21 locus were found in familial melanomas and melanoma cell lines; linkage

studies eventually led to the identification of the *p16/INK4a* gene as the candidate tumor-suppressor gene for familial melanoma.[32,33] The *p16/INK4a* gene encodes an inhibitor of the cyclin-dependent kinases CDK4 and CDK6 and leads to cell-cycle arrest at the G1 phase of the cell cycle. Because CDK4/CDK6 phosphorylates the retinoblastoma protein pRb and inactivates its tumor-suppressor function, this was considered a major mechanism of p16/INK4a tumor suppression in melanomas. Inherited mutations of the gene encoding the cell-cycle regulatory protein p16/INK4a or its associated cyclin-dependent kinase CDK4[34] predispose patients to melanoma.[35] Defects in the *p16/INK4a* gene or its associated kinase, *CDK4*, play a role in the development of a relatively small percentage of sporadic melanomas, and only approximately 20% of familial melanoma cases harbor *p16/INK4a* mutations, suggesting that most familial melanoma cases are associated with other genetic defects.[36] Expression of p16/INK4a is silenced in sporadic melanomas via epigenetic inactivation through promoter methylation[37]; however, this form of gene silencing seems to be activated in a limited number of primary tumors. Of note, in thin sporadic melanomas, loss of p16 expression is associated with disease progression, despite the low incidence of loss of heterozygosity at the *p16/INK4a* locus, *p16/INK4a* intragenic mutations, and *p16/INK4a* promoter methylation (<10% in lesions thinner than 4 mm).[38-40] This suggests that alternative mechanisms exist to allow for decreased expression of p16/INK4a in these early lesions. Other mechanisms of p16/INK4a inactivation in melanoma are under investigation, including transcriptional repression of the p16/INK4a promoter itself. An area of interest is the potential role of Id helix-loop-helix transcription factors in melanoma initiation. In general, high Id expression levels are found in proliferative, undifferentiated cells, a feature that is characteristic of tumor cells.[41] Id genes have been identified as potential proto-oncogenes because overexpression of Id proteins in primary cells promotes cellular immortalization.[42,43] Id gene expression is also elevated in various tumor cell lines as well as a broad spectrum of primary human tumors.[44] In situ evaluations have shown a correlation between tumor invasiveness, aggressiveness, and progression and Id expression. Recently, Id1 was shown to be a repressor of the familial melanoma gene *p16/INK4a*,[45,46] and early studies of primary melanocytic lesions showed that Id1 expression correlated with decreased p16/INK4a expression in early melanomas that were confined to a radial growth phase. In addition, later stages of melanoma that did not express Id1 had sustained genetic mutations that inactivated the *p16/INK4a* gene. The data suggest that Id1 transcriptional repression of *p16/Ink4a* may represent one of the earliest mechanisms of dysregulation of *p16/INK4a* expression, resulting in melanoma initiation, and that Id1 expression may be a useful marker for malignant disease in melanocytic lesions of questionable malignant potential.[47] Large-scale studies are underway to determine the utility of Id1 expression in melanocytic lesions as both a marker of malignant disease and an independent predictor of clinical outcome.

Ras/Raf and the MAP Kinase Pathway

Although mutations of *RAS* genes are uncommon in human melanomas, mouse models of melanoma suggest that activation of this pathway in conjunction with inactivation of the p16/INK4a tumor-suppressor pathway is important for tumor development.[48] Recent studies supported the importance of this pathway in melanoma development because a genome-wide screen of alterations in *RAS* or its downstream effectors identified activating mutations of the serine/threonine kinase BRAF in 59% of melanoma cell lines and six of nine primary melanomas.[49] Most *BRAF* mutations identified (80%) were accounted for by a single amino acid substitution (V599E) that rendered the kinase constitutively active. Subsequent studies showed a similarly high incidence of activating *BRAF* mutations in benign nevi,[50] suggesting that activation of BRAF kinase may be an initiating event for melanocyte proliferation, but is unlikely to be an important mediator of malignant conversion to melanoma. Additional studies have not identified BRAF kinase germline mutations in large-scale evaluations of patients with familial melanomas,[51-53] suggesting that BRAF kinase activation does not significantly predispose patients to melanoma. Interestingly, studies of uveal melanomas did not identify activating mutations of *BRAF*, suggesting that high-frequency *BRAF* mutation is specifically targeted to cutaneous melanocytic lesions.[54,55] Evaluation of primary melanocytic lesions confirmed the high rate of activating BRAF kinase mutations in both benign and malignant lesions.[56,57] However, it was specifically noted that early, radial-growth-phase melanomas showed the lowest incidence of BRAF mutation (10%),[57] suggesting that BRAF kinase activation may not be necessary for malignant conversion of melanocytes. Because therapeutic targeting of tyrosine kinases has resulted in effective treatment for a variety of malignancies, there has been much excitement over the development of BRAF kinase inhibitors as treatments for melanoma.[58] A *raf* kinase inhibitor is under clinical investigation for a variety of solid tumors, and we await the results of studies in patients with melanoma.[59] Current data on BRAF kinase mutations in benign and malignant melanocytic lesions suggest that these mutations are not sufficient to induce malignant conversion of melanocytes to melanoma. However, activating mutations of BRAF or other genes within the MAP kinase pathway may be necessary for melanoma to develop. Thus, inhibition of BRAF kinase may be a useful therapeutic intervention when used in conjunction with other therapeutic modalities.

p53 and Melanoma

Unlike in other malignancies, alterations of the tumor-suppressor gene *p53* itself is infrequent in melanomas.[60] Interestingly, APAF-1, a downstream effector of p53 involved in induction of apoptosis, has been shown to be inactivated in metastatic melanomas,[61] whereas the p53 inhibitor HDM2 is overexpressed in early melanomas,[62,63] suggesting that p53 dysfunction in melanoma may be related to targeting of p53-associated molecules. Interestingly, the p16/INK4a gene has been shown to reside at a genetic locus that encodes a second tumor suppressor gene, p14/ARF. This gene functions through the p53 tumor-suppressor pathway; its role in melanoma development has not been well substantiated.[64]

Apoptotic Pathways and the Development of Melanoma

The process of apoptosis, or programmed cell death, is critical to cellular responses to stress and is a major pathway of cell death induced by radiation therapy and traditional chemotherapy. Melanoma cells can be resistant to therapies that have shown efficacy in other tumor types; this is related, in part, to their ability to evade normal apoptotic signals.[65] Over the last decade, the particular signaling cascades regulating apoptotic pathways have been delineated. The two major apoptotic pathways have been designated the "extrinsic pathway," which is induced on activation of cell-membrane-associated death receptors by their associated ligands, and the "intrinsic" pathway, which is dependent on mitochondrial membrane permeability in response to cellular stress signals. Both pathways result in activation of caspases that are critical effectors of apoptosis. Melanomas evade both intrinsic and extrinsic apoptotic pathways, critical determinants of tumor response to traditional cytotoxic therapies. The cytochrome c-associated factor Apaf-1 is downregulated in advanced melanomas and influences the death response of melanoma cells to cytotoxic agents.[61] In addition, Fas and TRAIL death receptors are downregulated by a variety of mechanisms, leading to impaired activation of the extrinsic apoptotic pathway.[65] Therapeutic strategies aimed at circumventing impaired apoptotic pathways in melanoma are likely to require multiple interventions to ensure the continued activation of effective death pathways, given the variety of resistance mechanisms present in melanoma cells.

Telomerase and Melanoma

Telomeres are the protective ends of chromosomes that maintain chromosome stability. They are composed of repetitive DNA sequences and associated binding proteins.[66,67] In most somatic cells, telomeres shorten with each cell division, allowing telomere length to potentially reveal information about the age and mitotic rate of the cell.[68] In human tumors, expression of telomerase, the ribonucleoprotein responsible for addition of telomeric repeats, is elevated in association with tumor progression, and telomere maintenance is considered critical for tumor development (reviewed in Maser and DePinho[69]). This has been the impetus for developing telomerase inhibitors as cancer therapeutics.[70] Previous studies showed that telomerase activity increases in association with tumor progression in cutaneous melanomas; however, telomere length generally decreases in association with malignant potential, and active telomerase function is usually a late event in tumorigenesis.[71] Thus, assessing telomere length in a tissue specimen may give some indication of malignant potential. Studies are underway to evaluate a new technique combining immunostaining with quantitative fluorescent in situ hybridization (Q-FISH) techniques as a precise method of measuring telomere length in situ in melanocytic lesions.[72] These studies will be used in conjunction with clinical data to determine the utility of telomere length assessments in melanocytic lesions for predicting patient outcome. In addition, because telomerase is activated in late-stage melanomas, but not in benign melanocytic lesions, clinical trials of telomerase inhibitors as treatments for advanced stages of melanoma may show therapeutic benefit when used in conjunction with other treatment modalities.

CLINICAL PRESENTATION AND PATIENT EVALUATION

The most important clinical feature of a cutaneous melanoma is change in the color, size, perimeter, or contour of a mole or pigmented skin lesion. Sometimes patients report an itching sensation around a mole, or may report an unusual sensation in a mole. Bleeding and gross ulceration are usually late symptoms of locally advanced melanoma. The mnemonic **ABCD** is used in order to recall that a biopsy should be prompted by changes in a skin lesion's shape, contour, color, or size (**A**symmetry, **B**order irregularity, **C**olor variegation, **D**iameter >6mm).

Melanoma can be described in five clinical growth patterns: superficial spreading melanoma (SSM), nodular melanoma (NM), lentigo maligna melanoma (LMM), acral lentiginous melanoma (ALM), and desmoplastic melanoma (DM). The clinical features, anatomic distribution, ethnic distribution, and etiology are distinctive. SSM is the most common type of cutaneous melanoma among the white population, is largely responsible for the increased incidence of melanoma over the last few decades, and may arise from a preexisting nevus over a period of months to a few years. The average age at diagnosis is 51 years, which is one to two decades earlier than that of LMM or ALM. SSM has a predominant radial growth phase, both clinically and histologically. These lesions are more common on the trunk of men and on the legs of women, and are typically larger than common benign moles, with asymmetry, notched or irregular borders, and multiple colors (brown, black, pink, and gray). NM is the second most common type of melanoma. It is similar to SSM in terms of age at diagnosis and anatomic distribution, but does not have a precursor radial growth phase. They are usually shiny, smooth nodules, often with a single color, usually black, dark brown, or bluish. Nodular melanomas usually are thicker and thus are diagnosed at a more advanced stage than SSM. The survival rates and prognosis for SSM and NM are virtually the same when matched for thickness and ulceration. Both SSM and NM appear to be associated with acute exposure to UVB irradiation in fair-skinned persons who tend to sunburn rather than suntan. SSM is more common in individuals living in areas with greater UVB exposure.

LMM occurs on chronically sun-exposed skin, especially the face and neck in older persons. More than 75% of such patients are older than 60 years of age, and they typically have a history of a slowly growing mole that has been present for a decade or more. Histologically, LMM lesions have a predominant radial growth phase, and there is associated solar elastosis of the surrounding skin as a result of chronic sun damage. These lesions are probably less aggressive in their metastatic behavior compared with other growth patterns, although this is controversial.

ALM is relatively uncommon. In contrast to SSM, NM, and LMM, which occur almost exclusively in fair-skinned persons, ALM can occur in any ethic group or in persons with any degree of skin pigmentation. They occur on the palms, soles of the feet, and nail beds. They tend to present as more locally advanced lesions. Even when accounting for their greater tumor thickness at presentation, they tend to be more aggressive in their behavior.

DM is an uncommon form of melanoma. Lesions are often nondescript papules, plaques, or nodules, and may be non-pigmented; the appearance of DM may be more suggestive of basal cell carcinoma or a verruca. DM often occurs in the head and neck area and can be associated with neurotropism. The biologic behavior of DM is like that of a soft tissue sarcoma, in that lesions can invade across fascia and along peripheral nerves. DM has a higher rate of local recurrence than the other common forms of melanoma.

The thickness of the primary tumor is the single most important prognostic and staging feature for patients with newly diagnosed primary melanoma. Therefore, appropriate biopsy of a suspicious lesion is critical for proper staging, and a full-thickness biopsy should always be done when melanoma is in the differential diagnosis. Excisional biopsy for small lesions is preferred. For larger lesions (≥2 cm in diameter), a 6-mm or larger punch biopsy specimen obtained from the most raised portion of the lesion may be appropriate. A deep "saucerization" shave can sometimes be acceptable, but a thin shave biopsy of suspicious lesions should be avoided because it may compromise histologic interpretation and proper measurement of thickness. An excisional biopsy scar should be oriented to be compatible with subsequent wide local excision should the lesion prove to be melanoma.

On initial presentation, a person with a newly diagnosed thin or intermediate-thickness melanoma rarely shows evidence of metastatic disease. Most melanoma metastases cause symptoms or can be discovered on physical examination. Appropriate evaluation of all patients with newly diagnosed melanoma includes a thorough history, a skin examination to search for other primary skin cancers, and examination of the regional node basins. For patients with a primary melanoma 1 mm or thicker, chest x-ray and liver enzymes, including lactic dehydrogenase (LDH) are reasonable screening tools. In patients with concerning findings on history and physical examination or abnormal findings on chest x-ray or liver function tests, further imaging studies are warranted.

Prognostic Features

In a multifactorial analysis of 13,581 patients with localized melanoma (either clinically or pathologically), the two most powerful and independent characteristics of the primary melanoma, among all of the prognostic variables analyzed, were tumor thickness and ulceration.[18] No other feature of the melanoma or the patient with localized melanoma had the predictive capability of these two factors. Other factors that were statistically significant prognostic factors were patient age, site of the primary melanoma, level of invasion, and sex.

Thickness

In virtually all studies analyzing the prognosis of patients with stage I and II melanoma using a Cox regression analysis, melanoma thickness is the strongest predictor of outcome. Increasing melanoma thickness correlates with increasing risk of local recurrence, regional metastasis, and distant metastasis, and with poorer melanoma-specific survival.[17,18,73] Melanoma thickness is a continuous variable for which there are no naturally occurring breakpoints that delineate different biologic risks for melanoma-specific mortality.

Ulceration

Ulcerated melanomas are a more biologically aggressive form of the disease, and are associated with a substantially increased risk of metastasis. In virtually every Cox regression analysis of prognostic factors that includes ulceration, melanoma ulceration portends a significantly worse prognosis and a higher risk of metastatic disease compared with nonulcerated melanomas of equivalent thickness.[18,74-76] Melanoma ulceration correlates with increased mitotic rate within a primary melanoma, further suggesting that this factor is associated with increased risk of metastatic behavior.

Level of Invasion

The level of dermal invasion has been viewed as a valuable prognostic factor for decades.[16,77] However, there is less reproducibility in this determination than for thickness, and when all of the prognostic factors are analyzed in a multifactorial fashion, the level becomes much less important than thickness and ulceration for melanomas thicker than 1 mm. However, among patients with thin (≤1 mm) melanoma, the level of invasion was more predictive of survival outcome than was tumor ulceration.[18,78]

Age

Although older patients have thicker melanomas and a higher incidence of ulcerated melanomas, age is an independent adverse prognostic factor, even after multivariate adjusts for these other factors.[18] There is a consistent and incremental decline in both 5- and 10-year survival rates with each decade increase of age. Many studies have shown that older patients have a lower survival rate, especially those older than 60 years of age.[75,79,80]

LABORATORY AND IMAGING STUDIES

Liver function tests, including LDH, are basic screening tools for metastatic disease. Isolated elevation of the serum alkaline phosphatase or LDH level can be evidence of metastatic disease in the correct clinical setting.[81,82] However, there is no universal agreement among clini-cians at major cancer centers about the utility of the tests for screening for metastases in patients with melanoma.

Extensive routine radiographic evaluation of asymptomatic patients with American Joint Committee on Cancer (AJCC) stage I, II, or III melanomas rarely shows metastases. Routine computed tomography (CT) or positron emission tomography (PET) scans are seldom of practical value. For most asymptomatic patients, a standard chest x-ray provides adequate basic radiologic screening. Patients who have concerning findings on screening history and physical examination or on chest x-ray or liver enzyme tests should undergo further evaluation.

For patients with suspected intra-abdominal or hepatic metastases based on abnormal findings on physical examination or abnormal liver chemistry findings, CT scan of the abdomen should be obtained.[83] Hypervascular metastases of the liver are typically scanned by multiple-phase imaging, including unenhanced phase, hepatic arterial phase, and portal venous phase. Magnetic resonance imaging (MRI) may also be used to detect melanin as manifested by a high signal on T1-weighted images. For specific symptoms or signs of bone disease, x-ray of the bone or a radionuclide bone scan should be obtained. Other than MRI, a bone scan is probably the most sensitive test to detect skeletal metastatic disease, but a careful history and directed radiographs are necessary to ensure that areas of uptake do not represent old trauma or inflammation.[84,85]

PET scans obtained with 2-[18fluorine]-fluoro-2-deoxy-D-glucose (18FDG) are steadily gaining acceptance as a tool for detecting metastatic melanoma and following the effects of therapy. Unlike conventional morphologic imaging, PET scanning is based on metabolic changes that could detect early metastatic disease in high-risk patients. Recent studies of PET with FDG reported a sensitivity of 78% to 100% in detecting metastatic melanoma.[86-88] False-positive findings have been observed in association with inflammatory responses and second primary or metastatic tumors.[86] False-negative scans in the presence of sizeable metastases are rare. Metastases 5 mm or less in diameter may not image well. Wagner and associates[89] reported that the sensitivity of PET with FDG for detection of metastatic melanoma in lymph nodes depends on sufficient tumor volume. PET with FDG begins to reliably detect metastatic tumor in lymph nodes at volumes greater than approximately 80 mm^3, but sensitivity decreases rapidly below this point.

STAGING CLASSIFICATION

The new staging system went into effect in January 2003.[90] The AJCC Melanoma Database consisted of a total of 30,450 patients with melanoma. Of this group, 17,600 patients (58%) had information available for all of the factors required for the proposed TNM classification and stage grouping.[18] Of the 17,600 patients included in this analysis, 12,837 (73%) had at least 5 years of follow-up information, 8633 (49%) had at least 10 years of follow-up, and 2485 (14%) had at least 20 years of follow-up. The data were merged from prospective databases of patients who did not receive any adjuvant systemic therapy and who had all quality control measures in place for data entry, pathology, and surgery. The current melanoma TNM categories are listed in Table 72-1, and the stage groupings are shown in Table 72-2. The 15-year survival curves for patients with stage I to IV melanoma are shown in Figure 72-1. The major changes in the new (2002) version compared with the previous (1997) version of the melanoma staging system are the distinction between clinical and pathologic staging of the regional nodes, the inclusion of information on the number of positive nodes and whether the nodes are microscopically or grossly positive, and the inclusion of histologic ulceration as a necessary part of the staging system.[19]

Clinical Staging

Patients with clinical stage I and II disease have invasive melanoma with no evidence of metastases at either regional or distant sites, based on clinical, radiologic, or

TABLE 72-1

AJCC TNM Definitions

Primary Tumor (T)

Tx: Unable to assess (e.g., shave biopsy or regressed melanoma)
T0: No evidence of primary tumor
Tis: Melanoma in situ
T1: 0.1–1.0 mm thick
  T1a: Without ulceration and level II/III
  T1b: With ulceration or level IV/V
T2: 1.01–2.0 mm thick
  T2a: Without ulceration
  T2b: With ulceration
T3: 2.01–4.0 mm thick
  T3a: Without ulceration
  T3b: With ulceration
T4: >4.0 mm thick
  T4a: Without ulceration
  T4b: With ulceration

Regional Lymph Nodes (N)

Nx: Cannot be assessed
N0: No regional lymph node metastasis
N1: Metastasis in one node
  N1a: Micrometastasis (clinically occult)
  N1b: Macrometastasis (clinically apparent)
N2: Metastasis in two to three nodes or in-transit metastases without nodal metastases
  N2a: Micrometastases
  N2b: Macrometastases
  N2c: In-transit satellite(s) metastasis-without metastasis in nodes
N3: Metastasis in four or more regional nodes, matted nodes, or in-transit metastasis or satellite(s), with metastasis in node(s)

Distant Metastases (M)

Mx: Cannot be assessed
M0: No distant metastasis
M1: Distant metastasis
  M1a: Skin, subcutaneous, or distant lymph node metastases
  M1b: Lung, metastases
  M1c: All other visceral metastases, or distant metastasis at any site with elevated serum lactic dehydrogenase

From AJCC, American Joint Commission on Cancer, AJCC Staging Manual, (6th ed.) New York; Springer, 2002.

TABLE 72-2

AJCC Pathologic Stage Grouping

Stage 0:	TisN0M0
Stage IA:	T1aN0M0
Stage IB:	T1bN0M0
	T2aN0M0
Stage IIA:	T2bN0M0
	T3aN0M0
Stage IIB:	T3bN0M0
	T4aN0M0
Stage IIC:	T4bN0M0
Stage IIIA:	T1–4aN1aM0
	T1–4aN2aM0
Stage IIIB:	T1–4bN1aM0
	T1–4bN2aM0
	T1–4aN1bM0
	T1–4aN2bM0
	T1–4a/bN2cM0
Stage IIIC:	T1–4bN1bM0
	T1–4bN2bM0
	Any T N3M0
Stage IV:	Any T, any N, M1

From AJCC American Joint Commission on Cancer, AJCC Staging Manual, 6th ed. New York; Springer, 2002.

laboratory evaluation. Patients with stage III melanoma have clinical or radiologic evidence of regional metastases in the regional lymph nodes or evidence of intralymphatic satellite or in-transit metastases. Clinical stage III groupings rely on clinical or radiologic assessment of the regional lymph nodes. This assessment is inherently difficult, especially with respect to assessing the presence and number of metastatic nodes. There are therefore no subgroup definitions of clinically staged patients with nodal or intralymphatic regional metastases. They are all categorized as having clinical stage III disease. Patients with clinical stage IV melanoma have metastases at a distant site and are not subgrouped.

Pathologic Staging

In contrast to clinical staging, there is greater accuracy in defining distinctive prognostic subgroups when it is possible to combine pathologic information about the primary melanoma with information about the regional lymph nodes (after sentinel or complete lymphadenectomy). Patients with pathologic stage I and II melanoma have no evidence of regional or distant metastases, based on absence of nodal metastases after careful pathologic examination of the regional lymph nodes and absence of distant metastases based on routine clinical and radiologic examination.

Patients with pathologic stage III melanoma have pathologic evidence of regional metastases, either in the regional lymph nodes or in intralymphatic sites. Quantitative classification of pathologic nodal status requires that pathologists perform a careful examination of the surgically resected nodal basin and report on the number of lymph nodes examined and the number of nodes involved with metastases. Also required is a determination of whether the nodes are microscopically or macroscopi-

Figure 72-1. Fifteen-year survival for stages I, II, III, and IV melanoma. For each curve n = the number of patients in the American Joint Committee on Cancer melanoma database used to calculate rates. Curve differences are all highly significant. (P < 0.0001). (From Balch CM, Buzaid AC, Soong, SJ, et al: Final version of the American Joint Committee on Cancer staging system for cutaneous melanoma. J Clin Oncol 2001;19:3635.)

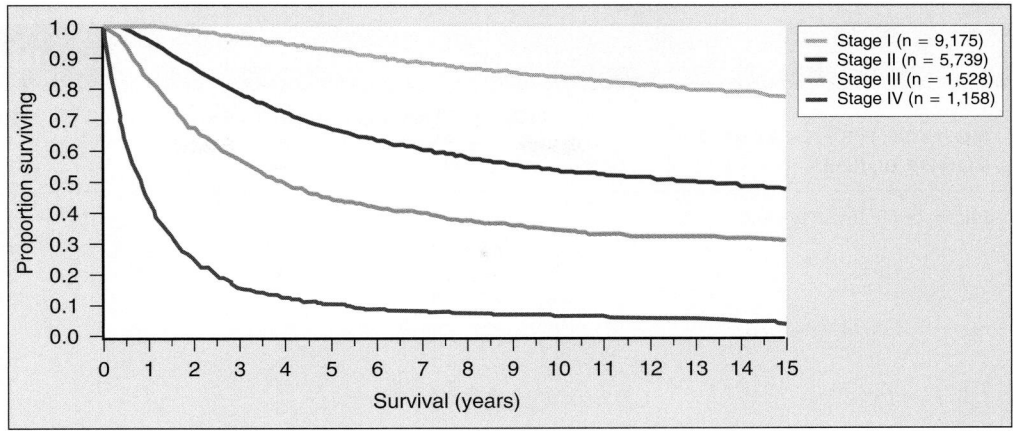

cally involved. Patients with pathologic stage IV melanoma have histologic documentation of metastases at one or more distant sites.

Clinical versus Pathologic Staging

The ability to stage patients more accurately with sentinel node evaluation has had a profound effect on staging, treatment planning, and the conduct of clinical trials of patients with melanoma.[91,92] With the widespread use of sentinel lymphadenectomy, there is considerable stage migration of patients previously staged as "node-negative" when these patients had undetected nodal metastases.[93,94] These patients with previously understaged stage III disease have shown the extraordinary heterogeneity of metastatic risk for stage III melanoma.[18,95] Significant differences were identified in the survival rates of patients with clinically staged melanoma compared with those whose nodal disease was staged pathologically. Survival differences between patients with clinically and pathologically staged disease were statistically significant among all T substages, except T4b. These results highlight the compelling prognostic value of knowing the nodal status as identified by lymphatic mapping and sentinel lymphadenectomy.

TNM Criteria

The primary criteria for the T classification are tumor thickness (measured in millimeters) and the presence of ulceration (determined histopathologically). In the new staging version, the T category thresholds of melanoma thickness are defined in even integers (i.e., 1.0, 2.0, and 4.0 mm), because they represent a statistical "best fit" and are most compatible with current thresholds in clinical decision-making.[73,96-98] A clinically convenient and widely used threshold of 1.0 mm or less is used for T1 melanomas. T2 melanomas are defined as those measuring 1.01 to 2.0 mm thick. T3 melanomas are defined as those 2.01 to 4.0 mm thick, and T4 melanomas are more than 4.0 mm thick. Melanoma ulceration heralds such a high risk for metastases that its presence implies a substantially worse prognosis of all such patients compared with patients with lesions of equivalent thickness without

ulceration. Survival rates for patients with an ulcerated melanoma are remarkably similar to those for patients with nonulcerated melanomas of the next highest T category.[73,99,100] The level of invasion, as defined by Wallace Clark, is an independent prognostic feature of "thin" (T1) melanomas, but not of thicker lesions.[16,18] As a result, the level of invasion is incorporated into the stage grouping definitions of T1 melanomas. In the cohort of T1 melanomas, the assignment of T1a is restricted to patients whose lesions meet three criteria: (1) lesion thickness of 1.0 mm or less; (2) absence of ulceration; and (3) depth of invasion limited to level II or III. T1b melanomas are defined as those with a thickness of 1.0 mm or less and with the more aggressive features of level IV or V, or with ulceration. All T2, T3, and T4 melanomas are defined according to the thickness and ulceration criteria as described previously, but not according to the level of invasion.

The definitions used for clinical and pathologic staging of stage III disease are more complicated than those used for the other stages because of the need to accommodate advances in staging of lymph node metastases. The marked diversity in the natural history of pathologic stage III melanoma is demonstrated by fivefold differences in 5-year survival rates for defined substages, ranging from 69% for patients with a nonulcerated melanoma (regardless of thickness) and a single clinically occult nodal metastasis (detected by sentinel or elective lymphadenectomy) to a low of 13% for patients with an ulcerated melanoma of any thickness and four or more clinically apparent nodal metastases documented by therapeutic lymphadenectomy (Table 72-3).[18]

The stage groupings for pathologic stage III melanoma use four criteria to assign patients with regional metastases to one of three groups, designated as stages IIIA, IIIB, and IIIC. Patients with pathologic stage IIIA disease have three or fewer microscopic (clinically occult) nodal metastases arising from a nonulcerated melanoma (T1-4aN1aM0 and T1-4aN2aM0). The 10-year survival rate for these patients is 60%. There are three subgroups of patients with pathologic stage IIIB disease that have equivalent survival rates: (1) those with three or fewer microscopic (clinically occult) nodes arising from an ulcerated primary melanoma (T1-4bN1aM0 and T1-4bN2aM0);

TABLE 72-3

Five-Year Survival Rates for Patients with Melanoma Who Have Nodal Metastases*

NO. POSITIVE NODES AND TUMOR BURDEN	NONULCERATED PRIMARY LESION		ULCERATED PRIMARY LESION	
	% ± SE	NO.	% ± SE	NO.
Microscopic Involvement				
I	69 ± 3.7	252	52 ± 4.1	217
2–3	63 ± 5.6	130	50 ± 5.7	111
≥4	27 ± 9.3	57	37 ± 8.8	46
Macroscopic Involvement				
I	59 ± 4.7	122	29 ± 5.0	98
2–3	46 ± 5.5	93	25 ± 4.4	109
≥4	27 ± 4.6	109	13 ± 3.5	104

SE, standard error.
*Stratified for nodal tumor burden, number of positive nodes, and ulceration of the primary lesion.
From Balch CM, Soong SJ, Gershenwald JE, et al: Prognostic factors analysis of 17,600 melanoma patients: Validation of the American Joint Committee on Cancer melanoma staging system. J Clin Oncol 2001;19:3622.

(2) those with three or fewer gross metastatic nodes and a nonulcerated primary (T1–4aN1bM0 and T1–4aN2bM0); and (3) those with satellite or in-transit metastases, but no evidence of nodal or distant metastases (T1–4 a/bN2cM0). Patients with stage IIIB disease have a 10-year survival rate of 52% to 54%. Patients with stage IIIC disease include the following groups: (1) those with four or more microscopic metastatic nodes and an ulcerated primary melanoma (T1–4bN2aM0); (2) those with three or more grossly involved nodes and a nonulcerated primary lesion (T1-4aN2bM0 and T1-4aN3M0); and (3) those with any combination of satellite or in-transit metastases and nodal metastases. The estimated 5-year survival rate for patients with stage IIIC disease is significantly lower, at 26%.[19]

In patients with distant metastases, the site (or sites) of metastasis and elevated serum levels of LDH are used to classify the M categories into three groups: M1a, M1b, and M1c. The 1-year survival rates range from 40% to 60%.[18] The site and number of metastases and elevated serum LDH levels are the factors that are most predictive of poor survival.[101-104] Patients with distant metastasis to the skin, subcutaneous tissue, or distant lymph nodes are categorized as M1a. Patients with metastasis to the lung are categorized as M1b, and have an "intermediate" prognosis when comparing 1-year survival rates.[102,105,106] Patients with metastases to all other visceral sites have a relatively worse prognosis, and are designated as M1c. When the serum LDH level is elevated above the upper limits of normal at the time of staging, patients are classified as M1c, regardless of the site of distant metastasis. Because the survival differences between the M categories are small, there are no subgroupings of stage IV melanoma.

PROGNOSIS

Patients with Primary Melanoma

In the multifactorial analysis of 13,581 patients with localized melanoma (either clinically or pathologically), the two most powerful and independent characteristics of the primary melanoma were tumor thickness and ulceration. No other feature of the melanoma or the patient had the predictive capability of these two factors. Other statistically significant prognostic factors were patient age, patient sex, site of the primary melanoma, and level of invasion.[18]

Patients with Regional Metastases

There are four major determinants of outcome for patients with pathologic stage III melanoma: (1) the number of metastatic lymph nodes; (2) the tumor burden, either microscopic (i.e., clinically occult and detected pathologically by sentinel node biopsy or elective lymphadenectomy) or macroscopic (i.e., clinically apparent by physical or radiologic examination and verified pathologically); (3) ulceration of the primary melanoma; and (4) satellite or in-transit metastases.[107-112] Table 72-2 shows the stage groupings for stage III melanoma. Figure 72-2 shows the survival rates for these patients.

Patients with Advanced Disease

In all studies analyzing prognosis in patients with distant metastases using a Cox regression analysis, the site of metastasis, the number of metastatic sites, and elevated serum LDH levels were the factors that were most predictive of poor survival.[113,114]

Site of Metastases

Patients with distant metastasis to the skin, subcutaneous tissue, or distant lymph nodes have a relatively better prognosis compared with patients with metastasis to another anatomic site.[74,113,115] Lung metastases are associated with better prognosis compared with other visceral sites.[18]

Number of Metastases

The number of metastases at distant sites is as an important prognostic factor.[101,102,105] There is significant

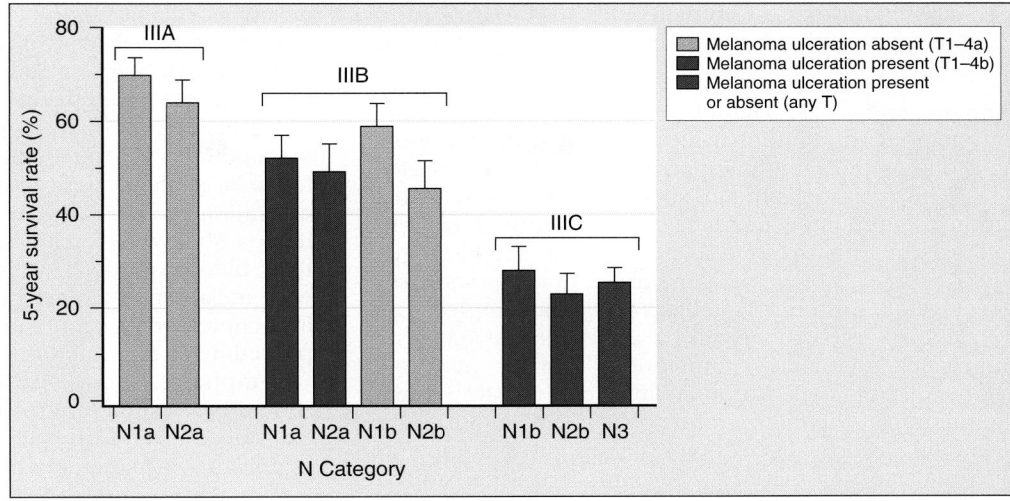

Figure 72-2. Five-year survival rates in the American Joint Committee on Cancer melanoma database showing different stage groupings for stage III melanoma. (From Balch CM, Buzaid AC, Soong SJ, et al: Final version of the American Joint Committee on Cancer staging system for cutaneous melanoma. J Clin Oncol 2001;19:3635.)

variability in the use of diagnostic tests to comprehensively search for distant metastases. Until the indications for testing and the types of tests used are better standardized, the number of metastases cannot reliably be used for staging purposes.

Elevated Lactic Dehydrogenase Level

Elevated serum LDH was among the independent factors most predictive of decreased survival in all published studies, even when the site of metastasis and the number of metastases were considered.[81,105,113,114] When an elevated serum LDH level is detected, the test should be repeated after more than 24 hours, because an elevated serum LDH level on a single determination can be falsely positive secondary to hemolysis or other factors.

PRIMARY TREATMENT

Locoregional Disease

Margins

Every primary melanoma requires wide local excision of the surrounding skin to maximize local control. Although the primary goal of wide excision is to decrease the risk of local and satellite recurrences, cosmesis and function should also be considered. Today, surgical excision is less radical than in most of the last century; the previously routine margins of 5 cm are no longer used. Primary invasive melanoma should be excised with a 1- to 2-cm minimum radial margin of normal-appearing skin around the biopsy site, with the margin determined by the anatomic site and the thickness of the melanoma. The World Health Organization (WHO) Melanoma Group randomized 612 patients with primary melanomas less than 2 mm thick to receive either 1-cm or 3-cm excisional margins. Only four local recurrences occurred, and all of these were in patients with primary melanomas between 1 and 2 mm thick that had been excised with a 1-cm margin. The two randomized groups did not differ significantly in either local recurrence rate or survival rate.[116] Thus a 1-cm margin is recognized as appropriate

for all thin (≤1 mm) melanomas, and is probably sufficient for many melanomas between 1 and 2 mm thick. The Intergroup Melanoma Trial reported a series of 486 patients with intermediate-thickness (1 to 4 mm) primary melanoma randomized to receive wide excision with either 2- or 4-cm margins. With a 15-year follow-up, local recurrence rates were the same in both groups. The 10-year overall survival rate was also the same.[117] The long-term results of the European multicenter trial of 2-cm vs. 5-cm margins for melanoma less than 2.1 mm thick have also shown no difference in local or distant recurrence with a median of 16 years of follow-up.[118]

For intermediate-thickness (1 to 4 mm) melanoma, wide excision with a measured 2-cm margin is appropriate for most patients. However, when melanoma occurs on anatomic sites where excision with a full 2-cm radial margin (e.g., hands and feet) is difficult, the widest possible margin up to 2 cm should used, without compromising function and avoiding a skin graft if possible. No prospective studies have been done to evaluate appropriate margins for thick (>4 mm) melanomas, but margins should be no less than 2 cm. Retrospective studies of patients with thick melanomas suggest that outcomes are similar for patients with margins of 2 cm or greater.[119]

In most cases, wide local excision can be done as an elliptical excision with primary closure. Excision is carried down to a plane between the superficial and the deep (muscular) fascia. Primary closure can often be facilitated by a length-to-width ratio of the ellipse of approximately 3:1 and by undermining the flaps to close the defect with an advancement flap if needed. In areas where the skin edges cannot be approximated primarily, a split-thickness skin graft or a rotational flap can be used to cover the defect. The skin graft donor site should be preferentially chosen outside the area of potential in-transit metastasis.

Difficult Sites

Ear. Primary melanoma of the ear can usually be treated with wedge excision. Primary closure is usually possible with acceptable cosmetic results. Complete amputation is used only for extensive involvement of the ear or for a local recurrence that is not amenable to wedge excision.

Fingers and Toes.

Fingers and Toes. Digital melanoma often requires amputation at the midphalanx proximal to the melanoma and follows the same margin recommendations as other sites. The great toe is the most common site of melanoma of the digits and generally requires amputation at the midproximal phalanx. Sufficient skin and soft tissue can often be saved on the plantar surface to allow soft tissue coverage of the stump. As long as the metatarsophalangeal joint is preserved there will be essentially no functional impairment with this amputation. Primary melanoma of the distal second through fifth toes usually requires amputation at the midproximal phalanx. Melanoma of the distal finger or nail bed typically requires amputation one phalanx proximal to the melanoma. Melanoma of the proximal finger or web space may be managed with soft tissue excision, with preservation of underlying tendon and bone and coverage with a full-thickness skin graft. For optimal preservation of function, patients with melanoma of the hand should be treated by a hand surgeon.

Sole of the Foot.

Sole of the Foot. Primary melanoma on the sole of the foot requires wide local excision down to the plantar fascia, with either skin graft or soft tissue coverage. When primary melanoma occurs on the instep, a split-thickness skin graft may be sufficient. On weight-bearing surfaces, the tendons should be preserved and a myocutaneous free flap can be used to provide optimal coverage.

Management of the Clinically Negative Regional Node Basin

The regional lymph nodes are the most common first site of metastasis of melanoma. The nodal status is of tremendous staging significance and has immediate implications for treatment. Sentinel node biopsy is a minimally invasive method used to evaluate the regional lymph nodes for clinically occult metastases. Sentinel node biopsy is performed based on the belief that metastasis will occur through specific lymphatic channels that involve the sentinel lymph node as the first site of metastasis. If the sentinel lymph node (or nodes) is free of disease, then the remaining (downstream) lymph nodes are likely to be free of metastases as well. In experienced hands, identification rates are greater than 95% and false-negative rates in reported series that included complete dissection are 0% to 2%.[120-122]

The Multicenter Selective Lymphadenectomy Trial is designed to determine whether the routine performance of sentinel node biopsy in patients with melanoma at least 1 mm thick is associated with improved survival compared with nodal observation. Results will not be available for a few more years. However, sentinel node biopsy is an accurate, minimally invasive way to stage patients with melanoma and affords the opportunity to identify node-positive patients at the earliest possible time so that they may be offered appropriate treatment. Sentinel node biopsy is appropriate in patients with newly diagnosed invasive melanoma who have a clinically negative regional node basin and no evidence of distant disease. It should be offered freely to patients with diagnosed primary melanoma 1 mm or deeper if that patient is motivated further treatment should the node be positive. Sentinel node biopsy should also be considered in patients with thin melanomas with poor prognostic features, such as Clark's level IV or V or evidence of ulceration, particularly in younger patients, who may have a somewhat greater risk of having positive nodes than older patients.[123] Clinically node-negative patients with melanoma who are being considered for later entry into clinical trials should undergo a sentinel node staging procedure at the time of primary melanoma excision.

Lymphatic mapping and sentinel node biopsy should be done before (or concurrently with) wide local excision, because the accuracy of the technique was established in patients who have not yet had wide local excision. Accurate detection of the sentinel node depends on mapping the lymphatic drainage from the skin directly next to the melanoma using the coordinated efforts of the surgeon and the nuclear medicine specialist. Radioisotope and blue dye are the two commonly used tracers, and many groups use both. Preoperative lymphoscintigraphy is vital to the success of sentinel node biopsy. All possible node basins should be scanned. With truncal or head and neck primary lesions, drainage often occurs to more than one node basin, and it is important to retrieve the sentinel node(s) from each node basin in which a sentinel node is identified.[120,122] Preoperative lymphoscintigraphy facilitates the identification of sentinel nodes that lie outside traditional node basins or at unexpected sites. Sentinel nodes have occasionally been identified at popliteal and epitrochlear sites and in the triangular intramuscular space in the back, at the supraclavicular fossa, and at internal mammary and paravertebral sites. Any sentinel node that is identified in an easily accessible site should be excised for pathologic review.

The sentinel node should be placed in formalin for permanent fixation. Frozen section analysis is discouraged because it inevitably wastes nodal tissue that might contain micrometastases. It is preferable to save the lymph node intact for permanent processing only, so that multiple sections can be taken with immunohistochemical stains (HMB-45, S-100, Melan-A) to look for microscopic evidence of disease. Immunohistochemical staining increases the node-positive rate by 10% to 12% over staining with hematoxylin and eosin alone.[120,124] In a large series of patients followed after negative findings on sentinel node biopsy, 8 of the 10 who had relapse in a previously mapped node basin had occult disease in the original sentinel node as shown by serial sectioning or immunohistochemical staining.[125] The risk of histologic node positivity is related to the thickness of the primary melanoma. In patients with lesions less than 0.76 mm thick, the chance of finding a positive sentinel node is minimal. For melanomas 0.76 to 1 mm thick, the chance of finding a metastatic sentinel node is 5% to 6%. For melanomas 1.1 to 1.5 mm thick, the chance is 7% to 8%. For melanomas 1.5 to 4.0 mm thick, the chance is 18% to 19%. For melanomas 4 mm or thicker, however, the chance is 29% to 34%.[122]

A number of groups have investigated the use of polymerase chain reaction (PCR) techniques for submicroscopic evaluation of sentinel nodes.[126,127] PCR for tyrosinase alone can be positive in the presence of cells other than melanoma, such as benign nevocytes and Schwann cells. The use of multiple markers may improve the specificity of PCR evaluation of sentinel nodes. The significance of sentinel nodes that are histologically and immunohistochemically negative, but positive by PCR, is being evaluated, and any conclusion on the routine use of this technique must await further research results.

If the sentinel node contains evidence of metastatic disease by routine histology, the patient must return for complete lymph node dissection and consideration of systemic adjuvant therapy. The treatment of patients with only PCR evidence of metastases is controversial and is the subject of ongoing trials, including the Sunbelt Melanoma Trial. Most patients today have a histologically negative sentinel node and are at lower risk of locoregional and systemic recurrence compared with patients with a positive sentinel node. Long-term recurrence rates are still being studied. However, with follow-up over several years, patients with a negative sentinel node appear to have a 2% to 6% risk of subsequent disease recurrence in the same node basin and therefore must remain in routine follow-up for the possibility of locoregional and distant recurrence.[128-130]

Management of Regional Nodal Metastases

Radical lymphadenectomy is standard treatment for all patients with regional nodal metastases. The goals of surgery include regional control of disease and improved survival. Patients who require lymphadenectomy include those who have histologically positive sentinel nodes and

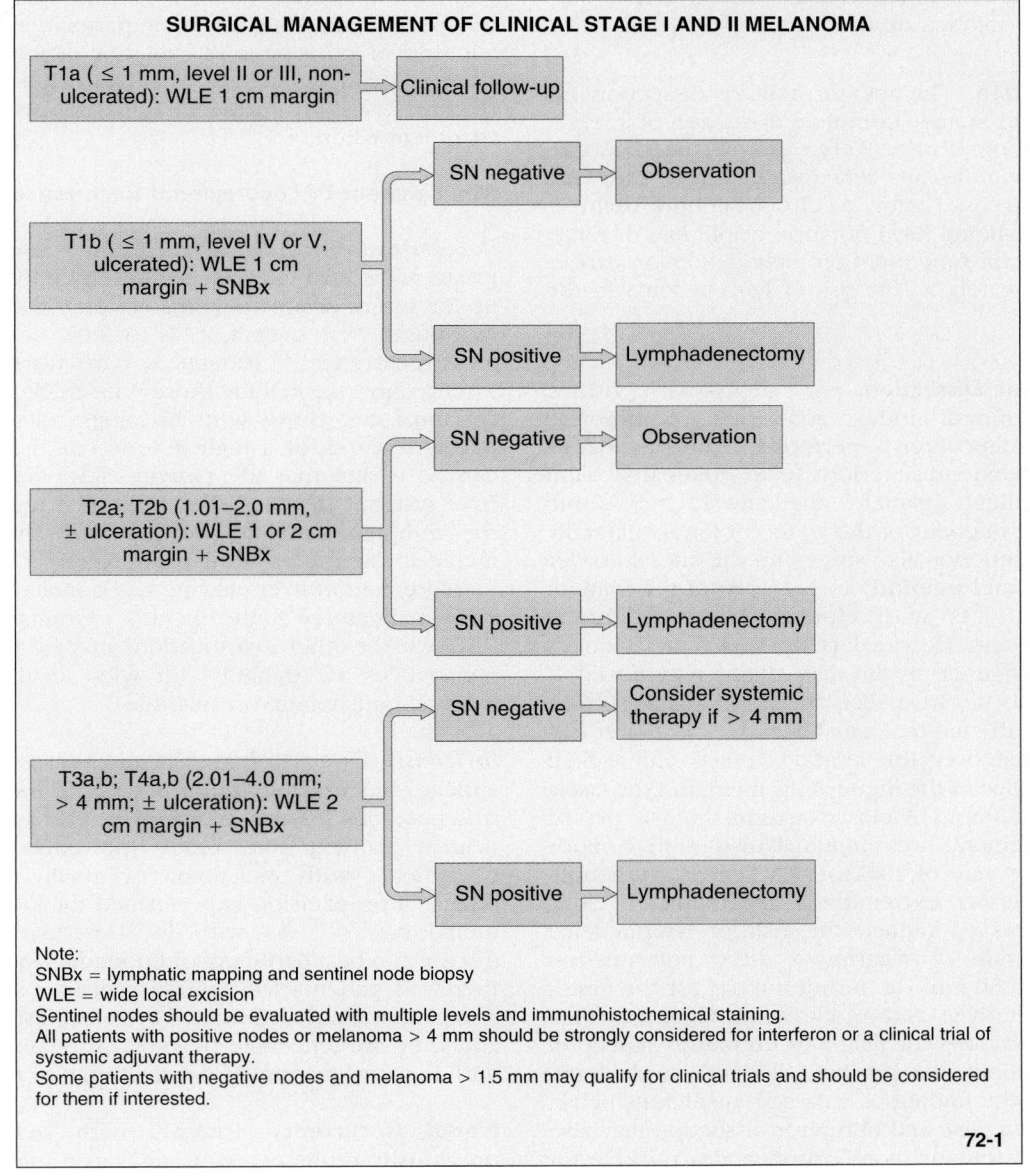

SURGICAL MANAGEMENT OF CLINICAL STAGE I AND II MELANOMA

T1a (≤ 1 mm, level II or III, non-ulcerated): WLE 1 cm margin → Clinical follow-up

T1b (≤ 1 mm, level IV or V, ulcerated): WLE 1 cm margin + SNBx
- SN negative → Observation
- SN positive → Lymphadenectomy

T2a; T2b (1.01–2.0 mm, ± ulceration): WLE 1 or 2 cm margin + SNBx
- SN negative → Observation
- SN positive → Lymphadenectomy

T3a,b; T4a,b (2.01–4.0 mm; > 4 mm; ± ulceration): WLE 2 cm margin + SNBx
- SN negative → Consider systemic therapy if > 4 mm
- SN positive → Lymphadenectomy

Note:
SNBx = lymphatic mapping and sentinel node biopsy
WLE = wide local excision
Sentinel nodes should be evaluated with multiple levels and immunohistochemical staining.
All patients with positive nodes or melanoma > 4 mm should be strongly considered for interferon or a clinical trial of systemic adjuvant therapy.
Some patients with negative nodes and melanoma > 1.5 mm may qualify for clinical trials and should be considered for them if interested.

72-1

those with clinically positive (and pathologically proven) regional nodes, with or without a history of melanoma. Any patient with clinically suspicious nodes should be evaluated with fine-needle aspiration if possible, followed by excisional biopsy if the results of fine-needle aspiration are indeterminate. Patients with biopsy-proven bulky nodal disease should be evaluated with baseline CT scans, a complete blood count, and measurement of liver enzymes, including LDH. Before the introduction of sentinel node biopsy and adjuvant therapy, patients with a single positive node who underwent complete node dissection had approximately a 40% chance of being alive and apparently free of disease at 10 years.[131] Patients with a single clinically occult or microscopic nodal metastasis detected by sentinel node biopsy have a 5-year survival rate of nearly 70%.[18]

As a general principle, lymphadenectomy should be anatomic. The nodal contents are excised in a single block of tissue within their surrounding fatty tissue, preserving motor nerves and muscle whenever possible. Perioperative antibiotics are used routinely.

Axillary Dissection. Therapeutic axillary dissection for melanoma should include complete dissection of levels I, II, and III. The long thoracic nerve and the thoracodorsal neurovascular bundle are left intact unless they are directly invaded by tumor. A closed-suction drain is placed. Patients should have no appreciable loss of range of motion or motor function. Complete dissection carries with it approximately a 10% risk of lymphedema in the upper extremity.

Inguinal and Iliac Dissection. For patients with positive inguinal or femoral nodes, anatomically complete inguinofemoral dissection is performed. The boundaries of the dissection extend superiorly to approximately 6 cm above the inguinal ligament, medially to the pubic tubercle and the midbelly of the adductor longus, laterally to the anterior superior iliac spine and the lateral border of the sartorius, and inferiorly to the apex of the femoral triangle. In patients with clinically detected nodal metastases, the femoral canal is opened and Cloquet's node (the lowest node in the iliac chain) is removed. If Cloquet's node is negative, iliac and obturator dissection is not done and the femoral canal is closed. The sartorius muscle is rotated over the femoral vessels and tacked in place to the edge of the inguinal ligament and the fascia of the adductor longus. A closed-suction drain is placed in the inguinofemoral area. Inguinal dissection wounds have an infection rate of 10% to 15%. The risk of lymphedema of the lower extremity is approximately 20%. Routine measures to reduce the risk of lymphedema include a program of wearing a fitted compression garment at 20 to 30 mm Hg during the day for the first 6 months postoperatively and leg elevation when possible.

Absolute indications for iliac and obturator dissection include the finding of a positive Cloquet's node intraoperatively and the finding of enlarged, suspicious pelvic nodes on CT scan. Iliac and obturator dissection may also be considered if four or more lymph nodes positive for

disease are found at the inguinofemoral level. The boundaries of the dissection are from the inguinal ligament inferiorly to the bifurcation of the common iliac vessels superiorly and to the obturator vessels medially.

Cervical Dissection. The extent of cervical lymphadenectomy depends on the location of the positive node and the presence of direct invasion into the structures of the neck. When a positive sentinel node is found, usually a functional neck dissection preserving the internal jugular vein, spinal accessory nerve, and sternocleidomastoid is appropriate. These structures should be sacrificed only if they are directly invaded by tumor.

Radiation Therapy. The risk of regional recurrence can sometimes be lowered by judicious use of radiation therapy in selected patients at particularly high risk, such as those with four or more positive nodes or nodal disease with extracapsular extension. Although there are no prospective studies showing superior outcome with the addition of postoperative radiation, a few retrospective studies strongly suggest that radiation may improve regional control in patients at particularly high risk for treatment failure.[132-134]

Management of Locoregional Recurrence

Local Recurrence. Local recurrence rates after appropriate wide local excision are low. With long-term follow-up of intermediate-thickness lesions in the Intergroup Melanoma Trial, overall, 2.1% to 2.6% of patients had a local recurrence.[117] Patients at particularly high risk for local recurrence include those with thick primary lesions (≥4 mm) and those with histologic ulceration, desmoplastic features, or a high mitotic rate. Local recurrence can be a sign that the patient either has or soon will have systemic disease. When local recurrence is detected, the minimal systemic workup that should be done includes careful physical examination, chest x-ray, and measurement of liver enzyme levels including LDH. If any abnormalities are found by this examination, CT scans, PET scan, or other investigations may be indicated. Local recurrences are treated with wide local excision with 1-cm margins whenever possible.

In-Transit Disease. In-transit metastases of melanoma appear as identifiable tumor nodules in the subcutaneous or cutaneous tissues between a primary site and its nearest draining node basin. Approximately 2% to 4% of patients with melanoma eventually have in-transit disease after excision is performed for localized primary melanoma.[135,136] As with local recurrence, in-transit disease can be a harbinger of impending systemic disease; therefore, patients with in-transit disease should undergo a staging evaluation. If limited in-transit lesions are present and they are amenable to excision, wide local excision with negative margins is the treatment of choice.

Nodal Recurrence. Patients with recurrence in a previously undissected node basin should undergo evaluation and complete node dissection, as described previously. Recurrence in previously dissected basin should be evaluated with a staging workup, including CT scans and measurement of liver enzymes, including LDH, and should undergo wide excision of the area of recurrence. Adjuvant radiation therapy can be considered as well.

Isolated Limb Perfusion. The indications for isolated limb perfusion in melanoma are limited. Limb perfusion with hyperthermia and melphalan has never been shown to be associated with improved survival, but has a role in securing local and regional control for patients with unresectable local recurrence or a large volume of in-transit disease. Still under study is the addition of tumor necrosis factor, which in some studies shows a suggestion of improved disease response.[137] However, the risk of regional toxicity is significant; isolated limb perfusion should be performed only in centers with experience with the technique, preferably in the setting of a clinical trial.[138] A technique of isolated limb infusion has been reported that is technically simpler and has reported responses similar to those of melphalan infusion.[139]

Systemic Adjuvant Therapy

The recently revised AJCC staging system for melanoma allows us to predict more accurately than ever an individual's chance of survival. Patients can be identified who have relapse rates of 50% or more.[90] Trials of adjuvant therapies for high-risk patients have been largely unsuccessful.[140] In 1996, based on a randomized trial showing a survival benefit of 1 year, high-dose interferon-alfa was approved by the U.S. Food and Drug Administration (FDA) as adjuvant therapy for patients with resected stage IIB (≥4 mm primary) or stage III (regional lymph node involvement) disease.[141] Subsequent randomized trials of high-dose interferon-alfa have shown a consistent disease-free survival benefit, but a less clear

SYSTEMIC TREATMENT

ADJUVANT THERAPY

Patients with primary melanoma 4 mm or thicker or with regional lymph node involvement should be considered for treatment with high-dose interferon after appropriate surgery because it is the only adjuvant treatment shown to improve disease-free survival and possibly overall survival. These patients may be offered enrollment in clinical trials of adjuvant therapies, either in a phase II setting or in a phase III trial with interferon or observation as a control. Standard therapy for patients with resected melanoma thinner than 4 mm and pathologically negative regional lymph nodes remains observation only. However, patients with ulcerated primary lesions thicker than 2 mm might be considered for high-dose interferon or a clinical trial, because their survival rate approaches 50%. Some adjuvant clinical trials enroll patients with melanoma as thin as 1.5 mm.

TREATMENT OF ADVANCED DISEASE

Because there is really no standard therapy for patients with metastatic melanoma, all patients should be considered for clinical trials. Patients with ECOG performance status of 0 and normal heart, lung, and kidney function should be offered high-dose IL-2, preferably in a high-dose IL-2–based clinical trials, because this therapy offers a 5% chance of achieving durable remission. Patients who do not meet the criteria for high-dose IL-2 therapy can be considered for clinical trials of less toxic new treatments. Patients without access to a trial can be offered either DTIC, with or without tamoxifen, or temozolomide, with or without thalidomide. Combination chemotherapy, such as Dartmouth or CVD, offers a slightly better chance of achieving durable remission than DTIC alone, and that biochemotherapy offers a slightly better chance of achieving durable remission than combination chemotherapy; however, patients must understand that this approach is unproven, and the chance of achieving durable remission with any of these treatment options is small.

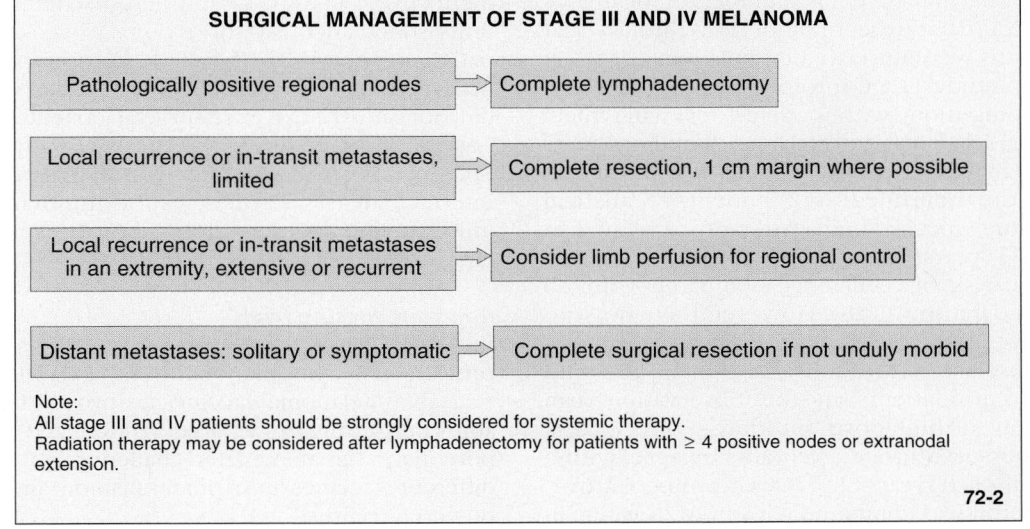

SURGICAL MANAGEMENT OF STAGE III AND IV MELANOMA

Pathologically positive regional nodes ⇒ Complete lymphadenectomy

Local recurrence or in-transit metastases, limited ⇒ Complete resection, 1 cm margin where possible

Local recurrence or in-transit metastases in an extremity, extensive or recurrent ⇒ Consider limb perfusion for regional control

Distant metastases: solitary or symptomatic ⇒ Complete surgical resection if not unduly morbid

Note:
All stage III and IV patients should be strongly considered for systemic therapy.
Radiation therapy may be considered after lymphadenectomy for patients with ≥ 4 positive nodes or extranodal extension.

72-2

overall survival benefit[142,143] The use of high-dose interferon remains controversial. A number of vaccines are in clinical trials for high-risk patients, but none have improved overall survival rates.

Early Adjuvant Therapy Trials

A variety of chemotherapeutic agents, including dacarbazine (DTIC)[144] and carmustine (BCNU),[145] showed no benefit in the adjuvant setting. The biologic agents Bacillus Calmette-Guérin[146] and interferon-gamma[147] did not improve survival in high-risk postoperative patients. A small, prospective, randomized study showed a survival benefit for patients who took megestrol acetate compared with control subjects.[148] One of four randomized studies of levamisole hydrochloride showed a survival benefit for patients in the treatment arm.[149] Nathan and Mastrangelo[140] published a comprehensive review of adjuvant therapy for melanoma through 1995.

High-Dose Interferon-Alfa-2b.

Three large published randomized trials evaluated 1 year of treatment with high-dose interferon-alfa-2b in high-risk patients. All three studies were conducted under the auspices of the Eastern Cooperative Oncology Group (ECOG). All defined high-risk patients as those with primary melanomas at least 4 mm thick or with regional lymph node involvement. The high-dose interferon dose schedule was the same in all three studies: interferon-alfa-2b, 20 million units/m^2 intravenously, Monday through Friday for 4 weeks, followed by 10 million units/m^2 subcutaneously, three times weekly for the remaining 11 months. In ECOG protocol 1684, the first trial, 287 patients were randomized to receive high-dose interferon or to receive no treatment after wide excision and regional lymph node dissection. In 1996, a statistically significant disease-free survival benefit (1.72 years vs. 0.98 years) and an overall survival benefit (3.82 years vs. 2.78 years) were seen in the interferon arm, at a median follow-up of 6.9 years.[141] The FDA then approved high-dose interferon for high-risk patients, as defined in this study. However, at a median follow-up of 12.6 years, the disease-free survival benefit persisted, but the overall survival benefit did not, with both arms now having an equal number of deaths.[150] Long-term survival data are confounded by the fact that many of the deaths were unrelated to melanoma.

The follow-up study, ECOG protocol 1690, involved a three-way randomization, with patients receiving high-dose interferon, low-dose interferon (3 million units subcutaneously three times a week for 2 years), or no therapy. The study enrolled 642 patients. Statistical analysis in this study focused on hazard ratios. At a median follow-up of 4.3 years, high-dose interferon led to a reduction in the risk of recurrence compared with no treatment (hazard ratio = 1.28). However, there was no difference in overall survival at 5 years, with a rate of 52% for high-dose interferon and a rate of 55% for no treatment.[143] Some patients in the observation arm eventually received high-dose interferon and had a surprisingly good survival rate, even after relapse, with a median survival of 6 years. In ECOG protocol 1694, high-dose interferon was compared with a GM2 vaccine in

the same defined patient population (primary lesion ≥4 mm thick or regional lymph node involvement), and 880 patients were enrolled. The Data Safety Monitoring Committee stopped the study early, and at a median follow-up of 16 months, a statistically significant disease-free survival benefit (hazard ratio = 1.47) and an overall survival benefit (hazard ratio = 1.52) were noted for the high-dose interferon arm. The estimated disease-free survival rate at 2 years for the patients receiving interferon was superior (62% vs. 49%), as was overall survival (78% vs. 73%).[142] Because there was no observation arm, it is impossible to know whether the vaccine was inferior or equivalent to no therapy. However, the fact that the survival curves were similar in the early portions of ECOG protocol 1684 (high-dose interferon vs. observation) and ECOG protocol 1694 (high-dose interferon vs. vaccine) supports the latter conclusion.

High-dose interferon is associated with a number of potential toxicities that necessitate dose reduction in approximately 75% of patients. Side effects include fatigue, anorexia, flulike symptoms, depression, liver abnormalities, and cytopenia. Patients require frequent blood draws, weekly for 4 weeks, and then monthly.[141] The treatment is expensive, and many insurers do not reimburse for home subcutaneous administration. Many patients are not candidates for high-dose interferon because of age or comorbid conditions.

The results of studies of high-dose interferon have generated much controversy.[150-152] Since the FDA approval of high-dose interferon in 1996, the treatment regimen has not been widely embraced by U.S. medical oncologists and has not been accepted at all by European practitioners.[150] There is a consistent disease-free survival benefit in all three studies that cannot be denied. However, the overall survival benefit faded in ECOG protocol 1684 and was never seen in ECOG protocol 1690. In ECOG protocol 1694, there is a survival benefit, but the follow-up time is still short.

Other Interferon Schedules.

A number of other interferon schedules have been evaluated in the adjuvant setting. High-dose interferon given for 3 months was ineffective.[153] Low-dose interferon schedules of 3 million units subcutaneously three times a week for 3 years for patients with stage III disease,[154] or for 18 months for patients with primary melanomas thicker than 1.5 mm,[155] did not show an overall survival benefit compared with observation. The European Organization for Research and Treatment of Cancer (EORTC) is currently studying intermediate-dose schedules of interferon, 10 million units subcutaneously three times a week for 12 or 24 months.[150]

Adjuvant Vaccine Trials

Increasing numbers of melanoma vaccines are in preclinical development and in phase I, II, and III clinical trials. No melanoma vaccine has proven beneficial in the adjuvant setting in a large randomized trial, but their potential is great. A major challenge is to test the many different vaccines in a timely fashion and in adequately powered trials.

Canvaxin (CancerVax, Carlsbad, CA) is an allogeneic whole-cell vaccine composed of three highly antigenic, irradiated melanoma cell lines. In a phase II trial, CancerVax appeared to improve survival compared with historical controls.[156] AVAX (AVAX Technologies, Philadelphia, PA), an autologous whole-cell melanoma vaccine modified by the hapten dinitrophenol and then irradiated, also improved survival in patients with stage III disease compared with historical control subjects.[157] Both of these vaccines are now in phase III trials.

Phase III Vaccine Trials. A small number of phase III vaccine trials have been completed. A vaccinia melanoma oncolysate vaccine did not improve outcome in patients with stage III melanoma.[158] In a large randomized trial, a vaccinia viral lysate of melanoma showed no benefit in patients with melanomas thicker than 4 mm or with regional lymph node involvement.[159] Melacine (Corixa Corp., Seattle, WA), a cell-lysate vaccine, was compared with observation by the Southwest Oncology Group (SWOG) in patients with melanomas 1.5 to 4 mm thick without lymph node involvement. No disease-free survival benefit was seen.[160] However, in a retrospective analysis, vaccinated patients who were positive for HLA-A2 or C3 had a disease-free survival rate of 77% compared with 64% for those who were observed.[161] In a study by Bystryn and colleagues,[162] polyvalent shed-antigen vaccine showed a survival benefit in a very small phase III trial that involved 38 patients with stage III disease, using a 2:1 randomization scheme. In ECOG protocol 1694, which was discussed earlier, the GM2 ganglioside vaccine was inferior to high-dose interferon at a relatively short median follow-up. This was a large, well-powered trial.[142] However, because there was no observation arm, it is impossible to know whether this ganglioside vaccine was equivalent to observation, or somehow detrimental to the patient.

Granulocyte-Macrophage Colony-Stimulating Factor

Granulocyte-macrophage colony-stimulating factor (GM-CSF) is a colony-stimulating factor approved by the FDA to speed neutrophil recovery after chemotherapy. It also promotes melanoma antigen presentation through activation of macrophages, monocytes, and dendritic cells.[163] GM-CSF was studied in 48 high-risk patients with melanoma (stage III with >4 positive lymph nodes or surgically resected stage IV with no evidence of disease). Their outcome was much better than that of historical control subjects. The median survival was 37.5 months for treated patients compared with 12.2 months for matched historical control subjects.[164] GM-CSF is now in phase III adjuvant therapy trials, either alone or with other immune modulators for patients with surgically resected stage IV melanoma and no evidence of disease. Some patients with stage IV melanoma who are disease-free after surgery do well and are good candidates for adjuvant therapy trials.[165]

Adjuvant Biochemotherapy

With the initial success of biochemotherapy in advanced disease,[166] it seemed logical to design a trial for the high-risk adjuvant setting. Intergroup trial S0008 is comparing three cycles of biochemotherapy with 1 year of high-dose interferon administration in very-high-risk patients with stage III disease (ulcerated primary lesion with regional lymph node involvement, grossly involved or clinically palpable nodes, matted nodes, two or more involved nodes, or satellite lesions). The study is open to accrual, although the disappointing, recently released data on biochemotherapy in patients with stage IV disease[167] casts doubt on the utility of this intensive, toxic approach in stage III disease.

Management of Advanced Disease

Diagnosis and Evaluation

When metastatic disease is suspected, the diagnosis should be pathologically confirmed whenever possible, because this knowledge drastically changes the prognosis and recommendations for appropriate therapy. Often this can be accomplished with a minimally invasive procedure, such as excisional biopsy, fine-needle aspiration, or core biopsy. Routine staining of the pathology slides plus immunohistochemical staining with S100, HMB-45, and Melan-A, if needed, should confirm the diagnosis of melanoma and differentiate it from other malignancies. In the rare circumstance in which it is necessary to differentiate clear cell sarcoma from melanoma, the presence of the t(12;22)(13;q13) translocation can be used to confirm the diagnosis of melanoma. Patients should be fully staged with appropriate imaging studies before therapy is initiated. All patients should undergo MRI scan of the brain, and CT scans of the chest, abdomen, and pelvis should be obtained. A PET scan is useful in clarifying questionable CT findings; its role as a primary staging study is being evaluated. Patients with bony symptoms should have a bone scan or plain x-rays.

Role of Surgery in Advanced Melanoma

Because highly effective chemotherapy is not available, surgery can be an effective palliative treatment for isolated metastases. Surgical excision of isolated metastatic melanoma can provide quick and effective palliation and in some cases long-term survival (>5 to 10 years).[168-170] Surgical candidates should be carefully selected. Surgery should be used only in cases of accessible lesions and when the risk of perioperative morbidity is acceptable. Isolated visceral metastases, especially brain and some lung metastases, are amenable to surgical therapy. The same is true for both symptomatic and asymptomatic gastrointestinal metastases and for many lesions in the skin, subcutaneous tissues, or distant lymph nodes. Liver metastases are associated with such a short survival time (2 to 4 months) that excision is usually not indicated.

Chemotherapy

DTIC as a single agent has been studied extensively in metastatic melanoma. In early studies by the Central Oncology Group (COG), DTIC had an overall response rate of 20%, with 5% of patients achieving complete responses.[171] Most of the patients responding to this treatment had nodal or cutaneous metastasis. Subsequent randomized studies showed objective response rates of

5% to 20%.[171,172] With modern antiemetic agents, DTIC is very well tolerated. Although multiple dosage schedules have been studied, 800 to 1000 mg/m^2 IV over 1 hour every 3 to 4 weeks is very convenient and at least as effective as any other schedule.[172] Unfortunately, DTIC has not been proven to provide a survival benefit compared with supportive care or other treatments. Temozolomide is an oral agent that was recently approved in the United States for the treatment of primary brain tumors, but not for melanoma. It can be thought of as DTIC in oral form, with much better central nervous system (CNS) penetration. In a phase II trial, temozolomide at a dose of 150 to 200 mg/m^2 PO on days 1 to 5 in a 28-day cycle had similar activity to DTIC, with a complete response rate of 5% and an overall response rate of 21%, with some responses in the CNS.[173] In a head-to-head comparison, the survival rates were similar (6.4 months for DTIC and 7.7 months for temozolomide).[174] Both agents are well tolerated and relatively convenient. The oral administration route for temozolomide is attractive to patients, but without FDA approval, it is not always adequately reimbursed by insurance. Temozolomide may be useful in small daily doses as a radiosensitizer when external beam radiation to the CNS is indicated.[175]

A long list of chemotherapeutic agents has shown low levels of activity in metastatic melanoma. These include the platinum coordination compound cisplatin[176] and carboplatin,[177] BCNU,[178] vindesine,[179] paclitaxel,[180] docetaxel,[181] and vinorelbine.[182] None has been shown to be superior as a single agent compared with DTIC in efficacy or in its toxicity profile. Two-drug combinations have not yet yielded superior results to single-agent DTIC. A small, randomized trial comparing DTIC with DTIC plus tamoxifen showed almost a doubling of the response rate with the addition of tamoxifen.[183] This result, however, was not confirmed in a follow-up study.[184] A three-drug combination of cisplatin, vinblastine (Velban), and DTIC showed encouraging early results in a phase III trial comparing the combination with single-agent DTIC,[185] but unpublished follow-up data showed no advantage to the combination.

Two combination chemotherapy regimens, BOLD and Dartmouth, showed great promise in the treatment of metastatic disease and became quite popular among clinicians during the 1980s and early 1990s. The BOLD regimen combined bleomycin, vincristine, lomustine, and DTIC. In a phase II trial, the objective response rate was greater than 40%.[186] However, in a phase III study, the response rate dropped down to the single digits and the regimen fell out of favor. In several single-institution studies of the Dartmouth regimen, which combined three alkylating agents (DTIC, BCNU, and cisplatin) with the antiestrogen agent tamoxifen, very high response rates of greater than 50% were consistently reported.[187] Of interest, in a single-institution study, when tamoxifen was removed from the regimen to minimize the risk of deep vein thrombosis, the response rate dropped precipitously.[188] However, in a randomized trial under the auspices of the National Cancer Institute of Canada, which compared the Dartmouth regimen with the Dartmouth regimen minus tamoxifen, there was no survival advantage with the addition of tamoxifen.[189] There were more objective responses in the tamoxifen group, particularly patients who would now be categorized as M1a. In an Intergroup study led by investigators at Memorial Sloan-Kettering Cancer Center, the Dartmouth regimen was compared with single-agent DTIC. In this large randomized study, there was no survival benefit seen with the Dartmouth regimen, although again there were more objective responses in the combination chemotherapy arm.[172] In a randomized trial comparing the Dartmouth regimen with Melacine (a melanoma cell-lysate vaccine) alone, the survival rate was equally poor in both regimens, although the vaccine was much less toxic than the Dartmouth regimen.[190]

Immunotherapy

Since the early 1980s, two biologic therapy agents, interferon-alfa (2a and 2b) and interleukin-2 (IL-2) have been extensively studied in patients with metastatic melanoma. In multiple studies of single-agent interferon-alfa in metastatic melanoma, the objective response rate was approximately 15%. With single-agent interferon, there are very few complete responses and a survival benefit has never been demonstrated. Most responses are in patients with soft tissue or lymph node involvement (M1a).[191,192] Higher, more toxic doses appear more active, but low, nontoxic doses (1 to 3 μm/m^2 subcutaneously) appear inactive in the metastatic setting.[192] There is no randomized clinical study showing a survival benefit when interferon is added to any single agent, such as DTIC[184] or IL-2,[193] or to any combination therapy regimen, including the BOLD[194] and Dartmouth regimens.[195]

IL-2, originally known as T-cell-derived growth factor, was first reported by Rosenberg and associates to have significant response rates in metastatic melanoma when given at high doses.[196] Its mechanism of action remains unclear; it activates several types of immune effector cells, including lymphokine-activated killer cells, natural killer cells, B and T lymphocytes, and macrophages. Its principal antimelanoma activity is believed to be mediated by the activation of melanoma-specific cytotoxic T cells.[197]

High-dose IL-2 has been extensively studied in metastatic melanoma. Two large series have been published using the high-dose schedule of 600,000 to 720,000 units/kg IV every 8 hours for 14 doses, originally described by Rosenberg and associates.[196] The National Cancer Institute reported an overall response rate of 18% and a complete response rate of 5%, with some of the responses being quite durable.[198] Similar results were reported by Atkins and associates[199] in 270 patients with metastatic melanoma. Of the 270 patients, 6% achieved complete responses and another 10% obtained partial responses. The striking finding in both studies was that some of the responses were very durable, with responses in some cases maintained for longer than 120 months. Adoptive immunotherapy with lymphokine-activated killer cells does not appear to improve the response rate seen with high-dose IL-2 alone.[200] The response rate with tumor-infiltrating lymphocytes and IL-2 was reported to be 40%, but this has not been confirmed in a phase III trial.[201]

High-dose IL-2 can cause substantial toxicity. The patient must be hospitalized for administration of the drug and subsequent close monitoring. Major side effects include fluid retention, renal failure, myocardial ischemia, and neurologic changes. Patients with underlying cardiac, renal, or pulmonary disease are not candidates for high-dose IL-2 therapy.[202] Patients with any risk factors for cardiac disease should have a normal cardiac stress thallium study before receiving high-dose IL-2. Many low-dose, alternative IL-2 regimens have been evaluated, including low-dose bolus administration, continuous infusion, and subcutaneous administration. Although these regimens are associated with less toxicity, none has shown a significant objective response rate and none has provided long-term remission. Polyethylene glycol modified–IL-2[203] and liposomal IL-2[204] have not shown any substantial clinical benefit.

Based on the in vitro synergy between IL-2 and interferon-alfa in metastatic melanoma, several clinical trials have been conducted combining the two agents. Activity was seen only with doses of IL-2 that required inpatient administration.[193] The hope that combined therapy with relatively nontoxic, low-dose, outpatient IL-2 and interferon would yield significant clinical activity in metastatic melanoma has not been realized.

Biochemotherapy

In the early 1990s, several investigators began to study intensive regimens that included combination chemotherapy and the biologic agents interferon and IL-2. Single-institution studies showed significant objective response rates. Richards and colleagues[205] combined BCNU, cisplatin, and DTIC with high-dose IL-2 and interferon in a sequential fashion and obtained an overall response rate of 55% and a complete response rate of 14%. Legha and colleagues[166] combined the cisplatin, vinblastine, and DTIC (CVD) chemotherapy regimen with continuous-infusion IL-2 and subcutaneous interferon, first sequentially, and then in a combined regimen, with all of the drugs given over a 5-day period and the cycle repeated every 3 weeks. The combined regimen consisted of cisplatin, 20 mg/m² IV on days 1 through 4; vinblastine, 1.5 mg/m² IV on days 1 through 4; DTIC, 800 mg/m² IV on day 1 only; IL-2, 9 million units/m² daily by continuous infusion on days 1 through 4; interferon, 5 million units/m² subcutaneously on days 1 through 5, and on days 7, 9, 11, and 13; and was repeated every 21 days. The authors reported an overall response rate of 64% and a complete response rate of 21%. The combined regimen seemed as active as the more protracted sequential regimen.

Two large single-institution randomized phase III studies have been reported comparing combination chemotherapy with biochemotherapy. The National Cancer Institute Surgery Branch compared a regimen of cisplatin, DTIC, and tamoxifen with the same regimen followed immediately by high-dose IL-2 and interferon. The overall response rate was higher in the biochemotherapy arm, but median survival was superior in the chemotherapy arm (15.8 vs. 10.7 months).[206] At M.D. Anderson Hospital, CVD was compared with CVD plus IL-2 and interferon given sequentially. The overall response rate and median survival rate were superior in the biochemotherapy arm (48% vs. 25% and 11.8 months vs. 9.5 months, respectively).[207]

The encouraging results reported in these studies led to a large randomized Intergroup study led by ECOG, Intergroup trial 3695.[167] This study compared CVD with the combined CVD, IL-2, and interferon regimen of Legha,[166] with several modifications, including reducing the dose of vinblastine by 25%, using prophylactic G-CSF, and limiting the number of chemotherapy cycles to four. This modified Legha biochemotherapy regimen was studied in a phase II trial and yielded an objective response rate of 48% and a complete response rate of 20% in 40 patients.[208] Intergroup trial 3695 was recently presented in abstract form. Between 1998 and 2002, the authors enrolled 416 patients. The patients could have no previous chemotherapy or treatment with IL-2. Sixty percent of the patients had received high-dose interferon before the development of metastatic disease and enrollment in the trial. The overall response rate was 17.1% in the biochemotherapy arm vs. 11.4% in the chemotherapy arm. Complete response rates were 3% in the biochemotherapy arm and 1.4% in the chemotherapy arm. Overall survival was equally poor in both arms, 8.7 months for biochemotherapy vs. 8.4 months for chemotherapy.[167]

The results of this large, well-done, randomized trial were obviously very disappointing. It may be that the reduction in the vinblastine dose and the lack of familiarity by physicians and nurses with the complex biochemotherapy regimen contributed to the low response rates in the cooperative group setting. However, the results show that biochemotherapy, as given in this trial, leads to very few durable responses and should not be considered a standard therapy. It is possible that when this study is published with a more detailed analysis, subsets of patients may be identified who are more likely to benefit from biochemotherapy, such as those who have an excellent performance status, low-volume disease, or no previous treatment with interferon. It seems unlikely that any variation of biochemotherapy currently being evaluated will prove superior to the regimen studied in Intergroup trial 3695.

O'Day and colleagues[209] explored the use of maintenance biotherapy for patients who achieved stable disease or partial remission with biochemotherapy. They treated 33 patients with a 1-year program consisting of IL-2, 1 million units/m² subcutaneously Monday through Friday; GM-CSF, 125 μg/m² subcutaneously, 2 weeks on and 2 weeks off; and seven, 2-day intravenous infusions of decrescendo IL-2. Five patients obtained complete remission and four achieved stable disease. The overall survival of the 33 patients was 18.5 months vs. 9.3 months for historical control subjects. Although the results are intriguing, in light of the low response rates to biochemotherapy reported in the Intergroup trial, it seems that only a very small number of patients would benefit from this approach.

New Therapies

The currently available treatments for metastatic melanoma are inadequate. In contrast, our understanding of immunology and the cellular biology of melanoma has increased rapidly in the last few years and is likely to continue to expand in the near future. A number of new and exciting treatment ideas are already in or about to enter early-phase clinical trials. We must encourage physicians and patients to take advantage of clinical trials in metastatic melanoma. The following is a survey of some new approaches to melanoma therapy that are in various stages of development.

Antiangiogenesis Agents. The use of antiangiogenesis agents in melanoma is being actively investigated, as it is in many other tumor types. Melanoma is a highly vascular tumor and should be a good target for such therapy. Interferon has antiangiogenesis activity, but it is not clear how much this activity contributes to its antimelanoma activity. Thalidomide by itself has limited activity in metastatic melanoma.[210] However, when Hwu and colleagues combined it with temozolomide, they obtained one complete response and four partial responses in 12 patients, including some with brain involvement.[211] They used a well-tolerated dosing schedule of temozolomide, 75 mg/m^2 PO, and thalidomide, 200 to 400 mg PO, each given daily for 42 days. A follow-up study is now underway. New antiangiogenesis agents in melanoma trials include thalidomide analogs,[212] anti-vascular endothelial growth factor,[213] and anti-alpha(v)beta3 integrin[214] agents.

Cytokines. A number of cytokines besides IL-2 are being investigated in metastatic melanoma. These agents include IL-1,[215] IL-4,[216] IL-12,[217] and IL-18.[218] They are being investigated in various cytokine combinations and as adjuvants to other immune therapy. None has proven beneficial for patients with melanoma.

Vaccines. The idea that a vaccine can very specifically activate the immune system against melanoma without significant toxicity is very appealing to both patients and physicians. Many melanoma vaccines are under preclinical and clinical evaluation; however, no melanoma vaccine has been proven to work in the adjuvant or metastatic setting in an adequately powered randomized trial. It seems most likely that vaccines will be of most benefit in the low-tumor-volume adjuvant setting or in the metastatic setting when combined with other therapies. A few studies looked at vaccines alone in metastatic disease. CancerVax, a whole-cell vaccine, induced remission in 23% of 40 patients in a phase II study.[156] Melacine, a cell-lysate vaccine, was compared with the Dartmouth chemotherapy regimen in a small, underpowered, phase III study. Overall survival rates were poor in both arms, 7.2 months for Dartmouth and 6.8 months for Melacine,[190] although Melacine was much less toxic. It would be interesting to know whether patients in the Melacine arm who were positive for HLA-A2 or C3 derived more benefit from the vaccine, as seemed to be true in the SWOG adjuvant study.[161]

Peptide vaccines have been intensely studied since the discovery of unique cancer-testis antigens (e.g., MAGE, BAGE) and melanoma-differentiation antigens (e.g.,

tyrosinase, gp100). Their genes code for small peptides, which are present on certain human leukoocyte antigen molecules on melanoma cells and elicit a specific cytotoxic T-cell response.[219] Many new melanoma-related peptides have been discovered. Clinical trials are exploring how best to administer these peptide vaccines, whether as a single peptide, with multiple peptides, with multiple peptides that sit on both human lymphocyte antigen class I and II molecules eliciting both a cytotoxic T-cell and a T-helper cell response,[220] with amino acid substitutions that augment their immunogenicity,[221] or with other biologic agents. Rosenberg and associates administered the gp100-209-2M peptide with high-dose IL-2 and obtained an objective response rate of 42% in 31 patients.[221] This therapy is now being evaluated in a multicenter randomized trial comparing high-dose IL-2 with this peptide vaccine plus high-dose IL-2. In another trial, patients who underwent unsuccessful treatment with IL-2 plus peptide were treated with nonmyeloablative doses of cyclophosphamide and fludarabine, followed by highly selected tumor-infiltrating lymphocytes and high-dose IL-2. Six of 13 patients obtained a major response.[222]

Targeted Therapies

G-3139 is an antisense oligonucleotide against BCL-2, which is expressed in 100% of melanoma cells. In a small phase I/II study in which it was administered with DTIC, there were some objective responses.[223] A large randomized trial comparing DTIC with DTIC plus G-3139 will soon be completing accrual. At least 50% of melanoma cells have tyrosine kinases targeted by imatinib mesylate (Gleevec; abl, PDGFr-alpha, PDGRr-beta, c-kit).[224] Preliminary results from a phase II trial using Gleevec, 800 mg daily, in patients with metastatic melanoma were disappointing.[225]

In a potentially important discovery, Davies and colleagues reported that 66% of metastatic melanoma cells contain a somatic point mutation of B-Raf in the Ras-Raf-MEK-ERK-MAP kinase pathway.[49] This mutation leads to an abnormal activated cytoplasmic serine/threonine kinase that can transform NIH3T3 cells.[49] This observation has been confirmed, and this mutation is also found in a high percentage of benign and dysplastic nevus cells.[50] Mutations of B-Raf may be involved in the progression, but not the initiation, of melanoma.[57] There is now an intense effort underway to find drugs that can reverse or bypass the effects of the B-Raf mutation. BAY-43-9006 is the first Raf kinase inhibitor to enter clinical trials. There have been a few early objective responses in a trial combining BAY-43-9006 with chemotherapy.[226]

Ending Treatment

Patients with a poor performance status, comorbid conditions, multiple brain metastases, or advanced age are unlikely to benefit from intensive systemic therapy. These patients may also experience more side effects from the currently available therapies than healthier patients. Providing comfort measures only may be a reasonable option in some patients with metastatic melanoma. Likewise, patients who undergo unsuccessful first-line therapy for metastatic melanoma should undergo a thoughtful assessment of their overall status before additional therapy is given.

Special Clinical Situations in Stage IV Disease

Solitary Metastasis

Occasionally, patients have a solitary metastatic lesion. There have been several reports of prolonged survival after surgical resection of solitary brain, lung, and liver metastases, regardless of whether patients also received postoperative adjuvant therapy.[227] A number of clinical trials exist for patients with stage IV melanoma and no evidence of disease, and patient enrollment should be strongly considered.

Brain Metastasis

Patients with brain metastases generally do poorly. Standard therapy is whole-brain irradiation, which offers some palliation. Patients with a solitary brain lesion and no disease elsewhere should strongly be considered for neurosurgical resection.[228] For patients with a solitary brain metastasis and responding or slowly growing disease elsewhere, consideration should still be given to neurosurgical resection, stereotactic radiosurgery,[229] or gamma-knife surgery. For patients with multiple brain metastases and a good performance status, consideration should be given to stereotactic radiosurgery or gamma-knife surgery, after whole-brain radiation.[230] With this approach, some patients can do well for a limited time.

TREATMENT COMPLICATIONS

Serious postsurgical complications are uncommon. The risks of bleeding and infection after surgery for melanoma are small and usually easily manageable. After sentinel node biopsy, some patients have a transient lymphocele at the site of node excision. The risk of lymphocele can be minimized by tying off the lymphatics during the sentinel node resection. If a lymphocele is large or painful, a simple office aspiration should provide adequate management. Small, asymptomatic lymphoceles can be observed and usually resolve on their own. Lymphedema has been reported in patients after sentinel node biopsy of the axilla and the inguinal area, but the incidence is low.[231]

Complete lymphadenectomy for regionally metastatic melanoma carries a risk of seroma, sensory loss, and lymphedema. A few patients have a seroma or prolonged drain output. Lymphedema is the most feared common complication of lymph node dissection and can occur after axillary or inguinal lymphadenectomy. The risk of lymphedema is low, and most cases are mild to moderate and controllable with diligent care.

FOLLOW-UP

Follow-up and Surveillance Plans

The hallmark of metastatic disease is a symptom complex that progresses in intensity or frequency. Among 261 patients with stage II or III melanoma who were followed prospectively by the North Central Cancer Treatment Group, symptoms signaled melanoma recurrence in 99 of the 145 patients (68%) who had a recurrence.[232] Physical examination detected recurrence in an additional 37 asymptomatic patients (26%). Altogether, 94% of recurrences were detected by history and physical examination. An abnormal chest x-ray identified only 9 of 145 recurrences (6%), and in no patient was an abnormal laboratory test the sole indicator of recurrent disease. Mooney and associates[233] assessed the effect of a surveillance program using physical examination, blood tests, and chest x-rays on 1004 patients with AJCC stage I or II cutaneous melanoma. Physical examination detected 72% of recurrences, constitutional symptoms indicated 17% of recurrences, and chest x-ray showed 11% of recurrences. Similarly, among the 373 patients followed in a surveillance program at the Yale Melanoma Unit, of the 78 patients who had recurrences, 34 (44%) were patient-detected and 25 (32%) were physician-detected on routine exam.[234] Thus, 76% of recurrences were diagnosed by a complete history and physical examination alone.

Diagnostic imaging remains crucial for tumor staging and for follow-up of patients with stage IV disease undergoing aggressive experimental treatments. Many imaging techniques are used to examine these patients, with CT scans currently used for staging and to guide diagnostic biopsies. However, there is no consensus about the optimal frequency or utility of CT scans. In some circumstances, false-positive lesions seen on CT scan can lead to further diagnostic tests or even biopsy of lesions that may be unrelated to the melanoma. CT scans of the chest are useful for evaluating suspected pulmonary, pleural, or mediastinal metastases.

However, even in patients with known distant metastases (stage IV disease), scans are best suited for cases in which the presence of additional metastases would alter the treatment plan or in which better definition of lesions is required for patient entry into a research protocol. A retrospective study conducted at the M.D. Anderson Cancer Center evaluated the value of CT scans in 89 patients with locoregional recurrence who were asymptomatic and had normal findings on chest x-rays and normal serum LDH levels.[235] In 71% of patients, CT scans yielded true-negative findings. True-positive findings were seen in only 7% of patients, and false-positive findings were seen in 22%. CT scans of the chest showed disease that was not visible on a chest x-ray film in only 1 of the 89 patients. CT scans of the abdomen or pelvis detected metastases in five patients. CT scans of the neck were performed in nine patients whose primary site had been the head or neck; in only one case did the scan show adenopathy that was not detectable on physical examination. The most common false-positive results were hypodense hepatic lesions, noncalcified pulmonary nodules, and hypodense splenic lesions. Obviously, positive findings on initial screening scans result in further imaging or invasive procedures, with their attendant costs and risks of morbidity. Of 57 CT scans and 25 MRI scans of the brain, none showed evidence of central nervous system metastases; this suggests that the yield of

MRI of the brain in this patient population is less than 10%. Interestingly, seven patients had brain metastases, and three did so within 6 months of a CT scan that showed normal findings.

For patients with suspected intra-abdominal or hepatic metastases based on abnormal findings on physical examination or abnormal liver chemistry results, a CT scan of the abdomen should be obtained. Hypervascular metastases of the liver are typically scanned by multiple-phase imaging, including the unenhanced phase, the hepatic arterial phase, and the portal venous phase. In general, imaging of the portal venous phase alone usually offers satisfactory lesion detection. Atypical melanoma metastases, however, may require all phases for optimal visualization. MRI scans may also be used to detect melanin, as manifested by a high signal on T1-weighted images. Contrast studies of the gastrointestinal tract, particularly an upper gastrointestinal series with small bowel follow-through, are indicated if there are signs of obstruction or gastrointestinal bleeding.

Brain, liver, and gallium radionuclide scans are not cost-effective for routine screening because of their low diagnostic yield.[84,236] However, x-rays of the bone and a radionuclide bone scan should be obtained if there are specific symptoms or signs of bony metastatic disease. Other than MRI, a bone scan is probably the most sensitive test for skeletal metastatic disease, but a careful history and directed x-rays are necessary to ensure that areas of uptake do not represent old trauma or inflammation.[85]

PET with FDG has a sensitivity of 78% to 100% in detecting metastatic melanoma. False-positive findings may be seen in patients with inflammatory processes, such as sarcoid, and in those with second primary tumors.[86-88] Wagner and associates[89] reported that the sensitivity of PET with FDG for detection of metastatic melanoma in lymph nodes depends on sufficient tumor volume. PET with FDG reliably detects metastatic tumor that forms a nodule of approximately 5 mm in lymph nodes, but sensitivity decreases rapidly for smaller lesions. PET can also be used to determine the need for further diagnostic procedures, such as radiologically guided needle biopsy of suspicious, accessible lesions. Although PET cannot detect micrometastases, it may be sufficient to observe patients with negative findings on PET, avoiding additional diagnostic procedures.

In a patient with symptoms, an abnormal finding on physical examination or laboratory tests, or an abnormal x-ray, the definitive diagnosis of metastatic melanoma can be made only by a biopsy. Excisional or needle biopsy is relatively easy to perform when the suspected metastasis is easily accessible. However, in many cases, x-rays are sufficient for a clinical diagnosis, especially if the metastases involve more than one site and the abnormality was absent on previous studies.

Unusual Problems

Unknown Primary Site

Patients can present with stage III or IV disease without a history of previously diagnosed melanoma. All of these patients should have a thorough skin examination, including the anal region. An eye examination is appropriate if the metastatic pattern is consistent with ocular melanoma. Often a primary site is not found. Sometimes patients provide a history of an unusual skin lesion arising and disappearing without biopsy or treatment, or a history of a skin lesion that was cauterized or frozen. Immunohistochemistry (S-100, HMB-45, Melan-A) is sometimes useful in confirming the pathology. Patients who appear to have only regional lymph node involvement should undergo only a potentially curative regional lymph node dissection just as any other patient with regional metastases. The patient should then be considered for systemic adjuvant therapy.

Ocular Melanoma

Ocular melanoma is rare. Although it can be morphologically similar to cutaneous melanoma, it behaves differently. It often metastasizes primarily to the liver. Sometimes the metastatic process moves relatively slowly. In addition, it appears to respond less often to chemotherapy and biologic therapy, although a review of the SWOG experience did not confirm this.[237] Most clinical trials for metastatic melanoma exclude patients with ocular melanoma. Some biologic correlates may explain these differences. There appears to be down-regulated human leukoocyte antigen expression on ocular melanoma cells,[238] and these cells do not appear to contain the recently described B-Raf mutation.[239] Although there were initial promising results using the BOLD plus interferon regimen in metastatic ocular melanoma, these results were not confirmed in a large trial.[240] Patients with primarily liver metastasis sometimes appear to benefit from chemoembolization[241] or liver perfusion.[242]

Mucosal Melanoma

Primary mucosal melanoma is also rare. Patients often have advanced disease at the time of initial diagnosis because primary sites in locations such as the gastrointestinal tract or sinuses make early detection difficult. A recent trial published in abstract form showed a surprisingly good response rate of 44% for biochemotherapy in 13 patients with metastatic anorectal melanoma.[243]

ISSUES FOR THE FUTURE

Today, most melanomas are found early and are thus very treatable. However, some melanomas are found when advanced, and even some thin melanomas eventually recur. There is no routinely reliable and successful way to treat patients with advanced disease. The most important ways to improve melanoma-related survival are prevention and early detection.

Although much progress has been made in identifying the molecular defects that are common to malignant melanocytic lesions, few of these discoveries have thus far been translated to effective therapies. It is expected that sequencing of the human genome and ready accessibility to laboratories of gene expression profiling will result in an explosion of information about the molecular events governing melanoma onset and progression. These data must be analyzed carefully and interpreted in a context that allows for clear definition of the altered pathways in the development and progression of melanoma. Ultimately, these discoveries will provide the framework for the design of targeted therapies for melanoma.

REFERENCES

1. Jemal A, Murray T, Samuels A, et al: Cancer statistics, 2003. CA Cancer J Clin 2003;53:5–26.
2. Swerdlow AJ: International trends in cutaneous melanoma. Ann N Y Acad Sci 1990;609:235–251.
3. Bulliard JL, Cox B, Semenciw R: Trends by anatomic site in the incidence of cutaneous malignant melanoma in Canada, 1969–93. Cancer Causes Control 1999;10:407–416.
4. Bliss JM, Ford D, Swerdlow AJ, et al: Risk of cutaneous melanoma associated with pigmentation characteristics and freckling: Systematic overview of 10 case-control studies. The International Melanoma Analysis Group (IMAGE). Int J Cancer 1995;62: 367–376.
5. Naldi L, Lorenzo Imberti G, Parazzini F, et al: Pigmentary traits, modalities of sun reaction, history of sunburns, and melanocytic nevi as risk factors for cutaneous malignant melanoma in the Italian population: Results of a collaborative case-control study. Cancer 2000;88:2703–2710.
6. Grulich AE, Bataille V, Swerdlow AJ, et al: Naevi and pigmentary characteristics as risk factors for melanoma in a high-risk population: A case-control study in New South Wales, Australia. Int J Cancer 1996;67:485–491.
7. Bataille V, Bishop JA, Sasieni P, et al: Risk of cutaneous melanoma in relation to the numbers, types and sites of naevi: A case-control study. Br J Cancer 1996;73:1605–1611.
8. Holly EA, Kelly JW, Shpall SN, et al: Number of melanocytic nevi as a major risk factor for malignant melanoma. J Am Acad Dermatol 1987;17:459–468.
9. Kraemer KH, Tucker M, Tarone R, et al: Risk of cutaneous melanoma in dysplastic nevus syndrome types A and B. N Engl J Med 1986;315:1615–1616.
10. Greene MH, Clark WH Jr, Tucker MA, et al: High risk of malignant melanoma in melanoma-prone families with dysplastic nevi. Ann Intern Med 1985;102:458–465.
11. Swerdlow AJ, English JS, Qiao Z: The risk of melanoma in patients with congenital nevi: A cohort study. J Am Acad Dermatol 1995;32:595–599.
12. Clark WH Jr, Elder DE, Guerry DT, et al: A study of tumor progression: The precursor lesions of superficial spreading and nodular melanoma. Hum Pathol 1984;15:1147–1165.
13. Gruber SB, Barnhill RL, Stenn KS, et al: Nevomelanocytic prolifer-ations in association with cutaneous malignant melanoma: A multivariate analysis. J Am Acad Dermatol 1989;21: 773–780.
14. Kruger S, Garbe C, Buttner P, et al: Epidemiologic evidence for the role of melanocytic nevi as risk markers and direct precursors of cutaneous malignant melanoma: Results of a case control study in melanoma patients and nonmelanoma control subjects. J Am Acad Dermatol 1992;26:920–926.
15. Tsao H, Bevona C, Goggins W, et al: The transformation rate of moles (melanocytic nevi) into cutaneous melanoma: A population-based estimate. Arch Dermatol 2003;139:282–288.
16. Clark WH Jr, From L, Bernardino EA, et al: The histogenesis and biologic behavior of primary human malignant melanomas of the skin. Cancer Res 1969;29:705–772.
17. Breslow A: Thickness, cross-sectional areas and depth of invasion in the prognosis of cutaneous melanoma. Ann Surg 1970;172:902–908.
18. Balch CM, Soong SJ, Gershenwald JE, et al: Prognostic factors analysis of 17,600 melanoma patients: Validation of the American Joint Committee on Cancer melanoma staging system. J Clin Oncol 2001;19:3622–3634.
19. Balch CM, Buzaid AC, Soong SJ, et al: Final version of the American Joint Committee on Cancer staging system for cutaneous melanoma. J Clin Oncol 2001;19:3635–3648.
20. Azzola MF, Shaw HM, Thompson JF, et al: Tumor mitotic rate is a more powerful prognostic indicator than ulceration in patients with primary cutaneous melanoma: An analysis of 3661 patients from a single center. Cancer 2003;97:1488–1498.
21. Ronan SG, Eng AM, Briele HA, et al: Thin malignant melanomas with regression and metastases. Arch Dermatol 1987;123: 1326–1330.
22. Barnhill RL, Fine JA, Roush GC, et al: Predicting five-year outcome for patients with cutaneous melanoma in a population-based study. Cancer 1996;78:427–432.
23. Egbert B, Kempson R, Sagebiel R: Desmoplastic malignant melanoma: A clinicohistopathologic study of 25 cases. Cancer 1988;62:2033–2041.
24. Carlson JA, Dickersin GR, Sober AJ, et al: Desmoplastic neurotropic melanoma: A clinicopathologic analysis of 28 cases. Cancer 1995;75:478–494.
25. Connelly J, Smith JL Jr: Malignant blue nevus. Cancer 1991;67:2653–2657.
26. Aloi F, Pich A, Pippione M: Malignant cellular blue nevus: A clinicopathological study of 6 cases. Dermatology 1996;192: 36–40.
27. Reed RJ, Ichinose H, Clark WH Jr, et al: Common and uncommon melanocytic nevi and borderline melanomas. Semin Oncol 1975;2:119–147.
28. Phillips ME, Margolis RJ, Merot Y, et al: The spectrum of minimal deviation melanoma: A clinicopathologic study of 21 cases. Hum Pathol 1986;17:796–806.
29. Chung EB, Enzinger FM: Malignant melanoma of soft parts: A reassessment of clear cell sarcoma. Am J Surg Pathol 1983;7:405–413.
30. Mrozek K, Karakousis CP, Perez-Mesa C, et al: Translocation t(12;22)(q13;q12.2-12.3) in a clear cell sarcoma of tendons and aponeuroses. Genes Chromosomes Cancer 1993;6:249–252.
31. Segal NH, Pavlidis P, Noble WS, et al: Classification of clear-cell sarcoma as a subtype of melanoma by genomic profiling. J Clin Oncol 2003;21:1775–1781.
32. Fountain JW, et al: Homozygous deletions within human chromosome band 9p21 in melanoma. Proc Natl Acad Sci USA 1992;89:10557–10561.
33. Cannon-Albright LA, et al: Assignment of a locus for familial melanoma, MLM, to chromosome 9p13-p22. Science 1992;258:1148–1152.
34. Zuo L, et al: Germline mutations in the p16INK4a binding domain of CDK4 in familial melanoma. Nat Genet 1996;12:97–99.
35. Platz A, Ringborg U, Hansson J: Hereditary cutaneous melanoma. Semin Cancer Biol 2000;10:319–326.
36. Albino AP, Fountain JW: Oncogenes and tumor suppressor genes in cutaneous malignant melanoma. Photochem Photobiol 1996;63:412–418.
37. Rocco JW, Sidransky D: p16(MTS-1/CDKN2/INK4a) in cancer progression. Exp Cell Res 2001;264:42–55.
38. Fujimoto A, Morita R, Hatta N, Takehara K, Takata M: p16INK4a inactivation is not frequent in uncultured sporadic primary cutaneous melanoma. Oncogene 1999;18:2527–2532.
39. Grover R, Chana JS, Wilson GD, Richman PI, Sanders R: An analysis of p16 protein expression in sporadic malignant melanoma. Melanoma Res 1998;8:267–272.
40. Reed JA, et al: Loss of expression of the p16/cyclin-dependent kinase inhibitor 2 tumor suppressor gene in melanocytic lesions correlates with invasive stage of tumor progression. Cancer Res 1995;55:2713–2718.
41. Israel MA, et al: Id gene expression as a key mediator of tumor cell biology. Cancer Res 1999;59:1726–1730.
42. Alani RM, et al: Immortalization of primary human keratinocytes by the helix-loop-helix protein, Id-1. Proc Natl Acad Sci USA 1999;96:9637–9641.
43. Nickoloff BJ, et al: Id-1 delays senescence but does not immortalize keratinocytes. J Biol Chem 2000;275:27501–27504.
44. Sikder HA, Devlin MK, Dunlap S, Ryu B, Alani RM: Id proteins in cell growth and tumorigenesis. Cancer Cell 2003;3:525–530.
45. Ohtani N, et al: Opposing effects of Ets and Id proteins on

p16Ink4a expression during cellular senescence. Nature 2001;409:1067–1070.

46. Alani RM, Young AZ, Shifflett CB: Id1 regulation of cellular senescence through transcriptional repression of p16/Ink4a. Proc Natl Acad Sci USA 2001;98:7812–7816.

47. Polsky D, Young AZ, Busam KJ, Alani RM: The transcriptional repressor of p16/Ink4a, Id1, is upregulated in early melanomas. Cancer Res 2001;61:6008–6011.

48. Chin L, et al: Essential role for oncogenic Ras in tumour maintenance. Nature 1999;400:468–472.

49. Davies H, et al: Mutations of the BRAF gene in human cancer. Nature 2002;417:949–954.

50. Pollock PM, et al: High frequency of BRAF mutations in nevi. Nat Genet 2003;33:19–20.

51. Lang J, Boxer M, MacKie R: Absence of exon 15 BRAF germline mutations in familial melanoma. Hum Mutat 2003;21:327–330.

52. Meyer P, Klaes R, Schmitt C, Boettger MB, Garbe C: Exclusion of BRAFV599E as a melanoma susceptibility mutation. Int J Cancer 2003;106:78–80.

53. Laud K, et al: BRAF as a melanoma susceptibility candidate gene? Cancer Res 2003;63:3061–3065.

54. Cohen Y, et al: Lack of BRAF mutation in primary uveal melanoma. Invest Ophthalmol Vis Sci 2003;44:2876–2878.

55. Edmunds SC, et al: Absence of BRAF gene mutations in uveal melanomas in contrast to cutaneous melanomas. Br J Cancer 2003;88:1403–1405.

56. Gorden A, et al: Analysis of BRAF and N-RAS mutations in metastatic melanoma tissues. Cancer Res 2003;63:3955–3957.

57. Dong J, et al: BRAF oncogenic mutations correlate with progression rather than initiation of human melanoma. Cancer Res 2003;63:3883–3885.

58. Druker BJ: Perspectives on the development of a molecularly targeted agent. Cancer Cell 2002;1:31–36.

59. Lee JT, McCubrey JA: BAY-43-9006 Bayer/Onyx. Curr Opin Investig Drugs 2003;4:757–763.

60. Papp T, Jafari M, Schiffmann D: Lack of p53 mutations and loss of heterozygosity in non-cultured human melanocytic lesions. J Cancer Res Clin Oncol 1996;122:541–548.

61. Soengas MS, et al: Inactivation of the apoptosis effector Apaf-1 in malignant melanoma. Nature 2001;409:207–211.

62. Polsky D, et al: HDM2 protein overexpression, but not gene amplification, is related to tumorigenesis of cutaneous melanoma. Cancer Res 2001;61,7642–7646.

63. Polsky D, et al: HDM2 protein overexpression and prognosis in primary malignant melanoma. J Natl Cancer Inst 2002;94:803–806.

64. Piepkorn M: Melanoma genetics: An update with focus on the CDKN2A(p16)/ARF tumor suppressors. J Am Acad Dermatol 2000;42:705–722; quiz 723–726.

65. Ivanov VN, Bhoumik A, Ronai Z: Death receptors and melanoma resistance to apoptosis. Oncogene 2003;22:3152–3161.

66. Blackburn EH: Structure and function of telomeres. Nature 1991;350:569–573.

67. de Lange T, Jacks T: For better or worse? Telomerase inhibition and cancer. Cell 1999;98:273–275.

68. Granger MP, Wright WE, Shay JW: Telomerase in cancer and aging. Crit Rev Oncol Hematol 2002;41:29–40.

69. Maser RS, DePinho RA: Connecting chromosomes, crisis, and cancer. Science 2002;297:565–569.

70. White LK, Wright WE, Shay JW: Telomerase inhibitors. Trends Biotechnol 2001;19:114–120.

71. Miracco C, et al: Evaluation of telomerase activity in cutaneous melanocytic proliferations. Hum Pathol 2000;31:1018–1021.

72. Meeker AK, et al: Telomere length assessment in human archival tissues: Combined telomere fluorescence in situ hybridization and immunostaining. Am J Pathol 2002;160:1259–1268.

73. Balch CM, Murad TM, Soong SJ, et al: A multifactorial analysis of melanoma: Prognostic histopathological features comparing Clark's and Breslow's staging methods. Ann Surg 1978;188:732–742.

74. Buzaid AC, Ross MI, Balch CM, et al: Critical analysis of the current American Joint Committee on Cancer staging system for cutaneous melanoma and proposal of a new staging system (see comments). J Clin Oncol 1997;15:1039–1051.

75. Balch CM, Soong S, Ross MI, et al: Long-term results of a multi-institutional randomized trial comparing prognostic factors and surgical results for intermediate thickness melanomas (1.0 to 4.0 mm). Ann Surg Oncol 2000;7:87–97.

76. Balch CM, Soong SJ, Milton GW, et al: A comparison of prognostic factors and surgical results in 1,786 patients with localized (stage I) melanoma treated in Alabama, USA, and New South Wales, Australia. Ann Surg 1982;196:677–684.

77. Morton DL, Davtyan DG, Wanek LA, Foshag LJ, Cochran AJ: Multivariate analysis of the relationship between survival and the microstage of primary melanoma by Clark level and Breslow thickness. Cancer 1993;71:3737–3743.

78. Mansson-Brahme E, Carstensen J, Erhardt K, et al: Prognostic factors in thin cutaneous malignant melanoma. Cancer 1994;73:2324–2332.

79. Balch CM, Soong SJ, Bartolucci A, et al: Efficacy of an elective lymph node dissection of 1 to 4 mm thick melanomas for patients 60 years of age and younger. Ann Surg 1996;224:255–266.

80. Austin PF, Cruse CW, Lyman G, Schroer K, Glass F, Reintgen D: Age as a prognostic factor in the malignant melanoma population. Ann Surg Oncol 1994;1:487–494.

81. Finck SJ, Giuliano AE, Morton DL: LDH and melanoma. Cancer 1983;51:840–843.

82. Amer MH, Al-Sarraf M, Vaitkevicius VK: Clinical presentation, natural history and prognostic factors in advanced malignant melanoma. Surg Gynecol Obstet 1979;149:687–692.

83. Kamel IR, Kruskal JB, Gramm HF: Imaging of abdominal manifestations of melanoma. Crit Rev Diagn Imaging 1998;39:447–486.

84. Muss HB, Richards F, Barnes PL, et al: Radionuclide scanning in patients with advanced malignant melanoma. Clin Nucl Med 1979;4:516–518.

85. Devereux D, Johnston G, Blei L, et al: The role of bone scans in assessing malignant melanoma in patients with stage III disease. Surg Gynecol Obstet 1980;151:45–48.

86. Holder WD, White RL, Zuger JH, et al: Effectiveness of positron emission tomography for the detection of melanoma metastases. Ann Surg 1998;227:764–769.

87. Eigtved A, Andersson AP, Dahlstrøm K, et al: Use of fluorine-18 fluorodeoxyglucose positron emission tomography in the detection of silent metastases from malignant melanoma. Eur J Nucl Med 2000;27:70–75.

88. Rinne D, et al: Primary staging and follow-up of high risk melanoma patients with whole-body 18F-fluorodeoxyglucose positron emission tomography. Cancer 1998;82:1664–1671.

89. Wagner JD, Schauwecker DS, Davidson D, et al: FDG-PET sensitivity for melanoma lymph node metastases is dependent on tumor volume. J Surg Oncol 2001;77:237–242.

90. Balch CM: AJCC Cancer Staging Manual, 6th ed. New York, Springer-Verlag, 2002.

91. Morton DL, Thompson JF, Essner R, et al: Validation of the accuracy of intraoperative lymphatic mapping and sentinel lymphadenectomy for early-stage melanoma: A multicenter trial. Multicenter Selective Lymphadenectomy Trial Group. Ann Surg 1999;230:453–463.

92. Gershenwald JE, Thompson W, Mansfield PF, et al: Multi-institutional melanoma lymphatic mapping experience: The prognostic value of sentinel lymph node status in 612 stage I or II melanoma patients. J Clin Oncol 1999;17:976–983.

93. Gershenwald JE, Prieto V, Colome-Grimmer MI, et al: The prognostic significance of microscopic tumor burden in 925 melanoma patients undergoing sentinel lymph node biopsy. Proc Am Soc Clin Oncol 2000;19:551a.

94. Yu LL, Flotte TJ, Tanabe KK, et al: Detection of microscopic melanoma metastases in sentinel lymph nodes. Cancer 1999;86:617–627.

95. Balch CM, Buzaid AC, Atkins MB, et al: A new American Joint Committee on Cancer staging system for cutaneous melanoma. Cancer 2000;88:1484–1491.

96. Buttner P, Garbe C, Bertz J, et al: Primary cutaneous melanoma: Optimized cutoff points of tumor thickness and importance of Clark's level for prognostic classification. Cancer 1995;75:2499–2506.

97. Haffner AC, Garbe C, Burg G, et al: The prognosis of primary and metastasizing melanoma: An evaluation of the TNM classification in 2,495 patients. Br J Cancer 1992;66:856-861.

98. Breslow A, Macht SD: Evaluation of prognosis in stage I cutaneous melanoma. Plast Reconstr Surg 1978;61:342-346.

99. Balch CM, Soong SJ, Murad TM, et al: A multifactorial analysis of melanoma: II. Prognostic factors in patients with stage I (localized) melanoma. Surgery 1979;86:343-351.

100. McGovern VJ, Shaw HM, Milton GW, et al: Ulceration and prognosis in cutaneous malignant melanoma. Histopathology 1982;6:399-407.

101. Eton O, Legha SS, Moon TE, et al: Prognostic factors for survival of patients treated systemically for disseminated melanoma. J Clin Oncol 1998;16:1103-1111.

102. Barth A, Wanek LA, Morton DL: Prognostic factors in 1,521 melanoma patients with distant metastases. J Am Coll Surg 1995;181:193-201.

103. Deichmann M, Benner A, Bock M, et al: S100-Beta, melanoma-inhibiting activity, and lactate dehydrogenase discriminate progressive from nonprogressive American Joint Committee on Cancer stage IV melanoma. J Clin Oncol 1999;17:1891-1896.

104. Franzke A, Probst-Kepper M, Buer J, et al: Elevated pretreatment serum levels of soluble vascular cell adhesion molecule 1 and lactate dehydrogenase as predictors of survival in cutaneous metastatic malignant melanoma. Br J Cancer 1998;78:40-45.

105. Balch CM, Soong SJ, Murad TM, et al: A multifactorial analysis of melanoma: IV. Prognostic factors in 200 melanoma patients with distant metastases (stage III). J Clin Oncol 1983;1:126-134.

106. Brand CU, Ellwanger U, Stroebel W, et al: Prolonged survival of 2 years or longer for patients with disseminated melanoma. Cancer 1997;79:2345-2353.

107. Balch CM: Cutaneous melanoma: Prognosis and treatment results worldwide. Semin Surg Oncol 1992;8:400-414.

108. Buzaid AC, Tinoco LA, Jendiroba D, et al: Prognostic value of size of lymph node metastases in patients with cutaneous melanoma. J Clin Oncol 1995;13:2361-2368.

109. Morton DL, Wanek L, Nizze JA, et al: Improved long-term survival after lymphadenectomy of melanoma metastatic to regional nodes: Analysis of prognostic factors in 1134 patients from the John Wayne Cancer Clinic. Ann Surg 1991;214:491-499; discussion 499-501.

110. Coit DG, Rogatko A, Brennan MF: Prognostic factors in patients with melanoma metastatic to axillary or inguinal lymph nodes: A multivariate analysis. Ann Surg 1991;214:627-636.

111. Drepper H, Biess B, Hofherr B, et al: The prognosis of patients with stage III melanoma. Cancer 1993;71:1239-1246.

112. Balch CM, Soong SJ, Murad TM, et al: A multifactorial analysis of melanoma: III. Prognostic factors in melanoma patients with lymph node metastases (stage II). Ann Surg 1981;193:377-388.

113. Manola J, Atkins M, Ibrahim J, et al: Prognostic factors in metastatic melanoma: A pooled analysis of Eastern Cooperative Oncology Group trials. J Clin Oncol 2000;18:3782-3793.

114. Sirott MN BD, Wong GYC, Tao YT, Chapman PB, Templeton MA, Houghton AN: Prognostic factors in patients with metastatic malignant melanoma: A multivariate analysis. Cancer 1993;72:3091-3098.

115. Unger JM, Flaherty LE, Liu PY, et al: Gender and other survival predictors in patients with metastatic melanoma on Southwest Oncology Group trials. Cancer 2001;91:1148-1155.

116. Veronesi U, Cascinelli N: Narrow excision (1-cm margin): A safe procedure for thin cutaneous melanoma. Arch Surg 1991;126:438-441.

117. Balch CM, Soong S, Ross MI, et al: Long-term results of a multi-institutional randomized trial comparing prognostic factors and surgical results for intermediate thickness melanomas (1.0 to 4.0 mm): Intergroup Melanoma Surgical Trial. Ann Surg Oncol 2000;7:87-97.

118. Khayat D, Rixe O, Martin G, et al: Surgical margins in cutaneous melanoma (2 cm versus 5 cm for lesions measuring less than 2.1-mm thick). Cancer 2003;97:1941-1946.

119. Heaton KM, Sussman JJ, Gershenwald JE, et al: Surgical margins and prognostic factors in patients with thick (>4 mm) primary melanoma. Ann Surg Oncol 1998;5:322-328.

120. Morton DL, Wen DR, Wong JH, et al: Technical details of intraoperative lymphatic mapping for early stage melanoma. Arch Surg 1992;127:392-399.

121. Reintgen D, Cruse CW, Wells K, et al: The orderly progression of melanoma nodal metastases. Ann Surg 1994;220:759-767.

122. Gershenwald JE, Thompson W, Mansfield PF, et al: Multi-institutional melanoma lymphatic mapping experience: The prognostic value of sentinel lymph node status in 612 stage I or II melanoma patients. J Clin Oncol 1999;17:976-983.

123. Bleicher RJ, Essner R, Foshag LJ, et al: Role of sentinel lymphadenectomy in thin invasive cutaneous melanomas. J Clin Oncol 2003;21:1326-1331.

124. Cochran AJ, Wen DR, Morton DL: Occult tumor cells in the lymph nodes of patients with pathological stage I malignant melanoma: An immunohistological study. Am J Surg Pathol 1988;12:612-618.

125. Gershenwald JE, Colome MI, Lee JE, et al: Patterns of recurrence following a negative sentinel lymph node biopsy in 243 patients with stage I or II melanoma. J Clin Oncol 1998;16:2253-2260.

126. Shivers SC, Li W, Lin J, et al: The clinical relevance of molecular staging for melanoma. Recent Results Cancer Res 2001;158:187-199.

127. Bostick PJ, Morton DL, Turner RR, et al: Prognostic significance of occult metastases detected by sentinel lymphadenectomy and reverse transcriptase-polymerase chain reaction in early-stage melanoma patients. J Clin Oncol 1999;17:3238-3244.

128. Cascinelli N, Belli F, Santinami M, et al: Sentinel lymph node biopsy in cutaneous melanoma: The WHO Melanoma Program experience. Ann Surg Oncol 2000;7:469-474.

129. Gadd MA, Cosimi AB, Yu J, et al: Outcome of patients with melanoma and histologically negative sentinel lymph nodes. Arch Surg 1999;134:381-387.

130. Vuylsteke RJ, van Leeuwen PA, Muller MG, et al: Clinical outcome of stage I/II melanoma patients after selective sentinel lymph node dissection: Long-term follow-up results. J Clin Oncol 2003;21:1057-1065.

131. Balch CM: Cutaneous melanoma: Prognosis and treatment results worldwide. Semin Surg Oncol 1992;8:400-414.

132. Stevens G, Thompson JF, Firth I, et al: Locally advanced melanoma: Results of postoperative hypofractionated radiation therapy. Cancer 2000;88:88-94.

133. Strom EA, Ross MI: Adjuvant radiation therapy after axillary lymphadenectomy for metastatic melanoma: Toxicity and local control. Ann Surg Oncol 1995;2:445-449.

134. Ballo MT, Strom EA, Zagars GK, et al: Adjuvant irradiation for axillary metastases from malignant melanoma. Int J Radiat Oncol Biol Phys 2002;52:964-972.

135. Essner R, Conforti A, Kelley MC, et al: Efficacy of lymphatic mapping, sentinel lymphadenectomy, and selective complete lymph node dissection as a therapeutic procedure for early-stage melanoma. Ann Surg Oncol 1999;6:442-449.

136. Roses DF, Harris MN, Rigel D, et al: Local and in-transit metastases following definitive excision for primary cutaneous malignant melanoma. Ann Surg 1983;198:65-69.

137. Fraker DL: Hyperthermic regional perfusion for melanoma and sarcoma of the limbs. Curr Probl Surg 1999;36:841-907.

138. Taber SW, Polk HC Jr: Mortality, major amputation rates, and leukopenia after isolated limb perfusion with phenylalanine mustard for the treatment of melanoma. Ann Surg Oncol 1997;4:440-445.

139. Lindner P, Doubrovsky A, Kam PC, et al: Prognostic factors after isolated limb infusion with cytotoxic agents for melanoma. Ann Surg Oncol 2002;9:127-136.

140. Nathan FE, Mastrangelo MJ: Adjuvant therapy for cutaneous melanoma. Semin Oncol 1995;22:647-661.

141. Kirkwood JM, Strawderman MH, Ernstoff MS, et al: Interferon alfa-2b adjuvant therapy of high-risk resected cutaneous melanoma: The Eastern Cooperative Oncology Group Trial EST 1684. J Clin Oncol 1996;14:7-17.

142. Kirkwood JM, Ibrahim JG, Sosman JA, et al: High-dose interferon alfa-2b significantly prolongs relapse-free and overall survival compared with the GM2-KLH/QS-21 vaccine in patients with resected stage IIB-III melanoma: Results of intergroup trial E1694/S9512/C509801. J Clin Oncol 2001;19:2370-2380.

143. Kirkwood JM, Ibrahim JG, Sondak VK, et al: High- and low-dose interferon alfa-2b in high-risk melanoma: First analysis of intergroup trial E1690/S9111/C9190. J Clin Oncol 2000;19:2444–2458.

144. Hill GJ II, Moss SE, Golomb FM, et al: DTIC and combination therapy for melanoma: III. DTIC (NSC 45388) Surgical Adjuvant Study COG PROTOCOL 7040. Cancer 1981;47:2556–2562.

145. Tranum BL, Dixon D, Quagliana J, et al: Lack of benefit of adjunctive chemotherapy in stage I malignant melanoma: A Southwest Oncology Group Study. Cancer Treat Rep 1987;71:643–644.

146. Veronesi U, Adamus J, Aubert C, et al: A randomized trial of adjuvant chemotherapy and immunotherapy in cutaneous melanoma. N Engl J Med 1982;307:913–916.

147. Meyskens FL Jr, Kopecky K, Samson M, et al: Recombinant human interferon gamma: Adverse effects in high-risk stage I and II cutaneous malignant melanoma. J Natl Cancer Inst 1990;82:1071.

148. Creagan ET, Ingle JN, Schutt AJ, et al: A prospective, randomized controlled trial of megestrol acetate among high-risk patients with resected malignant melanoma. Am J Clin Oncol 1989;12:152–155.

149. Spitler LE: A randomized trial of levamisole versus placebo as adjuvant therapy in malignant melanoma. J Clin Oncol 1991;9:736–740.

150. Punt CJ, Eggermont AM: Adjuvant interferon-alpha for melanoma revisited: News from old and new studie. Ann Oncol 2001;12:1663–1666.

151. Kirkwood JM, Sondak VK, Haluska FG, Ibrahim JG: Value of adjuvant interferon-alfa-2b therapy in high-risk melanoma: The case in favor. In DeVita VT, Hellman S, Rosenberg SA (eds): Progress in Oncology 2003. Sudbury, Mass, Jones and Bartlett, 2003, pp 373–390.

152. Spitler LE: Value of alpha interferon in adjuvant therapy for melanoma. In DeVita VT, Hellman S, Rosenberg SA (eds): Progress in Oncology 2003. Sudbury, Mass, Jones and Bartlett, 2003, pp 391–411.

153. Creagan ET, Dalton RJ, Ahmann DL, et al: Randomized, surgical adjuvant clinical trial of recombinant interferon alfa-2a in selected patients with malignant melanoma. J Clin Oncol 1995;13:2776–2783.

154. Cascinelli N, Belli F, MacKie RM, et al: Effect of long-term adjuvant therapy with interferon alpha-2a in patients with regional node metastases from cutaneous melanoma: A randomised trial. Lancet 2001;358:866–869.

155. Grob JJ, Dreno B, de la Salmoniere P, et al: Randomised trial of interferon alpha-2a as adjuvant therapy in resected primary melanoma thicker than 1.5 mm without clinically detectable node metastases: French Cooperative Group on Melanoma. Lancet 1998;351:1905–1910.

156. Morton DL, Foshag LJ, Hoon DS, et al: Prolongation of survival in metastatic melanoma after active specific immunotherapy with a new polyvalent melanoma vaccine. Ann Surg 1992;216:463–482.

157. Berd D, Maguire HC Jr, Schuchter LM, et al: Autologous hapten-modified melanoma vaccine as postsurgical adjuvant treatment after resection of nodal metastases. J Clin Oncol 1997;15:2359–2370.

158. Wallack MK, Sivanandham M, Balch CM, et al: Surgical adjuvant active specific immunotherapy for patients with stage III melanoma: The final analysis of data from a phase III, randomized, double-blind, multicenter vaccinia melanoma oncolysate trial. J Am Coll Surg 1998;187:69–77; discussion 77–99.

159. Hersey P, Coates AS, McCarthy WH, et al: Adjuvant immunotherapy of patients with high-risk melanoma using vaccinia viral lysates of melanoma: Results of a randomized trial. J Clin Oncol 2002;20:4181–4190.

160. Sondak VK, Liu PY, Tuthill RJ, et al: Adjuvant immunotherapy of resected, intermediate-thickness, node-negative melanoma with an allogeneic tumor vaccine: Overall results of a randomized trial of the Southwest Oncology Group. J Clin Oncol 2002;20:2058–2066.

161. Sosman JA, Unger JM, Liu PY, et al: Adjuvant immunotherapy of resected, intermediate-thickness, node-negative melanoma with an allogeneic tumor vaccine: Impact of HLA class I antigen expression on outcome, J Clin Oncol 2002;20:2067–2075.

162. Bystryn JC, Zeleniuch-Jacquotte A, Oratz R, et al: Double-blind trial of a polyvalent, shed-antigen, melanoma vaccine. Clin Cancer Res 2001;7:1882–1887.

163. Thomassen MJ, Barna BP, Rankin D, et al: Differential effect of recombinant granulocyte macrophage colony-stimulating factor on human monocytes and alveolar macrophages. Cancer Res 1989;49:4086–4089.

164. Spitler LE, Grossbard ML, Ernstoff MS, et al: Adjuvant therapy of stage III and IV malignant melanoma using granulocyte-macrophage colony-stimulating factor. J Clin Oncol 2000;18:1614–1621.

165. Essner R: Surgical treatment of malignant melanoma. Surg Clin North Am 2003;83:109–156.

166. Legha SS, Ring S, Eton O, et al: Development of a biochemotherapy regimen with concurrent administration of cisplatin, vinblastine, dacarbazine, interferon alfa, and interleukin-2 for patients with metastatic melanoma. J Clin Oncol 1998;16:1752–1759.

167. Atkins MB, Lee S, Flaherty LE, et al: A prospective randomized phase III trial of concurrent biochemotherapy (BCT) with cisplatin, vinblastine, dacarbazine (CVD), IL-2 and interferon alpha-2b (INF) versus CVD alone in patients with metastatic melanoma (E3695): An ECOG coordinated intergroup trial. Proc Am Soc Clin Oncol 2003;22:2847.

168. Karakousis CP, Velez A, Driscoll DL, et al: Metastasectomy in malignant melanoma. Surgery 1994;115:295–302.

169. Wong JH, Skinner KA, Kim KA, et al: The role of surgery in the treatment of nonregionally recurrent melanoma. Surgery 1993;113:389–394.

170. Wornom IL III, Smith JW, Soong SJ, et al: Surgery as palliative treatment for distant metastases of melanoma. Ann Surg 1986;204:181–185.

171. Hill GJ II, Krementz ET, Hill HZ: Dimethyl triazeno imidazole carboxamide and combination therapy for melanoma: IV. Late results after complete response to chemotherapy (Central Oncology Group protocols 7130, 7131, and 7131A). Cancer 1984;53:1299–1305.

172. Chapman PB, Einhorn LH, Meyers ML, et al: Phase III multicenter randomized trial of the Dartmouth regimen versus dacarbazine in patients with metastatic melanoma. J Clin Oncol 1999;17:2745–2751.

173. Bleehen NM, Newlands ES, Lee SM, et al: Cancer Research Campaign phase II trial of temozolomide in metastatic melanoma. J Clin Oncol 1995;13:910–913.

174. Middleton MR, Grob JJ, Aaronson N, et al: Randomized phase III study of temozolomide versus dacarbazine in the treatment of patients with advanced metastatic malignant melanoma. J Clin Oncol 2000;18:158–166.

175. Antonadou D, Paraskevaidis M, Sarris G, et al: Phase II randomized trial of temozolomide and concurrent radiotherapy in patients with brain metastase. J Clin Oncol 2002;20:3644–3650.

176. Song SY, Chary KK, Higby DJ, Henderson ES: Cisdiamminedichloride (II) in the treatment of metastatic malignant melanoma. Clin Res 1977;25:411.

177. Evans LM, Casper ES, Rosenbluth R: Phase II trial of carboplatin in advanced malignant melanoma. Cancer Treat Rep 1987;71:171–172.

178. Ramirez G, Wilson W, Grage T, et al: Phase II evaluation of 1,3-bis(2-chloroethyl-nitrosurea) (BCNU;NSC-409962) in patients with solid tumors. Cancer Chemother Rep 1972;25:787–790.

179. Retsas S, Newton KA, Westbury G: Vindesine as a single agent in the treatment of advanced malignant melanoma. Cancer Chemother Pharmacol 1979;2:257–260.

180. Legha SS, Ring S, Papadopoulos N, et al: A phase II trial of taxol in metastatic melanoma. Cancer 1990;65:2478–2481.

181. Einzig AI, Schuchter LM, Recio A, et al: Phase II trial of docetaxel (Taxotere) in patients with metastatic melanoma previously untreated with cytotoxic chemotherapy. Med Oncol 1996;13:111–117.

182. Feun LG, Savaraj N, Hurley J, et al: A clinical trial of intravenous vinorelbine tartrate plus tamoxifen in the treatment of patients with advanced malignant melanoma. Cancer 2000;88:584–588.

183. Cocconi G, Bella M, Calabresi F, et al: Treatment of metastatic

malignant melanoma with dacarbazine plus tamoxifen. N Engl J Med 1992;327:516–523.

184. Falkson CI, Ibrahim J, Kirkwood JM, et al: Phase III trial of dacarbazine versus dacarbazine with interferon alpha-2b versus dacarbazine with tamoxifen versus dacarbazine with interferon alpha-2b and tamoxifen in patients with metastatic malignant melanoma: An Eastern Cooperative Oncology Group study. J Clin Oncol 1998;16:1743–1751.

185. Buzaid AC, Leghas S, Winn R, et al: Cisplatin, vinblastine, and dacarbazine versus dacarbazine alone in metastatic melanoma: Preliminary results of a phase III Cancer Community Oncology Program trial. Proc Am Soc Clin Oncol 1993;12:389.

186. Seigler HF, Lucas VS Jr, Pickett NJ, et al: DTIC, CCNU, bleomycin and vincristine (BOLD) in metastatic melanoma. Cancer 1980;46:2346–2348.

187. Del Prete SA, Maurer LH, O'Donnell J, et al: Combination chemotherapy with cisplatin, carmustine, dacarbazine, and tamoxifen in metastatic melanoma. Cancer Treat Rep 1984;68:1403–1405.

188. McClay EF, Mastrangelo MJ, Sprandio JD, et al: The importance of tamoxifen to a cisplatin-containing regimen in the treatment of metastatic melanoma. Cancer 1989;63:1292–1295.

189. Rusthoven JJ, Quirt IC, Iscoe NA, et al: Randomized, double-blind, placebo-controlled trial comparing the response rates of carmustine, dacarbazine, and cisplatin with and without tamoxifen in patients with metastatic melanoma. National Cancer Institute of Canada Clinical Trials Group. J Clin Oncol 1996;14:2083–2090.

190. Mitchell MS, Von Eschen KB: Phase III trial of Melacine melanoma vaccine versus combination chemotherapy in the treatment of stage IV melanoma. Proc Am Soc Clin Oncol 1997;16:494a.

191. Krown SE, Burk MW, Kirkwood JM, et al: Human leukocyte (alpha) interferon in metastatic malignant melanoma: The American Cancer Society phase II trial. Cancer Treat Rep 1984;68:723–726.

192. Creagan ET, Ahmann DL, Green SJ, et al: Phase II study of recombinant leukocyte A interferon (rIFN-alpha A) in disseminated malignant melanoma. Cancer 1984;54:2844–2849.

193. Sparano JA, Fisher RI, Sunderland M, et al: Randomized phase III trial of treatment with high-dose interleukin-2 either alone or in combination with interferon alfa-2a in patients with advanced melanoma. J Clin Oncol 1993;11:1969–1977.

194. Vuoristo MS, Grohn P, Kellokumpu-Lehtinen P, et al: Intermittent interferon and polychemotherapy in metastatic melanoma. J Cancer Res Clin Oncol 1995;121:175–180.

195. Feun LG, Savaraj N, Moffat F, et al: Phase II trial of recombinant interferon-alpha with BCNU, cisplatin, DTIC and tamoxifen in advanced malignant melanoma. Melanoma Res 1995;5:273–276.

196. Rosenberg SA, Lotze MT, Muul LM, et al: Observations on the systemic administration of autologous lymphokine-activated killer cells and interleukin-2 in patients with metastatic melanoma. N Engl J Med 1985;313:1485.

197. Whittington R, Faulds D: Interleukin-2: A review of its pharmacological properties and therapeutic use in patients with cancer. Drugs 1993;46:446–514.

198. Rosenberg SA, Yang JC, White DE, et al: Durability of complete responses in patients with metastatic cancer treated with high-dose interleukin-2: Identification of antigens mediating response. Ann Surg 1998;228:307–319.

199. Atkins MB, Lotze MT, Dutcher JP, et al: High-dose recombinant interleukin 2 therapy for patients with metastatic melanoma: Analysis of 270 patients treated between 1985 and 1993. J Clin Oncol 1999;17:2105–2116.

200. Rosenberg SA: Immunotherapy of patients with advanced cancer using IL-2 alone or in combination with lymphokine activated killer cells. In DeVita VT, Hellman S, Rosenberg SA (eds): Important Advances in Oncology 1988. Philadelphia, JB Lippincott, 1988, pp 217–257.

201. Rosenberg SA, Yannelli JR, Yang JC, et al: Treatment of patients with metastatic melanoma with autologous tumor-infiltrating lymphocytes and interleukin 2. J Natl Cancer Inst 1994;86:1159–1166.

202. Schwartzentruber DJ: Interleukin-2: Clinical applications, principles of administration and management of side effects. In Rosenberg SA (ed): Biologic Therapy of Cancer, 3rd ed. Philadelphia, Lippincott Williams and Wilkins, 2000, pp 32–50.

203. Yang JC, Topalian SL, Schwartzentruber DJ, et al: The use of polyethylene glycol-modified interleukin-2 (PEG-IL-2) in the treatment of patients with metastatic renal cell carcinoma and melanoma: A phase I study and a randomized prospective study comparing IL-2 alone versus IL-2 combined with PEG-IL-2. Cancer 1995;76:687–694.

204. Adler A, Schachter J, Barenholz Y, et al: Allogeneic human liposomal melanoma vaccine with or without IL-2 in metastatic melanoma patients: Clinical and immunobiological effects. Cancer Biother 1995;10:293–306.

205. Richards JM, Mehta N, Ramming K, et al: Sequential chemoimmunotherapy in the treatment of metastatic melanoma. J Clin Oncol 1992;10:1338–1343.

206. Rosenberg SA, Yang JC, Schwartzentruber DJ, et al: Prospective randomized trial of the treatment of patients with metastatic melanoma using chemotherapy with cisplatin, dacarbazine, and tamoxifen alone or in combination with interleukin-2 and interferon alfa-2b. J Clin Oncol 1999;17:968–975.

207. Eton O, Legha SS, Bedikian AY, et al: Sequential biochemotherapy versus chemotherapy for metastatic melanoma: Results from a phase III randomized trial. J Clin Oncol 2002;20:2045–2052.

208. McDermott DF, Mier JW, Lawrence DP, et al: A phase II pilot trial of concurrent biochemotherapy with cisplatin, vinblastine, dacarbazine, interleukin 2, and interferon alpha-2B in patients with metastatic melanoma. Clin Cancer Res 2000;6:2201–2208.

209. O'Day SJ, Boasberg PD, Piro L, et al: Maintenance biotherapy for metastatic melanoma with interleukin-2 and granulocyte macrophage-colony stimulating factor improves survival for patients responding to induction concurrent biochemotherapy. Clin Cancer Res 2002;8:2775–2781.

210. Eisen T, Boshoff C, Mak I, et al: Continuous low dose thalidomide: A phase II study in advanced melanoma, renal cell, ovarian and breast cancer. Br J Cancer 2000;82:812–817.

211. Hwu WJ, Krown SE, Panagas KS, et al: Temozolomide plus thalidomide in patients with advanced melanoma. J Clin Oncol 2002;20:2610–2615.

212. Marriott JB, Clarke IA, Dredge K, et al: Thalidomide and its analogues have distinct and opposing effects on TNF-alpha and TNFR2 during co-stimulation of both CD4(+) and CD8(+) T cells. Clin Exp Immunol 2002;130:75–84.

213. Carson WE, Biber N, Shah K, et al: A phase II trial of recombinant humanized monoclonal anti-vascular endothelial growth factor (VEGF) antibody in patients with metastatic melanoma. Proc Am Soc Clin Oncol 2003;22:2873a.

214. Natali PG, Hamby CV, Felding-Habermann B, et al: Clinical significance of alpha(v)beta3 integrin and intercellular adhesion molecule-1 expression in cutaneous malignant melanoma lesions. Cancer Res 1997;57:1554–1560.

215. Triozzi PL, Kim JA, Martin EW, et al: Phase I trial of escalating doses of interleukin-1 beta in combination with a fixed dose of interleukin-2. J Clin Oncol 1995;13:482–489.

216. Olencki T, Finke J, Tubbs R, et al: Immunomodulatory effects of interleukin-2 and interleukin-4 in patients with malignancy. J Immunother Emphasis Tumor Immunol 1996;19:69–80.

217. Atkins MB, Robertson MJ, Gordon M, et al: Phase I evaluation of intravenous recombinant human interleukin 12 in patients with advanced malignancies. Clin Cancer Res 1997;3:409–417.

218. Nagai H, Hara I, Horikawa T, et al: Antitumor effects on mouse melanoma elicited by local secretion of interleukin-12 and their enhancement by treatment with interleukin-18. Cancer Invest 2000;18:206–213.

219. van der Bruggen P, Traversari C, Chomez P, et al: A gene encoding an antigen recognized by cytolytic T lymphocytes on a human melanoma. Science 1991;176:1643–1647.

220. Phan GQ, Touloukian CE, Yang JC, et al: Immunization of patients with metastatic melanoma using both class I- and class II-restricted peptides from melanoma-associated antigens. J Immunother 2003;26:349–356.

221. Rosenberg SA, Yang JC, Schwartzentruber DJ, et al: Immunologic and therapeutic evaluation of a synthetic peptide vaccine for the treatment of patients with metastatic melanoma. Nat Med 1998;4:321–327.

222. Dudley ME, Wunderlich JR, Robbins PF, et al: Cancer regression and autoimmunity in patients after clonal repopulation with antitumor lymphocytes. Science 2002;298:850–854.

223. Jansen B, Wacheck V, Heere-Ress E, et al: Chemosensitisation of malignant melanoma by BCL2 antisense therapy. Lancet 2000;356:1728–1733.

224. Preito VG, Zhang P, Eton OE: Expression of the tyrosine-kinase receptors c-kit, PDGFr-alpha, PDGFr-beta, abl, abl-related gene (ARG) in metastatic melanoma: Possible implications for therapy. Proc AACR 2002; 99a.

225. Wyman K, Atkins MB, Hubbard D, et al: A phase II trial of imatinib mesylate at 800 mg daily in metastatic melanoma: Lack of clinical efficacy with significant toxicity. Proc Am Soc Clin Oncol 2003;22:2865a.

226. Flaherty KT, Lee RJ, Humphries R, et al: Phase I trial of BAY 43-9006 in combination with carboplatin and paclitaxel. Proc Am Soc Clin Oncol 2003;22:2854a.

227. Karakousis CP, Velez A, Driscoll DL, et al: Metastasectomy in malignant melanoma. Surgery 1994;115:295–302.

228. Guazzo EP, Atkinson RL, Weidmann M, et al: Management of solitary melanoma metastasis of the brain. Aust N Z J Surg 1989;59:321–324.

229. Somaza S, Kondziolka D, Lunsford LD, et al: Stereotactic radiosurgery for cerebral metastatic melanoma. J Neurosurg 1993;79:661–666.

230. Douglas JG, Margolin K: The treatment of brain metastases from malignant melanoma. Semin Oncol 2002;29:518–524.

231. Wrone DA, Tanabe KK, Cosimi AB, et al: Lymphedema after sentinel lymph node biopsy for cutaneous melanoma: A report of 5 cases. Arch Dermatol 2000;136:511–514.

232. Weiss M, Loprinzi CL, Creagan ET, et al: Utility of follow-up tests for detecting recurrent disease in patients with malignant melanomas. JAMA 1995;274:1703–1705.

233. Mooney MM, Kulas M, McKinley B, et al: Impact on survival by method of recurrence detection in stage I and II cutaneous melanoma. Ann Surg Oncol 1998;5:54–63.

234. Poo-Hwu JJ, Ariyan S, Lamb L, et al: Follow-up recommendations for patients with American Joint Committee on Cancer Stages I–III malignant melanoma. Cancer 1999;86:2252–2258.

235. Buzaid AC, Tinoco L, Ross MI, et al: Role of computed tomography in the staging of patients with local-regional metastases of melanoma. J Clin Oncol 1995;13:2104–2108.

236. Evans RA, Bland KI, McMurtrey MJ, et al: Radionuclide scans not indicated for clinical stage I melanoma. Surg Gynecol Obstet 1980;150:532–534.

237. Flaherty LE, Unger JM, Liu PY, et al: Metastatic melanoma from intraocular primary tumors: The Southwest Oncology Group experience in phase II advanced melanoma clinical trials. Am J Clin Oncol 1998;21:568–572.

238. Krishnakumar S, Abhyankar D, Lakshmi SA, et al: HLA class II antigen expression in uveal melanoma: Correlation with clinicopathological features. Exp Eye Res 2003;77:175–180.

239. Cohen Y, Goldenberg-Cohen N, Parrella P, et al: Lack of BRAF mutation in primary uveal melanom. Invest Ophthalmol Vis Sci 2003;44:2876–2878.

240. Kivela T, Suciu S, Hansson J, et al: Bleomycin, vincristine, lomustine and dacarbazine (BOLD) in combination with recombinant interferon alpha-2b for metastatic uveal melanoma. Eur J Cancer 2003;39:115–120.

241. Mavligit GM, Charnsangavej C, Carrasco CH, et al: Regression of ocular melanoma metastatic to the liver after hepatic arterial chemoembolization with cisplatin and polyvinyl sponge. JAMA 1988;260:974–976.

242. Carroll NM, Alexander HR Jr: Isolation perfusion of the liver. Cancer J 2002;8:181–193.

243. Kim K, Hodges C, Papadopoulos O, et al: Biochemotherapy in patients with metastatic anorectal melanoma. Proc Am Soc Clin Oncol 2003;22:2883a.

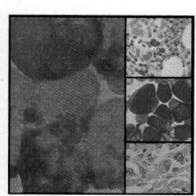

73

NONMELANOMA SKIN CANCERS: BASAL CELL AND SQUAMOUS CELL CARCINOMAS

Gary S. Wood

Mohammed Bagheri

Manish Gharia

Ellen Gordon

Paul O. Larson

Stephen N. Snow

SUMMARY OF KEY POINTS

INCIDENCE
- One million new cases of nonmelanoma skin cancer occur annually; 80% of cases are basal cell carcinoma (BCC), and 20% are squamous cell carcinoma (SCC).
- The incidence is increasing 2% to 3% per year.
- The incidence of SCC is 18- to 36-fold greater in organ transplant recipients than in other patients.

ETIOLOGY AND EPIDEMIOLOGY
- Ultraviolet radiation from sun exposure is a major risk factor and causes mutations in key genes.
- Hedgehog signaling pathway mutations are involved in the pathogenesis of BCC.
- p53 mutations are involved in the pathogenesis of both SCC and BCC and in the development of actinic keratosis, which is the precursor of SCC.

PATHOLOGY AND BIOLOGY
- There are several histopathologic subtypes of nonmelanoma skin cancer.
- The more infiltrative or poorly differentiated variants are more clinically aggressive. These variants include morpheaform BCC and spindle cell SCC.

CLINICAL FINDINGS
- BCC and SCC are found mainly on sun-exposed skin.
- Classic BCC is a pearly, telangiectatic, variably ulcerated nodule or a pale, sclerotic plaque.

- Classic SCC is a flesh-tone or red, variably keratotic, variably ulcerated nodule.

DIFFERENTIAL DIAGNOSIS AND STAGING
- The differential diagnosis includes amelanotic melanoma, kerato-acanthoma, cutaneous metastasis, cutaneous lymphoma, cutaneous lymphoid hyperplasia, adnexal tumor, Merkel cell carcinoma, and sebaceous gland carcinoma.
- BCC that is large, deep, or infiltrative may be locally aggressive and recurrent but metastasizes only rarely (<0.05%).
- SCC has a greater metastatic rate, especially when the tumor is large or deep, has perineural invasion, or is located on the dorsal aspect of the hands or on the lips, ears, penis, or sites of chronic infection, ulceration, or radiation.

PRIMARY THERAPY AND SALVAGE THERAPY
- Primary management of both BCC and SCC is surgical. Mohs surgery is preferred for ill-defined or aggressive lesions, because it allows microscopic control of tumor margins.
- Alternative therapies include various forms of physical destruction and radiation therapy. Interferons and inducers of interferons (e.g., imiquimod) are proving useful in selected cases.

- Retinoids, cyclo-oxygenase-2 inhibitors, and difluoromethylornithine are promising chemopreventive agents.
- Combinations of surgery, radiation therapy, and chemotherapy can be used to manage metastatic disease.

COMPLICATIONS
- Complications are principally related to local factors.
- Complications include local recurrence, destruction of adjacent structures, scarring, and loss of function.

PROGNOSIS
- Relative to most other forms of cancer, the overall prognosis for BCC and SCC is very good. There are only approximately 2000 deaths annually in the United States compared with approximately 1 million new cases diagnosed.
- Local recurrence is a problem for large, deep, or histologically infiltrative variants. SCC with these features may metastasize. The 5-year survival among patients with metastatic SCC is less than 50%.
- The rarer forms of nonmelanoma skin cancer have a significantly more aggressive clinical course than BCC and SCC. These include sebaceous carcinoma, Merkel cell carcinoma, dermatofibrosarcoma protuberans, and cutaneous angiosarcoma.

INTRODUCTION

Most nonmelanoma skin cancers (NMSCs) are basal cell carcinoma (BCC) or squamous cell carcinomas (SCC). However, several rarer forms of NMSC exist, including four malignant neoplasms discussed in this chapter: sebaceous gland carcinoma, Merkel cell carcinoma, angiosarcoma, and dermatofibrosarcoma protuberans. Each of these neoplasms is discussed separately after a summary of genetic alterations in BCC, SCC, and selected genodermatoses. Understanding the genetic basis of skin cancer is an important step in improving prognosis among patients with these neoplasms. Analysis of germline mutations in familial cancer syndromes and somatic mutations in sporadic skin cancers is providing new information that will facilitate the diagnosis of cutaneous malignant diseases and revolutionize their management.

GENETICS OF NONMELANOMA SKIN CANCER

Advances in molecular genetics have allowed for key advances in our understanding of NMSC, the most common cancer in the United States. Like visceral malignant neoplasms, cancer of the integument is caused by defects in the normal genetic code. These genomic defects are either germline mutations (those caused by inherited mutations) or somatic mutations (those caused by acquired mutations). Actual tumor formation, however, is a complicated process, usually requiring more than a single mutation and sometimes a combination of germline and somatic mutations. In addition, these cancerous cells are frequently altered in ways that help them escape detection by the host's immune system.

Tumor suppressor genes and oncogenes are two basic classes of genes that undergo mutations leading to skin cancer. Examples of tumor suppressor genes include the patched gene involved in development of BCC, p53 involved in development of SCC, and the xeroderma pigmentosum (XP) genes involved in development of BCC, SCC, and melanoma.[1-3] These genes can be further divided into tumor suppressor genes that directly participate in growth regulation, such as the patched and p53 genes, and those that participate indirectly and are called *caretaker genes*, such as the XP genes encoding DNA repair enzymes.

Oncogenes are the other class of genes contributing to skin cancer formation. These are generally growth-signaling molecules that once mutated can perpetually lead normal cells to become malignant cells by altering cellular growth. One example is the *ras* oncogene implicated in a number of skin cancers, including BCC, SCC, and melanoma.[4,5]

Sonic Hedgehog Pathway

The sonic hedgehog (Shh) pathway has been implicated in both hereditary and sporadic cases of BCC. These tumors are the most common of all skin cancers, with an estimated 1 million new cases per year.[6] In the Shh pathway, the transmembrane protein receptor for Shh, known as *patched1* (Ptch1), binds and inhibits another transmembrane protein called *smoothened* (Smoh).[7] Smoh is responsible for growth promotion, and binding by Ptch1 keeps this growth in check. However, when the soluble lipoprotein Shh binds Ptch1, this regulation is disrupted. Smoh is thus activated, and unregulated growth is promoted through downstream zinc-finger family transcription factors, such as gli1, gli2, and gli3.

The hedgehog pathway was originally elucidated in the fruit fly (*Drosophila melanogaster*), in which mutations in the gene cause segmental patterning defects, hence the name *patched*.[8] Involvement in human disease was found through analysis of nevoid BCC kindreds (Gorlin's syndrome, basal cell nevus syndrome).[9] Persons with this autosomal-dominant disease have odontogenic cysts, skeletal defects, palmar pits, various associated visceral tumors (medulloblastoma, meningioma, fibrosarcoma, cardiac fibroma, and ovarian fibroma), and multiple BCCs by a median age of 20 years. Early analyses mapped the defect to a tumor suppressor gene on chromosome 9q22-31.[10] This site proved to be the location of the Ptch1 gene. It was later elucidated that patients with nevoid BCC syndrome inherit one defective chromosome 9q region with loss of heterozygosity in the Ptch1 locus. Many BCCs from these patients show inactivation of the remaining Ptch1 gene through acquired somatic mutations, consistent with the view that the BCC phenotype develops once both alleles are nonfunctional. Thus *Ptch1* acts as a classic tumor suppressor gene in the skin. Mutations in *Ptch1* also are present in many sporadic BCCs, as are mutations in other Shh pathway genes, including *Smoh*, *Ptch2*, and *Shh*.[11]

p53 Mutations

The protein p53 is encoded by the TP53 gene on chromosome 17p and is an important regulator of cell proliferation, DNA repair, and apoptosis.[12] *p53* can act classically as a tumor suppressor gene or act in a dominant-negative role whereby abnormal, mutant p53 protein can bind normal p53 molecules and disrupt their function.

Inactivation of the p53 gene appears to play a principal role in the development of both premalignant actinic keratosis and SCC.[13] SCC is the second most common skin cancer, accounting for approximately 200,000 cases per year and 2000 deaths per year.[6] *p53* mutations causing SCC are ultraviolet (UV) induced, and many are pyrimidine alterations with CC to TT changes.[14] It appears that it is both the loss of the tumor suppressor ability of p53 and the ability of UV irradiation to affect induction of apoptosis by p53 that leads to tumor formation.[13]

Mutations of *TP53* have been implicated in development of sporadic BCC.[15] It appears that UV-induced alterations similar to those in SCC are involved in BCC induction. Many of the mutations are CC to TT or C to T alterations, consistent with UV damage.

Mutations of Caretaker Genes

Tumor suppressor genes involved in maintaining genomic integrity are called *caretaker genes*.[16] Examples of diseases associated with cutaneous malignant tumors and known defects in caretaker genes include XP, Bloom syndrome, Rothmund-Thomson syndrome, Werner's syndrome, and Muir-Torre syndrome.

The tumor suppressor genes involved in all of these familial syndromes have the common feature of being involved in an enzymatic DNA reparative process following a mutagenic insult. Defects in these genes inhibit the ability to repair genetic damage from naturally occurring events or environmental carcinogens such as UV radiation.

XP is a collection of autosomal-recessive disorders characterized by severe photosensitivity with onset of cutaneous malignant lesions at a very early age. BCC, actinic keratosis, SCC, and melanoma develop during the first decade of life in persons without adequate photo-protection. Mutations in seven genes have been implicated in different XP phenotypes. They are identified as complementation groups XPA through XPG and differ in severity of cutaneous neoplasia and frequency of neurologic delay.[17] All XP-associated genes encode proteins that are part of a DNA repair process known as *nucleotide excision repair*, which responds to UV-induced DNA damage.[3] These proteins recognize the damaged DNA, unwind the coiled DNA structure, and repair the damaged strand. Germline mutations in these genes result in defects in the repair process and their genomic caretaker role; however, actual tumor production is still caused by mutagenic inactivation of tumor suppressor genes such as p53 and activation of oncogenes such as *ras*.[18,19]

Rothmund-Thomson syndrome, Bloom syndrome, and Werner's syndrome all are rare autosomal-recessive disorders that have known defects in helicase genes and affect nucleotide excision repair. Like XP, these defects allow development of malignant skin lesions in affected patients. Rothmund-Thomson and Bloom syndromes both are marked by early onset of SCC; however, patients with Werner's syndrome appear to have only increased risk of melanoma. Other syndromes with helicase gene defects, such as Cockayne's syndrome and photosensitive trichothiodystrophy, have no associated increase in cutaneous malignant tumors. It is becoming clear that development of cutaneous malignant tumors is a complex process in which ability to repair DNA is but one part of an intricate pathway. It appears that other mutations in tumor suppressor genes and oncogenes, whether germline or somatic, are necessary to invoke a tumor phenotype, as seen in XP.

Muir-Torre syndrome (MTS) is an autosomal-dominant syndrome characterized by various sebaceous gland tumors and internal malignant lesions. The sebaceous gland tumors range from benign sebaceous adenoma to malignant sebaceous gland carcinoma predominantly on the face. Keratoacanthoma is another cutaneous neoplasm of variable malignant potential that has been reported in as many as 20% of MTS patients.[20]

In initial studies of MTS families, investigators identified linkage to chromosome 2p16.[21] In subsequent studies investigators identified germline mutations in the *h*MSH2 gene at that locus.[22] It appears that, like other caretaker genes, *h*MSH2 codes for a type of DNA mismatch repair enzyme involved in repairing errors in DNA replication that occur naturally at a low rate.

In cells that have this defect, the result is varying lengths of repetitive DNA sequences known as micro-satellite instability.[23] This microsatellite instability can result in functional gene mutations and has been observed in keratoacanthoma and sebaceous tumors from MTS patients.[24]

ras Oncogene

ras mutations have been implicated in development of sporadic BCC, premalignant actinic keratosis, and sporadic

BEST PRACTICES FOR PATIENT SCREENING AND TUMOR PREVENTION

A full-body skin examination is advised as part of an annual physical, especially for older adults or those with a family history of skin cancer. For those with a personal history of skin cancer, examination every 4 to 6 months is advised. For nonmelanoma skin cancer, special attention is paid to sites of previous skin cancer, changing or new skin lesions, and sun-exposed areas in general. Peripheral lymph nodes are palpated if there is a history of skin cancer with above average metastatic potential, such as squamous cell carcinoma of the lip.

Prevention of nonmelanoma skin cancer mainly involves protection from the sun. Suntans should be avoided because they are a sign of, and response to, UV damage. The skin should be protected with a combination of clothing and SPF 30 sunblock effective against both UV-A and UV-B wavelengths. Hats should have a 360-degree brim to protect the neck and ears as well as the face. Sunglasses that block UV light should be worn to protect the eyes, eyelids, and periorbital skin. Outdoor daylight activities are best restricted to the early morning, late afternoon, and early evening. The peak sunlight hours of 10 AM to 3 PM are best avoided by planning indoor activities during this period. The UV index is a daily rating of local UV intensity on a scale of 1 through 10. Although the scale can be useful in assessment of relative sun exposure risk, the best practice is always to follow the sun protection measures outlined previously. Protect children because sun-induced genetic damage begins in childhood, and most persons receive most of their lifelong sun exposure before adulthood. Retinoids, antioxidants, and cyclo-oxygenase-2 inhibitors may be beneficial for chemoprevention of nonmelanoma skin cancer.

WHEN AND HOW TO PERFORM BIOPSY

Unless logistical reasons preclude it, biopsy should be performed on all lesions suspected of being nonmelanoma skin cancer to establish the correct diagnosis, plan definitive therapy, and obtain prognostic information. The most important subjective symptoms can be summarized under the heading "change." The changes may be appearance of a new growth or a change in the size, shape, color, sensation (itch or pain), crusting, or bleeding of a preexisting lesion.

For most cases of nonmelanoma skin cancer, standard shave biopsy performed with a scalpel or razor blade is adequate. Well-differentiated squamous cell carcinoma and keratoacanthoma can be difficult to diagnose unless the deepest portions are included in the biopsy specimen because these often are the areas most likely to yield enough information for a diagnosis. Deep shave, punch, incisional, or excisional biopsy often is preferable to standard shave biopsy in these cases. For large or ill-defined tumors, it is frequently helpful to perform multiple mapping biopsies to identify the most biologically aggressive features, define margins, and plan treatment.

Specific Malignancies

SCC. They are among the most common mutations in human malignant disease.[25] ras proteins are small G-proteins responsible for transducing intracellular signaling. ras is activated only when guanosine triphosphate (GTP) is bound. The signal is attenuated by hydrolysis of GTP to guanosine diphosphate (GDP). Mutations in *ras* alter the rate of this hydrolysis, resulting in activated protein and promotion of cell growth and hence tumor growth. There is a class of proteins that shuts off *ras* by increasing GTP hydrolysis to GDP (GTPase-activating proteins, or GAPs).[26] There is evidence that alterations in GAPs are implicated in the development of sporadic BCC.

BASAL CELL CARCINOMA

Epidemiology and Pathogenesis

Basal cell carcinoma is the most common malignant tumor in the United States and in other areas with predominantly white populations. Approximately 900,000 cases per year are identified in the United States.[6] Australia has the highest incidence of skin cancer, the incidence of BCC being more than 2% among men and that of SCC being approximately 1% among men.[27] The incidence of BCC has increased over the past decades in a manner similar to the increase in melanoma. It is estimated that the incidence of NMSC is increasing 2% to 3% yearly.[28] One study, conducted in New Hampshire, showed an annual increase in incidence of SCC of approximately 10% and of BCC of approximately 5%.[29] Cumulative UV exposure and, more important, severe sunburn during childhood and adolescence are risk factors for BCC.[30] Other associated risk factors are Fitzpatrick skin types 1 and 2, red hair, freckling in childhood, family history of skin cancer, male sex, and Celtic ancestry.[31] BCC is more common in lighter-complexion African Americans than in darker persons.[32] Immunodeficiency secondary to acquired immunodeficiency syndrome or transplantation also is associated with increased risk of BCC. Other uncommon risk factors include exposure to arsenic and ionizing radiation, especially among patients who have received radiation for acne.

Keratin pattern and immunohistochemical results suggest the origin of BCC is the outer root sheath of the hair follicle below the isthmus.[33] The locally invasive characteristic of BCC could be related to the presence of abnormal hemidesmosome-anchoring fibril complex.[34] Genetic abnormalities and mutations are thought to play a major role in development of BCC, especially in inherited syndromes of BCC. Patients with XP cannot repair the UV-induced DNA mutations; therefore they are at increased risk of cutaneous carcinogenesis. Mutations in the hedgehog signaling pathway genes and p53 are important in the pathogenesis of sporadic BCC and those arising in patients with the nevoid BCC syndrome and XP.[11,13,35-37]

Clinical Manifestations

The most common location for BCC is the head and neck, especially the nose. BCC occurs on hair-bearing skin; mucosal surfaces are not involved. The major types of BCC

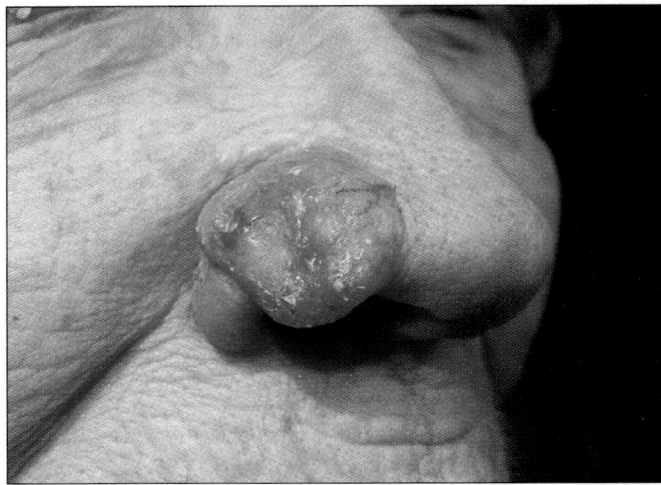

Figure 73-1. Typical presentation of basal cell carcinoma on the nose.

include nodular, pigmented, superficial, and morpheaform. The typical nodular BCC is a dome-shaped, pearly papule with a telangiectatic surface and translucent rolled borders (Fig. 73-1). The surface might become ulcerated (Fig. 73-2). In darker skinned individuals, especially African Americans, the more darkly pigmented BCC may be misdiagnosed as seborrheic keratosis or nodular melanoma. Superficial BCC is a well-demarcated erythematous scaly plaque with elevated borders that often occurs on the trunk or extremities. It might be confused with Bowen's disease or nummular eczema. The most difficult BCC to diagnose and manage is the morpheaform or sclerosing variant. This ill-defined, white, indurated plaque can be mistaken for a scar or localized patch of scleroderma and therefore is ignored by patient and physician, with resulting wide subclinical extension.

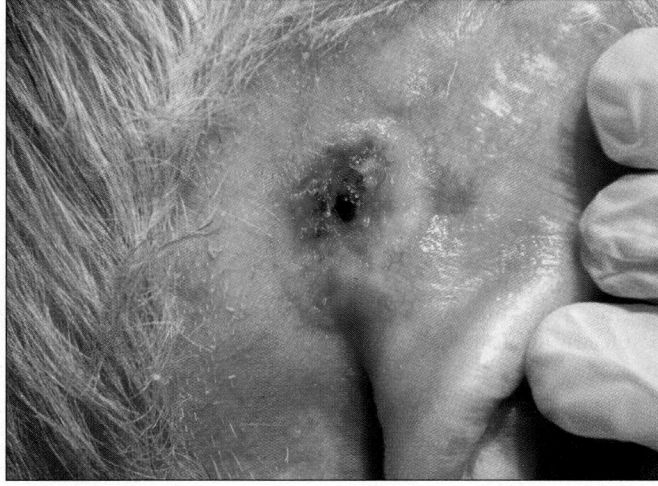

Figure 73-2. Ulcerated basal cell carcinoma with rolled borders on posterior ear.

Histopathology

In common nodular BCC, nodular masses of basaloid cells extend from the epidermis or outer root sheath into the dermis with surrounding connective tissue stroma (Fig. 73-3). A palisade arrangement of cells is present in the periphery. Sometimes as a result of tumor necrosis and disintegration, cystic spaces form. The surrounding stroma may retract from the tumor mass forming the typical lacunae, a sign that aids in diagnosis. In the pigmented type of BCC, large amounts of melanin are produced in the melanocytes that colonize the tumor. The many melanophages in the surrounding stroma also contribute to pigmentation. The superficial type of BCC exhibits multifocal small nests of basaloid tumor cells budding off the epidermis and adnexa. Morpheaform BCC

is different in that strands of tumor cells are embedded in a dense fibrous tissue stroma. These strands often extend in the deeper dermis. Micronodular BCCs contain small nodules of tumor cells that invade surrounding stroma. The morpheaform and micronodular types are generally the most locally invasive variants of BCC. It is common for BCCs to exhibit mixed histologic patterns of these various types. Even the less invasive variants may invade deeply when located in regions of embryonic fusion planes, such as around the nose and ears.

Treatment

BCC is rarely metastatic but can be locally invasive (Fig. 73-4). Therefore eradicating the primary tumor is the goal of therapy. Several treatment options are available,

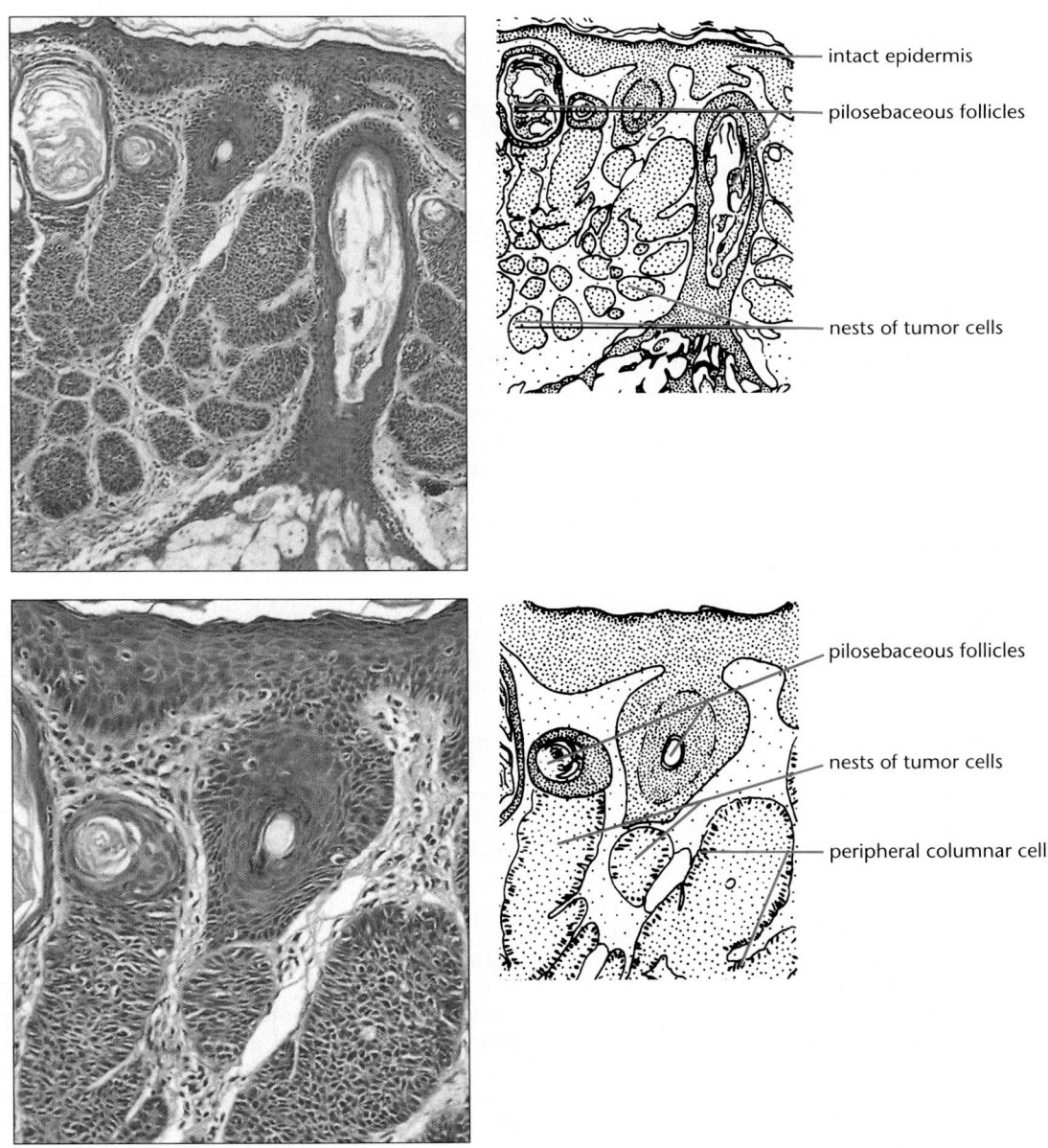

Figure 73-3. Histopathology of basal cell carcinoma. (From Skaria AK [ed]: Atlas of Diagnostic Oncology, 3rd ed. St. Louis, Mosby, 2003, p 374.)

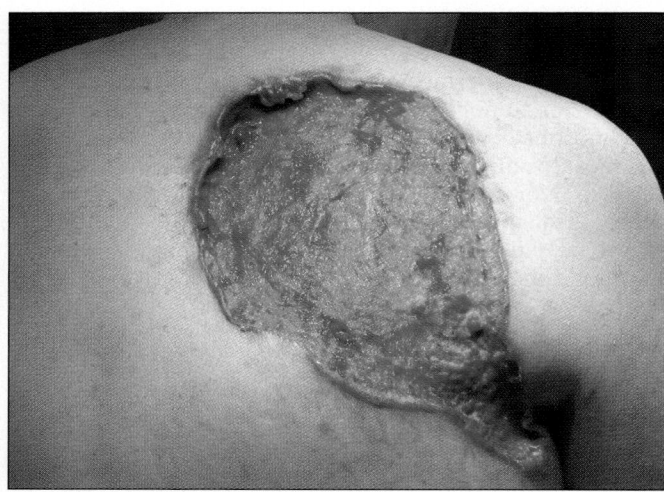

Figure 73-4. Basal cell carcinoma of 10 years' duration invading the scapula.

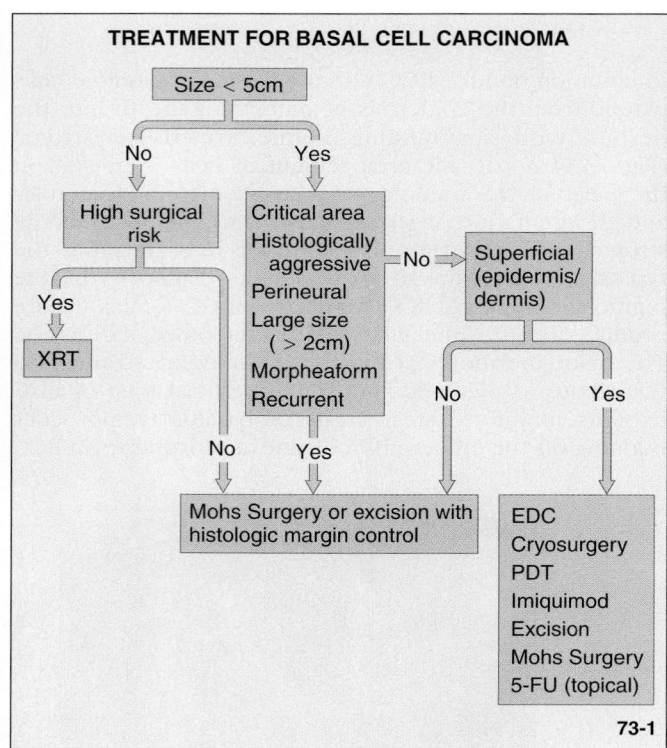

both surgical and nonsurgical. Selection depends on the tumor type, patient profile, size and location of tumor, recurrence, physician's experience, and patient preference. Surgical modalities include Mohs micrographic surgery, surgical excision, cryosurgery, and electrodesiccation and curettage.[31] Nonsurgical options include radiation therapy and photodynamic therapy.[38] Other treatment modalities, such as immunotherapy with intralesional interferon[39] and topical 5% imiquimod (Aldara),[40] chemotherapy with 5-fluorouracil,[41] and retinoids,[42] have been reported with variable success.

A systematic review of studies in which investigators reported recurrence rates of BCC after different treatment modalities showed that the mean 5-year-recurrence rates after Mohs surgery and surgical excision were approximately 1% and 5.3%, respectively.[43] Risk factors for BCC recurrence include greatest dimension larger than 2 cm, location in the midface (H zone) or ear, morpheaform or other aggressive histologic pattern, and long duration.[44] These tumors should be completely resected, preferably by Mohs technique or excision with margin control. Mohs surgery should be used in areas where preserving maximum tissue is important, such as eyelids, nose, and lips. It is also indicated for recurrent BCC and tumors with ill-defined clinical margins. If simple excision is used, the margin for excision should be at least 4 mm around tumors of 1 cm or less and 5 to 10 mm for tumors larger than 1 cm.[45] If there are contraindications to surgery, or the tumor is small and located on less critical sites such as the trunk, cryotherapy or electrodesiccation and curettage can be used with good outcome. Because of the less favorable long-term cosmetic results and possibility of secondary radiation-induced skin cancer, radiation therapy is best avoided in the care of relatively young patients. Very large or poorly controlled BCC may necessitate a coordinated approach of standard surgical excision, Mohs surgery, radiation therapy, and immunotherapy or chemotherapy.[46]

Prognosis and Follow-up Evaluation

The prognosis of BCC is generally good. Metastasis is rare, and tumor growth is slow. Two thirds of recurrences occur during the first 3 years after treatment.[47] The risk of development of another BCC is approximately 45% within 5 years.[48] The risk of development of another NMSC is associated with the number of previous NMSCs. In an Australian study of patients with three to nine previous NMSCs, the risk of development of a new cancer was 93%.[49] Patients treated for BCC need to be examined at least once a year for the first few years, preferably for 5 years after the last cancer was diagnosed. For patients with a history of multiple skin cancers, more frequent follow-up examinations are recommended. Photoprotection starting at a young age is advised to reduce the cumulative damage induced by the sun.

SQUAMOUS CELL CARCINOMA AND BOWEN'S DISEASE

Epidemiology and Pathogenesis

Squamous cell carcinoma is a malignant tumor of keratinocytes of the skin or mucosal surfaces. SCC has greater metastatic potential than BCC and causes most NMSC deaths. SCC can arise de novo or from a precursor such as actinic keratosis. Bowen's disease is an SCC in situ arising de novo. Bowen's disease that occurs on the glans penis or, rarely, the vulva is called *erythroplasia of Queyrat.* Bowen's disease can slowly progress to invasive SCC.

SCC is the second most common skin cancer in the United States, representing approximately 20% of cases of NMSC. Interestingly, SCC occurs more than BCC in blacks and Asians.[50] It is more common in men than women.[6] There are many risk factors for SCC, the most important being solar radiation. The incidence of SCC is increasing, especially on the head and neck area, because of exposure to sunlight.[51] SCC is thought to be correlated with recent (in the 10 years before diagnosis) chronic sunlight exposure[52] and cumulative sun exposure.[53] Phototherapy with PUVA (psoralen plus ultraviolet A) increases the risk of SCC. Other risk factors for SCC include fair skin, red hair, albinism, and Celtic origin. Nonsolar risk factors include exposure to chemicals (insecticides and herbicides),[54] arsenic, organic hydrocarbons, chronic thermal injury and scars, ionizing radiation, and chronic immunosuppression.[55] Risk of SCC increases 18 to 36 times in organ transplant patients.[56] This increase in risk correlates with the type of organ transplantation and elapsed time after transplantation. Heart transplant recipients have a higher risk of NMSC than kidney transplant recipients, possibly because of more intense immunosuppression.[57] Tobacco is a risk factor for oral SCC. Viruses, especially human papillomavirus, have been linked to epithelial malignant diseases, including SCC. The risk is especially high among patients with epidermodysplasia verruciformis, who have underlying immunodeficiency and can have SCC within human papillomavirus–infected warts.[55]

Carcinogens such as UV radiation, certain chemicals, and viruses play a role in the pathogenesis of SCC by damaging keratinocyte DNA and other cellular contents. It is known that UV radiation, especially UV-B, causes mutations in DNA of keratinocytes.[58] Early repair of these mutations is important for prevention of SCC. Patients with NMSC are thought to have decreased ability for DNA repair compared with controls, a condition that makes these patients more susceptible to the affects of UV radiation.[59] One example is the effect of UV radiation on DNA alterations in patients with XP who are genetically unable to repair these defects. UV radiation also causes cutaneous immunosuppression, weakening the host's immune response against tumor cells and promoting tumor growth.[60,61] Studies of SCC have shown that mutations in the p53 tumor suppressor gene are an early event.[2,62] Most of the mutations occur at dipyrimidine sequences, in the form of UV-induced cyclobutane pyrimidine dimers.[63] Development of SCC does not occur by a simple single step, but rather through a multistage process.[40] Conversion of susceptible keratinocytes to premalignant cells and then progression to carcinoma occurs as a result of successive genetic hits.[64] In the initiation stage of carcinogenesis, clonal expansion of premalignant cells occurs. The next stage is increased proliferation of premalignant cells and subsequent chromosomal aberrations. The final stage is conversion to SCC. DNA aneuploidy with a single peak was detected with flow cytometry in lesions of Bowen's disease, suggesting monoclonal proliferation of abnormal keratinocytes and a clonal basis for skin cancer.[65] Aberrant expression of P-cadherin and changes in expression of cytokeratins and transforming growth factors play a role in tumor progression.[66]

Clinical Manifestations

SCC occurs mainly on the head and neck area in whites, but in blacks there is no predilection for sun-exposed areas of the body.[67] SCC in situ may develop from premalignant lesions, such as actinic keratosis or arsenical keratosis. In whites most cases of SCC arise from actinic keratosis. These lesions can eventually spread beyond the epidermis and become invasive. Invasive SCC can arise from normal skin. It starts as a small, firm, dull red nodule that can undergo central ulceration. Sometimes if SCC arises from solar keratosis, adherent keratotic scale can be seen. If ignored, the lesion grows horizontally and vertically and can become fixed to the underlying tissue. The surface might become ulcerated with bleeding, malodorous exudate, or crust. The borders usually are elevated and firm. A fungoid lesion without ulceration occasionally is seen. SCC of the lower lip often arises from areas previously damaged by the sun (actinic cheilitis). Initially, local thickening of the vermillion border occurs and can progress to a noduloulcerative lesion (Fig. 73-5). Persistent subungual erythema with pain and swelling should alert the physician to the presence of SCC of the nail region. This form of SCC can be confused with warts (Fig. 73-6). SCC can arise from chronic ulcers, sinuses, scars, and chronic thermal damage.

Verrucous carcinoma is a distinct, slow-growing, low-grade type of SCC. The most common location is the plantar surface (epithelioma cuniculatum), but the lesions can occur on the buttocks, genitals (giant condyloma of Buschke and Loewenstein), face, oral cavity (oral florid papillomatosis), trunk, nails, and extremities. It grows as an exophytic verrucous mass. At clinical examination of the foot, the lesion can be mistaken for a plantar wart. It is locally aggressive and can penetrate into deep soft tissue or bone.

Bowen's disease often appears as a well-defined, single, red plaque with dry surface scaling. Lesions are slowly growing and asymptomatic and thus are ignored by many patients. The physician may initially manage the condition

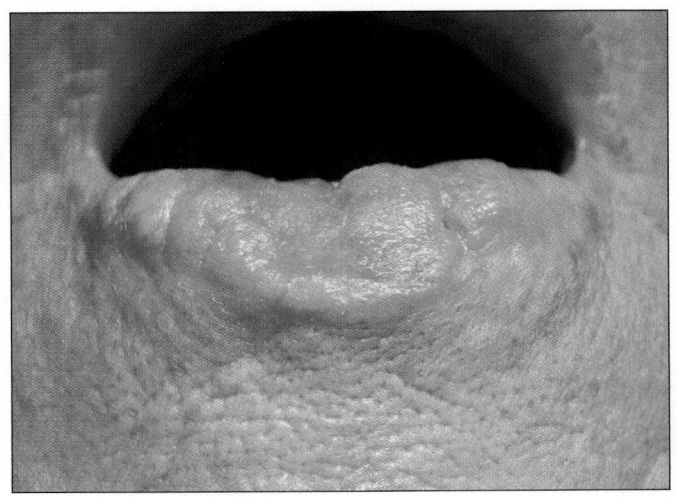

Figure 73-5. Squamous cell carcinoma of the lip of 5 years' duration.

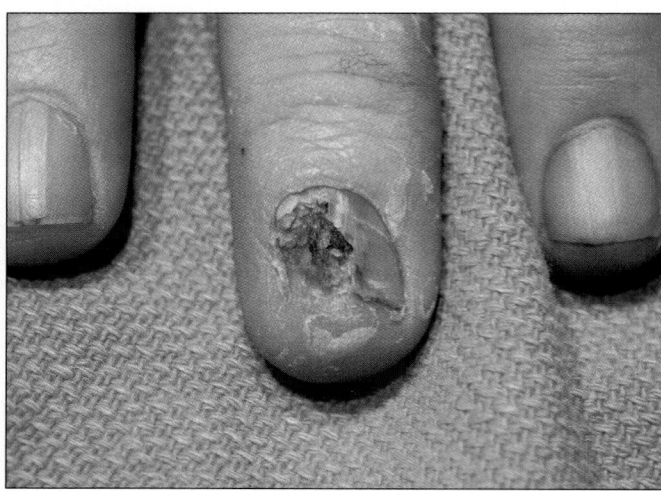

Figure 73-6. Squamous cell carcinoma of the nail bed. Patient was being treated for a wart.

as psoriasis or nummular eczema with no response. There is a 3% to 5% risk that Bowen's disease will progress into invasive SCC.[68] At clinical examination, erythroplasia of Queyrat resembles Bowen's disease but lacks dry superficial scale. Instead the surface is moist and smooth.

The risk of metastasis of SCC is variable, depending on the site and tumor characteristics. The deeper and larger the tumor, the higher is the likelihood of metastasis. Recurrent tumors are at high risk of metastasis. Lesions with perineural involvement have a 35% metastatic rate.[69] Among the different histologic types, desmoplastic SCC is most likely to metastasize.[70] The risk of metastasis of SCC derived from actinic keratosis is low (0.5%–3.7%) compared with that of SCC arising in radiation-induced SCC and chronic osteomyelitis (20% and 31%, respectively).[71,72] High-risk areas for metastasis include tumors arising from the dorsal aspect of the hands, lips, ears, and penis. For example, SCC of the lower lip has a 15% risk of

metastasis.[73] Bowen's disease and erythroplasia of Queyrat also have a low likelihood of metastasis, but once these conditions become invasive, the risk of metastasis increases significantly.

Histopathology

A deep shave or punch biopsy that includes the base of the tumor is needed to differentiate SCC in situ from invasive SCC. Bowen's disease is carcinoma in situ. The stratum corneum is thickened, and epidermis is hyperplastic with disordered maturation of keratinocytes. Mitotic figures, multinucleated keratinocytes, and dyskeratotic cells with hyperchromatic nuclei and eosinophilic cytoplasm are seen in the epidermis. Histologic examination of SCC shows masses of epidermal cells proliferating into the dermis (Fig. 73-7). Atypical squamous cells and mitotic figures are seen. The cells have abundant eosinophilic cytoplasm and large nuclei. Horn pearls, which are a result of keratinization of squamous cells, are seen. The dermis may show a marked inflammatory reaction. Spindle cell SCC is a rare variant composed of mainly spindle cells, but some squamous differentiation may be seen. Spindle cells have large vesicular nuclei and scant cytoplasm and intermingle with the collagenous stroma. Spindle cell SCC is poorly differentiated with numerous mitoses and deep invasion and requires immunohistochemical analysis for differentiation from other spindle cell tumors. Another uncommon histologic variant of SCC is acantholytic or adenoid SCC, seen more on the face and neck. There are nests of tumor cells, dyskeratotic cells, and central acantholysis forming pseudoglandular structures.

Treatment

The treatment options for SCC are similar to those for BCC; however, management needs to reflect the greater risk of metastasis among SCCs. The first step is to estimate peripheral and vertical extension of tumor cells. Tumors

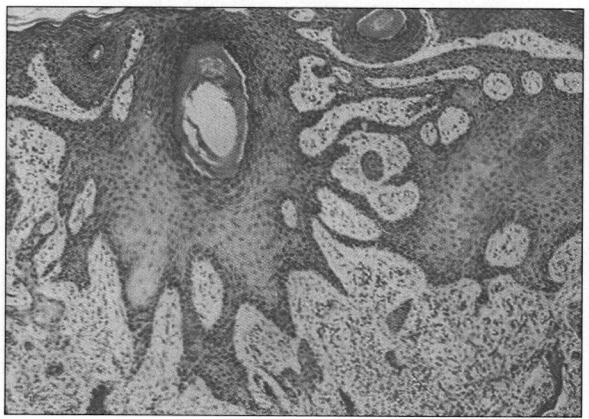
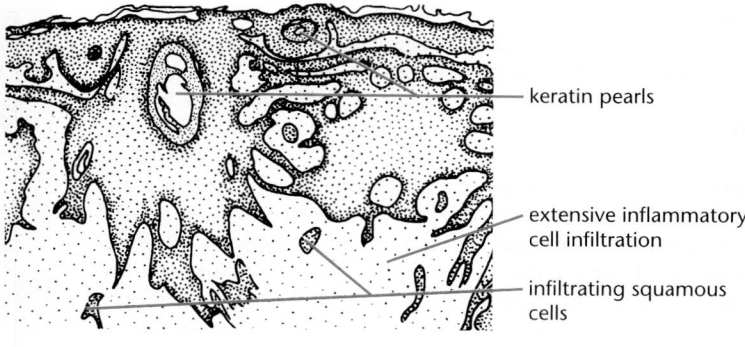

keratin pearls

extensive inflammatory cell infiltration

infiltrating squamous cells

Figure 73-7. Histopathology of squamous cell carcinoma. (From Skaria AK [ed]: Atlas of Diagnostic Oncology, 3rd ed. St. Louis, Mosby, 2003, p 376.)

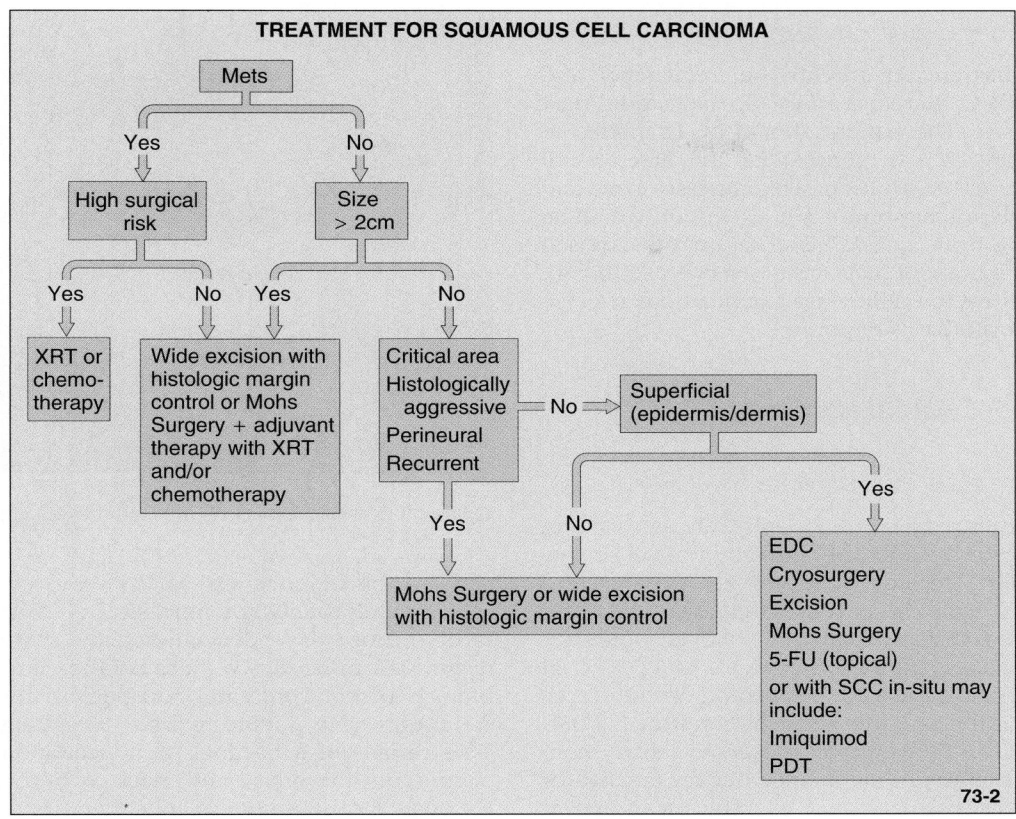

TREATMENT FOR SQUAMOUS CELL CARCINOMA

73-2

at high risk of local or distant spread are those larger than 2 cm in diameter or deeper than 6 mm, recurrent tumors, poorly differentiated tumors, and those with perineural invasion or arising in immunocompromised hosts.[74] Second, the patient needs evaluation for metastasis to the lymph nodes and other organs.

Destructive methods or surgical excision can be used for effective management of Bowen's disease. Small uncomplicated SCC (<1 cm) in low-risk locations frequently is managed with electrodesiccation and curettage. Cryotherapy is an alternative treatment. Simple surgical excision with margin control is commonly used for smaller tumors and those on the trunk and extremities. The recommended margin for low-risk SCC is 4 mm and for high-risk tumor is 6 mm.[75] The excision should include the subcutaneous fat. Mohs micrographic surgery is the therapy of choice for high-risk SCC or for tissue preservation when tissue sparing is cosmetically or functionally vital.[76] Aggressive or deeply invasive SCC is managed with deep surgical excision with margin control when practical. Mohs surgery can be helpful in delineating critical areas in massive tumors or tumors with ill-defined borders. SCC invading surrounding structures such as bone and cartilage must be excised. Tumors with neural or perineural involvement at high risk of recurrence should be completely excised, preferably with Mohs technique. High-risk tumors may require adjuvant therapy with radiation therapy[77] or chemotherapy.[78,79]

Radiation can be used as a primary choice of treatment. Usually 4000 cGy of radiation is given in 5 to 16 fractions. This form of treatment may be appropriate for elderly patients at high risk of surgical complications or other patients with contraindications to anesthesia or surgery. Radiation can be useful in the management of tumors on the eyelids, nose, ears, and lips when surgery is not practical. The disadvantages are cost, blind margin control, and prolonged treatment duration. The cure rate for tumors larger than 2 cm in greatest dimension is approximately 85% to 95%.[80] Radiation therapy is best avoided in the management of verrucous carcinoma and the care of younger patients because of poor long-term cosmetic results. SCC that has arisen from ulcers, scars, and radiated sites is best removed by margin-controlled surgery than by radiation therapy.

If lymph node metastasis has occurred, treatment is wide surgical resection of tumor with regional lymph node dissection with or without adjunctive radiation. However, elective lymph node dissection is not commonly performed in the absence of evidence of regional spread. Sentinel lymph node biopsy may be considered.[81]

For patients with Bowen's disease or advanced SCC, chemotherapy with isotretinoin alone or in combination with interferon α has been used with success.[82,83] Promising chemopreventive agents for lesions in the actinic keratosis/SCC spectrum include retinoids, cyclo-oxygenase-2 inhibitors, and difluoromethylornithine.

Prognosis and Follow-up Evaluation

SCC in general has greater potential for recurrence and metastasis than BCC; therefore follow-up evaluation must be more aggressive. The patient should be examined at close intervals (every 3–6 months) for the first several years, depending on the location, size, aggressiveness, and node status of the primary tumor. The exception would be small SCC arising from actinic keratosis on sun-exposed surfaces, where the rate of metastasis is very small (0.5%). In these patients, routine follow-up examinations every 6 to 12 months are all that is required.

SEBACEOUS CARCINOMA

Epidemiology and Pathogenesis

Sebaceous carcinoma is a rare, potentially devastating tumor derived from the adnexal epithelium of sebaceous glands. Principally, the tumor occurs in two different clinical scenarios: ocular sebaceous carcinoma (OSC) and extraocular sebaceous carcinoma.[84,85] OSC accounts for 0.2% to 0.8% of all eyelid tumors and 1% to 1.5% of all malignant tumors of the eyelid. Approximately 400 cases have been described in the English literature.[86] OSC affects women 1.5 times more frequently than men; however, a slight male preponderance occurs in cases of extraocular sebaceous carcinoma.[87-91] The mean age at diagnosis is 65 years (range, 40–60 years), but OSC has been reported in young children (12 years of age, after radiation therapy for retinoblastoma) and in persons as old as 90 years.[92,93] Sebaceous carcinoma appears to have a higher incidence in the Asian population.[92,94-96] This tumor has been associated with MTS, an autosomal dominant disorder of mismatch repair genes characterized by sebaceous tumors (benign and malignant) as well as other visceral malignant tumors.[20,97]

Clinical Manifestations

OSC typically manifests as a painless, slowly growing, yellowish papule (Fig. 73-8). The upper lid is affected two to three times more frequently than the lower lid. The tumor usually originates from the meibomian gland (sebaceous gland in the tarsus) or from a sebaceous gland of the eyelash (glands of Zeis).[91,93,98] Clinically, the signs can be subtle with only moderate lid thickening, eyelash alopecia, pale corneal changes, conjunctival injection, or thickening along the temporal or inferior temporal limbus.[87,98-100] There have been case reports of ipsilateral upper and lower eyelid involvement and bilateral upper and lower lid involvement.[86,99,101] The diagnosis is often elusive, because OSC is notorious for masquerading as more common ocular disorders, such as chalazion (most common), keratoconjunctivitis, blepharoconjunctivitis, SCC, BCC, granulomatous disorders, and benign neoplasms.[87,98-102] Initial recognition is 50% among ophthalmologists and only 18.6% among general practitioners.[103-105] Often there is a delay in diagnosis of 6 months to a year

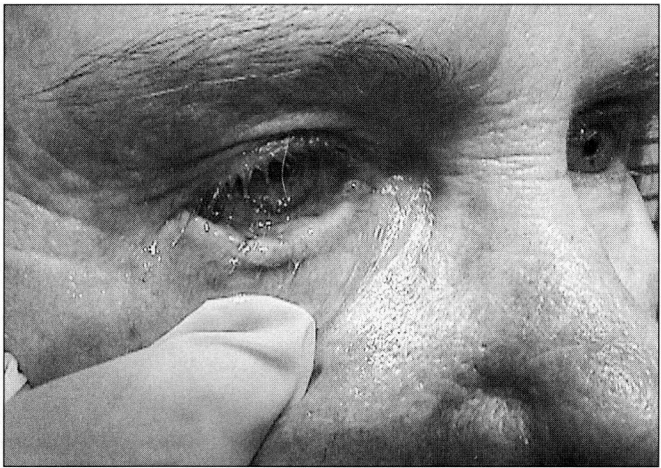

Figure 73-8. Ocular sebaceous carcinoma involving the lower eyelid.

and in some series up to 2.9 years, contributing to increased morbidity and mortality.[87,103] With regard to the rarer extraocular sebaceous gland carcinoma, initial diagnosis can be elusive because the clinical appearance often is pleomorphic and nonspecific and varies from a banal-appearing nodule to large ulcerating masses.[106-109] This variant of sebaceous gland carcinoma most often occurs on the head and neck region, reflecting the abundance of sebaceous glands there.

Histopathology

Full-thickness biopsy is needed to ensure adequate tissue sampling. Microscopic examination shows that OSC invades surrounding tissue by direct extension into the dermis or the overlying epithelium.[103,110,111] The tumor demonstrates epitheliotropic spread in 37% to 80% of cases. Atypical sebaceous cells have a pagetoid distribution within the conjunctival epithelium.[93,103] As many as 18% of cases of OSC may have multifocal regions of tumor involvement.[86]

There are basically two broad classification schemes with regard to light microscopic findings. Font[112] described three classes of tumor based on degree of differentiation: well differentiated, moderately well differentiated, and poorly differentiated. Others prefer to classify the tumor on the basis of growth pattern: lobular, comedocarcinoma, papillary, and mixed.[90] The intraepithelial neoplasia growth pattern and pagetoid spread are not addressed in this classification scheme. The histologic features are anaplastic cells with varying degrees of differentiation. Squamoid or basaloid features may be present.[87] Lobulated aggregates of basaloid cells usually contain irregular, hyperchromatic nuclei and vacuolated cytoplasm.[86,99,113,114] In cases of intraepithelial neoplasia, the epithelial pagetoid cells lack intercellular bridges and contain large hyperchromatic nuclei, prominent nucleoli, and abundant, pale-staining cytoplasm. Special stains, such as oil red O or Sudan black, often are helpful in delineating the atypical sebocytes; however, poorly differentiated tumors may not stain positively for lipids.[100,113] In addition, undifferentiated sebocytes often lack the foamy cytoplasm of their more differentiated counterparts and may resemble atypical SCC at standard hematoxylin and eosin staining.[87,99,113] Recognition of this particular biphasic nature of OSC is critical to appreciating the biologic behavior of this recalcitrant tumor. Ophthalmologists have known for years about the difficulty of assessing the tumor margins of this epitheliotropic neoplasm. It has been recommended that as many as nine mucosal biopsy specimens be obtained and mapped from the medial and lateral portions of the bulbar and palpebral conjunctiva of the upper and lower lids.[115,116]

Treatment

Evaluation of patients with known or suspected sebaceous gland carcinoma includes complete history with review of systems, family history and consideration of MTS, complete skin examination, and palpation of nodal basins and structures adjacent to the lesion. A chest radiograph, complete blood cell count, liver function tests, and electrolytes are recommended. If MTS is a consideration, colonoscopy is warranted.

Management of sebaceous gland carcinoma is primarily surgical, although there are a few reports of tumors managed primarily with radiation.[117] Given the paucity of cases, no randomized, controlled studies have been conducted to evaluate therapy. Traditionally, wide local excision with a margin of 4 to 6 mm of clinically normal tissue has been used.[87] Exenteration is recommended for extensive bulbar conjunctival involvement or evidence of orbital invasion.[91] Mohs micrographic surgery has had favorable outcome, achieving a nearly 90% 3-year cure rate and sparing the patient exenteration in several cases.[103] Some experts consider Mohs micrographic surgical technique the treatment of choice because it preserves the maximum amount of healthy tissue. This quality is especially crucial in the treatment of ocular tissue.[99,103,118-121] In addition, it allows for microscopic examination of all margins of the obtained tissue to ensure complete tumor eradication.

Local recurrence usually is the result of inadequate management of the primary tumor.[87] If the recurrent lesion is small enough, treatment can be repeated with Mohs micrographic surgery or local excision.[103] More extensive OSC tumor involvement usually necessitates exenteration.[105,114] Ophthalmologists have considered cryotherapy a useful modality in the management of epibulbar disease in a small subset of patients, and this therapy may be an alternative to exenteration.[95,122,123] Regional lymph node metastasis is managed by surgical resection and adjuvant radiation.

Prognosis and Follow-up Evaluation

Both OSC and extraocular sebaceous gland carcinoma are aggressive tumors that recur locally if inadequately managed and readily metastasize. Metastasis may occur through lymphatic vessels, and in the case of OSC, it is postulated to occur through the lacrimal and excretory systems.[87] Risk factors associated with poor prognosis include duration longer than 6 months; vascular or lymphatic involvement; orbital extension; poorly differentiated tumor morphology; multicentricity; pagetoid spread into the conjunctival epithelium, cornea, or skin; upper and lower lid involvement; and history of radiation.[92,93,99,103] In the past, 14% to 25% of patients reportedly had metastasis, most frequently involving regional nodal basins, followed by spread to the liver, lung, brain, and bones.[87,89-92] Because of increased index of suspicion, physician education, and earlier recognition with biopsy, the metastatic rate has decreased to 10% in some series.[103] Among industrialized countries, periocular mortality is reportedly 9% to 15%. Systemic disease is associated with a grave prognosis.

Follow-up care includes examining the patient on a regular basis, probably for the rest of his or her life. Given the complex issues in dealing with this aggressive tumor, patients are best served by being cared for in a tertiary care setting with a multidisciplinary approach. Physical examination, evaluation of the surgical site, and a low threshold for biopsy of suspicious lesions is a reasonable approach.

MERKEL CELL CARCINOMA

Epidemiology and Pathogenesis

Merkel cell carcinoma (MCC) is a rare aggressive tumor of unknown incidence. Fewer than 700 cases have been reported since the tumor was first described by Toker in 1972.[124,125] Many names have been ascribed to this neoplasm, including primary small cell carcinoma of the skin, trabecular carcinoma, APUDoma, neuroendocrine carcinoma, endocrine carcinoma, and primary undifferentiated tumor of the skin.[125-128]

MCC is a tumor that primarily affects elderly persons. Ninety percent of cases reported occur in patients older than 50 years, and the mean age at diagnosis is 69 years.[125,128,129] There does not appear to be a sex predilection.[130] More white persons than those of other races are affected; however, MCC has been reported among Asian and black persons.[131-135] MCC has been reported in association with BCC, SCC, a history of radiation, certain familial cancer syndromes, and immunosuppressed states.[111,132,136-139]

Clinical Manifestations

MCC often manifests as a painless, indurated, erythematous to violaceous nodule on sun-damaged skin, 50% of tumors arising on the head and neck.[124-129,132,140] Ten percent of these tumors are in the periocular areas (Fig. 73-9).[141] The extremities are the second most affected site, followed by the trunk.[126,131,142,143] MCC also has been reported in non–sun-exposed areas, such as the vulva, endocervix, penis, esophagus, bladder, and calvarium.[144-148] The overlying epidermis usually is

Specific Malignancies

III

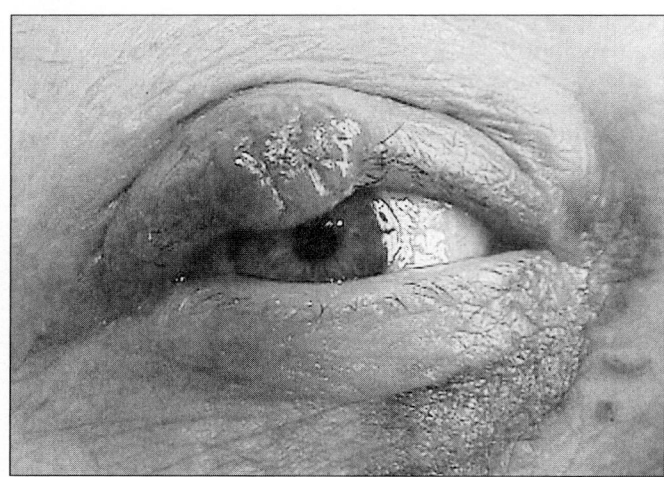

Figure 73-9. Merkel cell carcinoma involving the upper eyelid.

unremarkable; however, ulceration may be found.[127,132,149] In addition, there may be overlying or surrounding telangiectasis.[125] The clinical differential diagnosis includes BCC, SCC, amelanotic melanoma, lymphoma, and metastatic disease. The ultimate diagnosis is made on the basis of clinical appearance, histologic findings, and supporting immunohistochemical studies of the tissue subjected to biopsy.

Histopathology

MCC has a histologic appearance similar to that of other small cell neoplasms and must be differentiated from cutaneous metastatic lesions from carcinoid or small cell undifferentiated carcinoma of the lung.[125,127,132,149] The tumor cells are characteristically uniform in size, monomorphic, basophilic, and ovoid and measure up to 15 mm in diameter. The nuclei have finely dispersed chromatin with minimal surrounding cytoplasm.[127,132,149-151] Pathognomonic features include numerous mitotic figures, vesicular nuclei with essentially inconspicuous nucleoli, and apoptosis, especially when appreciated with certain architectural features.[125,127,152] The tumor involves the dermis, may extend into the subcutaneous fat or deeper, and usually spares the epidermis.[132] There may be a pagetoid pattern of epidermal spreading, which can mimic Bowen's disease, Paget's disease, extramammary Paget's disease, melanoma, and mycosis fungoides.[140,152] MCC also may have both squamous and adnexal differentiation.[128,151]

The architectural patterns of MCC have been classified into three separate groups: trabecular, intermediate cell, and small cell.[127] The trabecular pattern is the least common.[124,153,154] The cells are arranged in cords admixed among a fibrovascular background.[124,126,150] This pattern may be associated with pseudoglandular structures.[154,155] The tumor often involves tissue surrounding adnexal structures, such as hair follicles. More often, in the intermediate cell type, MCC displays large sheets or clusters of uniform cells with foci of necrosis.[126] The tumor also

can arise near adnexal structures and connect with the epidermis.[154,155] The cells in this pattern are less compact than those in the trabecular type. There often is a surrounding lymphocytic infiltrate.[125,152-156]

Finally, the small cell type of MCC arises in the dermis and appears as sheets of cells interrupted by strands of connective tissue.[154] Glandular or pseudoglandular structures are absent. The cells are round and small and may demonstrate "crush" artifact. It has been proposed that the intermediate cell type and the small cell type behave in a clinically more aggressive manner than the trabecular type.[154,155] Lymphatic invasion is frequently encountered and has negative prognostic implications.[127,132,153,154,156,157]

Immunohistochemical studies aid in the diagnosis of MCC and help to differentiate it from other tumors. A characteristic paranuclear dotlike pattern against cytokeratin 20 is probably the most useful immunohistochemical stain.[125,154,158,159] In addition, MCC stains positively for neuron-specific enolase (NSE).[126,150,154,158] However, NSE is not specific for MCC and cannot be relied on for differentiation of MCC from small cell carcinoma of the lung.[125,159] Chromogranin A and synaptophysin are specific for MCC but less sensitive than NSE. MCC also stains positively for epithelial membrane antigen and Ber-EP4.[125,150,159]

Treatment

When MCC is diagnosed, a detailed history should be obtained and a physical examination performed with emphasis on the skin and lymph nodes. Complete blood cell count and hepatic and renal function tests are reasonable. Evaluation of the chest, abdomen, and pelvis with computed tomography may be useful in differentiating MCC from metastatic small cell carcinoma and for initial staging.[140] Patients with MCC of the head and neck region need imaging for evaluation of draining nodal basins, especially if there is clinically evident lymphadenopathy.[125,140] Tumor staging is performed at clinical presentation.[160] Stage I disease is a primary tumor with no evidence of nodal involvement. Stage II disease equates to regional lymph node involvement. Stage III disease is defined by the presence of systemic metastasis.

Local disease is best managed by surgical excision to lower the tumor burden, and excision is followed by radiation.[129,131,140,156,160] Wide local excision of 2.5- to 3.0-cm margins is especially suitable for MCC of the trunk or extremity, being the historical standard.[125,129,131,140,156,160] The use of Mohs micrographic surgery for areas in which this goal would not be achievable, such as the face or neck, has been a logical extension of surgical therapy.[140,161] In addition to tissue conservation, the technique allows microscopic examination of all margins.[140,161]

Prophylactic or elective lymph node dissection (ELND) in all patients has been advocated by some surgeons.[125,126,160,162] Others suggest that sentinel lymph node biopsy for evaluation of draining lymph node basins would be a reasonable approach and avoid the morbidity of ELND.[125,163] Sentinel lymph node biopsy is best performed when the primary surgical site has been subjected to the least amount of manipulation. To date no studies have been conducted to compare the two methods. ELND currently is recommended for large primary tumors, head and neck lesions, small cell subtype, and evidence of vascular or lymphatic invasion.[126,129,131,143]

MCC is considered a radiosensitive tumor. Thus radiation therapy has been used as adjuvant primary treatment when surgery is not an option and for palliation.[129-132,140,160,162] Use of adjuvant external beam radiation therapy has been advocated by many authorities.[129,131] Current recommendations call for surgical management of the primary MCC followed by radiation to the primary site as well as the regional lymph node draining system.[131,132,140,162] Adjuvant chemotherapy has not been studied in a controlled manner. Many cytotoxic regimens have been used, including cyclophosphamide, methotrexate, 5-fluorouracil, cisplatin, etoposide, doxorubicin, procarbazine, dacarbazine, streptozocin, and nitrogen mustard.[128,129,164-167] Review of the literature on adjuvant chemotherapy has not demonstrated clear clinical benefit regarding relapse or survival.[133,136,160,166,167] Chemotherapy has been used for salvage therapy in patients with systemic disease.[137,160,165-167] Most regimens involve two or three drugs, and results are modest at best. No large, randomized studies have been conducted because of the rarity of MCC.

Prognosis and Follow-up Evaluation

MCC has been compared with malignant melanoma because of its similar aggressive behavior.[128,129,164,168] The local recurrence rate is 26% to 44% after primary treatment. As many as 30% of patients have regional lymph node involvement at the time of diagnosis with a 55% rate of regional lymph node relapse after treatment and a 34% to 49% rate of distant metastasis.[129,132,140,169,170] Survival rates reportedly are 68% for women and 36% for men at 3 years.[142,169] Given the relative rarity of the tumor, no large multicenter randomized trials have been conducted to assess stage, treatment modality, recurrence rate, and overall survival. There have been reports of patients with spontaneous resolution of MCC.[171-173]

Patients should be monitored closely for recurrence of locoregional or distant disease. Lymph node or distant metastatic disease has a uniformly grave prognosis; however, there may be a role for chemotherapy in prolonging survival. Almost all patients with metastatic disease eventually die of the disease.

DERMATOFIBROSARCOMA PROTUBERANS

Epidemiology and Pathogenesis

Dermatofibrosarcoma protuberans (DFSP) is an uncommon tumor of intermediate malignancy that arises in the dermis. It is a locally aggressive neoplasm with notoriously high recurrence rates even after wide local excision. In 1924, Darier and Ferrand[174] first described DFSP as a distinct clinicopathologic entity; however, it was Hoffman in 1925 who introduced the term *dermatofibrosarcoma protuberans.*[175]

DFSP constitutes less than 1% of all malignant tumors. The estimated incidence is 0.8% to 5 cases per 1 million persons per year.[176-179] The tumor commonly occurs between 20 and 50 years of age, rare cases occurring in young children.[180] In addition, there have been a few reported cases of congenital DFSP.[181-184] The sexes are affected equally; however, in some series there is a slight male preponderance.[176-178,181,185] Most reported cases of DFSP occur in white persons, but historically race rarely is mentioned.[176-178,186] DFSP also occurs in African Americans and Asians.[181,186,187]

DFSP is not known to have a genetic or familial predisposition.[188,189] The cause of DFSP is unknown. Chromosomal abnormalities consistent with a monoclonal origin have been found in several studies.[190,191] Most frequently, these abnormalities include ring 22 chromosomes, ring chromosomes containing chromosome 17 sequences, abnormal clones, and t(2;7) translocations.[191-194] Approximately 10% to 20% of patients report a history of antecedent trauma.[176,181,189,195,196] There have been reports of DFSP arising in multiple immunization sites, burn scars, and surgical scars.[186,197,198] DFSP has been associated with pregnancy as well as long-term arsenic exposure, acanthosis nigricans, and acrodermatitis enteropathica.[176,199-201]

Clinical Manifestations

DFSP usually manifests as a flesh-colored, firm, asymptomatic nodule or plaque (Fig. 73-10). The tumor is firm to palpation, and a subcutaneous component often is appreciated. There may be fixation to overlying skin but rarely to deeper structures. Lesions associated with pigment are known as *Bednar tumors.*[202] In addition to pigment, there may be red to violaceous erythema. Characteristically, DFSP initially manifests as a solitary nodule; however, there may be multiple primary lesions. The size typically ranges from 1 to 5 cm, but neglected lesions can be as large as 20 cm in diameter.[176,178,186] The lesion slowly enlarges in a relentless manner. Accelerated growth phases can result in nodularity or multiple outcroppings or protuberances. Ulceration occurs when the tumor erupts through the epidermis. Atypical clinical manifestations include sclerotic plaques with a morpheaform appearance.[203]

Approximately 50% to 60% of DFSP lesions occur on the trunk, 25% of those occurring on the chest and shoulders.[177,178,181,186] Twenty percent to 30% arise on the proximal aspects of the extremities.[178-181] Ten percent to 15% occur on the head and neck, the scalp being affected less than 5% of the time.[177,178,181,186] In rare instances, acral sites have been reported, mostly in young children and adolescents.[177,181,182,204] Often there is a delay in diagnosis given the indolent and nonspecific features of the tumor. DFSP often is mistaken for lipoma, deep-seated epidermal cyst, scar, hypertrophic scar, keloid, dermatofibroma, nodular fasciitis, and insect bite. The diagnosis is confirmed with biopsy and microscopic examination of the tissue.

Specific Malignancies

III

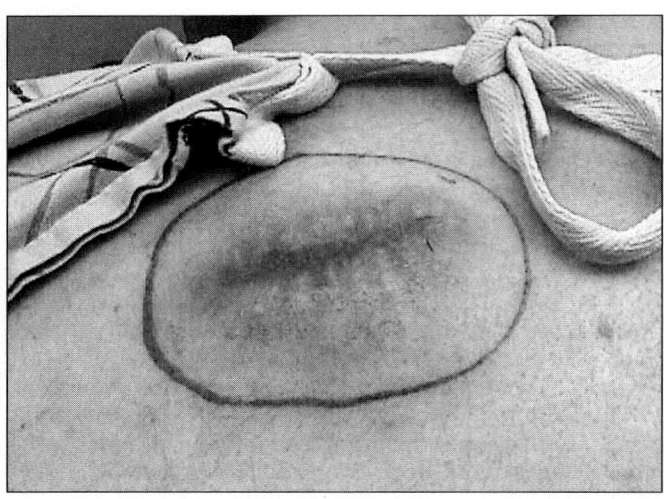

Figure 73-10. Dermatofibrosarcoma protuberans involving the back. Central linear scar from previous partial excision is encircled by ink to highlight clinical margins of the lesion.

Histopathology

The histologic features of DFSP often are easily recognized on low-power view. There is densely packed proliferation of monomorphic, bluish, spindle-shaped cells seated in and expanding the dermis. The overlying epidermis usually is normal appearing unless there has been invasion by the tumor. The central or nodular areas of the tumor demonstrate numerous spindle cells arranged in a characteristic "whirling, storiform or herring bone" configuration.[150] The lateral tumor margins have sharply pointed tumor cells and irregular strands dissecting between the native collagen bundles. Inferiorly, the DFSP cells invade downward within the fibrous septa that separate the adipose cells of the panniculus. The peripheral margins may have a deceptively bland appearance resembling normal collagen and making interpretation of tumor margins difficult.[178] Fascia, muscle, and underlying bone may be involved in longstanding lesions.[178,181,186,190] Histologic variants include DFSP with entirely myxomatous features (myxoid DFSP) and pigmented DFSP, also known as *Bednar tumor.*[202,205,206] This variant tends to occur more often in dark-skinned persons and accounts for approximately 1% to 5% of all cases of DFSP.[202] Bednar tumor has the characteristic storiform pattern of spindle cells admixed with a variable amount of melanin-laden dendritic cells. Immunohistochemical studies that may be helpful include positive staining for CD34, a human hematopoietic progenitor cell antigen. Unlike dermatofibroma, DFSP stains negatively for factor XIIIa.[150]

Treatment

After the diagnosis of DFSP has been confirmed, a complete history, review of systems, and physical examination with focus on the skin and structures contiguous with the tumor and palpation of lymph node basins are performed. Unless the physician suspects metastatic disease, extensive laboratory studies and radiologic investigation are not indicated.

The traditional mainstay of therapy for DFSP has been surgical resection, specifically wide local excision with a margin of 2 to 4 cm of normal-appearing skin.[186,207,208] Unfortunately, the biologic and histologic features of the tumor coupled with inability to clinically determine tumor margins account for exceptionally high recurrence rates with standard surgical therapy. Reported local recurrence rates are as high as 60% after standard surgical excision and 23% after wide local excision with margins greater than 4 cm.[207] Approximately 80% of local recurrences occur within 3 years.[176,186,191] Local recurrence after 10 years is rare but has been reported.[178,181] Mohs micrographic surgery has been receiving greater recognition as a useful method of management of DFSP.[207-216] The capability of microscopic examination of the entire specimen margins allows the surgeon to localize and excise the tumor in a precise manner. This method also allows for maximum conservation of tissue, a crucial factor in certain anatomic areas, such as the face, scalp, distal extremities, and genitalia. Results of several studies have suggested that Mohs micrographic surgery may be beneficial in the management of DFSP; however, few series have provided complete 5-year follow-up data.[207-216] At the University of Wisconsin, Madison, 36 patients with DSFP were treated with Mohs micrographic surgery. Of these, 29 participated in follow-up study for 5 or more years (range, 5 to 20 years). As of this writing, there have been no local recurrences or cases of regional metastasis.

Prognosis and Follow-up Evaluation

Although it is locally aggressive, DFSP rarely metastasizes. The overall rate of distant metastasis is approximately 5% and of regional metastasis is 1%.[185] In the past, the causes of the higher rate of metastasis were likely inclusion of malignant fibrohistiocytoma (MFH) in the database and degeneration of DFSP to a more sarcomatous subtype with its subsequent increased risk of metastasis.[217-219] MFH is now understood to be a totally different entity from DFSP. Its cellular morphologic characteristics and architecture have been clarified, and pathologists and dermatopathologists have reached consensus on the diagnostic criteria for MFH. The regional rate of metastasis of MFH is estimated to be greater than 50%.[150,216-218]

Recommendations for patient follow-up care include physical examination every 3 to 6 months postoperatively for 3 years and then annually for life. Particular attention to evaluation of surgical site, regional lymph node palpation, and a complete review of systems is appropriate.

CUTANEOUS ANGIOSARCOMA

Epidemiology and Pathogenesis

Cutaneous angiosarcoma (CAS) is a rare, highly malignant, potentially lethal tumor originating from the dermal vasculature endothelium. Elderly persons are most commonly affected, and there is a 2:1 male predominance.[220-223] White persons are affected most often, but CAS has been reported among other persons as well.[224,225] With the exception of CAS associated with lymphedema, the cause of CAS is uncertain. Cases have been associated with history of trauma, radiation, herpes zoster, fistula of chronic osteomyelitis, vinyl chloride and arsenic oxide exposure, and arteriovenous fistula sites in renal transplant recipients.[220,221,226-235] Ultraviolet light exposure does not appear to be an inciting factor. Only a minority of patients with CAS have temporally associated skin cancer.[222,223,236]

Clinical Manifestations

Principal clinical patterns include (1) CAS of the scalp and face, (2) CAS associated with chronic lymphedema most commonly following mastectomy (Stewart-Treves syndrome), and (3) radiation-associated angiosarcoma, which is the least common variant.[220,226] CAS of the scalp and face usually manifests as a painless, rapidly proliferating growth of the subcutaneous tissue plane (Fig. 73-11). CAS of this pattern occurs 50% of the time on the scalp and 30% of the time on the face or neck.[220-223,227,230,236] The tumor may be firm or spongy to palpation, the overlying skin surface smoothened because of tumor distention of the underlying structures.[237] An ill-defined area of dusky to violaceous erythema resembling a bruise or healing contusion often is present. The tumor infiltrates the surrounding tissues in a centrifugal and multifocal manner. As a result tumor involvement extends much farther than the clinical appearance of the margins. Multiple lesions may be separated by an isthmus of normal-appearing skin found at initial presentation if the primary tumor is more than 6 cm in diameter. Long-standing CAS may develop superimposed tumors and nodules. Ulceration and bleeding are not characteristic unless the CAS is larger than 10 cm in diameter. Misdiagnosis is common given the subtlety and nonspecific nature of the clinical findings. Initial differential diagnoses

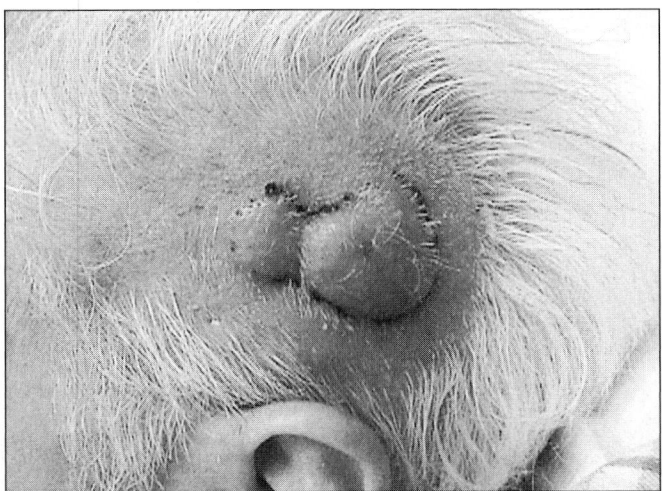

Figure 73-11. Cutaneous angiosarcoma involving the scalp. Ink highlights clinical margins of the lesion.

include cellulitis, nonspecific inflammatory changes, fungal infection, trauma, and hemangioma.[220,221,237] Reported atypical clinical scenarios include rosacea-like signs and symptoms, chronic edema of the eyelids, xanthelasma-like lesions, and even recurrent angioedema.[225,237,238]

In 1948, Stewart and Treves described six patients with postmastectomy chronic lymphedema in whom CAS developed in the affected extremity.[239] The estimated risk among postmastectomy patients who survive more than 5 years is approximately 0.5%.[240] The time interval between mastectomy and recognition of angiosarcoma ranges from 1 to 30 years with a mean duration of 10 years.[237] Clinically, the ipsilateral, upper inner aspect of the arm is a frequent site of early involvement. Less frequent are lesions distal to the elbow or on the chest wall that most often resemble a bruise or blotchy erythema. These color changes initially are attributed to trauma; however, rapid growth and induration often lead to ulceration and hemorrhage. Other causes of chronic lymphedema have been associated with development of angiosarcoma, including congenital lymphedema and postsurgical, post-traumatic, and infectious etiologic factors.[241-247]

Histopathology

Histologically, CAS has essentially three different cell growth patterns: (1) angiomatous or well differentiated with obvious vasoformative activity, (2) spindle cell with a range of differentiation, and (3) undifferentiated or highly anaplastic.[236,248] A single tumor may have all three growth patterns.[227,236,237,248] The well-differentiated variant (angiomatous) is characterized by recapitulation of atypical endothelial cells lining irregular vascular channels. These atypical vessels are located throughout the dermis, dissect through the collagen, and surround but do not invade the adnexal structures. With time there is infiltration into the subcutaneous fat, muscle, and fascia. This particular variant is often poorly recognized initially with frozen sections. The vessels do not contain red blood cells because hemolysis of the red blood cells during processing makes microscopic examination difficult. The spindle cell tumor variant forms dense cellular bundles that penetrate the dermis and underlying tissue.[236] Vascular channels are not easily recognized. The more anaplastic or undifferentiated CAS characteristically contains large, basophilic, pleomorphic polyhedral cells arranged in solid sheets or cords.[236,248] The dermis and subcutaneous structures often are occupied by tumor. Immunohistochemical stains for endothelium-related markers such as CD34 antigen, factor VIII–related antigen, or *Ulex europaeus agglutinin I* lectin binding may be helpful. Negative cytokeratin staining is helpful for differentiating CAS from carcinoma. Negative staining results for S-100 help to differentiate the tumor from melanoma.[237,248]

Treatment

Computed tomography and magnetic resonance imaging have not been extremely helpful unless there has been marked bony invasion.[249,250] Soft-tissue invasion of the tumor may be partially visualized, but the exact extent of the margins is poorly delineated because of the diffuse infiltrating nature of the tumor. Radiographic imaging is even more unreliable if the tumor is poorly appreciated microscopically. The peripheral margin of CAS may be partially assessed with random biopsies performed in a gridlike pattern circumferentially around the tumor.[236] Ideally, the biopsies should be full thickness of the skin and include the muscle and fascia if possible for complete assessment of the depth of the margin.

Traditional management of CAS has been wide local excision with a margin of 3 to 6 cm of normal-appearing skin. More recently, Mohs micrographic surgery with adjuvant radiation has been shown to produce favorable outcome.[236,251-253] The Mohs technique combines the benefits of both fresh-tissue and fixed-tissue technique. Well-localized lesions are good candidates for the fresh-tissue technique, because a microscope can be used for identification of the tumor and excision of the entire lesion. After excision, zinc chloride fixative paste may be applied circumferentially around the surgical skin edges to stimulate an immune response around the operative site.[252] The final defect is repaired with a flap or skin graft.

For scalp lesions, orthovoltage or electron beam radiation with a curvilinear delivery system is administered over the entire scalp in a swimming cap distribution.[254] The region from the eyebrows to the occipital nuchal line is included, and both auricular-temporal sulci are encompassed. The curvilinear delivery system distributes the radiation equally to all parts of the scalp simultaneously. Thus are avoided overlapping and under treatment of radiation sites that would otherwise accompany conventional flat-plate radiation when applied to curved surfaces, such as the scalp and forehead. Attention to these details of radiation treatment is essential because CAS is resistant to most forms of surgical therapy, and chemotherapy has not been reported effective.

Recurrence of CAS of the scalp usually is the result of inadequate treatment of the primary tumor.[222,236] Localized recurrence can be managed with radiation with a good response.[236,251] Management of regional lymph node metastasis is surgical resection and adjuvant radiation.[222,236] Systemic disease has a grave prognosis. Given the rarity of angiosarcoma, no single institution has enough experience to establish definitive treatment guidelines. Practical strategies include use of Mohs micrographic surgery combined with radiation, in the manner described earlier, for tumors less than 5 cm in diameter. For tumors larger than 5 cm, peripheral margin assessment (because of the multicentricity of the tumor spread), followed by orthovoltage or electron beam radiation should be considered.[236]

Prognosis and Follow-up Evaluation

The prognosis among patients with any form of angiosarcoma is uniformly poor. CAS of the scalp has an expected 5-year survival rate of less than 12%.[222] Histologic degree of differentiation, mitotic index, age, sex, location of primary lesion, and clinical appearance have no statistical bearing on survival. Tumor size has been found the only statistically significant indicator of prognosis. Lesions smaller than 5 cm correlate with improved survival at 5 years.[220] Another favorable indicator has been the presence of prominent lymphocytic infiltrate associated with the tumor. Local recurrence is common, and metastasis occurs hematogenously and through lymphatic vessels to the cervical lymph nodes, lungs, liver, and soft tissues.[222,224] There have been rare reports of spontaneous regression of CAS of the scalp and face.[255] Complete regression in one unreported case at the University of Wisconsin, Madison, was associated with frequent application of hot compresses.

Follow-up recommendations include frequent physical examinations with particular attention to the surgical site, contiguous structures, and palpation of lymph nodes. A complete review of systems, laboratory data, and radiologic studies should be performed as indicated. These patients are best treated in a tertiary care center with a multidisciplinary approach.

REFERENCES

1. Aszterbaum M, Rothman A, Johnson RL, et al: Identification of mutations in the human PATCHED gene in sporadic basal cell carcinomas and in patients with the basal cell nevus syndrome. J Invest Dermatol 1998;110:885-888.
2. Brash DE, Rudolph JA, Simon JA, et al: A role for sunlight in skin cancer: UV-induced p53 mutations in squamous cell carcinoma. Proc Natl Acad Sci USA 1991;88:10124-10128.
3. Bootsma D, Kraemer KH, Cleaver JE, Hoeijmakers JHJ: Nucleotide excision repair syndromes: Xeroderma pigmentosum, Cockayne syndrome, and trichothiodystrophy. In Vogelstein BV, Kinzier K (eds): The Genetic Basis of Human Cancer. New York, McGraw-Hill, pp 245-274.
4. van Elsas A, Zerp SF, van der Flier S, et al: Relevance of ultraviolet-induced N-ras oncogene point mutations in development of primary human cutaneous melanoma. Am J Pathol 1996;149:883-893.
5. van der Schroeff JG, Evers LM, Boot AJ, Bos JL: Ras oncogene mutations in basal cell carcinomas and squamous cell carcinomas of human skin. J Invest Dermatol 1990;94:423-425.
6. Miller DL, Weinstock MA: Nonmelanoma skin cancer in the United States: Incidence. J Am Acad Dermatol 1994;30:774-778.
7. Stone DM, Hynes M, Armanini M, et al: The tumour-suppressor gene patched encodes a candidate receptor for sonic hedgehog. Nature 1996;384:129-134.
8. Hahn H, Wicking C, Zaphiropoulous PG, et al: Mutations of the human homolog of Drosophila patched in the nevoid basal cell carcinoma syndrome. Cell 1996;85:841-851.
9. Wicking C, Berkman J, Wainwright B, Chenevix-Trench G: Fine genetic mapping of the gene for nevoid basal cell carcinoma syndrome. Genomics 1994;22:505-511.
10. Goldstein AM, Stewart C, Bale AI, Bale SJ, Dean M: Localization of the gene for the nevoid basal cell carcinoma syndrome. Am J Hum Genet 1994;54:765-773.
11. Johnson RL, Rothman AL, Xie J, et al: Human homolog of patched, a candidate gene for the basal cell carcinoma syndrome. Science 1996;272:1668-1671.
12. Parada LF, Land H, Weinberg RA, Wolf D, Rotter V: Cooperation between gene encoding p53 tumour antigen and ras in cellular transformation. Nature 1984;312:649-651.
13. Ziegler A, Jonason AS, Leffell DJ, et al: Sunburn and p53 in the onset of skin cancer. Nature 1994;372:773-776.
14. Dumaz N, Stary A, Soussi T, Daya-Grosjean L, Sarasin A: Can we predict solar ultraviolet radiation as the casual event in human tumours by analyzing the mutation spectra of the p53 gene? Mutat Res 1994;307:375-386.

15. Rady P, Scinicariello F, Wagner RF Jr, Tyring SK: P53 Mutations in basal cell carcinomas. Cancer Res 1992;52:3804–3806.

16. Tsao H. Genetics of nonmelanoma skin cancer. Arch Dermatol 2001;137:1486–1492.

17. Kraemer KH, Lee MM, Andrews AD, Lambert WC: The role of sunlight and DNA repair in melanoma and nonmelanoma skin cancer: The xeroderma pigmentosum paradigm. Arch Dermatol 1994;130:1018–1021.

18. Williams C, Ponten F, Ahmadian A, et al: Clones of normal keratinocytes and a variety of simultaneously present epidermal neoplastic lesions contain a multitude of p53 gene mutations in a xeroderma pigmentosum patient. Cancer Res 1998;58:2449–2455.

19. Daya-Grosjean L, Robert C, Drougard C, Suarez H, Sarasin A: High mutation frequency in ras genes of skin tumors isolated from DNA repair deficient xeroderma pigmentosum patients. Cancer Res 1993;53:1625–1629.

20. Cohen PR, Kohn SR, Kurzrock R: Association of sebaceous gland tumors and internal malignancy: The Muir-Torre syndrome. Am J Med 1991;90:606–613.

21. Peltomaki P, Aaltonen LA, Sistonen P, et al: Genetic mapping of a locus predisposing to human colorectal cancer. Science 1993;260:810–812.

22. Fishel R, Lescoe MK, Rao MR, et al: The human mutator gene homolog MSH2 and its association with hereditary nonpolyposis colon cancer. Cell 1993;75:1027–1038.

23. Honchel R, Halling KC, Schaid DJ, Pittelkow M, Thibodeau SN: Microsatellite instability in Muir-Torre syndrome. Cancer Res 1994;54:1159–1163.

24. Halling KC, Honchel R, Pittelkow MR, Thibodieau SN: Microsatellite instability in keratoacanthoma. Cancer 1995;76: 1765–1771.

25. Lieu FM, Yamanishi K, Konishi K, Kishimoto S, Yasuno H: Low incidence of H-ras oncogene mutations in human epidermal tumors. Cancer Lett 1991;59:231–235.

26. Friedman E, Gejman PV, Martin GA, McCormick F: Nonsense mutations in the c-terminal SH2 region of the GTPase activating protein (GAP) gene in human tumors. Nat Genet 1993;5:242–247.

Basal Cell Carcinoma and Squamous Cell Carcinoma

27. Diepgen TL, Mahler V: The epidemiology of skin cancer. Br J Dermatol 2002;146(suppl 61):1–6.

28. Marcil I, Stern RS: Risk of developing a subsequent nonmelanoma skin cancer in patients with a history of nonmelanoma skin cancer: A critical review of the literature and meta-analysis. Arch Dermatol 2000;136:1524–1530.

29. Karagas MR, Greenberg ER, Spencer SK, Stukel TA, Mott LA: Increase in incidence rates of basal cell and squamous cell skin cancer in New Hampshire, USA: New Hampshire Skin Cancer Study Group. Int J Cancer 1999;81:555–559.

30. Gallagher RP, Hill GB, Bajdik CD, et al: Sunlight exposure, pigmentary factors, and risk of nonmelanocytic skin cancer. I. Basal cell carcinoma. Arch Dermatol 1995;131:157–163.

31. Leffell DJ, Fitzgerald DA: Basal cell carcinoma. In Freedberg IM, Eisen AZ, Wolff Ketal (eds): Dermatology in General Medicine. New York, McGraw-Hill, 1999, pp 857–864.

32. Halder RM, Bang KM: Skin cancer in blacks in the United States. Dermatol Clin 1988;6:397–405.

33. Asada M, Schaart FM, de Almeida HL Jr, et al: Solid basal cell epithelioma (BCE) possibly originates from the outer root sheath of the hair follicle. Acta Derm Venereol 1993;73:286–292.

34. Korman NJ, Hrabovsky SL: Basal cell carcinomas display extensive abnormalities in the hemidesmosome anchoring fibril complex. Exp Dermatol 1993;2:139–144.

35. Shanley SM, Dawkins H, Wainwright BJ, et al: Fine deletion mapping on the long arm of chromosome 9 in sporadic and familial basal cell carcinomas. Hum Mol Genet 1995;4:129–133.

36. Bodak N, Queille S, Avril MF, et al: High levels of patched gene mutations in basal-cell carcinomas from patients with xeroderma pigmentosum. Proc Natl Acad Sci USA 1999;96:5117–5122.

37. Grossman D, Leffell DJ: The molecular basis of nonmelanoma skin cancer: New understanding. Arch Dermatol 1997;133:1263–1270.

38. Morton CA, Brown SB, Collins S, et al: Guidelines for topical photodynamic therapy: Report of a workshop of the British Photodermatology Group. Br J Dermatol 2002;146:552–567.

39. Kowalzick L, Rogozinski T, Wimheuer R, et al: Intralesional recombinant interferon beta-1a in the treatment of basal cell carcinoma: Results of an open-label multicentre study. Eur J Dermatol 2002;12:558–561.

40. Sterry W, Herrera E, Takwale A, et al: Imiquimod 5% cream for the treatment of superficial and nodular basal cell carcinoma: Randomized studies comparing low-frequency dosing with and without occlusion. Br J Dermatol 2002;147:1227–1236.

41. Romagosa R, Saap L, Givens M, et al: A pilot study to evaluate the treatment of basal cell carcinoma with 5-fluorouracil using phosphatidyl choline as a transepidermal carrier. Dermatol Surg 2000;26:338–340.

42. Levine N: Role of retinoids in skin cancer treatment and prevention. J Am Acad Dermatol 1998;39:S62–S66.

43. Thissen MR, Neumann MH, Schouten LJ: A systematic review of treatment modalities for primary basal cell carcinomas. Arch Dermatol 1999;135:1177–1183.

44. Randle HW: Basal cell carcinoma: Identification and treatment of the high-risk patient. Dermatol Surg 1996;22:255–261.

45. Wolf DJ, Zitelli JA: Surgical margins for basal cell carcinoma. Arch Dermatol 1987;123:340–344.

46. Robinson JK: Use of a combination of chemotherapy and radiation therapy in the management of advanced basal cell carcinoma of the head and neck. J Am Acad Dermatol 1987;17:770–774.

47. Rowe DE, Carroll RJ, Day CL Jr: Long-term recurrence rates in previously untreated (primary) basal cell carcinoma: Implications for patient follow-up. J Dermatol Surg Oncol 1989;15:315–328.

48. Marghoob A, Kopf AW, Bart RS, et al: Risk of another basal cell carcinoma developing after treatment of a basal cell carcinoma. J Am Acad Dermatol 1993;28:22–28.

49. Czarnecki D, Mar A, Staples M, Giles G, Meehan C: The development of non-melanocytic skin cancers in people with a history of skin cancer. Dermatology 1994;189:364–367.

50. Altman A, Rosen T, Tschen JA, et al: Basal cell epithelioma in black patients. J Am Acad Dermatol 1987;17:741–745.

51. Gallagher RP, Ma B, McLean DI, et al: Trends in basal cell carcinoma, squamous cell carcinoma, and melanoma of the skin from 1973 through 1987. J Am Acad Dermatol 1990;23:413–421.

52. Gallagher RP, Hill GB, Bajdik CD, et al: Sunlight exposure, pigmentation factors, and risk of nonmelanocytic skin cancer. II. Squamous cell carcinoma. Arch Dermatol 1995;131:164–169.

53. Vitasa BC, Taylor HR, Strickland PT, et al: Association of nonmelanoma skin cancer and actinic keratosis with cumulative solar ultraviolet exposure in Maryland watermen. Cancer 1990;65:2811–2817.

54. Gallagher RP, Bajdik CD, Fincham S, et al: Chemical exposures, medical history, and risk of squamous and basal cell carcinoma of the skin. Cancer Epidemiol Biomarkers Prev 1996;5:419–424.

55. Schwartz RA, Stoll HL: Squamous cell carcinoma. In Freedberg IM, Eisen AZ, Wolff K, et al (eds): Dermatology in General Medicine. New York, McGraw-Hill, 1999.

56. Gupta AK, Cardella CJ, Haberman HF: Cutaneous malignant neoplasms in patients with renal transplants. Arch Dermatol 1986;122:1288–1293.

57. Berg D, Otley CC: Skin cancer in organ transplant recipients: Epidemiology, pathogenesis, and management. J Am Acad Dermatol 2002;47:1–17.

58. Livneh Z, Cohen-Fix O, Skaliter R, Elizur T: Replication of damaged DNA and the molecular mechanism of ultraviolet light mutagenesis. Crit Rev Biochem Mol Biol 1993;28:465–513.

59. Alcalay J, Freeman SE, Goldberg LH, Wolf JE: Excision repair of pyrimidine dimers induced by simulated solar radiation in the skin of patients with basal cell carcinoma. J Invest Dermatol 1990;95:506–509.

60. Kripke ML: Immunologic mechanisms in UV radiation carcinogenesis. Adv Cancer Res 1981;34:69–106.

61. Ullrich SE: Modulation of immunity by ultraviolet radiation: Key effects on antigen presentation. J Invest Dermatol 1995;105(suppl 1):30S–36S.

62. Wang XM, McNiff JM, Klump V, Asgari M, Gasparro FP: An

unexpected spectrum of p53 mutations from squamous cell carcinomas in psoriasis patients treated with PUVA: Photochem Photobiol 1997;66:294–299.

63. Chen W, Barthelman M, Martinez J, Alberts D, Gensler HL: Inhibition of cyclobutane pyrimidine dimer formation in epidermal p53 gene of UV-irradiated mice by alpha-tocopherol. Nutr Cancer 1997;29:205–211.

64. Diem C, Runger TM: Processing of three different types of DNA damage in cell lines of a cutaneous squamous cell carcinoma progression model. Carcinogenesis 1997;18:657–662.

65. Kawara S, Takata M, Takehara K: High frequency of DNA aneuploidy detected by DNA flow cytometry in Bowen's disease. J Dermatol Sci 1999;21:23–26.

66. Wakita H, Shirahama S, Furukawa F: Distinct P-cadherin expression in cultured normal human keratinocytes and squamous cell carcinoma cell lines. Microsc Res Tech 1998;43:218–223.

67. Mora RG, Perniciaro C: Cancer of the skin in blacks. I. A review of 163 black patients with cutaneous squamous cell carcinoma. J Am Acad Dermatol 1981;5:535–543.

68. Kao GF: Carcinoma arising in Bowen's disease. Arch Dermatol 1986;122:1124–1126.

69. Goepfert H, Dichtel WJ, Medina JE, Lindberg RD, Luna MD: Perineural invasion in squamous cell skin carcinoma of the head and neck. Am J Surg 1984;148:542–547.

70. Petter G, Haustein UF. Squamous cell carcinoma of the skin: Histopathological features and their significance for the clinical outcome. J Eur Acad Dermatol Venereol 1998;11:37–44.

71. Sedlin ED, Fleming JL: Epidermal carcinoma arising in chronic osteomyelitic foci. J Bone Joint Surg Am 1963;45:827–837.

72. Martin H, Strong E, Spiro RH: Radiation-induced skin cancer of the head and neck. Cancer 1970;25:61–71.

73. Dinehart SM, Pollack SV: Metastases from squamous cell carcinoma of the skin and lip: An analysis of twenty-seven cases. J Am Acad Dermatol 1989;21:241–248.

74. Rowe DE, Carroll RJ, Day CL Jr: Prognostic factors for local recurrence, metastasis, and survival rates in squamous cell carcinoma of the skin, ear, and lip: Implications for treatment modality selection. J Am Acad Dermatol 1992;26:976–990.

75. Brodland DG, Zitelli JA: Surgical margins for excision of primary cutaneous squamous cell carcinoma. J Am Acad Dermatol 1992;27:241–248.

76. Weisberg NK, Bertagnolli MM, Becker DS: Combined sentinel lymphadenectomy and Mohs micrographic surgery for high-risk cutaneous squamous cell carcinoma. J Am Acad Dermatol 2000;43:483–488.

77. Shimm DS, Wilder RB. Radiation therapy for squamous cell carcinoma of the skin. Am J Clin Oncol 1991;14:383–386.

78. Merimsky O, Neudorfer M, Spitzer E, Chaitchik S: Salvage cisplatin and adriamycin for advanced or recurrent basal or squamous cell carcinoma of the face. Anticancer Drugs 1992;3:481–484.

79. Cartei G, Cartei F, Interlandi G, et al: Oral 5-fluorouracil in squamous cell carcinoma of the skin in the aged. Am J Clin Oncol 2000;23:181–184.

80. Freeman RG, Knox JM, Heaton CL: The treatment of skin cancer: A statistical study of 1,341 skin tumors comparing results obtained with irradiation, surgery, and curettage followed by electrodesiccation. Cancer 1964;17:535–538.

81. Cherpelis BS, Marcusen C, Lang PG: Prognostic factors for metastasis in squamous cell carcinoma of the skin. Dermatol Surg 2002;28:268–273.

82. Lippman SM, Parkinson DR, Itri LM, et al: 13-cis-retinoic acid and interferon alpha-2a: Effective combination therapy for advanced squamous cell carcinoma of the skin. J Natl Cancer Inst 1992;84:235–241.

83. Toma S, Palumbo R, Vincenti M, et al: Efficacy of recombinant alpha-interferon 2a and 13-cis-retinoic acid in the treatment of squamous cell carcinoma. Ann Oncol 1994;5:463–465.

Sebaceous Gland Carcinoma

84. Wolfe JT, Yeates RP, Wick MR, et al: Sebaceous gland carcinoma of the eyelid: Errors in clinical and pathologic diagnosis. Am J Surg Pathol 1984;8:597–606.

85. Wick MR, Goellner JR, Wolfe JT, et al: Adnexal carcinomas of the skin. II. Extraocular sebaceous carcinomas. Cancer 1985;56:1163–1172.

86. Jakobiec FA, To KW: Sebaceous tumors of ocular adnexa. In Albert DM, Jakobiec FA, Azar DT, Gragoudas ES (eds): Principles and Practice of Ophthalmology. Philadelphia, WB Saunders, 2000, pp 3382–3402.

87. Nelson BR, Hamlet KR, Gillard M, Railan D, Johnson TM: Continuing medical education: Sebaceous carcinoma. J Am Acad Dermatol 1995;33:1–15.

88. Straatsma BR: Meibomian gland tumors. Arch Ophthalmol 1956;56:71–93.

89. Doxanas MT, Green WR: Sebaceous gland carcinoma: A review of 40 cases. Arch Ophthalmol 1984;102:245–249.

90. Rao NA, McLean JW, Zimmerman LE: Sebaceous carcinoma of the eyelid and caruncle: Correlation of clinicopathologic features and prognosis. In Jakobiec FA (ed): Ocular and Adnexal Tumors. Birmingham, UK, Aesculapius, 1978, pp 461–476.

91. Rao NA, Hidayat AA, McLean JW, et al: Sebaceous carcinoma of the ocular adnexa: A clinicopathologic study of 104 patients with five year follow-up data. Hum Pathol 1982;13:113–122.

92. Boniuk M, Zimmerman LE: Sebaceous carcinoma of the eyelids, eyebrow, caruncle and orbit. Trans Am Acad Ophthalmol Otolaryngol 1968;72:619–642.

93. Yount AB, Bylund D, Pratt SG, Greenway HT: Mohs micrographic excision of sebaceous carcinoma of the eyelids. J Dermatol Surg Oncol 1994;20:523–529.

94. Tan KC, Lee ST, Cheah ST: Surgical treatment of sebaceous carcinoma of the eyelids with clinic-pathological correlation. Br J Plast Surg 1991;44:117–121.

95. Ni C, Searle SS, Kuo PK: Sebaceous cell carcinomas of the ocular adnexa. Int Ophthalmol Clin 1982;22:23–61.

96. Ni C, Kuo PK: Meibomian gland carcinoma: A clinicopathologic study of 156 cases with long-period follow up of 100 cases. Jpn J Ophthalmol 1979;23:388–401.

97. Cohen PR, Kohn SR, Davis DA, Kurzrock R: Muir-Torre syndrome. Dermatol Clin 1995;13:79–89.

98. Gurin DM, Rapini R: Aggressive sebaceous carcinoma of the eyelid: An elusive diagnosis. Cutis 1993;52:40–42.

99. Spencer JM, Nossa R, Tse DT, Sequeira M: Sebaceous carcinoma of the eyelid treated with Mohs micrographic surgery. J Am Acad Dermatol 2001;44:1004–1009.

100. Loeffler KU, Perlman JI: Diffuse intraepithelial sebaceous carcinoma of the conjunctiva. Br J Ophthalmol 1997;81:168–170.

101. Rumelt S, Hogan NR, Rubin PA, Jakobiec FA: Four-eyelid sebaceous cell carcinoma following irradiation. Arch Ophthalmol 1998;116:1670–1672.

102. Dzubow LM: Sebaceous carcinoma of the eyelid: Treatment with Mohs surgery. J Dermatol Surg Oncol 1985;11:40–44.

103. Snow SN, Larson PO, Lucarelli MJ, Lemke BN, Madjar DD: Sebaceous carcinoma of the eyelids treated by Mohs micrographic surgery: Report of nine cases with review of the literature. Dermatol Surg 2202;28:623–631.

104. Zurcher M, Hintschich CR, Garner A, Brunce A, Collin JR: Sebaceous carcinoma of the eyelid: A clinicopathological study. Br J Ophthalmol 1998;82:1049–1055.

105. Khan JA, Doane JF, Grove AS: Sebaceous and meibomian carcinomas of the eyelid: Recognition, diagnosis, and management. Ophthal Plast Reconstr Surg 1991;7:61–66.

106. Jensen ML: Extraocular sebaceous carcinoma of the skin with visceral metastases: Case report. J Cutan Pathol 1990;17:117–121.

107. Motley RJ, Douglas-Jones AF, Holt PJ: Sebaceous carcinoma: An unusual cause of a rapidly enlarging rhinophyma. Br J Dermatol 1991;124:283–284.

108. Rulon DB, Helwig EB: Cutaneous sebaceous neoplasms. Cancer 1974;33:82–102.

109. Rinaggio J, McGuff HS, Otto R, Hickson C: Postauricular sebaceous carcinoma arising in association with nevus sebaceus. Head Neck 2002;24:212–216.

110. Mohs FE, Blanchard L: Microscopically controlled surgery for extramammary Paet's disease. Arch Dermatol 1979;115:706–708.

111. Snow SN, Larson PO, Hardy S, et al: Merkel cell carcinoma of the skin and mucosa: Report of 12 cutaneous cases with 2 cases arising from the nasal mucosa. Dermatol Surg 2001;27:165–170.

112. Font RL: Eyelids and lacrimal drainage system. In Spencer WH (ed): Ophthalmic Pathology: An Atlas and Textbook, 3rd ed. Philadelphia, WB Saunders, 1986, pp 2169-214.

113. Bentley TJ, Koranda FC, Miller LM: Histologic evaluation of horizontal frozen sections: Improved staining and special staining techniques. J Dermatol Surg Oncol 1982;8:466-472.

114. Folberg R, Whitaker DC, Tse DT, Nerad JA: Recurrent and residual sebaceous carcinoma after Mohs' excision of the primary lesion. Am J Ophthalmol 1987;103:817-823.

115. Putterman AM: Conjunctival map biopsy to determine pagetoid spread. Am J Ophthalmol 1986;102:87-90.

116. Pardo FS, Wang CC, Albert D, et al: Sebaceous carcinoma of the ocular adnexa: Radiotherapeutic management. Int J Radiat Oncol Biol Phys 1989;17:643-647.

117. Rapini RP: Comparison of methods for checking surgical margins. J Am Acad Dermatol 1990;23:288-294.

118. Cottel WI, Bailin PL, Albom MJ, et al: Essential of Mohs micrographic surgery. J Dermatol Surg Oncol 1988;14:11-13.

119. Hruza G: Mohs micrographic surgery. Otolaryngol Clin North Am 1990;23:845-864.

120. Mohs FE: Chemosurgery: Microscopically controlled surgery for skin cancer—past, present and future. J Dermatol Surg Oncol 1978;4:41-54.

121. Lisman RD, Jakobiec FA, Small P: Sebaceous carcinoma of the eyelids: The role of adjuvant cryotherapy in the management of conjunctival pagetoid spread. Ophthalmology 1989;96:1021-1026.

122. Kass LG: Role of cryotherapy in treating sebaceous carcinoma of the eyelid. Ophthalmology 1990;97:2-3.

123. Yeates RP, Waller RR: Sebaceous carcinoma of the eyelid: Pitfalls in diagnosis. Ophthalmic Plast Reconstr Surg 1985;1:435-442.

Merkel Cell Carcinoma

124. Toker C. Trabecular carcinoma of the skin. Arch Dermatol 1972;105:107-110.

125. Gruber S, Wilson L: Merkel cell carcinoma. In Maloney ME, Miller SJ (eds): Cutaneous Oncology: Pathophysiology, Diagnosis, and Management. Boston, Blackwell, 1998.

126. Brissett AE, Olsen KD, Kasperbauer JL, et al: Merkel cell carcinoma of the head and neck: A retrospective case series. Head Neck 2002;10:982-987.

127. Haag M, Glass LF, Fenske NA: Merkel cell carcinoma: Diagnosis and treatment. Dermatol Surg 1995;21:669-683.

128. Gollard R, Weber R, Kosty MP, Greenway HT, Massullo V, Humberson C. Merkel cell carcinoma: Review of 22 cases with surgical, pathologic and therapeutic considerations. Cancer 2000;88:1842-1851.

129. Hitcock CL, Bland KI, Laney RG III, Franzini D, Harris B, Copeland EM III: Neuroendocrine (Merkel cell) carcinoma of the skin: Its natural history, diagnosis and treatment. Ann Surg 1988;207:201-207.

130. Pitale M, Sessions R, Husain S: An analysis of prognostic factors in cutaneous neuroendocrine carcinoma. Laryngoscope 1992;102:244-249.

131. Shaw JH, Rumball E: Merkel cell tumour: Clinical behaviour and treatment. Br J Surg 1991;78:138-142.

132. Silva EG, Mackay B, Goepfert H, et al: Endocrine carcinoma of the skin (Merkel cell carcinoma). Pathol Annu 1984;19:1-30.

133. Sharma D, Flora G, Grunberg SM: Chemotherapy of metastatic Merkel cell carcinoma: Case report and review of the literature. Am J Clin Oncol 1991;14:166-169.

134. Anderson LL, Phipps TJ, McCollough ML: Neuroendocrine carcinoma of the skin (Merkel cell carcinoma) in a black. J Dermatol Surg Oncol 1992:18:375-380.

135. Kuppuswami N, Sivarajan KM, Hussein L, et al: Merkel cell tumor in pregnancy: A case report. J Reprod Med 1991;36:613-615.

136. Saadi Ak, Danks JJ, Cree IA, Collin JR: Merkel cell tumour: Case reports and review. Orbit 1999;18:45-52.

137. Meland NB, Jackson IT: Merkel cell tumor: Diagnosis, prognosis and management. Plast Reconstr Surg 1986;77:632-638.

138. Sibley RK, Dehner LP, Rosai J: Primary neuroendocrine (Merkel cell) carcinoma of the skin. I. A clinicopathologic and ultrastructural study of 43 cases. Am J Surg Pathol 1985;9:95-108.

139. Chen KT: Merkel's cell (neuroendocrine) carcinoma of the vulva. Cancer 1994;73:2186-2191.

140. Best TJ, Metcalfe JB, Moore RB, Nguyen GK: Merkel cell carcinoma of the scrotum. Ann Plast Surg 1994;33:83-83.

141. Yang GC, Schneck MJ, Hayden RE, Gupta PK: Merkel cell tumor-like endocrine carcinoma associated with the submandibular gland: Report of case with cytologic, immunohistochemical, electron microscopic and flow cytometric studies. Acta Cytol 1994;38:742-746.

142. Canales LI, Parker A, Kadakia S: Upper gastrointestinal bleeding from Merkel cell carcinoma. Am J Gastroenterol 1992;87:1464-1466.

143. Collins MK, Cameron FG: Solitary regional bony recurrence in Merkel cell carcinoma. Australas Radiol 1993;37:277-278.

144. Catlett JP, Todd WM, Carr ME Jr: Merkel cell tumor in an HIV-positive patient. Va Med Q 1992;119:256-258.

145. Boyle F, Pendelbury S, Bell D: Further insights into the natural history and management of primary cutaneous neuroendocrine (Merkel cell) carcinoma. Int J Radiat Oncol Biol Phys 1995;31:315-323.

146. Grosh WW, Giannone L, Hande KR, Johnson DH: Disseminated Merkel cell tumor: Treatment with systemic chemotherapy. Am J Clin Oncol 1987;10:227-230.

147. Lentz SR, Krewson L, Zutter MM: Recurrent neuroendocrine (Merkel cell) carcinoma of the skin presenting as marrow failure in a man with systemic lupus erythematosus. Med Pediatr Oncol 1993;21:137-141.

148. Formica M, Basolo B, Funaro L, et al: Merkel cell carcinoma in a renal transplant recipient [letter]. Nephron 1994;68:399.

149. Ratner D, Nelson BR, Brown M, Johnson TM: Merkel cell carcinoma [review]. J Am Acad Dermatol 1993;29:143-156.

150. Lever WF, Schaumburg-Lever G: Histopathology of the Skin, 7th ed. Philadelphia, JB Lippincott, 1990.

151. Frigerio B, Capella C, Eusbi V, et al: Merkel cell carcinoma of the skin: The structure and origin of normal Merkel cells. Histopathology. 1983;7:229-249.

152. Leboit PE, Crutcher WA, Shapiro PE: Pagetoid intraepidermal spread in Merkel cell (primary neuroendocrine) carcinoma of the skin. Am J Surg Pathol 1992;16:584-592.

153. Gould VE, Dardi LE, Memoli VA, Johannessen JV: Neuroendocrine carcinomas of the skin: Light microscopic, ultrastructural, and immunohistochemical analysis. Ultrastruct Pathol 1980;1:499-509.

154. Gould VE, Moll R, Moll I, Lee J, Franke WW: Biology of disease. Neuroendocrine (Merkel) cell of the skin: Hyperplasias, dysplasias, and neoplasms. Lab Invest 1985;52:334-353.

155. Tang CK, Nedwich A, Toker C, Zaman ANF: Unusual cutaneous carcinoma with features of small cell (oat cell-like) and squamous cell carcinomas. Am J Dermatopathol 1982;4:537-548.

156. Pilotti S, Rilke F, Lombardi L: Neuroendocrine (Merkel cell) carcinoma of the skin. Am J Surg Pathol 1982;6:243-254.

157. Sidhu GS, Feiner H, Flotte TJ, et al: Merkel cell neoplasms: Histology, electron microscopy, biology and histogenesis. Am J Dermatopathol 1980;2:101-119.

158. Leong AS, Phillips GE, Pieterse AS, Milios J: Criteria for the diagnosis of primary endocrine carcinoma of the skin (Merkel cell type): A histological, immunohistochemical and ultrastructural study of 13 cases. Pathology 1986;18:393-399.

159. Tope WD, Sargueza OP: Merkel cell carcinoma: Histopathology, immunohistochemistry, and cytogenetic analysis. J Dermatol Surg Oncol 1994;20:648-652.

160. Yiengpruksawan A, Coit DG, Thaler HT, et al: Merkel cell carcinoma. Prognosis and management. Arch Surg 1991;126:1514-1519.

161. Wick MR, Goellenr JR, Scheithauer BW: Primary neuroendocrine carcinoma of the skin (Merkel cell tumor): A clinical, histological and ultrastructural study of 13 cases. Am J Clin Pathol 1983;79:6-13.

162. Hanke CW, Conner AC, Temofeew RK, Lingeman RE: Merkel cell carcinoma. Arch Dermatol 1989;125:1096-1100.

163. Bayrou O, Avril MF, Charpentier MD, et al: Primary neuroendocrine carcinoma of the skin: Clinicopathologic study of 18 cases. J Am Acad Dermatol 1991;24:198-207.

164. Safai B: Management of skin cancer. In Devita VT Jr, Hellman S, Rosenberg SA (eds): Principles and Practice of Oncology. Philadelphia, JB Lippincott, 1997, p 1905.

165. O'Rourke MGE, Bell JR: Merkel cell tumor with spontaneous regression. Dermatol Surg Oncol 1986;12:994-997.

166. Kayashima KI, Ono T, Johno M, Kojo Y, Yamashita N, Matsunaga W: Spontaneous regression in Merkel cell (neuroendocrine) carcinoma of the skin. Arch Dermatol 1991;127:550-553.

167. Duncan WC, Tschen JA: Spontaneous regression of Merkel cell (neuroendocrine) carcinoma of the skin. J Am Acad Dermatol 1986;12:653-654.

168. Mohs FE: Chemosurgery: Microscopically Controlled Surgery for Skin Cancer. Springfield, Ill, Charles C Thomas, 1978.

169. Goepfert H, Remmler D, Silva E, Wheeler B: Merkel cell carcinoma (endocrine carcinoma of the skin) of the head and neck. Arch Otolaryngol 1984;110:707-712.

170. Kurul S, Mudun A, Aksakal N, Aygen M: Lymphatic mapping for Merkel cell carcinoma. Plast Reconstr Surg 2000;105:680-683.

171. Feun LG, Sararaj N, Legha SS, Silva EG, Benjamin RS, Burgess MA: Chemotherapy for metastatic Merkel cell carcinoma. Cancer 1988;62:683-685.

172. Redmond J III, Perry J, Sowray P, Vukelja SJ, Dawson N: Chemotherapy of disseminated Merkel-cell carcinoma. Am J Clin Oncol 1991;14:305-307.

173. Queirolo P, Gipponi M, Peressini A, et al: Merkel cell carcinoma of the skin: Treatment of primary, recurrent, and metastatic disease—review of clinical cases. Anticancer Res 1997;17:673-678.

Dermatofibrosarcoma Protuberans

174. Darier J, Ferrand M: Dermatofibromes progressifs et recidivants ou fibrosarcomes de la peau. Ann Dermatol Syphiliga 1924;5:545-562.

175. Hoffman E: Veher das knollentribende fibrosarkam der haut (dermatofibrosarcoma protuberans). Dermatol Z 1925;43:1-28.

176. Bendix-Hansen K, Myhre-Jensen D, Haae S: Dermatofibrosarcoma protuberans: A clinicopathological study of nineteen cases and a review of world literature. Scand J Plast Reconstruct Surg Hand Surg 1983;17:247-252.

177. Burkhardt BR, Soule EH, Winkelmann RK, et al: Dermatofibrosarcoma protuberans: Study of fifty-six cases. Am J Surg 1966;111:638-644.

178. Pack GT, Tabah EJ: Dermatofibrosarcoma protuberans: A report of 39 cases. Arch Surg 1951;62:391-411.

179. Chaung TY, Su WPD, Muller SA: Incidence of T cell lymphoma and other rare skin cancers in a defined population. J Am Acad Dermatol 1990;23:254-256.

180. Gloster HM: Dermatofibrosarcoma protuberans. J Am Acad Dermatol 1996;35:355-374.

181. Taylor HB, Helwig EB: Dermatofibrosarcoma protuberans: A study of 115 cases. Cancer 1962;15:717-725.

182. McKee PH, Fletcher CD: Dermatofibrosarcoma protuberans in infancy and childhood. J Cutan Pathol 1991:18:241-246.

183. Schuarez LW: Congenital dermatofibrosarcoma protuberans of the hand. Hautl 1977;9:182-186.

184. Annessi G, Cimisan A, Girolomoni G, et al: Congenital dermatofibrosarcoma protuberans. Pediatr Dermatol 1993;10:40-42.

185. Rutgers EJ, Kroon BR, Albus-Lutter LE, et al: Dermatofibrosarcoma protuberans: Treatment and prognosis. Eur J Surg Oncol 1992;18:241-248.

186. McPeak C, Cruz T, Nicastri A: Dermatofibrosarcoma protuberans: An analysis of 86 cases, five with metastases. Ann Surg 1967;166:803-816.

187. Bang KM, Halder RM, White JE, et al: Skin cancer in black Americans: A review of 126 cases. J Natl Med Assoc 1987;79:51-58.

188. Costa OG: Progressive recurrent dermatofibrosarcoma (Darier-Ferrand): Anatomoclinical study. Arch Dermatol 1946;54:432-454.

189. McMaster PE: Sarcomatoid fibroma of the skin (progressive and recurring dermatofibroma). Ann Surg 1934;99:338-347.

190. Cook TF, Fosko SW: Unusual cutaneous malignancies. Semin Cutan Med Surg 1998;17:114-132.

191. Allan AE, Tsou HC, Harrington A, et al: Clonal origin of dermatofibrosarcoma protuberans. J Invest Dermatol 1993;100:99-102.

192. Pedeutour F, Simon MP, Minoletti F, et al: Ring 22 chromosomes in dermatofibrosarcoma protuberans are low level amplifiers of chromosome 17 and 22l sequences. Cancer Res 1995;55:2400-2403.

193. Mandahl N, Heim S, Willen H, et al: Supernumerary ring chromosome as the sole cytogenetic abnormality in a dermatofibroarcoma protuberans. Cancer Genet Cytogenet 1990;49:273-275.

194. Bridge JA, Neff JR, Sanberg AA:. Cytogenetic analysis of dermatofibrosarcoma protuberans. Cancer Genet Cytogenet 1990;49:199-202.

195. Bashara NE, Jules K, Potter G: DFSP: 4 years after local trauma. J Foot Surg 1992;31:160-165.

196. Barnes L, Coleman JA, Johnson JT: Dermatofibrosarcoma protuberans of the head and neck. Arch Otolaryngol 1984;110:398-404.

197. Coard K, Branday JM, LaGrenade L: Dermatofibrosarcoma protuberans: A 10 year clinicopathological review of an uncommon tumor. West Indian Med J 1994;43:130-133.

198. Morman MR, Lin RY, Petrozzi JN: Dermatofibrosarcoma arising in a site of multiple immunizations. Arch Dermatol 1979;115:1453.

199. Schneidman D, Belizaire R: Arsenic exposure followed by the development of dermatofibrosarcoma protuberans. Cancer 1986;58:1585-1587.

200. Shelley WB: Malignant melanoma and dermatofibrosarcoma in a 60- year-old patient with a life long history of acrodermatitis enteropathica. J Am Acad Derm 1982;6:63-66.

201. Melezea M, Duorsky C: Acanthosis nigracans bei dermatofibrosarcoma protuberans mit multplen hautmetastasen. Hautarzt 1957;8:54.

202. Dupree WB, Langloss JW, Weiss SW: Pigmented dermatofibrosarcoma protuberans (Bednar tumor): A pathologic, ultrastructural and immunohistochemical study. Am J Surg Pathol 1985;9:630-639.

203. Page EH, Assaad DM: Atrophic dermatofibroma and dermatofibrosarcoma protuberans. J Am Acad Dermatol 1987;17:947-950.

204. Sagi A, Ben-Yakar Y, Mahler D: A ten-year-old boy with dermatofibrosarcoma protuberans of the face. J Dermatol Surg Oncol 1987;13:82-83.

205. Hess K, Hanke CW, Estes NC, et al: Chemosurgical reports: Myxoid dermatofibrosarcoma protuberans. J Derm Surg Oncol 1985;11:268-271.

206. Zamecnik M, Michal M: Myxoid variant of dermatofibrosarcoma protuberans with fibrosarcomatous areas. Zentralbl Pathol 1993;139:373-376.

207. Gloster HM, Harris KR, Roenigk RK: A comparison between Mohs micrographic surgery and wide surgical excision for the treatment of dermatofibrosarcoma protuberans. J Am Acad Dermatol 1996;35:82-87.

208. Jimenez FJ, Grichnik JM, Buchanan MD, Clark RE: Immunohistochemical margin control applied to Mohs micrographic surgical excision of dermatofibrosarcoma protuberans. J Dermatol Surg Oncol 1994;20:687-689.

209. Peters CW, Hanke CW, Pasarell HA, Bennett JE: Chemosurgical reports: Dermatofibrosarcoma protuberans of the face. J Dermatol Surg Oncol 1982;10:823-826.

210. Parker TL, Zitelli JA: Surgical margins for excision of dermatofibrosarcoma protuberans. J Am Acad Dermatol 1995;32:233-236.

211. Robinson JK: Dermatofibrosarcoma protuberans resected by Mohs surgery (chemosurgery): A 5 year prospective study. J Am Acad Dermatol 1985;12:1093-1098.

212. Hobbs ER, Wheeland RG, Bailin PL, Rayz JL, Yetman RJ: Treatment of dermatofibrosarcoma protuberans with Mohs micrographic surgery. Ann Surg 1980;287:102-107.

213. Dawes KW, Hanke CW: Dermatofibrosarcoma protuberans treated with Mohs micrographic surgery: Cure rates and surgical margins. Dermatol Surg 1996:22:530-534.

214. Ratner D, Thomas CO, Johnson TM, et al: Mohs micrographic surgery for the treatment of dermatofibrosarcoma protuberans. J Am Acad Dermatol 1997;37:600-613.

215. Haycox CL, Odland PB, Olbricht SM, Casey B: Dermatofibrosarcoma protuberans (DFSP): Growth characteristics based on

tumor modeling and a review of cases treated with Mohs micrographic surgery. Ann Plast Surg 1997;38:246–251.

216. Rockley PF, Robinson JK, Magid M, Goldblatt D: Dermatofibrosarcoma protuberans of the scalp: A series of cases. J Am Acad Dermatol 1989;21:278–283.

217. Mohs FE: Chemosurgery: Microscopically Controlled Surgery for Skin Cancer. Springfield, Ill, Charles C Thomas, 1978, pp 250–255.

218. Enzinger FM, Weiss SW: Soft tissue tumors, 2nd ed. St. Louis, Mosby, 1988.

219. Ding J, Hashimoto H, Enjoji M: Dermatofibrosarcoma protuberans: A clinicopathological review with emphasis on fibrosarcomatous areas. Am J Surg Pathol 1992;16:921–925.

Angiosarcoma

220. Maddox JC, Evans HC: Angiosarcoma of the skin and soft tissue: A study of 44 cases. Cancer 1981;48:1907–1921.

221. Hodgkinson DJ, Soule EH, Woods J: Cutaneous angiosarcoma of the head and neck. Cancer 1979;144:1106–1113.

222. Holden CA, Spittle MF, Wilson Jones E: Angiosarcoma of the face and scalp, prognosis and treatment. Cancer 1987;59:1046–1057.

223. Wilson Jones E: Malignant vascular tumors. Clin Exp Dermatol 1976;1:287–312.

224. Simon SI, Sika JV, Lynfield YL: Angiosarcoma of the scalp. J Dermatol Surg Oncol 1980;11:935–937.

225. Tay YK, Ong BH: Cutaneous angiosarcoma presenting as recurrent angio-edema of the face. Br J Dermatol 2000;143:1346–1348.

226. Smith L, Buzdar AU, Rusch V, et al: Post-mastectomy angiosarcoma: Case report and review of the literature. Tex Med 1984;80:43–44.

227. Rosai J, Sumner H, Kostianovsky M, Perez-Mesa C: Angiosarcoma of the skin. Hum Pathol 1976;7:83–109.

228. Farr H, Carandang C, Huvos A: Malignant vascular tumors of the head and neck. Am J Surg 1970;120:501–504.

229. Mehregan A, Usndek H: Malignant angioendothelioma. Arch Dermatol 1976;112:1565–1567.

230. Panje W, Moran W, Bostwick D: Angiosarcoma of the head and neck: Review of 11 cases. Laryngoscope 1986;96:1381–1384.

231. Haustein U: Angiosarcoma of the face and scalp. Int J Dermatol 1991;30:851–856.

232. Bennett R, Keller J, Ditty J: Hemangiosarcoma subsequent to radiotherapy for hemangioma in infancy. J Dermatol Surg Oncol 1978;4:881–883.

233. Ward C, Buchanan R: Hemangiosarcoma following irradiation of a hemangioma of the face. J Maxillofac Surg 1977;5:164–166.

234. Narula A, Vallis M, El-Silimy O: Radiation induced angiosarcoma of the nasopharynx. Eur J Surg Oncol 1986;12:147–152.

235. Kibe Y, Kishimoto S, Katoh N, Yasuno H, Yasmara T, Oka T: Angiosarcoma of the scalp associated with renal transplantation. Br J Dermatol 1997;136:752–756.

236. Bullen R, Larson PO, Landeck AE, et al: Angiosarcoma of the head

and neck managed by a combination of multiple biopsies to determine tumor margin and radiation therapy: Report of three cases and review of the literature. Dermatol Surg 1998;24:1105–1110.

237. Requena L, Sangueza OP: Cutaneous vascular proliferations. III. Malignant neoplasms, other cutaneous neoplasms with significant vascular component and disorders erroneously considered vascular neoplasms. J Am Acad Dermatol 1998;38:143–175.

238. Mentzel T, Kutzner H, Wollina U: Cutaneous angiosarcoma of the face: Clinicopathologic and immunohistochemical study of a case resembling rosacea clinically. J Am Acad Dermatol 1998;38:387–340.

239. Stewart FW, Treves N: Lymphangiosarcoma in post-mastectomy lymphedema. Cancer 1948;1:64–81.

240. Shirger A: Postoperative lymphedema: Etiologic and diagnostic factors. Med Clin North Am 1962;46:1045–1050.

241. Alessi E, Sala F, Berti E: Angiosarcoma in lymphedematous limbs. Am J Dermatolpathol 196;8:371–378.

242. Offori TW, Platt CC, Stephens M, et al: Angiosarcoma in congenital hereditary lymphedema (Milroy's disease): Diagnostic beacons and review of the literature. Clin Exp Dermatol 1992;18:174–177.

243. Kirchmann TT, Smoller BR, McGuire J: Cutaneous angiosarcoma as a second malignancy in a lymphedematous leg in a Hodgkin's disease survivor. J Am Acad Dermatol 1994;31:861–866.

244. Goette DK, Detlefs RL: Postirradiation angiosarcoma. J Am Acad Dermatol 1985;12:922–926.

245. Girard C, Johnson WC, Graham J: Cutaneous angiosarcoma. Cancer 1970;26:868–883.

246. Muller R, Hajdu SI, Brennan MF: Lymphangiosarcoma associated with chronic filarial lymphedema. Cancer 1987;59:179–183.

247. Scully RE, Mark EJ, McNeely WF, et al: Case records of the Massachusetts General Hospital, weekly clinicopathological exercises: Case 18-1993—a 57- year old man with chronic lymphedema and enlarging purple cutaneous nodules of the leg. N Engl J Med 1993;328:1337–1343.

248. Lever WF, Schaumburg-Lever G: Histopathology of the Skin, 7th ed. Philadelphia, JB Lippincott, 1990, pp 708–711.

249. Stewart NJ, Prithard DJ, Nascimento AG, et al: Lymphangiosarcoma following mastectomy. Clin Orthop 1995;320:135–141.

250. Lewis JJ, Brennan MF: Soft tissue sarcomas. Curr Probl Surg 1996;33:817–872.

251. Golden DJ, Kim YA: Angiosarcoma of the scalp treated with Mohs micrographic surgery. J Dermatol Surg Oncol 1993;19:156–158.

252. Mikhail G, Kelly A: Malignant angioendothelioma of the face. J Dermatol Surg Oncol 1977;3:181–183.

253. Clayton BD, Leshin B, Hithcock MG, Marks M, White WL: Utility of rush paraffin-embedded tangential sections in the management of cutaneous neoplasms. Dermatol Surg 2000;26:671–678.

254. Graham W, Bogardus C: Angiosarcoma treated with radiation therapy alone. Cancer 1981;48:912–914.

255. Cerroni L, Peris K, Legge A, Chimenti S: Angiosarcoma of the face and scalp: A case report with complete spontaneous regression. J Dermatol Surg Oncol 1991;17:539–542.

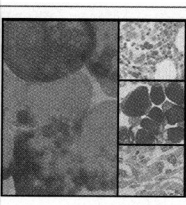

74

CANCER OF THE ENDOCRINE SYSTEM

Ronald J. Weigel

John S. Macdonald

Daniel Haller

I. Ross McDougall

SUMMARY OF KEY POINTS

THYROID CANCER

Incidence
17,200 cases per year

Types
- Follicular cell
- Differentiated (papillary follicular variants)
- Undifferentiated (anaplastic)
- Parafollicular cell (medullary)
- Connective tissue (lymphoma, sarcoma)
- Miscellaneous metastases (breast, lung, kidney, melanoma)

Presentation and Diagnosis
- Mass in the neck
- Mass noted on ultrasound, computed tomography, magnetic resonance imaging by chance
- Abnormal cervical lymph nodes
- Differentiate primary thyroid cancer, lymphoma, benign nodule, other causes of enlarged lymph nodes
- Tissue diagnosis required usually by fine needle aspiration
- Ultrasound identifies cysts likely to be benign
- Scintiscan distinguishes functioning nodules with a low likelihood of cancer

Treatment
- Thyroid resection (lobectomy or total thyroidectomy)
- ^{131}I for differentiated tumors
- External beam irradiation—palliative
- Chemotherapy—palliative

ADRENOCORTICAL CANCER

Incidence
Rare (2 cases per 1 million)

Clinical Features
- Abdominal mass, metastases
- Virilization in females
- Cushing's syndrome
- Feminization in males (rare)
- Hyperaldosteronism (rare)

Diagnosis
- Imaging techniques: computed tomography and magnetic resonance imaging of upper abdomen
- Biochemical: Increased urinary steroid excretion (functional tumors)

Treatment
- Radical adrenalectomy for localized tumor
- Antihormonal therapy—palliative
- Chemotherapy—palliative

MALIGNANT PHEOCHROMOCYTOMA

Incidence
Rare

Diagnosis
- Episodic hypertension
- May be familial
- May be part of MEN-2a or MEN-2b

Biochemical
- Vanillylmandelic acid, metanephrine, and catecholamine in urine
- Serum catecholamine measurements

Imaging
- Computed tomographic and magnetic resonance imaging scans
- Metaiodobenzylguanidine (MIBG) radionuclide scanning

Treatment
- Surgical resection of localized disease with preoperative α-blockade
- Palliative α- and β-adrenergic blockade

PARATHYROID CARCINOMA

Incidence
Rare

Diagnosis
- Refractory hypercalcemia
- Mass in neck

Imaging
- Sestamibi
- Imaging may be unecessary

Treatment
- En bloc resection of cancer and involved structures and ipsilateral lobe of thyroid
- Radiation—palliative only
- Chemotherapy—(dacarbazine)
- Therapy for hypercalcemia (etidronate, gallium nitrate)—palliative

CARCINOID TUMORS

Incidence
- Clinical disease: 7 to 13 cases per 1 million
- Autopsy: 6500 per 1 million

Diagnosis
- Nonfunctional bowel obstruction
- Abdominal pain
- Carcinoid syndrome (diarrhea, flushing, hypotension)

Imaging Techniques
- Computed tomographic scan of the abdomen
- Contrast radiography study with small bowel follow-through
- Enteroscopy (investigational)

Special Diagnostic Techniques
- Urinary 5-hydroxyindoleacetic acid (5-HIAA) measurement
- Radiolabeled sandostatin imaging

Treatment
- Complete surgical resection (curative)
- Partial surgical resection (palliative)
- Tumor embolization (palliative)
- Somatostatin analog
- Antiserotonin agents
- Antihistamines
- Anticholinergics
- Streptozotocin + 5-FU chemotherapy; 30% partial response

PANCREATIC ISLET CELL TUMORS

Incidence
1 case per 100,000

SUMMARY OF KEY POINTS—cont'd

Diagnosis
- Pancreatic mass
- Metastatic disease
- Varies with hormone produced

Imaging Techniques
- Computed tomographic scan of the abdomen
- Ultrasound of abdomen
- Endoscopic ultrasound
- Celiac angiography
- Intraoperative ultrasound

Special Diagnostic Techniques
- Plasma hormone assays
- Selective venous catheterization for hormonal levels

Treatment
- Complete surgical resection (curative)
- Partial surgical resection (palliative)
- Tumor embolization (palliative)

- Antihormonal therapy
- Somatostatin analog (for most hormonal excess syndromes)
- H_2-blockers, Na/K pump inhibitors (for gastrinoma)
- Insulin antagonists (for insulinoma)
- Chemotherapy: doxorubicin/streptozotocin 60% response rate

INTRODUCTION

Cancers of the endocrine glands are uncommon. Of the 19,000 endocrine cancers diagnosed annually in the United States, nearly 18,000 are thyroid cancers.[1] Endocrine tumors—both benign and malignant—although infrequent, present challenges in diagnosis and treatment. Cancers of the thyroid generally do not alter thyroid function, but abnormal hormone secretion can cause the earliest symptoms or signs in cancers of the other endocrine glands. Abnormal plasma levels of the hormone can be useful in monitoring the effects of therapy, and specific inhibitors of hormone biosynthesis or activity can palliate symptoms significantly without having any effect on tumor growth. Diagnosing and treating endocrine cancers requires oncologists, endocrinologists, surgeons, and other subspecialists to work together. The aim of this chapter is to provide a clear and practical guide to the diagnosis and management of endocrine tumors.

THYROID CANCER

Thyroid cancer is the most common tumor of the endocrine system. The biologic behavior of the various histologic types of thyroid neoplasms varies greatly. Approximately 18,000 cases of thyroid cancer are diagnosed in the United States annually. There are about 1200 deaths annually.[1] These data demonstrate the lack of aggressive growth of most thyroid cancers. In particular, papillary cancer, the most common type in the United States, has an excellent prognosis.

Etiology

It has been clearly documented that external radiation to the cervical region is a cause of thyroid cancer. This association has been recognized in patients who had thymic irradiation in childhood, in patients who had irradiation for acne in teenage years, and in patients with cancer such as Hodgkin's disease who received neck irradiation.[2-5] There is an increase in children who received irradiation to the scalp.[6] Reports from Israel of children who received scalp irradiation to treat ringworm have shown an increase in thyroid cancer compared to siblings and age-matched nonirradiated control subjects.[4] Retrospective phantom studies demonstrate that radiation doses as low as 9 rad could be incriminated as the cause of cancer in these children.

In addition, children exposed to radioactive fallout from Chernobyl have shown an increase in thyroid cancer, as will be discussed.[7-8] The radiation doses that were originally blamed were in the range of 1 to 10 Gy, but with the evidence in patients with Hodgkin's disease doses as high as 40 Gy are potentially carcinogenic.[9] In laboratory animals, combining radiation with an increased thyroid-stimulating hormone (TSH) increases the potential risk.[10] The lag time from radiation exposure to diagnosis of cancer is usually 10 to 20 years; however, periods from 5 to 50 years have been reported. Epidemiologic studies show that between 7% and 9% of patients who received 5 to 10 Gy external radiation develop thyroid cancer.[11] About 20% have a palpable abnormality; therefore, about one third of these nodules are cancers. It is now rare for patients to be given external radiation to the neck for benign disease, so this association should become rare. Patients treated for cancer are in general followed closely, and careful palpation of the neck and measurement of TSH annually is advisable. Radiation to the thyroid from internal sources and diagnostic or therapeutic doses of ^{131}I have not been associated with an increased incidence of thyroid cancer. However, the recent epidemics of childhood thyroid cancers in Belarus and the Ukraine have a clear connection with the massive release of radionuclides, including radioisotopes of iodine from the Chernobyl reactor.[12] These patients were almost all children at the time of exposure, and there was internal radiation to the thyroid from ^{131}I and other shorter-lived radionuclides of iodine. There was also exposure to external radiation and probably internal radiation from ^{137}Cs. The etiology of these cancers is probably multifactorial, but the data must cause us to reconsider the risks from internal radiation.

There is increasing evidence of genetic alterations in some thyroid cancers, especially in Chernobyl survivors.[13,14] Familial nonmedullary thyroid cancer is now recognized as a true phenomenon, and we have

TABLE 74-1

Histologic Classification of Thyroid Cancers and Their Incidence

TUMOR HISTOLOGY	INCIDENCE (%)
Differentiated carcinomas	81–87
Papillary	
Follicular variant of papillary	
Follicular and Hürthle cell	
Medullary	6–8
Anaplastic	5
Lymphoma	1–5
Metastatic	<1

experience with 14 families with two or more members with thyroid cancer.[15] There is an association of familial thyroid cancer and both Gardner's and Cowden's syndromes.[16]

Because of varied incidences of thyroid cancer in different ethnic groups, the role of an environmental factor or factors must be considered. A higher incidence of papillary cancer is found in regions with high dietary iodine intake such as the Pacific rim and Iceland.[17] In contrast, follicular cancer is more prevalent in iodine-deficient countries.

Classification and Prognosis

The most common thyroid cancers are papillary carcinoma and mixed papillary and follicular carcinoma[18,19] (Table 74-1; Fig. 74-1A and B), the latter of which are also classified as papillary carcinomas. Occult cancers have been reported in 10% to 30% of autopsy series; they are small (<1 cm) and have little clinical significance.[20]

Death from papillary cancer is rare, and in most reports nodal metastasis does not adversely influence prognosis.[21] Recent series, however, have demonstrated slightly lower survival rate with locoregional nodal metastases.[22,23] The prognosis in intrathyroidal papillary carcinoma depends on the age of the patient and size of the tumor; when the cancer is less than 5 cm in diameter, the prognosis is excellent.[24,25] Lymph node metastases can occur, but even in patients with nodal metastases only a small percentage of patients die of thyroid cancer. The situation in older patients with larger, more aggressive papillary cancers is different. In patients with local invasion and cancers that cannot be totally resected, the recurrence rate and mortality rate are higher.[24] Death can result from local invasion and extensive metastases; nevertheless, the overall death rate from papillary cancer is low (<10%).[26]

In summary, the prognosis for papillary cancer is better in the young and in those with cancers smaller than 2 cm

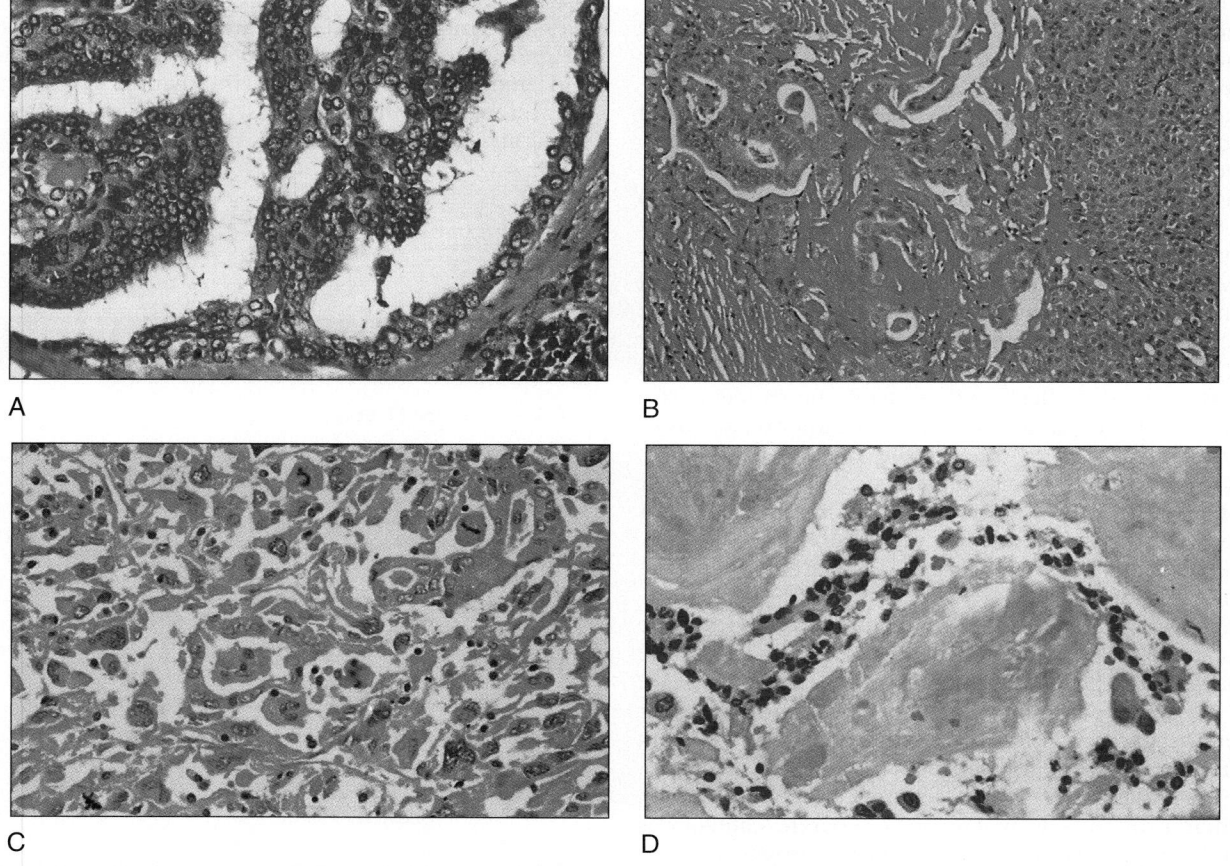

A   B

C   D

Figure 74-1. Histologic patterns of thyroid cancer. **A,** Papillary carcinoma. **B,** Pure follicular carcinoma. **C,** Anaplastic carcinoma. **D,** Medullary carcinoma.

Specific Malignancies

III

that are intrathyroidal and have no evidence of distant spread. The presence of metastases to lymph nodes has not been a negative prognostic factor in most series, although some series have reported increased recurrence and mortality rates for node-positive patients. Based on simple criteria such as the age of the patient, the size of the primary cancer, and whether local invasion or distant metastases are found, it is possible to determine the prognosis at presentation. Scoring systems such as AGES (age, grade of cancer, extrathyroidal spread, and size), MACIS (metastases, age, complete excision, invasion, and size) are examples of these approaches.[27] The TNM system also stresses the importance of age at time of presentation. In patients under 45 years of age, those without distant metastases are all stage I, and those with distant metastases are stage II.

Pure follicular carcinoma (see Fig. 74-1B) carries a poorer prognosis.[28,29] Even when the disease appears confined to the thyroid gland, 5% to 15% of patients will ultimately die of cancer, although survival is measured in decades. Lymph node metastases are seen less frequently than with papillary cancers of similar size. Approximately 50% of follicular cancers demonstrate intrathyroidal spread.[30] Prognosis[31] in follicular carcinoma depends on the size of the cancer, the amount of capsular and vascular invasion, and patient age. Cancers with good prognoses are smaller than 4 cm. If such a tumor occurs without marked local vascular invasion in a patient under 50 years of age, the prognosis is excellent. In older patients, thyroid carcinomas are more aggressive and have a poorer prognosis.

The incidence of anaplastic carcinoma appears to be decreasing and now represents less than 10% of thyroid malignancies[32,33] (Fig. 74-1C). This apparent decrease may be secondary to improved techniques to differentiate thyroid lymphoma and medullary carcinoma (Fig. 74-1D) from true anaplastic thyroid cancer. It is apparent that a proportion of patients with anaplastic cancers are emigrants from countries where goiter is common and the anaplastic cancer probably has arisen from a more differentiated cancer that went undiagnosed for many years. In some cases there is a spectrum from papillary to anaplastic cancer indicating that anaplastic cancers arise from more differentiated lesions,[34] and earlier diagnosis of the latter also plays a role in the reduced incidence. Anaplastic carcinomas usually occur in persons older than 60 years. These carcinomas are highly malignant and typically cause death within 6 months, either by local invasion or by distant metastases. Cure of anaplastic carcinoma is rare.[35]

Hürthle cell tumors of the thyroid are derived from the follicular cell.[36] Both carcinomas and adenomas of Hürthle cell origin have been described. Hürthle cell cancers are often classified with follicular cancer. As with follicular cancer, the differentiation of Hürthle cell adenoma from carcinoma is vascular, or capsular invasion in the latter. However, Hürthle cell cancers seldom concentrate iodine, and their prognosis is worse, so a separate category is justified. Adenomas have an excellent prognosis with resection, and less than 2.5% are subsequently found to demonstrate malignant behavior.[37,38] Large (>2 cm)

malignant tumors have a recurrence rate of 21% to 59% after surgical resection.[39] Because of differences in biology and behavior of thyroid cancers, assigning prognosis to an individual patient may be difficult. Byar and associates examined the significance of several variables on survival.[40] Age, gender, cell type, clinical extent of cancer, lymph node status, and number of metastatic sites had prognostic significance but were not all independent variables. However, a prognostic index that mirrored actual data was developed. Thus, in the "best" group (i.e., young patients with small localized differentiated tumors), 5-year survival rate was approximately 95%, whereas in the "worst" group, containing many patients with anaplastic carcinoma, the 5-year survival rate was less than 5%. These data agree with those from many other large series. To achieve uniformity in assessing results of therapy, it is important that a single tumor, node, metastasis (TNM)[41] and clinical staging system be used. Tables 74-2 and 74-3 outline the most recent iteration of staging systems for thyroid cancer. It should be noted that this system takes into account not only the effect of histologic type (papillary/follicular, medullary, anaplastic) on staging but also the negative prognostic effect of advancing age on stage and prognosis in differentiated thyroid neoplasms.

Primary lymphoma of the thyroid is not common. It usually occurs in an older woman with untreated Hashimoto's thyroiditis.[42] The condition characteristically presents as a rapidly growing thyroid mass with compressive symptoms and signs and sometimes causes pain. Diagnosis can often be made by fine-needle aspiration and immunophenotyping of the lymphocytic aspirate. Treatment usually consists of chemotherapy and sometimes radiation therapy.

TABLE 74-2

TNM Classification of Malignant Tumors of the Thyroid Gland

Primary Tumor (T Stage)

TX	Tumor cannot be assessed
T0	No clinical evidence of tumor
T1	Tumor ≤1 cm
T2	Tumor >1 cm and <4 cm
T3	Tumor ≥4 cm
T4	Tumor extending beyond thyroid capsule

Regional Lymph Nodes (N Stage)

N0	No palpable nodes
N1	Regional nodal metastases
	N1a Ipsilateral nodes
	N1b Contralateral, bilateral, or mediastinal nodes

Distant Metastases (M Stage)

MX	Metastases cannot be assessed
M0	No evidence of distant metastases
M1	Distant metastases present

Adapted from American Joint Committee on Cancer Manual for the Staging of Cancer. Philadelphia, JB Lippincott, 1988.

TABLE 74-3

Clinical Staging of Thyroid Cancer

Medullary			
Stage I	T1	N0	M0
Stage II	T2	N0	M0
Stage III	Any T	N1	M0
Stage IV	Any T	Any N	M1

Undifferentiated—All Cases Stage IV
Papillary or Follicular

Patients <45 yr of Age			Patients >45 yr of Age		
Stage I	Any T	Any N	M0	T1	N0	M0
Stage II	Any T	Any N	M1	T2	N0	M0
Stage III				T3, T4	N0	M0
Stage IV				Any T	Any N	M1

Adapted from American Joint Committee on Cancer Manual for the Staging of Cancer. Philadelphia, JB Lippincott, 1988.

Diagnosis

Despite extensive experience with thyroid neoplasms, diagnostic recommendations continue to evolve.[43] In a patient presenting with a thyroid nodule, history and physical examination are important, because a history of radiation exposure to the head and neck or a family history of thyroid cancer should increase the clinician's suspicion of thyroid cancer. In younger patients, a solitary nodule is more likely to be cancerous. The solitary nodule is more likely to be malignant than a multinodular goiter, and a history of recent painless growth is suggestive of cancer. Malignant nodules tend to be harder, and fixation to underlying structure is suggestive not only of cancer but also of a poorer prognosis. The presence of enlarged cervical nodes also increases the likelihood that a thyroid nodule is malignant. Table 74-4 categorizes the risk factors for a variety of clinical characteristics of thyroid nodules. Patients with nodules demonstrating high-risk characteristics should be referred for surgical resection.

Laboratory Tests

Except for measurement of calcitonin in the diagnosis of medullary carcinoma, assessment of plasma levels of thyroid hormones has limited value in the diagnosis of thyroid cancer. Serum thyroglobulin (Tg) levels can be elevated in patients with cancer, but this test is not specific, and similar increases are seen in benign thyroid disorders. However, serum thyroglobulin is an important test in the follow-up of patients who have undergone thyroid resection for differentiated thyroid cancer. A level greater than 10 ng/mL is a reliable indicator of locally recurrent or metastatic disease[44] and could predict the need for ablative doses of ^{131}I; undetectable values (<0.5 ng/mL) especially after TSH stimulation greatly reduce the need for further imaging studies to detect presumptive metastases.[45]

In patients who are hyperthyroid with a nodule, scanning with ^{123}I is advised; hyperfunctional or "hot" nodules are rarely malignant.[46] The exception to this dogma is a functioning nodule in a child. This nodule has

a higher risk of being a cancer.[47] In contrast, patients with Graves' disease can have a nonfunctioning nodule, which can be malignant and should be investigated by fine needle aspiration.[48] In euthyroid patients, fine needle aspiration is the best first test.[49] Although "hot" nodules are rarely malignant, approximately 10% to 20% of "cold" nodules are malignant. Thyroid radionuclide imaging therefore has limited efficacy in reliably distinguishing between benign and malignant abnormalities. Differentiated thyroid cancers will trap iodine but are less efficient at concentrating iodine than the normal thyroid gland. Therefore, iodine uptake in a thyroid cancer can be typically demonstrated only after all normal thyroid tissue has been ablated and TSH level is allowed to rise. There can be biochemical, quantitative, and intracellular positional alterations in the sodium iodide symporter (NIS) in thyroid cancer cells.[50]

Ultrasonography may be useful in distinguishing among cysts, cystic tumors, and solid tumors.[49] Small cysts are unlikely to be cancerous, but all cysts should be aspirated and the aspirate examined cytologically. Aspiration of a benign cyst will often suffice both for diagnosis and for therapy, whereas fluid tends to reaccumulate in a cystic cancer. Because a malignant tumor of the thyroid may present as a solid, cystic, or mixed lesion, ultrasonography alone is not diagnostic.[51]

Needle biopsy, particularly fine needle aspiration, is the diagnostic procedure of choice for thyroid nodules in

TABLE 74-4

Risk Factors for Malignancy in Nodular Thyroid

FACTOR	LOW RISK ⟶ HIGH RISK				
	1	2	3	4	5
Age					
Elderly				•	
Child				•	
Sex					
Male				•	
Female		•			
Low-dose radiation in childhood					•
Family history		•			
Cystic mass	•				
Solid mass				•	
Multiple masses		•			
Solitary mass			•		
Growing mass			•		
Stable mass		•			
Hot scan	•				
Cold scan			•		
Warm scan		•			
Fine needle aspiration (−)		•			
Fine needle aspiration (+)				•	
Associated cervical adenopathy				•	
Complete resolution to thyroid suppression	•				
Partial resolution to thyroid suppression			•		
No response to suppression				•	

Modified from Sessions RB, Diehl WL: Thyroid cancer and related nodularity. In Myers E, Suen J (eds): Cancer of the Head and Neck, 2nd ed. New York, Churchill Livingstone, 1981, p 766.

euthyroid patients.[49] When the result of biopsy is clearly positive or clearly negative, the decision regarding surgery, or no surgery, can be made confidently.[52-54] However, a negative fine needle biopsy or cutting needle biopsy does not ensure that a thyroid mass is not malignant (false negative rate, 1% to 5%), and clinical concern and careful follow-up will dictate the decision to proceed to resection. High-resolution ultrasound to accurately perform fine needle aspiration is being utilized on a routine basis. The common indications for ultrasound-guided fine needle aspiration are for biopsy of nonpalpable or difficult to palpate nodules, for previously failed fine needle aspiration, and for nodules incidentally identified during neck imaging for other reasons. Ultrasound-guided fine needle aspiration has been shown to result in improved cancer diagnosis on significantly smaller nodules compared to fine needle aspiration performed by palpation.[55]

Treatment

Treatment of thyroid cancer includes surgery, ^{131}I radiation, and suppression with thyroid hormone.[56,57] Rarely, external-beam therapy has also been employed.

Surgery of the Thyroid

Debate continues concerning the optimal surgical treatment of well-differentiated thyroid carcinoma. Preoperatively, the surgeon often does not know definitively whether a thyroid nodule is cancer and must make a decision concerning the extent of operation based upon clinical judgment. Young patients with small, well-encapsulated tumors that appear benign on frozen section, with a normal contralateral lobe, can be treated with lobectomy. A history of neck irradiation, the presence of contralateral disease, and cytologic or histologic findings suggestive of malignancy influences the decision to perform a total or near-total thyroidectomy. In addition, the location of the parathyroid glands and recurrent nerve can influence the extent of lobectomy on the contralateral lobe. When a diagnosis of thyroid carcinoma is clear, a total or near-total thyroidectomy is preferred.[58-60] The rationale for this decision is based on several facts related to the biology of thyroid carcinoma. First, thyroid cancer can often be multicentric, and resection of the contralateral lobe often identifies malignancy. Second, a total thyroidectomy can be performed safely with low morbidity rate. Patients with thyroid carcinoma will be treated with thyroid replacement postoperatively, regardless of whether an adequate, normal-functioning thyroid is left intact. Resection of the entire gland facilitates both the use of radioiodine postoperatively and the use of thyroglobulin levels as a tumor marker. Because papillary cancer often metastasizes to regional lymph nodes, a midneck dissection on the ipsilateral side is performed at resection. Follicular cancer rarely demonstrates lymph node metastases, and a midneck dissection is not justified on a routine basis during thyroidectomy. Modified neck dissection is advocated only in instances of obvious nodal metastases involving the lateral cervical nodes.

Debate continues as to whether recurrence and fatality are influenced by the extent of surgery.[61,62] A study by Nguyen and associates[63] showed that for low-risk patients total thyroidectomy gave identical results as lobectomy. Shaha and associates[64] reported 1038 patients with thyroid carcinoma, 465 of which were in the low-risk group. Mean follow-up period was for 20 years. Their study did demonstrate significant improvement in local recurrence comparing lobectomy with lesser operations. However, results for lobectomy compared to total thyroidectomy failed to achieve significance, with local recurrence of 4% versus 1% ($P = 0.1$) and overall failure of 13% versus 8% ($P = 0.06$). However, these studies did demonstrate a trend for total thyroidectomy giving superior results when compared to lobectomy. The work by Sanders and Cady[25] did not demonstrate a difference in survival comparing total thyroidectomy and lobectomy in low-risk patients. Of particular interest is the study by Wanebo and associates,[65] who examined extent of operation for low-risk, intermediate-risk, and high-risk groups. Their work failed to demonstrate any difference in survival with extent of operation in all risk groups.

Other studies have demonstrated improved outcome with total thyroidectomy. The study by Samaan and associates[66] examined 1599 patients with well-differentiated thyroid carcinoma and reported improvement in recurrence for total thyroidectomy compared to lesser operations. The study by DeGroot and associates[24] demonstrated a decreased recurrence rate for total thyroidectomy compared to lobectomy and a significant improvement in mortality rate. Mazzaferri and Jhiang[23] reported their study of 1355 patients with a mean follow-up of 15.7 years. They reported significant improvements in recurrence rate (26% vs. 40%; $P < 0.002$) and mortality rate (6% vs. 9%; $P = 0.02$) comparing total thyroidectomy with lesser procedures. Loh and associates[67] reported 700 patients with mean follow-up period of 11.3 years. They report significant improvement in recurrence and mortality rates with total thyroidectomy or near-total thyroidectomy compared to lesser operations, particularly for advanced tumors.

A thyroidectomy begins with the patient anesthetized in the supine position with the neck in extension (Fig. 74-2). A Kocher collar incision is made and dissection is carried out through the platysma. Superior and inferior flaps are raised by dissection in the avascular plane deep to the platysma muscle. Strap muscles can be divided in the midline. It is rarely necessary to transect either the strap muscles or the sternocleidomastoid muscle. The thyroid lobe is exposed using blunt dissection. Occasionally, it is necessary to resect en bloc regions of muscle invaded by tumor. The recurrent nerve is identified by careful dissection in the region of the inferior thyroid artery. Once the nerve is identified, branches of the superior pole vessels are ligated as they enter the gland. Similarly, inferior pole vessels are individually ligated and the thyroid is dissected off the trachea, being careful not to injure the recurrent nerve. The parathyroid glands should be sought and left with their blood supply intact. Occasionally, a parathyroid gland is devascularized; after confirmation of identity by frozen section, this gland can be reimplanted into the sternocleidomastoid muscle. The contralateral lobe should always be exposed to

Figure 74-2. Thyroidectomy. **A,** The patient is placed with the neck in extention. The thyroid is approached through a Kocher collar incision, which is commonly made approximately 2.0 cm superior to the sternal notch. **B,** The strap muscles are divided in the midline to expose the thyroid gland. **C,** The strap muscles are retracted laterally and the thyroid is retracted medially, exposing the structures of the midneck. The recurrent laryngeal nerve can be seen lying within the tracheosophageal groove. **D,** The superior pole vessels are individually clamped and ligated as they enter the thyroid gland. Inferior thyroid vessels, as well as the thyroid (IMA) vessels, are individually suture ligated. **E,** The dissection is completed by dissection of the thyroid gland off the trachea. The isthmus is then transected and can be oversewn with a suture for hemostatis.

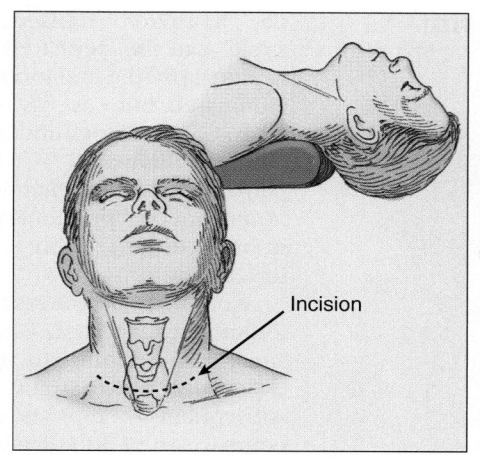

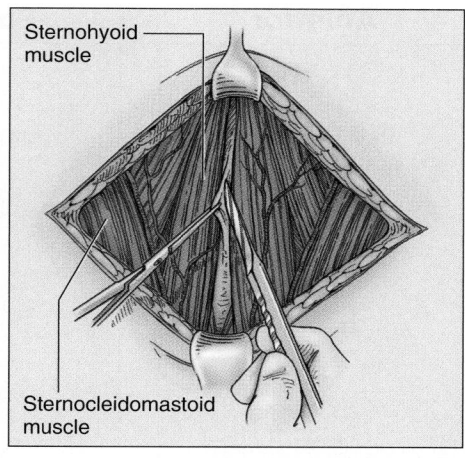

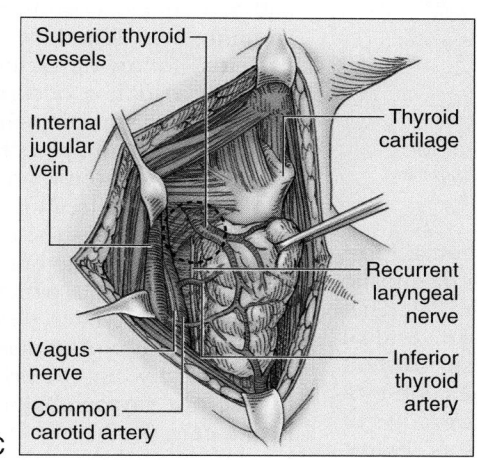

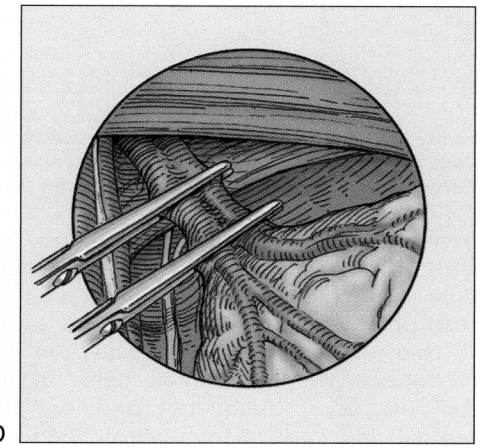

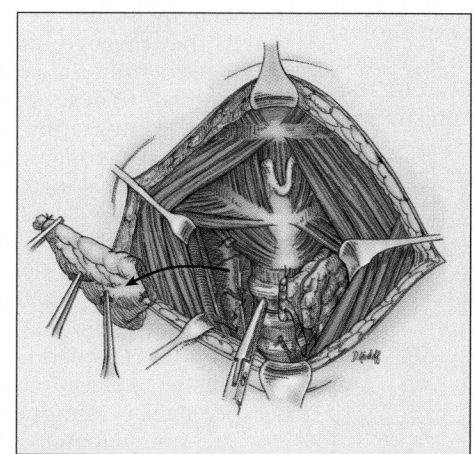

examine for gross pathologic processes. A total thyroidectomy is completed by performing the contralateral lobectomy in a fashion identical to the ipsilateral lobe. Occasionally, to preserve the blood supply to the parathyroid glands, it is reasonable to perform a subcapsular dissection of the contralateral lobe, leaving a small area of thyroid in the region of the parathyroid gland. This procedure is referred to as a near-total thyroidectomy.

Radiation Therapy

Metastatic tumors shown to accumulate ^{131}I warrant treatment with 100 to 200 mCi of ^{131}I. Radioiodine treatment is accomplished by discontinuing thyroid hormone replacement and allowing the patient to become hypothyroid, with resultant TSH stimulation of metastases to achieve increased uptake of ^{131}I. Figure 74-3 shows an example of a radionuclide scan in a patient with pulmo-

Anterior   ## Posterior

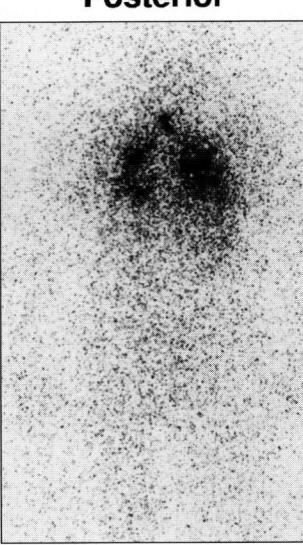

Figure 74-3. [131]I scan in patient with metastatic papillary thyroid cancer demonstrating diffuse pulmonary metastases from papillary thyroid carcinoma. Anterior and posterior views are shown.

nary metastases from papillary thyroid carcinoma. Most authorities obtain a whole-body scan with a diagnostic dose of ^{131}I, or ^{123}I before treatment with [131]I. That scan provides information about the quantity of residual thyroid tissue and the presence of local or distant metastases. The information helps in the selection of the appropriate therapeutic dose of [131]I. Knowledge of normal and variants of normal distributions of iodine help ensure that interpretation of the scan is not a "false" positive.[57] In Figure 74-4 a whole-body scan shows metastases in cervical lymph nodes. In contrast, Figure 74-5 shows uptake in the mediastinum indicating the thymus, not nodal metastasis. Following administration

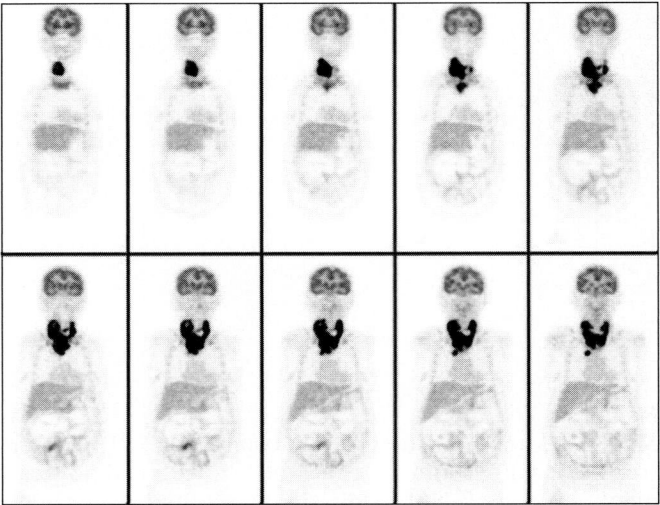

Figure 74-4. PET scan of a 75-year-old woman with anaplastic cancer of the thyroid. Images were acquired 1 hour after intravenous injection of ^{18}F-fluorodeoxyglucose (15 mCi). There is intense uptake of FDG in the undifferentiated cancer.

of ^{131}I, thyroid replacement therapy is restarted. This cycle can be repeated at 6- to 12-month intervals. Residual thyroid and locally invasive thyroid cancer can be eliminated, but success is related to extent of thyroidectomy.[68-70] Similarly, functioning metastases in lymph nodes can be eliminated[71-73]; however, when the nodes are palpable it is recommended that they be removed.[74] Small homogeneous pulmonary metastases can be cured, but in bulky distant lesions, especially in the skeleton, cure is infrequent.[43,75]

A number of controversial topics are related to radioiodine therapy. First, Park and associates[76] showed in a small number of patients that large diagnostic doses, especially 5 to 10 mCi, can "stun" the thyroid, and subsequent therapy is not trapped as expected. In a comparison of 300 diagnostic scans made with 2 mCi ^{131}I and subsequent post-therapy whole-body scans, possible stunning was found in only 2%.[77] In two of the four patients follow-up scan was negative, so stunning probably had not occurred. Second, is it necessary to conduct a diagnostic whole-body scan? Because of the report of Park and associates, some physicians prescribe ^{131}I therapy without a prior diagnostic scan. This practice could result in treating patients who do not require therapy, and it begs the question of what dose should be prescribed, and whether it is the same for all patients. Third, how should patients who have a negative diagnostic scan but have elevated thyroglobulin be treated? A small number of patients have been treated with large doses of ^{131}I when the prior diagnostic scan was negative, but serum thyroglobulin was elevated.[78] The rationale is that cells producing thyroglobulin can trap enough ^{131}I to expect a therapeutic effect. These patients are then followed by serum Tg measurement and are re-treated when the thyroglobulin remains high. The authors prefer to identify the source of Tg by alternative imaging procedures.[79] These procedures can include positron emission tomography (PET), sestamibi, tetrofosmin, ultrasound, and computed tomographic (CT) and magnetic resonance imaging (MRI) scans. Our preference is for PET scan.[80] Figure 74-6 is an example of a PET scan, which was performed to stage the extent of an anaplastic cancer and is presented to demonstrate the superb resolution. If the PET scan is positive, it is followed by either CT or MRI scan for additional anatomic information. The lesion can then be removed or treated by a defined amount of external-beam radiation depending on its site. Ultrasound has been used intraoperatively to identify small lesions that are not palpable at operation.[81] Adverse effects of radiation are minimal. Some patients develop swelling of the salivary glands, which can be reduced or prevented by having them suck lemon candy. Leukemia has been reported to occur following repeated doses of ^{131}I and at shorter intervals than is currently advised.[82] Although there are reports of pulmonary fibrosis developing when uptake in pulmonary metastases was extensive, the risk of dying from pulmonary metastases is significantly greater. Radiation safety precautions are necessary. The patient should be kept isolated until the body load of ^{131}I is reduced. This approach requires consultation among the patient, the family, and a nuclear medicine physician.

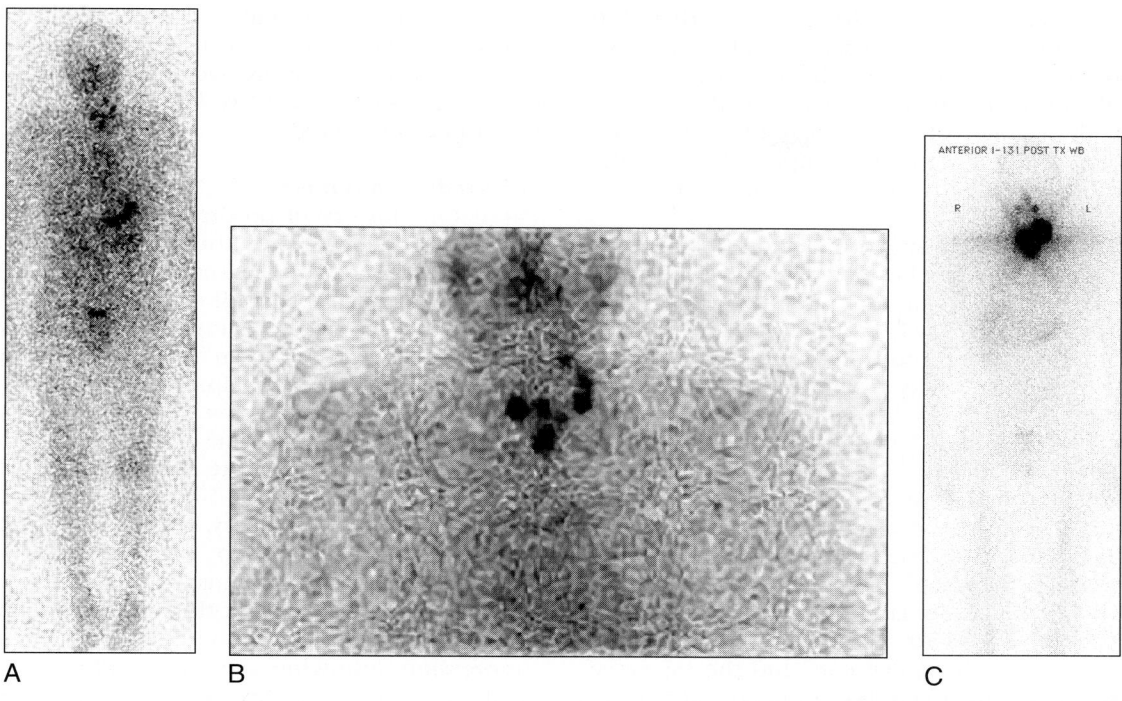

Figure 74-5. Left panel shows whole-body scan acquired 24 hours after 2 mCi ^{123}I. The middle panel is a spot view of the neck and chest. There are several areas of uptake indicative of residual thyroid and functioning metastases in cervical lymph nodes. The right panel is a posttherapy scan made 7 days after 150 mCi ^{131}I. There is intense uptake in the region, but the resolution is not as good as with ^{123}I. There is faint uptake in the liver on the posttreatment scan due to metabolism of radioiodinated thyroid hormones at that site.

The authors prefer this treatment to be conducted early in the management so that the timing of discontinuation of thyroid hormone, low-iodine diet, scan, and therapy can be coordinated.

Some studies have examined the use of recombinant human TSH (rhTSH) as an alternative protocol in preparation for ^{131}I treatment. Treatment with rhTSH has been shown to induce increased Tg and improved uptake of iodine in a manner similar to induction of hypothyroidism.[83] However, in a recent study of 127 patients in which rhTSH and thyroid hormone withdrawal were compared, induction of hypothyroidism was found to be superior to rhTSH.[84] Patients treated under rhTSH protocol do avoid the symptoms associated with hypo-

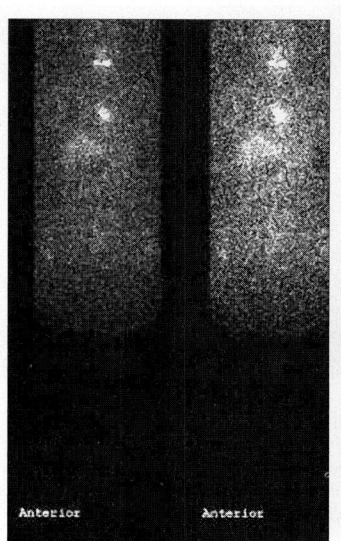
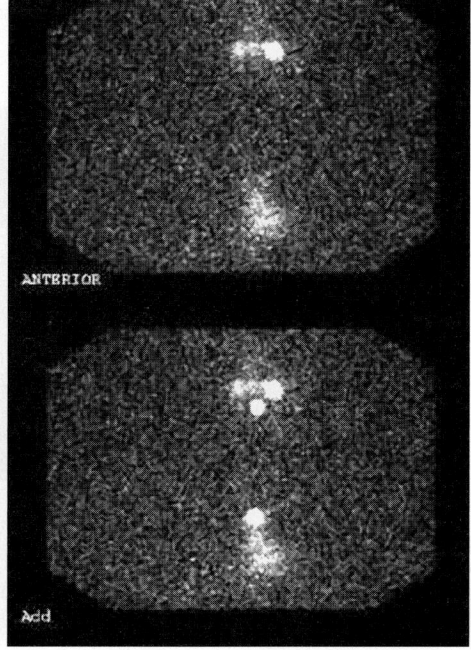

Figure 74-6. Left panel shows whole-body scans of a patient who had total thyroidectomy and ^{131}I for thyroid cancer. The right panels are spot views of the neck and chest. The lower panel has markers at the chin and mid sternum to help anatomical interpretation. She was treated with a second dose of ^{131}I because of an elevated Tg level. The posttreatment scan shows no uptake of ^{131}I in the neck, but there is physiologic uptake in the salivary glands and uptake in the mediastinum. The mediastinal uptake is characteristic of the thymus and is a potential false positive finding.

thyroidism. We have used rhTSH in more that 160 patients and found it can replace withdrawal scans provided both the scan and Tg are obtained. The average TSH is well above 100 IU/mL. RhTSH treatment was preferred in all but one patient compared to withdrawal of thyroid hormone.[85] In addition, improvement in the treatment protocol with rhTSH may result in improved efficacy.[86]

Although ^{131}I is the mainstay of radiation treatment of thyroid carcinoma, external-beam radiation also plays a role in the treatment of this disease.[87,88] Persistent or recurrent thyroid cancer may fail to take up ^{131}I, especially tumors that recur after multiple radioactive iodine treatments. Extremely bulky tumors may fail to be completely controlled with ^{131}I, and the treatment of anaplastic thyroid cancer[89] almost always includes external-beam treatment.

The treatment of the thyroid tumor bed involves treating both sides of the neck and the upper mediastinum. Minimal residual disease (positive surgical margins or small gross residual in an ^{131}I-negative tumor) can be treated with 60 Gy, while larger amounts of disease will require doses of 65 to 70 Gy. Because the target volume wraps around the spinal cord and the tolerance of that structure is only 45 Gy, the dosimetry of thyroid bed irradiation is extraordinarily challenging. Figure 74-7 illustrates the type of complex radiation therapy performed for this disease.

Use of Thyroid Preparations for Suppression of TSH

Differentiated thyroid cancers respond to TSH by growing, producing, and secreting Tg and by trapping more iodine. Conversely, suppression of TSH can slow or reverse growth and lower Tg. Some reports suggest that thyroxine suppression of TSH decreases recurrence after thyroid resection for differentiated carcinomas.[90] When using the strategy of "TSH suppression," it is important to follow plasma TSH levels to ensure an adequate thyroxine dose. In patients who have been adequately treated by surgery or radioiodine and who have no clinical evidence of disease, a negative ^{131}I scan, and undetectable Tg, it is debatable whether suppressed TSH adds any benefit, and side effects such as anxiety, bone loss, and arrhythmias have to be considered.

Postirradiation Tumors

The natural history of postirradiation thyroid carcinoma has been reviewed by Roundebush and DeGroot.[91] Patients tend to be younger (mean age, 28 years) and have a higher incidence of multifocal tumors. This study and others[2] have led to the following treatment recommendations for persons known to have been exposed to ionizing radiation. When palpation of the neck is normal, the patient is followed by careful clinical examination at yearly intervals. The value of a thyroid scan has not been proved. When a discrete nodule is noted, fine needle aspiration is indicated, and if the result is suspicious, the patient is referred to surgery. In the case of small benign nodules clinical follow-up with or without thyroid hormone is appropriate. Shimaoka[92] noted that exogenous thyroid caused shrinkage of the nodules in about 50% of cases, and Schneider and associates[93] reported that thyroid suppression following partial resection reduced the incidence of recurrent disease.

Schneider and associates,[94] reporting on a large surgical experience with postirradiation thyroid carcinoma, found results similar to those noted for spontaneous thyroid cancers. Because many glands have multifocal disease, the surgeon usually cannot perform lobectomy for an apparent single nodule, and in general, when there is preoperative suspicion of thyroid cancer, total or near-total thyroidectomy is advised. In the study by Schneider and associates,[94] the likelihood of nodules developing in the remnant following subtotal thyroidectomy was 36%. The risks of total thyroidectomy (i.e., damage to the laryngeal nerve and hypoparathyroidism) must be balanced against the slow growth of papillary carcinoma and the potential for cure.[2]

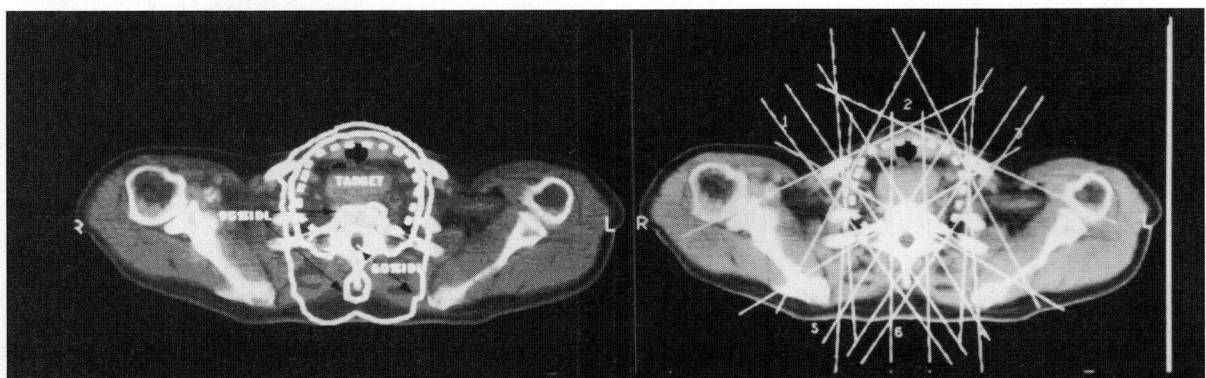

Figure 74-7. External beam radiation for thyroid carcinoma can be quite complex. On the left, the target for this bulky thyroid carcinoma is illustrated in the dashed line. The high-dose volume (95% dose line) encompasses this target while avoiding the spinal cord. The radiosensitive spinal cord is in the 60% isodose line, which permits delivery of doses up to 70 Gy with this plan. On the right is a superimposition of the six cross-firing fields that are used to create this dose distribution. The fields either avoid the spinal cord or include a lead block to shadow the spinal cord, protecting it from the high-dose radiation. The treatment planning and dosimetry of thyroid carcinoma treatment is one of the most complex challenges in radiation oncology.

Chemotherapy

Cytotoxic drug treatment for metastatic thyroid cancer has not been extensively evaluated. The largest experience is with anaplastic carcinomas, which have high growth rates and a very poor prognosis. Doxorubicin is the most active single agent in both medullary and nonmedullary carcinomas of the thyroid.[89,95] In a report from the Southwest Oncology Group, the combination of doxorubicin and cisplatin resulted in an objective response in 27% of 41 patients.[96] A similar trial reported by the Southeastern Cancer Study Group, however, failed to document this level of activity, with only 2 partial responses in 22.[97]

MEDULLARY CARCINOMA OF THE THYROID

Medullary thyroid carcinoma (MTC) arises from the parafollicular C cells,[59] which are part of the amine precursor uptake decarboxylation (APUD) system, rather than thyroid epithelial cells (see Fig. 74-1D). Medullary thyroid carcinoma accounts for 6% to 10% of all thyroid cancers. It can occur sporadically or in a familial form, either as part of multiple endocrine neoplasia type 2 (MEN-2) or as a familial MTC without MEN association. The gender distribution is approximately equal. The tumor is unilateral in most sporadic cases and bilateral and multifocal in familial cases.[98-100]

Diagnosis

Any thyroid nodule could be MTC; however, a family history of MTC, pheochromocytoma, hyperparathyroidism, or other manifestations of MEN-2 increases this likelihood. Plain film radiography of the neck may be useful. In the series reported by Keiser and associates,[101] tumor calcification was present in 35% of patients. Lymph nodes are frequently enlarged clinically and at surgery are pathologically involved in two thirds of patients.[102] Amyloid deposition between the spindle-shaped tumor cells is characteristic of MTC. The presence of calcitonin messenger RNA (mRNA) has been used to diagnose MTC when the histologic type is unclear.[103] The molecular diagnosis of MEN-2 is discussed later in this chapter.

The parafollicular C cells secrete calcitonin, a peptide hormone that inhibits bone resorption. Calcitonin secretion is stimulated by calcium infusion. In patients with MTC, the basal calcitonin level is elevated above normal[104] and can be further increased with infusion of calcium and pentagastrin. The few cases of MTC that exhibit normal basal plasma calcitonin levels demonstrate an exaggerated response to calcium and pentagastrin.[104,105]

The excessive calcitonin secretion does not appear to exert any metabolic effect. In the familial form, the associated parathyroid hyperplasia is an independent manifestation of the MEN syndrome inasmuch as it may precede MTC.[79] MTC tumors may also contain large quantities of histaminase[106] and dopa-decarboxylase,[107] neither of which produces any clinical syndrome. Serum histaminase is increased in many patients with metastatic disease, and its presence suggests metastases.[108] The diarrhea that occasionally accompanies the syndrome has been attributed in some studies to prostaglandin secretion,[109] but other investigators have not found this association.[104]

MTC is one cancer in which it is possible to recognize the precancerous state. In the familial form, C-cell hyperplasia occurs prior to the development of carcinoma.[110] It is thus incumbent on the physician to measure basal and stimulated calcitonin levels in all family members of an MTC patient. Stimulation tests performed with calcium or pentagastrin predicted MTC in 12 members of one family, 11 of whom had no clinical evidence of disease.[111,112] Similarly, Jones and Sisson[113] were able to identify eight children, whose disease was diagnosed by appropriate testing, who were members of a family with the MEN-2 syndrome. Because mutations in the *ret* proto-oncogene

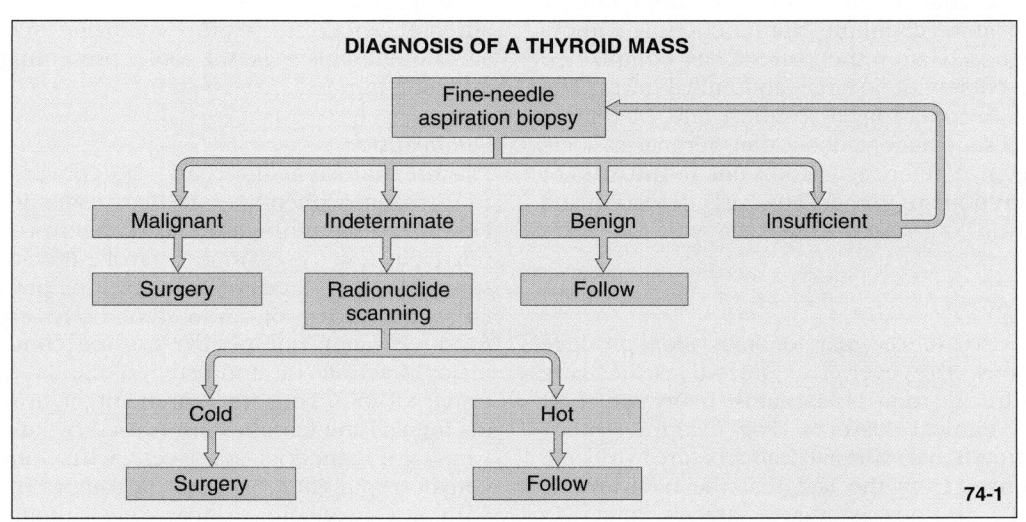

DIAGNOSIS OF A THYROID MASS

Fine-needle aspiration biopsy → Malignant → Surgery

Indeterminate → Radionuclide scanning → Cold → Surgery; Hot → Follow

Benign → Follow

Insufficient → (return to Fine-needle aspiration biopsy)

74-1

have now been established in MEN-2, family members can be screened at birth so that affected members can be offered early thyroidectomy.[114]

Treatment

Treatment of MTC is surgical excision. Since the cancer is often multifocal, surgery should include total thyroidectomy with complete resection of cervical and parasternal nodes.[115] Deftos and Stein[116] have reported that ^{131}I treatment is occasionally a useful adjunct to surgery when a calcitonin-secreting remnant is identified following total thyroidectomy; however, subsequent studies have failed to show any benefit from [131]I.[100] The cancer per se does not trap iodine. Because pheochromocytomas occur in the MEN-2 syndrome, it is necessary to exclude their presence in MTC patients, as thyroid surgery in a case with an undetected pheochromocytoma could be disastrous. An identified pheochromocytoma should be removed first and the patient given time to recover before the MTC is excised. Others advocate adrenalectomy and thyroidectomy at the same operation.

The clinical course in cases with metastatic MTC is variable. Death due to lung, liver, or bone metastases may occur quite quickly. However, it is not uncommon for patients with MTC to be relatively asymptomatic, even with large tumor burden. Many patients may be debilitated by intractable diarrhea,[104,109] which correlates with plasma calcitonin levels of greater than 20 ng/mL and which may be palliated by cytoreductive surgery[117] or the somatostatin analog octreotide.[118]

ADRENOCORTICAL CANCER

Adrenocortical carcinoma is infrequent, representing less than 0.2% of all cancers,[119] and has an incidence of only 2 per 1 million population.[120] Adrenal cancer may develop at any age[119,121] but most frequently appears in middle age. Hormonally functional tumors are slightly more common in women, and nonfunctioning tumors are more frequent in men. Although both functioning and nonfunctioning adrenal tumors occur, steroid-producing tumors[119,121] are more common. Nonfunctioning tumors are usually diagnosed after the patient has complained of pain or presents with a large abdominal mass. The combination of retroperitoneal location and inefficient steroid biosynthesis makes it likely that adrenal cancers will attain a large size before symptoms due to the mass or to hormonal secretion are noted. Thus, early detection and cure are unlikely.[119,121]

Clinical Features

Adrenocortical carcinomas may or may not produce steroid hormones. However, the steroid-synthesizing potential of adrenal tumors explains many of their laboratory and clinical features. For example, many women with functional adrenal cancers are virilized. This finding derives from the fact that the biosynthetic pathway to C19 steroids is almost always intact in

TABLE 74-5

Clinical Syndromes Produced by Adrenocortical Cancer and Their Frequency	
SYNDROME	**FREQUENCY (%)**
Virilization and Cushing's syndrome	50
Virilization	25
Cushing's syndrome	20
Feminization	<5
Precocious puberty	<5
Hypokalemia alkalosis	<5
Hypoglycemia	<5

functioning adrenal cancers, resulting in high urinary 17-ketosteroid (17-KS) excretion. Because adult men cannot be "hypervirilized," excessive androgen synthesis will not be clinically apparent in them unless urinary 17-KS or plasma androgens are measured. However, women are easily virilized, and this detection bias may account to some extent for the apparent predominance of functional tumors in women. Table 74-5 lists the hormonal syndromes produced by adrenal cancer, with estimates of their frequency. Specific diagnostic features of these syndromes are described in the following paragraphs.

Cushing's Syndrome
The characteristic[121] endocrine abnormality of Cushing's syndrome is an increase of plasma 11-deoxycortisol and its urinary metabolite. Cushing's syndrome may be a paraneoplastic syndrome associated with ectopic adrenocorticotropic hormone (ACTH) production by solid tumors. However, in such cases, virilization is rare. Virilization in association with Cushing's syndrome almost always indicates adrenal cancer,[122] because urinary 17-KS secretion ranges from 100 to 1000 mg/day—considerably higher than that produced by ectopic ACTH.

Virilization
Virilization is caused by testosterone, which is synthesized peripherally from adrenal androstenedione and dihydroepiandrosterone. It is the excess urinary 17-KS resulting from metabolism of these steroids that helps distinguish adrenal cancer from other virilizing syndromes. Occasionally, hirsutism is the only presenting feature with virilizing tumors.

Feminization
Plasma androstenedione may be converted peripherally to estrogen, a phenomenon that results in gynecomastia. Feminization with adrenal cancer is unusual. The relatively few cases in the world literature have been summarized.[123] Rates of aromatization are low; therefore, large quantities of androstenedione are required to produce significant plasma estrone concentrations. The major fraction of androstenedione is metabolized to urinary 17-KS. Thus, measurement of urinary 17-KS will distinguish the feminization caused by adrenal carcinoma from the gynecomastia seen with human chorionic gonadotropin (hCG)-producing tumors of the testis and with hCG-producing cancer. One should also be aware

that prepubertal adrenal cancers have been reported to produce hCG in quantities large enough to cause a positive result in pregnancy testing.

Precocious Puberty

In children, precocious puberty or virilization may be an important and presenting clinical finding because androgens are the predominant products of adrenal cancer secretion. Isosexual precocious puberty in boys and virilization in girls are usual. A few cases of feminizing adrenal cancer causing isosexual precocious puberty have been reported in girls.[124]

Sodium Retention and Hypokalemic Alkalosis

Rarely patients with adrenal cancer will present with the picture of primary hyperaldosteronism. Most patients with Conn's syndrome have either idiopathic hyperaldosteronism (IHA) or an aldosterone-producing adenoma (APA). Carcinomas that secrete aldosterone are rare, although a syndrome of mineralocorticoid excess may be caused by secretion of deoxycorticosterone.[122,125,126] In this situation, urinary 17-KS is high, and the tumor is generally much larger than the APA.

Hypoglycemia

As with other large mesenchymal tumors in the abdomen, adrenal cancer may cause hypoglycemia. Measurement of plasma insulin levels will rule out insulin-secreting tumors as a cause of hypoglycemia.

Diagnosis

The diagnosis of adrenal cancer depends upon clinical suspicion, urinary and plasma biochemical tests, and diagnostic imaging studies. The most useful imaging tests are CT scan, ultrasonography, and MRI. The size of the adrenal mass is important because in masses larger than 6 cm, the incidence of cancer has been reported to be 35% to 98%.[127] The CT scan also defines local extent of cancer, thereby facilitating surgical planning. Evidence of calcification in an abdominal mass on CT scan or plain abdominal film suggests adrenal carcinoma. MRI scanning can define the presence or absence of regional extension and influence the decision in regard to resectability. The characteristics of the adrenal mass on T_2-weighted MRI scanning can be useful in distinguishing adenomas and pheochromocytoma from carcinomas or metastatic cancer to the adrenal gland.[128,129] Iodocholesterol imaging is not useful[130] because steroid synthesis rates are low.

Pathology

Adrenal cancers are frequently large and can weigh more than 100 g. They can be locally invasive into kidney, liver, and large blood vessels, with the inferior vena cava involved in many cases of right adrenal tumors. Grossly, the tumor is yellow to tan, with areas of necrosis and hemorrhage.

Cytologically, it may be difficult to distinguish carcinoma from adenoma.[131,132] The tumor cells vary in configuration from spindle-shaped in less differentiated cancers to large polyhedral cells with abundant eosinophilic cytoplasm. Mitoses can be rare; some variation in nuclear morphology may be evident in both adenomas and carcinomas. Capsular invasion or blood vessel invasion is the most reliable sign of cancer. The diagnosis of malignancy of a completely resected adrenal tumor, however, may be made only in retrospect by the finding of metastatic disease many years later. Patterns of steroid secretion cannot be predicted by histologic or histochemical characteristics of adrenal neoplasms.

Primary Treatment and Prognosis

The only curative therapy for adrenal cancer is aggressive en bloc resection of the primary tumor including the ipsilateral kidney.[133] This approach is attempted only in patients who have relatively limited cancers deemed to be potentially resectable.[134] Even with this approach, adrenocortical cancer is[100] highly lethal, with a 5-year survival rate of 20% to 30%.[135] Fifty percent of patients have metastatic disease at diagnosis. In patients with incurable adrenal carcinoma, suffering from symptoms secondary to tumor bulk or hormone excess, partial resection of tumor may offer significant palliation. In a minority of cases, the course may be indolent, with metastases developing over a period of 5 to 10 years. Metastases occur in lung, liver, and peritoneum, but uncommonly involve brain or bone.

Therapy for Metastatic Disease

Antihormonal Therapy

Some patients suffer more symptoms of hormonal excess than from tumor bulk. In them, antihormonal therapy can be useful. Metyrapone, an inhibitor of the 11β-hydroxylation step in cortisol biosynthesis, has been reported to be useful in the management of individual cases of Cushing's syndrome of adrenal carcinoma. However, it has proved largely ineffective in patients with metastatic disease.[136] Chemical confirmation of its effectiveness requires direct measurement of plasma cortisol. Urinary concentration of 17-OH steroids cannot be used to assess the efficacy of metyrapone, because the drug produces elevation in urinary 11-deoxycortisol, and therefore elevation in 17-hydroxycorticosteroids (17-OHCS), even though it decreases plasma cortisol.

Aminoglutethimide, an anticonvulsant that causes adrenal insufficiency, has been used in the treatment of adrenal carcinoma.[137] It is an effective palliative treatment in Cushing's syndrome secondary to adrenocortical carcinoma, adenoma, and ectopic ACTH production by extra-adrenal carcinoma, with the potential for rapid and sustained suppression of corticosteroid synthesis.[138,139] Because the drug may alter extra-adrenal metabolism of cortisol, measurement of urinary 17-OHCS excretion alone may overestimate the effectiveness of therapy; plasma cortisol concentration is a more reliable index of drug efficacy.[140] The usual clinical dose is within the range of 1 to 2 g/day. Significant adverse effects include anorexia, dermatitis, somnolence, ataxia, and decreased thyroid function.

Antineoplastic Therapy

In animals, the drug *o,p′*-DDD (mitotane) induced adrenocortical necrosis. Studies also demonstrated that mitotane was capable of inhibiting steroidogenesis.[141-143] Mitotane was initially evaluated in the 1960s.[144] In 138 cases of adrenal cancer evaluated, 17-KS and 17-hydroxycorticosteroid excretion was decreased by 50% in 70% of cases. A minimum of 4 weeks of therapy was required to ensure an adequate trial of therapy. Although steroid secretion was frequently improved with mitotane, tumor regression was uncommon, occurring in only 34% of cases with measurable disease. The mean duration of antitumor response was 10 months. Although objective response correlated with increased survival, hormonal response did not. The prognosis in women was better than in men; 52% of women and 38% of men survived for 4 years following diagnosis, with median survival times of 56 and 19 months, respectively.[144] Complete regression of tumors was not achieved.

Other investigators have also reported experience with mitotane. Libitz and associates[145] reported 115 patients with adrenal carcinoma treated with mitotane between 1965 and 1969. The measurable disease response in this series was 61%, with a steroid excretion response of 89%. The improved response rate in this series is attributed to a shorter median time between diagnosis and treatment with mitotane. Nader and associates[146] reported only a 19% remission rate in 77 patients. These results are likely secondary to differences in patient selection.

Most patients treated with mitotane have experienced some degree of toxicity when the dosage was increased to the therapeutic range of 8 to 10 g/day. In general, the toxic reactions are mild, consisting of anorexia, nausea, vomiting, or diarrhea. Neuromuscular toxicity develops in 40% to 60% of patients, usually in the form of lethargy and somnolence. Vertigo and dermatologic toxicity are observed in 15%. Leukopenia and liver function abnormalities are rare.[144,145] Plasma mitotane levels may be useful in preventing toxicity.[147] With successful treatment of a functioning tumor, a substantial number of patients will develop signs of adrenal insufficiency.

In summary, it is reasonable to expect objective rates of tumor regression following mitotane therapy in approximately 25% of cases.[121,144] The median duration of remission is 1 year, although some remissions have lasted longer than 3 years. Dosage regimens vary. Most clinicians initially administer 10 g/day, reducing the dose gradually to 1 to 2 g/day as regression is obtained. Diminution in size of metastases is rarely apparent before 6 weeks, although laboratory evidence of decreased steroid production may be noted earlier. Prolonged regression has been reported,[110] and an apparent cure was seen with combined use of mitotane and 5-fluorouracil (5-FU).[148]

Very few chemotherapeutic agents other than mitotane have been evaluated in adrenocortical carcinoma in other than anecdotal experiences. Partial responses have been reported with doxorubicin.[149,150] Cisplatin has caused tumor regression in four patients, three of whom had previously received mitotane adjuvant therapy.[151] In two reports of only six patients, the combination of etoposide and cisplatin was reported to produce a

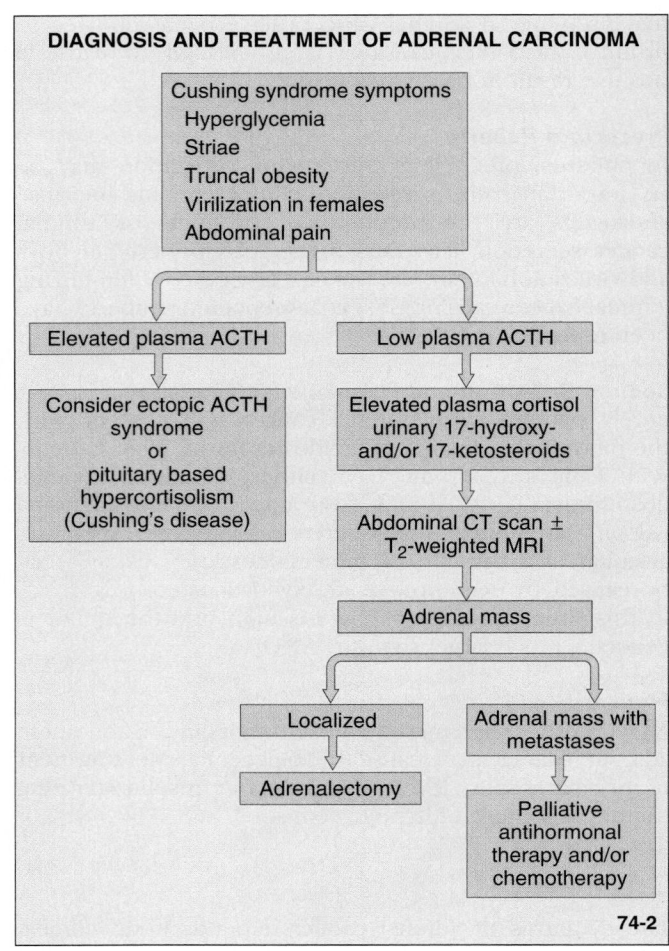

DIAGNOSIS AND TREATMENT OF ADRENAL CARCINOMA

Cushing syndrome symptoms
Hyperglycemia
Striae
Truncal obesity
Virilization in females
Abdominal pain

→ Elevated plasma ACTH → Consider ectopic ACTH syndrome or pituitary based hypercortisolism (Cushing's disease)

→ Low plasma ACTH → Elevated plasma cortisol urinary 17-hydroxy- and/or 17-ketosteroids → Abdominal CT scan ± T₂-weighted MRI → Adrenal mass

Adrenal mass → Localized → Adrenalectomy

Adrenal mass → Adrenal mass with metastases → Palliative antihormonal therapy and/or chemotherapy

74-2

response in five or six cases.[152,153] One patient had a complete response lasting 1 year. There has been recent interest in the use of suramin, a growth factor inhibitor, as therapy for adrenocortical carcinoma. In a Phase I study in 21 heavily pretreated patients, three cases developed partial response to suramin.[154-156] The role of suramin requires further definition, particularly because this drug may be associated with significant neurotoxicity. Owing to the rarity of adrenocortical carcinoma, all patients with this disease should be considered candidates for clinical trials. New classes of drugs—taxanes, campto-thecins, for example—have not been tested in adrenal carcinomas.

Surgical Approach to the Adrenal Gland

The surgical approach to the adrenal gland is influenced by the type of adrenal tumor. The two main approaches are posterior through the bed of the 12th rib, and a transabdominal approach. The posterior approach is usually indicated for small cortical adenomas, whereas an abdominal incision is employed for malignant adrenal tumors or pheochromocytomas. Recently, several series have been described in which adrenal tumors have been resected using laparoscopy.[157-158] Laparoscopic adrenalectomy has been reported by a number of institutions with excellent results. Although the laparoscopic approach to adrenalectomy has gained acceptance at a number of institutions, it is a more expensive technique and the advantage compared to a posterior approach has yet to be demonstrated.[159]

Adrenocortical Adenomas

Current techniques of adenoma localization permit a unilateral posterior approach to adrenocortical adenomas. This approach has several advantages over an abdominal approach, including a lower complication rate, avoidance of postoperative ileus, and shorter hospital stay. The adrenal gland is approached through a posterior incision, as shown in Figure 74-8. The gland is approached through the bed of the 12th rib, and the kidney is retracted inferiorly to expose the adrenal gland. These incisions are well tolerated, and much of the postoperative care is dictated by the metabolic consequences of removing the hormonally active adenoma.

Pheochromocytoma

Surgical treatment of resectable pheochromocytoma requires careful preoperative preparation. α-Adrenergic blocking agents are administered to inhibit the effects of excess norepinephrine secretion. Phenoxybenzamine is a selective α-adrenergic blocking agent, administered in an oral dose of 20 to 40 mg two to four times daily. Titration of the dose is performed by following physiologic parameters. Prazosin has also been successfully employed in the preoperative setting. β-Adrenergic blockers (e.g., propranolol) are added to control tachycardia as a sequela of excess epinephrine secretion. After adequate pharmacologic control and correction of fluid and electrolyte imbalance have been achieved, surgical resection is performed.

Intraoperative control of blood pressure can be maintained using short-acting intravenous medications such as nitroprusside. Careful physiologic monitoring during the operation is mandatory. The surgical approach is through the abdomen, and a chevron incision is often used, as

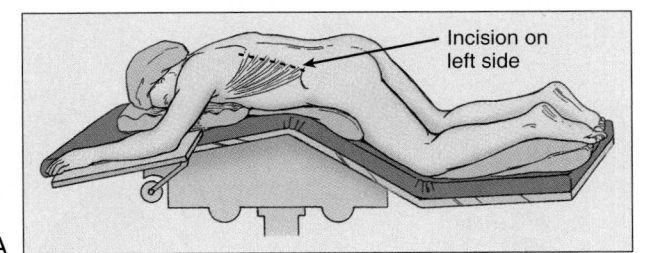

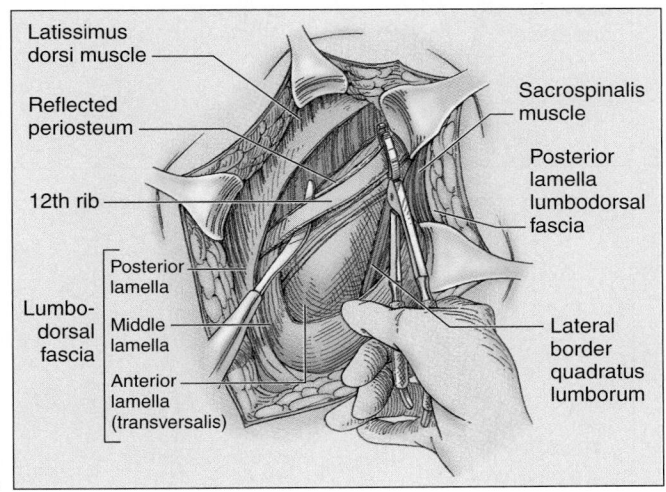

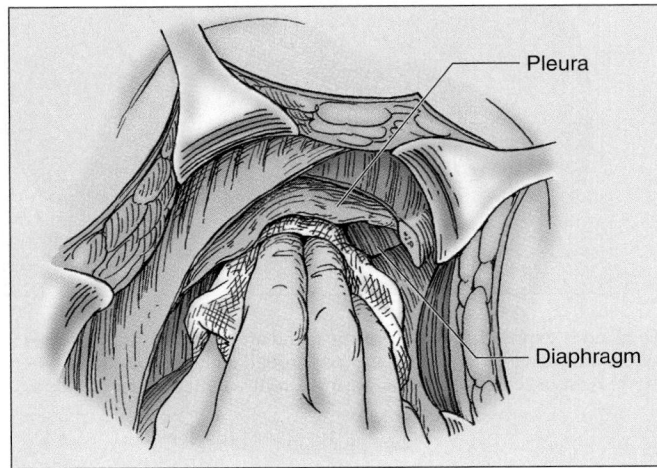

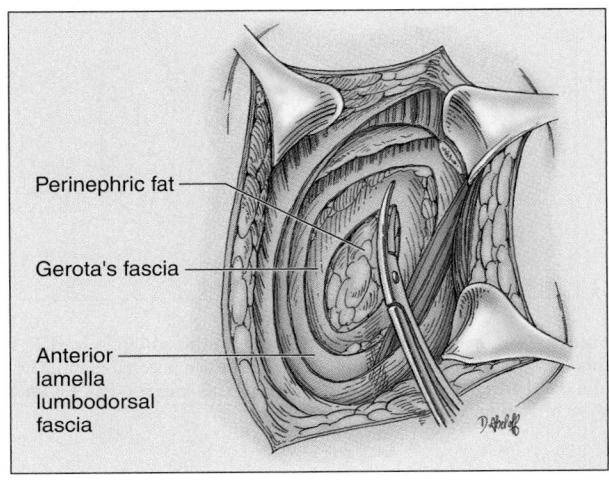

Figure 74-8. Posterior approach to the adrenal gland. **A,** The patient is placed in a jack-knife prone position and a curvilinear incision is made in the flank. **B,** The 12th rib is removed subperiosteally, exposing the lumbodorsal fascia. **C,** The pleura is swept superiorly using a gauze-covered finger. **D,** The diaphragm is transected, exposing Gerota's fascia, which is then opened. *Continued*

Specific Malignancies

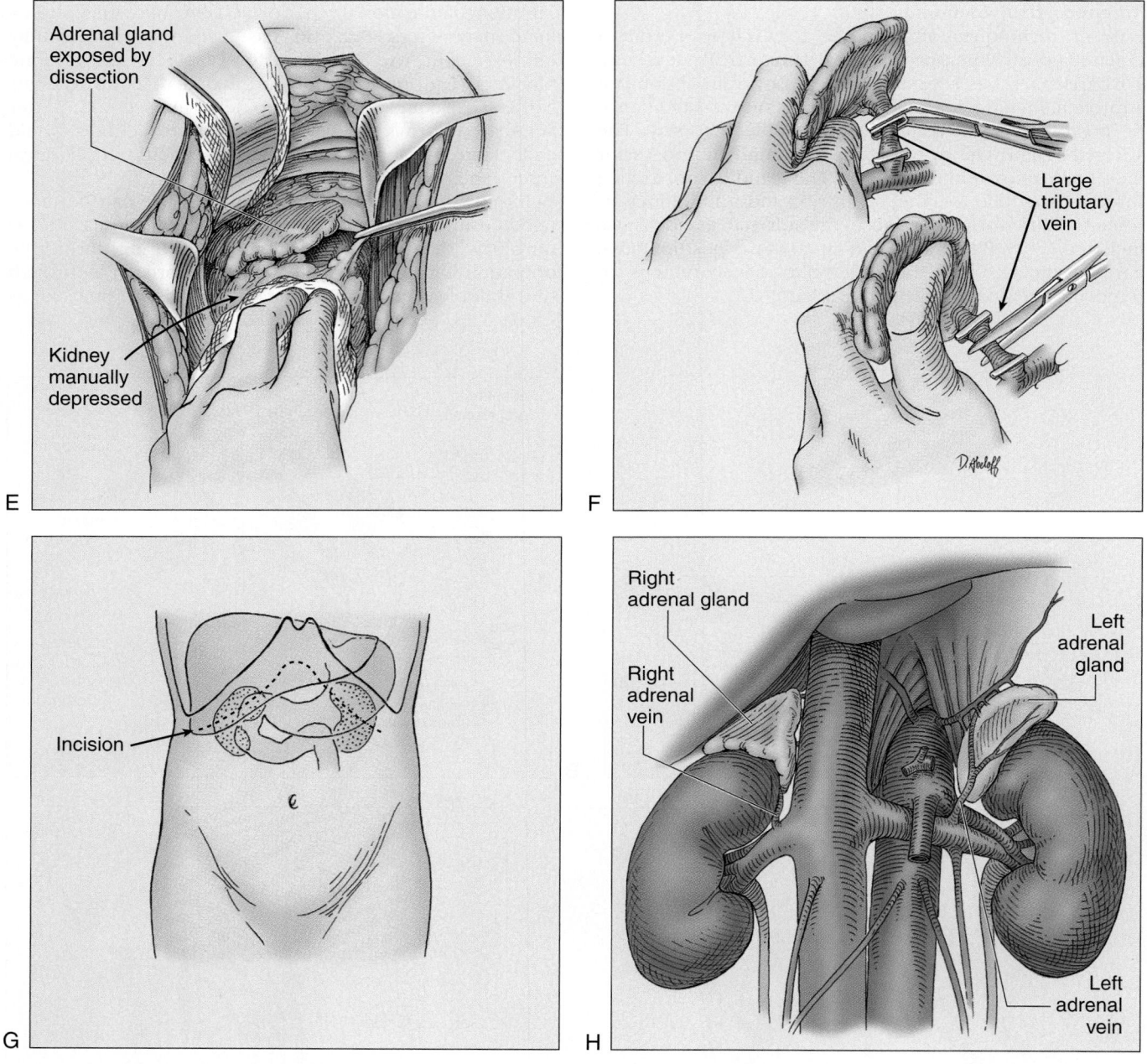

Figure 74-8, *cont'd.* Posterior approach to the adrenal gland. **E,** The adrenal gland is exposed. **F,** Vessels of the gland are ligated with hemoclips and then transected. **G,** Abdominal approach to the adrenal gland: The adrenal glands can be commonly approached through a chevron incision. When unilateral adrenal exploration is required, this incision can be limited to either a right or left subcostal. **H,** Basic anatomy of the adrenal glands as shown from an anterior approach.

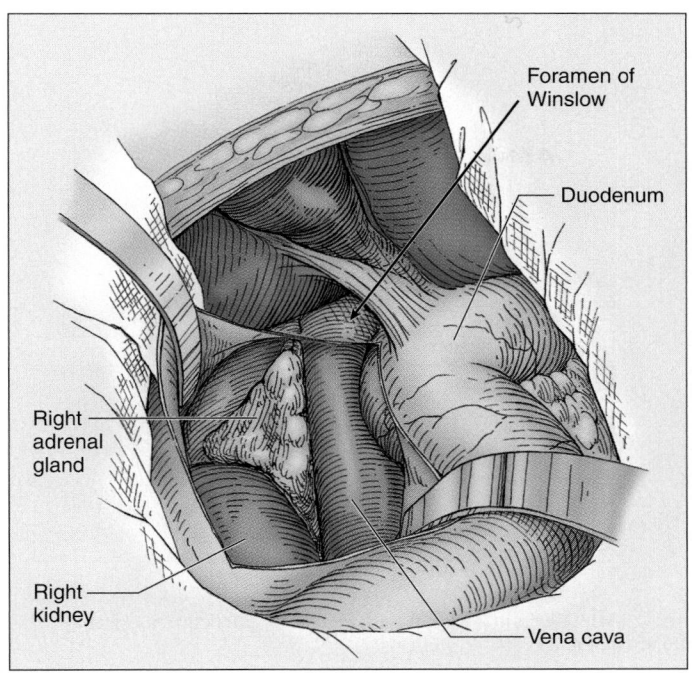
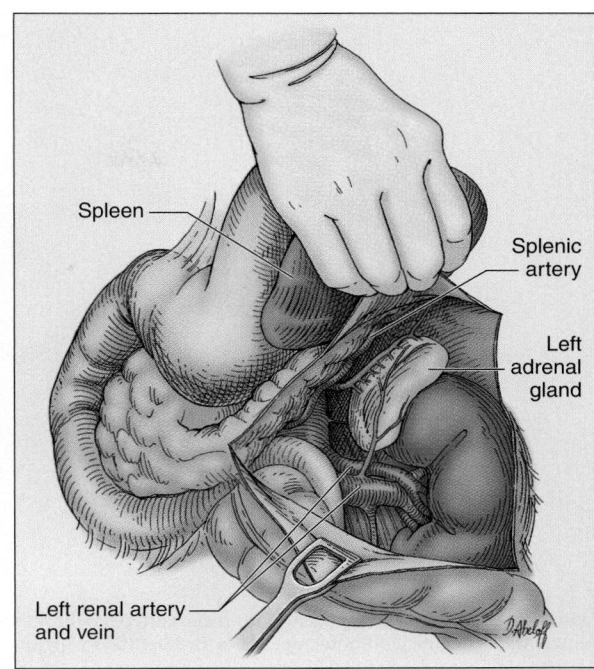

Figure 74-8, *cont'd.* Abdominal approach to the adrenal gland. **I,** The right adrenal gland can be exposed by performing a Kocher maneuver and retracting the duodenum to the left. This allows good exposure of the right adrenal gland. **J,** Exposure of the left adrenal gland in the retroperitoneum is accomplished by mobilizing the spleen and retracting the spleen and stomach medially.

shown in Figure 74-8G–J. On the right, a Kocher maneuver mobilizes the duodenum and exposes the adrenal gland. On the left, the spleen is mobilized; Gerota's fascia is then opened to expose the left adrenal gland.

MALIGNANT PHEOCHROMOCYTOMA

Ten percent of pheochromocytomas are malignant,[160] and malignancies are reported more commonly in tumors arising in extra-adrenal sites (25% to 40%). It is not clear whether malignancy occurs more frequently in familial pheochromocytoma; however, patients with familial pheochromocytoma more often have bilateral tumors.

Pheochromocytomas are also a component of MEN-2a and MEN-2b.[161] These syndromes are discussed in detail later in this chapter. When pheochromocytomas develop in the MEN syndromes, they are frequently bilateral. The pathologic diagnosis of malignancy can be difficult, because pleomorphism, nuclear atypia, and abundant mitotic figures are seen in benign tumors.[162] Even capsular invasion can be seen in benign tumors, although invasion of adjacent tissues indicates malignancy. Recent data suggest that flow cytometry can be useful in determining malignancy.[163] Malignant pheochromocytomas can be nonfunctional.

Diagnosis

Functioning malignant pheochromocytomas exhibit the same secretory pattern as benign tumors. The diagnosis is made by finding elevated catechols or catechol metabolites in the urine or plasma, or both. Urinary metanephrines are useful in diagnosing functional pheochromocytomas,[163] but the results may be falsely negative. The single most useful screening test is analysis of a 24-hour urine for vanillylmandelic acid (VMA), metanephrine, and catecholamines. Plasma catecholamine can also be elevated.[164] Oral clonidine will not reduce elevated plasma catechols to normal levels in patients with pheochromocytoma.[165] The clonidine suppression test is therefore highly useful in distinguishing pheochromocytoma from other causes of hypertension associated with elevated plasma catecholamine levels. Angiography has been largely superseded by CT and MRI scanning for tumor localization. Van Heerden and associates[166] reported that both techniques are highly accurate in localizing tumor at all sites, obviating other more invasive diagnostic procedures such as angiography and selective venous sampling for catecholamine levels.

Another useful technique for localization is radionuclide scanning with ^{131}I-MIBG, which concentrates in adrenergic tissues. The MIBG scan has proved to have a sensitivity of 87%[167] and a specificity of 96%.[168] An MIBG scan is shown in Figure 74-9.

Course and Treatment

Complete surgical resection[169] after careful preoperative preparation with α- and β-blocking agents is curative in localized pheochromocytoma. Malignant pheochromocytoma metastasizes to lung, brain, and bone. Metastatic disease generally progresses slowly. However, life-threatening complications due to secretory products can

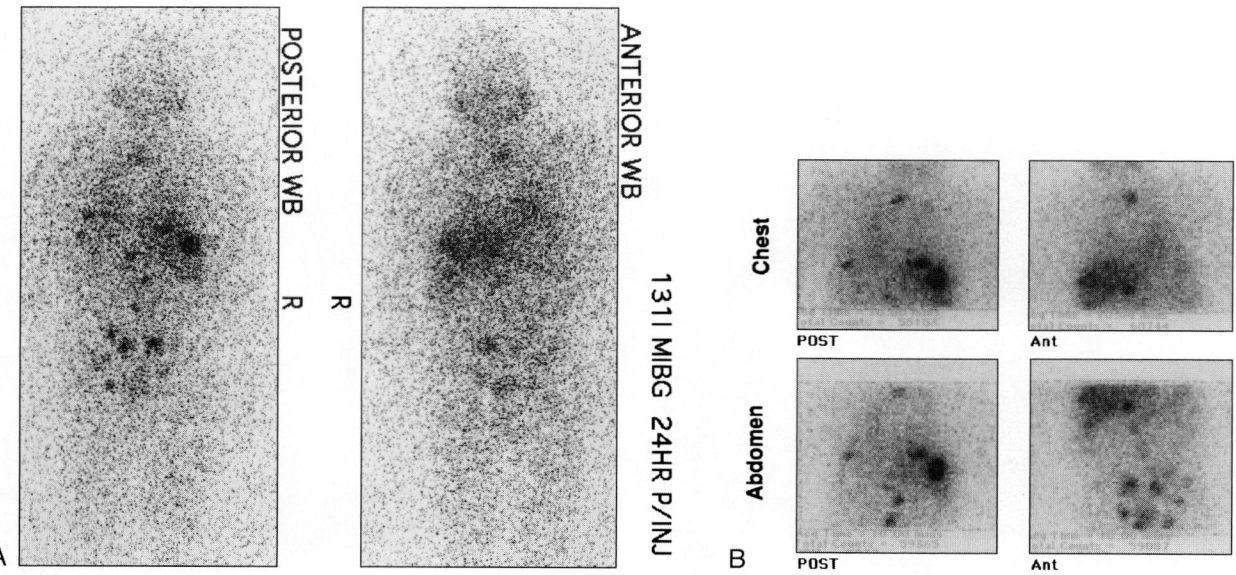

Figure 74-9. MIBG scan in patient with metastatic pheochromocytoma. **A,** ^{131}I-MIBG scan in a patient with metastatic pheochromocytoma demonstrates hepatic and bony metastasis. **B,** Magnified view of chest and abdomen.

develop over a period of many years. Survival for up to 20 years has been noted.[169]

Modern therapy for inoperable metastatic disease uses the same strategies employed in preparing a patient with primary pheochromocytoma for surgery.[23] Blockade of α-adrenergic receptors is accomplished with phenoxybenzamine; a gradual increase in dose can be required as disease advances. β-Adrenergic blockade may be of

additional benefit but should always follow establishment of α-adrenergic blockade. Otherwise, the absence of the vasodilating effects of the β-adrenergic receptors can precipitate severe hypertension. Surgery and radiation have palliative roles in treating metastatic disease; surgical reduction of metastatic tumors can decrease catecholamine secretion and result in symptomatic improvement. The results of chemotherapy are mainly anecdotal. How-

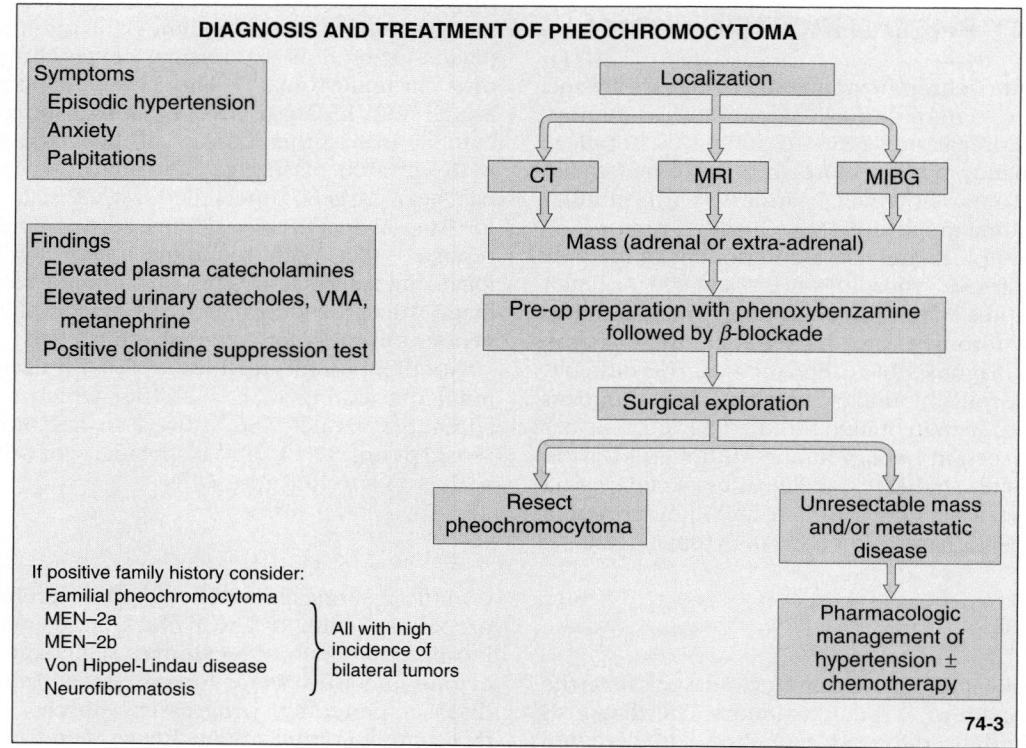

ever, a series of 14 patients treated with a combination of cyclophosphamide, vincristine, and dacarbazine (DTIC)[170] has been reported. The rates of biochemical response and measurable cancer reduction were 79% and 57%, respectively. Median duration of response was greater than 20 months. Other chemotherapy agents including streptozotocin, doxorubicin, and carmustine (BCNU) have not been effective.[171] Some studies have suggested a therapeutic value of ^{131}I-MIBG.[172-174]

PARATHYROID CARCINOMA

Parathyroid carcinoma is one of the rarest of cancers. Shantz and Castleman[175] reported the largest study of such cases. These investigators described 487 cases of hyperparathyroidism, of which only 70 (14%) were documented to be parathyroid carcinoma. The total number of reported cases is about 100. In most series parathyroid carcinoma accounts for about 1% of cases of hypercalcemia and hyperparathyroidism. The prevalence in Japan is higher.

Data concerning the possible origin of parathyroid carcinoma from preexisting abnormalities are rare. For example, transition to carcinoma from hyperplasia in patients with MEN-1 and MEN-2 syndromes does not appear to occur. However, parathyroid carcinoma has been reported to have developed in patients with familial hyperparathyroidism,[176] suggesting that transition from hyperplasia to cancer can take place.

Diagnosis

Almost all cases of parathyroid carcinoma are associated with hypercalcemia, and about 70% have values greater than 14 mg/dL, which is rare in benign hyperparathyroidism. The disease is usually diagnosed at surgery for hyperparathyroidism. No unequivocal diagnostic tests distinguish benign parathyroid neoplasms from carcinomas, although plasma calcium[177] concentration tends to be higher in carcinoma than in adenoma or hyperplasia. Evidence of a neck mass[177] or intraoperative finding of invasion of neck structures also suggests the presence of cancer.

The histologic pattern of parathyroid cancer shows frequent mitosis and blood vessel invasion. In one study, these features and a trabecular pattern with thick fibrous bands were considered characteristic[177] of malignancy and helped to distinguish cancer from benign hyperplasia or adenoma. As with many endocrine tumors, it may be difficult to differentiate benign from malignant tumors by histologic features alone.

Natural History

The 5-year survival rate of patients with parathyroid carcinoma varies between 29% and 44%,[177,178] and the 10-year survival rate averages 20%. A smaller, more recent study has been reported, however, with an 89% (eight of nine cases) survival rate at a median follow-up period of 6 years.[179] Although parathyroid cancer metastasizes to lung, bone, and liver in about 20% of patients, metastatic disease is less frequently a cause of morbidity and death than is the severe hypercalcemia associated with this disease.

Management

When parathyroid carcinoma is recognized at surgery, careful en bloc excision of the cancer and involved structures is indicated.[179] This tumor does not generally metastasize via the lymphatics; therefore, radical neck dissection is not warranted. Careful dissection without tumor spill is important because local recurrence has been demonstrated. Local recurrence occurs in about two thirds of patients, in some due to intraoperative seeding. If hypercalcemia persists or recurs after surgery, an attempt should be made to locate the metastasis using selective venous catheterization and measurement of hormone levels in the event other diagnostic modalities fail. Prolonged remission of hypercalcemia has been reported after resection of metastases.[180]

Nonsurgical treatment of recurrent or metastatic parathyroid cancer is disappointing. Radiation therapy has not been of significant value in treating primary or recurrent neck disease, although it may have some palliative benefit in controlling pain in bone metastases. Cytotoxic chemotherapy has been tested only infrequently, but it appears that dacarbazine has some activity in this disease.[181,182] Essentially, all patients with incurable parathyroid cancer require control of hypercalcemia. Diphosphonates, mithramycin, and calcitonin have been only marginally effective. It appears that the more recently developed pharmacologic therapies for hypercalcemia (etidronate[183] and gallium nitrate[184]) may be more effective in the palliative management of the severe hypercalcemia associated with parathyroid cancer.

MULTIPLE ENDOCRINE NEOPLASIA

MEN syndromes are characterized by the familial occurrence of endocrine neoplasms in various sites. MEN syndromes are inherited as autosomal dominant with high penetrance, variable expressivity, and pleiotropic expression. The neoplasms[110,185] of the MEN syndromes may be either benign or malignant. Manifestations of MEN-1, MEN-2a, and MEN-2b are summarized in Table 74-6. Steiner and associates[186] were the first to characterize MEN-1 and MEN-2.

MEN-1

MEN-1 syndrome is a disorder of three glands: parathyroid, pancreatic islet cells, and pituitary. Recently, the disease gene for MEN-1, menin, has been localized to the long arm of chromosome 11.[187] Menin has been reported to be a nuclear protein of still undefined function.[188]

Clinical Features
Parathyroid hyperplasia is the most frequently noted abnormality.[189] Next in frequency are pancreatic islet

TABLE 74-6

Syndromes of Multiple Endocrine Neoplasia

MEN-1	MEN-2
Pituitary tumors	MEN-2a and -2b
Eosinophilic adenoma (acromegaly)	Medullary carcinoma of
Prolactinoma	the thyroid
Nonfunctional tumors	Pheochromocytoma
ACTH-secreting tumors	MEN-2a
Hyperparathyroidism	Hyperparathyroidism
Pancreatic tumors	MEN-2b
Most common	Mucosal neuromas
Gastrinoma	Marfanoid habitus
Insulinoma	Typical facies
Pancreatic polypeptide-secreting	Bowel abnormalities
tumor	
Glucagonoma	
VIPoma	
GRFoma	

ACTH, adrenocorticotropic hormone; MEN-2a, -2b, multiple endocrine neoplasia types 2a, 2b.

tumors. Adenomas of the pituitary gland are noted in 50% to 80%[189,190] of MEN-1 cases. When pituitary adenomas are functioning, prolactin is the most common hormone produced.[191] Acromegaly caused by growth hormone–secreting adenomas occurs in approximately 25% of adenomas.[192] Cushing's syndrome secondary to pituitary adenoma is uncommon. Approximately 80% of cases of MEN-1 will have functional pancreatic islet cell tumors.[191] Islet cell tumors represent the most common cause of death in patients with MEN-1, with 60% of deaths resulting from ulcer disease or problems caused by islet cell tumors.[192]

A wide spectrum of pancreatic islet cell tumors can occur in MEN-1. In a comprehensive review,[192] pancreatic tumors were present in 100 of 122 MEN-1 patients with the following frequency: gastrinoma (64%), insulinoma (24%), glucagonoma (3%), and nonfunctioning tumor (9%). Rare cases of secretion of vasoactive intestinal peptide (VIP) and other peptides were observed. Forty-two percent of the gastrinomas were malignant, and 25% of the insulinomas were malignant. This finding is in contradistinction to sporadic insulinomas, in which only 10% are malignant. Pancreatic polypeptide (commonly), α- and β-hCG (less commonly), and other peptides such as ACTH may be elevated in MEN-1 patients and may serve as tumor markers. The adrenal cortex may be abnormal in about one third of cases,[189] usually with hyperplasia associated with pituitary adenomas producing ACTH. Rarely, a pancreatic tumor[194] may ectopically produce ACTH. Clinical Cushing's syndrome is uncommon. Bronchial carcinoids may occur in approximately 5% of cases.

Surgery

Management of MEN-1 first requires an awareness of the existence of the syndrome. Because almost all these patients will eventually manifest hyperparathyroidism,[189] continued surveillance of serum calcium is necessary. Parathyroidectomy is usually curative. In cases in which

all four glands are enlarged, complete resection with forearm implantation is the preferred treatment. However, parathyroid hyperplasia can be limited to one or a few glands. In this case, it is preferred to resect the abnormal glands and to obtain a biopsy of the normal-appearing parathyroids. The location of these normal glands should be marked with nonabsorbable suture. If possible, all parathyroid tissue on one side of the neck should be removed to avoid the need for repeat bilateral neck exploration. Detectable pituitary tumors may be treated with bromocriptine or are occasionally removed by trans-sphenoidal resection. The management of pancreatic islet cell tumors is described elsewhere in this chapter.

MEN-2

MEN-2 syndrome was initially reported by Sipple[195] in 1961. MEN-2 tumors include MTC, pheochromocytoma, and adenoma or hyperplasia of the parathyroid glands. When mucosal neuromas with or without marfanoid habitus are present as part of a distinctive syndrome, the designation is MEN-2b. Parathyroid disease is rare in MEN-2b. Specific MEN-2a[196,197] and MEN-2b[198] gene defects map to different regions of the *ret* proto-oncogene in the centromeric region of chromosome 10. More than 70% of pheochromocytomas occurring with MEN-2 are bilateral. These tumors may be derived from a hyperplastic adrenal medulla,[161] yet be benign, although carcinomas may occur in the same family. This progression from hyperplasia to tumor is similar to the progression noted in MTC.

Clinical Features

The clinical presentation of patients with MEN-2 can be dictated by any of the three neoplasms seen in the syndrome. However, all patients with MEN-2 have medullary carcinoma of the thyroid. In reviews of MEN-2a, pheochromocytoma was seen in 21% to 41% of patients, and parathyroid hyperplasia or adenoma was present in 17% to 60%.[199] All patients had medullary carcinoma of the thyroid.[101,200] In a series of patients with MEN-2b, all had medullary carcinoma, and 60% developed pheochromocytomas.[201] In general, MEN-2b tends to be a more rapidly progressive clinical entity because the medullary carcinoma of the thyroid that develops in this syndrome has a more aggressive course than that seen in MEN-2a.

Patients suspected of having MEN-2 syndrome should be screened for medullary carcinoma of the thyroid, pheochromocytoma, and hyperparathyroidism. The most effective way to screen for medullary carcinoma of the thyroid is to initially measure plasma calcitonin levels. All patients with medullary carcinoma of the thyroid will have either elevated basal plasma calcitonin levels or elevation after pentagastrin and calcium infusion stimulation tests.[202] The appropriate screening tests for pheochromocytoma include measuring urinary levels of epinephrine, norepinephrine, VMA, and metanephrines as described previously. When these tests are abnormal, tumor localization studies including MRI and abdominal CT scanning should be undertaken. When there is biochemical evidence of pheochromocytoma with a negative CT scan, MIBG scan may be useful. MIBG concentrates in pheochromocytoma cells, permitting tumor detection by scintigraphy.[203]

Surgery

Management of patients with MEN-2 syndromes is primarily surgical. The surgical treatment of medullary carcinoma is total thyroidectomy, as the tumor is always bilateral. Central lymph node dissection should also be performed. In patients with MEN-2a, the parathyroid gland should be resected and implanted into the forearm. Patients with pheochromocytoma should undergo pre-operative α-adrenergic blockade with phenoxybenzamine.[201,203] After adequate α-blockade has been obtained, β-blockers may be added if the patient has significant tachycardia, although in many instances β-blockade is not needed.

Postoperatively, patients with resected MTC may be followed with serum calcitonin levels. This measurement is a sensitive marker for recurrence of disease. Likewise, appropriate urinary catecholamine studies will demonstrate recurrence of pheochromocytoma. Because MEN-2 syndromes exhibit autosomal dominance, it is important to evaluate family members of patients with documented MEN-2 for presence of the syndrome. Genetic analysis for inheritance of the allele containing the mutant *ret* gene will identify family members likely to develop MEN. Family members who have not inherited the disease allele require no further evaluation. Genetically affected members can be offered early thyroidectomy.

CARCINOID TUMORS

Carcinoid is an English translation of a term used by German pathologists to describe a carcinoma-like tumor that behaves less aggressively than carcinomas.[204] Although their malignant potential was noted,[205] other unique characteristics of the tumors were described. They arise from enterochromaffin cells[205-207] in the gastrointestinal tract and lung. Enterochromaffin cells take up and reduce silver. Silver staining documented the argyrophilic nature of carcinoid tumors, ultimately leading to their being described as neoplasms of the diffuse endocrine or APUD system.[208] Other tumors of the APUD system include medullary carcinoma of the thyroid, pheochromocytoma, and pancreatic endocrine tumors. Newer immunohistochemical techniques including neuron-specific enolase (NSE)[209,210] and chromogranin A[211-212] hormone assays have allowed further characterization of the synthesis and secretion of neuroendocrine peptides by carcinoid cells. The knowledge that these neoplasms have common characteristics as defined by the APUD concept is important in understanding the production of polypeptides as from pancreatic islet cell tumors.

Carcinoid tumors have typically been classified as originating in foregut (lung and upper gastrointestinal tract to the jejunum), midgut, (ileum and appendix), and hindgut (colon and rectum). The origin of carcinoid tumors may in part explain the ectopic hormone secretion and syndromes related to primary tumor site.[213]

About 85% of carcinoid tumors develop in the gastrointestinal tract, usually the appendix. In one report, 44% of carcinoids were appendiceal, accounting for more than three fourths of all tumors in that organ.[214] In the same series, the intestine (19%), rectum (15%), and lung (10%) were also frequent sites. Carcinoids account for one third of tumors in the small intestine. Carcinoids of the appendix are commonly incidental findings. The majority are smaller than 1.0 cm and are cured by surgical resection. In the Mayo Clinic series,[215] no tumor of 1.0 cm or less recurred after resection. Therefore, appendectomy alone is adequate treatment. With the uncommon large appendiceal carcinoid, a true cancer operation (e.g., right hemicolectomy) can be required. Carcinoids of the rectum are similar to appendiceal carcinoids and are typically small and are best treated with conservative local measures.

Carcinoids of the small intestine are the most clinically important tumors because of their frequency of presentation, their more advanced stage at diagnosis, and their association with the carcinoid syndrome. The largest and most carefully followed series of patients with small bowel carcinoid has been reported from the Mayo Clinic,[215] where 183 consecutive cases have been followed for a median period of 15 years. Approximately 40% of the tumors occurred within 2 feet of the ileocecal valve, with very few in the proximal small intestine. Thirty-five percent of patients had more than one lesion, and most primary tumors were 2.0 to 4.0 cm in diameter. More than 80% of patients with resectable primary tumors were free of disease at 20 years. Overall survival rate in these patients was similar to that of an age- and sex-matched control group. Of the 72 patients who had resected regional node metastases, one half experienced recurrence by 16 years, with continued evidence of relapse after that time. Patients who had unresectable abdominal metastases and hepatic metastases fared least well, with median survival rates of 5 and 3 years, respectively. These data confirm that, even with advanced disease, carcinoid tumors tend to have a relatively indolent course. Goblet cell or adenoid carcinoid tumors may be more aggressive than typical gastrointestinal carcinoids.

Clinical Pathology

Carcinoid tumors are usually readily identified microscopically.[216] Immunohistochemical staining is performed to identify and classify these tumors.[217] In addition to immunohistochemical staining to reveal specific tumor-produced peptides, other semispecific markers including NSE[187,189] and chromogranin A[190] aid in diagnosis.

Carcinoid Syndrome

Many patients with metastatic carcinoid tumor will manifest the signs and symptoms of abnormal hormone production—the malignant carcinoid syndrome.[218,219] Serotonin (5-hydroxytryptamine, 5-HT), synthesized by the tumor from tryptophan and metabolized to 5-HIAA, which appears in the urine, is particularly important because urinary 5-HIAA levels are used to monitor the course of carcinoid syndrome. However, the relationship of serotonin levels to symptoms of the clinical carcinoid syndrome is uncertain.[215]

Carcinoid tumors also release the enzyme kallikrein,[220,221] which acts on α_2-globulin to produce bradykinin and its precursor, lysyl-bradykinin, both of which can induce flushing. Serotonin may be responsible for intestinal hypermotility and hypersecretion, but it probably does not cause the characteristic flushing that occurs with the carcinoid syndrome.[222] Vasodilation, which causes flushing, can be due to one or more substances released by the tumor cells, including bradykinin, tachykinins, and prostaglandins. The symptoms of the carcinoid syndrome vary in frequency. Flushing is most frequent, followed by diarrhea, heart disease, and bronchoconstriction.[215]

Flushing

Two types of flushing accompany the usual metastatic ileal carcinoid. One is red and diffuse, involving the face and upper body; it is of short duration and can be provoked by alcohol, excitement, emotional stress, and catecholamine release.[223] The other is more prolonged, produces venous dilation and a purplish hue, and can give rise to permanent dilation of facial veins and telangiectasia. This flush is more commonly precipitated by alcohol ingestion. Because infusion of serotonin does not cause either flush, it has been suggested that the kinins cause this symptom.[224] Brief flushes may be due to catecholamine-induced release of kallikrein; these flushes can be blocked effectively by α-adrenergic blocking agents.[225] Carcinoid of the foregut produces a more intense and erythematous flush, sometimes associated with itching, conjunctival suffusion, and facial edema suggestive of histamine. Occasionally, gastric carcinoids cause an urticarial reaction, which may be inhibited by the histamine H_1- and H_2-receptor antagonists diphenhydramine and cimetidine.[226]

Diarrhea

The diarrhea of carcinoid syndrome does not necessarily correlate with flushing. Diarrhea appears to be related to increased gut motility, rather than to secretion of fluids. Methysergide, a serotonin antagonist, is sometimes effective in treating or preventing diarrhea, hence the presumption that serotonin is directly responsible for this symptom. Infusion of serotonin produces intestinal dysmotility similar to that seen in the carcinoid syndrome.[227] Diarrhea of the carcinoid syndrome is rarely of high volume and, therefore, typically requires only mild palliative antidiarrheal therapy. Although abdominal cramping can be associated with this diarrhea, other possibilities for abdominal pain must be considered, including intermittent partial small bowel obstruction secondary to mesenteric fibrosis or bowel obstruction secondary to tumor bulk.

Heart Disease

The cardiac disease associated with the carcinoid syndrome is an endomyocardial fibrosis typically involving the right side of the heart, although left-sided lesions have been described.[186] Fibrotic deformation of the tricuspid and pulmonary valves usually leads to pulmonary stenosis and tricuspid insufficiency.[228,229] In the Mayo Clinic series, carcinoid heart disease was a late complication, with only 5 of 91 deaths identified as having a primary cardiac cause. In that series, most patients with heart disease had high levels of 5-HIAA as well as a lengthy history of carcinoid cardiac disease averaging more than 5 years.

Other,[215] relatively rarer, signs and symptoms are associated with carcinoid syndrome. Bronchoconstriction may occur in both pulmonary and extrapulmonary carcinoid and is usually associated with flushing. The classic triad of dermatitis, dementia, and diarrhea seen with pellagra has occasionally been identified. This syndrome is secondary to niacin deficiency as a result of shunting of dietary tryptophan from niacin synthesis to indole synthesis. This syndrome is rare, because of better overall nutrition in the population. It is treated with nicotinamide.

Diagnosis

The diagnosis of carcinoid tumor is by finding tumor or symptoms related to tumor bulk, biologically active peptides, or from urinary tumor markers.[230] Measurement of 5-HIAA is the most common and reproducible test for the presence of carcinoid syndrome. In most laboratories, the upper limit of normal for 24-hour urinary 5-HIAA excretion is 6 to 10 mg. In one study, 5-HIAA measurements were 100% specific and 73% sensitive for the presence of carcinoid syndrome.[231] Not all patients with carcinoid tumor have the associated syndrome, and the sensitivity of assays for detecting the presence of tumor alone is inadequate. Although markedly elevated 5-HIAA in the urine is remarkably specific for carcinoid tumor, a low-level false positive increase of 5-HIAA may be seen in patients with noncarcinoid tumor and after intake of certain foods (e.g., bananas, walnuts, and pecans) and medications (e.g., acetaminophen, salicylate, guaifenesin).[231-233] Also, 5-HIAA may be elevated to low abnormal levels (<30 mg) in patients with diarrhea or malabsorption from any cause. In addition to excellent specificity and high sensitivity, 5-HIAA measurement has a high level of consistency both in individual patients and among groups. In the Mayo Clinic series, the level of 5-HIAA excretion remained constant in a group of 85 patients in whom paired determinations were done during a 10-day period.[215] Moreover, in a given patient, the level of 5-HIAA secretion is a relatively accurate indicator of tumor bulk.[234] Recently, serum NSE and chromogranin A levels have been shown to correlate with the presence and natural history of gastrointestinal neuroendocrine tumors.[211,212] Recently, localization of carcinoid and islet cell tumors has been investigated by nuclear medicine techniques, including ^{123}I-MIBG and octreotide scan (Fig. 74-10).[235-237]

Treatment

Patient management depends not only on traditional methods of dealing with bulky disease and its manifestations, but also on management of associated medical

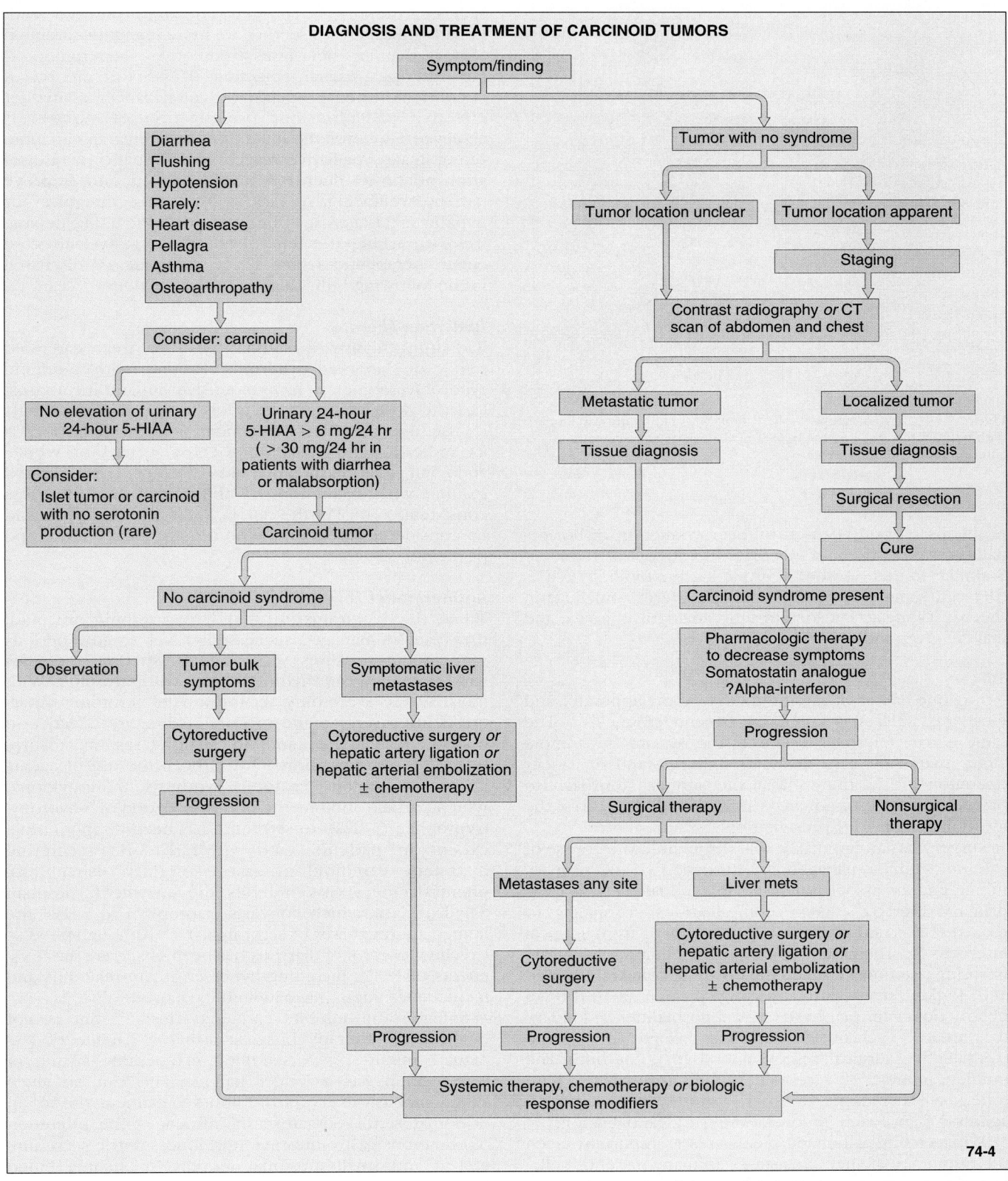

DIAGNOSIS AND TREATMENT OF CARCINOID TUMORS

Symptom/finding

Diarrhea
Flushing
Hypotension
Rarely:
Heart disease
Pellagra
Asthma
Osteoarthropathy

Consider: carcinoid

No elevation of urinary 24-hour 5-HIAA

Consider:
Islet tumor or carcinoid with no serotonin production (rare)

Urinary 24-hour 5-HIAA > 6 mg/24 hr (> 30 mg/24 hr in patients with diarrhea or malabsorption)

Carcinoid tumor

No carcinoid syndrome

Observation

Tumor bulk symptoms

Cytoreductive surgery

Progression

Symptomatic liver metastases

Cytoreductive surgery *or* hepatic artery ligation *or* hepatic arterial embolization ± chemotherapy

Tumor with no syndrome

Tumor location unclear

Tumor location apparent

Staging

Contrast radiography *or* CT scan of abdomen and chest

Metastatic tumor

Tissue diagnosis

Localized tumor

Tissue diagnosis

Surgical resection

Cure

Carcinoid syndrome present

Pharmacologic therapy to decrease symptoms Somatostatin analogue ?Alpha-interferon

Progression

Surgical therapy

Nonsurgical therapy

Metastases any site

Liver mets

Cytoreductive surgery

Cytoreductive surgery *or* hepatic artery ligation *or* hepatic arterial embolization ± chemotherapy

Progression

Progression

Progression

Systemic therapy, chemotherapy *or* biologic response modifiers

74-4

Specific Malignancies

III

Anterior   **Posterior**

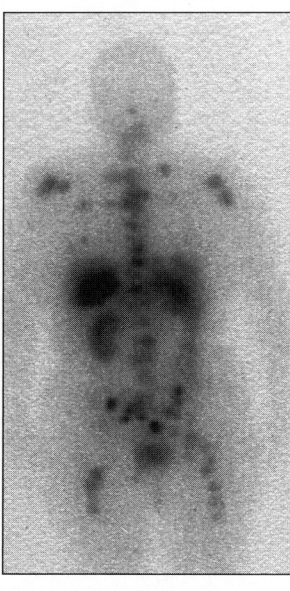
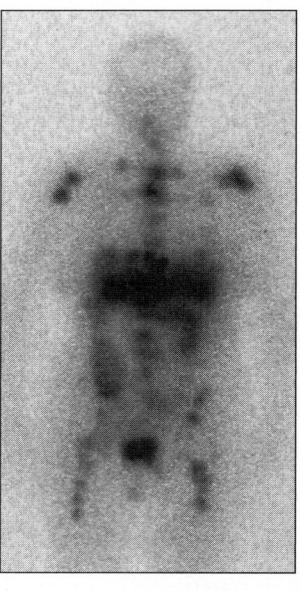

Figure 74-10. ^{111}In-octreotide scan. Patient with metastatic carcinoid with octreotide scan showing bony and visceral metastases with anterior and posterior views.

problems typically caused by overproduction of hormonally active peptides. In this regard, treatment of carcinoid is similar to that of other neuroendocrine tumors, such as islet cell tumors. For patients on long-term somatostatin therapy a long-acting somatostatin analog is effective and may be given monthly.[215]

Surgery
Nearly one half of all carcinoids arise in the appendix, and most are small and cured by appendectomy.[216,238] The same is true for small lesions of the rectum, but tumors larger than 2.0 cm in diameter require standard cancer operations.[239] It follows that the surgical approach to bronchial, gastric, or gonadal carcinoid will depend on the location and stage at presentation.

Surgery has an important role throughout the course of carcinoid tumor management. Resection of the primary tumor and of associated resectable nodal metastases is primary therapy.[239] Also, complications secondary to recurrent or residual carcinoid may benefit from surgical intervention. These tumors frequently elicit a mesenteric fibrosing reaction, in which the bowel becomes shortened and kinked, frequently causing partial small bowel obstruction. Pain or physiologic abnormalities secondary to partial bowel obstruction may be greatly relieved by palliative surgical resection or bypass, or both. The indolent course of carcinoid tumors mandates a high index of suspicion for such complications and an aggressive approach in considering surgical palliation.

Management of hepatic metastases is important given the frequency of such metastases. In many patients, bulky hepatic metastases constitute most of the tumor burden, so that tumor reduction may, at the least, diminish production of peptides that promote the carcinoid syndrome, as well as extend survival. Principles of surgical management of hepatic metastases are similar to those for islet cell tumors.[240] The indications to proceed with hepatic metastases resection are more liberal in carcinoid tumors than in metastases from other solid tumors.[241] For example, partial resection of hepatic metastases is contraindicated in metastatic colon cancer, as neither effective palliation nor prolongation of survival is achieved. However, the much longer survival in carcinoid tumor makes palliative resection of hepatic metastases appropriate to decrease tumor burden and improve patient well-being. A variety of cancer therapies for hepatic metastases may be attempted, including hepatic irradiation, hepatic embolization, and liver-directed chemotherapeutic agents. These therapies are discussed in the following individual treatment sections.

Radiation Therapy
Radiation therapy is seldom used to treat carcinoid tumor or carcinoid syndrome. Patients with carcinoid syndrome frequently have extensive hepatic metastases, and the dose-limiting toxicity of hepatic radiation limits its usefulness. Palliative treatment of bone metastases is an indication for radiation therapy. A trial of whole-abdomen radiation therapy (20 to 25 Gy)[242] yielded mixed results, with reduction of abdominal pain but less consistent control of the cancer. Radiation therapy should be considered in patients who require local control and palliation.[243]

Antihormonal Therapy
When the symptoms attributed to serotonin are mild, they can be managed successfully over lengthy periods with simple measures, such as administration of opiates and diphenoxylate hydrochloride with atropine. With more severe symptoms, the peripheral serotonin antagonists methysergide and cyproheptadine are effective in controlling diarrhea and, in some cases, malabsorption.[244,245] Another approach has been the use of agents known to inhibit serotonin synthesis. α-Methyldopa, which partially inhibits the decarboxylation of 5-hydroxytryptophan (5-HTP) to serotonin has been disappointing, except in patients with the rare 5-HTP–secreting metastatic carcinoid of gastric origin.[228] Parachlorophenylalanine (PCPA) inhibits the enzyme tryptophan 5-hydroxylase, which converts tryptophan to 5-HTP, the immediate precursor of serotonin.[246,247] Although good to excellent control of diarrhea has been observed, the toxic effects of PCPA, including hypersensitivity reactions and mental aberrations, have limited its clinical value.

Somatostatin inhibits carcinoid flush,[248] but is not practical for therapy because it has a half-life of less than 2 minutes.[249] A synthetic octapeptide analog of somatostatin has a longer half-life, and can be given subcutaneously every 8 to 12 hours to maintain the action of somatostatin. Somatostatin influences the inhibition of numerous gastrointestinal hormones, gastric secretion, gastric and small intestinal motility, splanchnic blood flow, pancreatic enzyme secretion, intestinal nutrient absorption, and gallbladder contractility.[250]

Somatostatin analog has two established uses in carcinoid tumors: chronic treatment of symptoms[251] such as diarrhea and flushing, and treatment of carcinoid crisis.[250] Kvols and associates,[251] in 1986, described the use of the somatostatin analog octreotide in therapy for carcinoid syndrome. Fifty-seven patients with carcinoid tumor and carcinoid syndrome were treated with daily doses of octreotide, ranging from 100 to 1127 µg (mean, 414 µg). Flushing was palliated in most patients, and diarrhea was adequately controlled in approximately 75%. Control of symptoms was usually associated with a decrease in the urinary 5-HIAA level, but reduction in tumor bulk was not consistently seen. The median duration of response to somatostatin analog was 4 months, with some patients escaping control quite early, yet in others response continued for more than 2 years. Increased doses of somatostatin may partially overcome resistance.[252] More recent studies have confirmed that somatostatin improves symptoms but has little effect on tumor regression.[337]

Somatostatin analog is generally well tolerated.[250,251] Minimal irritation at the injection site and alterations in bowel patterns have been observed. Fecal fat excretion may also increase, and aberrations in glucose tolerance resulting in hyperglycemia have been observed. Long-term therapy may predispose to the formation of gallstones; the drug promotes cholelithiasis by inhibition of cholecystokinin release and a resultant inhibition of gallbladder emptying. Approximately 50% of patients receiving chronic therapy will develop cholelithiasis and should, therefore, undergo elective cholecystectomy at the time of tumor debulking.[338]

Chemotherapy

Because the disease is indolent not much information is available on the role of chemotherapy.[258] Antineoplastic therapy may be called for in patients whose cancers are aggressive, with progressive liver metastases, signs of partial or impending complete intestinal obstruction, or severe symptoms of carcinoid syndrome uncontrollable by other methods. Controlled clinical trials have been difficult to carry out because of the rarity of the tumor, but cooperative study group trials have been useful in assessing tumor responsiveness.

Table 74-7 summarizes experience with cytotoxic drugs. During the 1970s, systemic therapy with single agents was reported, with 5-FU and streptozotocin shown to be active drugs.[259] The Mayo Clinic experience with more than 200 patients suggests that with single agents the response rates of greater than 10% were seen with only three adequately tested drugs: doxorubicin, 7 of 33 (21%); 5-FU, 5 of 19 (26%); and DTIC (dacarbazine), 2 of 15 (13%).[240]

Based on initial observations of patient response to 5-FU and streptozotocin, investigators at the Mayo Clinic studied that regimen and noted an overall response rate of 33% in 43 patients.[240] A larger series of patients was reported in a Phase III study by the Eastern Cooperative Oncology Group (ECOG)[235] comparing 5-FU plus streptozotocin to cyclophosphamide plus streptozotocin. Response rates for the two treatment arms were not

TABLE 74-7

Drug Treatment of Carcinoid Tumor

DRUG TREATMENT	RESPONSE RATE (%)	REFERENCES
Single Agents		
5-FU	26	240
Streptozotocin	30	235
Doxorubicin	21	240
DTIC	13	240
Combination Chemotherapy		
5-FU + streptozotocin	33	240
5-FU + streptozotocin	33	235
vs.		
5-FU + cyclophosphamide	26	235
5-FU + streptozotocin (lower dose)	23	255
5-FU + streptozotocin	16	256
vs.		
5-FU + Adriamycin	13	256
Biologic Response Modifiers		
Interferon		
Human leukocyte	47* (11)	258
Recombinant α	55†	258
Recombinant α	39* (20)	259
Octreotide	16‡	245
Octreotide	9‡	258

DTIC, dacarbazine; 5-FU, 5-fluorouracil; 5-HIAA, 5-hydroxyindoleacetic acid.
*Percentages in parentheses represent objective tumor regression. Overall percentages reflect decrease in 5-HIAA excretion and improvement in symptoms of carcinoid syndrome.
†Most responses were chemical, and not objective tumor regression.
‡Decreased 5-HIAA excretion demonstrated in more than 50% of cases. Objective tumor regression.

significantly different (33% vs. 26%, respectively), nor were there significant differences in overall survival. Assuming the 5-FU plus streptozotocin regimen to be standard, the ECOG subsequently reported their trial of this combination, with streptozotocin given less frequently to decrease toxicity, compared with doxorubicin alone.[255] Twenty-three percent of patients in each arm responded, further documenting doxorubicin activity.

Most recently, ECOG reported the results of their largest trial of combination chemotherapy.[256] This trial randomly allocated patients with measurable carcinoid tumors to the standard regimen of 5-FU plus streptozotocin (FS) and a new regimen of 5-FU and doxorubicin (FA). Patients who had either renal or heart disease making them ineligible for streptozotocin or doxorubicin-containing therapies were treated with DTIC. Of 208 patients who were eligible and analyzed for response and survival, FA and FS therapies were associated with response rates of 13% and 16%, respectively, in the randomized group. With DTIC, the response rate was approximately 10%, with no significant differences between previously treated and untreated patients. Although the response rates for FA and FS did not differ, there was a trend toward improved survival in the FS group. The median survival time of the group was 24 months, compared with 16 months for patient receiving FA ($P = 0.11$). This suggestive disparity between response rate and survival time may reflect the fact that reduction in tumor bulk has little correlation with survival in patients with an indolent disease such as carcinoid tumor. Alternatively, it may be true that survival is a better measure of tumor response, with inadequate determination of response by traditional techniques.

Because no highly effective chemotherapy regimen is available, it is clear that patients should be carefully selected for use of cytotoxic chemotherapy in metastatic carcinoid tumor and carcinoid syndrome. Less toxic and more effective palliative therapies for carcinoid syndrome should always be used initially, reserving chemotherapy for those patients who are significantly disabled by unresponsive hormonally related symptoms or those with refractory symptoms due to tumor bulk. Clinical trials of more recently available drugs (taxanes, gemcitabine, camptothecins) need to be carried out.

Interferon

Early clinical trials from Sweden suggested a role for low-dose human leukocyte interferon.[257] Subsequently, this group reported the results of three consecutive studies using interferon.[258] In the first study, involving 36 patients, an overall response rate of 47% was observed. In the second randomized trial, human leukocyte interferon was compared with FS. No response was observed in the 10 patients treated with chemotherapy, but 5 patients in the interferon-treated group did respond. In the third study, 20 patients were treated with recombinant interferon; an objective response rate of 55% was observed, with the bulk of responses being symptomatic or chemical responses manifested by a decrease in 5-HIAA, rather than by reduction in tumor bulk. As demonstrated in Table 74-7, objective regression of tumor bulk occurred in only 11% to 20% of cases. The Mayo Clinic subsequently reported the results of their Phase II trial of recombinant interferon-α (IFN-α) in 24 patients with malignant carcinoid syndrome.[259] Twenty percent of patients with measurable tumor experienced objective tumor regression, and 39% had a significant reduction in urinary 5-HIAA excretion. Flushing and diarrhea were transiently relieved, with objective responses lasting less than 2 months. The results suggest a limited role for this agent in treating carcinoid tumor. Clinical trials are currently being developed in which chemotherapy and interferons are being combined, although early results do not suggest additional benefit compared to single modalities.[260] Similarly, combinations of octreotide and IFN-α are being investigated to determine whether lower doses of interferon would be effective and whether the tachyphylaxis associated with octreotide could be overcome by the addition of interferon.[261] Patients with carcinoid tumors treated with interferon may develop a wide variety of autoimmune diseases, such as thyroid disease (thyrotoxicosis, hypothyroidism), pernicious anemia, and vasculitis.[262]

Hepatic-Directed Therapy

The results of surgical resection for hepatic metastases and anecdotal reports of hepatic and abdominal radiation in carcinoid tumors have already been described. The Mayo Clinic has investigated the role of hepatic arterial occlusion in metastatic carcinoid and islet cell tumors.[216] Significant improvement in symptoms and reduction in hepatic metastases were noted in 14 patients with carcinoid tumors, but the median length of response was less than 7 months. Mayo Clinic investigators have also examined the role of sequential hepatic arterial occlusion (HAO), followed by systemic chemotherapy with DTIC and doxorubicin alternating with the combination of 5-FU and streptozotocin in carcinoid tumors.[216,263] With 65 carcinoid cases treated, more than two thirds of all patients demonstrated objective regression with either HAO or HAO plus chemotherapy. The median duration of regression was longer in the groups receiving chemotherapy, but this trial was not randomized, and better-risk cases may have been selected for the chemotherapy plus HAO treatment. Other groups are investigating the role of selective hepatic arteriography with sequential hepatic arterial embolization or chemoembolization.[264-266] Significant reduction in the signs and symptoms associated with both carcinoid tumors[267] and islet cell tumors have been reported in the majority of patients so treated. In a study of 15 patients with advanced metastatic carcinoid tumors, hepatic artery chemoembolization improves symptoms and short-term quality of life.[336] Unfortunately, there is a paucity of data on the benefit of either intermittent or prolonged continuous hepatic arterial infusion of chemotherapeutic agents in patients with metastatic carcinoid tumors.

PANCREATIC ISLET CELL TUMORS

The advent of radioimmunoassay (RIA), immunofluorescence, and other techniques for identifying peptide hormones has expanded our knowledge of the prevalence and endocrine effects of islet cell tumors. A great percentage of islet cell tumors appear to remain asymptomatic and undiagnosed, as indicated by the high prevalence of these tumors in autopsy series (1500 per 100,000) compared with their low clinical incidence (1 per 100,000).[268]

The pancreatic islet contains α cells (glucagon), β cells (insulin), and δ cells (somatostatin), as well as enterochromaffin cells (serotonin). These cells are all part of the APUD system, and tumors so derived secrete a wide variety of polypeptides. Some of these peptides share the characteristics and functions of classic hormones: (1) their release follows a physiologic stimulus, (2) they have the ability to effect response in a distant organ, and (3) these effects are mimicked by exogenous infusion of the hormone. By contrast, some abnormal peptides produced by islet cell tumors have no known clinical hormonal effects.[269]

Clinically, in evaluating patients with islet cell tumors, it is important to understand that there appear to be two different types of patients with APUDomas. The first group consists of those patients who experienced their tumors singularly, in the absence of significant personal or family history of endocrine disorders. The second group includes those with clear evidence of an inherited predisposition to multiple neoplasia of the endocrine system in an autosomal dominant pattern. These MEN syndromes[195,270] have been described earlier.

As with carcinoid tumors, the approach to the patient with an islet cell tumor needs to be individualized, balancing management of the effects of hormone production with symptoms of tumor bulk. In any particular patient, one or the other management issue may predominate. Treatment should be directed not only by the presence of symptoms, but also by a consideration of the relatively lengthy natural history of islet cell tumors.

Diagnosis

Specific syndromes and diagnostic tests for each of the more common islet cell tumors are discussed separately. However, a few generally applicable principles should be understood. RIA[271] of peptides obtained by selective venous catheterization is most helpful in localizing tumors and may demonstrate the presence of metastatic spread, particularly in patients with gastrinomas (Zollinger-Ellison syndrome). CT scan and arteriography are particularly helpful in tumors greater than 1.0 cm in diameter. However, because many islet cell tumors and their metastases may be small, both procedures may be less sensitive than desired. As with most endocrine neoplasms, islet cell tumors have a rich vascularity, so that "tumor blush" can be seen on angiography. This sign may be a useful finding in differentiating between endocrine and nonendocrine gastrointestinal tumors. Ultrasonography is of some use in imaging both pancreatic primary tumors and hepatic metastases. Newer imaging techniques are therefore required for better diagnosis and staging. For example, MRI has been shown in some studies to be superior to contrast-enhanced CT scans for the identification of all islet cell tumors.[269] The mainstay of diagnosis remains the RIA to detect peptides secreted by these tumors: NSE and chromogranin.[211,212]

Insulinoma

The average age of presentation of insulinoma is in the mid-40s, and the sine qua non in diagnosing this syndrome is fasting or inappropriate hypoglycemia accompanied

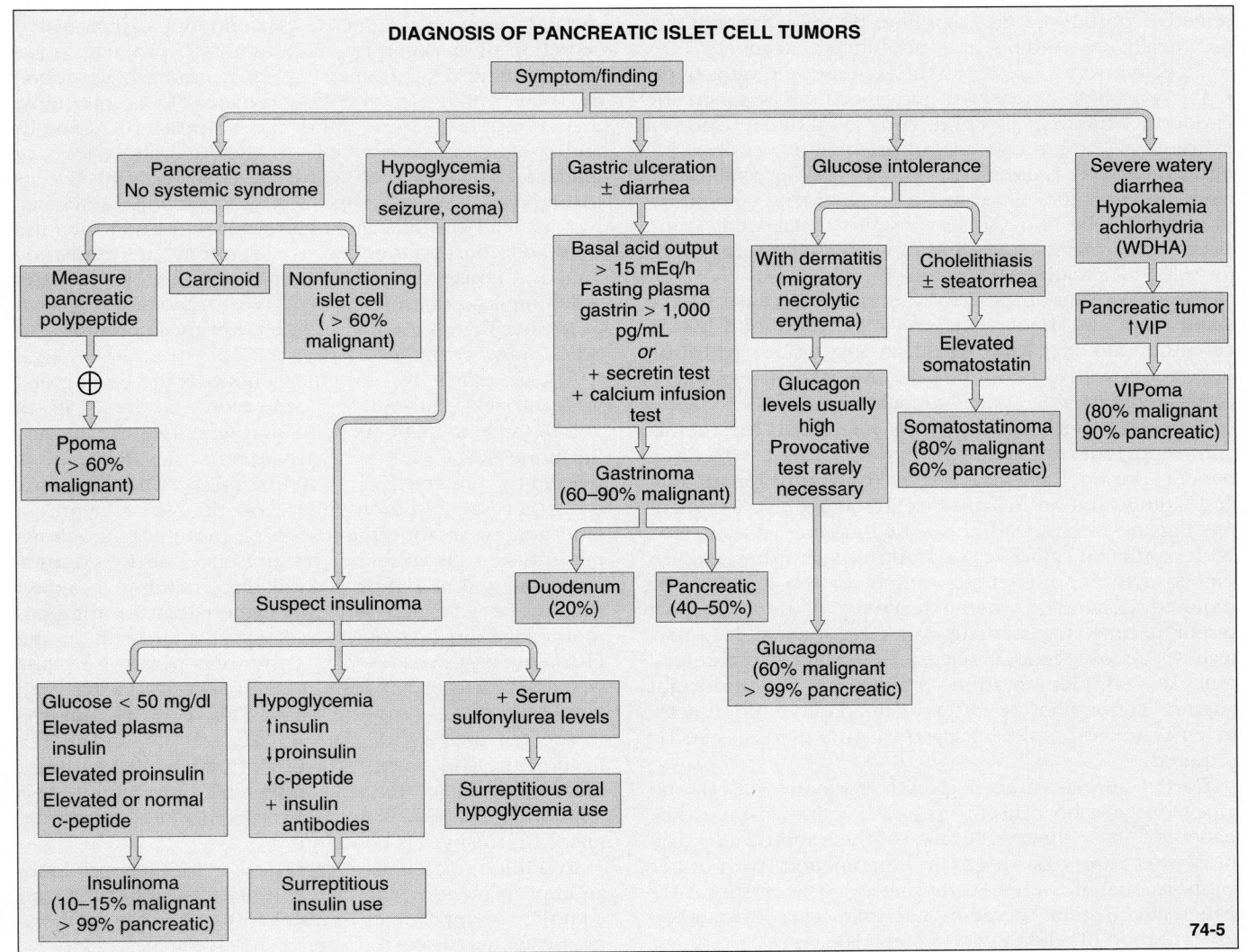

DIAGNOSIS OF PANCREATIC ISLET CELL TUMORS

74-5

by a relatively high plasma insulin level.[272,273] Other tests have been proposed, including a hypernormal response to tolbutamide, the response of plasma insulin to an infusion of calcium gluconate, and the ratio of proinsulin[273,274] to insulin in the plasma. The key to the diagnosis is a high index of suspicion.

Sporadic insulinomas are usually single and benign; about 10% are malignant.[275] Differentiation of benign from malignant is difficult from the pathologic features, but the presence of metastases defines malignancy. In patients with carcinoma, proinsulin may be increased in plasma[276] or circulating hCG.[277] In both malignant and benign insulinomas, jaundice may occur secondary to biliary tract obstruction from tumors in the head of the pancreas. The typical patient with symptoms of insulinoma has a single small benign pancreatic nodule. In atypical cases, with multiple primary endocrine tumors, including an insulinoma, one should suspect MEN-1 syndrome.[191] Because insulinomas are almost always confined to the pancreas, selective arteriography and portal venous sampling usually identify the lesion.[275] Endoscopic ultrasonography can be used to localize pancreatic endocrine tumors. Although such tumors have often been sought by pancreatic arteriography or selective portal venous sampling, these techniques are technically demanding and not always accurate. In a prospective series of 37 patients, endoscopic ultrasonography was highly sensitive and specific for pancreatic endocrine tumors, as confirmed by ultimate surgical excision.[278] The ultimate role of preoperative endoscopic ultrasonography is uncertain; until it is better established, many investigators continue to recommend abdominal ultrasonography and CT scan as the initial studies and reserve arteriography and intraoperative ultrasonography for selected situations.[279]

Surgical resection is usually curative because of the small size and benign nature of insulinomas. As in carcinoid tumor, partial resection may afford palliation in patients whose symptoms are disabling or cannot be controlled with nonsurgical modalities.

A patient with unresectable malignant insulinoma and recurrent episodes of hypoglycemia will often benefit, during the early stages, from appropriate diet and administration of an insulin antagonist. Frequent feedings between meals and at bedtime are administered with sufficient glucose to control symptoms. Adjustments in the carbohydrate content of the diet may be required, depending on the reactivity of the individual tumor, because the stimulus of a large glucose load may lead to an exaggerated release of insulin.[280] Parenteral glucose supplementation becomes an important adjunct in frequent or sustained hypoglycemic attacks; in emergencies, rapid injection of 50% glucose can be required.

Corticosteroids, human growth hormone (hGH), and glucagon have been useful palliative agents in individual patients.[281-284] However, because of their limited effectiveness, they are best used in combination with other antihormonal measures. Furthermore, glucagon stimulates pancreatic insulin secretion and may cause paradoxic exacerbation of a hypoglycemic episode.

A major advance in the palliation of malignant insulinoma came with the development of diazoxide. Its potent hyperglycemic properties, originally recognized during its use as an antihypertensive agent, have now been extended to the palliation of insulinoma and leucine-sensitive hypoglycemia of infancy.[285,286] Its principal action is to inhibit insulin release directly from the β cell.[265] It may also have an extrapancreatic hyperglycemic effect.[288] Diazoxide is administered orally in divided doses, ranging from 100 to 1000 mg/day. Although the plasma insulin level can often be reduced to a level that causes no symptoms, the tumor will continue to grow and metastasize if malignant, because diazoxide lacks anticancer activity. Diazoxide can cause edema, which can be corrected or prevented with a thiazide diuretic, which may also serve to reinforce the hyperglycemic effects.[273] Octreotide is valuable in the general management of all hormone-producing islet cell tumors. Octreotide reduces plasma insulin levels in at least 65% of patients with insulinoma.[289]

Glucagonoma

Glucagon from pancreatic α cells plays an important role in modulating serum glucose concentrations. Unregulated secretion of glucagon by α-cell tumors[290] produces a distinctive clinical syndrome.[291] A cutaneous rash, described as a necrotizing migratory erythema,[292] is the most characteristic feature. Mild insulin-resistant diabetes and weight loss attributable to the catabolic effects of glucagon are also seen. Glossitis, cheilosis, and venous thromboses can develop. Glucagon inhibits intestinal motility and the glucagonoma syndrome often includes ileus and constipation. Because symptoms are frequently mild and nonspecific, the tumor is often recognized late, when metastases are present.[291] Most tumors have grown to greater than 4.0 cm[293] in size at diagnosis, and 50% to 80% are metastatic.[293,294]

The diagnostic test for glucagonoma is the finding of a high plasma glucagon concentration (normal, 150 to 200 pg/mL). In patients with glucagonoma, the plasma hormone level is typically markedly elevated and is frequently greater than 1000 pg/mL.[294] The diagnosis is further suggested by failure of glucose to suppress glucagon, by an abnormal rise in plasma glucagon following infusion of arginine, by presence of hypoaminoacidemia, and if tumor is available, immunoperoxidase staining for glucagon. Reviews suggest that the tumor is more common in women and typically presents in the fifth and sixth decades.[295,296] Symptoms persist for many years before the diagnosis is made; survival, even with metastatic disease, may be lengthy. The primary tumor is in the tail or body of the pancreas in 50% and in the head of the pancreas in 8%; 42% of patients have diffuse involvement. The tumor is resectable for cure in less than one third of cases,[295] and recurrence after resection, mainly in the liver, is common.

In addition to surgical resection, octreotide produces an improvement of skin rash in up to 90% of patients and complete disappearance of rash in 30%.[289,297] Chemotherapeutic agents (discussed later) may have some activity.

Somatostatinoma

Somatostatin was first identified in pituitary cells, and a role in the regulation of growth hormone secretion was ascribed to it. Subsequently, it was recognized as a hormone of the islet δ cells. Somatostatin may serve as a paracrine regulator of other pancreatic islet cell hormones.[298] Inhibition of secretion of those hormones may account for some of the signs of somatostatinoma. In a review of 20 patients, 11 were noted to present with diabetes, 13 with gallbladder disease, and 7 with diarrhea.[299]

Somatostatinoma occurs most frequently in the head of the pancreas,[300] and as many as 80% of patients have evidence of metastases at diagnosis.[299] Somatostatinomas produce such common symptoms as diabetes and gallbladder disease; therefore, the clinician usually does not consider the diagnosis of somatostatinoma until late in the disease, at which time metastases are likely. Surgical resection is not usually curative.[299,301] Because of the relatively mild hormonally induced symptoms produced by somatostatin, octreotide does not have the same palliative benefit it has in other islet cell tumors. Cytoreductive surgery and chemotherapy may be the most appropriate palliative strategies.

Gastrinoma

Gastrin, the polypeptide hormone normally secreted by the G cell of the gastric antrum, stimulates gastric acid secretion. Tumors of the pancreatic or duodenal wall G cells are responsible for the signs and symptoms of Zollinger-Ellison syndrome, a disorder characterized by hypersecretion of gastrin. First described in 1955,[302] this syndrome is characterized by hypersecretion of gastric acid, severe peptic ulcer disease, and an islet cell tumor of the pancreas. It is estimated that less than 0.1% of patients with peptic ulcer disease have Zollinger-Ellison syndrome.[303]

The hallmark of the gastrinoma syndrome is recurrent peptic ulcer disease in spite of adequate medical or surgical treatment. Intermittent diarrhea, often with steatorrhea, may be present as a result of digestive enzyme inactivation in the small intestine by unbuffered gastric acid. All manifestations of the Zollinger-Ellison syndrome are secondary to hypersecretion of gastric acid.[304] A history of the MEN-1 syndrome has great significance, and gastrinoma may be present in up to 50% of these patients.[305] The combination of high gastric acid secretion and hypergastrinemia is strongly suggestive of gastrinoma, but this can also occur in patients with retained gastric antrum following surgery for peptic ulcer (antrectomy and Billroth II gastric resection) and following gastric outlet obstruction. Gastric rugal hypertrophy, multiple ulcers, or ulceration of the small bowel on radiographic studies suggests gastrinoma.[306]

In a review of 60 patients treated surgically for gastrinoma at Ohio State University, Ellison and associates[307] reported that the duration of ulcer symptoms prior to diagnosis averaged slightly more than 4 years. The incidence of MEN was 27%, and a primary tumor was detected in nearly 90% of cases. Gastrinoma can occur not only in the pancreas but also in extrapancreatic locations, including the duodenum, the stomach, and the retroperitoneal lymph nodes. More than one third of patients in the Ohio State series[307] had multiple tumors; metastatic disease in the liver was identified in 20% of patients.

The clinical diagnosis of Zollinger-Ellison syndrome has changed. Although the original case reports stressed the appearance of extensive and multiple gastric ulcers, a heightened index of suspicion and early detection have altered this pattern of disease presentation. The complete diagnosis of Zollinger-Ellison syndrome is based on four steps.[305] The first step is to identify fasting hypergastrinemia in association with a basal acid output greater than 15 mEq/hour. Generally, a gastrin level greater than 1000 pg/mL is pathognomonic. Less convincing elevations in fasting serum gastrin can be further evaluated by the secretin test, in which a peak level of serum gastrin higher than 200 pg/mL over the baseline following administration of secretin is considered diagnostic.[308] The remaining three steps include documentation of peptic ulcer disease, localization of the primary tumor, and assessment of benignancy versus malignancy.[309]

Localization of gastrinomas has been discussed extensively.[310,311] Techniques such as abdominal ultrasonography, CT scan, MRI, selective venous sampling for gastrin, and abdominal arteriography all have a role in the diagnosis and management of this disease. Because gastrinomas are so frequently malignant,[312,313] it is necessary to use every diagnostic modality to rule out metastatic disease before planning surgery.

The role of surgery in Zollinger-Ellison syndrome has changed over the past 20 years as a result of the introduction of RIA to diagnose hypergastrinemia and use of histamine H_2-receptor antagonists. The latter therapy has very significantly reduced the need to remove the end organ (the stomach); therefore, few patients will require surgical management to control the signs and symptoms of hypergastrinemia. In addition, gastrinomas are significantly less likely than insulinomas to be isolated, benign, or completely resectable. In a collected series of 457 surgical patients, only 69 (15%) were considered to have received surgery with curative intent.[307]

Ellison and associates[307] also analyzed 60 cases from their own institution to determine whether the introduction of the RIA for gastrinoma made earlier diagnosis more likely, with a higher possibility of curative resection. Before the introduction of the assay for serum gastrin levels, 15 of 25 (60%) patients underwent complete excision of all gross tumor. Of the 30 patients who underwent surgical treatment following availability of the assay, 18 (60%) had complete tumor resection. These results indicate no differences in rates of curative resection. However, resectability was associated with prolonged survival, with a 5-year survival rate of 69% in patients with resected tumor, compared with 38% in patients with unresectable disease. The 10-year survival rates were 38% and 9%, respectively. Nearly one half of the deaths were due to the effects of tumor and metastases. These data suggest, but do not prove, that earlier surgical intervention may prevent progression to the complications of bulky malignant tumor in some cases.

Medical management in gastrinoma is directed toward the hypersecretion of gastric acid. Before the introduction of histamine receptor antagonists, the only practical way to treat recurrent duodenal and jejunal ulcers was total gastrectomy. Cimetidine was reported to enhance recovery and make surgery less complicated, and to obviate surgery in some patients.[313] Histamine H_2-receptor antagonists alone or in combination with anticholinergic agents such as Pro-Banthine have been successful in producing long-term remissions of peptic ulcer disease complicating gastrinoma.[305] Second- and third-generation histamine H_2-receptor antagonists, such as ranitidine, famotidine, and the ion pump inhibitor omeprazole, have been reported to have progressively superior antisecretory activity, with few failures observed in patients who receive adequate doses.[314] Treatment for symptoms arising from tumor bulk from metastatic gastrinoma are discussed at the conclusion of this section.

Tumors Secreting Vasoactive Intestinal Peptide

In 1958, Verner and Morrison[315] described a syndrome of watery diarrhea, hypokalemia, and hypochlorhydria, and metabolic acidosis (the WDHA syndrome).[315] This syndrome is due to high circulating levels of vasoactive intestinal peptide secreted by a pancreatic islet tumor (VIPoma). Studies of VIP infusions in healthy volunteers have generally supported the concept that the diarrhea in VIPoma patients may be directly caused by elevated circulating levels of vasoactive intestinal polypeptide.[316] Because most patients with this syndrome have metastatic disease at presentation, usually to the liver, management is mainly medical, with chemotherapy or somatostatin analog. Surgical resection is rarely curative.[314] As with carcinoid tumors and other islet cell tumors, however, in patients with locally unresectable disease or those with hepatic metastases, surgical cytoreduction may improve symptom control.

Surgical Management

Pancreatic islet cell tumors are a challenging problem for the endocrine surgeon. Most are sporadic, but they can also occur as part of the MEN-1 syndrome. Patients with MEN-1 usually develop multicentric tumors that often preclude the ability to perform a curative resection. The commonly occurring islet cell tumors secrete gastrin, insulin, glucagon, pancreatic polypeptide, or somatostatin. These tumors can have profound physiologic effects; even in cases in which complete resection is not possible, tumor debulking may be indicated to alleviate the physiologic effects of hormone secretion. The surgical management of the commonly encountered pancreatic islet cell tumors is briefly discussed.

Gastrinoma

Gastrinomas occur within the pancreas or are found submucosally within the duodenum. Approximately 75% are malignant, with liver metastases a common finding.

CT scan is the best method to evaluate patients for resection. Patients with solitary tumors can be treated with enucleation or distal pancreatectomy; however, a Whipple's resection should be avoided. Duodenal tumors can be locally resected from the wall of the duodenum. Occasionally, localized metastases can be resected to control excess gastric secretion. Patients with unresectable gastrinoma whose acid secretion cannot be controlled medically require a total gastrectomy with esophagojejunostomy.

Insulinoma

Approximately 75% of insulinomas are solitary benign tumors. Preoperative evaluation begins with a CT scan. Small tumors that cannot be found by CT scan may be localized preoperatively with transhepatic portal venous sampling. Rarely, these techniques will establish a diagnosis of nesidioblastosis, which can be treated surgically by subtotal pancreatectomy. Patients with an insulinoma that cannot be localized preoperatively should undergo exploratory laparotomy. The entire pancreas should be exposed by a generous Kocher maneuver, entered through the lesser sac. Intraoperative ultrasound is very helpful in localizing small tumors and as an aid to avoid ductal injury during enucleation. After enucleation, the pancreatic surface is closed, and the area should be drained because of the possibility of pancreatic fistula.

Medical Management

Somatostatin Analog

The somatostatin analog octreotide is as useful in the treatment of syndromes associated with ectopic hormone production in islet cell tumors as it is in treatment of carcinoid tumors. In 1985, Santangelo and associates[317] described a single patient with life-threatening pancreatic cholera, successfully controlled by the synthetic somatostatin analog. A later series of patients from the Mayo Clinic[318] significantly supplemented these data; in this series, 24 patients with islet cell tumor were treated. The response to somatostatin analog was prompt and palliated symptoms. However, the median duration of response was only 2.5 months, with only 2 of 24 patients continuing to benefit beyond 1 year. Also, in a review of 66 cases[289] treated with octreotide, only 8 (12%) showed any indication of objective tumor response. The short duration of response and meager incidence of objective tumor regression suggest that somatostatin analog in the treatment of metastatic islet cell tumors has a more limited role than in carcinoid tumors.

Interferon

As somatostatin analog was being shown to be useful in patients with pancreatic cholera, the first reports of the use of interferon in such patients appeared.[319] In the initial report, two patients with the therapy-resistant pancreatic cholera syndrome were successfully treated with human leukocyte interferon, with reduction in tumor mass in one of the patients. Extending these observations, Swedish investigators reported on 22 patients treated with human leukocyte interferon, with an objective response rate of 77% and a median duration of response of 8.5 months.[258] Most of these responses were documented by decreased hormone production. Only 6 of 22 (27%) cases had objective reduction in tumor bulk. Further evaluation of interferon, with and without chemotherapy, is warranted. The mechanism of action of interferon in islet cell and carcinoid tumors is unknown.

Chemotherapy

As with carcinoid tumors, the use of cytotoxic chemotherapy in a patient with an islet cell tumor is not a first choice for therapy.[268] Chemotherapy is generally attempted in patients with symptoms due to tumor bulk that may not be palliated by cytoreductive surgery or in patients with uncontrolled syndromes of hormone excess. In contrast to carcinoid tumors, islet cell carcinomas are generally more responsive to chemotherapy. The first chemotherapeutic drug to elicit significant attention in the treatment of islet cell tumors was the antitumor antibiotic streptozotocin. This drug has a diabetogenic action in some animals that is correlated with selective uptake of the drug by pancreatic β cells.[268,320] In 1975, Kahn and associates[321] described two patients with pancreatic cholera and islet cell carcinoma successfully treated with intra-arterial streptozotocin. Subsequently, a number of chemotherapeutic drugs were identified as having activity in islet cell tumors (Table 74-8).

With the identification of 5-FU as a potentially useful drug in these tumors,[322] combination chemotherapy also began to be investigated. In a phase II trial of the combination of 5-FU and streptozotocin, six objective responses were noted in eight patients. In 1980 a larger study from the ECOG was reported, in which streptozotocin alone was compared with streptozotocin plus 5-FU in advanced islet cell carcinomas.[323] The combination was superior to streptozotocin alone in overall rate of response (63% versus 13%). These responses

were generally of long duration and yielded meaningful improvements in performance status and symptoms. The median survival time of patients receiving the combination was 26 months compared with 16.5 months in the group receiving streptozotocin alone. The combination was associated with a higher degree of nausea and vomiting, myelosuppression, and nephrotoxicity. With the identification of doxorubicin as a potentially useful drug in islet cell tumors,[324] the ECOG also piloted a randomized trial in which doxorubicin plus streptozotocin was compared with the earlier standard of 5-FU plus streptozotocin.[218] The results from this study[325] demonstrate that the doxorubicin plus streptozotocin combination produced objective response in 69% of cases, with a median duration of response in excess of 20 months and a median survival time of 2.2 years. This regimen is superior to the 5-FU plus streptozotocin combination both in tumor response and in survival. A study of 12 patients with islet cell carcinomas treated with the combination streptozotocin, doxorubicin, and 5-FU reported a 54% response.[338] However, these were partial responses and no complete responses were found.

A number of other chemotherapy drugs have demonstrated activity in islet cell tumors. Chlorozotocin, an analog of streptozotocin, has been shown to be less nephrotoxic but more myelosuppressive than the parent drug. In phase II trials of chlorozotocin, responses were significant when it was used alone or with 5-FU.[326,327] Unfortunately, chlorozotocin is no longer being produced. DTIC also has activity in islet cell tumors, and this agent is undergoing a prospective clinical trial by the ECOG. Other agents of interest include etoposide and cisplatin, which are active in various neuroectodermally derived tumors. The combination of etoposide and cisplatin has been shown to have activity in small cell lung cancer, and a recent trial demonstrates that more than 60% of anaplastic carcinoid and islet cell tumors respond to this combination, whereas well-differentiated tumors do not respond.[328] A phase II trial with DTIC, 5-FU, and leucovorin reported an overall response rate of 27%; however, 50% of the patients had carcinoid tumors which, as a subset, demonstrated particularly poor response.[334]

Liver-Directed Therapy

As is the case with carcinoid tumor, islet cell tumors frequently result in predominantly hepatic metastases, and reduction in tumor bulk in the liver may significantly influence hormone production and quality of life. For that reason, resection of hepatic metastases is warranted in selected patients. The use of hepatic radiation has been reported only anecdotally. Of two patients treated at the National Cancer Institute, one patient with a VIPoma had significant resolution of watery diarrhea for 25 months; the other, with gastrinoma, had significant diminution in abdominal pain and of gastrin levels.[329] Endocrine and tumor response to hepatic arterial occlusion with or without chemotherapy can be impressive. The Mayo Clinic experience[216,263] documents, in 46 patients with islet cell tumors, that a large proportion of cases had complete disappearance of tumor-related symptoms. Eighty percent to 90% of cases had some degree of

TABLE 74-8

▨ Chemotherapy for Islet Cell Tumors		
DRUG TREATMENT	**RESPONSE RATES (RANGE 36%–62%)**	**REFERENCES**
Single agents		
Streptozotocin	45	26
Doxorubicin	20	324
DTIC	9	216
Chlorozotocin	53	326
Combination chemotherapy		
Streptozotocin + 5-FU	63	323
Streptozotocin + doxorubicin	69	324
Streptozotocin + 5-FU + doxorubicin	40	330
Streptozotocin + 5-FU + doxorubicin	54	333
DTIC + 5-FU + leucovorin	27	335

DTIC, dacarbazine; 5-FU, 5-fluorouracil.

response. Chemotherapy in addition to hepatic arterial occlusion improved the duration of response, but this was not a randomized comparison. However, both objective tumor responses and hormonal regressions were frequent, and the increased activity of chemotherapy in these tumors supports the use of systemic therapy with or without HAO techniques. The use of cryosurgery for treatment of hepatic metastases that are resistant to chemotherapy has also been reported.[335] This approach has been reported to be effective in treating symptoms, but effect on survival has not been demonstrated.

REFERENCES

1. Landis SH, Murray T, Bolden S, Wingo PA: Cancer statistics, 1998. CA Cancer J Clin 1998;48:6.
2. DeGroot LJ: Radiation-Associated Thyroid Carcinoma. Orlando, Grune & Stratton, 1976.
3. Tucker MA, Meadows AT, Merris-Jones P, et al: Therapeutic radiation at young age, linked to secondary thyroid cancer. Proc Am Soc Clin Oncol 1986;5:211.
4. Ron E, Modan B, Preston D, et al: Thyroid neoplasia following low-dose radiation in childhood. Radiol Res 1989;120:516.
5. Shore RE, Hildreth N, Dvoretsky P, et al: Thyroid cancer among persons given x-ray treatment in infancy for an enlarged thymus gland. Am J Epidemiol 1993;137:1068.
6. Carroll RJ, Schafer DW, Lubin JH, Ron E, Stovall M: Thyroid cancer after scalp irradiation: A reanalysis accounting for uncertainty in dosimetry. Radiat Res 2000;154:721, discussion 723.
7. Tuttle RM, Becker DV: The Chernobyl accident and its consequences: Update at the millennium. Semin Nucl Med 2000;30:133.
8. Cetta F, Montalto G, Petracci M, Fusco A: Thyroid cancer and the Chernobyl accident. Are long-term and long distance side effects of fall-out radiation greater than estimated? J Clin Endocrinol Metab 1997;82:2015.
9. Hancock SL, Cox RS, McDougall IR: Thyroid diseases after treatment of Hodgkin's disease. N Engl J Med 1991;325:599.
10. Doniach I: Experimental induction of tumours of the thyroid by radiation. Br Med Bull 1958;14:181.
11. McDougall IR: Radiation and the thyroid. In McDougall IR (ed): Thyroid Disease in Clinical Practice. London, Chapman & Hall, 1992, p 304.
12. Fraker DL: Radiation exposure and other factors. Endocr Surg 1995;75:365.
13. Fugazzola L, Pierotti MA, Vigano E, Pacini F, Vorontsova TV, Bongarzone I: Molecular and biochemical analysis of RET/PTC4, a novel oncogenic rearrangement between RET and ELE1 genes, in a post-Chernobyl papillary thyroid cancer. Oncogene 1996;13:1093.
14. Elisei R, Romei C, Vorontsova T, et al: RET/PTC rearrangements in thyroid nodules: Studies in irradiated and not irradiated, malignant and benign thyroid lesions in children and adults. J Clin Endocrinol Metab 2001;86:3211.
15. Kwok C, McDougall IR: Familial differentiated carcinoma of the thyroid: Report of 5 families. Thyroid 1995;5:395-397.
16. Carlisle M, McDougall IR: Familial differentiated carcinoma of the thyroid. In Biersack HJ, Grunwald F (eds): Thyroid Cancer in the Year 2000. New York, Springer, 2001, p 77.
17. Horn-Ross P, Morris JS, Lee M, et al: Iodine and thyroid cancer risk among women in a multiethnic population. Cancer Epidemiol Biomarkers Prevention 2001;10:979.
18. Maffaferi FL: Papillary thyroid carcinoma: Factors influencing prognosis and current therapy. Semin Oncol 1987;14:315.
19. Merino MJ: Variant forms of thyroid carcinoma. In Robbins J (moderator): Thyroid Cancer: A Lethal Endocrine Neoplasm. Ann Intern Med 1991;115:133.
20. Martinez-Tello FJ, Martinez-Cabruja R, Fernandez-Martin J, et al: Occult carcinoma of the thyroid. Cancer 1993;71:4022.
21. Sessions RB, Davidson BJ: Thyroid cancer. Med Clin North Am 1993;77:517.
22. Scheumann GFW, Gimm O, Wegener G, et al: Prognostic significance and surgical management of locoregional lymph node metastases in papillary thyroid cancer. World J Surg 1994;18:559.
23. Mazzaferri EL, Jhiang SM: Long-term impact of initial surgical and medical therapy on papillary and follicular thyroid cancer. Am J Med 1994;97:418.
24. DeGroot LJ, Kaplan EL, McCormick M, Straus FH: Natural history, treatment, and course of papillary thyroid carcinoma. J Clin Endocrinol Metab 1990;71:414.
25. Sanders LE, Cady B: Differential thyroid cancer: Reexamination of risk groups and outcome of treatment. Arch Surg 1998;133:419.
26. Norton JA, Levin B, Jensen RT: Cancer of the endocrine system. In DeVita VT, Hellman S, Rosenberg SA (eds): Cancer Principles and Practice of Oncology, 4th ed. Philadelphia, JB Lippincott, 1993.
27. Hay ID BE, Goellner JR, Ebersold JR, Grant CS: Predicting outcome in thyroid carcinoma: Development of a reliable prognostic scoring system in a cohort of 1779 patients surgically treated at one institute during 1940 through 1989. Surgery 1993;114:1050.
28. Russell WO, Ibanex ML, Clark RL, White EC: Follicular (organoid) carcinoma of the thyroid gland. Report of 84 cases in thyroid cancer. UICC Monogr Series 1969;12:14.
29. Schlumberger MJ: Papillary and follicular thyroid carcinoma. N Engl J Med 1998;338:297.
30. Iida F, Yonekura M, Miyakawa M: Study of intraglandular dissemination of thyroid cancer. Cancer 1969;24:764.
31. Brennan MD, Bergstrahl EJ, van Heerden JA, McConahey WM: Follicular thyroid cancer treated at the Mayo Clinic: 1946 through 1970. Initial manifestations, pathologic findings, therapy and outcome. Mayo Clin Proc 1991;66:11.
32. Tollefson HR, DeCosse JJ: Papillary carcinoma of the thyroid: Recurrence in the thyroid gland after initial treatment. Am J Surg 1983;1066:728.
33. Van Heerden JA, Groh MA, Grant CS: Early postoperative morbidity after surgical treatment of thyroid carcinoma. Surgery 1986;101:224.
34. Matias-Guiu X, Cuatrecasas M, Musulen E, Prat J: p53 expression in anaplastic carcinomas arising from thyroid papillary carcinomas. J Clin Pathol 1994;47:337.
35. Ain KB: Management of undifferentiated thyroid cancer. Baillieres Best Pract Res Clin Endocrinol Metab 2000;14:615.
36. Grant CS: Operative and postoperative management of the patient with follicular and Hürthle cell carcinoma. Surg Clin North Am 1995;75:395.
37. Heppe H, Armin A, Calandm DB, et al: Hürthle cell tumors of the thyroid gland. Surgery 1985;98:1162.
38. Arganini M, Behar R, Wu TC, et al: Hürthle cell tumors: A twenty-five year experience. Surgery 1986;100:1108.
39. Gundry SR, Burhey RE, Thompson NW, Lloyd R: Total thyroidectomy for Hürthle cell neoplasm of the thyroid. Arch Surg 1983;118:529.
40. Byar DP, Green SB, Dot P, et al: A prognostic index for thyroid carcinoma. A study of the EORTC thyroid cancer cooperative group. Eur J Cancer Clin Oncol 1979;15:1033.
41. Harmer MT: Application of the TNM classification rules to malignant tumors of the thyroid gland. In Thyroid Cancer. UICC Monograph Series 1969;12:64.
42. Belal AA, Allam A, Kandil A, et al: Primary thyroid lymphoma: A retrospective analysis of prognostic factors and treatment outcome for localized intermediate and high grade lymphoma. Am J Clin Oncol 2001;24:299.
43. Macdonald JS: Thyroid carcinoma. In Schein PS (ed): Decision Making in Oncology. New York, BC Decker, 1988, p 88.
44. Barsano CP, Skosey C, DeGroot LJ, Refetoff S: Serum thyroglobulin in the management of patients with thyroid cancer. Arch Intern Med 1982;142:763.
45. Haugen BR, Ridgway EC, McLaughlin BA, McDermott MT: Clinical comparison of whole-body radioiodine scan and serum thyroglobulin after stimulation with recombinant human thyrotropin. Thyroid 2002;12:37.
46. Miller JM, Hamburger JI: The thyroid scintigram. I. The hot nodule. Radiology 1965;84:66.

47. Nagai GR PW, Basso L, Cisco JA, McDougall IR: Scintigraphically hot nodules and thyroid cancer. Clin Nucl Med 1987;6:123.

48. Belfiori A, Garofalo MR, Giuffrida D, Runello F, Filetti S, Fiurmana A: Increased aggressiveness of thyroid cancer in patients with Graves' disease. J Endocrinol Metabol 1990;70:830–835.

49. Mazzaferri EL: Management of a solitary thyroid nodule. N Engl J Med 1993;328:553.

50. Chung JK: Sodium iodide symporter: Its role in nuclear medicine. J Nucl Med 2002;43:1188.

51. Ashcraft MW, Van Herle AJ: Management of thyroid nodules. Head Neck Surg 1981;3:216.

52. Gershengom MC, McClung MR, Chu EW, et al: Fine-needle aspiration cytology in the preoperative diagnosis of thyroid nodules. Ann Intern Med 1977;87:256.

53. Lowhagen T, Granberg PO, Lundell G, et al: Aspiration biopsy cytology (ABC) in nodules of the thyroid gland suspected to be malignant. Surg Clin North Am 1979;59:3.

54. VanHerle AJ, Rich P, Ljung BM, et al: The thyroid nodule. Ann Intern Med 1982;96:221.

55. Carmeci C, Jeffrey RB, McDougall IR, et al: Ultrasound-guided fine-needle aspiration biopsy of thyroid masses. Thyroid 1998;8:283.

56. Schlumberger MJ: Papillary and follicular thyroid carcinoma. N Engl J Med 1998;338:297.

57. Carlisle M, Lu C, McDougall IR: The interpretation of ^{131}I scans in the evaluation of thyroid cancer, with an emphasis on false positive findings. Nucl Med Commun 2003;24:715.

58. Soh EY, Clark OH: Surgical considerations and approach to thyroid cancer. Thyroid Cancer 1996;25:115.

59. Weigel RJ: Advances in the diagnosis and management of well-differentiated thyroid cancer. Curr Opin Oncol 1996;8:37.

60. Orsenigo E, Beretta E, Veronesi P, et al: Total thyroidectomy in the treatment of thyroid cancer. Eur J Surg Oncol 1995 ;21:478.

61. Stephenson BM, Wheeler MH, Clark OH: The role of total thyroidectomy in the management of differentiated thyroid cancer. Curr Opin Gen Surg 1994;6:53.

62. Patwardhan N, Cataldo T, Braverman LE: Surgical management of papillary cancer. Endocr Surg 1995;75:449.

63. Nguyen KV, Dilawari RA: Predictive value of AMES scoring system in selection of extent of surgery in well differentiated carcinoma of thyroid. Am Surg 1995;61:151.

64. Shaha AR, Shah JP, Loree TR: Low-risk differentiated thyroid cancer: The need for selective treatment. Ann Surg Oncol 1997;4:328.

65. Wanebo H, Coburn M, Teates D, Cole B: Total thyroidectomy does not enhance disease control or survival even in high-risk patients with differentiated thyroid cancer. Ann Surg 1998;227:912.

66. Samaan NA, Schultz PN, Hickey RC, et al: The results of various modalities of treatment of well differentiated thyroid carcinoma: A retrospective review of 1599 patients. J Clin Endocrinol 1992;75:714.

67. Loh K-C, Greenspan FS, Gee L, et al: Pathological tumor-node-metastasis (pTNM) staging for papillary and follicular thyroid carcinomas: A retrospective analysis of 700 patients. J Clin Endocrinol Metab 1997;82:3553.

68. Arad E, O'Mara RE, Wilson GA: Ablation of remaining functioning thyroid lobe with radioiodine after hemithyroidectomy for carcinoma. Clin Nucl Med 1993;18:662.

69. Samuel AM, Rajashekharrao B: Radioiodine therapy for well-differentiated thyroid cancer: A quantitative dosimetric evaluation for remnant thyroid ablation after surgery. J Nucl Med 1994;35:1944.

70. DiRusso G, Kern KA: Comparative analysis of complications from I-131 radioablation for well-differentiated thyroid cancer. Surgery 1994;116:1024.

71. Pacini F, Cetani F, Miccoli P, et al: Outcome of 309 patients with metastatic differentiated thyroid carcinoma treated with radioiodine. World J Surg 1994;18:600.

72. Lin J-D, Kao P-F, Chao T-C: The effects of radioactive iodine in thyroid remnant ablation and treatment of well differentiated thyroid carcinoma. Br J Radiol 1998;71:307.

73. Leeper RD: The effect of ^{131}I therapy on survival of patients with metastatic papillary or follicular thyroid carcinoma. J Clin Endocrinol Metab 1973;36:1143.

74. Coburn M, Teates D, Wanebo HJ: Recurrent thyroid cancer: Role of surgery versus radioactive iodine (I^{131}). Ann Surg 1994;219:587.

75. Hindie E, Melliere D, Lange F, et al: Functioning pulmonary metastases of thyroid cancer: Does radioiodine influence the prognosis. Eur J Nucl Med Mol Imaging 2003;30:974.

76. Park HM, Park YH, Zhou XH: Detection of thyroid remnant/metastasis without stunning: An ongoing dilemma. Thyroid 1997;7:277.

77. McDougall IR: 74 MBq radioiodine ^{131}I does not prevent uptake of therapeutic doses of ^{131}I (i.e., it does not cause stunning) in differentiated thyroid cancer. Nucl Med Commun 1997;18:505.

78. Pineda JD, Lee T, Ain K, et al: Iodine-131 therapy for thyroid cancer patients with elevated thyroglobulin and negative diagnostic scan. J Clin Endocrinol Metab 1995;80:1488.

79. McDougall IR: ^{131}I treatment of ^{131}I negative whole body scan, and positive thyroglobulin in differentiated thyroid carcinoma: what is being treated? Thyroid 1997;7:669.

80. McDougall IR, Davidson J, Segall GM: Positron emission tomography of the thyroid, with an emphasis on thyroid cancer. Nucl Med Commun 2001;22:485.

81. Karwowski J, Jeffrey RB, McDougall IR, Weigel RJ: Intraoperative ultrasonography improves identification of recurrent thyroid cancer. Surgery 2002;132:924.

82. Pochin EE: Leukaemia following radioiodine treatment of thyrotoxicosis. BMJ 1960;2:1545.

83. Meier CA, Braverman LE, Ebner SA, et al: Diagnostic use of recombinant human thyrotropin in patients with thyroid carcinoma (phase I/II study). J Clin Endocrinol Metab 1994;78:188.

84. Ladenson PW, Braverman LE, Mazzaferri EL, et al: Comparison of administration of recombinant human thyrotropin with withdrawal of thyroid hormone for radioactive iodine scanning in patients with thyroid carcinoma. N Engl J Med 1997;337:888.

85. McDougall I, Weigel RJ: Recombinant human thyrotropin in the management of thyroid cancer. Curr Opin Oncol 2001;13:39.

86. Robbins RJ, Larson SM, Sinha N, et al: A retrospective review of the effectiveness of recombinant human TSH as a preparation for radioiodine thyroid remnant ablation. J Nucl Med 2002;43(11):1482.

87. Farahati J, Reiners C, Stuschke M, et al: Differentiated thyroid cancer. Cancer 1996;77:172.

88. Tsang RW, Brierley JD, Simpson WJ, et al: The effects of surgery, radioiodine, and external radiation therapy on the clinical outcome of patients with differentiated thyroid carcinoma. Cancer 1998;82:375.

89. Tennvall J, Lundell G, Hallquist A, et al, and the Swedish Anaplastic Thyroid Cancer Group: Combined doxorubicin, hyperfractionated radiotherapy, and surgery in anaplastic thyroid carcinoma. Cancer 1994;74:1348.

90. Cady B, Sedwick CE, Meissner WA, et al: Changing clinical, pathology treatment and survival pattern in differentiated thyroid carcinoma. Surgery 1976;184:541.

91. Roundebush CP, DeGroot LJ: The natural history of radiation-associated thyroid cancer. In DeGroot LJ (ed): Radiation-Associated Thyroid Carcinoma. Orlando, Grune & Stratton, 1977.

92. Shimaoka K: Suppressive therapy with thyroid hormones. In DeGroot LJ (ed): Radiation-Associated Thyroid Carcinoma. Orlando, Grune & Stratton, 1977.

93. Schneider AG, Favus MJ, Stachura ME, et al: Incidence, prevalence and characteristics of radiation-induced thyroid cancer. Am J Med 1978;64:243.

94. Schneider AB, Recant W, Pinsky SM, et al: Radiation-induced thyroid cancer. Ann Intern Med 1986;105:405.

95. Kvols LK, Buck M: Chemotherapy of endocrine malignancies: A review. Semin Oncol 1987;14:343.

96. Shimaoka K, Schoenfeld DA, Lerner H: A randomized trial of Adriamycin versus Adriamycin plus cisplatinum in patients with thyroid cancer. Proc Am Soc Clin Oncol 1983;2:168.

97. Williams SD, Birch R, Einhom LH: Phase II evaluation of doxorubicin and cisplatin in advanced thyroid cancer. Cancer Treat Rep 1986;70:405.

98. Williams ED: Histogenesis of medullary carcinoma of the thyroid. J Clin Pathol 1966;19:114.

Specific Malignancies

III

99. Hill CS Jr, Ibanez ML, Samaan NA, et al: Medullary (solid) carcinoma of the thyroid gland: an analysis of the MD Anderson Hospital experience with patients with the tumor, its special features and its histogenesis. Medicine (Baltimore) 1973;52:141.

100. Moley JF: Medullary thyroid cancer. Surg Clin North Am 1995;75:405.

101. Keiser HR, Beaven MA, Doppman J, et al: Sipple's syndrome: Medullary thyroid carcinoma, pheochromocytoma and parathyroid disease. Ann Intern Med 1973;78:561.

102. Williams ED, Brown CL, Doniach I: Pathological and clinical findings in 67 cases of medullary carcinoma of the thyroid. J Clin Pathol 1966;19:103.

103. Chin WW, Goodman RH, Jacobs JW, et al: Medullary thyroid carcinoma identified by cell-free translation of tumor messenger ribonucleic acid in a patient with neck mass and syndrome of etopic adrenocorticotropin. J Clin Endocrinol Metab 1981;52:572.

104. Melvin KEW, Tashjian AH Jr: Studies in familial (medullary) thyroid carcinoma. Recent Progr Horm Res 1972;28:399.

105. Alexander HR, Norton JA: Biology and management of medullary thyroid carcinoma of the parafollicular cells. Ann Intern Med 1991;115:133.

106. Baylin SB, Beaven MA, Engelman K, Sjoerdsma A: Elevated histaminase activity in medullary carcinoma of the thyroid. N Engl J Med 1970;283:1239.

107. Atkins E, Beaven MA, Keiser JR: Dopa decarboxylase in medullary carcinoma of the thyroid. N Engl J Med 1973;289:545.

108. Baylin SB, Beaven MA, Keiser HR, et al: Serum histaminase and calcitonin levels in medullary carcinoma of the thyroid. Lancet 1972;1:455.

109. Williams ED, Karim SMM, Sandlet M: Prostaglandin secretion by medullary carcinoma of the thyroid. Lancet 1968;1:22.

110. Wolfe HJ, Melvin KEW, Cervi-Skinner SJ, et al: C-cell hyperplasia preceding medullary thyroid carcinoma. N Engl J Med 1973;289:437.

111. Gagel RF, Melvin KEW, Tashjian AH Jr, et al: Natural history of familial medullary thyroid carcinoma-pheochromocytoma syndrome and identification of preneoplastic stages by screening studies: Five year report. Trans Assoc Am Physicians 1975;87:177.

112. Miller HH, Melvin KEW, Gibson JM, Tashjian AH Jr: Surgical approach to early familial medullary carcinoma of the thyroid. Am J Surg 1972;123:438.

113. Jones BA, Sisson JE: Early diagnosis and thyroidectomy in multiple endocrine neoplasia, type 2b. J Pediatr 1983;102:219.

114. Wells S Jr, Chi DD, Toshima K, et al: Predictive DNA testing and prophylactic thyroidectomy in patients at risk for multiple endocrine neoplasia type 2A. Ann Surg 1994;220:237.

115. Kallinowski F, Buhr HJ, Meybier H, et al: Medullary carcinoma of the thyroid—Therapeutic strategy derived from fifteen years of experience. Surgery 1993;114:491.

116. Deftos LJ, Stein MF: Radioiodine as an adjunct to the surgical treatment of medullary thyroid carcinoma. J Clin Endocrinol Metab 1980;50:967.

117. Chen H, Roberts JR, Ball DW, et al: Effective long-term palliation of symptomatic, incurable metastatic medullary thyroid cancer by operative resection. Ann Surg 1998;227:887.

118. Jerkins TW, Sacks HS, O'Dorisio TM, et al: Medullary carcinoma of the thyroid, pancreatic nesidioblastosis and microadenosis, and pancreatic polypeptide hypersecretion: A new association and clinical and hormonal responses to long-acting somatostatin analog SMS 201-995. J Clin Endocrinol Metab 1987;64:1313.

119. Hutter AM Jr, Kayhoe DE: Adrenal cortical carcinoma. Am J Med 1966;41:572.

120. National Cancer Institute Monograph: Third National Cancer Surgery: Incidence Data, Vol 41 (DHEW Pub NIH75-787). Bethesda, National Cancer Institute, 1975.

121. Lipsett MG, Ross GT, Hertz R: Clinical and pathophysiologic aspects of adrenocortical carcinoma. Am J Med 1963;35:374.

122. Bertagna C, Orth DN: Clinical and laboratory findings and results of therapy in 58 patients with adrenocortical tumors admitted to a single medical center (1951–1978). Am J Med 1981;71:855.

123. Gabrilove JL, Sharma DC, Wotiz HH, Doffman R: Feminizing adrenal cortical cancers in the male: A review of 52 cases including a case report. Medicine (Baltimore) 1965;44:37.

124. Wohltmann H, Mathurl RS, Williamson HP: Sexual precocity in a female infant due to feminizing adrenal carcinoma. J Clin Endocrinol Metab 1980;50:186.

125. Crane MG, Harris JJ: Desoxycorticosterone secretion rates in hyperadrenocorticism. J Clin Endocrinol Metab 1966;26:1135.

126. Grim CE, Ganguly A, Yum MN, et al: Hyperaldosteronism due to unsuspected adrenal carcinoma: Discovery during investigation of hypertension in a young woman. J Urol 1981;126:783.

127. Ross NS, Aron DC: Hormonal evaluation of the patient with an incidentially discovered adrenal mass. N Engl J Med 1990;323:1401.

128. Doppman JL, Reinig JW, Dwyer AJ, et al: Differentiation of adrenal masses by magnetic resonance imaging. Surgery 1987;102:1018.

129. Reinig JW, Doppman JL, Dwyer AJ, et al: Distincting between adrenal adenomas and metastases using MR imaging. J Comput Assist Tomogr 1985;9:898.

130. Schteingart DE, Seabold JE, Gross MD, Swanton DP: Iodocholesterol adrenal tissue uptake and imaging in adrenal neoplasm. J Clin Endocrinol Metab 1981;52:1156.

131. MCCorkell SJ, Miles NL: Fine-needle aspiration of catecholamine-producing adrenal masses. A possibly fatal mistake. Am J Roentgenol 1985;145:113.

132. Casola G, Nicolet V, Van Sonnenberg E, et al: Unsuspected pheochromocytomas: Risk of blood pressure alternations during percutaneous adrenal biopsy. Radiology 1986;159:733.

133. Cohn K, Gortesman L, Brennan M: Adrenocortical carcinoma. Surgery 1986;100:1170.

134. Hough AJ, Hollifield JW, Page DL, et al: Prognostic factors in adrenal cortical tumors. A mathematical analysis of clinical and morphologic data. Am J Clin Pathol 1979;72:390.

135. Luton JP, Cerdas S, Billaud L, et al: Clinical features of adrenocortical carcinoma. Prognostic factors and the effect of mitotane therapy. N Engl J Med 1990;322:1195.

136. Daniels H, Van Amstel WJ, Schopman W, Van Dommelen C: Effect of metopirone in a patient with adrenocortical carcinoma. Acta Endocrinol (Copenh) 1963;44:346.

137. Cash R, Brough AJ, Coehn MNP, Satoh PS: Aminoglutethimide (Elipten, Ciba) as an inhibitor of adrenal steroidogenesis: Mechanism of action and therapeutic trial. J Clin Endocrinol Metab 1967;27:1239.

138. Gorden P, Becker CE, Levey GS, Roth J: Efficacy of aminoglutethimide in the ectopic ACTH syndrome. J Clin Endocrinol Metab 1968;28:921.

139. Schteingart DE, Cash R, Coon JW: Aminoglutethimide and metastatic adrenal cancer. JAMA 1966;198:1007.

140. Fishman LM, Liddie GW, Island DP, et al: Effects of amino-glutethimide on adrenal function in man. J Clin Endocrinol Metab 1967;27:481.

141. Cueto C, Brown JH: Biological studies on an adrenocorticolytic agent and the isolation of the active components. Endocrinology 1958;62:334.

142. Nichols J, Henninger G: Studies on DDD, 2,2-bis(para-chlorophenyl)-1,1' dichloroethane. Exp Med Surg 1957;15:310.

143. Vilar P, Tullner WW: Effects of o,p'DDD on history and 17-hydroxycorticosteroids output of the dog adrenal cortex. Endocrinology 1959;65:80.

144. Hutter AM, Kayhoe DE: Adrenal cortical carcinoma: Results of treatment with o,p'DDD in 138 patients. Am J Med 1966;41:581.

145. Lubitz JA, Freeman L, Okun R: Mitotane use in inoperable adrenal cortical carcinoma. JAMA 1973;223:1109.

146. Nader S, Hickey RC, Sellin RV, Samaan NA: Adrenal cortical carcinoma. Cancer 1983;52:707.

147. Van Slooten H, Moolenaar AJ, Van Seters AP, Smeenk D: The treatment of adrenocortical carcinoma with o,p'DDD: prognostic simplifications of serum level monitoring. Eur J Cancer Clin Oncol 1984 ;20:47.

148. Ostuni JA, Roginski MS: Metastatic adrenal cortical carcinoma: Documented cure with combined chemotherapy. Arch Intern Med 1975;135:1257.

149. Decker RA, Elson P, Hogan TF, et al: Eastern Cooperative Oncology Group Study 1989: Mitotane and adriamycin in patients with advanced adrenocortical carcinoma. Surgery 1991;110:1006.

150. Hag MM, Legha SS, Samaan NA, et al: Cytotoxic chemotherapy in adrenal cortical carcinoma. Cancer Treat Rep 1980;64:909.

151. Tattersall MHN, Lander H, Bain B, et al: Cis-platinum treatment of metastatic adrenal carcinoma. Med J Aust 1980;1:419.

152. Johnson DH, Creco A: Treatment of metastatic adrenal cortical carcinoma with cisplatin and etoposide (VP-16). Cancer 1986;58:2198.

153. Hesketh PJ, McCaffrey RP, Finkel HE, et al: Cisplatin-based treatment of adrenocortical carcinoma. Cancer Treat Rep 1987;71:222.

154. Stein CA, LaRocca RV, Thomas R, et al: Suramin: An anticancer drug with a unique mechanism of action. J Clin Oncol 1989;7:499.

155. Allolio B, Reincke M, Afit W, et al: Suramin for treatment of adrenocortical carcinoma. Lancet 1989;1:277.

156. LaRocca RV, Stein CA, Danesi R, et al: Suramin in adrenal cancer: Modulation of steroid hormone production, cytotoxicity in vitro and clinical antitumor effect. J Clin Endocrinol Metab 1990; 71:497.

157. Gagner M, Pomp A, Heniford BT, et al: Laparoscopic adrenalectomy: Lessons learned from 100 consecutive procedures. Ann Surg 1997;226:238.

158. Filipponi S, Guerrieri M, Arnaldi G, et al: Laparoscopic adrenalectomy: A report on 50 operations. Eur J Endocrinol 1998;138:548.

159. Thompson GB, Grant CS, van Heerden JA, et al: Laparoscopic versus open posterior adrenalectomy: A case-control study of 100 patients. Surgery 1997;122:1132.

160. Manger WM, Gifford RW Jr: Pheochromocytoma. New York, Springer, 1977.

161. Carney A, Sizemore GW, Ty SG: Bilateral adrenal medullary hyperplasia in multiple endocrine neoplasia, type 2. The precursor of bilateral pheochromocytoma. Mayo Clin Proc 1975;50:3.

162. Symington T, Goodall AL: Studies in phaechromocytoma. I. Pathological aspects. Glasgow Med J 1953;34:75.

163. Sheps SG, Jiang NJ, Klee GG, et al: Recent developments in the diagnosis and treatment of pheochromocytoma. Mayo Clin Proc 1990;65:88.

164. Bravo EL, Tarazi RC, Grifford RW Jr, Stewart BH: Circulating and urinary catecholamines in pheochromocytoma: Diagnostic and pathophysiologic implications. N Engl J Med 1979;301:682.

165. Bravo EL, Tarazi RC, Fouad FM, et al: Clonidine-suppression test: A useful aid in the diagnosis of pheochromocytoma. N Engl J Med 1981;305:623.

166. Van Heerden JA, Sheps SG, Hamberger B, et al: Pheochromocytoma: Current status and changing trends. Surgery 1982; 91:363.

167. Shapiro B, Copp JE, Sisson JC, et al: Iodine-131 metaiodobenzylguanidine for the locating of suspected pheochromocytoma: experience in 400 cases. J Nucl Med 1985;26:576.

168. Swenson SJ, Brown MJ, Sheps SG, et al: Use of ^{131}I-MIBG scintigraphy in the evaluation of suspected pheochromocytoma. Mayo Clin Proc 1985;60:299.

169. Remine WH, Chong GC, VanHeerden JA, et al: Current management of pheochromocytoma. Ann Surg 1974;179:740.

170. Averbuch SD, Steakley CS, Young RC, et al: Malignant pheochromocytoma: Effective treatment with a combination of cyclophosphamide, vincristine and dacarbazine. Ann Intern Med 1988;109:267.

171. Brennan MF, Keiser HR: Persistent and recurrent pheochromocytoma: The role of surgery. World J Surg 1982;6:397.

172. Pujol P, Bringer J, Faurous P, Jaffiol C: Metastatic phaeochromocytoma with a long-term response after iodine-131 metaiodobenzylguanidine therapy. Eur J Nucl Med 1995;22:382.

173. Troncone L, Rufini V: ^{131}I-MIBG therapy of neural crest tumours. Anticancer Res 1997;17:1823.

174. Loh KC, Fitzgerald PA, Matthay KK, et al: The treatment of malignant pheochromocytoma with iodine-131 metaiodobenzylguanidine (^{131}I-MIBG): A comprehensive review of 116 reported patients. J Endocrinol Invest 1997;20:648.

175. Shantz A, Castleman B: Parathyroid carcinoma: A study of 70 cases. Cancer 1973;31:600.

176. Dinnen JS, Greenwood RH, Jones JH, et al: Parathyroid carcinoma in familial hyperparathyroidism. J Clin Pathol 1977;30:966.

177. Wang C, Gaz RD: Natural history of parathyroid carcinoma. Diagnosis, treatment and results. Am J Surg 1985;149:522.

178. Shane E, Bilezikian JP: Parathyroid carcinoma. A review of 62 patients. Endocr Rev 1982;3:218.

179. Cohn K, Silverman M, Corrado J, Sedgewick C: Parathyroid carcinoma: The Lahey Clinic experience. Surgery 1985;98:1095.

180. Flye MW, Brennan MF: Surgical resection of metastatic parathyroid carcinoma. Ann Surg 1981;193:425.

181. Bukowski RM, Sheclef L, Cunningham J, Esselstyn C: Successful combination chemotherapy for metastatic parathyroid carcinoma. Arch Intern Med 1984;144:399.

182. Calandra DB, Chejfec G, Foy BK, et al: Parathyroid carcinoma: Biochemical and pathologic response to DTIC. Surgery 1984;96:1132.

183. Singer FR, Ritch PS, Lad TE, et al: Treatment of hypercalcemia of malignancy with intravenous etidronate. Arch Intern Med 1991;151:471.

184. Warrell RP Jr, Israel R, Frisone M, et al: Gallium nitrate for acute treatment of cancer-treated hypercalcemia: A randomized, double-blind comparison to calcitonin. Ann Intern Med 1988;108:669.

185. Lips CJM, Minder WH, Leo JR, et al: Evidence of multicentric origin of the multiple endocrine neoplasia syndrome type 2A (Sipple's syndrome) in a large family in the Netherlands. Am J Med 1978;64:568.

186. Steiner EL, Goodman AD, Powers RS: Study of a kindred with pheochromocytoma, medullary thyroid carcinoma, hyperparathyroidism and Cushing's disease. Multiple endocrine neoplasia, type II. Medicine (Baltimore) 1968;47:371.

187. Chandrasekharappa SC, Guru SC, Manickam P, et al: Positional cloning of the gene for multiple endocrine neoplasia-type 1. Science 1997;276:404.

188. Guru SC, Goldsmith PK, Burns AL, et al: Menin, the product of the MEN1 gene, is a nuclear protein. Proc Natl Acad Sci USA 1998;95:1630.

189. Ballard HS, Frame B, Hartsock R: Familial multiple endocrine adenoma—Peptic ulcer complex. Medicine (Baltimore) 1964;43:481.

190. Eberle F, Grun R: Multiple endocrine neoplasia type I. Adv Intern Med Pediatr 1981;5:76.

191. Bone HG: Diagnosis of multiglandular endocrine neoplasias. Clin Chem 1990;36:711.

192. Eberle FM, Grun R: Multiple endocrine neoplasia, type I (MEN I). Ergeb Inn Med Kinderheilkd 1981;46:75.

193. Jensen RT, Norton JA: Pancreatic endocrine tumors. In Fordtran JS, Sleisinger MH, Feldman M, Scharschmidt B (eds): Gastrointestinal Diseases: Pathophysiology, Diagnosis and Management. Philadelphia, WB Saunders, 1992.

194. Maton PN, Gardner JE, Jensen RT: The incidence and etiology of Cushing's syndrome in patients with Zollinger-Ellison syndrome. N Engl J Med 1986;315:1.

195. Sipple JH: The association of pheochromocytoma with carcinoma of the thyroid. Am J Med 1961;31:163.

196. Mulligan LM, Kwok JB, Healey CS, et al: Germ-line mutations of the RET proto-oncogene in multiple endocrine neoplasia type 2A. Nature 1993;363:458.

197. Donis-Keller H, Dou S, Chi D, et al: Mutations in the RET proto-oncogene are associated with MEN 2A and FMTC. Hum Mol Genet 1993;2:851.

198. Eng C, Smith DP, Mulligan LM, et al: Point mutation within the tyrosine kinase domain of the RET proto-oncogene in multiple endocrine neoplasia type 2B and related sporadic tumours. Hum Mol Genet 1994;3:237.

199. Howe JR, Norton JA, Wells SA Jr: Prevalence of pheochromocytoma and hyperparathyroidism in multiple endocrine neoplasia type 2A: Results of long-term follow-up. Surgery 1993;114:1070.

200. Grun R, Eberle F: Multiple endocrine neoplasia, type I (NEMI). Ergeb Inn Med Kinderheildk 1981;46:151.

201. Wells SA Jr: Multiple endocrine neoplasia type II: Recent results. Cancer Res 1990;18:71.

202. Melvin KEW, Miller HH, Tashijian AH Jr: Early diagnosis of medullary carcinoma of the thyroid by means of calcitonin assay. N Engl J Med 1971;285:1115.

203. Shapiro B, Fig LM: Management of pheochromocytoma. Endocrinol Metab Clin North Am 1989;18:443.

204. Oberndoffer S: Karzinoide tumeren des Dunn darms. Frankf Z Pathol 1907;426.

205. Ransom WB: A case of primary carcinoma of the ileum. Lancet 1890;2:1020.

206. Masson P: Carcinoid (argentaffin-cell tumours) and nerve hyperplasia of appendicular mucosa. Am J Pathol 1982;4:181.

207. Kultschiuky N: Zur frage ueber den bau des darmkanals. Arch Mikrosk Anat 1987;49:7.

208. Peame AGE: The cytochemistry and ultrastructure of polypeptide hormone-producing cells of the APUD series and the embryologic, physiology, and pathologic implications of the concept. J Histochem Cytochem 1969;12:303.

209. Wilander E, Scheibenpflug L, Eriksson B, Oberg K: Diagnostic criteria of classical carcinomas. Acta Oncol 1991;30:469.

210. Wilander E: Diagnostic pathology of gastrointestinal and pancreatic neuroendocrine tumors. Acta Oncol 1989;28:363.

211. D'Alessandro M, Mariani P, Lomanto D: Serum neuron-specific enolase in diagnosis and follow-up of gastrointestinal neuroendocrine tumors. Tumor Biol 1992;13:352.

212. Schurmann G, Raeth U, Wiedenmann B: Serum chromogranin A in the diagnosis and follow-up of neuroendocrine tumors of the gastroenteropancreatic tract. World J Surg 1992;16:697.

213. Williams ED, Sandler M: The classification of carcinoid tumors. Lancet 1963;1:283.

214. Godwin DJ: Carcinoid tumor: An analysis of 2837 cases. Cancer 1975;36:560.

215. Rubin J, Ajani J, Schirmer W, et al: Octrietoid acetate long acting formulation versus octrietoid. J Clin Oncol 1999;17:600.

216. Moertel CG: An odyssey in the land of small tumors. J Clin Oncol 1987;5:1502.

217. Creutfeldt W, Stockmann E: Carcinoids and carcinoid syndrome. Am J Med 1987;82:4.

218. Grimelius L, Wilander E: Silver impregnation and other non-immunocytochemical staining methods. In Polak JM, Bloom SR (eds): Endocrine Tumors. Edinburgh, Churchill Livingstone, 1985, p 95.

219. Thorson A, Bjork G, Bjorkman G, Waldenström J: Malignant carcinoid of the small intestine with metastases to the liver, valvular disease of the right heart (pulmonary stenosis and tricuspid regurgitation without septal defect), peripheral vasomotor symptoms, bronchoconstriction and an unusual type of cyanosis. Am Heart J 1954;47:795.

220. Pemow B, Waldenström J: Paroxysm flushing and other symptoms caused by 5-hydroxytryptamine and histamine in patients with malignant tumor. Lancet 1954;2:951.

221. Oats JA, Melman K, Sjoerdsma M, et al: Release of a kinin peptide in the carcinoid syndrome. Lancet 1964;2:514.

222. Oates JA, Pettinger WA, Doctor RB: Evidence for the release of bradykinin in the carcinoid syndrome. J Clin Invest 1966;45:173.

223. Richter G, Stockmann F, Conlon JM, Creutzfeldt W: Serotonin release into blood after food and pentagastrin. Gastroenterology 1986;91:612.

224. Robertson JIS, Peart WS, Andrews TM: The mechanism of facial flushes in the carcinoid syndrome. Q J Med 1962;31:103.

225. Grahame-Smith DG: The Carcinoid Syndrome. London, Heinemann, 1972.

226. Adamson AK, Grahame-Smith DG, Peart WS, Starr M: Pharmacological blockade of carcinoid flushing provoked by catecholamines and alcohol. Lancet 1969;2:293.

227. Roberts JL II, Marney SR Jr, Oates JA: Blockade of the flush associated with metastatic gastric carcinoid by combined histamine H_1 and H_2 receptor antagonists. N Engl J Med 1979;300:236.

228. Mengel CE: Therapy of the malignant carcinoid syndrome. Ann Intern Med 1965;62:587.

229. Roberts WB, Sjoerdsma A: The cardiac disease associated with carcinoid syndrome (carcinoid heart disease). Am J Med 1964;36:5.

230. Lundin L: Carcinoid heart disease. Acta Oncol 1991;30:499.

231. Macdonald JS, Metcalfe MS: Carcinoid tumor. In Schein PS (ed): Decision Making in Oncology. New York, BC Decker, 1988, p 94.

232. Feldman JM: Carcinoid tumor and syndrome. Semin Oncol 1987;15:237.

233. Feldman JM, Lee EM: Serotonin content of foods. Effect on urinary excretion of 5-hydroxyindoleacetic acid. J Clin Nutr 1985;2:639.

234. Feldman JM, Butler SS, Chapman BA: Interference with measurement of 3-methoxy-4-hydroxymandelic acid and 5-hydroxyindoleacetic acid by reducing metabolites. Clin Chem 1974;20:607.

235. Moertel CG, Hanley HA: Combination chemotherapy trial for metastatic carcinoid tumor and the malignant carcinoid syndrome. Cancer Clin Trials 1979;2:327.

236. Bomanji E, Ur E, Mather S, et al: A scintigraphic comparison of iodine-123 metaiodobenzylguanidine and an iodine-labeled somatostatin analog (TYRG-octreotide) in metastatic carcinoid tumors. J Nucl Med 1992;33:112.

237. Kvols LK, Brown ML, O'Connor MK: Evaluation of a radiolabeled somatostatin analog (PD octreotide) in the detection and localization of carcinoid and islet cell tumors. Radiology 1993;187:129.

238. Moertel CG, Dockerty MB, Judd ES: Carcinoid tumors of the vermiform appendix. Cancer 1968;21:270.

239. Thompson GB, van Heerden JA, Martin JK, et al: Carcinoid tumors of the gastrointestinal tract: Presentation, management and prognosis. Surgery 1985;98:1054.

240. Moertel CG: Treatment of the carcinoid tumor and the malignant carcinoid syndrome. J Clin Oncol 1983;1:727.

241. Martin JK, Moertel CG, Adson MA: Surgical treatment of functioning metastatic carcinoid tumors. Arch Surg 1983;118:537.

242. Keane TJ, Rider WD, Hatwood AR, et al: Whole abdominal radiation in the management of metastatic gastrointestinal carcinoid tumors. Int J Radiat Oncol Biol Phys 1981;7:1519.

243. Schupak KD, Wallnet KE: The role of radiation therapy in the treatment of locally unresectable or metastatic carcinoid tumors. Int J Radiat Oncol Biol Phys 1993;20:439.

244. Brown RE, Hill SR Jr, Berry KW, Bing RJ: Studies on several possible antiserotonin compounds in the functioning carcinoid syndrome. Clin Res 1960;8:61.

245. Melmon KL, Sjoerdsma A, Oates JA, Laster L: Treatment of malabsorption and diarrhea of the carcinoid syndrome with methylsergide. Gastroenterology 1965;48:18.

246. Engelman K, Sjoerdsman A: Inhibition of catecholamine biosynthesis in man. Circ Res Suppl 1966;1:104.

247. Sjoerdsma A, Livenberg W, Engelman K, et al: Serotonin now: Clinical implications of inhibiting its synthesis with parachlorophenylalanine. Ann Intern Med 1970;73:607.

248. Frolich JC, Bloomgarden ZT, Oates JA, et al: The carcinoid flush: Provocation by pentagastrin and inhibition by somatostatin. N Engl J Med 1976;299:1055.

249. Kvoh LK: The carcinoid syndrome: A treatable malignant disease. Oncology 1988;2:33.

250. Grosman I, Simon D: Potential gastrointestinal uses of somatostatin and its synthetic analogue octreotide. Am J Gastroenterol 1990;85:1061.

251. Kvols LK, Moertel CG, O'Connell MJ: Treatment of the malignant carcinoid syndrome with a long-acting somatostatin analogue. N Engl J Med 1986;315:663.

252. Wynick D, Anderson JV, Williams SJ, Bloom SR: Resistance of metastatic pancreatic endocrine tumors after long-term treatment with the somatostatin analogue octreotide (SMS 201-995). Clin Endocrinol 1989;30:385.

253. Moertel CG, Sauer WG, Doekerry MG, Baggentoss AH: Life history of the carcinoid tumor of the small intestines. Cancer 1961;14:901.

254. Schein PS, LeLellis R, Kahn CR, et al: Current concepts and management of islet cell tumors. Ann Intern Med 1973;79:239.

255. Engstrom PF, Lavin PT, Folsch E: Streptozotocin plus fluorouracil versus doxorubicin therapy for metastatic carcinoid tumors. J Clin Oncol 1984;2:1255.

256. Hailer DG, Schutt A, Dayal Y, et al: Chemotherapy for metastatic carcinoid tumor: An ECOG phase II–III trial. Proc Am Soc Clin Oncol 1990;9:102.

257. Oberg K, Funa K, Alm G: Effects of leukocyte interferon on clinical symptoms and hormonal levels in patents with midget carcinoid tumors and the carcinoid syndrome. N Engl J Med 1983;309:129.

258. Oberg K, Eriksson B: Medical treatment of neuroendocrine gut and pancreatic tumors. Acta Oncol 1989;28:425.

259. Moertel CG, Rubin J, Kvols LK: Therapy of metastatic carcinoid tumor and the malignant carcinoid syndrome with recombinant leukocyte A interferon. J Clin Oncol 1989;7:865.

260. Janson E, Ronnblom L, Ahlstrom H: Treatment with alpha-interferon versus alpha-interferon in combination with streptozotocin and doxorubicin in patients with malignant carcinoid tumors: A randomized trial. Ann Oncol 1992;3:635.

261. Janson E, Ahlstrom H, Andersson T: Octreotide and interferon alfa: A new combination for the treatment of malignant of carcinoid tumours. Eur J Cancer 1992;28A:1647.

262. Rönnblom LE, Alm GV, Öberg KE: Autoimmunity after alpha interferon therapy for malignant carcinoid tumors. Ann Intern Med 1993;115:178.

263. Moertel CG, Johnson CM, McKusick MA: The management of patients with advanced carcinoid tumors and islet cell carcinomas. Ann Intern Med 1994;120:302.

264. Hall JT, Wallace S, Carrasco CH: Gastrointestinal and pancreatic endocrine tumors. Ballieres Clin Endocrinol Metab 1989;3:121.

265. Ruszniewski P, Rougier P, Roche A: Hepatic arterial chemoembolization in patients with liver metastases of endocrine tumors. Cancer 1992;71:2624.

266. Hazarizadeh H, Ivancey K, Mueller C: Effective palliative treatment of metastatic carcinoid tumors with intra-arterial chemotherapy/chemoembolization combined with octreotide acetate. Am J Surg 1992;163:1479.

267. Maton PN, Hodgson HJF: Carcinoid tumors and the carcinoid syndrome. In Bouchier JAD, Allan RN, Hodgson HJF, Keighly MRB (eds): Textbook of Gastroenterology. London, Ballierre-Tindall, 1984, p 620.

268. Schein PS, Kahn R, Gotden P, et al: Streptozotocin for malignant insulinomas and carcinoid tumors. Arch Intern Med 1973;132:555.

269. O'Dorisio TM, Vinik AL: Pancreatic polypeptide and mixed polypeptide producing tumors of the gastrointestinal tract. In Cohen S, Sobway RD (eds): Hormone-Producing Tumors of the Gastrointestinal Tract. New York, Churchill Livingstone, 1985, p 117.

270. Wermer P: Genetic aspects of adenomatosis of endocrine glands. Am J Med 1954;16:363.

271. Jensen RT, Norton JA: Pancreatic endocrine tumors. In Yamada T, Alpers DH, Owyang C, et al (eds): Textbook of Gastroenterology. Philadelphia, JB Lippincott, 1991, p 1912.

272. Boden G: Insulinoma and glucagonoma. Semin Oncol 1987;14:253.

273. Fajans SS, Vinik AL: Insulin-producing islet cell tumors. Endocrinol Metab Clin North Am 1989;18:45.

274. Grunberger G, Weiner JL, Silverman R, et al: Factitious hypoglycemia due to surreptitious administration of insulin: Diagnosis, treatment and long-term follow-up. Ann Intern Med 1988;108:252.

275. Comis R, Norton JA, Doppman JL: Insulinoma. In Go VLW, Gardner JD (eds): The Exocrine Pancreas: Biology, Pathobiology and Diseases. New York, Raven Press, 1986.

276. Alsever RN, Roberts JP, Gerber JG, et al: Insulinoma with low circulating insulin levels: The diagnostic value of proinsulin measurements. Ann Intern Med 1975;82:347.

277. Kahn CR, Rosen SW, Weintmub BD, et al: Ectopic production of chorionic gonadotropin and its subunits by islet cell tumors. N Engl J Med 1977;297:565.

278. Rosch T, Lightdale C, Botet J: Localization of pancreatic endocrine tumors by endoscopic ultrasonography. N Engl J Med 1992;326:1721.

279. Doppman J: Pancreatic endocrine tumors—The search goes on. N Engl J Med 1992;326:1770.

280. Power L: A glucose-responsive insulinoma. JAMA 1969;207:893.

281. Landau BR, Levine HJ, Hertz R: Prolonged glucagon administration in a case of hyperinsulinemia due to disseminated islet cell carcinoma. N Engl J Med 1958;259:286.

282. Mahon WA, Mitchell ML, Steinke J, Raben MS: Effect of human growth hormone on hypoglycemia states. N Engl J Med 1962;267:1179.

283. Marks V, Rose FC: Hypoglycemia. Oxford, Blackwell, 1965.

284. Roth H, Their S, Segal S: Zinc glucagon in the management of refractory hypoglycemia due to insulin-producing tumor. N Engl J Med 1966;274:493.

285. Dollery CT, Pentecost BL: Drug-induced diabetes. Lancet 1962;2:735.

286. Graber AL, Porte E Jr, Williams RH: Clinical use of diazoxide and mechanisms for its hyperglycemic effects. Diabetes 1966;15:143.

287. Basabe J, Lopey N, Viktora J, Wolff F: Studies of insulin secretion in the perfused rat pancreas. Diabetes 1970;19:271.

288. Gierchsky KE, Halse J, Mathisen W, et al: Endocrine tumors of the pancreas. Scand J Gastroenterol 1980;15:129.

289. Maton PN: The use of the long-acting somatostatin analogue, octreotide in patients with islet cell tumors. Gastroenterol Clin North Am 1989;18:897.

290. Mallinson CN, Bloom SR, Warin AP, et al: A glucagonoma syndrome. Lancet 1974;2:1.

291. Friesen SR: Tumors of the endocrine pancreas. N Engl J Med 1982;306:580.

292. Wilkinson DS: Necrolytic migratory erythema with carcinoma of the pancreas. Trans St Johns Hosp Dermatol Soc 1973;59:244.

293. Guillausseau PJ, Gauillausseau C, Villet R, et al: Les glucagonomas: Aspect cliniques, biologiques, anatomopathologiques et therapeutiques (revue general de 130 cas). Gastroenterol Clin Biol 1982;6:1029.

294. Stacpoole PW: The glucagonoma syndrome: Clinical features, diagnosis, and treatment. Endocrinol Rev 1981;2:437.

295. Higgins GA, Recant L, Fischman AB: The glucagonoma syndrome: Surgically curable diabetes. Am J Surg 1979;137:142.

296. Stacpoole PW, Jaspan J, Kasselberg AG, et al: A familial glucagonoma syndrome. Genetic, clinical and biochemical features. Am J Med 1981;70:1017.

297. Dunne MJ, Elton R, Fletcher T, et al: Somatostatin and gastroenteropancreatic endocrine tumors: Therapeutic characteristics. In O'Dorisio TM (ed): Somatostatin in the Treatment of GEP Endocrine Tumors. Berlin, Springer, 1987, p 93.

298. Yamada T, Chiha T: Somatostatin. In Makhlouf GN (ed): The Gastrointestinal System: Handbook of Physiology. Bethesda, American Physiological Society, 1979, p 431.

299. Boden G, Shimoyama R, Somatostatinoma. In Cohen S, Solow RD (eds): Hormone-Producing Tumors of the Gastrointestinal Tract. New York, Churchill Livingstone, 1985, p 85.

300. Krejs GJ, Orci L, Conlon M, et al: Somatostatinoma syndrome (biochemical, morphological and clinical features). N Engl J Med 1985;301:285.

301. Konomi K, Chijiiwa K, Katsuta T, Yamaguchi K: Pancreatic somatostatinoma 1990a: A case report and review of the literature. J Surg Oncol 1990;43:259.

302. Zollinger RM, Ellison EH: Primary peptic ulceration of the jejunum: associated with islet cell tumors of the pancreas. Ann Surg 1955;142:709.

303. Grossman MI (ed): Peptic Ulcer. Chicago, Year Book Medical, 1980, p 141.

304. Jensen RT, Doppman JL, Gardner JD: Gastrinoma. In Go VLM, Brooks FA, DiMagno EP, et al (eds): The Exocrine Pancreas: Biology, Pathobiologic and Disease. New York, Raven, 1986, p 727.

305. Jensen RT, Gardner JD, Raufman JP, et al: Zollinger-Ellison syndrome: Current concepts and management. Ann Intern Med 1983;98:59.

306. Isenberg JI, Walsh JH, Grossman MI: Zollinger-Ellison syndrome. Gastroenterology 1973;65:140.

307. Ellison EC, Carey LC, Sparks J, et al: Early surgical treatment of gastrinoma. Am J Med 1987;82:17.

308. McGuigan JE, Wolfe MM: Secretin injection test in the diagnosis of gastrinoma. Gastroenterology 1980;79:1324.

309. McCarthy DM, Jensen RT: Zollinger-Ellison syndrome-current issues. In Cohen S, Soloway RD (eds): Hormone-Producing Tumor of the Gastrointestinal Tract. New York, Churchill Livingstone, 1985.

310. Jensen RT, Maton PN: Zollinger-Ellison syndrome. In Gustavsson S, Kumar D, Graham DY (eds): The Stomach. London, Churchill Livingstone, 1991, p 341.

311. Wolfe MM, Jensen RT: Zollinger-Ellison syndrome. Current concepts in diagnosis and management. N Engl J Med 1987;317:1200.

312. Bonfils S, Landor JH, Mignon M, Hervir P: Results of surgical management in 92 consecutive patients with Zollinger-Ellison syndrome. Ann Surg 1981;194:692.

313. Zollinger RM, Ellison EC, Fabri PJ, et al: Primary peptic ulcerations of the jejunum associated with islet cell tumors: Twenty-five year appraisal. Ann Surg 1980;192:422.

314. Jensen RT, Collers MT, McArthur KE: Comparison of the effectiveness of ranitidine and cimetidine in inhibiting acid secretion in patients with gastric hypersecretory states. Am J Med 1985;77:90.

315. Verner JV, Morrison AB: Islet cell tumor and a syndrome of refractory watery diarrhea and hypokalemia. Am J Med 1958;25:374.

316. Kane MG, O'Dorisio TM, Krejs GL: Intravenous VIP infusion causes secretory diarrhea in man. N Engl J Med 1983;309:1501.

317. Santangelo WC, O'Dorisio TM, Kim JG, et al: Pancreatic cholera syndrome: Effects of a synthetic somatostatin analog on intestinal water and ion transport. Ann Intern Med 1985;103:363.

318. Kvols HM, Buck M, Moertel LG, et al: Treatment of metastatic islet cell carcinoma with a somatostatin analogue (SMS-201-995). Ann Intern Med 1987;107:162.

319. Oberg K, Lindstrom H, Alm G, et al: Successful treatment of therapy-resistant pancreatic cholera with human leucocyte interferon. Lancet 1985;1:725.

320. Anderson T, Schein PS, McMenamin MG, Cooney DA: Streptozotocin diabetes, correlation with extent of depression of pancreatic islet nicotinamide adenine dinucleotide. J Clin Invest 1974;54:672.

321. Kahn CR, Levy AG, Gardner JD, et al: Pancreatic cholera: Beneficial effects of streptozotocin. N Engl J Med 1975;292:941.

322. Moertel CG: Clinical management of advanced gastrointestinal cancer. Cancer 1975;36:675.

323. Moertel CG, Hanley JA, Johnson LA: Streptozotocin alone compared with streptozotocin plus fluorouracil in the treatment of advanced islet-cell carcinoma. N Engl J Med 1980; 303:1189.

324. Moertel CG, Lavin PT, Hahn RG: Phase II trial of doxorubicin therapy for advanced islet cell carcinoma. Cancer Treat Rep 1982;66:1567.

325. Moertel CG, Lefkopoulou M, Lipsitz S, et al: Streptozotocin-doxorubicin, streptozotocin fluorouracil, or chlorozotocin in the treatment of advanced islet-cell carcinoma. N Engl J Med 1992;326:519.

326. Bukowski RM, McCracken JD, Balanzak SP, et al: A phase II study of chlorozotocin in islet cell carcinoma. A Southwest Oncology Group Study. Cancer Chemother Pharmacol 1983;11:48.

327. Bukowski R, Tangen C, Lee R: Phase II trial of chlorozotocin and fluorouracil in islet carcinoma: A Southwest Oncology Group Study. J Clin Oncol 1992;10:1914.

328. Moertel CG, Kvols LK, O'Connell MJ, Rubin J: Treatment of neuroendocrine carcinomas with combined etoposide and cisplatin. Cancer 1991;68:227.

329. Tochner ZA, Kinsella TJ, Glatstein E: Hepatic irradiation in the management of metastatic hormone-secreting tumors. Cancer 1985;56:20.

330. Von Schrenck T, Howard JM, Doppman JL, et al: Prospective study of chemotherapy in patients with metastatic gastrinoma. Gastroenterology 1988;94:1326.

331. Sessions RB, Diehl WL: Thyroid cancer and related nodularity. In Myers E, Suen J (eds): Cancer of the Head and Neck, 2nd ed. New York, Churchill Livingstone, 1981, p 766.

332. American Joint Committee on Cancer Manual for the Staging of Cancer. Philadelphia, JB Lippincott, 1988.

333. Rivera E, Ajani JA: Doxorubicin, streptozotocin, and 5-fluorouracil chemotherapy for patients with metastatic islet-cell carcinoma. Am J Clin Oncol 1998;21:36.

334. Ollivier S, Fonck M, Bécouarn Y, Brunet R: Dacarbazine, fluorouracil, and leucovorin in patients with advanced neuroendocrine tumors. Am J Clin Oncol 1998;21:237.

335. Bilchik AJ, Sarantou T, Foshag LJ, et al: Cryosurgical palliation of metastatic neuroendocrine tumors resistant to conventional therapy. Surgery 1997;122:1040.

336. Drougas JG, Anthony LB, Blair TK, et al: Hepatic artery chemoembolization for management of patients with advanced metastatic carcinoid tumors. Am J Surg 1998;175:408.

337. Di Bartolomeo M, Bajetta E, Buzzoni R, et al: Clinical efficacy of octreotide in the treatment of metastatic neuroendocrine tumors. Cancer 1996;77:402.

338. Trendle MC, Moertel CG, Kvols LK: Incidence and morbidity of cholelithiasis in patients receiving chronic octreotide for metastatic carcinoid and malignant islet cell tumors. Cancer 1997;79:830.

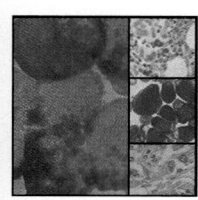

CANCER OF THE LUNG: NSCLC AND SCLC

John C. Ruckdeschel

Ann G. Schwartz

Gerold Bepler

Lynn Coppage

Fulvio Lonardo

Omer Kucuk

Harvey I. Pass

Henry Wagner

Antoinette J. Wozniak

Shirish M. Gadgeel

SUMMARY OF KEY POINTS

NON–SMALL CELL LUNG CANCER

Incidence

- Approximately 80% of 170,000 new cases a year of lung cancer in North America are non–small cell lung cancer.
- The most frequent types are adenocarcinoma, squamous cell carcinoma, and large cell anaplastic.

Differential Diagnosis

- Small cell carcinoma of the lung, carcinoid, carcinoma or sarcoma metastatic to the lung, various infections, sarcoidosis.

Staging Evaluations

- History and physical examination, routine hematologic and biochemical testing.

IMAGING

- Computed tomography scan (with contrast) evaluating lungs, mediastinum, liver, and adrenals.
- Positron emission tomography.
- If patient has locally advanced or metastatic disease, add magnetic resonance imaging of brain. If positron emission tomography is not available, add bone scan.
- Mediastinal node evaluation:
  - If disease is in early stage (I, II) and positron emission tomography of mediastinum is negative, proceed directly to surgery. If positron emission tomography is positive, proceed to biopsy depending on node location.
    - Cervical mediastinoscopy.
    - Mediastinotomy.
    - Transesophageal endoscopic ultrasound.
    - Bronchoscopy.

- If disease is clinically more advanced, use the least invasive biopsy procedure from the foregoing list. At surgery, all nodal areas need to be sampled at minimum.

Primary Therapy

- For stages I and II disease:
  - Surgery is often curative.
  - No clear advantage to pre- or postoperative therapy.
- For stage IIIA disease:
  - Preoperative chemotherapy for limited extent IIIA appears promising, but it is less clear whether preoperative chemotherapy plus radiation is effective as a preoperative approach except for Pancoast tumors.
- For stage IIIB disease:
  - Chemotherapy combined with radiation seems superior to radiation alone; there is some evidence that concurrent therapy is better than sequential, but increased toxicity limits this approach in frail patients.
  - Clinical trials of new approaches should be a high priority.
- For stage IV disease:
  - Primary chemotherapy with any of several "doublets" improves both the quality and quantity of life. Patients who are IIIB (wet) with a malignant pleural effusion should be treated as having stage IV disease.
  - There is no advantage for triplet therapy, and there are lesser results for single-agent therapy.
  - There is a clear need for more clinical trials at this stage.

Second- or Third-line Therapy

- Local recurrence after surgery should be treated with combined chemotherapy and radiation after complete restaging.
- Progression after chemotherapy is now well treated with several agents or regimens if patient sustains a good performance status. Clinical trials are sorely needed here.
- Newer targeted therapies could play an increasing role in second- or third-line therapy.

SMALL CELL LUNG CANCER

Incidence

- Small cell lung cancer accounts for approximately 15% of new cases a year of lung cancer, with the incidence dropping.
- Subtypes include oat cell, intermediate cell, and combined small cell and squamous cell carcinoma or adenocarcinoma.

Differential Diagnosis

- Non–small cell lung cancer, lymphoma, metastases from other small cell tumors, sarcoidosis, or infection.

Staging Evaluation

- History and physical examination, routine histologic and biochemical testing.
- Imaging:
  - Computed tomography scan (with contrast) evaluating lungs, mediastinum, liver, and adrenals.
  - Brain evaluation (magnetic resonance imaging preferred).
  - If there are signs or symptoms of advanced disease, a bone scan is required.
  - Positron emission tomography scans remain investigational.

SUMMARY OF KEY POINTS—*cont'd*

- Mediastinal node evaluation is generally not required unless as a convenient site for biopsy.
- A major task is defining the presence or absence of M_1 disease.
  - If peripheral smear or hemogram is abnormal, add bone marrow biopsy if no other site of metastatic disease has been confirmed.

Therapy
- Limited disease:
  - Provide concurrent chemotherapy and radiation to the intrathoracic disease.
  - Provide prophylactic cranial irradiation in complete responders.
- Extensive disease:
  - Use chemotherapy with etoposide or irinotecan and cisplatin or carboplatin (up to four to six cycles).
  - There is no evidence for effectiveness of triplets, dose intensification, or late intensification.

- Research studies are a clear priority given the lack of progress in this arena.
- Recurrent disease:
  - No clearly effective second-line therapy exists; any of several chemotherapies offer short-term benefit.
  - Research protocols are a preferred choice for patients at this stage.

INTRODUCTION

Lung cancer is a contemporary scourge that is the direct result of the substantial increase in tobacco consumption during the last century. Currently, it is estimated to account for 171,900 new cases in men and women in 2003 and 157,200 deaths annually.[1] It kills more men than prostate, colorectal and pancreatic cancer combined and as many women as breast and colorectal cancer combined.[1] It occupies a unique role in the pantheon of human cancers in that it is often considered a preventable cancer and hence one for which the victim is blamed. It also occurs most commonly in the setting of the older adult smoker who has significant pulmonary and cardiac morbidity in addition to the presence of a lung cancer.

There is, however, a general concurrence that this disease is amenable to earlier detection and that more aggressive pursuit of smoking cessation techniques would continue the downward trend we are seeing in incidence. The key molecular events in the genesis of lung cancer are not yet fully elucidated, and the linkages between the inflammatory response and pulmonary carcinogenesis are unclear. Nonetheless, it appears that the disease we call "lung cancer" might in fact represent several diseases, all of which originate in the pulmonary epithelium.

Unlike the molecular origins of lung cancer, the evaluation and clinical management of lung cancer have demonstrated a convergence of approaches and outcomes leading to very little distinction between the various histologies. In particular, the previously cited differences between small cell and non–small cell lung cancer have essentially disappeared.

EPIDEMIOLOGY

In 2002, an estimated 169,400 new lung cancers were diagnosed in the United States, second only to prostate cancer in males and breast cancer in females.[2] Lung cancer deaths, estimated to be 154,900 in 2002, remain the most frequent cause of cancer-related death in the United States. Although men have seen declines in incidence and mortality rates in the last ten years associated with reduction in smoking, this is not the case for women, among whom these rates continue to increase. Average annual age-adjusted incidence and mortality rates per 100,000 for the period 1995-1999 in the United States were 79.8 and 64.2, respectively, for white men, 120.6 and 97.0 for black men, 51.4 and 38.5 for white females, and 53.1 and 41.1 for black females. Worldwide geographic variation corresponds most closely to variations in smoking patterns. Survival after a lung cancer diagnosis has changed little, with overall five-year relative survival increasing only slightly from 12.4% for 1974-1976 diagnoses to 14.7% for 1992-1998 diagnoses. Five-year relative survival is as high as 48.5% for localized stage cancers, but only 15% of all lung cancers are diagnosed at this earliest stage.

Although cancers of the lung have proven difficult to diagnose early and treat successfully, the cause of most of these cancers is well known. Ninety percent of lung cancer incidence in males and 79% in females can be attributed to cigarette smoking.[3] The association between cigarette smoking and lung cancer was reported in case-control studies conducted as early as the 1950s.[4-6] Subsequent cohort studies provided additional evidence of increased risk of death from lung cancer as smoking amount increased, with an approximately 20-fold increased risk among those smoking two or more packs per day.[7-9] Although most initial studies focused on men, similar and sometimes higher risks of lung cancer are reported for women smokers.[10,11] To further support the causal role for smoking, those who quit smoking reduce their risk of developing lung cancer over time.[12] The largest declines in risk after quitting are seen in younger smokers and those with shorter duration of use.[13,14] In addition, lung cancer risk is increased approximately twofold in cigar and pipe smokers and approximately 30% in nonsmokers exposed to passive smoke.[15]

The importance of tobacco smoke as a cause of lung cancer often makes the study of other risk factors difficult because of the possibility of serious confounding by tobacco smoke exposure. Associations between dietary factors and lung cancer have been equivocal. Diets rich in fruits and vegetables have been associated with a 10%–50% reduction in risk of lung cancer.[16] A protective effect (on the order of 30%–80%) for β-carotene or total carotenoids has been shown in a number of observational studies; however, two large randomized intervention trials of β-carotene supplementation demonstrated a significant increase in lung cancer risk in the treated groups.[16-19] Occupational exposures to asbestos, radon, mustard gas, polycyclic hydrocarbons, chloromethyl ethers, chromium, nickel, and inorganic arsenic have also been associated with increased lung cancer risk.[20-28]

Given the strong and consistent associations between tobacco smoke and other environmental exposures and lung cancer risk, lung cancer has long been considered a disease determined solely by environmental exposures. Yet, even with the high risks attributable to cigarette smoking, only 10%–15% of all smokers develop lung cancer, and 10%–15% of all lung cancers occur among nonsmokers, suggesting that some individual differences in susceptibility to lung carcinogens could be inherited.[29]

Familial risk of lung cancer was first reported in the 1960s with the observation that the number of deaths due to lung cancer was higher among relatives of patients with lung cancer than among relatives of controls.[30] A number of other studies since then have demonstrated a familial component to lung cancer risk, with an approximately twofold risk associated with family history.[31-36] Additional studies have demonstrated familial aggregation of lung cancer even after adjustment for exposure to cigarette smoke, other risk factors among relatives, and the age structure of the family. Ooi and colleagues[37] reported a 2.4-fold increased risk of lung cancer among relatives of lung cancer cases compared with relatives of spouse controls after adjusting for age, sex, smoking history, and occupational exposures for each relative. Schwartz and coworkers[38] reported excess risk of lung cancer after adjustment for each relative's age, sex, race, smoking status, occupation, industry, and history of other lung diseases, in first-degree relatives of nonsmoking patients with lung cancer 40–59 years of age (RR = 6.1; 95% CI 1.1–33.4).

The role of inherited susceptibility of lung cancer is suggested by these findings of familial aggregation over and above that associated with familial clustering of smoking habits and adjustments for family size and structure. Two of the studies just described went on to demonstrate statistical evidence of inheritance of a major gene consistent with Mendelian codominant inheritance. In one study, the pattern of lung cancer occurrence in families of persons dying from lung cancer was consistent with Mendelian codominant inheritance of a rare autosomal gene with variable age at onset.[39] In the other study, families of nonsmoking patients with lung cancer age 40–59 years provided evidence for a Mendelian codominant gene, with significant modifying effects of smoking and chronic bronchitis.[40] These studies suggest that the pattern of cancer occurrence in some families is consistent with Mendelian inheritance of a rare major gene, particularly when onset is early.

A single gene for lung cancer has not yet been identified. Lung cancer has been shown to occur, on occasion, in Li-Fraumeni families, in which it is associated with inherited p53 mutations.[41] The existence of common susceptibility genes for lung cancer also is supported by findings of moderate familial aggregation. Candidate susceptibility genes include those associated with carcinogen metabolism and DNA repair. In general, association studies of these polymorphisms have yielded conflicting results. Conclusions from these studies have been limited by the low frequency of some polymorphisms in the population, variability in allele frequencies by ethnicity (thereby requiring well matched case-control studies), the potential for heterogeneity by histologic type of lung cancer, and variation in risk associated with level of exposure to tobacco smoke. Evidence for an association between *CYP1A1* polymorphisms and risk of lung cancer has come primarily from studies in Japanese populations (with risks increased more than twofold) and more recently, in a population in Hawaii, which included Caucasians, Japanese, and Hawaiians.[42,43] Other studies have reported no genetic associations.[44-47] In a pooled analysis from 22 case-control studies, a 2.4-fold increased risk was seen in Caucasians for the homozygous MspI polymorphism in *CYP1A1*.[48] Variants of *CYP2E1* have not been associated with increased risk of lung cancer in a number of studies.[44,46,49] A study in Hawaii, however, reported a tenfold decrease in risk of lung cancer in individuals homozygous for the rare variant alleles.[43] Several meta-analyses have shown moderate associations between lung cancer risk and *GSTM1* deficiency. Observed risk (OR) of 1.13 (95% CI 1.04–1.25), 1.41 (95% CI 1.23–1.61), and 1.17 (95% CI 1.07–1.27) have been reported.[50-52] Polymorphisms in *GSTT1* and *GSTP1* have been associated with lung cancer risk in combination with other genotypes.[53-58]

Individual variability in DNA repair capacity might contribute to inherited susceptibility to lung cancer, with individuals who are unable to repair DNA damage (or who do so at a slower rate) accumulating mutations that might modulate risk. Increased numbers of bleomycin or BPDE-induced breaks have been associated with a 4.3- and 7.3-fold increased risk of lung cancer, respectively.[59] Mutagen sensitivity has been shown to be correlated with DNA repair capacity.[60] Amino acid substitution variants have been identified in a number of DNA repair genes (*OGG1*, *ERCC1*, *XPD*, *XPF*, *XRCC3*, and *XRCC1*).[61,62] Studies of these polymorphisms and risk of lung cancer have shown moderate risks with polymorphisms in *OGG1*, *XRCC1*, and *XPD*.[62]

Additional large-scale studies are needed to more clearly define the gene-gene and gene-environment interactions that drive susceptibility to lung cancer in an effort to identify those individuals at highest risk. Identifying these individuals will lead to targeted screening practices for early detection. In the long term, prevention in the form of reducing the rate at which individuals start to smoke and increasing quitting rates is still the surest way to reduce morbidity and mortality from this disease.

BIOLOGY OF LUNG CANCER

The term *lung cancer* comprises all malignant neoplasms of the lung. Different entities of lung cancer are currently defined by histopathologic criteria that are based mainly on distinct light microscopic characteristics. The four major histologic types are adenocarcinoma, squamous cell carcinoma, large cell carcinoma, and small cell carcinoma, which together account for 85%-90% of all lung cancers. The remaining 10%-15% entities include adenosquamous carcinomas, adenoid cystic carcinomas, mucoepidermoid carcinomas, carcinoid tumors, malignant mesotheliomas, and other rarer types. Thus, lung cancer is not a homogeneous disease. Because light microscopic features are a major "phenotype" as a result of expression and processing of genes that are collectively controlled by the "genotype," it is clear that the biology of lung cancer must be highly complex and diverse.

Most lung cancers are epithelial tumors. Because of similar clinical characteristics, adeno-, squamous, and large cell carcinomas are collectively referred to as non–small cell lung carcinomas (NSCLC). This term arose to contrast these tumors from small cell carcinoma, which grows, invades, and metastasizes rapidly, resulting in a patient's death within a few months if left untreated. Carcinoid of the lung, another epithelial tumor, is slow growing with rare or delayed metastatic spread. Yet, morphologic and immunohistologic features of this tumor resemble those of small cell carcinoma rather than non–small cell carcinoma, which again underlines the biologic complexity and diversity of lung cancer.[63] On the other hand, electron microscopic, molecular biologic, and immunohistochemic characteristics of NSCLC have revealed features that are shared with small cell carcinoma and carcinoids. These findings suggest that some features are common to all lung cancers and argues for the hypothesis that all epithelial lung cancers arise from a common stem cell in the bronchial epithelium. The observed phenotypic diversity is then a result of a preexisting commitment of the cell to undergo a specific differentiation before malignant transformation. It further suggests that abrogation or alteration of a minimal set of cellular functions could account for the transformation of benign bronchial epithelial cell into malignancy.

The specific events that trigger malignant transformation of bronchoepithelial cells are unknown.[64,65] Based on epidemiologic investigations, however, it is clear that exposure to environmental carcinogens, such as those found in tobacco smoke or asbestos fibers, induce or facilitate the transformation (extrinsic component).[66] The contribution of the extrinsic carcinogen on transformation is modulated by genetic variations in genes (intrinsic component) that affect aspects of carcinogen metabolism, such as the conversion of procarcinogens to carcinogens and their subsequent inactivation.[67] These genetic variations occur at relatively high frequency in the population. Their contribution to an individual's lung cancer risk is generally low; because of their population frequency, however, their overall impact on lung cancer risk could be high. Epidemiologic studies further suggest that a familial predisposition to lung cancer exists that is independent of tobacco smoke exposure. This is likely the result of an autosomal recessive gene, whose loss of function could confer a high relative risk for lung cancer to an individual, much like the contribution of *BRCA1* to breast cancer risk. The identification of chromosomal loci for lung cancer susceptibility genes has been difficult, however, because the familial risk is obscured by environmental factors.[36,37,68]

An alternate approach has been to search for somatic genome alterations in lung cancer. Somatic alterations have mainly lead to the identification of so-called "modulator" genes rather than classical tumor suppressor genes. Molecular genetic investigations have used cell lines, short-term cell cultures, freshly resected lung cancers, and pathologic specimens as sources for chromosomes and DNA. Chromosomal segments and loci implicated in lung cancer are numerous. They are summarized in Table 75-1 together with the putative gene of importance, its function, and the reported frequencies of genomic alterations.

The histologic sequence of events that leads to the various forms of lung cancer is not well understood, and it could be different for the various histopathologic entities.[69-72] Current knowledge suggests that squamous cell carcinoma arises in an ordered progression that includes squamous metaplasia and carcinoma in situ (CIS). Precursor lesions of adenocarcinoma remain obscure, largely because this type of cancer arises predominantly in the peripheral airways of the lung, which are inaccessible by bronchoscopy. Atypical adenomatous hyperplasia is occasionally seen in airways of patients with adenocarcinoma and could be a precursor lesion. Small cell carcinoma might arise from neuroendocrine hyperplasia, but evidence in support of this hypothesis is scarce.

Premalignant lesions of the lung have been investigated for molecular alterations of several chromosomal regions on a limited number of specimens.[73] Microdissected specimens derived from normal, hyperplastic, metaplastic, dysplastic, and CIS, as well as invasive neoplastic foci of patients with lung cancer, were studied for gene mutations, promotor hypermethylation, and allele loss. Results obtained to date suggest that allele loss on chromosome 3p is the earliest event, followed by allele loss/hypermethylation on chromosome 9p and subsequently on chromosome 8p.[74] Loss of heterozygosity (LOH) at the *p53* gene locus (17q13.1) is relatively rare (10%) and occurs predominantly at the dysplasia or CIS stage.[72] Point mutations in the *p53* gene, however, have been observed in morphologically normal bronchial epithelium obtained from the airways of patients with lung cancer.[75] In contrast, K-*ras* gene mutations were found only in CIS.[76]

Investigations of LOH for chromosome 3p markers in normal-appearing epithelium adjacent to carcinomas revealed allele loss in these "normal" cells. The regions of 3p allele loss were associated with the histologic type of lung cancer—namely, large deletions in small cell carcinoma and more limited deletions in NSCLC. One might thus conclude that chromosome 3p allele loss is more a marker of environmental exposure and perhaps an indicator of the ultimately arising tumor type rather than a marker indicating tumor progression. In addition, these results could indicate that lung cancers can arise directly from "normal" epithelium without morphologic intermediates (hyperplasia-metaplasia-dysplasia-CIS).

In patients with lung cancer who are smokers or ex-smokers, morphologically normal-appearing bronchial mucosa frequently harbors molecular clonal abnormalities.[64] In a study by Park and associates,[64] 218 microdissected specimens from 19 patients who underwent

TABLE 75-1

Chromosomal Loci and Genes Frequently Altered in Lung Cancer

CHROMOSOME	LOCUS	PUTATIVE GENE	FUNCTION OF GENE AND FREQUENCY OF ALTERATION
2q33	PYNH24	?	35% LOH in NSCLC, 30% in SCLC
3p12.3	D3S1274	DUTT1	NCAM-related protein, involved in cell-cell recognition; no mutations known in lung cancer, 50% LOH in NSCLC, 98% LOH in SCLC
3p14.2	D3S1300	FHIT	Could be involved in hydrolysis of dinucleoside polyphosphates; 75% of NSCLC do not express the FHIT protein, 50% LOH in NSCLC, 98% LOH in SCLC
3p21.3	D3S1235	UBE1L	Ubiquitin-activating enzyme homologue; not completely inactivated in lung cancer but expressed at relatively low levels, 50% LOH in NSCLC, 98% LOH in SCLC
3p22–24	D3S1537	?	50% LOH in NSCLC, 98% LOH in SCLC
3p26.3	D3S1307	VHL	Regulates gene transcription by interaction with elongation factors; not inactivated in lung cancer, 50% LOH in NSCLC, 98% LOH in SCLC
4p15.1–15.3	D4S1546	?	50% LOH in SCLC and mesothelioma, 20% in NSCLC
4q25–26	D4S194	?	60% LOH in SCLC and mesothelioma, 30% in NSCLC
4q33–34	D4S408	?	80% LOH in SCLC and mesothelioma, 35% in NSCLC
5q21	APC	APC	Cell adhesion; LOH in 30% of NSCLC, no mutations in lung cancer
6p21	D6S105	?	45% LOH in SCLC
6q26–27	D6S264	M6P/IGF2R	Receptor involved in activation of TGF-α and degradation of IGF-2; mutations in lung cancers not reported, 45% LOH in SCLC
8p21–22	D8S136	TRAIL-R2	TNF-related apoptosis-inducing ligand receptor; mutated in 10% of NSCLC, LOH in 40% of NSCLC
9p21	D9S1758	p16^{INK4a}	Cyclin-dependent kinase inhibitor; inactivated in 70% of NSCLC, <10% in SCLC
10q25.3–26.1	D10S587	DMBT1	Unknown function; very low or absent expression in 45% of NSCLC
11p13	CAT	?	16%–38% LOH in lung cancer
11p15.5	D11S4932	RRM1	Regulatory subunit of ribonucleotide reductase; no mutations in coding region known in lung cancer, >85% LOH in SCLC, >60% in NSCLC
11p15.5	HRAS	?	35% LOH in lung cancer
11q22.2	D11S1647	PPP2R1B	Regulatory subunit of serine/threonine phosphatase 2A; mutations detected in 15% of lung cancers, 70% LOH in cell lines
11q23.1	D11S1792	ATM	Protein kinase, involved in intra S-phase DNA damage checkpoint regulation; mutations in lung cancer not reported, 70% LOH in cell lines
13q14.3	D13S133	Rb	Regulates activity of transcription factors; inactivated in >90% of SCLC, rarely in NSCLC
17p13.1	D17S786	p53	Multifunctional transcription factor; mutated in 75% of SCLC and 35%–50% of NSCLC; mutational hot spots are in exons 5–8
6p21		α-tubulin	Chromosome segregation, locomotion, others; mutated in 33% of NSCLC
8q24		c-myc	Transcription factor; amplified in 7% of NSCLC
1p32		L-myc	Transcription factor; amplified in 2% of NSCLC
2q23–24		N-myc	Transcription factor; amplified in <1% of NSCLC
12p11–12		Kras	G-protein; mutated in 25%–30% of adenocarcinomas; 85% of mutations are in codon 12; codons 13 and 61 less frequently altered
18q21		bcl2	Inhibits apoptosis; expressed in 35% of NSCLC
7p11		c-erbB1	p170 EGF receptor with tyrosine kinase activity; highly expressed in 65% of NSCLC
17q21		c-erbB2	p185^{neu}, EGFR-related tyrosine kinase transmembrane protein; highly expressed in 15% of NSCLC

surgical resection for lung cancer were investigated for LOH. Each specimen consisted of 200 adjacent epithelial cells, and the specimens were obtained from cross-sections of lobar, segmental, or subsegmental bronchi with partial or completely intact bronchial epithelium as close as possible to the surgical resection margin. Of these specimens, 195 had histologically normal or slightly abnormal epithelium, and 23 had dysplastic epithelium. All specimens were investigated for LOH with 12 microsatellite markers. Ten markers were specific for chromosome 3p loci, one was specific for 9p21, and one was specific for 17q13.1. Microdissected stromal cells or lymphocytes from the same slides served as a source of constitutional DNA. One-third (32%) of the "normal" specimens showed molecular anomalies, as did half (52%) of the dysplastic specimens. The approximate size of individual "clonal patches" was estimated to be 90,000 cells, and the molecular anomalies detected in separate patches within a given patient were heterogeneous. In contrast, molecular anomalies from different sites of the tumor from a given patient appeared to be homogenous. The authors estimated that one-third of the entire respiratory surface epithelium could be molecularly abnormal in patients with lung cancer.[64] The fate of morphologicly or molecularly abnormal areas is currently an intense area of research. Available data suggest that 58% of dysplastic lesions spontaneously regress, 39% remain unchanged, and 3% progress to CIS. Preliminary data also suggest that 86% of molecularly abnormal regions spontaneously regress, while "normal" regions might display molecular changes on repeat biopsies over time.

Malignant transformation is generally thought to arise from a series of somatic genetic events.[77] These events can occur spontaneously or be triggered by chemicals or ionizing radiation. The result is loss of DNA integrity,

Specific Malignancies

III

for instance, in the form of mutations, deletions, or translocations. As already mentioned, the rate at which this occurs is a function of dose and chemistry of the agent and the organism's ability to process it. Once the DNA modification has occurred, intracellular mechanisms become activated that serve to restore DNA integrity.[78] These mechanisms require that the DNA modification be detected, removed, and repaired. This process requires a complex interplay of a multitude of genes, many of which have polymorphisms (inherited DNA sequence variations or mutations) that affect the functional activity of their respective gene products. As a result, lung cancer risk is modified by the existence of polymorphisms in DNA repair genes, with higher risk resulting from less efficient repair. In addition, these genes are highly likely to affect the therapeutic efficacy of chemotherapy and radiation. In terms of treatment efficacy, however, genetic variants with low repair capacity are likely to be beneficial for patients.

If DNA damage is too extensive for repair, cells have the ability to commit suicide (apoptosis or programmed cell death).[79] This mechanism exists in all multicellular organisms and appears to serve organismal integrity. Thus, cells with irreparable DNA damage are not given the opportunity to damage the organism through aberrant growth. Individual variations in genes involved in apoptosis are thus likely to affect lung cancer risk, its malignant potential, and its response to therapy.

Proliferation is a *sine qua non* for cancer.[80] For proliferation to occur, cells must progress through the cell cycle, which includes DNA replication and mitosis. Physiologically, proliferation of bronchoepithelial cells is required to replace cells lost at the lumen and to repair epithelial damage caused by environmental influences. To control proliferation in response to tissue damage, a complex system of intercellular communication has evolved that includes epithelial cells, stroma, and inflammatory cells.[81] The vehicles of communication are growth factors, cytokines, peptides, lipids, and the respective membrane receptors. Their functions include induction and suppression of not only of proliferation but also of migration, contact inhibition, and apoptosis. DNA replication must occur during each cycle of proliferation, resulting in the duplication of over one billion base pairs in a matter of hours. This is accomplished at high fidelity by the replication machinery. Mistakes do occur, however, and are sensed and repaired through induction of so-called checkpoints. Formation of cancer, and perhaps even of premalignant lesions in the bronchoepithelial layer, might further trigger tissue damage responses, which are likely to contribute to tumor progression. Finally, reactive oxygen species that are generated during inflammation can result in DNA damage. It is thus plausible that individual variations in any of the genes involved in intercellular communication and signal processing are contributory to lung cancer risk, phenotype, and response to treatment.

Survival of patients with lung cancer is predominantly a function of disease stage, and it declines with increasing stage.[82] The current paradigm is that patients with NSCLC can be cured only by surgery, which is feasible in the 30% of patients who initially present in early stages of the disease. But even in this group with a "favorable" stage of lung cancer, the majority will ultimately succumb to recurrent disease.

Several lines of evidence suggest that metastatic dissemination of NSCLC has already occurred at the earliest stages of the disease in at least two-thirds of the patients. These findings include the following items:

1. Locoregional control of lung cancer can be achieved by surgery and/or radiation; yet more than 70% of relapses in patients with stage I disease (a single primary tumor located within one lobe of the lung without microscopic evidence for disease in hilar or mediastinal lymph nodes) occur at distant sites.[83]
2. Approximately 9% of relapses occur more than five years after initial treatment.[84]
3. The size of the primary tumor in patients with stage IA disease (tumors ≤3 cm in diameter without visceral pleural involvement) does not appear to affect survival.[85]
4. Chemotherapy given before surgery (neoadjuvant chemotherapy) in an effort to eliminate or reduce submicroscopic systemic disease was shown recently to be of some benefit in patients with stage I and II disease and had earlier been shown to be effective in resectable stage III disease.[86-88]
5. It appears that approximately 30% of patients with stage I disease and 60% with stage II disease have submicroscopic involvement of mediastinal lymph nodes by molecular analyses.[89]
6. Evidence for circulating cancer cells in the peripheral blood has been reported for patients at all stages of the disease.[90,91]

These data suggest that the metastatic ability of lung cancers is determined early on during the carcinogenic process. Identification of individual genes that determine this metastatic ability and an understanding of their function in pathways and systems that are required for migration, invasion, adhesion, and proliferation are crucial to intervene effectively in this process at the earliest point in time.

The discovery and validation of reliable markers predictive of relapse, response to therapy, and poor outcome from lung cancer have long been pursued by investigators with the goal of guiding clinicians in selecting treatment for patients. Over the last decade, several parameters potentially predictive of poor survival have been reported. The most promising include microvessel density, submicroscopic metastases, metabolic activity, mutations in oncogenes and tumor suppressor genes, expression of extracellular matrix proteinases and inhibitors, expression of proteins involved in cellular proliferation, genomic alterations, and expression of genes involved in chemotherapeutic efficacy.[92-112] All of these published reports are descriptive investigations, in which phenotypic parameters—for instance, the level of expression of a certain protein or the absence or presence of a specific gene mutation—were compared with the phenotypic parameter of interest, namely survival. Because survival, response to therapy, disease stage, and metastatic spread are closely related measures of tumor aggressiveness, it is plausible that any of these parameters or combinations thereof will become important for therapeutic decisions in the near future.

One future approach to improve patient outcome is tailored therapy based on individualized phenotypic or genotypic tumor characteristics. Even though the concept of patient-specific individualized therapy is novel, therapeutic intervention tailored according to a tumor phenotype is not new, and it has evolved over many decades. Among the various carcinomas, different therapies are used for those arising in the bladder, breast, colon, and lung. Except for leukemias and selected lymphomas, however, treatment is not currently based on molecular characteristics. In the treatment of lung cancer, an earlier attempt to use in vitro drug testing of freshly resected NSCLC specimens and SCLC cell lines established from cytologic material at the time of primary intervention as a tool to determine the best therapeutic combination of agents at recurrence, unfortunately did not prove successful.[113,114] Recent technological advances in mutation detection and quantitation of gene expression in minute clinical specimens herald the advent of clinical therapeutic decisions based on the intra-tumoral expression of specific therapeutic targets and/or characteristics. Examples of such targets might include:

- Enzymes specifically inhibited by chemotherapeutic agents (ribonucleotide reductase, topoisomerase I);
- Structural proteins (β-tubulin);
- Enzymes that lead to the inactivation of chemotherapeutic agents (glutathione-S-transferases, UDP-glucuronosyl transferases); or
- Enzymes that lead to reversal of those agents' effects (repair of DNA adducts by DNA damage repair enzymes).

A therapeutic decision that leads to an effective and clinically meaningful benefit for a specific patient, however, is unlikely to result from knowledge regarding a single parameter (e.g., level of RNA expression) or a single molecular determinant (e.g., topoisomerase I). This is a result of the complex intracellular cross-talk and feedback among the various molecules and pathways that control proliferation, migration, and survival—the key characteristics of cancer cells.

PATHOLOGIC ASPECTS OF LUNG CANCER

Clinical-Pathologic Aspects of Lung Cancer

Age at Presentation

Lung cancer is a disease of the middle-aged and elderly: 90% of cases occur between the ages of 40 and 80.[115] The incidence of lung cancer increases with the duration and intensity of smoking, and the age at presentation reflects a long latency period between exposure to smoking and development of cancer.[116] From a clinical standpoint, this latency suggests the existence of a "window of

opportunity" within which early cancer might be detected and virtually cured.

Lung cancers arising in patients younger than 40 years of age tend to occur more frequently among women and are characterized by a predominance of adenocarcinomas.[117-120] The reason for this gender predilection among young nonsmokers is not known. The hypotheses proposed by some authors—that women have a higher susceptibility to lung cancer and that lung cancer is linked to glutathione transferase polymorphism—have not been accepted unanimously.[121-126]

Etiology and Epidemiology

Smoking is the main, although not the only, etiologic factor of lung cancer. An estimated 5%–20% of lung cancers arise in association with exposure to other respiratory carcinogens, including asbestos.[127] Only an estimated 10% of heavy smokers develop lung cancer.[14,128] An estimated 20% of lung cancers arise in nonsmokers, and only 20% of these can be attributed to passive smoking.[116,129] These data stress the importance of the interaction of environmental exposure with other factors in the pathogenesis of lung cancer. Notably, diet has been proposed to be one of these factors, and the "usual suspects" (fruit and vegetables) have been proposed to have a protective effect against the development of lung cancer in both smokers and nonsmokers; this effect has been linked to a protective effect against mutations of nutrients.[130-136]

The existence of a genetic predisposition to lung cancer has been demonstrated by its occurrence within familial settings and by an association with gene polymorphism affecting mythochondrial oxidase phase I and detoxification, phase II genes.[137] The biologic rationale underlying the wide variations in the risk of developing lung cancer among smokers remains to be elucidated.[138] From a clinical standpoint, the absence of reliable clinical markers that can identify smokers who are at highest risk for developing lung cancer poses a significant challenge to the development of early detection programs.[139] Spirometry is a good screening tool, however, as heavy smokers with COPD have a significantly higher risk of lung cancer.[140] Molecular analysis of tissue is an invaluable tool for early detection, but the quest for a reliable and effective marker of risk continues.[141] Adenocarcinoma (Aca) is the most common histotype of lung cancer (Table 75-2). From 1973 to 1994, a much larger increase in the incidence of lung cancer was observed for women than for men.[142] Whether this increase suggests a higher gender-related risk of cancer for women or merely reflects changing smoking patterns remains controversial.[124,125,143] The overall increased incidence of Aca that has occurred since the 1960s has been correlated with the introduction of filter tips in cigarettes.[144,145] Different histopathologic types of lung cancer have different associations with cigarette smoking, and this association is the highest for squamous cell carcinoma (SqCC) and small cell carcinoma (SCC) (Table 75-3). The largest proportion of carcinomas arising in nonsmokers are Aca (18%), followed by large cell undifferentiated carcinoma (LCU) (7%), whereas only 1% of SCC cases and 2% of SqCC cases arise among nonsmokers.[146] Among patients with Aca, an even higher

Specific Malignancies

III

TABLE 75-2

Lung Cancer: Incidence of Different Histotypes		
HISTOTYPE	**SEER 1983–1987 (N = 59,620)**	**HARPER/KCI 1991–1999 (N = 2464)**
Adenocarcinoma	32%	37%
Squamous cell carcinoma	30%	28%
Large cell undifferentiated	18%	16%
Small cell carcinoma	10%	14%
Other	10%	4%

proportion of nonsmokers is reported in patients having the bronchiolo-alveolar (BAC) subtype (30%). The highest odds for contracting lung cancer conferred by smoking are for the squamous and small cell types, and this association persists even after smoking cessation.[122,147] We (and others) have observed that among nonsmokers, women and the Aca histotype are overrepresented.[148,149] In a series of 2464 lung cancer cases seen at Harper Hospital in Detroit, Michigan from 1991 to 1999, 60% of lung cancers arising in smokers occurred in males and 40% in females. The largest percentage of these patients (34%) had diagnoses of Aca, followed by SqCC at 30%. In contrast, 68% of lung cancers arising in nonsmokers occurred in females; 70% of these patients had diagnoses of Aca, while 8% had SqCC.

Human papillomavirus (HPV) infection is an etiologic factor in the rare cases of SqCC of the lung that arise in the setting of laryngeal papillomatosis.[150] HPV, including high-risk serotypes, has been detected in approximately 20% of patients with lung cancers; whether it constitutes a cofactor in the development of such cancers outside the setting of laryngeal papillomatosis, however, is not clear.[151]

Tissue Diagnosis of Lung Cancer

A tissue diagnosis of malignancy is necessary for appropriate treatment of lung cancer. Analysis of the cells present in sputum (sputum cytology) is the only non-invasive procedure for obtaining tissue. The others include transthoracic sampling of the lung, yielding either cells (fine-needle aspiration) or tissue (needle biopsy), and diagnostic procedures performed during bronchoscopy. These include washing and brushing (yielding cytologic specimens) and biopsy (bronchial or transbronchial)

yielding tissue. Differences in the anatomic distribution of lung cancer dictate differences in the sensitivity of these diagnostic techniques. Thus, the sensitivity of sputum cytology alone is the highest for central lesions (i.e., SqCC and SCC) and decreases significantly for peripherally located lesions (i.e., Aca and LCU).[152,153] The addition of washing and brushing to sputum cytology increases its sensitivity in detecting peripheral lesions.[154-156] Bronchoscopy-based techniques, including washing, brushing, and bronchial and transbronchial biopsy, allow a diagnosis in more than 70% of cases; the remaining cases require transthoracic sampling.[157] Most cases in which fine-needle aspiration is required to yield a diagnosis of malignancy are Aca and LC.[158] The sensitivity of bronchial biopsy is the highest for endobronchial lesions. Transthoracic aspiration (TTA) has the highest sensitivity (90%) in detecting peripheral lesions, followed respectively by brushing, transbronchial biopsy, and washings. The sensitivity of TTA decreases for lesions smaller than 2 cm in diameter. The estimated overall accuracy for distinguishing between small cell and non–small cell histotype with these techniques is 98%.[153]

Pathology of Lung Cancer

Classification

Tumors arising in the lung are classified on the bases of biologic behavior and differentiation. They entail epithelial, soft tissue, and mesothelial tumors and lymphoproliferative disorders. These are further divided into benign and malignant entities. Here we will focus on carcinomas, which are primary malignant tumors of epithelial origin and constitute the most common type of primary malignancy arising in this organ. Table 75-4 lists the entities included in this category, as recognized in the most recent classification.[159]

Anatomic Distribution

As depicted in Table 75-5, a distinctive association of different subtypes with specific lung compartments exists. SqCC and SCC are predominantly central, while LCU and Aca are predominantly peripheral. This differential distribution reflects differences in the cell of origin, as documented for the two histotypes (SqCC and Aca) for which precursor lesions are known. SqCC arises predominantly from the respiratory mucosa of lobar and

TABLE 75-3

Histologic Subtypes of Lung Cancer in Smokers and Nonsmokers	
HISTOLOGIC SUBTYPE	**SMOKERS (%)**
Squamous cell carcinoma	98.0
Adenocarcinoma	82
Small cell carcinoma	99
Large cell carcinoma	93

Modified from Colby TV, Kon MN, Travis WD: Tumors of the lower respiratory tract. In Rosai J (ed): Atlas of Tumor Pathology, 3rd series. Washington DC, AFIP, 1994.

TABLE 75-4

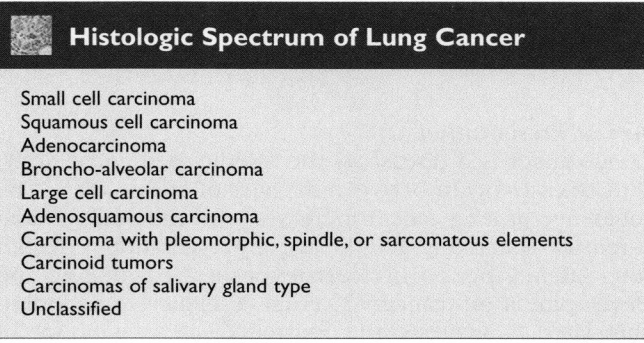

Histologic Spectrum of Lung Cancer
Small cell carcinoma
Squamous cell carcinoma
Adenocarcinoma
Broncho-alveolar carcinoma
Large cell carcinoma
Adenosquamous carcinoma
Carcinoma with pleomorphic, spindle, or sarcomatous elements
Carcinoid tumors
Carcinomas of salivary gland type
Unclassified

TABLE 75-5

Chest Radiographic Finding at Presentation According to Cancer Histotype

RADIOGRAPHIC FEATURE	SQUAMOUS CELL CARCINOMA (%)	ADENOCARCINOMA (%)	SMALL CELL CARCINOMA (%)	LARGE CELL UNDIFFERENTIATED CARCINOMA (%)
Nodule ≤4 cm	14	46	21	18
Peripheral location	29	65	26	61
Central location	64	5	74	42
Hilar/perihilar mass	40	17	78	32
Hilar adenopathy	38	19	61	32
Mediastinal adenopathy	5	9	14	10

Modified from Miller WE: Roentgenographic manifestations of lung cancer. In Strauss MJ (ed): Lung Cancer: Clinical Diagnosis and Treatments, 2nd ed. New York, Grune and Stratton, 1983.

segmental bronchi. In contrast, Aca arises from bronchioles and terminal alveolar units. Thus, the histotypes that are more prone to give clinical presentations secondary to the effect of the primary tumor are those that are either located centrally and/or involve the hilum (i.e., SCC and SqCC) or those that have an inordinate propensity for chest wall invasion (i.e., LC). Aca is the histotype that least commonly manifests with clinical signs secondary to local invasion.[160]

Precursor Lesions

The presence of preinvasive lesions is well recognized only for SqCC and Aca. Precursors for neuroendocrine neoplasms are not recognized, with the exception of a rare primary form of neuroendocrine hyperplasia (diffuse idiopathic pulmonary neuroendocrine cell hyperplasia) that is associated with bronchiolar fibrosis, which is regarded as a precursor of carcinoid tumors in this particular setting.[159] In contrast, the histologic precursors of SqCC and of Aca are well characterized morphologicly, and their molecular features are increasingly becoming recognized. The following scheme sketches the current view of the pathogenesis of SqCC:

Normal bronchial mucosa → Squamous metaplasia → Low-grade dysplasia → High-grade dysplasia → Invasive SqCC

Morphologic evidence that the pathogenesis of human SqCC includes progression through squamous metaplasia and bronchial dysplasia dates back to the early 1900s.[161,162] The first study to systematically characterize the morphologic changes occurring in the bronchial mucosa in association with cigarette smoke, however, was published by Auerbach and associates in 1957.[163] This seminal study was based on the microscopic examination of the entire bronchial tree, by serial sections, in 117 necropsies. It was the first to establish a relation between smoking and bronchial dysplasia and to link the degree of dysplasia with the duration and amount of cigarette smoke exposure. These observations predicted a progression from low- to high-grade dysplasia to invasive carcinoma, which was later directly observed to occur in a cohort of patients at risk followed prospectively by sputum cytology during a mass screening program.[164] This

latter study also showed that a long time interval separates the occurrence of dysplasia from the onset of invasive carcinoma. The clinical implication of this finding was that detection and treatment of a preinvasive lesion in this time window might prevent the progression of the lesion to an overt malignancy. This hypothesis was tested in a multi-institutional trial in the 1970s using both cytology and x-ray.[165]

The morphologic criteria to consider in this progression are degree of differentiation and cytologic grade. In squamous metaplasia, the lowest step in this progression, the native ciliated bronchial epithelium is replaced by squamous epithelium. This shows progressive and orderly maturation from basal cells (the stem cells of bronchial mucosa) to terminally differentiated, anucleated squamous cell. Increasing degrees of dysplasia, arising in the setting of preexisting squamous metaplasia, are characterized by an expansion of the replicative component within the epithelium at the expense of the superficial, differentiated component. In increasing degrees of dysplasia (i.e., low, moderate, severe, CIS), an increasing area of the epithelium is replaced by dysplastic cells characterized by high nuclear/cytoplasmic (N/C) ratios, variation in size and shape (pleomorphism), and a high proliferative rate. In CIS, the highest preinvasive grade, dysplastic cells occupy the full thickness of the epithelium, and apical maturation into differentiated squames is either absent or negligible.[146,159] Increasing molecular abnormalities in genes controlling cell cycle progression parallel these morphologic changes. These include overexpression of p53, Cyclin D1, and Cyclin E and chromosomal losses at 3p, 9q, and 5q loci, including the coding regions of the FHIT, p15, and 16 genes.[54]

The following scheme summarizes the current view of the pathogenesis of Aca:

Normal terminal bronchioles/alveoli → Atypical adenomatous hyperplasia → Invasive Aca

The view that noninvasive proliferations involving terminal bronchioles and alveoli constitute the precursors of overt Aca is supported by the following findings:[166]

1. Areas of pneumocyte hyperplasia are frequently seen adjacent to invasive Aca.[167-170]

2. A morphologic spectrum of intra-alveolar proliferative lesions showing increasing cytologic atypia can be identified; these include areas showing transitional growth patterns between noninvasive and invasive proliferations.[171-176]

3. Increasing positivity in p53 and K-*ras* positivity and proliferative rates are observed in this morphologic spectrum, supporting biologically the contention that they constitute steps in neoplastic progression.[177-181]

4. A similar spectrum can be reproduced in animal models of lung carcinogenesis.[182,183]

These changes take place in the peripheral lung, perturbing the morphology of normal alveoli. Normal alveolar sacs, through which gas exchanges take place, are thin membranes made up of the flattened, elongated cytoplasm of alveolar type I pneumocytes, juxtaposed through a shared basement membrane to endothelial cells. In atypical adenomatous hyperplasia (AAH), an increase in the number and cytologic grade (increasing N/C ratio, pleomorphism) of the pneumocytes of the alveolar lining takes place. In parallel, the alveolar septa become progressively thickened secondary to fibrosis. The alveolar surface becomes irregular and shaggy, being progressively replaced by enlarged pneumocytes with prominent nuclei and voluminous cytoplasm. The extent of lung involvement, together with the degree of cytologic atypia, set BAC apart from AAH. Whereas the latter is found only in microscopic foci and by definition is smaller than or equal to 5 mm, BAC either can be present in microscopic foci (usually associated with invasive Aca) or can form discrete single or multiple masses large enough to be identifiable by x-ray.[146,159,171] Because in BAC the basement membrane is not breached, it has been proposed that it be regarded as the peripheral equivalent of bronchial carcinoma in situ (i.e., Aca in situ).[167,171,173,184] Invasion of the septa sets preinvasive lesions and the BAC growth pattern apart from Aca. Progressive destruction and remodeling of the alveolar outline takes place in the transition from noninvasive to invasive proliferations.[176] Thus, transitional growth patterns still show some preservation of the alveolar outline, which is obliterated in overt Aca. It has been proposed that the cell of origin of Aca is the type II alveolar pneumocyte. This cell type makes up the stem cells of the alveolar epithelium and is physiologically responsible for the production of surfactant. It plays a crucial role in tissue remodeling and proliferation in both inflammatory and non-neoplastic processes in the peripheral lung and thus is "at the crossroads of inflammation, fibrogenesis and neoplasia."[185]

Major Histotypes of Lung Cancer

Squamous Cell Carcinoma
SqCC (Figs. 75-1 and 75-2) is defined by its ability to show squamous differentiation, highlighted by keratinization and/or intercellular bridges.[159] Keratinization is characterized by the intracytoplasmic accumulation of intermediate filaments and the progressive reduction of the N/C ratio, culminating in the formation of squames—elongated

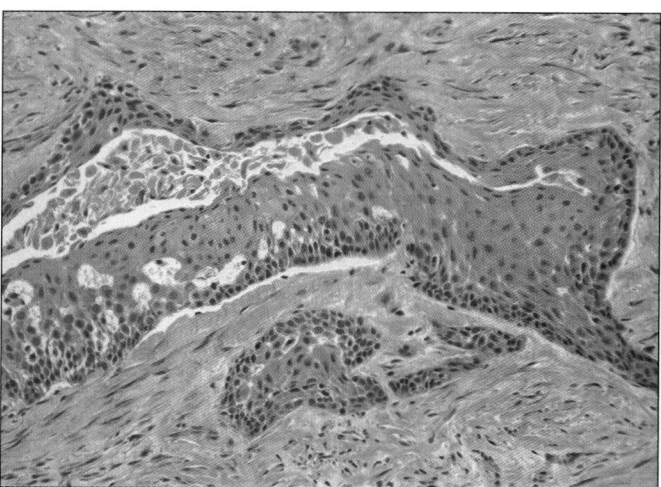

Figure 75-1. Well differentiated squamous cell carcinoma. Tumor nest shows a gradient of differentiation from the periphery to the center. Notice a rim of basaloid cells at the base of the tumor nest. Proceeding towards the center, cells with progressively lower N/C ratios are present. At the center of the tumor nest, there is accumulation of anucleated squames, with impending cavitation.

or spindly cells with deeply eosinophilic cytoplasm and absent or inconspicuous nuclei. Intercellular bridges are characterized by light microscopy as thin, intercellular striations that correspond ultrastructurally to the presence of desmosomes between interlocking cytoplasmic projections of adjacent cells. The same gradient of differentiation that is observed in normal squamous epithelia is reproduced in SqCC. This typically grows in nests featuring an undifferentiated component of basaloid cells at the periphery, with progressive differentiation toward the center. The center of tumor nests is often occupied by accumulating squames mixed with apoptotic and necrotic debris and cavitated. SqCC, even when small

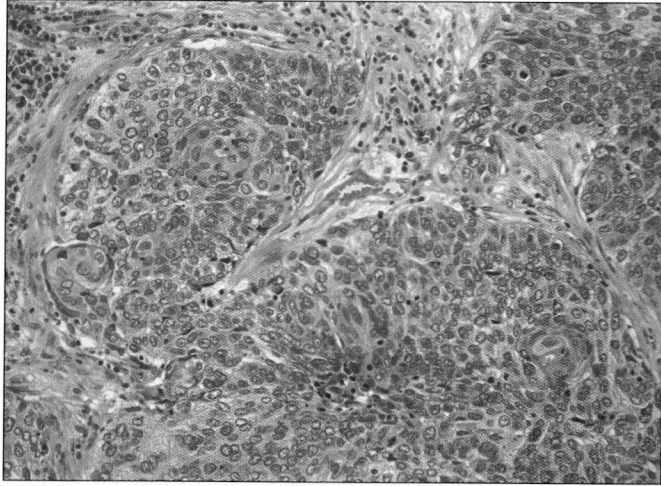

Figure 75-2. Poorly differentiated squamous cell carcinoma. Tumor nests show a predominance of undifferentiated, basaloid-type cells. Squamous differentiation is only focal and represented by nests showing keratinization.

in size, can cavitate; overall, cavitation is seen in one-third of cases.[146] The ratio of the different cell types and the degree of cytologic atypia dictates the grade of the lesion. Notably, the presence of intracellular mucin is not uncommonly detected in SqCC when mucin stains are performed. Similarly, evidence of neuroendocrine differentiation can be highlighted by special techniques in about one-quarter of patients with SqCC.[186] Heterogeneity is common in lung cancer by light microscopy examination, and it is even more common when special techniques and/or electron microscopy are used.[187] Although this phenomenon might be responsible for a high rate of interobserver variability in the classification of lung cancer, it has been proposed that it could also reflect the origin of lung cancers from a multipotent cell that can differentiate along different lineages.[188,189]

SqCC is typically bronchocentric.[190] Studies of early Sq Cca have revealed that SqCC could have a "crawling" growth pattern extending predominantly along the mucosal surface of bronchi, or that it could have a predominantly infiltrating pattern, penetrating the bronchial wall.[191] SqCC can also be entirely entirely exophytic and endobronchial.[192] These different growth patterns underlie the existence of major biologic differences in local invasiveness and natural history among cases of SqCC. The well-differentiated papillary variant is also characterized by a predominantly or exclusively exophytic growth pattern associated with low-grade histology and a favorable outcome.[192] A subset of papillary SqCC cases arise in the setting of recurrent laryngeal papillomatosis.[193] Poorly differentiated variants include the basaloid types, which are characterized by a predominance of poorly differentiated cell types, mimicking the basal cells of normal squamous epithelium.[194,195]

Adenocarcinoma

Adenocarcinoma (Aca) (Fig. 75-3) is a malignant epithelial tumor with glandular differentiation or mucin production by the tumor cells, showing acinar, papillary, or bronchiolo-alveolar growth patterns. Alternatively, it can be solid with mucin production, or it can demonstrate a mixture of these patterns.[159]

At the architectural level, glandular differentiation manifests itself in the arrangement of cells around central lumens, for example, in the acini of exocrine glands. At the single-cell level, glandular differentation is highlighted by the ability of tumor cells to manufacture secretory molecules. These are either mucins or molecules normally produced by Clara cell and/or type II pneumocytes, such as the 10 Kda-Clara cell protein or surfactant molecules, as demonstrated by immunohistochemistry, electron microscopy, and, recently, by high-throughput gene profiling.[196–200] Aca typically arises in the peripheral lung and can be associated with puckering of the overlying pleura, and/or it can grow into the pleural surfaces, mimicking the growth pattern of mesothelioma. The microscopic growth pattern allows distinction among the acinar, papillary, and solid subtypes. The acinar subtype is characterized by well-formed glandular structures that mimic the acini of exocrine glands. Papillary Aca, characterized by fibrovascular cores along which tumor

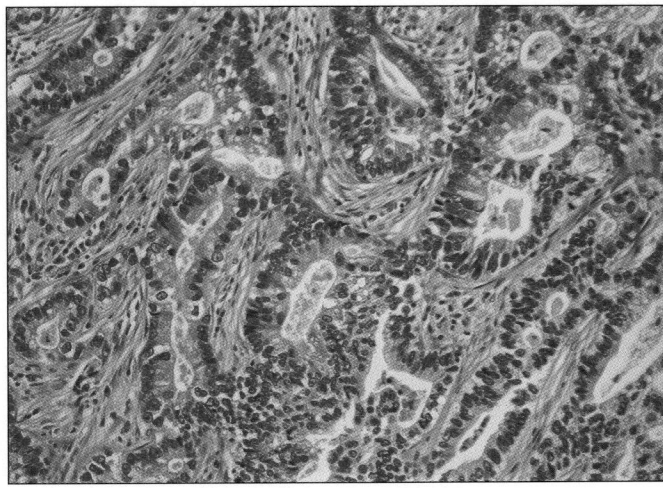

Figure 75-3. Well differentiated adenocarcinoma. Neoplastic cells have a palisaded arrangement around central lumens, forming acinar structures that are separated by fibrotic stroma.

cells grow, is reported as a distinct subtype with better prognosis than the conventional types. It bears more morphologic similarity to BAC than to conventional Aca.[201] The solid type is characterized by growth of tumor cells in large nests, without formation of intercellular glandular lumens but with glandular differentiation at the cellular level, characterized by intracellular accumulation of mucin.[159]

Signet cell Aca is a variant characterized by the presence of tumor cells with large amounts of cytoplasmic mucin which displaces the nucleus focally and confers on cells a resemblance to goblets, as is often found in primary gastric carcinoma.[202] Another variant is well differentiated fetal Aca, a rare tumor of young adults, characterized by the presence of vacuolated, embryonic-type malignant epithelium.[203]

One subtype of Aca with distinct clinical, radiologic, and pathologic features, including the weakest association with smoking among all lung cancers, is BAC (Table 75-3; Fig. 75-4).[171,204,205] The defining feature of this neoplasm is the growth of neoplastic cells along intact alveolar septa, in the absence of stromal invasion, such that the overall alveolar architecture of lung is preserved. BAC is subdivided in two types, mucinous and nonmucinous, depending on the appearance of its constituent cells.[146,159] BAC presents frequently as a small, peripheral lesion that is asymptomatic and has a slow growth rate and is often discovered incidentally. A typical but uncommon presentation of the mucinous subtype is an ill-defined area of pneumonia-like consolidation. BAC, particularly the mucinous subtype, is characterized by a propensity for multifocality, evident either at presentation or at follow-up. It has been proposed that this phenomenon reflects multifocal carcinogenesis rather than aerogenous spread of a single clone.[206] The presence in conventional Aca of areas showing a focal growth pattern of BAC is very common; however, the designation of BAC is warranted only for lesions having this growth pattern exclusively, and

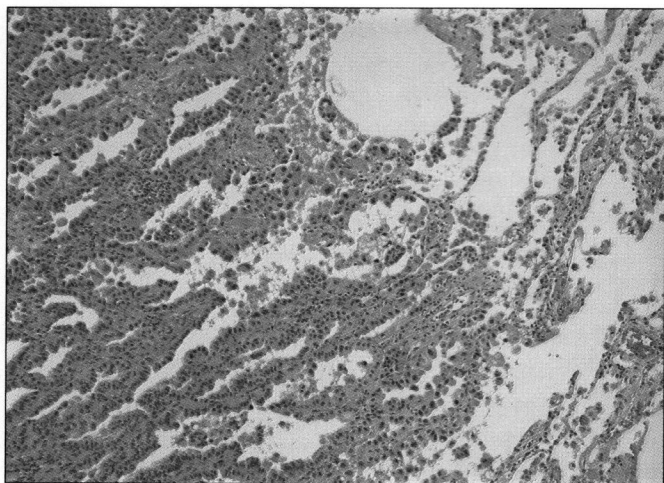

Figure 75-4. Bronchioloalveolar carcinoma. Typical growth pattern, characterized by growth of neoplastic cells along intact septa, with preservation of alveolar outline.

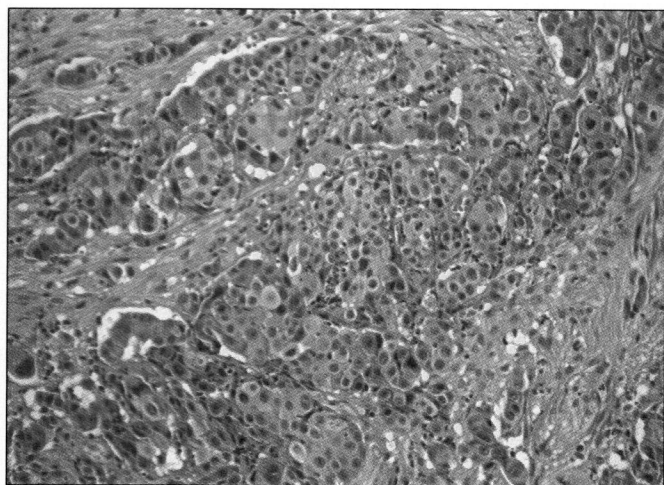

Figure 75-5. Large cell undifferentiated carcinoma. Large neoplastic cells have a large amount of eosinophylic cytoplasm, grow in cohesive nests, and show no evidence of squamous, glandular, or neuroendocrine differentiation.

the presence of any foci of invasion is incompatible with this diagnosis.[159]

Primary Aca of the lung does not have pathognomonic morphologic features and can be indistinguishable from metastases. This applies not only to ordinary Aca but also to BAC, the appearance of which (particularly the mucinous type) can be indistinguishable form metastatic gastrointestinal and ovarian carcinomas.[146,207] Immunohistochemistry is a valid aid to this differential, as the subset of keratins expressed differs among different sites.[208-211] Thyroid transcription factor-1 (TTF-1) has been shown to be a sensitive marker of lung Aca, with higher sensitivity than surfactant molecules in detecting primary Aca of the lung, and with good specificity, as outside the lung it is expressed only in thyroid neoplasms and nonpulmonary small cell carcinoma.[212-214]

Large Cell Undifferentiated Carcinoma

Large cell undifferentiated carcinoma (LCU) (Fig. 75-5) is an undifferentiated malignant tumor that lacks both the cytologic features of SCC and glandular or squamous differentiation. The cells typically have large nuclei, prominent nucleoli, and a moderate amount of cytoplasm. The term *large cell carcinoma* describes a specific variant of NSCLC and thus is not a synonym of non–small cell lung carcinoma (NSCLC), contrary to what is commonly implied in clinical parlance. Because its diagnosis is one of exclusion, thorough sampling is necessary for a correct diagnosis. LCU typically presents as a large and often necrotic lesion. It is more commonly located in the periphery of the lung and not unusually invades the pleura at presentation. Neoplastic cells are of large size and have ample clear or eosinophilic cytoplasm; nuclei are large with prominent nucleoli. The cells grow in solid and often discohesive sheets with prominent cell borders.

Varying amounts of hemorrhage and necrosis are often present, as is likewise the case with high-grade malignant tumors. A prominent chronic or acute inflammatory

infiltrate can be present, and polymorphonuclear leukocytes (PMNs) can be found within the cytoplasm of neoplastic cells (emperipolesis).[144,159] A variant of LCU is lymphoepithelioma-like carcinoma. This tumor is characterized by large tumor cells with prominent nucleoli growing in cohesive sheets, surrounded by an extensive lymphocytic infiltrate. Similarities with analogous tumors arising in the nasopharynx include not only morphologic features but also a high rate of Epstein-Barr virus (EBV) infection.[215,216]

Small Cell Carcinoma

Small cell carcinoma (SCC) (Fig. 75-6) is a tumor formed by cells with very high N/C ratios, a scant rim of cytoplasm, and finely granular nuclear chromatin with absent

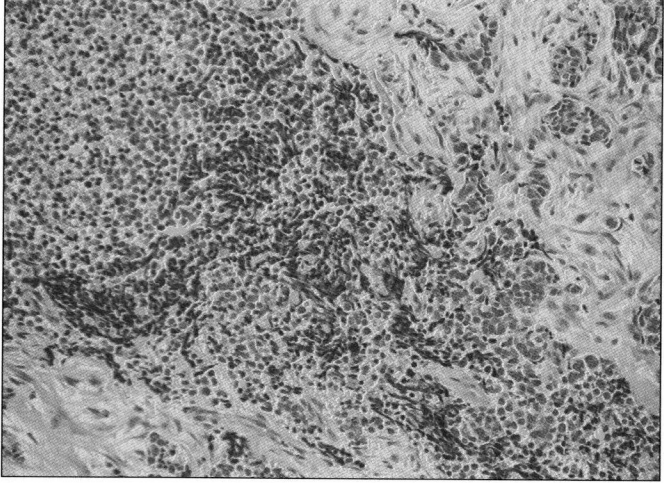

Figure 75-6. Small cell carcinoma. Tumor cells are of small size, with large nuclei with finely dispersed chromatin and a small rim of cytoplasm. Tumor forms variably sized nets surrounded by desmoplastic stroma and displays smearing (crush artifact) and extensive necrosis.

or very rare nucleoli. Cells are round to spindly, often exhibit molding, crush artifact, and extensive necrosis, and display an exceedingly high proliferative rate. Cells grow in nests, usually separated by desmoplastic stroma.

SCC is the type of lung cancer that has the highest association with smoking, almost never arising in the absence of a smoking history (see Table 75-3). It is predominantly located centrally in the lung and arises mostly in association with large bronchi. A mismatch might be found between the size of the primary lesion and its biologic behavior, such that disseminated metastases might be seen in presence of very small or even clinically undetectable primary lesions.[146] SCC is characterized by its ability to produce substances with neurohormonal activity, and to be associated with antibodies that produce a large spectrum of paraneoplastic syndromes and are directed against neural and muscle antigens.[217] Distinction of SCC into different morphologic subtypes has proven of no clinical relevance and is no longer recognized in the most recent WHO classification of lung tumors.[159,218,219] The typical appearance of SCC is seen in small biopsies, as the neoplasm is usually not resected.

The diagnosis can be challenging, particularly when extensive crush artifact is present, justifying differential diagnosis with normal and neoplastic crushed lymphocytes. In addition, SCC must be distinguished from neuroendocrine lesions of lesser histologic grade (including carcinoids) that have similar cytologic and architectural features but do not display the necrosis and high mitotic activity of SCC.[220] Diagnosis rests on morphologic, light microscopic features alone according to World Health Organization (WHO) recommendation, as the tumor is consistently keratin positive, but 20% or more patients can be negative for neuroendocrine markers.[159,221] Notably, because this malignancy is rarely resected, the appearance pathologists are most familiar with is that seen in transbronchial biopsies. Many of the most helpful diagnostic morphologic features of SCC, however—namely, crush artifact and small cell size—are artifacts generated by this procedure and are not present in resected lesions.

To demonstrate the epithelial nature of the cells (as is often the goal of transbronchial biopsies), immunohistochemic stain with keratin and leukocyte common antigen is advisable. This is especially the case when extensive crush artifact is present and areas with preservation of cytology are rare.

Ultrastructurally, neurosecretory granules are present in most, but not all, cases.[146] The most important differential diagnosis is with NSCLC, and such distinction has interobserver reproducibility among pathologists in more than 95% of cases.[222]

SCC can be present in association with NSCLC and large cell neuroendocrine carcinoma (LCNE), either at presentation or after treatment.[223,224] In the latter setting, it is not clear whether the finding of a non–small cell component reflects the effect of therapy or a sampling error.

Carcinoid Tumor

Carcinoid tumor constitutes a low-grade tumor with neuroendocrine differentiation. It is characterized by typical architectural and cytologic features. Carcinoid tumor is typically an indolent tumor. It is most often asymptomatic at presentation and has an excellent prognosis, rarely being a cause of mortality.[225,226] Symptoms at presentation are more common for tumors that are located centrally and include hemoptysis, dyspnea, and postobstructive pneumonia secondary to bronchial obstruction.[225]

Morphologically, carcinoid tumor is the prototype of neuroendocrine tumors. Tumor cells are characterized by a relatively low N/C ratio, with a prominent rim of eosinophilic or amphophylic granular cytoplasm, and they have typical nuclear features. The chromatin is fine and homogeneously dispersed in a "salt and pepper" pattern, with absent or very small nucleoli. The tumor cells are arranged in nests tightly juxtaposed to a rich capillary network, to form insular, trabecular, pseudoglandular, or organoid patterns. The neuroendocrine differentiation is highlighted by strong immunoreactivity of tumor cells for neuroendocrine markers, including synaptophysin and chromogranin. Utrastructurally, numerous neuroendocrine secretory granules are evident.[146,159]

Central carcinoid tumor can undermine the bronchial mucosa or can grow as exophytic, endobronchial masses. Along with primary mucoepidermoid and adenoid cystic carcinoma of bronchi, central carcinoid tumor enters endoscopically and pathologically into the differential diagnosis of bronchocentric tumors. Carcinoid tumors are usually covered by an intact bronchial mucosa with focal squamous metaplasia.[227] "Tumorlets" describe small peripheral carcinoid tumors, which usually are discovered incidentally.[228] Many morphologic variants of carcinoid tumor are described, among them a spindle cell variant that prompts differential diagnosis with primary and metastatic spindle cell neoplasms, including sarcomas.[229,230]

Atypical carcinoids (AC) are characterized by a much more aggressive behavior than typical carcinoid tumor, including a higher incidence of lymph node metastases and a worse prognosis, intermediate between that of carcinoid tumor and that of SCC.[231-233] The tumor is characterized morphologically by a growth pattern similar to that of carcinoid tumor and similar cytologic features; however, these occur in association with "necrosis and/or mitoses exceeding 2/10 high-power fields."[159] Necrosis occurs usually as punctate, comedo-like foci, and mitotic figures usually far exceed the 2/10 hpf range.

Other Tumors with Neuroendocrine Differentatiation

The family of major tumors showing evidence of neuroendocrine differentiation is indicated in Table 75-6. In addition to SCC, carcinoid tumor, and Aca, LCNE and

TABLE 75-6

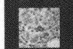 **Major Lung Cancer Types with Neuroendocrine Differentiation**

Typical carcinoid
Atypical carcinoid
Large cell neuoroendocrine carcinoma
Small cell carcinoma
Non–small cell carcinoma with focal neuroendocrine differentiation

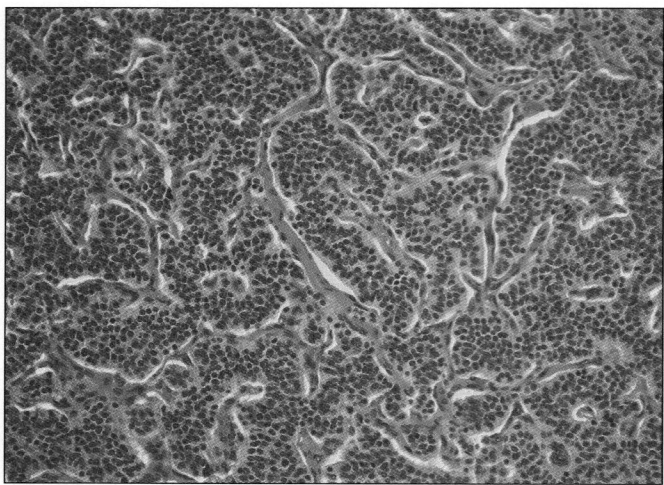

Figure 75-7. Carcinoid tumor. Tumor cells have stipled chromatin and conspicuous eosinophylic cytoplasm. They are arranged in insular/trabecular nests, juxtaposed to a rich capillary network.

NSCLC also demonstrate focal evidence of neuroendocrine differentiation. This probably reflects the pluripotent nature of cells involved in carcinogenesis that are able to differentiate along different lines. Evidence for this phenomenon is exhaustive, including common expression of molecular markers in tumors of different histotypes (i.e., TTF-1, expressed in a high percentage of both SCC and Aca) and the existence of great heterogeneity within NSCLC, not infrequently showing differentiation along multiple lines.[234-236] In contrast, LCNE is a distinctive morphologic entity that has intermediate prognosis between SCC and AC.[232] Cells in LCNE are larger than in SCC; the N/C ratio is lower than in SCC; and the nucleus has coarse chromatin, usually with prominent nucleoli (Figs. 75-7 and 75-8). Typical findings of SCC, such as molding, smearing, and spindling are not present;

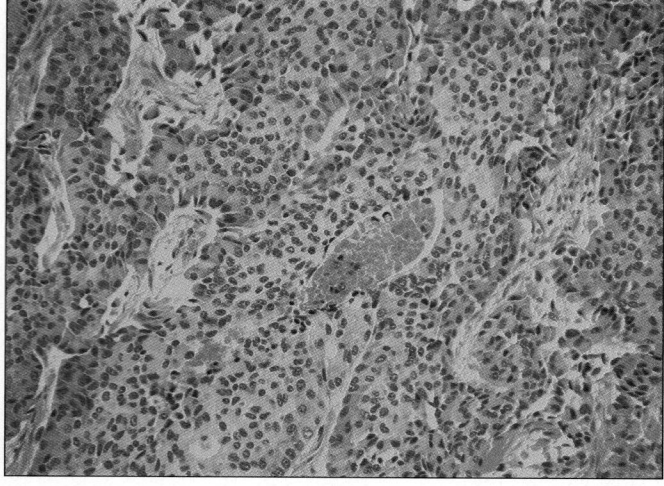

Figure 75-8. Atypical carcinoid. Cells have nuclei with fine, stipled chromatin and a large amount of eosinophylic cytoplasm. They are arranged in large nests, showing central, comedo-type necrosis.

however, immunohistochemic and ultrastructural studies reveal neuroendocrine differentiation.[237]

Relation of Tumor Histotype to Prognosis

Overall, SqCC Aca, LCU, and SCC have increasingly worse prognoses.[238] The tendencies of different histotypes for local, regional, and distant spread differ. SqCC has a higher propensity for local or regional spread relative to AC, SCC, and LCU, which, in contrast, have a higher propensity for distant spread, including to the central nervous system.[144,238] SCC has a distinctly worse prognosis, when untreated, than does NSCLC.[146] Whether the histotype constitutes a prognostic parameter independent of stage in NSCLC is controversial, however. Thus, the better prognosis of SqCC could reflect its more frequent presentation at a more limited stage.[239] A more favorable outcome of SqCC vs. Aca is reported by many authors, particularly for stages I and II disease, but this finding has not been confirmed universally.[239-242] A reduced number of recurrences has also been described for squamous vs. nonsquamous histology.[241,243] Differences in survival between NSCLC histotypes are nonsignificant in the more advanced stages, although an intrinsic limit of such studies is the limited follow-up available for these patients, who have a very limited overall survival.[238] On the other hand, a definite survival advantage has been described for BAC over other histotypes, adding to the unique clinical and morphologic features of this subtype of lung cancer.[146,244]

Relation of Histotype to Molecular Alterations

Different lung cancer histotypes have different sets of molecular alterations. K-ras mutations are most common in Aca and almost never occur in SqCC or in the entire spectrum of neuroendocrine neoplasms, including carcinoid tumor, Aca, and LCNE.[245-247] Rb deletions are infrequent in NSCLC but very common in SC, where they occur frequently in association with p53 mutations.[248] An inverse association has been found between Rb and p16 abnormalities, supporting the concept that molecular alterations within the same pathway are redundant and are not selected for during carcinogenesis.[249-251] K53 mutations are common across the spectrum of lung tumors, with the highest frequency observed in SqCC and SCC.[248] Interestingly, the type and spectrum of p53 mutations arising in nonsmokers are different than those that occur in smokers, the latter having a predominance of G-C transversions over G-T transitions.[252,253] Deletions of Chromosome 3p14 are common in lung cancers and are associated with loss of the fragile histidine triad (FHIT) gene.[254] FHIT acts as a tumor suppressor and is involved in apoptosis.[255,256] FHIT losses are common in both NSCL and SCC but are more common in SqCC than in Aca and are associated with smoking.[247,257-259] It has been proposed that FHIT deletion represents a marker of cigarette smoke-induced molecular damage.[257]

The spectrum of NE tumors that includes (in order of increasing histologic grade and increasingly worse prognosis) carcinoids, atypical carcinoids, LCNE, and SCC,

TABLE 75-7

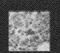
Symptoms of Lung Cancer Related to Local Tumor Growth

Due to Central Tumor Growth

Cough
Wheeze or stridor
Postobstructive pneumonia (fever, productive cough)
Dyspnea with "obstructive" pattern on testing
Hemoptysis
Poorly localized, dull pain

Due to Peripheral Tumor Growth

Pleuritic or chest wall pain
Dyspnea with a "restrictive" pattern on testing
Pleural effusion
Cough

is reproduced at the molecular level by a spectrum of increasing molecular alterations, as determined by loss of heterozygosity or immunohistochemistry.[247,260]

Clinical Presentation

The fundamental biology of lung cancer growth leads to the assumption that the cancer we ultimately see clinically has been present for a decade or more and that the fundamental issue of whether it has metastasized has been determined far in advance of our ability to detect the disease. Although this "preordained" behavior of lung cancer might guide the outcome for many patients, the fact that there are recognizable and reproducible differences in cure rates for patients with microscopic vs. clinically evident mediastinal node involvement and the fact that patients with stage IIIA or IIIB non–small cell lung cancer or small cell lung cancer can be cured speaks to the need for the earliest possible detection and intervention for patients with lung cancer.

Lung cancer can metastasize to virtually any organ in the body and hence can present with a myriad of symp-

TABLE 75-8

Symptoms of Lung Cancer Due to Regional Spread

Nerve Entrapment Syndromes

Horner's syndrome (enopthalmos, meiosis, ptosis), cervical
   sympathetic nerves
Diaphragmatic paralysis—phrenic nerve
Hoarseness—recurrent laryngeal nerve on the left
Ulnar pain with vasomotor changes—8th cervical and 1st thoracic
   nerves

Vascular Involvement

Venous distension and swelling of the face, neck, upper chest—
   superior vena cava
Tamponade, heart failure, arrythmias—pericardial involvement

Direct Invasion or Nodal Spread to the Mediastinum

Dysphagia-esophageal compression or invasion
Dyspnea, stridor due to tracheal involvement
Dyspnea due to pleural effusion
Broncho-esophageal fistula

toms. These are often described as a set of symptoms that are due to local, regional, or distant spread of the cancer (Tables 75-7, 75-8, and 75-9). Unfortunately, this classification does not take into account the clinical confusion that arises due to the overlap in symptoms among lung cancer, chronic obstructive pulmonary disease, coronary artery disease, and osteoarthritis. Rather than try to interpret the scores of symptoms that can be evident in lung cancer, it is more helpful to understand the common presentations of the disease, as these are often missed in clinical practice. There are at least nine generally recognizable patterns of lung cancer presentation (Table 75-10).

The Asymptomatic Pulmonary Nodule
Historically, the lesions known as asymptomatic pulmonary nodules were discovered at the time of an incidental chest x-ray taken for other reasons, although the

TABLE 75-9

Lung Cancer Symptoms Due to Metastatic Disease

Central Nervous System—Brain

Headache or change in pattern of chronic headaches
Unexplained nausea/vomiting
Blurred vision
Diplopia
Confusion or change in mentation
Focal weakness
Seizures—Jacksonian or grand mal
Ataxia

Central Nervous System—Spinal Cord

Back pain localizing over the spine
Radicular back pain
Ataxia
Bowel or bladder dysfunction
Paraparesis or paraplegia
Sensory loss—paresthesias or loss of positional sense

Central Nervous System—Leptomeninges

Change in mental status
Isolated cranial nerve dysfunction
Nondermatomal pain syndromes
Headache
Visual disturbances
Nausea/vomiting
Bowel or bladder dysfunction

Bone

Back pain
Long bone pain
Rib pain
Pathologic fractures

Liver

Right upper quadrant fullness/pain
Early satiety
Hectic fevers with no infectious etiology

Adrenal Gland

Flank pain
Adrenal hypofunction (Addison's disease)—rare

Other Sites

GI tract—nausea/vomiting, epigastric pain
Skin—subcutaneous nodules, breast masses
Choroid—blurred vision

TABLE 75-10

 Common Clinical Presentations of Lung Cancer

Asymptomatic pulmonary nodule
Change in "smoker's cough"
Nonpurulent "pneumonia" in an adult
Persistent upper respiratory infection
Hemoptysis
Hoarseness
Signs and symptoms of metastatic disease
Signs and symptoms of a paraneoplastic syndrome
Carcinoma of unknown primary site

tendency to miss these lesions is significant. The tendency to limit routine preoperative chest x-ray screening for cost reasons might in fact have lessened the number of early cancers found. Currently, there is a well-established algorithm for assessing these lesions.[261,262] The advent of spiral computed tomographic (CT) scanning for the early detection of lung and other cancers has led to a marked increase in the discovery of these early lesions.[263,264] There is an ongoing, contentious debate about the use of spiral CT screening for lung cancer, but the number of patients getting the scans continues to increase.[265] We will discuss the issues of screening later in this chapter, but suffice it to say that there will be a significant increase in patients who present with small, growing nodules. It is the presence of a growing lesion that offers the most compelling grounds for intervention, as the routine removal of all newly discovered lesions would result in excessive cost and morbidity.

Change in "Smoker's Cough"

There is clearly a coalescence of psychological, physical, and social factors that compel an individual to continue smoking despite the overwhelming evidence of the harm this habit causes.[266] There are an estimated 46 million adult smokers in the United States and an even larger number of former smokers who remain at increased risk of lung cancer on a long-term basis.[138,267] Many of these smokers and former smokers have what they refer to as a "smoker's cough," generally described as a nonproductive cough due to chronic irritation of the pulmonary tree. The fact that it has been present for many of the years during which they have been smoking leads to a certain fatalistic attitude that this is a necessary but essentially harmless consequence of smoking, and it is often not reported in their regular review of symptoms. Its presence is, therefore, likely underestimated. Lung cancer patients across the board are said to present with cough 73% of the time, but this symptom includes many infection-related sources as well.[268] Primary care physicians would do well to query for any such change in a baseline cough and order a relatively prompt chest x-ray, especially if the smoking history has been prolonged or there is evidence of a positive family history for lung cancer.

Nonpurulent Pneumonia in an Adult

Nonpurulent pneumonia is a relatively common presentation for patients with lung cancer. They might also have one or more of the symptoms of local or regional spread of lung cancer (see Tables 75-7 and 75-8), or they might just feel run down or fatigued. A chest x-ray or physical examination reveals consolidation in a lobar pattern, and the patient is diagnosed with "walking pneumonia." We have seen many lung cancer patients who state that they had no symptoms of fever, chills, or sputum production and yet were treated for several weeks to several months for "pneumonia." These patients clearly warrant more aggressive management. We recommend, at the least, a follow-up chest x-ray for resolution, but we often will progress to CT scan or bronchoscopy in the presence of a long history of cigarette smoking, current or not.

Persistent Upper Respiratory Infection

Persistent upper respiratory infection is probably the most common nonmetastatic presentation of lung cancer. Patients often describe coming down with the "flu" followed by a visit to the urgent care center, emergency room, or primary physician that results in a prescription for antibiotics without a chest x-ray. Clinical improvement is followed by prompt recurrence of symptoms, and if the patient is lucky enough to have a regular physician who notes this pattern, he or she is sent for further evaluation. Unfortunately, many patients seek intermittent care, and so the process is repeated several times, leading to a delay of several months in diagnosis.

Hemoptysis

The presence of blood in the sputum is often seen as a presenting sign in lung cancer patients (incidence, approximately 30%). The most common cause of hemoptysis is active bronchitis, not lung cancer, but the presence of blood is considered a grave finding by most patients, and they regularly seek medical care for it.[269]

Hoarseness

Adults who present with persistent hoarseness in the absence of an acute or recent upper respiratory infection are frequently misdiagnosed. We have seen many patients who have had "full" otolaryngology evaluations, including CT scan of the neck and laryngoscopy, only to be told they have a partially or fully paralyzed vocal cord, and then no thoracic imaging is done. The unfortunate route of the left recurrent laryngeal nerve down under the aortic arch makes it a frequent victim of local nodal invasion or compression, with resulting hoarseness.

Signs and Symptoms of Metastatic Disease

Whether the metastases are regional or disseminated, symptoms originating from them are the most common presenting sign for patients with lung cancer (see Tables 75-8 and 75-9). There are four major sites to which lung cancer tends to metastasize—the brain, bone, liver, and adrenals—and evaluation of all of these sites is critical to staging a patient with lung cancer accurately. There are several syndromes that should be recognizable to most physicians and lead to a prompt diagnosis. These include neck vein distension and facial swelling (superior vena cava syndrome), Horner's syndrome, persistent headache or visual changes, new onset confusion, new back or bone pain, and right upper quadrant pain and fullness.[270,271] The presence of any of these in a current or prior smoker should lead to an immediate diagnostic work-up to preserve quality of life while the diagnosis and therapy of an underlying lung cancer is being planned and executed. It is not the intention of this chapter to list or describe every sign or symptom related to lung cancer, but rather to stress those that are seen with some frequency.

Paraneoplastic Syndromes

There is an array of paraneoplastic syndromes that are either systemic or organ specific (Table 75-11). Several are critical to making a diagnosis of cancer in a timely fashion and should be recognized in most primary care settings. These include anorexia/cachexia, clubbing and other signs of hypertrophic pulmonary osteoarthropathy, hypercalcemia (usually seen with squamous cell lung cancers), hyponatremia (usually seen with small cell anaplastic lung cancer), dermatomyositis, and migratory venous thrombosis (Trousseau's syndrome).[272-279] Uncommon paraneoplastic syndromes involving the central and peripheral nervous systems, bone marrow, skin, kidneys, and gastrointestinal tract are rarely assessed early in the course of a lung cancer diagnosis.

TABLE 75-11

Common Paraneoplastic Syndromes Associated with Lung Cancer

Endocrine

Hypercalcemia (ectopic PTH)
Cushing's syndrome (ectopic ACTH)
SIADH (ectopic antidiuretic hormone)
Carcinoid syndrome (ectopic serotonin)
Gynecomastia (ectopic beta-HCG)

Neurologic

Eaton-Lambert syndrome
Optic neuritis
Subacute cerebellar degeneration
Progressive multifocal leukoencephalopathy
Autonomic neuropathy

Musculoskeletal

Polymyositis
Clubbing
Pulmonary hypertrophic osteoarthropathy

Hematologic

Anemia of chronic disease
Leukemoid reactions
Thrombocytosis
Thrombocytopenia
Hypercoagulable state (Trousseau's syndrome, marantic endocarditis, or DIC)

Cutaneous

Dermatomyositis
Hyperkeratosis
Acanthosis nigricans
Hyperpigmentation

Miscellaneous

Nephrotic syndrome
Anorexia/cachexia
Vasoactive intestinal peptide secretion with severe diarrhea

Carcinoma of Unknown Primary Site

The presentation of patients with a supraclavicular node or mediastinal nodes, brain metastasis, or bone metastasis, who do not have an obvious source of their cancer, is a common feature in clinical practice. The extent to which a full work-up should ensue, assuming a "negative chest CT for a parenchymal lesion," is hotly debated.[280]

Diagnostic Radiology

A significant percentage of patients presenting with non–small cell lung cancer will have inoperable disease at the time of presentation. It has been estimated that 26% of patients have mediastinal lymph node involvement and that as many as 49% have distant metastatic disease.[281] It is the goal of noninvasive staging to determine, efficiently and accurately, which patients are candidates for potentially curative surgical resection. Standard imaging modalities have included the plain chest radiograph, CT scanning, magnetic resonance imaging (MRI), bone scintigraphy, and ultrasonography. Endoscopic ultrasound (EUS), though less widely available, is a valuable tool in characterizing selected lymph node stations. An exciting newer modality, based on metabolic rather than anatomic characteristics, is positron emission tomography (PET).

Chest Radiograph

Frequently, it is an abnormality on the posteroanterior and lateral chest radiograph that heralds the diagnosis of bronchogenic carcinoma. A pulmonary parenchymal nodule or mass is the most common presentation of lung cancer, and peripheral carcinomas are easier to detect than those that are central in location. When a central, obstructing lesion is present, secondary signs such as lobar atelectasis or unresolving pneumonia might be the chest radiographic manifestation, rather than visualization of the primary tumor. Though the plain chest radiograph is considered relatively insensitive as a staging modality, it can detect the presence of mediastinal and/or hilar lymphadenopathy, pleural effusion, or involvement of the bony thorax. In the unusual circumstance (i.e., when a patient is severely debilitated or desires no treatment), further imaging might not be indicated.

Computed Tomography

Computed tomography (CT) scanning is the anatomic imaging modality of choice and is performed in virtually all patients with suspected or known lung cancer. In most centers, the patient is scanned from the lung apices through the adrenal glands or liver. Though the administration of intravenous contrast material is not mandatory, it facilitates the distinction of lymph nodes or tumor from vascular structures and is therefore employed readily.[282] The examination should be viewed in standard lung, soft tissue, and bone windows for accurate interpretation. Oral gastrointestinal contrast is not required for assessment of the liver and adrenals.

CT is useful in evaluating the primary tumor for size, characteristics, and location. It has limited accuracy in diagnosing mediastinal and/or chest wall invasion.[283-286] Invasion of mediastinal or other intrathoracic soft tissue or

Specific Malignancies

vascular structures can be better assessed by magnetic resonance imaging (MRI), and this is one of the few indications for MRI in the intrathoracic evaluation of lung cancer.[284,285] Hilar and mediastinal lymph nodes can be assessed for size (see the discussion to follow) and for the presence of calcification or central fat (signs favoring benignity) or necrosis (more indicative of malignancy). The presence of satellite pulmonary nodules, pleural or pericardial effusion, or chest wall abnormalities might necessitate further evaluation. Additionally, unsuspected hepatic or adrenal lesions might be detected and require correlation with PET or biopsy.

It is important to recognize that CT is not a reliable noninvasive modality for staging the mediastinum. Multiple studies in the 1990s evaluating the sensitivity and specificity of CT with regard to lymph node size and malignancy found that, regardless of size threshold employed, there were significant false positive and false negatives when compared with the "gold standard" of mediastinoscopy or surgical sampling.[285-289] Enlarged lymph nodes could be hyperplastic or, conversely, normal sized nodes could contain malignant cells. The majority of these studies have used a short-axis measurement of 1 cm or greater as the size criterion for abnormal. When a short axis of 1.5 cm or 2.0 cm has been utilized, there was improved specificity but a reduction in sensitivity. Toloza and colleagues[290] evaluated 20 studies (3438 patients total) for accuracy of CT in staging the mediastinum. There was notable heterogeneity of the individual studies. In all but three instances, a short axis of 1 cm or greater was considered abnormal. The pooled sensitivity was 57%, and the pooled specificity was 82%. It is unlikely that these percentages will change significantly, even with the improved resolution of the newer multichannel CT scanners.

Despite these limitations, CT continues to play an essential role in staging the mediastinum in patients with bronchogenic carcinoma. In conjunction with PET, the lymph node stations with the highest likelihood of being malignant can be identified, thus guiding the most appropriate means of lymph node sampling. For example, right paratracheal and precarinal lymph nodes can generally be biopsied by cervical mediastinoscopy, while aorticopulmonary and subcarinal lymph nodes are amenable to biopsy by endoscopic guided fine needle aspiration or a mediastinotomy.

Magnetic Resonance Imaging

Magnetic resonance imaging (MRI), like CT, is an imaging modality that is based on anatomic rather than biologic features. It currently has a limited role in the noninvasive staging of bronchogenic carcinoma but may be used to evaluate for vascular or vertebral body invasion with suspected T4 tumors or to assess the integrity of the brachial plexus in patients with a Pancoast tumor. Due to poorer spatial resolution and motion artifact, it is less sensitive than CT in evaluation of the pulmonary parenchyma.

The literature suggests that the overall accuracy of MRI in detecting mediastinal metastases is comparable to that of CT.[284,285] It has the theoretic advantage of multiplanar

imaging. There are, however, some disadvantages of MRI when compared with CT. Foci of nodal calcification are less likely to be detected on MRI, and a cluster of normal size lymph nodes might appear as a coalescent nodal mass, resulting in false positive readings.

Endoscopic Ultrasound

Endoscopic ultrasound (EUS), particularly in conjunction with guided fine-needle aspiration (FNA), is emerging as an accurate method of staging the mediastinum. It owes its accuracy to high resolution and ability to characterize lymph nodes smaller than 1 cm. Sonographic features that suggest malignancy include round shape, sharp margins, and hypoechoic texture.[291] EUS is most effective in evaluating subcarinal (station 7), aorticopulmonary window (station 5), and paraesophageal (station 8) lymph nodes.[291] Pretracheal and precarinal lymph nodes cannot be visualized well through the air-containing trachea.

EUS examination is minimally invasive and should be performed by a skilled endosonographer with the patient under conscious sedation. When suspicious lymph nodes are present, ultrasound-guided FNA is routinely performed. Accuracies of 82%–84% for EUS alone and 91%–96% for combined EUS-FNA have been reported.[292-294]

In patients with potentially resectable tumors who have suspicious findings on CT or PET in stations 5, 7 or 8, EUS-FNA is the preferred method for tissue confirmation.[291] Currently, EUS is less widely available than the other staging modalities.

Positron Emission Tomography

In contrast to the foregoing examinations, which are based on anatomic features, positron emission tomography (PET) is a physiologic imaging modality that relies on metabolic alterations of tumor cells (i.e., increased glucose uptake and a higher rate of glycolysis).[153] F-fluoro-deoxy-D-glucose (FDG) is a radiolabeled glucose analog that accumulates within neoplastic cells at a more rapid rate than in normal tissues. After phosphorylation, it is not further metabolized and remains trapped in cells. Accumulation of the radioisotope is identified using a PET camera, and images are generated from the skull base to the pelvic floor. In most centers, the lower extremities are not routinely imaged. Evaluation for neoplasm is limited in organs that normally accumulate FDG at higher than background levels, such as the brain, heart, muscles, and kidneys. Non-neoplastic processes, including granulomatous and inflammatory disease, can accumulate FDG and produce spurious results.

Compared with CT, PET has less precise anatomic resolution. The lower limit of resolution of PET is 1–1.2 cm. Localization of an abnormality on PET is optimized by visually correlating with a concurrent diagnostic CT scan. In some centers, PET and CT images can be fused by means of postacquisition software. State of the art "in-line" systems that combine a clinical PET camera and a helical CT scanner in one machine are just becoming available. A recent study suggests that reader confidence and accuracy are improved with this system.[295]

Uptake greater than the background activity of the mediastinum is considered abnormal. A standard uptake

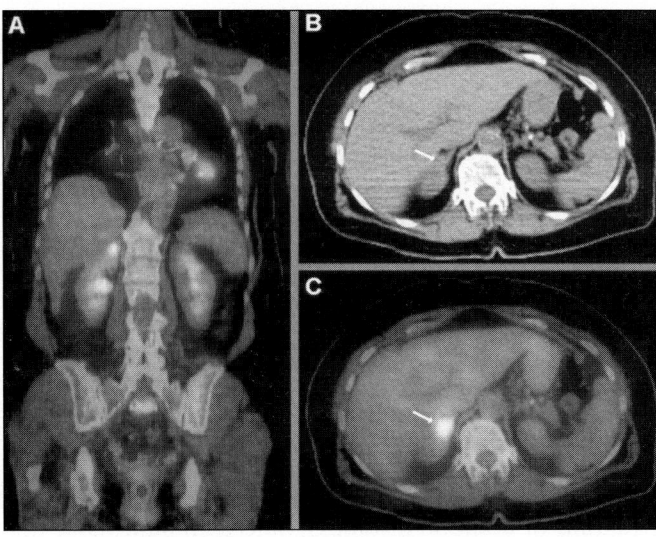

Figure 75-9. A and **C,** PET/CT scans demonstrate right adrenal mass. **B,** Less well-delineated on CT scan.

value (SUV) greater than 2.5% is often cited in the literature as a criterion for abnormality; however, there is overlap between neoplastic and non-neoplastic uptake values.[296,297] Some carcinomas—particularly bronchiolo-alveolar cell carcinoma—exhibit low or no discernible uptake. Though the majority of primary tumors demonstrate intense focal uptake, PET cannot assess reliably for direct mediastinal or chest wall invasion due to limited resolution capabilities.

PET is more accurate than CT in staging the mediastinum in patients with non–small cell lung cancer. In two meta-analyses, the sensitivity of PET for nodal staging was 84%–88%, and the specificity was 89%–92%.[290,298] False positive results occur in lymph nodes with reactive hyperplasia or silico-anthracosis, and thus tissue diagnosis should be obtained before a patient is deemed inoperable. When the PET scan is negative for mediastinal nodal involvement, however, preoperative mediastinoscopy is not routinely indicated, as the negative predictive values of the two methods are comparable.[299]

In several studies, it has been shown that PET detects distant metastatic disease in 10%–12% of patients whose metastases were not demonstrated by standard imaging (Figs. 75-9 and 75-10).[298-300] In the study by Pieterman and coworkers,[299] the overall sensitivity and specificity for distant metastases were 82% and 93%, respectively. The sensitivity and specificity of PET for skeletal metastases appear to exceed those of bone scintigraphy.[301] On the other hand, false negative results can occur in the presence of distal appendicular metastases if the lower extremities are not imaged. Similarly, PET has a significantly higher positive predictive value for detection of adrenal metastases than does CT. In contrast, the sensitivity for detecting central nervous system (CNS) metastases is limited by the normal accumulation of FDG in the brain. Therefore, PET should not replace conventional imaging (contrast-enhanced CT or MRI) for routine staging of the brain.

Diagnostic Radiology: Conclusion

FDG PET is the most powerful noninvasive staging tool currently available. PET and CT are complimentary imaging modalities, providing information at both molecular and anatomic levels. Despite improved accuracy, however, a significant percentage of false positives due to acute inflammation or granulomatous disease warrants histopathologic confirmation before a patient is "up-staged" and denied potentially curative surgery. Given the current evidence, a negative PET scan obviates the need for mediastinoscopy before surgery. PET detects unsuspected distant metastatic disease in fully 10% of patients and appears to be more accurate than bone scintigraphy in evaluating for skeletal metastases. In patients with clinically suspected brain metastases, standard imaging with contrast-enhanced CT or (preferably) MRI should be performed.

SCREENING

Although lung cancer screening is being rediscovered due to advances in technology, it remains controversial. The choice of the proper target (i.e., high-risk) population, the choice of central or peripheral screening, the appropriate algorithm for patient follow-up once an abnormality has been detected, and the timing and magnitude of the intervention are some of the unresolved issues.

Historical Perspective

In the 1970s and 1980s, after Saccomanno[164] described the use of exfoliated cytology in the early detection of lung cancer as an extension of the idea of aerodigestive

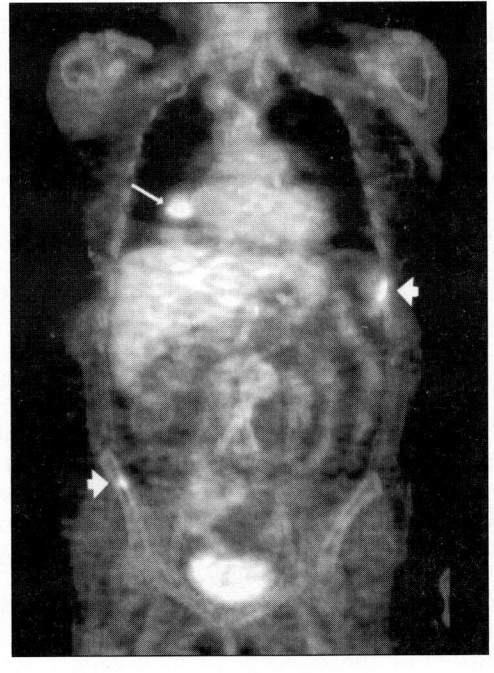

Figure 75-10. PET/CT scan demonstating right lung mass and two areas of bone metastasis, both asymptomatic.

field cancerization, the National Cancer Institute sponsored a study of 10,000 high-risk volunteers at Memorial Sloan Kettering and Johns Hopkins, and of another 10,000 high-risk volunteers at the Mayo Clinic.[165,302,303] A fourth study was performed in Czechoslovakia, and was similar to the Mayo Clinic study.[304] These trials were designed to investigate the efficacy of lung cancer screening using a combination of chest x-ray and conventional sputum cytology. The participants were all male smokers over 45 years of age who had a smoking history of at least one pack per day. In the Johns Hopkins and Memorial Sloan Kettering trials, both experimental and control participants had annual screening chest radiography, and the experimental arm had sputum cytology every four months. These trials were designed to address the incremental benefit of sputum cytology analysis rather than chest radiographs per se. Although they found that sputum analysis did not influence outcome favorably, these studies achieved survival rates among all groups three times higher than predicted by epidemiologic data.

The Mayo Lung Trial mandated a prevalence screening with chest x-ray and sputum cytology followed by randomization to radiographs and sputum cytology every 4 months or annually. The Czechoslovakian study, a 3-year study with 3-year follow-up, also began with a prevalence screen that then randomization to a screened or control group, and the control group was told not to get either radiograph or cytology during the 3-year study period. In both the Mayo and Czech studies, more lung cancers were found in the screened group, and there was a tendency toward earlier stage at diagnosis, resectability, and survival for the screened group. Five-year survival for the control group in the Mayo Study was 15% compared with 33% in the screened group.[305] Both studies demonstrated increases in cumulative lung cancer incidence in the experimental group above that of control groups. This led to significant improvements for the experimental groups in case fatality (*#cancer deaths / # individuals with cancer*) but not into significant reductions in lung cancer mortality (*# cancer deaths / # individuals screened*).

Lead-time bias, length bias, and overdiagnosis have been used to potentially explain the differences between lung cancer mortality and earlier stage at diagnosis, improved resectability, and survival of the screened.[306-308] Lead-time bias operates when the timing of diagnosis between screening and nonscreening cases is not adjusted—that is, earlier detection could result in longer survival from the time of diagnosis even if death is not delayed. Length bias occurs when conditions are not adjusted for the rate of cancer progression and the screening examination purportedly detects slow-growing cancers. In other words, the slower the growth of the neoplasm, the longer it is present without symptoms, and the greater the likelihood of detection. Overdiagnosis bias refers to the phenomenon of detecting a lung cancer that would otherwise have remained subclinical before death from other causes.

Supporters of the concept of lung cancer screening have argued that these original trials were flawed. Arguments include the following:

1. The researchers did not include a "no-screening" study arm, and thus no determination of true efficacy could be made.
2. The sample size of these studies was inadequate because both the Mayo Lung Project and the Czechoslovakian studies were powered to detect a 50% reduction in lung cancer mortality in the screened group compared with the control group. In contrast, the power to detect a smaller but clinically meaningful effect, such as a 10% reduction in mortality, was much lower (only 0.21 and 0.16, respectively).[265,309,310]

Present Screening Initiatives

Independent of the arguments regarding fatality, mortality, and bias, there has been a realization by the medical community that the efficacy of lung cancer screening should be investigated in a research setting. The rapid evolution of computed tomographic techniques and the development of potential molecular markers for the classification of high-risk sputa have led to collaborative groups to enroll patients on either radiographic, sputum-based, or combination programs for lung cancer screening. All lung cancer screening programs are based on the premise that high-risk populations must be chosen to have any hope of cost effectiveness, and in addition to the technologic evolution alluded to previously, there has been a greater refinement of the demographics of the individuals at high risk for lung cancer who could be candidates for enrolling in lung cancer screening programs.

High-Risk Populations

Smokers and Former Smokers

Tobacco consumption is the most important risk factor for lung cancer, and 85% of lung cancer deaths are attributable to smoking.[311] Although there are fewer people smoking, the incidence of lung cancer remains significant due to the risk among older former smokers, and it is estimated that about 40% of all new lung cancers occur in former smokers.[312] The risk of lung cancer is influenced by duration of smoking, the number of cigarettes smoked per day, and the age at which a smoker stopped smoking (i.e., the longer one lives after cessation of smoking, the greater the risk for developing lung cancer). Likewise, the greater the consumption of tobacco as measured by pack-years, the greater the risk that one will develop lung cancer. It has been estimated that a 60-year-old individual with a 10-pack-year smoking history will have a lung cancer prevalence of 0.5%. This is contrasted with the individual who has a greater than 20-pack-year consumption (2% prevalence) or a current 30-pack-year smoker (prevalence of 4%). Former 30-pack-year smokers who quit before the age of 50 have approximately a 2% lung cancer prevalence. Lung cancer prevalence is also influenced by the presence of airway obstruction. For individuals smoking 30–40-pack-years or more with airflow obstruction–defined by FEV1/FVC less than 70% and an FEV1 less than 70% predicted—the risk of lung cancer is three- to fourfold higher than for individuals with normal airflow.[313] This risk is illustrated by the finding of a 3% prevalence of stage I lung cancer found on CT scan in patients with pulmonary emphysema undergoing evaluation for either lung transplantation or lung volume reduction surgery.[314]

Previously Resected Aerodigestive Malignancies

Individuals with previously surgically treated stage I NSCLC or head and neck primary neoplasms are at increased risk for the development of a new primary lung cancer. It has been estimated from published studies on treatment outcomes that the approximate rate of developing a new primary lung cancer after undergoing curative-intent therapy for a NSCLC is 1%–2% per patient per year and that new primary lung cancers can develop up to 20 years after the original cancer has been treated.[315-317] Roentgenographically cured occult lung cancers detected by sputum cytology also have an especially high rate of metachronous tumors, approaching 11% at five years with an incidence per patient-year of surveillance of 2.2%.[318] The incidence of a second primary tumor in patients treated for squamous cell carcinoma of the aerodigestive tract can be as high as 16.2%, with 6.4% being synchronous and 9.8% being metachronous.[319] Metachronous tumors are most likely in the lung (57%), placing these patients in one of the highest-risk categories for the development of lung cancer.[319]

Present Screening Efforts

Chest X-Ray

The National Cancer Institute initiated a large, randomized controlled screening trial using chest radiographs for lung cancer screening as part of the Prostate-Lung-Colorectal-Ovarian (PLCO) trial. One of the objectives of the trial, which is ongoing, was to determine whether screening reduces lung cancer-specific mortality by at least 10% relative to unscreened groups.[320] This trial remains under analysis at this writing.

Low-Dose Helical CT Scanning of the Chest

Nonrandomized Approaches. Two different groups of Japanese investigators have reported the results of screening male smokers greater than 50 years of age.[321] The Japanese Anti-Lung Cancer Association screened approximately 26,000 patients from 1975 to 1993 with chest radiography and sputum cytology and added spiral CT scanning to the regimen in 1993. Significantly more cancers were detected in the CT era (36 over a 5-year period) compared with the pre-CT era (43 over the course of 18 years), and 81% of the CT-screened lung cancers were stage IA compared with 42% in the pre-CT era. There was a striking increase in the 5-year survival, from 48% to 82%. The CT era for the other reported series began in 1996, when a single-spiral CT prevalence scan was performed in 3967 of 5483 persons aged 40–74 years who had previously been screened with yearly chest x-rays and sputum cytologic screening. Among the 223 individuals with abnormal findings, 19 cancers were detected. Similar to the other Japanese study, 84% of these

were found to be stage I.[322,323] The addition of CT scanning increased the rate of lung cancer diagnosis by approximately 12-fold.

In the United States, the Early Lung Cancer Action Project (ELCAP) was initiated in 1993 and experimentally screened a cohort of 1000 high-risk persons using a non-comparative design in which a single cohort was recruited for baseline and annual repeat CT screening. The aims of ELCAP were to define the frequency with which malignancy was found in screen-detected nodules and the frequency with which malignant nodules were curable.[324] The volunteers were aged 60 years or older, with at least 10-pack-years of cigarette smoking and no previous cancer, who were medically fit to undergo thoracic surgery. Chest radiographs and low-dose CT were done for each participant, with the diagnostic/interventional investigation of screen-detected noncalcified pulmonary nodules by short-term, high-resolution CT follow-up dictated primarily by size of the nodule. Noncalcified nodules were detected in 233 participants (23% [95% CI 21–26]) by low-dose CT at baseline, compared with 68 participants (7% [5–9]) by chest radiography. Malignant disease was detected in 27 patients (2.7% [1.8–3.8]) by CT and in seven paitents (0.7% [0.3–1.3]) by chest radiography, and stage I malignant disease was detected in 23 (2.3% [1.5–3.3]) and four patients (0.4% [0.1–0.9]), respectively. Of the 27 CT-detected cancers, 26 were resectable. Biopsies were done on 28 of the 233 participants with noncalcified nodules; 27 had malignant noncalcified nodules and one had a benign nodule. Another three individuals underwent biopsy against the ELCAP recommendations; all had benign noncalcified nodules. No participant had thoracotomy for a benign nodule.[325]

At the time of the follow-up report, which concentrated on annual repeat screening, a total of 1184 annual repeat screenings had been performed.[326] A positive result from the screening test was defined as one to six newly detected, noncalcified pulmonary nodules with interim growth. Among the 1184 repeat CT screenings, the test result was positive in 30 patients (2.5%). In 2 of these 30 cases, the individual died (of an unrelated cause) before diagnostic work-up, and the nodule(s) resolved in another 12 individuals. In the remaining 16 individuals, the absence of further growth was documented by repeat CT in eight individuals, and further growth was documented in the remaining eight individuals. All eight individuals with further nodular growth underwent biopsy, and malignancy was diagnosed in seven. Six of these seven malignancies were non–small cell carcinomas (five of which were stage IA and one of which was stage IIIA), and the one small cell carcinoma was found to be of limited stage. The median size of these malignancies was 8 mm. In another two subjects, symptoms prompted the interim diagnosis of lung carcinoma. Neither of these malignancies was nodule-associated but rather was endobronchial; one was a stage IIB non–small cell carcinoma and the other was a small cell carcinoma of limited stage. The data from the ELCAP experience will be pooled with that of two initiatives that are outgrowths of the original ELCAP—the New York ELCAP (NY-ELCAP) and the International

Specific Malignancies

III

Early Lung Cancer Action Program (I-ELCAP). These efforts share the same set of principles and protocol, as well as the ELCAP Web-based management and data-recording system and its associated teaching files.[326]

The Mayo Clinic also has also reported its experience in evaluating CT-based lung screening in a prospective cohort study of 1520 individuals aged 50 years or older who had smoked for 20 or more pack-years.[327] Participants underwent three annual low-dose CT examinations of the chest and upper abdomen. Two years after baseline CT scanning, 2832 uncalcified pulmonary nodules were identified in 1049 participants (69%). Forty cases of lung cancer were diagnosed: 26 at baseline (prevalence) CT examinations and 10 at subsequent annual (incidence) CT examinations. CT alone depicted 36 cases; sputum cytologic examination alone revealed two. There were two interval cancers. The mean size of the non–small cell cancers detected at CT was 15.0 mm. The stages were as follows: IA, 22 patients; IB, three patients; IIA, four patients; IIB, one patient; IIIA, five patients; IV, one patient; limited small cell tumor, four patients. Twenty-one (60%) of the 35 non–small cell cancers detected at CT were stage IA at diagnosis.

Present Randomized Studies. The National Cancer Institute and the American College of Radiology Intervention Network are sponsoring a multicenter, randomized controlled trial of 88,000 individuals at high risk of developing lung cancer to determine whether screening with low-dose helical CT can reduce lung cancer-specific mortality relative to chest radiographs. High risk is defined by age 55–74 years with a current or previous heavy smoking history equaling at least 30-pack-years; former smokers must have quit within the preceding 15 years. The experimental group will undergo screening with low-dose helical CT. The control group will undergo screening with chest radiographs. Both groups will be screened annually for at least two incidence screens, and both groups will complete quality-of-life questionnaires. The primary endpoint of the trial is lung cancer-specific mortality. Intermediate endpoints will include the following:

- All-cause mortality;
- Surgical stage at diagnosis;
- Use of medical resources;
- The impact of screening on quality of life and psychologic effects; and
- The economic consequences of helical CT screening.

Sputum Cytology Screening

There was no benefit to adding sputum cytology to annual chest radiographs in the NCI randomized studies conducted at Memorial Sloan Kettering and the Johns Hopkins Oncology Center. Only 25% of existing cancers were discovered by sputum cytology among subjects randomized to dual screening, and sputum was the only means of detection in 15% of the cases.[328,329] This finding might have been due in part to the relatively low risk for lung cancer in the study population. It is possible that some of the sputum-discovered carcinomas could not be visualized on initial bronchoscopy, while in other cases

the lesion initially was subtle or distal to the larger airways accessible to the fiberoptic bronchoscope that was used at the time of the study. Nevertheless, the patients with squamous cell carcinomas had a 90% 5-year survival and echoed previous data from Martini and associates.[84,330]

Among the basic problems with sputum cytology studies for lung cancer are their low sensitivity (65%) and their inability to detect peripheral cancers with the same sensitivity as seen with centrally occurring squamous or small cell lung cancers.[331] Moreover, studies designed to screen patients for sputum abnormalities require huge numbers of subjects. From 1993 to 2001, the Colorado Lung SPORE examined the sputa of 2005 high-risk subjects (30-pack-years or greater consumption and FEV1 <70%) at baseline and annually. A total of 81 lung cancers were detected, and for patients with moderate or more severe atypia, the lung cancer incidence rate was 3.21 with a hazard ratio of 2.76. Time to development of lung cancer after the finding of moderate or severe atypia was 5–20 months.[332]

To be successful as a population-screening tool, sputum cytology sensitivity must be improved, as elaborated by Gazdar and Minna.[333] Several approaches to meeting this goal are under investigation:

1. Immunostaining of abnormal epithelial cells.
2. Computer-assisted image analysis of exfoliated sputum cells.
3. Polymerase chain reaction-based assays to detect changes in dominant and recessive oncogenes.
4. Genetic epidemiology markers to more precisely define at-risk populations of current and former smokers.

Tockman and colleagues[334] have reported that an antibody to heterogeneous nuclear ribonucleoprotein (hnRNP) could improve the accuracy of preclinical lung cancer detection. HnRNP is overexpressed in exfoliated airway cells as a prelude to the development of lung cancer. In a background of normal appearing airway cells, abnormal staining for hnRNP with the antibody can be performed by quantitative densitometry of immunostained slides. In separate, ongoing prospective studies, sputum has been collected annually from patients with stage I resected non–small cell lung cancer who are at high-risk of developing a second primary lung cancer and from Yunnan tin miners at high risk of primary lung cancer. These two prospective studies predicted accurately that 67% and 69%, respectively, of those with hnRNP up-regulation in their sputum would develop lung cancer in the first year of follow-up.[334] Other investigators are quantitating malignancy-associated changes by computer assisted image analysis to report nuclear distribution of DNA in histologically normal cells adjacent to preinvasive or invasive cancers. In a retrospective analysis, malignancy-associated changes in sputum cytology were able to identify correctly 74% of subjects who later developed lung cancer.[335] Other molecular markers that are being examined in sputum include microsatellite alterations, methylation changes, and point mutations in p53 and ras genes.[73,336-339]

The detection of sputum atypia and subsequent identification of the source of cells demand improvements in endoscopic visualization. Only 30%–40% of carcinomas in situ are visible to an experienced endoscopist on conventional bronchoscopy. Autofluorescence bronchoscopy is now being used with greater frequency as a technology complementary to sputum screening to provide targeted biopsies of dysplastic lesions.[340] The technique is based on the observation that when the bronchial surface is illuminated by a blue light (405 nm–442 nm), such as light from a helium-cadmium laser, there is a progressive reduction in the fluorescence intensity as the tissue becomes more abnormal, especially in the green wavelength band of the autofluorescence spectrum. The marked reduction in fluorescence intensity (up to a tenfold decrease in the green wavelength band and an approximately fivefold decrease in the red wavelength band) in precancerous and cancerous tissue is thought to be due to a combination of an increase in the thickness of the bronchial epithelium, a very slight increase in blood content in the area of the submucosa of the lesion, and a loss of fluorophore concentration or fluorescence quantum yield.[341] A multicenter clinical trial of 173 subjects with known or suspected lung cancer was performed in which conventional bronchoscopy was followed by fluorescence examination. The relative sensitivity of both examinations vs. conventional bronchoscopy alone was 6.3 for intraepithelial neoplastic lesions and 2.71 when invasive carcinomas were also included.[342]

LUNG CANCER PREVENTION

Lung cancer is the leading cause of cancer-related death in the United States and is projected to reach epidemic levels in the world during the 21st century, largely due to increasing tobacco use in the developing countries.[343] Mortality from this disease could be reduced greatly through the identification of persons at high risk for cancer and the development of effective interventions to inhibit or reverse carcinogenesis in the lungs. The success of this strategy depends on the identification of efficacious preventive interventions and on the validation of biomarkers that can identify persons at high risk or at the earliest stages of lung cancer development. These biomarkers could also be used to monitor the efficacy of the intervention agent.

Mortality from lung cancer could be reduced by the implementation of innovative risk reduction strategies because the risk factors for this disease are well established. Tobacco use and a low dietary intake of vegetables and fruits have been identified as important modifiable risk factors.[6,344] Consequently, lung cancer should be preventable through implementation of strategies to decrease tobacco use and increase dietary vegetable and fruit intake. In addition to tobacco prevention and diet modification, there could be a role for chemopreventive agents that modulate the pathways of lung carcinogenesis. Chemopreventive agents are nutritional or pharmaceutic compounds that may prevent cancer by altering cellular metabolism or cell cycle regulatory genes and decreasing cell proliferation and DNA damage. Currently, there are no chemopreventive compounds with proven efficacy for lung cancer; however, a variety of compounds are under investigation as potential chemopreventive agents.

Biomarkers and Risk Assessment

Development of chemopreventive strategies in lung cancer requires the efficient identification of high-risk populations. Cigarette smoking is clearly the primary factor leading to lung cancer, with estimates of relative risk ranging from 10- to 30-fold in comparison with the lifetime nonsmoker. Not all individuals who are exposed to tobacco smoke develop cancer, however, and the latency phase for the development of lung cancer is long, measuring approximately 20–30 years from the beginning of regular smoking exposure.[345]

Biomarkers could help in identifying high-risk cohorts for small, efficient phase II chemoprevention trials by allowing selection of small numbers of high-risk subjects and a relatively short time scale for intervention. Examples of biomarkers that are potentially practical for current application in lung cancer chemoprevention trials include RAR-β, p53, EGFR, cyclin D1, and genetic markers such as micronuclei from chromosomal damage, chromosomal polysomy, chromosomal deletions (3p, 5q, 9p, 11q, 13q, 17p), metabolites of cycloxygenase and lipoxygenase pathways, and methylation of p16 and other genes.

Belinsky and coworkers[73] have investigated genes inactivated by aberrant cytosine-guanosine (CpG) island methylation as candidate biomarkers for early detection of lung cancer. They demonstrated that aberrant methylation of the p16 and O^6-methylguanine-DNA methyltransferase (MGMT) promoters can be detected in DNA from sputum in 100% of patients with squamous cell carcinoma (SCC) up to 3 years before clinical diagnosis.[346] Moreover, the prevalence of these markers in sputum from cancer-free, high-risk subjects approximates lifetime risk for lung cancer.[346] Thus, DNA methylation might be useful as a biomarker to identify potential subjects for lung cancer prevention trials. CpG island methylation is an epigenetic modification of DNA associated with the silencing of gene transcription.[347] CpG island hypermethylation is detected at distinct chromosomal loci in many types of human cancer.[348] Methylation at CpG islands provides an alternative mechanism to mutation in inactivating tumor suppressor genes (TSG). A role for gene silencing in cancer development was substantiated when methylation of promoter CpG islands was implicated as one mechanism for inactivation of TSG and critical regulatory genes that included von Hippel-Lindau, estrogen receptor, $p16^{INK4a}$, E-cadherin, HIC-1, MGMT, DAP-Kinase, and TIMP-3.[349-356]

The p16 gene is inactivated predominantly by aberrant promoter methylation in SCC and adenocarcinoma with a frequency of 45%–70%.[73,351] In the rat, most adenocarcinomas (94%) induced by the tobacco-specific carcinogen, NNK, were hypermethylated at the p16 gene promoter, and this methylation change was detected frequently in precursor lesions, adenoma, and hyperplasia.[73] The p16 gene was coordinately methylated in 75% of carcinoma in situ (CIS) lesions adjacent to SCCs harboring this change.

Moreover, the frequency of this event increased during disease progression from basal cell hyperplasia (17%) to squamous metaplasia (24%) to CIS lesions (50%).

DAP-kinase is a serine/threonine, microfilament-bound kinase recently shown to be involved in apoptosis induced by γ-interferon-, TNF-α-, and Fas.[357,358] Loss of function of this kinase could significantly affect de novo and induced cellular apoptosis. The incidence of DAP-kinase promoter hypermethylation was 23% in a limited study of 22 cases of NSCLC.[359] Methylation was seen in both SCC and adenocarcinoma and occurred independently of tumor stage. A recent study focused on stage I NSCLC reported DAP-kinase methylation in 40% of tumors.[355] In addition, DAP-kinase was found to suppress oncogenic transformation of primary embryonic fibroblasts by activating p53 in a p19^{ARF}-dependent manner.[359] This finding suggests that DAP-kinase could play an important role in an early checkpoint to eliminate premalignant cells during cancer development.

The MGMT gene codes for a repair protein that removes mutagenic adducts from O^6-guanine in DNA. The failure to repair these adducts can lead to base mispairing, whereby the O^6-methylguanine pairs with thymine during replication, leading to the conversion of guanine-cytosine to adenine-thymine pairs in DNA. These GC-to-AT transition mutations are seen in activation of the K-*ras* oncogene and inactivation of the p53 TSG.[360,361] Recent studies also have demonstrated that loss of expression of this gene is due to aberrant methylation within the promoter region.[355] Aberrant methylation of the p16 and MGMT promoters was detected in DNA from sputum in 100% of patients with SCC up to 3 years before clinical diagnosis.[346] Moreover, the prevalence of these markers in sputum from cancer-free, high-risk subjects approximates lifetime risk for lung cancer.[362]

The cells exfoliated within sputum might reflect field cancerization in the airways that can ultimately develop into SCC. Mao and colleagues[363] reported the detection of K-*ras* mutations in sputum from patients with adenocarcinoma of the lung. In addition, DNA present in nanogram quantities in serum could be used to detect molecular changes.[364] Tumor DNA is also found in serum, and the serum of cancer patients shows approximately a fourfold enrichment of free DNA compared with that of control subjects.[365] Several studies have identified microsatellite alterations in the plasma and serum DNA of patients with head and neck carcinoma and small cell lung cancer.[366,367] In addition, p53 and ras gene mutations have been detected in the plasma and serum of patients with colorectal and pancreatic carcinomas.[368,369] Esteller and coworkers[359] detected aberrant DNA methylation in serum from patients with NSCLC. Assaying for methylation of p16, DAP-kinase, MGMT, and glutathione S-transferase P1, 15 of 22 NSCLCs (68%) were found to contain at least one inactivated gene. In the primary tumors with methylation, 11 of 15 samples (73%) also had abnormal methylated DNA in the matched serum samples, while none of the patients with nonmethylated tumors had positive serum. Abnormal promoter methylation in serum was also found at all tumor stages. Although DNA released into serum comes from organs throughout the body, the detection of

methylation of critical cancer genes in serum might still be useful for cancer diagnosis or the detection of disease recurrence. In support of this hypothesis, a recent study of head and neck cancer found that in 50 patients in whom methylation of at least one gene (p16, MGMT, or DAP-kinase) was detected, the same methylation pattern was detected in 42% of the corresponding sera.[370] Methylation was not seen in the sera of patients whose tumors did not contain this change.

Chemopreventive Compounds

Retinoids and Carotenoids

Retinoids are among the best-studied agents in human chemoprevention. The natural retinoids are vitamin A-related compounds and are important for growth, reproduction, vision, and epithelial cell differentiation. It is this latter characteristic that prompted the research efforts directed at the chemoprevention of lung cancer and other epithelial malignancies. Precursors of retinoids are carotenoids, which constitute a class of more than 600 compounds found predominantly in fruits and vegetables. Their role in cancer chemoprevention remains controversial, showing cancer-preventive effects in some situations, although pharmacologic doses in large clinical trials have shown neutral or sometimes detrimental effects.

Carotenoids have been reported to have a number of biologic actions, including important antioxidant activity and enhancement of immune function. The mechanisms for these actions are not well characterized, however.[371-373] Many of these compounds can quench singlet oxygen through a physical reaction in which the energy of the excited oxygen is transferred to the carotenoid. In addition to singlet oxygen, these compounds are also thought to quench oxygen free radicals. A strong body of work has linked oxygen free radicals to carcinogenesis; thus, there is considerable interest in antioxidant compounds and antioxidant activity as a mechanism for cancer prevention.[371,374] Antioxidant activity might not be responsible for the chemopreventive effects of carotenoids, however. In addition, various carotenoids have been reported to affect various growth regulatory pathways.[375,376]

Retinoids play an important role in maintainance of growth, differentiation, and apoptosis of various epithelial tissues. They also play a regulatory role in the activation of cytokines and the extracellular matrix. Most effects of these compounds are mediated by the interactions of their nuclear receptors.[377] These receptors belong to the superfamily of receptors that mediate the effects of many compounds, including steroid and thyroid hormones, vitamin D, prostaglandins, and drugs that activate peroxisomal proliferation.[378] Nuclear retinoic acid receptors (RAR) and retinoid receptors (RXR) play a role in mediating the effects of retinoids.[377,379] Each receptor contains α, β, and γ subtypes, and several of these subclasses have multiple isoforms, leading to great biologic diversity.[379-381] Retinoid receptors are active only as dimers, and different receptor dimerizations confer effector specificity to different cells. For example, RAR-α is expressed in most tissues, RAR-β is expressed only in some organs, and RAR-γ is expressed predominantly in the skin. Each of these receptors is thought to bind to specific response elements, named retinoic acid response elements (RARE), which govern the expression of genes and modify posttranslational mechanisms.[377,379]

The tissue patterns of retinoid receptor expression can change. Of all the receptor types, RAR-β displays the most marked changes between normal and abnormal tissue, selectively decreasing in expression with progressive cellular atypia and transformation, which suggests that loss of RAR-β expression could be important in tumor development.[382,383] Lotan and associates[384,385] found that mRNA expression of RAR-β was suppressed in more than 50% of oral and lung premalignant lesions, in dysplastic lesions adjacent to cancer, and in malignant oral and lung carcinomas. After three months of high-dose isotretinoin therapy, RAR-β expression increased from 40% to 90%. Furthermore, up-regulation of RAR-β was associated with a clinical response, indicating that RAR-β up-regulation might be one way by which retinoid compounds inhibit neoplastic cell growth.

Systemic therapy with retinoids is limited by the toxicities that result from activation of several signaling pathways. These toxicities include varying severity of cheilitis, facial erythema, dry and peeling skin, photosensitivity, and reversible elevation of hepatic enzymes and serum lipids.[386,387] Some of these toxicities can be ameliorated by the concomitant use of α-tocopherol without loss of retinoid activity.[388] Current efforts are concentrating on the development of receptor-selective retinoids targeting RAR-α, RAR-β, RAR-γ, RXR, and pan-agonists.[389]

Selenium

Several mechanisms have been proposed by which selenium could prevent cancer development. These include reducing oxidative damage through interactions with the antioxidant enzyme glutathione peroxidase and inhibition of 5-lipoxygenase (5-LO).[347,390–392] In addition, selenium might act as a demethylating agent through the inhibition of cytosine DNA-methyltransferase, a family of proteins responsible for maintenance and de novo methylation of CpG dinucleotides.[393]

Animal model studies have shown that inorganic and organic selenium compounds are effective at inhibiting chemical carcinogenesis at both the initiation and postinitiation stages.[347,390,394] Geographic studies have suggested that an inverse relationship exists between selenium status and cancer incidence. A study examining the ecologic relationship of environmental selenium levels and county levels of cancer mortality revealed that cancer mortality rates were significantly lower for total cancer in counties with intermediate or high selenium levels compared with counties having low selenium levels.[395] Recently, Clark and colleagues[396] conducted a double-blinded, randomized, placebo-controlled cancer prevention trial in patients with a history of basal cell or squamous cell carcinoma of the skin. A total of 1312 subjects received L-selenomethionine (200 μg/day, orally) or placebo for a mean of 4.5 years, with up to 6.4 years of follow-up. Although the primary endpoint of skin cancer prevention was negative, secondary endpoints revealed a significant protection for cancers of the lung (relative risk [RR], 0.54), prostate (RR, 0.37), colon (RR, 0.42), and esophagus (RR, 0.33). This significant protection against lung cancer led to the implementation of ECOG 5597, an intergroup study for prevention of second primary tumors in patients with stage I non–small cell lung cancer.

Reactive oxygen species stimulate 5-LO activity, while selenium-dependent peroxidases inhibit it.[391,392,397] For example, Weitzel and Wendel[391] observed that selenium-deficient rat basophilic leukemia cells demonstrated less than 1% of control glutathione peroxidase activity and and less than 35% of phospholipid hydroperoxide-glutathione peroxidase activity. Upon stimulation, these cells released an eightfold amount of lipoxygenase metabolites compared with controls. The addition of 0.25 μg/mL selenium to selenium-deficient cells restored control phospholipid hydroperoxide-glutathione peroxidase activity within eight hours, whereas restoration of glutathione peroxidase activity required seven days. Resupplemented cells released control amounts of 5-lipoxygenase metabolites, indicating that restoration of phospholipid hydroperoxide-glutathione peroxidase activity is associated with a selenium-adequate leukotriene metabolism. Werz and Steinhilber[392] also demonstrated that suppression of cellular 5-lipoxygenase activity in cell lines is selenium dependent. Selenium also acts as a demethylating agent through the inhibition of cytosine DNA-methyltransferase.[393]

Lipoxygenase Inhibitors

Eicosanoids derived from the arachidonic acid cascade have been implicated in the pathogenesis of cancer and metastasis. Although most attention has focused on prostaglandins and other cyclooxygenase (COX)-derived metabolites, accumulating evidence suggests that lipoxygenase (LO) metabolic products such as leukotrienes (LT) and hydroxyeicosatetraenoic (HETE) acids also exert profound biologic effects on the development and progression of human cancers. For example, 12-LO mRNA expression has been well documented in many types of solid tumors, including prostate, colon, and epidermoid carcinomas.[398,399]

12(S)-HETE is a critical intracellular signaling molecule, stimulating protein kinase C (PKC) and eliciting the biologic actions of many growth factors and cytokines that regulate transcription factor activation and induction of oncogenes or other gene products needed for neoplastic cell growth.[400–402] Examples of some implicated genes include EGF, FGF, PDGF, TNF, GM-CSF, IL-1, and IL-3.[403–407] These data imply that LO products might play important roles in modulating cancer development, and that compounds interfering with the production of LO metabolites or antagonizing the signaling functions of LO products could be effective in preventing cancer.

Two studies have found that lipoxygenase inhibitors have chemopreventive activity in animal models of lung carcinogenesis. Moody et al[408] and Rioux and Castonguay[409] showed that oral intake of LO inhibitors NDGA, MK 886, and A 79175 significantly reduced the multiplicity of NNK-induced lung tumors in A/J mice. The

LO inhibitor A 79175 also reduced tumor incidence. In one of the studies, aspirin also reduced tumor multiplicity; the combination of aspirin and A 79175 (inhibiting both the COX and LO pathways) synergistically lowered tumor incidence and multiplicity. These results strongly suggest that 5-LO pathway inhibitors could have chemopreventive activity in the lung.

Supporting evidence links 5-LO metabolites with lung cancer cell growth. Studies conducted by Avis and coworkers[410] on human lung cancer cell lines found that 5-LO is stimulated by autocrine growth factors, gastrin-releasing peptide, and insulin-like growth factor (IGF), which stimulate the production of 5-HETE. 5-HETE, in turn, stimulates the growth of lung cancer cells, whereas 5-LO inhibitors NDGA, AA-861, and MK-886 decrease proliferation. Expression of 5-LO and 5-LO–activating protein (FLAP) mRNA by lung cancer cell lines was confirmed using RT-PCR, and 5-LO mRNA was identified in samples of human lung cancer tissue, both small cell and NSCLC. Studies relevant to lung cancer development demonstrated that LO mediated oxidation of carcinogens such as benzidine, *o*-dianisidine, and others; this effect could be blocked by the LO inhibitors NDGA and esculetin.[411] In addition, rat lung LO oxidizes the lung carcinogen benzo(*a*)pyrene, and LO expression in human lung has been reported by multiple investigators.[412-414]

Clinical Trials

Two large randomized trials have studied chemoprevention of primary lung cancer. The Alpha-Tocopherol Beta Carotene (ATBC) trial used a 2 × 2 factorial design to test alpha-tocopherol and β-carotene in 29,133 male Finnish chronic smokers ages 50–69.[18] Subjects were randomized to one of four groups for 5 to 8 years:

1. β-carotene alone (20mg/day),
2. α-tocopherol alone (50mg/day),
3. β-carotene plus α-tocopherol, or
4. Placebo

Contrary to the study hypothesis, subjects receiving β-carotene either alone or in combination with α-tocopherol had a statistically significant 18% higher incidence of lung cancer (RR = 1.18; 95% confidence interval [CI] 1.03–1.36) and an 8% increase in total mortality (RR = 1.08; 95% CI 1.01–1.16) compared with subjects receiving placebo. Supplementation with α-tocopherol was associated with no effect on lung cancer events.

The harmful effect of β-carotene was found in another major trial, the Beta-Carotene and Retinol Efficacy Trial (CARET).[19] In this trial, 18,314 smokers, former smokers, and workers exposed to asbestos were randomized to β-carotene (30 mg/day) plus retinol (25,000 IU/day) or placebo. The primary endpoint was lung cancer incidence. The CARET trial was terminated early when interim results indicated that the supplement group developed lung cancer more frequently compared with the placebo group. In the intervention group, lung cancer incidence increased by 28% (RR = 1.28; 95% CI 1.04–1.57), and total mortality increased by 17% (RR = 1.17; 95% CI 1.03–1.33).

These surprising results were contradictory to prior epidemiologic data, which strongly suggested an association between dietary β-carotene intake and a decreased risk of lung cancer. Another large study, however, showed no detrimental effect of β-carotene supplementation.[415] The Physician's Health Study, a randomized, double-blind, placebo-controlled trial among 22,071 male physicians aged 40–84 years, tested the effects of β-carotene and aspirin in prevention of cancer and cardiovascular disease. The use of supplemental β-carotene showed no significant effect on total cancer incidence (1273 treated subjects vs. 1293 in the placebo group [RR 0.98]), lung cancer incidence, or mortality rate during a 12-year follow-up period.

Recent studies provide a biologic explanation for the adverse interaction between tobacco smoke and β-carotene that occurred in the ATBC and CARET trials. The unexpected result might be due in part to a paradoxic pro-oxidant effect of high concentrations of β-carotene in the presence of high oxygen tension.[416] In the lungs, where the oxygen tension is high, β-carotene at high concentrations could lead to oxidative DNA damage and a higher incidence of cancer. In addition, Paolini and associates[417] have found that β-carotene in rat lung produces a powerful booster effect on phase I carcinogen-bioactivating enzymes (including activators of polycyclic aromatic hydrocarbons) and postulate that the harmful effects observed in the trials might be due to the cocarcinogenic properties of β-carotene and its ability to generate oxidative stress. The compound has also been described as an enhancer of cell transforming activity of carcinogens (benzo[a]pyrene) and cigarette smoke condensate on BALB/c 3T3 cells, inducing p53-dependent enzymes and oxygen-centered radical formation.[418] Wang and colleagues[419] reported that oxidative metabolites of β-carotene resulting from the interaction between high concentrations of β-carotene and tobacco smoke could inhibit retinoid signaling, increasing activating protein-1 (AP-1) production and thus increasing lung tumorigenesis in ferrets. Additionally, it has been shown that β-carotene oxidation products and oxygen-reactive species generated by β-carotene pro-oxidant activity can convert benzo(a)pyrene to mutagenic forms.[420]

In some chemoprevention trials, precancerous changes in bronchial epithelium were used as study endpoints. Three trials used bronchial metaplasia in histologic studies of bronchoscopic biopsies or sputum samples. The first trial tested isotretinoin vs. placebo for the reversal of metaplasia in bronchial biopsy specimens and found a substantial reduction in metaplasia in both groups (19 [54%] of 35 drug-treated subjects and 20 [58.8%] of 34 placebo-treated subjects).[421] Complete reversal of metaplasia was noted in nine subjects from each group. Therefore, isotretinoin given 1 mg/kg/day had no impact on reversal of metaplasia in the isotretinoin group. In a similarly designed trial of fenretinide in 70 participants, no benefit was shown.[422] A comparable conclusion was reached in a randomized trial of etretinate for the reversal of metaplasia interpreted from sputum samples.[423] Of the 138 participants in this study who completed 6 months of treatment or placebo, 32.4% of the 71 treated patients and 29.8% of patients in the placebo group experienced improvement or reversal of sputum cytology metaplasia.

Atypical cells in sputum were used as an endpoint in two randomized clinical trials. Treatment with β-carotene plus retinol for 58 months resulted in no significant reduction in the prevalence of sputum atypia or cytologic progression in 755 asbestos workers.[424] Heimburger et al[425] initially reported a significant improvement in sputum atypia after 4-month folic acid and vitamin B_{12} supplementation compared with placebo (P = .02), but re-analysis of the data showed no statistically significant difference between the two groups.[426]

Three phase III studies evaluated retinoids in the prevention of lung second primary tumor (SPT). The rationale for testing retinoids in this setting came from head and neck chemoprevention studies showing that these agents significantly reversed oral premalignancy and prevented lung SPT in patients with cured head and neck cancers. In the first study, the adjuvant effect of high-dose retinyl palmitate (300,000 IU/day) was evaluated in 307 patients with stage I lung cancer, randomly assigned to treatment or placebo after surgery.[427] After a follow-up of 46 months, the percentage of patients with recurrence or SPT was 37% in the intervention arm and 48% in the placebo arm. Eighteen patients in the treated group and 29 patients in the control group developed SPTs (P = 0.045). On the other hand, in a large multicenter study, the European Study on Chemoprevention with Vitamin A and N-Acetylcysteine (EUROSCAN), there was no benefit of chemoprevention in patients with curatively treated lung and head and neck cancers.[428] The trial used a 2 × 2 factorial design to study the efficacy of retinyl palmitate and the antioxidant N-acetyl-cysteine. There were 2592 randomized and eligible patients, approximately 1000 of whom had lung cancer. No differences were observed between treatment and control arms for SPT (P = 0.54), event-free survival (P = 0.750), or long-term survival (P = 0.925).

An Intergroup trial involving NCI-supported Cooperative Oncology groups studied the efficacy of isotretinoin in the prevention of SPT after stage I non–small cell lung cancer.[429] In this randomized, double-blind, placebo-controlled trial, more than 1000 participants received 3 years of intervention and 4 years of follow-up. There were no statistically significant differences between the two arms with respect to time to SPT (RR = 1.08; 95% CI 0.78–1.49), recurrence (RR = 0.99; 95% CI 0.76–1.29), or mortality (RR = 1.07; 95% CI 0.84–1.35). The SPT rate was 3.9% per year and was exceeded by the recurrence rate (6.2%) even in T1N0 patients. A post hoc analysis found that isotretinoin was harmful in current smokers and beneficial in never-smokers. Mortality and recurrence rates were increased in current smokers but were decreased in never-smokers in the isotretinoin arm compared with the placebo arm.

Mayne and coworkers[430] conducted a randomized trial of supplemental β-carotene in the prevention of SPT and recurrence in patients with curatively treated early-stage head and neck cancers. Patients were randomly assigned to receive 50 mg of β-carotene per day or placebo and were followed for up to 7.5 years. After a median follow-up of over 4 years, there was no difference between the two groups in the time to failure (RR = 0.90; 95% CI 0.56–1.45), SPT of head and neck (RR = 0.69; 95% CI 0.39–1.25), or lung (RR = 1.44; 95% CI 0.62–3.39).

SURGICAL STAGING

Bronchoscopic Techniques Including Transbronchial Needle Aspiration Biopsy

Bronchoscopy, besides visualizing obvious endobronchial tumor or airway distortion, can play a key role in the staging of lung cancer. Carinal biopsy alone in the presence of an endobronchial tumor, especially if it is central, can have a yield as high as 5%.[431] Bronchoscopy also can detect other lesions unsuspected in the airway, and fluorescence bronchoscopy is being evaluated not only for finding occult lesions but also for defining margins of resection of the bronchus that could influence staging (i.e., proximity to the carina).[432] Transbronchial needle aspiration (TBNA) can be used to assess mediastinal adenopathy, including paratracheal, subcarinal, hilar, and aorticopulmonary window nodes. A variety of needles (usually 1.3 cm in length) can be used for transbronchial, transtracheal, or transcarinal aspiration, and the best results are achieved with larger-gauge (18- or 19-gauge) needles.[433,434] Inadequate insertion of the needle in the tissue of interest is the most common problem with the transbronchial needle mediastinal aspirations and can lead to false-negative biopsies without securing lymph nodal tissue. Aspiration of paratracheal lesions is difficult because of the angle of penetration and needle length, and the needle must be anchored between tracheal rings before an attempt is made to advance it. The yield is improved with at least seven passes with the TBNA needle, and in all cases, a cytopathologist should assess the adequacy of cellularity at the time of the procedure.[435] In a recent review of the literature regarding the accuracy of TBNA of the mediastinum in patients with lung cancer, the sensitivity was determined to be 76%, with a specificity of 96%. False positives can be decreased by avoiding the primary tumor before sampling the mediastinal nodes, to prevent contamination of the bronchoscope channel by tumor cells. The accuracy of TBNA could improve in the future with the addition of endobronchial ultrasound.

Endo-esophageal Ultrasound Fine-Needle Aspiration

The advent of endoscopic ultrasound has made possible excellent visualization of the mediastinum, particularly the left mediastinal lymph nodes and the subcarinal space.[294,435–438] Endo-esophageal ultrasound fine-needle aspiration (EUS-FNA) is usually performed in the outpatient setting with conscious sedation. Because the esophagus lies posteriorly and to the left of the trachea and is in proximity to the lymph nodes between these two structures, lymph node levels 5, 7, 8, and possibly 9 are accessible. Right-sided levels 2, 4, and the pretracheal space are not accessible with EUS-FNA. Wiersema and

Specific Malignancies

III

TABLE 75-12

STAGE	FEATURES
Tx	Tumor proved by the presence of malignant cells in bronchopulmonary secretions but not visible roentgenographically or bronchoscopically, or any tumor that cannot be assessed, as in a retreatment staging
T0	No evidence of primary tumor
TIS	Carcinoma in situ
T1	A tumor 3 cm or less in greatest dimension, surrounded by lung or visceral pleura and without evidence of invasion proximal to a lobar bronchus at bronchoscopy
T2	A tumor more than 3 cm in greatest dimension, or a tumor of any size that either invades the visceral pleura or has associated atelectasis or obstructive pneumonitis extending to the hilar region; at bronchoscopy, the proximal extent of demonstrable tumor must be within a lobar bronchus or at least 2 cm distal to the carina; any associated atelectasis or obstructive pneumonitis must involve less than an entire lung
T3	A tumor of any size with direct extension into the chest wall (including sulcus tumors), diaphragm, or the mediastinal pleura of pericardium without involving the heart, great vessels, trachea, esophagus, or vertebral body, or a tumor in the main bronchus within 2 cm of the carina without involving the carina
T4	A tumor of any size with invasion of the mediastinum or involving the heart, great vessels, trachea, esophagus, vertebral body, or carina or the presence of malignant pleural effusion
N0	No demonstrable metastasis to regional lymph nodes
N1	Metastasis to lymph nodes in the peribronchial or ipsilateral hilar region, or both, including direct extension
N2	Metastasis to ipsilateral mediastinal lymph nodes and subcarinal lymph nodes
N3	Metastasis to contralateral mediastinal lymph nodes, contralateral hilar lymph nodes, ipsilateral or contralateral scalene or supraclavicular lymph nodes
M0	No (known) distant metastasis
M1	Distant metastasis present—specify sites

TNM Staging System for Lung Cancer

associates[439] recently reported that EUS-FNA was superior to TBNA in the diagnosis of mediastinal metastases in NSCLC. The needle is guided by real-time ultrasonography, and the adequacy of the cytologic aspirate should be confirmed on site. EUS-FNA can also detect malignancy in normal-sized lymph nodes and has changed the staging of patients with normal-sized lymph nodes from 18% to 42%. The sensitivity and specificity are low in this situation due to the necessity to perform many aspirations of different sites to increase the yield.

Invasive Surgical Staging of the Mediastinum

Mediastinoscopy and Mediastinotomy

In 1949, Daniels described the technique of scalenes node biopsy, and in 1954, Harken described the visualization of the anterior mediastinum using the Jackson laryngoscope. Carlens revised the instrumentation for these by using a cervical mediastinoscope, which allowed superior access to the contralateral mediastinal nodes, thereby providing a method for preresectional determination of operability. Led by Pearson, the thoracic surgical group in Toronto was the first to perform mediastinoscopy in the preresectional staging of NSCLC, and they convincingly demonstrated the prognostic significance of positive lymph nodes identified at mediastinoscopy. Based on the relationship between prognosis and the level of lymph node involvement, Naruke and colleagues developed a thoracic lymph node map that illustrates the location of various lymph nodes. This map, now uniformly employed by thoracic oncologists, was revised most recently in 1997 by Mountain[82] and Dressler. Each lymph node is assigned to a specific nodal station (N0, N1, N2, or N3) representing

a prognostic subgroup or stage. In 1986 and subsequently in 1997, Mountain introduced and modified a new international staging system in which the extent of nodal spread serves as the principal prognostic determinant. Multiple reports have validated the prognostic value of this staging system (Tables 75-12, 75-13, and 75-14).

Overview of Invasive Surgical Staging

The method by which the mediastinum is explored depends on the site of the lesion. Cervical mediastinoscopy involves an initial digital exploration palpating suspicious nodes, followed by placement of the scope to visualize and biopsy the appropriate lymph nodes. The N2 (levels 4, 7) and N3 nodal stations (2, scalenus), with the exception of the aortic nodes (levels 5 and 6), the

TABLE 75-13

Staging of Lung Cancer

1987 TNM STAGING		1997 TNM STAGING	
Stage I	T1N0M0	Stage Ia	T1N0M0
	T2N0M0	Stage Ib	T2N0M0
Stage II	T1N1M0	Stage IIa	T1N1M0
	T2N1M0	Stage IIb	T2N1M0
			T3N0M0
Stage IIIA	T3N0M0	Stage IIIa	T1–3N2M0
	T3N1M0		T3N1M0
	T1–3N2M0		
Stage IIIB	Any TN3M0	Stage IIIb	T4* Any NM0
	T4N3M0		Any TN3M0
Stage IV	Any T Any NM1	Stage IV	Any T Any NM1†

*T4, includes ipsilobar satellite nodules.
†M1, includes extralobar satellite nodules.

TABLE 75-14

Estimated Survival Following Complete Surgical Resection

STAGE GROUPING		ESTIMATED 5-YEAR SURVIVAL FOLLOWING COMPLETE SURGICAL RESECTION (%)
0	TisN0M0	100
IA	T1N0M0	75
IB	T2N0M0	55
IIA	T1N1M0	50
IIB	T2N1M0	40
	T3N0M0	
IIIA	T1–3N2M0	15
	T3N1M0	35
IIIB	T1–3N3M0	5–10
	T4 Any NM0	5–10
IV	Any T, Any N, M1 (Solitary M1)	5–10

inferior pulmonary ligament nodes (level 9), and the para-esophageal nodes (level 8), are accessible for biopsy using this technique. Lee and Ginsberg[440] have emphasized the importance of combining standard cervical mediastino-scopy with exploration of the scalenus fat pad in patients with central nonsquamous tumors. Extended cervical mediastinoscopy is a technique that combines cervical mediastinoscopy with mediastinoscopic evaluation of the subaortic space as a single procedure. More commonly, the subaortic space is approached using the Chamberlain procedure, which permits the surgeon to palpate the subaortic extrapleural space directly and biopsy the lymph nodes in this region. Video-assisted thoracoscopic surgery (VATS), a minimally invasive surgical technique, is an alternative method to assess not only levels 5 and 6 but also the paraesophageal (level 8) and pulmonary ligament (level 9) nodes. Whether a surgeon surgically stages the ipsilateral and the contralateral mediastinal nodes in a patient with lung cancer is increasingly being dictated by the use of PET scanning. When PET scanning is not available, staging of the contralateral side usually is defined by nodal size on computed tomography.

Indications for Surgical Staging by Mediastinoscopy or Mediastinotomy

Numerous studies have addressed the role of noninvasive evaluation of the mediastinum, primarily by computed tomography (covered elsewhere in this chapter). Among patients with lung cancer, enlarged mediastinal lymph nodes detected by CT could prove to be benign on pathologic examination, and the histologic verification of disease dictates the appropriate protocol or off-protocol therapy for the patient. Mediastinal nodal enlargement by CT is, therefore, an absolute indication for mediastino-scopy. For patients with mediastinal nodes of any size, the documentation of metabolic activity within single nodes or in multiple nodal basins in an individual with suspected lung cancer is also an indication for surgical staging of the suspicious mediastinum. For patients whose eligibility criteria require documentation of mediastinal disease, as in randomized or nonrandomized trials of induction

therapy for loco-regional lung cancer, mediastinal biopsy is mandated.

Several lung cancer situations are associated with a sufficiently high risk of mediastinal nodal spread that the presence of any one of them in a patient with known or suspected primary lung carcinoma warrants preresec-tional mediastinoscopy, even if the CT scan shows no mediastinal adenopathy. A large mass or a lesion of any size located within the inner one-third of the lung field, especially if it is an adenocarcinoma or large cell carcinoma, correlates with an increased incidence of N2 nodal spread despite the finding of a normal mediastinum on CT scan. Because of the tendency for left lower lobe lesions to spread contralaterally, some centers recommend biopsy of bilateral mediastinal nodes, including subcarinal (level 7) and right and left tracheobronchial angle (stations 10R, 10L) nodes. A needle biopsy specimen of an apparent stage I lesion that reveals SCLC cytology warrants mediastinoscopy, which, if devoid of cancer cells and after further systemic staging, could justify resection and post resection adjuvant therapy.

Evidence of vocal cord palsy or hoarseness represents another indication for cervical mediastinoscopy. The left recurrent laryngeal nerve could be compromised by enlargement of the aortic nodes, resulting in ipsilateral vocal cord hemiparesis.

Results of Mediastinoscopy and Mediastinotomy

In a review of more than 5687 patients undergoing mediastinoscopy between 1983 and 1999, the overall sensitivity of standard cervical mediastinoscopy was 81%, with a negative predictive value of 91%. Extended cervical mediastinoscopy used in combination with standard cervical mediastinoscopy increased the overall sensitivity by 17%–44% and improved negative predictive value by 10%–20% when compared directly with standard mediastinoscopy. The Chamberlain procedure or anterior mediastinotomy had a sensitivity of 63%–86%, and its negative predictive value remains high, whether it is performed alone (89%–100%) or in combination with standard cervical mediastinoscopy (89%–92%).[441]

Complications of Mediastinoscopy/Mediastinotomy

Because of the risk of bleeding, the surgeon must always aspirate by needle any structure before biopsying it. Blood vessels are occasionally incorrectly identified as nodes; this can occur with bronchial vessels, the azygos vein, branches of the pulmonary artery near the region of the right tracheobronchial nodes, and other structures that might be adherent to biopsied lymph nodes. Hemostasis is usually obtained with electrocautery and packing. In the rare situation of significant bleeding, the mediastinoscope should not be removed, because direct tamponade is facilitated by the location of the scope near the source of hemorrhage. Packing with hemostatic materials and gauze packs for 5 minutes is the appropriate first attempt to achieve hemostasis. Damage to the main pulmonary artery, the aortic arch, or the innominate artery will likely require prompt operative exploration through an ipsilateral thoracotomy or median sternotomy. If thoracotomy is necessary, it should be

Specific Malignancies

III

performed on the side of the lung lesion to allow pulmonary resection after hemostasis has been achieved. Complications of mediastinoscopy, however, are rare and include recurrent nerve injury, pneumothorax, and arrhythmias. A left-sided mediastinotomy can be associated with local pain from resection of the second costal cartilage, and with injury to the internal mammary artery, pulmonary artery, pulmonary vein, phrenic nerve, and left recurrent laryngeal nerve. Nevertheless, several reports document the safety of mediastinoscopy and mediastinotomy, with mortalities of 0%–0.3% and morbidities of 1%–2.3%.[442]

Intraoperative Staging at the Time of Resection

There is controversy regarding whether complete ipsilateral mediastinal nodal dissection as opposed to minimal or more extensive hilar and mediastinal lymph nodes sampling has greater efficacy in determining intraoperative stage, and whether the degree of the dissection influences prognosis. A cadre of thoracic surgeons in North America and Japan feel that mediastinal lymph node dissection is important for both accurate staging and overall survival.[443-446]

Detection of Occult Disease by Type of Lymphadenectomy

A number of investigators have evaluated the extent of mediastinal biopsy necessary to obtain accurate staging information. Bollen and colleagues[447] found that systematic sampling of mediastinal lymph nodes was as successful as mediastinal lymph node dissection in identifying N2 disease (discovery ratio 2.7; CI 1.04–4.2). These authors described more injuries to the recurrent nerve with lymph node dissection when compared with historic controls and documented that lymph node dissection lengthens the operation. Izbicki and coworkers[448] conducted a randomized prospective trial with 182 patients comparing systemic mediastinal lymph node sampling to mediastinal lymph node dissection and found that the number of N2-positive levels was greater among the patients who underwent complete dissection, although the percentage of patients found to have N1 or N2 disease was not significantly different between the two study arms. There was no difference in blood loss or blood replacement.[448] A similar study was conducted by Sugi and associates;[449] in 115 patients with clinical T1N tumors that were less than 2 cm in diameter, mediastinal metastases were found in 13% of each group. From these data, it appears that systematic lymph node dissection is no more accurate than mediastinal dissection for staging NSCLC.

Survival and the Type of Lymphadenectomy

Whether regional lymph node sampling or complete ipsilateral lymphadenectomy affects long-term survival is unclear. There has been no long-term study of the effects of a complete mediastinal lymphadenectomy. The retrospective study by Funatsu and colleagues,[450] however, has shown that 5-year survival was significantly better in 64 patients who underwent a lymph node sampling when compared with 61 patients who underwent radical mediastinal lymphadenectomy. Conversely, in a series of 151 patients at Memorial Sloan-Kettering Cancer Center who had positive mediastinal lymph nodes, a 30% 5-year survival was observed as one of the highest in the current literature with mediastinal lymphadenectomy.[451] In the randomized trial by Izbicki and associates[448] comparing mediastinal node sampling with mediastinal lymphadenectomy, no increase in morbidity or mortality for lymphadenectomy was found, and there were no differences in survival. This trial, however, was underpowered to show differences in locoregional recurrence or survival.

The Intergroup Trial 0115 of adjuvant therapy in patients with completely resected stages II and IIIA NSCLC had the patients stratified by the type of lymph node dissection before participation (dissection vs. sampling). Of 373 eligible patients accrued to the study, 187 underwent sampling, and 186 underwent dissection. Although no significant difference in stage distribution was observed between patients receiving the two surgical procedures, complete dissection identified significantly more levels of N2 disease and was associated with improved survival with right-sided NSCLC when compared with systematic sampling.[452]

Wu and coworkers[453] recently presented the results of the largest randomized trial to date that compared the two techniques. In this study of 471 eligible patients with stages I–IIIA NSCLC followed up for up to 10 years after resection, complete dissection was associated with significant improvement in survival (59 months median survival for the complete dissection group vs. 34 months for the group undergoing sampling). Significant differences in survival were present for all pathologic stages of disease, and on multivariate analysis, the type of lymph node dissection was found to be an independent predictor of survival.

SURGICAL TREATMENT OF LUNG CANCER

General

Complete surgical resection of localized lung cancer offers patients the best chance for cure. Surgery as the entire treatment package or as part of the therapy should be considered for stages I, II, IIIa, and selected cases of IIIb disease. For stages I and II, there is really no controversy regarding a surgical role. The more controversial aspects of surgery in lung cancer for stages I and II include the management of screen-detected or occult lung cancer, the role of limited resections, the role of mediastinal node dissection for these stages, and the use of preoperative or postoperative therapies. For stage IIIa disease, the primary role of surgery is loosely connected to multiple factors, not the least of which include the technique and timing of the investigation of involved mediastinal lymph node disease, characteristics of this "discovered" mediastinal lymph node disease, residual, viable tumor in lymph nodes after induction therapy, and the safety of surgical resection after induction therapy. It is generally agreed that there are limited instances of surgical efficacy for Stage IIIb disease; in particular, surgery is contradicted for tumors with extensive local invasion of mediastinal, vascular, or boney structures in the absence of viable tumor in lymph nodes.

Selection of the Surgical Candidate

The operative mortality rates for resection of lung cancer average 4%, with lobectomy having a mortality of 3% and pneumonectomy a mortality of 7%–9%.[454] The most common causes of death include pneumonia and respiratory failure (41%), myocardial infarction (14%), empyema and bronchoplueral fistula (11%), hemorrhage (7%), and pulmonary embolus (6%). Surgical selection should not be defined by chronologic age but by compulsive functional correlation of the cardiopulmonary reserve with the age of the patient. In a recent review of the literature, the mortality of pulmonary resection for lung cancer in patients 70–79 years or 80 years or greater was 6% and 8%, respectively.[454] It has been suggested in some reports that for patients in their seventh decade or older, the mortality for lobectomy is 4%–7%, while for pneumonectomy it is approximately 14%–16%.[454-456] These rates are obviously higher than for younger patients and likely are more a function of comorbidity than of age alone. Accordingly, in all ages of patients selected for pulmonary resection, thorough preoperative functional assessment should be performed.

Preoperative Pulmonary Assessment

Preoperative arterial oxygen saturation of less than 90% has been associated with an increased risk of postoperative complications, and hypercapnea ($PaCO_2$ >45 mmHg) has been an exclusion criterion for lung resection.[457-459]

The generally accepted guidelines for preoperative FEV_1 for lobectomy and pneumonectomy are values greater than 1.5 liters and 2 liters, respectively, and in all cases the maximum voluntary ventilation (MVV) should be greater than 50% of predicted.[460] Preoperative diffusing capacity of the lung for carbon monoxide (DLCO) has also been linked to postresection morbidity and mortality. For pneumonectomy and lobectomy, a preoperative DLCO of greater than 60% and 50% are recommended for pneumonectomy and lobectomy, respectively. The risk of pulmonary complications also increases with DLCO of less than 80%.[461] It is felt that the predicted postoperative (ppo) DLCO could be a more sensitive indicator of mortality after standard resection, with a mortality of 25% among patients with ppo-DLCO% of less than 50% and a mortality of 33% for those with a ppo-DLCO% of 40% of less.[462] In general, patients with an FEV_1 greater than 80% of predicted, a DLCO greater than 80% of predicted, and no significant cardiac history are suitable for pneumonectomy.[458]

Postoperative Prediction of Lung Function

The ability to predict postoperative lung function after resection further defines pulmonary risk principally by using nuclear medicine perfusion scans and recently quantitative CT.[463-466] A quantitative radionuclide perfusion scan measures the relative function of each lung. In general, the threshold for postoperative FEV_1 for surgical resection is between 0.7 and 0.8 liters.[467,468] It is difficult to predict the absolute cut-off for surgical resection and predicted postoperative FEV_1 by percentage of normal, but a group of studies have suggested increased morbidity with a postoperative FEV_1 that is less than 40% of normal.[464,469] Moreover, a predicted postoperative DLCO below 40% is also associated with increased morbidity.[461,464,470]

Exercise Testing

Stair climbing has been used historically to gauge an individual's cardiopulmonary conditioning. In general, lobectomy candidates were expected to climb three flights of stairs, and indeed this ability correlates with an FEV_1 of greater than 1.7 L. Pneumonectomy patients who could climb five flights of stairs have an FEV_1 greater than 2 L.[471,472]

Formal cardiopulmonary exercise testing (CPET) with the measurement of oxygen consumption has also been used to stratify for the risk of perioperative complications. Patients with a preoperative oxygen consumption of greater than 20 mL/kg/minute are not at increased risk of complications or death, while those with measurements of less than 10 mL/kg/minute are at high risk for postoperative complications.[460,470,473-476]

SPECIFIC MANAGEMENT OF LUNG CANCER STAGES

Stage I: Early-stage Occult Lung Cancer (Tx, T1SN0M0)

Occult lung cancer is defined as tumor in an asymptomatic patient without radiographic or bronchoscopic findings. With the advent of sputum screening programs in high-risk individuals, it is expected that the number of individuals detected with abnormal cells on sputum cytology will increase. Occult lung cancer is also found in patients who have had a previous aerodigestive malignancy and are undergoing surveillance endoscopies. The majority of these lesions, even if they represent carcinoma in situ or microinvasive cancer, require lobectomy (70%), and between 1% and 4% have synchronous lung cancers.[477,478] The 5-year survival of patients treated with surgery for these early lesions approaches 90%.[479,480] Nevertheless, because the majority of these occult lung cancers invade the bronchial wall but do not involve the lymphatics and because there is a finite risk of acquiring a second lung cancer, lung preservation techniques for therapy could play an important role in this population of patients. Moreover, a cohort of these patients are unable to tolerate resectional therapy. Decisions about the appropriateness of endobronchial lung sparing techniques should be based on the depth of invasion of these lesions, information which derives from bronchosopic evaluation of their size and shape (i.e., <10 mm); superficial lesions have invasion in fewer than 5% of cases, while polypoid lesions invade up to 27% of the time.[481]

Lung-preserving endobronchial therapies include photodynamic therapy, brachytherapy, electrocautery, cryotherapy, and neodymium-yttrium-garnet (Nd-Yag) laser therapy.[482,483] Photodynamic therapy, in which the lesion is ablated using a wavelength-specific photo-activating drug known as Photofrin II, can accomplish a complete response in these early lesions in 75% of cases, with a recurrence rate of approximately 30%. Efficacy is directly related to the size of the lesion, with lesions smaller than 1 cm yielding the best results.[483] Similar results are achieved with electrocautery, endobronchial iridium-based brachytherapy, and (most recently) cryotherapy.[484-486]

At present, whenever possible, surgical treatment is indicated for early-stage disease and for all in situ lesions that persist after nonsurgical endobronchial therapies.

Stage I Lung Cancer (T1, T2N0M0)

For lung cancers limited to the hemithorax without lymph node involvement, and with tumor extension no further than the visceral pleura, surgical excision is the treatment of choice in physiologically sound individuals. When there is no medical contraindication to operative intervention, patients with stage IA and B should have complete surgical excision of the tumor with negative margins by a surgeon who is trained, board certified, and performs a sufficient number of operations per year. If negative surgical margins are not achieved, additional local therapies should be considered, including re-operation or radiotherapy. The use of adjuvant and induction therapies, specifically for the T2 subset, is discussed in another section of this chapter.

The 5-year survival of patients with pathologic stage IA and IB disease is 70% and 55%, respectively, independent of the histology of the tumor. Tumor differentiation and vascular invasion, however, seem to be significant prognostic factors. On average, about one-third of the patients with stage I lung cancer will have recurrence, with two-thirds of these recurrences being systemic and one-third local. Approximately 5% of patients with stage I lung cancer will develop a second primary cancer at the rate of 2% per year.[487]

The controversies regarding the management of stage IA and IB lung cancer include the issue of whether an anatomic resection should be preferred over wedge resection or less than a lobar anatomic resection (i.e., segmentectomy) and the role of lymphadenectomy at the time of resection. Limited resection as a compromise procedure in patients with poor pulmonary reserve carries a 5-year survival of 50%.[487] A 6%–24% risk of local recurrence was reported in earlier studies using wedge or segmental resection for stage I non–small cell lung cancer, along with a 5-year survival of 55%–93% when the procedures is performed in noncompromised individuals.[488-492]

A prospective, randomized controlled trial by the Lung Cancer Study Group, in which 247 patients were assigned to either lesser resection or lobectomy, revealed that the lung cancer recurrence rate was 75% greater in the limited resection group due to a tripling of local tumor recurrence. This same group experienced a 50% increase in cancer death.[493]

The issues regarding mediastinal node dissection and nodal sampling have been described in the staging portion of this chapter. There is, in fact, an ongoing American College of Surgeons Oncology Group (ACOSOG) study in which patients with N0 or N1 (less than hilar) non–small cell carcinoma are randomized to mediastinal lymph node sampling or complete lymphadenectomy. Conventional wisdom until this trial is complete is that all patients having surgical resection for lung cancer should have intraoperative systematic surgical mediastinal lymph node evaluation for accurate pathologic staging.[494]

Stage II Lung Cancer

T1-T2N1M0

Among patients with pathologic stage II lung cancers, approximately 80% have N1 disease and 20% have T3N0 disease.[82,495] For patients found to have intraparenchymal nodal involvement (without mediastinal node involvement), approximately 1%–5% are stage IIA and 15%–25% are stage IIB.[496] The 5-year survival of patients with pathologic stage II (N1) disease is 40%, with the survival of T1N1 disease being 15% higher than that for T2N1 patients.[496-499] Patients with squamous stage II lung cancers have approximately a 15% better 5-year survival than those with adenocarcinoma, and the most common sites of recurrence in all N1-involved patients are systemic rather than local sites.[500,501] The roles of induction and adjuvant therapy for N1-involved patients is discussed elsewhere in this chapter.

Treatment of Stage II NSCLC: T3 Category

T3 tumors are those that invade the chest wall, diaphragm, or mediastinum (mediastinal pleura, pericardium, phrenic nerve, azygous vein, or right or left pulmonary artery), or that have proximity (<2 cm) to the carina and involve the mainstem bronchus. They represent approximately 10% of all resected NSCLC or 5% of all NSCLC, and the T3N0 category predominates.[82,495] The ability to accomplish complete resection with central T3 tumors is more difficult than with peripheral T3 tumors of the chest wall. Because the 5-year survival of patients with T3N2 NSCLC is low, and because central tumors are more likely to have occult N2 metastases, mediastinoscopy should be performed in patients with T3 central tumors before resection.

Chest Wall T3 Disease

Forty percent of T3 tumors have involvement of the parietal pleura, chest wall muscle, or rib. The 5-year survival for completely resected T3N0 chest wall patients is approximately 50%–60%, with the prognosis depending on completeness of resection, nodal involvement, and depth of invasion.[501,502] The majority of thoracic surgeons feel that if, on exploration of the chest, the tumor is found to invade the parietal pleura or deeper, the preferred surgical technique is complete en bloc resection of the tumor plus chest wall with a minimum of 2 cm of normal chest wall in all directions beyond the tumor. The morbidity of operations incorporating en bloc resection of T3 (chest wall) tumors is similar to that of operations in which an extrapleural resection is performed.[501,503,504]

There are no data to justify postoperative radiotherapy for patients who have undergone complete resection of T3 (chest wall) NSCLC. The few studies that address postoperative radiotherapy in patients who have undergone an incomplete resection of T3 (chest wall) NSCLC did not identify a survival advantage in this group either.[502,505]

Pancoast (Superior Sulcus) Tumors

Henry Pancoast was the first to describe the constellation of symptoms associated with a tumor in the apex of the lung. Invasion of the first rib with associated involvement of the brachial plexus and stellate ganglion create the classic Pancoast Syndrome (rib erosion, shoulder pain radiating down the arm, Horner's syndrome). The majority of these tumors are adenocarcinomas, and a greater than 90% success rate in establishing a diagnosis is performed with fine-needle aspiration. In the absence of mediastinal nodal involvement, the overwhelming problem with these tumors is local control. Poor prognostic factors for a superior sulcus tumor include mediastinal nodal involvement, the presence of a Horner's syndrome, vertebral body invasion, and great vessel involvement.

Shaw and Paulson[506] were the first to describe curative resection of this disease, but many clinicians forget that even in the original paper, the only patients who had long-term survival were those with no evidence of mediastinal nodal involvement. Until recently, the standard of care for a documented superior sulcus tumor was radiotherapy of 3000–4500 cGy followed by en bloc resection of the involved lung, chest wall, and (frequently) the T1 nerve root. With this approach, approximately 66% of patients can have a complete resection, and the 5-year survival for completely resected patients is 40%. A minority of patients in the surgical series have mediastinal nodal involvement or have evidence of T4 disease.[507] Unfortunately, disease recurs locally in approximately 45% of resected patients, and disease recurs systemically in approximately 25% of patients, chiefly in the brain. The new standard of care for Pancoast tumors involves concurrent chemoradiation therapy followed by surgical resection. Initial results for 95 patients eligible for surgery in the Southwest Oncology Group Trial 9416 (Intergroup Trial 0160) using this approach revealed an operative mortality of 2.4% and a 92% complete resection rate. A pathologic complete response or minimal microscopic disease was seen in 65% of thoracotomy specimens. The 2-year survival was 55% for all eligible patients and 70% for patients who had a complete resection.[508]

Mediastinal T3 Disease

In the majority of cases of mediastinal invasion of the pleura, pericardium, or fat, an en bloc resection of the mediastinal tissue can be accomplished if the contact with the mediastinal fat or pericardium is over a small area (often discovered only at the time of surgery). The average

5-year survival of such patients is 25%.[508] Patients with mediastinal invasion usually have other major structures involved or concomitant mediastinal lymph node disease.[510,511]

Proximal Airway Involvement T3 Disease

Tumors within 2 cm of the carina can be resected by pneumonectomy, but in most of the series reported—especially with those tumors arising from the upper lobes and extending into the main bronchus—a sleeve resection is performed with preservation of the normal distal lung. In fact, patients with mainstem bronchial involvement are usually reported in series of sleeve resections, often mixed in with other stages. The range of 5-year survival in reported series varies from 12% to 40%.[512-515] No randomized trials comparing sleeve lobectomy with pneumonectomy have been reported in the literature. In single-institution reports comparing pneumonectomy with sleeve resection, the complication rate and mortalities were increased in the pneumonectomy patients, but survival of the two techniques was equivalent. The survival of patients with proximal airway disease is influenced by the ability to perform a a complete resection (35% vs. 18% 5-year survival, complete vs. incomplete resection, respectively) and the presence of mediastinal nodal involovment (45% 5-year survival for N0 disease vs. 37% for N1, and 0% for N2).[509,516,517] Although these studies are limited by their retrospective method and small numbers of patients, the authors agree with the conclusions of these articles that sleeve lobectomy is preferable to pneumonectomy whenever a complete pathologic resection can be obtained using bronchoplastic techniques.

Locally Advanced Lung Cancer: Stages IIIA and B

Stage IIIA (N2) Disease

Stage IIIA disease encompasses a T3N1 tumor or N2 nodal spread. The 5-year survival of patients with T3N1 disease is approximately 22%, and the finding of T3N1 disease is usually confirmed after resection of suspected T3N0 disease.

The role of surgery for N2 disease is much more complicated due to the heterogeneity of N2 scenarios in clinical presentation, treatment, and prognosis. Ruckdeschel[518] has classified N2 tumors into four subsets (IIIA$_{1-4}$), and the timing and role of surgery varies among these subsets.

Surgery for Incidental N2 Disease (Stage IIIA$_{1-2}$)

Despite careful preoperative staging that includes CT scan, positron emission tomography (PET), and mediastinoscopy, as many as one-fourth of patients will be found at thoracotomy to have metastases to mediastinal N2 lymph nodes (stage IIIA$_1$); some of these metastases are discovered by surprise a number of days postoperatively, on the final pathologic examination of the surgical specimen. In other patients, metastases will be found on intraoperative frozen-section examination of mediastinal nodes (stage IIIA$_2$). For patients with an occult, single-station mediastinal node metastasis recognized at thoracotomy in whom a complete resection of the nodes and primary tumor is technically possible, most thoracic surgeons proceed with the planned lung resection and a mediastinal lymphadenectomy. If a complete resection is not possible or there is multistation or bulky nodal disease or extracapsular nodal disease, then the planned lung resection should be aborted. These patients can then be considered for induction therapies and (potentially) re-exploration at the conclusion of their chemotherapy with or without radiotherapy. Although incomplete resection rarely results in long-term survival, collected results indicate that surgery alone in stage IIIA disease (N2 disease) is associated with a 14%–30% 5-year survival. The best survival is seen in cases with minimal N2 disease and complete resection.[444,519-525]

If, before thoracotomy, metastatic disease is found in the N2 nodes at mediastinoscopy, further surgery at that time should be avoided.[526] If appropriate, induction therapy first is more advantageous, followed later in selected patients by definitive surgical resection of the primary lung cancer along with as complete a mediastinal lymphadenectomy as possible. The role of postoperative adjuvant therapy in this situation will be covered elsewhere in the chapter.

Potentially Resectable N2 Disease (Stage IIIA$_3$)

With the development of chemotherapeutic agents that demonstrate significant activity against lung cancer and the development of modern radiotherapy techniques, studies have suggested that combining chemotherapy and/or radiotherapy followed by surgery in selected stage IIIA patients could offer therapeutic benefit. The poor survival rates with surgery alone in N2 disease, even with adjuvant postoperative chemotherapy or radiotherapy, has led to efforts at giving initial nonsurgical (radiotherapy and/or chemotherapy) therapy first, often to convert the unresectable tumor to resectable and to improve long-term survival. Patients considered for such approaches include those with enlarged (>1.0 cm short-axis diameter) N2 nodes (IIIA$_3$) on chest CT. Mediastinoscopy should generally be performed in this setting to document that these nodes actually contain metastatic tumor, as approximately 40% of moderately enlarged nodes could be benign, especially if there is an associated recent pneumonitis.

Prognostic Factors Related to N2 Disease

Adverse prognostic factors associated with positive mediastinal nodes include extracapsular spread of tumor, multiple levels of involved lymph nodes, bulky enlarged nodes, and the size of the primary tumor.[507,523,524,527] There is controversy regarding whether involvement of the higher, superior mediastinal nodes (nodes found positive that are generally available for biopsy at mediastinoscopy) portends a worse prognosis than a negative mediastinoscopy result in patients who nevertheless are found to have positive nodes at thoracotomy.[526] Multiple studies have found that metastatic disease to the subcarinal lymph nodes adversely affects prognosis compared with metastases to other lymph nodes.[519,521,523,525,528-532] It is generally believed that multistation nodal disease has a worse prognosis than single-station disease.

Surgical Considerations in Stage IIIA$_3$

Patients must be restaged carefully after induction therapy in consideration of a surgical exploration. Liberal use of radiographic examinations, including MRI of the brain, should be encouraged. Because persistent viable disease in lymph nodes is associated with a poor prognosis, either repeat mediastinoscopy or transesophageal ultrasound-guided biopsy of mediastinal nodes should be considered if suspicious areas persist in radiographic studies. Moreover, lymph-node dissection with liberal use of frozen sections should be performed at the inception of the exploration. In the phase II Southwestern Oncology Group trial of induction chemoradiotherapy followed by surgery in stage IIIA and IIIB disease, there was complete pathologic clearance of tumor in 22% of resection specimens, with an overall 3-year survival of 27%.[533-535] But it is of particular interest that the patients with a complete pathologic clearing of residual disease had a 30-month median survival compared with a median survival of 10 months for those with residual tumor in the lymph nodes (p = 0.0005). A more recent study by Bueno and associates[536] emphasized the importance of residual nodal disease after induction therapy in stage IIIA tumors. In their study, long-term survival was stratified by nodal status after induction therapy and lung resection; 28% of patients downstaged to pathologic N0 had a 35.8% 5-year survival, whereas the remainder of patients with residual nodal disease at surgery had only a 9% 5-year survival. These and other studies suggest that surgical resection should be avoided after induction therapy in patients who have definite, biopsy-proven residual tumor in the mediastinal nodes.

Although the use of neoadjuvant chemotherapy and/or radiotherapy appears to have potential advantages in the treatment of locally advanced lung cancer, concern has been raised in numerous publications about the perceived and real increase in morbidity and mortality related to subsequent lung resections. So far, in trials of surgery with induction chemotherapy for early, more minimal bulk disease, there has been no difference in overall post-operative mortality rates compared with the surgery-alone control arms.[86,88,537] Pulmonary complications and deaths due to pulmonary causes during the postoperative time period are the greatest concerns after induction therapy, and collectively, mortality rates are probably greater than reported in the literature after surgery alone. In particular, events such as extensive pneumonitis (usually culture-negative), acute respiratory distress syndrome (ARDS), and bronchopleural fistula are associated with high mortality in the postoperative period. Pulmonary morbidity and mortality rates are often quoted to be greater after induction regimens with chemoradiation therapy than after induction chemotherapy alone. A careful review of all the literature available discloses great variability, however. Postoperative mortality rates were reported after MVP- or VP-containing induction chemotherapy (3.1%–17%, including some cases of ARDS), after second-generation induction chemoradiation therapy (4%–15%), and after induction chemoradiation therapy with hyperfractionation (5%–7%). The specific type of mortal postoperative event might differ according to whether radiotherapy was included with induction chemotherapy, although this issue is not fully resolved. Moreover, the degree of pulmonary resection (i.e., pneumonectomy, especially on the right) is associated with higher morbidity and mortality rates.[538] The preoperative DLCO could be the most important screen for the risk of serious postoperative pulmonary complications; this hypothesis is being studied prospectively in the current North American Intergroup phase III trial in N2 disease.

Unresectable N2 Disease (Stage IIIA₄)

In general, patients with lymph nodes larger than 2 cm in short-axis diameter measured by CT, who have extranodal involvement, multistation disease along with groups of multiple involved smaller lymph nodes, are considered to have bulky, unresectable disease. These patients are referred for protocols involving chemoradiation if they are functionally fit to tolerate the therapy.

Stage IIIB Disease

Stage IIIB disease includes patients with T4 or N3 lesions. In the majority of cases, this is an unresectable situation, and patients are referred for chemotherapy with or without radiotherapy.

T4 Tumors

Tumor extension into major structures that usually preclude resection, including trachea, carina, superior vena cava, aorta, intrapericardial pulmonary artery, esophagus, or vertebral bodies, is classified as T4. Malignant pleural effusion and the presentation of multiple nodules (satellitosis) of lung cancer within one lobe are also classified as T4. Unlike lesions with tracheal involvement or malignant effusions, however, "T4" lesions are considered resectable by most clinicians based on satellite lesions if the disease is otherwise confined to the lobe or lung in question and would not change the planned operation.

Carinal Resection. The operative mortality at selected centers that perform carinal resection ranges from 4%–30%, with an average of approximately 18%.[512,539-543] Five-year survivals average 26% and are usually reserved for patients who have no lymph node involvement. The operation entails pneumonectomy with tracheal sleeve resection and direct anastomosis of the trachea to the contralateral main stem bronchus. The most common complications are ARDS and bronchial dehiscence, and the use of radiotherapy is reserved for postoperative patients with involved margins. There is concern regarding the use of radiotherapy preoperatively in these patients due to a higher rate of bronchial dehiscences and airway complications.

Superior Vena Cava. The superior vena cava (SVC) is occasionally involved by primary tumor extension, either focally or over its length. Partial resection with patching of gortex or pericardium has been performed and has resulted in long-term survival. More extensive replacement with ribbed gortex grafts or resection with bypass from the innominate artery to the atrium are associated with 5-year survivals as high as 30% in the absence of involved mediastinal nodes.[544-549] Preoperative distinction of SVC invasion by the tumor itself (T4) or by level 4 lymph nodes can be difficult, and this is an important classifier because long-term survival is not seen with N2-associated SVC resection.

Invasion of Myocardium, Aorta, and Esophagus. Surgical resection resulting in complete excision of the primary tumor is usually not possible when mediastinal organ invasion is present. Limited invasion of the atrial wall can occasionally be completely resected with the hope of an occasional cure, but en bloc resection of the lung with part of the involved aorta or esophagus is rarely associated with long-term survival.[510,511,550-554] Completeness of resection and nodal status are weak predictors of prognosis in this situation.

Vertebral Body. Selected centers, using a combined thoracic surgical, neurosurgical, or orthopedic approach, have performed multiple resections of involved vertebrae either totally or on portions of the vertebral body.[555-558] These resections are not performed en bloc and require internal stabilization of the spinal column.[557] The best results have been reported for extended resections of superior sulcus tumors.[557]

Malignant Pleural Effusion. When pleural effusions are associated with patients with documented lung cancer, aggressive attempts should be made to document malignant cells. If thoracentesis is unrevealing in an otherwise resectable individual with a pleural effusion and lung cancer, thoracoscopy should be performed.[559] Conversely, approximately 10% of patients who undergo a resection for lung cancer will be found to have malignant cells in a pleural lavage performed at the time of the thoracotomy, and the positivity has been correlated with the T status of the patient and nonsquamous histology. A positive pleural cytology on lavage is associated with a poorer prognosis.[560-569] These findings could redefine future strategies in patients having resection for lung cancer, but at present there are no data to justify surgical resection if a patient has a known cytologically positive pleural effusion.

Satellite Nodules. A satellite nodule is a secondary tumor nodule in the same lobe as the primary cancer having histology identical to that of the primary tumor. The overall 5-year survival of patients having resection for satellite nodules in the same lobe is 54%–70% if there are no lymph nodes involved. For all patients with satellite nodules, the 5-year survival independent of lymph node status is approximately 35%.[570-572] Alternative mechanisms independent of lymphatic spread are postulated for these nodules, and for patients with a preoperative staging workup that reveals no evidence of metastases or mediastinal involvement either by PET or invasive staging, surgery is the preferred treatment despite these patients' tendency to a poorer prognosis.

N3 Disease. Despite a number of papers from Japan advocating radical bilateral lymphadenectomy for lung cancer, there is little enthusiasm for surgical resection of N3 disease that presents as either contralateral mediastinal or supraclavicular involvement.[444,573,574] Poor 2-year survivals of 25% for N3 disease despite an 82% complete resection rate after chemoradiation therapy has generally given surgeons pause in the evaluation of this cohort of patients, even after induction therapy.[533,542] In fact, in the SWOG protocol of N3 chemoradiation therapy and surgery, all patients identified as having N3 contralateral mediastinal disease failed to have long-term survival. Supraclavicular involvement, treated by chemoradiotherapy and resection of the intrathoracic disease, had a 2-year survival of 35%.[534]

Surgical Management of Stage IV Disease

Pulmonary Nodules

It is virtually impossible to tell whether a solitary nodule that appears synchronously in a different lobe as a documented primary lung cancer is a metastasis (M1) or a synchronous lung cancer without molecular classification. Approximately one-third of multiple primary lung cancers are synchronous, and approximately 30% of these are discovered at thoracotomy. The majority are squamous cell carcinomas, and in 50% of the cases of synchronous lung cancers, the histology is the same as the primary lung cancer. The 5-year survival of resected patients with synchronous lung cancers is between 10% and 20%.[575] In any discussion of multiple nodules, either synchronous or metachronous, the issue of whether the nodule is a metastasis is a difficult one unless one is dealing confidently with multicentric bronchoalveolar carcinoma. This is probably why the 5-year survival in series that reportedly resected pulmonary metastases from lung cancer is identical to that of survival of "synchronous" lung cancers (approximately 20%).[576,577]

Brain Metastases. Brain metastases account for more than 25% of all recurrences in patients with lung cancer and are seen in up to 55% of patients at autopsy.[578,579] The brain is the first site of recurrence after resection of lung cancer in approximately 20% of such cases.[580] Risk of brain metastasis is associated with histology (metastases from adenocarcinoma being more frequent than from squamous cell carcinoma) and increasing stage, and the majority of metastases occur within the first year after resection.[580] Approximately 14%–44% of all brain metastases are thought to be resectable.[581] Nearly half of the patients with brain metastases have solitary lesions on CT scan. When such patients are symptomatic, the median survival without therapy is 1 month. Steroids and whole-brain irradiation can offer effective palliation of symptoms but only increase survival to 6 months.[582]

Approximately one-third of patients with both brain metastases and lung cancer present synchronously, and two-thirds present metachronously. The most important prognostic determinants of increased survival after resection of brain metastases in lung cancer are whether a complete resection of the primary tumor can be performed, the absence of systemic metastases, female gender, age younger than 60 years, and supratentorial lesion.[583] When a solitary brain metastasis is resected and these criteria are present, the 5-year survival approaches 20%. There is controversy regarding whether palliative resection of brain metastases is of benefit, with most studies having a 2-year survival of approximately 20% after resection or radiosurgery.[584] It is recognized that excision of a brain metastasis followed by radiotherapy is superior to radiotherapy alone in prolonging survival (9.2 months vs. 3.4 months), in preventing local recurrence, and in providing better quality of life.[585]

Adrenal Metastases. About one-third of patients having autopsy for bronchogenic carcinoma are found to have adrenal metastases, and isolated adrenal metastases occur in 2%–4% of patients with NSCLC.[586-589] Routine use of preoperative upper abdominal CT scanning reveals adrenal masses in about 10% of patients, and these can be further evaluated with MRI or PET scanning.[590] There are very few studies in the literature regarding the efficacy of resection of isolated adrenal metastases in lung cancer, and the 5-year survival of 23% is probably related to stage of the primary tumor, with longer survivals among patients with stage I and II disease.[588,591-594]

PRE- AND POSTOPERATIVE THERAPY FOR STAGES I, II, AND IIIA DISEASE

Surgery remains the standard of care and the best therapy that has a potential for cure in patients with early-stage non–small cell lung cancer (NSCLC). Unfortunately, only about one-third of patients present with potentially resectable disease. Prognosis in closely linked to pathologic stage, which is definitively established at the time of surgery.[82] It is therefore of utmost importance that thorough intraoperative staging is done with lymph node sampling and/or dissection as noted in the section on staging. Prognostic determinants include tumor size, lymph node involvement (number of nodes, site of involvement, extracapsular extension), and histology.[240,595]

Because surgery is an imperfect therapy for localized NSCLC, there have been a number of clinical trials using postoperative radiation therapy and/or adjuvant chemotherapy in an attempt to reduce both local and distant recurrences and thereby improve patient survival.

Postoperative Radiation Therapy

Many of the randomized trials that assessed postoperative radiotherapy used both radiotherapy that was inferior to current techniques and unsophisticated staging procedures that were far less accurate than those currently available. Two studies randomized node-negative patients to receive postoperative radiotherapy vs. observation.[596,597] Both studies demonstrated inferior survival for the irradiated group. An additional trial by Dautzenberg and colleagues[598] yielded similar results. A few trials have assessed postoperative irradiation in patients with N1 disease. Unfortunately, these patients are often grouped together with other patients who have different stages of disease, making data interpretation difficult. In a Lung Cancer Study Group trial (LCSG 773), patients with stages II and III squamous cell carcinoma were randomly assigned to receive radiotherapy or no further treatment.[599] Seventy-five percent of the patients had N1 disease. The treatment was biologically active with virtually no local recurrences in the treated group, but there was no impact on survival. A meta-analysis from the Medical Research Council (MRC) Lung Cancer Working Party examined the results from nine randomized trials comparing surgery alone with surgery plus postoperative radiation therapy.[600] For patients with all disease stages, there was a survival rate decrement of 7% that was most pronounced in early-stage (N1) patients.

A number of trials have examined postoperative therapy in patients with N2 disease. In LCSG 773, a subgroup analysis of the N2 patients indicated that there was a reduction in the overall recurrence rate for those with N2 tumors, but this did not translate into improved overall survival.[599] In the trials documented by Dautzenberg and colleagues,[598] there was also no improvement in survival for the treated patients, and there was actually an increase in the rate of non–cancer-related deaths in those randomized to postoperative radiotherapy. Conflicting results were seen in a randomized trial by the MRC.[601] There was a trend toward lower local recurrence and improved survival in N2 patients treated with postoperative radiotherapy. The MRC meta-analysis suggested neither survival decrement nor improvement for the administration of postoperative radiation therapy in the N2 setting.[601]

In summary, there is currently no evidence to support postoperative radiation therapy in stage I and II NSCLC patients, who have been resected completely. In patients with completely resected N2 disease, the evidence is more controversial. The use of postoperative radiotherapy in this setting must take into consideration the risks vs. benefits for the individual patient. Additional studies are needed to focus on prognostic factors that could identify the patients who are at risk for local recurrence and who might ultimately benefit from postoperative radiotherapy. Our current practice is to offer postoperative radiation when the resection is incomplete, when there is extracapsular extension, or when margins are close.

Adjuvant Trials

The need for adjuvant chemotherapy after surgical resection was recognized early in lung cancer treatment. During the 1960s and 1970s, a number of studies on this subject appeared, primarily using alkylating agents as adjuvant chemotherapy. The University Surgical Adjuvant Lung Project Cooperative Group and the Veterans Administration Surgical Adjuvant Group both examined

intrapleural and intravenous nitrogen mustard in the perioperative period.[602,603] The Veterans group also studied cyclophosphamide, cyclophosphamide alternating with methotrexate, and combination therapy with CCNU (lomustine) and hydroxyurea. In all these trials, there was no difference in disease-free or overall survival for the treated patients. Long-term follow-up data were published on a study that randomized more than 700 patients to receive either oral chemotherapy with busulfan or cyclophosphamide, or placebo.[604] After 15 years, there was no survival advantage for the treated patients. Adjuvant immunotherapy employing intrapleural BCG (bacillus Calmette-Guerin) postoperatively was effective in a single-institution trial but was not confirmed in the LCSG trial (LCSG771) (Table 75-15).[604-615] Other biologic and immunologic agents have been tested, with no positive results.

Many of the early adjuvant trials not only used inactive agents but also were fraught with trial design problems, particularly with regard to adequate surgical staging. In the late 1970s, the Lung Cancer Study Group (LSCG) was formed to confirm the intriguing results with intrapleural BCG. Patients who were enrolled on LSCG adjuvant trials underwent rigorous mediastinal node sampling at surgery, which allowed for proper stratification and survival analyses. The first adjuvant trial, LCSG 772, randomized patients with completely resected, stage II and III, nonsquamous NSCLC to eitherreceive CAP (cyclophosphamide, doxorubicin, cisplatin) chemotherapy for 6 months or intrapleural BCG and oral levamisole for 18 months (see Table 75-1).[606] The disease-free survival was significantly better for the patients treated with chemotherapy. Median survival and 2-year survivals were also improved, although the difference was not statistically significant. In the next trial, LCSG 791, patients with incompletely resected tumors (including highest sampled node as positive) were randomized between CAP plus radiation and radiation alone.[607] Again, the median survival was 7 months longer for the chemotherapy patients, but the survival curves converged at 2.5 years. In the third adjuvant trial, LCSG 801, completely resected patients received four courses of CAP chemotherapy or no additional treatment.[608] Difficulty was encountered in delivering all of the courses of chemotherapy. There was no improvement in median or long-term survival for the treated patients. A study from Finland randomized resected patients to six courses of CAP or no additional treatment.[609] Both disease-free survival and long-term survival (10-year survival, 61% vs. 48%, respectively) favored the treatment group. It should be noted that there were imbalances among the patient characteristics —for example, more patients on the observation arm required a pneumonectomy, an indication of more advanced disease. When the statistics were adjusted, the survival differences were no longer significant.

The results of a large Intergroup trial (Int 0115, ECOG 3590) were published recently by Keller and coworkers.[612] Patients with completely resected stages II and IIIA disease were randomized to receive cisplatin/etoposide for four cycles plus concurrent radiotherapy (50.4 Gy over 6 weeks), or radiotherapy alone. Patients

Specific Malignancies

III

TABLE 75-15

Adjuvant Chemotherapy Trials in NSCLC

TRIAL	NO. OF PATIENTS	TREATMENT	SURVIVAL MEDIAN (MO)	LONG-TERM
LCSG 772[606]	62	CAP	23.5	40%, 2 yr
	68	BCG, levamisole	16	30%, 2 yr
LCSG 791[607]	78	CAP + RT	20	40%, 2 yr
	86	RT	13	32%, 2 yr
LCSG 801[608]	136	CAP	76	73%, 2 yr; 56%, 5 yr
	133	—	76	80%, 2 yr; 52%, 5 yr
Niiranen[609]	54	CAP	—	67%, 5 yr; 61%, 10 yr
	56	—	—	56%, 5 yr; 48%, 10 yr
MSKCC[610]	36	VP + RT	16	31%, 2 yr; 17%, 5 yr
	36	RT	19	44%, 2 yr; 30%, 5 yr
Ohta[611]	90	VP	31	35%, 5 yr
	91	—	37	41%, 5 yr
E 3590[612]	246	EP + RT	38	50%, 3 yr; 33%, 5 yr
	242	RT	39	52%, 3 yr; 39%, 5 yr
Imaizumi[614]	155	CAUFT	—	62%, 5 yr
	154	—	—	58%, 5 yr
Wada[615]	109	CVUFT	—	61%, 5 yr
	103	UFT	—	64%, 5 yr
	98	—	—	49%, 5 yr

CAP, cyclophosphamide, doxorubicin, cisplatin; CAUFT, cyclophosphamide, doxorubicin, uracil + tegafur; CVUFT, cyclophosphamide, vindesine, uracil + tegafur; EP, etoposide, cisplatin; RT, radiotherapy; VP, vindesine, cisplatin.

were stratified by weight loss, histology, stage, and lymph node sampling vs. dissection. Toxicity rates were higher for the combined modality treatment, especially with regard to neutropenia and esophagitis, but there was no corresponding increase in toxic deaths. Only two-thirds of the patients on the chemoradiotherapy arm were able to complete their treatment. There was no difference found in disease-free, median, or long-term survivals between the study arms.

There have been a number of interesting Japanese studies using tegafur plus (UFT) or minus (FT) uracil.[613-615] FT is an oral 5-fluorouracil derivative, and the addition of uracil increases the tissue half-life of 5-fluorouracil. In the first trial, completely resected patients were randomized to receive mitomycin, cyclophosphamide, and UFT or surgery alone.[613] No difference in survival was seen in this study. The next randomized trial used postoperative cisplatin, doxorubicin, and UFT in patients with resected stages I, II, and IIIA.[614] The chemotherapy was well tolerated, and the majority of the treatment was delivered. Initial study analysis did not reveal a survival advantage for the chemotherapy, but an imbalance was discovered, with more patients having advanced disease assigned to the treatment arm. On re-analysis, there was a significant difference in overall and disease-free survival rates favoring the adjuvant chemotherapy. A third trial randomized patients to receive cisplatin, vindesine, and UFT, UFT alone, or no adjuvant treatment.[615] Once again there was good treatment tolerance and a significant increase in survival for the UFT group. The results of the UFT adjuvant studies are intriguing, and there has been interest in pursuing additional trials in North America.

Current and Ongoing Adjuvant Trials

The adjuvant trials to date have had mixed results, thus making it difficult to determine the advantage of chemotherapy in the postoperative setting. A large meta-analysis published in the British Medical Journal evaluated the impact of chemotherapy on survival in various stages of NSCLC.[616] Data were retrieved from 14 adjuvant trials. The use of alkylating agents for adjuvant chemotherapy was detrimental; however, the absolute benefit from cisplatin-based chemotherapy was 3% at 2 years and 5% at 5 years. This might appear to be a trivial improvement, but differences as small as these have resulted in a change in practice patterns for other disease sites.

Many adjuvant studies that have recently been completed or are ongoing still employ cisplatin-based chemotherapy. The results of the Adjuvant Lung Project Italy (ALPI) were presented at ASCO in 2002.[617] Twelve hundred patients with stages I, II, and IIIA NSCLC were randomized postoperatively to receive either MVP (mitomycin, vindesine, cisplatin) or no treatment. There was no statistically significant difference in overall or event-free survival between the study arms. In a subset of patients, the significance of p53, KI67 and K-ras were evaluated, but none of these variables were prognostic for survival. In the Big Lung Trial (BLT), patients with various stages of NSCLC were randomized to receive or not receive cisplatin-based chemotherapy in addition to their primary therapy (surgery, radiotherapy, best supportive care).[618] Preliminary results of the patients who received adjuvant chemotherapy after surgery were reported at ASCO 2003. There was no evidence for a survival benefit in the chemotherapy group. The National Cancer Institute of Canada (NCIC) completed an adjuvant study, JBR10, with the participation of several U.S. cooperative groups. Patients with stages IB and II disease were randomized to receive cisplatin/vinorelbine or surgery alone. Tissue was collected to assess prognostic markers; results from this trial should be reported in the near future. The Cancer and Leukemia Group B (CALGB) is currently conducting a trial in resected stage IB patients, in which carboplatin/paclitaxel is being used as adjuvant chemotherapy. The International Adjuvant Lung Cancer Trial (IALT) is the largest adjuvant trial ever conducted. This trial was designed to assess the impact of three to four cycles of cisplatin-based chemotherapy on postoperative patients with stages I, II, and IIIA NSCLC.[619] The results of this trial were presented in abstract form at the Plenary Session of ASCO 2003, and a 4.5% overall survival benefit was reported for postoperative chemotherapy.

The lack of benefit in many trials for standard chemotherapy in postoperative patients has spurred the study of novel agents in this setting. A Japanese group randomized 400 patients with resected stage I squamous cell carcinoma to ubenimex vs. placebo.[620] Ubenimex (Bestatin) is an aminopeptidase inhibitor. There was a significant improvement in 5-year survival (81.5% vs. 74%) for the treated group. The NCIC, in conjunction with several cooperative groups from the United States, has just initiated an adjuvant trial using the epidermal growth factor inhibitor, ZD1839 (gefitinib) in patients with stages IB, II, and IIIA NSCLC.

Preoperative Chemotherapy in Early-stage NSCLC

There is still a significant recurrence of disease in early-stage NSCLC patients after curative surgical resection. As discussed previously, the results of trials that deliver chemotherapy in the adjuvant setting after surgery have been disappointing and have not consistently resulted in improved survival. There have been several randomized trials comparing primary surgery with induction chemotherapy followed by surgery in patients with stage IIIA NSCLC.[86-88] In some of these trials, there was a significant improvement in survival for patients who received induction chemotherapy before surgery. Because of these results, interest has arisen in designing studies to evaluate the role of induction therapy before surgery in earlier-stage lung cancer patients. There could be some advantages to preoperative (as opposed to postoperative) delivery of chemotherapy, including tumor downstaging and early control of micrometastases, but definitive confirmation in animal models is lacking, and the only true test of the hypothesis in human cancer—the pre- vs. postoperative use of cyclophosphamide and doxorubicin in resected breast cancer—showed no difference in outcomes between the two study arms.[621] Patients might, however, be more tolerant of and compliant with chemotherapy in the preoperative setting compared with postoperative chemotherapy, in which treatment delivery poses a problem.

Depierre et al[86] reported the results of a trial that randomized patients with stages IB, II, and IIIA disease to receive induction chemotherapy with mitomycin, ifosfamide, and cisplatin before surgery or surgery alone. More than 300 patients were enrolled in the study, and 188 of these had stage I or II disease. The pathologic complete response rate was 11%. There was a nonsignificant improvement in median survival of 11 months for patients at all stages who received preoperative chemotherapy. On further analysis, the survival benefit was primarily for patients with stages I and II disease. Postoperative morbidity was increased in the combined-modality treatment arm (6.7% vs. 4.5% for patients receiving surgery alone). There was a significant decrease in distant metastases and an increase in the length of disease-free survival for the patients treated with chemotherapy.

The BLOT (Bimodality Lung Oncology Team) trial was a multi-institutional phase II study that employed the commonly used drug combination, carboplatin and paclitaxel, as preoperative treatment in early-stage lung cancer patients.[622,623] Ninety-four patients with stages T2N0, T1-2N1, and T3N0-1 NSCLC received two cycles of preoperative chemotherapy followed by three cycles postoperatively in patients who had a complete resection. The response rate for the induction chemotherapy was 56%. Ninety-four percent of the patients underwent resection, and 86% had a complete resection. The pathologic complete response rate was only 6%, and 5-year survival was 46%. The preoperative delivery of chemotherapy was feasible and did not increase postoperative complications. Only 45% of the patients were able to receive the postoperative treatment, and this experience was comparable to that of other surgical adjuvant trials. Based on these study results, there is a current phase III North American Intergroup trial comparing surgery alone with induction chemotherapy (carboplatin and paclitaxel) followed by surgery. The patient eligibility criteria are similar to the BLOT trial, but the patients randomized to chemotherapy will receive three treatment cycles only as induction therapy before surgery. In addition to this study, there are several planned or ongoing trials with a similar design that will attempt to answer the same questions.

Induction Chemotherapy and/or Radiotherapy in Stage IIIA Disease

As mentioned in the previous section, the interest in giving preoperative chemotherapy to earlier-stage NSCLC patients arose from prospective randomized trials that compared primary surgery with induction chemotherapy and surgery in stage IIIA NSCLC.[87,88] Initial induction trials utilized radiotherapy before surgery. These studies were done before more sophisticated staging techniques became available, and patients with both early and later disease stages were included in the patient mix. The LSCG conducted a study in which pathologically staged IIIA(N2) patients received 44 Gy preoperatively.[623] The results were disappointing, with only two pathologic complete responses and a median survival of 12 months. Currently, it is not felt that induction therapy with radiation alone is appropriate.

TABLE 75-16

Selected Phase II Trials of Induction Chemotherapy for Stage IIIA NSCLC

					SURVIVAL	
TRIAL	**NO. OF PATIENTS**	**CHEMO**	**RR (%)**	**CRR (%)**	**MEDIAN (MO)**	**LONG-TERM**
MSKCC[624,625]	136	MVP	78	65	19	17%, 5 yr
Toronto[627]	55	MVP	71	51	21	34%, 5 yr
LCSG 881[632]	28	MVP	46	68	12	—
CALGB 8935[628]	74	VP	64*	62	15	23%, 3 yr
Dana Farber[629]	34	PFL	65	62	18	—

CRR, complete resection rate; F, 5-fluorouracil (continuous infusion); L, leucovorin ; M, mitomycin; P, cisplatin; RR, response rate; V, vinblastine.
*Includes stable disease.

The next series of trials conducted during the 1980s primarily consisted of a number of phase II trials, usually using cisplatin-based chemotherapy with or without radiotherapy as induction treatment before surgery. The results of a selected number of trials using preoperative chemotherapy are listed in Table 75-16.[625-629] Three of these studies employed MVP (mitomycin, vinblastine, cisplatin) chemotherapy.[624-627] The majority of these trials treated patients with bulky N2 disease, and all of the studies required pathologic documentation of the disease stage. The response rate to chemotherapy varied from 46% to 78% and complete resection was achieved in were 51%–68% of patients. Postoperative or intraoperative radiotherapy was given in all of the studies except for LCSG 881.[623] Pathologic complete response rates of 0%, 5%, and 11% were reported in the CALGB, Toronto, and Memorial Sloan-Kettering studies, respectively.[624-627] The postoperative mortality rates were variable, with the highest rate (17%) found in the LSCG trial. The mortality rates for the other trials ranged from 0%–8%, although it was often not clear whether presurgical mortality from chemotherapy was included in the results of these primarily surgical trials. The median survivals were also variable, ranging from 12 months to 21 months. The local regional recurrence rate was about 25%; in the Memorial Sloan-Kettering trial at least, recurrence affected primarily those patients who did not have a complete resection. Although postoperative radiotherapy was given in a number of these trials, its delivery was variable.

A number of trials using chemoradiation as induction therapy are listed in Table 75-17.[542,628-635] The eligibility criteria for these trials were more varied and did not always require documentation of N2 disease. They could include patients with T3N0 and/or T3N1 disease as in the Rush, Tufts, and CALGB studies.[631,633-635] SWOG 8805[542,630] required pathologic proof of N2, N3, and T4 disease. Stage IIIB patients were included in all of the trials except the CALGB study. The response to treatment was somewhat higher than with surgery alone (56%–92%, including stable disease in some studies), as would be expected with the inclusion of radiotherapy as part of the induction therapy. This was also true of the pathologic complete response rates, which were 16%, 21%, and 27% in the LCSG, SWOG, and Rush studies.[632] It is interesting to note that in the SWOG study, 46% of the patients with stable disease after induction treatment had pathologic complete responses or rare microscopic tumor foci, indicating that clinical assessment by computed tomography can be misleading. The operative mortality rates in these trials were not increased by the addition of radiotherapy to the induction regimen and varied from 4% to 15%. The trials that excluded the favorable disease

TABLE 75-17

Randomized Trials of Induction Chemoradiotherapy for Stage IIIA NSCLC

						SURVIVAL	
TRIAL	**NO. OF PATIENTS**	**CHEMO**	**RT (Gy)**	**RR (%)**	**CRR (%)**	**MEDIAN (MO)**	**LONG-TERM**
SWOG 8805[629,630]	126	EP	45	59	71	15	20%, N2, 6 yr 22%, IIIB, 6 yr
Rush-Presbyterian[631]	85	PF ± E	40 (split)	92*	71	22	31%, 3 yr
LCSG 852[632]	85	PF	30	56	52	13	—
CALGB[633,634]	41	PVF	30	64*	61	16	22%, 7 yr
Tufts[635]	55	EP	59	69*	76	20	73%, N2, 3 yr 32%, IIIB, 3 yr

CRR, complete resection rate; E, etoposide; F, 5-fluorouracil; P, cisplatin; RR, response rate; RT, radiotherapy; V, vinblastine.
*Includes stable disease.

categories of T3N0 or T3N1 had the lowest median survivals (13 and 15 months). In the SWOG study, the incidence of local relapse at 11% was lower than in the chemotherapy-only induction studies, possibly as a result of the use of radiotherapy as part of the induction regimen.[630] A significant number of relapses in the brain were again reported.

The SWOG study was unique in that it included a large proportion (40%) of patients in the T4 and N3 categories. The median 2- and 3-year survivals were virtually identical for the IIIA(N2) and IIIB patients. In a long-term follow-up, the 6-year survival for the T4N0-1 subgroups was 49%, while the patients with N2 or N3 disease had an 18% 6-year survival. SWOG subsequently conducted another trial (9019) in patients with stage IIIB disease.[636] Patients were given the same induction therapy as in SWOG 8805, but instead of surgery, they received additional radiotherapy to 61 Gy and two additional cycles of chemotherapy. The overall survival for the stage IIIB patients in this study was consistent with the results for the same patients on SWOG 8805. For the T4N0-1 subgroup, the 2-year survival was 33% in study 9019 compared with 64% in study 8805. This historical comparison suggests that surgery might be beneficial for this particular subgroup of patients.

Some of the induction trials listed in Tables 75-16 and 75-17 assessed a number of potential predictors of overall survival. Methods of analyses and factors analyzed were not consistent across all the trials. Response to induction treatment was not a significant predictor of outcome, possibly because of the lack of correlation between CT restaging and the pathologic findings at resection. Some of the predictors of better outcome included lack of N2 or N3 disease, complete resection, pathologic complete response after induction therapy, and the clearance of N2 or N3 disease. Nodal downstaging was the only significant factor in the multivariate analysis of SWOG 8805. The 3-year survival of patients who had pathologic

clearance of their mediastinal nodes was 41%, compared with 3-year survival of only 11% for patients with persistent disease. These results could have major implications with regard to selecting candidates for surgery after induction therapy.

Randomized Trials of Surgery with or without Induction Therapy

There have been several randomized trials involving induction therapy; these are listed in Table 75-18.[86-88,622,637-639] These trials suffer from small numbers of patients and major imbalances in important prognostic variables. All the trials use cisplatin-based induction chemotherapy, but the radiotherapy is given at a variety of time points, including as induction therapy before surgery in the CALGB study.[639]

The NCI study reported by Pass and colleagues[637] was stopped because of slow accrual. The patients on this study had more advanced N2 disease, and the investigators found no statistical difference between the treatment arms. The Japanese trial also included patients with bulky mediastinal disease, and again there was no advantage demonstrated for induction therapy.[638]

The studies by Rosell and coworkers[87] and Roth and associates[88] were closed early because of major survival differences at the interim analyses. In both studies, mediastinal lymph node biopsy was not required if clinical staging of the mediastinum was negative. In the Roth and associates[88] trial, 40% of the patients on the surgery-alone treatment arm had stage IIIB or IV disease after surgery, compared with 11% of the patients on the induction chemotherapy arm, possibly accounting for the inferior survival for patients receiving surgery alone. On the Rosell and coworkers[87] trial, the patients were better balanced for clinical prognostic factors; however, on the surgery-alone arm, more patients had mutations of the K-*ras* gene and aneuploid tumors compared with patients on the

TABLE 75-18

Randomized Trials of Surgery with or without Induction Therapy

AUTHOR	NO. OF PATIENTS	TREATMENT	SURVIVAL MEDIAN	SURVIVAL LONG-TERM
Pass[637]	13	EP/Surg	28.7	42%, 3 yr
	14	Surg/RT	15.6	18%, 3 yr
Rosell[87]	30	MIP/Surg/RT	26	30%, 3 yr
	30	Surg/RT	8	0
Roth[88]	28	CEP/Surg	64	56%, 3 yr
	32	Surg	11	15%, 3 yr
Depierre[86]	179	MIP/Surg/± MIP, RT	37	43.9%, 4 yr
	176	Surg/± RT	26	35.3%, 4 yr
Yoneda[638]	83 (total)	VdP + RT/Surg	—	37%, 2 yr
		Surg	—	40%, 2 yr
Elias[639]	23	EP/Surg/EP/RT	19	—
	24	RT/Surg/RT	23	—

E, etoposide; I, ifosfamide; M, mitomycin; P, cisplatin; RT, radiotherapy; Vd, vindesine.
Data is for all patients stages I, II, IIIA.

induction arm. Because both of these factors have been associated with a poorer prognosis in NSCLC, they conceivably could have affected the survival outcome on the surgery-alone arm.

A small CALGB study reported by Elias and colleagues[639] assessed the role of induction chemotherapy or radiotherapy followed by surgery in patients with N2 disease. Postoperative therapy was also given—chemotherapy and radiation on the induction chemotherapy arm and additional radiotherapy on the other study arm. Median survival was lower on the induction chemotherapy arm, but the study was small, and the results were not statistically significant.

The French trial by Depierre and coworkers[86] was described earlier in the section on preoperative chemotherapy for early-stage NSCLC. Patients with N0 and N1 disease were included on the study. One hundred sixty-seven N2 patients were included in the trial. The overall survival favored the chemotherapy study arm, but the results were not statistically significant. In a subset analysis, the benefit of induction chemotherapy was significant for the patients with N0-1 disease but not for the patients with N2 disease. The authors suggested that this could be due to the inclusion of patients with bulky N2 disease.

Despite the deficiencies of these randomized trials, there is a suggestion that induction treatment might be beneficial. Future trials should be designed with better patient selection and incorporate more sophisticated imaging techniques for staging.

Superior Sulcus Tumors

Superior sulcus tumors are a unique subset of NSCLC. These are challenging tumors to treat because they routinely involve the brachial plexus, vertebrae, and subclavian vasculature. The historical approach to treatment was usually surgical resection followed by radiation until it was discovered that preoperative radiation facilitated resection of these tumors.[506] Radiotherapy consisted of 30–40 Gy followed 4 weeks later by surgery. Five-year survival ranged from 15% to 50%. A review of the experience with 225 patients at Memorial Sloan-Kettering is the largest series published to date.[630] Survival was most closely related to the T and N stages. Complete resection was possible in 64% of patients with T3N0 staging and in 39% of patients with T4N0 staging, and locoregional relapse was the most common site of recurrence.

Induction chemoradiotherapy before surgery proved to be feasible in a number of trials in locally advanced NSCLC. Rusch and associates[508,641] reported the results of Intergroup Trial 0160 (SWOG 9416), which tested the use of induction chemoradiotherapy and surgery in the treatment of superior sulcus tumors. Patients with pathologically staged T3-4N0 disease received concurrent cisplatin, etoposide, and radiation (45 Gy) followed by surgery and additional chemotherapy postoperatively. One hundred eleven patients were entered in the study, and 92% completed induction treatment. Eighty-eight of 95 eligible patients underwent thoracotomy, and 92% had a complete resection. The postoperative mortality was 2.4%. The pathologic response was high, with 66% of the

patients having a pathologic complete response or minimal residual disease. Median and 5-year overall survivals were 33 months, 41% for all patients and 71 months, 53% after complete resection. The resectability rate and survival, even for patients with T4 tumors, was improved compared with historical controls. A new intergroup trial is being planned that will include docetaxel consolidation therapy postoperatively.

CURRENT TREATMENT TRENDS

From the data available thus far, it appears that induction chemotherapy with or without radiation followed by surgery is a feasible approach to the treatment of patients with locally advanced NSCLC. There are many questions that need to be answered, however, and many of the current trials are attempting to tackle some of the more controversial issues.

Surgery can be done with acceptable postoperative mortality in patients who have received induction therapy. The question that needs to be answered pertains to patient selection for this mode of therapy. It is suggested that certain patient subgroups (i.e., T3-4, N0-1, minimal N2) benefit from this approach, but it is unclear whether it is appropriate treatment for all patients with stage III disease. There are two intergroup trials that are attempting to address the role of surgery in patients with N2 disease. The North American Intergroup Trial 0139, developed by SWOG, compares trimodality therapy (induction treatment as in SWOG 8805) to chemoradiotherapy alone.[642] This trial was presented at ASCO 2003 and demonstrated a clear time-to-progression benefit for the surgical arm but no clear improvement in overall survival in the initial analysis. The second study is an EORTC Intergroup trial that randomizes patients to either radiotherapy or surgery after three cycles of a cisplatin-containing regimen as induction treatment.

A number of new drugs have come into the treatment of NSCLC in the last decade (Table 75-19). These newer agents are being incorporated into induction regimens in phase II trials to assess efficacy and safety. Toxicity data are of particular importance if these drugs are combined with radiotherapy because a number of them are potent radiosensitizers. A Swiss group recently published an example of a study employing a newer induction regimen.[643] A multicenter phase II study investigated neoadjuvant docetaxel-cispatin before surgery in N2 NSCLC patients. Ninety patients were on the trial, and 66% responded to chemotherapy. Nineteen percent of the patients who were resected had a pathologic complete response. Downstaging to N0-1 was good prognostically and resulted in prolonged event-free and overall survival. The median survival for the entire group was 27.6 months and 33 months for the resected patients. It is anticipated that more data will be emerging regarding the use of these newer chemotherapy agents. It is likely that future studies also will incorporate the use of the new molecularly-targeted agents.

Another focus of investigation has been the use of various radiotherapy techniques. A West German group

TABLE 75-19

Chemotherapy Agents for the Treatment of Non–small Cell Lung Cancer

BEFORE 1990	AFTER 1990
Platinums	Vinorelbine
Cisplatin	Taxanes
Carboplatin	Docetaxel
Cyclophosphamide	Paclitaxel
Epipodophyllotoxins	Gemcitabine
Etoposide	Camptothecans
Teniposide	Irinotecan
5-Fluorouracil	Topotecan
Methotrexate	
Mitomycin C	
Doxorubicin	
Ifosfamide	
Vinca alkaloids	
Vinblastine	
Vindesine	

has been employing hyperfractionated radiotherapy as part of their induction schema.[644] In a phase II trial in patients with bulky locally advanced disease, chemotherapy (etoposide and cisplatin) and twice-daily radiation were administered before surgery. Sixty percent of patients with stage IIIA disease and 45% of patients with stage IIIB disease were resected. The pathologic complete response rate was 26%, and postoperative mortality (7%) was not increased compared with other trials. The somewhat low 5-year survivals (32% IIIA, 26% IIIB) were probably reflective of the patient selection for this trial. There is currently an ongoing study in Germany that is designed to test whether hyperfractionated radiation as part of the induction is better than induction chemotherapy alone.

It is important to note that the brain is a frequent site of treatment failure in many of the patients on these trials. In the West German trial just described, prophylactic cranial radiation (PCI) was mandated during the later half of the study because of the high incidence of brain relapse.[645] PCI significantly reduced brain recurrences and prolonged survival for those patients who had responded to treatment. A Radiation Therapy Oncology Group (RTOG) study is currently ongoing and is designed to assess the utility of PCI in patients who undergo aggressive, potentially curative treatment for locally advanced NSCLC. It should be noted, however, that an earlier LCSG analysis showed that in only 3% of resected patients with lung cancer would disease be expected to recur both initially and exclusively in the brain.[580]

Radiation and Chemotherapy for Patients with Locally Advanced Non–Small Cell Lung Cancer

Introduction

Locally advanced non–small cell lung cancer refers to a heterogeneous group of patients with disease that is either technically unresectable or in whom the likelihood of cure with surgery is felt to be so low as to not warrant the risks of surgery. Distant metastases cannot be detected, although they are suspected to be present in the majority of these patients. Whereas some 20 years ago these patients were typically treated with single-modality therapy (usually radiation and often to only modest palliative doses), recent clinical investigations clearly have shown that combined chemotherapy and radiation therapy is superior to either single modality and that a proportion of these patients might be cured with nonsurgical therapy. Current research strategies focus on developing better ways to image the radiation target and deliver dose to what is typically highly irregular and moving volume, developing drugs that more selectively and actively target tumor cells while sparing normal tissue, and rationally sequencing these two modalities to achieve the greatest therapeutic gains.

Although the past several decades have seen modest improvements in treatment outcomes for patients with locally advanced disease (largely though the demonstration of improved survival by combining systemic chemotherapy with thoracic radiation), overall survival for patients with unresectable disease (primarily stages IIIA and IIIB) remains at only about 10% at 5 years. There is increasing realization that not only does systemic adjuvant therapy for patients with apparently localized disease need to be emphasized but also that local control is a prerequisite for long-term survival, and that local control has often not been attained with conventional radiation therapy. Several recent trials and meta-analyses have convincingly demonstrated the value of thoracic irradiation in increasing long-term survival in patients with both SCLC and NSCLC.[646,647]

Studies conducted in the 1970s by the RTOG compared various dose schedules and found a modest improvement in 2-year survival by increasing dose from 40 Gy over 4 weeks to 60 Gy over 6 weeks, although long-term survival was not improved.[648] The analysis of these trials reported "failure to observe local progression" as a surrogate for local control. With early death of patients from distant metastatic disease, often before local failure could manifest itself, as well as difficulty in distinguishing between local persistence or recurrence and fibrosis, it is not surprising that local recurrences were in the range of 50%. These results led to a period of overoptimism about the effectiveness of radiation therapy in NSCLC and the erroneous belief that all that was needed for therapeutic improvement was better systemic therapy.

Considering that the ability of radiation therapy to control local disease is a function of local tumor bulk, it is hardly surprising that a dose of 60 Gy, which is appropriate for treating true vocal cord tumors measuring several millimeters, is insufficient for controlling a lung tumor measuring several centimeters, the volume of which could be a thousand-fold greater. The TNM staging system does not explicitly include tumor volume and is thus not well suited for classifying tumors treated nonsurgically. Several recent studies have reported a clear correlation between tumor volume and treatment outcome (in terms of both local control and survival) in patients treated with definitive radiotherapy or chemoradiotherapy.[649-651]

Reassessment with more appropriate actuarial assessment of local control (as distinct from crude absence of local failure) has indicated that long-term local control has been less than 10% in NSCLC.[652,653] Furthermore, several recent trials for patients with unresectable (predominantly stages IIIA and IIIB) NSCLC have shown that, despite the predominantly distant pattern of relapse, more aggressive local treatment that improves local control also can produce statistically significant and clinically meaningful improvements in survival. The EORTC compared split-course radiotherapy as a single modality with radiotherapy and the addition of either daily or weekly cisplatin.[654] The use of this concurrent radiosensitizing chemotherapy had no effect on the rate of development of distant metastases but significantly improved both local control and overall survival. Furuse and colleagues[655] have reported a randomized trial comparing sequential vs. concurrent chemoradiation for patients with stage III NSCLC. The concurrent schedule resulted in better local control and overall survival but no significant differences in systemic relapse. A phase III trial conducted by the RTOG similarly showed improved local control and median survival using concurrent rather than sequential administration or radiation and chemotherapy, although a third arm of the trial using BID radiotherapy with concurrent chemotherapy had the best local control but not the best survival.[656] Saunders and coworkers[657] conducted a prospective trial comparing conventionally fractionated radiotherapy with a continuous accelerated schedule (CHART), which delivered 57.6 Gy in 36 fractions over the course of 2.5 weeks. The accelerated regimen produced significantly improved local control and overall survival (Fig. 75-11).

Although these studies support the concept that improvement in local control for patients with locally advanced NSCLC can lead to statistically significant and clinically worthwhile improvements in survival, not all trials have confirmed this. One of the more striking discrepancies between improvement in local control and survival came in the Lung Cancer Study Group (LCSG) trial of adjuvant postoperative mediastinal radiation therapy for patients with resected stage II and III squamous cell carcinoma of the lung. The addition of postoperative mediastinal irradiation almost eliminated local recurrence as a first event from 20% in the control group to 1% in the treated group but had no significant effect on disease-free or overall survival.[658] In a disease such as lung cancer, in which both distant metastases and intercurrent disease account for a large number of deaths, the correlation between local control and survival can be expected to be less close than in diseases such as malignant gliomas or cancer of the head and neck, in which local events dominate survival. Our search for improvement in the treatment of stage III NSCLC ought not be a competition between local and systemic treatment modalities but rather a search for mutually effective combinations of the two.

Escalation of Radiation Dose, Physical and Biologic

The inadequate local control achieved with doses of 60–65 Gy suggests that dose escalation could be a useful strategy in treating lung cancer. With conventional approaches to treatment planning limited by ability to define target volume and deliver treatment, typical treatment plans for patients with stage IIIA or IIIB NSCLC involved treatment with opposed anterior and posterior beams to doses of 40–45 Gy followed by treatment with opposed oblique or lateral beams for an additional 20–25 Gy and a total dose in the range of 65 Gy. Simply increasing dose by giving additional fractions (and increasing overall treatment time) has several theoretic disadvantages. First, there are major constraints on conventional dose escalation imposed by the tolerance doses of surrounding normal tissues. The situation is particularly difficult in that the typical lung tumor with mediastinal node metastases is in proximity to both parallel and serial normal tissues. Although there are relatively absolute constraints to dose to the spinal cord (a serial organ with critical function), the lung clearly tolerates ablation of portions with relative impunity but shows marked volume dependence of toxicity. The esophagus occupies a more complex position in that acute toxicity (pain, mucositis) appears to be volume-dependent (length and circumference), while late strictures are more related to dose to any given segment; the esophagus thus behaves like a parallel organ for acute toxicity and like a serial organ for late toxicity.[659–661] Particularly if one adopts the philosophy of electively treating the full mediastinum for patients with any N_2 involvement, it rapidly becomes difficult to dose-escalate while protecting normal organs. Secondly, there is increasing evidence that protraction of treatment time, either by breaks or by extending a continuous treatment course, is deleterious to local control.[662] Increases in the proliferative rate of surviving tumor clonogens during a course of fractionated treatment offset gains potentially achieved from increasing the total dose. In this setting,

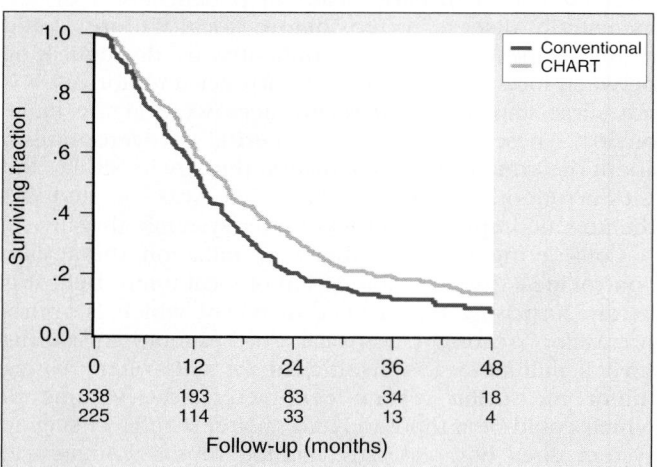

Figure 75-11. Randomized comparison of conventionally fractionated radiation therapy and continuous hyperfractionated accelerated radiation therapy (CHART) in patients with non-small cell lung cancer. (From Saunders M, et al: Continuous hyperfractionated accelerated radiotherapy [CHART] versus conventional radiotherapy in non–small-cell lung cancer: A randomised multicentre trial. Lancet 1997;350:161.)

more benefit would be obtained by shortening the overall treatment time. With conventional planning, such acceleration of treatment is invariably associated with in increase in acute toxicities (particularly mucositis), although late esophageal and other toxicities are not necessarily increased.[657]

In addition to inadequate dose, conventional radiation therapy of NSCLC has frequently failed to cover the target volume adequately. In a retrospective review of patients treated on CALGB protocol 8433, Boxwala and Rosenman[663] found that tumor was either missed or at the field edge in about one-quarter of cases. Even in the absence of dose escalation, adequate coverage of gross disease should result in better local control and survival. Some further improvement in conventionally planned treatment might also come from a better understanding of tumor volume (as seen on CT scan) and of the anatomic extent of microscopic tumor infiltration of surrounding lung tissue. Giraud and coworkers[664] prospectively compared tumor extension as seen on CT and in resection specimens of patients with lung tumors and found that the extent of microscopic infiltration varied by histology and was not necessarily encompassed by 1 cm margins around grossly visible disease.

Three-dimensional conformal radiation therapy (3D-CRT) should be regarded as a tool, or better as a set of tools, which can potentially permit delivery of higher doses of radiation therapy to properly defined target volumes while sparing critical normal tissues. It is not an end in itself. The achievement of elegant isodose curves and dose-volume histograms without demonstration of clinical benefit (improved local control, reduced acute or late normal tissue toxicity, median or landmark survival) might be a stimulating academic activity but does not necessarily constitute clinical progress. Demonstration of the overall validity of the physical techniques and biologic assumptions that underpin the development and current implementation of 3D-CRT awaits the performance and mature analysis of randomized clinical trials that can test these, either in combination or one by one, against the current standards of practice.[665,666]

The potential benefits of three-dimensional treatment planning and delivery are, therefore, improved coverage of the target volume with better protection of normal tissues. In a disease such as lung cancer, in which local control has historically been poor, the first effort will be to explore higher doses and/or accelerated fractionation while maintaining an acceptable level of acute and late complications. In other diseases in which local control is satisfactory with current techniques, the benefits from conformal treatment could come more from a reduction in toxicity.

The current approach to 3D-CRT in NSCLC includes at least three distinct domains, each theoretically separate but often interdependent in their clinical applications. These three domains include target delineation, choice of biologically relevant target, and dose escalation.

Treatment Planning

The process of treatment planning begins with the choice of anatomic position the patient will assume during imaging studies (e.g., CT and PET) used for both target delineation and treatment. The position should be one that minimizes placement of normal tissues in the radiation beams, is reasonably comfortable for the patient, and is accurately reproducible on a day-to-day basis. Particularly for treatment using multiple radiation beams and requiring precise positioning, the use of a variety of immobilization devices is common. For lung, external plastic casts or vacuum-locked bags of styrofoam beads are widely used. There is little uniformity, however, with regard to immobilization techniques, and relatively little research has been done to document their value.[667-672]

After the patient has been positioned and immobilized, radiographic studies (almost always a CT scan) are obtained with the patient in the treatment position. For lung tumors, scans are typically obtained every 4–5 mm through the target volume and every 8–10 mm throughout the remainder of the thorax. The administration of intravenous contrast during the planning CT is helpful in distinguishing mediastinal nodes from vessels, although it modestly perturbs electron density measurements used in tissue inhomogeneity calculations. In addition to the anatomic information from CT, there is burgeoning interest in using functional data from studies such as MRI, PET scanning, or radio-labeled antibody imaging, and technologies have been developed to fuse images obtained from multiple modalities.[673]

After the acquisition of this anatomic dataset, the physician, dosimetrist, or physicist must outline on each CT image the boundaries of tumor and normal organ volumes. Although this process has been partially automated in distinguishing boundaries between structures with greatly differing CT Hounsfield numbers, this is largely limited to normal tissue contouring. The determination of the target volume still requires detailed clinical input, is highly labor intensive, and is subject to substantial interobserver variability, especially in distinguishing peripheral extensions of the tumor from distal atelectasis.

Choice of Target Volume

The choice of target volume has been a contentious issue in lung cancer radiation therapy for many years. The predominant philosophy of the 1970s and 1980s was to treat large volumes encompassing both known primary and nodal disease plus one or more additional nodal echelons. Such elective nodal irradiation (ENI) was thought to be important in controlling tumors that grew in a stepwise Halstedian manner, spreading first to regional lymph nodes and only then to distant sites. Treatment protocols by the RTOG during that time routinely included the supraclavicular nodes and contralateral hilar nodes for patients with N_2 NSCLC. In the early 1980s, a move to reduce ENI began, with elimination of supraclavicular nodal irradiation in a number of clinical trials in both NSCLC and SCLC. Failure in unirradiated nodes was infrequent (only about 5% in these trials), and supraclavicular ENI has been abandoned in recent trials of the North American Cooperative groups.

The recognition that locoregional failure occurs predominantly in areas of known macroscopic disease has lent further impetus to reduce target volumes to facilitate dose escalation. The current philosophy of a number of groups that have been instrumental in implementing 3D-CRT for lung cancer can be summarized as follows:

1. Include all areas of known disease as visualized on imaging studies or ascertained by surgical staging procedures. Although this principle might seem straightforward, distinguishing between tumor and atelectatic lung on planning CT scans is not an easy task or one on which there is much consistency among radiation oncologists.[674]

2. Treat all areas of known disease to the same dose. Although in theory bulkier disease might require higher doses for control, we have not defined doses that are routinely capable of controlling more moderate but macroscopic disease (e.g., 2 cm NSCLC). When local nodal disease is controlled routinely, escalation of dose to the primary tumor only would be reasonable (assuming that the primary is larger than the nodal mass, which is not always the case, especially with small peripheral adenocarcinomas and extensive mediastinal adenopathy).

3. Do not intentionally irradiate other nodal sites, neither next-echelon nodes nor lymphatic pathways connecting the primary tumor with sites of known nodal involvement. In practice, many of these "elective" nodal stations will receive substantial dose even when not explicitly included in the target volume.[675] This exclusion is based on the argument that the inclusion of systemic chemotherapy should be adequate to control both microscopic nodal and systemic disease. If it is not, the patient is likely to die of systemic metastases and would not have benefited clinically from controlling microscopic nodal disease with irradiation.

Although this is a reasonable and internally consistent set of arguments, the true optimal target volume for patients with known involvement of mediastinal nodes remains unknown and has not been well studied in prospective trials. A major issue pertains to adjuvant irradiation of nodes in stations not demonstrably involved. It is increasingly recognized, however, that the use of such large target volumes greatly limits the ability to escalate the dose delivered to known disease.

Schraube and colleagues[676] have reported a series of 20 patients with locally advanced NSCLC whose radiotherapy treatments were planned using both 2D and 3D technology. Target volumes included known primary and nodal disease and electively treated mediastinal nodes. Although 3D planning gave better coverage of the target volume, dose to normal lung and NTCP were not reduced. The authors doubted that significant dose escalation would be possible if large elective volumes were to be treated.

McGibney and coworkers[677,678] investigated the role of 3D planning in considering patients treated with the accelerated CHART regimen. They studied 18 patients with stages IB through IIIB (15 of 18 had stage III) NSCLC and generated plans according to three different approaches.

1. Conventional 2D with inclusion of ENI (as had been used in the original CHART regimen);
2. 2D plans without ENI; and
3. 3D plans without ENI.

They found that coverage of the primary tumor volume (PTV) was suboptimal with either of the 2D approaches and improved only with 3D planning without ENI. The percentage of the PTV receiving greater than 95% of the prescribed dose was 87.38% for conventional 2D and 88.5% for 2D without ENI, compared with 100% for 3D without ENI. The use of 3D planning significantly reduced doses to the spinal cord, heart, and esophagus but did not improve lung sparing. This would suggest that acute tolerance (where esophagitis is often the limiting toxicity, both for accelerated radiotherapy schedules and for concurrent chemoradiation) might be more favorably impacted than long-term ability to dose escalate if late effects are limited by pulmonary toxicity.

The true incidence of microscopic involvement of normal-sized nodes has been evaluated in several recent studies. In general, CT staging using a size cutoff of 1.0 cm for the short axis of lymph nodes is reported to have approximately a 25% false-negative rate. Although involved nodes are, as a group, larger than uninvolved nodes, there is substantial overlap between the groups and substantial false-positive and -negative rates using CT scanning for nodal staging.[679] In a series of 348 patients with clinical N_0 NSCLC undergoing surgical resection, Sawyer and associates[680] were able to define four discrete risk groups for occult nodal involvement based on histologic grade, tumor location, and tumor size. For the lowest-risk group (well differentiated peripheral tumors), the risk was 15.6%, while it rose to as high as 64.8% for patients with central tumors greater than 3 cm in size (see Table 75-3). Giraud and associates[681] have described development of a software program, based on published surgical staging series and recent data on the sensitivity and specificity of CT and PET staging, to calculate the probability of involvement of each of the ATS nodal stations based on radiographic findings and tumor histology. Even for small peripheral tumors such as might be found by spiral CT-based screening programs, only those below 1 cm in size can reliably be considered to be without nodal metastases (Tables 75-20 and 75-21).[682,683]

The clinically important question, however, is not how often nodes are involved but rather how often are they the sole cause of clinical failure. Several retrospective series have reported a very low (<5%) incidence of isolated nodal failure among patients with clinical stage I and II NSCLC treated with radiation to the primary tumor volume only.[684,685] Local failure and distant metastatic disease dominate patterns of failure. Until such time as these are no longer problems, any incremental gains in survival achieved by elective irradiation of microscopically involved regional nodes, either in medically inoperable early-stage or stage III disease, are likely to be minimal. Furthermore, to the extent that chemotherapy is able to eradicate small volumes of systemic disease, as evidenced by the improved long-term and median survivals in several trials of radiation therapy alone or

TABLE 75-20

	Likelihood of Regional Lymph Node or Local Recurrence Involvement in Resected N_0 NSCLC	
RISK GROUP	**CHARACTERISTICS**	**N1/N2 OR LOCAL RECURRENCE (%)**
Low	Bronchoscopy (−) Grade 1/2	15.6
Low/Intermediate	Bronchoscopy (−) Grade 3/4	35.6
High/Intermediate	Bronchoscopy (+) CT size <3 cm	41.7
High	Bronchoscopy (+) CT size >3 cm	68.4

Data from Sawyer T, et al: Tumor and patient characteristics that are predictive of subclinical nodal involvement in patients with non–small cell lung cancer (NSCLC) without nodal enlargement or preoperative chest CT. Proc Am Radium Soc 1998;39.

preceded by induction chemotherapy, it might also be able to sterilize occult nodal disease. It should be noted that these trials, which indicated a reduction of distant failure, gave chemotherapy in full dose and on an intermittent schedule.[686,687] Trials using daily or weekly low-dose chemotherapy, while also showing survival gain, appear to have achieved this goal more from enhanced local control than from effective suppression of extrathoracic disease.[654] The details of combining radiation and chemotherapy will become increasingly important as we attempt to reduce radiation target volumes and increase dose, and schedules that combine local radiosensitizing effects with the systemic adjuvant effects of chemotherapy might prove to be most effective.

Treatment Delivery: Multiple Sessions and Moving Targets

The initial concerns in developing reproducible treatment setups in 3D-CRT planning and delivery have concentrated on assuring reproducibility of patient positioning and anatomic setup in relatively static organs such as the prostate. Issues of intrinsic positional uncertainty, variation in positioning for imaging, treatment planning, and treatment delivery are common to 3D-CRT approaches for all disease sites. Treatment of lung cancer adds the issue of physiologic motion of the target volume with the cardiac and respiratory cycles. Although these issues are not fully resolved, several strategies have been developed to address them. One set of approaches entails treating the

TABLE 75-21

	Histologic Involvement of Regional Nodes in Peripheral cT1No NSCLC				
AUTHOR	**TUMOR DIAMETER (CM)**	**N0**	**N1**	**N2**	**TOTAL**
Konaka[682]	≤1.0	19 (100%)	0	0	19
	>1.0 ≤ 1.5	43 (86%)	4	3	50
	>1.5 ≤ 2.0	80 (78%)	6	16	102
Miller[683]	≤1.0	93 (93%)	5	2	100

patient at a fixed phase of the respiratory cycle, either by voluntary breath holding at deep inspiration or by the use of mechanical ventilation to limit the degree of inspiration when the treatment beam is turned on.[688-690] A second approach allows the patient to breath freely but gates the treatment beam on and off to allow treatment only in a limited portion of the respiratory cycle. This portion is generally determined by external markers of respiration, such as airflow of position of markers located on the external chest surface. Such free-breathing approaches could be more acceptable than breath-holding ones to patients who are already dyspneic or anxious.

Both of these approaches attempt to limit the effect of organ motion by limiting the amount of motion during the time of treatment. Alternatively, one could allow free motion of the tumor but track it accurately in real time with imaging devices mounted on the treatment accelerator and dynamically adjust the position of the treatment beam relative to the patient to follow the tumor motion. In some systems, this strategy requires placement of radio-opaque fiducial markers within the tumor to allow accurate tracking. Several prototype devices for such treatment have been developed and their use described in treatment of medically inoperable patients with small peripheral lung tumors.[691,692] The general applicability of such approaches to larger tumors is questionable, however, as not only the position but also the shape of the tumor will change with the respiratory cycle, making a simple tracking approach unsatisfactory. An additional concern arises from the decreased lung density achieved with the deep inspiration-breath-holding techniques. With reduced lung density, there is a larger distance of electron disequilibrium with resultant underdosing of tumor at tumor-lung interfaces. Several groups have shown (using Monte Carlo dose calculations) that such inhomogeneities can reach clinically significant levels in the range of 8%–18% and are worse with small field sizes and higher photon beam energies (e.g., 15 mV vs. 6 mV).[693,694] Such considerations must be taken into account in attempts to deal with respiratory motion.

Clinical Experience

Several centers have published results of early therapeutic trials of 3D-CRT for patients with NSCLC. As these generally represent results from a period during which therapeutic techniques were in evolution, radiation doses often spanned a wide range as clinicians became more comfortable with dose escalation strategies. These studies also use variable mixtures of patients with early-stage but medically inoperable disease (stages I and II) and those with bulky stage IIIA or IIIB disease. Thus, all of these series should be viewed as works in progress rather than as definitive assessments of the clinical value of 3D-CRT (Table 75-22).

Hayman and colleagues[695,696] and Hazuka[697] have reported a dose-escalation trial in which the dose for a particular patient was determined in part by the calculated normal tissue complication probability (based on lung volume without accounting for regional variations in lung function). Target volumes included only gross disease plus margin without ENI. For patients in the

TABLE 75-22

Selected Large Trials of Conformal Radiation Therapy for NSCLC

AUTHOR	NO. OF PATIENTS	STAGE	DOSE (GY) (MEDIAN)	MEDIAN SURVIVAL (MO)	2-YEAR SURVIVAL (%)	LOCAL CONTROL AT 2 YEARS (%)	COMMENTS
Rosenman[719]	62	IIIA/B	60–74 [74]	24	50	—	Phase I-II trial with 32 patients treated to 74 Gy. Treated elective nodal sites
Armstrong[698]	28	I/II: 4 IIIA: 12 IIIB: 12	52.2–72 [70.2]	15.7	32	—	Phase I dose escalation trial
Sibley[703]	37	IIIA: 18 IIIB: 19	60–70 [66]	19.5	37	23	Phase I dose escalation
Graham[675]	70	I: 15 II: 7 IIIA: 36 IIIB: 12	60–74 [69]	16.5	33	—	Phase I dose escalation. Treated elective nodal sites
Hazuka[697]	88	I/II: 19 IIIA: 44 IIIB: 25	60–74	24	37	49	Phase I. No elective nodal radiation

low-risk group, doses have been escalated to 84 Gy without excessive pulmonary or other toxicity. Failure in nonirradiated adjacent nodes has not been observed.

Armstrong and McGibney[698] at the Memorial Sloan-Kettering Cancer Center are conducting a dose-escalation trial, also using conventional fractionation. Preliminary reports are encouraging for survival despite adverse patient clinical characteristics. For the sake of continuing dose escalation, the researchers have found it necessary to eliminate ENI and to target only known primary and nodal disease.

At Washington University, Graham and colleagues[675] have performed several trials of 3D-CRT with dose escalation to 74 Gy. Their initial approach was to begin with fairly traditional treatment planning approaches using the tools of 3D-RTP for evaluation of tumor coverage and normal tissue dose-volume histograms. Unlike some other groups, they have tended to avoid noncoplanar beam arrangements, feeling that these add little to treatment effectiveness and result in little lung sparing.

The group at the University of Pittsburgh, to limit lung dose, has advocated a technique that relies heavily on beams that are unopposed and might be noncoplanar.[699] Their approach relies heavily on the use of coplanar but nonopposing beams, which treat large amounts of lung to low dose (from one beam only) but limit the volume of beam overlap to the immediate vicinity of the tumor. Preliminary data on 31 patients indicates acceptable acute toxicity, although target doses were not escalated above 65 Gy.[699] Derycke and coworkers[701,702] have developed a somewhat similar approach using multiple parasaggital beams with intensity modulation; this approach gives good sparing of both lung and spinal cord and could be amenable to the development of class solutions, which simplify the treatment planning process somewhat.

Sibley and associates[703] have reported their experience with treatment of patients with stage III NSCLC using 3D-CRT to total doses of 66Gy. With a median survival of 19.5 months and 2-year survival of 37%, their results

with radiotherapy as a single modality compare favorably to or surpass those reported with combined-modality approaches.[704] Caution should be taken in comparing single-institution with cooperative group experiences. The researchers also found that despite this favorable survival, local control of tumor was poor, with only 23% of patients free of local progression at 2 years.

Issues for Consideration and Future Development

Most current data on lung tolerance are based on patients with either Hodgkin's disease or cancer of the lung. These two groups differ substantially in terms of median age, smoking history, and probable survival, and data from the two groups might not be entirely comparable. The techniques of radiation therapy used on the patients from whom these data have been derived were typically classic opposed fields—either AP-PA or obliques. The typical beam arrangement in conformal planning for stage III NSCLC or limited SCLC produces dose distributions that are much more conformal for the high-dose volume but might treat larger volumes of lung tissue to lower doses (e.g., >20 Gy) that are usually satisfactorily tolerated. How well such large-volume, modest-dose irradiation will be tolerated in the context of sequential or concurrent chemotherapy is not well characterized and will be a challenge for current and future clinical trials. Particularly with drugs that are radiation sensitizers (e.g., gemcitabine), caution should be applied before assuming that full-dose chemotherapy and full-dose radiation can be safely combined.[704]

The esophagus could well emerge as a dose-limiting organ in chest radiotherapy. Because of its proximity to mediastinal lymph nodes, it is frequently difficult, if not impossible, to establish a significant dose differential between nodal metastases and adjacent esophagus. Elimination of ENI will reduce the length of esophagus irradiated but not necessarily the maximum dose. Both of these factors have been correlated with toxicity.[659,660] The use of concurrent chemotherapy (and possibly anterior chemotherapy as well) worsens acute esophagitis with as yet not well characterized effects on late tolerance.

An alternative approach to conformal radiation therapy with photon beams involves the use of other radiation beams having intrinsic physical advantages in dose distribution. This approach has been most studied for proton beams. The relative lack of side scatter and controllable depth of penetration in tissue (with most energy being deposited in the region of the Bragg peak) theoretically allow substantial reductions in dose delivered to normal tissues. At present, proton beams optimized for clinical radiation therapy are available only in a small number of institutions worldwide. Little has been published to date on their use in patients with lung cancer, but preliminary data are encouraging, and several recently commissioned clinical proton beam facilities will provide additional information on this approach.[705]

It has long been recognized that there is an interdependent relation between staging of cancer and its treatment. Staging is of greatest importance in a setting of partially effective therapies. With no effective therapy, staging is irrelevant, and a therapy effective regardless of disease extent does not require a complex staging system. The ongoing modifications of the TNM staging system for lung cancer, both in its official rubric and in multiple suggested ad hoc modifications, is reflective of the current changes in lung cancer therapy. The present staging system was derived primarily from data on surgically treated patients and reflects this heritage.[82] Particularly for the T component, proximity to unresectable normal structures is given more importance than size. Although this makes sense surgically, it does not accord with well established radiobiologic principles relating tumor volume and probability of achieving local control. The only explicit consideration of tumor size is in the distinction between T_1 and T_2 lesions using a 3-cm cutoff. A 1-cm peripheral tumor involving visceral pleura, however, would be staged as T_2, while a 2.9-cm tumor without pleural involvement would be staged as T_1. Martel and colleagues[706] have examined tumor volume in patients with NSCLC receiving 3D-CRT and have shown that total tumor volume is not correlated with stage but that for patients without nodal involvement, it is strongly correlated with survival. Several other groups have reported similar findings.[650-651] One caution here is that the reproducibility of tumor volume measurements made from planning CT scans by several physicians is rather poor.[707,708]

Functional Imaging

Initial approaches to 3D-CRT have focused on the optimization of anatomic dose distribution. It has been realized that this was not optimum and that conventional CT imaging did not give important information on tissue type and function. Over the past several years, the growing ability to combine images obtained by various technologies such as CT with MRI or PET has become increasingly available. Such tools can be valuable both for evaluating adequacy of coverage of the tumor and in selecting treatment plans based on effect of normal tissue function in addition to normal tissue volume.[709]

PET scanning with ^{18}F-fluorodeoxyglucose has become widely used in the management of patients with a variety of malignancies over the past several years. For NSCLC, PET has shown considerable promise in several domains:

1. PET scanning has greater sensitivity and specificity in detecting mediastinal nodal metastases than does CT scanning, and a combination of the two modalities is currently the state of the art for noninvasive mediastinal staging.[294]

2. Whole-body PET scanning can reveal otherwise undetected extrathoracic metastatic disease in a substantial proportion of patients with locally advanced (typically stage III) disease who otherwise are thought to be candidates for potentially curative chemoradiation. Such detection is of high prognostic value and will guide therapy for individual patients.[710-712] It will also appear to improve the survival outcomes of patients for both those remaining in stage III and those migrating to stage IV, when compared with historical controls. The influence of such stage migration on survival of patient subsets (the so-called "Will Rogers effect") must be taken into account when introducing any new mode of tumor staging and/or classification.

3. The functional information obtained with PET scanning can be combined with the anatomic data from CT to aid in target volume delineation and treatment planning for radiation therapy. There is a rapid proliferation of reports on the effect of such combined information on treatment planning. There has been considerable variation between series in exactly how the CT and PET information were obtained and combined in the planning process. In the simplest models, the physician had access to the PET images while drawing the target volume on the planning CT; any fusion was performed in his or her head. In a second generation of trials, formal attempts of image fusion using internal anatomic references and/or external fiducial markers have been described. Most recently, the availability of dual-purpose imaging machines, which perform both CT and PET imaging in the same study session, are being investigated. Great care must be taken in fusing images obtained with the patient in somewhat different imaging positions, none of which might correspond precisely with the treatment position unless rigorous care is made to ensure consistent patient immobilization. Tumor motion with the respiratory and cardiac cycles, a factor we are just beginning to grapple with in "four-dimensional radiotherapy," becomes an even greater complexity when the times required for CT and PET image set acquisition differ by several orders of magnitude. The application of respiratory gating to PET image acquisition for RT planning is in its infancy.[713]

Despite these significant complexities and potential problems, however, the early investigations of including PET data in RT planning for NSCLC have shown two general themes:

1. The mediastinal component of the gross tumor volume (GTV) increases as nodes normal by CT size criteria are shown to be highly glucose avid on PET.

2. The primary tumor component of the GTV often decreases as densities peripheral to central obstruction tumors are interpreted (if cold on PET) as atelectasis rather than tumor.[714]

Such interpretations remain somewhat subjective and could well be influenced by choice of SUV threshold for interpretation.[715]

The final domain in which PET could be useful in managing patients with NSCLC is in assessing response to treatment. It has been recognized for some time that the measurement of tumor response to radiation therapy or chemoradiation by CT does not correlate well with long-term treatment outcome.[716] Several recent studies have suggested that posttreatment PET scan response is much more predictive of ultimate tumor control and patient outcome.[717] It is not known, however, what the optimal interval after chemotherapy of chemoradiation for such imaging might be. Particularly after radiation therapy, inflammatory changes in normal lung can complicate PET interpretation and yield false positive studies.

In addition to CT, MRI, and PET, a burgeoning number of newer functional imaging techniques are on the horizon and can provide potentially important information for radiation therapy planning.[718,719] These techniques might allow in situ noninvasive measurement of tumor hypoxia, proliferation rate, apoptosis, expression of a variety of surface receptors, and other parameters of interest.[720-722] If we can acquire such maps of biologic function reliably and correlate them with anatomic structure, the ability to differentially direct radiation dose to areas of greater tumor burden or functional radioresistance will usher in a new era of treatment optimization based on radiobiology in addition to physics.[723] Although this promises to be a daunting task, it offers the possibility of truly individualized therapy.

Cost-effectiveness of 3D-CRT

The development of conformal radiotherapy is occurring at a time when the cost of all medical procedures is coming under heavy scrutiny and new, often costly, technologies are being required to justify themselves by producing demonstrably better outcomes. For conformal radiotherapy, these outcomes could be either a reduction of the incidence of acute or late complications (and the costs of managing these) or improved survival outcomes if the dose escalation allowed by conformal therapy results in improved local control and survival. Clinical trials designed to assess these issues are currently being performed in several common disease sites, including NSCLC.

Several authors have investigated the economic aspects of conformal radiotherapy.[724-727] Although the initial cost of purchasing new hardware and software for treatment planning and delivery can be high, the greater ongoing expense is likely to be associated with the greater time and effort associated with conformal planning. Hohenberg and Sedlmayer[725] found in a survey of German radiotherapy facilities that had begun conformal planning that the number of hours spent per case doubled during the initial period of adoption of the new technologies.

Increases were seen for physician, dosimetrist, and physicist time. After about a year, the time requirements fell off and plateaued at about 150% of that required for conventional planning. Although improved technologies such as automated contouring of target and normal tissue volumes might improve the picture somewhat, it is clear that 3D planning is and will remain labor intensive. The implementation of intensity-modulated radiotherapy, an outgrowth of 3D-CRT, will further increase time and resource requirements.[728]

Combining Radiation and Chemotherapy

In planning to combine radiation and chemotherapy, several distinct strategies, which differ both in logistics and in intended mechanism of interaction between the modalities, can be envisioned and have been investigated. In the absence of stumbling over a highly effective and nontoxic regimen, which is unlikely to happen, attention to the details of such combined modality therapy could be our best near-term strategy for making modest but clinically worthwhile improvements in treatment efficacy. As implemented to date, the three primary modes of combining radiation and chemotherapy in NSCLC have been:

1. Sequential, with no temporal overlap of modalities. The intent of combining modalities in this fashion would be to take advantage of spatial cooperation between a local and a systemic treatment modality while avoiding the enhanced normal tissue toxicities associated with concurrent treatment (see Table 75-23). In view of the high frequency of occult systemic disease in patients with stage IIIA/IIIB NSCLC, it has seemed most reasonable to start with systemic (induction) chemotherapy and follow it with thoracic radiation (and possibly postirradiation chemotherapy as well) (Table 75-23).[686,687,729-732]
2. Concurrent administration of radiation and chemotherapy, with both given using conventional fractionation and dosage schedules (Table 75-24).[733,734]
3. Concurrent administration of radiation and chemotherapy, with chemotherapy given at reduced doses but greater frequency to maximize local radiation sensitization (Table 75-25).[654,735,736]

Limitations of Present Studies of Combined-modality Therapy

In evaluating the results of recent trials of combined chemoradiation for patients with stage IIIA/IIIB NSCLC and the conclusions derived from them, a number of caveats should be kept in mind:

1. Staging often did not include CT scanning. Several series have suggested that 15% or more of patients with apparent stage IIIA/IIIB NSCLC have evidence of stage IV disease on PET scan. As routine staging techniques improve, so will treatment outcomes for patients with apparently localized disease, even in the absence of improvements in treatment efficacy.
2. Radiation treatment planning and delivery in all of the cited phase II trials and in the majority of single-institution and cooperative group phase II trials have

TABLE 75-23

Randomized Trials of Radiation Therapy versus Induction Chemotherapy Followed by Radiation Therapy

	N	MEDIAN SURVIVAL (MO)	2-YR SURVIVAL	5-YR SURVIVAL	P
LeChevalier[686]	353	12/10	21/14	12/4	.02
Brodin[729]	330	9/9	–/–	–/–	NS
Sause[687]	303	14/11	32/19	8/5	.04
Mattson[730]	238	11/10	19/17	–/–	NS
Miller[731]	229	9/9	13/18	4/3	NS
Dillman[732]	155	14/10	26/13	17/6	.01

used, at best, CT-based 2D planning. Information based on PET scanning was included neither directly nor indirectly in treatment planning, and 3D planning and verification was not employed. Although the precise importance of such omissions will depend in part on the extent of "elective" irradiation (the more generous the elective volume, the more forgiving the plan will be of omission of areas of tumor from the intended treatment volume), such coverage will be gained at the expense of unnecessary irradiation of normal tissue.

3. Essentially all studies of combined chemoradiation have used radiation doses of 65 Gy or less, and many have used 60 Gy or less. These doses, stemming historically from the RTOG trial (which compared doses of 40, 50, and 60 Gy), have been fairly standard, at least in the United States, despite clear evidence that they produce long-term control in only a small proportion of patients (10%–15%). Conclusions about optimal treatment effectiveness and toxicity of combined-modality therapy, if based on such clearly inadequate radiation doses, might well be difficult to generalize to higher radiation doses or biologically more effective fractionation schedules.

4. Although many of the prospective trials have been stratified appropriately by TNM stage group, none have been stratified by tumor volume. Several recent studies have reported that tumor volume (often as measured during 3D treatment planning) could be a better predictor of local control and survival than TNM staging. Because the TNM system was derived initially

from surgically treated patients and does not explicitly include tumor volume, whereas the ability of radiation to control disease depends on the number of tumor clonogens (which logically should be a function of tumor volume), such an observation is biologically reasonable. Several efforts are underway to develop volume-based staging systems for patients with lung cancer (both NSCLC and SCLC) who are treated with radiation therapy or chemoradiation.

5. Of the five randomized trials that have compared sequential and concurrent chemoradiation (Table 75-26), only one (Furuse and associates[737]) has been published in full with adequate follow-up. This trial used very low-radiation doses (56 Gy in 28 fractions) in both treatment arms, with the radiation given in split-course fashion in the concurrent arm and as a continuous course in the sequential arm. The RTOG 94-10 trial has been reported in abstract.[656] Although it showed an overall superiority in median survival for the concurrent arm as opposed to the sequential treatment arm, further analysis should give some hesitancy in accepting this conclusion at face value. First, of the two concurrent chemoradiation arms in this trial, only one gave results superior to sequential therapy. The third arm, which used both BID radiotherapy to 69.6 Gy and more frequent chemotherapy

TABLE 75-24

Randomized Trials of Radiation Therapy versus Radiation Therapy and Concurrent Intermittent Chemotherapy

STUDY	N	MEDIAN SURVIVAL (MO)	2-YR SURVIVAL	5-YR SURVIVAL	P
Jeremic[733]	117				
RT		8	25	5	NS
RT + EC q2wk		13	27	16	
Blanke[734]	215				
RT		10	13	2	NS
RT + P q3wk		11	18	5	

EC, etoposide/carboplatin; P, cisplatin.

TABLE 75-25

Randomized Trials of Radiation Therapy versus Radiation Therapy and Daily Chemotherapy

	N	MEDIAN SURVIVAL (MO)	2-YR SURVIVAL	5-YR SURVIVAL	P
Schaake-Koning[654]	210				
RT		12	13	2	
RT + P daily		12	26	10	.009
Trovo[735]	146				
RT		10	14	—	NS
RT + P daily		10	14	—	
Jeremic[736]	135				
RT		14	26	9	.02
RT + EC daily		22	43	23	

EC, etoposide/carboplatin; P, cisplatin.

TABLE 75-26

Randomized Comparisons of Sequential and Concurrent Chemoradiation in Patients with Locally Advanced NSCLC

TRIAL	NO. OF PATIENTS	CHEMO	RADIATION DOSE (GY)	MEDIAN SURVIVAL (MO)	ACTUARIAL SURVIVAL (%)	STATISTICS	COMMENTS
Furuse[737]	314	MVP	56 SEQ 56 CON	13 17	9 19 (2-yr)	P = 0.04	Improved local control in concurrent arm despite split-course RT
Curran[656] (RTOG)	400	VP	63 SEQ 63 CON	14.6 17.1	18 26 (3-yr)	P = 0.04	Third arm with concurrent BID RT and DDP/VP16 was not statistically superior to sequential arm
GLOT[739]	212	NP PE/NP	66 SEQ 66 CON	13.9 15.6	24 36 (2-yr)	NS	Different chemotherapy regimens in the two arms
Zatloukal[740]	102	NP	60 SEQ 60 CON	13 20.4	—	P = 0.02	RT delayed until after 4 cycles of chemotherapy in sequential arm
LAMP[741]	178	TC	63 SEQ 63 CON	13 17.2	31 35 (2-yr)	NS	Randomized phase II trial without planned comparison between arms

MVP, mitomycin-C/vindesine/cisplatin; NP, vinorelbine/cisplatin; PE/NP, cisplatin/etoposide during RT, navelbine/cisplatin after RT; TC, paclitaxel/carboplatin; VP, vinblastine/cisplatin.

(cisplatin on days 1 and 8, oral etoposide on days 1 through 5 and days 8 through 12 during each cycle), had better local control than either of the other arms but had a median survival intermediate between the other two arms and was not superior to that of the sequential arm. Although late toxicities were not recorded as greater in this arm, it could be that such toxicities account in part for the poorer survival despite better local control.[739-741]

A second puzzling observation in this trial is that the benefit of the concurrent over the sequential arm was seen only in the subset of elderly patients. Subset analysis of prior RTOG studies by age had suggested that patients age 70 and above had not benefited from combined chemoradiation compared with radiation therapy alone. In this trial, however, median survival for the 80% of patients below age 70 did not differ for the concurrent and sequential arms (15.5 and 15.7 months, respectively), while for the 20% of patients age 70 or above, there was a striking difference (22.4 months vs. 10.8 months) favoring concurrent therapy.[747] These results are puzzling and counterintuitive and are not readily explained.

There are other complicating factors in the remaining trials. Different chemotherapy regimens were used in the two arms of the GLOT trial.[739] In the Czech study, radiotherapy was delayed in the sequential arm until completion of all (four or six) cycles of chemotherapy.[740] This strategy of delayed consolidation radiation has not been effective in SCLC, and there is little reason to favor it in NSCLC. The CALGB and RTOG trials, which showed benefit to sequential chemoradiation over radiation therapy alone, used a brief (6-week) induction period rather than more protracted chemotherapy before starting chest irradiation. Finally, the LAMP trial was a randomized

phase II trial which was not designed to make internal comparisons between its three arms but rather to compare each arm with the results of the sequential chemoradiation arm of RTOG 88-08, which had a median survival of 13.8 months.[741]

It is difficult at this time to make a robust conclusion that concurrent chemoradiation is better than the sequential use of these two modalities. There does tend to be a trend favoring concurrent therapy, at least for intermediate-term survival (2 to 3 years), but the gains are modest and obtained at the cost of greater acute toxicity, even in trials limited to patients of good performance status and limited weight loss.

If concurrent chemoradiation is better than sequential treatment, it would appear from analysis of patterns of failure that this is due primarily to better local control. This appears to be the case at least in the Western Japan Lung Group trial reported by Furuse[655] and in RTOG 94-10.[656] This then raises the question of whether such improvement in local control is better obtained by combining sensitizing chemotherapy with conventionally low-dose radiation therapy or by radiation dose escalation, either by extending conventional fractional fractionation to higher total dose or by adopting more innovative fractionation regimens, such as the accelerated CHART or HART regimens or the concurrent boost strategies that have been used in head and neck cancers. It could be that a strategy of sequential chemoradiation—in which the overall duration of treatment is kept short by accelerated fractionation of radiation and shortened chemotherapy cycle time with the use of hematopoetic growth factors—would be highly effective while avoiding some of the acute mucosal toxicities seen with concurrent treatment.

The Eastern Cooperative Oncology Group initiated a phase III trial evaluating this concept of induction chemotherapy followed by accelerated radiation therapy in EST 2597. Patients with stage IIIA/IIIB NSCLC were randomized to receive two cycles of induction chemotherapy with carboplatin and paclitaxel followed by either conventional radiation therapy (64 Gy in 32 fractions over 6.5 weeks) or an accelerated regimen of 57.6 Gy in 36 fractions over 2.5 weeks, with three fractions given per treatment day 5 days a week. This trial accrued more slowly than expected and was closed before meeting its initially planed accrual goal. Preliminary results suggest a benefit for the HART arm, with a median survival of 21 months, compared with a median survival of 12 months in the arm with conventional fractionation.[742] Analysis of patterns of failure and consideration of a larger trial to confirm these provocative results are underway.

Brain Metastases in Locally Advanced NSCLC

Brain metastases are common in lung cancer. Recognition that patients with SCLC who were responding to systemic therapy still failed in the brain led to the hypothesis that the CNS represented a pharmacologic sanctuary site, as had been previously demonstrated in acute lymphoblastic leukemia. After several decades of controversy and a large number of relatively underpowered randomized trials, it has now been established that the use of prophylactic cranial irradiation (PCI) in SCLC patients who have achieved a complete response to induction therapy prolongs survival significantly.[743] A similar situation could be present for patients with locally advanced NSCLC. As local and systemic therapy have become modestly more effective and as median survivals have improved from about 10 months with radiation therapy alone to 18 months with various combinations of chemotherapy and radiation therapy, brain metastases, either as a sole site or as part of systemic relapse, have been reported with increasing frequency. Several small randomized trials, as well as comparison of cohorts of patients treated with or without PCI, have suggested reductions in CNS failure without clear effects on survival. These have all been small studies, however, in which an improvement in survival on the order of that seen in SCLC (about 5% at 3 years) would not easily be detectable. Second, these trials generally did not limit PCI to patients in complete or even partial response to treatment of their intrathoracic disease; in some cases, PCI was given at the outset of all therapy. This is quite different from the situation in the SCLC meta-analysis, in which randomization to PCI was performed only in complete (albeit in some studies only by chest x-ray (CXR) responders. In an attempt to remedy these shortcomings, the RTOG recently launched a trial for patients with stage IIIA/IIIB NSCLC who have completed locoregional therapy and have at least stable disease. Patients will be randomized to PCI (30 Gy in 15 fractions) or observation. Although the inclusion of patients with less than a complete response (preferable by PET scan) could dilute the apparent benefits of PCI that might be observed, the accrual requirements of the study, with a sample size of 1068, argued against too restrictive entry criteria.

Current Treatment Trends: Conclusions

Present technology represents a major improvement in treatment delivery compared with 20 years ago and can deliver conventional doses much more accurately. The first developmental generation of technologies and clinical trials has shown the feasibility of applying 3D-CRT technology to the treatment of patients with lung cancer. What now remains is the evaluation of the clinical utility of these technologies in large clinical trials. Two approaches can reasonably be taken. In the first, more conservative approach, 3D-CRT will be used to assure better tumor coverage and normal tissue protection while maintaining conventional dose and fractionation regimens. It is currently a topic of considerable controversy whether this approach ought to be compared with current conventional therapy or with large-volume treatment.

A more challenging set of trials will investigate whether the escalation of radiation dose from the current 65 Gy "standard" to doses in the range of 80–100 Gy produces clinically useful improvements in local control and survival. In this setting, the desire to avoid major protraction of overall treatment time and to reduce the amount of normal tissue receiving the full fraction size will likely lead to the adoption of some form of accelerated fractionation, with fraction sizes to the PTV increasing from the present 1.8–2.0 Gy standard to 2.5–3.0 Gy or more, or to treatment acceleration by the use of multiple fractions per day as in the CHART, HART, or CHARTWEL regimens.

Some elements of 3D-CRT, such as improved visualization ensuring that the planned target volume is actually being covered, are so intuitively beneficial that they do not require large-scale validation in clinical trials. Other aspects of 3D-CRT—particularly the assumption that higher radiation doses are necessarily better—are better considered as promising hypotheses. To avoid a backlash by reimbursement agencies and the public, careful evaluation of the true costs and benefits of 3D-CRT in lung cancer and at other tumor sites should be a priority in this decade.

As systemic therapy improves, the clinical importance of achieving local disease control will increase. The current efforts to better define the appropriate target volume and deliver effective doses of radiation to it will have their greatest payoff in such a context of combined-modality therapy.

TREATMENT OF METASTATIC NON–SMALL CELL LUNG CANCER

The treatment of metastatic NSCLC remains a challenge. Nearly 50% of lung cancer patients present with advanced or stage IV disease and are incurable with currently available treatment. The mainstay of treatment for this group of patients is systemic chemotherapy.

Through the 1980s, there was a great deal of pessimism regarding the treatment of patients with metastatic NSCLC, as even with treatment, 1-year survivals rarely rose above 20%. During this same time period, there were several randomized trials comparing different chemotherapy regimens with best supportive care. The results were variable, but in two studies there was a statistically significant prolongation of survival for the patients treated with chemotherapy.[744,745] These trials did not address the quality of life of the patients, nor did they evaluate the palliation of symptoms with chemotherapy.

The Non–Small Cell Lung Cancer Collaborative Group published a meta-analysis assessing the benefit of chemotherapy in advanced disease.[746] Eleven trials were included, eight of which used cisplatin-based chemotherapy. There was a 1.5-month increase in median survival and an absolute increase in 1-year survival of 10% (to 20%) for cisplatin-treated patients. Older combinations using alkylating agents were actually detrimental. The Southwest Oncology Group (SWOG) did an analysis of their database to assess survival determinants in patients with advanced disease.[747] Cisplatin-based chemotherapy was an independent predictor of improved outcome. An ECOG analysis of "long-term survivors" of treatment for metastatic NSCLC demonstrated that 1-year survival was a better surrogate for clinical effectiveness than median survival and confirmed the poor outcome of patients with performance status 2 disease.[748]

In the early 1980s, the results with chemotherapy were less than optimal, and it was unclear whether there was any survival advantage for patients undergoing treatment. The drugs that were used routinely (usually in combination) are listed in Table 75-19, and there was a plethora of phase 2 studies suggesting benefit for one or another regimen. A number of randomized trials showed no significant benefit for one treatment over another.[749-751] It is interesting to note that in one Eastern Cooperative Group (ECOG) phase III trial, carboplatin, despite a dismal response rate of 9%, had a significantly longer median survival as a single agent than a popular combination, MVP (mitomycin, vinblastine, cisplatin).[750]

At the end of the 1980s, it could be said that treatment with cisplatin-based chemotherapy provided a modest survival advantage for patients with advanced NSCLC. It was also clear that improvement in survival, particularly

1-year survival, was a better outcome measurement for trial design than was improvement in response rate. There was no cisplatin-based combination that was demonstrated as superior, but the combination of etoposide and cisplatin became a de facto standard.

Chemotherapy in the 1990s

In the decade of the 1990s, a number of new chemotherapeutic agents became available, and several of them had activity as single agents (15%–20% response rate) in NSCLC (see Table 75-19). These new agents have been incorporated into a number of phase III trials. The results of some of these trials will be discussed in this section.

Cisplatin versus Combination Chemotherapy

Cisplatin has been the basis of combination chemotherapy for NSCLC; therefore, it was logical to combine the newer agents with cisplatin. Prior cisplatin-based combinations with vinca alkaloids, mitomycin, and so on usually produced better response rates than single-agent chemotherapy but did not consistently improve survival.[750] This observation led to a number of randomized trials that compared cisplatin with cisplatin and new-agent combinations (Table 75-27).[752-755] In three of the four trials, the cisplatin and new-agent combinations proved to be significantly superior to single-agent cisplatin.[752,753,755] The median and 1-year survivals were also very consistent across the studies and established these new-agent combinations as the basis for future clinical trials. A European trial failed to confirm a survival advantage of paclitaxel plus cisplatin compared with cisplatin alone.[754] Questions have been raised about the ethics of these trials, given that cisplatin as a single agent was not and is not a "standard" treatment for metastatic NSCLC, but nonetheless the agents were approved.

Tirapazamine is a novel bioreductive agent that has selective cytotoxicity against hypoxic cells. When combined with cisplatin in a randomized clinical trial, tirapazamine had activity similar to the other new

TABLE 75-27

				SURVIVAL	
AUTHOR	**TREATMENT**	**NO. OF PATIENTS**	**RESPONSE (%)**	**MEDIAN**	**1-YR (%)**
Wozniak[752]	Cis	209	12	6 mo	20
	Cis + Vnr	206	26*	8 mo*	36*
Sandler[753]	Cis	263	9	7.6 mo	28
	Cis + Gem	260	31*	9 mo*	39
Gatzemeier[754]	Cis	206	17	37 wks	35
	Cis + Pac	202	26*	35 wks	32
Von Pawel[755]	Cis	219	14	28 wks	22.5
	Cis + Tira	219	27*	35 wks	34*

Randomized Trials of Cisplatin versus Cisplatin–New Agent Combinations

Cis, cisplatin; Gem, gemcitabine; Pac, paclitaxel; Tira, tirapazamine; Vnr, vinorelbine.
*P < 0.05.

TABLE 75-28

Randomized Trials of Single New Agents versus New Agent–Platinum Combinations

AUTHOR	TREATMENT	NO. OF PATIENTS	RESPONSE (%)	SURVIVAL MEDIAN	1-YR (%)
LeChevalier[756]	Vnr	206	14	31 wks	30
	Vin + Cis	200	19†	32 wks†	27
	Vnr + Cis	206	30*	40 wks *	35*
Depierre[757]	Vnr	119	16	32 wks	—
	Vnr + Cis	121	43*	33 wks	—
Lilenbaum[758]	Pac	277	17	6.7 mo	33
	Pac + Carbo	284	29*	8.8 mo*	37
Sederholm[759]	Gem	170	11.5	9 mo	32
	Gem + Carbo	164	30*	10 mo	44*
Georgoulias[760]	Doc	145	20	8 mo	40
	Doc + Cis	158	36*	10 mo	45

Carbo, carboplatin; Cis, cisplatin; Doc, docetaxel; Gem, gemcitabine; Pac, paclitaxel; Vin, vindesine; Vnr, vinorelbine.
*Significant compared to single agent.
†Vnr + Cis compared with Vin + Cis

drugs.[755] It remains an investigational agent and is still being evaluated in a variety of clinical trials in combination with chemotherapy and/or radiation therapy.

New-Agent versus New Agent-Platinum Combinations

From the early phase II and III trials, it was clear that the new chemotherapeutic agents were active in the treatment of NSCLC and appeared to have toxicity profiles that were well tolerated by the majority of patients. A number of randomized trials addressed the issue of whether these new agents could stand on their own as effective treatment when compared with platinum-based combination chemotherapy. This discussion is limited to phase III trials, and they are represented in Table 75-28.

A French study by LeChevalier and coworkers[756] compared single-agent vinorelbine to vinorelbine plus cisplatin and the European standard of vindesine plus cisplatin. In this trial, the combination of cisplatin and vinorelbine was superior to the single agent and to another cisplatin-containing regimen. It was interesting that vinorelbine as a single agent was equivalent to the cisplatin/vindesine combination. Another French study by Depierre and associates,[757] which was conducted at the same time, did not confirm these data. Although there was a significant improvement in time to progression and response rate for the cisplatin/vinorelbine combination, overall survival was not improved (32 weeks vs. 33 weeks).

The other three studies are very recent and were all presented at the annual meeting of the American Society of Clinical Oncology (ASCO) in 2002.[758–760] Two of the trials utilize carboplatin instead of cisplatin in combination.[758,759] This has been the trend in clinical practice because of the general consensus that carboplatin has a better toxicity profile. The Cancer and Leukemia Group B (CALGB) trial, presented by Lilenbaum and associates[758] at the plenary session, demonstrated a better response rate and median survival for the combination of paclitaxel and carboplatin. The 1-year survival was not significantly improved, however. The authors indicate that survival could have been influenced by second-line chemotherapy. In the Sederholm study,[759] response rate and 1-year survival were superior for the gemcitabine plus carboplatin study arm compared with gemcitabine alone. In the trial by Georgoulias and colleagues,[760] however, the combination of docetaxel and cisplatin had a better response rate, but survival was not improved significantly for the combination therapy versus single agent docetaxel.

Comparison of Platinum-based Combinations

With many platinum-based combinations shown to have demonstrative clinical activity in NSCLC, two questions remained to be answered:

1. Were the new-agent combinations better than the old platinum-based treatments?, and
2. Was one new agent-platinum combination superior to another?

Again, the discussion will be limited to phase III trials that attempt to answer these questions. These trials are listed in Table 75-29.

The initial five trials, as compiled in Table 75-29, represent comparisons between "old" platinum-based combinations and those containing newer agents.[761–765] The Eastern Cooperative Group (ECOG) conducted a trial (ECOG 5592) that compared what was considered standard therapy (cisplatin plus etoposide) to cisplatin plus paclitaxel at 135 mg/m^2 (24-hour infusion) or cisplatin plus dose-intense paclitaxel at 250 mg/m^2 (24-hour infusion) plus granulocyte colony-stimulating-factor.[761] When the data from the two taxane-containing arms were combined, the response rate and survival were

Specific Malignancies

III

TABLE 75-29

Randomized Trial of Platinum-based Combinations

AUTHOR	TREATMENT	NO. OF PATIENTS	RESPONSE (%)	SURVIVAL	
				MEDIAN (MO)	1-YR (%)
Bonomi[761]	Cis/VP-16	193	12.4	7.6	32
	Cis/Pac	190	25.3*	9.5*	37*
	Cis/Pac (high dose)	191	27.7*	10.1*	40*
Giaccone[762]	Cis/Ten	162	28	9.9	41
	Cis/Pac	155	40†	9.7	43
Belani[763]	Cis/VP-16	179	14	9.1	37
	Carbo/Pac	190	22	7.7	32
Crino[764]	Mito/Ifex/Cis	152	26	9.6	34
	Cis/Gem	155	38†	8.6	33
Lopez-Cabrerizo[765]	Cis/VP-16	65	21.9	7	26
	Cis/Gem	69	40.6†	8.7	32
Kelly[766]	Cis/Vnr	202	28	8.1	36
	Carbo/Pac	206	25	8.6	38
Schiller[767]	Cis/Pac	303	21	7.8	31
	Cis/Gem	301	22	8.1	36
	Cis/Doc	304	17	7.4	31
	Carbo/Pac	299	17	8.1	34
Rodriguez[768]	Cis/Vnr	405	25	9.9	41
	Cis/Doc	408	32	11.3‡	46
	Carbo/Doc	405	24	10.4	41

Carbo, carboplatin; Cis, cisplatin; Doc, docetaxel; Gem, gemcitabine; Ifex, ifosfamide; Mit, mitomycin C; Pac, paclitaxel; Ten, teniposide; Vnr, vinorelbine; VP, 16-etoposide.
*Significant with paclitaxel arms combined.
†Significant.
‡Significant compared with Cis/Vnr.

significantly superior to cisplatin plus etoposide. The high-dose paclitaxel arm had a slightly better outcome compared with the low-dose paclitaxel, but the toxicities, particularly neurotoxicity, outweighed any potential benefits. On this study, quality of life (QOL) was analyzed using the Functional Assessment of Cancer Therapy-Lung (FACT-L) instrument, and no difference was seen between the treatment arms. In a European study reported by Giaccone and coworkers,[762] cisplatin/teniposide was compared with cisplatin/paclitaxel (175 mg/m² over 3 hours). There was a higher response for paclitaxel/cisplatin but a lack of survival benefit. The QOL was also analyzed on this study using the EORTC QLQ-C30 and LC-13 instruments, and the scores favored the paclitaxel-containing arm.

In the oncology community, the combination of paclitaxel and carboplatin had become the standard treatment based on promising phase II data and the relative ease of administration of the combination, particularly with the replacement of cisplatin by carboplatin. An industry-sponsored study that has only been published as an abstract compared cisplatin/etoposide to carboplatin/paclitaxel.[763] The response rate was higher for carboplatin/paclitaxel, and the toxicities were lower, indicating that this was a more tolerable regimen. These outcomes did not translate into improved survival, however. Again, the potential role of second-line chemotherapy was not addressed. Two European trials compared gemcitabine/cisplatin to either cisplatin/etoposide or MIC (mitomycin, ifosfamide, cisplatin).[764,765] In both of these studies, response rates were better for the new drug/cisplatin

combination. There was a trend for better 1-year survival that did not reach statistical significance.

The last three trials in Table 75-29 deal with the comparison between new drug-platinum combinations.[766-768] SWOG 9509 compared cisplatin/vinorelbine, the standard arm obtained from SWOG 9308 (cisplatin vs. cisplatin/vinorelbine), to the community standard of carboplatin/paclitaxel.[766] The response rate and survival results for the two regimens were equivalent. The toxicity profiles were different, with more neutropenia and gastrointestinal toxicity for cisplatin/vinorelbine and more neuropathy with carboplatin/paclitaxel. The QOL analysis was no different between the two study arms. A pharmacoeconomic analysis was also done and showed that the carboplatin/paclitaxel regimen was more expensive by more than $8000.[769] The increased expense was related primarily to drug cost (a factor now moot, as the drug has come off patent). SWOG, therefore, chose carboplatin/paclitaxel as its new standard because it was felt to be better tolerated and easier to combine with other drugs based on the delivered dose-intensity. Schiller and associates[767] reported a much-awaited trial, ECOG 1594, at the ASCO plenary session in 2001. In this large randomized trial of 1200 patients, three platinum-new drug combinations were compared with the reference treatment of cisplatin/paclitaxel (135 mg/m² over 24 hours) obtained from their previous trial, ECOG 5592. The results were disappointing in that no one regimen emerged as clearly superior. The only significant difference in survival was an improvement in median time to progression of 4.2 months for cisplatin/gemicitabine compared with 3.4

months for cisplatin/paclitaxel. The toxicity profiles were different depending on the regimen. Carboplatin/paclitaxel had the least number of grade 3–5 toxicities.

Another 1200-patient industry-sponsored trial compared the standard treatment of cisplatin/vinorelbine to docetaxel combined with either cisplatin or carboplatin. Cisplatin/docetaxel had a significantly better median survival (11.3 months vs. 9.9 months) and 2-year survival (21% vs.14%) than did cisplatin/vinorelbine.[768] The carboplatin/ docetaxel combination was not inferior to cisplatin/vinorelbine. The study was not designed to compare the two-docetaxel combinations. The QOL analysis indicated that the docetaxel-containing regimens were better tolerated then cisplatin/vinorelbine.[770]

Other Strategies

The phase III trials in advanced NSCLC have not been able to identify a superior platinum-based combination. There have been other treatment strategies whose goals have been to increase efficacy. One consideration has been to increase the dose of the active drugs. Because cisplatin had been associated with improved survival in this disease, there have been attempts at cisplatin dose intensification. A European Organization for Research on Treatment of Cancer (EORTC) trial randomized patients to receive cisplatin at either 120 mg/m^2 or 60 mg/m^2 in combination with etoposide in advanced NSCLC.[771] No difference in response rate or survival between the two study arms was observed. SWOG also evaluated cisplatin dose intensity by randomizing patients to receive cisplatin 50 mg/m^2 (days 1 and 8 every 28 days), high-dose cisplatin 100 mg/m^2 (days 1 and 8 every 28 days), or high-dose cisplatin plus mitomycin.[772] The dose-intense regimens were more toxic and did not result in increased survival.

In later years, ECOG 5592 (see Bonomi and associates[761]; Table 75-29) increased the paclitaxel dose from 135 mg/m^2 (24-hour infusion) to 250 mg/m^2 (24-hour infusion) combined with cisplatin and had an outcome similar to those of the other trials. It appears that dose intensification is not an appropriate strategy with currently available chemotherapy, as there is no dose-response relationship and because increasing dose does not overcome resistance.

Given that a number of new drugs had been added to the armamentarium, another strategy in the 1990s had been to increase the number of drugs used. A number of phase II trials showed promising results and acceptable safety with triplet therapy. The Spanish Lung Cancer Group Trial (GEPC/98-02) employed a three-drug regimen (cisplatin, gemcitabine, vinorelbine, and a sequential doublet (gemcitabine, vinorelbine/vinorelbine, ifosfamide) and compared them to cisplatin/gemcitabine.[773] The results of this phase III trial indicated that there was increased toxicity but no survival advantage for the triplet therapy. SWOG 9806 was a randomized phase II trial that evaluated platinum-based doublets followed sequentially by a taxane.[774] The obvious advantage to this approach is that there is no dose attenuation because the three drugs are not given at the same time. Unfortunately, the survival

on this trial was no better than that seen in the large trials comparing platinum-based-doublets, indicating that this approach to drug diversity does not increase efficacy.

Because the current goal in the treatment of advanced NSCLC is palliation, an important strategy has been to decrease toxicity without sacrificing efficacy. One approach has been to eliminate platinum altogether and use two new agents in combination. Numerous phase II trials have evaluated non–platinum-containing regimens using the new drugs in various combinations. An EORTC phase III trial compared cisplatin/pactlitaxel with cisplatin/gemcitabine and paclitaxel/gemcitabine, a non-platinum regimen.[775] The paclitaxel/gemcitabine arm had acceptable toxicity but inferior survival that did not reach statistical significance when compared with the reference arm of cisplatin/paclitaxel (6.9 months vs. 8.1 months, median survival; 26.5% vs. 35.5%, 1-year survival). Other trials are currently being done to evaluate whether non-platinum regimens are appropriate first-line therapy for advanced NSCLC.

There has been an interest in changing drug scheduling to reduce toxicity, one example of which would be weekly chemotherapy. Most of the studies utilizing this approach have been with the taxanes.[776,777] Weekly schedules usually reduce hematologic toxicities but do not eliminate other adverse effects, such as neuropathy and asthenia. Weekly administration might make it easier to combine certain drugs and to integrate them with radiotherapy.

Another area of clinical research involves the important issue of treatment duration. Smith and colleagues[778] reported a trial in patients with advanced NSCLC who were randomized to three vs. six cycles of MVP (mitomycin, vinblastine, cisplatin). Median survival (6 months vs. 7 months) and 1-year survival (22% vs. 25%) were no different between the treatment arms. QOL was, in certain aspects, better for patients randomized to only three courses of treatment, further indicating that there was no clinical advantage to continuing chemotherapy beyond three courses. A recently reported study by Socinski and coworkers[779] randomized patients to receive four cycles of carboplatin/paclitaxel or continuous treatment until progression. This study showed no overall benefit in survival (median survival, 6.6 vs. 8.5 months; 1-year survival, 28% vs. 34%), response rates (22% vs. 24%) or QOL for continuing treatment beyond four cycles. A French trial treated more than 500 patients with MIP (mitomycin, ifosfamide, cisplatin) and than randomized the responders to vinorelbine maintenance or observation.[780] Maintenance therapy did not increase survival but did increase toxicity. On the basis of these trials, it is clear that there is no advantage to continuing treatment to disease progression. Residual tumor is likely to be drug resistant, and at this point it might be better to opt for a more efficacious second-line treatment or a novel drug.

Second-line Treatment

The most recent ASCO guidelines indicated that there was no efficacious second-line treatment for advanced NSCLC. Because patients with advanced NSCLC are living longer and maintaining their performance status, there has been an unmet need for second-line chemotherapy. Many of the new agents (paclitaxel, gemcitabine, vinorelbine) have observed second-line activity in small phase II trials, but the majority of these drugs have not been examined rigorously in larger studies.

Docetaxel is the most established agent in this clinical setting. A number of encouraging phase II trials led to two large studies. Shepherd and associates[781] reported the results of a phase III trial that randomized patients to receive docetaxel 100 mg/m² or best supportive care. Midway through the study, the dose of docetaxel was reduced to 75 mg/m² because of a higher toxic death rate in the chemotherapy arm of the study. Eligibility criteria included patients who had received platinum-based chemotherapy but could not have been treated previously with taxanes. Time to progression (10.6 weeks vs. 6.7 weeks) and median survival (7.0 months vs. 4.6 months) was longer for the docetaxel patients. One-year survival (37% vs. 11%) significantly favored the patients who received docetaxel 75 mg/m² compared with the corresponding best supportive care patients. All QOL parameters favored the docetaxel-treated patients. In a second trial, Fossella and colleagues[782] randomized patients to receive docetaxel 100 mg/m² or docetaxel 75 mg/m² vs. vinorelbine or ifosfamide. Eligibility criteria were similar to the previous study, with the exception that patients could have received prior paclitaxel. Colony-stimulating factor was allowed to maintain drug dose. The docetaxel patients had a longer time to progression, but there were no significant differences between treatment groups with regard to overall survival. One-year survival, however, was significantly better for the patients treated with docetaxel 75 mg/m² as opposed to the control arm treatment (32% vs. 19%). In both studies, the patients who were refractory to platinum did not do well, but in the Fossella[782] trial, prior exposure to paclitaxel did not affect survival. These were the first randomized phase III trials to demonstrate a survival advantage for second-line chemotherapy in the treatment of patients with advanced NSCLC. At ASCO 2003, a phase III study comparing pemetrexed to docetaxel in patients with recurrent NSCLC was presented. Pemetrexed was just as efficacious and less toxic than docetaxel when used in this setting.[783]

Chemotherapy in the Elderly Patient

Elderly people (≥70 years) represent nearly 40% of all lung cancer patients. In the future, this number is likely to increase because the population is aging and cancer incidence increases with age. This population can be uniquely challenging because of the many comorbidities associated with aging. The Elderly Lung Cancer Vinorelbine Italian Study Group trial (ELVIS) was the first randomized study designed for elderly lung cancer patients (Table 75-30).[784] Patients were randomized to receive single-agent vinorelbine vs. best supportive care. The primary goal of the study was an improvement in quality of life. Treatment with chemotherapy significantly improved survival when compared with supportive care (1-year survival, 32% vs. 14%, respectively). The vinorelbine patents had improvements in all aspects of QOL and had a reduction in cancer-related symptoms with acceptable toxicity. Frasci and coworkers[785] reported the results of another trial comparing vinorelbine with vinorelbine/gemcitabine. The study was terminated early because of the significant improvement in survival for the combination therapy. It is interesting to note that the vinorelbine patients did much worse than expected and the patients who received both drugs did just as well as the vinorelbine patients on the ELVIS study. A third Italian study, the Multicenter Italian Lung Cancer Study (MILES), randomized patients to receive vinorelbine, gemcitabine, or vinorelbine/gemcitabine.[786] There was no survival advantage for the combination of the two agents compared with the single-drug therapy. The results with single-agent vinorelbine were similar to what was seen in the ELVIS study. It is unclear why the MILES trial results are contrary to those of the Frasci study. Docetaxel, on a weekly schedule, has been evaluated in the elderly in a phase II trial.[787]

The accepted standard of treatment for patients with advanced NSCLC is a platinum–based combination. There are no phase III trials that prospectively assess the efficacy and safety of combination chemotherapy in the elderly. In a retrospective analysis, Langer and associates[788] evaluated the outcomes for elderly patients treated on ECOG 5592. Fifteen percent of the patients were ≥70 years of age. There were no major differences between age

TABLE 75-30

Trials Involving the Elderly

TRIAL	NO. OF PATIENTS	TREATMENTS	RESPONSE RATE (%)	MEDIAN SURVIVAL (WK)	1-YR SURVIVAL (%)
ELVIS[784]	80	Vnr	20	28	32
	81	BSC	—	21	14
Frasci[785]	60	Vnr	15	18	13
	60	Vnr Gem	22	29	30
MILES[786]	233	Vnr	18.5	37	41
	233	Gem	17.3	28	26
	232	Vnr Gem	20	32	31

BSC, best supportive care; Gem, gemcitabine; Vnr, vinorelbine.

groups (≥70 years vs. <70 years) with regard to response and survival. The elderly patients had more hematologic and neuropsychiatric toxicities. Nineteen percent of the patients enrolled in SWOG 9308 and 9509 were 70 years or older.[789] There appeared to be a trend toward an inferior outcome for the elderly, but in the multivariate analysis, age did not affect survival. The older patients had more hematologic toxicity and tolerated the carboplatin/paclitaxel better than vinorelbine/cisplatin. In the previously described trial assessing duration of treatment with carboplatin/paclitaxel, 29% of the patients were elderly.[779,780] These patients did just as well as their younger counterparts with regard to both survival and toxicity. It is clear that the "fit" elderly can tolerate combination chemotherapy. Elderly patients in general are underrepresented in clinical trials and should not be denied enrollment on the basis of age alone. More studies are necessary to assess the influence of various comorbidities on the elderly patient's ability to tolerate cancer treatment.

Strategies for the New Millenium

The number of clinical trials in NSCLC have increased exponentially over the last decade because of the availability of new chemotherapeutic agents. There is currently a large number of new drugs with unique molecular targets that are being evaluated in numerous clinical trials.

The members of the epidermal growth factor receptor (EGFR) family have been the focus for new drug development. HER2/*neu* (ErbB-2) is a transmembrane glycoprotein with tyrosine kinase activity that belongs to the ErbB family and shares sequence homology with EGFR. HER2/*neu* has become important as a prognostic indicator and a therapeutic target in breast cancer patients. About 25% of NSCLC patients have 2+ or greater expression of HER2/*neu*, but only 6%–8% have 3+ overexpression.[790] Adenocarcinomas have the highest degree of expression. Less than 10% of patients with NSCLC have true gene amplification. Trastuzumab is a monoclonal antibody to HER2 and is approved for use in breast cancers that overexpress the HER2 protein.[791] A number of phase II trials have been completed combining trastuzumab with chemotherapy.[792] Gatzemeier and colleagues[793] reported a randomized phase II trial of gemcitabine/cisplatin ± trastuzumab in NSCLC patients overexpressing HER2. The results of this study indicated that there was no benefit for the additon of trastuzumab to chemotherapy in patients with advanced NSCLC. Considering the fact that very few patients strongly express HER2 and/or have gene amplification, it is not surprising that there is a lack of efficacy for this approach.

EGFR is a recognized modulator of the malignant process, and its aberrant expression or activation in tumor tissue has been associated with a poor prognosis in NSCLC and other solid tumors.[794] A number of new agents inhibit this target, including monoclonal antibodies such as IMC-C225, and small-molecule tyrosine kinase inhibitors (ZD1839 and OSI-774).[795] ZD1839 or gefitinib is the agent farthest along in clinical development. In phase I trials, ZD1839 was investigated in a variety of tumors that express EGFR-TK.[796] One hundred patients with refractory NSCLC were treated, and ten had a partial response. Diarrhea was the dose-limiting toxicity, and a frequent side effect was an acneiform rash. Because of the promising antitumor activity in phase I studies, randomized global and U.S.-based trials were conducted to evaluate two doses of ZD1839 as second- or third-line therapy in patients with advanced NSCLC. The IDEAL-1 trial randomized patients who had received at least one platinum-based chemotherapy to 250 or 500 mg/day of ZD1839.[797] The response rates were 18% and 19%, respectively, and the disease control rate was 54% and 51%, respectively (response + stable disease rates). Rapid improvement was seen in cancer-related symptoms, and patients tolerated the drug well, with side effects that were similar to those seen in the phase I trials.[798] The IDEAL-2 trial was conducted in the United States.[799,780] The patients had two or more previous treatments that contained platinum and docetaxel. All the patients had cancer-related symptoms, and a higher percentage were performance status 2. The response rates were 12% for 250 mg/day and 9% for 500 mg/day, with symptom improvement rates of 43% and 35%, respectively. Treatment outcomes were better for women and for patients with adenocarcinoma and bronchioalveolar histologies. These were the first large randomized trials to show activity for an EGFR inhibitor in patients with advanced NSCLC who had exhausted their treatment options.

The next logical step in the development of ZD1839 was to combine it with chemotherapy. Two large trials (1000 patients per study) were developed that randomized patients to receive chemotherapy plus ZD1839 250 mg/day or 500 mg/day or placebo. In the INTACT-1 trial, the chemotherapy was cisplatin/gemcitabine, and in the INTACT-2 trial, carboplatin/paclitaxel was used.[801,802] Both trials were presented at the ESMO meeting in 2002. Unfortunately, there was no survival benefit for the addition of ZD1839 to chemotherapy for either trial. As of May, 2003, the FDA had approved ZD1839 for use as a third-line therapy based on the phase II results.

Many new drugs are currently under investigation in a number of trials. There is a great interest in anti-angiogenesis agents. A monoclonal antibody to vascular endothelial growth factor (VEGF) has been used in combination with carboplatin/paclitaxel in chemo-naïve patients with NSCLC.[803,804] There was a trend toward better survival for patients who received the anti-VEGF and chemotherapy. Because there were several incidences of life-threatening pulmonary hemorrhage in patients with squamous histology, ECOG is currently conducting a phase III trial of carboplatin/paclitaxel with or without anti-VEGF in NSCLC patients with nonsquamous histology.

Other agents that are of interest include the matrix metalloproteinase inhibitors, antisense oligonucleotides, farnesyl-transferase inhibitors, and COX-2 inhibitors. This list by no means is all-inclusive but rather represents an example of some of the new targeted agents that are being evaluated in clinical trials and is indicative of a new direction for clinical research in lung cancer.

Specific Malignancies

III

SMALL CELL LUNG CANCER

Small cell lung cancer (SCLC) differs from NSCLC in several biologic, clinical, and therapeutic aspects, although the improvements in outcome for non–small cell lung cancer have blurred many of the clinical outcome differences. SCLC has a larger growth fraction, grows more rapidly, and more often has disseminated disease at diagnosis. The disease is characterized by large central tumors, and very few patients are asymptomatic at diagnosis. SCLC has a response rate of 60%–80% to initial combination chemotherapy, but despite such high response rates, the overall long-term (5-year) survival is less than 10%.

Staging

The TNM staging system is typically not used in patients with small cell lung cancer because surgical resection is rarely considered once the diagnosis is established, but most lung cancer clinical trialists would prefer that this system be used.[82] SCLC patients are staged according to the two-stage classification originally developed by the Veterans Administration Lung Cancer Study Group, which categorizes patients into limited- or extensive-stage disease (Table 75-31).[805] Limited-stage disease is typically limited to one hemithorax with hilar and mediastinal lymph nodes that can be included in a single radiation port. Extensive-stage disease is beyond the boundaries just defined.

Although this simple staging system has gained acceptance due to its easy applicability, there are areas of controversy. These pertain to ipsilateral pleural effusions, contralateral mediastinal nodes, and supraclavicular (ipsilateral or contralateral) nodes. Many limited-stage disease clinical trials have excluded patients with involvement of these areas, particularly patients with ipsilateral pleural effusions. Analysis of large series has failed to identify a difference in survival attributable to presence of isolated pleural effusions. A SWOG analysis of outcome of patients with small cell lung cancer demonstrated that the survival of patients with isolated pleural effusion without evidence of systemic metastases was nearly identical to that of patients with limited-stage disease, even if the

pleural effusion contained malignant cells.[806] It is important to realize that only a small minority of patients with limited-stage disease have isolated pleural effusions; therefore, it could be difficult to detect true differences in survival.

In 1989, the International Association for the Study of Lung Cancer recommended that limited-stage disease should include hilar, ipsilateral, contralateral mediastinal, and ispsilateral supraclavicular lymph nodes and ipsilateral pleural effusions, irrespective of whether the effusion is positive or negative for malignant cells.[807] The Association based these conclusions on the observation that the outcomes of these patients are similar to that of patients with limited disease and superior to that of patients with extensive-stage disease. The primary implication of limited-stage disease is the inclusion of radiation therapy in the management. Clinical judgment should be used in selecting patients for combined-modality therapy, especially early concurrent chemotherapy and radiation. It is not unreasonable to begin chemotherapy in patients with pleural effusion or supraclavicular or contralateral mediastinal lymph nodes and to initiate combined-modality therapy based on patients' clinical progressions and responses.

Staging Procedures

The primary objectives of staging procedures are to define the stage of the disease and to evaluate patient's symptoms properly (Tables 75-32 and 75-33). It is appropriate to terminate staging procedures once extensive stage has

---

TABLE 75-32

Staging Procedures in SCLC

Mandatory

History and physical examination

Laboratory

Complete blood count, electrolytes, liver functions, LDH
  CT scan of the thorax (that includes liver and adrenals)
Brain evaluation (MRI preferred)

Required in Certain Patients

Bone scan
Bone marrow aspirate and biopsy (rare)

Investigational

PET scans

TABLE 75-31

Definition of Limited and Extensive Stage for Patients with Small Cell Lung Cancer[805]

STAGE	PERCENT
Limited	30–40
Disease confined to one hemithorax with or without ipsilateral or contralateral mediastinal or supraclavicular lymph node metastasis and with or without ipsilateral pleural effusions independent of cytology	
Extensive	
Any disease at sites beyond the definition of limited disease	60–70

TABLE 75-33

Sites of Metastases in Patients Presenting with Small Cell Lung Cancer

SITE	PERCENT
Liver	30
Bone	25
Bone marrow	20
Brain	10
Extrathoracic lymph nodes	5
Subcutaneous masses	5

been established in a patient. One possible exception is the evaluation of the brain for metastatic disease.

Initial evaluation of all patients should include medical history, a physical examination, review of the histopathology specimen, complete blood count, and biochemical tests that include evaluation of electrolytes, liver function, BUN, creatinine, and LDH. All patients should undergo CT scan evaluation of the chest that includes the adrenals and liver. CT scanning is superior to chest radiographs in evaluating the tumor extent and mediastinal involvement. CT scans are also necessary in patients with limited-stage disease to plan the radiation fields.

Brain is a common site of metatstatic disease in SCLC. In patients who are being considered for thoracic radiation or surgery, brain imaging should be performed to rule out asymptomatic metastases. MRI with contrast enhancement is more sensitive in detecting brain metastases than are CT scans, particularly with regard to posterior fossa lesions.[808,809] MRI scans are also helpful in differentiating cerebral metastases from other brain lesions.

Bone marrow is involved in about 20% of patients with small cell lung cancer at the time of initial diagnosis but is seldom the only site of metastatic disease. Though bone marrow biopsies were routinely performed for staging SCLC patients in the past, many investigators have reported that a bone marrow examination changes the stage in fewer than 5% of SCLC patients. The general agreement is that a bone marrow examination is not required in patients with normal blood counts.[810-812] Almost 40% of patients have bone involvement on a radionuclide bone scan at diagnosis, but again, it is uncommon for bone to be the sole site of metastatic disease. A bone scan is essential in patients deemed to have limited-stage disease, as bone scans can reveal bony metastases in asymptomatic patients.

The role of Positron Emission Tomography (PET) scans in SCLC patients has been reported recently in studies with small numbers of patients. Hauber and colleagues,[813] in a preliminary report, observed that PET scans detected all disease found by other staging procedures. Schumacher and coworkers[814] reported on the use of PET scans among 26 SCLC patients for initial staging. PET scans upstaged seven patients from limited-stage disease to extensive disease, and all of the sites suspicious for tumor involvement on other staging modalities were also detected on PET scans. In the same study, six patients underwent PET scans after therapy. In one patient, PET scan suggested residual viability in the primary tumor when other staging studies did not detect any residual tumor. Another study has reported similar results, with 2 of 18 patients being upstaged by PET scans. These studies suggest that PET scans could be helpful in staging SCLC patients. The greatest utility of PET scans is likely to be in selecting patients for combined-modality therapy and possibly for restaging patients. All of the above studies are small, however, and the data regarding the utility of PET scans in SCLC is limited.

Paraneoplastic Syndromes

Paraneoplastic syndromes are more common in SCLC than in NSCLC. Many of the paraneoplastic syndromes are mediated by the production of peptide hormones or antibodies. The types of syndromes associated with SCLC are different from the ones observed in NSCLC. Thus, hypertrophic osteoarthropathy and hypercalcemia are uncommon in SCLC, while SIADH, Cushing's syndrome, or neurologic syndromes are by far more common in SCLC than NSCLC.

Approximately 15% of SCLC patients present with hyponatremia, but only 5% of the patients are symptomatic for this condition. Ectopic production of arginine vasopressin causes hyponatremia and SIADH.[16] In some SCLC patients who do not have evidence of vasopressin production, hyponatremia is a result of atrial natriuretic factor (ANF) production.[815-817] Cushing's syndrome is clinically apparent in about 5% of SCLC patients. Ectopic production of adrenocorticotropic hormone (ACTH) precursors is present in many SCLC tumors.[818-820] There appears to be a defect in converting these precursors to ACTH in a majority of the tumors.[821] Some studies have suggested limited survival in patients with hyponatremia and Cushing's syndrome.[820,822-824]

Multiple neurologic syndromes have been observed with SCLC. These appear to be mediated by autoantibodies directed against neural tissue.[825] The most common syndrome is Lambert-Eaton syndrome, which is characterized by proximal muscle weakness. The syndrome is a result of antibodies directed against voltage-gated channels, interfering in the release of acetylcholine from cholinergic fibers.[826,827] Other neurologic syndromes observed are subacute peripheral neuropathy, encephalomyelitis, cerebellar ataxia, retinopathy, and necrotizing myelopathy.[825,828-832] These syndromes can occur before the diagnosis of SCLC, and the neurologic paraneoplastic syndromes might not improve with treatment for SCLC.

Prognostic Factors

Although the simple staging system provides worthwhile prognostic information, analyses of large databases from several cooperative groups have identified subgroups of patients with both limited- and extensive-stage disease who have different outcomes. Such classification of patients could be helpful in prognosticating for individual patients and in the accurate stratification of patients enrolling in clinical trials. Many studies have analyzed prognostic factors in SCLC (Table 75-34).[823,833-838] Overall, 33 prognostic variables influencing survival have been investigated in these reports. Four variables that are common to all studies are age, gender, performance status, and disease stage. Performance status reflects the overall extent of the disease and is also predictive of tolerance of the patient to therapeutic modalities. Lactate dehydrogenase (LDH) is another variable that is found to be an independent prognostic factor for survival. LDH is elevated in about 70% of patients with extensive disease and in 40% of patients with limited stage disease and correlates well with both stage of disease and response to treatment.[839] In patients with extensive-stage disease, patients with a single site of metastasis have significantly longer survival than patients with multiple sites; in fact, their survival could be similar to that of patients with

TABLE 75-34

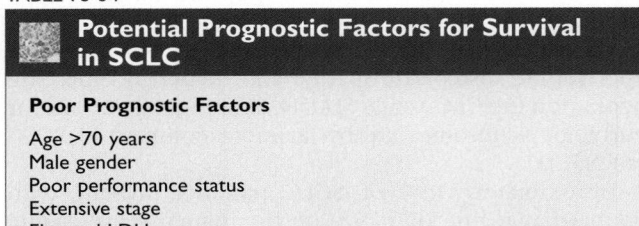

Potential Prognostic Factors for Survival in SCLC

Poor Prognostic Factors

Age >70 years
Male gender
Poor performance status
Extensive stage
Elevated LDH
Multiple metastatic sites

TABLE 75-35

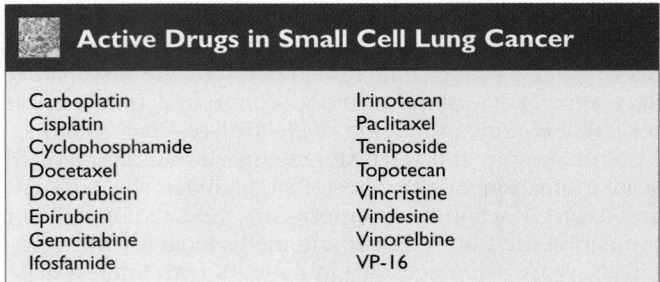

Active Drugs in Small Cell Lung Cancer

Carboplatin	Irinotecan
Cisplatin	Paclitaxel
Cyclophosphamide	Teniposide
Docetaxel	Topotecan
Doxorubicin	Vincristine
Epirubicin	Vindesine
Gemcitabine	Vinorelbine
Ifosfamide	VP-16

limited-stage disease. Patients with specific metastatic sites (e.g., brain and liver) have a worse prognosis.

Albain and colleagues,[834] in an analysis of the Southwest Oncology Group (SWOG) database, found good performance status, age less than 70 years, female gender, white race, and normal LDH as significant favorable predictors of survival in patients with limited-stage SCLC. Combined-modality therapy was also a strong predictor of survival. In extensive-stage SCLC, the presence of a single metastatic site and a normal LDH were favorable predictors of survival. Based on these analyses, patients could be classified into four groups with distinct survival outcomes. The best survival occurred in young patients with limited disease without effusion and a normal LDH. The poorest survival occurred in patients with extensive-stage disease and an elevated LDH.

Treatment

Therapy of SCLC has evolved over the years due to a better understanding of the biology of the disease and thanks to clinical data that has been generated through the years. Autopsy studies have shown that visceral metastases are common even in patients with limited-stage SCLC. In an autopsy study of patients who underwent potentially curative surgery and died of

unrelated causes shortly after surgery, 63% had visceral metastases.[840] These and other autopsy studies suggest the need for systemic therapy in most patients with SCLC.

Initially, surgery was the treatment of choice for all lung cancers, including SCLC. The Medical Research Council (MRC) in the United Kingdom conducted a study randomizing SCLC patients to radiation therapy alone or surgery alone. The study demonstrated a modest superiority of radiation therapy over surgery. Only 5% of patients were alive at 5 years, and all of the surviving patients were on the radiation arm.[841] Based on such autopsy and clinical studies, surgery alone is no longer considered as a therapeutic option for SCLC patients unless the patient is found to have a true T1N0 lesion.

Chemotherapy

The first studies evaluating chemotherapy in SCLC were conducted in the 1960s. Green and coworkers[842] found that three courses of single-agent cyclophosphamide improved survival over placebo in patients with extensive-stage SCLC.[842] Since then, a number of agents have been evaluated in SCLC patients and found to be active (Table 75-35). After the initial evaluation of anthracyclines and alkylators (which produced a response rate of 40%–50%), the platinum analogs and epipodophyllotoxins

RECOMMENDED TREATMENT STRATEGIES

LIMITED STAGE
Cisplatin 75mg/m² on day 1
Etoposide 100 mg/m² days 1-3
Concurrent chest radiation therapy
In patients with complete response recommend prophylactic cranial radiation (PCR)

EXTENSIVE STAGE
Good Performance Status
Cisplatin 60-90 mg/m² over 1 to 3 days or Carboplatin 300 mg/m² on day 1
and
Etoposide 80-120 mg/m² on days 1-3

Cyclophosphamide 1000 mg/m² day 1
and
Doxorubicin 45 mg/m2, day 1
and
Vincristine 2 mg, day 1
CAV alternating with EP
Cisplatin 60 mg/m² on day 1
and
Irinotecan 60 mg/m² on days 1, 8, 15, every 28 days

EXTENSIVE STAGE
Poor Performance Status
Cisplatin/Carboplatin and etoposide
Carboplatin
Carboplatin and gemcitabine

were introduced in the 1980s and demonstrated similar single-agent response rates. Subsequently, in the 1990s, taxanes, camptothecins, and gemcitabine have been evaluated and have demonstrated activity in SCLC.

Prior therapy and response to it appear to be important prognostic factors in predicting response to a new agent. Thus, responses are higher in previously untreated patients compared with sensitive relapse patients (progression-free survival of ≥3 months after completion of chemotherapy), which in turn are higher than in patients with refractory relapse. Based on retrospective analyses, a new agent is deemed active in SCLC if the response rates are higher than 10% in refractory patients, 20% or higher in patients with sensitive relapse, and about 30% in previously untreated patients.[843,844] Ettinger on behalf of the ECOG[845] and Evans and colleagues for NCIC[846] addressed ethical concerns about the appropriateness of enrolling previously untreated patients with extensive-stage SCLC, who are likely to derive benefits from systemic chemotherapy, on clinical trials evaluating new agents. These studies found that the overall survival and response rates of patients enrolled on clinical trials were reasonable irrespective of the activity of the new drug.

Combination Chemotherapy. Despite the partial responses observed, the overall results with single-agent therapy in SCLC are poor. In a retrospective review, 70% response rates were observed with combination chemotherapy, while the response rates with single-agent therapy were only 20%.[847] Survival was also longer in patients receiving combination chemotherapy. Multidrug combinations were developed and compared with single-agent cyclophosphamide in randomized studies and were found to be better.[848] The combination of cyclophosphamide, doxorubicin, and vincristine (CAV) evolved from these and subsequent studies and became a standard for many years.[849]

In the 1980s, VP-16 was identified as an active drug for the treatment of SCLC. The schedule of administration appears to influence the activity of VP-16. Bolus administration of VP-16 for 3 to 5 days every 3 weeks is superior to one bolus dose or infusion of VP-16 over 24 hours or 72 hours.[850-853] With the introduction of VP-16, several modifications of the CAV regimen that included VP-16 were evaluated. Modest improvements were observed when VP-16 was substituted for doxorubicin or vincristine.[854,855] Five randomized studies have evaluated the addition of VP-16 to CAV.[856-860] Greater hematologic toxicity was observed with the addition of VP-16 in all of these studies. In only one of the five studies was a very slight improvement in response duration and survival observed with the addition of VP-16.[857]

As single agents, cisplatin and carboplatin demonstrate response rates of 15% in previously treated patients and of about 60% in untreated patients.[861] Based on individual activity of cisplatin and VP-16 in SCLC, preclinical synergistic activity between the agents, and efficacy of the combination in other diseases, the combination of cisplatin and VP-16 (EP) was evaluated in SCLC. In patients previously treated with CAV, the combination of

EP produced a response rate of 55%, and in previously untreated patients the response rate was 86%.[862-864] Prospective randomized studies demonstrated comparable efficacy between EP and CAV, though the toxicity was less with EP.[865,866] Based on these results, EP became an alternative to CAV as part of a front-line regimen in the treatment of SCLC. In a meta-analysis of randomized trials comparing cisplatin regimens with a noncisplatin regimen, patients randomized to cisplatin-based regimens had a higher probability of response and survival.[867] Mascaux and coworkers[868] conducted a detailed analysis of the role of EP in the treatment of SCLC. They analyzed data of 36 trials conducted between 1980 and 1998. The authors concluded that regimens that included VP-16 and cisplatin showed a survival benefit with a high level of significance.

Carboplatin has been compared with cisplatin in combination with VP-16 and produces a similar response rate and survival. Phase II studies of carboplatin and VP-16 produced a response rate of 73%–93% in patients with limited-stage SCLC and 50%-85% in patients with extensive-stage disease.[869] The Hellenic Oncology Group randomized 147 patients to VP-16 at 100 mg/m^2 given on days 1 through 3 with either cisplatin at 50 mg/m^2 given on days 1 and 2, or carboplatin at 300 mg/m^2 given on day 1.[870] The cycles were administered every 3 weeks. Patients with limited-stage disease received radiation therapy after the third cycle. The median survival was similar in the two arms (12.5 months in the cisplatin/VP-16 arm and 11.8 months in the carboplatin/VP-16 arm). Patients who received carboplatin and etoposide experienced significantly less toxicity. Nausea and vomiting, nephrotoxicity, neurotoxicity, leukopenia, infection, and mucositis were reported less frequently for patients in the carboplatin arm. Grade 2/3 nausea and vomiting occurred in 75% of patients receiving etoposide and cisplatin, while nausea and vomiting occurred in only 25% of patients receiving etoposide and carboplatin (p = 0.0001). Patients assigned to the carboplatin arm had fewer hospitalizations.

A recent Japanese trial compared the combination of cisplatin and irinotecan with cisplatin and etoposide.[871] Patients were randomized to receive cisplatin at 60 mg/m^2 on day 1 with irinotecan at 60 mg/m^2 on days 1, 8, and 15 or cisplatin 80 mg/m^2 and VP-16 at 100 mg/m^2 on days 1, 2, and 3. The cisplatin and irinotecan combination was administered every 4 weeks, and the cisplatin and etoposide combination was given every 3 weeks. Both regimens were administered for four cycles. The trial was terminated at planned interim analyses, as the patients on the cisplatin and irinotecan arm had a clear survival advantage. The cisplatin and irinotecan arm had a superior response rate (84% vs 68%, p = 0.02), progression-free survival (6.9 months vs. 4.8 months, p = 0.003), and median survival (12.8 months vs. 9.4 months, p = 0.002). SWOG is currently conducting a trial to confirm the results of this Japanese study.

Multi-agent Chemotherapy. The addition of a third drug to the combination of cisplatin and etoposide has been investigated in multiple trials. The Hoosier Oncology

Group evaluated the addition of ifosfamide to cisplatin and VP-16. One hundred seventy-one patients with extensive-stage SCLC were randomized to the triplet combination or the doublet of cisplatin and etoposide.[872] A small but significant benefit in both median survival (9.0 months vs. 7.3 months) and 2-year survival (13% vs. 5%) was observed with the addition of ifosfamide. Greater myelotoxicity was observed in the ifosfamide arm. A smaller study that included patients with both limited- and extensive-stage disease showed no benefit to the addition of ifosfamide.[873]

Mavroudis and colleagues[874] compared the addition of paclitaxel to etoposide and platinum (TEP) with standard EP. The study was terminated early due to a higher number of toxic deaths with the three-drug regimen. Despite longer time to progression with TEP, the overall survival was not different between the treatment arms. Niell and associates[875] reported similar results for the CALGB in another phase III randomized study evaluating the addition of paclitaxel to standard EP. There are other multi-agent combinations that have been evaluated. Currently, there is no consistent evidence of benefit to the addition of a third drug to the standard combination of etoposide and platinum.

Duration of Therapy and Maintenance Therapy. Until the 1980s, patients were treated with multiple cycles of chemotherapy, often for the entire duration of the patients' lives. Randomized studies were conducted to address both the issue of duration of the initial chemotherapy and the value of maintenance chemotherapy (Table 75-36).

Many randomized studies have addressed the issue of continuing chemotherapy in patients responding to initial chemotherapy. Two studies did report a benefit to the use of maintenance chemotherapy. Mauler and associates[876] reported for the CALGB on a trial that randomized patients who achieved complete responses after induction therapy to six additional cycles of chemotherapy or observation. Among the 46 patients with limited-stage SCLC, survival was improved in patients who received maintenance therapy. Cullen and colleagues[877] evaluated maintenance CAV vs. no further therapy in patients after six cycles of induction CAV. Sixty-one patients with extensive-stage disease had a survival advantage with maintenance therapy. A third study reported by the Medical Research Council of Britain demonstrated a survival advantage, in a subset analysis, for patients who had achieved complete remission to the initial induction chemotherapy.[878] None of the other studies showed a survival advantage to the use of maintenance therapy. Patients treated on the maintenance chemotherapy suffered from increased toxicities. Also, it was observed that patients not receiving maintenance therapy were

TABLE 75-36

Randomized Trials of Chemotherapy with or without Maintenance Chemotherapy in Small Cell Lung Cancer

STUDY	NO. OF PATIENTS	NO. OF RANDOMIZED PATIENTS	LD AND/OR ED	CHEMOTHERAPY	MEDIAN SURVIVAL	P VALUE
Maurer et al[876]	258	57	Both	C CM CMV CM (HD) C with LCV +/– maintenance treatment with same chemotherapy	16.9 v 6.8 mo (LD)	.01
Cullen et al[877]	309	93	Both	VAC X 6 VAC X 6 + VAC X 8	372 v 259 d (ED)	.006
Byrne et al[981]	66	66	LD	EP/CMV X 3 EP/CMV X 3 + CMV X 6	19.2 mo 14.1 mo	.05
Bleehen et al[986]	497	265	Both	CEMV X 6 CEMV X 12	29 wk 35 wk	.27
Bleehen et al[879]	458	458	Both	ECMV X 3 ECMV X 6 EI X 6	7.4 mo 8.6 mo 8.8 mo	NS
Ettinger et al[982]	577	86	ED	CAV or CAV/Hem X 6–8 +/– maintenance treatment with same chemotherapy	NA	.90/.13
Lebeau et al[983]	320	79	Both	LCAE X 6 LCAE X 12	332 d 244 d	.41
Giaccone et al[984]	687	585	ED	CAE X 5 CAE X 12	288 d 275 d	.70
Beith et al[985]	202	129	Both	EP X 4 EP X 4 then CAV X 10	52 wk 54 wk	.72
Shevlin et al[987]	225		NA	EIMV X 3 EIMV X 6	307 dys 313 dys	
Spiro et al[880]	289		Both	CEV X 4 CEV X 8	38 wks 38–42 wks	NS

A, doxorubicin; C, cyclophosphamide; E, etoposide; Hem, hexamethymelamine; I, ifosfamide; L, lomustine; M, methotrexate; P, platinum; V, vincristine.

more likely to respond to salvage chemotherapy. Thus, at the current time it does not appear that maintenance chemotherapy provides a survival advantage, and it reduces the quality of life.

A number of studies have addressed the issue of minimum number of chemotherapy cycles. The Medical Research Council randomized 458 patients to either three or six cycles of combination etoposide, cyclophosphamide, methotrexate, and vincristine (ECMV) or six cycles of ifosfamide and etoposide. There was no statistical difference in survival between the three arms, although the study was not sufficiently powered to rule out a small survival advantage for the arms with six cycles of chemotherapy.[879] Spiro and coworkers[880] randomized 610 patients to four or eight cycles of cyclophosphamide, etoposide, and vincristine, with a further randomization at disease progression to second-line chemotherapy (methotrexate and doxorubicin) or no salvage therapy. There was no difference in response rate between patients receiving four cycles and eight cycles. The only group of patients who had an inferior survival was the group who received four cycles of chemotherapy but no chemotherapy at disease progression.

Based on the observation that topotecan has activity in relapsed SCLC, ECOG evaluated the benefit of topotecan in patients responding to initial chemotherapy. Patients who had a response or stable disease after four cycles of etoposide and cisplatin were randomized to four cycles of topotecan or observation. Though there was a slight prolongation of progression-free survival with topotecan, the overall survival was no different between the two arms.[881]

Based on the foregoing data, four to six cycles of chemotherapy represents adequate induction chemotherapy for SCLC patients. Maintenance chemotherapy or continuing chemotherapy beyond four to six cycles is more likely to produce toxicity without prolonging survival. It is possible that in the subset of patients with complete response to induction chemotherapy, there could be a benefit from maintenance chemotherapy. The available data is inadequate to make any firm conclusions regarding this subset.

Alternating Non–cross-resistant Chemotherapy. Based on the initial high response rate and the subsequent high rate of relapse, investigators have theorized that clones of cells present in tumors are resistant or less sensitive to initial chemotherapy. Optimal antitumor activity could be achieved with multiple active agents, administered simultaneously, which affect all the clones of cells within the tumor. Drug toxicity limits such an approach, however. The mathematical model proposed by Goldie and Coldman[882] suggests that rapid alternation of non–cross-resistant regimens could maximize tumor kill while limiting drug toxicity. Most of the studies that evaluated this concept have compared CAV with CAV alternating with EP (Table 75-37). The combination of etoposide and cisplatin does demonstrate a response rate of 50% in patients who have previously received CAV, suggesting that EP is potentially non–cross-resistant to CAV. Thus,

TABLE 75-37

Alternating Non–Cross-Resistant Chemotherapy Phase III Trials

REFERENCE	NO. OF PATIENTS	CHEMO	MS (MO)	P-VALUE
Evans[883]	289	CAV	8.0	
		CAV/PE	9.6	0.03
Fukuoka[866]	142	CAV	8.7	
		EP	8.3	
		CAV/EP	9.0	0.898
Roth[865]	437	CAV	8.6	
		EP	8.3	
		CAV/EP	8.1	0.425
Postmus[988]	143	CDE	7.6	
		CDE/VIMCA	8.7	0.243

A, doxorubicin; C, Cytoxan; CA, carboplatin; E, etoposide; I, ifosfamide; M, MESNA; P, cisplatin; V, vincristine.

it is feasible to affect many more clones of cancer cells by alternating between these two regimens, which could lead to better outcomes. The National Cancer Institute in Canada (NCIC) evaluated six cycles of CAV with CAV alternating with EP, for a total of six cycles in patients with extensive-stage SCLC.[883] The response rate (80% vs. 63.2%, p < 0.002) and survival (9.6 months vs. 8.0 months, p = 0.003) was better in the patients who received the alternating regimen. The presence of EP in the experimental arm, rather than the concept of alternating regimens, might have contributed to the superiority of this treatment. Southeastern Cancer Study Group (SECSG) compared EP, CAV, and alternating EP and CAV in patients with extensive-stage SCLC. Response rates and survival were almost identical for all three regimens.[865]

Fukuoka and associates[866] conducted a randomized study that included patients with both limited- and extensive-stage SCLC, evaluating CAV, EP, and CAV alternating with PE. In patients with limited disease, radiation therapy was administered after the completion of chemotherapy. The overall survival was modestly better with the alternating regimen (CAV/EP, 11.8 months; EP, 9.9 months; CAV, 9.9 months; p = 0.056). When the study was analyzed by stage, there was no difference in survival among the three arms in patients with extensive-stage disease; however, there was a significant survival advantage for the alternating regimen in patients with limited-stage disease (CAV/EP, 16.8 months; EP, 11.7 months p = 0.023; CAV, 12.4 months, p = 0.014).

These studies suggest that there is no benefit to the use of alternating regimens in patients with extensive-stage disease. In the study by Fukuoka and associates,[866] benefit for patients with limited-stage disease was observed with the use of alternating regimens. Radiation therapy was delivered in this study after the completion of chemotherapy, however. It is unclear whether alternating regimens would prove beneficial in patients with limited-stage disease over the standard therapy of concurrent EP chemotherapy and radiation. The lack of benefit from the alternating regimens could be related to the lack of true non–cross-resistant regimens, as no higher than

Specific Malignancies

III

50% response is observed as salvage therapy with any of the regimens. Appropriate testing of the Goldie and Coldman[882] hypothesis requires identification of truly non–cross-resistant drugs.

Dose Intensification

Preclinical tumor models suggest a steep dose-response curve for most chemotherapeutic drugs. It is therefore hypothesized that drug resistance might be overcome by escalating the dose intensification of the drugs. This can be achieved either by escalating the drug dosages or by delivering the drugs more frequently. The limiting factor to dose intensification is the toxicities from the drug. In the late 1970s, Cohen and colleagues[884] conducted a randomized study comparing standard-dose cyclophosphamide, methotrexate, and lomustine or higher dose of cyclophosphamide and lomustine and standard-dose methotrexate. These investigators observed both a higher overall response rate and a prolonged survival in the high-dose arm. The dosages used in the standard-dose arm would be considered inadequate by current standards. Nonetheless, the results of this study spurred interest in dose intensification.

Dose Intensification by Increasing Dose.

Several studies have explored the concept of increasing the dose of the drugs (Table 75-38). The Southeast Cancer Study Group evaluated higher-dose cyclophosphamide and doxorubicin in the CAV regimen compared with standard-dose CAV in patients with extensive-stage disease. The overall response rates (higher-dose CAV 63%, CAV 53%) and median survival duration (higher-dose CAV 29.3 weeks, CAV 34.7 weeks) were statistically not different in the two arms. The higher-dose arm demonstrated substantially higher toxicity.[885] Figueredo and coworkers,[886] in a randomized study evaluating escalation of the same drugs in the CAV regimen, observed similar results.

Ihde and associates[887] explored dose escalation of etoposide and cisplatin in patients with extensive-stage disease. Patients on the standard arm received etoposide, 80 mg/m^2 per day for 3 days and cisplatin, 80 mg/m^2 on day 1. On the higher-dose arm, patients received etoposide, 80 mg/m^2 per day for 5 days and cisplatin, 27 mg/m^2 per day for 5 days. There was no difference in

the two arms with respect to response rates (85% and 81%, respectively) or median survival (12 and 11 months, respectively). Higher myelosuppression was observed in the high-dose arm.

These results contrast with results reported by Arriagada and colleagues.[888] They randomized 105 patients with limited stage SCLC to standard-dose cisplatin, etoposide, cyclophosphamide, and doxorubicin alternating with thoracic radiation or the same treatment plan except for a 20% higher dose of cyclophosphamide and cisplatin in the first cycle only. The response rate and the overall survival were higher in the higher-dose group. It is accepted that split-course radiation might compromise the results from radiation therapy. It is unclear whether the higher-dose treatment arm from the Arriagada study, in which the radiation was split course, would be better than the standard treatment plan of cisplatin and etoposide given concurrently with radiation therapy.

Dose Intensification by Increasing Dose Density.

Dose intensification can also be achieved by shortening the interval between cycles (Table 75-39). Steward and coworkers[889] conducted a randomized study with a 2 × 2 factorial design, with randomization to six cycles of vincristine, cyclophosphamide, carboplatin, and etoposide given every 3 or 4 weeks and a second randomization to GM-CSF or placebo. Patients with both limited- and extensive-stage SCLC were included in the study. Radiation therapy was at the discretion of the treating physician, and the actual number of patients who received radiation therapy is unclear. GM-CSF did not reduce the complications from myelosuppression, nor did it impact on survival. On the other hand, the 3-week treatment arm had a superior median (443 and 351 days) and 2-year survival (33% and 18%) compared with the 4-week treatment arm. Similar improvement in survival rates were reported by the British Medical Research Council in a study comparing adriamycin, cyclophosphamide, and etoposide given every 3 weeks or 2 weeks with the use of G-CSF.[890]

EORTC evaluated dose intensification with weekly multiagent chemotherapy (doxorubicin, etoposide, cyclophosphamide, vincristine, cisplatin, and methotrexate)

TABLE 75-38

Randomized Trials of Dose Intensification by Increasing Dose					
STUDY	**NO. OF PATIENTS**	**LD AND/OR ED**	**CHEMOTHERAPY**	**MEDIAN SURVIVAL**	**P VALUE**
Johnson[885]	298	ED	hd CAV	34.7 wks	>0.05
			sd CAV	29.3 wks	
Figueredo[886]	103	Both	hd AVC	9 mo	NS
			sd AVC	7 mo	
Ihde[887]	90	ED	hd EP	11.4 mo	.68
			sd EP	10.7 mo	
Arriagada[888]	105	LD	hd CDPE	18 mo	0.02
			sd CDPE	14 mo	

ED, extensive disease; LD, limited disease.

TABLE 75-39

Randomized Trials of Dose Intensification by Increasing Dose Density

STUDY	NO. OF PATIENTS	LD AND/OR ED	CHEMOTHERAPY	MEDIAN SURVIVAL	P VALUE
Steward[889]	300	Both	O-ICaE every 3 wks (GM-CSF) V-ICaE every 4 wks	443 351 d	.0014
Thatcher[890]	403	Both	DCE every 2 wks DCE every 3 wks	47% at 1 yr 39% at 1 yr	.04
Sculier[891]	233	ED	Multidrug—3 weekly DCE—3 weekly	49 wks 43 wks	NS
Murray[892]	219	ED	CODE, weekly CyDO/EP, every 3 wks	0.98 yr 0.91 yr	NS
Furuse[893]	227	ED	CODE, GCSF CyDO/EP, every 3 wks	11.6 mo 10.9	NS
Ardizzoni[894]	244	Both	CyDE, GCSF, every 2 wks CyDE, every 3 wks	52 wks 52 wks	0.885

C, cisplatin; Ca, carboplatin; Cy, cyclophosphamide; D, doxorubicin; E, etoposide; ED, extensive disease; I, ifosfamide; LD, limited disease; Multidrug, doxorubicin, etoposide, cyclophosphamide, cisplatin, vindesine, vincristine, methotrexate; O, vincristine.

compared with cyclophosphamide, doxorubicin, and etoposide given every 3 weeks[891] There was no difference in the median or overall survival. The relative delivered dose intensity of the drugs common to both arms was actually lower in the weekly regimen due to treatment delays.

Canadian investigators reported encouraging results from a pilot study of a weekly regimen called CODE (cisplatin, vincristine, doxorubicin, and etoposide). Based on these promising results, NCIC and SWOG conducted a study comparing the CODE regimen with alternating CAV/EP in patients with extensive-stage SCLC.[892] A twofold increase in dose intensity was achieved in the CODE arm, as patients received slightly higher cumulative dosages of the four drugs and the treatment was completed in 9 weeks instead of 18 weeks. The progression-free survival or the overall survival was no better in the CODE arm, and ten patients died during chemotherapy in the CODE arm compared with one death in the control arm. Japanese investigators conducted a similar study but included G-CSF in the CODE arm.[893] Again there was no difference in survival, but despite the inclusion of G-CSF, the neutropenic fever rate was higher in the CODE arm compared with the control arm.

EORTC conducted a study in which the experimental arm had both dose increase as well as increased dose density. The standard arm received cyclophosphamide, doxorubicin, and etoposide at standard dosages every 3 weeks, while the experimental arm had about a 25% increase in the dosages of all three drugs, which were administered every 2 weeks with the use of G-CSF. The actual delivered dose intensification was 70% higher in the experimental arm. Despite greater toxicity in the dose-intensified arm, there was no difference in survival.[894]

Based on these trials, it does not appear that there is consistent benefit from dose intensification for patients with extensive-stage SCLC. As far as patients with limited-stage disease are concerned, the data suggests that it is important not to compromise on the drug dosages. It is unclear whether there is any benefit from intensifying the dosages beyond maximally tolerated dose. None of the dose-intensification trials have included concurrent radiation therapy, as toxicity precludes concurrent therapy when the dosages are intensified. It is therefore unclear whether the dose intensification strategies provide a benefit over and above standard concurrent etoposide and platinum chemotherapy and radiation.

High-dose Chemotherapy with Bone Marrow Transplant

One of the limiting factors in dose-intensification strategies is that very few achieve greater than a twofold increase in dose intensity, due primarily to hematologic toxicity. It is feasible to achieve higher dose intensification with cellular support such as bone marrow transplant (BMT). Small studies have addressed the issue of using BMT either as initial therapy or as late intensification in patients with SCLC. BMT has also been evaluated in patients with relapsed SCLC (Table 75-40).

Fourteen studies have reported on 52 patients with SCLC who received BMT in either relapsed or refractory disease.[895] Complete and partial responses were observed in 19% and 37% of patients, respectively, but the median response durations were only 2 to 3 months. A total of 103 patients with SCLC treated with high-dose therapy with BMT as the initial treatment have been reported.[896-901] Despite an impressive 42% complete response rate, the relapse-free, 2-year, and overall survival rates are comparable to those for patients treated with conventional chemotherapy. BMT as initial therapy for SCLC patients is challenging, as these patients are likely to have impaired performance status, resulting in high mortality rates and limiting the transplant dosages. Also, patients are more likely to have contamination of their bone marrow with tumor cells.

Specific Malignancies

III

TABLE 75-40

High Dose Intensification with BMT for SCLC

PATIENT	NO. OF PATIENTS	CR (%)	DF (%)	TOXIC DEATH (%)
Relapsed/refractory disease	52	19	0	13
Initial treatment	103	43	7	6
First PR/SD	189	42	8	11
ED	25		16	8
LD	85		38	1

Late intensification in patients responding to induction therapy has been evaluated in more patients than induction BMT. Humblet and colleagues[902] have conducted the only randomized study evaluating the concept of late intensification with BMT in patients with SCLC. The study randomized patients to five cycles of conventional chemotherapy followed by one cycle of either high-dose or conventional dose of cyclophosphamide, etoposide, and carmustine. Of 101 patients who entered the trial, 45 were eligible for randomization to high dose or conventional dose. Even though the relapse-free survival was higher in the high-dose arm (28 weeks vs. 10 weeks, p = 0.002), the overall survival was no different (68 weeks vs. 55 weeks, p = 0.13). Four patients (18%) died during the high-dose therapy. There are other small studies that have evaluated this concept with some success. Nonetheless, the small numbers, selection of good performance status, and relatively young patients in these studies limit proper interpretation of this data.

Despite the early promise of high-dose chemotherapy with autologous transplant, delivery of this therapy in patients with SCLC has severe limitations. Based on the expected aging of patients with lung cancer (particularly patients with SCLC), the relevance of this therapy is questionable. Many of the small studies of high-dose chemotherapy with cellular support were conducted with techniques that would be considered inadequate by current standards, however. With the improvement in supportive care and in transplantation techniques (introduction of stem cell transplant) in recent years, it could be feasible to limit the therapy-induced mortality and morbidity. It remains unclear whether a subset of younger patients undergoing dose intensification with cellular support by current standards might derive prolongation of survival.

Treatment of Elderly and Poor Performance Status Patients

Approximately 40%–50% of patients with lung cancer are above the age of 70 years.[1] With the population aging, this percentage is likely to increase. Also, SCLC is more typically associated with prolonged and heavy exposure to smoking. Therefore, the percentage of elderly patients with lung cancer who have SCLC is expected to increase over the next few years. Elderly patients are more likely to have poorer performance status and greater comorbid-

ity.[903,904] This has prompted the use of less aggressive therapy in these patients. In lung cancer trials, elderly patients have been significantly underrepresented; therefore, extrapolation of the available data to this population is limited.[905,906] Based on retrospective analysis, it is clear that elderly patients with good performance status and adequate organ function have outcomes similar to those for younger patients.[907,908] Greater toxicity, particularly hematologic, has been observed among elderly patients. It is therefore important to focus on the performance status of the patient rather than the age. Nonetheless, data for patients over the age of 80 years is very limited, and careful therapeutic decisions are crucial for these patients.

Among patients with poor performance status, concerns about tolerability of combination chemotherapy have lead to attempts at development of less toxic regimens. Single-agent oral etoposide, administered for 5 or 14 or 21 days, was evaluated as a "gentler" form of therapy.[909-912] The response rate ranged from 50% to 80%. These results led to two randomized studies evaluating oral etoposide as first-line therapy in patients with poor performance status. The British Medical Research Council conducted a trial comparing oral etoposide (50 mg twice daily for 10 days) with two IV combinations: etoposide with vincristine, and CAV.[912] The overall response rates were similar, but the survival data favored the IV arms of the study (183 days vs. 130 days, p = 0.03). Palliative effects were similar between the two arms of the study. A second British trial comparing oral etoposide (100 mg twice daily for 5 days) and CAV/EP among elderly or poor patients with extensive-stage SCLC and poor performance status found similar results.[913] Another trial compared single-agent carboplatin to CAV, with carboplatin demonstrating response rates, palliation of symptoms, and survival similar to those for the combination regimen.[914] Recently, results of a trial comparing carboplatin/gemcitabine with cisplatin/etoposide in patients with poor performance status were presented. The gemcitabine arm had more hematologic toxicity but less nonhematologic toxicity. Response rates and overall survival were similar between the two arms.[915] Several other less intensive regimens have been developed for patients with SCLC who have poor performance status; these regimens also incorporate thoracic radiation in patients with limited-stage disease.[916-920]

The foregoing data suggests that almost all patients with SCLC should be considered for chemotherapy because it provides symptom palliation and survival benefits. There does not appear to be a benefit to the use of oral etoposide over combination chemotherapy in patients with poor performance status. Introduction of newer agents, such as gemcitabine, could make it even more feasible to administer chemotherapy in poor-performance status patients with SCLC.

Relapsed SCLC

Despite high initial response rates, the response duration in patients with SCLC is usually short, with median progression-free survival of 4 months in extensive-stage

TABLE 75-41

Chemotherapy in Relapsed SCLC

	RESPONDERS/EVALUABLE (%)	
	SR	RD
Topotecan[922,923,996]	30/168 (18)	6/75 (8)
Irinotecan[924,925,997]	18/63 (28)	1/28 (3)
Docetaxel[929,998]	9/47 (19)*	
Paclitaxel[928]		7/24 (29)
Gemcitabine[932]		5/38 (14)
Vinorelbine[930,931]	7/41 (17)	0/8 (0)

*No data on sensitive and resistant disease.

disease and 12 months in limited-stage disease. Studies conducted in relapsed SCLC have revealed that two factors are predictive of response to further chemotherapy.[910,920,921] These are response to prior chemotherapy and progression-free survival from the previous chemotherapy. Lack of response to prior chemotherapy and/or progression-free survival of less than 3 months since the previous chemotherapy predicted for lack of response to salvage chemotherapy. Performance status and extent of disease at presentation were not predictive of response to salvage chemotherapy.

In reviewing results of clinical trials, it is important to consider whether the patients had sensitive relapse (patients who responded to prior chemotherapy and had progression-free intervals of greater than 3 months since last chemotherapy) or refractory disease. Multiple single-agent and combination chemotherapy trials have been conducted (Tables 75-41 and 75-42). Most trials, however, with the exception of trials of the topoisomerase I inhibitors topotecan and irinotecan, are small.

Both topotecan and irinotecan produce a response rate of about 24% in sensitive relapse patients but appear to be ineffective in patients with refractory disease, with response rates of less than 10%.[922-925] The median survival with both these agents is in the range of 5 to 7 months. Topotecan's activity in patients with sensitive relapse has been evaluated in randomized studies. In a large multicenter study, patients with a progression-free interval of greater than 60 days since the previous chemotherapy were randomized to topotecan or CAV (Table 75-43). The response rate and progression-free survival were quite similar, but the palliation of symptoms appeared to be better with single-agent topotecan.[926] Oral topotecan has been compared with IV topotecan in this setting and found to be equally efficacious.[927]

Oral etoposide induces responses in about 50% of patients whose disease recurs after treatment with regimens that included IV etoposide.[910] In one small study, paclitaxel demonstrated promising results in patients with refractory relapse.[928] Other single agents evaluated in patients with relapsed SCLC include docetaxel, gemcitabine, and vinorelbine.[929-932] The observed response rates

TABLE 75-42

Combination Chemotherapy in Relapsed SCLC

STUDY	REGIMEN	RESPONDERS/EVALUABLE (%)		MEDIUM SURVIVAL (WKS)
		SR	RD	
Masuda[990]	Irinotecan/etoposide	14/20 (70)	3/4 (75)	39
Ando[989]	Irinotecan/cisplatin	10/12 (83)	8/10 (80)	36+
Ardizzoni[992]	Topotecan/cisplatin	8/28 (28)	4/24 (17)	NR
Groen[991]	Paclitaxel/carboplatin		25/34 (73)*	31
Domine[993]	Gemcitabine/paclitaxel	8/13 (60)	7/18 (40)	NR
Hainsworth[994]	Gemcitabine/vinorelbine	3/28 (10)	0/17 (0)	22
Kosmas[995]	Paclitaxel/ifosfamide/cisplatin	10/13 (77)	14/20 (70)	28

RD, refractory disease; SR, sensitive relapse.
*Response not reported separately for SR and RD.

TABLE 75-43

Topotecan versus CAV in Sensitive Relapse Small Cell Lung Cancer

	RESPONDERS/ EVALUABLE (%)	PFS/MS (WK)	NEUTROPENIA	GRADE 4 THROMBOCYTOPENIA	ANEMIA
Topotecan	26/07 (25)	13.25	38	10	18
CAV	19/04 (18)	12/25	51	2	7

PFS/MS, progression-free survival/median survival.
Data from von Pawel J, Schiller JN, Shepherd FA, et al: Topotecan versus cyclophosphamide, doxorubicin, and vincristine for the treatment of recurrent small cell lung cancer. J Clin Oncol 1999;17:658.

appear to be similar to those for topotecan, but the numbers of patients in these trials are too small to make firm conclusions.

Combination chemotherapy has also been evaluated in patients with relapsed SCLC (see Table 75-42). Many of these trials have reported intriguing results, particularly in refractory disease. It remains to be determined, however, whether combination chemotherapy provides an advantage over single-agent chemotherapy as salvage therapy. One possible exception is the use of the original induction regimen in patients who relapse more than 6 months after the completion of chemotherapy. Such an approach has been associated with good response rate and prolonged remissions.[933]

SCLC patients with sensitive relapse should be considered for salvage chemotherapy at the time of progression. It is unclear from the current data whether patients with refractory disease derive any benefit from conventional chemotherapy. These patients, more than any others, should be considered for innovative clinical trials.

Combined-modality Therapy in Limited-stage Disease

Long-term survival with chemotherapy alone is uncommon (approximately 7%) in patients with limited-stage disease. Very early on, it was noted that impressive regressions of SCLC could be induced by radiotherapy. As stated previously, these observations lead to a randomized study comparing radiation therapy and surgery in SCLC patients who had operable disease.[841] The median survival was 28.5 weeks in the surgery arm and 43 weeks in the radiation arm (p = 0.04). The 5-year survival was 4% in the radiation arm and 1% in the surgery arm (the only patient who survived in the surgery arm refused surgery and opted for radiation). The results of this study should be viewed with caution, as the study was conducted during an era when modern staging techniques were unavailable; this could have lead to imbalance between the two arms. The standard of therapy for SCLC has since shifted away from surgery to thoracic radiation.

Integration of radiation therapy with chemotherapy in patients with limited-stage SCLC has been evaluated in multiple trials. Two meta-analyses have been published that have analyzed these trials.[934,935] The endpoints evaluated in the two meta-analyses differed slightly, and the study by Pignon and colleagues[934] contained updated information on the patients from the individual trial investigators. Because the studies evaluated by the two meta-analyses were the same, however, the conclusions were similar. The survival benefit from the addition of radiation becomes evident 15 months after the start of treatment. At 3 years, there is an absolute 5% survival advantage with the addition of radiation (14.3% vs. 8.9%). The relative risk of death in the combined-modality group was 0.86 (95% CI 0.78–0.94, p = 0.001). The local control rate was also significantly improved with the addition of radiation (23% vs. 48%, p = 0.0001). Most of the studies included in these meta-analyses included chemotherapy regimens other than cisplatin/etoposide. It is well docu-

mented that the safety of combining cisplatin/etoposide with radiation is markedly better than the older regimens, which included cyclophosphamide, nitrosoureas, and anthracyclines. It is therefore possible that the extent of benefit from combined modality therapy in patients with limited-stage SCLC could be better than that reported in the meta-analyses.

Subgroup analysis conducted indicated that gender and performance status did not affect the relative risk of death. Age was a significant factor with regard to survival, however. Almost all of the survival benefit observed was among patients younger than 55 years. The relative risk of death in favor of combined-modality therapy was 0.72 (95% CI 0.56–0.93) in patients younger than 55 years, while it was 1.07 (95% CI 0.70–1.64) for patients older than 70 years. These differences could also be related to the use of older regimens in combination with radiation. It is quite likely that the excess toxicity observed with the older regimens when combined with radiation could be more pronounced in the elderly. Recent data contradicts lack of benefit in the elderly patients observed in the meta-analyses. Yuen and associates[907] compared the outcomes for the elderly patients (>70 years) with those for the younger patients in the intergroup study, evaluating the concept of twice-daily radiation. Response rates (88% vs. 80%, p = 0.11), event-free survival rate (5 years, 19% vs 16%), and duration of response were similar between the two groups. The overall survival rates were slightly better among the younger patients (22% vs. 16%, p = 0.05). This finding probably was related to the higher fatal toxicity observed in the elderly (10% vs. 1%, p = 0.01) and to a higher proportion of patients with poor performance status in the elderly group (10% vs. 4%). Quon and associates[908] reported similar results after analyses of two NCIC studies, and they did not find any difference in survival based on age. These data suggest that in appropriately selected elderly patients, combined-modality therapy is beneficial.

Timing of Radiation Therapy

It is well recognized that the metastatic potential and drug resistance of a tumor increase over time. Experimental animal models also have suggested that there is accelerated tumor repopulation after cancer therapeutic modalities such as chemotherapy and radiation. Based on these theoretical reasons, it is felt that integration of all effective modalities early in the treatment of the tumor is likely to provide improved outcomes (Table 75-44). The concern about concurrent chemotherapy and radiation is that it is clearly more toxic than sequential therapy.

At least six randomized trials have addressed the issue of early or delayed radiation therapy.[936-942] Two of these studies have shown benefit for early radiation therapy.[936,942] In the study conducted by NCIC, all patients received alternating CAV/EP. Patients were randomized to early radiation, starting with the first cycle of EP (week 3) or late radiation, starting with the last cycle of EP (week 15). Median survival was 21.2 months in the early arm and 16 months in the late arm, while the 5-year survival rates were 22% in the early arm and 13% in the late arm.[940]

TABLE 75-44

Randomized Clinical Trials of Early versus Late Radiotherapy in SCLC

TRIAL	TYPE	START TIME		NO. OF PATIENTS		MEDIAN (MO)		5-YEAR (5%)		
		EARLY	LATE	EARLY	LATE	EARLY	LATE	EARLY	LATE	P
CALGB[937,938]	CEVA	Week 1	Week 9	125	145	13.04	14.54	6.6	12.8	NS
Aarhus[940]	CAV/EP (RT given with EP): total of 8 chemo cycles	Weeks 1 & 3	Weeks 18 & 23	99	100	10.7	12.9	10.0	10.0	NS
Hellenic Group[939]	Carbo/E: total 6 cycle	Week 1	Week 9	42	39	17.5	17	22.0	13.0	NS
NCIC[936]	CAV/EP: total 6 cycles	Week 3	Week 15	155	153	21.2	16.0	22.0	13.0	.013
Yugoslavian[942]	Carbo/EP-daily carbo/E during RT and an additional 4 cycles of EP	Week 1	Week 6	52	51	34	26	30	15	.027
JCOG[941]	EP: total 4 cycles	Week 1	Week 15	114	114	27.2	19.7	23.7	18.3	.097

A, doxorubicin; C, cyclophosphamide; Carbo, carboplatin; E, etoposide; P, cisplatin; V, vincristine.

Jeremic and colleagues[942] reported similar results when they compared early radiation (starting at week 1) in combination with carboplatin/etoposide vs. late radiation (starting at week 6) combined with the same chemotherapy. Five-year survival rates were 30% in the early arm and 15% in the late arm. A third study reported by the Japanese Clinical Oncology Group demonstrated survival benefit in the early radiation arm, but this did not reach statistical significance (5-year survival 23.7% vs. 18.3%, p = 0.097).[941]

Three studies have demonstrated similar survival among patients receiving early and late radiation. CALGB conducted a study randomizing patients to cyclophosphamide, etoposide, vincristine, and doxorubicin alone or the same chemotherapy combined with radiation starting in week 1 or the same chemotherapy with radiation starting at week 9.[139,140] Patients in the radiation arms did better than in the chemotherapy-alone arm, but there was no difference in survival between the two radiation arms (5-year survival 6.6% for the early group vs. 12.8% for the delayed group, p = NS). Patients in the early arm received an unplanned 50% dose attenuation of the chemotherapy drugs due to myelosuppression. The Aarhus Lung Cancer Group and the Hellenic Group reported similar negative results.[939,940]

Among all the studies that demonstrated no benefit for early radiation, the 5-year survival rates are in the range of 10%, while the 5-year survival rates in the positive studies are in the range of 25%. This raises the concern that patient populations in the negative trials might have poorer prognoses, which could be related to lower performance status or lack of modern staging procedures in any of these studies, leading to incorrect staging of these patients. Based on the available data in SCLC and on the emerging data in NSCLC, it is felt that radiation therapy should be integrated in the treatment of limited-stage SCLC at the earliest time feasible. In good performance status and appropriately staged patients, "early" could mean with the first cycle of chemotherapy. In patients with poor performance status or in patients who are awaiting completion of the staging procedures, on the other hand, radiation therapy could be initiated soon after the first cycle.

Radiation Therapy Dose and Fractionation

Data available on the appropriate dose of radiation therapy in SCLC is quite limited. Only one prospective study has evaluated the issue of radiation dose.[943] Patients in this study were randomized to 25 Gy in 10 fractions or 37.5 Gy in 15 fractions, delivered as consolidation therapy after six cycles of induction chemotherapy. The higher radiation dose resulted in a better progression-free survival, but the overall survival was no different. In a retrospective analysis of 154 patients treated from 1974 to 1986 at the Massachusetts General Hospital, a reduction in the local control rate was observed, from 79% with 30 Gy to 37% with 50 Gy.[944] No significant difference was noted when the dose was increased from 40 Gy to 50 Gy. Arriagada and coworkers[945] reviewed the data of phase II studies conducted by the French Cancer Center's Lung Group and found that an increase in dose from 45 Gy to 65 Gy did not improve the local control rate. Lack of benefit for the higher dose in these studies could be related to the prolonged time over which the dose was delivered, as radiation was delivered alternating with chemotherapy. It appears that a minimum of 40 Gy should be delivered to obtain benefits from radiation therapy. It is unclear whether a higher dose of radiation combined with cisplatin/etoposide administered without split-course therapy can achieve better local control and better survival.

Altered fractionation has generated much interest based on certain cellular observations. Late-responding normal tissues, such as microvasculature and neurons, are sensitive to the dose per fraction.[946] Thus, toxicity is less in these tissues for the same total dose if delivered in multiple small fractions rather than in single large fractions each day. On the other hand, in vitro data suggests that there is no "shoulder" to survival of SCLC cells in response to irradiation.[947,948] This data implies that

SCLC cells are unable to repair damage from even low levels of radiation, resulting in cell kill. The other issue that supports altered fractionation is accelerated repopulation after radiation therapy.[949] Multiple small fractions each day, therefore, can induce greater tumor kill, as they would limit tumor repopulation and minimize late toxicity with lower dose per fraction. Most normal tissues are able to repair the damage from low doses in 4 to 6 hours. Therefore, only two or three fractions are possible each day.

This concept of altered fractionation was tested in an intergroup study that randomized patients to 45 Gy in 25 fractions over 5 weeks or 45 Gy delivered in twice-daily 1.5 Gy fractions over 3 weeks.[950] Patients in both arms received concurrent cisplatin and etoposide. The accelerated radiation arm demonstrated a significant improvement in survival, with 5-year survivals of 26% compared with 16% (p = 0.04) in patients who received conventional fractionation. Intrathoracic failure rate was higher for patients in the conventional fractionation arm (52% vs. 36%, p = 0.06). The rate of esophagitis, toxicity not influenced by dose per fraction, was higher in the twice-daily arm (26% vs. 11%, p = 0.001). The other phase III study comparing twice-daily to once-daily radiation was conducted by the North Central Cancer Treatment Group (NCCTG).[951] This trial differed in two major ways from the intergroup study. The radiation therapy in both arms was administered starting with the fourth cycle. The other difference was that the patients in the hyperfractionated arm received radiation therapy in split course, with a planned 2-week break after 24 Gy, while the control arm received the radiation therapy without a break. In this study, there was no difference in survival between the twice-daily radiation arm and the control arm of conventional radiation. It is quite likely that the delayed start of the radiation and split-course therapy in the experimental arm lead to negative results.

Most radiation oncologists plan to deliver 60–64 Gy, in single daily fractions of 1.8 Gy, to patients with limited-stage SCLC. Currently, it is unclear whether twice-daily radiation to a dose of 45 Gy is superior to conventional fractionation to a dose of 64 Gy. Twice-daily radiation does have practical limitations, such as greater time commitment on the part of the patient. Such considerations have limited the wider use of the twice-daily radiation treatment plans.

Prophylactic Cranial Radiation and Brain Metastases

Brain metastases are a substantial source of morbidity and mortality in patients with SCLC. In earlier studies, the observed rate of brain metastases was 20%. With the introduction of better imaging modalities, rates as high as 50% have been reported at 2 to 3 years. Chemotherapeutic agents have limited efficacy in preventing brain metastases, as they are unable to cross the blood-brain barrier. This observation led to the proposal of prophylactic cranial irradiation to prevent brain metastases.[952] Early studies of prophylactic cranial radiation (PCI) suggested a reduction in brain metastases, but there did not appear to be a survival benefit. Further, the benefits observed with PCI were limited, in these early studies, to patients who had complete remission after induction therapy.[953]

Seven randomized trials of PCI, one of which is unpublished, were conducted in SCLC patients who had achieved a complete.[743,954-958] All studies reported a reduction in brain metastases in patients receiving PCI, and it was highly significant in two of these trials. Survival was consistently better in the PCI arms when it was reported, but such improvement did not attain statistical significance. Because many of these studies were too small to detect an improvement in survival, a meta-analysis of all of these trials was conducted to better understand the utility of PCI.[959] The Prophylactic Cranial Irradiation Overview Collaborative Group analyzed the results of the seven trials conducted in patients with complete remission. The analysis showed a statistically significant survival advantage to PCI, with a relative risk of death of 0.84 (95% CI 0.73-0.97) that translated into an absolute survival advantage of 5.4% at 3 years. There was a 54% proportional reduction in the incidence of brain metastases. The dose used in the individual trials varied, and the meta-analysis demonstrated a significant trend toward a lower rate of brain metastases with higher doses of PCI. Early PCI (less than 6 months from the start of induction therapy) appeared to be beneficial over late PCI in terms of reducing brain metastases.

Crossen and colleagues[960] conducted another meta-analysis that included all published trials, irrespective of whether PCI was given after CR. The study did not detect an improvement in survival when trials of up-front PCI were included (HR 0.94, 95% CI 0.87-1.02), but when studies in of PCI in completely responding patients were analyzed independently, there was a significant reduction in mortality with PCI (HR 0.82, 95% CI 0.71-0.96).

Neurocognitive toxicity is a major concern with PCI. The neurocognitive deficits have been observed for 6 to 24 months after irradiation.[961] This toxicity increases with increasing radiation fraction size, total dose, and volume of brain radiated. Toxicity also is higher when PCI is administered in conjunction with chemotherapy. Most of the reports that have detailed neuro-cognitive toxicity of PCI are from nonrandomized studies and retrospective analyses. Also, many of these reports did not include pretherapy neuro-cognitive assessments.

Van Oosterhout and Komaki have published small prospective series of PCI.[961,962] Baseline neurocognitive test results were worse in patients with SCLC than in matched controls. There was no significant neuro-psychologic impairment observed at 5 to 20 months after PCI. Both Arriagada and coworkers[953] and Gregor and associates[954] conducted prospective trials evaluating PCI. In both studies, baseline impairment of neurocognitive function was observed in a majority of the patients. Follow-up neurologic testing revealed neither a deterioration in neurocognitive function with PCI nor a difference between the patients who received PCI and those who did not. CALGB did find worsening of neurocognitive function after PCI, but in this study, PCI was administered concurrently with chemotherapy.[963]

In summary, PCI does appear to be beneficial in patients with SCLC who are in complete remission. In prospective studies, PCI does not appear to increase neurocognitive dysfunction for at least 2 years after PCI. PCI should not be administered concurrently with chemotherapy, as it appears to increase neurocognitive dysfunction. The optimum dose of PCI is unclear, but based on retrospective analyses, a dose higher than 20 Gy appears to be effective.

Whole-brain radiation remains the standard of care for the treatment of brain metastases. Systemic chemotherapy might be beneficial in patients with SCLC who have brain metastases, however. Kristensen and associates[964] reviewed 12 patient series published between 1981 and 1990. The overall response rate to chemotherapy in patients with brain metastases was 76%. In patients who have asymptomatic brain metastases without evidence of increased intracranial pressure, systemic chemotherapy may be initiated, with radiation therapy delivered after the completion of chemotherapy. Recent data suggest that topoisomerase I inhibitors might achieve better cerebrospinal fluid levels than other chemotherapy drugs. It is unclear whether the use of these agents in the treatment of SCLC will reduce the incidence of brain metastases or improve antitumor efficacy in the brain.

Surgery in SCLC

Many reports and retrospective reviews conducted in the 1950s and 1960s showed poor outcomes in SCLC patients treated with surgery alone. This was confirmed by a randomized study conducted by the British Medical Research Council that compared surgery to radiation therapy.[841] As stated previously, the results of the surgical treatment were inferior. Despite these results and the subsequent success with concurrent chemotherapy and radiation, surgery has been performed in patients with very early-stage SCLC

Surgical therapy in resectable, limited-stage SCLC has resulted in 5-year survival of 12% to 43%.[964-968] In patients who receive adjuvant chemotherapy after surgery, these results appear to be better, with 5-year survival rates ranging from 14% to 64%. There are no prospective randomized studies that have been conducted to address the issue of adjuvant chemotherapy. Based on the available reports and on the propensity of SCLC to metastasize, however, adjuvant chemotherapy is recommended. Postoperative radiation should also be considered if nodal disease (particularly N2 disease) is documented.

Appropriate staging of the patients is extremely crucial. Pathologic staging of the mediastinum should be performed before surgical resection. In a series from the Royal Brompton Hospital, the introduction of mediastinal evaluation improved the long-term survival rates of patients treated with surgery.[966] Apart from the routine noninvasive tests, patients being considered for surgery might potentially benefit from PET scanning; however, no data exists regarding the utility of PET scans in patients with SCLC who are being considered for surgery. In general, surgery should be considered only for patients with stage I and stage II SCLC.

Phase II studies of surgery after either induction chemotherapy or chemoradiation therapy have been reported. Five-year survival rates greater than 30% have been reported. There is one randomized study that addressed this issue and was conducted in North America and Europe.[968] All patients received five cycles of induction CAV chemotherapy. Patients who achieved a response were then randomized to surgery or no surgery. Both arms received radiation and PCI. Among the 328 patients randomized to preoperative induction therapy, 217 (66%) had a response. Of these 217, only 146 were randomized. Median survival of patients in the surgical arms and the nonsurgical arms were similar (15.4 months vs. 18.6 months, p = 0.78). Thus, the role of surgery in patients who have received induction chemotherapy or chemotherapy and radiation is uncertain.

Investigational Agents

The encouraging response rates observed with chemotherapy in SCLC led to expectations of producing high cure rates in this disease; however, many attempts at improving the outcomes of SCLC with traditional chemotherapy agents and radiation therapy have failed. Advances in molecular biology over the last few years have lead to the recognition of certain molecular abnormalities in SCLC that contribute to the progression of this disease. It is possible that agents that target these molecular abnormalities might improve upon the current standards of SCLC without causing significant toxicity. Some of the agents that have been tested are discussed in the sections that follow.

Matrix Metalloproteinase Inhibitors

Matrix metalloproteinases (MMPs) are extracellular enzymes that degrade connective tissue and play an important role in bone development and wound healing. These enzymes are upregulated in cancer cells, and they appear to be important in cancer cell invasion, metastasis, and angiogenesis.[969,970] MMP inhibitors (MMPIs) have been developed as potential anticancer agents. Marimastat was one of the first MMPIs developed and tested in patients with SCLC. Two phase III studies of marimastat in patients with SCLC as maintenance therapy after the completion of chemotherapy have been conducted. The results of one study have been reported.[971] In this study, conducted by the National Cancer Institute of Canada and EORTC, there was no difference in survival between patients on marimastat and patients on placebo. In addition, marimastat adversely impacted the quality of life. The second study was conducted in the United States, but the results are not available. A second MMPI BAY 12-9566 was tested similarly but was closed early due a shorter survival observed among patients receiving the experimental agent during an interim analysis.

Tyrosine Kinase Inhibitors

Tyrosine kinases (TKs) are enzymes associated with transmembrane growth receptors. These growth receptors and the associated TKs are overexpressed in many cancers and are involved in cancer cell growth, invasion, angiogenesis, and antiapoptosis. C-Kit is a growth receptor that appears to have a role in SCLC proliferation. Some studies have reported c-kit expression in 70% of patients with SCLC, though other studies have found lower expression.[972-976] Imatinib mesylate inhibits the TK associated with c-kit, and this inhibition has demonstrated therapeutic benefits in gastrointestinal stromal tumors. Imatinib has shown growth inhibition of SCLC cell lines, and this inhibition correlates with inhibition of c-kit TK.[977] A phase II study of imatinib in SCLC patients has been reported.[976] Nineteen patients who were either chemotherapy naive or had sensitive relapse were treated with imatinib; no responses were observed. In retrospective analyses, only four patients had c-kit positive tumor. Other studies are evaluating imatinib in combination with chemotherapy and as maintenance therapy after chemotherapy. Newer drugs that more potently inhibit c-kit are currently undergoing testing. Other TKs, such as c-met, are also being considered as potential targets.

Antibody-based Therapy

In vitro data suggests that peptides such as gastrin releasing peptide can participate in an autocrine growth loop in SCLC.[978] Thus, targeting such peptides could have therapeutic effect in SCLC. Monoclonal antibody 2A11 was shown to inhibit the binding of gastrin releasing peptide to cellular receptors, with growth inhibition of SCLC in preclinical models.[979] In a phase II study of previously treated patients with SCLC, one of 12 evaluable patients responded completely. Four patients had stable disease. Further testing has been halted due to production issues. Similar antibodies are being evaluated against targets such as cell surface antigen NKH-1.

Antisense Bcl-2. Bcl-2 is commonly overexpressed in SCLC. Bcl-2 inhibits apoptosis and might contribute to chemotherapy resistance. This is particularly important in refractory or relapsed tumors. Antisense oligonucleotides inhibit the translation of mRNA and thus suppress cellular protein levels. Genasense is a bcl-2 antisense oligonucleotide. Rudin and colleagues[980] treated 12 patients with refractory SCLC with a combination of genasense and paclitaxel. No objective responses were observed, but 2 of the 12 patients had stable disease. Further evaluation of this agent is ongoing.

REFERENCES

1. Jemal A, Murray T, Samuels A, et al: Cancer Statistics, 2003. CA Cancer J Clin 2003;53:5.
2. Ries LAG, Eisner MP, Kosary CL, Hankey BF, Miller BA, Clegg L, Edwards BK (eds): SEER Cancer Statistics Review, 1973–1999. Bethesda, MD, National Cancer Institute, http://seer.cancer.gov/csr/1973_1999/, 2002.
3. Surgeon General: Reducing the health consequences of smoking: 25 years of progress. Washington, DC: US Government Printing Office, 1989.
4. Doll R, Hill AB: A study of the aetiology of carcinoma of the lung. Br Med J 1952;2:1271.
5. Levin ML, Goldstein H, Gerhardt PR: Cancer and tobacco smoking: A preliminary report. JAMA 1950;143:336.
6. Wynder E, Graham E: Tobacco smoking as a possible etiologic factor in bronchiogenic carcinoma: A study of six hundred and eighty-four cases. JAMA 1950;143:329.
7. Hammond EC: Smoking in relation to the death rates of one million men and women. Natl Cancer Inst 1966;19:127.
8. Doll R, Peto R, Wheatley K, et al: Mortality in relation to smoking: 40 years' observations on male British doctors. Br Med J 1994;309:901.
9. McLaughlin JK, Hrubec Z, Blot WJ, et al: Smoking and cancer mortality among US veterans: A 26 year followup. Intl J Cancer 1995;60:190.
10. Zang EA, Wynder EL: Differences in lung cancer risk between men and women: Examination of the evidence. J Natl Cancer Inst 1996;88:183.
11. Risch HA, Howe GR, Jain M, et al: Are female smokers at higher risk for lung cancer than male smokers? Am J Epidemiol 1993;138:281.
12. IARC. Tobacco smoking: Monographs on the evaluation of carcinogenic risk of chemicals to man, Vol 38. Lyon, France, International Agency for Research on Cancer, 1986.
13. Lubin JH, Blot WJ, Berrino F, et al: Patterns of lung cancer risk according to type of cigarette smoked. Intl J Cancer 1984;33:569.
14. Halpern MT, Gillespie BW, Warner KE: Patterns of absolute risk of lung cancer mortality in former smokers. J Natl Cancer Inst 1993;85:457.
15. Surgeon General: The health consequences of involuntary smoking. Washington, DC: US Government Printing Office, 1986.
16. World Cancer Research Fund (WCRF): Lung. In: Food, Nutrition and the Prevention of Cancer: A Global Perspective (Part II, Cancers, Nutrition and Food). Washington, DC, American Institute for Cancer Research, 1997.
17. Albanes D: Beta-carotene and lung cancer: A case study. Am J Clin Nutr 1999;69:1345s.
18. ATBCCP Study Group (Alpha-Tocopherol, Beta-Carotene Cancer Prevention Study Group): The effect of vitamin E and beta-carotene on the incidence of lung cancer and other cancers in male smokers. N Engl J Med 1994;330:1029.
19. Omenn GS, Goodman GE, Thornquist M, et al: Effects of combination of beta-carotene and vitamin A on lung cancer and cardiovascular disease. N Engl J Med 1996;334:1150.
20. McDonald JC, McDonald AD: Epidemiology of asbestos-related lung cancer. In Antmand K, Aisner J (eds): Asbestos-related malignancy. Orlando, Fl, Grune & Stratton, 1987, pp 31–55.
21. Samet JM: Radon and lung cancer. J Natl Cancer Inst 1989;81:745.
22. Wada S, Miyanishi M, Nishimoto Y, et al: Mustard gas as a cause of respiratory neoplasm in man. Lancet 1968;1:1161.
23. Redmond CK: Cancer mortality among coke oven workers. Env Health Persp 1983;52:67.
24. Pasternack BS, Shore RE, Albert RE: Occupational exposure to chloromethyl ethers. J Morphol 1977;19:74.
25. Alderson MR, Tattan NS, Bidstrup L: Health of workmen in the chromate producing industry in Britain. Br J Industr Med 1981;38:117.
26. Doll R: Report of the International Committee on Nickel Carcinogenesis in Man. Scand J Work Env Health 1990;16:1.
27. Grimsrud TK, Berge SR, Haldorsen T, et al: Exposure to different forms of nickel and risk of lung cancer. Am J Epidemiol 202;156:1123.
28. Blot WJ, Fraumeni JF Jr: Arsenic and lung cancer. In Samet J (ed): The Epidemiology of Lung Cancer. New York, Marcell Dekker, 1994, pp 207–218.
29. Mattson ME, Pollack ES, Cullen JW: What are the odds that smoking will kill you? Am J Public Health 1987;77:425.
30. Tokuhata GK, Lilienfeld AM: Familial aggregation of lung cancer in humans. J Natl Cancer Inst 1963;30:289.
31. Samet J, Humble C, Pathak D: Personal and family history of respiratory disease and lung cancer risk. Am Rev Resp Dis 1986;134:466.
32. Wu AH, Yu MC, Thomas DC, et al: Personal and family history of lung disease as risk factors for adenocarcinoma of the lung. Cancer Res 1988;48:7279.
33. Shaw GL, Falk RT, Pickle LW, et al: Lung cancer risk associated with cancer in relatives. J Clin Epidemiol 1991;44:429.
34. Osann KE: Lung cancer in women: The importance of smoking, family history of cancer, and medical history of respiratory diseases. Cancer Res 1991;51:4893.

35. Wu AH, Fontham ETH, Reynolds P, et al: Family history of cancer and risk of lung cancer among lifetime nonsmoking women in the United States. Am J Epidemiol 1996;143:535.

36. Bromen K, Pohlabeln H, Jahn I, et al: Aggregation of lung cancer in families: Results from a population based case-control study in Germany. Am J Epidemiol 2000;152:497.

37. Ooi WL, Elston RC, Chen VW, et al: Increased familial risk for lung cancer. J Natl Cancer Inst 1986;76:217.

38. Schwartz AG, Yang P, Swanson GM: Familial risk of lung cancer among nonsmokers and their relatives. Am J Epidemiol 1996;144:554.

39. Sellers TA, Bailey-Wilson JE, Elston RC, et al: Evidence for Mendelian inheritance in the pathogenesis of lung cancer. J Natl Cancer Inst 1990;82:1272.

40. Yang P, Schwartz AG, McAllister AE, et al: Lung cancer risk in families of nonsmoking probands: Heterogeneity by age at diagnosis. Genet Epidemiol 1999;17:253.

41. Malkin D, Li FP, Strong LC, et al: Germ line p53 mutations in a familial syndrome of breast cancer sarcomas and other neoplasms. Science 1990;250:1233.

42. Kawajiri K, Nakachi K, Imai K, et al: Identification of genetically high risk individuals to lung cancer by DNA polymorphisms of the cytochrome P450IA1 gene. FEBS 1990;263:131.

43. LeMarchand L, Sivaraman L, Pierce L, et al: Associations of CYP1A1, GSTM1, and CYP2E1 polymorphisms with lung cancer suggest cell type specificities to tobacco carcinogens. Cancer Res 1998;58:4858.

44. Sugimura H, Hamada GS, Suzuki I, et al: CYP1A1 and CYP2E1 polymorphisms and lung cancer, a case-control study in Rio de Janeiro, Brazil. Pharmacogenetics 1995;5:S145.

45. Tefre T, Ryberg D, Haugen A, et al: Human CYP1A1 (cytochrome P_1450) gene: Lack of association between the MspI RFLP and incidence of lung cancer in a Norwegian population. Pharmacogenetics 1991;1:20.

46. Hirvonen A, Husgafvel-Pursianinen K, Antilla S, et al: Metabolic cytochrome P450 genotypes and assessment of individual susceptibility to lung cancer. Pharmacogenetics 1992;2:259.

47. Shields PG, Caporaso NE, Falk RT, et al: Lung cancer, risk, and a CYP1A1 genetic polymorphism. Cancer Epidemiol Biom Prev 1993;2:481.

48. Vineis P, Veglia F, Benhamou S, et al: CYP1A1 T^{3796} C polymorphism and lung cancer: A pooled analysis of 2,451 cases and 3,358 controls. Intl J Cancer 2003;104:650.

49. Watanabe J, Yang JP, Eguchi H, et al: An RsaI polymorphism in the CYP2E1 gene does not affect lung cancer risk in a Japanese population. Japan J Cancer Res 1995;86:245.

50. Houlston RS: Glutathione S-transferase M1 status and lung cancer risk: A meta-analysis. Cancer Epidemiol Biom Prev 1999;8:675.

51. McWilliams JE, Sanderson BJS, Harris EL, et al: Glutathione S-transferase MI (GSTM1) deficiency and lung cancer risk. Cancer Epidemiol Biom Prev 1995;4:589.

52. Benhamou S, Lee WJ, Alexandrie A-K, et al: Meta- and pooled analysis of the effects of glutathione S-transferase M1 polymorphisms and smoking on lung cancer risk. Carcinogenesis 2002;23:1343.

53. Kelsey KT, Spitz MR, Zuo Z-F, et al: Polymorphisms in the glutathione S-transferase class mu and theta genes interact and increase susceptibility to lung cancer in minority populations. Cancer Causes Control 1997;8:554.

54. Jourenkova N, Reinikanen M, Bouchardy C, et al: Effects of glutathione S-transferase GSTM1 and GSTT1 genotypes on lung cancer risk in smokers. Pharmacogenetics 1997;7:515.

55. Sunaga N, Kohno T, Yanagitani N, et al: Contribution of the *NQO1* and *GSTT1* polymorphisms to lung adenocarcinoma susceptibility. Cancer Epidemiol Biom Prev 2002;11:730.

56. Risch A, Wikman H, Thiel S, et al: Glutathione-S-transferase M1, M3, T1 and P1 polymorphisms and susceptibility to non-small-cell lung cancer subtypes and hamartomas. Pharmacogenetics 2001;11:757.

57. Stucker I, Hirvonen A, de Waziers I, et al: Genetic polymorphisms of glutathione S-transferases as modulators of lung cancer susceptibility. Carcinogenesis 2002;23:1475.

58. Miller DP, Liu G, De Vivo I, et al: Combination of the variant genotypes of *GSTP1, GSTM1* and *p53* are associated with an increased lung cancer risk. Cancer Res 2002;62:2819.

59. Amos CI, Xu W, Spitz MR: Is there a genetic basis for lung cancer susceptibility? Recent Results Cancer Res 1999;151:3.

60. Wei Q, Spitz MR, Gu J, et al: DNA repair capacity correlates with mutagen sensivity in lymphoblastoid cell lines. Cancer Epidemiol Biom Prev 1996;5:199.

61. Shen MR, Jones IM, Mohrenweiser H: Nonconservative amino acid substitution variants exist at polymorhic frequency in DNA repair genes in healthy humans. Cancer Res 1998;58:604.

62. Goode EL, Ulrich CM, Potter JD: Polymorphisms in DNA repair genes and associations with cancer risk. Cancer Epidemiol Biom Prev 2002;11:1513.

63. Gould EV, Linnoila RI, Memoli VA, et al: Neuroendocrine cells and neuroendocrine neoplasms of the lung. Pathol Ann 1983;18:287.

64. Park IW, Wistuba II, Maitra A, et al: Multiple clonal abnormalities in the bronchial epithelium of patients with lung cancer. J Natl Cancer Inst 1999;91:1863.

65. Pitterle DM, Jolicoeur EMC, Bepler G: Hot spots for molecular genetic alterations in lung cancer. In Vivo 1998;12:643.

66. Schuller H: Mechanisms of smoking-related lung and pancreatic adenocarcinoma development. Nature Rev 2002;2:455.

67. Bepler G: Lung cancer epidemiology and genetics. J Thorac Imag 1999;14:228.

68. Gauderman W, Morrison J, Carpenter C, et al: Analysis of gene-smoking interaction in lung cancer. Genet Epidemiol 1997;14:199.

69. Auerbach O, Stout AP, Hammond EC, et al: Changes in bronchial epithelium in relation to cigarette smoking and relation to lung cancer. N Engl J Med 1961;265:253.

70. Becker KL, Gazdar AF: The Endocrine Lung in Health and Disease. Philadelphia, WB Saunders, 1984.

71. Nakanishi K: Alveolar epithelial hyperplasia and adenocarcinoma of the lung. Arch Pathol Lab Med 1990;114:363.

72. Wistuba I, Behrens C, Milchgrub S, et al: Sequential molecular abnormalities are involved in the multistage development of squamous cell lung carcinoma. Oncogene 1999;18:643.

73. Belinsky S, Nikula K, Palmisano W, et al: Aberrant methylation of p16(INK4a) is an early event in lung cancer and a potential biomarker for early diagnosis. Proc Natl Acad Sci USA 1998;95:11891.

74. Wistuba II, Behrens C, Virmani AK, et al: Allelic losses at chromosome 8p21-23 are early and frequent events in the pathogenesis of lung cancer. Cancer Res 1999;59:1973.

75. Franklin W, Gazdar A, Haney J, et al: Widely dispersed p53 mutation in respiratory epithelium. A novel mechanism for field carcinogenesis. J Clin Invest 1997;100:2133.

76. Sugio K, Kishimoto Y, Virmani AK, et al: K-ras mutations are a relatively late event in the pathogenesis of lung carcinomas. Cancer Res 1994;54:5811.

77. Nowell PC: The clonal evolution of tumor cell populations. Science 1974;194:23.

78. Hoeijmakers JHJ: Genome maintenance mechanisms for preventing cancer. Nature 2001;411:366.

79. Schmitt CA: Senescence, apoptosis and therapy. Nature Rev 2003;3:286–295.

80. Evan GI, Vousden KH: Proliferation, cell cycle and apoptosis in cancer. Nature 2001;411:342.

81. Gabay C, Kushner I: Acute-phase proteins and other systemic responses to inflammation. N Engl J Med 1999;340:448.

82. Mountain C: Revisions in the international system for staging lung cancer. Chest 1997;111:1710.

83. Jaklitsch MT, Strauss GM, Healey EA, et al: An historical perspective of multi-modality treatment for resectable non-small cell lung cancer. Lung Cancer 1995;12:S17.

84. Martini N, Ginsberg R: Treatment of stage I and II disease. In Aisner J, Arriagada R, Green M, Martini N, Perry M (eds): Comprehensive Textbook of Thoracic Oncology. Baltimore, Williams & Williams, 1996, pp 339–350.

85. Patz EF Jr, Rossi S, Harpole DH Jr, et al: Correlation of tumor size and survival in patients with stage IA non-small cell lung cancer. Chest 2000;117:1568.

86. Depierre A, Milleron B, Moro-Sibilot D, et al: Preoperative chemotherapy followed by surgery compared with primary surgery in resectable stage I (Except T1N0), II, and IIIa non-small-cell lung cancer. J Clin Oncol 2002;20:247.

87. Rosell R, Gomez-Codina J, Camps C, et al: Randomized trial comparing preoperative chemotherapy plus surgery with surgery alone in patients with non-small-cell lung cancer. N Engl J Med 1994;330:153.

88. Roth JA, Fosella F, Komake R, et al: A randomized trial comparing perioperative chemotherapy and surgery with surgery alone in resectable stage IIIA non-small cell lung cancer. J Natl Cancer Inst 1994;86:673.

89. Martini N, Kris MG, Gralla RJ, et al: The effects of preoperative chemotherapy on the resectability of non-small cell lung carcinoma with mediastinal lymph node metastases (N2 M0). Ann Thorac Surg 1988;45:370–379.

90. Peck K, Sher Y, Shih J, et al: Detection and quantitation of circulating cancer cells in the peripheral blood of lung cancer patients. Cancer Res 1998;58:2761.

91. Aloia T, Bepler G, Harpole D, et al: Integration of peripheral blood biomarkers with computed tomography to differentiate benign from malignant pulmonary opacities. Cancer Detect Prev 2001; 25:336.

92. Harpole D, Richards W, Herndon J, et al: Angiogenesis and molecular biologic sub-staging in patients with stage I non-small cell lung cancer. Ann Thorac Surg 1996;61:1470.

93. Pantel K, Izbicki J, Passlick B, et al: Frequency and prognostic significance of isolated tumour cells in bone marrow of patients with non-small cell lung cancer without overt metastases. Lancet 1996;347:649.

94. Vansteenkiste J, Stroobants S, Dupont P, et al: Prognostic importance of the standardized uptake value on ^{18}F-fluoro-2-deoxy-glucose-positron emission tomography scan in non-small-cell lung cancer: An analysis of 125 cases. J Clin Oncol 1999;17:3201.

95. Slebos RJ, Hruban RH, Dalsio O, et al: Relationship between K-*ras* oncogene activation and smoking in adenocarcinoma of the human lung. J Natl Cancer Inst 1991;83:1024.

96. Carbone D, Mitsudomi T, Chiba I, et al: p53 immunostaining positivity is associated with reduced survival and is imperfectly correlated with gene mutations in resected non-small cell lung cancer. A preliminary report of LCSG 871. Chest 1994;106(Suppl):377S.

97. Fukuyama Y, Mitsudomi T, Sugio K, et al: K-ras and p53 mutations are an independent unfavourable prognostic indicator in patients with non-small-cell lung cancer. Br J Cancer 1997;75:1125.

98. Brambilla E, Moro D, Gazzeri S, et al: Alterations of expression of rb, p16(INK4A) and cyclin D1 in non-small cell lung carcinoma and their clinical significance. J Pathol 1999;188:351.

99. Volm M, Rittgen W: Cellular predictive factors for the drug response of lung cancer. Anticancer Res 2000;20:3449.

100. Schiller JH, Adak S, Feins RH, et al: Lack of prognostic significance of p53 and K-*ras* mutations in primary resected non-small cell lung cancer on E4592: A laboratory ancillary study on an Eastern Cooperative Oncology Group prospective randomized trial of postoperative adjuvant therapy. J Clin Oncol 2001;19:448.

101. Robert C, Bolon I, Gazzeri S, et al: Expression of plasminogen activator inhibitors 1 and 2 in lung cancer and their role in tumor progression. Clin Cancer Res 1999;5:2094.

102. Simony J, Pujol JL, Radal M, et al: In situ evaluation of growth fraction determined by monoclonal antibody Ki-67 and poidy in surgically resected non-small cell lung cancers. Cancer Res 1990;50:4382.

103. Greatens T, Niehans G, Rubins J, et al: Do molecular markers predict survival in non-small-cell lung cancer. Am J Respir Crit Care Med 1998;157:1093.

104. Graziano S, Kern J, Herndon J, et al: Analysis of neuroendocrine markers, HER2 and CEA before and after chemotherapy in patients with stage IIIA non-small cell lung cancer: A Cancer And Leukemia Group B study. Lung Cancer 1998;21:203.

105. Mehdi SA, Etzell JE, Newman NB, et al: Prognostic significance of Ki-67 immunostaining and symptoms in resected stage I and II non-small cell lung cancer. Lung Cancer 1998;20:99.

106. Lavezzi AM, Santambrogio L, Bellaviti N, et al: Prognostic significance of different biomarkers in non-small cell lung cancer. Oncol Rep 1999;6:819.

107. Shiba M, Kohno H, Kakizawa K, et al: Ki-67 immunostaining and other prognostic factors including tobacco smoking in patients

with resected non-small cell lung carcinoma. Cancer 2000;89:1457.

108. Ramnath N, Hernandez FJ, Tan DT, et al: MCM2 is an independent predictor of survival in patients with non-small-cell lung cancer. J Clin Oncol 2001;19:4259.

109. Bepler G, Gautam A, McIntyre LM, et al: Prognostic significance of molecular genetic aberrations on chromosome segment 11p15.5 in non-small-cell lung cancer. J Clin Oncol 2002;20:1353.

110. Lord RV, Brabender J, Gandara D, et al: Low ERCC1 expression correlates with prolonged survival after cisplatin plus gemcitabine chemotherapy in non-small cell lung cancer. Clin Cancer Res 2002;8:2286.

111. Simon G, Sharma A, Smith P, et al: Increased ERCC1 expression predicts for improved survival in resected patients with non-small cell lung cancer. Eur J Cancer 2002;38(Suppl 7):S15.

112. Rosell R, Scagliotti G, Danenberg KD, et al: Transcripts in pre-treatment biopsies from a three-arm randomized trial in metastatic non-small-cell lung cancer. Oncogene 2003;22:3548–3553.

113. Gazdar AF, Steinberg SM, Russell EK, et al: Correlation of in vitro drug-sensitivity testing results with response to chemotherapy and survival in extensive-stage small cell lung cancer: A prospective clinical trial. J Natl Cancer Inst 1990;82:117.

114. Shaw GL, Gazdar AF, Phelps R, et al: Correlation of in vitro drug sensitivity testing results with response to chemotherapy and survival: Comparison of non-small cell lung cancer and small cell lung cancer. J Cell Biochem 1996;24(Suppl):173.

115. Travis WD, Travis LB, Devesa SS: Lung cancer. Cancer 1995;75(Suppl 1):191–202.

116. Minna JD, Pass H, Gladstein E, et al: Cancer of the Lung. In De Vita VT, Hellman S, Rosenberg SA (eds): Cancer: Principles and Practice of Oncology. Philadelphia, Lippincott, 1988, p 591.

117. Skarin AT, Herbst RS, Leong TL, et al: Lung cancer in patients under 40. Lung Cancer 2001;32:255.

118. Kreuzer M, Kreienbrock L, Gerken M, et al: Risk factors for lung cancer in young adults. Am J Epidemiol 1998;147:1028.

119. Kreuzer M, Kreienbrock L, Muller KM, et al: Histologic types of lung carcinoma and age at onset. Cancer 1999;85:1958.

120. Liu NS, Spitz MR, Kemp BL, et al: Adenocarcinoma of the lung in young patients: The MD Anderson experience. Cancer 2000;88:1837.

121. Baldini EH, Strauss GM: Women and lung cancer: Waiting to exhale. Chest 1997;112:229S.

122. Khuder SA, Mutgi A: Effect of smoking cessation on major histologic types of lung cancer. Chest 2001;120:1577.

123. Dresler CM, Fratelli C, Babb J, et al: Gender differences in genetic susceptibility for lung cancer. Lung Cancer 2000;30:153.

124. Jemel A, Travis WD, Tarone RE, et al: Lung cancer rates convergence in young men and women in the United States: Analysis by birth cohort and histologic type. Int J Cancer 2003;105:1001.

125. Kreuzer M, Bofferra P, Whitley E, et al: Gender differences in lung cancer risk by smoking: A multicenter case-control study in Germany and Italy. Br J Cancer 2000;82:227.

126. Charloux A, Quoix E, Wolkove N, et al: The increasing incidence of lung adenocarcinoma: reality or artifact? A review of the epidemiology of lung adenocarcinoma. Int J Epidemiol 1997;26:14.

127. Shottenfeld, D: Etiology and epidemiology of lung cancer. In Pass HI, et al (eds): Lung Cancer: Principles and Practice, 2nd ed. Philadelphia, Lippincott Williams & Wilkins, 2000, p 368.

128. Villeneuve PJ, Mao Y: Lifetime probability of developing lung cancer, by smoking status. Canada. Can J Public Health 1994;85:385.

129. Parkin DM, Sasco AJ: Lung cancer: Worldwide variation in occurrence and proportion attributable to tobacco use. Lung Cancer 1993;9:1.

130. Neuhouser ML, Patterson RE, Thornquist MD, et al: Fruits and vegetables are associated with lower lung cancer risk only in the placebo-arm of the beta carotene and retinal efficacy trial (CARET). Cancer Epidemiol Biom Prev 2003;12:350.

131. Axelsson G, Rylander R: Diet as a risk for lung cancer: A Swedish case-control study. Nutr Cancer 2002;44:145.

132. Wright ME, Mayne ST, Swanson CA, et al: Dietary carotenoids,

vegetables and lung cancer risk in women: The Missouri women's health study. Cancer Causes Control 2003;14:85.

133. Jansen MC, Bueno de Mesquita HB, Rasanen L, et al: Cohort analysis of fruit and vegetable consumption in European men. Int J Cancer 2001;92:913.

134. Kalandidi A, Katsouyanni K, Voropoulu N, et al: Passive smoking and diet in the etiology of lung cancer among non-smokers. Cancer Causes Control 1990;1:15.

135. Hu J, Mao Y, Dryer D, et al: Canadian Cancer Registries Research Group. Risk factors for lung cancer among Canadian women who never smoked. Cancer Dect Prev 2002;26:129.

136. Nyberg F, Hou SM, Pershagen G, et al: Dietary fruit and vegetables protect against somatic mutation in vivo, but low or high intake of caroteinoids does not. Carcinogenesis 2003;24:689.

137. Schwartz A: Genetic susceptibility to lung cancer. In: Pass HI, et al (eds): Lung Cancer: Principles and Practice, 2nd ed. Philadelphia, Lippincott Williams & Wilkins, 2000, p 389.

138. Bach PB, Kattan MW, Thornquist MD, et al: Variations in lung cancer risk among smokers. J Natl Cancer Inst 995;470, 2003.

139. Petty TL: The early diagnosis of lung cancer. Dis Mon 2001;47:204.

140. Petty TL: The predictive value of spirometry. Identifying patients at risk for lung cancer in a hospital setting. Postgrad Med 1997; 101:128.

141. Brambilla C, Fievert F, Jeanmart M, et al: Early detection of lung cancer: Role of biomarkers. Eur Resp J Suppl 2003;39:36S.

142. Reis LA (ed): SEER Cancer Statistic Review, 1973-1994. Bethesda Md, National Cancer Institute, Publ No 97-2789, 1997.

143. Khudar SA: Effect of cigarette smoking on major histopathological types of lung cancer. Lung Cancer 2001;31:139.

144. Boring CC, Squires TS, Tong T: Cancer Statistics. CA Cancer J Clin 1993;43:7.

145. Thun MJ, Lally CA, Flannery JT, et al: Cigarette smoking and changes in the histopathology of lung cancer. J Natl Cancer Inst 1997;89:1580.

146. Colby TV, Koss MN, Travis WD: Tumors of the lower respiratory tract. In Rosai J (ed): Atlas of Tumor Pathology, 3rd series, Fascicle 13. Washington DC, AFIP, 1994.

147. Barbone F, Bovenzi M, Cavallieri F, et al: Cigarette smoking and histologic type of lung cancer in me. Chest 1997;112:1474.

148. Morabia A, Wynder EL: Cigarette smoking and lung cancer cell types. Cancer 1991;68:2074.

149. Toyooka S, Maruyama R, Toyooka KO, et al: Smoke exposure, histologic type and geography related differences in the methylation profile of non-small cell lung cancer. Int J Cancer 2003;103:153.

150. Cook JR, Hill DA, Humphrey PA, et al: Squamous cell carcinoma arising in recurrent papillomatosis with pulmonary involvement: Emerging common pattern of clinical features and human papillomavirus serotype association. Mod Pathol 2002;13:914.

151. Syrjanen KJ: HPV infection and lung cancer. J Clin Pathol 2002;55:885.

152. Pilotti S, Rilke F, Gribaudi G, et al: Sputum cytology for the diagnosis of lung cancer. Acta Cytolo 1982;26:661.

153. Schreiber G, McCrory DC: Performance characteristics of different modalities for diagnosis of suspected lung cancer: Summary of published evidence. Chest 2003;123:115S.

154. Truong LD, Underwood RD, Greenberg SD, et al: Diagnosis and typing of lung carcinoma by cytopathologic methods: A review of 108 cases. Acta Cytol 1985;29:379.

155. Fennessy JJ, Kittle CF: The role of bronchial brushing in the decision for thoracotomy. J Thorac Cardiovasc Surg 1973;66:541.

156. Johnston WW, Elso CE: Respiratory tract. In Bibbo M (ed): Compendium of Diagnostic Cytology. Philadelphia, WB Saunders, 1991, p 320.

157. Arroglia AC: The role of bronchoscopy in lung cancer. Clin Chest Med 1993;14:87.

158. Johnston WW: Fine needle aspiration vs. sputum and bronchial material in the diagnosis of lung cancer: A comparative study of 168 patients. Acta Cytol 1988;32:163.

159. Travis WD, Colby TV, Corrin B, et al: Histological Typing of Lung and Pleural Tumors, 3rd edition. Series: WHO International Classification of Tumors. Berlin, Springer-Verlag, 1999.

160. Cohen JH: Signs and symptoms of lung cancer. Oncol 1974;1:183.

161. Lindberg K: Uber die formale genese des lungenkrebses. Arb. a.d. path d.Univ. Helsingfors 1935;9:1-40.

162. Gray SH, Cordonnier J: Early carcinoma of the lung. Ann Surg 1925;136:1618.

163. Auerbach O, Gere JB, Forman JB, et al: Changes in the bronchial epithelium in relation to smoking and cancer of the lung. New Engl J Med 1957;3:97.

164. Saccomanno G, Archer VE, Auerbach O, et al: Development of carcinoma of the lung as reflected in exfoliated cells. Cancer 1974;33:256.

165. Frost JK, Ball WC Jr, Levin ML, et al: Early lung cancer detection: results of the initial (prevalence) radiological and cytologic screening in the John Hopkins Study. Am Rev Respir Dis 1984;130:549.

166. Colby T, Wistuba I, Gazdar A: Precursors of pulmonary neoplasia. Adv Hum Pathol 1998;5:205.

167. Meyer EC, Liebow AA: Relationship of interstitial pneumonia honeycombing and atypical epithelial proliferation to cancer of the lung. Cancer 1965;18:322.

168. Miller RR, Nelems B, Evans G, et al: Glandular neoplasia of the lung. A proposed analogy to colonic tumors. Cancer 1988;61: 1009.

169. Rao SK, Fraire AE: Alveolar cell hyperplasia in association with adenocarcinoma of lung. Mod Pathol 1995;8:165.

170. Bennett DE, Sasser WF, Ferguson TB: Adenocarcinoma of the lung. A clinico-pathological study of 100 cases. Cancer 1969;23:431.

171. Liebow AA: Bronchioloalveolar carcinoma. Adv Int Med 1960;10:329.

172. Kern WH, Jones JC, Chapman ND: Pathology of bronchogenic carcinoma in long-term survivors. Cancer 1968;21:772.

173. Bennett DE, Sasser WF: Bronchiolar carcinoma: a valid clinopathologc entity? A study of 300 cases. Cancer 1969;24:876.

174. Miller RR, Nelems B, Evans G, et al: Glandular neoplasia of the lung. A proposed analogy to colonic tumors. Cancer 1988;61:1009.

175. Carey FA, Wallace WAH, Fergussin, et al: Alveolar atypical hyplerpasia in association with primary pulmonary adenocarcinoma: A clinico-pathological study of 10 cases. Thorax 1992;47:1041.

176. Eto T, Suzuki H, Honda A, et al: The changes of the stromal elastotic framework in the growth of peripheral lung adenocarcinomas Cancer 1996;77:646.

177. Kerr KM, Carey FA, King G, et al: Atypical alveolar hyperplasia: Relationship with pulmonary adenocarcinoma, p53 and c-erbB-2 expression. J Pathol 1994;174:249.

178. Hua Z, Zheng J, Weiss LM, et al: K-ras and p53 mutations occur very early in adenocarcinoma of the lung. Am J Pathol 1994;144:303.

179. Kitamura H, Kameda Y, Nakamura N, et al: Proliferative potential and p53 overexpression in precursor and early stage lesions of bronchioloalveolar lung carcinoma. Am J Surg Pathol 1995;146:876.

180. Westra WH, Baas IO, Hruban RH, et al: K-ras oncogene activation in atypical alveolar hyperplasia of the human lung. Cancer Res 1996;56:2224.

181. Slebos R, Baas, IO, Clement MJ, et al: p53 alterations in atypical alveolar hyperplasia of the human lung. Hum Pathol 1998;29:801.

182. Kitamura H, Inayama Y, Shibagaki T, et al: Preneoplastic changes of xenotransplanted human distal airway epithelium induced by systemic administration of 4 nitroqinoline-1-oxide to host nude mice. Carcinogenesis 1991;12:2023.

183. Monobe Y, Manabe T: Morphologic changes and proliferative activity of alveolar epithelium in mouse treated with urethan. Virchows Archiv 1995;425:583.

184. Berkheiser SW: Carcinoma in situ of the lung of peripheral (bronchiolar) origin. Am J Clin Pathol 1996;46:315.

185. Saffiotti U: Alveolar type II cells at the crossroad of inflammation, fibrogenesis, and neoplasia. Am J Pathol 1996;149:1423.

186. Gatter KC, Dunhill MS, Heryet A, et al: Human lung tumors: Does intermediate filament co-expression correlate with other morphologic or immunohistochemical features? Histopathology 1985;9:805.

187. Vollmer RT, Greenberg SD, MCGravan MH, et al: Lung cancer heterogeneity: A blinded and randomized study of 100 consecutive cases. Hum Pathol 1985;16:569.

188. Dunnil MS, Gatter KC: Cellular heterogeneity in lung cancer. Histopathology 1986;10:461.

189. Yessner R: Spectrum of lung cancer and ectopic hormones. Pathol Annu 1978;13:217.

190. Johnston WW, Frable WJ: The cytopathology of respiratory tract. A review. Am J Pathol 1976;84:372.

191. Nagamoto N, Saito Y, Suda H, et al: Relationship between length of longitudinal extension and maximal depth of transmural invasion in roentgenographically occult squamous cells carcinoma of the bronchus (non polypoid type). Am J Surg Pathol 1989;13:11.

192. Dulmet-Brender E, Jaubert F, Huchon G: Exophytic endobronchial epidermoid cell carcinoma. Cancer 1986;57:1358.

193. Runckel D, Kessler S: Bronchogenic squamous carcinoma in non–irradiated juvenile laryngo-tracheal papillomatosis. Am J Surg 1986;4:293.

194. Brambilla E, Moro D, Veale D, et al: Basal cell(basaloid) carcinoma of the lung: A new morphologic and phenotypic entity with separate prognostic significance. Hum Pathol 1992;23:993.

195. Brambilla E, Moro D, Gazzeri S, et al: Alterations of Rb and cyclin D1 in NSLC and their prognostic significance. J Pathol 1999; 188:34.

196. Shimosato H: Pulmonary neoplasms. In Sternberg S (ed): Diagnostic Surgical Pathology, New York, Raven Press, 1994, p 1045.

197. Kitamura, H, Kameda Y, Ito T, et al: Cytodifferentiation of atypical adenomatous hyperplasia and bronchioloalveolar lung carcinoma: Immunohistochemical and ultrastructural studies. Virchow Archiv 1997;431:415.

198. Linnoila R, Jensen SM, Steinberg SM, et al: Peripheral airway cell marker expression in non-small cell carcinoma. Am J Clin Pathol 1992;97:233.

199. Bhattacharjee AB, Richards WG, Staunton J, et al: Classification of human lung carcinomas by mRNA expression profiling reveals distinct adenocarcinoma sub classes. Proc National Acad Sci USA 2001;98:13790.

200. Garber ME, Troyanskaya OG, Schluen K, et al: Diversity of gene expression in adenocarcinoma of the lung. Proc National Acad Sci USA 2001;98:13784.

201. Silver SA, Askin FB: True papillary carcinoma of the lung. A distinct clinicopathological entity. Am J Surg Pathol 1997;21:43.

202. Kish JK, Ro JY, Ayala AG, et al: Primary mucinous adenocarcinoma of the lung with signet ring cells: A histochemical comparison with signet-ring cell carcinomas of other sites. Hum Pathol 1989;20:1097.

203. Koss MN, Hochholzer L, O'Leary T: Pulmonary blastomas. Cancer 1991;67:2368.

204. Berkeiser SW: The prognostic significance of lung cancer of peripheral origin. Dis Chest 1962;42:392.

205. Watson WL, Farpour AF: Terminal bronchiolar or alveolar cell cancer of the lung. Cancer 1966;6:776.

206. Barsky SH, Grossman DA, Ho JH, et al: The multifocality of bronchioloalveolar carcinoma and implications of a multiclonal origin. Mod Pathol 1994;7:633.

207. Cassiere SG, McLain DA, Brooks E, et al: Metastatic carcinoma of the pancreas simulating primary bronchogenic carcinoma. Cancer 1980;46:2319.

208. Harlamert HA, Bejarano PA, Baughman RP, et al: Thyroid transcription factor-1 and cytokeratins 7 and 20 in pulmonary and breast carcinoma. Acta Cytol 1988;42:1328.

209. Rubin BP, Skarin AT, Rizk M, et al: Use of cytokeratins 7 and 20 in determining the origin of metastatic carcinoma of unknown primary, with special emphasis on lung cancer. Eur J Cancer 2001;10:77.

210. Duval JV, Savas L, Banner BF: Expression of cytokeratins 7 and 20 in crinomas of the extrahepatic biliary tract, pancreas and gallbladder. Arch Patol Lab Med 2000;124:1196.

211. Chu P, Weiss LM: Cytokeratin 7 and 20 expression in epithelial neoplasms: A survey of 435 cases. Mod Pathol 2000;13:962.

212. Kaufman O, Dietel M: Thyroid transcription factor-1 is the superior immunohistochemical marker for pulmonary adenocarcinomas and large cell carcinomas compared to surfactant proteins A and B. Histopathology 2000;36:8.

213. Cheuk W, Kwan MY, Chan JK: Immunostaining for thyroid transcription factor 1 and cytokeratin 20 aids in the distinction of small cell carcinoma from Merkel cell carcinoma, but non-pulmonary from extra-pulmonary small cell carcinoma. Arch Pathol Lab Med 2001;125:228.

214. Agoff SN, Lamps LW, Philip AT, et al: Thyroid TTF-1 is expressed in extrapulmonary small cell carcinomas, but not in other neuroendocrine tumors. Mod Pathol 2000;13:238.

215. Chang YL, Shih JY, Lee YC: New apects in clinico pathologic and oncogene studies of 23 pulmonary lymphoepithelioma-like carcinomas. Am J Surg Pathol 2002;26:715.

216. Castro CY, Sotrowski CY, Barrios R, et al: Relationship between Epstein-Barr virus and lymphoepithelioma-like carcinoma of the lung: A clinicopathology study of 6 cases and review of the literature. Hum Pathol 2001;32:863.

217. Kraut M, Wozniak A: Clinical presentation. In Pass HI, et al (eds): Lung Cancer: Principles and Practice, 2nd ed. Philadelphia, Lippincott Willams & Wilkins, 2000, p 522.

218. Bepler G, Neumann K, Holle R, et al: Clinical relevance of histologic subtyping in small cell lung cancer. Cancer 1989;64:74.

219. Hirsch FR, Osterlind K, Hansen HH: The prognostic significance of histopathologic subtyping of small cell carcinoma of the lung according to the WHO classification. A study of 375 consecutive patients. Cancer 1983;52:2144.

220. Warren WH, Memoli VA, Jordan AG, et al: Re-evaluation of pulmonary neoplasms resected as small cell carcinomas. Cancer 1990;65:1003.

221. Guinee D Jr, Jaffe E, Kingma D, et al: The spectrum of immunohistochemical staining of small cell carcinoma in specimens from transbronchial and open-lung biopsies. Am J Clin Pathol 1994;102:406.

222. Vollmer RT, Birch R, Ogden L, et al: Separation of small-cell from NSCLC. The SWOG pathologists' experience. Arch Pathol Lab Med 1984;108:792.

223. Fraire AE, Johnson EH, Yessner R, et al: Prognostic significance of histopathologic subtype and stage in small cell lung cancer. Hum Pathol 1992;23:520.

224. Sehested M, Hirsch FR, Ostrelind K, et al: Morphologic variations of small cell lung cancer. A histopathologic study of pretreatment and posttreatment specimens in 104 patients. Cancer 1986;57:804.

225. McCaughan BC, Martini N, Bains MS: Bronchial carcinoids. Review of 142 patients. J Thorac Cardiovasc Surg 1985;89:8.

226. Warren WH, Gould VE: Long term follow-up of classical carcinoid tumors. Clinicopathological observations. Scand J Thorac Cardiovasc Surg 1990;24:125.

227. Rosai J: Ackermann's Surgical Pathology. St Louis, Mo, Mosby, 1996.

228. Ranchod M: The histogenesis and development of pulmonary tumorlets. Cancer 1977;39:1135.

229. Wise WS, Bonder D, Aikawa M, et al: Carcinoid tumor of lung with varied histology. Am J Surg Pathol 1992;6:261.

230. Ranchod M, Levine GD: Spindle-cell carcinoid tumors of the lung. A clinicopathological study of 35 cases. Am J Surg Pathol 1980;4:315.

231. Arrigoni MG, Woolner LB, Bernatz PE: Atypical carcinoid tumors of the lung. J Thorac Cardiovasc Surg 1972;64:413.

232. Beasley MB, Thunnissen FB, Brambilla E, et al: Pulmonary atypical carcinoids: Predictors of survival in 106 cases. Hum Pathol 2000;31:1255.

233. Skuladottir H, Hirsch FR, Hansen HH, et al: Pulmonary neuroendocrine tumors: Incidence and prognosis of histologic subtypes. A population based study in Denmark. Lung Cancer 2002;37:127.

234. Cheuk W, Kwan MY, Suster S, et al: Immunostaining for TTF-1 and cytokeratin 20 aids in the distinction of small cell carcinoma from Merkel Cell Carcinoma, but not pulmonary from extrapulmonary small cell carcinomas. Arch Pathol Lab Med 2001;125:228.

235. Chejfec G, Capella C, Solcia E, et al: Amphicrine cells, dysplasia, and neoplasia. Cancer 1985;56:2683.

236. Hammar S, Bockus D, Remington F, et al: The unusual spectrum of neuroendocrine lung neoplasms. Ultrastruc Pathol 1989;13:515.

237. Travis WD, Linnoila RI, Tsokos MG, et al: Neuroendocrine tumors of the lung with proposed criteria for Large Cell Neuroendocrine Carcinoma. Am J Surg Pathol 1991;15:529.

238. Rosenthal SA, Curran WJ Jr: The significance of histology in non-small cell lung cancer. Cancer Treat Rev 1990;17:409.

239. Coy P, Elwood JM, Coldman AJ: Clinical indications of prognosis in unresected lung cancer. Chest 1981;80:453.

240. Mountain CF, Lukeman JM, Hammar SP, et al: Lung cancer classification: The relationship of disease extent to cell type to survival in clinical trials populations. J Surg Oncol 1987;35:147.

241. Gail MH, Eagan RT, Feld R, et al: Prognostic factors in patients with resected stage I non small cell lung cancer. A report from the Lung Cancer Study Group. Cancer 1984;54:1802.

242. Ludwig Lung Cancer Study Group. Patterns of failure in patients with resected Stage I and II non small-cell lung carcinoma of the lung. Ann Surg 1987;205:67.

243. Lung Cancer Study Group: Post operative T1 N0 no small-cell lung cancer. Squamous versus non squamous recurrences. J Thorac Cardiovasc Surg 1987;94:349.

244. Travis WD, Travis LB, Devesa SS: Lung cancer. Cancer 1995;75:191.

245. Wistuba II, Gazdar AF, Minna JD: Molecular genetics of lung carcinoma. Semin Oncol 2001;28:3.

246. Hirsch FR, Franklin WA, Veve R, et al: HER-2/neu overexpression in malignant lung tumors. Semin Oncol 2003;29:51.

247. Onuki N, Wistuba II, Travis WD, et al: Genetic changes in the spectrum of neuroendocrine lung tumors. Cancer 1999;85:600.

248. Salgia R, Skarin AT: Molecular abnormalities in lung cancer. J Clin Oncol 1998;16:1207.

249. Kratzke RA, Greatens TM, Rubins JB, et al: Rb and p16 expression in resected non-small cell lung tumors. Cancer Res 1996;56:3415.

250. Otterson GA, Kratzke RA, Coxon A, et al: Absence of p16 protein is restricted to the subset of lung cancers that retains wildtype Rb. Oncogene 1994;9:3375.

251. Kashiwabara K, Oyama T, Sano T, et al: Correlation between methylation status of the p16/CDK2gene and the expression of p16 and Rb proteins in primary non-small cell lung cancers. Int J Cancer 1998;79:215.

252. Gealy R, Zhang L, Siegfried JM, et al: Comparison of mutations in the p53 and K-Ras genes in lung carcinomas from smoking and nonsmoking women. Cancer Epidemiol Biom Prev 1999;8:297.

253. Hernandez-Boussard TM, Hainaut P: A specific spectrum of p53 mutations in lung cancer from smokers: Review of mutations compiled in the IARC p53 database. Environ Health Perspect 1998;106:385.

254. Wistuba II, Maitra A, Carrasco R, et al: High resolution chromosome 3p allelotyping of human lung cancer and preneoplastic/preinvasive bronchial epithelium reveals multiple, discontinuous sites of 3p allele loss and three regions of frequent breakpoints. Cancer Res 2000;60:1949.

255. Siprashvili Z, Sozzi G, Barnes LD, et al: Replacement of FHIT in cancer cells suppresses tumorigenicity. Proc Natl Acad Sci USA 1997;94:13771.

256. Sard L, Accornero P, Tornielli S, et al: The tumor suppressor FHIT is involved in the regulation of apoptosis and in cell cycle control. Proc Natl Acad Sci USA 1999;96:8489.

257. Veronese ML, Sozzi G, Huebner K, et al: The role of the FHIT gene in the pathogenesis of lung cancer. In Pass HI, et al (eds): Lung Cancer: Principles and Practice, 2nd ed. Philadelphia, Lippincott Williams & Wilkins, 2000, p 156.

258. Sozzi G, Sard L, De Gregorio L, et al: Association between cigarette smoking and FHIT gene alterations in lung cancer. Cancer Res 1997;57:2121.

259. Nelson HH, Wiencke JK, Gunn L, et al: Chromosome 3 p14 alterations in lung cancer: Evidence that the FHIT exon deletion is a target of tobacco carcinogenesis. Cancer Res 1998;58:1804.

260. Rusch VW, Klimstra DS, Venkatraman ES: Molecular markers help characterize neuroendocrine tumors. Ann Thorac Surg 1996; 62:798.

261. Quekel LGBA, Kessels AGH, Goei R, et al: Miss rate of lung cancer on the chest radiograph in clinical practice. Chest 1999;115:720.

262. Gambhir SS, Shepherd JE, Shah E, et al: Analytical decision model for the cost-effective management of solitary pulmonary nodules. J Clin Oncol 1998;6:2113.

263. Henschke CI, McCauley DI, Yankelovitz DF, et al: Early Lung Cancer Action Project: overall design and findings from baseline screening. Lancet 1999;354:99.

264. Kaneko M, Eguchi K, Ohmatsu H, et al: Peripheral lung cancer: Screening and detection with low dose spiral CT versus radiography. Radiology 1996;201:798.

265. Patz EF, Goodman PC, Bepler G: Screening for lung cancer. N Engl J Med 2000;343:1627.

266. Barendredgt J, Bonneux L, van der Maas PJ: The health care cost of smoking. N Engl J Med 1997;337:1052.

267. Bartecchi CE, MacKenzie TD, Schrier RW: The human costs of tobacco use. N Engl J Med 1994;330:907.

268. Hyde L, Hyde CI: Clinical manifestations of lung cancer. Chest 1974;65:299.

269. Braunwald E: Cough and hemoptysis. In Wilson JD, Braunwald E, Isselbacher K, et al (eds): Principles of Internal Medicine, 12th ed. New York, McGraw-Hill, 1991, p 219.

270. Lochridge SK, Knibbe WP, Doty DB: Obstruction of the superior vena cava. Surgery 1979;85:14.

271. McCoy BP: Apical pulmonary adenocarcinoma with contralateral hyperhidrosis. Arch Dermatol 1981;117:659.

272. Beutler B, Cerami A: Cachectin and tumor necrosis factor as two sides of the same biologic coin. Nature 1986;320:584.

273. Nelson KA, Walsh, D, Sheehan FA: The cancer-anorexia syndrome. J Clin Oncol 1994;12:213.

274. Hansen-Flaschen J, Nordberg J: Clubbing and hypertrophic osteoarthropathy. Clin Chest Med 1987;8:287.

275. Stenseth JH, Clagett OT, Woolner LB: Hypertrophic pulmonary osteoarthropathy. Dis Chest 1967;52:62.

276. Ralston SH, Gallacher SJ, Patel U, et al: Cancer-associated hypercalcemia: Morbidity and mortality. Ann Intern Med 1990;112:499.

277. List AF, Hainsworth JD, Davis BW, et al: The syndrome of inappropriate secretion of anti-diuretic hormone in small cell cancer of the lung. J Clin Oncol 1986;4:1191.

278. Sigurgeirsson B, Lindelhof B, Edhag O, et al: Risk of cancer in patients with dermatomyositis or polymyositis: a population based study. N Engl J Med 1992;326:363.

279. Sack GH, Levin J, Bell WR: Trousseau's syndrome and other manifestations of chronic disseminated coagulopathy in patients with neoplasms: Clinical, pathophysiologic and therapeutic features. Medicine 1977;56:1.

280. Doyle LA, Aisner J: Clinical presentation of lung cancer. In Roth RA, Ruckdeschel JC, Weisenburger TH (eds): Thoracic Oncology. Philadelphia, WB Saunders, 1989, pp 52–76.

281. Jemel A, Thomas A, Murray T, et al: Cancer statistics 2002. Cancer J Clin 2002;52:23.

282. Patz E, Erasmus, J, McAdams H, et al: Lung cancer staging and management: Comparison of contrast enhanced and nonenhanced helical CT of the thorax. Radiology 1999;212:56.

283. Pennes D, Glazer G, Wimbish K, et al: Chest wall invasion by lung cancer: Limitations of CT evaluation. Am J Roentgenol 1985;144:507.

284. Martini N, Heelan R, Westcott J, et al: Comparative merits of conventional, computed tomographic and magnetic resonance imaging in assessing mediastinal involvement in surgically confirmed lung carcinoma. J Thorac Cardiovasc Surg 1985;90:639.

285. Webb W, Gatsonis C, Zerhouni E, et al: CT and MR imaging in staging non-small cell bronchogenic carcinoma: Report of the radiology diagnostic oncology group. Radiology 1991;178:705.

286. Glazer H, Kaiser L, Anderson D: Indeterminate mediastinal invasion in bronchogenic carcinoma: CT evaluation. Radiology 1989;173:37.

287. McCloud T, Bourgoin P, Greenberg R, et al: Bronchogenic carcinoma: Analysis of staging in the mediastinum with CT by correlative lymph node mapping and sampling. Radiology 1992;182:319.

288. Staples C, Muller N, Miller R, et al: Mediastinal lymph nodes in bronchogenic carcinoma: Comparison between CT and mediastinoscopy. Radiology 1988;167:367.

289. Quint L, Francis I, Wahl R, et al: Preoperative staging of non-small cell carcinoma of the lung: Imaging methods. Am J Roentgenol 1995;164:1349.

290. Toloza E, Harpole L, McCrory D: Noninvsive staging of non-small cell lung cancer, a review of the current evidence. Chest 2003;123(1S):137.

291. Gress F, Savides T, Sandler A, et al: Endoscopic ultrasonography, fine-needle aspiration biopsy guided by endoscopic ultrasonography, and computed tomography in the preoperative staging of non-small cell lung cancer: a comparison study. Ann Intern Med 1997;127:604.

292. Fritscher-Ravens A, Bohuslavizki K, Brandt L, et al: Mediastinal lymph node involvement in potentially resectable lung cancer. Chest 2003;123(2):442.

293. Larsen S, Krasnik M, Vilmann P, et al: Endoscopic ultrasound guided biopsy of mediastinal lesions has a major impact on patient management. Thorax 2002;57:98.

294. Silvestri G, Hoffman B, Reed C: One from column A: Choosing between CT, positron emission tomography, endoscopic ultrasound with fine needle aspiration, transbronchial needle aspiration, thoracoscopy, mediastinoscopy, and mediastinotomy for staging lung cancer. Chest 2003;123(2):333.

295. Hany T, Steinert H, Goerres G, et al: PET diagnostic accuracy: Improvement with in-line PET-CT system: Initial results. Radiology 2002;225:575.

296. Dewan N, Gupta N, Redepenning L, et al: Diagnostic efficacy of FDG-PET imaging in solitary pulmonary nodules: Potential role in evaluation and management. Chest 1993;104:997.

297. Knight S, Delbeke D, Stewart J, et al: Evaluation of pulmonary lesions with FDG-PET. Chest 1996;109:982.

298. Reske S, Kotzerke J: FDG-PET for clinical use: Results of the 3rd German Interdisciplinary Consensus Conference. Eur J Nucl Med 2001;28:1707.

299. Pieterman R, Van Putten J, Meuzelaar J, et al: Preoperative staging of non-small lung cancer with positron-emission tomography. N Eng J Med 2000;343(4):254.

300. Gdeedo A, Van Schill P, Corthouts B, et al: Prospective evaluation of computed tomography and mediastinoscopy in mediastinal lymph node staging. Eur Respir J 1997;10:1547.

301. Marom E, McAdams H, Erasmus J, et al: Staging non-small cell lung cancer with whole-body PET. Radiology 1999;212(3):803.

302. Melamed MR: Lung cancer screening results in the National Cancer Institute New York study. Cancer 2000;89:2356.

303. Fontana RS, et al: Early lung cancer detection: results of the initial (prevalence) radiologic and cytologic screening in the Mayo Clinic study. Am Rev Respir Dis 1984;130:561.

304. Kubik AK, Parkin DM, Zatloukal P: Czech Study on Lung Cancer Screening: Post-trial follow-up of lung cancer deaths up to year 15 since enrollment. Cancer 2000;89:2363.

305. Fontana RS: The Mayo Lung Project: A perspective. Cancer 2000; 89:2352.

306. Black WC: Should this patient be screened for cancer? Eff Clin Pract 1999;2:86.

307. Marcus PM: Lung cancer screening: An update. J Clin Oncol 2001; 19:83S.

308. Marcus PM, Prorok PC: Reanalysis of the Mayo Lung Project data: The impact of confounding and effect modification. J Med Screen 1999;6:47.

309. Eddy DM: Screening for lung cancer. Ann Intern Med 1989; 111:232.

310. Bailar JC III: Screening for lung cancer–where are we now? Am Rev Respir Dis 1984;130, 541.

311. Doll R, Peto R: Mortality in relation to smoking: 20 years' observations on male British doctors. BMJ 1976;2:1525.

312. Tong L, Spitz MR, Fukeger JJ, et al: Lung carcinoma in former smokers. Cancer 1996;78:1004.

313. Tockman MS, Anthonisen NR, Wright EC, et al: Airways obstruction and the risk for lung cancer. Ann Intern Med 1987;106:512.

314. Austin JH, Pearson GD, Thomasow B: CT screening for early stage lung cancer. Chest 2002;121:1725.

315. Johnson BE, Cortazar P, Chuste JP: Second lung cancers in patients successfully treated for lung cancer. Semin Oncol 1997;24:492.

316. Levi F, Randimibison L, Te VC, et al: Second primary cancers in patients with lung carcinoma. Cancer 1999;86:186.

317. Colice GL, Rubins J, Unger M: Follow-up and surveillance of the lung cancer patient following curative-intent therapy. Chest 2003;123:272S.

318. Saito Y, et al: Multicentricity in resected occult bronchogenic squamous cell carcinoma. Ann Thorac Surg 1994;57:1200.

319. Stoeckli SJ, Zimmermann R, Schmid S: Role of routine panendoscopy in cancer of the upper aerodigestive tract. Otolaryngol Head Neck Surg 2001;124:208.

320. Kramer BS, Gohagan J, Prorok PC, et al: A National Cancer Institute sponsored screening trial for prostatic, lung, colorectal, and ovarian cancers. Cancer 1993;71:589.

321. Kaneko M, et al: Computed tomography screening for lung carcinoma in Japan. Cancer 2000;89:2485.

322. Sone S, et al: Results of three-year mass screening programme for lung cancer using mobile low-dose spiral computed tomography scanner. Br J Cancer 2001;84:25.

323. Sone S, et al: Mass screening for lung cancer with mobile spiral computed tomography scanner. Lancet 1998;351:1242.

324. Henschke CI, Yankelevitz DF, Libby D, et al: CT screening for lung cancer: The first ten years. Cancer J 2002;8(Suppl 1):S47.

325. Henschke CI, et al: Early Lung Cancer Action Project: Overall design and findings from baseline screening. Lancet 1999;354:99.

326. Henschke CI, Yankelevitz DF, Smith JP, et al: Screening for lung cancer: the early lung cancer action approach. Lung Cancer 2002;35:143.

327. Swensen SJ, et al: Lung cancer screening with CT: Mayo Clinic experience. Radiology 2003;226:756.

328. Flehinger BJ, et al: Early lung cancer detection: Results of the initial (prevalence) radiologic and cytologic screening in the Memorial Sloan-Kettering study. Am Rev Respir Dis 1984;130:555.

329. Fontana RS, et al: Screening for lung cancer. A critique of the Mayo Lung Project. Cancer 1991;67:1155.

330. Melamed MR, et al: Detection of true pathologic stage I lung cancer in a screening program and the effect on survival. Cancer 1981;47:1182.

331. Bocking A, Biesterfeld S, Chatelain R, et al: Diagnosis of bronchial carcinoma on sections of paraffin-embedded sputum. Sensitivity and specificity of an alternative to routine cytology. Acta Cytol 1992;36:37.

332. Prindiville SA, Byers T, Hirsch FR, et al: Sputum cytological atypia as a predictor of incident lung cancer in a cohort of heavy smokers with airflow obstruction. Cancer Epidemiol Biomarkers Prev 2003 Oct;12(10):987.

333. Gazdar AF, Minna JD: Molecular detection of early lung cancer. J Natl Cancer Inst 1999;91:299.

334. Tockman MS, Mulshine JL, Piantadosi S, et al: Prospective detection of preclinical lung cancer: Results from two studies of heterogeneous nuclear ribonucleoprotein A2/B1 overexpression. Clin Cancer Res 1997;3:2237.

335. Ikeda N, MacAulay C, Lam S, et al: Malignancy associated changes in bronchial epithelial cells and clinical application as a biomarker. Lung Cancer 1998;19:161.

336. Ahrendt SA, Chow JT, Xu LH, et al: Molecular detection of tumor cells in bronchoalveolar lavage fluid from patients with early stage lung cancer [see comments]. J Natl Cancer Inst 1999;91:332.

337. Anderson M, Sladon S, Michaels R, et al: Examination of p53 alterations and cytokeratin expression in sputa collected from patients prior to histologic diagnosis of squamous cell carcinoma. J Cell Biochem 1996;25(Suppl):185.

338. Dai Y, Morishita Y, Mase K, et al: Application of the p53 and K-ras gene mutation patterns for cytologic diagnosis of recurrent lung carcinomas. Cancer 2000;90:258.

339. Mao L, Hruban RH, Boyle JO, et al: Detection of oncogene mutations in sputum precedes diagnosis of lung cancer. Cancer Res 1994;54:1634.

340. Sato M, Sakurada A, Sagawa M, et al: Diagnostic results before and after introduction of autofluorescence bronchoscopy in patients suspected of having lung cancer detected by sputum cytology in lung cancer mass screening. Lung Cancer 2001;32:247.

341. Lam S, Lam B, Petty TL: Early detection for lung cancer. New tools for casefinding. Can Fam Physician 2001;47:537.

342. Lam S, Kennedy T, Unger M, et al: Localization of bronchial intraepithelial neoplastic lesions by fluorescence bronchoscopy. Chest 1998;113:696.

343. Landis SH, Murray T, Bolden S, et al: Cancer statistics, 1998. CA Cancer J Clin 1998;48:6.

344. Stenmetz KA, Potter JD, Folsom AR: Vegetables, fruit, and lung cancer in the Iowa's Women's Health Study. Cancer Res 1993;53:536.

345. Loeb LA, Ernster VL, Warner KE, et al: Smoking and lung cancer: An overview. Cancer Res 1984;44:5940.

346. Palmisano WA, Divine KK, Saccomanno G, et al: Predicting lung cancer by detecting aberrant promoter hypermethylation in sputum. Cancer Res 2000;60:5954.

347. Laird PW, Jaenisch R: DNA methylation and cancer. Human Mol Gen 1993;3:1487.

348. deBustros A, Nelkin BD, Silverman A, et al: The short arm of chromosome 11 is a "hot spot" for hypermethylation in human neoplasia. Proc Natl Acad Sci USA 1988;85:5693.

349. Herman JG, Latif F, Yongkai W, et al: Silencing of the VHL tumor-suppressor gene by DNA methylation in renal carcinoma. Proc Natl Acad Sci USA 1994;91:9700.

350. Issa J-PJ, Ottaviano YL, Celano P, et al: Methylation of the oestrogen receptor CpG island links aging and neoplasia in human colon. Nature Genet 1994;7:536.

351. Merlo A, Herman JG, Mao L, et al: 5 CpG island methylation is associated with inactivation of the tumor suppressor CDKN/p16 in human tumors. Nature Med 1995;1:686.

352. Yoshiura K, Kanai Y, Ochiai A, et al: Silencing of the E-cadherin invasion-suppressor gene by CpG island methylation in human carcinomas. Proc Natl Acad Sci USA 1995;92:7416.

353. Makos MW, Biel MA, Deiry WE, et al: p53 activates expression of HIC-1, a new candidate tumour suppressor gene on 17p13.3. Nature Med 1995;6:570.

354. Esteller M, Hamilton SR, Burger PC, et al: Inactivation of the DNA repair gene O^6-methylguaine-DNA methyltransferase promoter hypermethylation is a common event in primary human neoplasia. Cancer Res 1999;59:793.

355. Tang X, Khuri FR, Lee JJ, et al: L. Hypermethylation of the death-associated protein (DAP) kinase promoter and aggressiveness in stage I non-small cell lung cancer. J Natl Cancer Inst 2000;92:1511.

356. Bachman KE, Herman JG, Corn PG, et al: Methylation-associated silencing of the tissue inhibitor of metalloproteinase-3 gene suggests a suppressor role in kidney, brain, and other human cancers. Cancer Res 1999;59:798.

357. Cohen O, Feinstein E, Kimchi A, et al: DAP-kinase is a Ca^{2+}/calmodulin-dependent, cytoskeletal-associated protein kinase, with cell death-inducing functions that depend on its catalytic activity. EMBO J 1997;16:998.

358. Cohen O, Inbal J, Kissil JL, et al: DAP-kinase participates in TNF-a and Fas-induced apoptosis and its function requires the death domain. J Cell Biol 1999;146:141.

359. Esteller M, Sanchez-Cespedes M, Rosell R, et al: Detection of aberrant promoter hypermethylation of tumor suppressor genes in serum DNA from non-small cell lung cancer patients. Cancer Res 1999;59:67.

360. Rodenhuis S: Ras oncogenes and human lung cancer. In Pass H, Mitchell J, Johnson D, Turrisi A (eds): Lung Cancer, Principles and Practice. New York, Lippincott Raven, 1996, p 73.

361. Greenblatt MS, Bennett WP, Hollstein M, et al: Mutations in the p53 tumor gene: Clues to cancer etiology and molecular pathogenesis. Cancer Res 1994;54:4855.

362. Law MR, Morris JK, Watt HC, et al: The dose-response relationship between cigarette consumption, biochemical markers and risk of lung cancer. Br J Cancer 1997;75(11):1690.

363. Mao L, Hruban RH, Boyle JO, et al: Detection of oncogene mutations in sputum precedes diagnosis of lung cancer. Cancer Res 1994;54:1634.

364. Steinman CR: Free DNA in serum and plasma from normal adults. J Clin Invest 1980;66:1391.

365. Shapiro B, Chakrabaty M, Cohn E, et al: Determination of circulating DNA levels in patients with benign or malignant gastrointestinal disease. Cancer 1983;51:2116.

366. Nawroz H, Koch W, Anker P, et al: Microsatellite alterations in serum DNA of head and neck cancer patients. Nature Med 1996;2:1035.

367. Chen X, Stroun M, Magnenat J-L, et al: Microsatellite alterations in plasma DNA of small cell lung cancer patients. Nature Med 1996;2:1033.

368. Hibi K, Robinson R, Wu L, et al: Molecular detection of genetic alterations in the serum of colorectal cancer patients. Cancer Res 1997;58:1405.

369. Mulcahy HE, Lyautey J, Lederrey C, et al: A prospective study of K-ras mutations in the plasma of pancreatic patients. Clin Cancer Res 1998;4:271.

370. Sanchez-Cespedes M, Esteller M, Wu L, et al: Gene promoter hypermethylation in tumors and serum of head and neck cancer patients. Cancer Res 2000;60:892.

371. Mavne ST, Lippman SM: Retinoids, carotenoids and micronutrients. In Devita VT, Hellman S, Rosenberg SA (eds): Cancer: Principles and Practice of Oncology, 6th ed. Philadelphia, Lippincott Raven, 1997, p 575.

372. Krinsky NI: Actions of carotenoids in biologic systems. Ann Rev Nutr 1993;13:561.

373. Peto R, Doll R, Buckley JD, et al: Can dietary b-carotene materially reduce human cancer rates? Nature 1981;290:201.

374. Floyd RA: Role of free radicals in carcinogenesis and brain ischemia. FASEB J 1990;4:2587.

375. Toba T, Shidoji Y, Fujii J, et al: Growth suppression and induction of heat-shock protein-70 by 9-cis beta-carotene in cervical dysplasia-derived cells. Life Sci 1997;61:839.

376. Muto Y, Fujii J, Shidoji Y, et al: Growth retardation in human cervical dysplasia-derived cell lines by beta-carotene through down-regulation of epidermal growth factor receptor. Amer J Clin Nutr 1995;62(Suppl 6):1535S.

377. Mangelsdorf DJ, Umesono K, Evans RM: The retinoid receptors. In Sporn MB, Roberts AB, Goodman DS (eds): The Retinoids: Biology, Chemistry and Medicine, 2nd ed. New York, Raven Press, 1994, p 319.

378. Mangelsdorf DJ, Thummel C, Beato M, et al: The nuclear receptor superfamily: The second decade. Cell 1995;83:835.

379. Chambon P: A decade of molecular biology of retinoic acid receptors. FASEB J 1996;10:940.

380. Zelent A, Mendelson C, Kastner P, et al: Differentially expressed isoforms of the mouse retinoic acid receptor beta are generated by usage of two promoters and alternative splicing. EMBO J 1991;10:71.

381. Napgal S, Zelent A, Chambon P: RAR-beta-4, a retinoic acid receptor isoform is generated from RAR-beta-2 by alternative splicing and usage of a CUG initiator codon. Proc Natl Acad Sci USA 1992;89:2718.

382. Xu XC, Roy JY, Lee JS, et al: Differential expression of nuclear retinoic acid receptors in normal, premalignant, and malignant head and neck tissues. Cancer Res 1994;54:3580.

383. Xu XC, Sozzi G, Lee JS, et al: Suppression of retinoic acid receptor beta in non-small-cell lung cancer in vivo: Implications for lung cancer development. J Natl Cancer Inst 1997;89:624.

384. Lotan R, Xu X-C, Lippman SM, et al: Suppression of retinoic acid receptor-b in premalignant oral lesions and its upregulation by isotretinoin. N Engl J Med 1995;332:1405.

385. Lotan R: Retinoids and chemoprevention of aerodigestive tract cancer. Cancer Metast Rev 1997;16:349.

386. Mariani L, Formelli F, De Palo G, et al: Chemoprevention of breast cancer with fenretinide (4-HPR): Study of long-term visual and opththalmologic tolerability. Tumori 1996;82:444.

387. Costa A, Formelli F, Chiesa F, et al: Prospects of chemoprevention of human cancers with the synthetic retinoid fenretinide. Cancer Res 1994;54:2032S.

388. Dimery IW, Hong WK, Lee JJ, et al: Phase I trial of alpha-tocopherol effects on 13-cis-retinoic acid toxicity. Ann Oncol 1997;8:85.

389. Singh DK, Lippman SM: Cancer chemoprevention part 1: Retinoids and carotenoids and other classic antioxidants. Oncol 1998;11:1643.

390. Reddy BS, Sugie S, Maruyama H, et al: Chemoprevention of colon carcinogenesis by dietary organoselenium, benzylselenocyanate, in F344 rats. Cancer Res 1987;47:5901.

391. Weitzel F, Wendel A: Selenoenzymes regulate the activity of leukocyte 5-lipoxygenase via the peroxide tone. J Biol Chem 1993;268:6288.

392. Werz O, Steinhilber D: Selenium-dependent peroxidases suppress 5-lipoxygenase activity in B-lymphocytes and immature myeloid cells. The presence of peroxidase-insensitive 5-lipoxygenase activity in differentiated myeloid cells. Eur J Biochem 1996;242:90.

393. Fiala ES, Staretz ME, Pandya GA, et al: Inhibition of DNA cytosine methyltransferase by chemopreventive selenium compounds, determined by an improved assay for cytosine methyltransferase and DNA cytosine methylation. Carcinogenesis 1998;19:597.

394. Tanaka T, Makita H, Kawabata K, et al: 1,4-Phenylenebis (methylene-selenocyanate exerts exceptional chemopreventive activity in rat tongue carcinogenesis. Cancer Res 1997;57:3644.

Specific Malignancies

III

395. Clark LC, Cantor KP, Allaway WH: Selenium in forage crops and cancer mortality in U.S. counties. Arch Environ Health 1991;46:37.

396. Clark LC, Combs GF, Turnbull BW, et al: Effects of selenium supplementation for cancer prevention in patients with carcinoma of the skin. JAMA 1996;276:1957.

397. Werz O, Szellas D, Steinhilber D: Reactive oxygen species released from granulocytes stimulate 5-lipoxygenase activity in a B-lymphocytic cell line. Eur J Biochem 2000;267:1263.

398. Honn KV, Tang DG, Gao X, et al: 12-Lipoxygenases and 12(S)-HETE: Role in cancer metastasis. Cancer Metastasis Rev 1994;13:365.

399. Chen YQ, Duniec ZM, Liu B, et al: Endogenous 12(S)-HETE production by tumor cells and its role in metastasis. Cancer Res 1994;54:1574.

400. Timar J, Raso E, Fazakas ZS, et al: Multiple use of a signal transduction pathway in tumor cell invasion. Anticancer Res 1996;16:3299.

401. Liu B, Maher RJ, Hannun YA, et al: 12(S)-HETE enhancement of prostate tumor cell invasion: Selective role of PKCα. J Natl Cancer Inst 1994;86:1145.

402. Liu B, Timar J, Howlett J, et al: Lipoxygenase metabolites of arachidonic and linoleic acids modulates the adhesion of tumor cells to endothelium via regulation of protein kinase C. Cell Regul 1991;2:1045.

403. Liu Y-W, Chen B-K, Chen C-J, et al: Epidermal growth factor enhances transcription of human arachidonate 12-lipoxygenase in A431 cells. Biochem Biophys Acta 1997;1344:38.

404. Dethlefsen SM, Shepro D, D'Amore PA: Arachidonic acid metabolites in bFGF-, PDGF-, and serum-stimulated vascular cell growth. Exp Cell Res 1994;21:262.

405. Schade UF, Ernst M, Reinke M, et al: Lipoxygenase inhibitors suppress formation of tumor necrosis factor in vitro and in vivo. Biochem Biophys Re Commun 1989;159:748.

406. Stenke L, Mansour M, Reizenstein P, et al: Stimulation of human myelopoiesis by leukotrienes B4 and C4: Interactions with granulocyte-macrophage colony-stimulating factor. Blood 1996;81:352.

407. Denzlinger C, Walther J, Wilmanns W, et al: Interleukin-3 enhances the endogenous leukotriene production. Blood 1993;81:2466.

408. Moody TR, Leyton J, Martinez A, et al: Lipoxygenase inhibitors prevent lung carcinogenesis and inhibit non-small cell lung cancer growth. Exp Lung Res 1998;24:617.

409. Rioux N, Castonguay A: Inhibitors of lipoxygenase: A new class of cancer chemopreventive agents. Carcinogenesis 1998;19:1393.

410. Avis IM, Jett M, Boyle T, et al: Growth control of lung cancer by interruption of 5-lipoxygenase-mediated growth factor signaling. J Clin Invest 1996;97:806.

411. Kulkarni AP, Cai Y, Richards IS: Rat pulmonary lipoxygenase: Dioxygenase activity and role in xenobiotic metabolism. Int J Biochem 1992;24:255.

412. Nemoto N, Takayama S: Arachidonic acid-dependent activation of benzo[a]pyrene to bind to proteins with cytosolic and microsomal fractions from rat liver and lung. Carcinogenesis 1984;5:961.

413. Hunter JA, Finkbeiner WE, Nadel JA, et al: Predominant generation of 15-lipoxygenase metabolites of arachidonic acid by epithelial cells from human trachea. Proc Natl Acad Sci USA 1985;82:4633.

414. Kumlin M, Dahlen S-E: Characteristics of formation and further metabolism of leukotrienes in the chopped human lung. Biochim Biophys Acta 1990;1044:201.

415. Hennekens CH, Buring JE, Manson JE, et al: Lack of effect of long-term supplementation with beta carotene on the incidence of malignant neoplasms and cardiovascular disease. N Engl J Med 1996;334:1145–1149.

416. Palozza P, Luberto C, Calviello G, et al: Antioxidant and pro-oxidant role of beta-carotene in murine normal and tumor thymocytes: Effects of oxygen partial pressure. Free Radic Biol Med 1997;22:1065.

417. Paolini M, Cantelli-Forti G, Perocco P, et al: Co-carcinogenic effect of β-carotene. Nature 1999;398:760.

418. Perocco P, Paolini M, Mazzulo M, et al: β-Carotene as enhancer of cell transforming activity of poweful carcinogens and cigarette-smoke condensate on BALB/c 3T3 cells in vitro. Mutat Res 1999;440:83.

419. Wang X-D, Liu C, Bronson RT, et al: Retinoid signaling and activator protein-1 expression in ferrets given β-carotene supplements and exposed to tobacco smoke. J Natl Cancer Inst 1999;91:60.

420. Salgo MG, Cueto R, Winston GW, et al: Beta carotene and its oxidation products have different effects on microsome-mediated binding of benzo(a)pyrene to DNA. Free Radic Biol Med 1999;26:162.

421. Lee JS, Lippman SM, Benner SE, et al: Randomized placebo-controlled trial of isotretinoin in chemoprevention of bronchial squamous neoplasia. J Clin Oncol 1994;12:937.

422. Kurie JM, Lee JS, Khuri FR, et al: N-(4-Hydroxyphenyl) retinamide in the chemoprevention of squamous metaplasia and dysplasia of the bronchial epithelium. Clin Cancer Res 2000;6:2973.

423. Arnold AM, Browman GP, Levine MN, et al: The effect of the synthetic retinoid etretinate on sputum cytology: Results from a randomized trial. Br J Cancer 1992;65:737.

424. McLarty JW, Holiday DB, Girard WM, et al: Beta-carotene, vitamin A, and lung cancer chemoprevention: Results of an intermediate endpoint study. Am J Clin Nutr 1995;62:1431S.

425. Heimburger DC, Alexander CB, Birch R, et al: Improvement in bronchial squamous metaplasia in smokers treated with folate and vitamin B12. Report of a preliminary randomized double-blind intervention trial. JAMA 1988;259:1525.

426. Lippman SM, Benner SE, Hong WK: Cancer chemoprevention. J Clin Oncol 1994;12:851.

427. Pastorino U, Infante M, Maioli M, et al: Adjuvant treatment of stage I lung cancer with high-dose vitamin A. J Clin Oncol 1993;11:1216.

428. van Zandwijk N, Dalesio O, Pastorino U, et al: EUROSCAN, a randomized trial of vitamin A and N-acetylcysteine in patients with head and neck cancer or lung cancer. For the European Organization for Research and Treatment of Cancer Head and Neck and Lung Cancer Cooperative Groups. J Natl Cancer Inst 2000;92:977.

429. Lippman SM, Lee JJ, Karp DD, et al: Randomized phase III intergroup trial of isotretinoin to prevent second primary tumors in stage I non-small-cell lung cancer. J Natl Cancer Inst 2001;93:605.

430. Mayne ST, Cartmel B, Baum M, et al: Randomized trial of supplemental β-carotene to prevent second head and neck cancer. Cancer Res 2001;61:1457.

431. Shure D, Fedullo PF, Plummer M: Carinal forceps biopsy via the fiberoptic bronchoscope in the routine staging of lung cancer. West J Med 1985;142:511.

432. Sutedja TG, et al: Autofluorescence bronchoscopy improves staging of radiographically occult lung cancer and has an impact on therapeutic strategy. Chest 2001;120:1327.

433. Shure D, Fedullo PF: Transbronchial needle aspiration in the diagnosis of submucosal and peribronchial bronchogenic carcinoma. Chest 1985;88:49.

434. Shure D, Fedullo PF: The role of transcarinal needle aspiration in the staging of bronchogenic carcinoma. Chest 1984;86:693.

435. Chin R Jr, et al: Transbronchial needle aspiration in diagnosing and staging lung cancer: How many aspirates are needed? Am J Respir Cri Care Med 2002;166:377.

436. Silvestri GA, et al: Endoscopic ultrasound with fine-needle aspiration in the diagnosis and staging of lung cancer. Ann Thorac Surg 1996;61:1441.

437. Wallace MB, et al: Endoscopic ultrasound-guided fine needle aspiration for staging patients with carcinoma of the lung. Ann Thorac Surg 2001;72:1861.

438. Devereaux B, Ciaccia D, Imperiale T: Clinical utility of endoscopic ultrasound guided FNA in the preoperative staging of non-small cell lung cancer in computerized tomography negative patients [abstract]. Gastroint Endosc 2001;53:AB557.

439. Wiersema M, Edell E, Midthun D: Prospective comparison of transbronchial needle aspirate (TBNA) and endosonography guided biopsy (EUS-FNA) of mediastinal lymph nodes in patients with known or suspected non small cell lung cancer [abstract]. Gastroint Endosc 2002;55:AB79.

440. Lee JD, Ginsberg RJ: Lung cancer staging: The value of ipsilateral scalene lymph node biopsy performed at mediastinoscopy. Ann Thorac Surg 1996;62:338.

441. Toloza EM, Harpole L, Detterbeck F, et al: Invasive staging of non-small cell lung cancer: A review of the current evidence. Chest 2003;123:157S.

442. Abolhoda A, Keller S: Surgical staging of the mediastinum. In Pass HI, Mitchell JB, Johnson DH, et al (eds): Lung Cancer: Principles and Practice, 2nd ed. Philadelphia, Lippincott Williams & Wilkins, 2000, pp 628–646.

443. Ishida T, et al: Strategy for lymphadenectomy in lung cancer three centimeters or less in diameter. Ann Thorac Surg 1990;50:708.

444. Naruke T: Significance of lymph node metastases in lung cancer. Semin Thorac Cardiovasc Surg 1993;5:210.

445. Martini N, Beattie EJ Jr: Results of surgical treatment in Stage I lung cancer. J Thorac Cardiovasc Surg 1977;74:499.

446. Noda M, Vogel RL, Hasson DM: Leukemia inhibitory factor suppresses proliferation, alkaline phosphatase activity, and type I collagen messenger ribonucleic acid level and enhances osteopontin mRNA level in murine osteoblast-like (MC3T3E1) cells. Endocrinology 1990;127:185.

447. Bollen EC, van Duin CJ, Theunissen PH, et al: Mediastinal lymph node dissection in resected lung cancer: Morbidity and accuracy of staging. Ann Thorac Surg 1993;55:961.

448. Izbicki JR, et al: Radical systematic mediastinal lymphadenectomy in non-small cell lung cancer: A randomized controlled trial. Br J Surg 1994;81:229.

449. Sugi K, et al: Systematic lymph node dissection for clinically diagnosed peripheral non-small-cell lung cancer less than 2 cm in diameter. World J Surg 1998;22:290.

450. Funatsu T, et al: Preoperative mediastinoscopic assessment of N factors and the need for mediastinal lymph node dissection in T1 lung cancer. J Thorac Cardiovasc Surg 1994;108:321.

451. Martini N, Flehinger BJ: The role of surgery in N2 lung cancer. Surg Clin North Am 1987;67:1037.

452. Keller SM, Adak S, Wagner H, et al: Mediastinal lymph node dissection improves survival in patients with stages II and IIIa non-small-cell lung cancer. Eastern Cooperative Oncology Group. Ann Thorac Surg 2000;70:358.

453. Wu Y, Huang ZF, Wang SY, et al: A randomized trial of systematic nodal dissection in resectable non-small cell lung cancer. Lung Cancer 2002;36:1.

454. Kiser AC, Detterbeck FC: Diagnosis and Treatment of Lung Cancer. In Detterbeck FC, Riverra MP, Sopcinski MA, Rosenman JG (eds): An Evidence-Based Guide for the Practicing Clinician. Philadelphia, WB Saunders, 2001, p 133.

455. Damhuis RA, Schutte PR: Resection rates and postoperative mortality in 7,899 patients with lung cancer. Eur Respir J 1996;9:7.

456. Yellin A, Hill LR, Lieberman Y: Pulmonary resections in patients over 70 years of age. Isr J Med Sci 1985;21:833.

457. Ninan M, et al: Standardized exercise oximetry predicts postpneumonectomy outcome. Ann Thorac Surg 1997;64:328.

458. Wyser C, et al: Prospective evaluation of an algorithm for the functional assessment of lung resection candidates. Am J Respir Crit Care Med 1999;159:1450.

459. Celli BR: What is the value of preoperative pulmonary function testing? Med Clin North Am 1993;77:309.

460. Bolliger CT, Perruchoud AP: Functional evaluation of the lung resection candidate. Eur Respir J 1998;11:198.

461. Ferguson MK, et al: Diffusing capacity predicts morbidity and mortality after pulmonary resection. J Thorac Cardiovasc Surg 1988;96:894.

462. Martinolich K, Rivera MP: Pulmonary assessment and treatment. In Detterbeck FC, Rivera, MP, Socinski MA, Rosenman JG (eds): Diagnosis and Treatment of Lung Cancer: An Evidence-based Approach for the Practicing Clinician. Philadelphia, WB Saunders, 2001, pp 113–132.

463. Giordano A, Calcagni ML, Meduri G, et al: Perfusion lung scintigraphy for the prediction of postlobectomy residual pulmonary function. Chest 1997;111:1542.

464. Pierce RJ, Copland JM, Sharpe K, et al: Preoperative risk evaluation for lung cancer resection: Predicted postoperative product as a predictor of surgical mortality. Am J Respir Crit Care Med 1994;150:947.

465. Wu MT, et al: Prediction of postoperative lung function in patients with lung cancer: Comparison of quantitative CT with perfusion scintigraphy. Am J Roentgenol 2002;178:667.

466. Bolliger CT, Wyser C, Roser H, et al: Lung scanning and exercise testing for the prediction of postoperative performance in lung resection candidates at increased risk for complications. Chest 1995;108:341.

467. Pate P, Tenholder MF, Griffin JP, et al: Preoperative assessment of the high-risk patient for lung resection. Ann Thorac Surg 1996;61:1494.

468. Olsen GN, Block AJ, Tobias JA: Prediction of postpneumonectomy pulmonary function using quantitative macroaggregate lung scanning. Chest 1974;66:13.

469. Bolliger CT, et al: Exercise capacity as a predictor of postoperative complications in lung resection candidates. Am J Respir Crit Care Med 195;151:1472.

470. Markos J, et al: Preoperative assessment as a predictor of mortality and morbidity after lung resection. Am Rev Respir Dis 1989;139:902.

471. Bolton JW, et al: Stair climbing as an indicator of pulmonary function. Chest 1987;92:783.

472. Olsen GN, Bolton JW, Weiman DS, et al: Stair climbing as an exercise test to predict the postoperative complications of lung resection. Two years' experience. Chest 1991;99:587.

473. Walsh GL, et al: Resection of lung cancer is justified in high-risk patients selected by exercise oxygen consumption. Ann Thorac Surg 1994;58:704.

474. Bolliger CT, et al: Pulmonary function and exercise capacity after lung resection. Eur Respir J 1996;9:415.

475. Brutsche MH, et al: Exercise capacity and extent of resection as predictors of surgical risk in lung cancer. Eur Respir J 2000;15:828.

476. Olsen GN, et al: Submaximal invasive exercise testing and quantitative lung scanning in the evaluation for tolerance of lung resection. Chest 1989;95:267.

477. Cortese DA, et al: Roentgenographically occult lung cancer. A ten-year experience. J Thorac Cardiovasc Surg 1983;86:373.

478. Fujimura S, et al: A therapeutic approach to roentgenographically occult squamous cell carcinoma of the lung. Cancer 2000;89:2445.

479. Koike T, et al: Surgical results for centrally-located early stage lung cancer. Ann Thorac Surg 2000;70:1176.

480. Bechtel JJ, Kelley WR, Petty TL, et al: Outcome of 51 patients with roentgenographically occult lung cancer detected by sputum cytogic testing: A community hospital program. Arch Intern Med 1994;154:975.

481. Konaka C, et al: Comparison of endoscopic features of early-stage squamous cell lung cancer and histologic findings. Br J Cancer 1999;80:1435.

482. Sheski FD, Mathur PN: Endoscopic treatment of early-stage lung cancer. Cancer Control 2000;7:35.

483. Mathur PN, Edell E, Sutedja T, et al: Treatment of early stage non-small cell lung cancer. Chest 2003;123:176S.

484. van Boxem TJ, et al: Radiographically occult lung cancer treated with fibreoptic bronchoscopic electrocautery: A pilot study of a simple and inexpensive technique. Eur Respir J 1998;11:169.

485. Perol M, et al: Curative irradiation of limited endobronchial carcinomas with high-dose rate brachytherapy. Results of a pilot study. Chest 1997;111:1417.

486. Deygas N, Froudarakis M, Ozenne G, et al: Cryotherapy in early superficial bronchogenic carcinoma. Chest 2001;120:26.

487. Jones DR, Detterbeck FC: Surgery for stage I non–small cell lung cancer. In Detterbeck FC, Rivera, MP, Socinski MA, Rosenman JG (eds): Diagnosis and Treatment of Lung Cancer: An Evidence Based Guide for the Practicing Clinician. Philadelphia, WB Saunders, 2001, pp 177–190.

488. Martini N, et al: Incidence of local recurrence and second primary tumors in resected stage I lung cancer. J Thorac Cardiovasc Surg 1995;109:120.

489. Jensik RJ, Faber LP, Kittle CF: Segmental resection for bronchogenic carcinoma. Ann Thorac Surg 1979;28:475.

490. Kodama K, Doi O, Higashiyama M, et al: Intentional limited resection for selected patients with T1 N0 M0 non-small-cell lung cancer: A single-institution study. J Thorac Cardiovasc Surg 1997;114:347.

491. Landreneau RJ, et al: Wedge resection versus lobectomy for stage I (T1 N0 M0) non-small-cell lung cancer. J Thorac Cardiovasc Surg 197;113:691.

Specific Malignancies

III

492. Miller JI, Haticher CR: Limited resection of bronchogenic carcinoma in the patient with marked impairment of pulmonary function. Ann Thorac Surg 1987;44:340.

493. Ginsberg RJ, Rubinstein LV: Randomized trial of lobectomy versus limited resection for T1 N0 non-small cell lung cancer. Ann Thorac Surg 1995;60:615.

494. Smythe WR: Treatment of stage I non-small cell lung carcinoma. Chest 2003;123:181S.

495. Naruke T, Tsuchiya R, Kondo H, et al: Prognosis and survival after resection for bronchogenic carcinoma based on the 1997 TNM-staging classification: The Japanese experience. Ann Thorac Surg 2001;71:1759.

496. Inoue K, et al: Prognostic assessment of 1310 patients with non-small-cell lung cancer who underwent complete resection from 1980 to 1993. J Thorac Cardiovasc Surg 1998;116:407.

497. Yano T, et al: Surgical results and prognostic factors of pathologic N1 disease in non-small-cell carcinoma of the lung. Significance of N1 level: lobar or hilar nodes. J Thorac Cardiovasc Surg 1994;107:1398.

498. van Rens MT, de la Riviere AB, Elbers HR, et al: Prognostic assessment of 2,361 patients who underwent pulmonary resection for non-small cell lung cancer, stage I, II, and IIIA. Chest 2000;117:374.

499. Adebonojo SA, Bowser AN, Moritz DM, et al: Impact of revised stage classification of lung cancer on survival: A military experience. Chest 1999;115:1507.

500. Martini N, Burt ME, Bains MS, et al: Survival after resection of stage II non-small cell lung cancer. Ann Thorac Surg 1992;54:460.

501. Harpole DH Jr, Healey EA, DeCamp MM Jr, et al: Chest wall invasive non-small cell lung cancer: Patterns of failure and implications for a revised staging system. Ann Surg Oncol 1996;3:261.

502. Ratto GB, Piacenza G, Frola C, et al: Chest wall involvement by lung cancer: Computed tomographic detection and results of operation. Ann Thorac Surg 1991;51:182.

503. Downey RJ, Martini N, Rusch VW, et al: Extent of chest wall invasion and survival in patients with lung cancer. Ann Thorac Surg 1999;68:188.

504. Magdeleinat P, Alifano M, Benbrahem C, et al: Surgical treatment of lung cancer invading the chest wall: Results and prognostic factors. Ann Thorac Surg 2001;71:1094.

505. Patterson GA, Ilves R, Ginsberg RJ, et al: The value of adjuvant radiotherapy in pulmonary and chest wall resection for bronchogenic carcinoma. Ann Thorac Surg 1982;34:692.

506. Shaw RR, Paulson DL, Kee JL: Treatment of the superior sulcus tumor by irradiation followed by resection. Ann Surg 1961;154:29.

507. Detterbeck FC, Jones DR, Rosenman JG: Pancoast tumors. In Detterbeck FC, Rivera MP, Socinski MA, Rosenman JG (eds): Diagnosis and Treatment of Lung Cancer: An Evidence Based Guide for the Practicing Clinician. Philadelphia, WB Saunders, 2001, pp 233–243.

508. Rusch VW, Giroux DJ, Kraut MJ, et al: Induction chemoradiation and surgical resection for non-small cell lung carcinomas of the superior sulcus: Initial results of Southwest Oncology Group Trial 9416 (Intergroup Trial 0160). J Thorac Cardiovasc Surg 2001;121:472.

509. Detterbeck FC, Kiser AC: T3 non–small cell lung cancer (stage IIB–IIIA) In Detterbeck FC, Rivera MP, Socinski MA, Rosenman JG (eds): Diagnosis and Treatment of Lung Cancer: An Evidence-Based Guide for the Practicing Clinician. Philadelphia, WB Saunders, 2001, pp 223–232.

510. Burt ME, Pomerantz AH, Bains BS, et al: Results of surgical treatment of stage III lung cancer invading the mediastinum. Surg Clin North Am 1987;67:987.

511. Martini N, Yellin A, Ginsberg RJ, et al: Management of non-small cell lung cancer with direct mediastinal involvement. Ann Thorac Surg 1994;58:1447.

512. Deslauriers J, Jacques LF: Sleeve pneumonectomy. Chest Surg Clin N Am 1995;5:297.

513. Deslauriers J: Lung cancer: Reconstruction of the trachea and bronchus. Nippon Kyobu Geka Gakkai Zasshi 1989;37(Suppl):53.

514. Deslauriers J, Gaulin P, Beaulieu M, et al: Long-term clinical and functional results of sleeve lobectomy for primary lung cancer. J Thorac Cardiovasc Surg 1986;92:871.

515. Vogt-Moykopf I, Toomes H, Heinrich S: Sleeve resection of the bronchus and pulmonary artery for pulmonary lesions. Thorac Cardiovasc Surg 1983;31:193.

516. Pitz CC, Brutel DR, Elbers HR, et al: Results of resection of T3 non-small cell lung cancer invading the mediastinum or main bronchus. Ann Thorac Surg 1996;62:1016.

517. Okada M, Tsubota N, Yoshimura M, et al: How should interlobar pleural invasion be classified? Prognosis of resected T3 non-small cell lung cancer. Ann Thorac Surg 1999;68:2049.

518. Ruckdeschel JC: Combined modality therapy of non-small cell lung cancer. Semin Oncol 1997;24:429.

519. Vansteenkiste JF, et al: Survival and prognostic factors in resected N2 non-small cell lung cancer: A study of 140 cases. Leuven Lung Cancer Group. Ann Thorac Surg 1997;63:1441.

520. Suzuki K, et al: The prognosis of surgically resected N2 non-small cell lung cancer: The importance of clinical N status. J Thorac Cardiovasc Surg 1999;118:145.

521. Watanabe Y, Hayashi Y, Shimizu Y, et al: Mediastinal nodal involvement and the prognosis of non-small cell lung cancer. Chest 1991;100:422.

522. Wada H, et al: Time trends and survival after operations for primary lung cancer from 1976 through 1990. J Thorac Cardiovasc Surg 1996;112:349.

523. Martini N, Flehinger BJ, Zaman MB, et al: Results of resection in non-oat cell carcinoma of the lung with mediastinal lymph node metastases. Ann Surg 1983;198:386.

524. Mountain CF: Surgery for stage IIIa-N2 non-small cell lung cancer. Cancer 1994;73:2589.

525. Goldstraw P, Mannam GC, Kaplan DK, et al: Surgical management of non-small-cell lung cancer with ipsilateral mediastinal node metastasis (N2 disease). J Thorac Cardiovasc Surg 1994;107:19.

526. Pearson FG, Delarue NC, Ilves R, et al: Significance of positive superior mediastinal nodes identified at mediastinoscopy in patients with resectable cancer of the lung. J Thorac Cardiovasc Surg 1982;83:1.

527. Rusch VW: Surgery for stage III non-small cell lung cancer. Cancer Control 1994;1:455.

528. Abe K, Kato N, Miki K, et al: Malignant mesothelioma of testicular tunica vaginalis. Int J Urol 2002;9:602.

529. Miller DL, McManus KG, Allen MS, et al: Results of surgical resection in patients with N2 non-small cell lung cancer. Ann Thorac Surg 1994;57:1095.

530. Naruke T, Suemasu K, Ishikawa S: Lymph node mapping and curability at various levels of metastasis in resected lung cancer. J Thorac Cardiovasc Surg 1978;76:832.

531. Conill C, Astudillo J, Verger E: Prognostic significance of metastases to mediastinal lymph node levels in resected non-small cell lung carcinoma. Cancer 1993;72:1199.

532. Okada M, Tsubota N, Yoshimura M, et al: Prognosis of completely resected pN2 non-small cell lung carcinomas: What is the significant node that affects survival? J Thorac Cardiovasc Surg 1999;118:270.

533. Rusch VW, Albain Ks, Crowley JJ, et al: Surgical resection of stage IIIA and stage IIIB non-small-cell lung cancer after concurrent induction chemoradiotherapy. J Thorac Cardiovasc Surg 1993;105:97.

534. Albain KS, et al: Concurrent cisplatin/etoposide plus chest radiotherapy followed by surgery for stages IIIA (N2) and IIIB non-small-cell lung cancer: Mature results of Southwest Oncology Group phase II study 8805. J Clin Oncol 1995;13:1880.

535. Albain KS: Induction chemotherapy with/without radiation followed by surgery in stage III non-small-cell lung cancer. Oncol (Huntingt) 1997;11:51.

536. Bueno R, et al: Nodal stage after induction therapy for stage IIIA lung cancer determines patient survival. Ann Thorac Surg 2000;70:1826.

537. Siegenthaler MP, et al: Preoperative chemotherapy for lung cancer does not increase surgical morbidity. Ann Thorac Surg 2001;71:1105.

538. Martin J, et al: Morbidity and mortality after neoadjuvant therapy for lung cancer: The risks of right pneumonectomy. Ann Thorac Surg 2001;72:1149.

539. Dartevelle P, Macchiarini P: Techniques of pneumonectomy. Sleeve pneumonectomy. Chest Surg Clin N Am 1999;9:407.

540. Dartevelle PG, Macchiarini P, Chapelier AR: 1986: Tracheal sleeve pneumonectomy for bronchogenic carcinoma: Report of 55 cases. Updated in 1995. Ann Thorac Surg 1995;60:1854.

541. Mezzetti M, et al: Personal experience in lung cancer sleeve lobectomy and sleeve pneumonectomy. Ann Thorac Surg 2002;73:1736.

542. Roviaro G, Varoli F, Romanelli A, et al: Complications of tracheal sleeve pneumonectomy: Personal experience and overview of the literature. J Thorac Cardiovasc Surg 2001;121:234.

543. Tsuchiya R, Goya T, Naruke T, et al: Resection of tracheal carina for lung cancer. Procedure, complications, and mortality. J Thorac Cardiovasc Surg 1990;99:779.

544. Dartevelle PG, Chapelier AB, Pastorino U, et al: Long-term follow-up after prosthetic replacement of the superior vena cava combined with resection of mediastinal-pulmonary malignant tumors. J Thorac Cardiovasc Surg 1991;102:259.

545. Inoue H, Shohtsu A, Koide S, et al: Resection of the superior vena cava for primary lung cancer: 5 years' survival. Ann Thorac Surg 1990;50:661.

546. Spaggiari L, Thomas P, Magdeleinat P, et al: Superior vena cava resection with prosthetic replacement for non-small cell lung cancer: Long-term results of a multicentric study. Eur J Cardiothorac Surg 2002;21:1080.

547. Spaggiari L, Regnard JF, Magdeleinat P, et al: Extended resections for bronchogenic carcinoma invading the superior vena cava system. Ann Thorac Surg 2000;69:233.

548. Takahashi T, et al: Extended resection for lung cancer invading mediastinal organs. Jpn J Thorac Cardiovasc Surg 1999;47:383.

549. Yoshimura H, et al: Lung cancer involving the superior vena cava: Pneumonectomy with concomitant partial resection of superior vena cava. J Thorac Cardiovasc Surg 1979;77:83.

550. Tsuchiya R, Asamura H, Kondo H, et al: Extended resection of the left atrium, great vessels, or both for lung cancer. Ann Thorac Surg 1994;57:960.

551. Nakahara K, et al: Extended operation for lung cancer invading the aortic arch and superior vena cava. J Thorac Cardiovasc Surg 1989;97:428.

552. Rice TW, Blackstone EH: Radical resections for T4 lung cancer. Surg Clin North Am 2002;82:573.

553. Shohtsu A, et al: Resection of lung cancer involving the heart and great vessels. Tokai J Exp Clin Med 1981;6:73.

554. Takahashi T, et al: Extended resection for lung cancer invading mediastinal organs. Jpn J Thorac Cardiovasc Surg 1999;47:383.

555. DeMeester TR, Albertucci M, Dawson PJ, et al: Management of tumor adherent to the vertebral column. J Thorac Cardiovasc Surg 1989;97:373.

556. Fadel E, et al: En bloc resection of non-small cell lung cancer invading the thoracic inlet and intervertebral foramina. J Thorac Cardiovasc Surg 2002;123:676.

557. Gandhi S, et al: A multidisciplinary surgical approach to superior sulcus tumors with vertebral invasion. Ann Thorac Surg 1999;68:1778.

558. Gokaslan ZL, et al: Transthoracic vertebrectomy for metastatic spinal tumors. J Neurosurg 1998;89:599.

559. Canto A, Fener G, Romagosa V, et al: Lung cancer and pleural effusion: Clinical significance and study of pleural metastatic locations. Chest 1985;87:649.

560. Buhr J, et al: The prognostic significance of tumor cell detection in intraoperative pleural lavage and lung tissue cultures for patients with lung cancer. J Thorac Cardiovasc Surg 1997;113:683.

561. Buhr J, Berghauser KH, Morr H, et al: Tumor cells in intraoperative pleural lavage. An indicator for the poor prognosis of bronchogenic carcinoma. Cancer 1990;65:1801.

562. Doki Y, et al: Does pleural lavage cytology before thoracic closure predict both patient's prognosis and site of cancer recurrence after resection of esophageal cancer? Surgery 2001;130:792.

563. Dresler CM, Fratelli C, Babb J: Prognostic value of positive pleural lavage in patients with lung cancer resection. Ann Thorac Surg 1999;67:1435.

564. Eagan RT, et al: Pleural lavage after pulmonary resection for bronchogenic carcinoma. J Thorac Cardiovasc Surg 1984;88:1000.

565. Hillerdal G, Dernevik L, Almgren SO, et al: Prognostic value of malignant cells in pleural lavage at thoracotomy for bronchial carcinoma. Lung Cancer 1998;21:47.

566. Ichinose Y, et al: Prognosis of non-small cell lung cancer patients with positive pleural lavage cytology after a thoracotomy: Results of the survey conducted by the Japan Clinical Oncology Group. Lung Cancer 2001;31: 37.

567. Kondo H, et al: Pleural lavage cytology immediately after thoracotomy as a prognostic factor for patients with lung cancer. Jpn J Cancer Res 1989;80:233–237.

568. Kotoulas C, et al: Prognostic significance of pleural lavage cytology after resection for non-small cell lung cancer. Eur J Cardiothorac Surg 2001;20:330.

569. Riquet M, et al: Visceral pleura invasion and pleural lavage tumor cytology by lung cancer: A prospective appraisal. Ann Thorac Surg 2003;75:353.

570. Carretta, A, et al: Therapeutic strategy in patients with non-small cell lung cancer associated to satellite pulmonary nodules. Eur J Cardiothorac Surg 2002;21:1100.

571. Deslauriers J, et al: Carcinoma of the lung. Evaluation of satellite nodules as a factor influencing prognosis after resection. J Thorac Cardiovasc Surg 1989;97:504.

572. Urschel JD, Urschel DM, Anderson TM, et al: Prognostic implications of pulmonary satellite nodules: Are the 1997 staging revisions appropriate? Lung Cancer 1998;21:83.

573. Watanabe Y, et al: Improved survival in left non-small-cell N2 lung cancer after more extensive operative procedure. Thorac Cardiovasc Surg 1991;39:89.

574. Watanabe Y, Ichihashi T, Iwa T: Median sternotomy as an approach for pulmonary surgery. Thorac Cardiovasc Surg 1988;36:227.

575. Detterbeck FC, Jones DR, Funkhouser WK: Satellite nodules and multiple primary cancers. In Detterbeck FC, Rivera MP, Socinski MA, Rosenman JG (eds): The Diagnosis and Treatment of Lung Cancer: An Evidence Based Approach for the Practicing Clinician. Philadelphia, WB Saunders, 2001, pp 437–449,

576. Shimizu N, Ando A, Date H, et al: Prognosis of undetected intrapulmonary metastases in resected lung cancer. Cancer 1993;71:3868.

577. Fukuse T, et al: Prognosis of ipsilateral intrapulmonary metastases in resected non-small cell lung cancer. Eur J Cardiothorac Surg 1997;12:218.

578. Magilligan DJ Jr, et al: Surgical approach to lung cancer with solitary cerebral metastasis: Twenty-five years' experience. Ann Thorac Surg 1986;42:360.

579. Galluzzi S, Payne PM: Brain metastases from primary bronchial carcinoma: A statistical study of 741 necropsies. Br J Cancer 1956;10:408.

580. Figlin RA, Piantadosi S, Feld R: Intracranial recurrence of carcinoma after complete surgical resection of stage I, II, and III non-small-cell lung cancer. N Engl J Med 1988;318:1300.

581. Nakagawa H, Miyawaki Y, Fujita T, et al: Surgical treatment of brain metastases of lung cancer: Retrospective analysis of 89 cases. J Neurol Neurosurg Psychiatry 1994;57:950.

582. Martini N: Rationale for surgical treatment of brain metastasis in non-small cell lung cancer. Ann Thorac Surg 1986;42:357.

583. Wronski M, Burt M: Results and prognostic factors of surgery in the management of non-small cell lung cancer with solitary brain metastasis. Cancer 1992;70:2021.

584. Patchell RA: The treatment of brain metastases. Cancer Invest 1996;14:169.

585. Patchell RA, Tibbs PA, Walsh JW, et al: A randomized trial of surgery in the treatment of single metastases to the brain. N Engl J Med 1990;322:494.

586. Luketich JD, Burt ME: Does resection of adrenal metastases from non-small cell lung cancer improve survival? Ann Thorac Surg 1996;62:1614.

587. Luketich JD, van Raemdonck DE, Ginsberg RJ: Extended resection for higher-stage non-small-cell lung cancer. World J Surg 193;17:719.

588. Schuchert MJ, Luketich JD: Solitary sites of metastatic disease in non-small cell lung cancer. Curr Treat Options Oncol 2003;4:65.

589. Oliver TW Jr, Bernardino ME, Miller JI, et al: Isolated adrenal masses in non-small-cell bronchogenic carcinoma. Radiology 1984;153:217.

590. Allard P, Yankaskas BC, Fletcher RH, et al: Sensitivity and specificity of computed tomography for the detection of adrenal metastatic lesions among 91 autopsied lung cancer patients. Cancer 1990;66:457.

591. Ayabe H, Tsuji H, Hara S, et al: Surgical management of adrenal metastasis from bronchogenic carcinoma. J Surg Oncol 1995;58:149.

592. Detterbeck FC, Jones DR, Kernstine KH, et al: Lung cancer. Special treatment issues. Chest 2003;123:244S.

593. Higashiyama M, et al: Surgical treatment of adrenal metastasis following pulmonary resection for lung cancer: comparison of adrenalectomy with palliative therapy. Int Surg 1994; 79:124.

594. Urschel JD, Finley RK, Takita H: Long-term survival after bilateral adrenalectomy for metastatic lung cancer: A case report. Chest 1997;112:848.

595. Feld R, Arriagada R, Ball DL, et al: Prognostic factors in non small cell lung cancer: A consensus report on lung cancer. Lung Cancer 1991;7:3.

596. Van Houtte P, Rocmans P, Smets P, et al: Postoperative radiation therapy in lung cancer: A controlled trial after resection of curative design. Int J Radiat Oncol Biol Phys 1980;6:983.

597. Lafitte JJ, Ribet ME, Prevost BM, et al: Postresection irradiation for T2 N0 M0 non-small cell lung carcinoma: A prospective randomized study. Ann Thorac Surg 1996;62:830.

598. Dautzenberg B, Arriagada R, Chammard AB, et al: A controlled study of postoperative radiotherapy for patients with completely resected non-small cell lung carcinoma. Groupe d'etude et de traitement des cancers bronchiques. Cancer 1999;86:265.

599. The Lung Cancer Study Group: Effects of postoperative mediastinal radiation on completely resected stage II and III epidermoid cancer of the lung. N Engl J Med 1986;315:1371.

600. PORT meta-analysis Trialists Group: Postoperative radiotherapy in non-small-cell lung cancer: Systemic review and meta-analysis of individual patient data from nine randomized controlled trials. Lancet 1998;352:257.

601. Stephens RJ, Girling DJ, Bleehen NM, et al: The role of postoperative radiotherapy in non-small-cell lung cancer: A multicentre randomized trial in patients with pathologically staged T1-2, N1-2, M0 disease. Br J Cancer 1996;74:632.

602. Slack NH: Bronchogenic carcinoma. Nitrogen mustard as a surgical adjuvant and factors influencing survival. University surgical adjuvant lung trial. Cancer 1970;25:987.

603. Higgins GA, Shields TW: Experience of the Veterans Administration surgical adjuvant group. In Muggia F, Rozencweig M (eds): Lung cancer: Progress in therapeutic research. New York, Raven, 1979, p 433.

604. Girling DJ, Stott H, Stephens RJ, et al: Fifteen–year follow-up of all patients in a study of postoperative chemotherapy for bronchial carcinoma. Br J Cancer 1985;52:867.

605. The Ludwig Lung Cancer Study (LLSCG): Immunostimulation with intrapleural BCG as adjuvant therapy in resected non-small cell lung cancer. Cancer 1986;58:2411.

606. Holmes EC, Gail M, for the Lung Cancer Study Group: Surgical adjuvant therapy for stage II and stage III adenocarcinoma and large-cell undifferentiated carcinoma. J Clin Oncol 1986;4:710.

607. Lad T, Rubinstein L, Sadeghi A, et al: The benefit of adjuvant treatment for resected locally advanced non-small cell lung cancer. J Clin Oncol 1988;6:9.

608. Feld R, Rubinstein L, Thomas PA, and the Lung Cancer Study Group: Adjuvant chemotherapy with cyclophosphamide, doxorubicin, and cisplatin in patients with completely resected stage I NSCLC. J Natl Cancer Inst 1993;85:299.

609. Niiranen A, Niitamo-Korhonen S, Kouri M, et al: Adjuvant chemotherapy after radical surgery for non-small cell lung cancer: A randomized study. J Clin Oncol 1992;10:1927.

610. Pisters KMW, Kris MG, Gralla RJ, et al: Randomized trial comparing postoperative chemotherapy with vindesine and cisplatin plus thoracic irradiation with irradiation alone in stage III (N2) NSCLC. J Surg Oncol 1994;56:236.

611. Ohta M, Tsuchiya R, Shimoyama M, et al: Adjuvant chemotherapy for completely resected stage III non-small cell lung cancer. J Thorac Cardiovasc Surg 1993;106:703.

612. Keller SM, Sudeshna A, Wagner H, et al: A randomized trial of postoperative adjuvant therapy in patients with completely resected stage II or IIIA non-small-cell lung cancer. N Engl J Med 2000;343:1217.

613. Kunishima K, Karasawa K, Imaizumi M, et al: A randomized controlled trial of postoperative adjuvant chemotherapy in non-small cell lung cancer [in Japanese]. Haigan 1992;32:481.

614. Imaizumi M and The Study Group of Adjuvant Chemotherapy for Lung Cancer (Chuba, Japan): A randomized trial of postoperative adjuvant chemotherapy in non-small cell lung cancer (the second cooperative study). Eur J Surg Oncol 1995;21:69.

615. Wada H, Hitomi S, Teramatsu T, et al: Adjuvant chemotherapy after complete resection in non-small cell lung cancer. J Clin Oncol 1996;14:1048.

616. Non-Small Cell Lung Cancer Collaborative Group: Chemotherapy in non-small cell lung cancer: A meta-analysis using updated data on individual patients from 52 randomized clinical trials. Br Med J 1995;311:899.

617. Tonato M, on behalf of the ALP/EORTC-LCG investigators: Final report of the Adjuvant Lung Project Italy (ALPI): an Italian/ EORTC-LCG randomised trial of adjuvant chemotherapy in completely resected non-small cell lung cancer (NSCLC). Proc Am Soc Clin Oncol 2002;21:290a.

618. Waller D, Fairlamb D, Gower N, et al: The Big Lung Trial (BLT): Determining the value of cislatin-based chemotherapy for all patients with non-small cell lung cancer (NSCLC). Preliminary results in the surgical setting. Pro Am Soc Clin Oncol 2003;22:632a.

619. Le Chevalier T, for the IALT Investigators: Results of the randomized International Adjuvant Lung Trial (IALT): Cisplatin-based chemotherapy (CT) vs no CT in 1867 patients (pts) with resected non-small cell lung cancer (NSCLC). Pro Am Soc Clin Oncol 2003;22:2a.

620. Kato H, Konaka C, Tsuboi M, et al: A randomized phase III study comparing Ubenimex (Bestatin®) versus placebo as postoperative adjuvant treatment in patients with stage I squamous cell lung cancer. Pro Am Soc Clin Oncol 2001;20:307a.

621. Fisher B, Brown A, Mamounan E, et al: Effect of preoperative chemotherapy on local-regional disease in women with operable breast cancer, findings from National Surgical Adjuvant Breast and Bowel Project B-18. J Clin Oncol 1997;15:2483.

622. Pisters KMW, Ginsberg RJ, Giroux DJ, et al: Induction chemotherapy before surgery for early-stage lung cancer: A novel approach. J Thorac Cardiovasc Surg 2000;119:429.

623. Pisters K, Ginsberg R, Giroux M, et al: Bimodality lung oncology team (BLOT) trial of induction paclitaxel/carboplatin in early stage non-small cell lung cancer (NSCLC): Long term followup of a phase II trial. Pro Am Soc Clin Oncol 2003;22:633a.

624. Wagner H Jr, Lad T, Piantadosi S, et al: Randomized phase II evaluation of preoperative radiation therapy and preoperative chemotherapy with mitomycin-C, vinblastine and cisplatin in patients with technically unresectable stage IIIA and IIIB non-small cell cancer of the lung. Lung Cancer 1991;7:157.

625. Martini N, Kris MG, Flehinger BJ, et al: Preoperative chemotherapy for stage IIIA(N2) lung cancer: The Sloan-Kettering experience with 136 patients. Ann Thorac Surg 1993;55:1365.

626. Pisters KMW, Kris MG, Gralla RJ, et al: Pathologic complete response in advanced non-small-cell lung cancer following preoperative chemotherapy: Implications for the design of future non-small-lung cancer combined modality trials. J Clin Oncol 1993;11:1757.

627. Burkes RL, Shepherd FA, Ginsberg RJ, et al: Induction chemotherapy with MVP in patients with stage IIIA(N2) unresectable non-small cell lung cancer: The Toronto experience. Proc Am Soc Clin Oncol 1994;13:327a.

628. Sugarbaker DJ, Herndon J, Kohman LJ, et al: Results of Cancer and Leukemia Group B Protocol 8935: A multi-institutional phase II trimodality trial for stage IIIA(N2) non-small-cell lung cancer. J Thorac Cardiovasc Surg 1995;109:473.

629. Elias AD, Skarin AT, Leong T, et al: Neoadjuvant therapy for surgically staged IIIAN2 non-small cell lung cancer. Lung Cancer 1997;17:147.

630. Albain K, Rusch V, Crowley J, et al: Long-term survival after concurrent cisplatin/etoposide plus chest radiotherapy followed by surgery in bulky, stages IIIA(N2) and IIIB non-small cell lung cancer: 6-year outcomes from Southwest Oncology Group Study 8805. Proc Am Soc Clin Oncol 1999;18:467a.

631. Faber LP, Kittle CK, Warren WH, et al: Preoperative chemotherapy and irradiation for stage III non-small cell lung cancer. Ann Thorac Surg 1989;47:669.

632. Weiden PL, Piantadosi S, for the Lung Cancer Study Group: Preoperative chemotherapy (cisplatin and fluorouracil) and radiation therapy in stage III non-small cell lung cancer: A phase II study of the LCSG. J Natl Cancer Inst 1991;83:266.

633. Strauss GM, Herndon JE, Sherman DD, et al: Neoadjuvant chemotherapy and radiotherapy followed by surgery in stage IIIA non-small-cell carcinoma of the lung: Report of a Cancer and Leukemia Group B phase II study. J Clin Oncol 1992;10:1237.

634. Strauss GM: Author update on neoadjuvant chemotherapy and radiotherapy followed by surgery in stage IIIA non-small-cell carcinoma of the lung: Report of a Cancer and Leukemia Group B Study. Class Papers Curr Comm 1997;2:159.

635. Law A, Daly B, Madsen M, et al: High incidence of isolated brain metastases following complete response in advanced non-small cell lung cancer; a new challenge. Lung Cancer 1997;18(Suppl 1):65.

636. Albain KS, Crowley JJ, Turrisi AT, et al: Concurrent cisplatin, etoposide, and chest radiotherapy in pathologic stage IIIB non-small-cell lung cancer: A Southwest Oncology Group phase II study, SWOG 9019. J Cllin Oncol 2002;20:3454.

637. Pass HI, Pogrebniak H, Steinberg SM, et al: Randomized trial of neoadjuvant therapy for lung cancer: Interim analysis. Ann Thorac Surg 1992;53:992.

638. Yoneda S, Hibino S, Gotoh I, et al: A comparative trial on induction chemoradiotherapy followed by surgery or immediate surgery for stage III NSCLC. Proc Am Soc Clin Oncol 1995;14:367a.

639. Elias ED, Herndon J, Kumar P, et al, for the Cancer and Leukemia Group B: A phase III comparison of "best loco-regional therapy" with or without chemotherapy for stage IIIA T1-3N2 non-small cell lung cancer. Proc Am Soc Clin Oncol 1997;16:448a.

640. Rusch VW, Parekh KR, Leon L, et al: Factors determining outcome after surgical resection of T3 and T4 lung cancers of the superior sulcus. J Thorac Cardiovasc Surg 2000;119:1147.

641. Rusch VW, Giroux M, Kraut M, et al: Induction chemoradiotherapy and surgical resection for non-small cell lung carcinomas of the superior sulcus (Pancoast tumors): Mature results of Southwest Oncology Group trial 9416 (Integroup trial 0160). Pro Am Soc Clin Oncol 2003;22:634a.

642. Albain KS, Scott CB, Rusch VR, et al: Phase III comparison of concurrent chemotherapy plus radiotherapy (CT/RT) and CT/RT followed by surgical resection for stage IIIA(pN2) non-small cell lung cancer (NSCLC): Initial results from intergroup trial 0139 (RTOG 93-09). Pro Am Soc Clin Oncol 2003;22:621a.

643. Betticher DC, Hsu S-F, Tötsch M, et al: Mediastinal lymph node clearance after docetaxel-cisplatin neoadjuvant chemotherapy is prognostic of survival in patients with stage IIIA pN2 non-small-cell lung cancer: A multicenter phase II trial. J Clin Oncol 2003;21:1752.

644. Eberhardt W, Wilke H, Stamatis G, et al: Preoperative chemotherapy followed by concurrent chemoradiation therapy based on hyperfractionated accelerated radiotherapy and definitive surgery in locally advanced non-small cell lung cancer: Mature results of a phase II trial. J Clin Oncol 1998;16:622.

645. Stuschke M, Eberhardt W, Pöttgen C, et al: prophylactic cranial irradiation in locally advanced non-small-cell lung cancer after multimodality treatment: Long-term follow-up and investigations of late neuropsychologic effects. J Clin Oncol 1999;17:2700.

646. Arriagada R, Pignond P, Ihde DC, et al: Effect of thoracic radiotherapy on mortality in limited small cell lung cancer. A meta-analysis of 13 randomized trials among 2,140 patients. Anticancer Res 1994;14:333.

647. Kubota K, Furuse K, Kawahara M, et al: Role of radiotherapy in combined modality treatment of locally advanced non-small cell lung cancer. J Clin Oncol 1994;12:1547.

648. Perez C, Pajak TF, Rubin P, et al: Long-term observations of the patterns of failure in patients with unresectable non-at-cell carcinoma of the lung treated with definitive radiotherapy. Cancer 1987;59:1874.

649. Willner J, Baier K, Caragiani E, et al: Dose, volume, and tumor control predictions in primary radiotherapy of non-small-cell lung cancer. Int J Radiat Oncol Biol Phys 2002;52:382.

650. Bradley J, Ieumwananonthachai N, Purdy JA, et al: Gross tumor volume, critical prognostic factor in patients treated with three-dimensional conformal radiation therapy for non-small-cell lung carcinoma. Int J Radiat Oncol Biol Phys 2002;52:49.

651. Etiz D, Marks LB, Zhou SM, et al: Influence of tumor volume on survival in patients irradiated for non-small-cell lung cancer. Int J Radiat Oncol Biol Phys 2002;53:835.

652. Arriagada R, LeChevalier T, et al: Effect of chemotherapy on locally advanced non-small cell lung carcinoma: A randomized study of 353 patients. Int J Radiat Oncol Biol Phys 1991;20:1183.

653. Arriagada R, Kramar A, LeChevalier T, et al: Competing events determining relapse-free survival in limited small-cell lung carcinoma. J Clin Oncol 1992;10:447.

654. Schaake-Koning C, et al: Effects of concomitant cisplatin and radiotherapy in inoperable non-small-cell lung cancer. N Engl J Med 1992;326:534.

655. Furuse K, et al: Impact of tumor control on survival in unresectable stage III non-small cell lung cancer (NSCLC) treated with concurrent thoracic radiotherapy (TRT) and chemotherapy (CT) [abstract]. Proc ASCO 2000;19:1893a.

656. Curran WJ, et al: Phase III comparison of sequential vs. concurrent chemoradiation for PTS with unresected Stage III non-small cell lung cancer (NSCLC): Initial report on Radiation Therapy Oncology Group (RTOG) 9410 [abstract]. Proc ASCO 2000;19:1891a.

657. Saunders M, et al: Continuous hyperfractionated accelerated radiotherapy (CHART) versus conventional radiotherapy in non-small-cell lung cancer: A randomised multicentre trial. Lancet 1997;350:161.

658. Weisenberger TH, Gail M: Effects of postoperative mediastinal radiation on completely resected stage II and stage III epidermoid cancer of the lung. New Engl J Med 1986;315:1377.

659. Choy H, et al: Esophagitis in combined modality therapy for locally advanced non-small cell lung cancer. Semin Radiat Oncol 1999;9(Suppl 1):90.

660. Maguire P, Sibley GS, Zhou SM, et al: Clinical and dosimetric predictors of radiation-induced esophageal toxicity. Int J Rad Oncol Biol Phys 1999;45:97.

661. Singh A, Lockett M, Bradley J: Predictors of radiation-induced esophageal toxicity in patients with non-small-cell lung cancer treated with three-dimensional conformal therapy. Int J Radiat Oncol Biol Phys 2003;55:337.

662. Withers H, Taylor J, Maciejewski B: The hazard of accelerated tumor clongen repopulation during radiotherapy. Acta Oncol 1988;27:131.

663. Boxwala A, Rosenman J: Retrospective reconstruction of three dimensional treatment plans from two dimensional planning data. Int J Radiat Oncol Biol Phys 1994;28:1009.

664. Giraud P, Antoine M, Larrouy A, et al: Evaluation of microscopic tumor extension in non-small-cell lung cancer for three-dimensional conformal radiotherapy planning. Int J Radiat Oncol Biol Phys 2000;48:1015.

665. Glatstein E: Intensity modulated radiation therapy: The inverse, the converse, and the perverse. Semin Radiat Oncol 2002;12:272.

666. Glatstein E: The return of the snake oil salesmen. Int J Radiat Oncol Biol Phys 2003;55:561.

667. Bentel G, Marks L, Krishnamurthy R: Impact of cradle immobilization on setup reproducibility during external beam radiation therapy for lung cancer. Int J Radiat Oncol Biol Phys 1997;38:527.

668. Booth J, Zavgorodni S, Set-up error and organ motion uncertainty: A review. Australas Phys Eng Sci Med 1999;22:29.

669. Halperin R, Roa W, Field M, et al: Setup reproducibility in Radiation therapy for lung cancer: A comparison between T-bar and expanded form immobilization devices. Int J Radiat Oncol Biol Phys 1999;43:211.

670. Mirimanoff RO: Imobilization devices in conformal radiotherapy for non-small cell lung cancer. In van Houte P (ed): Treatment Optimization for Lung Cancer: From Classical to Innovative Procedures. Paris, Elsevier, 1998, p 103.

671. Samson M, Van Sornsen de Kost JR, de Boer HC, et al: An analysis of anatomic landmark mobility and setup deviations in radiotherapy for lung cancer. Int J Radiat Oncol Biol Phys 1999;43:827.

672. Thilmann C, Adamietz IA, Mose S, et al: Which factors modify the reproducibility of patient positioning in the daily irradiation routine? Strahlenther Oncol 1997;173:422.

673. Chen T, Pellizari C, Vijaykumar S: Imaging: The basis for effective

therapy. In Meyer JL, Purdy JA (eds): Frontiers in Radiation Therapy and Oncology, vol 29. Basel, Switzerland, Karger, 1996, pp 31–42.

674. Giraud P, Elles S, Helfie S, et al: Conformal radiotherapy for lung cancer: Different delineation of the gross tumor volume (GTV) by radiologists and radiation oncologists. Radiother Oncol 2002;62:27.

675. Graham M, Purdy JA, Emami B, et al: 3-D conformal radiotherapy for lung cancer. The Washington University experience. Front Radiat Ther Oncol 1996;29:188.

676. Schraube P, Spahn U, Oetzel P, et al: Effect of 3D compared with 2D radiotherapy planning within a conventional treatment schedule of advanced lung cancer. Strahlenther Onkol 2000;176:32.

677. McGibney C, et al: The potential impact of 3-D conformal radiotherapy (3DCRT) on continuous hyperfractionated acelerated radiotherapy (CHART) for NSCLC [abstract]. Lung Cancer 1997;18(Suppl 1):486.

678. McGibney C, Holmberg O, Sinning JM, et al: Dose escalation of CHART in non-small cell lung cancer: Is three dimensional conformal radiation therapy really necessary? Int J Radiat Oncol Biol Phys 1999;45:339.

679. Prenzel K, et al: Lymph node size and metastatic infiltration in non-small cell lung cancer. Chest 2003;123:463.

680. Sawyer T, Bonner JA, Gould PM, et al: Predictors of subclinical nodal involvement in clinical stages I and II non-small cell lung cancer: implications in the inoperable and three-dimensional dose-escalation settings. Int J Radiat Oncol Biol Phys 1999;43:965–970.

681. Giraud P, et al: Estimation de la probabilite d'envaissement tumoral mediastinal: Une definition statistique du volume-cible anatomoclinique pour la radiotherapie conformationelle des cancers bronchiques non a petits cellules? Cancer Radiother 2001;6:725.

682. Konaka C, Ikeda N, Hiyoshi T, et al: Peripheral non-small cell lung cancers 2.0 cm or less in diameter: proposed criteria for limited pulmonary resection based upon clinicopathological presentation. Lung Cancer 1998;21(3):185.

683. Miller D, et al: Surgical treatment of non-small cell lung cancer 1 cm or less in diameter. Ann Thor Surg 2002;73:1545.

684. Hayakawa K, et al: Limited field irradiation for medically inoperable patients with peripheral stage I non-small cell lung cancer. Lung Cancer 1999;26:137.

685. Sibley G: Radiotherapy for patients with medically inoperable Stage I nonsmall cell lung carcinoma. Smaller volumes and higher doses. A review. Cancer 1998;82:433.

686. LeChevalier T, et al: Radiotherapy alone versus combined chemotherapy and radiotherapy in unresectable non-small-cell lung cancer. J Natl Cancer Inst 1991;83:417.

687. Sause W, Kolesar P, Taylor SIV, et al: Final results of phase III trial in regionally advanced unresectable non-small cell lung cancer: Radiation Therapy Oncology Group, Eastern Cooperative Oncology Group, and Southwest Oncology Group. Chest 2000;117:358.

688. Hanley J, et al: Deep inspiration breath-hold technique for lung tumors: The potential value of target immobilization and reduced lung density in dose escalation. Int J Radiat Oncol Biol Phys 1996;36(Suppl 18):188.

689. Rosenzweig K, Hanley J, Mah D, et al: The deep inspiration breath-hold technique in the treatment of inoperable non-small-cell lung cancer. Int J Radiat Oncol Biol Phys 2000;48:81.

690. Wong J, Sharpe MB, Jaffray DA, et al: The use of active breathing control (ABC) to reduce margin for breathing motion. Int J Radiat Oncol Biol Phys 1999;44:911.

691. Shimizu S, Shirato H, Ogura S, et al: Detection of lung tumor movement in real-time tumor-tracking radiotherapy. Int J Radiat Oncol Biol Phys 2001;51:304.

692. Uematsu M, Shioda H, Suda A, et al: Computer tomography-guided frameless stereotactic radiotherapy for stage I non-small-cell lung cancer: A 5-year experience. Int J Radiat Oncol Biol Phys 2001;51:666.

693. Yorke E, et al: Evaluation of deep inspiration breath-hold lung treatment plans with Monte Carlo dose calcuation. Int J Radiat Oncol Biol Phys 2002;53:1058.

694. Johnson H, Schreiber E, Cullip T, et al: Significant underdosing of small tumors or portions of tumor in lung cancer treatment [abstract]. Proc Annu Meet Am Soc Ther Radiol Oncol 2002;1072.

695. Hayman J, Martel MK, Ten Haken PK, et al: Dose escalation in non-small-cell lung cancer using three dimensional conformal radiation therapy: Update of a phase I trial. J Clin Oncol 2001;19:127.

696. Hayman J, et al: Dose escalation in non-small cell lung cancer (NSCLC) using conformal 3-dimensional radiation therapy (C3DRT): Update of a phase I trial. Proc Am Soc Clin Oncol 1999;18:A1772.

697. Hazuka M, Turrisi A III, Martel MK, et al: Dose-escalation in non-small cell lung cancer (NSCLC) using conformal 3-dimensional radiation treatment planning (3DRTP): Preliminary results of Phase I study [abstract 1119]. Proc Annu Meet Am Soc Clin Oncol 1994;13:293.

698. Armstrong J, McGibney C: The impact of three-dimensional radiation on the treatment of non-small cell lung cancer. Radiother Oncol 2000;56:157.

699. Greenberger J, et al: Development of a technique for three-dimensional conformal radiotherapy of lung cancer using a total lung dose-volume histogram computational algorithm. Radiat Oncol Invest Clin Basic Res 1996;3:243.

700. Greenberger J, Bahri S, Jett J, et al: Considerations in optimizing radiation therapy for non-small cell lung cancer. Chest 1998;113(Suppl):46S.

701. Derycke S, De Gersem WR, Van Duyse BB, et al: Conformal radiotherapy of stage III non-small cell lung cancer: A class solution involving non-coplanar intensity modulated beams. Int J Radiat Oncol Biol Phys 1998;41:771.

702. Derycke S, Van Duyse B, DeGersem W, et al: Non-coplanar beam intensity modulation allows large dose escalation in stage III lung cancer. Radiother Oncol 1997;45:253.

703. Sibley G, Mundt AJ, Shapiro C, et al: The treatment of stage III nonsmall cell lung cancer using high dose conformal radiotherapy. Int J Radiat Oncol Biol Phys 1995;33:1001.

704. Scalliet P, et al: Gemzar (gemcitabine) with thoracic radiotherapy —A phase II pilot study in chemo-naive patients with advanced non-small cell lung cancer (NSCLC). Proc ASCO 1998;17:1923A.

705. Bush D, Slater JD, Bonnet R, et al: Proton-beam radiotherapy for early-stage lung cancer. Chest 1999;116:1313.

706. Martel M, Strawderman M, Hazuka MB, et al: Volume and dose parameters for survival of non-small cell lung cancer patients. Radiother Oncol 1997;44:23.

707. Bowden P, Fisher R, MacManus M, et al: Measurement of lung tumor volumes using three-dimensional computer planning software. Int J Radiat Oncol Biol Phys 2002;53:566.

708. Caldwell C, Mah K, Ung Y: Observer variation in contouring gross tumor volume in patients with poorly defined non-small-cell lung tumors on CT: The impact of 18FDG-hybrid PET fusion. Int J Radiat Oncol Biol Phys 2001;51:823.

709. Munley M, Marks LB, Scarfone C, et al: Multimodality nuclear medicine imaging in three-dimensional radiation treatment planning for lung cancer: Challenges and prospects. Lung Cancer 1999;23:105.

710. Hicks R, Kalff V, McManus MP, et al: (18)F-FDG PET provides high-impact and powerful prognostic stratification in staging newly diagnosed non-small cell lung cancer. J Nucl Med 2001;42:1596.

711. Hicks R, MacManus M: 18F-FDG PET in candidates for radiation therapy: Is it important and how do we validate its impact? J Nucl Med 2003;44:30.

712. Seltzer M, Yap CS, Silverman DH, et al: The impact of PET on the management of lung cancer: The referring physician's perspective. J Nucl Med 2002;43:752.

713. Nehmeh S, Erdi YE, Ling CC, et al: Effect of respiratory gating on quantifying PET images in lung cancer. J Nucl Med 2002;43:877.

714. Nestle U, Walter K, Schmidt S, et al: 18F-deoxyglucose positron emission tomography (FDG-PET) for the planning of radiotherapy in lung cancer: High impact on patients with atelectasis. Int J Radiat Oncol Biol Phys 1999;44:593.

715. Black Q, et al: Defining a radiotherapy target with positron emission tomography [abstract]. Int J Radiat Oncol Biol Phys 2002;54:53S.

716. Werner-Wasik M, Xiao Y, Pequignot E, et al: Assessment of lung cancer response after nonoperative therapy: Tumor diameter, bidimensional product, and volume, a serial CT scan-based study. Int J Radiat Oncol Biol Phys 2001;51:56.

717. Kostakoglu L, Goldamith S: 18F-FDG PET evaluation of the response to therapy for lymphoma and for breast, lung, and colorectal carcinoma. J Nucl Med 2003;44:224.

718. Ling C, et al: Towards multidimensional radiotherapy (MD-CRT): Biologic imaging and biologic conformality. Int J Radiat Oncol Biol Phys 2000;47:551.

719. Rosenman J: Incorporating functional imaging information into radiation treatment. Semin Radiat Oncol 2001;11:83.

720. Popple R, Ove R, Shen S: Tumor control probability for selective boosting of hypoxic subvolumes, including the effect of reoxygenation. Int J Radiat Oncol Biol Phys 2002;54:921.

721. Pugsley J, Schmidt R, Vesselle H: The Ki-67 index and survival in non-small cell lung cancer: A review and relevance to positron emission tomography. Cancer J 2002;8:222.

722. Belhocine T, et al: Increased uptake of the apoptosis-imaging agent ^{99m}Tc recombinanant human annexin V in human tumors after one course of chemotherapy as a predictor of tumor response and patient prognosis. Clin Can Res 2002;8:2766.

723. Brahme A: Optimized radiation therapy based on radiobiologic objectives. Semin Rad Oncol 1999;9:35.

724. Grant WI, Woo S: Clinical and financial issues for intensity modulated radiation therapy delivery. Semin Radiat Oncol 1999;9:99.

725. Hohenberg G, Sedlmayer F: Costs of standard and conformal photon radiotherapy in Austria. Strahlenther Onkol 1999;175(Suppl 2):99.

726. Martin P, Dubray B: Les aspects économiques de la radiothérapie conformationnelle. Cancer Radiother 1999;3:437.

727. Panten A, et al: Times requirements in conformal radiotherapy treatment planning. Radiother Oncol 1999;51:211.

728. Wong T: Intensity-modulated radiation therapy. In: The Oncology Roundtable. Washington DC, Advisory Board, 2000, pp 1–14.

729. Brodin O, Nou E, Mercke C, et al: Comparison of induction chemotherapy before radiotherapy with radiotherapy only in patients with locally advanced squamous cell carcinoma of the lung. The Swedish Lung Cancer Study Group. Eur J Cancer 1993;11:900.

730. Mattson K, Holsti LR, Holsti P, et al: Inoperable non-small-cell lung cancer: Radiation with or without chemotherapy. Eur J Cancer Clin Oncol 1988;24:477.

731. Miller J, et al: Pancoast tumors: Improved survival with preoperative and postoperative radiotherapy. Ann Thorac Surg 1987;43:32.

732. Dillman R, Seagren SL, Propert KJ, et al: A randomized trial of induction chemotherapy plus high-dose radiation versus radiation alone in stage III non-small-cell lung cancer. N Engl J Med 1990;14:940.

733. Jeremic B, Shibamoto Y, Acimovic L, et al: Randomized trial of hyperfractioned radiotherapy with or without concurrent chemotherapy for stage III non-small cell lung cancer. J Clin Oncol 1995;13:452.

734. Blanke C, Ansari R, Mantiavadi R, et al: Phase III trial of thoracic irridation with or without cisplatin for advanced unresectable non-small cell lung cancer: A Hoosier Oncology Group protocol. J Clin Oncol 1995;13:1425.

735. Trovo M, Minatel E, Franchin G, et al: Radiotherapy versus radiotherapy enhanced by cisplatin in stage III non-small-cell lung cancer. Int J Radiat Oncol Biol Phys 1992;24:573.

736. Jeremic B, Shibamoto Y, Acimovic L, et al: Hyperfractionated therapy with or without concurrent low-dose daily carboplatin/etoposide for stage III non-small-cell lung cancer: A randomized study. J Clin Oncol 1996;14:1065.

737. Furuse K, et al: Phase III study of concurrent vs. sequential thoracic radiotherapy (RT) in combination with mitomycin (M), vindesine (V) and cisplatin (C) in unresectable stage III non-small cell lung cancer (NSCLC): Five-year median follow-up results [abstract]. Proc ASCO 1999;18:1770.

738. Langer C, et al: Elderly patients (pts) with locally advanced non-small cell lung cancer (LA-NSCLC) benefit from combined modality therapy: Secondary analysis of Radiation Therapy Oncology Group (RTOG) 94-10. Proc ASCO 2002;21:1193.

739. Pierre F, et al: A randomized phase III trial of sequential chemo-radiotherapy versus concurrent chemo-radiotherapy in locally advanced non-small cell lung cancer (NSCLC) (GLOT-GFPC NPC 95-01 study). Proc ASCO 2001;20:1246.

740. Zatloukal P, et al: Concurrent versus sequential radiochemotherapy with vinorelbine plus cisplatin (V-P) in locally advanced non-small-cell lung cancer. A randomized phase II study. Proc ASCO 2002;21:1159.

741. Choy H, et al: Preliminary report of locally advanced multimodality protocol (LAMP) ACR 427: A randomized Phase II study of three chemo-radiation regimens with paclitaxel, carboplatin, and thoracic radiation (TRT) for patients with locally advanced non-small-cell lung cancer (LA-NSCLC). Proc ASCO 2002;21:1160.

742. Belani C, Wang W, Johnson DH, et al: Induction chemotherapy followed by standard thoracic radiotherapy vs. hyperfractionated accelerated radiotherapy for patients with unresectable stage IIIA & B non-small cell lung cancer: Phase III study of the Eastern Cooperative Oncology Group (ECOG 2597) [abstract 2501]. Proc ASCO 2003.

743. Auperin A, Arriagada R, Pignon JP, et al: Prophylactic cranial irradiation for patients with small cell lung cancer in complete remission. N Engl J Med 1999;341:476.

744. Cormier Y, Bergeron D, La Forge J, et al: Benefits of polychemotherapy in advanced non-small-cell bronchogenic carcinoma. Cancer 1982;50:845.

745. Rapp E, Pater JL, William A, et al: Chemotherapy can prolong survival in patients with advanced non-small-cell lung cancer. A report of the Canadian Multicenter trial. J Clin Oncol 1988;6:633.

746. Non-small Cell Lung Cancer Collaborative Group: Chemotherapy in non-small cell lung cancer: A meta-analysis using updated data on individual patients from 52 randomized trials. BMJ 1995;311:899.

747. Albain KS, Crowley JJ, LeBlanc M, et al: Survival determinants in extensive-stage non-small-cell lung cancer: The Southwest Oncology Group experience. J Clin Oncol 1991;9:1618.

748. Finkelstein DM, Ettinger DS, Ruckdeschel JC: Long-term survivors in metastatic non-small-cell lung cancer: An Eastern Cooperative Group study. J Clin Oncol 1986;4:702.

749. Ruckdeschel JC, Finkelstein DM, Ettinger DS, et al: A randomized trial of the four most active regimens for metastatic non-small cell lung cancer. J Clin Oncol 1986;4:14.

750. Bonomi PD, Finkelstein DM, Ruckdeschel JC, et al: Combination chemotherapy versus single agents followed by combination chemotherapy in non-small cell lung cancer: A study of the Eastern Cooperative Group. J Clin Oncol 1989;7:1602.

751. Wieck JK, Crowley J, Natale RB, et al: A randomized trial of five cisplatin-containing treatments in patients with metastatic non-small-cell lung cancer: A Southwest Oncology Group study. J Clin Oncol 1991;9:1157.

752. Wozniak AJ, Crowley JJ, Balcerzak SP, et al: Randomized trial comparing cisplatin with cisplatin plus vinorelbine in the treatment of advanced non-small-cell lung cancer: A Southwest Oncology Group study. J Clin Oncol 1998;16:2459.

753. Sandler AB, Nemunaitis J, Denham C, et al: Phase III trial of gemcitabine plus cisplatin versus cisplatin alone in patients with locally advanced or metastatic non-small-cell lung cancer. J Clin Oncol 2000;18:122.

754. Gatzemeier U, von Pawel J, Gottfried M, et al: Phase III comparative study of high-dose cisplatin versus a combination of paclitaxel and cisplatin in patients with advanced non-small-cell lung cancer. J Clin Oncol 2000;18:3390.

755. Von Pawel J, von Roemeling R, Gatzemeier U, et al: Tirapazamine plus cisplatin versus cisplatin in advanced non-small-cell lung cancer: A report of the international CATAPULT I study group—cisplatin and tirapazamine in subjects with advanced previously untreated non-small-cell lung tumors. J Clin Oncol 2000;18:1351.

756. LeChevalier T, Brisgand D, Douillard J-Y, et al: Randomized study of vinorelbine and cisplatin versus vindesine and cisplatin versus vinorelbine alone in advanced non-small-cell lung cancer: Results of a European multicenter trial including 612 patients. J Clin Oncol 1994;12:360.

757. Depierre A, Chastang C, Quoix E, et al: Vinorelbine versus vinorelbine plus cisplatin in advanced non-small-cell lung cancer: A randomized trial. Ann Oncol 1994;5:37.

758. Lilenbaum RC, Herndon J, List M, et al: Single-agent (SA) versus combination chemotherapy (CC) in advanced non-small cell lung cancer (NSCLC): A CALGB randomized trial of efficacy, quality of life (QOL), and cost-effectiveness. Proc Am Soc Clin Oncol 2002;21:1a.

759. Sederholm C: Gemcitabine (G) compared with gemcitabine plus carboplatin (GC) in advanced non-small lung cancer (NSCLC): A phase III study by the Swedish Lung Cancer Group (SLUSG). Proc Am Soc Clin Oncol 2002;21:291a.

760. Georgoulias V, Ardavanis A, Agelidou M, et al: Preliminary analysis of a multicenter phase III trial comparing docetaxel (D) versus docetaxel/cisplatin (DC) in patients with inoperable advanced and metastatic non-small cell lung cancer. Pro Am Soc Clin Oncol 2002;21:291a.

761. Bonomi P, Kim KM, Fairclough D, et al: Comparison of survival and quality of life in advanced non-small cell lung cancer patients treated with two dose levels of paclitaxel combined with cisplatin versus etoposide with cisplatin: Results of an Eastern Cooperative Oncology Group Trial. J Clin Oncol 2000;18:623.

762. Giaccone G, Splinter TA, Debruyne C, et al: Randomized study of paclitaxel-cisplatin versus cisplatin-teniposide in patients with advanced non-small-cell lung cancer. J Clin Oncol 1998;16:2133.

763. Belani C, Natale R, Lee J, et al: Randomized phase III trial comparing cisplatin/etoposide versus carboplatin/paclitaxel in advanced and metastatic non-small cell lung cancer (NSCLC). Proc Am Soc Clin Oncol 1998;17:455a.

764. Crino L, Scagliotti GV, Ricci S, et al: Gemcitabine and cisplatin versus mitomycin, ifosfamide, cisplatin in advanced non-small-cell lung cancer: A randomized phase III study of the Italian Lung Cancer Project. J Clin Oncol 1999;17:3522.

765. Lopez-Cabrerizo MP, Cardenal F, Artal A: Gemcitabine plus cisplatin versus etoposide plus cisplatin in advanced non-small cell lung cancer: A randomized trial by the Spanish Lung Cancer Group. Lung Cancer 1997;18:10.

766. Kelly K, Crowley J, Bunn PA, et al: Randomized phase III trial of paclitaxel plus carboplatin versus vinorelbine plus cisplatin in the treatment of patients with advanced non-small cell lung cancer: a Southwest Oncology Group trial. J Clin Oncol 2001;19:3210.

767. Schiller JH, Harrington D, Belani CP, et al: Comparison of four chemotherapy regimens for advanced non-small-cell lung cancer. N Engl J Med 2002;346:92.

768. Rodriguez J, Pawel J, Pluzanska A, et al: A multicenter, randomized multicenter phase III study of docetaxel + cisplatin (DC) and docetaxel + carboplatin (DCB) vs. vinorelbine + cisplatin (VC) in chemotherapy-naïve patients with advanced and metastatic non-small cell lung cancer. Pro Am Soc Clin Oncol 2001;20:314a.

769. Ramsey SD, Moinpour CM, Lovato LC, et al: Economic analysis of vinorelbine plus cisplatin versus paclitaxel plus carboplatin for advanced non-small cell lung cancer. J Natl Cancer Inst 2002;94:291.

770. Gralla RJ, Rodrigues J, von Pawel J, et al: Prospective analysis of quality of life (QOL) in a randomized multinational phase III study comparing docetaxel (D) plus either cisplatin (C) or carboplatin (Cb) with vinorelbine plus cisplatin (VC) in patients with advanced non-small cell lung cancer (NSCLC). Pro Am Soc Clin Oncol 2002;21:300a.

771. Klastersky JP, Sculier J, Ravez P, et al: A randomized study comparing a high and standard dose of cisplatin in combination with etoposide in the treatment of advanced non-small cell lung cancer. J Clin Oncol 1986;4:1780.

772. Gandara DR, Crowley J, Livingston RB, et al: Evaluation of cisplatin intensity in metastatic non-small-cell lung cancer: A phase III study of the Southwest Oncology Group. J Clin Oncol 1993;11:873.

773. Alberola V, Camps C, Provencia M, et al: Cisplatin/gemcitabine (CG) vs cisplatin/gemcitabine/vinorelbine (CGV) vs sequential doublets of gemcitabine/vinorelbine followed by ifosfamide/vinorelbine (GV/IV) in advanced non-small cell lung cancer (NSCLC): Results of a Spanish Lung Cancer Group phase III Trial (GEPC/98-02). Proc Am Soc Clin Oncol 2001;20:308a.

774. Edelman MJ, Clark JI, Chansky K, et al: Randomized phase II trial of sequential chemotherapy in advanced non-small cell lung cancer (SWOG 9806): Carboplatin/gemcitabine (CARB/G) followed by paclitaxel (P) or cisplatin/vinorelbine (C/V) followed by docetaxel (D). Proc Am Soc Clin Oncol 2001;20:314a.

775. Van Meerbeeck JP, Smit EF, Lianes P, et al: An EORTC randomized phase III trial of three chemotherapy regimens in advanced non-small cell lung cancer. Proc Am Soc Clin Oncol 2001;20:308a.

776. Akerley W: Paclitaxel in advanced non-small cell lung cancer: An alternative high-dose weekly schedule. Chest 2000;117:152S.

777. Hainsworth JD, Burris HA, Erland J, et al: Phase I trial of docetaxel administered by weekly infusion in patients with advanced refractory cancer. J Clin Oncol 1998;16:2164.

778. Smith I, O'Brien M, Talbot D, et al: Duration of chemotherapy in advanced non-small-cell lung cancer: A randomized trial of three versus six courses of mitomycin, vinblastine, and cisplatin. J Clin Oncol 2001;19:1336.

779. Socinski MA, Schell M, Peterman A, et al: Phase III trial comparing a defined duration of therapy versus continuous therapy followed by second-line therapy in advanced-stage IIIB/IV non-small-cell lung cancer. J Clin Oncol 2002;20:11335.

780. Depierre A, Quoix E, Mercier M, et al: Maintenance chemotherapy in advanced non-small cell lung cancer (NSCLC): A randomized study of vinorelbine (V) versus observation (OB) in patients (Pts) responding to induction therapy (French Cooperative Oncology Group). Proc Am Soc Clin Oncol 2001;20:309a.

781. Shepherd FA, Dancey J, Ramlau R, et al: Prospective randomized trial of docetaxel versus best supportive care in patients with non-small-cell lung cancer previously treated with platinum-based chemotherapy. J Clin Oncol 2000;18:2095.

782. Fossella FV, DeVore R, Kerr RN, et al: Randomized phase III trial of docetaxel versus vinorelbine or ifosfamide in patients with advanced non-small-cell lung cancer previously treated with platinum-containing chemotherapy regimens. J Clin Oncol 2000;18:2354.

783. Hanna NH, Shepherd F, Rosell R, et al: A phase III study of pemetrexed vs docetaxel in patients with recurrent non-small cell lung cancer (NSCLC) who were previously treated with chemotherapy. Proc Am Soc Clin Oncol 2003;22:622a.

784. The Elderly Lung Cancer Vinorelbine Italian Study Group: Effects of vinorelbine on quality of life and survival of elderly patients with advanced non-small cell lung cancer. J Natl Cancer Inst 1999;91:66.

785. Frasci G, Lorusso V, Panza N, et al: Gemcitabine plus vinorelbine vs vinorelbine alone in elderly patients with advanced non-small-cell lung cancer. J Clin Oncol 2000;18:2536.

786. Gridelli C, Perrone F, Cigolari S, et al: The MILES (Multicenter Italian Lung Cancer in the Elderly Study) phase III trial: Gemcitabine + vinorelbine vs vinorelbine vs gemcitabine in elderly advanced NSCLC patients. Proc Am Soc Clin Oncol 2001;20:308a.

787. Hainsworth JD, Burris HA, Litchy S, et al: Weekly docetaxel in the treatment of elderly patients with advanced non small cell lung carcinoma. A Minnie Pearl Cancer Research Network phase II trial. Cancer 2000;89:328.

788. Langer C, Manola J, Bernardo P, et al: Cisplatin-based therapy for elderly patients with advanced non-small-cell lung cancer: Implications of Eastern Cooperative Oncology Group 5592, a randomized trial. J Natl Cancer Inst 2002;6:173.

789. Kelly K, Giarritta S, Hayes S, et al: Should older patients (pts) receive combination chemotherapy for advanced stage non-small cell lung cancer (NSCLC)? An analysis of Southwest Oncology trials 9509 and 9308. Proc Am Soc Clin Oncol 2001;20:329a.

790. Hensing TA, Socinski MA, Schell MJ, et al: Age does not alter toxicity of survival for patients (pts) with stage IIIB/IV non-small cell lung cancer (NSCLC) treated with carboplatin (C) and paclitaxel (P). Pro Am Soc Clin Oncol 2001;20:346a.

791. Hirsch FR, Franklin WA, Veve R, et al: HER2/neu expression in malignant lung tumors. Semin Oncol 2002;21:297a.

792. Azzoli CG, Krug LM, Miller VA, et al: Trastuzumab in the treatment of non-small cell lung cancer. Semin Oncol 2002;29(Suppl 4):59.

793. Gatzemeier U, Groth G, Hirsch V, et al: Gemcitabine/cisplatin alone and with trastuzumab (Herceptin) in patients with non-small cell lung cancer overexpressing HER2: results of a randomized phase II study. Proc Am Soc Clin Oncol 2002;21:297a.

794. Fontanini G, De Laurentiis M, Vignati S, et al: Evaluation of epidermal growth factor-related growth factors and receptors and of neoangiogenesis in completely resected stage I-IIIA non-small-cell lung cancer. Amphiregulin and microvessel count are

independent prognostic indicators of survival. Clin Cancer Res 1998;4:241.

795. Ritter CA, Arteaga CL: The epidermal growth factor receptor-tyrosine kinase: A promising therapeutic target in solid tumors. Semin Oncol 2003;30(Suppl 1):3.

796. Herbst RS, Maddox A-M, Rothenberg ML, et al: Selective oral epidermal growth factor receptor tyrosine kinase inhibitor ZD1839 is generally well-tolerated and has activity in non-small-cell lung cancer and other solid tumors: Results of a Phase I trial. J Clin Oncol 2002;20:3815.

797. Fukuoka M, Yano S, Giaccone G, et al: A multi-institutional randomized phase II trial of gefitinib for previously treated patients with advanced non-small cell lung cancer (The IDEAL 1 Trial). J Clin Oncol 2003;21:2237–2246.

798. Douillard J-Y, Giaccone G, Horai T, et al: Improvement in disease-related symptoms and quality of life in patients with advanced non-small-cell lung cancer (NSCLC) treated with ZD1839 ("Iressa") (IDEAL 1). Proc Am Soc Clin Oncol 2002;21:299a.

799. Kris MG, Natale RB, Herbst RS, et al: A phase II trial of ZD1839 ("Iressa") in advanced non-small cell lung cancer (NSCLC) patients who had failed platinum- and docetaxel-based regimens (IDEAL 2). Proc Am Soc Clin Oncol 2002;21:292a.

800. Natale RB, Skarin A, Maddox A-M, et al: Improvement in symptoms and quality of life for advanced non-small cell lung cancer patients receiving ZD1839 ("Iressa") in IDEAL 2. Proc Am Soc Clin Oncol 2002;21:292a.

801. Giaccone G, Johnson DH, Manegold C, et al: A phase III clinical trial of ZD1839 ("Iressa") in combination with gemcitabine and cisplatin in chemotherapy-naïve patients with advanced non-small cell lung cancer (INTACT-1). Ann Oncol 2002;13(Suppl 5):127.

802. Johnson DH, Herbst R, Giaccone G, et al: ZD1839 ("Iressa") in combination with paclitaxel and carboplatin in chemotherapy-naïve patients with advanced non-small cell lung cancer (NSCLC): Initial results from a phase III trial (INTACT-2). Ann Oncol 2002;13(Suppl 5):127.

803. DeVore R, Fehrenbacher L, Herbst R, et al: A randomized phase II trial comparing rhumab VEGF (recombinant humanized monoclonal antibody to vascular endothelial growth factor) plus carboplatin/paclitaxel (CP) to CP alone in patients with stage IIIB/IV NSCLC. Proc Am Soc Clin Oncol 2000;19:485a.

804. Johnson DH, DeVore R, Kabbinavar F, et al: Carboplatin (C) + paclitaxel (T) + rhuMab-VEGF (AVF) may prolong survival in advanced non-squamous lung cancer. Proc Am Soc Clin Oncol 2001;20:315a.

805. Zelen M: Keynote address on biostatistics and data retrieval. Cancer Chemother Reports 1973;4:31.

806. Livingston RB, McCracken JD, Trauth CJ: Isolated pleural effusion in small cell lung carcinoma: Favorable prognosis. A review of the Southwest Oncology Group experience. Chest 1982;81:208.

807. Stahel R, Aisner J, Gisberg R, et al: Staging and prognostic factors in small cell lung cancer. Lung Cancer 1989;5:119.

808. Sze G, Milano E, Johnson C, et al: Detection of brain metastases: Comparison of contrast-enhanced MR with unenhanced MR and contrast CT. Am J Neuroradiol 1990;11:785.

809. Davis PC, Hudgins PA, Peterman SB, et al: Diagnosis of cerebral metastases: Double dose delayed CT vs contrast-enhanced MR imaging. Am J Neuroradiol 1991;12:293.

810. Levitan N, Byrne RE, Bromer RH, et al: The value of the bone scan and bone marrow biopsy staging small cell lung cancer. Cancer 1985;56:652.

811. Campling B, Quirt I, DeBoer G, et al: Is bone marrow examination in small cell lung cancer really necessary? Ann Intern Med 1986;105:508.

812. Bezwoda WR, Lewis D, Livini N: Bone marrow involvement in anaplastic small cell lung cancer. Diagnosis, hematologic features, and prognostic implications. Cancer 1986;58:1762.

813. Hauber HP, Bohuslavizki KH, Lund CH, et al: Positron emission tomography in the staging of small cell lung cancer: A preliminary study. Chest 2001;119:950.

814. Schumacher T, Brink I, Mix M, et al: FDG-PET imaging for the staging and follow up of small cell lung cancer. Eur J Nucl Med 2001;28:483.

815. Campling BG, Sarda IR, Baer KA, et al: Secretion of atrial natriuretic peptide and vasopressin by small cell lung cancer. Cancer 1995;75:2442.

816. Johnson BE, Damodaran A, Rushin J, et al: Ectopic production and processing of atrial natriuretic peptide in a small cell lung carcinoma cell line and tumor from a patient with hyponatremia. Cancer 1997;79:35.

817. Johnson BE, Chute JP, Rushin J, et al: A prospective study of patients with lung cancer and hyponatremia of malignancy. Am J Respir Crit Care Med 1997;156:1669.

818. Abeloff MD, Trump DL, Baylin SB: Ectopic adrenocorticotropic (ACTH) syndrome and small cell carcinoma of the lung: Assessment of clinical implications in patients on combination chemotherapy. Cancer 1981;48:1082.

819. Lokich JJ: The frequency and clinical biology of the ectopic hormone syndromes of small cell lung cancer. Cancer 1982;50:2111.

820. Shepherd FA, Laskey J, Evans WK, et al: Cushing's syndrome associated with ectopic corticotropin production in small cell lung cancer. J Clin Oncol 1992;10:21.

821. Stewart MF, Crosby SR, Gibson S, et al: Small cell lung cancer cell lines secrete predominantly ACTH precursor peptides, not ACTH. Br J Cancer 1989;60:20.

822. Souhami RL, Bradbury I, Geddes DM, et al: Prognostic significance of laboratory parameters measured at diagnosis in small cell carcinoma of the lung. Cancer Res 1985;45:2878.

823. Osterlind K, Andersen PK: Prognostic factors in small cell lung cancer: Multivariate model based on 778 patients treated with chemotherapy with or without radiation. Cancer Res 1986;46:4189.

824. Dimopoulos MA, Fernandez JF, Samaan NA, et al: Paraneoplastic Cushing's syndrome as an adverse prognostic factor in patients who die early with small cell lung cancer. Cancer 1992;69:66.

825. Anderson NE, Rosenblum MK, Graus F, et al: Autoantibodies in paraneoplastic syndromes associated with small cell lung cancer. Neurology 1988;38:1391.

826. O'Neill JH, Murray NM, Newson-Davis J: The Lambert-Eaton myasthenic syndrome. A review of 50 cases. Brain 1988;111:577.

827. Sher E, Canal N, Piccolo G, et al: Specificity of calcium channel antibodies in Lambert-Eaton myasthenic syndrome. Lancet 1989;2:640.

828. Dalmau J, Graus F, Rosenblum MK, et al: Anti-Hu-associated paraneoplastic encephalomyelitis/sensory neuronopathy: A clinical study of 71 patients. Medicine 1992;71:59.

829. Keime-Guibert F, Graus F, Broet P, et al: Clinical outcome of patients with anti-Hu-associated encephalomyelitis after treatment of the tumor. Neurology 1999;53:1719.

830. Graus F, Keime-Guibert F, Rene R, et al: Anti-Hu associated paraneoplastic encephalomyelitis: Analysis of 200 patients. Brain 2001;124:1138.

831. Thirkill CE, Fitzgerald P, Sergott RC, et al: Cancer-associated retinopathy (CAR syndrome) with antibodies reacting with retinal, optic nerve, and cancer cells. N Eng J Med 1989;321:1589.

832. Ojeda VJ: Necrotizing myelopathy associated with malignancy. A clinicopathologic study of two cases and literature review. Cancer 1984;53:1115.

833. Cerny T, Blair V, Anderson H, et al: Pretreatment prognostic factors and scoring system in 407 small cell lung cancer patients. Int J Cancer 1987;15:146.

834. Albain KS, Crowley JJ, LeBlanc M, et al: Determinants of improved outcome in small cell lung cancer: An analysis of the 2,580-patient Southwest Oncology Group Database. J Clin Oncol 1990;8:1563.

835. Sagman U, Maki E, Evans WK, et al: Small-cell carcinoma of the lung: derivation of a prognostic staging system. J Clin Oncol 1991;9:1639.

836. Ihde DC, Makuch RW, Carney DN, et al: Prognostic implications of stage disease and sites of metastases in patients with small cell carcinoma of the lung treated with intensive combination chemotherapy. Am Rev Respir Dis 1981;123:500.

837. Yip D, Harper PG: Predictive and prognostic factors in small cell lung cancer: Current status. Lung Cancer 2000;28;173.

838. Maetsu I, Pastor M, Gomez-Codina J, et al: Pretreatment prognostic factors for survival in small cell lung cancer: A new prognostic index and validation of three known prognostic indices on 341 patients. Ann Oncol 1997;8:547.

839. Sagman U, Feld R, Evans WK, et al: The prognostic significance of pretreatment serum lactate dehydrogenase in patients with small-cell lung cancer. J Clin Oncol 1991;9:954.

840. Matthews MJ, Kanhouwa S, Pickren J, et al: Frequency of residual and metastatic tumor in patients undergoing curative surgical resection for lung cancer. Cancer Chemother Rep 1973;4:63.

841. Fox W, Scadding JG: Medical Research Council comparative trial of surgery and radiotherapy in for primary treatment of small-celled or oat-celled carcinoma of bronchus. Lancet 1973;2:63.

842. Green RA, Humphrey E, Close H, et al: Alkylating agents and bronchogenic carcinoma. Am J Med 1969;46:516.

843. Grant SC, Gralla RJ, Kris MG, et al: Single-agent chemotherapy trials in small-cell lung cancer, 1970 to 1990: The case for studies in previously treated patients. J Clin Oncol 1992;10:484.

844. Ettinger DS, Finkelstein DM, Abeloff MD, et al: Justification for evaluating new anticancer drugs in selected untreated patients with extensive-stage small-cell lung cancer: An Eastern Cooperative Oncology Group randomized study. J Natl Cancer Inst 1992;84:1077.

845. Ettinger DS: Evaluation of new drugs in untreated patients with small-cell lung cancer: Its time has come. J Clin Oncol 1990;8:374.

846. Evans WK, Eisenhauer EA, Cormier Y, et al: Phase II study of amonafide: Results of treatment and lessons learned from the study of an investigational agent in previously untreated patients with small-cell lung cancer. J Clin Oncol 1990;8:390.

847. Bunn PA Jr, Inde DC: Small cell bronchogenic carcinoma: A review of therapeutic results. In Livingston RB (ed): Lung Cancer, vol 1. Boston, Martinus Mihjoff, 1981, p 169.

848. Lowenbraun S, Bartolucci A, Smalley RV, et al: The superiority of combination chemotherapy over single agent chemotherapy in small cell lung carcinoma. Cancer 1979;44:406.

849. Livingston RB, Moore TN, Heilbrun L, et al: Small-cell carcinoma of the lung: Combined chemotherapy and radiation: A Southwest Oncology Group study. Ann Intern Med 1978;88:194.

850. Slevin ML, Clark PI, Joel SP, et al: A randomized trial to evaluate the effect of schedule on the activity of etoposide in small-cell lung cancer. J Clin Oncol 1989;7:1333.

851. Abratt RP, Willcox PA, de Groot M, et al: Prospective study of etoposide scheduling in combination chemotherapy for limited disease small cell lung carcinoma Eur J Cancer 1991;27:28.

852. Cavalli F, Sonntag RW, Jungi F, et al: VP-16-213 monotherapy for remission induction of small cell lung cancer: A randomized trial using three dosage schedules. Cancer Treat Rep 1978;62:473.

853. Maksymiuk AW, Jett JR, Earle JD, et al: Sequencing and schedule effects of cisplatin plus etoposide in small-cell lung cancer: Results of a North Central Cancer Treatment Group randomized clinical trial. J Clin Oncol 1994;12:70.

854. Hong WK, Nicaise C, Lawson R, et al: Etoposide combined with cyclophosphamide plus vincristine compared with doxorubicin plus cyclophosphamide plus vincristine and with high dose cyclophosphamide plus vincristine in the treatment of small-cell carcinoma of the lung: A randomized trial of the Bristol Lung Cancer Study Group. J Clin Oncol 1989;7:450.

855. Bunn PA Jr, Greco FA, Einhorn L: Cyclophosphamide, doxorubicin, and etoposide as first-line therapy in the treatment of small-cell lung cancer. Semin Oncol 1986;13:45.

856. Jackson DV Jr, Zekan PJ, Caldwell RD, et al: VP-16-213 in combination chemotherapy with chest irradiation for small cell lung cancer: A randomized trial of the Piedmont Oncology Association. J Clin Oncol 1984;2:1343.

857. Jackson DV Jr, Case LD, Zekan PJ, et al: Improvement of long-term survival in extensive small-cell lung cancer. J Clin Oncol 1988;6;1161.

858. Jett JR, Everson L, Therneau TM, et al: Treatment of limited-stage small-cell lung cancer with cyclophosphamide, doxorubicin, and vincristine with or without etoposide: A randomized trial of the North Central Cancer Treatment Group. J Clin Oncol 1990;8:33.

859. Messeih AA, Schweitzer JM, Lipton A, et al: Addition of etoposide to cyclophosphamide, doxorubicin, and vincristine for remission induction and survival in patients with small cell lung cancer. Cancer Treat Rep 1987;71:61.

860. Lowenbraun S, Birch R, Buchanan R, et al: Combination chemotherapy in small cell lung carcinoma. A randomized study of two intensive regimens. Cancer 1984;54:2344.

861. Smith IE, Harland SJ, Robinson BA, et al: Carboplatin: A very active new cisplatin analog in the treatment of small cell lung cancer. Cancer Treat Rep 1985;69:43.

862. Evans WK, Osoba D, Feld R, et al: Etoposide (VP-16) and cisplatin: An effective treatment for relapse in small-cell lung cancer. J Clin Oncol 1985;3:65.

863. Evans WK, Feld R, Osoba D, et al: VP-16 alone and in combination with cisplatinn in previously treated patients with small cell lung cancer. Cancer 1984;53:1461.

864. Evans WK, Shepherd FA, Feld R, et al: VP-16 and cisplatin as first line therapy for small-cell lung cancer. J Clin Oncol 1985;3:1471.

865. Roth BJ, Johnson DH, Einhorn LH, et al: Randomized study of cyclophosphamide, doxorubicin, and vincristine versus etoposide and cisplatin versus alternation of these two regimens in extensive stage small-cell lung cancer: A phase III trial of the Southeastern Cancer Study Group. J Clin Oncol 1992;10:282.

866. Fukuoka M, Furuse K, Saijo N, et al: Randomized trial of cyclophosphamide, doxorubicin, and vincristine versus cisplatin and etoposide versus alternation of these regimens in small-cell lung cancer. J Natl Cancer Inst 1991;83:855.

867. Pujol JL, Carestia L, Daures JP: Is there a case for cisplatin in the treatment of small-cell lung cancer? A meta-analysis of randomized trials of a cisplatin-containing regimen vs a regimen without this alkylating agent. Br J Cancer 2000;83:8.

868. Mascaux C, Paesmans M, Berghmans T, et al: A systematic review of the role of etoposide and cisplatin in the chemotherapy of small cell lung cancer with methodology assessment and meta-analysis. Lung Cancer 2000;30:23.

869. Bishop JF, Raghavan D, Stuart-Harris R, et al: Carboplatin (CBDCA, JM-8) and VP-16-213 in previously untreated patients with small-cell lung cancer J Clin Oncol 1987;5;1574.

870. Skarlos DV, Samantas E, Kosmidis P, et al: Randomized comparison of etoposide-cisplatin vs etoposide-carboplatin and irradiation in small-cell lung cancer. A Hellenic Co-operative Oncology Group study. Ann Oncol 1994;5:601.

871. Noda K, Nishiwaki Y, Kawahara M, et al: Irinotecan plus cisplatin compared with etoposide plus cisplatin for extensive small-cell lung cancer. N Eng J Med 2002;346:85.

872. Loehrer PJ, Ansary R, Gonin R, et al: Cisplatin plus etoposide with and without ifosfamide in extensive stage small-cell lung cancer: A Hoosier Oncology Group Study. J Clin Oncol 1995;13:2594.

873. Miyomoto H, Nakabayashi T, Isobe H, et al: A phase III trial of etoposide/cisplatin with or without added ifosfamide in small-cell lung cancer. Oncology 1992;49:431.

874. Mavroudis D, Papadakis E, Veslemes M, et al: A multicenter randomized clinical trial comparing paclitaxel-cisplatin-etoposide vs cisplatin-etoposide as first line treatment in patients with small-cell lung cancer. Ann Oncol 2001;12:463.

875. Niell HB, Herndon JE, Miller AA, et al: Randomized phase III intergroup trial (CALGB 9732) of etoposide (VP-16) and cisplatin (DDP) with or without paclitaxel (TAX) and G-CSF in patients with extensive stage small cell lung cancer (ED-SCLC). Proc Am Soc Clin Oncol 2002;21:293a.

876. Maurer LH, Tulloh M, Weiss RB, et al: A randomized combined modality trial in small cell carcinoma of the lung: Comparison of combination chemotherapy-radiation therapy versus cyclophosphamide-radiation therapy effects of maintenance chemotherapy and prophylactic whole brain irradiation. Cancer 1980;45:30.

877. Cullen M, Morgan D, Gregory W, et al: Maintenance chemotherapy for anaplastic small cell carcinoma of the bronchus: A randomized control trial. Cancer Chemother Pharmacol 1986;17:157.

878. Controlled trial of twelve versus six courses of chemotherapy in the treatment of small cell lung cancer. Report to the Medical Research Council by its Lung Cancer Working Party. Br J Cancer 1989;59:584.

879. Bleehen NM, Girling DJ, Machin D, et al: A randomized trial of three or six courses of etoposide cyclophosphamide methotrexate and vincristine or six courses of etoposide and ifosfamide in small cell lung cancer (SCLC). I: Survival and prognostic factors. Medical Research Council Lung Cancer Working Party Br J Cancer 1993;68:1150.

880. Spiro SG, Souhami RL, Geddes DM, et al: Duration of chemother-

apy in small cell lung cancer: A Cancer Research Campaign trial. Br J Cancer 1989;59:578.

881. Schiller JH, Adak S, Cella D, et al: Topotecan vs observation after cisplatin plus etoposide in extensive-stage small-cell lung cancer: E7593: A phase III trial of the Eastern Cooperative Oncology Group. J Clin Oncol 2001;19:2114.

882. Goldie JH, Coldman AJ: The genetic origin of drug resistance in neoplasms: Implications for systemic therapy. Cancer Res 1984;44:3643.

883. Evans WK, Feld R, Murray N, et al: Superiority of alternating non-cross-resistant chemotherapy in extensive small cell lung cancer. Ann Intern Med 1987;107:451.

884. Cohen MH, Creaven PJ, Fossieck BE Jr, et al: Intensive chemotherapy of small cell bronchogenic carcinoma. Cancer Treat Rep 1977;69:1007.

885. Johnson DH, Einhorn LH, Birch R, et al: A randomized comparison of high-dose versus conventional-dose cyclophosphamide, doxorubicin, and vincristine for extensive-stage small cell lung cancer: A phase III trial of the Southeastern Cancer Study Group. J Clin Oncol 1987;5:1731.

886. Figueredo AT, Hryniuk WM, Strautmanis I, et al: Co-trimoxazole prophylaxis during high-dose chemotherapy of small cell lung cancer. J Clin Oncol 1985;3:54.

887. Ihde DC, Mulshine JL, Kramer BS, et al: Prospective randomized comparison of high-dose and standard-dose etoposide and cisplatin chemotherapy in patients with extensive-stage small-cell lung cancer. J Clin Oncol 1994;12:2022.

888. Arriagada R, Le Chevalier T, Pignon JP, et al: Initial chemotherapeutic doses and survival in patients with limited small-cell lung cancer. N Eng J Med 1993;329:1848.

889. Steward WP, von Pawel J, Gatzemeier U, et al: Effects of granulocyte-macrophage colony stimulating factor and dose intensification of V-ICE in small cell lung cancer: A prospective randomized study of 300 patients. J Clin Oncol 1998;16:642.

890. Thatcher N, Girling DJ, Hopwood P, et al: Improving survival without reducing quality of life in small cell lung cancer patients by increasing the dose-intensity of chemotherapy with granulocyte colony stimulating factor support: Results of a British Medical Research Council multicenter randomized trial-Medical Research Council Lung Cancer Working Party. J Clin Oncol 2000;18:395.

891. Sculier JP, Paesmans M, Bureau G, et al: Multiple drug weekly chemotherapy versus combination regimen in small cell lung cancer: A phase III randomized study conducted by the European Lung Cancer Working Party. J Clin Oncol 1993;11:1858.

892. Murray N, Shepherd F, James K, et al: A randomized study of CODE versus alternating CAV/EP for extensive stage small cell lung cancer: An intergroup study of the National Cancer Institute of Canada Clinical Trials Group and the Southwest Oncology Group. J Clin Oncol 1999;17:2300.

893. Furuse K, Fukuoka M, Nishiwaki Y, et al: Phase III study of intensive weekly chemotherapy with recombinant human granulocyte colony-stimulating factor versus standard chemotherapy in extensive-disease small-cell lung cancer. The Japan Clinical Oncology Group. J Clin Oncol 1998;16:2126.

894. Ardizzoni A, Tjan-Heijnen VCG, Postmus PE, et al: Standard versus intensified chemotherapy with granulocyte colony-stimulating factor support in small-cell lung cancer: A prospective European Organization for Research and Treatment of Cancer-Lung Cancer Group phase III trial-08923. J Clin Oncol 2002;20:3947.

895. Elias A: Hematopoietic stem cell transplantation for small cell lung cancer. Chest 1999;116:531S.

896. Littlewood TJ, Bentley DP, Smith AP: High-dose etoposide with autologous bone marrow transplantation for small cell lung cancer. Eur J Respir Dis 1986;68:370.

897. Souhami RL, Hajichristou HT, Miles DW, et al: Intensive chemotherapy with autologous bone marrow transplantation for small cell lung cancer. Cancer Chemother Pharmacol 1989;24:321.

898. Lange A, Kolodziej J, Tomeczko J, et al: Aggressive chemotherapy with autologous bone marrow transplantation in small cell lung carcinoma. Archiv Immunol Therap Exp 1991;39:431.

899. Nomura F, Shimokata K, Saito H, et al: High dose chemotherapy with autologous bone marrow transplantation for limited small cell lung cancer. Jpn J Clin Oncol 1990;20:94.

900. Johnson DH, Hande KR, Hainsworth JD, et al: High dose etoposide

as single-agent chemotherapy for small cell carcinoma of the lung. Cancer Treat Rep 1983;67:957.

901. Spitzer G, Farha P, Valdivieso M. et al: High dose intensification therapy with autologous bone marrow support for limited small-cell bronchogenic carcinoma. J Clin 1986;Oncol 4:4.

902. Humblet Y, Symann M, Bosly A, et al: Late intensification chemotherapy with autologous bone marrow transplantation in selected small-cell carcinoma of the lung: A randomized study. J Clin Oncol 1987;5:1864.

903. Dajczman E, Fu LY, Small D, et al: Treatment of small cell lung carcinoma in the elderly. Cancer 1996;77:2032.

904. Shepherd FA, Amdemichael E, Evans WK, et al: Treatment of small cell lung cancer in the elderly. J Am Geriatr Soc 1994;42:64.

905. Jara C, Gomez-Aldaravi JL, Tirado R, et al: Small-cell lung cancer in the elderly—is age of a patient a relevant factor? Acta Oncol 1999;38:781.

906. Findlay MP, Griffin AM, Raghavan D, et al: Retrospective review of chemotherapy for small cell lung cancer in the elderly: Does the end justify the means? Eur J Cancer 1991;27:1597.

907. Yuen AR, Zou G, Turrisi AT, et al: Similar outcome of elderly patients in the intergroup 0096: Cisplatin, etoposide, and thoracic radiotherapy administered once or twice daily in limited stage small cell lung carcinoma. Cancer 2000;89:1953.

908. Quon H, Shepherd FA, Payne DG, et al: The influence of age on the delivery, tolerance, and efficacy of thoracic irradiation in the combined modality treatment of limited stage small cell lung cancer. Int J Radiat Oncol Biol Phys 1999;43:39.

909. Clark PI, Cottier B: The activity of 10-, 14-, and 21-day schedules of single-agent etoposide in previously untreated patients with extensive small cell lung cancer. Semin Oncol 1992;19(Suppl 14):36.

910. Johnson DH, Greco FA, Strupp J, et al: Prolonged administration of oral etoposide in patients with relapsed or refractory small cell lung cancer: A phase II trial. J Clin Oncol 1990;8:1613.

911. Carney DN, Grogan L, Smit EF, et al: Single-agent oral etoposide for elderly small cell lung cancer patients. Semin Oncol 1990;17(Suppl 2):49.

912. Girling D: Comparison of oral etoposide and standard intravenous multidrug chemotherapy for small-cell lung cancer: A stopped multicenter randomized trial. Medical Research Council Lung Cancer Working Party. Lancet 1996;348:563.

913. Souhami RL, Spiro SG, Rudd RM, et al: Five-day oral etoposide treatment for advanced small-cell lung: Randomized comparison with intravenous chemotherapy. J Natl Cancer 1997;Inst 89:577.

914. White SC, Lorigan P, Middleton MR, et al: Randomized phase II study of cyclophosphamide, doxorubicin, and vincristine compared with single-agent carboplatin in patients with poor prognosis small cell lung carcinoma. Cancer 2001;92:601.

915. James LE, Rudd R, Gower NH, et al: A phase III randomized comparison of gemcitabine/carboplatin (GC) with cisplatin/etoposide (PE) in patients with poor prognosis small cell lung cancer (SCLC). Proc Am Soc Clin Oncol 2002;21:293a.

916. Murray N, Grafton C, Shah A, et al: Abbreviated treatment for elderly, infirm, or non-compliant patients with limited-stage small-cell lung cancer. J Clin Oncol 1998;16:3323.

917. Westeel V, Murray N, Gelmon K, et al: New combination of the old drugs for elderly patients with small-cell lung cancer: A phase II study of the PAVE regimen. J Clin Oncol 1998;16:1940.

918. Evans WK, Radwi A, Tomiak E, et al: Oral etoposide and carboplatin. Effective therapy for elderly patients with small cell lung cancer. Am J Clin Oncol 1995;18:149.

919. Matsui K, Masuda N, Fukuoka M, et al: Phase II trial of carboplatin plus oral etoposide for elderly patients with small-cell lung cancer. Br J Cancer 1998;77:1961.

920. Giaccone G, Donadio M, Bonardi G, et al: Teniposide in the treatment of small-cell lung cancer: The influence of prior chemotherapy. J Clin Oncol 1997;15:2090.

921. Chute JP, Kelley MJ, Venzon D, et al: Retreatment of patients surviving cancer-free 2 or more years after initial treatment of small cell lung cancer. Chest 1996;110:165.

922. Ardizzoni A, Hansen H, Dombernowsky P, et al: Topotecan, a new active drug in the second-line treatment of small-cell lung cancer: A phase II study in patients with refractory and sensitive disease. J Clin Oncol 1997;15:2090–2096.

923. Perez-Soler R, Glisson BS, Lee JS, et al: Treatment of patients with small-cell lung cancer refractory to etoposide and cisplatin with the topoisomerase I poison topotecan. J Clin Oncol 1996;14:2785.

924. Masuda N, Fukuoka M, Kusunoki Y, et al: CPT-11: A new derivative of camptothecin for the treatment of refractory or relapsed small-cell lung cancer. J Clin Oncol 1992;10:1225.

925. Le Chevalier T, Ibrahim N, Chomy P, et al: A phase II study of irinotecan (CPT-11) in patients (pts) with small cell lung cancer (SCLC) progressing after initial response to first-line chemotherapy (CT). Proc Am Soc Clin Oncol 1997;16:450a.

926. von Pawel J, Schiller JH, Shepherd FA, et al: Topotecan versus cyclophosphamide, doxorubicin, and vincristine for the treatment of recurrent small-cell lung cancer. J Clin Oncol 1999;17:658.

927. von Pawel J, Gatzemeier U, Pujol JL, et al: Phase II comparator study of oral versus intravenous topotecan in patients with chemosensitive small-cell lung cancer. J Clin Oncol 2001;19:1743.

928. Smit EF, Fokkema E, Biesma B, et al: A phase II study of paclitaxel in heavily pretreated patients with small-cell lung cancer. Br J Cancer 1998;77:347.

929. Smyth JF, Smith IE, Sessa C, et al: Activity of docetaxel (Taxotere) in small cell lung cancer. The Early Clinical Trials Group of the EORTC. Eur J Cancer 1994;30A:1058.

930. Jassem J, Karnicka-Mlodkowska H, van Pottelsberghe M, et al: Phase II study of vinorelbine (Navelbine) in previously treated small cell lung cancer patients. Eur J Cancer 1993;29A:1720.

931. Furuse K, Kubota K, Kawahara M, et al: Phase II study of vinorelbine in heavily previously treated small cell lung cancer. Oncology 1996;53:169.

932. van der Lee I, Smit EF, van Putten JW, et al: Single-agent gemcitabine in patients with resistant small cell lung cancer. Ann Oncol 2001;12:557.

933. Postmus PE, Berendsen HN, Van Zandwijk N, et al: Retreatment with induction regimen in small cell lung cancer relapsing after an initial response to short term chemotherapy. Eur J Cancer Clin Oncol 1987;23:1409.

934. Pignon JP, Arriagada R, Ihde DC, et al: A meta-analysis of thoracic radiotherapy for small-cell lung cancer. N Eng J Med 1992;327:1618.

935. Warde P, Payne D: Does thoracic irradiation improve survival and local control in limited-stage small-cell carcinoma of the lung? A meta-analysis. J Clin Oncol 1992;10:890.

936. Murray N, Coy P, Pater JL, et al: Importance of timing for thoracic irradiation in the combined modality treatment of limited-stage small-cell lung cancer. The National Cancer Institute of Canada Clinical Trials Group. J Clin Oncol 1993;11:336.

937. Perry MC, Eaton WL, Propert KJ, et al: Chemotherapy with or without radiation therapy in limited small-cell carcinoma of the lung. N Eng J Med 1987;316:912.

938. Perry MC, Herndnon JE, Eaton WL, et al: Thoracic radiation therapy added to chemotherapy for small-cell lung cancer: An update of Cancer and Leukemia Group B study 8083. J Clin Oncol 1998;16:2466.

939. Skarlos DV, Samantas E, Briassoulis E, et al: Randomized comparison of early versus late hyperfractionated thoracic irradiation concurrently with chemotherapy in limited disease small-cell lung cancer. A randomized phase II study of the Hellenic Cooperative Oncology Group (HeCOG). Ann Oncol 2001;12:1231.

940. Work E, Nielsen OS, Bentzen SM, et al: Randomized study of initial versus late chest irradiation combined with chemotherapy in limited-stage small-cell lung cancer. Aarhus Lung Cancer Group. J Clin Oncol 1997;15:3030.

941. Takada M, Fukuoka M, Kawahara M, et al: Phase III study of concurrent versus sequential thoracic radiotherapy in combination with cisplatin and etoposide for limited-stage small-cell lung cancer: Results of the Japan Clinical Oncology Group study 9104. J Clin Oncol 2002;20:3054.

942. Jeremic B, Shibamoto Y, Acimovic L, et al: Initial versus delayed accelerated hyperfractionated radiation therapy and concurrent chemotherapy in limited small-cell lung cancer: A randomized study. J Clin Oncol 1997;15:893.

943. Coy P, Hodson I, Payne DG, et al: The effect of dose of thoracic irradiation on recurrence in patients with limited stage small cell lung cancer. Initial results of a Canadian multicenter randomized trial. Int J Radiat Oncol Biol Phys 1988;14:219.

944. Choi NC, Carey RW: Importance of radiation dose in achieving improved loco-regional tumor control in limited stage small-cell lung carcinoma: An update. Int J Radiat Oncol Biol Phys 1989;17:307.

945. Arriagada R, Kramar A, Le Chevalier T, et al: Competing events determining relapse-free survival in limited small-cell lung carcinoma. The French Cancer Centers Lung Group. J Clin Oncol 1992;10:447.

946. Peters L, Ang K: Unconventional fractionation schemas in radiotherapy. In DeVita VT, Hellman S, Rosenberg SA (eds): Important Advances in Oncology 1986. Philadelphia, JB Lippincott, 1986, p 269.

947. Brodin O, Lennartsson L, Nilsson S: Single-dose and fractionated irradiation of four human lung cancer cell lines in vitro. Acta Oncol 1991;30:967.

948. Morstyn G, Russo A, Carney D, et al: Heterogeneity in the radiation survival curves and biochemical properties of human lung cancer cell lines. J Natl Cancer Inst 1984;73:801.

949. Withers HR, Taylor JM, Maciejewski B: The hazard of accelerated tumor clonogen repopulation during radiotherapy. Acta Oncol 1988;27:131.

950. Turrisi AT, Kim K, Blum R, et al: Twice-daily compared with once-daily thoracic radiotherapy in limited small-cell lung cancer treated concurrently with cisplatin and etoposide. N Eng J Med 1999;340:265.

951. Bonner JA, Sloan JA, Shanahan TG, et al: Phase III comparison of twice-daily split-course irradiation versus once-daily irradiation for patients with limited stage small-cell lung carcinoma. J Clin Oncol 1999;17:2681.

952. Rosen ST, Makuch RW, Lichter AS, et al: Role of prophylactic cranial irradiation in prevention of central nervous system metastases in SCLC: Potential benefit restricted to patients in complete response. Am J Med 1983;74:615.

953. Arriagada R, Le Chevalier T, Borie F, et al: Prophylactic cranial irradiation for patients with small-cell lung cancer in complete remission. J Natl Cancer Inst 1995;87:183.

954. Gregor A, Cull A, Stephens RJ, et al: Prophylactic cranial irradiation is indicated following complete response to induction therapy in small cell lung cancer: Results of a multicenter randomized trial. Eur J Cancer 1997;33:1752.

955. Aroney RS, Aisner J, Wesley MN, et al: Value of prophylactic cranial irradiation given at complete remission in small cell lung carcinoma. Cancer Treat Rep 1983;67:675.

956. Ohonoshi T, Ueoka H, Kawahara S, et al: Comparative study of prophylactic cranial irradiation in patients with small cell lung cancer achieving complete response: A long-term follow-up result. Lung Cancer 1993;10:47.

957. Wagner H, Kim K, Turrisi A: A randomized phase III study of prophylactic cranial irradiation versus observation in patients with small cell lung cancer achieving a complete response: Final report of an incomplete trial by the Eastern Cooperative Oncology Group and Radiation Therapy Oncology Group (E3589/R92-01). Proc Am Soc Clin Oncol 1996;15:376.

958. Laplanche A, Monnet I, Santos-Miranda JA, et al: Controlled clinical trial of prophylactic cranial irradiation for patients with small-cell lung cancer in complete remission. Lung Cancer 1998; 21:193.

959. Meert AP, Paesmans M, Berghmans T, et al: Prophylactic cranial irradiation in small cell lung cancer: A systematic review of the literature with meta-analysis. BMC Cancer 2001;1:5.

960. Crossen JR, Garwood D, Glatstein E, et al: Neurobehavioral sequelae of cranial irradiation in adults. A review of radiation-induced encephalopathy J Clin Oncol 1994;12:627.

961. van Oosterhout AG, Boon PJ, Houx PJ, et al: Follow-up of cognitive functioning in patients with small cell lung cancer. Int J Radiat Oncol Biol Phys 1995;31:911.

962. Komaki R, Meyers CA, Shin DM, et al: Evaluation of cognitive function in patients with limited small cell lung cancer prior to and shortly following prophylactic cranial irradiation. Int J Radiat Oncol Biol Phys 1995;33:179.

963. Ahles TA, Silberfarb PM, Herndon J, et al: Psychologic and neuropsychologic functioning of patients with limited small-cell

lung cancer treated with chemotherapy and radiation therapy with or without warfarin: A study by the Cancer and Leukemia Group B. J Clin Oncol 1998;16:1954.

964. Kristensen CA, Kristjansen PE, Hansen HH: Systemic chemotherapy of brain metastases from small-cell lung cancer: A review. J Clin Oncol 1992;10:1498.

965. Shah S, Thompson J, Goldstraw P: Results of operation without adjuvant therapy in the treatment of small cell lung cancer. Ann Thorac Surg 1992;54:498.

966. Sorensen HR, Lund C, Alstrup P: Survival in small cell lung carcinoma after surgery. Thorax 1986;41:479.

967. Shore DF, Paneth M: Survival after resection of small cell carcinoma of the bronchus. Thorax 1980;35:819.

968. Lad T, Piantadosi S, Thomas P, et al: A prospective randomized trial to determine the benefit of surgical resection of residual disease following response of small cell lung cancer to combination chemotherapy. Chest 1994;106:320S–323S.

969. Nawrocki B, Polette M, Marchand V, et al: Expression of matrix metalloproteinases and their inhibitors in human broncho-pulmonary carcinomas. Quantificative and morphologic analyses. Int J Cancer 1997;72:556.

970. Michael M, Babic B, Khokha R, et al: Expression and prognostic significance of metalloproteinases and their tissue inhibitors in patients with small-cell lung cancer. J Clin Oncol 1999;17:1802.

971. Shepherd F, Giaccone G, Debruyne C, et al: Randomized double-blind placebo-controlled trial of marimastat in patients with small cell lung cancer (SCLC) following response to first-line chemo-therapy: An NCIC-CTG and EORTC study. Proc Am Soc Clin Oncol 2001;20:4a.

972. Sekido Y, Obata Y, Ueda R, et al: Preferential expression of c-kit protooncogene transcripts in small cell lung cancer. Cancer Res 1999;51:2416.

973. Hibi K, Takahashi T, Sekido Y, et al: Co-expression of the stem cell factor and the c-kit genes in small cell lung cancer. Oncogene 1991;6:2291.

974. Plummer H, Catlett J, Leftwich J, et al: C-myc expression correlates with suppression of c-kit proto-oncogene expression in small cell lung cancer cell lines. Cancer Res 1993;53:4337.

975. Rygaard K, Nakamura T, Spang-Thomsen M: Expression of the proto-oncogenes c-met and c-kit and their ligands, hepatocyte growth factor/scatter factor and stem cell factor in SCLC cell lines and xenografts. Br J Cancer 1993;67:37.

976. Johnson BE, Fisher B, Fisher T, et al: A phase II study of STI571 (Gleevec) for patients with small cell lung cancer. Proc Am Soc Clin Oncol 2002;21:293a.

977. Krystal GW, Honsawek S, Litz J, et al: The selective tyrosine kinase inhibitor STI571 inhibits small cell lung cancer growth. Clin Cancer Res 2000;6:3319.

978. Cuttitta F, Carney DC, Mulshine J, et al: Bombesin-like peptides can function as autocrine growth factors in human small-cell lung cancer. Nature 1985;316:823.

979. Kelley MJ, Linnoila I, Avis IL, et al: Antitumor activity of a monoclonal antibody directed against gastrin-releasing peptide in patients with small cell lung cancer. Chest 1997;112:256.

980. Rudin C, Otterson GA, George CM, et al: A phase I/II trial of genasense and paclitaxel in chemorefractory small cell lung cancer. Proc Am Soc Clin Oncol 2001;20:322a.

981. Byrne MJ, Van Hazel G, Trotter J, et al: Maintenance chemotherapy in limited small cell lung cancer: A randomized control clinical trial. Br J Cancer 1989;60:413.

982. Ettinger DS, Finkelstein DM, Abeloff MD, et al: A randomized comparison of standard chemotherapy versus alternating

chemotherapy and maintenance versus no maintenance therapy for extensive-stage small-cell lung cancer: A phase III study of the Eastern Cooperative Oncology Group. J Clin Oncol 1990;8:230.

983. Lebeau B, Chastang CL, Allard P, et al: Six vs twelve cycles for complete responders in small cell lung cancer. Definitive results of a randomized clinical trial. Eur Respir J 1992;5:286.

984. Giaccone G, Dalesio O, McVie GJ, et al: Maintenance chemotherapy in small-cell lung cancer: Long term results of a randomized clinical trial. J Clin Oncol 1993;11:1230.

985. Beith JM, Clarke SJ, Woods RL, et al: Long-term follow-up of a randomised trial of combined chemoradiotherapy induction treatment, with and without maintenance chemotherapy in patients with small cell carcinoma of the lung. Eur J Cancer 1996;32A:438.

986. Bleehen NM, Fayers PM, Girling DJ, et al: Controlled trial of twelve versus six courses of chemotherapy in the treatment of small-cell lung cancer. Br J Cancer 1989;60:413.

987. Shevlin P, Brown I, Muers M, et al: A randomised trial of three versus six courses of etoposide, ifosfamide, mesna and vincristine in small cell lung cancer. Lung Cancer 1997;18(Suppl 1):8.

988. Postmus PE, Smit EF, Kirkpatrick A, et al: Testing the possible non-cross resistance of two equipotent combination chemotherapy regimens against small-cell lung cancer: A phase II study of the EORTC Lung Cancer Cooperative Group. Eur J Cancer 1993;29A:204.

989. Ando M, Kobayashi K, Yoshioka H, et al: Weekly administration of irinotecan (CPT-11) plus cisplatin (CDDP) for refractory or relapsed small cell lung cancer (SCLC). Proc Am Soc Clin Oncol 2001;20:319a.

990. Masuda N, Matsui K, Negoro S, et al: Combination of irinotecan and etoposide for treatment of refractory or relapsed small-cell lung cancer. J Clin Oncol 1998;16:3329.

991. Groen HJM, Fokkema E, Biesma B, et al: Paclitaxel and carboplatin in the treatment of small-cell lung cancer patients resistant to cyclophosphamide, doxorubicin, and etoposide: A non-cross resistant schedule. J Clin Oncol 1999;17:927.

992. Ardizzoni A, Manegold C, Debruyne C, et al: European Organization for Research and Treatment of Cancer (EORTC) 08957 Phase II study of topotecan in combination with cisplatin as second-line treatment of refractory and sensitive small cell lung cancer. Clin Cancer Res 2003;9:143.

993. Domine M, Gonzalez J, Larriba S, et al: Gemcitabine and paclitaxel as second line treatment in small cell lung cancer (SCLC). A multicentric phase II study. Proc Am Soc Clin Oncol 2000.

994. Hainsworth JD, Burris HA, Erland JB, et al: Combination chemotherapy with gemcitabine and vinorelbine in the treatment of patients with relapsed or refractory small cell lung cancer: A phase II trial of the Minnie Pearl Cancer Research Network. Cancer Invest 2003;21:193.

995. Kosmas C, Tsavaris NB, Malamos NA, et al: Phase II study of paclitaxel, ifosfamide, and cisplatin as second line treatment in relapsed small-cell lung cancer. J Clin Oncol 2001;19:119.

996. Eckardt A, Depierre A, Ardizzoni A, et al: Pooled analysis of topotecan (T) in second-line treatment of patients (pts) with sensitive small cell lung cancer (SCLC). Proc Am Soc Clin Oncol 1997;16:452a.

997. DeVore RF, Blanke CD, Denham CA, et al: Phase II study of irinotecan (CPT-11) in patients with previously treated small cell lung cancer. Proc Am Soc Clin Oncol 1998;17:451a.

998. Samantas E, Klamouris C, Kalofonos H, et al: Phase II study with docetaxel in pretreated patients with small cell lung cancer. Ann Oncol 1998;9:104.

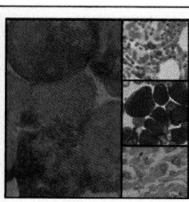

76 | Tumors of the Pleura and Mediastinum

Joseph Aisner

Chandra P. Belani

Seena C. Aisner

SUMMARY OF KEY POINTS

MALIGNANT PLEURAL MESOTHELIOMA

Epidemiology

- Malignant mesothelioma is a rare disease closely associated with asbestos exposure (all fiber types).
- Based on the prior use of asbestos, more than 8 million people are exposed and at risk in the United States.
- More than 3000 cases are estimated to be diagnosed in the United States annually, with the incidence still increasing.
- It is more likely seen in men; right side is more frequent.
- Three subtypes exist: epithelial, fibrosarcomatous, and mixed.

Differential Diagnosis

- The epithelial form must be distinguished from metastatic adenocarcinomas.
- To establish the diagnosis, a generous tissue biopsy or cell block is needed to perform a battery of tests, including histochemistry and immunohistochemistry.
- Immunohistochemistry can now be defining.
- Electron microscopy is often helpful; normal adjacent lung for fiber count is helpful.

Staging Evaluation

- Take a medical history, a complete occupational history, and perform a physical examination.
- Obtain CT scan of chest and abdomen and a PET scan to define the extent of disease and of mediastinal involvement.
- Focus on potential operability: CT scan of chest, bone scan, and pulmonary and cardiac function tests.
- Evaluation can be abbreviated if patient is not operable; CT scan is best to follow the disease.
- Use new TNM staging system.

Primary Therapy

- The role of therapeutic interventions is not well defined; consider referral to a specialty center.
- Assess symptoms carefully, and discuss risk-benefit ratio for any therapy.
- For operable disease, perform either pleural stripping with postoperative irradiation or extrapleural pneumonectomy. Role of adjuvant therapies is not certain.
- Intrapleural therapies are possible only in early disease.
- Consider radiation therapy to incision sites and needle traces to prevent growth.
- Use radiation therapy as a postoperative adjuvant or for symptom control.
- Chemotherapy: permetrexed (Alimta) plus cisplatin; high-dose methotrexate; gemcitabine plus cisplatin; new agents remain justified.

METASTATIC TUMORS OF THE PLEURA

Incidence

- Occurrence is related to the incidence of primary tumors.
- Metastases are most commonly seen with lung, breast, lymphoma, gastric, colon, melanoma, ovary, and prostate tumors.

Differential Diagnosis

- Cytology is often diagnostic of cell type—cell block for immunohistochemistry (adenocarcinoma vs. other). They should be distinguished from primary tumors, especially in high-risk individuals.
- Mucin positivity usually excludes mesothelioma.
- Primary source identification could help to define treatment for the underlying primary disease.

Staging

Metastatic disease, by definition (M1).

Primary Therapy

- Drain effusions for symptom control and treat the underlying primary neoplasm.
- For recurrent effusions, drain and sclerose using talc. Antibiotics (minocycline), chemotherapy (bleomycin), or biologics (corynebacterium parvum, [interferon {IFN} or IL-21]) are used also.

Secondary Therapies

For highly selected patients, consider pleurectomy if effusion is resistant and the prognosis is reasonable.

MEDIASTINAL NEOPLASMS

General

- Tumors are categorized or cataloged by anatomic compartments: anterior, middle, and posterior.
- Anterior compartment tumors are predominantly thymomas, lymphomas, and germ cell tumors.
- Middle compartment tumors are myxomas and malignant tumors and cysts of the heart and pericardium, including angiosarcomas, rhabdomyosarcomas, mesotheliomas, fibrosarcomas, lymphomas, extraskeletal osteosarcomas, neurogenic sarcomas, malignant teratomas, thymomas, leiomyosarcomas, liposarcomas, and synovial cell sarcomas.
- Posterior compartment tumors are neural crest tumors: peripheral neuroectodermal tumor (PNET), neuroblastoma, ganglioneuroma, pheochromocytoma, schwannoma, and neurofibroma.

SUMMARY OF KEY POINTS

TUMORS OF THE ANTERIOR MEDIASTINUM

Epidemiology

- Thymoma
  Twenty percent of all mediastinal tumors in adults have an equal male/female distribution, are most common in the fifth and sixth decades of life, and are more malignant in children; a possible association with Epstein-Barr virus (EBV) exists. Complications include myasthenia gravis, red cell aplasia, and hypogammaglobulinemia.
- Lymphoma
  Lymphomas commonly include Hodgkin's and non–Hodgkin's forms.
- Germ cell tumors
  Anterior mediastinal tumors form 1% of all germ cell neoplasms and are related to malignant transformation of mediastinal germinal elements. Malignant forms seen are predominantly similar to those of testicular germ cell tumors.

Differential Diagnosis

- Thymoma
  To establish diagnosis, a generous tissue biopsy is needed for special stains and definition of architecture. Subtypes include lymphocytic, epithelial, thymic carcinoma, and thymic carcinoid.
- Lymphoma
  To establish diagnosis, sufficient material is needed for flow cytometry for immunophenotyping. Tissue biopsy is helpful for special stains to define nodal architecture and cellular types. Flow and biopsy should be reviewed by a pathologist with experience in lymphomas.
- Germ cell tumors
  In the presence of appropriate biomarkers, fine-needle biopsy can establish diagnosis. Subtypes (seminomatous and nonseminomatous) could require more generous tissue samples in the absence of biomarkers.

Staging and Evaluation

- Thymoma
  Take history and perform physical examination, complete blood count, serum protein electrophoresis, and chest CT scan (role of MRI scans is not yet clear).

- Lymphoma
  Take history and perform physical examination. The remaining steps of staging and evaluation are described in the chapters on Hodgkin's and non–Hodgkin's lymphoma.
- Germ cell tumors
  Take history and perform physical examination, chest CT scan, α-fetoprotein (AFP), β-human chorionic gonadotropin (HCG), and lactate dehydrogenase (LDH).

Primary Treatment

- Thymoma
  Perform complete surgical resection. If residual disease exists after surgery, add radiation therapy. The role of chemotherapy is not established; if the tumor is nonresectable, use radiation therapy. The role of neoadjuvant therapies is not well defined.
- Lymphoma
  Therapeutic approaches are defined in the chapters on lymphoma.
- Germ cell tumors
  Therapeutic regimens generally follow the approaches outlined for poor-prognosis testicular germ cell tumors, with primary and secondary chemotherapy regimens and autologous bone marrow transplantation.

TUMORS OF THE MIDDLE MEDIASTINUM

Incidence

- These are all very rare tumors. More than half are benign atrial myxomas; malignant tumors of the heart are very rare.
- Malignant tumors can originate from or metastasize to the pericardium. Other mediastinal structures can be involved depending on site and histology. Too few cases of pericardial mesothelioma exist to draw any inferences about an association with exposure to asbestos.

Differential Diagnosis

- Myxomas are suspected from patterns of congestive failure or embolic disease; excisional biopsy is often based on angiographic studies.
- Malignant tumors can sometimes be biopsied through bronchoscopy or via thoracoscopy. Generous

amounts of tissue are often needed to define histology. Pathology experience with soft tissue tumors is usually helpful.

Staging and Evaluation

- A careful history and a physical examination are needed.
- Myxomas are best seen by cardiac catheterization. MRI might also be useful.
- Malignant tumors are best visualized by CT or MRI scan.

Primary Treatment

- Perform surgical excision of myxomas and soft tissue tumors; radiation therapy or chemotherapy have no defined role in the absence of metastases.
- Treat the underlying primary malignancy in the case of metastatic disease.

POSTERIOR MEDIASTINAL TUMORS

Incidence

- These are rare tumors mostly originating from the neural crest; others (rarely) include lymphoma and soft tissue tumors.

Differential Diagnosis

- Tumors are in two basic groups: (1) neuronal origin, including the nerve ganglion cells (neuroepithelioma, neuroblastoma, ganglioneuroblastoma, and ganglioneuroma) and neuroendocrine cells (e.g., pheochromocytoma, paraganglioma, and medullary thyroid carcinoma); and (2) neural sheath cells or Schwann cells, including schwannoma and neurofibroma.
- Most tumors are benign.
- Adequate tissue samples are needed to perform special stains, electron microscopy, and possible cytogenetics (peripheral neuroectodermal tumors).

Staging Evaluation

Perform CT scans; test for metanephrines in the case of labile hypertension.

Primary Treatment

- Perform surgical resection; local recurrence is likely with incomplete resection.
- Roles of radiation therapy and chemotherapy are not well defined.

PRIMARY TUMORS OF THE PLEURA

Introduction

Benign and malignant primary tumors of the pleura constitute a group of unusual and rare diseases. In contrast, metastases to the pleura are a relatively frequent manifestation of many cancers. The diagnosis and management of the benign and malignant tumors of the pleura are important but often difficult challenges for clinicians.

Primary tumors of the pleura can originate either from the surface of the mesothelium or from the submesothelium. These various rare tumors can present as either localized or diffuse and are categorized in Table 76-1. With the exception of the localized malignant soft tissue tumors, most of the localized tumors tend to behave in a benign manner, whereas the diffuse tumors tend to be more malignant in their behaviors. The usual approach to localized tumors is surgical excision, including the chest wall as needed. The role of adjunctive radiotherapy to augment local control is not well defined. For the localized soft tissue sarcomas, excision still remains the treatment of choice. In one review of 82 malignant localized tumors, 45% were cured by simple excision.[1] Because of the rarity of these tumors, studies of postoperative therapy are lacking, and there is no convincing evidence for the role of any adjunctive postoperative therapy.

Benign Mesothelioma

Benign (localized) tumors arising from the mesothelium have been described as arising from the pleura, the peritoneum, the tunica vaginalis testis, the atrioventricular (AV) node, the mediastinum, the liver, and the adrenal gland.[2-8] These tumors tend to grow to considerable size and produce symptoms by the effect of their mass, such

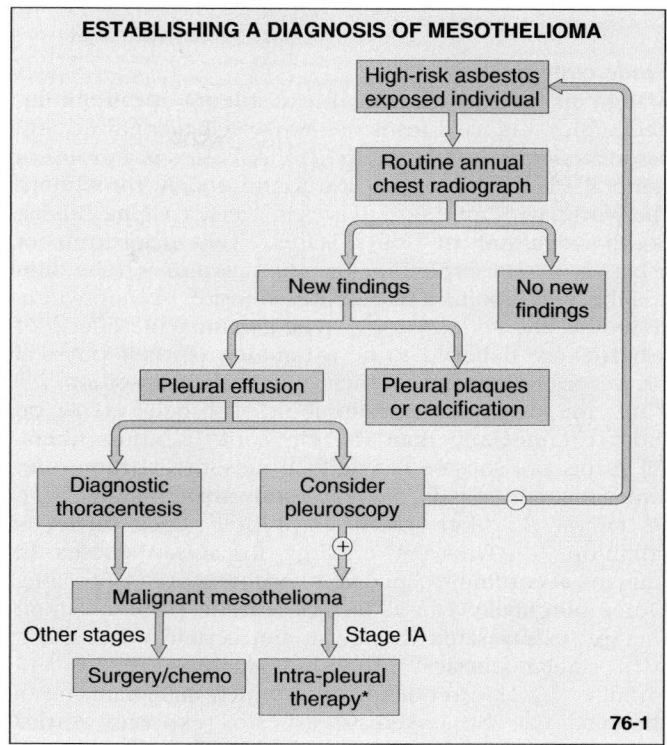

ESTABLISHING A DIAGNOSIS OF MESOTHELIOMA

76-1

as compression or blockage of adjacent structures. The most common approach to treatment is surgical excision. Local recurrences are prominent in cases of incomplete resection. These tumors are believed to originate from the mesothelial cells; however, there remains some uncertainty regarding the origin of AV node mesotheliomas, which might arise from submesothelial mesenchymal cells.

Benign fibrous tumors of the pleura are considerably less common than malignant mesotheliomas, although the age distribution is similar for both types of tumors.[9,10] The benign fibrous tumors can present as very large, pedunculated intrathoracic masses and are sometimes seen with hypertrophic pulmonary osteoarthropathy or serosanguinous effusions. These tumors are believed to arise from submesothelial fibrous tissue and have thus been called submesothelial fibromas, localized fibrous mesotheliomas, or solitary fibrous tumors of the pleura.[10-12] These tumors rarely invade the visceral pleura and therefore produce clear margins between the tumor and the compressed lung. Complete surgical resections are thus possible, although chest wall resections could be required. Local recurrences can be seen late and can result in fatality. In contrast to patients with malignant mesothelioma, there is no defined association of benign fibrous tumors of the pleura with asbestos exposure. Diagnostic imaging with either computed tomography (CT) or magnetic resonance imaging (MRI) scans tends to be highly suggestive of the tumor. Definitive diagnosis and exclusion of malignant mesothelioma must be based on histologic confirmation, however.[13]

TABLE 76-1

Classification of Tumors of the Pleura

LOCALIZED	DIFFUSE
Mesothelial (Pleural)	**Mesothelial(Pleural)**
Adenomatoid tumor	Epithelial malignant
Cystic mesothelioma	mesothelioma
Benign papillary mesothelioma	Tubulopapillary
Mesothelioma of the AV node	Nonglandular (solid)
	Sarcomatous (fibrous)
	Biphasic (mixed)
	Undifferentiated
Submesothelial (Subpleural)	**Submesothelial (Subpleural)**
Fibroma (localized mesothelioma)	Angiosarcoma
Fibrosarcoma (localized malignant fibrous mesothelioma)	
Angioma	
Angiosarcoma	

Specific Malignancies

III

Malignant Pleural Mesothelioma

Epidemiology

Malignant mesothelioma of the pleura, peritoneum, and tunica vaginalis testis are now well recognized and associated with asbestos exposure. Asbestos is a group of mineral silicate fibers that are found widely throughout the world, with mining activities in Canada, China, Russia, South Africa, and the United States.[14] Two major forms of asbestos exist: a serpentine form (chrysotile) and the thin, rodlike amphiboles (crocidolite, amosite, anthophyllite, tremolite, and actinolyte).[14,15] The carcinogenic effects of asbestos are believed to be a function of their physical properties rather than of their chemical composition.[15,16] Thus, the thin, rodlike amphiboles are believed to be more carcinogenic than the chrysotile asbestos fibers. All forms of asbestos can induce mesothelial tumors in experimental animals, however, and cross-contamination of chrysotile fibers with amphibole fiber forms is common.[16-19] Thus, an etiology for mesothelioma in humans according to specific fiber forms is not possible. Other potentially causal factors include prior radiation therapy, extravasated thoratrast, and certain other fibers with similar physical properties, such as zeolite and erionite.[20-31] The frequency with which malignant mesothelioma can be linked to asbestos exposure varies somewhat according to the geographic location. On the east and west coasts of the United States, the association approaches nearly 80%, whereas in the Midwestern states, the association is seen about 60% of the time.[32] Asbestos fibers separate easily to form numerous minute strands. The small, inhaled fibers, which are not cleared by muco-cilliary action, migrate distally through the endothelial lining and into the interstitial tissues, where they accumulate in the lower third of the lungs and then penetrate into the visceral pleura. The fibers are ingested by macrophages, which are often damaged in the process, leaking lysosomal enzymes, cytokines, superoxides, and other free radicals. The asbestos fibers thus produce inflammatory and fibrotic reactions.[33] The fibers can also carry absorbed carcinogens, which might contribute further to the carcinogenic process.

The number of asbestos-exposed individuals rose throughout most of the 20th century as a consequence of increased asbestos mining and use. Despite the large number of exposed individuals, mesothelioma remains a fairly rare cancer, leading some observers to argue that additional factors, such as accumulating genetic alterations or viruses, could contribute to the causation.[34] Advances in molecular technology now allow the identification of various oncogenes, tumor suppressor genes, and signaling pathways, which are perturbed in cases of mesothelioma.[34] One hypothesis suggests that Simian Virus 40 (SV-40) might play an important etiologic role. Based on experimental findings of SV-40–associated mesotheliomas in hamsters, several investigators performed polymerized chain reaction (PCR) analysis in human mesothelioma specimens and found SV-40 sequences in 40% to 50% of the specimens.[35-39] This hypothesis is of considerable concern, as there are as many as 32 million adults in the United States who were vaccinated with polio vaccine contaminated with infectious SV-40.[40] If this hypothesis is correct, malignant mesothelioma could become a far more common cancer, and further study of the molecular mechanisms of pathogenesis are needed urgently.

Current estimates suggest that about 3000 cases of mesothelioma are seen annually in the United States.[41,42] The exact incidence and death rate from malignant mesothelioma remain difficult to estimate due in part to the continued coding of mesothelioma as lung cancer. Before 1960, the existence of mesothelioma as a distinct pathological entity was still debated. In 1960, Wagner and colleagues[43] initially reported 33 cases and then added 14 additional cases of mesothelioma diagnosed in a South African crocidolite mining community, where patients were exposed to asbestos. Selikoff and coworkers[44] noted an association between asbestos exposure and mesothelioma among pipe fitters, and these observations were followed by reports of mesotheliomas among asbestos workers in other parts of the world.[45,46]

The incidence of mesothelioma has probably increased, due in part to the marked increased use of asbestos since World War II.[47,48] The incidence is expected to rise well into the 21st century, reflecting the large population of 8 million or more persons who are at risk due to asbestos exposure that occurred before the implementation of governmental regulations.[41,42,47]

Reflecting the association with asbestos exposure in the workplace, malignant mesothelioma is seen more frequently in men than in women. Furthermore, because of the long latent period in its development, the incidence rises with age, and the median age at presentation is greater than 65 years. Mesothelioma has been reported as a consequence of household exposure among family members of asbestos workers, however, and in young adults as a consequence of household or neighborhood exposure.[43,49-52] The risk of mesothelioma is thus not limited to those who are directly involved with the mining, milling, or application of asbestos but also extends to those who are in proximity to the use of the asbestos material or exposed to it when it is carried home in clothing or hair.

Clinical Presentation, Diagnosis, and Staging

Most commonly, signs and symptoms associated with pleural effusion, such as shortness of breath, dyspnea on exertion, or nonpleuritic chest wall pain, bring patients to medical attention. Fever of unknown origin and sweats are seen frequently. Declining performance status and weight loss are also common features at presentation.[53] Physical examination usually discloses unilateral shifting dullness, and chest roentgenograms show a large pleural effusion. Thrombocytosis, disseminated intravascular coagulation, thrombophlebitis, pulmonary emboli, and Coomb's positive hemolytic anemia have also been reported.[53-56] The median duration of survival ranges from 4 to 18 months in most reported series. Prognostic factors at presentation that are associated with a better survival include the following[53,56-59]:

- Younger age
- Good performance status

- Stage
- Epithelial histology
- Lack of chest pain
- Normal platelet count

The right side is involved more often than the left. Roentgenograms also might show evidence of asbestos exposure, such as pleural plaques or calcifications in the diaphragm, although asbestosis is not a necessary precondition. With the recent emphasis on asbestos-associated illness, increased surveillance occasionally identifies asymptomatic individuals with an incidental effusion on chest x-ray.[60] CT scans of the chest, however, are far more sensitive and are used to assess the extent of disease. Pleural thickening with involvement of the interlobar fissures and atelectasis are evident early on CT scan.[25,57,61-66] Initially, the shortness of breath and chest pain can be controlled with repeated thoracenteses and minor narcotics. Chest tube drainage and sclerosis usually fail to control the symptoms, however, once the fluid becomes loculated and the tumor obliterates the pleural space and traps the lung by encasement with progression of disease (Fig. 76-1).[67] Figure 76-2 outlines the natural progression and associated clinical findings of malignant pleural mesothelioma.

Mesothelioma predominantly invades adjacent organs and metastasizes late in the course of the disease. The tumor grows along thoracentesis, chest tube drainage, or thoracotomy tracts in 10% or more of cases.[67-69] Direct extension into esophagus, ribs, vertebrae, nerves, and the

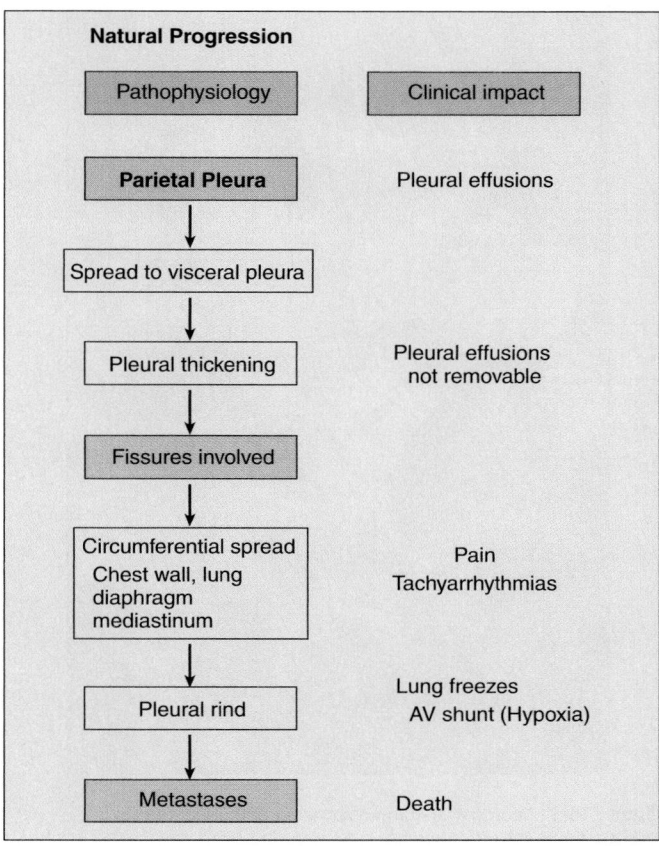

Figure 76-2. Outline of the progress of the natural history of malignant pleural mesothelioma and the approximate clinical events and findings at various stages of evolution.

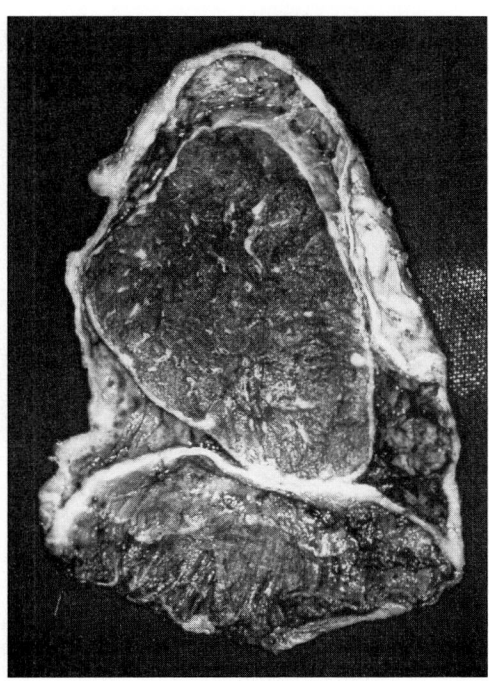

Figure 76-1. Resected lung showing thick rind of tumor encasing entire lung and trapping its function. Also illustrated is the extension of the pleural tumor into adjacent lung from the visceral pleura. Attempts to remove the visceral pleura would obviously leave residual tumor on the pulmonary surface. (Courtesy of SC Aisner, MD.)

superior vena cava can cause dysphagia, chest pain, cord compression, plexopathy, Horner's syndrome, or superior vena cava syndrome.[53,60] Direct extension also occurs commonly into the pulmonary parenchyma, the chest wall, into the mediastinum, and through the diaphragm into the abdominal cavity (Figs. 76-1 through 76-5). Mediastinal and cervical lymph nodes can also be involved. As the disease progresses, there is also loss of diaphragmatic and intercostal muscle movement, chest contraction, and scoliosis. Symptomatically, as the disease advances, patients complain of fatigue and dyspnea out of proportion to chest x-ray findings due to the shunting of poorly aerated blood in the trapped lung.

Most patients undergo repeated thoracenteses with negative or indeterminate cytology despite active tumor, as pleural effusions often produce atypical mesothelial cells. Needle biopsies might disclose tumor; however, pathologic distinction from adenocarcinoma can be difficult on the small specimens obtained. Thoracoscopy and pleuroscopy have been used with considerable success in obtaining adequate tissue samples.[70,71] Boutin and Rey[70] showed that thoracoscopy can be nearly 95% as accurate as diagnostic open thoracotomy. In early disease, discreet nodules and coalescent plaques are seen

Specific Malignancies

III

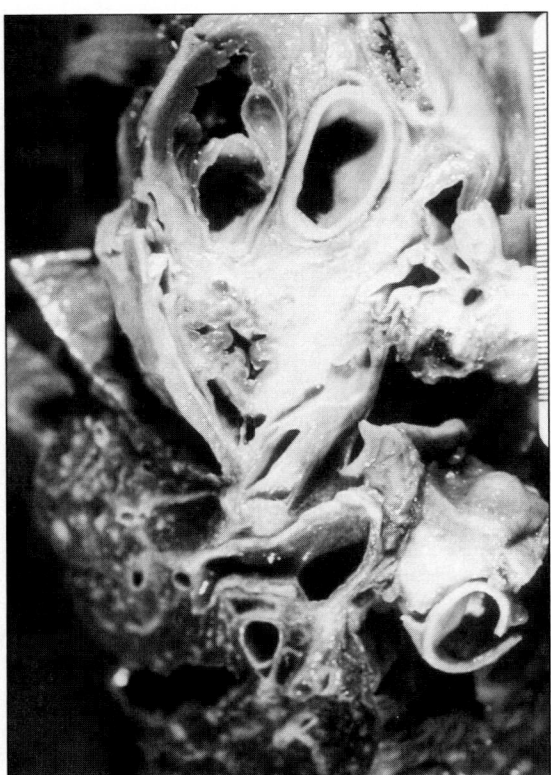

Figure 76-3. Necropsy specimen showing extension of the mesothelioma into the mediastinum, trapping heart, great vessels, and airways. (Courtesy of SC Aisner, MD.)

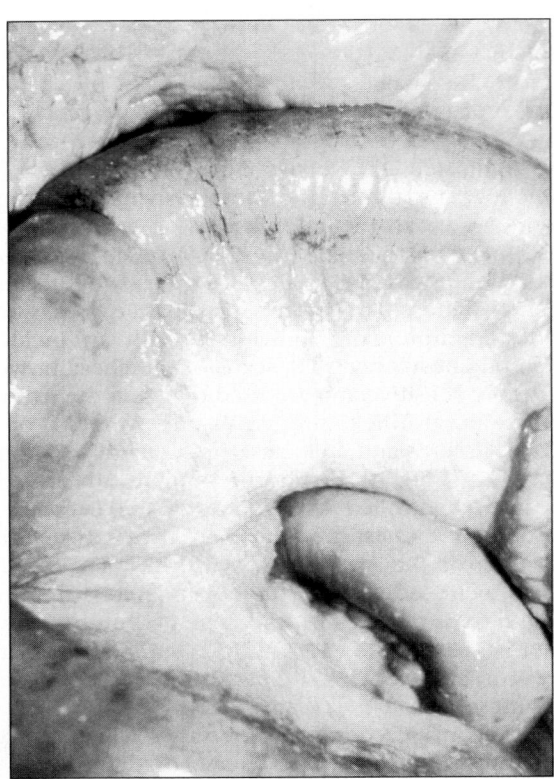

Figure 76-4. Necropsy illustration of extension of pleural mesothelioma through pores in diaphragm and invasion of abdominal contents as shown by the thick cake of tumor in the mesentery.

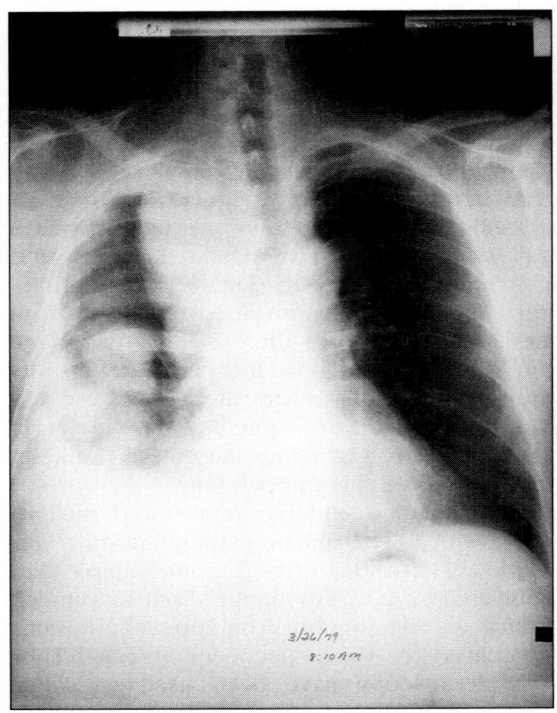

A

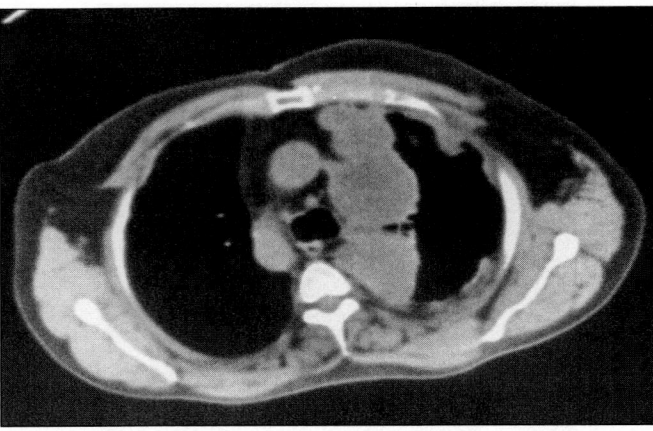

B

Figure 76-5. Right-sided mesothelioma. **A,** Conventional chest x-ray demonstrating right-sided pleural thickening haziness of the lung and obliteration of the border of the right side of the heart. **B,** CT image of chest showing right-sided pleural thickening and invasion of lung, mediastinum, and chest wall.

on the visceral and parietal pleura at the time of surgery. In more advanced disease, the pleural space is obliterated by a thick cake of tumor (see Fig. 76-1). Generous samples are usually taken for diagnosis. In view of the highly litigious nature of the disease, and although it is probably irrelevant, samples of uninvolved lung should also probably be obtained for counting asbestos fibers.[72]

Pathology

Three histologic subtypes of mesothelioma are usually described: epithelial, sarcomatous, and mixed (epithelial/sarcomatous).[72-76] The majority of mesotheliomas occur in the epithelial form, and these can exhibit papillary, solid, tubular, or vacuolated patterns. The sarcomatous form appears similar to a fibrosarcoma, with predominantly spindle-shaped or ovoid cells. The mixed or biphasic form demonstrates both epithelial and sarcomatoid elements. The finding of both elements on histology is usually diagnostic of malignant mesothelioma.

Metastatic adenocarcinoma from lung, breast, ovary, stomach, kidney, or prostate cancers can be difficult to distinguish grossly and histologically from epithelial mesothelioma. Histochemistry, immunocytochemistry, and electron microscopy can be helpful in this situation, however, and a panel of these tests is usually needed for diagnosis.[77-83] Periodic acid-Schiff stain (PAS) before and after diastase digestion is the most reliable histochemical staining method for making the distinction. Mucicarmine stains are rarely positive in mesothelioma, and a positive stain is highly suggestive evidence for adenocarcinoma. Alcian blue and colloidal-iron stains can also be helpful, as the disappearance of positive staining with hyaluronidase is considered characteristic of mesothelioma. Recent advances in the application of immunohistochemistry have permitted the identification of mesothelioma on tissue biopsies and cytology cell-blocks. Generally, mesotheliomas are cytokeratin positive and CEA negative. With the addition of several other immune markers, mesothelioma can now be differentiated from adenocarcinoma with greater ease.[77,78,83,84] Table 76-2 lists some of the differences seen among the various histochemical, immunohistochemical, and electron microscopy studies performed to distinguish mesothelioma from adenocarcinoma. The sarcomatous form should be distinguished from other soft-tissue sarcomas and localized fibrosarcoma. Carcinosarcomas also can demonstrate mixed sarcomatous and epithelial components but are seen predominantly as pulmonary parenchymal masses. Electron microscopy remains the major reference method for defining the diagnosis of malignant mesothelioma.[76,83-85] Polygonal cells with numerous long, slender branching surface microvilli, desmosomes, abundant tonofilaments, and intracellular lumen formation are the characteristic features of the epithelial form.[76,85] Elongated nuclei and abundant rough endoplasmic reticuli are found in the sarcomatoid variant.

Staging

Staging systems are usually developed to help define comparable groups for therapy and prognosis, and thus they provide a more accurate method for comparing results. To date, there is no uniformly accepted staging

TABLE 76-2

Histochemistry, Immunohistochemistry, and Electron Microscopy Findings Used to Distinguish Epithelial Malignant Mesothelioma from Adenocarcinoma

MARKER	MALIGNANT MESOTHELIOMA	ADENOCARCINOMA
Histochemistry		
Mucicarmine*	Rare	Frequent
PAS-diastase†	Rare	Frequent
Alcian blue with hyaluronidase‡	Frequent	Rare
Immunohistochemistry Antigens	**Involved (%)**	**Involved (%)**
Cytokeratin	100	100
CEA	<10	>95
Calretinin	>95	<10
LeuM1	<10	70–100
EMA	>80	100
CD34	<10	>70
CD15	<10	60–100
B72.3	<15	>80
Vimentin	40	<10
Electron Microscopy Findings		
Microvilli	Long, thin, branched, curved, interdigitated	Short, thick, not branched, straight, single
Mucin granules	None	+/–
Myelin figures	None	+/–
Core rootlets	None	+/–
Glycocalyx	None	+/–

*Mucicarmine stains for mucin production and neutral or weakly acidic mucopolysacharides.
‡Alcian blue stains for hyaluronic acid after pretreatment with hyaluronidase; positive, no stain.
†PAS-diastase: Periodic acid-Schiff stain with diastase digestion stains for neutral mucopolysaccharides.

system that accomplishes these goals in the staging of mesothelioma. The first staging system proposed by Butchart and colleagues[86] did not uniformly predict survival outcomes, did not provide tumor or organ invasion descriptions, and provided only vague statements about lymph node and chest wall involvement. Based on the large surgical experience at the Brigham and Women's Hospital and Dana Farber Cancer Institute, a clinical, postoperative staging system was proposed and is shown in Table 76-3.[87] After several attempts to develop a TNM-based staging system that considered the influence of regional lymph nodes and the extent of local invasion, the International Mesothelioma Interest Group (IMIG) organized a consensus TNM staging system, which forms the basis of the current AJCC Staging system (Table 76-4).[88]

Imaging Studies

Chest x-rays are usually obtained only after the patient first presents with shortness of breath or chest pain. Typically, a pleural effusion is found, prompting additional studies.[89] Pleural plaque or calcifications in the diaphragm might be seen and denote asbestos exposure, but these are found in less than 20% of patients with mesothelioma. These findings are thus sufficient, although not necessary to define asbestos exposure. CT scans are the most widely used imaging technique and can provide details of the extent of disease as it progressively encircles and traps the lung (see Figs. 76-1 and 76-2), extends into the fissures and along the pericardium, and invades the chest wall, diaphragm, and mediastinal structures.[66] The CT scan also can define enlarged mediastinal lymph nodes, a finding that carries an adverse prognosis. Other technologies have also been applied to imaging. MRI theoretically can improve differentiation between tumor and surrounding normal tissue. This could be of particular value in evaluation of penetration into the mediastinal structures, chest wall, and diaphragm. One small study, however, compared the staging information derived from CT and MRI scans and concluded that the two techniques offer approximately equivalent information.[90] Thus, both techniques are usually not necessary. In recent years, positron emission tomography (PET) scanning has offered the ability to identify tumors based on their metabolism of 18-F fluoro-deoxyglucose (FDG). This new technique

offers the ability to locate malignant lesions, and in one preliminary study, PET showed a slightly better detection of malignant mediastinal lymph nodes when compared with CT scans.[91] If this remains a consistent finding, then PET scanning could become a valuable adjunct to CT or MRI scanning.

Surgery

Because of the rarity of the disease and the highly selected nature of the patients entered into surgical trials, the

TABLE 76-3

Brigham and DFCI Revised Postoperative Staging System for Malignant Mesothelioma

STAGE	DEFINITION
I	Disease completely resected within the capsule of the parietal pleura without adenopathy: Ipsilateral pleura, lung, pericardium diaphragm, or chest wall disease limited to previous biopsy sites.
II	All of stage I with positive resection margin and/or intrapleural adenopathy.
III	Local extension into the chest wall or mediastinum; into the heart or through the diaphragm or peritoneum; or with extrapleural lymph node involvement.
IV	Distant metastatic disease.

TABLE 76-4

IMIG Staging of Mesothelioma

Primary Tumor and Extent (T)

Tx	Primary tumor cannot be assessed.
T0	No evidence of primary tumor.
T1	Tumor involves ipsilateral parietal pleura, with or without focal involvement of visceral pleura.
T1a	Tumor involves ipsilateral parietal (mediastinal, diaphragmatic) pleura. No visceral pleura involved.
T1b	Tumor involves ipsilateral parietal (mediastinal, diaphragmatic) pleura with focal involvement of visceral pleura.
T2	Tumor involves any of the ipsilateral pleural surfaces and one or more of the following: confluent visceral pleura and fissure, diaphragmatic muscle, ipsilateral lung parenchyma.
T3*	Tumor involves any of the ipsilateral pleural surfaces and one or more of the following: endothoracic fascia, mediastinal fat, solitary ipsilateral chest wall soft tissues, nontransmural invasion of the pericardium.
T4†	Tumor involves any of the ipsilateral pleural surfaces and one or more of the following: diffuse chest wall invasion, rib involvement, invasion through diaphragm, invasion through pericardium, positive pericardial effusion cytology, involvement of myocardium, involvement of any mediastinal organ, contralateral pleura, invasion of spine, or invasion of brachial plexus.

Lymph Nodes (N)

Nx	Regional lymph nodes cannot be assessed.
N0	No regional lymph node metastases.
N1	Metastases in ipsilateral bronchopulmonary or hilar lymph nodes.
N2	Metastases in subcarinal lymph nodes or in ipsilateral mediastinal or internal mammary lymph nodes.
N3	Metastases in contralateral mediastinal internal mammary, or hilar lymph nodes or any supraclavicular, or scalene lymph nodes.

Metastases (M)

Mx	Distant metastases cannot be assessed.
M0	No (known) distant metastases.
M1	Distant metastasis.

Stage Groupings

I	T1, N0, M0
IA	T1a, N0, M0
IB	T1b, N0, M0
II	T2, N0, M0
III	T1, T2, N1, M0
	T1, T2, N2, M0
	T3, N0, N1, N2, M0
IV	T4, any N, M0
	Any T, N3, M0
	Any T, Any N, M1

*T3 describes locally advanced but technically resectable disease.
†T4 describes locally advanced but technically unresectable disease.

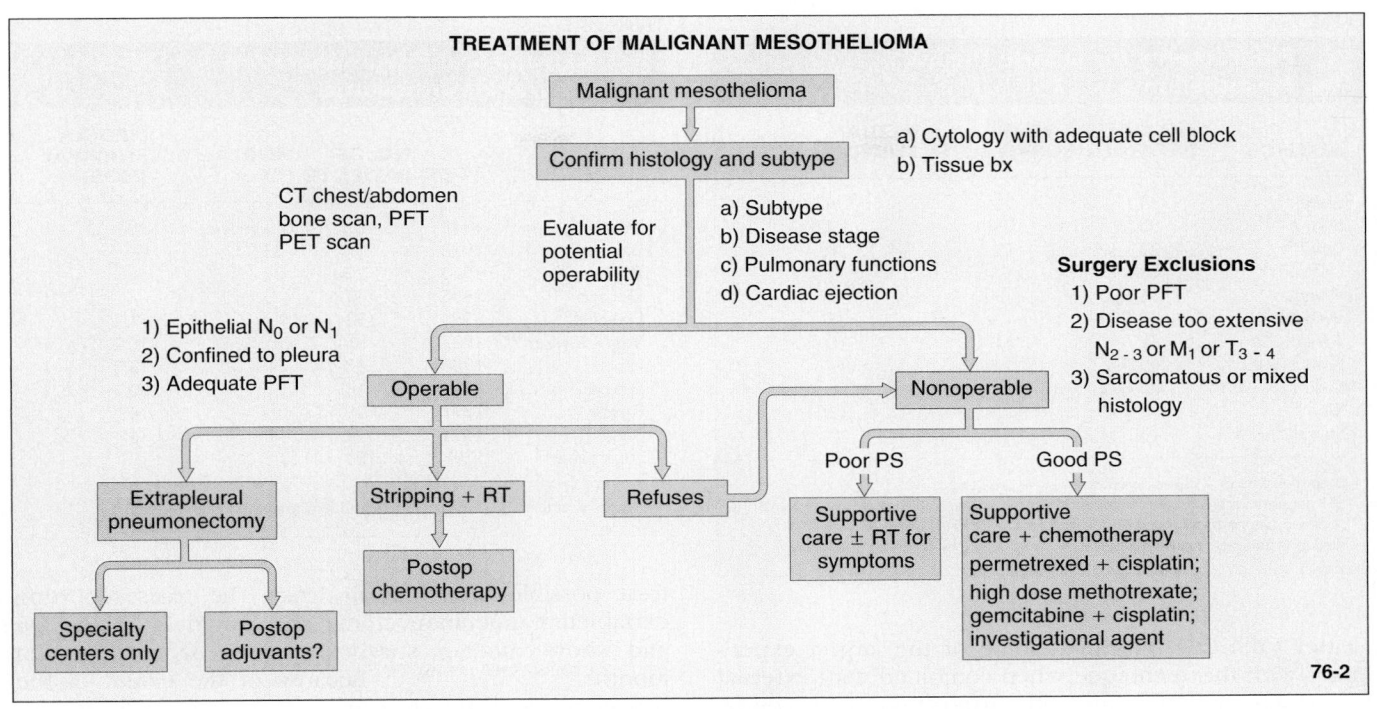

TREATMENT OF MALIGNANT MESOTHELIOMA

Malignant mesothelioma

Confirm histology and subtype

a) Cytology with adequate cell block
b) Tissue bx

Evaluate for potential operability

a) Subtype
b) Disease stage
c) Pulmonary functions
d) Cardiac ejection

CT chest/abdomen bone scan, PFT PET scan

Surgery Exclusions
1) Poor PFT
2) Disease too extensive
   N_{2-3} or M_1 or T_{3-4}
3) Sarcomatous or mixed histology

1) Epithelial N_0 or N_1
2) Confined to pleura
3) Adequate PFT

Operable

Nonoperable

Extrapleural pneumonectomy

Stripping + RT

Refuses

Poor PS

Good PS

Supportive care ± RT for symptoms

Supportive care + chemotherapy permetrexed + cisplatin; high dose methotrexate; gemcitabine + cisplatin; investigational agent

Specialty centers only

Postop adjuvants?

Postop chemotherapy

76-2

role of surgery in mesothelioma other than for biopsy remains controversial. Although pleurectomy can reduce the recurrence of effusions in most patients, surgery has little role in the palliative management of mesothelioma, and many clinicians advocate pleuradesis and supportive care.[58,92] With the recognition of the risk of disease in asbestos-exposed individuals, however, many patients are now found with earlier stages of mesothelioma, and such patients could have longer survival times. Thus, surgical excision could be a reasonable approach among patients who have their disease confined to the pleural space. Before considering aggressive surgery, bronchoscopy should be performed to define the anatomy and eliminate the possibility of endobronchial disease. Endobronchial tumor is likely to be a result of primary lung cancer rather than mesothelioma.[93] Because of the progressive nature of mesothelioma and the extent of surgery needed to eradicate the disease, any patient being considered for radical surgery must be able to withstand possible pneumonectomy and prolonged anesthesia. Careful evaluation of cardiac and pulmonary functions are thus critical.[94] For therapeutic approaches, three surgical techniques have been advocated: pleuradesis, pleurectomy (decortication), and extrapleural pneumonectomy (EPP). There are no comparative studies of these approaches, and patients treated are often highly selected for the various procedures. Thus, the studies of the different approaches often contain groups with highly different prognostic factors and so cannot be compared.

Pleuradesis is usually performed for palliation and is accomplished alone or with a partial pleurectomy by means of video-assisted thoracoscopic surgery (VATS) and the insufflation of sclerosing agents, such as talc.[95] This approach can control pleural effusions in about 90% of cases but does not offer any opportunity for cytoreduction of tumor. Advocates of this approach cite the lack of definitive data favoring more aggressive debulking procedures and the relative sparing of postoperative complications. This technique produces median survivals that recapitulate the natural history of the tumor, however, and it further complicates any subsequent attempt to perform a cytoreductive procedure.[95] Nevertheless, this approach could be the most appropriate for those with significant comorbid disease or those with adverse surgical prognostic factors.

Pleurectomy or decortication has been advocated by a number of investigators, and the median survivals in these series range from 6.7 to 21 months (Table 76-5).[58,92,96-106] This approach has also been used to control effusions (including cases of pleuradesis failure) and has achieved control of effusions in more than 80% of cases. With this technique, the pleura are stripped from the apex of the lung to the diaphragm, removing pericardium and parietal pleura in the course of dissection. Clean separation of lung and visceral pleura is often difficult because of the pattern of growth, and the diaphragmatic pleura usually cannot be completely resected. This eventually leads to a very high local recurrence rate. Chest tubes are placed to drain blood and to manage any possible bronchopleural fistulae. Operative mortality from pleurectomy is usually quite low (1.5%-5%), but complications include bronchopleural fistulae, hemorrhage, and subcutaneous emphysema. Of considerable interest is the impact of histological subtype on the outcome. In most surgical series in which subtype is specified, the median survival duration for the epithelial subtype is two- to threefold greater than for the sarcomatous form, and the mixed subtype shows an intermediate survival. Investigators at Memorial Sloan-Kettering Cancer

TABLE 76-5

Pleurectomy for Diffuse Pleural Mesothelioma

AUTHOR	NO. OF PATIENTS	2-YEAR SURVIVAL (%)	MEDIAN SURVIVAL (MOS)
Lewis[101]	4	25	6.7
Hilaris[98,99]	95*	35	12.6
Law[96,97]	28	32	20
DaValle[100]	23		11.2
Wanebo[102]	16(F)		11
Wanebo[102]	1(E)		21
Achatzy[103]	46	11	10
Brancatisano[92]	45		16
Rusch[104]	25		
Rice[105]	5		13†
Soysal[106]	100		

E, epithelial form; F, fibrosarcomatous form.
*41 patients received pleurectomy followed by external beam RT; 54 patients received pleurectomy followed by implant and external beam RT.
†Includes patients receiving pleurectomy and extrapleuropneumonectomy.

TABLE 76-6

Extrapleural Pneumonectomy for Diffuse Pleural Mesothelioma

AUTHOR	YEAR	NO. OF PATIENTS	MORTALITY (%)	MEDIAN SURVIVAL (MOS)
Worn[107]	1974	62	Unspecified	19
Bamler[108]	1976	17	23	—
Butchart[86]	1978	29	31	4
DeLaria[109]	1985	11	0	—
DaValle[100]	1986	33	9.1	11.2
Vogt-Moykopf[110]	1987	55	5.5	10.2
Faber[111]	1988	33	9.	13.5
Geroulanos[71]	1990	18	7	20
Rusch[112]	1991	20	15	10
Rice[105]	1994	10	–10	13*
Sugarbaker[87]	1999	183	3.8	19

*Includes patients with pleurectomy and extrapleural pneumonectomy.

Center (MSKCC) published some of the largest experiences with this technique when combined with external beam plus or minus interstitial irradiation, or in combination with postoperative intrapleural therapies and irradiation.[93,98,99] In their experience with 95 patients as listed in Table 76-5 (referenced as Hilaris and coworkers[98] and McCormack and associates[99]), a select group of 27 patients who had the epithelial subtype and who did not require an implant had a median survival of 22.5 months and a two-year survival rate of 41%. Wanebo and colleagues[102] also evaluated their surgical pleurectomy series by histologic subtype and found that those patients with the epithelial form had a better survival than those whose tumor showed the fibrosarcomatous form. The relatively poor results with a median of 6.7 months survival that were reported by Lewis and coworkers[101] were derived from an older group of patients. DaValle and associates[100] advocated the use of extrapleural pneumonectomy for patients with minimal invasion of the visceral pleura (free pleural space without tissue invasion) as an approach for possible cure, as the survival with pleurectomy was not striking (a median of 11.2 months). Although there are no studies that directly compare the various surgical approaches, the reported median survival for pleurectomy appears similar to the medians reported for even more aggressive surgical approaches.

Extrapleural pneumonectomy (EPP) is a more aggressive, extirpative procedure in which the parietal pleura, lung, pericardium, and diaphragm are resected en bloc. A graft to prevent herniation of the abdominal contents replaces the diaphragmatic defect. To prevent cardiac herniation, the right pericardium is also often reconstructed. A thoraco-abdominal approach allows for easier access for the resection of the diaphragm. DaValle and colleagues[100] advocated extrapleural dissection to the hilum, early entry into the pericardium retrosternally to accomplish intrapericardial pneumonectomy, and use of double-lumen anesthesia. With either approach, intercostal chest tubes are usually placed to drain blood, fluid, and

treat possible bronchial air leaks. The trials reporting extrapleural pneumonectomy are shown in Table 76-6 and show median survival ranging from 4 to 20 months.[71,86,87,100,105,107-112] Because of the extent of the procedure and the learning curve, the early studies showed postoperative mortality as high as 31%. With increasing experience, more recent studies demonstrate operative and postoperative mortality below 4%. Serious complications as high as 25% have been reported and include bronchial leaks, empyema, vocal cord paralysis, chylothorax, arrhythmias, and respiratory insufficiency.[108] Recent studies with careful preoperative screening have also reduced these postoperative complications.[87] The evolution of this approach is demonstrated in Table 76-6 by the increasing median survival and decreasing surgical mortality. Rusch and coworkers[112] reported a 2-year survival of 33% with a 10-month median survival in 20 patients, whereas Sugarbaker and associates[87] reported a 38% 2-year survival and 19-month median survival for those patients undergoing EPP. The surgical mortality reported in the two studies was 15% and 3.8%, respectively. These latter two studies are probably representative of modern selection criteria and contemporary surgical management. Both studies also offer the details of treatment failure sites. In contrast to the pleurectomy series, some of the reports of extrapleural pneumonectomy showed a small percentage of 5-year survivors. Although the degree of surgery, the selection criteria, and the possible stage shift biases preclude definitive statements, overview of the sites of treatment failure and long-term outcomes suggest that extrapleural pneumonectomy could alter the natural history of pleural mesothelioma.

Surgical Prognostic Factors

Results from both pleurectomy and EPP series suggest that certain pre- and postoperative factors carry important prognostic information that can help select appropriate surgical candidates. These factors include:

- Subhistologies (epithelial vs. other types)
- Preoperative tumor bulk

- Mediastinal lymph node involvement
- Resection margins
- Invasion beyond the pleural envelope

Among those studies that specify subhistology, nearly all show that patients with the sarcomatous and mixed forms of mesothelioma have a significantly worse disease-free and overall survival than those with the epithelial form.[87,102,105,113] These data strongly suggest that patients with sarcomatous or mixed subhistology should be offered palliative therapies such as pleuradesis and be spared the operative consequences of aggressive surgical procedures. Similarly, mediastinal lymph node involvement defines an adverse prognosis.[87,113] Because patients with mediastinal lymph node involvement have a significantly inferior survival, preoperative staging should probably assess the mediastinum. Whether this dictates a preoperative mediastinoscopy, or whether imaging techniques such as FDG PET scanning can provide adequate preoperative assessment, remains to be determined. Other factors that can predict survival include penetration through the diaphragm, extension to other extracapsular sites, and large preoperative tumor volume.[87,113] These surgical prognostic factors suggest that further revision of the staging systems could be required to better define which patients are most likely to benefit from surgical approaches. An alternative, postoperative, functional staging system based on the surgical experience at Brigham Hospital and Dana-Farber Cancer Institute is shown in Table 76-3.

Radiation Therapy

The role of radiation therapy in the definitive treatment of pleural mesothelioma remains uncertain, and radiation therapy alone for unresected disease produces inconsistent results for disease or symptom control. Because the pleura encompass the entire hemithorax, including the pericardium and diaphragm, tumorcidal doses of irradiation would likely cause significant organ toxicity to the lung, heart, and possibly the liver.[114] The types and severity of the complications depend in part on the dose, schedule, and type of radiotherapy. Other factors include the normal tissue included within the irradiation volume and the types of therapies being administered concurrently or immediately before radiotherapy. Among the various small studies of radiation therapy, some reported symptomatic improvement in a small fraction of the patients or control of effusions in a fraction of the patients.[68,96,97,115-118] Despite anecdotal reports of long-term survival after external beam irradiation or after intracavitary instillation of radioisotopes, most reviews of experience with radiation therapy suggest that the radiation therapy produces no significant effect on disease control or survival.[68,96,97,117,119-124] In addition, there is very little information regarding dose response or the effect of subhistology on radiation responsiveness or control.[68,117] Nevertheless, radiation therapy is used frequently for palliation of local pain. Despite the paucity of trials to prove its utility, radiation therapy has been added to surgical series with the aim of reducing the high incidence of local recurrence.[87]

Because the dose of radiation therapy needed to provide local control is directly related to the volume of irradiation, its addition to debulking (cytoreductive) surgical techniques has some rational basis.[125] The addition of radiation therapy to pleurectomy to reduce local recurrences has considerable appeal because of the high local recurrence observed with this surgical technique, and the addition of radiation therapy to EPP might also be better tolerated because the underlying lung has been removed. Its addition to EPP can also be rationalized on the basis of local recurrences, especially at the thoracotomy site. In one report, 21 Gy delivered in three fractions prevented the recurrence of tumor in the wound after thoracoscopy or thoracotomy in 24 patients, whereas in the researchers' prior experience, 61% of 33 patients not undergoing radiation developed tumors at the wound site.[126] Alberts and colleagues[123] compiled the treatment outcomes for 262 patients treated between 1965 and 1985 with either chemotherapy, radiotherapy (RT), both chemotherapy and RT, or decortication plus RT and chemotherapy. The median survival of 9.6 months was similar for all groups. Only a small group of patients treated with doxorubicin and irradiation with 10 Gy every 6 weeks for four courses appeared to show prolonged survival, with a median survival of 22.6 months.

Chemotherapy

Single Agents. In the past, the role of chemotherapy for malignant pleural mesothelioma was difficult to assess because of the small numbers of patients entered into individual chemotherapy trials, the pessimism regarding treatment, the difficulty in assessing response, and the bias associated with reporting predominantly positive results. Thus, much of the older data regarding single-agent and combination chemotherapy activity was derived from summary overviews of small pilot trials or from chemotherapy trials of soft-tissue sarcomas.[127] Over the last one to two decades, both the incidence and the accuracy of diagnosis have increased, thus permitting larger disease-specific trials to occur. The advent of CT and MRI have further allowed for assessment of response using rind thickness as a criterion. Table 76-7 shows the activity of various chemotherapy agents, based on trials of adequate size that include 14 or more patients.[128-181] At one time, the anthracyclines in general and doxorubicin specifically were considered to be the mainstay of chemotherapy for mesothelioma; however, adequately sized trials have shown that doxorubicin has only a modest activity (complete response + partial response) of 11%.[182] Epirubicin has a similar modest activity of 14%, and liposomal doxorubicin showed only 6% activity. Except for single, unconfirmed studies of detorubicin and pirorubicin, which are no longer available, the anthracyclines thus have only modest activity, and their use has essentially ceased. Among the alkylating agents, one trial of mitomycin C suggested an activity of 21%. The platinums (cisplatin and carboplatin) show only modest activity of 14% and 11%, respectively, but their value could reside in their ability to synergize with other agents. The campto-thecins, taxanes, and vincas have been disappointing as single agents. In contrast, the antimetabolites appear

TABLE 76-7

Response Rates for Adequately Evaluated* Single Agents in Malignant Mesothelioma

AGENT	NUMBER EVALUABLE	RESPONSE (%)[†]	REFERENCES
Anthracyclines			
Doxorubicin	66	9	128, 129
Detorubicin	35	26	130
Pirarubicin	35	22	131
Epirubicin	59	14	133, 193
Liposomal doxorubicin	72	5	134–136, 516
Mitoxantrone	62	5	137, 138
Menogaril	22	3	139
Alkylating Agents			
Cyclophosphamide	16	0	129
Ifosfamide	64	8	140–142, 144, 145
Mitomycin C	19	21	146
Platinums			
Cisplatin	295	14	147, 148
Carboplatin	88	11	150–152
Antimetabolites and Antifolates			
High-dose methotrexate	60	37	153
Trimetrexate	51	12	154
Edatrexate	20	25	155
Edatrexate + folinic acid	40	15	155
Pemetrexed	64	14	156
Antimetabolites, Other			
5-Fluorouracil	20	5	157
Capecitabine	26	4	158
Di deazafolic acid (CB3717)	18	6	159
Dihydro 5 azacytadine	56	7	160, 161
Gemcitabine	61	12	162–164
Camptothecins			
Topotecan	22	0	165
Irinotecan	28	0	166
Vincas and Related Compounds			
Vincristine	23	0	167
Vindesine	38	3	168, 169
Vinblastine	20	0	170
Etoposide (VP16)	111	3	171, 172
Taxanes			
Paclitaxel	60	0	173, 174
Docetaxel	50	8	175, 176
Miscellaneous			
M AMSA	19	1	178
AZQ	20	0	177
Onconase	105	5	179
Gefitinib	43	2	180
Imatinib	25	0	181

*Individual trial with 14 or more entries.
[†]Complete plus partial response.

to show some promise for further development. In particular, the antifolate compounds are of considerable interest. High-dose methotrexate was shown to have an appreciable response by Solheim and associates,[153] who reported a 37% response among 60 assessable patients. Vogelzang and colleagues[154] reported a 12% response for trimetrexate, while Kindler and coworkers[155] reported a 25% response with the new antifolate agent, edatrexate.

Another antifolate agent, pemetrexed, showed modest activity of 14% as a single agent but provided both improved response and improved survival when added to cisplatin, compared with the administration of cisplatin alone.[149,156] This class of agents is also of interest, as recent studies have shown enhanced folate expression in human mesotheliomas and potentially unique transport mechanisms for pemetrexed.[183,184]

Combination Chemotherapy. The vast majority of combination chemotherapy regimens tested with adequate sample size are either anthracycline- or platinum-based and are listed in Table 76-8. The various trials are difficult to compare because of issues concerning disease subgroups, pretreatment characteristics, and prior therapies. These make the survival data difficult to interpret, and for this reason, responses rather than survival are evaluated. Similar to the data on single agents, the early studies of combination chemotherapy suffered from small and often inadequate trials. More recent studies include more appropriate numbers of patients and modern response criteria, thus allowing for a better assessment of activity. Recently tested combination regimens are listed in Table 76-8.[57,149,185-215] For example, early composites of small doxorubicin combinations suggested reasonable responses and survival activity. One large study of doxorubicin plus cyclophosphamide with and without DTIC, however, showed a response rate of only 15%.[186] Three studies of doxorubicin plus cisplatin showed a composite response of 27%, but a large study of doxorubicin plus cisplatin showed only a 16% response rate.[190] One small trial of doxorubicin, cyclophosphamide, and cisplatin showed a response rate of 30%.[191] Overall, the

response data for the anthracycline-based combination regimens remains disappointing.

Most recent trials of combination chemotherapy are platinum based and show a somewhat greater response to therapy than prior combinations did. Whether this apparent improvement in response is an artifact of patient selection, earlier treatment, or better agents remains uncertain, but it is illustrated in the recent single-agent data for cisplatin, which was part of a randomized trial and showed a 16.7% response rate.[149] Unfortunately, models of mesothelioma have not yet been as helpful as one would hope in developing therapeutic strategies. An interesting model of human mesothelioma transplanted onto nude athymic mice suggested that the combination of cisplatin and mitomycin C is highly synergistic.[216] A prospective randomized phase II study by the Cancer and Leukemia Group B (CALGB) showed a response of 26% when the stable disease category was included, but the response rate declined to less than 20% if only objective criteria were considered.[190] Two combination chemotherapy regimens appear to show significant promise, and both focus on an antimetabolite plus cisplatin (see Table 76-8). Several phase II trials have shown reproducible responses for the combination of cisplatin and gemcita-

TABLE 76-8

Chemotherapy Combinations for Malignant Pleural Mesothelioma

COMBINATION	NO. OF PATIENTS	RESPONSE (%)*	REFERENCE
Anthracycline-based			
Doxorubicin + interferon	24	16	185
Doxorubicin + cyclophosphamide	36	11	186
Doxorubicin + cyclophosphamide + DTIC	60	17	197
Doxorubicin + ifosfamide	40	23	187, 188
Doxorubicin + cisplatin	59	16	189, 190
Doxorubicin + cisplatin + cyclophosphamide	23	30	191
Doxorubicin + 5-azacytidine	36	22	57
Doxorubicin + cisplatin + mitomycin-C	24	21	192
Epirubicin + ifosfamide	17	6	193
Epirubicin + interleukin-2	21	5	194
Platinum-based			
Cisplatin + interferon	55	32	195, 196
Cisplatin + vinblastine	20	25	198
Cisplatin + Dihydro 5 azacytadine	29	17	197
Cisplatin + irinotecan	15	27	199
Cisplatin + etoposide	25	24	200
Cisplatin + mitomycin C +	35	26	190
Cisplatin + mitomycin + vinblastine	39	20	201
Cisplatin + mitomycin + interferon	62	19	202, 203
Cisplatin + mitomycin + etoposide + fluoruracil	45	38	207
Cisplatin + gemcitabine	133	37	204–206, 208
Carboplatin + gemcitabine	50	26	209
Cisplatin +Pemetrexed	226	41	149
Carboplatin + interferon	14	7	210
Carboplatin + Pemetrexed	27	32	212
Oxaliplatin + raltitrexed	89	27	213
Oxaliplatin + vinorelbine +	26	23	211
Antifol-based			
High-dose methotrexate + interferon α	24	29	214
High-dose methotrexate + interferon α + δ	39	21	215

*Complete plus partial response.

bine, with potential schedule-dependent differences. The combination of cisplatin and pemetrexed showed activity in a phase I study and led to the large, randomized trial of this combination vs. cisplatin alone.[217] The response rate for this combination was 41.3% compared with 16.7% for cisplatin alone, and the combination showed significant superiority in terms of both time to progression and overall survival.[149] This observation led to the comment that this combination represents a new standard of therapy for malignant pleural mesothelioma and will clearly be the basis for comparison for new treatments.[218]

Intrapleural Therapy

Another approach to the treatment of pleural mesothelioma has been the instillation of therapeutic agents into the pleural space. Because mesothelioma develops superficially along pleural and peritoneal cavities, intracavitary instillation of chemotherapy, radioisotopes, or biologics potentially could treat the superficial disease. Anecdotal reports of prolonged survival with certain radioisotopes also has stimulated interest in this approach.[119,219] High intracavitary concentrations of chemotherapeutic agents potentially could capitalize on any dose-response relationships for the agents. This approach is limited, however, by the propensity of the pleural space to become progressively obliterated with advancing disease, and even in early disease the intracavitary chemotherapy penetrates only a very shallow level of the tumor. Thus intrapleural therapies have limited applications, only to either very early disease or post-debulking surgical procedures.

Cisplatin is the most extensively studied agent for intracavitary use.[220-223] Pharmacokinetic studies of its intracavitary use show that exposure and peak levels are much greater than for intravenous administration of cisplatin. This approach has not met with the same degree of success as has been seen with intraperitoneal administration of cisplatin for peritoneal mesothelioma.[222] The role of other agents, such as doxorubicin, cytosine arabinoside, and mitomycin-C by the intracavitary route, is not well established. Various permutations of this approach are currently under investigation, including hyperthermic perfusion.[224] Given the complexity of such maneuvers, it is unlikely that this approach will become well established unless a significant benefit occurs, which has yet to be demonstrated.

Biologic and Targeted Therapies

Another approach to treating mesothelioma has been the exploration of several biologic response modifiers, including the interferons, other cytokines such as IL-2, gene therapy, and vaccines.[69,195,225-237] Some of the various biological agents tested either systemically or intrapleurally are shown in Table 76-9. In addition, studies of cancer cell biology have identified various molecular targets that control growth and proliferation pathways; these studies have opened new vistas for therapeutic intervention. Tissue and molecular technology even offer the possibility of specifically phenotyping a given tumor for its molecular targets.

The interferons (IFNs) have been tested extensively because preclinical studies showed that malignant mesothelioma cell lines are susceptible to IFN-α alone and that this effect is enhanced in combination with other cytokines (e.g., IFN-γ and tumor necrosis factor [TNF]) and with chemotherapy.[237] Additionally, IFNs offer the possibility of improving immune recognition of the tumor. These data have served as the rationale for clinical trials with the IFNs (see Table 76-9), which mostly have been disappointing and have produced considerable systemic toxicities, including fever, nausea, vomiting, chill, mylagias, and anorexia. Intrapleural therapy also has produced some empyema. Intrapleural IFN-γ, however, is worthy of notice. Boutin and colleagues[238] performed pleuroscopy upon recognizing effusion in asbestos-exposed individuals and instilled IFN-g if tumor was identified. Pleuroscopy was repeated for subsequent evaluation. The overall response rate was 20%, but those patients with stage IA disease had a 45% response with eight confirmed complete responses and a prolonged disease-free survival. This data served as part of the impetus for the IMIG revision of the staging system.[88] Interleukin 2 (IL-2) was also shown to have an antiproliferative effect on mesothelioma cell lines.[237] Two small studies of intrapleural IL-2 produced responses of 55% and 19%, respectively (see Table 76-9), but showed considerable systemic toxicities.[233,234] The intramuscular administration of TNF plus IFN-γ and the intralesional administration of GM-CSF produced disappointing results and considerable toxicity (see Table 76-9).

The biological agents were also combined with chemotherapy, and the majority of these trials combined chemotherapy agents with IFN-α (see Table 76-8). Doxorubicin plus IFN-α produced a modest response with unaccept-

TABLE 76-9

Clinical Trials of Interferons and Other Cytokines in Malignant Mesothelioma				
AGENT	**ROUTE**	**NO. ENTERED**	**RESPONSE (%)**	**REFERENCE**
IFN-α	Systemic	38	11	225, 227
IFN-γ	Intrapleural	89	20	238
IFN-β	Systemic	14	0	228
IL-2	Intrapleural	58	41	229, 233, 234
IL-2 + LAK cells	Intrapleural	5	0	232
TNF + IFN-γ	Intramuscular	36	3	235
GM-CSF	Intralesional	14	7	236

able toxicity.[185] Two different doses of IFN-α plus 60 mg/[2] cisplatin produced responses of 25% and 30%, respectively.[195,196] The toxicities—which included nausea, vomiting, fever, anorexia, and asthenia—were unacceptable, however. Carboplatin plus IFN-α produced a 7% response, but the carboplatin was dosed by body surface area.[210] A trial of IFN-α plus mitomycin and cisplatin produced a 14% response (including 5% complete response) among 43 patients.[202,203] The combination of high-dose methotrexate and systemic IFN-α and IFN-γ produced a 29% response similar to that seen for high-dose methotrexate alone.[214,215] Given the significant systemic toxicities of this combined approach, further studies await better chemotherapy and biotherapy agents.

Gene Therapy. Another approach for biotherapeutics has been the use of gene therapies. Because early tumors are relatively localized, gene therapy via the pleuroscope has been tested by investigators at the University of Pennsylvania.[239] They used replication-defective adenovirus containing HSV-tk (a viral protein sensitive to gancyclovir) to test the concept that insertion of the HSV-tk genome into the tumor cells would make the transfected tumor cells (in contrast to normal mammalian cells) lethally susceptible to gancyclovir. Only a small percentage of screened patients were eligible, and 26 patients were treated intrapleurally with escalating doses of virus. Gene transfer was seen in 17 patients, humoral and cellular immune response were seen, and two patients achieved either a response or a prolonged disease-free survival. The median survival was 11 months, and further studies are in process, although the issues of generalized inflammatory responses remain of some concern. Other gene therapy approaches, such as inserting cytokines onto viral vectors and tumor vaccines, are also under development.[240]

Targeted Therapies. The identification of specific molecular targets that control tumor cell growth, replication, and metastases has led to the identification of agents that specifically target these molecular abnormalities. Antibodies and specific thymidine kinase inhibitors (TKIs) have been developed that target the epidermal growth factor receptor (EGFR), vascular endothelial growth factor (VEGF), and platelet-derived growth factor (PDGF). EGFR is overexpressed in many human epithelial tumors, including mesothelioma.[237] Interfering in this signaling pathway could influence growth, angiogenesis, and apoptosis. Inhibition of VEGF could also inhibit angiogenesis. PDGF is believed to be an important autocrine growth factor for growth of mesothelioma.[237] Thus interfering with this autocrine loop could inhibit growth. The initial trials of some of these agents, however, have so far shown disappointing results. Gefitinib, the EGFR TKI, was tested by the CALGB, and one response (2%) was seen among 43 patients.[180] Imatinib, the PDGF TKI, produced no responses among 25 patients.[181] Further testing with similar agents is ongoing, and the optimal use of these agents most likely depends on finding the correct biological indicators of the responses.

Combined-Modality Therapies

Another approach to the treatment of mesothelioma is to combine or sequence several treatment modalities to reduce both local and distant recurrences. Thus surgery, radiotherapy, chemotherapy, and biologics might be combined in various groupings. The accumulated experience with combined modalities is relatively limited.[57,87,98,99,102,105,241-246]

Because of the advanced stage of disease at presentation in the United States, most patients are not candidates for surgical resection. Thus, one possible approach is the use of chemotherapy with radiotherapy. There is, however, only limited experience with this approach, despite the recognized potential of many agents such as cisplatin to act as radiosensitizers. Doxorubicin plus radiotherapy was studied in two small trials.[57,241] A small subgroup of patients from the large series reported from South Africa was treated with doxorubicin and radiation therapy.[123] Compared with most of the patients in the report, this subgroup appeared to show a prolonged survival (median survival of 22.6 months). Conclusions about outcomes in a small, highly selected subgroup, however, is difficult at best.

Several trials have added either interstitial or external beam irradiation to pleurectomy as described in the earlier section on radiation therapy. Rusch[247] reviewed the multimodality experience at Memorial Sloan-Kettering. One hundred five patients underwent pleurectomy followed by interstitial and external beam irradiation. The median survival was 12.5 months, and those with early disease and epithelial histology demonstrated better survival. Another approach to postoperative irradiation is the use of photodynamic therapy (PDT) to the interior of the pleural or thoracic cavity. After a debulking procedure such as a pleurectomy or EPP, a diffusing solution is placed in the hemithorax, and a unique wavelength (usually red) light is used to activate the dye. Moskal and colleagues[248] treated 40 patients (24 with advanced disease) using surgical debulking and PDT. Although the median survival was 15 months for those who survived surgery, the patient with Butchard stage I disease survived for 36 months. Pass and coworkers[242] tested PDT as part of a complex, randomized, postoperative chemoimmunotherapy protocol. Sixty-three patients were randomized to receive cisplatin, tamoxifen, and IFN-α with or without PDT after maximal cytoreductive surgery. The two treatment arms were comparable in terms of local failure rate, time to progression, and median survival. Further studies using this approach do not seem likely.

Even among the patients in whom surgical resection is attempted in the United States, most usually have disease beyond the parietal pleura. Thus adjuvant therapies to improve local control and prevent systemic recurrence are often attempted. Rusch and coworkers[245] followed pleurectomy with intracavitary cisplatin and mitomycin-C to assess the pharmacokinetic behavior of these agents. The investigators observed a high intracavitary concentration of drug with adequate plasma levels and systemic chemotherapy toxic effects. Postoperative systemic cisplatin and mitomycin-C chemotherapy were also added subsequently. Thirty-six patients were enrolled; 28 underwent surgical debulking, and 23 went on to postoperative therapy. The median survival was 17 months. Rice and associates[105] used a similar approach for 19 patients, and the median survival was 13 months. A variation of this postoperative intrapleural therapy tested hyperthermic perfusion with cisplatin, cisplatin plus mitomycin, or cisplatin plus doxorubicin. Yellin and colleagues[249] tested hyperthermic perfusion with cisplatin in seven patients with mesothelioma. Monneuse and coworkers[250] used cisplatin plus mitomycin-C in 17 patients with mesothelioma, and van Ruth and associates[224] used cisplatin plus doxorubicin in 22 patients. Although these studies showed that this approach is feasible, the clinical complexity and toxicity remain difficult to justify on the basis of the early results.

Sugarbaker and coworkers[87] built a trimodality therapy program using extrapleural pneumonectomy followed first by various chemotherapy regimens (cyclophosphamide plus doxorubicin plus or minus cisplatin or carboplatin plus paclitaxel) and then by subsequent (or concurrent) external beam chest irradiation. One hundred eighty-three patients were entered into the sequential studies, and there were seven postoperative deaths. The median duration of survival (excluding the seven postoperative deaths) was 19 months. Epithelial histology, negative mediastinal lymph nodes, tumor confined to the pleural envelope, and negative resection margins were all highly favorable prognostic factors. This subset analysis led to the Dana Brigham/Farber postoperative staging system (see Table 76-3). The subgroup that satisfied these prognostic factors (Brigham/Farber stage I) had a median duration of survival of 51 months and 2- and 5-year survivals of 68% and 46%, respectively. These results again argue strongly for careful staging and preoperative patient selection.

METASTATIC TUMORS OF THE PLEURA

Introduction

Metastatic tumors in the pleura are far more common than primary pleural tumors. Clinically, patients with these tumors present in a manner similar to those who have primary tumors in the pleura, with effusions, dyspnea, cough, atelectasis, and (less often) pain and fever. Symptoms related to the primary site of tumor are seen in nearly half of the patients, and the prognosis with metastatic disease to the pleura is related most to the ability to control the underlying primary tumor. Compromised performance status and weight loss are adverse prognostic features. The pleura can be the site of metastases from many cancers, but the most common origins are tumors of the lung, breast, stomach, colon, ovary, prostate, and thyroid, and melanoma. Most often, the primary site of disease becomes clinically evident or is found easily after history, physical examination, and roentgenographic studies. In a small proportion of the presentations, the primary site of disease is not immediately obvious. In these circumstances, cytology, histopathology, and immunohistochemistry evaluation of the pleural fluid and pleural biopsies can be important in

suggesting an area of primary tumor.[251] On a statistical basis, cancers of the lung are most likely. If histology suggests an adenocarcinoma, then appropriate pathology diagnostic studies should be performed to exclude an epithelial form of malignant mesothelioma, as patients with early mesotheliomas could be candidates for various aggressive therapies. Exclusion of nonmalignant causes of the effusion (e.g., parapneumonic effusions, pulmonary embolism, congestive heart failure, etc.), or causes accompanying disease or its treatment (e.g., accompanying superior vena cava syndrome, accompanying trapped lung, chylothorax from lymphatic obstruction, etc.) can have important implications for therapy.

Symptom Management

The most effective means to deal with symptomatic pleural disease is to exercise effective treatment of the underlying disease. Many metastatic tumors are difficult to treat or are resistant to therapy, however; for this reason, palliative methods of symptom control are often needed. These approaches include radiation therapy for localized painful areas, therapeutic thoracentesis, sclerosis, or pleurodesis, and pleural resection in selected cases. The choice of therapeutic options needs to be based on a realistic appraisal of the patient's disease and its outcome, potential risks and benefits related to the choices, and a careful assessment of the goals of therapy.

For patients with symptomatic pleural effusion, the initial approach entails a diagnostic thoracentesis, obtaining sufficient material to define the presence of malignancy in the pleural space and perform the necessary pathology studies to help narrow the possible primary site if it is not clinically evident. If thoracentesis or small needle biopsies prove insufficient for diagnostic material, more aggressive surgical procedures for tissue would be needed. Thoracoscopy has proven quite useful in obtaining adequate material in this setting.[252,253] For subacute and chronic effusions, the diagnosis of malignancy can sometimes be difficult because of necrotic cellular debris and reactive mesothelial cells that might obscure the malignant cells. In these circumstances, freshly shed tumor cells in the fluid or needle biopsy of the pleura are most helpful. To obtain freshly shed cells, it might be necessary to repeat a thoracentesis in the recurrent effusion. Performing a complete thoracentesis (i.e., tap dry) also provides a potential therapeutic maneuver, as some effusions will not recur or will recur only slowly. Caution must be exercised when performing a thoracentesis to near dryness, however, as this approach increases the risk of pneumothorax, and removing a large effusion increases the risk of postexpansion pulmonary edema.[254,255] Draining the effusion to dryness might thus require multiple sequential attempts. If repeated thoracenteses are needed for symptom control, more aggressive procedures (e.g., pleurodesis or pleural resection) might be appropriate.

Pleural Sclerosis—Pleurodesis

One of the standard approaches in the treatment of recurrent symptomatic pleural effusions is to attempt to obliterate the pleural space by producing an irritation or inflammation of the pleural surfaces, thereby causing them to adhere. Techniques to accomplish this have included: repeated thoracentesis, chronic tube drainage, installation of various agents, or partial pleurectomy.[256-261] Many and various agents have been instilled into the pleural cavity to attempt a sclerosis (Table 76-10).[226,234,258,262-309] These agents included:

- Physical agent talc
- Radioisotopes P[32] or Au[198]
- Antibiotics tetracycline, minocycline, and doxycycline
- Antiparasitic agent quinacrine
- Variety of chemotherapy agents
- Biologic substances interferon-β, interleukin-2, and *Corynebacterium parvum*
- Steroids

The studies that report the results of intrapleural installations are often difficult to interpret, and considerable uncertainty remains about the use of many of these agents. The patients included in these reports often constitute a heterogeneous population with different underlying cancers and different prognostic factors, such as performance status and weight loss. In some reports, pleurodesis is performed with the first drainage procedure, whereas in other reports its use is limited to recurrent effusions. Another confounding factor resides in the definition of response to treatment. Although antitumor effects on measurable lesions are defined by uniform agreement as complete or partial responses, treatments of pleural effusions are not easily cataloged in any standardized manner. Chronic drainage can produce partial adhesions with subsequent loculations, so that the definitions of

partial response are difficult to assess. Time to recurrence of effusion, or percentage of patients without recurrence of effusion at some fixed time (usually 30 days) are the benchmarks used most often. Finally, there are considerable differences in the techniques used to obtain drainage and instill agents. Until recently, drainage was usually accomplished through a large-bore (28–32F) chest tube evacuated through a water seal by gravity or suction; however, effective drainage (and pleurodesis) via small-bore (10–12F) catheters has been described.[280,310-312] Thoracoscopic drainage and talc pleurodesis have also been studied extensively and have been shown to be highly effective in achieving control of effusions.[283-291,313-319] In the various comparison trials, talc appeared to be more effective than chest tube drainage alone, drainage plus bleomycin chemotherapy, or drainage plus low-dose bleomycin.[267,288,290,319,320] The timing can also vary from immediate instillation to waiting until the daily chest-tube drainage is less than 100 mL. The duration at which the pleura are exposed to the sclerosing agent can also vary, from several hours with periodic rotations to permanent inclusion. Despite all of the variables, most investigators feel that pleurodesis can provide relatively reproducible relief of recurrent symptoms and that talc is likely the most effective agent. The discomfort of the drainage technique and the side effects of the agents used for instillation are often of some concern in these symptomatic patients with advanced disease. Among the other agents tested, quinacrine was used with some modest success in the past; however, fever, pain, hypotension, hallucinations, and anecdotal reports of sudden death essentially removed this agent from use.[258,264-266] Radioactive isotopes such as P[32] and Au[198] have been used with

TABLE 76-10

Agents Utilized for Pleurodesis

INSTILLATION AGENTS	DOSE	NUMBER STUDIED	PERCENT CONTROL	COMPLICATIONS
Chest tube drainage alone[258]	—	69	55	Pain, fever
Nitrogen mustard[258]	—	—	52	Pain, fever, hypotension, nausea, vomiting myelosuppression
[198]Au or [32]P[262,263]	15 mCi	>100	55	Isolation, pain
Quinacrine[258,264-266]	—	128	80	Pain, fever, ARDS, sudden death
Tetracycline[267-276]	500mg (total)—20mg/kg	359	67	Pain, fever
Minocycline[277]	300 mg	7	86	Pain
Doxycycline[278-280]	500 mg	60	72	Pain
Methylprednisolone[281,282]	160–820 mg	10	60	None
Talc[283-291,315-319]	2.5–10 mg	>2000	~90	Pain, fever, ARDS
Bleomycin[273,275,288,292-295]	14–240 U	199	54	Pain, fever, nausea
Doxorubicin[274,296]	10–40 mg	55	24	Pain, fever, emesis, anorexia, mild count suppression
Fluorouracil[259]	2–3 gm	35	66	Mild leukopenia
Mitomycin-C[259]	8mg	27	41	Pain, fever, leukopenia
Cisplatin +cytarabine[297,298]	100 mg/m[2] +600 or 1200 mg	44	27	Pain, nausea, emesis, myelosuppression, cardiopulmonary
Etoposide[299]	150–300mg	10	0	Alopecia, emesis, malaise, myelosuppression
Corynebacterium parvum[295,300-306]	3.5–14 mg	169	76	Pain, fever, nausea, cough
Interferon-α[307,322]	50–75 million U	38	37	Flulike, fever, pruritis, myelosuppression
Interferon-β[226]	5–20 million U	32	37	Fever, pruritis
IL-2[234,308,309]		66	39	Fever, rash, pruritis, fluid retention, empyema
OK-432[323]	10 U	26	88	Fever, chills, pleuritic chest pain

some success.[262,263] These agents are difficult to use, however, in that the patients must be isolated during the period of use, and a supply of the isotopes was difficult to obtain for many years. Furthermore, a randomized study by Izbicki and colleagues[263] demonstrated that the use of P[32] was marginally superior to therapy by tube drainage alone.

Several antibiotics have been tested as sclerotic agents in the pleura and pericardium. The most common approach in the use of these agents includes a large-bore chest tube, drainage to less than 100 mL per day, and a short duration of exposure (e.g., 2 to 3 hours) with frequent body rotations, followed by drainage. Doses of tetracycline higher than 500 mg might have a greater success rate, but the mechanism of action is not clear. The hypothesis that the tetracycline-induced sclerosis is related to the pH of the antibiotic solution (such that the higher the dose, the lower the pH and the greater the effect) was essentially disproven in a comparative trial by Zaloznik and coworkers,[269] who compared tetracycline to a solution of similar pH and found a superior effect with the antibiotic. In the United States, parenteral forms of tetracycline are no longer available, and many investigators have substituted doxycycline. Whether a dose-response effect also occurs with doxycycline is currently unknown. Pain is a fairly significant side effect in the use of the antibiotics, and many clinicians add xylocaine into the pleural cavity before or during the instillation of the antibiotic. Xylocaine, however, is recognized as paralyzing both leukocytes and monocytes, and to the degree that these cells are helpful in the etiology of sclerosis, the effect of instilling the topical anesthetic on the effectiveness of sclerosis has not been studied adequately.[321]

Chemotherapeutic agents have also been used as intrapleural therapies with some success (see Table 76-10). Several agents that were used in the past (e.g., nitrogen mustard, which was associated with severe pain, nausea and vomiting, and significant blood count suppression) are no longer commonly instilled.[258] Similarly, doxorubicin produced both severe pain and systemic complications.[258] Ruckdeschel and coworkers[273] performed a randomized study of tetracycline vs. bleomycin and concluded that there appeared to be an advantage for the bleomycin, with less frequence recurrences of effusions. The pain associated with bleomycin was less severe than with tetracycline, although many patients experienced some febrile response. Bleomycin remains the most commonly used chemotherapeutic agent for sclerosis. Fluorouracil and mitomycin-C have also been tested in small numbers of patients with some success, although mitomycin-C was associated with significant myelosuppression.[259] Comparisons of talc with bleomycin, however, suggest a superiority of talc.[290,319,320]

Biologic agents have also been instilled into the pleural cavity as a means to treat recurrent effusions (see Table 76-10). Among this class of agents, *Corynebacterium parvum* has been the most extensively studied, with a control rate of about 75% in 169 patients.[295,300-306] Interferon-α produced a 37% response rate among 38 patients in two studies, its administration accompanied by

flulike symptoms of fever, chills, malaise, pain, nausea, and vomiting.[322] Interferon-β showed a similar 37% response among 32 patients, but only minimal side effects were reported.[226] Intrapleural administration of recombinant IL-2 was also tested for its ability to induce sclerosis and showed a 36% response rate among 66 patients.[234,308,309] The toxicities included fever, chills, rash, fluid retention, and empyema. OK-432 is a lyophilized derivative of *S. pyogenes*, which was tested in malignant pleural effusions based on its activity in malignant ascites. OK-432 was compared with mitomycin-C and found to have an 88% response among the 26 patients randomized to OK-432.[323] Fever, chills, and pleuritic chest pain were seen in 80% of patients, however.

A last option for the control of recurrent pleural effusions is the use of video-assisted thoracic surgery (VATS) thoracotomy and limited pleural stripping or pleurectomy, thereby achieving a mechanical form of pleurodesis. Although this procedure is highly successful in achieving control of pleural effusions, it is of limited potential application because of the high morbidity and mortality associated with it, even in experienced hands.[106,258] Martini and associates[324] found an 18% perioperative death rate and a 23% complication rate, although more recent studies suggest that the use of VATS can reduce these complications significantly.[260,261] Nevertheless, pleurectomy should be reserved for the unique ambulatory patient with an otherwise "good" prognosis whose effusion cannot be controlled with less aggressive techniques.

Future Studies

Although the therapy for metastatic effusions is difficult and the prognosis for patients with these metastases is poor, further studies are of some importance because of the symptoms involved, the cost of care, and the need to maintain quality of life as long as possible. Thus outpatient programs for pleural drainage and research into sclerosing agents with minimal side effects are important areas of development. Another area of further development includes the use of talc insufflation at the time of initial diagnosis, when the thoracoscope is used for intrapleural biopsies.

MEDIASTINAL TUMORS

General

The mediastinum is a complex space in the center of the chest, bounded by the thoracic inlet superiorly, the diaphragm inferiorly, the sternum anteriorly, the spine posteriorly, and the mediastinal pleura bordering each lung laterally. A number of tumors, both benign and malignant, are known to occur in this area, which is divided anatomically into anterior, middle, and posterior compartments, each extending from the thoracic inlet to the diaphragm. These tumors are often difficult to differentiate either clinically or with available imaging techniques. The anterior mediastinum encompasses the space between the sternum anteriorly and the anterior pericardium posteriorly and contains the thymus gland, lymph nodes, and mesenchymal tissues. The middle mediastinum contains the heart and great vessels, the trachea and esophagus, the vagus and phrenic nerves, and most of the mediastinal lymph nodes. Finally, the posterior mediastinum is bounded by the posterior aspect of the pericardium and trachea anteriorly and the vertebral bodies to the costovertebral sulci posteriorly, and it includes the paraspinal tissues along with sympathetic and peripheral nerves. Occasionally, a distinction is made for the superior mediastinum, which is part of the anterior mediastinum residing behind the manubrium sterni, extending from the suprasternal notch to the angle of Lewis.

Tumors of the mediastinum are usually categorized according to their specific histologic subtype and anatomical location. These are listed in Table 76-11. Only one third of all primary mediastinal masses are malignant, but they include a wide variety of neoplasms. The location and site of the tumor often provide valuable clues toward making a clinical diagnosis. The clinical presentation of these tumors is shown in Table 76-12.

Thymomas, lymphomas, and germ cell tumors constitute the majority of the anterior mediastinal masses. In a series of 41 patients with isolated anterior mediastinal masses, the pathological diagnosis was lymphoma in 13 patients, thymoma in 11, germ cell tumor in 6, carcinoid in 2, bronchogenic carcinoma in 2, and benign process in the remaining 7 patients.[325] The middle mediastinum is the site of lymphoid malignancies in addition to the neoplasms that are related to metastases from visceral organs (e.g., lung cancer). The majority of neurogenic

---

TABLE 76-11

Classification of Mediastinal Tumors by Location

Anterior Mediastinum

Thymoma
Thymic carcinoma
Thymic carcinoid
Mediastinal germ cell tumors
Hodgkin's disease
Non-Hodgkin's lymphoma

Middle Mediastinum

Angiosarcoma of heart
Rhabdomyosarcoma of heart
Fibrosarcoma
Mesothelioma of pericardium
Lymphoma
Malignant teratoma
Extraskeletal osteosarcoma
Thymoma
Liposarcoma

Posterior Mediastinum

Peripheral neuroepithelioma
Neuroblastoma
Ganglioneuroma
Ganglioneuroblastoma
Pheochromocytoma
Schwannoma
Neurofibroma

TABLE 76-12

Clinical Presentation of Mediastinal Neoplasms

Asymptomatic—approximately 50% discovered incidentally on imaging studies
Symptomatic
  Mass effect: cough, dyspnea, pain, dysphagia, hoarseness and stridor, Horner's syndrome
  Superior vena cava syndrome, cardiac tamponade, spinal cord compression
  Nonspecific symptoms: fever, night sweats, malaise, weight loss, anorexia
Specific manifestations: hypertension with catecholamine—producing neurogenic tumors, myasthenia gravis with thymomas

---

tumors are located in the posterior mediastinum. These generalizations according to anatomic site, however, are clinically helpful but not uniformly accurate because of the exceptions to these guidelines. A number of rare tumors, such as carcinoids, neoplasms of mesenchymal origin, melanomas, and undifferentiated carcinomas are known to occur in the mediastinum without any regular compartmental localization.

Substernal thyroid extends downward from the thyroid and does not arise in the mediastinum, although it can first present as a mass in the anterosuperior compartment and can result in symptoms due to compression of the structures in the thoracic inlet, such as the trachea, esophagus, superior vena cava, and other neurovascular structures.[326] Most substernal thyroids are benign, but occasionally carcinoma can be detected in the substernal goiter. Substernal thyroid can be detected by radioactive iodine scanning and is usually excised using a cervical approach, but in certain cases, median sternotomy could be required.

Approach to Obtaining Diagnostic Material

Transthoracic needle biopsy (aspiration biopsy or true-cut needle biopsy) of a mediastinal mass can be used to obtain tissue, and imaging techniques such as CT scan, MRI scan, fluoroscopy, or ultrasound have made these procedures safe and effective.[327-329] These small-volume biopsies are of value only in certain specific situations, however.[328-330] Because of the need to establish a definitive diagnosis, thymoma, lymphoma, and other neoplasms might not be categorized reliably by small tissue samples obtained by transthoracic needle aspiration and/or biopsy. In contrast, metastatic carcinoma and germ cell tumors can be diagnosed with a high degree of specificity and sensitivity (Table 76-13).[331] The pneumothorax rate with transthoracic needle biopsy varies from 11% to 34% in reported studies.[329,330] This procedure should not be performed if the lesion is suspected to be vascular or if the patient has a history of bleeding disorders or previous pneumonectomy.

When needle aspiration or biopsy is not feasible or is unlikely to yield sufficient material, mediastinoscopy or anterior mediastinotomy can provide adequate material for definitive histologic diagnosis, cell-surface marker

AN APPROACH TO THE DIAGNOSIS OF MEDIASTINAL TUMORS BY IMAGING STUDIES

CHEST RADIOGRAPH
Essential for diagnosis of mediastinal tumors

COMPUTED TOMOGRAPHY SCAN WITH CONTRAST
Imaging modality of choice and "gold standard" for noninvasive evaluation
Differentiates mediastinal masses from vascular and cystic lesions
Delineates the compartment involved
Defines the mass in relationship to adjacent tissues
Valuable in determining the best approach for diagnostic biopsy of the mediastinal mass

MAGNETIC RESONANCE IMAGING
Modality of choice for evaluating posterior and superior mediastinal masses, chest wall abnormalities, and diaphragmatic processes
Study of choice for detecting masses adjacent to the spinal cord and vertebral bodies
Defines the characteristics of neurogenic tumors and neural cysts
Defines intracardiac masses with gating studies
Unique image reconstruction with coronal and sagittal views
Avoids use of iodinated contrast and ionizing radiation

Might help to distinguish residual tumor from fibrosis
Should be reserved for specific situations described, until spatial resolution limitations are overcome

INTRAESOPHAGEAL ULTRASONOGRAPHY
Eliminates the lungs as a source of interference and is thus useful for imaging cysts

RAIDONUCLIDE SCANNING
I-scanning for thyroid neoplasms or goiter (must be performed before intravenous administration of contrast for CT because the iodine load will interfere with normal thyroid uptake of radioactive iodine)
I-labeled MIBG scanning for pheochromocytoma

DOUBLE ISOTOPE (TECHNETIUM AND THALLIUM) SUBTRACTION IMAGING FOR PARATHYROID TUMORS

GALLIUM SCANNING FOR LYMPHOMAS AND HODGKIN'S DISEASE

POSITRON EMISSION TOMOGRAPHY (PET) SCANNING FOR HODGKIN'S AND NON–HODGKIN'S LYMPHOMAS

studies, and flow cytometric and cytogenetic studies.[331] Thoracotomy has given way to VATS thoracoscopsy, which is increasingly being used for diagnosis and staging of mediastinal and intrathoracic masses.[332] Bronchoscopy and esophagoscopy are of limited value for mediastinal masses and should be reserved for patients with apparent involvement of the aerodigestive tract.

TUMORS OF THE ANTERIOR MEDIASTINUM

Thymoma

Thymoma is the most common cause of an anterior mediastinal mass in adults (Tables 76-11 and 76-14). Thymomas are derived from thymic epithelial cells

demonstrating a spectrum of histologic patterns that encompass both epithelial and lymphocytic components in varying proportions.[333] The epithelial cells are embryologically derived from the lower portion of the third pharyngeal pouch and are believed to be responsible for the neoplastic element in thymomas. The lymphocytes associated with both the normal thymus and thymomas are predmoninantly immature T lymphocytes and demonstrate TdT postivity.[334,335] Immunoglobulin and T-cell receptor gene studies failed to show genotypic evidence supporting the neoplastic nature of the lymphocytic component.[336]

Although thymomas initially were classified according to their proportion of epithelial and lymphocytic components, this classification repeatedly showed a lack of clinical relevance to patient response and survival.[337-339] In the mid-1980s, Marino and Muller-

TABLE 76-13

Transthoracic Needle Biopsy for Diagnosis of Anterior Mediastinal Masses					
ANTERIOR MEDIASTINAL MASS (FINAL DIAGNOSIS)	**THORACIC NEEDLE BIOPSY(%)**				
	NO. OF PATIENTS	**SENSITIVITY**	**POSITIVE PREDICTIVE**	**NEGATIVE SPECIFICITY**	**PREDICTIVE**
Thymoma	26	42	96	73	87
Lymphoma	28	71	94	77	92
Germ cell tumor	11	91	98	83	99
Metastatic carcinoma	33	70	100	100	90

Adapted from Herman SJ, Holub RV, Weisbrod GI, Chamberlain DW: Anterior mediastinal masses: utility of transthoracic needle biopsy. Radiology 180:167, 1991, with permission.

TABLE 76-14

Thymic Tumors

Thymoma
Thymic carcinoma
Thymic lymphoma
Thymic Hodgkin's disease
Thymic carcinoid
Thymic germ cell neoplasm
Thymic lipoma
Thymic cyst
Thymic myoid tumor
Thymic histiocytic tumor

Hermelink[340] revised this traditional classification based on the subtyping of tumors according to their microscopic resemblance to the normal thymic epithelial cells and thymic cortex. The 1999 WHO classification of thymomas further modified the Marino classification, adding thymic carcinoma to the classification schema, simplifying the terminology, and providing prognostic relevance.[341,342] Typically, thymomas are solid tumors covered by a thick, fibrous capsule. The cut section reveals tan fleshy lobulations divided by fibrous septae. Cystic degeneration, calcification, and hemorrhage may be seen.[333]

Histologically, thymomas are classified according to their cytologic appearance in association with the proportion of lymphocytes present.[333] These tumors are typically bland in appearance and can demonstrate mild to moderate cellular atypia. Thymic carcinomas, on the other hand, appear cytologically malignant with marked nuclear atypia and demonstrate a high correlation between cytologic malignancy and clinical outcome.[342]

The staging system used for thymoma as proposed by Masaoka is outlined in Table 76-15.[343] Tumor staging is considered to be the most significant prognostic factor in determining patient survival. Thymoma spreads via direct extension through its capsule into adjacent structures such as lung, mediastinal soft tissue, or pleura and can metastasize distantly. The extent of capsule invasion and

TABLE 76-15

Staging of Thymoma

STAGE	DEFINITION
I	Macroscopically, completely encapsulated; microscopically, no capsular invasion.
IIa	Macroscopic invasion into surrounding fatty tissues or mediastinal pleura.
IIb	Microscopic invasion into the capsule.
III	Macroscopic invasion into the neighboring organ (i.e., pericardium, great vessels, or lung).
IVa	Pleural or pericardial dissemination.
IVb	Lymphogenous or hematogenous metastases.

Modified from Masaoka A, Monden Y, Nakahara K, et al: Follow-up study of thymomas with special reference to their clinical stages. Cancer 1981;48:2485. © 1981 American Cancer Society, with permission.

the involvement of thoracic and extrathoracic structures determines the stage, which is correlated to the risk of recurrence and survival.[343,344] Thus extensive tissue sampling of the resected tumor is essential to define microscopic and macroscopic invasion through the fibrous capsule. Other prognostic factors include the completeness of excision, tumor size, histologic typing, involvement of the great vessels, and performance status.[345-348]

Epidemiology

Thymomas constitute 20% of all mediastinal masses in adults. In general, they occur with about the same frequency in males and females, and there is no predilection for a particular race or geographic distribution. They are most commonly seen in the fifth and sixth decades of life.[349,350] A recent study indicated that in thymoma found to have capsular invasion, there is a predilection for males and Asians or Pacific islanders.[351] Thymomas are extremely rare in children, but when they occur, they present as highly aggressive tumors with a high mortality rate.[352]

Clinical Manifestations

In 30% to 50% of cases, thymomas present as an asymptomatic anterosuperior mediastinal mass seen on a chest radiograph (Fig. 76-6A and B). When symptomatic, patients usually present with cough, chest pain, dyspnea, dysphagia, fever, weight loss, or anorexia.[350] A number of associated conditions are seen in patients with thymoma; these can include myasthenia gravis, red cell aplasia, hypogammaglobulinemia, polymyositis, and (rarely) systemic lupus erythematosus, rheumatoid arthritis, thyroiditis, hyperthyroidism, and other cytopenias.[353] When an anterior mediastinal mass is present with myasthenia gravis, red cell aplasia, or hypogammaglobulinemia, the diagnosis of thymoma is essentially established.

Myasthenia gravis (MG) is an acquired autoimmune disorder caused by circulating acetylcholine receptor antibodies, resulting in acetylcholine receptor deficiency at the motor end-plate.[354] Two thirds of the patients with MG have thymic lymphoid hyperplasia, and 8.5% to 15% have thymoma.[343,355] In keeping with this correlation, one third of the patients with thymoma have MG.[343,355,356] Thymomas with concurrent myasthenia gravis tend to be less aggressive tumors than those without this associated disorder, and histologically, the tumors tend to have a greater lymphocyte-to-epithelial cell ratio.[357,358] MG can involve the external ocular muscles selectively, with the patient presenting with diplopia and ptosis. When the other bulbar muscles are involved, the presenting symptoms can include difficulty with deglutition, slurred speech, and loss of facial expression. The general voluntary muscle system can be affected, either alone or with the involvement of the external ocular and bulbar muscles, resulting in fatigability of the limb muscles. The proximal muscles are more affected than the distal ones. In advanced cases, the weakness is universal, and the grade of dyspnea depends on the severity of the disease. Progression is most rapid during the first few years, and most deaths caused by MG occur within the first 3 years after diagnosis.[355]

The anticholinesterase test is usually diagnostic for MG. Administration of edrophonium results in rapid (although

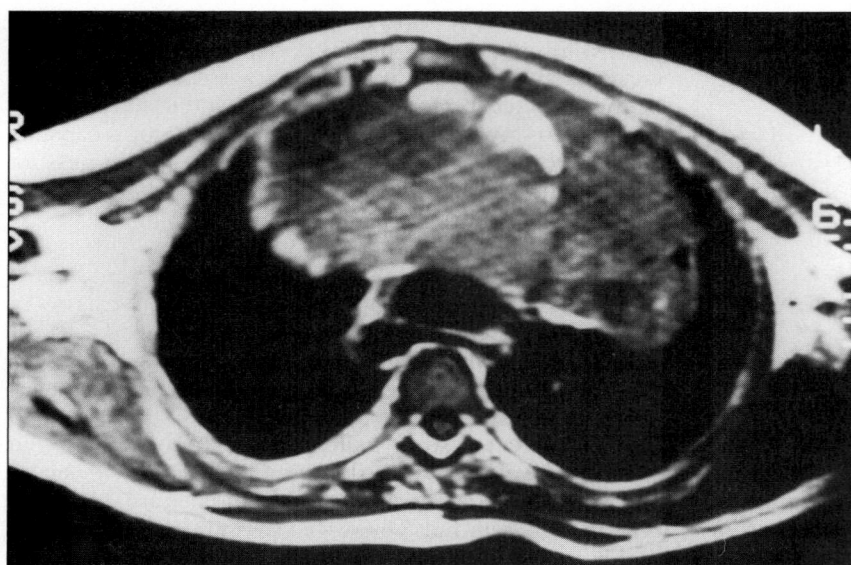

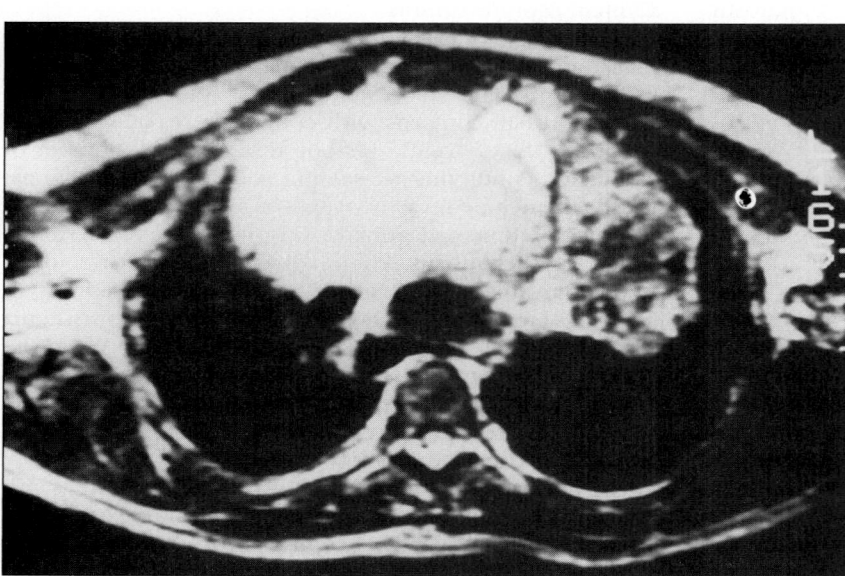

Figure 76-6. Anterior mediastinal mass—thymoma. **A,** Axial T_1-weighted MR image through the upper chest showing a large anterior mediastinal mass that extends laterally to both hemithoraces. **B,** Axial T_2-weighted image of the same mass, illustrating enhancement compatible with thymoma.

transient) clinical improvement, with objective response assessed by degree of ptosis, range of ocular movements, and the force of the hand grip. Electromyography performed with supramaximal stimulation of a motor nerve at 2 to 3 Hz results in progressive decrement of the amplitude of the evoked compound muscle action potential from the first to the fifth response. Other diagnostic studies include serologic tests for acetylcholine receptor antibody, C_3 localization of immune complexes at the end-plate in cryostat sections, and electrophysiologic studies of neuromuscular transmission.[359]

The initial current therapy of MG includes anticholinesterases and, alternately, prednisone. Pyridostigmine-bromide is widely used because of its longer duration of action and reduced muscarinic effects compared with neostigmine bromide.[360] The identification of thymoma in patients with MG represents an absolute indication for thymectomy. Although most patients experience some improvement in the thymoma-associated MG symptoms, complete remission of the associated MG symptoms can be expected in only a minority of patients.[361,362] Conversely, more than 75% of all patients with MG without thymoma show some improvement with thymectomy.[363] All thymus tissue, not only the thymoma, should be removed at the time of thymectomy, because residual thymus tissue can lead to persistence of the autoimmune disorder.[364] Other therapies for MG include immunosuppressive agents (e.g., azathioprine and plasmapheresis) in fulminant cases.

Red Cell Aplasia

Isolated red cell aplasia may be present in 5% to 10% of patients with thymoma. In this situation, there is an almost total absence of red cell precursors in the bone marrow and reticulocytes in the peripheral blood. One third of these patients also have reduced counts of both leukocytes and platelets. The exact etiology of this disorder is not known, but it has been reported to occur in patients together with MG and thymoma, which suggests an autoimmune mechanism.[365] Thymectomy in these patients results in improvement in approximately 30% of the patients.[366]

Hypogammaglobulinemia

Hypogammaglobulinemia is seen in about 5% of the patients with thymoma. Both cellular and humoral immunity are decreased in these patients. Only occasional remissions in hypogammaglobulinemia have been seen after thymectomy.[366]

Management of Thymoma

Surgical resection is the principal treatment modality for thymoma. All normal thymic tissue, including the perithymic fat, should be removed, especially if there is an associated autoimmune disease.[364] The usual surgical approach is by median sternotomy but can depend on the extent of the disease; more extensive resections might be required, including partial or total pneumonectomy or pericardiectomy.[367,368] Postoperative adjuvant radiation therapy is recommended for those patients found at the time of surgery to have invasive disease or thymic carcinoma, because such therapy leads to definite improvement in long-term survival, as shown by the results of randomized studies.[367] Patients with incompletely resected or unresectable disease are also candidates for radiation therapy. A dose of 30 to 60 Gy has been recommended. Even after whole mediastinal irradiation, recurrences are known to occur in the pleural cavity.[349,369] The role of radioisotope implants in areas of unresected tumor is not clear. Occasional responses of MG to radiation therapy have been noted in patients with persistent MG after thymectomy.[370]

Chemotherapy achieves only moderate responses for patients with recurrent or metastatic disease.[371] Agents with some degree of activity include cisplatin, doxorubicin, procarbazine, cyclophosphamide, ifosfamide, and corticosteroids. Only octreotide, cisplatin, and ifosfamide have completed phase II testing.[372-374] Anecdotal responses have also been reported to occur with corticosteroids.[375] Chemotherapy combinations generally produce higher response rates. Cisplatin-based combinations have been tested most extensively.[376-379] Fornasiero and colleagues[379] reported a 92% response rate in 37 patients with cisplatin, doxorubicin, vincristine, and cyclophosphamide. Loehrer and coworkers[372] reported a 50% response among 29 patients using cisplatin, doxorubicin, and cyclophosphamide. In another report, Park and associates[380] reported a 64% response rate with a similar regimen plus or minus prednisone. The EORTC reported a 56% response rate among 16 patients treated with cisplatin and etoposide, and the addition of ifosfamide was not beneficial.[381] A recent trial by Loehrer and colleagues[376] added ifosfamide to this regimen and demonstrated similar response rates. Thymic tumors have demonstrated a high uptake of indium-labeled octreotide (^{111}In-DTPA-D-Phe^1), which could be useful for imaging, but which in combination with prednisone has demonstrated complete and partial responses in patients with advanced disease.[372,382] These results indicate that thymoma could in fact be a chemosensitive tumor, and thus the role of chemotherapy in the adjuvant and neoadjuvant settings and in advanced disease needs to be further defined.

Thymic Carcinoma

Thymic carcinomas are epithelial neoplasms of the thymus that are characterized by a high degree of cytologic atypia. These tumors, unlike thymomas, express highly aggressive behavior and should thus be classified separately. Thymic carcinoma includes a heterogeneous group of neoplasms, of which more than half are undifferentiated carcinomas. Other tumor subtypes seen include squamous cell carcinoma, spindle cell carcinoma, lymphoepithelioma-like carcinoma, mucoepidermoid carcinoma, basaloid carcinoma, clear cell carcinoma, and adenoid cystic tumor.[383,384] Unlike their thymoma counterpart, thymic carcinomas lack immature T lymphocytes and are TdT negative.[385] Additionally, thymic carcinomas express the cytokeratin marker CD5, which is helpful in distinguishing these tumors from nonthymic epithelial malignancies.[386]

These tumors usually present in adult men and are seen only rarely in children. Symptoms include weight loss, shoulder discomfort, cough, and dyspnea. Paraneoplastic syndromes generally are not associated with thymic carcinoma. Well-differentiated thymic carcinoma has been reported in association with myasthenia gravis.[385] The spindle cell variety is generally an aggressive subtype, with mortality rates of up to 50% within 5 years reported.[383,387,388] There is increasing evidence that Epstein-Barr virus (EBV) might play a role in the development of a lymphoepithelioma-like carcinoma of the thymus gland, as is seen in nasopharyngeal carcinomas. EBV nuclease antigen has been detected in tumorous cells, and Southern blot analysis has demonstrated the EBV viral genome in the cells of thymic lymphoepithelioma-like carcinoma.[389] Although EBV-associated lymphoepitheliomas of the nasopharynx are often treated successfully, the thymic counterpart appears to have a poor prognosis, probably because it attains very large size before discovery.[383] Other forms of thymic carcinoma just mentioned are rare. Computed tomography usually shows an anterior mediastinal mass infiltrating along the pleura or mediastinum with necrosis or calcification.[390]

Thymic carcinomas are aggressive and highly lethal tumors. Usually, these patients present with advanced-stage disease and are candidates for multimodality treatment, including surgery, radiation therapy, and chemotherapy.[349,391] The combination of cisplatin, vinblastine, and bleomycin as used in the treatment of germ cell tumors has been applied to these neoplasms.[391]

Thymic Carcinoid

Thymic carcinoid arises from the neuroectodermal cells of foregut origin within the thymus and is an amine precursor uptake and decarboxylase (APUD) tumor, usually not associated with the classical carcinoid syndrome seen in carcinoids arising from the midgut.[392] These thymic carcinoids are usually locally invasive but can metastasize to bone, lymph nodes, skin, and liver.[393] In a large review of mediastinal thymic carcinoids, three groups of patients were identified:

1. Thymic carcinoid associated with Cushing's syndrome or other endocrinopathies (38%; age range 9–48 years).
2. Thymic carcinoid without other endocrinopathies (44.5%; age range 21–87 years).
3. Thymic carcinoid with multiple endocrine neoplasia, type I or II (17.5%; age range 30–46 years).[394]

Cushing's syndrome due to adrenocorticotropic hormone production by tumors is most often seen in children with thymic carcinoid.[395,396] In comparison with bronchial carcinoid tumors, thymic carcinoid tumors are a much less common cause of ectopic corticotropin syndrome.[397] Macroscopically, thymic carcinoids resemble thymomas but are usually not encapsulated. On histopathologic examination, thymic carcinoid is characterized by formation of tumor cells arranged into organoid clusters with tumor rosettes and ribbons. The vast majority of cells are positive for neuroendocrine markers such as chromagranin and synaptophysin, which are useful in confirming the diagnosis.[398] Wide excision of the thymus, when possible, is the mainstay of treatment.[393] The roles of postoperative radiation and chemotherapy is not known, but patients with unresectable or persistent tumors should probably be treated with radiation therapy. Control of hypercortisolism with metyrapone in patients with ectopic corticotropin syndrome is an important part of management.[396]

Mediastinal Germ Cell Tumors

Primary germ cell tumors constitute approximately 10% to 15% of all mediastinal neoplasms.[399] These tumors, though histologically similar to testicular neoplasms, are recognized as distinct entities with separate clinical and biological behaviors. They were initially thought to represent metastasis from occult testicular primary lesions based on the presence of testicular scars representing healed tumors.[400] Malignant transformation of germinal elements in the mediastinum without a primary gonadal tumor has now been well established, however, as isolated mediastinal metastasis from gonadal germ cell tumors rarely occurs. Autopsy series have failed to confirm the presence of either testicular occult primary tumors or fibrous scars in most of the cases with extragonadal germ cell tumors.[401,402] In addition to the mediastinum, other common sites of extragonadal germ cell tumors have been located along the body midline and identified in the pineal gland, sacrococcygeal region, and retroperitoneum.[403] This finding could be due to either abnormal migration of germinal elements to these areas during embryogenesis or their widespread distribution during early development.[404]

Epidemiology
The mediastinum is the most common site of extragonadal germ cell tumors in young adults.[405,406] They can be benign or malignant. The benign germ cell tumors show no predilection for sex, whereas the malignant mediastinal germ cell tumors occur almost exclusively in men.[407] The precise racial distribution of mediastinal germ cell tumors is unknown, unlike the distribution of gonadal germ cell tumors, which are seen most commonly among whites. There is some evidence that extragonadal germ cell tumors—especially mediastinal tumors—might occur with higher incidence among blacks and hispanics. The mediastinal nonseminomatous germ cell tumors have been recognized recently in association with Klinefelter's syndrome, with characteristic clinical features and cytogenetic abnormality 47XXY.[408] Whether the chromosomal abnormality seen in Klinefelter's syndrome plays a role in the development of these tumors is not known, but approximately 20% of patients with nonseminomatous germ cell tumors have Klinefelter's syndrome.[409] Systemic mast cell disease with circulating heparin-like anticoagulant has been reported in association with mediastinal germ cell neoplasms.[410] Acute nonlymphocytic leukemia and malignant histiocytosis are also known to occur in association with nonseminomatous mediastinal germ cell tumors; these are clearly not attributable to the therapy but seem to arise from a common progenitor.[411]

All histologic variants of germ cell tumors arise in extragonadal sites such as the mediastinum and are identical to those seen in the testes. This finding is compatible with the embryological concept that extragonadal germ cell tumors arise from primordial germ cells in the yolk sac or urogenital ridge that have failed to migrate into the scrotum. Benign teratomas are the most common germ cell tumors seen within the mediastinum, both in children and adults.[412,413] These tumors contain elements from all three germ layers: ectoderm, mesoderm, and endoderm. Seminoma is the most common malignant variety of germ cell tumor in the mediastinum, with an incidence of 40%.[414] Other subtypes include embryonal carcinoma, teratocarcinoma, choriocarcinoma, and endodermal sinus tumors, with pure and mixed forms of each type.[415] In a report of 11 cases of primary mediastinal germ cell tumors from a single institution, 4 were seminomas, 3 were mixed germ cell tumors, 2 were embryonal carcinomas, and 2 were teratocarcinomas.[416]

Clinical Presentation
The benign forms frequently do not give rise to any symptoms and are discovered incidentally on chest radiographs obtained for other reasons. If symptoms do occur, they are usually due to the enlarging mass in the anterior mediastinum.[413] On the other hand, almost all patients with malignant extragonadal germ cell tumors present with chest pain, cough, dyspnea, and constitutional symptoms such as fever, weight loss, and anorexia (Fig. 76-7A and B). Nonseminomatous tumors grow rapidly and metastasize early.[415] Occasionally, these patients develop superior vena cava syndrome or present with symptoms related to the site of metastasis, the most common of which are lungs, liver, bone, and brain.

The anterosuperior mediastinum is the most common site of mediastinal involvement, with rare presentation in the posterior compartment. Useful imaging studies

Figure 76-7. Anterior mediatinal mass—germ cell tumor. **A,** Unenhanced CT image of the chest at the level of the aortic arch showing a large anterior mediastinal mass that extends to the left to or through the chest wall. Note the extension of the pectoralis minor and the bulge of the pectoralis major anteriorly. Paratracheal adenopathy is evident on the right, as is a moderate left pleural effusion. **B,** T_1-weighted MR image at the same level, clearly demonstrating the extension of the mass into the chest wall.

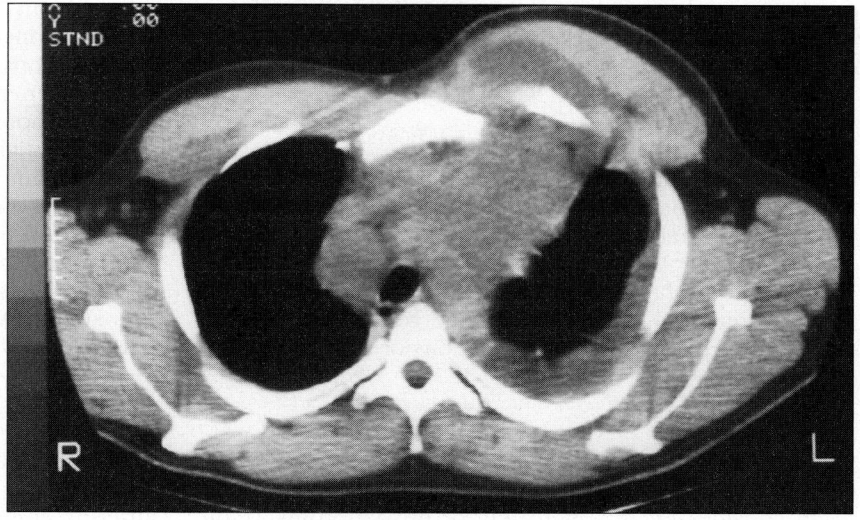

A

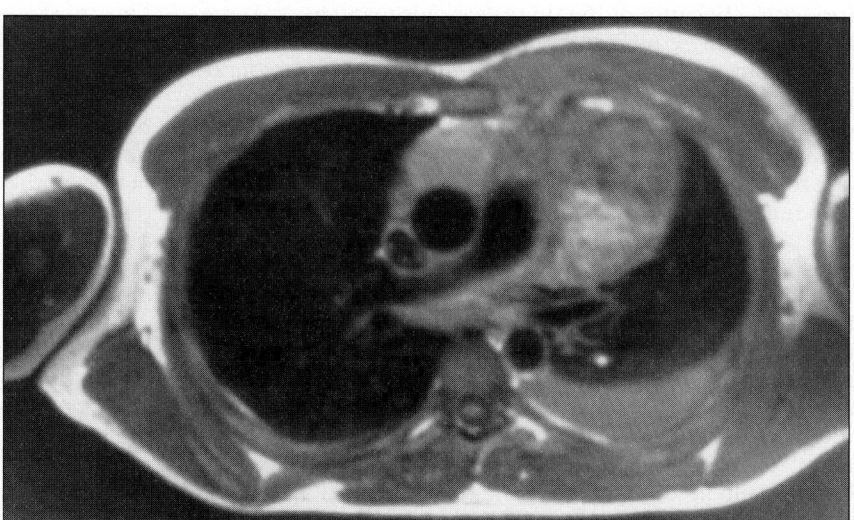

B

include chest radiographs and CT scans of the thorax to gauge the extent and characteristics of mediastinal involvement. Abdominal CT scans can detect the presence of liver metastasis or retroperitoneal disease. A testicular primary tumor should be suspected if significant retroperitoneal disease is found. Elevation of β subunit of human chorionic gonadotropin (HCG) and α-fetoprotein (AFP) suggest the malignant, nonseminomatous nature of these tumors. The incidence of elevated AFP is higher in patients with mediastinal, nonseminomatous germ cell tumors than in those with primary metastatic testicular tumors. Choriocarcinomas can produce both HCG and gynecomastia, which can be seen on initial presentation.[417] Elevation of lactic dehydrogenase is seen in 80% to 90% of patients with either seminomatous or nonseminomatous tumors. Serum markers, when present, are used both to assess response to treatment and to detect early recurrence.[418] Fluorescence in situ hybridization (FISH)

has permitted specific recognition of a genetic marker i(12p) for germ cell tumors.[419] The fluorescent signal at the centromere of the i(12p) is larger than that obtained from a normal chromosome 12 centromere using a probe specific for chromosome 12 centromeric DNA.[419] Presence of the i(12p) or excess 12p copy numbers tend to be associated with complete response to chemotherapy and long-term disease-free survival.[420]

Establishment of a definitive histopathological diagnosis is crucial for the management of these patients. The classic presentation is a young adult with an antero-superior mediastinal mass and a characteristic marker profile. Percutaneous imaging-guided fine-needle aspiration of the anterior mediastinal mass frequently establishes the diagnosis of germ cell neoplasms, but definitive tissue diagnosis is best obtained by parasternal mediastinotomy. If there is considerable risk involved with surgical intervention for diagnosis because of a patient's poor overall condition, and if there is a high index of suspicion with elevated markers, management can be initiated with chemotherapy without a diagnostic biopsy.[403]

Benign Mediastinal Germ Cell Tumors

Benign mediastinal teratomas are treated exclusively with surgical resection, which results in cure; there is no role for adjuvant therapies after surgical resection.[421] Lewis and coworkers[413] reported a series of 69 patients from the Mayo Clinic with benign mediastinal teratoma, of which 64 are long-term survivors. The five remaining patients died either from surgical complications or from unknown causes.

Mediastinal Seminoma

Mediastinal seminomas tend to be slow growing and can reach considerable size with few or no symptoms. Traditionally, the disease was treated with supradiaphragmatic irradiation because of the tumor's radiosensitivity.[422] Large masses might require large fields of irradiation, however, which can cause considerable compromise to surrounding organs. Several trials have thus tested the role of cisplatin-based chemotherapy and have found significant activity and long-term disease control.[403,423,424] Either approach offers the possibility of disease control. Depending on the individual characteristics of the patient and the comorbid diseases, small tumors might be considered for radiation therapy, whereas larger tumors would most likely be best treated with initial cisplatin-based chemotherapy. Surgical excision or management does not appear to play a role in the management of this disease.[403] Whether cisplatin-based chemotherapy or radiation therapy alone followed by chemotherapy at recurrence should be considered as the optimum treatment for mediastinal seminoma is still open to question; both result in comparable long-term survival rates. For patients who have bulky mediastinal disease or extramediastinal involvement, there is substantial evidence that cisplatin-based chemotherapy might be superior.

Mediastinal Nonseminomatous Germ Cell Tumors

Cisplatin-based chemotherapy is the cornerstone of management of mediastinal nonseminomatous germ cell tumors.[425-427] Overall, the prognosis of mediastinal nonseminomatous germ cell tumors is poor compared with that of their testicular counterparts, and they have the worst survival characteristics of all the nonseminomatous germ cell tumors.[428] In an old series from Memorial Sloan Kettering before the advent of cisplatin, only 5% of patients survived beyond 17 months with surgical resection followed by radiation therapy.[407] A French multicenter retrospective study reported a 53% 2-year projected survival rate and a median survival of 28 months for patients with mediastinal nonseminomatous germ cell tumor using cisplatin-based chemotherapy followed by resection of residual tumor, if present.[423] Complete response rates with cisplatin-based therapy have ranged from 50% to 70% in most series, with a long-term survival of approximately 50%.[426,427] Second-line chemotherapy combinations for patients with resistant or recurrent disease generally have yielded poor results.[429,430] These patients should thus be either entered into clinical trials with investigational agents in an effort to identify new active agents in this disease, or they should be treated with high-dose therapy followed by peripheral blood stem cell or autologous bone marrow transplantation.[431] Chemotherapy in general and salvage chemotherapy specifically tend to be less effective for the management of patients with mediastinal germ cell tumors than of patients with their testicular counterparts.[432]

Mediastinal Hodgkin's Disease

Approximately one half of the patients with Hodgkin's disease have mediastinal involvement, usually in the anterior compartment, either as a component of widespread disease or presenting solely as a mediastinal mass. The most common histologic subtype with mediastinal involvement is nodular sclerosis and is seen predominantly among young women.[433] The diagnosis is usually made from biopsy of a cervical lymph node and rarely requires biopsy of the mediastinal mass. The extent of mediastinal and pulmonary involvement can be gauged better with CT scan than with plain chest radiograph (Fig. 76-8A, B, and C).[434] The CT scan is also useful in planning the radiation fields. Approximately 40% of cases also have involvement in the form of hilar adenopathy and lung nodules. Pleural and pericardial effusions, though less common, are known to occur.[435] In cases of bulky mediastinal disease, acute tracheobronchial obstruction can occur during anesthesia.[436] Management of mediastinal Hodgkin's disease is based on the bulk of the tumor and the extent of parenchymal lung involvement.

Pulmonary extension significantly increases the risk of relapse and decreases the overall survival. In a study reported by the Baltimore Cancer Research Center (BCRC), small-volume mediastinal involvement with early-stage (stage I or II) Hodgkin's disease was treated successfully with upper-mantle radiotherapy alone.[437] For those with large mediastinal masses or pulmonary extension, radiotherapy alone was associated with 38% disease-free survival at 10 years, while combined chemotherapy and irradiation resulted in 88% disease-free survival at 10 years.[437] There was also an increased risk of relapse at the margin of the irradiation field when a "shrinking field technique" was used to decrease the incidence of pulmonary complications in patients with large mediastinal masses treated with radiation therapy alone. Although salvage chemotherapy can be useful in patients who fail to achieve a complete response to radiation therapy alone, the results are inferior when compared with combined-modality treatment. Combined-modality therapy was also superior to chemotherapy alone as reported in various studies for patients with large mediastinal masses due to Hodgkin's disease. Currently, therefore, the standard of care for patients with large mediastinal masses is combined chemotherapy and irradiation.

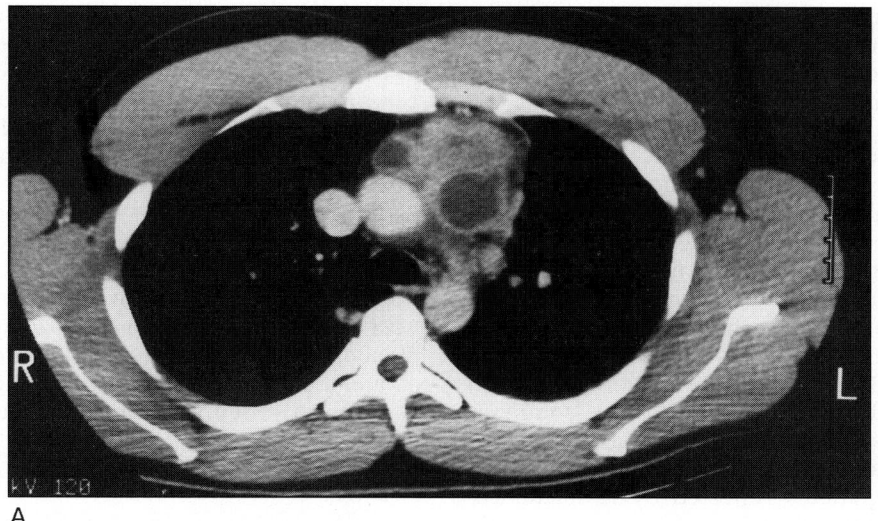

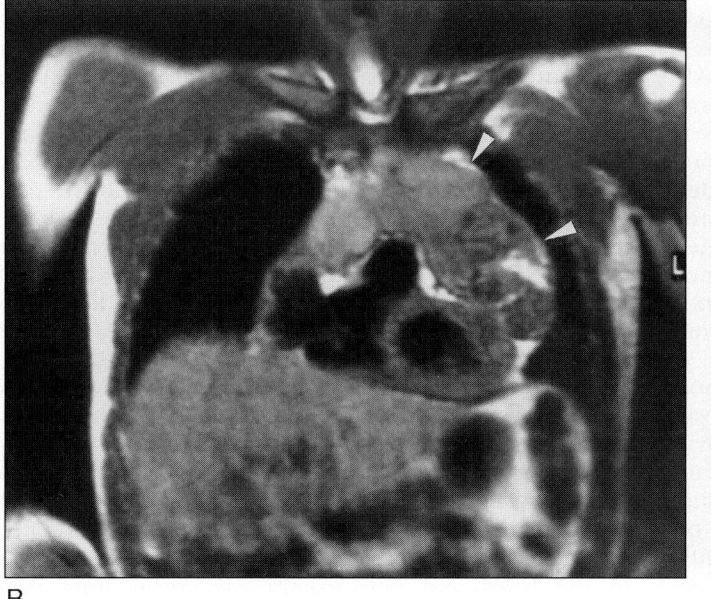

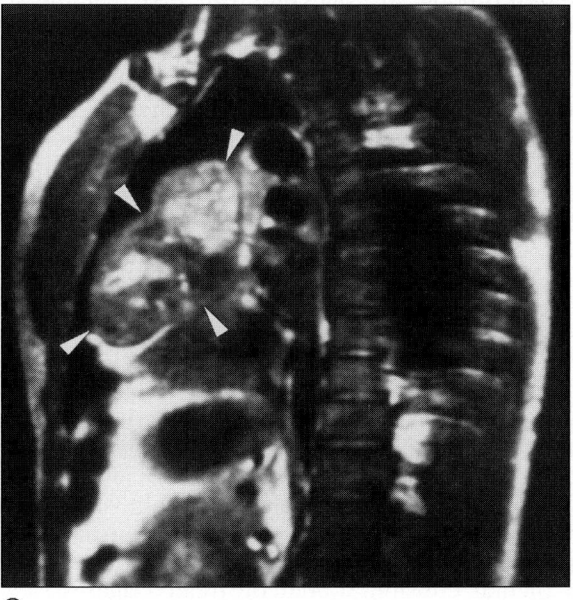

Figure 76-8. Anterior mediastinal mass—Hodgkin's disease. **A,** Enhanced CT image of the chest at the AP window showing a large mixed solid and cystic mass with extension to the left. **B,** Coronal T$_1$-weighted MR image of the chest showing the large mediastinal mass (*arrowheads*) with extension to the left. **C,** Sagittal T$_1$-weighted MR image of the chest showing the large mediastinal mass with areas of mixed signal corresponding to the mixed solid and cystic areas.

Gallium scans, including both CT and PET scans, have been used for detection of viable Hodgkin's disease in the mediastinum after chemotherapy or combined-modality therapy.[438-440] According to the results of a recent study, the value of these studies is limited in predicting disease sterilization, although a few patients have benefited from treatment modification due to abnormal activity seen on these scans.[439,440]

Mediastinal Non–Hodgkin's Lymphoma

Mediastinal non–Hodgkin's lymphomas have a wide clinical spectrum, ranging from nodal involvement as a part of generalized disease to bulky anterior mediastinal mass resulting in symptoms of compression of other structures such as the pericardium, heart, lungs, or great vessels (including the superior vena cava). The most common symptoms of bulky mediastinal disease include chest pain, dyspnea, sternal tenderness, superior vena caval compression syndrome, and pleural or pericardial effusions.[433,441] Constitutional symptoms such as fever, weight loss, and anorexia occur in 50% of patients and are associated with a poorer prognosis than disease without these symptoms.[442] In case of isolated mediastinal involvement, thoracotomy or mediastinotomy could be required for obtaining adequate diagnostic material. Complete staging evaluation is required, as extensive involvement of other organs is seen frequently. The two most common

Specific Malignancies

III

subtypes of non–Hodgkin's lymphoma seen predominantly in the mediastinum include diffuse large cell lymphoma (Category G & H according to the Working Formulation) and lymphoblastic lymphoma (Category I).

Diffuse large cell lymphoma (which includes large cell and immunoblastic lymphoma) can present as an anterior mediastinal mass. Mediastinal presentation is more common among young females, with a median age of about 30 years. The disease is usually bulky and extends from the mediastinum into contiguous structures such as pleura, pericardium, and lung. Pleural and pericardial effusions are known to occur in nearly one third of patients. Bone marrow and central nervous system involvement are usually not seen at presentation. These are predominantly B-cell neoplasms, with the dominant phenotype reported to be CD19+, CD22+, CD37+, CD21-, CD30-, CD10-, CD5-, and immunoglobulin negative.[443] In a large series of 57 patients reported by Kirn and co-workers,[444] 60% had large cell and 40% had immunoblastic histology. Among the patients who had lymphoma-cell immunophenotyping performed, 80% were found to have tumors of the B-cell type. Varying amounts of sclerosis were seen in the biopsy specimens of all patients. All patients received combination chemotherapy consisting of one of the following: CHOP (cyclophosphamide, doxorubicin, vincristine, and prednisone), M-BACOD (methotrexate, bleomycin, doxorubicin, cyclophosphamide, vincristine, and dexamethasone), MACOP-B (methotrexate, adriamycin, cyclophosphamide, vincristine, prednisone, and bleomycin), or C-MOPP (cyclophosphamide, vincristine, procarbazine, and prednisone). Among the 50 patients analyzed for relapse, 20 received subsequent radiation therapy. The overall 5-year survival was 50%, with a freedom from relapse of 45% at 5 years. The poor prognostic factors that predicted decreased survival included presence of pleural effusion, involvement of two or more extranodal sites, and a positive post-treatment gallium 67 scan. Most relapses were found to occur during the first 15 months. Bulk disease was not a predictor of relapse in the absence of pleural effusion. Thus patients with pleural effusion should be treated aggressively or should be considered for high-dose chemotherapy plus peripheral blood stems cell or autologous bone marrow transplantation because of their increased risk of relapse. The role of radiation therapy is controversial for patients with residual masses after chemotherapy, although a small subset might benefit from its use.

Lymphoblastic lymphoma is a distinct entity presenting as an anterior mediastinal mass in older children and young adults. It is predominantly seen in males and has a clinical and immunologic similarity to acute lymphoblastic leukemia. The cell of origin is the T cell or middle or late thymocyte in most of the cases, but rarely, it is of the pre-B cell or null cell types. Immunophenotyping reveals E rosette+, T6+, T4+, T8+, T1+, and T3+. On histopathology examination, cells have convoluted or nonconvoluted nuclei with fine chromatin without nucleoli. The histology-stained section gives a starry sky appearance. Staining with terminal deoxynucleotidyl transferase (TdT) is usually positive. Clinically, these cases present as a thymic mass with paracortical involvement of the thymus-dependent lymph nodes. There is a high incidence of meningeal spread and involvement of the bone marrow, peripheral blood, and testes. Cells obtained from cerebrospinal fluid should be stained with TdT.[445]

The management of lymphoblastic lymphoma is essentially similar to that of acute lymphoblastic leukemia. The response to chemotherapy is usually rapid.[446,447] Earlier regimens, such as CHOP, produced low complete remission rates and substantially fewer survivors.[448] Intrathecal therapy with or without craniospinal irradiation is applied early in the treatment course to prevent CNS relapse.[447-449] There is no evidence that radiotherapy in addition to chemotherapy improves survival, but it should be initiated if the patient is in severe distress and objective improvement is not seen quickly with chemotherapy.

TUMORS OF THE MIDDLE MEDIASTINUM

Malignant tumors of the heart and pericardium are rare entities. Approximately 75% of all cardiac tumors are benign, and more than half of these are myxomas (Fig. 76-9). Other malignant tumors and cysts of the heart and pericardium include angiosarcoma, rhabdomyosarcoma, mesothelioma, fibrosarcoma, lymphoma, extraskeletal osteosarcoma, neurogenic sarcoma, malignant teratoma, thymoma, leiomyosarcoma, liposarcoma, and synovial cell sarcoma.[450] In a recently reported series by Chen and coworkers,[451] 79 patients with cardiac tumors were seen at the Shanghai Institute from 1957 to 1988. Of these, 49 patients had benign and 30 had malignant tumors. All except two of the benign tumors were myxomas, and 86% of these were located in the left atrium. Among the 30 malignant tumors, 15 were secondary metastases, 3 were lymphomas, 2 were mesotheliomas, 2 were malignant myxoma, 1 was angiosarcoma, 1 was rhabdomyosarcoma, 1 was leiomyosarcoma, 1 was fibrosarcoma, and 4 were undiagnosed. Metastatic tumors to the heart and pericardium can result from direct extension from the mediastinal lymph nodes or by hematogenous dissemination of tumor. Metastatic renal cell carcinoma has been demonstrated to grow into the right atrium from the vena cava without myocardial infiltration, and occasionally, such tumors have been surgically resected.[452] The manifestations of cardiac and pericardial tumors are varied and depend on mass effect, local invasion, embolization, and systemic constitutional symptoms.[453] Pericardial involvement can result in severe substernal chest pain due to pericarditis with frequent effusion or tamponade (Fig. 76-10). Other manifestations include congestive heart failure, pulmonary hypertension, and dysrhythmias. Diagnostic procedures include echocardiography and CT of the chest in addition to chest radiographs and electrocardiograms.[453] CT with contrast can detect the intracavitary filling defect and its relationship to cardiac chambers and invasion. More recently, MRI has been used to localize intracardiac tumors, to assess their vascularity, and to distinguish them from cardiac metastasis.[454] Cardiac catheterization is able to detect

Figure 76-9. Middle mediastinal mass—Left atrial myxoma. Enhanced CT image through the heart showing a left atrial defect (*arrowheads*) with lower attenuation than the surrounding contrast-filled atria and ventricles.

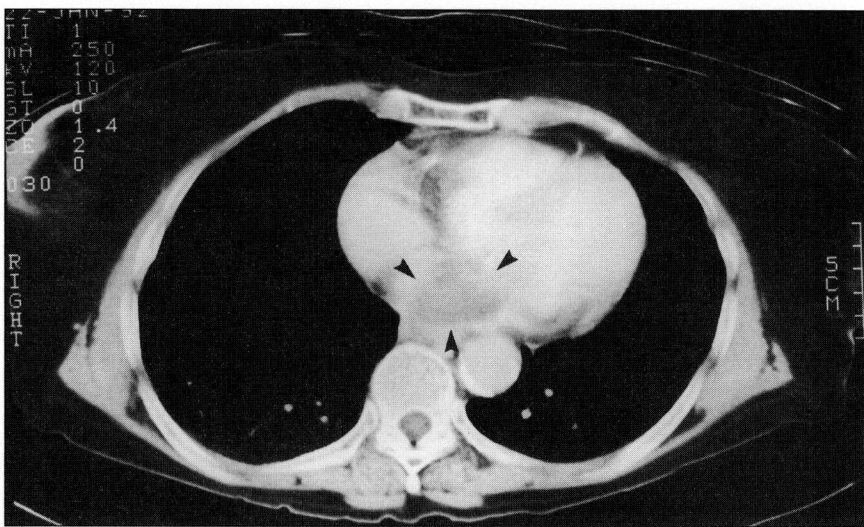

mass effects resulting in compression or deformity of various chambers, intracavitary filling defects, myocardial motion abnormalities, or pericardial effusion. Angiosarcoma and rhabdomyosarcoma are the two most common malignant cardiac tumors.[450,455,456] Microscopically, angiosarcomas contain foci of solid areas and spindle cells forming vascular channels while rhabdomyosarcomas contain rhabdomyoblasts, but in both types of tumors, there can be high degrees of anaplasia and pleomorphism with necrosis and hemorrhage. Most patients with malignant cardiac tumors survive less than a year from diagnosis. Local excision of intracardiac tumors might occasionally be successful, but usually the patients are left with residual disease.[457] Radiation and chemotherapy have been tried but are of limited value in these cases.

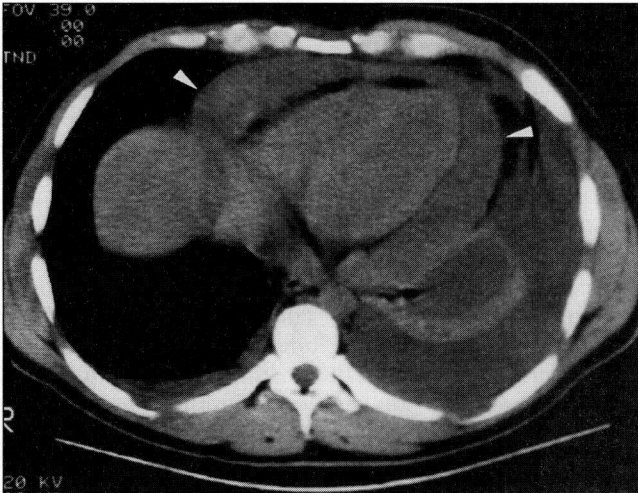

Figure 76-10. Middle mediastinal mass—Malignant pericardial effusion. Enhanced CT image showing a large pericardial effusion (*arrowheads*) and bilateral pleural effusions L > R. The collapsed left lower lobe is seen extending into the effusion at the left base.

Cardiac transplantation might result in improved survival in patients with inoperable cardiac tumors, but definitive data are lacking.

Malignant Mesothelioma of the Pericardium

Malignant mesothelioma originating on the pericardium is an exceptionally rare tumor; just over 100 cases (including children) have been reported in the literature.[458] Because of the rarity and age distribution of these tumors, asbestos exposure has not been associated in most of the reported cases. The clinical presentation can include mediastinal mass, pericardial effusion, congestive heart failure, or tamponade.[458-461] Diffuse involvement of the pericardium with invasion of myocardium and mediastinal structures is seen frequently. The diagnosis of this tumor is rarely made or suspected before surgery or autopsy.[462-464] Surgical excision is rarely complete, and most cases rapidly become fatal. The role of radiotherapy or chemotherapy is not known.

POSTERIOR MEDIASTINAL TUMORS

Malignant Neural Crest Neoplasms

The overall incidence of tumors arising from the neural crest is low, but they are the most common tumors found within the posterior mediastinum (Fig. 76-11).[465] The neurogenic tumors encompass a wide and complex spectrum of neoplasms that occur in both children and adults. These tumors can range in their usual clinical behavior from benign (schwannoma) to highly aggressive (neuroblastoma). They are frequently solitary and asymptomatic but can cause constitutional symptoms such as cough, dyspnea, and pain with tumor enlargement. Children are more likely than adults to present with malignant disease with metastasis. Mediastinal tumors

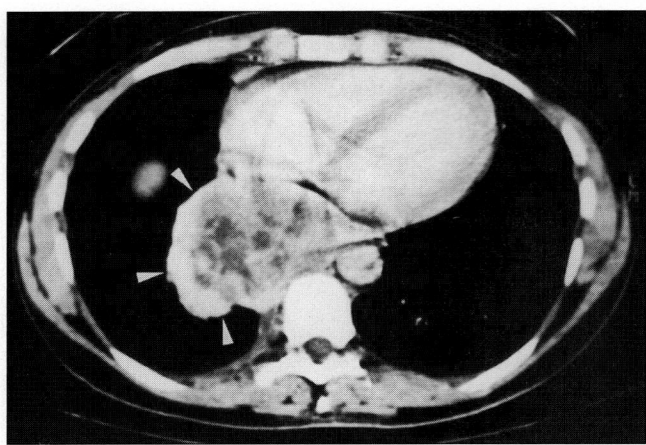

Figure 76-11. Posterior and middle mediastinal mass—Neurogenic tumor. Enhanced CT image of the lower chest just above the level of the diaphragm showing a large mass (*arrowheads*) in the posterior mediastinum extending to the middle mediastinum with variable CT attenuation. Comparison with prior unenhanced CT image showed a strong enhancement of the mass.

of the neural crest can be divided into two groups. One group of tumors arises from the neuronal cells, which include the nerve ganglion cells (ganglioneuroblastoma and ganglioneuroma) and the neuroendocrine cells (e.g., pheochromocytoma, paraganglioma). The second group arises from the neural sheath cells or the Schwann cells and includes schwannoma and neurofibroma.

Peripheral Primitive Neuroectodermal Tumor (Peripheral Neuroepithelioma, Askin Tumor, Extraosseous Ewing's Sarcoma)

Peripheral primitive neuroectodermal tumor (PNET) of the thorax can present either as a pleural-based mass or as a paraspinal posterior mediastinal mass. The clinical picture varies depending on the presence or absence of pleural effusion, rib destruction, or epidural spinal cord compression.[466] High fevers with other constitutional symptoms are usual accompaniments. These tumors usually occur in children or young adults and occur equally in males and females.[467] Histologically, these tumors are lobulated and have small, blue round cells with occasional rosettes. Electron microscopy reveals dense, neurosecretory granules and neurofilaments. The cells stain strongly for the antibody O-13, demonstrating membranous positivity.[468] PNETs might also stain for neuron-specific enolase, synaptophysin, and Leu-7. They demonstrate high levels of choline-acetyl transferase but are devoid of catecholamine enzymes seen in neuroblastomas, such as dopamine decarboxylase and tyrosine hydroxylase.[466,469] Cytogenetically, PNETs demonstrate a consistent pattern of chromosomal translocation: rcp (11;22) (q24;q12).[470] Whether the altered regulation of synthesis of the proteins encoded by the cellular proto-oncogenes at the site of chromosomal translocations

contribute to malignant transformation is not entirely clear.[471] Fluorescence in situ hybridization (FISH) probes directed at the EWS gene rearrangement can now be performed with accuracy on fixed and paraffin-embedded tissue.[472] In the past, a multimodality approach was used for the management of PNETs, but the median survival was only about 8 months despite the aggressive therapies. Radiotherapy (45–55 Gy) could produce shrinkage, but local recurrence was common. Metastases to the lung, bone, and bone marrow occurred with regularity.[473] Chemotherapy combinations of cyclophosphamide, doxorubicin, and vincristine (CAV) or CAV with actinomycin-D were used with some success, both as neoadjuvant therapy prior to local radiation therapy and wide surgical excision and to treat advanced metastatic disease.[466,474] High-dose chemotherapy with total body irradiation and autologous bone marrow transplantation was also attempted.[475] Recently, the combination of etoposide and cisplatin has shown somewhat better success in the treatment of this tumor, although large masses are still likely to recur and could require radiotherapy as part of combined modality therapy.[476]

Neuroblastoma, Ganglioneuroblastoma, and Ganglioneuroma

Neuroblastoma, ganglioneuroblastoma, and ganglioneuroma occur in children, although there are rare reports of these tumors arising in adults.[477–479] These tumors differ from each other only in terms of their degree of differentiation, with neuroblastoma being a high-grade, undifferentiated neoplasm and ganglioneuroma being a benign tumor possessing mature ganglion cells. Occasionally, these tumors present as masses in the posterior mediastinum rather than in their usual abdominal or widely disseminated presentation. When present in the thorax, these tumors are reported to have a better prognosis, possibly because of early detection due to the occurrence of symptoms.

Neuroblastoma

Neuroblastoma is the most frequent cause of mediastinal neurogenic mass in children and is a highly aggressive tumor thought to arise from primitive neural crest-derived cells called neuroblasts.[480,481] A thoracic presentation accounts for 15% of all cases of neuroblastoma, although it is seen predominantly in the very young. More than half of the patients with mediastinal presentation already have disseminated disease.[482] The most common sites of metastatic involvement include lymph nodes, bone, liver, and subcutaneous tissues. The signs and symptoms depend on the site of dissemination. Mediastinal neuroblastoma usually occurs in the posterior compartment and is usually seen as an incidental finding on a chest radiograph obtained for other reasons. Occasionally, patients can present with cough, dyspnea, malaise, and spinal cord compression. Bone marrow involvement is common. The presence of the opsoclonus polymyoclonus syndrome—characterized by acute cerebellar and truncal ataxia and dancing eyes—could indicate a favorable prognosis. Amplification of n-myc has been seen in neuroblastoma and is associated with early disseminated disease.[483,484] DNA content assessed by flow cytomety can also be clinically useful as a predictor of response in unresectable disease.[484] A number of specific genetic changes, including a deletion in the short arm of chromosome 1 (1p-) and abnormalities in chromosome 17, have marked neuroblastoma as a paradigm for the study of molecular changes and cancer.[485] Therapy usually consists of a multidisciplinary approach, with surgery for localized disease and chemotherapy being the mainstay of treatment for those with disseminated disease.

Pheochromocytoma

Pheochromocytoma is a tumor of the autonomic nervous system. It is a form of paraganglioma that both secretes and stores catecholamines. Extra-adrenal presentations are unusual, but the posterior mediastinum is the usual site of occurrence of intrathoracic pheochromocytoma. Pheochromocytomas have also been reported to occur in the middle mediastinum, with involvement of the cardiac atria and arch of the aorta.[486] The vast majority of all mediastinal pheochromocytomas are clinically benign but share histological similarities with their malignant counterparts.[487] Nuclear atypia and pleomorphism are the hallmarks of both benign and malignant tumors. Membrane-bound dense core neurosecretory granules (150–250 nm) are seen routinely with electron microscopy.[488] On immunohistochemical analysis, pheochromocytomas demonstrate neuron-specific enolase, chromagranin, synaptophysin, and corticotropin-like reactivity.[487,489,490] Metastatic disease is the only reliable benchmark for defining malignancy.[491] The malignant forms can also be locally aggressive and can metastasize to bone, lymph nodes, liver, lung, and brain. Clinically, patients with pheochromocytomas present with symptoms of catecholamine excess such as persistent hypertension, palpitation, headache, perspiration, orthostasis, chest pain, and constitutional symptoms.[492] Occasionally, cardiomyopathy can result from catecholamine excess. In addition to the usual diagnostic tests for mediastinal tumors, specific studies include measurement of urine and plasma catecholamines ^{131}I-MIBG [I-[131]-meta-iodobenzylguanidine], scintigraphy, and pharmacologic tests using provocative agents such as glucagon, tyramine histamine, or suppressive agents (e.g., phentolamine and clonidine).[493]

Pheochromocytomas are managed with surgical resection, which can result in cure in some cases. Pharmacologic adrenal blockage preoperatively is achieved with phenoxybenzamine and subsequent beta-adrenergic blockade with propranolol, while short-acting phentolamine is reserved for management if hypertension arises. α-methyl tyrosine is also used sometimes to decrease catecholamine synthesis. The 5-year survival of malignant mediastinal pheochromocytomas approaches 50%. The role of radiotherapy after surgical resection of malignant forms is not clear, although these tumors are relatively sensitive to radiation.[492] A number of chemotherapeutic agents have been tried for malignant pheochromocytoma with limited success; these include cyclophosphamide, vincristine, doxorubicin, dacarbazine, methotrexate, and streptozotocin.[494-496] Conceptually, ^{131}I MIBG with high specific activity could have a therapeutic role in the management of malignant pheochromocytomas.[493,497]

Schwannomas and Neurofibromas

Schwannomas and neurofibromas derive from neural sheath cells. Together, they form a group with the highest incidence among all mediastinal tumors in adults and are the most common tumors seen in association with Von Recklinghausen's disease.[498,499]

Schwannoma (Neurilemmoma) and Malignant Schwannoma

Schwannoma (neurilemmoma) is a benign, encapsulated nerve sheath tumor that is usually solitary except when seen in association with neurofibromatosis (NF-1).[500] Schwannomas arise from Schwann cells of the cranial, spinal, or peripheral nerves.[498] The lung and heart are other sites of intrathoracic involvement.[501,502] Schwannomas tend to be slow-growing tumors, usually in the right side of the upper posterior mediastinum, and they rarely extend into the intervertebral foramina. Clinically, they usually do not cause any symptoms until, in rare cases, there is involvement of the vagus or phrenic nerve. On histopathologic exam, these tumors demonstrate an alternating pattern of palisading spindle cells (Antoni A) and loose myxoid hypocellular areas with scattered spindle cells (Antoni B). Immunohistochemistry demonstrates strong S-100 positivity.[503] They can be treated with simple surgical resection without sacrificing neural structures.[504]

Malignant schwannomas or malignant peripheral nerve sheath tumors (MPNST) are aggressive spindle cell neoplasms most commonly arising from nerve trunks in the posterior mediastinum or in the vagus or other peripheral nerves. They rarely result from malignant transformation of their benign counterpart but can arise from either degeneration of neurofibroma in neurofibromatosis (NF-1) or within the field of prior radiation therapy.[505,506] On histologic examination, these malignant tumors demonstrate a variably cellular spindle cell and myxoid neoplasm. Mitotic figures are easily seen. Occasionally, mesenchymal elements such as fat, cartilage, bone, and muscle are seen in malignant schwannomas.[507,508] MRI and pathologic correlation showed that a non-homogeneous, high-intensity appearance of schwannomas on T$_2$-weighted images corresponded to alternating Antoni A and Antoni B areas, while a central, very high-intensity region was noted in areas of cystic degeneration.[508] Immunohistochemical studies show S-100 variable positivity.[509] Clinically, in addition to symptoms due to mass effect, patients can present with pain and constitutional symptoms such as fatigue, weight loss, anorexia, and occasionally fever. The tumor advances locally, invading nearby structures such as the heart, great vessels, and vertebral bodies, and it can extend into the intervertebral foramina. Lung, liver, bone, skin, and serous surfaces are common sites of metastases. Surgical resection is the primary treatment.[510] The role of adjuvant

Specific Malignancies

III

radiation therapy is not well defined. This family of malignant tumors tends to be very resistant to chemotherapy, although some anecdotal responses have been seen with novantrone plus vinblastine and the combination of cyclophosphamide, ifosfamide, doxorubicin, dacarbazine, and vincristine.[511,512]

Neurofibromas

Neurofibromas are also considered to originate from the Schwann cell and, like schwannomas, they are usually solitary masses except when seen in association with neurofibromatosis (NF-1), tuberous sclerosis, Sturg-Weber syndrome, or Von Hippel-Lindau disease.[513,514] They are slow-growing, benign tumors and can arise from any nerve. Clinically, they are usually asymptomatic until there is interspinal extension, resulting in signs of epidural cord compression. On histologic examination, the solitary forms are unencapsulated and consist of elongated wavy spindle cells separated by collagen and mucoid material. The plexiform variety, seen in patients with NF-1, involves expanded nerve trunks in a neurofibromatous background. Malignant transformation has been reported and is a serious complication of this disease.[498,515] On T_2-weighted magnetic resonance imaging, high-intensity regions in the periphery of neurofibromas correspond to myxoid degeneration, and curvalinear or nodular areas of low signal intensity correspond to collagenous fibrous tissue. On immunohistochemistry, neurofibromas show S-100 reactivity and demonstrate the presence of cholinesterase. Surgical resection is the treatment of choice.

REFERENCES

1. England DM, Hochholzer L, McCarthy MJ: Localized benign and malignant fibrous tumors of the pleura. A clinicopathologic review of 223 cases. Am J Surg Pathol 1989;13(8):640–658.
2. Antman K, Cohen S, Dimitrov NV, et al: Malignant mesothelioma of the tunica vaginalis testis. J Clin Oncol 1984;2(5):447–451.
3. de Klerk DP, Nime F: Adenomatoid tumors (mesothelioma) of testicular and paratesticular tissue. Urology 1975;6(5):635–641.
4. Fenoglio JJ Jr, Jacobs DW, McAllister HA Jr: Ultrastructure of the mesothelioma of the atrioventricular node. Cancer 1977;40(2):721–727.
5. Scully RE, Mark EJ, McNeely WF, et al: Case records of the Massachusetts General Hospital. Weekly clinicopathological exercises. Case 20-1997. A 74-year-old man with progressive cough, dyspnea, and pleural thickening. N Engl J Med 1997;336(26):1895–1903.
6. Balassiano M, Reichert N, Rosenman Y, et al: Localized fibrous mesothelioma of the mediastinum devoid of pleural connections. Postgrad Med J 1989;65(768):788–790.
7. Kottke-Marchant K, Hart WR, Broughan T: Localized fibrous tumor (localized fibrous mesothelioma) of the liver. Cancer 1989;64(5):1096–1102.
8. Simpson PR: Adenomatoid tumor of the adrenal gland. Arch Pathol Lab Med 1990;114(7):725–727.
9. Legha SS, Muggia FM: Pleural mesothelioma: Clinical features and therapeutic implications. Ann Intern Med 1977;87(5):613–621.
10. Briselli M, Mark EJ, Dickersin GR: Solitary fibrous tumors of the pleura: Eight new cases and review of 360 cases in the literature. Cancer 1981;47(11):2678–2689.
11. Dalton WT, Zolliker AS, McCaughey WT, et al: Localized primary tumors of the pleura: An analysis of 40 cases. Cancer 1979;44(4):1465–1475.
12. Scharifker D, Kaneko M: Localized fibrous "mesothelioma" of pleura (submesothelial fibroma): A clinicopathologic study of 18 cases. Cancer 1979;43(2):627–635.
13. Majoulet JF, Millant P, Bouillet P, et al: Radiologic aspect of benign pleural fibrous mesothelioma. Reports of 4 cases. Ann Radiol 1990;33(4–5):229–236.
14. Pooley FD: Mineralogy of asbestos: The physical and chemical properties of the dusts they form. Semin Oncol 1981;8(3):243–249.
15. Craighead JE, Mossman BT: The pathogenesis of asbestos-associated diseases. N Engl J Med 1982;306(24):1446–1455.
16. McDonald JC, Armstrong B, Case B, et al: Mesothelioma and asbestos fiber type. Evidence from lung tissue analyses. Cancer 1989;63(8):1544–1547.
17. Churg A, Wright JL: Fibre content of lung in amphibole- and chrysotile-induced mesothelioma: Implications for environmental exposure. IARC Sci Publ 1989;(90):314–318.
18. Gibbs AR, Griffiths DM, Pooley FD, et al: Comparison of fibre types and size distributions in lung tissues of paraoccupational and occupational cases of malignant mesothelioma. Br J Ind Med 1990;47(9):621–626.
19. Rogers AJ, Leigh J, Berry G, et al: Relationship between lung asbestos fiber type and concentration and relative risk of mesothelioma. A case-control study. Cancer 1991;67(7):1912–1920.
20. Antman KH, Corson JM, Li FP, et al: Malignant mesothelioma following radiation exposure. J Clin Oncol 1983;1(11):695–700.
21. Antman KH, Pomfret EA, Aisner J, et al: Peritoneal mesothelioma: Natural history and response to chemotherapy. J Clin Oncol 1983;1(6):386–391.
22. Horie A, Hiraoka K, Yamamoto O, et al: An autopsy case of peritoneal malignant mesothelioma in a radiation technologist. Acta Pathol Jpn 1990;40(1):57–62.
23. Jagirdar J, Frydman C, Sakurai H, et al: Mesothelial papillary proliferation of the pleura associated with radiation therapy: Does it have a role in the pathogenesis of mesothelioma? Mt Sinai J Med 1989;56(2):147–149.
24. Kawashima A, Libshitz HI, Lukeman JM: Radiation-induced malignant pleural mesothelioma. Can Assoc Radiol J 1990;41(6):384–386.
25. Lerman Y, Learman Y, Schachter P, et al: Radiation associated malignant pleural mesothelioma. Thorax 1991;46(6):463–464.
26. Dahlgren S: Effects of locally deposited colloidal thorium dioxide. Ann N Y Acad Sci 1967;145(3):786–790.
27. Maurer R, Egloff B: Malignant peritoneal mesothelioma after cholangiography with thorotrast. Cancer 1975;36(4):1381–1385.
28. Artvinli M, Baris YI: Malignant mesotheliomas in a small village in the Anatolian region of Turkey: An epidemiologic study. J Natl Cancer Inst 1979;63(1):17–22.
29. Rohl AN, Langer AM, Moncure G, et al: Endemic pleural disease associated with exposure to mixed fibrous dust in Turkey. Science 1982;216(4545):518–520.
30. Suzuki Y, Kohyama N: Malignant mesothelioma induced by asbestos and zeolite in the mouse peritoneal cavity. Environ Res 1984;35(1):277–292.
31. Gardner MJ, Saracci R: Effects on health of non-occupational exposure to airborne mineral fibres. IARC Sci Publ 1989;90:375–397.
32. Vogelzang NJ, Schultz SM, Iannucci AM, et al: Malignant mesothelioma. The University of Minnesota experience. Cancer 1984;53(3):377–383.
33. Rom WN, Travis WD, Brody AR: Cellular and molecular basis of the asbestos-related diseases. Am Rev Respir Dis 1991;143(2):408–422.
34. Carbone M, Kratzke RA, Testa JR: The pathogenesis of mesothelioma. Semin Oncol 2002;29:2–17.
35. Cicala C, Pompetti F, Carbone M: SV-40 induces mesotheliomas in hamsters. Am J Pathol 1993;142:1524–1533.
36. Carbone M, Pass HI, Rizzo P, et al: Simian virus like DNA sequences in human pleural mesotheliomas. Oncogene 1994;9:1781–1790.
37. Testa JR, Carbone M, Hirvonen A, et al: A multiinstitutional study confirms the presence and expression of simian virus 40 in human malignant mesotheliomas. Cancer Res 1998;58:4505–4509.

38. Jasani, B, Cristaudo A, Emri S, et al: Association of SV40 with human tumors. Semin Cancer Biol 2001;11:43-61.

39. Klein G, Powers A, Croce CM: Association of SV40 with human tumors. Oncogene 2002;21:1141-1149.

40. Kops SP: Oral polio vaccine and human cancer: A reassessment of SV40 based on legal documents. Anticancer Res 2000;20:4745-4750.

41. Enterline PE, Henderson VL: Geographic patterns for pleural mesothelioma deaths in the United States, 1968-81. J Natl Cancer Inst 1987;79(1):31-37.

42. Walker AM, Loughlin JE, Friedlander ER, et al: Projections of asbestos-related disease 1980-2009. J Occup Med 1983;25(5):409-425.

43. Wagner JC, Sleggs EA, Marchand P: Diffuse pleural mesothelioma and asbestos in the North Western Cape Province. Br J Ind Med 1960;17:260.

44. Selikoff IJ, Churg J, Hammond EC: Asbestos exposure and neoplasia. JAMA 1964;188:142.

45. Fowler DP: Exposures to asbestos arising from bandsawing gasket material. Appl Occup Environ Hyg 2000;15(5):404-408.

46. Newhouse ML, Thompson H: Mesothelioma of pleura and peritoneum following exposure to asbestos in the London area. Br J Ind Med 1965;22(4):261-269.

47. Connelly RR, Spirtas R, Myers MH, et al: Demographic patterns for mesothelioma in the United States. J Natl Cancer Inst 1987;78(6):1053-1060.

48. Spirtas R, Beebe GW, Connelly RR, et al: Recent trends in mesothelioma incidence in the United States. Am J Ind Med 1986;9(5):397-407.

49. Li FP, Lokich J, Lapey J, et al: Familial mesothelioma after intense asbestos exposure at home. JAMA 1978;240(5):467.

50. Anderson HA, Lilis R, Daum SM, et al: Household-contact asbestos neoplastic risk. Ann N Y Acad Sci 1976;271:311-323.

51. Risberg B, Nickels J, Wagermark J: Familial clustering of malignant mesothelioma. Cancer 1980;45(9):2422-2427.

52. Vianna NJ, Polan AK: Non-occupational exposure to asbestos and malignant mesothelioma in females. Lancet 1978;1(8073):1061-1063.

53. Antman KH: Clinical presentation and natural history of benign and malignant mesothelioma. Semin Oncol 1981;8(3):313-320.

54. De Pangher Manzini V, Brollo A, Bianchi C: Thrombocytosis in malignant pleural mesothelioma. Tumori 1990;76(6):576-578.

55. Wojtukiewicz MZ, Zacharski LR, Memoli VA, et al: Absence of components of coagulation and fibrinolysis pathways in situ in mesothelioma. Thromb Res 1989;55(2):279-284.

56. Antman K, Shemin R, Ryan L, et al: Malignant mesothelioma: Prognostic variables in a registry of 180 patients, the Dana-Farber Cancer Institute and Brigham and Women's Hospital experience over two decades, 1965-1985. J Clin Oncol 1988;6(1):147-153.

57. Chahinian AP, Pajak TF, Holland JF, et al: Diffuse malignant mesothelioma. Prospective evaluation of 69 patients. Ann Intern Med 1982;96(6 Pt 1):746-755.

58. Ruffie P, Feld R, Minkin S, et al: Diffuse malignant mesothelioma of the pleura in Ontario and Quebec: A retrospective study of 332 patients. J Clin Oncol 1989;7(8):1157-1168.

59. Schildge J, Kaiser D, Henss H, et al: Prognostic factors in diffuse malignant mesothelioma of the pleura. Pneumologie 1989;43(11):660-664.

60. Antman KH: Current concepts: Malignant mesothelioma. N Engl J Med 1980;303(4):200-202.

61. Grant DC, Seltzer SE, Antman KH, et al: Computed tomography of malignant pleural mesothelioma. J Comput Assist Tomogr 1983;7(4):626-632.

62. Alexander E, Clark RA, Colley DP, et al: CT of malignant pleural mesothelioma. AJR Am J Roentgenol 1981;137(2):287-291.

63. Kreel L: Computed tomography in mesothelioma. Semin Oncol 1981;8(3):302-312.

64. Mirvis S, Dutcher JP, Haney PJ, et al: CT of malignant pleural mesothelioma. AJR Am J Roentgenol 1983;140(4):665-670.

65. Leung AN, Muller NL, Miller RR: CT in differential diagnosis of diffuse pleural disease. Am J Roentgenol 1990;154(3):487-492.

66. Marom EM, Erasmus JJ, Pass HI, et al: The role of diagnostic imaging in malignant pleural mesothelioma. Semin Oncol 2002;29:26-35.

67. Elmes PC, Simpson JC: The clinical aspects of mesothelioma. Q J Med 1976;45(179):427-449.

68. Gordon W Jr, Antman KH, Greenberger JS, et al: Radiation therapy in the management of patients with mesothelioma. Int J Radiat Oncol Biol Phys 1982;8(1):19-25.

69. Boutin C, Viallat JR, Van Zandwijk N, et al: Activity of intrapleural recombinant gamma-interferon in malignant mesothelioma. Cancer 1991;67(8):2033-2037.

70. Boutin C, Rey F: Thoracoscopy in pleural malignant mesothelioma: A prospective study of 188 consecutive patients. Part 1: Diagnosis. Cancer 1993;72(2):389-393.

71. Geroulanos S, Lampe P, Hafner F, et al: Malignant pleural mesothelioma: diagnosis, therapy and prognosis. Schweiz Rundsch Med Prax 1990;79(12):361-367.

72. Churg A: Fiber counting and analysis in the diagnosis of asbestos-related disease. Hum Pathol 1982;13(4):381-392.

73. Hillerdal G: Malignant mesothelioma 1982: Review of 4710 published cases. Br J Dis Chest 1983;77:321-343.

74. Kannerstein M, Churg J, Magner D: Histochemistry in the diagnosis of malignant mesothelioma. Ann Clin Lab Sci 1973;3(3):207-211.

75. Kannerstein M, McCaughey WT, Churg J, et al: A critique of the criteria for the diagnosis of diffuse malignant mesothelioma. Mt Sinai J Med 1977;44(4):485-494.

76. Bolen JW, Thorning D: Mesotheliomas: A light- and electron-microscopical study concerning histogenetic relationships between the epithelial and the mesenchymal variants. Am J Surg Pathol 1980;4(5):451-464.

77. Corson J, Pinkus GS: Cellular localization patterns of keratin proteins in pleural mesothelioma and metastatic adenocarcinomas a diagnostic discriminant. Lab Invest 1991;64:114A.

78. Corson JM, Pinkus GS: Mesothelioma: profile of keratin proteins and carcinoembryonic antigen: An immunoperoxidase study of 20 cases and comparison with pulmonary adenocarcinomas. Am J Pathol 1982;108(1):80-87.

79. Said JW, Nash G, Lee M: Immunoperoxidase localization of keratin proteins, carcinoembryonic antigen, and factor VIII in adenomatoid tumors: Evidence for a mesothelial derivation. Hum Pathol 1982;13(12):1106-1108.

80. Said JW, Nash G, Tepper G, et al: Keratin proteins and carcinoembryonic antigen in lung carcinoma: An immunoperoxidase study of fifty-four cases, with ultrastructural correlations. Hum Pathol 1983;14(1):70-76.

81. Schlegel R, Banks-Schlegel S, McLeod JA, et al: Immunoperoxidase localization of keratin in human neoplasms: A preliminary survey. Am J Pathol 1980;101(1):41-50.

82. Ordonez NG: Value of calretinin immunostaining in differentiating epithelial mesothelioma from lung adenocarcinoma. Mod Pathol 1998;11(10):929-933.

83. Bedrossian CMW, Bonsib S, Moran CA: Differntial diagnosis between mesothlioma and adenocarcinoma: A multimodal appraoch based on ultrastructure and immunohistochemistry. Semin Diagnos Pathol 1992;9:124-135.

84. Ordonez NG, Mackay B: The role of immunohistochemistry and electron microscopy in distinguishing epithelial mesothelioma of pleura from adenocarcinoma. Adv Anat Pathol 1996;5:273-282.

85. Suzuki Y, Kannerstein M: Ultrastructure of human malignant diffuse mesothelioma. Am J Pathol 1976;85(2):241-262.

86. Butchart EG, Ashcroft T, Barnsley WC, et al: Pleuropneumonectomy in the management of diffuse malignant mesothelioma of the pleura. Experience with 29 patients. Thorax 1976;31(1):15-24.

87. Sugarbaker DJ, Flores RM, Jaklitsch MT, et al: Resection margins, extrapleural nodal status, and cell type determine postoperative long-term survival in trimodality therapy of malignant pleural mesothelioma: Results in 183 patients. J Thorac Cardiovasc Surg 1999;117(1):54-63; discussion 63-65.

88. Rusch VW: A proposed new international TNM staging system for malignant pleural mesothelioma. From the International Mesothelioma Interest Group. Chest 1995;108(4):1122-1128.

89. Wechsler RJ, Rao VM, Steiner RM: The radiology of thoracic malignant mesothelioma. Crit Rev Diagn Imaging 1984;20:283-310.

90. Heelan RT, Rusch VW, Begg CB, et al: Staging of malignant pleural mesothelioma: Comparison of CT and MR imaging. Am J Roentgenol 1999;172(4):1039-1047.

91. Benard F, Sterman D, Smith RJ, et al: Metabolic imaging of malignant pleural mesothelioma with fluorodeoxyglucose positron emission tomography. Chest 1998;114(3):713-722.

92. Brancatisano RP, Joseph MG, McCaughan BC: Pleurectomy for mesothelioma. Med J Aust 1991;154(7):455-457, 460.

93. Martini N, McCormack PM, Bains MS, et al: Pleural mesothelioma. Ann Thorac Surg 1987;43(1):113-120.

94. Rusch VW, Venkatraman E: The importance of surgical staging in the treatment of malignant pleural mesothelioma. J Thorac Cardiovasc Surg 1996;111(4):815-825; discussion 825-826.

95. Canto A, Guijarro R, Arnau A, et al: Videothoracoscopy in the diagnosis and treatment of malignant pleural mesothelioma with associated pleural effusions. Thorac Cardiovasc Surg 1997;45(1):16-19.

96. Law MR, Gregor A, Hodson ME, et al: Malignant mesothelioma of the pleura: A study of 52 treated and 64 untreated patients. Thorax 1984;39(4):255-259.

97. Law MR, Hodson ME, Turner-Warwick M: Malignant mesothelioma of the pleura: Clinical aspects and symptomatic treatment. Eur J Respir Dis 1984;65(3):162-168.

98. Hilaris BS, Nori D, Kwong E, et al: Pleurectomy and intraoperative brachytherapy and postoperative radiation in the treatment of malignant pleural mesothelioma. Int J Radiat Oncol Biol Phys 1984;10(3):325-331.

99. McCormack PM, Nagasaki F, Hilaris BS, et al: Surgical treatment of pleural mesothelioma. J Thorac Cardiovasc Surg 1982;84(6):834-842.

100. DaValle MJ, Faber LP, Kittle CF, et al: Extrapleural pneumonectomy for diffuse, malignant mesothelioma. Ann Thorac Surg 1986;42(6):612-618.

101. Lewis RJ, Sisler GE, Mackenzie JW: Diffuse, mixed malignant pleural mesothelioma. Ann Thorac Surg 1981;31(1):53-60.

102. Wanebo HJ, Martini N, Melamed MR, et al: Pleural mesothelioma. Cancer 1976;38(6):2481-2488.

103. Achatzy R, Beba W, Ritschler R, et al: The diagnosis, therapy and prognosis of diffuse malignant mesothelioma. Eur J Cardiothorac Surg 1989;3(5):445-447; discussion 448.

104. Rusch VW: Pleurectomy/decortication and adjuvant therapy for malignant mesothelioma. Chest 1993;103(4 Suppl):382S-384S.

105. Rice TW, Adelstein DJ, Kirby TJ, et al: Aggressive multimodality therapy for malignant pleural mesothelioma. Ann Thorac Surg 1994;58(1):24-29.

106. Soysal O, Karaoglanoglu N, Demiracan S, et al: Pleurectomy/decortication for palliation of malignant pleural mesothelioma: Results of surgery. Eur J Cardiothorac Surg 1997;11:210-213.

107. Worn H: Chances and results of surgery of malignant mesothelioma of the pleura (author's transl). Thoraxchir Vask Chir 1974;22(5):391-393.

108. Bamler KJ, Maassen W: The percentage of benign and malign pleura-tumors among the patients of a clinic of lung surgery with special consideration of the malign pleuramesothelioma and its radical treatment, including results of a diaphragma substitution of preserved dura mater (author's transl). Thoraxchir Vask Chir 1974;22(5):386-391.

109. DeLaria GA, Jensik R, Faber LP, et al: Surgical management of malignant mesothelioma. Ann Thorac Surg 1978;26(4):375-382.

110. Vogt-Moykopf I, Etspule W, Bulzebruck H: Das diffuse meligne pleuramesotheliom: Diagnostik, therapie und prognose. Z Herz Thorac Gefabchir 1987;1:67-77.

111. Faber LP: Surgical treatment of asbestos-related disease of the chest. Surg Clin North Am 1988;68(3):525-543.

112. Rusch VW, Piantadosi S, Holmes EC: The role of extrapleural pneumonectomy in malignant pleural mesothelioma. A Lung Cancer Study Group trial. J Thorac Cardiovasc Surg 1991;102(1):1-9.

113. Rusch VW, Venkatraman ES: Important prognostic factors in patients with malignant pleural mesothelioma, managed surgically. Ann Thorac Surg 1999;68(5):1799-1804.

114. Maasilta P: Deterioration in lung function following hemithorax irradiation for pleural mesothelioma. Int J Radiat Oncol Biol Phys 1991;20(3):433-438.

115. Ehrenhaft JL, Sensenig DM, Lawrence MS: Mesotheliomas of the pleura. J Thorac Cardiovasc Surg 1960;40:393-409.

116. Eschwege F, M Schlienger: Radiotherapy of malignant pleural mesotheliomas. Apropos of 14 cases irradiated at high doses. J Radiol Electrol Med Nucl 1973;54(3):255-259.

117. Ball DL, Cruickshank DG: The treatment of malignant mesothelioma of the pleura: Review of a 5-year experience, with special reference to radiotherapy. Am J Clin Oncol 1990;13(1):4-9.

118. Bissett D, Macbeth FR, Cram I: The role of palliative radiotherapy in malignant mesothelioma. Clin Oncol (R Coll Radiol) 1991;3(6):315-317.

119. Reichert R, Shermann CD: Prolonged survival in diffuse pleural mesothelioma treated with Au198. Cancer 1959;12:799-805.

120. Ratzer ER, Pool JL, Melamed MR: Pleural mesotheliomas. Clinical experiences with thirty-seven patients. Am J Roentgenol Radium Ther Nucl Med 1967;99(4):863-880.

121. Porter JM, Cheek JM: Pleural mesothelioma review of tumor histogenesis and report of 12 cases. J Thorac Cardiovasc Surg 1968;55(6):882-890.

122. Brady LW: Mesothelioma—the role for radiation therapy. Semin Oncol 1981;8(3):329-334.

123. Alberts AS, Falkson G, Goedhals L, et al: Malignant pleural mesothelioma: A disease unaffected by current therapeutic maneuvers. J Clin Oncol 1988;6(3):527-535.

124. Linden CJ, Mercke C, Albrechtsson U, et al: Effect of hemithorax irradiation alone or combined with doxorubicin and cyclophosphamide in 47 pleural mesotheliomas: A nonrandomized phase II study. Eur Respir J 1996;9(12):2565-2572.

125. Todoroki T, Suit HD: Effect of fractionated irradiation prior to conservative and radical surgery on therapeutic gain in a spontaneous fibrosarcoma of the C3H mouse. J Surg Oncol 1986;31(4):279-286.

126. Boutin C, Rey F, Viallat JR: Prevention of malignant seeding after invasive diagnostic procedures in patients with pleural mesothelioma. A randomized trial of local radiotherapy. Chest 1995;108(3):754-758.

127. Ong ST, Vogelzang NJ: Chemotherapy in malignant pleural mesothelioma. A review. J Clin Oncol 1996;14(3):1007-1017.

128. Lerner HJ, Schoenfeld DA, Martin A, et al: Malignant mesothelioma. The Eastern Cooperative Oncology Group (ECOG) experience. Cancer 1983;52(11):1981-1985.

129. Sorensen PG, Bach F, Bork E, et al: Randomized trial of doxorubicin versus cyclophosphamide in diffuse malignant pleural mesothelioma. Cancer Treat Rep 1985;69(12):1431-1432.

130. Colbert N, Vannetzel JM, Izrael V, et al: A prospective study of detorubicin in malignant mesothelioma. Cancer 1985;56(9):2170-2174.

131. Kaukel E, Koschel G, Gatzemeyer U, et al: A phase II study of pirarubicin in malignant pleural mesothelioma. Cancer 1990;66(4):651-654.

132. Magri MD, Veronesi A, Foladore S, et al: Epirubicin in the treatment of malignant mesothelioma: A phase II cooperative study. The North-Eastern Italian Oncology Group (GOCCNE)—Mesothelioma Committee. Tumori 1991;77(1):49-51.

133. Mattson K, Giaccone G, Kirkpatrick A, et al: Epirubicin in malignant mesothelioma: A phase II study of the European Organization for Research and Treatment of Cancer Lung Cancer Cooperative Group. J Clin Oncol 1992;10(5):824-828.

134. Skubitz KM: Phase II trial of pegylated-liposomal doxorubicin (Doxil) in mesothelioma. Cancer Invest 2002;20(5-6):693-699.

135. Oh Y, Perez-Soler R, Fossella FV, et al: Phase II study of intravenous Doxil in malignant pleural mesothelioma. Invest New Drugs 2000;18(3):243-245.

136. Steele JP, O'Doherty CA, Shamash J, et al: Phase II trial of liposomal doxorubicin in malignant pleural mesothelioma. Ann Oncol 2001;12:497-499.

137. Eisenhauer EA, Evans WK, Raghavan D, et al: Phase II study of mitoxantrone in patients with mesothelioma: A National Cancer Institute of Canada Clinical Trials Group Study. Cancer Treat Rep 1986;70(8):1029-1030.

138. van Breukelen FJ, Mattson K, Giaccone G, et al: Mitoxantrone in malignant pleural mesothelioma: A study by the EORTC Lung Cancer Cooperative Group. Eur J Cancer 1991;27(12):1627-1629.

139. Hudis CA, Kelsen DP: Menogaril in the treatment of malignant mesothelioma: A phase II study. Invest New Drugs 1992;10(2):103–106.

140. Andersen MK, Krarup-Hansen A, Martensson G, et al: Ifosfamide in malignant mesothelioma: A phase II study. Lung Cancer 1999; 24(1):39–43.

141. Falkson G, Hunt M, Borden EC, et al: An extended phase II trial of ifosfamide plus mesna in malignant mesothelioma. Invest New Drugs 1992;10(4):337–343.

142. Zidar BL, Metch B, Balcerzak SP, et al: A phase II evaluation of ifosfamide and mesna in unresectable diffuse malignant mesothelioma. A Southwest Oncology Group study. Cancer 1992;70(10):2547–2551.

143. Alberts AS, Falkson G, Van Zyl L: Malignant pleural mesothelioma: Phase II pilot study of ifosfamide and mesna. J Natl Cancer Inst 1988;80(9):698–700.

144. Icli F, Karaoguz H, Hasturk S, et al: Two dose levels of ifosfamide in malignant mesothelioma. Lung Cancer 1996;15(2):207–213.

145. Krarup-Hansen A: Studies concerning high dose ifosfamide to patients suffering from malignant mesothelioma. Lung Cancer 1996;16(1):101–102.

146. Bajorin D, Kelsen D, Mintzer DM: Phase II trial of mitomycin in malignant mesothelioma. Cancer Treat Rep 1987;71(9):857–858.

147. Zidar BL, Green S, Pierce HI, et al: A phase II evaluation of cisplatin in unresectable diffuse malignant mesothelioma: A Southwest Oncology Group Study. Invest New Drugs 1988;6(3):223–226.

148. Mintzer DM, Kelsen D, Frimmer D, et al: Phase II trial of high-dose cisplatin in patients with malignant mesothelioma. Cancer Treat Rep 1985;69(6):711–712.

149. Vogelzang NJ, Rusthoven JJ, Symanowski J, et al: Phase III study of pemetrexed in combination with cisplatin versus cisplatin alone in patients with malignant pleural mesothelioma. J Clin Oncol 2003;21(14):2636–2644.

150. Vogelzang NJ, Goutsou M, Corson JM, et al: Carboplatin in malignant mesothelioma: A phase II study of the Cancer and Leukemia Group B. Cancer Chemother Pharmacol 1990;27(3): 239–242.

151. Mbidde EK, Harland SJ, Calvert AH, et al: Phase II trial of carboplatin (JM8) in treatment of patients with malignant mesothelioma. Cancer Chemother Pharmacol 1986;18(3):284–285.

152. Raghavan D, Gianoutsos P, Bishop J, et al: Phase II trial of carboplatin in the management of malignant mesothelioma. J Clin Oncol 1990;8(1):151–154.

153. Solheim OP, Saeter G, Finnanger AM, et al: High-dose methotrexate in the treatment of malignant mesothelioma of the pleura. A phase II study. Br J Cancer 1992;65(6):956–960.

154. Vogelzang NJ, Weissman LB, Herndon JE II, et al: Trimetrexate in malignant mesothelioma: A Cancer and Leukemia Group B Phase II study. J Clin Oncol 1994;12(7):1436–1442.

155. Kindler HL, Belani CP, Herndon JE II, et al: Edatrexate (10-ethyl-deaza-aminopterin) (NSC #626715) with or without leucovorin rescue for malignant mesothelioma. Sequential phase II trials by the cancer and leukemia group B Cancer 1999;86(10):1985–1991.

156. Scagliotti G, Shin DM, Kindler HL, et al: Phase II study of ALIMTA (premetrexed disodium, MTA) single agent in patients with malignant pleural mesothelioma. Eur J Cancer 2001;37(Suppl 6): S20.

157. Harvey VJ, Slevin ML, Ponder BA, et al: Chemotherapy of diffuse malignant mesothelioma. Phase II trials of single-agent 5-fluorouracil and adriamycin. Cancer 1984;54(6):961–964.

158. Otterson GA, Herndon J, Watson D, et al: Capecitabine in malignant mesothelioma: a phase II trial by the Cancer and Leukemia Group B (CALGB 39807). Proc Am Soc Clin Oncol 2003;22:2778a.

159. Cantwell BM, Earnshaw M, Harris AL: Phase II study of a novel antifolate, N10-propargyl-5,8 dideazafolic acid (CB3717), in malignant mesothelioma. Cancer Treat Rep 1986;70(11): 1335–1336.

160. Dhingra HM, Murphy WK, Winn RJ, et al: Phase II trial of 5,6-dihydro-5-azacytidine in pleural malignant mesothelioma. Invest New Drugs 1991;9(1):69–72.

161. Vogelzang NJ, Herndon JE II, Cirrincione C, et al: Dihydro-5-azacytidine in malignant mesothelioma. A phase II trial demonstrating activity accompanied by cardiac toxicity. Cancer and Leukemia Group B. Cancer 1997;79(11):2237–2242.

162. van Meerbeeck JP, Baas P, Debruyne C, et al: A Phase II study of gemcitabine in patients with malignant pleural mesothelioma. European Organization for Research and Treatment of Cancer Lung Cancer Cooperative Group. Cancer 1999;85(12):2577–2582.

163. Kindler HL, Millard F, Herndon JE II, et al: Gemcitabine for malignant mesothelioma: A phase II trial by the Cancer and Leukemia Group B. Lung Cancer 2001;31(2–3):311–317.

164. Bischoff HG, Manegold C, Knopp M: Gemcitabine (Gemzar) may reduce tumor load and tumor associated symptoms in malignant pleural mesothelioma. Proc Am Soc Clin Oncol 1998;17:464a.

165. Maksymiuk AW, Marschke RF Jr, Tazelaar HD, et al: Phase II trial of topotecan for the treatment of mesothelioma. Am J Clin Oncol 1998;21(6):610–613.

166. Kindler HL, Herndon JE II, Vogelzang NJ: CPT-11 in malignant mesothelioma: A phase II trial by the Cancer and Leukemia Group B (CALGB 9733). Proc Am Soc Clin Oncol 2000;19:505a.

167. Martensson G, Sorenson S: A phase II study of vincristine in malignant mesothelioma—A negative report. Cancer Chemother Pharmacol 1989;24(2):133–134.

168. Kelsen D, Gralla R, Cheng E, et al: Vindesine in the treatment of malignant mesothelioma: A phase II study. Cancer Treat Rep 1983;67(9):821–822.

169. Boutin C, Irisson M, Guerin JC, et al: Phase II trial of vindesine in malignant pleural mesothelioma. Cancer Treat Rep 1987;71(2): 205–206.

170. Cowan JD, Green S, Lucas J, et al: Phase II trial of five day intravenous infusion vinblastine sulfate in patients with diffuse malignant mesothelioma: A Southwest Oncology Group study. Invest New Drugs 1988;6(3):247–248.

171. Sahmoud T, Postmus PE, van Pottelsberghe C, et al: Etoposide in malignant pleural mesothelioma: Two phase II trials of the EORTC Lung Cancer Cooperative Group. Eur J Cancer 1997;33(13): 2211–2215.

172. Tammilehto L, Maasilta P, Mantyla M, et al: Oral etoposide in the treatment of malignant mesothelioma. A phase II study. Ann Oncol 1994;5(10):949–950.

173. van Meerbeeck J, Debruyne C, van Zandwijk N, et al: Paclitaxel for malignant pleural mesothelioma: A phase II study of the EORTC Lung Cancer Cooperative Group. Br J Cancer 1996;74(6): 961–963.

174. Vogelzang NJ, Herndon JE II, Miller A, et al: High-dose paclitaxel plus G-CSF for malignant mesothelioma: CALGB phase II study 9234. Ann Oncol 1999;10(5):597–600.

175. Belani CP, Adak S, Aisner S, et al: Docetaxel for malignant mesothelioma: Phase II study of the Eastern Cooperative Oncology Group (ECOG 2595). Proc Am Soc Clin Oncol 1999;18:1829a.

176. Vorobiof DA, Rapoport BL, Chasen MR, et al: Malignant pleural mesothelioma: A phase II trial with docetaxel. Ann Oncol 2002;13(3):412–415.

177. Eagan RT, Frytak S, Richardson RL, et al: Phase II trial of diaziquone in malignant mesothelioma. Cancer Treat Rep 1986;70(3):429.

178. Falkson G, Vorobiof DA, Lerner HJ: A phase II study of m-AMSA in patients with malignant mesothelioma. Cancer Chemother Pharmacol 1983;11(2):94–97.

179. Mikulski SM, Costanzi JJ, Vogelzang NJ, et al: Phase II trial of a single weekly intravenous dose of ranpirnase in patients with unresectable malignant mesothelioma. J Clin Oncol 2002;20(1): 274–281.

180. Govindan R, Kratzke RA, Herndon JE, et al: Gefitinib in patients with malignant mesothelioma (MM): A phase II study by the Cancer and Leukemia Group B (CALGB 30101). Proc Am Soc Clin Oncol 2003;22:2535a.

181. Millward M, Parnis F, Byrne M, et al: Phase II trial of imatinib in patients with advanced pleural mesothelioma. Proc Am Soc Clin Oncol 2003;22:912a.

182. Yap BS, Benjamin RS, Burgess MA, et al: The value of adriamycin in the treatment of diffuse malignant pleural mesothelioma. Cancer 1978;42(4):1692–1696.

183. Bueno R, Appasani K, Mercer H, et al: The alpha folate receptor is

highly activated in malignant pleural mesothelioma. J Thorac Cardiovasc Surg 2001;121(2):225–233.

184. Wang Y, Zhao R, Chattopadhyay S, et al: A novel folate transport activity in human mesothelioma cell lines with high affinity and specificity for the new-generation antifolate, pemetrexed. Cancer Res 2002;62(22):6434–6437.

185. Upham JW, Musk AW, van Hazel G, et al: Interferon alpha and doxorubicin in malignant mesothelioma: A phase II study. Aust N Z J Med 1993;23(6):683–687.

186. Samson MK, Wasser LP, Borden EC, et al: Randomized comparison of cyclophosphamide, imidazole carboxamide, and adriamycin versus cyclophosphamide and adriamycin in patients with advanced stage malignant mesothelioma: A Sarcoma Intergroup Study. J Clin Oncol 1987;5(1):86–91.

187. Carmichael J, Cantwell BM, Harris AL: A phase II trial of ifosfamide/mesna with doxorubicin for malignant mesothelioma. Eur J Cancer Clin Oncol 1989;25(5):911–912.

188. Dirix LY, van Meerbeeck J, Schrijvers D, et al: A phase II trial of dose-escalated doxorubicin and ifosfamide/mesna in patients with malignant mesothelioma. Ann Oncol 1994;5(7):653–655.

189. Ardizzoni A, Rosso R, Salvati F, et al: Activity of doxorubicin and cisplatin combination chemotherapy in patients with diffuse malignant pleural mesothelioma. An Italian Lung Cancer Task Force (FONICAP) Phase II study. Cancer 1991;67(12):2984–2987.

190. Chahinian AP, Antman K, Goutsou M, et al: Randomized phase II trial of cisplatin with mitomycin or doxorubicin for malignant mesothelioma by the Cancer and Leukemia Group B. J Clin Oncol 1993;11(8):1559–1565.

191. Shin DM, Fossella FV, Umsawasdi T, et al: Prospective study of combination chemotherapy with cyclophosphamide, doxorubicin, and cisplatin for unresectable or metastatic malignant pleural mesothelioma. Cancer 1995;76(11):2230–2236.

192. Pennucci MC, Ardizzoni A, Pronzato P, et al: Combined cisplatin, doxorubicin, and mitomycin for the treatment of advanced pleural mesothelioma: A phase II FONICAP trial. Italian Lung Cancer Task Force. Cancer 1997;79(10):1897–1902.

193. Magri MD, Foladore S, Veronesi A, et al: Treatment of malignant mesothelioma with epirubicin and ifosfamide: A phase II cooperative study. Ann Oncol 1992;3(3):237–238.

194. Bretti S, Berruti A, Dogliotti L, et al: Combined epirubicin and interleukin-2 regimen in the treatment of malignant mesothelioma: A multicenter phase II study of the Italian Group on Rare Tumors. Tumori 1998;84(5):558–561.

195. Trandafir L, Ruffie P, Borel C, et al: Higher doses of alpha-interferon do not increase the activity of the weekly cisplatin-interferon combination in advanced malignant mesothelioma. Eur J Cancer 1997;33(11):1900–1902.

196. Soulie P, Ruffie P, Trandafir L, et al: Combined systemic chemoimmunotherapy in advanced diffuse malignant mesothelioma. Report of a phase I-II study of weekly cisplatin/interferon alfa-2a. J Clin Oncol 1996;14(3):878–885.

197. Samuels BL, Herndon JE II, Harmon DC, et al: Dihydro-5-azacytidine and cisplatin in the treatment of malignant mesothelioma: A phase II study by the Cancer and Leukemia Group B. Cancer 1998;82(8):1578–1584.

198. Tsavaris N, Mylonakis N, Karvounis N, et al: Combination chemotherapy with cisplatin-vinblastine in malignant mesothelioma. Lung Cancer 1994;11(3–4):299–303.

199. Nakano T, Chahinian AP, Shinjo M, et al: Cisplatin in combination with irinotecan in the treatment of patients with malignant pleural mesothelioma: A pilot phase II clinical trial and pharmacokinetic profile. Cancer 1999;85(11):2375–2384.

200. Planting AS, van der Burg ME, Goey SH, et al: Phase II study of a short course of weekly high-dose cisplatin combined with long-term oral etoposide in pleural mesothelioma. Ann Oncol 1995;6(6):613–615.

201. Middleton GW, Smith IE, O'Brien ME, et al: Good symptom relief with palliative MVP (mitomycin-C, vinblastine and cisplatin) chemotherapy in malignant mesothelioma. Ann Oncol 1998;9(3):269–273.

202. Tansan S, Emri S, Selcuk T, et al: Treatment of malignant pleural mesothelioma with cisplatin, mitomycin C and alpha interferon. Oncology 1994;51(4):348–351.

203. Metintas M, Ozdemir N, Ucgun I, et al: Cisplatin, mitomycin, and interferon-alpha2a combination chemoimmunotherapy in the treatment of diffuse malignant pleural mesothelioma. Chest 1999;116(2):391–398.

204. Byrne MJ, Davidson JA, Musk AW, et al: Cisplatin and gemcitabine treatment for malignant mesothelioma: A phase II study. J Clin Oncol 1999;17(1):25–30.

205. van Haarst JM, Baas P, Manegold C, et al: Multicentre phase II study of gemcitabine and cisplatin in malignant pleural mesothelioma. Br J Cancer 2002;86(3):342–345.

206. Nowak AK, Byrne MJ, Williamson R, et al: A multicentre phase II study of cisplatin and gemcitabine for malignant mesothelioma. Br J Cancer 2002;87(5):491–496.

207. Kasseyet S, Astoul P, Boutin C: Results of a phase II trial of combined chemotherapy for patients with diffuse malignant mesothelioma of the pleura. Cancer 1999;85(8):1740–1749.

208. Castagneto B, Zai S, Dongiovanni V, et al: Cisplatin and gemcitabine in malignant pleural mesothelioma: A phase II study. Proc Am Soc Clin Oncol 2003;22:2637a.

209. Favaretto AG, Aversa SM, Paccagnella A, et al: Gemcitabine combined with carboplatin in patients with malignant pleural mesothelioma: A multicentric phase II study. Cancer 2003;97(11):2791–2797.

210. O'Reilly EM, Ilson DH, Salz LB, et al: A phase II trial of interferon alpha-2a and carboplatin in patients with advanced malignant mesothelioma. Cancer Invest 1999;17:195–200.

211. Steele JP, Shamash J, Evans MT: Phase II trial of vinorelbine and oxaliplatin (VO) in malignant pleural mesothelioma (MPM). Proc Am Soc Clin Oncol 2001;20:335a.

212. Hugues A, Calvert P, Azzabi A, et al: Clinical and pharmacokinetic study of pemetrexed and carboplatin in patients with malignant pleural mesothelioma. J Clin Oncol 2002;20:3533–3544.

213. Fizazi K, Doubre H, Le Chevalier T, et al: Combination of raltitrexed and oxaliplatin is an active regimen in malignant mesothelioma: Results of a phase II study. J Clin Oncol 2003;21(2):349–354.

214. Halme M, Knuuttila A, Vehmas T, et al: High-dose methotrexate in combination with interferons in the treatment of malignant pleural mesothelioma. Br J Cancer 1999;80(11):1781–1785.

215. Brodin O, Knuutila A, Halme M, et al: Combined treatment of malignant mesothelioma of the pleura with high-dose methotrexate and interferon-alpha and gamma. Proc XII World Lung Cancer Congress 2000;XII:53a.

216. Chahinian AP, Norton L, Holland JF, et al: Experimental and clinical activity of mitomycin C and cis-diamminedichloroplatinum in malignant mesothelioma. Cancer Res 1984;44(4):1688–1692.

217. Thodtmann R, Depenbrock H, Dumez H, et al: Clinical and pharmacokinetic phase I study of multitargeted antifolate (LY231514) in combination with cisplatin. J Clin Oncol 1999;17(10):3009–3016.

218. Rusch VW: Pemetrexed and Cisplatin for malignant pleural mesothelioma: A new standard of care? J Clin Oncol 2003;21(14):2629–2630.

219. Rogoff EE, Hilaris BS, Huvos AG: Long-term survival in patients with malignant peritoneal mesothelioma treated with irradiation. Cancer 1973;32(3):656–664.

220. Casper ES, Kelsen DP, Alcock NW, et al: Ip cisplatin in patients with malignant ascites: Pharmacokinetic evaluation and comparison with the IV route. Cancer Treat Rep 1983;67(3):235–238.

221. Howell SB, Pfeifle CL, Wung WE, et al: Intraperitoneal cisplatin with systemic thiosulfate protection. Ann Intern Med 1982;97(6):845–851.

222. Markman M, Cleary S, Pfeifle C, et al: Cisplatin administered by the intracavitary route as treatment for malignant mesothelioma. Cancer 1986;58(1):18–21.

223. Markman M, Kelsen D: Efficacy of cisplatin-based intraperitoneal chemotherapy as treatment of malignant peritoneal mesothelioma. J Cancer Res Clin Oncol 1992;118(7):547–550.

224. van Ruth S, Baas P, Haas RL, et al: Cytoreductive surgery combined with intraoperative hyperthermic intrathoracic chemotherapy for stage I malignant pleural mesothelioma. Ann Surg Oncol 2003;10(2):176–182.

225. Christmas TI, Manning LS, Garlepp MJ, et al: Effect of interferon-alpha 2a on malignant mesothelioma. J Interferon Res 1993;13(1):9-12.

226. Rosso R, Rimoldi R, Salvati F, et al: Intrapleural natural beta interferon in the treatment of malignant pleural effusions. Oncology 1988;45(3):253-256.

227. Ardizzoni A, Pennucci MC, Castagneto B, et al: Recombinant interferon alpha-2b in the treatment of diffuse malignant pleural mesothelioma. Am J Clin Oncol 1994;17(1):80-82.

228. Von Hoff DD, Metch B, Lucas JG, et al: Phase II evaluation of recombinant interferon-beta (IFN-beta ser) in patients with diffuse mesothelioma: A Southwest Oncology Group study. J Interferon Res 1990;10(5):531-534.

229. Goey SH, Eggermont AM, Punt CJ, et al: Intrapleural administration of interleukin 2 in pleural mesothelioma: A phase I-II study. Br J Cancer 1995;72(5):1283-1288.

230. Sterman DH, Treat J, Litzky LA, et al: Adenovirus-mediated herpes simplex virus thymidine kinase/ganciclovir gene therapy in patients with localized malignancy: Results of a phase I clinical trial in malignant mesothelioma. Hum Gene Ther 1998;9(7):1083-1092.

231. Webster I, Cochrane JW, Burkhardt KR: Immunotherapy with BCG vaccine in 30 cases of mesothelioma. S Afr Med J 1982;61(8):277-278.

232. Robinson BW, Bowman RV, Manning LS, et al: Interleukin-2 and lymphokine activated killer cells in malignant mesothelioma. Eur Resp Rev 1993;3:220-222.

233. Astoul P, Picat-Joossen D, Viallat JR, et al: Intrapleural administration of interleukin-2 for the treatment of patients with malignant pleural mesothelioma: A Phase II study. Cancer 1998;83(10):2099-2104.

234. Astoul P, Viallat JR, Laurent JC, et al: Intrapleural recombinant IL-2 in passive immunotherapy for malignant pleural effusion. Chest 1993;103(1):209-213.

235. Smith JW, Urba WJ, Clark JW, et al: Phase I evaluation of recombinant tumor necrosis factor given in combination with recombinant interferon-gamma. J Immunother 1991;10:355-362.

236. Davidson JA, Musk AW, Wood BR, et al: Intralesional cytokine therapy in cancer: A pilot study of gm-CSF infusion in mesothelioma. J Immunother 1998;21:389-398.

237. Nowak AK, Lake RA, Kindler HL, et al: New approaches for mesothelioma: Biologics, vaccines, gene therapy, and other novel agents. Semin Oncol 2002;29:82-96.

238. Boutin C, Nussbaum E, Monnet I, et al: Intrapleural treatment with recombinant gamma-interferon in early stage malignant pleural mesothelioma. Cancer 1994;74(9):2460-2467.

239. Sterman DH, Kaiser LR, Albelda SM: Advances in the treatment of malignant pleural mesothelioma. Chest 1999;116(2):504-520.

240. Mukherjee S, Haenel T, Himbeck R, et al: Replication restricted vaccinia as a cytokine gene therapy vector in cancer: Persistent transgene expression despite antibody generation. Cancer Gene Ther 2000;7:663-670.

241. Sinoff C, Falkson G, Sandison AG, et al: Combined doxorubicin and radiation therapy in malignant pleural mesothelioma. Cancer Treat Rep 1982;66(8):1605-1607.

242. Pass HI, Temeck BK, Kranda K, et al: Phase III randomized trial of surgery with or without intraoperative photodynamic therapy and postoperative immunochemotherapy for malignant pleural mesothelioma. Ann Surg Oncol 1997;4(8):628-633.

243. Pass HI, Tochner Z, DeLaney T, et al: Intraoperative photodynamic therapy for malignant pleural mesothelioma. Ann Thorac Surg 1990;50(4):687-688.

244. Takita H, Dougherty TJ: Intracavitary photodynamic therapy for malignant pleural mesothelioma. Semin Surg Oncol 1995;11(5):368-371.

245. Rusch VW, Niedzwiecki D, Tao Y, et al: Intrapleural cisplatin and mitomycin for malignant mesothelioma following pleurectomy: Pharmacokinetic studies. J Clin Oncol 1992;10(6):1001-1006.

246. Calavrezos A, Koschel G, Husselmann H, et al: Malignant mesothelioma of the pleura. A prospective therapeutic study of 132 patients from 1981-1985. Klin Wochenschr 1988;66(14):607-613.

247. Rusch VW: Pleurectomy/decortication in the setting of multimodality treatment for diffuse malignant pleural mesothelioma. Semin Thorac Cardiovasc Surg 1997;9:367-372.

248. Moskal TL, Dougherty TJ, Urschel JD, et al: Operation and photodynamic therapy for pleural mesothelioma: 6-year follow-up. Ann Thorac Surg 1998;66:1128-1133.

249. Yellin A, Simansky DA, Paley M, et al: Hyperthermic pleural perfusion with cisplatin: Early clinical experience. Cancer 2001;92:2197-2203.

250. Monneuse O, Beaujard AC, Guibert B, et al: Long-term results of intrathoracic chemohyperthermia (ITCH) for the treatment of pleural malignancies. Br J Cancer 2003;88:1839-1843.

251. Mackay B, Ordonez NG: Pathological evaluation of neoplasms with unknown primary tumor site. Semin Oncol 1993;20(3):206-228.

252. Landreneau R, Dowling R, Hazelirgh S: Thoracoscopy for the diagnosis and treatment of intrathoracic malignancy. Proc Am Soc Clin Oncol 1992;11:291a.

253. Marchandise FX, Vandenplas O, Wallon J, et al: Thoracoscopy in the diagnosis and management of chronic pleural effusions. Acta Clin Belg 1993;48(1):5-10.

254. Ratliff JL, Chavez CM, Jamchuk A, et al: Re-expansion pulmonary edema. Chest 1973;64(5):654-656.

255. Trapnell DH, Thurston JG: Unilateral pulmonary oedema after pleural aspiration. Lancet 1970;1(7661):1367-1369.

256. Anderson CB, Philpott GW, Ferguson TB: The treatment of malignant pleural effusions. Cancer 1974;33(4):916-922.

257. Tiber C: Small chest tube for malignant pleural effusions. South Med J 1980;73(9):1291-1292.

258. Austin EH, Flye MW: The treatment of recurrent malignant pleural effusion. Ann Thorac Surg 1979;28(2):190-203.

259. Walker-Renard PB, Vaughan LM, Sahn SA: Chemical pleurodesis for malignant pleural effusions. Ann Intern Med 1994;120(1):56-64.

260. Waller DA, Morritt GN, Forty J: Video-assisted thoracoscopic pleurectomy in the management of malignant pleural effusion. Chest 1995;107(5):1454-1456.

261. Harvey JC, Erdman CB, Beattie EJ: Early experience with videothoracoscopic hydrodissection pleurectomy in the treatment of malignant pleural effusion. J Surg Oncol 1995;59(4):243-245.

262. Ariel IM, Oropeza R, Pack GT: Intracavitary administration of radioactive isotopes in the control of pleural effusion secondary to metastatic breast cancer. Eur J Clin Oncol 1966;22:1079-1088.

263. Izbicki R, Weyhing BT III, Baker L, et al: Pleural effusion in cancer patients. A prospective randomized study of pleural drainage with the addition of radioactive phsophorous to the pleural space vs. pleural drainage alone. Cancer 1975;36(4):1511-1518.

264. Stiksa G, Korsgaard R, Simonsson BG: Treatment of recurrent pleural effusion by pleurodesis with quinacrine. Comparison between instillation by repeated thoracenteses and by tube drainage. Scand J Respir Dis 1979;60(4):197-205.

265. Bayly TC, Kisner DL, Sybert A, et al: Tetracycline and quinacrine in the control of malignant pleural effusions. A randomized trial. Cancer 1978;41(3):1188-1192.

266. Taylor SA, Hooton NS, Macarthur AM: Quinacrine in the management of malignant pleural effusion. Br J Surg 1977;64(1):52-53.

267. Sorensen PG, Svendsen TL, Enk B: Treatment of malignant pleural effusion with drainage, with and without instillation of talc. Eur J Respir Dis 1984;65(2):131-135.

268. Wallach HW: Intrapleural tetracycline for malignant pleural effusions. Chest 1975;68(4):510-512.

269. Zaloznik AJ, Oswald SG, Langin M: Intrapleural tetracycline in malignant pleural effusions. A randomized study. Cancer 1983;51(4):752-755.

270. Gravelyn TR, Michelson MK, Gross BH, et al: Tetracycline pleurodesis for malignant pleural effusions. A 10-year retrospective study. Cancer 1987;59(11):1973-1977.

271. Sherman S, Grady KJ, Seidman JC: Clinical experience with tetracycline pleurodesis of malignant pleural effusions. South Med J 1987;80(6):716-719.

272. Landvater L, Hix WR, Mills M, et al: Malignant pleural effusion treated by tetracycline sclerotherapy. A comparison of single vs repeated instillation. Chest 1988;93(6):1196-1198.

273. Ruckdeschel JC, Moores D, Lee JY, et al: Intrapleural therapy for malignant pleural effusions. A randomized comparison of bleomycin and tetracycline. Chest 1991;100(6):1528-1535.

274. Kefford RF, Woods RL, Fox RM, et al: Intracavitary adriamycin nitrogen mustard and tetracycline in the control of malignant effusions: a randomized study. Med J Aust 1980;2(8):447-448.

275. Kessinger A, Wigton RS: Intracavitary bleomycin and tetracycline in the management of malignant pleural effusions: A randomized study. J Surg Oncol 1987;36(2):81-83.

276. Light RW, Wang NS, Sassoon CS, et al: Comparison of the effectiveness of tetracycline and minocycline as pleural sclerosing agents in rabbits. Chest 1994;106(2):577-582.

277. Hatta T, Tsubuota N, Yoshimura M, et al: Effect of intrapleural administration of minocycline on postoperative air leakage and maignant pleural effusions. Kyobu Geka 1990;43:283-289.

278. Muir JF, Defouilloy C, Ndarurinze S, et al: Use of intrapleural doxycycline via lavage-drainage in recurrent effusions of neoplastic origin. Rev Mal Respir 1987;4(1):29-33.

279. Mansson T: Treatment of malignant pleural effusion with doxycycline. Scand J Infect Dis Suppl 1988;53:29-34.

280. Patz, EF Jr, McAdams HP, Erasmus JJ, et al: Sclerotherapy for malignant pleural effusions: A prospective randomized trial of bleomycin vs doxycycline with small-bore catheter drainage. Chest 1998;113(5):1305-1311.

281. Buselmeier TJ, Simmons RL, Najarian JS, et al: Uremic pericardial effusion. Treatment by catheter drainage and local nonabsorbable steroid administration. Nephron 1976;16(5):371-380.

282. Bartal AH, Gazitt Y, Zidan G, et al: Clinical and flow cytometry characteristics of malignant pleural effusions in patients after intracavitary administration of methylprednisolone acetate. Cancer 1991;67(12):3136-3140.

283. Aelony Y, King R, Boutin C: Thoracoscopic talc poudrage pleurodesis for chronic recurrent pleural effusions. Ann Intern Med 1991;115(10):778-782.

284. Adler RH, Sayek I: Treatment of malignant pleural effusion: A method using tube thoracostomy and talc. Ann Thorac Surg 1976;22(1):8-15.

285. Pearson FG, MacGregor DC: Talc poudrage for malignant pleural effusion. J Thorac Cardiovasc Surg 1966;51(5):732-738.

286. Webb WR, Ozmen V, Moulder PV, et al: Iodized talc pleurodesis for the treatment of pleural effusions. J Thorac Cardiovasc Surg 1992;103(5):881-885; discussion 885-886.

287. Daniel TM, Tribble CG, Rodgers BM: Thoracoscopy and talc poudrage for pneumothoraces and effusions. Ann Thorac Surg 1990;50(2):186-189.

288. Fentiman IS, Rubens RD, Hayward JL: A comparison of intracavitary talc and tetracycline for the control of pleural effusions secondary to breast cancer. Eur J Cancer Clin Oncol 1986;22(9):1079-1081.

289. Aelony Y, King RR, Boutin C: Thoracoscopic talc poudrage in malignant pleural effusions: Effective pleurodesis despite low pleural pH. Chest 1998;113(4):1007-1012.

290. Hamed H, Fentiman IS, Chaudary MA, et al: Comparison of intracavitary bleomycin and talc for control of pleural effusions secondary to carcinoma of the breast. Br J Surg 1989;76(12):1266-1267.

291. Eselin J, Thompson DF: Talc in the treatment of malignant pleural effusion. Dicp 1991;25(11):1187-1189.

292. Bitran JD, Brown C, Desser RK, et al: Intracavitary bleomycin for the control of malignant effusions. J Surg Oncol 1981;16(3): 273-277.

293. Paladine W, Cunningham TJ, Sponzo R, et al: Intracavitary bleomycin in the management of malignant effusions. Cancer 1976;38(5):1903-1908.

294. Ostrowski MJ: Intracavitary therapy with bleomycin for the treatment of malignant pleural effusions. J Surg Oncol Suppl 1989;1:7-13.

295. Ostrowski MJ, Priestman TJ, Houston RF, et al: A randomized trial of intracavitary bleomycin and Corynebacterium parvum in the control of malignant pleural effusions. Radiother Oncol 1989;14(1):19-26.

296. Masuno T, Kishimoto S, Ogura T, et al: A comparative trial of LC9018 plus doxorubicin and doxorubicin alone for the treatment of malignant pleural effusion secondary to lung cancer. Cancer 1991;68(7):1495-1500.

297. Markman M, Cleary S, King ME, et al: Cisplatin and cytarabine administered intrapleurally as treatment of malignant pleural effusions. Med Pediatr Oncol 1985;13(4):191-193.

298. Rusch VW, Figlin R, Godwin D, et al: Intrapleural cisplatin and cytarabine in the management of malignant pleural effusions: A Lung Cancer Study Group trial. J Clin Oncol 1991;9(2):313-319.

299. Holoye PY, Jeffries DG, Dhingra HM, et al: Intrapleural etoposide for malignant effusion. Cancer Chemother Pharmacol 1990;26(2):147-150.

300. Webb HE, Oaten SW, Pike CP: Treatment of malignant ascitic and pleural effusion with Corynebacterium parvum. BMJ 1978;1(6109):338-340.

301. Rossi GA, Felletti R, Balbi B, et al: Symptomatic treatment of recurrent malignant pleural effusions with intrapleurally administered Corynebacterium parvum. Clinical response is not associated with evidence of enhancement of local cellular-mediated immunity. Am Rev Respir Dis 1987;135(4):885-890.

302. Millar JW, Hunter AM, Horne NW: Intrapleural immunotherapy with Corynebacterium parvum in recurrent malignant pleural effusions. Thorax 1980;35(11):856-858.

303. Felletti R, Ravazzoni C: Intrapleural Corynebacterium parvum for malignant pleural effusions. Thorax 1983;38(1):22-24.

304. McLeod DT, Calverley PM, Millar JW, et al: Further experience of Corynebacterium parvum in malignant pleural effusion. Thorax 1985;40(7):515-518.

305. Casali A, Gionfra T, Rinaldi M, et al: Treatment of malignant pleural effusions with intracavitary Corynebacterium parvum. Cancer 1988;62(4):806-811.

306. Hillerdal G, Kiviloog J, Nou E, et al: Corynebacterium parvum in malignant pleural effusion. A randomized prospective study. Eur J Respir Dis 1986;69(3):204-206.

307. Goldman CA, Skinnider LF, Maksymiuk AW: Interferon instillation for malignant pleural effusions. Ann Oncol 1993;4(2):141-145.

308. Viallat JR, Boutin C, Rey F, et al: Intrapleural immunotherapy with escalating doses of interleukin-2 in metastatic pleural effusions. Cancer 1993;71(12):4067-4071.

309. Yasumoto K, Ogura T: Intrapleural application of recombinant interleukin-2 in patients with malignant pleurisy due to lung cancer. A multi-institutional cooperative study. Biotherapy 1991;3(4):345-349.

310. Morrison MC, Mueller PR, Lee MJ, et al: Sclerotherapy of malignant pleural effusion through sonographically placed small-bore catheters. Am J Roentgenol 1992;158(1):41-43.

311. Parker LA, Charnock GC, Delany DJ: Small bore catheter drainage and sclerotherapy for malignant pleural effusions. Cancer 1989;64(6):1218-1221.

312. Thompson RL, Yau JC, Donnelly RF, et al: Pleurodesis with iodized talc for malignant effusions using pigtail catheters. Ann Pharmacother 1998;32(7-8):739-742.

313. Yim AP, Chan AT, Lee TW, et al: Thoracoscopic talc insufflation versus talc slurry for symptomatic malignant pleural effusion. Ann Thorac Surg 1996;62(6):1655-1658.

314. Kennedy L, Rusch VW, Strange C, et al: Pleurodesis using talc slurry. Chest 1994;106(2):342-346.

315. Boniface E, Guerin JC: Value of talc administration using thoracoscopy in the symptomatic treatment of recurrent pleurisy. Apropos of 302 cases. Rev Mal Respir 1989;6(2):133-140.

316. Ladjimi S, M'Raihi L, Djemel A, et al: Results of talc administration using thoracoscopy in neoplastic pleurisies. Apropos of 218 cases. Rev Mal Respir 1989;6(2):147-150.

317. Weissberg D, Ben-Zeev I: Talc pleurodesis. Experience with 360 patients. J Thorac Cardiovasc Surg 1993;106(4):689-695.

318. Sanchez-Armengol A, Rodriguez-Panadero F: Survival and talc pleurodesis in metastatic pleural carcinoma, revisited. Report of 125 cases. Chest 1993;104(5):1482-1485.

319. Zimmer PW, Hill M, Casey K, et al: Prospective randomized trial of talc slurry vs bleomycin in pleurodesis for symptomatic malignant pleural effusions. Chest 1997;112(2):430-434.

320. Hartman DL, Gaither JM, Kesler KA, et al: Comparison of insufflated talc under thoracoscopic guidance with standard tetracycline and bleomycin pleurodesis for control of malignant pleural effusions. J Thorac Cardiovasc Surg 1993;105(4):743-747; discussion 747-748.

321. Schiffer CA, Sanel FT, Young VB, et al: Reversal of granulocyte adherence to nylon fibers using local anesthetic agents: Possible application to filtration leukapheresis. Blood 1977;50(2): 213-225.

322. Davis M, Williford S, Muss HB, et al: A phase I-II study of recombinant intrapleural alpha interferon in malignant pleural effusions. Am J Clin Oncol 1992;15(4):328-330.

323. Luh KT, Yang PC, Kuo SH, et al: Comparison of OK-432 and mitomycin C pleurodesis for malignant pleural effusion caused by lung cancer. A randomized trial. Cancer 1992;69(3):674-679.

324. Martini N, Bains MS, Beattie EJ Jr: Indications for pleurectomy in malignant effusion. Cancer 1975;35(3):734-738.

325. Curreri AR, Gale JW: Mediastinal tumors. Arch Surg 1949;58:797.

326. Katlic MR, Wang CA, Grillo HC: Substernal goiter. Ann Thorac Surg 1985;39(4):391-399.

327. Link KM, Samuels LJ, Reed JC, et al: Magnetic resonance imaging of the mediastinum. J Thorac Imaging 1993;8(1):34-53.

328. Yang PC, Chang DB, Yu CJ, et al: Ultrasound-guided core biopsy of thoracic tumors. Am Rev Respir Dis 1992;146(3):763-767.

329. Weisbrod GL: Percutaneous fine-needle aspiration biopsy of the mediastinum. Clin Chest Med 1987;8(1):27-41.

330. Pearson FG: Mediastinal tumors. Diagnosis: Invasive techniques. Semin Thorac Cardiovasc Surg 1992;4(1):23-24.

331. Herman SJ, Holub RV, Weisbrod GL, et al: Anterior mediastinal masses: Utility of transthoracic needle biopsy. Radiology 1991;180(1):167-170.

332. Roviaro G, Varoli F, Nucca O, et al: Videothoracoscopic approach to primary mediastinal pathology. Chest 2000;117(4):1179-1183.

333. Dadmanesh F, Sekihara T, Rosai J: Histologic typing of thymoma according to the new World Health Organization classification. Chest Surg Clin N Am 2001;11(2):407-420.

334. Ito M, Taki T, Miyake M, et al: Lymphocyte subsets in human thymoma studied with monoclonal antibodies. Cancer 1988;61(2):284-287.

335. Chan WC, Zaatari GS, Tabei S, et al: Thymoma: An immunohisto-chemical study. Am J Clin Pathol 1984;82(2):160-166.

336. Katzin WE, Fishleder AJ, Linden MD, et al: Immunoglobulin and T-cell receptor genes in thymomas: Genotypic evidence supporting the nonneoplastic nature of the lymphocytic component. Hum Pathol 1988;19(3):323-328.

337. Bernatz PE, Harrison EG, Clagett OT: Thymoma: A clinico-pathologic study. Thorac Cardiovasc Surg 1961;42:424-444.

338. Gray GF, Gutowski WT III: Thymoma. A clinicopathologic study of 54 cases. Am J Surg Pathol 1979;3(3):235-249.

339. Pescarmona E, Rendina EA, Venuta F, et al: The prognostic implication of thymoma histologic subtyping. A study of 80 consecutive cases. Am J Clin Pathol 1990;93(2):190-195.

340. Marino M, Muller-Hermelink HK: Thymoma and thymic carcinoma. Relation of thymoma epithelial cells to the cortical and medullary differentiation of thymus. Virchows Arch A Pathol Anat Histopathol 1985;407(2):119-149.

341. Rosai J, Sobin LH: Histological typing of tumours of the thymus. WHO, International histologic classification of tumors. Berlin, Springer Verlag, 1999, p 65.

342. Chalabreysse L, Roy P, Cordier JF, et al: Correlation of the WHO schema for the classification of thymic epithelial neoplasms with prognosis: A retrospective study of 90 tumors. Am J Surg Pathol 2002;26(12):1605-1611.

343. Masaoka A, Monden Y, Nakahara K, et al: Follow-up study of thymomas with special reference to their clinical stages. Cancer 1981;48(11):2485-2492.

344. Okumura M, Ohta M, Tateyama H, et al: The World Health Organization histologic classification system reflects the oncologic behavior of thymoma: A clinical study of 273 patients. Cancer 2002;94(3):624-632.

345. Blumberg D, Port JL, Weksler B, et al: Thymoma: A multivariate analysis of factors predicting survival. Ann Thorac Surg 1995;60(4):908-913; discussion 914.

346. Regnard JF, Magdeleinat P, Dromer C, et al: Prognostic factors and long-term results after thymoma resection: A series of 307 patients. J Thorac Cardiovasc Surg 1996;112(2):376-384.

347. Okumura M, Miyoshi S, Takeuchi Y, et al: Results of surgical treatment of thymomas with special reference to the involved organs. J Thorac Cardiovasc Surg 1999;117(3):605-613.

348. Gripp S, Hilgers K, Wurm R, et al: Thymoma: Prognostic factors and treatment outcomes. Cancer 1998;83(8):1495-1503.

349. Thomas CR, Wright CD, Loehrer PJ: Thymoma: State of the art. J Clin Oncol 1999;17(7):2280-2289.

350. Patterson GA: Thymomas. Semin Thorac Cardiovasc Surg 1992;4(1):39-44.

351. Engels EA, Pfeiffer RM: Malignant thymoma in the United States: Demographic patterns in incidence and associations with subsequent malignancies. Int J Cancer 2003;105(4):546-551.

352. Spigland N, Di Lorenzo M, Youssef S, et al: Malignant thymoma in children: A 20-year review. J Pediatr Surg 1990;25(11):1143-1146.

353. Souadjian JV, Enriquez P, Silverstein MN, et al: The spectrum of diseases associated with thymoma. Coincidence or syndrome? Arch Intern Med 1974;134(2):374-379.

354. Drachman DB: Myasthenia gravis (second of two parts). N Engl J Med 1978;298(4):186-193.

355. Monden Y, Uyama T, Taniki T, et al: The characteristics of thymoma with myasthenia gravis: A 28-year experience. J Surg Oncol 1988;38(3):151-154.

356. Gerein AN, Srivastava SP, Burgess J: Thymoma: A ten year review. Am J Surg 1978;136(1):49-53.

357. Sassa K, Mizushima Y, Kusajima Y, et al: Clinical study on thymoma: Assessment of prognostic factors. Anticancer Res 1996;16(6B):3895-3900.

358. Quintanilla-Martinez L, Wilkins EW Jr, Ferry JA, et al: Thymoma—morphologic subclassification correlates with invasiveness and immunohistologic features: A study of 122 cases. Hum Pathol 1993;24(9):958-969.

359. Somnier FE, Trojaborg W: Neurophysiological evaluation in myasthenia gravis. A comprehensive study of a complete patient population. Electroencephalogr Clin Neurophysiol 1993;89(2):73-87.

360. Beekman R, Kuks JB, Oosterhuis HJ: Myasthenia gravis: Diagnosis and follow-up of 100 consecutive patients. J Neurol 1997;244(2):112-118.

361. Palmisani MT, Evoli A, Batocchi AP, et al: Myasthenia gravis associated with thymoma: Clinical characteristics and long-term outcome. Eur Neurol 1994;34(2):78-82.

362. Masaoka A, Yamakawa Y, Niwa H, et al: Extended thymectomy for myasthenia gravis patients: A 20-year review. Ann Thorac Surg 1996;62(3):853-859.

363. Blossom GB, Ernstoff RM, Howells GA, et al: Thymectomy for myasthenia gravis. Arch Surg 1993;128(8):855-862.

364. Rosenberg M, Jauregui WO, De Vega ME, et al: Recurrence of thymic hyperplasia after thymectomy in myasthenia gravis. Its importance as a cause of failure of surgical treatment. Am J Med 1983;74(1):78-82.

365. Bailey RO, Dunn HG, Rubin AM, et al: Myasthenia gravis with thymoma and pure red blood cell aplasia. Am J Clin Pathol 1988;89(5):687-693.

366. Rogers BH, Manligod JR, Blazek WV: Thymoma associated with pancytopenia and hypogammaglobulinemia. Report of a case and review of the literature. Am J Med 1968;44(1):154-164.

367. Bergh NP, Gatzinsky P, Larsson S, et al: Tumors of the thymus and thymic region: I Clinicopathological studies on thymomas. Ann Thorac Surg 1978;25(2):91-98.

368. Maggi G, Casadio C, Cavallo A, et al: Thymoma: Results of 241 operated cases. Ann Thorac Surg 1991;51(1):152-156.

369. Penn CR, Hope-Stone HF: The role of radiotherapy in the management of malignant thymoma. Br J Surg 1972;59(7):533-539.

370. Phillips TL, Buschke F: The role of radiation therapy in myasthenia gravis. Calif Med 1967;106(4):282-289.

371. Boston B: Chemotherapy of invasive thymoma. Cancer 1976;38(1):49-52.

372. Loehrer PJ, Wang W, Ettinger DS, et al: Phase II study of octreotide treatment in advanced or recurrent thymic malignancies. An Eastern Cooperative Oncology Group Study. Proc Am Soc Clin Oncol 2002;21:295a.

373. Bonomi PD, Finkelstein D, Aisner S, et al: EST 2582 phase II trial of cisplatin in metastatic or recurrent thymoma. Am J Clin Oncol 1993;16(4):342-345.

374. Highley MS, Underhill CR, Parnis FX, et al: Treatment of invasive thymoma with single-agent ifosfamide. J Clin Oncol 1999;17(9):2737-2744.

375. Almog C, Horowitz M, Burke M: Steroid therapy in inappropriate secretion of antidiuretic hormone due to malignant thymoma. Respiration 1983;44(5):382-386.

376. Loehrer PJ Sr, Kim K, Aisner SC, et al: Cisplatin plus doxorubicin

plus cyclophosphamide in metastatic or recurrent thymoma: Final results of an intergroup trial. The Eastern Cooperative Oncology Group, Southwest Oncology Group, and Southeastern Cancer Study Group. J Clin Oncol 1994;12(6):1164-1168.

377. Loehrer PJ Sr, Jiroutek M, Aisner S, et al: Combined etoposide, ifosfamide, and cisplatin in the treatment of patients with advanced thymoma and thymic carcinoma: An intergroup trial. Cancer 2001;91(11):2010-2015.

378. Loehrer PJ Sr, Chen M, Kim K, et al: Cisplatin, doxorubicin, and cyclophosphamide plus thoracic radiation therapy for limited-stage unresectable thymoma: An intergroup trial. J Clin Oncol 1997;15(9):3093-3099.

379. Fornasiero A, Daniele O, Ghiotto C, et al: Chemotherapy for invasive thymoma. A 13-year experience. Cancer 1991;68(1):30-33.

380. Park HS, Shin DM, Lee JS, et al: Thymoma. A retrospective study of 87 cases. Cancer 1994;73(10):2491-2498.

381. Giaccone G, Ardizzoni A, Kirkpatrick A, et al: Cisplatin and etoposide combination chemotherapy for locally advanced or metastatic thymoma. A phase II study of the European Organization for Research and Treatment of Cancer Lung Cancer Cooperative Group. J Clin Oncol 1996;14(3):814-820.

382. Palmieri G, Montella L, Martignetti A, et al: Somatostatin analogs and prednisone in advanced refractory thymic tumors. Cancer 2002;94(5):1414-1420.

383. Walker AN, Mills SE, Fechner RE: Thymomas and thymic carcinomas. Semin Diagn Pathol 1990;7(4):250-265.

384. Ritter JH, Wick MR: Primary carcinomas of the thymus gland. Semin Diagn Pathol 1999;16(1):18-31.

385. Chung DA: Thymic carcinoma—analysis of nineteen clinico-pathological studies. Thorac Cardiovasc Surg 2000;48(2):114-119.

386. Hishima T, Fukayama M, Fujisawa M, et al: CD5 expression in thymic carcinoma. Am J Pathol 1994;145(2):268-275.

387. Suster S, Rosai J: Thymic carcinoma. A clinicopathologic study of 60 cases. Cancer 1991;67(4):1025-1032.

388. Wick MR, Scheithauer BW, Weiland LH, et al: Primary thymic carcinomas. Am J Surg Pathol 1982;6(7):613-630.

389. Leyvraz S, Henle W, Chahinian AP, et al: Association of Epstein-Barr virus with thymic carcinoma. N Engl J Med 1985;312(20):1296-1299.

390. Lee JD, Choe KO, Kim SJ, et al: CT findings in primary thymic carcinoma. J Comput Assist Tomogr 1991;15(3):429-433.

391. Thomas CR Jr, Bonomi P: Mediastinal tumors. Curr Opin Oncol 1990;2(2):359-367.

392. Salyer WR, Salyer DC, Eggleston JC: Carcinoid tumors of the thymus. Cancer 1976;37(2):958-973.

393. Wick MR, Carney JA, Bernatz PE, et al: Primary mediastinal carcinoid tumors. Am J Surg Pathol 1982;6(3):195-205.

394. Wick MR, Scheithauer BW: Thymic carcinoid. A histologic, immunohistochemical, and ultrastructural study of 12 cases. Cancer 1984;53(3):475-484.

395. Gartner LA, ML Voorhess: Adrenocorticotropic hormone—producing thymic carcinoid in a teenager. Cancer 1993;71(1):106-111.

396. Aniszewski JP, Young WF Jr, Thompson GB, et al: Cushing syndrome due to ectopic adrenocorticotropic hormone secretion. World J Surg 2001;25(7):934-940.

397. Doppman JL, Pass HI, Nieman LK, et al: Corticotropin-secreting carcinoid tumors of the thymus: Diagnostic unreliability of thymic venous sampling. Radiology 1992;184(1):71-74.

398. Moran CA, and Suster S: Neuroendocrine carcinomas (carcinoid tumor) of the thymus. A clinicopathologic analysis of 80 cases. Am J Clin Pathol 2000;114(1):100-110.

399. Davis RD Jr, Oldham HN Jr, Sabiston DC Jr: Primary cysts and neoplasms of the mediastinum: Recent changes in clinical presentation, methods of diagnosis, management, and results. Ann Thorac Surg 1987;44(3):229-237.

400. Prym P: Spontanheilung lines bosartigen, wahscheinlich chorionephitheliomatosen gewach in laden. Virchows Arch A Pathol Anat Histopathol 1927;265:239.

401. Luna MA, Valenzuela-Tamariz J: Germ-cell tumors of the mediastinum, postmortem findings. Am J Clin Pathol 1976;65(4):450-454.

402. Lynch MJG, Blewett GL: Choriocarcinoma arising in the male mediastinum. Thorax 1953;8:157.

403. Hainsworth JD, Greco FA: Extragonadal germ cell tumors and unrecognized germ cell tumors. Semin Oncol 1992;19(2):119-127.

404. Friedman NB: The function of the primordial germ cell in extragonadal tissues. Int J Androl 1987;10(1):43-49.

405. Collins D, Pugh R: Classification and frequency of testicular tumors. Br J Urol 1964;36:11.

406. Kuhn MW, Weissbach L: Localization, incidence, diagnosis and treatment of extratesticular germ cell tumors. Urol Int 1985;40(3):166-172.

407. Martini N, Golbey RB, Hajdu SI, et al: Primary mediastinal germ cell tumors. Cancer 1974;33(3):763-769.

408. Nichols CR, Heerema NA, Palmer C, et al: Klinefelter's syndrome associated with mediastinal germ cell neoplasms. J Clin Oncol 1987;5(8):1290-1294.

409. Dexeus FH, Logothetis CJ, Chong C, et al: Genetic abnormalities in men with germ cell tumors. J Urol 1988;140(1):80-84.

410. Chariot P, Monnet I, LeLong F, et al: Systemic mast cell disease associated with primary mediastinal germ cell tumor. Am J Med 1991;90(3):381-385.

411. Nichols CR, Roth BJ, Heerema N, et al: Hematologic neoplasia associated with primary mediastinal germ-cell tumors. N Engl J Med 1990;322(20):1425-1429.

412. Dehner LP: Gonadal and extragonadal germ cell neoplasia of childhood. Hum Pathol 1983;14(6):493-511.

413. Lewis BD, Hurt RD, Payne WS, et al: Benign teratomas of the mediastinum. J Thorac Cardiovasc Surg 1983;86(5):727-731.

414. Knapp RH, Hurt RD, Payne WS, et al: Malignant germ cell tumors of the mediastinum. J Thorac Cardiovasc Surg 1985;89(1):82-89.

415. Nichols CR, Fox EP: Extragonadal and pediatric germ cell tumors. Hematol Oncol Clin North Am 1991;5(6):1189-1209.

416. Kiffer JD, Sandeman TF: Primary malignant mediastinal germ cell tumors: A study of eleven cases and a review of the literature. Int J Radiat Oncol Biol Phys 1989;17(4):835-841.

417. Kiffer JD, Sandeman TF: Primary malignant mediastinal germ cell tumours: A literature review and a study of 18 cases. Australas Radiol 1999;43(1):58-68.

418. Schultz SM, Einhorn LH, Conces DJ Jr, et al: Management of postchemotherapy residual mass in patients with advanced seminoma: Indiana University experience. J Clin Oncol 1989;7(10):1497-1503.

419. Mukherjee AB, Murty VV, Rodriguez E, et al: Detection and analysis of origin of i(12p), a diagnostic marker of human male germ cell tumors, by fluorescence in situ hybridization. Genes Chromosomes Cancer 1991;3(4):300-307.

420. Ilson DH, Motzer RJ, Rodriguez E, et al: Genetic analysis in the diagnosis of neoplasms of unknown primary tumor site. Semin Oncol 1993;20(3):229-237.

421. Wychulis AR, Payne WS, Clagett OT, et al: Surgical treatment of mediastinal tumors: A 40 year experience. J Thorac Cardiovasc Surg 1971;62(3):379-392.

422. Aygun C, Slawson RG, Bajaj K, et al: Primary mediastinal seminoma. Urology 1984;23(2):109-117.

423. Lemarie E, Assouline PS, Diot P, et al: Primary mediastinal germ cell tumors. Results of a French retrospective study. Chest 1992;102(5):1477-1483.

424. Giaccone G: Multimodality treatment of malignant germ cell tumours of the mediastinum. Eur J Cancer 1991;27(3):273-277.

425. Nichols CR: Mediastinal germ cell tumors. Clinical features and biologic correlates. Chest 1991;99(2):472-479.

426. Daugaard G, Rorth M, Hansen HH: Therapy of extragonadal germ-cell tumors. Eur J Cancer Clin Oncol 1983;19(7):895-899.

427. Einhorn LH, Donohue J: Cis-diamminedichloroplatinum, vinblastine, and bleomycin combination chemotherapy in disseminated testicular cancer. Ann Intern Med 1977;87(3):293-298.

428. Toner GC, Geller NL, Lin SY, et al: Extragonadal and poor risk nonseminomatous germ cell tumors. Survival and prognostic features. Cancer 1991;67(8):2049-2057.

429. Nichols CR, Saxman S, Williams SD, et al: Primary mediastinal nonseminomatous germ cell tumors. A modern single institution experience. Cancer 1990;65(7):1641-1646.

430. Harvey JC, Fleischman EH, Applebaum H: Resection of residual mediastinal germ cell masses with the Cavitron ultrasonic surgical aspirator. J Thorac Cardiovasc Surg 1991;102(3):425-426.

431. Broun ER, Nichols CR, Mandanas R, et al: Dose escalation study of high-dose carboplatin and etoposide with autologous bone marrow support in patients with recurrent and refractory germ cell tumors. Bone Marrow Transplant 1995;16(3):353-358.

432. Bokemeyer C, Hartmann JT, Fossa SD, et al: Extragonadal germ cell tumors: Relation to testicular neoplasia and management options. Apmis 2003;111(1):49-59; discussion 59-63.

433. Strickler JG, Kurtin PJ: Mediastinal lymphoma. Semin Diagn Pathol 1991;8(1):2-13.

434. Hopper KD, Diehl LF, Lesar M, et al: Hodgkin disease: Clinical utility of CT in initial staging and treatment. Radiology 1988;169(1):17-22.

435. Johnson DW, Hoppe RT, Cox RS, et al: Hodgkin's disease limited to intrathoracic sites. Cancer 1983;52(1):8-13.

436. Prakash UB, Abel MD, Hubmayr RD: Mediastinal mass and tracheal obstruction during general anesthesia. Mayo Clin Proc 1988;63(10):1004-1011.

437. Wiernik PH, Slawson RG: Hodgkin's disease with direct extension into pulmonary parenchyma from a mediastinal mass: A presentation requiring special therapeutic considerations. Cancer Treat Rep 1982;66(4):711-716.

438. Hagemeister FB, Fesus SM, Lamki LM, et al: Role of the gallium scan in Hodgkin's disease. Cancer 1990;65(5):1090-1096.

439. Cooper DL, Caride VJ, Zloty M, et al: Gallium scans in patients with mediastinal Hodgkin's disease treated with chemotherapy. J Clin Oncol 1993;11(6):1092-1098.

440. O'Doherty MJ, Macdonald EA, Barrington SF, et al: Positron emission tomography in the management of lymphomas. Clin Oncol (R Coll Radiol) 2002;14(5):415-426.

441. Adkins RB Jr, Maples MD, Hainsworth JD: Primary malignant mediastinal tumors. Ann Thorac Surg 1984;38(6):648-659.

442. Levitt LJ, Aisenberg AC, Harris NL, et al: Primary non-Hodgkin's lymphoma of the mediastinum. Cancer 1982;50(11):2486-2492.

443. al-Sharabati M, Chittal S, Duga-Neulat I, et al: Primary anterior mediastinal B-cell lymphoma. A clinicopathologic and immuno-histochemical study of 16 cases. Cancer 1991;67(10):2579-2587.

444. Kirn D, Mauch P, Shaffer K, et al: Large-cell and immunoblastic lymphoma of the mediastinum: Prognostic features and treatment outcome in 57 patients. J Clin Oncol 1993;11(7):1336-1343.

445. Braziel RM, Keneklis T, Donlon JA, et al: Terminal deoxynucleotidyl transferase in non-Hodgkin's lymphoma. Am J Clin Pathol 1983;80(5):655-659.

446. Coleman CN, Cohen JR, Burke JS, et al: Lymphoblastic lymphoma in adults: Results of a pilot protocol. Blood 1981;57(4):679-684.

447. Weinstein HJ, Cassady JR, Levey R: Long-term results of the APO protocol (vincristine, doxorubicin [adriamycin], and prednisone) for treatment of mediastinal lymphoblastic lymphoma. J Clin Oncol 1983;1(9):537-541.

448. Magrath IT, Janus C, Edwards BK, et al: An effective therapy for both undifferentiated (including Burkitt's) lymphomas and lymphoblastic lymphomas in children and young adults. Blood 1984;63(5):1102-1111.

449. Levine AM, Forman SJ, Meyer PR, et al: Successful therapy of convoluted T-lymphoblastic lymphoma in the adult. Blood 1983;61(1):92-98.

450. McAllister HA Jr: Primary tumors of the heart and pericardium. Pathol Annu 1979;14 Pt 2:325-355.

451. Chen HZ, Jiang L, Rong WH, et al: Tumors of the heart. An analysis of 79 cases. Chin Med J (Engl) 1992;105(2):153-158.

452. Choh JH, Gurney R, Shenoy SS, et al: Renal-cell carcinoma; removal of intracardiac extension with aid of cardiopulmonary bypass. N Y State J Med 1981;81(6):929-932.

453. Harvey WP: Clinical aspects of cardiac tumors. Am J Cardiol 1968;21(3):328-343.

454. Wann LS, Sampson C, Liu Y: Cardiac and paracardiac masses: Complementary role of echocardiography and magnetic resonance imaging. Echocardiography 1998;15(2):139-146.

455. Poole-Wilson PA, Farnsworth A, Braimbridge MV, et al: Angiosarcoma of pericardium. Problems in diagnosis and management. Br Heart J 1976;38(3):240-243.

456. Glancy DL, Morales JB Jr, Roberts WC: Angiosarcoma of the heart. Am J Cardiol 1968;21(3):413-419.

457. Poole GV Jr, Meredith JW, Breyer RH, et al: Surgical implications in malignant cardiac disease. Ann Thorac Surg 1983;36(4):484-491.

458. Eker R, Cantez T, Dogan O, et al: Pericardial mesothelioma. A pediatric case report. Turk J Pediatr 1989;31(4):305-309.

459. Taguchi T, Fujiwara Y, Ichiki H, et al: A case of malignant pericardial mesothelioma detected by gallium-67 scintigraphy. Kaku Igaku 1991;28(3):281-284.

460. Aggarwal P, Wali JP, Agarwal J: Pericardial mesothelioma presenting as a mediastinal mass. Singapore Med J 1991;32(3):185-186.

461. Pascual MA, Povar J, Munoz JR, et al: Pericardial mesothelioma: Apropos of a case. Rev Esp Cardiol 1989;42(8):559-561.

462. Dai RP: Primary pericardial mesothelioma: A report of four cases. Zhonghua Fang She Xue Za Zhi 1989;23(2):90-92.

463. Gurevich MA, Odinokova VA, Smirnov VB, et al: Clinico-morphological characteristics of pericardial mesothelioma. Sov Med 1991(1):8-11.

464. Torii T, Takasuga H, Mizushima M, et al: Primary malignant mesothelioma of the pericardium masquerading as malignant pleural mesothelioma: Report of an autopsy case and review of the reported cases in Japan as to its invasion to neighboring organs. Kokyu To Junkan 1989;37(9):1027-1032.

465. Carachi R, Campbell PE, Kent M: Thoracic neural crest tumors. A clinical review. Cancer 1983;51(5):949-954.

466. Hashimoto H, Enjoji M, Nakajima T, et al: Malignant neuroepithelioma (peripheral neuroblastoma). A clinicopathologic study of 15 cases. Am J Surg Pathol 1983;7(4):309-318.

467. Shimada H, Newton WA Jr, Soule EH, et al: Pathologic features of extraosseous Ewing's sarcoma: A report from the Intergroup Rhabdomyosarcoma Study. Hum Pathol 1988;19(4):442-453.

468. Weidner N, Tjoe J: Immunohistochemical profile of monoclonal antibody O13: Antibody that recognizes glycoprotein p30/32MIC2 and is useful in diagnosing Ewing's sarcoma and peripheral neuroepithelioma. Am J Surg Pathol 1994;18(5):486-494.

469. Triche TJ, Tsokos M, Linnoila RI, et al: NSE in neuroblastoma and other round cell tumors of childhood. Prog Clin Biol Res 1985;175:295-317.

470. Whang-Peng J, Triche TJ, Knutsen T, et al: Chromosome translocation in peripheral neuroepithelioma. N Engl J Med 1984;311(9):584-585.

471. Thiele CJ, McKeon C, Triche TJ, et al: Differential protooncogene expression characterizes histopathologically indistinguishable tumors of the peripheral nervous system. J Clin Invest 1987;80(3):804-811.

472. Kumar S, Pack S, Kumar D, et al: Detection of EWS-FLI-1 fusion in Ewing's sarcoma/peripheral primitive neuroectodermal tumor by fluorescence in situ hybridization using formalin-fixed paraffin-embedded tissue. Hum Pathol 1999;30(3):324-330.

473. Askin FB, Rosai J, Sibley RK, et al: Malignant small cell tumor of the thoracopulmonary region in childhood: A distinctive clinicopathologic entity of uncertain histogenesis. Cancer 1979;43(6):2438-2451.

474. Gonzalez-Crussi F, Wolfson SL, Misugi K, et al: Peripheral neuroectodermal tumors of the chest wall in childhood. Cancer 1984;54(11):2519-2527.

475. Miser JS, Steis RS, Longo DL, et al: Treatment of newly diagnosed high risk sarcoma and primitive neuroectodermal tumors (PNET) in children and young adults. Proc Am Soc Clin Oncol 1985;4:240.

476. Miser JS, Kinsella TJ, Triche TJ, et al: Treatment of peripheral neuroepithelioma in children and young adults. J Clin Oncol 1987;5(11):1752-1758.

477. Nagashima Y, Miyagi Y, Tanaka Y, et al: Adult ganglioneuroblastoma of the anterior mediastinum. Pathol Res Pract 1997;193(10):727-732; discussion 733.

478. Tateishi U, Hasegawa T, Makimoto A, et al: Adult neuroblastoma: Radiologic and clinicopathologic features. J Comput Assist Tomogr 2003;27(3):321-326.

479. Prece V, Bertagni A, Gallinaro L, et al: Neurogenic tumors of the mediastinum. Ann Ital Chir 2002;73(2):125-127.

480. Shields TW, Reynolds M: Neurogenic tumors of the thorax. Surg Clin North Am 1988;68(3):645-668.

481. Pizzo PA, Poplack DG: Principles and Practice of Pediatric Oncology, 4th ed. Philadelphia, Lippincott Williams & Wilkins, 2002, p 1692.

482. Grosfeld JL, Baehner RL: Neuroblastoma: an analysis of 160 cases. World J Surg 1980;4(1):29-37.

483. Schwab M, Alitalo K, Klempnauer KH, et al: Amplified DNA with limited homology to myc cellular oncogene is shared by human neuroblastoma cell lines and a neuroblastoma tumour. Nature 1983;305(5931):245–248.

484. Brodeur GM, Seeger RC, Schwab M, et al: Amplification of N-myc in untreated human neuroblastomas correlates with advanced disease stage. Science 1984;224(4653):1121–1124.

485. Brodeur GM: Neuroblastoma—clinical applications of molecular parameters. Brain Pathol 1990;1(1):47–54.

486. Vinken PJ, Bruyn GW: The Phakomatoses. Handbook of Clinical Neurology, vol 14. Amsterdam, North-Holland, 1973, p 821.

487. Lloyd RV, Shapiro B, Sisson JC, et al: An immunohistochemical study of pheochromocytomas. Arch Pathol Lab Med 1984;108(7):541–544.

488. Tannenbaum M: Ultrastructural pathology of adrenal medullary tumors. Pathol Annu 1970;5:145–171.

489. Lack EE: Pathology of Adrenal and Extra-adrenal Paraganglia. Major Problems in Pathology, vol 29. Philadelphia, WB Saunders, 1994, p 405.

490. Lack EE: Pathology of the Adrenal Glands. Contemporary Issues in Surgical Pathology, vol 14. New York, Churchill Livingstone, 1990, p 389.

491. Neville AM: The Adrenal Medulla. In Symington T (ed): Functional Pathology of the Human Adrenal Gland. Baltimore, Williams & Wilkens, 1969, pp 217–289.

492. Scott HW Jr, Reynolds V, Green N, et al: Clinical experience with malignant pheochromocytomas. Surg Gynecol Obstet 1982;154(6):801–818.

493. Fischer M, Vetter W, Winterberg B, et al: 131I-metaiodobenzylguanidine—a new agent for scintigraphic imaging and treatment of pheochromocytoma. Nuklearmedizin 1984;23(2):77–79.

494. Hamilton BP, Cheikh IE, Rivera LE: Attempted treatment of inoperable pheochromocytoma with streptozocin. Arch Intern Med 1977;137(6):762–765.

495. Feldman JM: Treatment of metastatic pheochromocytoma with streptozocin. Arch Intern Med 1983;143(9):1799–1800.

496. Keiser HR, Goldstein DS, Wade JL, et al: Treatment of malignant pheochromocytoma with combination chemotherapy. Hypertension 1985;7(3 Pt 2):118–124.

497. Shapiro B, Sisson JC, Shulkin BL, et al: The current status of radioiodinated metaiodobenzylguanidine therapy of neuro-endocrine tumors. Q J Nucl Med 1995;39 (4 suppl 1):55–57.

498. Brasfield RD, Das Gupta TK: Von Recklinghausen's disease: A clinicopathological study. Ann Surg 1972;175(1):86–104.

499. Bigner DD, McLendon RE, Bruner JM, et al: Russell and Rubinstein's Pathology of Tumors of the Nervous System, 6th ed. London, Oxford University Press, 1998.

500. Izumi AK, Rosato FE, Wood MG: Von Recklinghausen's disease associated with multiple neurolemomas. Arch Dermatol 1971;104(2):172–176.

501. Gautam HP: Pulmonary neurilemmoma. Br J Dis Chest 1970;64(3):176–178.

502. Gale AW, Jelihovsky T, Grant AF, et al: Neurogenic tumors of the mediastinum. Ann Thorac Surg 1974;17(5):434–443.

503. Fletcher CD: Solitary circumscribed neuroma of the skin (so-called palisaded, encapsulated neuroma). A clinicopathologic and immunohistochemical study. Am J Surg Pathol 1989;13(7):574–580.

504. Maiuri F, Donzelli R, Benvenuti D, et al: Schwannomas of the brachial plexus—diagnostic and surgical problems. Zentralbl Neurochir 2001;62(3):93–97.

505. Ducatman BS, Scheithauer BW, Piepgras DG, et al: Malignant peripheral nerve sheath tumors. A clinicopathologic study of 120 cases. Cancer 1986;57(10):2006–2021.

506. Sordillo PP, Helson L, Hajdu SI, et al: Malignant schwannoma—clinical characteristics, survival, and response to therapy. Cancer 1981;47(10):2503–2509.

507. Bojsen-Moller M, Myhre-Jensen O: A consecutive series of 30 malignant schwannomas. Survival in relation to clinico-pathological parameters and treatment. Acta Pathol Microbiol Immunol Scand 1984;92(3):147–155.

508. Sakai F, Sone S, Kiyono K, et al: Intrathoracic neurogenic tumors: MR-pathologic correlation. Am J Roentgenol 1992;159(2): 279–283.

509. Meis JM, Enzinger FM, Martz KL, et al: Malignant peripheral nerve sheath tumors (malignant schwannomas) in children. Am J Surg Pathol 1992;16(7):694–707.

510. Nambisan RN, Rao U, Moore R, et al: Malignant soft tissue tumors of nerve sheath origin. J Surg Oncol 1984;25(4):268–272.

511. Goldman RL, Jones SE, Heusinkveld RS: Combination chemotherapy of metastatic malignant schwannoma with vincristine, adriamycin, cyclophosphamide, and imidazole carboxamide: A case report. Cancer 1977;39(5):1955–1958.

512. Auersperg M, Us-Krasovec M, Zorc R, et al: Effectiveness of Novantrome and vinblastine in malignant schwannnoma. Proc. 4th Int Conf Adv Regional Can Ther, Berchtesgarten, FRG, Cyanamid-Lederle, 1989.

513. D'Agostino AN, Soule EH, Miller RH: Sarcomas of the peripheral nerves and somatic soft tissues associated with multiple neurofibromatosis. Cancer 1963;16:1015.

514. Thomas JV, Schwartz PL, Gragoudas ES: Von Hippel's disease in association with von Recklinghausen's neurofibromatosis. Br J Ophthalmol 1978;62(9):604–608.

515. Williams GD, Hoffman S, Schwartz IS: Malignant transformation in a plexiform neurofibroma of the median nerve. J Hand Surg 1984;9(4):583–587.

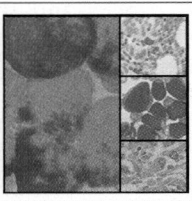

77

CANCER OF THE ESOPHAGUS

Lawrence R. Kleinberg

Arlene A. Forastiere

Richard F. Heitmiller

SUMMARY OF KEY POINTS

CLASSIFICATION
- Esophageal cancer is subdivided into the following four groups: epithelial tumors, metastatic tumors, lymphomas, and sarcomas.
- Cancers of epithelial origin, predominantly squamous cell and adenocarcinomas, are the most common, and other histologic types are rare.

INCIDENCE
- Within the United States, the incidence of esophageal cancer, in persons younger than 80 years, is 3.2 per 100,000 persons.
- Overall, the incidence is only slowly increasing; historically and internationally, squamous cell tumors are the most common histologic type; however, a dramatic increase in the prevalence of adenocarcinoma has been documented in the United States, United Kingdom, and western Europe.

PATHOGENESIS
- Exact etiology is unknown.
- The data support the hypothesis that epithelial tumors arise as a result of chronic irritation from a wide variety of sources, including gastric contents in chronic reflux and known carcinogens.
- A strong association of Barrett's esophagus and adenocarcinoma is

seen, but a benefit to screening endoscopy for those at risk for or with known Barrett's esophagus is unknown.

DIAGNOSIS AND STAGING
- Symptoms and demographics will strongly suggest the diagnosis.
- Endoscopy is the best screening examination.
- Diagnosis is made by endoscopy with cytology and biopsy of tumor.
- Transesophageal ultrasound can be used to assess T and N stage to guide optimal definitive therapy.
- Computed tomography (CT) of chest and abdomen is the best initial staging examination.
- Positron emission tomography (PET) scan may be useful in detecting additional cases of metastatic disease before costly and toxic definitive therapy.
- Additional studies include laparoscopy, thoracoscopy, bone scan, and CT of the brain when indicated by clinical circumstances.

TREATMENT
- Treatment of premalignant dysplasia is guided by grade of histology. Low-grade dysplasia should be closely followed by endoscopy. High-grade dysplasia is treated with esophagectomy, although close follow-up or endoscopic treatments may be appropriate for selected patients.

- Selection of appropriate treatment for carcinoma depends on tumor stage and patient performance status.
- Surgery is the best single-modality therapy for patients with localized disease (T1-3N0-1M0-1a).
- Combined chemoradiation leads to prolonged median survival and long-term survival compared with radiation alone, at the price of increased toxicity. This represents a potentially curative alternative to surgery and is appropriate for most unresectable T4NanyM0 lesions.
- Accumulating evidence suggests that combination therapy with neoadjuvant chemoradiation or chemotherapy followed by surgery may increase survival compared with surgery alone.
- Postoperative adjuvant chemotherapy or chemoradiation is less well studied.
- Endoscopic palliative therapy includes laser or electrical fulguration, photodynamic therapy (PDT), or stenting.
- Radiation therapy, with or without chemotherapy, may be used to palliate local symptoms.
- Chemotherapy may be used for metastatic disease, but response and duration of response are modest for most patients.

INTRODUCTION

Carcinoma of the esophagus is a devastating disease because of its poor survival outcome even with therapy, and because of its adverse affect on swallowing and therefore on the patient's quality of life. Although esophageal cancer continues to be an aggressive malignancy that usually is first seen in a locally advanced stage, significant progress has been made in the treatment

of this disease, including increased treatment options, decreased surgical morbidity and mortality, the development of more effective chemotherapies, and improvements in identifying patients at risk. These advances are resulting in incremental improvements in outcome, but considerable controversy remains about optimal management under individual scenarios. The emphasis of this chapter is on selecting the appropriate options in the curative and palliative management of esophageal cancer.

CLASSIFICATION AND LOCATION

A classification of esophageal cancers and the more frequent locations are presented here, because this information has a direct impact on the diagnosis and management of patients. Malignant esophageal cancer (Table 77-1) is classified based on histologic appearance and cellular origin, as follows: (1) epithelial tumors, (2) metastatic tumors, (3) lymphomas, and (4) sarcomas. Cancers of epithelial cell origin, predominantly squamous cell and adenocarcinomas, are the most common.

Squamous cell cancers usually occur in the middle third of the esophagus. In a collective review of more than 28,000 cases of squamous cell cancers, Postlethwait[1] estimated the ratio of upper, middle, and lower cancers to be 15:50:35, respectively. Adenocarcinomas, conversely, are most common in the lower third of the esophagus. In a collective review of 4783 cases of esophageal adenocarcinoma, Ming[2] noted an upper esophageal location in 4%, middle in 18%, and lower in 67%. Small cell cancers occur with equal frequency in the middle and lower thirds, with the upper third involved in fewer than 5% of cases.[3] Both malignant melanoma and choriocarcinoma, although rare, seem to be most common in the lower third. Esophageal sarcomas may occur anywhere along the esophagus.[4] No specific pattern of occurrence has been reported for patients with esophageal lymphomas or metastases.

INCIDENCE

Tumors of the esophagus other than squamous cell and adenocarcinoma are very rare. This chapter, therefore, focuses on the incidence of the more common esophageal squamous cell and adenocarcinomas. Epidemiologic data show that the incidence of esophageal cancer varies considerably from one country to another and often within a single country.[5] Such data emphasize the multi-factorial etiologies of esophageal cancer and the difficulties in determining trends in worldwide incidence. In many Western nations, including the United States, a growing number of studies document an increasing incidence of esophageal adenocarcinoma.[6,7] Yang and Davis[6] demonstrated a 74% increase in esophageal adenocarcinoma in white males between 1973 and 1982. In the same time interval, the authors showed no increase in squamous cell tumors in white males, and only a 30% increase in squamous cell cancers in black men and women. Pera and colleagues[8] reported a significant increase in the incidence of both esophageal and esophagogastric junction adenocarcinomas in Olmstead County, Minnesota. By contrast, during the same observation period, the incidence of esophageal squamous cell cancers actually decreased. Blot and associates[9] reported that the incidence of esophageal and esophagogastric adenocarcinoma between 1976 and 1987 increased at a rate exceeding that of skin melanoma, non-Hodgkin's lymphoma, and lung cancer. During the same study period, the incidence of squamous cancers remained unchanged. Vizcaino and coworkers[10] found that the incidence of adenocarcinoma of the esophagus in white males increased 8.6% per year on average from 1973 to 1995, whereas squamous cell carcinoma decreased at 1.5% per year. In African American males, the figures were 4.1% and –0.6%, respectively. Over this period, the incidence of adenocarcinoma was 1.5/100,000 in white men, 0.4/100,000 in African American men 0.3/100,000 in white women, and 0.1/100,000 in African American women. A similar increase in incidence of esophageal and esophagogastric adenocarcinoma was reported in the United Kingdom[11] and Western Europe.[12] The trend toward increased incidence of adenocarcinoma in Western nations has continued through the subsequent decade,[10,13] in marked contrast to the continued decrease in the incidence of adenocarcinoma of the noncardia areas of the stomach.

Heitmiller and Sharma[14] reviewed the prevalence of esophageal carcinoma at the Johns Hopkins Hospital from 1959 to 1994. They found that squamous cell cancers were the most common cell type overall. Adenocarcinoma, rare before 1978, began to increase in prevalence in 1979 and in 1992 and eventually exceeded the prevalence of squamous tumors. Adenocarcinoma continues to be the most common esophageal cancer at our institution and other tertiary care centers. Squamous cell cancers occur with equal frequency in white and black patients in this study, although some epidemiologic data suggest it may still occur more frequently in black men nationwide. The prevalence of squamous cell cancer in women has been steadily increasing since 1978 to 1979, perhaps because of tobacco-use patterns. The cause of this remarkable shift in esophageal cell type predominance to adenocarcinoma, occurring predominantly in white males, has yet to be determined. It cannot be explained simply on the basis of smoking and alcohol consumption habits. A proven association of esophageal adenocarcinoma and Barrett's esophagus (BE) exists in individuals with gastroesophageal reflux disease (GERD). However, many important issues remain unresolved, such as why

TABLE 77-1

Classification of Esophageal Cancer

Epithelial

Squamous cell
  Ordinary squamous cell
  Verrucous squamous cell
  Spindle cell (carcinosarcoma)
Adenocarcinoma
  Ordinary
  Adenoacanthoma
  Mucoepidermoid
  Adenoid cystic
Small cell
Melanoma
Choriocarcinoma

Metastatic Disease

Lymphoma
Sarcoma

Barrett's mucosa progresses to adenocarcinoma at all, why it tends to occur predominantly in white males, how long it takes for this progression to occur, and whether any therapy may affect this process. The association of BE and adenocarcinoma is discussed in more detail in the next section on pathogenesis.

Melanocytes are detected in esophageal mucosa in 2.5% to 11.5% of cases, depending on the assay used.[15,16] The incidence of malignant melanoma of the esophagus is 0.1%.[17] Small cell carcinoma accounts for 0.5% to 7.6% of all esophageal cancers.[18-20] Often these tumors are of mixed pathology. Sarcomas compose 0.5% of esophageal tumors.[21] Carcinomas arising elsewhere may involve the esophagus, either by direct extension (bronchogenic cancer) or by hematogenous (melanoma, testicular, prostatic, pancreatic) or lymphangiectatic spread (breast cancer).

PATHOGENESIS

The exact etiology of esophageal cancer is unknown. The data support the hypothesis that the more common epithelial tumors arise as a result of chronic irritation of the esophagus from a wide range of sources, including known carcinogens, and that the likelihood of developing cancer may be increased in patients with impaired host defenses. The pathogenesis of both nonepithelial and the less common epithelial esophageal cancers is unknown. The geographic, cultural, and demographic distribution of esophageal cancer varies widely. Whether this variance can be explained solely by environmental factors or whether a genetic component exists as well is conjectural. It is clear that some form of chronic esophageal irritation is important. The most commonly reported irritants include tobacco, alcohol, dietary factors, lye, radiation, and refluxed gastric contents.

Squamous Cell Carcinoma

Smoking is a proven etiologic factor in the development of squamous cell esophageal cancer for both men and women.[22-27] In their series, Choi and Kahyo[24] reported a dose-dependent relation between the amount of smoking and the risk of esophageal cancer. They also demonstrated that the risk of cancer decreases with smoking cessation. Smokeless tobacco products also have been shown to correlate with an increased risk of cancer of the mouth, larynx, throat, and esophagus.[28] Alcohol consumption potentiates the propensity for esophageal cancer in patients who smoke. It is not clear to what extent, if any, smoking contributes to the development of esophageal adenocarcinoma. In our review of patients undergoing esophagectomy for carcinoma, 71% of patients with adenocarcinoma and 91% of patients with squamous tumors were smokers.[29] Gray and colleagues[27] also reported that cigarette and alcohol use was lower in patients with esophageal or esophagogastric adenocarcinoma compared with patients with squamous tumors. They concluded that the recent increase in incidence of adenocarcinoma could not be explained on the basis of a concomitant increase in smoking and alcohol consumption in these patients. Numerous studies document the relation between alcohol consumption and squamous cell esophageal cancer.[24-27,30-32] The cancer risk appears to be dose related, and the risks from alcohol and smoking are additive.

Nutritional and dietary factors have been evaluated in an attempt to explain the worldwide variability in the incidence of esophageal cancer. Ghardirian and assoicates[33] reported that populations with the highest incidence of esophageal cancer shared dietary characteristics including a rapidly consumed high-starch diet with little or no fruits and vegetables. Many dishes consist of granular foods or foods that are served quite hot, both of which irritate the esophagus. Block and coworkers[34] reported that a diet rich in fruits was protective against esophageal cancer. Li and colleagues,[35] however, reviewed risk factors for patients in Linxian County, China, an area with one of the highest incidences of esophageal cancer, and did not note an increase in cancer in patients consuming low quantities of vegetables and fruits. Others have reported that dietary fungal contaminants may produce carcinogenic mycotoxins.[36]

Whether a connection exists between achalasia and cancer of the esophagus is an issue that is still debated. Aggestrup and associates[37] emphasized the considerable time interval between the onset of achalasia and the development of esophageal cancer. Furthermore, they argued that short follow-up studies evaluating the risk of cancer and achalasia underestimate the actual (and very real) risks.[38] In their series, 70% of patients in whom cancer developed were males, and all of the tumors were squamous, except in one patient with adenocarcinoma.[37]

Other factors associated with an increased risk of squamous cell esophageal cancer are lye ingestion, radiation therapy (RT), Plummer-Vinson syndrome, and previous head and neck squamous cancer. The interval between injury and the development of cancer may be considerable in patients who sustain lye ingestion or are irradiated.

Adenocarcinoma

The risk of adenocarcinoma has been increasing over the past several decades. The risk appears to be elevated in patients with GERD, most substantially in those who also have BE. Further study to identify those at highest risk and greater understanding of the molecular progression from BE through dysplasia on to malignancy may lead to effective strategies for screening or prevention. Currently, the benefits of screening those with GERD or BE are not well elucidated, although this approach is frequently utilized, with the goal of early detection. The progression from normal esophageal epithelium to BE to dysplasia and on to adenocarcinoma appears to be driven by chronic irritation, especially from GERD.

GERD itself has been investigated as a risk factor for esophageal adenocarcinoma. A population-based case-control study performed in Sweden[39] showed a relative risk of 7.7 for development of esophageal cancer in those with chronic reflux disease. With long-lasting and severe

Specific Malignancies

III

symptoms, the relative risk was 43.5. Similar increases in risk were not observed for esophageal squamous cell carcinoma or adenocarcinoma of the gastric cardia. Interestingly, the increased risk of esophageal carcinoma existed whether or not BE could be identified, leading the authors to speculate that GERD may cause esophageal adenocarcinoma by a mechanism independent of BE. An alternative explanation might be that the area of BE in these patients was overgrown by tumor. It remains controversial whether treating reflux in the setting of BE will significantly reduce or eliminate the risk of adenocarcinoma. The role of screening for BE is unknown. According to the American College of Gastroenterology practice guidelines, a one-time endoscopy may be prudent to rule out BE in patients with chronic GERD, especially in the highest-risk white male population.[40] However, specific criteria for selecting patients are not available.

A clear relation exists between BE and dysplasia and neoplasm. BE refers to a condition in which the normal stratified squamous mucosa is replaced by columnar-lined epithelium (CLE) that extends upward from the esophagogastric junction. Various lengths of esophagus may be involved. The condition is an acquired, metaplastic process that develops in response to an esophageal mucosal injury that heals in the setting of the inflammatory stimulus of continued GE reflux. BE may progress to dysplasia and then malignancy as the cells accumulate genetic changes.

The incidence of BE is not known, although reports range from 1% to 2% of the general population. A demonstrable association exist of BE, dysplasia, and esophageal adenocarcinoma. Miros and coworkers[41] prospectively followed up 81 patients with BE. In three patients, adenocarcinoma developed, two with antecedent high-grade and one with low-grade dysplasia. In no patient without dysplasia did adenocarcinoma develop. Tygat and colleagues[42] provided evidence that dysplasia is a prerequisite to adenocarcinoma, that low-grade dysplasia is potentially reversible, and that once the *threshold* of high-grade dysplasia is reached, it always progresses to invasive adenocarcinoma. The length of time for the progression from BE to adenocarcinoma is unknown. As the lifetime risk may be as high as 8% to 15% or 0.5% to 1% per 50 patient years, many advocate lifelong endoscopic surveillance for patients with Barrett's mucosa, with the goal of treating dysplastic changes and thereby reducing the risk of adenocarcinoma developing. Tumors discovered during surveillance appear to be earlier stage and therefore to have a higher chance of cure.[43,44] Still it is not certain whether a significant improvement in mortality is found with surveillance, as the risk of death from esophageal cancer is relatively low even in this high-risk population.[45,46]

Several centers reported results of planned screening endoscopy that suggest that progression of BE to esophageal cancer may be less common than originally thought, at least in the short term. A report of 55 patients[47] at Leicester General Hospital with median follow-up of 4.4 years demonstrated identification of adenocarcinoma in five patients, but in four of these five patients, the carcinoma was discovered because of urgent endoscopy

to evaluate deteriorating symptoms rather than on the annual study. In five additional patients, dysplasia developed, but it regressed in three and remained stable in another. Finally, 266 patients at the same institution were ineligible for the annual surveillance program because they were considered unfit for esophagectomy (which would be the therapy if an abnormality were detected), and only 1 of these patients died of esophageal cancer during the study period. In another series,[48] 60 patients with newly diagnosed BE were followed for a mean of 10 years, and esophageal cancer developed in only 2 patients (1 per 300 patient years). A Veterans Administration (VA) study[49] of patients requiring therapy for reflux disease found a 0.4% per patient year risk in patients with BE and 0.07% per year in those without BE. The uncertainty about the true incidence of esophageal adenocarcinoma has resulted in controversy about the benefits of an optimal interval for screening endoscopy. Those who advocate screening point out the increased risk of adenocarcinoma, whereas those who oppose point out that a low risk of death remains from esophageal cancer.[40] Given the observed incidence of progression to esophageal cancer and the lack of very long term follow-up in the available studies, a screening interval of 2 to 5 years may represent a prudent compromise.[40] The decision to screen should be based on a realistic assessment of the risks of esophageal cancer balanced against the patient's age and other comorbid conditions.[40]

Most patients in whom adenocarcinoma develops are found to have BE. Pera and associates[8] found Barrett's mucosa in 63.6% of their patients with adenocarcinoma. In our experience at Johns Hopkins, Barrett's mucosa was identified in 62.5% percent of patients undergoing esophagectomy for adenocarcinoma.[29] Some investigators believe that all esophageal adenocarcinoma arises from underlying BE and that when BE is not identified, it is because it has been *replaced* by the carcinoma. Indeed, Theisen and coworkers[50] reported that although BE was detected in only 75% on pretreatment endoscopy, it was "unmasked" in additional 22% in endoscopy done after neoadjuvant therapy, for a total incidence of 97%.[50]

Molecular genetics data support the hypothesis that a progression exists from BE to dysplasia to adenocarcinoma. Moskaluk and coworkers[51] performed immunohistochemical staining for p53, an important regulatory gene in cell-cycle control and apoptosis, and p21 WAF1 proteins, a gene that encodes a cyclin-dependent kinase inhibitor, in 98 adenocarcinoma esophagectomy specimens. The authors found similar p53 and p21 WAF1 expression in adenocarcinoma specimens with and without associated Barrett's mucosa, and they concluded that the molecular mechanisms of carcinogenesis for these two groups is the same. Wu and colleagues[52] investigated DNA replication errors and allelic losses of chromosomes 17p, 18q, and 5q in esophageal adenocarcinoma (without associated Barrett's mucosa), Barrett's adenocarcinoma, and Barrett's mucosa with dysplasia. More recently, Barrett and colleagues[53] have reported that alteration in p53 and p16 are generally seen throughout an area of Barrett's abnormality, suggesting that those were inherent in the original clonal development of BE.

Additional mutations involving loss of heterozygosity (LOH) at 5q, 13q, or 18q, occurring in no particular order, appeared important in the bifurcation into aneuploidy and on to progression into neoplasm.[53] Wong and coworkers[54] focused on the role of p16 inactivation and found that more than 85% of Barrett's clones had inactivation of one or both p16 genes by LOH (53%), hypermethylation (61%), or point mutation (15%). Interestingly, the incidence of other abnormalities, including 17p (p53) LOH, aneuploidy, or tetraploidy increased from 0 to 20% to 44% in patients observed to have p16 +/+, p16 +/-, and p16 -/- BE. In addition, the median length of Barrett's increased from 1.5 to 6.0 to 8.0 cm. This suggested that p16 may be an important step in the field change leading to BE and on to neoplasm.[54]

Promoter region hypermethylation is an epigenetic modification associated with gene inactivation that also may play an important role in the development of esophageal cancer. This process is important in development where hypermethylation is associated with inactivated genes in the X chromosome and also may be important in oncogenesis where hypermethylation can be associated with inactivation of tumor-suppressor genes, genes that suppress metastasis and angiogenesis, and genes that repair DNA. Methylation of DNA is catalyzed by DNA methyltransferase. A methyl group from S-adenosyl-methionine is transferred to cytosine to form 5-ethylcytosine, a process occurring mostly at CpG sites in the genome.

In esophageal adenocarcinoma, CpG-island methylation at CDKN2A has been implicated in the progression of BE to malignancy. Eads and associates[55,56] reported results for 31 normal esophagus specimens and 22 adenocarcinoma specimens. The following genes were observed to be methylated in a substantial portion of esophageal cancer specimens but less often in normal esophagus from the same patients (percentage tumor vs. percentage normal specimens): CDKN2a/p16 (41% vs. 0), ESR1 (86% vs. 0), MYOD1 (45% vs. 0), TIMP3 (86% vs. 19%), APC (68% vs. 3%), and CALCA (50% vs. 13%). In nine specimens of dysplasia, these genes were methylated in 22%, 89%, 67%, 56%, 78%, and 89%, respectively. Of note, APC was methylated in normal stomach in 12 of 12 specimens. MGMT was methylated in 55% of normal esophagus specimens, 73% of adenocarcinoma specimens, and 25% of stomach specimens.

Although much progress has occurred in unraveling the relation between Barrett's mucosa, dysplasia, and esophageal adenocarcinoma, still many unanswered questions remain, such as why Barrett's mucosa is seen in such a specific demographic pattern, and what is the trigger to initiate the progression to dysplasia and carcinoma.

Some evidence supports the hypothesis that impaired host defense increases the risk of developing esophageal cancer. Both vitamin and mineral deficiencies have been cited as explanations for the cancer rates seen in regions in which esophageal cancer is endemic. The risk of esophageal cancer is elevated in patients with pernicious anemia,[57] and Oka and coworkers[58] have documented immunosuppression in patients with BE.

DIAGNOSIS

Clinical Manifestation

The typical patient with squamous cell carcinoma of the esophagus is a man in the sixth or seventh decade who complains of difficulty swallowing and weight loss extending over a 3- to 6-month period. Cigarette and alcohol abuse are usually found in the patient's social history. More than 90% of patients with squamous cell cancers of the mid and upper thoracic esophagus will give this history. Pain on swallowing (odynophagia) and substernal or epigastric pain are less common complaints. The presence of Horner's syndrome, hoarseness from recurrent laryngeal nerve involvement, supraclavicular adenopathy, or a tracheoesophageal (TE) fistula indicates advanced, unresectable lesions.

The typical patient with an adenocarcinoma of the distal esophagus, GE junction, or cardia is first seen at a younger age (in the fifth or sixth decade) and is usually a white man from the middle or upper socioeconomic class. Significant weight loss at presentation is far less common than for the patient with a squamous cell cancer, and many patients with adenocarcinoma are overweight to obese. A history of cigarette or alcohol abuse (or both) may not be present. More often, a hiatal hernia leading to reflux and prolonged antacid use are reported.

Diagnostic Evaluation

A complaint of dysphagia should prompt the physician to obtain an endoscopy or barium esophagogram. The diagnosis is usually evident by the characteristic narrowing of the esophagus, but endoscopy and biopsy are essential for histopathologic diagnosis. Endoscopic biopsies and brushings of the lesion will yield the diagnosis in more than 90% of patients.[59,60] Multiple biopsies may be necessary to confirm the diagnosis of an invasive malignancy that is submucosal or necrotic.[59] A diagnosis of in situ carcinoma in the face of a large lesion seen on radiographic studies should not be accepted, and biopsy should be repeated.

Once the pathologic diagnosis is established, evaluation to determine the extent of disease should include a computed tomography (CT) scan of the chest and abdomen. The chest CT is useful for evaluating lung parenchyma and mediastinal structures.[61] Lymph nodes more than 1 cm in diameter with necrotic centers suggest metastatic involvement. The chest CT also is helpful for assessing aortic or pericardial involvement with tumor that would preclude esophagectomy. In contrast, the actual length of the esophageal lesion is better assessed on the barium esophagogram.

The accuracy of identifying metastases to the liver and celiac axis by abdominal CT depends on the bulk of the disease. Small liver metastases, peritoneal studding, and abdominal nodes will often be undetectable.[61-67] For squamous cell lesions of the upper and midthoracic esophagus, a CT scan of the upper abdomen that includes the liver and adrenals is sufficient. For the patient with an adenocarcinoma of the distal esophagus or cardia, a complete abdominal CT is necessary to visualize potential areas of nodal metastases. Cancers of this histologic type are more likely to metastasize early to periaortic lymph nodes. A complaint of back pain may signal the presence of enlarged retroperitoneal nodes.

Positron emission tomograghy (PET) scanning also may enable the identification of metastatic disease in patients who might otherwise inappropriately receive definitive local therapy. Prospective studies[68,69] demonstrated that PET will detect unsuspected metastatic disease in approximately 15% of patients after all other staging tests are completed, although it is not as useful as other techniques in identifying involved regional nodes. A 79-patient prospective study[68] found the specificity and sensitivity of PET for identifying stage IV disease was 90% and 74% versus 47% and 78% for the combination of CT and endoscopic ultrasonography (EUS), with the overall accuracy of identification of stage IV disease of 82% versus 64% ($P = .004$). More important, PET had additional value for the critical identification of stage IV disease. When added to CT and EUS, 22% of patients had a significant change in stage, with 15% upstaged to stage IV disease and 7% downstaged to a stage in which curative therapy would be appropriate. As more prospectively acquired data become available, the role of PET scanning will be further clarified.

A bone scan is recommended for patients with an elevated alkaline phosphatase level or symptomatic painful areas, although this may not be necessary when PET scan is performed. Bone metastases are infrequent as the initial site of metastases, but they do occur, more commonly in patients with adenocarcinoma. Evaluation for tracheal involvement with bronchoscopy is necessary for all middle- and upper-third lesions.

Accurate determination of the extent of disease has a major impact on such therapeutic issues as single-modality versus multimodality treatment or curative versus palliative intent, and therefore aggressive staging techniques are reasonable. A substantial literature now exists regarding transesophageal EUS, laparoscopy, and thoracoscopy. The greatest experience is with EUS.[70-76] In experienced hands, the depth of the primary tumor infiltration can be determined with an overall accuracy of 89%; overstaging occurs in 6% and understaging in 5%.[74,76] Nodal involvement can be determined with an overall accuracy of 81% (sensitivity, 95%; specificity, 50%).[70,74] EUS-guided fine-needle aspiration biopsy can distinguish benign from malignant lymph nodes with 92% accuracy when compared with surgery outcome.[73] EUS is not a reliable technique for diagnosing liver and peritoneal metastases because of the limited depth of penetration of ultrasound.[70]

The indications for invasive staging are not yet fully defined. Laparoscopic evaluation of abdominal lymph nodes can be achieved with minimal risks when a high yield of staging information is not obtainable with standard imaging studies. The staging accuracy of laparoscopy for nodal involvement exceeds 95%.[63-67,77,78] Unsuspected findings such as liver metastases or peritoneal studding that alter treatment and save the patient

from esophagectomy occur in 12% to 17% of patients studied.[63-66] Laparoscopy appears to be most useful for evaluating abdominal spread of disease in patients with distal third or GE junction T3 to T4 tumors. Thoracoscopy also has a high level of accuracy, 95%, in detecting regional nodal involvement compared with surgical staging.[63,79,80]

STAGING SYSTEM

Assessment of extent of disease is important at the time of initial diagnosis for determining optimal management, and after therapy is completed, for determining prognosis. In relation to research trials, accurate staging is critical for a meaningful interpretation of the study result and comparison with literature reports. In 1987, the tumor-node-metastasis (TNM) staging system for esophageal cancer developed by the American Joint Committee on Cancer (AJCC) was revised to consist of pathologic staging only, so that stage would more accurately reflect prognosis.[81,82] The current system is presented in Table 77-2.[83] Before that time, a preoperative clinical staging

TABLE 77-2

TNM Classification for Esophageal Cancer

Primary Tumor (T)

TX	Primary tumor
T0	No evidence of primary tumor
Tis	Carcinoma in situ
T1	Tumor invades lamina propria or submucosa
T2	Tumor invades muscularis propria
T3	Tumor invades adventitia
T4	Tumor invades adjacent structures

Regional Lymph Nodes (N)

Cervical esophagus (cervical and supraclavicular nodes)

NX	Regional lymph nodes cannot be assessed
N0	No regional lymph node metastasis
N1	Regional lymph node metastasis

Thoracic esophagus (nodes in the thorax, not those in cervical, supraclavicular, or abdominal areas)

N0	No nodal involvement
N1	Nodal involvement

Distant Metastasis (M)

MX	Distant metastasis cannot be assessed
M0	No evidence of distant metastasis
M1	Distant metastasis present

Stage Grouping

Stage 0	Tis	N0	M0
Stage I	T1	N0	M0
Stage IIA	T2	N0	M0
	T3	N0	M0
Stage IIIB	T1	N1	M0
	T2	N1	M0
Stage III	T3	N1	M0
	T4	Any N	M0
Stage IV	Any T	Any N	M1

system applied mainly to the primary tumor based on tumor length (T1, <5 cm; T2, >5 cm; T3, evidence of extraesophageal spread) and whether the tumor was circumferential or obstructing. Thus reports prior to 1988 often characterized patients at diagnosis by their "clinical" stage. Because depth of tumor and nodal involvement more accurately reflect outcome, preoperative staging using the length of the lesion provided a very crude determination of stage.

It is important to be aware of the change in the nature of the staging system in 1987 when comparing outcome in the older and newer literature. It is important also to be aware that although the current staging system is based on final histopathology, many patients are assigned a "clinical" stage before surgery in guiding the decision for preoperative therapy. In this situation, the criteria for preoperative staging may vary widely and depend on the tests used. This also can make comparing the results of trials quite difficult.

Many patients now receive preoperative therapies that effectively "downstage" the tumor so that the postoperative pathologic findings may not reflect the initial stage at diagnosis. This underscores the importance of accurately assessing the extent of local and regional disease before therapy is initiated. In determining response to preoperative therapies, a slight reduction in tumor size can lead to marked improvement in dysphagia. Furthermore, endoscopic biopsies after treatment overestimate pathologic complete response (CR) when compared with pathologic review of a resected specimen. An additional controversy is the proper approach to the patient with M1a stage disease. It is uncertain whether this is properly considered stage IV disease with no cure possible or whether a proportion of patients are curable. Patients with M1a disease are eligible for many clinical trials testing therapies for localized disease.

OVERVIEW: THE CHOICE OF THERAPY

The goal of any therapy to manage patients with esophageal cancer is to relieve symptoms (predominantly dysphagia) and to treat the underlying cancer. An ideal therapy would accomplish both, safely and effectively. Treatment options may be classified into potentially curative modalities and palliative methods. Which treatment is best for an individual patient is based on tumor staging and performance status. These options and the data supporting their use are summarized in Table 77-3. The important considerations are discussed later, and the data described in more detail in the relevant sections of this chapter.

Curative Therapy

For potentially curable patients, survival outcome with these different therapies as assessed by outcome reported in randomized trials is summarized in Table 77-4, which indicates that differences are somewhat marginal with currently available approaches. Although a true 10% to 15% difference in cure rate would be of major importance, it is impossible to draw firm conclusions by comparing arms across trials or with historical data. As the table indicates, survival with surgery, definitive chemoradiation, and adjuvant chemotherapy or chemoradiation does not clearly differ, although selection factors may have varied substantially. Radiation alone is rarely curative, and pre- or postoperative RT alone has never been shown to improve outcome in multiple randomized trials and therefore is not a focus of this chapter. Surgery remains the standard treatment for resectable tumors in fit patients. Some evidence, not considered to be definitive, indicates that preoperative chemoradiation or chemo-

TABLE 77-3

Options in the Definitive Therapy of Esophageal Carcinoma		
INDICATION	**RECOMMENDATION**	**EVIDENCE**
Surgery alone	Best single modality therapy. As yet no other options definitively proven to be superior	Long-term survival results well documented
Primary radiotherapy	Used only for patients who are not candidates for concurrent chemoradiation or with small early tumors	Long-term survival 0%–10% for locally advanced disease and 15%–25% for early disease. Randomized trials have demonstrated a survival and local control benefit when chemotherapy is added
Primary chemoradiotherapy	Appropriate choice for nonoperative management	Randomized trials have demonstrated 5-year survival of 9%–27%
Preoperative radiotherapy	No known benefit	5 randomized trials
Postoperative radiotherapy	No known benefit. Used for known residual disease	2 randomized trials
Preoperative chemoradiotherapy	Accepted alternative approach, although further data demonstrating a survival benefit are needed. Substantial local control benefit	Promising results in phase II trials. Mixed results in modestly powered randomized trials. A definitive large randomized U.S. intergroup trial closed with low accrual
Preoperative chemotherapy	Possible improvement in outcome	Mixed results in two large randomized trials
Postoperative chemoradiation	Benefits not assessed. Used for known residual disease	Very limited data. A randomized trial demonstrated possible benefit for distal lesions, although most patients in trial had gastric rather than GE junction tumors

GE, gastroesophageal.

TABLE 77-4

Results from Treatment Arms from Selected Recent Randomized Trials

	1 YR (%)	2 YR (%)	3 YR (%)	5 YR (%)	MEDIAN SURVIVAL (MO)	LOCAL FAILURE (%)
Surgery		37				
U.S. Intergroup[151]	60		26		16.1	59
MRC[152]		34			13.3*	37
Bossett[161]					18.6	
Walsh[162]	42	26	6		11*	
Urba[163]	58		16		17.6	52*
Hulscher (transhiatal)[123]				29	21.6	32
Hulscher (radical)[123]				39	24	31
Radiotherapy						
RTOG[206]	34	10	0	0	9.3*	68*
ECOG (surgery added in 24/56)[207]	33	12	8	7	9.2*	
Chemoradiotherapy						
RTOG[206]	52	36	30	26	14*	46*
RTOG (nonrandomized confirmatory group)[206]	62	35	26	14	16.7	58
ECOG (surgery added in 21/58)[207]	54	27	13	9	14.8*	
Preop Chemotherapy						
U.S. Intergroup[151]		35			14.9	58
MRC[152]		43			16.8*	27
Preop Chemoradiotherapy						
Walsh[162]	52	37	32		16*	
Bossett[161]					18.6	
Urba[163]	72		30		16.9	23*

Randomized trials included in table (further details in the text).
*Significant difference between respective arms in these trials.

therapy may improve on the results of surgery alone. Fewer data support postoperative administration of chemotherapy or chemoradiation, although this remains an area of investigational interest. Definitive chemoradiation is a potentially curative alternative to surgery and should be considered for unresectable inoperable lesions or for patients unable to tolerate a major surgical procedure. Given data that do not definitively demonstrate superiority for any of the available approaches for resectable disease, the decision about optimal management is complex and controversial.

Surgery as a single-modality therapy remains the standard therapy for localized esophageal cancer and is less toxic than combined-modality therapy. Surgery as a single modality is most appropriate for early lesions (stages I and IIa) or where toxicity is an important issue.

Preoperative chemoradiation remains controversial but is frequently used in treatment. Some data substantiate improved local control and suggest the possibility of a survival benefit (see Table 77-4) with this intensive multidisciplinary approach. An appropriately powered phase III randomized trial has not been conducted to validate this hypothesis, and smaller randomized trials have had mixed outcomes. This combined-modality therapy is quite toxic and should be used cautiously

in patients with poor performance status or comorbid conditions that increase the risk of toxicity. Conversely, the outcome with surgery alone is favorable for T1N0M0 lesions, so that we do not recommend neoadjuvant therapy when staging with EUS suggests such a very early lesion.

Preoperative chemotherapy is less toxic than preoperative chemoRT, and one randomized trial conducted by the Medical Research Council (MRC) suggested a survival benefit, whereas a similar U.S. Intergroup trial did not (see Table 77-4). Preoperative chemoradiation is more widely used, as it has a substantial local control benefit not observed with preoperative chemotherapy, providing a sound rationale for improved outcome and clinical benefit. Such a rationale does not as convincingly exist with preoperative chemotherapy alone, although it is reasonable to use this approach based on the results of the positive MRC trial.

Definitive chemoradiation is a curative alternative, which eliminates the operative risk, although the local control rate and possibly cure rate appear to be lower than that with surgery alone. When evaluating these results, however, it is important to consider selection biases that may be at work: Chemoradiation may be selected for patients with more advanced lesions, unresectable disease, or with significant intercurrent illness, a population less likely to achieve long-term survival. No direct comparative trials using a surgical control arm have been conducted.

The role of adjuvant therapy after surgical resection is less well studied. For patients undergoing surgery, limited randomized evidence indicates that postoperative chemoradiation may be appropriate for patients with resected GE junction lesions, but data are not available for other locations. Postoperative RT has not been beneficial, and postoperative chemotherapy has not been thoroughly studied, although all these options may be appropriate in selected cases. When surgical resection is used with microscopic or gross residual disease, postoperative chemoradiation should be considered based on an extrapolation from the data suggesting that chemoradiation is superior to radiation alone for definitive treatment of gross disease in newly diagnosed esophageal cancer.

Palliative Therapy Overview

For situations in which palliation rather than cure is the goal, several options exist. RT, with or without chemotherapy, is of palliative benefit in relieving local swallowing problems and symptoms of distant metastasis. However, endoscopic palliation including stent placement, laser therapy, and photodynamic therapy (PDT) may provide more immediate benefit in situations in which symptoms are severe; this does not commit the patient to a prolonged course of daily treatments. RT may be added to increase the durability of local palliation for patients who are likely to survive more than 3 to 6 months. It should be stressed that patients with locally advanced disease that is not resectable may be cured with chemoradiation, and those patients should be treated with palliative intent only when performance status is poor, disease is quite extensive, or the patient is judged unable to tolerate potentially curative chemoradiation.

For metastatic disease, chemotherapy is indicated with the goal of improving survival and preventing/treating symptoms at all locations. Given the modest response rate with available regimens, chemotherapy is not a reliable means of palliating substantial obstructive symptoms. Therefore chemotherapy alone may be the best choice when symptoms are mild or the disease is widespread, whereas consideration should be given to local palliative method in addition to chemotherapy when the symptoms are severe.

Endoscopic therapy is generally more appropriate for palliation or to relieve symptoms before definitive potentially curative therapy. Although endoscopic therapies have been investigated in the treatment of dysplasias and very early adenocarcinoma of the esophagus, the studies have involved a small number of patients, and long-term follow-up is limited. Therefore these approaches are not considered standard options in curative therapy, although they may be appropriate for some patients. The choice among the endoscopic options depends on the goals (i.e., stenting palliates but does not treat superficial tumors) and the available expertise.

DEFINITIVE TREATMENT OPTIONS

Surgery Alone

The precedent for resecting obstructing small or large bowel tumors, even in the setting of locally advanced disease, has been well established. The same principles apply to the management of patients with obstructing esophageal cancer. Local tumor control, with durable relief of dysphagia, is best accomplished surgically. This is especially true now that the surgical risks and length of hospitalization have decreased to acceptable figures.[84-89] Whether surgical resection is performed as the sole therapy, or as part of a combined approach, the surgical principles and techniques are the same. Concurrent chemotherapy and radiation without surgery is a potentially curative alternative for patients who refuse surgery, who are at high risk for surgery, who have unresectable tumors, or who have upper esophageal lesions for which resection may also require laryngectomy.

The standard operation to resect an esophageal cancer includes resecting the involved portion of esophagus, the proximal stomach, and the regional lymph nodes, as illustrated in Figure 77-1. The surgical resection is therefore properly termed a partial esophagogastrectomy with regional (or one-field) lymphadenectomy. The resected esophagus is replaced with the stomach or segments of the small or large intestine, which are mobilized as a vascularized pedicle and anastomosed to the remaining proximal esophagus (Fig. 77-2).

A number of incisional approaches are used to perform a partial esophagogastrectomy including the transhiatal, Ivor-Lewis, left thoracoabdominal, and three-incision techniques (Fig. 77-3). Other less common techniques are modifications of the approaches listed. The specific incisional approach used generally determines how much esophagus is removed and where the esophageal anastomosis will be located (see Fig. 77-1). In the past, proponents have argued in support of their preferred techniques, giving the impression that they were uniquely different procedures. All of the incisional techniques use partial esophagogastrectomy (except segmental esophagectomy with free jejunal grafting, which is discussed separately); the results reported are similar in terms of surgical morbidity and mortality. Survival is related to pathologic tumor stage. Prospective studies do not demonstrate a survival advantage related to the surgical esophagectomy technique.[90,91] The data continue to demonstrate no difference in morbidity, mortality, or survival between transthoracic and transhiatal esophagectomy approaches.[92] The only variables when performing a partial esophagogastrectomy are which incision(s) to use, the length of esophagus to resect, what to use to replace the esophagus, and which route through the chest this conduit will take.

Transhiatal Approach
Transhiatal esophagectomy (THE) is an increasingly popular surgical approach. With this technique, the

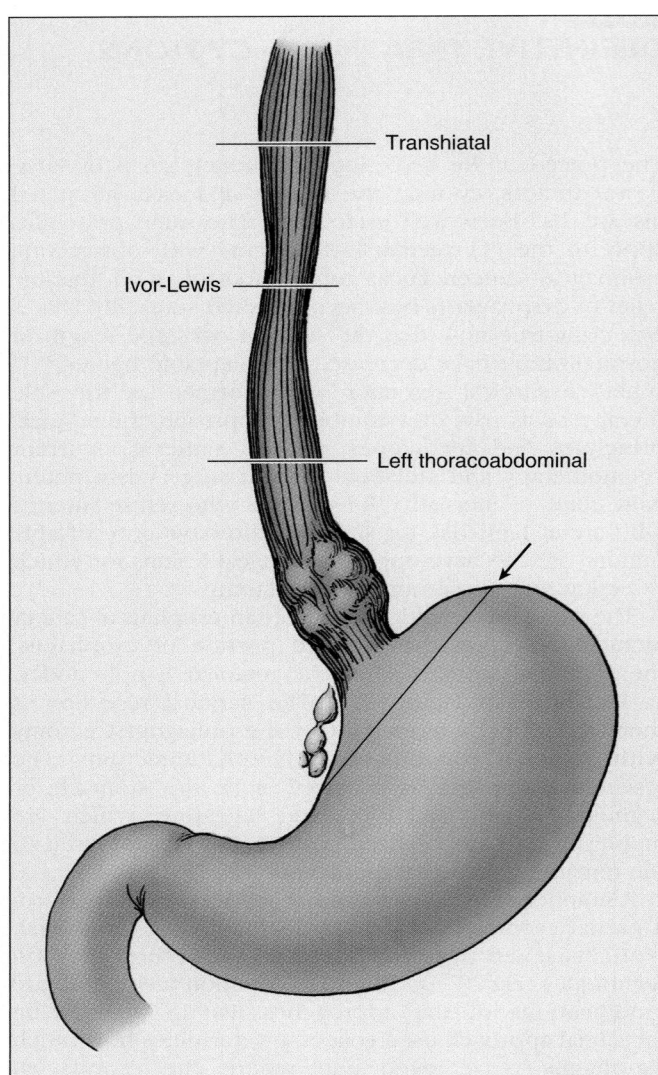

Figure 77-1. Regardless of the surgical approach used, a partial esophagogastrectomy is performed to resect esophageal tumors. Depending on the approach, different lengths of esophagus are removed. (From Heitmiller RF: Carcinoma of the esophagus. In Bayless TM [ed]: Current Therapy in Gastroenterology and Liver Disease, 4th ed. St. Louis, Mosby-Year Book, 1994, p 81, with permission.)

intrathoracic esophagus is mobilized distally through the esophageal hiatus and proximally through a cervical incision. The prevalence of adenocarcinoma has largely been responsible for the widespread use of the transhiatal approach. These tumors are invariably located in the distal esophagus near the esophagogastric junction, so they are readily accessible for direct-vision dissection through the hiatus. As well, the regional lymph nodes for these distal tumors are in the parahiatal and proximal lesser curvature regions, both accessible via laparotomy. The resected esophagus is then reconstructed by using stomach or long-segment colon, which are passed up into the neck as vascularized grafts to be anastomosed to the proximal cervical esophagus.[93-96] Although reports exist on the use of jejunum for long-segment esophageal replacement,

small bowel is generally not an option for esophageal replacement because of its mesenteric vascular anatomy, unless specialized techniques with vascular augmentation are used.[97] The esophageal-replacement conduit is passed through the chest into the neck by one of three routes: (1) subcutaneous, (2) substernal, or (3) posterior mediastinum. The posterior mediastinum is the preferred route when possible. The advantages of the THE include avoiding post-thoracotomy discomfort, wide proximal esophageal margin to ensure complete resection of tumor and Barrett's mucosa, cervical anastomosis where the consequences of anastomotic leak are minimized, and an esophageal reconstruction that results in an excellent quality of swallowing. It is well documented that the THE approach is acceptable for both benign and malignant esophageal diseases.[98,99] The disadvantages include inability to visualize middle or proximal third tumors, inability to perform intrathoracic regional lymphadenectomy, potential for injury to intrathoracic structures, and need for long-segment esophageal replacement. The technique is safe and well tolerated but associated with an incidence of ipsilateral recurrent nerve injury in 6%, major respiratory complications in 10%, pneumonia in 3%, and anastomotic leak rates of 0.8% to 8%. Mortality rates as low as none to 3% are reported in large series.[96,100]

Ivor-Lewis Approach

Partial esophagogastrectomy with an abdominal and right thoracotomy approach, also known as the Ivor-Lewis approach, was designed to optimize exposure of the intrathoracic esophagus, which passes through the upper two thirds of the chest along the right posterior mediastinum.[100] Once the involved intrathoracic esophagus is mobilized, a partial esophagogastrectomy is performed, and the esophagus is replaced by stomach, colon, or (less frequently) jejunum, which is passed into the chest along the esophageal bed, and anastomosed to the proximal esophagus, usually at or above the level of the azygos arch. The advantages of the technique are the excellent exposure of the mid to upper intrathoracic esophagus, and the disadvantages are related to the use of thoracotomy, with its potential for an intrathoracic esophageal anastomotic leak. Reported complications include respiratory problems in 11%, anastomotic leak in 3% to 7%, and wound infections in 5%. Operative mortality ranges from none to 4%.[84,87,101]

Left Thoracoabdominal Approach

The left thoracoabdominal approach uses a single incision extending from the left chest onto the abdomen; it provides excellent exposure of the lower third of the esophagus and left upper quadrant of the abdomen.[102] This technique is ideal for patients with tumors near the GE junction, especially when the extent of gastric invasion is unclear, because it yields superb exposure and maximizes reconstructive options of the lower third of the esophagus. Respiratory complications are the most common postoperative complication. At least some degree of atelectasis, usually involving the left lower lung, occurs in most patients. Pneumonia is reported to occur in none to 24% of cases. Anastomotic leakage occurs in

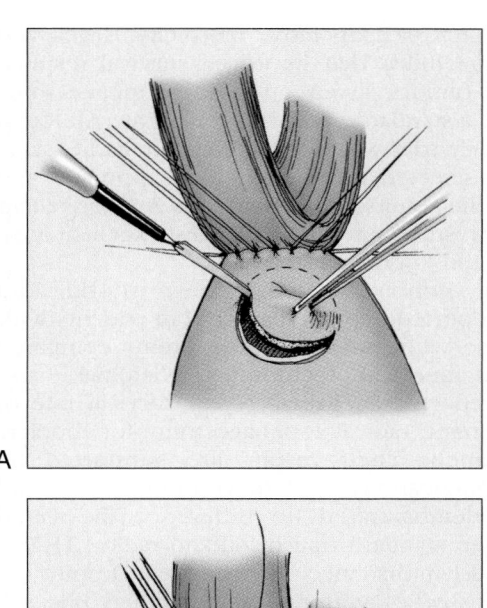

A

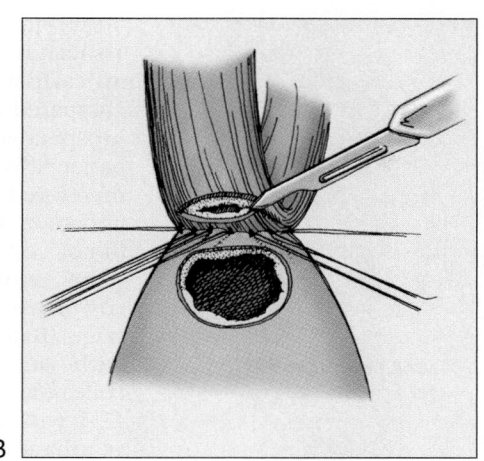

B

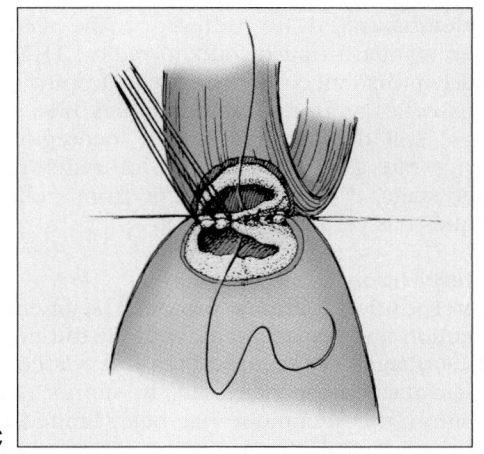

C

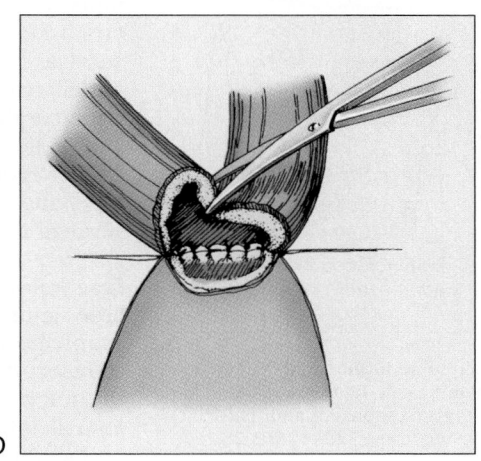

D

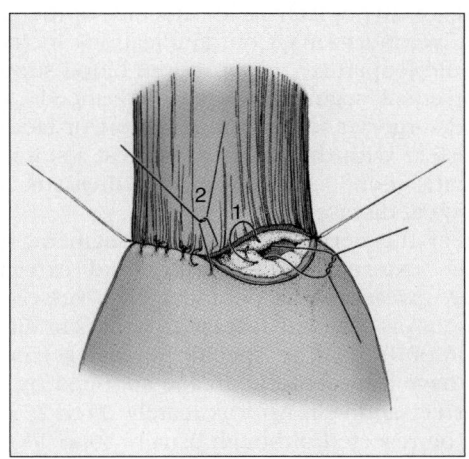

E

Figure 77-2. The inverting, two-layer, end-to-side esophagogastric anastomosis technique is illustrated. **A,** The outer posterior row consists of interrupted stitches approximating the esophageal muscularis to the seromuscular coat of the stomach. **B,** A gastric button is opened by using electrocautery, and the esophageal muscularis is sharply divided parallel to the posterior suture line. **C,** The inner posterior row approximates esophageal and gastric mucosa. **D,** The distal esophagus is sharply excised. **E,** The inner layer, which approximates esophagus to gastric mucosa, is continued anteriorly, inverting the stitches so that the knots are interluminal. The outer anterior layer is completed by sewing the esophageal muscularis to the seromuscular layer or stomach. (From Heitmiller RF: Results of standard left thoracoabdominal esophagogastrectomy. Semin Thorac Cardiovasc Surg 1992;4:314, with permission.)

none to 12% (mean, 3.7%) of cases. Other complications include atrial fibrillation in 10%, wound infection in 1.5% to 5.2%, and (infrequently) empyema and subphrenic abscess. The reported operative mortality is none to 6.2%.[103,104]

Multiple Incisions

Multiple-incision surgical approaches combine the incisional strategies of the standard techniques. Of these, the three-incision approach using a cervical incision (right

or left), right thoracotomy, and midline laparotomy, as described by McKeown,[105] is the most common, also referred to as the "three-incision," "three-hole," "total esophagectomy," or "modified McKeown" approach. It combines the exposure of the thoracotomy approach for esophageal mobilization or nodal dissection with the advantages of a cervical esophageal anastomosis. Outcome results with this technique are similar to those of other approaches, with reported mortality of 3% to 4%, and esophageal anastomotic leak rates of 5% or less.[106,107]

Specific Malignancies

III

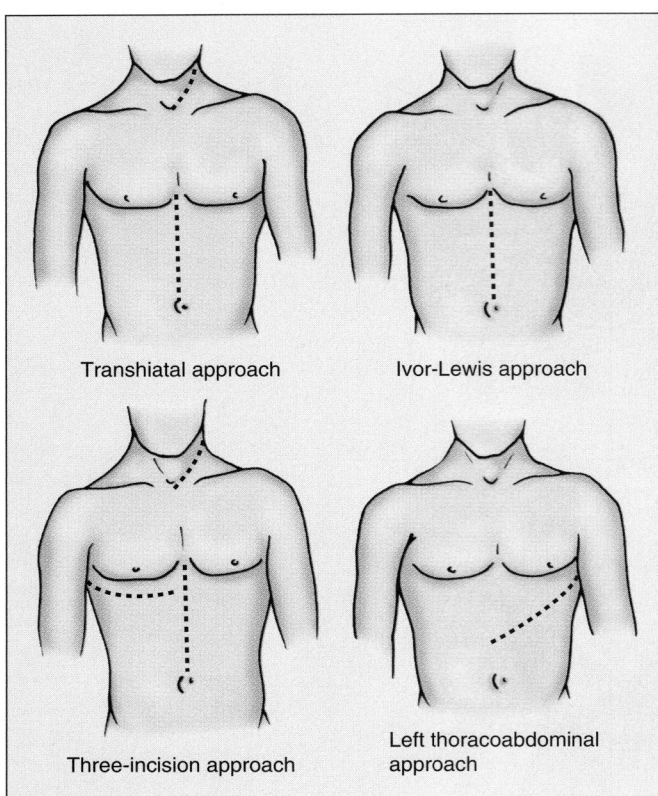

Transhiatal approach

Ivor-Lewis approach

Three-incision approach

Left thoracoabdominal approach

Figure 77-3. The different incisions used to perform partial esophagogastrectomy are depicted. (From Reichle RI, Fishman EK, Nison MS, et al: Evaluation of the post-surgical esophagus after partial esophagogastrectomy for esophageal cancer. Invest Radiol 1993;28:247, with permission.)

Radical Resection

The majority of patients with esophageal cancer are first seen with locally advanced (stage II and III) disease. In these patients, postsurgical survival results are poor. Two approaches attempt to improve survival in these patients. One involves the use of combination therapies, such as preoperative chemoradiation followed by surgery (to be discussed later), and the second involves adding an en bloc, wide-field lymphadenectomy to the standard esophagectomy technique. The esophagus has an extensive regional lymphatic drainage. Arbitrarily, the lymphatic drainage has been divided into three zones or fields—cervical, intrathoracic, and abdominal. Standard esophagectomy techniques involve regional, or one-field, lymphadenectomy. Radical approaches advocate two- or three-field lymphadenectomy in conjunction with esophageal resection and replacement. Hagen and colleagues[108] believe that proximal hemigastrectomy should also be included as part of an en bloc approach, using colon to replace the resected esophagus. Radical esophagectomy is more complex surgery than standard techniques. This is reflected in morbidity rates as high as 58%.[109] Nonetheless, 30-day mortality rates as low as 1.6% to 4.3% are reported.[108-111] Survival data using radical esophagectomy techniques are conflicting, and therefore it is unknown whether there is sufficient benefit to

outweigh the increased operative morbidity. Hagen and associates[108] concluded that improved survival resulted in early-stage tumors using en bloc esophagectomy compared with a standard transhiatal technique. Although prospective, their trial was not randomized. Earlier-stage patients were selected for the en bloc approach and therefore bias the results and conclusions. A more recent update of their results continues to suggest excellent local tumor control and improved survival.[112]

In another nonrandomized series, Altorki and coworkers[111] reported improved survival in patients with stage III disease with radical esophagectomy compared with standard surgical techniques. Nishimaki and colleagues[109] reported an overall 5-year survival rate of 41% with extended radical esophagectomy for thoracic esophageal cancer. Their results are supported by more recent publications.[113,114] In contrast, Bumm and coworkers[110] demonstrated no difference in overall survival between standard transhiatal and radical THE in which two-field lymphadenectomy is added. Despite the wide surgical dissection with radical techniques, Bhansali and colleagues[115] still documented a 21% locoregional cancer recurrence rate. The determination of which cell type and tumor stage, if any, will benefit from radical surgical techniques has yet to be resolved.

Free Jejunal Interposition

Free jejunal interposition permits proximal segmental esophageal resection and replacement, without the need to resect distal esophagus. For technical reasons related to the microvascular anastomosis necessary to support the jejunal interposition, this technique has been limited to replacement of the cervical esophagus for either esophageal, laryngeal, or hypopharyngeal cancers, or benign strictures (e.g., lye, radiation). Contraindications include factors that would jeopardize the proposed blood supply to the free intestinal segment, such as advanced age, previous carotid surgery, and cervical radiation, or factors that would interfere with the ability to harvest a suitable jejunal segment, such as peritoneal adhesions or inflammatory bowel disease.

In resection of the cervical esophageal segment, the branches of the external carotid artery and external jugular veins are preserved as potential host vessels. A segment of jejunum is selected at least 15 to 20 cm distal to the ligament of Treitz. The specific jejunal segment chosen should have a mesenteric arcade supplied by an adequate-size artery and vein. Approximately 20 to 25 cm of jejunum can be resected, although usually 10 to 15 cm is sufficient. The free jejunal segment is then transferred to the neck, where, in an isoperistaltic fashion, the proximal esophageal anastomosis is performed, the arterial and venous microvascular anastomosis carried out to the selected host vessels, and then the distal anastomosis completed.

With this technique, the reported graft survival rate is 85% to 95%, and the operative mortality is 5%. For those patients with successful grafting, 90% are reported to have an adequate swallowing quality. If graft failure occurs, a second attempt will be successful in 50% to 75% of cases.[116-118]

Minimally Invasive Esophagectomy

With the advent of minimally invasive surgical techniques, an interest has been shown in applying thorascopic and laparoscopic techniques to esophagectomy.[119] Certainly the techniques of gastric and esophageal mobilization have been well established for other complex minimally invasive surgeries. Minimally invasive esophagectomy required that these individual techniques be "spliced" together. Although a minimally invasive transhiatal approach can be used, most advocate video-assisted thoracoscopic (VATS) esophageal mobilization, followed by laparoscopic gastric mobilization, and the surgery completed with cervical esophagogastric anastomosis. A steep learning curve exists for these surgeries. Total length of hospitalization may be shortened somewhat. However, equipment costs and length of operative procedure may negate cost savings with this approach. Mortality rates of 4% to 7%, in experienced hands, are reported. Morbidity is 70% to 80%, and survival results have yet to be determined[120,121]; as minimally invasive techniques represent another form of incisional approach, survival should not be affected on the basis of this technique alone.

Survival with Surgery Alone

Survival after surgical resection is discussed separately from the description of individual techniques to emphasize the fact that postesophagectomy survival is a function of stage and not of surgical approach. Several points concerning postesophagectomy survival have now become quite clear. The first is that regardless of whether a thoracotomy or nonthoracotomy technique is used, cumulative postoperative survival is the same, at approximately 20% to 25%. This has been underscored most graphically by Muller and associates,[91] who reviewed the world literature to compare overall postesophagectomy survival by technique and showed no significant difference. Hulscher and coworkers[122] also reported a meta-analysis of the English language literature of the results of transthoracic and transhiatal resection of esophageal cancer, and this similarly demonstrated a higher risk of pulmonary morbidity and mortality with the transthoracic procedure, but a similar 5-year survival of approximately 20%. Subsequently, Hulscher and colleagues[123] reported the results of a randomized trial (see Table 77-4) comparing limited transhiatal resection with THE with extended en bloc lymphadenectomy for 220 patients with adenocarcinoma of the esophagus. No significant difference was found in survival or operative mortality, although postoperative pulmonary complications may have been somewhat higher with extended resection.

The second fact is that postoperative survival is stage related. Notably, the majority of patients considered for surgery are found to have stage III disease, and survival for these patients, even with surgery, is poor (approximately 10% to 15%). Hofstetter and associates[124] reported results for 1097 consecutive patients undergoing resection and compared outcome by stage for 1970 through 1985, 1986 through1996, and 1997 through 2001. Although median survival increased from 7 to 34 months, surgical mortality

decreased from 12% to 6%, and the R0 resection rate increased from 78% to 94%, no difference was found in survival by stage. Three-year survival rates through this period were 63%, 52%, and 44% for pathologic stage IIA and were 10%, 18%, and 6% for pathologic stage III. Multivariate analysis showed that survival was associated with complete resection and thorough preoperative staging, and that preoperative chemotherapy used in the later years was associated with increased complete resection. For T1 N0M0 adenocarcinoma of the esophagus,[125] survival at 5 and 10 years may be 77% and 68% after surgical resection.

New methods of pathological staging may improve ability to predict surgical outcome. Immunohistochemical staining may detect lymph node micrometastasis. In one study,[126] 62% of patients (adenocarcinoma and squamous cell carcinoma) with pathologic node-negative stage by conventional criteria had nodal disease, detected using monoclonal antibody Ber-EP4. This monoclonal antibody binds to certain glycoproteins found on epithelial tissues. The identification of micrometastatic nodal disease had a significant impact on survival. A somewhat lower incidence of micrometastatic disease was found by using anti-cytokeratin antibodies,[127-130] and the impact on survival was less clear. These techniques require validation in prospective trials, but may provide valuable prognostic information and allow selection of patients for adjuvant therapy.

The third point is that postsurgical survival is little influenced by whether there is squamous cell or adenocarcinoma. Holscher and coworkers[131] documented a postresection survival advantage *only* for patients with *stage I* adenocarcinoma. Salazar and colleagues[132] reported no difference in cumulative postoperative survival for patients with squamous cell carcinoma and adenocarcinoma. Finally, despite advances in surgical technique and results, postesophagectomy survival has remained remarkably stable over time. Wilkins[90] made this same point almost a decade ago after reviewing postoperative survival figures for the years 1952 to 1986. On the basis of his review, he queried as to whether surgery had "gone as far as it could go," and speculated that further improvement in survival figures would require combination therapy regimens that included systemic chemotherapy. As new systemic agents are developed, a differential response may be seen in adenocarcinoma and squamous cell carcinoma, which suggests that new agents will need to be evaluated separately in each histologic type.

Optimizing Surgical Outcome

Evidence-based surgery uses the treatment outcomes of cost, morbidity, mortality, and quality of life to help physicians, health care administrators, and hospitals determine the most appropriate setting and specific treatment for patient care. Evidence-based surgical techniques have consistently shown that increased provider experience improves patient outcome and reduces cost for complex surgeries. In terms of technical difficulty, length of stay, morbidity, and mortality, esophageal surgery is accepted to be complex gastrointestinal surgery. Gordon and associates[133] reported reduced hospital mortality, length of stay, and cost for a wide range of complex gastrointestinal (GI) procedures including esophagectomy. Zehr and coworkers[134] showed that the institution of standardized patient-care pathways, a product of the evidence-based surgery approach, reduced hospital cost for esophagectomies while keeping surgical mortality low (1.3%). Dimick and colleagues[135,136] documented the importance of surgical volume, hospital experience, and intensive care staffing in optimizing outcome after esophagectomy. These studies underscore the fact that even complex surgical procedures, such as esophagectomy, can be both effective therapy and cost-effective.

An important multi-institutional analysis[137] of outcome in Medicare patients for a variety of surgical procedures was published recently. A substantial difference in operative mortality exists based on number of esophagectomies per year at the institution. This varied from 23% for centers doing fewer than 2 cases per year down to 8.1% for high-volume centers performing more than 19 per year. The operative mortality rates reported in this series are higher than those reported in clinical trials, and this may relate not only to particular expertise of the study centers in esophageal cancer but also to patient selection for clinical research.

Combination Therapy Protocols, Including Surgery

Several combination-therapy protocols include surgery. Those protocols with the greatest published experience are covered in this chapter. One principle that remains constant for all of these protocols is that the surgical technique is not altered because of the combination therapy. The rationale for the combination therapy is not to alter the surgical technique or to change its morbidity and mortality. Rather, the nonsurgical therapy is added with the goal of improving postsurgical survival. Therefore, although not specifically stated in the ensuing reviews, the surgical techniques and principles are identical to those discussed under the section on surgery alone.

Chemotherapy Followed by Surgery

Numerous phase I and II trials of preoperative chemotherapy regimens known to be active in patients with metastatic disease were tested in newly diagnosed patients, and the results prompted two large randomized trials with differing results. Regimens tested in early phase I/II trials included cisplatin plus bleomycin,[138] cisplatin plus bleomycin plus vindesine,[139,140] and cisplatin plus methyl-glycosaminoglycan (GAG) plus vindesine[141] or vinblastine.[142] Later, Carey and associates[143-145] and Kies and coworkers[146] reported their results with preoperative cisplatin plus infusional 5-fluorouracil (5-FU). Two etoposide/cisplatin-containing regimens were studied in adenocarcinoma patients only.[147,148] Most of these studies administered two or three cycles of chemotherapy before resection. A barium esophagogram and CT scans were used to stage patients initially and were repeated before surgery to gauge response. The results of these pilot trials were quite similar, producing response in 40% to 60% of patients. Occasionally a pathologic CR was achieved; however, nearly all responses were partial. Median survivals varied from 8.5 to 23 months; in addition, two small randomized trials failed to demonstrate a benefit.[149,150]

The U.S. G-I Intergroup mounted a 467-patient randomized trial that compared (1) three courses of cisplatin, 100 mg/m², plus infusional 5-FU, 1000 mg/m², days 1 to 5 before surgery, and two courses after surgery (total, five courses), with (2) immediate surgery.[151] No benefit was demonstrated for the addition of chemotherapy in this trial (see Table 77-4), in which 45% had squamous cell carcinoma and 55% had adenocarcinoma. No differences were found in resectability or median, 1-, 2-, or 3-year survival rates between treatment groups and histologic types. The pathologic CR rate was 2.5%. Median and 2-year survivals with and without chemotherapy were 14.9 months and 35% versus 16.1 months and 37%. In both arms, approximately 60% of enrolled patients underwent a gross total resection (RO), and 17% had later local recurrence after RO resection for an ultimate 57% failure to control local disease. No differences were noted in surgical morbidity and mortality rates, which were 6% for both arms. Only 52% of eligible patients received one cycle, and 38%, both cycles of the planned postoperative therapy.

The MRC[152] conducted an 802-patient randomized trial, testing two cycles of cisplatin, 80 mg/m², and 5-FU, 1000 mg/m²/day continuous infusion for 4 days, given before resection of squamous cell or adenocarcinoma of the esophagus (see Table 77-4). Patients were required to have resectable tumor, although the staging evaluation was not proscribed by the study. Two thirds of patients had adenocarcinoma. Median survival was significantly improved from 13.3 to 16.8 months, with 2-year survival improved from 34% to 43%. No information about patterns of failure is available, but similar to the U.S. intergroup trial, 57% were able to undergo complete resection with negative margins. The effect of this well-tolerated chemotherapy regimen was similar regardless of histology, age, or sex. No immediate explanation for the difference between the results of this trial and the U.S. Intergroup trial is available, but may relate to the greater power, less rigorous staging, chance, or unknown differences between the populations in the two studies.

With the varying results of these two large randomized studies, the role of neoadjuvant chemotherapy remains controversial. Given the high local failure observed with neoadjuvant chemotherapy, combined chemotherapy and radiation before surgery is now a more active area of investigation. In the United States, preoperative chemotherapy is considered to be investigational, whereas in the United Kingdom, many oncologists consider this approach to be the standard of care.

Concomitant Chemotherapy and Radiation Therapy Followed by Surgery

Concomitant neoadjuvant chemotherapy and RT are frequently used in esophageal cancer, although the benefits have not been clearly demonstrated in the randomized trials that have been conducted to date. The rationale for neoadjuvant chemoradiation is that a high rate of both local and distant failure is seen with surgery alone (see Table 77-4).[151,153,154] The rate of complete resection with negative margins and ultimate local control do not appear to be substantially improved by the addition of chemotherapy alone.[151,152,154] The use of preoperative RT alone has been assessed in five fully reported[155-159] randomized trials and was not shown to be beneficial. Concurrent chemotherapy and RT results in tumor downstaging, with increased chance of resection of tumor with negative margins. Concurrent administration of chemotherapy and radiation takes advantage of the ability of some chemotherapy agents to potentiate the effects of RT on tumor cells. The agents that have been effective are generally those known to be radiosensitizers, such as 5-FU and cisplatin.

Five randomized trials of preoperative chemoradiation have been fully reported. The results of these trials are summarized in Table 77-5. Two trials, those of Nygaard and colleagues[157] and LePrise and associates,[160] used sequential chemotherapy and RT before surgery and failed to demonstrate any significant difference in median, disease-free, or overall survival. These are not discussed further here. The trials published by Bossett and coworkers,[161] Walsh and colleagues,[162] and Urba and associates[163] compared concomitant cisplatin-based chemotherapy and RT followed by immediate surgery. The trial reported by Walsh and coworkers[162] demonstrated a significant survival benefit. The single-institution University of Michigan trial reported by Urba demonstrated a local control but not a significant survival benefit, and the trial of Bossett and colleagues[161] demonstrated an improvement in disease-free survival but not overall survival. Interestingly, all three trials (see Table 77-4) observed similar 3-year survival rates for the combined treatment. However, the outcomes for the surgery arms varied and probably reflect differences in the patients enrolled in each trial. The details of these trials are described later.

The trial reported by Walsh[162] demonstrated improved survival in adenocarcinoma with concurrent 5-FU, 15 mg/kg on days 1 to 5 and 30 to 35; cisplatin, 75 mg/m² on days 7 and 37; and RT, 40-Gy in 15 fractions on days 1 to 19. Three-year survival was 32% versus 6%, and median survival was 16 months versus 11 months ($P = .01$). The CR rate for all patients enrolled in the preoperative therapy arm was 22%, and evidence was seen of nodal downstaging with 82% node positive in the surgery arm in contrast with 25% after neoadjuvant therapy ($P < .001$). This study has been criticized for its relatively small number of patients, poor results in the surgery-alone arm, and lack of uniform preoperative staging.

Urba and associates[163] reported results for patients randomized to surgery (generally THE) with or without preoperative therapy with cisplatin, 20 mg/m² on days 1 to 5, 17 to 21; vinblastine, 1 mg/m² on days 1 to 4, 17 to 20; 5-FU, 300 mg/m² on days 1 to 21; and RT, 1.5 Gy twice a day to 45 Gy. Median survival was 17.6 months with neoadjuvant therapy and 16.9 months with surgery alone, and 3-year survival was 30% versus 16%, respectively ($P = .18$). The gross total resection rate was in excess of 90% in both arms. The pathologic CR rate was 28% and did not differ significantly for adenocarcinoma or squamous cell carcinoma. Preoperative therapy reduced the incidence of local/regional failure as first disease recurrence from 39% versus 19%. Distant initial failure was approximately 60% in both arms. Operative mortality with THE was 4% with surgery alone and 2% after neoadjuvant therapy. This study did not have the power to detect a modest but significant improvement in survival, although it is noteworthy that 3-year survival was similar to the outcome of the trial reported by Walsh.[162]

Bossett and coworkers,[161] reporting the results of a French multicenter trial, found no difference in survival outcome with preoperative therapy, although a significant disease-free survival and local recurrence–free survival benefit were found. The patient population was limited

TABLE 77-5

Preoperative Chemotherapy and Radiation Therapy: Randomized Trials

AUTHOR	TREATMENT ARMS	MEDIAN (MO)	PERCENT SURVIVAL (YR)		
			1	2	3
Nygaard et al.[157]	S		13	9	
	Cisplatin/bleomycin + 35 Gy + surgery		23	17	
LePrise et al.[160]	S	10	47		14
	Cisplatin/5-FU + 35 Gy + surgery	10	46		19
Bossett et al.[161]	S	18.6	67	42	34
	Cisplatin + 37 Gy + surgery	18.6	69	48	37
Walsh et al.[162]	S	11	44	26	6
	Cisplatin/5-FU + 40 Gy + surgery	16	52	37	32
		$P = .01$			$P = .01$
Urba et al.[165]	S	17.5	58	39	16
	Cisplatin/5-FU/VBL + 45 Gy + surgery	16.3	70	42	32
					$P = .07$

5-FU, 5-fluorouracil; S, squamous cell carcinoma; VBL, vinblastine.

to those with stage I and II squamous cell carcinoma. The regimen was cisplatin, 80 mg/m^2 given 0 to 2 days before each set of RT treatments and the RT consisted of two 1-week courses of 18.5 Gy in five 3.7-Gy fractions beginning on days 1 and 22. Postoperative mortality was significantly worse, 12% versus 4%. This trial has been criticized because chemotherapy was often not administered on the same day as RT, the chemotherapy was less intensive than that in the other trials, and an unusual hypofractionated and split-course regimen of RT was used.

A U.S. Intergroup trial was initiated to assess the outcome definitively with neoadjuvant cisplatin and 5-FU chemotherapy with radiation in comparison with surgery alone. This trial was closed early as a result of poor accrual. Possible reasons include the existence of a strong bias among physicians about whether to use neoadjuvant therapy, lack of consensus about an optimal preoperative regimen, and patient resistance to randomization. It is not likely that this issue can be definitively examined in the United States.

In the absence of definitive randomized data, large phase II trials[164-184] may provide information relevant to appropriate use of this intensive approach and provide information that may guide future study. Phase II results with long-term follow-up are summarized in Table 77-6. The long-term results reported by Kleinberg and colleagues,[182] including patients treated with maximally tolerated regimens of cisplatin and protracted-infusion 5-FU, demonstrate that only limited further improvement in outcome with these agents is possible. Other studies have examined new regimens such as those containing paclitaxel, irinotecan, and oxaliplatin, but long-term data about survival outcome are not available. To the extent that these phase II trials have included patients with both squamous cell and adenocarcinoma, the outcome has generally been similar, although as newer regimens are developed, this may not be the case.

Rigorous staging of patients with EUS before neoadjuvant chemotherapy may in the future allow better selection for trimodality therapy, accurately excluding patients with early stage I disease, who may be treated with surgery alone or those with T4 lesions likely to be unresectable. In addition, the availability of accurate information about preoperative stage may allow more sensitive determination of response to preoperative therapy as measured by downstaging, although limited information is currently available to address this issue. Heath and associates[184] reported phase II results for patients staged with EUS: 69% were found to be downstaged at the time of surgery, and 19% were upstaged as a result of discovery of metastatic disease or regional nodes, in the context of a 25% histologic CR rate. Slater and coworkers[185] reported the incidence of downstaging based on EUS: 36% were downstaged in another trial, which had a 15% pathologic CR rate of patients treated with preoperative chemoradiation.

The recent randomized data demonstrated that the increase in surgical mortality after preoperative chemoradiation is modest, but controversy has remained about whether morbidity is increased. Doty and colleagues[186] reviewed the results of 120 patients treated with

TABLE 77-6

Selected Phase II Trials with Long-Term Follow-up

AUTHOR	NO. OF PATIENTS	ADENO* (%)	PREOPERATIVE CHEMOTHERAPY	RADIOTHERAPY	R0 (%)	CR (%)	MEDIAN SURVIVAL (MO)	5-YR SURVIVAL (%)
Forastiere et al., 1993[154]	43	48	Cisplatin, 20 mg/m^2/day 1–5, 17–21 Vinblastine, 1 mg/m^2/day 1–4, 17–20 5-FU, 300 mg/m^2/day 1–21	5-FU, 300 mg/m^2/day 1–21	84	24	29	34
Bedenne et al., 1998[†]	94	0	Cisplatin 20 mg/m^2/day 5-FU, 800 mg/m^2/day day 1–5, 22–26	30 Gy/10 fx, split course given, day 1–5, 22–26	82	20	17	23
Urba et al., 2000[163]	50	26	Cisplatin, 20 mg/m^2/day, 1–5, 17–21 Vinblastine 1 mg/m^2/day 1–4, 17–20 5-FU 300 mg/m^2/day 1–21	4500/30 fx/BID	90	28	17	22
Posner et al., 2001[‡]	44	75	5-FU, cisplatin, and interferon in varying schedules	4000/20 fx or 4500/30 fx BID	81	24	28	32
Kleinberg et al., 2003[182]	92	71	Cisplatin 20 or 26 mg/m^2/day, 1–5, 26–30 5-FU 225 or 300 mg/m^2/day 1–30	44 Gy/22 fx	87	37	35	40

CR, pathologic complete response; R, complete resection with negative margins.
*Patient had either adenocarcinoma (adeno) or squamous cell carcinoma.
†Bedenne L, Seitz JF, Milan C, et al: Cisplatin, 5-FU and preoperative radiotherapy in esophageal epidermoid cancer: Multicenter phase II FFCD 8804 study. Gastroenterol Clin Biol 1998;22:273–281.
‡Posner MC, Gooding WE, Lew JI, et al: Complete 5-year follow-up of a prospective phase II trial of preoperative chemoradiotherapy for esophageal cancer. Surgery 2001;130:620–628.

preoperative chemoradiation at Johns Hopkins Hospital. Surgical mortality was 1%. The complication rate was 59% for squamous cell carcinoma and 31.6% for adenocarcinoma. The primary difference in complication rate for squamous cell carcinoma, which tends to be more proximal, was an increased risk of pulmonary complications. These results are comparable to the mortality (2.2% to 9.0%) and morbidity (22% to 74%)[186] reported after surgery alone, suggesting that neoadjuvant therapy may be administered without significantly increasing the risk of surgery. Factors hypothesized as being important to optimizing surgical results after neoadjuvant chemoradiation were preoperative nutritional support, transhiatal approach with cervical anastomosis, and the use of standardized postoperative patient-care plans.

Based on these data, the use of neoadjuvant therapy is a rational strategy that clearly improves local control and may improve survival. Cisplatin- and 5-FU–based regimens are most commonly used, as long-term survival outcome of paclitaxel, docetaxel, and oxaliplatin and irinotecan-containing regimens are not yet available. These results also demonstrate that pathologic stage after neoadjuvant therapy is an important predictor of survival and may be useful in selecting patients for trials of novel adjuvant therapies such as cyclo-oxygenase-2 (COX-2) or epidermal growth factor receptor inhibitors. In addition, most trials of preoperative chemoRT have included only patients with resectable tumor. The role of preoperative therapy in converting tumors from unresectable to resectable is unknown, although recent reports demonstrated the feasibility of resection of some T4 tumors after neoadjuvant therapy.[187,188]

Assessment of Response to Neoadjuvant Therapy

Radiographic and endoscopic assessment of response has not proven accurate enough to allow this to serve as a selection criterion for proceeding to surgery, as post-treatment inflammatory changes and thickening are difficult to distinguish from tumor.[189-191] In one study, seven patients with pathologic CR at the time of surgery were staged by endoscopy and EUS as T4N1 (one patient), T3N1 (three patients), T2N1 (two patients), and T3N0 (one patient).[192] Several small studies evaluated whether change in metabolic activity was detected on PET scan comparing scans before therapy with scans during or after therapy. These studies demonstrated a general correlation with decreased metabolic activity and response, but the clinical utility of this observation requires prospective evaluation.[193-195] In a 39-patient prospective study at Sloan-Kettering Cancer Center, decrease in standardized uptake value of more than 60% was associated with improved 2-year disease-free survival (67% vs. 38%; P = NS),[196] whereas in a 40-patient trial at Technische Univsersitat Munich,[197] a 35% reduction was associated with improved tumor response (53% vs. 5%; $P < .001$), and median time to progression of 16 months vs. 9 months ($P = .01$), and overall survival (19 months vs. 13 months; $P = .04$). The ability of those techniques to determine who might benefit from proceeding with or omitting surgery by identifying complete responders who do not need surgery is unknown and is the subject of research.

Adjuvant Therapy

The role of postoperative therapy remains to be clarified. Several randomized trials have failed to demonstrate a benefit to postoperative RT,[198,199] although postoperative chemotherapy and postoperative chemoradiation remain areas of active investigation, with some limited data to support its use under select circumstances.

As discussed in the earlier sections, adjuvant chemotherapy has been poorly tolerated in patients who have received prior chemotherapy as part of neoadjuvant preoperative therapy or definitive chemoradiation. Only 54% completed the planned adjuvant chemotherapy after definitive cisplatin and 5-FU and radiation in RTOG 8501,[200] 58% received planned adjuvant taxol/cisplatin chemotherapy after neoadjuvant cisplatin and 5-FU chemoradiation,[184] and 38% after neoadjuvant cisplatin and 5-FU chemotherapy.[151] This limits the usefulness of this strategy in patients pretreated with surgery alone, although some evidence suggests that this approach may be useful after surgery alone.

Conversely, several retrospective studies suggested a benefit for postoperative chemoradiation after surgery alone.[201,202] A randomized intergroup trial[203] demonstrated a significant survival benefit when 5-FU, leucovorin, and RT are administered after resection of adenocarcinoma of the stomach or GE junction. In that trial, approximately 20% of the patients had tumor of the GE junction, and the remainder had gastric tumors. Therefore determining the applicability of the finding to patients with tumor involving primarily the GE junction will require further study. Nevertheless, median survival for the entire population in the study was improved from 27 months to 36 months (P = .005). Three-year survival was 50% versus 41%, and 3-year relapse-free survival was improved from 36% to 47%. Based on these limited data, it is reasonable to consider postoperative chemoradiation for patients after resection of stage II or III adenocarcinoma of the GE junction, but the issue is likely to remain controversial until more data applicable to this particular subset of patients are obtained. When incomplete resection is performed, definitive chemoradiation or palliative single-modality chemotherapy or RT may be considered, depending on the clinical circumstances.

Pathologic stage at the time of surgery was an important predictor of survival outcome that may be useful in the selection of high-risk patients for trials of adjuvant therapy. The relation of stage to survival outcome for patients treated with surgery alone was described earlier. Kleinberg and associates[182] reported that for patients treated with neoadjuvant therapy, survival also was closely related to pathologic stage at the time of surgical resection. Median survivals for patients with pathologic stage CR, I, IIA, IIB, III, and IV disease at the time of surgery were more than 5 years, more than 5 years, and 22, 13.5, 18, and 4.9 months, respectively.

Definitive Chemoradiation

Concurrent chemoradiation had been demonstrated in randomized trials to be a curative therapy and superior to RT alone. This approach represents a rational alternative to surgery for selected patients and should be used for unresectable disease. These trials demonstrate improved median survival and the possibility of long-term cure with the addition of concurrent chemotherapy. Although these studies primarily included patients with squamous cell carcinoma, combined chemoradiation also has become the standard approach for patients with adenocarcinoma who are candidates for definitive nonsurgical therapy. As there are likely significant selection criteria in patients who are selected for chemoradiation versus surgical trials, it is not possible to compare the outcome directly in terms of short-term morbidity and mortality, palliation, and survival. Radiation alone should be used only in potentially curable patients when they are not candidates for chemotherapy or surgery or if they refuse other treatments. Chemoradiation can result in long-term survival with T4 tumors at the price of significant risk of toxicity, such as tracheoesophageal fistula,[204] but patients with extensive unresectable nodal disease may be less likely to benefit from intensive local therapies.

The landmark trial, RTOG 8501,[200,205,206] established the role of concurrent chemoradiation in the therapy of locally advanced esophageal cancer (see Table 77-4). One hundred twenty-three patients were randomized to 64-Gy RT alone or 50-Gy RT with 5-FU, 1000 mg/m^2 on days 1 to 4, and cisplatin, 75 mg/m^2 on day 1 every 4 weeks during RT, and for two cycles every 3 weeks after RT. Eligibility criteria included localized (M0) esophageal cancer, as documented with CT scan of chest and abdomen, bone scan, and pan-endoscopy. Eighty-eight percent had squamous cell carcinoma. With the addition of chemotherapy, median survival was improved from 9.3 months to 14.1 months, and two-year survival was 10% versus 36%. Notably, although there were no 3-year survivors with RT alone, the 5-year survival with combined-modality therapy was 27%. Longer follow-up demonstrated 10-year survival of 20%, establishing combined chemoradiation as an alternative therapy for locally advanced, potentially curable esophageal cancer. Isolated locoregional persistent disease and failure as part of initial recurrence was reduced from 53% to 38%, whereas distant failure as part of initial failure was 30% versus 16% when chemotherapy was added. Although patients receiving combined-modality therapy had the expected increase in acute toxicities of therapy, no substantial increase was noted in long-term toxicities.

Because RTOG 8501 was closed early when a significant benefit was demonstrated on interim analysis, a confirmatory nonrandomized group of 69 patients was treated with the experimental combined-modality arm. Five-year survival for this group was 14%. The patterns of failure also were similar to those of the randomized group. In the randomized and confirmatory portions of the study, no difference in outcome was seen for the 15% of patients who had adenocarcinoma and the remainder with squamous cell carcinoma.

The Eastern Cooperative Oncology Group[207] conducted a trial comparing 60-Gy RT with 60-Gy RT given along with mitomycin C, 10 mg/m^2 on day 2, and 5-FU, 1000 mg/m^2/day for 4 days for squamous cell carcinoma of the esophagus (see Table 77-4). The results of this 135-patient study were confounded by the circumstance that patients could be selected for surgical resection after 40 Gy of RT was given. Thirty-eight percent were selected to have surgery. Nevertheless, median survival was improved from 9.2 to 14.8 months with the addition of chemotherapy. The 2- and 5-year survivals was 12% versus 27% and 7% versus 9%. Of note, no 3-year survivors who were treated with radiation alone did not also have surgery.

Long-term follow-up is available from a phase II trial at the National Cancer Institute of Milan[208] in 106 patients with squamous cell carcinoma of the esophagus treated with cisplatin, 100 mg/m^2 on day 1, and 5-FU, 1000 mg/m^2 on days 1 to 4 for two cycles with concurrent RT of 30 Gy in 15 fractions. Twenty-four of these patients also had surgery with complete resection. Overall survival was 22% at 5 years and 12% at 10 years, which did not differ whether or not surgery was added. These data confirm the curative potential of combined chemoradiation.

Salvage Therapy After Local Failure

The results of surgery for recurrence after definitive chemoradiation for esophageal cancer have been described for small selected groups of patients.[209-211] This intervention is associated with an increase in operative complications but also the possibility of long-term survival in these highly selected series. Prospective evaluation of the approach of concurrent chemoradiation with surgical salvage for recurrent/residual disease is needed. A significant barrier to the success of this approach is the difficulty of assessing response to chemoradiation with noninvasive techniques, described elsewhere in this chapter. Nevertheless, great interest exists in testing a therapeutic approach in which those having an apparent CR would have close follow-up with surgical salvage, if needed, rather than immediate surgery.

Similarly, only limited information is available about the results of RT for isolated local failure after surgical resection.[211] As combined chemoradiation is beneficial in gross disease when newly diagnosed esophageal cancer is present, we advocate this approach for the uncommon patient with isolated locoregional failure after full restaging evaluation. The RT dose may be limited to 45 Gy by the presence of a gastric pull-up in the treatment field.

Radiation Therapy Dose Selection

The RT dose required depends on the clinical circumstances. When RT alone is used as definitive treatment, a dose of 60 to 64 Gy should generally be used. This dose is limited by esophageal tolerance, as well as the need to limit RT dose to lung. The incidence of both early and late complications varies with total dose, administration of systemic chemotherapy, and volume of esophagus irradiated. Emami and coworkers[212] estimated the radiation dose (with conventional fractionation) that would lead to a 5% rate of clinical stricture or perforation within 5 years to be 60 Gy when one third of the esophagus is treated, 58 Gy if two thirds, and 55 Gy for all of the esophagus.

Dose escalation, when RT is used as a single modality, has been safely carried out by the addition of brachytherapy, although no clearly demonstrated benefit has been seen in survival or local control.[213-215] Nevertheless, it is reasonable to add brachytherapy in patients treated with RT alone in the uncommon situation in which the entirety of residual disease can be encompassed in the treated volume. The American Brachytherapy Society Clinical Research Committee has published guidelines[216] suggesting that a good candidate for brachytherapy has a tumor that is 10 cm or smaller confined to the thoracic esophagus and without regional nodes. When brachytherapy is used, the external-beam dose is generally limited to 45 to 50 Gy in 1.8- to 2.0-Gy fractions, followed by a high-dose-rate boost with two to three treatments of 5 Gy or followed by 1 low-dose-rate brachytherapy application of 20 Gy over a period of 24 to 48 hours. The dose is prescribed to 1 cm from the midpoint of the treatment catheter.

Given that local control is still not optimal with existing combined definitive chemoRT regimens, an interest has been indicated in intensifying the RT dose used in this therapeutic approach. When RTOG 8501, which demonstrated improved outcome with combined chemoradiation, was designed, the radiation dose for the combined-modality arm was reduced to 50 Gy from 64 Gy in the radiation-alone arm because of concerns about toxicity. However, other trials showed the feasibility of using higher radiation doses as part of combined-modality therapy. To investigate this question, the Intergroup Trial 0123[217] randomized patients to a dose of 50.4 Gy versus 64.8 Gy with two cycles of cisplatin, 75 mg/m^2 day 1, and 5-FU, 1000 mg/m^2/day, on days 1 to 4 during radiation and two adjuvant cycles. With the higher dose, no improvement was found in median survival (13.0 vs. 18.1 months), 2-year survival (31% vs. 40%), or control of local disease (44% vs. 48%). Use of intensified chemotherapy regimens or new agents also may ultimately play a role in improving outcome, but also can lead to substantially increased toxicity.[218] Therefore a dose of approximately 50 Gy with conventional fraction remains the standard when given with chemotherapy.

Another means of intensifying the local treatment is using preoperative RT (with chemotherapy) before surgery. In this setting, a dose of 44 to 45 Gy with conventional fractionation is used, followed by a 4- to 6-week interval before surgery. The isolated local failure rate is low, 0 to 15%,[182,219-222] and therefore escalating the dose of RT or further intensifying the local therapy beyond approximately 44 to 50 Gy at 1.8 to 2.0 Gy/day appears unlikely to improve outcome. Doses greater than 50 Gy are associated with increased surgical mortality,[223] and lower doses may be associated with increased local failure.[224] When postoperative RT is given, the dose should generally be limited to approximately 45 Gy to avoid injury to the gastric pull-up or interposed bowel.

Radiation Therapy Techniques

When RT is given, treatment fields extend a minimum of 5 cm above and below the radiographically identifiable lesion to account for microscopic or submucosal tumor extension. If definitive RT is used to doses more than 50 Gy, a reduction to a margin of 2 cm above and 2 cm below the tumor should be considered. A radial margin of 1.5 to 2.5 to the block edge should be used, but this may be limited posteriorly as needed to keep the spinal cord dose within tolerance. A three-field or four-field approach with an anterior and two posterior oblique off-cord fields with or without the addition of a fourth posterior field has become relatively standard in the treatment of esophageal cancer and allows high doses to be delivered to the tumor while limiting the radiation dose delivered to the spinal cord and lung. The dose delivered by the treatment fields should be weighted such that the maximal possible dose (that which delivers ≤45 Gy to the spinal cord) is delivered by the anterior or posterior fields, whereas only the remainder of the dose is delivered by the off-cord oblique fields to minimize dose delivered to the lung tissue. This beam arrangement also can be used for the treatment of upper esophageal tumors, as none of the beams enter laterally through the arms and shoulders. All fields can be treated from the first day of treatment, which has the advantage of delivering a lower fractional daily dose to uninvolved structures such as the lung, or treatment can begin with anteroposterior/posteroanterior (AP/PA) fields only, which may allow a quicker start to treatment while a formal plan is developed, allow more margin for error in daily patient setup, and decrease daily treatment time. Under the latter circumstance, the multifield plan is implemented later to protect the spinal cord and other critical structures. In all cases, care must be taken through careful dosimetry to keep the spinal cord dose within safe limits and to take account of varying thickness of the chest longitudinally. Wedges and compensators should be used as needed to maintain homogeneity of the RT dose distribution. The spinal cord should be limited to approximately 45 Gy, and the dose to lung tissue should be minimized. Care also must be taken to avoid an excess risk of cardiac toxicity when distal lesions are treated, which may necessitate giving a larger proportion of the radiation dose through oblique or lateral fields rather then through AP/PA portals, which generally treat more of the heart.

When advanced radiation techniques such as three-dimensional planning or intensity-modulated RT are used, the greater confidence in dosimetry may allow tighter margins with greater shielding of normal tissues. These techniques, although they may decrease normal tissue toxicity, are unlikely to improve outcome substantially, as marginal miss of the tumor has not been implicated as an important cause of treatment failure, dose escalation has not improved outcome, and the esophagus itself, rather than potentially shielded nearby normal structures, is generally the dose-limiting structure. Whether these techniques will reduce toxicity, improving the therapeutic ratio or resulting in better tolerance of combined-modality therapy, is unknown.[225,226]

Defining the extent of the tumor requires integration of data obtained from a variety of radiologic studies and procedures. Modern treatment techniques for planning esophageal RT involve the use of CT scans that depict the radial extension of the primary disease that cannot be visualized on barium studies. In addition, as barium also can underestimate the longitudinal extent of disease, all available data from endoscopy and ultrasound should be integrated into the planning process. The extent of nodal disease should be evaluated by CT scan and EUS. When appropriate, pathologic assessment of nodal disease can be obtained by ultrasound-guided needle biopsy or laparoscopy. It is unknown whether a benefit is found to elective treatment of clinically uninvolved supraclavicular nodes for proximal lesions. In situations in which spinal cord tolerance may be dose limiting, the patient should be treated in the prone position, which has been documented to increase the distance between the esophagus and the spinal cord by a mean of 1.3 to 1.9 cm, depending on the position along the thoracic esophagus.[227] Oral contrast administration at the time of simulation or CT simulation or both enhances visualization of the tumor and adds to the precision of treatment planning. This enhances the ability to deliver an adequate dose to the target while limiting the dose to the spinal cord. Consideration should be given to using immobilization devices to aid in ensuring uniform day-to-day patient positioning.

Radiation Therapy in Tracheoesophageal Fistula

The use of definitive or palliative RT in the setting of TE fistula has been controversial. Although TE fistula has historically been considered a contraindication to RT for fear that RT will worsen the fistula, mounting evidence indicates that RT can be beneficial and should not be withheld when it may be of palliative benefit. In a report from the Mayo Clinic,[228] lysis of tumor by RT could not be shown to be an important cause of TE fistula. In 22 patients in whom fistula developed after prior RT, recurrent tumor was the cause in all cases. For 10 patients irradiated with known TE fistula, the fistula did not worsen in any patients, and 6 of 10 had local disease controlled until the time of death from metastatic esophageal cancer.[228] Combined chemotherapy and RT also has been demonstrated to close fistula in four of five responders in one series.[229] The outcome appears to be improved with aggressive therapy rather than supportive care only.[230]

Toxicity of Radiotherapy

Patients will experience a marked esophagitis during radiation treatment, which clears within several weeks of the conclusion of therapy. Topical anesthetics, narcotics, and histamine (H_2) blockers are used to minimize discomfort during feeding. Oral nutritional supplements should be used to maintain nutritional state. Feeding tubes can be placed before therapy if necessary. Other grade III or greater early effects are uncommon but can include skin reactions, laryngeal toxicity (if in the treatment field), and pneumonitis. In RTOG 8501, toxicity with both radiation alone and combined chemoradiation therapy were prospectively collected. In 5% of patients treated with 60-Gy RT alone, grade III or greater esophagitis developed, whereas in 20% of those treated with concurrent chemoradiation therapy, these symptoms developed. Late esophageal toxicity was observed in 10 of 53 versus 11 of 51. Benign stricture is the most common serious late complication, reported to occur in 12% to

30% of curatively treated patients and can be treated with dilation,[231-233] although experience shows that most long-term strictures are associated with recurrent tumor rather than with the radiation. Decreased esophageal motility, delayed emptying, and reflux may occur.[233]

The toxicities with brachytherapy have not been well quantified. One series of 148 patients treated with external-beam RT of 60 Gy over a 6-week period, followed a week later by 12-Gy high-dose-rate brachytherapy in two fractions, demonstrated 28% ulceration, 10% stricture, and 6% fistula. Except for fistula, which was generally fatal, the other complications were rarely severe.[234] In RTOG 9207,[235] the concept of adding brachytherapy of 5 Gy for three high-dose-rate treatments to chemoradiation therapy (as in RTOG 8501) was tested, but the incidence of fistula was 6 of 35, and this approach is not recommended.

Brachytherapy for Palliation

Brachytherapy is useful in selected cases for palliative treatment of esophageal cancer and can be used in addition to, as an alternative to, or in patients previously treated with external-beam RT.[216] A catheter of 0.6 to 1 cm in width is inserted, and the lesion is treated with a 1- to 2-cm margin. The dose is generally prescribed at a distance of 1 cm from the radioactive sources, and dose fall-off beyond this range is rapid. Therefore only patients with symptoms resulting from tumor primarily confined to the esophageal wall and lumen itself can be given effective and durable palliation. High-dose-rate brachytherapy uses short applications of several minutes each, which are more convenient for the patient and do not require inpatient care. However, several applications are usually required, as fractionated treatment is thought to be safer. With low-dose-rate RT, in which treatment is given at 0.4 to 1.0 Gy/hr, treatment is given with one or two insertions of the applicator but over a 24- to 48-hour period. Although this approach does require overnight admission and prolonged esophageal intubation, fewer applications are needed, and the technology is more widely available.

Several palliative regimens have been recommended as appropriate by the American Brachytherapy Society Consensus Guidelines panel.[216] Palliation occurs in 50% to 90% of cases.[236-240] In previously untreated patients, a limited dose of external-beam RT (i.e., 30 Gy) can be followed by high-dose-rate brachytherapy (10 to 14 Gy in one or two fractions) or low-dose-rate brachytherapy (20 to 25 Gy in a single application over a 1- to 2-day period). Dysphagia was palliated by external-beam RT followed by brachytherapy in 90%[241] in one series, but the relative benefits of this approach compared with higher doses of external-beam RT alone are unknown. Conversely, brachytherapy alone can be used for palliation when life expectancy is short or when external-beam RT has been used in the past. Appropriate regimens include high-dose-rate treatment, 15 to 20 Gy in two to four applications, or low-dose-rate therapy, 25 to 40 Gy over a 1- to 2-day period. For poor-prognosis patients, high-dose-rate brachytherapy of 15 Gy in one session also may be an appropriate regimen, which also results in palliation in close to 70% of patients.[236,242]

These brachytherapy regimens are generally considered safe, although the rates of complications including acute esophagitis, ulceration, and stricture are not well quantified in palliatively treated patients. In patients who are treated curatively with 60-Gy external-beam RT followed by high-dose-rate brachytherapy of 12 Gy in two fractions, one series with routine endoscopic follow-up found a 50% incidence of esophageal ulceration that usually healed with conservative management and rarely became severe.[243] Brachytherapy along with chemotherapy or immediately after concurrent conventional chemoradiation therapy can result in an unacceptable rate of fistula formation.[235] Brachytherapy can be safely given several weeks after laser therapy and may improve the dysphagia-free interval,[244-246] whereas its role along with PDT is uncertain.

Swallowing Function and Palliative Radiation Therapy

Radiation can improve swallowing function in a significant proportion of patients. Radiation alone improves dysphagia in approximately 70% percent of patients,[247-249] and chemoradiation therapy improves dysphagia in 88%[232] of patients. Relief is not immediate but is often fast, with median time to maximal improvement of 4 weeks (range, 2 to 21 weeks). High doses of RT (with chemotherapy when appropriate) are generally required for effective palliation and should be used whenever life expectancy is greater than 3 months and Karnofsky performance status is 60 or greater. For patients treated with such aggressive palliative regimens, relief of dysphagia for the remaining lifetime occurs in 51%[250] to 67%[251] of patients. However, the results of RTOG 8501[200] indicate a substantial incidence of persistent or recurrent local disease, even in curatively treated patients, that no doubt translates into a significant incidence of local symptoms even under optimal circumstances. It also is noteworthy that the toxicity of therapy may transiently worsen swallowing before improvement. Palliative RT with or without chemotherapy may be used to prevent recurrence of swallowing difficulty after endoscopic palliative therapy such as stent placement or laser therapy.

Endoscopic Therapy

Endoscopic techniques to restore esophageal luminal patency are palliative procedures that should be used as sole therapy only in patients who are not candidates for curative therapy. However, endoscopic therapies are quite useful in providing symptom relief before definitive therapy for cancer and may make definitive therapy more easily tolerated. In rare situations with early-stage superficial tumors that have recurred after conventional therapies or for patients who are medically ineligible for conventional therapy, endoscopic therapies may be provided with curative intent, although the outcome data are limited.

Although the focus of endoscopic therapy has shifted from intubation with rigid funnel-shaped tubes to the use of expandable stents, and laser fulguration is being challenged by PDT, the principles of therapy have remained unchanged. The variables to be considered in selecting the most appropriate endoscopic method include cost, experience, tumor length, location and configuration, and the presence or absence of an esophagorespiratory fistula.

Rigid funnel tubes are not commonly used[252,253] anymore. The problem with these tubes stems from their rigid nature. Tube walls are thick, so a significant outer-to-inner diameter difference exists. The bigger the tube inserted, the better the expected swallowing result. Therefore the malignant stricture should be widened by dilatation or laser fulguration with the attendant risk of perforation, which is reported to occur in 4.9% to 19% of patients.[254-257] Once in place, the rigid tube is susceptible to erosion with hemorrhage or obstruction, which is reported to occur in 0 to 3.4%[255-267] and 4.4% to 12% of patients, respectively. Other reported complications include tube dislodgement in 1% to 10%, and aspiration pneumonia in 2.2% of patients.[255]

Self-expanding metallic stents (SEMSs) are compressible metal stents that were developed to improve the ease and safety of stent insertion. Initial SEMSs were uncovered and were associated with rapid tumor in-growth with stent obstruction. Up to 78% who survive for 4 or more months may require repeated intervention for palliation.[268] Newer SEMSs are covered with polyethylene, polyurethane, or silicone sheaths to delay or prevent in-growth of tumor, substantially reducing the need for repeated procedures.[269] SEMSs require less tumor dilatation for insertion, expand to greater luminal size than do standard rigid tubes, and have thin, nonbulky walls to minimize erosion and hemorrhage. SEMSs may be "stacked" one on top of another to manage tumor growth over the top of a previously placed expandable stent. Successful insertion of SEMSs is reported to occur in more than 90% of patients. Initial complications are less frequent and less morbid than are those reported with the use of rigid tubes. A series of 127 stent placements in 100 patients[268] resulted in no fatal complications, 1.6% pain necessitating removal, 3.1% inadequate deployment, 0.8% perforation, 7.9% food impaction, 11% severe reflux, and 8.7% stent migration requiring removal. Notably, in 2 of 16 patients who had placement of an expandable stent before chemoradiation, erosion developed through the esophagus. When the stent is placed at the GE junction, significant and uncomfortable reflux may result, although newer stents with antireflux valves may reduce this complication. Swallowing is improved in 88% to 100% of patients. In small series, SEMSs are effective in sealing esophagorespiratory fistula with low complication rates.[270] Patients generally do not tolerate having the top of the funnel near the cricopharyngeus because of the unpleasant foreign-body sensation, so esophageal intubation is often not an appropriate palliative strategy for cervical esophageal tumors. A retrospective comparison of self-expandable stent placement and palliative esophagectomy demonstrated palliation with stents that was as least as good as surgery over the limited survival period with less risk.[271]

Another means of providing palliation for patients with inoperable symptomatic obstructing esophageal cancer is endoscopic recannulation by using the neodymium:yttrium-aluminum-garnet (Nd:YAG) laser, or electrofulguration with a mono- or bipolar (BICAP) coagulating probe. Laser techniques use an endoscopically directed Nd:YAG laser probe to ablate the obstructing esophageal cancer directly. Although shorter lesions may be opened in one session, in general, more than one session is necessary to achieve the desired result. Repeated treatments are usually needed to maintain esophageal luminal patency. Successful improvements in swallowing symptoms have been reported in 64% to 100% of patients.[257] Success is related to the length of circumferential tumor.[257] For circumferential tumors longer than 4 cm, the number of endoscopic sessions needed increases, and the chance of success decreases. Endoscopic laser therapy is not recommended in the setting of an esophagorespiratory fistula. Complications include fevers, perforation, aspiration pneumonia, and later stricture formation. The reported procedural mortality ranges from 0 to 5%. Siegel and colleagues[262] reported improved survival in patients with squamous cell esophageal tumors treated with endoscopic laser therapy when compared with clinical stage–matched controls. The authors speculated that the survival advantage in the treated group may be due to tumor debulking, improved nutritional status, decrease in aspiration pneumonia, enhanced sense of well-being, and patient motivation. A randomized trial demonstrated that palliative RT reduces the need for repeated procedures for recurrent obstruction and may be warranted in patients with good performance status and limited disease, who may survive for a long period[272]—a concept that also may apply when other means of endoscopic palliation are used.

Electrofulguration techniques use either a monopolar probe or a BICAP. The monopolar probe directly coagulates the obstructing endoluminal tumor under endoscopic control. The BICAP tumor probe is passed through the narrowed esophageal lumen over a guidewire. The mechanism of action of the BICAP includes dilation of the narrowed lumen, tumor coagulation, hyperthermia, and tissue necrosis with delayed slough.[260] Because the BICAP probe coagulates blindly and circumferentially, it is not recommended for noncircumferential lesions, because injury to the normal esophageal mucosa may result in perforation. Comparisons of electrocoagulation (mono- or bipolar) with Nd:YAG laser techniques have shown comparable results in terms of morbidity, mortality, and relief of dysphagia.[260,261] Electrocoagulation is generally less costly than laser.

PDT is a technology that has generated a great deal of interest in the lay and scientific literature. This technique involves the administration of a chemical sensitizer, usually hematoporphyrin derivative or dihematoporphyrin ethers, that accumulates preferentially in the target tumor. The tumor is then exposed to a specific-wavelength low-power laser light that activates the accumulated sensitizing chemical, resulting in tumor necrosis mediated by production of singlet oxygen. Tumor cell death results from a photochemical and not a thermal effect, as with laser techniques. The clinical feasibility of using PDT to manage early or unresectable esophageal cancer is well documented.[273-276] PDT can be repeated to maintain tumor control. As the light generally will penetrate only several millimeters, this therapy is most useful for palliative benefit, as only superficial tumors would be treated in their entirety. One series with long-term follow-up[276] demonstrated that six of seven patients maintained controlled disease, with estimated 5-year survival of 62%. In another series with median follow-up of 19 months, superficial adenocarcinoma was ablated in 9 of 12 patients.[277] For more advanced tumors that are thicker or where lymph nodes are involved, PDT is not a potentially curative therapy and is used for palliation. Some studies document that PDT is at least equally effective to laser therapy in providing palliation to patients with esophageal cancer and is associated with a lower incidence of perforation.[264,275,278] Disadvantages of PDT relative to other methods of endoscopic palliation include a prolonged period of photosensitivity that may affect quality of life, the risk of post-treatment esophageal strictures, and significant cost (for both the laser and the chemical agents). The potential role of PDT in the therapy for BE is discussed in the section related to therapy for that condition. Newer agents for PDT may be developed to absorb wavelengths of light that will penetrate more deeply into tissue.

Argon plasma coagulation, which is generally less expensive than PDT, uses argon gas to cause thermal destruction of tissue. It generally penetrates only 3 mm and may be more useful in the therapy for superficial lesions or BE than for bulky obstructing lesions.[279]

Endoscopic mucosal resection is another means of treating superficial esophageal carcinoma. In general, a substance such as physiologic saline is injected into the submucosa to create a bleb, which may separate the submucosa from the mucosa. An electrocautery snare is then used to resect the elevated submucosa. This technique may be used for small superficial or microinvasive lesions, but more data are needed to demonstrate equivalence with conventional surgical therapy.[280,281]

Chemotherapy for Advanced Disease

In general, patients with metastatic or recurrent carcinoma of the esophagus have a large tumor burden and poor performance status. Chemotherapy responses in these patients tend to be very transient (several months) and thus have limited impact on survival. Many trials have small numbers of patients, and the response rates are variable, often influenced by the extent of prior treatment. When reported, palliation of symptoms may be minimal. Therefore the value of single-agent therapy is principally to identify active agents for further study in combination.

Table 77-7 summarizes the response rates to single agents (~15% to 30% complete plus partial response [CR + PR]). Only a few drugs have been adequately tested in patients with adenocarcinoma. Many of the data for older drugs such as bleomycin come from broad phase I and II trials with small numbers of esophageal cancer patients enrolled. Of the drugs tested to date, cisplatin, 5-FU, rinotecan, and paclitaxel appear to be the most active. Surprisingly, carboplatin showed little or no activity in three well-conducted trials for squamous cell carcinoma and adenocarcinoma histologic types.[282-284]

TABLE 77-7

Activity of Single-Agent Chemotherapy in Recurrent and Metastatic Disease

AGENT	HISTOLOGY	NO. OF TRIALS	EVALUABLE PATIENTS	PERCENT CR + PR (RANGE)
Bleomycin	S	7	80	15 (14–33)
5-Fluorouracil	S	1	26	15
Mitomycin-C	S	2	31	35 (14–42)
Doxorubicin (adriamycin)	S	2	33	18 (5–38)
Methotrexate	S	1	26	12
Cisplatin	S	4	86	23 (6–40)
Carboplatin	S,A	3	59	5 (0–14)
Vindesine	S	4	83	34 (11–46)
Methyl-GAG	S	1	23	17
Venorelbine	S	1	46	15
Paclitaxel	S,A	1	50	32
Gemcitabine	S,A	1	17	0
Docotaxel		2	22	18–28

A, adenocarcinoma; CR complete response; PR, partial response; S, squamous cell carcinoma.

With combination regimens (Table 77-8), CR and PR rates are higher than those reported for single agents, 25% to 40%, and responses are more durable, 3 to 6 months.[141,285-293] However, median survivals are generally 6 to 8 months, with some longer-term survival. Cisplatin plus 5-FU has been studied in patients with both adeno- carcinoma and squamous histologic types with similar response rates, in the 30% range. Irinotecan, paclitaxel, and docetaxel have been studied in combination regimens, and interest in seen in exploring the potential benefits of oxaliplatin. Whether these regimens improve on the outcome of standard 5-FU/cisplatin has not been assessed.

TABLE 77-8

Activity of Combination Chemotherapy in Recurrent and Metastatic Disease

CHEMOTHERAPY	HISTOLOGY	EVALUABLE PATIENTS	CR + PR (%)	REFERENCE
Cisplatin + bleomycin	S	17	17	138
Cisplatin + bleomycin + vindesine	S	51	31	139, 287
Cisplatin + bleomycin + methotrexate	S	40	30	288, 289
Cisplatin + methyl-GAG + vindesine	S	20	40	141
Cisplatin + methyl-GAG + vinblastine	S	36	11	290
Cisplatin + 5-FU	S	35	34	291
Cisplatin + 5-FU + allopurinol	S	37	35	292
Cisplatin + 5-FU + doxorubicin (adriamycin)	S	21	33	293
Folinic acid + 5-FU*	A	29	19	
Interferon-α + 5-FU†	S	37	37	
Interferon-α + 5-FU + cisplatin‡	S,A	15	50	
Cisplatin + VP-16§	A	65	48	
Paclitaxel + cisplatin + 5-FU‖	S,A	60	48	
Paclitaxel + cisplatin#	S,A	20	40	
Paclitaxel + cisplatin	S,A	38	44	297
Paclitxel + cisplatin	S,A	51	42	
Irinotecan + cisplatin¶	S,A	21	53	294
Irinotecan + cisplatin	A	36	58	295

A, adenocarcinoma; CR, complete response; 5-FU, 5-fluorouracil; GAG, glycosaminoglycan; S, squamous cell carcinoma.
*Kok TC, van der Gaast A, Splinter TA: 5-fluorouracil and folinic acid in advanced adenocarcinoma of the esophagus or esophago-gastric junction area: Rotterdam Esophageal Tumor Study Group. Ann Oncol 1996;7:533.
†Kelsen D, Lovett D, Wong J, et al: Interferon alfa-2a and fluorouracil in the treatment of patients with advanced esophageal cancer. J Clin Oncol 1992;10:269.
‡Kelson DP: A phase II trial of interferon alpha-2A, 5-fluorouracil, and cisplatin in patients with advanced esophageal carcinoma. Cancer 1995;75:2197.
§Kok TC, van der Gaast A, Splinter TA: Cisplatin and etoposide in oesophageal cancer: A phase II study: Rotterdam Oesophageal Tumour Study Group. Br J Cancer 1996;74:980.
‖Ilson DH, Jaffer A, Bhalla K, et al: Phase II trial of paclitaxel, fluorouracil, and cisplatin in patients with advanced carcinoma of the esophagus. J Clin Oncol 1998;16:1826.
#Costa F, Ilson D, Forastiere A, et al: Phase II study of paclitaxel and cisplatin in patients with advanced adenocarcinoma and squamous cell carcinoma of the esophagus [Abstract]. Am Soc Clin Oncol Proc 1997;16:930.
¶Polee MB, Eskens FA, van der Burg ME, et al: Phase II study of bi-weekly administration of paclitaxel and cisplatin in patients with advanced oesophageal cancer. Br J Cancer 2002;86:669–673.

Specific Malignancies

III

A phase II trial[294] of cisplatin, 30 mg/m^2, and irinotecan, 65 mg/m^2 weekly for 4 weeks followed by a 2-week rest, demonstrated a major response rate of 57% including 6% CR. Response rate was 52% in adenocarcinoma and 66% in squamous cell, with median duration of response of 4.3 months. Ninety percent (70% resolution) of patients with dysphasia had significant improvement in symptoms. Nine percent had grade 4 neutropenia, and 11% had grade 3 diarrhea. Ajani and associates[295] reported similar response rates with this regimen in a trial including untreated gastric and GE-junction tumors. Therefore irinotecan-based regimens are highly promising.

Taxol alone or with cisplatin has been demonstrated to have a high response rate in recurrent or metastatic esophageal cancer, with a response rate of 32% with taxol, 250 mg/m^2 every 21 days,[296] and a response rate of 40% (15% CR) with taxol, 90 mg/m^2 over a 3-hour period, and cisplatin, 50 mg/m^2 repeated every 14 days. In locally advanced esophageal carcinoma, a 47% response rate was seen with paclitaxel, 200 mg/m^2 over a 24-hour period, and cisplatin, 75 mg m^2 given twice.[297] Taxol, 200 mg/m^2, and carboplatin, AUC 5.0, demonstrated 44% response rate.[298] Paclitaxel,[299] 200 to 250 mg/m^2 over a 24-hour period on day 1, followed by cisplatin, 75 mg/m^2 on day 2 also has been evaluated in a phase II trial. PR occurred in 44% (46% with adenocarcinoma and 25% with squamous cell carcinoma) with median duration 3.9 months. With this regimen, grade 4 neutropenia occurred in 47%, 50% required hospitalization, and 11% died of therapy-related complications.

In summary, cisplatin plus infusion of 5-FU remains the most commonly used regimen for the treatment of either adenocarcinoma or squamous cell carcinoma of the esophagus. Whether oral fluoropyrimidines may be appropriately substituted, therefore making the therapy less burdensome to the patient and reducing the need for infusion catheters, is as yet not fully investigated. The identification of new active agents offers the potential for developing more effective therapies, and these are under investigation. We must investigate the role of new targeted therapies such as epidermal growth factor–receptor inhibitors, antiangiogenesis agents, and COX-2 inhibitors, which may enhance the efficacy of standard chemotherapy without substantially increasing toxicity. The goal of treatment for this patient group, palliation, should be the foremost consideration in planning therapy. Thus local therapies such as radiation therapy, stents, or laser endoscopy should be considered in addition to chemotherapy, depending on sites of disease and symptoms.

BARRETT'S ESOPHAGUS WITH HIGH-GRADE DYSPLASIA

Dysplasia in BE is a premalignant change that requires close follow-up or treatment. Generally low-grade dysplasia may be closely followed up with endoscopy, with esophagectomy only if progression to high-grade dysplasia occurs. The absence of high-grade dysplasia should be confirmed with extensive biopsy. Conversely, high-grade dysplasia[300] is frequently associated with adenocarcinoma at the time of diagnosis, or progression to adenocarcinoma may occur later. Therefore esophagectomy is currently standard for high-grade dysplasia to reduce the risk of adenocarcinoma. The long-term utility of close observation or endoscopic therapies such as PDT in preventing progression to fatal esophageal carcinoma is not known; these approaches should be used with caution in younger patients who are fit for surgery and are without other significant comorbidities.

Dysplasia in Barrett's mucosa refers to cytologic and histologic epithelial changes that are considered neoplastic. It does not refer to reactive or inflammatory epithelial changes, which are most commonly seen with esophagitis. Historically, it was thought that a minimum of 3 cm of CLE was required for the diagnosis of BE. These shorter lengths of CLE were considered to be normal variants and exempt from the complications of BE. Currently, it is accepted that no length of CLE is normal and that these short segments of BE (SSBE) are susceptible to all of the potential complications of BE including the development of dysplasia and adenocarcinoma. Therefore the significance of dysplasia and its management pertains to patients with SSBE as well. On the basis of mucosal architecture, epithelial morphology, and cytologic findings, dysplasia is classified as low, intermediate, and high grade. It is now generally accepted that dysplasia in BE precedes the development of invasive adenocarcinoma. Tygat and Hameeteman[301] illustrated that dysplasia is a prerequisite of adenocarcinoma, that low-grade dysplasia is potentially reversible, and that once the threshold of high-grade dysplasia is reached, it *always* progresses to invasive cancer. It is not clear what factors influence the time of progression from high-grade dysplasia to adenocarcinoma. As discussed in the earlier section on pathogenesis of adenocarcinoma, evidence exists that an accumulation of mutations or epigenetically mediated changes in expression of key genes may play an important role.

The diagnosis of Barrett's mucosa with dysplasia is made histologically by endoscopy with biopsies. Because of the significance of this diagnosis in terms of patient management, it is important that the diagnosis be confirmed by a pathologist experienced in this area, and second opinions should be obtained when needed.[302,303] Wang and coworkers[304] reported that dysplastic Barrett's mucosa has distinctive cytologic features, and therefore brush cytology should be considered in the endoscopic surveillance of these patients. Others confirmed that cytopathology plays a complementary role in evaluating dysplasia and adenocarcinoma in BE.[305,306]

Three options are available to manage patients with high-grade dysplasia. Heitmiller and colleagues[307] advocated prophylactic esophagectomy for patients with high-grade dysplasia, citing data showing that high-grade dysplasia is a premalignant condition in which no regression has been documented, and that occult invasive adenocarcinoma is found in 45% to 50% of patients who undergo esophagectomy with the diagnosis of high-grade dysplasia alone. In their series, operative mortality was 3.3%, occult invasive adenocarcinoma was found in 43%

of patients, and in five of these patients, the tumor was locally advanced stage. The authors emphasized that this aggressive surgical therapy is recommended only for patients who are suitable surgical candidates.

An alternative approach is close endoscopic surveillance. Advocates of this approach believe that rigorous biopsy procedures can distinguish high-grade dysplasia from adenocarcinoma, reducing the risk that therapy for invasive cancer will be inadvertently delayed while sparing many patients the need for esophagectomy. As the natural history of high-grade dysplasia is not well studied, advocates of endoscopic surveillance point out that adenocarcinoma may not develop for many years, and therefore this risk should be balanced against the immediate morbidity and mortality of esophagectomy. Others believe that high-grade dysplasia and invasive cancer cannot be accurately differentiated endoscopically, that the time course for progression from high-grade dysplasia to invasive adenocarcinoma is unknown, and that the risks of adenocarcinoma are too great to risk delay.[308]

The data to settle the controversy about optimal approach to high-grade dysplasia are not yet available. The data summarized later suggest a high enough risk that esophagectomy should be strongly considered. Levine and associates[309] reported an endoscopic biopsy protocol that they believe can accurately differentiate high-grade dysplasia from adenocarcinoma. Four-quadrant jumbo forceps biopsies were performed at 2-cm intervals, with additional specimens from any areas of known dysplasia. Based on their series of seven patients where follow-up surgery confirmed the absence of invasive cancer, the authors advocate endoscopic follow-up for patients with high-grade dysplasia alone. In their series, of 22 patients followed up in such a fashion for an average of 32 months (range, 4 to 67 months), in none has a known invasive adenocarcinoma developed. However, another group[310] used similar biopsy procedures before esophagectomy, and 10 of 38 were found to have unsuspected invasive adenocarcinoma in the surgical specimen. When high-grade dysplasia is followed up rather than treated, varying risk has been found in several recent large series. This incidence of adenocarcinoma has been reported to be 59% (5-year cumulative),[311] 32% (8-year follow-up),[312] and 16% over a period of 7.3 years.[313] The reason for the varying risks identified is unclear, although in the series with the smallest incidence, no confirmation of diagnosis of high-grade dysplasia was made by a central pathologist. Therefore, although intensive endoscopic surveillance may be a reasonable approach, a substantial portion of patients may have existing adenocarcinoma not detected on biopsy, or adenocarcinoma will develop over several years of follow-up.

A third option is endoscopic ablative therapy for high-grade dysplasia, although long-term data are unavailable. Therefore this may be most appropriate for patients who are not fit for surgery. Patients treated with PDT demonstrated 88% resolution of high-grade dysplasia and 78% resolution of low-grade dysplasia with PDT. The median follow-up was only 19 months.[277] Berenson and coworkers[314] recently reported that endoscopic argon laser photoablation of Barrett's mucosa, in conjunction with antacid therapy with omeprazole, resulted in squamous epithelial re-epithelialization. This therapeutic technique, although intriguing, requires further investigation, and whether such therapy will reduce the risk of adenocarcinoma is not known.

In summary, the standard management for low-grade dysplasia is close follow-up; for high-grade dysplasia, it is esophagectomy with close follow-up or endoscopic therapy appropriate under selected circumstances.

REFERENCES

1. Postlethwait RW: Squamous cell carcinoma of the esophagus. In Postlethwait RW (ed): Surgery of the Esophagus, 2nd ed. Norwalk, Conn., Appleton Century Crofts, 1986, p 369.
2. Ming S: Adenocarcinoma and other epithelial tumors of the esophagus. In Ming S, Goldman H (eds): Pathology of the Gastrointestinal Tract. Philadelphia, WB Saunders, 1992, p 459.
3. Ibrahim NB, Briggs JC, Corbishley CM: Extrapulmonary oat cell carcinoma. Cancer 1984;54:1645.
4. Choh JH, Khazei AH, Ihm HJ: Leiomyosarcoma of the esophagus: Report of a case and review of the literature. J Surg Oncol 1986;32:223.
5. Paymaster JC, Sanghvi LD, Gangadharan P: Cancer in the gastrointestinal tract in Western India. Cancer 1968;21:279.
6. Yang PC, Davis S: Incidence of cancer of the esophagus in the U.S. by histologic type. Cancer 1988;61:612.
7. Hesketh PJ, Clapp RW, Doos WG, Spechler SJ: The increasing frequency of adenocarcinoma of the esophagus. Cancer 1989;64:526.
8. Pera M, Cameron AJ, Trastek VF, et al: Increasing incidence of adenocarcinoma of the esophagus and esophagogastric junction. Gastroenterology 1993;104:510.
9. Blot J, Devesa SS, Kneller RW, Fraumen JF: Increasing incidence of adenocarcinoma of the esophagus and gastric cardia. JAMA 1991;265:128.
10. Vizcaino AP, Moreno V, Lambert R, Parkin DM: Time trends incidence of both major histologic types of esophageal carcinomas in selected countries, 1973–1995. Int J Cancer 2002;99:860–868.
11. Powell J, McConkey CC: Increasing incidence of adenocarcinoma of the gastric cardia and adjacent sites. Br J Cancer 1990;62:440.
12. Reed PI: Changing pattern of oesophageal cancer. Lancet 1991;338:178.
13. Botterweck AM, Schouten LJ, Volvics A, et al: Trends in incidence of adenocarcinoma of the oesophagus and gastric cardia in ten European countries. Int J Epidemiol 2000;29:645–654.
14. Heitmiller RF, Sharma R: Comparison of incidence and resection rates in patients with esophageal squamous cell carcinoma and adenocarcinoma. J Thorac Cardiovasc Surg 1996;112:130.
15. Tateishi R, Taniguchi H, Wade A, et al: Argyrophil cells and melanocytes in esophageal mucosa. Arch Pathol 1974;88:87.
16. De la Pava S, Nigogosyan G, Pickren JW, Cabrera A: Melanosis of the esophagus. Cancer 1963;16:48.
17. Chalkiadakis G, Wihlm JR, Morand G, et al: Primary malignant melanoma of the esophagus. Ann Thorac Surg 1985;39:472.
18. Briggs JC, Ibrahim NBN: Oat cell carcinoma of the oesophagus: A clinico-pathologic study of 23 cases. Histopathology 1983;7:261.
19. Doherty MA, McIntyre M, Arnott SJ: Oat cell carcinoma of the esophagus: A report of six British patients with a review of the literature. Int J Radiat Oncol Biol Phys 1984;10:147.
20. Nichols GL, Kelsen DP: Small cell carcinoma of the esophagus: The Memorial Hospital experience 1970–1978. Cancer 1989;64:1531.
21. Partyka EK, Sanowski RA, Kozarek RA: Endoscopic diagnosis of a giant esophageal leiomyosarcoma. Am J Gastroenterol 1981;75:132.
22. Newcomb PA, Carbone PP: The health consequences of smoking. Med Clin North Am 1992;76:305.

23. Hiyama T, Sato T, Yoshino K, et al: Second primary cancer following laryngeal cancer with special reference to smoking habits. Jpn J Cancer Res 1992;83:334.

24. Choi SY, Kahyo H: Effect of cigarette smoking and alcohol consumption in the etiology of cancers of the digestive tract. Int J Cancer 1991;49:381.

25. Francheschi S, Talamini R, Barra S, et al: Smoking and drinking in relation to cancers of the oral cavity, pharynx, larynx, and esophagus in Northern Italy. Cancer Res 1990;50:6502.

26. DeStefani E, Munoz N, Esteve J, et al: Mate drinking, alcohol, tobacco, diet, and esophageal cancer in Uruguay. Cancer Res 1990;50:426.

27. Gray JR, Coldman AJ, MacDonald WC: Cigarette and alcohol use in patients with adenocarcinoma of the gastric cardia or lower esophagus. Cancer 1992;69:2227.

28. Christen AG, McDonald JL Jr, Olson BL, Christen JA: Smokeless tobacco addiction: A threat to the oral and systemic health of the child and adolescent. Pediatrician 1989;16:170.

29. Heitmiller RF: Esophageal tumors. In Cameron JL (ed): Current Surgical Therapy, 5th ed. St. Louis, CV Mosby, 1995, p 45.

30. Adami HO, McLaughlin JK, Hsing AW, et al: Alcoholism and cancer risk: A population-based cohort study. Cancer Causes Control 1992;3:419.

31. Kato I, Nomura AM, Stemmermenn GN, Chyon PH: Prospective study of the association of alcohol with cancer of the upper aerodigestive tract and other sites. Cancer Causes Control 1992;3:145.

32. Van Cutsem E, Van Trappen G: Epidemiology and clinical aspects of esophageal cancer. J Belge Radiol 1991;74:365.

33. Ghardirian P, Ekoe JM, Thouez JP: Food habits and esophageal cancer: An overview. Cancer Detect Prev 1992;16:163.

34. Block G, Patterson B, Subar A: Fruit, vegetables, and cancer prevention: A review of the epidemiologic evidence. Nutr Cancer 1992;18:1.

35. Li JY, Ershow AG, Chen ZJ, et al: A case-control study of cancer of the esophagus and gastric cardia in Linxian. Int J Cancer 1989;43:755.

36. Liu GT, Qian YZ, Zhang P, et al: Etiological role of *Alternaria alternata* in human esophageal cancer. Chin Med J 1992;105:394.

37. Aggestrup S, Holm JC, Sorensen HR: Does achalasia predispose to cancer of the esophagus? Chest 1992;102:1013.

38. Chuong JJH, DuBovick S, McCallum RW: Achalasia as a risk factor for esophageal carcinoma: A reappraisal. Dig Dis Sci 1984;29:1105.

39. Lagergren J, Bergstrom R, Lindgren A, et al: Symptomatic gastroesophageal reflux as a risk factor for esophageal adenocarcinoma. N Engl J Med 1999;340:825-831.

40. Sampliner RE: Practice guidelines on the diagnosis, surveillance, and therapy of Barrett's esophagus. Am J Gastroenterol 2002;97:1888-1895.

41. Miros M, Kerlin P, Walker N: Only patients with dysplasia progress to adenocarcinoma in Barrett's esophagus. Gut 1991;32:1441.

42. Tygat GNJ, Hameeteman W: The neoplastic potential of columnar-lined (Barrett) esophagus. World J Surg 1992;16:302.

43. Corley DA, Levin TR, Habel LA, et al: Surveillance and survival in Barrett's adenocarcinomas: A population-based study. Gastroenterology 2002;122:633-640.

44. Van Sandick JW, Van Lanschott JJ, Kuiken BW, et al: Impact of endoscopic biopsy surveillance of Barrett's oesophagus on pathological stage and clinical outcome of Barrett's carcinoma. Gut 1998;43:216-222.

45. Lambert R: Barrett's oesophagus: Better left alone? Eur J Gastroenterol Hepatol 2001;13:627-630.

46. Volker F, Eckardt MD, Kanzler G, Bernhard G: Life expectancy and cancer risk in patients with Barrett's esophagus: A prospective controlled investigation. Am J Med 2001;111:33-37.

47. Macdonald CE, Wicks AC, Playford RJ: Final results from 10 year cohort of patients undergoing surveillance for Barrett's oesophagus: Observational study. BMJ 2000;321:1252-1255.

48. Eckardt VF, Kanzler G, Bernhard G: Life expectancy and cancer risk in patients with Barrett's esophagus: A prospective controlled investigation. Am J Med 2001;111:33-37.

49. Spechler SJ, Lee E, Ahnen, D, et al: Long-term outcome of medical and surgical therapies for gastroesophageal reflux disease. JAMA 2001;285:2331-2338.

50. Theisen J, Stein JH, Dittler HJ, et al: Preoperative chemotherapy unmasks underlying Barrett's mucosa in patients with adeno-carcinoma of the distal esophagus. Surg Endosc 2002;16:671-673.

51. Moskaluk CA, Heitmiller RF, Zuharak M, et al: p53 and p21 WAF1/CIP1/SDI1 gene products in Barrett esophagus and adenocarcinoma of the esophagus and esophagogastric junction. Hum Pathol 1996;27:1211.

52. Wu TT, Watanabe T, Heitmiller RF, et al: Genetic alterations in Barrett esophagus and adenocarcinoma of the esophagus and esophagogastric junction region. Am J Pathol 1998;153:287.

53. Barrett MT, Sanchez CA, Prevo LJ, et al: Evolution of neoplastic cell lineages in Barrett oesophagus. Nat Genet 1999;22:106-109.

54. Wong DJ, Paulson TG, Prevo LJ, et al: p16(INK4a) lesions are common, early abnormalities that undergo clonal expansion in Barrett's metaplastic epithelium. Cancer Res 2001;61:8284-8289.

55. Eads CA, Lord RV, Kurumboor SK, et al: Fields of aberrant CPG island hypermethylation in Barrett's esophagus and associated adenocarcinoma. Cancer Res 2000;60:5021-5026.

56. Eads CA, Lord RV, Wickramasinghe K, et al: Epigenetic patterns in the progression of esophageal adenocarcinoma. Cancer Res 2001;61:3410-3418.

57. Hsing AQ, Hanson LE, McLaughlin JK, et al: Pernicious anemia and subsequent cancer: A population-based cohort study. Cancer 1993;71:745.

58. Oka M, Attwood SE, Kaul B, et al: Immunosuppression in patients with Barrett's esophagus. Surgery 1992;112:112.

59. Kobayashi S, Kasugai T: Brushing cytology for the diagnosis of gastric cancer involving the cardia of the lower esophagus. Acta Cytol 1978;22:155.

60. Winawer SJ, Sherlock Belladonna JA, et al: Endoscopic brush cytology in esophageal cancer. JAMA 1975;232:1358.

61. Qunit LE, Glazer GM, Orringer MB, et al: Esophageal carcinoma: CT findings. Radiology 1985;155:171.

62. Becker CD, Barbier P, Porcellini B: CT evaluation of patients undergoing transhiatal esophagectomy for cancer. J Comput Assist Tomogr 1986;10:607.

63. Luketich JD, Schauer P, Landreneau R, et al: Minimally invasive surgical staging is superior to endoscopic ultrasound in detecting lymph node metastases in esophageal cancer. J Thorac Cardiovasc Surg 1997;114:817.

64. Bemelman WA, van Delden OM, van Lanschot JJ, et al: Laparoscopy and laparoscopic ultrasonography in staging of carcinoma of the esophagus and gastric cardia. J Am Coll Surg 1995;181:421.

65. Rau B, Hunerbein M, Reingruber B, et al: Laparoscopic lymph node assessment in pretherapeutic staging of gastric and esophageal cancer. Recent Results Cancer Res 1996;142:209.

66. Gouma DJ, de Wit LT, Nieveen van DE, et al: Laparoscopic ultrasonography for staging of gastrointestinal malignancy. Scand J Gastroenterol 1996;218:43.

67. Heath EI, Kaufman HS, Talamini MA, et al: The role of laparoscopy in preoperative staging of esophageal cancer. Surg Endosc 2000;14:495-499.

68. Flamen P, Lerut A, Van Cutsem E, et al: Utility of positron emission tomography for the staging of patients with potentially operable esophageal carcinoma. J Clin Oncol 2000;18:3202-3210.

69. Meltzer CC, Luketich JD, Friedman D, et al: Whole-body FDG positron emission tomographic imaging for staging esophageal cancer comparison with computed tomography. Clin Nucl Med 2000;25:882-887.

70. Heintz A, Mildenberger P, George M, et al: Endoscopic ultrasonography in the diagnosis of regional lymph nodes in esophageal and gastric cancer: Results of studies in vitro. Endosocpy 1993;25:231.

71. Botet JF, Lightdale CJ, Zauber AG, et al: Preoperative staging of esophageal cancer: Comparison of endoscopic US and dynamic CT (see comments). Radiology 1991;181:419.

72. Dittler HJ, Siewert JR: Role of endoscopic ultrasonography in esophageal carcinoma. Endoscopy 1993;25:156.

73. Wiersema M, Vilmann P, Giovannini G, et al: Endosonography-guided fine-needle aspiration biopsy: Diagnostic accuracy and complication assessment. Gastronintest Endosc 1996;112:1087.

74. Tio TL, Coene PPLO, den Hartog Jager FCA, Tytgat GNJ: Preoperative TNM classification of esophageal carcinoma by endosonography. Hepatogastroenterology 1990;37:376.

75. Tio TL, Cohen P, Coene PP: Endosonography and computed tomography of esophageal carcinoma. Gastroenterology 1989;96:1478.

76. Rice TW, Boyce GA, Sivall MV: Esophageal ultrasound and the preoperative staging of carcinoma of the esophagus. J Thorac Cardiovasc Surg 1991;101:536.

77. Krasna MJ: Advances in staging of esophageal carcinoma. Chest 1998;113(1 suppl):107S.

78. Van Delden OM, de Wit LT, Bemelman WA, et al: Laparoscopic ultrasonography for abdominal tumor staging: Technical aspects and imaging findings. Abdom Imaging 1997;22:125.

79. Krasna MJ, Flowers JL, Attar S, McLaughlin J: Combined thoracoscopic/laparoscopic staging of esophageal cancer. J Thorac Cardiovasc Surg 1996;111:800.

80. Luketich JD, Schauer PR, Meltzer CC, et al: Role of positron emission tomography in staging esophageal cancer. Ann Thorac Surg 1997;64:765.

81. Iizuka T, Isono K, Kakegawa T, et al: Parameters linked to ten-year survival in Japan of resected esophageal carcinoma. Chest 1989;96:1005.

82. Ellis FH Jr: Treatment of carcinoma of the esophagus and cardia. Mayo Clin Proc 1989;64:945.

83. American Joint Committee on Cancer: Manual for Staging of Cancer, 3rd ed. Philadelphia, JB Lippincott, 1988.

84. Mathisen DJ, Grillo HC, Wilkins EW, et al: Transthoracic esophagogastrectomy: A safe approach to carcinoma of the esophagus. Ann Thorac Surg 1988;45:137.

85. Barbier PA, Becker CD, Wagner HE: Esophageal carcinoma: Patient selection for transhiatal esophagectomy: A prospective analysis of 50 consecutive cases. World J Surg 1988;12:263.

86. Ellis FH, Gibb SP, Watkins E: Limited esophagogastrectomy for carcinoma of the cardia. Ann Surg 1988;208:354.

87. Mitchell RL: Abdominal and right thoracotomy approach as a standard procedure for esophagogastrectomy with low morbidity. J Thorac Cardiovasc Surg 1987;93:205.

88. Orringer MB: Transhiatal esophagectomy without thoracotomy for carcinoma of the thoracic esophagus. Ann Surg 1984;200:282.

89. Ellis FH Jr, Heatley GJ, Krasna MJ, et al: Esophagogastrectomy for carcinoma of the esophagus and cardia: A comparison of findings and results after standard resection in three consecutive eight-year intervals with improved staging criteria. J Thorac Cardiovasc Surg 1997;113:5.

90. Wilkins EW Jr: Perspective. In Delarue NC, Wilkins EW Jr, Wong J (eds): International Trends in General Thoracic Surgery, vol. 4. St. Louis, CV Mosby, 1988, p 440.

91. Muller JM, Erasmi H, Stelzner M, et al: Surgical therapy of oesophageal carcinoma. Br J Surg 1990;77:845.

92. Rentz J, Bull D, Harpole D, et al: Transthoracic versus transhiatal esophagectomy: A prospective study of 945 patients. J Thorac Cardiovasc Surg 2003;125:1114–1120.

93. Shriver CD, Burt M: Transhiatal esophagectomy. Semin Thorac Cardiovasc Surg 1992;4:307.

94. Orringer MB: Technical aids in performing transhiatal esophagectomy without thoracotomy. Ann Thorac Surg 1984;38:128.

95. Orringer MB: Transhiatal esophagectomy without thoracotomy for esophageal carcinoma. In Delarue NC, Wilkins EW Jr, Wong J (eds): International Trends in General Thoracic Surgery, vol. 4. St. Louis, CV Mosby, 1988, p 200.

96. Orringer MB: Surgical options for esophageal resection and reconstruction with stomach. In Baue AE, Geha AS, Hammond GL, et al (eds): Glenn's Thoracic and Cardiovascular Surgery, 6th ed. Stamford, Conn, Appleton & Lange, 1996, p 899.

97. Heitmiller EF, Gruber PJ, Swier P, Singh N: Long-segment substernal jejunal esophageal replacement with internal mammary vascular augmentation. Dis Esophagus 2000;13:240–242.

98. Orringer MB, Marshall B, Stirling MC: Transhiatal esophagectomy for benign and malignant disease. J Thorac Cardiovasc Surg 1993;105:265.

99. Davis E, Heitmiller RF: Esophagectomy for benign disease: Trends in surgical results and management. Ann Thorac Surg 1996;62:369.

100. Gillinov AM, Heitmiller RF: Strategies to reduce pulmonary complications after transhiatal esophagectomy. Dis Esophagus 1998;11:43.

101. Allen MS: Ivor Lewis esophagectomy. In Loop FD, Mathisen DJ (eds): Seminars in Thoracic and Cardiovascular Surgery. vol. 4. Philadelphia, WB Saunders, 1992, p 320.

102. Heitmiller RF: The left thoracoabdominal incision. Ann Thorac Surg 1988;46:250.

103. Shahian DM, Neptune WB, Ellis FH Jr: Transthoracic versus extrathoracic esophagectomy: Mortality, morbidity, and long-term survival. Ann Thorac Surg 1986;41:237.

104. Heitmiller RF: Results of standard left thoracoabdominal esophagogastrectomy. Semin Thorac Cardiovasc Surg 1992;4:314.

105. McKeown KC: Total three-stage esophagectomy for cancer of the oesophagus. Br J Surg 1976;63:259.

106. Swanson SJ, Sugarbaker DJ: The three-hole esophagectomy: The Brigham and Women's Hospital approach (modified McKeown technique). Chest Surg Clin North Am 2000;10:531–552.

107. Swanson SJ, Grondin SC, Sugarbaker DJ: Total esophagectomy: The Brigham and Women's Hospital approach. Oper Tech Thorac Cardiovasc Surg 1999;4:197–209.

108. Hagen JA, Peters JH, DeMeester TR: Superiority of extended en bloc esophagogastrectomy for carcinoma of the lower esophagus and cardia. J Thorac Cardiovasc Surg 1993;106:850.

109. Nishimaki T, Suzuki T, Suzuki S, et al: Outcomes of extended radical esophagectomy for thoracic esophageal cancer. J Am Coll Surg 1998;186:306.

110. Bumm R, Feussner H, Bartels H, et al: Radical transhiatal esophagectomy with two-field lymphadenectomy and endodissection for distal esophageal adenocarcinoma. World J Surg 1997;21:822.

111. Altorki NK, Girardi L, Skinner DB: En bloc esophagectomy improves survival for stage III esophageal cancer. J Thorac Cardiovasc Surg 1997;114:948.

112. Hagen JA, DeMeester SR, Peters JH, Chandrasoma P, DeMeester TR: Curative resection for esophageal adenocarcinoma: analysis of 100 en bloc esophagectomies. Ann Surg 2001;234:520–530.

113. Altorki N, Kent M, Ferrara C, Port J: Three-field lymph node dissection for squamous cell and adenocarcinoma of the esophagus. Ann Surg 2002;236:177–183.

114. Altorki N, Skinner D: Should en bloc esophagectomy be the standard of care for esophageal carcinoma? Ann Surg 2001;234:588–589.

115. Bhansali MS, Fujita H, Kakegawa T, et al: Pattern of recurrence after extended radical esophagectomy with three-field lymph node dissection for squamous cell carcinoma in the thoracic esophagus. World J Surg 1997;21:275.

116. Coleman JJ, Searles JM, Hester R: Ten years experience with the free jejunal autograft. Am J Surg 1987;154:394.

117. Jurkiewicz MJ: Reconstructive surgery of the cervical esophagus. J Thorac Cardiovasc Surg 1984;88:893.

118. Miller JI, Lee RB: Free jejunal interposition of the esophagus. Semin Thorac Cardiovasc Surg 1992;4:286.

119. Luketich JD, Schauer PR, Christie NA, et al: Minimally invasive esophagectomy. Ann Thorac Surg 2000;70:906–912.

120. Fernando HC, Luketich JD, Buenaventura PO, Perry Y, Christie NA: Outcomes of minimally invasive esophagectomy (MIE) for high-grade dysplasia of the esophagus. Eur J Cardiothorac Surg 2002;22:1–6.

121. Pierre AF, Luketich JD: Technique and role of minimally invasive esophagectomy for premalignant and malignant diseases of the esophagus. Surg Oncol Clin North Am 2002;11:337–350.

122. Hulscher JBF, Tijssen JGP, Obertop H, et al: Transthoracic versus transhiatal resection for carcinoma of the esophagus: A meta-analysis. Ann Thorac Surg 2001;72:306–313.

123. Hulscher JB, Van Sandick JW, DeBoer AG, et al: Extended transthoracic resection compared with limited transhiatal resection for adenocarcinoma of the esophagus. N Engl J Med 2002;347:1662–1669.

124. Hofstetter W, Swisher SG, Correa AM, et al: Treatment outcomes of resected esophageal cancer. Ann Surg 2002;236:376–384.

125. Rice TW, Blackstone EH, Goldblum JR, et al: Superficial adenocarcinoma of the esophagus. J Thorac Cardiovasc Surg 2001;122:1077–1090.

126. Hosch SB, Stoecklein NH, Pichlmeier U, et al: Esophageal cancer: The mode of lymphatic tumor cell spread and its prognostic significance. J Clin Oncol 2001;19:1970–1975.

127. Vazquez-Sequerros E, Wang L, Burgart L, et al: Occult lymph node metastases as a predictor of tumor relapse in patients with node-negative esophageal carcinoma. Gastroenterology 2002;122:1815–1821.

128. Sato F, Shimada Y, Li Z, et al: Lymph node micrometastasis and prognosis in patients with oesophageal squamous cell carcinoma. Br J Surg 2001;88:426–432.

129. Nakamura T, Ide H, Eguchi R, et al: Clinical implications of lymph node micrometastasis in patients with histologically node-negative (pN0) esophageal carcinoma. J Surg Oncol 2002;79:224–229.

130. Mueller JD, Stein HJ, Oyang T, et al: Frequency and clinical impact of lymph node micrometastasis and tumor cell microinvolvement in patients with adenocarcinoma of the esophagogastric junction. Cancer 2000;89:1874–1882.

131. Holscher AH, Bollschweiler E, Schneider PM, et al: Prognosis of early esophageal cancer: Comparison between adeno- and squamous cell carcinoma. Cancer 1995;76:178.

132. Salazar JD, Doty JR, Lin JW, et al: Does cell type influence postesophagectomy survival in patients with esophageal cancer? Dis Esophagus 1998;11:168.

133. Gordon TA, Bowman HM, Bass EB, et al: Complex gastrointestinal surgery: Impact of provider team experience on clinical and economic outcomes. J Am Coll Surg 1999;189:46.

134. Zehr KJ, Dawson PB, Yang SC, et al: Standardized clinical care pathways for major thoracic cases reduces hospital costs. Ann Thorac Surg 1998;66:914.

135. Dimick JB, Cattaneo SM, Lipsett PA, Pronovost PJ, Heitmiller RF: Hospital volume is related to clinical and economic outcomes of esophageal resection in Maryland. Ann Thorac Surg 2001;72:334–339.

136. Dimick JB, Pronovost PJ, Cowan JA, Lipsett PA: Surgical volume and quality of care for esophageal resection: Do high-volume hospitals have fewer complication? Ann Thorac Surg 2003;75:337–341.

137. Berkmeyer JD, Siewers AE, Finlayson EVA, et al: Hospital volume and surgical mortality in the United States. N Engl J Med 2002;346:1128–1137.

138. Coonley DJ, Baines M, Hilaris B, et al: Cisplatin and bleomycin in the treatment of esophageal carcinoma: A final report. Cancer 1984;54:2341.

139. Kelsen DP, Hilaris B, Coonley C, et al: Cisplatin, vindesine and bleomycin combination chemotherapy of local-regional and advanced esophageal carcinoma. Am J Med 1983;75:645.

140. Schlag P, Herrmann R, Raeth U, et al: Preoperative (neoadjuvant) chemotherapy in squamous cell cancer of the esophagus. Recent Results Cancer Res 1988;10:14.

141. Kelson DP, Fein R, Coonley C, et al: Cisplatin, vindesine and mitoguazone in the treatment of esophageal cancer. Cancer Treat Rep 1986;70:255.

142. Forastiere A, Gennis MK, Orringer M, et al: Cisplatin, vinblastine and mitoguazone chemotherapy for epidermoid and adenocarcinoma of the esophagus. J Clin Oncol 1987;5:1143.

143. Carey RW, Hilgenberg AD, Wilkins EW, et al: Preoperative chemotherapy followed by surgery with possible postoperative radiotherapy in squamous cell carcinoma of the esophagus: Evaluation of the chemotherapy component. J Clin Oncol 1986;4:697.

144. Hilgenberg AD, Carey RW, Wilkins EW, et al: Preoperative chemotherapy, surgical resection and selective postoperative therapy for squamous cell carcinoma of the esophagus. Ann Thorac Surg 1988;45:357.

145. Carey RW, Hilgenberg AD, Grillo HC, et al: Esophageal carcinoma: Long-term follow-up of patients treated by neo-adjuvant chemotherapy, surgery and possible postoperative radiation and/or chemotherapy (Abstract 404). Proc Am Soc Clin Oncol 1990;9:105.

146. Kies MS, Rosen ST, Tsang TK, et al: Cisplatin and 5-fluorouracil in the primary management of squamous esophageal cancer. Cancer 1987;60:215.

147. Ajani JA, Roth JA, Ryan B, et al: Evaluation of pre and postoperative chemotherapy for resectable adenocarcinoma of the esophagus or gastroesophageal junction. J Clin Oncol 1990;8:1231.

148. Ajani J, Roth J, Ryan B, et al: High-dose chemotherapy with GM-CSF for respectable adenocarcinoma of the esophagus (Abstract 472). Proc Am Soc Clin Oncol 1991;10:151.

149. Schlag P fur die CAO Studiengruppe Oesophaguscarcinom: Randomisierte Studie zur praoperativen Chemotherapic beim Plattenepithelcarcinom des Oesophagus. Chirurg 1992;63:709.

150. Roth JA, Pass HU, Flanagan MM, et al: Randomized clinical trials of preoperative and postoperative adjuvant chemotherapy with cisplatin, vindesine, and bleomycin for carcinoma of the esophagus. J Thorac Cardiovasc Surg 1988;96:242.

151. Kelsen DP, Ginsberg R, Pajak TF, et al: Chemotherapy followed by surgery compared with surgery alone for localized esophageal cancer. N Engl J Med 1998;339:1979–1984.

152. Medical Research Council: Surgical resection with or without preoperative chemotherapy in oesophageal cancer: A randomised controlled trial. Lancet 2002;359:1727–1733.

153. Wayman J, Bennett MK, Raimes SA, Griffin SM: The pattern of recurrence of adenocarcinoma of the oesophago-gastric junction. Br J Cancer 2002;86:1223–1229.

154. Forastiere AA, Orringer MB, Perez-Tamayo C, et al: Preoperative chemoradiation followed by transhiatal esophagectomy for carcinoma of the esophagus: Final report. J Clin Oncol 1993;11:1118–1123.

155. Gignoux M, Roussel A, Paillot B, et al: The value of preoperative radiotherapy in esophageal cancer: Results of a study of the EORTC. World J Surg 1987;11:426.

156. Arnott SJ, Duncan W, Kerr GR, et al: Low dose preoperative radiotherapy for carcinoma of the oesophagus: Results of a randomized clinical trial. Radiother Oncol 1992;24:108.

157. Nygaard K, Hagen S, Hansen HS, et al: Pre-operative radiotherapy prolongs survival in operable esophageal carcinoma: A randomized, multicenter study of pre-operative radiotherapy and chemotherapy: The second Scandinavian trial in esophageal cancer. World J Surg 1992;16:1104.

158. Launois B, Delarue D, Campion JP, et al: Preoperative radiotherapy for carcinoma of the esophagus. Surg Gynecol Obstet 1981;153:690.

159. Huang GJ, Gu XZ, Wang LJ, et al: Combined preoperative irradiation and surgery for esophageal carcinoma. In Delarue NC (ed): International Trends in General Thoracic Surgery, 1st ed. St. Louis, CV Mosby, 1988, p 315.

160. LePrise E, Etienne P, Meunier B, et al: A randomised study of chemotherapy, radiation therapy, and surgery versus surgery for localized squamous cell carcinoma of the esophagus. Cancer 1994;73:1779.

161. Bossett JF, Gignoux M, Triboulet JP, et al: Chemoradiotherapy followed by surgery compared with surgery alone in squamous-cell cancer of the esophagus. N Engl J Med 1997;337:161.

162. Walsh T, Noonan N, Hollywood D, et al: A comparison of multimodal therapy and surgery for esophageal adenocarcinoma. N Engl J Med 1996;335:462.

163. Urba S, Orringer M, Turrisi A, et al: Randomized trial of preoperative chemoradiation versus surgery alone in patients with locoregional esophageal carcinoma. J Clin Oncol 2001;19:305–313.

164. Steiger Z, Franklin R, Wilson RF, et al: Eradication and palliation of squamous cell carcinoma of the esophagus with chemotherapy, radiotherapy, and surgical therapy. J Thorac Cardiovasc Surg 1981;82:713.

165. Leichman L, Steiger Z, Seydel HG, et al: Preoperative chemotherapy plus radiation therapy for patients with cancer of the esophagus: Potentially curative approach. J Clin Oncol 1984;2:75.

166. Poplin E, Fleming T, Leichman L, et al: Combined therapies for squamous cell carcinoma of the esophagus: A Southwest Oncology Group Study (SWOG 8037). J Clin Oncol 1987;5:622.

167. Seydel HG, Leichman L, Byhardt R, et al: Preoperative radiation and chemotherapy for localized squamous cell carcinoma of the esophagus: An RTOG study. Int J Radiat Oncol Biol Phys 1988;14:33.

168. Forastiere AA, Orringer MB, Perez-Tamayo C, et al: Preoperative chemoradiation followed by transhiatal esophagectomy for carcinoma of the esophagus: Final report. J Clin Oncol 1993;11:1118–1123.

169. Bates BA, Detterbeck FC, Bernard SA, et al: Concurrent radiation therapy and chemotherapy followed by esophagectomy for localized esophageal carcinoma. J Clin Oncol 1996;14:156.

170. Forastiere A, Heitmiller RF, Lee D-J, et al: Intensive chemoradiation followed by esophagectomy for squamous cell and adenocarcinoma of the esophagus. Cancer J Sci Am 1997;3:144.

171. Naunheim KS, Petruska PJ, Roy TS, et al: Multimodality therapy for adenocarcinoma of the esophagus. Ann Thorac Surg 1995;59:1085.

172. Stahl M, Wilke H, Fink U, et al: Combined preoperative chemotherapy and radiotherapy in patients with locally advanced esophageal cancer: Interim analysis of a phase II trial. J Clin Oncol 1996;14:829.

173. Posner MC, Gooding WE, Landreneau RJ, et al: Preoperative chemoradiotherapy for carcinoma of the esophagus and gastroesophageal junction. Cancer J 1998;4:237.

174. Adelstein DJ, Rice TW, Becker M, et al: Use of concurrent chemotherapy, accelerated fractionation radiation, and surgery for patients with esophageal carcinoma. Cancer 1997;80:1001.

175. Lokich JJ, Sonneborn H, Anderson NR, et al: Combined paclitaxel, cisplatin, and etoposide for patients with previously untreated esophageal and gastroesophageal carcinomas. Cancer 1999;85:2347-2351.

176. Meluch AA, Hainsworth JD, Gray JR, et al: Preoperative combined modality therapy with paclitaxel, carboplatin, prolonged infusion 5-fluorouracil, and radiation therapy in localized esophageal cancer: Preliminary results of a Minnie Pearl Cancer Res Network phase II trial. Cancer J Sci Am 1999;5:84-91.

177. Adelstein DJ, Rice TW, Rybicki LA, et al: Does paclitaxel improve the chemoradiotherapy of locoregionally advanced esophageal cancer? A nonrandomized comparison with fluorouracil-based therapy. J Clin Oncol 2000;18:2032-2039.

178. Safran H, Gaissert H, Akerman P, et al: Paclitaxel, cisplatin, and concurrent radiation for esophageal cancer. Cancer Invest 2001;19:1-7.

179. Ajani JA, Komaki R, Putnam JB, et al: A three-step strategy of induction chemotherapy then chemoradiation followed by surgery in patients with potentially resectable carcinoma of the esophagus or gastroesophageal junction. Cancer 2001;92:279-286.

180. Bains MS, Stojadinovic A, Minsky B, et al: A phase II trial of preoperative combined-modality therapy for localized esophageal carcinoma: Initial results. J Thorac Cardiovasc Surg 2002;124:270-277.

181. Khushalani NI, Leichman CG, Proulx, G, et al: Oxaliplatin in combination with protracted-infusion fluorouracil and radiation: Report of a clinical trial for patients with esophageal cancer. J Clin Oncol 2002;20:2844-2850.

182. Kleinberg L, Knisely JP, Heitmiller R, et al: Mature survival results with preoperative cisplatin, protracted infusion 5-fluorouracil, and 44-Gy radiotherapy for esophageal cancer. Int J Radiat Oncol Biol Phys 2003;56:328-334.

183. Forastiere AA, Heitmiller RF, Lee DJ, et al: Intensive chemoradiation followed by esophagectomy for squamous cell and adenocarcinoma of the esophagus. Cancer J Sci Am 1997;3:144-152.

184. Heath EI, Burtness BA, Heitmiller RF, et al: Phase II evaluation of preoperative chemoradiation and postoperative adjuvant chemotherapy for squamous cell and adenocarcinoma of the esophagus. J Clin Oncol 2000;18:868-876.

185. Slater MS, Holland J, Faigel DO, et al: Does neoadjuvant chemoradiation downstage esophageal carcinoma? Am J Surg 2001;181:440-444.

186. Doty JR, Salazar JD, Forastiere AA, et al: Postesophagectomy morbidity, mortality, and length of hospital stay after preoperative chemoradiation therapy. Ann Thorac Surg 2002;74:227-331.

187. Ikeda K, Ishida K, Sato N, et al: Chemoradiotherapy followed by surgery for thoracic esophageal cancer potentially or actually involving adjacent organs. Dis Esophagus 2001;14:197-201.

188. Yano M, Tsujinaka T, Shiozaki H, et al: Concurrent chemotherapy (5-fluorouracil and cisplatin) and radiation therapy followed by surgery for T4 squamous cell carcinoma of the esophagus. J Surg Oncol 1999;70:25-32.

189. Isenberg G, Chak A, Canto MI, et al: Endoscopic ultrasound in restaging of esophageal cancer after neoadjuvant chemoradiation. Gastrointest Endosc 1998;48:158-163.

190. Giovannini M, Seitz JF, Thomas P, et al: Endoscopic ultrasonography for assessment of the response to combined radiation therapy and chemotherapy in patients with esophageal cancer. Endoscopy 1997;29:4-9.

191. Laterza E, deManzoni, G, Guglielmi A, et al: Endoscopic ultrasonography in the staging of esophageal carcinoma after preoperative radiotherapy and chemotherapy. Ann Thorac Surg 1999;67:1466-1469.

192. Beseth BD, Bedford R, Isacoff WH, et al: Endoscopic ultrasound does not accurately assess pathologic stage of esophageal cancer after neoadjuvant chemoradiotherapy. Am Surg 2000;66:827-831.

193. Kato H, Kuwano H, Nakajima M, et al: Usefulness of positron emission tomography for assessing the response of neoadjuvant chemoradiotherapy in patients with esophageal cancer. Am J Surg 2002;184:279-283.

194. Bjorn B, Weber W, Bauer M, et al: Neoadjuvant therapy of esophageal squamous cell carcinoma: Response evaluation by positron emission tomography. Ann Surg 2001;223:300-309.

195. Weber WA, Ott K, Becker K, et al: Prediction of response to preoperative chemotherapy in adenocarcinomas of the esophagogastric junction by metabolic imaging. J Clin Oncol 2001;19:3058-3065.

196. Downey RF, Akhurst T, Ilson D, et al: Whole body ^{18}FDG-PET and the response of esophageal cancer to induction therapy: Results of a prospective trial. J Clin Oncol 2003;21:428-432.

197. Weber WA, Ott K, Becker K, et al: Prediction of response to preoperative chemotherapy in adenocarcinomas of the esophagogastric junction by metabolic imaging. J Clin Oncol 2001;19:3058-3065.

198. Teniere P, Hay JM, Fingerhut A, et al: Postoperative radiation therapy does not increase survival after curative resection for squamous cell carcinoma of the middle and lower esophagus as shown by a multicenter controlled trial. Surgery 1991;173:123.

199. Fok M, Sham JST, Choy D, et al: Postoperative radiotherapy for carcinoma of the esophagus: A prospective, randomized controlled study. Surgery 1993;113:138.

200. Herskovic A, Martz K, Al-Sarraf M, et al: Combined chemotherapy and radiotherapy compared with radiotherapy alone in patients with cancer of the esophagus. N Engl J Med 1992;326:1593-1598.

201. Nyambi E, Kang HJ, Millikan K, et al: Integration of surgery in multimodality therapy for esophageal cancer. Am J Clin Oncol 1997;20:11.

202. Bedard EL, Inculet RI, Malthaner RA, et al: The role of surgery and postoperative chemoradiation therapy in patients with lymph node positive esophageal carcinoma. Cancer 2001;91:2423-2430.

203. Macdonald JS, Smalley SR, Benedetti J, et al: Chemoradiotherapy after surgery compared with surgery alone for adenocarcinoma of the stomach or gastroesophageal junction. N Engl J Med 2001;345:725-730.

204. Nishimura Y, Suzuki M, Nakamatsu K, et al: Prospective trial of concurrent chemoradiotherapy with protracted infusion of 5-fluorouracil and cisplatin for T4 esophageal cancer with or without fistula. Int J Radiat Oncol Biol Phys 2002;53:134-139.

205. Al-Sarraf M, Martz K, Herskovic A, et al: Progress report of combined chemoradiotherapy versus radiotherapy alone in patients with esophageal cancer: An intergroup study. J Clin Oncol 1997;15:277-284.

206. Cooper JS, Guo MD, Herskovic A, et al: Chemoradiotherapy of locally advanced esophageal cancer: Long-term follow-up of a prospective randomized trial (RTOG 85-01). Radiation Therapy Oncology Group. JAMA 1999;281:1623-1627.

207. Smith TJ, Ryan LM, Douglas HO Jr, et al: Combined chemoradiotherapy vs. radiotherapy alone for early stage squamous cell carcinoma of the esophagus: A study of the Eastern Cooperative Oncology Group. Int J Radiat Oncol Biol Phys 1998;42:269-276.

208. Bidoli P, Bajetta E, Stani SC, et al: Ten-year survival with chemotherapy and radiotherapy in patients with squamous cell carcinoma of the esophagus. Cancer 2002;94:352-361.

209. Meunier B, Raoul J, LePrise E, et al: Salvage esophagectomy after unsuccessful curative chemoradiotherapy for squamous cell cancer of the esophagus. Dig Surg 1998;15:224-226.

210. Swisher SG, Wynn P, Putnam JB, et al: Salvage esophagectomy for recurrent tumors after definitive chemotherapy and radiotherapy. J Thorac Cardiovasc Surg 2002;123:175–183.

211. Nemoto K, Ariga H, Kakuto Y, et al: Radiation therapy for loco-regionally recurrent esophageal cancer after surgery. Radiother Oncol 2001;61:165–168.

212. Emami B, Lyman J, Brown A, et al: Tolerance of normal tissue of therapeutic irradiation. Int J Radiat Oncol Biol Phys 1991;21:109.

213. Caspers RJL, Zwinderman AH, Griffioen G, et al: Combined external beam and low dose rate intraluminal radiotherapy in oesophageal cancer. Radiother Oncol 1993;27:7.

214. Sur RK, Deepinder PS, Sharma SC, et al: Radiation therapy of esophageal cancer: Role of high dose rate brachytherapy. Int J Radiat Oncol Biol Phys 1992;22:1043.

215. Hishikawa Y, Kurisu K, Tangiuchi M, et al: High-dose-rate intraluminal brachytherapy for esophageal cancer: 10 years experience in Hyogo College of Medicine. Radiother Oncol 1991;21:107.

216. Gasper LE, Subir N, Herskovic A, et al: American Brachytherapy Society (ABS) consensus guidelines for brachytherapy for esophageal cancer. Int J Radiat Oncol Biol Phys 1997;38:127.

217. Minsky BD, Pajak TF, Ginsbert RJ, et al: INT 0123 (Radiation Therapy Oncology Group 94-05) phase III trial of combined-modality therapy for esophageal cancer: High-dose versus standard-dose radiation therapy. J Clin Oncol 2002;20:1167–1174.

218. Minsky BD, Neuberg D, Kelsen DP, et al: Neoadjuvant chemotherapy plus concurrent chemotherapy and high-dose radiation for squamous cell carcinoma of the esophagus: A preliminary analysis of the phase II Intergroup trial 0122. J Clin Oncol 1996;14:149.

219. MacFarlane SD, Hill LD, Jolly PC, et al: Improved results of surgical treatment for esophageal and gastroesophageal junction carcinomas after preoperative combined chemotherapy and radiation. J Thorac Cardiovasc Surg 1988;95:415.

220. Kavanagh B, Anscher M, Leopold K, et al: Patterns of failure following combined modality therapy for esophageal cancer, 1984–1990. Int J Radiat Oncol Biol Phys 1992;24:633.

221. Gill PG, Denham JW, Jamieson GG, et al: Patterns of treatment failure and prognostic factors associated with the treatment of esophageal carcinoma with chemotherapy and radiotherapy either as sole treatment or followed by surgery. J Clin Oncol 1992;10:1037.

222. Whittington R, Coia LR, Haller DG, et al: Adenocarcinoma of the esophagus and esophago-gastric junction: The effects of single and combined modalities on the survival and patterns of failure following treatment. Int J Radiat Oncol Biol Phys 1990;19:593.

223. Kavanagh B, Anscher M, Leopold K, et al: Patterns of failure following combined modality therapy for esophageal cancer, 1984–1990. Int J Radiat Oncol Biol Phys 1992;24:633.

224. Herskovic A, Leichman L, Lattin P, et al: Chemo/radiation with and without surgery in the thoracic esophagus: The Wayne State experience. Int J Radiat Oncol Biol Phys 1998;15:655.

225. Nutting CM, Bedford JL, Cosgrove VP, et al: Intensity-modulated radiotherapy reduces lung irradiation in patients with carcinoma of the oesophagus. Front Radiat Ther Oncol 2002;37:128–131.

226. Nutting CM, Bedford JL, Cosgrove VP, et al: A comparison of conformal and intensity-modulated techniques for oesophageal radiotherapy. Radiother Oncol 2001;61:157–163.

227. Corn BW, Coia LR, Chu JCH, et al: Significance of prone positioning in planning treatment for esophageal cancer. Int J Radiat Oncol Biol Phys 1991;21:1303.

228. Gschossmann JM, Bonner JA, Foote RL, et al: Malignant tracheoesophageal fistula in patients with esophageal cancer. Cancer 1993;72:1513.

229. Ahmed HF, Hussain MA, Grant CE, Wadleigh RG: Closure of tracheoesophageal fistulas with chemotherapy and radiotherapy. Am J Clin Oncol 1998;21:177.

230. Alexander EP, Trachiotis GD, Lipman TO, Wadleigh RG: Evolving management and outcome of esophageal cancer with airway involvement. Ann Thorac Surg 2001;71:1640–1644.

231. O'Rourke MB, Tiver K, Bull C, et al: Swallowing performance after radiation therapy for carcinoma of the esophagus. Cancer 1988;61:2022.

232. Coia LR, Soffen EM, Schultheiss TE, et al: Swallowing function in patients with esophageal cancer treated with concurrent radiation and chemotherapy. Cancer 1993;71:281.

233. Coia LR, Myerson RJ, Tepper JE: Late effects of radiation therapy on the gastrointestinal tract. Int J Radiat Oncol Biol Phys 1995;31:1213.

234. Hishikawa Y, Kurisu K, Taniguchi N, et al: High-dose-rate intraluminal brachytherapy for esophageal cancer: 10 years experience in Hyogo College of Medicine. Radiother Oncol 1991;21:107.

235. Gaspar LE, Qian C, Kocha WI, et al: A phase I/II study of external beam radiation, brachytherapy and concurrent chemotherapy in localized cancer of the esophagus (RTOG 92-07): Preliminary toxicity report. Int J Radiat Oncol Biol Phys 1997;37:593.

236. Jager J, Langendijk H, Pannebakker M, et al: A single session of intraluminal brachytherapy in palliation of oesophageal cancer. Radiother Oncol 1995;37:237.

237. Fleischman EH, Kagan AR, Bellotti JE, et al: Effective palliation for inoperable esophageal cancer using intensive intracavitary radiation. J Surg Oncol 1990;44:234.

238. Sur RK, Deepinder PS, Sharma SC, et al: Radiation therapy of esophageal cancer: Role of high dose rate brachytherapy. Int J Radiat Oncol Biol Phys 1992;22:1043.

239. Sharma V, Mahantshetty U, Dinshaw KA, et al: Palliation of advanced/recurrent esophageal carcinoma with high-dose-rate brachytherapy. Int J Radiat Oncol Biol Phys 2002;52:310–315.

240. Sur RK, Levin CV, Donde B, et al: Prospective randomized trial of HDR brachytherapy as a sole modality in palliation of advanced esophageal carcinoma: An International Atomic Energy Agency study. Int J Radiat Oncol Biol Phys 2002;53:127–133.

241. Caspers RJL, Zwinderman AH, Griffioen G, et al: Combined external beam and low dose rate intraluminal radiotherapy in oesophageal cancer. Radiother Oncol 1993;27:7.

242. Rowland CG, Pagliero KM: Intracavitary irradiation in palliation of carcinoma of oesophagus and cardia. Lancet 1985;2:981.

243. Hishikawa Y, Izumi M, Kurisu K, et al: Esophageal ulceration following high-dose-rate intraluminal brachytherapy for esophageal cancer. Radiother Oncol 1993;28:252.

244. Sander R, Hagenmueller F, Sander C, et al: Laser versus laser plus afterloading with iridium-192 in the palliative treatment of malignant stenosis of the esophagus: A prospective, randomized, and controlled study. Gastrointest Endosc 1991;37:433.

245. Shmueli E, Srivastava E, Dawes PJDK, et al: Combination of laser treatment and intraluminal radiotherapy for malignant dysphagia. Gut 1996;38:803.

246. Spencer GM, Thorpe SM, Sargeant IR: Laser and brachytherapy in the palliation of adenocarcinoma of the oesophagus and cardia. Gut 1996;39:726.

247. Wara WM, Mauch PM, Thomas AN, Phillips TL: Palliation for carcinoma of the esophagus. Radiology 1976;121:717.

248. O'Rourke C, McNeil JR, Walker PJ, Bull CA: Objective evaluation of the quality of palliation in patients with oesophageal cancer comparing surgery, radiotherapy and intubation. Aust N Z J Surg 1992;62:922.

249. Hayter CRR, Huff-Winters C, Paszat L, et al: A prospective trial of short-course radiotherapy plus chemotherapy for palliation of dysphagia from advanced esophageal cancer. Radiother Oncol 2000;56:329–333.

250. Caspers RJ, Welvaart K, Verkes JR, et al: The effect of radiotherapy of dysphagia and survival in patients with esophageal cancer. Radiother Oncol 1988;12:15.

251. Coia LR, Engstrom PF, Paul AR, et al: Long-term results of infusional 5-FU, mitomycin-C, and radiation as primary management of esophageal carcinoma. Int J Radiat Oncol Biol Phys 1991;20:29.

252. Lishman AH, Dellipiani AW, Devlin HB: The insertion of oesophagogastric tubes in malignant esophageal strictures: Endoscopy or surgery? Br J Surg 1980;67:257.

253. Cusumano A, Ruol A, Seglin A, et al: Push-through intubation: Effective palliation in 409 patients with cancer of the esophagus and cardia. Ann Thorac Surg 1992;53:1010.

254. Lishman AH, Dellipiani AW, Devlin HB: The insertion of oesophagogastric tubes in malignant esophageal strictures: Endoscopy or surgery? Br J Surg 1980;67:257.

255. Cusumano A, Ruol A, Seglin A, et al: Push-through intubation: Effective palliation in 409 patients with cancer of the esophagus and cardia. Ann Thorac Surg 1992;53:1010.

256. Alderson D, Wright PD: Laser recanalization versus endoscopic intubation in the palliation of malignant dysphagia. Br J Surg 1990;77:1151.

257. Buset M, des Marez B, Baize M, et al: Palliative endoscopic management of obstructive esophagogastric cancer: Laser or prosthesis. Gastrointest Endosc 1987;124:225.

258. Portwood GL, Reed CE: Use of lasers and stents in malignant esophageal disease. In Franco KL, Putnam JB Jr (eds): Advanced Therapy in Thoracic Surgery. Hamilton, Ontario, BC, Decker, 1998, p 441.

259. Nava HR, Schuh ME, Nambisan R, et al: Endoscopic ablation of esophageal malignancies with the neodymium-YAG laser and electrofulguration. Arch Surg 1989;124:225.

260. Jensen DM, Machicado G, Randall G, et al: Comparison of low-power YAG laser and BICAP tumor probe for palliation of esophageal cancer strictures. Gastroenterology 1988;94:1267.

261. Suzuki H, Miho O, Watanabe Y, et al: Endoscopic laser therapy in the curative and palliative treatment of upper gastrointestinal cancer. World J Surg 1989;13:158.

262. Siegel HI, Laskin KJ, Dabezies MA, et al: The effect of endoscopic laser therapy on survival in patients with squamous cell carcinoma of the esophagus. J Clin Gastroenterol 1991; 13:142.

263. Marcon NE: Photodynamic therapy and cancer of the esophagus. Semin Oncol 1994;21(suppl 15):20.

264. Lightdale CJ, Jeier SK, Marcon NE, et al: Photodynamic therapy with porfimer sodium versus thermal ablation therapy with ND:YAG laser palliation of esophageal cancer. A multicenter randomized trial. Gastrointest Endosc 1995;42:507.

265. McCaughan JS Jr, Nims TA, Guy JT, et al: Photodynamic therapy for esophageal tumors. Arch Surg 1989;124:74.

266. Sibille A, Lambert R, Souquet J, et al: Long-term survival after photodynamic therapy for esophageal cancer. Gastroenterology 1995;108:337.

267. King MR, Pairolero PC, Trastek VF, et al: Ivor Lewis esophago-gastrectomy for carcinoma of the esophagus: Early and late functional results. Ann Thorac Surg 1987;44:119.

268. Christie NA, Buenaventura PO, Fernando HC, et al: Results of expandable metal stents for malignant esophageal obstruction in 100 patients: Short-term and long-term follow-up. Ann Thorac Surg 2001;71:1797–1802.

269. Song HY, Do YS, Han YM, et al: Covered, expandable esophageal metallic stent tubes: experiences in 119 patients. Radiol 1994;193:689–695.

270. Tomaselli F, Maier A, Sankin O, et al: Successful endoscopical sealing of malignant esophagotracheal fistulae by using a covered self-expandable stenting system. Eur J Cardiothorac Surg 2001;20:734–738.

271. Aoki T, Osaka Y, Takagi Y, et al: Comparative study of self-expandable metallic stent and bypass surgery for inoperable esophageal cancer. Dis Esophagus 2001;14:208–211.

272. Sargeant IR, Tobias JS, Blackman G, et al: Radiotherapy enhances laser palliation of malignant dysphagia: A randomised study. Gut 1997;40:362–369.

273. McCaughan JS Jr, Nims TA, Guy JT, et al: Photodynamic therapy for esophageal tumors. Arch Surg 1989;124:74.

274. Sibille A, Lambert R, Souquet J, et al: Long-term survival after photodynamic therapy for esophageal cancer. Gastroenterology 1995;108:337.

275. Lightdale CJ, Jeier SK, Marcon NE, et al: Photodynamic therapy with porfimer sodium versus thermal ablation therapy with Nd:YAG laser palliation of esophageal cancer: A multicenter randomized trial. Gastrointest Endosc 1995;42:507.

276. McCaughan JS Jr, Ellison EC, Guy JT, et al: Photodynamic therapy for esophageal malignancy: A prospective twelve-year study. Ann Thorac Surg 1996;62:1005–1009.

277. Overholt BF, Panjehpour M, Haydek JM: Photodynamic therapy for Barrett's esophagus: Follow-up in 100 patients. Gastrointest Endosc 1999;49:1–7.

278. Heier SK, Rothman KA, Heier LM, et al: Photodynamic therapy for obstructing esophageal cancer: Light dosimetry and randomized comparison with ND:YAG laser therapy. Gastroenterology 1995;109:63–72.

279. Ortner MA, Dorta G, Blum AL, Michetti P: Endoscopic interventions for preneoplastic and neoplastic lesions: Mucosectomy, argon plasma coagulation, and photodynamic therapy. Dig Dis 2002;20:167–172.

280. Lambert R: Endoscopic mucosectomy: An alternative treatment for superficial esophageal cancer. Recent Results Cancer Res 2000;155:183–192.

281. Sharma P, Ell C, May A, et al: Endoscopic mucosal resection of early cancer and high-grade dysplasia in Barrett's esophagus. Gastrointest Endosc 2000;118:670–677.

282. Sternberg C, Kelsen D, Dukeman M, et al: Carboplatin: A new platinum analog in the treatment of epidermoid carcinoma of the esophagus. Cancer Treat Rep 1985;69:1305.

283. Mannell A, Winters Z: Carboplatin in the treatment of oesophageal cancer. South Afr Med J 1989;76:213.

284. Queisser W, Preusser P, Mross KB, et al: Phase II evaluation of carboplatin in advanced esophageal carcinoma: A trial of the phase I/II study group of the Association for Medical Oncology of the German Center Society. Onkologie 1990;13:190.

285. Coonley DF, Bains M, Hilaris B, et al: Cisplatin and bleomycin in the treatment of esophageal carcinoma: A final report. Cancer 1984;54:2341.

286. Kelsen DP, Hilaris B, Coonley C, et al: Cisplatin, vindesine and bleomycin combination chemotherapy of local-regional and advanced esophageal carcinoma. Am J Med 1983;75:645.

287. Dinwoodie WR, Bartolucci M, Lyman GH, et al: Phase II evaluation of cisplatin, bleomycin, and vindesine in advanced squamous cell carcinoma of the esophagus: A Southeastern Cancer Study Group Trial. Cancer Treat Rep 1986;70:267.

288. DeBasi P, Salvagno L, Endrizi L, et al: Cisplatin, bleomycin and methotrexate in the treatment of advanced oesophageal cancer. Eur J Cancer Clin Oncol 1984;20:743.

289. Vogl SE, Greenwald E, Kaplan BH: Effective chemotherapy for esophageal cancer with methotrexate, bleomycin and cis-diamminedichloroplatinum II. Cancer 1981;48:2555.

290. Chapman R, Fleming TR, Van Damme J, et al: Cisplatin, vinblastine, and mitoguazone in squamous cell carcinoma of the esophagus: A Southwest Oncology Group Study. Cancer Treat Rep 1987;71:1185.

291. Iizuka T, Kakegawa T, Ide H, et al: Phase II study of CDDP + 5-FU for squamous esophageal carcinoma: JEOG co-operative study results (Abstract 496). Proc Am Soc Clin Oncol 1991;10:157.

292. DeBasi P, Sileni VC, Salvagno L, et al: Phase II study of cisplatin, 5-FU, and allopurinol in advanced esophageal cancer. Cancer Treat Rep 1986;70:909.

293. Gisselbrecht C, Calvo F, Mignot L, et al: Fluorouracil, Adriamycin and cisplatin combination chemotherapy of advanced esophageal carcinoma. Cancer 1983;52:974.

294. Ilson DH, Saltz L, Enzinger P, et al: Phase II trial of weekly irinotecan plus cisplatin in advanced esophageal cancer. J Clin Oncol 1999;17:3270–3275.

295. Ajani JA, Baker J, Pisters PW, et al: CPT-11 plus cisplatin in patients with advanced, untreated gastric or gastroesophageal junction carcinoma: Results of a phase II study. Cancer 2002; 94:641–646.

296. Ajani JA, Ilson DH, Daugherty K, et al: Activity of taxol in patients with squamous cell carcinoma and adenocarcinoma of the esophagus. J Natl Cancer Inst 1994;86:1086–1091.

297. Ilson DH, Forastiere A, Arquette M, et al: A phase II trial of paclitaxel and cisplatin in patients with advanced carcinoma of the esophagus. Cancer J 2000;6:316–323.

298. Philip PA, Zalupski MM, Gadgeel S, et al: A phase II study of carboplatin and paclitaxel in the treatment of patients with advanced esophageal and gastric cancer. Semin Oncol 1997; 24(6 suppl 19):S19–S86, S19–S88.

299. Ilson DH, Saltz L, Enzinger P, et al: Phase II trial of weekly irinotecan plus cisplatin in advanced esophageal cancer. J Clin Oncol 1999;17:3270–3275.

300. Spechler SJ: Clinical practice: Barrett's esophagus. N Engl J Med 2002;346836–842.

301. Tygat GNJ, Hameeteman W: The neoplastic potential of columnar-lined (Barrett) esophagus. World J Surg 1992;16:302.

302. Spechler SJ: Managing Barrett's esophagus. BMJ 2003; 326: 892–894.

303. Spechler SJ: Disputing dysplasia. Gastroenterology 2001;120: 1864–1868.

304. Wang HH, Doria MI Jr, Purohit-Buch S, et al: Barrett's esophagus: The cytology of dysplasia in comparison to benign and malignant lesions. Acta Cytol 1992;36:60.

305. Robey SS, Hamilton SR, Gupta PK, et al: Diagnostic value of cytopathology in Barrett's esophagus and associated carcinoma. Am J Clin Pathol 1988;89:493.

306. Geisinger KR, Teot LA, Richter JE: A comparative cytopathologic and histologic study of atypia, dysplasia, and adenocarcinoma in Barrett's esophagus. Cancer 1992;69:816.

307. Heitmiller RF, Redmond M, Hamilton SR: Barrett esophagus with high-grade dysplasia: An indication for prophylactic esophagectomy. Ann Surg 1996;224:66.

308. Reid BJ, Weinstein WM, Lewin KJ: Endoscopic biopsy can detect high-grade dysplasia or early adenocarcinoma in Barrett's esophagus without grossly recognizable neoplastic lesions. Gastroenterology 1988;94:81.

309. Levine DS, Haggitt RC, Blount PL, et al: An endoscopic biopsy protocol can differentiate high-grade dysplasia from early adenocarcinoma in Barrett's esophagus. Gastroenterology 1993;105:40.

310. Falk GW, Rice TW, Goldblum Jr, Richter JE: Jumbo biopsy forceps protocol still misses unsuspected cancer in Barrett's esophagus with high-grade dysplasia. Gastrointest Endosc 1999;49:170–176.

311. Reid BJ, Levine DS, Longton G, et al: Predictors of progression to cancer in Barrett's esophagus: Baseline histology and flow cytometry identify low- and high-risk patient subsets. Am J Gastroenterol 2000;95:1669–1676.

312. Buttar NS, Wang KK, Sebo TJ, et al: Extent of high-grade dysplasia in Barrett's esophagus correlates with risk of adenocarcinoma. Gastroenterology 2001;120:1630–1639.

313. Schnell TG, Sontag SJ, Chejfec G, et al: Long-term nonsurgical management of Barrett's esophagus with high-grade dysplasia. Gastroenterology 2001;120:1607–1619.

314. Berenson MM, Johnston TB, Markowitz NR, et al: Restoration of squamous mucosa after ablation of Barrett's esophageal epithelium. Gastroenterology 1993;10:1688.

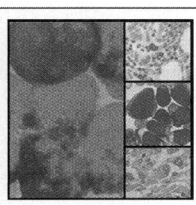

CANCER OF THE STOMACH

Leonard L. Gunderson
John H. Donohue
Steven R. Alberts

SUMMARY OF KEY POINTS

EPIDEMIOLOGY/PATHOLOGY

- For stomach cancer in the United States, the expected incidence in 2003 was 22,400 cases and 12,100 deaths.
- These cancers are usually adenocarcinomas.
- In the United States the site of origin is shifting as more proximal lesions are diagnosed.

BIOLOGIC CHARACTERISTICS

- Prognostic factors relate to tumor extent and include nodal involvement and extension beyond the gastric wall.
- Ploidy may be an independent prognostic factor.

STAGING EVALUATION

- Staging should always include history and physical examination, complete blood cell count, liver chemistries, chest film, upper gastrointestinal imaging, and endoscopy with biopsy and ultrasonography).
- Additional studies that may help define extragastric extent of disease include computed tomography (abdomen alone for gastric lesions; include chest for gastroesophageal junction lesions) and laparoscopy.

PRIMARY THERAPY

- Surgical resection is the primary therapy of resectable gastric cancers.
- Cure rates of 80% or higher are achieved only with early lesions (nodes negative, confined to mucosa or submucosa), which are uncommon in the United States.
- Role for extended node dissection has not been found in randomized trials.

ADJUVANT THERAPY

- Adjuvant therapy (chemotherapy, irradiation) is indicated on the basis of patterns of relapse and survival results with surgery alone (high incidence of locoregional relapse and distant metastases).
- Most Western chemotherapy trials are negative for both single and multiple drugs.
- Irradiation alone reduced locoregional relapse and improved overall survival in a Bejing trial of 370 patients testing preoperative irradiation versus surgery alone (5-year survival rate 30% versus 20%, $P = 0.009$).
- U.S. intergroup phase III trial of 556 patients found a survival benefit for

combined-modality postoperative irradiation plus chemotherapy versus surgery alone (3-year relapse-free survival rate 48% versus 31%, $P = 0.001$; 3-year overall survival rate 50% versus 41%, $P = 0.005$).

LOCALLY ADVANCED DISEASE

- Combined external irradiation (EBRT) plus chemotherapy or intraoperative irradiation (IORT) produced long-term survival in 10% to 20% of patients in most randomized and nonrandomized trials.
- Neoadjuvant chemotherapy studies reveal possible increase in resection rates but high incidence of locoregional relapse (IORT alone or with EBRT and chemotherapy to neoadjuvant chemotherapy regimens).

PALLIATION

- Palliative resection of gastric component of disease may be indicated.
- Multiple drug chemotherapy regimens have response rates of 30% to 50%, but most regimens do not affect survival.

INTRODUCTION

At the time of diagnosis, gastric cancers are localized and surgically resectable in approximately 50% of patients; however, regional nodal metastases or direct invasion of surrounding organs or structures are frequently encountered and preclude cure by surgery alone in many patients. Analyses of patterns of relapse after complete surgical resection demonstrate that subsequent relapse of cancer is common in both the tumor bed and nodal regions as well as systemically.

The standard of care for resectable gastric cancer for patients who can tolerate a surgical procedure is surgical resection. For patients with lower risk lesions (confined to

gastric wall, nodes negative; T1–2N0M0) adjuvant treatment is usually not recommended except in select instances. Because both local and systemic relapses are common after resection of high-risk gastric cancers (beyond wall, nodes positive, or both; T3–4N0, TanyN+), adjuvant treatment is indicated for these patients. The results of phase III trials that demonstrate a survival benefit for either preoperative irradiation or postoperative chemoradiotherapy versus surgery alone will be summarized and future trial designs will be discussed.

For patients with locally advanced disease that appears unresectable for cure, several treatment options appear to have a favorable impact on disease control and survival. These options include primary external beam irradiation (EBRT) plus concomitant chemotherapy, maximal resection plus intraoperative irradiation (IORT), and preoperative chemotherapy or chemoradiotherapy prior to resection. Results of these approaches will be summarized and future trial design will be discussed.

In the setting of metastatic disease, many active chemotherapy agents can produce meaningful response alone or in combination with other agents, but the duration of response is often limited. Trials now exist which demonstrate both a survival and quality of life benefit for multidrug chemotherapy versus best supportive care for patients with metastatic cancers.

EPIDEMIOLOGY AND ETIOLOGY

In 2003, cancer of the stomach had an expected incidence in the United States of 22,400 cases and an expected number of 12,100 deaths.[1] In spite of these significant figures, age-adjusted gastric cancer death rates have decreased dramatically in the United States since 1930 from approximately 28 to 2.3 in 100,000 females and from 38 to 5.2 in 100,000 males (Fig. 78-1). Of the 45 countries in which age-adjusted death rates for gastric cancer were compared for 2000 (Fig. 78-2), the United States ranked 45th for both males and females.[2] Kyrgyzstan ranked first for both males (47.0 in 100,000) and females (18.9 in 100,000).

The causes of the decline in the United States rates are incompletely understood, but environmental factors, chiefly dietary, are suspected. Within the United States, the lowest incidence is in whites, Chinese, and Filipinos, with a higher incidence in U.S. Japanese. However, epidemiologists have noted a significant decrease in incidence among migrants from high-incidence countries (such as Japan and Chile) to low-incidence countries. Although there is an overall reduction in gastric cancer incidence, there has been a steady rapid increase in the incidence of gastroesophageal junction and proximal gastric cancers.

Factors that have been associated with a higher incidence of gastric cancer include smoked or salted foods, foods contaminated with aflatoxin, low intake of fruits and vegetables, low socioeconomic status, and possibly a decreased use of refrigeration.[3,4] Possible occupational relationships include coal mining and rubber or asbestos workers. Precursor pathologic conditions include pernicious anemia, achlorhydria atrophic gastritis, gastric ulcers, and adenomatous polyps. Five to 10% of patients with pernicious anemia subsequently develop malignancy. Prior partial gastrectomy for benign gastric or duodenal ulcer disease produces an increased risk of subsequent malignancy in the gastric remnant with latency periods of 20 years or more.[5,6]

Several studies have shown a three- to sixfold increased risk of gastric cancer in patients with *Helicobacter pylori* infection versus those with no infection, but the precise role of this bacterium in the etiology of gastric cancer remains unknown.[79] A variety of bacterial, patient, and environment factors most likely act in combination to affect the development of gastric carcinoma. The increased association of *H. pylori* with gastric cancer seems to be mainly with distal gastric cancers and intestinal-type malignancy. Only a minority of *H. pylori* infected patients develop gastric cancer, and data do not yet exist on the effect of treatment of the *H. pylori* infection on subsequent malignancy.

PREVENTION AND EARLY DETECTION

Early detection would markedly improve the prognosis of gastric cancer in the United States, because surgical resection has a high cure rate with lesions limited to the mucosa or submucosa. However, the incidence of such early gastric cancers is less than 5% in most U.S. series. In Japan, the incidence of carcinomas confined to the mucosa or submucosa was only 3.8% in the 1955 to 1956 period. However, by 1966 the incidence of early lesions had increased to 34.5% because of vigorous screening procedures, leading to 5-year survival rates of 90.9% in this cohort of patients.[10] Although mass screening has been useful in Japan to detect early cancers, defined high-risk populations have not existed in the United States in the past to justify the expense of widespread screening endeavors. Whether screening of patients with *H. pylori* infection would be of value is not yet known. Individual practitioners should use upper gastrointestinal (GI) series and endoscopy to screen patients who have occupational or precursor risk factors or patients with persistent dyspepsia or gastroesophageal symptoms.

Germline mutations in the *CDH-1* gene, which encodes the E-cadherin protein, have recently been recognized in families with hereditary diffuse gastric adenocarcinoma. Carriers of these mutations have a 70% lifetime risk of developing gastric cancer. Several reports of prophylactic gastrectomy[11-13] have demonstrated the routine presence of microscopic intraepithelial carcinomas in patients having regular endoscopic surveillance that includes multiple random biopsies. Early total gastrectomy has been recommended for this small patient population because of the lack of effective early tumor detection by less aggressive techniques. Microscopic evaluation of the proximal and distal resection margins for complete removal of the gastric mucosa is necessary, because residual gastric mucosa can degenerate and result in a gastric cancer.[13]

PATHOLOGY

The terms gastric cancer and stomach cancer usually refer to adenocarcinoma, which accounts for 90% to 95% of all gastric malignancies. Other histologic types include lymphoma (usually intermediate- or high-grade histologic types), leiomyosarcoma, carcinoid, adenoacanthoma, and squamous cell carcinomas. The site of origin within the stomach has changed in frequency in the United States over recent decades, with more proximal lesions now being diagnosed and treated. The largest percentage of gastric cancers still arises within the atrum or distal stomach (around 40%), are least common in the body of the stomach (around 25%), and are of intermediate frequency in the fundus and esophagogastric junction (around 35%).[14]

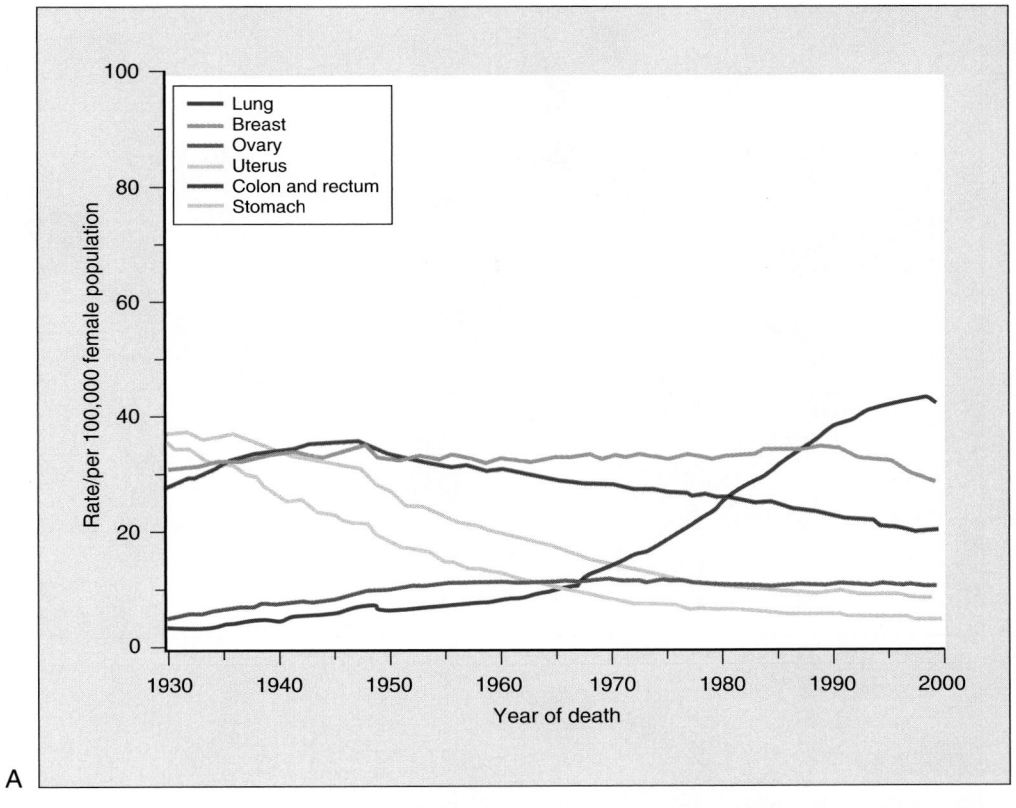

A

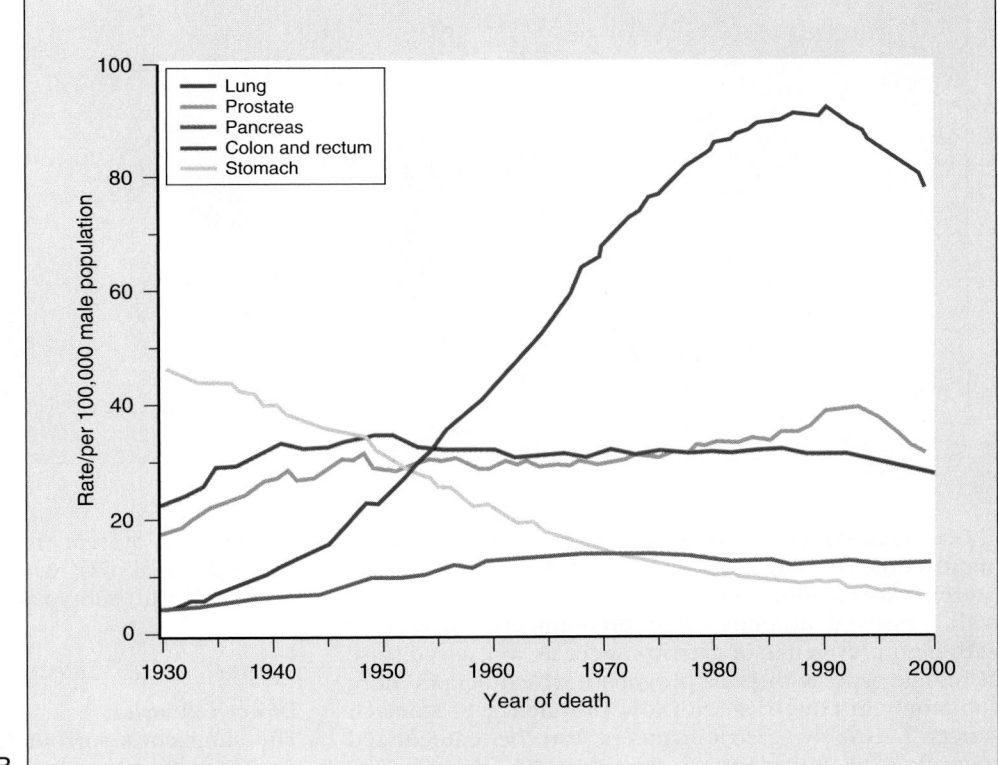

B

Figure 78-1. Age-adjusted (to U.S. 1970 standard population) cancer death rates in the United States from 1930 to 1999 in selected sites for females (**A**) and males (**B**). Females have a steady decrease in death rates for stomach, breast, and colorectal cancers. From 1960 to 1998, a continual increase in death rates occurred for lung cancer in females. For males, a similar decrease in death rates occurred with gastric cancer. An increase in death rates for lung cancer existed in males from 1930 to 1990 with a continual decrease during the 1990s. (Modified from Jemal A, Murray T, Samuels A, et al: Cancer statistics, 2003. CA Cancer J Clin 2003;53:5–26.)

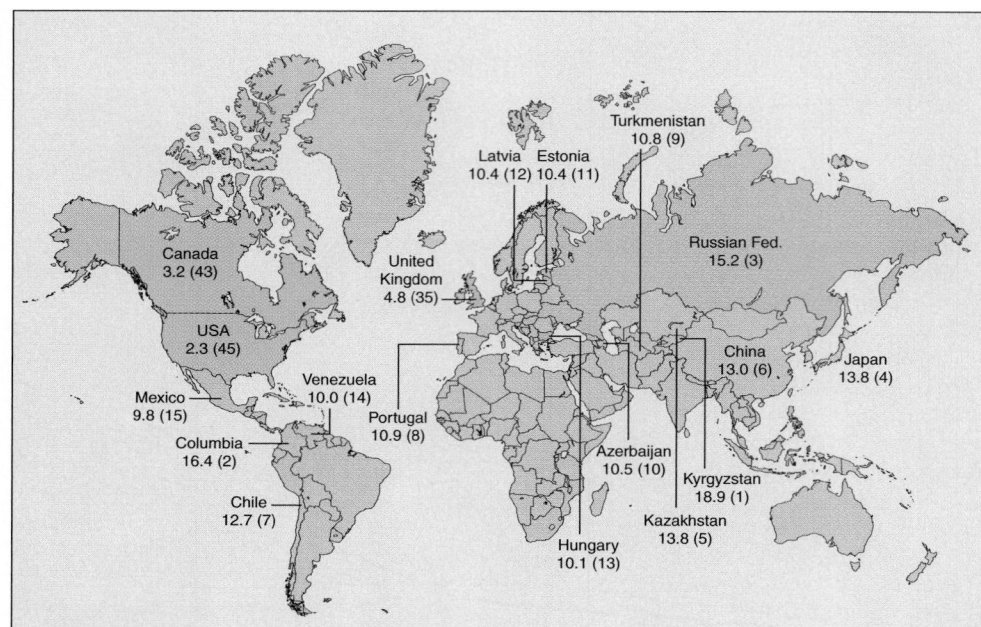

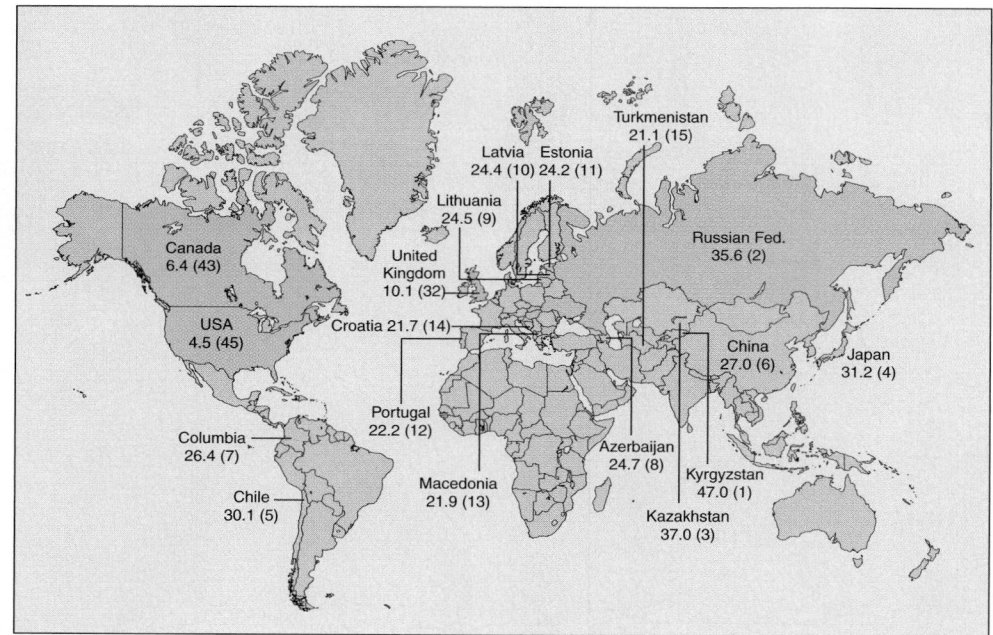

Figure 78-2. Age-adjusted (to World Health Organization world standard population) death rates for gastric cancer from 2000 in 45 countries for females **(A)** and males **(B)**. Rates in the United States, Canada, and United Kingdom are compared with selected countries, including the 15 countries with the highest death rates. (Data from Jemal A, Thomas A, Murray T, et al: Cancer statistics, 2002. CA Cancer J Clin 2002;52:23–47.)

Gastric carcinomas have been categorized by using both microscopic (Fig. 78-3) and gross pathologic features. The Lauren classification system includes an intestinal type with improved prognosis that predominates in regions with high prevalence of gastric cancer, as well as a diffuse histologic type, with poor prognosis, which occurs more commonly in countries with low prevalence of stomach cancer.[15] Grossly, gastric cancers can be categorized according to Borrmann's[16] five types: I, polypoid or fungating; II, ulcerating lesions surrounded by elevated borders; III, ulceration with invasion of the gastric wall; IV, diffusely infiltrating (linitis plastica); and V, unclassifiable. The Japanese Research Society for Gastric Cancer has a

classification system that divides lesions into protruded (I); superficial (II) with elevated (IIa), flat (IIb), and depressed (IIc) subtypes; and excavated (III) types.[17]

Pathways of Tumor Spread

Direct Extension

The stomach is surrounded by a number of organs and structures that can be involved once a lesion has extended beyond the gastric wall. These structures include the omenta, pancreas, diaphragm, transverse colon or mesocolon, duodenum, jejunum, spleen, liver, superior mesenteric and celiac vessels, abdominal wall, left adrenal gland,

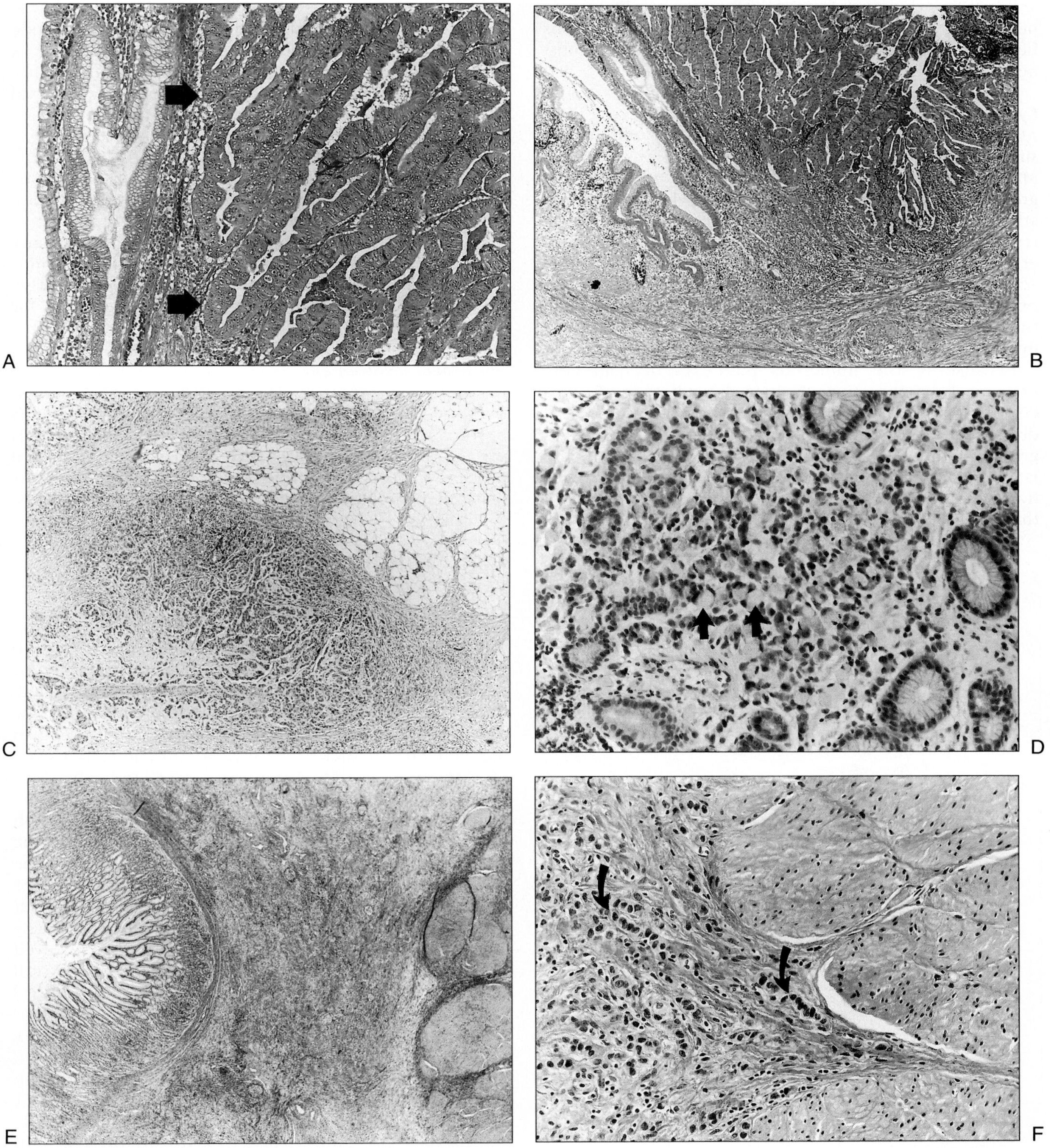

Figure 78-3. Photomicrographs demonstrating histopathologic features of gastric cancer. **A–C,** Gastric adenocarcinoma, intestinal type. **A,** The neoplasm shows complex gland formation (*arrows*). This type would be regarded as moderately differentiated or grade 2 in a four-grade system. (× 125.) **B,** This tumor infiltrates the superficial portion of the submucosa. Typical of intestinal type adenocarcinoma, the preexisting gastric epithelium is obliterated. (× 42.5.) **C,** This tumor extends into perigastric serosa and, in view of the more irregular gland formation, would be graded with grade 3 of 4. (× 42.5.) Diffuse-type gastric adenocarcinoma. **D,** Diffuse-type adenocarcinomas often contain signet cells (*arrows*). (× 225.) **E,** Linitis plastica. Note how the underlying mucosa, submucosa, and muscularis propria appear thickened but are otherwise intact, in contrast to intestinal type adenocarcinomas (**B**). (× 22.5.) **F,** Linitis plastica at high power. Neoplastic cells may be very subtle (*arrows*). This tumor extended to the peritoneal surface and had metastasized. (× 125.) (Courtesy of K. Batts, MD, Department of Pathology, Mayo Clinic, Rochester, MN.)

and kidney. Adherence from inflammatory conditions can mimic direct extension of tumor, but all adhesions between a gastric carcinoma and adjacent structures must be regarded as malignant.

Lymphatics

Abundant lymphatic channels are present within the submucosal and subserosal layers of the gastric wall. Microscopic or subclinical spread well beyond the visible gross lesion (intramural spread) occurs via these lymphatic channels. Accordingly, frozen sections of the gastric resection margins should be obtained intraoperatively to ensure that margins of resection are uninvolved microscopically. The submucosal lymphatic plexus is also prominent in the esophagus and the subserosal plexus in the duodenum, allowing both proximal and distal intramural tumor spread.

Because of the numerous pathways of lymphatic drainage from the stomach, it is difficult to perform a complete nodal dissection (Fig. 78-4). Although initial drainage is usually to lymph nodes along the lesser and greater curvatures (perigastric or N1 nodes using the Japanese Research Society for Gastric Cancer designation), primary node drainage includes nodes along all three branches of the celiac axis (common hepatic,

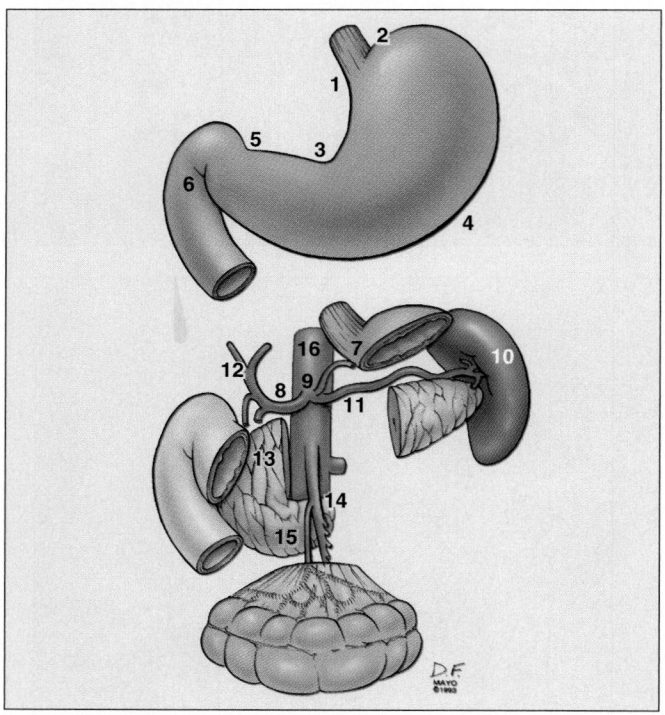

Figure 78-4. Classification and anatomic location of lymph node groups.[17] Involvement of nodes along the lesser or greater curvature (groups 1–6) constitutes N1 disease, and the celiac axis and its three branches are N2 (7–11), N3 (12–14), and N4 (15, 16). N1: 1, right paracardial; 2, left paracardial; 3, lesser curvature; 4, greater curvature; 5, suprapyloric; 6, infrapyloric. N2: 7, left gastric artery; 8, common hepatic artery; 9, celiac artery; 10, splenic hilus; 11, splenic artery. N3: 12, hepatic pedicle; 13, retropancreatic; 14, mesenteric root. N4: 15, middle colic artery; 16, para-aortic. (Reprinted by permission of the Mayo Foundation.)

splenic, left gastric) and the celiac artery itself (Japanese N2 nodes).[14] Node groups that are more distal include hepatoduodenal, peripancreatic, root of mesentery (N3), periaortic, and middle colic (N4). When proximal gastric lesions extend into distal esophagus, the paraesophageal nodal system is at risk for involvement.

Hematogenous Spread

For malignancies confined to the stomach, venous drainage is primarily to the liver via the portal system. At initial exploration, liver involvement is found in up to 30% of patients, predominantly as a result of hematogenous metastases but sometimes because of direct tumor extension. For lesions that extend proximally to involve the esophagus or posteriorly, the lung may be at risk for distant metastases.

Peritoneal Involvement

Because the stomach is an intraperitoneal organ, peritoneal dissemination is possible once a lesion extends beyond the gastric wall to a free peritoneal (serosal) surface. Peritoneal spread may initially be a localized process limited by surrounding organs and ligaments (gastrohepatic, gastrosplenic, and gastrocolic) and organs.

BIOLOGIC CHARACTERISTICS

Prognostic Factors

The most meaningful prognostic indicators relate to extent of tumor. With either hematogenous metastasis or peritoneal seeding, prognosis is almost uniformly fatal. Recent immunohistochemical analysis of bone marrow aspirates has shown the presence of tumor cells to be an independent predictor of adverse outcome; however, confirmatory studies have yet to be published.[18,19] Survival decreases with progressive direct tumor extension both within and beyond the gastric wall.[20,22] Lymph node involvement, per se, is not as important as the number and location of nodes.[21,23,24] Minimal lymph node involvement adjacent to the primary lesion results in the most favorable prognosis in node-positive patients, but even micrometastases in regional nodes may adversely impact survival.[25] The solitary finding of either involved lymph nodes or complete penetration of the gastric wall is usually not as ominous as the presence of both[20,23] (Table 78-1).

The tumor grade as well as gross and histologic pathologic appearance of the primary malignancy appear to provide some prognostic information, but none of these factors is a prognostic variable independent of the tumor stage. Prognosis is generally worse with higher grade and diffuse-type carcinomas, which usually present with higher pathologic stages of disease (see Fig. 78-3). Borrmann types I and II carcinomas have a relatively favorable 5-year survival rate, but patients with type IV tumors (linitis plastica) fare very poorly.[26,28]

Some investigators have suggested that tumors of the gastric cardia may have different epidemiologic factors than cancers of the distal stomach[29,30] and may exhibit

TABLE 78-1

Extent of Initial Disease versus Survival Rates in Stomach Cancer*

	5-YEAR SR (%)		>5-YR SR DISEASE-FREE (%) UNIVERSITY OF MINNESOTA REOPERATION SERIES
EXTENT OF DISEASE	DOCKERTY[20†]	KENNEDY[21]	
Lymph Nodes–			
Mucosa only	100	85	—
>Mucosa but within wall	61	52	—
Through wall	44	47	—
Lymph Nodes+			
Lymph node extent	15	—	19
Regional only	—	17	—
Nonregional	—	5	—
Extent of primary			
Within wall	—	—	40
Through wall	—	—	12

SR, survival rate.
*Compilation of data from various series.
†Percentages are only of patients who left the hospital.

different tumor biology.[31] The prognosis is worse for cardia lesions,[32,33] and flow cytometry reveals a greater incidence of aneuploidy when compared with tumors of the antrum and body.[34]

Flow cytometry provides valuable prognostic information for gastric cancer and may be an independent prognostic factor.[34,37] As noted previously, aneuploidy is associated with unfavorable tumor location such as the cardia[34,35] but is also associated with lymph node metastasis[35,37] and direct tumor extension.[37] Unfavorable DNA flow cytometry characteristics seem to relate closely to an unfavorable prognosis.[34,37] In one series in which multivariate analysis of DNA ploidy was analyzed with other known prognostic factors such as stage, age, and sex, DNA ploidy carried statistically significant independent prognostic information.[37]

The presence of several peptides including estrogen receptor,[38] epidermal growth factor receptor,[39] the e-erb-b2 protein,[40] and plasminogen activator inhibitor type 1[19] appears to affect prognosis adversely. The expression of epidermal growth factor receptor and high levels of epidermal growth factor correlate with a higher incidence of primary tumor infiltration, poor histologic differentiation, and linitis plastica. The pathophysiologic relationship between these peptide receptors and poor patient prognosis is not clear. Gastric cancers with class II major histocompatibility complex antigen expression (HLA-DR) have a better prognosis, but the loss of expression is not an independent prognostic factor.[41]

CLINICAL MANIFESTATIONS

Neither patient symptoms nor routine physical examination will lead to an early diagnosis of gastric cancer. The most common presenting symptoms and signs are loss of appetite, abdominal discomfort, weight loss, weakness (due to anemia), nausea and vomiting, and melena. The duration of symptoms is less than 3 months in nearly 40% of patients and longer than 1 year in only 20%.

EVALUATION OF THE PATIENT

Positive findings on physical examination are those of advanced disease. Findings may include an abdominal mass (representing the primary tumor, hepatic metastasis, or ovarian metastasis [Krukenberg's tumor]), remote node metastasis (left supraclavicular [Virchow's node]; periumbilical [Sister Mary Joseph node]; or left axillary [Irish's node]), ascites, or a rectal shelf (peritoneal seeding).

The diagnosis of gastric cancer is usually confirmed by upper gastrointestinal (UGI) endoscopy, or radiographs. Double-contrast radiographs may reveal small lesions limited to the superficial (inner) layers of the gastric wall. Endoscopy is now the preferred initial diagnostic test, because it allows direct tumor visualization, cytologic testing, and histologic biopsy that yields the diagnosis in 90% or more of patients with exophytic lesions. Ulcerated cancers and linitis plastica lesions may be harder to diagnose endoscopically, but multiple biopsies and washings enhance the probability of accurate diagnosis. Endoscopic ultrasonography (EUS) has a high degree of accuracy in determining depth of tumor invasion (i.e., does the lesion extend beyond the muscularis propria?) but is less accurate in detecting regional nodal metastasis.[42-44] Ultrasound-guided fine needle aspiration for cytologic test allows the assessment of regional lymph nodes and some distant metastatic sites (e.g., liver), further enhancing the ability of EUS to determine tumor stage and resectability.

The extent of disease at exploration or laparoscopy is usually more extensive than is suggested on UGI radiography or endoscopy. Abdominal CT scan is valuable in determining the abdominal extent of disease with regard to larger liver metastasis (1 cm or greater), involvement of celiac or periaortic nodes, or extragastric extension (may help determine which lesions extend to surgically unresectable structures). CT scan is of little value, however, in ruling out peritoneal metastases or small hepatic metastasis. Diagnostic laparoscopy allows visualization of small serosal or liver metastases and may give added information with regard to the amount of direct extension of the primary tumor. Distant (hematogenous) metastases should be ruled out with a chest radiograph, serum liver chemistries, and abdominal CT scan, or liver ultrasonography (we prefer CT scan to ultrasonography because of the additional information concerning regional nodal status, extragastric extent of disease, and extension within the distal esophagus). CT scans also provide valuable tumor localization information should irradiation be indicated. If a proximal gastric tumor extends to involve the esophagus, CT scan of the chest is useful in determining mediastinal node involvement or parenchymal lung metastases.

STAGING SYSTEM

With the development of laparoscopic general surgery, diagnostic laparoscopy is commonly used to assess for distant metastasis or unresectable locally advanced abdominal cancers. Several groups[45,48] have reported the use of laparoscopy in stomach cancer patients. Metastatic disease was documented laparoscopically in 35% to 40% of patients.[45,46,48] The sensitivity for metastases was 85% or greater[46,48] and this technique was particularly sensitive in detecting liver and peritoneal disease. Laparoscopy is more sensitive and accurate in staging patients with regard to intra-abdominal metastases than either ultrasound or CT scan.[46,47] Many surgeons now routinely perform laparoscopy in all gastric cancer patients who do not require palliation, to avoid nontherapeutic laparotomy.

The current TNM (tumor, lymph node, metastasis) staging system is depicted in Table 78-2.[49] Portions of this system[49] are compared in Table 78-3 with a modification of the Astler-Coller rectal system suitable for all alimentary tract carcinomas.[22] The modified Astler-Coller system is more inclusive with respect to degree of extension beyond the wall, but the TNM system has a better description of nodal involvement and level of gastric invasion in lesions confined to the wall. Several comparison studies, including some from Japan,[50,51] have shown better prediction of prognosis using the AJCC TNM system compared to other staging systems, including that of the Japanese Research Society for Gastric Cancer.

PRIMARY THERAPY AND RESULTS

Surgical Method

Surgical excision of the gastric and nodal components of disease remains the primary therapy for all potentially

TABLE 78-2

TNM Staging for Carcinoma of the Stomach*

STAGE	T	N	M
0	Tis	0	0
IA	1	0	0
IB	1	1	0
	2	0	0
II	1	2	0
	2a/b	1	0
	3	0	0
IIIA	2a/b	2	0
	3	1	0
	4	0	0
IIIB	3	2	0
IV	4	1–3	0
	1–3	3	0
	Any	Any	0

TNM definitions are as follows:
Tis   Carcinoma in situ; intraepithelial tumor without invasion of the lamina propria.
T1   Tumor invades lamina propria or submucosa.
T2   Tumor invades the muscularis propria (T2a) or the subserosa (T2b).
T3   Tumor penetrates the serosa (visceral peritoneum) without invasion of adjacent structures.
T4   Tumor invades adjacent structures.
N0   No regional lymph node metastasis.
N1   Metastasis in 1–6 regional nodes.
N2   Metastasis in 7–15 regional nodes.
N3   Metastasis in more than 15 regional nodes.
M0   No distant metastasis.
M1   Distant metastasis
*Metastasis to other intra-abdominal lymph nodes such as hepatoduodenal, retropancreatic, mesenteric, or para-aortic are considered distant metastasis within this system but are N3 or N4 in the Japanese Research Society Classification.

curable gastric carcinomas. Based on pathologic findings, the Japanese Research Society for Gastric Cancer has defined four categories of surgical resection: (1) absolute curative (no peritoneal or hepatic metastases, no serosal involvement, and a level of lymph nodes removed beyond those involved); (2) relative curative (same as 1 but nodal involvement to the level excised); (3) relatively noncurative (complete gross tumor excision but curative criteria not met); and (4) absolute noncurative (residual cancer).[17] Most curable tumors can be removed with adequate margins by subtotal gastrectomy; total gastrectomy is used when mandated by proximal cancer location or disease extent. Routine total gastrectomy does not improve survival by providing wider margins and eliminating multicentric disease but may increase the rates of patient morbidity and mortality. Two recent reports,[52,53] including a randomized study,[53] show similar probabilities and survival rates with subtotal and total gastrectomy. Surgical resection alone is an excellent treatment for gastric carcinomas limited to the mucosa or submucosa without nodal involvement (TIS or T1N0M0). These early gastric cancers now occur with an incidence of over 30% in Japan, but still less than 5% in the United States and other Western countries. At least one Japanese report showed similar excellent results for T2 cancers if lymph nodes were uninvolved.[54] For the more invasive gastric carcinomas, curative or palliative resection is indicated for

TABLE 78-3

Staging Systems for Gastric Carcinoma*

MODIFIED ASTLER-COLLER	TNM†	CHARACTERISTICS
A	TisN0	Nodes negative; lesion limited to mucosa
B1	T1–2N0	Nodes negative; extension of lesion beyond mucosa but still within gastric wall
B2	T3N0	Nodes negative; extension beyond the entire wall (including serosa if present) without adherence to or invasion of surrounding organs or structures
B3	T4N0	Nodes negative; beyond wall with adherence to of invasion or surrounding organs or structures
C1	Tis–2N1–3	Nodes positive; lesion limited to wall
C2	T3N1–3	Nodes positive; extension of lesion through the entire wall (including serosa)
C3	T4N1–3	Nodes positive; beyond wall with adherence to or invasion of surrounding organs or structures

*Comparison of TNM system with a modification of the Astler-Coller rectal system by Gunderson and Sosin.
†Also see Table 78-2.

50% to 60% of patients at the time of disease presentation, but only 25% to 40% of these patients will have potentially curative surgical procedures.

Only one prospective randomized trial[53] exists with regard to the extent of gastric resection, but extensive experience exists with various different surgical procedures, and appropriate generalizations can be made. The preferred treatment for lesions arising in the body or antrum of the stomach is a radical distal subtotal resection (Fig. 78-5). This removes approximately 80% of the stomach along with the first portion of the duodenum, the gastrohepatic and gastrocolic omenta, and the nodal tissue adjacent to the three branches of the celiac axis. Extensive

or proximal cancers will require a total gastrectomy to achieve an adequate proximal gastric margin (Fig. 78-6). Total gastrectomy does not seem advantageous when subtotal gastrectomy will provide a 5-cm clearance of the gross tumor.[52,54,57] The propensity for gastric carcinoma to spread via submucosal and subserosal lymphatics dictates the need for a 5-cm surgical resection margin of normal stomach beyond the visible lesion. It may be necessary to extend the resection to include some (or additional) esophagus or duodenum if frozen section pathologic evaluation of the surgical margins fails to confirm the adequacy of proximal and distal resection margins. If total gastrectomy is necessary, a splenectomy is sometimes

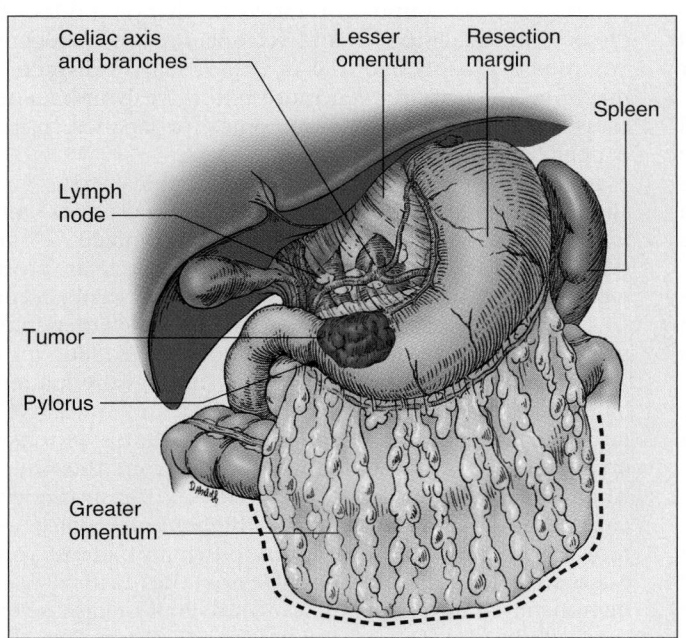

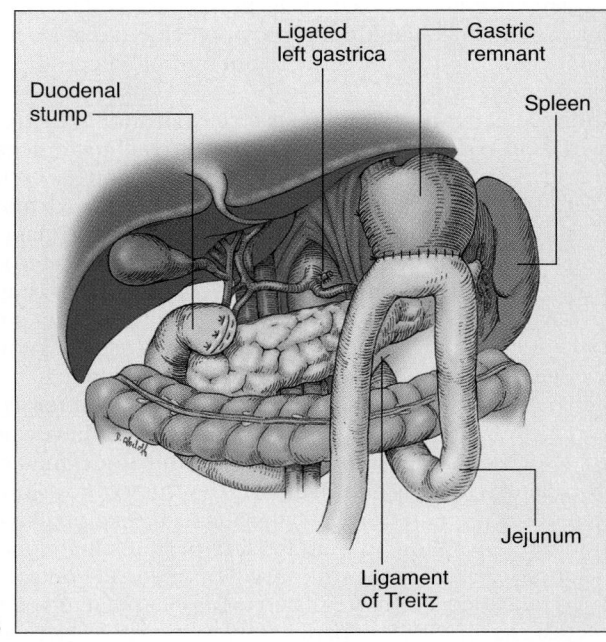

Figure 78-5. A, Radical subtotal gastrectomy. The extent of resection for this tumor of the antrum includes the distal 80% of the stomach, the lesser and greater omenta, the perigastric lymph nodes (Japan N1), and lymph nodes along the left gastric, celiac, and common hepatic arteries (Japan N2). **B,** Radical subtotal gastrectomy reconstruction. After closure of the duodenal stump and lesser curvature of the stomach, the gastric remnant and proximal jejunum are anastomosed end to side in an antecolic position. The spleen and distal pancreas have been left in situ.

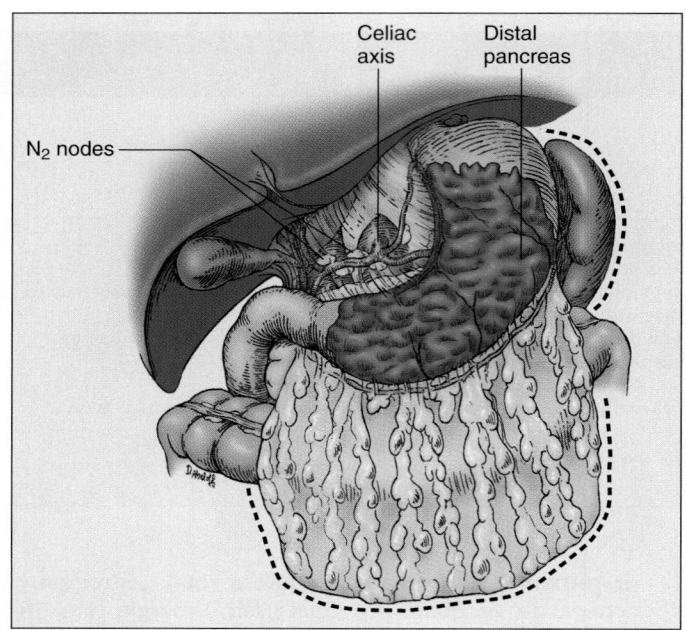 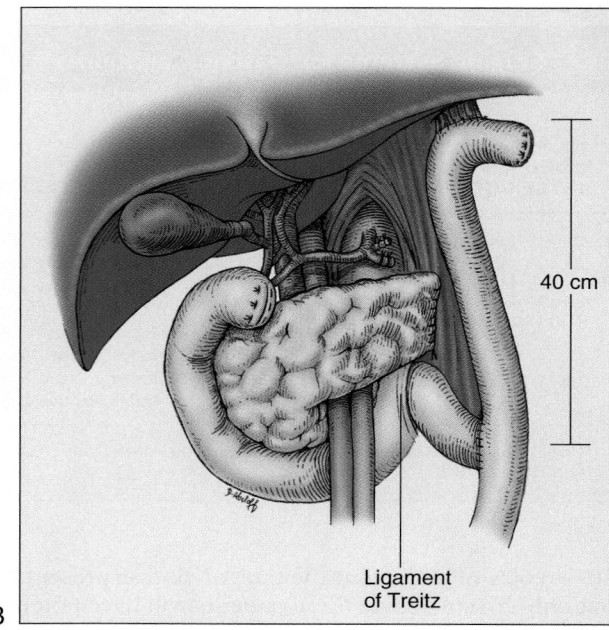

Figure 78-6. A, Radical total gastrectomy. A total gastrectomy is indicated for this extensive tumor of the stomach. Both omenta, the spleen, distal pancreas, and Japan N2 lymph nodes are to be included with the operative specimen. **B,** Radical total gastrectomy reconstruction. Although a variety of anastomoses and jejunal pouches have been described, no benefit appears to accrue from any approach, except to keep the biliary and pancreatic secretions away from the esophageal mucosa. The Cohn end-to-side Roux-en-Y esophagojejunostomy with a 40-cm limb is depicted.

performed, particularly in gastric cancers of the proximal third of the stomach, and tumors of the body near the greater curvature. These cancers are more apt to metastasize to lymph nodes in the splenic hilum that cannot be completely excised without a splenectomy. The value of routine splenectomy has not been addressed in prospective randomized trials. Retrospective Japanese[58,60] and American[61] data do not provide evidence of a survival benefit with this procedure, but rather suggest poorer outcome.

Direct spread beyond the gastric wall should be treated with en bloc extended resection to achieve negative margins of resection, if a curative resection is contemplated. Common examples of local tumor extension include involvement of the body or tail of the pancreas (treated by distal pancreatectomy and splenectomy), invasion of the transverse mesocolon (often requires transverse colectomy), and involvement of the spleen (splenectomy) or left lobe of the liver (usually requires wedge resection with a 1-cm or wider clearance).

The optimal extent of lymph node dissection for gastric cancer remains controversial. Several studies have shown that the presence and extent of lymph node metastasis correlate with the depth of primary tumor invasion.[61,64] Japanese surgeons universally advocate regional lymph node removal for all but in situ or intestinal mucosal tumors as a means to improve both local control and survival.[62] Because more distal nodes can be involved with metastasis in 11% of patients with negative perigastric nodes, a wider regional nodal dissection is deemed necessary for cure.[64] A recent study of sentinel lymph node biopsies in gastric cancer patients in Japan[65] demonstrated that 37% of tumors drained to N2 nodes, either in combination with N1 sentinel nodes (32%) or as the sole site of lymphatic drainage (5%). When performing a radical subtotal gastrectomy and omentectomy, all N1 and N2 nodes should be removed (D2 dissection) (see Fig. 78-4) (N1, perigastric nodes; N2, nodes along the left gastric, common hepatic, celiac, and splenic arteries). Some Japan surgeons routinely remove N3 lymph nodes (D3 dissection, usually portal and retropancreatic). A recently completed prospective trial of D2 versus D3 dissections may determine if an even more extensive lymphadenectomy will further enhance outcomes for Japanese gastric cancer patients.

Although several nonrandomized clinical trials have suggested that extended lymphadenectomies may improve survival,[60,66,71] other nonrandomized[72,73] and randomized trials[74,78] have not demonstrated an advantage. A large multicenter phase III study that accrued 711 curable gastric cancer patients in the Netherlands[75] provides objective data on the value of extended lymphadenectomy in gastric carcinoma. Among the patients having curative resections, morbidity[75,76] and mortality[75,77] rates were significantly higher with the more extensive nodal dissection. A randomized study from the United Kingdom that included 400 patients with gastric adenocarcinoma also demonstrated higher morbidity and mortality rates in the extended lymphadenectomy cohort.[78] Neither the Dutch[75] nor the British trial[79] demonstrated any improvement in overall or disease-free survival. In the Dutch study,[75] patients who did not undergo a splenectomy or distal pancreatectomy had an improvement in relapse-free survival (71% versus 59% at 5 years, $P = 0.02$). Splenectomy and pancreatectomy had significant adverse impact on survival in both trials.[75,79]

Any potential survival benefit seen with the extended node dissection performed in Japan may be due to the phenomenon of a shift in stage rather than superior surgery.[80,83] In Japan and the United States gastric resection specimens are handled quite differently.[84] Japan pathologists evaluated an average of 62 nodes in subtotal gastrectomy specimens and up to 100 in total gastrectomy cases, including lymph nodes less than 3 mm in diameter.[85] This number compares with an average of 12 and 13 nodes examined after subtotal and total gastrectomy, respectively, at Memorial Sloan-Kettering.[80] Two recent reports[81,82] have shown that patient survival after a curative operation significantly improves when more than 15 lymph nodes are pathologically examined. Failure to evaluate an adequate number of regional lymph nodes likely results in the understaging of many gastric cancer patients. N2 nodes cannot be defined as positive if they are not resected and examined; involvement of resected N1 nodes cannot be assessed if the specimen is not thoroughly evaluated by the pathologist. A small subset of Japanese patients with nodal metastasis to N3 or N4 lymph nodes may be salvaged by extended lymph node dissection.[60,86] Most patients with more than six lymph node metastases or with lymph node metastasis not adjacent to the primary tumor still have a very poor outcome[24]; however, extended lymph node dissection seems reasonable, because it can be performed by experienced surgeons without significantly increased surgical morbidity or mortality rates.[87,88]

Endoscopic laser surgery has been utilized in selected patients with early gastric cancer.[89] Small lesions (3 cm or less) that are not ulcerated, do not involve the submucosa, and are well differentiated infrequently have lymph node metastasis (<5%). Seventy to 75% of these select tumors can be completely removed endoscopically.[89,90] Although early gastric cancer may have a long natural history before progression, standard surgical resection rather than endoscopic removal is still preferable.[92] Irradiation plus chemotherapy should be considered as adjuvant therapy when the tumor is endoscopically treated.

Survival After Surgery Alone

Overall survival results with surgery alone remain poor, despite improved perioperative treatment, which has resulted in a substantial decline in postoperative mortality rate (median of 4.6% in the 1980s).[92] A large review from Europe reported excellent 5-year survival rate for early gastric cancer patients (83%) but a marked diminution in survival for more invasive cancers (31% for tumors of the antrum, 24% for the midstomach, and 16% for the cardia).[93] Excellent survival in excess of 90% has been achieved throughout the world with surgical resection of lesions confined to the mucosa or submucosa[54,94,97] (Table 78-4). In reports with lower 5-year survival rates for these early lesions, most of the deaths were due to non-cancer causes.[98,100] In contrast, for gastric cancers with deeper invasion or nodal involvement, survival decreases proportionally to the degree of invasion or involvement (see Table 78-4). When N1 or N2 nodes are involved, Western reports continue to show 5-year survival rates of

TABLE 78-4

Comparison of 5-Year Survivals Following Surgery for Gastric Carcinoma

TUMOR CLASSIFICATION	NODAL STATUS	5-YEAR SURVIVAL (%)	
		JAPAN	UNITED STATES
T1	N0	90	90
T2	N0	60	52
T3	N0	30	47
T4	N0	5	15
—	N1	53	20
—	N2	26	10
—	N3	10	—
—	N4	3	—

Modified from Noguchi Y, Imada T, Matsumoto A, et al: Radical surgery for gastric cancer. A review of the Japanese experience. Cancer 1989;64:2053.

10% to 30%,[101,102] whereas Japanese authors report 5-year surgical cure rates of 25% to 60% (versus <10% with N3 or N4)[60,103] (see Table 78-4). Although pathologic staging differences, different tumor biology, and more radical surgical extirpation have been proposed as explanations, the cause of the difference in U.S. and Japanese results with N1 or N2 disease remains uncertain. Even in the Orient half of all patients with more invasive gastric cancer die of their disease, a fact that underlies the need for new nonsurgical therapies.

Relapse Patterns After "Curative Resection"

Local regrowth or failure (LF) in the tumor bed and regional lymph nodes (RF) or distant failures (DF) via hematogenous (DM) or peritoneal (PS) routes are all common mechanisms of failure after "curative resection" in clinical,[104,105] reoperative,[22] and autopsy[106,110] series (Tables 78-5 and 78-6). For lesions of the esophagogastric

TABLE 78-5

Gastric Cancer—Patterns of Failure After "Curative" Resection (Reoperation and Autopsy Series)*

PATTERN OF FAILURE‡	UNIVERSITY OF MINNESOTA REOPERATION† (N = 107)		AUTOPSY (%)
	NO.	PERCENT	
Locoregional (LF-RF)	72	67	80–93
Peritoneal seeding (PS)	44	41	30–43
Localized	20	19	—
Diffuse	24	22	—
Distant metastases (DM)	24	22	49

*Data represent incidence in total patient group, any component.
†LF-RF, direct extension of tumor, lymphatic spread, or operative wound implant.
‡DM, distant metastases on hematologic basis; PS, abdominal involvement on basis of peritoneal seeding.

Specific Malignancies

III

TABLE 78-6

Gastric Cancer—Patterns of Locoregional Failure in Clinical, Reoperation, and Autopsy Series

	INCIDENCE—ANY COMPONENT							
	MGH[105] (CLINICAL) (N = 130)		U. MINN.[22] (REOPERATION) (N = 105)		MCNEER ET AL.[107] (AUTOPSY) (N = 92)		THOMSON AND ROBINS[109] (AUTOPSY) (N = 28)	
FAILURE AREA	NO.	(%)	NO.	(%)	NO.	(%)	NO.	(%)
Gastric bed	27	(21%)	58	(55%)	48	(52%)	19	(68%)
Anastomosis or stumps	33	(25%)	28	(27%)	55	(60%)	15	(54%)
Abdominal or stab wound	—	—	5	(5%)	—	—	—	—
Lymph node(s)	11	(8%)	45	(43%)	48	(52%)	—	—

From MacDonald JS, Steele G, Gunderson LL: Carcinoma of the stomach. In DeVita V, Hellman S, Rosenberg SA (eds): Principles and Practices of Oncology: 2nd ed. Philadelphia. JB Lippincott, 1989, p 675.

junction, both the liver and lungs are common sites of DM. With gastric lesions that do not extend to the esophagus, the initial site of DM is usually the liver, and many relapses could be prevented if an effectived "abdominal" therapy could be combined with treatment of the primary tumor and regional lymph nodes.

Locoregional failures occur commonly within the region of the gastric bed and nearby lymph nodes (see Table 78-6). Tumor relapse in anastomoses, the gastric remnant, or the duodenal stump is also frequently seen. In a University of Minnesota reoperative analysis,[22] locoregional failure occurred as the only evidence of relapse in 29% of the 86 patients with relapse (23% of the 105 evaluable patients at risk) and as any component of failure in 88%. More extensive operative procedures including routine splenectomy, omentectomy, and radical lymph node dissection neither improved survival[111] nor decreased the incidence of LF-RF[22] in the reoperative analysis. Subsequent relapse within the scope of the initial node dissection occurred in a high percentage of the patients even when radical node dissections were performed (removal of N1 and N2 with or without N3 nodes) (Table 78-7). This indicates the difficulty of obtaining a complete lymph node excision encompassing this anatomic location.

Patterns of failure by stage were analyzed in detail in a series of 130 patients who underwent resection performed with curative intent at the Massachusetts General Hospital.[105] Locoregional failure occurred as any component of failure in 49 patients (38%) and as the sole failure in 21 (16% of 130 patients at risk and 24% of the 88 patients with disease progression). The incidence of locoregional failure by stage was in excess of 35% for modified Astler-Coller stages B2 (T3N0), B3 (T4N0), C2 (T3N1–3), and C3 (T4N1–3). The sites at highest risk for locoregional failure included the gastric bed (27 of 130 patients, 21%) and the anastomosis or gastric remnant (33 of 130 patients, 25%). The true incidence of gastric

TABLE 78-7

Operative Method versus Patterns of Failure—Reoperation Series*,†

OPERATIVE PROCEDURES‡	NO. OF FAILURES/ TOTAL AT RISK	LOCOREGIONAL				PERITONEAL SEEDING				DISTANT METASTASES			
		ALONE		COMPONENT		ALONE		COMPONENT		ALONE		COMPONENT	
		NO.	(%)	NO.	(%)	NO.	(%)	NO.	(%)	NO.	(%)	NO.	(%)
Method 1 (pre-1950)	25/36	9	(25)	23	(64)	1	(3)	12	(33)	—		7	(19)
Method 2 (1950–1954)	29/32	6	(19)	24	(75)	1	(9)	17	(53)	3	(9)	9	(28)
Method 3 (1954 on)	26/37	8	(22)	23	(62)	1	(3)	15	(41)	2	(5)	7	(19)
Totals	80/105‡	23	(22)	70	(67)	3	(3)	44	(42)	5	(5)	23	(22)

*186 Patients with failure, 80 evaluable by all parameters.
†Data represent number of patients with failure; data in parentheses represent percent total group at risk who had complete follow-up.
‡Method 1 (pre-1950): subtotal or total gastrectomy, greater omentectomy, regional node dissection; method 2 (1950–1954): method 1 plus splenectomy, total omentectomy, additional node dissection regarding splenic, suprapancreatic, and central celiac axis; method 3 (1954 on): methods 1 and 2 plus extension of node dissection to porta hepatis and pancreaticoduodenal (intent: total lymph node dissection of all primary node areas equivalent to D2 or D3 dissection)
Modified from Macdonald JS, Steele G, Gunderson LL: Carcinoma of the stomach. In DeVita V, Hellman S, Rosenberg SA (eds): Principles and Practices of Oncology, 2nd ed. Philadelphia, JB Lippincott, 1989, p 765.

bed, regional lymph node, and peritoneal failures may be higher because this was neither a reoperative nor an autopsy series (see comparative findings in Tables 78-5 and 78-6). Some additional information on patterns of relapse by stage exist in both the University of Minnesota reoperation analysis[22] and the University of Washington autopsy analysis.[110] Although patterns of failure data are more accurate in such analyses, patient selection is biased.

All these data suggest that the development of an effective therapy for locoregional disease as an adjuvant to surgery could potentially benefit at least 20% of patients. However, effective systemic therapy is also essential to improve the outcome for resected high-risk gastric cancer patients.

ADJUVANT TREATMENT AFTER COMPLETE RESECTION—RESULTS

Adjuvant Systemic Chemotherapy

The results of surgery alone for resectable gastric cancer have already been presented and justify the evaluation of adjuvant chemotherapy with regard to systemic risks and survival. Although many active single agents exist and a number of drug combinations have been associated with response rates of 40% or more, randomized North American and European (Western) trials have generally failed to show positive survival findings for adjuvant chemotherapy.

The role of adjuvant chemotherapy for resected gastric cancer has been assessed in a number of clinical trials and in several meta-analyses. Each of the randomized clinical trials published to date have generally failed to show any clear long-term benefit beyond surgery alone (Table 78-8). However, differences in outcome have been noted between Western and Asian studies.

North American and European Studies

Initial trials in the United States were initiated by the Veterans Administration (VA) in 1957 testing *single agents*. Survival was not improved with the adjuvant use of either single-agent 5-fluorodeoxyuridine (FUDR) or triethylenethiophosphoramide (thiotepa) when compared with surgery alone.[115,116]

Subsequent protocols tested the value of nitrosourea-containing *multiple drug regimens*. 5-Fluorouracil (5-FU) and methyl-CCNU (MeCCNU) (lomustine), which had produced a response rate of 40% in prior trials of advanced gastric cancer, was examined as adjuvant therapy by three U.S. cooperative groups.[117] The first report came from the Gastrointestinal Tumor Study Group (GITSG) and demonstrated a survival advantage for the 71 patients assigned to combination chemotherapy when compared with an equal number of control patients assigned to surgery alone ($P < 0.03$).[118] Unfortunately, subsequent studies performed by the Eastern Cooperative Oncology Group (ECOG), and the VA could not confirm a survival advantage for patients treated with the same adjuvant chemotherapy.[119,120] In addition, a report from the Italian Gastrointestinal Tumor Study Group (IGTSG)

could not support the positive results of the GITSG study using 5-FU and MeCCNU either alone or combined with levamisole in the adjuvant setting.[121] A German study evaluated a different nitrosourea, BCNU (carmustine), in combination with 5-FU and also failed to demonstrate a survival advantage for postoperative chemotherapy.[122] Finally, the addition of doxorubicin (Adriamycin) to either 5-FU alone or with 5-FU and MeCCNU produced the same negative results.[123,124]

Following the reports of high response rates to 5-FU, Adriamycin, and mitomycin (FAM) in advanced gastric cancer, several studies with larger patient numbers were initiated to test the role of this promising regimen in the adjuvant setting. The International Collaborative Cancer Group (ICCG) could not detect a survival advantage for adjuvant FAM chemotherapy in their overall study population; however, some suggestive benefit was seen in a retrospective subset analysis of patients with T3 and T4 disease.[125] A study by the Southwest Oncology Group (SWOG) has not shown an advantage for the post-operative use of FAM.[126] An intensified version of FAM (FAM2) as surgical adjuvant therapy has been performed by the EORTC.[127] Although the time to progression was superior for FAM ($P = 0.020$), survival was not improved ($P = 0.295$) by this adjuvant chemotherapy approach. The second British Stomach Cancer Group (BSCG) trial (13 had stage IV disease) looked at the utility of adjuvant FAM following surgical resection and found no survival benefit in the treated patients.[129] Last, a group from Greece studied 5-FU, epirubicin, and mitomycin (FEM) compared to surgical control subjects. A trend toward improved survival in patients with histologic grade III tumor was observed ($P = 0.085$) but no statistically significant survival benefit for the entire study group was detected.[130]

The European Organization for Research and Treatment of Cancer (EORTC) and the International Collaborative Cancer Group (ICCG) conducted independent randomized phase III studies of either adjuvant FAMTX or FEMTX for patients undergoing resection of stomach cancer compared to surgery alone.[131] Both studies were closed by an independent data monitoring committee when they failed to reach accrual after having been open for 7 years. A pooled analysis of the two studies was performed given their similar design and treatment regimens. The combined analysis of the two regimens demonstrated that they both caused substantial toxicity, but had no significant effect on overall survival, the primary end point of both studies.

Other 5-FU-based combination chemotherapy regimens have been tested in the adjuvant setting. Huguier and colleagues could not demonstrate a survival benefit for the adjuvant use of 5-FU, vinblastine, and cyclophosphamide combination chemotherapy.[132] Rake and associates reported a small trial with 34 patients randomized to receive an induction course of 5-FU, cyclophosphamide, vincristine, and methotrexate followed by 6 weekly courses of 5-FU and mitomycin C.[133] Median survival was improved from 6 months in the surgical control subjects to 10 months for adjuvantly treated patients ($P = 0.034$). The BSCG similarly looked at a combination of 5-FU and mitomycin C alone or following an induction course of 5-FU, cyclophosphamide, vincristine, and methotrexate in

TABLE 78-8

Adjuvant Therapy for Gastric Cancer: North American and European Studies

AUTHOR (REF)	YEAR	REGIMEN	PATIENTS	SURVIVAL INTERVAL	PERCENT	P VALUE
Serlin[116]	1969	FUDR	110	3 yr	32.2	NS
		Control	129		34.2	
Dixon[115]	1971	Thiotepa	135	5 yr	34	NS
		Control	142		32	
Hugier[132]	1980	5-FU/VNB/CTX	27	5 yr	18	NS
		Control	26		16	
Schlag[122]	1987	5-FU	49	5 yr	42	NS
		Control	54		57	
GITSG[118]	1982	5-FU/MeCCNU	71	5 yr	50	<0.03
		Control	71		31	
Higgins[119]	1983	5-FU/MeCCNU	66	3.5 yr	37.8	0.88
		Control	68		38.9	
Engstrom[120]	1985	5-FU/MeCCNU	91	2 yr	57	0.73
		Control	89		51	
IGITSG[121]	1988	5-FU/MeCCNU	75	5 yr	~ 50	0.90
		5-FU/MeCCNU/Lev	69		~ 50	
		Control	69		~ 50	
Jakesz[135]	1988	5-FU/araC/Mito ± OK-432	53	5 yr	45	NS
		Control	34		34	
Coombes[125]	1990	FAM	133	5 yr	45.7	0.21
		Control	148		35.4	
Krook[123]	1991	5-FU/Adria	61	5 yr	32	0.88
		Control	64		33	
Grau[138]	1993	Mito	68	5 yr	41	<0.03
		Control	66		26	
Hallissey[129]	1994	5-FU/Adria/Mito	138	5 yr	19	0.69
		Control	145		20	
MacDonald[126]	1995	5-FU/Adria/Mito	93	5 yr	37	0.59
		Control	100		32	
Lise[127]	1995	5-FU/Adria/Mito	159	Med surv	42 mo	<0.30
		Control	155		36 mo	
Tsavaris[130]	1996	5-FU/Epirubicin/Mito	42	Med surv	42 mo	<0.25
		Control	42		39 mo	
Cirera[141]	1999	Mito/tegafur	76	5 yr	56	0.04
		Control	72		36	
Neri[140]	2001	5-FU/Epirubicin/LV	69	5 yr	30	<0.01
		Control	68		13	
Bajetta[142]	2002	EAP, 5-FU/LV	137	5 yr	52	0.87
		Control	137		48	

Adria, Adriamycin; araC, cytarabine; 5-FU, 5-fluorouracil; FUDR, 5-fluorodeoxyuridine; Lev, levamisole; MeCCNU, methyl-CCNU (lomustine); Med surv, median survival; Mito, mitomycin C; mo, months; NS, not significant; VNB, vinblastine; yr, year.

over 400 patients.[134] A large number of patients (80%) in this study, however, had residual disease following surgery. In the subset of patients who underwent complete resection, no benefit was derived from treatment with either chemotherapy regimen. Jakesz and colleagues tested the value of a combination regimen found effective in Japanese studies for advanced disease consisting of 5-FU, ara-C, and mitomycin C with or without the immunostimulant OK-432.[135] The 5-year survival rate was 45% for the treated patients and 29% for control subjects. This difference, however, was not statistically significant and the results are difficult to interpret given the small numbers available for analysis.

Of note, two other groups of investigators in Western countries have shown positive results for adjuvant systemic treatment, although the numbers of patients in these studies are small. A study from Spain involving 70 patients suggested a significant survival benefit for single-agent mitomycin at 5 and 10 years.[136,137] This trial has been extended to 134 patients with a median follow-up of 8.75 years and still shows a survival advantage for postoperative mitomycin ($P = 0.025$).[138] Interestingly, a recent adjuvant trial from Spain comparing mitomycin C and tegafur plus uracil showed no benefit for the treated patients versus surgical control subjects.[139] Neri and colleagues treated surgically resected node-positive patients with the addition of adjuvant epirubicin, 5-FU, and leucovorin (68 patients) and compared them to 69 surgery-alone control patients.[140] They noted a significant improvement in 5-year survival rate from 13% for the surgical control group to 30% for patients receiving adjuvant systemic treatment ($P < 0.01$).

From the preceding review it appears clear a vast majority of adjuvant systemic treatment trials in Western countries have failed to improve survival. Several problems in these adjuvant studies include small patient numbers, especially in the few positive studies, failure to control for prognostic factors, and the use of marginally effective chemotherapeutic regimens.

Asian Trials

Stomach cancer is a common disease in Japan, and a number of adjuvant studies have been performed using postoperative chemotherapy and chemoimmunotherapy following surgical resection. It should be noted, however, that most Japanese trials include patients with stages I to IV disease (Japanese Research Society for Gastric Cancer). Adjuvant trials in the United States would exclude patients with early (stage I) and advanced cancers (stage IV). Some Japanese studies either do not include surgical control subjects or are not prospectively randomized.[143,144] In addition, not all reports are available in the English language. The randomized trials that are published in English and include surgically treated control subjects are summarized in Table 78-9.

Imanaga and Nakazato[145] reviewed the early Japanese cooperative group experience with adjuvant systemic treatment in four studies involving over 2500 patients. Treatment included mitomycin C either alone or combined with other agents utilizing different routes and schedules. In their first study, mitomycin C was given intravenously twice a week for 5 weeks, with the first dose given on the day of surgery. Survival favored treated patients at 5 years (68% versus 54%). Subset analysis of this study showed particular benefit for treatment in stage II patients. In their second study, mitomycin C was given in higher doses on the day of surgery and the following day only. No survival advantage for the treated group was seen in this trial. The third study involved two treatment regimens in addition to a surgical control group. One group of patients received intraoperative mitomycin C into the hepatic artery, splenic artery, and peritoneal cavity followed by long-term oral cyclophosphamide. The second group received the intraoperative mitomycin C alone, and the third group surgery alone. No survival benefit was detected for either of the treated groups. The fourth trial also included three arms. One arm used mitomycin C twice a week. The second arm used twice-weekly mitomycin C, 5-FU, and cytosine arabinoside (MFC) for 5 weeks, and the third arm received surgery only. No advantage was seen for any of the treatments, but the study had only a short (3 years) period of follow-up at the time of publication.

Nakajima and colleagues have performed a series of four adjuvant studies for resected gastric cancer.[146] In their first study, mitomycin C was given on a twice-a-week

TABLE 78-9

Adjuvant Therapy of Gastric Cancer: Asian Studies

AUTHOR (REF)	YEAR	REGIMEN	PATIENTS	SURVIVAL		P VALUE
				INTERVAL	PERCENT	
Imanaga[145]	1977	Mito (5 weeks)	242	5 yr	68	Pos
		Control	283		54	
		Mito (2 days)	265	5 yr	60	Neg
		Mito IA/CTX	146		71/29	Neg
		Control	255		60	
		Mito IA	135	5 yr	68/36	Neg
		Control	152		73/41	
		Mito	197	3 yr	74	Neg
		Mito/5-FU/araC	208		69	Neg
		Control	217		69	
Nakajima[146]	1978	Mito	207	5 yr	52.2	Neg
		Control	223		43.5	
Nakajima[147]	1980	Mito	42	5 yr	64.3	Pos
		Mito/5-FU/araC	40		66.9	
		Control	38		50.0	
Ochiai[151]	1983	Mito/5-FU/araC	49	5 yr	NR	Pos
		Control	49			
Nakajima[148]	1984	Mito/5-FU/araC	73	5 yr	72.1	0.09
		Mito/5-FU/ftorafur/araC	76		65.5	
		Control	74		53.1	
Chou[150]	1994	Ftorafur	59	5 yr	53	<0.05
		Control	56		39	
Nakajima[149]	1999	Mito/5-FU/UFT	285	5 yr	86	0.17
		Control	288		83	

araC, cytarabine; CTX, cyclophosphamide; 5-FU, 5-fluorouracil; IA, intra-arterial; Mito, mitomycin C; NR, not recorded.

schedule for 5 weeks, but no survival benefit was seen for the whole cohort of patients. However, as in a similar study by Imanaga and Nakazato, a striking benefit was seen in the treatment of patients with involved serosa or advanced lymph node metastasis.[145] Nakajima and colleagues subsequently performed a three-arm adjuvant study in which patients were randomized to surgery alone, mitomycin C alone, or the combination of MFC.[147] Forty-two patients were entered in each arm of the study. At 5 years a survival benefit for MFC-treated patients was seen when compared with surgical control subjects. No significant benefit was seen for the mitomycin C arm. These same investigators studied the regimen of MFC followed by either long-term oral 5-FU or ftorafur compared with surgical subjects.[148] A significant survival benefit was seen for patients with stages I to III disease treated with MFC and oral 5-FU. In a fourth study, Nakajima and colleagues assessed the role of adjuvant mitomycin C and 5-FU followed by oral uracil and tegafur in patients undergoing complete resection for early stage gastric cancer.[149] When compared to a control group, adjuvant therapy for this group of patients showed no benefit over surgery alone.

Chou and coworkers performed a randomized trial of the oral 5-FU analog ftorafur compared to placebo. This demonstrated a significant 5-year survival for patients with stage III gastric cancer receiving ftorafur.[150]

Finally, Ochiai and colleagues conducted a trial that randomized patients to surgery alone, MFC chemotherapy, and MFC plus bacille Calmette-Guérin (BCG) cell wall skeleton. A benefit survival was demonstrated for the patients treated with chemoimmunotherapy.[151]

The foregoing data form the basis for the routine use of postoperative systemic therapy following the resection of gastric cancer in Japan. Currently, a common adjuvant regimen includes intravenous mitomycin C, 5-FU, and ara-C followed by the prolonged use of tegafur. Most current studies are examining issues of adding new drugs, intensifying the mitomycin dose, and the additive use of immunostimulants in addition to chemotherapy.[152-155]

Summary—Adjuvant Systemic Chemotherapy

The reason for the differences in outcomes between studies performed in Japan and those performed in Western countries is not clear. Nakajima has pointed out some of the features of Japanese trials that may contribute to positive trials with postoperative chemotherapy.[156] These include the initiation of systemic therapy in the immediate postoperative period, less postoperative tumor burden, and the use of mitomycin C. Some of the shortcomings of the studies include high exclusion rates, the frequent use of subset analysis, and the lack of surgical control subjects. It is noteworthy that only two small Western surgical adjuvant studies have ever shown a positive result using a mitomycin C regimen.[132,137] Others have speculated that the differences may be attributable to biologic differences in the cancers, different staging systems, or differences in adjuvant therapies used. In a detailed review of these issues Davis and Sano concluded that there are several plausible explanations including the rapid rise of gastroesophageal tumors in Western

countries, more aggressive surgery in Japan leading to stage migration, and heterogeneity of trials.[157] It is clear that further collaborative studies are needed.

Meta-Analysis of Adjuvant Trials

Many of the trials conducted to date have been underpowered to adequately assess any potential differences between the control and treatment arms in regard to overall survival. As such, several meta-analyses have been performed to better assess the use of adjuvant chemotherapy.

Since 1990 at least six meta-analyses have been published.[158-164] The two most recent meta-analyses both showed a significant survival advantage to the use of chemotherapy following surgical resection of gastric cancer. Seventeen randomized clinical trials were included in the meta-analysis conducted by Panzini and coworkers and involved 3118 patients.[158] The pooled odds ratio was 0.72 (95% CI, 0.62 to 0.84). The meta-analysis conducted by Janunger and associates included a slightly larger and somewhat different group of studies.[159] Altogether, 21 randomized clinical trials, involving 3962 patients, were included in the analysis. The pooled odds ratio from this study was 0.84 (95% CI, 0.74 to 0.96). In a subanalysis, Western and Asian studies were assessed separately. The meta-analysis of the Western studies did not show a benefit to adjuvant therapy with a pooled odds ratio of 0.96 (95% CI, 0.83 to 1.12), but the Asian studies did show evidence of benefit with an odds ratio of 0.58 (95% CI, 0.44 to 0.76). The conclusions of both meta-analyses urged caution in interpreting the apparent positive results. Many of the individual trials had small numbers of patients enrolled, used chemotherapy regimens of limited efficacy, and had an inadequate trial design.

Intraperitoneal Therapy

Some investigators have studied the use of postoperative *intraperitoneal chemotherapy* based on the pharmacokinetic advantage of intraperitoneal chemotherapy and the finding that many patients relapse in the peritoneum after surgical resection. A variety of phase II and III trials have been performed. Atiq and associates performed a phase II trial of adjuvant cisplatin and 5-FU combined with systemic 5-FU in 35 patients.[165] The peritoneal relapse rates in this trial appeared lower than other trials that have reported such results. This trial and other published phase II trials suggest that intraperitoneal therapy is tolerable.

Several phase III studies have evaluated the role of intraoperative or postoperative intraperitoneal therapy in patients undergoing potentially curative surgery. In an early study by Dixon and colleagues patients were randomized to surgery alone or to surgery followed by intraperitoneal thiotepa.[115] No significant difference in survival was seen between the two groups.

In a more recent study Sautner and coworkers examined the use of postoperative intraperitoneal cisplatin compared with surgery alone in a group of 67 patients.[166] Although the primary lesion was resected in each case, 21% of the patients had localized peritoneal carcinomatosis. No survival benefit was seen for the treated patients.

In a study from Japan 113 patients were randomized between surgery alone or intraoperative mitomycin C at the time of surgery.[167] For patients who underwent curative surgery intraperitoneal therapy led to a significant improvement in 2- and 3-year overall survival. No difference in survival was seen for patients with macroscopic peritoneal carcinomatosis.

In a single institution study from Korea 248 patients with clincial stage II or III gastric cancer were randomized to surgery alone or to receive intraperitoneal mitomycin C on day 1 and intraperitoneal 5-FU on days 2 to 5.[168] The final pathologic results showed that 103 of the 248 patients had either stage I or stage IV disease. When 5-year survival was calculated for the entire group no benefit to adjuvant therapy was seen ($P = 0.219$). In a subset analysis there did appear to be a survival benefit for patients with stage III disease.

The use of intraperitoneal therapy in the adjuvant setting remains investigational and requires further evaluation. Until further studies show clear benefit to this approach, the use of intraperitoneal therapy should be restricted to controlled clinical trials.

Adjuvant Irradiation

Postoperative Irradiation

Irradiation has only been minimally evaluated as the sole adjuvant treatment following complete surgical resection in randomized phase III trials (Table 78-10). Adjuvant external beam irradiation (EBRT) reduced locoregional failures when compared with the surgery-alone control arm in a British adjuvant trial, but no survival benefits were found.[128] Although phase III trials from Japan[168,169] and China[170] suggest some survival benefit for IORT versus a surgery-alone control arm, the advantage was found only in subset analyses. At the National Cancer Institute (NCI), Sindelar and associates[171] performed a small randomized trial of IORT versus external irradiation following complete surgical resection; this trial demonstrated improved local control with IORT but no survival benefit.[171] A surgery-alone control arm did not exist in the NCI trial. Phase II studies combining EBRT and IORT have been conducted in Pamplona (Spain), and the United States (by the Radiation Therapy Oncology Group [RTOG]) and are still under way in Lyon (France).

BSCG completed a prospectively randomized trial of surgery only versus postoperative FAM or irradiation (45 Gy in 25 fractions ± 5-Gy boost).[128] A total of 436 patients were randomized and followed for a minimum of 12 months; arms were well balanced with regard to prognostic factors. No patient survival differences by treatment arm were seen (median, 15 months). However, locoregional failure was documented in only 15 of 153 (10%) in the irradiation arm versus 39 of 145 (27%) in the surgery-alone arm, and 26 of 138 (19%) in the FAM group. Interpretation of the results is complicated by the inclusion of 93 patients (21%) with resection but gross residual disease (BSCG stage IVAi) and 78 (18%) with gross

total resection but microscopically positive resection margins. Neither group of patients would be candidates for current gastric surgical adjuvant trials in the United States. In addition, nearly one third of patients randomized to receive adjuvant treatment did not receive the assigned therapy. Of 153 patients randomized to the irradiation arm, only 104 (68%) received a dose of 40.5 Gy or more, and 36 (24%) received none. Only 62% of patients received six or more cycles of chemotherapy. The results in this study are similar to results seen in the adjuvant treatment of rectal cancer, in which adjuvant pre- and postoperative irradiation as a single adjuvant modality improve local control but do not increase patient survival in most trials, unless combined with chemotherapy.

Takahashi and Abe[169] reported results from a large Japanese trial in which 211 patients were randomized on the basis of day of hospital admission to receive either surgery only or surgery plus IORT (28 to 35 Gy). Five-year survival rates for Japanese stages II to IV were improved approximately 15% to 25% in the IORT group versus those treated with surgery alone (stage II, 84% versus 62%; stage III, 62% versus 37%; stage IV, 15% versus 0%). This magnitude of survival improvement correlates nicely with the approximately 20% of patients who fail only locoregionally after complete surgical resection. Although the data are intriguing, this method of randomization is susceptible to bias in treatment selection, and the trial failed to stratify for important prognostic factors.

In an analysis from Bejing, patients with stage III (serosal involvement or node-positive tumors) or stage IV (unresectable metastasis or adjacent organ involvement) disease were randomized to surgery alone or IORT (single dose, 25 to 40 Gy).[170] In their most recent report of 200 patients, a survival advantage with IORT was demonstrated for only stage III patients (65% versus 30% 5-year survival; 52% versus 22% 8-year survival; $P < 0.01$).

Preoperative Irradiation

Randomized trials testing preoperative irradiation have been performed in both Russia and China. All have reported a positive survival benefit when compared with surgery-alone control arms.

Three prospective randomized Russian trials have evaluated preoperative irradiation in potentially resectable gastric cancer.[172,174] The first trial randomly assigned 293 patients to receive either surgery alone, surgery after preoperative EBRT (20 Gy in four fractions), or surgery after the same EBRT plus daily hyperthermia. The survival rates at 3 and 5 years were improved in both irradiation arms compared with surgery alone, and the improvement with combined EBRT and hyperthermia was statistically significant at both 3 and 5 years.[172] The second trial compared preoperative EBRT (20 Gy) versus surgery alone in 279 patients. Three- and 5-year survival rates were increased, and no increase in operative morbidity was observed.[173] The third trial compared surgery alone versus preoperative EBRT (32 Gy with concomitant inhalation of 8% oxygen) plus surgery. A survival advantage was observed with preoperative treatment, and the resection rate was increased by 17%.[174] There are some methodologic uncertainties with all three of these

TABLE 78-10

Surgery ± Adjuvant Therapy for Resected Gastric or Esophagogastric Junction Cancer

TREATMENT	PATIENT NO.	SURVIVAL MEDIAN (MO)	SURVIVAL LONG-TERM* (%)	P VALUE	LOCAL-REGIONAL RELAPSE NO.	LOCAL-REGIONAL RELAPSE PERCENT	P VALUE	REF. NO.
Phase III Trials								
1. British Stomach Group (3 yr)		15						128,129
a. Surgery alone	145	—	20	—	39	27	—	—
b. Postop chemo	138	—	19	—	26	19	—	—
c. Postop EBRT	153	—	12	—	15	10	—	—
2. Japan – Surgery ± IOERT[†]	S IOERT 110 101		S IOERT					169
a. Stage I	43 24	—	93 vs 87%	—	—	—	—	—
b. Stage II	11 20	—	62 vs 84%	—	—	—	—	—
c. Stage III	38 30	—	37 vs 62%	—	—	—	—	—
d. Stage IV	18 27	—	0 vs 15%	—	—	—	—	—
3. China – Surgery ± IOERT[†]	100 100							170
a. Stage III (5 yr)	— —	—	30 vs 65%	<0.01	—	—	—	—
b. Stage III (8 yr)	— —	—	22 vs 52%	—	—	—	—	—
4. Mayo Clinic[‡]								180
a. Surgery alone	23	15	4	—	—	54	—	—
b. Postop EBRT + 5-FU	39	24	23	0.05	—	39	—	—
5. China-Beijing								175
a. Surgery alone	199	—	20	—	—	52		
b. Preop EBRT	171	—	30	0.009	—	39	<0.025	
6. U.S GI Intergroup (INT 0116)			(3-yr)			RFS (3-yr)		
a. Surgery alone	275	27	41			31		184,185
b. Postop EBRT + 5-FU leucovorin	281	36	50	0.005		48	0.001	
Phase II Trials								
1. MGH (gastric)								
a. Surgery alone	110	—	38 (B2, B3) 15 (C1–3)	—	46	42	—	105
b. Postop EBRT + chemo	14	24	43 (4 yr)	—	2	14	—	176
2. TJUH (gastric)								178
a. Total group T3, T4, or N+	120							
• Surgery alone	70	12	13		17/38	45	—	—
• Postop chemo, EBRT, both	50	19	17	<0.05	13/36	36	—	—
• Postop EBRT + chemo	20 of 50	19	21		3/16	19	—	—
b. T3/T4, N1/N2 (surg ± adjuv)	44, 30	9 vs 13	4 vs 22	0.04	—	—	—	—
3. U Penn (gastric or EG)[§]								179
a. Surgery alone	40	16	31 (2 yr)	—	31	75	—	
b. Postop EBRT	17	15	50 (2 yr)	—	4	24	—	
c. Postop EBRT + chemo	27	21	55 (2 yr)	—	4	15	—	
4. TJUH (EG junction)[∥]	S EBRT		S EBRT					182
Surgery ± EBRT + chemo	37 18	12 vs 20		—		74 vs 36	0.0014	—
a. T3, T4	— —	—	11 14	—		87 vs 47	0.0016	—
b. LN (–)	— —	—	42 100	—	—	—	—	—
c. LN (+)	— —	—	0 15	0.001		97 vs 14	0.0001	—
5. Mayo Clinic (gastric, EG) Postop EBRT ± chemo T3, T4 or N+	25	19	31 (4 yr)	—	5	20	—	181

Chemo, chemotherapy; EBRT, external beam irradiation; EG, esophagogastric; 5-FU, 5-fluorouracil; IOERT, intraoperative electron irradiation; LN, lymph nodes; MG-H Massachusetts General Hospital; postop; postoperative; preop, preoperative; RFS, relapse-free survival; S, surgery; TJUH, Thomas Jefferson University Hospital; U Penn, University of Pennsylvania.
*Long-term survival = 5-year data unless otherwise specified.
[†]Advantage to IOERT in subset analyses—Japan stages II–IV, China stage III (37% of patients).
[‡]Survival data based on intent to treat, relapse data on actual treatment.
[§]Long-term data = 2-year survival, negative margins.
[∥]Mehta, Mohuidden: ASTRO abstract. Int J Radiat Oncol Biol Phys 1994;30:272.

trials, and their applicability to Western gastric carcinoma is not clear.

A double-blind randomized trial from Bejing, conducted from 1978 to 1989, compared a surgery-alone control arm ($N = 199$) with preoperative EBRT plus surgery ($N = 171$) for patients with adenocarcinoma of the gastric cardia.[175] Irradiation was given with 8-MV photons or cobalt with anteroposterior-posteroanterior (AP-PA) fields to a dose of 40 Gy in 20 fractions of 2 Gy over 4 weeks. Surgery was performed 2 to 4 weeks after completion of irradiation. Both downstaging of disease and improvements in radical resection rates were found with the addition of preoperative EBRT (radical resection rates of 80% versus 62% with preoperative EBRT versus surgery alone).

Survival and locoregional disease control were improved in the patients assigned to preoperative EBRT versus surgery alone (see Table 78-10). The 5- and 10-year survival rates were 30% versus 20% and 20% versus 13%, respectively (*P* = 0.009 Kaplan-Meier log rank). The divergence in survival curves began in the first year of follow-up and persisted through 9 years. Local and regional disease control were also improved with combined-modality treatment with local relapse rates of 39% versus 52% (*P* < 0.025) and regional node relapse rates of 39% versus 54% (*P* < 0.05). The rate of distant metastases were the same at 24% versus 25%. The improvements in survival and disease control (locoregional) were accomplished with no increase in treatment-related morbidity or mortality rates (operative mortality 0.6% versus 2.5% with or without preoperative EBRT; intrathoracic leak rates were 1.8% and 4.2%, respectively).

In view of the survival advantage with or without disease control and radical resection rates demonstrated for preoperative EBRT in four published trials from Russia and China, such approaches need to be evaluated further in U.S. and European study groups. As suggested by the authors from the Bejing trial, factors to be evaluated include radiation dose escalation to 45 to 50 Gy (1.8- to 2.0-Gy fractions) and the addition of chemotherapy (maintenance, concomitant with EBRT).

Adjuvant Irradiation Plus Chemotherapy

Postoperative EBRT Plus Chemotherapy[176–185]

Phase II single-institution gastric cancer trials that show promise for combination postoperative adjuvant therapy have been reported from Massachusetts General Hospital (MGH),[176] Israel (Hadassah),[177] Thomas Jefferson University Hospital,[178] and the University of Pennsylvania.[179] Gunderson and associates,[176] from the MGH, reported a median survival time of 24 months and 4-year survival rate of 43% in 14 patients who had complete resection of tumors with extension beyond the wall, nodal involvement, or both. Patients received postoperative irradiation (45 to 52 Gy, 1.8 Gy/day) plus concomitant 5-FU-based chemotherapy. Subsequent locoregional relapse was documented in only 2 of the 14 (14%) in contrast to a 42% incidence in similar high-risk patients treated with surgery alone at MGH.[105] Median survival time and 4-year survival rate in the adjuvant chemoirradiation patients were 24 months and 43%. Investigators from Hadassah University reported on 25 patients with gross tumor resection, but at high risk for relapse, who were treated with irradiation (50 Gy over 7 weeks, 2 to 2.5 Gy per fraction with a 2-week split) and 5-FU on days 1 to 3 of each irradiation cycle plus 1 year of maintenance 5-FU.[177] High-risk factors included positive margins of resection in 7 of the 25 patients (28%) and positive nodes in 22 (88%). Median survival time was 33 months, and the 5-year actuarial survival rate was 40% (of the 13 survivors, 12 were disease-free). Local failure was documented in only 2 patients (8%). In the series from Thomas Jefferson University Hospital (TJUH), 120 patients had surgical resection but were at high risk for relapse because of

extension beyond the gastric wall, nodal metastases, or positive margins of resection.[178] Seventy patients had surgery alone and 50 received adjuvant therapy. Apparent improvements in local control as well as median and 5-year survival were noted with additional therapy. In those patients with negative resection margins, 2-year local control with surgery alone was 55% versus 93% with adjuvant irradiation with or without chemotherapy (*P* = 0.03). For patients with T3–4 tumors and lymph node involvement, median survival was 9 months versus 13 months (surgery alone or plus adjuvant treatment), and 5-year survival rate was 4% versus 22% (*P* = 0.03). In a University of Pennsylvania analysis, the incidence of local failure with surgery alone was 75% (31 of 40) versus 24% with adjuvant irradiation (4 of 17) and 15% with adjuvant irradiation plus chemotherapy (4 of 27).[179]

A prospective randomized trial conducted at the Mayo Clinic included 62 patients with poor-prognosis completely resected gastric cancers who were randomized to either surgery alone or surgery followed by irradiation (37.5 Gy in 24 fractions over 4 to 5 weeks) plus concomitant 5-FU (15 mg/kg, d 1-3 by IV bolus).[180] A non-stratified, prerandomization scheme was used with a 2:3 ratio favoring treatment. Informed consent was requested only of the 39 patients randomized to treatment. Ten of the 39 refused further therapy and were observed. When analyzed by intent to treat, the adjuvant arm had statistically significant improvement in both relapse-free and overall survival (overall 5-year survival 23% versus 4%; *P* < 0.05) (Tables 78-10 and 78-11). When patient outcome was compared by actual treatment received (29 adjuvant treatment, 33 surgery alone), 5-year survival rate still favored the adjuvant group (20% versus 12%), but the differences were not statistically significant in view of small patient numbers. As seen in Table 78-11 the 10 patients who refused assignment to adjuvant treatment had more favorable prognostic findings than the other two groups of patients. When the two groups with equally poor prognostic factors were compared, the 5-year overall survival rate was 20% versus 4%, with an advantage to those receiving adjuvant treatment (the survival data with adjuvant chemoradiotherapy parallel the high-risk TJUH gastric data with adjuvant chemoradiotherapy discussed in the prior paragraph and the GITSG adjuvant pancreas phase III trial that resulted in 19% versus 5% 5-year survival rate for adjuvant irradiation plus 5-FU versus surgery alone; *P* < 0.05).[183] When analyzed by treatment delivered, locoregional relapse was decreased with adjuvant treatment (54% incidence with surgery alone versus 39% with irradiation plus 5-FU).

In a recent retrospective Mayo Clinic analysis, 63 patients received postoperative EBRT plus or minus 5-FU[181] after resection of carcinoma of the stomach or gastroesophageal junction. Twenty-five of the 63 patients had complete resection with no residual disease but had high-risk factors for disease relapse (extension beyond gastric wall, 92% of patients; involved nodes, 92%; both high-risk factors, 84%). Concomitant 5-FU plus or minus leucovorin was given with EBRT in 84% of the 25 adjuvantly treated patients, but maintenance chemotherapy was given in only 20%. Locoregional control was

TABLE 78-11

	Randomized Gastric Adjuvant Trial at the Mayo Clinic (Surgery ± Irradiation + 5-FU)		
	ADJUVANT EBRT + 5-FU (%) (N = 29)	**SURGERY CONTROL (%) (N = 23)**	**REFUSED ADJUVANT (%) (N = 10)**
Pathologic Characteristics			
Cardia	55	56	30
Ulcerative	72	70	50
Grade 2	7	9	30
Grades 3, 4	93	91	70
	ADJUVANT EBRT + 5-FU (%)	**SURGERY ALONE (%)**	
Five-Year Survival			
Treatment intent (total patients)	(39)	(23)	
Overall	23	4 ($P <0.05$)	
Treatment delivered (total patients)	(29)	(33)	
Overall	20	12	
Disease-free	17	9	
Local Failure			
Treatment delivered	39	54	

EBRT, external-beam irradiation; 5-FU, 5-fluorouracil.
Modified from Moertel CG, Child DS Jr, O'Fallon JR, et al: Combined 5-fluorouracil and radiation therapy as a surgical adjuvant for poor prognosis gastric carcinoma. J Clin Oncol 1984;2:1249.

achieved in 20 of the 25 (80%) with median survival of 19 months. Four-year survival was 31% in spite of the very poor prognostic factors in these 25 patients.

Because of conflicting results in earlier small phase III studies, a confirmatory U.S. Gastrointestinal (GI) Intergroup trial (INT 0116) was initiated to evaluate postoperative combined 5-FU based chemotherapy and irradiation to the gastric bed and regional nodes versus surgery only in resected but high-risk gastric cancer patients.[184] Eligibility included patients with stages IB, II, IIIA, IIIB, and IV nonmetastatic adenocarcinoma of the stomach or gastroesophageal junction. After an en bloc resection, 556 patients were randomized to either surgery alone or postoperative combined modality therapy consisting of 45 Gy in 25 fractions plus concurrent 5-FU and leucovorin (4-day cycle on week 1, 3-day cycle on week 5) followed by two monthly 5-day cycles of 5-FU and leucovorin. Nodal metastases were present in 85% of patients. With median follow up period of 5-years, relapse-free survival at 3 years is 48% for adjuvant treatment and 31% for observation ($P = 0.001$); 3-year overall survival rate is 50% for treatment and 41% for observation ($P = 0.005$). The median overall survival in the surgery-only group was 27 months, as compared with 36 months in the chemoradiotherapy group. The median duration of relapse-free survival was 30 months in the chemoradiotherapy group and 19 months in the surgery-only group. Patterns of relapse were based on the site of first relapse only and were categorized as local, regional, or distant. Local recurrence occurred in 29% of the patients who relapsed in the surgery-only group and 19% of those who relapsed in the chemoradiotherapy patients. Regional relapse—typically abdominal carcinomatosis—was reported in 72% of those who relapsed in the surgery-only group and 65% of those who relapsed in the chemoradiotherapy patients. Extra-abdominal distant metastases was diagnosed in 18% of those who relapsed in the surgery-only patients and 33% of those who relapsed in the chemoradiotherapy patients. Treatment was tolerable, with 3 (1%) toxic deaths. Grade 3 and 4 toxicity occurred in 41% and 32% of cases, respectively.

The results of the large randomized phase III U.S. GI Intergroup trial (INT 0116) demonstrate a clear survival advantage to the use of postoperative chemoradiotherapy in resected high-risk patients.[184] Furthermore, the results strongly support the integration of postoperative chemoradiotherapy into the routine care of patients with curatively resected high-risk carcinoma of the stomach and gastroesophageal junction.

Quality control (QC) of irradiation field design in INT 0116 was conducted during the cycle of chemotherapy given prior to the start of concurrent chemoradiotherapy.[185] The upfront QC provided the mechanism to correct most of the major or minor deviations (35% incidence) in irradiation field design prior to the start of treatment, and resulted in only a 6.5% final major deviation rate. Utilization of upfront QC may have been a key factor in achieving a positive survival advantage for adjuvant chemoradiotherapy.

Preoperative EBRT Plus Chemotherapy

Randomized trials testing preoperative EBRT plus chemotherapy for gastric cancer alone have not yet been published, but the Walsh and associates trial for adenocarcinoma of the esophagus and gastric cardia certainly has relevance.[186] Patients were randomized to either immediate surgery (control arm) versus preoperative EBRT (40 Gy in 15 fractions), 5-FU (15 mg/kg/day continuous infusion [this is *approximately* equivalent to 600 mg/m^2] for 5 days, weeks 1 and 6), and cisplatin (75 mg/m^2 on the first day of each 5-FU infusion), followed by surgical resection 8 weeks after completion of EBRT plus chemotherapy. A highly significant difference in survival was observed with combined-modality therapy (intent to treat median survival time 16 versus 11 months, 3-year survival rate 32% versus 6%; P = 0.01; actual treatment median survival time, 32 versus 11 months; P = 0.001; 3-year survival rate 37% versus 7%; P = 0.006). A confirmatory intergroup trial was attempted in North America for either esophagus or esophagogastric junction cancers (squamous or adenocarcinoma); this trial was stopped owing to poor accrual.

Summary—Adjuvant Irradiation Alone or Plus Chemotherapy

In summary, although chemotherapy alone has not demonstrated significant benefit as adjuvant therapy for gastric cancer, both preoperative irradiation[175] and postoperative chemoradiotherapy[184,185] have been demonstrated to be superior to surgery alone for resectable gastric and gastroesophageal cancers in randomized phase III trials. Future preoperative irradiation trials should evaluate the addition of concurrent and maintenance chemotherapy. Postoperative chemoradiotherapy trials will evaluate more aggressive chemotherapy both as concurrent and maintenance components of treatment.

Irradiation Techniques

The irradiation field should include unresected or residual tumor or the tumor bed plus major nodal regions. The pattern of tumor bed and nodal failures in the reoperative series from the University of Minnesota is demonstrated in Figure 78-7A in conjunction with an idealized, shaped AP-PA irradiation portal that incorporates the areas of locoregional relapse.[22,187] The tumor bed and nodal volumes are reconstructed with the aid of preoperative and postoperative imaging studies and surgical clip placement. In Figure 78-7B the idealized AP-PA field is superimposed on the organs and structures that define irradiation tolerance.

Dose-limiting organs and structures in the upper abdomen are numerous (stomach, small intestine, liver, kidneys, and spinal cord). With properly shaped fields, doses of 45 to 50.4 Gy in 1.8- to 2.0-Gy fractions can be delivered to stomach and small intestine with a 5% or less

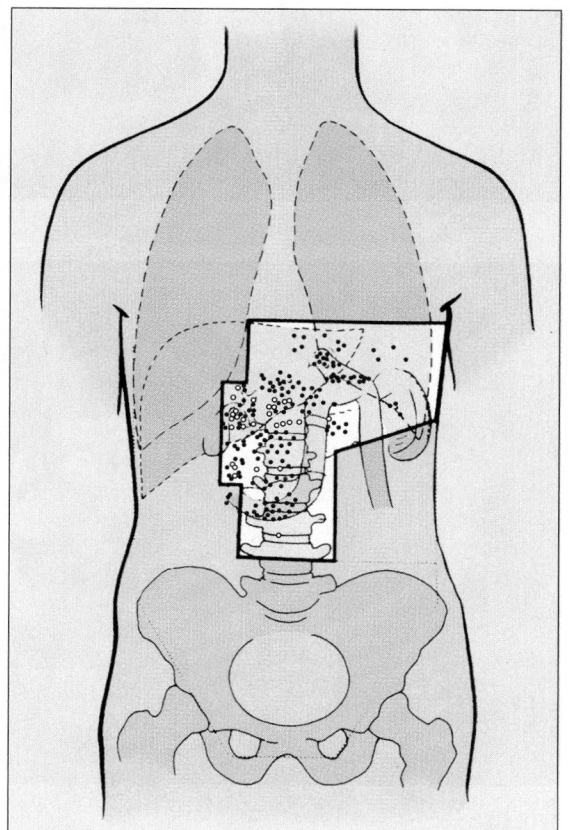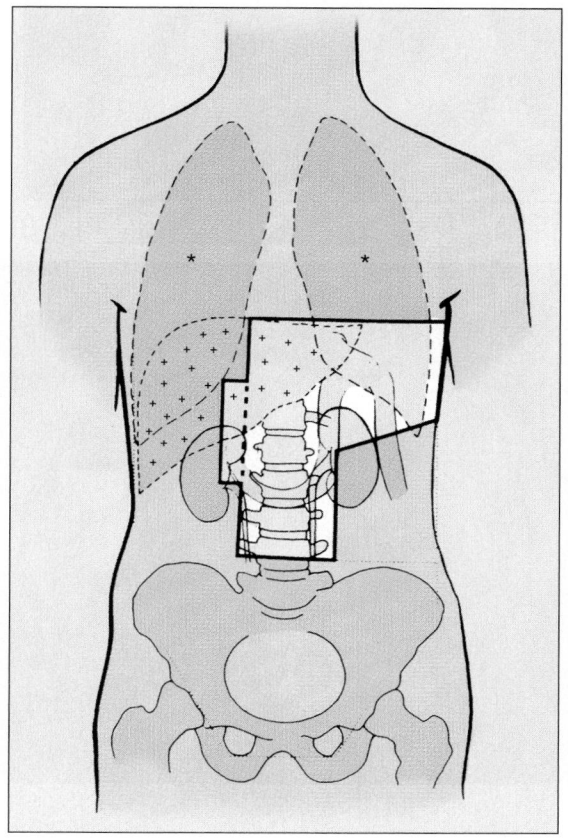

Figure 78-7. Patterns of failure in the University of Minnesota gastric cancer reoperative series with superimposed idealized irradiation fields **(A, B)** and relationship to dose-limiting organs or structures **(B)**. ●, local failures in surrounding organs or tissues; ○, lymph nodes failures; *, lung metastases; +, liver metastases. (From MacDonald JS, Steele G, Gunderson LL: Carcinoma of the stomach. In DeVita V, Hellman S, Rosenberg SA [eds]: Principles and Practices of Oncology, 2nd ed. Philadelphia, JB Lippincott, 1989, p 765.)

risk of severe toxicity.[188] In most patients a portion of both kidneys will be within the AP- PA treatment field, but at least two thirds to three fourths of one kidney should be excluded (can include entirety of both kidneys to the level of 20 Gy if necessary). For patients with proximal gastric cancers (Fig. 78-8), one half to two thirds of the left kidney can often be spared as a result of accurate field definition, which is aided by clip placement in the splenic hilum and porta hepatis. The pancreaticoduodenal nodal regions can be included while sparing 75% to 90% of the right kidney. However, for distal gastric lesions with narrow or positive duodenal resection margins, the duodenal circumference may need to be included as target

volume (Fig. 78-9). In such instances 50% or more of the right kidney is within the field, and two thirds to three fourths of the left kidney should be spared. Chronic renal problems are infrequent when these techniques are utilized.[176,189]

With esophagogastric junction or proximal gastric lesions, a 3- to 5-cm margin of distal esophagus should be within the irradiation field (see Fig. 78-8). If the lesion extends beyond the gastric wall with proximal lesions, a major portion of the left hemidiaphragm should be included. In either instance, Cerrobend blocks should be used to decrease the volume of irradiated heart (Figs. 78-8 through 78-10). Because doxorubicin (Adriamycin) may

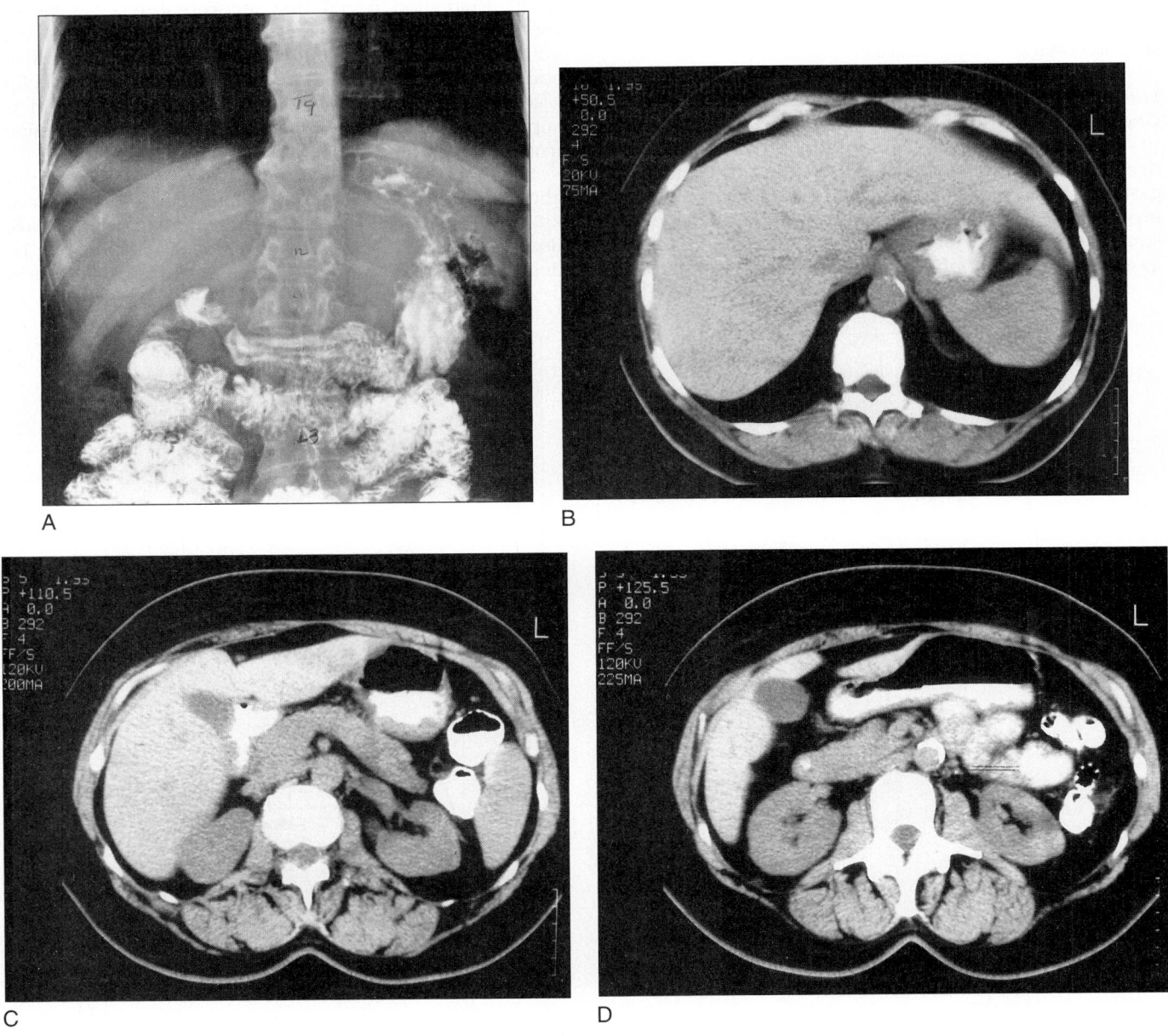

Figure 78-8. Postoperative irradiation fields based on preoperative radiographs following complete resection of a proximal gastric cancer (T3, N2, M0); patient was randomized to the irradiation chemotherapy arm on the intergroup gastric adjuvant study. **A–D**, Reconstruction of tumor bed/target volumes with preoperative upper gastrointestinal radiograph **(A)** and computed tomographic (CT) scans **(B, D)**. CT cuts demonstrated thickened gastric wall proximally **(B, C)** and normal thickness distally **(D)** as well as relationship of the stomach to surrounding organs including liver and spleen **(B)**. Liver, body and tail of pancreas, and splenic flexure **(C)**, and head of pancreas **(D)**.

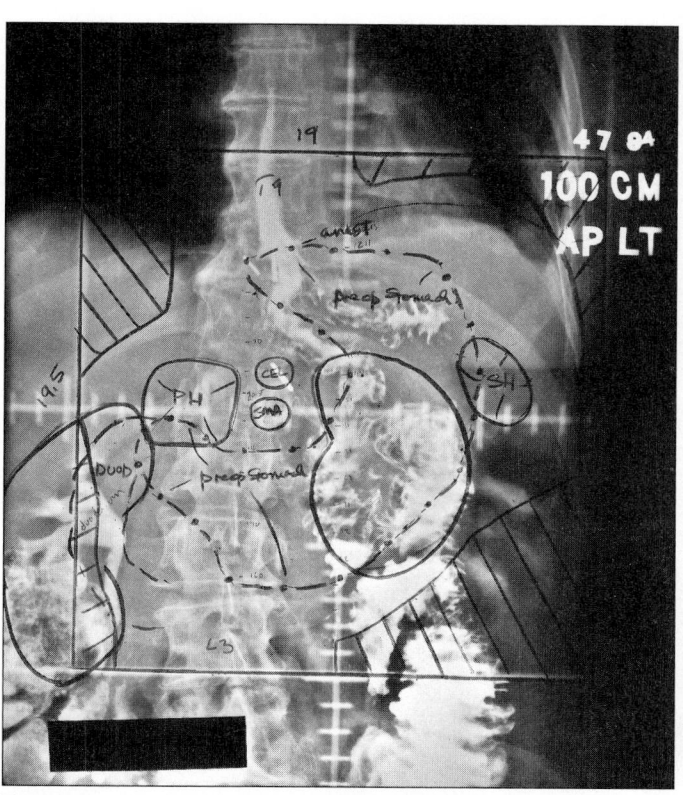

E

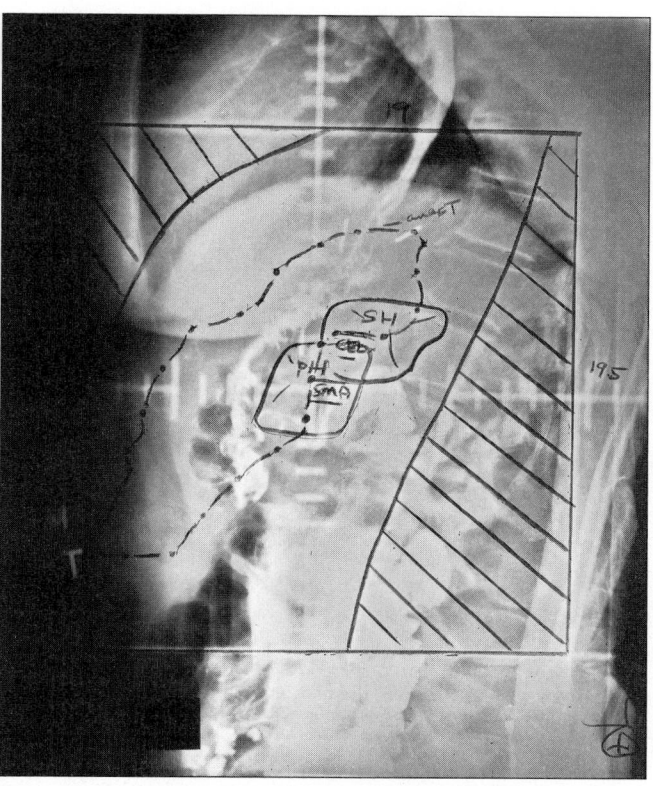

F

Figure 78-8, cont'd. Postoperative irradiation fields based on preoperative radiographs following complete resection of a proximal gastric cancer (T3, N2, M0); patient was randomized to the irradiation chemotherapy arm on the intergroup gastric adjuvant study. **E** and **F,** AP-PA irradiation field **(E)** with cross-hatched blocks encompasses all the left kidney but less than 20% of the right. Nodal groups at risk and preoperative gastric duodenal locations (–•–•) are demonstrated on the AP-PA and lateral **(F)** simulation fields. CEL, celiac; PH, porta hepatis; SH, splenic hilum; SMA, superior mesenteric artery.

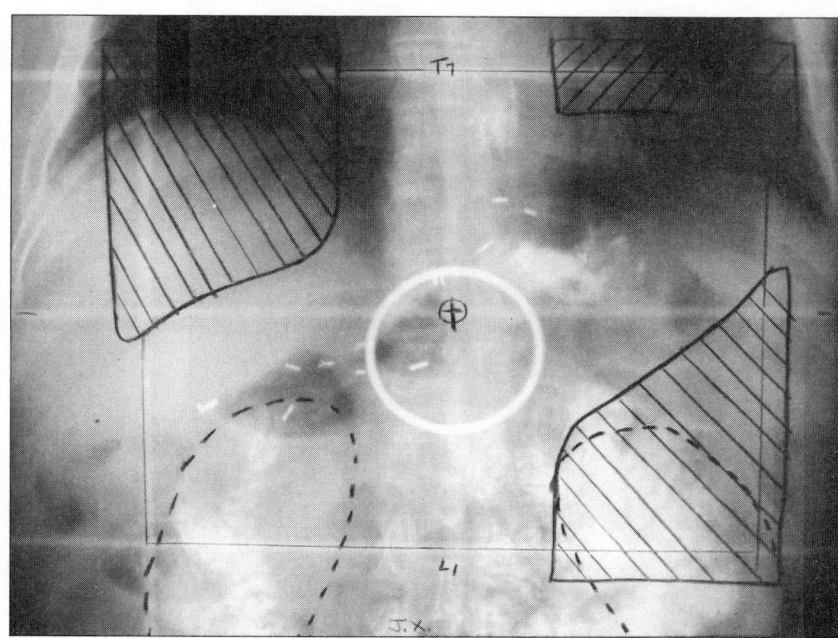

Figure 78-9. AP-PA irradiation fields for unresectable distal gastric cancer encompass around 50% of the right kidney. Because tumor extent was marked with clips at surgical exploration, shaped blocks (*cross-hatched*) could be used to spare the left kidney as well as a moderate amount of liver and some heart.

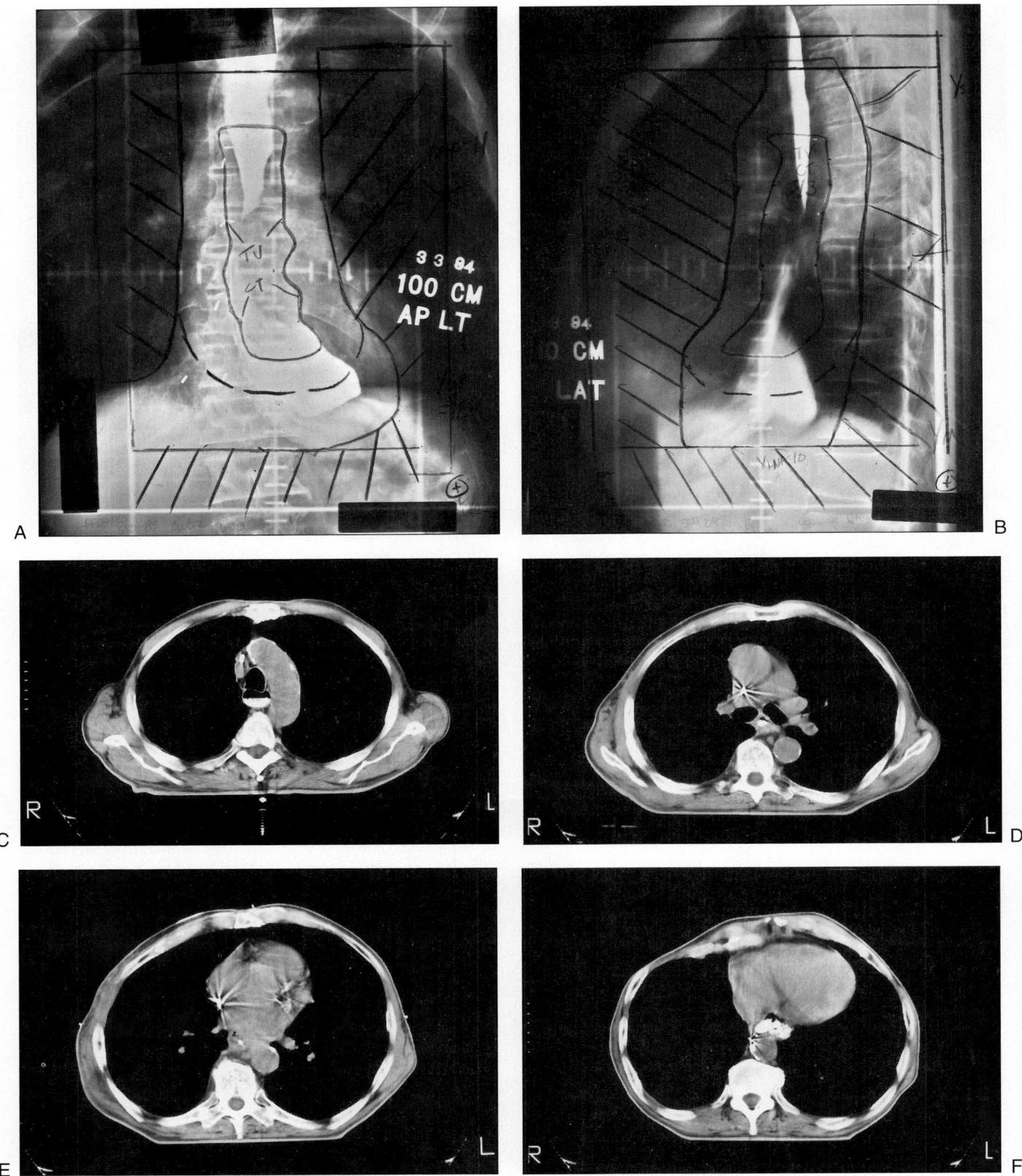

Figure 78-10. Irradiation fields **(A, B)** and computed tomographic (CT) scans **(C–F)** on patient with locally recurrent adenocarcinoma of the gastroesophageal junction found to be unresectable at exploration. The recurrent tumor volume (TV) is defined with a combination of contrast material given at the time of simulation of AP-PA **(A)** and lateral fields **(B)** and a treatment planning CT scan **(C–F)**. Normal wall thickness with intraluminal contrast material and air is seen on cuts taken above **(C)** and below **(F)** the recurrent lesion **(D, E)**; intervening cuts at the level of the carina **(D)** and below **(E)** demonstrate increased thickening of the wall with less contrast medium and air.

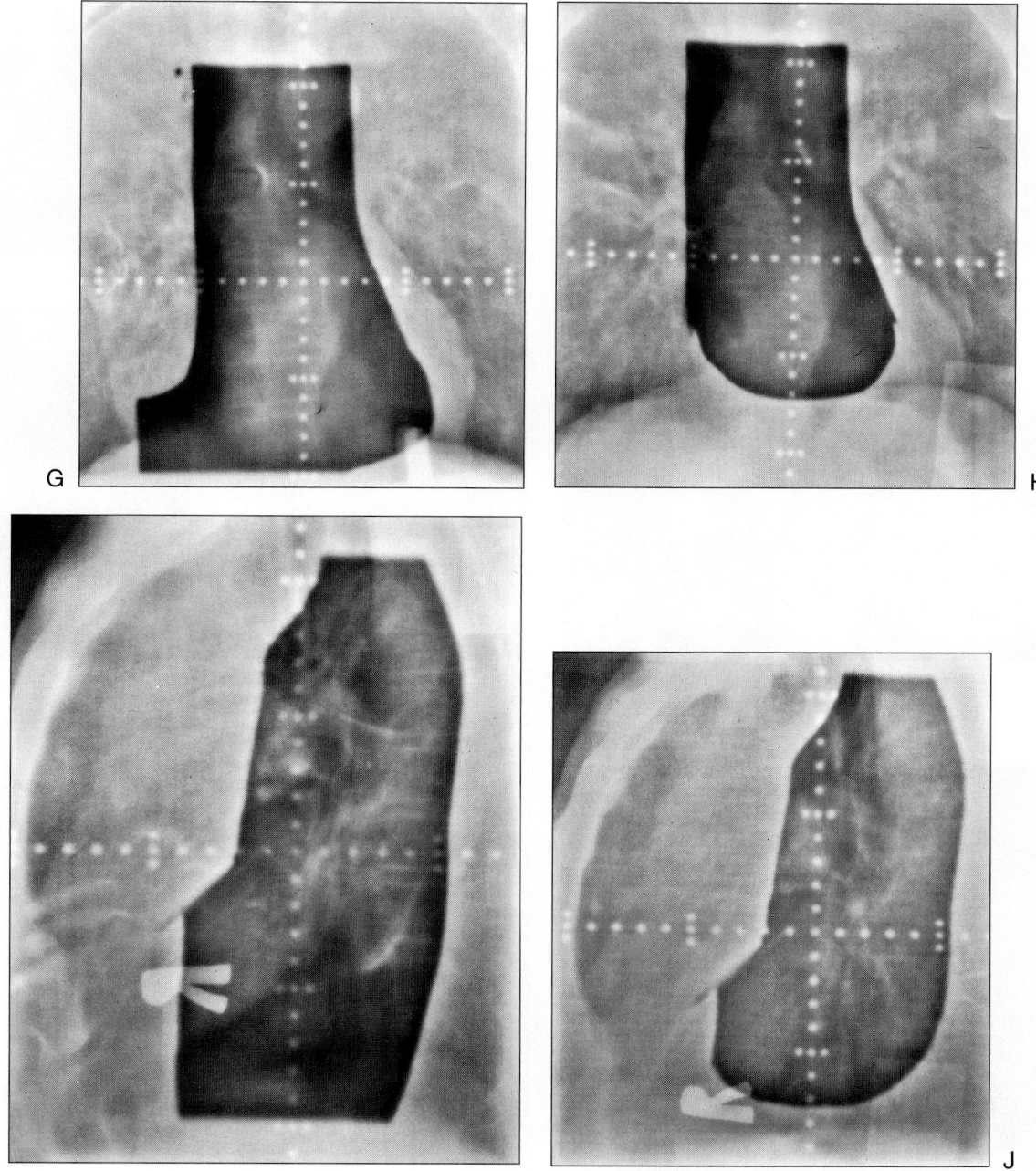

Figure 78-10, *cont'd.* AP-PA simulation **(A)** and port films **(G, H)** demonstrate a moderate amount of heart within the field. Lateral simulation **(B)** and port films **(I, J)** demonstrate the ability to spare some cardiac volume with appropriate use of blocks (*cross-hatched*).

be a component of multidrug chemotherapy regimens, cardiac exclusion is important, when technically feasible. With unresectable *primary* or *locally recurrent* lesions at the level of the esophagogastric junction, if moderate lateral extension is noted on a preoperative CT scan or operative clip placement, lateral or oblique fields can be used to decrease the volume of heart within the irradiation field (see Fig. 78-10).

More routine use of multiple field techniques should be considered when preoperative imaging exists to allow accurate reconstruction of target volumes (see Fig. 78-8).

Single institution data suggest that multiple field arrangements may produce less toxicity.[181] When patients are treated preoperatively, paired lateral fields are usually combined with AP-PA fields to achieve improve dose homogeneity (see Fig. 78-10). Dependent on the posterior extent of the gastric fundus, either oblique or more routine lateral portals can be used to deliver a 10 to 20 Gy component of irradiation to spare spinal cord or kidney. When lateral fields are used, liver and kidney tolerance limits the use of lateral fields to 20 Gy or less. With the wide availability of 3D treatment-planning systems, it may

Specific Malignancies

III

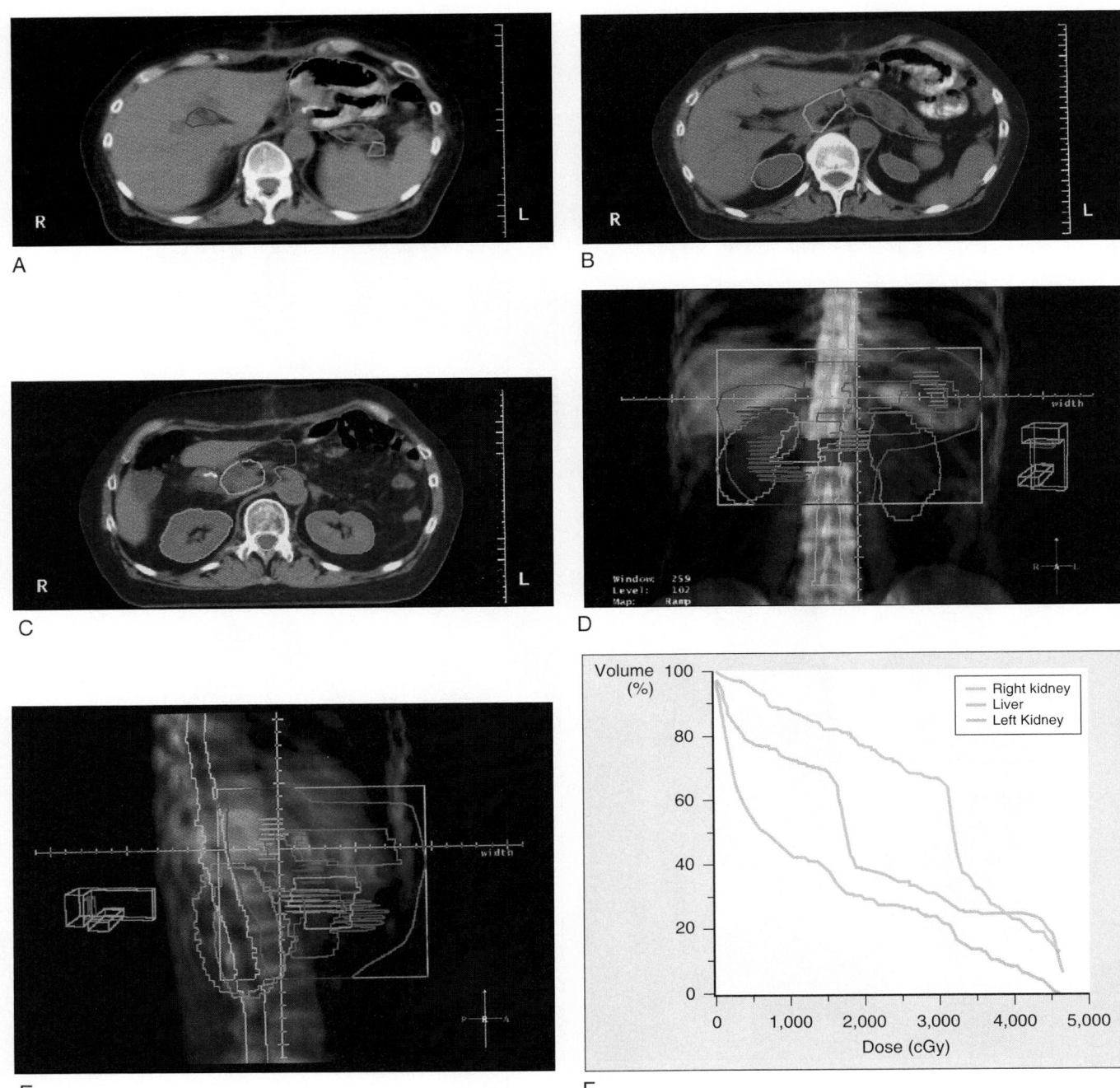

Figure 78-11. Optimized postoperative irradiation fields for patient with T3N2 antral primary tumor (see Table 78-14). **A–C,** Structures of interest were delineated at time of CT simulation. **D** and **E,** Irradiation fields were designed with the aid of digitally reconstructed radiographs (DRR). A dose volume histogram (DVH) was performed to be certain that appropriate volumes of liver and at least one kidney were excluded beyond certain dose levels. **A,** Gastric remnant (*lavender*) is demonstrated along with the body/tail of pancreas (*red-orange*), splenic hilum (*light green*), and porta hepatis (*dark blue*). **B,** Head of pancreas (*yellow*) and kidneys (*left—yellow green; right—yellow orange*) are delineated in addition to the body/tail of the pancreas. **C,** The celiac artery (*light blue*), antral tumor bed (*red*), and duodenum (*medium blue*) are shown together with the head of pancreas and kidneys. A four-field technique of AP (anteroposterior [**D**]), PA (posteroanterior), and paired lateral fields (**E**) was designed. The fields included the gastric remnant (*lavender*), tumor bed (*red*), head of pancreas (*yellow*), first and second part of the duodenum (*medium blue, cross-hatched*), pertinent nodal volumes (perigastric, pancreaticoduodenal, porta hepatic [*dark blue cross-hatched*], suprapancreatic), and the optional nodal volume of splenic hilum (*light green cross-hatched*). **D,** AP field (field margins as shown in *medium blue* exclude approximately two thirds of the left kidney while including approximately 90% of the right kidney). Exclusion of the optional splenic hilar nodes would not have allowed any additional sparing of the left kidney in view of the adjacency of the gastric remnant and the splenic hilum. **E,** Right lateral field demonstrated exclusion of the spinal cord (*turquoise*) along with substantial portions of both kidneys. **F,** The DVH, combining dose from all four fields, demonstrated that the dose volume of 20 Gy included about 30% of the left kidney versus approximately 75% of the right kidney. With regard to the liver, about 30% receives a dose of 30 Gy and about 25% receives a dose of 35 Gy and 40 Gy.

TABLE 78-12

General Guidelines of Impact of T and N Stage on Inclusion of Remaining Stomach, Tumor Bed, Nodal Sites Within Irradiation Fields

TN STAGE	REMAINING STOMACH*	TUMOR BED	NODES
T1–2 (not into subserosa) N0	N	N	N
T2N0–into subserosa[†]	Variable	Y	N
T3N0	Variable	Y	N
T4N0	Variable	Y	Variable
T1–2N+	Y	N	Y
T3–4N+	Y	Y	Y

*Inclusion of the remaining stomach is preferable in most patients if 2/3 of one kidney can be excluded. This is dependent on the extent of surgical resection and uninvolved margins (in cm).
[†]Posterior wall T2N0 lesions, or those that extend beyond muscularis propria, especially tumors located in the proximal or distal stomach, are at risk for local relapse. In addition, patients with low stage disease with close or positive surgical margins should be considered for treatment to the tumor bed.
From Tepper JE, Gunderson LL: Radiation treatment parameters in the adjuvant postoperative therapy of gastric cancer. Semin Radiat Oncol 2002;12:187.

be possible to target more accurately the high-risk volume and to use unconventional field arrangements to produce superior dose distributions. To accomplish this without marginal misses it will be necessary to both carefully define and encompass the various target volumes because use of oblique or noncoplanar beams could exclude target volumes that would be included in AP-PA fields or nonoblique four-field techniques (AP-PA and lateral).

In individual patients the idealized field needs to be modified depending on the surgical/pathologic extent of disease and site of the primary tumor.[190] The relative risk of nodal metastases at a specific nodal location is dependent on both the site of origin of the primary tumor and other factors including width and depth of invasion of the gastric wall. Tumors that originate in the proximal portion of the stomach and the GE junction have a higher propensity of spread to nodes in the mediastinum and pericardial region but a lower likelihood of involvement of nodes in the region of the gastric antrum, periduodenal area, and porta hepatis. Tumors that originate in the body of the stomach can spread to all nodal sites, but

have the highest likelihood of spreading to nodes along the greater and lesser curvature, near the location of the primary tumor mass. Tumors that originate in the distal stomach have a high likelihood of spread to the periduodenal, peripancreatic, and porta hepatis nodes, but they have a lower likelihood of spread to the nodes near the cardia of the stomach, the periesophageal and mediastinal nodes, or to the splenic hilar nodes (Fig. 78-11). Any tumor originating in the stomach has a high propensity of spread to nodes along the greater and lesser curvature, although they are most likely to spread to those sites in close anatomic proximity to the primary tumor mass.

Recently, guidelines for defining the clinical target volume for postoperative radiation fields have been developed based on location and extent of the primary tumor (T stage) and location and extent of known nodal involvement (N stage).[190] Table 78-12 presents general guidelines on the impact of T and N stages on inclusion of the remaining stomach (gastric remnant), tumor bed and nodal sites, and Tables 78-13 and 78-14 present treatment guidelines based on TN stage for two of the four primary

TABLE 78-13

Impact of Site of Primary Lesion and TN Stage on Irradiation Treatment Volumes for the EG Junction: General Guidelines

SITE OR PRIMARY AND TN STAGE	REMAINING STOMACH	TUMOR BED VOLUMES*	NODAL VOLUMES	TOLERANCE ORGANS OR STRUCTURES
EG junction	If allows exclusion of 2/3R kidney	T-stage dependent	N-stage dependent	Heart, lung, spinal cord, kidneys, liver
T2N0 with invasion of subserosa	Variable dependent on surgpath findings[†]	Medial L hemidiaphragm; adjacent body of pancreas	None or perigastric, periesophageal[‡]	
T3N0	Variable dependent on surgpath findings[†]	Medial L hemidiaphragm; adjacent body of pancreas	None or perigastric, periesoph, mediast, celiac[‡]	
T4N0	Preferable but dependent on surgpath findings[†]	As for T3N0 plus site(s) of adherence with 3–5 cm margin	Nodes related to site of adherence, +/– perigastric, perigastric, periesoph, mediast, celiac	
T1–2N+	Preferable	Not indicated for T1, as above for T2 into subserosa	Periesoph, mediast, prox perigastric, celiac	
T3–4N+	Preferable	As for T3, T4N0	As for T1–2N+ and T4N0	

*Use preop imaging (CT, barium swallow), surgical clips, and postop imaging (CT, barium swallow).
[†]For tumors with wide (>5 cm) surgical margins confirmed pathologically, treatment of residual stomach is optional, especially if this would result in substantial increase in normal tissue morbidity.
[‡]Optional node inclusion for T2–3N0 lesions if adequate surgical node dissection (D2 dissection) and at least 10–15 nodes examined pathologically.
From Tepper JE, Gunderson LL: Radiation treatment parameters in the adjuvant postoperative therapy of gastric cancer. Semin Radiat Oncol 2002;12:187.

TABLE 78-14

Impact of Site of Primary Gastric Lesion and TN Stage on Irradiation Treatment Volumes—Antrum/Pylorus/Distal Third of Stomach: General Guidelines

SITE OR PRIMARY AND TN STAGE	REMAINING STOMACH	TUMOR BED VOLUMES*	NODAL VOLUMES	TOLERANCE ORGANS OR STRUCTURES
Pylorus/distal third stomach	Yes but spare 2/3 of one kidney, usually left	T-stage dependent	N-stage dependent	Kidneys, liver, spinal cord
T2N0 with invasion of subserosa	Variable dependent on surgical pathologic findings†	Head of pancreas, (+/– body), 1st and 2nd duodenum	None or perigastric; optional pancreaticoduodenal, porta hepatis, celiac, suprapancreatic‡	
T3N0	Variable dependent on surgical-pathologic findings†	Head of pancreas (+/– body), 1st and 2nd duodenum	None or perigastric; optional pancreaticoduodenal, porta hepatis, celiac, suprapancreatic‡	
T4N0	Preferable but dependent on surgical-pathologic findings†	As for T3N0 plus site(s) of adherence with 3–5 cm margin	Nodes related to site(s) of adherence +/– perigastric, pancreaticoduodenal, porta hepatis, celiac, suprapancreatic	
T1–2N+	Preferable	Not indicated For T1	Perigastric, pancreatico-duodenal, porta hepatis, celiac, suprapancreatic; optional, splenic hilum	
T3–4N+	Preferable	As for T3, T4N0	As for T1–2N+ and T4N0	

*Use preoperative imaging (computed tomography, barium swallow), surgical clips, and postoperative imaging (computed tomography, barium swallow).
†For tumors with wide (>5cm) surgical margins confirmed pathologically, treatment of residual stomach is optional if this would result in substantial increased normal tissue morbidity.
‡Optional node inclusion for T2–3N0 lesions if adequate surgical node dissection (D2 dissection) and at least 10–15 nodes examined pathologically.
Tepper JE, Gunderson LL: Radiation treatment parameters in the adjuvant postoperative therapy of gastric cancer. Semin Radiat Oncol 2002;12:187.

sites (esophagogastric junction, proximal, mid-, and distal stomach). In general, for patients with node-positive disease, there should be wide coverage of tumor bed, remaining stomach, resection margins, and nodal drainage regions. For node-negative disease, if there is a good surgical resection with pathologic evaluation of at least 10 to 15 nodes, and there are wide surgical margins on the primary tumor (at least 5 cm), treatment of the nodal beds is optional. Treatment of the remaining stomach should depend on a balance of the likely normal tissue morbidity and the perceived risk of local relapse in the residual stomach.

LOCALLY ADVANCED DISEASE (UNRESECTABLE AND RESIDUAL): TREATMENT AND RESULTS

The term *locally advanced disease* has different interpretations depending on the author and institution. In our institution and for the purposes of this chapter, this term refers to primary cancers that the surgeon would not expect to resect with negative pathologic margins (i.e., locally unresectable for cure as determined at surgical exploration or as defined preoperatively with CT scan, endoscopic ultrasonography, laparoscopy, or other studies; locally recurrent cancers with no evidence of metastasis). Other authors use the term also to include lesions that are completely resected but have high-risk factors for local recurrence or distant metastasis (nodal involvement, extension beyond gastric wall, or both).

Surgical Aspects

The extent of the surgical procedures must be tempered by the knowledge that cure is at best improbable. Patients with symptomatic obstruction, hemorrhage, and ulceration, and some with perforation, can be successfully relieved of symptoms by even limited gastric resection. Radical subtotal or total gastrectomies may be indicated in some patients whose lesions cannot be completely resected with negative pathologic margins in order to achieve symptomatic palliation. Our own results with total gastrectomy in advanced gastric cancer showed good quality of life when this procedure was indicated for bulky or proximal tumors, but symptom relief was less likely for patients with linitis plastica.[191] Although adjacent organ resection should be undertaken if all gross tumor can be removed, it is rarely justified if residual tumor would remain. If sites of residual disease or adherence are judiciously marked with clips, postoperative irradiation plus chemotherapy can be delivered with greater accuracy.

Irradiation with or Without Chemotherapy

Although some patients in whom resection is not done have long-term survival using irradiation with or without chemotherapy, this approach is not a viable alternative to surgical resection plus adjuvant therapy as indicated, because the initial bulk of disease and the limited tolerance of the stomach and surrounding organs prevent a suitable therapeutic ratio between cure and complications. When locally advanced disease is diagnosed before surgical exploration, preoperative radiation would preferably be used in combination with chemotherapy (concomitant and maintenance) followed by restaging and an attempted resection of all gross primary and lymph node disease.

Irradiation Alone

The available literature suggests that adenocarcinoma of the stomach is radioresponsive. Wieland and Hymmen[192] used 60 Gy when feasible (1.5 to 2.0 Gy daily) with 11% (9 of 82) 3-year and 7% (5 of 72) 5-year survival rates. Takahashi[193] compared historical control subjects with patients who were unresectable or who had palliative procedures and received postoperative radiation (unknown if chemotherapy also used). The average survival time for the irradiated group was 9 to 10 months longer, with 74% 1-year (32 of 43) and 27% 2.5-year survival rates (12 of 43). Abe and Takahashi[168,169] reported 15% 5-year survival rate with a single dose of IORT (28 to 35 Gy) in a group of 27 patients with stage IV disease. Three of the four long-term survivors had proved residual disease after resection. In the same study, 18 stage IV patients were randomized to a surgery-alone control arm; the 5-year survival rate was 0%.

Irradiation Plus Chemotherapy

Most reports of combined irradiation and chemotherapy for gastric cancer involve patients with residual or unresectable primary disease, and most phase III trials in this setting show an advantage for combined-modality treatment over single-modality treatment. In a randomized series from the Mayo Clinic,[194,195] 5-FU was used during the first 3 days of irradiation in one half of the patients (irradiation, 35 to 37.5 Gy in 4 to 5 weeks; 5-FU, 15 mg/kg for 3 days, week 1 of irradiation). For the combined-treatment group, mean and overall survival was improved (13 months versus 5.9 months and 3 of 25 patients or 12% versus 0 of 23 patients surviving over 5 years) (Table 78-15). In a randomized study by the GITSG,[196,197] the combination of irradiation and 5-FU followed by maintenance 5-FU plus MeCCNU resulted in statistically superior long-term survival when compared with 5-FU MeCCNU alone (3- and 4-year survival rates of 18% versus 6% to 7%; $P < 0.05$). GITSG performed a second trial in which combined irradiation plus chemotherapy did not produce a survival advantage when compared with chemotherapy alone.[198] Because 46% of patients on the combined arm either did not receive full-course irradiation or had a major deviation in the delivery of the irradiation, the results are difficult to interpret. In a randomized EORTC trial of external irradiation with or without 5-FU, residual disease after resection was identified in 22 patients.[199] The three long-term survivors (14%) received both irradiation and 5-FU.

Data from nonrandomized single-institution or group analyses also suggest that the combination of external irradiation and chemotherapy may have an impact on

TABLE 78-15

Unresectable or Residual Gastric Cancer: Treatment Results

GROUP OR INSTITUTION	TREATMENT ARMS	EBRT DOSE/SCHEDULE (GY)	CHEMOTHERAPY	NO. OF PATIENTS	RESULTS (FAILURE PATTERNS AND SURVIVAL)
Randomized					
Mayo Clinic[194,195]	EBRT ± 5-FU	35–40/9–12 Gy/wk	5-FU 15 mg/kg, d 1–3, wk 1 EBRT	48	Increased SR for EBRT + 5-FU with mean SR 13 vs. 5.9 mo and 3/25 (12%) vs. 0/23 5-yr SR
GITSG[196,197] study 8274	CT ± EBRT	50/8 wk – 2 wk split after 25/3 wk	5-FU 500 mg/m², d 1–3, wk 1 + 6 EBRT; 5-FU + MeCCNU maintenance vs. 5-FU + MeCCNU	90	Advantage in long-term SR with EBRT + CT at 18% vs. 7% ($P < 0.05$)
Japan[169]	Operation ± IORT*	IORT, 28–40	None	110 operation 101 IORT	Increased 5-yr SR for 27 patients with IORT + operation for stage IV disease vs. 18 patients with operation alone (15% vs. 0%)
Nonrandomized					
MGH[176]	EBRT ± CT	45–55/5–6-1/2 wk	5-FU 500 mg/m², 3 d wk 1 EBRT ± maintenance FAM or 5-FU MeCCNU	32	Median SR res(m) 24 mo, res(g) 15 mo, unresected 14 mo; survival ≥30 mo, unresected 0%, residual after resection ~10%
Mayo Clinic[202]	EBRT ± CT ± IOERT	45–54/5–6-1/2 wk IOERT boost 13 patients	5-FU 500 mg/m² 3 d wk 1, 5 or 5-FU 400 mg/m² leucovorin 20 mg/m²	87	Median SR res(m) 17 mo, res(g) 9 mo, unresectable 12 mo, locally recurrent 10 mo; 4-year SR ≤9% res(m) and res(g) 18% unresectable or locally recurrent

CT, chemotherapy; EBRT, external-beam irradiation; GITSG, Gastrointestinal Tumor Study Group; IORT, intraoperative irradiation; MGH, Massachusetts General Hospital; res(m), microscopic residual; res(g), gross residual; SR, survival. For other abbreviations, see footnotes to Table 78-8 and 78-10.
*Treatment method based on date of hospitalization.

disease control and survival. In published series from the Mayo Clinic[200] and MGH,[176] long-term survival of 10% or more was demonstrated in patients who received external irradiation plus chemotherapy following subtotal surgical resection with residual disease (MGH) or with unresectable lesions. In a University of Pennsylvania analysis[179] of patients with unresected adenocarcinoma of the esophagogastric junction or esophagus, local control was better with combined- versus single-modality treatment (irradiation, 1 of 23 or 4%; chemotherapy, 0 of 8; irradiation plus chemotherapy, 11 of 21 or 52%). Median survival time with the combined-modality treatment was 10 months compared with 5 months for irradiation alone. In a Mayo Clinic NCCTG dose escalation pilot study, external irradiation was combined with 5-FU plus low-dose leucovorin (400 mg/m^2 and 20 mg/m^2, respectively, for 3 to 4 days, weeks 1 or 1 plus 5 of irradiation).[201] Two of six patients with locally advanced gastric cancer were alive and disease-free beyond 3 years.

Published analyses from both GITSG and MGH suggest an improvement in survival if partial resection with gross residual disease or gross total resection with microscopic residual can be accomplished. In the GITSG series 3-year survival rate was about 25% versus 10% in partially resected versus unresected patients.[191,192] In the MGH analysis, median survival with irradiation plus chemotherapy was 24 months for microscopic residual, 15 months with gross residual, and 14 months in unresected patients.[176] Four-year survival rate was 0% in unresected patients versus 10% in those with residual disease after maximal resection.

In the most recent Mayo Clinic analysis of irradiation plus or minus chemotherapy for gastric or esophagogastric cancers, an improvement in median survival was also suggested for patients with gross total resection but microscopic residual disease when compared with higher risk subsets of patients.[202] In this analysis, the results of irradiation or chemoirradiation were evaluated in 87 patients with either locally advanced primary or locally recurrent adenocarcinoma of the stomach or esophagogastric junction treated from July 1980 through January 1996 at the Mayo Clinic. Of those with primary lesions, 28 had unresectable disease, and 39 had resection but residual disease (microscopic, 28; gross, 10). An additional 21 presented with a local or regional relapse with no evidence of abdominal (liver, peritoneal) or extra-abdominal metastasis (lung, other). Chemotherapy with 5-FU (plus or minus leucovorin) was given during or following EBRT in 75% of the patients with microscopic residual disease and 92% of the other subgroups (concomitant with EBRT in 84%). An IOERT supplement to EBRT was given in 13 patients. Median survival time in primary cancer patients with microscopic residual was 16.7 months versus 9.2 months in patients with subtotal resection and gross residual or 12 months in those with unresectable disease. Patients who presented with local or regional relapse had a median survival of 10 months.

Prognostic factor analyses showed that long-term survival appeared slightly poorer in patients who had resection before irradiation or chemoradiotherapy in the latest Mayo Clinic analysis. Actuarial 4-year survival rate

was 0% versus 9% in patients with gross residual disease after partial resection (1 of 11 patients alive with no evidence of disease 2 years after treatment), 9% in those with microscopic residual after gross total resection, and 18% in patients with unresectable primary or locally recurrent cancers. The survival trends may be a reflection of both treatment sequence and higher irradiation dose; 12 of 13 patients with EBRT plus IOERT had unresectable primary or locally recurrent cancers. In the 21 patients with locally or regionally recurrent cancers, irradiation dose greater than 54 Gy had a trend for improved survival (median survival, 25.6 versus 5.5 months; $P = 0.06$). If patients with microscopic residual disease are excluded, an increase in the number of cycles of chemotherapy appeared to correlate with an improvement in median survival (less than two cycles – median survival 5.2 months versus 11.5 months with two or three cycles and 14.5 months with four or more cycles; $P = 0.014$).

Although problems with excess toxicity from combined chemoradiotherapy were encountered in the GITSG study,[191] such problems were minimal or non-existent in the MGH series of 46 patients.[176] In the latter series, 43 of 46 patients received both irradiation and chemotherapy, but shaped radiation portals and single fraction size of 1.8 Gy or less were utilized.

Neoadjuvant Chemotherapy with or Without Irradiation

The use of adjuvant preoperative (neoadjuvant) chemotherapy has been less well studied compared to adjuvant postoperative therapy. Due to the inability of adjuvant postoperative systemic therapy to prolong survival in surgically managed gastric cancer, several investigators have pursued the approach of neoadjuvant (preoperative) chemotherapy in an attempt to increase resectability and improve survival. These studies involve a mix of patients including surgically or clinically determined unresectable for cure patients, "locally advanced" (as defined by the study authors), and clinically operable patients. Some patients were staged clinically by a variety of methods, making it difficult to know which patients were truly resectable prior to neoadjuvant treatment. Table 78-16 summarizes the results of these reports. All but one of these studies are phase II protocols.

Unresectable Disease

One of the earliest reports of neoadjuvant systemic therapy came from Wilke and colleagues who examined the role of etoposide, Adriamycin (doxorubicin), and cisplatin (EAP) in a group of 34 patients with laparotomy-determined unresectable stomach cancer.[203] This study was prompted by their promising results with EAP in advanced disease (21% complete remission and 64% overall response rate).[204] Following exploratory laparotomy, patients were begun on EAP. Twenty patients (59%) who achieved a clinical response went on to a second-look operation followed by two additional courses of chemotherapy. Fifteen patients (44%) out of the original cohort could be resected. It is particularly noteworthy that five patients were pathologic complete responders (15% of

TABLE 78-16

Neoadjuvant Therapy for Gastric Cancer

AUTHOR	PATIENTS	REGIMEN	RESPONSE RATE (%)	EXPLORED (%)	RESECTED (%)	PATHOLOGIC CR (%)	MEDIAN SURVIVAL (MO)
Unresectable							
Wilke[203]	34	EAP	68	59	44	15	18
Plukker[206]	20	5-FU/MTX	30	70	40	0	9
Rosen[202]	19	EEP	42	53	37	0	NR
Facchini[208]	22	FAMTX	50	95	73	NR	NR
Lerner[209]	13	EAP	NS	38	8	8	NR
Roelofs[210]	14	FEMTX-P	50	36	29	0	NR
Yano[211]	13	FEMTXP	8	53	23	0	NS
	20	THP-FPLM	35	35	25	0	NS
Borderline Resectable, Locally Advanced							
Rougier[212]	30	5-FU/Plat	50	93	77	0	16
Fink[213]	30	EAP	57	90	80	0	17
Alexander[214]	22	5-FU/LV/IFL	36	91	59	NR	18
Kang[215]	53	EAP	NS	89	70	7	43
	54	Control		100	61	0	30
Resectable							
Ajani[216]	25	EFP pre/post	24	100	72	0	15
Ajani[217]	48	EAP pre/post	31	85	77	0	15.5
Stephens[218]	17	FAMB IA	65	100	NR	12	47.5
Kelsen[220]	56	FAMTX pre, 5-FU/ Plat IP post, 5-FU IV post	51	89	61	0	15.3
Crokes[221]	56	5-FU, LV, Plat pre; FUDR, Plat IP post	54	95	68	9	52
Songun[219]	27	FAMTX	30	100	56	7	13.1
	29	Control		100	62		12.8

CR, complete response; EAP, etoposide, doxorubicin, and cisplatin; EEP, epirubicin, etoposide, and cisplatin; EFP, etoposide, 5-FU, and cisplatin; FAMTX, 5-FU, Adriamycin, and methotrexate; FEMTX-P, 5-FU, epirubicin, methotrexate, and cisplatin; 5-FU, 5-fluorouracil; LV, leucovorin; IFL, interferon; Mtx, methotrexate; NR, not reported; Plat, cis-platinum; post, postoperatively; pre, preoperatively.

the original 34). Median survival in this phase II trial was 18 months for the entire study group. In an update of these data at an international gastrointestinal cancer symposium in Germany, results were reported in a series of 21 patients who had total resection after EAP chemotherapy for locally unresectable disease.[205] Fourteen of 21 patients had relapsed, and 11 of 14 had a local-regional component of disease (79% of relapses, 52% of group at risk).

Plukker and coworkers studied 20 patients with unresectable gastric cancer.[206] Seventeen of the patients had undergone laparotomy, and three patients were deemed unresectable on the basis of CT imaging. After receiving up to four courses of sequential 5-FU and high-dose methotrexate, 14 patients (70%) underwent attempted resection. Eight of 20 patients (40%) were found to be resectable for cure. Subsequent local relapse occurred in five of eight. There were no pathologic complete responders and the median survival for the entire group was 14 months. Similar results using etoposide, epirubicin, and cisplatin were reported by Rosen.[207]

Facchini and associates have studied neoadjuvant FAMTX in a group of 22 unresectable patients as judged by surgical or clinical staging.[208] Fifty percent of the patients were reported to have responded clinically,

most were explored, and 73% were resected for cure. The pathologic response rates and survival were not reported.

Two groups have studied the results of chemotherapy in patients with clinically unresectable disease. In both studies these patients were part of phase II studies of advanced disease. Lerner and associates reported a subset of 13 patients with unresectable disease that received EAP.[209] Five patients were subsequently explored and one patient was curatively resected with no tumor seen in the resected specimen. Roelofs and colleagues studied the regimen of sequential high-dose methotrexate and 5-FU alternating with epirubicin and cisplatin (FEMTX-P) in 50 patients, 14 with unresectable disease.[210] Seven patients responded, five were explored, and four were completely resected. No pathologic complete responses (CRs) were seen.

Yano and associates explored the use of two different multidrug regimens in a group of 33 patients. Salvage surgery was possible in 42% of the patients with a curative resection occurring in 24% of the patients.[211]

These seven trials of 155 patients with "unresectable" disease demonstrated that preoperative chemotherapy was feasible and resulted in clinical response rates of 30% to 68%. Curative resections were possible in as few as 8% or as many as 73% of patients. Most likely, this wide range of resectability reflects patient selection rather than superiority of any one regimen. Unfortunately, pathologic CRs were uncommon except for the Wilke study.

Borderline Resectable/Locally Advanced Disease

Three phase II studies have tested the use of preoperative systemic treatment in patients defined by the study authors as having "locally advanced" stomach cancer. Presumably this represents a mix of clinically resectable and unresectable or borderline resectable patients.

Rougier and colleagues treated 30 patients with two to three cycles of cisplatin and 5-FU before surgery.[212] Twenty-eight (93%) patients subsequently underwent laparotomy, and 23 (77%) were resected. Patients with T3 or N+ disease at surgery received up to three cycles of chemotherapy postoperatively. No pathologic complete responses were seen, and the overall median survival was 16 months.

EAP was studied in 30 patients by Fink and associates.[213] Over 50% of the patients were judged to have attained a clinical response. Eighty% were curatively resected. No pathologic CRs were seen and median survival was 17 months.

Alexander and associates used 5-FU, leucovorin, and interferon both pre- and postoperatively in 22 patients.[214] Most were explored and 59% had curative resection. Pathologic CRs were not reported and median survival was 17 months.

Kang and associates have presented an updated report of the only phase III trial of neoadjuvant chemotherapy in locally advanced or borderline resectable gastric cancer.[215] One hundred seven patients were randomized to receive two to three cycles of etoposide, 5-FU, and cisplatin (EFP) followed by surgery versus surgery alone. Of the 53 patients randomized to preoperative treatment, 47 (89%) were explored, and 37 (70%) were resected for cure. A 7% complete pathologic response rate was noted. In the control group of 54 patients, 100% were explored and 61% curatively resected. Median survival time was 43 months versus 30 months in favor of neoadjuvant treatment, but this difference did not reach statistical significance ($P = 0.114$).

In general, resectability rates were higher in this group of "locally advanced" or borderline resectable patients when compared to the unresectable group. It is likely that more patients in the studies defined as locally advanced disease were potentially resectable before neoadjuvant chemotherapy.

Resectable Disease

Several investigators have examined the role of neo-adjuvant chemotherapy in patients with clinically resectable disease. Ajani and colleagues have performed two phase II studies of preoperative chemotherapy in this setting. In their first study, 25 patients were treated with two cycles of EFP preoperatively.[216] Three cycles were administered postoperatively if a positive response to neoadjuvant treatment could be detected endoscopically or radiographically. All 25 patients underwent surgery, and 72% were resected for cure. No pathologic CRs were seen, and the median survival was 15 months overall. Following Wilke and coworkers' report of pathologic

complete response to EAP chemotherapy,[203] Ajani and associates treated 48 potentially curable patients with three cycles of preoperative EAP and two cycles following surgery if a response to preoperative treatment was observed.[217] Eighty-five percent of patients underwent exploration, and 77% were resectable. Although 12% of patients achieved a complete clinical response, no pathologic complete responders were seen. The overall median survival was 15.5 months. Unfortunately, in this group of resectable patients with potentially smaller tumor burdens, the impressive results obtained with neoadjuvant EAP in Wilke's study could not be reproduced.

One study has evaluated the use of preoperative intra-arterial therapy. Stephens reported on a group of 17 potentially resectable patients who received neoadjuvant intra-arterial 5-FU, Adriamycin, mitomycin C, and BCNU.[218] Sixty-five percent of patients attained a clinical response and all were explored. The number of completely resected patients was not detailed. Two (12%) patients had a pathologic CR and the mean survival time was 47.5 months.

One of the few randomized trials to assess the potential benefit of preoperative chemotherapy to surgery alone in potentially resectable patients failed to show any benefit.[219] In this Dutch study, patients were randomized to either FAMTX followed by surgery or surgery alone. Patients with T1 tumors, tumors arising from the gastric cardia or evidence of distant metastases were excluded from participation. The study was closed early due to poor accrual. However, analysis of the patients enrolled showed no benefit to rate of curative resectability, rate of relapse, or median survival.

Recently, other investigators have examined the utility of combining preoperative chemotherapy and post-operative treatment with intraperitoneal chemotherapy in view of the high peritoneal failure rate following resection of gastric cancer. Kelsen and associates studied 56 patients with high-risk (clinical T3–4) gastric cancer as determined by endoscopic ultrasound (EUS).[220] Patients received three cycles of neoadjuvant FAMTX. Following surgery, patients were treated with intraperitoneal 5-FU and cisplatin along with infusional 5-FU for three cycles. Fifty (89%) patients were explored and 34 (61%) resected for cure. Fifty-one percent were downstaged as determined by comparing the initial EUS and the final pathologic staging. No complete pathologic responses were observed and the median survival was 15.3 months. Crookes and colleagues have recently updated their promising results with a somewhat similar trial design.[221] Fifty-nine potentially resectable patients received two cycles of 5-FU, leucovorin, and cisplatin preoperatively, and two cycles of intraperitoneal 5-FUDR and cisplatin were given postoperatively to resected patients. Ninety-five percent of the patients underwent exploration, and 68% had a curative resection. The complete response rate pathologically was only 9%, but the median survival is estimated to be an impressive 52 months.

Summary

Preoperative systemic treatment may have certain advantages, such as the potential of reducing tumor bulk and increasing resectability. Micrometastatic disease may also be addressed earlier using this approach. Some investigators point to experimental models where surgical resection may serve as a stimulus for increased growth of residual disease.[222] Theoretically this stimulus to proliferate may lead to more spontaneous mutations and enhanced chemotherapy resistance. Finally, issues of altered vascular supply to tumor cells caused by surgery, which may compromise drug delivery, would be circumvented by a neoadjuvant approach. Potential negatives to preoperative treatment include toxicity, delay in definitive therapy, and possibly increased surgical morbidity and mortality rates.

The high response rates achieved with neoadjuvant chemotherapy are of interest, and this form of treatment will undoubtedly be the subject of further investigation over the next several years. To date, however, no survival advantage has been demonstrated in phase III trials, and neoadjuvant chemotherapy should be considered investigational. Resectability rates in neoadjuvantly treated patients seem higher than the median rate of 40% from several surgical studies, but the patients in these studies are highly selected. Except for the trials in which some patients were unresectable on the basis of prior exploration, the successful operations in these reports may not have been influenced by neoadjuvant chemotherapy. In general, pathologic complete response rates are low (≤15%), and no proof exists that clinically staged patients are made more resectable by such treatment. The impact of preoperative systemic treatment on survival is even less clear. The one randomized trial that has been reported shows a nonsignificant improvement in survival for neoadjuvant treatment in borderline resectable/locally advanced disease.[215] Newer technologies such as EUS may identify patients who will do poorly with standard therapy alone and would be reasonable candidates for future neoadjuvant studies.[39,40,207] The reports of combined systemic and intraperitoneal approaches are provocative and may warrant future phase III trials, as only through such studies will any impact on survival be determined.

In view of the high incidence of locoregional relapse in several series of patients resected after neoadjuvant chemotherapy for initially unresectable lesions, irradiation has been incorporated into the study design of recent trials for patients with high-risk factors. The study by Walsh and associates compared preoperative 5-FU and cisplatin plus radiotherapy followed by surgery (N = 58) versus surgery alone (N = 55) in patients with esophageal and gastric cardia adenocarcinoma.[186] Pathologic CR was found in 13 of 52 patients (25%) who had surgery after preoperative chemoradiotherapy. As noted earlier in this chapter, both median and long-term survival were improved with the preoperative treatment (P = 0.01). Thirty-five percent of the patients had lesions of the gastric cardia; however, there were more of these patients in the control group (42% versus 28%). The positive esophagus gastric cardia trial by Walsh and associates and high pathologic CRs in similar pilot studies with gastric cancer[223] led to a U.S. GI Intergroup confirmatory trial of neoadjuvant combined-modality therapy in carcinoma of the esophagus and gastroesophageal junction. This study was stopped because of inadequate accrual.

PALLIATION OF THE INCURABLE PATIENT

This section is limited to discussion of patients with proved hematogenous or peritoneal metastasis. Patients with locally unresected disease are occasionally cured and were discussed in the previous section (5-year survival rate of 5% to 20%).

Surgery

Surgical intervention in the patient with metastatic gastric cancer requires sound judgment. The underlying health and function (performance status) of the patient, the estimated duration of patient survival, and the nature of the symptoms must all be taken into account before deciding to proceed with an operation. Resection for palliation is generally better than bypass or intubation in appropriate selected patients, leading to better symptomatic relief and often longer survival.[224] Laparoscopic procedures, including subtotal gastrectomy, are feasible; however, reports of results are limited at present.[225,226] Obstructing lesions may be resected with excellent palliation, but endoluminal stents, endoscopic laser treatments, or gastrostomy tube placement should be considered for poor operative candidates. While significant hemorrhage from an ulcerating or necrotic polypoid tumor may be temporarily controlled by endoscopic techniques, stabilization and urgent surgical intervention should be undertaken when appropriate. A perforated gastric cancer usually presents as an emergency and may be unrecognized preoperatively. Aggressive treatment with gastric resection should be carried out in the fit patient, but pain control and hydration alone are preferable for the moribund or unfit patient.

Irradiation with or Without Chemotherapy

If palliative resection is not indicated in symptomatic patients with metastases, a shortened course of irradiation with or without 5-FU could be used (37.5 Gy in 15 fractions over 3 weeks), to be followed by systemic treatment. Patients who have proximal lesions with esophageal obstruction may be candidates for laser ablation instead of irradiation. If laser is successful in overcoming obstruction, patients could proceed directly to treatment with chemotherapy.

Chemotherapy

Traditional chemotherapy agents with reported response rates of 10% or higher include 5-FU, mitomycin C, doxorubicin, epirubicin, cisplatin, BCNU, methotrexate, etoposide, chlorambucil, and hydroxyurea.[141,227-230] More recently, a variety of new chemotherapy drugs have become available. Some have shown promising response rates in advanced gastric cancer including taxotere (23%), irinotecan (23%), and paclitaxel (17 to 21%).[231-233]

Multiple phase II trials of combination chemotherapy have built upon the promising activity seen with a variety of single agents. Many of the combinations have shown promising activity based on initial results, only to be shown to be less active and more toxic in subsequent phase II and III trials. It has therefore been important to interpret the results of initial phase II trials with caution. Nearly all the more frequently used combinations have included 5-FU. Some of the most popular regimens have been FAM, FAMTX, ELF, and more recently ECF.

The combination of 5-FU and a nitrosourea (MeCCNU or BCNU) represents one of the earliest studied regimens in advanced gastric cancer. While early response rates were encouraging, survival was not improved over single-agent 5-FU.[234,235]

In the early 1980s, the combination of FAM became widely used. MacDonald and colleagues reported a 42% response rate in 62 patients with advanced measurable gastric cancer.[236] Although the overall median survival time was a modest 5.5 months, the median survival time for responding patients was 12.5 months. Some were critical of this form of analysis; nevertheless, FAM became a popular regimen and was studied further.[237] Over 900 evaluable patients treated with FAM or modifications thereof have been reported, with response rates varying between 12% and 65% and with median survival times of 5 to 9 months.[238] Concern with the widespread use of FAM was raised, however, when randomized trials could not demonstrate a survival advantage versus 5-FU alone.[239-241]

The addition of cisplatin to 5-FU and Adriamycin (FAP) resulted in response rates of 53% in a Mayo Clinic phase II study.[242] Subsequent studies have yielded response rates ranging from 20% to 56%. A phase III study, however, could not show an advantage for FAP over 5-FU alone.[243]

In 1989, Preusser and coworkers reported interesting results for the combination of etoposide, Adriamycin, and cisplatin (EAP) in 67 patients with advanced gastric cancer.[204] The overall response rate was 64%, but more important, the CR rate was 21%. Follow-up phase II studies have shown response rates of 13% to 73%, with some authors reporting worrisome toxicity.[209] Interestingly, Preusser and colleagues developed a less toxic regimen for those medically unfit for EAP. This combination of etoposide, leucovorin, and 5-FU (ELF) produced a 53% response rate and a respectable 11-month median survival time.[244]

Multiple clinical trials have now evaluated the activity and tolerability of ELF.[245-247] These trials have generally shown overall survival in the range of 8 to 10 months and response rates of approximately 30%.

Sequential methotrexate and 5-FU followed by Adriamycin (FAMTX) has also been widely studied. A large phase II trial by Klein revealed a response rate of 58% and median survival time of 9 months.[248] Further studies of this regimen show response rates ranging from 12% to 41%.[249] When compared to FAM in a randomized study by the EORTC, FAMTX showed both superior response rates (41% versus 9%) and survival times (median, 42 weeks versus 29 weeks).[250] FAMTX has also been shown to be less toxic than EAP in a randomized trial.[251] In a more recent phase III trial by EORTC, FAMTX was compared

to ELF and to infusional 5-FU and cisplatin (FUP).[252] No difference was seen in overall response or median survival. Given the modest activity seen with these three regimens the authors suggested that other strategies should be pursued.

Investigators from Great Britain recently studied the regimen of epirubicin, cisplatin, and infusional 5-FU (ECF).[253] Initial results show a 71% response rate in 139 patients. A subsequent randomized phase III study showed superiority for ECF over FAMTX for both overall response rate (45% versus 21%) and median survival time (8.9 months versus 5.7 months).[254] In view of the promising results of this phase III trial, ECF has now become the standard regimen to which other newer regimens are frequently compared.

Another recently developed regimen includes the combination of cisplatin, epirubicin, leucovorin, and 5-FU (PELF).[255] PELF was compared to FAM in a study performed in Italy. Response rates were superior for PELF (43% versus 15%), but there was no improvement in survival.[256] An intensified weekly version of PELF with growth factor support showed a response rate of 62% and a median survival time of 11 months. The authors suggested the need for further study in the adjuvant setting.

Several recent phase II studies have evaluated non-5-FU-containing combinations. The response to combinations such as docetaxel and cisplatin, paclitaxel and cisplatin, and irinotecan and mitomycin C have been comparable to other 5-FU-containing regimens.[257-259]

Chemotherapy versus Supportive Care
Seven studies available in the literature address chemotherapy for advanced gastric cancer when compared to an untreated control group. The first three were reported before 1980 and the last four were reported after 1993.

Rake and colleagues studied 40 patients with incurable gastric cancer.[133] Patients were randomized to receive an induction course of 5-FU, methotrexate, cyclophosphamide, and vincristine followed by weekly 5-FU and mitomycin C. The median survival time in the control group was 2 months, which was not improved by treatment.

A large trial conducted by the West Midlands group was reported in 1973.[260] A total of 193 patients were randomized between 5-FU/MeCCNU and no treatment. The median survival time was reported as 22 weeks for control subjects and 25 weeks for those who received at least one 6-week course of chemotherapy. Patients who died in the first 2 months were excluded from these figures. Median survival, estimated from survival curves, is in the 8- to 10-week range for all the patients, with no apparent difference between the two groups. It is of interest that a quality-of-life (QOL) analysis was done in the West Midlands trial that was published in 1978. Pain, well-being, and performance status were assessed at 8 and 16 weeks. Results of this QOL analysis slightly favored the patients treated with chemotherapy, but few patient results were available for the 16-week time point.

Dent and colleagues reported a study looking at 76 patients with T4 or M1 disease and randomized patients between no treatment, localized radiotherapy, and thiotepa.[26] Median survival time (estimated from survival curves) for the three groups clusters was about 19 weeks ($P > 0.5$). There was no discernible improvement in QOL scores on a 13-point questionnaire, which was administered monthly.

In 1993, Murad and colleagues published a trial in which a modified FAMTX regimen was compared to supportive care in randomized fashion.[261] After the first 22 patients were entered, the trial was interrupted, as the treated patients were enjoying a significantly better outcome. The next 18 patients were assigned directly to treatment. Median survival time for all the treated patients was 10 months versus 3 months for the untreated control group ($P = 0.001$).

Pyrhonen and associates detailed a report of 41 patients randomized to 5-FU, epirubicin, and methotrexate (FEMTX) plus vitamins A and E, versus the same vitamins and best supportive care.[262] In the FEMTX group, 29% had an objective response and 33% had stable disease for longer than 2 months. In the control group, 20% exhibited stable disease. Median time to progression (5.4 months versus 1.7 months, $P = 0.0013$) and median survival time (12.3 months versus 3.1 months, $P = 0.006$) both favored treatment with FEMTX.

Glimelius and coworkers reported 61 patients randomized between chemotherapy with ELF or 5-FU/leucovorin compared to best supportive care.[263] Survival was improved in the treatment group (median 8 months versus 5 months; $P = 0.003$, adjusted) and QOL analysis also favored the treated patients ($P < 0.05$).

Finally, Park and colleagues performed a retrospective analysis of 409 patients with incurable gastric cancer; 202 were treated with a modified FAM regimen and 207 patients were not treated.[264] The 1-year survival rate was 34.1% for the patients treated with FAM versus 22.5% for the control group. Unfortunately, no details on how treatment decisions were made are available in their report.

Novel Agents

Given the limitations of chemotherapy other potential treatment options are being explored. The use of novel agents, either alone or in combination with chemotherapy, has been evaluated in several recent studies. In one of these studies the matrix metalloproteinase inhibitor marimastat was compared to a placebo in a double-blind randomized phase III trial.[265] A total of 369 advanced gastric cancer patients with no more than one prior 5-FU-based chemotherapy regimen were entered into the study. The median survival time (160 days versus 138 days) and the progression-free survival time (102 days versus 84 days) were significantly longer for patients receiving marimastat.

Summary

In summary, it is clear that chemotherapy may result in response rates of up to 50% or more in selected groups of patients with advanced gastric cancer.[141,227-230] Some evidence from recent small trials indicates that chemo-

therapy may prolong survival over patients managed with best supportive care.[262-264] However, median survival times have not clearly changed for treated patients over the last two decades. The intensity of more recent combination regimens has been increased, yet superiority over single-agent 5-FU has yet to be demonstrated. Some of these newer programs require hospitalization to administer.[254] It is not clear that there yet exists a standard treatment for advanced gastric cancer. Investigation of new agents and combinations must continue, and any "new standards" should be tested in controlled clinical trials looking at survival, QOL, and cost analysis end points.

THE FUTURE

Completely Resected Lesions

Many patients with gross complete resection of their gastric cancer are not cured with surgery alone. The final results of the British and Dutch multicenter trials evaluating the value of extended lymphadenectomy demonstrated that the procedure produced greater morbidity with no impact on survival. Because experienced surgeons have performed extended node dissection without significant increases in surgical morbidity or mortality rates,[87,88] use of the procedure is still reasonable in node-positive patients. Such patients will still be at high risk for local-regional and systemic relapse, however, and should receive postoperative chemoradiotherapy (Table 78-17).

With regard to replacement postoperative chemoradiotherapy trials, the U.S. GI Intergroup replacement phase III randomized trial will test 5-FU infusion versus bolus 5-FU leucovorin as the concurrent chemotherapy during EBRT, and will test ECF chemotherapy versus 5-FU leucovorin as the maintenance component of chemotherapy. A phase II trial tested the tolerance of the more aggressive infusion 5-FU and ECF regimen in a multicenter trial involving CALGB institutions together with Mayo Clinic Rochester and Mayo Clinic Scottsdale.[268] The irradiation treatment fields in both the phase II and successor phase III trials will be based on idealized field design related to site of the primary lesion and TN stage of disease.[190]

On the basis of encouraging results with preoperative chemotherapy and chemoradiotherapy for locally advanced or borderline resectable disease, future phase III studies should evaluate preoperative chemotherapy (alone or followed by postoperative chemoradiotherapy) and preoperative chemoradiotherapy in combination with resection for patients with potentially resectable lesions. A randomized phase II study is being conducted by RTOG to evaluate several combinations of preoperative chemoradiotherapy Because some of the newer chemotherapy drug combinations have CR rates of about 20%, the hope is that these regimens will lower systemic relapse rates more than previous combinations. This change has not yet been demonstrated in phase III trials.

TABLE 78-17

Treatment Algorithm for Gastric Cancer, Mayo Clinic Cancer Center

TNM EXTENT*	SURGERY	IRRADIATION (ALONE OR WITH CT)	CHEMOTHERAPY (CT)
T1–2N0M0	Radical subtotal gastrectomy and regional nodes	Not routinely recommended, except posterior wall T2N0M0	NR
T1–2N1–3M0; T3N0–3M0	Radical subtotal and regional nodes	Postop EBRT-CT, 45–50 Gy; evaluate preop EBRT-CT, gastric; *prefer preop EBRT-CT, GE jnctn†*	5-FU/leucovorin bolus wk 1, 5 – CCRT and maintenance (maint); evaluate alternate CCRT and maint CT (see T4)
T4N0–3M0	Radical subtotal and regional nodes; attempt en bloc resection, involved organ(s)	Preop EBRT-CT, 45–50 Gy; attempt resection and IOERT	5-FU-leucovorin, bolus wk 1, 5; evaluate alternate CCRT including infusion 5-FU; evaluate other maint CT (ECF, other)
T_{any}N_{any}M1	Palliative if feasible	Palliative CCRT if indicated	MACT; ICT phase I, II, or III

CCRT, concurrent chemoradiotherapy; EBRT, external beam irradiation; EBRT-CT, external beam irradiation + chemotherapy; ICT, investigational chemotherapy clinical trials; IOERT, intraoperative electron irradiation; MACT, multiagent chemotherapy; postop, postoperative; preop, preoperative; NR, not recommended.
*For TNM definitions, see Table 78-2.
†Prefer preop CRT for gastroesophageal junction cancer (GE jnctn) found to be T1–2N1–3M0 or T3N0–3M0 on EUS, as can usually design safer EBRT fields with preop CRT rather than postop CRT. If transhiatal resection is performed, keeping the reconstructed stomach in the mediastinal midline, postop CRT can be given more safely than if Ivor-Lewis resection is performed.

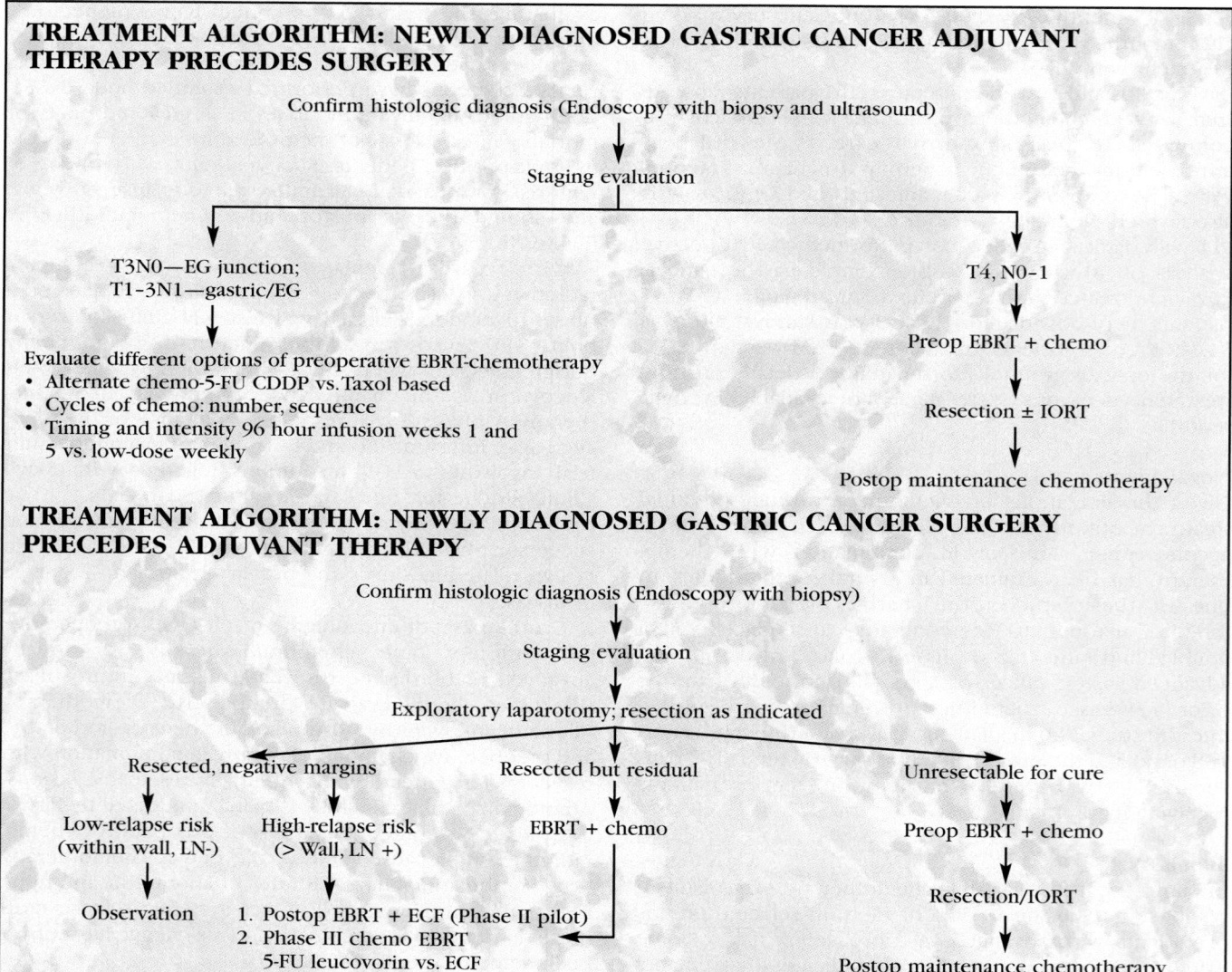

TREATMENT ALGORITHM: NEWLY DIAGNOSED GASTRIC CANCER ADJUVANT THERAPY PRECEDES SURGERY

Confirm histologic diagnosis (Endoscopy with biopsy and ultrasound)

Staging evaluation

T3N0—EG junction;
T1–3N1—gastric/EG

Evaluate different options of preoperative EBRT-chemotherapy
• Alternate chemo-5-FU CDDP vs. Taxol based
• Cycles of chemo: number, sequence
• Timing and intensity 96 hour infusion weeks 1 and 5 vs. low-dose weekly

T4, N0-1

Preop EBRT + chemo

Resection ± IORT

Postop maintenance chemotherapy

TREATMENT ALGORITHM: NEWLY DIAGNOSED GASTRIC CANCER SURGERY PRECEDES ADJUVANT THERAPY

Confirm histologic diagnosis (Endoscopy with biopsy)

Staging evaluation

Exploratory laparotomy; resection as Indicated

Resected, negative margins

Low-relapse risk (within wall, LN-)

Observation

High-relapse risk (> Wall, LN +)

1. Postop EBRT + ECF (Phase II pilot)
2. Phase III chemo EBRT 5-FU leucovorin vs. ECF

Resected but residual

EBRT + chemo

Unresectable for cure

Preop EBRT + chemo

Resection/IORT

Postop maintenance chemotherapy

Locally Advanced Disease (Unresectable for Cure)

For patients with locally advanced disease that appears unresectable for cure, it seems reasonable to build on existing positive segments of treatment data (EBRT plus chemotherapy, IORT, preoperative chemotherapy, preoperative chemoradiotherapy) plus patterns of relapse information. External irradiation plus chemotherapy or IORT with or without EBRT has controlled disease and produced long-term survival in 10% to 20% of patients in most single-institution analyses and randomized trials in patients with residual disease after resection. Neoadjuvant chemotherapy for unresectable disease has resulted in subsequent total resection of disease in 20% to 73% of patients in several European trials with EAP, FAMTX, or other regimens. However, the incidence of subsequent local regional relapse is significant, even after total resection. It would be of interest to merge these components of treatment together.

Following preoperative chemotherapy, patients with marginal gross total or subtotal resection with residual disease or resection but high-risk factors for relapse (beyond the gastric wall, nodes positive, or both) should be placed on studies that evaluate IORT, postoperative EBRT, or both in conjunction with concomitant and maintenance chemotherapy. For patients who are unresectable after preoperative (neoadjuvant) chemotherapy but still have localized tumor on the basis of preoperative staging (including laparoscopy) or exploratory laparotomy, EBRT plus concomitant chemotherapy should be given. Decisions regarding attempts at later resection with or without IORT could be individualized by institution.

An alternate approach is to initiate treatment with preoperative chemoradiotherapy followed by restaging, resection (with or without IORT), and postoperative maintenance chemotherapy. Questions to be addressed with this approach include whether to give several cycles of multiagent chemotherapy prior to initiating concomitant chemoradiotherapy versus start with concomitant chemoradiotherapy, how many cycles of chemotherapy to deliver, and which agents to give both with irradiation and as the systemic component of treatment.

Metastatic Disease

Although newer combination chemotherapy regimens have produced better response rates than single agents, survival has not been enhanced. Clearly, new drugs need to be tested in the treatment of advanced gastric cancer. The topoisomerase I inhibitors and taxanes are being evaluated presently. Alternative approaches such as biologicals, gene therapy, angiogenesis, and metastasis inhibitors are also being or will be evaluated in clinical trials.[259] Traditional phase II studies in advanced gastric cancer have included only patients with measurable indicator lesions. One approach to faster screening of new treatment regimens for future phase III trials in metastatic disease is to utilize survival end points, which allows entry of patients with advanced nonmeasurable disease. The

feasibility of this approach has recently been demonstrated in a phase II NCCTG trial.[260]

Given the limitations of chemotherapy, continued evaluation of novel agents, either alone or in combination with chemotherapy, is indicated. In one novel agent study previously discussed, the matrix metalloproteinase inhibitor marimastat was compared to a placebo in a double-blind randomized phase III trial of 369 advanced gastric cancer patients with no more than one prior 5-FU-based chemotherapy regimen.[265] Median survival and progression-free survival times were significantly longer for patients receiving marimastat, and therefore, further evaluation of this agent as earlier treatment in combination with chemotherapy is indicated.

Treatment Algorithm by TNM Disease Extent (see Table 78-17)

T1–2N0M0

Total surgical resection of the adenocarcinoma with a radical subtotal gastrectomy and reconstruction with gastrojejunostomy is recommended as standard treatment. Neither chemotherapy nor radiotherapy is routinely recommended as single modality adjuvants after resection. Patients with posterior wall T2N0M0 lesions should be evaluated for postoperative adjuvant chemoradiotherapy (see next discussion).

T1–2N1–3M0; T3N0–3M0

Postoperative chemoradiotherapy (CRT) is the preferred treatment based on demonstrated improvement in survival (disease-free and overall) when compared with a surgery-alone control arm in the phase III U.S intergroup trial (INT 0116).[184,185] This approach has become the standard of treatment in the United States for T2N1–3 and T3N0–3 lesions. Preoperative irradiation demonstrated a survival advantage over surgery alone in a phase III trial from Bejing[175] and serves as justification for an RTOG phase II randomized trial of preoperative chemoradiotherapy that is currently being conducted in patients with potentially resectable gastric cancer.

Our institutions prefer the use of *preoperative CRT for gastroesophageal junction cancers* found to be T1–2N1–3M0 or T3N0–3M0 on EUS, as we can usually design safer EBRT fields for preoperative CRT rather than postoperative CRT. If transhiatal resection is performed, keeping the reconstructed stomach in the mediastinal midline, postoperative CRT can be given more safely than if Ivor-Lewis resection is performed.

T4N0–3M0

Preoperative chemoradiotherapy followed by restaging, gross total resection (may include en bloc resection of adjacent organs), and intraoperative electron irradiation (IOERT) is recommended for potentially resectable T4N0–3 lesions. Postoperative chemoradiotherapy has also been used for completely resected lesions.

In locally unresectable T4N0–3M0 gastric cancers, preoperative or primary chemoradiotherapy or multiple drug chemotherapy can be utilized, preferably in the setting of controlled prospective clinical trials. For patients with good performance status, the treatment approach would preferably involve preoperative chemoradiotherapy, restaging and surgical resection with an attempt at marginal gross total resection and IOERT.

TanyNanyMI

Multidrug chemotherapy combinations are the preferred treatment for patients with metastatic cancers. Patients should be placed on controlled trials if available. Palliative irradiation can be used for painful metastatic lesions but is otherwise not indicated. Palliative resection may be indicated for patients with obstruction or bleeding, if total gastrectomy can be avoided.

Nutritional Support during Chemoradiotherapy

Many patients who receive preoperative chemoradio-therapy (with plans to proceed to surgical resection) or primary chemoradiotherapy may require parenteral or enteral hyperalimentation during treatment. This feeding may also be necessary in subsets of borderline perform-ance status patients who are candidates for postoperative chemoradiotherapy. Improvement in nutritional status may require stent placement during endoscopy, feeding jejunostomy, or percutaneous endoscopic gastrostomy (PEG) tube placement. Feeding jejunostomy may be preferable to PEG tube placement for patients receiving preoperative chemoradiotherapy, in order to preserve later use of the stomach for reconstruction.

CONCLUSIONS

In summary, gastric malignancies present a variety of challenges. Innovative combined-modality approaches will be required in order to improve survival with acceptable morbidity. This treatment may include combinations of EBRT plus chemotherapy, IORT, and resection for the local component of disease, systemic or intraperitoneal chemotherapy for the abdominal component, and systemic treatment (chemotherapy, other) for the extra-abdominal risks of relapse. For patients with metastatic disease, the availability of growth factors may allow more aggressive multidrug approaches.

REFERENCES

1. Jemal A, Murray T, Samuels A, et al: Cancer statistics 2003. CA Cancer J Clin 2003;53:5.
2. Jemal A, Thomas A, Murray T, Thun M: Cancer statistics 2002. CA Cancer J Clin 2002;52:23.
3. Coggon D, Barker DJP, Cole RB, Nelson M: Stomach cancer and food storage. J Natl Cancer Inst 1989;81:1178.
4. Howson CP, Hiyama T, Wynder EL: The decline in gastric cancer: Epidemiology of an unplanned triumph. Epidemiol Rev 1986;8:1.
5. Offerhaus GJA, Stadt J, Huibregtse K, et al: The mucosa of the gastric remnant harboring malignancy. Cancer 1989;64:698.
6. Lacaine F, Houry S, Huguier M: Stomach cancer after partial gastrectomy for benign ulcer disease. A critical analysis of epidemiological reports. Hepatogastroenterology 1992;39:4.
7. Parsonnet J, Friedman GD, Vanderstern DP, et al: *Helicobacter pylori* infection and the risk of gastric carcinoma. N Engl J Med 1991;325:1127.
8. Talley NJ, Zinmeister AR, Weaver A, et al: Gastric adenocarcinoma and *Helicobacter pylori* infection. J Natl Cancer Inst 1991;83:1734.
9. Fuchs CS, Mayer RJ: Gastric carcinoma. N Engl J Med 1995;333:32.
10. Prolla J, Kobayashi S, Kirsner J: Gastric cancer: some recent improvements in diagnosis based on the Japanese experience. Arch Intern Med 1969;124:238.
11. Chun YS, Lindor NM, Smyrk TC, et al: Germline E-cadherin gene mutations. Is prophylactic total gastrectomy indicated? Cancer 2001;92:181.
12. Huntsman DG, Carneiro F, Lewis FR, et al: Early gastric cancer in young, asymptomatic carriers of germline E-cadherin mutations. N Engl J Med 2001;344:1904.
13. Lewis FR, Mellinger JD, Hayashi A, et al: Prophylactic total gastrectomy for familial gastric cancer. Surgery 2001;130:612.
14. Hermann RE: Newer concepts in the treatment of cancer of the stomach. Surgery 1993;113:361.
15. Lauren P: The two histologic main types of gastric carcinoma: Diffuse and so-called intestinal type carcinoma. An attempt at a histological classification. Acta Pathol Microbiol Scand 1965;64:31.
16. Borrmann R: Geschwulste des Magens und Duodenums. In Henke F, Lanbarsch O (eds): Handbuch der Speziellen Pathologischen Anatomie and Histologie, Vol 4. Berlin, Julius Springer, 1926.
17. Japanese Research Society for Gastric Cancer: The general rules for the gastric cancer study in surgery and pathology. Part I. Clinical classification. Jpn J Surg 1981;11:127.
18. Jauch KW, Heiss MM, Gruetzner U, et al: Prognostic significance of bone marrow micrometastases in patients with gastric cancer. J Clin Oncol 1996;14:1810.
19. Heiss MM, Allgayer H, Gruetzner KU, et al: Clinical value of extended biologic staging by bone marrow micrometastases and tumor-associated proteases in gastric cancer. Ann Surg 1997;226:736.
20. Dockerty MB: Pathologic aspects of primary malignant neoplasms of the stomach. In ReMine WH, Priestley JT, Berkson J (eds): Cancer of the Stomach. Philadelphia, WB Saunders, 1964, p 173.
21. Kennedy BJ: TNM classification for stomach cancer. Cancer 1970;26:971.
22. Gunderson LL, Sosin H: Adenocarcinoma of the stomach: areas of failure in a reoperation series (second or symptomatic looks): Clinicopathologic correlation and implications for adjuvant therapy. Int J Radiat Oncol Biol Phys 1982;8:1.
23. Nagatomo T, Murakami E, Kondo K: Histologic criteria of serosal rupture and prognosis in gastric carcinoma. Cancer 1969;29:180.
24. Roder JD, Bottcher K, Busch R, et al: Classification of regional lymph node metastasis from gastric carcinoma. Cancer 1998;82:621.
25. Ishida K, Katsuyama T, Sugiyama A, Kawasaki S: Immunohisto-chemical evaluation of lymph node micrometastases from gastric carcinomas. Cancer 1997;79:1069.
26. Dent DM, Werner ID, Novis B, et al: Prospective randomized trial of combined oncological therapy for gastric carcinoma. Cancer 1979;44:385.
27. Maruta K, Shida H: Some factors which influence prognosis after surgery for advanced gastric cancer. Ann Surg 1968;167:313.
28. Tsukiyama I, Akine Y, Kajiura Y, et al: Radiation therapy for advanced gastric cancer. Int J Radiat Oncol Biol Phys 1988;15:123.
29. MacDonald WC, MacDonald JB: Adenocarcinoma of the esophagus and/or gastric cardia. Cancer 1987;60:1094.
30. Meyers WC, Damiano RJ, Postlethwait RW, Rotolo FS: Adeno-carcinoma of the stomach: Changing patterns over the last four decades. Ann Surg 1987;205:1.
31. Yamada Y, Kato Y: Greater tendency for submucosal invasion in fundic area gastric carcinomas than those arising in the pyloric area. Cancer 1989;63:1757.
32. Fein R, Kelsen DP, Geller N, et al: Adenocarcinoma of the esoph-agus and gastroesophageal junction: Prognostic factors and results of therapy. Cancer 1985;56:2512.
33. Hartley LC, Evans E, Windsor CJ: Factors influencing prognosis in gastric cancer. Aust NZ J Surg 1987;57:5.
34. Nanus DM, Kelsen DP, Niedzwiecki D, et al: Flow cytometry as a predictive indicator in patients with operable gastric cancer. J Clin Oncol 1989;7:1105.

35. Tsushima K, Nagorney DM, Cha SS, Reiman HM: Correlation of DNA ploidy, histopathology, stage, and clinical outcome in gastric carcinoma. Surg Oncol 1992;1:17.

36. Baba H, Korenaga D, Okamura T, et al: Prognostic significance of DNA content with special reference to age in gastric cancer. Cancer 1989;63:1768.

37. Korenaga D, Okamura T, Saito A, et al: DNA ploidy is closely linked to tumor invasion, lymph node metastasis, and prognosis in clinical gastric cancer. Cancer 1988;62:309.

38. Harrison JD, Morris DL, Ellis IO, et al: The effect of tamoxifen and estrogen receptor status on survival in gastric carcinoma. Cancer 1989;64:1007.

39. Sugiyama K, Yonemura Y, Miyazaki I: Immunohistochemical study of epidermal growth factor and epidermal growth factor receptor in gastric carcinoma. Cancer 1989;63:1557.

40. Yonemura Y, Ninomiya I, Ohoyama S, et al: Expression of e-erb B-2 oncoprotein in gastric carcinoma. Immunoreactivity for e-erb B-2 protein is an independent indicator of poor short-term prognosis in patients with gastric carcinoma. Cancer 1991;67:2914.

41. Hiton DA, West KP: An evaluation of the prognostic significance of HLA-DR expression in gastric carcinoma. Cancer 1990;66:1154.

42. Pollack BT, Chak A, Sivak MN Jr: Endoscopic ultrasonography. Semin Oncol 1996;23:336.

43. Wang J-Y, Hsieh J-S, Juang Y-S, et al: Endoscopic ultrasonography for preoperative locoregional staging and assessment of resectability in gastric cancer. Clin Imaging 1998;22:355.

44. Willis S, Truong S, Gribbritz S et al: Endoscopic ultrasonography in the preoperative staging of gastric cancer. Accuracy and impact on surgical therapy. Surg Endosc 2000;14:951.

45. Molloy RG, McCourtney JS, Anderson JR: Laparoscopy in the management of patients with cancer of the gastric cardia and oesophagus. Br J Surg 1995;82:352.

46. Stell DA, Carter CR, Stewart I, Anderson JR: Prospective comparison of laparoscopy, ultrasonography and computed tomography in the staging of gastric cancer. Br J Surg 1996;83:1260.

47. D'Ugo DM, Coppola R, Persiani R, et al: Immediately preoperative laparoscopic staging for gastric cancer. Surg Endosc 1996;10:996.

48. Burke EC, Karpeh MS Jr, Conlon KC, Brennan MF: Laparoscopy in the management of gastric adenocarcinoma. Ann Surg 1997;225:262.

49. Greene FL, Page DL, Fleming ID, et al: AJCC Cancer Staging Manual, 6th ed. New York, Springer Verlag, 2002, p 99.

50. Ichikura T., Tomimatsu S, Uefuji K, et al: Evaluation of the new American Joint Committee on Cancer/International Union against Cancer classification of lymph node metastasis from gastric carcinoma in comparison with the Japanese classification. Cancer 1999;86:553.

51. Hayashi H, Ochiai T, Suzuke T, et al: Superiority of a new UICC-TNM staging system for gastric carcinoma. Surgery 2000;127:129.

52. Bozzetti F, Marubini E, Bonfanti G, et al: Total versus subtotal gastrectomy. Surgical morbidity and mortality rates in a multicenter Italian randomized trial. Ann Surg 1997;226:613.

53. Harrison LE, Karpeh MS, Brennan MF: Total gastrectomy is not necessary for proximal gastric cancer. Surgery 1998;123:127.

54. Abe S, Yoshimura H, Nagaoka S, et al: Long-term results of operation for carcinoma of the stomach in T1/T2 stages: critical evaluation of the concept of early carcinoma of the stomach. J Am Coll Surg 1995;181:389.

55. Dupont JB Jr, Lee JR, Burton GR, et al: Adenocarcinoma of the stomach: Review of 1497 cases. Cancer 1978;41:941.

56. ReMine WH, Priestley JT, Berkson J: Cancer of the Stomach. Philadelphia, WB Saunders, 1964.

57. Serlin O, Keehn RJ, Higgins GA, et al: Factors related to survival following resection for gastric carcinoma. Cancer 1977;40:1318.

58. Sugimachi K, Kodama Y, Kumashiro R, et al: Critical evaluation of prophylactic splenectomy in total gastrectomy for stomach cancer. Gan To Kagaku Ryoho 1980;71:704.

59. Takahashi T, Sogabe K, Ichikawa J, et al: Examination of combined resection of the tail of the pancreas and spleen in advanced cancer of upper and mid stomach. In Proceedings of the 35th Meeting of the Japanese Research Society on Gastric Cancer, 1980.

60. Noguchi Y, Imada T, Matsumoto A, et al: Radical surgery for gastric cancer. A review of the Japanese experience. Cancer 1989;64:2053.

61. Wanebo HJ, Kennedy BJ, Winchester DP, et al: Role of splenectomy in gastric cancer surgery: Adverse effect of elective splenectomy on longterm survival. J Am Coll Surg 1997;185:177.

62. Iriyama K, Asukawa T, Koike H, et al: Is extensive lymphadenectomy necessary for surgical treatment of intramusocal carcinoma of the stomach? Arch Surg 1989;124:309.

63. Bolen T, Nakane Y, Okusa T, et al: Strategy for lymphadenectomy of gastric cancer. Surgery 1989;105:585.

64. Maruyama K, Gunven P, Okabayashi K, et al: Lymph node metastases of gastric cancer. General pattern in 1931 patients. Ann Surg 1989;210:596.

65. Kitagawa Y, Fujii H, Mukai M, et al: Radio-guided sentinel node detection for gastric cancer. Br J Surg 2002;89:604.

66. Douglass HO, Nava HR: Gastric adenocarcinoma: management of the primary disease. Semin Oncol 1985;12:32.

67. Kodama Y, Sugimachi K, Soejima K, et al: Evaluation of extensive lymph node dissection for carcinoma of the stomach. World J Surg 1981;5:241.

68. Okajima K: Surgical treatment of gastric cancer with specific reference to lymph node removal. Acta Med Okayama 1977;31:369.

69. Shiu MH, Moore E, Sanders M, et al: Influence of the extent of resection on survival after curative treatment of gastric carcinoma. Arch Surg 1987;122:1347.

70. Soja J, Ohyama S, Miyashita K, et al: A statistical evaluation of advancement in gastric cancer surgery with special reference to the significance of lymphadenectomy for cure. World J Surg 1988;12:398.

71. Otsuji E, Yamaguchi T, Sawai K, et al: Recent advances in surgical treatment have improved the survival of patients with gastric carcinoma. Cancer 1998;82:1233.

72. Kern KA: Gastric cancer: A neoplastic enigma. J Surg Oncol 1989;1(Suppl):34.

73. Haas CD, Mansfield CM, Leichman LP, et al: Combined non-simultaneous radiation therapy and chemotherapy with 5-FU, doxorubicin and mitomycin for residual localized gastric adenocarcinoma. A Southwest Oncology Group pilot study. Cancer Treat Rep 1983;67:421.

74. Dent DM, Madden MV, Price SK: Randomized comparison of R_1 and R_2 gastrectomy for gastric carcinoma. Br J Surg 1988;75:110.

75. Bonenkamp JJ, Hermans J, van de Velde CJH, for the Dutch Gastric Cancer Group: Extended lymph-node dissection for gastric cancer. N Engl J Med 1999;340:908.

76. Bonenkamp JJ, Songun I, Hermans J, et al: Randomized comparison of morbidity after D1 and D2 dissection for gastric cancer in 996 Dutch patients. Lancet 1995;345:745.

77. Sasako M: Risk factors for surgical treatment in the Dutch gastric cancer trial. Br J Surg 1997;84:1567.

78. Cuschieri A, Fayers P, Fielding J, et al: Postoperative morbidity and mortality after D_1 and D_2 resections for gastric cancer: Preliminary results of the MRC randomised controlled surgical trial. Lancet 1996;347:995.

79. Cushieri A, Weeden S, Fielding J, et al: Patient survival after D1 and D2 resections for gastric cancer: long-term results of the MRC randomized controlled surgical trial. Br J Cancer 1999;79:1522.

80. Brennan MF: Radical surgery for gastric cancer. A review of the Japanese experience. Cancer 1989;64:2063.

81. Karpeh MS, Leon L, Klimstra D, Brennen MF: Lymph node staging in gastric cancer: Is location more important than number? An analysis of 1038 patients. Ann Surg 2000;232:362

82. Hundahl SA, Phillips JL, Menck HR: The National Cancer Data Base report on poor survival of U.S. gastric carcinoma patients treated with gastrectomy. American Joint Committee on Cancer staging, proximal disease, and the "different disease" hypothesis. Cancer 2000;88:921.

83. Bunt AMG, Hermans J, Smit VTHBM, et al: Surgical/pathologic-stage migration confounds comparison of gastric cancer survival rates between Japan and Western countries. J Clin Oncol 1995;13:19.

84. Bunt AMG, Hermans J, van de Velde CJH, et al: Lymph node retrieval in a randomized trial on Western-type versus Japanese-type surgery in gastric cancer. J Clin Oncol 1996;14:2289.

85. Imada T, Noguchi Y, Abe M, et al: Lymph node metastases in gastric cancer. Eur Surg Res 1986;19(Suppl 1):90.

86. Douglass HO, Clark JL, Barcewicz P, et al: Importance of the R₂ lymph node dissection in the surgical treatment of gastric cancer. Proc Am Soc Clin Oncol 1989;8:101.

87. de Aretxabala X, Konishi K, Yonemura Y, et al: Node dissection in gastric cancer. Br J Surg 1987;74:770.

88. Smith JW, Shin MH, Kelsey L, Brennan MF: Morbidity of radical lymphadenectomy in the curative resection of gastric carcinoma. Arch Surg 1991;126:1469.

89. Miyata M, Yokoyama Y, Okoyama N, et al: What are the appropriate indications for endoscopic mucosal resection for early gastric cancer? Analysis of 256 endoscopically resected lesions. Endoscopy 2000;32:773.

90. Ono H, Kondo H, Gotoda T, et al: Endoscopic mucosal resection for treatment of early gastric cancer. Gut 2001;48:225.

91. Adachi Y, Mori M, Sujimachi K: Persistence of mucosal gastric carcinomas for 8 and 6 years in two patients. Arch Pathol Lab Med 1990;114:1046.

92. Macintyre DMC, Akoh JA: Improving survival in gastric cancer: Review of operation mortality in English language publications from 1970. Br J Surg 1981;78:773.

93. Heberer G, Teichmann RK, Krämling HJ, Günther B: Results of gastric resection for carcinoma of the stomach: The European experience. World J Surg 1988;12:374.

94. Green PH, O'Toole KM, Slonim D, et al: Increasing incidence and excellent survival of patients with early gastric cancer: Expression in a United States Medical Center. Am J Med 1998;85:658.

95. Itoh H, Oohata Y, Nakamura K, et al: Complete ten-year postgastrectomy follow-up of early gastric cancer. Am J Surg 1989;158:14.

96. Endo M, Habu H: Clinical studies of early gastric cancer. Hepatogastroenterology 1990;37:408.

97. de Dombral FT, Price AB, Thompson H, et al: The British Society of Gastroenterology early gastric cancer/dysplasia survey: An interim report. Gut 1990;3:115.

98. Gentsch HH, Groitl H, Geidl J: Results of surgical treatment of early gastric cancer in 113 patients. World J Surg 1981;5:103.

99. Farley DR, Donohue JH, Nagorney DM, et al: Early gastric cancer. Br J Surg 1992;79:539.

100. Jentschura D, Heubner C, Manegold BC, et al: Surgery for early gastric cancer: A European one-center experience. World J Surg 1997;21:845.

101. Majus WC, Damiano RJ Jr, Rotolo FS, et al: Adenocarcinoma of the stomach: Changing patterns over the last four decades. Ann Surg 1987;205:1.

102. Cady B, Rossi RL, Silverman ML, et al: Gastric adenocarcinoma: A disease in transition. Arch Surg 1989;124:303.

103. Nakamura K, Keyama T, Yao T, et al: Pathology and prognosis of gastric carcinoma. Findings in 10,000 patients who underwent primary gastrectomy. Cancer 1992;70:1030.

104. Papachristou DN, Fortner JG: Local recurrence of gastric adenocarcinomas after gastrectomy. J Surg Oncol 1981;18:47.

105. Landry J, Tepper J, Wood W, et al: Analysis of survival and local control following surgery for gastric cancer. Int J Radiat Oncol Biol Phys 1990;19:1357.

106. Horn RC: Carcinoma of the stomach. Autopsy findings in untreated cases. Gastroenterology 1955;29:515.

107. McNeer G, Vandenberg H, Donn FY, Bowden LA: A critical evaluation of subtotal gastrectomy for the cure of the stomach. Ann Surg 1957;134:2.

108. Stout AP: Pathology of carcinoma of the stomach. Arch Surg 1943;46:807.

109. Thomson FB, Robins RE: Local recurrence following subtotal resection for gastric carcinoma. Surg Gynecol Obstet 1952;95:341.

110. Wisbeck WA, Becker EM, Russell AH: Adenocarcinoma of the stomach: Autopsy observations with therapeutic implications for the radiation oncologist. Radiother Oncol 1986;7:13.

111. Gilbertson VA: Results of treatment of stomach cancer: An appraisal of efforts for more extensive surgery and a report of 1,938 cases. Cancer 1969;23:1305.

112. MacDonald JS, Steele G, Gunderson LL: Carcinoma of the stomach. In DeVita V, Hellman S, Rosenberg SA (eds): Principles and Practices of Oncology, 2nd ed. Philadelphia, JB Lippincott, 1989, p 765.

113. Moertel CG: Alimentary tract cancer. In Holland J, Frei E (eds): Cancer Medicine. Philadelphia, Lea & Febiger, 1982, p 1753.

114. O'Connell MJ: Current status of chemotherapy for advanced pancreatic and gastric cancer. J Clin Oncol 1985;3:1032.

115. Dixon WJ, Longmire WP, Holden J: Use of triethylenethio-phosphoramide as an adjuvant to the surgical treatment of gastric and colorectal carcinoma: Ten-year follow-up. Ann Surg 1971;173:26.

116. Serlin O, Wolkoff JS, Amadeo JM, Keehn RJ: Use of 5-fluorodeoxyuridine (FUDR) as an adjuvant to the surgical management of carcinoma of the stomach. Cancer 1969;24:223.

117. Moertel CG, Mittleman JA, Bakermeier RF, et al: Sequential and combination chemotherapy of advanced gastric cancer. Cancer 1976;38:678.

118. The Gastrointestinal Tumor Study Group: Adjuvant chemotherapy following resection for gastric cancer. Cancer 1982;49:1116.

119. Higgins GA, Amadeo JH, Smith DE, et al: Efficacy of prolonged intermittent therapy with combined 5-FU and methyl CCNU following resection for gastric carcinoma: Veterans Administration Surgical Oncology Group report. Cancer 1983;52:1105.

120. Engstrom PF, Lavin PT, Douglas HO, Brunner KW: Postoperative adjuvant 5-FU plus methyl CCNU therapy for gastric cancer patients: Eastern Cooperative Oncology Study Group 3275. Cancer 1985;55:1868.

121. Italian Gastrointestinal Tumor Study Group: Adjuvant treatments following curative resection for gastric cancer. Br J Surg 1988;75:1100.

122. Schlag P: Adjuvant chemotherapy in gastric cancer. World J Surg 1987;11:473.

123. Krook JE, O'Connell MJ, Wieand HS, et al: A prospective, randomized evaluation of intensive-course 5-fluorouracil plus doxorubicin as surgical adjuvant chemotherapy for resected gastric cancer. Cancer 1991;67:2454.

124. Estrada E, Lacave AJ, Valle M, et al: Methyl-CCNU, 5-fluorouracil and Adriamycin (MeFA) as adjuvant chemotherapy in gastric cancer. Proc Am Soc Clin Oncol 1988;7:358.

125. Coombes RC, Schein PS, Chilvers CE, et al: A randomized trial comparing adjuvant fluorouracil, doxorubicin, and mitomycin with no treatment in operable gastric cancer. J Clin Oncol 1990;8:1362.

126. MacDonald JS, Fleming TR, Peterson RF, et al: Adjuvant chemotherapy with 5-FU, Adriamycin, and mitomycin-C (FAM) versus surgery alone for patients with locally advanced gastric adenocarcinoma: a Southwest Oncology Group study. Ann Surg Oncol 1995;2:488.

127. Lise M, Nitti D, Marchet A, et al: Final results of a phase III clinical trial of adjuvant chemotherapy with the modified fluorouracil, doxorubicin, and mitomycin regimen in resectable gastric cancer. J Clin Oncol 1995;13:2757.

128. Allum WH, Hallissey MT, Ward LC, Hockey MS: For the British Stomach Cancer Group: A controlled, prospective, and randomised trial of adjuvant chemotherapy or radiotherapy in resectable gastric cancer: interim report. Br J Cancer 1989;60:739.

129. Hallissey MT, Dunn JA, Ward LC, et al: The second British Stomach Cancer Group trial of adjuvant radiotherapy or chemotherapy in resectable gastric cancer: Five-year follow-up. Lancet 1994;343:1309.

130. Tsavaris N, Tentas K, Dosmidis P, et al: A randomized trial comparing adjuvant fluorouracil, epirubicin, and mitomycin with no treatment in operable gastric cancer. Chemotherapy 1996;42:220.

131. Wils J, Nitti D, Guimaraes-Dos-Santos J, et al: Randomized phase III studies of adjuvant chemotherapy with FAMTX or FEMTX in resected gastric cancer. Pooled results of studies from the EORTC GI-group and the ICCG. Proc Am Soc Clin Oncol 2002;21:131a.

132. Hugier M, Destroyes JP, Baschet C, et al: Gastric carcinoma treated by chemotherapy after resection. A controlled study. Am J Surg 1980;139:197.

133. Rake MO, Mallinson CN, Cocking BJ, et al: Assessment of the value of cytotoxic therapy in the treatment of carcinoma of the stomach. Gut 1976;17:832.

134. Allum WH, Hallissey MT, Kelly KA: Adjuvant chemotherapy in operable gastric cancer. Five-year follow-up of first British Stomach Cancer Group trial. Lancet 1989;1:571.

135. Jakesz R, Dittrich C, Funovics J, et al: The effect of adjuvant chemotherapy in gastric carcinoma is dependent on tumor histology: 5-year results of a prospective randomized trial. Recent Results Cancer Res 1988;110:44.

136. Alcobendas F, Mills A, Estape J, et al: Mitomycin C as an adjuvant in resected gastric cancer. Ann Surg 1983;198:13.

137. Estape J, Grau JJ, Alcobendas F, et al: Mitomycin-C as an adjuvant treatment to resected gastric cancer. A 10-year follow-up. Ann Surg 1991;213:219.

138. Grau JJ, Estape J, Alcobendas F, et al: Positive results of adjuvant mitomycin-C in resected gastric cancer: A randomized trial on 134 patients. Eur J Cancer 1993;29A:340.

139. Carrato A, Diaz-Rubio E, Medrano J, et al: Phase III trial of surgery versus adjuvant chemotherapy with mitomycin C and tegafur plus uracil, starting within the first week after surgery for gastric adenocarcinoma. Proc Am Soc Clin Oncol 1995;14:198.

140. Neri B, Cini G, Andreoli F, et al: Randomized trial of adjuvant chemotherapy versus control after curative resection for gastric cancer: 5-year follow-up. Br J Cancer 2001;84:878.

141. Cirera L, Balil A, Batiste-Alentorn E, et al: Randomized clinical trial of adjuvant mitomycin plus tegafur in patients with resected stage III gastric cancer. J Clin Oncol 1999;17:3810.

142. Bajetta E, Buzzoni R, Mariani L, et al: Adjuvant chemotherapy in gastric cancer: 5-year results of a randomised study by the Italian Trials in Medical Oncology (ITMO) Group. Ann Oncol 2002; 13:299.

143. Maehara Y, Moriguchi S, Sakaguchi Y, et al: Adjuvant chemotherapy enhances long-term survival of patients with advanced gastric cancer following curative resection. J Surg Oncol 1990;45:169.

144. Inokuchi K, Hattori T, Taguchi T, et al: Postoperative adjuvant chemotherapy for gastric carcinoma. Analysis of data on 1805 patients followed for 5 years. Cancer 1984;53:2393.

145. Imanaga H, Nakazato H: Results of surgery for gastric cancer and effect of adjuvant mitomycin-C on cancer recurrence. World J Surg 1977;1:213.

146. Nakajima T, Fukami A, Ohashi I, Kajitani T: Long-term follow-up study of gastric cancer patients treated with surgery and adjuvant chemotherapy with mitomycin C. Int J Clin Pharmacol 1978; 16:209.

147. Nakajima T, Fukami A, Takagi K, Kajitani T: Adjuvant chemotherapy with mitomycin C, and with a multi-drug combination of mitomycin C, 5-fluorouracil and cytosine arabinoside after curative resection of gastric cancer. Jpn J Clin Oncol 1980;10:187.

148. Nakajima T, Takahashi T, Takagi K, et al: Comparison of 5-fluorouracil with Ftorafur in adjuvant chemotherapies with combined inductive and maintenance therapies for gastric cancer. J Clin Oncol 1984;2:1366.

149. Nakajima T, Nashimoto A, Kitamura M, et al: Adjuvant mitomycin and fluorouracil followed by oral uracil plus tegafur in serosa-negative gastric cancer: a randomised trial. Gastric Cancer Surgical Study Group. Lancet 1999;354:273.

150. Chou FF, Sheen-Chen SM, Liu PP, et al: Adjuvant chemotherapy for resectable gastric cancer: a preliminary report. J Surg Oncol Suppl 1994;57:239.

151. Ochiai T, Sato H, Hayashi R, et al: Postoperative adjuvant immunotherapy of gastric cancer with BCG-cell wall skeleton. Three- to six-year follow-up of a randomized clinical trial. Cancer Immunol Immunother 1983;14:167.

152. Niimoto M, Saeki T, Toi M, et al: Prospective randomized controlled study on bestatin in resectable gastric cancer. Third report. Jpn J Surg 1990;20:186.

153. Hattori T, Niimoto M, Toge T, et al: Effects of levamisole in adjuvant immunochemotherapy for gastric cancer: A prospective random-ized controlled study. Jpn J Surg 1983;13:480.

154. Niimoto M, Hattori T, Tamada R, et al: Postoperative adjuvant immunochemotherapy with mitomycin-C, futraful and PSK for gastric cancer. An analysis of data on 579 patients followed for five years. Jpn J Surg 1988;18:681.

155. Ochiai T, Sato H, Sato H, et al: Randomly controlled study of chemotherapy versus chemoimmunotherapy in postoperative gastric cancer patients. Cancer Res 1983;43:3001.

156. Nakajima T: Adjuvant chemotherapy for gastric cancer in Japan: Present status and suggestions for rational clinical trials. Jpn J Clin Oncol 1990;20:30.

157. Davis PA, Sano T: The difference in gastric cancer between Japan, USA and Europe: What are the facts? What are the suggestions? Crit Rev Oncol Hematol 2001;40:77.

158. Panzini I, Gianni L, Fattori PP, et al: Adjuvant chemotherapy in gastric cancer: A meta-analysis of randomized trials and a comparison with previous meta-analyses. Tumori 2002;88:21.

159. Janunger KG, Hafstrom L, Nygren P, et al: A systematic overview of chemotherapy effects in gastric cancer. Acta Oncol 2001;40:309.

160. Gianni L, Panzini I, Tassinari D, et al: Meta-analyses of randomized trials of adjuvant chemotherapy in gastric cancer. Ann Oncol 2001;12:1179.

161. Hermans J, Bonenkamp JJ, Boon MC, et al: Adjuvant therapy after curative resection for gastric cancer: Meta-analysis of randomized trials. J Clin Oncol 1993;11:1441.

162. Hermans J, Bonenkamp H: Meta-analysis of adjuvant chemotherapy in gastric cancer: A critical reappraisal. J Clin Oncol 1994;12:879.

163. Earle CC, Maroun JA: Adjuvant chemotherapy after curative resection for gastric cancer in non-Asian patients: Revisiting a meta-analysis of randomised trials. Eur J Cancer 1999;35:1059.

164. Mari E, Floriani I, Tinazzi A, et al: Efficacy of adjuvant chemotherapy after curative resection for gastric cancer: A meta-analysis of published randomised trials. A study of the GISCAD (Gruppo Italiano per lo Studio dei Carcinomi dell'Apparato Digerente). Ann Oncol 2000;11:837.

165. Atiq OT, Kelsen DP, Shiu MH, et al: Phase II trial of postoperative adjuvant intraperitoneal cisplatin and fluorouracil and systemic fluorouracil chemotherapy in patients with resected gastric cancer. J Clin Oncol 1993;11:425.

166. Sautner T, Hofbauer F, Depisch D, et al: Adjuvant intraperitoneal cisplatin chemotherapy does not improve long-term survival after surgery for advanced gastric cancer. J Clin Oncol 1994;12:970.

167. Takahashi T, Hagiwara A, Shimotsuma M, et al: Prophylaxis and treatment of peritoneal carcinomatosis: Intraperitoneal chemotherapy with mitomycin C bound to activated carbon particles. World J Surg 1995;19:565.

168. Yu W, Whang I, Suh I, et al: Prospective randomized trial of early postoperative intraperitoneal chemotherapy as an adjuvant to resectable gastric cancer. Ann Surg 1998;228:347.

169. Takahashi M, Abe M: Intraoperative radiotherapy for carcinoma of the stomach. Eur J Surg Oncol 1986;12:247.

170. Chen G, Song S: Evaluation of intraoperative radiotherapy for gastric carcinoma analysis of 247 patients. In Abe M, Takahashi M (eds): Proceedings of Third International IORT Symposium, Kyoto, Japan. New York, Pergamon Press, 1991, p 190.

171. Sindelar WF, Kinsella TJ, Tepper JE, et al: Randomized trial of intraoperative radiotherapy in carcinoma of the stomach. Am J Surg 1993;165:178.

172. Shchepotin IB, Evans SRT, Chorny V, et al: Intensive preoperative radiotherapy with local hyperthermia for the treatment of gastric carcinoma. Surg Oncol 1994;3:37.

173. Talaev MI, Starinskii VV, Kovalev BN, et al: Results of combined treatment of cancer of the gastric antrum and gastric body. Vopr Onkol 1990;36:1485.

174. Kosse VA: Combined treatment of gastric cancer using hypoxic radiotherapy. Vopr Onkol 1990;36:1349.

175. Zhang ZX, Gu XZ, Yin WB, et al: Randomized clinical trial combination on the preoperative irradiation and surgery in the treatment of adenocarcinoma of the gastric cardia (AGC) report on 370 patients. Int J Radiat Oncol Biol Phys 1998;42:929.

176. Gunderson LL, Hoskins B, Cohen AM, et al: Combined modality treatment of gastric cancer. Int J Radiat Oncol Biol Phys 1983;9:965.

177. Gez E, Sulkes A, Yablonsky-Peretz T, Weshler Z: Combined 5-fluorouracil (5-FU) and radiation therapy following resection of locally advanced gastric carcinoma. J Surg Oncol 1986;31:139.

178. Regine WF, Mohuidden M: Impact of adjuvant therapy on locally advanced adenocarcinoma of the stomach. Int J Radiat Oncol Biol Phys 1992;24:921.

179. Whittington R, Coia L, Haller DG, et al: Adenocarcinoma of the esophagus and esophagogastric junction: The effects of single

and combined modalities on the survival and patterns of failure following treatment. Int J Radiat Oncol Biol Phys 1990;19:593.

180. Moertel CG, Childs DS, O'Fallon JR, et al: Combined 5-fluorouracil and radiation therapy as a surgical adjuvant for poor prognosis gastric carcinoma. J Clin Oncol 1984;2:1249.

181. Henning GT, Schild SF, Stafford SL, et al: Results of irradiation or chemo-irradiation following resection of gastric adenocarcinoma. ASTRO abstracts 1997. Int J Radiat Oncol Biol Phys 2000; 46:589.

182. Mehta K, Mohuidden M: Improved local control with adjunctive therapy for cancers of the gastroesophageal junction. Int J Radiat Oncol Biol Phy 1994;30:272.

183. Kalser MH, Ellenberg SS: Pancreatic cancer: adjuvant combined radiation and chemotherapy following curative resection. Arch Surg 1985;120:899.

184. MacDonald JS, Smalley SR, Benedetti J et al: Chemoradiotherapy after surgery compared with surgery alone for adenocarcinoma of the stomach or gastroesophageal junction. N Engl J Med 2001;345:725.

185. Smalley SS, Gunderson L, Tepper J et al: Gastric surgical adjuvant radiotherapy consensus report: Rationale and treatment implementation. Int J Radiat Oncol Biol Phys 2002;52:282.

186. Walsh TN, Noonau N, Hollywood D, et al: A comparison of multimodal therapy and surgery in esophageal adenocarcinoma. N Engl J Med 1996;335:462.

187. Gunderson LL: Gastric cancer—Patterns of relapse after surgical resection. Semin Radiat Oncol 2002;12:150.

188. Gunderson LL, Martenson JA: Gastrointestinal tract radiation tolerance. In Vaeth JM, Meyer JL (eds): Radiation Tolerance of Normal Tissues, Vol 23. Basel, Karger, 1989, p 277.

189. Willett CG, Tepper JE, Orlow EL, Shipley WU: Renal complications secondary to radiation treatment of upper abdominal malignancies. Int J Radiat Oncol Biol Phys 1986;12:1601.

190. Tepper JE, Gunderson LL: Radiation treatment parameters in the adjuvant postoperative therapy of gastric cancer. Semin Radiat Oncol 2002;12:187.

191. Monson JRT, Donohue JH, McIlrath DC, et al: Total gastrectomy for advanced cancer. A worthwhile palliative procedure. Cancer 1991;68:1863.

192. Wieland C, Hymmen U: Megavoltage therapy for malignant gastric tumors. Strahlentherapie 1970;40:20.

193. Takahashi T: Studies on preoperative and postoperative telecobalt therapy in gastric cancer. Nipon Acta Radiol 1964;24:129.

194. Moertel CG, Childs DS Jr, Reitemeier RJ, et al: Combined 5-fluorouracil and supervoltage radiation therapy of locally unresectable gastrointestinal cancer. Lancet 1969;2:865.

195. Holbrook MA: Radiation therapy. Current concepts in cancer. Gastric cancer: Treatment principles. JAMA 1974;228:1289.

196. Schein PS, Novak J (for GITSG): Combined modality therapy (XRT-chemo) versus chemotherapy alone for locally unresectable gastric cancer. Cancer 1982;49:1771.

197. Chevalier TL, Smith FP, Harter WK, Schein PS: Chemotherapy and combined modality therapy for locally advanced and metastatic gastric carcinoma. Semin Oncol 1985;12:46.

198. The Gastrointestinal Tumor Study Group: The concept of locally advanced gastric cancer. Cancer 1990;66:2324.

199. Bleiberg H, Goffin JC, Dalesie O, et al: Adjuvant radiotherapy and chemotherapy in resectable gastric cancer. Eur J Surg Oncol 1989;15:535.

200. O'Connell MJ, Gunderson LL, Moertel CG, et al: A pilot study of intensive combined therapy for locally unresectable gastric cancer. Int J Radiat Oncol Biol Phys 1985;11:1827.

201. Moertel CG, Gunderson LL, Malliard JA, et al: Early evaluation of combined fluorouracil and leucovorin as a radiation enhancer for locally unresectable, residual or recurrent gastrointestinal carcinoma. J Clin Oncol 1994;12:21.

202. Henning GT, Schild SF, Stafford SL, et al: Results of irradiation or chemoirradiation for primary unresectable, locally recurrent or grossly incomplete resection of gastric adenocarcinomas. Int J Radiat Oncol Biol Phys 2000;46:109.

203. Wilke H, Preusser P, Fink U, et al: Preoperative chemotherapy in locally advanced and nonresectable gastric cancer: A phase II study with etoposide, doxorubicin, and cisplatin. J Clin Oncol 1989;7:1318.

204. Preusser P, Wilke H, Achterrath W, et al: Phase II study with the combination etoposide, doxorubicin, and cisplatin in advanced measurable gastric cancer. J Clin Oncol 1989;7:1310.

205. Wilke H, Preusser P, Fink U, et al: Neoadjuvant chemotherapy of primarily unresectable gastric cancer. In Proceedings of the International Conference on Biology and Treatment of Gastrointestinal Malignancies, Frankfurt, Germany, 1992.

206. Plukker JT, Mulder NH, Sleijfer D, et al: Chemotherapy and surgery for locally advanced cancer of the cardia and fundus: Phase II study with methotrexate and 5-fluorouracil. Br J Surg 1991;78:955.

207. Rosen HR, Scheithauer W, Jakesz R, et al: Epirubicin, etoposide, and cisplatin in the treatment of locally advanced, nonresectable gastric carcinomaresults of multicentric pilot study. GI Cancer 1995;1:49.

208. Facchini G, Tortoriello A, Caponigro F, et al: Neoadjuvant chemotherapy in locally advanced gastric cancer: Preliminary results of a phase II trial with a modified FAMTX combination. Oncol Rep 1995;2:727.

209. Lerner A, Gonin R, Stelle GD, et al: Etoposide, doxorubicin, and cisplatin chemotherapy for advanced gastric adenocarcinoma: results of a phase II trial. J Clin Oncol 1992;10:536.

210. Roelofs EJM, Wagener DJT, Conroy T, et al: Phase II study of sequential high-dose methotrexate and 5-fluorouracil alternated with epirubicin and cisplatin in advanced gastric cancer. Ann Oncol 1993;4:426.

211. Yano M, Shiozaki H, Inoue M, et al: Neoadjuvant chemotherapy followed by salvage surgery: Effect on survival of patients with primary noncurative gastric cancer. World J Surg 2002;26:1155.

212. Rougier P, Mahjoubi M, Lasser P, et al: Neoadjuvant chemotherapy in locally advanced gastric carcinoma phase II trial with combined continuous intravenous 5-fluorouracil and bolus cisplatin. Eur J Cancer 1994;30A:1269.

213. Fink U, Schuhmacher C, Stein HJ, et al: Preoperative chemotherapy for stage III-IV gastric carcinoma: Feasibility, response and outcome after complete resection. Br J Surg 1995;82:1248.

214. Alexander HR, Grem JL, Hamilton JM, et al: Thymidylate synthase protein expression. Association with response to neoadjuvant chemotherapy and resection for locally advanced gastric and gastroesophageal adenocarcinoma. Cancer J Sci Am 1995;1:49.

215. Kang YK, Choi DW, Im YH, et al: A phase III randomized comparison of neoadjuvant chemotherapy followed by surgery versus surgery for locally advanced stomach cancer. Proc Am Soc Clin Oncol 1996;15:215.

216. Ajani JA, Ota DM, Jessup JM, et al: Resectable gastric carcinoma. An evaluation of preoperative and postoperative chemotherapy. Cancer 1991;68:1501.

217. Ajani JA, Mayer RJ, Ota DM, et al: Preoperative and postoperative combination chemotherapy for potentially resectable gastric carcinoma. J Natl Cancer Inst 1993;85:1839.

218. Stephens FO, Adams BG, Crea P: Intra-arterial chemotherapy given preoperatively in the management of carcinoma of the stomach. Surg Gynecol Obstet 1986;162:370.

219. Songun I, Keizer HJ, Hermans J, et al: Chemotherapy for operable gastric cancer: Results of the Dutch randomised FAMTX trial. The Dutch Gastric Cancer Group (DGCG). Eur J Cancer 1999;35:558.

220. Kelsen D, Karpeh M, Schwartz G, et al: Neoadjuvant therapy of high-risk gastric cancer: A phase II trial of preoperative FAMTX and postoperative intraperitoneal fluorouracil-cisplatin plus intravenous fluorouracil. J Clin Oncol 1996;14:1818.

221. Crookes P, Leichman CG, Leichman L, et al: Systemic chemotherapy for gastric carcinoma followed by postoperative intraperitoneal therapy. Cancer 1997;79:1767.

222. Fink U, Stien HJ, Schuhmacher C, et al: Neoadjuvant chemotherapy for gastric cancer: Update. World J Surg 1995;19:509.

223. Ajani JA, Mansfield PF, Janjan N, et al: Preoperative chemoradiation therapy in patients with potentially resectable gastric carcinoma: A multi-institional pilot. Proc Am Soc Clin Oncol 1998;17:283a.

224. Ballesta-Lopez C, Bastida-Vila X, Catarci M, et al: Laparoscopic Billroth II distal subtotal gastrectomy with gastric stump suspension for gastric malignancies. Am J Surg 1996;171:289.

225. Smith JW, Brennan MF, Botet JF, et al: Preoperative endoscopic ultrasound can predict the risk of recurrence after operation for gastric carcinoma. J Clin Oncol 1993;11:2380.

226. Goh PMY, Alponat A, Mak K, Kum CK: Early international results of laparoscopic gastrectomies. Surg Endosc 1997;11:650.

227. O'Connell MJ: Current status of chemotherapy for advanced pancreatic and gastric cancer. J Clin Oncol 1985;3:1032.

228. Preusser P, Achterrath W, Wilke H, et al: Chemotherapy of gastric cancer. Cancer Treat Rev 1988;15:257.

229. Findlay M, Cunningham D: Chemotherapy of carcinoma of the stomach. Cancer Treat Rev 1993;19:29.

230. Wils J: The treatment of advanced gastric cancer. Semin Oncol 1996;23:397.

231. Sulkes A, Smyth J, Sessa C, et al: Docetaxel (Taxotere) in advanced gastric cancer: Results of a phase II clinical trial. Br J Cancer 1994;70:380.

232. Kambe M, Wakui A, Nakao I, et al: A late phase II study of irinotecan (CPT-11) in patients with advanced gastric cancer. Proc Am Soc Clin Oncol 1993;12:198.

233. Ajani JA, Fairweather J, Dumas P, et al: A phase II study of Taxol in patients with advanced untreated gastric carcinoma. Proc Am Soc Clin Oncol 1997;16:263a.

234. Kovach JS, Moertel CG, Schutt AJ, et al: A controlled study of combined 1,3-bis-(2-chloroethyl)-1-nitrosourea and 5-fluorouracil therapy for advanced gastric and pancreatic cancer. Cancer 1974;33:563.

235. Moertel CG, Engstrom P, Lavin PT, et al: Chemotherapy of gastric and pancreatic carcinoma. A controlled evaluation of combinations of 5-fluorouracil with nitrosoureas and lactones. Surgery 1979;85:509.

236. MacDonald JS, Schein PS, Wooley PV, et al: 5-Fluorouracil, doxorubicin, and mitomycin (FAM) combination chemotherapy for advanced gastric cancer. Ann Intern Med 1980;93:533.

237. Anderson JR, Cain KC, Gelber RD: Analysis of survival by tumor response. J Clin Oncol 1983;1:710.

238. MacDonald JS, Schnall SF: Adjuvant treatment of gastric cancer. World J Surg 1995;19:221.

239. Cullinan SA, Moertel CG, Fleming TR, et al: A comparison of three chemotherapeutic regimens in the treatment of advanced pancreatic and gastric carcinoma. Fluorouracil versus fluorouracil and doxorubicin versus fluorouracil, doxorubicin, and mitomycin. JAMA 1985;12:2061.

240. DeLisa V, Cocconi G, Tonato M, et al: Randomized comparison of 5-FU alone or combined with carmustine, doxorubicin, and mitomycin (BAFMi) in the treatment of advanced gastric cancer: A phase III trial of the Italian Clinical Research Oncology Group (GOIRC). Cancer Treat Rep 1986;70:481.

241. Kim NK, Park YS, Heo DS, et al: A phase III randomized study of 5-fluorouracil and cisplatin versus 5-fluorouracil, doxorubicin, and mitomycin C versus 5-fluorouracil alone in the treatment of gastric cancer. Cancer 1993;71:3813.

242. Moertel CG, Rubin J, O'Connell MJ, et al: A phase II study of combined 5-fluorouracil, doxorubicin, and cisplatin in the treatment of advanced upper gastrointestinal adenocarcinomas. J Clin Oncol 1986;4:1053.

243. Cullinan SA, Moertel CG, Wieand HS, et al: Controlled evaluation of three drug combination regimens versus fluorouracil alone for the therapy of advanced gastric cancer. J Clin Oncol 1994;12:412.

244. Stahl M, Wilke H, Preusser P, et al: Etoposide, leucovorin, and 5-fluorouracil (ELF) in advanced gastric carcinoma. Final results of a phase II study in elderly patients or patients with cardiac risk. Onkologie 1991;14:314.

245. Van Cutsem E, Filez L, Dewyspelaere J, et al: Etoposide, leucovorin and 5-fluorouracil in advanced gastric cancer: A phase II study. Anticancer Res 1995;15:1079.

246. Chiou TJ, Tung SL, Hsieh RK, et al: Phase II study of the modified regimen of etoposide, leucovorin and 5-fluorouracil for patients with advanced gastric cancer. Jpn J Clin Oncol 1998;28:318.

247. Au E, Koo WH, Tan EH, et al: A phase II trial of etoposide, leucovorin and 5-fluorouracil (ELF) in patients with advanced gastric cancer. J Chemother 1996;8:300.

248. Klein HO: Long-term results with FAMTX (5-fluorouracil, adriamycin, methotrexate) in advanced gastric cancer. Anticancer Res 1989;9:1025.

249. Meyerhardt JA, Fuchs CS: Chemotherapy options for gastric cancer. Semin Radiat Oncol 2002;12:176.

250. Wils JA, Klein HO, Wagner DJT, et al: Sequential high-dose methotrexate and fluorouracil combined with doxorubicin. A step ahead in the treatment of advanced gastric cancer: A trial of the European Organization for Research and Treatment of Cancer Gastrointestinal Tract Cooperative Group. J Clin Oncol 1991;9:827.

251. Kelsen D, Atiq OT, Saltz L, et al: FAMTX versus etoposide, doxorubicin, and cisplatin: A random assignment trial in gastric cancer. J Clin Oncol 1992;10:541.

252. Vanhoefer U, Rougier P, Wilke H, et al: Final results of a randomized phase III trial of sequential high-dose methotrexate, fluorouracil, and doxorubicin versus etoposide, leucovorin, and fluorouracil versus infusional fluorouracil and cisplatin in advanced gastric cancer: A trial of the European Organization for Research and Treatment of Cancer Gastrointestinal Tract Cancer Cooperative Group. J Clin Oncol 2000;18:2648.

253. Findlay M, Cunningham D, Norman A, et al: A phase II study in advanced gastroesophageal cancer using epirubicin and cisplatin in combination with continuous infusion 5-fluorouracil (ECF). Ann Oncol 1994;5:609.

254. Webb A, Cunningham D, Scarffe JH, et al: Randomized trial comparing epirubicin, cisplatin, and fluorouracil versus fluorouracil, doxorubicin, and methotrexate in advanced esophagogastric cancer. J Clin Oncol 1997;15:261.

255. Cocconi G, Mella M, Nironi S, et al: Fluorouracil, doxorubicin, and mitomycin combination versus PELF chemotherapy in advanced gastric cancer: A prospective randomized trial of the Italian Oncology Group for Clinical Research. J Clin Oncol 1994;12:2687.

256. Cascinu S, Labianca R, Alessandroni P, et al: Intensive weekly chemotherapy for advanced gastric cancer using fluorouracil, cisplatin, epi-doxorubicin, 6S-leucovorin, glutathione, and filgrastim: A report from the Italian Group for the Study of Digestive Tract Cancer. J Clin Oncol 1997;15:3313.

257. Ridwelski K, Gebauer T, Fahlke J, et al: Combination chemotherapy with docetaxel and cisplatin for locally advanced and metastatic gastric cancer. Ann Oncol 2001; 12:47.

258. Kornek GV, Raderer M, Schull B, et al: Effective combination chemotherapy with paclitaxel and cisplatin with or without human granulocyte colony-stimulating factor and/or erythropoietin in patients with advanced gastric cancer. Br J Cancer 2002;86:1858.

259. Yamao T, Shirao K, Matsumura Y, et al: Phase I-II study of irinotecan combined with mitomycin-C in patients with advanced gastric cancer. Ann Oncol 2001;12:1729.

260. Kingston RD, Ellis DJ, Powell J, et al: The West Midlands gastric carcinoma chemotherapy trial: Planning and results. Clin Oncol 1978;4:55.

261. Murad AM, Santiago FF, Petroianu A, et al: Modified therapy with 5-fluorouracil, doxorubicin and methotrexate in advanced gastric cancer. Cancer 1993;72:37.

262. Pyrhonen S, Kuitunen T, Nyandoto P, et al: Randomised comparison of fluorouracil, epidoxorubicin and methotrexate (FEMTX) plus supportive care with supportive care alone in patients with non-resectable gastric cancer. Br J Cancer 1995;71:587.

263. Glimelius B, Ekstrom K, Hoffman K, et al: Randomized comparison between chemotherapy plus best supportive care with best supportive care in advanced gastric cancer. Ann Oncol 1977;8:163.

264. Park JO, Chung HC, Cho JY, et al: Retrospective comparison of infusional 5-fluorouracil, doxorubicin, and mitomycin-C (modified FAM) combination chemotherapy versus palliative therapy in treatment of advanced gastric cancer. Am J Clin Oncol 1997;20:484.

265. Bramhall SR, Hallissey MT, Whiting J, et al: Marimastat as maintenance therapy for patients with advanced gastric cancer: A randomised trial. Br J Cancer 2002;86:1864.

266. Waters JS, Ross PJ, Popescu RA, et al: New approaches to the treatment of gastrointestinal cancer. Digestion 1997; 58:508.

267. Burch PA, Keppen MD, Wieand HS, et al: A North Central Cancer Treatment Group phase II trial of 5-FU and high dose levamisole in advance gastric cancer utilizing survival as the primary marker of therapeutic activity. Proc Am Soc Clin Oncol 1994;13:218.

268. Fuchs C, Fitzgerald TJ, Mamon H, et al: Postoperative adjuvant chemoradiation for gastric or gastroesophageal adenocarcinoma using epirubicin, cisplatin and infusional 5-fluorouracil (ECF) before and after 5-FU and radiotherapy: A multicenter pilot study. ASCO abstract #1029. J Clin Oncol 2003;22:257.

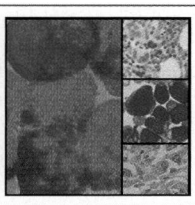

CANCER OF THE SMALL BOWEL

Alessandro Fichera

Fabrizio Michelassi

SUMMARY OF KEY POINTS

INCIDENCE
- Cancers of the small bowel are rare.
- These cancers account for less than 10% of all gastrointestinal tumors and less than 1% of all malignancies; apporoximately 5300 new cases are diagnosed each year, with 1100 cancer-related deaths.

ETIOLOGY AND EPIDEMIOLOGY
- Several factors explain the rarity of these tumors: rapid transit time of carcinogens; carcinogens diluted by gastric, biliary, and pancreatic secretions; small bowel flora being less metabolically active; detoxifying enzymes; immunosurveillance.
- Dietary risk factors for small bowel adenocarcinoma are similar to those for colorectal cancers.
- Increased incidence is seen in Crohn's disease, familial adenomatous polyposis, and hereditary nonpolyposis colorectal cancer and in patients with a prior history of radiation to the abdomen.

PATHOLOGY AND BIOLOGY
- About one third of all small bowel tumors are benign.
- Of the malignant lesions 45% are adenocarcinomas, 30% are carcinoids, 15% are lymphomas, and 10% are sarcomas and gastro-intestinal stromal tumors (GISTs).
- The majority of malignant lesions are located in the duodenum (50% to 60%), followed by the jejunum and ileum.
- Molecular markers for adenocarcinomas include: K-*ras*, p53, c-erbB-2, Ki-67, tenascin, CEA, and CA 19-9.
- For the diagnosis of GIST, KIT immunostaining has become the gold standard and the term *GIST* should apply only to tumors with KIT immunopositivity.

CLINICAL FINDINGS
- Symptoms, when they do occur, tend to be vague and nonspecific and are determined by the tumor's location, growth rate, and size.

STAGING
- Small bowel tumors are staged by the tumor–node–metastasis (TNM) staging system recently published by the American Joint Committee on Cancer (AJCC).
- Small bowel lymphomas are staged by the Ann Arbor system based on lymphatic and extralymphatic involvement on either side of the diaphragm.

PRIMARY THERAPY
- The treatment for localized resectable small bowel tumors is surgical excision with negative margins.
- Depending on the location of the tumor, specifically tailored surgical options are available.
- For primary small bowel lymphoma, para-aortic and mesenteric lymph node sampling, liver biopsy, and bone marrow biopsy should be performed upon surgical exploration.

PROGNOSIS
- Factors associated with poor prognosis for small bowel adenocarcinomas are advanced stage, poor tumor differentiation, extramural venous spread, and positive margins.
- Since the introduction of imatinib mesylate (Gleevec, Novartis), the reported overall or disease-specific 5-year survival rate is 28% to 60% among patients with malignant GISTs; the median disease-specific survival time is about 5 years for primary disease, and 10 to 20 months in recurrent or metastatic disease.

INCIDENCE

Although the small bowel accounts for 75% of the gastrointestinal length and 90% of its absorptive surface, neoplasms of this organ, both benign and malignant, are relatively rare. These tumors represent less than 10% of all gastrointestinal tumors, 1% to 3% of gastrointestinal malignancies, and 0.4% of all malignancies.[1,2] The annual incidence of small bowel cancer is about 5300 cases, with 1100 deaths related to small bowel cancer per year in the United States.[1] Malignant lesions have a slight male predominance[3]; benign tumors occur with roughly equal gender incidence.

Over the last decade, the incidence of two small bowel tumors, lymphomas and gastrointestinal stromal tumors (GISTs), has increased substantially. In the case of primary small bowel lymphomas, incidence in the United States has nearly doubled in the last two decades, due to the increased numbers of immunocompromised patients (i.e., those with acquired immunodeficiency syndrome [AIDS], rheumatoid arthritis, immune disorders in transplant recipients, or congenital immunodeficiency syndromes) and immigrants from third world countries.[4] In the case of GISTs, the recognition of the KIT protein (CD117) has changed the way spindle cell tumors of the gastro-intestinal tract are classified and has led to an increased awareness and recognition. As a consequence, in recent years, the annual incidence of new cases of GIST in the United States has greatly increased.

EPIDEMIOLOGY

The first reports of duodenal adenocarcinoma and small bowel sarcoma were published in the 18th and 19th centuries.[5] Since then many reports and reviews have been published based on autopsy data or single center series. The significance and relevance of these data are limited by the retrospective nature of these studies.

The National Cancer Data Base (NCDB), a joint project of the American College of Surgeons Commission on Cancer and the American Cancer Society, maintains data on as many as 60% of all cancer cases in the United States. It is the main source of epidemiologic data for all cancers, and it represents a particularly useful resource for rare neoplasms, such as small bowel malignancies. Howe and associates reviewed the database for nonampullary small bowel cancers and found 4995 cases for the period between 1985 and 1995.[6] The mean age at presentation was 65 years, with equal incidence in both genders. Upon presentation 32% had evidence of metastatic disease and 26% were locally advanced.[6]

Epidemiologic studies have identified several predisposing conditions associated with small bowel malignancies. Crohn's disease is associated with a 40- to 100-fold increase in relative risk.[7-14] Patients with familial adenomatous polyposis have a 50- to 300-fold increase in relative risk of developing proximal small bowel malignancy, specifically duodenal adenocarcinomas.[15,16] In a recent series, 57% of hereditary nonpolyposis colorectal cancer patients developed small bowel adenocarcinomas as the presenting neoplasm.[17] Other conditions such as blind loop syndrome,[18,19] Peutz-Jeghers syndrome,[20] celiac sprue,[21] neurofibromatosis, and IgA deficiency[18,19] have been associated with an increased risk of small bowel malignancy.

ETIOLOGY AND PATHOGENESIS

The disproportion between the rarity of malignant tumors of the small bowel in comparison to the size of its surface area suggests a significant sparing from or resistance to the development of malignancy. Indeed, several hypotheses, based on experimental animal models,[18,19] have postulated that carcinogens in the enteric content may be in contact with small bowel mucosa over a limited time due to the relatively rapid transit time or may be in a diluted and less carcinogenic form. The preponderance of small bowel adenocarcinomas in the duodenum suggests a role for bile or pancreatic secretions either as primary small bowel carcinogens or even as simple vectors for unknown carcinogens.[22] The fact that biliary diversion decreases the incidence of chemically induced small bowel malignancy in animal models supports a role for bile in small bowel carcinogenesis.[23]

Other specific characteristics of the small bowel microscopic and chemical environment might be responsible for the observed cancer resistance. The limited and metabolically inactive bacterial flora of the small bowel is likely unable to transform procarcinogens into their active metabolites,[24] especially in an alkaline milieu. In addition, the proximal small bowel secretes a number of enzyme systems (i.e., benzopyrene hydroxylase)[25,26] that detoxify carcinogens.

Finally, the presence of a high concentration of B cells and lymphocytes and high amounts of secretory immunoglobulin A (IgA) in the distal small bowel might constitute an effective local immunosurveillance system that prevents carcinogenesis and explains the rarity of distal small bowel neoplasms. This theory seems to be supported by the observation that immunocompromised patients (i.e., those with AIDS, rheumatoid arthritis, immune disorders in transplant recipients, or congenital immunodeficiency syndromes) have an increased incidence of lymphoma and Kaposi's sarcoma of the distal small bowel.

Dietary risk factors that have been involved in colorectal carcinogenesis have been looked at in patients with malignancies of the small bowel. High-caloric dietary intake in general and more specifically consumption of red meat, fat, and salt-cured smoked foods have been shown to increase the incidence of small bowel carcinoma in large population studies.[27-29] This similarity in risk factors explains the relatively high risk of synchronous or metachronous colorectal cancer in patients with a known small bowel malignancy.[30-33]

PATHOLOGY

Approximately one third of primary small bowel neoplasms are benign and two thirds are malignant. The most common benign tumors are leiomyomas and adenomas; less common lesions include inflammatory polyps, hemangiomas, lipomas, hamartomas (Peutz-Jeghers syndrome), and fibromas (Fig. 79-1).[19,20] These tumors can occur throughout the small bowel but tend to increase in frequency from proximal to distal, with the exception of adenomas, which occur with the highest frequency in the duodenum.

Leiomyomas arise from smooth muscle and can grow both intra- and extraluminally. They can often become very large before causing symptoms. On gross inspection, it is sometimes difficult to distinguish these lesions from their malignant counterparts. This distinction is made histologically with standard criteria including nuclear pleomorphism, increased mitosis, and the presence of necrosis, although, at times, even histologic examination may fail to unequivocally distinguish between benign and malignant lesions.

Adenomas are the next most common benign tumors of the small intestine. The duodenum is the most common site of involvement, and the lesion most commonly noted is the villous adenoma. These lesions tend to involve the region of the ampulla of Vater. They may present with obstructive jaundice and are easily diagnosed by upper endoscopy and biopsy. Up to 30% of these tumors may have a malignant degeneration. The risk of malignant

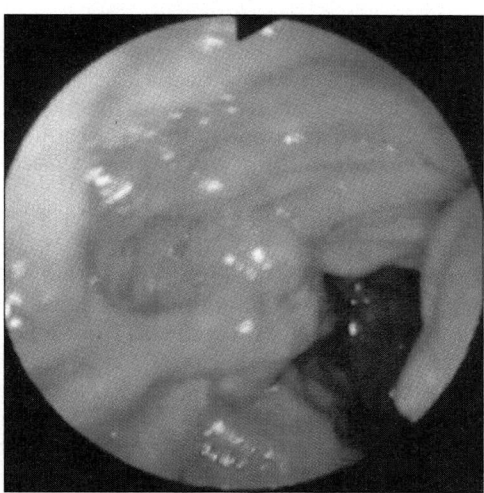

Figure 79-1. Hamartomatous polyp in Peutz-Jeghers syndrome. Endoscopic view shows a broad-based polyp in the duodenum in a patient with Peutz-Jeghers syndrome. These small intestinal polyps only rarely become malignant. This syndrome is an autosomal dominant condition that is also marked by deposits of melanin on the buccal mucosa, lips, and digits. Ovarian neoplasms arise in almost 5% of women with this syndrome. (Kulke H, Turner J, Skarin A: Cancer of the gastrointestinal tract. In Skarin A [ed]: Atlas of Diagnostic Oncology, 3rd ed. St. Louis, Mosby, 2003, p 113.)

degeneration in a significant proportion of patients poses challenges to treatment planning.

Malignant tumors tend to increase in frequency from proximal to distal, again with the exception of adenocarcinomas which are most frequent in the duodenum.[2,6,18,19,34,35] Adenocarcinoma is the most common histologic type (45%), followed by carcinoids (30%), lymphomas (15%), and sarcomas and GISTs (10%).[18,36,37] Pathologic staging is performed according to the American Joint Committee on Cancer (AJCC) tumor–node–metastasis (TNM) system.[38]

Most small bowel adenocarcinomas are solitary, sessile lesions, often appearing in association with adenomas. They are usually moderately to well differentiated and almost always positive for acid mucin. Most arise in the duodenum: Within the duodenum, 15% of these tumors are located in the first portion, 40% are in the second portion, and 45% are in the distal duodenum.[39,40] Most of these tumors are sporadic with the exception of the ones originating in the context of familial adenomatous polyposis. Presenting symptoms include epigastric and abdominal pain or discomfort, and possibly jaundice and gastric outlet obstruction, depending on the location of the tumor (Fig. 79-2). These symptoms and the accessibility of the duodenum and proximal small bowel to endoscopic modalities allow a relatively high rate of diagnosis and resectability.[41]

Carcinoid tumors are the most common endocrine tumors of the gastrointestinal system and the second most common malignancy involving the small bowel.[2,18,19,42,43] In the small bowel itself, carcinoids are the most common distal small bowel neoplasm. These neoplasms arise from enterochromaffin cells and are characterized by the ability to secrete many biologically active substances, including serotonin, bradykinin, dopamine, histamine, and 5-hydroxyindoleacetic acid (5-HIAA). They tend to be small (<2 cm) and submucosal in location, with a propensity for multicentricity. The most common classification for these tumors is based on embryologic derivation: foregut (stomach and pancreas), midgut (small bowel), and hindgut (colon and rectum). Their presentation depends largely on the hormones elaborated and on the site of origin.[42,43] The majority of these tumors (90% or more) are midgut primary cancers. Up to 40% of small bowel carcinoids are associated with a second gastrointestinal malignancy, and 30% are multicentric. A full evaluation of the small and large intestine is therefore warranted.[42,43]

The gastrointestinal tract is the most frequent site of extranodal lymphoma: within the gastrointestinal tract, the stomach is the most common site followed by the small bowel and the colon, respectively; within the small bowel, lymphomas parallel the distribution of lymphoid follicles, resulting in the ileum being the most common site of involvement.[2,18,19,36,44,45] These tumors may be primary or secondary as a manifestation of generalized involvement of systemic lymphoma. For the diagnosis of primary small bowel lymphomas there must be no peripheral or mediastinal lymphadenopathy, with a normal white blood cell count and differential, and the tumor must be predominantly in the gastrointestinal tract. When primary, they may be multifocal in as many as 15% of cases. Predisposing conditions include immunodeficiency conditions (i.e., AIDS, rheumatoid arthritis, and immune disorders in transplant recipients), Crohn's disease, and celiac disease.[14,18,19,21]

The five distinct clinical pathologic subtypes of primary small intestinal lymphoma are the adult Western type, the pediatric type, the immunoproliferative or Mediterranean type, enteropathy-associated (celiac sprue) T-cell

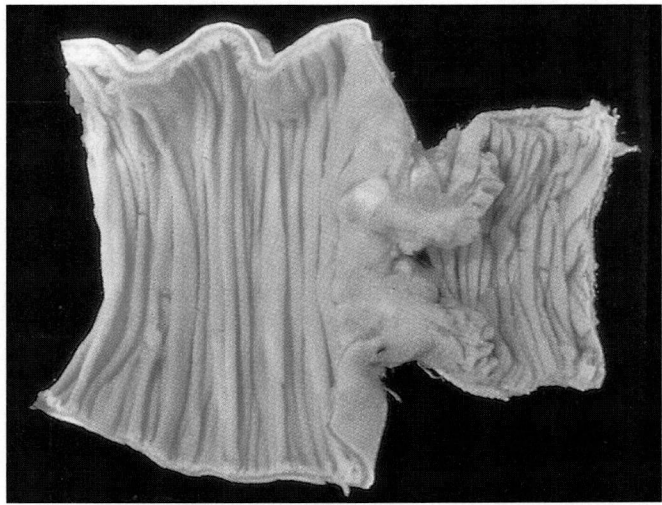

Figure 79-2. Adenocarcinoma of the jejunum causing annular constriction. (Kulke H, Turner J, Skarin A: Cancer of the gastrointestinal tract. In Skarin A [ed]: Atlas of Diagnostic Oncology, 3rd ed. St. Louis, Mosby, 2003, p 142.)

lymphoma, and Hodgkin's lymphoma.[4] The most common is the adult Western type, occurring in the sixth and seventh decades of life with a male predominance.[45]

Sarcomas make up only 10% of small bowel malignancies.[2,18,19,27,34] Overall, these tumors are located in the jejunum and ileum, are relatively slow growing, and are locally invasive. Their growth pattern is most commonly extramural; therefore, they rarely result in obstruction, but sometimes they present with free intra-abdominal bleeding from central tumor necrosis and peritoneal rupture. Owing to their insidious nature and growth pattern, more than three fourths of these tumors exceed 5 cm in diameter at the time of diagnosis. The most common histologic subtypes (in descending order of frequency) are GISTs (Fig. 79-3), leiomyosarcomas, fibrosarcomas, liposarcomas, and malignant schwannomas and angiosarcomas. Similar to sarcomas from other anatomic regions, small bowel sarcomas rarely metastasize to regional lymph nodes. Hematogenous dissemination tends to be the preferred route of distant spread, primarily to the liver, lungs, and bone. Peritoneal sarcomatosis is noted in later stages of the disease.

Mazur and Clark introduced the term GIST in 1983 to describe gastrointestinal nonepithelial stromal tumors that lack the immunohistochemical features of Schwann cells and did not have the characteristics of smooth muscle cells.[46] Malignant GIST is now considered the most common sarcoma of the gastrointestinal tract and accounts for about 5% of all small bowel malignancies.[47] Clinical, histopathologic, ultrastructural, and molecular biologic findings have clearly shown that GIST is a completely separate entity from leiomyoma and leiomyosarcoma. It is currently thought that GISTs originate from stem cells that differentiate toward the interstitial cells of Cajal (ICCs). ICCs arise from precursor mesenchymal cells and are the pacemaker cells of the gastrointestinal tract.[48] They intercalate between nerve fibers and muscle cells

and can be seen in the adult intestine in and around the myenteric plexus.[49] Both ICCs and GISTs express KIT protein, have similar ultrastructural features, and express the embryonic form of the heavy chain of smooth muscle myosin.[50,51] All these features support a common origin and the term *gastrointestinal pacemaker cell tumor* has been used to describe these lesions.[51]

KIT immunostaining has become the gold standard for the diagnosis of GIST, and the term *GIST* should apply only to tumors with KIT immunopositivity. In rare situations a GIST may be immunohistochemically inert, or after therapy with imatinib mesylate, KIT immunostaining may become negative.[52] Furthermore, a minority of GISTs lacks demonstrable KIT mutations, but KIT is nonetheless strongly activated. Such GISTs might contain KIT mutations, which are not readily detected by conventional screening methods, or alternately, KIT might be activated by nonmutational mechanisms. Most GISTs have non-complex cytogenetic profiles, often featuring deletions of chromosomes 14 and 22. Additional chromosomal aberrations are acquired as GISTs progress to higher histologic grade. These cytogenetic aberrations are undoubtedly important in GIST pathogenesis, but currently they do not play a key role as diagnostic adjuncts.[53]

To better characterize these tumors, other markers have been studied: About 60% to 70% of GISTs show immunopositivity for CD34, 30% to 40% for smooth muscle actin (SMA), and around 5% for S-100 protein. None of the latter antigens are therefore specific for GIST, but can help in the differential diagnosis in KIT-negative tumors. Desmin positivity in true KIT-positive GISTs is extremely uncommon (1% to 2% of cases) and is invariably focal, with positivity in only a small number of tumor cells.[52] The immunophenotype of true KIT-positive GISTs varies to some degree by location, with CD34 positivity seen most consistently in colorectal and esophageal lesions and SMA positivity seen most often in small bowel tumors.[54]

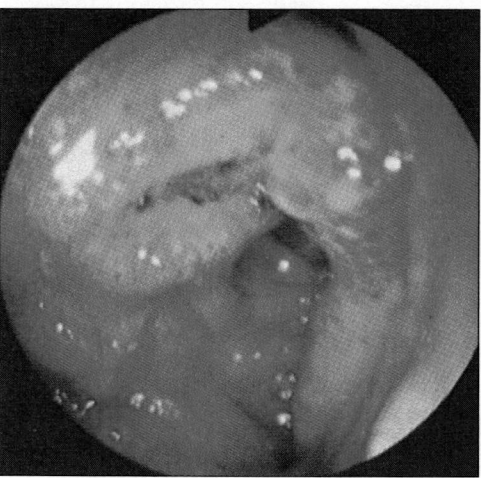

Figure 79-3. An endoscopic view of a malignant GIST of the duodenum. (Kulke H, Turner J, Skarin A: Cancer of the gastrointestinal tract. In Skarin A [ed]: Atlas of Diagnostic Oncology, 3rd ed. St. Louis, Mosby, 2003, p 142.)

BIOLOGY

There are similarities in the genetic makeup of small bowel and large bowel adenocarcinomas. *K-ras* mutations at codon 12 have been noted in duodenal adenocarcinomas, suggesting a possible pathogenetic role similar to that seen in pancreatic and colorectal cancer.[55] As shown in colorectal and other malignancies, overexpression of p53 in de novo small bowel adenocarcinomas has been associated with a worse prognosis.[56] Increased expression of c-erbB-2, Ki-67, and tenascin was associated with poorer survival rate in a small group of patients with duodenal adenocarcinomas.[57] Strong cytoplasmic carcinoembryonic antigen (CEA) staining has been described in small bowel adenocarcinomas.[58] Immunohistochemical staining for CEA, and to a lesser extent CA 19-9, is positive in the majority of ampullary and about half of nonampullary duodenal small bowel adenocarcinomas.[59] However, their independent prognostic value has not been established. The rarity of small bowel adenocarcinomas makes it difficult to carry out meaningful, large, prospective studies to assess the prognostic and clinical significance of these markers.

A recent major advance has been achieved by the recognition of the central role of activating KIT mutations in the pathogenesis of GISTs,[60–62] leading to expression of the KIT protein (CD117), a new and reliable phenotypic marker for these neoplasms.[51,63] Constitutive activation of the KIT receptor tyrosine kinase is a central pathogenetic event in most GISTs and generally results from point mutations, which involve either extracellular or cytoplasmic domains of the receptor. These mutations enable the KIT receptor to phosphorylate various substrate proteins, leading to activation of signal transduction cascades, which regulate cell proliferation, apoptosis, chemotaxis, and adhesion. KIT mutations can be broadly assigned to two groups, those that involve the "regulatory" regions responsible for modulating KIT enzymatic activity and those that involve the enzymatic region itself.[53]

CLINICAL PRESENTATION

The vast majority of patients with benign neoplasms are asymptomatic, whereas the vast majority of those with malignancies are symptomatic prior to diagnosis (Fig. 79-4). The most common presentation of benign tumors is intermittent episodes of acute crampy abdominal pain associated with intussusception, followed by chronic bleeding with iron deficiency anemia in up to 50% of patients.

Malignant lesions are generally associated with weight loss, due to delay in the establishment of a diagnosis. Symptoms, when they occur, tend to be vague and nonspecific. In general, most symptoms can be attributed to the location of the tumor, its rate of growth, and its size.[2,18,19,34,35] For example, tumors in the duodenum tend to be symptomatic at an earlier stage, presenting with pain, gastric outlet obstruction, or obstructive jaundice, whereas those in the jejunum or ileum may present at a later stage with obstructive symptoms. Obstruction in this setting tends to be progressive, compared to benign lesions, whose obstructive symptoms tend to be intermittent as they relate to episodes of intussusception. Bleeding and perforation (in up to 10%) may also occur, predominantly in lymphomatous lesions, but they can also be features of any malignant tumor because of ulceration or necrosis.

Carcinoid tumors produce symptoms secondary to hormone production, including hot flashes, bronchospasms, and arrhythmias. This constellation of symptoms, called carcinoid syndrome, occurs when the liver is not able to metabolize the active substances produced by the carcinoid tumor. This problem usually results when tumors are either bulky or metastatic or their venous drainage bypasses the liver.

LABORATORY AND IMAGING STUDIES

A high index of suspicion is required because of the nonspecificity of the signs and symptoms of these tumors. A correct preoperative diagnosis is made in only 50% of patients. Biochemical and hematologic studies are often not helpful. Iron deficiency anemia may be detected with chronic blood loss; elevated liver enzymes may be noted with periampullary lesions or hepatic metastases; elevated 24-hour urinary 5-hydroxyindoleacetic acid can be detected in more than 50% of patients with carcinoid tumors.

Radiographic contrast imaging modalities tend to be the most useful in the establishment of the diagnosis (Fig. 79-5). Plain films of the abdomen are generally not helpful and at best may demonstrate nonspecific signs of obstruction or a mass effect. Except for the duodenum and the very proximal jejunum, which can often be evaluated by endoscopy, the diagnosis of small intestinal neoplasms depends on contrast studies such as a small bowel follow-through or preferably enteroclysis. Small bowel follow-through is still the most commonly used method in most institutions in the evaluation of small bowel disease, although enteroclysis may be a superior imaging modality. In a recent study comparing the sensitivity and tumor detection rate of small bowel follow-through and enteroclysis, the sensitivity was 61% and 95%, respectively. The actual tumor detection rate was 33% for small bowel follow-through and 90% for enteroclysis.[64]

Computed tomography (CT), ultrasonography, and magnetic resonance imaging (MRI) are complementary to barium studies in the detection of small bowel neoplasms. Abdominal CT has a sensitivity of 50% to 80% in detecting the primary small bowel tumors and occasionally plays an important role in differentiating benign from malignant tumors. Additionally, CT is valuable in staging malignant tumors (presence or absence of hepatic metastases) and in providing important information related to local extent (presence or absence of local invasion, mesenteric implants, and metastatic lymph nodes). Contrast-enhanced abdominal CT examination and enteroclysis are truly complementary to each other. Enteroclysis provides optimal wall distention and displays mucosal pattern well;

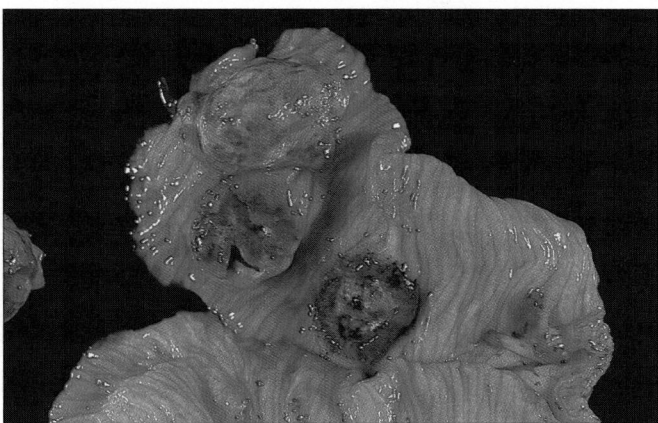

Figure 79-4. The small bowel is a frequent site for melanoma metastases. This resected jejunum contains multiple pigmented nodules, some with ulceration. (Kulke H, Turner J, Skarin A: Cancer of the gastrointestinal tract. In Skarin A [ed]: Atlas of Diagnostic Oncology, 3rd ed. St. Louis, Mosby, 2003, p 146.)

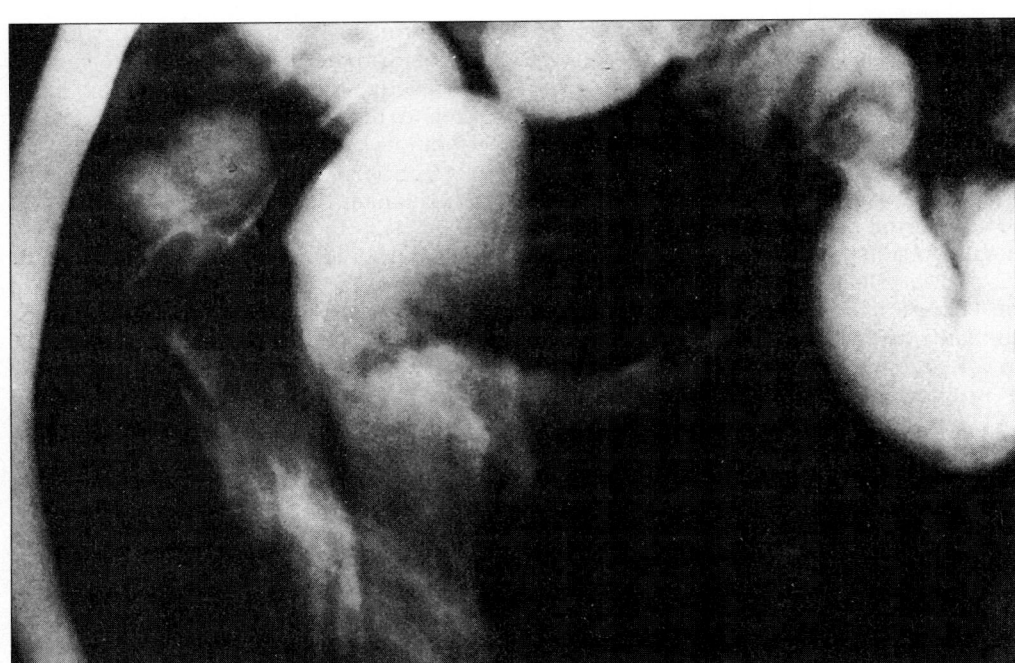

Figure 79-5. A barium contrast study of the small intestine demonstrating an annular constricting lesion that proved to be an adenocarcinoma of the ileum. (Kulke H, Turner J, Skarin A: Cancer of the gastrointestinal tract. In Skarin A [ed]: Atlas of Diagnostic Oncology, 3rd ed. St. Louis, Mosby, 2003, p 142.)

CT demonstrates the extraluminal component of the tumor and aids in the staging process.

Angiography, although helpful in diagnosing and localizing neoplasms of vascular origin, is rarely helpful in establishing or refining a diagnosis of small bowel malignancy. In rare cases angiographic demonstration of tumor neovascularity without contrast agent extravasation may be of diagnostic importance in patients with chronic occult bleeding when other diagnostic studies such as endoscopy and barium contrast have been negative.[65] By contrast, angiography is rarely beneficial in localizing bleeding tumors because the vast majority of such tumors bleed at a rate considerably below the limit of detection with this technique. Scintigraphy with technetium-labeled red blood cells may identify bleeding sites with blood loss rates as low as 0.1 mL per minute.

Sonde enteroscopy, by now only of historical interest,[66] involved intubation of the small bowel with a thin endoscope equipped with a balloon tip, inserted transnasally, and moved distally by way of peristalsis. Evaluation of the bowel occurred as the scope was withdrawn. This scope did not allow for biopsy or therapeutic intervention, the entire bowel lumen often was not visualized, and the duration of the procedure was on the order of 6 hours. This modality was used in the diagnostic workup of individuals who had had nondiagnostic contrast studies and upper and lower endoscopies.[67]

Enteroscopy is now available in a fiberoptic form, using conventional endoscopes or in a wireless form. Fiberoptic small bowel enteroscopy, or push enteroscopy, initially made use of a pediatric or adult colonoscope that was advanced orally.[68] Specialized scopes that can be used to visualize jejunum 100 cm or farther from the ligament of Treitz are now available. The bowel is evaluated as the endoscope is both advanced and withdrawn, and biopsy or cauterization can be done concomitantly through an accessory channel.

Wireless capsule endoscopy is a new technique that utilizes a miniature camera that is swallowed by the patient and records images as it progresses down the gastrointestinal tract. It offers the potential to examine the whole small intestine combined with the advantage of being painless. Using a miniature camera and a short focal length lens, images are obtained as the capsule progresses though the entire length of the intestine, without requiring air inflation. The capsule endoscope is propelled by peristalsis through the gastrointestinal tract. The video images are transmitted using radiotelemetry and are stored on a small portable recorder carried on a belt and subsequently downloaded for analysis. The system allows more than 7 hours of continuous recording of images of the gastrointestinal tract. The patients are free to continue their daily routine during the examination.[69] Animal studies using this modality have shown that capsule enteroscopy was as effective as enteroscopy in detecting beads in canine small intestine.[70] Recently, several human studies, usually looking at patients with occult gastrointestinal bleeding, have indicated that capsule endoscopy seems to be significantly superior to push enteroscopy in this group of patients,[71-74] and it is invariably preferred by patients undergoing both procedures.[69] A study by Costamagna[75] found wireless capsule endoscopy significantly superior to small bowel follow-through studies, if small bowel disease was suspected.

Fluorodeoxyglucose (labeled with fluorine-18) positron emission tomography (FDG-PET) has been shown to be highly sensitive to assess disease status in patients with GISTs. FDG-PET is used for preoperative staging, but more important, it can be used to assess response to therapy. Glucose uptake of GIST decreases within a few hours to a few days after the start of treatment with imatinib mesylate (Gleevec, Novartis), which can be verified by FDG-PET.[76] Furthermore in case of disease progression, increased areas of FDG uptake are observed by PET, often prior to the appearance of a mass on conventional imaging.[77] PET has also been advocated when a distinction between intratumoral bleeding and disease progression is necessary.

Limited information is available regarding the efficacy of diagnostic laparoscopy in the diagnosis and workup of small bowel neoplasms. At present, its usefulness may reside in obtaining staging information and determining resectability prior to formal laparotomy in the case of tumors of the duodenum, and in obtaining images and potentially in making tissue diagnoses when other imaging studies have failed to suggest an etiology. It is clear, however, that despite the currently available technology, the diagnosis of these tumors is difficult to establish preoperatively in a significant group of individuals. Laparotomy is often required for definitive diagnosis.

STAGING CLASSIFICATION

Radiologic staging is based mainly on the use of CT and MRI. Intraoperative assessment plays a role in clinical staging, especially when tumor cannot be resected. Metastatic involvement of the liver may be further evaluated by intraoperative ultrasonography. As far as pathologic staging, the TNM staging system has been recently revised by the American Joint Committee on Cancer (AJCC),[38] but no major changes have been implemented for small bowel neoplasms. The primary tumor is staged according to its depth of penetration and the involvement of adjacent structures or distant sites. There is no subdivision within the N category based on the number of nodes involved with tumor. Discontinuous hematogenous metastases or peritoneal metastases are coded as M1. Cancers of the small intestine can metastasize to most organs, especially the liver, or to the peritoneal surfaces. Involvement of the celiac nodes is considered M1 disease (Tables 79-1 and 79-2).

For small bowel lymphoma the most commonly used staging system is the Ann Arbor system, based on lymphatic and extralymphatic involvement on either side of the diaphragm (Table 79-3).

PROGNOSIS

Prognosis for small bowel adenocarcinoma is based on similar variables as for colorectal cancer, including stage, perineural and vascular invasion, grade, resectability, and surgical margins.[35,78–80] The majority of tumors have regional spread at time of diagnosis, and up to one fourth of patients have distant organ disease. Overall, the 5-year survival rate is 20% to 30% in most series. For resectable disease of the duodenum, the 5-year survival rate approaches 50%.[2,6,35,78–81]

It has been frequently postulated that a small bowel adenocarcinoma carries a worse prognosis in patients

TABLE 79-1

Definition of TNM Stages

Primary Tumor (T)

TX	Primary tumor cannot be assessed
T0	No evidence of primary tumor
TIS	Carcinoma in situ
T1	Tumor invades lamina propria or submucosa
T2	Tumor invades muscularis propria
T3	Tumor invades through the muscularis propria into the subserosa or into the nonperitonealized perimuscular tissue (mesentery or retroperitoneum) with extension 2 cm or less
T4	Tumor perforates the visceral peritoneum or directly invades other organs or structures (includes other loops of small intestine, mesentery, or retroperitoneum more than 2 cm, and abdominal wall by way of serosa; for duodenum only, invasion of pancreas)

Regional Lymph Nodes (N)

NX	Regional lymph nodes cannot be assessed
N0	No regional lymph node metastasis
N1	Regional lymph node metastasis

Distant Metastasis (M)

MX	Distant metastasis cannot be assessed
M0	No distant metastasis
M1	Distant metastasis

TABLE 79-2

Stage Grouping

STAGE	T	N	M
0	TIS	N0	M0
I	T1	N0	M0
	T2	N0	M0
II	T3	N0	M0
	T4	N0	M0
III	Any T	N1	M0
IV	Any T	Any N	M1

TABLE 79-3

Ann Arbor Staging System for Small Bowel Lymphoma

STAGE	CRITERIA
I	Involvement of a single nodal group (I) or a single extralymphatic organ or site (IE)
II	Involvement of more than one nodal group on the same side of the diaphragm (II) or a single extralymphatic site with one or more nodal groups on the same side of the diaphragm (IIE)
III	Involvement of nodes on both sides of the diaphragm (III) with or without involvement of extralymphatic sites (IIIE), spleen (IIIS), or both (IIIES)
IV	Diffuse involvement of viscera or bone marrow

Specific Malignancies

III

with Crohn's disease in comparison to the general population. Recent studies have demonstrated that in these patients survival correlates purely with stage of tumor at resection. In our series, no patient with regional or distant metastasis survived 5 years, in comparison with an 83% 5-year actuarial survival rate of patients with tumor confined to the intestinal wall. Mean survival time was 6 months for Crohn's disease patients with small bowel cancer in comparison with 65 months for Crohn's disease patients with large bowel cancer, reflecting a tendency toward more advanced lesions in the small bowel.[13]

The prognosis for carcinoid tumors with localized disease is excellent, with 5-year survival rates approaching 100% after resection. More than 90% of the symptomatic patients have metastatic disease at the time of surgical exploration. The likelihood of distant disease correlates closely with both the size of the primary lesion and the depth of invasion. For tumors larger than 1 cm, the risk of lymph node metastases is on the order of 2%; for 1- to 2-cm lesions, the incidence of lymph node involvement is approximately 50%; and 80% of tumors larger than 2 cm have positive nodes. Survival rates of up to 68% at 5 years have been reported when all gross metastatic disease, including hepatic metastases, is resected. For those unfortunate individuals with extensive unresectable disease, debulking has proved to be of some benefit in terms of symptomatic palliation. It is notable that the 5-year survival rate for unresectable disease is approximately 35% to 40%, reflecting the relatively indolent growth of these tumors.

Prognostic factors for primary small bowel lymphomas include higher grade, greater depth of tumor penetration, lymph node involvement, peritoneal disease, and distant metastases.[35,44,45] Overall 5-year survival rates range from 20% to 40% for all stages. Five-year survival rates of up to 60% have been reported for patients with resected localized low-grade tumors.[18]

Sarcomas tend to have an insidious growth pattern, more than three fourths of these tumors are larger than 5 cm at the time of diagnosis, and up to 50% of them are not resectable for cure when the diagnosis is established. Prognosis correlates most closely with grade, followed by stage.[82] Five-year survival rate after curative resection ranges from 60% to 80% for low-grade tumors and is no more than 20% for high-grade lesions.

Assessment of the malignant potential of a primary GIST lesion is difficult in many cases unless tumor spread can be documented beyond the organ of origin at the time of diagnosis. Historically, size has been used to assess tumor behavior. Although almost all small (<1 cm) GISTs are clinically benign and tumors larger than 5 cm in diameter are generally malignant, intermediate-size GISTs have uncertain malignant potential,[52] and no cut-off diameter predicts subsequent malignant behavior with certainty.[83]

In addition to size, mitotic rate has been used to predict tumor behavior. Tumors with more than five mitoses per 50 high-power fields (HPFs) are considered malignant and those with more than 20 to 50 mitoses per 50 HPFs are classified as high-grade malignancy.[49,84] However, a low mitotic count does not rule out malignancy with certainty.[85] Other factors that have shown prognostic value include presence of tumor necrosis, high cellularity, and pronounced pleomorphism; a high S-phase fraction and DNA aneuploidy in flow cytometry or image cytometry; a high Ki-67 score; proliferating cell nuclear-antigen expression; presence of telomerase activity;[37] incomplete surgical resection; tumor rupture at surgery;[86] and invasion of adjacent structures.

Recently *KIT* mutations have been shown to be an independent prognostic factor for patients with GISTs. Taniguchi and associates[87] have suggested that GISTs should be divided into mutation-positive and -negative subtypes, the prognosis being worse in patients with mutation-positive GISTs.

Precise data on long-term survival for patients with GISTs are difficult to provide owing to the introduction of an effective treatment strategy (imatinib mesylate) in clinical practice and the recognition of the KIT protein (CD117), which has changed the way spindle cell tumors of the gastrointestinal tract are classified. Prior to the introduction of imatinib mesylate, the available chemotherapeutic protocols were not effective against GISTs and the outcome of these patients was bleak.[88] Furthermore, until recently, studies on GISTs included tumors that are not presently classified as GISTs. It is, nevertheless, believed that the overall or disease-specific 5-year survival rate is 28% to 60% among patients with malignant GIST; the median disease-specific survival time is about 5 years for primary disease, and 10 to 20 months in recurrent or metastatic disease.[47,89] Most recurrences take place within 5 years of the primary diagnosis,[85] but in the slowly proliferating subset of GISTs and especially after therapy with imatinib mesylate, metastases can appear more than 10 years after the primary diagnosis.

The outcome of patients with metastatic malignancies to the small intestine (more commonly ovarian, colon, and lung cancers, renal cell carcinoma, and melanoma) is dismal despite palliative therapeutic intervention.

PRIMARY TREATMENT

Treatment of adenocarcinoma of the small intestine with localized disease is based on oncologic and anatomic principles. For duodenal lesions the availability of endoscopic ultrasound has allowed better preoperative staging,[90,91] and the availability of endoscopic resection techniques[92] has offered additional therapeutic options. Ultrasound-proved benign duodenal or ampullary adenomas can be resected endoscopically with excellent results. If associated with familial polyposis, chemoprevention with sulindac or cyclo-oxygenase-2 (COX-2) inhibitors may be beneficial.[93]

Invasive lesions of the first and second portion of the duodenum without major vessel involvement and distant spread are best treated by a pancreaticoduodenectomy (Whipple procedure). For tumors in the third or fourth portion of the duodenum segmental resection with regional lymphadectomy is indicated.[18,19,79-81] Debate persists about the optimal surgical management of early duodenal cancer. Although early reports suggest that an

TABLE 80-5

Basic Elements of Informed Consent for Germline DNA Testing[93]

- Information on the specific test being performed.
- Implications of a positive and negative result.
- Possibility that the test will not be informative.
- Options for risk estimation without genetic testing.
- Risk of passing a mutation or to children.
- Technical accuracy of the test.
- Fees involved in testing and counseling.
- Risks of psychological distress.
- Risks of insurance or employer discrimination.
- Confidentiality issues.
- Options and limitations of medical surveillance and screening after testing.

Counseling regarding the possible risks and benefits of cancer early detection and prevention modalities and a discussion of the basic elements of informed consent (Table 80-5) should be obtained before offering germline DNA testing. Genetic counselors in the past have not had much training in the cancer-related aspects of genetics because these clinical applications have developed only recently, so many are not yet experienced in the care of cancer patients. Alternatively, some specialist physicians (oncologists, gastroenterologists, etc.) could meet the needs of their patients by maintaining sufficient continuing education in molecular genetics, pedigree construction, and Bayesian analysis so that they can directly deliver the necessary counseling services or consult with other colleagues having expertise in cancer genetic testing.[93]

Screening and Surveillance Adjusted for Risk

In general, screening of asymptomatic individuals is appropriate when the disease can be treated more successfully at earlier stages when no symptoms are yet apparent, but it has increased risk for significant morbidity or mortality at later stages after clinically apparent symptoms have developed. Colon cancer screening after age 50 years certainly satisfies these criteria and has the most favorable cost-benefit ratio of any disease screening modality, with a cost affordable in most advanced societies of only $6000 per year of life saved.[94-97] Screening age and intervals should be adjusted to the level of risk based on the personal and family medical history. Patients with symptoms that suggest colon cancer need attention more promptly than screening protocols might indicate and should be offered an appropriate diagnostic evaluation.

Screening the General Population at Low-to-Average Risk

The American Gastroenterological Asssociation (AGA) and other groups recommend that "men/women at average risk should be offered options for screening for colorectal cancer and polyps beginning at age 50 years. They should be offered options for screening, with information about the advantages and disadvantages associated with each approach. If the result of a screening test is abnormal, physicians should recommend a complete structural examination of the colon and rectum by colonoscopy (or flexible sigmoidoscopy and double contrast barium enema if colonoscopy is not available."[97]

Fecal occult blood testing (FOBT) should be offered annually using a guaiac-based test with dietary restriction or an immunochemical test without dietary restriction. Two samples from each of three consecutive stools should be examined without rehydration. Patients with a positive test on any specimen should be followed up with colonoscopy.[97] The sensitivity of a single FOBT is low, detecting only about one third of cancers, but a program of repeated testing can detect the majority of cancers and result in an 18% to 21% reduction in colon cancer mortality according to strong evidence from randomized prospective clinical trials.[98-100] Disadvantages are the failure to detect many cancers and the particularly low sensitivity for polyps. Furthermore, most people who test positive by FOBT have bleeding from a source other than a tumor and will undergo the risk, discomfort, and cost of follow-up colonoscopy without any cancer prevention benefit.

Flexible sigmoidoscopy should be offered every five years, based on evidence of reduced mortality from four case-control studies and two randomized controlled trials.[101-106] When combined with FOBT, the FOBT should be done first, as if it is positive, a complete colon exam would be indicated.[107-109]

Colonoscopy should be offered every 10 years. The interval of ten years is based on the typical rate of progression from adenoma to cancer.[86,110] Although there are no studies evaluating whether screening colonoscopy alone reduces the incidence or mortality from colorectal cancer in people at average risk, several lines of evidence support the effectiveness of screening colonoscopy.[97] Colonoscopy has not only diagnostic but also therapeutic benefits, as it allows removal of adenomas and reduces the incidence of colorectal cancer, as demonstrated in two cohort studies of people with adenomatous polyps.[86,111] Colonoscopy examines more of the colon than sigmoidoscopy, and as expected, it has been proven to detect twice as many significant adenomas and cancers as sigmoidoscopy in two large prospective studies in which half of all patients with advanced proximal neoplasms had no distal colonic findings on sigmoidoscopy that would have prompted referral for a complete colon exam.[112,113])

Colonoscopy is the most frequent endoscopic procedure in this country and has dramatically changed the diagnosis, follow-up, and screening for colon cancer. Colonoscopy is performed with the patient receiving intravenous sedation and lying in the left lateral position. The scope is introduced through the rectum, and air insufflation helps identify the lumen as the scope is advanced gently. The sigmoid colon can present some difficulty, and navigating the scope with the colon is facilitated by a technique of pulling back and advancing. It might also be somewhat difficult to negotiate the angle of the hepatic flexure to get the scope down and into the cecum.

The most common complication is perforation, and this complication is best managed by emergent exploration and repair. Pedunculated polyps are removed using an electrocautery wire snare. The stalk is an extension of the normal mucosal epithelium, making it preferable to snare the polyp just below the head of the polyp rather than at the base. Electrocautery wire removal of sessile polyps is technically more demanding. Their removal may be facilitated by injecting a 1:200,000 epinephrine solution submucosally to elevate the polyp and decrease the risk of injury to the entire wall. It is generally necessary to remove sessile polyps in stages with several applications of the snare.

Colonic Polyps. The cecum and the low rectum are two areas where colonoscopy is known to be at risk for missing early polyps and cancers. Experienced endoscopists are well aware of this and spend extra time evaluating these areas. The low rectal area is best visualized by retroflexing the scope back on itself. It is imperative that the endoscopist document that the scope has reached the ileocecal valve. Colonic polyps of epithelial origin represent the vast majority of colon polyps and are the precursors of invasive cancer. They can be pedunculated with a nonadenomatous stalk, pedunculated with an adenomatous stalk, or sessile. The diagnosis of adenoma requires the presence of epithelial dysplasia.

Adenomatous Polyps (Tubular Adenomas). Adenomatous polyps are equally distributed through out the colon and are found at autopsy in roughly one third of adults. Their presence increases with age, and they have a familial predisposition. Most are asymptomatic and when found at the time of screening colonoscopy are usually less than 1 cm in diameter. There is an increased risk of cancer when the polyp is larger than 2 cm in diameter, when there is severe dysplasia, and when the pattern is more villous. Penetration of the muscularis mucosa by abnormal epithelial cells is the indication of malignancy. In general, as the polyp increases in size, there is a more villous component to its architecture, and such lesions may be termed villoglandular polyps or tubulovillous adenomas. Immunohistochemistry demonstrates carcinoembryonic antigen (CEA) localization in atypical sections. They are positive for keratin and may show overexpression of p53. Reactivity for bcl-2 is present in almost all polyps. Microadenomas or aberrant crypts, originally observed in experimental animals, are also seen in humans.

Villous Adenoma. Villous adenomas are distinct from adenomatous-type polyps and, although less common, are more often found in the distal colon and rectum. They can present with dehydration and hypokalemia. A villous adenoma is almost always an isolated lesion and can grow to considerable size. It has soft, frond-like growth with a wide base. The incidence of finding invasive cancer in a villous adenoma is variously reported at 30% to as high as 70%.

Screening Individuals with Moderately Increased Risk

Surveillance colonoscopy should be considered at more frequent intervals for patients who are at increased risk because they have been treated for colorectal cancer, have an adenomatous polyp diagnosed, have a disease that predisposes them to colorectal cancer (e.g., inflammatory bowel disease), or have a family history of colon polyps or cancer.[97]

Persons with first-degree relatives affected with colon cancer, or an adenoma after age 60 years, or two second-degree relatives affected by colon cancer should have screening exams of the same type and frequency as average risk but starting at age 40 years.[97]

Persons with two or more first-degree relatives with colon cancer or adenomatous polyps diagnosed at younger than age 60 years should have colonoscopy every five years beginning at age 40 or 10 years younger than the earliest diagnosis in the family, whichever comes first.[97]

Screening Individuals with High-Risk Familial Syndromes

Patients with more severe family history or syndromes, including FAP and HNPCC, require more frequent colon exams beginning at younger ages because of the earlier onset and higher frequency of cancers and polyps in individuals with an inherited or germline mutation.[114]

HNPCC. Colonoscopy exams for patients with HNPCC and their at-risk relatives has been proven an effective method for reducing the incidence and mortality of of colorectal cancer.[115] The incidence of cancer is reduced by more than half, presumably due to the removal of precursor polyps, when complete colonoscopy is begun at an early age and repeated at regular intervals.[116] Colonoscopy in HNPCC families generally should begin at least 5 to 10 years before the youngest age at cancer diagnosis in an affected family member, or no later than age 21 years. No guidelines or authorities recommend intervals longer than 3 years in HNPCC. The American Cancer Society guidelines recommend that colonoscopy for HNPCC screening be repeated every 2 years until age 40 and then annually.[117] Once a polyp or cancer has been detected, more frequent screening should be considered, perhaps every 6 to 12 months.

FAP. Screening is a well-established method of cancer prevention in FAP because polyposis can be diagnosed and colectomy completed long before cancer develops.[118] The mortality rate among those presenting themselves is 44%, compared with only 2% among relatives called up for screening.[119] In fact, appropriate screening could conceivably prevent all colon cancer in persons known to be at risk of FAP. To reach this goal, it is important to obtain an extensive family history and construct a pedigree chart to identify the earliest possible affected common ancestor for notification of all at-risk descendants (Fig. 80-7).

These relatives can then be referred for genetic counseling and testing, and exams can be recommended for early detection of the emergence of the phenotype of polyposis. Screening for FAP should be done by video-endoscopic rather than radiologic methods because of the usual small polyp size and because of the requirement to a few days after the start of treatment with imatinib mesylate (Gleevec, Novartis), which can be verified by FDG-PET.[76] Furthermore in case of disease progression, increased areas of FDG uptake are observed by PET, often prior to the appearance of a mass on conventional imaging.[77] PET has also been advocated when a distinction between intratumoral bleeding and disease progression is necessary.

Limited information is available regarding the efficacy of diagnostic laparoscopy in the diagnosis and workup of small bowel neoplasms. At present, its usefulness may reside in obtaining staging information and determining resectability prior to formal laparotomy in the case of tumors of the duodenum, and in obtaining images and potentially in making tissue diagnoses when other imaging studies have failed to suggest an etiology. It is clear, however, that despite the currently available technology, the diagnosis of these tumors is difficult to establish preoperatively in a significant group of individuals. Laparotomy is often required for definitive diagnosis.

STAGING CLASSIFICATION

Radiologic staging is based mainly on the use of CT and MRI. Intraoperative assessment plays a role in clinical staging, especially when tumor cannot be resected. Metastatic involvement of the liver may be further evaluated by intraoperative ultrasonography. As far as pathologic staging, the TNM staging system has been recently revised by the American Joint Committee on Cancer (AJCC),[38] but no major changes have been implemented for small bowel neoplasms. The primary tumor is staged according to its depth of penetration and the involvement of adjacent structures or distant sites. There is no subdivision within the N category based on the number of nodes involved with tumor. Discontinuous hematogenous metastases or peritoneal metastases are coded as M1. Cancers of the small intestine can metastasize to most organs, especially the liver, or to the peritoneal surfaces. Involvement of the celiac nodes is considered M1 disease (Tables 79-1 and 79-2).

For small bowel lymphoma the most commonly used staging system is the Ann Arbor system, based on lymphatic and extralymphatic involvement on either side of the diaphragm (Table 79-3).

PROGNOSIS

Prognosis for small bowel adenocarcinoma is based on similar variables as for colorectal cancer, including stage, perineural and vascular invasion, grade, resectability, and surgical margins.[35,78-80] The majority of tumors have regional spread at time of diagnosis, and up to one fourth of patients have distant organ disease. Overall, the 5-year survival rate is 20% to 30% in most series. For resectable disease of the duodenum, the 5-year survival rate approaches 50%.[2,6,35,78-81]

It has been frequently postulated that a small bowel adenocarcinoma carries a worse prognosis in patients

TABLE 79-1

Definition of TNM Stages

Primary Tumor (T)

TX	Primary tumor cannot be assessed
T0	No evidence of primary tumor
TIS	Carcinoma in situ
T1	Tumor invades lamina propria or submucosa
T2	Tumor invades muscularis propria
T3	Tumor invades through the muscularis propria into the subserosa or into the nonperitonealized perimuscular tissue (mesentery or retroperitoneum) with extension 2 cm or less
T4	Tumor perforates the visceral peritoneum or directly invades other organs or structures (includes other loops of small intestine, mesentery, or retroperitoneum more than 2 cm, and abdominal wall by way of serosa; for duodenum only, invasion of pancreas)

Regional Lymph Nodes (N)

NX	Regional lymph nodes cannot be assessed
N0	No regional lymph node metastasis
N1	Regional lymph node metastasis

Distant Metastasis (M)

MX	Distant metastasis cannot be assessed
M0	No distant metastasis
M1	Distant metastasis

TABLE 79-2

Stage Grouping

STAGE	T	N	M
0	TIS	N0	M0
I	T1	N0	M0
	T2	N0	M0
II	T3	N0	M0
	T4	N0	M0
III	Any T	N1	M0
IV	Any T	Any N	M1

TABLE 79-3

Ann Arbor Staging System for Small Bowel Lymphoma

STAGE	CRITERIA
I	Involvement of a single nodal group (I) or a single extralymphatic organ or site (IE)
II	Involvement of more than one nodal group on the same side of the diaphragm (II) or a single extralymphatic site with one or more nodal groups on the same side of the diaphragm (IIE)
III	Involvement of nodes on both sides of the diaphragm (III) with or without involvement of extralymphatic sites (IIIE), spleen (IIIS), or both (IIIES)
IV	Diffuse involvement of viscera or bone marrow

with Crohn's disease in comparison to the general population. Recent studies have demonstrated that in these patients survival correlates purely with stage of tumor at resection. In our series, no patient with regional or distant metastasis survived 5 years, in comparison with an 83% 5-year actuarial survival rate of patients with tumor confined to the intestinal wall. Mean survival time was 6 months for Crohn's disease patients with small bowel cancer in comparison with 65 months for Crohn's disease patients with large bowel cancer, reflecting a tendency toward more advanced lesions in the small bowel.[13]

The prognosis for carcinoid tumors with localized disease is excellent, with 5-year survival rates approaching 100% after resection. More than 90% of the symptomatic patients have metastatic disease at the time of surgical exploration. The likelihood of distant disease correlates closely with both the size of the primary lesion and the depth of invasion. For tumors larger than 1 cm, the risk of lymph node metastases is on the order of 2%; for 1- to 2-cm lesions, the incidence of lymph node involvement is approximately 50%; and 80% of tumors larger than 2 cm have positive nodes. Survival rates of up to 68% at 5 years have been reported when all gross metastatic disease, including hepatic metastases, is resected. For those unfortunate individuals with extensive unresectable disease, debulking has proved to be of some benefit in terms of symptomatic palliation. It is notable that the 5-year survival rate for unresectable disease is approximately 35% to 40%, reflecting the relatively indolent growth of these tumors.

Prognostic factors for primary small bowel lymphomas include higher grade, greater depth of tumor penetration, lymph node involvement, peritoneal disease, and distant metastases.[35,44,45] Overall 5-year survival rates range from 20% to 40% for all stages. Five-year survival rates of up to 60% have been reported for patients with resected localized low-grade tumors.[18]

Sarcomas tend to have an insidious growth pattern, more than three fourths of these tumors are larger than 5 cm at the time of diagnosis, and up to 50% of them are not resectable for cure when the diagnosis is established. Prognosis correlates most closely with grade, followed by stage.[82] Five-year survival rate after curative resection ranges from 60% to 80% for low-grade tumors and is no more than 20% for high-grade lesions.

Assessment of the malignant potential of a primary GIST lesion is difficult in many cases unless tumor spread can be documented beyond the organ of origin at the time of diagnosis. Historically, size has been used to assess tumor behavior. Although almost all small (<1 cm) GISTs are clinically benign and tumors larger than 5 cm in diameter are generally malignant, intermediate-size GISTs have uncertain malignant potential,[52] and no cut-off diameter predicts subsequent malignant behavior with certainty.[83]

In addition to size, mitotic rate has been used to predict tumor behavior. Tumors with more than five mitoses per 50 high-power fields (HPFs) are considered malignant and those with more than 20 to 50 mitoses per 50 HPFs are classified as high-grade malignancy.[49,84] However, a low mitotic count does not rule out malignancy with certainty.[85] Other factors that have shown prognostic value include presence of tumor necrosis, high cellularity, and pronounced pleomorphism; a high S-phase fraction and DNA aneuploidy in flow cytometry or image cytometry; a high Ki-67 score; proliferating cell nuclear-antigen expression; presence of telomerase activity;[37] incomplete surgical resection; tumor rupture at surgery;[86] and invasion of adjacent structures.

Recently *KIT* mutations have been shown to be an independent prognostic factor for patients with GISTs. Taniguchi and associates[87] have suggested that GISTs should be divided into mutation-positive and -negative subtypes, the prognosis being worse in patients with mutation-positive GISTs.

Precise data on long-term survival for patients with GISTs are difficult to provide owing to the introduction of an effective treatment strategy (imatinib mesylate) in clinical practice and the recognition of the KIT protein (CD117), which has changed the way spindle cell tumors of the gastrointestinal tract are classified. Prior to the introduction of imatinib mesylate, the available chemotherapeutic protocols were not effective against GISTs and the outcome of these patients was bleak.[88] Furthermore, until recently, studies on GISTs included tumors that are not presently classified as GISTs. It is, nevertheless, believed that the overall or disease-specific 5-year survival rate is 28% to 60% among patients with malignant GIST; the median disease-specific survival time is about 5 years for primary disease, and 10 to 20 months in recurrent or metastatic disease.[47,89] Most recurrences take place within 5 years of the primary diagnosis,[85] but in the slowly proliferating subset of GISTs and especially after therapy with imatinib mesylate, metastases can appear more than 10 years after the primary diagnosis.

The outcome of patients with metastatic malignancies to the small intestine (more commonly ovarian, colon, and lung cancers, renal cell carcinoma, and melanoma) is dismal despite palliative therapeutic intervention.

PRIMARY TREATMENT

Treatment of adenocarcinoma of the small intestine with localized disease is based on oncologic and anatomic principles. For duodenal lesions the availability of endoscopic ultrasound has allowed better preoperative staging,[90,91] and the availability of endoscopic resection techniques[92] has offered additional therapeutic options. Ultrasound-proved benign duodenal or ampullary adenomas can be resected endoscopically with excellent results. If associated with familial polyposis, chemoprevention with sulindac or cyclo-oxygenase-2 (COX-2) inhibitors may be beneficial.[93]

Invasive lesions of the first and second portion of the duodenum without major vessel involvement and distant spread are best treated by a pancreaticoduodenectomy (Whipple procedure). For tumors in the third or fourth portion of the duodenum segmental resection with regional lymphadenectomy is indicated.[18,19,79-81] Debate persists about the optimal surgical management of early duodenal cancer. Although early reports suggest that an endoscopic approach could be justified in early favorable lesions, long-term follow-up is still lacking,[94] and surgical resection is preferred in the good-risk patients. Palliative options for unresectable or metastatic duodenal carcinoma include gastrojejunostomy or biliary enteric bypass or endoscopic/interventional placement of stents to relieve the intestinal or biliary obstruction.

Adenocarcinoma of the jejunum and ileum is treated by wide excision, including areas of contiguous spread and the associated mesentery, with negative surgical margins.

Although only small series have been published, these tumors do not seem to respond to the conventional 5-FU-based chemotherapy regimens, and there is a radiation dose limitation due to small bowel toxicity. However, for palliation of chronic blood loss in patients with locally advanced unresectable duodenal carcinomas, radiotherapy may provide short-term benefit.

The mainstay of therapy for carcinoid tumors is radical surgical excision. In preparation for surgery a complete assessment of the entire gastrointestinal tract is warranted because up to 40% of midgut carcinoids are associated with a second gastrointestinal malignancy and 30% may be multicentric.[42,43] In addition, preemptive treatment with octreotide is indicated to prevent carcinoid crisis at the time of surgery. At surgery, wide en bloc resection including the draining mesentery is the standard approach,[18,19,42,43] particularly for small bowel carcinoid, because these lesions have the propensity to metastasize even when very small. Large lesions near the ampulla may require a pancreaticoduodenectomy for cure, and smaller lesions may be treated with either local excision or endoscopic resection with close endoscopic follow-up. Likewise, lesions of the terminal ileum or carcinoid tumors of the appendix larger than 2 cm require a formal right hemicolectomy for oncologic clearance of disease.

Treatment for advanced locoregional and distant disease includes both medical and surgical modalities. In one published study, after complete resection of all known disease a 73% actuarial 5-year survival rate was obtained, compared to 29% in patients that were deemed unresectable.[95] Therefore surgery should be indicated in patients with resectable metastatic disease for potential cure or at least meaningful palliation. Orthotopic liver transplantation (OLT) has been used in the treatment of metastatic neuroendocrine tumors to the liver.[96-99] In a recent report all patients had complete symptomatic response initially, but tumor recurrence was noted in 6 of 11 cases at a median of 11 months, with a mortality rate of 45%.[98] These discouraging results have limited the use of OLT for metastatic carcinoid tumors.

The role of multimodality therapy, including alpha-2b interferon and octreotide, for metastatic carcinoid remains limited.[100-102] Interferon seems to provide symptomatic control in up to 70% of patients with carcinoid syndrome[101] and to increase 5-year survival rates to 71% in patients who continued treatment for 1 year compared to 37% of those who stopped the treatment.[100] The addition of liver chemoembolization has not been shown to have a significant effect on survival in patients with metastatic disease to the liver[100,101] but may have a role in controlling or decreasing the symptoms associated with carcinoid

crisis. Octreotide has been effective in the treatment of patients with carcinoid syndrome by improving diarrhea in up to 83% of the patients and abolishing flushing and wheezing, but has no effect on survival.[102-104] In consideration of the slow growth rate of many carcinoid tumors, patients with distant metastatic disease can also undergo resection for debulking and palliation of symptoms.[95,105-107] For those unfortunate individuals with extensive unresectable disease, the indications for surgical intervention are limited to the occurrence of obstruction, perforation, and bleeding. Radiation therapy has not been proved to be effective in either the adjuvant or palliative setting.

Treatment of small bowel lymphoma requires conservative resections with para-aortic and mesenteric lymph node sampling, liver biopsy, and bone marrow biopsy performed for staging. Low-grade localized lesions are treated with resection alone, and for intermediate- and high-grade lesions resection and chemotherapy are recommended. Radiation is used only for palliation in poor performance patients.[45] This modality is associated with significant side effects, such as bowel necrosis, bleeding, and perforation, and is offered for palliation only to patients unfit for surgery or chemotherapy.

Surgical treatment for small bowel sarcomas consists of an en bloc resection with tumor-free margins. There is no role for extended lymphadenectomy in these tumors.[18,19,82] Hematogenous dissemination is the preferred route of metastatic spread to the liver, lungs, and bones. Carcinomatosis is noted in later stages of the disease. In the presence of metastatic disease, local excision or palliative bypass procedure might be indicated to prevent or ameliorate bleeding and obstruction. Furthermore, there is no clear benefit from chemoradiation therapy in the adjuvant setting, because radiation doses are limited owing to small bowel toxicity. In the presence of recurrent or metastatic disease partial response rates after palliative chemotherapy and radiation therapy have been reported in the 10% to 20% range, with minimal improvement in survival at best.

Treatment of localized GISTs is based on surgical resection. Usually a true tumor capsule does not exist, like in other soft tissue sarcomas, and the tumor should be removed en bloc with its pseudocapsule and margins of normal soft tissue or bowel.[108] In the presence of large lesions involving other organs, where an en bloc resection may be associated with significant morbidity, preoperative neoadjuvant use of imatinib mesylate may be entertained,[37] although at present data to support this practice are still lacking, pending results of the Radiation Therapy Oncology Group/American College of Radiology Imaging Network phase II study of imatinib mesylate in the neoadjuvant setting followed by surgery after 2 months of treatment.

At surgery an effort should be made to obtain tumor-free margins; several studies have shown better overall survival in patients who have undergone margin negative resections,[82,86,109] and this practice helps to avoid tumor violation or rupture, which is associated with increased risk of peritoneal implants.[82] Regional lymph node dissection is of unproved value and is not recommended.[108]

A significant breakthrough in the management of small bowel tumors and specifically GISTs has come from understanding the molecular and genetic makeup of these lesions. After the discovery that GISTs characteristically express the KIT protein, a transmembrane tyrosine kinase receptor for a stem cell factor, a specific tyrosine kinase inhibitor, imatinib mesylate (Gleevec, Novartis), has been introduced in clinical practice with partial response rates as high as 80% in advanced GISTs.[110] Studies are under way examining the potential benefit of giving imatinib mesylate after resection of primary GIST. The American College of Surgeons Oncology Group has two nationwide studies open for the study of imatinib mesylate in the adjuvant setting. The first is a phase II study for high-risk resected GIST. The second is a phase III study examining GISTs larger than 3 cm and randomizes patients to placebo or imatinib mesylate at 400 mg/day. In each study, the treatment is given for 1 year.

The role of surgery for recurrent or metastatic disease has been questioned since the introduction of imatinib mesylate.[111] Currently the standard of care for metastatic GIST is imatinib mesylate at a dose of 400 mg/day or 600 mg/day, the latter given in divided doses.[77] Few complete responses to imatinib mesylate have been observed, but the response rate is in the 60% to 80% range, a percentage better than any previously recommended chemotherapy regimen.[77] However, some evidence suggests that resection of metastasis may improve survival in selected patients with well to moderately differentiated GIST with isolated resectable metastasis and a disease-free interval of more than 12 months.[112,113] Surgery should still be considered in patients with bleeding or obstructive disease and after partial response to imatinib mesylate if the residual disease is deemed to be resectable.

Occasionally patients may appear to develop new metastatic disease, especially in the liver, while receiving imatinib mesylate, because such lesions often represent occult disease on the initial CT scan that becomes evident as the tumor mass necroses or changes density with decreased perfusion. Obviously, in these cases, it is important to continue treatment with imatinib mesylate. On the other hand, acquired clinical resistance to imatinib mesylate has been reported in chronic myeloid leukemia (CML)[114] and more recently in GISTs.[77] In CML, resistance to imatinib mesylate treatment is primarily associated with reactivation of BCR-ABL signal transduction.[114,115] This reactivation is caused by several different molecular mechanisms, including BCR-ABL gene amplification and single amino acid substitution.[114,115] The actual resistance mechanism to imatinib mesylate treatment in GIST is still unclear and is currently being studied. The proportion of GIST patients who will relapse after a response is not currently known.[37]

As imatinib mesylate is used more and more often in the treatment of GISTs, it is important to briefly review side effects and complications associated with its use. Recommended doses for imatinib mesylate are 400 to 600 mg/day, and tolerability has been reported for daily doses up to 800 mg. Most side effects are mild to moderate and include periorbital and lower extremity edema, nausea, muscle cramps, diarrhea, headache, dermatitis, fatigue, anemia, and neutropenia.[77] Grades 3 and 4 toxic effects occur in less than 30% of patients at the recommended dose of 400 to 600 mg/day.[77,116] Dramatic response to imatinib mesylate may be complicated by intratumoral bleeding in less than 5% of patients, sometimes resulting in free intraperitoneal or intraluminal bleeding requiring surgical exploration. Minor side effects usually resolve after cessation of treatment.[37] Drug interactions with warfarin and paracetamol have been reported and these combinations should be avoided.

FOLLOW-UP

In general, routine follow-up for small bowel cancers is accomplished with endoscopy and radiologic imaging. The only exception is GIST. As previously discussed, PET scan is used to follow tumor response to imatinib mesylate, to detect recurrence after either complete response to imatinib mesylate or after curative surgery, and to identify secondary resistance to imatinib mesylate before tumor progression on treatment. Data are still inconclusive regarding a survival advantage in patients followed with PET scan. The Radiation Therapy Oncology Group/American College of Radiology Imaging Network phase II study of imatinib mesylate in the neoadjuvant setting, involving pre- and post-treatment PET scan after biopsy confirmation of tumor, followed by surgery, should shed some light on the actual impact of PET scan on the management of these patients. Clinical resistance to imatinib mesylate poses a significant problem. Because we do not clearly know the mechanisms behind resistance to imatinib mesylate in GISTs, we do not know how to prevent or suppress this resistance. Furthermore, conventional chemotherapy regimens are not nearly as effective as imatinib mesylate, and long-term prognosis in patients who may have had an initial dramatic response and have become resistant is very poor.

CONCLUSIONS

Despite the remarkable advances in the imaging, classification, and treatment of small bowel cancer, much is still to be achieved. Capsule endoscopy, enteroclysis, endoscopic ultrasound, and PET scan have all improved our diagnostic ability, but differentiating diagnostic tools for earlier diagnosis of these rare malignancies are needed. Imatinib mesylate represents an innovative therapy, one of the first successful pharmacologic manipulations of the product of a constitutively activating mutation that derives pathogenesis of a solid tumor. As such, imatinib mesylate has an impact on the actual mechanism of cancer development and progression. However, many questions remain unanswered with this new drug: optimal duration of therapy, its role in the neoadjuvant or adjuvant setting, its role in combination therapy, and the overall long-term results. More important, the mechanisms behind acquired resistance to imatinib mesylate have to be further elucidated. Finally, combination therapy with conventional chemotherapy and other signal transduction inhibitors must be further investigated.

REFERENCES

1. Jemal A, Thomas A, Murray T, Thun M: Cancer statistics, 2002. CA Cancer J Clin 2002;52(1): 23–47.
2. North JH, Pack MS: Malignant tumors of the small intestine: A review of 144 cases. Am Surg 2000;66(1):46–51.
3. Stang A, Stegmaier C, Eisinger B, Stabenow R, Metz KA, Jockel KH: Descriptive epidemiology of small intestinal malignancies: The German Cancer Registry experience. Br J Cancer 1999;80(9):1440–1444.
4. Turowski GA, Basson MD: Primary malignant lymphoma of the intestine. Am J Surg 1995;169(4):433–441.
5. Coit DG: Cancer of the small intestine. In DeVita VT, Hellman S, Rosenberg SA (eds): Cancer. Principles and Practice of Oncology. Philadelphia, Lippincott-Raven, 1997, pp 1128–1143.
6. Howe JR, Karnell LH, Menck HR, Scott-Conner C: The American College of Surgeons Commission on Cancer and the American Cancer Society. Adenocarcinoma of the small bowel: Review of the National Cancer Data Base, 1985–1995. Cancer 1999;86(12): 2693–2706.
7. Greenstein AJ: Cancer in inflammatory bowel disease. Mt Sinai J Med 2000;67(3):227–240.
8. Greenstein AJ, Sachar D, Pucillo A, Kreel I, Geller S, Janowitz HD, Aufses A Jr: Cancer in Crohn's disease after diversionary surgery. A report of seven carcinomas occurring in excluded bowel. Am J Surg 1978;135(1):86–90.
9. Greenstein AJ, Sachar DB, Smith H, Janowitz HD, Aufses AH Jr: A comparison of cancer risk in Crohn's disease and ulcerative colitis. Cancer 1981;48(12):2742–2745.
10. Jaskowiak NT, Michelassi F: Adenocarcinoma at a strictureplasty site in Crohn's disease: Report of a case. Dis Colon Rectum 2001;44(2):284–287.
11. Ribeiro MB, Greenstein AJ, Heimann TM, Yamazaki Y, Aufses AH Jr: Adenocarcinoma of the small intestine in Crohn's disease. Surg Gynecol Obstet 1991;173(5):343–349.
12. Marchetti F, Fazio VW, Ozuner G: Adenocarcinoma arising from a strictureplasty site in Crohn's disease. Report of a case. Dis Colon Rectum 1996;39(11):1315–1321.
13. Michelassi F, Testa G, Pomidor WJ, Lashner BA, Block GE: Adenocarcinoma complicating Crohn's disease. Dis Colon Rectum 1993;36(7):654–661.
14. Collier PE, Turowski P, Diamond DL: Small intestinal adenocarcinoma complicating regional enteritis. Cancer 1985;55(3):516–521.
15. Jagelman DG, DeCosse JJ, Bussey HJ: Upper gastrointestinal cancer in familial adenomatous polyposis. Lancet 1988;1(8595): 1149–1151.
16. Offerhaus GJ, Giardiello FM, Krush AJ, Booker SV, Tersmette AC, Kelley NC, Hamilton SR: The risk of upper gastrointestinal cancer in familial adenomatous polyposis. Gastroenterology 1992;102(6): 1980–1982.
17. Rodriguez-Bigas MA, Vasen HF, Lynch HT, et al: Characteristics of small bowel carcinoma in hereditary nonpolyposis colorectal carcinoma. International Collaborative Group on HNPCC. Cancer 1998;83(2):240–244.
18. Martin RG: Malignant tumors of the small intestine. Surg Clin North Am 1986;66(4):779–785.
19. Ashley SW, Wells SA Jr: Tumors of the small intestine. Semin Oncol 1988;15(2):116–128.
20. Giardiello FM, Welsh SB, Hamilton SR, et al: Increased risk of cancer in the Peutz-Jeghers syndrome. N Engl J Med 1987; 316(24):1511–1514.
21. Trier JS: Celiac sprue. N Engl J Med 1991;325(24):1709–1719.
22. Ross RK, Hartnett NM, Bernstein L, Henderson BE: Epidemiology of adenocarcinomas of the small intestine: Is bile a small bowel carcinogen? Br J Cancer 1991;63(1):43–45.
23. Scudamore CH, Freeman HJ: Effects of small bowel transection, resection, or bypass in 1,2-dimethylhydrazine-induced rat intestinal neoplasia. Gastroenterology 1983;84(4):725–731.
24. Lowenfels AB: Why are small-bowel tumours so rare? Lancet 1973;1(7793):24–26.
25. Wattenberg LW: Studies of polycyclic hydrocarbon hydroxylases of the intestine possibly related to cancer. Effect of diet on benzpyrene hydroxylase activity. Cancer 1971;28(1):99–102.
26. Wattenberg LW: Carcinogen-detoxifying mechanisms in the gastrointestinal tract. Gastroenterology 1966;51(5):932–935.
27. Chow WH, Linet MS, McLaughlin JK, Hsing AW, Chien HT, Blot WJ: Risk factors for small intestine cancer. Cancer Causes Control 1993;4(2):163–169.
28. Lowenfels AB, Anderson ME: Diet and cancer. Cancer 1977; 39(4 suppl):1809–1814.
29. Lowenfels AB, Sonni A: Distribution of small bowel tumors. Cancer Lett 1977;3(1-2):83–86.
30. Brownstein EG: Multiple metachronous gastrointestinal carcinoma. Aust NZ J Surg 1981;51(5):446–450.
31. Hilbun BM, Block W: Primary malignant tumors of the small bowel. J Miss State Med Assoc 1987;28(7):169–171.
32. Honore LH: Metachronous primary carcinoma of small bowel following resected colorectal carcinoma: A report of three cases. J Surg Oncol 1980;14(4):341–346.
33. Neugut AI, Santos J: The association between cancers of the small and large bowel. Cancer Epidemiol Biomarkers Prev 1993;2(6):551-3.
34. Weiss NS, Yang CP: Incidence of histologic types of cancer of the small intestine. J Natl Cancer Inst 1987;78(4):653–656.
35. Cunningham JD, Aleali R, Aleali M, Brower ST, Aufses AH: Malignant small bowel neoplasms: Histopathologic determinants of recurrence and survival. Ann Surg 1997;225(3):300–306.
36. Chow JS, Chen CC, Ahsan H, Neugut AI: A population-based study of the incidence of malignant small bowel tumours: SEER, 1973–1990. Int J Epidemiol 1996;25(4):722–728.
37. Joensuu H, Fletcher C, Dimitrijevic S, Silberman S, Roberts P, Demetri G: Management of malignant gastrointestinal stromal tumours. Lancet Oncol 2002;3(11):655–664.
38. American Joint Committee on Cancer: Small intestine. In Green FL, et al (eds): Cancer Staging Manual. New York, Springer Verlag, 2002, pp 107–112.
39. Kerremans RP, Lerut J, Penninckx FM: Primary malignant duodenal tumors. Ann Surg 1979;190(2):179–182.
40. Spira IA, Ghazi A, Wolff WI: Primary adenocarcinoma of the duodenum. Cancer 1977;39(4):1721–1726.
41. Michelassi F, Erroi F, Dawson PJ, et al: Experience with 647 consecutive tumors of the duodenum, ampulla, head of the pancreas, and distal common bile duct. Ann Surg 1989;210(4):544–554; discussion 554–556.
42. Thompson GB, van Heerden JA, Martin JK Jr, Schutt AJ, Ilstrup DM, Carney JA: Carcinoid tumors of the gastrointestinal tract: Presentation, management, and prognosis. Surgery 1985;98(6): 1054–1063.
43. Moertel CG: Karnofsky memorial lecture. An odyssey in the land of small tumors. J Clin Oncol 1987;5(10):1502–1522.
44. Cooper BT, Read AE: Small intestinal lymphoma. World J Surg 1985;9(6):930–937.
45. Contreary K, Nance FC, Becker WF: Primary lymphoma of the gastrointestinal tract. Ann Surg 1980;191(5):593–598.
46. Mazur MT, Clark HB: Gastric stromal tumors. Reappraisal of histogenesis. Am J Surg Pathol 1983;7(6):507–519.
47. DeMatteo RP, Lewis JJ, Leung D, Mudan SS, Woodruff JM, Brennan MF: Two hundred gastrointestinal stromal tumors: Recurrence patterns and prognostic factors for survival. Ann Surg 2000; 231(1):51–58.
48. Lecoin L, Gabella G, Le Douarin N: Origin of the c-kit-positive interstitial cells in the avian bowel. Development 1996;122(3): 725–733.
49. Miettinen M, and Lasota J: Gastrointestinal stromal tumors: Definition, clinical, histological, immunohistochemical, and molecular genetic features and differential diagnosis. Virchows Arch 2001;438(1):1–12.
50. Sakurai S, Fukasawa T, Chong JM, Tanaka A, Fukayama M: Embryonic form of smooth muscle myosin heavy chain (SMemb/MHC-B) in gastrointestinal stromal tumor and interstitial cells of Cajal. Am J Pathol 1999;154(1):23–28.
51. Kindblom LG, Remotti HE, Aldenborg F, Meis-Kindblom JM: Gastrointestinal pacemaker cell tumor (GIPACT): Gastrointestinal stromal tumors show phenotypic characteristics of the interstitial cells of Cajal. Am J Pathol 1998;152(5):1259–1269.
52. Fletcher CD, Berman JJ, Corless C, et al: Diagnosis of gastrointestinal stromal tumors: A consensus approach. Hum Pathol 2002;33(5):459–465.

53. Heinrich MC, Rubin BP, Longley BJ, Fletcher JA: Biology and genetic aspects of gastrointestinal stromal tumors: KIT activation and cytogenetic alterations. Hum Pathol 2002;33(5):484–495.

54. Miettinen M, Sobin LH, Sarlomo-Rikala M: Immunohistochemical spectrum of GISTs at different sites and their differential diagnosis with a reference to CD117 (KIT). Mod Pathol 2000;13(10):1134–1142.

55. Younes N, Fulton N, Tanaka R, Wayne J, Straus FH 2nd, Kaplan EL: The presence of K-12 ras mutations in duodenal adenocarcinomas and the absence of ras mutations in other small bowel adenocarcinomas and carcinoid tumors. Cancer 1997;79(9):1804–1808.

56. Park SH, Kim YI, Park YH, et al: Clinicopathologic correlation of p53 protein overexpression in adenoma and carcinoma of the ampulla of Vater. World J Surg 2000;24(1):54–59.

57. Vaidya P, Yosida T, Sakakura T, Yatani R, Noguchi T, Kawarada Y: Combined analysis of expression of c-erbB-2, Ki-67 antigen, and tenascin provides a better prognostic indicator of carcinoma of the papilla of Vater. Pancreas 1996;12(2):196–201.

58. Blackman E, Nash SV: Diagnosis of duodenal and ampullary epithelial neoplasms by endoscopic biopsy: A clinicopathologic and immunohistochemical study. Hum Pathol 1985;16(9):901–910.

59. Yamaguchi K, Enjoji M, Tsuneyoshi M: Pancreatoduodenal carcinoma: A clinicopathologic study of 304 patients and immunohistochemical observation for CEA and CA19-9. J Surg Oncol 1991;47(3):148–154.

60. Lux ML, Rubin BP, Biase TL, et al: KIT extracellular and kinase domain mutations in gastrointestinal stromal tumors. Am J Pathol 2000;156(3):791–795.

61. Rubin BP, Fletcher JA, Fletcher CD: Molecular insights into the histogenesis and pathogenesis of gastrointestinal stromal tumors. Int J Surg Pathol 2000;8(1):5–10.

62. Hirota S, Isozaki K, Moriyama Y, et al: Gain-of-function mutations of c-kit in human gastrointestinal stromal tumors. Science 1998;279(5350):577–580.

63. Sarlomo-Rikala M, Kovatich AJ, Barusevicius A, Miettinen M: CD117: A sensitive marker for gastrointestinal stromal tumors that is more specific than CD34. Mod Pathol 1998;11(8):728–734.

64. Bessette JR, Maglinte DD, Kelvin FM, Chernish SM: Primary malignant tumors in the small bowel: A comparison of the small-bowel enema and conventional follow-through examination. AJR Am J Roentgenol 1989;153(4):741–744.

65. Rollins ES, Picus D, Hicks ME, Darcy MD, Bower BL, Kleinhoffer MA: Angiography is useful in detecting the source of chronic gastrointestinal bleeding of obscure origin. Am J Roentgenol 1991;156(2):385–388.

66. Berner JS, Mauer K, Lewis BS: Push and sonde enteroscopy for the diagnosis of obscure gastrointestinal bleeding. Am J Gastroenterol 1994;89(12):2139–2142.

67. Lewis BS, Kornbluth A, Waye JD: Small bowel tumours: Yield of enteroscopy. Gut 1991;32(7):763–765.

68. Chong J, Tagle M, Barkin JS, Reiner DK: Small bowel push-type fiberoptic enteroscopy for patients with occult gastrointestinal bleeding or suspected small bowel pathology. Am J Gastroenterol 1994;89(12):2143–2146.

69. Fritscher-Ravens A, Swain CP: The wireless capsule: New light in the darkness. Dig Dis 2002;20(2):127–133.

70. Appleyard M, Fireman Z, Glukhovsky A, et al: A randomized trial comparing wireless capsule endoscopy with push enteroscopy for the detection of small-bowel lesions. Gastroenterology 2000;119(6):1431–1438.

71. Lewis BS, Swain P: Capsule endoscopy in the evaluation of patients with suspected small intestinal bleeding: Results of a pilot study. Gastrointest Endosc 2002;56(3):349–353.

72. Appleyard M, Glukhovsky A, Swain P: Wireless-capsule diagnostic endoscopy for recurrent small-bowel bleeding. N Engl J Med 2001;344(3):232–233.

73. Iddan G, Meron G, Glukhovsky A, Swain P: Wireless capsule endoscopy. Nature 2000;405(6785):417.

74. Ell C, Remke S, May A, Helou L, Henrich R, Mayer G: The first prospective controlled trial comparing wireless capsule endoscopy with push enteroscopy in chronic gastrointestinal bleeding. Endoscopy 2002;34(9):685–689.

75. Costamagna G, Shah SK, Riccioni ME, et al: A prospective trial comparing small bowel radiographs and video capsule endoscopy for suspected small bowel disease. Gastroenterology 2002;123(4):999–1005.

76. Joensuu H, Dimitrijevic S: Tyrosine kinase inhibitor imatinib (STI571) as an anticancer agent for solid tumours. Ann Med 2001;33(7):451–455.

77. Demetri GD, von Mehren M, Blanke CD, et al: Efficacy and safety of imatinib mesylate in advanced gastrointestinal stromal tumors. N Engl J Med 2002;347(7):472–480.

78. Abrahams NA, Halverson A, Fazio VW, Rybicki LA, Goldblum JR: Adenocarcinoma of the small bowel: A study of 37 cases with emphasis on histologic prognostic factors. Dis Colon Rectum 2002;45(11):1496–1502.

79. Ouriel K, Adams JT: Adenocarcinoma of the small intestine. Am J Surg 1984;147(1):66–71.

80. Lowell JA, Rossi RL, Munson JL, Braasch JW: Primary adenocarcinoma of third and fourth portions of duodenum. Favorable prognosis after resection. Arch Surg 1992;127(5):557–560.

81. Barnes G Jr, Romero L, Hess KR, Curley SA: Primary adenocarcinoma of the duodenum: Management and survival in 67 patients. Ann Surg Oncol 1994;1(1):73–78.

82. Ng EH, Pollock RE, Munsell MF, Atkinson EN, Romsdahl MM: Prognostic factors influencing survival in gastrointestinal leiomyosarcomas. Implications for surgical management and staging. Ann Surg 1992;215(1):68–77.

83. Nishida T, Hirota S: Biological and clinical review of stromal tumors in the gastrointestinal tract. Histol Histopathol 2000;15(4):1293–1301.

84. Miettinen M, El-Rifai W, HL Sobin L, Lasota J: Evaluation of malignancy and prognosis of gastrointestinal stromal tumors: A review. Hum Pathol 2002;33(5):478–483.

85. Emory TS, Sobin LH, Lukes L, Lee DH, O'Leary TJ: Prognosis of gastrointestinal smooth-muscle (stromal) tumors: Dependence on anatomic site. Am J Surg Pathol 1999;23(1):82–87.

86. Chou FF, Eng HL, Sheen-Chen SM: Smooth muscle tumors of the gastrointestinal tract: Analysis of prognostic factors. Surgery 1996;119(2):171–177.

87. Taniguchi M, Nishida T, Hirota S, et al: Effect of c-kit mutation on prognosis of gastrointestinal stromal tumors. Cancer Res 1999;59(17):4297–4300.

88. Edmonson JH, Marks RS, Buckner, Mahoney MR: Contrast of response to dacarbazine, mitomycin, doxorubicin, and cisplatin (DMAP) plus GM-CSF between patients with advanced malignant gastrointestinal stromal tumors and patients with other advanced leiomyosarcomas. Cancer Invest 2002;20(5–6):605–612.

89. Conlon KC, Casper ES, Brennan MF: Primary gastrointestinal sarcomas: Analysis of prognostic variables. Ann Surg Oncol 1995;2(1):26–31.

90. Mukai H, Nakajima M, Yasuda K, Mizuno S, Kawai K: Evaluation of endoscopic ultrasonography in the pre-operative staging of carcinoma of the ampulla of Vater and common bile duct. Gastrointest Endosc 1992;38(6):676–683.

91. Yasuda K, Mukai H, Cho E, Nakajima M, Kawai K: The use of endoscopic ultrasonography in the diagnosis and staging of carcinoma of the papilla of Vater. Endoscopy 1988;20(Suppl 1):218–222.

92. Gersin KS, Heniford BT, Baradi H, Ponsky JL: Laparoendoscopic excision of a duodenal mass. Endoscopy 1999;31(5):398–400.

93. Bresalier RS: Chemoprevention comes to clinical practice: COX-2 inhibition in familial adenomatous polyposis. Gastroenterology 2000;119(6):1797–1798.

94. Yoshimoto T, Akahoshi K, Nakanishi K, Nawata H: Endoscopic removal of a pedunculated early duodenal cancer: Diagnostic value of endoscopic ultrasound. Acta Gastroenterol Belg 2002;65(1):52–54.

95. Chen H, Hardacre JM, Uzar A, Cameron JL, Choti MA: Isolated liver metastases from neuroendocrine tumors: Does resection prolong survival? J Am Coll Surg 1998;187(1):88–92; discussion 92–93.

96. Coperchini ML, Jones R, Angus P, Read A, Schmidt G, Zalcberg J: Liver transplantation in metastatic carcinoid tumour. Aust NZ J Med 1996;26(5):702–704.

97. Le Treut YP, Delpero JR, Dousset B, et al: Results of liver transplantation in the treatment of metastatic neuroendocrine tumors. A 31-case French multicentric report. Ann Surg 1997; 225(4):355-364.

98. Routley D, Ramage JK, McPeake J, Tan KC, Williams R: Orthotopic liver transplantation in the treatment of metastatic neuroendocrine tumors of the liver. Liver Transpl Surg 1995;1(2):118-121.

99. Frilling A, Rogiers X, Knofel WT, Broelsch CE: Liver transplantation for metastatic carcinoid tumors. Digestion 1994;55(Suppl 3): 104-106.

100. Jacobsen MB, Hanssen LE, Kolmannskog F, Schrumpf E, Vatn MH, Bergan A: Interferon-alpha 2b, with or without prior hepatic artery embolization: Clinical response and survival in mid-gut carcinoid patients. The Norwegian carcinoid study. Scand J Gastroenterol 1995;30(8):789-796.

101. Hanssen LE, Schrumpf E, Kolbenstvedt AN, Tausjo J, Dolva LO: Treatment of malignant metastatic midgut carcinoid tumours with recombinant human alpha2b interferon with or without prior hepatic artery embolization. Scand J Gastroenterol 1989;24(7): 787-795.

102. Diaco DS, Hajarizadeh H, Mueller CR, Fletcher WS, Pommier RF, Woltering EA: Treatment of metastatic carcinoid tumors using multimodality therapy of octreotide acetate, intra-arterial chemotherapy, and hepatic arterial chemoembolization. Am J Surg 1995;169(5):523-528.

103. Kvols LK, Moertel CG, O'Connell MJ, Schutt AJ, Rubin J, Hahn RG: Treatment of the malignant carcinoid syndrome. Evaluation of a long-acting somatostatin analogue. N Engl J Med 1986;315(11):663-666.

104. Vinik A, Moattari AR: Use of somatostatin analog in management of carcinoid syndrome. Dig Dis Sci 1989;34(3 suppl):14S-27S.

105. Lindell G, Ohlsson B, Saarela A, Andersson R, Tranberg KG: Liver resection of noncolorectal secondaries. J Surg Oncol 1998;69(2):66-70.

106. Dousset B, Saint-Marc O, Pitre J, Soubrane O, Houssin D, Chapuis Y: Metastatic endocrine tumors: Medical treatment, surgical resection, or liver transplantation. World J Surg 1996;20(7): 908-914; discussion 914-915.

107. Ahlman H, Westberg G, Wangberg B, et al: Treatment of liver metastases of carcinoid tumors. World J Surg 1996;20(2):196-202.

108. Pidhorecky I, Cheney RT, Kraybill WG, Gibbs JF: Gastrointestinal stromal tumors: Current diagnosis, biologic behavior, and management. Ann Surg Oncol 2000;7(9):705-712.

109. Crosby JA, Catton CN, Davis A, et al: Malignant gastrointestinal stromal tumors of the small intestine: A review of 50 cases from a prospective database. Ann Surg Oncol 2001;8(1):50-59.

110. Blanke CD, Eisenberg BL, Heinrich MC: Gastrointestinal stromal tumors. Curr Treat Options Oncol 2001;2(6):485-91.

111. Mudan SS, Conlon KC, Woodruff JM, Lewis JJ, Brennan MF: Salvage surgery for patients with recurrent gastrointestinal sarcoma: Prognostic factors to guide patient selection. Cancer 2000;88(1): 66-74.

112. Chen H, Pruitt A, Nicol TL, Gorgulu S, Choti MA: Complete hepatic resection of metastases from leiomyosarcoma prolongs survival. J Gastrointest Surg 1998;2(2):151-155.

113. Karakousis CP, Blumenson LE, Canavese G, Rao U: Surgery for disseminated abdominal sarcoma. Am J Surg 1992;163(6): 560-564.

114. Gorre ME, Mohammed M, Ellwood K, et al: Clinical resistance to STI-571 cancer therapy caused by BCR-ABL gene mutation or amplification. Science 2001;293(5531):876-880.

115. Mahon FX, Deininger MW, Schultheis B, et al: Selection and characterization of BCR-ABL positive cell lines with differential sensitivity to the tyrosine kinase inhibitor STI571: Diverse mechanisms of resistance. Blood 2000;96(3):1070-1079.

116. van Oosterom AT, Judson I, Verweij J, et al: Safety and efficacy of imatinib (STI571) in metastatic gastrointestinal stromal tumours: A phase I study. Lancet 2001;358(9291):1421-1423.

Specific Malignancies

III

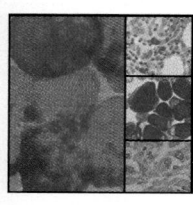

COLON CANCER

John E. Niederhuber

Carolyn E. Cole

Louise Grochow

Russell F. Jacoby

Fred T. Lee, Jr.

Margaret Mooney

Mark Ritter

SUMMARY OF KEY POINTS

EPIDEMIOLOGY

- Colon cancer is the fourth most common cancer worldwide, with about 450,000 new cases each year. In the United States in 2003, there were an estimated 105,500 new cases (49,000 male and 56,500 female).
- Five-year relative survival:
  - 63% U.S. white population
  - 53% U.S. black population
  - 41% European population
  - 30% Eastern European and China
  - The United States has seen a 0.6% decline in annual incidence over the past 10 years, with a 1.7% decrease in annual mortality.

ETIOLOGY

- 80% of colon cancer is sporadic and not associated with known hereditary genetic alterations.
- Age is a recognized risk factor, with 90% of cases occurring after 50 years of age.
- Inherited genetic variation increases risk in concert with dietary and environmental exposures.
- There is a two- to fourfold increased incidence among those with an affected first-degree relative (rel. risk ~1.72 for one relative; 2.75 for two or more). There is a direct correlation between increased body weight and development of colon cancer—concept of energy balance.
- Initiation with progression to adenoma and on to invasive carcinoma within the adenoma.
- At least two types of genetic instability have been observed in colon cancer development— chromosomal instability (~60% of colon cancer) and micro satellite instability.
- The APC tumor suppressor gene is defective in more than 80% of adenomatous polyps and colon cancers.

PREVENTION OF CANCER

- Flexible fiberoptic and video colonoscopy is the mainstay of prevention as well as a useful tool in diagnosis.
- Diagnosis of a specific hereditary syndrome requires the identification of a mutation that functionally inactivates or alters a gene known to cause the syndrome.
- A mutation is defined as a stable, heritable change in DNA inherited in an autosomally dominant manner.
- Colonic polyps of epithelial origin are precursors of invasive cancer.
- Familial syndromes include FAP, HNPCC, AAPC, JS, JP, and HMPS.
- Chemopreventive drugs such as COX-2 inhibitors may prevent polyps in high-risk patients.

DIAGNOSIS AND STAGING

- Colorectal cancer is often insidious in development, underlying the importance of screening.
- Fatigue, anemia, altered bowel function, and weight loss are frequent symptoms.
- Obstruction is the most common acute surgical problem (about 30% of left-sided lesions present with an obstruction).
- About 5% will have synchronous cancer. About 20%–40% will have synchronous polyps with cancer primary.
- Imaging used in staging includes CT, MRI, and PET.
- Intraoperative ultrasound is the most sensitive way to evaluate the liver.
- Most common site for synchronous metastases and elevated preoperative CEA.
- Tumor size is not as critical as depth of invasion and nodal status in determining prognosis.

SURGICAL TREATMENT

- En bloc resection of anatomically defined portions of colon with in-continuity draining nodes to root of mesocolon.
- Laparoscopic-assisted surgery is investigational; sentinel node mapping remains to be studied.
- Careful preparation of the bowel prior to surgery minimizes the risk or morbidity and mortality.
- Experienced surgeons and the use of high-volume hospitals improve the chance of good surgical outcome.

SURVEILLANCE

- 80% to 90% of recurrence after curative resection occurs within the first 2 or 3 years. Fewer than 5% of recurrences occur after 5 years.
- Recurrent disease is frequently isolated and surgically resectable— 35% of surgically managed metastatic disease results in a cure. A high percentage of first failures occur in the liver and are asymptomatic. Of those patients followed closely for evidence of recurrence, about 20% are candidates for surgery to clear metastases. They have 18.6% 5-year disease-free survival compared to only a 5.6% 5-year survival when metastatic disease is diagnosed because it has become symptomatic (patients who are not undergoing surveillance).
- Suggested surveillance:
  - Physician exam every three months for first two years and then every six months
  - CEA monitoring every three months
  - Colonoscopy one year postsurgery and then every three to five years
  - CT scan every three to four months

ADJUVANT THERAPY

- 50% to 60% of patients who undergo successful surgery for colon carcinoma have residual micrometastatic disease.

SUMMARY OF KEY POINTS—cont'd

- Systemic chemotherapy is given in an effort to clear micrometastatic disease and is routine for patients with nodal disease (Dukes' C). Adjuvant therapy is also used for selected Dukes' B2 patients.
- Recommended therapy is 6 months of 5-FU and leucovorin and results in a 16% difference in 5 years

disease-free survival compared to surgery-only patients.

MANAGEMENT OF METASTATIC DISEASE

- Chemotherapy with infusional 5-FU and leucovorin regimens in combination with irinotecan or oxaliplatin has prolonged median survival to more than 20 months.

- Additional trials have demonstrated advantages for both FOLFOX and IFL-bevacizumab compared with IFL.
- Capecitabine and cetuximab, as well as agents that are still investigational, provide a variety of available treatments that can be tailored to meet an individual patient's situation.

INTRODUCTION

Adenocarcinoma of the colon and rectum is one of the most common human malignancies. It is a major public health issue in developing and underdeveloped countries. In developed countries, thanks to screening, removal of neoplastic polyps, and advances in surgery, radiation and chemotherapy, there has been a small but persistent improvement in survival over the past two decades, improvements that have not yet been seen in the rest of the world. This chapter reviews progress in understanding the biology of colon cancer, the epidemiology and prevention of colon cancer, and its diagnosis and treatment. The chapter has been divided into eight sections pertaining to the following topics:

- Epidemiology and etiology of colon cancer
- Anatomy and physiology of the colon
- Prevention of colon cancer
- Diagnosis and staging of colon cancer
- Surgical treatment
- Outcomes of surgical treatment and the role of adjuvant therapy
- Medical oncology management of metastatic disease
- New horizons

EPIDEMIOLOGY AND ETIOLOGY OF COLON CANCER

The National Center for Health Statistics (NCHS), the American Cancer Society's *Cancer Facts and Figures-2003*, The National Cancer Data Base of the American College of surgeons, and the Surveillance, Epidemiology, and End Results Program (SEER) are good sources of information concerning the incidence and death rates for colon cancer among Americans.[1-4] For 2003, it is estimated that there will be 105,500 new cases of colon cancer in the United States (49,000 male and 56,500 female patients).

Worldwide, there are an estimated 450,000 new cases each year. SEER data predicts a five-year relative survival rate of 63% for the U.S. white population and 53% for black patients with colon cancer. European and Indian tumor registries report a significantly lower 5-year survival of 41% and 42%, respectively.[5] Even lower 5-year survival rates (approaching 30%) have been reported from Eastern Europe and China.

Over the past 10 years, the United States has witnessed a 0.6% decline in the annual incidence of colon cancer and a decrease of 1.7% in the annual mortality rate (Figs. 80-1 and 80-2). Although this is true for the United States and most countries in the western hemisphere, the incidence and mortality rate for colon cancer vary greatly throughout the world and even regionally within the United States. Worldwide, the incidence varies as much as 30-fold. The United States ranks 15th among 48 industrialized nations reporting colorectal cancer statistics. Mortality from colorectal cancer is characteristically higher in industrialized parts of the world, while lower colon cancer death rates have been reported in East Asia, Eastern Europe, and developing countries. There are geographic differences even within the United States, with a higher incidence in the northeast than in the south and southwest.

U.S. Cancer Burden 2003 Estimates	
1,344,100 cases	556,500 deaths
220,900 prostate	157,200 lung
211,300 female breast	57,100 colorectum
171,900 lung	39,800 breast
147,500 colorectum	30,000 pancreas
65,500 ovary and endometrial	28,900 prostate
57,400 bladder	23,400 NHL
54,200 melanomas	21,900 leukemia
53,400 NHL	14,400 liver and IHBD
31,900 kidney	14,300 ovary
30,700 pancreas	13,100 brain
30,600 leukemia	13,000 esophagus

Figure 80-1. U.S. Cancer Burden 2003 estimates of expected new cases and deaths in relation to other organ sites.

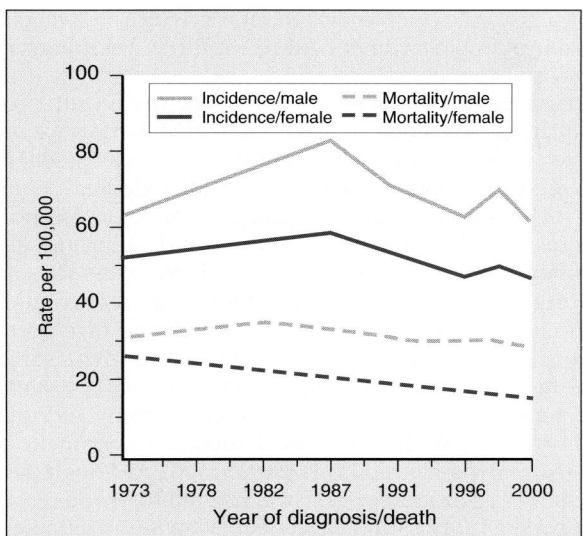

Figure 80-2. Decline in incidence and mortality of colorectal cancer in the United States from 1973–2000. The decline of new cases per year began in the mid 1980s first for women and then for men. The decline occurred in each stage with a recent increase in localized disease. The decline in mortality began for women before 1973 and for men in the mid 1980s.

Race is also a factor in the incidence of colon cancer. For example, the incidence of colon cancer per 100,000 in the U.S. population is 48.7 for blacks, 39.3 for whites, 26.5 for Hispanics, 32.0 for Asians and Pacific islanders, and 26.0 for Native Americans and Alaskan natives. Altogether, it is estimated that slightly fewer than 1,000,000 people in the United States carry a diagnosis of colon cancer.

It is generally agreed that 80% of colon cancer cases are sporadic and not associated with any known hereditary mutations. Age is certainly a risk factor. The risk of developing colorectal cancer begins to increase significantly after the age of 40 and rises sharply at ages 50 to 55 years. Ninety percent of cases of sporadic colon cancer occur after the age of 50.

Although our understanding of etiologic factors in colorectal cancer is still limited, lifestyle and dietary issues (e.g., decreased fiber intake and higher dietary fat consumption) could be important considerations. It is often postulated that this "western lifestyle" plus underlying genetic factors could be important variables to explain the disparity in incidence between geographic regions. Additionally, increases in longevity can vary considerably between population groups, which might also factor into observed geographic differences in colon cancer incidence. It has also been shown that individuals residing in a low-incidence country adopt a higher risk on their immigration to a high-risk country.[6]

In the United States, decreases in the incidence of colon cancer date to the mid-1980s. This decline in incidence and improvement in survival result from a combination of factors. Certainly, increased surveillance and endoscopic polypectomy have been important, but changes in dietary caloric intake, increased exercise, efforts to lower serum cholesterol, the daily use of low-dose aspirin, and decreases in tobacco use all have contributed. It is also important to note that there has been an apparent shift in the anatomic distribution of colon cancer, with fewer left-sided lesions and more right-sided cancers.

Colorectal cancer has been the most intensely studied of all human malignancies. Colon cancer, like other human malignancies, is a disease of dysregulated cell growth and cell death or apoptosis. The development of colon cancer is controlled by changes in specific growth-regulating genes and complicated by the ongoing evolution of these dysregulated cells during disease progression. In colon cancer in particular, the progression of allelic loss has been correlated with progression in malignancy.[7] In addition to inherited genetic variations that increase the risk of colorectal cancer significantly, dietary and other environmental factors appear to influence both the incidence and mortality from this disease by as much as tenfold. The importance of environmental factors and diet would appear to be major variables in carcinoma development. Jewish immigrants from Europe to Israel have a reported two- to threefold increase in risk over similar ethnic populations from North Africa or Asia. This risk equalized between groups after they immigrated to Israel.[8] Even if perceived ideal diets and lifestyles were adopted, however, colorectal cancer would remain a major public health problem, as vegetarians and groups that eschew alcohol and tobacco still have a substantial incidence of colorectal cancer, although it is lower than that in the general population.[9]

As noted previously, age factors also affect the incidence of colorectal cancer, which increases with advancing age. Although colorectal cancer can develop at an early age, occurrence under the age of 40 years accounts for less than 5% of diagnosed cases. Sex distribution of colorectal malignancy is nearly equal between male and female patients.

Familial history of colorectal malignancy does appear to affect overall risk and incidence. The majority of reports have demonstrated a two- to fourfold increased incidence of colorectal cancer among patients with affected first-degree relatives.[7,8] The relative risk for this group of patients is approximately 1.72 compared with patients without an affected first-degree relative.[9] This risk increases to 2.75 when two or more first-degree relatives are affected. In an additional study of first-degree relatives, St. John and colleagues[10] found a relative risk of 1.8 with one affected first-degree relative and a higher risk of 5.7 with two affected relatives. Planck and colleagues[11] analyzed a group of individuals in Sweden whose mothers were diagnosed with colon carcinoma or rectal cancer between 1958 and 1993. The children were born during the period 1941–1993, and the incidence of cancer was studied from 1961 to 1993. The expected Swedish incidence was used as a reference. There were several interesting findings. The cohort demonstrated significant increased risks of developing non-Hodgkin's lymphoma, colon cancer, and rectal cancer. The cancer risk was approximately threefold greater for those whose mothers were diagnosed under the age of 50 years. Maternal colon cancer implied an increased risk of both colon and rectal cancers in offspring, but a maternal history of rectal cancer showed an increased risk for rectal cancer but not colon cancer among their children.[11,12] As our understanding of genetic alterations involved in the pathogenesis of colorectal cancer has expanded, the implications of an interrelationship between lifestyle and genetic risk factors for the development of colorectal cancer have become apparent.

Dietary Factors

Dietary fat and fiber have been implicated as prime factors in the pathogenesis of colorectal cancer. Consumption of plant foods in general, and vegetables in particular, appears to be associated consistently with decreased cancer risk.[11,13] Clinical reports assessing the relationship between total caloric or fat intake and colorectal cancer have noted a significant correlation; however, poorly understood interactions between unrelated risk factors (e.g., genetic susceptibility, exposure to toxins such as ethanol or tobacco, and physical activity) and somewhat poorly defined dietary constituents (e.g., fiber, without regard to type) create serious limitations on the interpretation of such studies.

Epidemiologists also have found associations between dietary fat intake and colon cancer, with 12 of 13 studies demonstrating a direct correlation between fat intake and the incidence or mortality of colon cancer.[14] Two prospective studies of fat intake and colon cancer found an increased incidence with a high-fat diet.[15,16] In an epidemiological study of 98,464 nurses, 150 developed colon cancer, with a significant increase in the intake of total and animal fat by affected versus unaffected individuals.[17] Animal studies also have demonstrated an association between fat and malignancy. Nigro and coworkers[18] demonstrated an increased incidence of colon cancer among rats with 35% versus 5% beef fat intake. The mechanism between fat intake and activation of cellular proliferation, although hypothesized to be related to bile acids, is not fully understood.

Along with his observation of the role of dietary fiber in limiting benign disease in native Americans, Burkitt also noted that fiber might play a role in the development of colorectal cancer.[19] When this population's customary high-fiber diet was discontinued, an increase in colorectal cancer occurred. The role of dietary fiber in the pathogenesis of colorectal malignancy is debatable, however. Animal studies by Cruse and associates[20] and Nigro and colleagues[21] failed to demonstrate a protective effect of increased fiber intake in animals with a diet containing 5% to 30% fat. In contrast, Trock and coworkers[22] noted an inverse correlation between fiber intake and colorectal cancer in a detailed analysis of 12 studies examining the role of fiber in limiting tumor growth. Although dietary fiber intake should be considered along with other factors in the pathogenesis of colorectal cancer, the lack of supportive scientific data except for observational studies does not support a major role. Additionally, two large American cohort studies—the Nurses Health study, which involved 88,757 women followed for 16 years, and the Health Profession's Follow-up study, which included 47,325 men followed for 10 years—found no evidence to support a role for dietary fiber or fruit and vegetable consumption in reducing the risk for developing colon and rectal cancers.[22-26]

Terry and colleagues[27] reported the results of a population-based cohort study of 61,463 Swedish women followed for 9.6 years. They found only a weak association between increased dietary fruit and a decrease in the risk of colorectal cancer. Asano and McLeod[28] reported the results of a systematic review and meta-analysis of prospective random assignment trials to assess the effect of dietary fiber on the incidence or recurrence of colorectal adenomas and on the incidence of colorectal cancer. There were five studies involving 4349 subjects that met their rigorous inclusion criteria. The authors concluded that there was no evidence from randomized trials to suggest that increased dietary fiber intake will reduce polyps within a 4-year period. Although failing to show a correlation between high-fiber diet and a reduced risk of colorectal cancer, a high-fiber intake has been shown to reduce the risk of symptomatic colonic diverticuli, coronary artery disease, hypertension, and diabetes.[28] Oral calcium intake (1500–1800 mg daily) has been suggested as a potential agent to decrease the risk of colorectal cancer based on its ability in experimental models to inhibit hyperproliferation of colon epithelial cells induced experimentally by increased intraluminal levels of fatty acids or bile acids.[29] Supplements of dietary calcium have also been shown to decrease epithelial cell proliferation and migratory activity within the crypts of patients with a high risk for colorectal cancer.[30] It is postulated that calcium might act to precipitate cytotoxic surfactants within the colon.[31-33] Although epidemiologic and experimental findings have suggested that calcium supplementation could reduce hyperproliferative changes that underlie malignant transformation, a review of such case-control studies has not supported this concept.[34-36]

The possible function of antioxidant vitamins as free radical scavengers to reduce the risk of cancer has also been explored. In the Iowa Women's Health Study, vitamin E supplementation (but not vitamin A or C) was associated with a decreased risk.[37] In the Physician's Health Study, β-carotene supplementation did not reduce the incidence of colorectal cancer.[38] The Finnish chemoprevention study of vitamin E and β-carotene was also negative.[39] Only one of five studies of vitamin supplementation in patients with adenomas showed a reduction in recurrence.[40-44]

Several lines of evidence suggest that higher intake of folic acid could be beneficial in reducing the risk of colon cancer. For example, folic acid provides a methyl group required in the synthesis of methionine, used in DNA methylation and regulation of gene expression. Folic acid also provides a methyl group for the conversion of uracil to thyanine. Deficiencies in folic acid can cause uracil to replace thymine in DNA synthesis.[45]

If dietary consumption of fat, fiber, fruits, and vegetables cannot be related directly to a change in the risk for colon cancer, other environmental factors must be implicated to explain the greater than tenfold geographic differences in colon cancer risk. In searching for an explanation, there has been increasing evidence in recent years that such risks could be the result of energy balance. Although an accurate determination of the difference between energy intake and energy expenditure is not practical in large population studies, there are indirect measures such as body weight, changes in weight over time, lean body mass, and physical activity that can be measured. From such studies, there appears to be a direct correlation between increased body weight and colon cancer.[46-48]

Experimental evidence suggests that excess energy in the form of substantial weight gain results in the development of insulin resistance, with increased levels of circulating insulin, triglycerides, and nonesterified fatty acids. These changes provide a proliferative stimulus to colonic epithelial cells and expose the increased number of dividing cells to reactive oxygen intermediates.[49-51]

The excess levels of growth stimulants would presumably favor proliferation of colonic epithelial cells that already harbor defective cell-cycle control. In addition to stimulation of epithelial cell proliferation, there appears to be focal loss of normal epithelial cell barrier function. This focal loss of barrier causes a local inflammation and release of reactive oxygen intermediates. The result of these focal effects is the generation of aberrant crypt foci of proliferating cells. These cells begin to pile up at the luminal surface of the crypt, eventually becoming an adenoma. The steps in adenoma formation and the eventual transition from adenoma to cancer within the adenoma are dependent on a progressive activation of specific oncogenes and a concomitant loss of specific suppressor genes.

Whether genetic mutations are initiated during the earliest stage of aberrant crypt formation is unknown, but there could be a complex interaction between environmental factors (e.g., diet or energy balance) and ingestion of carcinogens. The relative importance of environmental vs. genetic factors shifts strongly toward underlying genetic alterations in individuals affected by hereditary conditions such as polyposis syndromes or hereditary nonpolyposis colon cancer (HNPCC).

Hereditary Colon Cancer Syndromes

Familial adenomatous polyposis (FAP) syndrome is one of three different hereditary colon cancer syndromes. FAP accounts for an estimated 1% to 2% of incident cases of colorectal cancer and is associated with the APC gene.[52] FAP has a high penetrance: Family members who inherit the mutant allele of the APC gene have a very high probability of developing invasive cancer. Identification requires a high level of suspicion based on family history that leads to genetic testing. The APC gene is a tumor suppressor gene and, therefore, when both alleles are defective, patients develop florid polyposis and subsequent invasive cancer. In general, the APC gene on one chromosome is inherited as a mutant defective allele from one of the parents. This mutation does not alter the function of the APC gene but instead leaves the patient at risk for a second mutation, which disrupts the function of the APC gene.[52] The normal APC allele becomes mutated in individual colon epithelial cells early in childhood, initiating the cancer process. This begins as hyperplasia, progresses to multiple polyposis, and

one or more polyps develop invasive cancer. A number of years and multiple additional genetic alterations in other target genes are required for the progression to invasive cancer. Invasive cancers in patients with FAP syndrome occur at an average age of 42 years.

HNPCC accounts for 4% to 6% of incident cases of colorectal cancer and has only a moderate penetrance of 30% to 70%. HNPCC is an autosomal dominant disorder. It is associated with other cancers and has been shown to be the result of mutations in mismatch repair (MMR) genes. Carriers of MMR mutations are estimated to have an 85% lifetime risk of colon neoplasia. In contrast to patients with FAP, patients with HNPCC do not have abnormal APC alleles and therefore do not develop extensive polyposis, making identification more difficult. Although their lesions are more commonly right sided, clinically they present identically to patients with sporadic colon carcinomas. It is only through careful family profiling of three generations of family that suspicion of HNPCC is generated.[53] Hereditary HNPCC has been defined clinically as a history of at least three affected family members involving two generations with at least one person diagnosed before age 50. Recently, it has been shown that HNPCC is caused by defective DNA mismatch repair genes. As stated previously, these patients develop colon polyps at a rate similar to the normal population because they do not harbor a defective APC gene. Once they develop a polyp, however, there is more rapid progression to cancer because of the presence of inherited mismatch repair gene defects. At least four genes in the mismatch repair group have been found to be associated with HNPCC. Replication error phenotype has also been associated in individual patients with the occurrence of multiple primary cancers.[53] Knowing the family members that harbor specific genetic abnormalities and the relative risk for cancer provides critical information to determine the need for surveillance and, in certain instances, the need for total proctocolectomy.

Genetic Alterations in Colorectal Carcinogenesis

The development of carcinoma occurs along a multistep pathway of events that has been outlined by Vogelstein and colleagues[54] and others in the now well recognized model for colorectal carcinogenesis.[53-60] This model describes a pathway of mutational activation of oncogenes and inactivation of tumor suppressor genes. More than nine genes are believed to be altered for carcinoma formation. The initial mutation probably occurs at the APC gene on chromosome 5q and involves inactivation the APC gene. The adenoma-to-cancer sequence is further activated by the K-ras oncogene. The final step involves loss or mutation of the p53 tumor suppressor gene on chromosome 17p. Multiple pathways from normal mucosa to carcinoma are not necessarily sequential but rather are an association of mutations that is characteristic of sporadic and inherited colorectal cancer.[54-58]

The molecular genetic model for colorectal tumorogenesis has been demonstrated to be a series of specific chromosomal and somatic genetic changes occurring as a sequential accumulation while the oncogenic process proceeds through initiation, promotion, and progression (Fig. 80-3).[56,59,60]

These genetic alterations include deletions and point mutations of tumor suppressor genes such as APC, p53, and DCC (deleted in colon cancer), as well as oncogenic mutations of KRAS.[56,60] In the case of the three tumor suppressor genes, both alleles must be lost or defective for phenotypic expression, where as with the proto-oncogenes, mutation in only one allele is needed for expression of the cancer phenotype. It is important to emphasize that thus far, investigations have failed to identify any one gene that is involved exclusively in all colon cancers.

At least two types of genetic instability are observed in colon cancer development. Chromosomal instability (CIN) is the path by which a majority (about 60%) of colon cancers evolve and is characterized by aneuploidy, multiple chromosomal rearrangements, and clonal heterogeneity.[56] Some 15% to 20% of colorectal cancers, however, develop through a different path, where there is a defective DNA mismatch repair system. This path is characterized by instability of repetitive sequences (e.g., DNA microsatellites) and is therefore referred to as the microsatellite instability (MSI) pathway. Tumors developing from defective mismatch repair genes hMLH1 and hMSH2 might also acquire somatic frameshift mutations of

coding repeats within other important cancer genes. For example, mutations are found in TGFβIIr, IGFR2, and BAX.

Studies of early, benign colon adenomas, however, have failed to reveal any evidence for generalized chromosomal or microsatellite instability (CIN or MSI) at these earliest stages of the oncogenic path.[53] This lack of evidence leads to the conclusion that neither of these forms of genomic instability is necessary for the formation of aberrant crypt foci and early adenomas.[61]

The APC tumor surpressor gene is defective in greater than 80% of adenomatous polyps and colon cancers. It is the most common defect and the one that appears earliest in the sequence of accumulated genetic alterations. In colorectal cancers, the majority of mutations in the APC tumor suppressor gene cause a truncation of the APC protein and, therefore, loss of function. The normal APC protein functions to degrade cytoplasmic β-catenin. This degradation occurs when β-catenin is bound to the APC/AXIN/GSK-3β complex. GSK-3β acts to phosphorylate β-catenin, leading to its being conjugated to the ubiquitin protein and degraded. β-catenin stability is regulated by diacylglycerol-independent protein kinase C-like kinase activity, which is required for β-catenin ubiquitination[62] (Fig. 80-4).

The absence of a functioning APC protein leads to the accumulation of β-catenin in the cytoplasm and its translocation to the nucleus. β-catenin plays an important

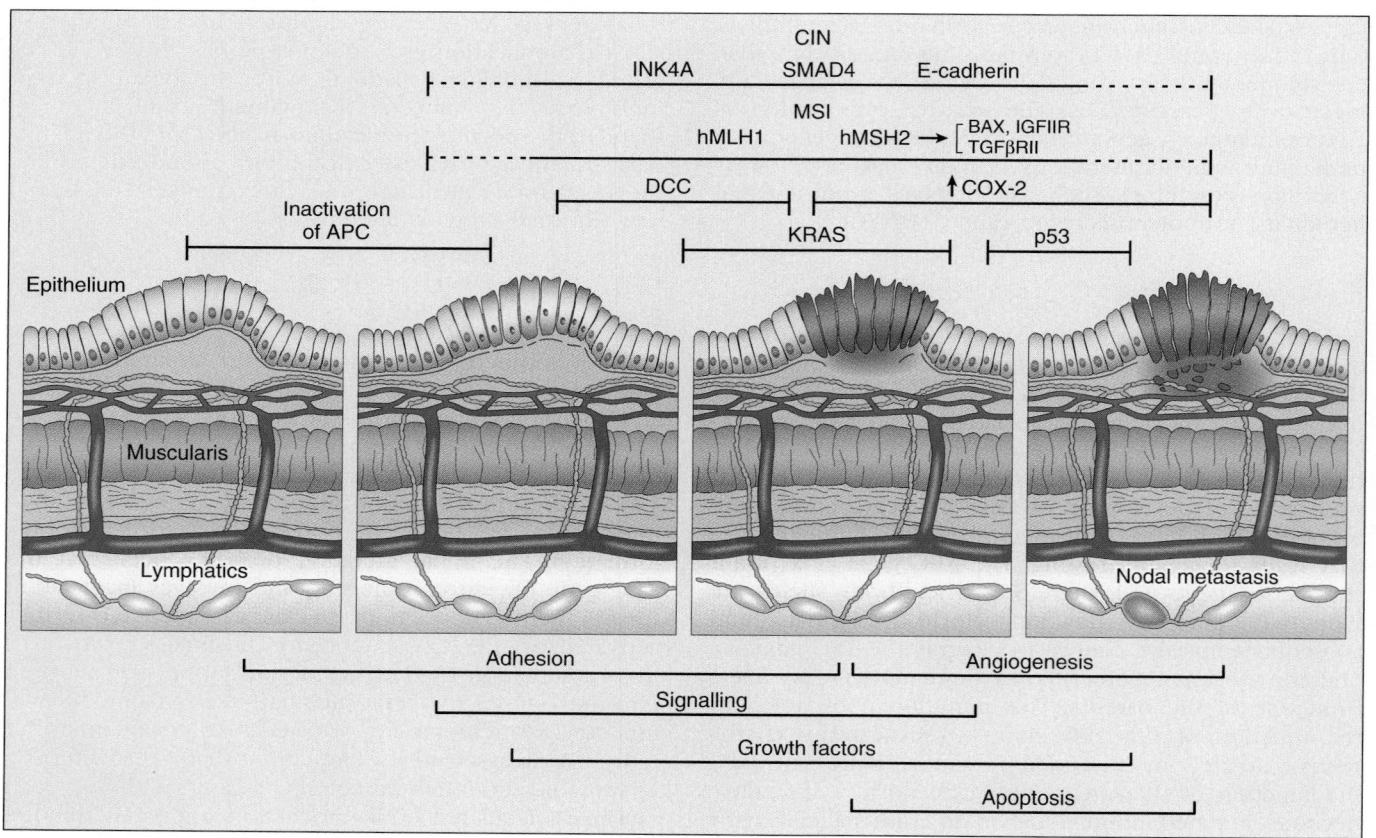

Figure 80-3. Adenoma-to-carcinoma sequence and the associated molecular alterations involved in colon cancer development.

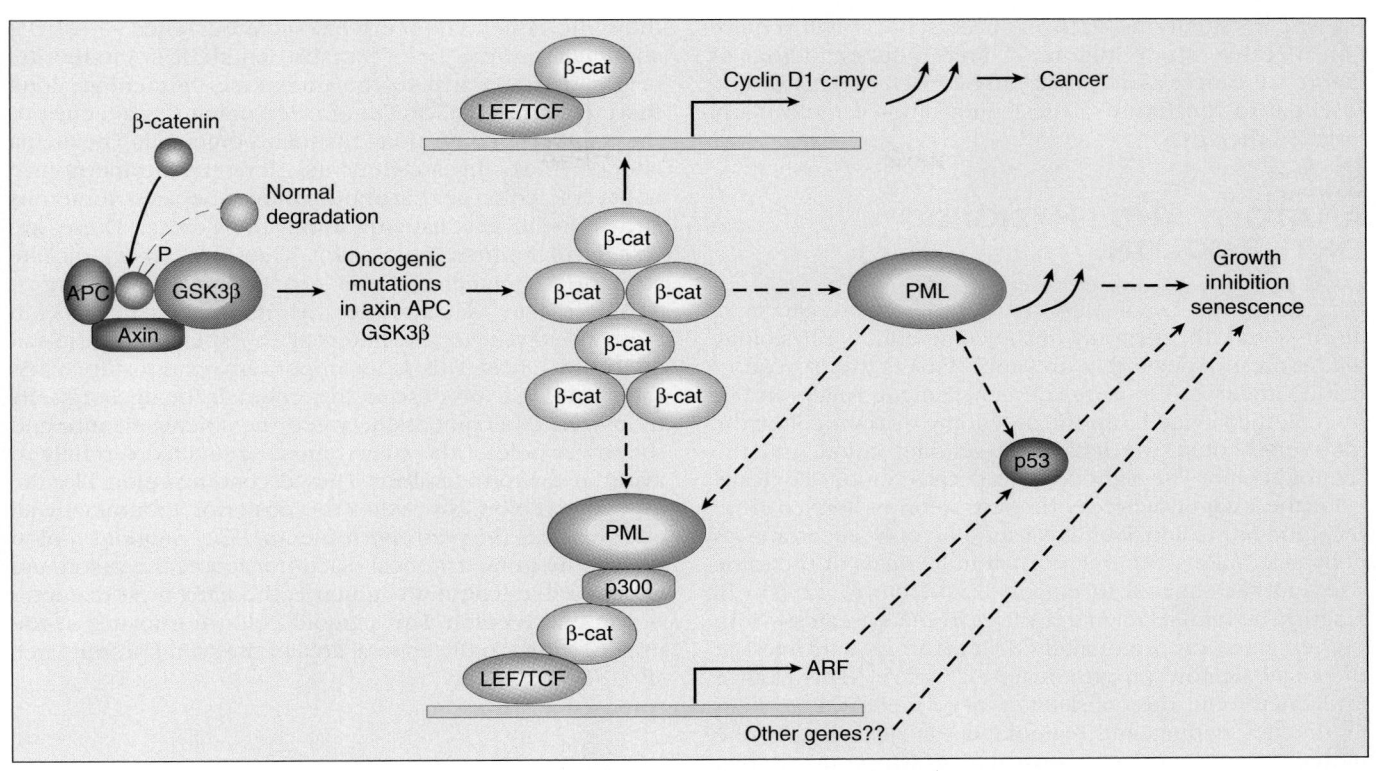

Figure 80-4. Molecular pathway for the oncogenic and tumor-suppressive effects caused by the activation of β-catenin (overexpression). In the normal colonic epithelial cell, β-catenin is phosphorylated by GSK-β after it is bound to the APC/Axin/GSK-3β complex. This leads to normal degradation of β-catenin. Oncogenic mutation of APC leads to failure to bind, phosphorylate, and degrade β-catenin. The result is increasing cytoplasmic concentrations of β-catenin which translocates to the nucleus and activates the LEF/TCF complex, in turn activating a number of target genes promoting cell proliferation. β-catenin induces expression of the PML gene and other pathways. (Adapted from Figure 6 in Shtutman M, Zlurinsky J, Oren M, Levina E, Ben-Ze'ev A: PML is a target gene of β-catenin and plakoglobin, and coactivates β-catenin-mediated transcription. Cancer Res 2002;62:5947–5954.)

role in cell-cell adhesion by linking cadherin receptors to the actin cytoskeleton. β-catenin is also related to the *Wnt* signaling pathway that determines cell fate, specifically during development. If *Wnt* signaling is activated and in turn activates the *Wnt* receptor, phosphorylation and inactivation of GSK-3β occurs, which then prevents GSK-3β from phosphorylating β-catenin.[63,64]

The nuclear accumulation of β-catenin causes it to complex with LEF/TCF (lymphocyte enhancer factor/T-cell factor). The β-catenin LEF protein complex can activate genes with TCF/LEF promoter recognition sites, including c-Myc, cyclinD1, PPARS, matrilysn, Fra-1, UPAR, c-Jun, PML, and gastrin. The results of this increase in β-catenin–induced transcription are stimulation of cell proliferation and inhibition of apoptosis.[65]

Deletions of 18q21 were described and DCC, a tumor suppressor gene, was identified at this chromosomal location. In addition, SMAD2 and SMAD4 genes involved in colon cancer are also positioned at 18q21.[55,65–69] SMAD2 is a receptor-regulated gene and is activated by TGFβ and activin signaling. It appears that its role in colon cancer is a late event, acting to accelerate progression in the later stages of invasive carcinogenesis.[70]

The p53 tumor suppressor gene located on chromosome 17 is the most commonly inactivated tumor suppressor (TS) in human malignancy. The normal p53 protein recognizes damaged DNA and acts to block the progression of the cell cycle to permit DNA repair. The p53 protein also can trigger apoptosis.

An interesting observation in FAP and other syndromes with polyps is the significant difference in the number of polyps that occur even within the same family. Using a mouse model of FAP, Dietrich and colleagues[71] were able to identify a modifying gene called MOM1 and show that it codes for phospholipase A2, which acts to inhibit the number of polyps.

Although investigations have focused on identifying the genetic alterations present in the adenoma to carcinoma model of colorectal cancer, recent work has suggested an alternative (but probably minor) path for colon cancer development. This alternative route evolves from hyperplastic polyps through serrated adenomas and is characterized by mutations in the BRAF kinase gene. Studies suggest that 3% to 10% of adenomas have BRAF mutations, compared with 30% to 60% having KRAS mutations. The term *serrated adenoma* has been used for hyperplastic polyps with serrated morphology that demonstrate dysplasia throughout the lesion.[72–74]

What is becoming clear, perhaps not unexpectedly, is the recognition that colorectal cancer is a heterogeneous disease made up of several genetically discrete subsets, each of which evolves through quite separate pathways

Specific Malignancies

III

of genetic alterations. Each of these subsets will require considerable study before a final understanding of colorectal cancer as a disease can be reached. This will be essential to the future of designing rational molecularly targeted therapy.

ANATOMY AND PHYSIOLOGY OF THE COLON

For the purposes of this chapter on colon cancer, a discussion of the anatomy of the colon and its physiology will address aspects that are important to the spread of colon cancer and its surgical management. Anatomically, the colon is divided into the ascending or right colon, the transverse colon, the left or descending colon, and the sigmoid colon. The right colon is derived embryologically from the midgut, whereas the left colon is derived from the hindgut. Colon length varies not only according to body size but also among normal individuals of the same size and is estimated to range from 91 cm to 125 cm in length. The luminal diameter varies from its greatest width at the cecum (approximately 8.5 cm) to its narrowest at the distal sigmoid (approximately 2.5 cm).[75] This change in diameter and the consistency of formed fecal content in the descending and sigmoid colon account for the frequent presentation of obstructive symptoms among patients with annular cancers in these colonic segments. The merging of the three taenia coli (from the Latin "tape") or longitudinal muscle bands into a continuous (encompassing) longitudinal muscle layer for the rectum at the pelvic peritoneal reflection marks the junction between the sigmoid colon and rectum.[76]

Three segments of the colon—the cecum, transverse colon, and sigmoid colon—are intraperitoneal. The ascending colon, hepatic flexure, splenic flexure, descending colon, and the beginning and end of the sigmoid colon are retroperitoneal structures. As a result, the surgical resection and the patterns of recurrence are greatly influenced by the location of the tumor within the colon and, for the segments that are retroperitoneal, by its position within the bowel at the primary site (e.g., primarily posterior in location versus on the anterior wall of the colon).

Although the beginning of the colon (cecum) and its appendix are largely intraperitoneal, the ascending colon and its mesocolon are fused to the posterior abdominal wall in a retroperitoneal position. It should be noted that the ileocecal valve at the junction of the ileum to the colon is actually formed by two reflected folds of the mucosal wall of the cecum. These folds unite and project further around the cecum as the frenulum. The opening of the appendix into the cecum is near the ileocecal valve.

Examination of the inner surface of the colon reveals the semilunar folds, the sacculations termed *haustrae*, and the longitudinal muscle bands or taenia. Lymphoid follicles are also visible on the luminal surface. As noted previously, the longitudinal muscle bands or taenia start at the base of the appendix and continue throughout the colon.

The hepatic flexure lies just below the right lobe of the liver and the gallbladder and overlies the lower pole of the right kidney. The transverse colon extends across the abdomen and can be of variable length. It is intraperitoneal and is attached to the transverse mesocolon along the taenia mesocolica. The greater omentum attaches to the transverse colon along the taenia omentalis. The taenia libera is free of any attachments. Along the intraperitoneal transverse colon and sigmoid colon, one sees numerous fatty appendages hanging from the serosa. These are called *appendices epiploicae*. They are small, sac-like structures containing fat and have no known function.

The splenic flexure lies, as its name suggests, in close proximity to the hilum of the spleen and the tail of the pancreas. This is an important relationship when the transverse or descending colon is being surgically mobilized. Attachments between the splenic flexure and the lower pole of the spleen must be divided carefully to avoid injury to the spleen. The descending colon, like the ascending colon, is fused to the posterior abdominal wall and lies in the retroperitoneum. The sigmoid colon begins the intraperitoneal distal portion of the colon and is of variable length. Its lumen is the narrowest diameter of the entire colon. The sigmoid colon terminates at the upper rectum in the general area of the sacral prominence (Fig. 80-5).

Vascular Supply to the Colon

The superior mesenteric vessels supply the cecum, the ascending colon, and a good portion of the transverse colon. The major branches of the superior mesenteric artery are the ileocolic artery supplying the ileocecal region, the right colic artery in support of the ascending colon, and the middle colic branch to the hepatic flexure and transverse colon. These vessels have extensive branching near the colon and contribute to the formation of the important marginal artery (marginal artery of Drummond). The veins accompanying these arteries drain back to the superior mesenteric vein and thence to the portal vein. It is this unique venous drainage to the liver that is believed to account for the high incidence (approximately 80%) of first-site metastatic failure in the liver for colon and rectal cancers.

The inferior mesenteric artery arises from the aorta and supplies the descending colon via the left colic artery. The marginal artery acts as a collateral vessel to link the branches of the superior mesenteric artery to the right colon with the arterial flow from the inferior mesenteric artery and its left colic artery. Distally, the inferior mesenteric artery gives rise to several sigmoid arteries and the superior rectal artery. Veins draining the left side accompany these arteries and drain via the inferior mesenteric vein to the splenic vein and thence to the portal vein. A patent, healthy marginal artery provides a measure of safety in performing resections of the colon by providing collateral arterial flow. These arteries and veins lie within the "leaves" of the mesocolon.

Lymphatics of the Colon

Lymphatics and nerves to the colon also lie within the mesocolon and follow the course of the arteries. The

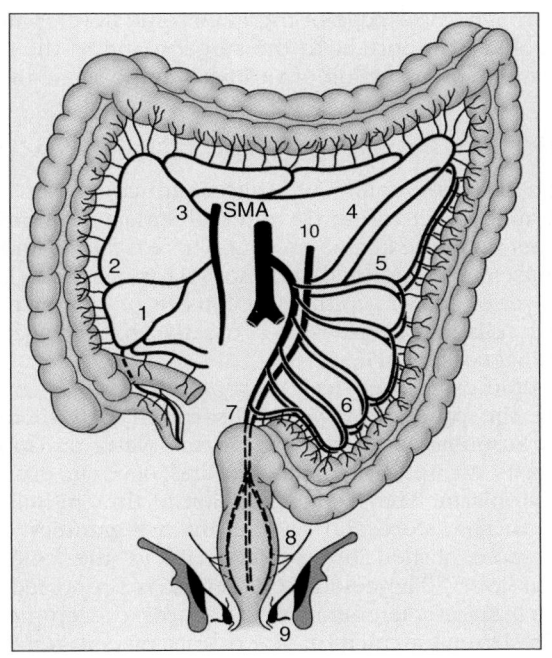
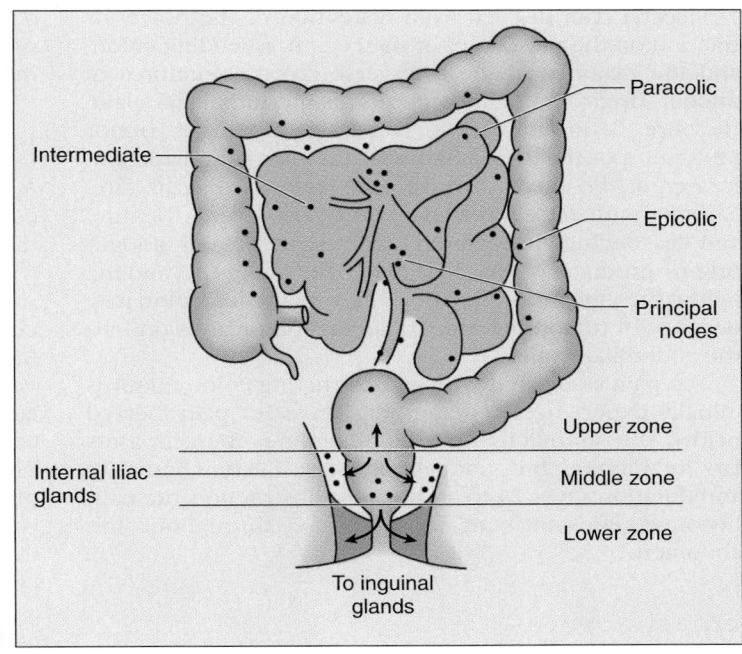

Figure 80-5. A, Arterial and venous supply of the colon. Branches of the superior mesenteric artery: (1) ileocolic, (2) right colic, (3) middle colic. Branches of the inferior mesenteric artery: (4) ascending left colic, (5) left colic, (6) sigmoid branches, (7) superior rectal artery, (8) middle rectal artery, (9) inferior rectal artery, (10) inferior mesenteric vein. **B,** Principal nodal drainage sites of the colon.

lymphatic channels originate in the lower lamina propria and along the muscularis mucosa of the wall of the colon. These channels drain into the extramural lymphatics. Cancer that is growing superficial to the level of the lamina propria has not been shown to have access to the lymphatic channels and therefore, has not been found to have metastatic potential.[77-79] The lymph nodes lie roughly along the vessels and are grouped as epicolic, paracolic (located along the marginal artery), the intermediate nodes along mesenteric vessels, and principal or central nodes at the junction with the superior mesenteric artery or, in the case of the inferior mesenteric artery, with the aorta.

All collecting lymph channels from the abdominal viscera, the abdominal wall, and lower extremities converge in an elongated sac (approximately 5 cm), known as the cisterna chyli. The cisterna chyli lies along the aorta, and a large afferent lymph channel proceeds from the cisterna superiorly through the aortic opening in the diaphragm along the right diaphragmatic crus. There are numerous communicating lymphatics between the larger channels, which could account for the observed "skipping" of metastases. Malignant cells might also pass through initial nodes before being trapped in more distant nodes. Lymph nodes also have an arterial supply and venous drainage a feature, which could play a role in metastatic spread to nodes as hematogenous metastases and account for unusual sites of node involvement that appear completely unrelated to direct drainage of lymph fluid from the original tumor.

Autonomic Innervation

The autonomic nervous system mediates control of colonic motor and secretory function and primary visceral sensation. The autonomic innervation includes both sympathetic and parasympathetic components. The preganglionic parasympathetic nerve fibers are quite long, extending from the brain stem to the colon wall, where they terminate within the myenteric and submucosal plexuses. In contrast, the first synapse of the sympathetic fibers can occur within the paravertebral ganglia, but most pass through the ganglion without synapsing. The sympathetic fibers are gathered into bundles know as the greater (fourth to tenth thoracic), the lesser (ninth to eleventh thoracic), the least (eleventh thoracic to the first lumbar), and the lumbar (second and third lumbar) splanchnic nerves. The splanchnic nerves (preganglionic fibers) pass to the preaortic ganglia, so named for the adjacent arterial trunks such as celiac and superior mesenteric ganglia and plexus. These preganglionic sympathetic fibers synapse within the preaortic ganglia. The postganglionic adrenergic fibers follow arteries to their effector organs in the wall of the colon.

An extensive network of fibers and ganglia cells lies within the submucosa and muscular walls of the colon. The intact mucosa of the colon is insensitive to direct stimuli. Sensory receptors in the colon wall react to stretching (as with gas) and to muscular spasm. The mesentery is sensitive to tugging or stretching. Impulses arising from these stimuli are sent over the autonomic (mainly sympathetic) afferent fibers.

Visceral pain derived from distention of the bowel or traction on the mesentery of the cecum, ascending colon, and the majority of the transverse colon (structures of midgut origin) initially presents as periumbilical pain. If there is inflammation, ischemia, or direct tumor infiltration of the abdominal wall, the pain is somatic and located at the site of involvement. Referred pain is rare. Pathology of the distal transverse colon, splenic flexure, and descending and sigmoid colon (structures of hindgut origin) produces visceral pain, initially along the midline below the umbilicus. Somatic pain from the left colon may occur with tumors, causing inflammation or invasion into the abdominal wall.

The pain associated with an obstructing colon tumor is initially experienced as cramping waves of pain located below the umbilicus. In the beginning, these spasms last for minutes but gradually increase in their intensity and duration. Over 24 to 48 hours of obstruction, the pain becomes constant and more diffuse throughout the abdomen.

Embryology

By the 6-week embryo stage, the midgut has formed and exists as a long intestinal loop in an elongated celomic cavity within the umbilical cord. At the beginning of the third month, the intestinal loop residing in the umbilical cord begins to rotate counterclockwise around the axis of the superior mesenteric artery. In doing so, the distal limb of the intestinal loop, consisting of the future cecum, terminal ileum and ascending colon, passes over and to the right of the future jejunum and ileum. With this twist, the superior mesenteric artery comes to cross in front of the duodenum. As the intestinal loop withdraws from the umbilical cord, the proximal limb leads the way and as a result pushes the distal colon to the left side of the abdomen. The cecum and terminal ileum migrate downward and to the right lower quadrant of the abdomen.

From this brief discussion, it is obvious that any interruption of this rotation can alter the position of certain segments of the colon. The most common is a high position of the cecum beneath the liver in the right upper abdomen. Earlier interruptions of rotation could find the colon remaining on the left side.

When the rotation process proceeds normally, the entire mesentery to the cecum and ascending colon become fused to the right posterior abdominal wall as a triangle with the apex at the base of the mesentery just above the emergence of the superior mesenteric artery. The upper section of this mesenteric triangle covers the second and third segments of the duodenum, which sweeps from right to left behind the superior mesenteric artery.

The mesentery of the transverse colon is retained, and the transverse colon develops an attachment horizontally with the greater omentum. Similar to the ascending colon, when the descending colon becomes fixed to the left posterior abdominal wall, its mesentery becomes part of the posterior wall. The sigmoid colon retains its redundancy and, therefore, a mesentery.

A thorough knowledge of the embryonic development of the colon is important to the surgeon and to the safe mobilization and resection of various colonic segments.

Microscopic Anatomy of the Normal Colon

A single layer of columnar epithelium comprises the colonic mucosa, covering the internal surface and lining the crypts along the lamina propria. There is a thin, underlying muscle layer termed the muscularis mucosae. The single layer of colonic epithelium consists of columnar or cuboidal cells and serves as a protective barrier against the luminal content (Fig. 80-6).

The epithelial layer has two functions. One is to facilitate the process of water absorption, and specific cells are responsible for colonic ion and water transport. These cells do not contain mucin and have an eosinophilic cytoplasm. The second function of the epithelium is to synthesize, store, and secrete mucous granules, and this is accomplished by Goblet cells in the colonic epithelial layer.[80] The colonic epithelium is supported by a thin basement membrane that anchors the epithelial cells. The basement membrane consists of collagen and other proteins and is permeable to absorbed or secreted ions, water, and proteins. One of the unique characteristics of the colon mucosa is the presence of crypts. The crypts have a somewhat heterogeneous population of epithelial

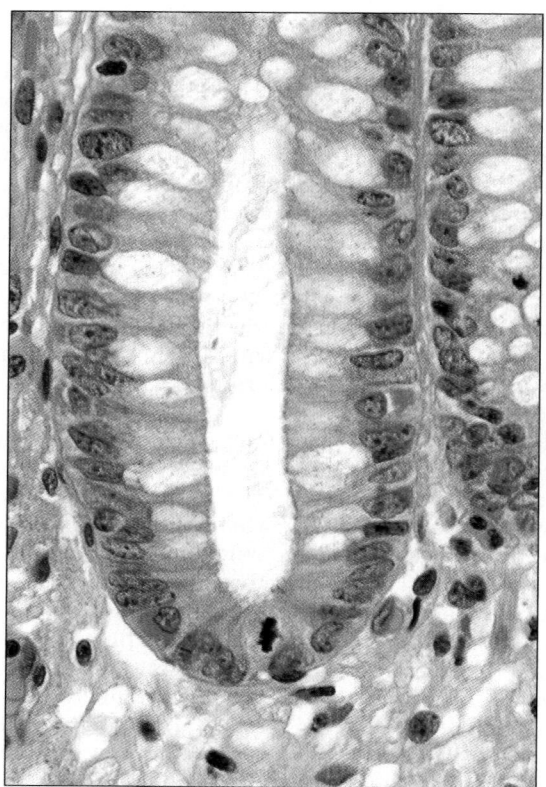

Figure 80-6. Normal colonic basal crypt epithelium. Among the absorptive cells and goblet cells are a mitotic figure and endocrine cells with basally oriented secretory granules. (From Sternberg SS: Histology for Pathologists. New York, Raven Press, 1992.)

cells. At the base of each crypt are undifferentiated stem or precursor cells. These cells are dividing and also migrating toward the surface epithelial layer. The crypts function to renew the surface epithelium, which is constantly being shed into the lumen or undergoing apoptotic death. As the cells move from the base of the crypt toward the lumen of the colon, they lose their ability to divide but continue to differentiate to become functionally mature. The upper 25% of the crypt represents such mature cells. Endocrine cells and Paneth cells are found in the bases of the crypts, but such cells are confined to the crypts of the cecum and proximal right colon.

The lamina propria extends from the basement membrane to the muscularis mucosae. It is composed of loose strands of collagen, and B-lymphoid cells are abundant. These B-cells produce immunoglobulins, mostly of IgA class. T-lymphocytes and macrophages are also found in the lamina propria, as are fibroblasts.

The muscularis mucosa is a thin layer of muscle that separates the superficial layers of epithelium and lamina propria from the deeper submucosa. Between the muscularis mucosae and the submucosa are found the neural plexus of Meissner and the deep submucosal neural plexus of Henle. The muscular layers of the colon include a circular inner layer of smooth muscle fibers and an outer longitudinal layer. Auerbach's neural plexus lies between the circular and longitudinal muscle layers. These muscle layers are covered by the serosa covering of the colon.

Physiology of the Colon

The colon functions to prepare the normal waste products left after digestion and absorption of nutrient food products for elimination in a controlled manner. Water is withdrawn through the colonic mucosa from the fluid stool entering the cecum and ascending colon. Both water and salt are absorbed as the right colon acts to reduce the daily liter of ileal liquid chyme to approximately 200 g of formed fecal matter. The left colon is responsible for storage and eventual explusion. The movement of fecal matter through the colon is regulated hormonally and neurally.

The mucosal lining of the colon keeps its surface coated with mucous to protect the epithelial cells from injury and to act as a lubricant. Mucus is produced by the tubular glands containing many goblet cells, and mucous production is controlled primarily by parasympathetic nerve fibers.

The colon has abundant bacterial flora, including *Eschericia coli, Aerobacter aerogenes, Clostridium welchii,* various lactobacilli, cocci, and yeast organisms. The flora is somewhat influenced by diet, being more gram-negative when the diet is primarily protein in nature and more gram-positive if the diet is mainly carbohydrates and green vegetables. Some of the colonic organisms synthesize vitamins of the B complex and vitamin K.

Carbohydrate-consuming bacteria within the lumen work on undigested carbohydrates and dietary fiber, producing short-chain fatty acids, flatus, and water. These short-chain fatty acids can be absorbed by colonic mucosal epithelial cells and can be a source of dietary calories.[81] Although these various bacteria reside in relative balance, the normal equilibrium of bacteria can be altered significantly by antibiotics, giving rise to an overgrowth of harmful bacteria such as *Clostridium difficile.*

Antibiotic-associated diarrhea occurs in an estimated 1% to 15% of individuals who are given broad-spectrum antimicrobic therapy. It is caused by an overgrowth of *Clostridium difficile* when the normal bacterial flora of the colonic mucosa is suppressed. *C. difficile* colonic infection generally causes cramping and mild diarrhea, but it can result in a more life-threatening pseudomembranous colitis. Patients with colon cancer or those receiving treatment for recurrent disease are frequently at risk for developing antibiotic-associated diarrhea. In such cases, the antibiotic should be stopped and the patient given vancomycin (250 mg every 6 hours orally for 7 days) or metronidazole (500 mg every 8 hours for 7 days). Treatment should be started when the diagnosis is suspected, before the results of a stool assay for *C. difficile* toxins are available.

PREVENTION OF COLON CANCER

The methods available now for the prevention of colon cancer provide some of the most cost-effective and practical opportunities for improving human health. Advances in understanding the genetics and pathogenesis of colon polyps and cancer have provided the knowledge needed to intervene effectively at earlier, more curable stages of tumor development. Flexible fiber-optic colonoscopy and video colonoscopy have proven to be exceptionally useful, not only for diagnosis of symptomatic patients (who more often have advanced disease) but also in a screening or surveillance mode for asymptomatic individuals. Routine colonoscopy has been shown to provide therapeutic benefit through early detection and removal of adenomatous polyps. Screening methods that target adenomas are particularly effective in reducing the incidence of colon cancer, because the benign adenoma is an early-stage cancer precursor and is the most frequent mode of colon tumor development in humans.[82] The hypothesis that adenomas are the major precursors to colon cancer is supported by several lines of evidence:[83-85]

- Molecular genetic alterations accumulate in association with adenoma-carcinoma progression, beginning with mutation of the APC gene pathway in adenomas.[53]
- Cancer foci often occur within adenomatous colon polyps.
- Cancer incidence increases proportionally to polyp size.
- Patient age at diagnosis with adenomas is approximately 5 years earlier than of diagnosis with colon carcinomas, not only for patients with familial polyposis but also in the general population.
- Cancer incidence is reduced by colonoscopic polypectomy, and adenoma incidence is reduced by chemopreventive medications.[86]

As research in genetics continues to discover inherited mutations causing disease, there will be further opportunities to develop preventive measures and treatments targeted against these specific molecular defects. Presymptomatic knowledge of an inherited cancer-predisposing mutation has the benefit of indicating a need for increased surveillance to allow earlier diagnosis at a curable stage. The public will probably demand genetic testing for cancer susceptibility: 83% of respondents to a random survey expressed a moderate to strong interest in such testing.

Genetic and Familial Risk Assessment

The process of evaluating a patient with suspected hereditary cancer should begin with a thorough family history and verification of pathological diagnoses to establish the most likely syndrome(s). Genetic counseling and informed consent are necessary before proceeding to molecular diagnostic testing, which should begin with a clearly affected member of the family. The diagnosis of a specific hereditary syndrome cannot be confirmed without identifying a mutation that functionally inactivates a gene known to cause the syndrome. If such a mutation can be identified in the index case, any other relatives at risk can then be tested, even if they are asymptomatic. Inheritance of the mutant allele would indicate a need for that relative to have intensive screening and preventive treatment, whereas inheritance of only normal alleles would indicate that only standard interventions similar to those used for the low-risk general population are sufficient.

A mutation is generally defined as a stable, heritable change in DNA. Mutations can be inherited and thus affect the entire organism and perhaps its progeny (germline mutations), or they can affect only a single clone of cells within the individual (somatic mutations). They range in magnitude from the entire genome (e.g., triploidy) to alterations of chromosomal structure (deletions, insertions, inversions, duplications, translocations of a portion of one chromosome to another) or single base changes (missense, nonsense, splice site, frameshift). Their functional impact can range from no effect at all (silent mutations) to a complete lack of gene function (null muations), decrease of function (hypomorphic mutations), or gain of a new function (neomorphic mutations). Because of adverse selective pressures, mutations causing a severe phenotype (a greatly increased risk for cancer at a young age) are probably much less frequent in the population than those with a milder effect. These milder, more common alleles are more difficult to detect by linkage analysis than are classic syndromes like familial adenomatous polyposis but could impact a much larger fraction of the population. Practically every human being has some mutations with potential clinical significance, but most of these are not detectable by current methods. Mutation analysis is also complicated by the fact that most disorders are not monogenic, but are determined by other major modifying genes and the environment (the latter etiologies are probably more likely for diseases with a later age of onset).

Almost all genes predisposing to cancer are inherited in an autosomal dominant manner. This might seem surprising at first glance, as tumor suppressor gene mutations generally inactivate a normal function and thus would be expected to act in a recessive manner on a cellular level. The seeming paradox is resolved by considering the fact that in an organism consisting of an extremely large number of cells with each carrying a heterozygous germline mutation, one or more cells is highly likely to develop somatic mutations inactivating the normal allele, and tumors will then almost invariably develop. For a single-gene (Mendelian) autosomal dominant disorder, any child of an affected person has a 50% chance of inheriting the disease allele. For children of two carriers of a recessive disorder, the risk of inheritance of the disease alleles is 25%.

The Mendelian probability is usually quite straightforward to calculate and represents the initial risk estimate available. It reflects the average population risk and is based on a pool of gametes that have an equal probability of carrying the disease or normal allele. In some cases, it is possible to obtain a more precise estimate of the actual personal risk of disease gene inheritance, which obviously is all or none for any one individual. For example, haplotype analysis using genetic markers within 5 centimorgans (cM) of the disease gene would be able to refine the risk estimates to approximately 5% versus 95%, and more closely linked markers (within 1 cM) would refine the risk estimates to 1% versus 99%. Direct detection of the disease mutation by DNA sequencing or other techniques can diagnose inheritance at the 0% versus the 100% level. These risks refer only to gene inheritance, of course, which is not the same as the risk of developing the disease unless penetrance and expressivity are both complete.

Mutations in genes often reveal themselves in some manner that can be recognized as a clinical characteristic or phenotype, but there might not be any easily observable phenotype prior to the development of cancer in some syndromes. Recognition of the tumor pattern among close relatives, followed by an extended family history and then confirmation of the pathological diagnoses, are the essential initial steps in the identification of new kindreds with cancer predisposition syndromes. Hereditary nonpolyposis colon cancer (HNPCC) was first recognized more than a century ago by Dr. Warthin, but not until many decades later was this same family and others studied by Dr. Henry Lynch, and the molecular basis of this syndrome was elucidated only recently. Hereditary cancer registries have now been established at several medical centers throughout the world to provide appropriate diagnosis and care for families with HNPCC and a variety of other syndromes. These centers provide multidisciplinary consulting teams with expertise in gastroenterology, genetics, oncology, pathology, and surgery.

An excellent example of risk assessment based on phenotype is the detection of the underlying abnormality that causes HNPCC, a form of genomic instability caused by mutations in DNA mismatch repair (MMR) genes. This phenomenon was discovered serendipitously in 1993, when microsatellite markers used for loss of heterozygo-

TABLE 80-1

Amsterdam Criteria for HNPCC[88]

- At least three affected relatives with verified colorectal cancer.
- At least two successive generations affected.
- At least one is a first-degree relative of the other two.
- At least one colon cancer <50 years of age.
- FAP is excluded.

sity (LOH) analyses were noted to have ubiquitous somatic variations in the number of repeat sequences. This variation in the number of repeat sequences caused unexpected shifts in the size of alleles in tumors as detected by gel electrophoresis and is known as microsatellite instability (MSI). Germline mutations in MMR genes have been linked to HNPCC and implicated in the pathogenesis of colon cancer. MSI testing is relatively inexpensive and could be a reasonable screening option prior to MMR gene mutation analysis. DNA from both normal and tumor tissue is needed for MSI analysis, as the phenotype is not observed in normal tissue and is recognized as a variation present only in the tumors. DNA for analysis can be obtained from either fresh or frozen tissue or from paraffin-embedded pathology specimens (even after many years, archival blocks retain sufficiently intact DNA). The incidence of germline mutations detected in MMR genes in HNPCC kindreds selected by MSI or linkage analysis was 70% but was only 25% in kindreds negative for MSI and linkage.[87]

Various phenotypic criteria (Tables 80-1, 80-2, and 80-3) have been developed during the past few years to guide genetic testing because DNA sequencing analysis is expensive and has a lower yield in unselected cases with suspected hereditary cancer. The Amsterdam criteria (see Table 80-1) were developed in 1991 to provide a clinical definition of HNPCC; they are also useful to select families for genetic testing of the DNA mismatch repair genes associated with this syndrome.[88-90] The Bethesda criteria

TABLE 80-2

Bethesda Criteria for Testing of Colorectal Tumors for Microsatellite Instability[89,90]

- Individuals with cancer in families that meet the Amsterdam criteria.
- Individuals with two HNPCC-related cancers, including synchronous and metachronous colorectal cancers or associated extracolonic cancers.
- Individuals with colorectal cancer and a first-degree relative with colorectal cancer and/or HNPCC-related extra-colonic cancer and/or a colorectal adenoma; one of the cancers diagnosed at age <45 years and the adenoma diagnosed at age <40 years.
- Individuals with colorectal cancer or endometrial cancer diagnosed at age <45 years.
- Individuals with right-sided colorectal cancer with an undifferentiated pattern (solid/cribiform) on histopathology diagnosed at age <45 years.
- Individuals with signet-ring type colorectal cancer diagnosed at age <45 years.
- Individuals with adenomas diagnosed at age <40 years.

TABLE 80-3

International Criteria for Determining Microsatellite Instability in Colorectal Cancer[90]

- The form of genomic instability associated with defective DNA mismatch repair in tumors is to be called microsatellite instability (MSI).
- A reference panel of five microsatellites (BAT 25, BAT 26, D5S346, D2S123, and D17S250) has been standardized and is recommended for future research in the field. Tumors may be characterized as high-frequency MSI (MSI-H) if two or more of the five markers show instability (i.e., have insertion/deletion mutations), low-frequency MSI (MSI-L) if only one of the five markers show instability, or microsatellite stable if none of the five markers is unstable.
- A unique clinical and pathologic phenotype has been identified for the MSI-H tumors, which comprise about 15% of colorectal cancers, whereas MSI-L and MSS tumors appear to be phenotypically similar. MSI-H tumors are found predominantly in the proximal colon, have unique histopathologic features, and are associated with a less aggressive clinical course than stage-matched MSI-L or MSS tumors. Preclinical models suggest the possibility that these tumors could be resistant to the cytotoxicity induced by certain chemotherapeutic agents. The implications of MSI-L are not yet clear.
- MSI can be measured in fresh or fixed tumor specimens equally well. Microdissection of pathologic specimens is recommended to enrich for neoplastic tissue, and normal tissue is required to document the presence of MSI.
- The Bethesda Guidelines, developed in 1996 to assist in the selection of tumors for microsatellite analysis, were endorsed.
- The spectrum of microsatellite alterations in noncolonic tumors was reviewed, and it was concluded that the foregoing recommendations apply only to colorectal neoplasms.

(see Table 80-2) were developed in 1996 specifically to provide guidelines to select tumors for MSI testing. The large number of studies reporting MSI in colorectal cancer and other extracolonic malignancies prior to 1998 lacked uniform criteria regarding which markers should be used and how many should be altered before a tumor is diagnosed with the instability phenotype.[89] A National Cancer Institute workshop in December 1997 (see Table 80-3) defined specific criteria and consensus guidelines for MSI testing.[90] Further indications for MSI testing could also be considered. These might include predicting differences in response to therapy related to the biology of this phenotype in the tumor itself, rather than implications at the level of organization of the patient or family regarding inherited cancer risk.

The impact that genetic test results can have on medical decisions and outcomes has made molecular diagnostics an important new component of standard medical practice for certain familial syndromes. Molecular diagnosis is potentially a powerful method of cancer risk assessment for individuals inheriting mutant alleles of genes that have been identified as causing cancer predisposition (Table 80-4). Mutation detection is commercially available for several colon cancer susceptibility genes, including APC, MSH2, MLH1. These tests usually cost several hundred dollars or more, and results might not be available for many weeks. Many other tests will be developed in the near future, but their availability does not necessarily imply that clinical indications, sensitivity,

TABLE 80-4

Genes with Germline Mutations Associated with Increased Colon Cancer Risk

HEREDITARY SYNDROME	CHROMOSOME	GENE(S)
Familial adenomatous polyposis	5q21	APC*
Juvenile polyposis	10q22	BMPR1A
	10q23	PTEN
	18q21	SMAD4
Cowden syndrome	10q23	PTEN
Peutz-Jeghers syndrome	19p13	STK11
Hereditary mixed polyposis	6q	unknown
Hereditary nonpolyposis	2p22	MSH2*
colon cancer	3p21	MLH1*
	2q31	PMS1
	7p22	PMS2
	14q24	MLH3(15)

*Mutation detection is commercially available, but availability does not imply that the sensitivity, specificity, or indications of such tests is known or validated.

or specificity are studied adequately and thoroughly validated. Any clinician ordering genetic tests should have a good understanding of all the complex issues involved (see for example, http://infonet.welch.jhu.edu/policy/ genetics/contents.html). There are several possible sources of error in genetic testing, including clinical misdiagnosis of the suspected syndrome, inaccurate representation of relationships on the pedigree, and sample misidentification or contamination.

Molecular diagnostic testing is increasingly being approved by many insurers and managed care organizations, as definitive negative results rule out disease inheritance and decrease the frequency of endoscopies for the otherwise necessary surveillance colonoscopies—which, because they are performed annually, eventually cost much more than the fee charged for the protein truncation assay. The specialists most frequently ordering this test are gastroenterologists (who account for 47% of patients), with only 18% of patients tested by medical geneticists and/or genetic counselors, and the remainder by a variety of other practitioners.[89] Consultation with a knowledgeable gastroenterologist, particularly one with a special interest in this problem who can counsel the patient appropriately and perform any necessary endoscopic procedures is important. Many physicians (32%) involved in the care of families with FAP are unfortunately unaware that a negative test in any patient is informative and useful only if a mutation has been detected in an affected relative.[89] Erroneously failing to institute endoscopic surveillance due to such a false-negative test result could have devastating future consequences if polyps and cancer are not diagnosed early. The quality of care for patients with hereditary polyp and cancer syndromes should be improved by referral to specialized centers or physicians familiar with the complexity and manifold ramifications of genetic testing.

Several commercial and university laboratories perform DNA sequencing analysis for genes such as BRCA1, MSH2, MLH1, and so forth (see Table 80-4). A blood sample is usually all that is needed to perform these genetic tests, as DNA can simply be extracted from leukocytes, or the leukocytes can be immortalized as a permanent source of DNA or RNA. The functional significance of a sequence variant is an important consideration for the proper interpretation of these test results and is more in doubt if the mutation has not been observed previously in other families. Web sites have been established to compile databases of mutations reported for some disease genes, such as ATM (http://www.vmmc.org/vmrc/atm.htm) or BRCA1 and BRCA2 (http://www.nchgr.nih.gov/dir/ Intramural-research/Lab-transfer/Bic/index.html). In general, because the most up-to-date and complete information is not available from any one database, consultation with one or more of the few clinicians and researchers who have a special interest in or focus on a particular syndrome should be obtained.

The strongly predisposing alleles are likely to be less frequent in the population than more common weaker alleles. An example of such a low-penetrance allele in the APC gene, I1307K, converts an AAATAAAA sequence to AAAAAAAA. Although this germline variant is not in itself a cause of disease, it is more vulnerable to somatic mutations that can inactivate the APC gene. It has been reported to be present in 6% of all Ashkenazi, compared with 10% of Ashkenazi with colon cancer. The utility of genetic screening for this I1307K allele, which carries only a modest increase in risk for colon cancer, is not clear.[91]

Linkage analysis can indicate which of several genes for a genetically heterogeneous syndrome might be mutated in a newly investigated family, particularly if these genes are located on different chromosomes and direct mutational analysis is expensive or difficult (e.g., MSH2 and MLH1 genes in HNPCC). Linkage analysis could also be useful in some families with disorders thought to be monogenic, if direct detection of a mutation is not possible by DNA sequencing or the protein truncation assay (e.g., APC). Linkage analysis may be used to make predictions about disease status if there are at least two or more family members with a confirmed clinical diagnosis available to participate in DNA testing, along with the individual in question and unaffected relatives. The pedigree in question should be reviewed by the testing laboratory, and informed consent should be obtained before submitting blood samples for analysis. Linkage analysis is performed using PCR markers or RFLP analysis. The pattern of highly polymorphic intragenic and flanking markers are compared with those of affected and unaffected family members. A pattern of inheritance indicating segregation of the affected haplotype is reported if evident.[92] In rare cases, a family is found to be "uninformative," which means that the affected allele cannot be distinguished from the unaffected allele, and no result can be reported.

The American Society of Clinical Oncology recommends cancer predisposition testing only if all of the following criteria are met:

1. The person has a strong family history of cancer or very early onset of disease.
2. The test can be interpreted adequately.
3. The results will influence the medical management of the patient or family member.[93]

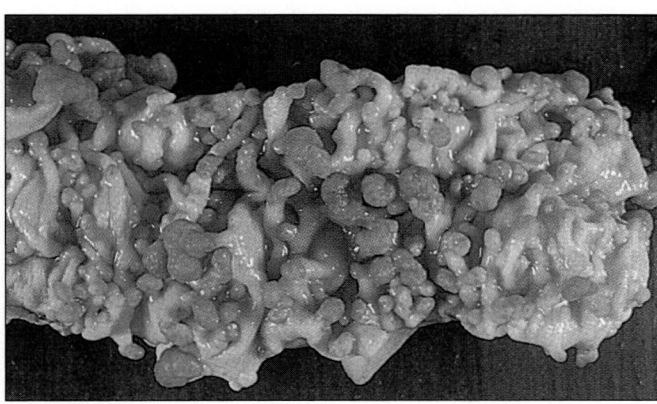

Figure 80-7. A segment of a large intestine covered with adenomatous polyps in a patient with familial adenomatous polyposis. The entire colon is covered with hundreds of polyps. (From Skarin AT, Shaffer K, Wieczorek T [eds]: Atlas of Diagnostic Oncology, 3rd ed, St. Louis, MO Mosby, Elsevier Science Limited, 2003, p 153.)

of histology to confirm the diagnosis of adenomas. Full colonoscopy should be done in anyone with polyposis that is already well developed at the time of initial diagnosis, because in such cases, larger polyps and malignancy could be present in the proximal colon. Flexible sigmoidoscopy is considered sufficient for scheduled screening of any descendants of a person with FAP, because those with the classic severe phenotype will develop numerous polyps throughout the colon. Annual examinations should begin by 10 to 12 years of age in anyone with a known deleterious mutation of the APC gene and in those for whom genetic testing has not been done or is uninformative or not definitively negative. Screening intervals can be increased with each decade of life after age 30 and transitioned to average-risk screening by age 50 if polyposis is not present.[114]

Attenuated Adenomatous Polyposis Coli (AAPC). Several families have been identified in which a smaller number of adenomas develop about 10 years later and with a more predominantly proximal colon distribution compared with classic FAP.[120,121] The lifetime colon cancer risk appears somewhat lower than with FAP and has been estimated at about 80%.[114] This attenuated phenotype is correlated with mutations at the extreme 5′ or 3′ ends or in exon 9 of the APC gene, in contrast to classic severe phenotype FAP, which tends to have mutations clustering in the middle exons of the APC gene.[121] Screening in AAPC should include complete colonoscopy of family members at risk, starting with early adulthood or 10 years younger than the earliest case of colon cancer in the family, and should be repeated about every 3 years; colonoscopy can be repeated more frequently if numerous polypectomies are required or to follow up sessile adenomas. Colonoscopy is needed because of the paucity of polyps and their possible proximal location.

Peutz-Jeghers Syndrome (PJS). Clinical diagnosis relies on examination of the mucocutaneous surfaces for typical melanin spots and on evaluation of the gastrointestinal tract for polyps. Mutations of the STK11 gene are found in about 60% of PJS families.[122,123] Upper and lower gastrointestinal endoscopy and small-bowel radiography are recommended. Colonoscopy should begin when there are symptoms, or screening colonoscopy should be started by age 25 if no symptoms occur and should be repeated at least every 3 years after a diagnosis is made.[124] Polypectomy is performed for any hemorrhagic or large polyps (>1 cm). Smaller polyps that are grossly suspicious should be biopsied or removed because of the associated cancer risk.

Juvenile Polyposis. Colonoscopy screening has been recommended starting in the late teens and should be repeated every 3 years, then increased to annual frequency after polyps occur. Colonoscopic polypectomy is often adequate therapy for a small number of polyps.[125,126] Colon exams could be needed sooner in anyone with symptoms or a genetic diagnosis. Mutations have been found in the SMAD4 gene in about 15% of families, and in the BMPR1A gene in about 38%, and in some other families another gene in that region of chromosome 10, the PTEN gene, is mutated.[114,127,128] Asymptomatic adult relatives should also be screened because of their increased risk of cancer, unless they test definitively negative for a deleterious mutation that accounts for JP in their family.[128]

Hereditary Mixed Polyposis Syndrome. Juvenile polyps often develop foci of adenomatous change, and hyperplastic polyps are quite common, so the occasional finding of these three types of histology in some patients with juvenile polyposis might not be unexpected.[129] Researchers at the Imperial Cancer Research Fund and St. Mark's Hospital in London, however, have described a large kindred with a tendency to develop colonic polyps of mixed histological types, and they named this the hereditary mixed polyposis syndrome (HMPS).[88] The earliest age at diagnosis of polyps in this HMPS kindred (with 42 affected members) was age 18 years, the median symptomatic presentation was age 40 years, and the median age at diagnosis of colon cancer was age 47 years. Typically, fewer than 15 polyps were found at colonoscopy. The characteristic lesion was an atypical juvenile polyp, some affected individuals had polyps of more than one histological type, and individual polyps sometimes had mixed histology. Linkage of mixed polyposis in this family to a locus on chromosome 6 and lack of linkage to the juvenile polyposis locus on chromosome 10 suggest that HMPS is distinct from juvenile polyposis.[84,102] No linkage was found to APC or to other known colon tumor genes, but until the underlying germline and somatic mutations in this family are described at the nucleotide level, it is uncertain whether HMPS is truly a separate disease.[84] Another family with HMPS identified in North America had polyps demonstrating allele loss at the same chromosome 6 locus that had been linked to HMPS in London, providing further evidence for this newly recognized polyposis syndrome.[103] Biennial colonoscopy has been recommended for surveillance because of an estimated 30% lifetime risk for colon cancer among affected individuals.

Hyperplastic Polyposis.

Hyperplastic Polyposis. Hyperplastic polyps are non-neoplastic mucosal elevations rarely larger than 5 mm that account for about half of the diminutive polyps found in the colon. The typical patient with a few small hyperplastic polyps has a cancer risk close to average; however, rare instances of adenomatous and carcinomatous change in these polyps have been described. An increased cancer risk could be associated with hyperplastic polyposis, defined as at least five hyperplastic polyps proximal to the sigmoid with at least two larger than 10 mm or more than 20 polyps of any size if distributed throughout the colon, or any number proximal to the sigmoid in a relative of an individual with HP.[114] Screening colonoscopy could be done every 1 to 3 years depending on the number of polyps.

Lymphoid Hyperplasia.

Lymphoid Hyperplasia. Normal lymphoid follicles range from 1 mm to 10 mm or larger in diameter but are larger and more numerous in younger individuals.[130] It appears that the prominent gastrointestinal lymphoid tissue of childhood often regresses with age. On the other hand, nodular lymphoid hyperplasia associated with common variable immunodeficiency and lymphoma is usually detected in older age groups. Nodular lymphoid hyperplasia, lymphoid hyperplasia of the terminal ileum, and normal lymphoid tissue must be differentiated from other polyposis conditions, especially FAP.[131] Confusion of lymphoid polyps with FAP has led to unnecessary colectomy in several patients. The terminal ileum of FAP patients likewise has been sometimes inappropriately resected during colectomy because of hyperplastic lymphoid tissue. Endoscopic or surgical biopsy should always precede surgical resection. Nodular lymphoid hyperplasia as an entity does not require therapy. It is most important to define associated diseases so that they can be treated and to differentiate hyperplastic lymphoid tissue from other conditions.

Chemoprevention Agents, Drugs, or Diet

Colorectal cancer is one of the most common malignancies in industrialized countries, but despite having some of the best opportunities for prevention, it remains the second leading cause of cancer death in the United States.[2,82] Although colon cancers are more often diagnosed at an earlier stage and are curable by surgery in patients diagnosed through screening programs, treatments currently available for patients presenting with symptomatic later-stage and metastatic colon carcinomas are generally unsatisfactory. Because most colon cancers arise from premalignant adenomatous polyps, secondary prevention by colonoscopic surveillance and polypectomy is possible but not feasible for all patients.[82,86,132] Thus, other primary prevention initiatives, such as the development of chemopreventive medications, could have important roles. Chemoprevention should particu-larly benefit populations with an increased risk for the development of colonic neoplasms, including patients with a family history of colon cancer and those who are at high risk of a second primary tumor because of a personal history of successfully treated adenomatous colonic polyps or cancer.[133-135] Analyses of germline DNA are now being used to a greater extent to diagnose individuals with significant genetic risk factors, and these persons will demand interventions such as chemoprevention.[114,115]

Preclinical studies in animal models, human epidemiologic data, and clinical trials in patients with adenomatous polyposis have consistently indicated that aspirin, NSAIDs, and other cyclo-oxygenase inhibitors have the greatest potential efficacy among current candidates for colon tumor chemopreventive agents.[136-141] Sulindac, an NSAID with prostaglandin inhibitory properties, has been shown in a number of studies to cause adenoma regression both in the rectums of FAP patients who have undergone subtotal colectomy with ileorectal anastomosis and in the colons of unoperated patients with FAP.[138,142-144] The NSAIDs are quite effective for inducing regression of adenomas in familial polyposis, but their significant side effects make the risk/benefit ratio somewhat unfavorable for preventing colon tumors in the general population.[99,114] Further studies will be necessary to determine whether NSAIDs prevent adenomas primarily through cyclooxygenase inhibition, and if so, the relative importance of COX-1 or COX-2 inhibition. Celecoxib, a specific COX-2 inhibitor, prevents adenomas in mice with FAP and in humans.[139,140] Celecoxib regresses adenomas rapidly without much toxicity, in contrast to other nonspecific inhibitors considered for colon cancer prevention that have significant gastrointestinal ulcer and bleeding toxicity related to their COX-1 inhibition, such as aspirin, sulindac, or piroxicam.

Although chemopreventive drugs should not be relied on as primary therapy for unoperated FAP, they could be useful as an adjunctive therapy. Effective polyp control might delay the need for eventual proctocolectomy or completion proctectomy and possibly reduce colon cancer risk in patients with FAP. Such drugs also can decrease the number of polypectomies that would otherwise be needed in patients who have had subtotal colectomy with ileorectal anastomosis. Duodenal polyps, however, are less responsive to therapy compared with colon polyps, so continued close surveillance of the peri-ampullary duodenum remains important in FAP.[139,140,145]

Because selective inhibitors of cycloxygenase-2 have less long-term toxicity than NSAIDs, coxib drugs might be useful for prevention of adenomas in the large number of patients who require polypectomy for sporadic polyps.

Environmental factors do not appear to be of primary importance in the pathogenesis of adenomas in FAP and are not likely to have as strong an effect on sporadic adenomas or cancer as NSAIDs or coxibs. Nonetheless, polyps have been observed to resolve in patients with FAP after subtotal colectomy, pregnancy, oral calcium, oral fiber, and oral sulindac.[41,61,146-148] There is evidence that a variety of factors naturally present within the lumen of the intestine also have an influence on adenoma growth. The complete deprivation of any intralumenal flow beginning with early development by surgically closing off an explant of fetal intestinal segment in polyposis mice results in the complete absence of any adenomas.[149] These intestinal explants remain sterile, suggesting that microbial flora might be important for tumor development. Bacterial flora could also promote tumor development in humans, as the ileal pouch of patients undergoing restorative proctocolectomy can develop numerous polyps, similar to the disease originally present in the colon.[150,151] Supporting this hypothesis, germ-free mice indeed have reduced numbers of tumors. Other factors must also be involved, however, as some tumors still develop.[152] The presence of bile has been implicated as another important factor because in humans with FAP, adenomas cluster in the periampullary region, where a high concentration bile flow enters the intestine.[150] Furthermore, surgical reimplantation of the bile duct shifts the location of carcinogen-induced tumors in rats.[153,154] The particular composition of bile seems to be important, as treatment of such animals with ursodeoxycholic acid inhibits formation of tumors.[155-159] Recent publications suggest that humans treated with ursodiol for primary sclerosing cholangitis in the setting of ulcerative colitis might indeed have decreased dysplasia and cancer.[160,161]

Surgical Prophylaxis Considered for Hereditary Syndromes

HNPCC

Segmental colectomy is typically performed to treat cancer in the initial patient in a family, particularly if the patient is not unusually young and has no family history to suggest a diagnosis of HNPCC. Among patients treated by segmental colectomy, the risk of a second (metachronous) cancer is 30% within 10 years and 50% within 15 years.[162,163] When the first colon cancer has been diagnosed in a person in whom the existence of HNPCC has been established by molecular diagnostic testing or by clinical criteria, either subtotal colectomy or (preferably) total proctocolectomy with ileoanal pouch anastomosis should be recommended. If only subtotal colectomy is done, there is a 1% annual risk of cancer in the remaining rectum, requiring continued frequent surveillance colonoscopy.[164] Colonoscopy screening is not needed after total proctocolectomy with ileoanal pouch anastomosis because that surgical procedure removes all of the colonic mucosa.

Prophylactic colectomy, according to guidelines of the American Gastroenterological Association, may be strongly considered for patients with an HNPCC mutation in whom adenomas are identified at an early age or whose adenomas show microsatellite instability. Prophylactic colectomy may also be considered in uaffected mutation carriers who are unwilling or unable to undergo periodic surveillance.

FAP

Colectomy at an appropriate time is necessary to prevent colon cancer in patients with FAP and should be considered whenever numerous adenomas emerge. Most centers prefer to wait until the child is fully grown if polyps remain small and relatively few in number, but delay is associated with some risk for cancer.[165] Colonoscopy should be performed if a delay longer than a few months is anticipated, then repeated every 6 to 12 months, depending on the size and number of polyps. Persons first screened at an older age might have more fully developed polyposis that requires more expeditious surgical intervention.

The surgical options include subtotal colectomy with ileorectal anastomosis, total proctocolectomy with ileostomy, and colectomy with mucosal proctectomy and ileoanal pouch as either a one- or two-stage procedure.[166-169] Proctocolectomy with ileostomy is rarely required unless cancer is already present in the distal rectum.

Subtotal colectomy with ileorectal anastomosis is a relatively simple procedure, with slightly less morbidity than the ileal pouch procedures, but it carries a serious risk of rectal neoplasia.[166] Because adenomas continue to develop in the retained rectum, sigmoidoscopy and polypectomy is needed at frequent intervals.[167] These patients have a 6% risk of rectal cancer within 20 years, increasing to a 55% risk by 30 years after surgery.[166] Thus, subtotal colectomy is a good option only for patients and families with few rectal adenomas, particularly for those with AAPC.[114]

Colectomy with mucosal proctectomy and ileoanal pouch is considered the procedure of choice in many centers because it allows complete removal of potentially neoplastic colonic and rectal mucosa with retained rectal sphincter function.[170,171] More frequent stools (five to six per day) are expected in most patients, but only a few have problems such as nighttime incontinence or sexual dysfunction.[167] An intermediate approach has been suggested that includes selecting patients with fewer rectal polyps for ileorectal anastomosis and then later revision to ileoanal pouch if warranted. This approach could become more attractive if sulindac and other nonsteroidal antiinflammatory drugs (NSAIDs) or selective cyclo-oxygenase-2 inhibitors such as celebrex adequately maintain polyp suppression in the rectum. Nonetheless, total colectomy with mucosal proctectomy and ileoanal pouch is the surest means of prevention for colorectal cancer.

Peutz-Jeghers Syndrome and Juvenile Polyposis

Surgery in PJS is indicated for removal of any polyps of the small intestine that are symptomatic or larger than 1 cm. Intraoperative small bowel endoscopy and polypectomy can be done during laparotomy.[172] Colectomy is indicated for carcinoma or advanced colonic polyps that are too large or numerous to control safely by colonoscopic polypectomy.[114,173-175] If subtotal colectomy is done instead of proctocolectomy, continued surveillance of the remaining rectum is necessary to remove recurrent polyps. Removal of the rectal mucosa with ileoanal pouch anastomosis additionally has been necessary in some patients because of continued symptoms after colectomy.[176,177] One group recommends that prophylactic colectomy to prevent cancer be strongly considered after 20 years of age if it has not already been necessary for medical problems.

DIAGNOSIS AND STAGING OF COLON CANCER

Colon cancer is usually quite insidious in its development. Asymptomatic patients are suspected of having colon cancer because of anemia or a positive fecal occult blood test found during routine physical exam. With increasing awareness of the benefits of screening colonoscopy, cancer could be discovered at the time of this exam. Symptomatic patients might relate episodes of bleeding per rectum (hematochesia) or increased frequency of bowel dysfunction—either constipation or diarrhea and/or vague abdominal discomfort. Weight loss is less common unless disease is advanced, but fatigue is frequent. On occasion, the degree of anemia can be severe enough to produce cardiac ischemic symptoms in patients with occult coronary artery disease and syncope, which leads to the finding of anemia and evidence of bleeding from the colon tumor. On occasion, patients present with hypokalemia secondary to diarrhea from large villous tumors producing excess mucous.

Fatigue and anemia are symptoms associated with right-sided lesions. Gross bright red blood per rectum, increasing constipation, and cramping abdominal pain are symptoms suggesting a left-sided lesion. Advanced tumors can present with symptoms indicative of extension to other organs, such as the bladder (pneumaturia). A perforated colon cancer must always be considered when the patient presents emergently with abdominal free air and diffuse peritonitis. At times, the emergent status presents the surgeon with the difficult task of differentiating between an inflammatory mass secondary to a perforated colon cancer of the sigmoid colon or upper rectum and a perforated diverticulitis. Obstruction, however, is the most common acute problem requiring emergency surgery for colon cancer (incidence of approximately 30%). Although obstruction almost always occurs secondary to the tumor obstructing the lumen, the tumor can cause intussusception in the adult.

The diagnosis of colon cancer is best established by colonoscopy. Colonoscopy provides direct visualization, a fairly accurate determination of location, and the opportunity to obtain tumor tissue for histologic evaluation. There are two issues to keep in mind during the course of evaluating the patient with suspected colon cancer. The first is the possibility of a second occult primary cancer (approximately 5%), and the second is the presence of additional polyps (approximately 20%–40% probability), which must be cleared or tattooed so they can be dealt with at the time of surgery. When it is not possible to complete colonoscopy to the ileocecal valve, air-contrast barium enema and virtual colonoscopy are options for completing the evaluation of the colon.

Laboratory Evaluation

The goal in preoperative evaluation of the patient newly diagnosed with colon cancer is to determine whether comorbid conditions exists that could affect perioperative morbidity and mortality. The standard laboratory evaluation includes a hemogram, evaluation of clotting capacity, liver injury and renal function tests, fasting blood sugar, electrolytes, a urinalysis, and measurement of carcinoembryonic antigen (CEA) level. Other laboratory studies are determined by a careful history of past medical problems and a thorough system review.

Imaging Modalities for Staging of Colon Cancer

The use of imaging for the staging of colon cancer can be divided into two broad categories: detection and staging of the primary tumor, and determination of the extent of metastatic disease. For the detection of the primary cancer and of polyps greater than 1.0 cm, conventional single- and double-contrast barium enema has been used for many years. With the advent of helical computed tomography (CT) scanning, CT colonography has been used for screening for polyps and other masses (Figs. 80-8, 80-9), and more recently, some investigators are examining techniques for magnetic resonance imaging (MRI) colonography. For the staging of potential extracolonic metastatic disease, ultrasound, CT, MRI, and positron emission tomography (PET) have been used with varying levels of success.[178,179]

Barium Enema. Until the advent of modern colonoscopy, barium enema was considered the mainstay for detection of large colonic polyps and colon cancer (Fig. 80-10). Single-contrast barium enema uses a continuous column of barium injected in a retrograde fashion, and double-contrast barium enema uses a thicker barium mixture that adheres to the colonic mucosa, resulting in a mucosal relief image. For small polyps, double-contrast studies are generally considered to have a higher sensitivity than single-contrast enemas.[180] Regardless of the technique, barium enema is not as sensitive or specific as colonoscopy for colonic pathology and should be chosen as the

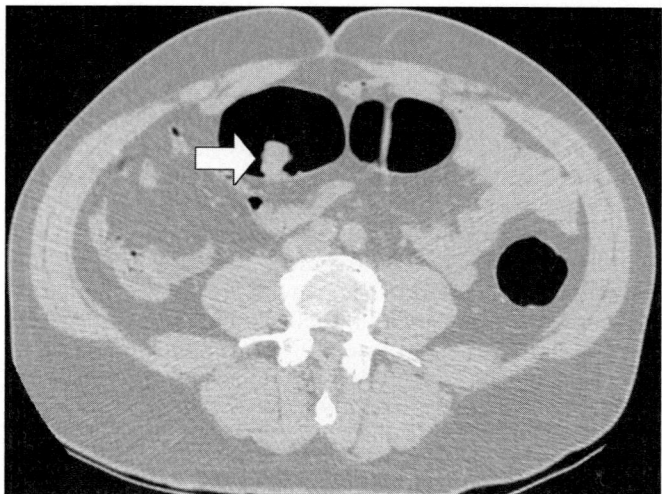

Figure 80-8. Nonenhanced CT image (source data for a virtual colon examination) demonstrates a large pedunculated polyp in the transverse colon (*arrow*). This was later proven to contain colon carcinoma.

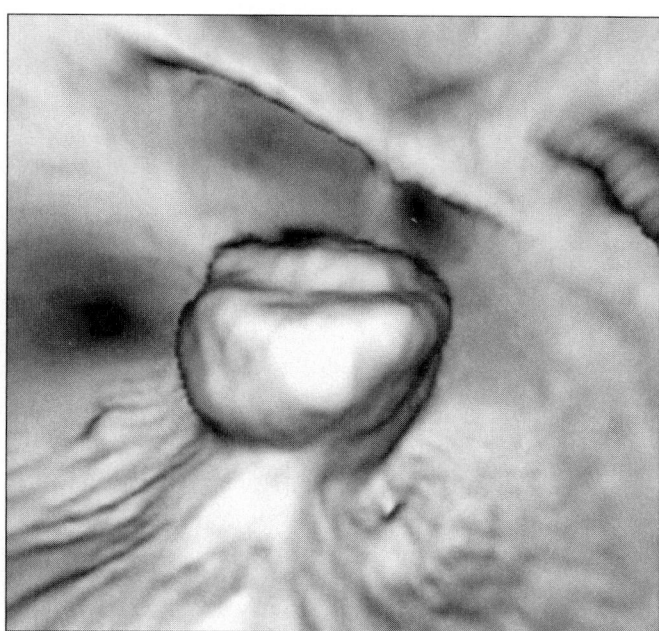

Figure 80-9. Surface-rendered three-dimensional reconstruction of the polyp seen in Figure 80-8. Primary three-dimensional image interpretation is now available. When combined with an appropriate software platform, "fly-through" examinations that mimic the views obtained by conventional video-assisted colonoscopy are now possible.

initial screening test only for patients in whom colonoscopy has failed, who are at high risk for complications from colonoscopy, or for whom colonoscopy is not available.[181] Barium enema has no role in determining the extent of colonic wall invasion by colon cancer, lymph node involvement, or distant disease in patients at high risk for metastases.

Ultrasound. Conventional transcutaneous ultrasound plays no role in the detection of primary colonic tumors. Because the liver can be imaged with varying degrees of success, however, ultrasound has been used to screen the liver for signs of metastatic disease in patients with known colon cancer. In addition, liver metastases often are found incidentally using sonography in patients presenting with vague gastrointestinal symptoms or for other reasons. In studies performed on North American patients, the sensitivity of hepatic ultrasound is not sufficient for it to be as a sole modality for screening or as a preoperative evaluation in patients who are to undergo hepatic metastectomy.[182,183] Ultrasound is the modality of choice for liver biopsy for most hepatic masses (Figs. 80-11, 80-12) due to its low cost, real-time imaging, and excellent needle-guidance systems.[184,185]

Intraoperative Ultrasound (Open and Laproscopic). Intraoperative ultrasound is considered the most sensitive and specific imaging test for detection of hepatic metastases from colon cancer (Figs. 80-13, 80-14). It is far more sensitive for the detection of metastatic lesions than inspection and palpation of the liver by the surgeon,

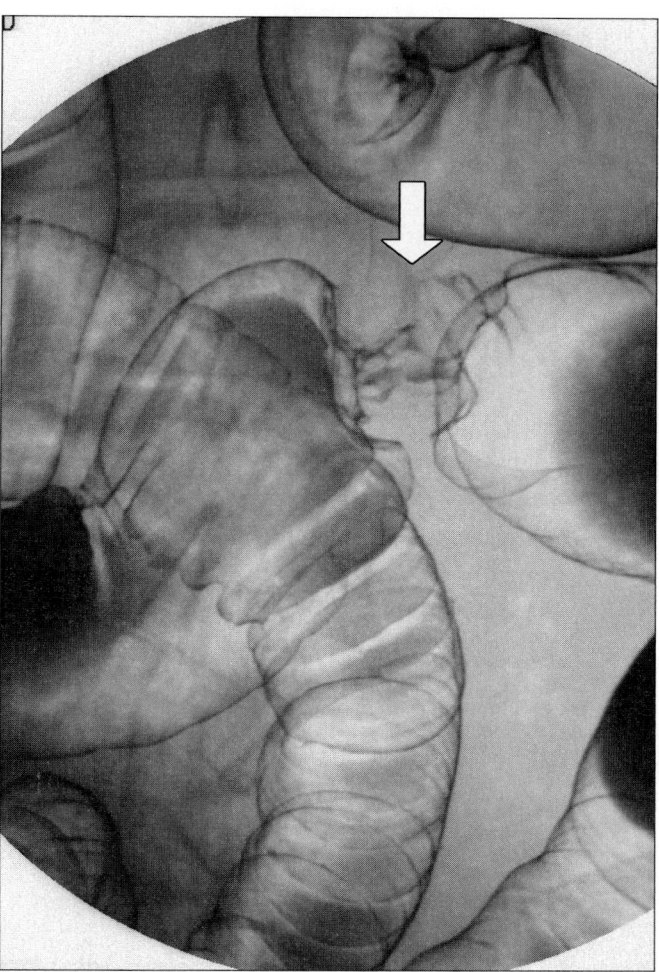

Figure 80-10. Double-contrast barium enema demonstrates circumferential luminal narrowing with mucosal destruction (*arrow*) due to colon carcinoma, the so-called "apple core" lesion.

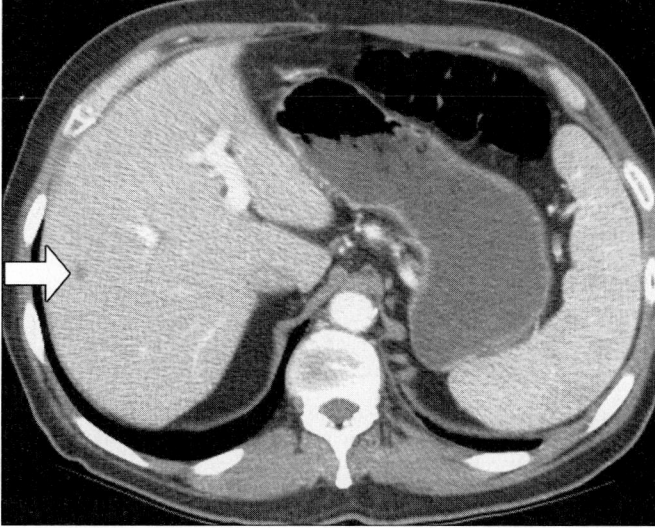

Figure 80-11. Helical CT image of the liver after intravenous contrast injection demonstrates a small right lobe metastatic tumor (*arrow*) from a primary colon cancer.

Specific Malignancies

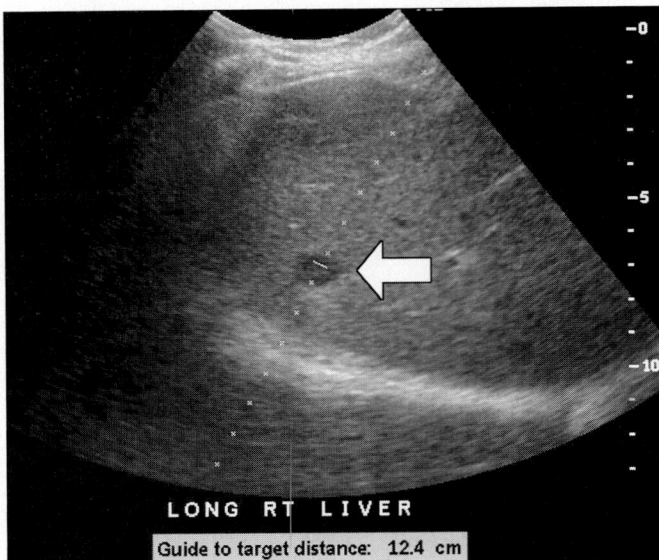

Figure 80-12. Ultrasound-guided biopsy of the liver lesion in Figure 80-11 (*arrow*). Note the needle guidance software that predicts the path of the biopsy needle before its deployment through a fixed guide. This procedure can also be performed "freehand" without the use of a guide. Ultrasound-guided biopsy has been found to be both efficient and cost-effective in comparison with other modalities due to the real-time capability and low cost of ultrasound.

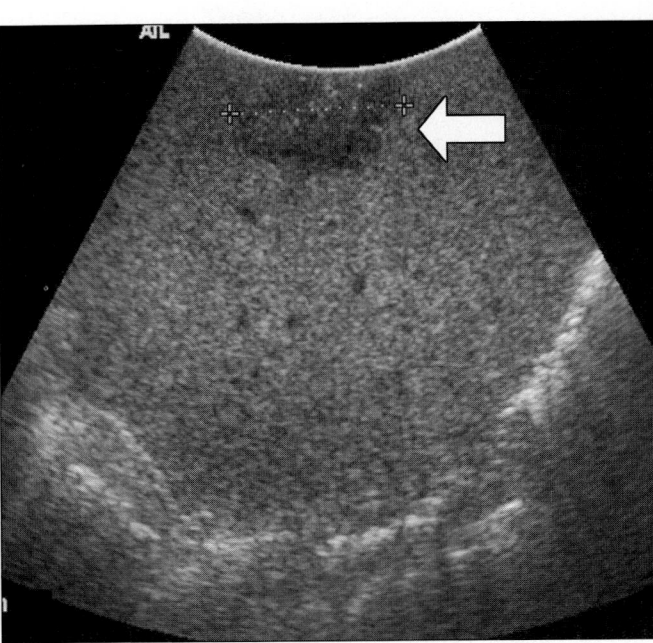

Figure 80-14. Intraoperative ultrasound (IOUS) of the right lobe liver metastasis seen in Figure 80-13. Note the high-quality ultrasound images that are possible with IOUS. Tumors as small as 3.0 mm are detected routinely with this technique.

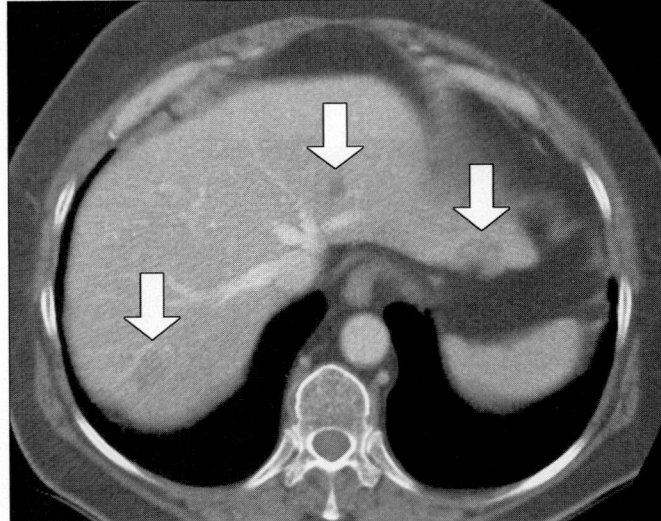

Figure 80-13. Helical CT image of the liver after intravenous contrast in a patient with known colon carcinoma. Three low-attenuation hepatic metastases are visible (*arrows*).

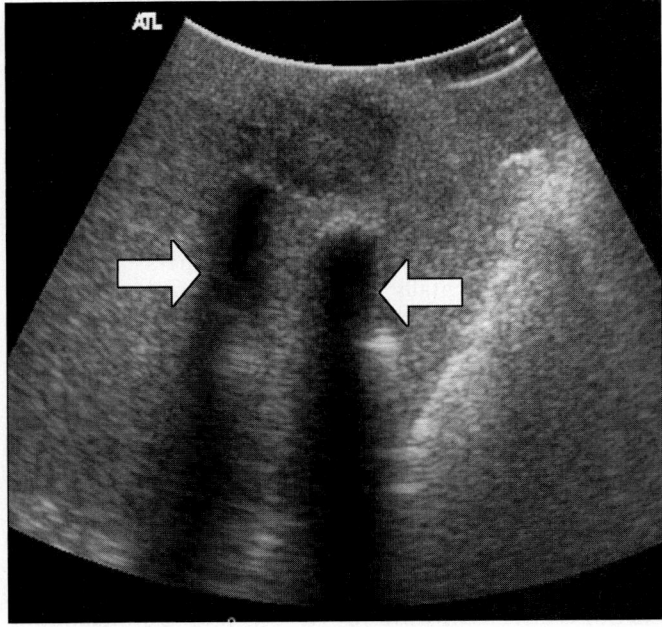

Figure 80-15. Intraoperative ultrasound of the liver during cryoablation. The right lobe hepatic metastasis in Figure 80-14 has undergone cryoablation with formation of an iceball superimposed over the tumor. Ice does not conduct sound, hence the lack of information from within the iceball and the posterior acoustic shadowing. Two cryoablation probes are also visible (*arrows*) with acoustic shadows.

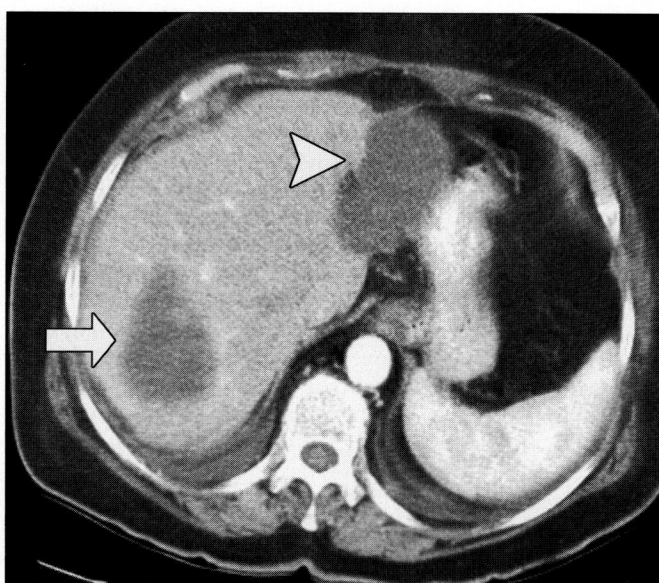

Figure 80-16. Helical CT image of the liver after intravenous contrast in the same patient shown in Figures 80-13 through 80-15. This postoperative image demonstrates a small hematoma after a left lobe hepatic resection (*arrowhead*) and typical postcryoablation changes of the right hepatic lobe tumor (*arrow*).

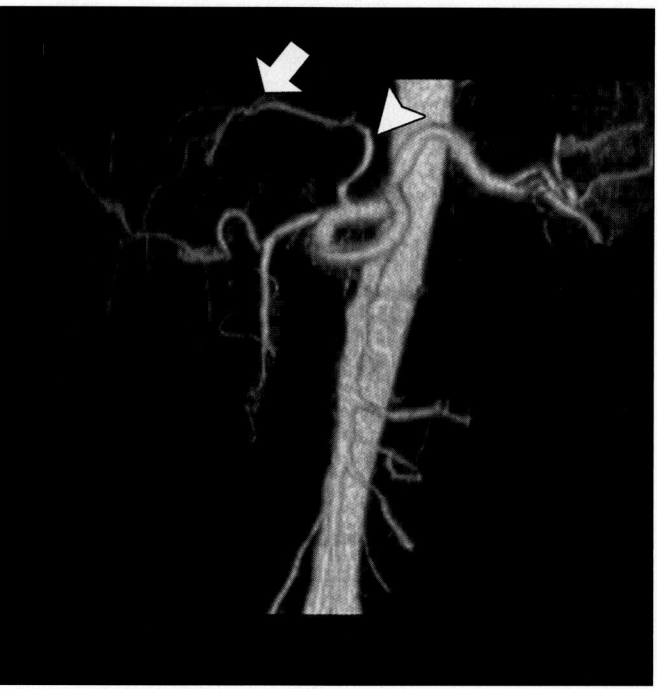

Figure 80-17. CT angiogram (CTA) of the abdominal vasculature shows a replaced left hepatic artery (*arrow*) arising from the left gastric artery (*arrowhead*). CTA can be a valuable preoperative screening tool to evaluate hepatic arterial, portal venous, and hepatic venous anatomy.

particularly for deep tumors.[186,187] Liver metastases as small as 3.0 mm can be detected routinely by intraoperative ultrasound.[188] Additional advantages of intraoperative ultrasound are its ability to guide biopsies of suspicious hepatic lesions and its use as an aid in both liver resection planning and guiding tumor ablation (e.g., cryoablation or radiofrequency ablation) (Figs. 80-15, 80-16). Intraoperative ultrasound has a very limited role in the evaluation of extrahepatic metastases from colon cancer because of the highly targeted nature of the examination. Occasionally, retroperitoneal lymph nodes and other metastatic deposits can be imaged, if specific abnormalities are noted on preoperative imaging or if an abnormality is noted during inspection and palpation of the abdomen.

Laproscopic ultrasound can be used for the same purposes as open intraoperative ultrasound of the liver. Due to lack of access to some areas of the liver, the sensitivity of laproscopic ultrasound appears to be slightly less than that of open intraoperative ultrasound, but it has the advantage of being a less invasive approach.[189] This is particularly useful in patients who have a high likelihood of unresectable liver disease or peritoneal disease, or in patients who are to undergo another minimally invasive treatment for known liver metastases, such as tumor ablation.

Computed Tomography (CT). Contrast-enhanced helical CT is considered the mainstay of preoperative imaging of colon cancer. CT combines a high sensitivity for the detection of liver metastases with availability, safety, and the ability to aid in the detection of peritoneal disease and metastatic lymph nodes. The sensitivity of CT is low, however, for abnormalities that adhere to peritoneal and visceral surfaces, such as peritoneal carcinomatosis. An added advantage of CT as a preoperative imaging modality for hepatic surgery is that CT angiography (CTA) can be obtained at the same time as a conventional diagnostic CT (Fig. 80-17). This can be important when screening for hepatic arterial and venous anomalies prior to hepatic resection, or if the surgeon is considering inserting a hepatic artery infusion pump. CTA is an excellent modality for determining the hepatic arterial, portal venous, and hepatic venous anatomy and for assessing variants of these vessels.[190]

CT technology recently has undergone major changes due to the introduction of multidetector row helical CT scanners. Currently, 16-channel scanners are in widespread clinical use. These scanners can reconstruct image data with thicknesses as low as 0.625 mm. Unfortunately, although the thin slices possible with multidetector row CT are likely to increase sensitivity for the detection of hepatic metastases, there is a paucity of data comparing single-detector row to multidetector row helical CT. Recent data for detection of colon cancer metastases using single-detector row CT demonstrate sensitivities on the order of 85% and specificity approaching 96%, but this sensitivity greatly decreases for metastases smaller than 1.0 cm.[191,192]

Magnetic Resonance Imaging (MRI). Compared with CT, MRI is probably slightly more sensitive and specific for detection and characterization of colon cancer metastases in the liver.[193,194] On the other hand, the long scan times, the relatively high degree of image artifacts, the lack of availability of MRI scanners and scan time, questions about

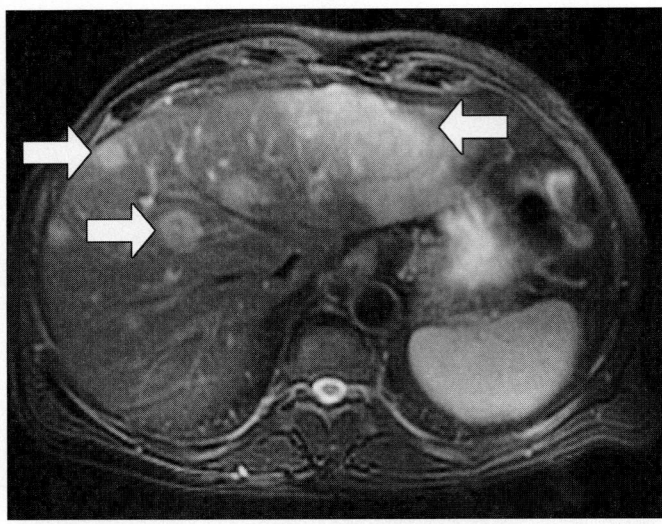

Figure 80-18. Axial MR (T2 with fat suppression) demonstrating rounded high-intensity metastatic lesions (*arrows*) throughout the liver in a patient with known colon cancer primary.

the ability of MRI to detect bowel abnormalities and other evidence of experitoneal disease, and the increased expense of MRI combine to limit the use of MRI for the routine preoperative staging of colon cancer. Indications for preoperative MRI (rather than or in addition to CT) for colon cancer include an inability to tolerate conventional iodinated contrast materials (renal insufficiency or allergies) and clarification of abnormalities detected at CT. Recently, gadolinium-enhanced fat saturation MRI, particularly when combined with delayed imaging, has shown promise in identifying even very thin, "sheet-like" peritoneal tumor involvement.[195] Most colon cancer metastases show high signal intensity on T2-weighted images compared with background liver (Fig. 80-18)

and low signal intensity on T1-weighted images. Rapid gradient-echo pulse sequences are now available that allow imaging of the entire liver in a single breath-hold. When combined with a bolus injection of gadolinium-based contrast agents, information similar to that derived from contrast-enhanced CT scanning can be obtained, which aids in lesion characterization. New liver-specific contrast materials recently have become available for clinical use. These agents are either based on targeting of hepatocytes (gadbenate dimglumine [Gd-BOPTA], gadoxetic acid [Gd-EOB], mangafodipir trisodium [Mn-DPDP]), or the reticuloendothelial cell system (superparamagnetic iron oxides [SPIO]).[196] Several studies have demonstrated increased sensitivities for the detection of liver metastases for MRI enhanced with these targeted agents, but their increased expense, complicated delivery methods, and lack of availability of MRI time have hampered routine use of these compounds.[194,195]

Fluorodeoxyglucose Positron Emission Tomography (FDG-PET). The advent of FDG-PET imaging has been a huge advance in triaging patients who are potential candidates for surgery. The main value of PET imaging has been in the detection of small-volume, extrahepatic metastatic disease. Compared with CT imaging, PET has a lower sensitivity for the detection of hepatic metastases but a higher sensitivity for extrahepatic metastases.[197] Therefore, many centers now use a combination of CT and PET scanning to stage patients prior to potential hepatic resection. This can be accomplished with dedicated PET/CT machines that decrease misregistration artifacts and allow precise localization of areas of increased glucose metabolism, or with CT and PET performed at different settings (Figs. 80-19, 80-20).[198] Overall, the sensitivity of PET for detecting recurrent tumor throughout the body is in the range of 92%.[199] In detection of extrahepatic disease, however, the increased sensitivity of PET com-

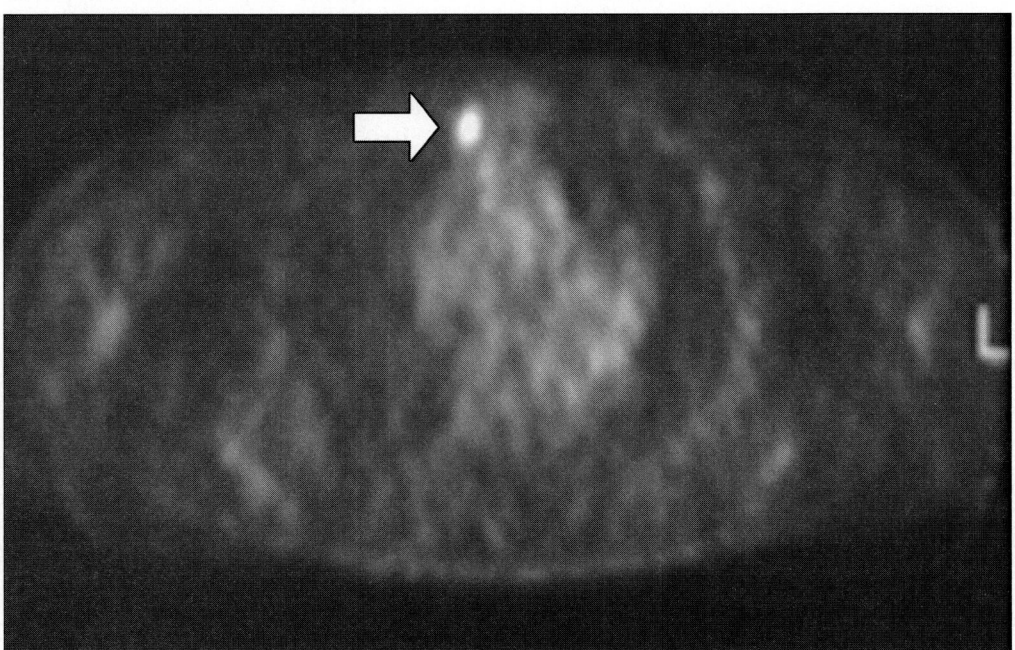

Figure 80-19. PET image of the chest in a patient with colon carcinoma. The patient was being evaluated for a hepatic resection. PET imaging unexpectedly showed a lesion in the chest wall (*arrow*), which changed management from hepatic metastectomy to systemic chemotherapy.

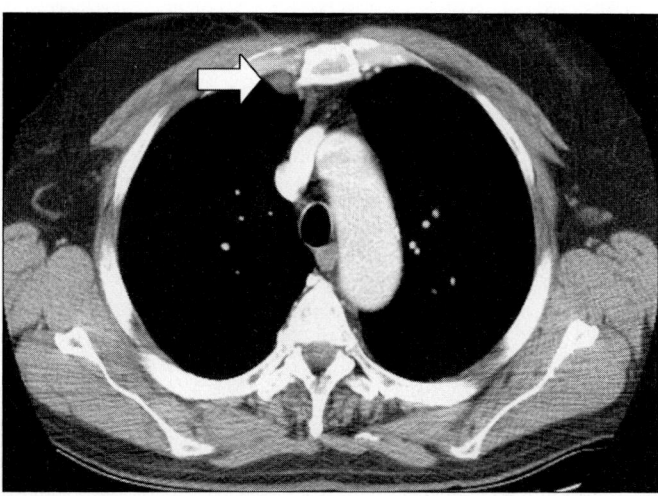

Figure 80-20. Helical CT image of the chest (same patient as in Fig. 80-19) demonstrates the small chest wall metastasis (*arrow*).

pared with CT often has changed patient management (29%–40% of cases).[200,201] Patients who might otherwise be considered candidates for potentially curative resection but who have retroperitoneal metastases identified by FDG-PET may be referred for systemic chemotherapy and spared the complications of surgical procedures that will not be curative.

Table 80-6 compares the various methods of imaging and their relative sensitivities with regard to the detection of hepatic metastases.[202]

Clinical Staging

The most widely used and accepted colorectal cancer staging system is the Astler-Coller modified Duke's system. This system is based on depth of tumor invasion into the colon wall, the number of regional lymph nodes with histologic evidence of metastases, and the presence or absence of distant disease.

The AJCC has modified the TNM staging system for colon cancer to reflect the prognostic factors more accurately. For example, unlike the majority of tumors, tumor size in colon cancer does not by itself affect the

TABLE 80-6

Sensitivity of Imaging for Detection of Hepatic Metastases	
MODALITY	**DETECTION RATE FOR INDIVIDUAL METASTASES (%)**
Transabdominal sonography	40–70
Noncontrast CT	50
Nonspiral contrast enhanced CT	60–75
Spiral contrast CT (single detector)	90–92
MRI	80–90
CT arterial portography	85–95
Intraoperative ultrasound	90–96

Adapted from Paulson EK: Evaluation of the liver for metastatic disease. Sem Liver Dis 2001;21(2):225–236.

patient's risk for developing recurrent disease. The new TNM staging system places an increased emphasis on the number of lymph nodes involved (Fig. 80-21; Table 80-7).

In colon cancer, the preoperative clinical staging is less important than the postsurgical final pathologic stage for managing the patient. The pathologic stage provides the best estimate of prognosis. Currently, "N" or nodal status is based on gross and standard histologic evaluation. The presence of micrometastases (≤0.2 mm) is noted, but the significance of such is not known. In a similar vein, although newer techniques for detecting occult metastasis by immunohistochemistry and polymerase chain reaction (PCR) have become available, their significance to determining prognosis remains to be evaluated. When such findings are available for a patient, they are noted as such on the pathology report but staged as N0.

Newer pathology techniques permit the identification of small numbers of cancer cells in lymph nodes, which are not evident by conventional histopathology. Both immunohistochemistry (IHC) for cytokeratin (which permits the analysis of anatomic location) and reverse transcriptase-polymerase chain reaction (RT-PCR) for cytokeratin RNA (which increases sensitivity) have been evaluated in small series to date. In a series of 200 patients, 122 of whom had histologically negative nodes, 43 patients (34%) had evidence of occult metastatic disease by K20 RT-PCR with an 81% 5-year survival, compared with 90% for those with negative lymph nodes diagnosed by both histology and PCR.[203] Only the six patients with negative histology and four or more nodes involved by PCR had a significantly worse outcome (50% 5-year survival). Using the less sensitive IHC for cytokeratin for 396 Dukes A and B patients, only 73 (18.3%) were positive; no correlation was identified with outcome, although the trend for all subgroups except the Dukes B (who received adjuvant therapy) was for a slightly worse outcome for patients with positive nodes.[204] Given the small number of patients in each trial and the difference in the techniques used, there is no clear evidence to date that more sensitive techniques for establishing tumors with the capacity to colonize lymph nodes signal a worse prognosis.[203,204]

M1 disease reflects tumor present in other organs within the body, peritoneal seeding, a positive peritoneal fluid cytology, and tumor cells found in the bone marrow. Involved lymph nodes outside the regional field (e.g., positive portahepatic or celiac axis nodes) are considered M1 disease.

The R classification is used to determine prognosis as it relates to the outcome of surgical resection of the primary tumor or surgical removal of recurrent disease. R0 denotes a complete resection with no known residual tumor. R1 indicates the presence of residual microscopic disease, and R2 refers to gross residual tumor being present after surgical resection.

Histopathology and Pathologic Staging

The final pathology report of a colon cancer specimen provides critical information regarding the location (with the assistance of the surgeon) of the primary tumor,

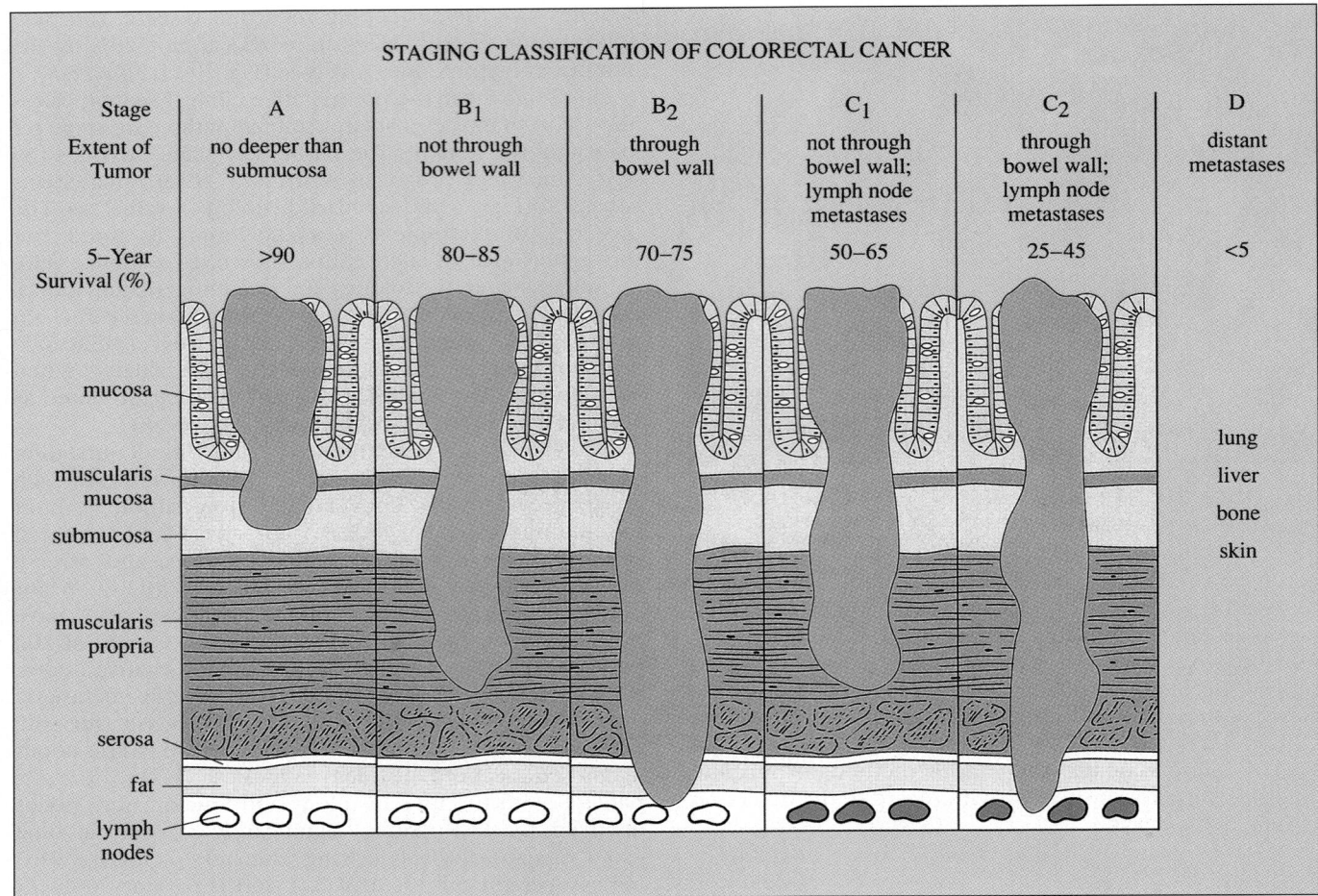

STAGING CLASSIFICATION OF COLORECTAL CANCER

Stage	A	B₁	B₂	C₁	C₂	D
Extent of Tumor	no deeper than submucosa	not through bowel wall	through bowel wall	not through bowel wall; lymph node metastases	through bowel wall; lymph node metastases	distant metastases
5–Year Survival (%)	>90	80–85	70–75	50–65	25–45	<5

Figure 80-21. **A,** Modified Duke's staging classification of colon cancer. Stages B3 and C3 (not shown) signify perforation or invasion of contiguous organs or structures (T4; see also Table 80-7). **B,** The TNM classification provides a more accurate staging system. (Adapted from Skarin AT, Shaffer K, Wieczorek T [eds]: Atlas of Diagnostic Oncology, 3rd ed, St. Louis, Mosby, Elsevier Science Limited, 2003, pp 155–156.)

whether there were satellite lesions or other adenomatous polyps, the size of the tumor, to what degree it was circumferential and whether it was obstructing. The report should define the length of margins related to the resected specimen. These gross descriptions are supported by the histopathology, which documents the type of tumor, the extent to which the tumor has invaded through the colon wall and into surrounding tissue, the tumor grade, and the status of regional lymph nodes. Numerous studies have shown that tumor size by itself is not a prognostic factor.

Most authors describe four macroscopic forms of colon cancer:

1. Ulcerative
2. Polypoid
3. Annular
4. Diffusely infiltrating

The ulcerating lesion is typically circular or oval with raised, rolled edges and having a deep central ulceration. This form of colon cancer is more likely to perforate, as the tumor invades deeply into the wall. Polypoid lesions are cauliflower in gross appearance. They are more commonly found in the right (ascending) colon, and some

evidence suggests that these exophytic lesions have a worse prognosis. Annular lesions, as their name implies, are circumferential in growth and tend to be ulcerated. They are more commonly found in the distal colon. Diffusely infiltrative lesions can infiltrate the bowel wall for a distance of 5 to 8 cm and are similar in their patterns of growth to gastric linitis plastica.

Colon cancers are generally graded as well differentiated, moderately differentiated, poorly differentiated, or undifferentiated (Fig. 80-22).[206]

Microscopically, the tumor could be invading all layers of the bowel wall. There is unusually a significant inflammatory response, and the tumor can be seen invading perineural spaces and into veins. Most colon cancers are mucin producing.[206] Colon adenocarcinoma is usually positive for keratin 20 and negative for keratin 7; this information can be helpful in determining whether a pulmonary lesion is metastatic colon cancer or a new primary lung adenocarcinoma.[207] Colon adenocarcinomas are also positive immunohistochemically for CEA, and the pattern of staining tends to be diffuse throughout the cell surface rather than focal. Antibiodies to CEA epitopes of group 1 and 2 are most sensitive for immunohistochemistry.[208] Essentially, all invasive colon cancers stain

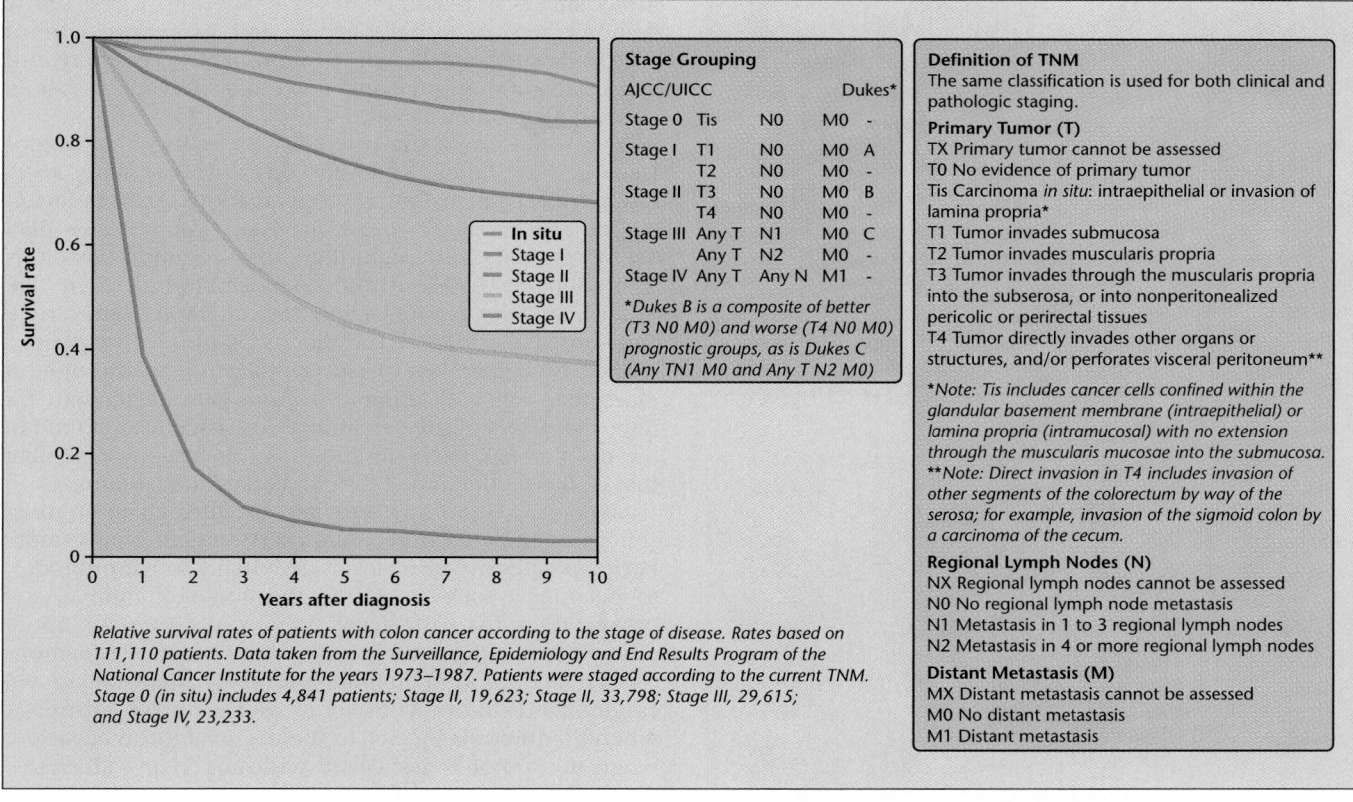

Relative survival rates of patients with colon cancer according to the stage of disease. Rates based on 111,110 patients. Data taken from the Surveillance, Epidemiology and End Results Program of the National Cancer Institute for the years 1973–1987. Patients were staged according to the current TNM. Stage 0 (in situ) includes 4,841 patients; Stage II, 19,623; Stage II, 33,798; Stage III, 29,615; and Stage IV, 23,233.

Figure 80-21, *cont'd.*

TABLE 80-7

Surgical Stage and Survival Rates in Colorectal Cancer

	AJCC/UICC CANCER STAGING*			COMPARISON TO DUKES AND MAC CLASSIFICATIONS	ASTLER, COLLER[†]	COMPARISON TO SEER	5-YEAR SURVIVAL RATES AFTER SURGICAL RESECTION ALONE[‡]
STAGE	**TUMOR**	**REGIONAL LYMPH NODES**	**DISTANT METASTASES**				
Stage 0	Tis	N0	M0	—	Limited to mucosa	In situ	
Stage I	T1	N0	M0	Dukes A; MAC A	Extending into submucosa	Localized	**Stage I** 85%–95%
	T2	N0	M0	Dukes A; MAC B1	Extending into muscularis propria	Localized	**Stage II** 60%–80%
Stage IIA	T3	N0	M0	Dukes B; MAC B2	Extending through muscularis propria	Regional	
Stage IIB	T4	N0	M0	Dukes B; MAC B3		Regional	
Stage IIIA	T1–T2	N1	M0	Dukes C; MAC C1	Limited to bowel wall with involved nodes	Regional	**Stage III** 30%–60%
Stage IIIB	T3–T4	N1	M0	Dukes C; MAC C2-C2	Extension through bowel wall with involved nodes	Regional	
Stage IIIC	Any T	N2	M0	Dukes C; MAC C1-C2-C3		Regional	
Stage IV	Any T	Any N	M1	—; MAC D	Distant metastases	Distant	**Stage IV** <5%

MAC, modified Astler-Coller.
*Greene FL, Page, DL, Fleming ID, et al (eds): Colon and rectum. In American Joint Committee on Cancer: AJCC Cancer Staging Manual, 6th ed. New York, Springer-Verlag, 2002, pp 113–119.
[†]Astler VB, Coller FA: The prognostic significance of direct extension of carcinoma of the colon and rectum. Ann Surg 1954;139:846.
[‡]Macdonald JS: Adjuvant therapy of colon cancer. CA Cancer J Clin 1999;49:202–219.

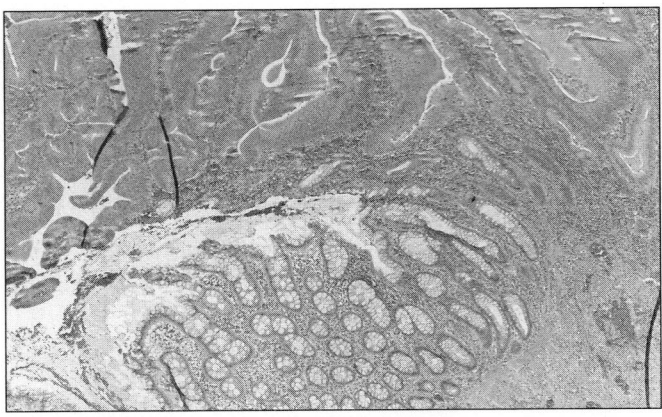

A

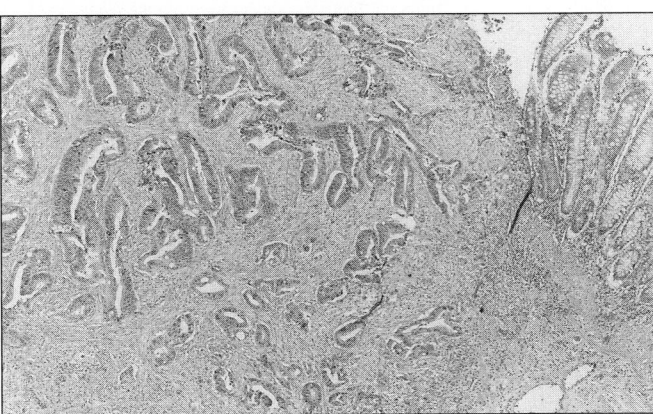

B

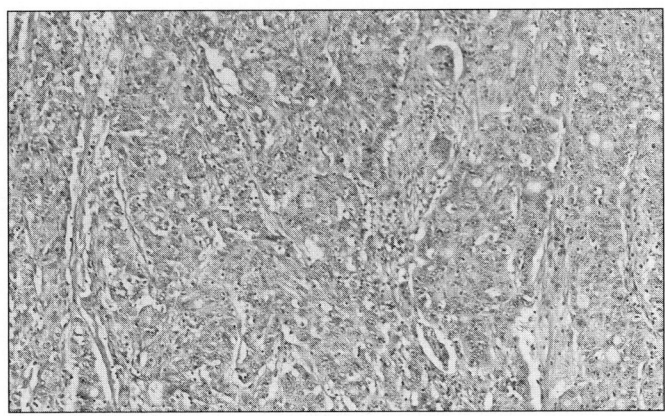

C

Figure 80-22. Histologic grades of colorectal cancer. **A,** Well-differentiated adenocarcinoma. **B,** Moderately differentiated adenocarcinoma. **C,** Poorly differentiated adenocarcinoma.

positive for tumor-associated glycoprotein (TAG-72) using monoclonal antibody B72.3. This glycoprotein is also present in a high percentage of hyperplastic and adenomatous polyps.[209]

Colon cancers frequently have a loss of blood group isoantigens and of HLA A, B, and C histocompatibility antigens.Often, they acquire blood group substance H. The cytoskeleton protein villen is present, along with increased expression of cathepsin B and the adhesion molecule E-cadherin. Molecular analysis consistently demonstrates mutation of p53 and overexpression of the associated abnormal protein. There is increased expression of the *c-myc* oncogene, and a few tumors show *ras* oncogene mutations.

It is well known that the gross margins of the tumor visualized at surgery or endoscopy correlate fairly accurately with the actual microscopic margins. Any significant degree of intramural spread of tumor occurs in less than 5% of patients. Although the most common histology is moderately differentiated adenocarcinoma, there are other histologic variants, including mucinous, signet ring, and squamous type.[206] The mucinous tumors are characterized by large lakes of extracellular mucin throughout more than half the tumor. Mucinous tumors account for only about 15% of the carcinomas and usually are found in the distal colon. Their prognosis is somewhat worse than that of the moderately differentiated adenocarcinomas.

Signet ring tumors are rare and are diffusely infiltrating, similar to their gastric counterparts. Signet ring tumors have a propensity to metastasize initially to lymph nodes, to peritoneal surfaces within the abdomen, and to the ovary rather than the liver. As a result, they are more difficult to manage and have a poor outcome. Squamous (or, as it is more commonly termed, adenosquamous) carcinoma is more commonly found as the histology when the tumor is located in the cecum and, on occasion, when the tumor is associated with underlying ulcerative colitis. There are other possible uncommon histologies, such as clear cell, rhabdoid morphology, basaloid (similar to cloacogenic carcinoma), choriocarcinomatous histology, and endocrine differentiation.[206] The latter includes neuroendocrine variants and a pulmonary-like small cell carcinoma. Carcinoid tumors have also been described as originating in the colon.

SURGICAL TREATMENT

Radical resection of the tumor-bearing segment of colon, with wide margins and removal of the lymphatic drainage of the tumor, is the standard for curative therapy. The extent of resection is determined by tumor size, location, histological grade, and tumor extension into the colon wall and into adjacent tissue or organs. Historically, resections of the colon for cancer have been quite radical with respect to the removal of the mesocolon-bearing draining lymphatics at risk for tumor spread. Studies, however, indicate that there is no major survival advantage by extended lymph node dissection.[210-213] Even so, limited segmental resections are indicated primarily when the surgery is deemed palliative.

Preoperative preparation of the colon to clear the colon of fecal matter and to reduce the quantity of bacteria within the colon are important to ensure a safe operation with minimal morbidity. For elective surgery, patients are placed on a liquid diet starting 3 days before scheduled surgery. For the last 24 hours of diet preparation, they are urged to take only clear liquids. The night prior to surgery, patients have an active mechanical bowel preparation to ensure optimal cleansing of the colon. Before surgery, they are given parenteral antibiotics.

PREPARATION OF BOWEL FOR ELECTIVE RESECTION

- Begin diet restriction to full liquids three days before scheduled surgery.
- Limit diet to clear liquids for 24 hours preceeding surgery.
- Admit patient to hospital 1 day before surgery for i.v. hydration.
- Administer metoclopramide, 10 mg intramuscularly or orally, 30 minutes before beginning mechanical bowel preparation.
- Administer D5/0.5 saline solution with 40 mg KCL intravenously at 100 mL/hour beginning 11 P.M. on the evening before surgery.
- Administer 1.5 L GI lavage solution four times hourly by mouth until stool is clear. Begin lavage at ~ 4 P.M. on the afternoon before surgery.
- Administer neomycin base orally 1 and 2 hours after completion of GI lavage (approximately 10 P.M.)
- Administer erythromycin base orally 1 and 2 hours after completion of GI lavage.
- Check serum potassium 2 hours after completion of GI lavage and at 6:00 A.M. preoperatively.
- Ensure that intravenous Cefotetan is available on call to the operating room.

Patients should be given intravenous hydration before surgery, preferably during the night of their mechanical bowel preparation. It might be necessary to modify the preparation of the colon if the tumor is large enough to cause partial obstruction.

It is important to use a suitable regimen to minimize the risk of deep venous thrombosis and thereby to reduce the likelihood of pulmonary embolism. We routinely use low-molecular-weight heparin and intermittent compression leggings during the perioperative period. Early ambulation is an important adjunct to heparin and compression.

The choice of placement of the incision is dependent on the location of the tumor and the surgeon's preference. I favor a midline or Para median incision for two reasons. First, it allows better access to the liver in case unexpected synchronous liver metastases are discovered, and second, it is not uncommon to reoperate such patients for recurrent tumor. A midline approach, in contrast to a transverse approach (incision) allows the surgeon to move up or down within the abdomen for future surgical therapy.

Once the abdomen is entered, the surgeon performs a thorough exploration of the abdomen to assess the extent of the tumor and to search for metastatic disease. The liver deserves special attention because it is most commonly the site of first failure, and approximately 10% to 15% of patients will have synchronous metastatic involvement of the liver. Intraoperative evaluation of the liver is generally accomplished by visual inspection and palpation. If there is any suspicion of liver metastasis based on preoperative CT scan, intraoperative ultrasound of the liver is performed and increases the frequency of detecting occult metastases.[186-188,214-218] The author pays particular attention to nodes in the porta hepatis, and if

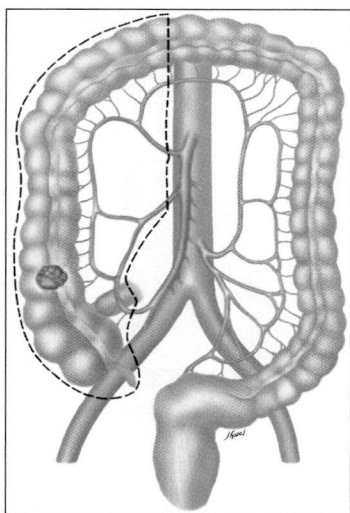

Figure 80-23. Right hemicolectomy resection margins for right colon carcinoma.

unusually large or suspicious nodes are found, they are sampled.

The four classic resections for colon cancer are depicted in Figures 80-23, 80-24, 80-25, and 80-26. A right hemicolectomy (see Fig. 80-23) is the standard approach for tumors involving the cecum and right colon. The mesocolon and its vascular structures are transected at the base of the mesocolon along the superior mesenteric artery. The ileocolic and right colic arteries are the branches of the superior mesenteric artery that are ligated, along with branches of the middle colic artery. The middle colic artery is usually preserved unless the tumor is located in the hepatic flexure of the colon. In this situation, the resection is extended to include the middle colic artery. For a right hemicolectomy, the ileum is divided approximately 10 cm from the ileocecal valve. Continuity of the bowel is re-established by anastomosis of the terminal ileum to the transverse colon. Although

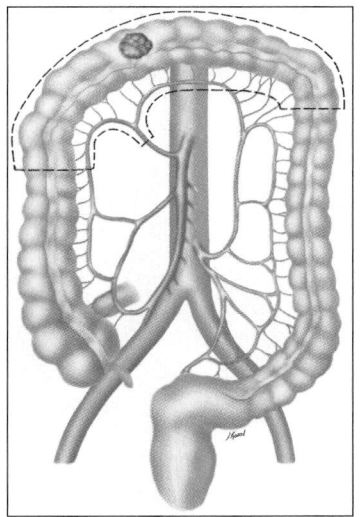

Figure 80-24. Transverse colon resection margins for transverse colon carcinoma.

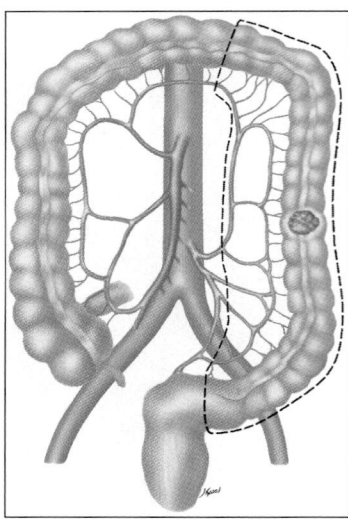

Figure 80-25. Left colon resection margins for left colon carcinoma.

the greater omentum is often removed in part or completely to facilitate resections of the right and transverse colon, there is no evidence that this measure improves survival.

Cancer involving the transverse colon requires mobilization of both the hepatic and splenic flexures. The middle colic artery is transected at the superior mesenteric artery (see Fig. 80-24). When the tumor is located in the splenic flexure region, the surgeon must be more concerned about adequate collateral blood supply through the marginal artery. This concern is increased in elderly patients with a history of significant vascular disease.

Tumors located in the left colon are managed by a left hemicolectomy. The inferior mesenteric artery is ligated near its origin on the aorta. The more distal the location of the cancer, the more mobilization of the upper rectum will be needed. It is almost always necessary to mobilize the splenic flexure. Cancers that involve the sigmoid

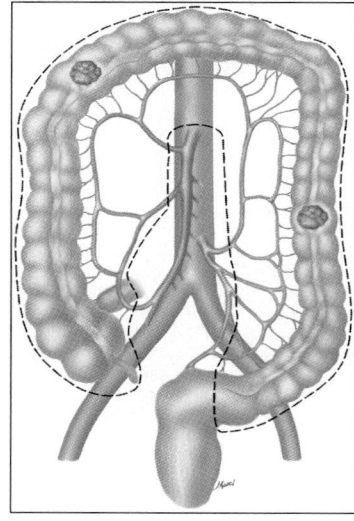

Figure 80-26. Resection margins for synchronous right colon and left colon carcinomas with reconstruction via ileorectostomy.

portion of the colon are resected by what is commonly termed an anterior sigmoid colon resection or a low anterior sigmoid resection. The more distal sigmoid tumors require resection of the upper rectum to achieve an adequate distal margin. It is always more difficult, in cases of left colon and sigmoid colon cancers, to determine an appropriate amount of colon and mesentery for resection. It is helpful to map the vascular structures draining the area of the tumor visually. There is increasing evidence that aggressive radical resections of the left colon provide no additional survival benefit.[211,213]

As noted, in colon surgery it is the arterial blood supply that usually dictates the extent of resection. The rule is to provide a minimum of 5 to 6 cm margin of colon in the resection. Evidence suggests, however, that it is rare to find colon cancer spread beyond 1.2 cm from the gross margin of the tumor. Figure 8-26 illustrates a subtotal colectomy and ileorectostomy. A subtotal colectomy may be required in patients harboring synchronous cancer in the right and left colon and patients presenting with colon cancer at a young age. Other indications for subtotal colectomy could include obstructing cancer, extensive diverticular disease, and a right colon lesion with extension into the sigmoid colon or similarly, a cancer of a redundant sigmoid colon that invades into the right colon.

Restoring Continuity

The restoration of bowel continuity is an important step in the procedure. Use of appropriate techniques for accomplishing the anastomosis minimizes the risks of abscess, sepsis, and the significant morbidity associated with a leak postoperatively. The anastomosis is performed either hand-sewn or using a stapling technique. There is little if any evidence that one technique is superior to the other. It is important to use surgical packs to isolate the anastomosis procedure from the rest of the abdomen until it is completed.

I use a separate set of instruments once the bowel is opened and discard these when I have completed the closure of the anastomosis. Schwab and colleagues[219] reported the results of an in vitro study comparing initial "bursting strength" for three different anastomosis techniques. These authors performed 10 hand-sutured anastomoses, 10 biofragmentable ring anastomosis, and 10 stapled anastomoses of fresh human colon harvested at time of colon cancer surgery. They measured the pressure required to burst the anastomosis and found no significant difference. They concluded that because there were no differences, hand-sutured anastomosis were certainly the least expensive and should remain the standard.

In prior years, some surgeons advocated a "no-touch technique" in removing colon cancer. This was based on the concern that manipulation of the tumor-bearing tissue before high ligation of the draining veins and lymphatics might increase the risk of metastasis. A study by Sales and coworkers[220] failed to show a survival benefit for rigorous application of the "no-touch" high ligation of vessel technique.

Occasionally, surgeons either use providone-iodine to irrigate a segment of colon during preparation for anastomosis or inflate the distal rectum and sigmoid colon to kill shed tumor cells within the lumen. Concern had existed regarding mucosal injury and absorption of iodine. Studies have shown that the elevated serum iodine levels that can occur with irrigation do not cause thyroid or bowel injury, and such irrigations can be performed with negligible risk.[221]

Surgical Management of Lymph Nodes in Colon Cancer

Lymph node metastases are the most important prognostic factors in colon cancer. As described previously in this chapter, colon resection has classically involved taking the mesocolon of the resected bowel at the origin of the vessels supplying the segment of colon to be removed. This ensures removal of the first level of lymph nodes (often called the epicolic and pericolic nodes) and the intermediate or second level of nodes in the resection when the vascular branches supplying the segment are taken at the SMA and IMA. The rationale for these more or less standard resections is based on the assumption that lymphatic tumor dissemination follows an orderly, sequential route of first order nodes, second order nodes, and so forth.

It is known, however, that metastases can be found in distant node groups—para-aortic, celiac, and porta hepatis—even when regional nodes appear to be normal. Supporting this observation is a report of administering 25-mci 99mTc-tagged fab–fragment–antibody to CEA before the patients underwent colon resection. Intraoperatively, a hand-held scintillation probe was used, and surgeons removed all nodes identified as suspicious. Seven of 20 patients were up-staged, and metastatic spread was found at distant sites of retroperitoneum and renal hilum.[222]

A concern, of course, is that therapeutic decisions are based heavily on lymph node status at the time of primary resection. Often, because of limitations of conventional surgical resection and pathological lymph node examination, the actual number of patients with involved nodes can be underestimated. In a recent report, investigators from the Fox Chase Cancer Center analyzed patient data from the intergroup trial INT-0089 to determine whether there was a relationship between survival and the number of nodes found by the pathologist. Regardless of the number of positive nodes, the researchers found that survival improved as more nodes were removed.[223]

To overcome this problem of distant node metastasis, there has been an effort to extend the well established techniques of sentinel lymph node mapping (SLN) for melanoma and breast cancer to colorectal cancer. A preliminary study of 20 patients used the intraoperative subserosal peritumoral injection of 1% lymphazurin 10 minutes before resecting the colon. The blue-stained supposed "sentinel node" was excised, frozen immediately, and examined by serial 200-μg samples using H & E staining. The sections were also subjected to immunohistochemical staining for the cytokeratin marker AE 1-AE3. Although there was difficulty in surgically identifying the stained SLN(s), the pathologist was able to find the SLN(s) in 90% of cases. The average number of SLN(s) was 3.9 nodes. The investigators believed that the status of 5 of the 20 patients changed from being node negative to node positive through this procedure.[224-227]

In another study, 35 patients with colon cancer had intraoperative SLN mapping using 1% isosulfan blue dye. SLN mapping identified the stained node in 25 patients (71%), and in 15 cases in which the SLN was negative, all other nodes were also found to be negative, yielding a 0% false-negative rate. The SLN was the only positive node in four (11%) of the 35 patients, and CAM 5.2 staining provided the only evidence of metastasis in four patients (11%).[225]

Clearly, SLN mapping has not reached a confidence level in colon cancer therapy sufficient to use it as standard of care. The incidence of false negatives is not 0%, and the SLN status cannot yet be used to select patients for more limited resection of the colonic mesentery.[226,227] Much more work is required to establish the role of SLN mapping in the staging and decision-making process defining overall treatment of such patients.

Several additional presentations of colon cancer deserve special comments; these are obstructing tumors, invasion into other organs, and perforation.

Surgical Management of Obstructing Colon Cancer

In a larger population of 4583 patients in the United Kingdom, obstruction was noted in 16%.[228,232] The obstructing tumor, as expected, occurred more frequently on the left side, with the spleenic flexure being the most common site (49%). Twenty-three percent of obstructions occurred in the descending colon and 23% in the right colon. Serpell and associates[229] reported a similar incidence of 16%, with 30% demonstrating symptoms and evidence of partial obstruction.

Malignant obstruction can present as a progression of symptoms associated with colon function, such as increasing frequency and severity of episodes of cramping abdominal pain or decreasing frequency of bowel evacuation leading to constipation and abdominal distention. It is not uncommon to have the patient present in the emergency room with the acute onset of symptoms. Diagnosis is confirmed by abdominal x-rays and CT scan. Carefully conducted colonoscopy to avoid dangerous distention of colon by air insufflation and barium contrast study could prove useful in localizing the tumor and clearing the colon of other polyps or synchronous cancer.[230]

There are several options for managing obstructing tumors, depending on their location. These include:

- Resection with proximal temporary colostomy and Hartmann's procedure (closed distal stump).
- Intraoperative lavage of colon, systemic antibiotics, and primary anastomosis.
- Subtotal colectomy with primary anastomosis.

A temporary colostomy and Hartmann's procedure require a second operation for colostomy take-down and restoration of bowel continuity. Although this is a safe approach, with approximately 10% morbidity, subsequent colostomy closure might not be feasible or advisable in the poor-risk patient and itself carries an additional risk of complications of 40%.[231,232]

The second approach, intraoperative colon lavage, is accomplished by placing a Foley catheter through the appendiceal stump and irrigating the preserved colon until it is mechanically clean. Although this procedure is time consuming, the overall morbidity is approximately only 10%, and the rate of anastomotic leak is quite low.[231,233,234]

The third approach, subtotal colectomy, has become more acceptable. It can be accomplished quickly, does not require a temporary colostomy, and has the advantage of removing any proximal synchronous lesions.[235-237] Wong and colleagues,[236] in an analysis of 35 patients undergoing subtotal colectomy for an obstructing cancer, found a significant incidence of proximal synchronous tumors in 32% of patients. Thus, patients with complete obstruction of their colon and dilated proximal colon might best be served by undergoing a subtotal colectomy. In general, less than 50% of obstructing lesions can be resected for cure, and review of 12 reports by Sugarbaker and coworkers[237] found a 5-year survival rate of only 40% for those patients resected for cure.

Surgical Management with Involvement of Adjacent Organs

When a cancer of the colon is adherent to the peritoneal surface of the abdominal wall, the area of contact should not be divided, even if it is suspected to be an adhesion. In more than 50% of patients, what appears to be an adhesion will involve direct invasion of the tumor into the peritoneum.[238] Surgically disrupting these sites of adherence could result in a spill of cancer cells within the peritoneal cavity, leading to an increase in intra-abdominal recurrence and a decrease in survival. Adjacent organs are usually partially resected or totally resected in continuity with the colon tumor. When the tumor involves the abdominal wall, a portion of the peritoneum and underlying muscle are resected by developing a 2 to 3 cm margin around the site of adherence. Such carefully performed resections can lead to a good outcomes in 20% to 50% of patients.[238] The redundant nature of the sigmoid colon frequently is responsible for involvement of the bladder by a sigmoid tumor. Fujisawa and colleagues[239] reported an analysis of 35 patients requiring some aspect of urologic surgery to accomplish a removal of their cancers. This group included 19 sigmoid cancers that involved 15 patients undergoing bladder-sparing partial cystectomy. An ileal conduit and ileal neobladder were needed in two patients.

Surgical Management of Perforated Colon Cancer

The frequency of colon cancer presenting as isolated acute perforation with peritonitis is low. But perforation combined with fistulation into an adjacent organ or into the retroperitoneum with the development of an abscess is estimated to be present in 6% to 8% of patients with colon cancer.[240] When the presentation is acute, with free air and diffuse peritonitis, an emergent surgery is required, and prognosis for long-term survival is poor. Sugarbaker and coworkers[237] found a 5-year survival rate of 7.3% for

free perforation and 41% for contained perforations. The risk of peritoneal seeding and the future development of carcinomatosis is reported to be approximately 20% for patients with perforation.[241]

Surgical Management of the Malignant Colon Polyp

A malignant colon polyp is defined as one in which there is invasion of the cancer beyond the muscularis mucosa. The surgeon must decide whether additional surgery following endoscopic polypectomy is indicated. The rationale for a resection of the portion of colon from which the polyp was removed is to minimize the risk of residual cancer at the site of polypectomy and to remove regional nodes at risk for metastatic spread. Factors that influence a decision to resect the colon are whether the cancer was well or poorly differentiated, whether there is evidence of vascular or lymphatic invasion, and whether there is good evidence that the polyp was removed completely. More often, it is the question of complete removal that dictates the decision.[242] Pedunculated polyps are easier to remove endoscopically and lend themselves to optimal histopathologic assessment of margins. The stalk of the pedunculated polyp often provides adequate margin.

Sessile polyps containing cancer are more problematic. They have a higher incidence of lymph node involvement —approximately 10% to 25%, compared with 3% for pedunculated polyps.[243] Unless there are significant comorbid conditions that preclude resection, it is safest to resect the segment of the colon in which a cancerous sessile polyp was found.[243] Extension of cancer to "Haggitt" level 3 in predunculated polyp is a good indicator for performing colon resection (Fig. 80-27).[244]

In dealing with malignant polyps, it is best to err on the side of overtreatment. Any polyp for which there is a question of adequate margin or angiolymphalic invasion should have a resection of the involved colon if the histology is grade 3. Identifying the correct segment to resect can be difficult at the time of surgery. Identification of the polyp site is facilitated by the endoscopist tattooing the site or by placing small metal chips at the polypectomy site. The histology of benign and malignant polyps is illustrated in Figure 80-28.

My approach is a limited segmental resection measuring 6 to 10 cm in either direction and including enough mesentery to provide assessment of the first level of draining lymph nodes. Often, this type of segmental resection can be accomplished by laproscopic or laproscopic assisted approaches.

Surgical Management of Synchronous Metastatic Disease

Synchronous metastatic disease is present in 10% to 15% of patients with a newly diagnosed colon cancer. The vast majority of such patients present with synchronous involvement of the liver. It is rare for patients to present with extensive peritoneal metastases or visceral metastases other than the liver. When the latter, more extensive, disease is found, the surgeon is faced with determining

Figure 80-27. A, Pedunculated polyp showing the distance by which the invasion in a pedunculated polyp would need to travel in the stalk before reaching the submucosa of the bowel wall. **B,** Sessile polyp; contrasted with pedunculated polyp. (From Haggitt RC, Glotzbach RE, Soffer EE, Wruble LD: Prognostic factors in colorectal carcinomas arising in adenomas: Implications for lesions removed by endoscopic polypectomy. Gastroenterology 1985;82:328–336.)

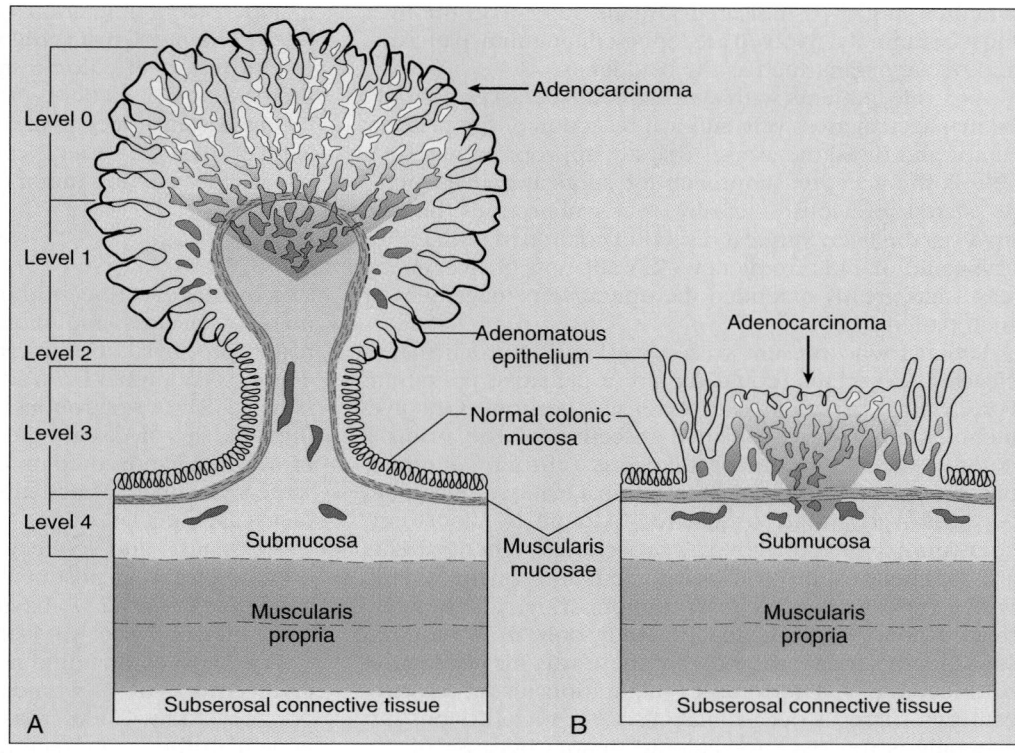

Figure 80-28. Adenomatous lesions of colon. **A,** In the premalignant neoplastic lesion, the muscularis mucosa is intact. **B,** In the malignant lesion, the musculares is obviously invaded by malignant epithelium. Malignant glands in the lymphatics are seen close to the base of the stalk. (From Skarin AT, Shaffer K, Wieczorek T [eds]: Atlas of Diagnostic Oncology, 3rd ed. St. Louis, MO, Mosby, Elsevier Science Limited, 2003, p 149.)

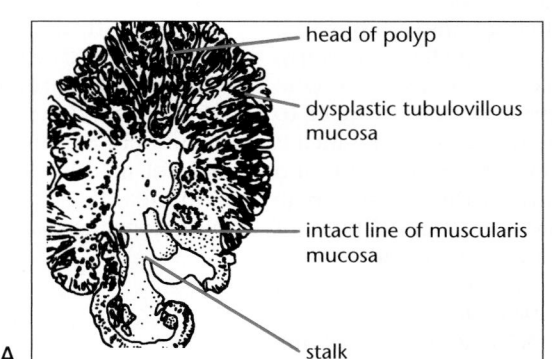

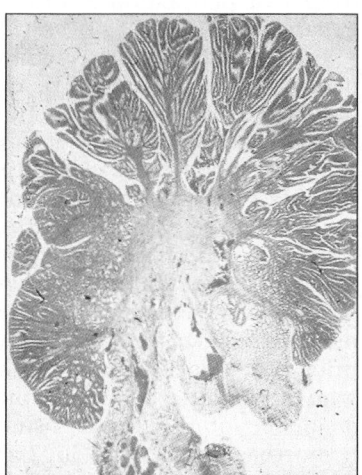

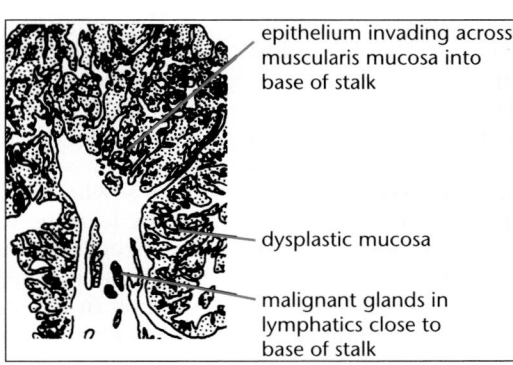

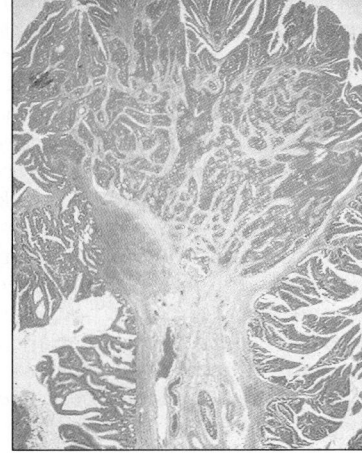

whether surgery is indicated. Organs other than the liver most commonly involved are kidney, duodenum, pancreas, and pelvic organs such as the bladder.

As a rule, patients with synchronous metastases should be managed aggressively. Surgical resection of the primary tumor and those metastases that are appropriately resectable is the accepted approach for surgical management. As stated previously, usually the synchronous disease involves the liver. Surgical resection combined with either cryogenic or radiofrequency (RF) ablation of liver metastases has greatly extended the operative management of such patients.

Patients who present with a metastatic burden that is clearly unresectable could require a palliative operation. For example, a patient with extensive peritoneal involvement could require palliative resection of the primary colon cancer to control bleeding (chronic anemia), obstructive symptoms, or perforation. Quality of life could be improved in an obstructed patient by ileostomy, colostomy, or intestinal bypass procedures. When patients are deemed to be truly advanced and asymptomatic with regard to their primary tumors, they can be safely treated nonoperatively. In one study, only 8.7% required subsequent surgery, and none of these was for perforation or bleeding.[245] Endoscopic fulguration using electrocautery or laser is occasionally used for rectal lesions but generally is too risky for colonic tumors because of the danger of perforation. Another option being explored is expandable stents.

Patients who present with synchronous, unresectable metastatic disease should be evaluated by a multidisciplinary team to establish the need for surgery, radiation, and/or chemotherapy, to ensure that a curative approach is not feasible, and to select appropriate palliative therapy. Patients who present with metastatic disease and who do not require resection of the primary colon cancer to address acute or subacute problems such as significant bleeding, impending obstruction, or perforation and abscess may receive chemotherapy as their initial treatment. A review of 82 patients who were treated without prior resection compared with 280 concurrent patients who did undergo resection showed no increased incidence of peritonitis, fistula formation, or intestinal hemorrhage, occurring in 2.4%, 3.7%, and 3.7% of unresected patients, respectively. Nor was there an increased incidence of obstruction, which occurred in 13.4% of the unresected and 13.2% of the resected patients.[246]

Several reports of endoscopically placed self-expanding stents suggest that these could have a palliative role for the obstructed patient who is not a candidate for surgery. In one report, stents were placed correctly in 37 patients. There were no immediate complications, but three stents dislodged within 1 week. The remaining patients were followed (median follow-up time, 7 months), and 28 patients (78%) had long-term restoration of luminal patency with disappearance of obstructive symptoms.[247]

Aviv and associates[248] reported placing 16 stents in 13 patients. Two attempted stent placements, one of which was introduced in a proximal transverse colon tumor, were not successful. There were minor postplacement complications in two patients, and late complications included stent migration (13%) and ingrowth of tumor (19%). The median survival was only 2 months.

In a report of colonic stent placement in 26 patients, there were 12 patients with colonic obstruction who received stent placement as a bridge to elective surgery. Nine of these 12 patients eventually had surgical resection of their obstructing tumor.[249]

Surgical Management of the Ovaries

The ovaries have been known as a site of both synchronous metastases and metachronous involvement. As a result, prophylactic oophorectomy at the time of initial colon resection has been advocated in the past to improve survival. The synchronous involvement of the ovaries as the sole site of disease, however, occurs in less than 5% of newly diagnosed colon cancer patients, and about the same percentage of patients will develop isolated ovarian metastases at a later time.

Sielezneff and colleagues[250] studied prophylactic oophorectomy in postmenopausal women and found an incidence of only 2.4% having ovarian metastases, with no difference in 5-year survival.

The Mayo clinic found no gross or microscopic ovarian involvement in 77 women randomized to prophylactic oophorectomy. There was no evidence of a survival benefit in the oophorectomy arm.[251] As a result, there is no evidence to support prophylactic oophorectomy, even in the postmenopausal patient.

Occasionally, the surgeon and pathologist will be confronted with a "Krukenberg's" tumor of the ovary that presents the dilemma of whether the cancer is primary ovarian with direct extension or metastasis to the colon or a colonic cancer extending to the ovary. Because very different chemotherapy regimens are used to treat these two primary cancers, it is important to diagnose them accurately. Serum markers CEA and CA125 are not very helpful in this situation, and careful histologic examination including immunohistochemistry by an experienced pathologist is essential.

Minimally Invasive Laparoscopic Colon Cancer Resection

Laparoscopically assisted colon resection was first described in 1991.[252] Its advantages, as with any minimally invasive procedure, are reduced pain, reduced impact on pulmonary function, more rapid return of bowel function, and less fatigue.[253,254]

The surgical approach is either completely laparoscopic or laparoscopically assisted colon resection with intra-peritoneal gas insufflation or mechanical abdominal wall lift. The anastomosis can be performed intraperitoneally using a double-staple technique, or extraperitoneally through a small (7–8 cm) incision to permit stapling or hand sewing the anastomosis.

The learning curve for laparoscopic colorectal surgery has been estimated to range from 20 to 70 cases. This presents a significant hurdle for the average general surgeon in this country, who performs only six to seven open colorectal resections annually.[255,256]

One of the concerns for laparoscopic surgery for cancer is the reported incidence (0%–21%) of port-site recurrences. The incidence of port-site recurrence appears to be related to operator experience. Schneider and associates[257] reported a study of port-site recurrences using a porcine model. The authors created a pneumo-peritoneum and injected 107 human HeLa cells, creating a xenogeneic tumor. The pigs were subjected to a laparoscopic sigmoid colon resection using four trocars. They tested preventive measures in nine animals, including trocar fixation, prevention of gas leaks, rinsing of instruments with povidone-iodine, rinsing of trocars before removal, peritoneal closure, and irrigation of port wounds with povidone-iodine. Tumor was found in 23 of 36 port sites in control animals and in only 5 of 36 port sites of animals in the prevention group. These results strongly supported the importance of high-quality technique in minimizing the risk of port-site recurrence.

Advantages of Laparoscopically Assisted Colon Resection
Short Term
- earlier return of bowel function (2 days vs. 4.5–5.0 days)
- shorter hospital stay (est. ~ 40% reduction in length of stay)
- fewer days of parenteral and oral analgesics
- earlier recovery
- fewer infections and wound complications

Long Term
- (?) fewer incisional hernias
- (?) lower risk of small bowel obstruction
- (?) less impact on immune function
- (?) better oncologic outcome

Several prospective randomized trials have been designed and implemented to test the hypothesis that disease-free survival and overall survival are equivalent for laparoscopic-assisted colectomy and standard open colectomy. To be appropriately powered, these trials require the enrollment of a large number of patients.[258]

The Clinical Outcome of Surgical Therapy (COST) study group reported that laparoscopically assisted colectomy (LAC) has emerged as the preferred minimally invasive technique for colon resections.[259] This group also confirms that LAC for colon cancer provides only minimal short-term quality-of-life benefits over open colectomy. As noted, there appears to be ample evidence that LAC is safe and that it accomplishes the same degree of colon resection in terms of margins, removal of lymph nodes, and mortality or morbidity as does open colon resection. Although technically equivalent, the data concerning local and distant recurrence and long-term survival await the completion of large prospective trials. One thing seems clear: the benefits of LAC will need to be significant to overcome the increased intraoperative expense.[260] For benign disease, however, LAC is the ideal approach.

Age as a Factor in Surgery of Colon Cancer

Although colon cancer is a major cause of morbidity and mortality in elderly people, it does occur in patients younger than 40 years of age. Although younger patients present with the same symptoms (abdominal pain, rectal bleeding, weight loss, changes in bowel habits), they are more likely to experience a delay in diagnosis and to present with stage III or IV disease. Survival by stage is comparable for the younger patients and those older than 40 years.[261] Some reports suggest that the younger population is less responsive to chemotherapy.[262]

Older patients are more likely to present with right-sided cancers and to have disease detected when it is less invasive than the younger than 40-years age group.[263] Elderly patients, as expected, are more likely to have comorbid conditions that increase their risk for surgery. Simmonds and coworkers[264] reported the results of a systematic review of published and aggregated data examining the outcomes of colorectal surgery in elderly patients. They grouped patients aged 65 to 74 years, 75 to 84 years, and older than 85 years and compared these groups to those younger than 65 years. They analyzed 28 studies that included 34,194 patients. Their review found that elderly patients had an increased risk of comorbid diseases, presented with later-stage disease, had a higher incidence of emergent surgery, and were at greater risk for having noncurative surgery when compared with the age group younger than 65 years.

As expected, postoperative morbidity and mortality increase with advancing age. Differences in cancer-specific survival, however, are much less dependent on increasing age. Thus, careful preoperative evaluation to diagnose comorbid conditions, so that these can be appropriately managed during surgery and the period of postoperative recovery, is important to providing a successful outcome. Elderly patients (older than 85 years of age) can anticipate a good survival and should be managed similarly to younger people when at all possible.

Managing Complications of Colon Cancer Surgery

The most common postoperative morbidity associated with colon cancer surgery is prolonged ileus. With open resection of the colon, the majority of patients have return of bowel function as manifested by the presence of bowel sounds on abdominal auscultation and the passage of flatus by 4½ to 5 days after surgery. For the majority of patients, postresection nasogastric decompression is not required. An exception is the patient presenting with significant obstruction or perforation. If the delay in return of function exceeds 7 to 10 days, there must be concern for an underlying cause. The surgeon must look for electrolyte imbalance, evaluate the level of narcotic use (ruling out excessive use), and search for evidence of intra-abdominal abscess or mechanical obstruction. Instituting nasogastric decompression is often indicated.

Anastomotic leaks are reported to be between 4% and 18%, but subclinical leaks could occur much more frequently.[265] Often, leaks can be managed by percutaneous drainage using CT or ultrasound guidance to place the drain tube. Larger leaks with anastomotic dehiscence and peritonitis require operative intervention, with closure of the anastomosis or resection of the anastomosis and proximal diverting colostomy or ileostomy.

Wound infections are dependent on preoperative preparation of the bowel for surgery, decreasing skin bacteria, and operative technique, all of which measures are designed to minimize bacterial contamination of the wound. The risk of wound infection after colon surgery is 3% to 16% for all presentations. For elective colon cancer resection performed under ideal circumstances and optimal bowel preparation (which accounts for the majority of cases), the risk of wound infection is less than 5%. When an infection occurs, the portion of the wound involved is opened to allow irrigation and twice daily packing. Wound dehiscence is uncommon and should raise suspicion of anastomotic leak. As might be expected, such dehiscence is significantly increased for patients undergoing emergency surgery for colon cancer.[266]

As with other major cancer operations, there has been interest in whether a surgeon's training, experience, and operative volume is important to patient outcome when undergoing colon resection for cancer. One such report involved a retrospective analysis of 15,427 admissions in northern Illinois undergoing segmental colon resection between 1994 and 1997. These surgeries were performed at 76 nonfederal hospitals and involved 514 surgeons. The authors determined inpatient mortality, complications of surgery, and hospital length of stay. They found that American Board of Surgery certification and increasing years of experience were associated with reduced mortality. Added colorectal certification and site of training did not factor significantly into the outcomes.[267] Other studies suggest that high volume colonic surgery performance by the surgeon and having the procedure at a high-volume hospital are important predictors of in-hospital outcome.[268]

Managing Uncommon Tumors of the Colon

More than 98% of the tumors of the large intestine are adenocarcinomas. The remaining 2% of colon tumors are lymphomas, leiomyosarcomas (including gastrointestinal stromal tumors [GIST]), carcinoids, and (rarely) nonpulmonary small cell cancer. Gastrointestinal stromal tumors (GIST) are tumors arising from the "pacemaker" cells located in the muscularis propria. These tumors tend to present as large masses within the colon but can extend to other organs.[269-271]

The peak incidence of stromal tumors of colon is in the fifth decade, with slightly more males than females being diagnosed. Pain is the most frequent presenting symptom.[272]

GIST tumors are managed by resection, and recurrences may be found in the peritoneal cavity and liver. The introduction of imatinib mesylate (STI-571, Gleevec) an inhibitor of tyrosine kinase activity of the c-kit proto-oncogene, has provided the first significant opportunity to treat this malignancy by means other than surgery.

Carcinoid tumors of the colon account for an estimated 6% of all gastrointestinal carcinoids, with more than half originating in the cecum. They almost never present as classic carcinoid syndrome but tend to be advanced, with

nodal involvement in 60% and liver metastases in 40% of patients. Carcinoid tumors tend to be indolent in their course, and although patients generally live more than five years (often with known disease), the overall survival is probably only 25% to 35% with standard treatment.[273]

Lymphomas are known to arise in the gastrointestinal tract, and the colon is the site of origin for approximately 15% of gastrointestinal lymphoma cases. They are extremely rare, accounting for less than 1% of colon malignancies, and to be accepted as the primary site, there must be no clinically detected peripheral adenopathy and no imaging evidence of disease in the chest, the peripheral blood smear and bone marrow analysis must be negative, and there must be no evidence of liver or spleen involvement. Malignant lymphoma of the colon has been found as a complication of ulcerative colitis. Both Hodgkins and non-Hodgkin's lymphoma have been diagnosed.[274] The majority of colon lymphomas are B-cell type and of intermediate- to high-grade histology. Treatment is often surgical resection, but systemic chemotherapy is the mainstay of long-term survival, and surgery might be better used for chemotherapy failures. Overall 5-year survival is usually cited to be approximately 50%. There have been a few case reports of multiple mucosal lymphomatous polyps affecting various lengths of colon that appear to be similar to the mucosa-associated lymphoid tissue (MALT) lymphoma seen in the stomach; treatment is three months of combination chemotherapy.[275] There are rare reports of mast cell sarcoma and clear cell sarcoma arising in the colon.[276,277]

Surgical Management of Tumors of the Appendix

An estimated 1% (0.9%–1.4%) of all appendectomy specimens contain a neoplasm. The majority of appendiceal tumors are carcinoids, while the remaining 10% to 20% are mucinous cyst adenocarcinoma, adenocarcinoma, lymphosarcoma, paraganglioma, and granular-cell tumors.[278-280] As expected, most present as acute appendicitis, and in some 40% of cases, the diagnosis is made after appendectomy.

If a mass in the appendix is encountered incidentally during the course of abdominal surgery, an appendectomy is performed with frozen-section analysis of the mass. Most masses prove to be benign mucoceles or very small carcinoids. When carcinoid tumors of the appendix are small (<1 cm in diameter), they may be treated adequately by standard appendectomy. If they are greater than 2 cm in size, the patient should have a right hemicolectomy.

Treatment of appendiceal adenocarcinoma is a right hemicolectomy. Mucinous cystadenocarcinoma can be very difficult to manage.[280] Treatment should be a right hemicolectomy and debulking of peritoneal implants.

Currently, the best results treating mucinous cystadenocarcinoma appear to be obtained with an aggressive combination of cytoreductive surgery, perioperative intraperiotneal chemohyperthermia, and early postoperative intraperitoneal chemotherapy.[281] These measures could provide 5-year and 10-year survival rates as high as 80% and 60%, respectively. If debulking is incomplete, the survival rates are markedly reduced to only 20% and 0%, respectively, and long-term survival cannot be achieved. This tumor can be indolent in its course, and patients commonly have multiple debulking surgeries before ultimately succumbing to their disease.

Managing Colon Cancer in the Pregnant Patient

The incidence of diagnosing a cancer of the colon during pregnancy is estimated to be less than 0.1%. It is interesting that pregnant women have a much higher incidence of rectal cancer (83%), compared with colon sites (17%). This is in contrast to nonpregnant women younger than 40 years of age, among whom the site distribution is 68% colon and 32% rectum.[282]

Certainly, any pregnant patient reporting rectal bleeding or having hemoccult positive stool on exam deserves careful evaluation to rule out cancer.[283]

OUTCOMES OF SURGICAL TREATMENT AND ROLE OF ADJUVANT THERAPY

Optimal Surveillance After Curative Resection

There are several aspects of the natural history of colon cancer that influence the approach to follow-up. For example, it is well-recognized that 80% to 90% of recurrences after curative resection are discovered within the first 2 to 3 years.[284-288] Fewer than 5% of all recurrences occur after 5 years. Furthermore, these recurrences are often isolated and, when resected completely, they provide about 35% of patients with a cure of their disease.[289,290] This is somewhat unique to colon cancer and clearly influences the frequency and method of postsurgical evaluation. It is also recognized that a high percentage of first failures occur in the liver and lung, which could, therefore, be asymptomatic at the time when they are detected by imaging.

In theory, early detection of recurrent disease can alter the long-term prognosis for an individual patient if the disease found is resectable (e.g., isolated liver or lung metastases) or if prompt treatment can alter the long-term prognosis. Patients who can undergo salvage surgery— approximately 20% of patients who are followed closely for recurrence—have an 18.6% 5-year disease-free survival, compared with only 5.6% of patients whose recurrences are identified by new symptoms.[291]

Surveillance strategies and inadequately powered trials of surveillance have been reviewed recently.[292] National Comprehensive Cancer Network (NCCN) practice guidelines recommendations for follow-up, using "evidence-based" medicine approaches, suggest the following measures:

- Physician visits every 3 months for the first 2 years, then at 6-month intervals until 5 years.
- CEA testing at 3-month intervals for 2 years, then every six months for 5 years.
- Colonoscopy 1 year postoperatively, then every 3 to 5 years.[293]

Web sites that maintain current recommendations are available: www.nccn.org and www.esmo.org.

For these reasons, patients are initially seen every three to four months for review of symptoms and examination. In addition, liver injury tests and serum CEA are obtained. Patients with suspicious symptoms, whether focal or constitutional, should undergo evaluation at the time they present. Constitutional symptoms include fatigue, decreased appetite, night sweats, and fever. Suspicious focal symptoms include early satiety, right-upper-quadrant or right shoulder pain, and crampy abdominal pain.

If complete colonoscopy was not achieved at the time of diagnosis, the first postoperative colonoscopy for the detection of synchronous disease and elimination of any additional polyps should be performed 6 months after surgery to permit complete healing of the anastomosis. Otherwise, colonoscopy is usually performed at yearly intervals for the first 2 years, then every third year, unless additional adenomatous polyps are identified or the patient is in a group genetically at high risk for rapid development of invasive malignancy (as discussed previously).

The controversial aspect of follow-up concerns the use of CT imaging and its associated expense. In practice, patients at greater risk (Dukes stage B2 and C patients) are candidates for regular CT imaging at many institutions although it is not included in evidence-based guidelines. The majority of these patients will already have made a significant personal investment in adjuvant therapy.

Those who argue against regular frequent follow-up base their conclusions on the estimate that only 10% of recurrences are isolated and amenable to surgical resection even with optimal surveillance.[294,295] This small percentage, and the lack of significant survival benefit from early institution of systemic therapy, make it difficult to justify the expense of frequent monitoring, especially with CT imaging.

Other analyses of prospectively followed cohorts of patients reached different conclusions, however.[291] A review of 1247 patients with resected stage II or III colon carcinoma followed in cooperative group trials identified recurrences in 548 patients, of whom 109 underwent a second surgical procedure with curative intent. Of the patients who went to surgery, 77 recurrences were identified by CEA or CT scan. The 5-year disease-free survival for all patients undergoing surgery with curative intent was 23%.

A second review from the University of Barcelona looked at the outcomes for 199 patients followed at 3-month intervals.[296] Of the 140 patients who underwent regular surveillance, 18 of the 56 patients with recurrence were operable, compared with only 3 of 28 patients with symptomatic recurrence. This difference also resulted in differences in long-term cancer-related deaths, with 51% of the nonscreened patients dying of cancer within 5 years of their original surgery, compared with 31% percent of the patients who underwent close follow-up. Obrand and Gordon[297] reported that 24% of their 146 patients with recurrence underwent attempts at re-resection, with a 47% 80-month survival rate (i.e., 17 of 146 patients with recurrence were reresectable with long-term survival).[297]

For patients with hereditary colon cancer syndromes who develop cancer, postoperative recommendations do not differ from those already described for screening these patients. For all other patients, recommendations for follow-up are described in the NCCN practice guidelines and in the 2000 update of guidelines agreed to by the American Society of Clinical Oncology.[293,298]

Carcinoembryonic Antigen in the Management of Patients with Colorectal Cancer

Carcinoembryonic antigen (CEA) is an oncofetal antigen first described by Gold and Freedman[299] in 1965. Although CEA is the most commonly used serum marker for malignancies of the gastrointestinal tract, it has never proved useful as a screening test for early cancers. Primary colorectal cancers are commonly CEA negative, even though 90% of tumors can be shown to produce CEA.[300,301] An explanation for this can be found in the fact that CEA produced by colorectal cancer (except for the very low rectal cancers) enters the portal venous circulation and is extracted on the first pass through the liver.[302] As a result, CEA is hypothetically a useful marker of systemic recurrence, even for patients who initially at time of diagnosis presented with normal levels (<5 µg/mL for normal individuals), because the venous drainage from the recurrence is into the systemic circulation. CEA can be modestly elevated in about 19% of smokers who do not have cancer and in 3% of the normal population.[303] These false elevations, however, are almost always less than 10 ng/mL and remain stable during serial testing, in contrast to CEA produced by recurrent tumor, where increasing values are evident over a period of months.[303,304]

When CEA levels are elevated preoperatively for the primary colorectal cancer, they predict a worse prognosis. The sensitivity of CEA as a monitoring test varies from 43% to 89%, with a specificity of 70% to 90%. Elevation of CEA in primary tumors correlates with Dukes stage (45% of C tumors and 25% of B tumors). Even though CEA predicts a worse prognosis, studies have not proved it to be useful in determining the need for adjuvant therapy.[305,306]

Persistent elevation of CEA 1 month postoperatively suggests the presence of occult metastatic disease and predicts for early development of measurable recurrence. For those patients with a normal preoperative CEA and patients whose CEA returns to normal within four to six weeks of the resection of their primary tumor, a CEA increase is often the first warning of metastatic disease. A significant and progressively increasing CEA is associated with 75% of patients with metastatic colorectal cancer.[310] Monitoring of CEA at intervals of 3 to 6 months is the single most effective method of detecting early failures. The benefit of monitoring, however, decreases after 2 years. Opponents of regular CEA monitoring argue that the gain in lives saved or significantly prolonged is quite small, perhaps only in the 1% to 3% range.[291,297] Those patients whose disease is detected by CEA and proved to have isolated recurrence (e.g., solitary hepatic metastasis), do achieve significant benefit, however (approximately 50% 2-year survival).[297]

CEA measurements during therapy of metastatic disease are quite helpful. A decrease to normal levels after metastectomy is a positive finding predicting a more favorable course. Similarly, during chemotherapy, a substantial fall in CEA occurs in patients with image-based responses. It is not, however, a substitute for appropriate tumor imaging. The ASCO Tumor Marker Panel recommends monitoring CEA every 2 to 3 months during chemotherapy treatment of metastatic disease if CEA is elevated initially.[298] If CEA increases in two consecutive occasions above baseline or lowest level during therapy, this usually indicates progression of disease; however, patients can develop modest elevations of CEA during adjuvant therapy in association with fatty infiltration of the liver. Intercurrent acute events such as pneumonia, hepatitis, and severe gastroenteritis can also produce modest, reversible elevations of CEA as high as 20 ng/mL.

Metastatic disease patterns for colon cancer include a 15% incidence of local recurrence as the first site of recurrence. Patients have a 36% chance of having liver metastasis as their first site of failure. Reviews of patients in large randomized trials (randomized to the surgery-only arm) confirm these patterns of recurrence.[310] The majority of patients who do recur develop recurrence within the first 3 years, providing a logical basis for less frequent screening visits after that period. Patients with nodal involvement have earlier recurrence than those without nodal involvement.

Evaluation of a Patient with Symptoms

Patients with recurrent cancer can present with very nonspecific symptoms, such as weight loss, malaise, fatigue, or night sweats. They can have focal pain complaints, right upper quadrant or right shoulder pain from liver metastases, or diffuse crampy abdominal pain and abdominal distension from peritoneal carcinomatosis, or pelvic or low back pain from pelvic recurrence. They can develop unilateral pedal edema or pleuritic chest pain from Trousseau's syndrome, with deep venous thrombosis or pulmonary emboli. Cough or dyspnea on exertion could indicate pulmonary metastases. Morning headache

---

SURVEILLANCE GUIDELINES

- Serum CEA performed every 3 months. 64% of recurrences detected first by CEA*
- Liver injury tests
- Colonoscopy following resection of primary 6 to 12 months after surgery and repeated every 3 years if no polyps are found.
- CT every 3 to 4 months for 2 years, then every 6 months through 5 years. This is controversial absent elevation in CEA (CT scan is first positive test in 11% of patients).

*Castells A, Bessa X, Daniels M, et al: Value of postoperative surveillance after radical surgery for colorectal cancer. Dis Colon Rectum 1998;41:714–724.

or focal neurologic complaints (from CNS metastases) or focal musculoskeletal pain (from bony metastases), although they are rarely the first signs of metastatic disease in patients with colorectal cancer, could suggest recurrence. New subcutaneous nodules, particularly at preexisting scar sites, can also be the first presentation of metastatic disease and are a more common physical finding than new lymphadenopathy in otherwise asymptomatic patients.

Patients with symptoms suggestive of recurrent disease should be assessed both with focal radiologic techniques (e.g., CT of the chest, abdomen, and pelvis), clinical chemistries, and serum CEA. The peritoneal surface is notoriously difficult to evaluate, however, and some patients with extensive, symptomatic peritoneal carcinomatosis can have false-negative CT scans because of the difficulty in evaluating this area. For patients with abdominal symptoms, CT scanning, newer MRI techniques, or FDG-PET scanning as discussed earlier for primary staging may suggest the diagnosis and direct further treatment.

Evaluation of a Patient with Findings on Screening Evaluations

In patients with CEA elevations at the time of initial resection, many clinicians obtain serial CEA measurements to aid in the early detection of potentially resectable recurrence. To trigger further evaluation, CEA should not only be above the normal limit but should have doubled in value twice. For the majority of patients, history, physical examination, and CT will identify the source of CEA elevation. Up to 10% of patients may have lesions identified that appear amenable to curative re-resection. When conventional evaluations do not reveal the source of CEA elevation, patients become, understandably, even more distressed than they were when informed that they could have recurrent disease.

Single photon emission computed tomography (SPECT) with radiotagged antibodies has been evaluated for its utility in identifying potentially resectable sites of recurrence. To date, immunoscintigraphy has not been shown to alter clinical outcomes, and its cost effectiveness is unproven.[311] Murine and humanized antibodies directed against tumor-associated antigens have been evaluated for their utility in identifying the site of disease recurrence in these patients.[312] ^{111}In-CYT-103, a murine monoclonal antibody targeting TAG-72, has been shown to be comparable to CT in sensitivity, although it did identify lesions in six patients with negative CT scans.[313] Immunoscintigraphy with ^{99m}Tc anti-CEA showed 20% greater sensitivity for pelvic and retroperitoneal disease.[314] In 173 patients with at least one tumor site that had been identified by CT scan, a totally monoclonal antibody, 88BV59, technetium scan was able to identify only 87% of the lesions (sensitivity 87%) but had a better specificity, with 57% of the lesions identified by SPECT actually representing malignancy at exploration.[315] In 29 patients with rising CEA and no apparent disease, 15 patients (68%) had true positive SPECT findings. Of all 43 lesions identified, only 10 were in the liver (where resection of limited disease may be curative), and the number of patients who had disease that was actually resectable

for possible cure was not stated. The authors point out, however, that use of CT alone results in an underestimate of disease extent in 41% of patients, compared with 27% underestimation for patients undergoing both procedures.[315] Given the limitations of SPECT scanning, despite the approval of two different preparations for this purpose, its utility at present is limited to identifying disease that is unlikely to be resectable (e.g., inapparent retroperitoneal adenopathy) to avoid futile attempts at surgical ablation of apparently limited metastatic disease.

In patients with a rising CEA and no apparent disease shown via CT, FDG-PET, or enhanced MRI, surgical exploration failed to find the source of the CEA elevation in 7 of 29 patients (25%) who proceeded to laparotomy.[316] In a series of patients undergoing resection for recurrent disease, however, more than half will actually have resectable disease at exploration.[296]

Patients with Potentially Resectable Recurrent Disease

When a suspicious lesion is identified by CT scan of an asymptomatic patient, further evaluation is directed at ascertaining the feasibility of curative resection. Thus, a solitary lesion in the liver or lung will precipitate spiral CT scan of the remainder of the thorax, abdomen, and pelvis or FDG-PET scan to identify any additional lesions that might preclude resection. In the absence of symptoms or signs of metastatic disease to the bone or brain, these sites are so rarely involved that radiologic evaluation is not undertaken. However, in patients where the suspicion of additional metastatic sites is high (i.e., liver metastasis within 1 year of the primary surgery in patient with multiple positive nodes), scanning with radioimmunoglobulin or PET scanning may suggest sites of additional disease that would mandate against an attempt at surgical resection.

In patients who have potentially resectable abnormalities identified by CT scan, 5% to 6% will have benign findings at laparoscopy.[316] PET scanning with fluorodeoxyglucose (FDG) could identify the site(s) of disease for 80% to 90% of these patients. Before PET scanning became available, surgical exploration for potentially resectable disease was undertaken in selected patients. At present, if no disease sites are identifiable in an asymptomatic patient, regular reevaluation at 3- to 6-month intervals is appropriate.

Additional imaging could be valuable for patients who appear to have potentially resectable liver metastases, to identify the 5% to 10% of patients who have extrahepatic disease and spare them the morbidity and expense of surgery (see Chapter 59). A second group who might benefit from more accurate assessment of the extent of disease consists of patients who will undergo reresection of recurrent rectal carcinoma, identifying those who might have a chance of benefiting from radical surgical resection.

Experienced cancer surgeons regularly evaluate patients with recurrence for their potential resectability. Patients with isolated, solitary metastasis in the liver or lung, in the absence of other life-limited illnesses, are widely considered to be candidates for resection.

Indications for Adjuvant Therapy

Surgical stage remains the most accurate predictor of survival. Table 80-7 shows the 5-year survival rates associated with stage after surgical resection for cure. Many additional risk factors have been proposed to refine prognosis.

Molecular Risk Factors

At present, all molecular risk factors remain the IIB category according to the College of American Pathologists.[317] Unfortunately, despite some studies analyzing data from larger patient populations, markers or combinations of markers that might identify patients who are more (or less) likely to benefit with current adjuvant therapy have not been identified. Many small series have explored additional prognostic factors for patients with colorectal carcinoma, including angiogenic factors such as VEGF and nitric oxide,[318,319] tumor aggression factors such as microsatellite instability or loss of heterozygosity of chromosome 18, proliferation measures such as Ki-67, survival measures such as p53, and factors related to chemotherapy effects such as thymidylate synthase (TS).[320-328]

Mutations in p53, frequently leading to overexpression of nonfunctional protein, have been associated in the laboratory with decreased sensitivity to several classes of chemotherapy, including DNA-damaging agents such as irinotecan and oxaliplatin.[325,326] There have been serious limitations in the assessment of p53 status from clinical samples, so that direct sequencing is rarely used and immunohistochemistry results only correlate with sequencing results in the 60% to 80% range.[323-324] The association of p53 overexpression with poor outcome has not been demonstrated consistently in clinical trials.[320,322]

Several studies have reported that patients with cancer overexpressing thymidylate synthase have a lower response rate to treatment with 5-FU.[321,322,326-330] Ichikawa and colleagues[331] evaluated both dihydropyrimidine dehydrogenase (DPD) expression (lower activity would result in decreased catabolism of 5-FU and greater exposure to active drug) and TS, finding that patients with low DPD and low TS had a median survival time of 16.3 months, compared with 8.4 months for patients with high DPD and high TS. Johnston and colleagues[332] found that the expression of TS as measured in primary tumors using TS106 antibody did not correlate with 5-FU activity in metastatic sites. Overexpression of TS, however, predicts for a poorer survival regardless of whether patients received adjuvant therapy, and formal tests for interaction with chemotherapy suggest that patients with differing levels of TS expression maintained benefit from adjuvant chemotherapy.[322]

McLeod and coworkers[333] obtained samples for pharmacogenomic analysis from 524 of 795 patients treated for metastatic colorectal carcinoma with IFL, FOLFOX, or IROX (see chemotherapy regimens discussed later in this chapter). They looked at panels relevant to 5-FU metabolism and variations in its targets of thymidylate synthase and MTHFR, and panels relevant to oxaliplatin metabolism, and excision repair (ERCC2 and XRCC1), and irinotecan metabolism (14 potential variants in all). Only ERCC2 K751Q (14% frequency) was correlated with response to treatment (p = 0.0052), and UGT1A1 7/7 was associated with neutropenia from irinotecan (7% frequency, p = 0.007). The only other statistically relevant association with response and time to progression was the thymidylate synthase variant 1494del, with a 47% frequency (p = 0.02).

Other recently proposed prognostic markers include the CpG island methylator phenotype, a phenotype observed in 20% to 40% of patients with colon cancers, which presumably is associated with transcriptional silencing of tumor suppressor genes.[334] Although CIMP-positive patients have a poorer survival if treated with surgery alone, there was a trend for improved survival of CIMP-positive patients who received adjuvant chemotherapy. Van Rijnsoever and colleagues hypothesize that the hypermethylated DNA status in CIMP-positive tumors could be a marker for aberrations in cellular folate and methyl group metabolism, rendering CIMP-positive cancers more sensitive to 5-FU. This proposal needs to be evaluated prospectively in a larger patient population.

History of Development of Adjuvant Treatment and Established Adjuvant Regimens

As many as 50% to 60% of patients who undergo "successful" surgery for colon carcinoma have residual micrometastatic disease, and clinically evident cancer will develop, either locally or at distant sites, within 5 years of surgery. Systemic treatment, known as adjuvant therapy and intended to reduce the risk of recurrence, is now widely recommended for patients with lymph node involvement (stage 3 or Dukes stage C), as well as patients with Dukes stage B2, although the absolute percentage benefit for B2 patients is quite small. There has been considerable variability regionally in both the United States and elsewhere in the use of adjuvant therapy after curative surgery. In Japan, adjuvant chemotherapy has been used for all patients except stage A; in the United States, on the other hand, it is used for patients with stage B2 rectal carcinoma (see Chapter 81) and is used selectively for patients with higher-risk B2 colon cancer. It is generally recommended for patients with lymph node involvement without other significant comorbidities. In Europe, in contrast, even patients with stage C (nodal involvement) did not receive routine adjuvant therapy until 1995.

The original trials of systemic chemotherapy after surgery for colorectal cancer were undertaken more than 40 years ago. Although some clinicians favored adjuvant therapy based on these early experiences, the studies were underpowered to identify the realistic benefits of such treatment.[335,336] Larger trials with more aggressive drug administration schedules were initiated in the 1970s and showed small but statistically significant benefits for adjuvant therapy. A small positive trial of levamisole, an antihelminthic agent with immunostimulatory properties, led to a series of large confirmatory trials. In contrast to the initial trial, these studies showed no benefit for levamisole as a single agent but did show benefits for

TABLE 80-8

Selected Early Randomized Trials of Adjuvant 5-FU-based Chemotherapy versus Observation Following Surgical Resection in Colon Cancer

STUDY TIME PERIOD COUNTRY	N	STAGE	TREATMENT REGIMENS	5-YEAR DFS (%)	P-VALUE	5-YEAR OS (%)	P-VALUE	COMMENTS	REF
INT 0035 [1984–1987] USA	929	Stage III	1. Observation 2. Levamisole 3. 5-FU-LEV	47 (3-yr) NR 63 (3-yr)	<0.0001 (1 vs 3)	55 (3-yr) NR 71 (3-yr)	0.007 (1 vs 3)	5-FU + LEV reduced recurrence rate by 40% and the death rate by 33%. No survival benefit was associated with LEV alone.	338 340
INT 0085 [1988–1989] USA	309	Stage II (high-risk) and Stage III	1. Observation 2. 5-FU-LV	58 74	0.004	63 74	0.01	5-FU plus LV for 6 months demonstrated a survival advantage over observation alone in patients with high-risk colon cancer	350
NSABP C-01 (1977–1983) USA	1,166	Stage II and III	1. Observation 2. 5-FU/Semustine/ Vincristine (MOF) 3. Bacille Calmette-Guérin	51 58 56	0.02 (1 vs 2) 0.09 (1 vs 3)	59 67 67	0.05 (1 vs 2) 0.03 (1 vs 3)	Survival advantage demonstrated for adjuvant chemotherapy for Dukes B and C (stage II and III) colon cancer	351 352
IMPACT-1 (1982–1993) (Meta-analysis of Trials from Italy France, Canada)*	1,526	Stage II and III	1. Observation 2. 5-FLU-LV	62 (3-yr) 71 (3-yr)	<0.0001	68 (3-yr) 74 (3-yr)	0.018	Long-term follow-up demonstrated a survival benefit for 5-FU-LV for patients with stage III cancer.	348 354 355

DFS, disease-free survival; 5-FU, 5-fluorouracil; LEV, levamisole; LV, leucovorin; NR, not reported; OS, overall survival.
*The three trials (GMO, NCIC-CTG, FFCD) included in this meta-analysis were those stopped prematurely when surgery alone control arms were no longer felt to be the standard of care in Dukes' C (stage III) disease.
Adapted from Chau I, Cunningham D: Chemotherapy in colorectal cancer: New options and new challenges. Br Med Bull 2002;64:159–180.

levamisole combined with 5-FU.[337,338] Selected early randomized trials of adjuvant regimens are listed in Table 80-8. Compared with 5-FU modified with folinic acid (leucovorin), however, 5-FU with levamisole was inferior, and it no longer is used in this setting (see later discussion). Subsequent trials have addressed the use of 5-FU with leucovorin on a variety of schedules and durations, and ongoing trials are exploring the use of oxaliplatin, irinotecan, capecitabine, celocoxib, immunotherapy, cetuximab, and bevacizumab in the adjuvant setting.

Adjuvant Treatment of Patients with Full-Thickness Bowel Wall Invasion and Negative Lymph Nodes (Stage II, T3N0M0, Dukes B2)

The role of adjuvant therapy for node-negative patients with disease extending through the bowel wall has not been established unequivocally, as many underpowered clinical trials have been published. Many current trials accrue these patients to trials of adjuvant therapy, but in numbers inadequate to establish the value of treatment definitively. Because surgery alone results in five-year disease-free survival of 75% to 80% for patients with B2 colon carcinoma, 3572 patients must be randomized to show a 4% improvement to 84% with 80% power.[339] Clinicians vary in their recommendations to patients, with many reserving adjuvant therapy for patients who have some adverse prognostic indicator, such as vascular or lymphatic invasion.

The same schedule of 5-FU and levamisole used for patients with lymph node involvement (see later discussion) was evaluated in patients with stage II colon cancer.[340] Although the recurrence rate was reduced by 31% in these patients (71% percent disease-free survival for the observation arm vs. 79% for patients receiving 5-FU/levamisole), there was no difference in overall survival (72% at 5 years). The lack of survival advantage was attributed in part to the unexplained occurrence of twice the number of noncancer-related deaths in the patients receiving adjuvant chemotherapy. It should be noted that these deaths also were not directly associated with treatment. In addition, six of seven patients who had surgically curable recurrences were in the surgery-only group.[340] This result was confirmed in a European study that showed a similar improvement in survival from 70% to 78%.[341] An Italian study comparing surgery alone with postoperative 5-FU and leucovorin (375 mg/m^2 plus 200 mg/m^2 daily for 5 days for the first week of each 4-week cycle for 6 months (six cycles of chemotherapy) showed a 21% reduction in mortality rate (23% to 20%). There was an 8% absolute difference in disease-free survival at 5 years (76% vs. 68% alive without recurrence). It should be noted that the 5-year disease-free survival in this study was somewhat inferior to other trials conducted during the same period.[342]

A single trial of autologous tumor cell vaccine augmented with bacille Calmette-Guérin (BCG) has also shown some disease free survival benefit for patients with B2 disease, although trials attempting to evoke immune responses to eradicate micrometastatic disease have not yet shown improvement in overall survival (see following discussion).[343]

A discussion of approaches to meta-analysis of the many inadequately powered trials has been undertaken.[344] Meta-analysis from four large trials conducted by the National Surgical Adjuvant Breast and Bowel Project has assessed the improvements in overall survival and disease-free survival to be comparable for patients with stage II tumors, from 82% to 88% (p = 0.08).[345] Another group, however, found a smaller (and also statistically non-significant) possible benefit in their meta-analysis, with a five-year overall survival of 80% for untreated and 82% for treated patients.[346] The results for the 318 B2 patients in the Intergroup trial of 5-FU plus levamisole vs post-operative observation also favored adjuvant therapy, but again the trial was too small to demonstrate a probability of false positive of less than 5%.[340]

There are several recently completed and ongoing clinical trials of adjuvant therapy that include patients with B2 colon carcinoma:

1. QUASAR 2 (Quick and simple and reliable) is comparing a regimen of 5-FU and leucovorin with one of capecitabine and irinotecan and has accrued patients with B2 and C colon cancer.
2. The EORTC/PETACC 4 trial is comparing FOLFIRI (irinotecan, infusional 5-fluorouracil, and leucovorin) with surgery alone.
3. NSABP C-07 included stage II patients comparing six weekly treatments with bolus 5-FU and leucovorin followed by a 2-week break, with or without oxaliplatin given every other week of treatment.
4. CALGB compared edrecolomab (17-1A monoclonal antibody) to observation.
5. VICTOR is comparing adjuvant therapy with rofecoxib versus placebo after definitive surgery (and chemotherapy).

Adjuvant Treatment of Patients with Lymph Node Involvement (Stage III, Dukes C)

Chemotherapy with 6 months of 5-FU and leucovorin after primary surgery is currently recommended for patients with colon carcinoma and nodal involvement to reduce the rate of cancer recurrence and prolong survival. Although adjuvant 5-FU and leucovorin is not universally useful to patients, an additional 10% to 20% percent of patients with nodal involvement are cured by post-operative adjuvant chemotherapy, and others have prolongation of disease-free survival, although they eventually relapse. Recently published trials have addressed the control of side effects, the appropriate duration of treatment, and the cost of treatment while maintaining the established value of postresection adjuvant therapy. Oral chemotherapy regimens, additional agents (including oxaliplatin, irinotecan, and cox-2 inhibitors) and immuno-modulation are being studied in the adjuvant setting.

The NSABP C-03 was the first trial to demonstrate the value of 5-FU and leucovorin in the adjuvant setting.[347] Those results were subsequently confirmed in additional large trials.[348-355] Table 80-9 summarizes selected randomized trials comparing various 5-FU-based adjuvant regimens. Early adjuvant trials were not sized adequately to detect survival differences as small as 10% to 15%, and chemotherapy was not widely prescribed postoperatively until a decade ago. Most of the early trials enrolled only 100 to 200 patients, a sample size that can only detect survival differences greater than 30%. The initial trials of 5-FU and levamisole, using a 5-day "loading dose" followed 1 month later by weekly 5-FU, showed absolute differences of 8%. A large confirmatory trial randomizing 929 patients reduced the recurrence rate by 40% and the death rate by 33%, resulting in 5-year disease-free survival rates of 47% compared with 35% in patients who underwent surgery alone or with levamisole.[338]

Because of the advances observed in patients with metastatic disease who were treated with fluorouracil modulated by leucovorin, this regimen has been evaluated widely in the adjuvant setting. The NSABP trial found similar improvements in disease-free and overall survival for 1 year of treatment with 5-FU (500 mg/m² weekly, for 6 out of 8 weeks) and leucovorin (500 mg/m²).[345,349] Meta-analysis of adjuvant trials of 6 months of 5-FU (370–400 mg/m² daily for 5 days in the first week of a 4-week cycle) with leucovorin (200 mg/m² daily for 5 days) also demonstrated improved disease-free and overall survival.[349]

Subsequent studies have evaluated the role of leucovorin and the duration of treatment in this setting. Patients undergoing 6 months of treatment with 5-FU (425 mg/m² daily for 5 days every fourth week) plus leucovorin (20 mg/m² daily for 5 days every fourth week) experienced a 16% absolute difference in 5-year disease-free survival compared with patients undergoing surgery only (74% vs. 58% disease-free survival at 5 years).[350] The overall 5-year survival difference was 11% to 74% for the patients receiving 5-FU plus leucovorin versus 63% for the control group. Six months of treatment with 5-FU and leucovorin produced 5-year survival rates comparable to 12 months of either 5-FU plus leucovorin or 5-FU plus levamisole. Six months of treatment with 5-FU plus levamisole appears to yield results inferior to those of the other regimens.[356]

A three-armed trial of 5-FU plus leucovorin (weekly intravenous bolus) versus 5-FU plus levamisole versus all three agents enrolled 2151 patients with Dukes B or C colon carcinoma. 5-FU with leucovorin, used for 6 months, resulted in a modest increase in disease-free survival at 5 years (65% vs. 60%, p = 0.04) and in overall survival (74% versus 70%, p = 0.07); levamisole added toxicity and resulted in lower (statistically insignificant) disease-free and overall survival.[357] The QUASAR trial randomized 4927 patients with stage II and III disease in a 2 × 2 trial of 5-FU and high-dose (175 mg) folinic acid versus low-dose (25 mg) folinic acid with either levamisole or placebo. This study demonstrated no benefit to the higher doses of folinic acid and no benefit for levamisole.[358] The INT0089 study compared 8 months of weekly 5-FU and leucovorin versus 6 months of 5-FU and leucovorin five times daily versus 12 months of 5-FU with levamisole versus 8 months of all three agents.[359]

TABLE 80-9

Selected Randomized Trials of Adjuvant Chemotherapy Comparing 5-FU–based Regimens in Colon Cancer

STUDY/ TIME PERIOD/ COUNTRY	STAGE	N	REGIMEN	5-YEAR DFS (%)	5-YEAR OS (%)	COMMENT (P-VALUES)
NSABP C-03 [1987–1988] US[347]	Stage II and III	1,080	1. 5-FU-HDLV (1 year) 2. 5-FU/Semustine/ Vincristine (MOF)	66 54	76 66	Both a DFS benefit (p=0.0004) and OS benefit (p=0.003) were noted for 5–FU-LV over the MOF regimen.
INT 0089 [1988] USA[359]	Stage II (high-risk Dukes 82) and Stage III	3,759	1. 5-FU-LEV (1 year) 2. 5-FU-LDLV (6 months) 3. 5-FU-HDLV (6 months) 4. 5-FU-LDLV + LEV (6 months)	56 59 60 60	63 66 65 67	5-FU-LDLV + LEV had improved DFS (p=0.014) and OS (p=0.007) compared to 5-FU-LEV. All other did not demonstrate any differences. 6 months of 5-FU-LV became the standard for adjuvant therapy.
NSABP C-04 [1989–1990] USA[357]	Stage II and III	2,151	1. 5-FU-HDLV (1 year) 2. 5-FU-LEV (1 year) 3. 5-FU-HDLV + LEV (1 year)	65 60 64	74 70 73	5-FU-HDLV was superior to 5-FU-LEV in DFS (p=0.04) and not significantly better for OS (p=0.07). The addition of LEV to 5-FU-HDLV was not beneficial.
NCCTG 894651 [NCCTG-NCIC] [1996] USA, Canada[356]	Stage II (Dukes B2) and Stage III	890	1. 5-FU-LEV (6 months) 2. 5-FU-LEV (1 year) 3. 5-FU-LDLV + LEV (6 months) 4. 5-FU-LDLV + LEV (1 year)	57 63 63 57	60 68 70 63	5-FU-LDLV + LEV for 6 months was superior to 5-FU + LEV for 6 months (p<0.01); however, there were no significant difference between 6 and 12 months of treatment with the same regimen
QUASAR [1994–1997] United Kingdom[358]	Stage II and III (2 by 2 factorial design)	4,927	1. 5-FU-LDLV + LEV (6 months) 2. 5-FU-LDLV + Placebo (6 months) 3. 5-FU-HDLV + LEV (6 months) 4. 5-FU-HDLV + Placebo (6 months)	64 (3-yr) HDLV arms 64 (3-yr) LDLV arms 63 (3-yr) LEV arms 65 (3-yr) placebo arms	70 (3-yr) HDLV arms 71 (3-yr) LDLV arms 69 (3-yr) LEV arms 72 (3-yr) placebo arms	No significant difference in DFS and OS between high-dose or low dose LV and no difference between LEV and placebo.
French National Study (1996–1999) France[360]	Stage II and II (2 by 2 factorial design)	905	1. Infusional LVFU2 (semi-monthly) (24 weeks) 2. Bolus 5FU-LV (monthly) (24 weeks) 3. Infusional LVFU2 (semi-monthly) (36 weeks) 4. Bolus 5FU-LV (monthly) (24 weeks)	73 (3-yr) LVFU2 arms 72 (3-yr) 5FU-LV arms 73 (3-yr) 24 wk arms 72 (3-yr) 36 wk arms	86 (3-yr) LVFU2 arms 88 (3-yr) 5FU-LV arms 87 (3-yr) 24 wk arms 83 (3-yr) 36 wk arms	No significant difference in DFS and CS between treatment arms but small trial size precluded demonstration of small advantages for one arm and LVFU2 was less toxic.
MOSAIC [1998–2001) Europe[361]	Stage II and III	2,246	1. LV5FU2 (de Gramont regimen) (6 months) 2. FOLFOX4 (6 months)	73 (3-yr) 78 (3-yr)	Results not yet available	3-year DFS benefit (p<0.01)

DFS, disease-free survival; 5-FU, 5-fluorouracil; FOLFOX4, oxaliplatin with infusional 5-fluorouracil (de Gramont regimen); HDLV, high-dose leucovorin; LDLV, low-dose leucovorin; LEV, levamisole; LV5FU2, de Gramont regimen of infusional 5-fluorouracil with leucovorin; OS, overall survival.
Adapted from Chau I, Cunningham D: Chemotherapy in colorectal cancer: New options and new challenges. Br Med Bull 2002;64:159–180.

Adjuvant infusional regimens of 5-FU have been evaluated in European studies and demonstrated to have efficacy similar to 5-day intravenous bolus regimens given monthly, but with reduced adverse effects.[360,362] An FULV2 regimen (leucovorin, 200 mg/m^2 over 2 hours, 5-FU intravenous bolus 400 mg/m^2, followed by 5-FU, 600 mg/m^2 over 22 hours on days 1 and 2) was compared with five times daily in the first of 4 weeks (leucovorin, 200 mg/m^2 intravenous bolus plus 5-FU, 400 mg/m^2 intravenous bolus for 5 days in the first week of a 4-week cycle), prescribed for either 24 or 36 weeks in a 2 × 2 factorial design. Nine-hundred five patients were followed for a median of 40 months.[360] The 48-hour infusional regimen was less toxic, and no difference in disease-free or overall survival was found between the arms, although the cohort size

precludes demonstrating small advantages for one arm. The PETACC2 study also has accrued patients with stage III cancer to LVFU2 versus 5-FU/LV, and meta-analysis of both trials may soon clarify the equivalence or superiority of these regimens. Protracted venous infusion of 5-FU at 300 mg/m^2/day for 12 weeks has been compared with 6 months of 5-FU/LV (5-FU, 425 mg/m^2 plus leucovorin, 20 mg/m^2 as intravenous bolus on days 1 through 5 repeated every 28 days) in a cohort of 716 patients with Dukes B2 or C colon cancer. Although overall survival at 3 years did not differ statistically between the study arms (83.2% vs. 87.9%), patients receiving 6 months of bolus therapy had worse relapse-free survival (68.6% vs. 80%) and greater toxicity, including increased neutropenia, diarrhea, and stomatitis.[362]

Adjuvant therapy regimens for colon carcinoma are generally well tolerated after individual dose adjustment. Treatment-related mortality has been found to be rare for 5-FU/LV regimens (0 of 317 and 0 of 869 patients in two studies, respectively), and only 18 deaths while on chemotherapy occurred among the 2151 patients treated in NSABP C-04.[347,357] On regimens using 5-FU at 425 mg/m^2 for 5 days, one third of patients will experience severe (grade 3 or 4) stomatitis, and one-quarter will have severe diarrhea. Grade 3 leukopenia occurs in 10% to 15% of patients and severe nausea in only 5% to 7%. On a weekly bolus schedule, hematologic toxicity occurs in fewer than 2% of patients, ataxia in 1%, and grade 3 or 4 diarrhea occurs in at least one course for 35% of patients, resulting in dose reductions.[357] About half of patients treated require dose reduction, with a reduction to 75% of baseline as the median adjustment. The percentage of the total prescribed dose that is actually given averages 70%, with 77% of patients completing all courses of therapy (excluding patients who die or have disease recurrence).[347] Dose reduction (either 4 days of treatment or reduced daily doses) usually abrogates the intensity of these side effects in subsequent cycles. When starting at a lower dose (375 mg/m^2), only 5% of patients experience grade 3 to 4 mucositis, while 4.5% experience severe diarrhea and 2.5% experience severe emesis. Transient grade 4 neutropenia occurs in 14%. If lower doses are used initially, however, physicians should consider dose escalations for those patients who have no side effects in the first cycle of treatment, as dose intensity of 5-FU has been correlated with activity against disease.

The National Cancer Institute-sponsored CALGB trial, which randomized 1263 stage III patients between irinotecan, 5-FU, and leucovorin (IFL) for 30 weeks versus 5-FU/LV weekly, was closed in April 2001 due to concerns about the 60-day all-cause mortality in the IFL arm.[363] This trial has subsequently not shown an advantage for the addition of irinotecan in the adjuvant setting. Attention to dose-adjustment recommendations and supportive care can minimize the adverse effects of 5-FU/LV on patient well being. In particular, close nursing observation is critical for the safety of these regimens and ensures that treatment breaks are initiated when patients experience mucositis or diarrhea. Patients who develop oral pain or diarrhea before receiving their fifth of five daily doses should not receive the final scheduled dose(s). It is important to assess any changes in the patient's bowel habits prior to administering weekly doses of 5-FU/LV. Persisting in the administration of a cell cycle-specific antimetabolite after diarrhea or mucositis has developed exposes proliferating crypt cells that have been recruited into S-phase to a drug specific for cells in S-phase and can result in more severe diarrhea and mucositis symptoms that could require hospitalization for management. Symptomatic measures could be helpful; for example, mucositis can be reduced by using oral ice chips for 30 minutes when 5-FU is administered by intravenous bolus.[364] Patients who experience moderate to severe diarrhea usually benefit symptomatically from loperamide administration but still require a treatment break, even if their symptoms are subsiding with supportive care. For the IFL regimen used in metastatic disease, excess deaths (2.5% vs. 0.8%) can be minimized (see later discussion).

Adjuvant trials that have recently completed accrual or are still in progress for patients with stage III colon cancer are listed in Table 80-10.[365] Table 80-11 summarizes selected adjuvant trials currently planned to evaluate newer agents such as bevacizumab and cetuximab in the adjuvant setting.

TABLE 80-10

Selected Randomized Trials of Adjuvant Chemotherapy in Colon Cancer That Have Closed Recently or Are Still in Progress*

STUDY/ COUNTRY	STAGE	N	REGIMEN	STATUS
CALGB-89803 USA	Stage III	1264	IFL 5-FU-LV (Roswell Park schedule)	Closed (Activated 4/15/1999). Preliminary results showed no difference in OS or failure-free. Survival between the two arms. Final results pending.
CALGB-9581 USA	Stage II	1738	Monoclonal antibody 17-1A Observation	Closed (Activated 5/31/1997). Final results pending.
NSABP C-07 USA	Stage II and III	2492	FLOX (oxaliplatin + bolus 5FU-LV) 5-FU-LV (Roswell Park schedule)	Closed (Activated 2/1/2000). Final results pending.
PETACC 2 Europe	Stage III	1600	High-dose infusional 5-FU (+/− LV) Standard bolus 5-FU-LV	Open (Activated 3/3/1999).
PETACC 3 Europe	Stage III	1794	CPT-11 with high-dose 5-FU-LV infusional regimen Same high-dose 5-FU-LV infusional regimen	Closed (Activated 1/1/2001). Final results pending.
VICTOR United Kingdom	Stage II and III	7000	Oral rofecoxib once daily for 2 years Oral rofecoxib once daily for 5 years Oral placebo once daily for 2 years Oral placebo once daily for 5 years	Open. Treatment starts after surgical resection alone or completion of adjuvant chemotherapy after surgical resection.
X-ACT Europe	Stage III	1987	Capecitabine (1,250 mg/m^2 bid days 1–14 q 3 wks) 5-FU-LV (Mayo Clinic schedule)	Closed (activated November 1998). Final results pending.

FLOX, Oxaliplatin, bolus 5-fluorouracil with leucovorin; 5-FU: 5-fluorouracil; IFL, irinotecan, bolus 5-fluorouracil with leucovorin; LV, leucovorin.
*As of December 2003.

TABLE 80-11

Selected Randomized Trials of Adjuvant Chemotherapy in Colon Cancer in Development

STUDY/ COUNTRY	STAGE	REGIMEN
ECOG-E5202 USA	Stage II (High-risk group defined by molecular markers)	mFOLFOX6 mFOLFOX6 + bevacizumab
N0147 USA	Stage III	FOLFIRI mFOLFOX6 mFOLFOX6 followed by FOLFIRI (trial may be amended to include cetuximab)
NSABP C-08 USA	Stage II and III	mFOLFOX6 mFOLFOX6 + bevacizumab
PETACC4 Europe/ EORTC	Stage II	Infusional 5-FU + Irinotecan (+/− LV) Observation

FOLFIRI, Irinotecan, infusional 5-fluorouracil with leucovorin; mFOLFOX6, Oxaliplatin, infusional 5-fluorouracil with leucovorin.
*As of December 2003.

Radiation Therapy

Although prospective randomized trials have defined the benefits of adjuvant chemotherapy for patients with high-risk colon cancer, the role of adjuvant radiation therapy for colon cancer has not been well defined. Adjuvant radiation therapy remains investigational, primarily because failure patterns after attempted curative resection tend to favor abdominal rather than local recurrence. Yet, although the overall incidence of local failure is 20% or less, there is evidence that the local failure risk can be significantly higher in certain subsets of patients, implying that a selective application of postoperative radiation therapy could provide benefit. Such subgroups might be identifiable based on information from various reports on patterns of failure.[1,366-370] Analysis of patients undergoing reoperation or autopsy indicates that patients with tumor adherence (T4) and/or lymph node involvement have increased local recurrence risk.[368,371] Gunderson and colleagues[368] found a 67% incidence of local regional failure in 24 patients with adherence to or invasion of surrounding structures, while Russell and coworkers[367] found a 69% incidence in a similar group of patients and a 30% incidence of local failure in patients with both regional nodal involvement and bowel wall penetration.

In addition to these pathologic factors, anatomic location has also been proposed to influence risk of local recurrence, presumably by compromising radial margins, although there is less consensus over this issue. Gunderson and colleagues[368] have suggested that lesions located in immobile areas such as the ascending and descending colon, particularly when posteriorly located, could have compromised margins of resection, a situation not likely to occur in mobile, intraperitoneal structures such as the sigmoid and transverse colon. But whereas

Willet and associates[366,370] also found differences in local recurrence rates by location, these patterns were not entirely consistent with the observations made in the previous study. Also, Minsky and associates[369] did not find differences in failure rates between regions of colon considered to be mobile or immobile, thus further calling into question the degree to which location and bowel mobility are predictive of local recurrence risk.

Overall, then, pathology rather than location remains the clearest predictor of local recurrence risk, with tumor adherence to abdominal structures and with bowel penetration in combination with nodal involvement predicting local recurrence risks that can reach or exceed 30%.

Role of Adjuvant Radiation Therapy

Although several randomized clinical trials have demonstrated that postoperative chemoradiotherapy decreases pelvic recurrence and increases survival in T3 or higher T stage and/or N-positive rectal cancer, no similar randomized trials exist in the case of colon cancer. Several single-institution studies, however, have indicated that postoperative irradiation reduces local failure.[370,372-377]

Willet and colleagues[370] have the largest and most definitive report. In this retrospective trial, 203 patients received postoperative radiation therapy (45 Gy plus a reduced-field boost to 50.4–54 Gy) with and without concurrent fluorouracil (5-FU) chemotherapy after resection of T3, T4, and T3/4, N-positive colon tumors. Of the 203 patients, 30 (15%) had residual local tumor after resection. The 173 remaining patients treated with adjuvant radiation therapy were compared with a historical control group of 395 patients undergoing surgery only. Improved local control and recurrence-free survival rates were seen for patients with T4 and T4, N-positive colon carcinoma treated with postoperative radiation therapy, compared with a similarly staged group of patients undergoing surgery only. In addition, irradiated patients whose tumors had an associated abscess or fistula formation had improved local control and recurrence-free survival rates compared with a similar group of patients undergoing surgery only. Finally, patients with residual local disease after subtotal resection still had a 37% 5-year disease free survival, indicating that a certain proportion of patients with residual disease can sometimes be salvaged. Treatment toxicities were acceptable, with 4.5% of patients developing bowel conditions requiring surgery. A 10-year update of this series again found increased control for adjuvantly treated T4 and T4, N-positive patients.[378] In this study, the nonrandomized addition of 5-FU chemotherapy did not alter local control, the rate of distant metastasis, or disease-free survival.

Another retrospective study from the University of Florida carried out in patients with locally advanced but completely resected colon cancer found a local control rate of 88%. A dose response was also found, with local control rate of 96% versus only 76% for patients receiving greater than or less than 50 Gy, respectively.[376] An additional retrospective study carried out in 103 patients with locally advanced colon cancer who received postoperative radiation therapy found 5-year actuarial local failure rates of 10%, 54%, and 79% in patients with no residual disease, microscopic disease, or gross residual disease after surgery, respectively.[377] In the 35 patients with gross residual disease, the addition of intraoperative radiotherapy to external beam reduced the local failure rate from 82% to 11%.

These retrospective studies strongly suggest that selected groups of patients with more locally advanced colon carcinoma could benefit from postoperative irradiation. Therefore, it became important to validate these retrospective findings in a prospective randomized trial. Given the proven benefit of adjuvant chemotherapy in node-positive colon cancer and its enhancement of radiation efficacy in rectal cancer, an Intergroup trial (INT 0130) was designed to compare adjuvant chemotherapy alone to chemotherapy plus radiation. This important trial was terminated early secondary to poor accrual, but a preliminary report on those patients accrued is available.[379] Patients with tumor adherence or invasion of surrounding structures or T3N1-2 tumors were randomized to one year of 5-FU plus levamisole with or without 45–50.4 Gy in 25 to 28 fractions. A total of 222 out of an original accrual goal of 400 patients were randomized and, of these, 189 were eligible for analysis. Grade 3 toxicities were slightly (but not significantly) higher in the radiation arm than in the nonradiation arm (43% vs. 37%, p = 0.30). With 2.9 years of follow-up in surviving patients, however, no differences were seen in survival or relapse rate, although the distribution of failures has not yet been reported.

In conclusion, several retrospective trials indicate that a subset of patients with high-risk, resected colon cancer benefit from the addition of adjuvant radiation therapy to the resected tumor bed. The one randomized trial that tested adjuvant radiation therapy did not, however, confirm a benefit, but the study was weakened by a failure to reach accrual goals. Therefore, adjuvant radiotherapy for colon cancer must continue to be regarded as investigational at this time. Its selective use would be reasonable, however, in those patients with positive margins or regional adherence to other structures whose risk of local recurrence is known to be high.

Hepatic and Whole Abdominal Irradiation

High rates of hepatic metastases and peritoneal failure have led to the investigation of adjuvant hepatic and whole abdominal radiotherapy. A phase III trial to explore the role of adjuvant hepatic irradiation was performed by the Gastrointestinal Tumor Study Group.[380] A total of 300 patients with resected T3, T4, or node-positive colon cancer were randomized to either observation or 21 Gy in 1.5-Gy fractions with concomitant 5-FU chemotherapy. Results of the study, however, indicated no therapeutic benefit for either survival or recurrence endpoints, with the liver recurrence rate remaining unchanged by the therapy.

Several nonrandomized studies of whole abdominal irradiation have been reported.[377,378,381] The largest study, a Southwestern Oncology Group phase I/II trial (SWOG 8572), reported on 41 patients who received 30 Gy whole abdominal irradiation with an additional 16 Gy tumor bed boost, along with concurrent, continuous infusional 5-FU.[381] Five-year disease-free and overall survival estimates were 58% and 67%, respectively, for all T3N1-2 patients. Seventeen percent of patients had severe toxicity and 7% had life-threatening toxicity of any kind. Although conclusions are difficult in the absence of randomized trials, patients in SWOG 8572 who received whole abdominal irradiation plus tumor bed irradiation with infusional 5-FU did demonstrate reduced tumor bed, liver, and peritoneal relapse rates when compared with patients treated in other studies who received either surgery alone or surgery plus chemotherapy.[381]

In conclusion, there is substantial retrospective data indicating that adjuvant radiation therapy to the tumor bed can decrease the risk of local recurrence after resection of colon cancer. Such findings have not been supported, however, by the findings of the only available randomized trial exploring this question, although its findings are preliminary and the study itself fell well short of accrual goals. In the absence of level III evidence, selective offering of adjuvant tumor bed radiotherapy is a reasonable approach for those patients with tumor pathologic features that give them high risk for recurrence. Intraoperative radiation therapy to achieve higher doses could play a role in patients with less-than-completely resected disease. Finally, the role for hepatic or whole abdominal irradiation remains highly investigational.

MEDICAL ONCOLOGY MANAGEMENT OF METASTATIC DISEASE

As noted previously, 50% of the 147,500 patients who are diagnosed with colorectal cancer in the United States will either present with or eventually develop disease recurrence.[382] Similar risks apply to the nearly 1,000,000 patients who will be diagnosed worldwide, as 492,000 deaths were estimated in 2000.[383] At the time of diagnosis of metastatic disease, the median survival was estimated to be 6 months without additional therapy. Chemotherapy regimens have increased that survival to 12 to 20 months.[384-392]

Assessment of the effect of treatment is a tenet of all medical care. For cancer, this assessment is usually made for an individual patient by measuring the area of lesions and establishing that no new lesions have developed since treatment was initiated. It is important that the baseline measurements be obtained within a short period before initiation of treatment (i.e., within one week and certainly within one month), as growth of disease before chemotherapy is initiated could otherwise be misinterpreted as progression. Clinical trials frequently reevaluate for efficacy at eight-week intervals. Response can be assessed by radiologic measurements (e.g., chest x-ray of lung lesions or CT of liver metastases). Other markers have also been used and generally correlate with cell kill and extended survival—50% decline in CEA, for example (see the discussion on carcinoembryonic antigen earlier in this chapter). Improvement in patient well being can also be an indication that treatment is containing the neoplastic process, although the placebo effect has been implicated in some improvements, particularly in pain assessment. Nonetheless, patients whose performance status improves and who gain weight on treatment in the absence of a change in measurable disease may be clinically benefiting from the treatment.

When evaluating a patient with colon cancer prior to therapy, CT of the chest, abdomen, and pelvis usually suffices to establish measurable disease. Because metastases to the brain and bone are rare (<10%) and tend to occur late in disease progression, only patients with symptoms such as headache and skeletal pain are evaluated with imaging of the brain or bone scan. Assessing hematopoietic function (with blood counts), liver injury, and renal function are included in all protocols before start of treatment.

Historically, alterations in overall survival were difficult to detect due to study size and the modest effect of single-agent 5-FU therapy. If only 33% of patients have substantial decrease in disease (partial or complete regression) and the responding patients have a true median survival of 18 months compared with 12 months for patients receiving only supportive care, and if the remaining 66% of patients receiving chemotherapy have no change in their 12-month survival, a randomized trial with 100 patients treated and 100 observed would show a 2-month difference in survival, with a P value of 0.1.

Response to chemotherapy is itself a prognostic factor for individual patients, albeit one that cannot be assessed until the treatment has been initiated. The availability of additional agents has increased the response rate and median survival. Current trials including irinotecan, oxaliplatin, and bevacizumab have shown improvements in overall survival. This, unfortunately, will complicate the evaluation of additional new agents being considered for a treatment indication for patients with colorectal cancer.

The quandary of patients who have definite tumor regression (partial regression assessed as greater than 50% decline in the area of lesions) but also a decline in functional status due to treatment-related morbidity is commonly faced in general oncology but has not generally been a problem for patients with colon cancer. Patients who have "failure to thrive" while receiving chemotherapy need to be reassessed carefully regarding the goals of treatment. Patients who are receiving potentially curative adjuvant therapy in a high-risk setting are balancing short-term toxicity against the possibility of a normal life span. In the setting of metastatic disease, in which cure is generally not feasible, both quality and quantity of life—usually assessed as adjusted quality-of-life years—has to be balanced. For many patients with symptomatic disease, even a minimal regression can be associated with improved quality of life (resolution of jaundice, return of appetite, increased performance status, diminished pain, absence of tumor fever, weight gain) at the cost of inconvenience and intermittent mild fatigue, nausea, and loose stools. Patients who are asymptomatic fall somewhere between two opposite ends of a spectrum in their approach to treatment. Some, possibly with unrealistic expectations of cure, want the most aggressive (i.e., toxic) approach available, hoping to maximize their survival and possibly be one of the few long-term survivors with un-resectable metastatic disease. Others are, understandably, reluctant to impair their currently excellent quality of life for the small chance that they might have a modestly longer survival if chemotherapy is initiated at the first evidence of recurrence.

As a tumor marker, CEA, although neither sensitive enough nor specific enough to be useful for screening, is helpful in monitoring the course of disease during and after treatment, particularly in patients with metastases that are not easily evaluated by current imaging technology, such as peritoneal carcinomatosis. Evidence of regression in patients with colon carcinoma is generally not rapidly apparent, even in the few patients who eventually have complete regression of measurable disease. Thus, reevaluation after 8 weeks of treatment, in the absence of signs or symptoms that suggest progression in the interval, is generally appropriate. Measurement of CEA earlier than this can result in false impressions of progression, as CEA can be released from dying tumor cells, and with its slow systemic clearance it could initially be elevated before eventually declining.

For the greater than 50% of patients who have measurable regressions with current chemotherapy regimens, response is durable for the majority, with the median time to progression after first-line therapy at 7 to 11 months (see later discussion). Even patients with less than 50% regression could have meaningful improvement in duration of survival with minimal symptoms.

5-Fluorouracil (5-FU) in the Treatment of Metastatic Colorectal Carcinoma

For the past 30 years, 5-FU has been used to treat patients with metastatic colorectal cancer,[393,394] but improved understanding of its pharmacology has led to steady improvements in the usefulness of treatment. Bolus intravenous administration of 5-FU was the standard of care until 1990. Compared with best supportive care, intravenously administered 5-FU might result in small improvements in survival duration.[395,396] Patients receiving chemotherapy also had a trend toward better quality of life (see later discussion).

Our understanding of the role of inhibition of thymidylate synthase and the cofactor, folinic acid, by the active metabolite of 5-FU, 5-FdUMP, reflects 5-FU's status as both the first "molecularly targeted agent" and as an outstanding example of the potential benefits of careful biochemical pharmacology research.[393,397,398] Improved understanding of the biochemistry of 5-FU and its congeners has permitted the development of more effective regimens.[385] To enhance the duration of thymidylate synthase inhibition, 5-FU can be given by continuous infusion or in conjunction with leucovorin (LV; also called folinic acid, FA) to improve the response rate.[385,398-403]

Infusion regimens permit the administration of higher doses of 5-FU while minimizing hematologic toxicity and reducing diarrhea. Meta-analysis of trials that compared infusional regimens (with or without leucovorin) also confirm the increase in response rate (22% vs. 14%) and modest increase in survival (12.1 vs. 11.3 months) that this approach provides.[404]

The intensity of treatment with fluorouracil has been well correlated with its activity in patients with advanced disease.[394] Patients with a lower 5-FU exposure (measured as the area under the concentration-versus-time curve, or AUC) were more likely to have disease progression even when treated with the same regimen.[405,406] In a multivariate analysis in patients with head and neck cancer, the exposure to 5-FU correlated with both response and with survival.[406] A meta-analysis of randomized trials comparing 5-FU alone with 5-FU and leucovorin has confirmed the improved response rates (23%) and median survival (10.5 months) provided by modulating 5-FU with LV.[407]

It is possible to use 5-FU without any side effects, but only at the cost of compromising its activity. On the other hand, patients with intolerable toxicity generally are receiving the highest drug exposures, and their doses can be reduced to produce acceptable quality of life while still providing enough drug to produce a predictable likelihood of benefit. This information is important to reassure patients who worry that dose reductions mandated by severe toxicity will compromise their chances of cure in the adjuvant setting. The corollary, however, is that patients who have minimal or no side effects when receiving 5-FU could have their doses increased as tolerated in subsequent courses.

Although few of these regimens have been compared directly in randomized trials, regimens that produce similar rates of moderate to severe toxicity produce similar response rates. The various regimens do differ in their dose-limiting toxicities and in respect to the time, cost, and technical demands for their delivery, although all can be provided in the outpatient setting.[420] Regimens that deliver 5 days of treatment every 3 to 4 weeks result in dose-limiting mucositis, diarrhea, and neutropenia. Weekly 5-FU/leucovorin regimens are generally limited by diarrhea. Continuous-infusion regimens are limited by hand-foot syndrome or mucositis and rarely result in severe diarrhea or neutropenia, but they do require placement of vascular access catheters. High-dose regimens

delivered over 24 to 48 hours of continuous infusion also can cause altered mental status or angina-like chest pain rarely seen in the other regimens, but the de Gramont 48-hour bolus and infusion regimens (Table 80-12) are generally well tolerated, with diarrhea and hand-foot syndrome generally dose limiting

Randomized Trials of 5-FU Regimens

In patients without prior therapy, 5-FU administered continuously intravenously as 750 mg/m^2/day for 7 out of 21 days was compared to administration of 500 mg/m^2/day via intravenous bolus for 5 days every 28 days (without leucovorin), with response rates of 26% versus 13%, respectively. Diarrhea and stomatitis were more common in the infusion group and would have been less prominent at lower daily doses without interruption.[400] In another four-arm randomized trial (477 patients) comparing conventional loading dose followed by weekly 5-FU (500 mg/m^2/day for 5 days followed by a 1-week break, then 600 mg/m^2 once a week, compared with infusional 5-FU at 300 mg/m^2/day), responses were seen in 18% of 153 patients versus in 28% of 159 patients.[402] Median time to progression overall was 5.1 months for the group receiving intravenous bolus adminstration versus 6.2 months for the group receiving continuous intravenous infusion.[402] Survival was 10.4 months for the intravenous bolus group and 13 months for the continuous intravenous infusion group; 6% of the patients were still alive at 3 years. These extended infusion regimens are much less likely to cause neutropenia (24% grade 4 for the intravenous bolus group versus 1% for the continuous intravenous infusion group). Hand-foot syndrome is seen in only 20% and infusion site infections in 14% of patients; 2% of patients have bacteremia.[401-421]

The de Gramont regimen of bolus followed by 48-hour infusions, for total FU doses of 2000 mg/m^2 every 2 weeks, has been evaluated with several modifications. The basic regimen is leucovorin, 200 mg/m^2 over 2 hours at 0 and 24 hours, with bolus 5-FU, 400 mg/m^2 after the 2 hours, at 2 and 26 hours, and then 600 mg/m^2 over the ensuing 22 hours, on both the first and second days. The first phase II trials reported a 38% response rate (2.5%

TABLE 80-12

	Commonly Used 5-FU and LV Regimens	
	REGIMEN	**INVESTIGATOR**
1	LV 20 mg/m^2 days 1–5, 5-FU 425 mg/m^2, d1–5, q4–5 wks (Mayo 5-FU/LV regimen).	Poon et al.[384]
2	LV infusion 500 mg/m^2 over 2 hrs, 5-FU IV bolus 600 mg/m^2 wkly X 6, then 2 wks rest (Roswell-Park regimen).	Petrelli et al.[386]
3	LV 200 mg/m^2 IV bolus, 5-FU 340-400 mg/m^2 IV infusion over 15 min., days 1-5; 21-day intervals between cycles (Machover regimen).	Machover et al.*
4	LV 200 mg/m^2 over 2 hrs followed by 5-FU IV bolus 400 mg/m^2 plus 5-FU 600 mg/m^2 over 22 hrs, days 1 and 2, q 2 wks (DeGramont regimen).	de Gramont et al.[401]
5	LV 500 mg/m^2 over 2 hrs followed by 5-FU 2600 mg/m^2 over 24 hrs weekly x 6 then 2 wks rest (AIO regimen).	Kohne et al.[388]
6	5-FU 3000 mg/m^2 over 48 hrs.	Diaz-Rubio et al.[387]
7	5-FU 250-300 mg/m^2/day continuous IV infusion for 6 wks, then 2 wks rest (Lokich regimen).	Lokich et al.[400]

*Machover D, Goldschmidt E, Chollet P, et al: Treatment of advanced colorectal and gastric carcinomas with 5-FU and high dose folinic acid. J Clin Oncol 1986;4:685–696.

complete remissions) with an overall median survival of 10.3 months, and 17 months median survival in patients with a response. More than 60% of patients treated at this dose had either no toxicity or minor side effects, and only 8% experienced grade 3 or 4 toxicity.[401,421] In a randomized trial compared with 5-FU 425 mg/m^2 plus leucovorin 20 mg/m^2 daily for 5 days out of 4 weeks (Mayo regimen), response rates were 14.4% (somewhat low for the Mayo regimen) versus 32.6% (GERCOD), with a 5-week improvement in median survival (56.8 weeks versus 62 weeks). The Mayo arm produced grade 3 to 4 toxicities in 24%, versus GERCOD reporting 11%, primarily neutropenia, diarrhea, and mucositis (7% grade 4 vs. 2%–3% for de Gramont).[401] Further dose escalation of the GERCOD regimen to 500 mg of leucovorin and 1500 to 2000 mg/m^2/day 5-FU resulted in toxicity equal to the Mayo regimen (grade 3 to 4 in 15%, 2% with grade 4 neutropenia, 5% with grade 3 to 4 diarrhea, 1% encephalopathy) and produced a similar response rate (34%, 101 patients), but with five complete responses and a median survival of 18 months. The median time to progression was 8 months.[401,422] Additional modulation with the addition of hydroxyurea did not produce a further increment in response rate.[423]

Current Combinations of 5-FU with New Classes of Agents for Colorectal Carcinoma

Although leucovorin modulation and infusion of 5-FU have resulted in improved response rates, for decades, colon carcinoma was not treated with combination chemotherapy. Clinical trials showed no advantage for combining either nitrosoureas (principally methyl-CCNU) mitomycin, cisplatin, or interferon with 5-FU. Over the past decade, two new classes of chemotherapy have been introduced into clinical use: the topoisomerase I inhibitor irinotecan (CPT-11, Camptosar-Pfizer) and the platinating agent oxaliplatin (Eloxatin, Sanofi-Synthelabo).

Irinotecan. Irinotecan is a prodrug catabolized to its much more potent, active form, SN-38, which interacts to stabilize topoisomerase I bound to DNA, resulting in DNA strand breaks. It was approved by the U.S. Food and Drug Administration (FDA) in 1997 for the treatment of patients with refractory colorectal cancer. The response rate for single-agent irinotecan is 32% in patients without prior therapy and 13% in patients with prior 5-FU therapy, with a median duration of response of 9 months.[424-426] The U.S. phase III trials used a schedule of 125 mg/m^2 weekly for 4 out of 6 weeks, and the European trials used 300 mg/m^2 once every 3 weeks. A randomized trial comparing these two schedules for patients with progression on 5-FU/LV confirmed that there was no difference in response rate, survival, or time to progression.[427] The type of serious toxicity differed between the two schedules: Grade 3 to 4 diarrhea was reported in 36% of patients treated weekly and in 19% of patients receiving the therapy every 3 weeks, while grade 3 to 4 neutropenia occurred in 29% of weekly and 34% of triweekly patients. Acute cholinergic symptoms and nausea were more common with the triweekly schedule.[427] Irinotecan alone is somewhat more toxic than 5-FU/LV regimens, producing severe or life-threatening neutropenia and diarrhea in one fourth to one third of patients. Despite the combination of neutropenia and diarrhea, neutropenic fever was unusual (4 of 121 patients, 3.3%).[424,425] Patients with prior radiation therapy are more likely to develop severe leucopenia. Diarrhea can generally be well controlled with the aggressive use of loperamide. During the infusion, irinotecan can produce nausea, vomiting, and cholinergic symptoms (sweating, cramping, nasal stuffiness, and acute diarrhea). Clinical experience with irinotecan has been reviewed by Rougier and Bugat.[425]

Irinotecan has been shown to improve survival in patients with disease progression on 5-FU/LV when compared with either best supportive care or infusional 5-FU.[428,429] Rougier and colleagues[428] reported a randomized trial of irinotecan versus fluorouracil by continuous infusion after fluorouracil failure in patients with metastatic colorectal cancer, and Cunningham and coworkers[429] reported a randomized trial of irinotecan plus supportive care versus supportive care alone after fluorouracil failure for patients with metastatic colorectal cancer. The trial comparing infusional therapy and irinotecan (350 mg/m^2) given every 3 weeks permitted sites to use their infusional regimen of choice—either the "de Gramont" bolus/46 hour infusion every 2 weeks, the "Lokich" continuous infusion, or the "AIO" 24-hour infusion weekly (see Table 80-8)—and demonstrated better response rates, progression-free survival (5.2 months vs. 2.9 months) and 1-year survival (54% vs. 32%) for the combination with irinotecan. For those patients with disease progression after initial 5-FU/LV treatment, median survival was 10.1 months, compared with 8.5 months for patients receiving infusion 5-FU.[428,429]

The overlapping dose-limiting toxicity, diarrhea, initially precluded delivering both 5-FU and irinotecan at full doses at maximal dose intensity. Many sequences were evaluated, and additional sequences continue to be evaluated.[430,431] Two combination regimens have been in widespread use: IFL and FOLFIRI.[408,409] IFL in comparison with 5-FU/LV bolus daily for 5 days resulted in significantly longer progression-free survival (median, 7.0 vs. 4.3 months; p = 0.004), higher response rate (39% vs. 21%, p < 0.001), and longer overall survival (median, 14.8 months vs. 12.6 months; p = 0.04).[408] Combining irinotecan with 48-hour infusional (de Gramont) schedules also improved time to progression (median, 6.7 months vs. 4.4 months; p < 0.001), response rate (35% vs. 22%, p < 0.005) and overall survival (median, 17.4 months vs. 14.1 months, p = 0.031).[409]

Careful screening of patients to ensure that they can tolerate IFL's potential for diarrhea and neutropenia, close monitoring during the first month of therapy, aggressive treatment of diarrhea, attention to symptoms and mandated dose adjustments, and institution of aggressive inpatient support (including antibiotics for patients who have neutropenia, diarrhea, and fever) are critical to minimizing mortality associated with this regimen. The life-threatening toxicity of IFL became evident in randomized trials for patients with both metastatic disease and in the adjuvant setting.[409,432] Early deaths on those trials were threefold higher compared with the other arms in the trials (2.5% vs. 0.8% and 3.5% vs 1.1%). Although these values appeared higher than the treatment-related death rate in the phase III IFL studies (0.2%–1.3%), it is consistent with the 60-day "all cause" mortality reported in Saltz's original publication.[407-411]

For patients without prior therapy for metastatic disease (first-line regimen), direct comparison of IFL with FOLFOX (see later) in an NCI-sponsored randomized trial conducted by the North Central Oncology Group with six initial arms found FOLFOX to produce superior response rates (38% vs 29%, p = 0.03), time to progression (8.6 months vs. 6.9 months, p = 0.0009) overall survival (18.1 months vs. 14.4 months, p = 0.004), and adverse event profile.[391]

Oxaliplatin. Although prior studies suggested that cisplatin in conjunction with 5-FU would enhance response rate and duration of response by altering DNA repair, clinical trials comparing the addition of cisplatin to 5-FU by continuous intravenous infusion showed insignificant improvement in response at the cost of substantial additional toxicity.[433] Oxaliplatin (trans-*l*-1,2 diaminocyclohexane oxaloplatinum), a novel diaminocyclohexane platinum complex, has greater in vitro activity than other platinum analogs.[434] Oxaliplatin has not only demonstrated synergistic cytotoxicity in vitro,[434-437] it also has clearly improved both progression-free and overall survival compared to IFL[391] and was approved by the U.S. FDA in 2002 for patients with colon cancer. Like cisplatin and carboplatin, this compound platinates DNA and forms DNA interstrand links and adducts that block DNA transcription and replication.[436,437]

The single-agent response rate for oxaliplatin is 10% in previously treated patients with colorectal cancer.[438,439] In patients without prior therapy, oxaliplatin as a single agent produces an 18% to 24% partial response rate, with a median time to progression of 6 months and a median survival of 13 to 14 months.[440,441]

Oxaliplatin's role in patients with disease refractory to 5-FU/LV was demonstrated by partial responses in 20 of 97 patients with documented progression on infusional 5-FU/LV who received the same initial regimen with oxaliplatin 85 mg/m^2—a response rate approximately double that for oxaliplatin as a single agent in second-line therapy. The median duration of response was 7.5 months.[410] The combination of continuous intravenous infusion 5-FU with oxaliplatin was shown to improve response rates compared with high-dose infusional 5-FU alone in several small trials, with response rates between 29% and 58%.[442-444]

Initial treatment for 420 patients with intravenously administered 5-FU2 LV 200 (de Gramont—5-FU bolus 400 mg/m^2/day for 2 days, followed by 22-hour infusion of 600 mg/m^2/day for 2 days administered every 2 weeks, with oxaliplatin 85 mg/m^2 on day 1 [FOLFOX]) was shown to be superior to LV5FU2, producing an improvement in progression-free survival from 6.2 months to 9 months, and improving the response rate from 22.3% to 50.7%. The study cohort was too small, however, to show

an improvement in overall survival (16.2 months vs. 14.7 months, p = 0.12).[445] Two phase II trials also were not designed to demonstrate improvements in survival (19.9 months and 19.4 months for chronomodulated 5-FU regimen and 16.2 vs. 14.7 months; p = 0.12 for the FOLFOX regimen).[445] The combination results in a 42% rate of grade 3 to 4 neutropenia, 12% grade 3/4 diarrhea, and 18% grade 3 neurotoxicity, which is the most common reason for discontinuing therapy.[445] When compared with a 5-day chronomodulated 5-FU infusion (700 mg/m^2/day given for 5 days, with peak dose delivered at 4 A.M.) with oxaliplatin, 125 mg/m^2 versus the same 5-FU/LV regimen, there was a difference in response rate (53% for the oxaliplatin/FU/LV vs. 16% for the 5-FU/LV) and in terms of progression-free survival (8.7 months vs. 6.1 months, p = 0.48).[446] This regimen also resulted in a 43% rate of grade 3 to 4 diarrhea, 13% moderate neuropathy, and less than 2% grade 4 neutropenia.[446]

The survival benefit provided by FOLFOX was definitively demonstrated in N9741, an NCI-sponsored cooperative group trial led by the North Central Cancer Treatment Group, which incorporated six different treatment arms. Time to progession for FOLFOX compared with IFL was 8.7 months versus 6.9 months (p = 0.0014), response rates were 45% versus 31%, and the overall survival was 19.5 months versus 15.0 months (p = 0.0001), unequivocally demonstrating that FOLFOX can prolong survival as first-line therapy for metastatic colon cancer.[391] A three-arm trial for second-line use of FOLFOX after disease progression on IFL found no response to infusional 5-FU (LV5FU2), a 1.3% response rate for oxaliplatin alone, and a 9% response rate for FOLFOX.[427]

A series of combinations of oxaliplatin on the background of de Gramont bolus and infusions of 5-FU/LV have been published, referred to collectively as FOLFOX 1–7. Table 80-13 lists selected combination regimens. The FOLFOX 4 regimen is inconvenient for patients and caregivers, requiring a second intravenous 2-hour infusion of leucovorin and 5-FU on the second day. FOLFOX 6 has yielded similar results as second-line therapy, with a response rate of 27% and a median survival of 10.9 months, and it is now commonly used in clinical trials.[411] In an effort to delay the onset of cumulative neurotoxicity that would result in discontinuation of treatment, a modified FOLFOX 6 (mFOLFOX 6) appears to maintain efficacy in phase II studies and is being used in several trials[447-449]

Oxaliplatin has also been combined with capecitabine, an oral prodrug producing 5-FU intracellularly (see later discussion). Oxaliplatin and capecitabine were given to 43 patients, with a response rate of 44%. Diarrhea was dose limiting, occurring in 28% of the patients.[416] The median overall survival was 20 months in this phase II study. Additional studies have been published, including both formal trials and institutional experiences.[417-419] Oxaliplatin (130 mg/m^2 on day 1) and capecitabine (1250 mg/m^2 twice daily on days 1–14 every 3 weeks) produced a partial response rate of 49% in 42 patients without prior therapy and in 15% of 26 patients with prior 5-FU.[419] Borner and colleagues[419] recommend a reduced dose of capecitabine (to 1000 mg/m^2 twice daily) for

TABLE 80-13

Commonly Used 5-FU–LV Chemotherapy Combination Regimens

REGIMEN	DOSES/SCHEDULE	REFERENCE
IFL	Irinotecan 125 mg/m^2 over 90 minutes day 1; LV 20 mg/m^2 IV bolus; 5-FU 500 mg/m^2 IV bolus weekly for 4 weeks followed by 2 week rest in a 6-week cycle	Saltz et al.[408]
FOLFIRI	Irinotecan 180 mg/m^2 in 90 minute infusion day 1; leucovorin 200 mg/m^2 IV over 2 hrs after irinotecan administration or concurrently with irinotecan in separate infusion line — day 1; 5-FU bolus 400 mg/m^2, followed by 5-FU 22-hr continuous infusion 600 mg/m^2 day 1 and day 2, q 2 weeks	Douillard et al.[409]
FOLFOX4*	Oxaliplatin 85 mg/m^2 over 120 minutes day 1; LV 200 mg/m^2 – 2 hr infusion — day 1 and day 2; 5-FU 400 mg/m^2 IV bolus plus 5-FU 600 mg/m^2 IV over 22 hrs — day 1 and day 2, q 2 weeks	Andre et al.[410]
FOLFOX6	Oxaliplatin 100 mg/m^2 over 120 minutes day 1; LV 400 mg/m^2 — 2 hr infusion — day 1; 5-FU bolus 400 mg/m^2 plus 2400 (to 3000) mg/m^2 46 hr (– 48 hr) infusion day 1, q 2 weeks	Maindrault-Goebel et al.[411]
mFOLFOX6	Oxaliplatin 85 mg/m^2 over 120 minutes day 1; l-LV 175 mg/m^2 — day 1; 5-FU bolus 400 mg/m^2 plus 2400 (to 2800) mg/m^2 — 46 hr – 48 hr infusion day 1, q 2 weeks	Braun et al.[413] Cheeseman et al.[412]
FOLFOX7	Oxaliplatin 130 mg/m^2 over 120 minutes day 1; LV 400 mg/m^2 — 2 hr infusion — day 1; 5-FU bolus 400 mg/m^2 plus 2400 mg/m^2 — 46-hr infusion day 1, q 2 weeks	Maindrault-Goebel et al.[414]
FLOX	LV 500 mg/m^2 IV over 2 hours; 5-FU 500 mg/m^2 IV bolus 1 hr after the infusion has begun; 5-FU and LV given weekly (days 1, 8, 15, 22, 29) for 6 weeks followed by a rest period; Oxaliplatin 85 mg/m^2 IV over 120 minutes before the 5-FU and LV (days 1, 15, 29). Repeat treatment begins 21 days after last dose previous cycle (1 cycle = 8 weeks) for a total of 3 cycles	Kuebler and de Gramont[415]
CAPOX	Oxaliplatin 120–130 mg/m^2 over 120 minutes day 1; capecitabine 1000–1250 mg/m^2 po bid days 1–14, q three weeks	Zenli et al.[416] Scheithauer et al.[417] Sumpter et al.[418] Borner et al.[419]
IROX	Oxaliplatin 85 mg/m^2 IV over 120 minutes day 1; irinotecan 200 mg/m^2 IV over 30 minutes day 1, q 3 weeks	Goldberg et al.[391]

*The doses of leucovorin used in the FOLFOX4 regimen may vary; some refer to d.l leucovorin and some to pure l-leucovorin.

patients with prior therapy. Two- and three-week courses were also explored in a randomized trial of either

- Oxaliplatin, 130 mg/m^2 on day 1 with capecitabine, 1000 mg/m^2 twice daily for 14 days of a 21-day cycle or
- Oxaliplatin, 85 mg/m^2 on day 1 with capecitabine, 1750 mg/m^2 twice daily for the first 7 of a 14-day cycle in 89 patients.

The biweekly regimen had a higher response rate (54.5% vs. 42.2%) and a longer progression-free survival (10.5 months vs. 6 months, p = 0.013). Overall survival was not reported because the median had not been reached.[417]

Delayed peripheral neuropathy and acute oral-pharyngeal dysesthesia occur in most patients receiving oxaliplatin and are particularly exacerbated by cold exposures.[391,440,450] The acute dysethesia can be quite disconcerting for patients if they have not been warned in advance. Patients can experience a "TMJ-like syndrome" when chewing; a sharp pain can occur with the first few bites and then abate quickly as the meal continues. Patients can also experience an acute dysesthesia during or shortly after drug infusion, which produces a sensation that they are not breathing, although their tidal volume and oxygenation remain normal. The sensation subsides quickly and is well addressed by forewarning the patient and providing reassurance. Grade 3 delayed neurotoxicity can present as a fine movement disturbance, as tingling or numbness in a peripheral sensory neuropathy, or as ataxia at an oxaliplatin median cumulative dose of 900 mg/m^2

(about 10 doses/20 weeks). The incidence increases from 10% of patients at 790 mg/m^2 to 50% at 1170 mg/m^2 to 75% of patients receiving 1560 mg/m^2. The likelihood that neurologic symptoms will regress after treatment is discontinued is inversely related to cumulative dose and severity of the neuropathy. Within 4 to 6 months, grade 1 to 2 neuropathy will have improved in 82% of patients and will have resolved entirely in 41% of patients by 6 to 8 months. The neurotoxicity of oxaliplatin has been reviewed recently.[451] Grade 3 or worse neutropenia occurs in 50% of patients receiving FOLFOX.[391] Other toxicities that are commonly reported are nausea and vomiting (which usually are well controlled with 5-HT3 antagonists), anemia, and infrequent diarrhea.

Orally Available Agents Producing 5-FU. Because extended exposure to short lived, cell-cycle–specific agents such as 5-FU is desirable, many attempts to provide 5-FU orally have been undertaken to eliminate extended infusion regimens and their requirements for indwelling lines and pump hardware. Efforts to develop oral cytotoxic agents are complicated by patient adherence to oral regimens, an issue not dealt with in many cancer treatment regimens.

Several approaches to overcoming the inconsistent and minimal absorption of oral 5-FU have been undertaken in the past decade, including agents that would inactivate the principal catabolic enzyme, dihydropyrimidine dehydrogenase (DHPD), such as eniluracil/5-FU or the uracil/tegafur combination, UFT,[452-455] and prodrugs such as capecitabine (Xeloda, Roche).[456]

Capecitabine. Capecitabine is a fluoropyrimidine carbamate that is adequately absorbed after oral dosing. It is metabolized by carboxyl esterase in the liver to 5'-deoxy-5-fluorocytidine, deaminated via cytidine deaminase in both liver and tumor tissue to 5'-deoxy-5-fluorouridine (5'-dFUR), and then further transformed by thymidine phosphorylase in tumors to 5-FU.[457,458] The final steps of anabolism to 5'FdUMP and binding in a ternary complex to TS in the presence of folinic acid are then identical to parenterally administered 5-FU. The relative concentration of 5-FU generated in tumors is eight- to 14-fold higher than the plasma concentrations.[457,458] These differentials, though substantial, are not as large as those in murine studies, which reported intracellular levels of 5-FU 16- to 35-fold higher than those produced by administration of 5-FU, with tissue levels 100- to 200-fold higher in tumors than in plasma or muscle, where the final conversion of 5'-dFUrd to 5-FUra does not occur.[458] Two phase III trials of capecitabine (1250 mg/m^2 twice daily for 2 weeks out of 3) in 602 and 605 patients with previously untreated metastatic colon cancer compared the oral regimen to the Mayo regimen (5 days of bolus 5-FU/LV every 28 days).[459-461] The overall response rate was 26% for capecitabine and 17% for 5-FU/LV (P < 0.002); the median time to progression was 4.3 to 5.2 months versus 4.3 to 4.7 months; and the overall survival was 13.2 to 12.5 months versus 12.1 to 13.3 months (combined, 12.9 months vs. 12.8 months).[443-445] Neither trial showed a statistically significant difference in any activity parameter except response rate. Adverse effects for capecitabine on this schedule are comparable to those for high-dose, 48-hour infusional 5-FU, with hand-foot syndrome prominent and occurring in 53% of patients (17% grade 3) and diarrhea occurring in 48%. Bilirubin elevations to grade 3 to 4 were reported in 28% of patients for capecitabine versus in 6% for 5-FU/LV, but less stomatitis (2% grade 3 to 4) and neutropenia (2.2% grade 3 to 4) were seen with capecitabine.[462] Because the Mayo five times daily regimen is also more toxic than continuous infusion or de Gramont 48 hour infusion, the significance of these toxicity differences is unclear.

Combinations of capecitabine with oxaliplatin have already been discussed in the section on oxaliplatin. The role of capecitabine in CAPOX versus FOLFOX will be compared in an NCI-sponsored trial led by the Southwest Oncology Group in a phase III 2 x 2 factorial design comparing CAPOX versus mFOLFOX6 with and without bevacizumab as first-line therapy.

Capecitabine as a single agent is currently being evaluated in the adjuvant setting: The X-ACT trial recruited nearly 2000 patients with Dukes C colon carcinoma, comparing capecitabine versus 5-FU/LV given for 5 days every 28 days.

Capecitabine adverse effects are comparable to those for infusional 5-FU regimens, although capecitabine is more likely than protracted continuous infusions to produce diarrhea. Dose-limiting toxicity is gastrointestinal, involving diarrhea, nausea, and vomiting. When capecitabine is used without any break, hand-foot syndrome, fatigue, and dizziness also occur. In combinations with oxaliplatin, neutropenia occurs in more than half of patients (rarely grade 4), and thrombocytopenia occurs in approximately one third.

DHPD Blocking Approaches. Another approach to providing 5-FU orally has been to block dihydropyrimidine dehydrogenase (DHPD), the principle metabolic enzyme, which is highly expressed in the gastrointestinal tract and results in the high first-pass clearance that normally stymies oral administration. Agents that block DHPD include eniluracil and 5-chloro-2,4-dihydroxypyridine (referred to as S1 when used in combination) and uracil itself. DHPD blockage could produce several significant advances over current therapeutic options:

- Because all patients are made DHPD deficient, the occasional patient with genetic absence of DHPD expression will not suffer life-threatening toxicity.
- Oral administration of 5-FU with DHPD blockage produces consistent 100% bioavailability.
- Consistent clearance rates, which would depend only on glomerular filtration rate (GFR), would produce more consistent toxicity, and dose adjustments for creatinine would be straightforward.
- The long half-life produces blood levels comparable to those for continuous infusion 5-FU, but without the need for intravenous access and ambulatory delivery pumps.
- Some tumors could be resistant on the basis of DHPD overexpression.[463]

Eniluracil (5-ethynyl uracil) is a novel compound that inhibits DHPD. The 5-FU prodrug tegafur [5-fluoro-1-(tetrahydro-2-furyl)-uracil] has been administered in combination with uracil by mouth (UFT) and in combination with both a DHPD-blocking agent (5-chloro-2,4-dihydroxypyridine) and potassium oxonate in the oral combination S-1.[464,465] Phase III trials of DHPD-blocking combinations, which were sized to demonstrate superiority compared with 5-FU/LV, have demonstrated similarity, if not equivalence. Two smaller trials of UFT versus Mayo FU/LV randomized 380 and 816 patients, respectively and reported equivalence, although for all parameters except toxicity UFT was slightly inferior.[466,467] Median survival was 12.4 months for UFT/LV and 13.4 months for 5-FU/LV (p = 0.630); response rate was 11.7% versus 14.5% (p = 0.232); and median time to progression was 3.5 months versus 3.8 months (p = 0.011). Although available throughout most of the world, UFT is not available in the United States. Similarly, although phase II trials of fixed doses of eniluracil/5-FU as first-line therapy showed activity similar to that of IV 5-FU/LV (13.2% response rate in first line) and a 10% response rate for second-line therapy,[468,469] phase III trial randomizing 981 patients showed inferior time to progression and survival compared with 5 days of 5-FU/LV on a 28-day cycle.[470] Trials to demonstrate equivalence in survival to meet U.S. FDA standards require enormous patient numbers and are not being pursued.

A Canadian analysis of the cost of administering UFT orally compared with intravenous infusion of 5-FU/LV (excluding the cost of the medications themselves) calculated that medical costs were reduced by 826

Canadian dollars per cycle ($C3221 for a course of treatment) and that patients were spared 5 hours per month in the oncology clinic.[471]

Other New Agents Directed at Thymidine Synthase

Raltitrexed. Establishing thymidylate synthase (TS) as a principal target for 5-FU and understanding its bio-chemistry has permitted the identification of other compounds that are potent, reversible TS inhibitors. Raltitrexed (Tomudex, AstraZeneca) is a quinazoline folate analog that is actively transported into cells and undergoes polyglutamylation, resulting in prolonged cytotoxic effects after a single dose. Overall, its efficacy and toxicity are comparable to those of 5-FU/leucovorin regimens, although its daily 3-week schedule reduces clinic visits.[472] Investigators have compared raltitrexed (3 mg/m² over 15 minutes, once every three weeks) with 5-FU/LV. Objective response rates were comparable, as was overall survival. Raltitrexed caused less mucositis. Mild reversible elevations in liver injury tests have also been noted. Grade 3 to 4 leukopenia was seen in 6% of patients, however, and diarrhea was seen in 10%. Fatigue (severe in 6%–18% of patients) and flulike symptoms also occur.[473] The phase II and III trials have recently been reviewed.[473-476] Raltitrexed, however, does not have clear benefit compared with 5-FU based regimens.[476-478] Evaluation of mechanisms of resistance have suggested that high expression of thymidylate synthase would interfere with either 5-FU or raltitrexed-based therapy. Although there has been a variety of technically problematic assessments of TS expression using different techniques, quantitation of TS mRNA with RT-PCR in 25 patients treated with ratltirexed distinguished a 5 out of 6 response rate in patients with TS below 4.1, compared with a 1 in 14 response rate for patients with higher TS expression.[479]

Pemetrexed. Pemetrexed (Alimta, LY231514, Eli Lilly Company) is a small molecule that inhibits both thymidylate synthase and other folate-dependent enzymes, such as DHFR and GARFT. It is avidly polyglutamated, as its pyrrolopyrimidine structure makes it an excellent substrate for folylpolyglutamate synthase.[480] Response rates in small phase II trials were 15% to 17% when it was used as first-line therapy.[481,482] No responses were seen in patients previously treated with both 5-FU and irinotecan.[483]

NEW HORIZONS

Molecularly Targeted Agents: EGFR

Four related receptor tyrosine kinases (ErbB1, ErbB2, ErbB3, ErbB4) are involved as heterodimers in proliferative signaling as both autocrine and paracrine mediators of the RAS/RAF/MAPK and PI3K/AKT pathways, among others. Each protein has extracellular, transmembrane, and intracellular ATP binding sites that present potential therapeutic targets. Monoclonal antibodies to the extra-cellular domain are presumed to act by preventing ligand binding and dimerization. Agents that mimic the intra-cellular ATP binding site interfere with the tyrosine kinase phosphorylation and downstream activation of proliferative networks. These interactions can produce cell-cycle arrest, potentiate apoptosis, and reduce angiogenesis, invasion, and metastases in the laboratory.[484,485]

ErbB1 (EGFR) is overexpressesd in 25% to 77% of colorectal cancers, and overexpression is associated with poor prognosis.[486] However, there is no evidence that overexpression is required for activity of EGFR-directed therapy. Overexpression of erbB2 (Her-2/neu), the target of trastuzumab (herceptin), is infrequent in colorectal carcinoma, resulting in very limited accrual of patients to a clinical trial of trastuzumab.

Cetuximab (C-225, IMC-C225, Erbitux) is a partially humanized (chimeric) IgG₁ antibody directed at EGFR. Binding of both natural ligands (EGF and TGF-α) is blocked, and ligand-induced activation of the tyrosine kinase is inhibited.[487] When used as a single agent in 57 patients with advanced disease refractory to chemotherapy, it had a response rate of 11%, and when used with irinotecan, it had a response rate of 19% in 139 patients whose tumors expressed EGFR.[488,489]

These results were verified in a randomized phase III trial performed in Europe, in which a total of 329 patients with metastatic colorectal cancer whose disease had progressed on a previous irinotecan-based therapy were randomized in a 2:1 manner to either cetuximab plus irinotecan or cetuximab alone. The response rate (primary endpoint of the study) in patients who received the combination was 23% compared with 11% in those who received cetuximab alone. The median time to progression was 4.1 months in the combination arm compared with 1.5 months in the single-agent arm. There was no difference in overall survival between the two arms; however, patients were allowed to cross over from the single-agent arm to the combination arm at progression.[490] In 2004, the U.S. FDA approved cetuximab for use in second-line treatment.

Adverse events related to cetuximab include the mechanism-associated acneiform skin rash, which occurs in 75% of patients but is grade 3 or 4 in only 15%, and allergic infusion reactions. Patients also can have fatigue, nausea, emesis, and diarrhea; one third of patients have these symptoms, with fewer than 10% at an intensity of grade 3 or 4.[491] An ongoing CALGB trial sponsored by the National Cancer Institute will evaluate first-line chemotherapy with or without cetuximab. Fully humanized anti-EGFR MAb or related compounds (ABX-EGF, EMD 72000) are also in early clinical development.

Gefinitib (ZD1839, Iressa), erlotinib (OSI-774, Tarceva), PKI-166, and GW2016 are small-molecule inhibitors of the phosphorylation of EGFR. These agents are dose limited by both the mechanism-specific acneiform rash and by diarrhea. As single agents, they have not produced responses in phase II trials in patients with refractory colorectal carcinoma.[492,493] The reasons for the difference in activity of the antibodies and small molecules in colon cancer is being explored actively, and combinations of novel agents are being evaluated.

Specific Malignancies

III

Antiangiogenic Approaches

Considerable evidence has been developed regarding the importance of angiogenesis in tumor growth and progression.[494] Vascular endothelial growth factor (VEGF) is a central regulator of normal and neoplastic angiogenesis. Increased expression of VEGF in patients with colorectal carcinoma has been associated with recurrence and poor prognosis.[495]

Bevacizumab (anti-VEGF, Avastin, Genentech) is a human monocolonal antibody directed at vascular endothelial grown factor (VEGF) as an antiangiogenic strategy. A phase II study of two doses of bevacizumab (5 mg/kg or 10 mg/kg every 2 weeks) with 5-FU and folinic acid (weekly) in patients without prior chemotherapy produced response rates of 40% in the low-dose arm, 24% in the high-dose arm, and 17% in the chemotherapy-alone arm; longer time to progression (9 months vs. 7.2 months vs. 5.2 months, respectively), and improved survival (21.5 months vs. 16.1 months vs 13.8 months, p = NS) were also noted. Only 2 of 22 patients treated with bevacizumab as second-line therapy after failure of chemotherapy alone had partial responses, and median time to progression for these patients was only 2 months.[496] This dose-ranging study preceded two large randomized phase III studies in colon cancer. Bevacizumab (5 mg/kg daily every other week with IFL, which was the "standard" first-line regimen at the time the study was initiated) was compared with IFL alone in 925 patients. Median survival was 20.3 versus 15.6 months, progression-free survival was 10.6 months versus 6.2 months, and response rate was 45% versus 35%, respectively.[392] An increased incidence of hypertension was observed on the bevacizumab arm of the study (11% vs. 2.3%), as was an increase in bowel perforation, but there was no statistically significant increase in grade 3 or 4 bleeding (2.5% vs. 3.1%) or thromboembolic events (16.1% vs. 19.3%). In 2004, the U.S. FDA approved bevacizumab in combination with 5-FU–based chemotherapy for first-line treatment. The role of bevacizumab has been evaluated in patients who previously had been given IFL in a complete but not yet mature trial sponsored by the NCI and conducted by ECOG. The trial randomized patients to FOLFOX plus bevacizumab versus FOLFOX versus bevacizumab alone. The bevacizumab-alone arm was closed early by the data safety monitoring committee for futility—there was no chance statistically that it would match the other arms. The NCI is also sponsoring a phase III trial led by SWOG, comparing mFOLFOX6 to CAPOX with or without bevacizumab in a 2 x 2 factorial design for patients with metastatic disease who had not previously received chemotherapy. Novartis is sponsoring a trial of FOLFOX4 with PTK737/ZK222584, an oral VEGF1 inhibitor, or placebo.

In common with most targeted therapies, and in contrast to the common expectations that such treatments will be as benign as low-dose aspirin, bevacizumab treatment is associated with adverse events, including hypertension (generally responsive to medical management but severe on rare occasions), thrombotic events (venous and arterial), bowel perforation, and dehiscence of wound healing by secondary intent. In patients with lung cancer, lethal hemoptysis has been reported; an increased rate of gastrointestinal bleeding can occur in patients with colon cancer; and other serious and life-threatening hemorrhages have been reported. Less serious events include epistaxis (grade 1 or 2), proteinuria with rare nephrotic syndrome, fever, headache, and rash.

Many additional antiangiogenic approaches are currently in early clinical development, including other agents directed at VEGF itself (VEGF-TRAP) and agents directed at the VEGFr, such as PTK787, ZD6474, and SU11248.

Immunologic Approaches to the Treatment of Colon Cancer

Attempts to activate lymphocytes and/or antibodies that would eliminate colon cancer have been undertaken for decades. Tumor-associated antigens present targets for these effector arms (which might be activated by enhancing the immunogenicity of the tumor-associated antigens) and by increasing the activity of the immune response. In the third in a series of adjuvant trials in patients with stage II and III disease, comparing vaccination with autologous tumor cells mixed with BCG for three weekly doses postoperatively in 412 patients, no improvement in disease-free or overall survival was evident.[497] In a phase II trial, the autologous tumor cell plus BCG approach was combined with 5-FU/LV to assess alterations in immunity; delayed-type hypersensitivity measured by induration decreased only from 20.3 mm to 18.4 mm.[498] Addition of a fourth vaccination at 6 months, when immunity was waning, was evaluated in a randomized trial involving 254 patients. This study was felt to have better quality control for the vaccine production (one facility was used and 98% of all vaccines met quality control specifications); 97% of all patients receiving vaccine developed induration greater than 5 mm by the third vaccination, compared with only 88% of the vaccines prepared and only 85% of the patients developing induration in the ECOG trial. Only 101 of 128 vaccination patients received all four vaccinations, however. Four-year disease-free survival was 70% versus 59% for those observed, but there was no difference in overall survival.[499]

Another strategy to breaking tolerance to tumor antigens is to use anti-idiotype antibodies that mimic the tumor-associated antigen and permit the immune system to generate anti-anti-idiotype antibodies that also recognize the tumor antigen. CeaVac (3H1 IgG) is an anti-idiotype murine monoclonal antibody to a murine antibody against CEA, and TriAb (11D10 IgG) is a murine anti-idiotype antibody to a murine antibody against HMFG (another tumor-associated antigen).[500] These are being evaluated in patients who have had resection of liver metastases as adjuvant therapy.

REFERENCES

1. http://www.cdc.gov/nchs/products/pubs/pubd/nvsr/49/49-13htm#49_11
2. American Cancer Society: Cancer Facts and Figures–2003,

American Cancer Society Surveillance Research, Atlanta, Ga. (http://www.cancer.org/downloads/STT/CAFF2003pwsecured.pdf)

3. http://www.facs.org/cancer/nedb/index.html

4. National Cancer Institute, Cancer Control and Population Sciences (http://surveillance.cancer.gov/statistics) and (http://seer.cancer.gov/faststats/htm/inc_colorect.html)

5. Parkin DM, Pisani P, Ferlay J: Global cancer statistics. CA Cancer J Clin 1999;49:33.

6. Kune S, Sune G, Watson L: The Melbourne Colorectal Cancer Study: Incidence findings by age, sex, site migrants and religion. Int J Epidemiol 1986;15:483–493

7. Solomon E, Voss R, Hall V: Chromosome 5 allele loss in human colorectal carcinomas. Nature 1987;328:616.

8. Rozen P, Lynch HT, Figer H, et al: Familial colon cancer in the Tel Aviv area and the influence of ethnic origin. Cancer 1987;60:2355.

9. Correa P, Haenszel W: The epidemiology of large bowel cancer. Adv Cancer Res 1978;26:1.

10. St John DJB, McDermott FT, Hoppes JL, et al: Cancer risk in relatives of patients with common colorectal cancer. Ann Intern Med 1993;118:785.

11. Planck M, Anderson H, Bladstrom A, Moller T, Wenngren E, Olsson H: Increased cancer risk in offspring of women with colorectal carcinoma: A Swedish register-based cohort study. Cancer 2000;89:741–749.

12. Steinmetz KA, Potter JD: Vegetables, fruits and cancer II. Mechanisms. Cancer Causes Control 1991;2:427.

13. Potter JD: Nutrition and colorectal cancer. Cancer Causes Control 1996;7:127.

14. Potter JD, Slattery ML, Bostick RM, et al: Colon cancer: A review of the epidemiology. Epidemiol Rev 1993;5:499.

15. Stemmermann GN, Nomura AM, Heilbrun LK: Dietary fat and the risk of colorectal cancer. Cancer Res 1984;44:4633.

16. Willett MD, Walter C, Stampfer MJ, et al: Relation of meat, fat and fiber intake to the risk of colorectal cancer. N Engl J Med 1990;323:164.

17. Willett C, Stampfer M, Colditz GA, et al: Relationship of meat, food and fiber intake to the risk of colon cancer in a study amongst women nurses. N Engl J Med 1990;323:164.

18. Nigro ND, Singh DV, Campbell RL, et al: Effect of dietary beef fat on intestinal cancer formation in rats. J Natl Cancer Inst 1990;54:439.

19. Burkitt DP: Epidemiology of cancer of the colon and rectum. Cancer 1971;28:313.

20. Cruse JP, Lewin MR, Clark CG: Failure of bran to protect against experimental colon cancer in rats. Lancet 1978;2:1278.

21. Nigro ND, Bull AW, Klopfer BA, et al: Effect of dietary fiber on intestinal carcinogenesis in rats. J Natl Cancer Inst 1979;62:1097.

22. Trock B, Lanza E, Greenwald P: Dietary fiber, vegetables, and colon cancer: Critical review and meta-analyses of the epidemiologic evidence. J Natl Cancer Inst 1990;82:650.

23. Fuchs CS, Giovannucci EL, Colditz GA, et al: Dietary fiber and the risk of colorectal cancer and adenoma in women. N Engl J Med 1999;340:169.

24. Michels KB, Edward G, Joshipura KJ, et. al. Prospective study of fruit and vegetable consumption and incidence of colon and rectal cancers. J Natl Cancer Inst 2000;92:1740–1752.

25. Thun M, Colle E, Namboodiri M, et. al. Risk factors for fatal colon cancer in a large prospective study. J Natl Cancer Inst 1992;84:1491–1500.

26. Platz E, Giovannucci E, Rimm E, et al: Dietary fiber and distal colorectal adenoma in men. Cancer Epidemiol Biomarkers Prev 1997;6:661–670.

27. Terry P, Giovannuci E, Michels KB, et al: Fruit, vegetables, dietary fiber, and risk of colorectal cancer J Natl Cancer Inst 2001;93(7):525–533.

28. Asano T, McLeod RS: Dietary fiber for the prevention of colorectal adenomas and carcinomas (Cochrane Review). Cochrane Library 2002;4.

29. Newmark HL, Lipkin M: Calcium, vitamin D and colon cancer. Cancer Res 1992;52(Suppl 1):2067–2070.

30. Rosen P, Fireman Z, Fine N, Wax Y, Ron E: Oral calcium suppresses increased rectal epithelialprolifertion of persons at risk of colorectal cancer. Gut 1989;30:650–655.

31. Van der Meer R, Lapre JA, Grovers MJ, Kleibeuker JH: Mechanisms of the intestinal effects of dietary fats and milk products on colon carcinogenesis [review]. Cancer Lett 1997;114:75–83.

32. Nagengast FM, Grubben MJAL, Munster IP: Role of bile acids in colorectal carcinogenesis [review]. Eur J Cancer 1995;31A:1067–1070.

33. Pence BC. Role of Calcium in colon cancer prevention: Experimental and clinical studies. Mutat Res 1993;290(1):87–95.

34. Bostick RM, Fosdick L, Wood JR, et al: Calcium and colorectal epithelial cell proliferation in sporadic adenoma patients: A randomized double blinded placebo controlled clinical trial. J Natl Cancer Inst 1995;87:1307.

35. Bergsma-Kadijk JA, Van't Veer P, Kampman E, Burema J: Calcium does not protect against colorectal neoplasia. Epidemiology 1996;7:590–597.

36. Martinez ME, Willet WC: Calcium, vitamin D, and colorectal cancer: A review of epidemiologic evidence. Cancer Epidemiol Biomarkers Prev 1998;7:163–168.

37. Bostick RM, Potter JD, McKenzie DR, et al: Reduced risk of colon cancer with high intake of vitamin E. Cancer Res 1993;53:4230.

38. Hennekens CH, Buring JE, Manson JE, et al: Lack of effect of long-term supplementation with beta carotene on the incidence of malignant neoplasm and cardiovascular disease. N Engl J Med 1996;34:1145.

39. Albanes D, Heinonen OP, Huttunen JK, et al: Effects of alpha tocopherol and beta carotene supplements on cancer incidence. Am J Clin Nutr 1995;S62:1427.

40. Bussey HJ, Decosse JJ, Deschner EE, et al: A randomized trial of ascorbic acid in polyposis coli. Cancer 1982;50:1434.

41. DeCosse JJ, Miller HH, Lesser JL: Effect of wheat fiber and vitamins C and E on rectal polyps in patients with familial adenomatous polyposis. J Natl Cancer Inst 1989;84:1290.

42. McKeown-Eyssen G, Holloway C, Jazmaji V, et al: A randomized trial of vitamins C and E in the prevention of recurrence of colorectal polyps. Cancer Res 1988;48:471.

43. Greenberg ER, Baron JA, Tosteson TD, et al: A clinical trial of antioxidant vitamins to prevent colorectal adenoma. N Engl J Med 1994;331:141.

44. Roncucci L, DiDonato P, Carati L, et al: Antioxidant vitamins or lactulose for prevention of the recurrence of colorectal adenomas. Dis Colon Rectum 1993;36:227.

45. Willett WC: Diet and cancer: One view at the start of the millenium. Cancer Epidemiol Biomarkers Prev 2001;10:3–8.

46. Martinez ME, Giovannucci E, Spiegleman D, Hunter DJ, Willett WC, Coldity GA: Leisure-time physical activity, body size, and colon cancer in women. Nurses Health Study Research Group. J Natl Cancer Inst 1997;89:948–955.

47. Caan BJ, Coates AO, Slattery AL, Potter JD, Quesenberry CP Jr, Edwards SM: Body size and the risk of colon cancer in a large case-control study. Int J Obes Relat Metab Disord 1998;22:178–184.

48. Platz EA, Willett WC, Colditz GA, Rimm EB, Spiegelman DL, Giovannucci EL: Proportion of colon cancer risk that might be preventable in a cohort of middle-aged US men. Cancer Causes Control 2000;11:579–588.

49. McKeown-Eyssen GE, Toronto Polyp Prevention Group: Insulin resistance and the risk of colorectal neoplasia. Cancer Epidemiol Biomarkers Prev 1996;5:235.

50. Kaaks R, Toniolo P, Akhmedkhanov A, et al: Serum C-peptide, IGF-I, IGF-binding proteins and risk of colorectal cancer in women. J Natl Cancer Inst 2000;92:34–42.

51. Schoen RE, Tangen CM, Kuller LH, et al: Increased blood glucose and insulin, body size, and incident colorectal cancer. J Natl Cancer Inst 1999;91:1147–1154.

52. Laken SJ, Petersen GM, Gruber SB, et al: Familial colorectal cancer in Ashkenazim due to a hypermutable tract in APC. Nat Genet 1997;17:79.

53. Brown SR, Finan PJ, Hall NR, Bishop DT: Incidence of DNA replication errors in patients with multiple primary cancers. Dis Colon Rectum 1998;41:765.

54. Vogelstein B, Feron E. Hamilton S, et al: Genetic alterations during colorectal-tumor development. N Engl J Med 1988;319:525–532.

55. Fearon ER, Cho KR, Nigro JM, et al. Identification of a chromosome 18q gene that is altered in colorectal cancers. Science 1990;247:49–56.

Specific Malignancies

III

56. Fearon E, Vogelstein B: A genetic model for colorectal tumorogenesis. Cell 1990;61:759–767.

57. Lengauer C, Kinzler KW, Vogelstein B: Genetic instability in colorectal cancers. Nature 1997;386:623–627.

58. Bodmer WR, Bailey DJ, Bodmer J, et al: Localization of the gene for familial adenomatosis polyposis on chromasome 5. Nature 1987;328:614–616.

59. Leppert M, Dobbs M, Scambler P, et al. The gene from familial polyposis coli maps to the long arm of chromosome 5. Science 1987;238:1411–1413.

60. Feeruhead NS, Wilidng JL, Bodmer WF: Advances in colorectal cancer. Br Med Bull 2002;64:27–43.

61. Haigies KM, Caya JG, Reichelderfer M, Dove WF: Intestinal adenomas can develop with a stable karyotype and stable microsatellites. Proc Natl Acad Sci USA 2002;99:8927–8931.

62. Orford K, Crockett C, Jensen JP, Weissman AM, Byers SW: Serine phosphorylation-regulated ubiquitination and degradation of B-catenin. J Biol Chem 1997;272:735–738.

63. Peifer M, Polakis P: Wnt signaling in oncogenesis and embryogenesis—a look outside the nucleus. Science 2000;287:1606–1609.

64. Cook D, Fry M, Hughes K, et al: Wingless inactivates glycogen synthase kinase-3 via an intracellular signaling pathway which involves a protein kinase C. Embo J 1996;15:4526–4530.

65. Mann B, Gelos M, Siedow A, et al: Target genes of beta-catenin–T cell-factor/lymphoid-enhancer-factor signaling in human colrecta carcinomas. Proc Natl Acad Sci USA 1999;96:1603–1608.

66. Keino-Masu K, Masu M, Itinck L, et al: Deleted in colorectal cancer (DCC) encodes a natrin receptor. Cell 1996;87:175–185.

67. Miyaki M, Iijima T, Komishi M, et al: Higher frequency of Smad4 gene mutation in human colorectal cancer with distant metastisis. Oncogene 1999;18:3098–3103.

68. Eppert K, Scherer SW, Ozcelik H, et al: MADR2 maps to 18q21 and encodes a TGF-β-regulated MAD-related protein that is functionally mutated in colorectal carcinoma. Cell 1996;86:543–552.

69. Takagi Y, Koumura H, Futamura M, et al: Somatic alteration of the SMAD-2 gene in human colorectal cancers. Br J Cancer 1998;78:1152–1155.

70. Hamamoto T, Beppa H, Okada H, et al: Compound disruption of Smad2 accelerates malignant progression of intestinal tumors in *Apc* knockout mice. Cancer Res 2002;62:5955–5961.

71. Dietrich WF, Lander ES, Smith JS, et al: Genetic identification of Mom-1, a major modifier locus affecting Min-induced intestinal neoplasia in the mouse. Cell 1993;75:631–639.

72. Hawkins NJ, Bariol C, Ward RL: The serrated neoplasia pathway. Pathology 2002;34:548–555.

73. Jass JR, Whitehall VL, Young J, Deggett BA: Emerging concepts in colorectal neplasia. Gastroenterology 2002;123:862–876.

74. Chan TL, Zhao W, Cancer Genome Project, Leung SY, Yuen ST: BRAF& KRAS mutations in colorectal hyperplastic polyps and serrated adenoma. Cancer Res 2003;63:4878–4881.

75. Warwick R, Williams PL: Gray's Anatomy, 35th British Ed. Philadelphia, WB Saunders, 1973.

76. Frazer ID, Condon RE, Schulte WJ, et al: Longitudinal muscle of muscularis externa in human and nonhuman primate colon. Arch Surg 1981;116:61.

77. Fenoglio CM, Kay GI, Lane N: Distribution of human colonic lymphatics in normal, hyperplastic, and adenomatous tissue: Its relationship to metastasis from small carcinoma in pedunculated adenomas, with two case reports. Gastroenterology 1973;64:51.

78. Okike N, Weiland LH, Anderson MJ, Adson MA: Stromal invasion of cancer in pedunculated adenomatous colorectal polyps. Arch Surg 1977;112:527.

79. Whitehead R: Rectal polyps and their relationship to cancer. Clin Gastroenterol 1975;4:545.

80. Shamsuddin AM, Phelps PC, Trump BF: Human large intestinal epithelium: Light microscopy, histochemistry, and ultrastructure. Hum Pathol 1982;13:790–830.

81. Roediger WEW: Role of anaerobic bacteria in the metabolic welfare of the colonic mucosa in men. Gut 1980;21:793–798.

82. Winawer SJ, Zauber AG, Stewart E: The natural history of colorectal cancer: Opportunities for intervention. Cancer 1991;67:1143–1149.

83. Jass JR: Do all colorectal carcinomas arise in preexisting adenomas? World J Surg 1989;13:45–51.

84. Jass JR: Evolution of hereditary bowel cancer. Mutat Res 1993;290:13–25.

85. Morson BC: The Pathogenesis of Colorectal Cancer. In Morson BC (ed): Major Problems in Pathology, vol 10. Philadelphia, WB Saunders, 1978, pp1–13.

86. Winawer SJ, Zauber AG, Ho MN, et al: Prevention of colorectal cancer by colonoscopic polypectomy. The National Polyp Study Workgroup. N Engl J Med 1993;329:1977–1981.

87. Fuchs CS, Giovannucci EL, Colditz GA, et al: A prospective study of family history and the risk of colorectal cancer. N Engl J Med 1994;331:1169.

88. Vasen HF: The International Collaborative Group on Hereditary Non-Polyposis Colorectal Cancer (ICG-HNPCC). Dis Colon Rectum 1991;34:424–425.

89. Rodriguez-Bigas MA, Boland CR, Hamilton SR, et al: A National Cancer Institute workshop on hereditary nonpolyposis colorectal cancer syndrome: Meeting highlights and Bethesda guidelines. J Natl Cancer Inst 1997;89:1758–1762.

90. Boland CR: A National Cancer Institute workshop on microsatellite instability for cancer detection and familial predisposition: Development of international criteria for the determination of microsatellite instability in colorectal cancer. Cancer Res 1998;58:5248–5257.

91. Giardiello FM, Brensinger JD, Petersen GM, et al: The use and interpretation of commercial APC gene testing for familial adenomatous polyposis. N Engl J Med 1997;336:823–827.

92. White RL: Excess risk of colon cancer associated with a polymorphism of the APC gene? Cancer Res 1998;58:4038–4039.

93. Anonymous statement of the American Society of Clinical Oncology: Genetic testing for cancer susceptibility, adopted on February 20, 1996. J Clin Oncol 1996;14:1730–1740.

94. Frazier AL, Colditz GA, Fuchs CS, Kuntz KM: Cost-effectiveness of screening for colorectal cancer in the general population. JAMA 2000;284:1954–1961.

95. Loeve F, Brown ML, Boer R, van Ballegooijen M, van Oortmarssen GJ, Habbema JD: Endoscopic colorectal cancer screening: A cost-saving analysis. J Natl Cancer Inst 2000;92:557–563.

96. Sonnenberg A, Delco F, Inadomi JM: Cost-effectiveness of colonoscopy in screening for colorectal cancer. Ann Intern Med 2000;133:573–584.

97. Winawer S, Fletcher R, Rex D, et al: Colorectal cancer screening and surveillance: Clinical guidelines and rationale—update based on new evidence. Gastroenterology 2003;124:544–560.

98. Hardcastle JD, Chamberlain JO, Robinson MH, et al: Randomised controlled trial of faecal-occult-blood screening for colorectal cancer. Lancet 1996;348:1472–1477.

99. Kronborg O, Fenger C, Olsen J, Jorgensen OD, Sondergaard O: Randomised study of screening for colorectal cancer with faecal-occult-blood test. Lancet 1996;348:1467–1471.

100. Mandel JS, Church TR, Ederer F, Bond JH: Colorectal cancer mortality: Effectiveness of biennial screening for fecal occult blood. J Natl Cancer Inst 1999;91:434–437.

101. Selby JV, Friedman GD, Quesenberry CP Jr, Weiss NS: A case-control study of screening sigmoidoscopy and mortality from colorectal cancer. N Engl J Med 1992;326:653–657.

102. Newcomb PA, Norfleet RG, Storer BE, Surawicz TS, Marcus PM: Screening sigmoidoscopy and colorectal cancer mortality. J Natl Cancer Inst 1992;84:1572–1575.

103. Muller AD, Sonnenberg A: Protection by endoscopy against death from colorectal cancer. A case-control study among veterans. Arch Intern Med 1995;155:1741–1748.

104. Kavanagh AM, Giovannucci EL, Fuchs CS, Colditz GA: Screening endoscopy and risk of colorectal cancer in United States men. Cancer Causes Control 1998;9:455–462.

105. Thiis-Evensen E, Hoff GS, Sauar J, Langmark F, Majak BM, Vatn MH: Population-based surveillance by colonoscopy: effect on the incidence of colorectal cancer. Telemark Polyp Study I. Scand J Gastroenterol 1999;34:414–420.

106. Single flexible sigmoidoscopy screening to prevent colorectal cancer: Baseline findings of a UK multicentre randomised trial. Lancet 2002;359:1291–1300.

107. Lieberman DA, Weiss DG: One-time screening for colorectal cancer with combined fecal occult-blood testing and examination of the distal colon. N Engl J Med 2001;345:555–560.

108. Berry DP, Clarke P, Hardcastle JD, Vellacott KD: Randomized trial of the addition of flexible sigmoidoscopy to faecal occult blood testing for colorectal neoplasia population screening. Br J Surg 1997;84:1274-1276.

109. Rasmussen M, Kronborg O, Fenger C, Jorgensen OD: Possible advantages and drawbacks of adding flexible sigmoidoscopy to hemoccult-II in screening for colorectal cancer. A randomized study. Scand J Gastroenterol 1999;34:73-78.

110. Hofstad B, Vatn M: Growth rate of colon polyps and cancer. Gastrointest Endosc Clin N Am 1997;7:345-363.

111. Citarda F, Tomaselli G, Capocaccia R, Barcherini S, Crespi M: Efficacy in standard clinical practice of colonoscopic polypectomy in reducing colorectal cancer incidence. Gut 2001;48:812-815.

112. Lieberman DA, Weiss DG, Bond JH, Ahnen DJ, Garewal H, Chejfec G: Use of colonoscopy to screen asymptomatic adults for colorectal cancer. Veterans Affairs Cooperative Study Group 380. N Engl J Med 2000;343:162-168.

113. Imperiale TF, Wagner DR, Lin CY, Larkin GN, Rogge JD, Ransohoff DF: Risk of advanced proximal neoplasms in asymptomatic adults according to the distal colorectal findings. N Engl J Med 2000;343:169-174.

114. Burt R, Jacoby RF: Polyposis syndromes. In Yamada T, Alpers DH, Laine L, Kaplowitz N, Onyang C, Powell OW (eds): Textbook of Gastroenterology, 4th ed. Philadelphia, Lippincott Williams & Wilkins, 2003, pp 1914-1939.

115. Lynch HT, Smyrk TC, Watson PT, et al: Genetics, natural history, tumor spectrum, and pathology of hereditary nonpolyposis colorectal cancer: An updated review. Gastroenterology 1993;104:1535-1549.

116. Jarvinen HJ, Aarnio M, Mustonen H, et al: Controlled 15-year trial on screening for colorectal cancer in families with hereditary nonpolyposis colorectal cancer. Gastroenterology 2000;118:829-834.

117. Anonymous: Colorectal cancer screening. ACS guidelines. CA Can J Clin 1999;49:4.

118. Heiskanen I, Luostarinen T, Jarvinen HJ: Impact of screening examinations on survival in familial adenomatous polyposis. Scand J Gastroenterol 2000;35:1284-1287.

119. Bjork JA, Akerbrant HI, Iselius LE, Hultcrantz RW: Risk factors for rectal cancer morbidity and mortality in patients with familial adenomatous polyposis after colectomy and ileorectal anastomosis. Dis Colon Rectum 2000;43:1719-1725.

120. Leppert M, Burt R, Hughes JP, et al: Genetic analysis of an inherited predisposition to colon cancer in a family with a variable number of adenomatous polyps. N Engl J Med 1990;322:904-908.

121. Spirio L, Olschwang S, Groden J, et al: Alleles of the APC gene: An attenuated form of familial polyposis. Cell 1993;75:951-957.

122. Jenne DE, Reimann H, Nezu J, et al: Peutz-Jeghers syndrome is caused by mutations in a novel serine threonine kinase. Nat Genet 1998;18:38-43.

123. McGarrity TJ, Kulin HE, Zaino RJ: Peutz-Jeghers syndrome. Am J Gastroenterol 2000;95:596-604.

124. Williams CB, Goldblatt M, Delaney PV: 'Top and tail endoscopy' and follow-up in Peutz-Jeghers syndrome. Endoscopy 1982;14:82-84.

125. Grotsky HW, Rickert RR, Smith WD, Newsome JF: Familial juvenile polyposis coli. A clinical and pathologic study of a large kindred. Gastroenterology 1982;82:494-501.

126. Giardiello FM, Hamilton SR, Kern SE, et al: Colorectal neoplasia in juvenile polyposis or juvenile polyps. Arch Dis Child 1991;66:971-975.

127. Zhou XP, Woodford-Richens K, Lehtonen R, et al: Germline mutations in BMPR1A/ALK3 cause a subset of cases of juvenile polyposis syndrome and of Cowden and Bannayan-Riley-Ruvalcaba syndromes. Am J Hum Genet 2001;69:704-711.

128. Jacoby RF, Schlack S, Sekhon G, Laxova R: Del(10)(q22.3q24.1) associated with juvenile polyposis. Am J Med Genet 1997;70:361-364.

129. Haggitt RC, Reid BJ: Hereditary gastrointestinal polyposis syndromes. Am J Surg Pathol 1986;10:871-887.

130. Nagasako K, Takemoto T: Endoscopy of the ileocecal area. Gastroenterology 1973;65:403-411.

131. Schwartz DC, Cole CE, Sun Y, Jacoby RF Diffuse nodular hyperplasia of the colon: Polyposis syndrome or normal variant? Gastroint Endosc 2003;58:630-632.

132. Vasen HF, Mecklin JP, Watson P, et al: Surveillance in hereditary nonpolyposis colorectal cancer: An international cooperative study of 165 families. DisColon Rectum 1993;36:1-4.

133. Kelloff GJ: Perspectives on cancer chemoprevention research and drug development. Adv Cancer Res 2000;78:199-334.

134. Kelloff GJ, Johnson JR, Crowell JA, et al: Approaches to the development and marketing approval of drugs that prevent cancer. Cancer Epidemiol Biomarkers Prev 1995;4:1-10.

135. Kelloff GJ, Malone WF, Boone CW, Sigman CC, Fay JR: Progress in applied chemoprevention research. Semin Oncol 1990;17:438-455.

136. Thun MJ, Namboodiri MM, Heath CW Jr: Aspirin use and reduced risk of fatal colon cancer. N Engl J Med 1991;325:1593-1596.

137. Marnett LJ, DuBois RN: COX-2: A target for colon cancer prevention. Annu Rev Pharmacol Toxicol 2002;42:55-80.

138. Giardiello FM, Hamilton SR, Krush AJ, et al: Treatment of colonic and rectal adenomas with sulindac in familial adenomatous polyposis. N Engl J Med 1993;328:1313-1316.

139. Jacoby RF, Seibert K, Cole CE, Kelloff G, Lubet RA: The cyclooxygenase-2 inhibitor celecoxib is a potent preventive and therapeutic agent in the min mouse model of adenomatous polyposis. Cancer Res 2000;60:5040-5044.

140. Steinbach G, Lynch PM, Phillips RK, et al: The effect of celecoxib, a cyclooxygenase-2 inhibitor, in familial adenomatous polyposis. N Engl J Med, 2000;342:1946-1952.

141. Lipkin SM: MLH3: A DNA mismatch repair gene associated with mammalian microsatellite instability. Nature Genet 2000;24:27-35.

142. van Stolk R, Sivak MV Jr, Petrini JL, Petras R, Ferguson DR, Jagelman D: Endoscopic management of upper gastrointestinal polyps and periampullary lesions in familial adenomatous polyposis and Gardner's syndrome. Endoscopy 1987;19(Suppl 1):19-22.

143. Labayle D, Fischer D, Vielh P, et al: Sulindac causes regression of rectal polyps in familial adenomatous polyposis. Gastroenterology 1991;101:635-639.

144. Rigau J, Pique JM, Rubio E, Planas R, Tarrech JM, Bordas JM: Effects of long-term sulindac therapy on colonic polyposis. Ann Intern Med 1991;115:952-954.

145. Nugent KP, Farmer KC, Spigelman AD, Williams CB, Phillips RK: Randomized controlled trial of the effect of sulindac on duodenal and rectal polyposis and cell proliferation in patients with familial adenomatous polyposis. Br J Surg 1993;80:1618-1619.

146. Feinberg SM, Jagelman DG, Sarre RG, et al: Spontaneous resolution of rectal polyps in patients with familial polyposis following abdominal colectomy and ileorectal anastomosis. Dis Colon Rectum 1988;31:169-175.

147. Stevenson JK, Reid BJ: Unfamiliar aspects of familial polyposis coli. Am J Surg 1986;152:81-86.

148. Lipkin M, Newmark H: Effect of added dietary calcium on colonic epithelial-cell proliferation in subjects at high risk for familial colonic cancer. N Engl J Med 1985;313:1381-1384.

149. Gould KA, Dove WF: Action of Min and Mom1 on neoplasia in ectopic intestinal grafts. Cell Growth Differ 1996;7:1361-1368.

150. Burt R, Jacoby RF: Polyposis syndromes. In Yamada T, Alpers DH, Laine L, Kaplowitz N, Onyang C, Powell OW (eds): Textbook of Gastroenterology, 4th ed. Philadelphia, Lippincott Williams & Wilkins, 2003, pp 1914-1939.

151. Stoltenberg RL: Neoplasia in ileal pouch mucosa after total proctocolectomy for juvenile polyposis: Report of a case. Dis Colon Rectum 1997;40:726-730.

152. Dove WF, Clipson L, Gould KA, et al: Intestinal neoplasia in the ApcMin mouse: Independence from the microbial and natural killer (beige locus) status. Cancer Res 1997;57:812-814.

153. Williamson RC, Bauer FL, Ross JS, Watkins JB, Malt RA: Enhanced colonic carcinogenesis with azoxymethane in rats after pancreaticobiliary diversion to mid small bowel. Gastroenterology 1979;76:1386-1392.

154. Williamson RC, Bauer FL, Terpstra OT, Ross JS, Malt RA: Contrasting effects of subtotal enteric bypass, enterectomy, and

Specific Malignancies

III

colectomy on azoxymethane-induced intestinal carcinogenesis. Cancer Res 1980;40:538–543.

155. Narisawa T, Fukaura Y, Terada K, Sekiguchi H: Inhibitory effects of ursodeoxycholic acid on N-methylnitrosourea-induced colon carcinogenesis and colonic mucosal telomerase activity in F344 rats. J Exp Clin Cancer Res 1999;18:259–266.

156. Narisawa T, Fukaura Y, Terada K, Sekiguchi H: Prevention of N-methylnitrosourea-induced colon tumorigenesis by ursodeoxycholic acid in F344 rats. Jpn J Cancer Res 1998;89:1009–1013.

157. Earnest DL, Holubec H, Wali RK, et al: Chemoprevention of azoxymethane-induced colonic carcinogenesis by supplemental dietary ursodeoxycholic acid. Cancer Res 1994;54:5071–5074.

158. Brasitus TA: Primary chemoprevention strategies for colorectal cancer: Ursodeoxycholic acid and other agents. Gastroenterology 1995;109:2036–2038.

159. Ikegami T, Matsuzaki Y, Shoda J, Kano M, Hirabayashi N, Tanaka N: The chemopreventive role of ursodeoxycholic acid in azoxymethane-treated rats: Suppressive effects on enhanced group II phospholipase A2 expression in colonic tissue. Cancer Lett 1998;134:129–139.

160. Tung BY, Emond MJ, Haggitt RC, et al: Ursodiol use is associated with lower prevalence of colonic neoplasia in patients with ulcerative colitis and primary sclerosing cholangitis. Ann Intern Med 2001;134:89–95.

161. Pardi DS, Loftus EV Jr, Kremers WK, Keach J, Lindor KD: Ursodeoxycholic acid as a chemopreventive agent in patients with ulcerative colitis and primary sclerosing cholangitis. Gastroenterology 2003;124:889–893.

162. Lynch HT, Harris RE, Lynch PM, Guirgis HA, Lynch JF, Bardawil WA: Role of heredity in multiple primary cancer. Cancer 1977;40: 1849–1854.

163. Mecklin JP, Jarvinen HJ: Clinical features of colorectal carcinoma in cancer family syndrome. Dis Colon Rectum 1986;29: 160–164.

164. Rodriguez-Bigas MA, Vasen HF, Pekka-Mecklin J, et al: Rectal cancer risk in hereditary nonpolyposis colorectal cancer after abdominal colectomy. International Collaborative Group on HNPCC. Ann Surg 1997;225:202–207.

165. Mills SJ, Chapman PD, Burn J, Gunn A: Endoscopic screening and surgery for familial adenomatous polyposis: Dangerous delays. Br J Surg 1997;84:74–77.

166. Rhodes M, Bradburn DM: Overview of screening and management of familial adenomatous polyposis. Gut 1992;33:125–131.

167. Nugent KP, Phillips RK: Rectal cancer risk in older patients with familial adenomatous polyposis and an ileorectal anastomosis: a cause for concern. Br J Surg 1992;79:1204–1206.

168. Jagelman DG: Ileorectal anastomosis—familial adenomatous polyposis. Hepatogastroenterology 1991;38:535–537.

169. Skinner MA, Tyler D, Branum GD, Cucchiaro G, Branum MA, Meyers WC: Subtotal colectomy for familial polyposis. A clinical series and review of the literature. Arch Surg 1990;125:621–624.

170. Dayton MT, Faught WE, Becker JM, Burt R: Superior results of ileoanal pull through (IAPT) in polyposis coli vs ulcerative colitis patients. J Surg Res 1992;52:131–134.

171. Hrabovsky EE, Watne AL, Carrier JM: Changing management in familial polyposis. Role of ileoanal endorectal pull-through. Am J Surg 1984;147:130–133.

172. van Coevorden F, Mathus-Vliegen EM, Brummelkamp WH: Combined endoscopic and surgical treatment in Peutz-Jeghers syndrome. Surg Gynecol Obstet 1986;162:426–428.

173. O'Riordan DS, O'Dwyer PJ, Cullen AF, McDermott EW, Murphy JJ: Familial juvenile polyposis coli and colorectal cancer. Cancer 1991;68:889–892.

174. Longo WE, Touloukian RJ, West AB, Ballantyne GH: Malignant potential of juvenile polyposis coli. Report of a case and review of the literature. Dis Colon Rectum 1990;33:980–984.

175. Jarvinen H, Franssila KO: Familial juvenile polyposis coli: Increased risk of colorectal cancer. Gut 1984; 25:792–800.

176. Grosfeld JL, West KW: Generalized juvenile polyposis coli. Clinical management based on long-term observations. Arch Surg 1986;121:530–530.

177. Golladay ES: Diffuse juvenile polyposis: Management by ileoendorectal pull-through. South Med J 1988;81:1571–1573.

178. Fenlon HM, Nunes DP, Schroy PC III, et al: A comparison of virtual and conventional colonoscopy for the detection of colorectal polyps. N Engl J Med 1999;341(20):1496–1503.

179. Pappalardo G, Polettini E, Frattaroli FM, et al: Magnetic resonance colonography versus conventional colonoscopy for detection of colonic endoluminal lesions. Gastroenterology 2000;119(2): 300–304.

180. Ott DJ, Chen YM, Glefand DW, Wu WC, Munitz HA: Single contrast vs double contrast barium enema in detection of colonic polyps. Am J Roentgenol 1986;146(5):993–996.

181. Winawer SJ, Stewart ET, Zauber AG, et al: A comparison of colonoscopy and double-contrast barium enema for surveillance after polypectomy N Engl J Med 2000;342(24):766–772.

182. Wernecke K, Rummeny E, Bongartz G, et al. Detection of hepatic masses in patients with carcinoma: Comparative sensitivities of sonography, CT, and MR imaging. Am J Roentgenol 1991;157(4): 731–739.

183. Kinkel K, Lu Y, Both M, Warren RS, Thoeni RF: Detection of hepatic metastases from cancers of the gastrointestinal tract by using noninvasive imaging methods (US, CT, MR imaging, PET): A meta-analysis. Radiology 2002;224(3):748–756.

184. Kliewer MA, Sheafor DH, Paulson EK, Helsper RS, Hertzberg BS, Nelson RC: Percutaneous liver biopsy: A cost-benefit analysis comparing sonographic and CT guidance. Am J Roentgenol 1999;173(5):1199–1202.

185. Sheafor DH, Paulson EK, Simmons CM, DeLong DM, Nelson RC: Abdominal percutaneous interventional procedures: Comparison of CT and US guidance. Radiology 1998;207(3):705–710.

186. Yu J, Zhong S: Intraoperative ultrasound for hepatic neoplasm during surgery. Chin Med Sci J 1999;14(3):170–173.

187. Staren ED, Gambla M, Deziel DJ, et al: Intraoperative ultrasound in the management of liver neoplasms. Am Surg 1997;63(7):591–596.

188. Kane RA, Hughes LA, Cua EJ, Steele GD, Jenkins RL, Cady B: The impact of intraoperative ultrasonography on surgery for liver neoplasms. J Ultrasound Med 1994;13(1):1–6.

189. Cozzi PJ, McCall L, Jorgensen JO, Morris DL: Laparoscopy vs open ultrasound of the liver: An in vitro study. HPB Surgery 1996;10: 87–89.

190. Takahashi S, Murakami T, Takamura M, et al: Multi-detector row helical CT angiography of hepatic vessels: Depiction with dual-arterial phase acquisition during single breath hold. Radiology 2002;222:81–88.

191. Kamel IR, Choti MA, Horton KM, et al: Surgically staged focal liver lesions: Accuracy and reproducibility of dual-phase helical CT for detection and characterization. Radiology 2003;227(3):752–757.

192. Valls C, Andía E, Sánchez A, et al: Hepatic metastases from colorectal cancer: Preoperative detection and assessment of resectability with helical CT. Radiology 2001;218:55–60.

193. Bluemke DA, Paulson EK, Choti MA, DeSena S, Clavien PA: Detection of hepatic lesions in candidates for surgery: Comparison of ferumoxides-enhanced MR imaging and dual-phase helical CT. AJR Am J Roentgen 2000;175(6):1653–1658.

194. Oudkerk M, Torres CG, Song B, et al. Characterization of liver lesions with mangafodipir trisodium–enhanced MR imaging: Multicenter study comparing MR and dual-phase spiral CT. Radiology 2002;223:517–524.

195. Low RN, Chen SC, Baron R: Distinguishing benign from malignant bowel obstruction in patients with malignancy: Findings at MR imaging. Radiology 2003;228(1):157–165.

196. Semelka RC, Helmberger TK: Contrast agents for MR imaging of the liver. Radiology 2001;218(1):27–38.

197. Tanaka T, Kawai Y, Kanai M, Taki Y, Nakamoto Y, Takabayashi A: Usefulness of FDG-positron emission tomography in diagnosing peritoneal recurrence of colorectal cancer. Am J Surg 2002; 184(5):433–436.

198. Delbeke D, Vitola JV, Sandler MP, et al: Staging recurrent metastatic colorectal carcinoma with PET. J Nucl Med 1997;38: 1196–1201.

199. Bar-Shalom R, Yefremov N, Guralnik L, et al: Clinical performance of PET/CT in evaluation of cancer: Additional value for diagnostic imaging and patient management. J Nucl Med 2003;44(8): 1200–1209.

200. Huebner RH, Park KC, Shepherd JE, et al: A meta-analysis of the literature for whole-body FDG PET detection of recurrent colorectal cancer. J Nucl Med 2000;41:1177–1189.

201. Desai DC, Zervos EE, Arnold MW, Burak WE Jr, Mantil J, Martin EW Jr: Positron emission tomography affects surgical management in recurrent colorectal cancer patients. Annal Surg Oncol 2003;10(1):59–64.

202. Paulson EK: Evaluation of the liver for metastatic disease. Semin Liver Dis 2001;21(2):225–236.

203. Merrie AE, van Rij AM, Dennett ER, Phillips LV, Yun K, McCall JL: Prognostic significance of occult metastases in colon cancer. Dis Colon Rectum 2003;46:221–31.

204. Fisher ER, Colangelo L, Wieand S, Fisher B, Wolmark N: Lack of influence of cytokeratin-positive mini micrometastases in "Negative Node" patients with colorectal cancer: Findings from the National Surgical Adjuvant Breast and Bowel Projects protocols R-01 and C-01. Dis Colon Rectum 2003;46:1021–1026.

205. Grinnell RS: The grade and prognosis of carcinoma of the colon and rectum. Ann Surg 1939;109:560.

206. Rosai J: Ackerman's Surgical Pathology, 8th ed. St Louis, MO, Mosby, 1996, pp 754–799.

207. Loy TS, Calaluce RD: Utility of cytokeratine immunostaining in separating pulmondary adenocarcinomas from colonic adenocarcinomas. Amer J Clin Pathol 1994;102:764–767.

208. O'Brien MJ, Zamcheck N, Burke B, et.al: Immunocytochemical localization of carcinoembryonic antigen in benign and malignant colo-rectal tissues. Assessment of diagnostic value. Amer J Clin Pathol 1981;75:283–290.

209. Listrom MB, Little JV, McKinley M, et al: Immunoreactivity of tumor-associated glycoprotein (TAG-72) in normal hyperplastic and neoplastic colon. Hum Pathol 1989;20:994–1000.

210. Busuttil RW, Foglia RP, Longmire WP: Treatment of carcinoma of the sigmoid colon and upper rectum. A comparison of local segmental resection and left hemicolectomy. Arch Surg 1977; 112:920.

211. Grinnell RS: Results of ligation of inferior mesenteric artery at the aorta in resections of carcinoma of the descending and sigmoid colon and rectum. Surg Gynecol Obstet 1965;170:1031.

212. Dwight RW, Higgins GA, Keehn RJ: Factors influencing survival after resection in cancer of the colon and rectum. Am J Surg 1969;117:512.

213. Pezim ME, Nicholls RJ: Survival after high or low ligation of the inferior mesenteric artery during curative surgery for rectal cancer. Am J Surg 1984;200:729.

214. Charnely RM, Morris DL, Dennison AR, et al: Detection of colorectal metastases using intraoperative ultrasonography. Br J Surg 1991;78:45.

215. Rafaelson SR, Kronborg O, Larsen C, Fenger C: Intraoperative ultrasounography in detection of hepatic metastases from colorectal cancer. Dis Colon Rectum 1995;38:355.

216. Nagorney DM: Diagnosis of liver metastases in colorectal cancer. World J Surg 1991;15:557.

217. Short note: Risk of extracolonic cancer in familial adenomatous polyposis. Br J Surg 1996;83:1121.

218. Rodriguez-Bigas MA, Mahoney MC, Karakousis CP, Petrelli NJ: Desmoid tumors in patients with familial adenomatous polyposis. Cancer 1994;74:1270.

219. Schwab R, Wessendorft S, Gutcke A, Becker P: Early bursting strength of human colon anastomosis—an in vitro study comparing current anastomosis techniques. Langenbecks Arch Surg 2002;286:507–511.

220. Sales JP, Wind P, Douard R, et al: Blood dissemination of colonic epithelial cells during no-touch surgery for rectosigmoid cancer. Lancet 1999;354:392.

221. Tsuoroda A, Shibusawa M, Kamiyama G, Takata M, Choh H, Kusano M: Iodine absorption after intraoperative bowel irrigation with providone-iodine. Dis Colon Rectum 2000;43:1127–1132.

222. Lechner P, Lind P, Snyder M, Haushohr H: Probe-guided surgery for colorectal cancer. Rec Results Cancer Res 2000;157: 272–280.

223. LeVoyer TE, Sigurdson ER, Hanlon AL, et al: Colon cancer survival is associated with increasing number of lymph nodes analyzed: A secondary survey of intergroup trial INT-0089. J Clin Oncol 2003;21:2912–2919.

224. Ben David Y, Latulippe JF, Younan RJ, et. al: Phase I study on sentinel lymph node mapping in colon cancer: A preliminary report. J Surg Oncol. 2002;79(Suppl 2):81–84.

225. Paramo JC, Summerall J, Wilson C, et.al: Intraoperative sentinel lymph node mapping in patients with colon cancer. Amer J Surg 2001;182:40–43.

226. Fitzgerald TL, Khalifa MA, Al Zahrani M, Law CH, Smith AJ: Ex vivo sentinel lymph node biopsy in colorectal cancer: A feasibility study; J Surg Oncol 2002 80:27–33.

227. Feig BW, Curley S, Lucci A, Hunt KK., et.al: A caution regarding lymphatic mapping in patients with colon cancer. Amer J Surg 2001;182:707–712.

228. Phillips KS, Hittinger R, Fry JS, Fielding LP: Malignant large bowel obstruction. Br J Surg 1985;72:296.

229. Serpell JW, McDermott FT, Katrivessis H, Hughes ESR: Obstructing carcinomas of the colon. Br J Surg 1989;76:965.

230. Passman MA, Pommier RF, Vetto JT: Synchronous colon primaries have the same prognosis as solitary colon cancers. Dis Colon Rectum 1996;39:329.

231. Deans GT, Krukowski ZH, Irwin ST: Malignant obstruction of the left colon. Br J Surg 1994;81:1270.

232. Porter JA, Salvati EP, Rubin RJ, Eisenstat TE: Complications of colostomies. Dis Colon Rectum 1989;32:299.

233. Konishi F, Muto T, Kanazawa K, et al: Intraoperative irrigation and primary resection for obstructing lesions of the left colon. Int J Colorectal Dis 1988;3:204.

234. Poon RTP, Law WL, Chu KW, Wong J: Emergency resection and primary anastomosis for left sided obstructing colorectal carcinoma in the elderly. Br J Surg 1998;85:1539.

235. Nyam DC, Leong AF, Ho YH, Seow-Choen F: Comparison between segmental left and extended right colectomies for obstructing left-sided colonic carcinomas. Dis Colon Rectum 1996;39:1000.

236. Wong SK, Eu KW, Lim SL, et al: Total colectomy removes undetected proximal synchronous lesions in acute left-sided colonic obstruction. Tech Coloproctol 1996;4:87.

237. Sugarbaker PH, Gunderson LL, Wittes RE: Colorectal cancer. In DeVita VT Jr, Hellman S, Rosenberg SA (eds): Cancer Principles and Practices of Oncology, 2nd ed. Philadelphia, JB Lippincott, 1985, p 795.

238. Gall FP, Tonak J, Altendorf A: Multivisceral resections in colorectal cancer. Dis Colon Rectum 1987;30:337.

239. Fujisawa M, Nakamura T, Ohno M, et.al: Surgical management of the urinary tract in patients with locally advanced colorectal cancer. Urology 2002;60:983–987.

240. Wolloch Y, Zer M, Lurie M, et al: Ischemic colitis proximal to obstructing carcinoma of the colon. Am J Protocal 1979;30:17.

241. Slanetz CA Jr: The effect of inadvertent intraoperative perforation on survival and recurrence in colorectal cancer. Dis Colon Rectum 1984;27:792.

242. Gordon MS, Cohen AM: Management of invasive carcinoma in pedunculated colorectal polyps. Oncology 1989;3:99.

243. Netzer P, Forster C, Biral R, et al: Risk factor assessment of endoscopically removed malignant colorectal polyps. Gut 1998;43:669.

244. Haggitt RC, Glotzbach RE, Soffer EE, Wruble LD: Prognostic factors in colorectal carcinoma arising in adenomas: Implications for lesions removed by endoscopic polypectomy. Gastroenterology 1985;82:328–336.

245. Scroggins CR, Mesyaely IM, Blansee CD, et al: Nonoperative management of primary colorectal cancer in patients with stage IV disease. Ann Surg Oncol 1999;6:651.

246. Tebbutt NC, Cattell E, Midgley R, Cunningham D, Kerr D: Systemic treatment of colorectal cancer. Eur J Cancer 2002 38:1000–1015.

247. Spinelli P, Mancini A: Use of self-expanding metal stents for palliation of recto sigmoid cancer. Gastrointest Endosc 2001; 53:203–206.

248. Aviv RI, Shymalan G, Watkinson A, Tibballs J, Ogunbaye G: Radiological palliation of malignant colonic obstruction. Clin Radiol 2002;57:347–351.

249. Dauphine CE, Tan P, Beart RW Jr, Vukasin P, Cohen H, Corman ML: Placement of self-expanding metal stents for acute malignant large bowel obstruction: A collective review with 33 references. Ann Surg Oncol 2002;9:574–579.

250. Sielezneff I, Salle E, Antoine K, et al: Simultaneous bilateral oophorectomy does not improve prognosis of postmenopausal women undergoing colorectal resection for cancer. Dis Colon Rectum 1997;40:1299.

Specific Malignancies

III

251. Young-Fadok TM, Wolff BG, Nivatvongs S, et al: Prophylactic oophorectomy in colorectal carcinoma. Preliminary results of a randomized prospective trial. Dis Colon Rectum 1998;41:277.

252. Jacobs M, Verdaja JC, Goldstein HS: Minimally invasive colon resection (laparoscopic colectomy) Surg Laparosc Endosc 1991;1:11-15.

253. Franklin ME, Ramos R, Rosenthal D, Schuessler W: Laproscopic colonic procedures. World J Surg 1993;17:56.

254. Schwenk W, Bohm B, Muller JM: Postoperative pain and fatigue after laparscopic or conventional colorectal resections a prospective randomized trail. Surg Endosc 1998;12:113-136.

255. Young L, Deane M, Monson JRT, Darzi A: Systemic review of laparoscopic surgery for colorectal malignancy. Surg Endosc 2001;15:1431-1439.

256. Lacy AM, Garcia-Valdccasas JC, Delegando S, et. al: Laparoscopy-assisted colectomy versus open colectomy for treatment of non-metastatic colon cancer: A randomized trial. Lancet 2002;359:2224-2229.

257. Schneider C, Jung A, Reymond MA, et al: Efficacy of surgical measures in preventing port-site recurrences in a porcine model. Surg Endosc 2001:15:121-125.

258. Hazebrook EJ, The Color Study Group: COLOR: A randomized clinical trial comparing laparoscopic and open resection for colon cancer. Surg Endosc 2002;16:948-953.

259. Weeks JC, Nelson H, Gelber S, Sargent D, Schroeder G Clinical Outcome of Surgical Therapy (COST) Study Group. Short-term quality-of-life outcomes following laparoscopic-assisted colectomy vs open colectomy for colon cancer: A randomized trial. JAMA 2002;287:321-328.

260. Rickard MJ, Bokey EL: Laparoscopy for colon cancer—a review with 97 references. Surg Oncol Clin N Am 2001;10:579.

261. Parramore JB, Wei JP, Yeh KA: Colorectal cancer in patients under forty: Presentation and outcome. Am Surg 1998;64:563.

262. Hansen RM, Ryan L, Anderson T, et al: Phase III study of bolus versus infusion fluorouracil with or without cisplatin in advanced colorectal cancer. J Natl Cancer Inst 1996;88:668.

263. Lichtman SM, Mandel F, Hoexter B, et al: Prospective analysis of colorectal carcinoma. Determination of an age-site and stage relationship and the correlation of DNA index with clinico-pathologic parameters. Dis Colon Rectum 1994;37:1286.

264. Simmonds P, Best L, Baughand C, et.al: Surgery for colorectal cancer in elderly patients: A systematic review. Lancet 2000;356:968-974.

265. Daly JM, DeCosse JJ: Complications in surgery of the colon and rectum. Surg Clin N Am 1983;63:1215-1231.

266. Smothers L, Hynan L, Fleming J: Emergency surgery for colon carcinoma. Dis Colon Rectum 2003;46:24-30.

267. Prystowsky JB, Bordage G, Feinglass JM: Patient outcomes for segmental colon resection according to surgeon's training, certification and experience. Surgery 2002;132:663-670.

268. Ko CY, Chang JT, Chaudhry S, Kominski G: Are high-volume surgeons and hospitals the most important predictors of inhospital outcome for colon cancer resection? Surgery 2002;132:268-273.

269. Akwari OE, Dozois RR, Weiland LH, Beahrs OH: Leimosarcoma of the small and large bowel. Cancer 1978;42:1375-1384.

270. Miettinen M, Sarlom-Rikala M, Sobin LH, Lasota J: Gastrointestinal stromal tumors and leiomyosarcomas in the colon: A clinicopathologic, immunohistochemical and molecular genetic study of 44 cases. Am J Surg Pathol 2000;24:1339-1352.

271. DeMettes RP, Lewis JJ, Leung D, et al: Two hundred gastrointestinal stromal tumors: Recurrence patterns and prognostic factors for survival. Ann Surg 2000;231:51-58.

272. Hatch KF, Blanchard DK, Hatch GF III, et al: Tumors of the appendix and colon. World J Surg 2000;24:430-436.

273. Ballantyou GH, Savoca PE, Flannery DT, Ahlman MH, Modlin I: Incidence and mortality of carcinoids of the colon. Data from Connecticut Tumor Registry. Cancer 1992;69:2400-2405.

274. Kumar S, Fend F, Quintanill-Martinez L: Epstein-Barr virus-positive primary gastrointestinal Hodgkins disease: Associated with inflammatory bowel disease and immunosuppression. Am J Surg Path 2000;24:66-73.

275. Breslin NP, Urbasnskis J, Shaffer EA. Mucosa-associate lyphoid tissue (MALT) lyphoma manifesting as multiple lymphomatous polyposis of the gastrointestinal tract. Am J Gastroenterol 1999;94:2540-2545.

276. Kojima M, Nakamura S, Itoh H, et al: Mast cell sarcoma with tissue eosinophilia arising in the ascending colon. Modern Pathol 1999;12:739-743

277. Fukudo T, Kakihara T, Babak K, Yamaki T, Yamaguchi T: Clear cell sarcoma arising in the transverse colon. Pathol Intl 2000;50:412-416.

278. Lyss AP: Appendiceal malignancies. Semin Oncol 1988;15:129-137.

279. Rutledge RH, Alexander JW: Primary appendiceal malignancies: Rare but important. Surgery 1992;111:244-250.

280. McCusker ME, Cote TR, Clegg LX, Sobin LH: Primary malignant neoplasms of the appendix: A population-based study from the surveillance, epidemiology and end-results program, 1978-1998. Cancer 2002;94:3307-3312.

281. Sugarbaker PH, Ronnett BM, Archer A, et al: Pseudomyxcoma peritonei syndrome. Adv Surg 1996;30:233-280.

282. Medich DS, Fazio VW: Hemorrhoids, anal fissure and carcinoma of the colon, rectum, and anus during pregnancy. Surg Clin N Am 1995;75:77-88.

283. Bernstein MA, Madoff RD, Caushaj PF: Colon and rectal cancer in pregnancy. Dis Colon Rectum 1993;36:172-178.

284. Olson RM, Perencevich NP, Malcolm AW, et al: Patterns of recurrence following curative resection of adenocarcinoma of the colon and rectum. Cancer 1980;45:2969.

285. Sugarbaker PH, Gianola FJ, Dwyer A, Neuman NR: A simplified plan for follow-up of patients with colon and rectal cancer supported by prospective studies of laboratory and radiologic test results. Surgery 1987;102:79.

286. Fantini GA, DeCosse JJ: Surveillance strategies after resection of carcinoma of the colon and rectum. Surg Gynecol Obstet 1990;171:267.

287. Makela J, Haukipuro K, Laitinen S, Kairaluoma MI: Surgical treatment of recurrent colorectal cancer. Five-year follow-up. Arch Surg 1989;124:1029.

288. Galandiuk S, Wieand HS, Moertel CG, et al: Patterns of recurrence after curative resection of carcinoma of the colon and rectum. Surg Gynecol Obstet 1992;174:27.

289. D'Angelica M, Brennan MF, Fortner JG, et al: Ninety-six five-year survivors after liver resection for metastatic colorectal cancer. J Am Col Surg 1997;185:554.

290. Jamison R, Donohue JH, Nagorney DM, et al: Hepatic resection of metastatic colorectal cancer results in cure for some patients. Arch Surg 1997;132:505.

291. Goldberg RM, Fleming TR, Tangen CM, et al: Surgery for recurrent colon cancer. Strategies for identifying resectable recurrence and success rates after resection. Ann Inter Med 1998;129:27-35.

292. Meyerhardt JA, Catalano PJ, Haller DG, et al: Influence of body mass index on outcomes and treatment-related toxicity in patients with colon carcinoma. Cancer 2003;98:484-495.

293. Benson AB III, Choti MA, Cohen AM, et al: National Comprehensive Cancer Network: NCCN practice guidelines for colorectal cancer. Oncology 2000 14:203-212.

294. Richard CS, McLeod RS: Follow-up of patients after resection for colorectal cancer: A position paper of the Canadian Society of Surgical Oncology and the Canadian Society of Colon and Rectal Surgeons. Can J Surg 1997;40:90.

295. Moertel CG, Fleming TR, Macdonald JR, et al: An evaluation of the carcinoembryonic antigen (CEA) test for monitoring patients with resected colon cancer. JAMA 1993;270:943.

296. Castells A, Bessa X, Daniels M: Value of postoperative surveillance after radical surgery for colorectal cancer: Results of a cohort study. Dis Col Rectum 1998;41:714.

297. Obrand DI, Gordon PH: Incidence and patterns of recurrence following curative resection for colorectal carcinoma. Dis Colon Rectum 1997;40:15.

298. Benson AB, Desch CE, Flynn PJ, et al: 2000 update of American Society of Clinical Oncology colorectal cancer surveillance guidelines. J Clin Oncol 2000;18:3586-3588.

299. Gold P, Freedman S: Demonstration of tumor-specific antigens in human colonic carcinomata by immunological tolerance and absorption techniques. J Exp Med 1965;121:439.

300. Gold P, Shuster J, Freeman SO: Carcinoembryonic antigen (CEA) in clinical medicine: Historical perspectives, pitfalls, and projections. Cancer 1978;42:1399.

301. Cutait R, Alves V, Lopez L, et al: Restaging of colorectal cancer based on CEA and cytokeratins. Dis Colon Rectum 1991;34:917.

302. Tabuchi Y, Deguchi H, Imanishi K, Saitoh Y: Comparison of carcinoembryonic antigen levels between portal and peripheral blood in patients with colorectal cancer. Correlation with histopathologic variables. Cancer 1987;59:1283.

303. Alexander JC, Silverman NA, Chretien PB: Effect of age and cigarette smoking on carcinoembryonic antigen levels. JAMA 1976;235:1975.

304. Mitchell EP: Role of carcinoembryonic antigen in the management of advanced colorectal cancer. Semin Oncol 1998;25:12.

305. Tate H: Plasma CEA in the post-surgical monitoring of colorectal carcinoma. Br J Cancer 1982;46:323.

306. Hall NR, Finan PJ, Stephenson BM, et al: The role of CA-242 and CEA in surveillance following curative resection for colorectal cancer. Br J Cancer 1994;70:549.

307. McCall JL, Black RB, Rich CA, et al: The value of serum carcinoembryonic antigen in predicting recurrent disease following curative resection of colorectal cancer. Dis Colon Rectum 1994;37:875.

308. Mayer RJ, Garnick MB, Steele GD Jr, Zamcheck N: Carcinoembryonic antigen (CEA) as a monitor of chemotherapy in disseminated colorectal cancer. Cancer 1978;42(Suppl 3):1428.

309. Reithmuller G, Holz E. Schlimok G, et al: Monoclonal antibody therapy for resected Dukes' C colorectal cancer: Seven year outcome of a multicenter randomized trial. J Clin Oncol 1998;16:1788.

310. Tominaga T, Sakabe T, Koyama Y, et al: Prognostic factors for patients with colon or rectal carcinoma treated with resection only. Five-year follow-up report. Cancer 1996;78:403.

311. Stocchi L, Nelson H: Diagnostic and therapeutic applications of monoclonal antibodies in colorectal cancer. Dis Col Rectum 1998;41:232.

312. Saunders TH, Mendes Ribeiro HK, Gleeson FV: New technologies for imaging colorectal cancer: The use of MRI, PET and radioimmunoscintigraphy for primary staging and follow-up. Br Med Bull 2002;64:81–99.

313. Collier BD, Abdel-Nabi H, Doerr RJ, et al: Immunoscintigraphy with In-111-labeled CYT-103 in the management of colorectal cancer. Comparison with CT. Radiology 1992;185:179.

314. Moffat FL Jr, Pinsky CM, Hammershaimb L, et al: Clinical utility of external immunoscintigraphy with the IMMU-4 technetium-99m Fab' antibody fragment in patients undergoing surgery for carcinoma of the colon and rectum: Results of a pivotal, phase III trial. The Immunomedics Study Group. J Clin Oncol 1996;14:2295.

315. Serafini AN, Klein JL, Wolff BG, et al: Radioimmunoscintigraphy of recurrent, metastatic or occult colorectal cancer with technetium 99m-labeled totally human monoclonal antibody 88BV59: Results of pivotal, phase III multicenter studies. J Clin Oncol 1998;16:1777.

316. Flanagan FL, Dehdashti F, Ogunbiyi OA, et al: Utility of FDG-PET for investigating unexplained plasma CEA elevation in patients with colorectal cancer. Ann Surg 1998;27:319.

317. Compton CC, Fielding LP, Burgart LJ, et al: Prognostic factors in colorectal cancer. College of American Pathologists Consensus Statement 1999. Arch Pathol Lab Med 2000;124:979–994.

318. Akbulut H, Altuntas F, Akbulut KG, et al: Prognostic role of serum vascular endothelial growth factor, basic fibroblast growth factor and nitric oxide in patients with colorectal carcinoma. Cytokine 2002;20:184–190.

319. Chin KF, Greenman J, Gardiner E, Kumar H, Topping K, Monson J: Pre-operative serum vascular endothelial growth factor can select patients for adjuvant treatment after curative resection in colorectal cancer. Br J Cancer 2000;83:1425–1431.

320. Watanabe T, Wu TT, Catalano PJ, et al: Molecular predictions of survival after adjuvant chemotherapy for colon cancer. N Engl J Med 2001;344:196–206.

321. Compton CC: Colorectal carcinoma: Diagnostic, prognostic, and molecular features. Mod Pathol 2003;16:376–388.

322. Allegra CJ, Paik S, Colangelo LH, et al: Prognostic value of thymidylate synthase, Ki-67, and p53 in patients with Dukes' B and C colon cancer: A National Cancer Institute-National Surgical Adjuvant Breast and Bowel Project collaborative study; J Clin Oncol 2003;21:241–250.

323. Hashimoto T, Tokuchi Y, Hayashi M, et al: p53 null mutations undetected by immunohistochemical staining predict a poor outcome with early-stage non-small cell lung carcinomas. Cancer Res 1999;59:5572–5577.

324. Logullo AF, de Moura RP, Nonogaki S, et al: A proposal for the integration of immunohistochemical staining and DNA-based techniques for the determination of TP53 mutations in human carcinomas. Diagn Mol Pathol 2000;9:35–40.

325. Magrini R, Bhonde MR, Hanski ML, et al: Cellular effects of CPT-11 on colon carcinoma cells: Dependence on p53 and hMLH1 status. Int J Cancer 2002;101:23–31.

326. Manic S, Gatti L, Carenini N, et al: Mechanisms controlling sensitivity to platinum complexes: Role of p53 and DNA mismatch repair. Curr Cancer Drug Targets 2003;3:21–29.

327. Allegra CJ, Parr AL, Wold LE, et al: Investigation of the prognostic and predictive value of thymidylate synthase, p53, and Ki-67 in patients with locally advanced colon cancer. J Clin Oncol 2002;20:1735–1743.

328. Johnston PG, Fisher ER, Rockette HE, et al: The role of thymidylate synthase expression in prognosis and outcome to adjuvant chemotherapy in patients with rectal cancer. J Clin Oncol 1994;12:2640–2647.

329. Lenz HJ, Danenberg KD, Leichman CG, et al: p53 and thymidylate synthase expression in untreated stage II colon cancer: Associations with recurrence, survival and site. Clin Cancer Res 1998;4:1227–1234.

330. Edler D, Glimelius M, Hallstrom M, et al: Thymidylate synthase expression in colorectal cancer: A prognostic and predictive marker of benefit from adjuvant fluorouracil based chemotherapy. J Clin Oncol 2002;20:1721–1728.

331. Ichikawa Y, Uetake H, Shirota Y, et al: Combination of dihydropyrimidine dehydrogenase and thymidylate synthase gene expressions in primary tumors as predictive parameters for the efficacy of fluoropyrimidine-based chemotherapy for metastatic colorectal cancer. Clin Cancer Res 2003;9:786–791.

332. Johnston PG, Benson AB III, Catalano P, Rao MS, O'Dwyer PJ, Allegra CJ: Thymidylate synthase protein expression in primary colorectal cancer: Lack of correlation with outcome and response to fluorouracil in metastatic disease sites. J Clin Oncol 2003;21:815–819.

333. McLeod HL, Sargent DJ, Marsh S, et al: Pharmacogenetic analysis of systemic toxicity and response after 5-fluorouracil (5FU)/CPT-11, 5FU/oxaliplatin (oxal), or CPT-11/oxal therapy for advanced colorectal cancer (CRC): Results from an intergroup trial. American Society of Clinical Oncology, Thirty-Ninth Annual Meeting; Abstract 1013, 2003.

334. Van Rijnsoever M, Elsaleh H, Joseph D, McCaul K, Iacopetta B: CpG island methylator phenotype is an independent predictor of survival benefit from 5-fluorouracil in stage III colorectal cancer. Clin Cancer Res 2003;9:2898–2903.

335. Grage TB, Moss SE: Adjuvant chemotherapy in cancer of the colon and the rectum: Demonstration of effectiveness of prolonged 5-FU chemotherapy in a prospectively controlled randomized trial. Surg Clin North Am 1981;61:1321.

336. Higgins GA, Dwight RW, Smith JV, et al: Fluorouracil as an adjuvant to surgery in carcinoma of the colon. Arch Surg 1971;102:339.

337. Laurie JA, Moertel CG, Fleming TR, et al: Surgical adjuvant therapy of large bowel carcinoma: An evaluation of levamisole and the combination of levamisole and fluorouracil. J Clin Oncol 1989;7:1447.

338. Moertel CG, Fleming TR, Macdonald JS, et al: Levamisole and fluorouracil for adjuvant therapy of resected colon carcinoma. N Engl J Med 1990;322:352–358.

339. Shrag D, Rifas-Shiman S, Saltz L, et al: Adjuvant chemotherapy use for medicare beneficiaries with stage II colon cancer. J Clin Oncol 2002;20:3999–4005.

340. Moertel CG, Fleming TR, Macdonald JS, et al: Intergroup study of fluorouracil plus levamisole as adjuvant therapy for stage II/Dukes' B2 colon cancer. J Clin Oncol 1995;13:2936–2943.

341. Taal BG, Van Tinteren H, Zoetmulder FA; NACCP group: Adjuvant 5FU plus levamisole in colonic or rectal cancer: Improved survival in stage II and III. Br J Cancer 2001;85:1437–1443.

342. Zaniboni A, Labianca R, Marsoni S, et al: GIVIO-SITAC 01: A randomized trial of adjuvant 5-fluorouracil and folic acid administered to patients with colon carcinomalong term results and evaluation of the indicators of health-related quality of life. Gruppo Italiano Valutazione Interventi in Oncologia. Studio Italiano Terapia Adiuvante Colon. Cancer 1998;82:2135.

343. Vermorken JB, Claessen AM, van Tinteren H, et al: Active specific immunotherapy for stage II and stage III human colon cancer: A randomised trial. Lancet 1999;353:345.

344. Buyse M, Piedbois P: Should Dukes' B patients receive adjuvant therapy? A statistical perspective. Semin Oncol 2001;28(Suppl 1):20–24.

345. Mamounas E, Wieand S, Wolmark N, et al: Comparative efficacy of adjuvant chemotherapy in patients with Dukes' B versus Dukes' C colon cancer: Results from four National Surgical Adjuvant Breast and Bowel Project adjuvant studies (C-01, C-02, C-03, and C-04). J Clin Oncol 1999;17:1349–1355.

346. International Multicentre Pooled Analysis of B2 Colon Cancer Trials (IMPACT B2) Investigators: Efficacy of adjuvant fluorouracil and folinic acid in B2 colon cancer. J Clin Oncol 1999;17:1356–1363.

347. Wolmark N, Rockette H, Fisher B, et al: The benefit of leucovorin-modulated fluorouracil as postoperative adjuvant therapy for primary colon cancer: Results from National Surgical Adjuvant Breast and Bowel Project protocol C-03. J Clin Oncol 1993;11:1879–1887.

348. International Multicentre Pooled Analysis of Colon Cancer Trials (IMPACT) Investigators: Efficacy of adjuvant fluorouracil and folinic acid in colon cancer. Lancet 1995;345:939.

349. Dube S, Heyen F, Jenicek M: Adjuvant chemotherapy in colorectal carcinoma: Results of a meta-analysis. Dis Colon Rectum 1997;40:35–41

350. O'Connell MJ, Mailliard JA, Kahn MJ, et al: Controlled trial of fluorouracil and low-dose leucovorin given for 6 months as postoperative adjuvant therapy for colon cancer. J Clin Oncol 1997;1:246.

351. Wolmark N, Fisher B, Rockette H, et al: Postoperative chemotherapy or BCG for colon cancer: Results from NSABP protocol C-01. J Natl Cancer Inst 188;80:30–36.

352. Wolmark N, Colangelo L, Wieand S: National Surgical Adjuvant Breast and Bowel Project trials in colon cancer. Semin Oncol 2001;28-9-13.

353. International Multicentre Pooled Analysis of Colon Trials (IMPACT) investigators: Efficacy of adjuvant fluorouracil and folinic acid in colon cancer. Lancet 1995;345:939–944.

354. Marsoni S: Efficacy of adjuvant fluorouracil and leucovorin in stage B2 and C colon cancer. International Multicenter Pooled Analysis of Colon Cancer Trials Investigators. Semin Oncol. 2001;28(1 Suppl 1):14–19.

355. Chau I, Cunningham D: Chemotherapy in colorectal cancer: New options and challenges. Br Med Bull 2002;64:159–180.

356. O'Connell MJ, Laurie JA, Kahn M, et al: Prospectively randomized trial of postoperative adjuvant chemotherapy in patients with high-risk colon cancer. J Clin Oncol 1998;16:295.

357. Wolmark N, Rockette H, Mamounas E, et al: Clinical trial to assess the relative efficacy of fluorouracil and leucovorin, fluorouracil and levamisole, and fluorouracil, leucovorin, and levamisole in patients with Dukes' B and C carcinoma of the colon: Results from National Surgical Adjuvant Breast and Bowel Project C-04. J Clin Oncol 1999;17:3553–3559.

358. QUASAR Collaborative Group: Comparison of flourouracil with additional levamisole, higher-dose folinic acid, or both, as adjuvant chemotherapy for colorectal cancer: A randomised trial. Lancet 2000 355:1588–1596.

359. Haller PG, Catalano JS, MacDonald RJ, et al: Fluorouracil (FU), Leucovorin (LV) and levamisone (LEV) adjuvant therapy for colon cancer: Five year final report of INT 0089. Proc Am Soc Clin Oncol 1998;1256a.

360. Andre T, Colin P, Louvet C, et al: Semimonthly versus monthly regimen of fluorouracil and leucovorin administered for 24 or 36 weeks as adjuvant therapy in stage II and III colon cancer: Results of a randomized trial. J Clin Oncol 2003;21:2896–2903.

361. de Gramont A, Banzi M, Navarro M, et al: Oxaliplatin/5-FU/LV in adjuvant colon cancer: Results of the international randomized Mosaic trial. Proc Am Soc Clin Oncol 2003;22:1015a.

362. Saini A, Norman AR, Cunningham D, et al: Twelve weeks of protracted venous infusion of fluorouracil (5-FU) is as effective as 6 months of bolus 5-FU and folinic acid as adjuvant treatment in colorectal cancer. Br J Cancer 2003;88:1859–1865.

363. Rothenberg JL, Meropol NJ, Poplin EA, et al: Mortality associated with irinotecan plus bolus fluoruracil/leucovorin: Summary findings of an independent panel. J Clin Oncol 2001;19:3801–3807.

364. Mahood DJ, Dose AM, Loprinizi CL, et al: Inhibition of 5-fluorouracil induced mucositis by oral cryotherapy. J Clin Oncol 1991;9:449.

365. Kerr D: Capecitabine/irinotecan in colorectal cancer: European early-phase data and planned trials. Oncology 2002;16(Suppl 14):12–15.

366. Willett C, Tepper JE, Cohen A, et al: Local failure following curative resection of colonic adenocarcinoma. Int J Radiat Oncol Biol Phys 1984;10:645–651.

367. Russell AH, Tong D, Dawson LE, et al: Adenocarcinoma of the proximal colon. Sites of initial dissemination and patterns of recurrence following surgery alone. Cancer 1984;53:360–367.

368. Gunderson LL, Sosin H, Levitt S: Extrapelvic colon—areas of failure in a reoperation series: implications for adjuvant therapy. Int J Radiat Oncol Biol Phys 1985;11:731–741.

369. Minsky BD, Mies C, Rich TA, et al: Potentially curative surgery of colon cancer: Patterns of failure and survival. J Clin Oncol 1988;6:106–118.

370. Willett CG, Fung CY, Kaufman DS, et al: Postoperative radiation therapy for high-risk colon carcinoma. J Clin Oncol 1993;11:1112–1127.

371. Welch JP, Donaldson GA: The clinical correlation of an autopsy study of recurrent colorectal cancer. Ann Surg 1979;189:496–502.

372. Kopelson G: Adjuvant postoperative radiation therapy for colorectal carcinoma above the peritoneal reflection. II. Antimesenteric wall ascending and descending colon and cecum. Cancer 1983;52:633–636.

373. Kopelson G: Adjuvant postoperative radiation therapy for colorectal carcinoma above the peritoneal reflection. I. Sigmoid colon. Cancer 1983;51:1593–1598.

374. Brenner HJ, Bibi C, Chaitchik S: Adjuvant therapy for Dukes C adenocarcinoma of colon. Int J Radiat Oncol Biol Phys 1983;9:1789–1792.

375. Shehata WM, Meyer RL, Jazy FK, et al: Regional adjuvant irradiation for adenocarcinoma of the cecum. Int J Radiat Oncol Biol Phys 1987;13:843–846.

376. Amos EH, Mendenhall WM, McCarty PJ, et al: Postoperative radiotherapy for locally advanced colon cancer. Ann Surg Oncol 1996;3:431–436.

377. Schild SE, Gunderson LL, Haddock MG, et al: The treatment of locally advanced colon cancer. Int J Radiat Oncol Biol Phys 1997;37:51–58.

378. Willett CG, Goldberg S, Shellito PC, et al: Does postoperative irradiation play a role in the adjuvant therapy of stage T4 colon cancer? Cancer J Sci Am 1999;5:242–247.

379. Martenson J, Willett CG, Sargent D, et al: A phase III study of adjuvant radiation therapy (RT), 5-flourouracil (5-FU), and Levamisole (LEV) vs 5-FU and LEV in selected patients with resected high risk colon cancer: Initial results of Int 0130. J Clin Oncol 1999;18:235a.

380. Group GTSG: Adjuvant therapy with hepatic irradiation plus fluorouracil in colon carcinoma. The Gastrointestinal Tumor Study Group. Int J Radiat Oncol Biol Phys 1991;21:1151–1156.

381. Estes NC, Giri S, Fabian C: Patterns of recurrence for advanced colon cancer modified by whole abdominal radiation and chemotherapy. Am Surg 1996;62:546–550.

382. Jemal A, Murray T, Samuels A, et al: Cancer statistics 2003. CA Cancer J Clin 2003;53:5–26.

383. Parkin DM, Bray F, Ferlay J, et al: Estimating the world cancer burden: Globocan 2000. Int J Cancer 2000;94:153–156.

384. Poon MA, O'Connell MJ, Moertel CG, et al: Biochemical modulation of fluorouracil: Evidence of significant improvement of survival and quality of life in patients with advanced colorectal carcinoma. J Clin Oncol 1989;7:1407–1418.

385. Machover D, Goldschmidt E, Chollet P, et al: Treatment of advanced colorectal and gastric carcinomas with 5-FU and high-dose folinic acid. J Clin Oncol 1986;4:685–696.

386. Petrelli N, Douglas HO, Herrera L, et al: The modulation of fluorouracil with leucovorin in metastatic colorectal carcinoma: A prospective randomized phase III trial. J Clin Oncol 1989;7:1419–1426.

387. Diaz-Rubio E, Aranda E, Matin M, et al: Weekly high-dose infusion of 5-fluorouracil in advanced colorectal cancer. Eur J Cancer 1990;26:727–729.

388. Kohne CH, Wilke PH, et al: Effective biochemical modulation by leucovorin of high-dose infusion fluorouracil given as a weekly 24-hour infusion: Results of a randomized trial in patients with advanced colorectal cancer. J Clin Oncol 1998;16:418–426.

389. Erlichman C, Fine S, Wong A, et al: The modulation of fluorouracil with leucovorin in metatstatic colorectal carcinoma: A prospective randomized phase III trial. J Clin Oncol 1989;7:1419–1426.

390. Cunningham D, Glimelius B: A phase III study of irinotecan (CPT-11) versus best supportive care in patients with metastatic colorectal cancer who have failed 5-fluorouracil therapy. V301 Study Group. Semin Oncol 1999;26(Suppl 5):6–12.

391. Goldberg RM, Sargent DJ, Morton RF, et al: A randomized controlled trial of fluorouracil plus leucovorin, irinotecan, and oxaliplatin combinations in patients with previously untreated metastatic colorectal cancer. J Clin Oncol 2004;22:23–30.

392. Hurwitz H, Fehrenbacher L, Cartwright T, et al: A Phase III trial of Bevacizumab (Avastin) in combination with bolus IFL (Irnotecan, 5-FU, Leucovorin) as first-line therapy in subjects with metastatic CRC: Efficacy results in arm 3 (5-FU/LV/BV) and other exploratory analyses [Abstract 2646]. Proc ASCO 2003.

393. Heidelberger CG, Chandari NK, Dannenberg P, et al: Fluorinated pyrimidines: A new class of tumor inhibitory compounds. Nature 1969;179:665.

394. Ansfield F, Klotz J, Nealon T, et al: A Phase III study comparing the clinical utility of four regimens of fluorouracil. Cancer 1977;39:34.

395. Scheithauer V, Rosen H, Kornek G-V, et al: Randomized comparison of combination chemotherapy plus supportive care with supportive care alone in patients with metastatic colorectal cancer. BMJ 1993;306:752.

396. Nordic Gastrointestinal Tumor Adjuvant Therapy Group: Expectancy or primary chemotherapy in patients with advanced asymptomatic colorectal cancer: A randomized trial. J Clin Oncol 1992;10:904.

397. Ullman B, Lee M, Martin DW, Santi DV: Cytotoxicity of 5′fluoro 2′deoxyuridine: Requirement for reduced folate cofactors and antagonism of methotrexate. Proc Natl Acad Sci USA 1978;75:980.

398. Machover D, Schwarzenberg L, Goldschmidt E, et al: Treatment of advanced colorectal and gastric adenocarcinomas with 5-fluorouracil combined with high dose folinic acid: A pilot study. Cancer Treat Rep 1982;66:1803.

399. Lokich JJ, Moore C: Chemotherapy associated palmar-plantar erythrodysesthesia syndrome. Ann Intern Med 1984;101:798.

400. Lokich JJ, Ahlgren JD, Gullo JJ, et al: A prospective randomized comparison of continuous infusion fluorouracil with a conventional bolus schedule in metastatic colorectal carcinoma. A Mid-Atlantic Oncology Program study. J Clin Oncol 1989;7:425.

401. de Gramont A, Bosset JF, Milan C, et al: Randomized trial comparing monthly low-dose leucovorin and fluorouracil bolus with bimonthly high-dose leucovorin and fluorouracil bolus plus continuous infusion for advanced colorectal cancer: A French Intergroup study. J Clin Oncol 1997;15:808.

402. Rougier P, Paillot B, LaPlance A, et al: 5-fluorouracil continuous intravenous infusion compared with bolus administration. Final results of a randomised trial in metastatic colorectal cancer. Eur J Cancer 1997;33:1789.

403. de Gramont A, Louvet C, Andre T, et al: A review of GERCOD trials of bimonthly leucovorin plus 5-FU 48-h continuous infusion in advanced colorectal cancer: Evolution of a regimen. Groupe d'Etude et de Rechereche sur les Cancers de l'Ovaire et Digestifs (GERCOD) Eur J Cancer 1998;34:619–626.

404. Meta-analysis Group in Cancer: Efficacy of intravenous continuous infusion of fluorouracil compared with bolus administration in advanced colorectal cancer. J Clin Oncol 1998;6:301–308.

405. Hillcoat BL, McCullock PB, Figuerado AT, et al: Clinical response and plasma levels of 5-fluorouracil in patients with colon cancer treated by drug infusion. Br J Cancer 1978;38:719.

406. Milano G, Etienne MC, Renée N, et al: Relationship between fluorouracil systemic exposure and tumor response and patient survival. J Clin Oncol 1994;12:1291.

407. Piedbois P, Michiels S for the meta analysis group in cancer: Survival benefits of 5-FU/LV over 5-FU bolus in patients with advanced colorectal cancer. An updated meta-analysis based on 2,751 patients [abstract]. Proc Am Soc Clin Oncol 2003;22:294.

408. Saltz LB, Cox JV, Blanke C, et al: Irinotecan plus fluorouracil and leucovorin for metastatic colorectal cancer. Irinotecan Study Group [comment]. N Engl J Med 2000; 343:905–914.

409. Douillard JY, Cunningham D, Roth AD, et al: Irinotecan combined with fluorouracil compared with fluorouracil alone as first-line treatment for metastatic colorectal cancer. A multicentre randomised trial [erratum appears in Lancet 2000;355:1372]. Lancet 2000;355:1041–1047.

410. Andre T, Bensmaine MA, Louvet C, et al: Multicenter phase II study of bimonthly high-dose leucovorin, fluorouracil infusion, and oxaliplatin for metastatic colorectal cancer resistant to the same leucovorin and fluorouracil regimen. J Clin Oncol 1999;17: 3560–3568.

411. Maindrault-Goebel F, Louvet C, Andre T, et al: Oxaliplatin added to the simplified bimonthly leucovorin and 5-fluorouracil regimen as second-line therapy for metastatic colorectal cancer (FOLFOX6). Eur J Cancer 1999;35:1338–1342.

412. Cheeseman SL, Joel SP, Chester JD, et al: A modified de Gramont regimen of fluorouracil alone and with oxaliplatin, for advanced colorectal cancer. Br J Cancer 2002;87:393–399.

413. Braun MS, Adab F, Bradley C, et al: Modified de Gramont with oxaliplatin in the first-line treatment of advanced colorectal cancer. Br J Cancer 2003;89:1155–1158.

414. Maindrault-Goebel F, de Gramont A, Louvet C, et al: High-dose intensity oxaliplatin added to the simplified bimonthly leucovorin and 5-fluorouracil regimen as second-line therapy for metastatic colorectal cancer (FOLFOX7). Eur J Cancer 2001;37: 1000–1005.

415. Keubler JP, de Gramont A: Recent experience with oxaliplatin or irinotecan combined with 5-fluorouracil and leucovorin in the treatment of colorectal cancer. Semin Oncol 2003;30(Suppl 15): 40–46.

416. Zeuli M, Nardoni C, Pino, MS, et al: Phase II study of capecitabine and oxaliplatin as first-line treatment in advanced colorectal cancer. Ann Oncol 2003;14:1378–1382.

417. Scheithauer W, Kornek GV, Raderer M, et al: Randomized multicenter phase II trial of two different schedules of capecitabine plus oxaliplatin as first-line treatment in advanced colorectal cancer. J Clin Oncol 2003;21:1307–1312.

418. Sumpter K, Harper-Wynne C, Cunningham D: Oxaliplatin and capecitabine chemotherapy for advanced colorectal cancer: A single institution's experience. Clin Oncol 2003;15:221–226.

419. Borner MM, Dietrich D, Stupp R, et al: Phase II study of capecitabine and oxaliplatin in first- and second-line treatment of advanced or metastatic colorectal cancer. J Clin Oncol 2002;20: 1759–1766.

420. Meta-analysis Group in Cancer: Toxicity of fluorouracil in patients with advanced colorectal cancer: Effect of administration schedule and prognostic factors. J Clin Oncol 1998;16: 3537–3541.

421. Becouarn Y, Brunet RC, Rouhier ML, et al: High dose folinic acid and 5-fluorouracil bolus and continuous infusion for patients with advanced colorectal cancer. Cancer 1995;76:1126.

422. Beerblock K, Rinaldi Y, Andre T, et al: Bimonthly high dose leucovorin and 5-fluorouracil 48 hour continuous infusion in patients with advanced colorectal cancer. Groupe d'Etude et de Recherce sur les Cancers de l'Ovaire dt Digestifs (GERCOD) Cancer 1997;79:1100.

423. de Gramont A, Louvet C, Bennamoun M, et al: Dual modulation of 5-fluorouracil with folinic acid and hydroxyurea in metastatic colorectal cancer. J Infus Chemother 1996;6:97.

424. Pitot HC, Wener DB, O'Connell MJ, et al: Phase II trial of irinotecan I patients with metastatic colorectal carcinoma. J Clin Oncol 1997;15:2910.

425. Rougier P, Bugat R: CPT-11 in the treatment of colorectal cancer: clinical efficacy and safety profile. Semin Oncol 1996;23(Suppl 3): 34.

426. Benson AB III, Goldberg RM: Optimal use of the combination of irinotecan and 5-fluorouracil. Semin Oncol 2003;30(Suppl 6): 68–77.

427. Rothenberg ML, Oza AM, Bigelow RH, et al: Superiority of oxaliplatin and fluorouracil-lucovorin complared with either therapy alone in patients with progressive colorectal cancer after irinotecan and fluorouracil-leucovorin: Interim results of a phase III trial. J Clin Oncol 2003;21:2059–2069.

428. Rougier P, Van Cutsem E, Bajetta E, et al: Randomized trial of irinotecan versus fluorouracil by continuous infusion after fluorouracil failure in patients with metastatic colorectal cancer {see comments}. Lancet 1998;352:1407.

429. Cunningham D, Pyrhonen S, James RD, et al: Randomized trial of irinotecan plus supportive care versus supportive care alone after fluorouracil failure for patients with metastatic colorectal cancer {see comments}. Lancet 1998;352:1413.

430. Comella P, Casaretti R, De Vita F, et al: Concurrent irinotecan and 5-fluorouracil plus levo-folinic acid given every other week in the first-line management of advanced colorectal carcinoma: A phase I study of the Southern Italy Cooperative Oncology Group. Ann Oncol 1999;10:915–921.

431. Bulusu VR: Irinotecan and 5-fluorouracil in colorectal cancer. Time for a pause. Eur J Cancer 1998;34:286–289.

432. Miller L, Emanuel D, Elfring G, et al: 60-day all cause mortality with first line irinotecan/fluorouracil/leucovorin (IFL) or fluorouracil/leucovorin (FL) for metastatic colorectal cancer [Abstract 515]. Proc Am Soc Clin Oncol 2002;21:129a.

433. Hansen RM, Ryan L Anderson T, et al: Phase III study of bolus versus infusional fluorouracil with or without cisplatin on advanced colorectal cancer. J Natl Cancer Inst 1996;88:668–674.

434. Raymond E, Chaney SG, Taama A, et al: Oxaliplatin: A review of preclinical and clinical studies. Ann Oncol 1998;9:1053–1071.

435. Goldberg R.: Oxaliplatin in colorectal cancer: Current studies [review]. Oncology 2000;14(Suppl 11):42–47.

436. Saris CP, van de Vaart PJ, Rietbroek RC, et al: In vitro formation of DNA adducts by cisplatin, lobaplatin and OXAL in calf thymus DNA in solution and in cultured human cells. Carcinogenesis 1996;17:2763–2769.

437. Woynarowski JM, Chapman WG, Napier C, et al: Sequence and region-specificity of OXAL adducts in naked and cellular DNA. Mol Pharmacol 1998;54:770–777.

438. Machover D, Diaz-Rubio E, deGramont A, et al: Two consecutive phase II studies of oxaliplatin (L-OHP) for treatment of patients with advanced colorectal carcinoma who were resistant to previous treatment with fluoropyrimidines. Ann Oncol 1996;7:95.

439. Levi F, Perpoint B, Garufi C, et al: OXAL activity against metastatic colorectal cancer. A phase II study of 5-day continuous venous infusion at circadian rhythm modulated rate. Eur J Cancer 1993;29A:1280–1284.

440. Diaz-Rubio E, Sastre J, Zaniboni A, et al: Oxaliplatin as single agent in previously untreated colorectal carcinoma patients: A phase II multicentric study. Ann Oncol 1998;9:105–108.

441. Becouran Y, Ychou M, Ducreux M, et al: Phase II trial of oxaliplatin as first-line chemotherapy in metastatic colorectal cancer patients. J Clin Oncol 1998;16:2739–2744.

442. Gerard B, Bleiberg H, Van Daele D, et al: Oxaliplatin combined to 5-fluorouracil and folinic acid: An effective therapy in patients with advanced colorectal cancer. Anticancer Drugs 1998;9:301.

443. Ducreux M, Louvet C, Bekradda M, Cvitkovic E: Oxaliplatin for the treatment of advanced colorectal cancer: Future directions [review]. Semin Oncol 1998;25:47.

444. Bleiberg H, de Gramont A: Oxaliplatin plus 5-fluorouracil: Clinical experience in patients with advanced colorectal cancer. Semin Oncol 1998;25(Suppl 5):32.

445. de Gramont A, Figer A, Seymour M, et al: Leucovorin and fluorouracil with or without oxaliplatin as first-line treatment in advanced colorectal cancer. J Clin Oncol 2000;18:2938–2947.

446. Giacchetti S, Perpoint B, Zidani, R: Phase III multicenter randomized trial of oxaliplatin added to chronomodulated fluorouracil-leucovorin as first-line treatment of metastatic colorectal cancer. J Clin Oncol 2000;18:136–147.

447. Kuebler JP, de Gramont A: Recent experience with oxaliplatin or irinotecan combined with 5-fluorouracil and leucovorin in the treatment of colorectal cancer. Semin Oncol 2003;30(Suppl 15): 40–46.

448. Braun MS, Adab F, Bradley C, et al: Modified de Gramont with oxaliplatin in the first-line treatment of advanced colorectal cancer. Br J Cancer 2003;89:1155–1158.

449. Maindrault-Goebel F, de Gramont A, Louvet C, et al: High-dose intensity oxaliplatin added to the simplified bimonthly leucovorin and 5-fluorouracil regimen as second-line therapy for metastatic colorectal cancer (FOLFOX7). Eur J Cancer 2001;37:1000–1005.

450. Gamelin E, Gamelin L, Bossi L, et al: Clinical aspects and molecular basis of oxaliplatin neurotoxicity: Current management and development of preventive measures. Semin Oncol 2002;29: 21–33.

451. Grothey A: Oxaliplatin safety profile: Neurotoxicity. Semin Oncol 2003;30(Suppl 15):5–13.

452. Schilsky RL, Levin J, West WH, et al: Randomized, open-label, phase III study of a 28-day oral regimen of eniluracil plus fluorouracil versus intravenous fluorouracil plus leucovorin as first-line therapy in patients with metastatic/advanced colorectal cancer. J Clin Oncol 2002;20:1519–1526.

453. Carmichael J, Popiela T, Radstone D, et al: Randomized comparative study of tegafur/uracil and oral leucovorin versus parenteral fluorouracil and leucovorin in patients with previously untreated metastatic colorectal cancer.[comment]. J Clin Oncol 2002;20:3617–3627.

454. Douillard JY, Hoff PM, Skillings JR, et al: Multicenter phase III study of uracil/tegafur and oral leucovorin versus fluorouracil and leucovorin in patients with previously untreated metastatic colorectal cancer [comment]. J Clin Oncol 2002;20:3605–3616.

455. Hoff PM, Saad ED, Ajani JA, et al: Phase I study with pharmacokinetics of S-1 on an oral daily schedule for 28 days in patients with solid tumors. Clin Cancer Res 2003;9:134–142.

456. Wagstaff AJ, Ibbotson T, Goa KL: Capecitabine: A review of its pharmacology and therapeutic efficacy in the management of advanced breast cancer. Drugs 2003;63;217–236.

457. Schuller J, Cassidy J, Dumont E, et al: Preferential activation of capecitabine in tumor following oral administration to colorectal cancer patients. Cancer Chemother Pharmacol 200;45:291–297.

458. Ishikawa T, Utoh M, Sawada N, et al: Tumor selective delivery of 5-fluorouracil by capecitabine, a new oral fluoropyrimidine carbamate, in human cancer xenografts. Biochem Pharmacol 1998;55:1091.

459. Van Cutsem E, Twelves C, Cassidy J, et al: Oral capecitabine compared with intravenous fluorouracil plus leucovorin in patients with metastatic colorectal cancer: Results of a large phase III study. J Clin Oncol 2001;19:4097–4106.

460. Twelves C, Xeloda Colorectal Cancer Group: Capecitabine as first-line treatment in colorectal cancer. Pooled data from two large, phase III trials. Eur J Cancer 2002;38(Suppl2):15–20.

461. Hoff PM, Ansari R, Batist G: Comparison of oral capecitabine versus intravenous fluorouracil as first-line treatment in 605 patients with metastatic colorectal cancer. J Clin Oncol 2001;19:2282–2292.

462. Cassidy J, Twelves C, Van Cutsem E, et al: Capecitabine Colorectal Cancer Study Group: First-line oral capecitabine therapy in metastatic colorectal cancer: A favorable safety profile compared with intravenous 5-fluorouracil/leucovorin. Ann Oncol 2002;13:566–575.

463. Diasio RB: Improving 5-FU with a novel dihydropyrimidine dehydrogenase inactivator. Oncology 1998;12(Suppl4):51.

464. Shirasaka T, Nakano K, Takechi T, et al: Antitumor activity of 1 M tegafur-0.4 M 5-chloro-2,4,-dihydroxypyridine-1 M potassium oxonate (S-1) against human colon carcinoma orthotopically implanted into nude rats. Cancer Res 1996;56:2602.

465. Tsunoda A, Shibusawa M, Tsunoda Y, et al: Antitumor effect of S-1 on DMH colon cancer in rats. Anticancer Res 1998;18: 1137.

466. Carmichael J, Popiela T, Radstone D, et al: Randomized comparative study of tegafur/uracil and oral leucovorin versus parenteral fluorouracil and leucovorin in patients with previously untreated metastatic colorectal cancer [comment]. J Clin Oncol 2002;20:3617-362

467. Douillard JY, Hoff PM, Skillings JR, et al: Multicenter phase III study of uracil/tegafur and oral leucovorin versus fluorouracil and leucovorin in patients with previously untreated metastatic colorectal cancer [comment]. J Clin Oncol 2002;20:3605–3616.

468. Marsh JC, Catalano P, Huang J, et al: Eastern Cooperative Oncology Group phase II trial (E4296) of oral 5-fluorouracil and eniluracil as a 28-day regimen in metastatic colorectal cancer [comment].Clin Colorectal Cancer 2002;2:43–50.

469. Leichman CG, Chansky K, MacDonald JS, et al: Biochemical modulation of 5-fluorouracil through dihydropyrimidine dehydrogenase inhibition: A Southwest Oncology Group phase II trial of eniluracil and 5-fluorouracil in advanced resistant colorectal cancer. Invest New Drugs 2002;20:419–424.

470. Schilsky RL, Levin J, West WH, et al: Randomized, open-label, phase III study of a 28-day oral regimen of eniluracil plus fluorouracil versus intravenous fluorouracil plus leucovorin as first-line therapy in patients with metastatic/advanced colorectal cancer. J Clin Oncol 2002;20:1519–1526.

471. Maroun J, Asche C, Romeyer F, et al: A cost comparison of oral tegafur plus uracil/folinic acid and parenteral fluorouracil for colorectal cancer in Canada. Pharmacoeconomics 2003;21: 1039–1051.

472. Van Cutsem E: Raltitrexed (Tomudex) in combination treatment for colorectal cancer: New perspectives. Eur J Cancer 1999;35(Suppl 1):1–2.

473. Zalcberg JR, Cunningham D, Van Cutsem E, et al: ZD1694: A novel thymidylate synthase inhibitor with substantial activity in the treated of patients with advanced colorectal cancer. Tomudex Colorectal Study Group. J Clin Oncol 1996;14:716.

474. Cunningham D: Mature results from three large controlled studies with raltitrexed ('Tomudex'). Br J Cancer 1998;77(Suppl2):15.

475. Gunasekara NS, Faulds D: Raltitrexed. A review of its pharmacologic properties and clinical efficacy in the management of advanced colorectal cancer. Drugs 1998;555:423.

476. Cunningham D, Zalcberg J, Maroun J, et al: Efficacy, tolerability and management of raltitrexed (Tomudex) monotherapy in patients with advanced colorectal cancer: A revier of phase II/III trials. Eur J Cancer 2002;38:478–486.

477. Maughan TS, James RD, Kerr DJ, et al: Comparison of survival, palliation, and quality of life with three chemotherapy regimens in metastatic colorectal cancer: A multicentre randomized trial [comment]. Lancet 2002;359:1555–1563.

478. Jackman AL, Kimbell R, Ford HE: Combination of raltitrexed with other cytotoxic agents: Rationale and preclinical observations. Eur J Cancer 1999;35(Suppl 1):S3–8.

479. Farrugia DC, Ford HE, Cunningham D, et al: Thymidylate synthase expression in advanced colorectal cancer predicts for response to raltitrexed. Clin Cancer Res 2003;9:792–801.

480. Shih C, Chen VJ, Gossett LS, et al: LY231514, a pyrrolo[2,3-d]pyrimidine-based antifolate that inhibits multiple folate-requiring enzymes. Cancer Res 1997;57:1116–1123.

481. Cripps C, Burnell M, Jolivet J: Phase II study of first-line LY231514 (multi-targeted antifolate) in patients with locally advanced or metastatic colorectal cancer: An NCIC Clinical Trials Group study. Ann Oncol 1999;10:1175–1179.

482. John W, Picus J, Blanke CD, et al: Activity of multitargeted antifolate (pemetrexed disodium, LY231514) in patients with advanced colorectal carcinoma: results from a phase II study. Cancer. 2000;88:1807–1813.

483. Hochster H: The role of pemetrexed in the treatment of colorectal cancer [review]. Semin Oncol. 2002;29(6 Suppl 18):54–56.

484. Mendelsohn J, Baselga J: Status of epidermal growth factor receptor antagonists in the biology and treatment of cancer [review]. J Clin Oncol. 2003;21:2787–2799.

485. Dancey J, Sausville EA: Issues and progress with protein kinase inhibitors for cancer treatment [review]. Nat Rev Drug Discov. 2003;2:296–313.

486. Baselga J: The EGFR as a target for anticancer therapy—focus on cetuximab [review]. Eur J Cancer. 2001;37(Suppl 4):S16–22.

487. Goldstein NI, Prewett M, Zuklys K, Rockwell P, Mendelsohn J: Biological efficacy of a chimeric antibody to the epidermal growth factor receptor in a human tumor xenograft model. Clin Cancer Res. 1995;1:1311–1318.

488. Saltz L, Rubin M, Hochster H, et al: Cetuximab (IMC-C225) plus irinotecan (CPT-11) is active in CPT-11-refractory colorectal cancer (CRC) that expresses epidermal growth factor receptor Proc ASCO 2001;21:504.

489. Saltz L: PROC AACR-NCI-EORTC. J Clin Invest 2001;68:559.

490. Cunningham D, Humblet Y, Siena S, et al: Cetuximab (C225) alone or in combination with irinotecan (CPT-11) in patients with epidermal growth factor receptor (EGFR)-positive, irinotecan-refractory metastatic colorectal cancer (MCRC) [Abstract #1012]. Proc Am Soc Clin Oncol 2003;22:252.

491. Needle MN: Safety experience with IMC-C225, an anti-epidermal growth factor receptor antibody. Semin Oncol 2002;29(5 Suppl 14):55–60.

492. Seymour L, Goss G, Stewart D, et al: A translational research study of ZD1839 at a dose of 750mg in patients with pretreated advanced or metastatic colorectal cancer: NCIC CTG IND.122 [Abstract]. Ann Oncol 2002;13(Suppl. 5), 73.

493. Townsley C, Major P, Siu LL: Phase II study of OSI-774 in patients with metastatic colorectal cancer [Abstract]. Eur J Cancer 2002;38(Suppl 7):179.

494. Kerbel R, Folkman J. Clinical translation of angiogenesis inhibitors. Nat Rev Cancer. 2002;2:727–739.

495. Tokunaga T, Oshika Y, Abe Y, et al: Vascular endothelial growth factor (VEGF) mRNA isoform expression pattern is correlated with liver metastasis and poor prognosis in colon cancer. Br J Cancer 1998;77:998-1002.

496. Kabbinavar F, Hurwitz HI, Fehrenbacher L, et al: Phase II, randomized trial comparing bevacizumab plus fluorouracil (FU)/leucovorin (LV) with FU/LV alone in patients with metastatic colorectal cancer. J Clin Oncol. 2003;21:60–65.

497. Harris JE, Ryan L, Hoover HC Jr, et al: Adjuvant active specific immunotherapy for stage II and III colon cancer with an autologous tumor cell vaccine: Eastern Cooperative Oncology Group Study E5283. J Clin Oncol. 2000;18:148–157.

498. Baars A, Claessen AM, Wagstaff J, et al: A phase II study of active specific immunotherapy and 5-FU/Leucovorin as adjuvant therapy for stage III colon carcinoma. Br J Cancer 2002;86:1230–1234.

499. Vermorken JB, Claessen AM, van Tinteren H, et al: Active specific immunotherapy for stage II and human colon cancer: A randomised trial. Lancet 1999 30;353:345–350.

500. Foon KA, John WJ, Chakraborty M, et al: Clinical and immune responses in resected colon cancer patients treated with anti-idiotype monoclonal antibody vaccine that mimics the carcinoembryonic antigen. J Clin Oncol 1999;17:2889–2895.

Specific Malignancies

III

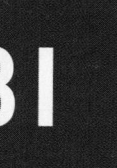
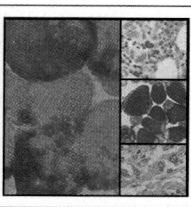

81 — CANCER OF THE RECTUM

William F. Regine

Nader Hanna

Philip DeSimone

Alfred M. Cohen

SUMMARY OF KEY POINTS

INCIDENCE

- The incidence of rectal cancer in the United States is 44 cases per 100,000 population for a total number of new cases annually of approximately 34,000.
- Since 1985, the incidence rate has been decreasing by 1.6% per year.
- The peak incidence of rectal cancer is during the fifth decade of life.
- Blacks have a 7% to 10% higher mortality rate from rectal cancer than whites.

CLINICAL PRESENTATION

Numerous clinical features suggest the presence of rectal cancer:

- Located approximately 12 cm from the anal verge
- Rectal bleeding, often bright red and on the surface of the stool
- Subtle changes in bowel habits
- Decreased caliber of stool; mucus in stool
- Sensation of fullness and tenesmus
- Increased straining during defecation
- Synchronous colon cancer (in 2% to 9% of patients with rectal cancer)

STAGING AND ASSESSMENT

- Careful rectal examination yields 67% to 84% accuracy in staging and should include pelvic examination for women and prostate examination in men.
- Rigid proctosigmoidoscopy provides the most accurate assessment of

distance, size, and position as well as tethering to surrounding structures.

- Colonoscopy or double-contrast barium enemas are used to assess anal sphincter function.
- Endorectal ultrasound can assess depth of invasion, nodal status, and malignant nodes.
- Magnetic resonance imaging (MRI) with endorectal coil is equivalent to ultrasound, and both are more sensitive and accurate than computed tomography alone. MRI is used to assess locally advanced or recurrent local disease. Computed tomography should be performed on all patients, even those with T1 stage disease.
- The liver is the most frequent site of distant spread, followed by lung, retroperitoneum, ovary, and peritoneal cavity.
- Carcinoembryonic antigen levels are often (95%) above 20 ng/mL. Prostate-specific antigen is assessed in men.

DIFFERENTIAL DIAGNOSIS

Differential diagnosis includes the following:

- Kaposi's sarcoma
- Inflammatory mass
- Developmental cysts
- Embryonic tumors (teratomas, chondromas, meningoceles)
- Sacral and presacral tumors (neurogenic tumors, liposarcomas, neurofibromatosis)

TREATMENT

- Goals of treatment are cure, local control, and quality of life.
- All retrorectal tumors should be resected, and preoperative biopsy must be avoided.
- Full-thickness local excision is indicated for T1 mucosal, submucosal, and early invasive cancer.
- For T1–T3 rectal adenocarcinomas, surgical procedures are low anterior resection, low colorectal or coloanal anastomosis, with J-pouch, and abdominoperineal resection, leaving at least 2 cm distal margin and clear lateral margins. With surgery, mortality rates are 1% to 7% and morbidity rates are 13% to 46%. Survival rate at 5 years is 74% to 87%.
- Optimal therapy for T3 tumors is sharp mesorectal excision combined with total mesorectal excision.
- The majority of N0 patients are cured by surgery and, for some selected patients, adjuvant multimodal therapy. Combined therapy cures 50% of N1 patients; 25% of tethered or fixed rectal cancers treated by neoadjuvant chemoradiotherapy are subsequently resected and cured.
- Of patients who die of rectal cancer, 25% fail with pelvic disease only.

INTRODUCTION

The pathology, biology, and etiology of colorectal cancer are discussed in Chapter 80. Although the incidence of distal (rectal and lower sigmoid) cancers has declined, with a concurrent increase in more proximal colon cancers, approximately one quarter of colorectal cancers are located in the rectum. For many years, almost all patients with rectal cancer underwent abdominoperineal

resection with a permanent colostomy. Today, this approach is rarely required. The successful treatment of patients with rectal cancer involves optimal surgical technique, and frequently adjuvant chemoradiotherapy. This combined modality approach will maximize cure, minimize the risk of a subsequent symptomatic local/pelvic recurrence, and maintain quality of life. Such multimodality approaches are applicable to patients with rectal cancers at or below the peritoneal reflection. This designation generally represents cancers below 12 cm from the anal verge. Tumors in the upper rectum or rectosigmoid are treated by surgical resection, and adjuvant therapy is based on the colon cancer paradigm.

EPIDEMIOLOGY

The incidence of rectal cancer in the United States is 44 cases per 100,000 population for a total number of new cases annually of approximately 34,000.[1] Since 1985, the incidence rate has been decreasing by 1.6% per year through 1997. A decrease in colon and rectal cancer incidence rates has been observed in males and females and all racial/ethnic groups. The incidence rate rises dramatically during the fifth decade of life. A study of 75,000 Medicare enrollees[2] observed that proximal colon cancers appear to be disproportionally high among elderly patients. Blacks have a higher mortality rate for colorectal cancer, which holds true for both rectal and colon cancers. In a 25-year period,[1] 1974–1999, the gap between the survival rates of blacks and whites increased from a difference of 5% to 11% for colon cancer and from 7% to 10% for rectal cancer.

The anatomic subsites of colorectal cancer have also been changing in the same 25-year period. The cancer incidence by anatomic subtype has shown that the incidence of rectal cancer has decreased from 9.6 cases per 100,000 population to 7.6 cases per 100,000 population.[3] This same finding has been reported in Japan[4] in a report that shows an increasing percentage of right-sided colon cancers and a continuous decline in percentage of rectal cancers in both sexes and at all ages. Sharpe[5] reported an observational study that showed a positive association between cigar smoking and cancer of the rectum. He also noted a weak positive association between cigarette smoking and cancer of the proximal colon. Cigarette use was not shown to be associated with rectal cancer.

CLINICAL PRESENTATION, EVALUATION, AND STAGING

Patients with rectal cancer can have a broad range of clinical presentations. Early symptoms suggestive of rectal carcinoma include rectal bleeding and subtle changes in bowel habits. Rectal bleeding is often mixed with stools or may coat the surface of the stool. It can be bright red and separate from the stools, and therefore is often mistakenly attributed to hemorrhoids. Bright red blood only on the tissue paper may be evaluated in a young person with proctosigmoidoscopy. All other types of bleeding, including presence of occult blood in the stools during routine physical examination or presence of iron deficiency anemia, warrant a more complete endoscopic evaluation. Increased frequency, decreased caliber of the stools, mucus with stools, or mucus diarrhea (particularly associated with large villous adenomas) is quite common. Advanced tumors induce a permanent sense of fullness and tenesmus and increased straining during defecation. Sacral or deep pelvic pain, sometimes radiating down the

perineum and thighs, occurs when the tumor invades the sacrum and the sacral plexus of nerves. Anal pain, initially on defecation and later continuous, may occur when low rectal cancer invades the anal canal. Incontinence supervenes when the anal sphincter is involved.

The importance of detailed history and a thorough physical examination cannot be overstressed. Comorbid conditions and the patient's physical habitus may preclude major surgery and influence the decision of adjuvant therapy. Physical examination should always include a digital rectal examination to feel for a mass, assess its location and mobility, and feel for enlarged extrarectal lymph nodes (50% accuracy). Depth of invasion and whether the tumor is tethered or fixed can also be assessed during rectal examination with 67% to 84% accuracy.[6,7] A careful pelvic examination in women and prostate assessment in men are essential. Rigid proctosigmoidoscopic examination of the rectum and the anus should follow. The distance of the tumor from the anal verge, anterior/posterior/lateral position, size, morphologic configuration, and extent of circumferential involvement are determined. Tumor mobility and tethering to surrounding structures are ascertained. If not obstructed, patients with rectal cancer should have a preoperative double-contrast barium enema or preferably a colonoscopy to assess for synchronous colon cancer (2% to 9%). Subjective and objective assessment of the patient's anal sphincter function is desirable. A weak or incompetent sphincter may favor a colostomy.

Endorectal ultrasound provides valuable preoperative staging (Fig. 81-1), including depth of tumor invasion into the rectal wall (89% to 92% accuracy,[8,9] 96% sensitivity, 90% specificity, 96% negative predictive value[10]) and nodal enlargement (79% sensitivity, 74% positive predictive value, 84% negative predictive value[11]), but confirmation of nodal metastasis with ultrasound guided needle biopsy is less reliable (77% accuracy, 71% sensitivity, 89% specificity, 92% positive predictive value and 62% negative predictive value[12]). Malignant nodes are differentiated

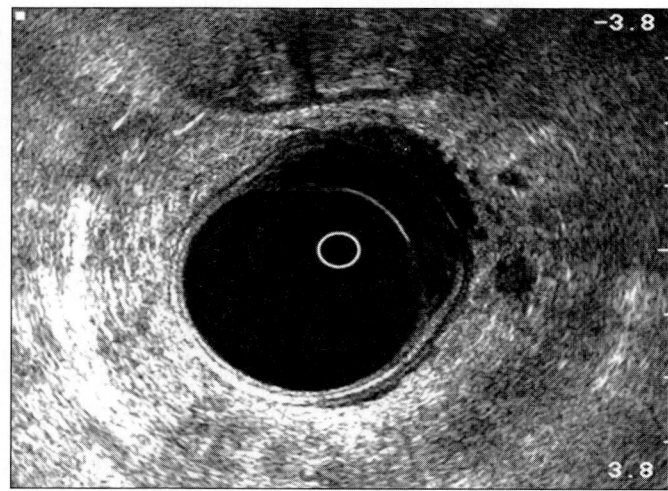

Figure 81-1. Endorectal ultrasound of T3N1 rectal cancer. (Provided by Dr. WD Wong, Memorial Sloan-Kettering Cancer Center.)

from reactive nodes by being hypoechoic, hypervascular, and irregular.[13,14] Both endorectal ultrasonography (EUS) and magnetic resonance imaging (MRI) with endorectal coil exhibited similar accuracy and were superior to conventional computed tomographic (CT) scans in preoperative assessment of depth of invasion and adjacent organ invasion.[15] This improved diagnostic staging information is essential when considering local treatment for rectal cancer, deciding selective use of preoperative chemoradiotherapy in locally advanced tumors, and choosing between an abdominoperineal and low anterior resection.

The liver is the most frequent site of metastasis, followed by the lung, retroperitoneum, ovary, peritoneal cavity, and rarely the adrenal glands. Contrast-enhanced CT scan of the abdomen and the pelvis is recommended in all patients with rectal cancer, excluding the very elderly and those with very early cancer such as cancer within a polyp or T1 rectal cancer. MRI is reserved for patients with locally advanced and recurrent rectal cancer requiring an exenterative procedure. A plain chest radiograph is useful and economical for screening for lung metastasis. Laboratory studies should be ordered as indicated by the patient's medical condition and anesthetic requirements. Measurement of carcinoembryonic antigen (CEA) level in combination with imaging can refine accuracy of preoperative assessment and overall prognosis and is useful if postoperative CEA monitoring is planned. Up to 95% of patients with advanced hepatic metastasis will have a CEA level above 20 ng/mL.[16] Normal preoperative CEA levels will identify patients who will not benefit from following CEA levels postoperatively. In men a prostate-specific antigen (PSA) level should be checked, particularly if the prostate gland is enlarged.

DIFFERENTIAL DIAGNOSIS

Kaposi's sarcoma of the rectum should be suspected in patients with acquired immunodeficiency syndrome (AIDS) presenting with unusual or atypical anorectal lesion. It is often associated with proctalgia (62%), hematochezia (50%), and diarrhea (50%).[17] Except for inflammatory masses, developmental cysts (such as dermoid, epidermoid, duplication, and tailgut cysts) and embryonic tumors (such as teratomas, chondromas, and meningoceles) are the most common retrorectal tumors. Other sacral and presacral tumors include neurogenic tumors, liposarcoma, and neurofibromatosis. Sacral pain and the sensation of fullness in the perirectal area are the commonest symptoms of retrorectal lesions.[18] Digital rectal examination is the most important diagnostic maneuver. Posteroanterior and lateral radiographs of the sacrum and CT scanning are the preferred methods for characterization and differential diagnosis of retrorectal masses. MRI may also aid in planning the operative approach. Barium enema evaluation will confirm the presence of mass effect. Proctoscopy, although indicated, is usually normal. All retrorectal lesions should be resected when diagnosed, even if they are asymptomatic and seem benign. Preoperative biopsy is generally not recom-

mended as it will not change the surgical need for resection and may contaminate the surgical field. Biopsy is reserved only for unresectable large retrorectal tumors.

SURGICAL TREATMENT OF RESECTABLE RECTAL CANCER

For most patients with early rectal cancer (T1–T3), surgical resection is the primary treatment modality. Sound surgical techniques and adjuvant therapy can improve outcomes and maximize local and overall cure rates. Tumors in the upper third of the rectum have their lowermost edge 12 cm from the anal verge. Anterior resection or low anterior resection is the primary surgical procedure. Middle and lower third rectal cancers can be treated with restorative proctectomy with colorectal or coloanal anastomosis or abdominosacral resection with similar results to those achieved with abdominoperineal resection and permanent colostomy.[19] Overall surgical success depends on ability to obtain a 2-cm distal margin, surgical expertise in obtaining clear lateral margins, and the patient's body habitus, pelvic width, prostate size, adequate collateral blood flow through the marginal artery, and associated colonic disease such as diverticulosis. Local approaches may be appropriate for patients with early rectal cancer within 8 cm from the anal verge or in those patients with major medical contraindications to radical surgery.

Local Treatment

Selection Factors
Selection factors for full-thickness local excision (FTLE) are the same or similar to those used for endocavitary radiation therapy (RT). This decision is therefore largely based on findings of digital rectal examination with increasing integration of use of transrectal ultrasound or MRI with endorectal coil.[12,15,20] Patients with T1 tumors without adverse pathologic features have a low incidence of local failure (5% to 10%) or lymph node involvement (<10%) with unfavorable pathologic features (lymphvascular invasion, high grade, deep submucosal invasion, signet ring cell, or colloid histology)[21–24] or evidence of tumor invasion into or through the muscularis propria[22,25,26]; the local recurrence rate is at least 17% and the risk of regional lymph node involvement is at least 10% to 15%.[21] In an analysis by the Massachusetts General Hospital of 40 patients who underwent local excision only, patients were categorized according to unfavorable clinical or pathologic features.[22] Among patients with T1 or T2 cancers following local excision Blumberg and associates reported positive lymph nodes in 10% of T1 and 17% of T2 cancers.[27] In addition, among the total group of 159 patients, the incidence increased with the presence of lymphatic and vascular invasion (14% without versus 33% with). Even among the 42 patients with the most favorable features (negative lymphatic and vascular space involvement, well or moderately differentiated T1 cancers) 7% were found to have lymph node involvement. The overall 5-year survival rate for the whole group was

65% with a locoregional recurrence rate of 27%. Hager and associates reported on a series of 20 patients with T2 rectal cancer for which local excision was performed and who were otherwise felt to be "low risk" (well to moderately differentiated, nonmucinous, no lymphvascular invasion, and negative margins) despite which the incidence of locoregional failure was still 17%.[25] Others have reported locoregional failure rates as high as 43% following either local or transanal excision in patients with T2 cancers.[28]

Local Approaches

Local approaches for treatment of early rectal cancer include transanal local excision, suprasphincteric posterior proctectomy (the Kraske procedure), transsphincteric posterior approaches (Bevan or York-Mason procedure), transanal endoscopic microsurgery (TEM), transanal fulguration, or local/contact radiation therapy (Papillon approach). The goal is to select patients with minimal risk of transmural and regional lymph node spread. The potential benefits of local excision for rectal cancer include reduced perioperative complications and preservation of anorectal, bladder, and sexual function. A mobile, well-differentiated, exophytic T1 lesion smaller than 2 cm is ideal. Larger, deeper lesions and those with high-grade or lymphatic and vascular invasion are treated by local excision only as a compromise strategy, primarily in medically unfit patients. Surgical excision for cure should always involve a full-thickness resection with negative margins, ideally attempting to remove perirectal lymph nodes if feasible.

Transanal excision is the technique most frequently used for local excision of rectal carcinomas. However, because of limitations in exposure, this procedure should be reserved principally for relatively small tumors (less than 3 cm in diameter) within 6 to 8 cm of the anal verge and generally limited to one quadrant of the rectal circumference. Although a 1-cm margin is ideal, a 5-mm margin of grossly normal mucosa beyond the edge of the tumor is more realistic. The rectal wall excision to the level of perirectal fat is performed with emphasis placed on a perpendicular dissection in order to prevent undermining and premature "coning-in," taking care to protect the vagina in females and the prostate in males. If feasible, perirectal fatty tissue should be included in order to attempt to detect nodal spread. Proper orientation of the specimen is maintained as it is pinned on a surface to facilitate accurate margin status and depth of invasion by the pathologist. Mortality rate is 0% to 2% and morbidity rate is 15% to 25%, usually mild.

Suprasphincteric posterior proctectomy (the Kraske procedure) and trans-sphincteric posterior approaches (Bevan or York-Mason procedure) have been used for lesions that are not suitable for a standard transanal approach. In husky males, transanal techniques are problematic and these posterior approaches are advantageous. In addition, lymph node excision may be facilitated by such procedures. The suprasphincteric or Kraske operation[29] facilitates wide resection of posterior or lateral lesions. This approach is performed with the patient in the prone jack-knife position. Once the suprasphincteric midline fascia (anococcygeal ligament)

has been divided, the pelvis is entered by dividing the levator muscle in the midline. The coccyx and a portion of S5 sacrum is removed with a rongeur. For a posterior lesion, the mesorectum is mobilized superiorly and laterally. The rectal wall with overlying fat is then excised with an intraluminal finger providing control of margins.

The York-Mason or the Bevan[30] operation is a posterior proctotomy combined with sphincter division. Exposure of anterior wall lesions is excellent. Closure of the proctotomy and sphincter must be meticulous. Diverting colostomy is not required. Both procedures are technically demanding and have a 1% to 5% mortality rate and an 18% to 34% morbidity rate.

Fulguration and intracavitary radiation are alternative local treatment options. Fulguration can be safely performed completely through the bowel wall. A ball-tip cautery with frequent curettage of charred material is required. Late delayed hemorrhage as the eschar sloughs occurs in 20% of patients. Fulguration should not be used near the vagina in women or the urethra in men. Local or contact radiation is available in relatively few centers. Low-energy (50-Kv) x-ray is applied through an operating (4-cm) proctoscope in doses of 3000 cGy every 3 to 4 weeks for three to four sessions. A small midposterior lesion is ideal for this treatment, but these lesions are usually amenable to excision.

Transanal endoscopic microsurgery (TEM) is a minimally invasive surgical technique introduced in 1984 by Buess. It incorporates a high-quality binocular operating system and pressure-regulated insufflation with continuous suction. Compared with conventional transanal resection, TEM provides superior intraoperative visualization and the ability to perform full-thickness excision of the tumor with clear margins, together with perirectal fat and adjacent lymph nodes[31,32] of tumors higher up in the rectum (4 to 18 cm from anal verge). The technique is not yet generally established because of the high cost, the necessary special instrumentation and tools, and the unusual technical aspects of the approach.[32-36] Treatment of cT2 rectal tumors with TEM combined with preoperative high-dose radiotherapy in 35 patients achieved similar survival to conventional open surgery.[37] Only minor postoperative complications occurred in five (14.3%) patients and included suture line dehiscence in three patients and stool incontinence in two patients. At a median follow-up period of 38 months, one patient presented with a local recurrence (2.85%) at 30 months of follow-up and four patients developed systemic metastasis (11.4%). The survival and local recurrence rates reported in that study led to a prospective multicenter randomized trial (the so-called Urbino trial) to evaluate the efficacy of local excision in T2 tumors preoperatively treated by chemotherapy and high-dose radiotherapy versus standard open treatment (low anterior resection or abdominoperineal resection).

Radical Resections

Sharp, total mesorectal excision with autonomic nerve preservation (TME) is the radical surgical technique of choice in conjunction with low anterior resection (LAR) or abdominoperineal resection (APR). Mortality rate is

1% to 7% and morbidity rate (including genitourinary dysfunction, fecal incontinence, and permanent colostomy) is 13% to 46%. Disabling recurrent disease is observed in 4% to 10%, and the 5-year survival rate is 74% to 87%.[38-42]

Surgical Issues in Radical Resections

Lateral Circumferential Margins and Total Mesorectal Excision. The ability to obtain a negative lateral circumferential margin is associated with a decreased risk of local recurrence.[43-46] In multivariate analysis, circumferential margin involvement was the most powerful predictor of local recurrence (hazard ratio 12.2) and of overall cancer mortality (hazard ratio 3.2) (Fig. 81-2). Heald and colleagues have advocated TME in conjunction with LAR or APR as the optimal surgical treatment for rectal cancer. This technique involves removal of the entire rectal mesentery, including that distal to the tumor, as an intact unit. Complete and distal TME is essential for clearance of any tumor deposits, which occur in 50% of T3 tumors with a maximal distal spread of 4 to 5 cm,[47] and is associated with increased frequency of local recurrence and decreased overall survival.[48,49]

Sharp mesorectal excision (SME) combined with TME provides optimal surgical strategy. In contrast to conventional blunt dissection techniques, SME facilitates nerve preservation, enables complete hemostasis, and emphasizes gentle handling to avoid tearing or disruption of the smooth outer surface of the mesorectum. Sharp TME has been shown to achieve a negative circumferential margin in 93% of resected specimens. Although no randomized trial of TME has been performed, TME has been evaluated prospectively in Sweden, where it has been introduced via a formal preceptorship-based training program. A 5-year prospective audit reveals a local recurrence rate of 7% following the addition of TME compared to a historical control rate of 23%.

Distal Mucosal Margin. The ability to perform sphincter preservation surgery is dictated by the requirements of a 2-cm distal margin rather than the traditional 5-cm margin.[70-74] Only 2.5% of patients (usually with poorly differentiated and node positive rapidly disseminating disease) had disease spread greater than 2 cm.[19] There is no correlation between risk of local recurrence and the extent of distal margin in excess of 2 cm.[50-55]

Proximal Extent of Lymph Node Dissection. Proximal lymph node dissection should extend just distal to the origin of the left colic artery. No evidence indicates a relationship between local recurrence and survival and dissection of deep iliac lymph nodes,[56] or high ligation of inferior mesenteric pedicle.[57,58] Patients with pathologically positive nodes along the inferior mesenteric artery have very low 5-year survival rates.[59,60]

Low Anterior Resection

The procedure involves complete mobilization of the descending colon and the rectum to the level of the levators. In LAR, the lateral rectal attachments containing the middle hemorrhoidal vessels are divided. Restorative options include side-to-end (Baker anastomosis) or end-to-end hand-sewn or stapled anastomosis. The use of the transanal intraluminal circular stapler allows the creation of very low anastomosis in the pelvis.

In ultra low resections, bowel continuity with colonic J-pouch have better bowel functional outcome compared to straight coloanal anastomosis[61-64] or coloplasty pouch[65] in prospective randomized trials. Successful creation of a pouch requires complete mobilization of the splenic flexure, high ligation of the inferior mesenteric artery and vein, and use of well-vascularized descending or sigmoid colon[66] free of diverticular disease. The length of the pouch can be either 5 or 10 cm with equal continence rates, defecation frequency, and urgency.[67,68] Excessive enlargement of the pouch can lead to evacuation difficulty.[69]

Sexual Function Preservation

Conventional resection for rectal cancer in men is associated with postoperative erectile impotence or retrograde ejaculation in 25% to 75% of cases. Postoperative sexual dysfunction is due to operative damage to the pelvic autonomic nerves and can be correlated with the extent of lateral pelvic dissection, late surgical scarring, and the early and late impact of chemoradiotherapy. Havenga and coworkers[70] have reviewed 19 studies (only three studies were prospective) of male sexual function after conventional resection for rectal

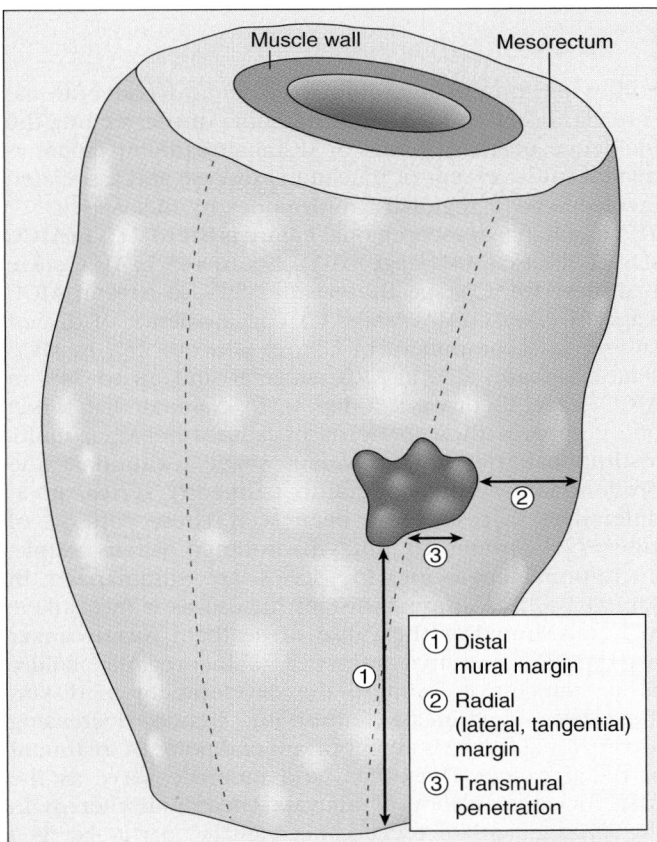

Muscle wall   Mesorectum

① Distal mural margin
② Radial (lateral, tangential) margin
③ Transmural penetration

Figure 81-2. Rectal cancer primary tumor margins.

Specific Malignancies

III

cancer. In most of these studies, sexual function was assessed using a questionnaire or an interview. Many studies excluded patients older than 60, 65, and 70 years of age at time of surgery. He correctly pointed out that comparison of results is very difficult owing to selection of patient groups, differences in operative techniques and adjuvant therapy, utilization of nonstandardized questionnaires, and cultural differences. When the difficulties of comparing retrospective studies are ignored and all data are taken collectively, the number of patients who developed complete erectile dysfunction is 25% for all patients: 34% after APR and 20% after LAR. Loss of ejaculation occurred in 16% of patients: 19% after APR and 33% after LAR. In his analysis of seven studies (mostly retrospective) regarding long-term sexual dysfunction after autonomic nerve sparing resection of rectal cancer, excellent results in male sexual function were achieved. In five Japanese studies, erection and ejaculation were maintained in 76% to 96% and 55% to 83% of male patients, respectively, when there was complete preservation of the pelvic autonomic nerves. In a study from Memorial Sloan-Kettering Cancer Center, 86% of male patients younger than 60 years of age and 67% of patients 60 years and older maintained ability to engage in intercourse.[40] A recent study by Mannaerts and associates[71] evaluated urologic and sexual morbidity following multimodality treatment for locally advanced primary and locally recurrent rectal cancer. The preoperative ability to have an orgasm was lost in 45% of patients after treatment of locally advanced primary and in 57% after treatment of locally recurrent cancer. Hanna and associates[72] recently reported their preliminary experience using intraoperative nerve stimulation and tumescence monitoring during TME to assess its ability to objectively demonstrate intact functional parasympathetic nerves in the pelvis at the completion of operative dissection. They correlated the ability to demonstrate intact nerves with clinical recovery and outcome of sexual function.

Abdominoperineal Resection

Many patients with cancers in the distal third of the rectum, and in particular patients with poor baseline anal function, still may require an APR. The rectum is mobilized down to the pelvic floor, the proximal bowel is divided, and the distal sigmoid colon is brought out as an end-colostomy in the left lower quadrant of the abdomen through the rectus sheath to minimize risk of subsequent hernia. A perianal elliptical incision is made to mobilize and deliver the anus and distal rectum. The levators are divided laterally and the specimen is removed. Anteriorly, the dissection in males is constrained by the urethra and prostate. A large urethral catheter facilitates identification and protection of the urethra. Mobilization is much easier in females, for the back wall of the vagina can be removed with the rectum, providing a particularly useful maneuver for clearing anterior tumors.

In nonirradiated patients, the pelvis can be left open and packed, with rapid granulations and secondary closure within 2 months. Radiated patients should all be closed primarily. In patients who received preoperative radiation therapy, the bowel may be allowed to prolapse

into the pelvis without consequence. However, in the remaining patients, an effort at excluding the small bowel from the pelvis is warranted to allow postoperative radiation therapy, although not always feasible. In women, the uterus may be retroverted into the pelvis with a single figure-of-eight suture to the midsacrum. In men and some women, the peritoneum may be reapproximated. Thin peritoneum may leave small defects, leading to a subsequent small bowel herniation and obstruction. An omental pedicle flap is ideal, but not always feasible. Absorbable mesh may be sutured with fine silk over the true pelvic inlet.

Laparoscopic Surgery

Laparoscopic surgery for curable rectal cancer is controversial and still considered investigational. Laparoscopic anterior resection with curative intent generates considerably more reservations than laparoscopic APR, which is technically much easier to perform. Data on the extent of lymphadenectomy, margins of resection, actuarial survival, and local recurrence rates have not been determined, and the current randomized trials of laparoscopic resection for colorectal cancer specifically exclude rectal cancer. The technique of laparoscopic TME is well described by Pikarsky and associates.[73] Reports suggest short-term gains of reduced pain, shortened hospital stay, accelerated activity, possible cost reduction, and improved cosmesis.[74] Hand-assisted laparoscopic surgery (HALS) is a new technique that has the potential to overcome many of the existing limitations of pure laparoscopy.[75]

Patterns of Failure

Following potentially curative standard/conventional surgical resection for adenocarcinoma of the rectum, the incidence of locoregional or distant treatment failure is related to the extent of transmural disease and associated involvement of regional lymph nodes by metastases.[76-83] The incidence of locoregional failure is 8% to 21% in AJCC stage I disease (MAC stage A/B1), 29% to 44% in AJCC stage II disease (MAC stage B2/B3), and 50% to 61% in AJCC stage III disease (MAC stage C). The incidence of distant failure (as a component of failure) is up to 28% in AJCC stage I disease, 47% in AJCC stage II, and up to 74% in AJCC stage III disease. It has been claimed that when one compares these patterns of failures between multi-institutional trial settings versus single-institutional and predominantly single-operator (surgeon) series, great differences in results can been seen. These patterns of failures according to multi-institutional versus single-institutional/single-operator series are summarized in Table 81-1.[76-83] Although distant metastasis is most likely to be attributed as the cause of death in rectal cancer patients, the potential influence of locoregional failure as an antecedent event to the development of distant metastases is clinically important. Hence, decreasing locoregional failure is an important end point of treatment in rectal cancer. These data and rationale serve as the basis for consideration of adjuvant chemoradiotherapy in the management of rectal cancer and, in particular, as a standard for AJCC stage II (MAC stage B2/B3) and stage III

TABLE 81-1

Patterns of Locoregional Recurrence and Overall Failure Following Standard/Conventional Surgery Alone for Rectal Cancer

MULTI-INSTITUTIONAL SERIES	N*	MAC STAGE	LR	OF
GITSC[76]	58	B/C	24%	44%
EORTC[77]	166	A–C	32%	41%
NSABP[78]	191	B/C	33%	58%

	STAGE I			STAGE II			STAGE III		
SINGLE INSTITUTION SERIES	N*	LR	OF	N	LR	OF	N	LR	OF
MDAH[79]	39	8%	18%	59	31%	47%	44	50%	70%
UT[80]	28	21%	28%	37	29%	45%	43	51%	74%
MSKCC[81]	47	14%	–	69	44%	–	52	61%	–

			MAC	
SINGLE INSTITUTION AND PREDOMINANTLY SINGLE OPERATOR SERIES		N*	STAGE	LR
Patel et al[82]		435	A-C	24%
Enker et al[83]		412	A–C	27%

EORTC, European Organization for Research and Treatment of Cancer, GITSC, Gastrointestinal Tumor Study Group; LR, locoregional recurrence; MDAH, M.D. Anderson Hospital; MSKCC, Memorial Sloan-Kettering Cancer Center; NSABP, National Surgical Adjuvant Breast and Bowel Project; OF, overall failure; UT, University of Texas.
*Number of patients.

disease (MAC stage C). It is important to note that limited retrospective data identify subsets of patients with stage I disease who may be considered for adjuvant therapy as well as subsets of patients with T3N0 disease who may not require adjuvant therapy.[84,85] Willett and associates identified a subset of patients with stage I disease who have an increased incidence of locoregional failure following an APR.[84] In an additional review of 117 patients with T3N0 disease, Willet and associates identified a favorable group of patients with moderately or well-differentiated cancers invading less than 2 mm into perirectal fat who had a 10-year actuarial locoregional failure rate of only 5% following surgery alone, as compared to 29% in T3N0 patients without these favorable features.[85]

As just described, locoregional recurrence rates as low as 4% have been reported with more optimal (TME) surgery.[86] In addition to potential selection bias, 18% to 58% of patients reported in TME series actually have received radiation therapy with or without chemotherapy.[45,87,88]

Radiation Sequencing Issues

Preoperative versus Postoperative Therapy: Potential Advantages and Disadvantages

Table 81-2 summarizes the advantages and disadvantages of preoperative (typically chemoradiotherapy) versus postoperative adjuvant therapy. The major advantages of preoperative therapy are tumor downstaging with increased resectability and sphincter preservation as well as a reduced incidence of acute toxicity. Adequate doses of radiation (>4000 Gy) can sterilize peripheral margins of disease.[83] Marginally resectable and unresectable tumors can undergo tumor shrinkage, making them amenable to curative surgical resection particularly within the confines of the ridged funnel-shaped bony pelvis, which often limits the potential for adequate circumferential margins of resection.[43,46] Preoperative therapy also allows tumors to be resected with limited longitudinal surgical margins, thereby extending the level to which sphincter-sparing procedures can be performed safely in the distal rectum.[89] These advantages in turn are associated with the potential for a significant reduction in a source of tumor spillage associated with locoregional recurrence of disease as well as a reduction of the dissemination during surgery of viable tumor cells increasing the risk for developing

TABLE 81-2

Advantages of Preoperative versus Postoperative Adjuvant Therapy*

ADVANTAGE	PREOPERATIVE THERAPY	POSTOPERATIVE THERAPY
Tumor downstaging	+	–
Increased tumor resectability	+	–
Increased sphincter preservation	+	–
Treatment based on operative/pathologic findings	–	+
Decreased locoregional recurrence	++	+
Increased survival	+	–

*Typically chemoradiation therapy.

distant metastatic foci. The potential therapeutic advantage of preoperative therapy (particularly radiation) with enhanced oxygenation prior to surgical disruption of tumor blood supply is well established.[90,91]

Preoperative therapy also has the potential advantage of reducing the risk of treatment of both chemotherapy- and radiation-related morbidity as compared to that seen with postoperative therapy.[92,93] Following surgical resection, adhesions often develop and cause loops of bowel to be fixed within the pelvis. These fixed bowel loops often show enhanced tissue reaction with associated bacterial invasion, increasing the risk of severe treatment-related complications. In the preoperative therapy setting small bowel is less likely to be fixed within the treatment field and thereby less prone to both acute and chronic treatment-related injury.

The major advantage of postoperative therapy is the ability to select patients at high risk for locoregional or distant disease recurrence based on pathologic staging of disease and operative findings. This also minimizes the potential of overtreating patients with either early disease (pathologic stage I) or metastatic disease. Other potential advantages include the avoidance of possible wound-healing problems associated preoperative therapy. Other-wise, studies have failed to demonstrate any increased potential for the development of disseminated disease during preoperative therapy and the subsequent waiting period prior to surgery.

Preoperative versus Postoperative Therapy: Results of Randomized Trials

The evaluation of the advantages or disadvantage of preoperative versus postoperative adjuvant therapy in the setting of a randomized trial has been limited, including a failed attempt of such a study in the United States closed early owing to poor patient accrual (Intergroup Study R1023). In a Swedish multicenter trial[91] comparing preoperative versus postoperative radiation in rectal and rectosigmoid carcinoma, 471 patients were randomized to 25.5 Gy in 5 to 7 days preoperatively versus 60 Gy in 8 weeks after surgery. The local recurrence rate was statistically lower after preoperative radiation (12%) than after postoperative radiation (21%, $P = 0.02$). This improvement was observed despite the relatively modest dose of preoperative radiation (25.5 Gy) compared to the postoperative radiation dose (60 Gy). There was no difference in survival between the two groups (43% versus 40%), with a minimum follow-up period of 3 years and a mean follow-up period of 6 years.

Other Sequencing Issues

Until the recent publication of the Lyon R90-01 randomized trial[94] the optimal timing of surgery following preoperative therapy in rectal cancer was based on hypothesis or retrospective data. This study randomized 201 patients with stage T2/T3, NX, M0 into two treatment groups: (1) the short-interval (SI) group, with surgery being performed within 2 weeks of completion of preoperative radiation therapy (39 Gy and 13 fractions) versus (2) the long-interval (LI) group, with surgery being performed within 6 to 8 weeks after completion

of preoperative radiation therapy. At a median follow-up time of 33 months there was no difference in morbidity, local recurrence, or short-term survival between the two groups. These findings along with the previously demonstrated findings that rectal cancers undergo slow tumor shrinkage over several months after radiation[95] lend further support to the rationale that a longer delay before surgery, particularly in locally advanced tumors, may be desirable to allow for maximal tumor regression prior to surgery.

Lee and associates reported the results of a phase III study of postoperative adjuvant therapy in stage II and III rectal cancer designed to define the optimal sequencing of chemotherapy and RT.[96] In this study 308 patients were randomized to early RT versus late RT. Patients received 45 Gy in 25 fractions of RT with 8 monthly cycles of 5-fluorouracil (5-FU)/leucovorin chemotherapy. RT began with the start of chemotherapy in the early RT group versus with the start of the third cycle of chemotherapy in the late RT group. With a median active follow-up of 37 months, disease-free survival rate was significantly improved in the early RT group as compared to the late RT group (81% versus 71% at 4 years; $P = 0.043$). This finding was associated with an increase in both distant and locoregional disease recurrence in the late RT group and with an overall recurrence rate of 17% in the early RT group versus 27% in the late RT group ($P = 0.047$). Although overall survival was not significantly different between the treatment arms, these results suggest that the timing of adjuvant postoperative RT can have a significant impact on the outcome of patients with rectal cancer.

ADJUVANT THERAPY

Postoperative Adjuvant Therapy

As previously discussed, the major advantage of post-operative therapy in rectal cancer is to base treatment on operative/pathologic staging (Table 81-3). Early studies instrumental in defining the role of postoperative adjuvant therapy for rectal cancer included the GITSG and the NCCTG studies.[76,97] The GITSG study randomized 202 patients who had undergone "curative" surgical resection for adenocarcinoma of rectum to one of four treatment arms: (1) surgery alone, (2) surgery + postoperative radiation (40 to 48 Gy over 4.5 to 5.5 weeks), (3) post-operative chemotherapy (5-FU + methyl-CCNU), or (4) postoperative combined chemoradiotherapy.[76] At a median follow-up time of 94 months for all survivors this study found a significant improvement in the long-term survival of patients receiving adjuvant postoperative chemoradiotherapy as compared to surgery alone (59% versus 44%, $P = 0.005$).[97] This improvement was associated with a significant reduction of locoregional recurrence from 24% with surgery alone to 11% with postoperative adjuvant chemoradiotherapy. However, this was also associated with the increase in overall "severe or worse" toxicity associated with adjuvant postoperative chemoradiotherapy.

Subsequent to the GITSG study, the NCCTG study

TABLE 81-3

Results of GITSG, NCCTG, and NSABP Studies Evaluating Postoperative Adjuvant Therapy for Rectal Cancer*

| TYPE OF THERAPY | GITSG[76] | | NCCTG[97] | | NSABP R-02[101] | |
	LR	5-YEAR SURVIVAL	LR	5-YEAR SURVIVAL	LR	5-YEAR SURVIVAL
Surgery alone	24%	44%	—	—	—	—
Radiation therapy	20%	50%	25%	48%	—	—
Chemotherapy	27%	50%	—	—	13%	~65%
Chemoradiotherapy	11%	59%	13%	57%	8%	~65%

GITSG, Gastrointestinal Tumor Study Group; LR, locoregional recurrence; NCCTG, North Central Cancer Treatment Group; NSABP, National Surgical Adjuvant Breast and Bowel Project.

randomized 204 patients with pathologic high-risk rectal carcinoma to surgery and postoperative radiation (45 to 50.4 Gy in 5 to 5.5 weeks) versus surgery + postoperative chemoradiotherapy utilizing 5-FU + methyl-CCNU, which both preceded and followed combined chemoradiotherapy.[98] At a median follow-up time of over 7 years there was a significant benefit in the adjuvant postoperative chemoradiotherapy group versus the postoperative radiation-alone group. This benefit was characterized by a significant reduction in locoregional recurrence rate, 25% versus 13% ($P = 0.036$); reduction in distant metastases, 46% versus 29% ($P = 0.011$); and improvement in overall 5-year survival rate, 57% versus 48% ($P = 0.0016$). These trials led to the 1990 NIH Consensus that recommended adjuvant treatment.[99]

An additional intergroup study evaluated the addition of biologic response modifiers, leucovorin and levamisole, as means of improving patient outcome; 1695 patients were entered on this three-arm phase III randomized trial, and at a median follow-up period of over 7 years there was no advantage to leucovorin or levamisole regimens over bolus 5-FU in the postoperative adjuvant chemoradiotherapy treatment of high-risk rectal cancer.[100] Meanwhile, the NSABP R-02 trial was in part designed to evaluate the effect of radiation on overall survival in the postoperative adjuvant setting. It also evaluated the potential modulation of 5-FU by leucovorin. The study randomized 694 patients to receive either postoperative adjuvant chemotherapy alone ($N = 348$) or postoperative chemoradiotherapy ($N = 346$). In addition, all female patients received 5-FU + leucovorin chemotherapy; male patients received either methyl-CCNU, vincristine, and 5-FU or 5-FU + leucovorin. This latter aspect of the study design was related to the enigmatic findings of the prior NSABP postoperative rectal adjuvant trial showing differences in outcome related to gender.[78] With surviving patients on the R-02 study being followed on average over 7 years, adjuvant postoperative radiation resulted in no beneficial effect on overall survival ($P = 0.89$). The cumulative incidence of locoregional relapse among patients being treated with chemotherapy alone was 13% as compared to 8% among those receiving postoperative adjuvant chemotherapy at 5 years ($P = 0.02$).[101]

Treatment Planning for Adjuvant Postoperative Pelvic Radiation

In the treatment planning for adjuvant postoperative pelvic radiation the risk of small bowel complications is high, especially following an APR with the associated empty pelvis syndrome, and thus, efforts to exclude small bowel is of critical importance. Treatment planning should involve patients being given presimulation small bowel contrast medium consisting of 100 mL of diluted barium by mouth at least 1 hour prior to simulation or CT-based treatment planning. The patient should be positioned prone on a modified "belly board" to allow displacement of small bowel internally rather than being pushed into the pelvis (Fig. 81-3). This displacement can be further maximized by giving patients explicit instructions to increase fluid intake to allow maximal distention of the bladder to further push small bowel out of the pelvis during actual treatment.

In patients who have undergone an APR the perineal scar should be marked and included within the radiation treatment fields with consideration of the addition of bolus depending on treatment distribution. For cancers arising in the mid- to proximal portion of the rectum, only the posterior half of the pelvis/presacral space needs to be included within the treatment field with the anterior border posterior to the symphysis. However, for patients with low-lying or distal rectal cancers, particularly those involving surrounding adjacent organs such as the prostate, bladder, uterus, and vagina, the anterior border should be placed anterior to the symphysis, in association with shaped alloyed blocks to maximize small bowel exclusion. Such technical considerations have been previously published in detail.[102-104]

Preoperative Adjuvant Therapy

In the early 1970s and 1980s a number of studies evaluated preoperative radiation therapy (no chemotherapy) for rectal cancer that primarily utilized relatively low doses (<35 Gy; Table 81-4).[105-109] The interpretation of these trials within the context of contemporary management requires some consideration. Eligibility criteria in these studies generally allowed all patients to be

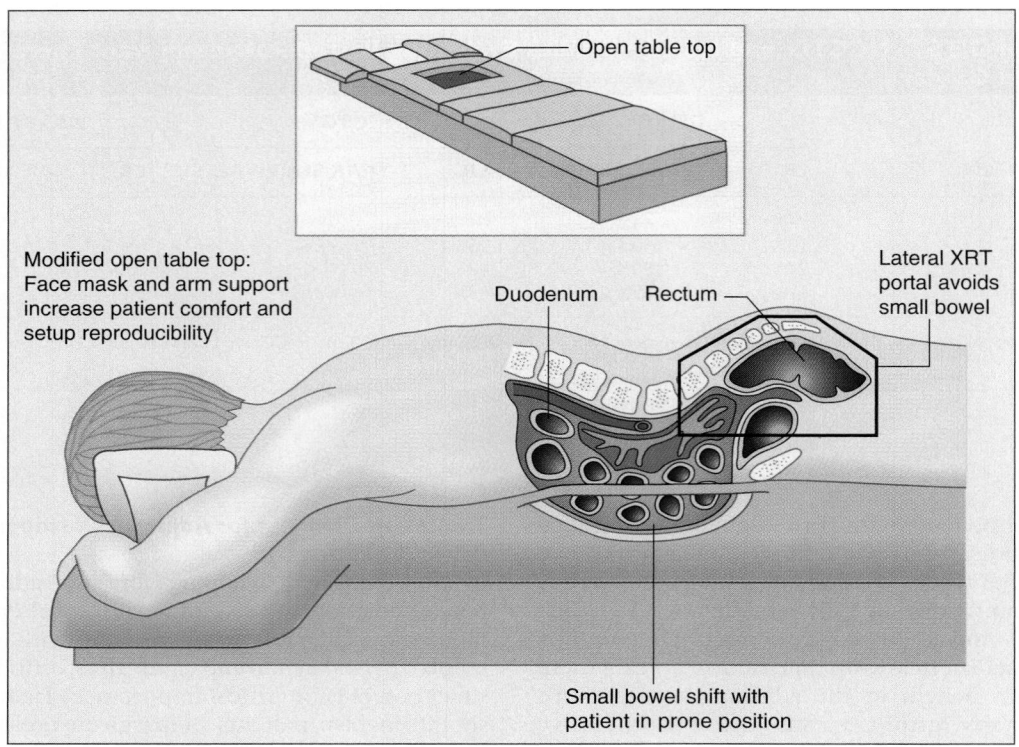

Figure 81-3. The belly board or open table-top device allows for maximal displacement of small bowel (with bladder distention) during radiation treatment. Example of lateral treatment portal is shown. The pubic bone is positioned just inferior to the edge of the opening. (From Mak AC, Rich TA, Schultheiss TE, Kavanagh B, Ota DM, Romsdahl MM: Late complications of postoperative radiation therapy for cancer of the rectum and rectosigmoid. Int J Rad Oncol Biol Phys 1994;28:597–603.)

entered, including those patients without imaging (e.g., CT scan or ultrasound) to rule out distant liver disease or those without transrectal ultrasound or MRI with endorectal coil to confirm extent of local transmural disease. In addition, there is great variance in fraction size used. Nevertheless, although there appears to be some benefit in local control, there was no improvement in survival.

In Europe, the EORTC completed a study[77] of moderate-dose preoperative radiation, 34.5 Gy in 19 days at 230 cGy per fraction followed by immediate surgical resection

TABLE 81-4

Rectal Cancer: Results of Low-Dose Preoperative Radiation Therapy			
RANDOMIZED STUDIES	**DOSE (GY)**	**RT***	**SURGERY***
Rider[105]	0.5	39%	35%
MRC[106]	0.5	42%	38%
	2.0	40%	38%
MSKCC[107]	2.0	52%	59%
VASOG I[108]	2.5	40%	32%
VASOG II[109]	3.15	35%	35%

MRC, Medical Research Council; MSKCC, Memorial Sloan-Kettering Cancer Center; RT, radiation therapy; VASOG, Veterans Administration Surgical Oncology Group.
*Five-year survival rates.

compared to surgery alone. The results of this study showed a significant improvement in locoregional control of disease with preoperative radiation (15% versus 35%, *P* = 0.003).

In a follow-up trial to their preoperative versus postoperative radiation trial, the Swedish group reported the results of a study evaluating 25 Gy in 5 days preoperatively (no adjuvant chemotherapy) versus surgery alone for resectable rectal cancer.[110] This trial is remarkable for being the first to demonstrate a survival benefit. After 5 years of follow-up, and randomly assigning 1168 patients, the overall 5-year survival rate was 58% in the preoperative radiation plus surgery group versus 48% in the surgery-alone group (*P* = 0.004). This was associated with a local recurrence rate of 11% in the preoperative radiation group versus 27% in the surgery-alone group (*P* < 0.001). In addition, this benefit was seen for all stages of disease compared with surgery alone, suggesting that the initial clinical stage of rectal cancer may not be as important as previously considered.

The Medical Research Council (MRC) rectal cancer working party staged a randomized trial of 40 Gy in 4 weeks preoperatively (no chemotherapy) versus surgery alone in only 279 patients with "potentially operable" locally advanced rectal cancer.[111] The results indicated a reduction in local recurrence (*P* = 0.04) and benefit in disease-free survival (*P* = 0.02) with use of preoperative radiation without a significant increase in overall survival (*P* = 0.10).

TABLE 81-5

Rectal Cancer: Results of High-Dose Preoperative Radiation Therapy

STUDY	NO. OF PATIENTS	DOSE (GY)	LOCAL RECURRENCE RATES		5-YEAR SURVIVAL RATES	
			RT (%)	SURGERY (%)	RT (%)	SURGERY (%)
Mendenhall et al[112]	71	3–4.5	8	—	71	41
Fortier et al[113]	60	4.5	16	40	52	48
Stevens et al[114]	57	5.6	0	—	53	38
Kodner et al[115]	112	4.5	2	—	86	—
Mohiuddin et al[120]	220	4.5–7	15	—	72	—

RT, radiation therapy.

In the United States several single-institution studies have examined the use of high-dose preoperative radiation (>40 Gy) and have reported lower recurrence rates with improved resectability and 5-year overall survival rates; some of these experiences are summarized in Table 81-5.[112-116] These results appear to be better than published results following surgery and postoperative adjuvant therapy. This benefit of preoperative radiation has been further substantiated with the results of a meta-analysis published by Camma and associates[110] (Fig. 81-4). This analysis involves 14 randomized controlled clinical trials of preoperative radiation (alone) followed by surgery versus surgery alone for "resectable" rectal cancers. It included a total of 6426 patients, 3081 of whom were treated with surgery alone. The meta-analysis found that the addition of preoperative radiation compared to surgery alone significantly reduced the 5-year overall mortality rate (odds ratio [OR] 0.84; 95% confidence

interval [CI], 0.72 to 0.98; $P = 0.03$) and cancer-related mortality rate (OR, 0.71; 95% CI, 0.61 to 0.82; $P < 0.001$). This reduction was associated with a significant reduction in local recurrence rate (OR, 0.49; 95% CI, 0.38 to 0.62; $P < 0.001$) without a significant reduction in the observed occurrence of distant metastases.

Neoadjuvant Radiation in Addition to Total Mesorectal Excision

Between 1996 and 1999 the Dutch Colorectal Cancer Group randomly assigned 1861 patients with "resectable" rectal cancer to preoperative radiation (5 Gy for 5 days) prior to TME versus TME alone.[117] The trial used rigid quality control measures, training, and standardization as a requirement for selected surgeons, as well as pathologists, who met such requirements for study participation. At a median follow-up period of approximately 2 years for surviving patients, the overall 2-year survival rates for

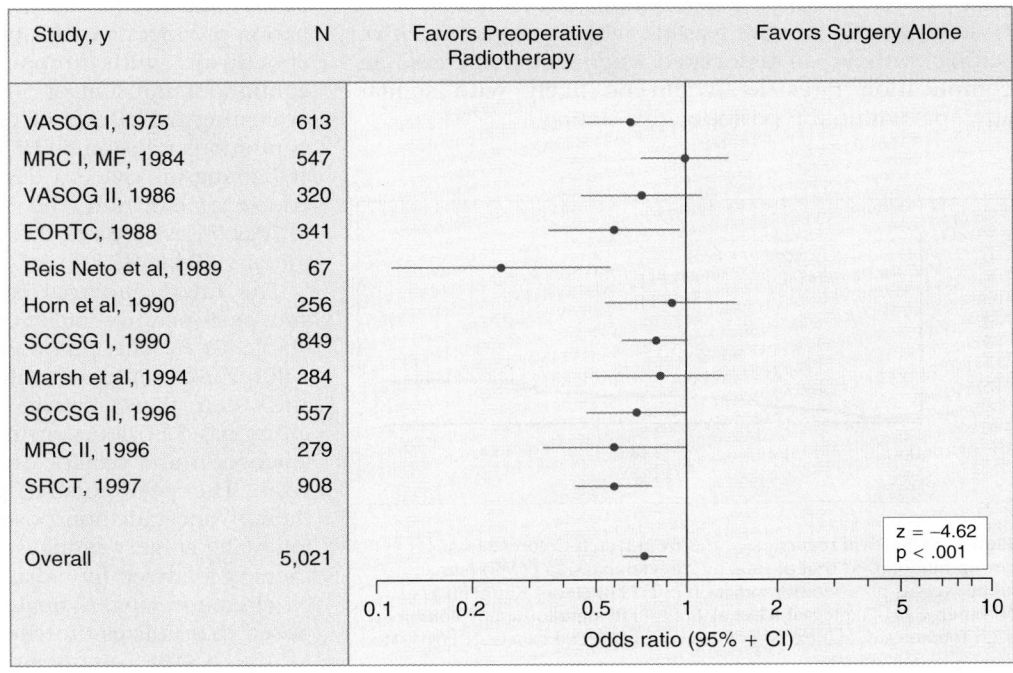

Figure 81-4. Results of meta-analysis of 11 randomized trials of preoperative radiation versus surgery alone for "resectable" rectal cancer. The odds ratio and 95% confidence interval (CI) for treatment effect on 5-year cancer-related mortality rate are shown on a logarithmic scale. (From Camma C, Giunta M, Fiorica F, Pagliaro L, Craxi A, Cottone M: Preoperative radiotherapy for resectable rectal cancer: A meta-analysis. JAMA 2000;284: 1008–1015.)

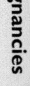

Specific Malignancies

III

the two treatment groups were essentially identical at approximately 82%. However, with this relatively early follow-up, preoperative radiation was associated with a significant reduction in the relative risk at 2 years of local recurrence compared to TME alone—2.4% in the preoperative radiation group versus 8.2% in the TME-alone group ($P < 0.001$); actuarial curves are shown in Figure 81-5. Actuarial analyses from the Dutch and the Swedish groups utilizing TME without adjuvant therapy suggest local failure rates in node-positive patients will likely remain in the 15% to 20% range at 5 years.

Whether the preoperative combined modality therapy as is currently used in this country with 5-FU-based chemotherapy is more effective than preoperative radiotherapy alone is unknown. This question is currently being addressed within an ongoing randomized EORTC trial. In the meantime, consideration of the use of pathologic response as a "surrogate" measure predictive of long-term outcome in rectal cancer patients has been suggested by a number of series.[111,118-120] Such a surrogate marker for survival or outcome could expedite evaluation of rapidly evolving novel preoperative combined modality/chemoradiotherapy combinations. This strategy is currently being utilized nationally by the RTOG in a randomized phase II trial evaluating preoperative 5-FU and hyperfractionated radiation versus preoperative 5-FU and CPT-11 with once-daily radiation in T3 and T4 rectal cancer patients and will be reviewed later. However, routine use of pathologic response following preoperative adjuvant therapy as a surrogate marker for outcome awaits further confirmation and long-term evaluation.[121]

Technical considerations in the preoperative setting are similar to those for postoperative radiation therapy. There is one major exception, however: the ability to dose escalate above 50 Gy (with its potential benefits,[122,123]) particularly in the locally advanced setting, by way of once- or twice-daily hyperfractionated radiation.[123-125] Dose escalation is more feasible within the preoperative setting without an associated exponential increase in complication rates, as would be likely with similar attempts within the postoperative setting.[123-125]

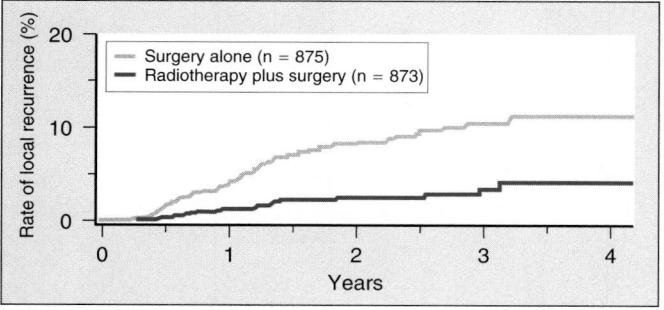

Figure 81-5. Local recurrence rates from Dutch Colorectal Cancer Group randomized trial of total mesorectal excision (TME) (surgery alone) versus preoperative radiation plus TME. (From Kapiteijn E, Marijnen CAM, Nagtegaal ID, et al: Preoperative radiotherapy combined with total mesorectal excision for resectable rectal cancer. N Engl J Med 2001;345:638–646.)

TABLE 81-6

Rectal Cancer: Clinical Staging

STAGE	DESCRIPTION	LOCATION*
I	Mobile: Free movement in all directions	A: >6 cm
II	Partially fixed (tethered): Movable in at least one direction (cephalocaudad or lateral)	B: 3–6 cm
III	Fixed: Immovable in any direction due to fixation (not size) or perforated, obstructed, deeply ulcerated	C: 0–3 cm
IV	Frozen pelvis: Invasion of pelvic sidewalls and/or sacrum—unresectable	D: <0 cm (i.e., into anal canal)

*Location as measured from the anorectal junction.

Adjuvant Therapy Based on Clinical Staging

Parameters include tumor fixation, distance from the anorectal junction, and the consideration/feasibility of sphincter preservation. Such parameters, along with modern imaging techniques (e.g., CT scan, transrectal ultrasound, or MRI with endorectal coil), can be integrated into use of a clinical staging system such as that previously published by Mohiuddin and associates (Table 81-6).[126] Clinical staging systems have been proposed by others.[127] Such a staging system can then be used to determine an optimal treatment strategy (utilizing pre- or postoperative therapy) for patients with rectal cancer.

Adjuvant Therapy Protocols

Three protocols are asking important questions: (1) NSABP R-04, (2) Intergroup Rectal Adjuvant Therapy E2301, and (3) RTOG R-0012. The NSABP trial is comparing preoperative radiation therapy and capecitabine ± epoetin-alfa with preoperative radiation therapy and continuous infusion of 5-FU ± epoetin-alfa. The study is evaluating the effects of capecitabine; is it equivalent to continuous infusion 5-FU? The capecitabine will be given at 825 mg/m^2 twice a day continuously throughout the course of radiation. The 5-FU will be given at 225 mg/m^2/day 7 days a week throughout the course of radiation therapy (Table 81-7).

The Intergroup trial is evaluating both preoperative and postoperative radiation therapy investigator choice (Table 81-8). The preoperative radiation therapy group will receive continuous infusion 5-FU followed by surgery and then three treatment regimens which include infusional 5-FU/leucovorin and CPT-11, infusional 5-FU/leucovorin and oxaliplatin versus bolus 5-FU and leucovorin. The postoperative group would receive chemotherapy and radiation postoperatively. The planned arms following surgery would be the same as for preoperative therapy followed by radiation therapy and then followed by chemotherapy. A single national agenda is being proposed that utilizes the chemotherapy and radiation arms of the NSABP preoperatively and then following the

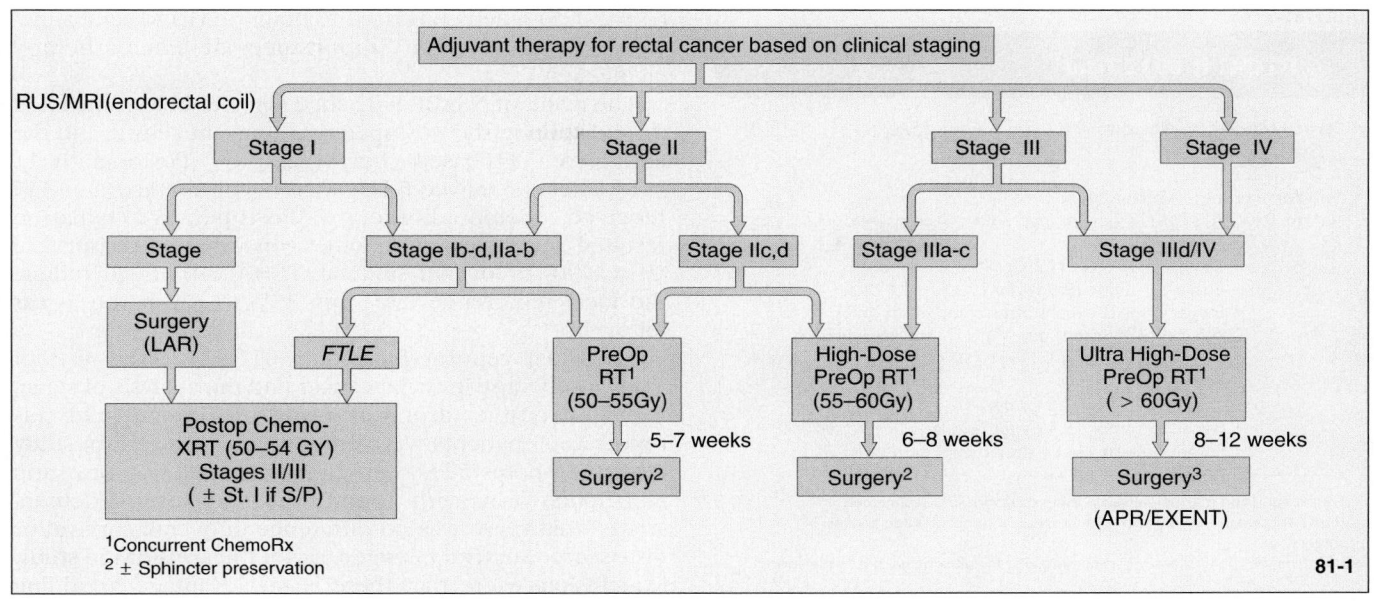

Adjuvant therapy for rectal cancer based on clinical staging

RUS/MRI(endorectal coil)

Stage I → Stage II → Stage III → Stage IV

Stage Ib-d,IIa-b ← Stage I → Stage IIc,d ← Stage II

Stage IIIa-c ← Stage III → Stage IIId/IV ← Stage IV

Stage → Surgery (LAR)

FTLE

PreOp RT¹ (50–55Gy) → 5–7 weeks → Surgery²

High-Dose PreOp RT¹ (55–60Gy) → 6–8 weeks → Surgery²

Ultra High-Dose PreOp RT¹ (> 60Gy) → 8–12 weeks → Surgery³ (APR/EXENT)

Postop Chemo-XRT (50–54 GY) Stages II/III (± St. I if S/P)

¹Concurrent ChemoRx
² ± Sphincter preservation

81-1

patients postoperatively into the three therapies of CPT-11, infusional 5-FU, and leucovorin; 5-FU and oxaliplatin; or leucovorin alone. The dosage of the postsurgical chemotherapy has not been fully developed. There is a question of using either bolus 5-FU with leucovorin or continuous 5-FU or capecitabine.

The third study, RTOG R-0012, is the first of a group of studies that will be performed utilizing present-day chemotherapy in the preoperative management of distal rectal carcinomas (Table 81-9). The lesions may be mobile,

T3 by endorectal ultrasound, or fixed T4 as defined as a clinical 4 on palpation. The two arms are as follows: Arm 1 is evaluated continuous-infusion 5-FU at 225 mg/m²/day 7 days a week until the completion of radiation therapy. The pelvic radiation therapy will be 45.6 Gy delivered at 1.2 Gy twice a day at 6-hour (or greater) intervals. Boost to the tumor will be at 9.6 Gy for T3 and 14.4 Gy for fixed tumors. Surgery will be performed at 4 to 10 weeks after the completion of radiation therapy. The second arm of the study is evaluating continuous infusion 5-FU daily for 5 days until the completion of radiation therapy plus CPT-11, 50 mg/m² once weekly for 4 weeks. The radiation therapy will be 45 Gy at 1.8 Gy per day. There will be a boost to the tumor of 4.5 Gy for T3 and 9 Gy for fixed T4 tumors. The surgery will be started at 4 to 10 weeks after radiation. This study is looking at the addition of twice-a-day radiation therapy to continuous infusion

TABLE 81-7

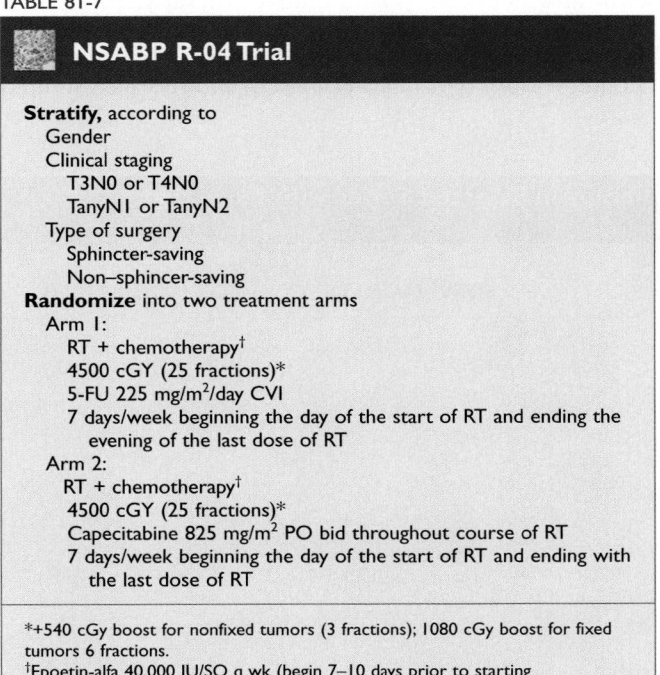

NSABP R-04 Trial

Stratify, according to
Gender
Clinical staging
T3N0 or T4N0
TanyN1 or TanyN2
Type of surgery
Sphincter-saving
Non–sphincer-saving
Randomize into two treatment arms
Arm 1:
RT + chemotherapy†
4500 cGY (25 fractions)*
5-FU 225 mg/m²/day CVI
7 days/week beginning the day of the start of RT and ending the evening of the last dose of RT
Arm 2:
RT + chemotherapy†
4500 cGY (25 fractions)*
Capecitabine 825 mg/m² PO bid throughout course of RT
7 days/week beginning the day of the start of RT and ending with the last dose of RT

*+540 cGy boost for nonfixed tumors (3 fractions); 1080 cGy boost for fixed tumors 6 fractions.
†Epoetin-alfa 40,000 IU/SQ q wk (begin 7–10 days prior to starting RT/chemotherapy).

TABLE 81-8

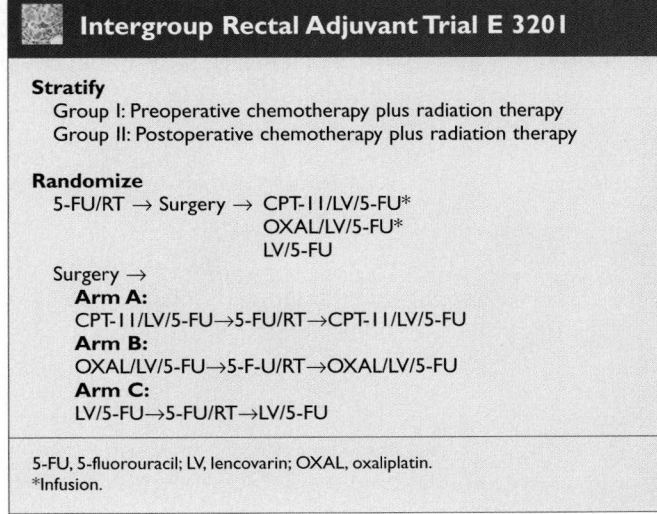

Intergroup Rectal Adjuvant Trial E 3201

Stratify
Group I: Preoperative chemotherapy plus radiation therapy
Group II: Postoperative chemotherapy plus radiation therapy

Randomize
5-FU/RT → Surgery → CPT-11/LV/5-FU*
                    OXAL/LV/5-FU*
                    LV/5-FU

Surgery →
Arm A:
CPT-11/LV/5-FU→5-FU/RT→CPT-11/LV/5-FU
Arm B:
OXAL/LV/5-FU→5-F-U/RT→OXAL/LV/5-FU
Arm C:
LV/5-FU→5-FU/RT→LV/5-FU

5-FU, 5-fluorouracil; LV, lencovorin; OXAL, oxaliplatin.
*Infusion.

TABLE 81-9

RTOG R-0012 Trial

Stratify, based on clinical staging
  Group 1: T3
  Group 2: T4
Randomize into two treatment arms
  Arm 1: CVI 5-FU (225 mg/m²/day, 7 days, 7 days/week, until completion of RT)
      + Pelvic RT 45.6 Gy (1.2 Gy bid, 6-h interval)
      + Boost to tumor (9.6 Gy for T3 and 14.4 Gy for fixed T4)*
      + Surgery+ 4–10 weeks after completion of RT
  Arm 2: CVI 5-FU (225 mg/m² day, M-F, 120 hr/week, until completion of RT) plus CTP-11 (50 mg/m², once weekly × 4 weeks)
      + Pelvic RT 45 Gy (1.8 Gy/day)
      + Boost to tumor (5.4 Gy for T3 and 9 Gy for fixed T4)*
      + Surgery† 4–10 weeks after completion of RT

*Boost radiation may be delivered using conformal 3D techniques.
†IORT (optional) may be delivered to areas of tumor fixation at time of surgery.
Maintenance chemotherapy is recommended for all patients after irradiation.

versus continuous infusion plus CPT-11 (50 mg/m² weekly for 4 weeks) in conventional radiation therapy. The importance of this study is that it is actually looking at, in a prospective manner, fixed tumors that are locally advanced and will give us greater understanding of upfront aggressive therapy for locally advanced tumors.

Chemotherapy

Chemotherapy has until recently played a supportive role in the management of rectal cancer. The results of recent studies will place more emphasis on the use of chemotherapy. O'Connell and coworkers[128] demonstrated that continuous-infusion 5-FU in the adjuvant setting significantly increased time to relapse by a decrease of 27% (P = 0.01) and decreased the death rates by 31%

(P = 0.005) when compared to bolus 5-FU and semustine; with this study the importance of chemotherapy changed.

The result of NSABP R-02 shed some doubt on the need for radiation in the postoperative adjuvant setting and the impact of 5-FU-based chemotherapy.[101] Postoperatively, 348 patients received 5-FU-based chemotherapy and 345 received chemoradiotherapy. Postoperative radiation resulted in no beneficial effect on disease-free survival (P = 0.90) or overall survival (P = 0.89). It did reduce the local recurrence rate from 13% to 8% at the 5-year follow-up.

The final report (Intergoup 0114) on the use of adjuvant therapy in rectal cancer and the analysis of stage, sex, and local control was made by Tepper.[100] In this report 1695 patients were entered into a three-arm study evaluating bolus 5-FU by itself, 5-FU plus leucovorin, and 5-FU/leucovorin with levamisole. The results demonstrated that there was no difference in overall survival or disease-free survival between any of the arms of the study. Conclusions were that there is no advantage to adding either leucovorin or levamisole to IV bolus 5-FU. The study demonstrated high rates of local relapse from 14% to 18%. This study was undertaken at a time when no data showed protracted infusion of 5-FU with radiation.

Adjuvant Therapy with Local Treatment

Standard therapy for resectable rectal cancer has been radical/conventional surgical resection (inclusive of the possibility of TME) with increasing integration of pre- or postoperative adjuvant therapy. In highly select patients this approach has often been challenged by use of more conservative local measures (Table 81-10).

Table 81-11 summarizes the results of local excision with and without postoperative therapy.[129-134] It is important to note that most series are retrospective, single-institution, with varying degrees of integration of chemotherapy (typically 5-FU-based) and relatively limited

TABLE 81-10

Local Excision of T1, T2 Lesions without Adjuvant Therapy in Selected Series with More than 50 Patients

REFERENCE	NO. OF PATIENTS (PER STAGE)	FOLLOW-UP TIME	LR	SURVIVAL RATE	SALVAGE SURGERY FOR ISOLATED LR
Paty et al*[175]	125 (T1=74, T2=51)	6.7 yr	T1=17% T2=26%	10-year OS: T1=74%, T2=72%	14/17
Mellgren et al[176]	108 (T1=69, T2=39)	4.4 yr	T1=21% T2=47%	5-year OS: T1=72%, T2=65%	24/27
Garcia-Aguilar et al[177]	83 (T1=55, T2=27)	54 mo	T1=18% T2=37%	5-year: T1=98%, T2=89%	17/20
Chakravarti et al[134]	52 (T1=44, T2=8)	52 mo	28%	5-year DFS: 66	NS
Steele et al[133]	59 (T1=59)	48 mo	T1=5%	6-year survival: 85	2/2
Kim and Madoff[178]	69 (T1=44, T2=25)	NS	T1=9% T2=28%	Cancer-specific 5-year Survival: 88%	NS
Hager et al[25]	59 (T1=39, T2=20)	33–40.5 mo	T1=8% T2=17%	5-year survival: T1=90%, T2=78%	NS

DFS, disease-free survival; LR, local recurrence; NS, not specified; OS, overall survival.
*In this series 16 patients received postoperative radiotherapy and 15 additional patients received postoperative 5-FU and radiotherapy; however, local and overall recurrence rates were similar in both groups.

TABLE 81-11

Local Excision for T1–T3 Rectal Cancer Plus Postoperative Adjuvant Therapy

SERIES	NO. OF PATIENTS	5-FU (%)	T3 (%)	FOLLOW-UP TIME	SURVIVAL RATES	INITIAL LOCAL CONTROL (SALVAGED WITH APR/ LOCAL FAILURES)
U. Florida[129]	45	4	2	2 yr (minimum)	88% 5-yr disease specific	89% (1/5)
Memorial Sloan-Kettering[130]	39	51	21	41 mo (median)	70% 5-yr actuarial	79% (5/8)
M.D. Anderson[19]	46	17	33	36 mo (median)	93% 3-yr overall	87% (–/4)
N.E. Deaconess[132]	48	54	10	41 mo (mean)	94% overall	92% (3/4)
CALGB[132]	51*	100	0	48 mo (median)	85% 6-yr actuarial	86% (4/7)
MGH[134]	47	55	0	51 mo (median)	74% 5-yr disease free	90% (5/9)

*Analysis is limited to the 51 of 110 patients with T2 disease who underwent a full-thickness local excision and received postoperative chemoradiotherapy.

follow-up.[129-133] Although these factors limit the degree with which results from these selective series can be reproduced within general practice and in the community, they at least suggest survival data comparable to that seen with radical or more conventional surgery alone for T1/T2, N0 rectal cancer.

Such results can now perhaps be felt to be reproducible in the general community setting with a greater degree of confidence given the results of the CALGB trial 8984. This trial was an Intergroup trial and is the only multi-institutional prospective phase II trial evaluating the outcome of local excision in patients with T1/T2 rectal cancers.[133] Study entry criteria included T1/T2 adeno-carcinomas which were more than 4 cm in diameter, encompassing less than 40% of the bowel wall circum-ference, being less than 10 cm from the dentate line, and having negative excisional margins. A total of 110 eligible patients were entered into the study. Of these patients, 59 had T1 adenocarcinoma and received no further therapy; 51 had T2 carcinomas and received external beam irradiation (54 Gy in 30 fractions at 5 days per week) and 5-FU (500 mg/m² IV days 1 to 3 and days 29 to 31) after full-thickness local excision (FTLE). It is interesting that 51 additional patients were also entered into the study but were later (postsurgery) found to be ineligible, most commonly due to (1) unclear/involved or uninterpretable surgical margins –(49%) (N = 25), (2) tumor stage above T2 –(25%) (N = 13), and (3) tumor diameter greater than 4 cm (24%) (N = 13). In addition, those who had excisions that were not felt to be "full thickness" were also considered ineligible –(10%) (N = 5). With a median follow-up period of 48 months the local failure rate was 3%, 6-year failure-free survival rate was 85%, and overall survival rate was 87% among the T1 patients; among the T2 patients the local failure rate was 14%, 6-year failure-free survival rate was 71%, and overall survival rate was 85%. Overall, 5 of the 9 local-only recurrences were able to be surgically salvaged (APR) without evidence of distant disease.

However, local failure seen beyond 5 years of treatment has been reported and is not uncommon.[134] Careful follow-up and review of long-term results of this treatment strategy are clearly required.

Complications of Adjuvant Therapy

Preoperative Versus Postoperative Therapy

Despite the survival advantage in select patients receiving adjuvant postoperative chemoradiotherapy, such treatment is associated with substantial toxicity. In the previously discussed GITSG trial, the incidences of greater than grade 3 toxicity in patients who received adjuvant postoperative chemoradiotherapy was 35% for nonhematologic effects and 26% for hematologic effects.[76] In the NCCTG trial greater than grade 3 toxicity among patients receiving postoperative adjuvant radiation therapy alone was limited to a 5% rate of diarrhea.[98] In comparison, among the treatment group receiving combined adjuvant postoperative chemoradiotherapy greater than grade 3 toxicity included a 41% rate of diarrhea and 33% rate of leukopenia. In both the GITSG and NCCTG trials, 35% of patients were unable to complete all planned cycles of chemotherapy due to toxicity. Also, in the NCCTG trial, an additional 25% refused to complete their therapy.

As previously discussed in the "Sequencing Issues in Adjuvant Therapy" section, preoperative therapy has the potential advantage of reducing the risk of treatment-related morbidity as compared to that seen with post-operative therapy.[92,93] In addition, it would appear that higher doses of chemotherapy can be delivered within the preoperative setting as compared to the postoperative setting. This is particularly evidenced in review of serial phase I studies of combined chemoradiotherapy performed at the Memorial Sloan-Kettering Cancer Center (MSKCC) in both the postoperative and preoperative setting with similar design.[135,136] With the doses of leuco-vorin and radiation remaining constant, the maximally tolerated dose of 5-FU was higher for the preoperative radiation therapy regimen.

Use of preoperative radiation, particularly high dose (>40 Gy) has raised some concerns regarding technical difficulty in surgical resection and delayed healing of abdominal and perineal wounds. As previously discussed, in both the Swedish and MRC trials postoperative mortality rate was not increased with the use of pre-operative radiation; and with use of the more conventionally fractionated preoperative MRC regimen (40 Gy at 2 Gy per fraction) there was no increase in postoperative or late complications.[137,138] Delay in wound healing has been implicated to be more likely associated with patients undergoing immediate surgical resection following preoperative radiation as compared to patients whose surgery was delayed 6 to 8 weeks. However, in the previously discussed Lyon R90-01 randomized trial of short-interval (2 weeks after completion of radiation therapy) versus long-interval (6 to 8 weeks after radiation therapy) time to resection, there did not appear to be a significant difference in perioperative morbidity and mortality rates.[94] It would appear that an increase in perioperative morbidity or delay of wound healing is more likely associated with use of higher dose per fraction, similar to the intensive short course of 25 Gy given in 5 fractions.[139,140]

General Acute Complications

The few complications occurring during adjuvant therapy in general include diarrhea with or without abdominal cramping, acute proctitis with or without tenesmus, bloody or mucous discharge, dysuria/cystitis, leukopenia, and thrombocytopenia. As previously discussed, although the addition of concurrent chemotherapy with radiation is associated with improved patient outcome, it also clearly increases the occurrences of these toxicities. Fortunately, these acute events are usually transient and resolve within a few weeks following the completion of therapy. The management of bowel-related toxicity usually involves the use of loperamide or diphenoxylate/atropine. Radiation proctitis can be treated with hydrocortisone foam or suppositories. Controlling bowel frequency will also help control the symptoms of proctitis. Bowel mucosa typically recovers within 1 to 3 months following completion of therapy.

Cystitis is due to the effects of radiation on the transitional cells lining the bladder. Symptoms include dysuria, frequency, urgency, and nocturia. An infectious process must be ruled out, particularly if symptoms occur early during the course of therapy or if bladder catheterization was performed for treatment planning. Infection should be treated with an antibiotic based on urine culture and antibiotic sensitivity. Urinary analgesics, such as pyridium, are helpful for dysuria. Bladder spasms may require antispasmodics such as flavoxate.

Perineal dermatitis is more common in patients being treated postoperatively after APR in which the inferior border of the radiation fields is extended to cover the perineal scar and in patients with low-lying rectal tumors being treated preoperatively. Concurrent chemotherapy and bolus over the scar can often exacerbate the reaction. Treatment should be aimed at controlling frequency of bowel movements, which tend to further exacerbate and irritate the perineal skin and reaction. Mild dermatitis can be treated with sitz baths and aloe wipes. More severe cases can be treated with nonmetallic skin creams.

General Long-Term Complications

Long-term complications include diarrhea, proctitis, small bowel obstruction (SBO), perineal and scrotal tenderness, urinary incontinence, and bladder atrophy/bleeding. In the MGH experience of 165 patients receiving 45 Gy postoperatively to the pelvis with a boost to the tumor bed to 50.4 Gy total, the incidence of long-term mild to moderate complications was 8% (4% transient and 4% persistent).[141] Persistent long-term complications were limited to proctitis (2%), delayed perineal wound healing (1%), and urinary incontinence (1%). The incidence of SBO requiring surgery was essentially equal in the patients who received radiation (6%) as compared to a historical control group of patients who were treated with surgery alone (5%).

Sphincter and Bowel Function

Radiation therapy can affect sphincter function; however, systematic, prospective data inclusive of uniformly treated patients with pretreatment baseline sphincter assessment are lacking. Two such studies reporting on the impact of postoperative therapy on long-term sphincter function utilized nonrandomized, nonblinded, and retrospective telephone survey methods. The report from the Mayo Clinic evaluated the impact of postoperative chemoradiotherapy utilizing conventional doses and techniques of pelvic radiation combined with 5-FU-based chemotherapy in comparison to a matched group of patients undergoing surgery alone.[142] In comparison to the 59 patients who underwent surgery alone, the 41 patients who received chemoradiotherapy had a significant increase in bowel movements, incontinence, urgency, and the need to wear pads. Paty and associates reported on sphincter function in a series of 81 patients following coloanal anastomosis. The 40 patients who received pre- or postoperative radiation therapy (with or without chemotherapy) following coloanal anastomosis had increased stool frequency and difficulty with evacuation compared with 41 patients undergoing surgery alone.[143]

In contrast to the preceding series Birnbaum and colleagues have reported on the prospective evaluation of both short-term and long-term impact of preoperative radiation on sphincter function.[144,145] All the patients were treated with conventional radiation techniques and doses and were assessed objectively with anal manometry with or without transrectal ultrasound. Radiation therapy had minimal effect on sphincter function in the 20 patients assessed for short-term results and the 10 patients assessed for long-term results.

MANAGEMENT OF LATE SIDE EFFECTS OF TREATMENT

Dietary modifications may be necessary for control of bowel function. Initially, a low-roughage diet may be helpful. After sphincter-saving rectal surgery, fecal urgency and frequency may be ameliorated with stool-bulking agents. Antispasmodic drugs may be required. Ultimately, a low-fat, high-fiber diet should be recommended. Anastomosis strictures may require dilation or cautery division. Small bowel obstruction, a late-occurring problem related to surgical scarring or radiation enteritis, necessitates surgery in 5% of patients. The need for continued advice about colostomy management, irrigation techniques, and prevention of skin irritation may necessitate consultation with an enterostomal therapist. Surgical castration or pelvic irradiation in premenopausal women leads to menopause with vaginal dryness with dyspareunia and general symptoms. Local and systemic estrogens may be helpful. Male impotence due to psychological and organic factors may require intervention. Papaverine injections, urethral prostaglandin drugs, and surgical implants can improve erectile function.

SPECIFIC RECTAL CANCER MANAGEMENT ISSUES

Management of Locally Advanced Rectal Cancer

Locally advanced rectal cancer is characterized by invasion through the muscle wall adherent to or invading surrounding structures, yet is confined to the pelvis. The accurate incidence of locally advanced rectal cancer is unknown and estimated at 5%.[146,147] Surgical resection within the context of a multimodality approach is essential for successful treatment outcome and control of symptoms. Surgery often involves TME with en bloc resection of contiguously involved structures to obtain negative margins of resection, which is essential to minimize risk of recurrence. At the time of surgery, thorough exploration to rule out metastatic disease is essential. The operative goal is complete resection with negative margins. Gross residual disease or microscopic margins has a negative impact on prognosis.[148] Adherent structures must be resected. Clinical distinction between benign adherence and malignant invasion is impossible, particularly if the patient received preoperative radiation. The most commonly resected organs in order are ovaries, uterus, vagina, and bladder.[149] Bladder preservation can be achieved with partial cystectomy with 2-cm margin. If the trigone is involved, total cystectomy with urinary diversion with ileal conduit or continent reservoir is required. The presence of positive bladder margins will adversely affect survival.[150]

M.D. Anderson Hospital (2000)[151] has reported on the institution's study of locally advanced tumors. Forty-five patients were evaluated. 5-FU was given at 300 mg/m^2 daily as a continuous infusion 5 days per week with radiation therapy. Radiation therapy was given as a concomitant boost using a three-field belly board technique. The boosts were given during the last week of therapy with a 6-hour intrafraction dose to the tumor plus 2- to 3-cm margin. The boost dose equaled 7.5 Gy per five fractions for a total dose of 52.5 Gy for 5 weeks to the primary tumor. Sphincter preservation was noted in 79% of the patients, and 31% of the patients achieved a pathologic complete response rate. Tumor downstaging was pathologically confirmed in 86% of the patients.

The University of Kentucky reported in 1999 that preoperative chemoradiotherapy was effective in the control of fixed distal rectal cancers.[125] Two chemotherapy regimens were studied (5-FU at 1000 mg/m^2 on the first

and fifth weeks of radiation days 1 to 4 and 28 to 32 and the continuous infusion 5-FU was 225 mg/m^2 for the duration of radiation). Two radiation arms were studied: 45 to 50 Gy and 55 Gy. Pathologic complete responses were noted more often in a continuous infusion and in radiation therapy when given in doses above 55 Gy. The analysis showed that 10% of the patients given bolus 5-FU achieved a complete response (CR) while 67% achieved a CR with continuous infusion. With higher-dose radiation therapy, 67% achieved a complete response with continuous infusion chemotherapy and none in the bolus 5-FU. Similar results were reported by Minsky[136] in 1991 and by Rich[152] in 1995. Rich at that time had the largest number of patients studied, 77 to be treated with continuous infusion 5-FU with a complete response rate being reported at 29% and a local recurrence for T3 lesions at 9%.

Data from the MGH, the Mayo Clinic, and the Memorial Sloan-Kettering Cancer Center have suggested the beneficial effect of intraoperative radiation therapy (IORT) (primarily, reducing the local recurrence rate to 10%), when combined with high-dose external beam radiation therapy (EBRT) and surgical resection in locally advanced primary rectal cancer. IORT is given in a single dose ranging from 10 to 20 Gy when given in patients who received preoperative EBRT and 20 to 40 Gy when given alone. The 5-year actuarial local control and disease-specific survival rates in patients receiving IORT correlate with extent of residual cancer (Table 81-12).[153] In a retrospective analysis by Sadahiro and associates,[154] survival, disease-free survival, and local recurrence-free survival in the intraoperative radiotherapy group were significantly more favorable than in the non-IORT group ($P = 0.01$, $P = 0.04$, and $P = 0.02$). Differences in survival were observed in stage II patients but not in stage I or stage III patients. There was no difference in the distant metastasis rate between the two groups. The results are less satisfactory for patients with recurrent rectal cancer, regardless of extent of resection.[155]

Pelvic exenteration and sacral resection for locally advanced primary rectal cancer have survival benefit if curative resection is possible. However, they are associated with high rates of morbidity. In a recent report by Yamada and coworkers,[156] the morbidity, reoperation, and mortality rates were 50%, 4.5%, and 0%, respectively. The overall 5-year survival rate for this group of patients

TABLE 81-12

5-Year Actuarial Local Control and Disease-Specific Survival Rates*

TREATMENT	LOCAL CONTROL RATE (%)	DISEASE-SPECIFIC SURVIVAL RATE (%)
Complete resection	89	63
Microscopic residual disease	68	40
Macroscopic residual disease	57	14

*For patients with locally advanced primary rectal cancer, receiving adjuvant and intraoperative radiation therapy.

Specific Malignancies

III

was 74.1% for Dukes' B and 47.4% for Dukes' C (difference not statistically significant).

Management of Rectal Cancer with Synchronous Distant Disease

Approximately 25% of the colorectal cancer patients present with synchronous metastasis. Patients with metastatic rectal carcinoma often present with symptomatic primary disease.[157] The symptoms referable to the primary disease area are anemia due to blood loss at the primary site, obstructive symptoms, and pelvic pain. Because pelvic pain is continuous and progressive, control of this pelvic disease is most important if one is to reach any goal in either curable patients or palliative means in incurable patients.

Two very important studies have helped to make decisions in patients with incurable rectal and colon cancer. Mahteme and coworkers[158] reported that palliative resection of the primary rectal tumor with incurable disease does not extend patient survival and does not benefit the patient's quality of life. Poor prognostic findings were lymph node involvement, peritoneal metastasis, and extensive hepatic involvement as defined by an elevation in liver function studies. Patients with distant metastasis and normal hepatic function had a slightly better prognosis.

Assersohn[159] showed similar prognostic metastatic site factors when utilizing 5-FU-based treatment. Patients with peritoneal, lung, and lymph node metastatic disease were least likely to respond, but single hepatic metastasis or locally advanced disease and normal serum albumin was more likely to respond.

M.D. Anderson Hospital[160] has reported on their experience of 80 patients who presented with synchronous distant metastasis from their rectal cancer. Two groups were evaluated. All patients received pelvic chemoradiotherapy and 25 were selected for surgery; 91% of the patients involved received 5-FU at 300 mg/m² for the length of the time of radiation to three fields. Those patients who were selected for surgery had isolated liver metastasis in 19 of 25 cases. Other means for selection were extent of disease, type of resection required, response to preoperative therapy, and response to systemic chemotherapy. Of the 80 patients, 68 (83%) presented with pelvic symptoms that included bleeding, obstruction, pelvic pain, and tenesmus. Of these 68 patients, 62 had a complete resolution of their symptoms. Only 5 of the 80 patients needed a colostomy for intraluminal progression or recurrent disease. In group one 10 patients had diverting colostomies, 5 pretreatment and 5 at time of progression or complication; in group two, 12 patients needed permanent colostomy, 10 from APR and 2 from recurrence. In group one, patients were treated without initial diverting colostomy (N = 50). The overall actuarial colostomy-free status for group one patients was 79% at 1 year. The overall 2-year survival rates were 11% and 46% for groups one and two, respectively (P > 0.001). If a colostomy was not performed at the start of treatment, 92% were colostomy-free at the time of death or last follow-up.

Management of Isolated Local/ Pelvic Failure

Typically, 55% to 80% of local recurrences present during the first 2 years after surgery. Several large reviews of outcome have identified an overall recurrence rate higher than 40% in rectal cancer, with pelvic recurrence the most common first site of relapse.[161] Among patients who relapse locally, half have isolated pelvic failure.[162,163] Two studies of patterns of recurrence in rectal cancer have demonstrated that local failure, without clinical evidence of distant metastases, accounts for about half the cancer-related deaths at 5 years. In a large series, reported by McDermott and associates,[164] 27% of rectal cancer deaths were attributable to isolated local relapse, and another 24% had combined local and systemic failure. In an autopsy series reported by Welch and Donaldson[165] 25% of patients had only local disease at the time of death, 50% had both local and systemic disease, and only 25% died of systemic metastases alone. On average, two thirds of patients with pelvic relapse after simple local excision of their tumor are able to undergo curative re-excision, whereas for more radical primary surgery, complete re-excision is usually possible in only 30% of patients.[166]

Low anterior resection also appears to result in a small number of central, anastomotic recurrences that are easy to detect and treat. Unfortunately, these relatively favorable lesions account for only 25% of locoregional relapses after anterior resection.[166] Most appear to arise in the residual mesorectum, and encroach on the lumen only secondarily, at a more advanced stage of their growth. Abdominoperineal resection (APR), the most extensive of the standard operations for rectal cancer, is apt to relapse with diffuse pelvic tumor or laterally situated masses invading the pelvic sidewall. Therefore, recurrence after APR has, in general, a poorer prognosis.[166,167]

PET scan can differentiate between recurrent tumors in the pelvis and scar. Bone scan to rule out osseous metastasis is indicated in the presence of musculoskeletal pain or if deep bony invasion in the pelvis is suspected. A positive bone scan, indicating that the tumor has penetrated the cortex of bone to invade the marrow, eliminates the possibility of curative resection. Pelvic MRI can be quiet helpful to evaluate local encroachment of the tumor on adjacent vascular structures as well as pelvic bony destruction. Other clinical and radiologic criteria of unresectability include unilateral or bilateral hydronephrosis,[168] sciatic nerve pain,[169] frozen pelvis, and unilateral leg edema.[170]

Treatment of clinically apparent local recurrence is palliative rather than curative for most patients. Although systemic chemotherapy and radiation offer effective palliation, surgery, when possible, remains the treatment of choice. Radical surgical treatment of recurrent rectal cancer offers excellent pain relief, improved quality of life, and in some cases significant prolongation of life.[171] Intraoperative radiation therapy and brachytherapy may also be used as an adjunct to surgical resection.[172]

In patients with posterior pelvic recurrence, near or adherent to the sacrum, even more radical surgery is required. APR with in-continuity sacrectomy or pelvic exenteration with in-continuity sacrectomy (composite or sacropelvic exenteration) may help highly selected younger patients. The technical aspects of the procedure with the expected outcomes and potential complications should be thoroughly discussed with the patient. The impact of sacropelvic resection on all facets of a patient's life is tremendous. Sexual function is severely affected, the bladder is usually replaced by an ileal conduit, and a colostomy is required. Wanebo has now reported on over 50 patients who underwent curative abdominosacral resection, with seemingly good palliation with excellent pain control and long-term survival in 31% of the patients.[173] These operative procedures have a formidable morbidity rate and a high mortality rate from hemorrhage or infection. Pearlman and associates[174] resected 21 patients with recurrent rectal cancer, and 18 had prior radiation. Twelve patients had complete abdominosacral exenteration. Of the 16 patients who had potentially curative surgery, 8 were free of recurrence at 6 to 48 months after the procedure. If tumor is adherent only to the distal sacrum, then rather than full-thickness sacrectomy, the anterior cortex can be removed. This procedure is quite simple from S4 down. The use of argon beam coagulation provides additional tumor destruction along the periosteum without the need for sacrectomy. Finally, intraoperative radiation therapy may replace or add to the bone resections for posterior pelvic recurrence.

ISSUES FOR THE FUTURE

Improved chemoradiotherapy therapy regimens may lead to such high clinical response rates that the "anal cancer" paradigm may be adopted. At present, most patients with clinical complete responses have microscopic residual tumor at resection. The biologic significance of these nests remains unclear. Because it is unlikely that patients will accept randomization between resection and observation, we should continue to capture data on a cohort of patients who decline radical surgery after neoadjuvant therapy. Correlative molecular markers and improved imaging (such as FDG-PET) may provide additional insight into which patients are likely to respond to neoadjuvant therapy, or if a complete clinical response is observed, which patients can be followed and could avoid radical surgery.

Improved chemotherapy concurrent with radiation therapy is under study, frequently capturing pathologic complete remission as an early surrogate end point. 5-FU infusion with CPT-11 or oxaliplatin is in trial. Comparing continuous intravenous infusion 5-FU with oral capecitabine is also an important issue. The use of recombinant erythropoietin is under study in a double-blind trial to evaluate anemia, intraoperative transfusion, and quality-of-life endpoints associated with adjuvant chemoradiotherapy.

Data are increasingly compelling that neoadjuvant therapy is more effective than postoperative treatment. This paradigm needs to be tested in patients selected for local excision. Ideally, this question should be assessed in a randomized trial of local excision comparing preoperative versus postoperative adjuvant therapy. If this is not feasible, a large multicenter trial of neoadjuvant therapy followed by local excision can be compared to the extensive published series of the postoperative paradigm. The goal should be to reduce local failure to less than 5%.

The more widespread adoption of more optimal surgical technique to minimize colostomy, positive radial margins, and autonomic nerve dysfunction is a challenge for the surgical community. The value of minimally invasive surgical approaches in the pelvis has been shown to be feasible in expert hands; whether these approaches reduce morbidity and are applicable to the general surgical community remains unclear.

SUMMARY

The goals in the treatment of rectal cancer are cure, local control, and maintainance of quality of life. A small subset of patients with mucosal, submucosal, or early invasive cancer can be treated by local excision. Adjuvant chemoradiotherapy may improve the outcomes in such patients. The majority of patients with invasive resectable rectal cancer require radical surgery. Optimal surgery for mid and low rectal cancer involves sharp pelvic dissection, total mesorectal excision, and for many patients, restorative J-pouch colorectal or coloanal reconstruction. Adjuvant chemoradiotherapy improves the local control and increases the overall cure, even with optimal surgery.

Optimizing quality of life involves not only avoidance of a permanent stoma, but utilization of an adequate-sized compliant neo-rectum. Preoperative, rather than postoperative, radiation-surgery sequencing may minimize the negative impact of radiation on late bowel function. Surgical identification and preservation of the sympathetic and parasympathetic autonomic nerves maximizes the likelihood that bladder and sexual function will be preserved.

Adjuvant radiation utilizes concurrent 5-FU-based chemotherapy. Continuous infusion 5-FU or bolus leucovorin modulated 5-FU are the two most common regimens. Phase II and III studies of capecitabine, CPT-11, and oxaliplatin are under way to further improve the therapeutic ratio. Molecular and pharmacogenomic assessments of each patient and the tumor may allow improved patient-specific adjuvant therapy.

The large majority of patients with node-negative rectal cancer are cured with surgery and the use of selective adjuvant multimodality therapy. Approximately half of node-positive patients will be cured with combined modality therapy. One quarter of patients with tethered or fixed rectal cancers treated with neoadjuvant chemoradiotherapy are subsequently resected and cured. Most cancer-related deaths are from distant disease, but three quarters of such patients also fail in the pelvis. One quarter of all rectal cancer patients who die of the cancer fail with pelvic disease only; this stresses the need for optimal surgery and adjuvant chemoradiotherapy to maximize local control.

REFERENCES

1. Greenlee RT, et al: Cancer statistics, 2001. CA Cancer J Clin 2001;51(1):15–36.
2. Cooper GS, et al: A national population-based study of incidence of colorectal cancer and age. Implications for screening in older Americans. Cancer 1995;75(3):775–781.
3. Hawk ET, Limburg PJ, Viner JL: Epidemiology and prevention of colorectal cancer. Surg Clin North Am 2002;82(5):905–941.
4. Takada H, et al: Changing site distribution of colorectal cancer in Japan. Dis Colon Rectum 2002;45(9):1249–1254.
5. Sharpe CR, Siemiatycki JA, Rachet BP: The effects of smoking on the risk of colorectal cancer. Dis Colon Rectum 2002;45(8): 1041–1050.
6. Bailey HR, et al: Local excision of carcinoma of the rectum for cure. Surgery 1992;111(5):555–561.
7. Taylor RH, Hay JH, Larsson SN: Transanal local excision of selected low rectal cancers. Am J Surg 1998;175(5):360–363.
8. Katsura Y, et al: Endorectal ultrasonography for the assessment of wall invasion and lymph node metastasis in rectal cancer. Dis Colon Rectum 1992;35(4):362–368.
9. Herzog U, et al: How accurate is endorectal ultrasound in the preoperative staging of rectal cancer? Dis Colon Rectum 1993;36(2):127–134.
10. Glaser F, Schlag P, Herfarth C: Endorectal ultrasonography for the assessment of invasion of rectal tumours and lymph node involvement. Br J Surg 1990;77(8):883–887.
11. Solomon MJ, McLeod RS: Endoluminal transrectal ultrasonography: Accuracy, reliability, and validity. Dis Colon Rectum 1993;36(2): 200–205.
12. Milsom JW, et al: Preoperative biopsy of pararectal lymph nodes in rectal cancer using endoluminal ultrasonography. Dis Colon Rectum 1994;37(4):364–368.
13. Hildebrandt U, Feifel G: Preoperative staging of rectal cancer by intrarectal ultrasound. Dis Colon Rectum 1985;28(1):42–46.
14. Beynon J, et al: Preoperative assessment of mesorectal lymph node involvement in rectal cancer. Br J Surg 1989;76(3):276–279.
15. Kim NK, et al: Comparative study of transrectal ultrasonography, pelvic computerized tomography, and magnetic resonance imaging in preoperative staging of rectal cancer. Dis Colon Rectum 1999;42(6):770–775.
16. Durdey P, Williams NS: Pre-operative evaluation of patients with low rectal carcinoma. World J Surg 1992;16(3):430–436.
17. Lorenz HP, et al: Kaposi's sarcoma of the rectum in patients with the acquired immunodeficiency syndrome. Am J Surg 1990; 160(6):681–682; discussion 682–683.
18. Hannon J, Subramony C, Scott-Conner CE: Benign retrorectal tumors in adults: The choice of operative approach. Am Surg 1994;60(4):267–272.
19. Williams NS: The rationale for preservation of the anal sphincter in patients with low rectal cancer. Br J Surg 1984;71(8):575–581.
20. Kwok H, Bissett IP, Hill GL: Preoperative staging of rectal cancer. Int J Colorectal Dis 2000;15(1):9–20.
21. Minsky BD, et al: Selection criteria for local excision with or without adjuvant radiation therapy for rectal cancer. Cancer 1989;63(7):1421–1429.
22. Willett CG, et al: Patterns of failure following local excision and local excision and postoperative radiation therapy for invasive rectal adenocarcinoma. J Clin Oncol 1989;7(8):1003–1008.
23. Willett CG, et al: Selection factors for local excision or abdominoperineal resection of early stage rectal cancer. Cancer 1994;73(11):2716–2720.
24. Nascimbeni R, et al: Risk of lymph node metastasis in T1 carcinoma of the colon and rectum. Dis Colon Rectum 2002;45(2):200–206.
25. Hager T, Gall FP, Hermanek P: Local excision of cancer of the rectum. Dis Colon Rectum 1983;26(3):149–151.
26. Biggers OR, Beart RW Jr, Ilstrup DM: Local excision of rectal cancer. Dis Colon Rectum 1986;29(6):374–377.
27. Blumberg D, et al: All patients with small intramural rectal cancers are at risk for lymph node metastasis. Dis Colon Rectum 1999;42(7):881–885.
28. Horn A, Halvorsen JF, Morild I: Transanal extirpation for early rectal cancer. Dis Colon Rectum 1989;32(9):769–772.
29. Wilson SE, Gordon HE: Excision of rectal lesions by the Kraske approach. Am J Surg 1969;118(2):213–217.
30. Mason AY: Transsphincteric approach to rectal lesions. Surg Annu 1977;9:171–194.
31. Buess G, et al: Technique and results of transanal endoscopic microsurgery in early rectal cancer. Am J Surg 1992;163(1):63–69; discussion 69–70.
32. Lezoche E, et al: Is transanal endoscopic microsurgery (TEM) a valid treatment for rectal tumors? Surg Endosc 1996;10(7):736–741.
33. Winde G, et al: Surgical cure for early rectal carcinomas (T1). Transanal endoscopic microsurgery vs. anterior resection. Dis Colon Rectum 1996;39(9):969–976.
34. Heintz A, Morschel M, Junginger T: Comparison of results after transanal endoscopic microsurgery and radical resection for T1 carcinoma of the rectum. Surg Endosc 1998;12(9):1145–1148.
35. Lezoche E, et al: Transanal endoscopic microsurgical excision of irradiated and nonirradiated rectal cancer. A 5-year experience. Surg Laparosc Endosc 1998;8(4):249–256.
36. Ambacher T, Kasperk R, Schumpelick V: [Effect of transanal excision on rate of recurrence of stage I rectal carcinoma in comparison with radical resection methods.] Chirurgia 1999;70(12):1469–1474.
37. Lezoche E, et al: Long-term results of patients with pT2 rectal cancer treated with radiotherapy and transanal endoscopic microsurgical excision. World J Surg 2002;26(9):1170–1174.
38. Heald RJ, Ryall RD: Recurrence and survival after total mesorectal excision for rectal cancer. Lancet 1986;1(8496):1479–1482.
39. Enker WE, et al: Safety and efficacy of low anterior resection for rectal cancer: 681 consecutive cases from a specialty service. Ann Surg 1999;230(4):544–552; discussion 552–554.
40. Havenga K, et al: Male and female sexual and urinary function after total mesorectal excision with autonomic nerve preservation for carcinoma of the rectum. J Am Coll Surg 1996;182(6):495–502.
41. Maas CP, et al: A prospective study on radical and nerve-preserving surgery for rectal cancer in the Netherlands. Eur J Surg Oncol 2000;26(8):751–757.
42. Nesbakken A, et al: Bladder and sexual dysfunction after mesorectal excision for rectal cancer. Br J Surg 2000;87(2):206–210.
43. Quirke P, et al: Local recurrence of rectal adenocarcinoma due to inadequate surgical resection. Histopathological study of lateral tumour spread and surgical excision. Lancet 1986;2(8514): 996–999.
44. Adam IJ, et al: Role of circumferential margin involvement in the local recurrence of rectal cancer. Lancet 1994;344(8924): 707–711.
45. de Haas-Kock DF, et al: Prognostic significance of radial margins of clearance in rectal cancer. Br J Surg 1996;83(6):781–785.
46. Ng IO, et al: Surgical lateral clearance in resected rectal carcinomas. A multivariate analysis of clinicopathologic features. Cancer 1993;71(6):1972–1976.
47. Hida J, et al: Lymph node metastases detected in the mesorectum distal to carcinoma of the rectum by the clearing method: Justification of total mesorectal excision. J Am Coll Surg 1997; 184(6):584–588.
48. Scott N, et al: Total mesorectal excision and local recurrence: A study of tumour spread in the mesorectum distal to rectal cancer. Br J Surg 1995;82(8):1031–1033.
49. Cawthorn SJ, et al: Extent of mesorectal spread and involvement of lateral resection margin as prognostic factors after surgery for rectal cancer. Lancet 1990;335(8697):1055–1059.
50. Williams NS, Dixon MF, Johnston D: Reappraisal of the 5 centimetre rule of distal excision for carcinoma of the rectum: A study of distal intramural spread and of patients' survival. Br J Surg 1983;70(3):150–154.
51. Shirouzu K, Isomoto H, Kakegawa T: Distal spread of rectal cancer and optimal distal margin of resection for sphincter-preserving surgery. Cancer 1995;76(3):388–392.
52. Vernava AM 3rd, et al: A prospective evaluation of distal margins in carcinoma of the rectum. Surg Gynecol Obstet 1992;175(4):333–336.
53. Heimann TM, et al: Local recurrence following surgical treatment of rectal cancer. Comparison of anterior and abdominoperineal resection. Dis Colon Rectum 1986;29(12):862–864.

54. Hojo K: Anastomotic recurrence after sphincter-saving resection for rectal cancer. Length of distal clearance of the bowel. Dis Colon Rectum 1986;29(1):11–14.

55. Pollett WG, Nicholls RJ: The relationship between the extent of distal clearance and survival and local recurrence rates after curative anterior resection for carcinoma of the rectum. Ann Surg 1983;198(2):159–163.

56. Glass RE, et al: The results of surgical treatment of cancer of the rectum by radical resection and extended abdomino-iliac lymphadenectomy. Br J Surg 1985;72(8):599–601.

57. Surtees P, Ritchie JK, Phillips RK: High versus low ligation of the inferior mesenteric artery in rectal cancer. Br J Surg 1990;77(6):618–621.

58. Pezim ME, Nicholls RJ: Survival after high or low ligation of the inferior mesenteric artery during curative surgery for rectal cancer. Ann Surg 1984;200(6):729–733.

59. Grinnell R: Results of ligation of inferior mesenteric artery at the aorta in resection of carcinoma of the descending and sigmoid colon and rectum. Surg Gynecol Obstet 1965;120:1031.

60. Hojo K, Koyama Y, Moriya Y: Lymphatic spread and its prognostic value in patients with rectal cancer. Am J Surg 1982;144(3):350–354.

61. Seow-Choen F: Colonic pouches in the treatment of low rectal cancer. Br J Surg 1996;83(7):881–882.

62. Hallbook O, et al: Randomized comparison of straight and colonic J pouch anastomosis after low anterior resection. Ann Surg 1996;224(1):58–65.

63. Hida J, et al: Indications for colonic J-pouch reconstruction after anterior resection for rectal cancer: Determining the optimum level of anastomosis. Dis Colon Rectum 1998;41(5):558–563.

64. Sailer M, et al: Randomized clinical trial comparing quality of life after straight and pouch coloanal reconstruction. Br J Surg 2002;89(9):1108–1117.

65. Ho YH, et al: Comparison of J-pouch and coloplasty pouch for low rectal cancers: A randomized, controlled trial investigating functional results and comparative anastomotic leak rates. Ann Surg 2002;236(1):49–55.

66. Heah SM, et al: Prospective, randomized trial comparing sigmoid vs. descending colonic J-pouch after total rectal excision. Dis Colon Rectum 2002;45(3):322–328.

67. Lazorthes F, et al: Prospective, randomized study comparing clinical results between small and large colonic J-pouch following coloanal anastomosis. Dis Colon Rectum 1997;40(12):1409–1413.

68. Hida J, et al: Functional outcome after low anterior resection with low anastomosis for rectal cancer using the colonic J-pouch. Prospective randomized study for determination of optimum pouch size. Dis Colon Rectum 1996;39(9):986–991.

69. Hida J, et al: Enlargement of colonic pouch after proctectomy and coloanal anastomosis: Potential cause for evacuation difficulty. Dis Colon Rectum 1999;42(9):1181–1188.

70. Havenga K, et al: Avoiding long-term disturbance to bladder and sexual function in pelvic surgery, particularly with rectal cancer. Semin Surg Oncol 2000;18(3):235–243.

71. Mannaerts GH, et al: Urologic and sexual morbidity following multimodality treatment for locally advanced primary and locally recurrent rectal cancer. Eur J Surg Oncol 2001;27(3):265–272.

72. Hanna NN, et al: Intraoperative parasympathetic nerve stimulation with tumescence monitoring during total mesorectal excision for rectal cancer. J Am Coll Surg 2002;195(4):506–512.

73. Pikarsky AJ, et al: Laparoscopic total mesorectal excision. Surg Endosc 2002;16(4):558–562.

74. Scheidbach H, et al: Laparoscopic abdominoperineal resection and anterior resection with curative intent for carcinoma of the rectum. Surg Endosc 2002;16(1):7–13.

75. Pietrabissa A, et al: Hand-assisted laparoscopic low anterior resection: Initial experience with a new procedure. Surg Endosc 2002;16(3):431–435.

76. Holyoke ED: Prolongation of the disease-free interval in surgically treated rectal carcinoma. Gastrointestinal Tumor Study Group. N Engl J Med 1985;312(23):1465–1472.

77. Gerard A, et al: Preoperative radiotherapy as adjuvant treatment in rectal cancer. Final results of a randomized study of the European Organization for Research and Treatment of Cancer (EORTC). Ann Surg 1988;208(5):606–614.

78. Fisher B, et al: Postoperative adjuvant chemotherapy or radiation therapy for rectal cancer: results from NSABP protocol R-01. J Natl Cancer Inst 1988;80(1):21–29.

79. Rich T, et al: Patterns of recurrence of rectal cancer after potentially curative surgery. Cancer 1983;52(7):1317–1329.

80. Mendenhall WM, Million RR, Pfaff WW: Patterns of recurrence in adenocarcinoma of the rectum and rectosigmoid treated with surgery alone: implications in treatment planning with adjuvant radiation therapy. Int J Radiat Oncol Biol Phys 1983;9(7):977–985.

81. Minsky BD, et al: Resectable adenocarcinoma of the rectosigmoid and rectum. I. Patterns of failure and survival. Cancer 1988;61(7):1408–1416.

82. Patel SC, Tovee EB, Langer B: Twenty-five years of experience with radical surgical treatment of carcinoma of the extraperitoneal rectum. Surgery 1977;82(4):460–465.

83. Enker WE, et al: En bloc pelvic lymphadenectomy and sphincter preservation in the surgical management of rectal cancer. Ann Surg 1986;203(4):426–433.

84. Willett CG, et al: Are there patients with stage I rectal carcinoma at risk for failure after abdominoperineal resection? Cancer 1992;69(7):1651–1655.

85. Willett CG, et al: Prognostic factors in stage T3N0 rectal cancer: Do all patients require postoperative pelvic irradiation and chemotherapy? Dis Colon Rectum 1999;42(2):167–173.

86. MacFarlane JK, Ryall RD, Heald RJ: Mesorectal excision for rectal cancer. Lancet 1993;341(8843):457–460.

87. Enker WE, et al: Total mesorectal excision in the operative treatment of carcinoma of the rectum. J Am Coll Surg 1995;181(4):335–346.

88. Arenas RB, et al: Total mesenteric excision in the surgical treatment of rectal cancer: A prospective study. Arch Surg 1998;133(6):608–611; discussion 611–612.

89. Marks G, Mohiuddin M, Rakinic J: New hope and promise for sphincter preservation in the management of cancer of the rectum. Semin Oncol 1991;18(4):388–398.

90. Hansen E, et al: Tumor cells in blood shed from the surgical field. Arch Surg 1995;130(4):387–393.

91. Pahlman L, Glimelius B: Pre- or postoperative radiotherapy in rectal and rectosigmoid carcinoma. Report from a randomized multicenter trial. Ann Surg 1990;211(2):187–195.

92. Frykholm G, Glimelius B, Pahlman L: Preoperative irradiation with and without chemotherapy (MFL) in the treatment of primarily nonresectable adenocarcinoma of the rectum. Results from two consecutive studies. Eur J Cancer Clin Oncol 1989;25(11):1535–1541.

93. Minsky BD, et al: Relationship of acute gastrointestinal toxicity and the volume of irradiated small bowel in patients receiving combined modality therapy for rectal cancer. J Clin Oncol 1995;13(6):1409–1416.

94. Francois Y, et al: Influence of the interval between preoperative radiation therapy and surgery on downstaging and on the rate of sphincter-sparing surgery for rectal cancer: The Lyon R90-01 randomized trial. J Clin Oncol 1999;17(8):2396.

95. Cummings BJ, et al: Radical external beam radiation therapy for adenocarcinoma of the rectum. Dis Colon Rectum 1983;26(1):30–36.

96. Lee JH, et al: Randomized trial of postoperative adjuvant therapy in stage II and III rectal cancer to define the optimal sequence of chemotherapy and radiotherapy: A preliminary report. J Clin Oncol 2002;20(7):1751–1758.

97. Douglass HO Jr, et al: Survival after postoperative combination treatment of rectal cancer. N Engl J Med 1986;315(20):1294–1295.

98. Krook JE, et al: Effective surgical adjuvant therapy for high-risk rectal carcinoma. N Engl J Med 1991;324(11):709–715.

99. NIH Consensus Conference: Adjuvant therapy for patients with colon and rectal cancer. JAMA 1990;264(11):1444–1450.

100. Tepper JE, et al: Adjuvant therapy in rectal cancer: Analysis of stage, sex, and local control—final report of intergroup 0114. J Clin Oncol 2002;20(7):1744–1750.

101. Wolmark N, et al: Randomized trial of postoperative adjuvant chemotherapy with or without radiotherapy for carcinoma of the rectum: National Surgical Adjuvant Breast and Bowel Project Protocol R-02. J Natl Cancer Inst 2000;92(5):388–396.

Specific Malignancies

III

102. Herbert SH, et al: Decreasing gastrointestinal morbidity with the use of small bowel contrast during treatment planning for pelvic irradiation. Int J Radiat Oncol Biol Phys 1991;20(4):835–842.

103. Mak AC, et al: Late complications of postoperative radiation therapy for cancer of the rectum and rectosigmoid. Int J Radiat Oncol Biol Phys 1994;28(3):597-603.

104. Minsky BD: Pelvic radiation therapy in rectal cancer: Technical considerations. Semin Radiat Oncol 1993;3(1):42–47.

105. Rider WD, et al: Preoperative irradiation in operable cancer of the rectum: Report of the Toronto trial. Can J Surg 1977;20(4):335-338.

106. The evaluation of low dose pre-operative X-ray therapy in the management of operable rectal cancer; results of a randomly controlled trial. Br J Surg 1984;71(1):21–25.

107. Stearns MW Jr, et al: Preoperative roentgen therapy for cancer of the rectum and rectosigmoid. Surg Gynecol Obstet 1974;138(4):584–586.

108. Roswit B, Higgins GA, Keehn RJ: Preoperative irradiation for carcinoma of the rectum and rectosigmoid colon: Report of a National Veterans Administration randomized study. Cancer 1975;35(6):1597–1602.

109. Higgins GA, et al: Preoperative radiation and surgery for cancer of the rectum. Veterans Administration Surgical Oncology Group Trial II. Cancer 1986;58(2):352–359.

110. Camma C, et al: Preoperative radiotherapy for resectable rectal cancer: A meta-analysis. JAMA 2000;284(8):1008–1015.

111. Chen ET, et al: Downstaging of advanced rectal cancer following combined preoperative chemotherapy and high dose radiation. Int J Radiat Oncol Biol Phys 1994;30(1):169–175.

112. Mendenhall WM, et al: Does preoperative radiation therapy enhance the probability of local control and survival in high-risk distal rectal cancer? Ann Surg 1992;215(6):696–705; discussion 705–706.

113. Fortier GA, et al: Dose response to preoperative irradiation in rectal cancer: Implications for local control and complications associated with sphincter sparing surgery and abdominoperineal resection. Int J Radiat Oncol Biol Phys 1986;12(9):1559–1563.

114. Stevens KR Jr, Allen CV, Fletcher WS: Preoperative radiotherapy for adenocarcinoma of the rectosigmoid. Cancer 1976;37(6):2866–2874.

115. Kodner IJ, et al: Preoperative irradiation for rectal cancer. Improved local control and long-term survival. Ann Surg 1989;209(2):194–199.

116. Mohiuddin M, Marks G: High dose preoperative irradiation for cancer of the rectum, 1976–1988. Int J Radiat Oncol Biol Phys 1991;20(1):37–43.

117. Kapiteijn E, et al: Preoperative radiotherapy combined with total mesorectal excision for resectable rectal cancer. N Engl J Med 2001;345(9):638–646.

118. Janjan NA, et al: Prognostic implications of response to preoperative infusional chemoradiation in locally advanced rectal cancer. Radiother Oncol 1999;51(2):153–160.

119. Kaminsky-Forrett MC, et al: Prognostic implications of downstaging following preoperative radiation therapy for operable T3-T4 rectal cancer. Int J Radiat Oncol Biol Phys 1998;42(5):935–941.

120. Mohiuddin M, et al: Prognostic significance of postchemoradiation stage following preoperative chemotherapy and radiation for advanced/recurrent rectal cancers. Int J Radiat Oncol Biol Phys 2000;48(4):1075–1080.

121. Onaitis MW, et al: Complete response to neoadjuvant chemoradiation for rectal cancer does not influence survival. Ann Surg Oncol 2001;8(10):801–806.

122. Suwinski R, Taylor JM, Withers HR: Rapid growth of microscopic rectal cancer as a determinant of response to preoperative radiation therapy. Int J Radiat Oncol Biol Phys 1998;42(5):943–951.

123. Ahmad NR, Marks G, Mohiuddin M: High-dose preoperative radiation for cancer of the rectum: Impact of radiation dose on patterns of failure and survival. Int J Radiat Oncol Biol Phys 1993;27(4):773–778.

124. Mohiuddin M, et al: Reirradiation for rectal cancer and surgical resection after ultra high doses. Int J Radiat Oncol Biol Phys 1993;27(5):1159–1163.

125. Mohiuddin M, et al: Preoperative chemoradiation in fixed distal rectal cancer: Dose time factors for pathological complete response. Int J Radiat Oncol Biol Phys 2000;46(4):883–888.

126. Mohiuddin M, Marks G: Adjuvant radiation therapy for colon and rectal cancer. Semin Oncol 1991;18(5):411–420.

127. Myerson RJ, et al: Pretreatment clinical findings predict outcome for patients receiving preoperative radiation for rectal cancer. Int J Radiat Oncol Biol Phys 2001;50(3):665–674.

128. O'Connell MJ, et al: Improving adjuvant therapy for rectal cancer by combining protracted-infusion fluorouracil with radiation therapy after curative surgery. N Engl J Med 1994;331(8):502–507.

129. Mendenhall WM, et al: Conservative treatment of rectal adenocarcinoma with endocavitary irradiation or wide local excision and postoperative irradiation. J Clin Oncol 1997;15(10):3241–3248.

130. Wagman R, et al: Conservative management of rectal cancer with local excision and postoperative adjuvant therapy. Int J Radiat Oncol Biol Phys 1999;44(4):841–846.

131. Ota D: M.D. Anderson Cancer Center experience with local excision and multimodality therapy for rectal cancer. Surg Oncol Clin North Am 1992;1:17–152.

132. Bleday R, et al: Prospective evaluation of local excision for small rectal cancers. Dis Colon Rectum 1997;40(4):388–392.

133. Steele GD Jr, et al: Sphincter-sparing treatment for distal rectal adenocarcinoma. Ann Surg Oncol 1999;6(5):433–441.

134. Chakravarti A, et al: Long-term follow-up of patients with rectal cancer managed by local excision with and without adjuvant irradiation. Ann Surg 1999;230(1):49–54.

135. Minsky BD, et al: Phase I trial of postoperative 5-FU, radiation therapy, and high dose leucovorin for resectable rectal cancer. Int J Radiat Oncol Biol Phys 1992;22(1):139–145.

136. Minsky BD, et al: Preoperative high-dose leucovorin/5-fluorouracil and radiation therapy for unresectable rectal cancer. Cancer 1991;67(11):2859–2866.

137. Improved survival with preoperative radiotherapy in resectable rectal cancer. Swedish Rectal Cancer Trial. N Engl J Med 1997;336(14):980–987.

138. Medical Research Council Rectal Cancer Working Party: Randomised trial of surgery alone versus radiotherapy followed by surgery for potentially operable locally advanced rectal cancer. Lancet 1996;348(9042):1605–1610.

139. Holm T, et al: Postoperative mortality in rectal cancer treated with or without preoperative radiotherapy: Causes and risk factors. Br J Surg 1996;83(7):964–968.

140. Holm T, et al: Adjuvant preoperative radiotherapy in patients with rectal carcinoma. Adverse effects during long term follow-up of two randomized trials. Cancer 1996;78(5):968–976.

141. Tepper JE, et al: Postoperative radiation therapy of rectal cancer. Int J Radiat Oncol Biol Phys 1987;13(1):5–10.

142. Kollmorgen CF, et al: The long-term effect of adjuvant postoperative chemoradiotherapy for rectal carcinoma on bowel function. Ann Surg 1994;220(5):676–682.

143. Paty PB, et al: Long-term functional results of coloanal anastomosis for rectal cancer. Am J Surg 1994;167(1):90–94; discussion 94–95.

144. Birnbaum EH, et al: Early effect of external beam radiation therapy on the anal sphincter: A study using anal manometry and transrectal ultrasound. Dis Colon Rectum 1992;35(8):757–761.

145. Birnbaum EH, et al: Chronic effects of pelvic radiation therapy on anorectal function. Dis Colon Rectum 1994;37(9):909–915.

146. Lopez MJ, Monafo WW: Role of extended resection in the initial treatment of locally advanced colorectal carcinoma. Surgery 1993;113(4):365–372.

147. Devine RM, Dozois RR: Surgical management of locally advanced adenocarcinoma of the rectum. World J Surg 1992;16(3):486–489.

148. Izbicki JR, et al: Extended resections are beneficial for patients with locally advanced colorectal cancer. Dis Colon Rectum 1995;38(12):1251–1256.

149. Orkin BA, et al: Extended resection for locally advanced primary adenocarcinoma of the rectum. Dis Colon Rectum 1989;32(4):286–292.

150. Talamonti MS, et al: Locally advanced carcinoma of the colon and rectum involving the urinary bladder. Surg Gynecol Obstet 1993;177(5):481–487.

151. Janjan NA, et al: Prospective trial of preoperative concomitant boost radiotherapy with continuous infusion 5-fluorouracil for locally advanced rectal cancer. Int J Radiat Oncol Biol Phys 2000;47(3):713–718.

152. Rich TA, et al: Preoperative infusional chemoradiation therapy for stage T3 rectal cancer. Int J Radiat Oncol Biol Phys 1995;32(4):1025–1029.

153. Willett CG: Intraoperative radiation therapy. Int J Clin Oncol 2001;6(5):209–214.

154. Sadahiro S, et al: Intraoperative radiation therapy for curatively resected rectal cancer. Dis Colon Rectum 2001;44(11):1689–1695.

155. Lindel K, et al: Intraoperative radiation therapy for locally advanced recurrent rectal or rectosigmoid cancer. Radiother Oncol 2001;58(1):83–87.

156. Yamada K, et al: Pelvic exenteration and sacral resection for locally advanced primary and recurrent rectal cancer. Dis Colon Rectum 2002;45(8):1078–1084.

157. August DA, Ottow RT, Sugarbaker PH: Clinical perspective of human colorectal cancer metastasis. Cancer Metastasis Rev 1984;3(4):303–324.

158. Mahteme H, et al: Prognosis after surgery in patients with incurable rectal cancer: A population-based study. Br J Surg 1996;83(8):1116–1120.

159. Assersohn L, et al: Influence of metastatic site as an additional predictor for response and outcome in advanced colorectal carcinoma. Br J Cancer 1999;79(11–12):1800–1805.

160. Crane CH, et al: Effective pelvic symptom control using initial chemoradiation without colostomy in metastatic rectal cancer. Int J Radiat Oncol Biol Phys 2001;49(1):107–116.

161. Pilipshen SJ, et al: Patterns of pelvic recurrence following definitive resections of rectal cancer. Cancer 1984;53(6):1354–1362.

162. Cass AW, Million RR, Pfaff WW: Patterns of recurrence following surgery alone for adenocarcinoma of the colon and rectum. Cancer 1976;37(6):2861–2865.

163. Rao AR, et al: Patterns of recurrence following curative resection alone for adenocarcinoma of the rectum and sigmoid colon. Cancer 1981;48(6):1492–1495.

164. McDermott FT, et al; Local recurrence after potentially curative resection for rectal cancer in a series of 1008 patients. Br J Surg 1985;72(1):34–37.

165. Welch JP, Donaldson GA: The clinical correlation of an autopsy study of recurrent colorectal cancer. Ann Surg 1979;189(4):496–502.

166. Hoffman JP, et al: Isolated locally recurrent rectal cancer: A review of incidence, presentation, and management. Semin Oncol 1993;20(5):506–519.

167. Willett CG, et al: Intraoperative electron beam radiation therapy for recurrent locally advanced rectal or rectosigmoid carcinoma. Cancer 1991;67(6):1504–1508.

168. Rodriguez-Bigas MA, Herrera L, Petrelli NJ: Surgery for recurrent rectal adenocarcinoma in the presence of hydronephrosis. Am J Surg 1992;164(1):18–21.

169. Steele G Jr: Standard postoperative monitoring of patients after primary resection of colon and rectum cancer. Cancer 1993;71(12 suppl):4225–4235.

170. Ketcham AS: The management of recurrent rectal carcinoma. Can J Surg 1985;28(5):422–424.

171. Tschmelitsch J, et al: Survival after surgical treatment of recurrent carcinoma of the rectum. J Am Coll Surg 1994;179(1):54–58.

172. Lowy AM, et al: Preoperative infusional chemoradiation, selective intraoperative radiation, and resection for locally advanced pelvic recurrence of colorectal adenocarcinoma. Ann Surg 1996;223(2):177–185.

173. Wanebo HJ, et al: Pelvic resection of recurrent rectal cancer: Technical considerations and outcomes. Dis Colon Rectum 1999;42(11):1438–1448.

174. Pearlman NW, Stiegmann GV, Donohue RE: Extended resection of fixed rectal cancer. Cancer 1989;63(12):2438–2441.

175. Paty PB, et al: Long-term results of local excision for rectal cancer. Ann Surg 2002;236(4):522–529; discussion 529–530.

176. Mellgren A, et al: Is local excision adequate therapy for early rectal cancer? Dis Colon Rectum 2000;43(8):1064–1071; discussion 1071–1074.

177. Garcia-Aguilar J, et al: Local excision of rectal cancer without adjuvant therapy: A word of caution. Ann Surg 2000;231(3):345–351.

178. Kim DG, Madoff RD: Transanal treatment of rectal cancer: Ablative methods and open resection. Semin Surg Oncol 1998;15(2):101–113.

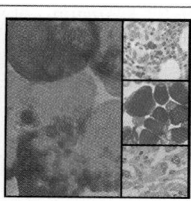

CANCER OF THE ANAL CANAL

Uzma Malik

Mohammed Mohiuddin

INTRODUCTION

Cancer of the anal canal is an uncommon malignancy, accounting for approximately 1.5% to 2% of all cancers of the lower alimentary tract in the United States.[1] The risk of anal canal cancer seems to be increasing, with its association with human papilloma virus and human immunodeficiency virus, and although approximately 4000 new cases per year are expected, it is still considered one of the more curable cancers.

ANATOMY

The anal canal is a 4-cm-long structure that passes downward and backward from the rectal ampulla (level of pelvic floor) to the anus (anal verge). The proximal border of the anal canal clinically corresponds to the anal sphincter at the level of the puborectalis muscle (palpable as the anorectal ring on digital rectal examination). This is where the rectum enters the puborectalis sling, made by fibers from both sides. The distal end of the anal canal is at the level of the anal verge, where the groove between the internal sphincter and the subcutaneous part of the external sphincter is palpable. This is also the level of the squamous-mucocutaneous junction and the perianal skin. At the dentate or pectinate line, which is a line that corresponds to the anal valves and anal sinuses, a zone of transitional mucosa is often present. This is defined as the zone interposed between uninterrupted colorectal-type mucosa above and uninterrupted squamous epithelium below.[2] Distal to the dentate line, the anal canal is lined by nonkeratinizing squamous epithelium, which merges with perianal skin (true epidermis). This junction has historically been called *anal verge* or *anal margin*. It follows that two distinct categories of tumors arise in the anal region. Tumors that develop from mucosa (columnar, transitional, or squamous) are true *anal canal cancers*, whereas tumors that arise from skin at or distal to the squamous-mucocutaneous junction are termed *anal margin tumors* (Fig. 82-1).

Lymphatic drainage of anal cancers depends on the location of the primary tumor. Tumors below the dentate line drain to superficial inguinal nodes, with some communication to femoral nodes and to the external iliac nodes. Tumors that originate above the dentate line drain to internal pudendal, hypogastric, and obturator nodes of the internal iliac system. The most proximal portion of the canal drains to perirectal and superior hemorrhoidal lymph nodes of the inferior mesenteric system.[3]

EPIDEMIOLOGY

The annual incidence of anal canal cancer in the United States is 0.47 per 100,000 in white men and 0.69 per 100,000 in white women.[4] More than 85% of cases diagnosed are in non-Hispanic whites. Approximately 4000 cases of anal canal cancer are predicted this year.[5] Overall, the risk of anal cancer is increasing.[6] The median age at diagnosis is 62 years, although more cases are being seen in younger human immunodeficiency virus (HIV)-positive patients.

Women more commonly have lesions above the dentate line, whereas distal anal canal cancers tend to be somewhat more common in men. Marked predominance is noted in females, and the preferential location is the posterior wall of the anal canal.[7] Anal canal incidence is higher in urban compared with rural populations.[8]

ETIOLOGY AND RISK FACTORS

The incidence of anal cancer and its precursor lesions (such as anal intraepithelial neoplasia) is increasing in HIV-positive patients.[9] The absolute risk in acquired immunodeficiency syndrome (AIDS) patients is 1 per 1000. Increased risk is found in young homosexual males, irrespective of HIV status. This suggests anal sexual activity as an etiologic factor.[10] Association with HIV positivity may be the consequence of chronic immunosuppression, which in itself has also been associated with an increased risk of anal canal cancer. This has been demonstrated along with vulvar cancer in renal transplant patients.[11] Human papilloma virus (HPV) is a sexually transmitted agent that also has been implicated and, of all the known subtypes, HPV-16, -18, -31, -33, and -35 have been associated with malignancy or high-grade dysplasia.[12] HPV-6 and HPV-11 have been associated with benign genital condylomata. An association of other infectious agents with anal cancer has been suggested, such as syphilis and gonorrhea in men[13] and chlamydia and herpes simplex type 2 in both men and women.[14] It appears that cancers of the genital tract and anal cancer share some common etiologic factors.[15] An association between anal cancer and the number of sexual partners has been shown in

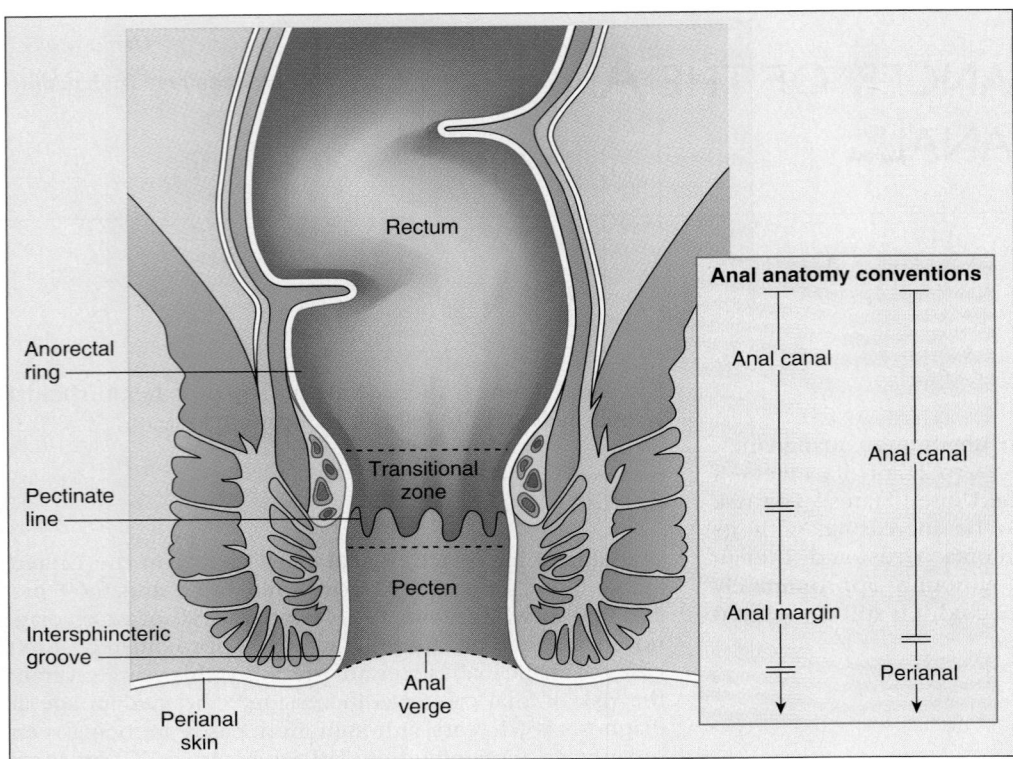

Figure 82-1. Anatomy of the anal region.

women,[14] and anal cancer patients are more likely to have a prior diagnosis of cervical intraepithelial neoplasia.[15]

Smoking and anal cancer have been associated by some studies, positively correlated with the number of cigarettes smoked per day and the duration for which a patient had been a smoker.[16]

The presence of benign conditions leading to the development of anal cancer also has been suggested.[17] An association with anal fistulae, perianal abscesses, fissures, and hemorrhoids has been reported. This may be as a result of the chronic inflammation and irritation associated with these conditions. However, this may not be a clear-cut association, as there is evidence that the risk of anal canal cancer is the highest during the first year after diagnosis of the benign condition, and this decreases after 5 years with an almost 10-fold reduction, suggesting that patients with benign conditions may actually have had undiagnosed anal malignancy as a cause of their symptoms.[18]

Molecular alterations also may play an important role in anal canal cancer causation. Alterations in the expression of wild-type p53 protein have been demonstrated.[19] As mentioned previously, cancers of the anus and cervix appear to have similar etiology, and approximately 80% of squamous cell cancers of the cervix contain a subtype of HPV, whereas most anal canal squamous cell cancers that lack HPV have a p53 mutation. Patients who have cervix cancer that contains HPV DNA tend to have a better prognosis,[19] perhaps because tumor DNA damaged by ionizing radiation is left unrepaired because of the

absence of wild-type p53. Therefore it is possible that anal cancers also are more susceptible to radiation if functional p53 protein is absent. This was shown in results from the Radiation Therapy Oncology Group (RTOG) 8704 study. These suggested that tumors with overexpression of p53 had a worse outcome than did those with normal or absent expression. Overexpression of the c-*myc* oncogene also has been implicated in the pathogenesis of squamous cell cancers of the anal region.[20]

SCREENING, EARLY DETECTION, AND PREVENTION

Screening efforts in high-risk patients include physical examination, anal pap smear, and anoscopy if the pap smear is abnormal. High-grade squamous intraepithelial lesion (HSILs) may be a precursor to invasive anal cancer, which may be detected by cytologic smears or anoscopy and biopsy, as the specificity of anal cytology for the detection of HSIL is low.[21] This screening should not undermine efforts at prevention, which should include educating the general population to the risks associated with sexually transmitted infections, especially HPV, and anogenital cancers. Prevention efforts also may include development of a prophylactic vaccine, treatment of HPV infection with development of antiviral agents, delayed onset of sexual intercourse, and cessation of smoking. These are recommendations by The National Institutes of Health Consensus Panel of 1996.[22]

NATURAL HISTORY

Anal cancer is predominantly a locoregional disease with possible direct extension to surrounding tissues and lymphatic dissemination to inguinal and pelvic nodes, with hematogenous distant metastasis being a relatively rarer occurrence. Anal canal cancers constitute 75% of all the lesions, and only 25% are anal margin tumors.

Local spread may be present in approximately 50% of cancers at diagnosis, with involvement of the anal sphincter or surrounding soft tissues.[23] Extension to the rectum and perianal skin also may occur. Invasion of the vaginal septum is more common than invasion of the prostate gland because of the presence of Denonvillier's fascia in men, which acts as a barrier.[24]

Lymphatic drainage is dependent on the anatomic location of the primary tumor. Tumors that arise distal to the dentate line drain to inguinal lymph nodes (superficial and deep), and those above the dentate line spread primarily to the internal iliac system, and from more proximal lesions, spread occurs to the inferior mesenteric group. The regional nodes are considered to be inguinal (superficial and deep femoral), internal iliac, and perirectal (anorectal, perirectal, and lateral sacral). All other nodal groups represent sites of distant disease. Involvement of inguinal nodes is directly proportional to the size and extent of the primary tumor. Overall this risk may be about 10% at diagnosis but may increase to 20% for tumors larger than 4 cm, and with T4 disease, this may be as high as 60%.[25] A suggestion is found in the literature about lymph nodal metastasis not being directly related to tumor size.[26]

Distant metastasis may occur to any organ, but those most frequently involved are the liver and lungs. Overall, distant metastases are relatively rare, as anal canal cancer tends to be a locoregional process. At diagnosis, only 5% to 10% will have distant disease. After curative reatment, the risk of distant diseases varies between 10% and 30% and depends on the initial T stage.[27] The risk of distant metastasis also increases with the number of regional nodes involved.[23]

CLINICAL PRESENTATION AND DIAGNOSIS

Most patients with anal cancer are first seen with bleeding. Approximately 30% experience pain or the sensation of a rectal mass.[28] A common concern in most anal neoplasms is the delay that often occurs in diagnosis because of confusion with more common benign conditions. Thus the clinician must maintain a high index of suspicion when evaluating lesions of the anal canal and margin.[29]

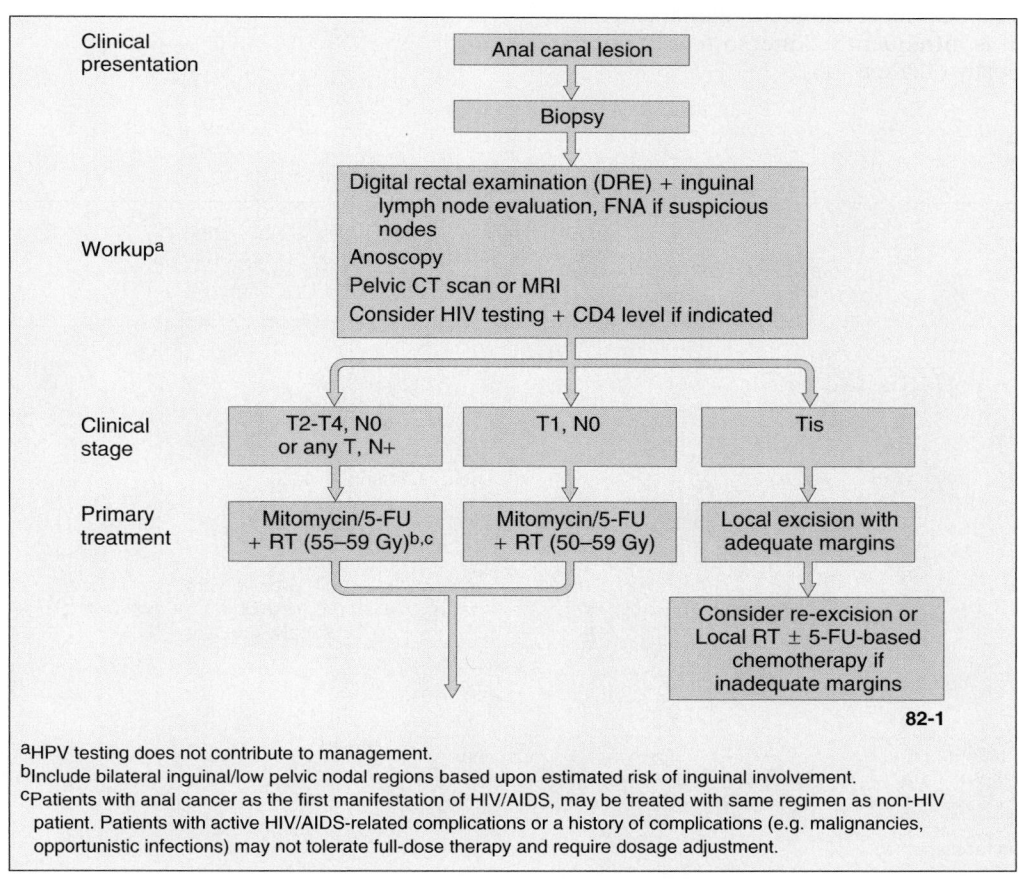

82-1

aHPV testing does not contribute to management.
bInclude bilateral inguinal/low pelvic nodal regions based upon estimated risk of inguinal involvement.
cPatients with anal cancer as the first manifestation of HIV/AIDS, may be treated with same regimen as non-HIV patient. Patients with active HIV/AIDS-related complications or a history of complications (e.g. malignancies, opportunistic infections) may not tolerate full-dose therapy and require dosage adjustment.

An interval of 4 to 6 months may occur between onset of symptoms and diagnosis in up to 50% of patients. A thorough evaluation of any patient with a lesion in the anal canal is, therefore, recommended. This includes a digital rectal examination, palpation of inguinal nodes, and an anoscopic visual examination with biopsy of suggestive lesions, including enlarged lymph nodes, which may be caused by tumor or reactive hyperplasia in as many as 50% of palpable nodes. The anal cancer need not be excised at the time of biopsy. Computed tomography (CT) scan or magnetic resonance imaging (MRI) is done to assess pelvic and suggestive inguinofemoral nodes. Rectal ultrasound is an accurate means of determining the depth of penetration of the tumor into the anal wall. It also serves to visualize local lymph nodes. CT scan of the abdomen and pelvis and chest radiograph are recommended to assess locoregional and distant disease. HIV testing also is suggested in patients with risk factors such as sexual history and drug-abuse history. Carcinoembryonic antigen (CEA) level may be elevated in 20% of cases but is rarely requested, as no clinical benefit in patient management is found by obtaining this information.[30]

STAGING

Staging for anal canal caners in based on the AJCC (American Joint Committee on Cancer) TNM staging. The TNM classification for tumors is based on clinical and/or pathologic examination as well as results of radiographic studies. The latter assess local and locoregional extension. Surgical excision is infrequently done, so few tumors are staged pathologically (Table 82-1).

DIAGNOSTIC WORKUP FOR CANCER OF THE ANAL CANAL

ESSENTIAL
History
Physical examination
　　Regional lymph nodes
　　Adjacent organs for direct invasion
　　Anogenital areas for concurrent malignancies
Proctoscopy
Biopsy of primary tumor
Fine-needle aspiration biopsy or simple excision of
　　enlarged inguinal nodes
Chest radiograph
CT of abdomen and pelvis
Liver and renal chemistry
Complete blood cell count
HIV antibodies, if risk factors present

USEFUL
Colonoscopy or air-contrast barium enema (to exclude other sources of lower gastrointestinal tract bleeding)

BIPEDAL LYMPHANGIOGRAPHY

Choa KS, Perez CA, Brady LW (eds): Radiation Oncology Management Decisions. Philadelphia, Lippincott Williams & Wilkins, 1999, p 411.

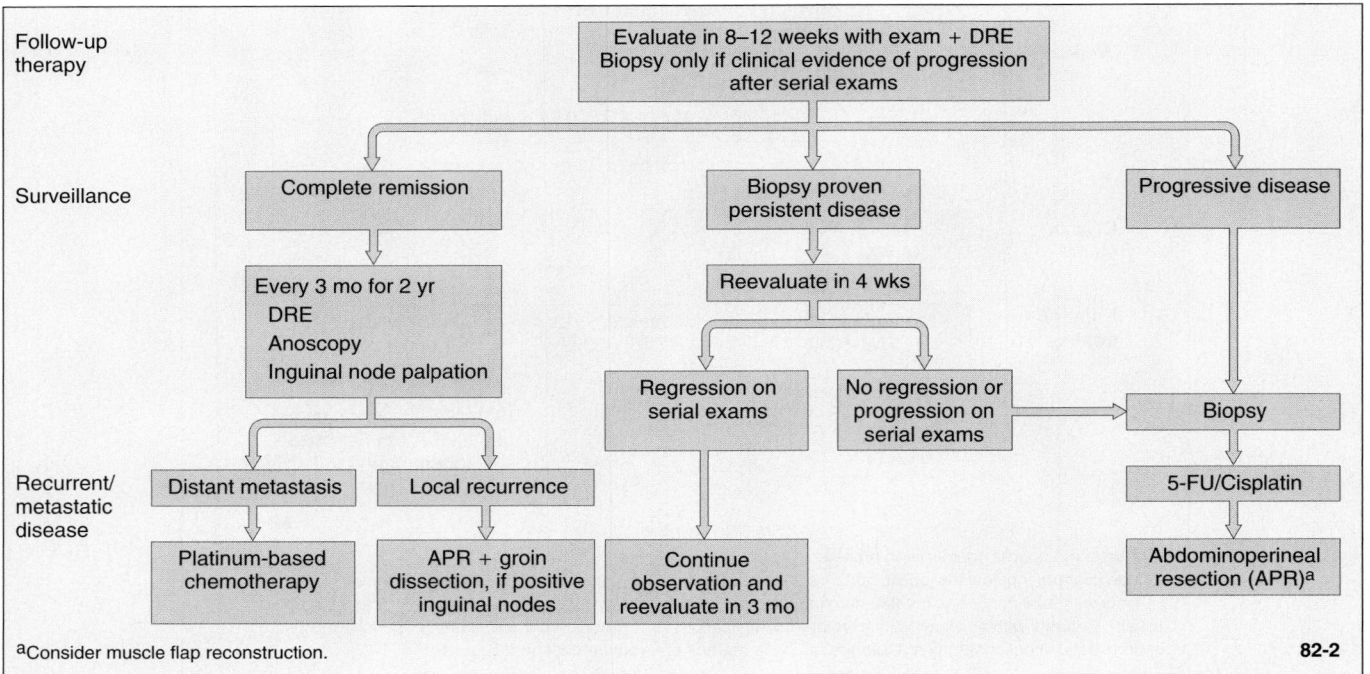

^aConsider muscle flap reconstruction.

82-2

TABLE 82-1

Definition of TNM

Primary Tumor (T)

TX	Primary tumor cannot be assessed
T0	No evidence of primary tumor
Tis	Carcinoma in situ
T1	Tumor ≤2 cm in greatest dimension
T2	Tumor >2 cm but ≤5 cm in greatest dimension
T3	Tumor >5 cm in greatest dimension
T4	Tumor of any size invades adjacent organ(s) (e.g., vagina, urethra, bladder)*

Regional Lymph Nodes (N)

NX	Regional lymph nodes cannot be assessed
N0	No regional lymph node metastasis
N1	Metastasis in perirectal lymph node(s)
N2	Metastasis in unilateral internal iliac and/or inguinal lymph node(s)
N3	Metastasis in perirectal and inguinal lymph nodes and/or bilateral internal iliac and/or inguinal lymph nodes

Distant Metastasis (M)

Stage Grouping

Stage 0	Tis	N0	M0
Stage I	T1	N0	M0
Stage II	T2	N0	M0
	T3	N0	M0
Stage IIIA	T1	N1	M0
	T2	N1	M0
	T3	N1	M0
	T4	N0	M0
Stage IIIB	T4	N1	M0
	Any T	N2	M0
	Any T	N3	M0
Stage IV	Any T	Any N	M1

MX, distant metastasis cannot be assessed; M0, no distant metastasis; M1, distant metastasis.
*Direct invasion of the rectal wall, perirectal skin, subcutaneous tissue, or the sphincter muscle(s) is not classified as T4.

WHO CLASSIFICATION OF CARCINOMA OF THE ANAL CANAL*

Squamous cell carcinoma
Adenocarcinoma
   Rectal type
   Of anal glands
   Within anorectal fistula
Mucinous adenocarcinoma
Small cell carcinoma
Undifferentiated carcinoma

---

*Note: The term carcinoma, NOS (not otherwise specified) is not part of the WHO classification.

HISTOPATHOLOGY

The staging system applies to all carcinomas arising in the anal canal, including carcinomas that arise within anorectal fistulae. Melanomas, carcinoid tumors, and sarcomas are excluded from this staging system. Most carcinomas of the anal canal are squamous cell carcinomas. The World Health Organization (WHO) classification of the types and subtypes of carcinomas of the anal canal follows: The terms transitional cell and cloacogenic carcinoma have been abandoned because these tumors are now recognized as nonkeratinizing types of squamous cell carcinoma.[31]

TREATMENT OF ANAL CANCER

Carcinoma of the anal canal is a chemoradiotherapy-sensitive tumor and therefore is often a curable cancer, with anal preservation in 65% to 75% of patients. Significant advances have occurred over the past years in its treatment. The treatment of anal canal cancer has changed from radical surgery to organ-sparing chemotherapy and radiotherapy and is one of the success stories in recent oncologic management. This principle also has served as a model for treatment of other types of malignancy.

Surgery

Surgical treatment was the primary therapy 15 to 20 years ago, but it has been replaced by sphincter-sparing therapy with combination chemoradiotherapy. Surgical therapy is now used most often as the method of salvage.

Surgical treatment, when it was used as a primary therapy, required an abdominoperineal resection (APR). This consisted of wide local excision of the anus, including the levator ani muscles and contents of the ischiorectal fossa. The operation results in a permanent colostomy as well as loss of sexual function in most patients. Overall, 5-year survival rates were approximately 50% after curative APR for anal canal cancer, with slightly better results of 55% to 71% in more recent series.[32-37] Despite reasonable survival rates, local recurrence continues to remain a significant cause of treatment failure. A review of 118 cases treated at the Mayo Clinic showed an overall survival rate of 70% and local recurrence rate of 40% (including patients with inguinal node recurrence). Local recurrence was a component of failure in more than 80% of patients who relapsed.[33] Frost and colleagues[34] reported an overall survival of 62% with a 45% rate of failure in the pelvic and/or inguinal lymph nodes. Because of the high morbidity associated with inguinal lymph node dissection and risks outweighing benefits with the procedure, prophylactic groin dissection is not recommended. Surgery alone should be considered only for lesions of the anal margin in which the sphincter can be spared. The results of several major surgical reviews are summarized in Table 82-2.

Tumor size, depth of invasion, and presence of inguinal or pelvic lymph nodes have been shown to have prognostic significance in terms of higher risk of local recurrence and worse survival.[23,32-36] A large series from Memorial Sloan Kettering Hospital demonstrated survivals of 63%, 55%, and 40% for T1, T2 and T3 lesions, respectively. The corresponding local recurrence rates were 16%, 35%, and 56%. Furthermore, patients with

Specific Malignancies

TABLE 82-2

Results of Abdominoperineal Resection for Anal Cancer

AUTHOR	YEARS	NO. OF PATIENTS	LOCAL RECURRENCE (%)	SURVIVAL (%)
Dillard et al. [32]	1940–1957	40	—	45
Boman et al. [33]	1950–1976	118	40	70
Frost et al. [34]	1954–1979	132	27 (pelvic)	62
			18 (inguinal)	
Greenall et al. [35]	1950–1978	103	—	55
Pintor et al. [36]	1948–1984	118	—	62

superficial invasion of the anal sphincter had a 79% survival rate compared with 52% with deep muscle invasion.[35] Another review by Pintor and associates[36] demonstrated 60% survival in patients with T1 and T2 lesions compared with 54% for T3 and T4 disease. In a series from the Mayo Clinic, tumors confined to the anal epithelium and subepithelial connective tissues did not recur, whereas those invading the anal sphincter recurred in approximately one fourth of the cases, and those invading adjacent pelvic tissues recurred in almost half the cases. Survival is affected by inguinal node metastases, with 5-year survival rate of only 18%.[35]

APR is rarely used as initial therapy. However, it remains a useful procedure for salvage after sphincter-preserving therapy and for management of complications related to conservative therapy.[37]

Radiotherapy

Radiotherapy has been used for treatment of anal cancers since the early 1900s, especially in Europe, whereas surgery was the treatment of choice in the United States. Most series have demonstrated survival rates in the order of 45% to 65%. As with surgery, better outcomes have been seen with smaller tumors and patients with negative inguinal lymph nodes.[38-40]

In a series from the Institut Curie between 1968 and 1979, the 5-year overall survival rate was 59% (70% for tumors <4 cm, 57% for those between 4 and 6 cm, and 33% for those >6 cm). Correspondingly, sphincter function was retained in 76% and 57% of cases for tumors smaller than 4 cm and from 4 to 6 cm. Likelihood of survival and local recurrence also depended on the tumor's circumferential size. For tumors with a circumferential involvement of 25% and 50%, survival rates of 71% and 61%, respectively, were demonstrated. However, this decreased to 19% with 75% or more circumferential involvement. Local recurrence was 16%, 28%, and 100%, respectively.[38] Local control and survival rates from retrospective series of radiation alone are summarized in Table 82-3.

Complications of radiotherapy may result in the need for colostomy in 2% to –10% of patients.[38-44] Overall, results with a definitive course of radiotherapy are similar to, if not better than, results with surgery, especially for tumors smaller than 4 cm in diameter.[45] Radiotherapy allows sphincter preservation, making it a more preferred option compared with surgery.

Excellent results also have been obtained by using external beam and interstitial radiation in combination. Papillon and Montbaron[44] treated 222 patients with external beam radiation consisting of 30 to 42 Gy, followed 2 months later with an interstitial implant using Ir-192 to deliver 15 to 20 Gy. Five-year survival was 65%. Tumors smaller than 4 cm had a 76% survival rate compared with 58% for larger lesions. Sphincter preservation was achieved in 82% and 70%, respectively.[44]

Combined-Modality Treatment

Combined-modality therapy was described initially by Nigro and coworkers[46] This was a preoperative regimen inspired by reports that 5-fluorouracil (5-FU) potentiated the effects of radiotherapy on gastrointestinal tumors.[47] This regimen consisted of delivering 30 Gy in 15 fractions to the primary tumor and pelvic lymph nodes with concurrent 5-FU (1000 mg/m^2 as 4-day continuous infusion) and mitomycin-C (MMC; 15 mg/m^2 bolus injection) chemotherapy, and APR 6 weeks after completion of the protocol.[48,49] However, promising early results suggested that surgery may not be necessary. The series of Nigro and colleagues[46] included 31 patients who underwent surgery and 73 who were treated with chemoradiotherapy alone. Twenty-two of the 31 surgical specimens had no evidence of disease (NED) pathologically, and with long-term follow-up, the NED rate of 79% for the surgical patients compared with 82% NED for the combined-modality patients. Overall death rate was 6% for tumors smaller than 4 cm and 26% for those larger than 4 cm.

Subsequent to the Wayne State Protocol of Nigro and associates, Cummings and coworkers[50] performed a series of sequential prospective nonrandomized studies at The Princess Margaret Hospital in Canada, evaluating radiation alone, radiation and concomitant 5-FU, and radiation with 5-FU and MMC. The best results were observed with both 5-FU and MMC along with radiation therapy. Cummings and colleagues[41] compared 30 patients treated with chemoradiation with 25 patients treated previously with similar doses and techniques of radiotherapy alone. Local control was 93% in the combined group, with no difference between continuous and split-course regimens, and 60% in the radiotherapy-alone group. Overall survival was 70% in both groups. The RTOG confirmed these results in a phase II trial with the same chemotherapy and a total radiation dose of 40.8 Gy at 1.8 Gy per fraction.

TABLE 82-3

Results of Irradiation Alone for Anal Cancer

AUTHOR	SCHEMA	NO. OF PATIENTS	T-STAGE/ SIZE	LOCAL RECURRENCE (%)	SURVIVAL (%)	FUNCTIONING ANUS (%)
Cummings et al.[41]	45–50 Gy, 2.5 Gy/day	51	0	43	59	77
Salmon et al.[38]	60–65 Gy	158	<4 cm	—	70	76
			4–6 cm	—	57	57
			>6 cm	—	33	—
Eschwege et al.[39]	60–65 Gy, 6–12 weeks	64	T1 and T2	9	72	91
			T3 and T4	30	35	50
Papillon and Montbarbon[44]	30–42 Gy/10 fractions rest 2 mo 15–20 Gy/ implant	159	<4 cm	11	76	82
			>4 cm	27	58	70
Schlienger et al.[40]	40–45 Gy/4–5 wk, rest 4–6 wk	T1 and T2	29	85	55	
		T3a	26	75	55	
	15–20 Gy/perineal boost	T3b	39	65	55	
		T4	43	59	55	
Martenson and Gunderson[42]	47–67 Gy, 5.5–7 weeks	18	T1–2 (17 pt) T3 (1 pt)	10	86	
Dobrowsky[43]	45–70 Gy, 4–7 wk	23	Unknown	18	65	
Doggett et al.[45]	45–76 Gy, 4.5–8 wk	35	1.3–4.5 cm	23	92	

Patients with smaller tumors of less than 3 cm had a 2-year disease-free survival of 77% compared with 53% for large tumors. Local control was also tumor size dependent: 84% for smaller lesions and 66% for larger tumors. Investigators suggested higher radiation doses for larger tumors.[51-54]

The rate of sphincter preservation also appears to be higher in patients treated with combined-modality therapy; 85% to 100% was reported by several authors.[41,52,54-56] However, no definite evidence was found of a survival benefit with the combined-modality approach, but local control and colostomy-free survival are definitely improved with the combination of chemotherapy and radiotherapy. The need for chemotherapy in addition to radiation has been established by two well-done randomized trials. Table 82-4 summarizes a number of series consisting of treatment with radiation and chemotherapy, the latter using 5-FU and MMC, as initially described by Nigro. Most show good survival and local control rate in the range of 60% to 90%.

Following up in a trial from Princess Margaret Hospital,[57] the EORTC (European Organization for Research and Treatment of Cancer) and the UKCCR (United Kingdom Coordination Committee and Cancer Research) have done two randomized studies comparing radiation alone with concomitant radiation therapy and 5-FU/MMC

TABLE 82-4

Results of Combined Modality Therapy for Anal Cancer

AUTHOR	SCHEMA	NO. OF PATIENTS	T-STAGE/ SIZE	LOCAL RECURRENCE (%)	SURVIVAL (%)
Cummings et al.[41,57]	RT, 50–60 Gy in 20–30 fx 5-FU, days 1–4, repeat at beginning of each RT course, MMC, day 1	69	—	14	—
Nigro et al.[48,49]	RT, 30 Gy/15 fx 5-FU days 2–6 MMC, day 1	104	—	—	82
Leichman et al.[51]	RT, 30 Gy/15 fx 5-FU, MITO-C	45		16	76
Sischy et al.[52]	RT-60 Gy in 33 fx 5-FU days 2–5 MMC, day 2	29	—	10	—
Flam et al.[53]	RT, 41–50 Gy/fx 5-FU, MITO-C	30	—	3	90
Sischy et al.[54]	RT, 40 Gy in 24 fx 5-FU days 2–5, days 28–31 MMC, day 2	79	<3 cm >3 cm	16 38	85 68
Tveit et al.[55]	RT, 50 Gy/fx 5-FU, MITO-C	24	—	17	58
Zucali et al.[56]	RT, 54 Gy in 30 fx 5-FU, days 1–5 MMC, day 1	38	—	32	84

5-FU, 5-fluorouracil; MMC, mitomycin C; RT, radiation therapy.

TABLE 82-5

Results of EORTC and UKCCR Trials Comparing Radiation Alone with Radiation and Chemotherapy

STUDY	N	COMPLETE RESPONSE (%)	3-YEAR LOCAL CONTROL (%)	3-YEAR OVERALL SURVIVAL
EORTC, 1987–1994[58]	103			
RT	52	54	55	64
RT plus 5-FU, MMC	51	80	69	69
P	—	.02	.02	.17
UKCCR, 1987–1981[59]	577			
RT	285	30	39	58
RT plus 5-FU, MMC	292	39	61	65
P	—	.08	<.0001	.25

EORTC, European Organization for Research and Treatment of Cancer; 5-FU, 5-fluorouracil; MMC, mitomycin C; RT, radiation therapy; UKCCR, United Kingdom Coordination Committee and Cancer Research.

chemotherapy.[58,59] Results of these two trials at a median follow-up of 42 months are outlined in Table 82-5.

In the EORTC trial, a locally advanced primary tumor (T3/T4) or regional lymph node involvement was required for eligibility. Any stage of disease was eligible for the UKCCR trial. Initial radiotherapy consisted of 45 Gy to the pelvis in both trials, but the boost was different. In the EORTC trial, 20-Gy boost was delivered to partial responders 6 weeks after completion of therapy, and complete responders received 15 Gy. In the UKCCR trial, a 15- to 25-Gy boost was given to those who had a more than 50% response, and those who had a less than 50% response underwent surgery. Chemotherapy was 5-FU, 750 mg/m^2/24hr on days 1 to 5 and 29 to 33, with a single 15-mg/m^2 dose of MMC on day 1 in the EORTC trial. In the UKCCR trial, 5-FU was 1000 mg/m^2/24hr on days 1 to 4 and 29 to 32 or 750 mg/m^2/24hr on days 1 to 5 and 29 to 33, with a single 12-mg/m^2 dose of MMC. The complete response rate 6 weeks after boost radiotherapy was 80% versus 54%, favoring the combined-modality arm in the EORTC trial. A trend toward a higher complete response rate also was reported in the UKCCR trial. However, this was measured 6 weeks after induction therapy, as opposed to 6 weeks after completion of all therapy, as was done in the EORTC trial. Although local control was low in the UKCCR study at 39% at 3 years, it should be noted that their definition of failure was less than 50% tumor reduction at 6 weeks after 45 Gy to the pelvis. Local control was significantly better in both trials in the combination arms, but no impact was seen on survival.[58,59]

The need for MMC in combined modality therapy of anal cancers was evaluated in a randomized U.S. RTOG/ECOG trial (RTOG 87-04/ECOG 1289). This was the first study comparing two methods of chemoradiotherapy in patients with anal cancer. One arm used 5-FU alone with radiotherapy, and the other arm used 5-FU and MMC with radiotherapy.[60] (Results of this study are summarized in Table 82-6). The addition of MMC was associated with fewer colostomies, higher local control, and disease-free survival, but a significantly greater risk grade of 4 or 5 toxicity in 26% of patients compared with 7%. Survival was slightly higher in the arm containing MMC, but this was not statistically significant. Disease-free survival was 73% versus 51%, favoring the MMC-containing arm.

5-FU was administered at 1000 mg/m^2/day as a continuous infusion for 4 days beginning on days 1 and 28 of radiotherapy. MMC was administered at 10 mg/m^2 IV bolus on day 1 of each 5-FU course. Two of the four treatment-related deaths on the MMC arm were believed to be due to failure to follow protocol dosage-reduction guidelines for the second MMC dose.

TABLE 82-6

Results of RTOG-ECOG Trial (Radiation and 5-Fluorouracil ± Mitomycin C)

TREATMENT ARM	NO. OF PATIENTS	TOTAL RT DOSE (GY)	NEGATIVE 4 TO 6 WK BIOPSY (%)	LOCAL CONTROL AT 4Y (%)	COLOSTOMY RATE AT 4Y (%)	COLOSTOMY-FREE SURVIVAL AT 4Y (%)	DISEASE-FREE SURVIVAL AT 4Y (%)	OVERALL SURVIVAL AT 4Y (%)	GRADE 4–5 TOXICITY (%)
RT plus 5-FU	145	45–50.4	85	66	22	59	51	67	8
RT plus 5-FU, MMC	146	45–50.4	92	84	9	71	73	76	26
P	—	—	.135	.0008	.002	.014	.003	.31	≤.001

ECOG, Eastern Cooperative Oncology Group; 5-FU, 5-fluorouracil; MMC, mitomycin C; RTOG, Radiation Therapy Oncology Group.

TABLE 82-7

Response Rates to Cisplatin-Containing Chemotherapy

AUTHOR	NO. OF PATIENTS	CHEMOTHERAPY	COMPLETE AND PARTIAL RESPONSES			DESCRIPTION
			CR	PR	OVERALL	
Mahjoubi et al.[75]	20	CDDP, 5-FU	2	9	11 (55%)	Locally recurrent and/or metastatic
Brunet et al.[76]	22	CDDP, 5-FU	6	13	18 (82%)	Primary tumors: neoadjuvant therapy

CDDP, cis-diaminedichloro platinum; 5-FU, 5-fluorouracil.

FUTURE DIRECTIONS

5-FU and cisplatin have resulted in significant antitumor activity in patients with metastatic anal carcinoma.[61,62] This combination has generated great interest, with a number of reports demonstrating response rates ranging from 55% to 82%. Table 82-7 summarizes some of these series.

This is currently being investigated in a RTOG study. This compares external-beam radiotherapy (EBRT) with 5-FU/MMC with two courses of induction 5-FU and cisplatin, followed by concurrent EBRT plus 5-FU and cisplatin. The hypothesis is that induction chemotherapy in the experimental arm may reduce the tumor bulk before concurrent chemoradiation and thereby provide better local control and colostomy-free survival. An additional two cycles of chemotherapy may positively affect on the distant metastatic rate.[63]

RADIOTHERAPY TECHNIQUES

Patients are treated with photon energy of 6 MV or greater for pelvic fields. In the past, large anteroposterior/posteroanterior (AP/PA) fields were used to treat the area of primary disease and inguinal nodes comprehensively. This is still an appropriate technique. However, alternate-field arrangements also have been used. One such technique suggests that supplementary inguinal node radiation be given, preferably with electrons. In this alternate technique, initial pelvic fields include AP/PA fields to include the pelvis, anus, perineum, and inguinal lymph nodes. The lateral inguinal nodes should be treated with the AP field but not the PA field to minimize radiation dose to the femoral head and neck. The posterior field should extend 2 cm lateral to the sciatic notch and should be designed to treat the primary tumor and pelvic nodes. Electron fields are designed to treat the lateral inguinal nodes not included in the posterior field (Fig. 82-2). The superior border of the initial pelvic fields starts at L_5/S_1 and is dropped to the level of the inferior border of the sacroiliac (SI) joints at 36 Gy (Fig. 82-3). The inferior border includes the anus with at least a 2.5 cm margin. The initial dose is 36 Gy at 1.8 Gy per fraction. This is calculated to midplane from the anterior and posterior pelvic fields. Dose to inguinal nodes is calculated, as these do not receive a contribution from the initial posterior pelvic field, which is not as wide as the anterior photon field. The remaining dose is supplemented with electrons

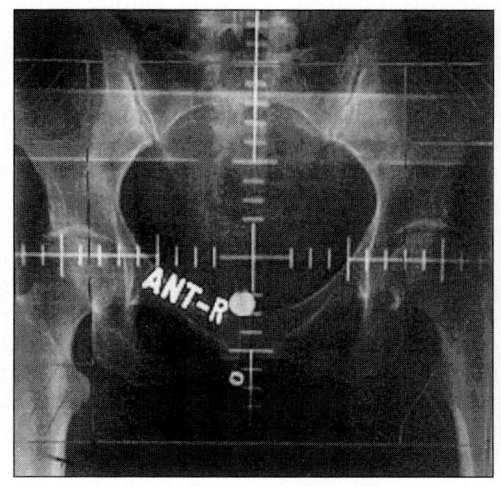
A

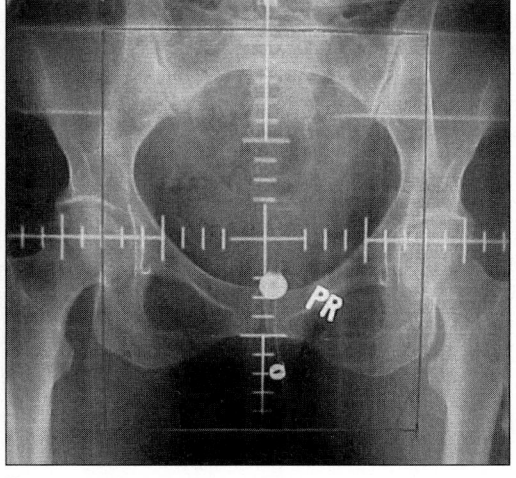
B

Figure 82-2. A, Initial anterior photon fields (*solid line*) and supplementary electron fields to boost dose to lateral inguinal nodes (*dotted line*).
B, Initial pelvic posterior photon field.

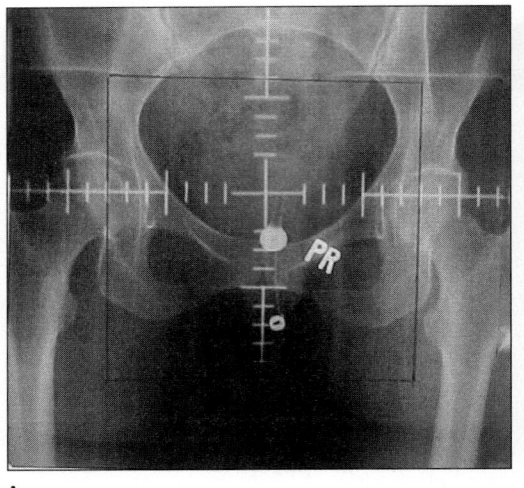 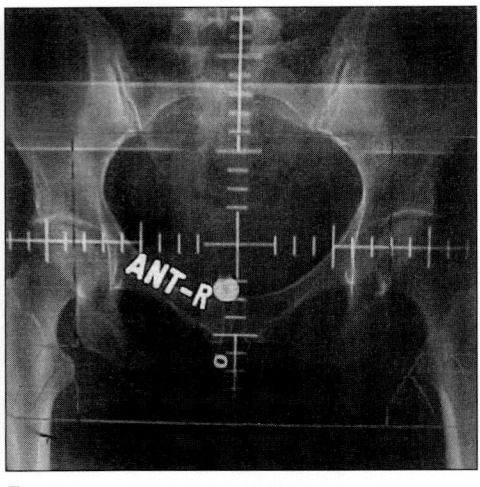

A   B

Figure 82-3. A, Posterior pelvic field with superior border at level of inferior SI joints. **B,** Anterior pelvic field reduction when superior border is brought down to inferior border of SI joints.

to make up to 180 cGy per day (typically, inguinal nodes are situated at 3 cm).

Another method of treatment uses a three-field technique as for rectal cancer, with posterior and two lateral fields. The posterior field is large enough to include the lateral inguinal nodes. The dose to the inguinal nodes is calculated and is typically about one third of the contribution from the PA field. The remaining dose is supplemented with inguinal electron fields.

It is not yet known whether escalating radiation doses to more than 45 to 50 Gy in combined-modality therapy will result in greater benefit. Analysis from the Massachusetts General Hospital, the University of Kansas, the University of Maryland, and M.D. Anderson Cancer Center suggests a benefit in local control with higher radiation doses of 54 to 66 Gy.[64-68] A benefit with higher radiation dose also was suggested in the RTOG-8704/ECOG 1289 trial.[60] This issue is being investigated currently in the ongoing RTOG 9811 study. After 45 Gy, an additional boost of 10 to 14 Gy is an option for residual disease.[63] A phase II RTOG study, RTOG 9208, unfortunately demonstrated a high incidence of colostomies of 23% with a dose of 59.4 Gy with 5-FU and MMC.[69] This

complication rate was thought to be related to a planned treatment break. A subsequent RTOG pilot trial, however, showed only an 11% colostomy rate with no treatment break.[70]

SIDE EFFECTS/RADIATION COMPLICATIONS

Anal function is maintained in 65% to 80% of patients after combined-modality treatment.[63] Late complications may result in loss of anal function, and colostomies may be needed in 2% to 10% of patients.[64] APR is usually done for disease recurrence.

Acute toxicity may be significant with radiation and chemotherapy. The severity of toxicity may be influenced by fraction size and the type of chemotherapy. Fraction size was found to be a contributing factor by Cummings and associates[60] at the Princess Margaret Hospital. The incidence of toxicity was decreased by about 50% when fraction size was decreased from 250 cGy to 200 cGy or when a planned treatment break was given. The type of chemotherapy in the RTOG/ECOG trial also determined the severity of toxicity. With 5-FU and MMC, 26% of patients experienced grade 4 or 5 toxicity compared with only 7% in the 5-FU–alone arm.[60]

In the short term, most patients experience significant perineal skin reactions, often with confluent moist desquamation, such that a treatment break becomes obligatory during most treatment courses. Other reactions may include fatigue, nausea, vomiting, diarrhea, dysuria, rectal and vaginal irritation, and possible bleeding secondary to proctitis, cystitis, and vaginitis. The latter are slightly less common.

Late complications may consist of perineal fibrosis, telangiectasia, and intermittent bleeding from the anorectal region or bladder/vagina. Other late complications may include hyper- or hypopigmentation of the skin,

---

COMBINED MODALITY TREATMENT FOR SQUAMOUS CELL CANCER OF ANAL CANAL

CHEMOTHERAPY
5-FU, 1000 mg/m^2/24 h continuous infusion IV for 96 h, starting days 1 and 28
Mitomycin-C, 10 mg/m^2 IV bolus days 1 and 28

RADIATION THERAPY
45 Gy in 25 fractions to pelvis ± boost to residual disease to total dose of 54 to 59.6 Gy

pruritus, and atrophy of the skin. Edema of the genitals or lower extremities also may occur. A possibility exists of long-term alteration of bowel function, fecal incontinence, and fistula formation requiring colostomy. Other rare complications may include painful nonhealing ulcers of the skin or anal mucosa, strictures of the anus or vagina, and osteoradionecrosis of the femoral head or neck.

Patients with comorbid conditions that would compromise tolerance to combined therapy or specifically chemotherapy may best be treated with radiation alone. This may include patients who may not be able tolerate chemotherapy, as well as HIV-positive patients who have a CD4 count of less than 200. In our experience, patients whose CD4 counts are more than 200 can be treated effectively and without an increased risk of toxicity or complications with the usual combined-modality approach, and no alteration to dose or chemotherapeutic agents need be made.

PROGNOSIS

Prognosis is directly dependent on the size of the primary tumor and the likelihood of lymphatic spread of the cancer. Tumors 2 cm or smaller are cured in 80% of cases, whereas those 5 cm or larger are cured in fewer than 50% of cases. Tumor regression after radiotherapy may be slow and may take up to 36 weeks, with a median time to tumor regression of 12 weeks from start of therapy. The majority of recurrences occur within 2 years of treatment.[50] Routine biopsies of regressing or clinically absent tumor are not recommended. Further radiation-dose supplementation may be beneficial, but this is controversial. The supposed benefit of extra radiation dose as salvage therapy may be the result of continued slow tumor regression and may not necessarily be related to the increased radiation. However, this is still not absolutely clear and continues to be investigated. Biopsy may be considered after 12 weeks if evidence of progressive disease is found. Additional chemotherapy with 5-FU and cisplatin and APR may be considered for tumor persistence or recurrence.

SUMMARY

In summary, squamous cell carcinoma of the anal canal is a disease best managed by a multidisciplinary approach. Optimal treatment is combined chemotherapy and radiotherapy. The recommended chemotherapeutic agents are 5-FU, delivered at a dose of 1000 mg/m^2 /24 hr by a continuous IV infusion for 96 hours, starting on days 1 and 28. MMC is 10 mg/m^2 IV, days 1 and 28. It should be kept in mind that MMC can cause delayed thrombocytopenia, and platelet levels should be monitored before the second dose. Radiation therapy consists of 45 Gy in 25 fractions to the pelvis over a 5–week period. The upper border of the field is reduced at a dose of 36 Gy. The issue of boost radiation for residual disease at the completion of the larger pelvic field is controversial. Some data suggest that local control is better with the addition of a boost. However, the risk of complications with a higher incidence

of colostomy rate also has been reported. This issue is currently under investigation in the RTOG 9811 protocol, which is a phase III randomized study of 5-FU, MMC, and EBRT versus 5-FU, cisplatin, and radiotherapy. This protocol permits a 10- to 14-Gy boost, 2 Gy/fx, to a reduced field after the larger pelvic fields of 45 Gy in 25 fractions for T3 and T4 or node-positive lesions, as well T2 lesions with residual disease after 45 Gy. As clear evidence exists in the literature of poor local control with T3 and higher lesions of only 50%, it is reasonable to prescribe a higher dose to lesions that are T3 or larger. Our recommendation and current practice is to treat more extensive disease with a dose of 59.6 Gy to a field 2.5 cm around the area of the anal canal malignancy. This field reduction is done after 45 Gy to the pelvis.

Cisplatin is currently not a standard chemotherapeutic agent for the treatment of anal canal cancer. In the future, however, it may play a larger role. Cisplatin and 5-FU chemotherapy has been used by a number of investigators.[68] Rich and coworkers[68] treated 21 patients with 5-FU, at a dose of 250 mg/m^2/day, and cisplatin, 4 mg/m^2/day. These were both delivered by infusion 5 days a week along with radiotherapy of 54 to 55 Gy. Local control was 89%. However, patients receiving 5-FU alone along with similar radiation showed a local control of only 73%.[68]

Doci and colleagues[71] also reported on the results of a phase II trial of 35 patients. Local recurrence with the cisplatin arm was 6% versus 24% with the mitomycin-containing arm. Cisplatin, however, is subject to investigation in its role for the treatment of anal canal cancer and now is not recommended for standard treatment. It is, however, often considered for metastatic disease, in which situation further 5-FU and mitomycin or cisplatin made be used. It also may be considered for patients whose medical conditions preclude the safe use of MMC. AIDS patients in whom standard doses of chemoradiotherapy may be too toxic may tolerate 5-FU and cisplatin as a safer alternative.[72,73]

Patients who do not respond to chemoradiotherapy usually are treated with an APR. Further chemotherapy consisting of 5-FU and cisplatin is often considered. Zelnick and colleagues[74] reported on 30 patients who were treated with APR after chemoradiotherapy for recurrent or persistent anal canal cancer. Seventy seven percent of tumors that were smaller than 5 cm with negative nodes were disease free 37 months after APR. However, none of the lesions larger than 5 cm was free of disease.[74]

Tumors of the anal margin or perianal region are treated much as are skin cancers. Our treatment recommendation is local excision. However, if the tumor were large enough such that it required an APR, we would recommend treatment as for an anal canal cancer with combination chemoradiotherapy. Most of the lesions in this area, however, are small enough that a simple excision is sufficient therapy.

Adenocarcinoma of the anal canal also can occur, arising from anal ducts. This is a fairly uncommon entity. In general, these patients are treated with preoperative chemoradiotherapy followed by an APR. The chemotherapy used in this situation is 5-FU, appropriate for adenocarcinoma, with radiotherapy fields appropriate for anal canal cancer. Treatment is governed mainly by the cell type.

Anal canal cancer is a rare entity. Interest in tumors in this area has increased in the recent past because of increased incidence. It is a curable disease with combined chemoradiotherapy, in which significant advances have occurred recently in its management. The selection of therapy for each patient requires the cooperative effort of many physicians, including radiation oncologists, medical oncologists, surgeons, and gastroenterologists.

REFERENCES

1. Jemal A, Thomas A, Murray T, et al: Cancer statistics. CA Cancer J Clin 2002;52;23–47.
2. Fenger C: The Anal transitional zone. Acta Pathol Microbiol Immunol Scand 1987;289 (Suppl):1–42.
3. Chao KS, Perez C, Brady L: Anal canal. In Chao KS, Perez C, Brady L (eds): Radiation Oncology Management Decisions. Philadelphia, Lippincott Williams & Wilkins, 1999, p 409.
4. Myerson RJ, Karnell LH, Menck HR: The National Cancer Data Base Report on Carcinoma of the Anus. Cancer 1997;80:805–815.
5. American Cancer Society: Cancer Facts and Figures 2003. Atlanta, American Cancer Society, p 4.
6. Landis SH, Murray T, Bolden S, Wingo PA: Cancer statistics. CA Cancer J Clin 1998;48:6.
7. Ghavamzadeh M, Widgren S: Carcinoma of the anal canal: Anatomical study of 21 cases. Schweiz Med Wochenschr 1979;109: 646–652.
8. Frisch M, Melbye M, Moller H: Trends in incidence of anal cancer in Denmark. BMJ 1993;306:419.
9. Melbye M, Cote TR, Kessler L, et al: High incidence of anal cancer among AIDS patients. Lancet 1994;343:636.
10. Melbye M, Rabkin C, Frisch M, Biggar RJ: Changing patterns of anal cancer incidence in the United States, 1940-1989. Am J Epidemiol 1994;139:772.
11. Penn I: Cancers of the anogenital region in renal transplant recipients: Analysis of 65 cases. Cancer 1986;58:611.
12. Zaki SR, Judd R, Coffield LM, et al: Human papilloma virus infection and anal carcinoma: Retrospective analysis by in situ hybridization and the polymerase chain reaction. Am J Pathol 1992;140:1345.
13. Daling JR, Weiss NS, Klopfenstein LL, et al: Correlates of homosexual behavior and the incidence of anal cancer. JAMA 1982;247:1988.
14. Hassanein R, Fishback J, Behbehani A, et al: Anal cancer in women. Gastroenterology 1988;95:107.
15. Melbye M, Sprogel P: Aetiological parallel between anal cancer and cervical cancer. Lancet 1991;338:657.
16. Daling JR, Sherman KJ, Hislop TG, et al: Cigarette smoking and the risk of anogenital cancer. Am J Epidemiol 1992;135:180.
17. Singh R, Nime F, Mittleman A: Malignant epithelial tumors of the anal canal. Cancer 1981;48:411.
18. Frisch M, Olsen JH, Bautz A, Melbye M: Benign anal lesions and the risk of anal cancer. N Engl J Med 1994;331:300.
19. Crook T, Wrede D, Tidy JA, Mason WP, Evans DJ, Vousden KH: Clonal p53 mutation in primary cervical cancer: association with human papilloma virus: Negative tumors. Lancet 1992;339:1070 –1073.
20. Ogunbiyi OA, Scholefield JH, Rogers K, et al: C-myc oncogene expression in anal squamous neoplasia. J Clin Pathol 1993;46:23.
21. de Ruiter A, Carter P, Katz DR: A comparison between cytology and histology to detect anal intraepithelial neoplasia. Genitourin Med 1994;70:22.
22. National Institutes of Health: Cervical Cancer: NIH consensus statement. J Natl Cancer Inst Monogr 1996;14:vii-xix.
23. Boman BM, Moertel CG, O'Connell, et al: Carcinoma of the anal canal: A clinical and pathological study of 188 cases. Cancer 1984;54:114.
24. Stearns MW Jr, Urimacker C, Sternberg SS, et al: Cancer of the anal canal. Curr Probl Cancer 1980;4:1.
25. Salmon RJ, Zafrani B, Labib A, et al: Prognosis of cloacogenic and squamous cancers of the anal cancer. Dis Colon Rectum 1986;29:336.
26. Wade DS, Herrera L, Castillo NB, Petrelli NJ: Metastases to the lymph nodes in epidermoid carcinoma of the anal canal studied by a clearing technique. Surg Gynecol Obstet 1989;169:238–242.
27. Luna-Perez P, Fernandez A, Labastida S, Lira-Puerto V, Vazquez-Curiel JA, Herrera L: Patterns of recurrence in squamous cell carcinoma of the anal canal. Arch Med Res 1995;26:213–219.
28. Tanum G, Tveit K, Karlsen KO: Diagnosis of anal carcinoma: Doctor's finger still the best? Oncology 1991;48:383.
29. Moore HG, Guillem JG: Anal neoplasms. Surg Clin North Am 2002;82:1233–1251.
30. Tanum G, Stenwig AE, Bormen OP, Tveit KM: Carcinoembryonic antigen in anal carcinoma. Acta Oncol 1992;31:333.
31. AJCC: Cancer Staging Manual, 6th ed. New York, Springer Verlag, 2002. 126–127.
32. Dillard BM, Spratt JS, Ackermann LV, Butcher HR: Epidermoid cancer of anal margin and canal. Arch Surg 1963;86772–777.
33. Bowman BM, Moertel CA, O'Connell MJ, et al: Carcinoma of the anal canal: A clinical and pathologic study of 188 cases. Cancer 1984;54:114–125.
34. Frost DB, Richards PC, Montagne ED, Giacco GG, Martin RB: Epidermoid cancer of the ano-rectum. Cancer 1984;53:1285–1293.
35. Greenall MJ, Quan SHQ, Urmacher C, DeCosse J: Treatment of epidermoid carcinoma of the anal canal. Surg Gynecol Obstet 1985;161:509–516.
36. Pintor MP, Northover HMA, Nicholss RJ: Squamous cell carcinoma of the anus at one hospital from 1948-1984. Br J Surg 1989;76: 806–810.
37. Gordon PH: Squamous cell carcinoma of the anal canal. Surg Clin North Am 1988;68:1391.
38. Salmon RJ, Fenton J, Asselain B, et al: Treatment of epidermoid anal cancer. Am J Surg 1984;147:43–8.
39. Eschwege F, Lasses P, Chavy A, et al: Squamous cell carcinoma of the anal canal: Treatment by external beam irradiation. Radiother Oncol 1985;3:145–150.
40. Schlienger M, Krzisch C, Pene F, et al: Epidermoid carcinoma of the anal canal treatment results and prognostic variables in a series of 242 cases. Int J Radiol Oncol Biol Phys 1989;17:1141–1151.
41. Cummings BJ, Thomas GF, Keane TJ et al: Primary radiation therapy in the treatment of anal canal carcinoma. Dis Colon Rectum 1982;25:778–782.
42. Martenson JA Jr, Gunderson LL: External radiation therapy without chemotherapy in the management of anal cancer. Cancer 1993;71:1736.
43. Dobrowsky W: Radiotherapy of epidermoid anal cancer. Br J Radiol 1989;62:53–58.
44. Papillon J, Montbarbon JF: Epidermoid carcinoma of the anal canal. Dis Colon Rectum 1987;30:324.
45. Doggett HSW, Green JP, Cantril ST: Efficacy of radiation therapy alone for limited squamous cell carcinoma of the anal canal. Int J Radiat Oncol Biol Phys 1988;15:1069.
46. Nigro ND, Seydel HG, Considine B, et al: Combined preoperative radiation and chemotherapy for squamous cell carcinoma of the anal canal. Cancer 1983;51:1826.
47. Haghbin M, Hinson EJ, Sischy B. Anal cancer. In Dobelbower R (ed): Gastrointestinal Cancer: Radiation Therapy. Berlin, Springer-Verlag, 1990, pp 217–246.
48. Nigro ND, Vaitkevicius VK, Considine B: Combined therapy for cancer of the anal canal. Dis Colon Rectum 1974;17:354–356.
49. Nigro ND: An evaluation of combined therapy of squamous cell cancer of the anal canal. Dis Colon Rectum 1984;27:763–766.
50. Cummings BJ, Keane TJ, O'Sullivan B, et al: Epidermoid anal cancer: Treatment by radiation alone or by radiation and 5-fluorouracil with and without mitomycin C. Int J Radiat Oncol Biol Phys 1991;21:1115.
51. Leichman L, Nigro N, Vatikevicius V, et al: Cancer of the anal canal: Model for preoperative adjuvant combined modality therapy. Am J Med 1985;78:211–216.
52. Sischy B: The use of radiation therapy combined with chemotherapy in the management of squamous cell carcinoma of the anus and marginally resectable adenocarcinoma of the rectum. Int J Radiat Oncol Biol Phys 1985;11:1587–1593.

53. Flam MS, John MJ, Mowry PA, et al: Definitive combined modality therapy of carcinoma of the anus: a report of 30 cases including results of salvage therapy in patients with residual disease. Dis Colon Rectum 1987;30:495–502.

54. Sischy B, Dossett RLS, Krall JM, et al: Definitive irradiation and chemotherapy for radiosensitization in management of anal carcinoma: Interim report a RTOG 83–14. J Natl Cancer Inst 1989;84:850–856.

55. Tveit KM, Karlsen KO, Fossa SD, et al: Primary treatment of carcinoma of the anus by combined radiotherapy and chemotherapy. Scand J Gastroenterol 1989;24:1243.

56. Zucali R, Doci R, Borubelli L: Combined chemotherapy: Radiotherapy for anal cancer. Int J Radiat Oncol Biol Phys 1990;19:1221–1223.

57. Cummings BJ, Keane TJ, O'Sullivan B, Wong CS, Catton CN: Epidermoid anal cancer: treatment by radiation alone or by radiation and 5-fluorouracil with and without mitomycin-C. Int J Radiat Oncol Biol Phys 1991;21:115–125.

58. Bartelink H, Roelofson F, Eschwege F, et al: Concomitant radiotherapy and chemotherapy is superior to radiotherapy alone in the treatment of locally advanced anal cancer: Results of a phase III randomized trial of the European Organization for Research and Treatment of Cancer Radiotherapy and Gastrointestinal Cooperative Groups. J Clin Oncol 1997;15:2040.

59. UKCCR Anal Cancer Working Party: Epidermoid anal cancer: Results from the UKCCR randomized trial of radiotherapy alone versus radiotherapy, 5-fluorauracil and mitomycin. Lancet 1996;348:1049.

60. Flam M, Madhu J, Pajak TF, et al: Role of mitomycin in combination with fluorouracil and radiotherapy, and of salvage chemoradiation in the definitive non-surgical treatment of epidermoid carcinoma of the anal canal: Results of a phase III randomized intergroup study. J Clin Oncol 1996;14:2527.

61. Carey RW: Regression of pulmonary metastases from cloacogenic carcinoma after cisplatinum/5-fluorouracil treatment. J Clin Gastroenterol 1984;6:257–259.

62. Ajani JA, Carrasco CH, Jackson DE, Wallace S: Combination of cisplatin plus fluoropyrimidine chemotherapy effective against liver metastases from carcinoma of the anal canal. Am J Med 1989;87:221–224.

63. RTOG 98-11: A phase III randomized study of 5-fluorouracil, mitomycin-c, and radiotherapy versus 5-fluorouracil, cisplatin and radiotherapy in carcinoma of the anal canal.

64. Hughes LL, Rich TA, Delclos L, et al: Radiotherapy for anal cancer: Experience from 1979 – 1987. Int J Radiat Oncol Biol Phys 1989;17:1153.

65. Allal AS, Mermillod B, Roth AD, et al: The impact of treatment factors on local control in T2, T3 anal carcinomas treated by radiotherapy with or without chemotherapy. Cancer 1997;79:2329.

66. Constantinou EC, Daly W, Fung CY, et al: Time-dose considerations in the treatment of anal cancer. Int J Radiat Oncol Biol Phys 1997;39:651.

67. Nish SS, Smalley SR, Elman AT, et al: Conservative therapy for anal carcinoma: An analysis of prognostic factors: Proc ASTRO 1991. Int J Radiat Oncol Biol Phys 1991;suppl 1:224.

68. Rich TA, Ajani JA, Morrison WH, et al: Chemoradiation therapy for anal cancer; radiation plus continuous infusion 5-fluorouracil with or without cisplatin. Radiother Oncol 1993;27:209–215.

69. John M, Pajak T, Flam M, et al: Dose escalation in chemoradiation for anal cancer: Preliminary results of RTOG 92-08. Cancer J Sci Am 1996;2:205.

70. John M, Pajak T, Kreig R, et al: Dose escalation without split-course chemoradiation for anal cancer: Results of a phase II RTOG study. Int J Radiat Oncol Biol Phys 1997;39(suppl 2):203.

71. Doci R, Zucali R, La Monica G, et al: Primary chemoradiotherapy with fluorouracil and cisplatin for cancer of the anus: Results in 35 consecutive patients. J Clin Oncol 1996;14:3121.

72. Holland JM, Swift PS: Tolerance of patients with human immunodeficiency virus and anal carcinoma to treatment with combined chemotherapy and radiation therapy. Radiology 1994;193:251.

73. Peddada AV, Smith DE, Rao AR, et al: Chemotherapy and low dose radiotherapy in the treatment of HIV infected patients with carcinoma of the anal canal. Int J Radiat Oncol Biol Phys 1997;37:1101.

74. Zelnick RS, Haas PA, Ajlouni M, et al: Results of abdominal perineal resections for failures after combinations chemotherapy and radiation therapy for anal canal cancers. Dis Rectum 1992;35:574.

75. Mahjoubi M, Sadek H, Francois E, et al: Epidermoid and carcinoma: Activity of cisplatin and continuous infusion 5-FU in metastatic and or local recurrent disease. Proc ASCO 1989;8:157.

76. Brunet R, Sadek H, Vignoud J, et al: Cisplatin and 5-FU for the neoadjuvant treatment of epidermoid anal canal carcinoma. Proc ASCO 1990;9:104.

Specific Malignancies

III

LIVER AND BILE DUCT CANCER

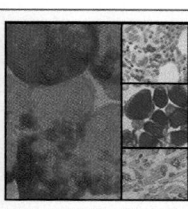

Sharon Weber

Eileen M. O'Reilly

Ghassan K. Abou-Alfa

Leslie Blumgart

SUMMARY OF KEY POINTS

INCIDENCE

- Hepatocellular cancer is one of the most common solid organ malignancies worldwide, with up to 1 million cases per year. This high incidence relates to its common association with cirrhosis from either alcohol or hepatitis B or C.
- Cholangiocarcinoma and gallbladder cancer are less common hepatobiliary malignancies.

ETIOLOGY AND EPIDEMIOLOGY

- The primary risk factor for hepatocellular cancer is underlying cirrhosis.
- Although several associated risk factors occur for gallbladder cancer and cholangiocarcinoma, most tumors occur as a sporadic event.

PATHOLOGY AND BIOLOGY

- All of these tumors are primarily adenocarcinomas. Because the majority of patients are first seen with advanced disease, only a small proportion are amenable to curative resection.
- Hilar cholangiocarcinoma has a propensity for local invasion that makes definitive treatment challenging.

CLINICAL FINDINGS

- Although patients with cholangiocarcinoma or gallbladder cancer may have jaundice, the majority of patients with liver neoplasms are asymptomatic.
- Patients with cirrhosis are often incidentally discovered to have hepatocellular cancer because of an elevated α-fetoprotein (AFP) level or a liver mass found at the time of routine screening.

DIFFERENTIAL DIAGNOSIS

Differential diagnosis includes secondary hepatic malignancies or benign neoplasms such as focal nodular hyperplasia, hemangioma, or adenoma.

PRIMARY THERAPY AND SALVAGE THERAPY

- Primary treatment for liver and bile duct neoplasms is complete surgical resection. In patients with unresectable disease, few effective alternative treatments are available.
- Patients with nonresectable disease are candidates for experimental therapy, liver function and performance status permitting.

PROGNOSIS

- Overall survival for all patients with these tumors is less than 5%. However, the 5-year survival for patients with resectable disease is approximately 30% to 50%.
- Unfortunately, even after complete resection, the disease recurs in the majority of patients.

HEPATOCELLULAR CANCER

Introduction

Hepatocellular cancer (HCC) is a leading solid organ malignancy worldwide due to its common etiology from chronic liver damage due to hepatitis or cirrhosis. Curative treatment includes complete surgical resection, although even after definitive resection, recurrence is common. Treatment of unresectable disease is limited. Greek mythology is abundant with references to the liver organ that relate to both life and death. In the *Iliad*, Achilles slew Tros with a sword in his liver. On the summit of Mt. Caucasus, Prometheus, the Greek legend, was tormented day and night by a giant eagle tearing at his constantly regenerating liver.[1] Daily we are humbled by the might of both primary and secondary liver malignancies, yet daily we savor the living legend of Prometheus's liver that has allowed modern medicine and surgery to affect these challenging cancers.

Epidemiology

HCC accounts for 6% of all cancers worldwide. It is the fifth most common malignancy in the world[2] with an estimate of a half million cases per year, and a mortality rate equivalent to its incidence. These estimates must be looked at in context of a specific geographic area and be interpreted accordingly. About 80% of the cases worldwide arise in the developing countries of Southeast Asia and sub-Saharan Africa.[3] The etiology of the disease differs in different parts of the world. In broad categories, in developing countries, the risk factors for developing HCC are mainly due to chronic hepatitis B virus (HBV) infection and aflatoxin B1 food contamination. This is in contrast to the etiologic factors in the developed world, which include alcohol and hepatitis C virus (HCV) infection, with the latter becoming increasingly prevalent. With local etiologic factors being guided by local customs and behaviors, some emerging reports show the incidence rates to be declining in some developing areas of the world,[4] while increasing in some developed countries.[5,6]

In essence, the world's incidence of HCC can be divided into three categories: high, intermediate, and low. Southeast Asia and sub-Saharan Africa dominate the highest incidence regions of liver cancer in the world. However, caution is required in accepting this fact, as few cancer registries in developing countries use the International Classification of Diseases (ICD)-O (oncology) coding system that is dependent on an accurate histologic diagnosis.[7] The highest incidence of liver cancer in the world is in Thailand; however, these rates reflect an exceptionally high incidence of cholangiocarcinoma[8] due to infestation with the liver fluke *Opisthorchis viverrini*.[9] In many high-incidence regions, the carrier state for hepatitis begins in infancy because of vertical transmission between mother and child. In all populations, males are affected at a higher frequency than are females. It is important to note that this high incidence can move along with the migration patterns of certain ethnic groups. For instance, the incidence rate of liver cancer is 23.9 among the Korean population of Los Angeles, compared with a low incidence of 1.1 among the white population of New Mexico.[3] Additionally, the incidence may vary in certain regions because of the higher prevalence of other risk factors. This is exemplified in the differing incidence rate in European men that ranges from 1.6 in the Netherlands to 18.2 in Trieste, Italy.

The intermediate-incidence category includes South America, even though certain pockets of the country have a higher incidence (e.g., Port Alegre, Brazil, with a rate of 8.3/100,000).[3] Southern Europe accounts for most of the remaining world regions with an intermediate incidence of HCC.

North America, although still categorized as a low-incidence region, has had a dramatic increase in the incidence of HCC primarily due to an increasing incidence of HCV infection. El-Serag[10] reviewed records of 1605 patients diagnosed with HCC between 1993 and 1998 in 171 Veterans Administration (VA) hospitals. They noted a threefold increase in the age-adjusted rates for HCC associated with HCV from 2.3/100,000 between 1993 and 1995 to 7.0/100,000 between 1996 and 1998. Oceania and Northern Europe provide the remainder of the contribution to the low-incidence category.

Etiology and Pathogenesis

Sixty percent to eighty percent of patients first seen with HCC have cirrhosis from associated liver parenchymal disease, most often due to chronic viral hepatitis from either hepatitis B or hepatitis C. The risk for development of HCC in the setting of hepatitis B–related cirrhosis is approximately 0.5% per year,[11] whereas development of HCC in the setting of hepatitis C may occur in as many as 5% of cirrhotic patients per year.[12]

The management of this disease is made more difficult because of the underlying liver disease. In one study in which patients with underlying liver disease with small (<3 cm) HCCs were followed up, death occurred solely because of hepatic failure in 20%.[13]

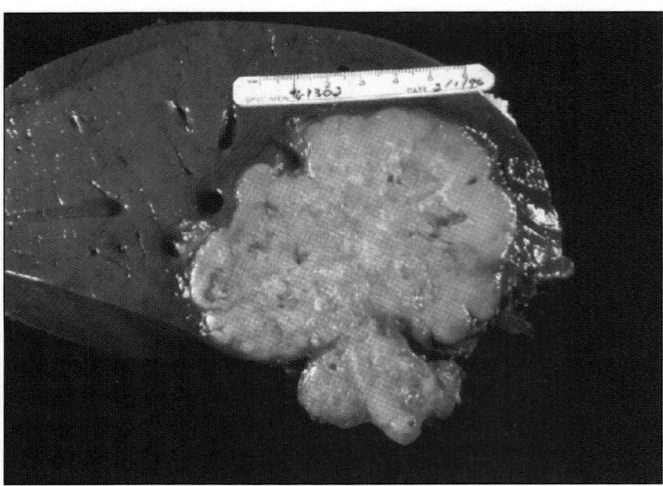

Figure 83-1. Gross image of hepatocellular cancer demonstrates large mass lesion.

Pathology

The most common form of HCC is an adenocarcinoma, which may be unifocal or multifocal at presentation. These tumors can reach a large size before they are detected (Fig. 83-1). HCC has a strong propensity for vascular invasion, which is clearly a poor prognostic sign. More unusual forms of this tumor include a mixed hepatocellular-cholangiocarcinoma pattern and a fibrolamellar variant, which arises in the setting of normal liver function.

Biology

HCC can metastasize to lung and bone late in its course, but for many patients, the tumor is a local-regional issue. Commonly, even after complete curative resection, tumor recurs in the liver, because of the common inciting event of prolonged damage to the hepatocytes from hepatitis or cirrhosis.

Clinical Presentation and Patient Evaluation

Most patients with HCC have few symptoms until very late in the disease, when tumors are at an advanced stage. Patients may have malaise, anorexia, abdominal pain, abdominal fullness due to ascites or mass effect, or weight loss. Because the majority of cases of HCC occur in patients with underlying cirrhosis, any worsening of hepatic function in a previously diagnosed cirrhotic patient must result in an evaluation for occult HCC. After a liver lesion is discovered, patients should be asked about a history of hepatitis, ethanol abuse, or family history of metabolic diseases such as hemochromatosis or α-1–antitrypsin deficiency, all of which are risk factors for HCC.

Laboratory and Imaging Studies

Screening Tests
An accurate screening test for patients with risk factors for HCC is extremely important in discovering the disease

at an early, potentially resectable stage. However, because the majority of patients with HCC have underlying liver dysfunction from cirrhosis, routine liver function tests are poor screening tests for the presence of HCC. Serum α-fetoprotein (AFP) level is one relatively sensitive screening test for the presence of HCC. An AFP level of greater than 20 ng/mL in a patient with a liver mass is highly sensitive but has poor specificity for the diagnosis of HCC.[14-16] AFP levels greater than 500 are diagnostic of HCC, and an AFP level greater than 2000 is a poor prognostic indicator, with no 5-year survivors in this group.[17] Interestingly, racial differences may exist in the level of AFP expression, with a lower sensitivity in African Americans compared with non–African Americans.[14]

Although AFP is the most widely used screening and diagnostic test for HCC, serum concentration levels of des-γ-carboxy prothrombin (DCP) and *Lens culinaris* agglutinin-reactive fraction (AFP-L3) also are useful tumor markers for the diagnosis of HCC.[18,19] In a prospective study evaluating all three tumor markers in 90 patients with viral hepatitis, the sensitivity and specificity by using the panel of markers was significantly higher than by using any one alone (>80% sensitive and specific, panel of tumor markers).[18] Okuda and colleagues[20] correlated outcome with seropositivity for these markers and found that HCC patients who were seropositive for AFP-L3 but seronegative for DCP demonstrated clinicopathologic features of more advanced HCC compared with those who were seropositive for DCP alone. In addition, this group found that seropositivity for AFP alone was associated with less advanced HCC compared with seropositivity for DCP alone.[21]

Screening ultrasound for patients with cirrhosis has been widely used and found to be effective in high-risk patients, although the interval between screening examinations remains controversial. The sensitivity and specificity of screening ultrasound in high-risk patients is approximately 75% and 90%, respectively.[16,22] In one recent study in Taiwan with a high endemic hepatitis B infection rate, screening ultrasound was found to decrease the mortality from HCC compared with that in patients found to have HCC by other means.[23] This is likely because of the ability to detect suggestive lesions at an earlier stage. Unfortunately, because of the generalized acceptance of screening ultrasound in high-risk patients, no randomized prospective trial has been performed to assess the effect of screening ultrasound on disease-specific mortality. In addition, because of geographic differences in mean body mass index, clear differences occur in the ability of radiologists to detect liver lesions with ultrasound.

Screening patients with cirrhosis or hepatitis B or C is critical, because it has been found that occult HCC discovered as a result of screening with AFP or ultrasound is more likely to be resectable, and patients have both a lower operative mortality and higher 5-year survival than do patients with clinically detected HCC.[24]

Diagnostic Tests

All patients with suspected HCC should also have hepatitis serologies tested, including hepatitis B surface

TABLE 83-1

Child-Pugh Classification for Assessing the Degree of Liver Impairment			
CRITERIA	**1 POINT**	**2 POINTS**	**3 POINTS**
Bilirubin	<2	2–3	>3
Albumin	>3.5	2.8–3.5	<2.8
Prothrombin time (seconds greater than normal)	1–3	4–6	>6
Ascites	None	Mild	Moderate
Encephalopathy	None	Mild	Moderate

By adding the points based on each patient's factors, a Child-Pugh A is 5–6 points; B, 7–9 points; C, 10–15 points.

antigen and hepatitis C *polymerase chain reaction* (PCR). Depending on the degree of underlying liver damage from fibrosis, the liver function tests and prothrombin time may be abnormal. An assessment of liver function should be performed; the most commonly used assessment with the most widespread availability is the Child-Pugh score (Table 83-1).

Radiologic assessment of HCC is extremely important in making the diagnosis and deciding which treatment modality is appropriate. Although ultrasound is widely available and therefore is often the first imaging study used to examine the liver in a patient suspected of have an HCC, ultrasound is a poor test for characterizing liver lesions in patients with cirrhosis, where regenerating nodules can often be mistaken for tumor. On ultrasound, HCC will typically have a thin halo, lateral shadows, and posterior echo enhancement.

A more useful imaging test is dynamic computed tomography (CT). In the early phase, the tumor is hyperdense because of its increased vascularity (Fig. 83-2). In later phases, the tumor becomes hypodense as contrast washes out of the lesion. Magnetic resonance imaging (MRI) is becoming more frequently used as an imaging modality for evaluation of HCC. On MRI, HCC appears to be low in intensity on T_1-weighted images, and intermediate in intensity on T_2-weighted images. MRI also can be useful in distinguishing HCC from benign lesions such as hemangiomas and regenerating nodules. Because of the

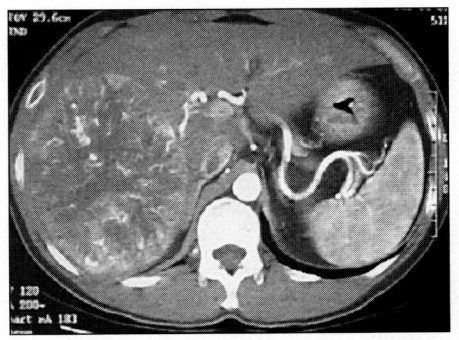

Figure 83-2. Dynamic computed tomography scan of a hypervascular right lobe hepatocellular cancer. (Courtesy of Spiros Hiotis, MD, New York University School of Medicine.)

propensity for extension into and along major vasculature, contrast-enhanced CT or MRI is particularly useful to image portal and hepatic veins. In addition, contrast-enhanced images provide critical information about multifocality, resectability, and presence of extrahepatic disease.

On imaging with CT or MRI, three growth patterns of HCC are seen—invading, pushing, or hanging. In the invading pattern, the tumor grows into structures in its path, whereas in the pushing pattern, the tumor may move structures such as major blood vessels as it grows. Finally, the tumor may grow largely removed from the liver in a hanging pattern, sometime attached to the liver by a relatively small stalk. Another common feature of HCC is its ability to invade vascular structures, such as the inferior vena cava (Fig. 83-3) or portal vein (PV; Fig. 83-4). The tumor thrombus, which is actually an extension of the tumor itself into the vasculature, can be well seen on contrast-enhanced CT or MRI. The classic appearance is a mass within the vasculature, which fills and expands the lumen.

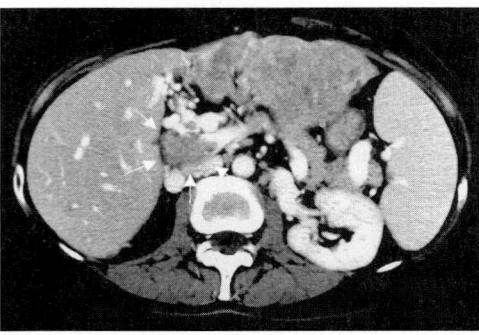

Figure 83-4. Large left lobe hepatocellular carcinoma with vascular invasion into the portal vein, demonstrated by the classic finding of tumor thrombus filling and expanding the main portal vein (*arrows*), with cavernous transformation of the portal vein.

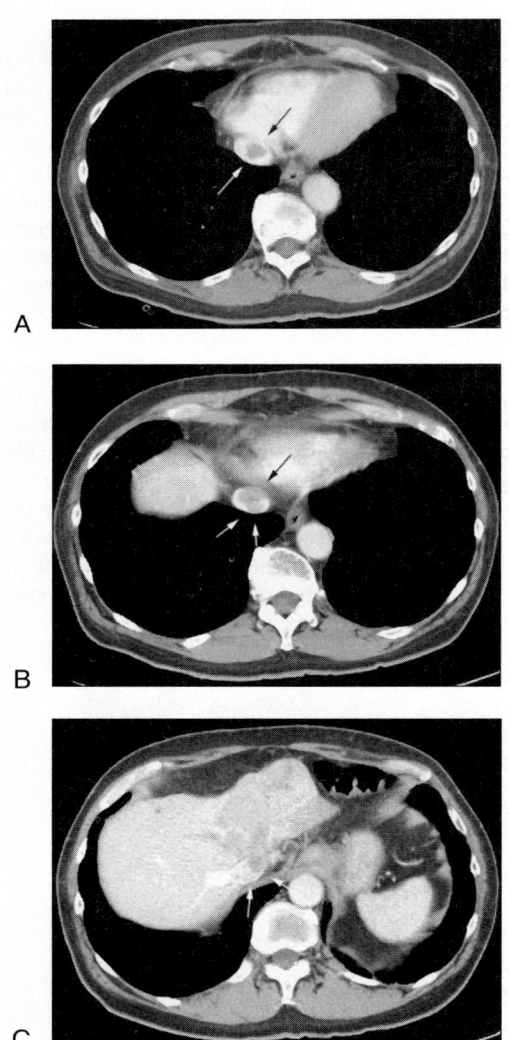

Figure 83-3. A–C, Left lobe hepatocellular cancer with tumor invasion into the inferior vena cava (*arrows*).

The angiographic appearance of HCC can be even more diagnostic because HCC is characteristically hypervascular. However, because the study is invasive, it is difficult to recommend it routinely for diagnostic purposes. Angiography is often used for therapeutic reasons in embolizing HCC with thrombotic agents with or without chemotherapy, and often detects small tumors not seen on other imaging modalities.

Although fluorodeoxyglucose–positron emission tomography (FDG-PET) imaging has been found to be useful in a variety of tumors, its use in HCC has been disappointing, with significantly lower SUV (standardized uptake value) for HCC compared with that for metastatic tumor or other primary liver tumors[25] and an accuracy of 20% to 50%.[26,27] Thus FDG-PET currently has no proven role in the staging of patients with either primary or recurrent HCC.

Staging Classification

The American Joint Committee on Cancer (AJCC) sixth edition staging classification uses size, presence of vascular invasion, lymph node status, and metastatic disease as prognosticators of outcome (Table 83-2). Several important changes have been incorporated into the new tumor-node-metastasis (TNM) staging system. First, all solitary tumors without vascular invasion, regardless of size, are classified as T1 because of similar prognosis. Second, all solitary tumors with vascular invasion, again independent of size, are combined with multiple tumors 5 cm or smaller and classified as T2 because of a similar prognosis. Third, multiple tumors larger than 5 cm and tumors with evidence of major vascular invasion are combined and classed as T3 because of a similarly poor prognosis. Fourth, stage IV refers to metastatic disease only. The subcategories IVA and IVB have been eliminated.

Prognosis

Outcome

Overall survival after liver resection or transplantation has been reported from numerous investigators (Table 83-3). In patients with unresectable disease, the survival is

TABLE 83-2

Staging System for Hepatocellular Carcinoma Including Intrahepatic Bile Ducts

STAGE	TUMOR	NODES	METASTASIS
I	T1	N0	M0
II	T2	N0	M0
IIIA	T3	N0	M0
IIIB	T4	N0	M0
IIIC	Any T	N1	M0
IV	Any T	Any N	M1

Definition of TNM

Primary Tumor (T)

TX Primary tumor cannot be assessed
T0 No evidence of primary tumor
T1 Solitary tumor without vascular invasion
T2 Solitary tumor with vascular invasion; or multiple tumors, none >5 cm
T3 Multiple tumors >5 cm, or tumor involving a major branch of the portal or hepatic vein(s)
T4 Tumor(s) with direct invasion of adjacent organs other than the gallbladder or with perforation of the visceral peritoneum

Regional Lymph Nodes (N)

NX Regional lymph nodes cannot be assessed
N0 No regional lymph node metastasis
N1 Regional lymph node metastasis

Distant Metastasis (M)

MX Presence of distant metastasis cannot be assessed
M0 No distant metastasis
M1 Distant metastasis

From Greene FL: AJCC Cancer Staging Manual, 6th ed. New York, Springer-Verlag, 2002.

dismal, with a median survival less than 12 months even with chemotherapy.[28,29]

Patterns of Recurrence

At 5 years after resection of HCC, the recurrence rate has been reported to be between 30% and 60%.[30-32] Cirrhotic patients have recurrence at a much greater rate than do noncirrhotics. The liver is the first site of recurrence in up to 90% of these patients.[30,33,34] Other common sites of metastases include lung, adrenal glands, other intra-abdominal spread, and bones.[35] It is uncommon for patients to have isolated extrahepatic recurrences.[35]

TABLE 83-3

Results of Hepatic Resection for Hepatocellular Carcinoma in the Noncirrhotic Patient

INSTITUTION	N	OPERATIVE MORTALITY (%)	SURVIVAL 1-YR	SURVIVAL 3-YR	SURVIVAL 5-YR
Pittsburgh, 1991[40]	59	12 (90 d)	81	60	44
Shimane Univ, 1993[30]	52	6	87	66	55
MSKCC, 1999[22]	54	4	83	58	42
Beujon Hospital, 2002[29]	58	3	95	78	50

The most well-accepted risk factors for recurrence include tumor size,[31] vascular invasion,[31,34,36,37] and high preoperative AFP.[31] Other risk factors include tumor differentiation,[37] tumor rupture,[38] and cirrhosis,[34,38,39] particularly when stratified for the size of the tumor.[31] Interestingly, multifocal HCC has been found to be a risk factor for recurrence in few studies.[40,41] Some suggestion exists that outcome after resection is improved in patients with HCC associated with hepatitis B compared with those with hepatitis C.[42]

Primary Treatment

Resection

Partial Hepatectomy. Surgical excision by partial or total hepatectomy represents the only potentially curative therapy for hepatocellular carcinoma. Resectability for any hepatic tumor, including HCC, is dependent on the patient's ability to withstand a major surgical intervention, absence of extrahepatic disease, and anatomic resectability. The results of surgical resection are influenced greatly by the preoperative liver functional status. Cirrhosis adversely influences surgical outcome in many ways, and often is the only determinant that results in an unresectable status. Because the liver parenchyma in cirrhotics is fibrotic and firm, retraction and isolation of intraparenchymal vessels is hazardous for the surgeon, and makes hemorrhage a particular concern during resection of HCC. Patients with cirrhosis also are likely to have thrombocytopenia from hypersplenism, further exacerbating the potential for hemorrhage. Finally, cirrhosis is associated with decreased regenerative capacity, increasing the risk of liver failure after partial resections. For these reasons, hepatic resection for patients with cirrhosis carries a significantly higher operative risk than the risk for noncirrhotic patients, and typically patients with cirrhosis and HCC are better served with transplantation if indications regarding tumor size and number are met.

Outcome after resection in noncirrhotic patients is excellent; partial hepatic resection can be performed with less than a 5% operative mortality and is associated with a 5-year survival in excess of 30% (see Table 83-3). For noncirrhotic patients with resectable HCC, therefore, surgical resection represents the treatment of choice. However, the adverse influence of cirrhosis on surgical outcome is well documented by clinical data, as the operative mortality is more than 10% even at large-volume centers (Table 83-4). Nevertheless, cirrhotic patients who survive the operation have a 5-year survival of approximately 30% (see Table 83-4).

Thus patient selection for surgery depends primarily on hepatic function. Over the years, many complex methods of evaluating liver function have been tested to assist in patient selection. Assessment by Child-Pugh classification (see Table 83-1) remains the most useful and most widely used in Western series, although the indocyanine green (ICG) retention rate is used commonly in Asia. Few surgeons are willing to perform hepatic resection for patients with Child-Pugh C liver status, and operative

TABLE 83-4

Results of Hepatic Resection for Hepatocellular Carcinoma in Cirrhotic Patients

INSTITUTION	N	OPERATIVE MORTALITY (%)	SURVIVAL		
			1-YR	3-YR	5-YR
Keio University, 1990[170]	80	9	82	60	45
Shimane Medical University, 1993[30]	177	12	77	43	21
MSKCC, 1999[22]	100	5	77	47	37
Beujon Hospital, 2002[29]	168	10	78	55	34

mortality may be as high as 30% for patients with Child-Pugh B cirrhosis. These patients are clearly better served with transplantation if they meet accepted criteria. Therefore most surgeons will consider resection only for patients with Child-Pugh A liver function reserve.

HCC has a great propensity for vascular extension, and the presence of tumor thrombus within the main PV or vena cava (see Figs. 83-3 and 83-4) is an ominous sign and should be regarded as a contraindication to resection. Liver resections accompanied by portal venous tumor thrombectomies are unlikely to yield long-term survival. Multiple lesions do not preclude surgical resection,[31,39,43] because 5-year survival can still be expected to be between 20% and 30%.[31,39]

Total Hepatectomy and Transplantation. Total hepatectomy and liver transplantation is an attractive option for the patient with cirrhosis and cancer, because it may potentially cure both the underlying liver disease and the tumor. Generally well-accepted indications for liver transplant are Child-Pugh B or C patients with single HCC smaller than 5 cm in size, or fewer than three tumors all smaller than 3 cm. With these criteria, the most recent series have found a 5-year survival of approximately 70% with a 15% chance for recurrence (Table 83-5). In comparing the results of transplantation with those of resection, one must remember the inherent selection

bias of choosing not only those patients with small HCCs that have a better prognosis, but additionally, the bias of transplanting only those patients whose cancer has not progressed while waiting for an organ. Thus the patients that receive liver transplants are those with a less aggressive natural history. This is demonstrated by a recent intention-to-treat analysis, which found "drop-out from waiting list" to be the sole survival predictor.[44] This study found that the 2-year survival rate of patients evaluated for transplantation was reduced from 84% to 54% during two separate time periods in which the waiting time increased markedly, and therefore more patients were excluded from transplantation because of progression of disease. Survival was significantly worse for patients on the transplant list than for patients who were the best candidates for resection.[44] In addition, a recent article evaluated the outcome of patients undergoing liver resection with tumors that fit the criteria for liver transplantation. In this selected group of patients, overall survival at 5 years was 70%, similar to outcome after liver transplantation.[32]

In practice, many obstacles limit the applicability of transplantation to a large number of patients worldwide. The greatest obstacle is the lack of available organs for transplant. Some U.S. centers report long waiting times, with the number of patients being excluded from transplant while on the waiting list because of progression of disease nearly equal to that of those that receive transplant.[45] In Asian countries where the need for donor organs is greater, social and cultural obstacles are found for organ donation, and thus livers are in even greater shortage than in the United States. In addition, because of organ scarcity, it is vital that a thorough cost-effectiveness analysis be performed to compare results after liver transplantation for benign versus malignant disease.

The costs associated with the transplantation procedure also are a major obstacle. Although perioperative morbidity and mortality are declining, in most centers, mortality is still substantial. Table 83-5 summarizes some of the published data, including only relatively recent trials with more than 50 patients. It is clear that operative mortality can be as high as 10% to 20%,[46,47] and recurrence rates as high as 50%[48] in these series.[40] However, for patients with liver dysfunction, total hepatectomy with liver transplantation represents the only potentially

TABLE 83-5

Results of Total Hepatectomy with Orthotopic Hepatic Transplantation for Hepatocellular Carcinoma

INSTITUTION	N	FOLLOW-UP (MO)	OPERATIVE MORTALITY (%)	RECURRENT HCC (%)	SURVIVAL		
					1-YR	3-YR	5-YR
Pittsburgh, 1991[40]	105		14 (90 d)	43	66	39	36
Hopital Paul Brousse, 1993[34]	60		5		75	47	
Mount Sinai, 1995[37]	57		19 (90 d)	5	75	65	NR
Hannover, 1997[171]	124	36			83	77	76
Barcelona, 1998[38]	58	31	14 (90 d)		84	74	74
Humboldt University, 2001[172]	120	49	2	17	90		71

NR, not reported.

curative option, because few of these patients will tolerate major hepatectomy. To demonstrate this point, in non-cirrhotic HCC, survival is similar after hepatectomy or transplantation, whereas in patients with cirrhotic HCC, survival was significantly improved after transplantation compared with hepatectomy at each TNM stage.[49]

Long-term results of HCC treated with transplantation also are related to extent of original liver involvement, with the best results reported in patients with small HCC discovered incidentally during transplantation performed for cirrhosis.[50] Clearly large tumor size and the presence of vascular invasion are associated with a high risk for recurrence after transplantation.[40,51,52]

Recently several authors reported the results of living donor–related liver transplantation (LDLT) for HCC. Because this procedure requires a right hepatectomy in a healthy donor, concerns have been expressed about the safety and ethical implications of this procedure. In addition, sporadic reports of deaths in donors from the United States and abroad have intensified these concerns. In one of the largest series reporting the results of LDLT in 71 patients, with approximately 40% due to HCC, the mean waiting time to transplant was markedly reduced from 414 (cadaveric organ) to 83 days (living-related), with a recurrence rate was 15%.[53] To summarize, patients without liver dysfunction and HCC should be considered for resection, whereas patients with HCC arising in the setting of Child-Pugh B/C cirrhosis should be referred for transplantation.

Hepatic Artery Embolization. Because a large majority of patients have liver-only disease that is technically unresectable, other forms of therapy are needed for HCC. Because these tumors are so intensely vascular and are fed primarily by the hepatic artery (HA), embolization of the feeding arterial vessels has been shown to be one possible treatment option for these patients. A recent randomized controlled trial (RCT) compared patients with Child-Pugh A or B cirrhosis with unresectable HCC who were randomized to chemoembolization versus embolization versus conservative treatment. The trial was stopped early because of the survival advantage of chemoembolization, with 2-year survival of 63% compared with 27% for control and 50% for embolization.[54] In addition, in a prior RCT performed by these same investigators, no difference in survival was noted for embolization compared with conservative treatment.[55] Lee and colleagues[56] assessed the benefits of transcatheter arterial chemoembolization compared with standard hepatic resection in an Asian population of 182 patients. Both groups received initial chemoembolization with Lipiodol CT. Ninety-one patients subsequently undergoing surgery and 91 who refused surgery were allocated to serial chemoembolizations. The authors' observations were interesting in that chemo-embolization appeared to be as effective as resection in the population of patients with locally advanced liver tumors with adequate liver function. Thus it appears that chemoembolization is a potentially viable option for patients with both unresectable and resectable disease, and additionally, it may have an advantage over conservative treatment.

Cryosurgery. Cryoablation is becoming an increasingly popular method for treating HCC. In this modality, probes that are cooled by liquid nitrogen or argon are introduced into tumors, followed by freezing under ultrasound guidance until adequate volume of tumor plus a 1-cm margin has been treated (Fig. 83-5). Cryosurgery has great theoretical advantage in the treatment of tumors in cirrhotic patients, in that very little nonmalignant parenchyma is damaged; thus patients with cirrhosis are still often candidates for the procedure. In addition, this technique is useful for treating bilobar tumors, whether with cryosurgery alone or with cryosurgery plus resection.[57]

The major disadvantage is the need for general anesthesia and laparotomy, because this technique cannot be performed percutaneously. In addition, some tumors are not treatable with cryosurgery, primarily because of size, because it is clear the complications increase as more tumor volume is destroyed. A number of published series clearly demonstrated the safety of such an ablative approach in experienced hands.[57,58]

Radiofrequency Ablation. Radiofrequency ablation (RFA) is an excellent alternative to cryosurgery and offers the advantage of percutaneous as well as intraoperative application (Fig. 83-6). Some authors have suggested that both the complication rate and recurrence rate after RFA are lower than that after cryosurgery.[58] However, no true prospective comparative trials exist. The disadvantage of RFA is that it is difficult to monitor under real-time US guidance, unlike cryosurgical ablation, because no distinct demarcation can be seen between viable tissue and RF-ablated tissue.

In the largest study of RFA in patients with cirrhosis and HCC (Child-Pugh class A, 50; B, 31; C, 29), 110 patients were treated. The complication rate was 13%, with local recurrence developing in only 4% at a follow-up of 19 months, although in a large number of patients, recurrent disease developed at other sites within the liver.[59] Of note, although it is possible to perform RFA percutaneously, clearly a greater number of tumors are incompletely ablated percutaneously, when compared with open RFA.[59] One of the additional advantages of RFA is that it is useful in treating those patients with recurrent disease.[60] Finally, a recent cost analysis of patients undergoing treatment for HCC while waiting for transplantation showed a survival advantage for the use of percutaneous treatments.[61]

Ethanol Injection. Percutaneous ethanol injection is a highly effective treatment for small HCC, with a 3-year survival of 60%[62] and a 5-year survival of 45%.[63] In this technique, absolute alcohol is injected into liver tumors percutaneously under CT or US guidance, which results in tissue necrosis (Fig. 83-7).[64] Tumors that are amenable to ethanol injection include those smaller than 4 cm and usually fewer than four. This method may be curative for small lesions, but trials comparing this technique with other methods of ablation are needed.

In one of the only studies comparing ethanol injection with RFA for patients with small HCCs, effective tumor

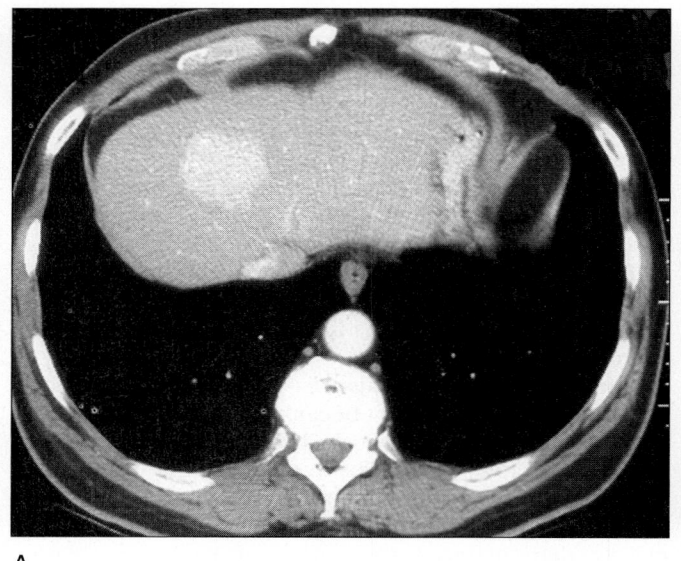

A

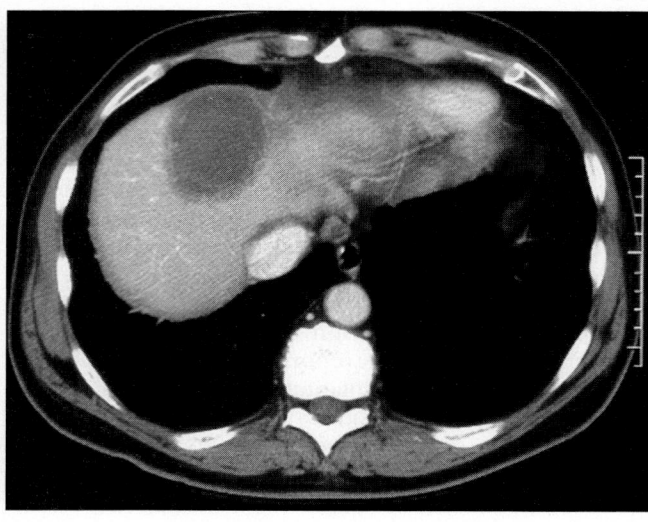

B

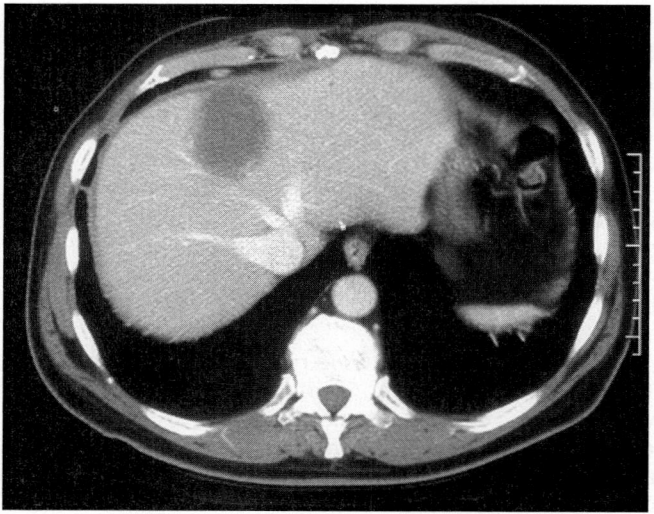

C

Figure 83-5. Cryoablation of hepatocellular carcinoma. **A,** Precryoablation image. **B** and **C,** Cryolesion 1 month after ablation demonstrates central necrosis and no evidence of recurrent tumor.

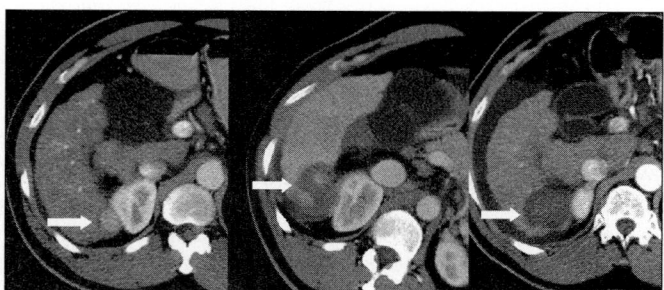

Figure 83-6. Percutantous radiofrequency ablation (RFA) of hepatocellular carcinoma in a high-risk patient with advanced cirrhosis, demonstrating the pre-RFA image (*left panel*) and post-RFA images (*middle, right panels*).

necrosis occurred by using either technique, but RFA required fewer treatments to achieve that effect (1.2 sessions, RFA, vs. 4.8 sessions, ethanol). However, more complications occurred in the patients undergoing RFA.[65] Thus treatment decisions for these patients should be individualized.

Microwave Ablation. Ablation of liver tumors by using percutaneous microwave coagulation is a relatively new technique that will require further prospective trials before widely adapting the technique to patients with HCC. The advantages of this technique are the higher temperatures it can achieve in a shorter time and the ability to use multiple probes. In a preliminary study, the survival for patients with primary disease and recurrent HCC was 47% (5-year) and 50% (4-year), respectively.[57]

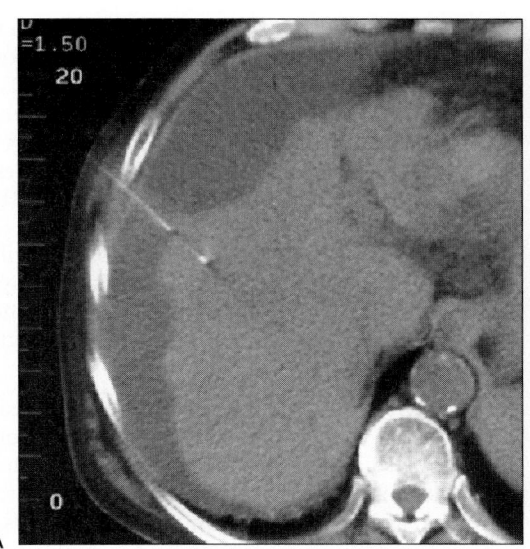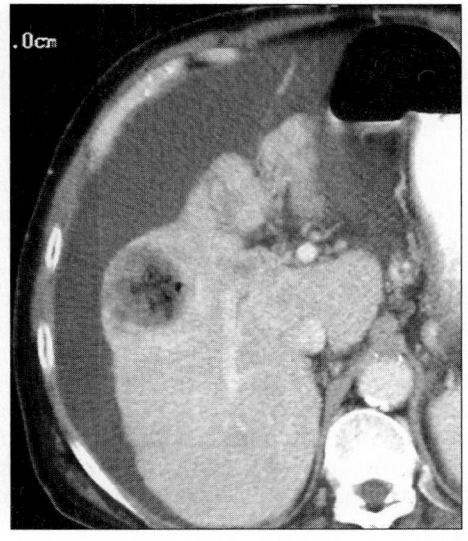

Figure 83-7. A, Percutaneous needle placement under noncontrast computed tomography (CT) for alcohol ablation of small hepatocellular carcinoma in a cirrhotic patient with ascites. **B,** Postablation contrast-enhanced CT scan.

Chemotherapy. Two major challenges exist with respect to chemotherapy administration in HCC. First, the inherent resistance of HCC to chemotherapy, and second, underlying liver function, which may be the major determinant of prognosis in patients with HCC.[66,67] The low efficacy may relate to the overexpression of multidrug-resistant genes and TP53 gene mutations, which are frequent in advanced HCC.[68-70] However, for patients with locally unresectable and extrahepatic disease, those with underlying poor liver function, or the medically unfit, chemotherapy may represent the only potentially viable treatment option. A theoretical argument can be made for considering chemotherapy in the adjuvant setting. For those patients who undergo potentially curative surgery, the risk of recurrence is high; therefore even drugs that have a modest impact on established disease may confer significant benefit when administered in an adjuvant setting. Many issues complicate chemotherapy and its assessment of benefit in HCC: (1) a majority of patients have significant underlying liver dysfunction in the context of cirrhosis or chronic hepatitis, (2) most drugs are tested in advanced-stage HCC in trials with small patient numbers, and (3) quantitating chemotherapy response in HCC is fraught with methodologic difficulties. To date no single chemotherapy drug or combination has been clearly demonstrated to affect either overall survival or quality of life; however, some of the newer drug combinations offer some promise in this regard and indeed pathologic complete remissions have been observed after systemic chemotherapy, suggesting that the true role of chemotherapy in HCC remains to be defined.[66]

Multiple single-agent therapies have been assessed in HCC. Historically anthracyclines have been considered to have the highest single-agent activity, with response rates ranging in the 10% to 79% range; however, more recent studies demonstrate response rates of about 10% to 20%.[71]

One small randomized trial of doxorubicin versus supportive care demonstrated a modest impact in median survival from 7 to 11 weeks for the anthracycline[72]; however, several other randomized studies failed to confirm this benefit.[73] Concerns with regard to anthracycline administration in HCC include the fact that many patients have significant liver dysfunction, which can compromise drug dosing and enhance the potential for toxicity. One approach to overcoming the frequently encountered systemic toxicity of anthracyclines in HCC is to use compounds with anticipated low systemic toxicity [e.g., long-circulating polyethylene glycol–coated (pegylated) liposomal doxorubicin]. A small phase II study of liposomal doxorubicin in HCC demonstrated a partial response rate of 10% and an overall median survival of 3 months in 40 patients.[74] Notably, three patients with cirrhosis died of infection in the absence of neutropenia. The authors concluded that although patients with HCC had a lower initial serum concentration of the drug, a larger volume of distribution, and more rapid clearance, compared with patients with normal liver function, pegylated liposomal doxorubicin did not appear to have a greater advantage over standard anthracyclines. A further small study by Dangoor and associates[75] was terminated early after no responses were seen with pegylated doxorubicin in the first 16 patients, confirming the limited activity of this drug in advanced HCC. Of the other newer single agents, irinotecan and gemcitabine have been disappointingly relatively inactive in HCC.[76-78]

Combination chemotherapy regimens have consistently demonstrated modestly higher response rates over single-agent therapy, in the 20% to 30% range in many studies.[79-86] One of the more promising, but toxic combinations is the PIAF regimen, initially published by Leung and coworkers.[81] This combination uses cisplatin, interferon alpha-2b, doxorubicin, and 5-fluorouracil (5-FU). The initial phase II report was provocative, noting a high partial response rate of 26%, and of the patients with a baseline elevation of AFP, 42% had a greater than 50% decline in AFP with treatment. Additionally, nine patients were able to undergo surgery, and in four, no evidence of viable tumor was noted at the time of surgery. Of concern was the high rate of myelosuppression and mucositis, and two treatment-related deaths occurred in the context of neutropenic infection. In further publications, the authors more clearly identified which patients are most likely to benefit from PIAF therapy.[87,88] These patients included those without cirrhosis, a low level of bilirubin, and a positive hepatitis C serology. Poor prognostic factors predictably included high Okuda stage, presence of cirrhosis, and vascular involvement. Clearly the PIAF regimen must be assessed in the context of a large randomized study before its merits can be judged. Such a study is currently under way in Hong Kong comparing PIAF with single-agent doxorubicin in advanced HCC. Additionally, the role of PIAF as neoadjuvant therapy must be defined.

Considerable interest has been expressed in developing chemoimmunotherapy combinations for HCC based on modest single-agent activity of interferon alfa-2b in HCC, as well as the possible preventive role of HCC in patients with HBV- or HCV-related cirrhosis. Additionally, recombinant interferon has been shown to enhance the cytotoxicity of fluoropyrimidine therapy, possibly via effects on a critical enzyme in fluoropyrimidine metabolism, thymidine phosphorylase. Patt and colleagues[83] conducted a phase II trial of 5-fluorouracil and recombinant interferon alfa-2b in HCC on the basis that it would prove to be a tolerable combination for patients with cirrhosis. Five (62.5%) of eight patients with fibrolamellar HCC (no underlying cirrhosis) and four (14.3%) of 28 with HCC responded, and an overall survival of 19.5 months was observed. Toxicities were predictable and included stomatitis, fatigue, and myelosuppression. This regimen has been suggested as a viable combination for patients with cirrhosis-related HCC in which more intensive drug combinations (e.g., PIAF) may not be well tolerated.

Intra-arterial Infusion Chemotherapy. Investigators also examined the role of hepatic arterial chemotherapy for HCC.[31,32] The drug regimens examined are usually based on either doxorubicin, cisplatin, or mitomycin-C. The optimal drug combination to be administered intra-arterially is not known. In one recent series, intra-arterial floxuridine (FUDR), mitomycin, and subcutaneous alpha-interferon were administered to patients with HCC,[33] and a response in six of the ten highly selected patients was observed. In a second more recent trial, Murata and colleagues[89] assessed intra-arterial cisplatin and 5-FU as well as epirubicin. The authors concluded superiority for cisplatin and 5-FU, even for patients with PV tumor thrombus. Ando and colleagues[90] observed similar results for a low-dose cisplatin and 5-FU combination in a known poor-prognostic group of patients with advanced HCC and PV tumor thrombus. Although these results in aggregate are encouraging, the high risks of general anesthesia and laparotomy in patients with advanced liver dys-

function, as well as the risks of chemotherapy in patients who have liver dysfunction and thrombocytopenia, are likely to limit the feasibility of intra-arterial chemotherapy to a very small group of selected patients with HCC. One small prospective randomized trial from Hong Kong has assessed the adjuvant role of intra-arterial cisplatin and Lipiodol in resected patients with HCC.[91] Patients were randomized to either a single dose of intra-arterial cisplatin and Lipiodol or to four doses administered every 3 months. Although toxicity was not a significant issue, no significant difference was noted in either disease-free or overall survival rates between the two groups.

Hormone and Vitamin Therapy. In past years, enthusiasm has been seen for using hormonal therapy in HCC, particularly with tamoxifen and anti-androgens. Part of the rationale for using tamoxifen relates to in vitro data demonstrating inhibition of HCC cells positive for estrogen receptors.[92] However, a majority of HCC cells are estrogen receptor negative. Early trials of tamoxifen suggested a survival advantage[93]; however, more recent data in the context of randomized trials have not supported the early enthusiasm for hormonal therapy.[94,95] In one large, 329-patient, randomized placebo-controlled study[96] conducted in the Asia-Pacific region of high-dose tamoxifen (120 mg/day) versus lower-dose tamoxifen (60 mg/day) versus placebo in the treatment of inoperable HCC, investigators observed no improvement in survival or quality of life for either of the tamoxifen-containing arms over placebo, and noted a higher death rate for the high-dose tamoxifen group. This trial provides definitive proof of the lack of benefit for tamoxifen therapy in advanced HCC. Octreotide, a long-acting somatostatin derivative, has been compared with observation in several small random-assignment trials.[97-99] Part of the rationale relates to the octreotide's potent in vitro anti-antigenosis and antiproliferative effects against HCC xenografts.[100] In one study, a survival advantage was demonstrated for octreotide[97]; however, in a more recent study, no survival advantage was found for the long-acting form of octreotide.[98] Another interesting approach has been to assess the activity of vitamin D analogues in HCC. The rationale relates to induction of differentiation and cancer cell line growth inhibition in vivo and in vitro for vitamin D analogues as well as the overexpression of the vitamin D receptor in hepatocytes and in HCC cells.[101,102] In a preliminary dose-titration study of seocalcitol,[103] a vitamin D analogue, several durable complete responses were observed (29 and 36 months). Expectedly, the main toxicity was hypercalcemia. The authors speculated that, given the activity in bulk HCC, it is possible that it may have a role in the adjuvant setting in the context of a minimal residual disease state.

Adjuvant Therapy. A compelling rationale considers adjuvant therapy for HCC based on the high rate of intra- and extrahepatic recurrence after potentially curative resections, as well as the development of second primary tumors within the diseased liver. A meta-analysis of three prospective randomized trials of adjuvant systemic chemotherapy versus observation after resection in a Japanese population of 108 patients by using a variety of systemic chemotherapy regimens concluded a lack of benefit for chemotherapy on either disease-free or overall survival.[104] A concern in patients with cirrhosis, postoperative chemotherapy resulted in a significantly worse disease-free and overall survival.[104] However, Schwartz and associates[105] conducted a larger meta-analysis of 13 randomized trials, 3 involving systemic adjuvant therapy, 4 assessing the role of HA chemoembolization, and 6 assessing a variety of other therapeutic agents. The overall conclusion was similar in that neither systemic or intra-arterial–based chemotherapy nor chemoembolization has been shown to improve overall or disease-free survival after resection compared with no treatment. Reservations with regard to the quality of the data included small-sized trials in patients with heterogeneous underlying liver function and a lack of documented effect for many of the agents tested in a more advanced disease setting.

One provocative study from Hong Kong assessed a single-dose treatment of intra-arterial iodine-131–labeled Lipiodol as adjuvant therapy compared with observation for patients with hepatitis B–related HCC. The study was terminated early after 43 patients were enrolled when an interim analysis demonstrated a marked difference in survival for the treated group, 57.2 versus 13.6 months. The 3-year survival rate for the adjuvantly treated group was 86.4%, and 46.3% in the control group. In an updated report of an additional 57 nonrandomized patients treated with adjuvant iodine 131–labeled Lipiodol, the same investigators reported a 50% five-year overall survival and a 38% disease-free survival. Further larger randomized trials are needed for iodine-131–labeled Lipiodol in broader patient groups with HCC the better to understand its utility. One additional small study of iodine-131–labeled Lipiodol in patients with unresectable disease noted a decline in AFP levels and tumor bulk reduction in 50% of patients and suggested that further assessment of this approach also is warranted in advanced unresectable disease.

Overexpression of cyclo-oxygenase-2 (COX-2) has been clearly associated with oncogenesis in colorectal cancer. Given that COX-2 also is overexpressed in HCC, especially in early well-differentiated tumors,[106] and that completed in vitro studies have shown that both NS-398 and sulindac, COX-2 inhibitors, effectively inhibit growth of human HCC cell lines, further studies are eagerly awaited. These agents may find an application in both the adjuvant and chemoprevention settings for HCC.

Both new-drug development and drug assessment are complicated subjects in HCC. Drug development in HCC is hampered by the fact that the liver remains the major organ of activation and inactivation of many drugs. As previously noted, a "standard of care" in HCC is doxorubicin, which may require significant attenuation in a majority of patients with HCC because of elevated bilirubin and liver dysfunction. This issue underscores the problem of new-drug development in HCC. One option that is sometimes considered is to conduct a disease-specific phase I trial of a new agent in HCC. This may be a way to bring new drugs quickly to the clinical arena for this disease.

Response assessment is another critical area in the interpretation of both chemotherapeutic and novel therapy trials in HCC. Difficulties include delineation of margins of tumor on CT or MRI scans, lack of reproducibility between radiologists, lack of incorporation of AFP declines into currently used response-assessment systems, and lack of dynamic-imaging approaches. With newer imaging modalities, it is possible that functional tumor imaging (e.g., the percentage of viable tumor in total tumor mass), may prove to be a more reliable method of assessing treatment response. For now, these approaches are investigational, and it remains to be seen how and whether they will be integrated into day-to-day practice.

To summarize, no randomized chemotherapy trial has been clearly shown to affect either duration or quality of life in HCC. Promising approaches include the PIAF regimen, although its role remains to be defined. However, clearly the future is focused on novel-drug development in this disease.

Novel Therapies. The rapid development of targeted therapies and the lack of effective chemotherapeutic agents for hepatocellular carcinoma have made the evaluation of many different novel therapies along the signal-transduction pathway a natural second step. At the cell surface, ligand binding to different cell receptors is the first event in a multistep cascade that leads to further cell duplication. This phenomenon can go unchecked against multiple feedback mechanisms, leading to oncogenesis, or a disease of deranged intracellular signaling. The epidermal growth factor receptor (EGFr) is a well-studied therapeutic target. C225 (cetuximab, Erbitux) has been tested against several tumors and has shown promise; however, this does not seem to be the case in HCC. Although it has not been tested clinically, the role of EFGr in HCC is debated, with several authors reporting no difference in expression of EGFr with noncancerous diseased liver tissues, whereas Kiss and coworkers[107] reported overexpression in 17% of HCC cases. Her-2/neu overexpressed was found to be rare in human HCC tissues, suggesting no role for trastuzumab (Herceptin), a monoclonal antibody against Her-2/neu, in this disease. Other tyrosine kinase inhibitors including ZD1839 (gefitinib; Iressa), and OSI-774 (erlotinib; Tarceva) have not been formally tested in HCC. Although the data to date suggest no role for anti-EGFr molecules in HCC, clinical trials assessing their role in the subset of HCCs overexpressing EGF may still be warranted. Hepatocyte growth factor (HGF), and its receptor c-met, have been found to be overexpressed in 33% and 20%, respectively, in human HCC. An effective targeted therapy against cytokine HGF or its epithelial receptor c-met does not yet exist; this target might carry some promise in the treatment of HCC.

Downstream, and on the other side of the cellular membrane, lies the Ras-anchoring protein, which has been the subject of intense studies. Ras mutations are overexpressed in a multitude of solid tumors including HCC. The rate-limiting, or anchoring to the cell membrane, is a post-translational farnesylation of a cytosine residue located at the carboxyl terminus of Ras. Several farnesylation inhibitors have been studied, including simvastatin and pravastatin. In their latest study, Kawata and colleagues[108] demonstrated (in a randomized study of standard therapy with or without pravastatin in advanced HCC) a survival advantage for the group of patients who received pravastatin as part of their treatment. Other potential modalities to block Ras activity includes CAAX box peptidomimetic farnesyltransferase inhibitors, and geranylgeranlytransferase inhibitors. However, none has been formally tested in HCC. Downstream from Ras, Raf is another promising target that now is the subject of extensive study. Raf-1 may be important in neoplastic transformation of hepatocytes. In HCV infection, HCV core proteins result in high basal activity of Raf-1, which results in sustained response to EGF by hepatocytes, resulting in increasing possibility of neoplastic transformation. This, in addition to reported evidence of response in a phase I study, led to a phase II study currently analyzing the activity of BAY 43-9006 in HCC.

The signal-transduction pathway continues to regulate cellular proliferation up to the nuclear membrane. Reaching the nucleus, the cell-cycle transitional points are under control of the cyclin-dependent kinases. Flavopiridol causes cell-cycle arrest in both growth phases (G_1 and G_2) of the cell cycle[109] by inhibiting CDK. Although single-agent flavopiridol has not been tested in HCC, encouraging results have been observed in a phase I study of irinotecan combined with flavopiridol by Shah and associates.[110] Two patients with HCC in this trial remained on study for longer than 1 year, suggesting that further assessment of this combination in HCC is warranted.

As previously mentioned, evaluating response in HCC is a complex and difficult task. A dynamic assessment may become increasingly important in this era of newly discovered targeted therapies in which their oncologic action may not be easily quantitated in two-dimensional tumor shrinkage on CT or MRI scans.

Other than the signal-transduction pathway, antiangiogenesis remains a very appealing concept for novel therapeutics, particularly given the new data reported on bevacizumab in colorectal cancer. Bevacizumab will undoubtedly be studied in HCC, both as a single agent and in combination with other novel therapeutics and cytotoxics. While we are awaiting such trials, the only data available on an antiangiogenic drug is from a phase II trial of thalidomide by Schwartz and coworkers,[111] who observed a minimal response rate of 6% in advanced HCC. The future is indeed exciting with regard to novel therapeutics in HCC, but as yet no targeted therapy has a defined role in the treatment of HCC.

Outcome of Treatment of Recurrence

Because patients with recurrence of HCC may be amenable to potentially curative resection, detecting early recurrences is extremely important. Multiple series have shown that recurrent resectable HCC can result in 5-year survival between 20% and 82%.[33,112-115] In addition, repeated liver resection in this group is safe, as demonstrated by one study that found no difference in blood loss, operative time, and incidence of complications when comparing repeated liver resections with first-time resections.[113] Therefore in patients found to have medical fitness for surgery, adequate liver reserve, and technically resectable tumors, repeated hepatic resection is the therapy of choice. In patients who are not candidates for surgery, percutaneous RFA, microwave ablation, and ethanol injection are effective methods to treat recurrent liver disease.[60,63,116] In addition, transcatheter arterial embolization (TAE) also has been considered a useful therapy for recurrent HCC.

TREATMENT OF HEPATOCELLULAR CARCINOMA

Patients with tumors suggestive of HCC based on known risk factors (hepatitis or alcohol use) and/or preoperative contrast-enhanced imaging undergo serologic testing for AFP. In patients with elevated AFP and surgically resectable lesions, definitive treatment is then performed. In patients with known risk factors and a new liver lesion found on axial imaging, we pursue definitive treatment without biopsy. Only in patients in whom the diagnostic imaging is not classic for HCC and the AFP is normal would we consider biopsy of these lesions. This is for two main reasons: suggestive lesions must be dealt with surgically regardless of biopsy results, and a small, but real, risk of needle-track seeding exists.*†‡

Evaluation of liver functional reserve is by using the Child-Pugh classification. Preoperative staging evaluation is performed by using abdomen and pelvis contrast-enhanced biphasic CT with thin sections (5 mm) of the liver. Patients with disease limited to the liver undergo treatment according to the accompanying algorithm.

Patients are not considered surgical candidates if they have high medical risk that precludes surgery. Selected patients with bilobar tumors may be treated with either multiple segmental resections or a combination of resection and ablation. Selected patients with isolated portal vein involvement may be considered candidates for hepatectomy with concomitant portal vein resection.

Patients with unresectable disease not amenable to alcohol injection or percutaneous RFA are first considered for embolization. We attempt to place patients who are not candidates for embolization in clinical trials, particularly because response to traditional systemic chemotherapy is so poor.

---

*Druand F, Regimbeau JM, Belghiti J, et al: Assessment of the benefits and risks of percutaneous biopsy before surgical resection of hepatocellular carcinoma. J Hepatol 2001;35:254-258.

†Kim SH, Lim HK, Lee WJ, Cho JM, Jang HJ: Needle-tract implantation in hepatocellular carcinoma: Frequency and CT findings after biopsy with a 19.5-gauge automated biopsy gun. Abdom Imaging 2000;25:246-250.

†Takamori R, Wong LL, Dang C, Wong L: Needle-tract implantation from hepatocellular cancer: Is needle biopsy of the liver always necessary? Liver Transpl 2000;6:67-72.

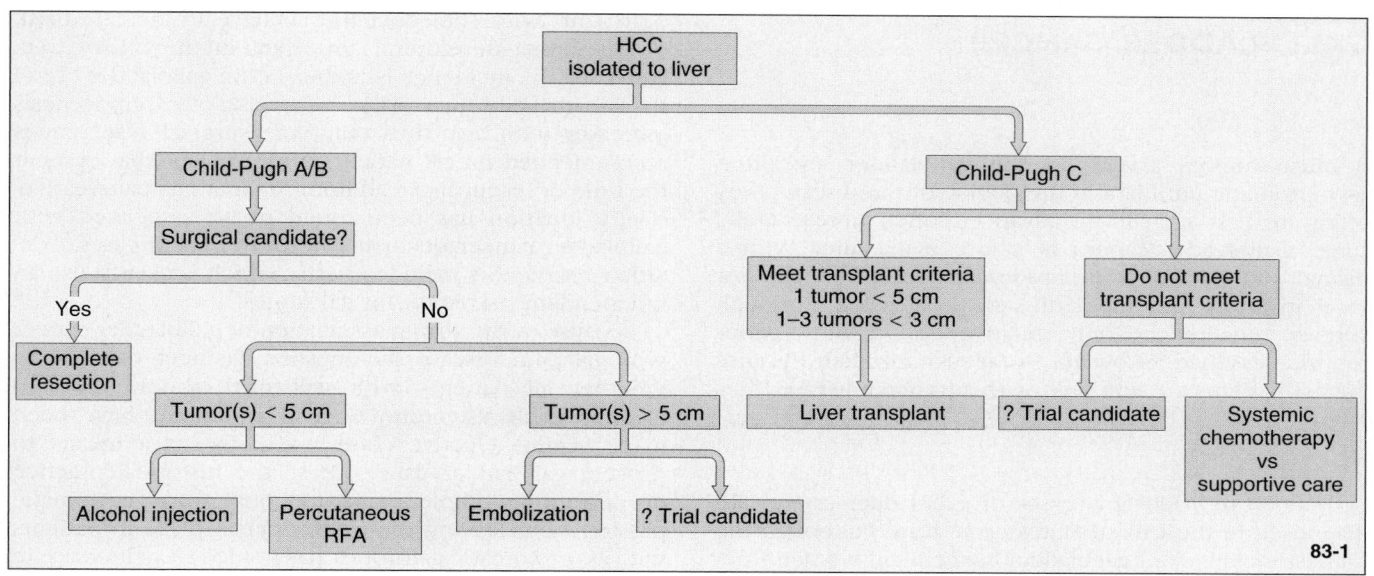

83-1

Treatment Complications

After resection, postoperative morbidity occurs in 40% of patients, consisting primarily of transient hepatic insufficiency, intra-abdominal abscess or biloma, gastrointestinal (GI) bleeding, and cardiopulmonary complications.[31] Postoperative mortality ranges from 3% to 12% in most series (see Tables 83-3 and 83-4). After transplantation, the 90-day mortality is approximately 15% (see Table 83-5).

Follow-up

After surgical treatment of HCC, scheduled follow-up is extremely important to evaluate for recurrent disease, which can occur in up to two thirds of patients after potentially curative resection. Many patients with recurrent disease will actually be manifesting metachronous second primaries, which occur in cirrhotic patients because the entire liver is affected. These recurrent or new hepatomas can be treated effectively only if discovered early.

Associated Medical Conditions

Follow-up also must aim to prevent and treat complications of associated parenchymal disease, which is common in this patient population. Patients may need treatment for alcoholism, whereas patients with hemochromatosis should be treated for iron overload. Most important, patients should be treated to prevent the complications of portal hypertension, because it is estimated that up to one fourth of patients who die after diagnosis of liver cancer succumb to GI bleeding from portal hypertension.[117]

Recommended Follow-up

The routine follow-up of a patient after resection of HCC should include an office visit 2 to 3 weeks after hospital discharge. Liver function tests, as well as tumor markers, are assessed. For classic HCC, the tumor marker is AFP,[118]

whereas for the fibrolamellar variant of HCC, it may be neurotensin or other markers[119,120] that were elevated in the serum before resection. A postoperative return of tumor markers to normal should result in routine follow-up.

The routine follow-up consists of office visits every 3 months with history, examination, and measurement of liver function tests and tumor markers. Patients should be asked about symptoms of worsening portal hypertension or liver failure and symptoms of biliary obstruction, including itching or changes in stool or urine color, primarily because a significant proportion of patients die of liver failure, not HCC.[13] New-onset right upper quadrant pain or bone pain should prompt investigation by appropriate radiologic examinations. Physical examination should evaluate for new masses, worsening ascites, and jaundice. Patients also should be followed up with contrast-enhanced abdominal CT every 6 months, with a chest radiograph obtained yearly. Five years after resection, office visits should be reduced to every 6 months.

Issues for the Future

Because the incidence of HCC is increasing, it is imperative that improved screening tests be developed to improve the sensitivity and specificity for detecting HCC. Some authors have suggested that a more sensitive means to detect recurrence may be evaluating the serum for the presence of AFP messenger RNA (mRNA) by reverse-transcription PCR. In this study, the postoperative presence of AFP mRNA was an independent prognostic factor for HCC.[121] Molecular studies to assess genes associated with a high risk of recurrence have shown promise in preliminary studies but require further evaluation.[122-124] Clearly, it would be helpful if the molecular characterization of specific genes associated with an increased risk for developing HCC also could help either early detection or prevention of the disease.[125]

GALLBLADDER CANCER

Introduction

Because tumors arising in the gallbladder are often asymptomatic until late in the course of the disease, they often are first seen in an advanced, often unresectable, stage. Gallbladder cancer is a rare malignancy with a dismal outlook due to its insidious onset, propensity for local invasion, and rapid disease progression. Although surgery remains the only curative option, most series report a less than 5% overall 5-year survival, likely because 40% of patients are first seen with advanced disease.[126]

Epidemiology

Only 6000 to 7000 new cases of gallbladder cancer are diagnosed in the United States each year,[127] although the highest incidence of gallbladder cancer is in women from La Paz, Bolivia (15.5 cases/100,000).[128] Attesting to the rarity of this lesion, after routine screening abdominal ultrasound examinations in asymptomatic patients in Japan, only 19 (0.01%) of 194,767 were found to have gallbladder cancer.[129]

Gallbladder cancer is more common in women than in men in all populations, and in some geographic areas, the rates are three times higher for women. Incidence increases with age in all populations.[126,128] Some geographic areas have a high incidence of gallbladder cancer, including South America and India. A high incidence also is found in North American Native Americans and Mexican Americans. The geographic variability clearly correlates with populations that have a higher rate of gallstone formation.[128] To strengthen this association further, the mortality rate from gallbladder cancer has been inversely correlated with cholecystectomy rates in Chile, a high-incidence region.[130]

Etiology and Pathogenesis

Although an increased risk of gallbladder cancer exists with cholelithiasis, in fewer than 0.5% of patients with gallstones does gallbladder cancer subsequently develop.[131] However, up to 85% of patients with gallbladder cancer are found to have gallstones.[132,133] The association of gallstones with carcinoma is probably related to chronic inflammation. Larger stones, greater than 3 cm, are associated with a 10-fold increased risk of cancer.[134]

Besides gallstones, the other main associated risk factors include chronic infections of the gallbladder and environmental exposure to specific chemicals such as thorium dioxide (Thorotrast). Thorotrast is a radiologic contrast medium that emits alpha particles, thus causing prolonged exposure to internal alpha-particle radiation when it was administered systemically. A study conducted in Sweden found that the incidence rates for cancer at all sites was increased three times over that in the general population, with the largest increase in primary liver and gallbladder cancer.[135]

Patients with choledochal cysts have an increased risk of carcinoma developing anywhere in the biliary tree. However, the incidence is higher in the gallbladder (12%) than in the bile duct (5%).[136] The risk of carcinogenesis increases with age; thus complete surgical resection is recommended for all patients with choledochal cysts at the time of diagnosis. In addition, anomalous pancreaticobiliary junction has been found to be associated with gallbladder cancer, occurring in up to 65% of cases.[137,138] Other risk factors include obesity, which is clearly also an independent risk factor for gallstones.[139]

Because of the strong association of gallbladder cancer with gallstone disease, the question has been raised as to whether all patients with gallstones should undergo elective cholecystectomy. Several arguments have been made against elective cholecystectomy as a means to prevent gallbladder cancer. First, the historical practice of performing cholecystectomy only for symptomatic patients, thus leaving the gallbladder in place in patients with asymptomatic gallstones, has not led to an increase in the prevalence of gallbladder cancer over time. Second, epidemiologic studies have found that the 20-year risk of developing cancer in patients with gallstones is less than 0.5% for the overall population and 1.5% for high-risk groups.[131] Thus routine cholecystectomy for asymptomatic gallstones due to concern for future increased risk of gallbladder cancer does not appear to be warranted.

One higher-risk subset of patients with gallbladder disease is the population with "porcelain gallbladder," a calcified gallbladder wall. Historically, it was thought that the incidence of gallbladder cancer in patients with porcelain gallbladder was as high as 25% to 60% (Fig. 83-8). Because of this, it was previously thought that all patients with calcification of the gallbladder wall should undergo open cholecystectomy, even if they were asymptomatic. More recently, however, this association has been challenged by the finding that fewer than 20% of

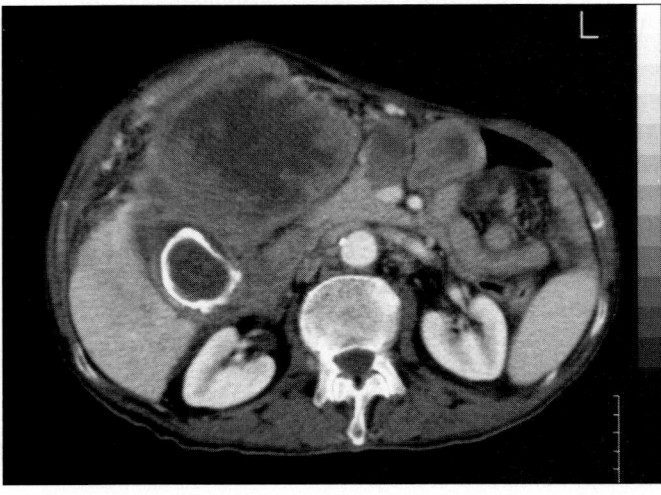

Figure 83-8. Porcelain gallbladder demonstrated on computed tomography scan with concentric calcification of the gallbladder wall. A large gallbladder cancer is present in association with the porcelain gallbladder.

patients with diffuse calcified gallbladder wall are found to have cancer.[133] Interestingly, Stephen and colleagues[140] recently reported a retrospective analysis of more than 25,000 gallbladder specimens and subdivided those patients with calcified gallbladders into two types: those with complete intramural calcification and those with selective mucosal calcification. Although a significant increase in the incidence of gallbladder cancer was found in patients with selective mucosal wall calcification (7%; odds ratio, 13.89), no patients with diffuse intramural calcification were found to have cancer.[140] Finally, another recent retrospective review found 15 porcelain gallbladders among more than 10,000 specimens examined, and none had gallbladder cancer.[141] The results of these studies indicate that the risk of gallbladder cancer in patients with porcelain gallbladder appears to have been greatly overestimated, and therefore cholecystectomy should be performed only in patients with either selective calcification of the gallbladder wall or other findings causing concern for carcinoma on preoperative studies.

Pathology

More than 80% of gallbladder cancers are adenocarcinomas; several histologic subtypes exist, including papillary, nodular, and tubular. Papillary tumors, which grow predominantly into the gallbladder lumen, have an improved prognosis compared with the other subtypes.[126] Poor prognostic signs in gallbladder cancer include grade[126,142] and vascular invasion.[126] The most important prognostic sign may be lymph node status,[143] although 5-year survivors with nodal involvement have been documented.[144] Fewer than 5% of cases are squamous cell carcinomas, with the remaining 10% being anaplastic lesions including small cell carcinoma, which has a particularly virulent course, but which may be responsive to cisplatin-based chemotherapy.

Limited information exists regarding the genetic changes in gallbladder cancer. The most widely reported gene abnormalities associated with gallbladder cancer include p53,[145] K-ras,[145,146] and CDKN2 (9p21) mutations.[146,147] The finding that patients with an anomalous pancreaticobiliary junction have a greater frequency of K-ras mutations has led investigators to believe that reflux of pancreatic enzymes into the biliary tree may contribute to the development of cancer.[146] Because of our limited knowledge of the sequence of molecular changes, no detectors of early disease or of risk assessment are known. Clearly this area needs improvement, particularly in areas in which it is endemic.

Biology

Gallbladder cancer spreads via the lymphatic and venous drainage. Because of drainage of the cholecystic veins directly into the adjacent liver, these tumors often involve hepatic parenchyma, most often portions of segments IV and V that directly abut the gallbladder fossa. The rapid spread of gallbladder cancer has been thought to be partially due to its thin wall and discontinuous muscle layer. In addition, the portion of the gallbladder in direct contact with the liver has no serosa; thus direct liver invasion is common. Lymphatic spread is first to the cystic duct (Calot's) node, then to pericholedochal and hilar nodes, and finally to peripancreatic, duodenal, periportal, celiac, and superior mesenteric artery nodes. Nodal disease in the porta hepatis often causes common bile duct (CBD) obstruction and resultant jaundice, which is the first clinical symptom in 30% of patients. Jaundice also may be caused by tumors arising in the gallbladder infundibulum, which may spread directly to the cystic duct and common hepatic duct. Although peritoneal metastases are frequent, distant extraperitoneal metastases are not.

Clinical Presentation and Patient Evaluation

In patients with signs or symptoms, abdominal pain consistent with biliary colic or acute cholecystitis is most common, followed by jaundice.[148] The majority of patients are found to have gallbladder cancer during evaluation for possible cholelithiasis or choledocholithiasis. Patients also may first be seen with weight loss, anorexia, or an increase in abdominal girth secondary to ascites. Physical findings include right upper quadrant (RUQ) tenderness or a palpable mass, hepatomegaly, and ascites. Because of its nonspecific presentation, gallbladder cancer is not diagnosed preoperatively in more than half the cases. In patients with jaundice and identified to have a diagnosis of gallbladder cancer, in the absence of a stone causing jaundice, the majority of the patient group will be found to have unresectable disease.

Laboratory and Imaging Studies

Laboratory tests are usually normal, except in patients with jaundice who have elevated liver function tests consistent with biliary obstruction. No reliable screening tests are available to evaluate patients at increased risk for gallbladder cancer.

Imaging evaluation often reveals an asymmetrically thickened gallbladder wall (Fig. 83-9) or a mass within or replacing the gallbladder on US examination. Because polyps and carcinoma can have an echogenicity similar to that of the gallbladder wall, these lesions are often difficult to distinguish. This is even more difficult when

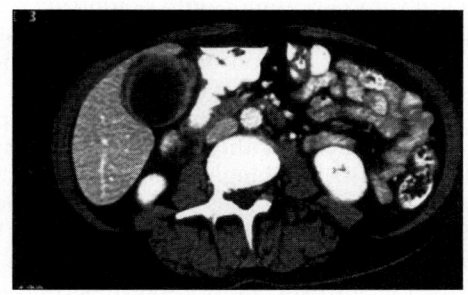

Figure 83-9. Computed tomographic scan demonstrating asymmetric thickening of the gallbladder wall, a classic finding for gallbladder carcinoma.

Specific Malignancies

III

inflammation is present from gallstones. At times, US can visualize invasion of the liver, adjacent adenopathy, and a dilated biliary tree. The ability of US to differentiate benign from neoplastic disease is enhanced by using endoscopic US, and it may be more specific than CT or MRI.[149-151]

A dynamic contrast-enhanced CT scan may identify a gallbladder mass or invasion into the liver parenchyma or adjacent organs. The classic finding in a patient with gallbladder cancer is asymmetric thickening of the gallbladder wall (see Fig. 83-9). The sensitivity and specificity of contrast-enhanced CT in diagnosing neoplastic lesions is close to 90%.[152] However, staging of gallbladder carcinoma with CT is limited by poor sensitivity in identifying nodal spread.[153]

In patients who are jaundiced, direct cholangiography may be useful to delineate extent of biliary involvement as well as to palliate symptoms of biliary obstruction. A mid–bile duct obstruction not due to gallstones is gallbladder cancer, until proven otherwise (see Fig. 83-2). More recently, with the improvements in MRI technology, magnetic resonance cholangiopancreatography (MRCP) has evolved into a single, noninvasive imaging modality that allows complete assessment of biliary, vascular, hepatic parenchymal, and nodal involvement, as well as involvement of adjacent organs (see Fig. 83-3); thus this modality may be helpful in selected cases.[154-156]

Staging Classification

The AJCC TNM staging system (Table 83-6) reflects prognostic characteristics of tumor depth, regional nodal disease, or distant spread. Gallbladder cancers frequently spread to the liver, which is involved in 70% of patients at the time of surgical evaluation. The gallbladder differs histologically from the rest of the GI tract in that it lacks a muscularis mucosa and submucosa. Thus the gallbladder wall is composed of (1) a single layer of columnar cells, the mucosa, and lamina propria; (2) a fibromuscular layer; (3) a perimuscular, subserosal layer containing lymphatics and neurovascular structures; and (4) a serosal surface, except where the gallbladder is embedded in the liver.[157] Because lymphatics are present in the subserosal layer only, tumors invading less than the full thickness of the muscular layer have minimal risk of nodal spread.

Several changes have recently been incorporated into the AJCC staging system (6th edition, 2002); specifically, the T and N classifications have been simplified to try to separate locally invasive tumors into potentially resectable (T3) and unresectable (T4) tumors. The distinction between T3 and T4 based on depth has been abolished. Lymph node metastasis is now classified as stage IIB, and stage IIA refers to resectable tumors with no lymph node involvement. In line with other pancreaticobiliary malignancies, the stage III grouping refers to locally advanced, unresectable disease, and stage IV indicates metastatic disease. Stage I includes tumors invading into but not through the muscular layer of the gallbladder. In stage II disease, invasion into the perimuscular, subserosal layer is found, without spread to the liver and without nodal disease. Stage III and stage IV disease are as previously defined.

TABLE 83-6

AJCC Staging System for Gallbladder Carcinoma

STAGE	TUMOR	NODES	METASTASIS
0	Tis	N0	M0
IA	T1	N0	M0
IB	T2	N0	M0
IIA	T3	N0	M0
IIB	T1	N1	M0
	T2	N1	M0
	T3	N1	M0
III	T4	Any N	M0
IV	Any T	Any N	M1

Definition of TNM

Primary Tumor (T)

TX	Primary tumor cannot be assessed
T0	No evidence of primary tumor
Tis	Carcinoma in situ
T1	Tumor invades the lamina propria or muscle layer
	T1a Tumor invades the lamina propria
	T1b Tumor invades the muscle layer
T2	Tumor invades the perimuscular connective tissue; no extension beyond the serosa or into the liver
T3	Tumor perforates the serosa (visceral peritoneum) and/or directly invades the liver and/or one other adjacent organ or structure (e.g., stomach, duodenum, colon, pancreas, omentum, or extrahepatic bile ducts)
T4	Tumor invades main portal vein or hepatic artery or invades multiple extrahepatic organs or structures

Regional Lymph Nodes (N)

NX	Regional lymph nodes cannot be assessed
N0	No regional lymph node metastasis
N1	Regional lymph node metastasis

Distant Metastasis (M)

MX	Presence of distant metastasis cannot be assessed
M0	No distant metastasis
M1	Distant metastasis

From Greene FL: AJCC Cancer Staging Manual, 6th ed. New York, Springer-Verlag, 2002.

Prognosis

The 5-year survival rate of all patients with gallbladder cancer is less than 5% in most series, with a median survival of 6 months.[158,159] This is primarily because most patients are first seen with unresectable disease. Of those patients undergoing resection, survival is dependent on depth of penetration and nodal status. Large series have shown that the overall 5-year survival rate after resection is 40%.[158] Near 100% survival is reported after simple cholecystectomy for T1 disease, whereas T2 and T3 tumors without nodal disease have a 5-year survival of more than 50%.[143,144,160-163] Node positivity is an ominous finding, with only a few series reporting 5-year survivors.[144]

Primary Treatment

It is clear that the only curative option in patients with gallbladder cancer is complete surgical resection. It is essential for optimal patient care that patients with

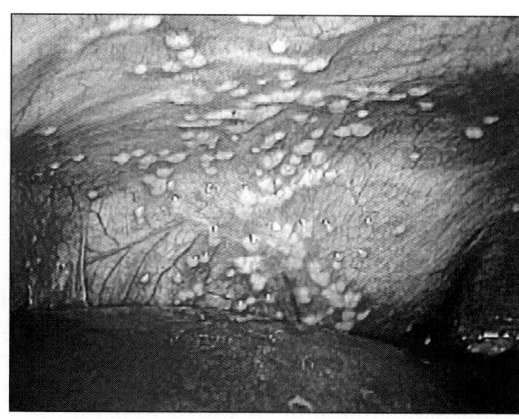

Figure 83-10. Intraoperative photograph during staging laparoscopy demonstrating occult peritoneal metastases on the inferior surface of the right diaphragm.

gallbladder cancer be recognized before laparoscopic cholecystectomy is performed, because of the risk of port-site seeding and bile spillage.[148,163]

Role of Staging Laparoscopy

Because a large percentage of patients have been found to have occult unresectable disease at the time of exploration, several authors have investigated the use of initial staging laparoscopy for this disease.[159,163-166] Because gallbladder cancer has such a propensity to spread intra-abdominally, laparoscopy is ideal for detection of intra-abdominal metastases. This is demonstrated by the fact that up to 50% of patients are found to have unresectable disease at the time of laparoscopy (Fig. 83-10).[159] Patients who are detected to have unresectable disease at laparoscopy can begin other forms of therapy earlier and may undergo the procedure as an outpatient. Particularly because patients with unresectable disease have a median survival of only 6 months, the importance of quality of life and time out of the hospital cannot be overemphasized.

Cholecystectomy with or Without Partial Hepatectomy

Gallbladder cancer results in rapid local progression and death unless it can be curatively resected. In a collected

review of 5836 patients with gallbladder cancer, the overall mean survival was between 2 and 5 months, whereas the 5-year survival was 4%.[131] The 5-year survival of patients undergoing resection with curative intent was 17%. Of the 2115 patients with unresectable tumors, only a single 5-year survivor was found.[131] Although surgical resection represents the treatment of choice and the only potentially curative therapy available, resection is possible in only 25% of patients at presentation because of the advanced nature of the disease.[131]

The operation of choice must be tailored to the depth of penetration of the tumor (Table 83-7). For tumors limited to the muscular layer of the gallbladder (T1), near-universal agreement exists that simple cholecystectomy is adequate.[144,167-169] T1 tumors have not yet invaded the subserosal layer, which contains lymphatics, and therefore lymphadenectomy is not required. Attesting to the fact that early gallbladder carcinoma is completely curable, simple cholecystectomy has resulted in near 100% survival when early cancer is an incidental finding after elective cholecystectomy.[170]

Difficulty can arise at the time of surgery in evaluating polypoid lesions of the gallbladder as either benign or early gallbladder cancer. Although it appears that frozen-section diagnosis is fairly reliable in distinguishing whether lesions are malignant or benign (95% accurate), the accuracy in correctly assessing depth of invasion is only 70%.[171] Thus it may be difficult at the time of surgery to determine the extent of resection. Because of this, pursuing a more aggressive resection if the depth of invasion is in doubt is important for adequate tumor clearance.[172]

The extent of surgical resection for T2 or greater tumors is controversial, with recommendations ranging from simple cholecystectomy to radical excision including hepatectomy. Whereas it is clear that major hepatic resection can be performed safely with a mortality of less than 5% (see Table 83-7),[143,144,158,168,169] it has not been universally accepted that more aggressive resections improve survival. For advanced local disease, some groups have advocated radical resections including hepatectomy and pancreatectomy. To understand the rationale for extensive resections, one must understand that the usual pattern of spread for gallbladder cancer is by either direct extension or nodal spread. Direct extension to the adjacent liver parenchyma often occurs first, followed by

TABLE 83-7

	T1 OR T2 TUMORS		**T3 OR T4 TUMORS**	
	SIMPLE CHOLECYSTECTOMY (%)	RADICAL CHOLECYSTECTOMY (%)	SIMPLE CHOLECYSTECTOMY (%)	RADICAL CHOLECYSTECTOMY (%)
INSTITUTION				
University of Virginia, 1982[28]	33	—	3	13
Tohoku University, 1987[20]	57	100	0	23
Hamamatsu University, 1989[26]	—	100	—	15
Mayo Clinic, 1990[21]	—	—	0	29
Nigata University, 1992[23]	—	72	—	37

Five-year Survival after Resection for Gallbladder Cancer

adjacent organ involvement, including duodenum, colon, and stomach (see Fig. 83-2). Because most cases are diagnosed late in their course, lymphatic spread of gallbladder cancer also is very common, often involving nodes in the porta hepatis, peripancreatic region, celiac axis, and the aortocaval nodal basins in more advanced cases.

Because the gallbladder is not surrounded by serosa where it is attached to the liver in the gallbladder fossa, even T2 tumors (full-thickness invasion of the muscular layer into the perimuscular connective tissue, but not into the serosa) may invade into the normal plane of dissection in the gallbladder fossa during simple cholecystectomy. Therefore T2 tumors cannot be completely removed with cholecystectomy alone, and a radical cholecystectomy, with resection of a 1- to 2-cm rim of normal liver around the gallbladder fossa, is the minimum resection that is required. Many authors, however, have found that segmental resection of segments 4b and 5 of the liver, which abut the gallbladder fossa, results in a more anatomically controlled dissection with less blood loss.[17] An additional part of the definitive surgical treatment is regional lymphadenectomy, because about half the patients with T2 tumors are found to have nodal spread after resection.[143] Dissection of lymph nodes should include all tissue from the bifurcation of the hepatic ducts to the distal CBD. Proponents of this approach advocate liver resection on the basis that it is the only way to obtain an adequate margin on the hepatic side of the gallbladder, and resection of the regional nodes allows the best chance for complete tumor clearance. For all of these reasons, simple cholecystectomy is inadequate for T2 or greater tumors. When segment 4b/5 resections have been performed in patients with T2 tumors, it has increased the 5-year survival from 25% to 40% after simple cholecystectomy to 70% to 100% after radical resection.[143,144,161,167,168,170]

For T3 and T4 lesions, a high likelihood is found of intraperitoneal and hematogenous spread and significant morbidity of the radical procedures that are often necessary for excision of local disease. However, in patients with disease limited to the gallbladder, recent series support an aggressive approach to resection (Tables 83-7 and 83-8). For T3 tumors, segment 4b/5 resection is warranted to clear the hepatic bed of tumor completely. Local recurrence after resection of more advanced

gallbladder cancer usually occurs in segment 4, 5, or 8, because of the venous drainage of the gallbladder into intrahepatic right portal branches (66% of patients), left portal branches (6%), or both right and left branches (28%).[162] Therefore for complete excision of T4 tumors, an extended right hepatectomy (segments 4, 5, 6, 7, and 8) is most often necessary because of the deeper invasion into the liver. With aggressive resection, long-term survival can be achieved for stage III or IV patients.[143,144,160,168,169,173]

Surgical exploration should be performed for all patients with no medical contraindications. If a T1 tumor is suspected, a cholecystectomy and biopsy of regional nodes should be performed after thorough examination of the abdominal cavity for any signs of tumor dissemination. The pathology and depth of penetration should be confirmed by frozen section, and the procedure terminated if a T1 tumor with negative margins is confirmed. For T2 lesions, either a radical cholecystectomy (wedge resection of the hepatic bed) or a segment 4b/5 resection with lymphadenectomy should be performed.[143] For T3 lesions, a segment 4b/5 resection or extended right hepatectomy is performed. Finally, for T4 lesions, a more radical excision of the liver, such as extended right hepatectomy, usually must be performed for adequate tumor clearance.

Location of the tumor is important in determining the extent of resection. If the tumor arises in the gallbladder infundibulum, the CBD is often involved with tumor, either by direct extension or by external invasion of the hepatoduodenal ligament. In this case, an extended liver resection and removal of a portion of the CBD should be performed. In addition, clearly all patients with jaundice will require resection of the CBD to clear the tumor. Reconstruction is then performed by roux-en-Y hepaticojejunostomy. Tumor arising in the fundus of the gallbladder, however, can be treated with limited hepatic resection without excision of the CBD. To clear the lymph nodes in the porta hepatis, complete lymphadenectomy should be performed by skeletonizing the CBD, HA, and PV.

Incidentally or Laparoscopically Discovered Gallbladder Cancer

Gallbladder cancer is often discovered during pathologic examination after cholecystectomy for presumed benign

TABLE 83-8

Results after Radical Resection for Gallbladder Cancer

INSTITUTION	MORTALITY	NUMBER RESECTED	STAGE III–IV (%)	FIVE-YEAR SURVIVAL (%)
Hamamatsu University, 1989[26]	0	15	87	25
Mayo Clinic, 1990[21]	2	42	40	33
Japan Multicenter, 1991[22]	5	1686	50	51
Nigata University 1992[23]	0	40	53	65
Kyushu University, 1994[29]	0	32	75	53
MSKCC, 1996[25]	0	23	78	58

gallstone disease. Since the popularization of laparoscopic cholecystectomy in the past decade, an increasing number of patients with gallbladder cancer are found incidentally. Particularly in patients with bile spillage at the time of surgery, laparoscopic resection in patients with unknown gallbladder cancer may convert potentially curable early gallbladder cancer into incurable disease.[163] However, because radical resection remains the only possibility for cure, patients with T2 or greater tumors without signs of distant disease should be offered repeated resection to eradicate all disease. At the time of surgery, excision of laparoscopic port sites also should be performed because of the well-documented history of port-site seeding, even if they appear grossly normal.[170,174-176]

Patients first seen with incidentally discovered gallbladder cancer after laparoscopic cholecystectomy present the surgeon with multiple technical challenges. Postoperative inflammation is often found in the RUQ, hindering distinction of tumor from normal tissue. Determination of gross ductal or nodal involvement by tumor is always difficult at the time of reoperation. In addition, postoperative fibrosis often encases the right HA, which crosses behind the bile duct in most patients. For all of these reasons, a second operation for incidentally discovered gallbladder cancer often requires an extended right hepatectomy along with excision of the extrahepatic biliary tree and periductal lymphatic tissues. This resection allows adequate excision of the lymphatic tissues at the confluence of the bile ducts, greater confidence of a negative margin on the bile duct, and permits biliary reconstruction to only one side of the liver. The disadvantage is that a large portion of normal liver parenchyma is sacrificed, and, consequently, transient postoperative liver dysfunction is common. Although patients with incidentally discovered gallbladder cancer may be more difficult to resect curatively, no difference is noted in the overall survival between patients initially treated with noncurative resection and then re-explored for definitive resection, and those patients undergoing initial curative resection.[158]

When a patient has T1 gallbladder cancer discovered after simple cholecystectomy, the pathology must be reviewed to determine if the entire gallbladder has been removed and if the cystic duct margin is clear of tumor. If the cystic duct margin is positive, the patient requires local bile duct excision at a minimum. If all margins are negative, no further therapy is warranted. However, if the tumor is proven to be T2 or greater, the patient should undergo a radical resection if no evidence of extrahepatic disease is discovered. Patients with a known or suspected early gallbladder carcinoma should not undergo laparoscopic cholecystectomy. Rather, open exploration and cholecystectomy should be performed.

Adjuvant Therapy and Treatment of Advanced Gallbladder Cancer

Adjuvant Therapy

Adjuvant therapy for biliary tract (gallbladder and cholangiocarcinoma) remains a controversial and unproven consideration. Very few randomized trials have been conducted, and those that have are notable for (1) small patient numbers and (2) inclusion of patients with several malignancies (e.g., gallbladder and cholangiocarcinoma, ampullary, and sometimes pancreatic malignancies), in aggregate, limiting the statistical power and validity of the conclusions. Given the relative rarity of these malignancies in the United States, large-scale randomized trials are feasible only in the context of a multi-institutional or co-operative group setting.

One recent prospective randomized phase III trial by Takada and associates[177] of adjuvant chemotherapy with 5-fluorouracil and mitomycin-C versus surgery alone for resected patients with pancreaticobiliary malignancies offers some interesting results. A total of 508 patients were randomized from 31 centers over a 6-year period, including 140 with gallbladder cancer. Of 112 evaluable gallbladder cancer patients, the 5-year survival rate was significantly better in the adjuvant group, 26%, versus the control group of 14% ($P = .0367$). Similarly, the 5-year disease-free survival rate of 20.3% versus 11.6% ($P = .021$) favored the adjuvantly treated group. Significantly improved body weight also was observed in the adjuvantly treated gallbladder population. For the other malignancies assessed in this trial, pancreas, bile duct, and ampulla of Vater cancers, no benefits with regard to disease-free and overall survival were observed.[178] This trial suggests that adjuvant chemotherapy may offer benefit for patients with resected gallbladder cancer; however, replication in a larger-scale setting is required before definitive conclusions can be drawn.

Given that a majority of gallbladder cancers recur with both local and systemic disease, a logical approach is to consider combined chemoradiation in the adjuvant setting. Kresl and coworkers[179] recently reported on the Mayo Clinic retrospective experience of adjuvant 5-FU chemotherapy and external-beam radiation in patients with resected gallbladder cancer. Patients with completely resected (negative margins) gallbladder cancer who received adjuvant chemoradiotherapy had a 5-year survival rate of 64%, suggesting a favorable outcome compared with historical data for complete resection without additional treatment (~33%). Again, large-scale prospective trials of postoperative adjuvant chemoradiation are needed to determine the true merits of such an approach. Investigational questions with regard to adjuvant therapy include incorporating drugs with greater systemic activity than the fluoropyrimidines (e.g., gemcitabine) into an up-front adjuvant setting, as well as trying to define further the role of local-radiation modalities (e.g., brachytherapy) in the adjuvant context.

Metastatic Disease. A majority of studies assessing the role of chemotherapy in gallbladder cancer include patients with cholangiocarcinoma. To date, chemotherapy has not been shown to affect definitively the quality of life or overall survival in either of these malignancies. However, the studies that have been conducted have been small scale and mostly single institution. Older drugs such as 5-fluorouracil has a reported single-agent response rate of about 10%.[180,181] Capecitabine, an oral tumor-activated fluoropyrimidine, looks interesting in biliary tract malignancies, with a preliminary response rate of 50% in nonoperable gallbladder cancer and 6% in cholangiocarcinomas in a phase II trial.[182] Of the newer single agents, gemcitabine is the drug with the greatest potential. Gemcitabine is a nucleoside analogue prodrug, which is activated by intracellular phosphorylation. It is a Food and Drug Administration (FDA)-approved drug for locally advanced and metastatic pancreatic adenocarcinoma.[183,184] Several studies of biliary tract malignancies have been conducted.[185-188] Gallardo and colleagues[187] treated 25 patients with locally advanced or metastatic gallbladder cancer with gemcitabine on a conventional weekly schedule. Nine (36%) partial responses and a median survival of 30 weeks were observed in this phase II trial from Chile. In another study by Raderer and associates,[185] conducted in 19 patients (4 gallbladder, 15 cholangiocarcinoma), 3 (16%) partial responses were observed. A natural next step is to combine gemcitabine with other potentially active agents in gallbladder cancer. Malik and coworkers[189] from Pakistan observed one complete response and six (55%) partial responses in a small trial of gemcitabine and cisplatin in advanced gallbladder cancer. Several other preliminary reports from India[190] and Argentina[191] suggest activity for a cisplatin-gemcitabine combination; however, further data are needed to better define the utility of this combination. Kuhn and colleagues[192] assessed a gemcitabine-docetaxel combination in patients with advanced biliary tract malignancies. Of the 43 patients treated, 9% had a partial response, and an overall median survival of 11 months was observed. No obvious benefit appears for this combination over single-agent gemcitabine. For the other taxane, paclitaxel, minimal activity has been reported in advanced biliary tract cancers.[193]

Other newer agents assessed in biliary tract cancers include the topoisomerase-1 inhibitor, irinotecan. Fishkin and associates[194,195] observed two (9%) responses in 21 patients, with 25% of patients experiencing significant GI and hematologic toxicity. Sanz-Altamira and colleagues[196] reported similar results with two (8%) responses in 25 patients with unresectable gallbladder and bile duct cancers and a median survival of 10 months. At present, enrollment of patients with advanced gallbladder cancer remains a high priority.

Small cell carcinoma of the gallbladder must be recognized as a disease that should be primarily treated with chemotherapy.[197,198] Occasional complete and sometimes durable responses have been reported with cisplatin-based therapy, analogous to chemotherapy used for small cell lung cancer.[199] More typically after initial responses, these cancers progress with a virulent, often refractory course.

Novel Therapies. Given the traditionally poor response rates and unclear impact on either quality of life or survival from chemotherapy,[200,201] the focus in identifying new agents in biliary tract malignancies must be based around a greater understanding of the genetics and molecular pathogenesis of gallbladder cancer. Such an approach may lead to the identification of novel targets as well as pave the way for a more sophisticated approach to identifying who is at risk for developing this cancer and ultimately screening and early detection, which is likely to represent one of the few strategies that may affect the long-term outcome of this cancer. Along the signal-transduction pathway, therapeutic targets are abundant; but their potential has not been verified. EGFr and c-erb-B2 expression has been observed in gallbladder carcinoma.[202-205] C-erb-B2 and p53 protein expression has been associated with neoplastic progression and a poorer prognosis in gallbladder cancer, potentially providing therapeutic targets.[206,207] Platelet-derived growth factor (PDGF) has been expressed in the bile of patients with gallbladder cancer.[208] STI-571 has been preliminarily tested in gallbladder, based on this observation. Definitive data are awaited. In addition, activation of mitogen-activated protein kinase (MAP kinase) and upregulation of COX-2 levels have been observed in mice models of gallbladder cancer.[209-212] These mice models provide an opportunity to identify and test new treatment targets. Such concepts are beginning to be tested in the context of ongoing clinical trials. Speculatively, COX-2 over-expression may offer an opportunity to potentiate traditional cytotoxic agents in the advanced disease setting or indeed to offer the possibility for a chemo-preventive approach for a population of patients deemed to be at high risk of gallbladder cancer.

Treatment Complications

Larger series of patients treated with definitive surgical resection have shown complication rates of 28% and mortality of 0% to 4%.[148,158,160] The most common post-operative complications include intra-abdominal abscess or biloma, or other infectious complications such as pneumonia or wound complications.[148]

Follow-up

The most common sites of recurrence after resection of gallbladder cancer include carcinomatosis, intrahepatic metastases, or nodal recurrence in the retroperitoneum. Jaundice is a common sign, but patients with recurrence also may have ascites due to carcinomatosis. For most tumors, local recurrence is found synchronous with diffuse intra-abdominal spread. Therefore surgical treatment of recurrence has little potential for cure. If recurrent disease is found after resection, prognosis is exceedingly poor, with death occurring secondary to biliary sepsis or liver failure within months of diagnosis.

The main goal of follow-up after resection of gallbladder cancer is to provide palliation for symptomatic recurrences. The main symptoms associated with recurrence requiring palliation are pruritus or cholangitis associated with jaundice, or bowel obstruction associated with carcinomatosis. Additional goals of follow-up are to detect benign complications of surgical treatment such as biliary stricture. When jaundice or cholangitis is the presenting symptom of possible recurrence, a nonsurgical palliative approach using percutaneous transhepatic cholangiogram (PTC) and stenting is usually favored unless a benign postsurgical stricture is suspected. Because of the rapid growth of tumor in patients with recurrence, the hospitalization and recovery time from a surgical bypass is usually not justified for recurrences resulting in biliary obstruction.

The routine follow-up of a patient after resection of gallbladder cancer includes office visits every 3 months with physical examination and measurement of liver function tests. Although CA 19-9 may be elevated in patients with gallbladder cancer, the sensitivity and specificity are poor[213] and thus should not be used for screening patients for recurrence. Because an asymptomatic recurrence of gallbladder cancer has only limited treatment options, overaggressive use of imaging studies is not warranted. Therefore the use of imaging studies should be individualized.

Issues for the Future

Clearly, improving our ability to recognize early gallbladder cancer in high-risk geographic areas would have an important impact on outcome in these patients. This will likely require improvements in understanding the sequential molecular changes associated with gallbladder cancer. Other improvements in screening programs in high-risk areas, which could result in prophylactic cholecystectomy, would likely be beneficial.[128]

CANCER OF THE BILE DUCT

Introduction

One of the most technically difficult surgical resections is in those patients with Klatskin tumors, bile duct tumors arising in the hepatic hilus, or hilar cholangiocarcinoma. Bile duct cancers can arise at other sites, including within the liver (intrahepatic cholangiocarcinoma) and below the biliary bifurcation but above the pancreas (mid–bile duct cholangiocarcinoma). Distal cholangiocarcinoma involves that portion of the bile duct within the pancreas, which requires pancreaticoduodenectomy and is discussed in Chapter 84. The location of the tumor affects prognosis as well as the potential for curative resection.

Resection of biliary neoplasms, particularly hilar cholangiocarcinoma, often requires radical resections and complex biliary reconstructions that have only recently become safe in routine practice. Surgery also may offer effective palliation for these cancers by providing biliary bypass for jaundiced patients with unresectable tumors. Because patients are often diagnosed late in their course and because complex operative techniques are required for potentially curative resection, these tumors represent one of the greatest challenges for definitive treatment. Adding to this is the fact that no proven effective options exist for adjuvant treatment.

Epidemiology and Pathogenesis

The overall incidence of hilar cholangiocarcinoma in the United States is 1.0/100,000 per year, although other geographic regions such as Israel and Japan have higher rates.[214] The incidence of intrahepatic cholangiocarcinoma in the United States is approximately 0.7/100,000, with a similar mortality. During the last 30 years, it appears that both the incidence and mortality in the United States are increasing.[215]

Cholangiocarcinoma is a rare cancer that arises from the biliary epithelium and occurs in fewer than 4500 patients in the United States each year.[216] Cholangiocarcinomas arise slightly more often in men,[217] with a male/female ratio of 1.3:1, with an average age between 50 and 70 years. Risk factors for this disease include primary sclerosing cholangitis, ulcerative colitis, choledochal cysts, and biliary tract infection, either with *Clonorchis* or in chronic typhoid carriers.[218] Treating patients with cholangiocarcinoma arising from one of these underlying conditions is challenging.[219] Some industrial chemicals such as nitrosamines, dioxin, asbestos, and polychlorinated biphenyls also have been implicated in the pathogenesis of cholangiocarcinoma.[214] Although some suggest an increased risk of cholangiocarcinoma arising after transduodenal sphincteroplasty,[220] it is difficult to distinguish whether this is due to the surgical intervention or to the underlying disease leading to sphincteroplasty.

Pathology

Similar to gallbladder cancer, hilar cholangiocarcinoma tends to invade locally. More than 95% of these tumors are adenocarcinomas. They are morphologically described as nodular, which is the most common, scirrhous, diffusely infiltrating, or papillary. Histologic subtypes include acinar, ductular, trabecular, alveolar, and papillary. Papillary tumors (Fig. 83-11) appear to have an improved outcome. Much less frequent bile duct tumors include cystadeno-

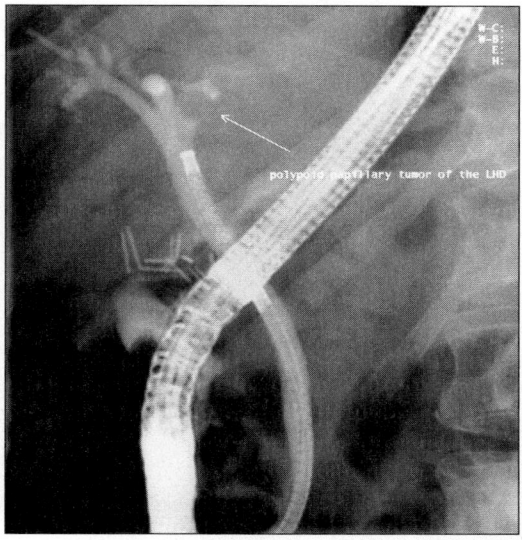

Figure 83-11. Endoscopic retrograde cholangiopancreatography (ERCP) with a filling defect in the left bile duct, which was biopsy-proven papillary cholangiocarcinoma.

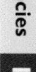

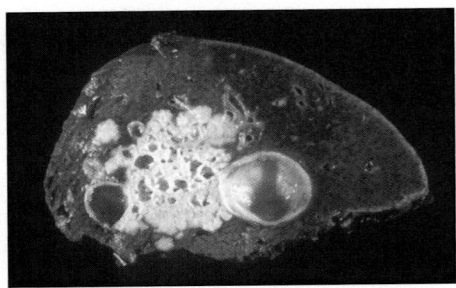

Figure 83-12. Gross image of resected intrahepatic cholangicarcinoma reveals solid and cystic components to the tumor.

carcinomas, hemangioendotheliomas, and mucoepidermoid carcinomas. Perineural invasion is clearly a poor prognostic sign.[221]

In patients with intrahepatic cholangiocarcinoma, negative prognostic signs include vascular invasion, multiple tumors, positive margin, large size, and lymph node metastases.[222-225] These tumors can be either sclerotic, mass-like lesions (Fig. 83-12) or cystic lesions (Fig. 83-13).

Historically, cholangiocarcinomas have been classified according to their location in the upper (60%), middle (15% to 20%), or lower third (15% to 20%) of the bile duct. Middle-third lesions arise between the cystic duct and the superior border of the duodenum. Lower-third lesions are found below the superior border of the duodenum but above the ampulla. The problem with this classification is that the anatomic landmarks are somewhat arbitrary and not clinically useful. Many mid–bile duct obstructions due to malignancy are the result of gallbladder cancer. Even when the obstruction is truly secondary to a mid–bile duct cholangiocarcinoma, very few of these tumors are amenable to treatment by local excision of the bile duct. A more useful classification may be to divide these lesions into upper-half or lower-half tumors, based on the location of the cystic duct as it enters the common duct, in the case of normal

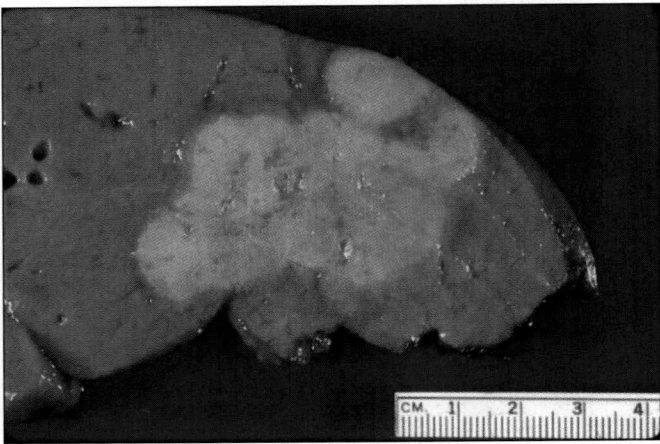

Figure 83-13. Gross image of resected intrahepatic cholangicarcinoma reveals sclerotic, solid mass.

anatomy. The usefulness of this classification scheme is that it allows the surgeon to delineate whether a hepatic or pancreatic resection will be required for clearance of tumor.

Biology

Because hilar cholangiocarcinomas arise in the bile duct, which is in close approximation to the PV, the tumor often causes PV occlusion as it enlarges. This results in lobar atrophy on the ipsilateral side. In addition to local invasion, nodal metastases occur frequently. Intrahepatic cholangiocarcinoma, unless arising in a location near the hilus, less commonly results in local invasion.

Clinical Presentation and Patient Evaluation

The vast majority of patients with hilar cholangiocarcinoma are first seen with painless jaundice, though mild RUQ pain, pruritus, anorexia, malaise, and weight loss also may be reported. Cholangitis is the presenting symptom in 10% to 30% of patients. Some patients have cancer discovered on evaluation for otherwise asymptomatic elevations of alkaline phosphatase (AP) and γ-glutamyl transferase (GGT).

Patients with intrahepatic cholangiocarcinoma are usually asymptomatic. Many patients are found to have a liver tumor present on cross-sectional imaging obtained for other reasons. Many of these patients will have a biopsy showing adenocarcinoma without a known primary. The standard evaluation in these patients should include tumor markers to rule out an elevated carcinoembryonic antigen (CEA) or AFP level, upper and lower endoscopy to evaluate for a GI source, CT scan to assess for a primary in the GI tract or pancreas, and, in women, a mammogram. If no site of primary disease is found, in the majority of patients, the diagnosis is intrahepatic cholangiocarcinoma.

Laboratory and Imaging Studies

Laboratory evaluation usually reveals elevated bilirubin or alkaline phosphatase and GGT consistent with biliary obstruction in patients with hilar cholangiocarcinoma or a mid–bile duct lesion. Other laboratory tests are usually normal. In patients with intrahepatic cholangiocarcinoma, laboratory evaluation is usually normal.

A variety of imaging tests are available to assess patients with hilar cholangiocarcinoma. Abdominal US is noninvasive, easily available, and inexpensive, and thus is commonly used as a first imaging modality. The advantage of US is that is can quickly establish the level of biliary obstruction. Cross-sectional imaging with intravenous contrast–enhanced CT scan is probably the most easily accessible and provides the most staging information. CT scans frequently reveal dilated intrahepatic biliary ducts with a normal, collapsed gallbladder and, depending on the level of the tumor, a nondilated or partially dilated extrahepatic biliary tree (see Fig. 83-5). In addition, the presence of hilar adenopathy can be assessed. PV patency

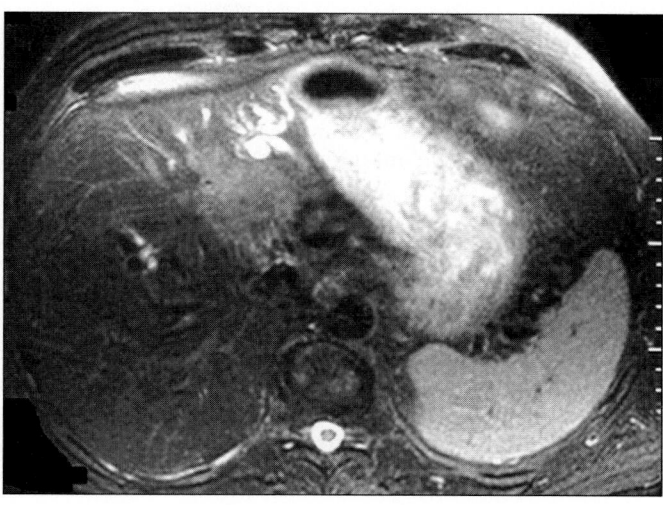
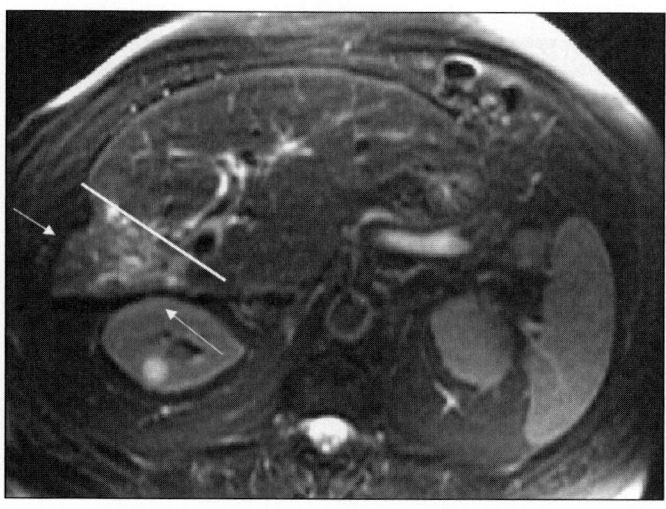

A

B

Figure 83-14. Lobar atrophy in the liver due to portal venous invasion by cholangiocarcinoma. Magnetic resonance imaging demonstrates **(A)** left lobar atrophy and **(B)** right lobe atrophy (*arrows; line* marks delineation between right and left lobes).

can be determined with US or helical CT. In addition, signs of hepatic lobar atrophy should be sought (Fig. 83-14), because this is associated with a high incidence of ipsilateral PV involvement by tumor. MRCP offers the potential of evaluating parenchymal, vascular, biliary, and nodal involvement with a single noninvasive examination.[225-227] Frequently it is possible to visualize the tumor itself with MRI (see Figs. 83-6 and 83-7).

In most centers, direct cholangiography is used to evaluate the extent of biliary involvement and provide palliation for jaundice. Endoscopic retrograde cholangiopancreatography (ERCP) has little role to play in high biliary obstruction because opacification of the proximal biliary tree is difficult. However, ERCP can be effectively used to image more distal lesions. At the time cholangiography is performed, some authors advocate the routine preoperative placement of biliary drainage catheters to aid in intraoperative identification of the bile ducts.[229,230] Others have found a higher incidence of infectious complications[231] and mortality[232] and a longer hospital stay[233] after preoperative placement of biliary drainage catheters. The difficulty in making the decision regarding preoperative stenting is that many patients are severely symptomatic because of jaundice and pruritus and thus require palliation; thus if a delay occurs in operative intervention, many patients require palliation.

In many cases, it is difficult to obtain pathologic confirmation of cholangiocarcinoma except in very advanced cases, even with the use of biliary brushings and cytology obtained at the time of direct cholangiography. For the majority of cases, patients are offered surgical therapy based on clinical suspicion and radiographic appearance.

In patients with intrahepatic cholangiocarcinoma, cross-sectional imaging with CT scan is usually sufficient. Tumors may be mass-like or may have cystic areas (see Figs. 83-12 and 83-13).

Staging Classification

The AJCC TNM staging system for bile duct cancers is described in Table 83-9. Cholangiocarcinomas occurring at the hepatic hilus are commonly referred to as hilar cholangiocarcinomas. These tumors have been further classified into four types, based on the modified Bismuth-Corlette classification (see Fig. 83-4).[234] To attempt to incorporate clinically important indicators of resectability, some preoperative staging systems incorporate imaging features consistent with advanced disease, such as hepatic lobe atrophy or PV involvement.[235] Most important, with the increasing acceptance of major hepatic resection for these tumors, these systems attempt to define whether ipsilateral involvement occurs alone, because tumors with bilateral extension past the primary biliary radicles are not resectable.

In the sixth edition of the AJCC TNM staging for extrahepatic bile duct cancer, several changes have been incorporated. The T and N classifications have been simplified. T1 is now classified as invasion of the subepithelial fibromuscular connective tissue. T2 is defined as invasion beyond the wall of the bile duct. Involvement of branches of the PV, HA, or liver is termed T3. Invasion of the main PV, common HA, and/or regional organs is now termed T4. In line with other hepatobiliary tract malignancies, stage III now signifies locally advanced, unresectable disease, and stage IV denotes metastatic disease.

Prognosis

Prognosis After Resection for Hilar Cholangiocarcinoma
Unfortunately, the prognosis for all patients with hilar cholangiocarcinoma is limited by the fact that as many as 90% of patients are unresectable at the time of presentation.[217] In addition, of those patients submitted to

TABLE 83-9

AJCC Staging System for Extrahepatic Bile Duct Carcinoma

STAGE	TUMOR	NODES	METASTASIS
0	Tis	N0	M0
IA	T1	N0	M0
IB	T2	N0	M0
IIA	T3	N0	M0
IIB	T1	N1	M0
	T2	N1	M0
	T3	N1	M0
III	T4	Any N	M0
IV	Any T	Any N	M1

Definition of TNM

Primary Tumor (T)

TX	Primary tumor cannot be assessed
T0	No evidence of primary tumor
Tis	Carcinoma in situ
T1	Tumor confined to bile duct histologically
T2	Tumor invades beyond the wall of the bile duct
T3	Tumor invades the liver, gallbladder, pancreas, and/or unilateral branches of the portal vein or hepatic artery
T4	Tumor invades any of the following: main portal vein or its branches, common hepatic artery, or other adjacent structures (e.g., colon, stomach, duodenum, abdominal wall)

Regional Lymph Nodes (N)

NX	Regional lymph nodes cannot be assessed
N0	No regional lymph node metastasis
N1	Regional lymph node metastasis

Distant Metastasis (M)

MX	Presence of distant metastasis cannot be assessed
M0	No distant metastasis
M1	Distant metastasis

From Greene FL: AJCC Cancer Staging Manual, 6th ed. New York, Springer-Verlag, 2002.

surgery with curative intent, up to 50% of the tumors are unresectable.[236,237] In patients with unresectable disease, the median survival is less than 1 year.[233] The immediate causes of death in these patients are hepatic failure or cholangitis related to tumor growth and inadequate drainage of the biliary tree.[238] In patients amenable to curative resection, the median survival is 35 months with a 5-year survival of 10% to 30%.[229,236,239-244] The results of major studies on resection of hilar cholangiocarcinoma are summarized in Table 83-10. Surgical resection provides not only improved survival but also improved quality of life.[245] The greatest risk factors for recurrence include the presence of positive margins[236,245,246] and node-positive tumors.[247,248]

Prognosis After Resection for Intrahepatic Cholangiocarcinoma

In patients with intrahepatic cholangiocarcinoma, expected 3-year survival as high as 60% has been reported,[159,249] with 5-year survival of 30% to 45%.[237] Patients with unresectable disease have a median survival of 12 months.[224,250] Thus completely resected intrahepatic cholangiocarcinoma appears to have an improved prognosis over proximal (hilar) cholangiocarcinoma.

Primary Treatment

Proximal (Hilar) Cholangiocarcinoma

Untreated, the majority of patients with bile duct cancers die within a year of diagnosis.[233] Surgical excision is the clearly the treatment of choice, as no other therapies have the potential for cure. The objectives of surgical management for patients with cholangiocarcinoma include both complete removal of tumor and adequate biliary drainage. It has become clear over the last three decades that curative treatment of tumors involving the upper half of the bile duct depends on aggressive excision that often requires a major liver resection.[236,244] Until as recently as one decade ago, treatment of hilar cholangiocarcinomas was associated with mortality as high as 30%.[234,239,251,252] Recently, major improvements in the safety of these operations has been demonstrated by multiple investigators, and resection of hilar tumors now results in mortality of less than 10%, even when liver resections are required.[234,239,246,251]

Assessment of Resectability and Surgical Procedure. Surgical exploration is often the only means of assessing resectability. Because of the potential morbidity of a laparotomy with no therapeutic benefit, staging laparos-

TABLE 83-10

Results after Resection for Hilar Cholangiocarcinoma

AUTHOR	N	PERCENTAGE RESECTED	POSTOPERATIVE MORTALITY (%)	FIVE-YEAR SURVIVAL (%)	SURVIVAL (MO) MEAN	SURVIVAL (MO) MEDIAN
Iwasaki, 1986[241]	46	22	0	20	—	25
Iida, 1987[242]	41	56	4	30	—	8
Cameron, 1990[229]	96	55	2	8	—	18
Hadjis, 1990[240]	131	21	7	12	25	—
Altaee, 1991[239]	70	21	—	19	—	12
Baer, 1993[251]	48	44	4	23	34	—
Nagorney, 1993[246]	79	15	5	16	—	13
McMasters, 1997[243]	91	44	0	26	—	22
Burke, 1998[235]	69	43	7	45		40

copy has been advocated to save patients from unnecessary laparotomy. In patients with hilar cholangiocarcinoma, up to 25% of patients will benefit from staging laparoscopy because of detection of occult extrahepatic disease.[159] Laparoscopy is a very sensitive means of detecting peritoneal metastases or additional intrahepatic disease through the use of laparoscopic US, but is less sensitive in detecting nodal metastases.[159]

Hilar cholangiocarcinoma is considered unresectable because of both local factors and metastatic spread. Clearly patients with disease outside the liver, including most commonly peritoneal or intrahepatic metastases, are not amenable to curative resection. Local factors that make these tumors unresectable include invasion of the main PV or both the right and left PVs or HAs and tumor extension into second-order biliary radicals of both right and left hepatic lobes. By contrast, tumors extending into second- or third-order biliary radicles on one side of the liver without vascular involvement can be resected with curative outcome.

The goals of surgical management for cholangiocarcinomas are both eradication of tumor and establishment of adequate biliary drainage. Tumors of the biliary confluence are particularly difficult to treat because symptoms often appear late in the course of disease when the lesion has already involved adjacent structures, including the PV or adjacent hepatic parenchyma. Complete resection, therefore, requires biliary and hepatic resection and often major vascular reconstruction. Therefore it is not surprising that, in the past, the surgical therapy for proximal biliary malignancies consisted mainly of biliary-enteric bypass as palliation for jaundice and cholangitis. The therapeutic approach to hilar cholangiocarcinoma was largely nihilistic, because of difficulty in delineating the extent of disease and the technical challenge of complete resection for such lesions.

Over the last decade, surgical approaches have become more aggressive, as demonstrated by the increasing number of hepatic resections that have been performed for bile duct cancers.[234,236,239,251,252] Recent improvements in US, CT, and MRI have greatly facilitated preoperative evaluation and staging of cholangiocarcinoma. This has allowed improved patient selection and surgical planning.

The location and local extension of tumor dictates the extent of resection, with most lesions requiring an extended right or left hepatectomy for complete excision. Caudate resection is often required because of direct extension into caudate biliary radicles or parenchyma.[234-236,240] CBD excision and portal lymphadenectomy also are essential for tumor clearance.

Surgical Treatment of Unresectable Hilar Cholangiocarcinoma.

For patients with unresectable hilar cholangiocarcinomas, significant improvement in quality of life can occur with surgical bypass, because most patients are symptomatic with pruritus due to jaundice. Palliative bypass can be performed in several ways. A partial excision of the left lateral segment and biliary-enteric anastomosis to the left hepatic duct (Longmire procedure) was used commonly in the past, but more recent, less complicated surgical techniques do not require hepatic parenchymal transection. One technique involves biliary decompression through the left duct, approached through the round ligament, a segment III bypass. In this position, a long anastomosis can be performed from the segment III duct to a jejunal limb, because of the horizontal course of the duct in this location. Although less commonly used, the right hepatic duct can be approached at the base of the gallbladder fossa. This is technically more difficult and results in a higher rate of late bypass failure.[253]

Nonoperative palliative biliary decompression can be accomplished with percutaneous or endoscopic stenting, depending on the level of obstruction. Proximal lesions are usually approached percutaneously with placement of expandable stents or drainage catheters (see Fig. 83-9). Internal stents result in fewer electrolyte abnormalities and improvement in patient comfort, although morbidity and mortality occurs in up to 30% of patients, and stent occlusion is common.[254-256] A significant risk of cholangitis is found with external and internal drainage, occurring in more than 90% of patients with metallic expandable internal stents in one series.[255] Bleeding and bile leaks also are frequent complications. More recent techniques such as photodynamic therapy have been used to palliate biliary obstruction and may hold some promise for the future.[257]

Because patients with unresectable disease have a short median survival, patients who are clearly unresectable on preoperative imaging should undergo percutaneous internal or external drainage. In patients who are explored and found to be unresectable, surgical bypass offers the advantage of fewer episodes of cholangitis and stent obstruction, with an improved quality of life.[253] In some series, surgical bypass for unresectable patients is the only biliary drainage procedure ever required by a patient with unresectable disease.

Intrahepatic Cholangiocarcinoma

Patients with intrahepatic cholangiocarcinoma typically are first seen with single liver lesions. Standard treatment with anatomically based hepatic resection is the procedure of choice. Because these tumors are frequently asymptomatic, fewer issues occur with palliative management.

Treatment of Advanced Bile Duct Cancers

Chemotherapy. To date, no chemotherapeutic regimen has consistently shown activity against cholangiocarcinoma. Many of the issues that pertain to chemotherapy trials in gallbladder cancer are directly relevant to the interpretation of trials for cholangiocarcinomas. Studies performed to date have typically been small, single-institution trials, including patients with both gallbladder and bile duct cancers.[181]

Although 5-FU–based chemotherapy is often offered to patients with unresectable disease, the likelihood of response is less than 10%. Capecitabine as a single agent may have some modest activity in cholangiocarcinomas.[258] The use of mitomycin-C and doxorubicin

Specific Malignancies

(Adriamycin), in combination with 5-FU, has resulted in combined response rates of less than 30%, with higher toxicity than 5-FU alone.[120] No proven role exists for adjuvant chemotherapy alone in the treatment of cholangiocarcinoma.

Multiple other single agents and combinations have been assessed. Of the newer drugs, gemcitabine, analogous to the situation in gallbladder cancer, shows some promise. A small phase II study of docetaxel in unresectable cholangiocarcinoma demonstrated minimal activity and moderate toxicity.[259] Kubicka and associates[76] assessed the activity of single-agent gemcitabine in 23 patients with advanced bile duct cancer and 20 patients with HCC. A response rate of 30% (seven partial responses) was observed in the cholangiocarcinoma group and only 5% in the HCC group. The authors concluded that gemcitabine was ineffective in HCC but had a possible palliative role in bile duct cancers.

In advanced biliary malignancies, various chemotherapeutic combinations have been assessed. Patt and coworkers[260] conducted a phase II trial of cisplatin, interferon alpha-2b, doxorubicin, and 5-FU (PIAF) in patients with unresectable biliary tract cancers. Forty-one patients were treated (22 cholangiocarcinoma, 19 gallbladder). The overall response rate was 21%, with a response rate of 9.5% in the bile duct population and 35% in the gallbladder group noted. Toxicities were moderate, mostly hematologic, GI, and fatigue. The authors concluded limited efficacy in bile duct cancer but suggested a role in the treatment of gallbladder cancer. Sanz-Altamira and coworkers[261] conducted a phase II study of 5-FU, leucovorin, and carboplatin in patients with advanced biliary tract cancer. A response rate of 21% was noted with acceptable toxicity. In a French trial,[262] a phase II assessment of 5-FU, leucovorin, and cisplatin combination resulted in a 34% objective response rate in 29 patients with advanced biliary malignancies, again suggesting potential utility of the combination.

To summarize, single-agent chemotherapy has elicited disappointing results in advanced biliary tract malignancies, with response rates ranging from 5% to 20%. Even newer agents such as paclitaxel, gemcitabine, and irinotecan have response rates in the 0 to 20% range.[76,193,196] Combination chemotherapy has yielded modestly higher response rates in the 20% to 30% range at the extent of higher toxicity and has an unclear impact on median and overall survival. No large randomized phase III trials and only a small number of phase II trials have been completed in biliary tract cancers to better answer the true role of cytotoxic systemic chemotherapy.

Intra-arterial Chemotherapy. Intra-arterial chemotherapy administration for unresectable hepatobiliary malignancies remains an attractive concept. The rationale relates to the natural history of biliary tract malignancies with a high propensity for locoregional as well as systemic failure. The experience of this approach in cholangiocarcinomas is limited. Several small trials have demonstrated interesting response rates with acceptable toxicity in selected patient populations.[263,264] In a small pilot

trial by Cantore and colleagues[263] 10 patients with cholangiocarcinoma were treated with intrahepatic epirubicin and cisplatin, as well as with systemic infusional 5-FU. A 70% response rate was noted, and 55% of patients were alive at 2 years. Further trials are currently under way to better understand the role of intra-arterial chemotherapy in cholangiocarcinoma and other biliary tree malignancies.

Radiation Therapy. In cases of unresectable cholangiocarcinoma, the use of external-beam radiation therapy has been explored.[121-124] No study has clearly demonstrated efficacy for this modality. Anecdotal reports of long-term survivors after external-beam radiation therapy show that some individuals may benefit from such treatment, but this must be weighed against the potential complications such as duodenal or bile duct stenosis and duodenitis. The most encouraging results involve use of intraoperative[122-125] or interstitial radiation.[118,123,126] Our current practice is to use combined interstitial radiation and external beam radiation in unresectable cases after palliative bypass. In patients who are resected, adjuvant radiation therapy as a single modality has not been shown to increase quality of life or survival.[127] Crane and colleagues[265] undertook a retrospective review of a single-institution experience of chemoradiation in patients with unresectable cholangiocarcinoma. Fifty-two patients with locally advanced cholangiocarcinomas were treated with radiation with or without concurrent chemotherapy. The authors observed a 72% occurrence of local failure as the site of first failure. In 15% of patients, metastatic disease developed. The conclusion was that the reason for treatment failure in a majority of patients was local tumor progression. The future recommendation was to incorporate novel radiosensitizing cytotoxics or biologics or both with high-dose conformal radiation.[266]

Novel Therapies. Given the limitations of standard therapy, clearly a major niche exists for the development of novel therapeutics in bile duct cancers. Along the signal-transduction pathway, the level of EGRr expression reported in cholangiocarcinoma has been variable.[267,268] Whereas Cheifetz and associates[269] reported no expression in cholangiocarcinoma, Ito and coworkers[267] found a correlation between EGFr expression and aggressiveness of the disease. As in gallbladder cancer, PDGF was found to be expressed and present at high levels in ampullary cancers and cholangiocarcinomas.[208] Further down along the signal-transduction pathway, the Fas receptor and Fas ligand have been recognized as key steps in apoptosis induction.[270,271] Laboratory data suggested antitumor activity of an ant-Fas receptor antibody in human tumors.[270,272] Shimonishi and colleagues[273] observed variable expression of Fas ligand in cholangiocarcinoma, again suggesting possible therapeutic application.

In vitro work with the somatostatin analogue, octreotide, demonstrated antiproliferative activity in several cholangiocarcinoma cell lines, suggesting possible therapeutic application for octreotide.[274,275] Other novel approaches include development of an adenoviral vector therapy with tumor-restrictive gene expression for cholangiocarcinoma.[275] Ongoing studies are assessing the diagnostic and therapeutic value of a radioactive-labeled chimeric monoclonal antibody against a G250 cell-surface antigen, which is expressed in about two thirds of patients with biliary tract cancers.[275]

Along with hepatocellular cancer and gallbladder cancer, the future in treating cholangiocarcinomas will be novel therapeutics and targeting of features unique to these malignancies and most likely a combination of these approaches with currently available cytoreductive therapies.

Treatment Complications

Attesting to the difficult management of patients with hilar cholangiocarcinoma, the complication rate is as high as 50% to 60%.[236,276] The majority of these complications are infectious, partially due to biliary obstruction with resultant biliary stenting. In many series, treatment of hilar cholangiocarcinoma with aggressive resection results in a perioperative mortality of approximately 5% to 10%.[236]

Fewer postoperative complications are expected from surgical procedures for patients with intrahepatic cholangiocarcinoma, because these operations are usually more straightforward and do not usually require bile duct resection. The overall complication rate is approximately 20% to 30%, with a mortality of less than 3%.[224,225,244,246,276]

Follow-up

The most likely site of recurrence after resection of a hilar cholangiocarcinoma is locally within the bile duct, regional lymph nodes, or liver. For patients with intrahepatic cholangiocarcinoma, the most common site of recurrence is within the liver or regional nodes.[224,277] Therapy for recurrence is palliative, because curative surgical re-excision is usually impossible because of the challenging anatomic location and the radical procedures that are required for resection of the primary tumor. Therefore the goal of follow-up is diagnosis of symptomatic recurrences to direct the palliative therapy and diagnosis of benign complications of surgical treatment such as biliary strictures. The main symptoms of recurrence that demand palliation are pruritus or cholangitis associated with jaundice. For biliary drainage to relieve jaundice or cholangitis, either surgical drainage[255] or drainage by PTC can be effective.[278] Endoscopic drainage has little role in the relief of jaundice in patients who have had roux-en-Y biliary reconstruction. For limited recurrences, intraluminal brachytherapy, or external beam radiation therapy[279] may improve palliation and, potentially, survival.

Routine follow-up consists of office visits every 3 months with physical examination and measurement of liver function tests. Although an increasing alkaline phosphatase is a good indicator of evolving biliary obstruction, patients recovering from liver resection and biliary obstruction may have persistent elevations of alkaline phosphatase. However, in up to 10% of patients

with biliary surgical reconstruction, a benign anastomotic stricture may develop. Most patients with recurrence or a benign stricture will have jaundice or cholangitis. Because a low likelihood of effective therapy exists for recurrences, the routine use of tumor markers is not recommended, although a fair percentage of biliary malignancies will express CEA or CA 19-9. The routine use of imaging studies to follow up patients with cholangiocarcinoma after resection should be limited for the same reasons.

Issues for the Future

The only known curative therapy for intra- and extrahepatic bile duct cancers is surgery. No proven role has been found for adjuvant chemotherapy alone or adjuvant combined chemoradiation, although further studies are needed to define fully the role of these therapies. Continued assessment of new drugs, novel radiosensitizers, and biologic agents is warranted. A better understanding of the molecular pathogenesis and genetics of bile duct cancers may lead to new therapeutic and ultimately preventive strategies for high-risk populations.

REFERENCES

1. Chen TS, Chen PS: The myth of Prometheus and the liver. J R Soc Med 1994;87:754–755.
2. Parkin DM, Pisani P, Ferlay J, et al: Estimates of the worldwide incidence of 25 major cancers in 1990. Int J Cancer 1999;80: 827–841.
3. McGlynn KA, Tsao L, et al: International trends and patterns of primary liver cancer. Int J Cancer 2001;94:290–296.
4. Jin F, Devesa SS, et al: Cancer incidence trends in urban Shanghai, 1972–1994: An update. Int J Cancer 1999;83:435–440.
5. Taylor-Robinson SD, Foster GR, et al: Increase in primary liver cancer in the UK, 1979–94. Lancet 1997;350:1142–1143.
6. Deuffic S, Poynard T, et al: Trends in primary liver cancer. Lancet 1998;351:214–215.
7. Gerard-Marchant R: Coding of tumorous lesions in anatomopathology. Ann Anat Pathol (Paris) 1976;21:381–386.
8. Vatanasapt V, Martin N, et al: Cancer incidence in Thailand, 1988–1991. Cancer Epidemiol Biomarkers Prev 1995;4:475–483.
9. Kullavanijaya P, Tangkijvanich P, et al: Current status of infection-related gastrointestinal and hepatobiliary diseases in Thailand. Southeast Asian J Trop Med Public Health 1999;30:96–105.
10. El-Serag HB: Hepatocellular carcinoma: An epidemiologic view. J Clin Gastroenterol 2002;35(5 suppl 2):S72–S78.
11. Beasley RP: Hepatitis B virus: The major etiology of hepatocellular carcinoma. Cancer 1988;61:1942–1956.
12. DiBisceglie AM, Simpson LH, Lotze MT, Hoofnagle JH: Development of hepatocellular carcinoma among patients with chronic liver disease due to hepatitis C viral infection. J Clin Gastroenterol 1994;19:222–226.
13. Ebara M, Hatano R, Fukuda H, Yoshikawa M, Sugiura N, Saisho H: Natural course of small hepatocellular carcinoma with underlying cirrhosis: A study of 30 patients. Hepatogastroenterology 1998;45(suppl 20):18–20.
14. Nguyen MH, Garcia RT, Simpson PW, Wright TL, Keeffe EB: Racial differences in effectiveness of alpha-fetoprotein for diagnosis of hepatocellular carcinoma in hepatitis C virus cirrhosis. Hepatology 2002;36:410–417.
15. Poon TC, Mok TS, Chan AT, et al: Quantification and utility of monosialylated alpha-fetoprotein in the diagnosis of hepatocellular carcinoma with nondiagnostic serum total alpha-fetoprotein. Clin Chem 2002;48:1021–1027.
16. Sherman M, Peltekian KM, Lee C: Screening for hepatocellular

carcinoma in chronic carriers of hepatitis B virus: Incidence and prevalence of hepatocellular carcinoma in a North American urban population. Hepatology 1995;22:432–438.

17. Billingsley KG, Jarnagin WR, Fong Y, Blumgart LH: Segment-oriented hepatic resection in the management of malignant neoplasms of the liver. J Am Coll Surg 1998;187:471–481.

18. Shimizu A, Shiraki K, Ito T, et al: Sequential fluctuation pattern of serum des-gamma-carboxy prothrombin levels detected by high-sensitive electrochemiluminescence system as an early predictive marker for hepatocellular carcinoma in patients with cirrhosis. Int J Mol Med 2002;9:245–250.

19. Sato Y, Nakata K, Kato Y, et al: Early recognition of hepatocellular carcinoma based on altered profiles of alpha-fetoprotein. N Engl J Med 1993; 328:1802–1806.

20. Okuda H, Nakanishi T, Takatsu K, et al: Clinicopathologic features of patients with hepatocellular carcinoma seropositive for alpha-fetoprotein-L3 and seronegative for des-gamma-carboxy prothrombin in comparison with those seropositive for des-gamma-carboxy prothrombin alone. J Gastroenterol Hepatol 2002;17:772–778.

21. Okuda H, Nakanishi T, Takatsu K, et al: Comparison of clinicopathological features of patients with hepatocellular carcinoma seropositive for alpha-fetoprotein alone and those seropositive for des-gamma-carboxy prothrombin alone. J Gastroenterol Hepatol 2001;16:1290–1296.

22. Pateron D, Ganne N, Trinchet JC, et al: Prospective study of screening for hepatocellular carcinoma in Caucasian patients with cirrhosis. J Hepatol 1994;20:65–71.

23. Chen TH, Chen CJ, Yen MF, et al: Ultrasound screening and risk factors for death from hepatocellular carcinoma in a high risk group in Taiwan. Int J Cancer 2002;98:257–261.

24. Tang ZY, Yu YQ, Zhou XD, Yang BH, Ma ZC, Lin ZY: Subclinical hepatocellular carcinoma: An analysis of 391 patients. J Surg Oncol Suppl 1993;3:55–58.

25. Iwata Y, Shiomi S, Sasaki N, et al: Clinical usefulness of positron emission tomography with fluorine-18-fluorodeoxyglucose in the diagnosis of liver tumors. Ann Nucl Med 2000;14:121–126.

26. Trojan J, Schroeder O, Raedle J, et al: Fluorine-18 FDG positron emission tomography for imaging of hepatocellular carcinoma. Am J Gastroenterol 1999;94:3314–3319.

27. Verhoef C, Valkema R, de Man RA, Krenning EP, Yzermans JN: Fluorine-18 FDG imaging in hepatocellular carcinoma using positron coincidence detection and single photon emission computed tomography. Liver 2002;22:51–56.

28. Fuchs CS, Clark JW, Ryan DP, et al: A phase II trial of gemcitabine in patients with advanced hepatocellular carcinoma. Cancer 2002;94:3186–3191.

29. Itamoto T, Nakahara H, Tashiro H, et al: Hepatic arterial infusion of 5-fluorouracil and cisplatin for unresectable or recurrent hepatocellular carcinoma with tumor thrombus of the portal vein. J Surg Oncol 2002;80:143–148.

30. Imaoka S, Sasaki Y, Masutani S, et al: Palliative surgical treatment for recurrent and non-resectable hepatocellular carcinoma. Hepatogastroenterology 1993;40:342–346.

31. Fong Y, Sun RL, Jarnagin W, Blumgart LH: An analysis of 412 cases of hepatocellular carcinoma at a Western center. Ann Surg 1999;229:790–799.

32. Poon RT, Fan ST, Lo CM, Liu CL, Wong J: Intrahepatic recurrence after curative resection of hepatocellular carcinoma: Long-term results of treatment and prognostic factors. Ann Surg 1999;229: 216–222.

33. Arii S, Teramoto K, Kawamura T, et al: Characteristics of recurrent hepatocellular carcinoma in Japan and our surgical experience. J Hepatobiliary Pancreat Surg 2001;8:397–403.

34. Hanazaki K, Kajikawa S, Shimozawa N, et al: Survival and recurrence after hepatic resection of 386 consecutive patients with hepatocellular carcinoma. J Am Coll Surg 2000;191: 381–388.

35. Lo CM, Lai EC, Fan ST, Choi TK, Wong J: Resection for extrahepatic recurrence of hepatocellular carcinoma. Br J Surg 1994;81:1019–1021.

36. Poon RT, Fan ST, Ng IO, Wong J: Significance of resection margin in hepatectomy for hepatocellular carcinoma: A critical reappraisal. Ann Surg 2000;231:544–551.

37. Poon RT, Fan ST, Ng IO, Lo CM, Liu CL, Wong J: Different risk factors and prognosis for early and late intrahepatic recurrence after resection of hepatocellular carcinoma. Cancer 2000;89: 500–507.

38. Belghiti J, Regimbeau JM, Durand F, et al: Resection of hepatocellular carcinoma: A European experience on 328 cases. Hepatogastroenterology 2002;49:41–46.

39. Nagasue N, Kohno H, Chang YC, et al: Liver resection for hepatocellular carcinoma: Results of 229 consecutive patients during 11 years. Ann Surg 1993;217:375–384.

40. Schlitt HJ, Neipp M, Weimann A, et al: Recurrence patterns of hepatocellular and fibrolamellar carcinoma after liver transplantation. J Clin Oncol 1999;17:324–331.

41. Kawasaki S, Makuuchi M, Miyagawa S, et al: Results of hepatic resection for hepatocellular carcinoma. World J Surg 1995;19: 31–34.

42. Roayaie S, Haim MB, Emre S, et al: Comparison of surgical outcomes for hepatocellular carcinoma in patients with hepatitis B versus hepatitis C: A Western experience. Ann Surg Oncol 2000;7:764–770.

43. Bismuth H, Chiche L, Adam R, Castaing D, Diamond T, Dennison A: Liver resection versus transplantation for hepatocellular carcinoma in cirrhotic patients. Ann Surg 1993;218:145–151.

44. Llovet JM, Fuster J, Bruix J: Intention-to-treat analysis of surgical treatment for early hepatocellular carcinoma: Resection versus transplantation. Hepatology 1999;30:1434–1440.

45. Bruix J, Llovet JM: Prognostic prediction and treatment strategy in hepatocellular carcinoma. Hepatology 2002;35:519–524.

46. Schwartz ME, Sung M, Mor E, et al: A multidisciplinary approach to hepatocellular carcinoma in patients with cirrhosis. J Am Coll Surg 1995;180:596–603.

47. Llovet JM, Bruix J, Fuster J, et al: Liver transplantation for small hepatocellular carcinoma: The tumor-node-metastasis classification does not have prognostic power. Hepatology 1998;27:1572–1577.

48. Klintmalm GB: Liver transplantation for hepatocellular carcinoma: A registry report of the impact of tumor characteristics on outcome. Ann Surg 1998;228:479–490.

49. Iwatsuki S, Starzl TE, Sheahan DG, et al: Hepatic resection versus transplantation for hepatocellular carcinoma. Ann Surg 1991;214:221–228.

50. Haug CE, Jenkins RL, Rohrer RJ, et al: Liver transplantation for primary hepatic cancer. Transplantation 1992;53:376–382.

51. Iwatsuki S, Dvorchik I, Marsh JW, et al: Liver transplantation for hepatocellular carcinoma: A proposal of a prognostic scoring system. J Am Coll Surg 2000;191:389–394.

52. Roayaie S, Frischer JS, Emre SH, et al: Long-term results with multimodal adjuvant therapy and liver transplantation for the treatment of hepatocellular carcinomas larger than 5 centimeters. Ann Surg 2002;235:533–539.

53. Gondolesi G, Munoz L, Matsumoto C, et al: Hepatocellular carcinoma: A prime indication for living donor liver transplantation. J Gastrointest Surg 2002;6:102–107.

54. Llovet JM, Real MI, Montana X, et al: Arterial embolisation or chemoembolisation versus symptomatic treatment in patients with unresectable hepatocellular carcinoma: A randomised controlled trial. Lancet 2002;359:1734–1739.

55. Bruix J, Llovet JM, Castells A, et al: Transarterial embolization versus symptomatic treatment in patients with advanced hepatocellular carcinoma: Results of a randomized, controlled trial in a single institution. Hepatology 1998;27:1578–1583.

56. Cha C, Lee FT Jr, Rikkers LF, Niederhuber JE, Nguyen BT, Mahvi DM: Rationale for the combination of cryoablation with surgical resection of hepatic tumors. J Gastrointest Surg 2001;5:206–213.

57. Lee HS, Kim KU, Yoon JH, et al: Therapeutic efficacy of transcatheter arterial chemoembolization as compared with hepatic resection in hepatocellular carcinoma patients with compensated liver function in a hepatitis B virus-endemic area. J Clin Oncol 2002;20:4459–4465.

58. Pearson AS, Izzo F, Fleming RY, et al: Intraoperative radiofrequency ablation or cryoablation for hepatic malignancies. Am J Surg 1999;178:592–599.

59. Curley SA, Izzo F, Ellis LM, Nicolas VJ, Vallone P: Radiofrequency ablation of hepatocellular cancer in 110 patients with cirrhosis. Ann Surg 2000;232:381–391.

60. Nicoli N, Casaril A, Marchiori L, Mangiante G, Hasheminia AR: Treatment of recurrent hepatocellular carcinoma by radio-frequency thermal ablation. J Hepatobiliary Pancreat Surg 2001;8: 417–421.

61. Llovet JM, Mas X, Aponte JJ, et al: Cost effectiveness of adjuvant therapy for hepatocellular carcinoma during the waiting list for liver transplantation. Gut 2002;50:123–128.

62. Livraghi T, Bolondi L, Lazzaroni S, et al: Percutaneous ethanol injection in the treatment of hepatocellular carcinoma in cirrhosis: A study on 207 patients. Cancer 1992;69:925–929.

63. Tanikawa K, Majima Y: Percutaneous ethanol injection therapy for recurrent hepatocellular carcinoma. Hepatogastroenterology 1993;40:324–327.

64. Shiina S, Tagawa K, Unuma T, et al: Percutaneous ethanol injection therapy for hepatocellular carcinoma: A histopathologic study. Cancer 1991;68:1524–1530.

65. Livraghi T, Goldberg SN, Lazzaroni S, Meloni F, Solbiati L, Gazelle GS: Small hepatocellular carcinoma: Treatment with radio-frequency ablation versus ethanol injection. Radiology 1999;210:655–661.

66. Leung TW, Johnson PJ: Systemic therapy for hepatocellular carcinoma. Semin Oncol 2001;28: 514–520.

67. Johnson PJ: Hepatocellular carcinoma: Is current therapy really altering outcome? Gut 2002;51:459–462.

68. Bonin S, Pascolo L, et al: Gene expression of ABC proteins in hepatocellular carcinoma, perineoplastic tissue, and liver diseases. Mol Med 2002;8:318–325.

69. Park JG, Lee SK, et al: MDR1 gene expression: Its effect on drug resistance to doxorubicin in human hepatocellular carcinoma cell lines. J Natl Cancer Inst 1994;86:700–705.

70. Park NH, Chung YH, et al: Close correlation of p53 mutation to microvascular invasion in hepatocellular carcinoma. J Clin Gastroenterol 2001;33:397–401.

71. Nerenstone S, Friedman M: Medical treatment of hepatocellular carcinoma. Gastroenterol Clin North Am 1987;16:603–612.

72. Lai EC, Lo CM, et al: Postoperative adjuvant chemotherapy after curative resection of hepatocellular carcinoma: A randomized controlled trial. Arch Surg 1988;133:183–188.

73. Mathurin P, Rixe O, et al: Overview of medical treatments in unresectable hepatocellular carcinoma: An impossible meta-analysis [review article]? Aliment Pharmacol Ther 1998;12:111–126.

74. Hong RL, Tseng YL: A phase II and pharmacokinetic study of pegylated liposomal doxorubicin in patients with advanced hepatocellular carcinoma. Cancer Chemother Pharmacol 2003;51:433–438.

75. Dangoor A, Ranson M, et al: Treatment of Inoperable Hepatocellular Carcinoma (HCC) with Pegylated Liposomal Doxorubicin: A Phase II Study. Chicago, American Society of Clinical Oncology, 2003.

76. Kubicka S, Rudolph KL, et al: Phase II study of systemic gemcitabine chemotherapy for advanced unresectable hepatobiliary carcinomas. Hepatogastroenterology 2001;48:783–789.

77. O'Reilly EM, Stuart KE, et al: A phase II study of irinotecan in patients with advanced hepatocellular carcinoma. Cancer 2001;91:101–105.

78. Yang TS, Lin YC, et al: Phase II study of gemcitabine in patients with advanced hepatocellular carcinoma. Cancer 2000;89: 750–756.

79. Falkson G, MacIntyre JM, et al: Primary liver cancer: An Eastern Cooperative Oncology Group Trial. Cancer 1984;54:970–977.

80. Bobbio-Pallavicini E, Porta C, et al: Epirubicin and etoposide combination chemotherapy to treat hepatocellular carcinoma patients: A phase II study. Eur J Cancer 1997;33:1784–1788.

81. Leung TW, Patt YZ, et al: Complete pathological remission is possible with systemic combination chemotherapy for inoperable hepatocellular carcinoma. Clin Cancer Res 1999;5: 1676–1681.

82. Patt YZ, Yoffe B, et al: Low serum alpha-fetoprotein level in patients with hepatocellular carcinoma as a predictor of response to 5-FU and interferon-alpha-2b. Cancer 1993;72:2574–2582.

83. Patt YZ, Hassan MM, et al: Phase II trial of systemic continuous fluorouracil and subcutaneous recombinant interferon alfa-2b for treatment of hepatocellular carcinoma. J Clin Oncol 2003;21: 421–427.

84. Tanioka H, Tsuji A, et al: Combination chemotherapy with continuous 5-fluorouracil and low-dose cisplatin infusion for advanced hepatocellular carcinoma. Anticancer Res 2003;23(2C): 1891–1897.

85. Komorizono Y, Kohara K, et al: Systemic combined chemotherapy with low dose of 5-fluorouracil, cisplatin, and interferon-alpha for advanced hepatocellular carcinoma: A pilot study. Dig Dis Sci 2003;48:877–881.

86. Porta C, Moroni M, et al: 5-Fluorouracil and d,l-leucovorin calcium are active to treat unresectable hepatocellular carcinoma patients: Preliminary results of a phase II study. Oncology 1995;52: 487–491.

87. Lau WY, Leung TW, et al: Preoperative systemic chemoimmunotherapy and sequential resection for unresectable hepatocellular carcinoma. Ann Surg 2001;233:236–241.

88. Leung TW, Tang AM, et al: Factors predicting response and survival in 149 patients with unresectable hepatocellular carcinoma treated by combination cisplatin, interferon-alpha, doxorubicin and 5-fluorouracil chemotherapy. Cancer 2002;94:421–427.

89. Murata K, Shiraki K, et al: Low-dose chemotherapy of cisplatin and 5-fluorouracil or doxorubicin via implanted fusion port for unresectable hepatocellular carcinoma. Anticancer Res 2003;23(2C):1719–1722.

90. Ando E, Tanaka M, et al: Hepatic arterial infusion chemotherapy for advanced hepatocellular carcinoma with portal vein tumor thrombosis: Analysis of 48 cases. Cancer 2002;95:588–595.

91. Kwok PC, Lam TW, et al: Randomized controlled trial to compare the dose of adjuvant chemotherapy after curative resection of hepatocellular carcinoma. J Gastroenterol Hepatol 2003;18: 450–455.

92. Pignata S, Daniele B, et al: Endocrine treatment of hepatocellular carcinoma: Any evidence of benefit? Eur J Cancer 1998;34:25–32.

93. Farinati F, Salvagnini M, et al: Unresectable hepatocellular carcinoma: A prospective controlled trial with tamoxifen. J Hepatol 1990;11:297–301.

94. Castells A, Bruix J, et al: Treatment of hepatocellular carcinoma with tamoxifen: A double-blind placebo-controlled trial in 120 patients. Gastroenterology 1995;109:917–922.

95. Bruix J, Sherman M, et al: Clinical management of hepatocellular carcinoma: Conclusions of the Barcelona-2000 EASL conference, European Association for the Study of the Liver. J Hepatol 2001;35:421–430.

96. Chow PK, Tai BC, et al: High-dose tamoxifen in the treatment of inoperable hepatocellular carcinoma: A multicenter randomized controlled trial. Hepatology 2002;36:1221–1226.

97. Kouroumalis E, Skordilis P, et al: Treatment of hepatocellular carcinoma with octreotide: A randomised controlled study. Gut 1998;42:442–447.

98. Yuen MF, Poon RT, et al: A randomized placebo-controlled study of long-acting octreotide for the treatment of advanced hepatocellular carcinoma. Hepatology 2002;36:687–691.

99. Samonakis DN, Moschandreas J, et al: Treatment of hepatocellular carcinoma with long acting somatostatin analogues. Oncol Rep 2002;9:903–907.

100. Jia WD, Xu GL, et al: Octreotide acts as an antitumor angiogenesis compound and suppresses tumor growth in nude mice bearing human hepatocellular carcinoma xenografts. J Cancer Res Clin Oncol 2003;129:327–334.

101. Miyaguchi S, Watanabe T: The role of vitamin D3 receptor mRNA in the proliferation of hepatocellular carcinoma. Hepatogastroenterology 2000;47:468–472.

102. Sahpazidou D, Stravoravdi P, et al: Significant experimental decrease of the hepatocellular carcinoma incidence in C3H/Sy mice after long-term administration of EB1089, a vitamin D analogue. Oncol Res 2003;13:261–268.

103. Dalhoff K, Dancey J, et al: A phase II study of the vitamin D analogue seocalcitol in patients with inoperable hepatocellular carcinoma. Br J Cancer 2003;89:252–257.

104. Ono T, Yamanoi A, et al: Adjuvant chemotherapy after resection of hepatocellular carcinoma causes deterioration of long-term prognosis in cirrhotic patients: Metaanalysis of three randomized controlled trials. Cancer 2001;91:2378–2385.

105. Schwartz JD, Schwartz M, et al: Neoadjuvant and adjuvant therapy for resectable hepatocellular carcinoma: Review of the randomised clinical trials. Lancet Oncol 2002;3:593–603.

106. Koga H, Sakisaka S, et al: Expression of cyclooxygenase-2 in human hepatocellular carcinoma: Relevance to tumor dedifferentiation. Hepatology 1999;29:688–696.

107. Kiss A, Wang NJ, et al: Analysis of transforming growth factor (TGF)-alpha/epidermal growth factor receptor, hepatocyte growth factor/c-met, TGF-beta receptor type II, and p53 expression in human hepatocellular carcinomas. Clin Cancer Res 1997;3:1059–1066.

108. Kawata S, Nagase T, et al: Modulation of the mevalonate pathway and cell growth by pravastatin and d-limonene in a human hepatoma cell line (Hep G2). Br J Cancer 1994;69:1015–1020.

109. Kaur G, Stetler-Stevenson M, et al: Growth inhibition with reversible cell cycle arrest of carcinoma cells by flavone L86-8275. J Natl Cancer Inst 1992;84:1736–1740.

110. Shah MA, Kortmansky J, et al: A Phase I/Pharmacologic Study of Weekly Sequential Irinotecan (CPT) and Flavorpiridol (F). Chicago, American Society of Clinical Oncology, 2002.

111. Schwartz JD, Lehrer D, et al: Thalidomide in Hepatocellular Cancer (HCC) with Optional Interferon-alpha upon Progression. Chicago, American Society of Clinical Oncology, 2003.

112. Itamoto T, Katayama K, Fukuda S, et al: Percutaneous microwave coagulation therapy for primary or recurrent hepatocellular carcinoma: Long-term results. Hepatogastroenterology 2001;48:1401–1405.

113. Sugimachi K, Maehara S, Tanaka S, Shimada M, Sugimachi K: Repeat hepatectomy is the most useful treatment for recurrent hepatocellular carcinoma. J Hepatobiliary Pancreat Surg 2001;8:410–416.

114. Nakajima Y, Ko S, Kanamura T, et al: Repeat liver resection for hepatocellular carcinoma. J Am Coll Surg 2001;192:339–344.

115. Kakazu T, Makuuchi M, Kawasaki S, et al: Repeat hepatic resection for recurrent hepatocellular carcinoma. Hepatogastroenterology 1993;40:337–341.

116. Zhou XD, Yu YQ, Tang ZY, et al: Surgical treatment of recurrent hepatocellular carcinoma. Hepatogastroenterology 1993;40:333–336.

117. Okuda K, Ohtsuki T, Obata H, et al: Natural history of hepatocellular carcinoma and prognosis in relation to treatment: Study of 850 patients. Cancer 1985;56:918–928.

118. Belghiti J, Di CI, Ferreira LL, Bezeaud A, Sauvanet A, Fekete F: Prognostic value of pre- and postoperative alpha-fetoprotein in the follow-up of patients with surgically-treated hepatocellular carcinoma. Minerva Chir 1993;48:25–28.

119. Read D, Shulkes A, Fernley R, Simpson R: Characterization of neurotensin (6-13) from an hepatic fibrolamellar carcinoma. Peptides 1991;12:887–892.

120. Warnes TW, Smith A: Tumour markers in diagnosis and management. Baillieres Clin Gastroenterol 1987;1:63–89.

121. Ijichi M, Takayama T, Matsumura M, Shiratori Y, Omata M, Makuuchi M: Alpha-fetoprotein mRNA in the circulation as a predictor of postsurgical recurrence of hepatocellular carcinoma: A prospective study. Hepatology 2002;35:853–860.

122. Cheung ST, Chen X, Guan XY, et al: Identify metastasis-associated genes in hepatocellular carcinoma through clonality delineation for multinodular tumor. Cancer Res 2002;62:4711–4721.

123. Liu LX, Jiang HC, Liu ZH, et al: Integrin gene expression profiles of human hepatocellular carcinoma. World J Gastroenterol 2002;8:631–637.

124. Li Y, Li Y, Tang R, et al: Discovery and analysis of hepatocellular carcinoma genes using cDNA microarrays. J Cancer Res Clin Oncol 2002;128:369–379.

125. Blum HE: Molecular targets for prevention of hepatocellular carcinoma. Dig Dis 2002;20:81–90.

126. Henson DE, Albores-Saavedra J, Corle D: Carcinoma of the gallbladder: Histologic types, stage of disease, grade, and survival rates. Cancer 1992;70:1493–1497.

127. Diehl AK: Epidemiology of gallbladder cancer: A synthesis of recent data. J Natl Cancer Inst 1980;65:1209–1214.

128. Lazcano-Ponce EC, Miquel JF, Munoz N, et al: Epidemiology and molecular pathology of gallbladder cancer. CA Cancer J Clin 2001;51:349–364.

129. Okamoto M, Okamoto H, Kitahara F, et al: Ultrasonographic evidence of association of polyps and stones with gallbladder cancer. Am J Gastroenterol 1999;94:446–450.

130. Chianale J, Valdivia G, Del Pino G, Nervi F: Gallbladder cancer mortality in Chile and its relation to cholecystectomy rates: An analysis of the last decade. Rev Med Chil 1990;118:1284–1288.

131. Piehler JM, Crichlow RW: Primary carcinoma of the gallbladder. Surg Gynecol Obstet 1978;147:929–942.

132. Nervi F, Duarte I, Gomez G, et al: Frequency of gallbladder cancer in Chile, a high-risk area. Int J Cancer 1988;41:657–660.

133. Roa I, Araya JC, Villaseca M, et al: Preoplastic lesions and gallbladder cancer: An estimate of the period required for progression. Gastroenterology 1996;111:232–236.

134. Diehl AK: Gallstone size and the risk of gallbladder cancer. JAMA 1983;250:2323–2326.

135. Nyberg U, Nilsson B, Travis LB, Holm LE, Hall P: Cancer incidence among Swedish patients exposed to radioactive Thorotrast: A forty-year follow-up survey. Radiat Res 2002;157:419–425.

136. Funabiki T, Matsubara T, Ochiai M, et al: Surgical strategy for patients with pancreaticobiliary maljunction without choledochal dilatation. Keio J Med 1997;46:169–172.

137. Wang HP, Wu MS, Lin CC, et al: Pancreaticobiliary diseases associated with anomalous pancreaticobiliary ductal union. Gastrointest Endosc 1998;48:184–189.

138. Tanaka K, Ikoma A, Hamada N, Nishida S, Kadono J, Taira A: Biliary tract cancer accompanied by anomalous junction of pancreaticobiliary ductal system in adults. Am J Surg 1998;175:218–220.

139. Zatonski WA, Lowenfels AB, Boyle P, et al: Epidemiologic aspects of gallbladder cancer: A case-control study of the SEARCH Program of the International Agency for Research on Cancer. J Natl Cancer Inst 1997;89:1132–1138.

140. Stephen AE, Berger DL: Carcinoma in the porcelain gallbladder: A relationship revisited. Surgery 2001;129:699–703.

141. Towfigh S, McFadden DW, Cortina GR, et al: Porcelain gallbladder is not associated with gallbladder carcinoma. Am Surg 2001;67:7–10.

142. Yamamoto M, Nakajo S, Tahara E: Carcinoma of the gallbladder: The correlation between histogenesis and prognosis. Virchows Arch 1989;414:83–90.

143. Bartlett DL, Fong Y, Fortner JG, Brennan MF, Blumgart LH: Long-term results after resection for gallbladder cancer: Implications for staging and management. Ann Surg 1996;224:639–646.

144. Shirai Y, Yoshida K, Tsukada K, Muto T, Watanabe H: Radical surgery for gallbladder carcinoma: Long-term results. Ann Surg 1992;216:565–568.

145. Wistuba II, Sugio K, Hung J, et al: Allele-specific mutations involved in the pathogenesis of endemic gallbladder carcinoma in Chile. Cancer Res 1995;55:2511–2515.

146. Matsubara T, Sakurai Y, Sasayama Y, et al: K-ras point mutations in cancerous and noncancerous biliary epithelium in patients with pancreaticobiliary maljunction. Cancer 1996;77:1752–1757.

147. Wistuba II, Albores-Saavedra J: Genetic abnormalities involved in the pathogenesis of gallbladder carcinoma. J Hepatobiliary Pancreat Surg 1999;6:237–244.

148. Fong Y, Brennan MF, Turnbull A, Colt DG, Blumgart LH: Gallbladder cancer discovered during laparoscopic surgery: Potential for iatrogenic tumor dissemination (see comments). Arch Surg 1993;128:1054–1056.

149. Hirooka Y, Naitoh Y, Goto H, et al: Contrast-enhanced endoscopic ultrasonography in gallbladder diseases. Gastrointest Endosc 1998;48:406–410.

150. Sugiyama M, Xie XY, Atomi Y, Saito M: Differential diagnosis of small polypoid lesions of the gallbladder: The value of endoscopic ultrasonography. Ann Surg 1999;229:498–504.

151. Mizuguchi M, Kudo S, Fukahori T, et al: Endoscopic ultrasonography for demonstrating loss of multiple-layer pattern of the thickened gallbladder wall in the preoperative diagnosis of gallbladder cancer. Eur Radiol 1997;7:1323–1327.

152. Shinkai H, Kimura W, Muto T: Surgical indications for small polypoid lesions of the gallbladder. Am J Surg 1998;175:114–117.

153. Ohtani T, Shirai Y, Tsukada K, Muto T, Hatakeyama K: Spread of gallbladder carcinoma: CT evaluation with pathologic correlation. Abdom Imaging 1996;21:195–201.

154. Soto JA, Barish MA, Yucel EK, Siegenberg D, Ferrucci JT, Chuttani R: Magnetic resonance cholangiography: Comparison with endoscopic retrograde cholangiopancreatography (see comments). Gastroenterology 1996;110:589-597.
155. Demachi H, Matsui O, Hoshiba K, et al: Dynamic MRI using a surface coil in chronic cholecystitis and gallbladder carcinoma: Radiologic and histopathologic correlation. J Comput Assist Tomogr 1997;21:643-651.
156. Schwartz LH, Coakley FV, Sun Y, Blumgart LH, Fong Y, Panicek DM: Neoplastic pancreaticobiliary duct obstruction: Evaluation with breath-hold MR cholangiopancreatography. Am J Roentgenol 1998;170:1491-1495.
157. Cotran RS, Kumar V, Robbins S: Robbins Pathologic Basis of Disease. Philadelphia, WB Saunders, 1989.
158. Fong Y, Jarnagin W, Blumgart LH: Gallbladder cancer: Comparison of patients presenting initially for definitive operation with those presenting after prior noncurative intervention. Ann Surg 2000; 232:557-569.
159. Weber SM, DeMatteo RP, Fong Y, Blumgart LH, Jarnagin WR: Staging laparoscopy in patients with extrahepatic biliary carcinoma: Analysis of 100 patients. Ann Surg 2002;235:392-399.
160. Nakamura S, Sakaguchi S, Suzuki S, Muro H: Aggressive surgery for carcinoma of the gallbladder. Surgery 1989;106:467-473.
161. Wanebo HJ, Castle WN, Fechner RE: Is carcinoma of the gallbladder a curable lesion? Ann Surg 1982;195:624-631.
162. Wanebo HJ, Vezeridis MP: Carcinoma of the gallbladder. J Surg Oncol Suppl 1993;3:134-139.
163. Weiland ST, Mahvi DM, Niederhuber JE, Heisey DM, Chicks DS, Rikkers LF: Should suspected early gallbladder cancer be treated laparoscopically? J Gastrointest Surg 2002;6:50-56.
164. Barbot DJ, Marks JH, Feld RI, Liu JB, Rosato FE: Improved staging of liver tumors using laparoscopic intraoperative ultrasound. J Surg Oncol 1997;64:63-67.
165. Bhargava DK, Sarin S, Verma K, Kapur BM: Laparoscopy in carcinoma of the gallbladder. Gastrointest Endosc 1983;29:21-22.
166. Dagnini G, Marin G, Patella M, Zotti S: Laparoscopy in the diagnosis of primary carcinoma of the gallbladder: A study of 98 cases. Gastrointest Endosc 1984;30:289-291.
167. Ouchi K, Owada Y, Matsuno S, Sato T: Prognostic factors in the surgical treatment of gallbladder carcinoma. Surgery 1987;101: 731-737.
168. Donohue JH, Nagorney DM, Grant CS, Tsushima K, Ilstrup DM, Adson MA: Carcinoma of the gallbladder: Does radical resection improve outcome? Arch Surg 1990;125:237-241.
169. Ogura Y, Mizumoto R, Isaji S, Kusuda T, Matsuda S, Tabata M: Radical operations for carcinoma of the gallbladder: Present status in Japan. World J Surg 1991;15:337-343.
170. Shirai Y, Yoshida K, Tsukada K, Muto T: Inapparent carcinoma of the gallbladder: An appraisal of a radical second operation after simple cholecystectomy. Ann Surg 1992;215:326-331.
171. Yamaguchi K, Chijiiwa K, Saiki S, Shimizu S, Tsuneyoshi M, Tanaka M: Reliability of frozen section diagnosis of gallbladder tumor for detecting carcinoma and depth of its invasion. J Surg Oncol 1997;65:132-136.
172. Yamaguchi K, Tsuneyoshi M: Subclinical gallbladder carcinoma. Am J Surg 1992;163:382-386.
173. Chijiiwa K, Tanaka M: Carcinoma of the gallbladder: An appraisal of surgical resection. Surgery 1994;115:751-756.
174. Fong Y, Brennan MF, Turnbull A, Colt DG, Blumgart LH: Gallbladder cancer discovered during laparoscopic surgery: Potential for iatrogenic tumor dissemination (see comments). Arch Surg 1993;128:1054-1056.
175. Drouard F, Delamarre J, Capron JP: Cutaneous seeding of gallbladder cancer after laparoscopic cholecystectomy. N Engl J Med 1991;325:1316.
176. Pezet D, Fondrinier E, Rotman N, et al: Parietal seeding of carcinoma of the gallbladder after laparoscopic cholecystectomy (see comments). Br J Surg 1992;79:230.
177. Takada T, Amano H, et al: Is postoperative adjuvant chemotherapy useful for gallbladder carcinoma? A phase III multicenter prospective randomized controlled trial in patients with resected pancreaticobiliary carcinoma. Cancer 2002;95:1685-1695.
178. Hanazaki K: Systemic chemotherapy following non-curative resection may increase survival for people with gall bladder carcinoma, but not carcinomas of the pancreas, bile duct or ampulla of Vater. Cancer Treat Rev 2003;29:135-137.
179. Kresl JJ, Schild SE, et al: Adjuvant external beam radiation therapy with concurrent chemotherapy in the management of gallbladder carcinoma. Int J Radiat Oncol Biol Phys 2002;52:167-175.
180. Falkson G, MacIntyre JM, et al: Eastern Cooperative Oncology Group experience with chemotherapy for inoperable gallbladder and bile duct cancer. Cancer 1984;54:965-969.
181. Yee K, Sheppard BC, et al: Cancers of the gallbladder and biliary ducts. Oncology (Huntingt) 2002;16:939-946, 949; discussion 949-950, 952-953, 956-957.
182. Lozano RD, Patt YZ, et al: Oral Capecitabine (Xeloda) for the Treatment of Hepatobiliary Cancers (Hepatocellular Carcinoma, Cholangiocarcinoma, and Gallbladder Cancer). Chicago, American Society of Clinical Oncology, 2000.
183. Rothenberg ML, Moore MJ, et al: A phase II trial of gemcitabine in patients with 5-FU-refractory pancreas cancer. Ann Oncol 1996;7:347-353.
184. Burris HA III, Moore MJ, et al: Improvements in survival and clinical benefit with gemcitabine as first-line therapy for patients with advanced pancreas cancer: A randomized trial. J Clin Oncol 1997;15:2403-2413.
185. Raderer M, Hejna MH, et al: Two consecutive phase II studies of 5-fluorouracil/leucovorin/mitomycin-C and of gemcitabine in patients with advanced biliary cancer. Oncology 1999;56: 177-180.
186. Gallardo J, Fodor M, et al: Efficacy of gemcitabine in the treatment of patients with gallbladder carcinoma: A case report. Cancer 1998;83:2419-2421.
187. Gallardo JO, Rubio B, et al: A phase II study of gemcitabine in gallbladder carcinoma. Ann Oncol 2001;12:1403-1406.
188. Teufel A, Lehnert T, et al: Chemotherapy with gemcitabine in patients with advanced gallbladder carcinoma. Z Gastroenterol 2000;38:909-912.
189. Malik IA, Aziz Z, et al: Gemcitabine and cisplatin is a highly effective combination chemotherapy in patients with advanced cancer of the gallbladder. Am J Clin Oncol 2003;26:174-177.
190. Doval DC, Sekhon JS, et al: Chemotherapy in biliary tract carcinomas: Results in India. Semin Oncol 2002;29(6 suppl 20):46-50.
191. Carraro S, Servienti PJ, et al: Gemcitabine and Cisplatin in Locally Advanced or Metastatic Gallbladder and Bile Duct Adenocarcinoma. Chicago, American Society of Clinical Oncology, 2001.
192. Kuhn R, Hribaschek A, et al: Outpatient therapy with gemcitabine and docetaxel for gallbladder, biliary, and cholangio-carcinomas. Invest New Drugs 2002;20:351-356.
193. Jones DV Jr, Lozano R, et al: Phase II study of paclitaxel therapy for unresectable biliary tree carcinomas. J Clin Oncol 1996;14: 2306-2310.
194. Fishkin P, Alberts S, et al: Irinotecan (CPT-11) in Patients (Pts) with Advanced Gallbladder (GB) Carcinoma (CA): A North Central Cancer Treatment Group (NCCTG) phase II study. Chicago, American Society of Clinical Oncology, 2001.
195. Alberts SR, Fishkin PA, et al: CPT-11 for bile-duct and gallbladder carcinoma: A phase II North Central Cancer Treatment Group (NCCTG) study. Int J Gastrointest Cancer 2002;32:107-114.
196. Sanz-Altamira PM, O'Reilly E, et al: A phase II trial of irinotecan (CPT-11) for unresectable biliary tree carcinoma. Ann Oncol 2001;12(4):501-504.
197. Moskal TL, Zhang PJ, et al: Small cell carcinoma of the gallbladder. J Surg Oncol 1999;70:54-59.
198. Maitra A, Tascilar M, et al: Small cell carcinoma of the gallbladder: A clinicopathologic, immunohistochemical, and molecular pathology study of 12 cases. Am J Surg Pathol 2001;25:595-601.
199. Fujii H, Aotake T, et al: Small cell carcinoma of the gallbladder: A case report and review of 53 cases in the literature. Hepatogastroenterology 2001;48:1588-1593.
200. Hejna M, Zielinski CC: Nonsurgical management of gallbladder cancer: Cytotoxic treatment and radiotherapy. Expert Rev Anticancer Ther 2001;1:291-300.
201. Misra S, Chaturvedi A, et al: Carcinoma of the gallbladder. Lancet Oncol 2003;4:167-176.

202. Valerdiz-Casasola S: Expression of epidermal growth factor receptor in gallbladder cancer. Hum Pathol 1994;25:964–965.

203. Lee CS, Pirdas A: Epidermal growth factor receptor immuno-reactivity in gallbladder and extrahepatic biliary tract tumours. Pathol Res Pract 1995;191:1087–1091.

204. Yukawa M, Fujimori T, et al: Expression of oncogene products and growth factors in early gallbladder cancer, advanced gallbladder cancer, and chronic cholecystitis. Hum Pathol 1993;24:37–40.

205. Zhou YM, Li YM, et al: Significance of expression of epidermal growth factor (EGF) and its receptor (EGFr) in chronic cholecystitis and gallbladder carcinoma. Ai Zheng 2003;22:262–265.

206. Kim YW, Huh SH, et al: Expression of the c-erb-B2 and p53 protein in gallbladder carcinomas. Oncol Rep 2001;8:1127–1132.

207. Boudny V, Murakami Y, et al: Expression of activated c-erbB-2 oncogene induces sensitivity to cisplatin in human gallbladder adenocarcinoma cells. Anticancer Res 1999;19:5203–5206.

208. Su WC, Shiesh SC, et al: Expression of oncogene products HER2/Neu and Ras and fibrosis-related growth factors bFGF, TGF-beta, and PDGF in bile from biliary malignancies and inflammatory disorders. Dig Dis Sci 2001;46:1387–1392.

209. Ghosh M, Kawamoto T, et al: Cyclooxygenase expression in the gallbladder. Int J Mol Med 2000;6:527–532.

210. Grossman EM, Longo WE, et al: The role of cyclooxygenase enzymes in the growth of human gall bladder cancer cells. Carcinogenesis 2000;21:1403–1409.

211. Kiguchi K, Carbajal S, et al: Constitutive expression of ErbB-2 in gallbladder epithelium results in development of adenocarcinoma. Cancer Res 2001;61:6971–6976.

212. Asano T, Shoda J, et al: Expressions of cyclooxygenase-2 and prostaglandin E-receptors in carcinoma of the gallbladder: Crucial role of arachidonate metabolism in tumor growth and progression. Clin Cancer Res 2002;8:1157–1167.

213. Kim HJ, Kim MH, Myung SJ, et al: A new strategy for the application of CA19-9 in the differentiation of pancreaticobiliary cancer: Analysis using a receiver operating characteristic curve. Am J Gastroenterol 1999;94:1941–1946.

214. Pitt HA, Dooley WC, Yeo CJ, Cameron JL: Malignancies of the biliary tree. Curr Probl Surg 1995;32:1–90.

215. Patel T: Increasing incidence and mortality of primary intrahepatic cholangiocarcinoma in the United States. Hepatology 2001;33:1353–1357.

216. Longmire WP Jr: Tumors of the extrahepatic biliary radicles. Curr Probl Cancer 1976;1:1–45.

217. Henson DE, Albores-Saavedra J, Corle D: Carcinoma of the extrahepatic bile ducts: Histologic types, stage of disease, grade, and survival rates. Cancer 1992;70:1498–1501.

218. de Groen PC, Gores GJ, LaRusso NF, Gunderson LL, Nagorney DM: Biliary tract cancers. N Engl J Med 1999;341:1368–1378.

219. Kaya M, de Groen PC, Angulo P, et al: Treatment of cholangiocarcinoma complicating primary sclerosing cholangitis: The Mayo Clinic experience. Am J Gastroenterol 2001;96:1164–1169.

220. Hakamada K, Sasaki M, Endoh M, Itoh T, Morita T, Konn M: Late development of bile duct cancer after sphincteroplasty: A ten- to twenty-two-year follow-up study. Surgery 1997;121:488–492.

221. Bhuiya MR, Nimura Y, Kamiya J, et al: Clinicopathologic studies on perineural invasion of bile duct carcinoma. Ann Surg 1992;215:344–349.

222. Yamamoto M, Takasaki K, Yoshikawa T: Lymph node metastasis in intrahepatic cholangiocarcinoma. Jpn J Clin Oncol 1999;29:147–150.

223. El Rassi ZE, Partensky C, Scoazec JY, Henry L, Lombard-Bohas C, Maddern G: Peripheral cholangiocarcinoma: Presentation, diagnosis, pathology and management. Eur J Surg Oncol 1999;25:375–380.

224. Weber SM, Jarnagin WR, Klimstra D, DeMatteo RP, Fong YM, Blumgart LH: Intrahepatic cholangiocarcinoma: Resectability, recurrence pattern, and outcomes. J Am Coll Surg 2001;193:384–391.

225. Valverde A, Bonhomme N, Farges O, Sauvanet A, Flejou JF, Belghiti J: Resection of intrahepatic cholangiocarcinoma: A Western experience. J Hepatobiliary Pancreat Surg 1999;6:122–127.

226. Soto JA, Barish MA, Yucel EK, Siegenberg D, Ferrucci JT, Chuttani R: Magnetic resonance cholangiography: Comparison with endoscopic retrograde cholangiopancreatography (see comments). Gastroenterology 1996;110:589–597.

227. Demachi H, Matsui O, Hoshiba K, et al: Dynamic MRI using a surface coil in chronic cholecystitis and gallbladder carcinoma: Radiologic and histopathologic correlation. J Comput Assist Tomogr 1997;21:643–651.

228. Schwartz LH, Coakley FV, Sun Y, Blumgart LH, Fong Y, Panicek DM: Neoplastic pancreaticobiliary duct obstruction: Evaluation with breath-hold MR cholangiopancreatography. Am J Roentgenol 1998;170:1491–1495.

229. Cameron JL, Pitt HA, Zinner MJ, Kaufman SL, Coleman J: Management of proximal cholangiocarcinomas by surgical resection and radiotherapy. Am J Surg 1990;159:91–97.

230. Nakayama T, Ikeda A, Okuda K: Percutaneous transhepatic drainage of the biliary tract: Technique and results in 104 cases. Gastroenterology 1978;74:554–559.

231. Hochwald SN, Burke EC, Jarnagin WR, Fong Y, Blumgart LH: Association of preoperative biliary stenting with increased postoperative infectious complications in proximal cholangiocarcinoma. Arch Surg 1999;134:261–266.

232. McPherson GA, Benjamin IS, Hodgson HJ, Bowley NB, Allison DJ, Blumgart LH: Pre-operative percutaneous transhepatic biliary drainage: The results of a controlled trial. Br J Surg 1984;71:371–375.

233. Pitt HA, Gomes AS, Lois JF, Mann LL, Deutsch LS, Longmire WP Jr: Does preoperative percutaneous biliary drainage reduce operative risk or increase hospital cost? Ann Surg 1985;201:545–553.

234. Bismuth H, Nakache R, Diamond T: Management strategies in resection for hilar cholangiocarcinoma. Ann Surg 1992;215:31–38.

235. Burke EC, Jarnagin WR, Hochwald SN, Pisters PW, Fong Y, Blumgart LH: Hilar cholangiocarcinoma: Patterns of spread, the importance of hepatic resection for curative operation, and a presurgical clinical staging system. Ann Surg 1998;228:385–394.

236. Jarnagin WR, Fong Y, DeMatteo RP, et al: Staging, resectability, and outcome in 225 patients with hilar cholangiocarcinoma. Ann Surg 2001;234:507–517.

237. Nakeeb A, Pitt HA, Sohn TA, et al: Cholangiocarcinoma: A spectrum of intrahepatic, perihilar, and distal tumors. Ann Surg 1996;224:463–473.

238. Ottow RT, August DA, Sugarbaker PH: Treatment of proximal biliary tract carcinoma: An overview of techniques and results. Surgery 1985;97:251–262.

239. Altaee MY, Johnson PJ, Farrant JM, Williams R: Etiologic and clinical characteristics of peripheral and hilar cholangiocarcinoma. Cancer 1991;68:2051–2055.

240. Hadjis NS, Blenkharn JI, Alexander N, Benjamin IS, Blumgart LH: Outcome of radical surgery in hilar cholangiocarcinoma. Surgery 1990;107:597–604.

241. Iwasaki Y, Okamura T, Ozaki A, et al: Surgical treatment for carcinoma at the confluence of the major hepatic ducts. Surg Gynecol Obstet 1986;162:457–464.

242. Iida S, Tsuzuki T, Ogata Y, Yoneyama K, Iri H, Watanabe K: The long-term survival of patients with carcinoma of the main hepatic duct junction. Cancer 1987;60:1612–1619.

243. McMasters KM, Tuttle TM, Leach SD, et al: Neoadjuvant chemoradiation for extrahepatic cholangiocarcinoma. Am J Surg 1997;174:605–608.

244. Kosuge T, Yamamoto J, Shimada K, Yamasaki S, Makuuchi M: Improved surgical results for hilar cholangiocarcinoma with procedures including major hepatic resection. Ann Surg 1999;230:663–671.

245. Blumgart LH, Hadjis NS, Benjamin IS, Beazley R: Surgical approaches to cholangiocarcinoma at confluence of hepatic ducts. Lancet 1984;1:66–70.

246. Nagorney DM, Donohue JH, Farnell MB, Schleck CD, Ilstrup DM: Outcomes after curative resections of cholangiocarcinoma. Arch Surg 1993;128:871–877.

247. Reding R, Buard JL, Lebeau G, Launois B: Surgical management of 552 carcinomas of the extrahepatic bile ducts (gallbladder and periampullary tumors excluded): Results of the French Surgical Association Survey. Ann Surg 1991;213:236–241.

248. Klempnauer J, Ridder GJ, von Wasielewski R, Werner M, Weimann A, Pichlmayr R: Resectional surgery of hilar cholangiocarcinoma: A multivariate analysis of prognostic factors. J Clin Oncol 1997;15: 947–954.

249. Lieser MJ, Barry MK, Rowland C, Ilstrup DM, Nagorney DM: Surgical management of intrahepatic cholangiocarcinoma: A 31-year experience. J Hepatobiliary Pancreat Surg 1998;5: 41–47.

250. Berdah SV, Delpero JR, Garcia S, Hardwigsen J, Le Treut YP: A western surgical experience of peripheral cholangiocarcinoma. Br J Surg 1996;83:1517–1521.

251. Baer HU, Stain SC, Dennison AR, Eggers B, Blumgart LH: Improvements in survival by aggressive resections of hilar cholangiocarcinoma. Ann Surg 1993;217:20–27.

252. Bengmark S, Ekberg H, Evander A, Klofver-Stahl B, Tranberg KG: Major liver resection for hilar cholangiocarcinoma. Ann Surg 1988;207:120–125.

253. Jarnagin WR, Burke E, Powers C, Fong Y, Blumgart LH: Intrahepatic biliary enteric bypass provides effective palliation in selected patients with malignant obstruction at the hepatic duct confluence. Am J Surg 1998;175:453–460.

254. Glattli A, Stain SC, Baer HU, Schweizer W, Triller J, Blumgart LH: Unresectable malignant biliary obstruction: Treatment by self-expandable biliary endoprostheses. HPB Surg 1993;6: 175–184.

255. Kuvshinoff BW Armstrong JG, Fong Y, et al: Palliation of irresectable hilar cholangiocarcinoma with biliary drainage and radiotherapy. Br J Surg 1995;82:1522–1525.

256. Lee BH, Choe DH, Lee JH, Kim KH, Chin SY: Metallic stents in malignant biliary obstruction: Prospective long-term clinical results. Am J Roentgenol 1997;168:741–745.

257. Rumalla A, Baron TH, Wang KK, Gores GJ, Stadheim LM, de Groen PC: Endoscopic application of photodynamic therapy for cholangiocarcinoma. Gastrointest Endosc 2001;53:500–504.

258. Stemmler J, Heinemann V, et al: Capecitabine as second-line treatment for metastatic cholangiocarcinoma: A report of two cases. Onkologie 2002;25:182–184.

259. Pazdur R, Royce ME, et al: Phase II trial of docetaxel for cholangiocarcinoma. Am J Clin Oncol 1999;22:78–81.

260. Patt YZ, Hassan MM, et al: Phase II trial of cisplatin, interferon alpha-2b, doxorubicin, and 5-fluorouracil for biliary tract cancer. Clin Cancer Res 2001;7:3375–3380.

261. Sanz-Altamira PM, Ferrante K, et al: A phase II trial of 5-fluorouracil, leucovorin, and carboplatin in patients with unresectable biliary tree carcinoma. Cancer 1998;82: 2321–2325.

262. Taieb J, Mitry E, et al: Optimization of 5-fluorouracil (5-FU)/ cisplatin combination chemotherapy with a new schedule of leucovorin, 5-FU and cisplatin (LV5FU2-P regimen) in patients with biliary tract carcinoma. Ann Oncol 2002;13:1192–1196.

263. Cantore M, Rabbi C, et al: Intra-arterial hepatic chemotherapy combined with continuous infusion of 5-fluorouracil in patients with metastatic cholangiocarcinoma. Ann Oncol 2002;13:1687–1688.

264. Tanaka N, Yamakado K, et al: Arterial chemoinfusion therapy through an implanted port system for patients with unresectable intrahepatic cholangiocarcinoma: Initial experience. Eur J Radiol 2002;41:42–48.

265. Crane CH, Macdonald KO, et al: Limitations of conventional doses of chemoradiation for unresectable biliary cancer. Int J Radiat Oncol Biol Phys 2002;53:969–974.

266. Macdonald KO, Crane CH: Palliative and postoperative radiotherapy in biliary tract cancer. Surg Oncol Clin North Am 2002;11:941–954.

267. Ito Y, Takeda T, et al: Expression and clinical significance of the erbB family in intrahepatic cholangiocellular carcinoma. Pathol Res Pract 2001;197:95–100.

268. Yoon JH, Higuchi H, et al: Bile acids induce cyclooxygenase-2 expression via the epidermal growth factor receptor in a human cholangiocarcinoma cell line. Gastroenterology 2002;122:985–993.

269. Cheifetz RE, Davis NL, et al: An animal model of benign bile-duct stricture, sclerosing cholangitis and cholangiocarcinoma and the role of epidermal growth factor receptor in ductal proliferation. Can J Surg 1996;39:193–197.

270. Pickens A, Pan G, et al: Fas expression prevents cholangiocarcinoma tumor growth. J Gastrointest Surg 1999;3:374–381, discussion 382.

271. Ahn EY, Pan G, et al: IFN-gamma upregulates apoptosis-related molecules and enhances Fas-mediated apoptosis in human cholangiocarcinoma. Int J Cancer 2002;100:445–451.

272. Que FG, Phan VA, et al: Cholangiocarcinomas express Fas ligand and disable the Fas receptor. Hepatology 1999;30:1398–1404.

273. Shimonishi T, Isse K, et al: Up-regulation of Fas ligand at early stages and down-regulation of Fas at progressed stages of intrahepatic cholangiocarcinoma reflect evasion from immune surveillance. Hepatology 2000;32:761–769.

274. Tan CK, Podila PV, et al: Human cholangiocarcinomas express somatostatin receptors and respond to somatostatin with growth inhibition. Gastroenterology 1995;108:1908–1916.

275. Zhao B, Zhao H, et al: Cholangiocarcinoma cells express somatostatin receptor subtype 2 and respond to octreotide treatment. J Hepatobiliary Pancreat Surg 2002;9:497–502.

276. Nimura Y, Kamiya J, Kondo S, et al: Aggressive preoperative management and extended surgery for hilar cholangiocarcinoma: Nagoya experience. J Hepatobiliary Pancreat Surg 2000;7: 155–162.

277. Kaczynski J, Hansson G, Wallerstedt S: Incidence, etiologic aspects and clinicopathologic features in intrahepatic cholangiocellular carcinoma: A study of 51 cases from a low-endemicity area. Acta Oncol 1998;37:77–83.

278. Polydorou AA, Cairns SR, Dowsett JF, et al: Palliation of proximal malignant biliary obstruction by endoscopic endoprosthesis insertion. Gut 1991;32:685–689.

279. Shiina T, Mikuriya S, Uno T, et al: Radiotherapy of cholangiocarcinoma: The roles for primary and adjuvant therapies. Cancer Chemother Pharmacol 1992;31(suppl):S115–118.

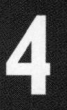
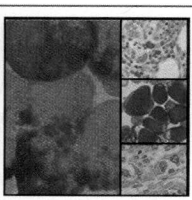

CARCINOMA OF THE PANCREAS

Jeffrey A. Drebin

SUMMARY OF KEY POINTS

INCIDENCE
- There were approximately 30,000 new pancreatic cancer cases in the United States in 2003.
- There were approximately 29,000 deaths from pancreatic cancer in the United States in 2003.
- Pancreatic cancer is the fourth leading cause of cancer deaths for both men and women.

PATHOLOGY
- Adenocarcinomas make up 90% of pancreatic cancer.
- Less than 5% are endocrine tumors.
- Less than 5% are cystic tumors.

CLINICAL PRESENTATION
- Two thirds of pancreatic tumors are located in the head of the pancreas; presentation includes vague pain, weight loss, and jaundice.
- One third of pancreatic tumors are in the body or tail; presentation includes epigastric and/or back pain, weight loss, and evidence of metastatic disease.

STAGING EVALUATION
- Triple phase helical CT scan is performed on all patients.
- Cholangiography is used for severe jaundice if the patient is not scheduled for immediate surgical exploration or as the result of equivocal findings on the CT scan.
- Endoscopic ultrasound with biopsy is used for atypical lesions.
- Fine needle aspiration biopsy is performed prior to palliative treatment if the lesion is unresectable.
- MRI, angiography, and PET scans are used in selected cases.
- There is no need for preoperative tissue diagnosis for resectable lesions.
- Laparoscopic staging may decrease the necessity of laparotomy for unresectable lesions.

THERAPY
- Surgical resection of the tumor (10%–15% of all tumors are resectable; 70%–80% of tumors staged preoperatively as resectable are resected) is performed.
- Adjuvant chemoradiation is given.

PALLIATION
- Endoscopic or percutaneous transhepatic biliary stents are used.
- Operative gastric and/or biliary bypass in performed on selected patients.
- Alcohol celiac plexus block is used.
- Chemoradiation is used for locally advanced unresectable lesions.
- Chemotherapy is used for metastatic disease.

SURVIVAL
- "Curative" surgical resection gives a median survival of 18 months and a 5-year survival of approximately 20%. New adjuvant approaches may substantially improve these results.
- Survival of patients with unresectable lesions is 4–8 months, with less than 20% surviving for 1 year.

INTRODUCTION

Pancreatic adenocarcinoma is one of the most lethal malignancies, with an overall 5-year disease-free survival rate on the order of 1% to 2%. Most pancreatic cancers are not diagnosed until locally advanced or regionally disseminated disease has developed that is not amenable to curative surgical resection. Chemotherapy and radiation therapy have only modest benefit in this disease, and typical survival is on the order of 6 months. Among those patients with apparently resectable disease who undergo surgical exploration, between 20% and 40% percent are found to be unresectable. Even those pancreatic cancer patients who have a margin-negative resection have a 5-year disease-free survival of less than 30%, and in approximately half of patients surviving 5 years, the cancer will relapse between years 6 and 10. Thus the treatment of pancreatic cancer remains a challenge to the surgical, radiation, and medical oncologist.

In recent years, a number of positive developments have occurred in the management of pancreatic cancer. Improvements in the preoperative staging of pancreatic cancer have reduced the number of patients undergoing laparotomy for what proves to be unresectable disease. Advances in surgical technique and perioperative management allow pancreatic cancer resections to be performed with very low mortality and tolerable morbidity. Patients after resection, even when not cured, appear to have a substantially longer survival than do patients managed with other modalities, and thus at a minimum receive substantial palliation and extension of survival. Furthermore, evolving approaches to adjuvant chemoradiation therapy may substantially improve long-term survival after an attempted curative resection.

For patients who are first seen with unresectable disease, an appropriate focus has been placed on optimizing quality of life. Nonoperative methods of relieving obstructive jaundice avoid the need for laparotomy in most patients. Appreciation of the importance of palliating pain is of great benefit to those patients who are not potentially curable. Furthermore, new approaches to chemotherapy offer the hope of extending both quality and quantity of life in many patients. This chapter reviews current approaches to the management of patients with pancreatic cancer.

INCIDENCE

Pancreatic carcinoma is a relatively uncommon malignancy. Approximately 28,000 new cases are diagnosed annually in the United States, comprising 2% of all cancer diagnoses. However, because the annual death rate from pancreatic cancer approximates its incidence, pancreatic cancer is a fairly common cause of cancer mortality in the United States. Carcinoma of the pancreas ranks fifth behind carcinomas of the lung, colorectum, breast, and prostate as a cause of cancer deaths.[1-3] Because of the relative rarity of breast cancer in men and the nonexistence of prostate cancer in women, pancreatic cancer is the fourth most common cause of cancer death in both men and in women, accounting for approximately 6% of cancer deaths overall.

The incidence of pancreatic carcinoma has increased three- to fourfold in the 20th century, but appears to have leveled off in recent decades. This most likely reflects both improvements in the accuracy of diagnostic techniques such as computed tomography (CT) scanning and a genuine increase in incidence. The risk of developing pancreatic cancer increases with age;[1,4] it has been estimated that this risk increases two- to threefold for each decade of life after age 40 years. Whereas patients typically are first seen in their 60s and 70s, patients in their 40s and 50s are not uncommon; pancreatic cancer is rarely seen in patients younger than 30 years.

EPIDEMIOLOGY

Adenocarcinoma of the pancreas has traditionally been viewed as occurring more commonly in men than in women (relative risk, 1.5:1), although recent data suggest that relative risk in women is approaching that seen in men,[1,3] perhaps because of increased tobacco use by women in the latter half of the 20th century. In the United States, pancreatic cancer occurs more frequently in blacks than in whites (relative risk, 2:1) and may be somewhat less common in Asians than in whites (relative risk, 0.7:1). Worldwide incidence rates are highest in industrialized countries and lowest in African and Asian countries,[1,5] suggesting that environmental factors linked to a "Western lifestyle" substantially increase the risk of pancreatic cancer. The high incidence rates observed in African-Americans as opposed to the low rates observed in African countries also argue strongly for the role of environmental

TABLE 84-1

Risk Factors for Pancreatic Cancer

PROVEN RISK FACTORS	RELATIVE INCREASE IN RISK
Cigarette smoking	2- to 3-fold
Industrial chemical exposure	3- to 5-fold
Chronic pancreatitis	2- to 10-fold
Diabetes mellitus	2- to 3-fold
Obesity	2- to 3-fold
Unproven or Disproven Risk Factors	
Coffee consumption	
Alcohol consumption	

as opposed to hereditary factors in the etiology of most pancreatic cancers.

Environmental Risk Factors

Studies of environmental factors linked to the development of pancreatic carcinoma have identified a number of agents that may play a role in pancreatic carcinogenesis, as summarized in Table 84-1.[1,6-25] Cigarette smoking significantly increases the risk of this form of cancer, as it does for a variety of other tumors. Certain industrial solvents, particularly those used in metal refining, have been linked to the development of pancreatic cancer. Dietary factors also play a role. Dietary fat intake and obesity clearly increase the risk of developing pancreatic cancer, whereas vitamin C intake and consumption of fruits and vegetables may decrease the risk of pancreatic cancer. Although alcohol consumption does not appear to be a risk factor for the development of pancreatic cancer, chronic pancreatitis almost certainly is.[8] Consumption of coffee and other caffeinated beverages, which had been suggested to be a risk factor based on early studies, appears to be unrelated to the development of pancreatic cancer.

Perhaps the most controversial risk factor is diabetes. About 15% of patients with pancreatic cancer become diabetic in the 6 months preceding the diagnosis of their cancer. This most likely reflects local alterations in pancreatic function resulting from an occult tumor rather than rapid development of cancer after the onset of diabetes. However, when patients in whom diabetes develops within 2 years of their diagnosis of pancreatic cancer are excluded, an approximately twofold increased risk is found for the development of pancreatic cancer among patients with long-standing diabetes.[9]

PATHOLOGY AND TUMOR BIOLOGY

If one excludes stromal tissue, nerves, and lymphatics, three principal cell types are seen in the pancreas: ductal cells, acinar cells, and endocrine cells (Fig. 84-1). Adenocarcinomas with a duct cell morphology compose the vast majority (>90%) of pancreatic neoplasms. Although ductal adenocarcinoma of the pancreas is the most

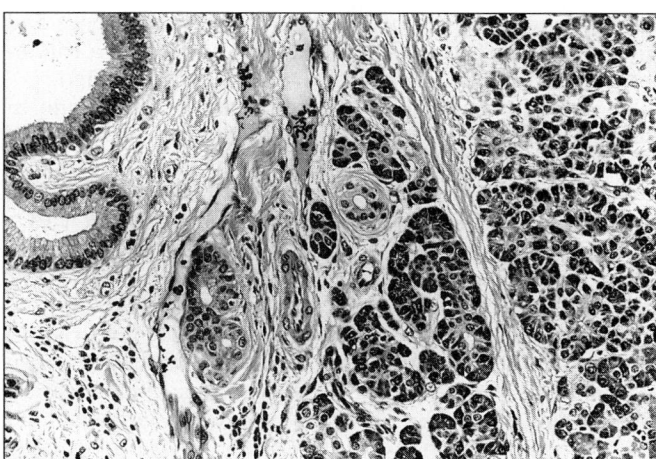

Figure 84-1. Section of normal pancreas showing exocrine glands on the right and a portion of the wall of the large duct on the left. Note the regularity of the ductal lining epithelium. (H&E, × 200)

common pancreatic tumor, a variety of other benign and malignant pancreatic tumors have been described, as shown in Table 84-2. Most other malignant pancreatic lesions, such as acinar cell carcinomas and cystadenocarcinomas, appear to be less biologically aggressive than pancreatic adenocarcinomas and have a somewhat better prognosis. In contrast, adenosquamous cancers of the pancreas are particularly lethal, with few 1-year survivors and essentially no 5-year survivors.[26]

Pancreatic malignancies arise in the head of the pancreas approximately 75% of the time, with the remainder of lesions being distributed evenly in the body and tail of the gland.

It is important to note that nonpancreatic tumors of the distal bile duct, duodenum, and ampulla of Vater, although much less common than pancreatic adenocarcinoma, comprise almost one third of resectable tumors in the

TABLE 84-2

Histologic Classification of Pancreatic Tumors

Benign Tumors

Serous cystadenoma
Mature cystic teratoma

Tumors of Indeterminate Malignancy

Mucinous tumors of the pancreas
Intraductal tumors
Solid and papillary tumors
Neuroendocrine tumors

Malignant Tumors of Pancreatic Origin

Ductal adenocarcinoma
Acinar cell carcinoma
Adenosquamous carcinoma
Anaplastic carcinoma
Cystadenocarcinoma
Pancreaticoblastoma
Small cell carcinoma

TABLE 84-3

Staging for Pancreatic Cancer

Primary Tumor (T)

TX	Primary tumor cannot be assessed
T0	No evidence of primary tumor
TI	Tumor <2 cm
T2	Tumor >2 cm, confined to the pancreas
T3	Tumor extends locally beyond the pancreas
T4	Tumor involves celiac or superior mesenteric arteries

Lymph Nodes (N)

NX	Regional lymph nodes cannot be assessed
N0	No regional lymph node metastasis
NI	Regional lymph node metastasis

Distant Metastases (M)

MX	Presence of distant metastasis cannot be assessed
M0	No distant metastasis
MI	Distant metastasis

Stage Grouping

IA	TI, N0, M0
IB	T2, N0, M0
IIA	T3, N0, M0
IIB	TI–3, NI, M0
III	T4, N0–I, M0
IV	TI–4, N0–I, MI

region of the pancreatic head. Furthermore, these tumors tend to be biologically less aggressive than pancreatic carcinomas, with 5-year disease-free survival after resection ranging from 30% to 50%.[27-29] It can be difficult, if not impossible, to distinguish these tumor types from routine adenocarcinoma of the pancreas based on endoscopic, radiologic, or needle cytology criteria. Only histologic sectioning of a resected tumor mass can accurately classify the specific tumor type in some circumstances.

Pancreatic adenocarcinomas tend to be aggressive tumors that disseminate early and tend to follow similar patterns of metastatic spread in most patients. Local invasion into adjacent structures is frequently seen, with encasement of the superior mesenteric/portal vein and the superior mesenteric artery representing a common event that may preclude resection. Spread to regional lymphatics is common, as is metastasis to the liver via the portal vein. Spread to peritoneal surfaces (carcinomatosis) is frequently seen in advanced disease, as are lung metastases.

The pathologic staging of pancreatic cancer has recently been revised and is based on the extent of tumor involvement of local and distant structures, as shown in Table 84-3. Stage I tumors are limited to the pancreas. Stage II tumors are regionally invasive, without involvement of the celiac or superior mesenteric arteries, but may involve regional lymph nodes. Stage I and II tumors are considered potentially amenable to resection with curative intent. Stage III lesions are defined by direct involvement of the celiac or superior mesenteric arteries, and stage IV lesions are defined by the presence of distant metastases. Patients with stage III and IV disease are generally not considered resectable for cure, although this view has recently been challenged for selected patients with isolated liver metastases.[30,31]

Cystic Neoplasms

Cystic neoplasms of the pancreas can be divided into benign tumors and malignant tumors (cystadenocarcinomas).[26] Benign cystic tumors can be further divided, on the basis of radiologic factors and by analysis of cyst fluid, into lesions with little predilection to become malignant, termed *serous cystadenomas* and those with a significant risk of malignant degeneration, termed *mucinous cystic neoplasms*. Although previously classified as either benign mucinous cystadenomas or malignant cystadenocarcinomas, the term mucinous cystic neoplasm is preferred because of the malignant potential of all mucinous cystic tumors, as evidenced by the frequent identification of cystadenocarcinoma in patients suspected of harboring a mucinous cystadenoma.

Cystadenocarcinomas of the pancreas are less biologically aggressive than pancreatic adenocarcinomas, with a high cure rate after complete resection. Because even serous cystadenomas can be locally invasive,[3] an aggressive approach to the removal of most serous cystadenomas as well as of all mucinous tumors of the pancreas is justified. In contrast, mucinous tumors of the pancreas are less predictable in their biologic behavior, with some malignant tumors remaining indolent for months to years. They may be locally or regionally invasive without forming metastases. When mucinous tumors of the pancreas do disseminate, they tend to form peritoneal implants but rarely develop liver or lung metastases.

A related but distinct lesion is the intraductal papillary mucinous neoplasm (IPMN).[26] This disorder is an abnormality of the pancreatic duct in which all or part of the pancreatic duct epithelium becomes dysplastic, and it may degenerate to overt malignancy. Typically the entire pancreatic duct is ectatic and mucus filled, giving a characteristic appearance when evaluated at endoscopic retrograde cholangiopancreatography (ERCP). Because of their predilection to harbor carcinoma in situ and even areas of invasive carcinoma, surgical resection of IPMNs may require total pancreatectomy in some patients. No consensus now exists on appropriate follow-up for patients who have undergone partial pancreatectomy for IPMNs.

GENETICS

Molecular Genetics

Research performed over the last several decades has demonstrated that the development of malignancy is a multistep process in which distinct oncogenes are activated and tumor-suppressor genes inactivated in a clonal population of cells. This process ultimately gives rise to a cell population that is resistant to molecular mechanisms that normally regulate cell proliferation and programmed cell death.[32] Molecular events underlying the development of pancreatic cancer have been studied extensively, and a number of alterations in oncogenes and tumor-suppressor genes that are thought to play a role in the development of this disease have been identified.[33-38] Common abnormalities include activating mutations in the K-*ras* oncogene (which occur in more than 90% of pancreatic cancers), overexpression of the HER2-neu oncogene (seen in 50% to 70% of pancreatic cancers), and loss of expression of the CDKN2, p53, and DPC4 tumor-suppressor genes (seen in 100%, 70%, and 50% of pancreatic cancers, respectively).

The identification and characterization of histologically distinct premalignant precursor lesions that give rise to pancreatic adenocarcinomas, termed *pancreatic intraepithelial neoplasms* (PanINs), suggest that the activation of oncogenes and loss of tumor-suppressor genes occurs in a stepwise fashion. Activation of the K-*ras* oncogene is seen in very early preneoplastic lesions (PanIN1s) and even in secretions of patients with chronic pancreatitis and no known pancreatic cancer.[26] Similarly, HER2-neu overexpression is frequently seen in early intraepithelial neoplasms. In contrast, loss of the CDKN2, p53, and DPC4 tumor-suppressor genes appears to be a relatively late event in tumorigenesis, seen in more advanced preneoplastic (PanIN2 and PanIN3) and frankly neoplastic lesions.

Familial Pancreatic Cancer

Although the majority of pancreatic cancers appear to be sporadic, approximately 5% of pancreatic malignancies are seen in patients with a familial history of pancreatic cancer.[39] Among patients with two first-degree relatives with pancreatic cancer, the relative risk of developing pancreatic cancer is increased 18-fold. In patients with three or more affected relatives, the increased risk is 57-fold. Such data strongly support the notion that familial pancreatic cancer is a real entity.

An additional unknown percentage of pancreatic cancers may reflect the presence of an overall cancer family syndrome that is less strikingly specific for the pancreas. For example, it has been shown that among a subset of kindreds with the familial atypical mole malignant melanoma syndrome (FAMM), approximately a 20-fold increased risk occurs for the development of pancreatic cancer,[38] although the relative risks for other forms of cancer are not substantially increased. Molecular analysis has demonstrated that this subset of FAMM patients has a germ-line alteration in the CDKN2 tumor-suppressor gene.[38] Similarly, patients at risk for breast cancer as a result of inherited BRCA2 gene abnormalities also have a risk of pancreatic cancer at least tenfold higher than that of the general population.[32,40] Other familial syndromes associated with an increased risk of pancreatic cancer include the hereditary nonpolyposis colon cancer syndrome, familial adenomatous polyposis, and ataxia telangiectasia. Furthermore, the hereditary pancreatitis syndrome, caused by a mutation in the trypsinogen gene, carries a 40% to 70% risk of pancreatic cancer. Thus genetic factors, although of variable penetrance, clearly play a role in the predisposition to pancreatic cancer development in many patients.

DIAGNOSIS

Signs and Symptoms

Patients with pancreatic cancer often are vaguely unwell for a number of months before the development of overt symptoms that lead to the diagnosis of their illness. Common signs and symptoms of pancreatic cancer are summarized in Table 84-4. Although the development of "painless jaundice" is often thought of as a typical presenting feature of patients with pancreatic cancer, most patients have mild to moderate abdominal pain. The presence of back pain is a particularly ominous symptom, which may reflect retroperitoneal nerve invasion by tumor.

The development of obstructive jaundice is related to the anatomic location of the primary tumor. It is almost universal in tumors of the pancreatic head but is quite rare in patients with primary tumors of the pancreatic tail. Liver function tests should be performed to distinguish obstructive jaundice from a primary hepatocellular process such as hepatitis. Patients with severe obstructive jaundice may have some degree of associated coagulopathy from hepatic dysfunction. Coagulation parameters should be tested in all jaundiced patients, and those with coagulation abnormalities should receive preoperative vitamin K and/or perioperative fresh-frozen plasma.

The presence of weight loss is relatively common. This may reflect duodenal obstruction by tumor, an as yet poorly understood inhibitory effect of pancreatic cancer on gastric motility, and/or effects of tumor-related cytokines on host metabolism. Except in extremely malnourished patients, aggressive preoperative or perioperative nutritional support, or both, of pancreatic cancer patients has not been shown to be of benefit.[3]

Findings on physical examination are often nonspecific.[3] Jaundice is common, as noted earlier, but not specific for the presence of a malignancy. The presence of a palpable pancreatic mass or gallbladder (Courvoisier's sign) is uncommon and usually is observed only in thin patients. Hepatomegaly due to liver congestion or the presence of metastatic disease is similarly seen in the minority of patients at the time of initial diagnosis.

Radiologic Evaluation

Patients suspected of having a pancreatic malignancy are generally evaluated by thin-cut, contrast-enhanced computerized tomographic (CT) scanning. This is of use in identifying the tumor mass as well as in assessing the liver for metastasis. Vascular involvement of superior mesenteric vein, portal vein, and celiac and superior mesenteric arteries also can be determined by CT scanning (Fig. 84-2). Ultrasonography is useful in identifying the primary tumor mass (Fig. 84-3), particularly in the pancreatic head, but is less sensitive than CT and provides less information regarding local and regional dissemination. Magnetic resonance imaging has not proven superior to CT scanning for assessment of the primary tumor, metastatic disease, or vascular encasement. Occasional patients with CT findings suggestive but not diagnostic of vascular encasement may benefit from preoperative visceral angiography, although improvements in CT methods, particularly the use of dynamic contrast infusion and spiral techniques, have largely supplanted angiography.

Positron emission tomography using [^{18}F]fluorodeoxyglucose (FDG-PET) has not proved useful in the diagnosis or staging of pancreatic cancer. Initial hopes that FDG-PET would distinguish chronic pancreatitis from pancreatic neoplasia have not been supported in clinical studies.[41] Furthermore, FDG-PET misses a substantial number of lymph node metastases and peritoneal metastases.[42] Most important, the addition of FDG-PET to CT-based diagnostic algorithms appears rarely to alter subsequent diagnostic or therapeutic maneuvers. Whether PET technology using agents that detect cell proliferation rather than cell metabolism will improve these results is currently under evaluation.

Patients with a pancreatic mass on CT and no evidence of metastatic disease or vascular encasement require no further testing and can be taken to the operating room for surgical resection. At the time of definitive surgery, a laparoscopic evaluation of resectability may be performed, as discussed later. It is not necessary to obtain a preoperative tissue diagnosis. Indeed, because of the frequent presence of a dense reactive stroma surrounding small islands of cancer cells, cytologic assessment of pancreatic malignancies is notoriously inaccurate, rendering absence of malignant cells on percutaneous or endoscopic biopsy of little value in patient management. An additional concern with percutaneous techniques is the possibility of tumor dissemination as a result of the biopsy process, as has been suggested in some studies.[43]

Endoscopic Retrograde Cholangiopancreatography

Patients with jaundice but no mass on CT are generally evaluated with ERCP. This may reveal an irregular or tapering biliary stricture characteristic of an obstructing periampullary tumor (Fig. 84-4). Sometimes the biliary stricture is seen in conjunction with a pancreatic duct

TABLE 84-4

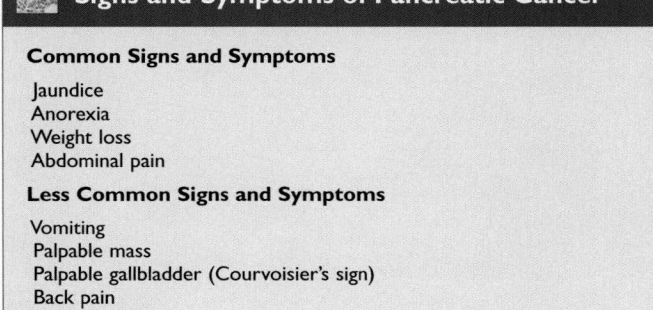

Signs and Symptoms of Pancreatic Cancer

Common Signs and Symptoms

Jaundice
Anorexia
Weight loss
Abdominal pain

Less Common Signs and Symptoms

Vomiting
Palpable mass
Palpable gallbladder (Courvoisier's sign)
Back pain
Splenomegaly
Constipation
Thrombophlebitis (Trousseau's sign)

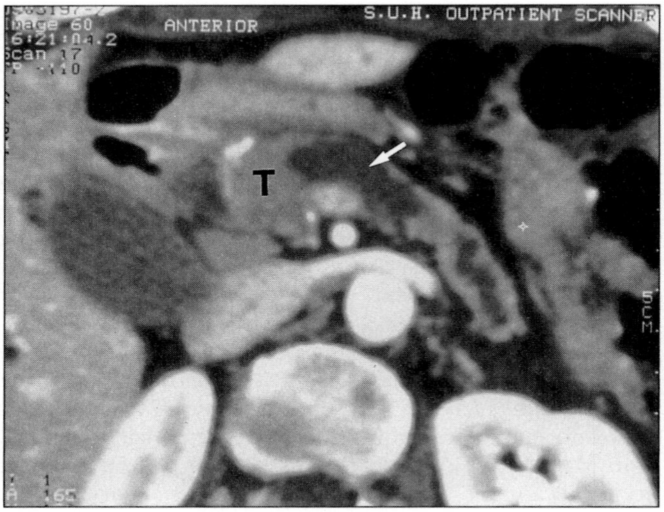

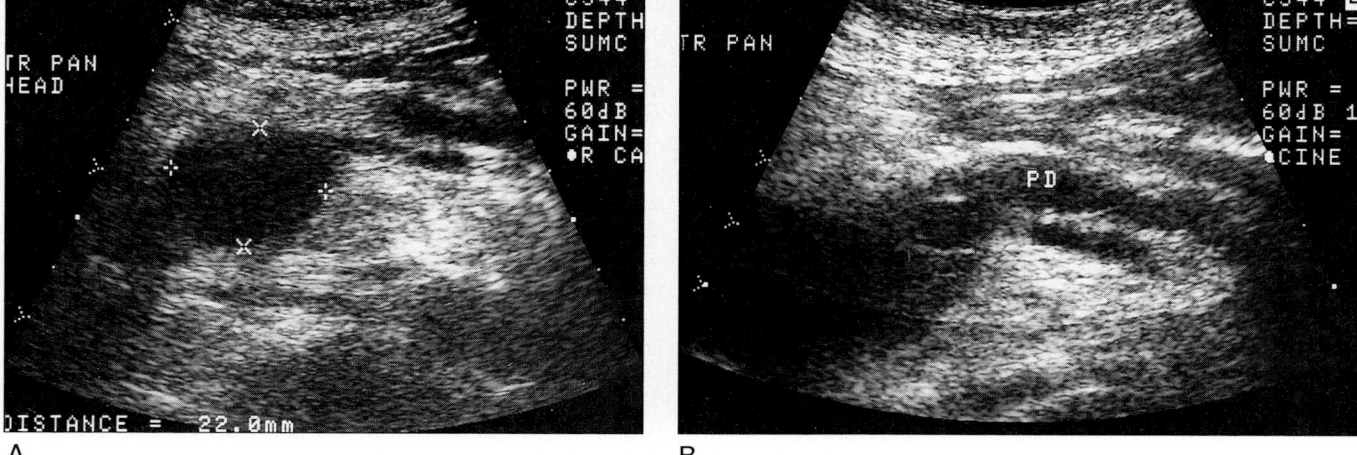

Figure 84-2. Dynamic computed tomography (CT) studies of resectable and unresectable pancreatic tumors. **A,** Dynamic CT revealing a dilated pancreatic duct (*arrow*) and mass in the head of the pancreas (*T*). No evidence is seen of vascular involvement suggesting that no local factors prevent resection of this lesion. **B,** A different patient shown here with a dynamic CT study illustrating tumor encasement of the celiac artery. **C,** Encasement of the superior mesenteric artery.

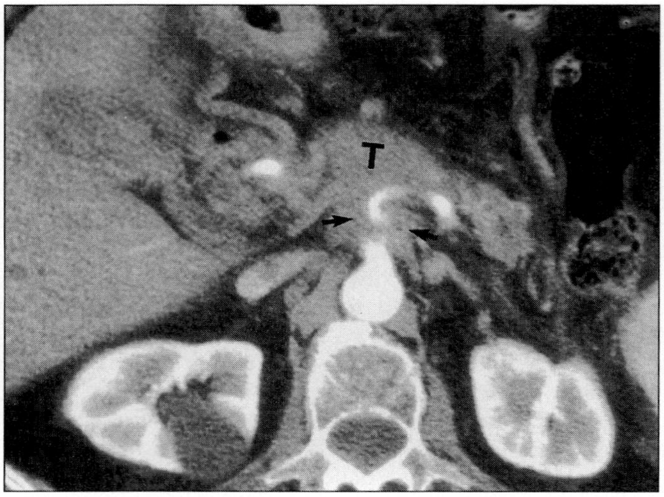

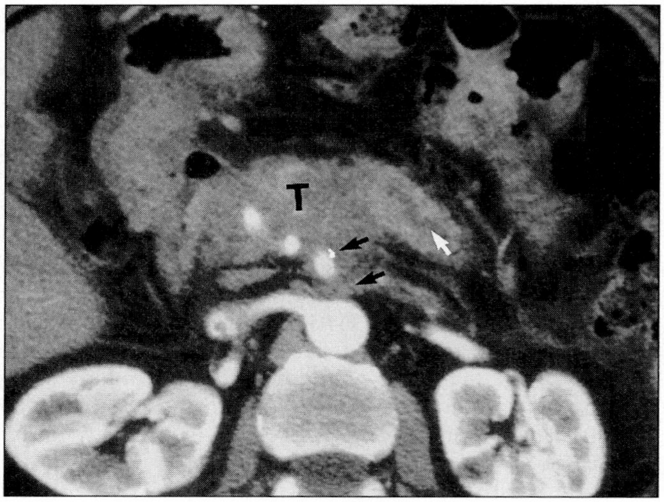

Figure 84-3. A, Untrasonographic examination of a mass in the head of the pancreas. The pancreatic mass is hypoechoic compared with normal parenchyma and is easily discernible from the surrounding normal pancreatic tissue. **B,** Tranverse ultrasonographic image of the body of the pancreas in the same patient shows marked pancreatic duct dilation.

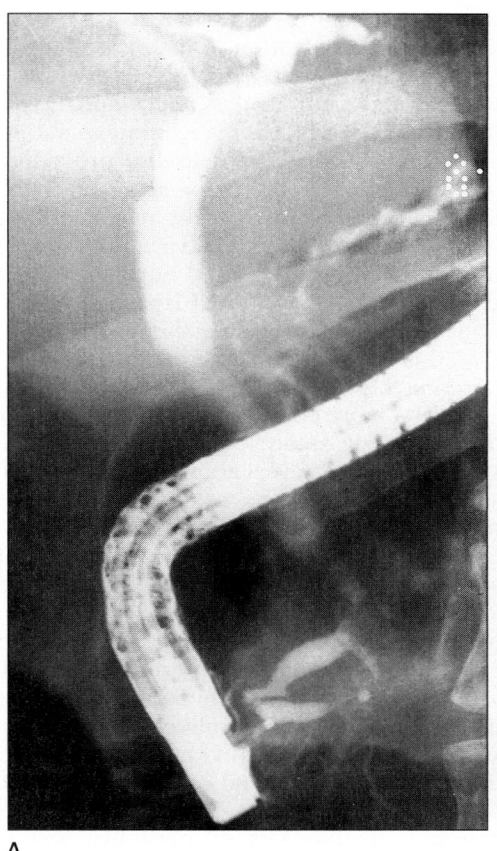 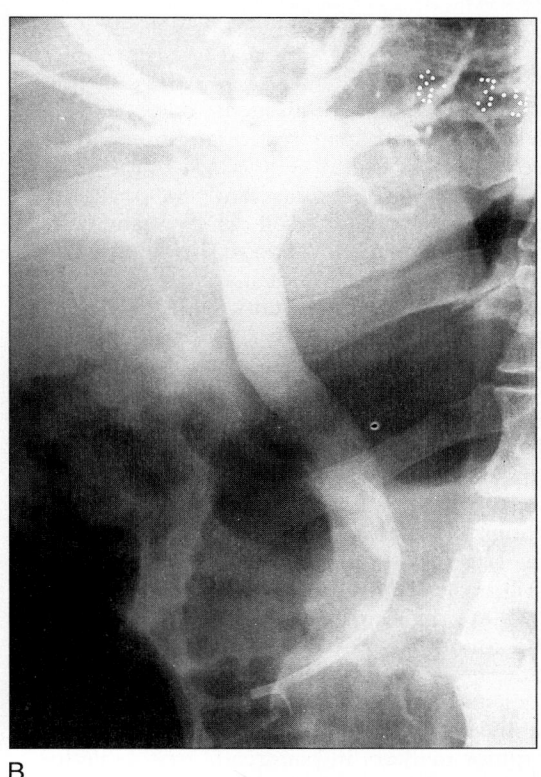

A   B

Figure 84-4. A, Endoscopic retrograde cholangiopancreatography illustrating distal common bile duct obstruction of the "knee" of the distal bile duct. This study also illustrates occlusion of the main pancreatic duct. **B,** This same patient has had a biliary stent placed endoscopically for palliation of jaundice.

stricture—the "double duct" sign—which is highly suggestive of the presence of a malignancy. Irregular strictures of the pancreatic duct also may be seen in patients with pancreatic carcinoma. Such endoscopic findings, even in the absence of a pancreatic mass on CT scanning, justify proceeding to surgical resection. Endoscopic brushings and biopsies may confirm the presence of a pancreatic neoplasm but have a relatively high false-negative rate, as discussed earlier. An aggressive surgical approach to patients with suggestive biliary strictures, particularly in those patients without a history of gallstone disease, will often result in removal of tumors at a relatively early stage.

The risks and benefits of decompressing the biliary tree before resecting a pancreatic cancer remain controversial.[44-47] Although the rationale for relieving obstructive jaundice and normalizing liver function before surgery is clear, several randomized prospective trials have failed to show a benefit of preoperative biliary stenting by ERCP or percutaneous techniques. Furthermore, a nontrivial incidence of complications is found in patients who undergo stenting before resection, and the presence of an endoscopically placed stent appears to increase the risk of postoperative morbidity, particularly the development of infectious complications, in patients undergoing pancreaticoduodenectomy.[47]

Probably the critical factor in deciding whether preoperatively to decompress a jaundiced patient who will definitely be taken for surgical exploration is the interval to surgery. If the patient can be operated on in a few days and is not symptomatic from jaundice, it may be best to proceed directly to surgery. If there will be a delay in scheduling surgery or if the patient is extremely symptomatic from jaundice, it may be best to stent the patient, both for comfort and to minimize the risk of cholangitis.

Endoscopic Ultrasonography

Another important endoscopic technique that has begun to play a major role in the diagnosis and staging of patients with pancreatic malignancies is endoscopic ultrasonography (EUS). EUS can assess tumor size, portal and mesenteric vascular involvement, and regional nodal involvement. EUS also can obtain tissue samples for histologic analysis from virtually all pancreatic lesions and from suggestive lymph nodes located close to the stomach and duodenum. It has the advantage of not requiring a general anesthetic and can be performed outside an operating suite with mild sedation. As in all sonographic procedures, the quality of clinical information achieved with EUS is highly operator dependent. Furthermore, EUS cannot evaluate lesions, such as peritoneal metastases, which are located at sites distant from the lumen of the gastrointestinal tract.

Tumor Markers

A number of tumor-associated antigens detectable in the serum of patients with pancreatic carcinoma have been described, the most useful being CA19-9.[48] CA19-9 is a mucin-associated carbohydrate antigen produced by normal pancreatic cells, as well as by pancreatic carcinoma cells. CA19-9 can be detected in serum and pancreatic juice. As with other tumor markers, the use of CA19-9 in the management of patients with pancreatic cancer is plagued by problems related to sensitivity and specificity. Small tumors often fail to produce enough CA19-9 to be detectable above the accepted serum threshold of 35 units/mL. Non-neoplastic disorders of the pancreas and biliary tract, particularly pancreatitis, are associated with elevations of CA19-9, which may reach several hundred units per milliliter. Patients with CA19-9 levels in the thousands almost definitely have pancreatic cancer but are generally quite symptomatic from their tumors, which are often unresectable. Thus little use is found for CA19-9 in screening asymptomatic populations. A role may be found for postoperative monitoring of CA19-9 in patients after tumor resection, but in the absence of effective therapy for recurrent disease, this also is of questionable value except in research protocols.

Analysis of tumor markers in pancreatic cyst aspirates may be of use in distinguishing pseudocysts from cystic neoplasms and in separating serous cystadenomas from mucinous tumors if radiologic criteria alone are inadequate. Interestingly, CA19-9 levels in cyst aspirates are of little use in separating these different lesions. However, it has been shown that analyzing the combination of amylase, carcinoembryonic antigen, CA-125, and tissue polypeptide antigen allows fairly accurate separation among the different cystic lesions of the pancreas.[49,50] These studies are particularly useful in the elderly or medically frail patient in whom resection of a cystic lesion of the pancreas poses an unusually high risk. When cyst-fluid analysis suggests a low likelihood of malignancy, such high-risk patients can be managed without surgery.

Laparoscopic Staging

The development of laparoscopic staging procedures is a significant advance in the preoperative staging of patients with pancreatic cancer and other periampullary tumors.[43,51-54] Among patients that appear to have a resectable pancreatic cancer based on spiral CT scanning techniques, a 20% to 30% incidence is seen of either locally advanced disease or of small hepatic or peritoneal implants, undetected by radiologic imaging, which preclude curative resection. With advances in nonoperative palliation of advanced disease, particularly improvements in biliary stenting, as discussed later, no need may be found for formal laparotomy in patients with disease not amenable to curative resection. Avoiding unnecessary laparotomy is an important goal of palliating patients

with advanced disease, which may be facilitated by laparoscopic evaluation.

Simple laparoscopy and biopsy allows the evaluation of visceral and peritoneal surfaces and may reveal disease undetectable by other techniques. Patients may then avoid unnecessary open surgical procedures if adequate palliation of jaundice can be achieved with percutaneous or transhepatic biliary stent placement. Staging laparoscopy, with frozen-section evaluation of biopsy specimens if necessary, can be carried out in 15 to 20 minutes and can be followed by formal laparotomy and tumor resection under the same anesthetic. Available data suggest that this technique alone can reduce the incidence of unresectable disease at laparotomy by more than 50%.[52,54]

Several more complex techniques may further enhance the utility of laparoscopic staging. Laparoscopic ultrasonography can reveal abnormalities beneath the visceral surfaces and, with the use of flow Doppler techniques, may identify vascular encasement or occlusion.[51,52] Conlon and colleagues described a more thorough laparoscopic staging of periampullary tumors, including pathologic evaluation of celiac, periportal, and peripancreatic lymph nodes.[53] Finally, the assessment of occult disease by cytologic assessment of peritoneal washings obtained at laparoscopy may further define patients with tumor dissemination who are unlikely to benefit from extensive surgical resection.[43] It is worth noting, however, that all of these techniques extend operative time and may require several days to obtain a definitive diagnosis in the case of lymph node biopsies or peritoneal cytology. Surgeons favoring these approaches often perform laparoscopic staging procedures and definitive resections under separate anesthetics, with a corresponding increase in cost and patient morbidity. The precise role of these more complex procedures will no doubt be determined in the coming years.

THERAPY

Surgical Resection

For patients with potentially resectable pancreatic malignancies, defined as those that have not yet metastasized to distant sites, encased the portal or superior mesenteric veins, or invaded the roots of the celiac or superior mesenteric arteries, surgical resection remains the best hope for achieving prolonged disease-free survival. Most resectable tumors occur in the head of the pancreas and are resected by pancreaticoduodenectomy (Whipple procedure). This procedure was initially described as a two-stage operation,[55] although it fairly rapidly evolved into a one-stage procedure.[56] Although individual surgeons perform this procedure differently, in all cases, the head of the pancreas, distal bile duct, and most of the duodenum and proximal jejunum are resected en bloc. In many cases, the entire duodenum, as well as the gastric antrum, are included with the resection specimen. Reconstruction involves the performance of pancreatic, biliary, and gastric or duodenal anastomoses to the remaining jejunum. A schematic drawing of a pancreaticoduodenectomy with distal gastrectomy (classic Whipple procedure) or with pylorus preservation and reconstruction is shown in Figure 84-5.

Pancreaticoduodenectomy is a demanding technical operation, requiring meticulous dissection around portal and mesenteric blood vessels and three distinct anastomoses; the morbidity and mortality associated with the Whipple procedure can be significant. Indeed, in the mid-1970s, it was seriously questioned whether patients with resectable pancreatic malignancies might be better managed with palliative bypass procedures.[57-59] Over the past several decades, however, a steady improvement has occurred in the results reported after pancreaticoduodenectomy with regard to morbidity and mortality, with a corresponding improvement in long-term survival of patients with resected tumors.

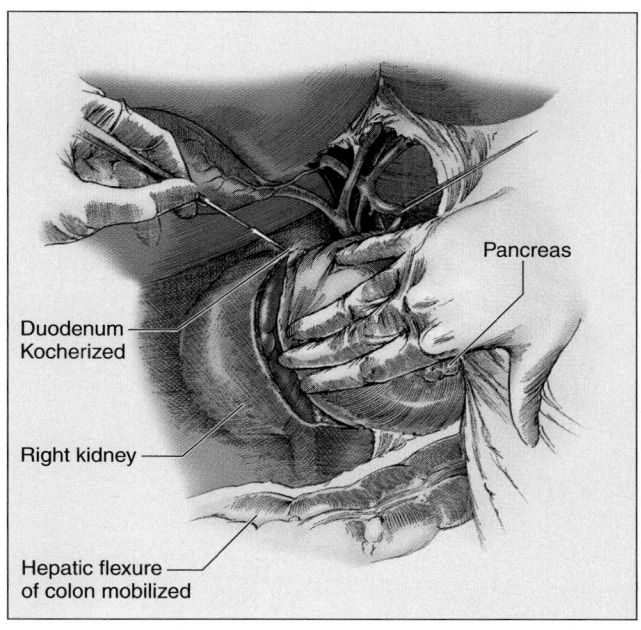

A

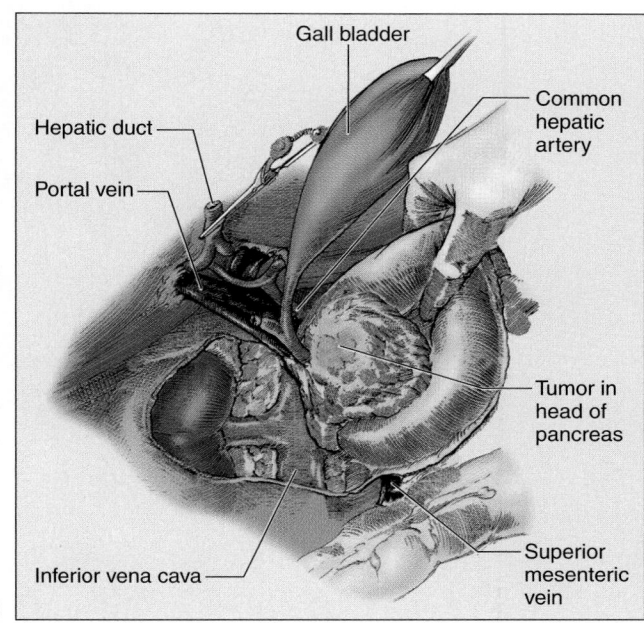

B

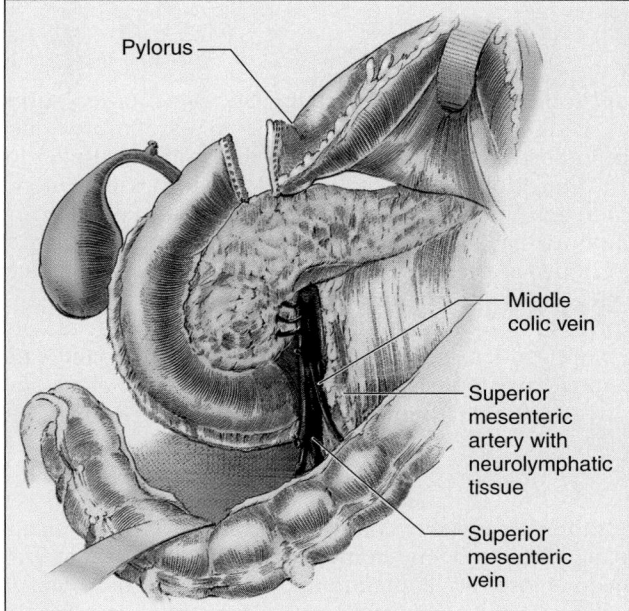

C

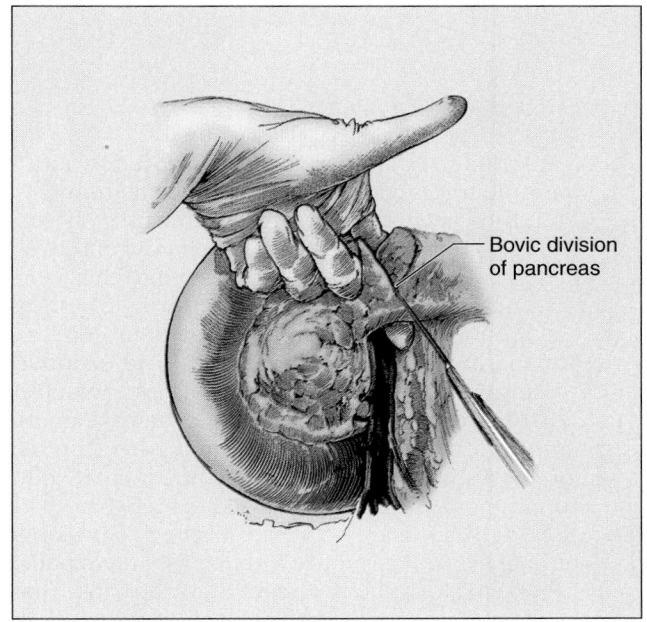

D

Figure 84-5. Pancreaticoduodenectomy. **A,** Kocherization of the duodenum is illustrated as an early step in this procedure. **B,** The head of the pancreas and duodenum are free from the retroperitoneum and the common hepatic duct, and the gastroduodenal artery has been divided. **C,** The gastroduodenal artery and the first portion of the duodenum are divided. **D,** After dissection under the neck of the pancreas, the body of the pancreas is divided as illustrated.

Continued

Specific Malignancies

III

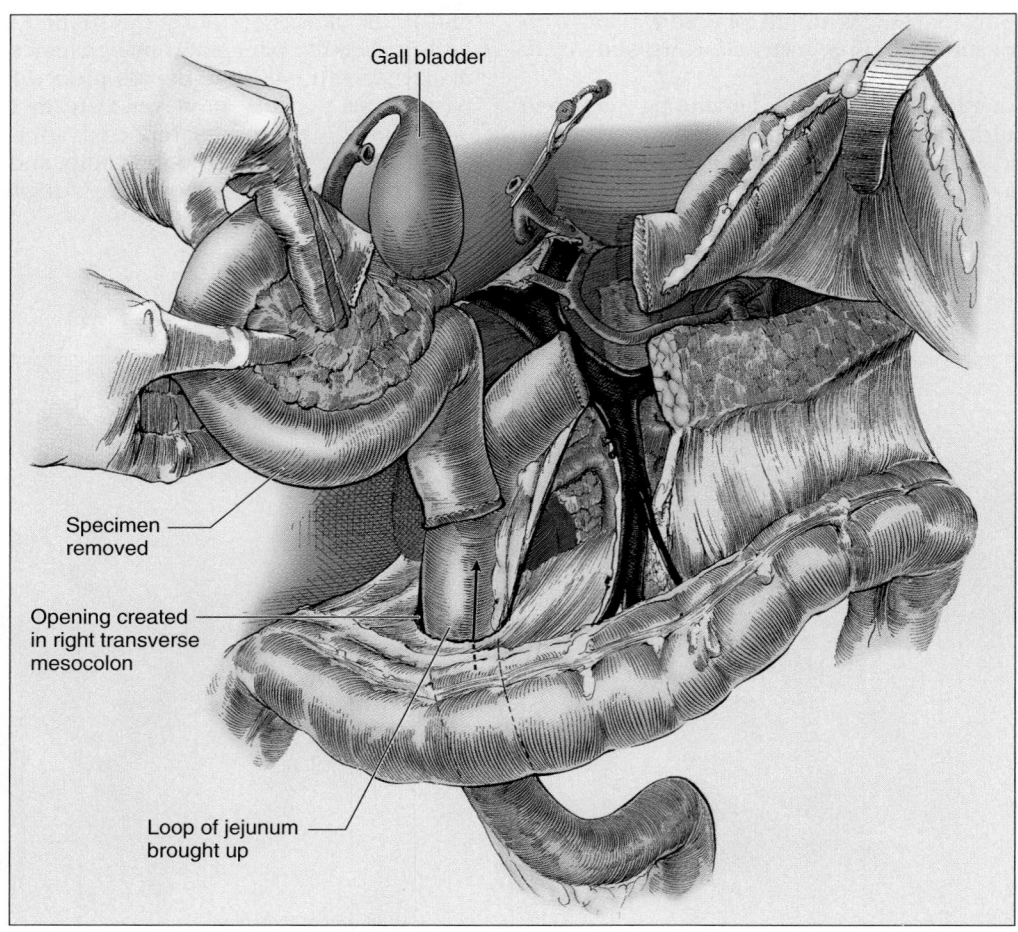

Gall bladder

Specimen
removed

Opening created
in right transverse
mesocolon

Loop of jejunum
brought up

E

Figure 84-5, *cont'd.* Pancreaticoduodenectomy. **E,** Removal of the pancreaticoduodenectomy specimen, illustrating the common hepatic duct, duodenum, and the residual pancreas. The proximal jejunum brought through the transverse mesocolon will be used for reconstruction.

Perioperative Mortality

A steep decline in the perioperative mortality rate of patients undergoing pancreaticoduodenectomy has been noted in recent years.[60] During the past 30 years, postoperative mortality rates have declined from 20% to less than 5% in many institutions around the world. Near-zero mortality rates, which we define as 2% or less, are being reported with increasing frequency in case series numbering more than 100 patients. These mortality rates are so low that many hundreds of cases would be required to determine precise mortality rates. Nonetheless, it is safe to make the general statement that extremely low mortality rates are now the norm for pancreaticoduodenectomies performed in specialized centers.

The reason(s) for the precipitate decline in perioperative mortality rates is not completely understood. It appears, in part, to reflect concentration of pancreaticoduodenectomy procedures at high-volume centers;[61-64] low-volume centers still have perioperative mortality rates of 15% to 20% in national surveys.[63,64] The observed improvement in perioperative mortality in high-volume centers is no doubt multifactorial and parallels a general

decline in operative mortality seen for other surgical procedures. Other contributing factors are improvements in intensive care, diagnostic and interventional radiology, and nutritional support. Prophylaxis and management of infection, venous thromboembolism, and gastrointestinal hemorrhage also have improved greatly during this period. As a result, postoperative cardiopulmonary complications and gastrointestinal hemorrhage, which used to be fairly common, have been sharply reduced. Other complications, such as disruption of the pancreaticojejunal anastomosis, which were often fatal 30 years ago, now lead to death infrequently.[65]

Morbidity

Although mortality rates have improved significantly, pancreaticoduodenectomy remains a procedure in which major morbidity is common. Complication rates are difficult to evaluate because no uniformly adopted method exists of reporting or even defining complications. Additionally, some series provide numbers of complications, whereas others report the number of patients with complications. Despite these limitations, it is apparent that some complications, such as pulmonary embolism, gastrointestinal bleeding, pneumonia, and myocardial infarction are much less common today than in the past.

Improvements in surgical technique have reduced the incidence of leakage at biliary-enteric anastomoses (biliary fistula) to less than 5% in many series.[60] In contrast, leakage at the pancreaticoenteric anastomosis (pancreatic fistula) is still a major complication of pancreaticoduodenectomy, occurring in 10% to 20% of patients in most series.[60] In reported case series, much improvement in the incidence of this complication has not occurred over the years. For most surgeons, the pancreaticoenteric anastomosis continues to be the weak point of the operation, leakage being most common when the pancreatic duct is small and the gland very soft. However, in the current era, leakage at the pancreaticojejunostomy generally leads to an increased length of hospital stay but rarely to reoperation or death.[65]

Probably the most common postoperative complication seen in patients undergoing pancreaticoduodenectomy is delayed gastric emptying. Although not well understood, it is thought that disruption of enterogastric signaling after duodenectomy is responsible for the gastric motility problems so frequently seen. Although it once was thought to be more common in patients undergoing pylorus preservation,[66] randomized studies have demonstrated that delayed emptying is equally common in patients undergoing classic Whipple resection with hemigastrectomy.[67] Delayed gastric emptying is seen in more than 20% of patients and may range in severity from mild nausea and inability to eat, to persistent vomiting requiring nasogastric suction for days to weeks after surgery. Problems with gastric emptying are rarely life threatening but can significantly prolong postoperative hospitalization. A randomized prospective trial of erythromycin demonstrated modest but statistically significant benefits in improving gastric emptying after pancreaticoduodenctomy, presumably through the effects of erythromycin on motilin receptors.[68]

Long-Term Survival after Surgical Resection

With improvements in perioperative morbidity and mortality, some improvement in 5-year survival rates has been noted for patients undergoing pancreaticoduodenectomy for pancreatic cancer. Five-year survival rates after Whipple resection for ampullary, bile duct, and duodenal malignancies have always been reasonable, ranging from 30% to 50% in most series, whereas resection of a mucinous tumor of the pancreas results in 5-year survival rates of more than 75%. In contrast, the long-term survival of patients with pancreatic adenocarcinoma has generally been extremely poor. A recent review of the world literature dating back over the past 50 years suggests that the overall 5-year survival of patients after attempted curative resection for adenocarcinoma of the pancreas is on the order of 4%.[69] Furthermore, some of these patients had recurrence beyond 5 years, suggesting that they had not been cured by resection of their tumors.

Several large case series from high-volume centers suggest that better long-term results are now being obtained, with up to 20% of patients with documented pancreatic adenocarcinoma surviving 5 years after resection.[70,71] In patients with negative resection margins, small tumors, and no evidence of lymph node metastases, the results may be even better, with more than 40% of such patients expected to survive 5 years. It is important to note, however, that these survival curves are based on actuarial rather than actual survival, and not all recent series have noted such results. Those who believe that results have improved point to improvements in diagnosis, surgical technique, and the use of adjuvant chemotherapy and radiation therapy as possible contributing factors.

Technical Aspects of Pancreaticoduodenectomy

Variations in pancreaticoduodenectomy technique between experienced surgeons are the rule, and multiple approaches can be reviewed in surgical atlases and texts. However, certain strategic aspects to the successful performance of this operation are worth emphasizing. Probably first and foremost is that this is not an operation that should be carried out by surgeons who do pancreatic surgery on an infrequent basis. Studies from multiple centers have demonstrated a strong relation between surgical volume and outcome in patients undergoing pancreaticoduodenectomy.[61-64] The statewide mortality rates in Maryland and New York and the national Medicare data base show remarkably similar findings, with mortality three- to fivefold higher in patients undergoing surgery at low-volume centers, defined as doing fewer than five cases per year, compared with centers doing 20 or more cases per year. A significant fraction of pancreaticoduodenectomies are still performed in low-volume centers,[72] which may account for the higher mortality reported in national surveys as opposed to reported rates at high-volume centers. Other specific technical issues are discussed later.

Total Pancreatectomy

One of the oldest controversies regarding resection of pancreatic tumors in the periampullary region was between a classic Whipple-type pancreaticoduodenectomy with preservation of the pancreatic body and tail and a total pancreatectomy. Advocates of total pancreatectomy claimed that the more extensive resection offered the opportunity to resect extensive or multifocal disease and more thoroughly removed potentially involved peripancreatic nodes.[73,74] In addition, by completely removing the pancreas, it was not necessary to perform a pancreaticoenteric anastomosis, eliminating the risk of a postoperative pancreatic fistula.

Patients undergoing total pancreatectomy did uniformly develop diabetes, which was frequently quite brittle and difficult to control. Furthermore, it was shown that pancreatic carcinomas are rarely multifocal[75] and that a total pancreatectomy per se does not remove a significantly greater number of the lymph nodes to which periampullary tumors are likely to metastasize.[76] Improvement in our ability to prevent or manage pancreatic anastomotic leaks has changed this once-dreaded complication into one that is rarely a cause of mortality.[65,77] Finally, analysis of a number of studies of partial and total pancreatectomy for periampullary tumors failed to show a benefit for total pancreatectomy and suggested an equivalent or inferior outcome when compared with a Whipple-type pancreaticoduodenectomy. Thus total pancreatectomy has been largely discredited as an operation for pancreatic tumors, except for those relatively rare cases in which direct tumor extension into the body and tail of the pancreas, or the presence of an extensive intraductal papillary mucinous neoplasm involving the entire pancreatic duct, makes a total pancreatectomy the only way to excise the primary neoplasm completely.

Regional Pancreatectomy

Based on careful study of the patterns of local and lymphatic metastases in pancreatic carcinoma, Fortner's group at The Memorial Sloan-Kettering Cancer Center championed a more extensive operation for cancers arising in the pancreatic head, which they termed *regional pancreatectomy*.[78] This operation removed not only the pancreatic mass (with either a total or subtotal pancreatectomy) but also included resection and reconstruction of the superior mesenteric vein–portal vein confluence and an extensive en bloc regional lymph node dissection.[79] In some patients, resection and reconstruction of the superior mesenteric artery or hepatic artery were performed as well.

Fortner recently summarized his experience with this procedure in 56 patients,[79] which demonstrated a near universal occurrence of major morbidity and a 30-day surgical mortality of more than 5%. In addition, it appears that several other patients survived more than 30 days but succumbed to surgical complications after a continuous postoperative hospitalization in excess of thirty days. Long-term survival in patients undergoing this procedure was closely related to tumor size, with an estimated 33% 5-year survival in patients with tumors smaller than 2.5 cm in diameter and a 12% survival in patients with tumors ranging from 2.5 to 5.0 cm; no patients with larger tumors survived 5 years. The survival figures obtained with regional pancreatectomy are not significantly better than those reported with the standard Whipple-type pancreaticoduodenectomy,[60] whereas the morbidity and mortality are clearly greater.

Sindelar and colleagues at The National Cancer Institute also found the regional pancreatectomy to be associated with a significantly greater morbidity and mortality than is standard pancreaticoduodenectomy.[80] Furthermore, they analyzed the sites of tumor recurrence in patients undergoing regional pancreatectomy and found that in the majority of patients, both locoregional recurrence and evidence of distant metastases developed.[81] Thus the more radical operation was not successful in providing better local control or survival when compared with pancreaticoduodenectomy.

Although few surgeons now perform the regional pancreatectomy as originally conceived by Fortner, two of its principles (portal vein resection and extensive regional lymph node resection) are being carried out elsewhere and may have a role in selected patients. These are discussed individually later.

Portal Vein Resection

Among the many factors complicating resection of cancers arising in the head of the pancreas is the close proximity of major vessels in the porta hepatis, particularly the portal vein. In a number of studies, tumor involvement of the portal vein has been associated with a poor outcome.[82,83] This may reflect a difference in the biology of such tumors, with tumors that are more aggressive and destined to do poorly being more likely to invade the portal vein. In contrast, it also is possible that portal vein invasion is simply a consequence of where the tumor anatomically arises, and that if it can be adequately resected with negative margins, such patients may do as well as patients undergoing resection who do not have portal vein involvement. Although somewhat controversial, the current data favor the latter conclusion.

The first reports of superior mesenteric vein–portal vein resection for periampullary tumors date to the 1950s. However, only recently have large series of patients undergoing portal vein resection been reported.[84,85] Results from both M.D. Anderson and Memorial Sloan-Kettering suggest that patients undergoing en bloc resection of the portal vein have a morbidity and mortality comparable to those of patients undergoing a standard pancreaticoduodenectomy. Analysis of resected specimens from patients whose tumors had invaded the portal vein suggest that these tumors are no more likely to have positive lymph nodes or to be aneuploid than are tumors that did not invade the portal vein.[84] Thus vein invasion does not appear to reflect a difference in tumor biology and most likely is the unfortunate result of tumor anatomy.

Although the recent data are not completely mature with regard to survival in patients undergoing portal vein resection, preliminary analysis of these studies suggests that patients undergoing portal vein resection and reconstruction who have negative surgical margins do no worse than patients in whom the portal vein is uninvolved.[83-85] It seems reasonable to conclude that in patients with tumors involving the portal vein that are otherwise resectable with negative margins, en bloc resection of the portal vein is warranted.

From a technical standpoint, resection of the portal (or superior mesenteric) vein can be relatively simple or quite complex. Involvement of a small segment of the side wall of the vein can be locally resected, followed by primary venorrhaphy. Longer or more circumferential involvement generally requires segmental vein resection. Reconstruction can often be carried out with primary anastomosis if the resected segment is shorter than 2 to 3 cm and the anastomosis can be performed without undue tension. Resection of longer segments generally requires interposition grafting by using autologous vein. Either the saphenous vein, femoral vein, or the internal jugular vein can be used in reconstruction of the portal/superior mesenteric vein and can generally be harvested unilaterally without significant morbidity.

It is important to note that some situations still exist in which portal/superior mesenteric vein involvement can be an indication of unresectability. Circumferential involvement (encasement) of the portal or superior mesenteric veins, and particularly occlusion of the portal vein with resulting mesenteric venous hypertension, render resection exceedingly difficult if not impossible, in most circumstances. Tumors that encase the portal vein often invade or encase the superior mesenteric artery as well. We do not perform pancreaticoduodenectomy in patients whose preoperative staging demonstrates encasement of the portal or superior mesenteric veins, a position taken at other high-volume centers as well.[84,85]

Extended Lymphadenectomy

Periampullary malignancies frequently metastasize to lymph nodes beyond the limits of a standard pancreatico-duodenectomy.[76] In an effort to eradicate regional nodal disease before the development of distant metastases, a number of groups have championed the performance of an extended lymphadenectomy in addition to the standard pancreaticoduodenectomy.[86,87] This procedure involves the wide resection of lymphatic tissue from the celiac axis to the iliac bifurcation, including resection of nodal tissues between the portal vein and the superior mesenteric artery; resection of the portal vein–superior mesenteric vein confluence is often included and renders this portion of the case simpler from a technical point of view.

The Japanese have aggressively adopted this technique, and a number of series demonstrate favorable results compared with historical controls or concurrent patient populations that received a standard pancreaticoduo-denectomy.[88,89] However, other series have not shown such a difference.[90] In analyzing the results of multiple series of patients undergoing pancreaticoduodenectomy with extended lymph node dissection, it was concluded that the perioperative morbidity and mortality, as well as 5-year survival results, were not different from the results of the standard Whipple-type pancreaticoduodenec-tomy.[87,91] In part, this no doubt reflects the fact that, as in other malignancies, lymph node metastases reflect a more advanced stage of disease, in which systemic spread beyond the boundaries of possible resection has occurred. A prospective randomized trial of extended lymphadenectomy is clearly needed to determine whether this procedure is of benefit to patients with periampullary malignancies.

Pylorus Preservation

Traverso and Longmire introduced the pylorus-preserving pancreaticoduodenectomy in an effort to minimize complications of the procedure related to the hemi-gastrectomy, specifically dumping, marginal ulceration, and bile reflux gastritis.[92] The pylorus-preserving Whipple procedure preserves the entire stomach and pylorus, as well as the proximal 3 to 6 cm of duodenum, which is anastomosed to the jejunum to restore gastrointestinal continuity. Although this portion of duodenum is occasionally invaded by tumor, in many cases, it can be preserved without apparent compromise of the tumor margin. Studies have confirmed preservation of pyloric function with resulting decreases in dumping and enterogastric reflux.[93]

Surgeons critical of pylorus preservation raise a number of arguments, however. The incidence of marginal ulceration is quite low in the era of H_2-receptor blockers and proton pump inhibitors. Furthermore, delayed gastric emptying, which can occur after either pylorus-preserving or classic Whipple resection, is thought by some to be more common after pylorus preservation,[66] although this view is not supported by randomized studies.[67] Finally, the adequacy of pylorus preservation as a cancer operation has never been formally demonstrated in a randomized study. It must be noted, however, that available data from case series do not suggest a markedly different 5-year survival among patients with pancreatic tumors undergoing either type of pancreaticoduodenectomy.[3]

Improvements in Pancreaticoenteric Anastomosis

As mentioned earlier, leakage at the pancreaticoenteric anastomosis remains a significant source of morbidity. Furthermore, this complication was reported in one large series to double the average postoperative hospital stay from 2 to 4 weeks.[77] Different types of pancreatico-jejunostomies have been performed in an effort to minimize leakage from this anastomosis; most are variations on one of two very different techniques. The first approach, the so-called intussuscepting or "dunking" anastomosis, is performed by mobilizing the body of the pancreas 3 to 4 cm off the underlying splenic vein and then invaginating the cut end of the pancreas into the open end of the jejunal limb, which is sutured around the pancreas. This anastomosis is not dependent on the size of the pancreatic duct, although it may be technically difficult in certain circumstances, particularly when the pancreas is quite thick. A variation of this technique is to intussuscept the pancreas into the stomach.[77]

The alternative approach, the duct-to-mucosa anasto-mosis, is performed by anastomosing the cut edges of the pancreatic duct to the intestinal mucosa via a small defect in the jejunum, by using fine absorbable sutures. A reinforcing layer of sutures between the pancreatic capsule and the jejunal serosa is commonly placed to take tension off of the anastomosis. This anastomosis is satisfying from a physiologic viewpoint, but may be technically quite difficult in the presence of a nondilated pancreatic duct or a soft pancreas. Pancreatic fistula rates in series using either the duct-to-mucosa technique or the intussuscepting technique appear to be equivalent, and both are widely performed. A number of factors undoubtedly play a role in the success of pancreatico-enteric anastomoses.

Recently a number of reports suggesting that the incidence of pancreatic fistula development could be reduced to less than 5% have appeared in the surgical literature.[94,95,96] Although a number of distinct operative approaches have been used to achieve these remarkable results, several of the studies have championed the performance of a meticulous duct-to-mucosa anastomosis

Specific Malignancies

III

with fine absorbable suture under loupe magnification. Although it may be impossible to prevent completely the development of pancreatic fistulae after pancreatico-duodenectomy, it appears that the incidence of this complication can be substantially reduced. A number of studies have looked at the utility of somatostatin analogues such as octreotide in preventing the development of pancreatic fistulae. Although somatostatin analogues have proven effective in some European studies of patients undergoing a range of pancreatic surgical procedures,[97,98] these studies did not show a significant benefit in the subset of patients undergoing pancreatico-duodenectomy. Furthermore, several randomized trials of octreotide in patients undergoing Whipple resections in the United States have failed to demonstrate any benefit from the prophylactic use of this agent to prevent pancreatic fistula.[99,100] Octreotide also is expensive and, when administered subcutaneously, uncomfortable for patients. Its use to prevent pancreatic fistula development in the postoperative period cannot be recommended.

Distal Pancreatectomy

Patients with adenocarcinoma of the pancreas involving the body or tail of the pancreas are generally not symptomatic until their tumors have reached an advanced stage and thus are rarely resectable at the time of diagnosis. Furthermore, the long-term outcome after attempted surgical resection of more distal pancreatic adenocarcinomas is poor.[101,102] Probably the one subset of patients most likely to benefit from distal pancreatectomy are those with mucinous tumors of the pancreas. These tumors have a high cure rate after surgical resection and thus warrant aggressive surgical measures regardless of their size or anatomic location.

Distal pancreatectomy is a less daunting technical undertaking than pancreaticoduodenectomy, involving en bloc resection of the spleen and pancreatic tail. As with the Whipple procedure, it is critical to achieve an adequate resection margin, in this case, the proximal pancreatic margin and the retroperitoneal margin; peripancreatic tissue should be widely mobilized from the retroperitoneum to ensure removal of adjacent lymphatic tissue. Distal pancreatectomy is generally performed by mobilizing the pancreatic tail (along with the spleen in most cases) and proceeding medially (retrograde) toward the pancreatic neck. Recently the performance of this procedure from the pancreatic neck outward (antegrade) has been proposed as an approach to optimizing the retroperitoneal margin.[103] Whether this difference in technique will improve long-term outcomes is uncertain.

Adjuvant and Neoadjuvant Therapy

The modest success of surgical resection in producing long-term survival of patients with pancreatic tumors has led to a number of studies using chemotherapy and radiation therapy in an effort to diminish local and systemic recurrence after surgery. The classic study of adjuvant therapy for pancreatic carcinoma was performed by the Gastrointestinal Tumor Study Group (GITSG). This study prospectively randomized patients undergoing resection with curative intent to either no additional therapy or combined-bolus 5-fluorouracil (5-FU) and external-beam radiation therapy. Despite small numbers of patients in each arm of the study, a significant difference in outcome was observed between the two groups, with treated patients surviving 20 months, versus 11 months for untreated controls.[104] The GITSG subsequently completed a confirmatory trial in a larger patient population.[105]

Case series from several institutions, although non-randomized, also support a beneficial role for adjuvant 5-FU chemotherapy and radiation therapy in patients undergoing resection of pancreatic carcinomas.[106] In contrast, a multiinstitutional study conducted in Europe (ESPAC-1) suggested that chemoradiation was of no benefit after resection of pancreatic or other peri-ampullary tumors.[107] However, this study had substantial methodologic flaws that bring its findings into question. Additional multiinstitutional studies, in both the United States and Europe, are currently evaluating the benefit of postoperative chemoradiation after pancreatic cancer resection.

Recently, a single-institution phase II chemoradiation adjuvant study by Picozzi and colleagues, with a combination of 5-FU, cis-Platinum, and α-interferon as radiation sensitizers, demonstrated a remarkable improvement in median and 5-year survival (>36 months and ~50%, respectively) in a cohort of patients after surgical resection.[108] Although only 53 patients were treated, this result was so striking that an independent review panel from the American College of Surgeons Oncology Group evaluated charts and slides on treated patients to be certain that patients in this series did have pancreatic adenocarcinoma and that no selection bias existed that might account for the favorable outcome of treated patients. The review panel found no reason to question the conclusions of the phase II study; several single-institution trials are ongoing, with a multiinstitutional trial about to open enrollment. If the improvement in survival is verified by these studies, this adjuvant regimen will be one of the most striking advances in the treatment of pancreatic cancer.

Neoadjuvant Chemotherapy and Radiation Therapy

Recently several groups reported results from studies of preoperative neoadjuvant therapy in patients with periampullary tumors.[109,110] Such therapy is theoretically attractive from several perspectives. Shrinking of the primary tumor mass may make technical aspects of surgical resection easier. Data from animal experiments suggest that such therapy may reduce the incidence of tumor dissemination at the time of surgery. Furthermore, up to one third of eligible patients may fail to receive postoperative adjuvant therapy in a timely fashion because of the development of postoperative complications.

Against these advantages must be weighed several disadvantages, however. Significant tumor shrinkage has been rarely seen in neoadjuvant trials. More common is the development of local or distant disease progression, precluding curative resection, which has been noted with disturbing frequency. Furthermore, the effects of preoperative radiation and chemotherapy on surgical healing and complications such as biliary and pancreatic fistulae have not been established. It is our belief that postoperative adjuvant fluorouracil and external beam radiation therapy should be considered standard therapy and should be offered to all patients except for those participating in clinical trials. Given the limited benefit of such therapy, enrollment in clinical trials of novel adjuvant and neoadjuvant regimens should be encouraged.

MANAGEMENT OF PATIENTS WITH LOCALLY ADVANCED OR METASTATIC DISEASE

Downstaging

A substantial fraction of pancreatic cancer patients are first seen with locally advanced disease, either encasement of the superior mesenteric or portal veins or involvement of the celiac or superior mesenteric arteries, which precludes curative resection. This has led to a number of studies attempting to use chemoradiation to "downstage" the patient's tumor and permit a margin-negative surgical resection.[111,112] Unfortunately the results of these studies have generally been poor, with none to 10% of patients achieving sufficient tumor shrinkage to permit surgical resection; survival after resection also may be more limited than that usually seen after pancreaticoduodenectomy (unpublished results).

Radiation Therapy

Pancreatic cancer is a relatively radioresistant malignancy, with doses in excess of 7000 centiGray (cGy) required to eradicate all viable tumor cells.[113] Unfortunately the tolerances of surrounding tissues, including liver, stomach, kidney, and small bowel, do not permit this dose to be achieved clinically. Efforts to boost the tumor radiation dose by using brachytherapy or intraoperative radiation therapy in combination with external beam radiation have succeeded in decreasing local recurrence but have not substantially affected survival because of the development of metastatic disease outside the radiation field.[114-117] Radiation therapy does play a role in the adjuvant treatment of patients after resection, as described earlier, and can modestly extend survival in patients with advanced disease.[118] Furthermore, radiation therapy can substantially ameliorate pain in patients with disseminated disease.[119]

Chemotherapy for Advanced Disease

Chemotherapy for pancreatic cancer has had a minimal impact on the survival of patients with advanced disease.[119] For many years, 5-FU–based therapy, either as a single agent or in combination with other drugs, was the principal treatment strategy used in patients with advanced pancreatic cancer. Although a number of studies suggested that such therapy resulted in a modest survival advantage compared with that in patients receiving supportive care alone, the gains were quite modest.

The development and approval of gemcitabine as a first-line agent for the treatment of advanced pancreatic cancer represents an advance in both the therapeutic armamentarium and the approach to identifying agents of benefit to patients with this disease. Because of the problems with dense tumor stroma, it was considered probable that some patients who benefited from therapy might not show classic criteria for partial response: a 50% decrease in the perpendicular diameters of a radiologically detectable tumor mass. Therefore a new set of "clinical benefit response" criteria was developed.

By using these clinical benefit response criteria, it was demonstrated in a prospective randomized study that gemcitabine resulted in substantial clinical benefit in approximately 25% of patients as compared with fewer than 5% of patients who received 5-FU.[120] This study also demonstrated a modest, but statistically significant extension of median survival in patients receiving gemcitabine (5.4 vs. 4.3 months; $P < .05$). Furthermore, the fraction of patients surviving more than 1 year was approximately ninefold higher in the gemcitabine group (18% vs. 2%). It is worth noting that the fraction of patients achieving a partial radiologic response in this study was less than 5% and was not significantly different in the two treatment groups. Thus this study has not only identified an agent that improves the quality and the quantity of life for patients with advanced pancreatic cancer, but it has also demonstrated the limitations of traditional radiologic measures of tumor response and the importance of alternative criteria in testing novel agents for the treatment of patients with pancreatic cancer.

The identification of gemcitabine as an active agent in pancreatic cancer has led to the study of additional regimens using single-agent gemcitabine on different dosing schedules[121] or gemcitabine-based combinations.[119] Although additional studies are ongoing, it appears that gemcitabine-based combination therapies may be modestly more active in terms of median survival than is single-agent gemcitabine, but at the cost of increased toxicity. Even with the application of more potent gemcitabine-based combination therapies, survival of longer than 1 year is uncommon in patients with advanced disease.

The emerging development of molecularly targeted therapeutics offers the hope of more potent and less toxic approaches to treatment of pancreatic cancer. A number of novel agents are currently in phase II trials in pancreatic cancer, either alone or in combination with gemcitabine.[122] These include antisense compounds targeting the BCL2 cell-survival protein, agents that block ras function (such as farnesyl-transferase inhibitors), monoclonal antibodies and drugs that inhibit tumor angiogenesis, and a number of distinct signal-transduction inhibitors including monoclonal antibodies to the epidermal growth factor (EGF) receptor and HER2/neu protein, as well as chemical inhibitors of signaling kinase cascades. It is hoped that one or more of these agents will have substantially greater activity in pancreatic cancer patients and may thus represent a real advance in the management of patients with this disease.

Specific Malignancies

III

Palliative Management of Patients with Advanced Disease

Modern approaches to surgical management of pancreatic carcinoma and the use of adjuvant therapy have made pancreatic resection safer and more effective. Such therapy has resulted in significant extension of survival for many patients. However, long-term eradication of disease is still the exception among patients with pancreatic carcinoma undergoing attempted curative resection. Furthermore, only 10% to 20% of patients with pancreatic carcinoma are first seen at an early enough stage to be eligible for resection. Thus the vast majority of patients with pancreatic cancer either have advanced disease, or it develops in the setting of tumor recurrence. For physicians involved in the palliative management of patients with advanced pancreatic cancer, a number of important issues must be addressed.

Palliation of Pain

Advanced pancreatic cancer can be extremely painful, and most patients experience moderate or severe pain in the course of their illness. Pancreatic malignancies commonly invade neural and perineural tissues. Invasion of neural structures in the retroperitoneum by the growing pancreatic tumor mass is associated with a steady, unrelenting pain, which can be psychologically devastating. In the management of such patients, important aspects include the use of long-acting analgesics in appropriate doses and consideration for celiac plexus ablation. Whereas the use of long-acting oral or topical narcotic preparations should be well understood by all physicians that care for patients with advanced cancer, the use of celiac plexus blockade is less often appreciated.

Probably the best study of celiac plexus ablation was performed by Lillemoe and colleagues.[123] They randomized patients with unresectable disease, who were undergoing laparotomy for palliative biliary and gastric bypass, to receive injections of either 50% alcohol or saline into the celiac ganglia bilaterally. The study was carried out in a double-blind, prospective fashion, and outcomes of interest included pain, narcotic use, and survival among treated patients. This study convincingly demonstrated that patients undergoing chemical splanchnicectomy had significant relief of pain and required less narcotic use than did patients receiving saline. The benefit of such therapy appeared to last for 4 to 6 months. In the subset of patients with moderate to severe pain at the time of treatment, a statistically significant survival advantage was seen among those treated with alcohol injection. Celiac plexus block can be easily and safely performed at the time of a palliative surgical bypass procedure, and it also can be performed percutaneously, with or without CT guidance, in patients who have no other indication for laparotomy.

Palliation of Jaundice

Most patients with tumors of the periampullary region are first seen with jaundice. Although pancreaticoduodenectomy is an effective method of relieving jaundice, most patients have disease too extensive for attempted curative surgical resection. Multiple approaches exist to the management of jaundice in such patients, including endoscopic and percutaneous biliary stent placement and surgical biliary bypass. Several trials compared surgical with nonsurgical approaches to biliary tract obstruction.[124] In general, these trials demonstrated a lower initial morbidity among those undergoing nonoperative stenting. However, the stent-occlusion rates were significantly higher than the failure rates of surgical biliary bypass, resulting in more frequent bouts of cholangitis and the need for multiple procedures over time in patients managed nonoperatively.

The greater long-term morbidity among stented patients was thought to be approximately equivalent to the greater short-term morbidity among patients undergoing surgical bypass, leading to the conclusion that the treatments were approximately equivalent. It has been suggested that patients with a relatively short life expectancy due to extensive disease, and those with increased operative risk due to other medical problems, might be best managed with biliary stenting. In contrast, patients thought to have less extensive disease and to be reasonable operative candidates might benefit more from surgical biliary bypass.[124]

The development of expandable wall stents has changed this treatment algorithm. Wall stents can be placed endoscopically or percutaneously, but unlike older stent technology, wall stents have a significantly longer time to stent failure. In one recent study, it was demonstrated that the stent occlusion rate among patients receiving wall stents was less than 30% at 10 months.[125] Because the median survival of patients with advanced pancreatic cancer ranges from 4 to 8 months and rarely exceeds 1 year, most patients receiving a wall stent will be adequately palliated for life. The rare patients who outlive the functional life of a wall stent can generally be restented by endoscopic or percutaneous techniques. Our practice, therefore, is to spare patients with unresectable pancreatic tumors the morbidity and mortality of surgical biliary bypass in favor of wall stent placement.

It is worth noting that, at times, surgical biliary bypass is preferred. The most common is when a patient undergoing laparotomy for attempted curative resection is found to have unresectable disease. In such cases, it is our practice to perform surgical gastric and biliary bypass as well as an intraoperative chemical splanchnicectomy. Another group of patients who benefit from surgical biliary bypass are those with duodenal obstruction at the time of diagnosis. Such patients generally require laparotomy for creation of a gastrojejunostomy and should have a surgical biliary bypass under the same anesthetic. The precise type of biliary bypass created is largely a choice of the operating surgeon. Choledochojejunostomy to a defunctionalized jejunal loop is the preferred approach to surgical biliary bypass, but cholecystojejunostomy may be an acceptable alternative, except in cases in which the tumor is encroaching on the cystic duct.

Palliation of Gastric Outlet Obstruction

Approximately 15% of patients with periampullary tumors have symptoms of gastric outlet obstruction at the time of diagnosis, and in another 20% to 30% of patients, symptomatic duodenal obstruction will develop in the course of their disease. Surgical gastrojejunostomy is the preferred approach to palliating such patients. When carcinomatosis involving the small bowel also is present, it is our practice to place a gastrostomy tube along with performing surgical bypass of the gastric and/or intestinal obstruction. In patients with carcinomatosis, almost invariably, a reobstruction forms in a matter of weeks, and the presence of a gastrostomy tube can greatly facilitate terminal care by avoiding the need for nasogastric suction in most patients.

SUMMARY

Pancreatic cancer is a particularly virulent neoplasm. Most patients are first seen with disease that is too advanced to permit an attempt at curative resection, and in most patients who undergo resection, tumor will eventually recur. Radiation and chemotherapy are of only modest benefit in extending survival in patients with unresectable tumors. However, a number of advances have been made, including enhanced understanding of the molecular mechanisms leading to pancreatic carcinogenesis, improvements in staging, optimization of surgical techniques, and improvements in adjuvant therapy for patients with resectable disease and a focus on effective palliation for patients with more advanced disease. It is hoped that our understanding of molecular mechanisms will lead to the development of more effective targeted therapeutics for the treatment of patients with this disease.

SUGGESTED READINGS

1. Howe GR: Epidemiology of cancer of the pancreas. In Cameron JL (ed): Pancreatic Cancer London, BC Decker, 2001, pp 1-12.
2. Bell RH Jr: Neoplasms of the exocrine pancreas. In Bell RH, Rikkers LF, Mulholland MW (eds): Digestive Tract Surgery: A Text and Atlas. Philadelphia: Lippincott-Raven Publishers, 1996, pp 849-878.
3. Drebin JA, Strasberg SM: Carcinoma of the pancreas and tumors of the periampullary region. In Winchester DP, Jones RS, Murphy GP (eds): Cancer Surgery for the General Surgeon. Philadelphia, Lippincott Williams & Wilkins, 1999, pp 195-211.
4. Parkin DM, Muir CS, Whelan SL, et al: Cancer incidence in five continents, Vol VI. Lyon, International Agency for Research on Cancer, 1992, p 301.
5. Akoi K, Ogawa H: Cancer of the pancreas: International mortality trends. World Health Stat Q 1978;31(1):2-27.
6. Fuchs CS, Colditz GA, Stampfer MJ, et al: A prospective study of cigarette smoking and the risk of pancreatic cancer. Arch Intern Med 1996;156(19):2255-2260.
7. Ahlgren JD: Epidemiology and risk factors in pancreatic cancer. Semin Oncol 1996;23(2):241-250.
8. Lowenfels AB, Maisonneuve P, Cavallini G, et al: Pancreatitis and the risk of pancreatic cancer. International Pancreatitis Study Group. N Engl J Med 1993;328(20):1433-1437.
9. Gullo L, Pezzilli R, Morselli-Labate AM: Diabetes and the risk of pancreatic cancer. Italian Pancreatic Cancer Study Group. N Engl J Med 1994;331(2):81-84.
10. Zheng W, McLaughlin JK, Gridley G, et al: A cohort study of smoking, alcohol consumption and dietary factors for pancreatic cancer. Cancer Causes Control 1993;4:477-482.
11. Kalapothaki V, Tzonou A, Hsieh CC, Toupadaki N, Karakatsani A, Trichopoulos D: Tobacco, ethanol, coffee, pancreatitis, diabetes mellitus, and cholelithiasis as risk factors for pancreatic carcinoma. Cancer Causes Control 1993;4:375-382.
12. Friedman GC, Van den Eeden SK: Risk factors for pancreatic cancer: An exploratory study. Int J Epidemiol 1993;22:30-37.
13. Kahn H: The Dorn study of smoking and mortality among U.S. veterans: Report on eight and one-half years of observation. Natl Cancer Inst Monogr 1966;19:1-125.
14. Chyou PH, Nomura AM, Stemmermann GN: A prospective study on the attributable risk of cancer due to cigarette smoking. Am J Public Health 1992;82:37-40.
15. Lyon JL, Mahoney AW, French TK, Moser R Jr: Coffee consumption and the risk of cancer of the exocrine pancreas: A case control study in a low-risk population. Epidemiology 1992;3:164-170.
16. Adami HO, McLaughlin JK, Hsing AW, et al: Alcoholism and cancer risk: A population-based cohort study. Cancer Causes Control 1992;3:419-425.
17. Kato I, Nomura AM, Stemmermann GN, Chyou PH: Prospective study of the association of alcohol with cancer of the upper aerodigestive tract and other sites. Cancer Causes Control 1992;3:145-151.
18. Bueno de Mesquita HG, Maisonneuve P, Moerman CJ, Runia S, Boyle P: Lifetime consumption of alcoholic beverages, tea and coffee and exocrine carcinoma of the pancreas: A population-based case-control study in the Netherlands. Int J Cancer 1992;50:514-522.
19. Gold EB, Goldin SB: Epidemiology of and risk factors for pancreatic cancer. Surg Oncol Clin North Am 1998;7:67-91.
20. Mack TM, Peters JM, Yu MC, Hanisch R, Wright WE, Henderson BE: Pancreas cancer is unrelated to the workplace in Los Angeles. Am J Ind Med 1985;7:253-266.
21. Gold EB, Gordis L, Diener MD, et al: Diet and other risk factors for cancer of the pancreas. Cancer 1985;55:460-467.
22. Kalapothaki V, Tzonou A, Hseih CC, et al: Nutrient intake and cancer of the pancreas: A case-control study in Athens, Greece. Cancer Causes Control 1993;4:383-389.
23. Olsen GW, Mandel JS, Gibson RW, Wattenburg LN, Schuman LM: Nutrients and pancreatic cancer: a population-based case-control study. Cancer Causes Control 1991;2:291-297.
24. Mack TM, Yu MC, Hanisch R, Henderson BE: Pancreas cancer and smoking, beverage consumption and past medical history. J Natl Cancer Inst 1986;76:49-60.
25. Hsing AW, Hansson LE, McLaughlin JK, et al: Pernicious anemia and subsequent cancer: A population-based cohort study. Cancer 1993;71:745-750.
26. Wilenitz RE, Hruban RH: Pathology of pancreatic cancer. In Cameron JL (ed): Pancreatic Cancer. London, B.C. Decker, 2001, pp 37-66.
27. Fong Y, Blumgart LH, Lin E, Fortner JG, Brennan MF: Outcome of treatment for distal bile duct cancer. Br J Surg 1996;83(12):1712-1715.
28. Rose DM, Hochwald SN, Klimstra DS, Brennan M: Primary duodenal adenocarcinoma: A ten-year experience with 79 patients. J Am Coll Surg 1996;183(2):89-96.
29. Talamini MA, Moesinger RC, Pitt HA, et al: Adenocarcinoma of the ampulla of Vater. A 28-year experience. Ann Surg 1977;225:590-599.
30. Lillemoe KD, Cameron JL, Yeo CJ, Taylor AS, Nakeeb A, et al: Pancreaticoduodenectomy. Does it have a role in the palliation of pancreatic cancer? Ann Surg 1996;223:718-725; discussion 725-728.
31. Howard JM: Pancreaticoduodenectomy (Whipple resection) with resection of hepatic metastases for carcinoma of the exocrine pancreas. Arch Surg 1997;132:1044.
32. Kern SE, Hruban RH: Molecular genetics of adenocarcinoma of the pancreas. In Cameron JL (ed): Pancreatic Cancer. London, B.C. Decker, 2001, pp 13-24.
33. Almoguera C, Shibata D, Forrester K, Martin J, Arnheim N, Perucho M: Most human carcinomas of the exocrine pancreas contain mutant c-K-ras genes. Cell 1988;53:549-554.
34. Day JD, Digiuseppe JA, Yeo C, et al: Immunohistochemical evaluation of HER-2/neu expression in pancreatic adenocarcinoma and pancreatic intraepithelial neoplasms. Hum Pathol 1996;27(2):119-124.

35. Abbruzzese JL, Evans DB, Raijman I, et al: Detection of mutated c-Ki-ras in the bile of patients with pancreatic cancer. Anticancer Res 1997;17(2A):795–801.

36. Caldas C, Hahn SA, da Costa LT, et al: Frequent somatic mutations and homozygous deletions of the p16 (MTS1) gene in pancreatic adenocarcinoma. Nat Genet 1994;8:27–32.

37. Redston MS, Caldas C, Seymour AB, et al: p53 mutations in pancreatic carcinoma and evidence of common involvement of homocopolymer tracts in DNA microdeletions. Cancer Res 1994;54(11):3025–3033.

38. Goldstein AM, Fraser MC, Struewing JP, et al: Increased risk of pancreatic cancer in melanoma-prone kindreds with p16INK4 mutations. N Engl J Med 1995;333(15):970–974.

39. Hruban RH, Offerhaus GJA, Kern SE: Familial pancreatic cancer. In Cameron JL (ed): Pancreatic Cancer. London, B.C. Decker, 2001, pp 25–36.

40. Kern SE: Advances from genetic clues in pancreatic cancer. Curr Opin Oncol 1998;10:74–80.

41. Kasperk RK, Riesener KP, Wilms K, Schumpelick V: Limited value of positron emission tomography in treatment of pancreatic cancer: Surgeon's view. World J Surg 2001;25(9):1134–1139.

42. Kalady MF, Clary BM, Clark LA, et al: Clinical utility of positron emission tomography in the diagnosis and management of periampullary neoplasms. Ann Surg Onc 2002;9(8):799–806.

43. Warshaw AL: Implications of peritoneal cytology for staging of early pancreatic cancer. Am J Surg 1991;161:26–30.

44. Pitt HA, Gomes AS, Lois JF, Mann LL, Deutsch LS, Longmire WP Jr: Does preoperative percutaneous biliary drainage reduce operative risk or increase hospital cost? Ann Surg 1985;201:545–553.

45. Lygidakis NJ, van der Heyde MN, Lubbers NJ: An evaluation of preoperative biliary drainage in the surgical management of pancreatic head carcinoma. Acta Chir Scand 1987;153:665–668.

46. Lai ECS, Mok, FPT, Fan ST, et al: Preoperative endoscopic drainage for malignant obstructive jaundice. Br J Surg 1994;81:1195–1198.

47. Povoski SP, Karpeh MS Jr., Conlon KC, et al: Association of preoperative biliary drainage with postoperative outcome following pancreaticoduodenectomy. Ann Surg 1999;23(2):131–142.

48. Safi F, Roscher R, Beger HG: The clinical relevance of the tumor marker CA 19-9 in the diagnosing and monitoring of pancreatic carcinoma. Bull Cancer 1990;77:83–91.

49. Lewandrowski KB, Southern JF, Pins MR, Compton CC, Warshaw AL: Cyst fluid analysis in the differential diagnosis of pancreatic cysts: A comparison of pseudocysts, serous cystadenomas, mucinous cystic neoplasms and mucinous cystadenocarcinoma. Ann Surg 1993;217(1):41–47.

50. Yang JM, Southern JF, Warshaw AL, Lewandrowski KG: Proliferation tissue polypeptide antigen distinguishes malignant mucinous cystadenocarcinomas from benign cystic tumors and pseudocysts. Am J Surg 1996;171(1):126–129.

51. John TG, Greig JD, Carter DC, Garden OJ: Carcinoma of the pancreatic head and periampullary region: Tumor staging with laparoscopy and laparoscopic ultrasound. Ann Surg 1995;221:165–170.

52. Callery MP, Strasberg SM, Doherty GM, Soper NJ, Norton JA: Staging laparoscopy with laparoscopic ultrasonography: Optimizing resectability in hepatobiliary and pancreatic malignancy. J Am Coll Surg 1997;185(1):33–39.

53. Conlon KC, Dougherty E, Klimstra DS, Coit DG, Turnbull AD, Brennan MF: The value of minimal access surgery in the staging of patients with potentially resectable peripancreatic malignancy. Ann Surg 1996;223:134–140.

54. Vollmer C, Drebin JA, Middleton WD, et al: Utility of staging laparoscopy in subsets of peripancreatic and biliary malignancies. Ann Surg 2002;235:1–7.

55. Whipple AO, Parsons WB, Mullins CR: Treatment of carcinoma of the ampulla of Vater. Ann Surg 1935;102:763–776.

56. Trimble IR, Parsons JW, Sherman CP: A one-stage operation for the cure of carcinoma of the ampulla of Vater and head of the pancreas. Surg Gynecol Obstet 1941;73:711–722.

57. Shapiro TM: Adenocarcinoma of the pancreas: A statistical analysis of bypass vs. Whipple resection in good risk patients. Ann Surg 1975;182:715–721.

58. Crile G: The advantages of bypass operations over radical pancreatoduodenectomy in the treatment of pancreatic carcinoma. Surg Gynecol Obstet 1970;130:1049–1053.

59. Hertzberg J: Pancreatico-duodenal resection and by-pass operation in patients with carcinoma of the head of the pancreas, ampulla, and distal end of the common duct. Acta Chir Scand 1974;140:523–527.

60. Strasberg SM, Drebin JA, Soper NJ: Evolution and current status of the Whipple procedure: An update for gastroenterologists. Gastroenterology 1997;113:983–994.

61. Gordon TA, Burleyson GP, Tielsch JM, Cameron JL: The effects of regionalization on cost and outcome for one general high-risk surgical procedure. Ann Surg 221(1): 1995;43–49.

62. Lieberman MD, Kilburn H, Lindsey M, Brennan MF: Relation of perioperative deaths to hospital volume among patients undergoing pancreatic resection for malignancy. Ann Surg 1995;222:638–645.

63. Birkmeyer JD, Siewers AE, Finlayson EV, et al: Hospital volume and surgical mortality in the United States. N Engl J Med 2002;346(15):1128–1137, 2002.

64. Birkmeyer JD, Stukel TA, Siewers AE, Goodney PP, Wennberg DE, Lucas FL: Surgeon volume and operative mortality in the United States. N Engl J Med 2003;349(22):2117–2127.

65. Cullen JJ, Sarr MG, Ilstrup DM: Pancreatic anastomotic leak after pancreaticoduodenectomy: Incidence, significance and management. Am J Surg 1994;168:295–298.

66. Warshaw AL, Torchiana DL: Delayed gastric emptying after pylorus preserving pancreaticoduodenectomy. Surg Gynecol Obstet 1985;160:1–4.

67. Stojadinovic A, Hoos A, Brennan MF, Conlon KC: Randomized clinical trials in pancreatic cancer. Surg Onc Clin N Am 2002;11(1):207–229.

68. Yeo CJ, Barry MK, Sauter PK, et al: Erythromycin accelerates gastric emptying after pancreaticoduodenectomy. Ann Surg 1993;218:229–238.

69. Gudjonsson G: Carcinoma of the pancreas: Critical analysis of costs, results of resections, and the need for standardized reporting. J Am Coll Surg 1995;181:483–503.

70. Yeo CJ, Cameron JL, Lillemoe KD, et al: Pancreaticoduodenectomy for cancer of the head of the pancreas. 201 patients. Ann Surg 1995;221(6):721–731; discussion 731–733.

71. Trede M, Schwall G, Saeger HD: Survival after pancreatoduodenectomy. 118 consecutive resections without an operative mortality. Ann Surg 1990;21(4):447–458.

72. Janes RH Jr, Niederhuber JE, Chmiel JS, et al: National patterns of care for pancreatic cancer. Results of a survey by the Commission on Cancer. Ann Surg 1996; 223:261–272.

73. VanHeerden JA, McIlrath DC, Ilstrup DM, Weiland LH: Total pancreatectomy for ductal adenocarcinoma of the pancreas: An update. World J Surg 1988;12:658–662.

74. Brooks JR, Brooks DC, Levine JD: Total pancreatectomy for ductal cell carcinoma of the pancreas. Ann Surg 1989;209:405–410.

75. Kloppel G, Lohse T, Bosslet K, Ruckert K: Ductal adenocarcinoma of the head of the pancreas: Incidence of tumor involvement beyond the Whipple resection line. Pancreas 1987;2:170–175.

76. Cubilla AL, Fortner J, Fitzgerald, PJ: Lymph node involvement in carcinoma of the pancreas area. Cancer 1978;41:880–887.

77. Yeo CJ, Cameron JL, Maher MM, et al: A prospective randomized trial of pancreaticogastrostomy versus pancreaticojejunostomy after pancreaticoduodenectomy. Ann Surg 1995;222(4):580–588; discussion 588–592.

78. Fortner JG: Regional pancreatectomy for cancer of the pancreas, ampulla, and other related sites. Ann Surg 1984;199:418–425.

79. Fortner JG, Klimstra DS, Senie RT, Maclean BJ: Tumor size is the primary prognosticator for pancreatic cancer after regional pancreatectomy. Ann Surg 1996;223:147–153.

80. Sindelar WF: Clinical experience with regional pancreatectomy for adenocarcinoma of the pancreas. Arch Surg 1989;124:127–132.

81. Johnstone PA, Sindelar WF: Patterns of disease recurrence following definitive therapy of adenocarcinoma of the pancreas using surgery and adjuvant radiotherapy: Correlations of a clinical trial. Int J Radiat Oncol Biol Phys 1993;27:831–834.

82. Cameron JL, Crist DW, Sitzmann JV et al: Factors influencing

survival after pancreaticoduodenectomy for pancreatic cancer. Am J Surg 1991;161:120-124; discussion 124-125.

83. Furukawa H, Kosuge T, Mukai K, et al: Helical computed tomography in the diagnosis of portal vein invasion by pancreatic head carcinoma. Arch Surg 1998;133:61-65.

84. Fuhrman GM, Leach SD, Staley CA, et al: Rationale for en bloc vein resection in the treatment of pancreatic adenocarcinoma adherent to the superior mesenteric-portal vein confluence. Ann Surg 1996;223:154-162.

85. Harrison LE, Klimstra DS, Brennan MF: Isolated portal vein involvement in pancreatic adenocarcinoma. A contraindication for resection? Ann Surg 1996;224(3):342-347.

86. Pedrazzoli S, DiCarlo V, Dionigi R, et al: Standard versus extended lymphadenectomy associated with pancreatoduodenectomy in the surgical treatment of adenocarcinoma of the head of the pancreas: A multicenter, prospective, randomized study. Ann Surg 1998;228(4):508-517.

87. Yeo CJ, Cameron JL, Lillemoe KD, et al: Pancreaticoduodenectomy with or without distal gastrectomy and extended retroperitoneal lymphadenectomy for periampullary adenocarcinoma, part 2: Randomized controlled trial evaluating survival, morbidity and mortality. Ann Surg 2002;236(3):355-366.

88. McFadden DW, Reber HA: Cancer of the pancreas: Radical resection—supporting view. Adv Surg 1994;27:257-272.

89. Ishikawa O, Ohhigashi H, Sasaki Y, et al: Practical usefulness of lymphatic and connective tissue clearance for carcinoma of the head of the pancreas. Ann Surg 1988;208:215-220.

90. Satake K, Nishiwaki H, Yokomatsu H, et al: Surgical curability and prognosis for standard versus extended resection for T1 carcinoma of the pancreas. Surg Gynecol Obstet 1992;175:259-265.

91. Yeo CJ, Cameron JL: Arguments against radical (extended) resection for adenocarcinoma of the pancreas. Adv Surg 1994;27:273-284.

92. Traverso LW, Longmire WP: Preservation of the pylorus in pancreaticoduodenectomy. Surg Gynecol Obstet 1978;146: 959-962.

93. Williamson RC, Bliouras N, Cooper MJ, Davies ER: Gastric emptying and enterogastric reflux after conservative and conventional pancreatoduodenectomy. Surgery 1993;114(1):82-86.

94. Howard JM: Pancreatojejunostomy: Leakage is a preventable complication of the Whipple resection. J Am Coll Surg 1997;184:454-457.

95. Strasberg SM, Drebin JA, Mokadam NA, et al: Prospective trial of a blood supply-based technique of pancreaticojejunostomy: Effect on anastomotic failure in the Whipple procedure. J Am Coll Surg 2002;194:746-758; discussion 759-760.

96. Peng S, Mou Y, Cai X, Peng C: Binding pancreaticojejunostomy is a new technique to minimize leakage. Am J Surg 2002;183(3): 283-285.

97. Montorsi M, Zago M, Mosca F, et al: Efficacy of octreotide in the prevention of pancreatic fistula after elective pancreatic resections: A prospective, controlled, randomized clinical trial. Surgery 1995;117(1):26-31.

98. Friess H, Berger HG, Sulkowski U, et al: Randomized controlled multicentre study of the prevention of complications by octreo-tide in patients undergoing surgery for chronic pancreatitis. Br J Surg 1995;82(9):1270-1273 [erratum 1996;83(1):126].

99. Lowy AM, Lee JE, Pisters PW, et al: Prospective, randomized trial of octreotide to prevent pancreatic fistula after pancreatico-duodenectomy for malignant disease. Ann Surg 1997;226(5): 632-641.

100. Yeo CJ, Cameron JL, Lillemoe KD, et al: Does prophylactic octreotide decrease the rates of pancreatic fistula and other complications after pancreaticoduodenectomy? Results of a prospective randomized placebo-controlled trial. Ann Surg 2000;232(3):419-429.

101. Brennan MF, Moccia RD, Klimstra D: Management of adeno-carcinoma of the body and tail of the pancreas. Ann Surg 1996;223(5):506-511.

102. Nordback IH, Hruban RH, Boitnott JK, Pitt HA, Cameron JL: Carcinoma of the body and tail of the pancreas. Am J Surg 164:26-31, 1992.

103. Strasberg SM, Drebin JA, Linehan DL: Radical antegrade modular pancreatosplenectomy. Surgery 2003;133:521-527.

104. Kalser MH, Ellenberg SS: Pancreatic cancer: Adjuvant combined radiation and chemotherapy following curative resection. Arch Surg 1985;120:899-903.

105. Gastrointestinal Tumor Study Group: Further evidence of effective adjuvant combined radiation and chemotherapy following curative resection of pancreatic cancer. Cancer 1987;59: 2006-2010.

106. Yeo CJ, Cameron JL, Sohn TA, et al: Six hundred fifty consecutive pancreaticoduodenectomies in the 1990s: Pathology, complications, outcomes. Ann Surg 1997;226:248-260.

107. Neoptolemos JP, Dunn JA, Stocken DD, et al: Adjuvant chemoradiotherapy and chemotherapy in resectable pancreatic cancer: A randomised controlled trial. Lancet 2001;358: 1576-1585.

108. Picozzi VJ, Kozarek RA, Traverso LW: Interferon-based adjuvant chemoradiation therapy after pancreaticoduodenectomy for pancreatic adenocarcinoma. Am J Surg 2003;185(5):476-480.

109. Spitz FR, Abbruzzese JL, Lee JE, et al: Preoperative and postoperative chemoradiation strategies in patients treated with pancreaticoduodenectomy for adenocarcinoma of the pancreas. J Clin Oncol 1997;15(3):928-937.

110. Hoffman JP, Lipsitz S, Pisansky T, Weese JL, Solin L, Benson AB 3rd: Phase II trial of preoperative radiation therapy and chemotherapy for patients with localized, resectable adenocarcinoma of the pancreas: an eastern cooperative oncology group study. J Clin Oncol 1997;16:317-323.

111. Coia L, Hoffman J, Scher R, et al: Preoperative chemoradiation for adenocarcinoma of the pancreas and duodenum. Int J Rad Onc Biol Phys 1994;30(1):161-167.

112. White RR, Hurwitz HI, Morse MA, et al: Neoadjuvant chemoradiation for localized adenocarcinoma of the pancreas. Ann Surg Oncol 2001;8(10):758-765.

113. Bastidas JA, Poen JC, Niederhuber JE: Pancreas. In Abeloff MD, Armitage JA, Lichter AS, Niederhuber JE (eds): Clinical Oncology, 2nd ed, Philadelphia, Churchill Livingstone, 2000, pp 1749-1783.

114. Gotoh M, Monden M, Sakon M, et al: Intraoperative irradiation in resected carcinoma of the pancreas and portal vein. Arch Surg 1992;127:1213-1215.

115. Staley CA, Lee JE, Cleary KR, et al: Preoperative chemoradiation, pancreaticoduodenectomy, and intraoperative radiation therapy for adenocarcinoma of the pancreatic head. Am J Surg 1996;171:118-124; discussion124-125.

116. Hiraoka T, Uchino R, Kanemitsu K, et al: Combination of intraoperative radiation with resection of the cancer of the pancreas. Int J Pancreatol 1990;7:201-207.

117. Zerbi A, Fossati V, Parolini D, et al: Intraoperative radiation therapy adjuvant to resection in the treatment of pancreatic cancer. Cancer 1994;73:2930-2935.

118. Blackstock AW, Cox AD, Tepper JE: Treatment of pancreatic cancer: Current limitations, future possibilities. Oncology 1996;10:301-307; discussion 308-323.

119. el Kamar FG, Grossbard ML, Kozuch PS: Metastatic pancreatic cancer: Emerging strategies in chemotherapy and palliative care. Oncologist 2003;8:18-34.

120. Burris HA 3rd, Moore MJ, Andersen J, et al: Improvement in survival and clinical benefit with gemcitabine as first-line therapy for patients with advanced pancreatic cancer: A randomized trial. J Clin Oncol 1997;15:2403-2413.

121. Tempero M, Plunkett W, Ruiz Van Haperen V, et al: Randomized phase II comparison of dose-intense gemcitabine: Thirty-minute infusion and fixed dose rate infusion in patients with pancreatic adenocarcinoma. J Clin Onc 2003;21(18):3402-3408.

122. Von Hoff DD, Bearss D: New drugs for patients with pancreatic cancer. Curr Opin Oncol 2002;14:621-627.

123. Lillemoe KD, Cameron JL, Kaufman HS, Yeo CIJ, Pitt HA, Sauter PK: Chemical splanchnicectomy in patients with unresectable pancreatic cancer: a prospective randomized trial. Ann Surg 1993;217:447-455; discussion 456-457.

124. Lillemoe KD, Pitt HA: Palliation: Surgical and otherwise. Cancer 1996;78(3 Suppl):605-614.

125. Neuhaus H, Hagenmuller F, Griebel M, Classen M: Percutaneous cholangioscopic or transpapillary insertion of self-expanding biliary metal stents. Gastrointest Enodsc 1991;7(1):31-37.

Specific Malignancies

III

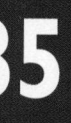 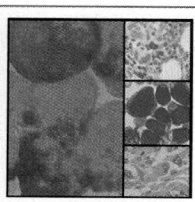

35

Wayne B. Harris

Jonathan W. Simons

KIDNEY AND URETER

SUMMARY OF KEY POINTS

RENAL CELL CARCINOMA

Incidence
- More than 30,000 new cases of adenocarcinoma of the kidney in the United States.
- Histologic classifications: clear cell (conventional), chromophobe (granular), papillary, sarcomatoid, mixed histology.

Differential Diagnosis
Renal cyst, renal adenoma, angiomyolipoma, oncocytoma and other benign tumors, xanthogranulomatous pyelonephritis, renal infarct, and metastasis from a distant primary.

Staging Evaluation
Staging requires a complete history and physical examination, hemogram, chemistries. Radiologic procedures potentially include intravenous pyelogram (IVP), sonogram, magnetic resonance imaging (MRI), and computed tomography (CT) scan of the thorax and abdomen.

Primary Therapy
- Radical nephrectomy (open or laparoscopic).
- High-dose interleukin-2 (IL-2) or subcutaneous interferon-α ± IL-2.
- Thalidomide.
- Investigational strategies including immunotherapy (e.g., cytokine, gene and vaccine therapies), antiangiogenesis, or cytotoxic therapies.

INTRODUCTION

Renal cell carcinoma (RCC) accounts for about 2% of adult malignancies. Tumors that arise in the kidney exhibit a variety of histologic patterns that may be benign or malignant. Some benign tumors of the kidney such as oncocytomas may be confused with RCC. Other tumors of benign histology include angiomyolipomas, fibromas, lipomas, lymphangiomas, and hemangiomas.

Historically, RCC was widely known as *hypernephroma*. The term was coined by Grawitz in 1883 and reflected his belief that these tumors arise from the adrenal gland. Although some continue to use the term *hypernephroma*, the appropriate description of the most common type of kidney cancer is *renal cell adenocarcinoma*.

RCC exists in sporadic and hereditary forms. The sporadic form of the disease usually is first seen in the fifth decade or later in life. It has been said that RCC often appears clinically with a classic triad of symptoms that include hematuria, flank pain, and an abdominal mass. This clinical presentation is the exception rather than the rule, however, with an increasing numbers of tumors being detected incidentally while imaging the abdomen for other clinical indications. The uncommon familial forms of RCC are seen in disorders such as von Hippel-Lindau (VHL) disease and tuberous sclerosis.

RISK FACTORS FOR SPORADIC RENAL CELL ADENOCARCINOMA: SMOKING, OBESITY, AND HYPERTENSION

Smoking, obesity, and hypertension have been shown to be independent risk factors for kidney cancer.[1] This is the conclusion of a large study of 363,992 Swedish men who received at least one physical examination between 1971 and 1992 and who were followed up until death or until the end of 1995. Fifty-two percent of the men were current or former smokers. The mean body mass index (BMI) for all men was 24.5 ± 3.1, with a mean systolic blood pressure of 140 ± 18 mm Hg and a mean diastolic pressure of 84 ± 13 mm Hg. Seven hundred fifty-nine cases of RCC were diagnosed during the follow-up period and 136 cases of renal pelvis cancer.

The relative risk [with 95% confidence intervals (CIs)] for RCC was 1.3 (CI, 1.0 to 1.6) for former smokers and 1.6 (CI, 1.3 to 1.9) for current smokers. The relative risk for renal pelvis cancer was even higher at 1.6 (CI, 0.9 to 3.1) for former smokers and 3.5 (CI, 2.1 to 5.8) for current smokers. With regard to obesity, patients with a BMI in the highest eighth of the cohort had a relative risk of 1.9 (CI, 1.3 to 2.7) when compared with the leanest subgroup. Hypertension was confirmed as a third risk factor for RCC. A clear dose-response relation was identified for the diastolic pressure, but not for the systolic. The risk of RCC for men with a diastolic pressure of 90 mm Hg or more was more than double the risk for men with a diastolic pressure of less than 70 mm Hg. No increased risk for renal pelvis cancer was identified for either BMI or hypertension. The most consistently reported occupational risk factor for RCC is asbestos exposure; however, current environmental regulations have made this a risk factor of diminishing importance.[2,3]

Patients with end-stage renal disease (ESRD) have an increased incidence of RCC when compared with the general population. Patients receiving prolonged dialysis tend to develop acquired renal cystic disease (ARCD), possibly as a result of disordered proliferation within the native kidney. In these patients, the tumors are often bilateral and multifocal, with a papillary histology.[4] For this reason, these patients should be monitored regularly with renal ultrasound. Bilateral nephrectomy should be performed in patients with ESRD who are diagnosed with RCC.

INCIDENCE OF RENAL CELL CARCINOMA

The incidence of RCC is increasing in the United States. The increasing incidence of RCC has been attributed to the widespread use of imaging modalities such as computed tomography, ultrasonography, and magnetic resonance.[5] A parallel worldwide increase has occurred in kidney cancer.[6] This conclusion is supported by data from a multinational study of 23 ethnic populations including 6 from Asia, 2 from Oceania, 10 from Europe, and 5 from the Americas. Data were included in the study if the source documents were found to be sufficiently complete for analysis, based on a review of selected cancer registries from 20 countries. Sufficient data were not available from Africa and were therefore not analyzed or included in the study. Separate data for renal parenchyma and renal pelvis cancers were available for only 14 of the 23 regions. All rates were age adjusted to the world-standard population. The study spanned five 5-year periods from 1973 to 1992. Percentage changes in incidence rates were computed by using the relative difference between the time periods of 1973 to 1977 and 1988 to 1992. For the 1988 to 1992 time period, the incidence rates were highest in France (16.1/100,000 man-years and 7.3/100,000 woman-years) and lowest in India (2.0 and 0.9, respectively). Rates increased among men and women in all regions and ethnic groups, with few exceptions, mostly in Scandinavian countries. The largest percentage increases were for men in Japan and women in Italy. The incidence trends may result from increases in the prevalence of risk factors and in the use of diagnostic imaging.

The increases in incidentally detected RCC and the associated stage migration falsely lengthen current survival times relative to historic controls. In a single-institution Italian study of 1092 patients, incidental detection of RCC has increased from 13.0% in 1982 to 1983 to 59.2% in 1996 to 1997. A corresponding decrease in stage

was found at the time of diagnosis, grade, and percentage of metastases. Of the patients who underwent conservative surgery, 80.4% (82 of 102 patients) had incidental RCC.[7]

PATHOLOGY

The kidneys' location in the retroperitoneum allows many RCCs to become quite large before clinical detection. The kidney is surrounded by Gerota's fascia, which serves to some degree as a barrier to tumor extension. A pseudocapsule of compressed renal tissue usually surrounds these tumors, with larger tumors frequently showing signs of hemorrhage and necrosis. Cystic areas are often present, representing sites of previous necrosis. The tumors are usually unilateral but may be bilateral in 2% to 4% of cases.[8] These tumors tend to grow into the renal vein and may form a tumor thrombus that extends into the vena cava and even the right atrium. Vascular involvement is present in 4% to 10% of patients at the time of presentation.[9]

Historically, adult RCC was divided into two subtypes: "clear cell carcinoma" and "granular cell carcinoma." The current classification system for renal cortical epithelial neoplasms includes the following categories: conventional (clear cell), chromophobe, papillary, and collecting duct carcinoma.[10] Tumors may be composed of mixed histologic subtypes, and each subtype may feature high-grade sarcomatoid characteristics. Nevertheless, sarcomas, adenomas, and renal medullary carcinomas are not included in this classification system. The conventional histologic pattern is the most common, characterized by large clear cells with abundant cytoplasm. The chromophobe pattern is granular with abundant mitochondria. The papillary or tubulopapillary variant may represent a different type of tumor, because they tend to be smaller with fewer anaplastic features.

The most widely used grading system for RCC is the nuclear grading system developed by Fuhrman and colleagues.[11] This system assigns a grade from I to IV, based on nuclear size, roundness, and other morphologic features such as the prominence of nucleoli and the presence or absence of clumped chromatin. Patients with tumors of high Fuhrman grade tend to have poorer clinical outcomes.

A relatively obscure variant of RCC is the cystic variant, which appears to have a favorable prognosis with surgical resection. Histologic classifications of cystic RCC include RCC with cystic necrosis, multilocular RCC, and unilocular RCC. In a Japanese study of 21 patients with incidentally found cystic RCC, the 5-year disease-specific survival of multilocular cystic RCC ($n = 9$) and RCC with cystic necrosis ($n = 11$) were 100% and 80%, respectively, after radical or partial nephrectomy. Nineteen of 21 cystic tumors were of clear cell or conventional histology.[12]

GENETICS

A molecular signature of RCC is the inactivation of a critical gene on the short arm of chromosome 3.

Figure 85-1. Example of expression profiling of renal epithelial neoplasm with complementary DNA microarrays.

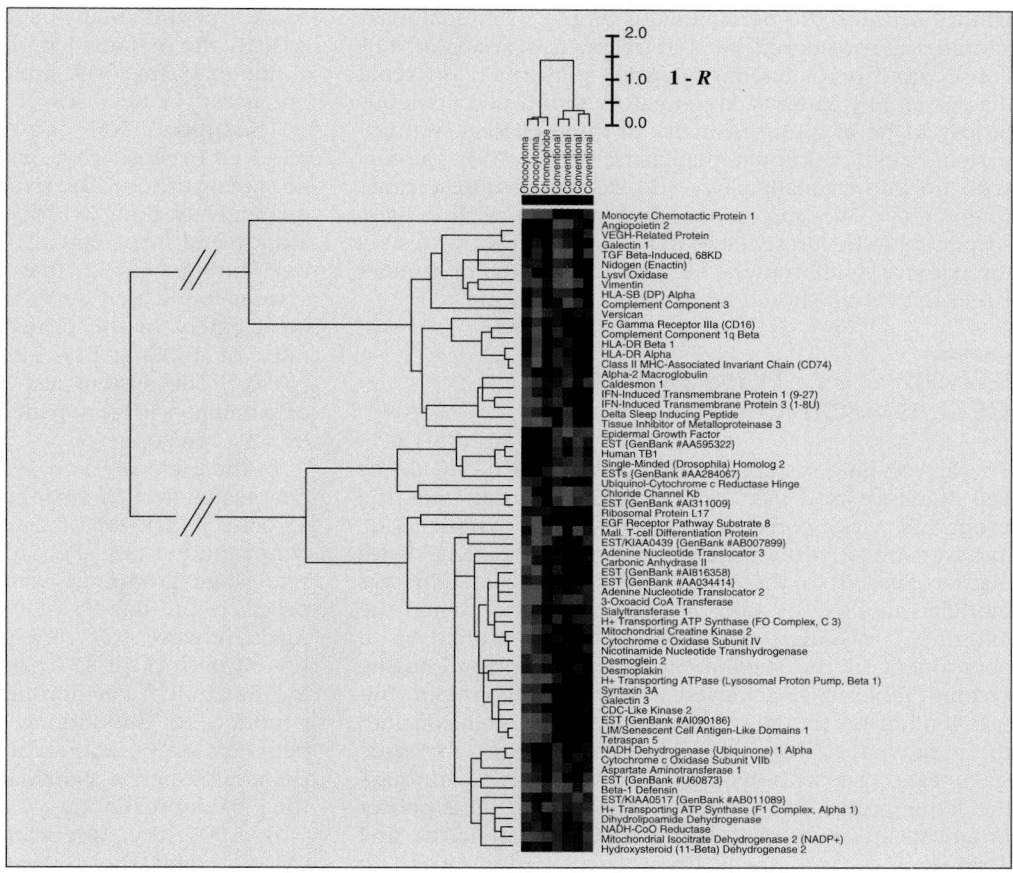

Mutations that inactivate the VHL gene occur in 50% or more of sporadic RCCs and are the cause of hereditary clear cell renal carcinoma. The consequences of VHL mutations are under intensive study and are likely to disclose key pathways in the pathogenesis of kidney cancer. The VHL protein, pVHL, is involved in degrading key proteins in cancer initiation and progression. pVHL normally targets the transcription factor hypoxia-inducible factor-1 (HIF-1 gene) for polyubiquitination and subsequent proteolysis. Mutations in VHL permit abnormal levels of HIF-1 accumulation in the tumor cell. Restoration of pVHL function in VHL(-/-) mutant renal carcinoma cells suppresses their ability to form tumors experimentally by reducing HIF-1 levels. HIF-1 and the genes it regulates in tumor angiogenesis, invasion, and cell survival in hypoxia have become central targets for genetic medicine drug discovery in RCC in the past 3 years.

Analysis of mutations in exon 3 of the VHL gene may be useful in refining the diagnostic criteria for conventional RCC versus chromophobe RCC with clear cells.[13] Single-strand conformational polymorphism (SSCP) has been used to identify mutations in the VHL gene in RCCs of various histologic subtypes. The cohort (*n* = 67) included cases of conventional or clear cell (*n* = 24), chromophobe (*n* = 14), papillary (*n* = 14), and oncocytomas (*n* = 15). Thirteen of the 14 VHL gene mutations identified were novel. Interestingly, no mutations were found in the papillary or oncocytoma subtypes. Mutations in exon 3 appeared to favor conventional RCC with a more aggressive phenotype.

Expression profiling of renal epithelial neoplasms with complementary DNA (cDNA) microarrays also may be used to identify novel molecular markers with potential diagnostic utility (Fig. 85-1). A comparison of the expression profiles of 7075 genes has been reported for four conventional and one chromophobe RCC as well as two oncocytomas.[14] Conventional RCCs were found to underexpress mitochondrial and distal nephron genes and were distinguished from chromophobe RCC and oncocytomas by overexpression of vimentin and class II major histocompatibility complex–associated molecules. Vimentin was found to be a sensitive and specific marker for conventional RCC. Parvalbumin was detected primarily in chromophobe RCC and oncocytomas. Gene-profiling experiments such as these should lead to improvements in the basic understanding of renal tumor pathogenesis.

DIAGNOSIS OF RENAL CELL CARCINOMA

Nephrectomy is the most effective therapy for RCC that is confined to the kidney and should be used both diagnostically and therapeutically in most patients who are candidates for this type of surgery. However, in certain

Specific Malignancies

III

clinical settings, the percutaneous biopsy of a renal mass should be considered. In a retrospective study of 115 consecutive percutaneous biopsies performed on renal masses in 113 patients, investigators found percutaneous biopsy to be of high sensitivity in three clinical settings: patients with a known malignancy (n = 55), patients with no known malignancy and suspected unresectable tumor (n = 36), and nonsurgical patients with a mass suspected to be a resectable RCC (n = 8). Negative results for patients with tumors of 3 cm or smaller or tumors larger than 6 cm should be viewed with caution.[15]

STAGING SYSTEMS FOR RENAL CELL CARCINOMA

The first staging system for RCC was proposed by Flocks and Kadesky in 1958.[16] These authors noted that the prognosis was worse for patients with lymph node involvement or distant metastasis than for patients with disease limited to the kidney. This staging system was modified in 1969 by Robson and colleagues[17] when the extent of vascular involvement was included as a component of the staging process. The Robson staging system (Table 85-1) achieved worldwide recognition but was limited by the fact that tumors with extension into the renal vein or vena cava were grouped into the same stage as those with lymph node metastases, although the latter group was later recognized to have a poorer prognosis. In an effort to address this limitation, the first TNM staging system for RCC was developed in 1978.[18] In the TNM system, tumors are characterized on the basis of the degree of local extension of the tumor at the primary site (T), the involvement of regional lymph nodes (N), and the presence or absence of distant metastases (M). The addition of numbers to each of the TNM components allows one more precisely to categorize the extent of malignant disease at the primary, lymph node, and metastatic sites, respectively. The classification may be clinical (cTNM) or pathological (pTNM). Clinical TNM classification is based on findings at physical examination, imaging, endoscopy, and biopsy. Pathological TNM classification is based on the surgical resection of tissue sufficient to establish the highest pT, pN, and pM

TABLE 85-1

STAGE	FEATURES
Robson Classification of Renal Cell Carcinoma	
I	Tumor is confined to the kidney; perinephric fat, renal vein, and regional nodes show no evidence of malignancy
II	Tumor involves the perinephric fat, but is confined within Gerota's fascia; renal vein and regional nodes show no evidence of malignancy
III	Tumor involves the renal vein or regional nodes, with or without involvement of the vena cava or perinephric fat
IV	Distant metastases secondary to renal cell carcinoma are present at the time of diagnosis, or tumor histologically involves contiguous visceral structures

categories and entails microscopic evaluation. In the case of RCC, the regional lymph nodes are defined as the hilar, abdominal para-aortic, and paracaval nodes. Laterality does not affect N categories.

The initial TNM classification system was not well received because it was cumbersome and used nonspecific staging criteria. The size of the primary was determined qualitatively along with enlargement or deformity of the kidney and involvement of the renal pelvis. A retrospective study (n = 252) that was conducted to validate this system found that survival was most dependent on the local extent of the primary, with 5-year overall survival rates of 100% (pT1), 91% (pT2), 58% (pT3), and 25% (pT4).[19] The system also resulted in poor stratification of patients, with few patients in the pT1 (n = 7) and pT4 (n = 9) categories.

In the 1987 revision of the TNM system, a value of 2.5 cm was chosen to distinguish pT1 from pT2 tumors, and an entirely new set of criteria was introduced to evaluate lymph node status. Perhaps most important, comprehensive stage groupings were introduced to define more precisely the impact of TNM characteristics on survival. Again, however, very few patients were stratified to stage I, with only 11 of 872 patients classified in this category in one study.[20] Furthermore, a study of 337 RCC tumors confined to the kidney found no survival difference between stage I and stage II tumors at the 2.5-cm break point, although a significant difference was identified at the 7.5-cm breakpoint.[21]

In 1997, the American Joint Committee on Cancer (AJCC)[22] and the International Union Against Cancer (UICC)[23] published an updated version of the TNM system. The result of this international collaboration was a more uniform categorization of RCC based on improved clinical evaluation and management. In this version, the breakpoint between pT1 and pT2 was increased from 2.5 cm to 7.0 cm. In addition, the requirement for the T3a classification was more precisely defined as invasion of the adrenal gland by direct extension of the tumor or invasion of perinephric fat. The subcategories of venous tumor extension (pT3) were revised so that venous tumor extension above the diaphragm was classified as T3c, whereas venous tumor extension limited to the vena cava below the diaphragm was classified as T3b. This reflected the decreased adverse prognostic significance of venous tumor extension alone. The classification of lymph node metastasis also was simplified to include involvement of a single lymph node (N1) or multiple lymph nodes (N2), with the stipulation that four to eight nodes should be analyzed before assigning the pN0 classification. An excellent review documents the historical development of staging systems for RCC through 1997.[24]

VALIDATION OF THE 1997 TUMOR-NODE-METASTASIS SYSTEM

In 2002, the AJCC published the sixth edition of the AJCC Cancer Staging Manual.[25] The manual was developed in close collaboration with the UICC to refine further the uniform staging system to bring worldwide consistency to cancer staging. In the case of RCC (Table 85-2), the key change was to subdivide T1 lesions into T1a and T1b. The rationale was based on evidence from studies of patients undergoing partial nephrectomy, a procedure commonly used for tumors that are 4 cm or smaller. It has been reported that patients who receive partial nephrectomy for RCC tumors smaller than 4 cm have equivalent survival to those undergoing radical nephrectomy.[26] In a separate study of 485 patients undergoing nephron-sparing surgery for RCC and a mean follow-up of 47 months, patients were divided into four groups based on the size of the primary.[27] Patients in group 1 (tumors <2.5 cm) and group 2 (tumors 2.5 to 4.0 cm) had equivalent survival, although

TABLE 85-2

The 2002 American Joint Committee on Cancer TNM Classification of Renal Tumors

T, N, M	FEATURES
Primary Tumor (T)	
TX	Primary tumor cannot be assessed
T0	No evidence of primary tumor
T1	Tumor ≤7 cm in greatest dimension, limited to the kidney
T1a	Tumor ≤4 cm in greatest dimension, limited to the kidney
T1b	Tumor >4 cm but ≤7 cm in greatest dimension, limited to the kidney
T2	Tumor >7 cm in greatest dimension, limited to the kidney
T3	Tumor extends into major veins or invades adrenal gland or perinephric tissues but not beyond Gerota's fascia
T3a	Tumor directly invades adrenal gland or perirenal and/or renal sinus fat but not beyond Gerota's fascia
T3b	Tumor grossly extends into the renal vein or its segmental (muscle containing) branches or vena cava below the diaphragm
T3c	Tumor grossly extends into vena cava above diaphragm or invades the wall of the vena cava
T4	Tumor invades beyond Gerota's fascia
Regional Lymph Nodes (N)*	
NX	Regional lymph nodes cannot be assessed
N0	No regional lymph node metastasis
N1	Metastasis in a single regional lymph node
N2	Metastasis in more than one regional lymph node
Distant Metastasis (M)	
MX	Distant metastasis cannot be assessed
M0	No distant metastasis
M1	Distant metastasis
Histopathologic Grading (G)	
GX	Grade of differentiation cannot be assessed
G1	Well differentiated
G2	Moderately differentiated
G3–4	Poorly differentiated/undifferentiated

STAGE	GROUPING		
I	T1a, T1b	N0	M0
II	T2	N0	M0
III	T1	N1	M0
	T2	N1	M0
	T3a, T3b, T3c	N0, N1	M0
IV	T4	N0, N1	M0
	Any T	N2	M0
	Any T	Any N	M1

*Laterality does not affect the N classification.

survival was significantly greater for groups 1 and 2 than for group 3 (tumors 4 to 7 cm) and group 4 (tumors >7 cm). These findings were similar to those previously published in a separate series of 394 patients.[28]

THE NATURAL HISTORY OF RENAL CELL CARCINOMA

Unfortunately, only about 40% of patients with RCC have disease confined to the kidney, and roughly 25% of patients will have metastatic disease at the time of diagnosis. In general, patients with metastatic or recurrent disease have a median survival of approximately 12 to 18 months.

PARANEOPLASTIC SYNDROMES OF RENAL CELL CARCINOMA

The association of RCC with paraneoplastic syndromes is well established. Paraneoplastic erythrocytosis occurs in 3% to 10% of patients with RCC, whereas anemia has been reported in more than 28% of patients.[29] Paraneoplastic erythrocytosis in RCC has been recently defined at the molecular level. The high circulating levels of erythropoietin that drive the syndrome in the bone marrow are derived from direct secretion from the renal cancer cells. These tumors are VHL gene mutated, and thus HIF-1 levels in the tumor are supraphysiologically increased. Normally, HIF-1 is a transcription factor that turns on the expression of the erythropoietin gene by binding to key DNA sequences called hypoxia response elements (HREs) under hypoxia, but in this case, because of the mutation of the VHL gene in the RCC, erythropoietin can be secreted independent of venous oxygen tension or hematocrit. Surgical resection of the VHL mutant primary tumor removes the HIF-1 erythropoietin secretion source and can restore a normal hematocrit.

The pathogenesis of the anemia in RCC is not known, although it is likely multifactorial and does not appear to be related to bleeding or bone marrow replacement by metastasis. Thrombocytosis, defined as any platelet count greater than $400,000/mm^3$, has been associated with decreased cancer-specific survival in patients who have undergone nephrectomy with curative intent for early-stage disease.[30]

Hypercalcemia of malignancy may occur in RCC through a variety of mechanisms including the expression of parathyroid hormone–related protein by the cancer cells (most common), increased local osteolytic activity, and prostaglandin mediation. Nephrectomy ameliorates the hypercalcemia only temporarily in a subgroup of patients.[31]

SURGICAL APPROACHES FOR LOCALIZED DISEASE

Laparoscopic radical nephrectomy has gained popularity in recent years because it is less invasive, resulting in abbreviated periods of convalescence when compared with open surgery. Transabdominal and retroperitoneal approaches have been used in conjunction with removal of an intact, fractionated, or morcellated specimen (dissected into smaller dimensions within a sack-like device). A retrospective Japanese study of 100 patients with tumors smaller than 5 cm in diameter revealed a longer mean operative time (5.2 vs. 3.3 hours; $P < .001$), less mean blood loss (255 vs. 512 mL; $P < .001$), and a shorter time to completion of convalescence (23 vs. 57 days; $P < .001$) for patients treated with laparoscopic radical nephrectomy ($n = 60$) rather than open radical nephrectomy ($n = 40$). No significant difference was found in the 5-year disease-free survival of patients who had laparoscopy (95.5%) and those who underwent open nephrectomy (97.5%).[32]

Cytoreductive radical nephrectomy is commonly performed in patients with metastatic RCC before administering systemic interleukin-2 (IL-2). In this setting, laparoscopic techniques that use tumor morcellation reduce surgical trauma and allow resection of larger tumors. In patients with metastatic disease, the precise delineation of local invasiveness and the possibility of surgically mediated tumor dissemination are not primary concerns. Laparoscopic techniques offer the possibility of lower morbidity and faster recovery, to minimize the delay in starting treatment with high-dose IL-2.

In a pilot study conducted at the National Institutes of Health, patients with metastatic RCC underwent either open radical nephrectomy ($n = 19$) or laparoscopic cytoreductive nephrectomy ($n = 11$). Of the group treated laparoscopically, six tumors were removed with morcellation, and five tumors were removed as intact specimens. The median tumor diameter in this group was 9 cm. Patient characteristics were similar for the patients who had the open procedure or laparoscopy with or without morcellation. The median time to treatment with IL-2 was shortest in the morcellation group (37 days) without evidence of port seeding.[33] These preliminary findings warrant further study.

Hand-assisted laparoscopic radical nephrectomy (HALRN) may minimize the need for conversion to an open procedure or re-exploration. In a retrospective study of 18 HALRNs and 18 open radical nephrectomies, the patients undergoing HALRN had shorter hospital stays, returned to work earlier, and returned to a 100% normal status earlier than patients undergoing open radical nephrectomy, with no open procedure or re-exploration required.[34]

Cryosurgery for Renal Cell Carcinoma

Renal cryosurgery is a technique that is being developed for small renal tumors as an alternative to nephron-sparing surgery, with the goal of reducing the morbidity of open partial nephrectomy. Standard cryoprobes of 3 to 8 mm can cause rupture of the renal capsule and parenchyma, resulting in significant bleeding. The use of multiple 1.5-mm cryoprobes under intraoperative real-time ultrasound guidance may decrease the risk of bleeding and make this technique a more feasible approach.[35]

Nephron-Sparing Surgery

Traditionally, indications for nephron-sparing surgery for the treatment of RCC have included conditions such as unilateral renal agenesis, horseshoe kidney, or bilateral RCC in which radical nephrectomy would leave the patient anephric, resulting in the need for immediate dialysis. Additional indications have included unilateral RCC with a diseased contralateral kidney that is at risk for severe compromise in future function. Examples of these conditions include diabetes, hypertensive nephrosclerosis, renal artery stenosis, renal calculi, and chronic pyelonephritis. Evidence from a retrospective, single-institution, case-controlled analysis of data from the University of California–Los Angeles (UCLA) Kidney Cancer Program suggests that these indications may be expanded to include patients with T1 lesions, as established by the 1997 TNM classification system. This study compared 146 patients treated at UCLA Medical Center with partial nephrectomy between 1980 and 1997 with 125 patients treated with radical nephrectomy between 1986 and 1997. The cancer-specific survival for patients with T1 lesions (<7 cm) was similar for those treated with either radical nephrectomy or partial nephrectomy, whereas cancer-specific survival for patients undergoing partial nephrectomy for T2 lesions was significantly less than that for those who had radical nephrectomy.[36]

The standard for surgical margins in patients undergoing nephron-sparing surgery for RCC has been set arbitrarily at 1 cm, although this point has not been assessed rigorously. In a retrospective analysis of 67 cases ($n = 55$, open; $n = 12$, laparoscopic), the mean tumor size was 3.0 cm. With a mean follow-up period of 60 months, one of the seven patients with positive margins had died of metastatic disease, and one was alive with systemic recurrence. Of the patients who had negative margins of less than 1 mm, 2 of 11 were alive with metastatic disease. Of the remainder of the patients with negative margins greater than 1 mm ($n = 49$), all were alive without evidence of recurrence.[37] The optimal margin distance remains to be determined, although it would appear that this may be less than 1 cm.

A retrospective Austrian study of two approaches ($n = 32$, retroperitoneal; $n = 19$, transperitoneal) for wedge resections of small exophytic renal neoplasms reported that all procedures were finished laparoscopically without the need for conversion to an open procedure. No local or distant recurrences were noted with a mean follow-up of 34.2 months. Complications occurred in five patients, including a transient pneumothorax with spontaneous resolution in one patient, three cases of urinary leakage (one requiring open surgery), and one case of late hemorrhage requiring open reintervention on postoperative day 1. Negative surgical margins were achieved in all 51 patients. The difficulty with either of these approaches is that no current imaging modality can effectively determine whether the entire carcinoma has been destroyed.[38]

Patients with a solitary or remnant kidney should periodically undergo formal assessment for hyperfiltration nephropathy. Hyperfiltration nephropathy results from increased pressure in the glomeruli of the remaining kidney, resulting in proteinuria, glomerulosclerosis, and further nephron loss, leading to decreased glomerular filtration rates and progressive renal insufficiency. A low-protein diet and therapy with an angiotensin-converting enzyme (ACE) inhibitor should be initiated if proteinuria of more than 150 mg per 24 hours is documented in an attempt to preserve renal function.[39]

Surveillance after Complete Resection: Sporadic Renal Cell Carcinoma

The appropriate schedule of surveillance of cancer patients after definitive surgery is controversial. Because RCC is generally recognized as an aggressive malignancy, protocols for postsurgical radiologic imaging have tended to be intensive. The most common sites of recurrence include lung, bone, liver, and brain, although RCC can recur in almost any anatomic site. Skeletal metastases tend to occur somewhat later than recurrences at other locations. An important consideration in determining the appropriate frequency of surveillance imaging after surgery is the ability to provide curative or palliative salvage therapy. Because improved survival can be achieved for certain subsets of patients with recurrent disease, an active approach to surveillance is warranted. For instance, patients with solitary metachronous metastases who are treated aggressively with surgical resection have a 5-year survival rate of 20% to 44%.[40-43] Extended survival (21 to 136 months) also can be achieved in as many as 33% of patients who undergo resection of an isolated local recurrence in the retroperitoneum.[44,45]

Follow-up imaging of cancer patients after curative therapy has been challenged on the basis of survival benefit and cost effectiveness.[46] Recent strategies for surveillance have been based on three retrospective analyses of stage-based protocols after radical nephrectomy. The first study was based on data from a single institution ($n = 137$) using a TNM staging system that predated the 1997 classification.[47] Recurrence rates were as follows: none for patients with pT1 disease ($n = 19$; median follow-up, 44 months); 15% for patients with pT2 disease ($n = 82$; median time to recurrence, 29.5 months); and 53% ($n = 36$; median time to recurrence, 22 months). T1 lesions in this study were smaller than 2.5 cm, and similar low recurrence rates appear to be maintained in subsequent studies for local lesions that are smaller than 4 cm.

A second major study ($n = 286$) used the 1997 TNM classification system[48] and reported the following recurrence rates: 7% ($n = 8$) for patients with pT1 disease (earliest diagnosis, 30 months after nephrectomy); 27% ($n = 17$) for patients with pT2 disease; and 40% ($n = 43$) for patients with pT3 disease (11 occurring within 6 months of surgery). In this study, 64% of recurrences were not accompanied by symptoms, including 90% of pulmonary metastases detected by routine chest radiography. In spite of the low yield, the authors recommended computed tomography (CT) scans in asymptomatic high-risk patients (pT2 and pT3) at 24 and 60 months. Appropriate radiologic and laboratory studies should be pursued in symptomatic patients.

In the third study ($n = 161$) the 1997 TNM system also was used.[49] This study also evaluated the contribution of DNA ploidy to risk of recurrence, retrospectively. The following recurrence rates were reported: 7% for patients for pT1 disease (median time to recurrence, 43 months); 14% for patients with pT2 disease (median time to recurrence, 29 months); and 67% for patients with pT3 disease (median time to recurrence, 18 months). All patients with lesions smaller than 5 cm remained disease free. DNA ploidy had no effect on rates of recurrence in patients with pT3 disease, whereas in 11 (17%) of 64 patients, aneuploid primary pT1 and pT2 tumors recurred.

Recommendations for surveillance after nephron-sparing surgery have been made on the basis of a retrospective study of 327 patients at The Cleveland Clinic with a median follow-up of 55 months with the pre-1997 TNM classification system.[50] The stage-specific local recurrence rates were as follows: none for pT1 disease (0 of 68), 2% for pT2 disease (3 of 151), 8.2% for pT3a disease (5 of 61), and 10.6% for pT3b disease (5 of 47). About half of the patients with local recurrences also had distant metastases. Again, pT1 disease in this system refers to patients with primary tumors of smaller than 2.5 cm. The authors recommend that all patients with T1, T2, and T3 disease receive an annual evaluation with a history and physical examination, liver-function tests, serum creatinine, calcium, and alkaline phosphatase levels. No surveillance radiography is recommended for patients with T1 disease. A yearly chest radiograph is recommended for patients with T2 and T3 disease. A CT of the abdomen and pelvis is recommended every 2 years for patients with T2 disease. Patients with T3 disease should receive CT scans of the abdomen and pelvis every 6 months for 2 years and every 2 years thereafter.

Lifelong surveillance is necessary for patients with RCC. Late recurrence is arbitrarily defined as a recurrence that occurs more than 10 years after nephrectomy. Recurrences may occur in sporadic RCC as much as 45 years after initial surgical resection.[51] The appropriate intensity of follow-up after 5 years remains to be established. However, approximately 85% of recurrences will take place in the first 3 years after resection of the primary.[52]

Surveillance after Complete Resection: VHL/Familial Renal Cell Carcinoma

Patients with VHL or other familial forms of RCC are at extremely high risk for local recurrence after nephron-sparing surgery and require close lifelong surveillance. More than 80% of patients with VHL disease treated with nephron-sparing surgical resection will have a recurrence in the ipsilateral kidney within 10 years, and lesions will develop in the contralateral kidney if they have not done so already.[53] This is because multiple microscopic lesions are present throughout the kidneys despite the grossly normal appearance of the parenchyma.[54] A diagnosis of VHL disease should be considered in any patient with early-onset or multifocal RCC or RCC in conjunction with the following: (1) a history of visual or neurologic symptoms, (2) a family history of blindness, central nervous system (CNS) tumors, or RCC; or (3) coexisting pancreatic cysts, epididymal lesions, or inner ear tumors.[55,56]

Standard recommendations for surveillance in patients with VHL include (1) CT of the abdomen and pelvis every 6 months, (2) annual physical and ophthalmologic evaluations, (3) estimation of urinary catecholamines every 1 to 2 years, (4) magnetic resonance imaging (MRI) of the CNS every 2 years, and periodic auditory examinations. Molecular genetic and clinical screening should be offered to appropriate family members based an autosomal dominant pattern of inheritance.[53,56,57]

CYTOREDUCTIVE NEPHRECTOMY FOR PATIENTS WITH METASTATIC RENAL CELL CARCINOMA

The role of nephrectomy in patients with metastatic disease at the time of diagnosis has long been the subject of debate. A general consensus exists that noncurative nephrectomy is appropriate when symptoms produced by the primary tumor require palliation, in addition to a growing consensus that nephrectomy is appropriate in patients who wish to receive treatment with high-dose IL-2 or the benefit of other cytokine therapies. The Southwest Oncology Group (SWOG) conducted a randomized study in which patients who were acceptable candidates for nephrectomy either underwent radical nephrectomy followed by therapy with interferon (IFN)-α-2b ($n = 120$) or received IFN-α-2b alone ($n = 121$). The primary endpoint was survival, with objective response as the secondary endpoint. The patients were stratified by SWOG performance status (0 or 1), the presence or absence of lung metastases only, and the presence or absence of at least one measurable metastatic lesion in the region not to be resected. After randomization, patients either underwent immediate radical nephrectomy followed by IFN-α-2b or were immediately given IFN-α-2b without surgery. During the 3-day induction period, the IFN-α-2b was given subcutaneously at a dose of 1.25 million IU/m^2 body surface area (BSA) 3 days before, 2.5 million IU/m^2 2 days before, and 3.75 million IU/m^2 1 day before initiating full-dose therapy. IFN-α-2b was then continued at full doses on a Monday/Wednesday/Friday schedule until disease progression. The median survival was 11.1 months for patients who received nephrectomy plus IFN-α-2b and 8.1 months for patients who received IFN-α-2b alone. This difference in median survival was found to be significant with two-sided P values ($P = 0.05$) and to be independent of performance status, metastatic site, or the presence or absence of a measurable metastatic lesion. Nonetheless, it is difficult to interpret these data in light of the poor median survival seen in both treatment arms of this study.[58]

RESECTION OF METASTASES IN RCC

Resection of solitary metastases from RCC is associated with improved survival, although the selection criteria

---

SPECIAL CONSIDERATIONS FOR THE CLINICIAN

- Cytoreductive nephrectomy for metastatic disease should be considered for patients who are candidates for high-dose IL-2 therapy
- Monitor thyroid function after IL-2
- The development of antithyroid antibodies after cytokine therapy may correlate with survival benefit
- Late recurrence >5 years, ≥7%
- Life-long follow-up clinically indicated if family history
- Resection of solitary metastases may confer significant survival benefit
- Hematuria often does not occur
- PLTS >400,000, poorer prognosis at any stage
- Erythrocytosis: ectopic RCC erythropoietin is a VHL mutant/HIF-1α syndrome.

---

have been poorly defined. This issue was addressed in a retrospective, single-institution analysis of patients with recurrent RCC ($n = 278$) at the Memorial Sloan-Kettering Cancer Center (MSKCC).[59] Recurrent disease was defined as solitary if it recurred within the resected renal bed or if one organ system or site was involved. Multiple unilateral lesions in the lung were considered a solitary site of metastasis. Bilateral lung involvement or recurrence in two or more sites was considered multiple. Surgery for metastatic disease was considered curative if metastases were curatively resected and noncurative if gross tumor was left behind. Of the 278 patients who underwent initial curative nephrectomy, recurrence was solitary in 155 patients and multiple in 123 patients, with a median time to first recurrence of 25 months. The overall 5-year survival rate of patients who underwent curative resection for the first recurrence was 44% ($n = 141$), 14% for those who received noncurative resection ($n = 70$), and 11% for those who were treated nonsurgically ($n = 67$). Favorable predictors of survival by multivariate analysis included a single site of first recurrence, curative resection of the first metastasis, a disease-free interval of more than 12 months, and a metachronous presentation with recurrence. Curative resection of isolated metastases to glandular tissue (thyroid, salivary gland, pancreas, adrenal, ovary) was associated with the best 5-year overall survival (63%), followed by resection of isolated lung metastases (54%). Resection of solitary brain metastases, however, was associated with poor outcome, with an 18% 5-year overall rate. The 5-year overall survival of 46% and 44%, respectively, for patients who underwent second ($n = 62$) or third curative resection ($n = 22$) of subsequent metastases after initial curative metastectomy was not significantly different from that of patients who received only initial curative metastectomy (44%; $n = 141$). Thus patients who undergo complete resection of metastatic disease to a solitary site after a disease-free interval of longer than 12 months may experience long-term survival. As with previous reports, complete resection is the important factor rather than the number of sites resected, even in patients who have undergone prior metastectomy.

SPONTANEOUS REGRESSION IN PATIENTS WITH METASTATIC RENAL CELL CARCINOMA

Spontaneous regression is a well-documented although infrequent phenomenon in patients with metastatic RCC. Perhaps the best documentation of spontaneous regression of RCC was reported by the Canadian Urologic Oncology Group in a study of IFN-γ-1b, although this was not the intent of the study.[60] This prospective, multicenter, placebo-controlled clinical trial of recombinant IFN-γ-1b was conducted at 17 centers across Canada. All patients in this trial ($n = 197$) had biopsy-proven metastatic RCC and had undergone nephrectomy or angioinfarction at least 3 weeks before enrollment. Clinical responses were independently confirmed by a blinded central review committee. Of the patients who could be evaluated ($n = 181$), 91 received IFN-γ-1b ($60 \mu g/m^2$) subcutaneously each week, and 90 received placebo. The overall response rate was 4.4% for the IFN group and 6.6% in the placebo group, with no differences in time to disease progression or survival. This carefully conducted study confirms that spontaneous regressions are an infrequent occurrence in RCC. Spontaneous regression does not represent spontaneous cure, however, nor does it appear to convey a survival advantage.

ADJUVANT CYTOKINE THERAPY AFTER NEPHRECTOMY

Adjuvant therapy after nephrectomy is still investigational. One randomized, multicenter prospective study has been reported on the efficacy of adjuvant IFN-α-2b given after nephrectomy to patients with Robson stages II and III RCC.[61] Patients randomized to receive IFN-α-2b were treated with a dose of 6 million IU intramuscularly 3 times per week for 6 months starting within 1 month of surgery. Patients in the observation arm who relapsed were treated with IFN-α-2b, 10 million IU intramuscularly, 3 times per week, or best available treatment at the time of relapse. Treatment groups were well matched at baseline for patient and tumor characteristics. No significant differences were observed in the overall or event-free survival of patients randomized to observation ($n = 124$) and patients receiving IFN-α-2b ($n = 123$). Relapses occurred in 38 (30.6%) control patients and 51 (41.5%) of the patients treated adjuvantly after a median follow-up period of 62 months. The overall probability of survival at 5 years was estimated by the Kaplan-Meier method to be .665 for the control group and .660 for the treated group. This study does not support the routine use of adjuvant IFN-α-2b after nephrectomy. A recently analyzed and reported phase III study of IFNα-NL as adjuvant treatment for resectable RCC by the Eastern Cooperative Oncology Group (ECOG)/Intergroup showed that adjuvant treatment with IFN did not contribute to survival or relapse-free survival.[62] Enrollment in adjuvant therapy clinical trials is to be encouraged.

PROGNOSTIC FACTORS FOR RENAL CELL CARCINOMA

Clinicians who care for patients with RCC have long been aware that the TNM staging system alone is inadequate for accurate prognosis. Some patients with local disease succumb to aggressive disease progression within a few months of diagnosis, whereas the clinical course of others with recurrent or metastatic disease is much more indolent and may extend beyond 10 years without specific intervention.

Histologic subtyping with routine light-microscopic hematoxylin and eosin–based examination has been found to have prognostic utility. In one series of 405 cases from a single institution, the 5-year disease-specific survival was 100%, 86%, 76%, and 24% for chromophobe, papillary, conventional, and unclassified subtypes, respectively. If sarcomatoid change was present, the 5-year disease-specific survival was 35%.[63]

The UCLA Integrated Staging System (UISS) was developed for the purpose of improving the prognostic accuracy of the 1997 TNM staging system by incorporating clinical variables.[64] The study was based on the analysis of patients treated at a single institution between 1989 and 1999 ($n = 661$). All patients underwent radical or partial nephrectomy, and most patients with metastatic disease were treated with recombinant IL-2–based immunotherapy within the context of 11 clinical trials. The median follow-up was 37 months. The study group was restricted to patients with complete data sets ($n = 477$), although the survival of the excluded group ($n = 184$) was not significantly different from that of the study group ($P = .4$). Patients with papillary tumors ($n = 42$) showed a trend toward improved prognosis that did not achieve statistical significance, whereas patients with sarcomatoid ($n = 45$) and collecting-duct tumors ($n = 3$) had worse prognosis. Survival for patients with clear cell and chromophobe histologies was similar. The UISS uses five stratification groups (I through V) that incorporate variables commonly used in clinical practice, including 1997 TNM stage, ECOG performance status, and Fuhrman grade. The projected 5-year survival by the UISS group was as follows: I (94%), II (67%), III (39%), IV (23%), and V (0%). The system appears to be internally valid, based on a subsequent assessment of 1154 patients in the UCLA Kidney Cancer Database compared with the original 477 patients used to develop the system.[65] These data have been used to develop a mathematical model, $S_t = S_b{}^c$, the better to predict individual survival by using an exponential formula that incorporates the relative risk of multiple variables to form a single probability for patients with M0 and M1 disease.[66] S_t is survival at a given point in time; S_b is baseline survivorship given in the form of a fraction between 0 and 1; and c = $e^{(\beta 1 + \beta 2 + \beta 3 + ... + \beta n)}$, where b is (the coded Cox explanatory variable value) × (the Cox coefficient – "the boot strap value"). The system and the equation must be validated prospectively by using external data sets.

The original UCLA integrated staging system has since been modified so that patients are grouped into two general categories: those with nonmetastatic disease at the time of diagnosis and those with metastatic disease.[67] Each category is then divided into high-, intermediate-, and low-risk subcategories, based on the 1997 TNM staging system, the Fuhrman grade, and the ECOG performance status. These factors allow one to establish a patient's risk group and clarify prognosis quickly. Surprisingly, patients with high-risk nonmetastatic disease had rates of disease-specific survival at 8 years similar to those with low-risk metastatic disease (~40% vs. 35%, respectively).

Some caveats are important to keep in mind when applying the UCLA algorithm. All patients in the study ($n = 814$) underwent nephrectomy before receiving immunotherapy, including those with metastatic disease. The immunotherapy consisted of IFN-α or IL-2, with or without an experimental biologic agent. No patient received thalidomide. A variety of surgical techniques were used, and patients with bilateral disease were excluded from the study. Although prospective external validation is required, the UCLA algorithm may become a useful tool in clinical trial design for patients with RCC.

A retrospective, single-institution review of 24 consecutive clinical trials conducted at MSKCC by using cytokines or chemotherapy for the treatment of advanced RCC ($n = 670$) identified a small subgroup of patients ($n = 30$) who were long-term survivors after nephrectomy and treatment with IFN-α, IL-2, or surgical resection of metastasis.[68,69] The five most prominent negative prognostic factors that were identified by multivariate analysis included low Karnofsky performance status (<80%), elevated lactate dehydrogenase (>1.5 the upper limit of normal), low serum hemoglobin (below the lower limit of normal), high corrected serum calcium (>10 mg/dL), and absence of nephrectomy. Patients with zero risk factors were assigned a favorable risk status; those with one to two risk factors, an intermediate risk status; and those with three or more risk factors, a poor risk status. All long-term survivors in this study were of either good- or intermediate-risk groups. The median survival of patients in all risk categories approximately doubled after treatment with cytokine therapy versus chemotherapy.

The MSKCC and UCLA prognostic systems are similar in several ways. First, both systems are based on a series of consecutive clinical trials for RCC conducted at single institutions [24 trials ($n = 670$) vs. 11 trials ($n = 814$), respectively]. Second, good performance status was found to correlate with lower risk in both systems. Third, cytoreductive nephrectomy for metastatic disease before immunotherapy was found to confer a more favorable prognosis (MSKCC) or was used as standard therapy (UCLA) in both systems.

A report on the risk of metachronous contralateral recurrence of RCC after initial diagnosis has been published based on an analysis of data in the Surveillance, Epidemiology, and End Results database from 1973 to 1997.[70] A review of the records of 43,483 patients with a first diagnosis of RCC identified 40,049 patients who had no synchronous disease in the contralateral kidney. Of the patients who initially had no contralateral disease, a contralateral recurrence subsequently developed in 155 (0.4%). Analysis included stratification by tumor stage and

demographic factors, with a median follow-up of 2.25 years (range, 0.08 to 24.9 years). Calendar year–specific and race-specific incidence rates were used to minimize bias. The relative risk of recurrence in the contralateral kidney was significantly higher for black men than for white men in the first 5 years of follow-up. The authors concluded that the frequency of imaging of the contralateral kidney should not be altered beyond 10 years because the relative rates of recurrence were constant over time, with the exception of black men within 5 years of the initial diagnosis. Known environmental factors for RCC such as smoking, obesity, and hypertension may contribute to the higher incidence of metachronous RCC in black men, because the incidence of these risk factors is higher in black men than in white men, although supportive data are lacking. Neither sex nor tumor stage was identified as a factor that should modify the frequency of surveillance of the contralateral kidney. Confirmation by testing of an independent data set is needed before a general recommendation can be made to increase the frequency of surveillance for black men in the first 5 years of follow-up.

HIGH-DOSE INTERLEUKIN-2 FOR ADVANCED DISEASE

High-dose IL-2 has resulted in objective response rates of 15% to 17% in patients with RCC and durable complete response rates of approximately 6%.[71,72] The treatment was approved by the U.S. Food and Drug Administration (FDA) in 1992 for patients with metastatic RCC or melanoma to be administered as an IV bolus at 600,000 IU/kg every 8 hours, as tolerated. A dose of 720,000 IU/kg also is frequently used. Currently, most patients receive about 8 doses in the first cycle as opposed to 13 doses in earlier reports. As a result, treatment-related mortality is almost nonexistent when high-dose IL-2 is administered by physicians who adhere strictly to the pretreatment screening criteria and when patients are monitored by properly trained nurses who are prepared to initiate therapeutic intervention in a timely manner according to carefully established guidelines.[73,74]

Pretreatment screening for high-dose IL-2 includes pulmonary-function tests and cardiac evaluation with an exercise tolerance or stress thallium test in patients older than 50 years (Table 85-3). An MRI of the brain is required. If brain lesions are present, they must be successfully removed by surgery or radiosurgery and have no evidence of recurrence for a minimum of 3 months before consideration of high-dose IL-2. Treatment should be delayed 1 to 2 weeks if patients have used steroids in any form or if an infection is identified. Steroids negate the effectiveness of cytotoxic T lymphocytes and should be avoided unless they are required for the treatment of a life-threatening event. Patients taking antihypertensives should discontinue these medications 24 hours before starting high-dose IL-2 therapy. A triple-lumen central line must be placed on admission and removed before discharge with each cycle of therapy to diminish the risk of infection.

TABLE 85-3

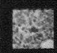

Pretreatment Screening Guidelines for High-Dose Interleukin-2

Physical Examination

No major cardiac, pulmonary, or renal disease

Infections

No infections (respiratory, urinary tract, intravenous, etc.) in the last 7 days

Medications

No use of steroids (systemic, topical, or inhalational) in the last 7 to 14 days
Discontinue antihypertensives 24 hr before high-dose interleukin-2 (IL-2)

Electrocardiogram

Normal or unchanged for patients who have received IL-2

Laboratory Studies

Comprehensive metabolic profile. Serum creatinine, ≤1.6 mg/dL. Serum bilirubin, ≤1.6 mg/dL
Complete blood count

Imaging

Brain magnetic resonance imaging (Brain metastases must be adequately treated with no recurrence for 3 months before therapy)
Computed tomography C/A/P
Chest radiograph (no infiltrates or effusions)

Functional Studies

Pulmonary function tests (FEV1 and FVC >65% of predicted)
Stress thallium (for patients younger than 50 years or with family history of heart disease)

Patients experience a broad range of toxicities when receiving high-dose IL-2. Some patients experience few toxicities, whereas others experience sudden and severe toxicities that may be life threatening. These toxicities can affect many organ systems and include flulike symptoms, vascular leak syndrome, as well as cardiovascular, pulmonary, renal, gastrointestinal, hematologic, neurologic, and dermatologic toxicities. Autoimmune phenomena also may be observed. Infectious complications are minimized by the use of prophylactic antibiotics. Guidelines for monitoring patients receiving high-dose IL-2 are given in Table 85-4.

Typically patients will experience fever and chills within several hours of the first or second dose, along with mild to moderate hypotension and tachycardia secondary to decreased systemic vascular resistance. Oliguria is generally noted within the first 24 hours, requiring intravenous (IV) fluids to restore urine output. Edema, weight

TABLE 85-4

Guidelines for Monitoring Patients Receiving High-Dose Interleukin-2

PARAMETER	PRESSORS NOT IN USE	PRESSORS IN USE OR ICU
Vital signs	Every 4 hr	Every hour
Intake and output	Every 4 hr	Every hour
Weight	Daily	Daily
Mental status	Every 8 hr	Every 8 hr
IV Site	Every 8 hr (change peripheral IV every 3 days)	Every 8 hr
Laboratory values		
CBC	Daily	Twice daily
Electrolytes, BUN, Cr, Glu	Daily	Twice daily
ALT, AST, total bilirubin	Daily	Daily
Ca^{2+}, Mg^{2+}, phosphorus	Daily	Daily
PT, PTT	Daily after day 2	Daily
Total CK	Daily	Daily
TSH, Free T$_4$	Each cycle	Each cycle
Urinalysis	Each cycle	Each cycle
ECG	Each cycle	Each cycle
CXR	Each cycle	Each cycle

SYSTOLIC BP	BASELINE	THERAPEUTIC TARGET
	<100 mm Hg	>80 mm Hg
	100–200 mm Hg	>85 mm Hg
	>120 mm Hg	>90 mm Hg

ALT, alanine aminotransferase; AST, aspartate aminotransferase; BP, blood pressure; BUN, blood urea nitrogen; CK, creative kinase; Cr, creatinine; CXR, chest radiograph; ECG, electrocardiogram; Glu, glucose; ICU, intensive care unit; IV, intravenous; PT, prothrombin time; PTT, partial thromboplastin time; TSH, thyroid-stimulating hormone.

gain, and pulmonary congestion are manifestations of the capillary leak syndrome and are typically progressive throughout the course of treatment, requiring the judicious use of IV fluids and pressors after the first 24 hours. Other symptoms such as nausea, vomiting, and diarrhea usually become more prominent toward the end of a course of therapy. When infections occur, they are typically bacterial and are thought to occur as a result neutrophil dysfunction caused by IL-2. Neuropsychiatric side effects of IL-2 may be subtle and include confusion and visual hallucinations. Frequent neuropsychiatric assessments are required, and true alterations require immediate termination of therapy.

The most prominent laboratory abnormalities noted in patients receiving high-dose IL-2 include a progressive increase in serum creatinine, total bilirubin, and coagulation parameters in conjunction with a decrease in the platelet count. These abnormalities and clinical symptoms are usually reversible within 2 to 3 days after the termination of treatment.

No dose reductions of IL-2 are used. IL-2 doses are delayed whenever necessary to allow sufficient symptomatic recovery. A delay of 24 hours or more typically results in the discontinuation of a cycle of IL-2. The decision to delay or discontinue a cycle of high-dose IL-2 therapy is based on a series of relative and absolute

stopping criteria. Guidelines for discontinuing therapy with high-dose IL-2 are given in Table 85-5. Physical examination and thorough review of these criteria are required before the administration of each dose of IL-2.

In the post-therapy assessment period, vital signs must be monitored until the patient is stable, and continue monitoring input and output until the patient is discharged. Laboratory tests should be monitored daily until abnormalities plateau and begin to normalize. Intravenous fluids should be discontinued as soon as possible, typically within 8 hours of the last IL-2 dose. IV fluids should not be reinstated unless severe diarrhea occurs or the patient's weight decreases to less than the admission weight. Aggressive diuretic therapy is generally initiated when the patient's blood pressure stabilizes while not taking pressors, with a target urine output of 200 mL/hr. Acetaminophen, indomethacin, and H_2 blockers are usually continued for up to 24 hours after the last dose of IL-2.

The patient should receive supportive care until toxic symptoms and laboratory abnormalities stabilize and pressors have been discontinued. Patients are usually discharged within 3 days of stopping high-dose IL-2. Imaging studies to assess response to therapy are typically obtained after the second treatment when all laboratory abnormalities and clinical symptoms have resolved.

TABLE 85-5

Relative and Absolute Stopping Criteria for High-Dose Interleukin-2

SYSTEM	RELATIVE CRITERIA	ABSOLUTE CRITERIA
Cardiac	Sinus tachycardia, 120–130 beats/min	Sustained sinus tachycardia, >130 that persists after correcting any hypotension, fever, and stopping dopamine ECG changes of ischemia Atrial fibrillation Supraventricular tachycardia Ventricular arrhythmias (frequent PVCs, bigeminy, tachycardia) Elevated CPK-MB
Dermatologic		Moist desquamation
Gastrointestinal	Diarrhea, 1000 cc/shift Ileus or abdominal distention Bilirubin, >7.0 mg/dL	Diarrhea, 1000 cc/shift × 2 Severe abdominal distension affecting breathing or severe abdominal pain
Hemodynamic	Maximum neosynephrine, 1–1.5 µg/kg/min	Maximum neosynephrine, 1.5–2.0 µg/kg/min
Hemorrhagic	Guaiac-postive sputum, emesis, stool Platelets, 30–50,000/mm^3	Frank blood in sputum, emesis, stool Platelets, <30,000/mm^3
Infectious		Strong suspicion or documented
Musculoskeletal	Weight gain 15% Extremity tightness	Extremity paresthesias
Neurologic	Vivid dreams Emotional lability	Mental status changes not reversible in 2 hr Disorientation Hallucination
Pulmonary	Resting shortness of breath 3–4 L O$_2$ NC for sat. ≥95% Rales 1/3 up chest	>4 L O$_2$ by NC for sat. ≥95% 40% O$_2$ mask for sat. ≥95% Endotracheal intubation Moist rales $^1/_2$ up chest Pleural effusion requiring tap or chest tube while on therapy
Renal	Urine 80–160 mL/shift Urine 10-20 mL/hr Creatinine, 2.5–2.9 mg/dL	Urine <80 mL/shift Urine <10 mL /hr Creatinine, ≥3.0 mg/dL

CPK, creatine phosphokinase; ECG, electrocardiogram; NC, nasal catheter; PVC, premature ventricular contraction.

HIGH-DOSE INTERLEUKIN-2 VERSUS SUBCUTANEOUS INTERLEUKIN-2 REGIMENS

Although the symptoms of high-dose IL-2 may be quite severe, they are almost always self-limited and reversible. Most patients receive the treatment 2 or 3 times over the course of 4 to 6 weeks. This is an important point when helping patients choose between a subcutaneous outpatient regimen and a more intense high-dose regimen. Clearly the side effects of outpatient subcutaneous regimens of IL-2 are relatively less intense, but they are significant, and responsive patients must continue therapy indefinitely, along with the long-term side effects of flu-like symptoms and fatigue. Although it is true that durable clinical complete responses will occur in only about 1 of 20 patients receiving high-dose IL-2, they rarely occur when IL-2 is administered subcutaneously.

OUTPATIENT REGIMENS OF INTERFERON-α2, INTERLEUKIN-2, OR BOTH FOR ADVANCED RENAL CELL CARCINOMA

Currently, no randomized phase III trial demonstrates a survival benefit for combination therapy compared with treatment with IFN-α-2a or IL-2 alone in patients with advanced RCC.

CYTOKINES WITH CHEMOTHERAPY FOR ADVANCED RENAL CELL CARCINOMA

A multicenter phase II trial of IL-2, IFN-α-2a, and continuous-infusion 5-fluorouracil (5-FU) was conducted to determine whether the combination would produce a response rate greater than 20%.[75] During the induction phase of 10 weeks, the cytokines were administered subcutaneously each Monday, Wednesday, and Friday at a dose of 18 million IU (IL-2) and 9 million IU (IFN-α-2a) for 8 weeks. The 5-FU (750 mg/m^2) was infused over a 30-minute period each Monday for 8 weeks. Doses were reduced to 9 million IU (IL-2) and 6 million IU (IFN-α-2a) for patients with cytokine toxicities of grades 3 or 4. The dose of 5-FU was reduced by 50% for grades 3 or 4 hematologic toxicity. A 2-week break was given at the end of the induction period, followed by maintenance therapy of 2-week treatment cycles and 3-week rest periods for a maximum of seven cycles. Of the 62 patients who participated in the study, only 17 received maintenance therapy because of severe toxicity. The overall objective response rate at the end of the induction period was 19% [1 complete response (CR), 11 partial responses (PRs)]. Response rates of greater than 20% were not observed in this study.

A multicenter phase II trial of IL-2, IFN-α-2a, and continuous-infusion 5-FU has been reported by the Groupe Français d'Immunothérapie.[76] The regimen was administered in 8-week cycles: IL-2 was delivered subcutaneously at a dose of 9 million units daily for 6 days during weeks 1, 3, 5, and 7. IFN-α-2a also was delivered subcutaneously at a dose of 6 million IU on days 1, 3, and 5 of weeks 1, 3, 5, and 7. A continuous infusion of 5-FU was administered at a daily dose of 600 mg/m^2 on days 1 through 5 of weeks 1 and 5. Nearly all patients enrolled in this trial ($n = 111$) were assessable for toxicity ($n = 110$) and response ($n = 105$). The median survival for all patients in the study was 12 months (357 days). The overall objective response rate of 1.8% was much lower than those that had previously been reported. This discrepancy cannot be explained by significant differences in patient population, although the previous protocols used a variety of regimens in which the cytokines were given intravenously as well as subcutaneously. Thus the efficacy of regimens combining IL-2, IFN-α-2a, and 5-FU has yet to be clearly established.

CHEMOTHERAPY FOR ADVANCED RENAL CELL CARCINOMA

Conventional cytotoxics generally offer little benefit to patients with RCC. The response rates for a wide variety of chemotherapeutic agents in phase II trials have generally been in the range of 6% to 20%. Although these responses are durable on occasion, no improvement in median survival has been reported.[77] In a review of 83 trials of a variety of chemotherapeutic regimens published from 1983 to 1993, Yagoda and colleagues[78] reported a 6% overall response rate for 4093 patients with advanced RCC.

Data from a multi-institutional phase II trial of gemcitabine and 5-FU suggest that this regimen could be active for patients with advanced RCC and warrant further investigation.[79] Gemcitabine (600 mg/m^2) was infused over a 30-minute period on days 1, 8, and 15. 5-FU was administered as a continuous infusion at a dose of 150 mg/m^2/d via a permanent catheter on days 1 to 21 of a 28-day cycle. Most patients (34 of 41) had received prior chemotherapy or immunotherapy. For the 39 assessable patients, the objective response rate was 17% with no CR and seven PRs. The median overall survival for the entire cohort was 11.6 months. Five of the seven patients with PRs had undergone nephrectomy and prior therapy with an IL-2–based regimen. Responses were seen in a variety of metastatic sites including lung, lymph node, renal fossa, and liver. The observation that median progression-free survival (28.7 weeks) was significantly longer than that of the historic control of a similar cohort of patients treated on phase II studies at the University of Chicago (8 weeks) requires prospective confirmation.

INTERLEUKIN-2, INTERFERON-α-2A, AND 13-*CIS*-RETINOIC ACID

A multicenter phase II trial of IL-2, IFN-α-2a, and 13-*cis*-retinoic acid (13-CRA) found this combination to be feasible in the outpatient setting with modest efficacy.[80]

The therapy included IL-2 administered subcutaneously at a fixed dose of 11 million IU, given 4 days per week (generally Monday through Thursday) for 4 weeks. IFN-α-2a or IFN-α-2b was given at a fixed dose of 9 or 10 million IU subcutaneously 2 days per week (generally Monday and Thursday) for 4 weeks. Cytokine therapy was discontinued for 2 weeks at the end of each 6-week cycle. 13-CRA was administered orally at a daily dose of 1 mg/kg (rounded to the nearest 20 mg) for 6 weeks. Of the patients enrolled ($n = 49$), 48 were assessable for toxicity and response. Eight objective responses were observed (1 CR, 7 PRs) for an objective response rate of 17%. The overall median survival was 74 weeks (17.1 months). Phase III confirmation of these data is needed.

A multi-institutional phase III study of patients with metastatic RCC ($n = 284$) conducted by ECOG compared patients randomized to receive IFN-α-2a ($n = 145$) or IFN-α-2a plus oral 13-CRA ($n = 139$).[81] Subcutaneous IFN-α-2a was administered daily at a dose of 3 million units with dose escalation every 7 days as tolerated (nonhematologic toxicity less than grade 2, hematologic toxicity less than grade 3) in increments of 3 million units to a maximum daily dose of 9 million units in both arms of the study. Patients randomized to combination therapy received oral 13-CRA at a dose of 1 mg/kg/d in two divided doses, rounded to the nearest 10 mg, plus IFN-α-2a. Stratification factors included center (MSKCC vs. ECOG), lung-only disease, prior nephrectomy, and Karnofsky Performance Status (KPS; 70% or 80% vs. 90%). Response rates and survival did not significantly improve with the addition of 13-CRA to IFN-α-2a. Complete and partial responses were 1 and 8 for the IFN-α-2a–alone arm and 5 and 11 for the IFN-α-2a plus 13-CRA arm. The median overall survival for all patients was 15 months. There were significant declines in compliance with both regimens from 81% and 86% at baseline to 24% and 39% at 52 weeks for IFN-α-2a alone vs. IFN-α-2a plus 13-CRA, respectively. The observed enhancement in duration of response and improved progression-free survival may indicate that 13-CRA lengthens the duration of response in the small subset of patients with MRCC whose tumors are sensitive to IFN-α-2a.

PREDICTORS OF RESPONSE TO CYTOKINE THERAPY

Reversible thyroid dysfunction and a transient induction of thyroid autoantibodies occurs in up to 60% of patients with metastatic RCC treated with IL-2 alone or in combination with IFN-α or lymphokine-activated killer cells. It has been proposed that cytokine-induced hypothyroidism correlates with more favorable tumor responses. To examine this hypothesis, a retrospective, single-institution study was performed on patients treated at the Medizinische Hochschule Hannover in Hannover, Germany.[82] Cases of unselected patients with metastatic RCC ($n = 329$) treated with subcutaneous IL-2 and IFN-α-2 were reviewed. All patients were treated with 8-week cycles of subcutaneous IL-2 and IFN-α-2 with ($n = 247$) or without IV 5-fluorouracil ($n = 82$). IL-2 was administered at 20 million IU/m² 3 times per week in weeks 1 and 4 and at 5 million IU/m² 3 times per week in weeks 2 and 3. IFN-α-2 was administered at 6 million U/m² once per week in weeks 1 and 4, three times per week in weeks 2 and 3, and increased to 10 million U/m² 3 times per week in weeks 5 through 8. The dose of 5-FU was not reported. After 8 weeks of therapy, 60 patients were found to be thyroid autoantibody positive. Thyroid dysfunction (either hyper- or hypothyroidism) was diagnosed in 65% of these patients, whereas 68% of the thyroid autoantibody-negative patients were euthyroid. The median survival for all 329 patients was 22 months. The median survival had not yet been reached for the thyroid-autoantibody–positive patients with no difference in survival noted between patients with cytokine-induced thyroid autoantibodies ($n = 35$) and those with preexisting thyroid autoimmunity ($n = 25$). Although no association with other autoimmune phenomena was observed, human leukocyte antigen (HLA)-phenotype analysis of a subgroup of 70 patients revealed a correlation of HLA class I antigen Cw7 expression with prolonged survival ($P = .009$). Prospective confirmation is needed of these provocative preliminary data.

SECOND-LINE CYTOKINE THERAPY AFTER FAILURE OF FIRST-LINE CYTOKINES

Because nearly all patients with metastatic RCC will progress while receiving first-line therapy, it is important to know the effectiveness of second-line therapy. This issue has been addressed in a prospective randomized crossover trial conducted by the Groupe Français d'Immunothérapie. Enrollment in the crossover trial required prior enrollment in the Cancer Renal Cytokines (CRECY) trial conducted by the same group. The CRECY trial compared the effectiveness of IL-2 alone (arm 1) or IFN-α-2a alone (arm 2) to a combination of both cytokines (arm 3). Patients who received IL-2 ($n = 132$) or IFN-α-2a ($n = 146$) were offered treatment with the other cytokine at time of progression. However, participation in the crossover trial was dependent on patients meeting the criteria for receiving intravenous IL-2. One hundred seventy-two patients did not meet these criteria and were therefore excluded. IL-2 infusions were carried out via a central line and administered continuously over 5 days at a dose of 18 million IU/m²/day for four cycles. IFN-α-2a was administered subcutaneously at a dose of 18 million IU/day 3 times a week for 10 weeks as induction therapy, followed by an additional 13 weeks of maintenance therapy. Of the 113 patients who participated in the crossover trial and were assessable for response, 65 went on to receive IL-2, whereas 48 received IFN-α-2a. No CRs were seen in either group. One patient who switched to IFN-α-2a had a PR, as did three patients who switched to IL-2. No difference in median survival was noted between patients who received first-line IL-2 (19 months) or IFN-α-2a (18 months) and the 113 patients who participated in the crossover (19 months) or the 140 patients who received first-line combination therapy (17 months).[83]

TREATMENT OF ADVANCED RENAL CELL CARCINOMA: INVESTIGATIONAL APPROACHES

IMMUNOTHERAPY CLINICAL TRIALS
- Dendritic cell vaccines with defined RCC antigens/ whole cell
- If allogeneic match: PBSC/BMT clinical trial
- Cytokines (IL-2) + vaccine/adoptive therapy
- T cells

ANTIANGIOGENESIS CLINICAL TRIALS
- Anti-VEGF targeted therapies
- Antineovessel molecules (e.g., thalidomide/neovast)

TARGETED THERAPIES OF FUTURE
- Anti-VHL mutation drug discovery
- Anti-ATK-1 drug discovery
- Anti-HIF-1 signaling activation inhibitors (e.g., CCI-779 [TOR Inhibitors])

TUMOR-INFILTRATING LYMPHOCYTES WITH INTERLEUKIN-2 FOR METASTATIC DISEASE

Tumor-infiltrating lymphocytes (TILs) are found in high numbers in RCC tumors. Preclinical and clinical data suggest that TILs and IL-2 may act synergistically to activate the cellular immune response, resulting in tumor regression. Furthermore, TILs can be expanded ex vivo in the presence of IL-2 to yield predominantly T lymphocytes. A phase I/II pilot study of 55 patients treated at UCLA with nephrectomy followed by TILs plus low-dose IL-2 via continuous IV infusion (2 million IU/m^2/day) revealed a 43% overall survival rate at 2 years after radical nephrectomy.

Based on these promising early data, a prospective, randomized, multicenter, placebo-controlled study was conducted by using this approach.[84] Of 178 patients enrolled, 160 were randomized to TILs plus IL-2 ($n = 81$) or IL-2 alone ($n = 79$). Patients were treated with one to four cycles of 5 million IU/m^2/day of IL-2 via continuous IV infusion for 4 days per week for 4 weeks. One treatment cycle consisted of 4 weeks of treatment and 2 weeks of rest. CD8$^+$ TILs (5×10^7 to 3×10^{10}) were administered as a single infusion. Patients in the control group were allowed to cross over at the time of progression. Twenty randomized patients received no form of treatment because of complications of nephrectomy. Only 39 of the 72 patients eligible to receive TILs plus IL-2 actually received TILs because the others did not have sufficient numbers of viable cells. Overall objective responses were 9.9% for the TILs plus IL-2 group and 11.4% for the IL-2 control group, with corresponding 1-year survival rates of 55% and 47%, respectively. The study was terminated early for lack of efficacy and significant life-threatening toxicities. The use of immune cell therapy or adoptive immunotherapy for investigational treatment of RCC was

technically limited in the case of TILs. The cumbersome nature of the procedures in the laboratory and lack of standardization in each patient preparation was due to the number of manipulations in the sterile hoods and heterogeneity of necrosis in the tumors themselves in preparing TILs. The dosing of TILs itself was difficult to control. However, with the development of further biotechnologies for closed-system, autologous immune cell and tumor cell separations, additional approaches are warranted in academic centers. Of particular interest is the use of specific T-cell subsets that recognize proven RCC-associated tumor-associated antigens (TAAs).

ANGIOGENESIS INHIBITORS FOR ADVANCED RENAL CELL CARCINOMA

Tumor growth beyond a few cubic millimeters cannot occur without the induction of a new vascular supply. Inhibiting the development of new blood vessels (antiangiogenesis) is a potential approach to cancer therapy—particularly RCC. The discovery of the VHL gene–HIF-1 connection in kidney cancers has further intensified interest in drug development for approaches aimed at the disruption of angiogenesis in the treatment of RCC. Vascular endothelial growth factor (VEGF) is so far the best-characterized proangiogenic factor. It is virtually ubiquitous in human tumors, and higher levels have been correlated with more aggressive disease in kidney cancer. VEGF-A is a potent stimulator of angiogenesis because its binding to VEGF receptors has been shown to promote endothelial cell migration and proliferation, two vital features required for the development of new tumor-induced blood vessels. In addition, VEGF-A increases vascular permeability, which also may contribute to angiogenesis and tumor growth. HIF-1 regulates the activation of VEGF gene expression. Several approaches are being taken to block the VHL/HIF-1/VEGF axis. Of these, clinical experience with the humanized anti–VEGF-A monoclonal antibody bevacizumab (Avastin, rhuMAb-VEGF; Genentech, South San Francisco, CA) has been encouraging. Clinical efficacy of antiangiogenic therapy with bevacizumab is being evaluated in several controlled trials in RCC. The National Cancer Institute has placed a high priority on development of antiangiogenesis agents in RCC. Clinicians should be evaluating options for enrollment of their kidney cancer patients in phase I through phase III trials for antiangiogenesis agents.

A multi-institutional phase II study of the fumigillin analog TNP-470 has been reported in patients who had previously been treated for metastatic RCC.[85] TNP-470 was the first specific antiangiogenesis agent to undergo widespread clinical testing in RCC. In this study, TNP-470 was administered 3 times weekly as an IV bolus over 1 hour at a dose of 60 mg/m^2. Patients were enrolled at five institutions, with the initial week of therapy being administered in the outpatient area of the parent institution. Subsequent weeks of therapy were administered in the patients' homes if no significant toxicities were observed in the first week. Of the patients enrolled in the study ($n = 33$), most had received at least one prior therapy that included IL-2 and/or IFN-a ($n = 30$), and some had received chemotherapy as well ($n = 9$). One objective response was observed, yielding an objective response rate of 3%. Cerebellar symptoms were common, as well as a variety of psychiatric symptoms including abnormal dreams, anxiety, depression, emotional lability, insomnia, nervousness, and somnolence. Other schedules of administration or other formulations of this agent may be found to be more effective.

Data on the role of thalidomide in the treatment of advanced RCC are preliminary. The rationale for the use of thalidomide to treat advanced RCC is based in part on the fact that it is known to be an angiogenesis inhibitor in vivo.[86] Because RCCs are typically quite vascular tumors and the VHL protein is known to stabilize VEGF, and because thalidomide has shown antitumor activity in patients with refractory multiple myeloma in which bone vascularization is a prominent feature, trials of thalidomide for advanced RCC have been patterned after the early studies in multiple myeloma. Since the initial report by Eisen and colleagues in 1999,[87] most published data to date remain in abstract form, as summarized by Motzer and others.[88] The progression-free survival ranged from more than 3 months to 6 or more months with target daily doses of thalidomide ranging from 100 mg to 1200 mg. The aggregate response rates for the six clinical trials (four ongoing) were modest among the patients that were assessable for response ($n = 144$), with no complete responses reported, although PRs ($n = 8$; 5.6%) and stable disease ($n = 59$; 41.0%) were observed.

Stable disease in RCC is not easy to assess as drug effect, but some patients will respond to thalidomide after having failed to respond to IL-2 or IFN-α. Patients being treated with thalidomide must be monitored closely for drowsiness, fatigue, rash, constipation, and peripheral neuropathy. Because constipation may be severe, all patients should take a stool softener or gentle laxative such as senna to maintain regular bowel movements. All patients should be assessed for hypothyroidism at baseline with a thyroid-stimulating hormone (TSH) level determined before treatment and every 2 months thereafter while taking thalidomide. On occasion, severe bradycardia may require that therapy with thalidomide be discontinued. A causative role for hypothyroidism has not been definitively established for thalidomide-induced bradycardia.

THALIDOMIDE PLUS INTERFERON-α

Unexpected toxicity has been reported in at least one trial of thalidomide in combination with IFN-α-2a, resulting in the closure of a phase II study after accruing only 13 patients.[89] In this trial, the IFN-α-2a was administered at a dose of 9 million IU subcutaneously 3 times per week after a single introductory dose of 4.5 million IU. Thalidomide was begun 2 weeks later at an initial dose of 100 mg each evening and escalated monthly in 100-mg increments to a maximum dose of 400 mg. Five patients experienced serious adverse events including visual disturbances ($n = 4$) in conjunction with complex partial

seizures ($n = 1$), transient right arm numbness and loss of speech ($n = 1$), perioral tingling, facial numbness, with a left-sided headache ($n = 1$), and significant depression ($n = 1$). CT scans revealed no evidence of cerebrovascular events or intracranial metastases. In a fifth patient, Stevens-Johnson syndrome developed at a thalidomide dose of 200 mg and resolved on discontinuing the study drugs and treatment with corticosteroids. It is of interest to note that a phase III trial being conducted by the ECOG with IFN-α-2b with or without thalidomide continues to accrue without reports of similar toxicities.

NONMYELOABLATIVE ALLOGENEIC PERIPHERAL-BLOOD STEM CELL TRANSPLANTATION

Inducing antitumor T cells from "graft versus tumor" manipulations has some promise in RCC. Nonmyeloablative allogeneic peripheral-blood stem cell transplantation is a promising new approach to the treatment of metastatic RCC. It was first reported in 1999 to induce the complete resolution of IFN-α-2b–resistant pulmonary metastases in a patient who had undergone nephrectomy for stage III disease.[90] These so-called "minitransplants" use nonmyeloablative low-dose preparative regimens and allogeneic peripheral-blood stem cell transplantation to exploit the graft-versus-tumor effect of allogeneic T lymphocytes. A follow-up study of 19 patients conducted at the U.S. National Institutes of Health confirmed that sustained regression of metastatic RCC is achievable in patients who were refractory to prior therapy.[91] In this study, all patients were required to have an HLA-identical sibling or a sibling with a mismatch at a single HLA locus to serve as a donor. Patients were excluded if they had bone metastases alone, active brain metastases, or hypercalcemia. The preparative regimen included cyclophosphamide (60 mg/kg) on day 7 and day 6 before transplantation. Intravenous fludarabine (25 mg/m^2) was administered daily on days 5 to 1 before transplantation. For the two patients who received a transplant from a donor with a mismatch at a single HLA locus, intravenous antithymocyte globulin (40 mg/kg) was administered daily on days 5 to 2 before transplantation. Cyclosporine was used to prevent rejection of the graft and graft-versus-host disease (GVHD). Intravenous cyclosporine (3 mg/kg) was administered daily, starting on day 4 before transplantation. Oral cyclosporine (5 mg/kg twice daily) was substituted as tolerated. The allograft was infused into the recipient on day 0 without removal of donor T cells. Stem cell donors received 10 µg/kg granulocyte colony-stimulating factor subcutaneously each day for 5 or 6 days with leukapheresis of mobilized peripheral-blood stem cells starting on day 5 and repeated on days 6 and 7 as needed to obtain the target dose of more than 5×10^6 CD34 cells per kilogram of the recipient's weight.

Decisions regarding discontinuation of cyclosporine and lymphocyte infusions after transplantation were dependent on the rate of donor T-cell chimerism in peripheral blood. Rapid and complete engraftment of donor immune cells is associated with an increased risk for GVHD.[90] Patients with 100% donor T-cell chimerism in the peripheral blood on post-transplant day 30 took cyclosporine to day 60, followed by a 25% taper every 10 days until it was discontinued on day 100 if GVHD had not developed. For patients with mixed donor-recipient lymphoid chimerism on day 30, the cyclosporine was rapidly tapered over a 2-week period because the risk of GVHD was low. Three monthly infusions of escalating doses of donor lymphocytes were given to patients who did not have complete donor T-cell chimerism after the cyclosporine taper was complete. Chimerism was assessed weekly until complete T-cell chimerism, GVHD, or disease regression occurred. Patients with stable or progressive disease after discontinuation of cyclosporine and who had no grade III or IV GVHD were eligible to receive up to three monthly donor lymphocyte infusions (DLIs) in escalating doses (5×10^6, 1×10^7, and 5×10^7 CD3 T cells). Patients who failed to respond to DLIs and patients with severe GVHD were eligible to receive subcutaneous IFN-α or IL-2.

Ultimately this approach, although very promising, will have limited application because of the requirement for HLA-matched siblings to serve as donors. Methods for further enhancing the graft-versus-tumor effect while minimizing the GVH effect are needed.

CLINICAL TRIAL DESIGN FOR PATIENTS WITH RCC

Heterogeneity of treatment protocols is a significant complicating factor in interpreting the results of clinical trials for RCC. Progression-free and overall survival of patients treated with IFN-α has been proposed as a standard of comparison for new phase II and III clinical investigations.[92] Stratification based on the UCLA algorithm of low, intermediate, and high risk for patients with nonmetastatic and metastatic disease should provide a basis for distinguishing the therapeutic effects from outcomes that simply reflect the natural history of the disease.[67]

MANAGING BONE METASTASES

Although RCC is generally resistant to standard radiation therapy (XRT), a short course of XRT can be quite helpful as a palliative measure when RCC metastasizes to bone. Bisphosphonate therapy with zoledronate should be initiated once bone metastases have been identified and administered indefinitely on a monthly basis. Humoral hypercalcemia of malignancy usually occurs in the absence of extensive bone metastases and should be treated with either pamidronate or zoledronate.

VACCINE STRATEGIES FOR RENAL CELL CARCINOMA

Many cancer vaccines are in various stages of preclinical and clinical development. These vaccines are based on the hypotheses that TAAs are inherently weakly immunogenic or functionally nonimmunogenic and that effective vaccines will enhance the efficacy of presentation of TAAs to the immune system, resulting in dramatically increased activation of host T cells. To "break tolerance" against TAAs is the common purpose of antigen presentation by vaccination. Several well-characterized TAAs in RCC have been cloned from patient's tumors and mapped in the human genome. The complete "set" of TAAs in RCC is a subject of ongoing research.

One approach to vaccine therapy for patients with RCC involves the use of heat-shock protein peptide complex 96 (HSPPC-96). This complex consists of Hsp-96, gp96, and an array of gp-associated cellular peptides. The collection of gp96-associated peptides is representative of the antigenic peptide pool within a given cell and varies between normal cells and tumor cells. Immunization with purified HSPPC-96 is specific for the individual as well as the tumor type and has produced protective T-cell immunity against a variety of tumors in animal models.[93] More data on the clinical efficacy of this approach in the adjuvant setting should become available when the results of an international, multicenter, double-blind, phase III trial of patients with resected stage III RCC are reported.

Other strategies for the development of cancer vaccines include (1) identifying novel TAAs for RCC-reactive cytotoxic T lymphocytes, (2) improving modes of antigen delivery and antigen presentation by using dendritic cells, (3) enhancing antigen immunogenicity (e.g., alternating vaccine prime and boost, enhancing T-cell costimulation, and engineering amino acid sequences in peptide TAAs), (4) improving systemic T-cell dissemination, (5) enhancing destruction of tumor cells (effector phase), (6) improving T-cell memory, and (7) enhancing the adaptive response to tumor variants (e.g., use of cytokines as vaccine adjuvants). Thus multiple hurdles must be overcome before the promise of cancer vaccines as adjuvant therapy becomes a reality for patients with RCC.

Agents Approved for Fast-Track Clinical Development

CCI-779 is an mTOR (mammalian target of rapamycin) inhibitor that received fast-track development status from the FDA in March 2002. The drug targets mTOR, a protein kinase that plays a key role in cell growth. mTOR activates HIF-1 and other key genes, drives signaling to VEGF expression, and is a rational new target for genetic medicines against RCC. Preliminary data suggest that CCI-779 may have clinical activity against kidney and breast cancers. The drug reportedly is well tolerated, with rash as the most common side effect. The FDA fast-track program is designed to facilitate development and expedite review of new drugs or biologicals that are intended to treat serious or life-threatening conditions and that demonstrate the potential to address unmet medical needs. The fast-track designation does not guarantee, however, approval or expedited approval of any product.

Neovastat is an aqueous extract of shark cartilage that received fast-track designation by the FDA on October 16,

2002, for the treatment of RCC. Neovastat is a promising oral agent that exhibits a variety of anticancer properties including inhibition of angiogenesis. Preliminary data from a prospective, randomized, double-blind, placebo-controlled, phase III clinical trail were reported at ASCO 2003.[94] These data suggest that this agent has an acceptable toxicity profile with a trend toward enhanced survival, although a final determination cannot be established until the data mature.

TREATMENT OF KIDNEY CANCERS WITH NONCONVENTIONAL HISTOLOGIES

Sarcomatoid RCC is a poorly differentiated form of RCC that is associated with poor prognosis. A retrospective, single-institution study of 31 consecutive patients treated in the UCLA Kidney Cancer Program from 1990 to 1997 revealed that patients treated with regimens that included high-dose IL-2 ($n = 9$) had improved survival relative to patients who had surgery alone ($n = 6$) or immunotherapy with low-dose IL-2 ($n = 5$), dendritic cell vaccines ($n = 1$), or a combination of IFN-a, TILs, and low-dose IL-2 ($n = 9$). The relative risk of death was 10.4 times higher for patients not receiving high-dose IL-2 therapy ($n = 22$) after adjusting for age, sex, and percentage of sarcomatoid tumor.[95]

A retrospective, single-institution study of metastatic RCC reviewed data on patients in the MSKCC clinical trials database ($n = 286$), surgery database ($n = 1166$), and pathology database ($n = 357$) treated from 1985 to 2001.[96] A variety of non–clear cell histologies were identified including collecting duct ($n = 26$), chromophobe ($n = 12$), papillary ($n = 18$), and tumors that could not be classified for specific histology ($n = 8$). The patients who received systemic therapy ($n = 43$) were treated with 86 different forms of therapy including 37 cytokine-based regimens, with only two PRs observed. The median overall survival for this group was 9.4 months. Patients with chromophobe histology had a longer overall median survival (29 months) than did patients with collecting duct (11 months) or papillary histologies (5.5 months). No data were presented on patients with sarcomatoid histology.

Renal medullary carcinoma is a rare form of kidney cancer that occurs almost exclusively in blacks with sickle cell (SC) trait or hemoglobin SC disease.[97] In a report of 34 patients from the Armed Forces Institute of Pathology, none of the tumors was found to be confined to the kidney at the time of nephrectomy, with most having metastasized when first discovered. The mean duration of life after surgery was 15 weeks. No reports on therapeutic intervention are available at this time for review.

Collecting duct RCC is a rare and aggressive neoplasm of the distal collecting duct system for which there is no established therapy. In a case report, a 37-year-old woman with metastatic collecting duct RCC had 80% reduction in her tumor burden including complete regression of lymph node metastases and significant shrinkage of the primary after treatment with paclitaxel and carboplatin. The patient was subsequently rendered free of disease by nephrectomy without evidence of recurrence at 20 months of follow-up.[98] Thus chemotherapy with paclitaxel/carboplatin and surgery should be considered for patients with metastatic collecting duct RCC.

SUMMARY

RCC is being detected with increasing frequency in the United States and worldwide. The risk factors that have been identified to date for sporadic RCC include smoking, obesity, and hypertension, along with the hereditary patterns of VHL disease and tuberous sclerosis. Recent advances in molecular classification of RCC with techniques such as DNA microarray analysis with laser capture of single malignant cells and comparative genomic hybridization should allow targeted therapies to be developed for specific histologic subtypes. The list is expanding, but new targets include VHL, HIF-1, VEGF, and mTOR.

Surgical resection remains the principal therapeutic modality when RCC is confined to the kidney. Surgical techniques continue to be refined through the growing use of laparoscopic procedures that result in less morbidity while maintaining comparable therapeutic outcomes. Angioinfarction may be used preoperatively to reduce bleeding at the time of nephrectomy when primary tumors are large. Patients at high risk for recurrence after nephrectomy include those with positive lymph nodes, extension beyond Gerota's fascia, or extension into the renal vein or vena cava. Overall survival is influenced by stage, performance status, Fuhrman grade, and histologic subtype (sarcomatoid or collecting duct).

Adjuvant cytokine therapy for resected stage II or III disease does not appear to be effective. Cytoreductive nephrectomy for patients with metastatic disease may enhance responsiveness to high-dose IL-2 and make the primary tumor available for use in clinical trials that utilize patient-specific vaccines. Metastectomy is considered acceptable if all disease can be resected, and in some instances, this may be curative. Patients with advanced disease and who are in excellent physical condition should consider treatment with high-dose IL-2. Subcutaneous regimens with IL-2 and IFN-a, with or without 5-FU, induce overall response rates that are similar to those with high-dose IL-2, but durable CRs are observed even more infrequently. Second-line cytokine therapy and chemotherapy are generally ineffective for advanced RCC, although new combinations with gemcitabine warrants further study.

Allogeneic peripheral-blood stem cell transplantation can induce high CR rates in patients with advanced RCC, although most patients experience the morbidity of grade 3 or 4 GVHD, which can be permanently crippling and life threatening. Patients should receive this therapy only in the context of carefully conducted clinical trials. Patients with bone metastases should receive monthly bisphosphonate therapy with zoledronic acid to decrease the incidence of new bone lesions and pathologic fractures. On occasion, metastatic RCC will follow an indolent

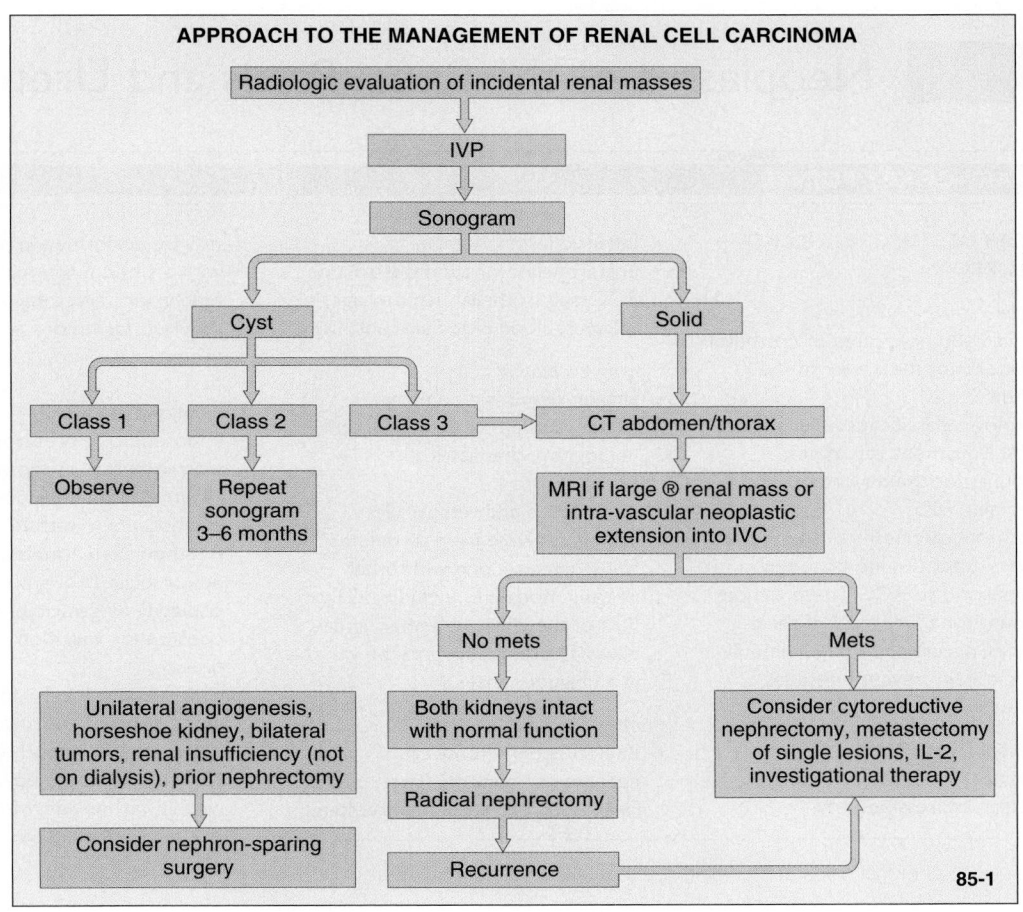

APPROACH TO THE MANAGEMENT OF RENAL CELL CARCINOMA

Radiologic evaluation of incidental renal masses

IVP

Sonogram

Cyst — Solid

Class 1 — Class 2 — Class 3 → CT abdomen/thorax

Observe

Repeat sonogram 3–6 months

MRI if large ® renal mass or intra-vascular neoplastic extension into IVC

No mets — Mets

Unilateral angiogenesis, horseshoe kidney, bilateral tumors, renal insufficiency (not on dialysis), prior nephrectomy

Both kidneys intact with normal function

Consider cytoreductive nephrectomy, metastectomy of single lesions, IL-2, investigational therapy

Consider nephron-sparing surgery

Radical nephrectomy

Recurrence

85-1

clinical course, and patients will remain asymptomatic without specific intervention with stable disease or even spontaneous remission. Other patients may have recurrence more than 20 years after resection of the primary. Strong physician encouragement of patient participation in clinical trials of newer agents, especially those targeting angiogenesis, should be a widely practiced standard of care. More effective and less toxic therapies for patients with advanced RCC are on the horizon of clinical development, but patient awareness and participation in controlled clinical trials will dictate the pace of progress.

Wayne B. Harris
Jonathan W. Simons

Neoplasms of the Renal Pelvis and Ureter

SUMMARY OF KEY POINTS

CANCER OF THE URETER AND RENAL PELVIS

Incidence
- About 2400 new cases of urothelial carcinoma of the ureter in the United States.
- Histologic classifications: urothelial (90%). Squamous carcinoma accounts for the majority of the remaining 10%.
- Urothelial carcinoma of the upper urinary tract is quite uncommon in comparison to RCC. These tumors account for 5% to 10% of renal tumors, occurring most commonly in the sixth and seventh decades of life.

Differential Diagnosis
- Extrinsic masses: parapelvic cyst, vascular impressions.

- Intrinsic lesions: benign ureteropelvic junction obstruction, RCC, suburothelial hemorrhage, calculus, blood clot, malacoplakia.

Staging Evaluation
- Staging requires a complete history and physical examination, hemogram, chemistries, urinalysis.
- Intravenous and retrograde pyelography are used to define filling defects along with other imaging modalities including CT or MRI of the chest, abdomen, and pelvis. Ureteroscopy may be valuable in ambiguous cases.

Primary Therapy
- Radical nephrectomy or nephroureterectomy (open or laparoscopic). Partial nephrectomy

may be performed in patients with a single functioning kidney.
- Nephroureterectomy is not always required for lesions of the distal ureter.

Secondary Therapies
- Endoscopic or ureteroscopic laser electrocautery in the vicinity of recurrence and bleeding; systemic chemotherapy with MVAC [methotrexate, vinblastine, doxorubicin (Adriamycin), and cisplatin] or gemcitabine and cisplatin for palliation of metastatic disease.
- Unresectable locally advanced urothelial carcinoma: possible postoperative radiotherapy with or without chemotherapy such as weekly carboplatin with paclitaxel.

INTRODUCTION

Urothelial (transitional cell) carcinoma may occur at any site in the upper urinary tract including the renal pelvis and ureter. These tumors occur most commonly in adults older than 40 years. The incidence is two- to threefold higher in men than in women. The lesions are often multifocal and occur more often in patients with a history of urothelial carcinoma of the bladder.

Cigarette smoking is a significant risk factor for urothelial carcinoma, as is occupational exposure to chemicals or petrochemicals.[99] Other less common risk factors include analgesic abuse, particularly phenacetin abuse, and a form of progressive interstitial inflammation endemic in Eastern Europe, known as Balkan nephritis, that results in renal failure.[100] Areas of endemic schistosomiasis have an incidence of carcinoma of the bladder that may involve the ureters. Chronic infection and stones may result in squamous carcinoma of the renal pelvis, presumably on the basis of chronic irritation.

Arsenic-contaminated water has been implicated as a contributing factor in the unusually high incidence of upper urinary tract urothelial carcinoma in Taiwan, although a retrospective review of tumor location (renal pelvis vs. ureter vs. urinary bladder) reports that the incidence appears to be high throughout the country and not limited to the southern regions where the contaminated water is found.[101] The presence of upper-tract disease in this study was associated with more aggressive clinical behavior in patients with early-stage disease.

CLINICAL PRESENTATION AND DIAGNOSIS

Roughly 75% of patients with urothelial carcinoma have microscopic or gross hematuria. Diagnosis is made on the basis of urine cytology, intravenous pyelography, and cystoscopy. In a study of 52 renal pelvic washings for which tissue confirmation was available, the sensitivity and specificity of the cytologic diagnosis of high-grade urothelial carcinoma was reported at 89% and 97%, with a positive predictive value of 93%. Two of 37 cases of high-grade urothelial carcinoma were reported as negative by this method.[102] One report asserted that the ratio of RNA isoforms of CD44 may serve as a novel prognostic predictor and indicator of extent of urothelial carcinoma.[103] Although the isoform designated CD44v8-10 can scarcely be detected in normal tissues, robust expression is often detected in specimens containing urothelial carcinoma. In this study, voided urine samples were analyzed from patients with urothelial carcinoma ($n = 150$) and patients with benign disease ($n = 50$). The mean ratio of CD44v8-10 to standard CD44 was significantly higher in urinary exfoliated cells of patients with invasive urothelial carcinoma relative to those with superficial urothelial carcinoma. Furthermore, patients who underwent complete resection for invasive urothelial carcinoma and who had an elevated ratio of CD44v8-10 to standard CD44 had significantly lower disease-free survival than did patients with a normal ratio.

PATHOLOGY

The vast majority of upper tract tumors are urothelial carcinomas (>90%), some of which are papillary. Squamous cell carcinomas account for most in the remainder of the patients and are often associated with staghorn calculi, chronic infection, and poor renal function. Uncommon histologic types include epidermoid carcinoma and adenocarcinoma. Often serum carcinoembryonic antigen (CEA) is elevated, and this biomarker can be useful in monitoring response to treatment.

STAGING

Clinical staging usually includes radiographic imaging with intravenous and/or retrograde pyelography. CT scanning is useful for assessing regional lymph nodes. Ureteroscopic visualization of the tumor is preferred and may allow tissue biopsy. If tissue biopsy is not feasible, urine cytology may help determine the grade. The presence or absence of concomitant disease in the bladder does not alter the staging of the renal pelvis and ureter. When metastatic disease is present and tumors are present in the upper and lower tract, the tumor of highest grade or stage is presumed to have contributed to the nodal or distant metastasis. Pathologic staging is dependent on determining the extent of invasion by the primary tumor.

The AJCC 2002 TNM classification of neoplasms of the renal pelvis and ureter (Table 85-6) applies only to carcinomas. Papilloma is excluded. As in the TNM classification of neoplasms of the kidney, regional lymph nodes for the renal pelvis are defined as the hilar, abdominal para-aortic, and paracaval lymph nodes. The same regional nodes are assigned to the ureter, in addition to the intrapelvic nodes. Laterality does not affect the N classification.

Some evidence indicates that the pattern of invasion of pathologic T3 lesions has prognostic significance. In a retrospective Japanese study of patients with pT3 disease ($n = 70$), extensive parenchymal involvement was the strongest prognostic indicator of decreased cause-specific survival ($P = .0004$; hazard ratio, 5.59). Lesions without extensive invasion had a prognosis similar to that of lower-stage disease. The authors suggest that patients with pT3 disease be subclassified into two separate entities for prognostic purposes, those with and without extensive parenchymal invasion.[104]

RADICAL NEPHROURETERECTOMY

Urothelial carcinoma of the upper urinary tract is often treated with nephroureterectomy, in which the kidney and ureter are resected along with a cuff of bladder tissue

TABLE 85-6

 The 2002 American Joint Committee on Cancer TNM Classification of Tumors of the Renal Pelvis and Ureter

T, N, M	FEATURES
Primary Tumor (T)	
TX	Primary tumor cannot be assessed
T0	No evidence of primary tumor
Ta	Papillary noninvasive carcinoma
Tis	Carcinoma in situ
T1	Tumor invades the subepithelial connective tissue
T2	Tumor invades the muscularis
T3	*(For renal pelvis only)* Tumor invades beyond muscularis into peripelvic fat or the renal parenchyma
	(For ureter only) Tumor invades beyond muscularis into periureteric fat
T4	Tumor invades adjacent organs or through the kidney into the perinephric fat
Regional Lymph Nodes (N)*	
NX	Regional lymph nodes cannot be assessed
N0	No regional lymph node metastasis
N1	Metastasis in a single lymph node, ≤2 cm in greatest dimension
N2	Metastasis in a single lymph node, >2 cm but ≤5 cm in greatest dimension; or multiple lymph nodes, none >5 cm in greatest dimension
N3	Metastasis in a lymph node more than >5 cm in greatest dimension
Distant Metastasis (M)	
MX	Distant metastasis cannot be assessed
M0	No distant metastasis
M1	Distant metastasis
Histopathologic Grading (G)	
GX	Grade cannot be assessed
G1	Well differentiated
G2	Moderately differentiated
G3–4	Poorly differentiated or undifferentiated

STAGE		GROUPING	
0a	Ta	N0	M0
0is	Tis	N0	M0
I	T1	N0	M0
II	T2	N0	M0
III	T3	N0	M0
IV	T4	N0	M0
	Any T	N1, N2, N3	M0
	Any T	Any N	M1

*Laterality does not affect the N classification.

surrounding the ureteral orifice. Appropriate regional nodes should be sampled. If the distal ureter is involved or if renal function is compromised, more conservative surgical procedures may be warranted.

LAPAROSCOPIC NEPHRECTOMY AND OTHER LESS INVASIVE PROCEDURES

Selected patients with small renal tumors may benefit from the decreased morbidity of radical laparoscopic nephroureterectomy. Techniques that require the kidney to be morcellated into small fragments are problematic, however, because they severely compromise the ability to stage the tumor accurately. A novel transvesical needle-scopic technique that allows the specimen to be extracted intact appears to have outcomes comparable to those of traditional open procedures, with significantly less morbidity.[105] More limited surgical options include endoscopic resection via ureteroscope, percutaneous procedures, as well as laser or electrocautery coagulation or vaporization. These procedures may leave little or no tissue for histologic evaluation.

CHEMOTHERAPY FOR ADVANCED UROTHELIAL CARCINOMA

Common palliative chemotherapy regimens for treating metastatic urothelial carcinoma use platinum-containing compounds. Phase II data indicate that treatment with MVAC [methotrexate/vinblastine/doxorubicin (Adriamycin)/cisplatin] and gemcitabine/cisplatin is associated with median survivals of about 12 months. The median survival for paclitaxel/carboplatin has been reported at approximately 10 months. MVAC is clearly a more toxic regimen, whereas paclitaxel/carboplatin is the least toxic. Because many patients with metastatic urothelial carcinoma have had a prior nephroureterectomy, regimens containing cisplatin may be contraindicated if significant compromise in renal function is present. None of these therapies has been tested in randomized phase III trials.

Gemcitabine and docetaxel have been recently identified to be active agents in advanced urothelial carcinoma in phase II trials.[106] Docetaxel is given at a dose of 40 mg/m^2 over a 1-hour period followed by gemcitabine, 800 mg/m^2, over a 30-minute period, both IV on days 1 and 8. Cycles were repeated every 21 days until disease progression or a maximum of six cycles. This generated a response rate of 17% (90% confidence interval, 7% to 33%). One patient achieved a CR. The median overall survival of the group was 7.7 months. Toxicities were moderate, with granulocytopenia, anorexia, and fatigue being the most common. Responses in visceral, lymph node, and soft tissue sites can be observed. The combination of gemcitabine and docetaxel has the potential to palliate a subset of previously treated patients with an excellent performance status and will be undergoing additional clinical evaluation.

SUMMARY

Urothelial carcinoma of the upper urinary tract is environmentally induced, often by cigarette exposure and industrial carcinogens. Drug development has been oriented toward regimens used in bladder cancer. Treatment with gemcitabine and docetaxel should be considered for palliation in appropriate patients.

REFERENCES

1. Chow W-H, Gridley G, Fraumeni JF Jr, Jarvholm B: Obesity, hypertension, and the risk of kidney cancer in men. N Engl J Med 2000;343:1305-1311.
2. Selikoff U, Hammond EC, Seidman H: Mortality experience of insulation workers in the United States and Canada 1943-1976. Ann NY Acad Sci 1979;330:91-116.
3. Smith AH, Shearn VI, Wood R: Asbestos and kidney cancer: The evidence supports a causal association. Am J Ind Med 1989;16:159-166.
4. Bretan PN, Busch MP, Hricak H, Williams RD: Chronic renal failure: A significant risk factor in the development of acquired renal cysts and renal cell carcinoma: Case reports and review of the literature. Cancer 1986;57:1871-1879.
5. Chow W-H, Devessa SS, Warren JL, Fraumeni JF Jr: Rising incidence of renal cell cancer in the United States. JAMA 1999;281:1628-1631.
6. Mathew A, Devesa SS, Fraumeni JF Jr, Chow W-H: Global increases in kidney cancer incidence, 1973-1992. Eur J Cancer Prev 2002;11:171-178.
7. Luciani LG, Cestari R, Tallarigo C: Incidental renal carcinoma: Age and stage characterization and clinical implications: Study of 1092 patients (1982-1997). Urology 2000;56:58-62.
8. Moertel CG, Dockerty MB, Baggenstoss AH: Multiple primary multiple malignant neoplasms, III: Tumors of multicentric origin. Cancer 1961;14:238.
9. Pritchett TR, Lieskovsky G, Skinner DG: Extension of renal cell carcinoma into the vena cava: Clinical review and surgical approach. J Urol 1986;135:460.
10. Storkel S, Eble JN, Adlakha K, et al: Classification of renal cell carcinoma: Workgroup No. 1. Union Internationale Contre le Cancer (UICC) and the American Joint Committee on Cancer (AJCC). Cancer 1997;80:987-989.
11. Fuhrman SA, Lasky LC, Limas C: Prognostic significance of morphologic parameters in renal cell carcinoma. Am J Surg Pathol 1982;6:655-663.
12. Koga S, Nishikido M, Hayashi T, Matsuya F, Saito Y, Kanetake H: Outcome of surgery in cystic renal cell carcinoma. Urology 2000;56:67-70.
13. Barnabas N, Amin MB, Pindolia K, Nanavati R, Amin MB, Worsham MJ: Mutations in the von Hippel-Lindau (VHL) gene define differential diagnostic criteria in renal cell carcinoma. J Surg Oncol Suppl 2002;80:52-60.
14. Young AN, Amin MB, Moreno CS, et al: Expression profiling of renal epithelial neoplasms. Am J Pathol 2001;158:1639-1651.
15. Rybicki FJ, Shu KM, Cibas ES, Fielding JR, vanSonnenberg E, Silverman SG: Percutaneous biopsy of renal masses: Sensitivity and negative predictive value stratified by clinical setting and size of masses. Am J Roentgenol 2003;180:1281-1287.
16. Flocks RH, Kadesky MC: Malignant neoplasms of the kidney: an analysis of 353 patients followed five years or more. J Urol 1958;79:196-201.
17. Robson CJ, Churchill BM, Anderson W: The results of radical nephrectomy for renal cell carcinoma. J Urol 1969;101:297-301.
18. Harmer M: TNM Classification of Malignant Tumors, 3rd ed. Geneva, International Union Against Cancer, 1978.
19. Bassil B, Dosoretz DE, Prout GR Jr: Validation of the tumor, nodes and metastasis classification of renal cell carcinoma. J Urol 1985;134:450-454.
20. Hermanek P, Schrott KM: Evaluation of the tumor, nodes, and metastases classification of renal cell carcioma. J Urol 1990;144:238-244.
21. Guinan P, Saffrin R, Struhldreher D, et al: Renal cell carcinoma: comparison of the TNM and Robson stage groupings. J Surg Oncol 1995;59:186-189.
22. Flemming ID, Cooper JS, Henson DE, et al: AJCC Cancer Staging Manual, 5th ed. Philadelphia, Lippincott-Raven, 1997, pp 231-232.
23. Guinan P, Sobin LH, Algaba F, et al: TNM staging of renal cell carcinoma. Cancer 1997;80:992-993.
24. Gettman MT, Blute ML: Update on pathologic staging of renal cell carcinoma. Urology 2002;60:209-217.
25. Greene FL, Page DL, Fleming ID, et al (eds): AJCC Cancer Staging Handbook, 6th ed. New York, Springer-Verlag, 2002, pp 361-365.
26. Lee CT, Katz J, Shi W, Gthaler HT, Reuter VE, Russo P: Surgical management of renal tumors 4 cm or less in a contemporary cohort. J Urol 2000;163:730-736.
27. Hafez KS, Fergany AF, Novick AC: Nephron sparing surgery for localized renal cell carcinoma: Impact of tumor size on patient

survival, tumor recurrence and TNM staging. J Urol 1999;162: 1930–1933.

28. Lerner SE, Hawkins CA, Blute ML, et al: Disease outcome in patients with low stage renal cell carcinoma treated with nephron sparing or radical surgery. J Urol 1996;155:1868–1873.

29. Chisolm GD: Paraneoplastic syndromes: Introduction in renal tumors. In Proceedings of the First International Symposium on Kidney Tumors. New York, AR Liss, 1982, pp 277–282.

30. O'Keefe SC, Marshall FF, Issa MM, Harmon MP, Petros JA: Thrombocytosis is associated with a significant increase in the cancer specific death rate after radical nephrectomy. J Urol 2002;168:1378–1380.

31. Walther MM, Patel B, Choyke PL, et al: Hypercalcemia in patients with metastatic renal cell carcinoma: Effect of nephrectomy and metabolic evaluation. J Urol 1997;158:733–739.

32. Ono Y, Kinukawa Y, Hattori R, et al: Laparscopic radical nephrectomy for renal cell carcinoma: A five-year experience. Urology 1999;53:280–286.

33. Walther MM, Lyne JC, Libutti SK, Linehan WM: Laparoscopic cytoreductive nephrectomy as preparation for administration of systemic interleukin-2 in the treatment of metastatic renal cell carcinoma: A pilot study. Urology 1999;53:496–501.

34. Nakada SY, Fadden P, Jarrard DF, Moon TD: Hand-assisted laparoscopic radical nephrectomy: Comparison to open radical nephrectomy. Urology 2001;58:517–520.

35. Pantuck AJ, Zisman A, Cohen J, Belledegrun A: Cryosurgical ablation of renal tumors using 1.5-millimeter, ultrathin cryoprobes. Urology 2002;59:130–133.

36. Belldegrun A, Tsui K-H, deKernion JB, Smith RB: Efficacy of nephron-sparing surgery for renal cell carcinoma: Analysis based on the new 1997 tumor-node-metastasis staging system. J Clin Oncol 1999;17:2868–2875.

37. Piper NY, Bishoff JT, Magee C, et al: Is a 1-cm margin necessary during nephron-sparing surgery for renal cell carcinoma? Urology 2001;58:849–852.

38. Jeschke K, Peschel R, Wakonig J, Schellander L, Bartsch G, Henning K: Laparoscopic nephron-sparing surgery for renal tumors. Urology 2001;58:688–692.

39. Brenner B: Hemodynamically mediated glomerular injury and progressive nature of kidney disease. Kidney Int 1983;23: 647–655.

40. O'Dea M, Zincke H, Utz D, et al: The treatment of renal cell carcinoma with solitary metastases. J Urol 1975;114:836–838.

41. Middleton R: Surgery for metastatic renal cell carcinoma. J Urol 1967;97:973–977.

42. Klugo R, Detmres M, Stiles R, et al: Aggressive versus conservative management of stage 4 renal cell carcinoma. J Urol 1977;118:244–246.

43. Golimbu M, Al-Askari S, Tessler A, et al: Aggressive treatment of metastatic renal cancer. J Urol 1986;136:805–807.

44. Esrig D, Ahlering T, Lieskovsky G, et al: Experience with fossa recurrence of renal cell carcinoma. J Urol 1992;147:1491–1494.

45. Tanguay S, Pisters L, Lawrence D, et al: Therapy of locally recurrent renal cell carcinoma after nephrectomy. J Urol 1996;155:26–29.

46. Edelman M, Meyers F, Siegel D: The utility of follow-up testing after curative cancer therapy. J Gen Intern Med 1997;12:318–331.

47. Sandock D, Sefiel A, Resnick M: A new protocol for the followup of renal cell carcinoma based on pathologic stage. J Urol 1995;154:28–31.

48. Levy D, Slaton J, Swanson D, et al: Stage specific guidelines for surveillance after radical nephrectomy for local renal cell carcinoma. J Urol 1998;159:1163–1167.

49. Ljunberg B, Alamdari R, Rasmuson T, et al: Follow-up guidelines for nonmetastatic renal cell carcinoma based on the occurrence of metastases after radical nephrectomy. BJU Int 1999;84:405–411.

50. Hafez K, Novick A, Campbell S: Patterns of tumor recurrence and guidelines for followup after nephron sparing surgery for sporadic renal cell carcinoma. J Urol 1997;157:2067–2070.

51. Tapper H, Klein H, Rubenstein W, et al: Recurrent renal cell carcinoma after 45 years. Clin Imaging 1997;21:273–275.

52. Rabinovitz RA, Zelefsky MJ, Gaynor JJ, Fuks Z: Patterns of failure following surgical resection of renal cell carcinoma: Implications for adjuvant local and systemic therapy. J Clin Oncol 1994;12: 206–212.

53. Steinbach F, Novick A, Zincke H, et al: Treatment of renal cell carcinoma in von Hippel-Lindau disease: A multicenter study. J Urol 1995;153:1812–1816.

54. Walther MM, Lubensky IA, Venzon D, et al: Prevalence of microscopic lesions in grossly normal renal parenchyma from patients with von Hippel-Lindau disease, sporadic renal cell carcinoma and no renal disease: Clinical implications. J Urol 1995;154:2010–2014; discussion, 2014–2015.

55. Maher EWK Jr: von Hippel-Lindau disease. Medicine 1997;76: 381–391.

56. Neuman HP, Zbar B: Renal cysts, renal cancer and von Hippel-Lindau disease. Kidney Int 1997;51:16–26.

57. Zbar B, Kaelin W, Maher E, et al: Third International Meeting on von Hippel-Lindau disease. Cancer Res 1999;59:2251–2253.

58. Flanigan RC, Salmon SE, Blumenstein BA, et al: Nephrectomy followed by interferon-alfa-2b compared with interferon alfa-2b alone for metastatic renal-cell cancer. N Engl J Med 2001;345: 1655–1659.

59. Kavolius JP, Mastorakos DP, Pavlovich C, Russo P, Burt ME, Brady MS: Resection of metastatic renal cell carcinoma. J Clin Oncol 1998;16:2261–2266.

60. Gleave ME, Elhilali M, Fradet Y, et al: Interferon-gamma-1b compared with placebo in metastatic renal-cell carcinoma. N Engl J Med 1998;338:1265–1271.

61. Pizzocaro G, Piva L, Colavita M, et al: Interferon adjuvant to radical nephrectomy in Robson stages II and III renal cell carcinoma: A multicentric randomized study. J Clin Oncol 2001;19:425–432.

62. Messing EM, Manola J, Wilding G, et al: Phase III study of interferon alfa-NL as adjuvant treatment for resectable renal cell carcinoma by the Eastern Cooperative Oncology Group/Intergroup. J Clin Oncol 2003;21:1214–1222.

63. Amin MB, Amin MB, Tamboli P, et al: Prognostic impact of histologic subtyping of adult renal epithelial neoplasms: an experience of 405 cases. Am J Surg Pathol 2002;26:281–291.

64. Zisman A, Pantuck AJ, Dorey F, et al: Improved prognostication of renal cell carcinoma using an integrated staging system. J Clin Oncol 2001;19:1649–1657.

65. Zisman A, Pantuck AJ, Figlin RA, Belldegrun AS: Validation of the UCLA integrated staging system for patients with renal cell carcinoma. J Clin Oncol 2001;20:3792–3793.

66. Zisman A, Pantuck AJ, Dorey F, et al: Mathematical model to predict individual survival for patients with renal cell carcinoma. J Clin Oncol 2002;20:1368–1374.

67. Zisman A, Pantuck AJ, Wieder J, et al: Risk assessment and clinical outcome algorithm to predict the natural history of patients with surgically resected renal cell carcinoma. J Clin Oncol 2002;20: 4559–4566.

68. Motzer RJ, Mazumdar M, Bacik J, et al: Survival and prognostic stratification of 670 patients with advanced renal cell carcinoma. J Clin Oncol 1999;17:2530–2540.

69. Motzer RJ, Mazumdar M, Bacik J, Russo P, Berg WJ, Metz EM: Effect of cytokine therapy on survival for patients with advanced renal cell carcinoma. J Clin Oncol 2000;18:1928–1935.

70. Rabanni F, Herr HE, Almahmeed T, Russo P: Temporal change in risk of metachronous contralateral renal cell carcinoma: Influence of tumor characteristics and demographic factors. J Clin Oncol 2002;20:2370–2375.

71. Rosenberg SA, Yang JC, White DE, Steinberg SM: Durability of complete responses in patients with metastatic cancer treated with high-dose interleukin-2: Identification of the antigens mediating response. Ann Surg 1998;228:307–319.

72. Fisher RI, Rosenberg SA, Fyfe G: Long-term survival update for high-dose recombinant interleukin-2 in patients with renal cell carcinoma. Cancer J Sci Am 2000;6(suppl 1):S55–S57.

73. Mekhail T, Wood L, Bukowski R: Interleukin-2 in cancer therapy: Uses and optimum management of adverse effects. BioDrugs 2000;14:299–318.

74. Schwartzentruber DJ: Guidelines for the safe administration of high-dose interleukin-2. J Immunother 2001;24:287–293.

75. Tourani J-M, Pfister C, Berdah J-F, et al: The Subcutaneous Administration Proleukin Program Cooperative Group: Outpatient treatment with subcutaneous interleukin-2 and interferon alfa administration in combination with fluorouracil in patients with metastatic renal cell carcinoma: Results of a sequential

Specific Malignancies

III

nonrandomized phase II study. J Clin Oncol 1998;16:2505–2513.

76. Ravaud A, Audhuy B, Gomez F, et al, and the Groupe Français d'Immunothérapie: Subcutaneous interleukin-2, interferon alfa-2a, and continuous infusion of fluorouracil in metastatic renal cell carcinoma: A multicenter phase II trial. J Clin Oncol 1998;16: 2728–2732.

77. Motzer RJ, Vogelzang NJ: Chemotherapy for renal cell carcinoma. In: Raghavan D, Scher, HI, Leibel SA, Lange P (eds): Principles and Practice of Genitourinary Oncology. Philadelphia, Lippincott-Raven, 1997, pp 885–896.

78. Yagoda A, Abi-Rached B, Petrylak D: Chemotherapy for advanced renal cell carcinoma: 1983-1993. Semin Oncol 1995;22:42–60.

79. Rini BI, Vogelzang NJ, Dumas MC, Wade JL III, Taber DA, Stadler WM: Phase II trial of weekly intravenous gemcitabine with continuous infusion fluorouracil in patients with metastatic renal cell cancer. J Clin Oncol 2000;18:2419–2426.

80. Stadler WM, Kuzel T, Dumas M, Vogelzang NJ: Multicenter phase II trial of interleukin-2, interferon-a, and 13-cis-retinoic acid in patients with metastatic renal-cell carcinoma. J Clin Oncol 1998;16:1820–1825.

81. Mozter RJ, Murphy BA, Bacik J, et al: Phase III trial of interferon-a2a with or without 13-cis-retinoic acid for patients with advanced renal cell carcinoma. J Clin Oncol 2000;18:2972–2980.

82. Franzke A, Peest D, Probst-Kepper M, et al: Autoimmunity resulting from cytokine treatment predicts long-term survival in patients with metastatic renal cell carcinoma. J Clin Oncol 1999;17:529–533.

83. Escudier B, Chevreau C, Lasset C, et al: Cytokines in metastatic renal cell carcinoma: Is it useful to switch to interleukin-2 or interferon after failure of a first treatment? J Clin Oncol 1999;17:2039–2043.

84. Figlin RA, Thompson JA, Bukowski RM, et al: Multicenter, randomized, phase III trial of CD8+ tumor-infiltrating lymphocytes in combination with recombinant interleukin-2 in metastatic renal cell carcinoma. J Clin Oncol 1999;17:2521–2529.

85. Stadler WM, Kuzel T, Shapiro C, Sosman J, Clark J, Volgelzang NJ: Multi-institutional study of the angiogenesis inhibitor TNP-470 in metastatic renal cell carcinoma. J Clin Oncol 1999;17:2541–2545.

86. D'Amato RJ, Loughman MS, Flynn J: Thalidomide is an inhibitor of angiogenesis. Proc Natl Acad Sci USA 1994;91:4082–4085.

87. Eisen T, Boshoff C, Sapunar F, et al: Continuous low-dose thalidomide: A phase II study in advancer melanoma, renal cell, ovarian and breast cancer. Br J Cancer 1999;82:812–817.

88. Motzer RJ, Berg W, Ginsberg M, et al: Phase II trial of thalidomide for patients with advanced renal cell carcinoma. J Clin Oncol 2002;20:302–306.

89. Nathan PD, Gore ME, Eisen TG: Unexpected toxicity of combination thalidomide and interferon-alfa-2a treatment in metastatic renal cell carcinoma. J Clin Oncol 2002;20:1429–1430.

90. Childs RW, Clave E, Tisdale J, Plante M, Hensel N, Hensel J: Successful treatment of metastatic renal cell carcinoma with a nonmyeloablative allogeneic peripheral-blood progenitor-cell transplant: Evidence for a graft-versus-tumor effect. J Clin Oncol 1999;17:2044–2049.

91. Childs R, Chernoff A, Contentin N, et al: Regression of metastatic renal-cell carcinoma after nonmyeloablative allogeneic peripheral-blood stem-cell transplantation. N Engl J Med 2000;343:750–758.

92. Motzer RJ, Bacik J, Murphy BA, Russo P, Mazumdar M: Interferon-alfa as a comparative treatment for clinical trials of new therapies against advanced renal cell carcinoma. J Clin Oncol 2002;20: 289–296.

93. Caudill MM, Li Z: HSPPC-96: A personalized cancer vaccine. Expert Opin Biol Ther 2001;1:539–547.

94. Escudier B, Venner P, Buckowski R, et al: Phase III trial of neovastat in metastatic renal cell carcinoma patients refractory to immunotherapy [abstract 844]. ASCO 2003;22:211.

95. Cangiano T, Liao J, Naitoh J, Dorey F, Figlin R, Belldegrun A: Sarcomatoid renal cell carcinoma: Biologic behavior, prognosis, and response to combined surgical resection and immunotherapy. J Clin Oncol 1999;17:523–528.

96. Motzer RJ, Bacik J, Mariani T, Russo P, Mazumdar M, Reuter V: Treatment outcome and survival associated with metastatic renal cell carcinoma of non-clear-cell histology. J Clin Oncol 2002;20: 2376–2381.

97. Davis CJ Jr, Mostofi FK, Sesterhenn IA: Renal medullary carcinoma. Am J Surg Pathol 1995;19:1–11.

98. Gollob JA, Upton MP, DeWolf WC, Atkins MB: Long-term remission in a patient with metastatic collecting duct carcinoma treated with taxol/carboplatin and surgery. Urology 2001;58:1058i–1058iii.

99. Jansen OM, Knudsen JB, McLaughlin JK, et al: The Copenhagen case-control study of renal pelvis and ureter cancer: Role of smoking and occupational exposures. Int J Cancer 1988; 41:557.

100. Steffens J, Nagel R: Tumours of the renal pelvis and ureter: Observations in 170 patients. Br J Urol 1988;61:277.

101. Yang MH, Chen KK, Yen CC, et al: Unusually high incidence of upper urinary tract urothelial carcinoma in Taiwan. Urology 2002;59:681–687.

102. Witte D, Truong LD, Ramzy I: Transitional cell carcinoma of the renal pelvis: The diagnostic role of pelvic washings. Am J Clin Pathol 2002;117:444–450.

103. Miyake H, Eto H, Arakawa S, Kamidono S, Hara I: Overexpression of CD44V8-10 in urinary exfoliated cells as an independent prognostic predictor in patients with urothelial cancer. J Urol 2002;167:1282–1287.

104. Yoshimura K, Arai Y, Fujimoto H, et al: Prognostic impact of extensive parenchymal invasion pattern in pT3 renal pelvic transitional cell carcinoma. Cancer 2002;94:3150–3156.

105. Gill IS, Sung GT, Hobart MG, et al: Laparoscopic radical nephroureterectomy for upper tract transitional cell carcinoma: The Cleveland Clinic experience. J Urol 2000;164:1513–1522.

106. Dreicer R, Manola J, Schneider DJ, et al: Phase II trial of gemcitabine and docetaxel in patients with advanced carcinoma of the urothelium. Cancer 2003;97:2743–2747.

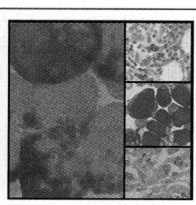

36

CARCINOMA OF THE BLADDER

James Montie

David C. Smith

Howard Sandler

SUMMARY OF KEY POINTS

INCIDENCE

- Bladder cancer accounts for 4% of all cancers in the United States with an estimated 57,400 cases and 12,500 deaths in 2003. The male-to-female ratio is 3:1.
- Risk increases with advancing age, with 70% of male bladder cancers and 75% of female bladder cancers occurring in individuals over the age of 65 years.

EPIDEMIOLOGY AND RISK FACTORS

- Cigarette smoking is an established cause of bladder cancer, accounting for half of male and one third of female bladder cancers in Western populations.
- Quitting smoking is associated with a dramatic drop in risk of bladder cancer.
- Occupational chemical exposure associated with bladder cancer includes arylamines and derivatives (also found in cigarette smoke), *O*-toluidine, and benzidine-based dyes; those at risk include painters, truck drivers, and drill press operators.
- Long-term cyclophosphamide therapy increases the risk for bladder cancer probably by as much as 30-fold.
- Schistosomiasis and spinal cord injury are associated with increased risk for squamous cell carcinoma of the bladder.

CLINICAL PRESENTATION

The primary symptom of bladder cancer is hematuria; 20% to 30% of patients will have symptoms of frequency, urgency, and dysuria.

DIAGNOSIS

- Cystoscopy with transurethral resection (TUR) is the mainstay of diagnosis.
- Upper tract imaging is necessary to detect additional urothelial tumors and obstruction.

PATHOLOGY AND STAGING

- Almost all bladder cancers are urothelial (transitional cell) in origin. Most present with a papillary growth pattern: flat carcinoma in situ (CIS) or a solid nodular tumor are other forms.
- At diagnosis, approximately one third of cases are noninvasive (Ta/TIS), one third are minimally invasive (T1), and another third are more deeply invasive (T2 and beyond).
- Grade and stage are strong prognostic factors and primary determinants of therapy.

THERAPY

- Most bladder cancers recur in the bladder, but can be managed with a combination of TUR and intravesical chemotherapy or immunotherapy.
- Few low-grade cancers progress (invade the bladder wall), but high-grade cancers have greater risk.
- Bacillus Calmette-Guérin (BCG) vaccine is the most effective agent for treating high-grade lesions, resulting in decreased progression and potentially increased survival.
- Most muscle-invasive cancers are not cured by TUR alone.
- Radical cystectomy with urinary diversion is the most effective means to eliminate the cancer.

- Orthotopic diversion with a neobladder provides improved rehabilitation by allowing volitional voiding.
- Pelvic recurrence rates, as well as distant metastases, in patients with locally advanced cancer remain disappointingly high.
- Radiation therapy combined with an aggressive TUR and a chemotherapeutic radiation sensitizer, such as cisplatin, may allow bladder preservation.
- Preoperative radiation has not been demonstrated to be consistently effective.
- Systemic chemotherapy for urothelial cancers is rapidly evolving.
- Traditional regimens, such as MVAC (methotrexate, vinblastine, doxorubicin, and cisplatin), have not produced durable results, and toxicity is high.
- New agents, such as paclitaxel and gemcitabine, are active and combinations of these agents with platinum-based compounds have comparable response rates with substantially less toxicity.
- Neoadjuvant chemotherapy prior to cystectomy is supported by increasing evidence, particularly in patients with locally advanced (T3b) tumors.
- Less data are available on the degree of benefit for adjuvant chemotherapy. Treatments must be individualized based on risk, benefits, and patient preference.

BACKGROUND AND INCIDENCE

Bladder cancer is a disease with a wide spectrum of risk to the patient. Well-differentiated, papillary tumors rarely present a threat of death or loss of the bladder to the patient. High-grade cancers are commonly lethal and treatment may greatly alter urinary and sexual function. The physician and patient often face difficult decisions about undertreatment and overtreatment. The initiation of intravesical therapy or cystectomy depends heavily on clinical judgment. Even experienced clinicians often find it difficult to separate the appropriate cystectomy patient from one in whom it may be unnecessary at one extreme or futile at the other. The integration of recently available effective and less toxic systemic chemotherapy as well as radiation therapy remains a challenge. Substantial progress in the delivery of bladder cancer care is clearly evident in the last two decades, but fundamental uncertainties in management decisions persist.

EPIDEMIOLOGY AND RISK FACTORS

Bladder cancer represents approximately 5% in men (fifth most common neoplasm) and 3% in women (eighth most common neoplasm) of new cases of cancer in the United States.[1] In 2003, there were an estimated 57,400 cases, including in men and in women. The age-adjusted incidence in the United States is 32 per 100,000 men and 8 per 100,000 women.[2] The historic male-female ratio of 3:1 may be decreasing related to smoking patterns in women.[1] There were an estimated 12,500 deaths from bladder cancer in 2003 (in men and in women). Bladder cancer incidence and mortality rate strongly increase with age and will be an increasing problem as the population becomes more elderly. Based on 1994 data, 70% of male cases and 74% of female cases were individuals 65 years of age or older.[3] Bladder cancer incidence rates continue to increase with age, cresting at a rate of 317.2 per 100,000 for men age 85 years of age and older.[3] Death rates reflect this age dependence with 83% of male and 87% of female bladder cancer deaths found in those 65 years of age and older. Death rates have decreased in the 1990–1995 period (–0.3%) based on SEER data, but to a lesser degree than the 1973–1990 interval (–1.8%).[4]

Most bladder cancers are noninvasive or minimally invasive at the time of diagnosis. Based on 1993 National Cancer Database data collected from a sampling from 2100 hospitals in the United States, 32.5% of cases were noninvasive (Ta) and 29% were minimally invasive (T1), and 80% were localized in the pelvis.[5] Using SEER data, 74% were localized in the pelvis at diagnosis. Women are slightly more likely to be diagnosed with advanced stages than men.[5,6] African Americans have a diminished survival overall and stage-for-stage compared to Caucasians.[7] Incidence of familial transitional cell carcinoma is uncertain, although some data support a familial form.[2,8]

Defined risk factors account for an estimated 80% of all bladder cancer cases.[9] In Western populations, cigarette smoking may account for approximately 50% of bladder cancer patients.[10] Zeegers and associates performed a meta-analysis of 43 epidemiologic studies on smoking characterisitics for bladder cancer risk and concluded that current cigarette smokers have an approximately threefold higher risk of urinary tract cancers than nonsmokers.[11] The carcinogenic effect of cigarette smoking is related to dose as well as the type of tobacco used. Black (air-cured) tobacco carries a higher risk than blond (flue-cured) tobacco, most likely because of higher concentrations of the known carcinogens arylamines.[10] Quitting smoking is associated with a drop in the risk of bladder cancer, regardless of type of tobacco.[10-12] The age

at which one begins smoking also carries an associated risk; those starting at a younger age have an increased risk for bladder cancer, even 10 to 15 years after quitting. Cigarette filters do not provide protection. The molecular mechanisms are likely based on exposure to the carcinogens 4-aminobiphenyl and 2-naphthylamine in cigarette smoke, possibly with modulation based on metabolic phenotype which governs noninducible enzymes in the liver under autosomal dominant control. The carcinogens are metabolized in the liver by N-acetylation; "slow" acetylators are homozygous for the slow acetylator gene and at higher risk for bladder cancer.[10]

Data from the U.S. National Bladder Cancer Study on Occupation and Bladder Cancer suggest that population-attributable risks for occupation in Caucasian men range from 21% to 25%.[13] Occupational bladder cancer remains a public health issue around the world. Leather and rubber workers are at increased risk, but this risk is decreasing as workplace exposure diminishes. New higher-risk occupations, such as painters, truck drivers, primary aluminum workers, and metal machinery workers are becoming evident.[13] There is a positive trend for increased risk associated with increasing duration of employment, particularly longer than 10 years.[13]

Several medications increase bladder cancer risk as use and exposure increase. Chronic phenacetin use increases risk of transitional cell carcinoma (TCC) of the bladder and the renal pelvis. Long-term oral cyclophosphamide use increases the risk for bladder cancer by as much as 30-fold.[14] In a cohort of 145 patients treated with cyclophosphamide for Wegener's granulomatosis, the incidence of bladder cancer was 5% at 10 years and 16% at 15 years.[14] Patients present with gross or microscopic hematuria, cytologic examination may not always be a reliable screening tool, and the cancers are often highly aggressive.[15]

An upper tract TCC is highly associated with bladder cancer. Of patients with either renal pelvic or ureteral TCC, 40% will have a bladder cancer at some point in the course of their disease; thus, surveillance cystoscopy is appropriate and necessary.

Chronic irritation of the bladder is associated with bladder cancer, typically squamous cell carcinoma (SCC) rather than TCC. Schistosomiasis is also highly associated with development of SCC of the bladder and remains a major public health problem in endemic areas even though a true causal link is not established.[16,17] Spinal cord injury patients with chronic or recurrent urinary tract infections, particularly with indwelling catheters, are at increased risk for bladder cancer at 16 to 20 times that of the general population.[18] Periodic cystoscopy is advocated in spinal cord injury patients after more than 10 years following the injury.[18]

CLINICAL PRESENTATION

The classic symptom of bladder cancer is hematuria, usually gross and painless, but occasionally only microscopic. Some patients (20% to 30%) may have primarily "irritable" bladder symptoms of frequency, urgency, and dysuria, particularly in patients with carcinoma in situ of the bladder. It is remarkably common that patients still present to a urologist with a substantial delay in diagnosis, which may be either patient- or physician-driven, because of attributing the hematuria to an infection or a stone without proper investigation. Gross hematuria requires a urologic evaluation. One study suggests that microscopic hematuria may be present years before the detection of the bladder cancer, and thus may be a predictor of bladder cancer.[19]

More advanced local disease causes pelvic pain, bladder outlet obstruction, or flank pain secondary to an obstructed upper tract. Extensive pelvic disease can cause rectal obstruction, lymphedema of the extremities, and deep venous thrombosis from compression of iliac veins.

Screening for bladder cancer has not been widely advocated or tested owing to a relatively low prevalence of the disease. In a study of asymptomatic men 50 years of age and older, Messing and colleagues provide data that a simple, repeated test of the urine with a chemical reagent dipstick for microhematuria detects bladder cancer.[20] In addition, they suggest that screening can detect cancers in earlier stage with resultant reduced disease-related mortality rate. A randomized trial in a high-risk population would be necessary to confirm the effectiveness and value of such screening.

DIAGNOSIS AND NATURAL HISTORY

The mainstay of detection of bladder cancer is cystoscopy. Most diagnostic cystoscopies are now done in an outpatient setting using a 16F flexible cystoscope (approximately the caliber of a small Foley catheter) and local intraurethral lidocaine for topical anesthesia. A flexible instrument with excellent optics substantially decreases discomfort of the procedure, particularly in men. Most bladder cancers appear grossly as a papillary, exophytic tumor, and low-grade tumors have a reliable, characteristic appearance.[21,22] A higher grade, invasive cancer may appear as erythema and edema of the mucosa with distortion of the bladder wall. If an abnormality is visualized in the bladder, an outpatient transurethral resection (TUR) or biopsy is done with anesthesia. This TUR is diagnostic, important for staging, and often therapeutic as the only treatment needed.[21] An examination under anesthesia to identify a pelvic mass or induration of the bladder is important in many cases. Occasionally, patients require a brief hospital admission after the procedure for hematuria, urinary retention, or bladder perforation.

During the evaluation of hematuria or after the diagnosis of bladder cancer is established, imaging of the upper urinary tract collecting system is essential. An intravenous pyelogram (IVP), retrograde pyelogram, or computed tomographic (CT) or magnetic resonance (MR) urogram identifies additional urothelial tumors and obstruction of the upper tract due to bladder cancer.[23] With typical papillary tumors, 2% to 4% of patients have or will develop an upper tract tumor. Patients with carcinoma in situ may have a substantially greater risk for

upper tract cancers. Imaging of the bladder with an IVP, CT scan, or ultrasonography can demonstrate a bladder cancer as a "filling defect" displacing contrast material or urine.

The natural history of bladder cancer is such that recurrences in the bladder are the rule (in 50% to 75% of patients), and prognostic factors governing risk for recurrence and progression are discussed later in detail.[24] Propensity for recurrences requires surveillance of the bladder at defined intervals. The mainstay of surveillance is cystoscopy, which is easily performed as an outpatient procedure with local anesthesia. If the cystoscopy is likely to be positive and require biopsy or resection, general or regional anesthesia is necessary. The classical follow-up protocol for patients without recurrence entails cystoscopy at 3-month intervals for 1 year, 4-month intervals during the second year, 6-month intervals for years 3 and 4, and then annually. This regimen is excessive in many patients at low risk for recurrence and very low risk for progression and can be altered by lengthening the intervals between cystoscopies more quickly.[25,26] The results of the first cystoscopy 3 months after the initial diagnostic resection often sets a precedent for the future recurrence pattern.[25]

Bladder cancer requires lifelong follow-up consisting of cystoscopy and periodic imaging of the upper tracts because recurrences may occur late, even after prolonged disease-free intervals.[26,27] Supplemental diagnostic aids in addition to or in place of an "invasive" cystoscopy are attractive. A test performed on a voided urine sample would be ideal. Unfortunately, no test in the urine can currently replace cystoscopy for either detection or follow-up.[28,29] Research is expanding on urinary markers for detection, but performance remains disappointing.[30]

Urinary cytologic examination plays an important role in detection and monitoring of bladder cancer and has stood the test of time.[31] Cytologic testing is particularly effective in patients with carcinoma in situ manifested by irritable symptoms and nonspecific inflammatory changes on visual cystoscopic examination. In these cases, cytologic examination may be the most important test to alert the physician to the presence of the cancer. However, in the aggregate, cytologic examination has substantial limitations in detection of bladder cancer; the sensitivity is approximately 60% and specificity is 70% to 80%.[30] Urine cytologic assessment is subjective, has considerable interobserver variability, and depends on an adequate number of cells in the specimen; also, interpretation can be influenced by collection method and cellular preservation techniques. As one may anticipate, cytologic testing is extremely valuable for detection and follow-up of high-grade lesions populated by cells with substantial abnormal morphologic characteristics. On the other hand, low-grade cancers in which the cells often closely resemble normal bladder epithelial cells have a low detection rate by cytologic test with a sensitivity as low as 10% to 40%. It is important to provide the cytologist with relevant clinical history, such as whether the specimen was a voided urine sample or a specimen obtained with a catheter or cystoscope and whether the patient has had prior therapy, such as intravesical bacillus

Calmette-Guérin (BCG) vaccine or external radiation therapy. Methods to improve cytologic assessment using immunostaining, either with Lewis-X antigen or cytokeratin 20, are also under exploration.[32,33]

Several urinary tests are now approved by the FDA (Food and Drug Administration) as aids for the detection or monitoring of bladder cancer. However, their clinical utility remains uncertain.[29,34] The ideal test fulfills at least one of two requirements: (1) it is highly sensitive so that a cytoscopy could be avoided or (2) it identifies patients with occult mucosal disease not visualized at cystoscopy, allowing a better assessment of treatment response or identification of a recurrence earlier. No test currently available consistently performs these functions well enough.

The first urine assay available for bladder cancer detection, the BTA test identifies a bladder tumor antigen.[35] The original BTA test detected basement membrane complexes and was attractive as a point-of-service urine test that gave immediate results. Initial trials demonstrate possible superiority over urinary cytologic testing, but cytologic accuracy in these trials was less than commonly accepted. Newer assays, termed *BTA stat* and *BTA TRAK*, aim to improve performance and are FDA-approved as well.[35,36] BTA stat is a qualitative measure of human complement factor H protein, whereas BTA TRAK is a quantitative measure. The results appear promising, but are no longer easy to use.[36] Urinary nuclear matrix protein (NMP-22) is approved by the FDA for detection of occult or rapidly recurring disease after a TUR and may perform better than cytologic examination as a diagnostic tool.[37] Higher NMP-22 levels correlated with cancer with a favorable receiver operating characteristic (ROC) curve, but experience is limited. Aura Tek fibrin degradation products measure urinary fibrinogen and fibrinogen degradation products and was also purported to outperform cytologic examination, and had an attraction as a dipstick type assay at point of service that was easy to use, but is no longer commercially available.[30,38] Several other tests are under development to capitalize on the shedding of malignant cells or proteins into the urine. More than 300 proteins shed into the urine of bladder cancer patients have been detected.[39] Several nuclear matrix proteins are present in bladder cancer but not in normal urothelium.[40] Antigens associated with bladder cancer, such as M344 and DD23, are potential detection targets.[30,41] Measurements of the urinary level of hyaluronic acid and hyaluronidase have shown promising results.[29] Telomerase is an enzyme responsible for maintenance of the chromosome-end telomere, which is commonly active in cancer. A polymerase chain reaction (PCR)-based telomeric repeat amplification protocol (TRAP) assay on urine yielded a high sensitivity, but special collection techniques may be required.[42,43] Other molecular studies, such as fluorescent in situ hybridization (FISH) of centromere probes for abnormalities of chromosomes 3, 7, 17, and band 9p21 are under way.[44]

A study of three bladder tumor markers in urine (NMP22, BTA stat test, and urinary bladder cancer [UBC] antigen test for fragments of cytokeratin 8 and 18) and bladder wash cytologic test by Boman and colleagues demonstrated that no combination of the studies could reliably replace surveillance cystoscopy, primarily because most recurrences are small.[45] Similarly, "virtual cystoscopy" with multiplanar computerized tomography did not provide comparable sensitivity to cystoscopy, even when a catheter was inserted into the bladder to improve visualization.[46] The use of deoxyribonucleic acid flow cytometry or image analysis may improve results slightly over cytology but not to a sufficient degree to warrant incorporation into general use.[47] Bladder "washings" to obtain a larger cellular yield improve sensitivity of cytology and is commonly used in the follow-up of bladder cancer patients.[47]

In summary, cystoscopy remains a requirement for the diagnosis of bladder cancer. Cytology is widely available and particularly valuable in high-grade cancers. Newer urinary diagnostic tests are fascinating, but as yet not practically helpful.

PATHOLOGY AND NATURAL HISTORY

An appreciation of the growth pattern and histology of bladder cancer is essential for appropriate treatment decisions. Most bladder cancers are epithelial in origin and 95% of epithelial tumors demonstrate transitional cell histology.[5] Grade and depth of invasion (stage) are both independent prognostic variables. A complete review of bladder cancer pathology is beyond the scope of this discussion, but certain aspects are crucial. A superb current review by Grignon is available.[48]

An important consensus on the terminology of urothelial tumors by members of the International Society of Urological Pathology is currently available[49] (Table 86-1). These recommendations will likely be widely incorporated into the description of bladder cancers and clinicians must be cognizant of the changes. A consensus statement was necessary because of considerable confusion regarding the definition of a papilloma and poor reproducibility of grading, with a preponderance of cases falling into the intermediate grade category. Nevertheless, the acceptance and use of the new classification remain a concern.[50]

A basic aspect of terminology is preference for the more precise term *urothelial* to describe the epithelium as opposed to *transitional*. The term *superficial* is also imprecise and is discouraged.[49] A "papilloma" is an exophytic papillary growth lined by urothelium of normal thickness and cytologic appearance. Defined as such, it is a rare, benign condition. A "papillary urothelial neoplasm of low malignant potential" has minimal cytologic and architectural abnormalities but is an important entity because of a propensity for recurrent lesions, occasionally of higher grade. "Papillary urothelial carcinoma, low grade" is composed of overtly neoplastic cells and may invade in a small percentage of cases. "Papillary urothelial carcinoma, high grade" is disorganized by both cytologic and architectural abnormalities. No subclassification is proposed but comment may be made if there is marked cytologic anaplasia. High-grade papillary lesions that are originally noninvasive may progress in 15% to 40% of cases.

TABLE 86-1

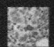

International Society of Urological Pathology Consensus Classification

Normal

Normal urothelium*

Hyperplasia

Flat urothelial hyperplasia
Papillary urothelial hyperplasia

Flat Urothelial Lesions with Atypia

Reactive (inflammatory) atypia
Atypia of unknown clinical significance
Dysplasia (low-grade intraurothelial neoplasia)
Carcinoma insitu (high-grade intraurothelial neoplasia)†

Papillary Urothelial Neoplasms

Urothelial papilloma
Inverted urothelial papilloma
Papillary urothelial neoplasm of low malignant potential
Papillary urothelial carcinoma, low grade
Papillary urothelial carcinoma, high grade

Invasive Urothelial Neoplasms

Urothelial carcinoma with lamina propria Invasion
Urothelial carcinoma with muscularis propria (detrusor muscle)
   invasion

---

*May include cases formerly diagnosed as "mild dysplasia."
†Includes cases with "severe dysplasia."
Rasmussen HH, Orntaft TF, Wolf H, Celis JE: Towards a comprehensive database of proteins from the wine of patients with bladder cancer. J Urol 1996;155(6): 2113–2119.

Carcinoma in situ (CIS) (high-grade intraurothelial neoplasia) represents an entity worthy of special attention. CIS is defined as high-grade (anaplastic) carcinoma confined to the epithelium growing in a flat, disordered, nonpapillary configuration and is likely underdiagnosed.[49] CIS can be focal (one area), multifocal, or diffuse. Diffuse CIS is often characterized by irritable voiding symptoms of frequency, urgency, and dysuria, but smaller volume disease may be asymptomatic. The gross appearance of CIS is a slightly raised, reddened, velvety mucosa, occasionally with associated edema. Smaller areas of CIS not associated with underlying bladder inflammation may not be so apparent cystoscopically and it is common for a urologist to underestimate the extent of mucosal disease. The mechanism of mucosal spread of CIS is poorly understood, but a substantial portion of cases have involvement of the prostatic urethra, prostatic ducts, seminal vesicles, or distal ureters with an important implication that intravesical treatments will likely fail.[51] Extension into von Brunn's nests is not uncommon and must be distinguished from invasion. Lastly, intercellular cohesiveness is frequently disturbed such that segments of the mucosa may be denuded.

STAGING

An experienced urologist recognizes the gross differences between well and poorly differentiated cancers. Also, it is often easily apparent whether or not the lesion is grossly invasive. Nevertheless, the confirmation of depth of invasion relies on the pathologic examination of the resected tissue. Adequate tissue must be provided to the pathologist for proper interpretation of depth of invasion. Cold-cup biopsies of the tumor have an advantage of avoiding cautery artifact and are useful for sampling mucosa, but a TUR is the common method to remove the cancer as completely as possible and provide tissue to the pathologist.[21] In general, sampling of the muscle beneath the papillary tumor is necessary to exclude muscle invasion (with the possible exception of an extremely well-differentiated, grossly noninvasive lesion). Carcinoma in situ has the propensity for the mucosa to become denuded, leaving only the appearance of "chronic cystitis" in the underlying stroma. When CIS is suspected, special care is needed to minimize mucosal trauma during the biopsy process. Cytologic examination of the urine is particularly helpful in this setting.

The staging of bladder cancer greatly influences treatment decisions. The American Joint Committee on Cancer (AJCC) 2002 TNM staging classification is recommended (Table 86-2).[52] The 2002 system retains the modifications initially described in 1997 by (1) placing all tumors invading muscularis propria into the T2 category (T2a superficial muscle, T2b deep muscle) and (2) segregating tumors outside the bladder into microscopic (T3a) and macroscopic (T3b). In practice, the clinical differentiation between T2a and T2b based on a TUR only is difficult and arbitrary and is barely reliable on a cystectomy specimen.[49] In addition, the segregation of prognosis becomes most evident when comparing organ confined (≤T2) versus extravesical (≥T3a) disease. CIS in the prostatic urethra or ducts does not decrease survival but prostatic stromal invasion does, thus justifying classification as T4a.

Using large data sets from hospitals either in the United States or Germany, the stage at diagnosis is typically Ta or TIS in 30% to 35% of cases, T1 in 25% to 30%, and T2 and higher in 30% to 35%.[5,52]

However, the microscopic assessment of depth of invasion is subject to interobserver variability, exemplified by an alteration in stage observed in 18% of cases when reviewed at a single referral center.[53]

The staging of bladder cancer, along with the grade, provides the basis for most treatment decisions. Non-invasive cancers (Ta and TIS) represent a biologically

TABLE 86-2

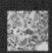

Primary Tumor Staging of Bladder Cancer

Ta: Noninvasive papillary carcinoma
T1: Tumor invades lamina propria
T2: Tumor invades muscle
     T2a: Invades superficial muscularis propria
     T2b: Invades deep muscularis propria
T3: Tumor invades perivesical tissue
     T3a: Microscopic perivesical fat invasion
     T3b: Macroscopic perivesical fat invasion (extravesical mass)
T4a: Invades adjacent organs (uterus, ovaries, prostate stoma)
T4b: Invades pelvic wall, abdominal wall

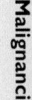

Specific Malignancies

III

different tumor from those demonstrating invasion (T1 and greater). T1 cancers are often lumped together with Ta as "superficial" cancers, but these tumors frequently behave differently with respect to recurrence rates, risk for later invasion into the muscle, and response to intravesical therapy.[24,54] Use of the imprecise term *superficial* tumor should be discouraged.[49,55]

Ta, grade 1 and 2 (low-grade) tumors have a propensity for recurrence but a low risk for progression to muscle invasion. The later recurrence risk is dependent on several factors. Multiple tumors (≥3) and larger cancers (>2 cm) are predictive of more recurrences.[24,56] A recurrence at the time of first cystoscopy heralds a pattern of more recurrences.[24] Progression to muscle invasion is seen in only 5% to 10% of patients.[56,57] Thus the goal of therapy primarily is to decrease or eliminate recurrences. Intravesical therapy should be reserved for patients demonstrating a need for treatment based either on the initial characteristics or more commonly on the recurrence pattern evident.

Disease invading the lamina propria represents a more dangerous disease (low or high grade, T1). Such disease has a higher recurrence rate *and* a substantial progression rate of 30% to 50% in spite of therapy.[54,56] Incomplete resection may lead to understaging, and a repeat TUR 6 to 8 weeks after the initial resection may identify such patients earlier.[56,58] The risk for understaging is particularly high as 60% in patients in whom no muscle was evident in the specimen demonstrating lamina propria invasion.[31] The risk for death due to progression is as high as 30% of patients with long follow-up.[54,56] Thus, the goal of therapy for such patients with high-grade cancers must be *complete* elimination of the cancer; simply reducing the recurrence rate will be insufficient in the long term.

Increasing evidence (although not all consistent) indicates that the depth of penetration into the lamina propria is important.[49] The mucularis mucosa (MM) is a discontinuous band of muscle fibers in the lamina propria. Invasion deep to the MM causes a higher risk for later muscularis propria invasion.[57] Orientation of the specimen often makes precise interpretation of the depth of invasion difficult. A measurement of the histologic depth of invasion into the lamina propria has been proposed but has not been widely accepted.[59]

Imaging studies of the bladder contribute minimally to the staging of bladder cancer. However, imaging of the upper tracts with an IVP, retrograde pyelogram, or CT scan is essential at the time of diagnosis. The practical information obtained from pelvic imaging leaves much to be desired.[60] CT scanning is the study applied most commonly, but understandably cannot differentiate non-invasive disease from small volume muscle-invading cancers. Also, the depth of muscle invasion cannot be reliably differentiated (Fig. 86-1). Bulkier tumors with gross invasion of perivesical fat are reliably visualized on CT, but the incremental information gained over that provided by a cystoscopy and examination under anesthesia is poorly quantified. In addition, CT imaging commonly occurs after the diagnostic/therapeutic TUR, which then distorts the bladder wall and surrounding tissue. Nevertheless, the appearance of a mass in the bladder wall and perivesical fat generally predicts a large

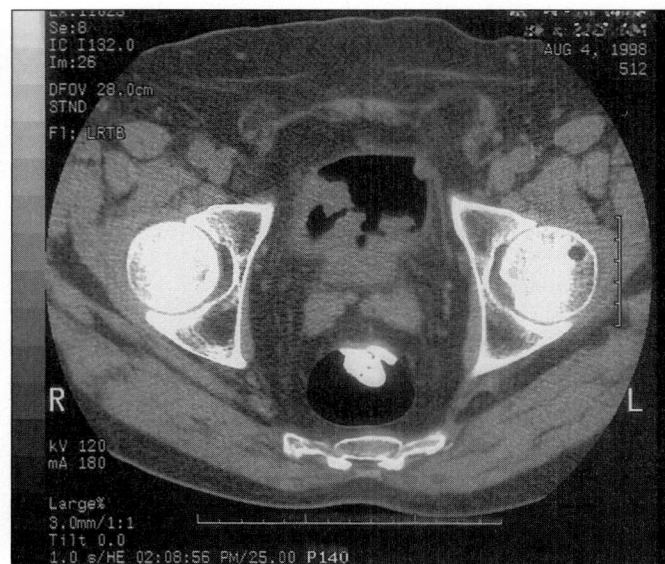

Figure 86-1. Pelvic computed tomographic (CT) scan which demonstrates multiple exophytic bladder cancers with thickening of bladder wall on right. Muscle invasion is certainly suspected, but depth of invasion is uncertain.

volume tumor with a worse prognosis. The presence of a palpable mass on examination under anesthesia portends a poor response to external radiation therapy and the presence of T3 disease at cystectomy corresponds to a diminished survival.

CT scan identifies large, probably malignant lymph nodes, but not all abnormal nodes harbor cancer, especially if the scan is done soon after a TUR. Percutaneous biopsy of an abnormal lymph node to confirm cancer is necessary prior to major treatment decisions.

MRI provides some advantages over CT scanning with multiplanar projections.[61,62] However, this somewhat better demonstration of the tumor is offset by greater expense and inconvenience to the patients. Evolving refinements in CT data manipulation allow image display in different planes as well, further diminishing any incremental benefit of MRI over CT scan. Positron emission tomography (PET) is theoritically attractive in evaluating bladder cancer, but despite some promising preliminary studies, it remains largely used in an investigative setting.[63]

Studies necessary to search for metastases in patients with invasive bladder cancer are not standardized.[64] Common sites of metastases from bladder cancer are regional lymph nodes, lungs, liver, and bone. A chest x-ray and abdominal/pelvic CT scan are in essence part of standard practice, although the clinical utility of such studies are poorly quantified. Bone scans are not routinely obtained unless a clinical suspicion has arisen because of bone pain or an elevated alkaline phosphatase level.

MOLECULAR BIOLOGY

There is little doubt that stage and grade provide the current most important prognostic confirmation for bladder cancer. However, heterogeneity of growth characteristics as well as staging inaccuracies contribute to the uncertainty of risk for an individual patient. Much hope rests on molecular biologic characterization of tumor findings to aid treatment decisions. As yet, no molecular characteristics are sufficiently reliable to dictate a conservative or aggressive deviation from traditional therapy. However, mounting evidence suggests that individual or several combined molecular events may be sufficient to tell the clinician that intravesical therapy may not work, early invasive (T1) cancers are likely to be particularly aggressive, some local cancers are at greater risk to metastasize, and finally some metastatic cancer may be more or less likely to respond to systemic chemotherapy.

A large number of genetic alterations occur in bladder cancers, and some may correlate with clinical behavior.[65] Noninvasive Ta tumors have fewer genetic alterations than invasive cancers and are commonly at 9q, 9p, 1p, and the Y chromosome.[66] Invasive cancers, T1 and higher, have many more genetic abnormalities and the challenge is to both categorize the gene abnormalities and correlate with functional alterations in the cell. Fundamental cell cycle regulators p53 and Rb appear to be particularly important in bladder cancers, and some authors suggest treatment

decisions will be influenced by the functional status of these markers in the near future.[67-72] Increase of accumulation of p53 protein correlates with greater risk for progression in T1 disease (even when depth of invasion in the lamina propria is considered).[73,74] The interaction between p53 and Rb may be important and abnormalities in both proteins may have an additive prognostic effect.[53-55] For more deeply invasive disease, a p53 abnormality may increase risk for metastases after cystectomy.[75] The relationships between these cell cycle regulators and other markers of growth is complex and interactive. Proto-oncogenes c-erb B-1, epidural growth factor receptor (EGFR) and HER-2/neu, proliferation markers Ki-67 and M1B-1, and the apoptosis inhibitor bcl-2 all may relate to progression of urothelial tumors.[76,77] Although preliminary data are provocative, prospective studies confirming the value of molecular markers for treatment decisions are only from single institutions; multicenter trials with molecular studies performed at a single reference center are in progress. However, uncertainties persist about methodologic issues, such as reproducibility and variability of p53 immunohistochemistry between institutions and the ideal method to

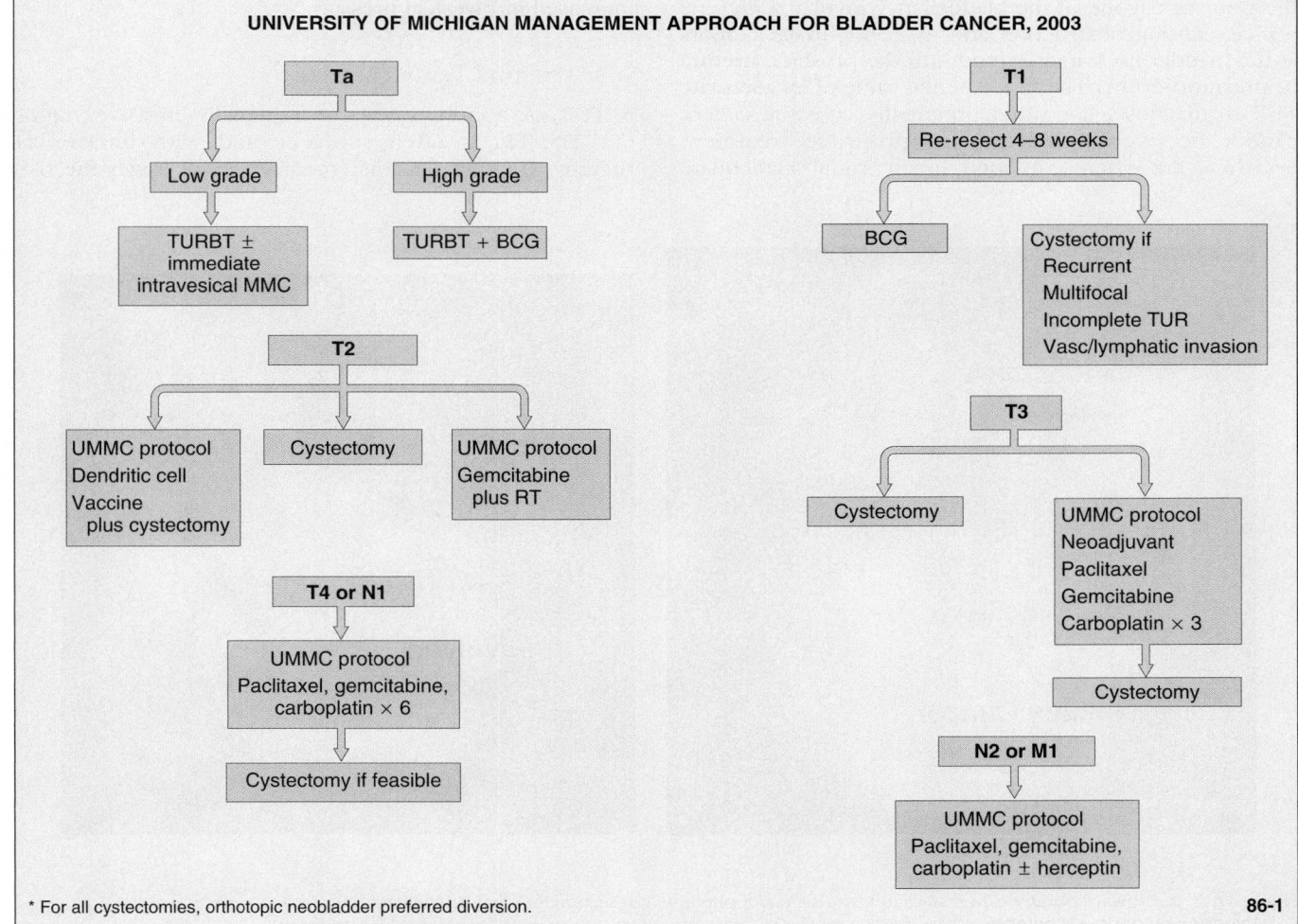

UNIVERSITY OF MICHIGAN MANAGEMENT APPROACH FOR BLADDER CANCER, 2003

* For all cystectomies, orthotopic neobladder preferred diversion.

86-1

identify abnormalities of p53.[78] Thus a urologist or oncologist currently cannot rely on molecular markers to guide a decision on timing of cystectomy for T1 disease or use of adjuvant chemotherapy.

THERAPY

The common papillary, noninvasive growth pattern of most bladder cancers makes them amenable to TUR. TUR as primary therapy has attractive low rates for immediate complications and long-term morbidity.[21] However, the multifocal and recurrent nature of bladder cancer emphasizes the limitations of TUR as an isolated modality. Because TUR is the mainstay of bladder cancer therapy, proficiency of TUR is presumed for all urologists, but the procedure is more difficult than commonly appreciated[21] (Fig. 86-2). Data from the European Organization for the Research and Treatment of Cancer (EORTC) suggest that the quality of a TUR by individual surgeons may influence recurrence rates.[79] Tumors may range from a few millimeters to many centimeters. The location of the cancer at the dome or anterior wall makes the resection considerably more difficult and increases the risk for incomplete resection or perforation of the bladder. Tumors in the obese patient are also more difficult to resect. Tumors on the floor or trigone of the bladder may involve a ureteral orifice, causing obstruction and hydronephrosis. Tumors at the bladder neck may extend into the prostatic urethra or prostatic stroma. The fundamental value of an adequate TUR to diagnose, stage, and potentially cure the cancer cannot be overemphasized. Inappropriate treatment decisions are often grounded in an initial inadequate TUR. For most cancers, the TUR should include sampling of the muscularis propria of the bladder at the base of the bladder.

For noninvasive (Ta) or minimally invasive (T1) cancers, a TUR is often sufficient to eradicate individual lesions. If there are multiple tumors, a large tumor (greater than 5 cm), recurrent tumors, or adjacent carcinoma in situ, TUR alone is less likely to provide durable cancer elimination. Another important prognostic factor for recurrence is the findings of the first cytoscopy 2 to 3 months after the initial resection.[25] If additional tumors are present, then the probability of continuing recurrences is as high as 80%.

At the time of the TUR, the urologist can commonly estimate if the cancer is high or low grade and if gross muscle invasion is present (see Fig. 86-1).[21,22] The presence of an invasive, palpable mass at the time of the TUR is an important indicator of gross extravesical (T3b) disease and is an adverse prognostic factor.

A long-term consequence of repeated TUR may be fibrosis of the bladder wall causing a small capacity bladder. This process can take a period of 5, 10, or more years to become evident and can be accelerated by intravesical treatments or radiation therapy. Symptoms of a small capacity bladder are frequency, urgency, and nocturia; bilateral hydronephrosis may occur due to increased intravesical pressure.

Intravesical Treatments

A TUR of a noninvasive or minimally invasive tumor (Ta, TIS, T1) is often supplemented with intravesical therapy to either decrease recurrences or lower the risk

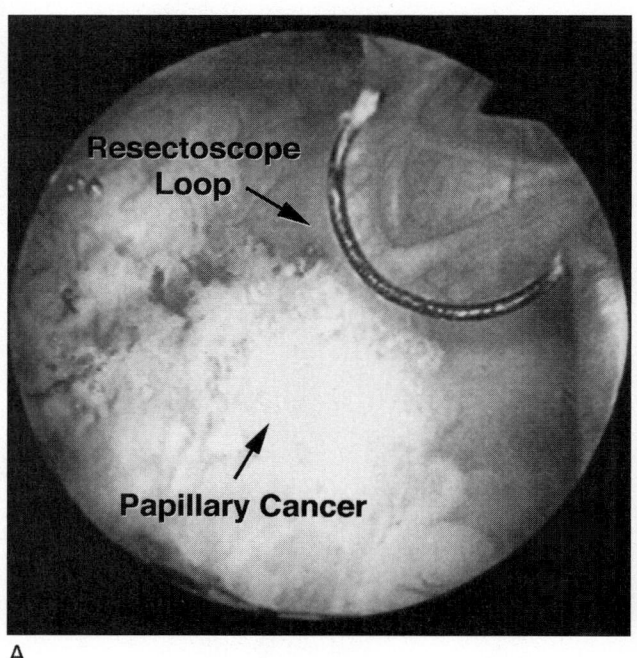

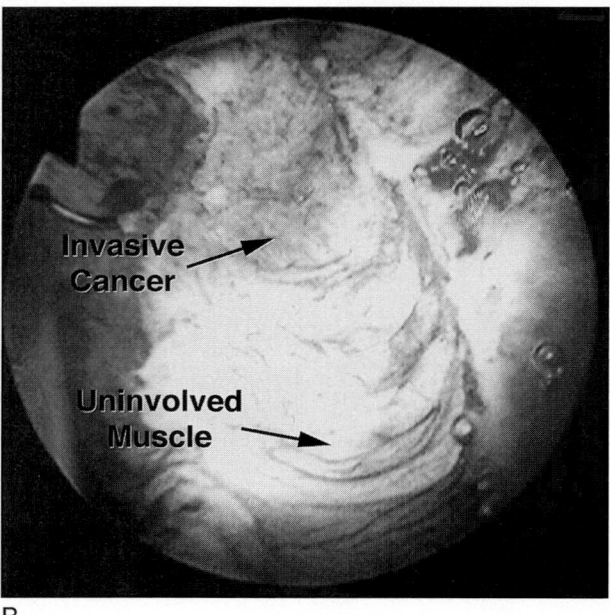

A

B

Figure 86-2. A, Papillary bladder cancer in right lower aspect of photo with resection loop poised to begin transurethral resection. **B,** Demonstration of grossly uninvolved muscularis propria (*bottom*) and cancer grossly invading the bladder wall (*top*).

of progression to a more invasive cancer. Introduced in the 1950s, intravesical treatments are based either on the cytotoxic effects of the agent or an immunologic response.[80] Treatments are commonly administered on a weekly or monthly schedule by inserting a catheter into the bladder, emptying the bladder of urine, instilling the medication, and then emptying the bladder after 2 hours either by voluntary voiding or catheterization. Much of the literature on the results of extravesical treatments is flawed owing to poorly designed studies with small numbers of patients, heterogenous patient populations with varying risk for relapse, and poorly defined outcomes.[81] Data suggest intravesical chemotherapy with mitomycin C, doxorubicin, ethoglucid, epirubicin, or thiotepa may reduce recurrence rate (the number of positive cystoscopies), but has no impact on progression (development of muscle-invading disease) rate.[80,82-85] The current most commonly used chemotherapeutic intravesical agent in the United States is mitomycin, which has few systemic or local side effects because of its high molecular weight and minimal systemic absorption. Recent animal and human studies have suggested efforts aimed at enhancing mitomycin efficacy by increasing the concentration, decreasing urine volume during treatment, and urine alkalinization to stabilize the drug.[86] Thiotepa is used less commonly now than previously because of marginal efficacy, although it causes relatively few local symptoms; life-threatening hematologic toxicity from bone marrow suppression is possible with chronic use.

Noteworthy but as yet unexplained is the observation that most agents selected for topical therapy are generally ineffective systemically and effective systemic agents, such as cisplatin, methotrexate, or vinblastine, are ineffective intravesical treatments. However, in a recent, small trial of intravesical gemcitabine in BCG refractory patients, 7 of 18 patients had an apparent complete response.[87]

Urologists have historically overused intravesical treatments, treating some patients at very low risk for recurrence or prolonging treatment when it was minimally beneficial.[81] In general, patients should have either a high-grade Ta, TIS, or T1 cancer or frequently recurrent low-grade cancers. There are several mechanisms for recurrence of bladder cancers. Incomplete resection, implantation of tumor cells to spatially separate sites, or mucosal migration of carcinoma in situ can all occur. Immediate intravesical therapy consisting of a single dose of a chemotherapeutic agent instilled in the bladder within 24 hours of the resection is designed to interfere with the implantation process. Randomized studies using either mitomycin C or thiotepa support such a strategy, and use is increasing.[84]

The current most efficacious, although somewhat more toxic intravesical, therapy available is BCG vaccine, an attenuated strain of live TB organisms.[55,80,88] Surprisingly, of all the strategies employing BCG treatment for a wide variety of cancers, intravesical BCG has stood the test of time and has been proved to increase patient survival by diminishing progression rates to invasive cancers. The mechanism of BCG effect is unknown, but contact between live BCG organisms and the tumor plus an intact host immune response is necessary. The dose and schedule are empirically derived; the most common protocol uses 120 mg intravesically weekly for 6 weeks. A reinduction with another 6 weeks of therapy may be beneficial partial responders.

Approximately 70% to 80% of patients with carcinoma in situ alone or carcinoma in situ associated with a resected papillary tumor will have a complete response to BCG.[89-91] In a landmark randomized trial, Herr and colleagues demonstrated a significant decrease in the need for a cystectomy and decreased death rate from bladder cancer when BCG + TUR was compared with TUR alone.[91] BCG is also more effective than mitomycin C (20 mg/dose) and doxorubicin.[88,89,92] Finally, maintenance BCG for complete responders, using a schedule of one weekly dose for 3 weeks administered every 6 months for approximately 2 to 3 years, is superior to a 6-week induction cycle only.[55,93] Monthly maintenance BCG is not effective, particularly due to a high dropout rate from bladder toxicity.[94] Nevertheless, the ideal amount of BCG required to obtain the highest and most durable response is variable; some patients respond to half the originally recommended dose, some patients obtain a complete response with only the 6-week induction course, and others cannot tolerate intravesical BCG because of local bladder or systemic symptoms.[93-95]

The drawbacks of BCG are common local bladder symptoms and rare, but potentially serious, systemic complications.[96,97] Dysuria, frequency, a flulike syndrome with fever, and some degree of hematuria are seen for approximately 24 hours in the majority of patients treated with BCG.[55,98] Such symptoms are self-limiting, and persistence beyond 48 hours causes concern for active *Mycobacterium* infection. Prophylactic isoniazid does not appear to decrease the frequency of side effects, but may be of value for persisting but non-life-threatening symptoms.[99] Deaths have occurred secondary to overwhelming BCG sepsis, and aggressive antibacterial therapy, possibly with steroids, is necessary.[55,97] Severe systemic symptoms are more likely if treatment is initiated too soon after a large TUR or if there is a traumatic catheterization at the time of instillation of the BCG.

Although BCG is highly effective initially, the durability raises some concerns. Early failure at 6 months is ominous, and more aggressive treatment is generally needed.[98] Later relapse after many years of a disease-free state can occur in the bladder, upper tracts, or prostate in 20% to 40% of patients.[51,54,91,100,101] Continued surveillance of patients with previous CIS requires cystoscopy, upper tract imaging, and cytologic testing. The presence of p53 nuclear protein in the persisting cancer may be a particularly ominous indication of the aggressive nature of cancer.[102,103]

Many other agents are available or under testing as intravesical treatments for bladder cancer, but none are comparable to BCG. Interferon-alpha has been extensively studied but confirmed beneficial role is still uncertain.[104] More promising but yet unconfirmed results have been suggested with a combination of interferon and low-dose BCG.[105] High-dose vitamins, garlic, and the immune activator keyhole limpet hemocyanin (KLH) are among the more intriguing agents with data to suggest a benefit.[106-108]

Treatment of Invasive Cancers

Historically, bladder cancers were segregated into "superficial" and "invasive" cancers. The inclusion of T1 cancers into the "superficial" category is not necessarily inaccurate, but is biologically unsound because T1 cancers have already demonstrated the machinery necessary to penetrate the basement membrane and thus access angiolymphatic spaces and the deeper muscle, and potentially to metastasize.[58,109] T1 cancers represent the early part of the spectrum of invasive cancers and thus have a somewhat better prognosis than more deeply invading cancers. The classical paradigm of treatment of T1 cancers was endoscopic management with or without intravesical therapy until muscle invasion was found and then a cystectomy was recommended. Such a strategy has not proved consistently to be wise because when muscle invasion was discovered and the patient subjected to a cystectomy, the chance of survival was certainly no better than that for an individual presenting with a muscle-invading cancer, implying some decrement in survival for those progressing to muscle invasion while under observation.[110,111] Thus the last decade has witnessed an increased respect for the danger posed by such tumors, prompting some to favor early cystectomy as opposed to more conservative approaches, such as TUR and intravesical therapy.[112] T1 cancers have a molecular phenotype more typical of lethal cancers, and the urologist's biggest worry is underestimation of the extent of the disease, thereby leaving cancer remaining in the lamina propria (or muscle) which will be undertreated.[75,113,114] Early re-resection by TUR of the site of a T1 lesion is worthwhile to assure accurate staging and complete excision.[115] After such is accomplished, intravesical agents, such as BCG, may treat the rest of the mucosa, which likely harbors incipient cancers.[114]

Traditionally, muscle-invading cancers have prompted the need for more aggressive local therapy, such as cystectomy or definitive external radiation therapy, in addition to TUR.

Transurethral Resection Alone

Historically, TUR was used as long as possible to treat muscle-invading cancers because of the severe morbidity of cystectomy. As cystectomy became safer, TUR alone was employed more selectively but with admirably good results. An oft-quoted figure of approximately 50% 5-year survival rate is not substantially different from cystectomy results in large series.[116,117] However, the patients treated with TUR alone were often selected by a second TUR at a referral institution that did not demonstrate any residual disease, indicating the initial TUR removed the cancer entirely.[117] The comparison of survival of such selected patients with smaller cancers to the entire group of patients undergoing a cystectomy is inappropriate; indeed, the good survival rate of these TUR-only patients may have been even better had they had an immediate cystectomy. Circumstantial evidence to support such an expectation exists in the survival data of patients with small volume muscle-invading disease at cystectomy in

which the 5-year survival rate is in the range of 60% to 80%.[118-120] Nevertheless, some patients are cured by a TUR alone, based on the survival data, absence of recurrence in bladder, and a P0 (no residual cancer) in a cystectomy specimen.[26] Selection of patients cured with TUR alone or who may have only a small volume of residual disease, making cure possible with the addition of radiation with or without chemotherapy, is the perplexing dilemma. One can hope that molecular markers predicting responsiveness to either radiation therapy or chemotherapy would be particularly helpful in such a setting. Because of the inherent uncertainty of the completeness of the TUR, it is rarely used alone for muscle-invading cancers if the patient is medically fit for aggressive treatments.

Partial Cystectomy

As illustrated in the preceding discussion, removal of a portion of the bladder wall may cure a patient in whom the cancer is confined to the segment removed. A 50% 5-year survival rate is reported for partial cystectomy, similar to cystectomy and TUR alone.[121] However, important selection criteria are evident, which may be best summarized as the patient has a "single tumor in space and time." The patients who are ideal candidates for a partial cystectomy have a single tumor with no or minimal carcinoma in situ cancer at a site amenable to a partial cystectomy, and do not have a history of previous multifocal bladder cancers. In general, only about 5% of patients with muscle-invading cancers meet such criteria.

Partial cystectomy is best accomplished by removal of the overlying peritoneum along with the involved bladder wall; high posterior and anterior wall locations of the cancer are better suited for partial cystectomy than other sites.[121] If too much of the bladder is excised, the patient can be left with a small capacity bladder with poor function. The impetus for partial cystectomy is diminishing in view of better functional results of total cystectomy followed by orthotopic neobladder formation, as discussed later.

Total Cystectomy

The current most effective local therapy for potentially lethal bladder cancer is total cystectomy.[122] The term *radical cystectomy* implies removal of the bladder and prostate in men, and uterus and anterior vaginal wall in women, as well as a pelvic lymphadenectomy. The rationale for removal of the prostate in men is the historical observation of a 40% to 50% pelvic recurrence rate in cystectomy series from 40 to 50 years ago when the prostate was left in situ, but also the more relevant and recent identification of carcinoma in situ in the prostatic urethra or ducts in 30% to 40% of men undergoing cystectomy.[123] Such disease would be left behind if the prostate was not removed entirely. However, the concept of preservation of the prostate in selected patients has been proposed.[124] Removal of the uterus and anterior vaginal wall in women provides a greater soft tissue margin of normal tissue, but also may be necessary only for larger, posterior wall or trigonal cancers. Currently, cystectomy in men almost always includes resection of the prostate, whereas in women the extent of removal of adjacent organs is based more on the local extent of the tumor.[125]

If cystectomy is the most efficacious treatment to control bladder cancer, why is it not used exclusively as the sole treatment? The reason is the undeniable morbidity from cystectomy imposed by the risk of the operation and the long-term impact on urinary and sexual function.

Cystectomy has historically been the most dangerous operation performed by a urologist. Mortality rates after cystectomy in the 1940s were in the 40% to 50% range. In the last 50 years, steady progress is evident such that the mortality rate has now been reduced to 1% to 3%.[119,122,125] Previously in the United States and still in some segments of the world, cystectomy was reserved only for the young and healthy, with older patients (>70 years of age) being relegated to less effective therapies.[126] It is now clear that cystectomy can be done safely in patients of all ages when attention to perioperative care of comorbid disease is emphasized.[118,126,127] A higher operative morality rate in older patients (>80 years of age) of 3% to 5% is evident, but defensible when the potential ineffectiveness of alternative therapies in this population is considered and when the risk imposed by the cancer is greatest in the short term. For a relatively healthy 80-year-old, the greater risk in the ensuing 3 to 4 years is the invasive bladder cancer rather than general cardiovascular concerns. Thus there is a growing appreciation that an expedient cystectomy in the relatively healthy elderly person offers the greatest potential for tumor control and successful rehabilitation when compared with external radiation therapy or chemotherapy in which optimal intensity of the treatment may not be deliverable.

The therapeutic results of cystectomy can be evaluated by two parameters: pelvic recurrence rate and survival, a reflection of local recurrences and systemic disease. Pelvic recurrence rates after cystectomy are approximately 10% to 20% and clearly depend on clinical stage.[119] Large cancers, clinical T3b, may have a pelvic recurrence rate as high as 25%, and thus additional strategies may be necessary to specifically address this failure site in such patients.[128] Preoperative radiation therapy is not beneficial to the entire group of cystectomy patients, but some data suggest a possible role for preoperative radiation in the subset of T3b patients at higher risk for local recurrence.[128,129] Neoadjuvant or adjuvant chemotherapy needs additional investigation in this patient subset and is discussed later.

Survival after cystectomy is dependent largely on pathologic stage.[74,119] Grade is an important overall prognostic factor; most patients coming to cystectomy have grade III or poorly differentiated cancers, so the discriminatory value is lost. However, pathologic stage is clearly relevant. The overall 5-year survival rate after cystectomy is 50%. However, it is more evident now that an apparent cut point of organ-confined (≤T2b, muscle-invading) disease has a substantially better prognosis than extravesical disease (≥T3a) as reflected in the newer staging system.[130]

Lymphatic metastases are a strong predictor of relapse, but again a spectrum of risk is evident, and some patients are cured by surgery alone in the face of positive lymph nodes.[119,131,132] Both the extent of the nodal metastases and the pathologic stages of bladder cancer are important variables; a single positive microscopic lymph node involvement associated with organ-confined disease (≤T2b) has a 5-year survival rate of up to 50%. Greater volume of nodal metastases and more extensive local disease progressively increase the risk of later metastases, such that involvement of multiple pelvic lymph nodes associated with a T3b cancer may only have a 10% 5-year survival rate with surgery alone. Increasing evidence supports the therapeutic value of a pelvic lymphadenectomy, particularly in patients with lower stage local disease in whom micrometastases may be present, but cure is still possible and particularly when a sufficiently complete pelvic node dissection was accomplished.[131] The traditional pelvic lymphadenectomy has a superior limit bounded by the bifurcation of the common iliac artery; however, some advocate a more extensive dissection up to the aortic bifurcation.[119,131,132] Standarization of the limits of a pelvic node dissection is needed and data suggest a sufficient number of nodes must be removed for the therapeutic benefit to be realized.[132]

Improvements in perioperative care fueled the decrease in operative mortality rate evident in the last few decades.[119,133] Of note, recent data suggest that comorbidity may also negatively impact cancer control and survival after cystectomy.[134] A major etiologic factor for bladder cancer, cigarette smoking, also contributes to greater risk for cardiovascular and pulmonary disease, with attendant increased risk for postoperative complications. Optimization of pulmonary and cardiac function preoperatively, as well as aggressive perioperative monitoring, are valuable adjuncts. Prevention of a complication and recognition of a complication early in its evolution (congestive heart failure before an arrhythmia or myocardial infarction or deep venous thrombosis before a pulmonary embolism) reduces morbidity. A perioperative "care pathway" in which anticipated milestones for care are articulated and incorporated into the care delivery is beneficial for the resident staff, nursing caregivers, outpatient support personnel, and the patient.[135] Not only are costs diminished, but deviations from the anticipated quality of care become quickly evident and are opportunities for improvement.

Urinary Diversion

After cystectomy, the urinary system must be reconstructed to preserve renal function and to keep the patient dry. The mainstay of urinary diversion since 1951 has been the ileal conduit, in which a 15- to 20-cm isolated segment of small bowel drains urine from the ureters to the skin; urine flows directly from the stoma of the bowel into a collecting pouch that adheres to the skin around the stoma.[136] Although considerable adjustment is necessary, ultimate return to usual activities is anticipated, including walking, exercising (including swimming), and social events.[137] Improved quality of appliances and stomal care by enterostomal therapists lessens the risk for urinary leakage or "accidents" and improves confident rehabilitation. Nevertheless, the presence of a stoma and the need for an external collecting device have a negative impact on body image, possibly disabling some patients.[138] In the early 1980s, continent cutaneous reservoirs became available with the advantage of not needing an external collecting pouch, but a disadvantage remaining of requiring an abdominal stoma that was catheterized every 4 to 6 hours by the patient to empty an internal reservoir configured from the bowel.[139] Such reservoirs were initially plagued by a reoperation rate of 20% to 50% to obtain continence, easy catheterization, and adequate reservoir function. Ultimately, the ileal colic reservoir termed the *Indiana pouch* became the most popular surgical procedure with a reoperation rate of less than 10%.[140] Nevertheless, the higher complication rate and continued need for intermittent catheterization offset the marginal benefit of avoiding a collecting device to many patients and surgeons.

Later in the 1980s, experience increased with an internal, orthotopic urinary reservoir termed a *neobladder*. Most urologists and patients believe the neobladder to be a substantial improvement in rehabilitation of urinary function by allowing volitional urination with continence and excellent preservation of renal function in both men and women.[140,141] Refinements in the operation providing an adequate size and detubularized bowel segment reconfigured into a spherical shape now allow reliable reservoir formation with minimal increase in operative time and no increase in postoperative complications, even in patients with more comorbid medical conditions[119,142] (Fig. 86-3). Patient satisfaction appears to be better, although the quality of life studies are difficult to interpret because of unavoidable selection biases inherent in the choice of urinary diversion.[137,138]

Selection of patients for neobladder urinary diversion depends on characteristics of both the cancer and the patient. Because the bowel reservoir is anastomosed to the urethra, patient selection should identify those patients with a low risk for a urethral recurrence. No or minimal involvement of the prostatic urethra in men and absence of involvement of the bladder neck in women is needed, both with a negative margin at the time of surgery.[143,144] Such practices select patients with a risk of urethral recurrence of only 2% to 3%.[145] Even with ideal selection, the remant urothelium remains at some risk for further urothelial cancer and as such must be monitored.[145] Advanced local disease is not necessarily a contraindication to orthotopic diversion because adjuvant treatments, such as radiation or chemotherapy, can also be administered as necessary. From a patient perspective, motivation to endure some initial frustration with the function of the reservoir until it enlarges and tolerance for

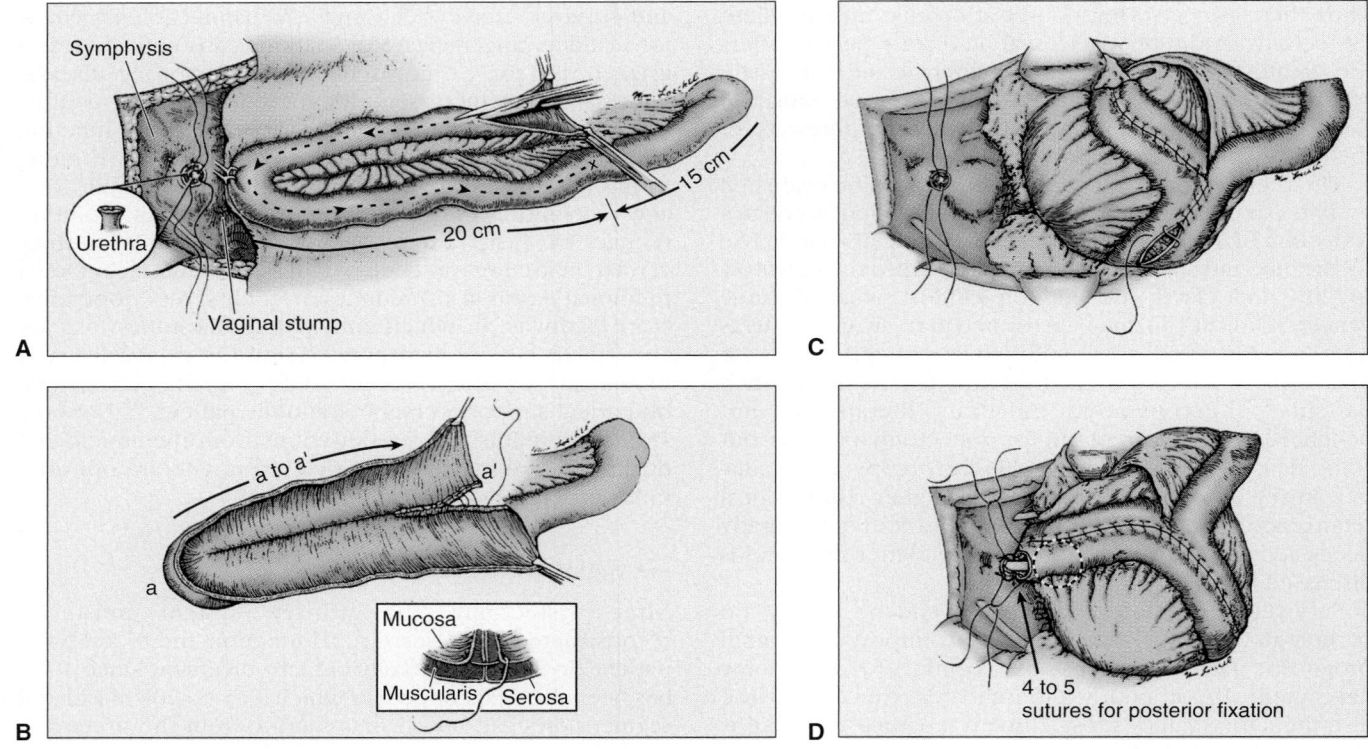

Figure 86-3. Neobladder construction in a female using Studer reservoir. **A,** Urethral stump is shown at left of drawing. A segment of ileum is isolated from continuity and opened on the antimesenteric border for approximately 45 cm. **B,** Posterior walls of adjacent limbs are anastomosed to form the "back" wall of the reservoir. **C,** Anterior wall of the reservoir closed to detubularize the segment and give a spherical shape. **D,** After completion of construction of the neobladder, the dependent portion on left is anastomosed to the urethra. The ureters are anastomosed to the afferent limb which protrudes superiorly. (From Montie JE: Orthotopic bladder replacement in women. In Webster GD (ed): Urinary Diversion: Scientific Foundation and Clinical Practice. Oxford, Blackwell Scientific Publications, 1995.)

potential nocturnal incontinence are both necessary. For many elderly patients who are frail and sedentary, the ileal conduit remains the best choice because of the quickest and easiest rehabilitation.[136] Adequate renal function of a serum creatinine level less than 2.5 to 3 mg/mL to prevent postoperative electrolyte abnormalities, as well as normal preoperative bowel function, are necessary for orthotopic diversion. Lifelong follow-up is necessay to monitor upper tracts and the metabolic and functional consequences of the diversion.[146]

The functional benefits of neobladder formation in both men and women have potentially lessened the pressure to delay cystectomy until absolutely necessary, and some authors have suggested such a strategy will improve overall survival results.[147] Also, bladder preservation strategies using combinations of TUR, chemotherapy, and external radiation therapy provide a smaller incremental gain in the functional preservation that must be measured against the risk of incomplete elimination of the cancer.[148] However, it must be stressed that the neobladder does not reproduce entirely normal bladder function, with some persisting annoyance of many patients with nocturnal enuresis and stress incontinence in a few.[138] Maturation of the neobladder takes several months following surgery, and patient expectations must accommodate such an adjustment period.

Interference with sexual function in men after cystectomy and urinary diversion remains problematic. A "nerve-sparing" dissection, which preserves the neurovascular bundles containing microscopic nerves, which innervate the corpora cavernosa, is feasible.[120] Even in highly selected patients, return of even adequate erectile function is seen in only 20% to 40% of men. Continued refinement in techniques is necessary. Measures to assist erections, such as alprostadil or viagra, will help in some, but experience is currently limited. The emotional adjustment after a very large operation, changes in body image, and concern about cancer recurrence all contribute to alterations in health-related quality of life (HR QOL) concerns.[138] No widely accepted, validated measurement tool for HR QOL is yet available for postcystectomy patients and is sorely needed.

Radiation Therapy

Preoperative Radiotherapy

Preoperative radiotherapy (RT) has a long history of use in bladder cancer treatment, although it is not currently employed frequently. The purported benefit has been a decreased risk of local failure following the combination of RT and radical cystectomy compared with radical cystectomy alone.[149,150] The available data are difficult to interpret but generally confirm that preoperative RT results in significant downstaging. This downstaging occurs when doses of 40 to 50 Gy are used preoperatively rather than short courses of RT followed within a few days by radical cystectomy. The data through 1985 has been summarized well by Parsons and Million who comprehensively reviewed the literature and suggested that, in addition to causing tumor downstaging and decreasing the local failure rate, preoperative radiotherapy results in

a 15% to 20% increase in the 5-year survival rate compared with cystectomy alone.[151] Nevertheless, a more contemporary randomized study did not demonstrate an overall survival benefit compared with cystectomy alone.[129]

Given the problems with comparing retrospective reviews and the methodologic problems with the available prospective clinical trials, it seems clear that published data are insufficient to either confirm or refute the hypothesis that preoperative RT results in a survival advantage compared with radical cystectomy alone. However, assuming that a decrease in local recurrences, and the potential morbidity which local failures bring, is beneficial, there may be a role for preoperative RT in some bladder cancer patients.

M.D. Anderson Hospital has supplied data that shed light on this issue. This institution had a policy for full-dose, preoperative RT between 1960 and 1983, after which time a change in treatment philosophy occurred and preoperative RT was no longer used. Thus both treatments were used for large numbers of patients at a single facility. In 1988, a report on pelvic failures for patients treated without preoperative RT described a failure rate of only 6% (10 of 178 patients).[152] However, this was a crude failure rate, not an actuarial estimate, and the follow-up period was relatively short (median, 22.5 months). Also, the patients were staged pathologically, rather than clinically, and patients who did not complete the surgical resection were excluded. Naturally, patients who are candidates for preoperative RT are staged only clinically. So, this report is unable to define the pelvic failure rate for clinically staged, high-risk patients, meaning those with tumor extension through the bladder wall.

In a later report from Cole and colleagues compared the preoperative RT patients treated between 1960 and 1983 to the more modern patients treated with radical cystectomy only, many of whom received adjuvant chemotherapy.[153] In this review, the 5-year actuarial pelvic failure rate for clinical T3b disease was substantially reduced from 28% without preoperative RT to 9% with preoperative RT. No significant difference in pelvic failure was observed for T2 and T3a patients. The 28% failure rate with surgery alone for T3b patients is similar to that reported earlier by Greven for clinically staged T3 patients (39%).[154] Thus, for locally advanced disease, surgery alone has a substantial pelvic failure rate and, despite the high rate of distant failure, an argument can be made in favor of preoperative RT and perhaps this issue should be studied further in future clinical trials.

Palliative Therapy

Radiotherapy is often used to palliate locally advanced bladder cancer, particularly when gross hematuria, not amenable to local surgical procedures, is causing clinical problems. Usually, this situation is treated with a shorter course (hypofractionation) of RT than is used for the definitive treatment of potentially curative disease. In bladder cancer, like many other malignancies that have bleeding as a symptomatic manifestation, hematuria is generally well controlled. Control of other local urinary symptoms is not as good, with control of dysuria and urinary frequency approximately 25%. It is expected that some acute RT effects will occur during a course of therapy, but they are generally mild, if multiple treatment fields and customized blocks are created to spare normal tissues.

Jose and others from the Royal Marsden Hospital performed a phase II study evaluation of a palliative, hypofractionation regimen consisting of either 5 or 6 weekly fractions of 6 Gy each for a total dose of 30 to 36 Gy; 65 poor performance status patients with median age of 81 years were enrolled. Median survival time was just 35 weeks, but 23 of 37 patients who were evaluated cystoscopically at 3 months had a complete response. In addition, although nocturia was rarely improved, most patients had symptomatic control of hematuria, frequency, and dysuria.[155]

Duchesne and associates recently reported the results of an international, multicenter, randomized trial of two palliative radiotherapy regimens for bladder cancer; 500 patients were entered and were randomized to receive either 35 Gy in 10 fractions over 2 weeks or 21 Gy in 7 fractions over 1 week on alternating weekdays. To be eligible, patients were either medically unable to tolerate cystectomy (64%) or had advanced disease (T4b, N1, or M1) (36%). Median age was 80 years. The median survival time was 7.5 months. Of 272 patients available for assessment at 3 months, 68% had improvement in at least one bladder cancer symptom by at least one grade without worsening of any other symptoms. There were no differences between the two regimens for either survival or symptom control.

Recent trials thus confirm older data indicating that radiotherapy can play an important role in ameliorating local symptoms from inoperable or unresectable bladder cancer.

Bladder Preservation Using Radiotherapy with or Without Chemotherapy

Organ preservation approaches, using RT as one of the treatment modalities, have been applied to several malignant diseases. Given the potential disruption in lifestyle associated with radical bladder surgery, there has been strong motivation for exploring bladder-conserving techniques and decades of experience to draw on. Early attempts using RT for preservation focused on RT as the sole modality of treatment with surgery reserved for salvage treatment; more recent studies have used concurrent chemotherapy agents to increase the efficacy of RT.

Bladder preservation using RT as the only treatment modality, with surgery reserved for salvage of local, nonmetastatic recurrences has been compared to radical cystectomy in randomized trials. Although differences in 5-year survival rates have been detected in these studies, which favor early cystectomy, the differences are small and generally do not reach statistical significance.

Bloom and colleagues reported for the Institute of Urology, London, the 5-year results of a randomized trial of preoperative pelvic RT (40 Gy) and radical cystectomy versus RT only (60 Gy) for patients with T3 bladder cancer.[156] Nearly 200 patients were randomized. The 5-year survival rate was 38% for the immediate cystectomy

arm and 29% for the RT alone arm ($P = 0.2$). Although salvage cystectomy was not part of the planned protocol therapy, 18 patients underwent this salvage treatment with 60% 5-year survival rate for this subset. This study completed patient accrual in 1975, and it is unclear how relevant it is to today's patients, given changes in staging evaluation and improvements in surgical and radiotherapeutic techniques over the past 25 years. Nevertheless, it remains interesting that the survival rate differences are small enough to be due to chance alone, despite the higher risk of local recurrence in the RT-alone group. Tumors that recur locally after RT may serve as markers for lesions that tend to recur distantly. Thus local recurrence may not adversely affect the overall survival rate.

In a more recent study, Sell and colleagues performed a randomized trial with treatment arms similar to the Bloom study (preoperative RT and radical cystectomy versus RT with surgical salvage), and which randomized patients between 1983 and 1986. The results are remarkably similar to the Bloom report: 5-year survival rate is 29% for immediate surgery versus 23% for RT alone ($P = $ NS). In this study, 28% of the RT patients underwent salvage surgery.[157]

Thus RT, as a sole modality, has an appreciable 5-year survival rate in the treatment of invasive bladder cancer, although the local control rate is only approximately 25% to 50% at 5 years. Favorable prognostic factors for patients who are treated with RT alone include papillary morphology, extensive TUR, lack of ureteral obstruction, and higher pretreatment hemoglobin level.[158,159]

As discussed fully elsewhere in this chapter, chemotherapy has become a highly useful treatment for bladder cancer, and approaches combining active agents with RT to improve bladder conservation have proliferated. Strategies have included the use of concurrent RT and 5-FU; concurrent RT and intra-arterial cisplatin; concurrent 5-FU, cisplatin, and large dose per fraction RT; and, more recently, concurrent paclitaxel.[160-164] However, most interest has been on the use of RT with concurrent cisplatin, with or without the use of neoadjuvant chemotherapy to address the issue of systemic disease.[165-167] Most of these strategies employ an aggressive TUR prior to conservative therapy and this stage is considered to be an important component of therapy.

A recent update of results from Massachusetts General Hospital (MGH) summarizing the results of sequential clinical trials employing TURBT, chemotherapy, and radiotherapy for bladder preservation illustrates the outcome with this approach.[166] Most commonly, this group has used neoadjuvant chemotherapy with MCV (methotrexate, cisplatin, and vinblastine) up front for two cycles followed by RT. However, as mentioned later, the use of neoadjuvant therapy in this setting is debatable. Regardless of the use of neoadjuvant chemotherapy, concurrent chemotherapy and RT is used and a dose of 39.6 Gy with two courses of concurrent cisplatin (70 mg/m^2 or 100 mg/m^2) was the most frequent regimen. At this point in the treatment regimen—two thirds through the radiotherapy—patients are restaged. Those with tumors sensitive to treatment, as demonstrated by a complete response (negative biopsies and negative urinary cytologic test), continue with additional concurrent cisplatin and RT to a total dose of 64.8 Gy. Patients with less than a CR go on to radical cystectomy. Others who perform bladder-sparing treatment forgo the intra-RT tumor assessment and perform a restaging shortly after the completion of the full dose of radiotherapy, with salvage surgery performed on incomplete responders.[168]

Results of treatment for 190 patients with the MGH approach reveal a 5-year survival rate of 54% and a 10-year survival rate of 36%.[169] Of the surviving patients, 73% (46% of the total) have an intact bladder at 5 years. Bladder function after TURBT, chemotherapy, and RT is reported to be good, although studies carefully examining quality of life issues in this patient population are lacking.[170] However, in a large German series of 282 consecutive patients treated with RT alone (*N* = 98) or RT and concurrent cisplatin or carboplatin (*N* = 184), only 3 patients underwent a cystectomy for poor bladder function or radiation cystitis.[171]

Of note, approximately 25% of patients who achieve a complete response when treated with bladder-sparing approaches subsequently develop noninvasive recurrences, and the long-term outcome of these patients remains of some concern. Zietman and coworkers. have examined the results of 32 patients who developed noninvasive recurrences.[172] These cancers were usually carcinoma in situ and usually occurred at the site of the original tumor. Of the 32, 27 were treated conservatively and the irradiated bladder tolerated this therapy well; 10 ultimately required salvage cystectomy. In general, what was observed was that the noninvasive recurrences that occur after RT-containing, bladder-sparing approaches could be managed with conventional intravesical therapies.

As mentioned earlier, the role of the neoadjuvant chemotherapy as a part of bladder preservation has come into question. This component of treatment was added to provide additional downstaging and also to address the potential for subclinical metastatic disease. However, this chemotherapy also added to the acute morbidity of treatment. The RTOG recently reported on a randomized study that compared the approach described above, with two cycles of MCV prior to concurrent cisplatin/RT, to a treatment arm that had no pre-RT MCV.[173] With a median follow-up of 5 years, no significant difference in survival was detected. Thus, although systemic relapse is an important component of treatment failure, it is not clear yet how to decrease the probability of this event in patients undergoing a modern bladder preservation approach.

The RTOG continues to evaluate and refine bladder preservation strategies. An active RTOG study (RTOG 0233) is assessing the tolerability and efficacy of two regimens in a randomized phase II trial. Patients receive radiosensitization with cisplatin and either 5-FU or paclitaxel. Adjuvant systemic therapy is then delivered with gemcitabine, cisplatin, and paclitaxel. Future studies will examine the role of newer chemotherapy agents, such as docetaxel and gemcitabine as radiosensitizers in bladder preservation approaches, and at present, bladder preservation using TURBT, chemotherapy, and RT should

be considered a method that is still being enhanced. However, it is clear that for selected patients, this conservative approach is a feasible technique to achieve both tumor eradication and organ preservation.

Chemotherapy

Adjuvant and Neoadjuvant Chemotherapy

Advances in surgery and radiation therapy have markedly improved the treatment of invasive transitional cell carcinoma, providing improved local control while decreasing the morbidity and fatality associated with therapy. Despite these advances, a large proportion of patients with muscle-invasive disease will develop metastases accounting for much of the morbidity and almost all the deaths associated with this disease. These metastatic lesions are presumably due to the presence of disseminated disease at the time of local therapy. The development of chemotherapeutic agents and regimens with activity in the setting of metastatic transitional cell carcinoma, along with the demonstrated efficacy of both neoadjuvant and adjuvant chemotherapy in other diseases, has prompted considerable interest in these strategies for the treatment of transitional cell carcinoma.

Both approaches aim to improve the overall mortality rate associated with bladder cancer by treating in the setting of minimal metastatic disease. The hope is that the disease will be more susceptible to therapy while the patients are more tolerant of associated side effects. Adjuvant therapy is given following definitive local therapy, and neoadjuvant chemotherapy is given prior to local treatment. Several reviews have pointed out the advantages and disadvantages to these approaches.[174-176] In the case of adjuvant therapy, the decision to proceed with treatment can be based on the pathologic stage as dictated by the findings at cystectomy. Criteria can be defined for patient eligibility, and the population enrolled on trials can be fairly uniform. The disadvantage, however, is that definitive local therapy may render some patients either unable or unwilling to undergo adjuvant therapy due to complications associated with the procedure. Patients may develop overt metastatic disease while recovering from their definitive local therapy, which may render the advantage of adjuvant therapy moot.

Neoadjuvant chemotherapy therapy, by contrast, delivers treatment at the earliest possible time. It allows assessment of the chemotherapeutic responsiveness of the primary tumor, which has been shown to be a prognostic indicator for response.[177] In addition, tumors that may initially be judged to be unresectable may be rendered resectable by neoadjuvant therapy. Neoadjuvant therapy also allows maximal delivery of chemotherapy because vascular beds have not been disrupted by either surgery or radiation. The disadvantages of neoadjuvant therapy are that it must be based on clinical staging criteria, which frequently overstate the extent of disease when compared to pathologic review, and that a significant proportion of patients will receive treatment when they do not need chemotherapy.

Although both neoadjuvant and adjuvant therapy are attractive in concept, major problems have arisen in the study of these approaches. To date there is suggestive, but no definitive, evidence that either approach improves overall survival of patients with bladder cancer.

Adjuvant Chemotherapy

Adjuvant chemotherapy of transitional cell carcinoma has been the subject of several single-institution randomized trials. Unfortunately, no multicenter randomized study has ever been conducted. The largest study is a retrospective analysis from M.D. Anderson Hospital.[178] This study reports the results of a treatment algorithm in which high-risk patients with good performance status were offered adjuvant chemotherapy, while those with low risk or contraindications to therapy were observed. A total of 339 patients who underwent cystectomy were stratified into high-risk and low-risk groups based on the presence of nodal involvement, extravesical spread, direct extension to the pelvic viscera, or vascular or lymphatic invasion. A total of 71 patients were treated with cisplatin, doxorubicin, and cyclophosphamide (CISCA), with most patients (75%) receiving five courses of treatment. The remaining patients in the high-risk population either had medical contraindications to therapy, were not offered adjuvant chemotherapy, or refused. Patients receiving chemotherapy had a 5-year survival rate of 70%, while those in the high-risk group that did not receive treatment had a 5-year survival rate of only 37%. The selection bias inherent in this nonrandomized sample makes any comparison between the two high-risk groups somewhat tenuous, owing to the imbalance in prognostic factors between the two groups. As an example, a higher frequency of lymphatic/vascular invasion was present in patients who were not offered chemotherapy.

The first report of a prospective randomized trial of modern combination chemotherapy versus observation was published by Skinner and coworkers.[179] From a cystectomy population of 498 patients, they determined that 160 were eligible for adjuvant chemotherapy by pathologic criteria. These patients had pathologic stage III or IV disease or lymph node positive transitional cell carcinoma. Patients with nodal involvement above the aortic bifurcation were excluded. Sixty-nine additional patients were ineligible for various reasons, including age, prior malignancy, and other medical conditions, leaving a total of 91 patients who participated in the study. Chemotherapy consisting of cisplatin, doxorubicin, and cyclophosphamide was initiated 6 weeks following cystectomy with a plan to administer four cycles of treatment. Forty-four patients were randomized to the chemotherapy arm. Eleven subsequently refused therapy, and four received only one cycle of therapy. In 17 of the 33 patients who received chemotherapy, the treatment was modified on an individual basis using a human tumor cloning assay. Sixteen of these 17 patients received cisplatin. Time to disease progression was significantly delayed in the chemotherapy arm ($P = 0.011$), although there was no significant difference in overall survival ($P = 0.0999$). Subset analysis did show a survival benefit for the single node-positive group, but this group consisted of only 7 patients in the chemotherapy group with 17 in the control group. It is not clear if the patients randomized to chemotherapy in the single-node positive group actually received treatment and if they did, what they received or how much. This group, however, is the only one which has a survival benefit, and weighs heavily into the reported overall survival benefit reported in the abstract of the study ($P = 0.0062$) using a stratified measure. These methodologic problems, in terms of design and statistical interpretation, have engendered much criticism of this study. The study does suggest that there is a benefit to adjuvant chemotherapy, but does not provide definitive evidence in terms of overall survival.

Similar problems, in terms of study design and chemotherapy administration, were seen in a randomized trial reported by Stockle and associates.[180] Patients were treated with either methotrexate, vinblastine, doxorubicin, and cisplatin (MVAC), or a similar regimen with epirubicin substituted for the doxorubicin (MVEC). This study closed early after accruing only 49 patients, owing to a significant benefit in terms of time to recurrence for the patients receiving chemotherapy. Twenty-six patients were randomized to chemotherapy; only 18 actually received treatment. Three of the 18 patients who received chemotherapy relapsed, compared with 18 of the 22 in the observation arm. A subsequent follow-up report, which included a nonrandomized cohort, confirmed a delay in the time to recurrence, but there was no analysis of overall survival.[181] It is also unclear from the reports whether patients in the observation arm received chemotherapy at relapse, which could have had a significant effect on the overall survival in the control group.

Freiha reported the results of a more recent trial in which 50 patients were randomized to either adjuvant cisplatin, methotrexate, and vinblastine (CMV) chemotherapy or observation.[182] Twenty-five patients were randomized to receive chemotherapy; of these, 24 actually received treatment, with 22 completing all four planned cycles. Thirteen patients in the CMV arm subsequently developed disease recurrence, and 20 in the observation arm did. With a median follow-up of more than 5 years, the adjuvant chemotherapy group demonstrated a significant improvement in disease-free survival, with a median of 37 months versus 12 months in the observation arm ($P = 0.01$). The difference in overall survival did not reach statistical significance, although the median survival in the adjuvant group was 63 months compared to 36 months for the observation group ($P = 0.32$). The authors speculated that this difference may be due to the fact that patients received effective chemotherapy at relapse.

The results of these studies are summarized in Table 86-3. Despite the widespread use of adjuvant chemotherapy for invasive transitional cell carcinoma, we still do not have definitive evidence of benefit in terms of overall survival. This is primarily due to the limited number of patients entered on the randomized studies reported to date, resulting in too few patients being treated and followed to detect a difference in overall survival. Only 75 patients have actually received chemotherapy on the three randomized trials reported to date; the conclusions that can be drawn from such small studies are extremely limited. The improved disease-free survival in patients treated with adjuvant chemotherapy on the

TABLE 86-3

Adjuvant Combination Chemotherapy Trials

AUTHOR REFERENCE	ARMS	NO. OF PATIENTS (RECEIVING CHEMOTHERAPY)	RESULTS
Logothetis[178]	Nonrandomized trial	339 (71)	Improved survival in chemotherapy group
Skinner[179]	PAC	44 (33)	Improved disease-free survival in chemotherapy group; survival advantage for single-node positive group
	Observation	46	
Stockle[180]	MVAC or MVEC	26 (18)	Halted early with improved disease-free survival in chemotherapy group
	Observation	23	
Freiha[182]	CMV	25 (24)	Improved disease-free survival in chemotherapy group
	Observation	25	

CMV, cisplatin, methothexate, rinblastine; MVAC, methothexate, vinblastine, doxorubicin, cisplatin; MVEC, methothexate, vinblastine, epirubicin, cisplatin; PAC, cyclophosphamide, doxorubicin, cisplatin.

trials provides a tantalizing hint that this approach may result in a higher cure rate for this disease. Proof of the benefit of adjuvant chemotherapy will require a multi-center randomized trial with appropriate sample size, and clinical trials designed to address this question should be the first priority for these patients. In the absence of such a trial, adjuvant chemotherapy will remain of uncertain benefit.

These hints of activity led investigators at M.D. Anderson Hospital to address the question in a different way.[183] They randomized 140 patients with high-risk resectable bladder cancer to receive either two cycles of neoadjuvant MVAC followed by surgery and three additional cycles of adjuvant therapy, or surgery followed by five cycles of MVAC. Only 65% of the patients received at least four cycles of chemotherapy because of a variety of reasons, but chiefly because of toxicity. There was no difference in overall survival in the two groups, suggesting that the timing of chemotherapy is not a major factor in determining its impact. The design of this study does not allow evaluation of the overall efficacy of chemotherapy in either setting, but two observations emerged confirming prior findings that have potential impact on future trials. First, a high rate of clinical understaging in terms of nodal involvement and lymphatic or vascular invasion on the initial resection specimen is correlated with this finding. Second, tumor downstaging by neoadjuvant therapy is associated with a high rate of long-term survival. Both factors are critically important in the design of future neoadjuvant trials.

Neoadjuvant Chemotherapy

Despite the theoretic advantages cited for this approach, neoadjuvant chemotherapy also remains an investigational tool. As with adjuvant chemotherapy, the primary reason is that large multicenter trials with the potential provide definitive evidence of benefit have have only recently been completed. Neoadjuvant chemotherapy has been used in a multitude of single agent trials and is fairly commonly administered in the community setting.[120] Chemotherapy has been used alone, concurrently with radiation therapy, sequentially, or alternating with radio-therapy. Most of these trials used cisplatin either singly or in combination, with pathologic complete response rates reported from 0% to 96%. The wide range of response rates points to the major problems in interpreting this data. Case selection is based entirely on clinical criteria, and biologic markers of invasive metastatic potential were unknown at the time these studies were designed and conducted. Most of the studies enrolled patients who had undergone TUR in their bladder tumor and may, therefore, have been in complete response at the time they were treated. At least a fraction of these patients may actually have been cured by their local therapy. Finally, the initial workup of patients enrolled on these studies varied widely, with some of the studies being conducted prior to the incorporation of modern diagnostic techniques into the eligibility criteria. Some of the early studies may well have included patients with early metastatic disease resulting in a significant impact on the survival data. Finding any conclusion from these nonrandomized studies is extremely difficult.

Seven randomized studies have been completed. Most of these studies have been relatively small and failed to show a definitive benefit for neoadjuvant chemotherapy. A total of 845 patients were enrolled on five phase III trials completed in the late 1980s using primarily cisplatin alone as the chemotherapy regimen.[184-187] These trials were the subject of a meta-analysis, published in 1995, which used individual patient data from 479 of the patients.[188] Two of these trials tended to favor chemotherapy, while two showed no benefit. The fifth and largest trial, which provided no individual patient data for the meta-analysis, enrolled 325 patients and used a combination of cisplatin and doxorubicin. This trial favored chemotherapy.[184] The overall survival curves for the meta-analysis showed no statistically significant benefit to chemotherapy ($P = 0.33$).

Two large studies have recently reported their results. The largest randomized trial of neoadjuvant therapy was conducted in Europe by the Medical Research Council (MRC) and the EORTC.[189] The study was designed to detect a difference in survival of 10% or greater with the use of chemotherapy. A total of 975 patients were enrolled, with patients randomized to receive CMV every 3 weeks for three cycles, or no chemotherapy prior to a previously selected definitive local therapy. The definitive local therapy was either radical cystectomy, full-dose external beam radiotherapy, or preoperative radiotherapy followed by cystectomy. The study was designed to detect an absolute increase of at least 10% in the 3-year survival rate. Four hundred eighty-nine patients were randomized to receive chemotherapy, and 486 received local therapy alone. A total of 484 underwent cystectomy, 414 received radiotherapy, and 77 were treated with combined radiotherapy and surgery. A comparison of the cystectomy plus chemotherapy patients to those who were treated with cystectomy alone showed a 21% improvement in the pathologic complete response rate at cystectomy in the patients receiving chemotherapy. At 3 years the overall survival rate was 55.5% for the chemotherapy arm and 50% in the no chemotherapy arm ($P = 0.075$). The chemotherapy therefore failed to demonstrate the anticipated 10% improvement in overall survival at this time. Further analysis as this trial matures is anticipated.

In the United States, results of an Intergroup randomized trial of MVAC plus cystectomy versus cystectomy alone have been reported.[190] This trial randomized 317 patients enrolled over 11 years. By intention to treat analysis, the median survival of the combination arm of therapy was 77 months compared to 46 months in the cystectomy alone arm. At 5 years 43% of the subjects in the cystectomy alone arm were still alive while 57% of those who received combined modality therapy survived ($P = 0.06$). Improved survival was associated with pathologic complete response in the cystectomy specimen. There were significantly more patients with no residual disease at operation in the combination therapy arm (38% versus 15%, $P < 0.001$). These data have been the subject of considerable debate.[191,192] The results of both the Intergroup and EORTC/MRC trials suggest that there may be a benefit to neoadjuvant chemotherapy, but at present, this remains an investigational approach.

Chemotherapy for Metastatic Disease

Urothelial carcinoma has long been known to be a chemotherapy-sensitive malignancy. Single-agent phase II trials conducted in the 1970s identified cisplatin and methotrexate as the most active agents with response rates of approximately 30%.[193] Doxorubicin, 5-fluorouracil, vinblastine, vincristine, and mitomycin C were all shown to have single-agent response rates of approximately 15%. These phase II trials provided the basis for the development of combination regimens such as CMV (cisplatin, methotrexate, and vinblastine), CISCA (cisplatin, cyclophosphamide, and doxorubicin), and MVAC (methotrexate, vinblastine, doxorubicin, and cisplatin).

In phase II trials CMV demonstrated an overall response rate of 56%, with a complete response rate of 28%, and a median survival time of 8 months.[194] In multiple phase II and III trials, CISCA showed response rates ranging from 13% to 78%, with a complete response rate ranging from 9% to 39%.[195-197] The median survival time for this regimen was on the order of 12 months. MVAC was developed at Memorial Sloan-Kettering Cancer Center, and initial results of the phase II trial were reported in 1985.[198] The subsequent update in 1989, with 121 evaluable patients,

showed an overall response rate of 72%, with a complete clinical response rate to chemotherapy alone of 18%.[199] An additional 11 patients were rendered disease-free by surgery following chemotherapy. The median survival time for the entire group was 13.3 months, and only 20% of the patients were long-term disease-free survivors. MVAC was subsequently compared to CISCA in a phase III randomized trial.[200] The combined complete and partial response rate was significantly better for patients treated with MVAC (65% versus 46%) as was the overall survival time (median 11 months versus 10 months). Based on these studies MVAC has emerged as the standard therapy for metastatic transitional cell carcinoma, although it has never been compared head-to-head with CMV.

Despite the encouraging early results, MVAC has not proved to be curative therapy for transitional cell carcinoma, nor has the high response rate been replicated in the cooperative group or community setting. A randomized trial comparing MVAC to single-agent cisplatin showed an overall response rate to MVAC of 39%, with only 13% complete responses.[201] Median survival time for the patients receiving MVAC was 12.5 months, similar to prior studies, but a recent update showed that only 4% of patients were alive at 5 years.[202]

Several attempts have been made to improve both the toxicity profile and response rate of MVAC. Even at standard doses, MVAC is a highly toxic regimen and a majority of patients are unable to receive the full prescribed dose over sequential cycles. Use of colony-stimulating factors has yielded mixed results in terms of allowing patients to receive standard therapy. An initial trial of prophylactic granulocyte colony-stimulating factor (GCSF) with MVAC showed an overall reduction of the days of significant neutropenia along with a decrease in the incidence of febrile neutropenia and mucositis.[203] However, a similar trial using granulocyte-macrophage colony-stimulating factor (GMCSF) showed that this effect was transient and that the growth factor failed to have an significant impact for subsequent cycles of therapy.[202] Efforts to improve the efficacy of the regimen have focused primarily on the use of dose-escalated MVAC. Initial enthusiasm for this approach was based on the observation of responses in up to 40% of patients with disease refractory to prior systemic chemotherapy including standard dose MVAC.[204] Subsequent trials have shown no improvement in response rates compared to a conventional dose MVAC, but a marked increase in toxicity.[205-208] One of the trials conducted by the Eastern Cooperative Oncology Group was halted early due to a 40% incidence of febrile neutropenia and a 23% death rate due to treatment-related complications.[205] The most recent use of this approach was conducted by the EORTC.[206] This trial demonstrated that high-dose MVAC given on an every 2 weeks schedule with GCSF had markedly increased complete and overall response rates when compared to standard MVAC. Median time to progression and 2-year progression-free survival times favored the high-dose arm, but the trial did not demonstrate the 50% improvement in median overall survival it was designed to detect. Toxicities were roughly equivalent in the two arms of the study, slightly favoring the high-dose arm, presumably due to the use of the GCSF. To date dose escalation of MVAC has not demonstrated a significant benefit to patients.

The toxicity and relatively limited efficacy of MVAC has prompted a search for new agents and combinations. Several agents have emerged from this search, including gallium nitrate, ifosfamide, and the folate antagonist trimetrexate.[207,209-211] Each of these agents have shown significant activity in the phase II trials, although they have been largely abandoned in subsequent trials. The two most promising agents to emerge are paclitaxel and gemcitabine. Both show significant activity as single agents. A phase II trial of paclitaxel was conducted by the Eastern Cooperative Oncology Group in patients who had receive no prior chemotherapy or radiotherapy.[212] Using a 24-hour continuous infusion of 250 mg/m^2 every 3 weeks along with GCSF, 11 patients out of 26 (42%) showed evidence of response, with 7 patients (27%) achieving a complete response. Paclitaxel was then combined with carboplatin in a phase I-II trial.[213] With a target area under the curve (AUC) for carboplatin of 6 mg/mL/minute and paclitaxel at 225 mg/m^2, the overall objective response rate was 50%. An nearly identical response rate of 52% was documented in a phase II trial of paclitaxel at 200 mg/m^2 over 3 hours, followed by carboplatin at a target AUC of 5 mg/mL/minute every 3 weeks.[214] These results prompted further investigation in the cooperative group setting. The Southwest Oncology Group used this regimen in previously untreated patients.[215] The overall response rate was only 21%. The Eastern Cooperative Oncology Group evaluated the combination in patients with renal insufficiency and demonstrated an overall response rate of 24%.[216] The combination was well tolerated in both trials, but the low response rate has discouraged further development.

The activity of gemcitabine was originally demonstrated in an Italian phase I trial in which 15 patients with metastatic bladder cancer were enrolled.[217] One complete response and three partial responses were seen for an overall response rate 27%. Of note is the fact that responses were seen in hepatic metastases as well as lung nodules, which are sites where conventional chemotherapy is relatively ineffective for transitional cell carcinoma. Confirmatory trials were conducted in the United States and Canada.[218,219] Patients received gemcitabine at 1200 mg/m^2 weekly for 3 weeks, with a 1-week rest period. Overall response rates were 28% in the U.S. trial and 24% in the Canadian trial. Both trials reported relatively minimal toxicity and these trials serve as a basis for the incorporation of gemcitabine into combination chemotherapy regimens. A recent trial combined gemcitabine with cisplatin (GC).[220] The initial regimen called for cisplatin at a dose of 100 mg/m^2 on day 1 and gemcitabine at 1000 mg/m^2 on days 1, 8, and 15 out of a 28-day cycle. Significant myelosuppression was seen in the original patients enrolled on this trial, resulting in a subsequent dose reduction of the cisplatin to 75 mg/m^2. Thirteen complete and 18 partial responses were seen in 47 patients enrolled, for an overall response rate of 66% in this multicenter trial. A Canadian trial using the same regimen demonstrated a nearly identical response rate.[221]

Responses were seen in hepatic and bone metastases on both trials. A similar trial in Europe demonstrated an overall response rate of 42%.[222] Based on these results, this regimen was compared to MVAC in a randomized multicenter trial being conducted in Europe and North America.[223] Four hundred five patients were randomized between the two therapies. Overall survival times (median: GC 13.8 months, MVAC 14.8 months) and response rates (GC 49.4%, MVAC 45.7%) were similar in the study arms, but patients receiving GC had much less severe toxicity despite receiving much more therapy. Although this study was not designed to demonstrate that GC was equivalent to MVAC, it does appear that efficacy is roughly similar with markedly less toxicity.

The next major questions under investigation are whether taxanes can add to the efficacy of therapy for advanced disease, and what the role of targeted therapy is in metastatic urothelial cancer. A large international intergroup trial comparing GC and GC plus paclitaxel is now under way. Ongoing phase II trials are assessing the prevalence of Her2 overexpression in metastatic urothelial cancer and the toxicity and efficacy of adding trastuzumab to combination chemotherapy for this disease.[224] It is hoped that these studies will open the door to new regimens for the treatment of this disease.

These new regimens hold significant promise both in terms of efficacy and increased tolerability. In assessing a patient with metastatic transitional cell carcinoma for chemotherapy, toxicity is a major consideration. In general, patients with bladder cancer are older and may have significant comorbidity. At this point therapy is not curative and the impact of toxicity on quality of life is significant. This situation is particularly true with MVAC, although the newer regimens also can be associated with significant toxicity in patients with poorer performance status. The responses seen in visceral metastatic sites, which are usually less responsive to chemotherapy, are encouraging, but these agents should be used with caution in patients with borderline performance status.

REFERENCES

1. Jemal A, Thomas A, Murray T, Thun M: Cancer statistics, 2002 [comment]. [erratum appears in CA Cancer J Clin 2002;52(2): 119] CA Cancer J Clin 2002;52(1):23-47.

2. Kiemeney LA, Schoenberg M: Familial transitional cell carcinoma [comment]. J Urol 1996;156(3):867-872.

3. Yancik R, Ries LA: Cancer in older persons. Magnitude of the problem. How do we apply what we know? Cancer 1994; 74(7 suppl):1995-2003.

4. Wingo PA, Ries LA, Rosenberg HM, Miller DS, Edwards BK: Cancer incidence and mortality, 1973-1995: A report card for the U.S. Cancer 1998;82(6):1197-207.

5. Fleshner NE, Herr HW, Stewart AK, Murphy GP, Mettlin C, Menck HR: The National Cancer Data Base report on bladder carcinoma. The American College of Surgeons Commission on Cancer and the American Cancer Society. Cancer 1996;78(7): 1505-1513.

6. Mungan NA, Kiemeney LA, van Dijck JA, van der Poel HG, Witjes JA: Gender differences in stage distribution of bladder cancer. Urology 2000;55(3):368-371.

7. Prout GR Jr, Wesley MN, Greenberg RS, et al: Bladder cancer: Race differences in extent of disease at diagnosis. Cancer 2000;89(6): 1349-1358.

Specific Malignancies

III

8. Plna K, Hemminki K: Familial bladder cancer in the National Swedish Family Cancer Database. J Urol 2001;166(6):2129-2133.

9. Burch JD, Rohan TE, Howe GR, et al: Risk of bladder cancer by source and type of tobacco exposure: A case-control study. Intl J Cancer 1989;44(4):622-628.

10. Vineis P, Martone T: Molecular epidemiology of bladder cancer. Ann Ist Super Sanita 1996;32(1):21-27.

11. Zeegers MP, Tan FE, Dorant E, van Den Brandt PA: The impact of characteristics of cigarette smoking on urinary tract cancer risk: A meta-analysis of epidemiologic studies. Cancer 2000;89(3):630-639.

12. Aveyard P, Adab P, Cheng KK, Wallace DM, Hey K, Murphy MF: Does smoking status influence the prognosis of bladder cancer? A systematic review. Br J Urol Intl 2002;90(3):228-239.

13. Silverman DT, Levin LI, Hoover RN, Hartge P: Occupational risks of bladder cancer in the United States: I. White men. J Natl Cancer Inst 1989;81(19):1472-1480.

14. Talar-Williams C, Hijazi YM, Walther MM, et al: Cyclophosphamide-induced cystitis and bladder cancer in patients with Wegener granulomatosis [comment]. Ann Intern Med 1996;124(5):477-484.

15. Fernandes ET, Manivel JC, Reddy PK, Ercole CJ: Cyclophosphamide associated bladder cancer—A highly aggressive disease: Analysis of 12 cases. J Urol 1996;156(6):1931-1933.

16. Ghoneim MA, el-Mekresh MM, el-Baz MA, el-Attar IA, Ashamallah A: Radical cystectomy for carcinoma of the bladder: Critical evaluation of the results in 1,026 cases. J Urol 1997;158(2):393-399.

17. Zhang ZF, Steineck G: Epidemiology and etiology of bladder cancer. Philadelphia, Lippincott Raven, 1997.

18. Navon JD, Soliman H, Khonsari F, Ahlering T: Screening cystoscopy and survival of spinal cord injured patients with squamous cell cancer of the bladder [comment]. J Urol 1997;157(6):2109-2111.

19. Friedman GD, Carroll PR, Cattolica EV, Hiatt RA: Can hematuria be a predictor as well as a symptom or sign of bladder cancer? Cancer Epidemiol Biomarkers Prevention 1996;5(12):993-996.

20. Messing EM, Young TB, Hunt VB, et al: Comparison of bladder cancer outcome in men undergoing hematuria home screening versus those with standard clinical presentations. Urology 1995;45(3):387-396; discussion 96-97.

21. Shelfo SW, Brady JD, Soloway MS: Transurethral resection of bladder cancer. Urol Clin North Am 1997;5:1.

22. Herr HW, Donat SM, Dalbagni G: Correlation of cystoscopy with histology of recurrent papillary tumors of the bladder. J Urol 2002;168(3):978-980.

23. Caoili EM, Cohan RH, Korobkin M, et al: Urinary tract abnormalities: Initial experience with multi-detector row CT urography [comment]. Radiology 2002;222(2):353-360.

24. Fitzpatrick JM: Superficial bladder carcinoma. Factors affecting the natural history. World J Urol 1993;11(3):142-147.

25. Fitzpatrick JM, West AB, Butler MR, Lane V, O'Flynn JD: Superficial bladder tumors (stage pTa, grades 1 and 2): The importance of recurrence pattern following initial resection. J Urol 1986;135(5):920-922.

26. Thompson RA Jr, Campbell EW Jr, Kramer HC, Jacobs SC, Naslund MJ: Late invasive recurrence despite long-term surveillance for superficial bladder cancer. J Urol 1993;149(5):1010-1011.

27. Cookson MS, Herr HW, Zhang ZF, Soloway S, Sogani PC, Fair WR: The treated natural history of high risk superficial bladder cancer: 15-year outcome. J Urol 1997;158(1):62-67.

28. Wiener HG, Mian C, Haitel A, Pycha A, Schatzl G, Marberger M: Can urine bound diagnostic tests replace cystoscopy in the management of bladder cancer? J Urol 1998;159(6):1876-1880.

29. Lokeshwar VB, Soloway MS: Current bladder tumor tests: Does their projected utility fulfill clinical necessity? J Urol 2001;165(4):1067-1077.

30. Grossman HB: New methods for detection of bladder cancer. Semin Urol Oncol 1998;16(1):17-22.

31. Gregoire M, Fradet Y, Meyer F, et al: Diagnostic accuracy of urinary cytology, and deoxyribonucleic acid flow cytometry and cytology on bladder washings during followup for bladder tumors. J Urol 1997;157(5):1660-1664.

32. Pode D, Golijanin D, Sherman Y, Lebensart P, Shapiro A: Immunostaining of Lewis X in cells from voided urine, cytopathology and ultrasound for noninvasive detection of bladder tumors [comment]. J Urol 1998;159(2):389-392; discussion 93.

33. Klein A, Zemer R, Buchumensky V, Klaper R, Nissenkorn I: Expression of cytokeratin 20 in urinary cytology of patients with bladder carcinoma [comment]. Cancer 1998;82(2):349-354.

34. Badalament RA: Is the role of cystoscopy in the detection of bladder cancer really declining? [comment] J Urol 1998;159(2):399-400.

35. Sarosdy MF, deVere White RW, Soloway MS, et al: Results of a multicenter trial using the BTA test to monitor for and diagnose recurrent bladder cancer [comment]. J Urol 1995;154(2 Pt 1):379-383; discussion 83-84.

36. Ellis WJ, Blumenstein BA, Ishak LM, Enfield DL: Clinical evaluation of the BTA TRAK assay and comparison to voided urine cytology and the Bard BTA test in patients with recurrent bladder tumors. The Multi Center Study Group. Urology 1997;50(6):882-887.

37. Stampfer DS, Carpinito GA, Rodriguez-Villanueva J, et al: Evaluation of NMP22 in the detection of transitional cell carcinoma of the bladder [comment][erratum appears in J Urol 1998;159(5):1650]. J Urol 1998;159(2):394-398.

38. Johnston B, Morales A, Emerson L, Lundie M: Rapid detection of bladder cancer: A comparative study of point of care tests [comment]. J Urol 1997;158(6):2098-2101.

39. Rasmussen HH, Orntoft TF, Wolf H, Celis JE: Towards a comprehensive database of proteins from the urine of patients with bladder cancer. J Urol 1996;155(6):2113-2119.

40. Getzenberg RH, Konety BR, Oeler TA, et al: Bladder cancer-associated nuclear matrix proteins. Cancer Res 1996;56(7):1690-1694.

41. Fradet Y: Phenotypic characterization of bladder cancer. Eur Urol 1998;33(suppl 4):5-6.

42. Kavaler E, Landman J, Chang Y, Droller MJ, Liu BC: Detecting human bladder carcinoma cells in voided urine samples by assaying for the presence of telomerase activity. Cancer 1998;82(4):708-714.

43. Linn JF, Lango M, Halachmi S, Schoenberg MP, Sidransky D: Microsatellite analysis and telomerase activity in archived tissue and urine samples of bladder cancer patients. Intl J Cancer 1997;74(6):625-629.

44. Halling KC, King W, Sokolova IA, et al: A comparison of cytology and fluorescence in situ hybridization for the detection of urothelial carcinoma. J Urol 2000;164(5):1768-1775.

45. Boman H, Hedelin H, Holmang S: Four bladder tumor markers have a disappointingly low sensitivity for small size and low grade recurrence. J Urol 2002;167(1):80-83.

46. Song JH, Francis IR, Platt JF, et al: Bladder tumor detection at virtual cystoscopy. Radiology 2001;218(1):95-100.

47. van der Poel HG, Boon ME, van Stratum P, et al: Conventional bladder wash cytology performed by four experts versus quantitative image analysis. Modern Pathol 1997;10(10):976-982.

48. Grignon DJ: Bladder Neoplasms. In Eble JN, Bostwick D (eds): Urological Surgical Pathology. New York: Mosby Year Book, 1996, pp 214-305.

49. Epstein JI, Amin MB, Reuter VR, Mostofi FK: The World Health Organization/International Society of Urological Pathology consensus classification of urothelial (transitional cell) neoplasms of the urinary bladder. Bladder Consensus Conference Committee [comment]. Am J Surg Pathol 1998;22(12):1435-1448.

50. Grignon DJ, Murphy WM: Classification of urothelial neoplasms: One, two, three, and around we go. Urol Oncol 2001;158:1895.

51. Montie JE, Wojno K, Klein E, Pearsall C, Levin H: Transitional cell carcinoma in situ of the seminal vesicles: 8 cases with discussion of pathogenesis, and clinical and biological implications. J Urol 1997;158(5):1895-1898.

52. Greene FL, et al (eds): Urinary bladder. In AJCC Cancer Staging Manual Sixth Edition. New York, Springer Verlag, 2002, pp 335-340.

53. Fischer CG, Waechter W, Kraus S, Fuentecilla Perez E, Weidner W, Dudeck J: Urologic tumors in the Federal Republic of Germany: Data on 56,013 cases from hospital cancer registries. Cancer 1998;82(4):775-783.

54. Coblentz TR, Mills SE, Theodorescu D: Impact of second opinion

pathology in the definitive management of patients with bladder carcinoma. Cancer 2001;91(7):1284–1290.

55. Herr HW: Tumour progression and survival in patients with T1G3 bladder tumours: 15-year outcome [comment]. Br J Urol 1997;80(5):762–765.

56. Smith JA Jr, Labasky RF, Cockett AT, Fracchia JA, Montie JE, Rowland RG: Bladder cancer clinical guidelines panel summary report on the management of nonmuscle invasive bladder cancer (stages Ta, T1 and TIS). The American Urological Association [comment]. J Urol 1999;162(5):1697–1701.

57. Kiemeney LA, Witjes JA, Heijbroek RP, Verbeek AL, Debruyne FM: Predictability of recurrent and progressive disease in individual patients with primary superficial bladder cancer. J Urol 1993;150(1):60–64.

58. Holmang S, Hedelin H, Anderstrom C, Holmberg E, Johansson SL: The importance of the depth of invasion in stage T1 bladder carcinoma: A prospective cohort study [comment]. J Urol 1997;157(3):800–803; discussion 804.

59. Herr HW, Reuter VE: Progression of T1 bladder tumors: Better staging or better biology? [comment] Cancer 1999;86(6):908–912.

60. Cheng L, Bostwick DG: Progression of T1 bladder tumors: Better staging or better biopsy? Cancer 1999;47:324; available from C:\WINNT\Profiles\tderry\Desktop\Bladder Ca Copy Copy.enl.

61. Herr HW: Routine CT scan in cystectomy patients: Does it change management? [erratum appears in Urology 1996;47(5):785]. Urology 1996;47(3):324–325.

62. Persad R, Kabala J, Gillatt D, Penry B, Gingell JC, Smith PJ: Magnetic resonance imaging in the staging of bladder cancer. Br J Urol 1993;71(5):566–573.

63. Tachibana M, Baba S, Deguchi N, et al: Efficacy of gadolinium-diethylenetriaminepentaacetic acid-enhanced magnetic resonance imaging for differentiation between superficial and muscle-invasive tumor of the bladder: A comparative study with computerized tomography and transurethral ultrasonography. J Urol 1991;145(6):1169–1173.

64. Hofer C, Kubler H, Hartung R, Breul J, Avril N: Diagnosis and monitoring of urological tumors using positron emission tomography. Eur Urol 2001;40(5):481–487.

65. Montie JE: Follow-up after cystectomy for carcinoma of the bladder. Urol Clin North Am 1994;21(4):639–643.

66. Czerniak B, Li L, Chaturvedi V, et al: Genetic modeling of human urinary bladder carcinogenesis. Genes Chromosomes Cancer 2000;27(4):392–402.

67. Sauter G, Moch H, Mihatsch MJ, Gasser TC: Molecular cytogenetics of bladder cancer progression. Eur Urol 1998;33(suppl 4):9–10.

68. Cordon-Cardo C: Cell cycle regulators as prognostic factors for bladder cancer. Eur Urol 1998;33(suppl 4):11–12.

69. Grossman HB, Liebert M, Antelo M, et al: p53 and RB expression predict progression in T1 bladder cancer. Clini Cancer Res 1998;4(4):829–834.

70. Cote RJ, Dunn MD, Chatterjee SJ, et al: Elevated and absent pRb expression is associated with bladder cancer progression and has cooperative effects with p53. Cancer Res 1998;58(6):1090–1094.

71. Cordon-Cardo C, Zhang ZF, Dalbagni G, et al: Cooperative effects of p53 and pRB alterations in primary superficial bladder tumors. Cancer Res 1997;57(7):1217–1221.

72. Smith ND, Rubenstein JN, Eggener SE, Kozlowski JM: The p53 tumor suppressor gene and nuclear protein: Basic science review and relevance in the management of bladder cancer. J Urol 2003;169(4):1219–1228.

73. Lorenzo-Romero JG, Salinas-Sanchez AS, Gimenez-Bachs JM, et al: Prognostic implications of p53 gene mutations in bladder tumors. J Urol 2003;169(2):492–499.

74. Hermann GG, Horn T, Steven K: The influence of the level of lamina propria invasion and the prevalence of p53 nuclear accumulation on survival in stage T1 transitional cell bladder cancer. J Urol 1998;159(1):91–94.

75. Sarkis AS, Dalbagni G, Cordon-Cardo C, et al: Nuclear overexpression of p53 protein in transitional cell bladder carcinoma: A marker for disease progression. J Natl Cancer Inst 1993;85(1):53–59.

76. Esrig D, Elmajian D, Groshen S, et al: Accumulation of nuclear p53 and tumor progression in bladder cancer [comment]. N Engl J Med 1994;331(19):1259–1264.

77. Vollmer RT, Humphrey PA, Swanson PE, Wick MR, Hudson ML: Invasion of the bladder by transitional cell carcinoma: Its relation to histologic grade and expression of p53, MIB-1, c-erb B-2, epidermal growth factor receptor, and bcl-2. Cancer 1998;82(4):715–723.

78. Popov Z, Hoznek A, Colombel M, et al: The prognostic value of p53 nuclear overexpression and MIB-1 as a proliferative marker in transitional cell carcinoma of the bladder. Cancer 1997;80(8):1472–1481.

79. Kraggerud SM, Jacobsen KD, Berner A, et al: A comparison of different modes for the detection of p53 protein accumulation. A study of bladder cancer. Pathol Res Pract 1997;193(7):471–478.

80. Brausi M, Collette L, Kurth K, et al: Variability in the recurrence rate at first follow-up cystoscopy after TUR in stage Ta T1 transitional cell carcinoma of the bladder: A combined analysis of seven EORTC studies. Eur Urol 2002;41(5):523–531.

81. Lamm DL, Riggs DR, Traynelis CL, Nseyo UO: Apparent failure of current intravesical chemotherapy prophylaxis to influence the long-term course of superficial transitional cell carcinoma of the bladder. J Urol 1995;153(5):1444–1450.

82. Kilbridge KL, Kantoff P: Intravesical therapy for superficial bladder cancer: Is it a wash? [comment] J Clin Oncol 1994;12(1):1–4.

83. Kurth K, Tunn U, Ay R, et al: Adjuvant chemotherapy for superficial transitional cell bladder carcinoma: Long-term results of a European Organization for Research and Treatment of Cancer randomized trial comparing doxorubicin, ethoglucid and transurethral resection alone. J Urol 1997;158(2):378–384.

84. Pawinski A, Sylvester R, Kurth KH, et al: A combined analysis of European Organization for Research and Treatment of Cancer, and Medical Research Council randomized clinical trials for the prophylactic treatment of stage TaT1 bladder cancer. European Organization for Research and Treatment of Cancer Genitourinary Tract Cancer Cooperative Group and the Medical Research Council Working Party on Superficial Bladder Cancer. J Urol 1996;156(6):1934–1940, discussion 40–41.

85. Tolley DA, Parmar MK, Grigor KM, et al: The effect of intravesical mitomycin C on recurrence of newly diagnosed superficial bladder cancer: A further report with 7 years of follow up. J Urol 1996;155(4):1233–1238.

86. Ali-el-Dein B, el-Baz M, Aly AN, Shamaa S, Ashamallah A: Intravesical epirubicin versus doxorubicin for superficial bladder tumors (stages pTa and pT1): A randomized prospective study. J Urol 1997;158(1):68–73; discussion 73–74.

87. Au JL, Badalament RA, Wientjes MG, et al: Methods to improve efficacy of intravesical mitomycin C: Results of a randomized phase III trial [comment]. J Natl Cancer Inst 2001;93(8):597–604.

88. Dalbagni G, Russo P, Sheinfeld J, et al: Phase I trial of intravesical gemcitabine in bacillus Calmette-Guerin-refractory transitional-cell carcinoma of the bladder [comment]. J Clin Oncol 2002;20(15):3193–3198.

89. Bohle A, Jocham D, Bock PR: Intravesical bacillus Calmette-Guerin versus mitomycin C for superficial bladder cancer: A formal meta-analysis of comparative studies on recurrence and toxicity. J Urol 2003;169(1):90–95.

90. Lamm DL, Blumenstein BA, Crawford ED, et al: A randomized trial of intravesical doxorubicin and immunotherapy with bacille Calmette-Guerin for transitional-cell carcinoma of the bladder. N Engl J Med 1991;325(17):1205–1209.

91. Herr HW, Schwalb DM, Zhang ZF, et al: Intravesical bacillus Calmette-Guerin therapy prevents tumor progression and death from superficial bladder cancer: Ten-year follow-up of a prospective randomized trial. J Clin Oncol 1995;13(6):1404–1408.

92. Davis JW, Sheth SI, Doviak MJ, Schellhammer PF: Superficial bladder carcinoma treated with bacillus Calmette-Guerin: Progression-free and disease-specific survival with minimum 10-year followup. J Urol 2002;167(2 Pt 1):494–500; discussion 501.

93. Lamm DL, Blumenstein B, Crawford ED, et al: Randomized intergroup comparison of bacillus Calmette-Guerin immunotherapy and mitomycin C chemotherapy prophylaxis in superficial transitional cell carcinoma of the bladder. Urol Oncol 1995;1:119.

94. Lamm DL, Blumenstein B, Sardosdy M, et al: Significant long-term patient benefit with BCG maintenance therapy: A Southwest Oncology Group study. J Urol 1997;157:213.

95. Badalament RA, Herr HW, Wong GY, et al: A prospective randomized trial of maintenance versus nonmaintenance intravesical bacillus Calmette-Guerin therapy of superficial bladder cancer. J Clin Oncol 1987;5(3):441–449.

96. Hurle R, Losa A, Ranieri A, Graziotti P, Lembo A: Low dose Pasteur bacillus Calmette-Guerin regimen in stage T1, grade 3 bladder cancer therapy [comment]. J Urol 1996;156(5):1602–1605.

97. Lamm DL, van der Meijden PM, Morales A, et al: Incidence and treatment of complications of bacillus Calmette-Guerin intravesical therapy in superficial bladder cancer. J Urol 1992;147(3):596–600.

98. Rawls WH, Lamm DL, Lowe BA, et al: Fatal sepsis following intravesical bacillus Calmette-Guerin administration for bladder cancer. J Urol 1990;144(6):1328–1330.

99. Merz VW, Marth D, Kraft R, Ackermann DK, Zingg EJ, Studer UE: Analysis of early failures after intravesical instillation therapy with bacille Calmette-Guerin for carcinoma in situ of the bladder. Br J Urol 1995;75(2):180–184.

100. Vegt PD, van der Meijden AP, Sylvester R, Brausi M, Holtl W, de Balincourt C: Does isoniazid reduce side effects of intravesical bacillus Calmette-Guerin therapy in superficial bladder cancer? Interim results of European Organization for Research and Treatment of Cancer Protocol 30911. J Urol 1997;157(4):1246–1249.

101. Herr HW, Cookson MS, Soloway SM: Upper tract tumors in patients with primary bladder cancer followed for 15 years. J Urol 1996;156(4):1286–1287.

102. Herr HW: Extravesical tumor relapse in patients with superficial bladder tumors. J Clin Oncol 1998;16(3):1099–1102.

103. Lacombe L, Dalbagni G, Zhang ZF, et al: Overexpression of p53 protein in a high-risk population of patients with superficial bladder cancer before and after bacillus Calmette-Guerin therapy: Correlation to clinical outcome. J Clin Oncol 1996;14(10):2646–2652.

104. Ick K, Schultz M, Stout P, Fan K: Significance of p53 over-expression in urinary bladder transitional cell carcinoma in situ before and after bacillus Calmette-Guerin treatment. Urology 1997;49(4):541–546; discussion 46–47.

105. Belldegrun AS, Franklin JR, O'Donnell MA, et al: Superficial bladder cancer: The role of interferon-alpha.[erratum appears in J Urol 1998;160(4):1444] J Urol 1998;159(5):1793–1801.

106. Punnen SP, Chin JL, Jewett MA: Management of BCG refractory superficial bladder cancer: Results with intravesical BCG and interferon combination therapy. Canad J Urol 2003;10:1790.

107. Lamm DL, Riggs DR, Shriver JS, vanGilder PF, Rach JF, DeHaven JI: Megadose vitamins in bladder cancer: A double-blind clinical trial. J Urol 1994;151(1):21–26.

108. Riggs DR, DeHaven JI, Lamm DL: Allium sativum (garlic) treatment for murine transitional cell carcinoma. Cancer 1997;79(10):1987–1994.

109. Jurincic-Winkler C, Metz KA, Beuth J, Sippel J, Klippel KF: Effect of keyhole limpet hemocyanin (KLH) and bacillus Calmette-Guerin (BCG) instillation on carcinoma in situ of the urinary bladder. Anticancer Res 1995;15(6B):2771–2776.

110. Dutta SC, Smith JA Jr, Shappell SB, Coffey CS, Chang SS, Cookson MS: Clinical under staging of high risk nonmuscle invasive urothelial carcinoma treated with radical cystectomy. J Urol 2001;166(2):490–493.

111. Herr HW, Sogani PC: Does early cystectomy improve the survival of patients with high risk superficial bladder tumors? J Urol 2001;166(4):1296–1299.

112. Yiou R, Patard JJ, Benhard H, Abbou CC, Chopin DK: Outcome of radical cystectomy for bladder cancer according to the disease type at presentation. Br J Urol Intl 2002;89(4):374–378.

113. Freeman JA, Esrig D, Stein JP, et al: Radical cystectomy for high risk patients with superficial bladder cancer in the era of orthotopic urinary reconstruction. Cancer 1995;76(5):833–839.

114. Yoshimura I, Kudoh J, Saito S, Tazaki H, Shimizu N: p53 gene mutation in recurrent superficial bladder cancer. J Urol 1995;153(5):1711–1715.

115. Pansadoro V, Emiliozzi P, Defidio L, et al: Bacillus Calmette-Guerin in the treatment of stage T1 grade 3 transitional cell carcinoma of the bladder: Long-term results. J Urol 1995;154(6):2054–2058.

116. Dalbagni G, Herr HW, Reuter VE: Impact of a second transurethral resection on the staging of T1 bladder cancer. Urology 2002;60(5):822–824; discussion 24–25.

117. Solsona E, Iborra I, Ricos JV, Monros JL, Casanova J, Calabuig C: Feasibility of transurethral resection for muscle infiltrating carcinoma of the bladder: Long-term followup of a prospective study. J Urol 1998;159(1):95–98; discussion 98–99.

118. Herr H: Uncertainty and outcome of invasive bladder tumors. Urol Oncol 1996;2:92.

119. Figueroa AJ, Stein JP, Dickinson M, et al: Radical cystectomy for elderly patients with bladder carcinoma: An updated experience with 404 patients. Cancer 1998;83(1):141–147.

120. Stein JP, Lieskovsky G, Cote R, et al: Radical cystectomy in the treatment of invasive bladder cancer: Long-term results in 1,054 patients. J Clin Oncol 2001;19(3):666–675.

121. Schoenberg MP, Walsh PC, Breazeale DR, Marshall FF, Mostwin JL, Brendler CB: Local recurrence and survival following nerve sparing radical cystoprostatectomy for bladder cancer: 10-year followup [comment]. J Urol 1996;155(2):490–494.

122. Wood DP Jr: Partial cystectomy. Urol Clin North Am 1997;5:79.

123. Petrovich Z, Baert L, Boyd SD, et al: Management of carcinoma of the bladder. Am J Clin Oncol 1998;21(3):217–222.

124. Wood DP Jr, Montie JE, Pontes JE, VanderBrug Medendorp S, Levin HS: Transitional cell carcinoma of the prostate in cystoprostatectomy specimens removed for bladder cancer. J Urol 1989;141(2):346–349.

125. Vallancien G, Abou El Fettouh H, Cathelineau X, Baumert H, Fromont G, Guillonneau B: Cystectomy with prostate sparing for bladder cancer in 100 patients: 10-year experience. J Urol 2002;168(6):2413–2417.

126. Chang SS, Cole E, Cookson MS, Peterson M, Smith JA Jr: Preservation of the anterior vaginal wall during female radical cystectomy with orthotopic urinary diversion: technique and results. J Urol 2002;168(4 Pt 1):1442–1445.

127. Leibovitch I, Avigad I, Ben-Chaim J, Nativ O, Goldwasser B: Is it justified to avoid radical cystoprostatectomy in elderly patients with invasive transitional cell carcinoma of the bladder? Cancer 1993;71(10):3098–3101.

128. Stroumbakis N, Herr HW, Cookson MS, Fair WR: Radical cystectomy in the octogenarian. J Urol 1997;158(6):2113–2117.

129. Hall CM, Dinney CP: Radical cystectomy for stage T3b bladder cancer. Semin Urol Oncol 1996;14(2):73–80.

130. Smith JA Jr, Crawford ED, Paradelo JC, et al: Treatment of advanced bladder cancer with combined preoperative irradiation and radical cystectomy versus radical cystectomy alone: A phase III intergroup study. J Urol 1997;157(3):805–807; discussion 807–808.

131. Greene FL: Urinary Bladder. Philadelphia, Lippincott Raven, 2002.

132. Vieweg J, Gschwend JE, Herr HW, Fair WR: Pelvic lymph node dissection can be curative in patients with node positive bladder cancer. J Urol 1999;161(2):449–454.

133. Herr HW, Bochner BH, Dalbagni G, Donat SM, Reuter VE, Bajorin DF: Impact of the number of lymph nodes retrieved on outcome in patients with muscle invasive bladder cancer. J Urol 2002;167(3):1295–1298.

134. Cookson MS, Chang SS, Wells N, Parekh DJ, Smith JA Jr: Complications of radical cystectomy for nonmuscle invasive disease: Comparison with muscle invasive disease [comment]. J Urol 2003;169(1):101–104.

135. Miller DC, Taub DA, Dunn RL, Montie JE, Wei JT: The impact of co-morbid disease on cancer control and survival following radical cystectomy [comment]. J Urol 2003;169(1):105–109.

136. Koch MO, Seckin B, Smith JA Jr: Impact of a collaborative care approach to radical cystectomy and urinary reconstruction. J Urol 1995;154(3):996–1001.

137. Montie JE: Ileal conduit diversion after radical cystectomy. Pro. Urology 1997;49(5):659–662.

138. Hara I, Miyake H, Hara S, et al: Health-related quality of life after radical cystectomy for bladder cancer: A comparison of ileal conduit and orthotopic bladder replacement. Br J Urol Intl 2002;89(1):10–13.

139. Bjerre BD, Johansen C, Steven K: Health-related quality of life after cystectomy: Bladder substitution compared with ileal conduit diversion. A questionnaire survey [comment]. Br J Urol 1995;75(2):200–205.

140. Stein JP, Freeman JA, Esrig D, et al: Complications of the afferent antireflux valve mechanism in the Kock ileal reservoir [comment]. J Urol 1996;155(5):1579-1584.

141. Wilson TG, Moreno JG, Weinberg A, Ahlering TE: Late complications of the modified Indiana pouch [comment]. J Urol 1994;151(2):331-334.

142. Turner WH, Bitton A, Studer UE: Reconstruction of the urinary tract after radical cystectomy: The case for continent urinary diversion. Urology 1997;49(5):663-667.

143. Parekh DJ, Clark T, O'Connor J, et al: Orthotopic neobladder following radical cystectomy in patients with high perioperative risk and co-morbid medical conditions. J Urol 2002;168(6):2454-2456.

144. Iselin CE, Robertson CN, Webster GD, Vieweg J, Paulson DF: Does prostate transitional cell carcinoma preclude orthotopic bladder reconstruction after radical cystoprostatectomy for bladder cancer? J Urol 1997;158(6):2123-2126.

145. Hautmann RE: Complications and results after cystectomy in male and female patients with locally invasive bladder cancer. Eur Urol 1998;33(suppl 4):23-24.

146. Stenzl A, Bartsch G, Rogatsch H: The remnant urothelium after reconstructive bladder surgery. Eur Urol 2002;41(2):124-131.

147. Gerharz EW, Turner WH, Kalble T, Woodhouse CR: Metabolic and functional consequences of urinary reconstruction with bowel. Br J Urol Intl 2003;91(2):143-149.

148. Hautmann RE, Paiss T: Does the option of the ileal neobladder stimulate patient and physician decision toward earlier cystectomy? J Urol 1998;159(6):1845-1850.

149. Montie JE: Against bladder sparing: Surgery. J Urol 1999;162(2):452-455; discussion 55-57.

150. Smith JA Jr, Batata M, Grabstald H, Sogani PC, Herr H, Whitmore WF Jr: Preoperative irradiation and cystectomy for bladder cancer. Cancer 1982;49(5):869-873.

151. Parsons JT, Million RR: Planned preoperative irradiation in the management of clinical stage B2-C (T3) bladder carcinoma. Intl J Radiat Oncol Biol Physics 1988;14(4):797-810.

152. Wishnow KI, Dmochowski R: Pelvic recurrence after radical cystectomy without preoperative radiation. J Urol 1988;140(1):42-43.

153. Cole CJ, Pollack A, Zagars GK, Dinney CP, Swanson DA, von Eschenbach AC: Local control of muscle-invasive bladder cancer: Preoperative radiotherapy and cystectomy versus cystectomy alone. Intl J Radiat Oncol Biol Physics 1995;32(2):331-340.

154. Greven KM, Spera JA, Solin LJ, Morgan T, Hanks GE: Local recurrence after cystectomy alone for bladder carcinoma. Cancer 1992;69(11):2767-2770.

155. Jose CC, Price A, Norman A, et al: Hypofractionated radiotherapy for patients with carcinoma of the bladder. Clin Oncol (R Coll Radiol) 1999;11(5):330-333.

156. Bloom HJ, Hendry WF, Wallace DM, Skeet RG: Treatment of T3 bladder cancer: Controlled trial of pre-operative radiotherapy and radical cystectomy versus radical radiotherapy. Br J Urol 1982;54(2):136-151.

157. Sell A, Jakobsen A, Nerstrom B, Sorensen BL, Steven K, Barlebo H: Treatment of advanced bladder cancer category T2, T3 and T4a. A randomized multicenter study of preoperative irradiation and cystectomy versus radical irradiation and early salvage cystectomy for residual tumor. DAVECA protocol 8201. Danish Vesical Cancer Group. Scand J Urol Nephrol Suppl 1991;138:193-201.

158. Greven KM, Solin LJ, Hanks GE: Prognostic factors in patients with bladder carcinoma treated with definitive irradiation. Cancer 1990;65(4):908-912.

159. Gospodarowicz MK, Hawkins NV, Rawlings GA, et al: Radical radiotherapy for muscle invasive transitional cell carcinoma of the bladder: Failure analysis. J Urol 1989;142(6):1448-1453; discussion 53-54.

160. Rotman M, Aziz H, Porrazzo M, et al: Treatment of advanced transitional cell carcinoma of the bladder with irradiation and concomitant 5-fluorouracil infusion. Intl J Radiat Oncol Biol Physics 1990;18(5):1131-1137.

161. Russell KJ, Boileau MA, Higano C, et al: Combined 5-fluorouracil and irradiation for transitional cell carcinoma of the urinary bladder [comment]. Intl J Radiat Oncol Biol Physics 1990;19(3):693-699.

162. Eapen L, Stewart D, Danjoux C, et al: Intraarterial cisplatin and concurrent radiation for locally advanced bladder cancer. J Clin Oncol 1989;7(2):230-235.

163. Housset M, Maulard C, Chretien Y, et al: Combined radiation and chemotherapy for invasive transitional-cell carcinoma of the bladder: A prospective study. J Clin Oncol 1993;11(11):2150-2157.

164. Nichols RC Jr, Sweetser MG, Mahmood SK, et al: Radiation therapy and concomitant paclitaxel/carboplatin chemotherapy for muscle invasive transitional cell carcinoma of the bladder: A well-tolerated combination. Intl J Cancer 2000;90(5):281-286.

165. Kachnic LA, Kaufman DS, Heney NM, et al: Bladder preservation by combined modality therapy for invasive bladder cancer. J Clin Oncol 1997;15(3):1022-1029.

166. Tester W, Caplan R, Heaney J, et al: Neoadjuvant combined modality program with selective organ preservation for invasive bladder cancer: Results of Radiation Therapy Oncology Group phase II trial 8802. J Clin Oncol 1996;14(1):119-126.

167. Shipley WU, Zietman AL, Kaufman DS, Althausen AF, Heney NM: Invasive bladder cancer: Treatment strategies using transurethral surgery, chemotherapy and radiation therapy with selection for bladder conservation. Intl J Radiat Oncol Biol Physics 1997;39(4):937-943.

168. Dunst J, Rodel C, Zietman A, Schrott KM, Sauer R, Shipley WU: Bladder preservation in muscle-invasive bladder cancer by conservative surgery and radiochemotherapy. Semin Surg Oncol 2001;20(1):24-32.

169. Shipley WU, Kaufman DS, Zehr E, et al: Selective bladder preservation by combined modality protocol treatment: Long-term outcomes of 190 patients with invasive bladder cancer. Urology 2002;60(1):62-67; discussion 67-68.

170. Caffo O, Fellin G, Graffer U, Luciani L: Assessment of quality of life after cystectomy or conservative therapy for patients with infiltrating bladder carcinoma. A survey by a self-administered questionnaire. [erratum appears in Cancer 1996 Nov 1;76(9):2037] Cancer 1996;78(5):1089-1097.

171. Sauer R, Birkenhake S, Kuhn R, Wittekind C, Schrott KM, Martus P: Efficacy of radiochemotherapy with platin derivatives compared to radiotherapy alone in organ-sparing treatment of bladder cancer. Intl J Radiat Oncol Biol Physics 1998;40(1):121-127.

172. Zietman AL, Grocela J, Zehr E, et al: Selective bladder conservation using transurethral resection, chemotherapy, and radiation: Management and consequences of Ta, T1, and Tis recurrence within the retained bladder. Urology 2001;58(3):380-385.

173. Shipley WU, Winter KA, Kaufman DS, et al: Phase III trial of neoadjuvant chemotherapy in patients with invasive bladder cancer treated with selective bladder preservation by combined radiation therapy and chemotherapy: Initial results of Radiation Therapy Oncology Group 89-03 [comment]. J Clin Oncol 1998;16(11):3576-3583.

174. Herr HW: Neoadjuvant chemotherapy for invasive bladder cancer. Semin Surg Oncol 1989;5(4):266-271.

175. Scher HI: Chemotherapy for invasive bladder cancer: Neoadjuvant versus adjuvant. Semin Oncol 1990;17(5):555-565.

176. Dirix LY, Van Oosterom AT: Neoadjuvant and adjuvant therapy for invasive bladder tumors. Eur J Cancer 1991;27(3):326-330.

177. Schultz PK, Herr HW, Zhang ZF, et al: Neoadjuvant chemotherapy for invasive bladder cancer: Prognostic factors for survival of patients treated with M-VAC with 5-year follow-up [comment]. J Clin Oncol 1994;12(7):1394-1401.

178. Logothetis CJ, Johnson DE, Chong C, et al: Adjuvant cyclophosphamide, doxorubicin, and cisplatin chemotherapy for bladder cancer: An update. J Clin Oncol 1988;6(10):1590-1596.

179. Skinner DG, Daniels JR, Russell CA, et al: The role of adjuvant chemotherapy following cystectomy for invasive bladder cancer: A prospective comparative trial. J Urol 1991;145(3):459-464; discussion 64-67.

180. Stockle M, Meyenburg W, Wellek S, et al: Advanced bladder cancer (stages pT3b, pT4a, pN1 and pN2): Improved survival after radical cystectomy and 3 adjuvant cycles of chemotherapy. Results of a controlled prospective study. J Urol 1992;148(2 Pt 1):302-306; discussion 306-307.

181. Stockle M, Meyenburg W, Wellek S, et al: Adjuvant polychemo-therapy of nonorgan-confined bladder cancer after radical cystectomy revisited: Long-term results of a controlled

Specific Malignancies

III

prospective study and further clinical experience. J Urol 1995; 153(1):47–52.

182. Freiha F, Reese J, Torti FM: A randomized trial of radical cystectomy versus radical cystectomy plus cisplatin, vinblastine and methotrexate chemotherapy for muscle invasive bladder cancer [comment]. J Urol 1996;155(2):495–499; discussion 499–500.

183. Millikan R, Dinney C, Swanson D, et al: Integrated therapy for locally advanced bladder cancer: Final report of a randomized trial of cystectomy plus adjuvant M-VAC versus cystectomy with both preoperative and postoperative M-VAC [comment]. J Clin Oncol 2001;19(20):4005–4013.

184. Raghavan D, Grundy R, Greenaway TM, et al: Pre-emptive (neo-adjuvant) chemotherapy prior to radical radiotherapy for fit septuagenarians with bladder cancer: age itself is not a contraindication. Br J Urol 1988;62(2):154–159.

185. Rintala E, Hannisdahl E, Fossa SD, Hellsten S, Sander S: Neoadjuvant chemotherapy in bladder cancer: A randomized study. Nordic Cystectomy Trial I. Scand J Urol Nephrol 1993;27(3):355–362.

186. Martinez-Pineiro JA, Gonzalez Martin M, Arocena F, et al: Neoadjuvant cisplatin chemotherapy before radical cystectomy in invasive transitional cell carcinoma of the bladder: A prospective randomized phase III study. J Urol 1995;153(3 Pt 2):964–973.

187. Coppin CM, Gospodarowicz MK, James K, et al: Improved local control of invasive bladder cancer by concurrent cisplatin and preoperative or definitive radiation. The National Cancer Institute of Canada Clinical Trials Group. J Clin Oncol 1996;14(11):2901–2907.

188. Does neoadjuvant cisplatin-based chemotherapy improve the survival of patients with locally advanced bladder cancer: A meta-analysis of individual patient data from randomized clinical trials. Advanced Bladder Cancer Overview Collaboration. Br J Urol 1995;75(2):206–213.

189. Neoadjuvant cisplatin, methotrexate, and vinblastine chemotherapy for muscle-invasive bladder cancer: A randomised controlled trial. International collaboration of trialists [comment]. [erratum appears in Lancet 1999;354(9190):1650]. Lancet 1999;354(9178):533–540.

190. Grossman HB, Natale RB, Tangen CM, Speights VO, Vogelzang, NJ, Trump DL, et al: Neoadjuvant chemotherapy plus cystectomy compared with cystectomy alone for locally advanced bladder cancer. N Engl J Med 2003;349(9):859–866.

191. Bajorin DF: Plenary debate of randomized phase III trial of neoadjuvant MVAC plus cystectomy versus cystectomy alone in patients with locally advanced bladder cancer. J Clin Oncol 2001;19(18 suppl):17S–20S.

192. Sternberg CN, Parmar MK: Neoadjuvant chemotherapy is not (yet) standard treatment for muscle-invasive bladder cancer. J Clin Oncol 2001;19(18 suppl):21S–26S.

193. Yagoda A: Chemotherapy of urothelial tract tumors. Cancer 1987;60(3 suppl):574–575.

194. Harker WG, Meyers FJ, Freiha FS, et al: Cisplatin, methotrexate, and vinblastine (CMV): An effective chemotherapy regimen for metastatic transitional cell carcinoma of the urinary tract. A Northern California Oncology Group study. J Clin Oncol 1985;3(11):1463–1470.

195. Logothetis CJ, Samuels ML, Ogden S, et al: Cyclophosphamide, doxorubicin and cisplatin chemotherapy for patients with locally advanced urothelial tumors with or without nodal metastases. J Urol 1985;134(3):460–464.

196. Khandekar JD, Elson PJ, DeWys WD, Slayton RE, Harris DT: Comparative activity and toxicity of cis-diamminedichloroplatinum (DDP) and a combination of doxorubicin, cyclophosphamide, and DDP in disseminated transitional cell carcinomas of the urinary tract. J Clin Oncol 1985;3(4):539–545.

197. Troner M, Birch R, Omura GA, Williams S: Phase III comparison of cisplatin alone versus cisplatin, doxorubicin and cyclophosphamide in the treatment of bladder (urothelial) cancer: A Southeastern Cancer Study Group trial. J Urol 1987;137(4):660–662.

198. Sternberg CN, Yagoda A, Scher HI, et al: Preliminary results of M-VAC (methotrexate, vinblastine, doxorubicin and cisplatin) for

transitional cell carcinoma of the urothelium. J Urol 1985;133(3):403–407.

199. Sternberg CN, Yagoda A, Scher HI, et al: Methotrexate, vinblastine, doxorubicin, and cisplatin for advanced transitional cell carcinoma of the urothelium. Efficacy and patterns of response and relapse. Cancer 1989;64(12):2448–2458.

200. Logothetis CJ, Dexeus FH, Finn L, et al: A prospective randomized trial comparing MVAC and CISCA chemotherapy for patients with metastatic urothelial tumors [comment]. J Clin Oncol 1990;8(6): 1050–1055.

201. Loehrer PJ Sr, Einhorn LH, Elson PJ, et al: A randomized comparison of cisplatin alone or in combination with methotrexate, vinblastine, and doxorubicin in patients with metastatic urothelial carcinoma: A cooperative group study [comment]. [erratum appears in J Clin Oncol 1993;11(2):384] J Clin Oncol 1992;10(7):1066–1073.

202. Saxman SB, Propert KJ, Einhorn LH, et al: Long-term follow-up of a phase III intergroup study of cisplatin alone or in combination with methotrexate, vinblastine, and doxorubicin in patients with metastatic urothelial carcinoma: A cooperative group study. J Clin Oncol 1997;15(7):2564–2569.

203. Gabrilove JL, Jakubowski A, Scher H, et al: Effect of granulocyte colony-stimulating factor on neutropenia and associated morbidity due to chemotherapy for transitional-cell carcinoma of the urothelium. N Engl J Med 1988;318(22):1414–1422.

204. Logothetis CJ, Dexeus FH, Sella A, et al: Escalated therapy for refractory urothelial tumors: Methotrexate-vinblastine-doxorubicin-cisplatin plus unglycosylated recombinant human granulocyte-macrophage colony-stimulating factor. J Natl Cancer Inst 1990;82(8):667–672.

205. Loehrer PJ Sr, Elson P, Dreicer R, et al: Escalated dosages of methotrexate, vinblastine, doxorubicin, and cisplatin plus recombinant human granulocyte colony-stimulating factor in advanced urothelial carcinoma: An Eastern Cooperative Oncology Group trial. J Clin Oncol 1994;12(3):483–488.

206. Sternberg CN, de Mulder PH, Schornagel JH, et al: Randomized phase III trial of high-dose-intensity methotrexate, vinblastine, doxorubicin, and cisplatin (MVAC) chemotherapy and recombinant human granulocyte colony-stimulating factor versus classic MVAC in advanced urothelial tract tumors: European Organization for Research and Treatment of Cancer Protocol no. 30924. J Clin Oncol 2001;19(10):2638–2646.

207. Seidman AD, Scher HI, Gabrilove JL, et al: Dose-intensification of MVAC with recombinant granulocyte colony-stimulating factor as initial therapy in advanced urothelial cancer [comment]. J Clin Oncol 1993;11(3):408–414.

208. Logothetis CJ, Finn LD, Smith T, et al: Escalated MVAC with or without recombinant human granulocyte-macrophage colony-stimulating factor for the initial treatment of advanced malignant urothelial tumors: Results of a randomized trial. J Clin Oncol 1995;13(9):2272–2277.

209. Seligman PA, Crawford ED: Treatment of advanced transitional cell carcinoma of the bladder with continuous-infusion gallium nitrate. J Natl Cancer Inst 1991;83(21):1582–1584.

210. Witte RS, Elson P, Bono B, et al: Eastern Cooperative Oncology Group phase II trial of ifosfamide in the treatment of previously treated advanced urothelial carcinoma. J Clin Oncol 1997;15(2): 589–593.

211. Witte RS, Elson P, Khandakar J, Trump DL: An Eastern Cooperative Oncology Group phase II trial of trimetrexate in the treatment of advanced urothelial carcinoma. Cancer 1994;73(3):688–691.

212. Roth BJ, Dreicer R, Einhorn LH, et al: Significant activity of paclitaxel in advanced transitional-cell carcinoma of the urothelium: A phase II trial of the Eastern Cooperative Oncology Group. J Clin Oncol 1994;12(11):2264–2270.

213. Vaughn DJ, Malkowicz SB, Zoltick B, et al: Paclitaxel plus carboplatin in advanced carcinoma of the urothelium: An active and tolerable outpatient regimen. J Clin Oncol 1998;16(1):255–260.

214. Redman BG, Smith DC, Flaherty L, Du W, Hussain M: Phase II trial of paclitaxel and carboplatin in the treatment of advanced urothelial carcinoma. J Clin Oncol 1998;16(5):1844–1848.

215. Small EJ, Lew D, Redman BG, et al: Southwest Oncology Group Study of paclitaxel and carboplatin for advanced transitional-cell

carcinoma: The importance of survival as a clinical trial end point. J Clin Oncol 2000;18(13):2537-2544.

216. Vaughn DJ, Manola J, Dreicer R, See W, Levitt R, Wilding G: Phase II study of paclitaxel plus carboplatin in patients with advanced carcinoma of the urothelium and renal dysfunction (E2896): A trial of the Eastern Cooperative Oncology Group. Cancer 2002;95(5):1022-1027.

217. Pollera CF, Ceribelli A, Crecco M, Calabresi F: Weekly gemcitabine in advanced bladder cancer: A preliminary report from a phase I study. Ann Oncol 1994;5(2):182-184.

218. Stadler WM, Kuzel T, Roth B, Raghavan D, Dorr FA: Phase II study of single-agent gemcitabine in previously untreated patients with metastatic urothelial cancer. J Clin Oncol 1997;15(11):3394-3398.

219. Moore MJ, Tannock IF, Ernst DS, Huan S, Murray N: Gemcitabine: A promising new agent in the treatment of advanced urothelial cancer. J Clin Oncol 1997;15(12):3441-3445.

220. Kaufman D, Raghavan D, Carducci M, et al: Phase II trial of gemcitabine plus cisplatin in patients with metastatic urothelial cancer. J Clin Oncol 2000;18(9):1921-1927.

221. Moore MJ, Winquist EW, Murray N, et al: Gemcitabine plus cisplatin, an active regimen in advanced urothelial cancer: A phase II trial of the National Cancer Institute of Canada Clinical Trials Group. J Clin Oncol 1999;17(9):2876-2881.

222. von der Maase H, Andersen L, Crino L, Weinknecht S, Dogliotti L: Weekly gemcitabine and cisplatin combination therapy in patients with transitional cell carcinoma of the urothelium: A phase II clinical trial. Ann Oncol 1999;10(12):1461-1465.

223. von der Maase H, Hansen SW, Roberts JT, et al: Gemcitabine and cisplatin versus methotrexate, vinblastine, doxorubicin, and cisplatin in advanced or metastatic bladder cancer: Results of a large, randomized, multinational, multicenter, phase III study [comment]. J Clin Oncol 2000;18(17):3068-3077.

224. Jimenez RE, Hussain M, Bianco FJ Jr, et al: Her-2/neu overexpression in muscle-invasive urothelial carcinoma of the bladder: Prognostic significance and comparative analysis in primary and metastatic tumors. Clin Cancer Res 2001;7(8):2440-2447.

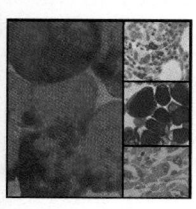

William G. Nelson

H. Ballentine Carter

Theodore L. DeWeese

Gopal Bajaj

Travis L. Thompson

Mario A. Eisenberger

PROSTATE CANCER

SUMMARY OF KEY POINTS

INCIDENCE

- Prostate cancer is the most commonly diagnosed life-threatening cancer in men (220,900 cases and 28,900 deaths in 2003)
- Small prostate cancers are present in 29% of men between ages 30 and 40 years and 64% of men between ages 60 and 70 years
- The lifetime risk of a prostate cancer diagnosis is 1 in 6, and the risk of dying of prostate cancer is 1 in 30
- Age, family history, diet and lifestyle, and ethnicity are risk factors for prostate cancer development

MOLECULAR PATHOGENESIS

- Germline mutations in *RNASEL* and *MSR1*, encoding proteins that function in host responses to infections, appear responsible for some cases of hereditary prostate cancer
- An inflammatory lesion, termed *proliferative inflammatory atrophy* (PIA), may be an early precursor to prostate cancer
- Somatic inactivation of *GSTP1*, encoding a carcinogen-detoxification enzyme, may initiate prostatic carcinogenesis by increasing the vulnerability of prostate cells to damage mediated by oxidant and electrophilic carcinogens
- Defects in the functions of *NKX3.1*, *PTEN*, and *CDKN1B* are common in prostate cancer cells

PREVENTION

- The type 2 5α-reductase inhibitor finasteride reduced the overall number of prostate cancers, but may have increased the number of high-grade prostate cancers, in a large randomized clinical trial (PCPT)
- The antioxidants selenium and vitamin E are under scrutiny in a large randomized clinical trial (SELECT) for prevention of prostate cancer

SCREENING AND DIAGNOSIS

- Prostate cancer screening, by using serum prostate-specific antigen (PSA) and digital rectal examination, detects prostate cancers early, when the disease is clinically localized to the prostate gland
- Transrectal ultrasound (TRUS)-guided core needle biopsies are used to diagnose prostate cancer
- Stage, histologic grade (Gleason score), and serum PSA levels are prognostic factors

TREATMENT OF LOCALIZED DISEASE

- Treatment options include watchful waiting, anatomic radical retropubic prostatectomy, external-beam radiation therapy, and brachytherapy
- Adjuvant androgen suppression can improve survival for some men with prostate cancer treated with external-beam radiation therapy

- A progressive increase in the serum PSA after treatment indicates prostate cancer recurrence
- Depending on the approach used, side effects associated with treatment of localized prostate cancer can include erectile dysfunction, irritative voiding symptoms or difficulties with urinary control, and rectal irritation
- Radiation therapy can be used to treat local prostate cancer recurrences after radical prostatectomy

TREATMENT OF ADVANCED DISEASE

- Androgen suppression, most often accomplished with the use of luteinizing hormone–releasing hormone (LHRH) agonists, with or without antiandrogens, is the most commonly used treatment
- Side effects can include loss of libido, hot flashes, gynecomastia, and loss of lean muscle mass and bone density
- Progressive androgen-independent cancer can be treated with systemic chemotherapy; clinical trials are under way to assess the impact of chemotherapy on prostate cancer survival
- Other agents, including bisphosphonates, signal transduction–modulating agents, immunotherapy, and gene therapies, also are under scrutiny in clinical trials

INTRODUCTION

In 2003, an estimated 220,900 prostate cancer diagnoses will be made in the United States, accompanied by an estimated 28,900 prostate cancer deaths.[1] Beginning around 1994 to 1996, with widespread use of serum prostate-specific antigen (PSA) testing and digital rectal examination for prostate cancer screening, and with increased treatment of clinically localized prostate cancer with surgery or radiation therapy, age-adjusted prostate cancer death rates have decreased steadily.[1] Although this trend might indicate a beneficial impact of prostate cancer screening or early prostate cancer treatment or both on prostate cancer mortality, mass screening of the general population for prostate cancer remains controversial.[2,3] One challenge for prostate cancer screening is the prevalence of the disease in the United States: Autopsy series have revealed small prostate cancers in as many as 29% of men between ages 30 and 40 years and 64% of men between ages 60 and 70 years.[4] Obviously, not all of these men are at risk for symptomatic or life-threatening prostate cancer progression. Many such men, if diagnosed with prostate cancer, may be at greater risk for treatment-associated morbidity. Currently, for U.S. men, the lifetime risk of a diagnosis of prostate cancer is about 1 in 6, whereas the lifetime risk of death of prostate cancer is on the order of 1 in 30.[1] Over the past two decades, treatment approaches for men with prostate cancer have changed dramatically, with improvement in established prostate cancer treatments and the introduction of new prostate cancer treatment approaches. Now men diagnosed with prostate cancer often face a bewildering array of treatment choices. Clearly, the physicians that care for these men must weigh the risks of prostate cancer progression against the potential for side effects from treatment, in the context of other health risks and life choices, to best use the current collection of treatments for the greatest benefit. To aid physicians who care for men with prostate cancer, this chapter provides an overview of prostate cancer etiology, biology, screening, detection, diagnosis, prevention, and treatment.

PROSTATE ANATOMY AND FUNCTION

The prostate is a male sex accessory gland that surrounds the urethra and contributes secretions to the ejaculate (Fig. 87-1). Located in the pelvis, the prostate sits adjacent to the bladder and rectum, is surrounded incompletely by a thin capsule composed of collagen, elastin, and smooth muscle, and at the apex of the gland, forms part of the urethral sphincter apparatus.[5] Nerves to the corpora cavernosa of the penis, needed for penile erection, travel through fascia along the posterolateral surface of the prostate. These nerves can be recognized as a neurovascular bundle by urologists and preserved during radical prostatectomy to minimize postoperative sexual dysfunction.[6,7] The prostate parenchyma has been divided into three zones that can be seen by transrectal ultrasonography (TRUS) and recognized readily by surgical pathologists examining radical prostatectomy specimens: a central zone, surrounding the ejaculatory ducts and accounting for some 25% of the prostate; a transition zone, near the prostatic urethra, with 10% of prostate tissue normally; and a peripheral zone, with the bulk of prostate tissue encompassing posteriolateral region of the prostate (Fig. 87-2).[8,9]

In addition to developing cancer, the prostate also frequently manifests benign enlargement (benign prostatic hyperplasia or BPH) and chronic or recurrent inflammation (prostatitis). Like prostate cancer, each of these conditions can elevate the serum PSA, confounding the use of serum PSA testing for prostate cancer screening.[10] When present, BPH is usually located near the prostatic urethra (in the transition zone), whereas prostate cancer, as well as the prostate cancer precursor lesion, prostatic intraepithelial neoplasia (PIN), usually arises in the periphery (the peripheral zone). Prostatic inflammation, although often prominent in the peripheral zone, can be seen throughout the prostate. Remarkably, although prostate cancer, BPH, and prostatitis all commonly afflict U.S. men and can be simultaneously present in a single prostate gland, mechanistic associations of the

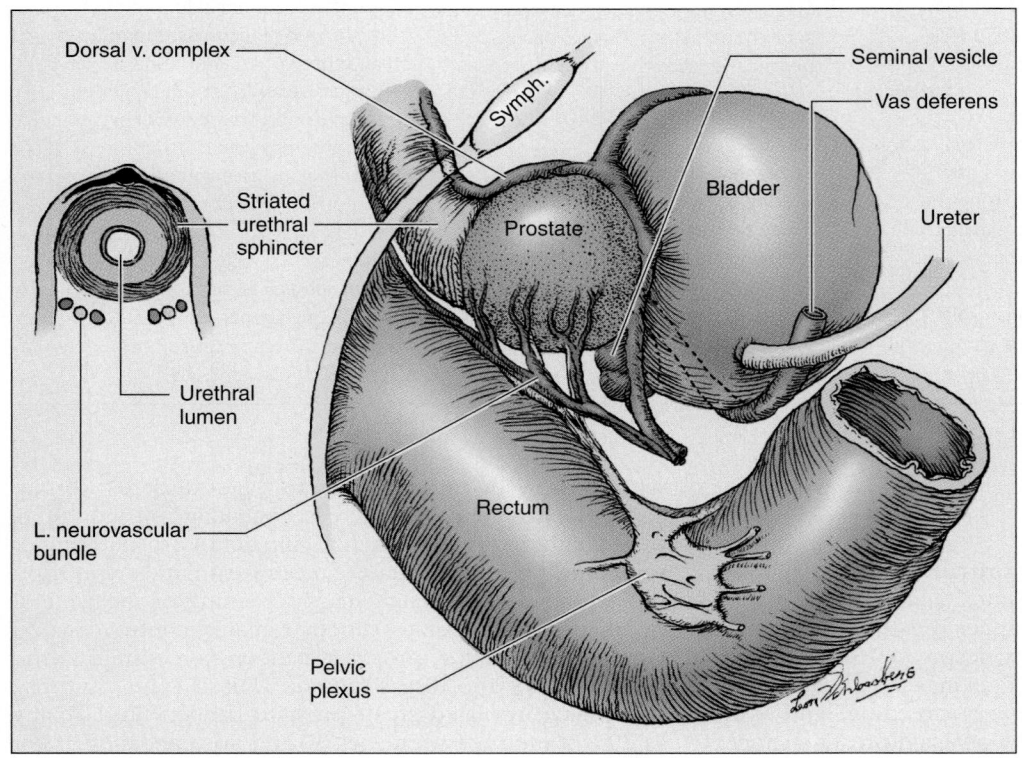

Figure 87-1. The anatomy of the prostate: rectum, bladder, dorsal vein complex, striated urethral sphincter, pelvic plexus, and neurovascular bundle.

Figure 87-2. Zones of the prostate. The peripheral zone, comprising 70% of the prostate gland, is the site of the origin of ≥70% of prostate cancers; the central zone, approximately 25% of the prostate gland, gives rise to only 1% to 5% of prostate cancers; and the transition zone, ~5% to 10% of the prostate gland, gives rise to 20% of prostate cancers and is the site of origin of benign prostatic hyperplasia (BPH). (From Green DR, Shabsign R, Scardino PT: Urological ultrasonography. In Walsh PC, Rettic AB, Stamey CA, Vaughan ED Jr [eds]: Campbells's Textbook of Urology, 6th ed. Philadelphia, WB Saunders, 1992, with permission.)

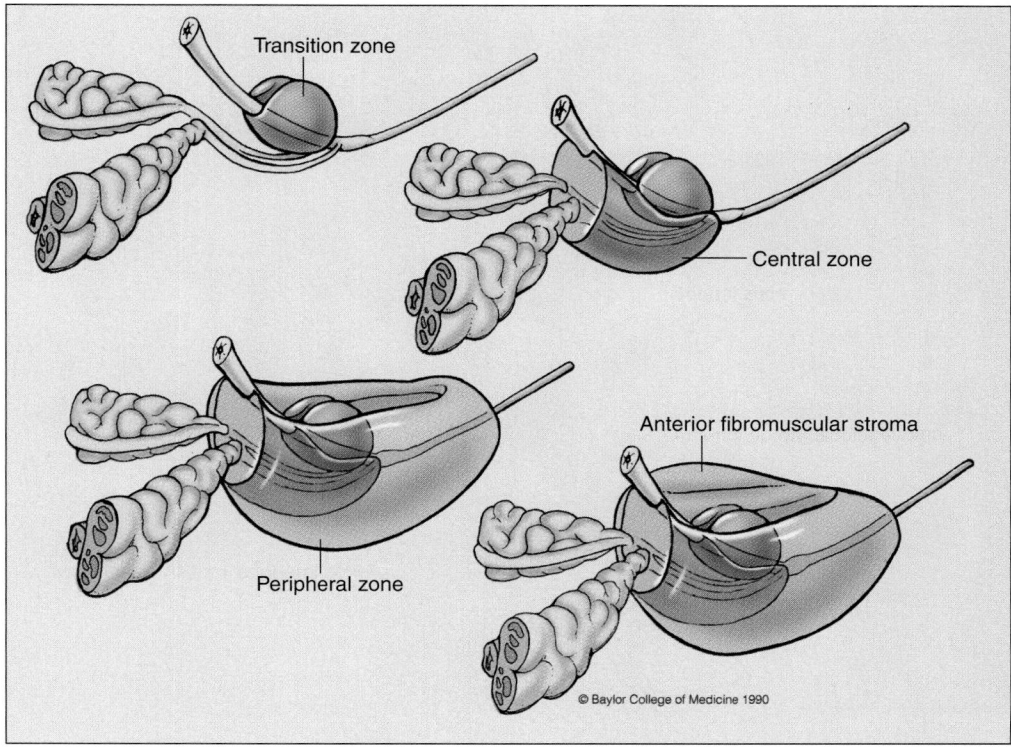

three diseases have been difficult to demonstrate. The prostate requires androgenic hormones and an intact androgen receptor for normal growth and development. In the prostate, the major circulating androgenic hormone, testosterone, produced by Leydig cells in the testes on stimulation by luteinizing hormone (LH), is converted by 5α-reductase (nicotinamide-adenine dinucleotidephosphate[11]–dependent Δ⁴-3-ketosteroid 5α-oxidoreductase) to 5α-dihydrotestosterone (DHT).[12] DHT, a more potent androgen than testosterone, binds to intracellular androgen receptors, alters androgen-receptor conformation to promote dissociation from chaperone proteins, triggers androgen-receptor dimerization and transport into the cell nucleus, and activates the expression of selected target genes.[13,14] Stereotypically, androgen-receptor target genes are characterized by the presence of androgen response element (ARE) DNA sequences within the transcriptional regulatory region, permitting direct binding and transactivation by the androgen receptor.[15] For genes like PSA, which are activated by the androgen receptor selectively in prostate cells, and not in cells of other tissues, the transcriptional regulatory region also contains additional DNA sequences (prostate-specific enhancer or PSE) conferring prostate-specific expression.[16] The normal prostate epithelium is composed of basal epithelial cells, characterized by the expression of cytokeratins K5 and K14, and p63, columnar secretory epithelial cells, which express the androgen receptor, PSA, cytokeratins K8 and K18, prostate-specific membrane antigen (PSMA), and prostate-specific acid phosphatase (PSAP), and rare neuroendocrine cells, which

secrete chromogranin A, neuron-specific enolase, and synaptophysin (Fig. 87-3).[17-19] The basal epithelial cell compartment likely contains pluripotent prostatic stem cells, capable of self-renewal proliferation and of differentiation.[17] In contrast, columnal secretory cells, specialized to produce secretions for the ejaculate, are terminally differentiated, particularly under the influence of androgenic hormones. The prostate epithelium is in turn supported by a stroma containing fibroblasts, smooth muscle cells, nerves, and blood vessels. Stromal cells, which also express the androgen receptor, secrete polypeptide growth factors, such as keratinocyte growth factor (KGF) that contribute to the regulation of epithelial homeostasis via a paracrine signaling mechanism.[20,21] Abnormal stromal/epithelial interactions, with disordered regulation of epithelial cell proliferation and differentiation, may contribute to the pathogenesis of both prostate cancer and BPH.[22]

Prostate cancer cells and PIN cells arise from the prostatic epithelium. Even though transformed, such cells typically retain many of the phenotypic attributes characteristic of differentiated columnar secretory cells, including the expression of androgen receptor, PSA, PSMA, and PSAP. Prostate cancers reminiscent of basal epithelial cells are exceptionally rare; prostate cancers with features of neuroendocrine cells are somewhat more common.[23] However, unlike normal columnar epithelial cells, neoplastic prostate epithelial cells are capable of proliferation. This has led to the concept that the target cell for neoplastic transformation in the prostate may be an "intermediate" cell, in transit from a basal epithelial stem

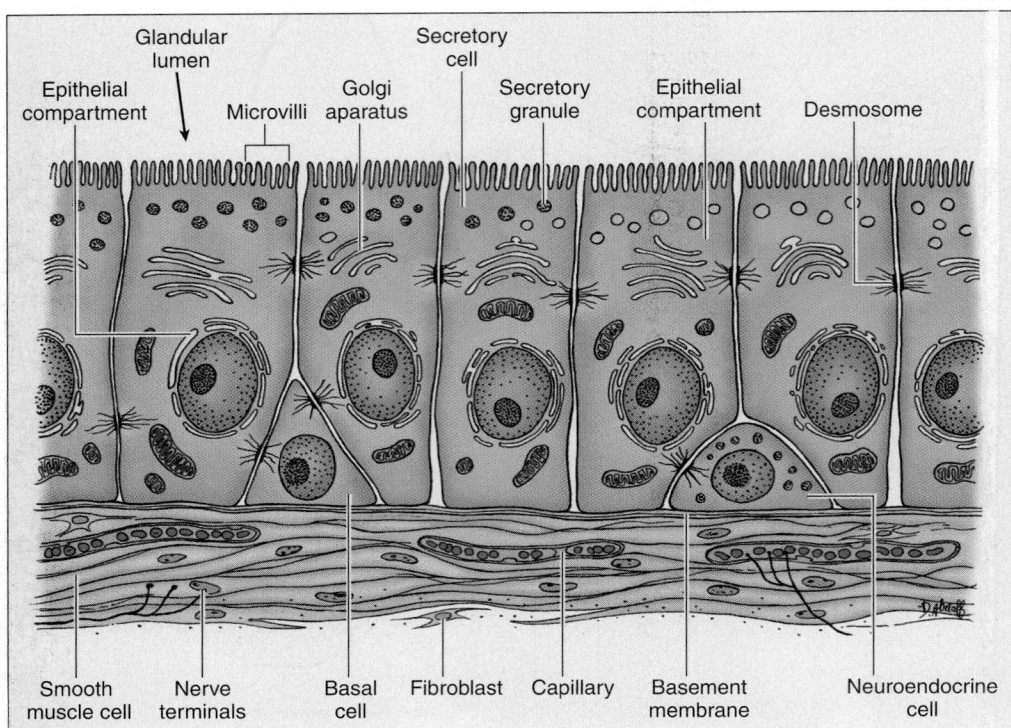

Figure 87-3. The prostate epithelium.

cell to a differentiated columnar secretory epithelial cell, with properties of both stem cells and differentiated cells.[17,19] Another feature of neoplastic prostate epithelial cells, as compared with normal basal or columnar secretory cells, is that the neoplastic cells appear to use androgen-receptor signaling not only for differentiation, but also for proliferation, as most prostate cancer cells tend, at least initially, to display some dependence on androgens for maintenance of growth and survival.[24] Ultimately, in life-threatening prostate cancer, prostate cancer cells escape from the prostate gland, proliferate in lymph nodes, in bones, and in other organs, and become less and less dependent on androgenic hormones.

THE ETIOLOGY OF PROSTATE CANCER

Genetic Predisposition to Prostate Cancer

Familial clusters of prostate cancer have been recognized since at least 1956, when Morganti and colleagues[25] reported that men with prostate cancer were more likely to have relatives with prostate cancer than were men without a prostate cancer diagnosis. In a study conducted more that three decades later, when detailed family histories were collected from men with prostate cancer and their spouses, the men with prostate cancer were more likely to have a brother or father with prostate cancer.[26] Furthermore, the presence of one, two, or three affected family members appeared to increase the risk of prostate cancer to first-degree relatives by 2-, 5-, and 11-fold, respectively, whereas the risk to more distant relatives was only marginally increased.[26] Similar findings

have been reported in a number of additional studies.[27-32] In addition, several twin studies, comparing the tendency for concordant prostate cancer development between monozygotic twins, sharing all of their genes, and dizygotic twins, sharing half of their genes, have hinted at a significant contribution of hereditary to prostate cancer.[33-36] In one study of 44,788 pairs of twins in Sweden, Denmark, and Finland,[33] 42% of the prostate cancer cases (with a 95% confidence interval of 29% to 50%) were attributed to heredity. In principle, familial clustering of prostate cancer cases could be a result of inherited susceptibility genes, shared exposure to carcinogenic stresses, or to some sort of detection or diagnosis bias (e.g., the brother of a man diagnosed with prostate cancer may be more likely to pursue screening for prostate cancer). To discriminate these possibilities, several complex segregation analyses tested the mode of prostate cancer inheritance in familial prostate cancer clusters. In one study, rare autosomal dominant prostate cancer genes were predicted to account for as many as 43% of prostate cancer cases before age 55 years, and some 9% of all prostate cancer cases.[37] In another study, an additional X-linked gene also appeared to be responsible for inherited prostate cancer in certain families.[38] Mendelian inheritance of prostate cancer risk was further supported by the results of a genome-wide screen of polymorphic DNA markers at approximately 10-cM resolution (the human genome encompasses ~3300 cM), featuring 66 families with three or more first-degree relatives diagnosed with prostate cancer, or with two or more brothers with prostate cancer diagnoses made at age 55 years or younger.[39] The analysis identified seven regions of linkage (LOD score, >1), at chromosomal positions 1q24-25,

1q33-42, 4q26-27, 5p12-13, 7p21, and 13q31-33; the chromosomal region 1q24-25, linked to prostate cancer with an LOD score of 2.75, has been designated the locus of the *HPC1* gene.[39] In addition to *HPC1*, the loci attracting the greatest interest thus far have been *PCAP* at 1q42-43,[40] *CaPB* at 1p36,[41] *HPCX* at Xq27-28,[42] *HPC20* at 20q13,[43] *ELAC2/HPC2* at 17p,[44] and *MSR1* at 8p22-23.[45]

Genetic mapping studies have identified *RNASEL* and *MSR1* as potential prostate cancer susceptibility genes.[46,47] *RNASEL*, a candidate *HPC1*, encodes a latent endoribonuclease component of an interferon-inducible 2′,5′-oligoadenylate–dependent RNA decay pathway that functions to degrade viral and cellular RNA on viral infection.[48-52] The evidence that *RNASEL* mutations might predispose to hereditary prostate cancer development included the finding that four brothers with prostate cancer in one prostate cancer family were found to carry *RNASEL* alleles with a base substitution $795^{G \to T}$, predicted to result in the conversion of a glutamic acid codon to a termination codon at amino acid position 265 ($aa256^{glu \to X}$), and that four of six brothers with prostate cancer in another prostate cancer family were found to carry *RNASEL* alleles with a base substitution $3^{G \to A}$, affecting the initiator methionine codon ($aa1^{met \to ile}$).[46] In addition, in a case-control study, a common polymorphic variant *RNASEL* allele with a base substitution $1385^{G \to A}$, encoding a less active enzyme (with an amino acid change $aa462^{arg \to glu}$), was correlated with increased prostate cancer risk ($P = .011$).[53] In this study, the polymorphic *RNASEL* allele accounted for as many as 13% of all prostate cancer cases. *MSR1* encodes subunits of a trimeric class A macrophage scavenger receptor capable of binding bacterial lipopolysaccharide and lipoteichoic acid, and oxidized high- and low-density serum lipoproteins (oxidized HDL and LDL).[54] For *MSR1*, not only have mutations been linked to prostate cancer susceptibility in some prostate cancer families, but one mutant allele, encoding a receptor subunit polypeptide with an $aa293^{arg \to X}$ expected to have "dominant negative" function, also has been detected in ~3% of non-*HPC* prostate cancer cases but only 0.4% of unaffected men ($P < .05$).[47,55] The identification of *RNASEL* and *MSR1* as candidate prostate cancer susceptibility genes has intensified interest in the possibility that infection or inflammation or both might contribute to the pathogenesis of human prostate cancer. In mice, targeted disruption of *RnaseL* leads to increased diminished interferon-α activity and increased susceptibility to viral infection,[56] whereas targeted disruption of *Msr-A* leads to increased vulnerability to infection with *Listeria monocytogenes, Staphylococcus aureus, Escherichia coli*, and herpes simplex virus type 1.[54,57-59]

Androgenic hormones are necessary for prostate growth and development. Thus it is not surprising that polymorphic variants of genes involved in androgen action, like *AR, CYP17*, and *SRD5A2*, may affect prostate cancer risk. Polymorphic polyglutamine (CAG) repeats, varying in length from 11 to 31 amino acids,[60] and polymorphic polyglycine (GGC) repeats, varying in length from 10 to 22 amino acids, have been described for *AR*. For the polyglutamine repeats, androgen receptors with shorter repeats may possess increased transcriptional

trans-activation activity.[61-64] African Americans, who have higher prostate cancer risks than Asians, also have shorter androgen-receptor polyglutamine repeats. Furthermore, genetic epidemiology analyses have correlated high prostate cancer risk with short androgen-receptor polyglutamine repeats.[65-69] Variations in androgen-receptor polyglycine repeats also may affect prostate cancer risk.[65,68-70] *SRD5A2*, encoding the type 2 5α-reductase, the enzyme that generates DHT from testosterone in the prostate, has several polymorphic variants.[71,72] Some variant alleles encoding enzymes with increased activity have been associated with increased prostate cancer risk and with poor prostate cancer prognosis.[71,73] 5α-Reductase variants also may respond differently to inhibition by finasteride, used to treat BPH and under scrutiny as a prostate cancer prevention drug.[11,74] *CYP17*, encoding cytochrome P450c17α, an enzyme that functions to synthesize sex steroids, also has polymorphic variants. One variant allele, with a T→C transition in the transcriptional regulatory region of the gene that creates an Sp1 transcription factor recognition site, has been subjected to both population and genetic linkage analyses for association with prostate cancer, with inconsistent results.[75-81]

Prostate Cancer Epidemiology

Accumulated epidemiologic evidence implicates the environment as the major contributor to the development of most prostate cancers. Prostate cancer incidence and mortality display wide geographic variation, with high rates of prostate cancer incidence and mortality in the United States and Western Europe, and low prostate cancer risks more characteristic of Asia.[82] African Americans in the United States have very high prostate cancer risks.[83] The geographic variation in prostate cancer incidence and mortality can best be explained by lifestyle influences, as Asian immigrants to North America typically adopt higher prostate cancer risks.[84-86] The key aspect of lifestyle in the United States most likely responsible for high prostate cancer incidence and mortality is the diet, generally rich in animal fats and meats and poor in fruits and vegetables. In the Health Professions Follow-up Study, a prospective cohort study involving 51,529 men, total fat intake, animal fat intake, and consumption of red meats were associated with increased risks of prostate cancer development.[87] Red meat consumption was similarly correlated with prostate cancer risks in the Physicians Health Study[88] and in a large cohort study in Hawaii.[89] The cooking of red meats at high temperatures, or on charcoal grills, is known to lead to the formation of both heterocyclic aromatic amine and polycyclic aromatic hydrocarbon carcinogens.[90-93] Ingestion of 2-amino-1-methyl-6-phenylimidazopyridine (PhIP), one of the heterocyclic amine carcinogens that appear in "well-done" red meats, leads to prostate cancer in rats.[94,95] Consumption of dairy products also appears to increase prostate cancer risks, an effect that may be more attributable to calcium intake than to dietary fat or protein.[96]

Consumption of vegetables and antioxidant micronutrients reduces prostate cancer risks. High intake of tomatoes, which contain lycopene, and of cruciferous

Specific Malignancies

III

vegetables, which contain sulforaphane, may protect against prostate cancer development.[97,98] Lycopene likely prevents prostate cancer development by acting as an antioxidant. As part of a recent clinical trial, men were provided tomato sauce–based pasta dishes for 3 weeks before radical prostatectomy for prostate cancer.[99] For these men, tomato consumption was associated with increased lycopene levels in the blood and in the prostate, with decreased oxidative genome damage in leukocytes and in prostate cells, and with a reduction in serum PSA.[99] Sulforaphane, a compound that can prevent cancer in animals by triggering induction of carcinogen-detoxification enzymes, also can act as an antioxidant.[100-103] In addition to lycopene and sulforaphane, other antioxidants, such as the micronutrients vitamin E and selenium, also may reduce prostate cancer risks.[104-106] A clinical trial of supplementation with vitamin E and selenium to prevent prostate cancer (the SELECT Trial), involving a planned 32,400 men, has just been initiated.[107] The consistent finding of a protective effect of various antioxidants against prostate cancer development suggests that oxidative stresses might contribute to prostatic carcinogenesis. Oxidants can be generated by metabolic processes, by a number of different exposures, and by inflammation.[108,109] Androgens, necessary for normal prostate development and function, have been reported to increase oxidant production in prostate cancer cells.[110,111]

Prostate Inflammation, Proliferative Inflammatory Atrophy, and Prostate Cancer

Chronic or recurrent inflammation is known to play a causative role in the development of many human cancers, including cancers of the liver, esophagus, stomach, large intestine, and bladder. Inflammatory changes have been recognized in prostate tissues for many years, leading to speculation that inflammation might contribute in some way to prostate cancer development.[112] However, over the past few years, evidence has accumulated in support of a more critical role for prostatic inflammation in the pathogenesis of prostate cancer. Inflammatory changes are present in almost all radical prostatectomy specimens from men with prostate cancer. Because inflammation in the prostate is not usually associated with symptoms, the prevalence of prostate inflammation is not known, and the association with prostate cancer has been difficult to test.[113,114] A syndrome of irritative voiding symptoms and pelvic pain, perhaps attributable to inflammation near the prostatic urethra, is reported by some 9% or more of men between ages 40 and 79 years, with as many as 50% of such men having more than one episode by age 80 years.[115] Most episodes of symptomatic prostatitis are not clearly attributable to specific infectious agents. Even so, sexually transmitted infections do appear to increase prostate cancer risks.[116,117] Nonetheless, if prostate infection and inflammation lead to prostate cancer, the mechanism does not appear likely to involve direct transformation of prostate epithelial cells by microbial DNA. Instead, the production of microbicidal oxidants by inflammatory cells, such as

superoxide, nitric oxide, and peroxynitrite, may promote prostate cancer development by triggering cell and genome damage.[118,119] Increased production of oxidants by inflammatory cells in the prostate may be why decreased prostate cancer risk has been associated with intake of a variety of antioxidants or of nonsteroidal anti-inflammatory drugs, and why *RNASEL* and *MSR1*, the two prostate cancer susceptibility genes identified thus far, encode proteins that function in host responses to infections.[46,47,54,56,97,104-106,120-122]

Despite these provocative hints, the contribution of prostate inflammation to prostatic carcinogenesis has been difficult to assess. However, in 1999, De Marzo and associates[123] provided the most compelling linkage of prostate inflammation to prostate cancer by proposing that a prostate lesion, termed *proliferative inflammatory atrophy* (PIA), might be a precursor to PIN and to prostate cancer (Fig. 87-4). Areas of the prostate containing epithelial cells that do not fully differentiate into columnar secretory cells have long been recognized as focal atrophy lesions by prostate pathologists.[112,124] The term *PIA* has been used to describe those focal atrophy lesions that contain proliferating epithelial cells, are associated with chronic inflammation, and are often located adjacent to PIN lesions or prostate cancers or both.[123,125-127] The epithelial cells in PIA lesions typically express high levels of stress-response polypeptides such as GSTP1, GSTA1, and cyclo-oxygenase 2 (COX-2).[123,128,129] Loss of GSTP1 expression in rare PIA lesions, attributable to de novo *GSTP1* CpG island hypermethylation, may lead to the development of PIN and prostate cancer.[125,130,131]

The hypothesis that inflammation might promote prostate cancer development offers new challenges to prostate cancer epidemiology, to the search for prostate cancer susceptibility genes, and to the molecular pathogenesis of prostate cancer. Although prostatic inflammation is common in regions of the world with high prostate cancer risks, whether regions of the world with low prostate cancer risks have less prostatic inflammation has

---

PROSTATE INFLAMMATION AND PROSTATE CANCER

Several lines of evidence have stimulated a renewed interest in the notion that prostate infection or inflammation or both may contribute to the development of prostate cancer. First, two of the inherited susceptibility genes so far identified for prostate cancer, *RNASEL* and *MSR1*, encode proteins that function in host responses to infection. Second, a new candidate prostate cancer precursor lesion, proliferative inflammatory atrophy (PIA), appears to arise as a consequence of prostate inflammation. Third, prostate cancer cells typically acquire defects in genes, like *GSTP1*, that encode enzymes that defend against cell and genome damage inflicted by oxidants, such as those elaborated by inflammatory cells. Finally, epidemiologic and early clinical trial data suggest that consumption of a variety of different antioxidants, including selenium, vitamin E, and lycopene, may protect against prostate cancer development.

Figure 87-4. Proliferative inflammatory atrophy (PIA) as a precursor to prostatic intraepithelial neoplasia (PIN) and prostate cancer. (From Nelson WG, DeMarzo AM, Isaacs WB: Prostate cancer. N Engl J Med 2003;349: 366–381, with permission.)

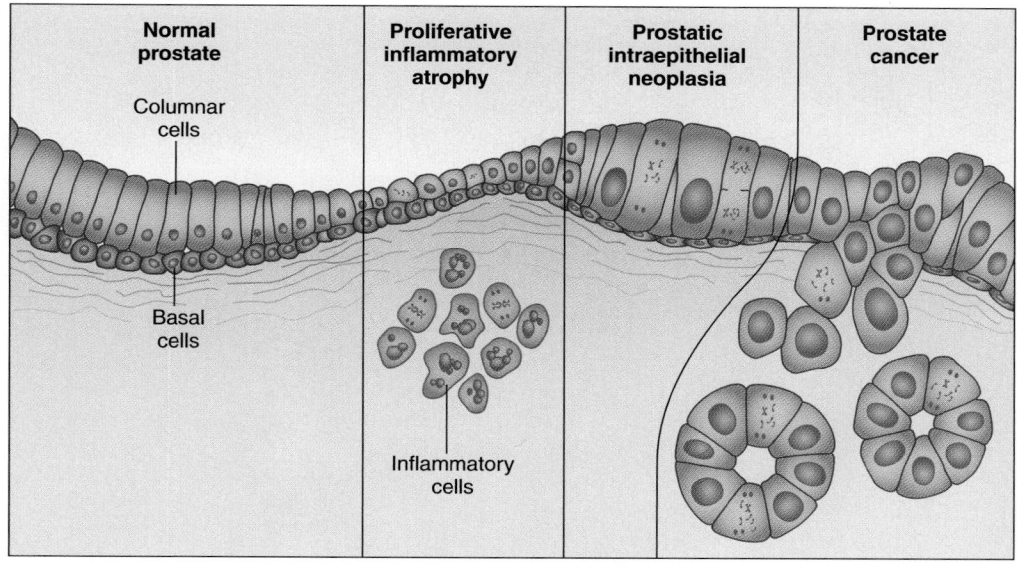

not been determined. New strategies for assessing the presence and extent of PIA and of prostate inflammation may be needed. Perhaps new biomarkers of prostate inflammation, assayable in blood, urine, or prostate fluid, can be developed for use in epidemiology studies. In addition, polymorphic genes encoding regulators of immune responses likely must be systematically evaluated for prostate cancer risk associations. As for prostate cancer pathogenesis, PIA lesions, appearing to arise in response to prostatic inflammation, may be precursors to PIN or prostate cancer or both. However, whether prostatic inflammation is initiated in response to a prostatic infection or to some other provocation has not been ascertained. Finally, whether prostate cancer risks can be reduced by therapeutically attenuating prostate inflammation must tested in clinical trials.

THE MOLECULAR PATHOGENESIS OF PROSTATE CANCER

Somatic Genome Alterations in Prostate Cancer Cells

Prostate cancer cells typically contain a plethora of somatic genome alterations, including gene mutations, gene deletions, gene amplifications, chromosomal rearrangements, and changes in DNA methylation (Fig. 87-5). In the United States, prostate cancer diagnoses are typically made in men between ages 60 and 70 years, whereas small prostate cancers have been detected at autopsy in nearly 30% of men between ages 30 and 40 years.[4] Thus the somatic genome changes present in prostate cancers have often accumulated over many decades. The acquisition of somatic genome changes in the prostate may be influenced by lifestyle as well: Although small prostate cancers have been detected at autopsy in men from geographic regions with low prostate cancer mortality,

these small prostate cancers are usually present in only much older men.[132-134] In the United States, prostates removed at radical prostatectomy for prostate cancer usually contain more than one prostate cancer lesion (Fig. 87-6). Several techniques, including karyotyping, fluorescence in situ hybridization (FISH), comparative genome hybridization, and loss-of-heterozygosity analyses, have been used to catalog somatic genome changes in prostate cancers. Often these analyses reveal different chromosomal abnormalities in different cancer cases, in different cancer lesions in the same cancer case, and in different areas within the same cancer lesion. The most commonly reported chromosomal abnormalities are gains at 7p, 7q, 8q, and Xq, and losses at 8p, 10q, 13q, and 16q.[135] Gains of 8q and losses of 7q, 8p, 13q, and 16q have been reported in association with recurrent, progressive prostate cancer.[136-140] The propensity to develop such a heterogeneous collection of somatic genome lesions over so many years, and in a manner so sensitive to environment and lifestyle, suggests strongly that prostate cancers likely arise as a consequence of either prolonged or recurrent exposure to genome-damaging stresses, defective protection against genome damage, or some combination of both processes. The resultant genomic instability may be the reason some prostate cancers progress to threaten life. Although most prostate cancers initially respond well to therapeutic reductions in circulating androgens, the cancers ultimately become androgen independent, a process likely resulting from selection of preexisting variant androgen-independent cancer cell clones, spontaneously generated through the acquisition of critical somatic genome changes.[141-143]

Hypermethylation of CpG island sequences encompassing the regulatory region of *GSTP1*, encoding the π-class glutathione *S*-transferase (GST) is the most common somatic genome change yet reported for prostate cancer.[130,144-146] GSTs catalyze the detoxification of carcinogens, and of other reactive chemical species,

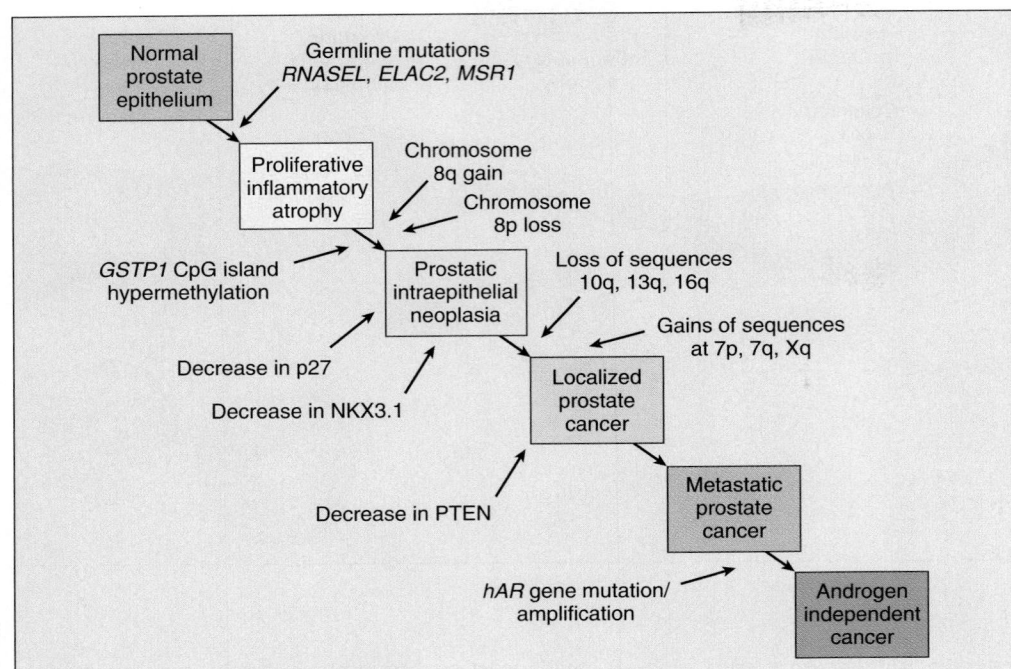

Figure 87-5. The molecular pathogenesis of prostate cancer.

through conjugation with the intracellular scavenger glutathione. In mice, targeted disruption of π-class GST genes leads to increased skin tumors after treatment with the carcinogen dimethylbenzanthracene (DMBA).[147,148] Similarly, human prostate cancer cells devoid of *GSTP1* appear especially vulnerable to genome damage mediated by exposure to *N*-OH-PhIP, the charred-meat carcinogen that causes prostate cancer when fed to rats, and by exposure to oxidant stresses.[94,95,149] In the normal prostate epithelium, *GSTP1* is present in basal cells, but not in columnar secretory cells, although the enzyme can be induced in columnar epithelial cells subjected to genome-damaging stresses. In contrast, the enzyme is almost never present in prostate cancer cells. For more than 90% of prostate cancer cases, this absence of *GSTP1* expression in prostate cancer cells can be attributed to hypermethylation of *GSTP1* CpG island sequences, a somatic genome change that prevents *GSTP1* transcription.[130] Absence of *GSTP1* expression and *GSTP1* CpG island hypermethylation also may be characteristic of cells composing PIN lesions, thought to be precursors to prostate cancer.[131] The mechanism by which hypermethylated *GSTP1* CpG island alleles arise during prostatic carcinogenesis remains to be elucidated. Nonetheless, prostate cells carrying inactivated *GSTP1* genes appear to enjoy some sort of selective growth advantage early during the development of prostate cancer. *NKX3.1* encodes a prostate-specific homeobox gene essential for normal prostate development that may be a target for somatic loss on chromosome 8p21.[150,151] *NKX3.1* has been shown to bind DNA and to repress *PSA* expression through interactions with a prostate-derived Ets transcriptional trans-activator.[152,153] Mice carrying one or two disrupted *Nkx3.1* alleles manifest prostatic epithelial hyperplasia and dysplasia.[154,155] In men, loss of

8p21 DNA sequences occurs early during prostatic carcinogenesis, with 63% of PIN lesions, and more than 90% of prostate cancers, showing loss of heterozygosity at polymorphic 8p21 marker sequences in one report.[156] However, although mapping studies have indicated that *NKX3.1* lies within a common region of deletion, encompassing 2 megabases at 8p21, for prostate cancer, molecular pathology analyses have not yet established *NKX3.1* as a somatic target for inactivation during prostatic carcinogenesis, principally because no somatic *NKX3.1* mutations, accompanying allelic losses, have been identified.[157-159] Nonetheless, loss of *NKX3.1* expression does appear to accompany prostate cancer progression. In one study, absence of *NKX3.1* was reported for 20% of PIN lesions, 6% of low-stage prostate cancers, 22% of high-stage prostate cancers, 34% of androgen-independent prostate cancers, and 78% of prostate cancer metastases.[160]

PTEN, a tumor-suppressor gene encoding a phosphatase active against both proteins and lipid substrates, appears to be a common target for somatic alteration during prostate cancer progression.[161-169] *PTEN* is an inhibitor of the phosphatidylinositol 3′-kinase/protein kinase B (PI3K/Akt) signaling pathway needed for cell cycle progression and cell survival.[170-173] Although *PTEN* is expressed by normal prostate epithelial cells and by cells present in PIN lesions, the expression of *PTEN* is often diminished in prostate cancers, with many prostate cancers containing collections of neoplastic cells with no *PTEN*.[174] *PTEN* defects have been found in a wide variety of cancers and cancer cell lines.[164] For prostate cancer, a number of somatic *PTEN* alterations have been reported, including homozygous deletions, loss of heterozygosity, mutations, and probable CpG island hypermethylation.[168,169,175-177] However, despite common losses of 10q

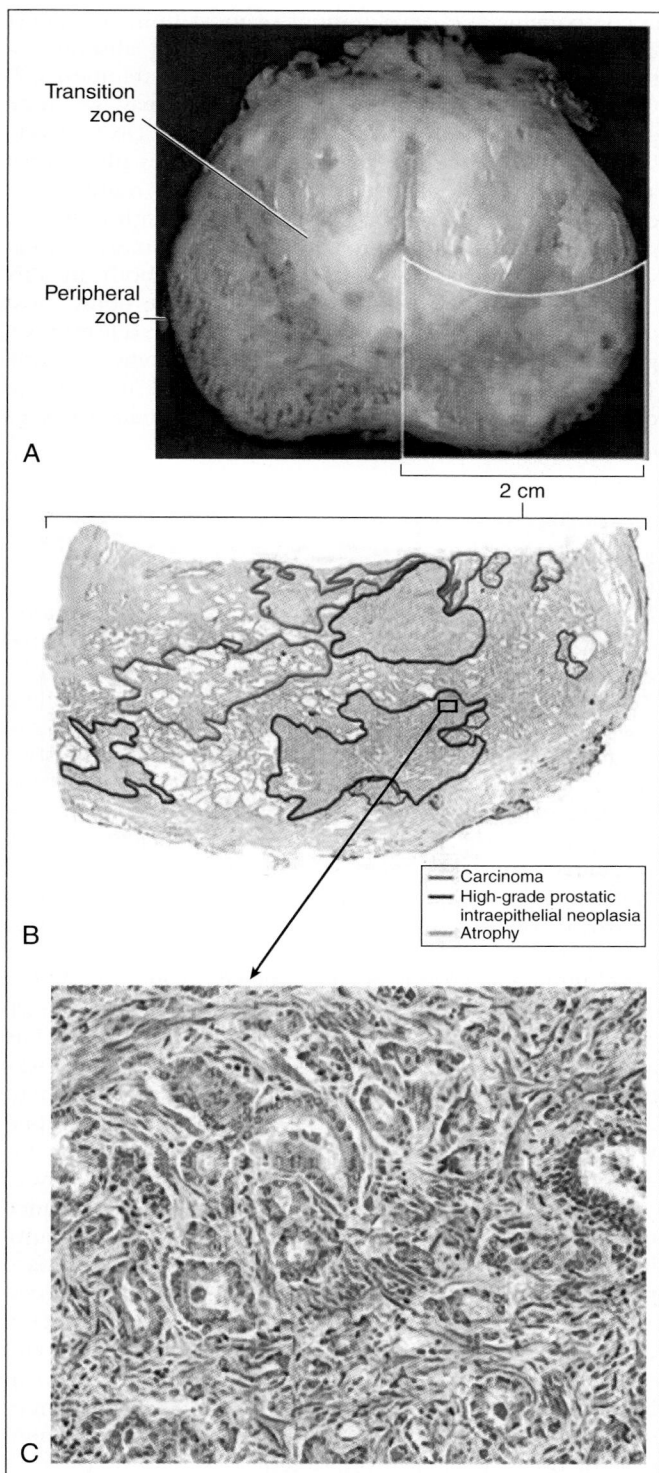

Transition zone

Peripheral zone

A

2 cm

B

Carcinoma
High-grade prostatic intraepithelial neoplasia
Atrophy

C

Figure 87-6. Multiple foci of prostate cancer, and the prostate cancer precursor lesions, in the peripheral zone of the prostate. (From Nelson WG, DeMarzo AM, Isaacs WB, et al: Prostate cancer. N Engl J Med 2003;349:366–381, with permission.)

sequences near *PTEN* in prostate cancers, somatic mutations at the remaining *PTEN* alleles are not as frequent. In a study of prostate cancer metastases recovered at autopsy, somatic *PTEN* alterations were even more common than in primary prostate cancers, and a significant heterogeneity in *PTEN* defects in different metastatic deposits from the same patient also was evident.[169] Haploinsufficiency for *PTEN* may contribute to the phenotype of transformed cells in the prostate. *Pten*[+/-] mice display prostatic hyperplasia and dysplasia, and crosses of *Pten*[+/-] mice with *Nkx3.1*[+/-] mice have revealed that *Pten*[+/-]*Nkx3.1*[+/-] mice and *Pten*[+/-]*Nkx3.1*[-/-] mice develop lesions reminiscent of human PIN.[178-180] *Pten* also appears to influence prostate cancer progression in mice. When *TRAMP* mice, which carry SV40 T-antigen under the control of a prostate-specific promoter and develop prostate cancer, were crossed with *Pten*[+/-] mice, *Pten*[+/-] *TRAMP* progeny had a poorer survival from prostate cancer than did *Pten*[+/+]*TRAMP* littermates.[181]

Defective regulation of p27, a cyclin-dependent kinase inhibitor encoded by *CDKN1B*, also may accompany prostatic carcinogenesis.[182-187] In PIN cells and prostate cancer cells, p27 levels are almost always diminished, although the mechanism(s) for the reduction in p27 levels appear complex: Somatic loss of DNA *CDKN1B* sequences at 12p12-13 have been reported for only 23% of localized prostate cancers, 30% of prostate cancer lymph node metastases, and 47% of distant prostate cancer metastases.[188] In place of *CDKN1B* gene alterations, p27 polypeptide levels may be lowered indirectly by inadequate *PTEN* repression of the PI3K/Akt signaling pathway.[171,173,189-191] In this way, low p27 levels may be as much a result of loss of *PTEN* function as of *CDKN1B* alterations. The critical contribution of *PTEN* to epithelial growth regulation in the prostate is evident in mice, where disruption of *Cdkn1b* alleles leads to prostatic hyperplasia, and *Pten*[+/-]*Cdkn1b*[-/-] mice develop prostate cancer by age 3 months.[185,192]

Metastatic prostate cancer is almost always treated with androgen deprivation, antiandrogens, or a combination of androgen deprivation and antiandrogens.[193-195] However, despite such treatment, androgen-independent prostate cancer cells eventually emerge and progress to threaten life. Curiously, in these cells, androgen-receptor expression and androgen-receptor signaling remain intact despite the absence of androgens.[24,196-198] Somatic alterations of *AR* have been reported for many prostate cancers, especially for androgen-independent prostate cancers.[24,199-212] *AR* amplification, accompanied by high-level expression of androgen receptors, may promote the growth of androgen-independent prostate cancer cells by increasing the sensitivity of the cells to low androgen levels.[200] *AR* mutations, encoding androgen receptors with altered ligand specificity, also have been detected; for some of the mutant androgen receptors, even antiandrogens can act as agonist ligands.[213-215] When 44 mutant androgen receptors from prostate cancers were evaluated for transcriptional regulatory capabilities, 16% of the receptors had lost transcriptional activation activity, 45% of the receptors had gained some transcriptional regulatory ability, 32% of the receptors maintained some partial

Specific Malignancies

III

transcriptional modulatory activity, and the remaining 7% behaved like wild-type receptors.[216] In addition to somatic *AR* gene changes, androgen-independent prostate cancer cells with wild-type androgen receptors may activate androgen-receptor signaling even in the absence of androgens, through post-translational modifications of the androgen receptor or androgen-receptor coactivators or both in response to other growth factor–signaling pathways.[24,217-220]

Changes in Gene Expression in Prostate Cancers

Alterations in gene expression in prostate cancers have been cataloged by using complementary DNA (cDNA) microarray technologies.[221-232] Among the many genes exhibiting over- or underexpression in prostate cancers, the products of at least two genes appear consistently increased, and the product of a third gene appears to become elevated during androgen-independent progression. *Hepsin*, located at 19q11-13.2, encodes a transmembrane serine protease, expressed at high levels in many normal tissues.[233] The contribution of *Hepsin* to the prostate cancer phenotype has not been discerned. Antisense oligonucleotides targeting *Hepsin* messenger RNA (mRNA) have been reported to retard the growth of hepatoma cells, but *Hepsin*[-/-] mice develop normally, exhibit normal liver regeneration, and have no striking phenotype.[234-236] α-Methylacyl-coenzyme A (CoA) racemase (AMACR), a mitochondrial and peroxisomal enzyme that acts on pristanoyl-CoA and C27-bile acyl-CoA substrates to catalyze the conversion of *R*- to *S*-stereoisomers to permit metabolism by β-oxidation, has been reported to be overexpressed in almost all prostate cancers.[237,238] Germline *AMACR* mutations have been reported to lead to adult-onset neuropathy.[239] Immunohistochemistry studies, which have revealed that AMACR is occasionally present in normal prostate cells, increased in PIN cells, and further elevated in prostate cancer cells, have prompted the use of antibodies against AMACR as tools for prostate cancer diagnosis by surgical pathologists.[238,240,241] The polycomb protein enhancer of zeste homolog 2 (EZH2), a transcriptional regulatory protein, is elevated in metastatic androgen-independent prostate cancer.[242] The mechanism by which EZH2 contributes to prostate cancer progression has not been established. However, elevated EZH2 expression in primary prostate cancers portends a poor prognosis.[242]

Telomere Shortening During Prostatic Carcinogenesis

Telomeres, containing repeat DNA sequences at the termini of chromosomes, protect against loss of chromosome sequences during genome replication.[243,244] DNA ends tend to shorten each generation as a consequence of bidirectional DNA synthesis (the "end-replication" problem); the telomere repeat sequences serve as templates for the enzyme telomerase, which can extend the chromosome termini and maintain chromosome integrity through cell division.[243,245] Growth dysregulation

accompanying the development of most human cancers tends to lead to cell proliferation in the absence of telomerase and to shortened chromosome telomeres.[244] Critically shortened telomere sequences may promote genome instability by increasing illegitimate DNA recombination.[246,247] Mice carrying disrupted genes needed for a functioning telomerase show increased numbers of cancers, especially when crossed to mice with defective p53 genes.[248] In the prostate, short telomere repeat sequences appear characteristic of cells both in PIN lesions and in prostate cancer.[249-251] At some point, most cancer cells activate the expression of telomerase, providing some maintenance of chromosome termini. Telomerase expression has been detected in prostate cancers, but not at high levels in normal prostate tissues or in BPH.[249]

THE PREVENTION OF PROSTATE CANCER

The high lifetime risks of prostate cancer development, the morbidities associated with treatment of established prostate cancer, and the inability to eradicate life-threatening metastatic prostate cancer offer compelling reasons for prostate cancer prevention. In addition, epidemiology data, indicating a dominant role for lifestyle factors in prostate cancer development, suggest that prostate cancer risk modification may be feasible, if only through lifestyle modification. Also, because prostatic carcinogenesis takes many decades, a broad window of opportunity may exist to change lifestyle in an effort to retard prostate cancer development. Clearly, although the specific lifestyle factors fostering prostate cancer development have not been conclusively identified, it is likely that consumption of a diet rich in fruits, vegetables, and antioxidant micronutrients, and poor in saturated fats and "well-done" red meats, may significantly reduce risks of prostate cancer development, and of the development of other diseases characteristic of life in the developed world. Nonetheless, as the etiology of prostate cancer is better understood, new opportunities for prostate cancer prevention will arise. For example, if prostate inflammation contributes to prostate cancer development, anti-inflammatory drugs might be considered candidate prostate cancer prevention drugs. For drugs to be developed and tested for prostate cancer prevention, randomized clinical trials, capable of assessing both drug safety and drug efficacy, will be required.[252] Ideally, such trials can be targeted at men with a high risk for prostate cancer development, analogous to women thought to be at high risk for breast cancer development identified by the Gail model.[253] Thus far, two classes of agents, 5α-reductase inhibitors and antioxidant micronutrients, have been subjected to large randomized clinical trials.

The Prostate Cancer Prevention Trial

In the Prostate Cancer Prevention Trial (PCPT), the propensity for the type 2 5α-reductase inhibitor finasteride to reduce the prevalence of prostate cancer in healthy men age 55 years and older when given for 7 years was tested.[74] Finasteride, which has been marketed both for BPH and for alopecia, was known to have few worrisome side effects and to lower the serum PSA in some men with prostate cancer.[254,255] 5α-Reductase inhibitors had shown promising activity in preventing prostate cancer development or prostate cancer progression or both in animal models.[256-258] However, the effects of finasteride on prostate cancer development in various clinical trials have not been as encouraging. In one randomized placebo-controlled trial, in which finasteride was used to treat BPH (N = 3040), 4.7% of men treated with finasteride and 5.1% of men treated with placebo were ultimately diagnosed with prostate cancer (P = .7).[259] In another randomized trial (N = 52), 30% of men with an elevated serum PSA but no cancer on an initial prostate biopsy that were given finasteride for 12 months had cancer on a subsequent prostate biopsy versus 4% of men who did not receive finasteride.[260] In this small trial, finasteride also had little beneficial activity in men with PIN.[260] For PCPT, 18,882 men with a PSA of 3.0 ng/mL or less and a normal digital rectal examination were randomized to treatment with finasteride (5 mg/day) or to placebo.[74] While on study, men with a PSA elevation or an abnormal rectal examination were subjected to prostate biopsy; in addition, at the end of the treatment period, a prostate biopsy was planned for all of the men in the trial. The Data and Safety Monitoring Committee for PCPT closed the study 15 months before the anticipated completion, with some 9060 men evaluable for the presence of prostate cancer.[74] Prostate cancer was detected in 18.4% of the men treated with finasteride versus 24.4% of men receiving placebo (P < .001).[74] Of concern, however, high-grade prostate cancers appeared more commonly associated with finasteride treatment than with placebo (6.4% vs. 5.1%).[74] This may mean that finasteride prevents or treats low-grade cancers better than high-grade cancers. Some 37% of men treated with finasteride, versus 29% of men receiving placebo (P < .001), discontinued treatment, usually citing side effects of reduced ejaculate volume, erectile dysfunction, loss of libido, and gynecomastia.[74] These mixed results, a reduction in overall prostate cancer prevalence, but an increase in high-grade prostate cancers, associated with finasteride treatment, make recommendations for healthy men who want to reduce their prostate cancer risks very difficult. A large clinical trial testing the effects of dutasteride, an inhibitor of both type 1 and type 2 5α-reductases used to treat BPH, on prostate cancer development has just been initiated.[261]

The Selenium and Vitamin E Cancer Prevention Trial

Epidemiologic studies have provided compelling evidence that intake of selenium and of vitamin E might diminish prostate cancer risks.[262-268] In addition, two clinical trials have provided further evidence for protection against prostate cancer by consumption of these antioxidant micronutrients.[104-106,147,269] In one of the studies, men and women (N = 1312) with a history of non-melanoma skin cancer were treated with 200 μg selenized

brewer's yeast, or a placebo, daily to ascertain whether selenium consumption might decrease the risk of a second skin cancer.[105] Although selenium supplementation failed to prevent new skin cancers, a reduced risk of prostate cancer was evident for men receiving selenium supplements, particularly men with low-baseline selenium levels.[104,105,269] In the other study, α-tocopherol, β-carotene, the combination of α-tocopherol and β-carotene, or placebo were administered to male smokers (N = 29,133) in Finland for lung cancer prevention.[147] Again, although neither of the supplements appeared to prevent lung cancer, a reduced risk of prostate cancer was evident for men receiving α-tocopherol.[106,147] A prospective, randomized, placebo-controlled clinical trial of selenium and vitamin E (SELECT; N > 32,400) was initiated in 2001 to test the ability of the antioxidant micronutrients to prevent prostate cancer.[270] Selenium (200 μg selenomethionine), α-tocopherol (400 mg), the combination of selenium and α-tocopherol, or neither, will be given to men randomized to four different treatment groups by using a 2 × 2 factorial design, for 7 to 12 years.[270] The trial subjects will be men, age 55 years or older (50 years or older for African Americans), with an unremarkable digital rectal examination and a serum PSA of 4 ng/mL or less.[270] Until the SELECT results are available, it will be difficult to make definitive recommendations about micronutrient supplementation to prevent prostate cancer. Nonetheless, the limited data available from epidemiology studies and early clinical trials suggest that men with low blood levels of the micronutrients tend to be at the highest risk for prostate cancer development, and that micronutrient supplementation might be most effective at preventing prostate cancer if given to such men.[263,264,268,269] For this reason, perhaps a supplementation strategy designed to correct antioxidant micronutrient deficiencies might ultimately prove generally safe and effective. The risks and benefits of high doses of antioxidant micronutrients, or other supplements, are not known.

PROSTATE CANCER SCREENING, DIAGNOSIS, AND STAGING

Clinical Evaluation

The staging system for prostate cancer includes the results of imaging studies of the prostate [transrectal ultrasound or magnetic resonance imaging (MRI)] in the stage assignment (Table 87-1).

Prostate cancer rarely causes symptoms early in the course of the disease because the majority of adenocarcinomas arise in the periphery of the gland (the peripheral zone) distant from the urethra. The presence of symptoms attributable to prostate cancer suggests locally advanced or metastatic disease. With progressive growth of prostate cancer into the urethra, or into the bladder neck, lower urinary symptoms of obstruction (e.g., urinary hesitancy, decreased force of urine stream, intermittency) and irritation (e.g., urinary frequency, nocturia, urgency, urge incontinence) can occur. Local progression of prostate

TABLE 87-1

TNM and AUA Staging Systems

TNM Staging System

Primary Tumor (T)
- TX   Primary tumor cannot be assessed
- T0   No evidence of primary tumor
- T1   Clinically inapparent tumor neither palpable nor visible by imaging
  - T1a   Tumor incidental histologic finding in ≤5% of tissue resected
  - T1b   Tumor incidental histologic finding in >5% of tissue resected
  - T1c   Tumor identified by needle biopsy (e.g., because of elevated PSA)
- T2   Tumor confined within prostate*
  - T2a   Tumor involves one half of a lobe or less
  - T2b   Tumor involves more than one half of lobe, but not both lobes
  - T2c   Tumor involves both lobes†
- T3   Tumor extends through the prostate capsule
  - T3a   Unilateral extracapsular extension
  - T3b   Bilateral extracapsular extension
  - T3c   Tumor invades seminal vesicle(s)
- T4   Tumor is fixed or invades adjacent structures other than seminal vesicles
  - T4a   Tumor invades bladder neck, external sphincter, or rectum
  - T4b   Tumor invades levator muscles or is fixed to pelvic wall, or both

Node (N)
- NX   Regional lymph nodes cannot be assessed
- N0   No regional node metastasis
- N1   Metastasis in single lymph node, ≤2 cm
- N2   Metastasis in a single node, >2 cm but ≤5 cm
- N3   Metastasis in a node >5 cm

Metastasis (M)
- MX   Presence of metastasis cannot be assessed
- M0   No distant metastasis
- M1   Distant metastasis
  - M1a   Nonregional lymph node(s)
  - M1b   Metastasis in bone(s)
  - M1c   Metastasis in other site(s)

AUA Staging System

- Stage A   Clinically unsuspected disease
  - A1   Focal carcinoma, well differentiated
  - A2   Diffuse carcinoma, usually poorly differentiated
- Stage B   Tumor confined to prostate gland
  - B1   Small, discrete nodule of one lobe of gland
  - B2   Large or multiple nodules or areas of involvement
- Stage C   Tumor localized to periprostatic area
  - C1   Tumor outside prostate capsule, estimated weight ≤70 g, seminal vesicles uninvolved
  - C2   Tumor outside prostate capsule, estimated weight >70 g, seminal vesicles involved
- Stage D   Metastatic Prostate cancer
  - D1   Pelvic lymph node metastases or ureteral obstruction causing hydronephrosis, or both
  - D2   Bone, soft tissue, organ, or distant lymph node metastases

AUA, American Urological Association; PSA, prostate-specific antigen; TNM, tumor-node-metastasis.
*Invasion into the prostatic apex or into (but not beyond) the prostatic capsule is not classified as T3, but as T2.
†Tumor found in one or both lobes by needle biopsy but not palpable or visible by imaging is classified T1c.

cancer and obstruction of the ejaculatory ducts can result in hematospermia and a decrease in the ejaculate volume. Extension of prostate cancer outside the prostate capsule can damage the branches of the pelvic plexus (neurovascular bundle) responsible for innervation of the corpora cavernosa and cause erectile dysfunction. Metastatic cancer involving the axial or appendicular skeleton can lead to bone pain, or through replacement of the bone marrow, can cause pancytopenia. Lower-extremity edema can result from cancerous involvement of the pelvic lymph nodes and compression of the iliac veins. Less common consequences of metastatic disease include malignant retroperitoneal fibrosis from dissemination of cancer cells along the periureteral lymphatics, paraneoplastic syndromes from ectopic hormone production by small cell variants of adenocarcinoma, and disseminated intravascular coagulation (DIC).

Although men with prostate cancer can have voiding symptoms suggesting locally advanced cancer, or signs and symptoms suggesting metastatic cancer, currently more than 90% of men diagnosed with prostate cancer are initially detected as a result of digital rectal examination (DRE) abnormalities or of serum PSA elevations.[271]

Digital Rectal Examination

In men with early-stage prostate cancers, physical findings, if present, are usually limited to an abnormal DRE, used for both diagnosis and staging. Palpable areas of induration or asymmetric firmness of the gland suggests the presence of prostate cancer, but these findings also can be caused by prostate inflammation (especially granulomatous prostatitis), by BPH, and by prostatic stones. DRE has only fair reproducibility in the hands of experienced examiners.[272] When used alone for detection of prostate cancer, DRE misses from 23% to 45% of the cancers that are subsequently detected by prostate biopsies done for serum PSA elevations or for TRUS abnormalities.[273-275] In addition, prostate cancers detected by DRE are at an advanced pathologic stage in more than 50% of men.[276,277]

The positive predictive value of DRE (the fraction of men who have prostate cancer if the DRE is abnormal) is dependent on age, race, and PSA level (Table 87-2).[278,279] African American race, older age, and higher PSA levels are associated with a higher positive predictive value for DRE.[279] The positive predictive value of a suggestive DRE was 5%, 14%, and 29% in white men, and 8%, 37%, and 50% in black men, with PSA levels of 0 to 1.0, 1.1 to 2.5, and 2.6 to 4.0 ng/mL, respectively. The positive predictive value of a suggestive DRE ranged from 33% to 83% in men with PSA levels of 3.0 to 9.9 ng/mL or more.[273-275,280-284] A prostate biopsy is generally recommended for men with an abnormality on DRE that is suggestive of prostate cancer regardless of the PSA level.

Serum Prostate-Specific Antigen

PSA is a member of the human kallikrein gene family of serine proteases encoded by genes located on chromosome 19.[285,286] A component of the ejaculate, PSA

TABLE 87-2

Positive Predictive Value of DRE and PSA in a Multicenter Screening Trial

DRE	PSA	PPV (%)
Abnormal	Any	21.4
Any	PSA >4	31.5
	4–10	26.1
	>10	52.9
Normal	PSA >4	24.4
Abnormal	PSA <4	10.0
	4–10	40.8
	>10	69.1

DRE, digital rectal examination; PPV, positive predictive value; PSA, prostate-specific antigen.
Modified from Catalona WJ, Richie JP, Ahmann FR, et al: Comparison of digital rectal examination and serum prostate specific antigen in the early detection of prostate cancer: Results of a multicenter clinical trial of 6,630 men. J Urol 1994; 151:1283, with permission.

is produced by columnar secretory cells in the prostate. PSA expression is regulated by androgens, becoming detectable in serum at puberty, accompanying increases in luteinizing hormone and testosterone.[287–289] In the absence of prostate cancer, serum PSA levels increase with age and prostate volume and are generally higher in African Americans (Fig. 87-7). Cross-sectional population data suggest that the serum PSA increases 4% per milliliter of prostate volume, and that 30% and 5% of the variance in PSA can be accounted for by prostate volume and age, respectively.[290] African Americans without prostate cancer have higher serum PSA values than do whites.[291,292]

Serum PSA elevations likely occur as a result of disruption of the normal prostate architecture, permitting PSA to diffuse into the prostate parenchyma and gain access to the circulation. This can occur in the setting of both benign and malignant prostate diseases (prostatitis, BPH, and prostate cancer) and as a result of prostate manipulation (prostate massage and prostate biopsy).[293] Whereas the presence of some type of prostate disease is the most important determinant driving elevation of the serum PSA, an increased serum PSA is not specific for prostate cancer.[294,295] Furthermore, not all men with prostate disease have elevated serum PSA levels. Treatments targeting the prostate gland (for BPH or for prostate cancer) can reduce serum PSA by decreasing the number of prostatic epithelial cells capable of producing PSA and by decreasing the amount of PSA produced by each cell. Modulation of sex steroid hormone levels for treatment of BPH or prostate cancer, radiation therapy for prostate cancer, and surgical ablation of prostate tissue for BPH or prostate cancer can all lead to decreases in serum PSA. 5α-Reductase inhibitors, like finasteride (Proscar; Merck and Company), reduce PSA levels by 50% after 12 months of treatment.[296] Thus for men treated with finasteride for 12 months or more, the serum PSA level is one half of a "true" PSA value. Interpretation of serum PSA values should always take into account the presence of prostate disease, previous diagnostic procedures, and prostate-targeted treatments.

Numerous studies have documented the validity of serum PSA testing as a strategy for assessing the risk that prostate cancer is present.[274] Routine use of serum PSA testing increases the detection of prostate cancer over that with DRE, improves the predictive value of the DRE for cancer, and tends to detect prostate cancers at an early stage. Evaluation of prostate cancer detection methods in both screened and nonscreened populations of men has shown that the serum PSA value is the test with the highest positive predictive value for prostate cancer. If the serum PSA is elevated, a greater proportion of men will be found to have cancer at biopsy as compared with an abnormality detected by DRE or TRUS.[273,275] The serum PSA value is directly correlated with prostate cancer risk.[274] In addition, the use of serum PSA determinations augments the predictive value of DRE for prostate cancer.[273–275,278,297]

Serum PSA testing increases the lead time for prostate cancer diagnosis. For this reason, the use of serum PSA testing for prostate cancer screening results in the detection of prostate cancers that are more often confined to the prostate, as compared with cancers discovered by DRE alone. Data from longitudinal population studies using frozen serum samples suggest a lead time of around 5 years with PSA testing using a 4.0-ng/mL cutoff.[298,299] A simulation model based on the results of a screening trial has estimated a lead time of more than a decade.[300] The most effective method for early detection of prostate cancer is the combined use of DRE and serum PSA testing. When DRE and the serum PSA are used as screening tests for prostate cancer, detection rates are higher with serum PSA determinations than with DRE alone, and highest with a combination of both tests.[275,278,283] Because DRE and serum PSA determinations are not always simultaneously abnormal in the presence of prostate cancer, the tests are complementary when used for prostate cancer detection. Experts disagree on the use of DRE for screening when PSA levels are very low, because in that setting, the DRE has a relatively poor positive predictive value.

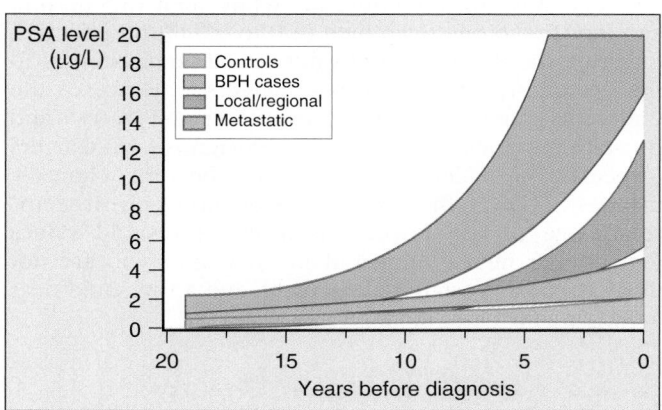

Figure 87-7. Longitudinal increases in serum prostate-specific antigen levels in men with and without prostate cancer. (From Fromter HB, Pearson JD, Metter EJ, et al: Longitudinal evaluation of prostate-specific antigen levels in men with and without prostate disease. JAMA 1992;267:2215, with permission.)

The widespread use of PSA for early detection of prostate cancer has stimulated efforts to improve the sensitivity (correct identification of men with prostate cancer in a population of men with the disease) and specificity (correct identification of men without prostate cancer in a population of men without the disease) of the test. Altering the serum PSA threshold value used to trigger prostate biopsy, adjusting the PSA level for the prostate volume (the PSA "density"[301-308]), monitoring the rate of change in serum PSA values over time (the PSA "velocity"[309-311]), and the selective assay of various molecular forms of PSA in the serum[10,312] have all been evaluated as methods of distinguishing prostate cancer from BPH and other prostate diseases.

Prostate-Specific Antigen Threshold for Prostate Biopsy

The choice of a serum PSA threshold value or "cut point," above which further evaluation to rule out prostate cancer (by prostate biopsy) should be recommended, is controversial.[313,314] A PSA serum threshold of 4.0 ng/mL has been most commonly used; however, some experts have recommended the use of lower threshold values to avoid missing important prostate cancers and to increase the likelihood that prostate cancers are detected at a curable stage.[315,316] The 95th percentile of serum PSA values among "healthy" populations of men, carefully screened to exclude prostate cancer, has been used to establish age- and race-specific serum PSA ranges.[290,292] Because serum PSA values tend to increase with age and because older men are more likely to have prostate enlargement that leads to serum PSA elevations, lower PSA thresholds for younger men and higher PSA thresholds for older men have been suggested to improve the sensitivity of PSA testing for younger men and the specificity of PSA testing for older men. The identified serum PSA threshold values for detecting 95% of prostate cancers among men age 40 to 50 years are lower than 4.0 ng/mL, but for men age 50 to 69 years (the primary target group for most early prostate cancer detection at present), the threshold values are very close to 4.0 ng/mL for white men (3.5 ng/mL) and for African American men (4.0 to 4.5 ng/mL). Clearly, lowering the PSA threshold value for all men will lead to the detection of more prostate cancers.[315] However, the tradeoff is an increase in unnecessary serum PSA tests and prostate biopsies[278,317,318] and overdiagnosis of cancers (especially in older men) that may become clinically manifest.[300] Given the current state of knowledge, it seems reasonable to use lower serum PSA threshold values for younger men (younger than 50 years) who are not likely to have prostate enlargement, and a threshold near 4.0 ng/mL for older men.

Prostate-specific Antigen "Density"

Benson and coworkers[303,304] suggested that adjusting serum PSA values for prostate size, by calculating the PSA "density," the quotient of the serum PSA (in ng/mL) and the prostate volume (in mL as estimated by TRUS), might help distinguish between men with serum PSA

TABLE 87-3

Age-specific Reference Ranges for Serum PSA and PSA Density

AGE RANGE (YR)	SERUM PSA (ng/mL)	PSA DENSITY (ng/mL)
40–49	0.0–2.5	0.0–0.10
50–59	0.0–3.5	0.0–0.12
60–69	0.0–4.5	0.0–0.14
70–79	0.0–6.5	0.0–0.16

PSA, prostate-specific antigen.
From Osterling J, Jacobsen S, Klee G, et al: Free, complexed, and total serum prostate specific antigen: The establishment of appropriate reference ranges for their concentrations and ratios using newly developed immunofluorometric assays (IFMA). J Urol 1995;154:1090 with permission.

elevations due to BPH versus those caused by prostate cancer (Table 87-3). A correlation between PSA "density," and the presence of prostate cancer has been documented: A PSA "density" of 0.15 or greater has been proposed as a trigger for recommending prostate biopsy in men with serum PSA levels between 4 and 10 ng/mL and no suspicion of prostate cancer on DRE or TRUS.[305,306,319] The utility of PSA "density" determinations for prostate cancer detection has not been confirmed in all studies.[320,321] Although PSA "density" may be an imperfect predictor of prostate cancer, it does appear to provide an additional tool for prostate cancer risk assessment when elevated serum PSA levels are in the intermediate range (4 to 10 ng/mL), aiding in the identification of which men may need prostate biopsy, and helping to ascertain which men with a persistently elevated serum PSA may need repeated prostate biopsies.[322]

The major source of serum PSA in men without prostate cancer is the transition zone epithelium, not the epithelium of the peripheral zone.[323] Because BPH represents an enlargement of the transition zone, and because serum PSA levels are largely a reflection of transition zone volume in men with BPH, adjusting the serum PSA for transition zone volume has been proposed to help in distinguishing BPH from prostate cancer.[324]

Prostate-specific Antigen "Velocity"

Substantial variability in PSA levels is found for individual men subjected to repeated serum PSA determinations.[309,311,325,326] Changes in serum PSA levels can be adjusted (corrected) for the elapsed time between the measurements, a concept known as PSA "velocity" or the rate of change in serum PSA.[309] Men with prostate cancer manifest a higher rate of increase in serum PSA than do men without prostate cancer (see Fig. 87-7).[309] Rate of increase in serum PSA was found to be a specific marker for the presence of prostate cancer in a study using stored blood samples in which 72% of men with prostate cancer, but only 5% of men without prostate cancer, had a PSA "velocity" of more than 0.75 ng/mL per year when the PSA was between 4 and 10 ng/mL.[309] In a prospective screening study, the prostate cancer detection rate was 47% among men with a PSA "velocity" greater than 0.75 ng/mL per year versus 11% among men with a PSA velocity less than 0.75 ng/mL per year.[310] In addition, several studies have found that fewer than 5% of men without prostate cancer have a PSA velocity more than 0.75 ng/mL per year (the 95th percentile for PSA "velocity"), supporting the concept that rate of increase in PSA may be a specific marker for the presence of prostate cancer.[311,327,328] The minimal duration of follow-up over which changes in serum PSA should be monitored to best use PSA "velocity" for prostate cancer detection has been calculated to be 18 months.[310,311,327] Furthermore, the use of at least three serum PSA determinations to determine the average rate of change in serum PSA appears to optimize the accuracy of PSA "velocity" for cancer detection.[309,311] PSA "velocity" threshold values have not been determined for men with serum PSA levels less than 4.0 ng/mL.

Molecular Forms of Prostate-specific Antigen

PSA in the bloodstream circulates in both bound and unbound forms. Most of the detectable PSA in the serum (65% to 90%) is bound to α_1-antichymotrypsin, whereas the rest (10% to 35%) remains unbound or "free."[329,330] The assays used primarily for prostate cancer detection and monitoring detect both "free" and "complexed" PSA, providing a determination of the "total" serum PSA. Newer assays that can distinguish free and complexed serum PSA have been more recently developed and approved by the U.S. Food and Drug Administration (FDA) for use in the early detection of prostate cancer.

In general, men with prostate cancer have a greater fraction of serum "total" PSA that is bound to α_1-antichymotrypsin, and a commensurately lower fraction of "total" PSA that is free, than do men without prostate cancer.[331-334] This difference is thought to be due to the differential expression of PSA isoforms by cells in the transition zone (the zone of origin for BPH) tissue as compared with the peripheral zone (the zone where most prostate cancers arise) tissue.[335-338] The percentage of free serum PSA appears most useful in distinguishing men with and without prostate cancer in the setting of "total" serum PSA levels between 4 and 10 ng/mL (Table 87-4). In a prospective multi-institutional study of men aged 50 to 75 years with serum PSA levels of 4 to 10 ng/mL and a nonsuggestive DRE, a free serum PSA less than 25% detected 95% of prostate cancers while avoiding 20% of unnecessary biopsies.[339] In this study, the risk of prostate cancer varied markedly for different percentages of free serum PSA values, ranging from 8% when the free PSA was more than 25% to 56% when the free PSA was less than 10%. It has been suggested that use of free serum PSA determinations can reduce unnecessary biopsies, while maintaining the sensitivity for prostate cancer detection, even when "total" serum PSA is in the range of 2.6 to 4.0 ng/mL.[340] Most urologists use free serum PSA determinations to help make decisions about the need for a repeated biopsy in a man with a persistently elevated serum PSA and previous negative prostate biopsies, where the possibility of a missed prostate cancer may be a concern. Of interest, like the percentage of free serum PSA, measurement of "complexed" serum PSA, by using a

TABLE 87-4

Probability of Cancer Based on PSA and Percent of FPSA Results

PSA	PROBABILITY OF CANCER (%)	FPSA (%)	PROBABILITY OF CANCER (%)
0–2 ng/mL	1	0–10	56
2–4 ng/mL	15	10–15	28
4–10 ng/mL	25	15–20	20
>10 ng/mL	>50	20–25	16
		>25	8

DRE, digital recta examination; FPSA, free prostate-specific antigen; PSA, prostate-specific antigen.
Men with nonsuspicious DRE results, any age: % FPSA can stratify risk for men with PSA between 4 and 10 ng/mL.
Modified from Catalona WJ, Partin AW, Slawin KM, et al: Use of the percentage of free prostate-specific antigen to enhance differentiation of prostate cancer from benign prostatic disease: A prospective multicenter clinical trial. JAMA 1998; 279:1542, with permission.

single assay, has been shown to have higher specificity for the detection of prostate cancer than the use of serum "total" PSA alone at a fixed sensitivity.[341,342] Therefore it may be possible to use a single assay that detects "complexed" serum PSA, rather than two assays ("total" serum PSA and free serum PSA), needed for determination of percentage of free serum PSA.

Transrectal Ultrasound–Guided Prostate Biopsy

TRUS is not an accurate method for localizing early prostate cancer and is not recommended for use in prostate cancer screening.[273,343] The primary role of TRUS in prostate cancer detection and diagnosis is to ensure accurate sampling of prostate tissue by prostate biopsies in men suspected of harboring cancer based on serum PSA levels and DRE.[274] This is best accomplished by targeting peripheral zone lesions that appear hypoechoic by TRUS for biopsy, along with performing systematic sampling biopsies of areas without hypoechoic lesions in the prostate periphery.[344] Biopsies of the transition zone are recommended for men undergoing repeated prostate biopsies for persistently elevated serum PSA levels when a missed cancer is suspected.[345] The optimal biopsy technique, including the number and placement of biopsies for tissue procurement that will minimize the chance of missing a relevant cancer, remains controversial.[346,347] Nonetheless, the best evidence available suggests that biopsies placed more laterally within the peripheral zone of the prostate may be important to exclude prostate cancer in men with elevated serum PSA values and a nonsuggestive DRE. TRUS-guided prostate biopsies are performed routinely with an 18-gauge needle fired from a spring-loaded gun through a port mounted on the ultrasound probe. It is common practice to administer a fluoroquinolone antibiotic, and for patients to give themselves a cleansing enema, before the biopsy procedure. In a randomized, placebo-controlled trial, injection of a local anesthetic around the periphery of the prostate was shown to reduce the discomfort associated with prostate biopsy.[348] Major complications from TRUS-guided prostate biopsies are rare: In a series of 5802 prostate biopsies, although hematuria and hematospermia were present after 22.6% and 50.4% of the procedures, respectively, only 3.5% of men had fever, 0.4% of men had urinary retention, and 0.5% of men required hospitalization, mostly for treatment of postbiopsy infections.[349]

Screening for Prostate Cancer

Prostate cancer screening as a means of reducing prostate cancer mortality by earlier detection and treatment remains controversial.[350] The PLCO (Prostate, Lung, Colon, Ovary) Trial of the National Cancer Institute and the ERSPC (European Randomized Study of Screening for Prostate Cancer) are ongoing randomized trials designed to address this controversy.[351] No organization endorses universal or mass screening for prostate cancer. The U.S. Preventive Services Task Force (USPSTF) has recently concluded that the evidence is insufficient to recommend for or against routine screening for prostate cancer by using serum PSA determinations or DRE antigen (see U.S. Preventive Services Task Force. Screening for Prostate Cancer: Recommendations and Rationale. December 2002. Agency for Healthcare Research and Quality, Rockville, MD. http://www.ahrq.gov/clinic/3rduspstf/prostatescr/prostaterr.htm[352]). The American Academy of Family Physicians, American Cancer Society, American College of Physicians–American Society of Internal Medicine, American Medical Association, and American Urologic Association recommend that physicians discuss with patients the potential benefits and possible harms of PSA screening, consider patient preferences, and individualize the decision to screen for prostate cancer (see the American Cancer Society guidelines for the early detection of cancer: update of early detection guidelines for prostate, colorectal, and endometrial cancers; see also: Update 2001—testing for early lung cancer detection, CA Cancer J Clin 2001 Jan–Feb;51(1):38–75, accessed at http://www.cancer.org on 25 October 2002; Clinical guideline part III: screening for prostate cancer, American

College of Physicians, Ann Intern Med 1997;126:480–484, Report 9 of the Council on Scientific Affairs (A-00), American Medical Association, Screening and Early Detection of Prostate Cancer, June 2001, available at http://www.ama-assn.org/ama/pub/article/2036-2928.html, accessed March 1, 2001; and Prostate-specific antigen (PSA) best practice policy, American Urological Association (AUA), Oncology (Huntingt) 2000;14(2):267–272, accessed at http://www.auanet.org on October 25, 2002).

In the absence of randomized trials, some researchers have used computer simulations that model the natural history of prostate cancer to consider the potential benefits of prostate cancer screening,[353,354] to estimate lead times and rates of overdiagnosis (the detection of clinically insignificant cancers) attributable to attempts at prostate cancer screening,[300,355] and to propose optimal prostate screening strategies.[318,356] Results from some of these model studies have suggested only a minimal benefit of prostate cancer screening in terms of lives saved, especially after adjusting for quality of life. This conclusion has been questioned, with concerns that (1) the prostate cancer progression rates used to model the natural history of the prostate cancer were unrealistically low, leading to an underestimate of a prostate cancer screening benefit; (2) the models focused on only a single screening event, rather than on repeated screening, to ascertain effects on prostate cancer mortality; and (3) the utility weights (used to calculate "quality-adjusted life years" saved by screening) assigned to the development of progressive metastatic prostate cancer, for which no treatment exists, and treatment-associated side effects, such as incontinence after radical prostatectomy, for which effective treatment is available, were inappropriate. Nonetheless, the computer simulations of prostate cancer screening estimate lead times for prostate cancer diagnosis of 6 to 12 years and overdiagnosis rates of 30% to 50%, increasing with subject age at the time of screening. When different screening strategies have been compared by using computer simulations, with the assumption that prostate cancer screening provides some sort of benefit, annual screening does not appear to be necessary. Furthermore, screening of relatively young men, who may derive a greater benefit from effective prostate cancer treatment, may be more cost effective. Longitudinal data from a cohort study of aging and from prostate cancer screening trials also support the notion that screening can be conducted less often than once a year, preserving the ability to detect curable prostate cancer while reducing unnecessary testing.[357,358] If screening is ultimately determined to be an effective strategy for reducing prostate cancer deaths, the frequency of screening should be determined by the baseline serum PSA level, a strong predictor of prostate cancer risk.[298,357,358]

Histopathology of Prostate Cancer

Microscopic analysis of prostate tissue by a surgical pathologist is needed for the diagnosis of prostate cancer, for determining prostate cancer stage after prostatectomy, and for histologic grading, by the assignment of a Gleason score, to predict the behavior of prostate cancer. The

---

POPULATION SCREENING FOR PROSTATE CANCER

No data definitively demonstrate whether prostate cancer screening saves lives. Nonetheless, the use of serum prostate-specific antigen (PSA) testing, along with digital rectal examination (DRE), to screen men for prostate cancer, detects prostate cancers at very early stages of progression. As a result, prostate cancers discovered by screening are more likely to be treated with curative intent through surgery or radiation therapy. The major concern about prostate cancer screening is the potential for overdiagnosis of prostate cancers that would be unlikely to pose a threat for morbidity or mortality. For these reasons, screening approaches for prostate cancer remain in evolution, with the optimal screening test (serum PSA vs. other molecular forms of PSA), the optimal screening population (younger vs. older men), and the optimal screening interval yet to be determined.

majority of prostate cancers are adenocarcinomas, although other types of cancers can appear. Most often, prostate cancer diagnoses are made using by core-needle biopsy specimens, which sample small amounts of prostate tissue. For many prostate cancer cases, needle biopsies contain only small numbers of prostate cancer cells among more plentiful noncancerous glands. Several prostate conditions, including acute, chronic, or granulomatous prostate inflammation, epithelial atrophy, and PIN, exhibit histologic features that mimic some of those present in prostate cancers.[359] Thus prostate cancers can be difficult to recognize in needle biopsy specimens and difficult to distinguish from other prostate abnormalities. Most experienced prostate pathologists use a combination of architectural, cytologic, and ancillary findings to make a diagnosis of prostate cancer on needle biopsy.[359-361] In addition, because normal prostate glands, but not glands present in prostate cancers, contain basal epithelial cells, immunohistochemical staining for basal epithelial cell markers, such as cytokeratins K5 and K14, can be used to help distinguish benign from malignant glands in prostate tissue samples.[362,363] Immunohistochemical staining for AMACR, a prostate cancer biomarker discovered through cDNA microarray transcriptome profiling, can aid in prostate cancer diagnosis.[238,240,241] Neither of these immunohistochemistry reagents perfectly distinguishes prostate cancer: the absence of basal epithelial cell markers is not always diagnostic of prostate cancer, and AMACR expression is absent in some prostate cancers and present in PIN.[359] For all of these reasons, second-opinion interpretations of prostate biopsy findings, especially when foci of atypical glands suggestive of cancer are identified, are often helpful.

High-grade PIN, a lesion characterized by the proliferation of malignant-appearing prostate epithelial cells within the confines of otherwise normal glandular structures, is identified in about 5% of men subjected to prostate biopsies.[364,365] The evidence that high-grade PIN is a likely precursor to prostate cancer includes the findings that (1) high-grade PIN is more commonly present in prostates that also contain prostate cancer, (2) that high-grade PIN and prostate cancer both tend to arise in the peripheral zone of the prostate and are often directly contiguous, and (3) that high-grade PIN and prostate cancer express similar biomarkers and share many somatic genome abnormalities.[366,367] The notion that high-grade PIN lesions might be prostate cancer precursors has stimulated interest in possibly treating men with high-grade PIN to prevent prostate cancer.[367] Unfortunately, the natural history of individual high-grade PIN lesions is not known. Furthermore, high-grade PIN lesions, which can be recognized only by sampling prostate biopsies, are not easily monitored. These limitations have hindered the use of high-grade PIN as a response surrogate for cancer-prevention drug development. Because high-grade PIN is not currently treated, the major significance of the finding of high-grade PIN, in the apparent absence of prostate cancer, by prostate biopsy is that prostate cancer may have been missed by the prostate-sampling strategy used for the biopsy procedure. As serum PSA screening was first introduced, men with an elevated serum PSA and high-grade PIN by prostate biopsy seemed to have as high as a 50% chance of having prostate cancer when subjected to repeated prostate biopsies.[365] With more widespread adoption of serum PSA screening strategies for men with an elevated serum PSA, the chance that a second set of prostate biopsies will detect prostate cancer after an initial diagnosis of high-grade PIN on a first set of prostate biopsies has decreased to 23% to 35%, only slightly greater than the 20% chance that repeated prostate biopsies will detect prostate cancer even in the absence of an initial diagnosis of high-grade PIN.[368-370] Of interest, unlike prostate cancer, prostate inflammation, or BPH, PIN lesions are not thought to perturb prostate architecture enough to elevate the serum PSA.[371,372] Recently, increasing attention has been afforded the notion that PIA lesions might be precursors to PIN or prostate cancer or both. Like PIN, PIA lesions tend to arise in the peripheral zone of the prostate, where prostate cancers arise, and some PIA cells acquire somatic genome alterations reminiscent of prostate cancer cells.[123,126] At present, men with PIA lesions are not subjected to any kind of treatment, and presence of PIA on an initial prostate biopsy is not thought to predict the detection of prostate cancer on repeated biopsy. The major significance of PIA to the diagnosis of prostate cancer by prostate biopsy may be a propensity for such lesions occasionally to exhibit features that mimic prostate cancer.[359]

The most frequently used approach to histologic grading of prostate cancer is the application of Gleason scoring.[373] The Gleason grade refers to architectural prostate cancer patterns, numbered 1 (well differentiated) to 5 (poorly differentiated). Because prostate cancers are often heterogeneous, Gleason scoring (sometimes referred to as the "combined" Gleason grade) is accomplished by adding the Gleason grade of the most abundant pattern to the Gleason grade of the second most abundant pattern (e.g., a Gleason score of 4 + 3 = 7). The Gleason score, when applied by an expert pathologist, is one of the best tools available for predicting the outcomes of men treated with radical prostatectomy or with radiation therapy; prostate cancers with Gleason scores of 8 to 10 are much more likely to recur after primary treatment than are prostate cancers with Gleason scores of 2 to 6.[374,375] Furthermore, for prostate cancers with a Gleason score of 7, Gleason 4 + 3 = 7 appears more correlated with prostate cancer recurrence than does Gleason 3 + 4 = 7. One challenge presented by Gleason grading is the variability in Gleason scores assigned the same prostate cancers by different pathologists.[376,377] To address this challenge, Internet educational tools have been developed by expert pathologists to improve the fidelity of Gleason scoring by community pathologists.[378] Because Gleason scoring applies pattern grades to the architecture of cancer within the prostate, metastatic prostate cancers detected by biopsies of metastatic deposits are not assigned a Gleason score.

Evaluation of the Extent of Prostate Cancer

The extent of prostate cancer is correlated with tumor stage, Gleason score (the sum of two Gleason grades), and

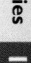

Specific Malignancies

III

serum PSA level.[379] Nomograms, incorporating clinical stage, estimated by using DRE findings, the serum PSA level, and the Gleason score, have been shown to be capable of predicting both prostate cancer extent (when compared with the pathologic stage evident at the time of prostate surgery) and the long-term outcome after primary tumor treatment.[380-382] D'Amico and colleagues[382] suggested that men with prostate cancer can be stratified into low risk (stages T1c to 2a, serum PSA <10 ng/mL, and Gleason score of ≤6); intermediate risk (stage T2b, or serum PSA between 10 and 20 ng/mL, or Gleason score of 7); and high risk (stage T2c, or serum PSA >20 ng/mL, or Gleason score of ≥8) groups, reporting that the fraction of men free of prostate cancer 10 years after radical prostatectomy is significantly different for the risk categories: 83% of men with low-risk prostate cancer, 46% of men with intermediate-risk prostate cancer, and 29% of men with high-risk prostate cancer.[382] When undertaken before initiating prostate cancer treatment, risk stratification of men with prostate cancer aids in counseling such men about the expected outcome of aggressive local prostate cancer treatment, providing estimates of the chance that local treatments might be curative.

Radiographic Imaging

Although computed tomography (CT) scanning is used routinely by radiation oncologists for prostate cancer treatment planning, no imaging technique available today has been proven to add additional useful information when used to evaluate the extent of prostate cancer in men with low- and intermediate-risk disease.[383] TRUS and MRI give the most accurate definition of prostatic architecture and anatomy, but current imaging technologies do not provide very precise assessments of cancer extent within the prostate or the presence of microscopic foci of prostate cancer that have escaped the confines of the prostate gland. Radionuclide bone scans detect metastatic prostate cancer in fewer than 1% of men with a serum PSA value of 20 ng/mL or less and are not recommended for the initial evaluation of men with low- or intermediate-risk prostate cancer.[384] Positron emission tomography (PET) has not yet been found to be useful in the evaluation of men with prostate cancer and has no place in the prostate cancer staging.[385] New imaging technologies, including three-dimensional color Doppler, contrast-enhanced color Doppler, magnetic resonance spectroscopy, and high-resolution MRI with magnetic nanoparticles have great potential for improving the assessment of local and distant prostate cancer extent.[383,386] Cross-sectional imaging of the pelvis, by CT scan or MRI, for the purpose of detecting lymph node metastases, and radionuclide bone scans for the detection of bony metastases, should be reserved for men with high-risk prostate cancer.

[111In]capromab penditide, a radioimmunoconjugate featuring a monoclonal antibody to an intracellular domain of prostate-specific membrane antigen (PSMA; ProstaScint, Cytogen Corporation) has been approved by the U.S. FDA for use in the evaluation of men for treatment of clinically localized prostate cancer. Some evidence indicates that when [111In]capromab pendetide immunoscintigraphy is used in combination with other pretreatment prostate cancer staging tools, the predictive value for presence of lymph node metastases increases.[387] However, this scan is not being used routinely today for assessment of prostate cancer extent, in large part because of frequent difficulties in scan interpretation and because of the lack of scan sensitivity, even among men with fairly high-risk prostate cancer.[388,389]

Serum Biomarker Assays and "Molecular" Staging

Increases in serum PSA and in serum prostatic acid phosphatase (PSAP)[390] correlate directly with the extent (stage) of prostate cancer disease. As described earlier, the serum PSA is a useful tool for the preoperative assessment of prostate cancer extent, especially when considered along with other pretreatment parameters. Radioimmunoassays for PSAP appear more sensitive, but less specific, than enzymatic assays, when used to detect serum PSAP as a marker of advanced prostate cancer. Several studies have documented a correlation between the presence of advanced prostate cancer and elevations of serum PSAP.[391-393] Elevated serum PSAP values and serum PSAP levels in the upper half of the normal range portend a high likelihood (>80%) of extraprostatic cancer.[392,393] However, normal serum PSAP levels are not very predictive of the absence of extraprostatic disease. For men thought to have clinically localized prostate cancer based on the results of serum PSA, DRE, and Gleason score, serum PSAP testing rarely adds additional information.[394] In the PSA era, the use serum PSAP testing for prostate cancer staging has declined substantially, giving way to the use of serum PSA testing.[293] "Molecular" staging for prostate cancer refers to the detection of circulating prostate cancer cells, either directly, with centrifugation/immunostaining methods,[395] or indirectly, by identifying mRNA species, like those encoding PSA or PSMA, characteristically expressed by epithelial cells from the prostate.[396] To detect mRNAs, reverse transcriptase–polymerase chain reaction (RT-PCR) methods, capable of astonishing sensitivity, are typically used. Of course, a "positive" RT-PCR test for *PSA* mRNA in a peripheral blood specimen might indicate the presence of circulating prostate epithelial cells that may be either normal or neoplastic; the hope is that, in the right clinical context, the detection of prostate cells in the bloodstream may provide some prognostic information. RT-PCR for *PSA* mRNA in the blood has been reported to be more predictive of pathologic prostate cancer stage when compared with other pretreatment predictors such as serum PSA and Gleason score,[397] and to be an independent predictor of disease-free survival after treatment.[398] However, as many as one in four men with localized prostate cancer who underwent radical prostatectomy for cancer confined to the prostate had "positive" RT-PCR assays for *PSA* mRNA in blood specimens in one study.[397] These men would be denied aggressive treatment if the presence of circulating prostate cells indicated the presence of distant blood-borne prostate cancer metastases. In another study, 7% of men without prostate cancer exhibited "positive" RT-PCR assays for *PSA* mRNA in blood.[399] The relation between circulating prostate cancer cells, regardless of how they are detected, and the development of metastatic prostate cancer is not well understood, but it is likely that the formation of metastatic prostate cancer deposits in bone and at other sites may be a relatively inefficient process, and that dissemination of prostate cancer cells into the bloodstream may be necessary, but not sufficient, for metastasis.[396,400] Until the predictive value of a "positive" RT-PCR assay for *PSA* mRNA in the blood has been established for a cohort of men with long-term follow-up after treatment for clinically localized prostate cancer, the assay will remain an investigational test.

THE TREATMENT OF LOCALIZED PROSTATE CANCER

Selection of Treatment Approach

Men thought to have localized prostate cancer face a number of treatment choices, including watchful waiting, radical prostatectomy, interstitial brachytherapy, and external-beam radiation therapy. Not all of these treatment approaches are appropriate for every man with prostate cancer. The different treatment approaches tend to be associated with different potential side effects. Men diagnosed with prostate cancer may have other medical conditions that can increase the chance or severity of such side effects. Prognostic factors, including prostate cancer stage, Gleason score, and serum PSA, are used to stratify men into low-, intermediate-, and high-risks groups for prostate cancer recurrence after treatment, providing some guidance as to likely treatment efficacy. Age and life expectancy also should be considered in treatment selection. Some prostate cancers exhibit a very indolent natural history. Many older men likely die with such cancers, rather than as a result of them. The increased use of serum PSA for prostate cancer screening and early detection, particularly if applied to older men, may tend to overdiagnose such cancers. In contrast, young, healthy men with more-aggressive prostate cancers may benefit from early prostate cancer detection and definitive treatment.

Over the past two decades, both surgery and radiation therapy for prostate cancer have improved dramatically, providing effective local control of cancer in the prostate while reducing the threat of side effects. At this point, the optimal treatment approach for men with localized prostate cancer who are appropriate candidates for surgery and radiation therapy has not been fully resolved. Comparisons between the treatment approaches remain difficult because no randomized clinical trials tested differences in treatment outcomes. Furthermore, historical data offer only limited assistance in choosing between surgery and radiation therapy because each approach has improved in the time since most men were treated in case series with long-term follow-up data, and because most men treated in the past with radiation therapy

tended to be older, to have more substantial comorbidities, and to have more aggressive (higher stage and grade) prostate cancers.

The 2003 National Comprehensive Center Cancer Network (NCCN) guidelines for the management of clinically localized prostate cancer reflect the needed consideration of both life expectancy and the risk for prostate cancer recurrence in making treatment recommendations.[401] In these guidelines, men with a life expectancy of less than 10 years and low-risk prostate cancer (defined as stage T1 or T2, a Gleason score of 2 to 6, and a serum PSA value of ≤10 ng/mL) are recommended for watchful waiting or for radiation therapy, whereas men with a life expectancy of more than 20 years and low-risk prostate cancer would be recommended for radical prostatectomy or for radiation therapy. Men with longer than 10-year life expectancy and intermediate-risk prostate cancer (stage T2b to T2c, Gleason score of 7, or serum PSA between 10 and 20 ng/mL) also are recommended for radical prostatectomy or radiation therapy. Men with a life expectancy of more than 5 years and high-risk cancer (stage T3a to T3b, Gleason score 8 to 10, or serum PSA >20 ng/mL) are recommended for radiation therapy and some sort of adjuvant androgen-deprivation therapy, or in certain specific cases, for radical prostatectomy. No adjuvant chemotherapy has been shown to benefit men with clinically localized prostate cancer.

Watchful Waiting (Conservative or Expectant Management)

Even when it was detected before widespread use of serum PSA for prostate cancer screening, the natural history of localized prostate cancer treated conservatively

---

TREATMENT OF MEN WITH CLINICALLY LOCALIZED PROSTATE CANCER

Men with localized prostate cancer have several treatment options, including watchful waiting, radical prostatectomy, interstitial brachytherapy, and external-beam radiation therapy. Age, life expectancy, and medical history, as well as prostate cancer prognostic factors, such as stage, Gleason score, and serum PSA, are typically used to guide treatment recommendations. For example, men with a life expectancy of less than 10 years and low-risk prostate cancer (defined as stage T1 or T2, a Gleason score of 2 to 6, and a serum PSA value of 10 ng/mL or less) are often counseled to consider watchful waiting or radiation therapy, whereas men with a life expectancy of more than 20 years and low-risk prostate cancer might be offered radical prostatectomy or radiation therapy. Men with greater than 10-year life expectancy and intermediate-risk prostate cancer (stage T2b to T2c, Gleason score of 7, or serum PSA between 10 and 20 ng/mL) are usually referred for radical prostatectomy or radiation therapy. Men with a life expectancy of more than 5 years and high-risk cancer (stage T3a to T3b, Gleason score 8 to 10, or serum PSA >20 ng/mL) tend to be candidates for radiation therapy, administered along with adjuvant androgen-deprivation therapy.

Specific Malignancies

III

TABLE 87-5

Cancer-specific Mortality Rates

GLEASON SUM	AGE (YR)			
	50–59	60–64	65–69	70–74
2–4	4%	5%	6%	7%
5	6%	8%	10%	11%
6	18%	23%	27%	30%
7	70%	62%,	53%	42%
8–10	87%	81%	72%	60%

Probability of dying of prostate cancer within 15 years of diagnosis in men with clinical stage prostate cancer treated conservatively.
Modified from Albertsen PC, Hanley JA, Gleason DF, et al: Competing risk analysis of men aged 55 to 74 years at diagnosis managed conservatively from clinically localized prostate cancer. JAMA 1998;280:975, with permission.

was characterized by slow progression of the disease, with few deaths within 10 years but a substantial risk of death at 15 years, especially for men with Gleason combined scores of 6 or greater (Table 87-5).[402,403] Thus most men with life expectancies beyond 10 years are thought to be candidates for curative therapy (Table 87-6). No long-term studies of conservatively managed patients with prostate cancers detected by serum PSA screening are available. However, several observations suggest that conservative management may be a very reasonable option for selected men with prostate cancers diagnosed after serum PSA screening. First, the lead time for prostate cancer diagnosis using serum PSA screening has been estimated to be 6 to 12 years.[300,355] Second, among men with palpable (stage T2) disease that was not detected with serum PSA screening, 8 years of follow-up were required to demonstrate an absolute difference in prostate cancer–specific survival of 7% in a randomized trial of surgery versus conservative management that showed an advantage for surgical treatment.[404] Thus only a small minority of men with palpable prostate cancer benefit from surgery at 8 years. For men diagnosed with nonpalpable prostate cancer with serum PSA screening, with a lead time of 6 to 12 years, it seems unlikely that most

TABLE 87-6

Life Expectancy of Men (All Races) in the United States of America, by Age

AGE (YR)	LIFE EXPECTANCY (YR)	
	1989	2000
50	26.4	27.9
55	22.3	23.8
60	18.5	19.9
65	15.1	16.3
70	12.1	13.0
75	9.4	10.1
80	7.1	7.6
85	5.3	5.6

From Arias E: United States life tables, 2000. Natl Vital Statistics Rep 2002;51:1–42, with permission.

men age 70 years and older will derive much benefit from aggressive treatment. Such men should be offered watchful waiting as an alternative to surgery or radiation therapy. In addition, some younger men who are thought to have small-volume prostate cancer also may not benefit from aggressive treatment.

With the adoption of serum PSA screening, an estimated 20% to 30% of men detected with nonpalpable prostate cancer (stage T1c) appear to have small-volume cancers (≤0.5 mL) that are not poorly differentiated.[277,405] Given the long natural history of prostate cancer, and the high rates of prostate cancer overdiagnosis (detection of cancer that would not have been detected without PSA testing) with serum PSA screening, especially for older men, watchful waiting should be considered in selected men with nonpalpable, serum PSA–detected, non–poorly differentiated (Gleason score of ≤6) prostate cancers.

Most watchful-waiting approaches have involved periodic general follow-up with initiation of palliative treatment as needed for symptomatic prostate cancer progression or for the appearance of cancer metastases.[406] However, the ability to use serum PSA as a biomarker for prostate cancer activity has led to newer approaches with which older men who are thought to harbor small-volume prostate cancers are followed up more closely, with initiation of aggressive treatment with curative intent when appropriate. The challenges for these approaches are to identify men with small-volume disease who may be candidates for such an approach, and to identify which triggers can be used to change the management strategy from conservative to curative.

Epstein and associates[277] presented criteria for identifying men with small-volume cancers. In their analyses, if the serum PSA "density" was less than 0.15 and no adverse pathologic findings were detected by prostate needle biopsy (Gleason score ≤6, fewer than three biopsy cores containing prostate cancer, and ≤50% involvement of any biopsy core with prostate cancer), at the time of radical prostatectomy, 79% of such men had tumors of 0.5 mL or less that were organ confined and were not high grade. In contrast, if the PSA density was 0.15 or greater, or if any adverse needle-biopsy findings were present (Gleason score ≥7, more than two biopsy cores containing prostate cancer, or >50% involvement of any biopsy core with prostate cancer), 83% of men had prostate cancers that were larger than 0.5 mL, cancers that were not confined to the prostate, or cancers that were high grade at radical prostatectomy. The predictive value of these criteria was subsequently confirmed in a prospective study.[407] When the criteria were used to identify a cohort of men (median age, 67 years) with small-volume prostate cancer for a watchful-waiting program, featuring serial serum PSA determinations and DREs as well as yearly surveillance prostate biopsies, some 30% of the men followed up for more than a year had adverse findings on surveillance biopsies that prompted a recommendation for curative treatment.[407] Nevertheless, 90% of the men found to have adverse prostate biopsy findings in this cohort were still thought to have curable prostate cancer when treatment was recommended.[407] The absence of prostate cancer on subsequent surveillance biopsies was strongly correlated with absence of adverse pathology findings on future surveillance biopsies, but serum PSA determinations (including "free" PSA and PSA "velocity") were not helpful in predicting the future appearance of adverse pathology.[407] Thus watchful waiting, conducted with curative intent, may be a reasonable approach for selected men older than 65 years with a high likelihood of harboring small-volume prostate cancer based on serum PSA and prostate biopsy criteria.

Radical Prostatectomy

Radical prostatectomy is used to treat men with clinically localized prostate cancer who have a life expectancy of at least 10 years. Although no specific or universally accepted age limits exist for radical prostatectomy, the life expectancy of men older than 70 to 75 years is low enough that few men in this age range undergo radical prostatectomy.[408] Clearly, men with uncontrolled or acute medical conditions are not candidates for surgery. Previous pelvic surgery or radiation therapy, which can lead to increased complications, are relative contraindications to radical prostatectomy.[409,410] Preoperative assessment of men for radical prostatectomy typically includes a history and physical examination, hematology studies, serum electrolyte studies (with a serum creatinine determination), a urinalysis, coagulation studies, and an electrocardiogram. Surgery for prostate cancer is usually delayed for 6 to 8 weeks after prostate needle biopsy to permit resolution of hematoma caused by the biopsy procedure. In anticipation of surgery, men avoid aspirin, nonsteroidal anti-inflammatory agents, or high doses of vitamin E that might promote excess bleeding. Some men bank blood for possible transfusion if necessary.[411,412] Anesthesia for radical prostate surgery has been provided by using general, spinal, and epidural approaches; however, most surgeons today prefer regional anesthesia, which has been reported to be associated with less blood loss and a lower risk for pulmonary emboli.[411,413]

The most common radical prostatectomy performed today uses a retropubic approach that has been perfected to permit better removal of all cancer in the prostate and to better preserve anatomic structures essential for erectile function and urinary control.[6,7,414] Other surgical procedures for removal of the prostate gland include radical perineal prostatectomy and laparoscopic approaches to radical prostatectomy.[415-417] The radical retropubic prostatectomy proceeds by performance of a staging pelvic lymphadenectomy; division of puboprostatic ligaments; identification, ligation, and division of the dorsal vein complex to control blood loss; division of the urethra; identification and preservation of the neurovascular bundles needed for penile erection (unless wide excision of a neurovascular bundle is necessary for cancer control); division of the bladder neck and resection of the seminal vesicles; and construction of a urethrovesical anastomosis to provide urinary continence.[418] The most common intraoperative complication is hemorrhage, although blood loss greater than 1000 mL is uncommon for most procedures.[418] Much less frequently, the obturator nerve can be injured during the pelvic lymphadenectomy,

a ureter can be injured near the bladder, or the rectum can be injured during the dissection of the apex of the prostate gland.[418,419] In the immediate postoperative period, complications include deep venous thrombosis and pulmonary emboli.[420] The operative mortality (death within 30 days) for radical prostatectomy is around 0.2%.[418]

Urinary Continence after Radical Prostatectomy

Urinary incontinence rates after radical prostatectomy vary greatly in different reports, with incontinence rates as high as 31% for men in the general population who underwent radical prostatectomy and as low as 10% or less for men who underwent radical prostatectomy at centers of excellence.[421-424] Some of the variation in reported incontinence rates may be attributable to differences in definitions of incontinence (stress incontinence vs. more severe difficulties with urinary control), differences in the time after surgery when urinary continence was assessed (urinary control can improve over as long as a year after surgery), and differences in whether incontinence was reported by treating surgeons in case series or by patients in survey questionnaires. However, surgical technique likely has significant consequences for urinary control after radical prostatectomy. Both the striated urinary sphincter musculature and the smooth muscle surrounding the urethra can be injured during surgery.[418] Postoperative strictures at the site of the vesicourethral anastomosis also can affect control of urination.[425] Such strictures can be dilated, if necessary, to improve urination. Avoidance of such injuries, accompanied by modifications of the urethrovesical anastomosis, has led to improved urinary control rates by expert surgeons.[426,427] In the best case series, as many as 95% of men are completely dry 2 years after radical prostatectomy, and as many as 98% of men report no significant urinary problems.[424,428] Men with persistent or severe urinary incontinence after radical prostatectomy can be treated with periurethral collagen injections or with placement of an artificial urinary sphincter.[429,430]

Erectile Function after Radical Prostatectomy

Most men subjected to radical prostatectomy before 1982 were rendered impotent by the procedure. At that time, Walsh and Donker[6] meticulously assessed the anatomy of the nerves traversing the lateral surface of the prostate en route to the corpora cavernosa of the penis, discerning the close proximity of the nerves to vascular structures (the neurovascular bundles) visible at the time of radical prostatectomy. This revelation led Walsh and coworkers[7] to propose a modification of the radical prostatectomy procedure to preserve the neurovascular bundles in an effort to maintain postoperative erectile function. Wide adoption of this modification has led to improvements in sexual potency rates after radical prostatectomy. As many as 91% of young men (younger than 50 years) with good preoperative erectile function and low-stage prostate cancers who undergo an anatomic radical

Specific Malignancies

III

prostatectomy with preservation of both neurovascular bundles can expect recovery of potency after surgery.[431] Improvement in sexual function after surgery tends to occur gradually over at least 24 months.[424,432] Poor recovery of erectile function after surgery is correlated with increasing age (75% of men aged 50 to 60 years, 58% of men aged 60 to 70 years, and 25% of men 70 years or older were potent after radical prostatectomy in one series), poor potency before surgery, advanced prostate cancer stage (with capsular penetration or seminal vesicle invasion), and excision of neurovascular bundles.[431,433] Population studies have confirmed these predictors of erectile dysfunction after radical prostatectomy, with as many as 60% of men reporting impotence after surgery and some 42% reporting that poor sexual function was a significant problem.[422] In the best case series, 86% of men were able to have erections sufficient for sexual intercourse by 18 months.[424] Interposition grafts, from the sural nerve, have been used in attempts to repair nerves severed when wide excision of neurovascular bundles was required during radical prostatectomy, but the effectiveness of this procedure has been questioned.[434,435] Many men use suldenafil citrate (Viagra; Pfizer, Inc.) to improve sexual function after radical prostatectomy.[436]

Control of Prostate Cancer with Radical Prostatectomy

Radical prostatectomy is an effective means of treating localized prostate cancer. In a randomized trial ($N = 695$ men) comparing radical prostatectomy with watchful waiting, the odds ratio for death due to prostate cancer for men treated with surgery was 0.50 (with a 95% confidence interval of 0.27 to 0.91, $P = .02$; Fig. 87-8).[404] After surgery, serum PSA levels should decrease to undetectable levels. A persistently detectable serum PSA

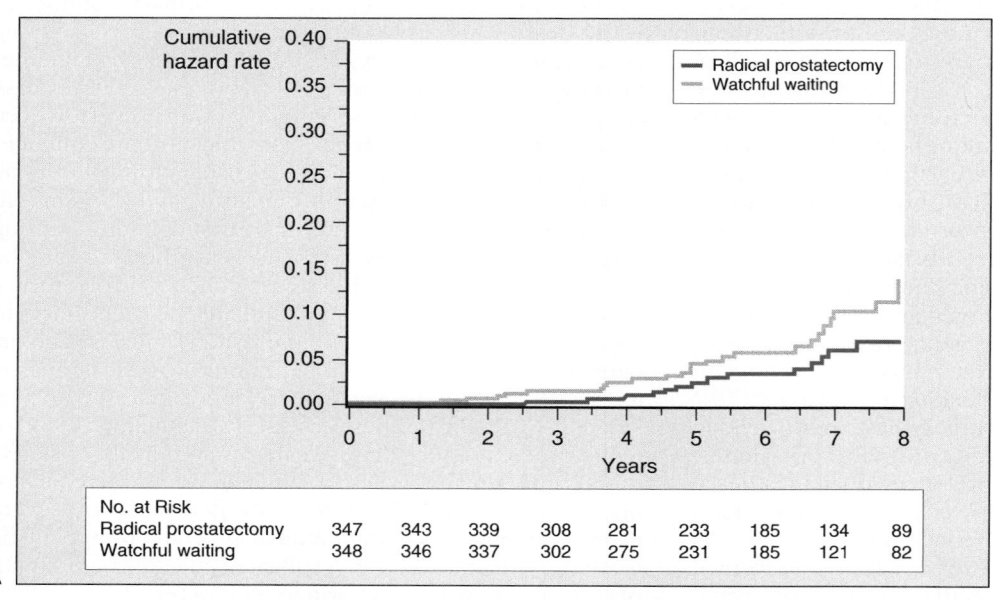

No. at Risk								
Radical prostatectomy	347	343	339	308	281	233	185	134	89
Watchful waiting	348	346	337	302	275	231	185	121	82

A

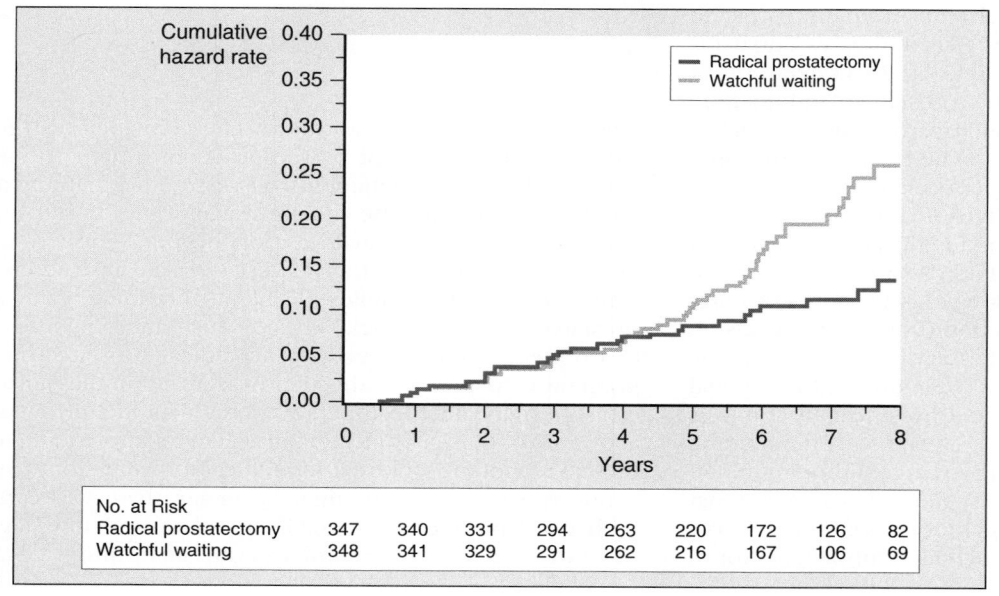

No. at Risk								
Radical prostatectomy	347	340	331	294	263	220	172	126	82
Watchful waiting	348	341	329	291	262	216	167	106	69

B

Figure 87-8. Results of a randomized clinical trial of radical prostatectomy versus watchful waiting. **A,** Cumulative hazard rates of prostate cancer death. **B,** Cumulative hazard rates of prostate cancer metastasis. (From Holmberg L, Bill-Axelson A, Helgesen F, et al: A randomized trial comparing radical prostatectomy with watchful waiting in early prostate cancer. N Engl J Med 2002;347:781–789, with permission.)

TABLE 87-7

Actuarial Probability (%) of Freedom from Progression 5 Years after Radical Prostatectomy for cT1–2 NXMO Prostate Cancer According to Clinical Stage, Gleason Sum in the Biopsy Specimen, Preoperative PSA, and Pathologic Stage

	PARTIN ET AL.[380]	CATALONA AND SMITH[441]	ABBAS ET AL.[442]
No. of Patients	894	925	1359
Clinical Stage			
T1a	100	89*	87*
T1b	91		
T1c	100	99	89
T2a	87		
T2b	71	85†	74‡
T2c	69		
Gleason Score	98	91	90
2–4	92	⎫	⎫ 84‖
6	85	⎬ 89	⎬ 58
7	62	⎭	⎭ 53
8–10	46	74	
Preoperative PSA (ng/mL)			
0–4.0	92	95	95
4.1–10.0	83	93	84
10.1–20.0	56		
>20	45	71¶	68¶
Pathologic Stage			
Organ-confined	97	91	94
Capsular penetration			74
Seminal vesicle invasion	47	—	40
Positive lymph nodes	15	—	16

PSA, prostate-specific antigen.
*T1a and T1b combined.
†T2a, T2b, and T2c combined.
‡Gleason sum 5–7.
‖Gleason sum 5–6.
¶Preoperative PSA >10.0.
Modified from Eastham JA, Scardino PT: Radical prostatectomy for clinical stage T1 and T2 prostate cancer. In Vogelzang NJ, Scardino PT, Shipley WU, Coffey DS (eds): Comprehension Textbook of Genitourinary Oncology. Baltimore, Williams & Wilkins, 1966, p 741, with permission.

after radical prostatectomy most often reflects the presence of disseminated cancer, occasionally indicating an incomplete resection of prostate tissues. After the serum PSA has declined to an undetectable level after radical prostatectomy, the subsequent detection of PSA in the serum always indicates prostate cancer recurrence, preceding clinically significant prostate cancer progression by as many as 6 years or more.[437] Most modern case series examining outcomes of men with prostate cancer treated with radical prostatectomy feature the serum PSA as a surrogate biomarker for recurrence of prostate cancer. In such series, some 80% of men remain free of prostate cancer recurrence by 5 years after surgery (Table 87-7).[438–442] In multivariate statistical analyses, the risk of serum PSA recurrence after radical prostatectomy has been correlated with clinical stage, Gleason score in prostate biopsies, and serum PSA values determined preoperatively, and with pathologic stage and Gleason score in the resected prostate specimen, determined postoperatively.[380,381]

Radiation Therapy

Radiation therapy has been used in the management of prostate cancer for nearly a century. After Roentgen's discovery of the x-ray in 1895,[443] and the isolation of radium by Pierre and Marie Curie in 1898,[444] several pioneering physicians began treating prostate disorders, including prostate cancer, with radiation. In 1910, Paschkis and Tittinger inserted radium into the prostatic urethra with a cystoscope in what may be the first use of radiation for prostate cancer. Not long after, Hugh Hampton Young[445] from Johns Hopkins reported the relatively large experience of treating prostate cancer patients with urethral and rectal radium "applicators." These and other early studies revealed that even when radiation was applied in this crude manner, it could improve symptoms and kill prostate cancer. However, treatment was technically difficult for the physician and uncomfortable for the patient. In 1928, the first report on the use of externally delivered low-energy kilovoltage radiation for prostate cancer was proffered by Barringer.[446] The associated dosimetry was not well worked out, and thus men were treated until their skin turned red. These types of low-energy radiation machines were used until cobalt machines became available and provided the first opportunity to treat more deeply seated tumors in the body. The first reported series of prostate cancer patients treated with ^{60}Co therapy was by George and colleagues[447] in 1965 and featured men with unresectable disease. It also was during this time (beginning in the late 1950s) that the megavoltage linear accelerator was being developed at Stanford University.[448] The pioneering work of Bagshaw, Kaplan, Del Regato, and others ushered in the modern era of radiation therapy for prostate cancer by offering the possibility of cure with radiation therapy in this disease.[449,450] Now men with prostate cancer have several different radiotherapeutic options, each of which can be used with very high precision and with great effectiveness. The integration of computer-based technology for the design of three-dimensional conformal treatment plans and use of high-energy accelerators with sophisticated dynamic shielding allows men with prostate cancer to be treated with high doses of radiation while sparing surrounding normal tissues. In addition, the development of permanently implantable radioactive sources, along with the use of real-time imaging and treatment planning, also has provided the opportunity for sophisticated prostate brachytherapy techniques resulting in safe and efficacious treatment of men with prostate cancer.

Traditionally, men with prostate cancer referred for radiation therapy tended to be older, to be in poorer health, and to have higher-risk, more advanced tumors than those patients treated surgically. As such, results of using less sophisticated radiation therapy techniques were less than optimal, raising concerns that radiation therapy might not be as effective as radical prostatectomy. However, with long-term results obtained across a broad range of patients, it is now clear that radiation therapy for prostate cancer provides excellent disease-free survival, comparable with that of radical prostatectomy for men at similar risk of prostate cancer recurrence. In this section, a brief description of how men are evaluated and risk-stratified for radiation therapy is provided, followed by a description of treatment techniques and a review of treatment outcomes for men with low-, intermediate-, and high-risk prostate cancer. The use of radiation therapy to treat local prostate cancer recurrences after radical prostatectomy also is reviewed.

Conventional External-Beam Radiotherapy for Localized Prostate Cancer

For more than three decades, external-beam radiotherapy and radical prostatectomy have been widely used for the definitive management of clinically localized prostate cancer. Although no large randomized trials in North America or Europe have directly compared the two treatment modalities, retrospective comparisons are plentiful, but limited by the tendency of older men with higher-stage prostate cancer to have been treated with suboptimal radiation doses and techniques. In general, the conventional techniques used standard radiation fields, based on bony pelvic landmarks, to define the region of clinical interest for a dose range of 65 to 70 Gy delivered to the prostate. Commonly, a four-field pelvic box with custom cerrobend blocking was used to treat the prostate, seminal vesicles, and proximal lymphatic drainage. These fields were treated to a dose of 45 to 50 Gy in 1.8- to 2.0-Gy fractions. The prostate and sometimes the seminal vesicles, plus a safety margin, were then boosted to 65 to

70 Gy. Cerrobend blocking was used to shield, if possible, the posterior wall of the rectum, anal canal, and any small bowel. In spite of its limitations, this version of external-beam radiation therapy was fairly effective: Although overall survival numbers were generally higher for men treated with radical prostatectomy (often younger and healthier men), cause-specific survival rates were not significantly different.[451] In an analysis of pathologically staged men with stage A2-B prostate cancer treated as part of Radiation Therapy Oncology Group (RTOG) Trial 77-06, 5- and 10-year survival rates, 87% and 63%, respectively, were comparable to those of age-matched controls without prostate cancer.[452] The prostate cancer–specific survival was 86%, which was similar to the outcomes of some surgical series.[453,454]

With the ready availability of serum PSA testing, current outcome comparisons focus on PSA as a marker of prostate cancer recurrence after primary treatment ("PSA relapse"–free survival). An increasing serum PSA level after radiotherapy for prostate cancer is correlated with the appearance of progressive or metastatic prostate cancer on further follow-up.[455] Furthermore, the rate of serum PSA increase may help distinguish between a local or distant treatment failure. Men with slow rates of serum PSA increases are more likely to have local prostate cancer recurrences, whereas men with rapid serum PSA increases appear more likely to have distant prostate cancer metastates.[456] In 1997, the American Society for Therapeutic Radiology and Oncology (ASTRO) issued a consensus statement establishing the definition of recurrence after radiation therapy as three consecutive increases in serum PSA levels ("biochemical" treatment failure) with determinations made at least 3 months apart.[457] Before these criteria were formulated, treatment outcomes in different studies and case series were difficult to compare because of the lack of uniformity in defining treatment failure.[458-464] Pretreatment serum PSA levels are particularly predictive of radiation treatment outcome (Table 87-8). In a case series of men (N = 461) with stage T1 to T2 prostate cancer treated at M.D. Anderson Cancer Center, 5-year PSA relapse-free survival rates for men with pretreatment PSA levels of less than 4 ng/mL, 4 to 10 ng/mL, 10 to 20 ng/mL, and more than 20 ng/mL were 91%, 69%, 62%, and 38%, respectively.[461] In another study, Zietman and associates[465] reported 4-year PSA relapse-free survival of 65% for pretreatment PSA level of less than 15 ng/mL and 6% for patients with more than 15 ng/mL. The routine monitoring of serum PSA to detect cancer recurrence after primary treatment spurred interest in escalating radiation doses to improve cancer control.

Toxicity of Conventional External-Beam Radiation Therapy

Dose escalation with conventional external-beam radiotherapy has been limited by the toxicity of treatment (Table 87-9). Most men experience dysuria or diarrhea or both during the course of prostate cancer therapy, but these symptoms generally resolve weeks after completion of treatment. Long-term sequelae of conventional external-

TABLE 87-8

Rates of PSA Relapse-free Survival for Men Treated with External-beam Radiation Therapy According to Pretreatment Serum PSA Levels

SERIES	PRETREATMENT SERUM PSA (ng/mL)										
	<4	4–10	<10	<13	>13	10–20	>20	10–30	>30	20–50	>50
Cleveland Clinic	100%	65%									
Eastern Virginia Medical School	69%	57%				56%	20%				
Mayo Clinic				92%	58%						
M.D. Anderson Cancer Center	84%	66%				49%	11%				
Massachusetts General Hospital	82%	44%				30%				8%	0%
Stanford			65%			72%				28%	17%
William Beaumont Hospital	90%	54%				27%	14%				

Adapted from Horwitz EM, Hanks GE: External beam radiation therapy for prostate cancer. CA Cancer J Clin 2000;50:349–375, with permission.

beam radiotherapy (i.e., delivered without the use of conformal techniques) were reviewed in an analysis of 1020 patients treated in RTOG trials 75-06 and 77-06.[466] The incidence of late grade 3 or 4 urinary complications, such as hematuria, cystitis, bladder contracture, or urethral stricture, was 7.7%, with surgical intervention needed for 0.5%. Grade 3 or 4 rectal complications, such as bleeding, ulceration, proctitis, rectal/anal stricture, or chronic diarrhea, were seen in 3.3%, with surgery for bowel obstruction or perforation needed in 0.6%. Notably, the risk of complications was significantly higher when doses larger than 70 Gy were administered by these nonconformal techniques.

Data on the incidence of erectile dysfunction after external-beam radiotherapy has been widely variable. Sexual function has many facets that are difficult to evaluate or quantify. A commonly used qualitative definition of sexual potency is the ability to achieve spontaneous erections sufficient for intercourse. Although potency rates after radical prostatectomy have increased with use of nerve-sparing techniques, the mechanism of radiation-related erectile dysfunction appears unrelated to the neurovascular bundles. Zelefsky and Eid[467] specifically

addressed this topic by performing duplex ultrasound studies before and after prostaglandin injection to stimulate erections in a men with radiation-related erectile dysfunction. A diminished peak penile blood flow rate (<25 mL/min) was evident in 63% of such men, with abnormal distensibility of the corpora cavernosa in 32%. Thus the primary mechanism of radiation therapy–associated impotence may be vascular damage rather than nerve damage. Fisch and coworkers[468] demonstrated a correlation between incidence of erectile dysfunction after radiotherapy and radiation dose to the vascular penile bulb. Men receiving more than 70 Gy to more than 70% of the bulb of the penis are at greatest risk of experiencing radiation therapy–associated erectile dysfunction. A steady decline in potency rates over time is characteristic of men treated with external-beam radiation therapy. In a large series (N = 434) of men treated with radiation therapy at Stanford University, 86% of the men remained potent at 15 months after treatment, but only 50% were potent 6 years later, and only 30% maintained erectile function for the remainder of their lives.[469] Sildenafil administration resulted in improvement of erectile function in 74% of men with radiation therapy–associated erectile dysfunction in a study at Memorial Sloan-Kettering Cancer Center.[470] Men that do not respond to sildenafil may respond to intracavernosal prostaglandin injections.

Second malignancy after definitive radiotherapy for prostate cancer is an infrequent occurrence. Using data from the Surveillance, Epidemiology, and End Results (SEER) program cancer registry, Brenner and colleagues[471] compared second malignancy risks for men (N = 51,584) who received radiotherapy for prostate cancer from 1973 to 1993 versus men (N = 70,539) who underwent radical surgery during the same time period, finding a small, but significant, increase in second malignancy attributable to radiation treatment. The most common radiation-induced tumors were carcinomas of the bladder and rectum, and sarcoma. The absolute risk of second malignancy for men treated with radiotherapy was 1 in 290. For survivors more than 10 years after treatment, the risk increased to 1 in 70.

TABLE 87-9

Radiation Therapy Oncology Group Criteria for Late Morbidity after Radiation Therapy

GRADE	CRITERIA
1	Minor symptoms requiring no treatment
2	Symptoms responding to simple outpatient management, lifestyle not affected
3	Distressing symptoms altering patient's lifestyle Hospitalization for diagnosis or minor surgical intervention (such as urethral dilatation) may be required
4	Major surgical intervention (such as laparotomy, colostomy, cystectomy) or prolonged hospitalization
5	Fatal complication

Three-Dimensional Conformal Radiotherapy

The advent of CT-based simulation and treatment planning and the innovation of multileaf collimators in modern linear accelerators have allowed increased precision and accuracy in radiotherapy. Three-dimensional reconstructions of acquired CT images are generated, and target volumes (e.g., prostate and seminal vesicles) are delineated. Critical structures (e.g., bladder and rectum) to be avoided also are contoured. Computerized treatment-planning software allows the iterative process of designing beam arrangements that will deliver a prescribed dose to the regions of interest and minimize dose to a given volume of a critical organ. Target volumes and normal organs are visualized in three dimensions (permitting the so-called "beam's eye view," a portrayal of the target area as if looking straight down the path of the radiation beam). Computerized multileaf collimators shape each individual beam to conform to the shape of the target in the "beam's eye view." The treatment-planning system generates a dose-volume histogram for a selected treatment plan, a graphic description of the relation between dose administered and volume of an organ that is receiving a given dose (Fig. 87-9). This allows an objective assessment of the anticipated performance of a proposed radiation-treatment plan. As these technologies became clinically available in the 1990s, they have been used in dose-escalation studies in prostate cancer.

The profound effect of radiation dose escalation on treatment outcomes for prostate cancer has been demonstrated through work from several institutions.[472-475] Men with intermediate-risk prostate cancer (serum PSA values of 10 to 20 ng/mL) may benefit most from dose escalation.[472,475] However, in a large cohort of men (N = 1100) treated with three-dimensional conformal radiotherapy (3D-CRT) at Memorial Sloan-Kettering Cancer Center, a significant benefit of dose escalation was evident regardless of the pretreatment PSA.[473,474] Initially, men with prostate cancer were treated with conventional radiation dose levels of 64.8 to 70.2 Gy by using 3D-CRT techniques, and then the radiation dose was increased to as high as 86.4 Gy. At a median follow-up of 60 months, PSA relapse-free survivals for men with low-risk prostate cancer treated to radiation doses of 64.8 to 70.2 Gy versus 81 Gy were 77% and 98%, respectively.[474] Men with intermediate- and high-risk prostate cancers also showed significant improvement.

Will improved treatment outcomes from 3D-CRT, evidenced by reduced numbers of men with prostate cancer relapses detected as an increasing serum PSA, result in improvements in disease-free survival, freedom from distant metastasis, or overall survival? A randomized dose-escalation trial detected a substantial improvement in prostate cancer control rates for men with prostate cancer, especially men with a pretreatment PSA greater than 10 ng/mL (Fig. 87-10).[472,476] This study involved the stratification of men (N = 305) with stage T1 to T3 prostate cancer to undergo treatment to a total dose of either 70 Gy with conventional radiotherapeutic techniques, or 78 Gy with a six-field 3D-CRT boost after the delivery of an initial 46 Gy. Results revealed a freedom-from-PSA relapse of 64% and 70% at 6 years for the 70-Gy and 78-Gy groups, respectively (P = .03). Men who had a pretreatment PSA greater than 10 ng/mL were found to have the most significant benefit from radiation dose escalation, with freedom-from-PSA relapse rates of 62% for the 78-Gy arm and 43% for the 70-Gy arm (P = .01), a benefit not seen for men with a pretreatment PSA of 10 ng/mL or less. Overall survival was not significantly different between the two radiation doses, but a trend toward an improved freedom from distant metastasis was evident in men treated in the 78-Gy arm, 98% versus 88% at 6 years (P = .056).

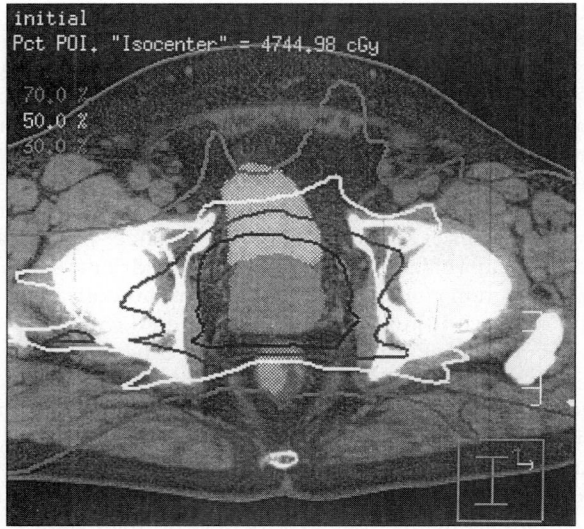

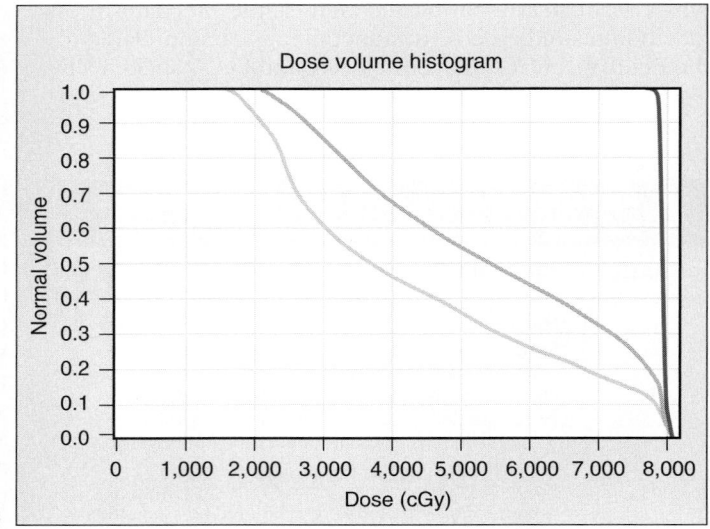

Figure 87-9. Intensity-modulated radiation therapy (IMRT). **A,** A representative axial computed tomography slice from a man with low-risk prostate cancer treated by using a seven-field IMRT plan: The isodose distribution is displayed. *Dark inner line,* prescription isodose curve. **B,** The IMRT treatment plan shown as a dose/volume histogram: The curves form the left to right represent bladder, rectum, and prostate.

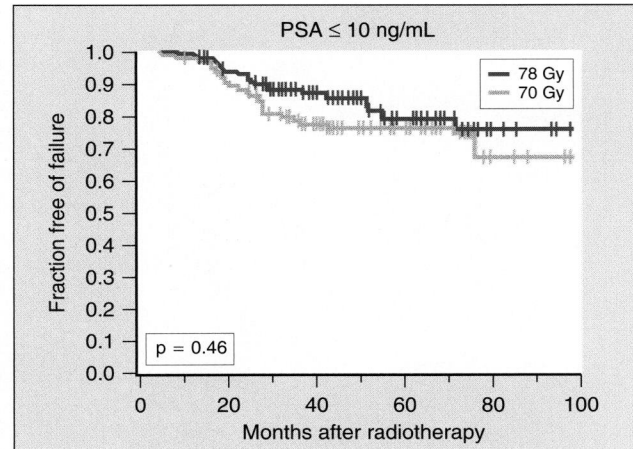

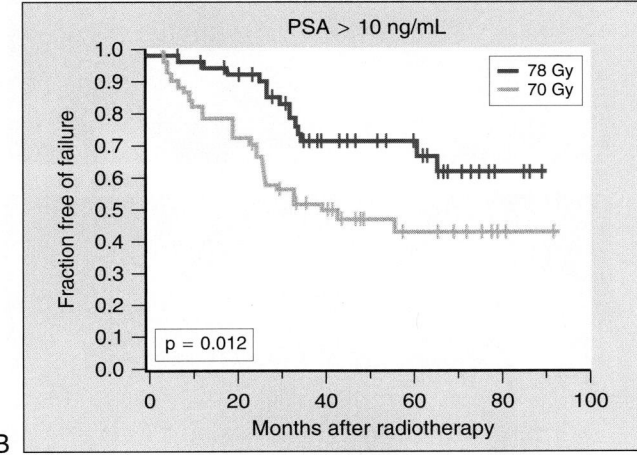

Figure 87-10. Kaplan-Meier actuarial probability of relapse-free survival after radiation therapy for prostate cancer, stratified by radiation dose (78 Gy vs. 70 Gy). **A,** Men with favorable-prognosis prostate cancer (serum prostate-specific antigen, ≤10 ng/mL). **B,** Men with poorer-prognosis prostate cancer (serum prostate-specific antigen, 10 ng/mL). (From Pollack A, Zagars GK, Starkschall G, et al: Prostate cancer radiation dose response: Results of the M.D. Anderson phase III randomized trial. Int J Radiat Oncol Biol Phys 2002;53:1097–1105, with permission.)

Toxicity of Three-Dimensional Conformal Radiotherapy

Although the use of 3D-CRT was intended to minimize the effects of high-dose radiation on normal tissues, increased late toxicities have been noted with escalating radiation doses used in 3D-CRT.[475,477] In the Fox Chase case series, the 5-year incidence of grade 3 or 4 rectal toxicity at a dose of 75 to 76 Gy was 8%.[475] However, after the anterior rectal wall was shielded to keep the dose to this region under 72 Gy, grade 3 or 4 rectal toxicity was evident in only 2%. From the M.D. Anderson dose-escalation case series, men who received more than 70 Gy to 30% or more of the defined rectal volume had a significantly higher risk of rectal toxicity.[478] Zelefsky and associates[477] reported a 1.2% actuarial risk of grade 3 or higher rectal toxicity by 5 years with 3D-CRT. Grade 2 rectal bleeding was seen among 17% of men who received 75.6 Gy or

more as compared with 6% for men receiving 64.8 to 70.2 Gy. Furthermore, even if the rectum was completely shielded in each field above a dose of 72 Gy, grade 2 rectal bleeding was seen in 15% of men. As for urinary toxicity with 3D-CRT, urethral strictures have been observed in 1.5% of treated men, with a 4% incidence of stricture in men with a history of previous transurethral resection of the prostate (TURP). Grade 3 hematuria appears in as many as 0.5% of men, with grade 2 hematuria in 13% of men treated to a dose of 75.6 Gy or higher and 4% of men treated to lower total doses. Urinary incontinence is rare after treatment with 3D-CRT (<0.2%, with 2% in the setting of a prior TURP).[479]

Intensity-Modulated Radiation Therapy

Intensity-modulated radiation therapy (IMRT) equipment and treatment-planning software have become increasingly available, with the technology attracting interest from both academic and community cancer centers for the treatment of a variety of malignancies. The largest experience with IMRT to date has been in the treatment of prostate cancer. Through inverse planning, IMRT allows identification of the region to be treated along with surrounding critical normal organs so that radiation dose and volume goals can be prescribed for each target and structure. The treatment-planning software then derives an optimized dose distribution by modifying the number, orientation, and intensity of the beams across the designated volume. This is in contrast to 3D-CRT, where beam arrangement and field shapes must be designed manually to accomplish radiation dose/volume goals, a task that typically requires multiple time-consuming iterations. In a case series ($N = 772$) of men with clinically localized prostate cancer treated with IMRT at Memorial Sloan-Kettering Cancer Center, a reduction in late rectal toxicity was seen in comparison to 3D-CRT.[480] Most of the men (698 of the 772) were treated to a total dose of 81 Gy, while the remainder received 86.4 Gy. With a median follow-up of 24 months, actuarial rate of grade 2 or higher rectal bleeding at 3 years was 4%, and only 0.5% of men experienced any grade 3 rectal toxicity (no grade 4 rectal toxicity was seen). However, despite the increased conformality of incident radiation and the decreased bladder volumes receiving high radiation doses, no improvement was found in late urinary toxicity with IMRT versus 3D-CRT, with 15% of men having late grade 2 urinary toxicity. Because this may be the result of high-dose radiation to the urethra, decreasing urethral doses for men with prostate cancer limited to the peripheral zone of the prostate may be a means of reducing late urinary toxicity with IMRT, but better diagnostic imaging is necessary to identify such cancers.

One concern with IMRT techniques, in general, is the potential for inadequate treatment at the margins of radiation fields with increasingly conformal radiation-dose delivery. However, preliminary treatment-outcome data obtained thus far with IMRT appear similar to those with 3D-CRT, with 3-year actuarial PSA relapse-free survival rates, using ASTRO consensus criteria, for men with low-, intermediate-, and high-risk prostate cancer of 92%, 86%, and 81%, respectively.[480] It should be noted that planning target volume (PTV) definitions for IMRT are often the same as those used with 3D-CRT. If tighter PTV definitions are to be used, better prostate immobilization and localization techniques are likely needed. This strategy is currently being investigated in several centers with the use of electronic portal imaging (EPI), a real-time treatment setup verification system, and of B-Mode Acquisition and Targeting (BAT), an ultrasound-based real-time localization system.[481]

Brachytherapy

Prostate brachytherapy refers to the implantation of radioactive sources into the prostate under TRUS guidance. In principle, brachytherapy offers an attractive means for radiation dose escalation and conformality in the treatment of clinically localized prostate cancer. Modern prostate brachytherapy techniques that use ultrasound or CT-based targeting, a perineal template for precise seed implantation, and computerized treatment planning have gained in popularity over the past 10 years (Fig. 87-11). For the patient with prostate cancer, this option may be most convenient, allowing a rapid return to normal lifestyle and activity. A typical brachytherapy procedure is performed in 2 hours, often under spinal anesthesia, and does not require an overnight hospital stay. Before the procedure, an ultrasound- or CT-based volume study is performed and a preplan is formulated, specifying three-dimensional seed distribution to deliver a prescribed dose to the prostate and a periprostatic margin. Typically, peripherally biased seed distributions provide a relatively lower dose to the urethra. In the operating room, with the spinal or general anesthesia and with Foley catheter in place, the patient is placed in the dorsal lithotomy position, a TRUS of the prostate volume is registered to approximate the prostate volume obtained from a preprocedure study (some centers use real-time intraoperative treatment planning systems to make adjustments to optimize the dose distribution because the prostate volume may be slightly different from that of the preplan), hollow needles are guided into the prostate through the perineum by using a template, and radioactive sources are deposited in the prostate according to the plan as the needles are withdrawn (through use of the Mick applicator or with seeds strewn on ribbons with equal spacing). Post-treatment CT scans are then routinely done to evaluate the quality of the implant procedure.[482]

Thus far, every use of permanent brachytherapy for prostate cancer reported has been a retrospective analysis of a case series from a single institution. Comparisons among these series, or with results from external-beam radiotherapy or radical prostatectomy, are fraught with difficulty due to the lack of uniformity in reporting of patient selection and treatment outcomes criteria. Additionally, implantation techniques, isotopes, dosimetry, and operator experience vary widely between prostate cancer brachytherapy series. Many practitioners have recommended brachytherapy for men with low-risk prostate cancer, but have added supplementary external-

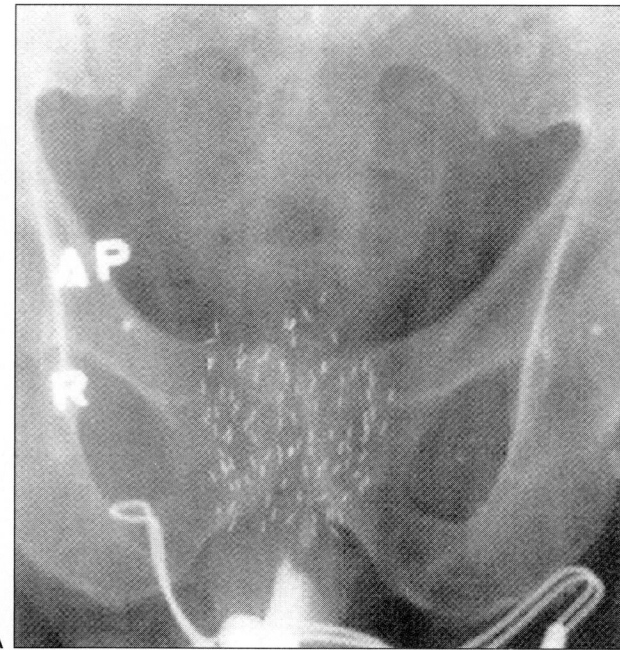

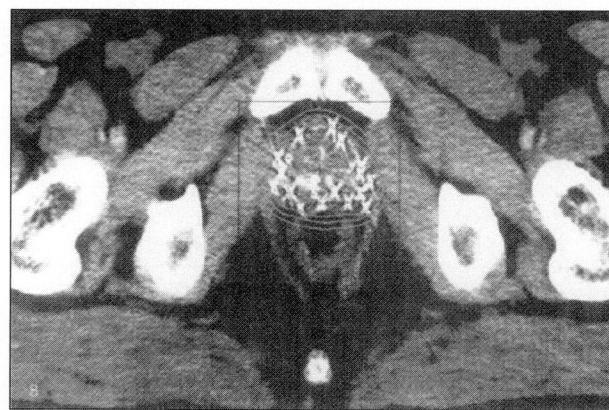

Figure 87-11. Interstitial brachytherapy for prostate cancer. **A,** Radiograph obtained after implantation of radioactive seeds. **B,** Computed tomography image showing radioactive seed location within prostate. (From Speight JL, Roach M III: Imaging and radiotherapy of the prostate. Radiol Clin North Am 2000;38:159–177, with permission.)

beam radiotherapy to brachytherapy for men with prostate cancer at higher risk for extraprostatic extension. Combinations of brachytherapy and external-beam radiotherapy also have been advocated for use in all men with clinically localized prostate cancer.[483] In 1999, the American Brachytherapy Society recommended that brachytherapy using radioactive iodine or palladium might be appropriate for men with prostate cancer of clinical stage T1 to T2a, with a serum PSA of 10 ng/mL or less, and a Gleason score 6 or less, and that supplemental external-beam radiotherapy should be added for men with higher-risk disease.[484] This recommendation was based in part on inferior outcomes reported for men with high-risk prostate cancer treated with brachytherapy.[485] It is possible that favorable outcomes may be achieved even in some men with prostate cancer and some high-risk features through the use of generous periprostatic treatment margins at the time of implant or the use of supplemental external-beam therapy or both.[486-488]

In the absence of a prospective randomized trial, the routine use of prostate brachytherapy in the treatment of clinically localized prostate cancer has been criticized because of lack of long-term follow-up data (Table 87-10). Currently, three series are reporting long-term results with brachytherapy.[489-491] Ragde and coworkers[491] reported 12-year treatment results from a group of 229 men with T1 to T3 prostate cancer who underwent ^{125}I or [103]Pd implantation. Men with low-risk prostate cancer ($n = 147$) in this case series were treated with brachytherapy alone, whereas men with high-risk prostate cancer ($n = 82$) received external-beam radiation therapy followed by implant. The PSA relapse-free survival was 66% for men with low-risk prostate cancer and 79% for men with high-risk prostate cancer. In light of subsequent superior results in men with low-risk prostate cancer treated with brachytherapy alone, a possible explanation for the poor performance of brachytherapy alone in this case series is that significant refinement of technique and treatment planning has occurred since many of these men were treated.[485,489,490,492-496] In another case series, men with low-risk prostate cancer treated in 1986 through 1987 exhibited a significantly worse progression-free survival (PFS) than did men treated in 1988 through 1990.[490]

The addition of supplemental external-beam radiotherapy to brachytherapy remains somewhat controversial. Davis and colleagues[497] examined the radial distance of extraprostatic extension of prostate cancer and found it to be almost always 5 mm or less, which would be within a typical brachytherapy dose distribution. Thus generous periprostatic margins in brachytherapy planning may obviate the need for supplemental external-beam radiotherapy. Proponents of combination therapy point to the advantage of higher biologic doses and the ability to smooth out cold spots inherent with brachytherapy, the so-called "spackle effect." It will be important to determine the incremental benefit of supplemental external-beam radiotherapy in each risk group, as the addition of this therapy nearly doubles the cost of treatment.[498] Relative contraindications to the use of prostate brachytherapy are large prostate size, preimplant obstructive urinary symptoms, history of prior TURP, and the presence of perineural prostate cancer invasion on prostate biopsy. Large prostate size has been perceived to be associated with a higher risk of urinary morbidity after implant and with unsuitability for implant due to pubic arch interference. Men with a prostate volume of greater than 50 mL have been either counseled against brachytherapy or placed on androgen-deprivation therapy in an attempt to reduce gland size.[499] Nonetheless, the implantation of large prostates with radioactive seeds has been described with acceptable morbidity.[499,500] In one case series, postimplant dosimetry quality was found to be independent of prostate size or use of androgen-deprivation therapy.[500] The use of the extended dorsal lithotomy position and steering of needles around the pubic arch increases the fraction of men that can be implanted with radioactive seeds by experienced radiation oncologists.[492] The correlation of preimplantation obstructive urinary symptoms and postimplantation urinary obstruction is not resolved. Terk and associates[501] reported that a high International Prostate Symptom Score (I-PSS), a measure of obstructive urinary symptoms, predicted postimplant urinary retention. With the use of alpha-blockers before and after implant procedures, others have noted no association between preimplant I-PSS and urinary obstruction.[502] A prospective study examining preimplant urinary flow rate and postvoid residual, in addition to I-PSS, showed no association of obstructive urinary symptoms with postimplant urinary retention or long-term urinary function.[503] TURP is thought to be a relative contraindication to prostate brachytherapy, as it has been associated with unacceptably high rates of urinary incontinence.[504] This could possibly be attributable to seed-loading approaches that result in a high central dose to the TURP defect. However, by using a peripheral source loading approach to limit dose to the TURP defect to 110% of the prescription dose, the incidence of urinary incontinence may be reduced.[505]

TABLE 87-10

PSA Relapse-free Survival after Interstitial Brachytherapy as Monotherapy for Prostate Cancer

SERIES	RECURRENCE RISK			PRETREATMENT PSA (ng/mL)			
	LOW RISK	INTERMEDIATE RISK	HIGH RISK	0–4	4–10	10–20	>20
Blasko et al. (N =197)				98%	90%	89%	80%
Blasko et al. (N = 230)	92%	82%	65%	90%	87%	80%	67%
Brachman et al. (N = 695)				88%	70%	50%	35%
D'Amico et al. (N = 66)	85%	35%	0*				
Grimm et al. (N = 125)				95%	78%	88%	55%
Potters et al. (N = 493)	92%	74%	55%				
Zelefsky et al. (N = 226)	88%	77%	38%	96%	84%	62%†	

*Projected.
†Pretreatment prostate-specific antigen (PSA), >10 ng/mL.
Adapted from Merrick GS, Wallner KE, Butler WM: Permanent interstitial brachytherapy for the management of carcinoma of the prostate gland. J Urol 2003;169:1643–1652, with permission.

TABLE 87-11

Physical Differences between ^{125}I and ^{103}Pd Radioactive Seeds		
	^{125}I	^{103}PD
Year introduced	1965	1986
Photon energy (keV)	28	21
Half-life (days)	59.4	17
Initial dose rate (for monotherapy)	7 cGy/hr	18–20 cGy/hr
RBE	1.4	1.9

RBE, relative biologic effectiveness.

Finally, because prostate cancers exhibiting perineural invasion have been shown to be associated with inferior outcome in radical prostatectomy series, this adverse prognostic finding will likely also be associated with inferior outcome from brachytherapy.[506] Curiously, in one case series, no difference in brachytherapy treatment outcome attributable to the presence of perineural invasion was evident.[507] A phenomenon peculiar to prostate brachytherapy that deserves mention is the so-called "PSA spike." With a time of onset between 12 and 30 months after implantation, approximately one third of men with prostate cancer treated with brachytherapy will experience a transient increase in serum PSA.[508] This spike may be due to radiation-associated prostatitis that compromises prostate architecture, permitting more PSA to appear in the serum. Notably, such "PSA spikes" portend no worse long-term outcome.

Another controversy for prostate brachytherapy concerns the choice of isotope and use of androgen-deprivation therapy. The most common sources in use today are ^{125}I and ^{103}Pd (Table 87-11). Thus far, no compelling data support the superiority of one isotope or the other. It has been hypothesized that the higher initial dose rate of ^{103}Pd might be advantageous for the treatment of cancers with a relatively low α/β ratio (more radio-resistant) like prostate cancer; however, retrospective data for prostate cancer have been inconclusive.[509] A prospective randomized trial directly comparing ^{125}I with ^{103}Pd for prostate cancer brachytherapy is ongoing. The majority of experience with prostate brachytherapy has been with permanent low-dose-rate (LDR) implants. Several centers have collected experience with temporary high-dose-rate (HDR) implants for prostate cancer brachytherapy.[510-512] Although this treatment approach is not widely used, the available results appear comparable to those of permanent brachytherapy for clinically localized prostate cancer. HDR approaches have a theoretical advantage over LDR brachytherapy for the treatment of cancers with a low α/β ratio that approximates that of normal tissue. That is, higher biologically equivalent radiation dose (BED) with HDR implants could be delivered with similar rates of morbidity as compared with LDR implants. Therefore HDR implants would seem to be ideal for prostate cancer. Further study is needed to validate this theory.

Androgen-deprivation therapy has been used with prostate cancer brachytherapy both to reduce the size of the prostate gland and to improve outcomes. Most prostate glands exhibit some decrease in volume after 3 months of androgen-deprivation therapy, with an average 30% to 40% reduction, and little further volume decreases.[513] About 10% of prostate glands will show no volume reduction at all in response to androgen deprivation. Decreasing the size of the prostate may reduce pubic arch interference in selected men. Blank and coworkers[514] reported that men treated with androgen-deprivation therapy tended to have smaller prostates that required less seed implants. However, at this point, no data suggest that smaller prostate volumes correlate with reduced early or late morbidity from brachytherapy. Furthermore, although prospective randomized trials have demonstrated improved survival in those men with locally advanced prostate cancer treated with external-beam radiotherapy and androgen-deprivation therapy, it is not clear that these results can be extrapolated to men treated with brachytherapy. A retrospective matched-pair analysis of men ($N = 60$) with prostate cancer treated at Memorial Sloan-Kettering Cancer Center showed no benefit for the addition of androgen-deprivation therapy to brachytherapy for men with low-, intermediate-, or high-risk prostate cancers.[515]

Toxicity of Brachytherapy

The short- and long-term sequelae of brachytherapy for prostate cancer differ from those of external-beam radiotherapy and radical prostatectomy (Tables 87-12 and 87-13). Kleinberg and colleagues[516] described the morbidity outcomes of the early Memorial Sloan-Kettering Cancer Center experience with permanent transperineal brachytherapy, reporting that the most common side effects were nocturia and dysuria (80% and 48%, respectively, 2 months after implantation). By 12 months after implantation, these figures had declined (to 45% and 20%). More recent assessments have focused on post-implant urinary retention, which has been observed in 3% to 14% of men and usually lasts 1 week or less.[496,501,502,517-519] The most bothersome late complications of prostate cancer brachytherapy are urethral stricture and urinary incontinence. Ragde and associates[520] reported a 5.1% incidence of urinary incontinence in men treated with

TABLE 87-12

Urinary Morbidity Associated with Prostate Brachytherapy			
SERIES	**GRADE 2**	**GRADE 3**	**URINARY RETENTION**
Brown et al. ($N = 87$)	37%	6%	6%
Lee et al. ($N = 91$)	Not specified	Not specified	12%
Stokes et al. ($N = 142$)	23%	8%	Not specified
Storey et al. ($N = 206$)	Not specified	Not specified	11%
Zelefsky et al. ($N = 248$)	55%	3%	3%

TABLE 87-13

Rectal Morbidity Associated with Prostate Brachytherapy				
SERIES	**BLEEDING**	**ULCERATION**	**FISTULA**	**COLOSTOMY**
Benoit et al. (N = 2124)	Not specified	1%	1.8%	0.7%
Merrick et al. (N = 45)	9%	0	0	0
Snyder et al. (N = 212)	10%	0	0	0
Zelefsky et al. (N = 248)	9%	0.4%	0.4%	0.4%

prostate cancer brachytherapy and followed up for 7 years; each of the men with incontinence had a history of TURP. Urethral stricture appeared in 14.4% of the men. Others also have seen an increased incidence of urinary incontinence in the setting of a history of TURP.[521] In a cohort study of Medicare beneficiaries (N = 2124) who were treated with brachytherapy, urinary incontinence was noted in 6.6%, and bladder outlet obstruction requiring intervention was found in 8.3%.[522]

Rectal morbidity after brachytherapy includes change in bowel habits, rectal bleeding or ulceration, and fistula. Kleinberg and coworkers[516] reported that 25% of men treated with prostate cancer brachytherapy had a change in bowel habits within 2 months of implant. By 12 months after implant, no patient had grade 2 or higher rectal symptoms. The 3-year actuarial incidence of rectal bleeding was 31%, and the incidence of ulceration was 16%. With more operator experience, rates of rectal complications subsequently declined: an update of the Memorial Sloan-Kettering Cancer Center experience revealed only a 9% incidence of rectal bleeding.[496] Among Medicare beneficiaries, rectal injury not requiring colostomy was reported in 5.1% of men treated with prostate cancer brachytherapy, whereas colostomy was required in 0.3%.[522] Radiation proctitis was reported in 2.2%, fistula in 1.8%, and ulceration in 1.1%.[522] Generally, the onset of late rectal complications is within 3 years of implant. Conservative measures will generally result in spontaneous resolution of bleeding. As popularity of prostate brachytherapy for clinically localized prostate cancer grew in the 1990s, a commonly cited advantage of the treatment modality was a lower incidence of treatment-associated erectile dysfunction compared with that of external-beam radiotherapy or radical prostatectomy. Undoubtedly, this selling point tipped the scales in favor of brachytherapy for many men faced with selecting a treatment for early-stage prostate cancer. For instance, Stock and colleagues[523] reported a 2-year potency rate of 94% after implant, whereas Wallner and associates[524] reported a 3-year potency rate of 86%. Studies with longer follow-up, however, have shown a continued decrease in sexual potency over time. With more long-term follow-up in other case series, only 57% of men retained potency at 5 years.[496] Even Stock and coworkers[525] subsequently reported a 6-year potency rate of 59% in their case series. Notably, their study found that 70% of men with normal erectile function before implant retained potency at 6 years, whereas men with "erectile function sufficient for intercourse" but suboptimal erections had only a 34%

6-year potency rate. In postimplant dosimetry studies, Merrick and colleagues[507] demonstrated that dose to the penile bulb correlated with postimplant erectile dysfunction. In the majority of men who retained potency, the dose delivered to 50% of the penile bulb was less than 50 Gy. Potentially, this knowledge may result in improved morbidity outcomes with technical attention to this dose threshold. Erectile dysfunction is not the sole complication of prostate brachytherapy with the potential to affect sexual quality of life, however, with reports of hematospermia in 28%, orgasmalgia in 15%, and alteration in the intensity of orgasm in 38%.[526] These side effects tend to be transient in most men.

Recently, health-related quality-of-life instruments have become available to evaluate morbidity outcomes for prostate cancer treatments. A prospective study of health-related quality-of-life outcomes in men treated with brachytherapy, external-beam radiotherapy, or radical prostatectomy was recently reported.[527] Men treated with external-beam radiotherapy did not show significant changes in health-related quality of life after completion of treatment. Men treated with brachytherapy and radical prostatectomy had significant decreases in health-related quality of life within the first month after treatment. By 12 months after treatment, health-related quality of life had returned to baseline in each of the three treatment groups.

Proton Beam Radiotherapy

Although only available at a few centers worldwide, proton-beam therapy for prostate cancer has provoked interest. The unique physical properties of protons make them ideal for the treatment of disease in close proximity to critical strictures. Specifically, protons deposit the majority of their energy at the very end of their linear tracks, a phenomenon termed the *Bragg peak*. The dose falls off very rapidly at depths beyond the Bragg peak. This is particularly useful in the treatment of prostate cancer, to minimize rectal and bladder dose. Investigators from Loma Linda University reported their experience treating men (N = 319) with T1 to T2 prostate cancer and pretreatment serum PSA of 15 ng/mL or less.[528] Men were treated with protons alone to 74 cobalt Gray equivalents (CGE) or with photons to 45 Gy followed by proton boost to 75 CGE. The 5-year PSA relapse-free survival was 88%. No severe complications of therapy were seen. The 3-year actuarial incidence of grade 2 urinary symptoms was 5%, and grade 2 rectal symptoms were found in 6%. Currently, proton-beam IMRT is being investigated in an attempt to improve on these excellent results.

Adjuvant Endocrine Therapy and Radiation Therapy for Low-Risk Localized Prostate Cancer

Androgen-deprivation therapy has been found to improve survival in randomized trials of men with high-risk prostate cancer treated with external-beam radiation therapy (Fig. 87-12).[529-531] The role of androgen-deprivation therapy in men with low-risk prostate cancer is unknown. D'Amico and associates[532] reported results of a large retrospective study (N = 1586) of men treated with 3D-CRT plus or minus androgen-deprivation therapy for low-risk, intermediate-risk, and high-risk prostate cancer. In this study, the median radiation dose was 70.2 Gy, and androgen-deprivation therapy was used for 276 of the men for 2 months before radiation therapy, during treatment, and for 2 months after treatment was completed. With a median follow-up of 51 months, the 5-year PSA relapse-free survival for men with low-risk prostate cancer was 92% with the addition of androgen-deprivation therapy versus 84% without (P = .09). Men with intermediate- and high-risk prostate cancer also fared significantly better when given androgen-deprivation therapy. RTOG Trial 94-08, which completed accrual in 2001, has been designed to ascertain whether men with stage T1b to T2 prostate cancer and a serum PSA of 20 ng/mL or less benefit from the addition of "complete androgen blockade" given for 4 months before and concomitant with external-beam radiation therapy.

Adjuvant Endocrine Therapy and Radiation Therapy for Intermediate- and High-Risk Localized Prostate Cancer

Men with intermediate-risk prostate cancer (clinical stage T2b, Gleason score of 7, or PSA ranging from 10 to 20 ng/mL) fall at a breakpoint of defined prognostic subgroups in many case series reporting treatment

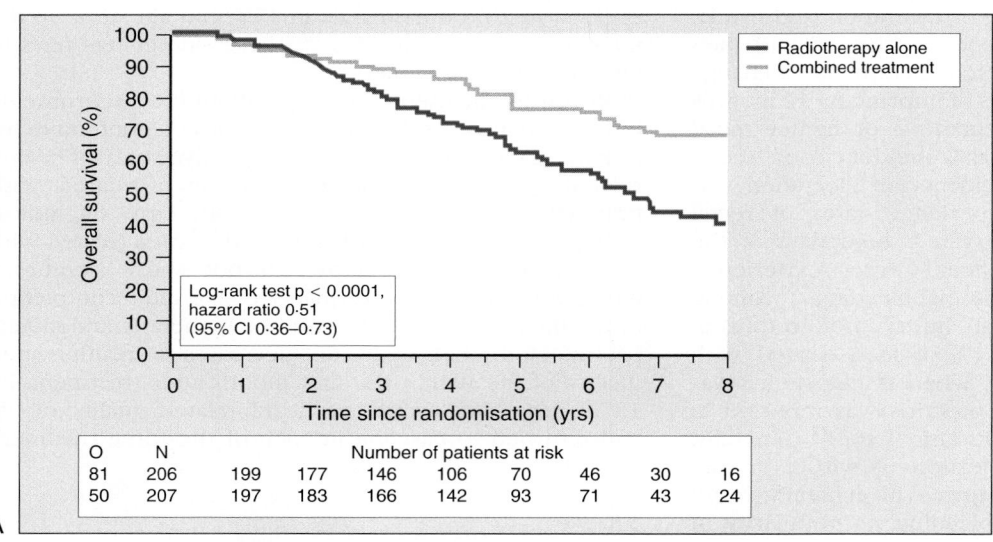

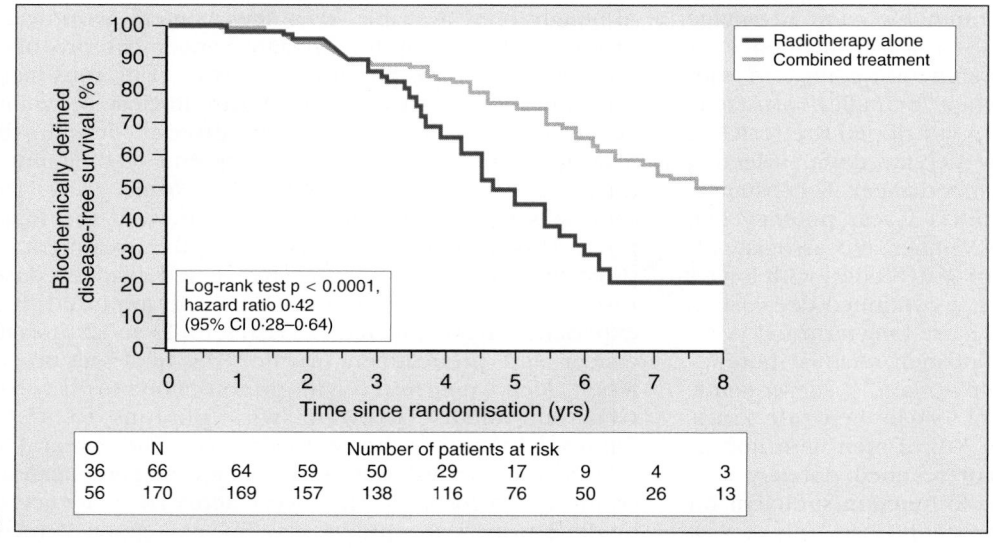

Figure 87-12. Kaplan-Meier estimates of survival for men with prostate coancer from a prospective randomized clinical trial comparing a combination of androgen-deprivation therapy (goserelin acetate for a total of 3 years with cyproterone acetate for 1 month) and radiation therapy versus radiation therapy alone. **A,** Overall survival. **B,** Relapse-free. O, number of deaths; N, number of subjects. (From Bolla M, Collette L, Blank L et al: Long-term result with immediate androgen suppression and external irradiation in patients with locally advanced prostate cancer [an EORTC study]: A phase II randomized trial. Lancet 2002;360:103–106, with permission.)

outcomes, making treatment recommendations difficult. Although dedicated phase III trials evaluating the role and technique of radiotherapy with this group of men have not been performed, intermediate-risk men are often included in studies of radiation treatment for men with both low-risk prostate cancer and more advanced disease. Radiotherapeutic options for men with intermediate-risk prostate cancer range from external-beam radiation therapy, prostate brachytherapy, to a combination of both modalities. The need for adjuvant androgen-deprivation therapy in this subset of men is debatable, but a potential benefit can be inferred from phase III clinical trials and single-institution case series.

High-risk prostate cancer (clinical stage T2c to T4, Gleason score of 8 to 10, or serum PSA >20 ng/mL) is usually treated with androgen-deprivation therapy in conjunction with radiation therapy. The optimal duration and sequencing of androgen-deprivation therapy, however, remains to be determined. Brachytherapy, usually in conjunction with both androgen-deprivation therapy and external-beam radiation therapy, also has been used to treat men with high-risk prostate cancer.

Adjuvant Endocrine Therapy and Radiation Therapy for Locally Advanced Prostate Cancer

Combined-modality treatment, using androgen-deprivation therapy in conjunction with external-beam radiation therapy, takes advantage of separate and noncompeting modes of cell death, such that cells that can survive the insult of one modality cannot survive the other or the additive/synergistic properties of the two.[533-536] Androgen-deprivation therapy has been used along with radiation therapy for many years in an attempt to modify the outcome of men with stage C (T3) prostate cancer. Historically, the rationale for this treatment approach was that these men had an inferior outcome when compared with men with earlier stage prostate cancer treated with radiation therapy. In addition, the tumors were often quite bulky, and it was thought that a course of cytoreductive therapy might provide a more favorable geometry for external irradiation.[537] However, the use of androgen-deprivation therapy in combination with radiation was not universally accepted throughout the 1970s and 1980s. Radiation therapy techniques were improving, and the results from early case series exploring the benefit of androgen-deprivation therapy before or during radiation therapy or both were often negative.[538,539] In the early 1980s, two case series reported encouraging results with the use of androgen-deprivation therapy and external-beam radiation therapy to treat men with locally advanced prostate cancer.[537,540] Pilepich and coworkers[541] also found that men with histologically unfavorable prostate cancers who had been treated with androgen-deprivation therapy and external-beam radiation therapy as part of the RTOG 75-06 trial exhibited similar disease-free survival and overall survival rates as did men with more favorable prostate cancers who did not receive androgen-deprivation therapy along with radiation therapy. More recently, phase III clinical trials have established the local

control and survival benefits of androgen-deprivation therapy given along with external-beam radiation therapy for locally advanced prostate cancer. The advantage of androgen-deprivation therapy before irradiation, as opposed to starting both androgen-deprivation therapy and external-beam radiation therapy together, has never been established by a head-to-head comparison. RTOG 86-10 was a randomized phase III clinical trial of external-beam radiation therapy alone (standard treatment arm) versus neoadjuvant and concomitant total androgen suppression and external-beam radiation therapy (experimental treatment arm).[542,543] Eligible men had bulky (>25 cm^2) locally advanced prostate cancer (stage T2b to T4, N0 to N1, M0). Men randomized to receive total androgen suppression were treated with goserelin acetate, 3.6 mg every 28 days, and flutamide, 250 mg 3 times daily for 2 months before the start of, and during, radiation therapy. Standard radiation techniques were used, with 45 Gy delivered to the pelvis followed by a 20- to 25-Gy boost to the prostate. Extended fields were used to treat the lymph nodes when they were involved. A total of 471 men were enrolled and randomized to one of the two treatment arms. Analysis of the trial results revealed that men treated with total androgen suppression and radiation had a significant improvement in local control at 5 years compared with those men treated with radiation only ($P < .001$). A recent update of this trial, with a median follow-up over 6 years, continues to report a statistically significant difference in the 5-year probability of local treatment failure (22% vs. 35%, $P = .004$) as well as an increase in both disease-free survival (33% vs. 21%, $P = .004$) and cause-specific mortality (23% vs. 31%, $P = .05$), when considering the entire group, in favor of combined treatment. In subset analyses, an improvement in overall survival was noted for those men with Gleason score 2 to 6 prostate cancer (70% vs. 52%, $P = .015$), in favor of combined treatment.[542] This improvement in overall survival was not seen when evaluating all men in the study. This has several possible explanations. It is possible that an overall survival benefit for men may not exist when total androgen suppression is added in this fashion and/or in this patient population as a whole. However, it is important to note that this study was limited in that it did not routinely obtain serum PSA levels from all men before entry, a parameter now recognized to be an extremely important prognostic factor and indicator of disease extension. Therefore a large number of men likely had elevated serum PSA levels in the range frequently associated with a high risk for micrometastatic prostate cancer. The study also included men with node-positive disease, also recognized to be a poor risk factor, for which the value of any treatment modality to overall survival can be debated. Nonetheless, this was an important study, performed in a rigorous fashion, and revealing important and measurable benefits attributable to the addition of androgen-deprivation therapy to external-beam radiation therapy for these men with prostate cancer.

The RTOG 85-31 Trial also targeted men with loco-regionally advanced prostate cancer, including men who had undergone radical prostatectomy and were identified at pathologic examination as being at high risk.[531,544]

The aim of this phase III trial was to evaluate the role of long-term adjuvant androgen suppression in men with high-risk prostate cancer. Men enrolled on the trial who underwent definitive radiation were those with clinical stage T3 (>25 cm^2), or T1 to T2 disease and radiographic or histologic lymph node involvement. Men were eligible after prostatectomy if prostate cancer with capsular penetration and positive surgical margins or with seminal vesicle involvement was found. A total of 945 evaluable men were enrolled and followed up for a median of 4.5 years. Conventional radiotherapy techniques were used to deliver a total dose of 44 to 46 Gy to the whole pelvis with a boost of 20 to 25 Gy to the prostate or postoperative prostatic fossa for a total dose of 65 to 70 Gy. Androgen-deprivation therapy was accomplished by using goserelin acetate, 3.6 mg monthly beginning the last week of radiation therapy. Actuarial projections at 5 years revealed 84% of men receiving adjuvant androgen deprivation versus 71% of men on the observation arm remained without evidence of local recurrence (P < .0001). The corresponding figures for freedom from distant metastases and disease-free survival were 83% versus 70% (P < .001) and 60% and 44% (P < .0001). The 5-year survival rate for the entire population was 75% on the adjuvant androgen-deprivation arm versus 71% on the observation arm (P = .52). However, in men with prostate cancers with a Gleason score of 8 to 10, a statistically significant difference in actuarial 5-year survival of 66% versus 55% favoring the adjuvant androgen-deprivation arm was evident (P = .03). A recent update of this trial with a median follow-up of 5.6 years confirmed the statistically significant improvement in both absolute and cause-specific survival for adjuvant androgen deprivation given with external-beam radiation therapy.[544]

Bolla and colleagues[529,530] published results of the European Organization for Research and Treatment of Cancer (EORTC) 22863 trial. This phase III trial enrolled 415 men with stage T3 to T4 prostate cancer of any grade or stage T1 to T2 World Health Organization (WHO) grade 3 prostate cancer with no evidence of nodal or metastatic disease. Men were randomized to receive either external-beam radiation therapy alone (control arm) or androgen-deprivation therapy plus external-beam radiation therapy (experimental arm). Androgen deprivation consisted of oral cyproterone acetate, 50 mg 3 times daily for 4 weeks before radiation, and goserelin acetate, 3.6 mg started on the first day of radiation and continued every month for 3 years. Radiation therapy was delivered as 50 Gy to prostate and regional lymph nodes, followed by a 20-Gy boost to the prostate, for a total prostate dose of 70 Gy. A total of 401 men were studied, with a median follow-up of 45 months. Overall survival at 5 years for the entire population was 79% in the androgen-deprivation therapy plus external-beam radiation therapy arm and 62% in the external-beam radiation therapy alone arm (P = .001). The local recurrence-free survival was 97% for men treated with androgen-deprivation therapy plus external-beam radiation therapy versus 77% for men treated with external-beam radiation therapy alone (P < .001). The relapse-free survival was reported to be 85% for combined treatment and 48% for radiation alone (P < .001). A recent update of this trial, at a median follow-up of 66 months, confirmed the durability of these initial results with 5-year overall survival of 78% versus 62%, favoring the androgen-deprivation therapy plus external-beam radiation therapy arm (P = .0002).[530] Five-year relapse-free survival also continued to favor the combination treatment (74% vs. 40%). The RTOG 92-02 Trial, which completed accrual in 2000, is a phase III prospective randomized trial of androgen-deprivation therapy plus external-beam radiation therapy for men with locally advanced prostate cancer.[545] This study compared the efficacy of short-term androgen deprivation, as was administered in RTOG 86-10, with that of long-term androgen deprivation, similar to that used in the EORTC 22863 trial. A total of 1554 men with locally advanced prostate cancer stage T2c to T4 with serum PSA less than 150 ng/mL were enrolled in the trial and followed up for a median of 4.8 years. All men received 4 months of goserelin acetate and flutamide, 2 months before and during radiation therapy. Men were then randomized either to receive no further therapy (short-term androgen deprivation) or to be treated with goserelin acetate for an additional 24 months (long-term androgen deprivation). Radiation dose was 65 to 70 Gy to the prostate and 44 to 50 Gy to pelvic nodes. At 5 years, the long-term androgen-deprivation group showed significant improvement in disease-free survival of 54% versus 34% (P = .0001), in clinical local progression of 6.2% versus 13% (P = .0001), and in freedom from distant metastasis of 11% versus 17% (P = .001). Five-year overall survival was not significantly different between the two treatment arms (78% vs. 79%). Subset analyses were performed for direct comparison of this trial with both the EORTC 22863 and RTOG 85-31 studies. The first subset included men with high-risk prostate cancer defined by clinical stage T3 to T4 or stage T2 with a Gleason score of 8 to 10 for comparison with the results reported by Bolla and associates.[529,530] No overall survival difference (77% vs. 80%) was noted at 5 years, but a significant advantage in disease-free survival for long-term androgen deprivation of 90% versus 86% (P = .03). A second subset included all men with Gleason 8 to 10 prostate cancer for comparison with results from RTOG 85-31.[543] Five-year overall survival (80% vs. 69%, P = .02) and disease-free survival (90% vs. 78%, P = .007) were significantly better with long-term androgen deprivation.

The results of RTOG 92-02 have helped to establish the superiority of more protracted courses of androgen-deprivation therapy for men with high-risk or locally advanced disease. The optimal sequencing of androgen-deprivation therapy and radiation, however, has come into question. To date, it is not known whether the effects of androgen-deprivation therapy on prostate cancer control were merely additive to the tumoricidal effects of radiation or were synergistic, providing an enhancement of tumor killing. Of interest in this regard, RTOG 94-13 trial compared whole-pelvic radiation with prostate-only radiation and neoadjuvant and concomitant androgen-deprivation therapy, given 2 months before and 2 months during radiation therapy, with adjuvant androgen-deprivation therapy, given after completion of radiation treatment for 4 months.[546] A total of 1295 men with prostate cancer and an estimated risk of lymph node involvement of more than 15% were randomized to one of the four treatment arms. No difference in outcome was found for neoadjuvant versus adjuvant androgen-deprivation therapy; however, this may be confounded by a lead-time bias because the follow-up time for men on the neoadjuvant arm is 2 months longer than that on the adjuvant arm. When comparing all four of the treatment arms, a PFS advantage was seen for the whole-pelvis radiation therapy plus neoadjuvant and concomitant androgen-deprivation therapy arm versus the other three arms (61% vs. 45%, 49%, and 47%, respectively; P = .005). The follow-up (median, 59.5 months) is too short to detect adequately a difference in overall survival.

Risk of Pelvic Lymph Node Involvement and Determination of Radiation Field Size

Considerable effort has been directed at defining the optimal radiation-treatment volumes for men with prostate cancer. Men with high-risk prostate cancer are of particular interest in this regard, as no universally accepted standard of care exists for this group of men with a defined risk of pelvic lymph node involvement. The rationale for prophylactic irradiation of pelvic lymph nodes is based on well-established surgical data that predict a rate of lymph node positivity ranging from 5% to 50% for men with prostate cancer and one or more high-risk features.[547] Since the advent of 3D-CRT and its progressive refinement into more accurate dose-delivery techniques, the debate over whether to treat pelvic nodes has intensified. Because a potentially higher risk of complications may be associated with whole-pelvis irradiation, it would be considered desirable not to treat such a large radiation portal if it were not beneficial. The RTOG 77-06 trial found no advantage to pelvic radiation for men with T1/T2 prostate cancer.[548] However, this study included men estimated to be at low risk for lymph node involvement, including some proven to be pathologically lymph node negative. RTOG 76-05, which randomized men with T3/T4 disease to pelvis-only versus pelvic and para-aortic radiation therapy, also failed to detect an advantage for the extended radiation-treatment field.[549] This trial has often been misinterpreted as suggesting that no role exists for radiation of pelvic nodes in men with prostate cancer, although it really examined only the efficacy of para-aortic radiation.

More recently, results of the phase III randomized RTOG 94-13 trial have provided further insight into the use of larger radiation fields.[546] The details of the study were described earlier. In brief, the study featured a 2 × 2 factorial design comparing whole-pelvic radiation with prostate-only radiation (and neoadjuvant and concomitant androgen-deprivation therapy with adjuvant androgen-deprivation therapy). Whole-pelvis radiation therapy consisted of a conventional four-field technique with a minimum field size of 16 × 16 cm treated to a maximum dose of 50.4 Gy. An additional 19.8 Gy was then delivered to the prostate by using a conedown boost technique. Prostate-only radiation therapy was limited to the prostate and seminal vesicles, with a maximum field size of 11 ×

11 cm to a total dose of 70.2 Gy. Four-year PFS was 56% for whole-pelvic radiation therapy compared with 46% for prostate-only radiation therapy (P = .014), with no difference in overall survival. No significant difference was seen in immediate or late gastrointestinal or genitourinary toxicities between the two treatment approaches.

Postprostatectomy Adjuvant Radiation Therapy

Pathologic features that portend a higher risk of local recurrence are common after radical prostatectomy.[550] A positive surgical margin is associated with an approximately 50% risk of prostate cancer recurrence.[465,550-553] Other features associated with recurrence are extracapsular extension, seminal vesicle invasion, and Gleason score of 7 or greater. Several retrospective series have now demonstrated improved PSA relapse-free survival with the addition of adjuvant radiation therapy after radical prostatectomy in men with these risk factors (Table 87-14).[554-556] In one study, some men (N = 52) with pathologic stage T3N0 prostate cancer and an undetectable postoperative serum PSA received adjuvant radiation therapy to a median dose of 64.8 Gy, whereas others with the same characteristics (N = 97) underwent no further treatment.[554] In a matched-pair analysis, the 5-year freedom-from-PSA relapse rate was 89% in the adjuvant radiation therapy group versus 55% for treatment with surgery alone (P < .01). Taylor and coworkers[556] recently summarized the M.D. Anderson Cancer Center experience of men (N = 75) with prostate cancer and adverse pathologic features who had an undetectable PSA after prostatectomy that were treated with radiation to a median dose of 60 Gy. The 5-year freedom-from-PSA relapse rate for these men was 88%. Those with seminal vesicle involvement had a 5-year freedom-from-PSA relapse rate of only 65%, as compared with 94% for men without seminal vesicle involvement. In the largest reported case series to date (N = 423), men with pathologic stage T3N0 prostate cancer were treated with adjuvant radiation therapy to a median dose of 48 Gy with a median follow-up of 7 years.[555] For these men, the serum PSA was less than 0.05 ng/mL in 69% at 5 years and in 51% at 10 years. Overall survival at 5 and 10 years was 92% and 73%, respectively. By multivariate analysis, seminal vesicle involvement and Gleason score of 7 or higher portended worse treatment outcome, with less than 20% free-from-PSA relapse at 10 years.

Salvage Radiotherapy after Radical Prostatectomy

Salvage radiotherapy refers to the use of radiation therapy after prostatectomy in the setting of recognized prostate cancer recurrence. As many as 27% to 53% of men who undergo radical prostatectomy for prostate cancer will have a detectable PSA within 10 years of surgery.[437] Subsequently, approximately 25% of men who undergo radical prostatectomy will be treated with salvage radiation therapy for recurrent prostate cancer.[557] In the setting of persistent or increasing serum PSA after radical

TABLE 87-14

Salvage Radiation Therapy for Men with a Persistently Elevated or Rising Serum PSA after Radical Prostatectomy

SERIES	RADIATION DOSE (GY)	FOLLOW-UP (MO)	DISEASE FREE (%)	PROGNOSTIC FACTORS
Allison et al. (N = 14)	65	35–56	64	
Anscher et al. (N = 89)	66	48	53	Dose, >65 Gy
Cadeddu et al. (N = 57)	64	40	20	
Catton et al. (N = 59)	60	44	5–30	Pre-RT PSA, <2 ng/mL; Gleason score
Coetzee et al. (N = 15)	66–70	33	20	
Crane et al. (N = 41)	60	55	24	Pre-RT PSA, <2.7 ng/mL
Do et al. (N = 60)	64.8	36	55	Pre-RT PSA, <1 ng/mL; no perineural invasion
Egawa et al. (N = 32)	58.7	35	34	Time to postoperative relapse, >12 mo
Forman et al. (N = 47)	66	36	64	Pre-RT PSA, <2 ng/mL; SV or LN involvement
Garg et al. (N = 78)	66	25	64	Pre-RT PSA, <2 ng/mL
Hudson et al. (N = 21)	60	13	29	
Kaplan et al. (N = 39)	60–70	27	44	
Katz et al. (N = 115)	66.6	42	46	Negative/close margins, absence of extracapsular extension, SV involvement
Keisch et al. (N = 10)	60	5	50	
Lange et al. (N = 42)	60	22	38	
Link et al. (N = 25)	60	18	32	Pre-RT PSA, <1.1 ng/mL
McCarthy et al. (N = 37)	60–65	33	54	
Medini et al. (N = 40)	59.5	>60	27	
Morris et al. (N = 48)	60–64	32	47	
Nudell et al. (N = 69)	68	35	53	Preoperative PSA, <20 ng/mL
Partin et al. (N = 20)	65	24	10	
Peschel et al. (N = 39)	61.2	37	27	
Pisansky et al. (N = 166)	64	52	46	Pre-RT PSA; Gleason score; SV involvement
Schild et al. (N = 46)	64	37	50	Pre-RT PSA, <1.1 ng/mL; dose, >64 Gy
Song et al. (N = 61)	66.6	36	48	Pre-RT PSA, <1 ng/mL; Gleason score
Taylor et al. (N = 71)	70	35	66	Time to post-op PSA increase
Valicenti et al. (N = 34)	64.8	32	59	Pre-RT PSA, <2 ng/mL; dose, >64.8 Gy

LN, lymph node; PSA, prostate-specific antigen; RT, radiation therapy; SV, seminal vesicle.
From Song DY, Thompson TL, Ramakrishnan V, et al: Salvage radiotherapy for rising or persistent PSA after radical prostatectomy. Urology 2002;60:281–287, with permission.

prostatectomy, it is important to rule out distant metastatic prostate cancer with bone scan, chest radiography, and CT scan of the abdomen and pelvis, before the initiation of salvage radiation therapy. Partin and colleagues[558] correlated the rate of serum PSA increase with likelihood of local versus distant relapse after surgery. A serum PSA increase of 0.75 ng/mL/yr was associated with local recurrence. In 1999, an ASTRO consensus panel concluded that treatment of men with local prostate cancer recurrence after radical prostatectomy who had a pre–radiation therapy serum PSA of less than 1.5 ng/mL was more likely to be successful.[559] In addition, doses greater than 64 Gy were recommended in the salvage setting. Several studies have demonstrated a Gleason score greater than 7 to be associated with a low likelihood of successful salvage after prostate cancer recurrence after prostatectomy.[460,560-562] Cadeddu and associates[560] reported no men free of PSA relapse treated with salvage radiation therapy after prostatectomy for prostate cancer with Gleason scores of 8 or higher.[62] Similarly, Song and coworkers[562] found only 2 of 14 men with a Gleason score of 8 or higher to be prostate cancer free at the time of analysis. These results indicate that men with recurrent prostate cancer and a Gleason score of 8 or greater are unlikely to benefit from salvage radiation therapy because of the likelihood of microscopic systemic prostate cancer

metastases. In the Memorial Sloan-Kettering series of salvage 3D-CRT, four independent predictors of PSA relapse after salvage radiation therapy were identified: preradiation therapy PSA more than 0.6 ng/mL, "negative" surgical margins, Gleason score 8 and higher, and seminal vesicle involvement.[563] Men with no risk factors, one risk factor, two risk factors, and three to four risk factors had PSA relapse-free survivals at 4 years of 94%, 55%, 21%, and 0, respectively. In a case series from M.D. Anderson Cancer Center, a distinction was made between men treated with salvage radiation therapy for persistently elevated serum PSA after prostatectomy versus men treated for a delayed increase in serum PSA after surgery: the 5-year freedom-from-PSA relapse rates were 43% and 78%, respectively.[556] These data may aid in the selection of men who may or may not benefit from salvage radiation therapy for prostate cancer recurrence after radical prostatectomy.

The role of androgen-deprivation therapy concomitant with radiation therapy given as an adjuvant to surgery or as salvage for prostate cancer recurrence after surgery has not been established. In the RTOG 85-31 trial, a subgroup of men with pathologic T3N0 prostate cancer who underwent radical prostatectomy received adjuvant radiation therapy to a dose of 60 to 65 Gy and then were randomized to immediate androgen deprivation or androgen deprivation initiated at the time of PSA relapse.[564] At 5 years, 65% of men treated with immediate androgen deprivation versus 42% of men treated with delayed androgen deprivation were free of PSA relapse. No prospective trials examined the addition of androgen-deprivation therapy to salvage radiation therapy for local prostate cancer recurrence after prostatectomy. Taylor and colleagues[556] reported a benefit to the addition of androgen-deprivation therapy to salvage radiation therapy in a retrospective case series. In this series, adjuvant androgen-deprivation therapy was given to men who received salvage radiation therapy for a median duration of 24 months. At 5 years, 81% of men receiving androgen-deprivation therapy (vs. 54% not treated with androgen deprivation) were free of PSA relapse. In contrast, Song and associates[562] reported identical median disease-free survivals of 26 months for men treated with or without concurrent androgen-deprivation therapy along with salvage radiation therapy for prostate cancer recurrence. The 1999 ASTRO Consensus Panel concluded that insufficient evidence existed to support routine use of androgen-deprivation therapy with postprostatectomy radiation therapy.[559]

Toxicity of Postprostatectomy Radiation Therapy

In general, men receiving radiation therapy after prostatectomy experience little in the way of additional morbidity.[565] The incidence of urinary incontinence does not seem to be increased, and erectile function does not seem to be worsened in men treated with adjuvant radiation therapy after prostatectomy.[566,567] Bastasch and coworkers[568] reported that 100% of men who were potent after nerve-sparing radical prostatectomy remained potent after adjuvant IMRT.

SYSTEMIC TREATMENT OF METASTATIC CANCER

Natural History of Metastatic Prostate Cancer

Over the past decade, widespread and routine clinical use of serum PSA testing has changed not only screening and diagnosis of prostate cancer, but also virtually all aspects of prostate cancer management.[569,570] Current estimates of prostate cancer incidence by stage illustrate a major prostate cancer stage migration with a categorical shift toward less advanced cancer at the time of diagnosis. Similarly, outcome data from large cohorts and from contemporary large-scale prospective randomized clinical trials reveal that time-to-progression and survival from prostate cancer have changed substantially over the past decade. Previously collected outcome data must be scrutinized and considered in the context of more contemporary findings before making treatment recommendations or designing new clinical trials. For example, for men with newly diagnosed metastatic prostate cancer who have not received androgen-suppression therapy (stage D2 disease; sometimes referred to as "hormone naïve"), randomized

prospective trials conducted before the serum PSA testing era have consistently shown a median time-to-progression ranging between 12 and 18 months, and a median survival ranging between 24 and 30 months. Men with limited metastatic prostate cancer (appendicular skeleton or nonvisceral soft tissue metastases or both) tended to have a median survival of 52 months, whereas men with extensive bony metastases or visceral disease or both had a median survival of 24 months. The distribution of men with prostate cancer according to extent of disease in the earlier studies typically included as many as 80% with extensive metastatic disease, whereas more contemporary studies often have fewer than 50% of men in this category. In a recent case series, the median metastasis-free survival of men with recurrent prostate cancer after radical prostatectomy at the Johns Hopkins Hospital who underwent routine yearly follow-ups, with serial serum PSA determinations and bone scans, from the time of biochemical relapse after surgery, was more than 6 years.[437] One explanation for the relatively long survival of these men may be that the overwhelming majority of the men in whom distant metastasis developed had limited metastatic disease, most likely due to an increased lead time in diagnosis of metastatic prostate cancer resulting from intensive follow-up featuring serum PSA assays.

This lead-time effect also is apparent in men with prostate cancer progression after initial androgen-deprivation therapy. The survival of androgen-independent (sometimes called "hormone refractory") men with prostate cancer in chemotherapy trials conducted over a decade ago ranged between 6 and 12 months, whereas in more contemporary studies, median survival has ranged between 15 and 20 months. Furthermore, a large and increasing proportion of men with metastatic prostate cancer who progress after initial androgen-deprivation therapy are first identified because of increasing serum PSA values without other evidence of prostate cancer progression. Not unexpectedly, survival for men with serum PSA increases as the only manifestation of prostate cancer progression is significantly longer than that for men with evidence of radiologic and/or clinical progression (new findings on physical examination or cancer-related symptoms or both) in addition to increasing serum PSA levels. A number of prognostic models for men with metastatic prostate cancer, both before and after androgen-deprivation therapy, have been reported. The models consistently identified similar prostate cancer features and host factors as independent predictors for a variety of adverse outcomes (Table 87-15).[571] However, in view of the lead-time effect of prostate cancer recurrence or progression recognized by serum PSA increases evident in comparison to prostate cancer recurrence or progression defined more conventionally (by using clinical and radiological criteria), new prognostic models incorporating serum PSA progression may be needed.

Endocrine Approaches to Prostate Cancer Treatment

The dependence of prostate cancer cells on androgens for growth and differentiation has been has been well

TABLE 87-15

Prognostic Factors for Men with Androgen-Independent Prostate Cancer Treated with Chemotherapy

PROGNOSTIC FACTOR	SIGNIFICANCE
Performance status	Definite: seen in virtually all studies
Baseline hemoglobin	
Liver metastases (metastasis to other visceral sites)	Possible: seen in some studies (associations detected by using multivariate
Baseline serum acid phosphatase, alkaline phosphatase,	analysis of uncontrolled clinical trials; not shown to be correlated
lactate dehydrogenase	with survival in randomized trials)
Time from initiation of androgen-deprivation therapy to initiation	
of chemotherapy	
Response to chemotherapy (reduction in measurable cancer	
deposits and/or ≥50% decline in serum PSA for ≥4 wk)	
Baseline serum PSA	
Extent of disease (on bone scan)	Equivocal: more data needed
Continuation of androgen-deprivation therapy	

PSA, prostate-specific antigen.

recognized for at least five decades.[572] Testosterone, produced by Leydig cells in the testes on stimulation by LH, is converted to DHT by the action of 5α-reductase.[12] DHT, a more potent androgen than testosterone, binds to intracellular androgen receptors to activate the expression of target genes.[13,14] Androgen-deprivation therapy for prostate cancer involves maneuvers that reduce circulating testosterone to levels around or below levels present in castrated men (<50 ng/mL). Forced reduction of testosterone levels by castration, or via gonadal suppression, triggers a wave of apoptosis in both normal and neoplastic prostate cells, with few or no immediate effects on non-androgen target tissues, providing one of the most

effective systemic palliative treatments known for solid organ cancers. Unfortunately, despite the magnitude of the initial beneficial treatment response, prostate cancer inexorably evolves to androgen independence.[24] No therapeutic maneuver has been shown to prevent this sequence of progression.

Strategies for Androgen Deprivation

Currently, a general consensus holds that a reduction in testosterone produced by the testes represents the best standard approach to androgen-deprivation therapy for prostate cancer. This can be accomplished by surgical removal of the testis (bilateral orchiectomy), by inhibition of the synthesis and release of pituitary gonadotropins by gonadotropin hormone–releasing hormone analogs (GnRH or LHRH analogs and LHRH antagonists), or by the administration of pharmacologic doses of estrogens (Fig. 87-13).

Bilateral orchiectomy results in a rapid decline of testosterone to 5% to 10% of normal values and remains the treatment of choice for severely symptomatic patients; although the suppression of testosterone production associated with LHRH analogs is comparable to that with bilateral orchiectomy, the nadir of serum testosterone levels is not reached until after 3 to 4 weeks of treatment. The LHRH analogs, highly potent LHRH agonists, initially stimulate LH release by the pituitary, but on prolonged administration, subsequently suppress LH and testosterone production.[573,574] Thus LHRH analog treatment also is associated with an initial increase in LH and in serum testosterone in virtually all patients. This brief elevation of testosterone levels has been reported to be associated with a flare of the prostate cancer, manifested by an increase in pain in symptomatic patients, or by more worrisome consequences of prostate cancer progression, including epidural cord compression and urinary obstruction.[575] Longer-acting depot preparations of LHRH analogs (administered monthly, every 3 or 4 months, or yearly) are available for clinical use. Clinical trials comparing bilateral orchiectomy with a

SYSTEMIC TREATMENT OF MEN WITH METASTATIC PROSTATE CANCER

Androgen-deprivation therapy, usually accomplished through the administration of luteinizing hormone–releasing hormone (LHRH) agonists, remains the standard treatment approach for men with symptomatic metastatic prostate cancer. In certain cases, antiandrogens are used to prevent the flare reaction associated with initiating LHRH-agonist treatment.

With the widespread use of serum prostate-specific antigen (PSA) testing as a monitoring tool for prostate cancer relapse after surgery or radiation therapy, a major new challenge has confronted physicians who treat patients with prostate cancer: many men with recurrent prostate cancer have no symptoms attributable to the disease and no evident metastatic cancer deposits that can be detected by radiographic imaging. Which of these men should be considered for treatment and when should treatment be initiated? Although these issues have not been fully resolved, available data indicate that the time between surgery or radiation therapy and PSA relapse, the Gleason score at the time of primary treatment, and the PSA doubling time are predictive of the risk and timing of overt metastatic prostate cancer. Men at high risk for progressive metastatic prostate cancer are likely the best candidates for systemic treatment.

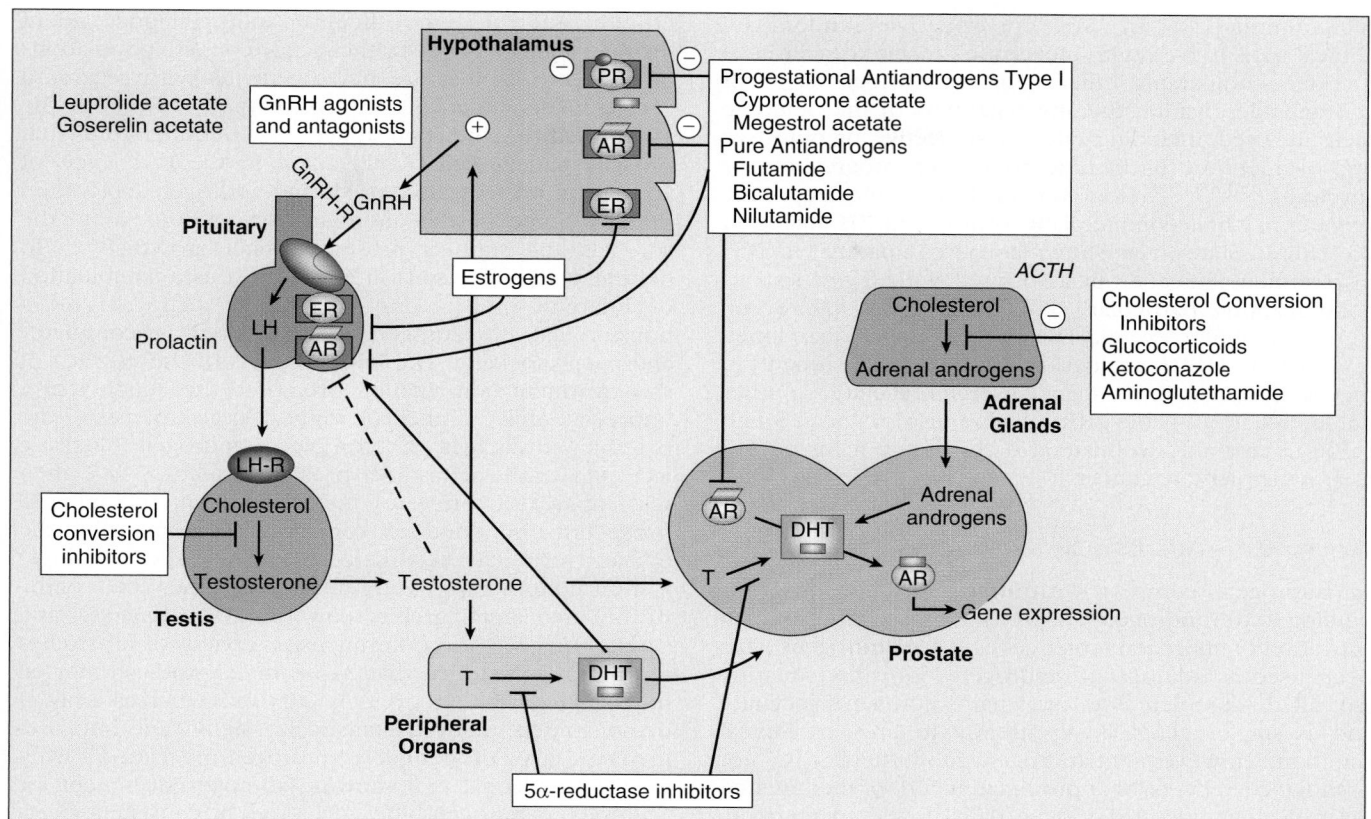

Figure 87-13. Sites of action of different treatments that affect androgen action.

variety of LHRH analogs have revealed comparable short-term and long-term efficacy in patients with metastatic prostate cancer. Because of convenience and the ability to avoid surgery, LHRH analogs have become the most widely used method for reducing serum testosterone. New LHRH antagonists have been introduced to achieve a reduction in serum testosterone without the brief flare associated with initial stimulation of pituitary gonadotropin secretion and testicular androgen production associated with LHRH analogs. These agents appear to be generally as effective as LHRH analogs, achieving a faster suppression of gonadal androgen production to the castrate range with comparable long-term sustained reductions of serum testosterone and no evidence of flare reactions.[576] The efficacy of LHRH antagonists as treatments for prostate cancer, in comparison to bilateral orchiectomy or to LHRH analogs, has not been fully evaluated. Nonetheless, because LHRH agonists can rapidly reduce the serum testosterone, like bilateral orchiectomy, these agents may well offer an attractive alternative to LHRH analogs for the treatment of men with symptomatic prostate cancer for whom a flare reaction might threaten significant morbidity.

The administration of pharmacologic doses of synthetic estrogens represented the earliest strategy for drug treatment of prostate cancer.[577] Initial studies using diethylstilbestrol (DES) revealed a dose-dependent suppression of serum testosterone to the castrate range. When used

for prostate cancer progression, DES provided clinical benefits comparable to those achieved with bilateral orchiectomy. In a clinical trial conducted by the Veterans Administration Cooperative Urological Research Group (VACURG Study 1), men with prostate cancer treated with DES had a prostate cancer–specific survival comparable to that of men treated with bilateral orchiectomy.[577,578] However, men in this study treated with DES (at a 5-mg daily dose) had a high incidence of cardiovascular deaths.[579] A subsequent clinical trial (VACURG Study 2) evaluated different daily doses of DES (0.2 mg, 1.0 mg, and 5.0 mg) versus placebo.[577,578] Results suggested that the 1.0-mg daily DES dose was as effective as the 5.0-mg daily dose in terms of prostate cancer deaths, but was associated with a lower incidence of fatal cardiovascular complications. Subsequent analyses of men treated with DES at a daily dose of 1 mg revealed that testosterone was often not adequately suppressed, especially in younger patients with initially normal gonadal function.[577,578,580] All of these findings led to recommendation that DES, at a 3-mg daily dose (known to result in effective long-term suppression of testosterone comparable to that of bilateral orchiectomy), constituted an effective prostate cancer treatment, although the safety and efficacy of this DES dose, relative to lower or higher doses, remain untested in prospective randomized clinical trials. With the ready availability of LHRH analogs, synthetic estrogens are not commonly used for prostate cancer treatment.

Specific Malignancies

III

Accumulated data from prospective randomized clinical trials in men with metastatic prostate cancer have revealed comparable efficacy of the various forms of androgen-deprivation therapy, regardless of the outcome measure used, including rates of subjective or objective improvement or both, time to cancer progression, or survival.[572,578,581-586] However, in 1984, after leuprolide acetate, the first commercially available LHRH analog in the United States, was shown to be comparable to DES in treatment efficacy but associated with fewer serious complications, particularly congestive heart failure and thromboembolic events, DES was virtually abandoned in favor of LHRH analogs for the initial treatment of metastatic prostate cancer. Goserelin acetate, another commercially available LHRH analog, also has been found to be comparable to bilateral orchiectomy in men with metastatic prostate cancer.

Antiandrogens and 5α-Reductase Inhibitors

Antiandrogens compete with androgenic hormones for binding to the androgen receptor, blocking transcriptional activation of androgen target genes.[24] Antiandrogens have been used as adjuncts to androgen-deprivation therapy (so-called "complete" or "maximal" androgen blockage) and as single agents, in an attempt to preserve sexual function. However, antiandrogen monotherapy is not without side effects: In approximately 50% of men treated with bicalutamide at a 150-mg daily dose, gynecomastia develops, and although libido can often be maintained, fewer men remain potent.[587] Bicalutamide monotherapy has been reported to provide similar survival outcomes as bilateral orchiectomy in men with nonmetastatic advanced prostate cancer (stage T3 and T4).[587] Nonetheless, antiandrogens used alone appear inferior to androgen-deprivation therapy in prospective randomized clinical trials in men with metastatic prostate cancer.[587] The efficacy of antiandrogens used earlier in the natural history of prostate cancer (as adjuvant therapy for men with high-risk prostate cancer treated with radical prostatectomy or as treatment for men with an increasing serum PSA after failure of cancer control with primary therapy) remains to be established. Flutamide, bicalutamide, and nilutamide are the nonsteroidal antiandrogens available currently in the United States.

Although DHT is a more potent androgen than testosterone, 5α-reductase inhibitors have not been found to be particularly effective in the treatment of metastatic prostate cancer when used alone.[255] A combination of the type 2 5α-reductase inhibitor finasteride and the nonsteroidal antiandrogen flutamide has been explored in clinical trials; the results obtained do not suggest any striking advantage for combination treatment.[588] Dutasteride, an inhibitor of both type 1 and type 2 5α-reductases, has not been fully tested against prostate cancer.

"Complete" Androgen Blockade

A substantial amount of basic research has been devoted to enhancing the understanding of critical mechanisms involved in the hormonal control of prostate cancer growth and the emergence of androgen-independent prostate cancer.[24] Prostate cancers contain populations of cancer cells that are heterogeneous with regard to androgen dependency and sensitivity.[141,143,589,590] In the 1980s, Labrie and colleagues[591,592] hypothesized that prostate cancer cells could adapt to the low levels of androgens present after or during androgen-deprivation therapy. Some of the androgens are produced by the adrenals and support prostate cancer growth.[591,592] To neutralize the effects of adrenal androgens, a combination of bilateral orchiectomy (or LHRH analogs) and a nonsteroidal antiandrogen was promoted as "complete" androgen blockade. The initial reports of the efficacy of this treatment combination prompted the conduct of a unprecedented number of clinical trials to assess the possible advantages of "complete" androgen blockade for men with metastatic prostate cancer: 7987 men with metastatic prostate cancer were entered into 27 prospective randomized clinical trials comparing the efficacy of bilateral orchiectomy (or LHRH analogs) alone (monotherapy) with almost every possible combination of bilateral orchiectomy (or LHRH analogs) and antiandrogens.[195] A comprehensive review of all studies reported has revealed that 24 of the 27 studies reported no significant differences in survival, whereas only 3 demonstrated modest, statistically significant improvements in favor of "complete" androgen blockade.[195] Even for the occasional trial showing an apparent benefit for "complete" androgen blockade, a lack of consistency was found when considered in the context of other trials. For example, flutamide resulted in a survival advantage in one trial in combination with an LHRH analog, whereas nilutamide did not, whereas nilutamide resulted in a survival advantage in one trial in combination with bilateral orchiectomy, whereas flutamide did not. For each of the trials hinting at a benefit for "complete" androgen blockade, at least one, and as many as five, similarly designed trials were without any evidence for the benefit. Taken together, the large collection of clinical trial data testing the efficacy of "complete" androgen blockade suggests that any potential benefit of "complete" androgen blockage is likely minimal and of negligible clinical significance.

The first published large-scale prospectively randomized clinical trial was the National Cancer Institute (NCI)-sponsored trial INT-0036.[194] Men (N = 603) with stage D2 prostate cancer were randomly assigned to receive daily subcutaneous injections (1 mg/day) of leuprolide acetate and the nonsteroidal antiandrogen flutamide versus leuprolide acetate and placebo. The median overall survival with "complete" androgen blockade was 36 months, whereas the median survival with monotherapy was 28 months (P = .035). Although the NCI INT-0036 trial clearly showed a benefit to the treatment combination, several explanations other than the "complete" androgen-blockage hypothesis have been proffered to account for the trial results. One argument was that the difference in favor of combination treatment could have been an attenuation of the LHRH analog flare reaction by the antiandrogen.[593] In support of this contention, men randomized to receive combination treatment exhibited a trend toward more favorable pain control, improvement in performance status, and reduction in PSAP, as compared with men treated with monotherapy, evident during the first 12 weeks of treatment.[194] However, this notion is not supported by the results of another study that discerned no difference in survival between men randomized to receive leuprolide acetate with 2 weeks of flutamide treatment versus leuprolide acetate alone.[594] A second argument for the superiority of combination treatment in the NCI INT-0036 trial was that noncompliance with the daily leuprolide acetate injection regimen might result in inadequate gonadal suppression, providing the opportunity for an advantage for the combination of daily leuprolide and flutamide. Because routine evaluations of serum testosterone were not included in the study, this argument could not be effectively excluded. To address these issues, a confirmatory trial, using bilateral

orchiectomy rather than leuprolide acetate for androgen deprivation, was conducted (the NCI INT-0105 trial).

Bilateral orchiectomy represents the optimal method of reducing testosterone for testing the "complete" androgen-blockade hypothesis because it is not associated with a flare reaction or compliance difficulties. The NCI INT-0105 clinical trial prospectively randomized men ($N = 1387$) with stage D2 prostate cancer to treatment with bilateral orchiectomy with flutamide versus bilateral orchiectomy with a placebo (Fig. 87-14).[193] The trial was designed to have sufficient power to detect a 25% or better advantage in survival attributable to combination treatment. However, at a median follow-up time of approximately 50 months, and with 70% of deaths occurring by the date of final analysis, the trial failed to detect a survival advantage to "complete" androgen blockade, finding a median

Figure 87-14. Results of a randomized clinical trial of orchiectomy plus flutamide versus orchiectomy plus placebo for men with metastatic prostate cancer. **A,** Overall survival. **B,** Overall survival, stratified by extent of disease. **C,** Progression-free survival stratified by extent of disease. (From Eisenberger MA, Blumenstein BA, Crawford ED et al: Bilateral orchiectomy with or without flutamide for metastatic prostate cancer. N Engl J Med 1998;339:10036–10042, with permission.)

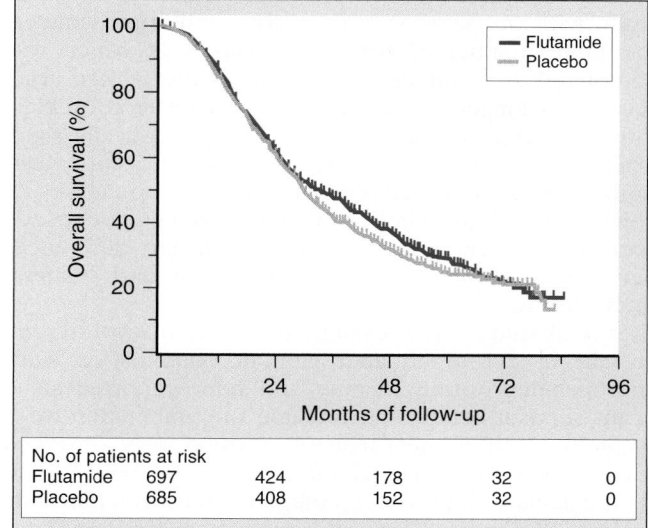

A

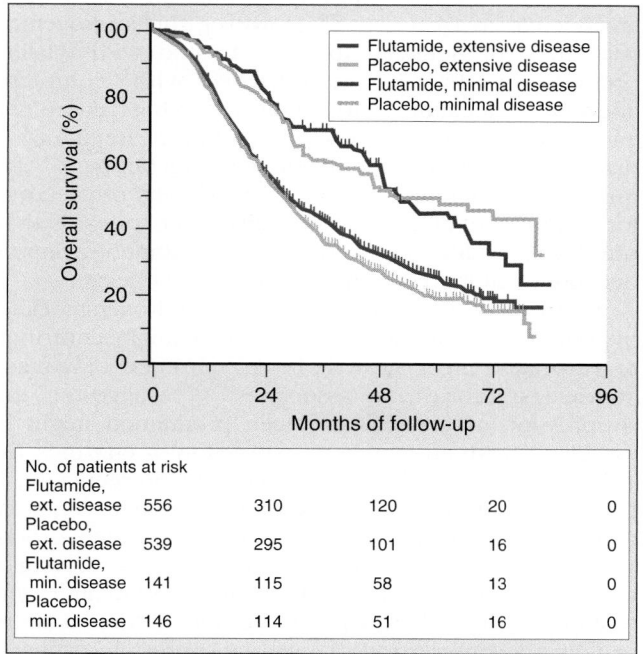

B

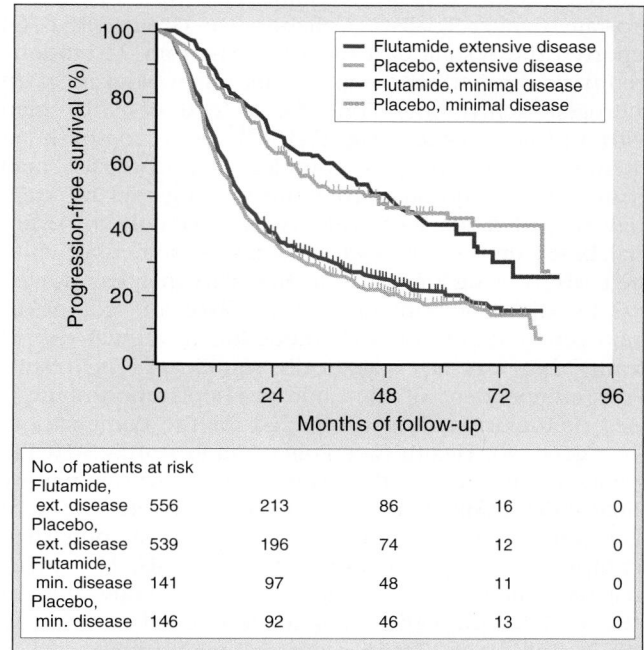

C

Specific Malignancies

III

survival of 33 months for men treated with combination therapy versus 30 months for men treated with orchiectomy alone (hazard ratio, 0.91 for combination treatment, with a 90% confidence interval of 0.81 to 1.01; $P = .14$). Although a slightly greater fraction of men in the bilateral orchiectomy ± flutamide trial (20%) than in the leuprolide ± flutamide trial (13%) had minimal metastatic prostate cancer, men in the two trials otherwise were very similar with regard to age and other demographic features.[193,194]

The EORTC conducted a clinical trial ($N = 327$) comparing goserelin acetate plus flutamide with bilateral orchiectomy in men who mostly had stage D2 prostate cancer.[595-598] Although an initial analysis of trial results, at a median follow-up time of 30 months, had disclosed no significant survival differences, a later analysis showed a 7-month improvement in median survival ($P = .04$) in favor of combination treatment. The Danish Prostatic Cancer Group (DAPROCA) conducted a virtually identical study, with the same treatment arms and approximately the same number of patients.[599] This trial, which was completed at about the same time as the EORTC trial, revealed a longer overall survival with bilateral orchiectomy, although the difference was not statistically significant.[599] The reason for the discordant results is not clear: Both studies recruited similar patient populations. A combined analysis of both studies, undertaken to enhance statistical power, failed to detect significant differences between "complete" androgen blockade and bilateral orchiectomy.[600]

Several studies have examined the use of cyproterone acetate, a steroid antiandrogen, in combination with androgen-deprivation therapy, and none reported significant survival benefits attributable to combination treatment.[601-605] In a meta-analysis, a trend was observed toward decreased survival for men treated with cyproterone acetate as part of a "complete" androgen-blockade regimen.[606] The use of cyproterone acetate for "complete" androgen blockade is not recommended. In 1995, the Prostate Cancer Trialists' Collaborative Group (PCTCG) reported the results of a meta-analysis from 22 randomized trials comparing "complete" androgen blockade with androgen deprivation alone for a total of 5710 men with prostate cancer (Fig. 87-15).[607] To accomplish an intention-to-treat analysis, complete data for each man treated were requested from the investigators for each trial. Hazard ratios were calculated separately for every trial, based on the raw data, and then combined for all of the trials by using log-rank statistics. This analysis revealed a 2.1% difference in survival in favor of "complete" androgen blockade (a 6.4% reduction in annual risk of death) that was not statistically significant. The results were independent of the androgen-deprivation strategy used or the antiandrogen selected for the combination. The Agency for Health Care Policy and Research [AHCPR; results published on the Web (http://www.ahcpr.gov/clinic/index.html#evidence, AHCPR report No.99-E012)] also conducted a meta-analysis based on all published "complete" androgen-blockade clinical trials. This meta-analysis found no difference in 2-year survival rates (hazard ratio, 0.970, with a 95% confidence interval of 0.866 to 1.087). Only 10 of 27 trials reported 5-year survival data, in

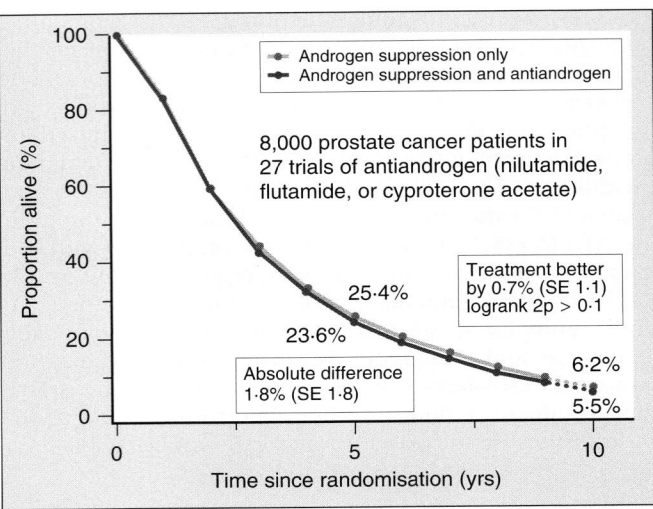

Figure 87-15. A meta-analysis of survival from metastatic prostate cancer with maximal androgen blockade versus androgen deprivation alone. (From Prostate Cancer Trialists Cooperative Group: Maximum androgen blockade in advanced prostate cancer: An overview of the randomised trial. Lancet 2000;355:1491–1498, with permission.

addition to the 2-year survival figures, and the combined results of these 10 trials suggested a minimal 5-year survival difference in favor of "complete" androgen blockade of uncertain clinical significance (hazard ratio, 0.871, with a 95% confidence interval of 0.805 to 0.9887).

Androgen-deprivation therapy and antiandrogens are associated with a number of side effects, whether given alone or in combination, including hot flashes, loss of libido, loss of bone and muscle mass, fatigue, anemia, gynecomastia, and other symptoms. When the impact of such side effects was prospectively evaluated and compared with the beneficial impact of treatment, by using a quality-of-life questionnaire, men treated as part of the NCI INT-0105 trial reported an improvement in quality of life attributable to treatment.[608] However, the improvement was more pronounced for men treated with bilateral orchiectomy than for men treated with "complete" androgen blockade, with men receiving "complete" androgen blockade reporting of a higher frequency of diarrhea and worsening emotional functioning.[608] The quality-of-life benefit resulting from bilateral orchiectomy for treatment of metastatic prostate cancer appeared to be offset by the addition of antiandrogen treatment, primarily because of an increased incidence of side effects.

A key feature of the "complete" androgen-blockade hypothesis was that adrenal androgens might contribute to prostate cancer growth in the absence of gonadal androgens. Labrie and associates[609,610] suggested that suppression of gonadal androgen production might be associated with an increased expression of enzymes, like 17β-hydroxysteroid dehydrogenase and 5α-reductase, in the prostate and elsewhere, capable of converting weak adrenal androgens (androstenedione and dehydroepiandrosterone) into testosterone and DHT, attributing as much as 30% to 50% of the intracellular pool of androgens to adrenal origin. At this point, the role of adrenal androgens in the progression of metastatic prostate cancer is not established. Conversely, new insights into the diverse molecular mechanisms associated with prostate cancer progression in the face of androgen-deprivation therapy, with myriad alterations in androgen-receptor function, activation of cell proliferation, loss of the apoptosis, increase in tumor angiogenesis, modulation of tumor invasion and metastasis by the extracellular matrix, and maintenance of immune tolerance, have suggested that considerable heterogeneity exists in the androgen-independent prostate cancer phenotype.[24] With all of these mechanisms possibly contributing to androgen-independent prostate cancer progression, it is not entirely surprising that the "complete" androgen-blockade treatment approach proposed by Labrie and coworkers[591] was not associated with a clinically significant survival benefit.

The Optimal Timing for Initiation of Androgen-Deprivation Therapy

Although a general belief holds that immediate initiation of androgen-deprivation therapy for men with metastatic prostate cancer may improve quality of life, no compelling evidence exists of a reduction in survival resulting from deferring treatment until time of symptomatic progression. Effects of the timing of androgen-deprivation therapy on the survival of men with metastatic prostate cancer has become a more critical issue recently, since an increasing number of men are recognized to have recurrent or metastatic prostate cancer very early because of increases in the serum PSA. The VACURG Study 1, testing the benefits of androgen-deprivation therapy achieved by administration of DES, even though conducted decades ago, provides valuable insights into the effect of timing of androgen-deprivation therapy on survival from metastatic prostate cancer. In the trial, men with advanced prostate cancer were randomized to initial treatment with bilateral orchiectomy plus a 5-mg daily dose of DES, bilateral orchiectomy plus a placebo, 5 mg DES per day alone, or placebo alone, with results indicating no significant differences in survival among the different treatment groups.[577,578] However, men in the placebo arm that were subsequently crossed over to another treatment arm at the time of progression had a survival comparable to that of men initially treated in one of the other treatment arms, suggesting that immediate initiation of androgen-deprivation therapy was without marked benefit.

The Medical Research Council also evaluated immediate versus deferred androgen-deprivation therapy for advanced prostate cancer.[611] In their study, men with prostate cancer (N = 934 men; 434 men with and 500 men without prostate cancer metastasis) were randomized either to early androgen deprivation or to androgen deprivation initiated for symptomatic prostate cancer progression. Follow-up procedures were not strictly defined in the trial, relying on the discretion of the treating physicians, and 5% of the men who died of prostate cancer never received androgen-deprivation therapy, whereas 10% of the men were not treated until they had a pathologic bone fracture or spinal cord compression. Using death from prostate cancer as a study endpoint for the men who had metastatic prostate cancer, no

significant difference was detected between the early (65% prostate cancer deaths) versus late treatment groups (69% prostate cancer deaths). In an initial report of trial results, the group of men with nonmetastatic prostate cancer appeared to have fewer deaths (32%) when treated with early androgen-deprivation therapy than when treatment was delayed (49%). However, of the men in this group who died in the delayed-treatment arm, 54% never received endocrine therapy. In a more recent report, reflecting greater follow-up time, no statistically significant differences were evident for men with prostate cancer treated with early versus delayed androgen-deprivation therapy.

The Eastern Cooperative Oncology Group carried out a randomized prospective trial of immediate androgen-deprivation therapy versus observation in men (N = 98) who underwent radical prostatectomy and were found to have lymph node metastases.[612] After a median of 7.1 years of follow-up, a significant difference in survival, favoring immediate androgen-deprivation therapy, was detected. This finding was surprising because a fairly large difference in survival was evident within a relatively short period of observation. In the trial, prostate cancer–specific survival in the observation group was 78% at 5 years. This is quite low compared with rates seen in men with prostate cancer and microscopic lymph node metastasis treated with radical prostatectomy alone. Furthermore, in a nonrandomized case series (N = 790) from the Mayo Clinic, representing the largest retrospective collection of data on men with lymph node–positive prostate cancer treated with radical prostatectomy, with almost three decades of follow-up, a survival advantage in favor of immediate androgen deprivation was seen only for men with prostate cancers that were diploid, and this survival advantage did not become apparent until 10 years after surgery.[613] In that case series, men with aneuploid prostate cancers and lymph node metastases subjected to radical prostatectomy did not appear to benefit from immediate adjuvant androgen-deprivation therapy. When men with diploid prostate cancers (N = 57) were treated similarly and followed up for 10 years, no improvement in survival was attributable to adjuvant androgen-deprivation therapy, but at 15 years of follow-up, 14 men with diploid prostate cancers were alive, 12 who had received early androgen-deprivation therapy and 2 who had not (83.2% ± 4.1% vs. 48.5% ± 13%). Thus the finding of a benefit to early androgen-deprivation therapy was based on the experience with 14 men of 790 men with lymph node–positive prostate cancer who underwent radical prostatectomy. Why are the ECOG study results, indicating a benefit for early androgen-deprivation therapy, different from other data suggesting only a marginal benefit to immediate initiation of treatment? In an editorial that accompanied publication of the ECOG study findings, one concern raised was that this study never realized its projected accrual goal of 240 patients.[614] This may be critically important because the outcome of patients with prostate cancer nodal metastasis is extremely variable and difficult to predict. This problem could have been minimized if a sufficient number of men with prostate cancer were randomized to the different treatment arms. Unfortunately, the ECOG trial was relatively small and might have been affected by imbalances of factors that were not identified at the time the study began. In support of this concern, the fact that 50% of the men in the observation arm had progressed by 5 years, with 22% deaths, suggested that this control group most likely represented a collection of men with poor-risk or high-grade prostate cancers or both.[612]

Intermittent Androgen-Deprivation Therapy

Intermittent androgen-deprivation therapy has the promise of reducing the impact of treatment-associated side effects while still maintaining some benefits from treatment. Additionally, findings from one group of animal model studies suggested that intermittent reductions in testosterone levels, versus continuous androgen deprivation, might actually delay prostate cancer progression to androgen independence.[615] In these preclinical experiments, androgen-dependent cancers carried subcutaneously in mice were treated with bilateral orchiectomy once the tumors grew to 3 g. After the tumors had regressed 30%, they were transplanted into intact mice and then treated again with bilateral orchiectomy once the tumors had again grown to 3 g. This treatment cycle was continued until the cancer became androgen independent. For comparison, mice carrying 3-g cancers were treated with a single cycle of androgen deprivation. Remarkably, androgen-independent cancer progression occurred 51 days after one-time bilateral orchiectomy versus 147 days for mice cycled through intermittent androgen deprivation. The mechanism for this difference, attributed to a superiority of intermittent androgen deprivation as cancer treatment, has not been fully elucidated. However, other preclinical animal-model studies have yielded conflicting results. When rats carrying a transplantable androgen-dependent prostate cancer were treated with immediate bilateral orchiectomy, with continuous high- or low-dose DES, or with intermittent high- or low-dose DES, rats treated with androgen deprivation continuously survived 38% to 50% longer than rats treated with intermittent androgen deprivation.[616] These uncertainties from preclinical studies suggest that the clinical use of intermittent deprivation therapy should be carefully evaluated in well-designed clinical trials before routine use in clinical practice. The efficacy and safety of intermittent versus continuous androgen deprivation is currently under scrutiny in clinical trials.

"Second-Line" Endocrine Treatment

During the past several years, it has become evident that men with prostate cancer progression after initial androgen-deprivation therapy are a heterogeneous group with varying degrees of residual sensitivity to hormonal manipulations. Kelly and colleagues[617,618] described the "flutamide-withdrawal" syndrome, later found also to be associated with other antiandrogens, characterized by an improvement seen in 20% to 25% of men on discontinuation of antiandrogen treatment. This phenomenon occurred both for men who were initially treated with "complete" androgen blockade and for men who had received antiandrogens at some other time. The clinical observation of an "antiandrogen withdrawal" syndrome prompted a renewed interest in the biology of the androgen receptor in prostate cancer cells.[619] A variety of AR alterations have been described in prostate cancers progressing after initial hormone manipulations; *AR* mutations, encoding androgen receptors with altered ligand specificity, also have been detected for which antiandrogens can act as agonists.[213,214,216]

The agents reported to cause beneficial treatment responses (a decrease in the serum PSA or other response) after adequate androgen-deprivation treatment include bicalutamide (20% to 24%), megestrol acetate (8% to 13%), DES (26% to 66%), ketoconazole with hydrocortisone (27% to 63%), and glucocorticoids alone (18% to 22%).[625] PC-SPES, a multicomponent herbal mixture with estrogenic properties, also has been reported to produce treatment responses in men with androgen-independent prostate cancer.[621] However, many PC-SPES lots were contaminated with prescription drugs, including DES, coumadin, and indomethacin, and as a result, PC-SPES is no longer available.[622] In general, responses to second-line hormonal manipulations are usually brief, with median durations of benefit ranging between 3 and 4 months. An ongoing ECOG study will compare the role of the second-line combination of ketoconazole with hydrocortisone versus the chemotherapy combination of estramustine plus taxotere for men with androgen-independent, nonmetastatic prostate cancer and an increasing serum PSA after initial androgen-deprivation treatment.

Clinical Approach to Men with Androgen-Independent Prostate Cancer

Most men with androgen-independent prostate cancer demonstrate an increasing PSA as the first manifestation of prostate cancer progression after androgen deprivation. In a prospective evaluation of men ($N = 282$) who had received first-line androgen-deprivation therapy and had cancer progression, an increase in serum PSA levels occurred approximately 6 months before any other clinical (radiologic or bone scan) evidence of worsening cancer.[623] However, for men initially treated with androgen deprivation based only on an increasing serum PSA (and no clinical evidence of prostate cancer metastases), the time interval between subsequent serum PSA increases, indicating androgen-independent prostate cancer progression, and the appearance of clinically significant metastases is not known. However, the serum PSA level at initial presentation, the rate of serum PSA increase, the Gleason score at the time of prostate biopsy or surgery, the clinical stage at presentation, and the response to androgen-deprivation treatment are likely of prognostic significance.[624] When the appearance of androgen-independent prostate cancer is suspected for men treated with androgen-deprivation therapy, a determination of the serum testosterone (to ensure that androgen deprivation has been adequately accomplished), serum PSA, PSAP, and alkaline phosphatase, hematology and serum chemistry studies, radiographic imaging (including a bone scan), and a history and physical examination are often undertaken.

TABLE 87-16

Single-Agent Chemotherapy Activity in Phase II Clinical Trials for Androgen-Independent Prostate Cancer (Before Serum PSA Was Used to Monitor Treatment Effect)

DRUG	RESPONSES
Cyclophosphamide (Carter, 1975)	8/57 (14%)
Doxorubicin (O'Bryan, 1973; O'Bryan, 1977; Scher, 1984; Torti, 1983	13/88 (14.5%)
Estramustine phosphate (Mittleman, 1976; Kuss, 1980; Veronesi, 1982)	15/86 (17%)
Cisplatin (Yagoda, 1979; Merrin, 1979; Rossof, 1979; Qasi, 1983; Moore, 1986)	24/146 (13.5%)
Mitoxantrone (Osborne, 1983; Raghavan, 1986)	3/64 (5%)
Vinblastine (Yagoda, 1993; Logothetis, 1983)	8/39 (21%) (response rate unclear in one trial)
5-Fluorouracil (Eisenberger, 1988)	<20%

PSA, prostate-specific antigen.
Adapted from Eisenberger MA: Chemotherapy for prostate carcinoma. NCI Monogr 1988;7:151–163, and from Eisenberger et al: A reevaluation of nonhormonal cytotoxic chemotherapy in the treatment of prostatic carcinoma. J Clin Oncol 1985;3:827–841, with permission.

For years it has been suggested that discontinuation of androgen deprivation in men who have not undergone bilateral orchiectomy may adversely affect prostate cancer progression and survival.[625] The administration of exogenous testosterone and its derivatives is known to produce a significant prostate cancer flare with severe pain, and neurologic, urologic, and coagulation complications in a small proportion of men.[626-628] In a retrospective analysis of men ($N = 205$) with androgen-independent prostate cancer who were treated with chemotherapy, men with prior bilateral orchiectomy, versus men treated with gonadal androgen suppression that was discontinued at least 4 weeks before chemotherapy, did not appear different with respect to prostate cancer progression and survival.[629] Of course, many of the men treated with gonadal suppression likely never achieved normal serum androgen levels. Until the issue of whether discontinuation of gonadal suppression might compromise survival

from androgen-independent prostate cancer has been resolved, maintenance of gonadal androgen suppression is recommended. Because stopping antiandrogen treatment at the time of prostate cancer progression can result in decreases in serum PSA levels, and in occasional symptomatic benefits or objective improvements in soft tissue and bone metastasis, men taking antiandrogens along with androgen-deprivation therapy should be encouraged to discontinue these agents for at least 4 to 8 weeks before considering other treatment maneuvers.[630]

Systemic Chemotherapy

The conduct and evaluation of clinical trials for men with metastatic prostate cancer are almost always confounded by significant methodologic challenges concerning the assessment of treatment benefit (Tables 87-16 to 87-18). The most common site of prostate cancer metastasis is

TABLE 87-17

Single-Agent Chemotherapy Activity in Phase II Clinical Trials for Androgen-Independent Prostate Cancer (Using Serum PSA for Monitoring Treatment Efficacy)

DRUG	RESPONSES	RESPONSE CRITERIA
Cyclophosphamide		
(VonRoemeling, 1992)	4/13 (30%)	PSA decline (but measurable responses also seen)
(Abell, 1995)	6/20 (33%)	
(Smith, 1992)	6/10 (primarily >50%)	
Paclitaxel (Taxol)		
(Roth, 1992)	1/23 (4%)	Measurable disease
	6/12 (50%)	PSA decline >50%
(Ahmed, 1997)	2/4 (50%)	PSA decline and measurable responses
Mitoxantrone		
(Rearden, 1995)	4/14 (29%)	1 measurable response; 3 subjective improvements; none had >50% decline in PSA
Vinorelbine		
(Oudard, 1999)	19/47 (40%)	50% decline in PSA
Estramustine phosphate		
(Yagoda, 1991)	9/42 (21%)	>50% decline in PSA
5-Fluorouracil		
(Kuzel, 1993)	0/18 (0)	No objective measurable responses or >50% PSA decline
Etoposide		
(Hussain, 1994)	2/24 (8%)	1 had >50% decline in PSA; 1 had a measurable response
Carboplatin		
(Canobbio, 1993)	3(2)/25 (12%)	3 had >50% PSA declines; 2 had measurable responses

PSA, prostate-specific antigen.

TABLE 87-18

Phase II Clinical Trials for Androgen-Independent Prostate Cancer with Selected Chemotherapy Drug Combinations

REGIMEN	≥50% DECLINE IN SERUM PSA	MEASURABLE RESPONSES
Estramustine phosphate (10 mg/kg/day p.o. in 3 divided doses for 6–7 wk) + Vinblastine (4 mg/m² /IV/wk)	13/24 (54%) 22/36 (61%) (Hudes, 1992)	2/5 (40%) 1/7 (14%)
Estramustine phospate (15 mg/kg/day p.o. for 3 wk) + Etoposide (50 mg/m²/day p.o. for 3 wk)	29/42 (69%) (Pienta, 1994)	9/18 (50%)
Estramustine phosphate (600 mg/m² p.o./day) + Paclitaxel (120–140 mg/m² by 96-hr infusion)	10/17 (59%) (Hudes, 1995)	3/6 (50%)
Estramustine phosphate (280 mg p.o. 3x/day on days 1–5 every 3 wk) + Docetaxel (70 mg/m² on day 2 every 3 wk) or	23/35 (74%) (Petrylak, 2000)	4/7 (57%)
Estramustine phosphate (280 mg p.o. every 6 hr for 5 doses every 3 wk) + Docetaxel (70 mg/m² every 3 wk) or	(13/29 (45%) (Sinibaldi, 2000)	3/13 (23%)
Estramustine phosphate (420 mg p.o. for 4 doses, then 280 mg p.o. for 5 doses 3x/day every 3 wk) + Docetaxel (35 mg/m² on day 2 every 3 wk)	13/18 (72%) (Copur, 2000)	4/8 (50%)
Estramustine phosphate (280 mg p.o 3x/day for 14 days every 3 wk) + Etoposide (100 mg/day for 14 days every 3 wk) + Paclitaxel (135 mg/m² over 1 hr on day 2 every 3 wk)	26/40 (65%) (Smith, 1999)	10/22 (46%)
Estramustine phosphate (280 mg 3x/day days 1–3 weekly for 8 wk then every other week for ≤26 wk) + Vinorelbine (15–20 mg/m² on day 2 weekly for 8 wk then every other week for ≤26 wk)	15/21 (71%) (Sweeny, 2000)	1/8 (13%)
Doxorubicin (40 mg/m² IV every 3 wk) + Cyclophosphamide (800–2000 mg/m² every 3 wk) + G-CSF (5 mg/kg/day)	12/29 (41%) (Small, 1995)	4/12 (33%)
Mitoxantrone (12 mg/m² IV every 3 wk) + Prednisone (10 mg p.o. daily)	5/23 (22%) (Moore, 1994)	1/7 (14%)
Ketoconazole (1200 mg p.o. daily) + Doxorubicin (20 mg/m² by 24-hr infusion weekly) + Hydrocortisone (30 mg p.o. daily)	21/39 (55%) (Sella, 1994)	7/12 (58%)

G-CSF, granulocyte–colony-stimulating factor; PSA, prostate-specific antigen.

bone, with many men manifesting diffuse osteoblastic bone lesions that cannot be measured reliably by current methods to permit treatment-response determinations. The presence of soft tissue or visceral metastases, which can be subjected to serial "bidirectional" measurements, is uncommon and still frequently associated with dominant bone metastases, compromising a full evaluation of response to treatment.[631] Of all the clinical, laboratory, and radiographic parameters available, those most correlated with survival from metastatic prostate cancer are baseline functional status (performance status) and pretreatment hemoglobin levels. The contribution of pretreatment serum PSA level and extent of cancer involvement by bone scan (number of lesions or pattern of lesion distribu-tion) have not been consistently associated with outcome thus far.

Although changes in serum PSA levels are often used to assess the therapeutic effects of chemotherapy for men with androgen-independent prostate cancer, a more precise definition of the significance of such serum PSA changes will require scrutiny in phase III trials specifically designed to address this issue. Data derived from multi-variate analyses of uncontrolled clinical trials involving men with androgen-independent prostate cancer have demonstrated that a 50% or greater decline in serum PSA from baseline values, for a period of 4 weeks or longer, is strongly correlated with survival, prompting this criterion to be monitored as a surrogate for therapeutic efficacy.[632-634] In other analyses, the magnitude of serum PSA decline indicating treatment benefit has not been clear, arguing against serum PSA determinations as the sole indicator of treatment effect for prostate cancer drug development.[635] In preclinical studies, various agents appear to be able to reduce PSA expression or secretion, without affecting prostate cancer growth.[636,637] PSA changes have not yet been shown to correlate with survival in randomized phase III trials of chemotherapy for men with androgen-independent prostate cancer, although this may be more a consequence of the absence of a contemporary phase III trial demonstrating a chemotherapy treatment benefit than a problem with the predictive utility of serum PSA decreases. Cognizant of these issues, workers have proposed consensus guidelines concerning the use of serum PSA determinations in clinical trials.[633] Clearly, in addition to serum PSA, new validated biomarkers are needed to improve the efficiency of new drug development for men with androgen-independent prostate cancer. Most of chemotherapy drugs available have been tested as single agents in men with androgen-independent prostate cancer (see Tables 87-16 to 87-18).[638,639] However, data from different phase II clinical trials of chemotherapy for prostate cancer are often very difficult to compare. For example, clinical trials of drugs conducted before the late 1980s, in contrast to more recent studies, tended not have monitored serum PSA changes. Thus it is likely that some of the men in the earlier clinical trials who were considered nonresponders may have been classified as having a response or stable disease if serum PSA determinations were performed, underestimating response rates.[640,641] Because some amount of PSA decline can often be seen on administration of agents like estramustine phosphate, which has estrogenic activity, or of corticosteroids, which are often given along with taxanes to prevent or minimize anaphylactic reactions or fluid retention, more recent trials may overestimate response rates. Furthermore, men referred for more recent chemotherapy trials were often recognized to have androgen-independent prostate cancer, based on a serum PSA determination, and tend to have less advanced or symptomatic prostate cancer than did men in the earlier trials. This lead-time effect is also important for survival data reported for these men, with the current survival of men with androgen-independent prostate cancer at least 12 to 18 months as opposed to 6 to 12 months, as described earlier.[638,639] Finally, the lead-time effect for men with androgen-independent prostate cancer also results in less cancer-associated anemia, renal dysfunction, symptoms, and decline in functional status, making men in contemporary clinical trials generally better candidates for chemotherapy than were men in earlier trials. Modest single-agent activity with the bifunctional alkylating agent cyclophosphamide, with reported responses in approximately 10% to 20% of men with androgen-independent prostate cancer, has long been recognized. In more contemporary trials, cyclophosphamide, whether given orally or at high doses intravenously, has been reported to have an even higher level of anticancer activity.[642-644] Despite their utility for many other cancers, doxorubicin, fluorouracil, and cisplatin have been found to have only minimal benefits when given as single agents to men with androgen-independent prostate cancer. The combination of doxorubicin and ketoconazole does appear to have significant anticancer activity. Mitroxantrone, a semisynthetic anthracenedione, has been reported to provide subjective improvement to androgen-independent prostate cancer despite minimal evidence of objective anticancer activity.[645-647] In a prospective randomized clinical trial, mitoxantrone and prednisone, when compared with prednisone alone, demonstrated a significant beneficial impact on pain and quality of life, but not on survival (Table 87-19).[648] Nonetheless, this trial provided justification for approval by the U.S. FDA of the combination of mitoxantrone and prednisone for treatment of symptomatic men with androgen-independent prostate cancer.

Estramustine phosphate, a nitrogen mustard derivative of estradiol-17β-phosphate, has demonstrated limited activity against androgen-independent prostate cancer as a single agent. In prospective randomized trial for men with androgen-independent prostate cancer, estramustine phosphate, given at a daily oral dose of 560 mg, failed to show superiority to placebo for palliation or for survival.[649] In laboratory studies, the cytotoxic mechanism of action for estramustine phosphate was found to involve interference with microtubular function and binding to nuclear matrix structures within cancer cells.[650-652] To enhance the cytotoxicity of estramustine phosphate, the agents have been combined with other drugs targeting microtubules, including vinblastine, paclitaxel, docetaxel, and vinorelbine, and drugs, such as etoposide, targeting DNA topoisomerase II, a component of the nuclear matrix.[653] Several of these clinical trials of estramustine combinations have revealed promising preliminary evidence of anticancer activity. Of all the combinations, the greatest attention has been afforded those that feature docetaxel, an agent that appears to have significant activity in men with androgen-independent prostate cancer when used alone,[654-656] as well as with estramustine phosphate.[657] Single-agent docetaxel, at two different dose/schedules (weekly or every 3 weeks), and a combination of docetaxel with estramustine phosphate are in current phase III clinical trials testing whether these regimens offer any improvement over the combination of mitoxantrone and prednisone for men with androgen-independent prostate cancer.[658]

Neuroendocrine Prostate Cancer

Neuroendocrine transformation of prostate cancer has been reported for a number of men with advanced androgen-independent prostate cancer.[659,660] The implications of neuroendocrine transformation are that such cells have a number of different properties from those of adenocarcinoma cells, often including the absence of androgen receptors and PSA production, and presence of a variety of peptide growth factors and growth-factor receptors, such as bombesin/gastrin-releasing-peptide antagonist, somatostatin, chromogranin-A, serotonin, and parathyroid-hormone–related protein. Not surprisingly, the clinical behavior of neuroendocrine prostate cancer is

TABLE 87-19

Prospective Randomized Clinical Trials of Chemotherapy for Androgen-Independent Prostate Cancer

REGIMEN	MEDIAN SURVIVAL	COMMENTS
Cyclophosphamide vs.	47 wk	More men on the chemotherapy arms had stable disease; difference in survival not statistically significant
5-Fluorouracil vs.	44 wk	
No chemotherapy	38 wk	
Estramustine phosphate vs.	26 wk	
Streptozotocin vs.	25 wk	As above
No chemotherapy	24 wk	
Cyclophosphamide vs.	27 wk	Survival difference not significant
Dacarbazine vs.	40 wk	
Procarbazine	31 wk	
Estramustine + prednimustine vs.	37 wk	As above
Prednimustine	36 wk	
Cyclophosphamide vs.	41 wk	High rate of men not evaluable; survival differences are not statistically significant
Semustine vs.	22 wk	
Hydroxyurea	19 wk	
Estramustine vs.	26 wk	As above
Vincristine vs.	27 wk	
Estramustine + vincristine	32 wk	
Estramustine vs.	43 wk	As above
Methotrexate vs.	37 wk	
Cisplatin	33 wk	
Mitoxantrone + prednisone vs.	9–10 mos	Improved control of pain and prolongation of time to symptomatic progression in favor of the combination
Prednisone	(no difference)	
Mitoxantrone + hydrocortisone vs.	12.3 mo	38% vs. 22% PSA response; quality of life not significantly different, but pain better controlled
Hydrocortisone	12.6 mo	
Suramin + hydrocortisone vs.	9–10 mo	33% vs. 16% PSA response; pain control and time-to-pain progression significantly better with suramin; toxicity modest
Placebo + hydrocortisone	(no difference)	
Estramustine + vinblastine vs.	11.9 mo	PSA response 25% vs. 3%
Vinblastine	9.2 mo	
Estramustine vs.	38 wk	As above
Cisplatin vs.	28 wk	
Estramustine + cisplatin	40 wk	
Doxorubicin vs.	29 wk	Survival differences not statistically significant
5-Fluorouracil	24 wk	
CAF vs.	25 wk	As above
5-Fluorouracil	34 wk	
Cyclophosphamide + doxorubicin vs.	27 wk	No difference in survival
Hydroxyurea	28 wk	
Estramustine vs.	34 wk	Survival differences not statistically significant
Placebo	24 wk	

CAF, cyclophosphamide/doxorubicin/fluorouracil; PSA, prostate-specific antigen.

quite different from that of prostatic adenocarcinoma, with more frequent visceral and soft tissue metastases, osteolytic bone metastases, hypercalemia, brain metastases, and explosive growth and progression in the absence of an increasing serum PSA. If neuroendocrine transformation of prostate cancer is suspected, biopsy of cancer deposits is recommended. Often, small cell prostate cancer or a poorly differentiated cancer expressing neuroendocrine markers will be evident.[660] Treatment of prostate cancer with neuroendocrine transformation is usually similar to that attempted for other neuroendocrine cancers (e.g., small cell carcinoma of the lung), using combinations of cisplatin or carboplatin and etoposide.[661]

New Approaches to Prostate Cancer Treatment

For men with recurrent or metastatic prostate cancer, although androgen-deprivation therapy offers significant benefits, when prostate cancer progresses to androgen independence, no treatments have been shown to improve survival. For this reason, men with progressive metastatic cancer should be considered for participation in clinical trials of new treatments. An expanding portfolio of new treatment approaches for prostate cancer has emerged over the past decade. Several new agents have reached advanced clinical development.

One exciting new area concerns the targeted treatment of bony metastases from prostate cancer. For men with prostate cancer bone metastases, zoledronic acid (Zometa), a potent bisphosphonate, has been shown to reduce the appearance of skeletal complications in a prospective randomized clinical trial (from 44.2% to 33.2%; $P = .021$).[662] Zoledronic acid also has been found to reduce bone loss associated with androgen-deprivation therapy in a randomized clinical trial.[663] With these data, zoledronic acid has now been approved by the U.S. FDA, and many men with metastatic prostate cancer now receive the drug. Another strategy focusing on prostate cancer bone metastases involves the combination use of ^{89}Sr, a bone-targeted radiopharmaceutical used to palliate painful bony metastases, and doxorubicin.[664,665] In a provocative clinical trial, men with androgen-independent prostate cancer and bone metastases ($N = 72$) who had responded to an induction chemotherapy regimen were randomized to receive doxorubicin versus doxorubicin with ^{89}Sr as consolidation treatment.[665] The findings were an improvement in survival from a median of 16.8 months (with a range of 4.4 to 34.2 months) for chemotherapy alone versus 27.7 months (4.9 to 37.7 months) for combined treatment ($P = .0014$). These observations have stimulated further interest in the pathophysiology of prostate cancer bone metastasis, and in identifying new molecular targets for modulation of behavior of prostate cancer cells at bony sites.[666-669] Other new treatments under active clinical development include various vaccine immunotherapies for prostate cancer,[670-673] replication-restricted cytolytic adenoviruses,[674] endothelin A–receptor antagonists,[675,676] and vitamin D analogs.[677]

SUMMARY

Although mortality from prostate cancer has declined over the past few years, demographic trends, such as the general aging of the population, suggest that prostate cancer will remain one of the most common health threats for men in the developed world. Widespread implementation of prostate cancer screening, using the serum PSA, has resulted in a changing character of prostate cancer at its initial presentation, with younger men being diagnosed at earlier prostate cancer stages than ever before. The use of serum PSA testing for disease-activity monitoring has changed the character of prostate cancer throughout the rest of its natural history, with healthier men having less prostate cancer at later stages of the disease than ever before. These changes have put new demands on improving prostate cancer treatment, whether minimizing the morbidity of local prostate cancer treatment or increasing the efficacy of systemic prostate cancer treatment. In the very near future, large clinical studies of prostate cancer prevention, of the benefits of prostate cancer screening, of systemic adjuvant therapies given along with primary local prostate cancer treatment, of systemic chemotherapy for androgen-independent prostate cancer, and of a variety of new agents will provide new insights of critical importance to prostate cancer care. Ultimately, new biomarkers, new imaging strategies, and new prevention and treatment approaches may hold the secret to eradicating prostate cancer morbidity and mortality.

REFERENCES

1. Jemal A, Murray T, Samuels A, Ghafoor A, Ward E, Thun MJ: Cancer statistics, 2003. CA Cancer J Clin 2003;53:5-26.
2. Hankey BF, Feuer EJ, Clegg LX, et al: Cancer surveillance series: Interpreting trends in prostate cancer. I. Evidence of the effects of screening in recent prostate cancer incidence, mortality, and survival rates. J Natl Cancer Inst 1999;91:1017-1024.
3. Bartsch G, Horninger W, Klocker H, et al: Prostate cancer mortality after introduction of prostate-specific antigen mass screening in the Federal State of Tyrol, Austria. Urology 2001;58:417-424.
4. Sakr WA, Grignon DJ, Crissman JD, et al: High grade prostatic intraepithelial neoplasia (HGPIN) and prostatic adenocarcinoma between the ages of 20-69: An autopsy study of 249 cases. In Vivo 1994;8:439-443.
5. Brooks JD: Anatomy of the lower urinary tract and male genitalia. In Walsh PC (ed): Campbell's Urology. Philadelphia, Saunders, 2002, pp 41-80.
6. Walsh PC, Donker PJ: Impotence following radical prostatectomy: Insight into etiology and prevention. J Urol 1982;128:492-497.
7. Walsh PC, Lepor H, Eggleston JC: Radical prostatectomy with preservation of sexual function: Anatomical and pathological considerations. Prostate 1983;4:473-485.
8. McNeal JE: The zonal anatomy of the prostate. Prostate 1981;2:35-49.
9. McNeal JE: Normal histology of the prostate. Am J Surg Pathol 1988;12:619-633.
10. Polascik TJ, Oesterling JE, Partin AW: Prostate specific antigen: A decade of discovery—what we have learned and where we are going. J Urol 1999;162:293-306.
11. Makridakis NM, di Salle E, Reichardt JK: Biochemical and pharmacogenetic dissection of human steroid 5 alpha-reductase type II. Pharmacogenetics 2000;10:407-413.
12. Steers WD: 5alpha-Reductase activity in the prostate. Urology 2001;58(6 suppl 1):17-24.
13. Brinkmann AO, Blok LJ, de Ruiter PE, et al: Mechanisms of androgen receptor activation and function. J Steroid Biochem Mol Biol 1999;69:307-313.
14. Chang CS, Kokontis J, Liao ST: Molecular cloning of human and rat complementary DNA encoding androgen receptors. Science 1988;240:324-326.
15. Roche PJ, Hoare SA, Parker MG: A consensus DNA-binding site for the androgen receptor. Mol Endocrinol 1992;6:2229-2235.
16. Schuur ER, Henderson GA, Kmetec LA, Miller JD, Lamparski HG, Henderson DR: Prostate-specific antigen expression is regulated by an upstream enhancer. J Biol Chem 1996;271:7043-7051.
17. De Marzo AM, Nelson WG, Meeker AK, Coffey DS: Stem cell features of benign and malignant prostate epithelial cells. J Urol 1998;160:2381-2392.
18. Parsons JK, Gage WR, Nelson WG, De Marzo AM: p63 protein expression is rare in prostate adenocarcinoma: Implications for cancer diagnosis and carcinogenesis. Urology 2001;58:619-624.
19. van Leenders G, Dijkman H, Hulsbergen-van de Kaa C, Ruiter D, Schalken J: Demonstration of intermediate cells during human prostate epithelial differentiation in situ and in vitro using triple-staining confocal scanning microscopy. Lab Invest 2000;80:1251-1258.
20. Peehl DM, Rubin JS: Keratinocyte growth factor: An androgen-regulated mediator of stromal-epithelial interactions in the prostate. World J Urol 1995;13:312-317.
21. Planz B, Wang Q, Kirley SD, Lin CW, McDougal WS: Androgen responsiveness of stromal cells of the human prostate: Regulation of cell proliferation and keratinocyte growth factor by androgen. J Urol 1998;160:1850-1855.
22. Marker PC, Donjacour AA, Dahiya R, Cunha GR: Hormonal, cellular, and molecular control of prostatic development. Dev Biol 2003;253:165-174.
23. Oesterling JE, Hauzeur CG, Farrow GM: Small cell anaplastic carcinoma of the prostate: A clinical, pathological and immunohistological study of 27 patients. J Urol 1992;147:804-807.
24. Feldman BJ, Feldman D: The development of androgen-independent prostate cancer. Nat Rev Cancer 2001;1:34-45.
25. Morganti G, Gianferrari L, Cresseri A, Arrigoni G, Lovati G: Recherches clinicostastisiques et genetiques sur les neoplasies de la prostate. Acta Genet 1956;6:304-305.
26. Steinberg GD, Carter BS, Beaty TH, Childs B, Walsh PC: Family history and the risk of prostate cancer. Prostate 1990;17:337-347.
27. Lesko SM, Rosenberg L, Shapiro S: Family history and prostate cancer risk. Am J Epidemiol 1996;144:1041-1047.

28. Ghadirian P, Howe GR, Hislop TG, Maisonneuve P: Family history of prostate cancer: A multi-center case-control study in Canada. Int J Cancer 1997;70:679–681.

29. Glover FE Jr, Coffey DS, Douglas LL, et al: Familial study of prostate cancer in Jamaica. Urology 1998;52:441–443.

30. Rodriguez C, Calle EE, Miracle-McMahill HL, et al: Family history and risk of fatal prostate cancer. Epidemiology 1997;8:653–657.

31. Whittemore AS, Wu AH, Kolonel LN, et al: Family history and prostate cancer risk in black, white, and Asian men in the United States and Canada. Am J Epidemiol 1995;141:732–740.

32. Spitz MR, Currier RD, Fueger JJ, Babaian RJ, Newell GR: Familial patterns of prostate cancer: A case-control analysis. J Urol 1991;146:1305–1307.

33. Lichtenstein P, Holm NV, Verkasalo PK, et al: Environmental and heritable factors in the causation of cancer: Analyses of cohorts of twins from Sweden, Denmark, and Finland. N Engl J Med 2000;343:78–85.

34. Page WF, Braun MM, Partin AW, Caporaso N, Walsh P: Heredity and prostate cancer: A study of World War II veteran twins. Prostate 1997;33:240–245.

35. Ahlbom A, Lichtenstein P, Malmstrom H, Feychting M, Hemminki K, Pedersen NL: Cancer in twins: Genetic and nongenetic familial risk factors. J Natl Cancer Inst 1997;89:287–293.

36. Gronberg H, Damber L, Damber JE: Studies of genetic factors in prostate cancer in a twin population. J Urol 1994;152:1484–1487.

37. Carter BS, Beaty TH, Steinberg GD, Childs B, Walsh PC: Mendelian inheritance of familial prostate cancer. Proc Natl Acad Sci USA 1992;89:3367–3371.

38. Monroe KR, Yu MC, Kolonel LN, et al: Evidence of an X-linked or recessive genetic component to prostate cancer risk. Nat Med 1995;1:827–829.

39. Smith JR, Freije D, Carpten JD, et al: Major susceptibility locus for prostate cancer on chromosome 1 suggested by a genome-wide search. Science 1996;274:1371–1374.

40. Berthon P, Valeri A, Cohen-Akenine A, et al: Predisposing gene for early-onset prostate cancer, localized on chromosome 1q42.2-43. Am J Hum Genet 1998;62:1416–1424.

41. Gibbs M, Stanford JL, McIndoe RA, et al: Evidence for a rare prostate cancer-susceptibility locus at chromosome 1p36. Am J Hum Genet 1999;64:776–787.

42. Xu J, Meyers D, Freije D, et al: Evidence for a prostate cancer susceptibility locus on the X chromosome. Nat Genet 1998;20:175–179.

43. Berry R, Schroeder JJ, French AJ, et al: Evidence for a prostate cancer-susceptibility locus on chromosome 20. Am J Hum Genet 2000;67:82–91.

44. Tavtigian SV, Simard J, Teng DH, et al: A candidate prostate cancer susceptibility gene at chromosome 17p. Nat Genet 2001;27:172–180.

45. Xu J, Zheng SL, Hawkins GA, et al: Linkage and association studies of prostate cancer susceptibility: Evidence for linkage at 8p22-23. Am J Hum Genet 2001;69:341–150.

46. Carpten J, Nupponen N, Isaacs S, et al: Germline mutations in the ribonuclease L gene in families showing linkage with HPC1. Nat Genet 2002;30:181–184.

47. Xu J, Zheng SL, Komiya A, et al: Germline mutations and sequence variants of the macrophage scavenger receptor 1 gene are associated with prostate cancer risk. Nat Genet 2002;32:321–324.

48. Silverman RH, Jung DD, Nolan-Sorden NL, Dieffenbach CW, Kedar VP, SenGupta DN: Purification and analysis of murine 2-5A-dependent RNase. J Biol Chem 1988;263:7336–7341.

49. Jacobsen H, Czarniecki CW, Krause D, Friedman RM, Silverman RH: Interferon-induced synthesis of 2-5A-dependent RNase in mouse JLS-V9R cells. Virology 1983;125:496–601.

50. Floyd-Smith G, Slattery E, Lengyel P: Interferon action: RNA cleavage pattern of a (2'-5')oligoadenylate–dependent endonuclease. Science 1981;212:1030–1032.

51. Clemens MJ, Williams BR: Inhibition of cell-free protein synthesis by pppA2'p5'A2'p5'A: A novel oligonucleotide synthesized by interferon-treated L cell extracts. Cell 1978;13:565–572.

52. Zhou A, Hassel BA, Silverman RH: Expression cloning of 2-5A-dependent RNAase: A uniquely regulated mediator of interferon action. Cell 1993;72:753–765.

53. Casey G, Neville PJ, Plummer SJ, et al: RNASEL Arg462Gln variant is implicated in up to 13% of prostate cancer cases. Nat Genet 2002;32:581–583.

54. Platt N, Gordon S: Is the class A macrophage scavenger receptor (SR-A) multifunctional? The mouse's tale. J Clin Invest 2001;108:649–654.

55. Dejager S, Mietus-Snyder M, Friera A, Pitas RE: Dominant negative mutations of the scavenger receptor: Native receptor inactivation by expression of truncated variants. J Clin Invest 1993;92:894–902.

56. Zhou A, Paranjape J, Brown TL, et al: Interferon action and apoptosis are defective in mice devoid of 2',5'-oligoadenylate–dependent RNase L. EMBO J 1997;16:6355–6363.

57. Suzuki H, Kurihara Y, Takeya M, et al: A role for macrophage scavenger receptors in atherosclerosis and susceptibility to infection. Nature 1997;386:292–296.

58. Peiser L, Gough PJ, Kodama T, Gordon S: Macrophage class A scavenger receptor–mediated phagocytosis of *Escherichia coli*: Role of cell heterogeneity, microbial strain, and culture conditions in vitro. Infect Immun 2000;68:1953–1963.

59. Thomas CA, Li Y, Kodama T, Suzuki H, Silverstein SC, El Khoury J: Protection from lethal gram-positive infection by macrophage scavenger receptor–dependent phagocytosis. J Exp Med 2000;191:147–156.

60. Edwards A, Hammond HA, Jin L, Caskey CT, Chakraborty R: Genetic variation at five trimeric and tetrameric tandem repeat loci in four human population groups. Genomics 1992;12:241–253.

61. Chamberlain NL, Driver ED, Miesfeld RL: The length and location of CAG trinucleotide repeats in the androgen receptor N-terminal domain affect transactivation function. Nucleic Acids Res 1994;22:3181–3186.

62. Kazemi-Esfarjani P, Trifiro MA, Pinsky L: Evidence for a repressive function of the long polyglutamine tract in the human androgen receptor: Possible pathogenetic relevance for the (CAG)n-expanded neuronopathies. Hum Mol Genet 1995;4:523–527.

63. Irvine RA, Ma H, Yu MC, Ross RK, Stallcup MR, Coetzee GA: Inhibition of p160-mediated coactivation with increasing androgen receptor polyglutamine length. Hum Mol Genet 2000;9:267–274.

64. Beilin J, Ball EM, Favaloro JM, Zajac JD: Effect of the androgen receptor CAG repeat polymorphism on transcriptional activity: Specificity in prostate and non-prostate cell lines. J Mol Endocrinol 2000;25:85–96.

65. Hsing AW, Gao YT, Wu G, et al: Polymorphic CAG and GGN repeat lengths in the androgen receptor gene and prostate cancer risk: A population-based case-control study in China. Cancer Res 2000;60:5111–5116.

66. Hakimi JM, Schoenberg MP, Rondinelli RH, Piantadosi S, Barrack ER: Androgen receptor variants with short glutamine or glycine repeats may identify unique subpopulations of men with prostate cancer. Clin Cancer Res 1997;3:1599–1608.

67. Giovannucci E, Stampfer MJ, Krithivas K, et al: The CAG repeat within the androgen receptor gene and its relationship to prostate cancer. Proc Natl Acad Sci USA 1997;94:3320–3323.

68. Stanford JL, Just JJ, Gibbs M, et al: Polymorphic repeats in the androgen receptor gene: Molecular markers of prostate cancer risk. Cancer Res 1997;57:1194–1198.

69. Irvine RA, Yu MC, Ross RK, Coetzee GA: The CAG and GGC microsatellites of the androgen receptor gene are in linkage disequilibrium in men with prostate cancer. Cancer Res 1995;55:1937–1940.

70. Platz EA, Giovannucci E, Dahl DM, et al: The androgen receptor gene GGN microsatellite and prostate cancer risk. Cancer Epidemiol Biomarkers Prev 1998;7:379–384.

71. Makridakis NM, Ross RK, Pike MC, et al: Association of mis-sense substitution in SRD5A2 gene with prostate cancer in African-American and Hispanic men in Los Angeles, USA. Lancet 1999;354:975–978.

72. Makridakis N, Ross RK, Pike MC, et al: A prevalent missense substitution that modulates activity of prostatic steroid 5alpha-reductase. Cancer Res 1997;57:1020–1022.

73. Nam RK, Toi A, Vesprini D, et al: V89L polymorphism of type-2, 5-alpha reductase enzyme gene predicts prostate cancer presence and progression. Urology 2001;57:199–204.

74. Thompson IM, Goodman PJ, Tangen CM, et al: The influence of finasteride on the development of prostate cancer. N Engl J Med 2003;349:215–224.

75. Stanford JL, Noonan EA, Iwasaki L, et al: A polymorphism in the CYP17 gene and risk of prostate cancer. Cancer Epidemiol Biomarkers Prev 2002;11:243–247.

76. Kittles RA, Panguluri RK, Chen W, et al: Cyp17 promoter variant associated with prostate cancer aggressiveness in African Americans. Cancer Epidemiol Biomarkers Prev 2001;10:943–947.

77. Haiman CA, Stampfer MJ, Giovannucci E, et al: The relationship between a polymorphism in CYP17 with plasma hormone levels and prostate cancer. Cancer Epidemiol Biomarkers Prev 2001;10:743–748.

78. Habuchi T, Liqing Z, Suzuki T, et al: Increased risk of prostate cancer and benign prostatic hyperplasia associated with a CYP17 gene polymorphism with a gene dosage effect. Cancer Res 2000;60:5710–5713.

79. Gsur A, Bernhofer G, Hinteregger S, et al: A polymorphism in the CYP17 gene is associated with prostate cancer risk. Int J Cancer 2000;87:434–437.

80. Wadelius M, Andersson AO, Johansson JE, Wadelius C, Rane E: Prostate cancer associated with CYP17 genotype. Pharmacogenetics 1999;9:635–639.

81. Lunn RM, Bell DA, Mohler JL, Taylor JA: Prostate cancer risk and polymorphism in 17 hydroxylase (CYP17) and steroid reductase (SRD5A2). Carcinogenesis 1999;20:1727–1731.

82. Hsing AW, Tsao L, Devesa SS: International trends and patterns of prostate cancer incidence and mortality. Int J Cancer 2000;85:60–67.

83. Reddy S, Shapiro M, Morton R Jr, Brawley OW: Prostate cancer in black and white Americans. Cancer Metastasis Rev 2003;22:83–86.

84. Whittemore AS, Kolonel LN, Wu AH, et al: Prostate cancer in relation to diet, physical activity, and body size in blacks, whites, and Asians in the United States and Canada. J Natl Cancer Inst 1995;87:652–661.

85. Haenszel W, Kurihara M: Studies of Japanese migrants. I. Mortality from cancer and other diseases among Japanese in the United States. J Natl Cancer Inst 1968;40:43–68.

86. Shimizu H, Ross RK, Bernstein L, Yatani R, Henderson BE, Mack TM: Cancers of the prostate and breast among Japanese and white immigrants in Los Angeles County. Br J Cancer 1991;63:963–966.

87. Giovannucci E, Rimm EB, Colditz GA, et al: A prospective study of dietary fat and risk of prostate cancer. J Natl Cancer Inst 1993;85:1571–1579.

88. Gann PH, Hennekens CH, Sacks FM, Grodstein F, Giovannucci EL, Stampfer MJ: Prospective study of plasma fatty acids and risk of prostate cancer. J Natl Cancer Inst 1994;86:281–286.

89. Le Marchand L, Kolonel LN, Wilkens LR, Myers BC, Hirohata T: Animal fat consumption and prostate cancer: A prospective study in Hawaii. Epidemiology 1994;5:276–282.

90. Gross GA, Turesky RJ, Fay LB, Stillwell WG, Skipper PL, Tannenbaum SR: Heterocyclic aromatic amine formation in grilled bacon, beef and fish and in grill scrapings. Carcinogenesis 1993;14:2313–2318.

91. Morgenthaler PM, Holzhauser D: Analysis of mutations induced by 2-amino-1-methyl-6-phenylimidazo[4,5-b]pyridine (PhIP) in human lymphoblastoid cells. Carcinogenesis 1995;16:713–718.

92. Knize MG, Salmon CP, Mehta SS, Felton JS: Analysis of cooked muscle meats for heterocyclic aromatic amine carcinogens. Mutat Res 1997;376:129–134.

93. Lijinsky W, Shubik P: Benzo(a)pyrene and other polynuclear hydrocarbons in charcoal-broiled meat. Science 1964;145:53–55.

94. Stuart GR, Holcroft J, de Boer JG, Glickman BW: Prostate mutations in rats induced by the suspected human carcinogen 2-amino-1-methyl-6-phenylimidazo[4,5-b]pyridine. Cancer Res 2000;60:266–268.

95. Shirai T, Sano M, Tamano S, et al: The prostate: A target for carcinogenicity of 2-amino-1-methyl-6-phenylimidazo[4,5-b]pyridine (PhIP) derived from cooked foods. Cancer Res 1997;57:195–198.

96. Chan JM, Stampfer MJ, Ma J, Gann PH, Gaziano JM, Giovannucci EL: Dairy products, calcium, and prostate cancer risk in the Physicians' Health Study. Am J Clin Nutr 2001;74:549–554.

97. Gann PH, Ma J, Giovannucci E, et al: Lower prostate cancer risk in men with elevated plasma lycopene levels: Results of a prospective analysis. Cancer Res 1999;59:1225–1230.

98. Cohen JH, Kristal AR, Stanford JL: Fruit and vegetable intakes and prostate cancer risk. J Natl Cancer Inst 2000;92:61–68.

99. Chen L, Stacewicz-Sapuntzakis M, Duncan C, et al: Oxidative DNA damage in prostate cancer patients consuming tomato sauce-based entrees as a whole-food intervention. J Natl Cancer Inst 2001;93:1872–1879.

100. Zhang Y, Kensler TW, Cho CG, Posner GH, Talalay P: Anticarcinogenic activities of sulforaphane and structurally related synthetic norbornyl isothiocyanates. Proc Natl Acad Sci USA 1994;91:3147–3150.

101. Zhang Y, Talalay P, Cho CG, Posner GH: A major inducer of anticarcinogenic protective enzymes from broccoli: Isolation and elucidation of structure. Proc Natl Acad Sci USA 1992;89:2399–2403.

102. Dinkova-Kostova AT, Talalay P: Persuasive evidence that quinone reductase type 1 (DT diaphorase) protects cells against the toxicity of electrophiles and reactive forms of oxygen. Free Radic Biol Med 2000;29:231–240.

103. Gao X, Dinkova-Kostova AT, Talalay P: Powerful and prolonged protection of human retinal pigment epithelial cells, keratinocytes, and mouse leukemia cells against oxidative damage: The indirect antioxidant effects of sulforaphane. Proc Natl Acad Sci USA 2001;98:15221–15226.

104. Clark LC, Dalkin B, Krongrad A, et al: Decreased incidence of prostate cancer with selenium supplementation: Results of a double-blind cancer prevention trial. Br J Urol 1998;81:730–734.

105. Clark LC, Combs GF Jr, Turnbull BW, et al: Effects of selenium supplementation for cancer prevention in patients with carcinoma of the skin: A randomized controlled trial: Nutritional Prevention of Cancer Study Group [published erratum appears in JAMA 1997;277:1520]. JAMA 1996;276:1957–1963.

106. Heinonen OP, Albanes D, Virtamo J, et al: Prostate cancer and supplementation with alpha-tocopherol and beta-carotene: Incidence and mortality in a controlled trial. J Natl Cancer Inst 1998;90:440–446.

107. Hoque A, Albanes D, Lippman SM, et al: Molecular epidemiologic studies within the Selenium and Vitamin E Cancer Prevention Trial (SELECT). Cancer Causes Control 2001;12:627–633.

108. Ames BN, Gold LS, Willett WC: The causes and prevention of cancer. Proc Natl Acad Sci USA 1995;92:5258–5265.

109. Jackson AL, Loeb LA: The contribution of endogenous sources of DNA damage to the multiple mutations in cancer. Mutat Res 2001;477:7–21.

110. Ripple MO, Henry WF, Rago RP, Wilding G: Prooxidant-antioxidant shift induced by androgen treatment of human prostate carcinoma cells. J Natl Cancer Inst 1997;89:40–48.

111. Ripple MO, Henry WF, Schwarze SR, Wilding G, Weindruch R: Effect of antioxidants on androgen-induced AP-1 and NF-kappaB DNA-binding activity in prostate carcinoma cells. J Natl Cancer Inst 1999;91:1227–1232.

112. Gardner WA, Bennett BD: The prostate overview: Recent insights and speculations. In Weinstein RS, Garnder WA (eds): Pathology and Pathobiology of the Urinary Bladder and Prostate. Baltimore, Williams & Wilkins, 1992, pp 129–148.

113. Giovannucci E: Medical history and etiology of prostate cancer. Epidemiol Rev 2001;23:159–162.

114. Hoekx L, Jeuris W, Van Marck E, Wyndaele JJ: Elevated serum prostate specific antigen (PSA) related to asymptomatic prostatic inflammation. Acta Urol Belg 1998;66:1–2.

115. Roberts RO, Lieber MM, Rhodes T, Girman CJ, Bostwick DG, Jacobsen SJ: Prevalence of a physician-assigned diagnosis of prostatitis: The Olmsted County Study of Urinary Symptoms and Health Status Among Men. Urology 1998;51:578–584.

116. Hayes RB, Pottern LM, Strickler H, et al: Sexual behaviour, STDs and risks for prostate cancer. Br J Cancer 2000;82:718–725.

117. Dennis LK, Dawson DV: Meta-analysis of measures of sexual activity and prostate cancer. Epidemiology 2002;13:72–79.

118. Xia Y, Zweier JL: Superoxide and peroxynitrite generation from inducible nitric oxide synthase in macrophages. Proc Natl Acad Sci 1997;94:6954–6958.

119. Eiserich JP, Hristova M, Cross CE, et al: Formation of nitric

oxide-derived inflammatory oxidants by myeloperoxidase in neutrophils. Nature 1998;391:393–397.

120. Roberts RO, Jacobson DJ, Girman CJ, Rhodes T, Lieber MM, Jacobsen SJ: A population-based study of daily nonsteroidal anti-inflammatory drug use and prostate cancer. Mayo Clin Proc 2002;77:219–225.

121. Nelson JE, Harris RE: Inverse association of prostate cancer and non-steroidal anti-inflammatory drugs (NSAIDs): Results of a case-control study. Oncol Rep 2000;7:169–170.

122. Norrish AE, Jackson RT, McRae CU: Non-steroidal anti-inflammatory drugs and prostate cancer progression. Int J Cancer 1998;77:511–515.

123. De Marzo AM, Marchi VL, Epstein JI, Nelson WG: Proliferative inflammatory atrophy of the prostate: Implications for prostatic carcinogenesis. Am J Pathol 1999;155:1985–1992.

124. Franks LM: Atrophy and hyperplasia in the prostate proper. J Pathol Bacteriol 1954;68:617–621.

125. Putzi MJ, De Marzo AM: Morphologic transitions between proliferative inflammatory atrophy and high-grade prostatic intraepithelial neoplasia. Urology 2000;56:828–832.

126. Shah R, Mucci NR, Amin A, Macoska JA, Rubin MA: Postatrophic hyperplasia of the prostate gland: Neoplastic precursor or innocent bystander? Am J Pathol 2001;158:1767–1773.

127. Ruska KM, Sauvageot J, Epstein JI: Histology and cellular kinetics of prostatic atrophy. Am J Surg Pathol 1998;22:1073–1077.

128. Zha S, Gage WR, Sauvageot J, et al: Cyclooxygenase-2 is up-regulated in proliferative inflammatory atrophy of the prostate, but not in prostate carcinoma. Cancer Res 2001;61:8617–8623.

129. Parsons JK, Nelson CP, Gage WR, Nelson WG, Kensler TW, De Marzo AM: GSTA1 expression in normal, preneoplastic, and neoplastic human prostate tissue. Prostate 2001;49:30–37.

130. Lin X, Tascilar M, Lee WH, et al: GSTP1 CpG island hypermethylation is responsible for the absence of GSTP1 expression in human prostate cancer cells. Am J Pathol 2001;159:1815–1826.

131. Brooks JD, Weinstein M, Lin X, et al: CG island methylation changes near the GSTP1 gene in prostatic intraepithelial neoplasia. Cancer Epidemiol Biomarkers Prev 1998;7:531–536.

132. Shiraishi T, Watanabe M, Matsuura H, Kusano I, Yatani R, Stemmermann GN: The frequency of latent prostatic carcinoma in young males: The Japanese experience. In Vivo 1994;8:445–447.

133. Yatani R, Shiraishi T, Nakakuki K, et al: Trends in frequency of latent prostate carcinoma in Japan from 1965–1979 to 1982–1986. J Natl Cancer Inst 1988;80:683–687.

134. Yatani R, Chigusa I, Akazaki K, Stemmermann GN, Welsh RA, Correa P: Geographic pathology of latent prostatic carcinoma. Int J Cancer 1982;29:611–616.

135. Elo JP, Visakorpi T: Molecular genetics of prostate cancer. Ann Med 2001;33:130–141.

136. Dong JT, Chen C, Stultz BG, Isaacs JT, Frierson HF Jr: Deletion at 13q21 is associated with aggressive prostate cancers. Cancer Res 2000;60:3880–3883.

137. Elo JP, Harkonen P, Kyllonen AP, Lukkarinen O, Vihko P: Three independently deleted regions at chromosome arm 16q in human prostate cancer: Allelic loss at 16q24.1-q24.2 is associated with aggressive behaviour of the disease, recurrent growth, poor differentiation of the tumour and poor prognosis for the patient. Br J Cancer 1999;79:156–160.

138. Takahashi S, Shan AL, Ritland SR, et al: Frequent loss of heterozygosity at 7q31.1 in primary prostate cancer is associated with tumor aggressiveness and progression. Cancer Res 1995;55:4114–4119.

139. Nupponen NN, Kakkola L, Koivisto P, Visakorpi T: Genetic alterations in hormone-refractory recurrent prostate carcinomas. Am J Pathol 1998;153:141–148.

140. Takahashi S, Qian J, Brown JA, et al: Potential markers of prostate cancer aggressiveness detected by fluorescence in situ hybridization in needle biopsies. Cancer Res 1994;54:3574–3579.

141. Isaacs JT, Coffey DS: Adaptation versus selection as the mechanism responsible for the relapse of prostatic cancer to androgen ablation therapy as studied in the Dunning R-3327-H adenocarcinoma. Cancer Res 1981;41:5070–5075.

142. Isaacs JT, Wake N, Coffey DS, Sandberg AA: Genetic instability

143. Craft N, Chhor C, Tran C, et al: Evidence for clonal outgrowth of androgen-independent prostate cancer cells from androgen-dependent tumors through a two-step process. Cancer Res 1999;59:5030–5036.

144. Millar DS, Ow KK, Paul CL, Russell PJ, Molloy PL, Clark SJ: Detailed methylation analysis of the glutathione S-transferase pi (GSTP1) gene in prostate cancer. Oncogene 1999;18:1313–1324.

145. Lee WH, Morton RA, Epstein JI, et al: Cytidine methylation of regulatory sequences near the pi-class glutathione S-transferase gene accompanies human prostatic carcinogenesis. Proc Natl Acad Sci USA 1994;91:11733–11737.

146. Nelson WG, De Marzo AM, DeWeese TL: The molecular pathogenesis of prostate cancer: Implications for prostate cancer prevention. Urology 2001;57(4 suppl 1):39–45.

147. The Alpha-Tocopherol, Beta Carotene Cancer Prevention Study Group. The effect of vitamin E and beta carotene on the incidence of lung cancer and other cancers in male smokers. N Engl J Med 1994;330:1029–1035.

148. Henderson CJ, Smith AG, Ure J, Brown K, Bacon EJ, Wolf CR: Increased skin tumorigenesis in mice lacking pi class glutathione S-transferases. Proc Natl Acad Sci USA 1998;95:5275–5280.

149. Nelson CP, Kidd LC, Sauvageot J, et al: Protection against 2-hydroxyamino-1-methyl-6-phenylimidazo[4,5-b]pyridine cytotoxicity and DNA adduct formation in human prostate by glutathione S-transferase P1. Cancer Res 2001;61:103–109.

150. Bieberich CJ, Fujita K, He WW, Jay G: Prostate-specific and androgen-dependent expression of a novel homeobox gene. J Biol Chem 1996;271:31779–31782.

151. Sciavolino PJ, Abrams EW, Yang L, Austenberg LP, Shen MM, Abate-Shen C: Tissue-specific expression of murine Nkx3.1 in the male urogenital system. Dev Dyn 1997;209:127–138.

152. Steadman DJ, Giuffrida D, Gelmann EP: DNA-binding sequence of the human prostate-specific homeodomain protein NKX3.1. Nucleic Acids Res 2000;28:2389–2395.

153. Chen H, Nandi AK, Li X, Bieberich CJ: NKX-3.1 interacts with prostate-derived Ets factor and regulates the activity of the PSA promoter. Cancer Res 2002;62:338–340.

154. Bhatia-Gaur R, Donjacour AA, Sciavolino PJ, et al: Roles for Nkx3.1 in prostate development and cancer. Genes Dev 1999;13:966–977.

155. Abdulkadir SA, Magee JA, Peters TJ, et al: Conditional loss of Nkx3.1 in adult mice induces prostatic intraepithelial neoplasia. Mol Cell Biol 2002;22:1495–1503.

156. Emmert-Buck MR, Vocke CD, et al: Allelic loss on chromosome 8p12-21 in microdissected prostatic intraepithelial neoplasia. Cancer Res 1995;55:2959–2962.

157. He WW, Sciavolino PJ, Wing J, et al: A novel human prostate-specific, androgen-regulated homeobox gene (NKX3.1) that maps to 8p21, a region frequently deleted in prostate cancer. Genomics 1997;43:69–77.

158. Ornstein DK, Cinquanta M, Weiler S, et al: Expression studies and mutational analysis of the androgen regulated homeobox gene NKX3.1 in benign and malignant prostate epithelium. J Urol 2001;165:1329–1334.

159. Voeller HJ, Augustus M, Madike V, Bova GS, Carter KC, Gelmann EP: Coding region of NKX3.1, a prostate-specific homeobox gene on 8p21, is not mutated in human prostate cancers. Cancer Res 1997;57:4455–4459.

160. Bowen C, Bubendorf L, Voeller HJ, et al: Loss of NKX3.1 expression in human prostate cancers correlates with tumor progression. Cancer Res 2000;60:6111–6115.

161. Wu X, Senechal K, Neshat MS, Whang YE, Sawyers CL: The PTEN/MMAC1 tumor suppressor phosphatase functions as a negative regulator of the phosphoinositide 3-kinase/Akt pathway. Proc Natl Acad Sci USA 1998;95:15587–15591.

162. Li J, Yen C, Liaw D, et al: PTEN, a putative protein tyrosine phosphatase gene mutated in human brain, breast, and prostate cancer. Science 1997;275:1943–1947.

163. Steck PA, Pershouse MA, Jasser SA, et al: Identification of a candidate tumour suppressor gene, MMAC1, at chromosome 10q23.3 that is mutated in multiple advanced cancers. Nat Genet 1997;15:356–362.

164. Teng DH, Hu R, Lin H, et al: MMAC1/PTEN mutations in primary tumor specimens and tumor cell lines. Cancer Res 1997;57: 5221-5225.

165. Myers MP, Pass I, Batty IH, et al: The lipid phosphatase activity of PTEN is critical for its tumor suppressor function. Proc Natl Acad Sci USA 1998;95:13513-13518.

166. Myers MP, Stolarov JP, Eng C, et al: P-TEN, the tumor suppressor from human chromosome 10q23, is a dual-specificity phosphatase. Proc Natl Acad Sci USA 1997;94:9052-9057.

167. Maehama T, Dixon JE: The tumor suppressor, PTEN/MMAC1, dephosphorylates the lipid second messenger, phosphatidylinositol 3,4,5-trisphosphate. J Biol Chem 1998;273: 13375-13378.

168. Cairns P, Okami K, Halachmi S, et al: Frequent inactivation of PTEN/MMAC1 in primary prostate cancer. Cancer Res 1997;57:4997-5000.

169. Suzuki H, Freije D, Nusskern DR, et al: Interfocal heterogeneity of PTEN/MMAC1 gene alterations in multiple metastatic prostate cancer tissues. Cancer Res 1998;58:204-209.

170. Furnari FB, Huang HJ, Cavenee WK: The phosphoinositol phosphatase activity of PTEN mediates a serum-sensitive G1 growth arrest in glioma cells. Cancer Res 1998;58:5002-5008.

171. Li DM, Sun H: PTEN/MMAC1/TEP1 suppresses the tumorigenicity and induces G1 cell cycle arrest in human glioblastoma cells. Proc Natl Acad Sci USA 1998;95:15406-15411.

172. Ramaswamy S, Nakamura N, Vazquez F, et al: Regulation of G1 progression by the PTEN tumor suppressor protein is linked to inhibition of the phosphatidylinositol 3-kinase/Akt pathway. Proc Natl Acad Sci USA 1999;96:2110-2115.

173. Sun H, Lesche R, Li DM, et al: PTEN modulates cell cycle progression and cell survival by regulating phosphatidylinositol 3,4,5,-trisphosphate and Akt/protein kinase B signaling pathway. Proc Natl Acad Sci USA 1999;96:6199-6204.

174. McMenamin ME, Soung P, Perera S, Kaplan I, Loda M, Sellers WR: Loss of PTEN expression in paraffin-embedded primary prostate cancer correlates with high Gleason score and advanced stage. Cancer Res 1999;59:4291-4296.

175. Wang SI, Parsons R, Ittmann M: Homozygous deletion of the PTEN tumor suppressor gene in a subset of prostate adenocarcinomas. Clin Cancer Res 1998;4:811-815.

176. Gray IC, Stewart LM, Phillips SM, et al: Mutation and expression analysis of the putative prostate tumour-suppressor gene PTEN. Br J Cancer 1998;78:1296-1300.

177. Whang YE, Wu X, Suzuki H, et al: Inactivation of the tumor suppressor PTEN/MMAC1 in advanced human prostate cancer through loss of expression. Proc Natl Acad Sci USA 1998;95: 5246-6250.

178. Podsypanina K, Ellenson LH, Nemes A, et al: Mutation of Pten/Mmac1 in mice causes neoplasia in multiple organ systems. Proc Natl Acad Sci USA 1999;96:1563-1568.

179. Di Cristofano A, Pesce B, Cordon-Cardo C, Pandolfi PP: Pten is essential for embryonic development and tumour suppression. Nat Genet 1998;19:348-355.

180. Kim MJ, Cardiff RD, Desai N, et al: Cooperativity of Nkx3.1 and Pten loss of function in a mouse model of prostate carcinogenesis. Proc Natl Acad Sci USA 2002;99:2884-2889.

181. Kwabi-Addo B, Giri D, Schmidt K, et al: Haploinsufficiency of the Pten tumor suppressor gene promotes prostate cancer progression. Proc Natl Acad Sci USA 2001;98:11563-11568.

182. Yang RM, Naitoh J, Murphy M, et al: Low p27 expression predicts poor disease-free survival in patients with prostate cancer. J Urol 1998;159:941-945.

183. Cheville JC, Lloyd RV, Sebo TJ, et al: Expression of p27kip1 in prostatic adenocarcinoma. Mod Pathol 1998;11:324-328.

184. Cote RJ, Shi Y, Groshen S, et al: Association of p27Kip1 levels with recurrence and survival in patients with stage C prostate carcinoma. J Natl Cancer Inst 1998;90:916-920.

185. Cordon-Cardo C, Koff A, Drobnjak M, et al: Distinct altered patterns of p27KIP1 gene expression in benign prostatic hyperplasia and prostatic carcinoma. J Natl Cancer Inst 1998;90:1284-1291.

186. Guo Y, Sklar GN, Borkowski A, Kyprianou N: Loss of the cyclin-dependent kinase inhibitor p27(Kip1) protein in human prostate cancer correlates with tumor grade. Clin Cancer Res 1997;3:2269-2274.

187. De Marzo AM, Meeker AK, Epstein JI, Coffey DS: Prostate stem cell compartments: Expression of the cell cycle inhibitor p27Kip1 in normal, hyperplastic, and neoplastic cells. Am J Pathol 1998;153: 911-919.

188. Kibel AS, Faith DA, Bova GS, Isaacs WB: Loss of heterozygosity at 12p12-13 in primary and metastatic prostate adenocarcinoma. J Urol 2000;164:192-196.

189. Graff JR, Konicek BW, McNulty AM, et al: Increased AKT activity contributes to prostate cancer progression by dramatically accelerating prostate tumor growth and diminishing p27Kip1 expression. J Biol Chem 2000;275:24500-24505.

190. Gottschalk AR, Basila D, Wong M, et al: p27Kip1 is required for PTEN-induced G1 growth arrest. Cancer Res 2001;61:2105-2111.

191. Nakamura N, Ramaswamy S, Vazquez F, Signoretti S, Loda M, Sellers WR: Forkhead transcription factors are critical effectors of cell death and cell cycle arrest downstream of PTEN. Mol Cell Biol 2000;20:8969-8982.

192. Di Cristofano A, De Acetis M, Koff A, Cordon-Cardo C, Pandolfi PP: Pten and p27KIP1 cooperate in prostate cancer tumor suppression in the mouse. Nat Genet 2001;27:222-224.

193. Eisenberger MA, Blumenstein BA, Crawford ED, et al: Bilateral orchiectomy with or without flutamide for metastatic prostate cancer. N Engl J Med 1998;339:1036-1042.

194. Crawford ED, Eisenberger MA, McLeod DG, et al: A controlled trial of leuprolide with and without flutamide in prostatic carcinoma. N Engl J Med 1989;321:419-424.

195. Laufer M, Denmeade SR, Sinibaldi VJ, Carducci MA, Eisenberger MA: Complete androgen blockade for prostate cancer: What went wrong? J Urol 2000;164:3-9.

196. Amler LC, Agus DB, LeDuc C, et al: Dysregulated expression of androgen-responsive and nonresponsive genes in the androgen-independent prostate cancer xenograft model CWR22-R1. Cancer Res 2000;60:6134-6141.

197. Mousses S, Wagner U, Chen Y, et al: Failure of hormone therapy in prostate cancer involves systematic restoration of androgen responsive genes and activation of rapamycin sensitive signaling. Oncogene 2001;20:6718-6723.

198. van der Kwast TH, Schalken J, Ruizeveld de Winter JA, et al: Androgen receptors in endocrine-therapy-resistant human prostate cancer. Int J Cancer 1991;48:189-193.

199. Visakorpi T, Hyytinen E, Koivisto P, et al: In vivo amplification of the androgen receptor gene and progression of human prostate cancer. Nat Genet 1995;9:401-406.

200. Koivisto P, Kononen J, Palmberg C, et al: Androgen receptor gene amplification: A possible molecular mechanism for androgen deprivation therapy failure in prostate cancer. Cancer Res 1997;57:314-319.

201. Haapala K, Hyytinen ER, Roiha M, et al: Androgen receptor alterations in prostate cancer relapsed during a combined androgen blockade by orchiectomy and bicalutamide. Lab Invest 2001;81:1647-1651.

202. Marcelli M, Ittmann M, Mariani S, et al: Androgen receptor mutations in prostate cancer. Cancer Res 2000;60:944-949.

203. Taplin ME, Bubley GJ, Shuster TD, et al: Mutation of the androgen-receptor gene in metastatic androgen-independent prostate cancer. N Engl J Med 1995;332:1393-1398.

204. Taplin ME, Bubley GJ, Ko YJ, et al: Selection for androgen receptor mutations in prostate cancers treated with androgen antagonist. Cancer Res 1999;59:2511-2515.

205. Tilley WD, Buchanan G, Hickey TE, Bentel JM: Mutations in the androgen receptor gene are associated with progression of human prostate cancer to androgen independence. Clin Cancer Res 1996;2:277-285.

206. Veldscholte J, Ris-Stalpers C, Kuiper GG, et al: A mutation in the ligand binding domain of the androgen receptor of human LNCaP cells affects steroid binding characteristics and response to anti-androgens. Biochem Biophys Res Commun 1990;173:534-540.

207. Schoenberg MP, Hakimi JM, Wang S, et al: Microsatellite mutation (CAG24Æ18) in the androgen receptor gene in human prostate cancer. Biochem Biophys Res Commun 1994;198:74-80.

208. Suzuki H, Akakura K, Komiya A, Aida S, Akimoto S, Shimazaki J: Codon 877 mutation in the androgen receptor gene in advanced prostate cancer: Relation to antiandrogen withdrawal syndrome. Prostate 1996;29:153-158.

Specific Malignancies

III

209. Suzuki H, Sato N, Watabe Y, Masai M, Seino S, Shimazaki J: Androgen receptor gene mutations in human prostate cancer. J Steroid Biochem Mol Biol 1993;46:759-765.

210. Newmark JR, Hardy DO, Tonb DC, et al: Androgen receptor gene mutations in human prostate cancer. Proc Natl Acad Sci USA 1992;89:6319-6323.

211. Gaddipati JP, McLeod DG, Heidenberg HB, et al: Frequent detection of codon 877 mutation in the androgen receptor gene in advanced prostate cancers. Cancer Res 1994;54:2861-2864.

212. Evans BA, Harper ME, Daniells CE, et al: Low incidence of androgen receptor gene mutations in human prostatic tumors using single strand conformation polymorphism analysis. Prostate 1996;28:162-171.

213. Tan J, Sharief Y, Hamil KG, et al: Dehydroepiandrosterone activates mutant androgen receptors expressed in the androgen-dependent human prostate cancer xenograft CWR22 and LNCaP cells. Mol Endocrinol 1997;11:450-459.

214. Veldscholte J, Voorhorst-Ogink MM, Bolt-de Vries J, van Rooij HC, Trapman J, Mulder E: Unusual specificity of the androgen receptor in the human prostate tumor cell line LNCaP: High affinity for progestagenic and estrogenic steroids. Biochim Biophys Acta 1990;1052:187-194.

215. Culig Z, Hobisch A, Cronauer MV, et al: Mutant androgen receptor detected in an advanced-stage prostatic carcinoma is activated by adrenal androgens and progesterone. Mol Endocrinol 1993;7:1541-1550.

216. Shi XB, Ma AH, Xia L, Kung HJ, de Vere White RW: Functional analysis of 44 mutant androgen receptors from human prostate cancer. Cancer Res 2002;62:1496-1502.

217. Sadar MD, Gleave ME: Ligand-independent activation of the androgen receptor by the differentiation agent butyrate in human prostate cancer cells. Cancer Res 2000;60:5825-5831.

218. Craft N, Shostak Y, Carey M, Sawyers CL: A mechanism for hormone-independent prostate cancer through modulation of androgen receptor signaling by the HER-2/neu tyrosine kinase. Nat Med 1999;5:280-285.

219. Hobisch A, Eder IE, Putz T, et al: Interleukin-6 regulates prostate-specific protein expression in prostate carcinoma cells by activation of the androgen receptor. Cancer Res 1998;58:4640-4645.

220. Nazareth LV, Weigel NL: Activation of the human androgen receptor through a protein kinase A signaling pathway. J Biol Chem 1996;271:19900-19907.

221. Dhanasekaran SM, Barrette TR, Ghosh D, et al: Delineation of prognostic biomarkers in prostate cancer. Nature 2001;412:822-826.

222. Luo JH, Yu YP, Cieply K, et al: Gene expression analysis of prostate cancers. Mol Carcinog 2002;33:25-35.

223. Stamey TA, Warrington JA, Caldwell MC, et al: Molecular genetic profiling of Gleason grade 4/5 prostate cancers compared to benign prostatic hyperplasia. J Urol 2001;166:2171-2177.

224. Welsh JB, Sapinoso LM, Su AI, et al: Analysis of gene expression identifies candidate markers and pharmacological targets in prostate cancer. Cancer Res 2001;61:5974-5978.

225. Magee JA, Araki T, Patil S, et al: Expression profiling reveals hepsin overexpression in prostate cancer. Cancer Res 2001;61:5692-5696.

226. Luo J, Duggan DJ, Chen Y, et al: Human prostate cancer and benign prostatic hyperplasia: Molecular dissection by gene expression profiling. Cancer Res 2001;61:4683-4688.

227. Waghray A, Schober M, Feroze F, Yao F, Virgin J, Chen YQ: Identification of differentially expressed genes by serial analysis of gene expression in human prostate cancer. Cancer Res 2001;61:4283-4286.

228. Nelson PS, Han D, Rochon Y, et al: Comprehensive analyses of prostate gene expression: Convergence of expressed sequence tag databases, transcript profiling and proteomics. Electrophoresis 2000;21:1823-1831.

229. Xu J, Stolk JA, Zhang X, et al: Identification of differentially expressed genes in human prostate cancer using subtraction and microarray. Cancer Res 2000;60:1677-1682.

230. Walker MG, Volkmuth W, Sprinzak E, Hodgson D, Klingler T: Prediction of gene function by genome-scale expression analysis: Prostate cancer-associated genes. Genome Res 1999;9:1198-1203.

231. Huang GM, Ng WL, Farkas J, et al: Prostate cancer expression profiling by cDNA sequencing analysis. Genomics 1999;59:178-186.

232. Rhodes DR, Barrette TR, Rubin MA, Ghosh D, Chinnaiyan AM: Meta-analysis of microarrays: Interstudy validation of gene expression profiles reveals pathway dysregulation in prostate cancer. Cancer Res 2002;62:4427-4433.

233. Tsuji A, Torres-Rosado A, Arai T, et al: Hepsin, a cell membrane-associated protease: Characterization, tissue distribution, and gene localization. J Biol Chem 1991;266:16948-16953.

234. Torres-Rosado A, O'Shea KS, Tsuji A, Chou SH, Kurachi K: Hepsin, a putative cell-surface serine protease, is required for mammalian cell growth. Proc Natl Acad Sci USA 1993;90:7181-7185.

235. Yu IS, Chen HJ, Lee YS, et al: Mice deficient in hepsin, a serine protease, exhibit normal embryogenesis and unchanged hepatocyte regeneration ability. Thromb Haemost 2000;84:865-870.

236. Wu Q, Yu D, Post J, Halks-Miller M, Sadler JE, Morser J: Generation and characterization of mice deficient in hepsin, a hepatic transmembrane serine protease. J Clin Invest 1998;101:321-326.

237. Schmitz W, Albers C, Fingerhut R, Conzelmann E: Purification and characterization of an alpha-methylacyl-CoA racemase from human liver. Eur J Biochem 1995;231:815-822.

238. Jiang Z, Woda BA, Rock KL, et al: P504S: A new molecular marker for the detection of prostate carcinoma. Am J Surg Pathol 2001;25:1397-1404.

239. Ferdinandusse S, Denis S, Clayton PT, et al: Mutations in the gene encoding peroxisomal alpha-methylacyl-CoA racemase cause adult-onset sensory motor neuropathy. Nat Genet 2000;24:188-191.

240. Rubin MA, Zhou M, Dhanasekaran SM, et al: Alpha-methylacyl coenzyme A racemase as a tissue biomarker for prostate cancer. JAMA 2002;287:1662-1670.

241. Luo J, Zha S, Gage WR, et al: Alpha-methylacyl-CoA racemase: A new molecular marker for prostate cancer. Cancer Res 2002;62:2220-2226.

242. Varambally S, Dhanasekaran SM, Zhou M, et al: The polycomb group protein EZH2 is involved in progression of prostate cancer. Nature 2002;419:624-629.

243. McEachern MJ, Krauskopf A, Blackburn EH: Telomeres and their control. Annu Rev Genet 2000;34:331-358.

244. Maser RS, DePinho RA: Connecting chromosomes, crisis, and cancer. Science 2002;297:565-569.

245. Greider CW, Blackburn EH: Identification of a specific telomere terminal transferase activity in Tetrahymena extracts. Cell 1985;43:405-413.

246. O'Hagan RC, Chang S, Maser RS, et al: Telomere dysfunction provokes regional amplification and deletion in cancer genomes. Cancer Cell 2002;2:149-155.

247. Hackett JA, Feldser DM, Greider CW: Telomere dysfunction increases mutation rate and genomic instability. Cell 2001;106:275-286.

248. Chin L, Artandi SE, Shen Q, et al: p53 deficiency rescues the adverse effects of telomere loss and cooperates with telomere dysfunction to accelerate carcinogenesis. Cell 1999;97:527-538.

249. Sommerfeld HJ, Meeker AK, Piatyszek MA, Bova GS, Shay JW, Coffey DS: Telomerase activity: A prevalent marker of malignant human prostate tissue. Cancer Res 1996;56:218-222.

250. Meeker AK, Gage WR, Hicks JL, et al: Telomere length assessment in human archival tissues: Combined telomere fluorescence in situ hybridization and immunostaining. Am J Pathol 2002;160:1259-1268.

251. Meeker AK, Hicks JL, Platz EA, et al: Telomere shortening is an early somatic DNA alteration in human prostate tumorigenesis. Cancer Res 2002;62:6405-6409.

252. Prevention of cancer in the next millennium: Report of the Chemoprevention Working Group to the American Association for Cancer Research. Cancer Res 1999;59:4743-4758.

253. Gail MH, Brinton LA, Byar DP, et al: Projecting individualized probabilities of developing breast cancer for white females who are being examined annually. J Natl Cancer Inst 1989;81:1879-1886.

254. Andriole G, Lieber M, Smith J, et al: Treatment with finasteride following radical prostatectomy for prostate cancer. Urology 1995;45:491-497.

255. Presti JC Jr, Fair WR, Andriole G, et al: Multicenter, randomized, double-blind, placebo controlled study to investigate the effect of finasteride (MK-906) on stage D prostate cancer. J Urol 1992;148:1201–1204.

256. Homma Y, Kaneko M, Kondo Y, Kawabe K, Kakizoe T: Inhibition of rat prostate carcinogenesis by a 5alpha-reductase inhibitor, FK143. J Natl Cancer Inst 1997;89:803–807.

257. Tsukamoto S, Akaza H, Imada S, et al: Chemoprevention of rat prostate carcinogenesis by use of finasteride or casodex. J Natl Cancer Inst 1995;87:842–843.

258. Esmat AY, Refaie FM, Shaheen MH, Said MM: Chemoprevention of prostate carcinogenesis by DFMO and/or finasteride treatment in male Wistar rats. Tumori 2002;88:513–521.

259. Andriole GL, Guess HA, Epstein JI, et al: Treatment with finasteride preserves usefulness of prostate-specific antigen in the detection of prostate cancer: Results of a randomized, double-blind, placebo-controlled clinical trial. PLESS Study Group. Proscar Long-term Efficacy and Safety Study. Urology 1998;52:195–201.

260. Cote RJ, Skinner EC, Salem CE, et al: The effect of finasteride on the prostate gland in men with elevated serum prostate-specific antigen levels. Br J Cancer 1998;78:413–418.

261. Roehrborn CG, Boyle P, Nickel JC, Hoefner K, Andriole G: Efficacy and safety of a dual inhibitor of 5-alpha-reductase types 1 and 2 (dutasteride) in men with benign prostatic hyperplasia. Urology 2002;60:434–441.

262. Hardell L, Degerman A, Tomic R, Marklund SL, Bergfors M: Levels of selenium in plasma and glutathione peroxidase in erythrocytes in patients with prostate cancer or benign hyperplasia. Eur J Cancer Prev 1995;4:91–95.

263. Chan JM, Stampfer MJ, Ma J, Rimm EB, Willett WC, Giovannucci EL: supplemental vitamin E intake and prostate cancer risk in a large cohort of men in the United States. Cancer Epidemiol Biomarkers Prev 1999;8:893–899.

264. Brooks JD, Metter EJ, Chan DW, et al: Plasma selenium level before diagnosis and the risk of prostate cancer development. J Urol 2001;166:2034–2038.

265. Kristal AR, Stanford JL, Cohen JH, Wicklund K, Patterson RE: Vitamin and mineral supplement use is associated with reduced risk of prostate cancer. Cancer Epidemiol Biomarkers Prev 1999;8:887–892.

266. Helzlsouer KJ, Huang HY, Alberg AJ, et al: Association between alpha-tocopherol, gamma-tocopherol, selenium, and subsequent prostate cancer. J Natl Cancer Inst 2000;92:2018–2023.

267. Nomura AM, Lee J, Stemmermann GN, Combs GF Jr: Serum selenium and subsequent risk of prostate cancer. Cancer Epidemiol Biomarkers Prev 2000;9:883–887.

268. Yoshizawa K, Willett WC, Morris SJ, et al: Study of prediagnostic selenium level in toenails and the risk of advanced prostate cancer. J Natl Cancer Inst 1998;90:1219–1224.

269. Duffield-Lillico AJ, Dalkin BL, Reid ME, et al: Selenium supplementation, baseline plasma selenium status and incidence of prostate cancer: An analysis of the complete treatment period of the Nutritional Prevention of Cancer Trial. BJU International 2003;91:608–612.

270. Klein EA, Thompson IM, Lippman SM, et al: SELECT: The next prostate cancer prevention trial. Selenium and Vitamin E Cancer Prevention Trial. J Urol 2001;166:1311–1315.

271. Paquette EL, Sun L, Paquette LR, Connelly R, McLeod DG, Moul JW: Improved prostate cancer-specific survival and other disease parameters: Impact of prostate-specific antigen testing. Urology 2002;60:756–759.

272. Smith DS, Catalona WJ: Interexaminer variability of digital rectal examination in detecting prostate cancer. Urology 1995;45:70–74.

273. Ellis WJ, Chetner MP, Preston SD, Brawer MK: Diagnosis of prostatic carcinoma: The yield of serum prostate specific antigen, digital rectal examination and transrectal ultrasonography. J Urol 1994;152:1520–1525.

274. Cooner WH, Mosley BR, Rutherford CL Jr, et al: Prostate cancer detection in a clinical urological practice by ultrasonography, digital rectal examination and prostate specific antigen. J Urol 1990;143:1146–1152.

275. Catalona WJ, Richie JP, Ahmann FR, et al: Comparison of digital rectal examination and serum prostate specific antigen in the early detection of prostate cancer: Results of a multicenter clinical trial of 6,630 men. J Urol 1994;151:1283–1290.

276. Thompson IM, Rounder JB, Teague JL, Peek M, Spence CR: Impact of routine screening for adenocarcinoma of the prostate on stage distribution. J Urol 1987;137:424–426.

277. Epstein JI, Walsh PC, Carmichael M, Brendler CB: Pathologic and clinical findings to predict tumor extent of nonpalpable (stage T1c) prostate cancer. JAMA 1994;271:368–374.

278. Schroder FH, van der Maas P, Beemsterboer P, et al: Evaluation of the digital rectal examination as a screening test for prostate cancer. Rotterdam section of the European Randomized Study of Screening for Prostate Cancer. J Natl Cancer Inst 1998;90: 1817–1823.

279. Carvalhal GF, Smith DS, Mager DE, Ramos C, Catalona WJ: Digital rectal examination for detecting prostate cancer at prostate specific antigen levels of 4 ng./ml. or less. J Urol 1999;161: 835–839.

280. Catalona WJ, Smith DS, Ratliff TL, et al: Measurement of prostate-specific antigen in serum as a screening test for prostate cancer. N Engl J Med 1991;324:1156–1161.

281. Brawer MK, Chetner MP, Beatie J, Buchner DM, Vessella RL, Lange PH: Screening for prostatic carcinoma with prostate specific antigen. J Urol 1992;147:841–845.

282. Labrie F, Dupont A, Suburu R, et al: Serum prostate specific antigen as pre-screening test for prostate cancer. J Urol 1992;147:846–851.

283. Littrup PJ, Lee F, Mettlin C: Prostate cancer screening: Current trends and future implications. CA Cancer J Clin 1992;42: 198–211.

284. Kranse R, Beemsterboer P, Rietbergen J, Habbema D, Hugosson J, Schroder FH: Predictors for biopsy outcome in the European Randomized Study of Screening for Prostate Cancer (Rotterdam region). Prostate 1999;39:316–322.

285. McCormack RT, Rittenhouse HG, Finlay JA, et al: Molecular forms of prostate-specific antigen and the human kallikrein gene family: A new era. Urology 1995;45:729–744.

286. Diamandis EP, Yousef GM, Clements J, et al: New nomenclature for the human tissue kallikrein gene family. Clin Chem 2000;46: 1855–1858.

287. Young CY, Montgomery BT, Andrews PE, Qui SD, Bilhartz DL, Tindall DJ: Hormonal regulation of prostate-specific antigen messenger RNA in human prostatic adenocarcinoma cell line LNCaP: Cancer Res 1991;51:3748–3752.

288. Henttu P, Liao SS, Vihko P: Androgens up-regulate the human prostate-specific antigen messenger ribonucleic acid (mRNA), but down-regulate the prostatic acid phosphatase mRNA in the LNCaP cell line. Endocrinology 1992;130:766–772.

289. Vieira JG, Nishida SK, Pereira AB, Arraes RF, Verreschi IT: Serum levels of prostate-specific antigen in normal boys throughout puberty. J Clin Endocrinol Metab 1994;78:1185–1187.

290. Oesterling JE, Jacobsen SJ, Chute CG, et al: Serum prostate-specific antigen in a community-based population of healthy men: Establishment of age-specific reference ranges. JAMA 1993;270:860–864.

291. Fowler JE Jr, Bigler SA, Kilambi NK, Land SA: Relationships between prostate-specific antigen and prostate volume in black and white men with benign prostate biopsies. Urology 1999;53: 1175–1178.

292. Morgan TO, Jacobsen SJ, McCarthy WF, Jacobson DJ, McLeod DG, Moul JW: Age-specific reference ranges for prostate-specific antigen in black men. N Engl J Med 1996;335:304–310.

293. Stamey TA, Yang N, Hay AR, McNeal JE, Freiha FS, Redwine E: Prostate-specific antigen as a serum marker for adenocarcinoma of the prostate. N Engl J Med 1987;317:909–916.

294. Wang MC, Papsidero LD, Kuriyama M, Valenzuela LA, Murphy GP, Chu TM: Prostate antigen: A new potential marker for prostatic cancer. Prostate 1981;2:89–96.

295. Ercole CJ, Lange PH, Mathisen M, Chiou RK, Reddy PK, Vessella RL: Prostatic specific antigen and prostatic acid phosphatase in the monitoring and staging of patients with prostatic cancer. J Urol 1987;138:1181–1184.

296. Guess HA, Heyse JF, Gormley GJ: The effect of finasteride on prostate-specific antigen in men with benign prostatic hyperplasia. Prostate 1993;22:31–37.

Specific Malignancies

III

297. Hammerer P, Huland H: Systematic sextant biopsies in 651 patients referred for prostate evaluation. J Urol 1994;151:99-102.

298. Gann PH, Hennekens CH, Stampfer MJ: A prospective evaluation of plasma prostate-specific antigen for detection of prostatic cancer. JAMA 1995;273:289-294.

299. Carter HB, Pearson JD: Prostate-specific antigen velocity and repeated measures of prostate-specific antigen. Urol Clin North Am 1997;24:333-338.

300. Draisma G, Boer R, Otto SJ, et al: Lead times and overdetection due to prostate-specific antigen screening: Estimates from the European Randomized Study of Screening for Prostate Cancer. J Natl Cancer Inst 2003;95:868-878.

301. Babaian RJ, Fritsche HA, Evans RB: Prostate-specific antigen and prostate gland volume: Correlation and clinical application. J Clin Lab Anal 1990;4:135-137.

302. Littrup PJ, Kane RA, Williams CR, et al: Determination of prostate volume with transrectal US for cancer screening. I. Comparison with prostate-specific antigen assays. Radiology 1991;178:537-542.

303. Benson MC, Whang IS, Olsson CA, McMahon DJ, Cooner WH: The use of prostate specific antigen density to enhance the predictive value of intermediate levels of serum prostate specific antigen. J Urol 1992;147:817-821.

304. Benson MC, Whang IS, Pantuck A, et al: Prostate specific antigen density: A means of distinguishing benign prostatic hypertrophy and prostate cancer. J Urol 1992;147:815-816.

305. Bazinet M, Meshref AW, Trudel C, et al: Prospective evaluation of prostate-specific antigen density and systematic biopsies for early detection of prostatic carcinoma. Urology 1994;43:44-51.

306. Rommel FM, Agusta VE, Breslin JA, et al: The use of prostate specific antigen and prostate specific antigen density in the diagnosis of prostate cancer in a community based urology practice. J Urol 1994;151:88-93.

307. Djavan B, Zlotta AR, Remzi M, et al: Total and transition zone prostate volume and age: How do they affect the utility of PSA-based diagnostic parameters for early prostate cancer detection? Urology 1999;54:846-852.

308. Djavan B, Zlotta A, Kratzik C, et al: PSA, PSA density, PSA density of transition zone, free/total PSA ratio, and PSA velocity for early detection of prostate cancer in men with serum PSA 2.5 to 4.0 ng/mL. Urology 1999;54:517-522.

309. Carter HB, Pearson JD, Metter EJ, et al: Longitudinal evaluation of prostate-specific antigen levels in men with and without prostate disease. JAMA 1992;267:2215-2220.

310. Smith DS, Catalona WJ: Rate of change in serum prostate specific antigen levels as a method for prostate cancer detection. J Urol 1994;152:1163-1167.

311. Carter HB, Pearson JD, Waclawiw Z, et al: Prostate-specific antigen variability in men without prostate cancer: Effect of sampling interval on prostate-specific antigen velocity. Urology 1995;45:591-596.

312. Mikolajczyk SD, Marks LS, Partin AW, Rittenhouse HG: Free prostate-specific antigen in serum is becoming more complex. Urology 2002;59:797-802.

313. Carter HB: A PSA threshold of 4.0 ng/mL for early detection of prostate cancer: The only rational approach for men 50 years old and older. Urology 2000;55:796-799.

314. Catalona WJ, Ramos CG, Carvalhal GF, Yan Y: Lowering PSA cutoffs to enhance detection of curable prostate cancer. Urology 2000;55:791-795.

315. Catalona WJ, Smith DS, Ornstein DK: Prostate cancer detection in men with serum PSA concentrations of 2.6 to 4.0 ng/mL and benign prostate examination: Enhancement of specificity with free PSA measurements. JAMA 1997;277:1452-1455.

316. Krumholtz JS, Carvalhal GF, Ramos CG, et al: Prostate-specific antigen cutoff of 2.6 ng/mL for prostate cancer screening is associated with favorable pathologic tumor features. Urology 2002;60:469-473.

317. Catalona WJ, Hudson MA, Scardino PT, et al: Selection of optimal prostate specific antigen cutoffs for early detection of prostate cancer: Receiver operating characteristic curves. J Urol 1994;152:2037-2042.

318. Ross KS, Carter HB, Pearson JD, Guess HA: Comparative efficiency of prostate-specific antigen screening strategies for prostate cancer detection. JAMA 2000;284:1399-1405.

319. Seaman E, Whang M, Olsson CA, Katz A, Cooner WH, Benson MC: PSA density (PSAD): Role in patient evaluation and management. Urol Clin North Am 1993;20:653-663.

320. Catalona WJ, Richie JP, deKernion JB, et al: Comparison of prostate specific antigen concentration versus prostate specific antigen density in the early detection of prostate cancer: Receiver operating characteristic curves. J Urol 1994;152:2031-2036.

321. Brawer MK, Aramburu EA, Chen GL, Preston SD, Ellis WJ: The inability of prostate specific antigen index to enhance the predictive the value of prostate specific antigen in the diagnosis of prostatic carcinoma. J Urol 1993;150:369-373.

322. Keetch DW, McMurtry JM, Smith DS, Andriole GL, Catalona WJ: Prostate specific antigen density versus prostate specific antigen slope as predictors of prostate cancer in men with initially negative prostatic biopsies. J Urol 1996;156:428-431.

323. Lepor H, Wang B, Shapiro E: Relationship between prostatic epithelial volume and serum prostate-specific antigen levels. Urology 1994;44:199-205.

324. Kalish J, Cooner WH, Graham SD Jr: Serum PSA adjusted for volume of transition zone (PSAT) is more accurate than PSA adjusted for total gland volume (PSAD) in detecting adenocarcinoma of the prostate. Urology 1994;43:601-606.

325. Prestigiacomo AF, Stamey TA: Physiological variation of serum prostate specific antigen in the 4.0 to 10.0 ng/ml range in male volunteers. J Urol 1996;155:1977-1980.

326. Riehmann M, Rhodes PR, Cook TD, Grose GS, Bruskewitz RC: Analysis of variation in prostate-specific antigen values. Urology 1993;42:390-397.

327. Kadmon D, Weinberg AD, Williams RH, Pavlik VN, Cooper P, Migliore PJ: Pitfalls in interpreting prostate specific antigen velocity. J Urol 1996;155:1655-1657.

328. Lujan M, Paez A, Sanchez E, Herrero A, Martin E, Berenguer A: Prostate specific antigen variation in patients without clinically evident prostate cancer. J Urol 1999;162:1311-1313.

329. Stenman UH, Leinonen J, Alfthan H, Rannikko S, Tuhkanen K, Alfthan O: A complex between prostate-specific antigen and alpha 1-antichymotrypsin is the major form of prostate-specific antigen in serum of patients with prostatic cancer: Assay of the complex improves clinical sensitivity for cancer. Cancer Res 1991;51:222-226.

330. Lilja H, Christensson A, Dahlen U, et al: Prostate-specific antigen in serum occurs predominantly in complex with alpha 1-antichymotrypsin. Clin Chem 1991;37:1618-1625.

331. Leinonen J, Lovgren T, Vornanen T, Stenman UH: Double-label time-resolved immunofluorometric assay of prostate-specific antigen and of its complex with alpha 1-antichymotrypsin. Clin Chem 1993;39:2098-2103.

332. Christensson A, Bjork T, Nilsson O, et al: Serum prostate specific antigen complexed to alpha 1-antichymotrypsin as an indicator of prostate cancer. J Urol 1993;150:100-105.

333. Lilja H: Significance of different molecular forms of serum PSA: The free, noncomplexed form of PSA versus that complexed to alpha 1-antichymotrypsin. Urol Clin North Am 1993;20:681-686.

334. Stenman UH, Hakama M, Knekt P, Aromaa A, Teppo L, Leinonen J: Serum concentrations of prostate specific antigen and its complex with alpha 1-antichymotrypsin before diagnosis of prostate cancer. Lancet 1994;344:1594-1598.

335. Mikolajczyk SD, Millar LS, Wang TJ, et al: "BPSA," a specific molecular form of free prostate-specific antigen, is found predominantly in the transition zone of patients with nodular benign prostatic hyperplasia. Urology 2000;55:41-45.

336. Mikolajczyk SD, Millar LS, Wang TJ, et al: A precursor form of prostate-specific antigen is more highly elevated in prostate cancer compared with benign transition zone prostate tissue. Cancer Res 2000;60:756-759.

337. Mikolajczyk SD, Grauer LS, Millar LS, et al: A precursor form of PSA (pPSA) is a component of the free PSA in prostate cancer serum. Urology 1997;50:710-714.

338. Chen Z, Chen H, Stamey TA: Prostate specific antigen in benign prostatic hyperplasia: Purification and characterization. J Urol 1997;157:2166-2170.

339. Catalona WJ, Partin AW, Slawin KM, et al: Use of the percentage of free prostate-specific antigen to enhance differentiation of

prostate cancer from benign prostatic disease: A prospective multicenter clinical trial. JAMA 1998;279:1542–1547.

340. Roehl KA, Antenor JA, Catalona WJ: Robustness of free prostate specific antigen measurements to reduce unnecessary biopsies in the 2.6 to 4.0 ng/ml range. J Urol 2002;168:922–925.

341. Djavan B, Remzi M, Zlotta AR, et al: Complexed prostate-specific antigen, complexed prostate-specific antigen density of total and transition zone, complexed/total prostate-specific antigen ratio, free-to-total prostate-specific antigen ratio, density of total and transition zone prostate-specific antigen: Results of the prospective multicenter European trial. Urology 2002;60(4 suppl 1):4–9.

342. Horninger W, Cheli CD, Babaian RJ, et al: Complexed prostate-specific antigen for early detection of prostate cancer in men with serum prostate-specific antigen levels of 2 to 4 nanograms per milliliter. Urology 2002;60(4 suppl 1):31–35.

343. Flanigan RC, Catalona WJ, Richie JP, et al: Accuracy of digital rectal examination and transrectal ultrasonography in localizing prostate cancer. J Urol 1994;152:1506–1509.

344. Hodge KK, McNeal JE, Terris MK, Stamey TA: Random systematic versus directed ultrasound guided transrectal core biopsies of the prostate. J Urol 1989;142:71–74.

345. Liu IJ, Macy M, Lai YH, Terris MK: Critical evaluation of the current indications for transition zone biopsies. Urology 2001;57:1117–1120.

346. Babaian RJ, Toi A, Kamoi K, et al: A comparative analysis of sextant and an extended 11-core multisite directed biopsy strategy. J Urol 2000;163:152–157.

347. Terris MK: Extended field prostate biopsies: Too much of a good thing? Urology 2000;55:457–460.

348. Berger AP, Frauscher F, Halpern EJ, et al: Periprostatic administration of local anesthesia during transrectal ultrasound-guided biopsy of the prostate: A randomized, double-blind, placebo-controlled study. Urology 2003;61:585–588.

349. Raaijmakers R, Kirkels WJ, Roobol MJ, Wildhagen MF, Schröder FH: Complication rates and risk factors of 5802 transrectal ultrasound-guided sextant biopsies of the prostate within a population-based screening program. Urology 2002;60:826–830.

350. Frankel S, Smith GD, Donovan J, Neal D: Screening for prostate cancer. Lancet 2003;361:1122–1128.

351. de Koning HJ, Auvinen A, Berenguer et al: Large-scale randomized prostate cancer screening trials: Program performances in the European Randomized Screening for Prostate Cancer trial and the Prostate, Lung, Colorectal and Ovary cancer trial. Int J Cancer 2002;97:237–244.

352. Harris R, Lohr KN: Screening for prostate cancer: An update of the evidence for the U.S. Preventive Services Task Force. Ann Intern Med 2002;137:917–929.

353. Krahn MD, Mahoney JE, Eckman MH, Trachtenberg J, Pauker SG, Detsky AS: Screening for prostate cancer: A decision analytic view. JAMA 1994;272:773–780.

354. Barry MJ, Fleming C, Coley CM, Wasson JH, Fahs MC, Oesterling JE: Should Medicare provide reimbursement for prostate-specific antigen testing for early detection of prostate cancer? IV. Estimating the risks and benefits of an early detection program. Urology 1995;46:445–461.

355. Etzioni R, Penson DF, Legler JM, et al: Overdiagnosis due to prostate-specific antigen screening: Lessons from U.S. prostate cancer incidence trends. J Natl Cancer Inst 2002;94:981–990.

356. Etzioni R, Cha R, Cowen ME: Serial prostate specific antigen screening for prostate cancer: A computer model evaluates competing strategies. J Urol 1999;162:741–748.

357. Carter HB, Epstein JI, Chan DW, Fozard JL, Pearson JD: Recommended prostate-specific antigen testing intervals for the detection of curable prostate cancer. JAMA 1997;277:1456–1460.

358. Hugosson J, Aus G, Lilja H, Lodding P, Pihl CG, Pileblad E: Prostate specific antigen based biennial screening is sufficient to detect almost all prostate cancers while still curable. J Urol 2003;169:1720–1723.

359. DeMarzo AM, Nelson WG, Isaacs WB, Epstein JI: Pathological and molecular aspects of prostate cancer. Lancet 2003;361:955–964.

360. Epstein JI: Diagnostic criteria of limited adenocarcinoma of the prostate on needle biopsy. Hum Pathol 1995;26:223–229.

361. Baisden BL, Kahane H, Epstein JI: Perineural invasion, mucinous fibroplasia, and glomerulations: Diagnostic features of limited cancer on prostate needle biopsy. Am J Surg Pathol 1999;23:918–924.

362. Hedrick L, Epstein JI: Use of keratin 903 as an adjunct in the diagnosis of prostate carcinoma. Am J Surg Pathol 1989;13:389–396.

363. Wojno KJ, Epstein JI: The utility of basal cell-specific anti-cytokeratin antibody (34 beta E12) in the diagnosis of prostate cancer: A review of 228 cases. Am J Surg Pathol 1995;19:251–260.

364. McNeal JE, Bostwick DG: Intraductal dysplasia: A premalignant lesion of the prostate. Hum Pathol 1986;17:64–71.

365. Wills ML, Hamper UM, Partin AW, Epstein JI: Incidence of high-grade prostatic intraepithelial neoplasia in sextant needle biopsy specimens. Urology 1997;49:367–373.

366. Haggman MJ, Macoska JA, Wojno KJ, Oesterling JE: The relationship between prostatic intraepithelial neoplasia and prostate cancer: Critical issues. J Urol 1997;158:12–22.

367. O'Shaughnessy JA, Kelloff GJ, Gordon GB, et al: Treatment and prevention of intraepithelial neoplasia: An important target for accelerated new agent development. Clin Cancer Res 2002;8:314–346.

368. Davidson D, Bostwick DG, Qian J, et al: Prostatic intraepithelial neoplasia is a risk factor for adenocarcinoma: Predictive accuracy in needle biopsies. J Urol 1995;154:1295–1299.

369. O'Dowd GJ, Miller MC, Orozco R, Veltri RW: Analysis of repeated biopsy results within 1 year after a noncancer diagnosis. Urology 2000;55:553–559.

370. Kronz JD, Allan CH, Shaikh AA, Epstein JI: Predicting cancer following a diagnosis of high-grade prostatic intraepithelial neoplasia on needle biopsy: Data on men with more than one follow-up biopsy. Am J Surg Pathol 2001;25:1079–1085.

371. Ronnett BM, Carmichael MJ, Carter HB, Epstein JI: Does high grade prostatic intraepithelial neoplasia result in elevated serum prostate specific antigen levels? J Urol 1993;150:386–389.

372. Alexander EE, Qian J, Wollan PC, Myers RP, Bostwick DG: Prostatic intraepithelial neoplasia does not appear to raise serum prostate-specific antigen concentration. Urology 1996;47:693–698.

373. Gleason DF, Mellinger GT: Prediction of prognosis for prostatic adenocarcinoma by combined histological grading and clinical staging. J Urol 1974;111:58–64.

374. Epstein JI, Partin AW, Sauvageot J, Walsh PC: Prediction of progression following radical prostatectomy: A multivariate analysis of 721 men with long-term follow-up. Am J Surg Pathol 1996;20:286–292.

375. Green GA, Hanlon AL, Al-Saleem T, Hanks GE: A Gleason score of 7 predicts a worse outcome for prostate carcinoma patients treated with radiotherapy. Cancer 1998;83:971–976.

376. Allsbrook WC Jr, Mangold KA, Johnson MH, et al: Interobserver reproducibility of Gleason grading of prostatic carcinoma: Urologic pathologists. Hum Pathol 2001;32:74–80.

377. Allsbrook WC Jr, Mangold KA, Johnson MH, Lane RB, Lane CG, Epstein JI: Interobserver reproducibility of Gleason grading of prostatic carcinoma: General pathologist. Hum Pathol 2001;32:81–88.

378. Kronz JD, Silberman MA, Allsbrook WC, Epstein JI: A web-based tutorial improves practicing pathologists' Gleason grading of images of prostate carcinoma specimens obtained by needle biopsy: Validation of a new medical education paradigm. Cancer 2000;89:1818–1823.

379. Partin AW, Yoo J, Carter HB, et al: The use of prostate specific antigen, clinical stage and Gleason score to predict pathological stage in men with localized prostate cancer. J Urol 1993;150:110–114.

380. Partin AW, Kattan MW, Subong EN, et al: Combination of prostate-specific antigen, clinical stage, and Gleason score to predict pathological stage of localized prostate cancer: A multi-institutional update. JAMA 1997;277:1445–1451.

381. Han M, Partin AW, Zahurak M, Piantadosi S, Epstein JI, Walsh PC: Biochemical (prostate specific antigen) recurrence probability following radical prostatectomy for clinically localized prostate cancer. J Urol 2003;169:517–523.

382. D'Amico AV, Whittington R, Malkowicz SB, et al: Predicting prostate specific antigen outcome preoperatively in the prostate specific antigen era. J Urol 2001;166:2185–2188.

383. Purohit RS, Shinohara K, Meng MV, Carroll PR: Imaging clinically localized prostate cancer. Urol Clin North Am 2003;30:279-293.

384. Oesterling JE: Using PSA to eliminate the staging radionuclide bone scan: Significant economic implications. Urol Clin North Am 1993;20:705-711.

385. Hofer C, Kubler H, Hartung R, Breul J, Avril N: Diagnosis and monitoring of urological tumors using positron emission tomography. Eur Urol 2001;40:481-487.

386. Harisinghani MG, Barentsz J, Hahn PF, et al: Noninvasive detection of clinically occult lymph-node metastases in prostate cancer. N Engl J Med 2003;348:2491-2499.

387. Polascik TJ, Manyak MJ, Haseman MK, et al: Comparison of clinical staging algorithms and 111indium-capromab pendetide immunoscintigraphy in the prediction of lymph node involvement in high risk prostate carcinoma patients. Cancer 1999;85:1586-1592.

388. Ponsky LE, Cherullo EE, Starkey R, Nelson D, Neumann D, Zippe CD: Evaluation of preoperative ProstaScint scans in the prediction of nodal disease. Prostate Cancer Prostatic Dis 2002;5:132-135.

389. Elgamal AA, Troychak MJ, Murphy GP: ProstaScint scan may enhance identification of prostate cancer recurrences after prostatectomy, radiation, or hormone therapy: Analysis of 136 scans of 100 patients. Prostate 1998;37:261-269.

390. Heller JE: Prostatic acid phosphatase: Its current clinical status. J Urol 1987;137:1091-1103.

391. Whitesel JA, Donohue RE, Mani JH, et al: Acid phosphatase: Its influence on the management of carcinoma of the prostate. J Urol 1984;131:70-72.

392. Bahnson RR, Catalona WJ: Adverse implications of acid phosphatase levels in the upper range of normal. J Urol 1987;137:427-430.

393. Oesterling JE, Brendler CB, Epstein JI, Kimball AW Jr, Walsh PC: Correlation of clinical stage, serum prostatic acid phosphatase and preoperative Gleason grade with final pathological stage in 275 patients with clinically localized adenocarcinoma of the prostate. J Urol 1987;138:92-98.

394. Burnett AL, Chan DW, Brendler CB, Walsh PC: The value of serum enzymatic acid phosphatase in the staging of localized prostate cancer. J Urol 1992;148:1832-1834.

395. Ts'o PO, Pannek J, Wang ZP, Lesko SA, Bova GS, Partin AW: Detection of intact prostate cancer cells in the blood of men with prostate cancer. Urology 1997;49:881-885.

396. Moreno JG, Croce CM, Fischer R, et al: Detection of hematogenous micrometastasis in patients with prostate cancer. Cancer Res 1992;52:6110-6112.

397. Katz AE, Olsson CA, Raffo AJ, et al: Molecular staging of prostate cancer with the use of an enhanced reverse transcriptase-PCR assay. Urology 1994;43:765-775.

398. de la Taille A, Olsson CA, Buttyan R, et al: Blood-based reverse transcriptase polymerase chain reaction assays for prostatic specific antigen: Long term follow-up confirms the potential utility of this assay in identifying patients more likely to have biochemical recurrence (rising PSA) following radical prostatectomy. Int J Cancer 1999;84:360-364.

399. Shariat SF, Gottenger E, Nguyen C, et al: Preoperative blood reverse transcriptase-PCR assays for prostate-specific antigen and human glandular kallikrein for prediction of prostate cancer progression after radical prostatectomy. Cancer Res 2002;62:5974-5979.

400. Ellis WJ, Pfitzenmaier J, Colli J, Arfman E, Lange PH, Vessella RL: Detection and isolation of prostate cancer cells from peripheral blood and bone marrow. Urology 2003;61:277-281.

401. Scherr D, Swindle PW, Scardino PT: National Comprehensive Cancer Network guidelines for the management of prostate cancer. Urology 2003;61(2 suppl 1):14-24.

402. Albertsen PC, Hanley JA, Gleason DF, Barry MJ: Competing risk analysis of men aged 55 to 74 years at diagnosis managed conservatively for clinically localized prostate cancer. JAMA 1998;280:975-980.

403. Chodak GW, Thisted RA, Gerber GS, et al: Results of conservative management of clinically localized prostate cancer. N Engl J Med 1994;330:242-248.

404. Holmberg L, Bill-Axelson A, Helgesen F, et al: A randomized trial comparing radical prostatectomy with watchful waiting in early prostate cancer. N Engl J Med 2002;347:781-789.

405. Humphrey PA, Keetch DW, Smith DS, Shepherd DL, Catalona WJ: Prospective characterization of pathological features of prostatic carcinomas detected via serum prostate specific antigen based screening. J Urol 1996;155:816-820.

406. Wilt TJ, Brawer MK: The Prostate Cancer Intervention Versus Observation Trial: A randomized trial comparing radical prostatectomy versus expectant management for the treatment of clinically localized prostate cancer. J Urol 1994;152:1910-1914.

407. Carter HB, Walsh PC, Landis P, Epstein JI: Expectant management of nonpalpable prostate cancer with curative intent: Preliminary results. J Urol 2002;167:1231-1234.

408. Arias E: United States life tables, 2000. Natl Vital Stat Rep 2002;51:1-38.

409. Rogers E, Ohori M, Kassabian VS, Wheeler TM, Scardino PT: Salvage radical prostatectomy: Outcome measured by serum prostate specific antigen levels. J Urol 1995;153:104-110.

410. Tefilli MV, Gheiler EL, Tiguert R, et al: Salvage surgery or salvage radiotherapy for locally recurrent prostate cancer. Urology 1998;52:224-229.

411. Peters CA, Walsh PC: Blood transfusion and anesthetic practices in radical retropubic prostatectomy. J Urol 1985;134:81-83.

412. O'Hara JF Jr, Sprung J, Klein EA, Dilger JA, Domen RE, Piedmonte MR: Use of preoperative autologous blood donation in patients undergoing radical retropubic prostatectomy. Urology 1999;54:130-134.

413. Shir Y, Raja SN, Frank SM, Brendler CB: Intraoperative blood loss during radical retropubic prostatectomy: Epidural versus general anesthesia. Urology 1995;45:993-999.

414. Walsh PC: Anatomic radical prostatectomy: Evolution of the surgical technique. J Urol 1998;160:2418-2424.

415. Weldon VE, Tavel FR, Neuwirth H, Cohen R: Patterns of positive specimen margins and detectable prostate specific antigen after radical perineal prostatectomy. J Urol 1995;153:1565-1569.

416. Weldon VE, Tavel FR, Neuwirth H: Continence, potency and morbidity after radical perineal prostatectomy. J Urol 1997;158:1470-1475.

417. Abbou CC, Salomon L, Hoznek A, et al: Laparoscopic radical prostatectomy: Preliminary results. Urology 2000;55:630-634.

418. Walsh PC: Anatomic radical retropubic prostatectomy. In Walsh PC (ed): Campbell's Urology. Philadelphia, WB Saunders, 2002, pp 3107-3130.

419. Borland RN, Walsh PC: The management of rectal injury during radical retropubic prostatectomy. J Urol 1992;147:905-907.

420. Cisek LJ, Walsh PC: Thromboembolic complications following radical retropubic prostatectomy: Influence of external sequential pneumatic compression devices. Urology 1993;42:406-408.

421. Fowler FJ Jr, Barry MJ, Lu-Yao G, Roman A, Wasson J, Wennberg JE: Patient-reported complications and follow-up treatment after radical prostatectomy. The National Medicare Experience: 1988-1990 [updated June 1993]. Urology 1993;42:622-629.

422. Stanford JL, Feng Z, Hamilton AS, et al: Urinary and sexual function after radical prostatectomy for clinically localized prostate cancer: The Prostate Cancer Outcomes Study. JAMA 2000;283:354-360.

423. Steiner MS, Morton RA, Walsh PC: Impact of anatomical radical prostatectomy on urinary continence. J Urol 1991;145:512-514.

424. Walsh PC, Marschke P, Ricker D, Burnett AL: Patient-reported urinary continence and sexual function after anatomic radical prostatectomy. Urology 2000;55:58-61.

425. Geary ES, Dendinger TE, Freiha FS, Stamey TA: Incontinence and vesical neck strictures following radical retropubic prostatectomy. Urology 1995;45:1000-1006.

426. Steiner MS: Continence-preserving anatomic radical retropubic prostatectomy. Urology 2000;55:427-435.

427. Walsh PC, Marschke PL: Intussusception of the reconstructed bladder neck leads to earlier continence after radical prostatectomy. Urology 2002;59:934-938.

428. Walsh PC: Radical prostatectomy for localized prostate cancer provides durable cancer control with excellent quality of life: A structured debate. J Urol 2000;163:1802-1807.

429. Montague DK, Angermeier KW: Postprostatectomy urinary incontinence: The case for artificial urinary sphincter implantation. Urology 2000;55:2-4.

430. Smith DN, Appell RA, Rackley RR, Winters JC: Collagen injection

therapy for post-prostatectomy incontinence. J Urol 1998;160: 364-367.

431. Quinlan DM, Epstein JI, Carter BS, Walsh PC: Sexual function following radical prostatectomy: Influence of preservation of neurovascular bundles. J Urol 1991;145:998-1002.

432. Rabbani F, Stapleton AM, Kattan MW, Wheeler TM, Scardino PT: Factors predicting recovery of erections after radical prostatectomy. J Urol 2000;164:1929-1934.

433. Walsh PC, Epstein JI, Lowe FC: Potency following radical prostatectomy with wide unilateral excision of the neurovascular bundle. J Urol 1987;138:823-827.

434. Kim ED, Scardino PT, Hampel O, Mills NL, Wheeler TM, Nath RK: Interposition of sural nerve restores function of cavernous nerves resected during radical prostatectomy. J Urol 1999;161:188-192.

435. Walsh PC: Nerve grafts are rarely necessary and are unlikely to improve sexual function in men undergoing anatomic radical prostatectomy. Urology 2001;57:1020-1024.

436. Zippe CD, Jhaveri FM, Klein EA, et al: Role of Viagra after radical prostatectomy. Urology 2000;55:241-245.

437. Pound CR, Partin AW, Eisenberger MA, Chan DW, Pearson JD, Walsh PC: Natural history of progression after PSA elevation following radical prostatectomy. JAMA 1999;281:1591-1597.

438. Pound CR, Partin AW, Epstein JI, Walsh PC: Prostate-specific antigen after anatomic radical retropubic prostatectomy: Patterns of recurrence and cancer control. Urol Clin North Am 1997;24:395-406.

439. Trapasso JG, deKernion JB, Smith RB, Dorey F: The incidence and significance of detectable levels of serum prostate specific antigen after radical prostatectomy. J Urol 1994;152:1821-1825.

440. Zincke H, Oesterling JE, Blute ML, Bergstralh EJ, Myers RP, Barrett DM: Long-term (15 years) results after radical prostatectomy for clinically localized (stage T2c or lower) prostate cancer. J Urol 1994;152:1850-1857.

441. Catalona WJ, Smith DS: 5-year tumor recurrence rates after anatomical radical retropubic prostatectomy for prostate cancer. J Urol 1994;152:1837-1842.

442. Hull GW, Rabbani F, Abbas F, Wheeler TM, Kattan MW, Scardino PT: Cancer control with radical prostatectomy alone in 1,000 consecutive patients. J Urol 2002;167:528-534.

443. Roentgen WK: Proceedings of the Wurzburg Phisico-Medical Society, 1895.

444. Curie MS: Recherches sur les substances radioactives. Faculte des Sciences de Paris pour obtenir le grade de docteur es science physiques, 2nd ed. Paris, Gauthier-Villars, 1904.

445. Young HH, Frontz WA: Some new methods in the treatment of carcinoma of the lower genito-urinary tract with radium. J Urol 1917;1:505-541.

446. Barringer BS: Phases of the pathology, diagnosis and treatment of cancer of the prostate. J Urol 1928:407-411.

447. George FW, Carlton CE, Dykhuizen RF, Dillon JR: Cobalt-60 telecurietherapy in the definitive treatment of carcinoma of the prostate: A preliminary report. J Urol 1965;93:102-109.

448. Kaplan HS, Bagshaw MA: The Stanford medical linear accelerator. III. Application to clinical problems of radiation therapy. Stanford Med Bull 1957;15:141-151.

449. Bagshaw MA, Kaplan HS, Sagerman RH: Linear accelerator super-voltage radiotherapy. VII. Carcinoma of the prostate. Radiology 1965;85:121-129.

450. Del Regato JA: Radiotherapy in the conservative treatment of operable and locally inoperable carcinoma of the prostate. Radiology 1967;88:761-766.

451. Fowler JE Jr, Braswell NT, Pandey P, Seaver L: Experience with radical prostatectomy and radiation therapy for localized prostate cancer. J Urol 1995;153:1026-1031.

452. Hanks GE, Asbell S, Krall JM, et al: Outcome for lymph node dissection negative T-1b, T-2 (A-2, B) prostate cancer treated with external beam radiation therapy in RTOG 77-06. Int J Radiat Oncol Biol Phys 1991;21:1099-103.

453. Elder JS, Jewett HJ, Walsh PC: Radical perineal prostatectomy for clinical stage B2 carcinoma of the prostate. J Urol 1982;127: 704-706.

454. Gibbons RP, Correa RJ Jr, Brannen GE, Mason JT: Total prostatectomy for localized prostatic cancer. J Urol 1984;131: 73-76.

455. Zagars GK: The prognostic significance of a single serum prostate-specific antigen value beyond six months after radiation therapy for adenocarcinoma of the prostate. Int J Radiat Oncol Biol Phys 1993;27:39-45.

456. Sartor CI, Strawderman MH, Lin XH, Kish KE, McLaughlin PW, Sandler HM: Rate of PSA rise predicts metastatic versus local recurrence after definitive radiotherapy. Int J Radiat Oncol Biol Phys 1997;38:941-947.

457. Consensus statement: Guidelines for PSA following radiation therapy. American Society for Therapeutic Radiology and Oncology Consensus Panel. Int J Radiat Oncol Biol Phys 1997;37:1035-1041.

458. Hanks GE, Hanlon AL, Pinover WH, Horwitz EM, Price RA, Schultheiss T: Dose selection for prostate cancer patients based on dose comparison and dose response studies. Int J Radiat Oncol Biol Phys 2000;46:823-832.

459. Keyser D, Kupelian PA, Zippe CD, Levin HS, Klein EA: Stage T1-2 prostate cancer with pretreatment prostate-specific antigen level < or = 10 ng/ml: Radiation therapy or surgery? Int J Radiat Oncol Biol Phys 1997;38:723-729.

460. Pisansky TM, Kozelsky TF, Myers RP, et al: Radiotherapy for isolated serum prostate specific antigen elevation after prostatectomy for prostate cancer. J Urol 2000;163:845-850.

461. Zagars GK, Pollack A, von Eschenbach AC: Prognostic factors for clinically localized prostate carcinoma: Analysis of 938 patients irradiated in the prostate specific antigen era. Cancer 1997;79: 1370-1380.

462. D'Amico AV, Whittington R, Malkowicz SB, et al: A multivariate analysis of clinical and pathological factors that predict for prostate specific antigen failure after radical prostatectomy for prostate cancer. J Urol 1995;154:131-138.

463. Kaplan ID, Cox RS, Bagshaw MA: Prostate specific antigen after external beam radiotherapy for prostatic cancer: Followup. J Urol 1993;149:519-522.

464. Horwitz EM, Vicini FA, Ziaja EL, et al: Assessing the variability of outcome for patients treated with localized prostate irradiation using different definitions of biochemical control. Int J Radiat Oncol Biol Phys 1996;36:565-571.

465. Zietman AL, Shipley WU, Coen JJ: Radical prostatectomy and radical radiation therapy for clinical stages T1 to 2 adenocarcinoma of the prostate: New insights into outcome from repeat biopsy and prostate specific antigen followup. J Urol 1994;152:1806-1812.

466. Lawton CA, Won M, Pilepich MV, et al: Long-term treatment sequelae following external beam irradiation for adenocarcinoma of the prostate: Analysis of RTOG studies 7506 and 7706. Int J Radiat Oncol Biol Phys 1991;21:935-939.

467. Zelefsky MJ, Eid JF: Elucidating the etiology of erectile dysfunction after definitive therapy for prostatic cancer. Int J Radiat Oncol Biol Phys 1998;40:129-133.

468. Fisch BM, Pickett B, Weinberg V, Roach M: Dose of radiation received by the bulb of the penis correlates with risk of impotence after three-dimensional conformal radiotherapy for prostate cancer. Urology 2001;57:955-959.

469. Bagshaw MA, Cox RS, Ray GR: Status of radiation treatment of prostate cancer at Stanford University. NCI Monogr 1988;7: 47-60.

470. Zelefsky MJ, McKee AB, Lee H, Leibel SA: Efficacy of oral sildenafil in patients with erectile dysfunction after radiotherapy for carcinoma of the prostate. Urology 1999;53:775-778.

471. Brenner DJ, Curtis RE, Hall EJ, Ron E: Second malignancies in prostate carcinoma patients after radiotherapy compared with surgery. Cancer 2000;88:398-406.

472. Pollack A, Zagars GK, Starkschall G, et al: Prostate cancer radiation dose response: Results of the M: D: Anderson phase III randomized trial. Int J Radiat Oncol Biol Phys 2002;53: 1097-1105.

473. Zelefsky MJ, Leibel SA, Gaudin PB, et al: Dose escalation with three-dimensional conformal radiation therapy affects the outcome in prostate cancer. Int J Radiat Oncol Biol Phys 1998;41:491-500.

474. Zelefsky MJ, Fuks Z, Hunt M, et al: High dose radiation delivered by intensity modulated conformal radiotherapy improves the outcome of localized prostate cancer. J Urol 2001;166:876-881.

Specific Malignancies

III

475. Hanks GE, Hanlon AL, Schultheiss TE, et al: Dose escalation with 3D conformal treatment: Five year outcomes, treatment optimization, and future directions. Int J Radiat Oncol Biol Phys 1998;41:501–510.

476. Pollack A, Zagars GK, Smith LG, et al: Preliminary results of a randomized radiotherapy dose-escalation study comparing 70 Gy with 78 Gy for prostate cancer. J Clin Oncol 2000;18:3904–3911.

477. Zelefsky MJ, Cowen D, Fuks Z, et al: Long term tolerance of high dose three-dimensional conformal radiotherapy in patients with localized prostate carcinoma. Cancer 1999;85:2460–2468.

478. Storey MR, Pollack A, Zagars G, Smith L, Antolak J, Rosen I: Complications from radiotherapy dose escalation in prostate cancer: Preliminary results of a randomized trial. Int J Radiat Oncol Biol Phys 2000;48:635–642.

479. Lee WR, Schultheiss TE, Hanlon AL, Hanks GE: Urinary incontinence following external-beam radiotherapy for clinically localized prostate cancer. Urology 1996;48:95–99.

480. Zelefsky MJ, Fuks Z, Hunt M, et al: High-dose intensity modulated radiation therapy for prostate cancer: Early toxicity and biochemical outcome in 772 patients. Int J Radiat Oncol Biol Phys 2002;53:1111–1116.

481. Chandra A, Dong L, Huang E, et al: Experience of ultrasound-based daily prostate localization. Int J Radiat Oncol Biol Phys 2003;56:436–447.

482. Speight JL, Roach M 3rd: Imaging and radiotherapy of the prostate. Radiol Clin North Am 2000;38:159–177.

483. Critz FA, Williams WH, Levinson AK, Benton JB, Holladay CT, Schnell FJ Jr: Simultaneous irradiation for prostate cancer: Intermediate results with modern techniques. J Urol 2000;164:738–741.

484. Nag S, Beyer D, Friedland J, Grimm P, Nath R: American Brachytherapy Society (ABS) recommendations for transperineal permanent brachytherapy of prostate cancer. Int J Radiat Oncol Biol Phys 1999;44:789–799.

485. D'Amico AV, Whittington R, Malkowicz SB, et al: Biochemical outcome after radical prostatectomy, external beam radiation therapy, or interstitial radiation therapy for clinically localized prostate cancer. JAMA 1998;280:969–974.

486. Blasko JC, Grimm PD, Sylvester JE, Cavanagh W: The role of external beam radiotherapy with I-125/Pd-103 brachytherapy for prostate carcinoma. Radiother Oncol 2000;57:273–278.

487. Merrick GS, Butler WM, Lief JH, Galbreath RW, Adamovich E: Biochemical outcome for hormone-naive patients with high-risk prostate cancer managed with permanent interstitial brachytherapy and supplemental external-beam radiation. Cancer J 2002;8:322–327.

488. Dattoli M, Wallner K, True L, et al: Prognostic role of serum prostatic acid phosphatase for 103Pd-based radiation for prostatic carcinoma. Int J Radiat Oncol Biol Phys 1999;45:853–856.

489. Blasko JC, Grimm PD, Sylvester JE, Badiozamani KR, Hoak D, Cavanagh W: Palladium-103 brachytherapy for prostate carcinoma. Int J Radiat Oncol Biol Phys 2000;46:839–850.

490. Grimm PD, Blasko JC, Sylvester JE, Meier RM, Cavanagh W: 10-year biochemical (prostate-specific antigen) control of prostate cancer with (125)I brachytherapy. Int J Radiat Oncol Biol Phys 2001;51:31–40.

491. Ragde H, Korb LJ, Elgamal AA, Grado GL, Nadir BS: Modern prostate brachytherapy: Prostate specific antigen results in 219 patients with up to 12 years of observed follow-up. Cancer 2000;89:135–141.

492. Merrick GS WK, Butler WM: Permanent interstitial brachytherapy for the management of carcinoma of the prostate gland. J Urol 2003;169:1643–1652.

493. Blasko JC, Wallner K, Grimm PD, Ragde H: Prostate specific antigen based disease control following ultrasound guided 125iodine implantation for stage T1/T2 prostatic carcinoma. J Urol 1995;154:1096–1099.

494. Brachman DG, Thomas T, Hilbe J, Beyer DC: Failure-free survival following brachytherapy alone or external beam irradiation alone for T1-2 prostate tumors in 2222 patients: Results from a single practice. Int J Radiat Oncol Biol Phys 2000;48:111–117.

495. Potters L, Cha C, Oshinsky G, Venkatraman E, Zelefsky M, Leibel S: Risk profiles to predict PSA relapse-free survival for patients undergoing permanent prostate brachytherapy. Cancer J Sci Am 1999;5:301–306.

496. Zelefsky MJ, Hollister T, Raben A, Matthews S, Wallner KE: Five-year biochemical outcome and toxicity with transperineal CT-planned permanent I-125 prostate implantation for patients with localized prostate cancer. Int J Radiat Oncol Biol Phys 2000;47:1261–1266.

497. Davis BJ, Pisansky TM, Wilson TM, et al: The radial distance of extraprostatic extension of prostate carcinoma: Implications for prostate brachytherapy. Cancer 1999;85:2630–2637.

498. Brandeis J, Pashos CL, Henning JM, Litwin MS: A nationwide charge comparison of the principal treatments for early stage prostate carcinoma. Cancer 2000;89:1792–1799.

499. Stone NN, Stock RG: Prostate brachytherapy in patients with prostate volumes > = 50 cm: Dosimetric analysis of implant quality. Int J Radiat Oncol Biol Phys 2000;46:1199–1204.

500. Merrick GS, Butler WM, Dorsey AT, Lief JH: Effect of prostate size and isotope selection on dosimetric quality following permanent seed implantation. Tech Urol 2001;7:233–240.

501. Terk MD, Stock RG, Stone NN: Identification of patients at increased risk for prolonged urinary retention following radioactive seed implantation of the prostate. J Urol 1998;160:1379–1382.

502. Merrick GS, Butler WM, Lief JH, Dorsey AT: Temporal resolution of urinary morbidity following prostate brachytherapy. Int J Radiat Oncol Biol Phys 2000;47:121–128.

503. Landis D, Wallner K, Locke J, et al: Late urinary function after prostate brachytherapy. Brachytherapy 2002;1:21.

504. Blasko JC, Ragde H, Grimm PD: Transperineal ultrasound-guided implantation of the prostate: Morbidity and complications. Scand J Urol Nephrol Suppl 1991;137:113–118.

505. Wallner K, Lee H, Wasserman S, Dattoli M: Low risk of urinary incontinence following prostate brachytherapy in patients with a prior transurethral prostate resection. Int J Radiat Oncol Biol Phys 1997;37:565–569.

506. Stone NN, Stock RG, Parikh D, Yeghiayan P, Unger P: Perineural invasion and seminal vesicle involvement predict pelvic lymph node metastasis in men with localized carcinoma of the prostate. J Urol 1998;160:1722–1726.

507. Merrick GS, Butler WM, Galbreath RW, Lief JH, Adamovich E: Perineural invasion is not predictive of biochemical outcome following prostate brachytherapy. Cancer J 2002;8:79–80.

508. Merrick GS, Butler WM, Wallner KE, Galbreath RW, Anderson RL: Prostate-specific antigen spikes after permanent prostate brachytherapy. Int J Radiat Oncol Biol Phys 2002;54:450–456.

509. Wallner K, Merrick G, True L, Cavanagh W, Simpson C, Butler W: I-125 versus Pd-103 for low-risk prostate cancer: Morbidity outcomes from a prospective randomized multicenter trial. Cancer J 2002;8:67–73.

510. Martinez AA, Pataki I, Edmundson G, Sebastian E, Brabbins D, Gustafson G: Phase II prospective study of the use of conformal high-dose-rate brachytherapy as monotherapy for the treatment of favorable stage prostate cancer: A feasibility report. Int J Radiat Oncol Biol Phys 2001;49:61–69.

511. Yoshioka Y, Nose T, Yoshida K, et al: High-dose-rate interstitial brachytherapy as a monotherapy for localized prostate cancer: Treatment description and preliminary results of a phase I/II clinical trial. Int J Radiat Oncol Biol Phys 2000;48:675–681.

512. Deger S, Boehmer D, Turk I, et al: High dose rate brachytherapy of localized prostate cancer. Eur Urol 2002;41:420–426.

513. Gleave ME, Goldenberg SL, et al: Randomized comparative study of 3 versus 8-month neoadjuvant hormonal therapy before radical prostatectomy: Biochemical and pathological effects. J Urol 2001;166:500–506.

514. Blank KR, Whittington R, Arjomandy B, et al: Neoadjuvant androgen deprivation prior to transperineal prostate brachytherapy: Smaller volumes, less morbidity. Cancer J Sci Am 1999;5:370–373.

515. Potters L, Torre T, Ashley R, Leibel S: Examining the role of neoadjuvant androgen deprivation in patients undergoing prostate brachytherapy. J Clin Oncol 2000;18:1187–1192.

516. Kleinberg L, Wallner K, Roy J, et al: Treatment-related symptoms during the first year following transperineal 125I prostate implantation. Int J Radiat Oncol Biol Phys 1994;28:985–990.

517. Brown D, Colonias A, Miller R, et al: Urinary morbidity with a modified peripheral loading technique of transperineal (125)i prostate implantation. Int J Radiat Oncol Biol Phys 2000;47:353–360.

518. Lee N, Wuu CS, Brody R, et al: Factors predicting for post-implantation urinary retention after permanent prostate brachytherapy. Int J Radiat Oncol Biol Phys 2000;48:1457–1460.

519. Storey MR, Landgren RC, Cottone JL, et al: Transperineal ^{125}iodine implantation for treatment of clinically localized prostate cancer: 5-year tumor control and morbidity. Int J Radiat Oncol Biol Phys 1999;43:565–570.

520. Ragde H, Blasko JC, Grimm PD, et al: Interstitial iodine-125 radiation without adjuvant therapy in the treatment of clinically localized prostate carcinoma. Cancer 1997;80:442–453.

521. Talcott JA, Clark JA, Stark PC, Mitchell SP: Long-term treatment related complications of brachytherapy for early prostate cancer: A survey of patients previously treated. J Urol 2001;166:494–499.

522. Benoit RM, Naslund MJ, Cohen JK: Complications after prostate brachytherapy in the Medicare population. Urology 2000;55: 91–96.

523. Stock RG, Stone NN, Iannuzzi C: Sexual potency following interactive ultrasound-guided brachytherapy for prostate cancer. Int J Radiat Oncol Biol Phys 1996;35:267–272.

524. Wallner K, Roy J, Harrison L: Tumor control and morbidity following transperineal iodine 125 implantation for stage T1/T2 prostatic carcinoma. J Clin Oncol 1996;14:449–453.

525. Stock RG, Kao J, Stone NN: Penile erectile function after permanent radioactive seed implantation for treatment of prostate cancer. J Urol 2001;165:436–439.

526. Merrick GS, Wallner KE, Butler WM: Management of sexual dysfunction after prostate brachytherapy. Oncology (Huntingt) 2003;17:52–62.

527. Lee WR, Hall MC, McQuellon RP, Case LD, McCullough DL: A prospective quality-of-life study in men with clinically localized prostate carcinoma treated with radical prostatectomy, external beam radiotherapy, or interstitial brachytherapy. Int J Radiat Oncol Biol Phys 2001;51:614–623.

528. Slater JD, Rossi CJ Jr, Yonemoto LT, et al: Conformal proton therapy for early-stage prostate cancer. Urology 1999;53:978–984.

529. Bolla M, Gonzalez D, Warde P, et al: Improved survival in patients with locally advanced prostate cancer treated with radiotherapy and goserelin. N Engl J Med 1997;337:295–300.

530. Bolla M, Collette L, Blank L, et al: Long-term results with immediate androgen suppression and external irradiation in patients with locally advanced prostate cancer (an EORTC study): A phase III randomised trial. Lancet 2002;360:103–106.

531. Pilepich MV, Caplan R, Byhardt RW, et al: Phase III trial of androgen suppression using goserelin in unfavorable-prognosis carcinoma of the prostate treated with definitive radiotherapy: Report of Radiation Therapy Oncology Group Protocol 85-31. J Clin Oncol 1997;15:1013–1021.

532. D'Amico AV, Schultz D, Loffredo M, et al: Biochemical outcome following external beam radiation therapy with or without androgen suppression therapy for clinically localized prostate cancer. JAMA 2000;284:1280–1283.

533. DeWeese TL, Song DY. Current evidence for the role of combined androgen suppression and radiation in the treatment of adenocarcinoma of the prostate. Urology 2000;55:169–174.

534. Joon DL, Hasegawa M, Sikes C, et al: Supraadditive apoptotic response of R3327-G rat prostate tumors to androgen ablation and radiation. Int J Radiat Oncol Biol Phys 1997;38:1071–1077.

535. Zietman AL, Prince EA, Nakfoor BM, Park JJ: Androgen deprivation and radiation therapy: Sequencing studies using the Shionogi in vivo tumor system. Int J Radiat Oncol Biol Phys 1997;38:1067–1070.

536. Pollack A, Ashoori F, Sikes C, et al: The early supra-additive apoptotic response of R3327-G prostate tumors to androgen ablation and radiation is not sustained with multiple fractions. Int J Radiat Oncol Biol Phys 2000;46:153–158.

537. Green N, Bodner H, Broth E, et al: Improved control of bulky prostate carcinoma with sequential estrogen and radiation therapy. Int J Radiat Oncol Biol Phys 1984;10:971–976.

538. Neglia WJ, Hussey DH, Johnson DE: Megavoltage radiation therapy for carcinoma of the prostate. Int J Radiat Oncol Biol Phys 1977;2:873–883.

539. van der Werf-Messing B, Sourek-Zikova V, Blonk DI: Localized advanced carcinoma of the prostate: Radiation therapy versus hormonal therapy. Int J Radiat Oncol Biol Phys 1976;1: 1043–1048.

540. Mukamel E, Servadio C, Lurie H: Combined external radiotherapy and hormonal therapy for localized carcinoma of the prostate. Prostate 1983;4:283–287.

541. Pilepich MV, Krall JM, Sause WT, et al: Prognostic factors in carcinoma of the prostate—analysis of RTOG study 75-06. Int J Radiat Oncol Biol Phys 1987;13:339–349.

542. Pilepich MV, Winter K, John MJ, et al: Phase III radiation therapy oncology group (RTOG) trial 86-10 of androgen deprivation adjuvant to definitive radiotherapy in locally advanced carcinoma of the prostate. Int J Radiat Oncol Biol Phys 2001;50:1243–1252.

543. Pilepich MV, Krall JM, al-Sarraf M, et al: Androgen deprivation with radiation therapy compared with radiation therapy alone for locally advanced prostatic carcinoma: A randomized comparative trial of the Radiation Therapy Oncology Group. Urology 1995;45:616–623.

544. Lawton CA, Winter K, Murray K, et al: Updated results of the phase III Radiation Therapy Oncology Group (RTOG) trial 85–31 evaluating the potential benefit of androgen suppression following standard radiation therapy for unfavorable prognosis carcinoma of the prostate. Int J Radiat Oncol Biol Phys 2001;49: 937–946.

545. Hanks GE, Lu JD, Machtay M, et al: RTOG protocol 92-02: A phase III trial of the use of long term androgen suppression following neoadjuvant hormonal cytoreduction and radiotherapy in locally advanced carcinoma of the prostate [abstract]. Int J Radiat Oncol Biol Phys 2000;48(suppl):112.

546. Roach M 3rd, DeSilvio M, Lawton C, et al: Phase III trial comparing whole-pelvic versus prostate-only radiotherapy and neoadjuvant versus adjuvant combined androgen suppression: Radiation Therapy Oncology Group 9413. J Clin Oncol 2003;21:1904–1911.

547. Partin AW, Mangold LA, Lamm DM, Walsh PC, Epstein JI, Pearson JD: Contemporary update of prostate cancer staging nomograms (Partin tables) for the new millennium. Urology 2001;58:843–848.

548. Asbell SO, Krall JM, Pilepich MV, et al: Elective pelvic irradiation in stage A2, B carcinoma of the prostate: Analysis of RTOG 77-06. Int J Radiat Oncol Biol Phys 1988;15:1307–1316.

549. Pilepich MV, Krall JM, Johnson RJ, et al: Extended field (periaortic) irradiation in carcinoma of the prostate: Analysis of RTOG 75-06. Int J Radiat Oncol Biol Phys 1986;12:345–351.

550. Kupelian PA, Katcher J, Levin HS, Klein EA: Stage T1–2 prostate cancer: A multivariate analysis of factors affecting biochemical and clinical failures after radical prostatectomy. Int J Radiat Oncol Biol Phys 1997;37:1043–1052.

551. Grossfeld GD, Tigrani VS, Nudell D, et al: Management of a positive surgical margin after radical prostatectomy: Decision analysis. J Urol 2000;164:93–99.

552. Anscher MS, Prosnitz LR: Multivariate analysis of factors predicting local relapse after radical prostatectomy: Possible indications for postoperative radiotherapy. Int J Radiat Oncol Biol Phys 1991;21:941–947.

553. Paulson DF: Impact of radical prostatectomy in the management of clinically localized disease. J Urol 1994;152:1826–1830.

554. Valicenti RK, Gomella LG, Ismail M, et al: The efficacy of early adjuvant radiation therapy for pT3N0 prostate cancer: A matched-pair analysis. Int J Radiat Oncol Biol Phys 1999;45:53–58.

555. Petrovich Z, Lieskovsky G, Stein JP, Huberman M, Skinner DG: Comparison of surgery alone with surgery and adjuvant radiotherapy for pT3N0 prostate cancer. BJU Int 2002;89:604–611.

556. Taylor N, Kelly JF, Kuban DA, et al: Adjuvant and salvage radiotherapy after radical prostatectomy for prostate cancer. Int J Radiat Oncol Biol Phys 2003;56:755–763.

557. Lu-Yao GL, Potosky AL, Albertsen PC, Wasson JH, Barry MJ, Wennberg JE: Follow-up prostate cancer treatments after radical prostatectomy: A population-based study. J Natl Cancer Inst 1996;88:166–173.

558. Partin AW, Pearson JD, Landis PK, et al: Evaluation of serum prostate-specific antigen velocity after radical prostatectomy to distinguish local recurrence from distant metastases. Urology 1994;43:649–659.

559. Cox JD, Gallagher MJ, Hammond EH, Kaplan RS, Schellhammer PF: Consensus statements on radiation therapy of prostate cancer: Guidelines for prostate re-biopsy after radiation and for radiation therapy with rising prostate-specific antigen levels after radical

prostatectomy: American Society for Therapeutic Radiology and Oncology Consensus Panel. J Clin Oncol 1999;17:1155.

560. Cadeddu JA, Partin AW, DeWeese TL, Walsh PC: Long-term results of radiation therapy for prostate cancer recurrence following radical prostatectomy. J Urol 1998;159:173–177.

561. Catton C, Gospodarowicz M, Warde P, et al: Adjuvant and salvage radiation therapy after radical prostatectomy for adenocarcinoma of the prostate. Radiother Oncol 2001;59:51–60.

562. Song DY, Thompson TL, Ramakrishnan V, et al: Salvage radiotherapy for rising or persistent PSA after radical prostatectomy. Urology 2002;60:281–287.

563. Katz MS ZM, Venkatraman ES: Predictors of biochemical outcome with salvage conformal radiotherapy after radical prostatectomy for prostate cancer. J Clin Oncol 2003;21:483–489.

564. Corn BW, Winter K, Pilepich MV: Does androgen suppression enhance the efficacy of postoperative irradiation? A secondary analysis of RTOG 85-31: Radiation Therapy Oncology Group. Urology 1999;54:495–502.

565. Thompson IM, Paradelo JC, Crawford ED, Coltman CA, Blumenstein B: An opportunity to determine optimal treatment of pT3 prostate cancer: The window may be closing. Urology 1994;44:804–811.

566. Van Cangh PJ, Richard F, Lorge F, et al: Adjuvant radiation therapy does not cause urinary incontinence after radical prostatectomy: Results of a prospective randomized study. J Urol 1998;159:164–166.

567. Formenti SC, Lieskovsky G, Skinner D, Tsao-Wei DD, Groshen S, Petrovich Z: Update on impact of moderate dose of adjuvant radiation on urinary continence and sexual potency in prostate cancer patients treated with nerve-sparing prostatectomy. Urology 2000;56:453–458.

568. Bastasch MD, Teh BS, Mai WY, et al: Post-nerve-sparing prostatectomy, dose-escalated intensity-modulated radiotherapy: Effect on erectile function. Int J Radiat Oncol Biol Phys 2002;54:101–106.

569. Partin AW, Hanks GE, Klein EA, Moul JW, Nelson WG, Scher HI: Prostate-specific antigen as a marker of disease activity in prostate cancer. Oncology (Huntingt) 2002;16:1218–1224.

570. Partin AW, Hanks GE, Klein EA, Moul JW, Nelson WG, Scher HI: Prostate-specific antigen as a marker of disease activity in prostate cancer. Oncology (Huntingt) 2002;16:1024–1038.

571. Eisenberger MA, Crawford ED, Wolf M, et al: Prognostic factors in stage D2 prostate cancer; important implications for future trials: Results of a cooperative intergroup study (INT.0036). The National Cancer Institute Intergroup Study #0036. Semin Oncol 1994;21:613–619.

572. Huggins C, Stevens RE, Hodges CV: Studies on prostate cancer. II. The effects of castration on advanced carcinoma of the prostate gland. Arch Surg 1941;43:209–222.

573. Auclair C, Kelly PA, Labrie F, Coy DH, Schally AV: Inhibition of testicular luteinizing hormone receptor level by treatment with a potent luteinizing hormone-releasing hormone agonist of human chorionic gonadotropin. Biochem Biophys Res Commun 1977;76:855–862.

574. Tolis G, Ackman D, Stellos A, et al: Tumor growth inhibition in patients with prostatic carcinoma treated with luteinizing hormone-releasing hormone agonists. Proc Natl Acad Sci USA 1982;79:1658–1662.

575. Thompson IM, Zeidman EJ, Rodriguez FR: Sudden death due to disease flare with luteinizing hormone-releasing hormone agonist therapy for carcinoma of the prostate. J Urol 1990;144:1479–1480.

576. Wong SL, Lau DT, Baughman SA, Menchaca D, Garnick MB: Pharmacokinetics and pharmacodynamics of abarelix, a gonadotropin-releasing hormone antagonist, after subcutaneous continuous infusion in patients with prostate cancer. Clin Pharmacol Ther 2003;73:304–311.

577. Cox RL, Crawford ED: Estrogens in the treatment of prostate cancer. J Urol 1995;154:1991–1998.

578. Byar DP, Corle DK: Hormone therapy for prostate cancer: Results of the Veterans Administration Cooperative Urological Research Group studies. NCI Monogr 1988;7:165–170.

579. Blackard CE, Doe RP, Mellinger GT, Byar DP: Incidence of cardiovascular disease and death in patients receiving

diethylstilbestrol for carcinoma of the prostate. Cancer 1970;26:249–256.

580. Kent JR, Bischoff AJ, Arduino LJ, et al: Estrogen dosage and suppression of testosterone levels in patients with prostatic carcinoma. J Urol 1973;109:858–860.

581. Leuprolide versus diethylstilbestrol for metastatic prostate cancer. The Leuprolide Study Group. N Engl J Med 1984;311:1281–1286.

582. Parmar H, Phillips RH, Lightman SL, Edwards L, Allen L, Schally AV: Randomised controlled study of orchidectomy vs long-acting D-Trp-6-LHRH microcapsules in advanced prostatic carcinoma. Lancet 1985;2:1201–1205.

583. Turkes AO, Peeling WB, Griffiths K: Treatment of patients with advanced cancer of the prostate: Phase III trial, zoladex against castration; a study of the British Prostate Group. J Steroid Biochem 1987;27:543–549.

584. Peeling WB: Phase III studies to compare goserelin (Zoladex) with orchiectomy and with diethylstilbestrol in treatment of prostatic carcinoma. Urology 1989;33(5 suppl):45–52.

585. Soloway MS, Chodak G, Vogelzang NJ, et al: Zoladex versus orchiectomy in treatment of advanced prostate cancer: A randomized trial: Zoladex Prostate Study Group. Urology 1991;37:46–61.

586. Fleischmann JD, Catalona WJ: Endocrine therapy for bladder outlet obstruction from carcinoma of the prostate. J Urol 1985;134:498–500.

587. Iversen P, Tyrrell CJ, Kaisary AV, et al: Bicalutamide monotherapy compared with castration in patients with nonmetastatic locally advanced prostate cancer: 6.3 years of followup. J Urol 2000;164:1579–1582.

588. Oh WK, Manola J, Bittmann L, et al: Finasteride and flutamide therapy in patients with advanced prostate cancer: Response to subsequent castration and long-term follow-up. Urology 2003;62:99–104.

589. Labrie F, Veilleux R: A wide range of sensitivities to androgens develops in cloned Shionogi mouse mammary tumor cells. Prostate 1986;8:293–300.

590. Sadi MV, Barrack ER: Image analysis of androgen receptor immunostaining in metastatic prostate cancer: Heterogeneity as a predictor of response to hormonal therapy. Cancer 1993;71:2574–2580.

591. Labrie F, Dupont A, Belanger A, et al: New approach in the treatment of prostate cancer: Complete instead of partial withdrawal of androgens. Prostate 1983;4:579–594.

592. Labrie F, Dupont A, Giguere M, et al: Advantages of the combination therapy in previously untreated and treated patients with advanced prostate cancer. J Steroid Biochem 1986;25:877–883.

593. Kuhn JM, Billebaud T, Navratil H, et al: Prevention of the transient adverse effects of a gonadotropin-releasing hormone analogue (buserelin) in metastatic prostatic carcinoma by administration of an antiandrogen (nilutamide). N Engl J Med 1989;321:413–418.

594. Bono AV, DiSilverio F, Robustelli della Cuna G, et al: Complete androgen blockade versus chemical castration in advanced prostatic cancer: Analysis of an Italian multicentre study: Italian Leuprorelin Group. Urol Int 1998;60(Suppl 1):18–24.

595. Keuppens F, Denis L, Smith P, et al: Zoladex and flutamide versus bilateral orchiectomy: A randomized phase III EORTC 30853 study: The EORTC GU Group. Cancer 1990;66(5 suppl):1045–1057.

596. Denis LJ, Carnelro de Moura JL, Bono A, et al: Goserelin acetate and flutamide versus bilateral orchiectomy: A phase III EORTC trial (30853) EORTC GU Group and EORTC Data Center. Urology 1993;42:119–129.

597. Keuppens F, Whelan P, Carneiro de Moura JL, et al: Orchidectomy versus goserelin plus flutamide in patients with metastatic prostate cancer (EORTC 30853): European Organization for Research and Treatment of Cancer-Genitourinary Group. Cancer 1993;72(12 suppl):3863–3869.

598. Denis LJ, Keuppens F, Smith PH, et al: Maximal androgen blockade: Final analysis of EORTC phase III trial 30853: EORTC Genito-Urinary Tract Cancer Cooperative Group and the EORTC Data Center. Eur Urol 1998;33:144–151.

599. Iversen P, Rasmussen F, Klarskov P, Christensen IJ: Long-term results of Danish Prostatic Cancer Group trial 86: Goserelin

acetate plus flutamide versus orchiectomy in advanced prostate cancer. Cancer 1993;72(12 suppl):3851–3854.

600. Suciu S, Sylvester R, Iversen P, Christensen I, Denis L: Comparability of prostate trials. Cancer 1993;72(12 suppl):3841–3846.

601. de Voogt HJ, Studer U, Schroder FH, Klijn JG, de Pauw M, Sylvester R: Maximum androgen blockade using LHRH agonist buserelin in combination with short-term (two weeks) or long-term (continuous) cyproterone acetate is not superior to standard androgen deprivation in the treatment of advanced prostate cancer: Final analysis of EORTC GU Group Trial 30843: European Organization for Research and Treatment of Cancer (EROTC) Genito-Urinary Tract Cancer Cooperative Group. Eur Urol 1998; 33:152–158.

602. Di Silverio F, Serio M, D'Eramo G, Sciarra F: Zoladex vs. Zoladex plus cyproterone acetate in the treatment of advanced prostatic cancer: A multicenter Italian study. Eur Urol 1990;18(Suppl 3):54–61.

603. Thorpe SC, Azmatullah S, Fellows GJ, Gingell JC, O'Boyle PJ: A prospective, randomised study to compare goserelin acetate (Zoladex) versus cyproterone acetate (Cyprostat) versus a combination of the two in the treatment of metastatic prostatic carcinoma. Eur Urol 1996;29:47–54.

604. Robinson MR, Smith PH, Richards B, Newling DW, de Pauw M, Sylvester R: The final analysis of the EORTC Genito-Urinary Tract Cancer Co-Operative Group phase III clinical trial (protocol 30805) comparing orchidectomy, orchidectomy plus cyproterone acetate and low dose stilboestrol in the management of metastatic carcinoma of the prostate. Eur Urol 1995;28:273–283.

605. Jorgensen T, Tveter KJ, Jorgensen LH: Total androgen suppression: Experience from the Scandinavian Prostatic Cancer Group Study No. 2. Eur Urol 1993;24:466–470.

606. Maximum androgen blockade in advanced prostate cancer: An overview of the randomised trials: Prostate Cancer Trialists' Collaborative Group. Lancet 2000;355:1491–1498.

607. Maximum androgen blockade in advanced prostate cancer: An overview of 22 randomised trials with 3283 deaths in 5710 patients: Prostate Cancer Trialists' Collaborative Group. Lancet 1995;346:265–269.

608. Moinpour CM, Savage MJ, Troxel A, et al: Quality of life in advanced prostate cancer: Results of a randomized therapeutic trial. J Natl Cancer Inst 1998;90:1537–1544.

609. Labrie F, Veilleux R, Fournier A: Low androgen levels induce the development of androgen-hypersensitive cell clones in Shionogi mouse mammary carcinoma cells in culture. J Natl Cancer Inst 1988;80:1138–1147.

610. Carmichael R, Belanger A, Cusan L, Seguin C, Caron S, Labrie F: Increased testicular 5 alpha-androstane-3 alpha, 17 beta-diol formation induced by treatment with [D-Ser (TBU) 6, des-Gly-NH2(10)] LHRH ethylamide in the rat. Steroids 1980;36:383–391.

611. Immediate versus deferred treatment for advanced prostatic cancer: Initial results of the Medical Research Council Trial: The Medical Research Council Prostate Cancer Working Party Investigators Group. Br J Urol 1997;79:235–246.

612. Messing EM, Manola J, Sarosdy M, Wilding G, Crawford ED, Trump D: Immediate hormonal therapy compared with observation after radical prostatectomy and pelvic lymphadenectomy in men with node-positive prostate cancer. N Engl J Med 1999;341:1781–1788.

613. Seay TM, Blute ML, Zincke H: Long-term outcome in patients with pTxN+ adenocarcinoma of prostate treated with radical prostatectomy and early androgen ablation. J Urol 1998;159: 357–364.

614. Eisenberger MA, Walsh PC: Early androgen deprivation for prostate cancer? N Engl J Med 1999;341:1837–1838.

615. Akakura K, Bruchovsky N, Goldenberg SL, Rennie PS, Buckley AR, Sullivan LD: Effects of intermittent androgen suppression on androgen-dependent tumors: Apoptosis and serum prostate-specific antigen. Cancer 1993;71:2782–2790.

616. Russo P, Liguori G, Heston WD, et al: Effects of intermittent diethylstilbestrol diphosphate administration on the R3327 rat prostatic carcinoma. Cancer Res 1987;47:5967–5970.

617. Kelly WK, Scher HI: Prostate specific antigen decline after antiandrogen withdrawal: The flutamide withdrawal syndrome. J Urol 1993;149:607–609.

618. Scher HI, Zhang ZF, Nanus D, Kelly WK: Hormone and

antihormone withdrawal: Implications for the management of androgen-independent prostate cancer. Urology 1996;47 (1A suppl):61–69.

619. Schellhammer PF, Venner P, Haas GP, et al: Prostate specific antigen decreases after withdrawal of antiandrogen therapy with bicalutamide or flutamide in patients receiving combined androgen blockade. J Urol 1997;157:1731–1735.

620. Oh WK: Secondary hormonal therapies in the treatment of prostate cancer. Urology 2002;60(3 suppl 1):87–92.

621. Small EJ, Frohlich MW, Bok R, et al: Prospective trial of the herbal supplement PC-SPES in patients with progressive prostate cancer. J Clin Oncol 2000;18:3595–3603.

622. Sovak M, Seligson AL, Konas M, et al: Herbal composition PC-SPES for management of prostate cancer: Identification of active principles. J Natl Cancer Inst 2002;94:1275–1281.

623. Eisenberger M, Crawford D, MacLeod D, Hussain M, Loehrer P, Blumenstein B: The prognostic significance of prostate specific antigen in stage D2 prostate cancer: Interim evaluation of intergroup 0105. Proc Am Soc Clin Oncol 1995;14:236.

624. Sinibaldi VJ, Garrett E, Rosenbaum E, et al: The outcome of androgen suppressed prostate cancer (PCa) patients after biochemical (PSA) relapse and no clinical/radiological evidence of metastasis (M0). Proc Am Soc Clin Oncol 2003;24:443.

625. Taylor CD, Elson P, Trump DL: Importance of continued testicular suppression in hormone-refractory prostate cancer. J Clin Oncol 1993;11:2167–2172.

626. Fowler JE Jr, Whitmore WF Jr: The response of metastatic adenocarcinoma of the prostate to exogenous testosterone. J Urol 1981;126:372–375.

627. Fowler JE Jr, Whitmore WF Jr: Considerations for the use of testosterone with systemic chemotherapy in prostatic cancer. Cancer 1982;49:1373–1377.

628. Manni A, Bartholomew M, Caplan R, et al: Androgen priming and chemotherapy in advanced prostate cancer: Evaluation of determinants of clinical outcome. J Clin Oncol 1988;6: 1456–1466.

629. Hussain M, Wolf M, Marshall E, Crawford ED, Eisenberger M: Effects of continued androgen-deprivation therapy and other prognostic factors on response and survival in phase II chemotherapy trials for hormone-refractory prostate cancer: A Southwest Oncology Group report. J Clin Oncol 1994;12:1868–1875.

630. Scher HI, Kelly WK: Flutamide withdrawal syndrome: Its impact on clinical trials in hormone-refractory prostate cancer. J Clin Oncol 1993;11:1566–1572.

631. Yagoda A: Cytotoxic agents in prostate cancer: An enigma. Semin Urol 1983;1:311–321.

632. Kelly WK, Scher HI, Mazumdar M, Vlamis V, Schwartz M, Fossa SD: Prostate-specific antigen as a measure of disease outcome in metastatic hormone-refractory prostate cancer. J Clin Oncol 1993;11:607–615.

633. Bubley GJ, Carducci M, Dahut W, et al: Eligibility and response guidelines for phase II clinical trials in androgen-independent prostate cancer: Recommendations from the Prostate-Specific Antigen Working Group. J Clin Oncol 1999;17:3461–3467.

634. Smith DC, Dunn RL, Strawderman MS, Pienta KJ: Change in serum prostate-specific antigen as a marker of response to cytotoxic therapy for hormone-refractory prostate cancer. J Clin Oncol 1998;16:1835–1843.

635. Sridhara R, Eisenberger MA, Sinibaldi VJ, Reyno LM, Egorin MJ: Evaluation of prostate-specific antigen as a surrogate marker for response of hormone-refractory prostate cancer to suramin therapy. J Clin Oncol 1995;13:2944–2953.

636. LaRocca RV, Cooper MR, Uhrich M, et al: Use of suramin in treatment of prostatic carcinoma refractory to conventional hormonal manipulation. Urol Clin North Am 1991;18:123–129.

637. Steiner MS, Seckin B, Anthony CT, Murphy B: Can prostate specific antigen levels and clinical response be used as a valid endpoint for chemotherapy efficacy in advanced prostate cancer. Proc Am Assoc Cancer Res 1995;36:209.

638. Eisenberger MA: Chemotherapy for prostate carcinoma. NCI Monogr 1988;7:151–163.

639. Eisenberger MA, Simon R, O'Dwyer PJ, Wittes RE, Friedman MA: A reevaluation of nonhormonal cytotoxic chemotherapy in the treatment of prostatic carcinoma. J Clin Oncol 1985;3:827–841.

640. Schmidt JD, Gibbons RP, Johnson DE, Prout GR, Scott WW, Murphy GP: Chemotherapy of advanced prostatic cancer. Evaluation of response parameters. Urology 1976;7:602–610.

641. Slack NH, Mittelman A, Brady MF, Murphy GP: The importance of the stable category for chemotherapy treated patients with advanced and relapsing prostate cancer. Cancer 1980;46:2393–2402.

642. Abell F, Wilkes J, Divers L, Huben R, Velagapudi S, Raghavan D: Oral cyclophosphamide for hormone-refractory prostate cancer. Proc Am Soc Clin Oncol 1995;14:213.

643. Von Roemiling R, Fisher HA, Horton J: Daily oral cyclophosphamide is effective in hormone-refractory prostate cancer: A phase I/II pilot study. Proc Am Soc Clin Oncol 1992;11:213.

644. Smith D, Vogelzang N, Goldberg H, Gockerman J, Winder E, Trump D: High-dose cyclophosphamide with granulocyte-macrophage colony stimulating factor in hormone-refractory prostate cancer. Proc Am Soc Clin Oncol 1992;11:213.

645. Osborne CK, Drelichman A, Von Hoff DD, Crawford ED: Mitoxantrone: Modest activity in a phase II trial in advanced prostate cancer. Cancer Treat Rep 1983;67:1133–1135.

646. Raghavan D, Bishop J, Woods J: Mitoxantrone: A non-toxic, moderately active agent for hormone resistant prostate cancer. Proc Am Soc Clin Oncol 1986;5:102.

647. Rearden T, Small E, Valone F, Carroll P, Ernest M, Wilkinson M: Phase II study of mitoxantrone for hormone refractory prostate cancer. Proc Am Soc Clin Oncol 1995;14:218.

648. Tannock IF, Osoba D, Stockler MR, et al: Chemotherapy with mitoxantrone plus prednisone or prednisone alone for symptomatic hormone-resistant prostate cancer: A Canadian randomized trial with palliative end points. J Clin Oncol 1996;14:1756–1764.

649. Iversen P, Rasmussen F, Asmussen C, et al: Estramustine phosphate versus placebo as second line treatment after orchiectomy in patients with metastatic prostate cancer: DAPROCA study 9002. Danish Prostatic Cancer Group. J Urol 1997;157:929–934.

650. Hudes G: Estramustine-based chemotherapy. Semin Urol Oncol 1997;15:13–19.

651. Hartley-Asp B, Kruse E: Nuclear protein matrix as a target for estramustine-induced cell death. Prostate 1986;9:387–395.

652. Kanje M, Deinum J, Wallin M, Ekstrom P, Edstrom A, Hartley-Asp B: Effect of estramustine phosphate on the assembly of isolated bovine brain microtubules and fast axonal transport in the frog sciatic nerve. Cancer Res 1985;45:2234–2239.

653. Pienta KJ, Lehr JE: Inhibition of prostate cancer growth by estramustine and etoposide: Evidence for interaction at the nuclear matrix. J Urol 1993;149:1622–1625.

654. Picus J, Schultz M: Docetaxel (Taxotere) as monotherapy in the treatment of hormone-refractory prostate cancer: Preliminary results. Semin Oncol 1999;26(5 suppl 17):14–18.

655. Friedland D, Cohen J, Miller R Jr, et al: A phase II trial of docetaxel (Taxotere) in hormone-refractory prostate cancer: Correlation of antitumor effect to phosphorylation of Bcl-2. Semin Oncol 1999;26(5 suppl 17):19–23.

656. Beer TM, Pierce WC, Lowe BA, Henner WD: Phase II study of weekly docetaxel in symptomatic androgen-independent prostate cancer. Ann Oncol 2001;12:1273–1279.

657. Petrylak DP, Macarthur RB, O'Connor J, et al: Phase I trial of docetaxel with estramustine in androgen-independent prostate cancer. J Clin Oncol 1999;17:958–967.

658. Hussain M, Petrylak D, Fisher E, Tangen C, Crawford D: Docetaxel (Taxotere) and estramustine versus mitoxantrone and prednisone for hormone-refractory prostate cancer: Scientific basis and design of Southwest Oncology Group Study 9916. Semin Oncol 1999;26(Suppl 17):55–60.

659. Logothetis CJ, Hoosein NM, Hsieh JT: The clinical and biological study of androgen independent prostate cancer (AI PCa). Semin Oncol 1994;21:620–629.

660. di Sant'Agnese PA: Neuroendocrine differentiation in carcinoma of the prostate. Diagnostic, prognostic, and therapeutic implications. Cancer 1992;70(1 suppl):254–268.

661. Frank S, Amsterdam A, Kelly W, et al: Platinum-based chemotherapy for patients with poorly differentiated hormone-refractory prostate cancer: Response and pathologic considerations. Proc Am Soc Clin Oncol 1995;14:232.

662. Saad F, Gleason DM, Murray R, et al: A randomized, placebo-controlled trial of zoledronic acid in patients with hormone-refractory metastatic prostate carcinoma. J Natl Cancer Inst 2002;94:1458–1468.

663. Smith MR, Eastham J, Gleason DM, Shasha D, Tchekmedyian S, Zinner N: Randomized controlled trial of zoledronic acid to prevent bone loss in men receiving androgen deprivation therapy for nonmetastatic prostate cancer. J Urol 2003;169:2008–2012.

664. Crawford ED, Kozlowski JM, Debruyne FM, et al: The use of strontium 89 for palliation of pain from bone metastases associated with hormone-refractory prostate cancer. Urology 1994;44:481–485.

665. Tu SM, Millikan RE, Mengistu B, et al: Bone-targeted therapy for advanced androgen-independent carcinoma of the prostate: A randomised phase II trial. Lancet 2001;357:336–341.

666. Corey E, Quinn JE, Bladou F, et al: Establishment and characterization of osseous prostate cancer models: Intra-tibial injection of human prostate cancer cells. Prostate 2002;52:20–33.

667. Mundy GR: Metastasis to bone: Causes, consequences and therapeutic opportunities. Nat Rev Cancer 2002;2:584–593.

668. Nelson JB, Nabulsi AA, Vogelzang NJ, et al: Suppression of prostate cancer induced bone remodeling by the endothelin receptor A antagonist atrasentan. J Urol 2003;169:1143–1149.

669. Uehara H, Kim SJ, Karashima T, et al: Effects of blocking platelet-derived growth factor-receptor signaling in a mouse model of experimental prostate cancer bone metastases. J Natl Cancer Inst 2003;95:458–470.

670. Small EJ, Fratesi P, Reese DM, et al: Immunotherapy of hormone-refractory prostate cancer with antigen-loaded dendritic cells. J Clin Oncol 2000;18:3894–3903.

671. Eder JP, Kantoff PW, Roper K, et al: A phase I trial of a recombinant vaccinia virus expressing prostate-specific antigen in advanced prostate cancer. Clin Cancer Res 2000;6:1632–1638.

672. Hwang LC, Fein S, Levitsky H, Nelson WG: Prostate cancer vaccines: Current status. Semin Oncol 1999;26:192–201.

673. Simons JW, Mikhak B, Chang JF, et al: Induction of immunity to prostate cancer antigens: Results of a clinical trial of vaccination with irradiated autologous prostate tumor cells engineered to secrete granulocyte-macrophage colony-stimulating factor using ex vivo gene transfer. Cancer Res 1999;59:5160–5168.

674. DeWeese TL, van der Poel H, Li S, et al: A phase I trial of CV706, a replication-competent, PSA selective oncolytic adenovirus, for the treatment of locally recurrent prostate cancer following radiation therapy. Cancer Res 2001;61:7464–7472.

675. Carducci MA, Padley RJ, Breul J, et al: Effect of endothelin-A receptor blockade with atrasentan on tumor progression in men with hormone-refractory prostate cancer: A randomized, phase II, placebo-controlled trial. J Clin Oncol 2003;21:679–689.

676. Carducci MA, Nelson JB, Bowling MK, et al: Atrasentan, an endothelin-receptor antagonist for refractory adenocarcinomas: Safety and pharmacokinetics. J Clin Oncol 2002;20:2171–2180.

677. Liu G, Oettel K, Ripple G, et al: Phase I trial of 1alpha-hydroxyvitamin D(2) in patients with hormone refractory prostate cancer. Clin Cancer Res 2002;8:2820–2827.

CANCER OF THE PENIS AND URETHRA

Daniel J. Culkin

Adam R. Metwalli

SUMMARY OF KEY POINTS

INCIDENCE

- The incidence of squamous cell carcinoma (SCC) of the penis is estimated at 1/100,000 in Western countries
- By contrast, the incidence has been estimated as high as 17% in Brazil and between 10% and 20% in Africa and Asia
- However, the overall incidence has been decreasing worldwide

ETIOLOGY/EPIDEMIOLOGY

- Neonatal circumcision appears to protect against penile carcinoma
- The risk of penile cancer is three times higher for both uncircumcised men and those circumcised after the perinatal period
- Hygiene, history of sexually transmitted disease, and sexual promiscuity may play an equal or greater role
- Factors that do appear to play a role in the development of penile carcinoma are ultraviolet radiation and cigarette smoking

PATHOLOGY/BIOLOGY

- More than 95% of primary penile tumors are SCCs
- Fewer than half of patients will have superficial disease at the time of diagnosis

CLINICAL FINDINGS

- Generally, penile carcinoma is a disease of older men
- Presentation can vary from an innocuous-appearing induration with slight erythema to an obviously malignant fungating penile tumor that leads to autoamputation
- Inguinal lymphadenopathy is a common finding at diagnosis

DIFFERENTIAL DIAGNOSIS/ STAGING

- Differential diagnosis of a penile lesion includes sexually transmitted diseases such as syphilis, chancroid, as well as penile leukoplakia, balanitis xerotica obliterans, erythroplasia of Queyrat/Bowen's disease, bowenoid papulosis, verrucous carcinoma, acquired immunodeficiency syndrome (AIDS)-related Kaposi's sarcoma, basal cell carcinoma of the penis, extramammary Paget's disease, melanoma of the penis, and secondary tumors of the penis from metastatic nongenital primary malignancies
- Current staging of penile carcinoma incorporates tumor invasion, local node involvement, and the presence of distant metastases [i.e., tumor-node-metastasis (TNM) staging]

PRIMARY THERAPY

- The foundation of therapy for penile carcinoma has been surgical excision of both the primary tumor and regional lymph nodes
- Organ-preserving techniques such as Mohs' micrographic surgery, radiation, or laser ablation into therapy should be considered for small T1 and T2 lesions
- Radiation therapy and interstitial brachytherapy for penile carcinoma are effective therapy for T1 lesions and for patients with well-differentiated T2 tumors
- Large tumors generally require a total penectomy or complete corporal body resection with a perineal urethrostomy
- Patients with T2 to T4 disease and clinically negative inguinal nodes should undergo a modified superficial inguinal lymphadenectomy

SALVAGE THERAPY

- Given the dismal long-term survival for patients with known pelvic nodal metastases, experimental protocols that include combinations of chemotherapy and radiation are advisable in this high-risk cohort
- Combination chemotherapy should contribute to multimodality approaches in the management of penile carcinoma
- Chemotherapeutic regimens can shrink bulky nodal disease to allow surgical resection

COMPLICATIONS

- The disfigurement after partial or radical penectomy has tremendous psychological impact on patients
- Postoperative sequelae of lymphadenectomy are lymphedema, deep venous thrombosis, and wound complications; the estimated morbidity of this procedure including all complications is less than 20%
- Chemotherapeutic complications include pneumonitis, hepatic insufficiency, myelosuppression, renal insufficiency, skin rashes, and sepsis
- Common radiation-induced complications are telangiectasias, urethral strictures, and meatal stenosis

PROGNOSIS

- The most important factors in prognosis and treatment of penile carcinoma are tumor grade, depth of invasion, and tumor location
- Low-grade and low-stage tumors have an excellent prognosis and long-term survival even with organ-preserving therapies such as radiation
- Patients without nodal involvement have an excellent 5-year survival rate of 95%, but only 81% of those with up to three positive nodes will be alive after the same period
- Patients with more than three malignant lymph nodes have a 50% mortality, and no patients with pelvic disease are alive at 5 years.

INTRODUCTION

Cancer of the penis is an uncommon tumor in North America and composes less than one half of 1% of all male malignancies. It is most common in the sixth decade of life. A delay of diagnosis for just 1 year can account for the high proportion of advanced disease (i.e., 30% of the new cases). Data reveal more than 95% of the lesions to be squamous cell carcinomas (SCCs); most start as a lesion on the glans penis or prepuce and typically progress from a superficial neoplasm to local invasion of the corpora cavernosa, with early metastases to the inguinal lymph nodes. Currently, the most important factor for long-term survival is the stage of the disease at the time of diagnosis. Early detection is the key to improving survival and quality of life for the patient.

EPIDEMIOLOGY

Geographic Variations

Penile carcinoma is exceedingly rare in North America and Scandinavia and is far more prevalent in South America, Asia, and Africa. The incidence of SCC of the penis is similar in Finland and is estimated at 1/100,000 (.0001) in Western countries.[1,2] By contrast, the incidence has been estimated as high as 17% in Brazil and between 10% and 20% in Africa and Asia.[3,4] Despite the geographic differences in number of new cases of penile carcinoma, the overall incidence has been decreasing worldwide.[2,5,6]

ETIOLOGY AND PATHOGENESIS

Several factors predispose a patient to penile carcinoma, such as an intact prepuce and poor hygiene. Neonatal circumcision appears to protect against penile carcinoma, as the incidence of this malignancy is essentially nil among those with neonatal circumcision.[7] Postperinatal circumcision does not appear to confer this protection, because the risk of penile cancer is three times higher for both uncircumcised men and those with postperinatal circumcision.[8] However, the protective effect of neonatal circumcision is debatable, because countries such as Finland and Denmark have a low rate of neonatal circumcision with a penile carcinoma incidence similar to that of North America, where the rate of neonatal circumcision is much higher.[6,9,10] To confound the debate further, in Israel, the rate of neonatal circumcision is nearly 100%; however, the incidence of penile carcinoma is closer to 1/1,000,000 than to 1/100,000.[11] Recent studies show the incidence of penile intraepithelial neoplasia to be quite high in neonatally circumcised men.[12] Ultimately, associated factors such as hygiene, history of sexually transmitted disease, and sexual promiscuity may play a role equal to or greater than that of neonatal circumcision in the etiology of male genital cancer.

Although the association of phimosis and penile carcinoma is well established,[13,14] the carcinogenesis of smegma and the bacteria *Mycobacterium smegmatis* are less likely to have a relevant role in the etiology of penile carcinoma.[15-17] Current investigations appear to implicate human papilloma virus (HPV) in the development of penile carcinoma. A study of SCCs of the penis showed that 71% had detectable strains of HPV.[18] A few similar studies among specimens from patients with penile carcinoma have revealed comparable levels of HPV DNA detection,[19,20] yet other larger studies have shown much lower detection rates of HPV DNA in penile cancer specimens.[8,21-24]

The association between penile carcinoma and other sexually transmitted diseases has not been established, nor has any substantive correlation been made between this disease and alcohol consumption or illicit drug use.[8] Furthermore, whereas the common perception is that penile carcinoma is confined to older men, nearly one fourth of U.S. patients are younger than 40 years at the time of diagnosis. Nearly 10% of these patients are younger than 30 years, and this pathology has been reported in the pediatric population as well.[25]

Factors that do appear to play a role in the development of penile carcinoma are ultraviolet radiation and cigarette smoking. The former is supported by the increased incidence of cases in men treated with ultraviolet phototherapy for psoriasis.[26] Several recent population-based studies found an increased incidence of penile carcinoma in smokers.[27]

PREVENTION AND EDUCATION

Many texts tout the protective effects of perinatal circumcision in the prevention of penile carcinoma, but it seems clear that the benefit is primarily due to facilitation of better hygiene. The very low incidence of penile carcinoma in countries such as Denmark and Finland where perinatal circumcision is uncommon supports the notion that proper hygiene and early education in these matters provides equal protection against this disease process. In situations in which hygiene may become an issue because of behavioral or neurologic disorders that limit self-care, perinatal circumcision may still be warranted.

PATHOLOGY

Penile carcinoma is merely one of many pathologic processes with visible dermatologic signs that may be identified on the genitals. Vigilance on the part of primary and secondary health care providers is essential to early diagnosis because of the many benign and premalignant lesions that may imitate or precede penile carcinoma. Interestingly, in a clinical correlation, Bezerra and colleagues[28] found HPV DNA in 30% of penile carcinoma specimens from 82 patients but demonstrated no significant difference in lymph node metastasis and 10-year survival between HPV-positive and HPV-negative groups. However, viral etiology may be significant, based on tumor subtype. Verruciform subtype of penile SCC appears to be more strongly associated with HPV infection and tends to display a less-aggressive clinical phenotype.[21,28] In addition, these findings suggest that different etiologic pathways may be relevant depending on the type of penile carcinoma diagnosed.

Leukoplakia

Leukoplakia is seen in diabetic men as perimeatal, blanched plaques or scaled areas that can extend into the urethral meatus. The microscopic appearance is consistent with acanthosis, parakeratosis, and hyperkeratosis and is often seen in close proximity to malignant lesions. Although this lesion may arise in response to recurrent inflammation or irritation, it is not proven to be a premalignant condition. Penile leukoplakia may be treated with surgical excision, laser ablation, irradiation, or topical treatments,[29-31] but any therapy must include careful follow-up for the development of possible malignancy, because the risk of malignant degeneration has been reported to be as high as 10% to 20%.[32] Successful therapy with bleomycin for extensive lesions has been reported.[33]

Balanitis Xerotica Obliterans

Balanitis xerotica obliterans (BXO) is lichen sclerosis et atrophicus (LSA) of the penis. First diagnosed in 1928, this disorder can affect the glans, prepuce, and/or urethra. Recent epidemiologic data suggest that the overall incidence is far less than 1% but that an increased incidence is noted among minority cohorts in the population and among men between the ages of 30 and 40 years.[34,35] BXO is associated with SCC of the penis in 2.3% to 5.8% of cases.[36,37] BXO is generally regarded as a benign lesion.[36,38,39] The natural history of BXO is highly variable, with some patients having an indolent chronic affliction that produces few early symptoms, whereas others may have diffuse disease only weeks after onset. Early cases of BXO often appear as areas of ivory-colored, sclerotic plaque on the glans or inner prepuce, and the patient may complain of pruritus. These lesions can be distinguished from leukoplakia clinically by the characteristic appearance of BXO, as well as histologically because of the fibrosis, epidermal atrophy, interface dermatitis, and dermal edema. Other symptoms may include painful erections or a burning sensation with erection, phimosis, or dysuria. If untreated, these lesions will spread and coalesce, becoming less pliable and more fibrotic. Sexual intercourse will often result in fissures, blisters, and bleeding. Continued progression of disease can result in contraction of the frenulum and/or fibrotic phimosis. Topical steroids or circumcision for advanced disease is recommended treatment for BXO.[36,40,41]

Carcinoma in Situ

Carcinoma in situ (CIS) of the genitals is classified by location of the lesion. A sharply demarcated, shiny, raised erythematous plaque of the glans or mucosal surface of the prepuce is called erythroplasia of Queyrat (EQ); whereas Bowen's disease (BD) describes the same histologic entity, seen as red, scaling patches on the keratinized genital surfaces such as the penile shaft, scrotum, or perineum.[42,43] Unlike those of BXO, these lesions are definitely premalignant or malignant and progress to SCC at a rate of 10% to 30%.[44-46] EQ and BD tend to be diseases of older men, with the most common diagnosis in the fifth decade. BD typically involves the epithelial cell layers of hair follicles, with a histologic appearance very similar to that of EQ. When found on the penis, this lesion often appears as a scaling plaque without notable erythema and signifies the presence of CIS. Only about 10% will progress to invasive carcinoma, a rate comparable to that of EQ.

Histologically these lesions demonstrate diffuse changes throughout the squamous epithelial cell layers, including keratinocyte hyperplasia, nuclear atypia with many mitoses, proliferation of enlarged hyperchromatic cells, multinucleated cells, and loss of polarity within most cells. Presence of inflammatory cell infiltration and increased density of microvasculature is common. Similar to invasive penile carcinoma, links to HPV infection have been investigated and have revealed a correlation with many of the same viral strains.[47] A small study of EQ identified DNA from HPV type 8 in every sample of penile CIS, whereas this viral DNA was not identified in any samples of BD lesions.[48] In addition, HPV type 16 was found in more than 80% of these samples.[48]

Bowenoid Papulosis

Bowenoid papulosis (BP) is markedly different from EQ and BD in presentation, demographics, and clinical course. Men who have BP are much younger than their EQ counterparts, with a mean age of almost 30 years.[49] These lesions are groups of scaling, erythematous papules typically seen on the keratinized skin of the penile shaft. Histologically the cellular morphology mimics that of CIS, but the keratinocytes tend to be slightly more differentiated than those seen in CIS. In addition, histologic sections of bowenoid papules demonstrate that the more atypical-appearing cells tend to be found among the top epithelial cell layers and in the upper portion of the sweat glands, which is the opposite of the histologic pattern that defines BD. Because of histologic similarities, a physician must combine the clinical presentation and the histologic findings to arrive confidently at the diagnosis.

Although the etiology of BP is still unclear, the viral etiology of BP been suggested by increasing evidence of an etiologic link to HPV subtypes (6, 11, 18, 42, 43, and 44).[50-55] This is further supported by the reported progression of BP to SCC in lesions with high-risk HPV strains (31 and 67).[56] Spontaneous regression also has been reported,[57,58] and BP is usually not considered a premalignant lesion by most physicians.[59,60]

Recent treatment for BP has consisted primarily of topical therapy including 5-fluorouracil (5-FU), imiqimod cream, and cidofovir in immunocompromised patients.[60-62] Historically these lesions have been surgically excised, and results with laser and other forms of ablative therapy have been mixed.[63,64] Often topical and extirpative therapy can be used in combination, with good results.

Buschke-Lowenstein Tumor

Commonly known as verrucous carcinoma or giant condyloma acuminatum, Buschke-Lowenstein (B-L) tumors are very similar in appearance to benign condyloma venereatum. Unlike their benign counterparts, B-L tumors tend to invade tissue and cause significant local damage. This can be seen histologically, as the rete pegs of these lesions are often seen penetrating deeply into surrounding tissue. This aggressive behavior is in contrast to the very-well-differentiated cells that compose B-L tumors; cellular anaplasia is very atypical in these specimens. Like many of these premalignant and benign genital lesions, a viral etiology appears to play a role in the development of this condition, as investigators have found associations with HPV strains 6 and 11.[65] Despite the local tissue destruction commonly found with these tumors, metastatic progression of the tumor does not occur; local control is the primary objective. This may require partial or total penectomy.[66] No large-scale trials of effective topical or radiation therapies have shown efficacy, and most data can be derived from isolated case reports of various treatment modalities.[67,68] A recently published report of B-L tumor regression after treatment with intralesional injections of interferon alpha suggests that local nonexcisional therapies that are directed at viral etiology may hold promise for future therapies.[69] By contrast, use of systemic chemotherapy with bleomycin, methotrexate, and cisplatin has been reported to achieve regression of B-L lesions; given the known toxicities of these agents, this approach is rarely, if ever, indicated for this disease.[70] Currently, CO_2 laser ablation seems to be the method of choice for local control of this lesion.[71,72] For very large lesions, staged laser ablation may in the long term provide an acceptable cosmetic result.

Nonsquamous Malignancies

Nonsquamous cell carcinoma of the penis is rare, and the tumors compose less than 5% of penile tumors. Of this small subset, the most common malignancy is sarcoma. Other histologic penile tumors that have been reported are melanoma, basal cell carcinoma, and lymphoma. With the increasing prevalence of human immunodeficiency virus (HIV) and acquired immunodeficiency syndrome (AIDS) patients, the incidence of Kaposi's sarcoma is increasing, particularly among sexually transmitted cases of HIV; genital lesions can be found in nearly 20% of patients with AIDS-related Kaposi's sarcoma. Only a very small percentage of these patients will initially have a penile lesion. The gross appearance is of erythematous nodules with sharp margins, found most often on the glans penis.[73] Standard therapy involves conservative measures such as local excision, laser ablation, or palliative radiation.[74]

Basal cell carcinoma of the penis most often can be found on the penile shaft, with only a fraction of cases reported on the prepuce or glans.[75] Appearance of this tumor on the scrotum or perineum is even less common.[76,77] The typical appearance of basal cell carcinoma of the penis is a well-circumscribed lesion with clear borders and central pitting. Given the slow rate of growth and lack of metastasis, local excision is often curative.[75,77,78]

In contrast, melanoma of the penis carries a very poor prognosis, with 40% of patients initially seen with regional lymph node metastasis.[79] Two of every three lesions are found on the glans. Wide, local excision with a 3- to 5-cm margin is the treatment of choice for lesions smaller than 1.5 mm Breslow depth.[80] Bilateral inguinal lymph node dissection has been the standard of care for lesions that penetrate more than 1.5 mm.[79] Despite the success of sentinel lymph node biopsy for melanoma in other anatomic locations, this technology has been unreliable for penile lesions. Sentinel lymph node studies for penile malignancy, discussed in detail later in the chapter, should be regarded cautiously. We continue to recommend bilateral lymph node dissection for penile melanoma lesions invading deeper than 1.5 mm.

Extramammary Paget's disease is a very rare penoscrotal neoplasm, and distinguishing this lesion from EQ or BD is clinically impossible. Histologically it is diagnosed by the presence of large, clear-staining cells with hypochromatic nuclei called Paget's cells within the epidermis. This disease is seen in older men and appears as a well-demarcated erythematous, eczematous lesion. Metastasis to regional lymph nodes occurs very rarely. The etiology of this disease is currently considered adenocarcinoma in situ of the epidermis, arising from pluripotent intraepidermal cells undergoing malignant transformation during apocrine differentiation.[81] Clinical suspicion for underlying genitourinary malignancies should be very high, because 16% to 33% of patients with penoscrotal Paget's disease have been found to have concurrent internal genitourinary carcinoma.[81-83] Historically, patients with extramammary Paget's disease were evaluated extensively for occult pulmonary and gastrointestinal malignancy; however, retrospective analysis of patients with penoscrotal Paget's disease reveals that 92% of those with associated malignancy have genitourinary pathology.[81] Treatment generally consists of wide local excision that typically requires coverage of the defect with skin grafting or tissue flaps.[81] Others suggest that Mohs micrographic surgery is the therapy of choice due to the very high incidence of positive margins with radical excision with standard surgical techniques.[84] Other nonexcisional treatments have been used, but these isolated reports do not provide enough data to evaluate these techniques for efficacy.[83] Recurrence is very common, and close follow-up is essential.

Other unusual tumors have been reported anecdotally and include penile schwannoma, plexiform neurofibroma, vascular hemangioendothelioma, leimyosarcoma, rhabdomyosarcoma, epitheliod sarcoma, Ewing's sarcoma, mucoepidermoid carcinoma, and synovial sarcoma.[85-92] Generally the prognosis for these tumors is similar to the reported outcomes of these malignancies when they are identified in more typical anatomic locations.

Metastatic Tumors

Secondary tumors of the penis from metastatic nongenital primary malignancies are rare, with only 460 cases reported.[93] Isolated metastases to the penis are most often found in the presence of advanced systemic carcinoma. Although nongenitourinary cancers metastasizing to the penis do occur, 75% result from primary genitourinary cancers.[94] The index of suspicion for penile metastasis should be high in patients with a known malignancy in whom priapism or a new penile lesion develops. The common presentation of penile metastases is multiple nodules along the penile skin with occasional ulcerations similar to a syphilitic chancre. These lesions typically are not painful, are associated with extensive involvement of the corpora cavernosa in almost 50% of patients, and commonly account for priapism.[95] The primary tumors that most frequently metastasize to the penis are prostate, bladder, urothelial, renal cell, testis, and rectal carcinomas.[93,95] An excellent review by Chan and associates[93] of metastatic carcinoma to the penis reveals that multiple treatment regimens have been used involving various combinations of hormonal therapy, surgery, irradiation, and chemotherapy, with equally variable outcomes. Most of these regimens appear to involve some effort toward systemic therapy combined with local palliation.

Invasive Squamous Cell Carcinoma

Pathology and Natural History

More than 95% of primary penile tumors are SCCs, and malignancy can arise in any location on the penis.[96] The lesions of the glans account for nearly half of squamous cell penile carcinomas; tumors of the prepuce account for more than 20% of penile SCCs; and almost 10% of patients will have lesions on both the glans and the foreskin.[96]

Metastasis of penile carcinoma occurs first in the superficial inguinal lymph nodes, and the risk of metastatic disease is related to tumor size. Small tumors found only on the glans or prepuce are rarely metastatic at diagnosis,[97] whereas large tumors that involve more than 75% of the penile shaft have a very high risk of nodal metastasis.[98,99]

Histologically these tumors have a hyperkeratotic dermis with cords of carcinoma cells extending into deeper tissue layers, with intercellular bridges, keratin, and keratin pearls prominent throughout the specimen. More than 50% of tumors that first arise on the penile shaft tend to be high-grade carcinoma, whereas only 10% of preputial SCCs demonstrate poorly differentiated histology.

A grading system based on histologic features was proposed by Broders[100] with grade I lesions demonstrating well-differentiated morphology with keratin pearls and prominent intercellular bridges. Tumors classified as grade II or III have greater nuclear atypia with increased mitotic activity and fewer keratin pearls. Grade IV histology is characterized by significant nuclear pleomorphism with many mitoses, lymphatic and perineural invasion, no keratin pearls, and necrosis (Fig. 88-1; see Table 88-2).

Other grading systems have been developed to improve the reproducibility of the Broders classification. Factors that influence grading in these systems are the number of mitotic cells per high-power field, degree of keratinization and cellular atypia, and the infiltration of inflammatory cells into the tumor. Each parameter is assigned a score, and these are then summed to give a grade. Application of this system revealed 80% survival among patients with low-grade tumors.[5] Another classification has demonstrated prognostic correlation and categorizes tumors based on superficial spread, vertical growth, verrucous features, and multicentricity. These categories revealed metastatic disease in 42% with superficial disease and 82% with vertical tumor growth.[101] None of the patients with verrucous carcinoma had nodal metastases, but one in three patients with multicentric disease had positive lymph nodes.[101] Other features studied for prognostic significance include ulcerative versus exophytic appearance; not surprisingly, the latter tends to be poorly differentiated with a higher incidence of metastatic disease than the former. Exophytic tumors have a high degree of keratinization on histologic examination, with cells that appear fairly well differentiated. Conversely, ulcerative penile malignancy more often has a poorly differentiated appearance and, as one might expect, has a higher incidence of lymph node involvement.[3,101] In

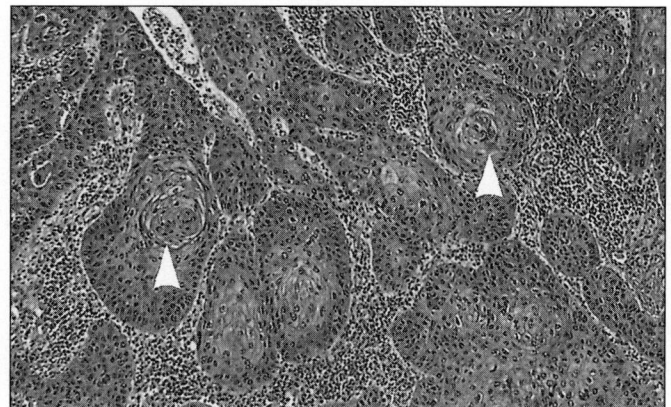

A

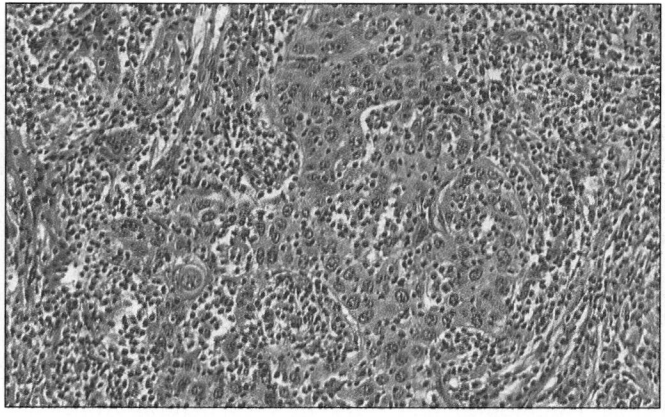

B

Figure 88-1. Squanomus cell carcinoma. **A,** Irregular nests of neoplastic cells invade the underlying tissue. Note the focci of keratinization (*arrows*). **B,** At the point of the deepest invasions, the squamous carcinoma cells are nonkeratinizing and exhibit considerable pleomorphism with large vascular nuclei. Note the associated intense inflammation often seen in invasive carcinoma.

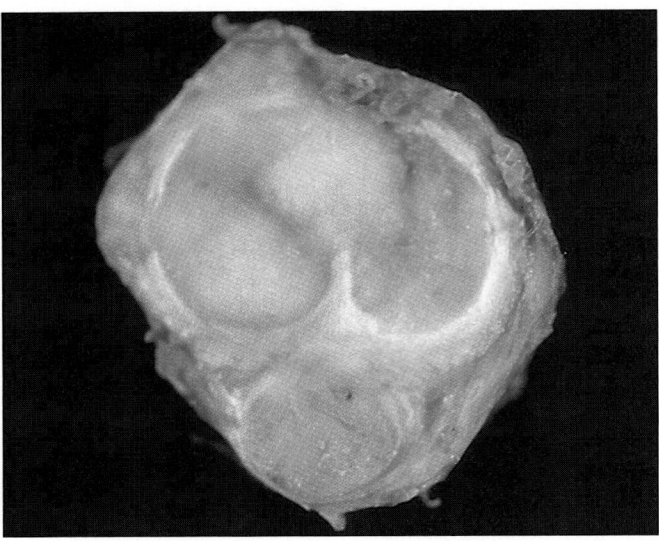

Figure 88-2. Squamous cell carcinoma. A cross section of the penile shaft illustrating replacement of the corpus cavernosum by tumor.

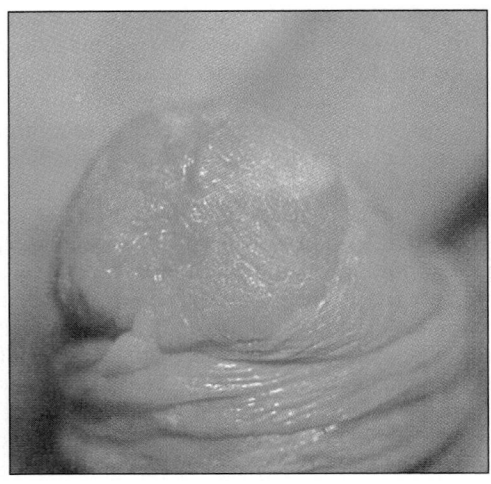

Figure 88-3. Carcinoma in situ. This lesion presents clinically as a well-demarcated, slightly elevated erythematous plaque. (Courtesy of KR Greer, MD, Charlottesville, VA.)

summary, tumor-grading systems and morphologic quantification have improved the ability to predict the presence of nodal metastases and tumor progression.

The natural history of this disease typically includes invasion and destruction of local tissues with continuous growth of the tumor, leading to the eventual invasion of the corpora and urethra (Fig. 88-2). Metastatic spread occurs as the tumor invades the lymphatic network of the prepuce and penile skin, which empties into the base of the penis and then fans to both inguinal node beds. This anatomy has complicated efforts to develop reliable sentinel node biopsy techniques. Once lymph has entered either superficial inguinal nodal chain, its drainage pattern is more predictable into the deep inguinal nodes found below the fascia lata and medial to the femoral vein. The lymphatic system for the glans, urethra, and corpus spongiosum also has a variable drainage to either the superficial or deep inguinal nodes. Lymphatic drainage from these structures very rarely goes to the external iliac lymph node complex. Metastatic disease in distant sites such as the liver, lungs, and bones is a late sign of advanced disease and has a dismal prognosis.[102] Fortunately, fewer than 5% of patients have evidence of distant metastases at diagnosis.[103,104] The variability of the lymphatic drainage accounts for a false-negative rate of 25% with the sentinel lymph node biopsy, but skip metastases do not occur within the superficial lymphatic drainage.

CLINICAL PRESENTATION AND DIFFERENTIAL DIAGNOSIS

Penile carcinomas may vary in presentation from the innocuous-appearing induration (Fig. 88-3) with slight erythema to the obviously malignant fungating penile tumor that leads to autoamputation (Fig. 88-4). Pruritus of the prepuce or a burning sensation may be an early

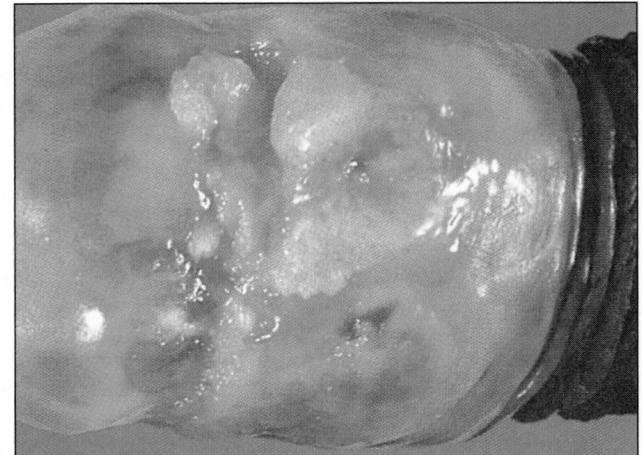

A

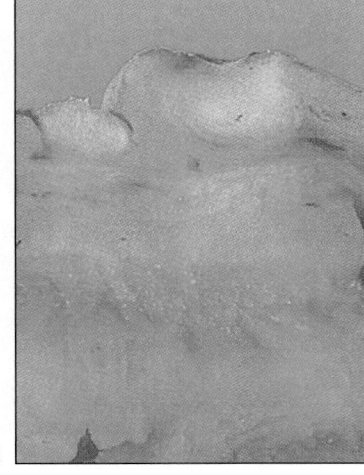

B

Figure 88-4. Squamous cell carcinoma. **A,** This resection specimen shows a small lesion arising in the coronal sulcus. **B,** Cut sections from the specimen demonstrated two small nodules of invasive tumor.

symptom of this tumor, and careful inspection may reveal a lesion on the prepuce or glans. This small ulceration may then progress to a papule or mass, which can be found in nearly half of cases. Phimosis may make early identification of these lesions difficult if not impossible, and patients often delay evaluation by a physician for an average of 1 year as a result.[105] A chronic malodorous discharge will often drain from under the prepuce, and further delay leads to bleeding from invasion as well as urethrocutaneous fistula.[25]

Nearly 60% of patients will have palpable inguinal lymph nodes, and many of these patients have concomitant infections that may be responsible for the inflammation of the inguinal nodes. This adenopathy may subside with appropriate antibiotic treatment. One in five patients also will have microscopic nodal metastasis.[102]

The differential diagnosis of a penile lesion includes sexually transmitted diseases such as the chancre of syphilis and chancroid. Benign lesions such as cutaneous horn, herpes virus, and condyloma acuminata also must be considered. In addition, the multitude of premalignant and malignant lesions noted in the previous section is among the diagnostic possibilities of a penile lesion.

STAGING AND PROGNOSIS

Although many historical staging systems have been used, current staging of penile carcinoma follows the American Joint Committee on Cancer (AJCC) system that incorporates tumor invasion, local node involvement, and the presence of distant metastases (TNM) to stratify patients based on prognosis[106] (Table 88-1). SCCs of the penis are graded by using the Broder scale to quantify the degree of tumor cell differentiation (Table 88-2). Half of all lesions are either grade I or II at initial diagnosis.

The importance of physical examination with a suspected penile malignancy cannot be overstated and requires a thorough evaluation. Physical findings such as the size and location of the tumor as well as the possibility of corporal involvement and palpable inguinal lymphadenopathy affect the ensuing treatment algorithm. The overall sensitivity and specificity of a careful physical examination of the inguinal region is poor,[107,108] and inflammatory changes may mimic tumor invasion of the corpora; magnetic resonance imaging (MRI) may improve detection of corporal tumor invasion.[109]

Clinical suspicion of penile malignancy and information gleaned from physical examination must be confirmed by histology. Aids for detection include tissue cultures and special stains to exclude infectious etiologies. Small lesions confined to the glans or foreskin can be sampled through circumcision or excisional biopsy, whereas in large lesions, biopsies are often performed at the time of definitive treatment, and initial diagnosis is made with frozen-section histology.

The management of inguinal lymphadenopathy has been controversial because of the morbidity of the lymph node dissection and the significant percentage of patients who do not have metastatic disease. Some investigators have proposed cytologic aspiration or computed tomo-

graphy (CT)-guided biopsy of suggestive nodes to aid in the decision to excise lymph nodes. Ultrasound guidance for needle aspiration of lymph nodes also can be performed, citing the ability of good ultrasonographers to show reliably the changes in nodal architecture such as hypoechogenicity or heterogeneity that suggest the presence of malignancy.[108] However, the considerable false-negative rate with aspiration cytology limits the clinical utility of this procedure.[110,111] As noted previously, the lack of predictable lymph drainage patterns also has limited the clinical application of sentinel lymph node biopsy for penile malignancy.[112]

TABLE 88-1

American Joint Committee Staging System for Penile Carcinoma (TNM Classification)

CLASSIFICATION	DESCRIPTION
Tumor	
TX	Primary tumor cannot be assessed
T0	No primary tumor
Tis	Carcinoma in situ
Ta	Noninvasive verrucous carcinoma
T1	Tumor invades subepithelial connective tissue
T2	Tumor invades corpus cavernosum or spongiosum
T3	Tumor invades urethra or prostate
T4	Tumor invades other adjacent structures
Node	
NX	Regional nodes cannot be assessed
N0	No regional lymph node metastases
N1	Metastasis in a single superficial inguinal node
N2	Metastasis in multiple or bilateral superficial inguinal nodes
N3	Metastasis in deep inguinal or pelvic lymph nodes; unilateral or bilateral
Metastasis	
MX	Distant metastases cannot be assessed
M0	No distant metastases
M1	Distant metastases

TABLE 88-2

Broaders Classification for Grading of Squamous Cell Carcinoma

GRADE	HISTOLOGIC FEATURES
I	Cells well differentiated with keratinization
	Prominent intercellular bridges
	Keratin pearls
II–III	Increased mitotic activity
	Fewer keratin pearls
IV	Marked nuclear pleomorphism
	Many mitoses
	Necrosis
	Lymphatic and perineural invasion
	Absence of keratin pearls
	Deeply invasive

From Lucia MS, Miller GJ: Histopathology of malignant lesions of the penis. Urol Clin North Am 1992;19:227.

IMAGING MODALITIES IN PENILE CARCINOMA

Many different imaging modalities have been used in the diagnosis and treatment of penile carcinoma, but none is widely accepted. Most often the best evaluation is a physical examination to determine the extent of the primary tumor. However, in the evaluation of the inguinal nodal packets, accurate imaging could potentially be useful because of the confounding lymphadenitis that is so common at the time of diagnosis. Computed tomography (CT) and magnetic resonance imaging (MRI) do not currently distinguish between the etiologies of the clinical lymphadenopathy. Nevertheless, these modalities may be helpful in assessing pelvic lymphadenopathy. Lymphoscintigraphy is currently experimental, and the anatomic variations of penile lymphatic drainage have resulted in unacceptably high false-negative rates for sentinel-node biopsy techniques. Ultrasound has been reported to distinguish between lymphadenopathy due to inflammation or infection and that caused by metastases. The ultrastructural changes caused by metastatic malignancy may be identifiable by exceedingly skilled ultrasonographers and radiologists; however, these techniques are not widely practiced and consequently have not been reliably reproduced at other centers. Certainly the most promising imaging for penile carcinoma appears to be ultrasound, and the most valuable information is gained from real-time rather than static images, but results are often operator dependent. Ultimately, imaging techniques currently contribute modestly to the initial evaluation of penile carcinoma, but several modalities hold promise for more accurate diagnosis in the future as technical advances are made.

Conservative approaches for the management of inguinal nodes have unacceptably high risks. The window of curability is evidenced by the fact that only 5% of patients with proven nodal metastases who are treated conservatively are still alive after 3 years, and patients with node-negative disease have a 77% 5-year survival rate.[113,114] The most important prognostic factor predicting nodal involvement is the depth of invasion of the primary tumor. Superficial disease, with T1 lesions, has a very low rate of metastases to the inguinal region. This is not true for penile carcinoma that has invaded Buck's fascia and involves the corpora; nearly half of patients with T2 disease will have histologically positive lymph nodes, and the percentage increases with increasing stage, so that more than two thirds of patients with T4 disease have nodal metastasis.[115]

Extent of nodal involvement also has prognostic significance because 5-year survival decreases in conjunction with increasing numbers of involved lymph nodes. Patients without nodal involvement have an excellent 5-year survival rate of 95%, but only 81% of those with up to three positive nodes will be alive after the same period. Patients with more than three malignant lymph nodes have a 50% mortality, and no patients with pelvic disease are alive at 5 years.[116] A meta-analysis of several series confirms these findings, with a 93% 5-year and 84% 10-year survival for node-negative patients, but only 62% to 65% survival for N1 and N2 patients over the same time span.[117]

Undoubtedly the most reliable method for determining regional node status is the inguinal lymphadenectomy. As noted previously, this invasive procedure is not without significant morbidity.[116,118,119] Consequently, efforts are being made to identify other methods of determining who will benefit most from the procedure to limit unnecessary morbidity. Some investigators have suggested that combining the tumor grade with the TNM staging provides better estimation of those at risk for nodal metastases.[115,120]

PRIMARY TREATMENT

Historically, the foundation of therapy for penile carcinoma has been surgical excision of both the primary tumor and regional lymph nodes. The impact of damage to or loss of the organ men closely associate with their standard of masculinity, as well as associated features such as the inability to stand while urinating, can be psychologically traumatic. Consequently, these patients must be counseled before surgery to minimize negative emotional and psychological reaction after surgery.[121] Furthermore, if medically feasible, attempts to incorporate into therapy the organ-preserving techniques such as Mohs micrographic surgery or laser ablation should be considered. Ongoing research to develop less-disfiguring treatments are being investigated to maintain or improve outcomes while minimizing the need for complete penile reconstruction.

Treatment of the Penile Tumor

Circumcision is an excellent form of therapy for small Tis or T1 lesions limited to the prepuce; intraoperative use of frozen-section pathology to determine negative surgical margins is critical to ensure an optimal result. When the malignancy is located on the glans or penile shaft, nonextirpative therapies should be explored in an effort to provide excellent opportunity for a cure without severe disfigurement. 5-FU also has been applied as a topical chemotherapy in the treatment of CIS of the penis with acceptable results.[122] Limitations include poor patient compliance due to the long course of therapy (3 to 7 weeks) and local skin irritation. The gold standard for these lesions is partial penectomy; with negative margins, the recurrence rate for this procedure is from none to 8%.[123,124] Other surgical techniques include limited local excision and Mohs' micrographic surgery. The former has an unacceptably high recurrence rate and should not be considered a viable treatment option.[114,123,124] Mohs' micrographic surgery requires microscopic inspection of surgical margins to enable complete excision of the lesion, and initial studies report an 80% cure rate at 5 years. This technique has be used in conjunction with other therapies to treat patients who refuse penectomy, with good results.[125] The complication rate for this therapy is very low.[126] This technique, however, typically requires multiple procedures and specially trained surgical staff.[127,128]

TREATMENT ALGORITHM FOR PENILE CARCINOMA

The treatment schematic for penile carcinoma begins with the initial assessment of the patient and the tumor itself. The initial arms of the treatment algorithm (see later discussion) depend on the method of obtaining a pathologic diagnosis; small lesions are likely to be completely excised, whereas large fungating tumors may undergo incisional biopsy to confirm the diagnosis. Once penile carcinoma has been established, the controversial questions then arise: For low-stage, small lesions (i.e., T1 and T2), is inguinal lymphadenectomy indicated and, if so, when? For high-stage lesions, do chemotherapy and/or radiation improve prognosis and surgical efficacy, and when should they be administered? Observation is appropriate for patients with small grade 1 lesions and clinically negative lymph nodes. For T1 and small T2 lesions with clinically negative inguinal nodes, higher-grade lesions may dictate the necessity for inguinal lymph node dissection. Between 20% and 80% of patients will have clinically negative nodes and pathologic evidence of metastatic disease; those patients with grade 2 or 3 tumors should undergo a superficial inguinal lymph node dissection. All patients with bulky T2 and any T3 to 4 tumor should undergo superficial lymph node dissection. Subsequent pelvic node dissection should be performed if more than two superficial nodes are identified. Pelvic lymphadenectomy is for staging purposes only; positive pelvic nodal status is not associated with any long-term survival in the literature.

Surgical Therapy in Advanced Penile Cancer

If the primary tumor is large enough to have infiltrated 75% of the penile shaft, it is unlikely that the required 2-cm margin will be achieved while leaving adequate penile length to urinate with sufficient hygiene. In such cases, a total penectomy or complete corporal body resection with a perineal urethrostomy is indicated. More-aggressive tumors that appear to invade the surrounding bony structures mandate local bone resection in addition to penectomy and perineal diversion.

The typical patient with advanced penile malignancy will often have associated infections that must be addressed as well as a lymph node beds that will require staging. Evaluation of the nodal involvement allows more accurate stratification of those patients whose malignancy is likely to recur with conventional therapy. Biopsies of bulky pelvic nodes can be performed with CT or ultrasound guidance or with open incisional techniques to confirm that radiographically abnormal nodes demonstrate malignant dissemination. The literature does not support any suggestion that pelvic lymphadenectomy is curative, but the pathological information from the dissection allows precise staging and identifies those patients who may benefit from adjuvant treatments. Given the dismal long-term survival for patients with known pelvic nodal metastases, experimental protocols that include combinations of chemotherapy and radiation are advisable in this high-risk cohort.

Superficial Inguinal Lymphadenectomy

Patients with T2 to T4 disease and clinically negative or minimally palpable inguinal nodes should undergo a modified superficial inguinal lymphadenectomy (ILND). Frozen-section pathology is a critical intraoperative tool to identify patients who need more extensive nodal excision. Several retrospective reviews have shown that the incidence of noncontiguous or "skip" metastases is almost negligible when fewer than two involved nodes are found in the superficial lymph node bed.[129-133] Consequently, if more than two lymph nodes are found to be involved with metastatic disease on frozen section, the lymph node dissection must be expanded to include the deeper lymph node chains as well. In addition, patients with T1 penile malignancy but poorly differentiated histology should be offered superficial ILND, given the higher incidence of nodal metastasis among patients with poorly differentiated primary tumors. Some controversy exists regarding the timing of ILND, but some data suggest a benefit to early intervention.[105] McDougal and colleagues[114] reported a 5-year survival rate of 83% in patients with clinically negative but pathologically malignant inguinal lymph nodes who underwent early lymphadenectomy, compared with only 43% of the patients who underwent delayed lymphadenectomy after initial surveillance.

Technical considerations for superficial ILND include preservation of the areolar adipose layer superficial to Scarpa's fascia, which decreases the likelihood of flap necrosis and epidermolysis; also, sparing the saphenous vein preserves lymphatic drainage. Anatomic boundaries of dissection are confined anteriorly by Scarpa's fascia and posteriorly by the fascia lata; the superior-inferior limits are from 2 cm cephalad to 10 cm caudad to the inguinal ligament. Careful adherence to proper surgical guidelines for superficial ILND are important because many series have demonstrated that this procedure also is an effective treatment for limited node metastases.[134-137] Furthermore, the modified superficial ILND appears to have refined the ILND, with resultant decrease in morbidity. The primary postoperative complication that results in debilitating morbidity is severe leg edema, which can occur in up to half of patients, with more than 30% having leg edema that is classified as severe.[137] However, modified dissection techniques have been developed, and more recent series have seen the overall percentage of patients with this complication decrease to fewer than 25%.[138-143] In some patients, the newfound pedal edema is self-limited, resolving within 6 months after treatment with support stockings. Morbidity from superficial lymph node excision also is commonly caused by wound seromas and infections, venous thromboembolism, and skin-flap necrosis.

Radical Inguinal Lymph Node Dissection

This procedure is currently performed essentially as it was originally described by Daseler and colleagues in 1948.[144] The limits of this dissection are from the sartorius muscle to the adductor longus in a lateral-to-medial direction, and from the inguinal ligament inferior to the apex of the femoral triangle. The initial incision of this dissection is through the tensor fascia lata over the adductor longus, with ligation of the greater saphenous vein and carried

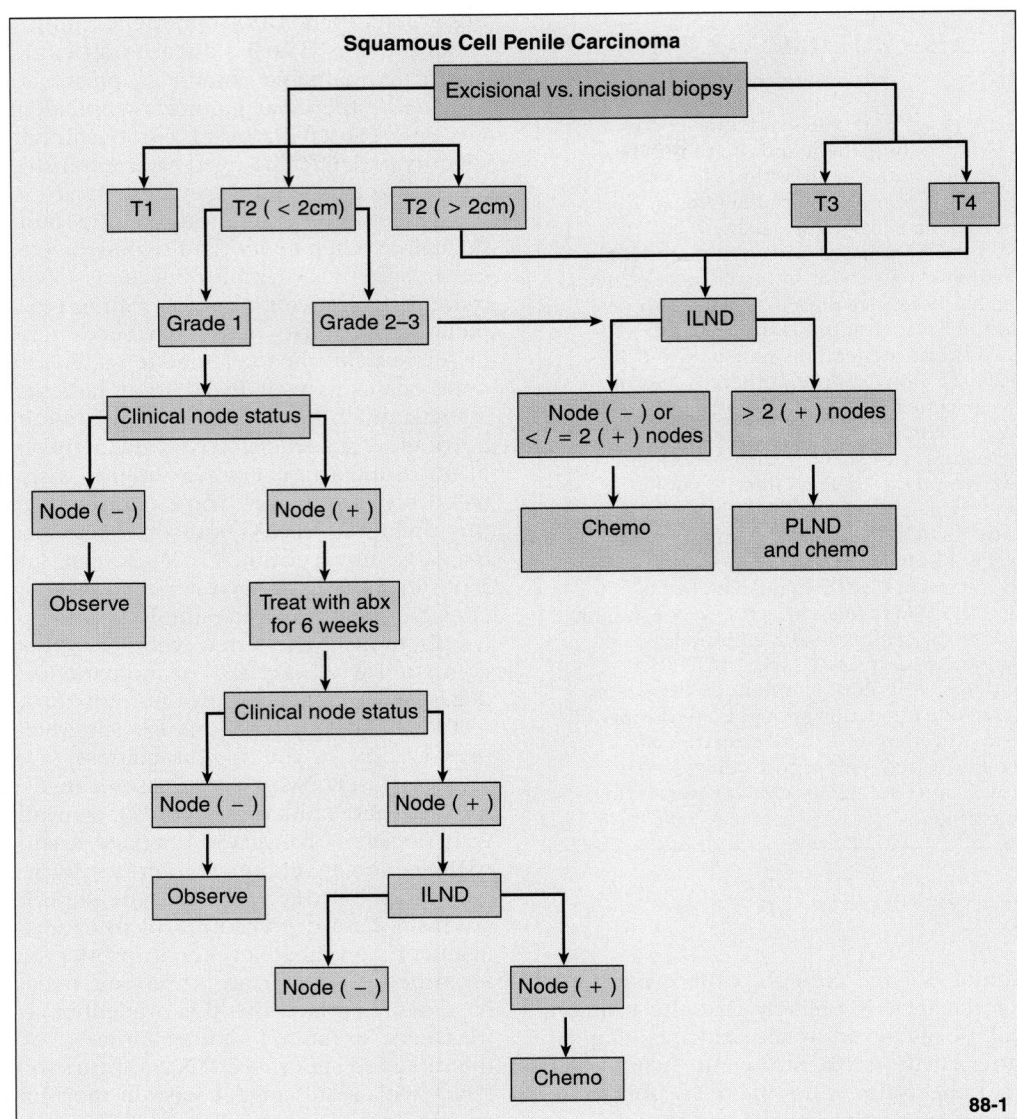

Squamous Cell Penile Carcinoma

Excisional vs. incisional biopsy

T1 — T2 (< 2cm) — T2 (> 2cm) — T3 — T4

Grade 1 — Grade 2–3 → ILND

Clinical node status

Node (−) → Observe

Node (+) → Treat with abx for 6 weeks

Clinical node status

Node (−) → Observe

Node (+) → ILND

Node (−)

Node (+) → Chemo

Node (−) or < / = 2 (+) nodes → Chemo

> 2 (+) nodes → PLND and chemo

88-1

medially to the border of the sartorius muscle. A requirement for the deep nodal dissection includes incision of the femoral vascular sheath to excise the extensive lymphatic networks that completely encase these vessels.

Reconstructive options to cover the exposed femoral vessels include rotation of a sartorius muscle flap, as previously mentioned. This procedure involves dissecting the sartorius tendon from the anterior superior iliac spine and suturing it to the inguinal ligament over the femoral vessels. Ulcerated and matted nodes often result in wide excision of the overlying skin with at least a 3-cm margin; rotated myocutaneous gracilis, rectus abdominis, or tensor fascia lata flaps can be used to augment coverage and assist healing. Local control of these advanced lymph nodes is critical because progression of the disease can lead to vascular erosion and hemorrhage. Surgical treatment often requires careful dissection and control of the femoral vessels; advanced and erosive disease may mandate resection of part or all of the femoral vein wall, as well as venous thrombectomy.

Pelvic Lymphadenectomy

This procedure may be done simultaneous with a superficial ILND or as a staged procedure; this dissection also has been performed laparoscopically.[145] This procedure excises the nodal chains from the common iliac vessels down to the internal and external perivascular iliac nodes and from the lateral pelvic side wall to the bladder medially. The posterior limit of dissection is the obdurator nerve. To date, pelvic lymphadenectomy has value only as a staging procedure, because the survival of patients with pelvic lymph node dissection is less than 5% 5-year survival.[146,147]

Chemotherapy for Advanced Penile Carcinoma

Single-Agent Therapy

Historically, chemotherapeutic agents have been applied in the treatment of advanced penile carcinoma in combination with surgical and/or radiation therapies. The most commonly used agents that have proven cytotoxic effects in penile carcinoma are bleomycin, methotrexate, and cisplatin. These drugs have been reported in several combinations in small series with variable doses and medication schedules. As single-agent chemotherapy, these medications have produced only modest results, with response rates of 10% to 15% (Table 88-3).[148-151] The vast majority of patients who showed any regression of disease had a partial response; in the report on methotrexate activity by Sklaroff and Yagoda,[149] the median duration of remission in partial responders was 3 months. However, two patients had durable responses that lasted more than 12 months. Investigation into cisplatin yielded similar results, with the duration of partial response a mere 1 to 3 months and a median survival of only 5 months.[151]

Combination Chemotherapy

The intent of combination chemotherapeutic regimens is to optimize cytotoxicity while increasing the range of activity of treatment and reducing the probability of inducing tumor drug resistance. In a small series, an 80% response rate with 40% complete response was achieved in five patients treated with cisplatin and 5-FU before lymphadenectomy.[152] Another small series had similar success with one complete response and five partial responses in six patients who subsequently underwent surgical or radiation treatments.[153] In this series, all six patients eventually had progression of their disease, but median time to progression was 1 year, and median survival was 16 months. However, a similar regimen with 5-FU and cisplatin resulted in only a 25% response rate

in eight patients.[154] The variability in outcomes may be a result of chance, given the small sample sizes in each study, or may be related to different modes of delivery of chemotherapeutic medicines or patient selection. Nevertheless, these results suggest that this combination has significant activity in the treatment of penile SCC despite the lack of a durable response.

Another trial of combination chemotherapy with cisplatin, bleomycin, and methotrexate resulted in a 72% response rate in 10 of 14 patients, with the vast majority having a partial response.[155] Patients underwent leuovorin rescue after treatment with methotrexate. The average duration of response was nearly 6 months, and one patient continued to be disease free at 2 years. In this study, a small percentage of patients received the bleomycin and cisplatin through locoregional infusion into pelvic arteries. In addition, Huang and coworkers[156] reported three of three responders with exclusively intra-arterial administration of all three agents. Reported toxicities were similar to those seen with single-agent treatment with these agents.

These results led to a larger multiinstitutional prospective study of methotrexate/bleomycin/cisplatin combination therapy in 45 patients by the Southwest Oncology Group (SWOG).[157] These investigators were able to achieve a 32.5% response rate, with 5 of 13 responders showing a complete response. However, this regimen also resulted in five patient deaths and grade 4 toxicities in more than 30% of participants. In addition, other adverse reactions included gastrointestinal complaints in 73%, hematologic complications in 60%, and mucosal toxicity in 31%.[157] The unacceptable level of toxicity prevented further clinical trials of this regimen.

TABLE 88-3

Selected Reports of Chemotherapy for Penile Cancer

DRUG AND REGIMEN	NO. OF PATIENTS	PERCENT RESPONSE (NO)	REFERENCE
Bleomycin			
3–20 mg/m^2/day continuous infusion or 10–30 mg/m^2 qd or qwk boluses	14	21% (4)	Ahmed, et al.[148]
Methotrexate			
Various treatment schedules or 250 mg/m^2 q2–4wk or 30–40 mg/m^2 qwk	8	38% (3)	Sklaroff, Yagoda[149]
	13	61% (8)	
Cisplatin			
70 or 120 mg/m^2 q21d or 50 mg/m^2 on day 1 and 8 q28d	14	21% (3)	Ahmed, et al.[150]
	26	15% (4)	
Cisplatin, Methotrexate, and Bleomycin			
75 mg/m^2 IV, 25 mg/m^2 × 2 doses, and 10 μ/m^2 × 2 doses	40	32.5% (13)	Haas, et al.[157]
Cisplatin and Interferon-α-2B			
20 mg/m^2 and 5 × 10^6 mU/m^2 IV qd × 5 d	12	75% (9)	Mitropoulos, Dimopoulos MA, et al.[160]
13-Cis-Retinoic Acid and Interferon-α-2a			
1 mg/kg PO qd × 8 wk and 3 mU/day SQ × 8 wk	16	6% (1)	Skeel, et al.*

*Skeel RT, Huang J, Manola J, et al: A phase II study of 13-cis-retinoic acid plus interferon alpha-2a in advanced stage penile carcinoma: An Eastern Cooperative Oncology Group Study (E3893). Cancer Invest 2003;21:41–46.

The combination of vincristine, bleomycin, and methotrexate was investigated in patients with advanced penile malignancy, and a 53.8% response rate was reported.[158] In 13 patients with bulky inguinal metastases that were deemed unresectable before chemotherapy, 5 had sufficient response to undergo postchemotherapy radical excision. Two of the 5 had long-term disease-free survival longer than 5 years. Toxicities were less severe than those with other regimens, with fever, cutaneous hyperpigmentation, and pulmonary fibrosis reported.

The activity of chemotherapeutic agents in treatment of advanced penile carcinoma indicates that combination chemotherapy should contribute to multimodality approaches in the management of penile carcinoma. As with chemotherapeutic investigations of other malignancies, identification of active combinations while minimizing toxicity remains the objective. More-intensive efforts must be made to refine combination chemotherapies for penile SCC.

Chemotherapy with Surgery

No large studies of preoperative chemotherapy in penile cancer patients exist, but reports of patients who have received chemotherapy before surgical treatment can be gleaned from the published literature on chemotherapy for advanced disease. In the published series on cisplatin-based chemotherapy, 40 patients with fixed inguinal nodes received chemotherapy and then subsequently underwent excisional surgery.[153-155,158-160] More than 70% of patients from these series showed some response to chemotherapy, with 32% demonstrating a durable response, and the treatment allowed complete resection of tumor in 15. Thirteen of these patients had long-term survival in excess of 12 months and as long as 10 years. Another study in 27 patients with T1 lesions resulted in 85% penile preservation after treatment with vinblastine, bleomycin, and methotrexate followed by surgical excision or ablation with CO_2 laser. Furthermore, 44% of those treated had no pathologic evidence of disease, and an additional 34% had partial response to this combination therapy.

In another small series, Pizzocaro and Piva[161] treated 12 patients with a postoperative adjuvant chemotherapy regimen consisting of vinblastine, methotrexate, and bleomycin. Only 1 of these 12 patients relapsed during median follow-up of 42 months. In addition, 5 patients with unresectable bulky inguinal disease were treated with this chemotherapeutic regimen. Subsequently, 3 patients who exhibited a partial response underwent radical lymphadenectomy and continued to be disease free at 20 to 72 months after surgery. Two minimal responders could not have radical surgery, and they died of the disease within 1 year. Encouraged by these findings, the same group then reported on 26 patients who had fixed inguinal nodes; 10 of these were treated with radiotherapy, with or without chemotherapy, and 16 received neoadjuvant chemotherapy. Radiotherapy resulted in only 1 patient who could later have lymphadenectomy, and all of these patients died of their disease within 3 years. In dramatic contrast, 9 (56%) of those who were treated with neoadjuvant chemotherapy responded sufficiently to have subsequent node excision, and 5 (31%) were found to be disease free on 5-year follow-up.[162]

Since then, Roth and associates[163] designed a more extensive adjuvant chemotherapeutic regimen including 5-FU, cisplatin, mitomycin, bleomycin, and methotrexate and treated eight patients with penile carcinoma, who received eight intra-arterial infusions over a 48-hour period. All but one patient had previous resection of disease with pathologic confirmation of nodal involvement or were found to have recurrence in the inguinal region on follow-up. Three patients had complete response, and three had partial response, with one demonstrating stable disease. Two of three patients with complete response had long-term disease-free survival for more than 5 years.

Clearly the use of chemotherapeutic regimens to enable patients with bulky nodal disease to undergo surgical resection or as an adjuvant after lymphadenectomy has been effective in some patients. Combining these small reports reveals that of the 83 patients who have received neoadjuvant chemotherapy before surgical resection, more than 70% demonstrated a response, and 65% had sufficient tumor regression to allow subsequent radical excision. These data tend to be hidden within other reports because no large-scale prospective trials have been designed to assess optimal timing and regimens for the adjuvant chemotherapeutic treatment of penile SCC in conjunction with surgical excision. Given the rarity of this disease in many countries, compiling enough cases to perform such a study is certainly a daunting task, which emphasizes the need for multi-institutional international collaboration to determine the optimal therapy for advanced disease.

Radiation Therapy in Penile Cancer

An alternative to topical or extirpative therapy for penile cancer is radiation therapy via interstitial brachytherapy or external beam radiation. Radiation therapy has been reported in many series as a single-agent treatment for both primary penile tumors and metastatic lymph node disease.[103,116,164-170] Crook and colleagues[171] reported the use of interstitial brachytherapy for penile carcinoma with a 93% disease-free rate for T1 and T2 lesions and a 100% cure rate for patients with well-differentiated tumors. This treatment has been the therapy of choice for small clinically localized penile cancer in France, with a 74% penile conservation rate and only 11% local failure for tumors smaller than 2 cm.[171] The success rates from other reports has varied from 65% to 80% for these superficial lesions.[135,137,167,169,172-174] Furthermore, salvage surgery can be curative in cases of postradiation-therapy recurrence.

In more advanced penile malignancy, treatment with radiation therapy has an unacceptably high rate of tumor recurrence of between 20% and 40%.[167,173,175] Furthermore, radiotherapy for tumors larger than 4 cc often results in a nonfunctional penis or significant active residual disease; both outcomes defeat the purposes of organ-preserving therapy, which are to treat the disease adequately while maintaining function.[169,174] In choosing radiation treatment rather than surgical extirpation of the primary lesion, the patient must realize that the tumor may progress to lymph nodes or distant metastases despite treatment, thus precluding the opportunity for cure. The complete response rate for external beam radiotherapy has been reported as 56%, with local failure rate of 40%.[116,164] Fortunately, in some cases, postradiation excision of local recurrence can provide local control. However, complicating the clinical situation are the tissue changes in response to radiation treatment that often lead to necrosis, which has a clinical appearance similar to residual tumor and may result in severe impairment of organ function. Nevertheless, given the undeniable activity of radiation therapy in penile carcinoma, particularly in early-stage disease, this modality will undoubtedly continue to be an integral part of integrated organ-sparing therapy for penile cancer.

Radiation therapy for low-stage and low-grade penile malignancy provides an effective therapy that has excellent organ preservation and cosmesis without compromising cure rates. Salvage surgery can be curative in those patients who relapse after radiotherapy. The critical component for this modality is tumor volume; radiation should not be offered for those patients with bulky tumors larger than 4 cc because the response rate is poor, and the complication rate is high, yet for small low-grade tumors, radiation should be considered a first-line therapy.

Chemotherapy with Radiation

Several small series of combination chemotherapy and radiation regimens demonstrate response rates superior to those reported for radiation therapy alone.[176-178] Modig and colleagues[176] found similar survival rates between 19 patients treated with bleomycin and radiation and a similar cohort of patients who underwent surgery. Most efforts in organ-preserving therapy have involved bleomycin and radiation because bleomycin is a known radiosensitizer, and most treated patients have had relatively low-stage tumors. A series of 47 patients with penile carcinoma ranging from T1 to T3 disease were treated with bleomycin and 45 or 58 Gy of radiation for a period of 5 to 6 weeks with little overall toxicity. Results from the two arms of this study demonstrated 2 (18%) of 7 patients treated with 45 Gy required further tumor excision, whereas 4 (10%) of 40 patients who received 58 Gy subsequently underwent surgical salvage.[179] However, smaller studies do not support these findings; 10 patients treated with a similar dose of bleomycin and 60-Gy external-beam radiation administered in three equal doses resulted in one treatment-related death with moderate to severe toxicity in 8 patients. Worse, only 4 patients ultimately achieved organ preservation.[180]

Unquestionably, the published literature supports the notion that penile SCC is sensitive to chemotherapy. No conclusive data exist to suggest that one chemotherapeutic regimen is superior to the myriad combinations that have been investigated, yet many other agents other than bleomycin, 5-FU, methotrexate, and cisplatin have not been evaluated for activity in the treatment of penile malignancy. In addition, the significant toxicity of the commonly used therapy of bleomycin, methotrexate,

and cisplatin and the heretofore unknown side effect profiles of other chemotherapeutic combinations demand further investigation into other regimens that ultimately have superior outcomes in terms of morbidity as well as response rate and overall mortality. Consequently, SWOG has begun preliminary evaluation of docetaxel in hopes of identifying biologically active agents with better side effect profiles.

TREATMENT COMPLICATIONS

Although the psychological impact of the disfigurement after partial or radical penectomy is undeniable, the surgical complications of these procedures rarely deviate from common postoperative problems. Postoperative sequelae of superficial ILND are lymphedema, deep venous thrombosis, and wound complications; the estimated morbidity of this procedure including all complications is less than 20%. The incidence of skin-flap necrosis has decreased dramatically with newer surgical techniques.

As would be expected, complications of the deeper nodal excision are more severe and frequent than those encountered with the superficial and modified procedures. In addition to flap necrosis and wound infections, postoperative morbidity can be caused by lower extremity and scrotal edema, lymphocele, and lymphorrhea, as well as seroma and thrombophlebitis.[116,124,136,168,181-183] Despite improvements in surgical techniques that have decreased the severity and incidence of complications by almost 50%, postoperative morbidity after deep inguinal lymphadenectomy continues to be a significant clinical problem.[142,184]

Chemotherapeutic Complications

Dose-dependent side effects of bleomycin were pneumonitis and pulmonary fibrosis, with elevated risk with dosing of more than 400 units.[149] Patients undergoing treatment with methotrexate most frequently had mucositis as the primary adverse reaction; infrequent side effects of methotrexate were pneumonitis, hepatic insufficiency, myelosuppression, renal insufficiency, skin rashes, and sepsis.[149] The most debilitating effect of cisplatin single-agent treatment was nausea and vomiting, which should be reasonably well controlled with antiemetic medications.[151] Other significant toxicities of cisplatin therapy were nephrotoxicity, which led to cessation of treatment in 8% of patients, as well as ototoxicity, myelosuppression, and neuropathy.[151]

The documented complications of the chemotherapeutic combination regimen of methotrexate/bleomycin/cisplatin resulted in 11% treatment-related mortality, primarily due to pulmonary complications, with an additional 17% of patients experiencing life-threatening toxicity.

Radiation Complications

Complications from radiation treatment for penile malignancy can vary from relatively benign and exceedingly common telangiectasias and catarrhal reactions seen in more than 90% of patients to more troublesome urethral strictures in 20% to 35% and meatal stenosis in 15% to 30%.[103,165,170] Penile chordee also can be a potential problem after radiation therapy.

FOLLOW-UP

The post-treatment evaluation of patients with penile carcinoma must be vigilant, particularly for patients who have not undergone inguinal lymphadenectomy. These patients should be seen and a careful physical examination performed every 2 to 4 months after primary therapy for the first year. The risk of developing palpable inguinal nodes after excision of the primary lesion is greatest in the first 6 months after treatment. However, longer delays in the development of clinically palpable disease mandate careful extended follow-up. A patient who has undergone radical penectomy must be disease free for at least 24 months at our institution before consideration of penile reconstruction is entertained. The cornerstone of follow-up evaluation is the physical examination for all patients with a history of penile malignancy. In experienced hands, inguinal ultrasonography may suggest changes in lymph node architecture before disease is clinically palpable. CT of the pelvis can be of benefit in patients who have undergone inguinal lymphadenectomy.

ISSUES FOR THE FUTURE

The gold standard of therapy for penile carcinoma remains early detection with local tumor control, if feasible. Treatment guidelines based on pathologic stage are shown in Table 88-4. Patients at high risk for relapse

TABLE 88-4

Stage-Based Guidelines for Treatment of Penile Carcinoma

PENILE CANCER TREATMENT GUIDELINES

pT1, pT2	Partial penectomy, superficial ILND, frozen-section confirmation, deep ILND if frozen-section evaluation of superficial nodes is positive
pT3	Total penectomy, superficial and deep ILND
T4	Initial treatment with neoadjuvant chemotherapy followed by salvage lymphadenectomy if possible
N2-N3	Enroll in postoperative adjuvant chemotherapy or radiation treatments

ILND, inguinal lymphadenectomy.

should strongly consider neoadjuvant therapy. Currently the small numbers in the reported series and the different combinations and administrations investigated limit the ability to draw firm conclusions about multimodality therapy for penile carcinoma. However, the data do suggest that preoperative administration of chemotherapy that includes cisplatin will enable 40% of patients with locoregional dissemination of malignancy to proceed with surgical resection with good probability of negative margins and will result in long-term disease-free survival in up to 20%. Other combinations such as vinblastine, bleomycin, and methotrexate do not appear to achieve comparable response rates. Combinations of bleomycin and radiotherapy seem to hold promise for organ-preserving treatment in carefully selected subjects.

Coordinated programs designed to improve patient education will aid in early detection as well as increase prevention, with the implementation of appropriate hygiene. Future studies should involve underdeveloped nations where penile carcinoma is more prevalent to improve the power of these investigative efforts.

Daniel J. Culkin
Adam R. Metwalli

Urethral Carcinoma

SUMMARY OF KEY POINTS

INCIDENCE
Fewer than 15 cases per year have been reported in the literature on average.

ETIOLOGY/EPIDEMIOLOGY
- The average patient first seen with primary urethral carcinoma is between ages 50 and 70 years.
- Various proposed etiologies have included a history of venereal disease, urethral stricture disease, chronic irritation, viral infection, cystitis glandularis, and parturition.
- The prevalence of strictures in this group of patients has been estimated at between 24% and 76%.

PATHOLOGY/BIOLOGY
- Nearly 60% of male urethral carcinoma occurs in the bulbomembranous urethra, one third of tumors in the pendulous urethra, and 7% in the prostatic urethra.
- Nearly half of female urethral tumors occur in the distal urethra.
- Nearly 80% of urethral malignancies are SCC, less than 15% are transitional cell carcinoma (TCC), and fewer than 5% are adenocarcinoma.

CLINICAL FINDINGS
- The predominant symptoms of male urethral malignancy can easily be mistaken for those of far more common and benign entities such as lower tract infections (prostatitis, urethritis, cystitis).

- Priapism and impotence can be presenting symptoms.
- The predominant male complaint is bladder outlet obstructive symptoms, whereas dysuria and bleeding are the primary symptoms among female patients with urethral carcinoma.

DIFFERENTIAL DIAGNOSIS/STAGING
- Urethral carcinoma must be differentiated from urethral stricture disease, prostatitis, urethritis, cystitis, and TCC of the bladder.
- As has been done with virtually all other cancers, a TNM system has been developed for staging urethral carcinoma.
- The histologic grade of the tumor has no significant value in predicting long-term survival.
- An examination under anesthesia can improve the accuracy of clinical staging, and CT and MRI can improve localization of the tumor and determine the extent of local invasion as well as pelvic lymphadenopathy.

PRIMARY THERAPY
- Distal urethral carcinoma in male patients should be treated essentially the same as distal penile carcinoma, with a partial penectomy with a 2-cm margin.
- Although superficial disease can be treated with transurethral resection, a very high rate of recurrence

should be anticipated with this therapy.
- Patients with tumor larger than 4 cm and those who received only external-beam radiation fared significantly worse than patients with smaller tumor bulk and recipients of brachytherapy.
- For high-stage urethral neoplasm, combination therapy involving chemotherapy, surgery, and radiation results in superior local control of disease with improved quality of life compared with surgical monotherapy.

SALVAGE THERAPY
- Distant metastatic disease from urethral carcinoma is treated with a multimodality approach that includes radiation, chemotherapy, and palliative surgery when indicated.
- Isolated metastases that cause significant pain can be treated with focal irradiation to relieve symptoms.

PROGNOSIS
- The most critical prognostic factors are the clinical stage at the time of diagnosis and the location of the primary tumor.
- The histologic grade of the tumor has no significant value in predicting long-term survival.
- Even with inguinal node metastases, long-term survival up to 5 years can be achieved when patients are rendered disease free.

INTRODUCTION

Urethral cancer is rare and is the only genitourinary malignancy that is diagnosed more frequently in women than in men. Since its identification and classification in the late 17th century by Thiaudierre, fewer than 15 cases per year have been reported. Because of this rare presentation, no large-scale series have been reported, and consensus therapeutic guidelines are lacking. Consequently, some investigators have called for standardization of management strategies so that series from different institutions can be compared more effectively.[185] For the most part, the obvious morphologic differences between the male and female urethras mandate that these be addressed as separate entities in this text.

ETIOLOGY AND EPIDEMIOLOGY

Although the average patient first seen with primary urethral carcinoma is between ages 50 and 70 years and tends to have poor long-term survival because the disease has disseminated at the time of diagnosis, it has been seen in children as young as 13 years as well as in the extremely elderly.[186,187] The etiology of urethral carcinoma is unknown. The proposed etiologies include venereal disease, urethral stricture disease, chronic irritation, viral infection, cystitis glandularis, coitus, and parturition.[188-194] Little or no evidence can be identified to verify these as "causes" for urethral carcinoma. Even though urethral stricture disease has been associated with 24% to 76% of urethral cancers, causality has not been proven.[188,195] Although about half have a history of venereal disease, no evidence supports that this contributes to the development of urethral carcinoma.[188,190] In addition, investigators have shown the presence of HPV strain 16 in SCCs of the urethra, which supports the notion that a history of sexually transmitted disease directly correlates with development of urethral carcinoma.[196,197]

ANATOMY

Male Urethra

The male urethra is divided into five distinct segments: prostatic, membranous, bulbous, pendulous or penile, and the fossa navicularis. The histologic characteristics of the urethra change from the prostatic urethra to the distal aspect of the urethra. The urothelium found in the prostatic urethra is the same as that found in the bladder with a transitional cell epithelium. The bulbar and pendulous urothelium is a pseudostratified columnar cell layer, whereas the fossa navicularis and meatus have a stratified squamous epithelium. What is described as the anterior urethra includes the fossa navicularis and the pendulous urethra. These portions of the urethra have the same lymphatic drainage as the glans and corpus spongiosum: the superficial and deep inguinal lymph nodes. The posterior urethra is composed of the bulbomembranous and prostatic segments of the urethra and drain into pelvic lymph nodes along the iliac and obturator lymphatics.[198,199]

Female Urethra

Given the significantly shorter length of the female urethra, only two histologic urothelial types are seen. The proximal portion is transitional epithelium; the distal 70% of the female urethra is stratified squamous epithelium. The lymphatic drainage is identical to that found in a male patient, despite the different histologic composition of the organ.[198,199]

PATHOLOGY AND NATURAL HISTORY

An organization of urethral carcinoma based on location of the tumor in male patients is often used. Nearly 60% of male urethral carcinoma occurs in the bulbomembranous urethra; one third of tumors originate in the pendulous urethra, whereas fewer than 10% of these malignancies are seen in the prostatic urethra.[200] The histologic types of

carcinoma also vary with location. Like penile malignancy, the vast majority of urethral malignancies are SCCs, fewer than one of four is transitional cell carcinoma (TCC), and fewer than 5% of urethral malignancies are adenocarcinomas.[200] Other histologic malignancies have been reported as primary urethral neoplasms, including melanoma, biologically active neuroendocrine carcinoid tumors, and sarcoma.[79,201-204]

Metastatic disease to the urethra has been reported; most cases are from advanced prostatic carcinoma.[205] Two cases each of renal cell carcinoma and Wilms' tumor metastasizing to the urethra have been reported, one of the former occurring 5 years after radical nephrectomy.[206-209]

Nearly half of urethral tumors occur in the distal female urethra. Although only 30% of the female urethra is squamous cell epithelium, almost 75% of tumors are SCCs. Adenocarcinoma and TCC compose nearly equal parts of the remaining 25% of these carcinomas.[197,210,211]

SCC in the urethra has focal keratinization and most often demonstrates good or moderate degrees of differentiation. The gross appearance of the malignancy is typically exophytic; however, advanced disease often has necrotic areas or obvious infiltration. Anaplastic or pleomorphic cellular features are sometimes present.[212] Others have reported multiple chromosomal abnormalities, although none correlates with those seen in TCC (alterations of chromosomes 9 and 17).[213] Furthermore, previously cited studies suggest an etiologic link between HPV 16 and SCC of the urethra.[196,197]

TCC of the urethra can occur at any point, but this histology is most common in the posterior portion of the urethra. The tumor histology of TCC of the urethra and of the bladder is similar; as such, these lesions can appear as papillary, infiltrative, or CIS. TCC of the posterior urethra is most often associated with concomitant TCC of the bladder.[214] Thus it is imperative to examine the bladder carefully when primary urethral TCC is initially diagnosed.

The etiology of urethral adenocarcinoma is theorized to be due to the malignant degeneration of the periurethral glandular elements, such as Cowper's glands.[214] This occurs in the bulbomembranous urethra and demonstrates anaplastic cells lining irregular glandular elements with significant mucin production. Some investigators have used different histologic stains to identify the tissue of origin for urethral adenocarcinoma. These efforts revealed that the multiple histologies and variable staining of these tumors indicate that urethral adenocarcinoma does not arise from a single periurethral tissue source, as some have previously suggested.

For example, four cases of signet-ring cell carcinoma, an unusual histologic variant of urethral adenocarcinoma, have been reported as a primary urethral malignancy; two of these stained strongly for carcinoembryonic antigen (CEA).[215] Furthermore, Murphy and colleagues[216] demonstrated that columnar/mucinous adenocarcinoma of the urethra reacts positively with antibodies to colonic epithelium, suggesting glandular origin of these cells. Baldi and associates[217] showed similar immunohistochemical and histologic staining patterns between urethral and colon adenocarcinomas. In other reports, this type of histology stained strongly for cytokeratins 7 and 20 and negative for prostate-specific antigen (PSA), suggesting an association with urethritis glandularis.[218] However, a cribriform histology did not stain for the same antibody but did demonstrate the presence of PSA.[216] An interesting study may have identified clues that help clarify the etiologic significance of these variable histologic markers; apparently paraurethral duct cells near the urethra strongly express CEA, whereas cells in the distal portions of the duct are positive for PSA and prostatic acid phosphatase (PAP),[219] yet, some urethral tumors arise from other tissue origins; clear cell variants in several of these studies were negative for both CEA and PSA.[216,220] Other reports suggest that the clear cell variant derives from nephrogenic metaplasia or müllerian duct remnants.[221-223] Prostatic adenocarcinomas can be found in the prostatic urethras of male patients, and similar-appearing tumors arise occasionally from the urethral meatus in women.[214] These tumors have been found to stain strongly for PSA and PAP in both men and women. Urethral diverticula occasionally develop aggressive clear cell adenocarcinomas, which have a tubuloacinar appearance similar to that of renal cell carcinoma. This tumor tends to metastasize early and has poor long-term survival rates as a result.[214]

The progression of urethral malignancies is from lymphatic, to vascular, and to local tissue invasion. SCCs tend to exhibit more aggressive local extension compared with transitional cell neoplasms, with rapid infiltration into the corpora and ultimately through the cutaneous layers. These tumors also grow along the length of the urethra and will extend through the genitourinary diaphragm to the bladder and rectum.[212] Given the predictable lymphatic drainage of the urethra, lymphatic metastases from the anterior urethra migrate first into the inguinal nodes, whereas posterior urethral tumors spread to the pelvic nodal chains. Whereas extensive local invasion and node metastases are common at presentation, distant metastatic disease to the liver, brain, and bones is seen in only 15% of patients.[224]

CLINICAL MANIFESTATIONS

The typical symptoms of urethral malignancy can easily be mistaken for those of far more common and benign entities such as lower tract infections (prostatitis, urethritis, cystitis) and stricture disease. Consequently, a very high index of suspicion is required to identify this disease. Common symptoms include urethral obstruction or palpable mass, discharge, and bleeding. Although unusual, priapism and impotence also have been reported as a presenting symptoms.[225,226] Identification of a periurethral abscess or fistula in an elderly patient warrants consideration of a possible malignant etiology in the absence of obvious causes. Approximately half of male patients with urethral tumors have obstructive symptoms, whereas most women complain of dysuria and bleeding.[211,227,228] Male patients will often exhibit noticeable symptoms earlier if the lesion arises in the distal urethra; lesions in the posterior urethra tend to be more insidious and typically are seen after a long delay.

Multiple courses of antibiotics for suspected infections or repeated interventions for stricture disease are common and contribute to the average delay of 5 to 6 months between onset of symptoms and diagnosis.[188,190] Consequently, 20% of patients will have nodal metastases at presentation, and another 15% will subsequently progress to metastatic disease during evaluation.[229]

LABORATORY AND IMAGING STUDIES

Primary Urethral Carcinoma

Women with distal urethral malignancy will often have a visible mass at the urethral meatus; in male patients, visible tumors are rare, but a palpable mass may be noted. Consequently, a thorough examination of the external genitalia and perineum is imperative, including careful palpation of both inguinal regions to identify adenopathy. Palpable nodes in the groin are valuable for staging and very likely signify regional metastases, because reactive inflammation and/or infection of inguinal nodes are rare in urethral carcinoma.

For accurate diagnosis, cystoscopy with deep biopsies is necessary because inflammation around the primary tumor is common and may obscure diagnosis if adequate amounts of tissue are not obtained. An examination under anesthesia also may be helpful to improve the accuracy of clinical staging, and localization of the tumor precisely can be achieved with a retrograde urethrogram. Other radiographic modalities such as CT or MRI may aid in the evaluation of pelvic lymphadenopathy, as well as help guide efforts to obtain biopsies of suggestive nodes. In several reports, pelvic MRI was used to demonstrate clearly tumor invasion of the bladder neck and anterior vaginal wall in women and corporal invasion in men.[215,225,230-232] MRI with surface coils has been proposed to improve visualization of tumors in the pendulous or preprostatic regions of the urethra.[233,234] In women, transvaginal ultrasound may be useful in defining local extent of urethral carcinoma.[235] These imaging modalities have not been evaluated prospectively for sensitivity because of the small number of cases to evaluate; a selection bias exists with these reports because the lesions tend to be relatively large tumors.

STAGING CLASSIFICATION

Several staging systems for urethral malignancy have been proposed, but none has been universally accepted or applied. As with virtually all other cancers, a TNM system has been developed by the AJCC to standardize classification of these tumors in both men and women[195] (Table 88-5).

The most critical prognostic factors are the clinical stage at the time of diagnosis and the location of the primary tumor.[188,190,236] The histologic grade of the tumor has no significant value in predicting long-term survival. Nearly one third of women with urethral carcinoma will have inguinal metastases; between 14% and 30% of

TABLE 88-5

AJCC TNM Staging System for Urethral Cancer

CLASSIFICATION	DESCRIPTION
Tumor	
TX	Primary tumor cannot be assessed
T0	No evidence of primary tumor
Tis	Carcinoma in situ
Ta	Noninvasive papillary, polypoid, or verrucous carcinoma
T1	Tumor invades subepithelial connective tissue
T2	Tumor invades periurethral musculature (corpus spongiosum or prostate)
T3	Tumor invades anterior vagina or bladder neck (corpus cavernosum or beyond prostate or bladder neck)
T4	Tumor invades other adjacent structures
Node	
NX	Regional lymph nodes cannot be assessed
N0	No regional lymph node metastases
N1	Metastasis in one superficial lymph node <2 cm in diameter
N2	Metastasis in one superficial lymph node >2 cm but <5 cm in diameter, or multiple nodal metastases all <5 cm
N3	Metastasis to a lymph node >5 cm in diameter
Metastasis	
MX	Distant metastasis cannot be assessed
M0	No distant metastasis
M1	Distant metastasis present

AJCC, American Joint Commission for Cancer; TNM, tumor/node/metastasis.

their male counterparts will have involved nodes at diagnosis.[188,190,237] With some of the very rare carcinoid tumors, survival appears to be related to tumor size, with better long-term prognosis with small tumors.[202-204] However, these tumors are simply case reports, with insufficient numbers to establish meaningful conclusions or valid treatment algorithms, nor does this trend apply to standard urethral adenocarcinoma.

PRIMARY TREATMENT AND PROGNOSIS

Male Urethral Cancer

Distal urethral carcinoma in male patients should be treated essentially the same as distal penile carcinoma, with a partial penectomy with a 2-cm margin. Again surgical consideration must be given to leaving a usable penile stump, or a perineal urethrostomy should be performed. For patients with N0 stage disease, most series show that half will still be alive 5 years after treatment.[188,190,199] Although Ta disease can be treated with transurethral resection, a very high rate of recurrence should be anticipated with this therapy.[238] Furthermore, understaging of patients may lead to inadequate treatment that is frequently fatal; consequently, meticulous evaluation of patients who are candidates for conservative

therapy is critical. Because of the physical and psychological impact of the disfigurement of radical penectomy, alternative techniques that limit resection have been proposed[61,62]; these efforts at subcutaneous penectomy should be viewed as more radical therapy and are not the standard of care because of the increased risk of relapse and disease progression. Organ-preserving surgery should not be used as monotherapy for high-stage urethral carcinoma; these techniques are more reasonable in conjunction with systemic adjuvant therapy to reduce the risk of local or disseminated recurrence.

Radiotherapy for Urethral Carcinoma

Typically, radiation for urethral carcinoma is reserved for patients who refuse surgical resection of their tumors, and long-term results have been variable.[226] A large series reporting the use of radiation therapy as primary treatment for varied histologic types of urethral cancer resulted in tumor recurrence in 21 of 34 patients, with 45% disease-specific survival at 7 years.[239] Patients with large tumor volume and those who received only external-beam radiation fared significantly worse than patients with smaller tumor bulk and recipients of brachytherapy.[239] In addition, patients with very large tumor volume tend to have a higher incidence of local wound problems after radiation therapy; thus this treatment modality is contraindicated for bulky tumors larger than 4 cc. Four patients who were deemed medically unfit to tolerate surgery or even interstitial brachytherapy were treated with both external-beam and intracavitary radiation for locally advanced urethral carcinoma. One patient died at 1 year of unrelated causes, and one remained disease free at 55 months' follow-up. The remaining two patients died of metastatic disease nearly 2 years after therapy. No debilitating urethral or pelvic complications such as strictures, fistulas, or necrosis were reported.[240] However, other sources demonstrate long-term survival rates of less than one in four for external-beam radiation for anterior urethral tumors at 5 years after treatment.[188]

Combination Regimens for Locally Advanced Urethral Carcinoma

The development of disseminated metastatic disease portends a grim prognosis; consequently, achieving local control is of paramount importance. However, surgical therapy alone is unlikely to eradicate advanced disease completely, regardless of the aggressiveness of the surgeon. Many investigators and clinicians are incorporating chemotherapy or radiation or both into the treatment protocol to improve the prospects of achieving local control.[241-244] Unfortunately, many of the reported series are understandably small. A compilation of the published reports reveals eight patients who were treated with radiation and differing combinations of chemotherapy, which resulted in prolonged survival in 75%; two died of causes unrelated to urethral carcinoma.[46,67,69,70]

Dalbagni and coworkers[245] recently reported the results of combination therapy with intraoperative radiation at very high doses after aggressive locoregional resection in six women with locally advanced disease. Four of these patients also underwent neoadjuvant or simultaneous platinum-based chemotherapy. Despite 50% disease-specific mortality within 2 years, they concluded that combination therapy results in superior local control of disease with improved quality of life as a consequence. These authors state unequivocally that surgical mono-therapy is inadequate treatment for high-stage urethral neoplasm. This sentiment echoes the conclusions of Gheiler and associates,[236] who reported a 42% overall survival among 12 patients with T3 disease or greater but observed a 60% survival among those who received multimodality treatment including chemotherapy and radiation. Table 88-6 shows the results of several recent reports of combination therapy for advanced urethral carcinoma.

Unfortunately, any broad conclusions cannot be drawn from these reports because of the different regimens and inconsistent doses of chemotherapy and radiation. However, these data do indicate that urethral carcinoma is chemosensitive and radiosensitive; further investigation is necessary with controlled randomized prospective trials.

Management of Lymph Nodes

Unlike penile carcinoma, palpable inguinal lymphadeno-pathy often indicates the presence of metastatic disease; inflammation and infection do not confuse the clinical picture in urethral carcinoma to the same degree as is the case in penile malignancy. Ilioinguinal lymph node resection in combination with urethrectomy can result in no evidence of residual disease; several series show survival up to 5 years when patients can be rendered disease free.[190,241-244]

Clinically benign inguinal nodes should be evaluated carefully throughout treatment of primary urethral carcinoma. The later development of inguinal lymph-adenopathy should lead to resection because patients may still benefit from delayed lymphadenectomy. Given the absence of documented benefit and the significant morbidity of inguinal lymphadenectomy, prophylactic lymphadenectomy should not be performed.[199,211] Initial reports of sentinel node biopsy for patients with urethral carcinoma have had mixed results. The M.D. Anderson Cancer Center experience with this technique to screen patients with clinically benign inguinal regions resulted in positive nodes in two of nine patients.[241] Both patients underwent radical inguinal lymphadenectomy and adjuvant chemotherapy with durable long-term survival. One patient demonstrated distant metastatic recurrence nearly 4 years later. For tumors in the distal anterior urethra, for which the lymph consistently drains into the inguinal nodes, sentinel lymph node techniques may eventually limit unnecessary inguinal dissections and identify patients who will benefit from additional systemic therapies.

TABLE 88-6

Reports of Combination Therapy for Advanced Urethral Carcinoma

REFERENCE	NUMBER	SURGERY	RADIATION	CHEMOTHERAPY	OUTCOME	FOLLOW-UP (MO)
Dalbagni et al.[245]	6	Anterior pelvic extenteration	High-dose iridium-192 intraoperatively	4/6 received platinum-based chemotherapy	2/6 Disease-free 3/6 Distant mets 2/6 Local recurrence	12–47
Hakenberg et al.*	3	Urethrectomy and ILND	No	Platinum-based chemotherapy	3/3 Complete remission	4–47
Kent et al.[251]	1	Transurethral resection with delayed ILND	No	6 courses of MVAC w/salvage paclitaxel, methotrexate, cisplatin, 5-FU, INF-α	1/1 Disease free	39
Gheiler et al.[236]	10	6/10, pelvic exenteration 3/10, no surgery 1/10, urethrectomy	Yes	Yes	5/10 Disease free 3/10 Local recurrence 2/10 Dead w/distant mets	5–46
Lee[230]	1	No	External-beam radiation, 4000 cGy	Cisplatin and 5-FU	1/1 Disease free	70
Oberfield et al.†	2	No	45 Gy of external-beam radiation	Mitomycin and 5-FU	2/2 Disease free	18–48
Dinney et al.[241]	8	4/8, partial penectomy 1/8, local resection 1/8, pelvic exenteration	2/8 60–66 Gy external-beam radiation	Yes	6/8, Disease free 2/8, Local recurrence, 1 alive w/disease at 44 mo, 1 died of disease at 8 mo	16–156

5-FU, 5-fluorouracil; ILND, inguinal lymphadenectomy; mets, metastasis; MVAC, methotrexate, vincristine, doxorubicin, (Adriamycin), cisplatin.
*Hakenberg OW, Franke HJ, Froehner M, Wirth MP: The treatment of primary urethral carcinoma—the dilemmas of a rare condition: Experience with partial urethrectomy and adjuvant chemotherapy. Onkologie 2001;24:48–52.
†Oberfield RA, Zinman LN, Leibenhaut M, Girshovich L, Silverman ML: Management of invasive squamous cell carcinoma of bulbomembranous male urethra with coordinated chemoradiotherapy and genital preservation. Br J Urol 1996;78:573–578.

Distant Metastases

Most patients with distant metastatic disease from urethral carcinoma are treated with a multimodality approach that includes radiation, chemotherapy, and palliative surgery when indicated. Naturally, the severity of the symptoms, the long-term prognosis, and the performance status of the patient influence the aggressiveness of surgical intervention. Isolated metastases that cause significant pain can be treated with focal irradiation to relieve symptoms.[226]

In Conjunction with Transitional Cell Carcinoma of the Bladder

Male patients who undergo a radical cystectomy without urethrectomy for treatment of transitional carcinoma of the bladder have a less than 15% chance of recurrence in the urethral stump.[214,246] TCC recurrence in the retained urethral remnant typically occurs within 5 years of cystoprostatectomy, although it has been diagnosed as long as 15 years after initial resection of primary bladder disease.[247-249] Malignant infiltration of the prostatic urethra with TCC increases the likelihood of urethral recurrence[246]; urethral barbotage washings and cytology examination are an effective screening tool for recurrence.[250] Even in the presence of a negative cytology, urethral discharge or bleeding should prompt cystoscopic evaluation to rule out recurrence. Physicians involved in postoperative care of these patients should have a very low threshold for treatment, which historically has been delayed urethrectomy. An organ-preserving alternative to urethrectomy has been reported by Kent and colleagues,[251] who treated a 42-year-old man with invasive TCC of the urethra with methotrexate, vinblastine, doxorubicin (Adriamycin), and cisplatin (MVAC) chemotherapy with good response. Subsequent recurrence of inguinal lymphadenopathy was treated with salvage chemotherapy and resection of superficial, deep, and pelvic nodes; the patient remained disease free with maintenance of potency and fertility more than 3 years after treatment. In summary, neoadjuvant chemotherapeutic regimens designed for TCC of the bladder also apply to treatment of urethral recurrences.

TREATMENT COMPLICATIONS

The complications of urethrectomy are rare but include penile edema as well as hematomas and infection. Surgical excision of distal urethral lesions in the female patient may result in incontinence. The technique for ilioinguinal lymphadenectomy is the same for both penile and urethral carcinomas; consequently, the complications are the same and were previously discussed in the penile carcinoma section. The use of radiation to provide local tumor control for primary urethral malignancy has been documented; however, morbidity is problematic because of the development of urethral strictures, penile atrophy, bowel obstruction, fistula formation, incontinence, and chronic edema.

FOLLOW-UP

The post-treatment evaluation of patients with urethral carcinoma must be as vigilant as that for penile malignancy. These patients should be seen and a careful physical examination performed every 4 to 6 months after primary therapy for 2 years. The cornerstone of follow-up evaluation is the physical examination with careful evaluation of both inguinal regions and the operative site. Careful history taking with emphasis on weight loss, discharge, and localized pain is important. In experienced hands, inguinal ultrasonography may suggest changes in lymph node architecture before disease is clinically palpable. CT of the pelvis can be of benefit in patients who have undergone inguinal lymphadenectomy.

ISSUES FOR THE FUTURE

Given the rarity of this disease process, it is unlikely that large series will ever be compiled with standardized protocols to provide meaningful algorithms for the treatment of primary urethral carcinoma. In all likelihood, basic science investigations at the molecular level will allow clinicians to recognize similarities between various histologic types of urethral carcinoma and more common tumors, which may help direct future therapies. Based on the few published series, further investigation into the effectiveness, morbidity, and long-term survival profile for radiation and chemotherapeutic treatments is warranted. In addition, sentinel lymph node technology is currently experimental, but may prove useful because of the more predictable lymphatic drainage of the anterior urethra.

REFERENCES

1. Pukkala E, Weiderpass E: Socio-economic differences in incidence rates of cancers of the male genital organs in Finland, 1971-95. Int J Cancer 2002;102:643.
2. Vatanasapt V, Martin N, Sriplung H, et al: Cancer incidence in Thailand, 1988-1991. Cancer Epidemiol Biomarkers Prev 1995;4:475.
3. Ornellas AA, Seixas AL, Marota A, et al: Surgical treatment of invasive squamous cell carcinoma of the penis: Retrospective analysis of 350 cases. J Urol 1994;151:1244.
4. Percy CL, Miller BA, Gloeckler Ries LA: Effect of changes in cancer classification and the accuracy of cancer death certificates on trends in cancer mortality. Ann N Y Acad Sci 1990;609:87.
5. Maiche AG, Pyrhonen S, Karkinen M: Histological grading of squamous cell carcinoma of the penis: A new scoring system. Br J Urol 1991;6-7:522.
6. Frisch M, Friis S, Kjaer SK, et al: Falling incidence of penis cancer in an uncircumcised population (Denmark 1943-90). BMJ 1995;31-1:1471.
7. Schoen EJ, Baker JC, Colby CJ. et al: Cost-benefit analysis of universal tandem mass spectrometry for newborn screening. Pediatrics 2002;110:781.
8. Maden C, Sherman KJ, Beckmann AM, et al: History of circumcision, medical conditions, and sexual activity and risk of penile cancer. J Natl Cancer Inst 19932;85:19.
9. Fleiss PM: Re: The detection of human papillomavirus deoxyribonucleic acid in intraepithelial, in situ, verrucous and invasive carcinoma of the penis. J Urol 1996;155:2034.

10. Lansimies E: penile cancer and routine newborn circumcision uncommon in Finland. Pediatrics 2000;105:36.

11. Schoen EJ: Response of Dr Esko Lansimies to penile carcinoma. Pediatrics 2000;105:e36.

12. Malek RS, Goellner JR, Smith TF, et al: Human papillomavirus infection and intraepithelial, in situ, and invasive carcinoma of penis. Urology 1993;42:159.

13. Tsen HF, Morgenstern H, Mack T, et al: Risk factors for penile cancer: Results of a population-based case-control study in Los Angeles County (United States). Cancer Causes Control 2001;12:267.

14. Brinton LA, Li JY, Rong SD, et al: Risk factors for penile cancer: results from a case-control study in China. Int J Cancer 1991;47:504.

15. Van Howe RS: Re: The detection of human papillomavirus deoxyribonucleic acid in intraepithelial, in situ, verrucous and invasive carcinoma of the penis. J Urol 1996;155:2035; author reply 2035.

16. Reddy C, Baruah I: Carcinogenic action of human smegma. Arch Pathol 1963;75:414.

17. Pratt-Thomas H, Heins H, Latham E, et al: The carcinogenic effect of human smegma: An experimental study. Cancer 1956;9:671.

18. Picconi MA, Eijan AM, Distefano AL, et al: Human papillomavirus (HPV) DNA in penile carcinomas in Argentina: Analysis of primary tumors and lymph nodes. J Med Virol 2000;61:65.

19. Sarkar FH, Miles BJ, Plieth DH, et al: Detection of human papillomavirus in squamous neoplasm of the penis. J Urol 1992; 147:389.

20. Carter JJ, Madeleine MM, Shera K, et al: Human papillomavirus 16 and 18 L1 serology compared across anogenital cancer sites. Cancer Res 2001;61:1934.

21. Rubin MA, Kleter B, Zhou M, et al: Detection and typing of human papillomavirus DNA in penile carcinoma: Evidence for multiple independent pathways of penile carcinogenesis. Am J Pathol 2001;159:1211.

22. Gregoire L, Cubilla AL, Reuter VE, et al: Preferential association of human papillomavirus with high-grade histologic variants of penile-invasive squamous cell carcinoma. J Natl Cancer Inst 1995;87:1705.

23. Wiener JS, Effert PJ, Humphrey PA, et al: Prevalence of human papillomavirus types 16 and 18 in squamous-cell carcinoma of the penis: A retrospective analysis of primary and metastatic lesions by differential polymerase chain reaction. Int J Cancer 1992;50:694.

24. Cupp MR, Malek RS, Goellner JR, et al: The detection of human papillomavirus deoxyribonucleic acid in intraepithelial, in situ, verrucous and invasive carcinoma of the penis. J Urol 154:1024.

25. Burgers JK, Badalament RA, Drago JR: Penile cancer: Clinical presentation, diagnosis, and staging. Urol Clin North Am 1992;19:247.

26. Stern RS: Genital tumors among men with psoriasis exposed to psoralens and ultraviolet A radiation (PUVA) and ultraviolet B radiation: The Photochemotherapy Follow-up Study. N Engl J Med 1990;322:1093.

27. Hellberg D, Valentin J, Eklund T, et al: Penile cancer: Is there an epidemiological role for smoking and sexual behaviour? Br Med J (Clin Res Ed) 1987;295:1306.

28. Bezerra AL, Lopes A, Landman G, et al: Clinicopathologic features and human papillomavirus DNA prevalence of warty and squamous cell carcinoma of the penis. Am J Surg Pathol 2001;25:673.

29. Kuzaka B, Szymanska K, Suleiman W: [YAG:Nd laser cw in treatment of precancerous states of the penis]. Pol Tyg Lek 1996;51:98.

30. Bissada NK: Conservative extirpative treatment of cancer of the penis. Urol Clin North Am 1992;19:283.

31. Grossman HB: Premalignant and early carcinomas of the penis and scrotum. Urol Clin North Am 1992;19:221.

32. Schellhammer PF, Jordan GH, Robey EL, et al: Premalignant lesions and nonsquamous malignancy of the penis and carcinoma of the scrotum. Urol Clin North Am 1992;19:131.

33. Sakoda R, Oka M, Nakashima K: Leukoplakia of the penis: Bleomycin treatment. Br J Urol 1978;50:355.

34. Kizer WS, Prarie T, Morey AF: Balanitis xerotica obliterans: Epidemiologic distribution in an equal access health care system. South Med J 2003;96:9.

35. Das S, Tunuguntla HS: Balanitis xerotica obliterans: A review. World J Urol 2000;18:382.

36. Depasquale I, Park AJ, Bracka A: The treatment of balanitis xerotica obliterans. BJU Int 2000;86:459.

37. Nasca MR, Innocenzi D, Micali G: Penile cancer among patients with genital lichen sclerosis. J Am Acad Dermatol 1999;41:911.

38. Giannakopoulos X, Basioukas K, Dimou S, et al: Squamous cell carcinoma of the penis arising from balanitis xerotica obliterans. Int Urol Nephrol 1996;28:223.

39. Pride HB, Miller OF III, Tyler WB: Penile squamous cell carcinoma arising from balanitis xerotica obliterans. J Am Acad Dermatol 1993;29:469.

40. Bunker CB: Topics in penile dermatology. Clin Exp Dermatol 2001;26:469.

41. Kiss A, Csontai A, Pirot L, et al: The response of balanitis xerotica obliterans to local steroid application compared with placebo in children. J Urol 2001;165:219.

42. Queyrat L: Erythroplasie du gland. Soc Franc Dermatol Syphilol 1911;22:378.

43. Bowen J: Precancerous dermatoses: A review of two cases of chronic atypical epithelial proliferation. J Cutan Dis 1912;30:241.

44. Micali G, Innocenzi D, Nasca MR, et al: Squamous cell carcinoma of the penis. J Am Acad Dermatol 1996;35:432.

45. Mikhail GR: Cancers, precancers, and pseudocancers on the male genitalia: A review of clinical appearances, histopathology, and management. J Dermatol Surg Oncol 1980;6:1027.

46. Graham JH, Helwig EB: Erythroplasia of Queyrat: A clinicopathologic and histochemical study. Cancer 1973;32:1396.

47. Mitsuishi T, Sata T, Iwasaki T, et al: The detection of human papillomavirus 16 DNA in erythroplasia of Queyrat invading the urethra. Br J Dermatol 1998;138:188.

48. Wieland U, Jurk S, Weissenborn S, et al: Erythroplasia of Queyrat: coinfection with cutaneous carcinogenic human papillomavirus type 8 and genital papillomaviruses in a carcinoma in situ. J Invest Dermatol 2000;115:396.

49. Patterson JW, Kao GF, Graham JH, et al: Bowenoid papulosis: A clinicopathologic study with ultrastructural observations. Cancer 1986;57:823.

50. Papadopoulos AJ, Schwartz RA, Lefkowitz A, et al: Extragenital bowenoid papulosis associated with atypical human papillomavirus genotypes. J Cutan Med Surg 2002;6:117.

51. Purnell D, Ilchyshyn A, Jenkins D, et al: Isolated human papillomavirus 18-positive extragenital bowenoid papulosis and idiopathic CD4+ lymphocytopenia. Br J Dermatol 2001;144:619.

52. Pala S, Poleva I, Vocatura A: The presence of HPV types 6/11, 16/18, 31/33/51 in bowenoid papulosis demonstrated by DNA in situ hybridization. Int J STD AIDS 2000;11:823.

53. Olhoffer IH, Davidson D, Longley J, et al: Facial bowenoid papulosis secondary to human papillomavirus type 16. Br J Dermatol 1999;140:761.

54. Park KC, Kim KH, Youn SW, et al: Heterogeneity of human papillomavirus DNA in a patient with bowenoid papulosis that progressed to squamous cell carcinoma. Br J Dermatol 1998;139:1087.

55. Gross G, Hagedorn M, Ikenberg H, et al: Bowenoid papulosis: Presence of human papillomavirus (HPV) structural antigens and of HPV 16-related DNA sequences. Arch Dermatol 1985;121:858.

56. Yoneta A, Yamashita T, Jin, HY, et al: Development of squamous cell carcinoma by two high-risk human papillomaviruses (HPVs), a novel HPV-67 and HPV-31 from bowenoid papulosis. Br J Dermatol 2000;143:604.

57. Barnes RD, Sarembock LA, Abratt RP, et al: Carcinoma of the penis: The Groote Schuur Hospital experience. J R Coll Surg Edinb 1989;34:44.

58. Eisen RF, Bhawan J, Cahn TH: Spontaneous regression of bowenoid papulosis of the penis. Cutis 1983;32:269.

59. Su CK, Shipley WU: Bowenoid papulosis: A benign lesion of the shaft of the penis misdiagnosed as squamous carcinoma. J Urol 1997;157:1361.

60. Petrow W, Gerdsen R, Uerlich M, et al: Successful topical immunotherapy of bowenoid papulosis with imiquimod. Br J Dermatol 2001;145:1022.

61. Snoeck R, Van Laethem Y, De Clercq E, et al: Treatment of a bowenoid papulosis of the penis with local applications of cidofovir in a patient with acquired immunodeficiency syndrome. Arch Intern Med 2001;161:2382.

62. Redondo P, Lloret P: Topical imiquimod for bowenoid papulosis in an HIV-positive woman. Acta Derm Venereol 2002;82:212.

63. Lassus J, Happonen HP, Niemi KM, et al: Carbon dioxide (CO_2)-laser therapy cures macroscopic lesions, but viral genome is not eradicated in men with therapy-resistant HPV infection. Sex Transm Dis 1994;21:297.

64. Tschanz C, Salomon D, Skaria A, et al: Vulvodynia after CO_2 laser treatment of the female genital mucosa. Dermatology 2001;202:371.

65. Coldiron BM, Jacobson C: Common penile lesions. Urol Clin North Am 1988;15:671.

66. Gersh I: Giant condyloma acuminata (carcinoma-like condylomata or Bushke-Loewenstein tumors) of the penis. J Urol 1953;69:164.

67. Persky L, deKernion J: Carcinoma of the penis. CA Cancer J Clin 1986;36:258.

68. Kraus FT, Perezmesa C: Verrucous carcinoma: Clinical and pathologic study of 105 cases involving oral cavity, larynx and genitalia. Cancer 1966;19:26.

69. Gomez De La Fuente E, Castano Suarez E, Vanaclocha Sebastian F, et al: Verrucous carcinoma of the penis completely cured with shaving and intralesional interferon. Dermatology 2000;200:152.

70. Ilkay AK, Chodak GW, Vogelzang NJ, et al: Buschke-Lowenstein tumor: Therapeutic options including systemic chemotherapy. Urology 1993;42:599.

71. Frega A, Stentella P, Tinari A, et al: Giant condyloma acuminatum or Buschke-Lowenstein tumor: Review of the literature and report of three cases treated by CO_2 laser surgery: A long-term follow-up. Anticancer Res 2002;22:1201.

72. Perisic Z, Popovic Lazic J, Terzic B, et al: Condylomata gigantea in anal and perianal region: Surgical and CO(2) laser treatment. Arch Gynecol Obstet 2003;267:263.

73. Casado M, Jimenez F, Borbujo J, et al: Spontaneous healing of Kaposi's angiosarcoma of the penis. J Urol 1988;139:1313.

74. Wishnow KI, Johnson DE: Effective outpatient treatment of Kaposi's sarcoma of the urethral meatus using the neodymium:YAG laser. Lasers Surg Med 1988;8:428.

75. Smith HR, Black MM: Basal cell carcinoma of the penis. Br J Dermatol 1999;140:361.

76. Nahass GT, Blauvelt A, Penneys NS: Metastases from basal cell carcinoma of the scrotum. J Am Acad Dermatol 1992;26:509.

77. Betti R, Bruscagin C, Inselvini E, et al: Basal cell carcinomas of covered and unusual sites of the body. Int J Dermatol 1997;36:503.

78. Fegen JP, Beebe D, Persky L: Basal cell carcinoma of the penis. J Urol 1970;104:864.

79. Begun FP, Grossman HB, Diokno AC, et al: Malignant melanoma of the penis and male urethra. J Urol 1984;132:123.

80. Stillwell TJ, Zincke H, Gaffey TA, et al: Malignant melanoma of the penis. J Urol 1988;140:72.

81. Park S, Grossfeld GD, McAninch JW, et al: Extramammary Paget's disease of the penis and scrotum: Excision, reconstruction and evaluation of occult malignancy. J Urol 2001;166:2112.

82. Chanda JJ: Extramammary Paget's disease: Prognosis and relationship to internal malignancy. J Am Acad Dermatol 1985;13:1009.

83. Zollo JD, Zeitouni NC: The Roswell Park Cancer Institute experience with extramammary Paget's disease. Br J Dermatol 2000;142:59.

84. Schoenberger B, Loening S: Editorial comment: Extramammary Paget's disease of the penis and scrotum. J Urol 2001;166:2117.

85. Sasso F, Delicato G, Gentile G, et al: Primary synovial sarcoma of the penis. J Urol 2002;168:633.

86. Toh KL, Tan PH, Cheng WS: Primary extraskeletal Ewing's sarcoma of the external genitalia. J Urol 1999;162:159.

87. Layfield LJ, Liu K: Mucoepidermoid carcinoma arising in the glans penis. Arch Pathol Lab Med 2000;124:148.

88. Leviav A, Devine PC, Schellhammer PF, et al: Epithelioid sarcoma of the penis. Clin Plast Surg 1988;15:489.

89. Parsons MA, Fox M: Malignant fibrous histiocytoma of the penis. Eur Urol 1988;14:75.

90. Planz B, Brunner K, Kalem T, et al: Primary leiomyosarcoma of the epididymis and late recurrence on the penis. J Urol 1998;159:508.

91. Rasbridge SA, Parry JR: Angiosarcoma of the penis. Br J Urol 1989;63:440.

92. Sacker AR, Oyama KK, Kessler S: Primary osteosarcoma of the penis. Am J Dermatopathol 1994;16:285.

93. Chan PT, Begin LR, Arnold D, et al: Priapism secondary to penile metastasis: A report of two cases and a review of the literature. J Surg Oncol 1998;68:51.

94. Razi SS, Gottenger EE, Garcia RL, et al: An unusual case of a metastatic lesion to the penis. J Urol 2000;163:908.

95. Abeshouse B, Abeshouse G: Metwastatic tumors of the penis: A review of the literature and a report of two cases. J Urol 1961;86:99.

96. Sufrin G, Huben R: Benign and malignant lesions of the penis. In Gillenwater JY, Grayhack JT, Howards SS, et al (eds): Adult and Pediatric Urology, 3rd ed. St. Louis, Mosby-Year Book, 1996, p 2014.

97. Mukamel E, deKernion JB: Early versus delayed lymph-node dissection versus no lymph-node dissection in carcinoma of the penis. Urol Clin North Am 1987;14:707.

98. Fraley EE, Zhang G, Sazama R, et al: Cancer of the penis: Prognosis and treatment plans. Cancer 1985;55:1618.

99. Staubitz W, Melbourne H, Oberkircher O: Carcinoma of the penis. Cancer 1955;8:371.

100. Broders AC: Carcinoma: Grading and practical applications. Arch Pathol Lab Med 1926;2:376–381.

101. Cubilla AL, Barreto J, Caballero C, et al: Pathologic features of epidermoid carcinoma of the penis: A prospective study of 66 cases. Am J Surg Pathol 1993;17:753.

102. Beggs J, Spratt J: Epidermoid carcinoma of the penis. J Urol 1966; 91:166.

103. el-Demiry MI, Oliver RT, Hope-Stone HF, et al: Reappraisal of the role of radiotherapy and surgery in the management of carcinoma of the penis. Br J Urol 1984;56:724.

104. Salaverria JC, Hope-Stone HF, Paris AM, et al: Conservative treatment of carcinoma of the penis. Br J Urol 1979;51:32.

105. Hardner GJ, Bhanalaph T, Murphy GP, et al: Carcinoma of the penis: Analysis of therapy in 100 consecutive cases. J Urol 1972;108:428.

106. Fleming I, Cooper J, Henson D, et al: AJCC Cancer Staging Manual. Philadelphia, JB Lippincott, 1997.

107. Lopes A, Hidalgo GS, Kowalski LP, et al: Prognostic factors in carcinoma of the penis: Multivariate analysis of 145 patients treated with amputation and lymphadenectomy. J Urol 1996;156:1637.

108. Horenblas S: Lymphadenectomy for squamous cell carcinoma of the penis, Part 1: Diagnosis of lymph node metastasis. BJU Int 2001;88:467.

109. Vapnek JM, Hricak H, Carroll PR: Recent advances in imaging studies for staging of penile and urethral carcinoma. Urol Clin North Am 1992;19:257.

110. Horenblas S, Van Tinteren H, Delemarre JF, et al: Squamous cell carcinoma of the penis: Accuracy of tumor, nodes and metastasis classification system, and role of lymphangiography, computerized tomography scan and fine needle aspiration cytology. J Urol 1991;146:1279.

111. Kulkarni JN, Kamat MR: Prophylactic bilateral groin node dissection versus prophylactic radiotherapy and surveillance in patients with N0 and N1-2A carcinoma of the penis. Eur Urol 1994;26:123.

112. Pettaway CA, Pisters LL, Dinney CP, et al: Sentinel lymph node dissection for penile carcinoma: the M.D. Anderson Cancer Center experience. J Urol 1995;154:1999.

113. Theodorescu D, Russo P, Zhang ZF, et al: Outcomes of initial surveillance of invasive squamous cell carcinoma of the penis and negative nodes. J Urol 1996;155:1626.

114. McDougal WS, Kirchner FK Jr, Edwards RH, et al: Treatment of carcinoma of the penis: The case for primary lymphadenectomy. J Urol 1986;136:38.

115. Solsona E, Iborra I, Ricos JV, et al: Corpus cavernosum invasion and tumor grade in the prediction of lymph node condition in penile carcinoma. Eur Urol 1992;22:115.

116. Ravi R: Correlation between the extent of nodal involvement and survival following groin dissection for carcinoma of the penis. Br J Urol 1993;72:817.

117. Horenblas S: Lymphadenectomy for squamous cell carcinoma of the penis, Part 2: The role and technique of lymph node dissection. BJU Int 2001;88:473.

118. Johnson DE, Lo RK: Complications of groin dissection in penile cancer. Experience with 101 lymphadenectomies. Urology 1984;24:312.

119. Yamada Y, Gohji K, Hara I, et al: Long-term follow-up study of penile cancer. Int J Urol 1998;5:247.

120. McDougal WS: Carcinoma of the penis: Improved survival by early regional lymphadenectomy based on the histological grade and depth of invasion of the primary lesion. J Urol 1995;154:1364.

121. Opjordsmoen S, Fossa SD: Quality of life in patients treated for penile cancer. A follow-up study. Br J Urol 1994;74:652.

122. Goette DK, Carson TE: Erythroplasia of Queyrat: treatment with topical 5-fluorouracil. Cancer 1976;38:1498.

123. Horenblas S, van Tinteren H, Delemarre JF, et al: Squamous cell carcinoma of the penis, II: Treatment of the primary tumor. J Urol 1992;147:1533.

124. Skinner DG, Leadbetter WF, Kelley SB: The surgical management of squamous cell carcinoma of the penis. J Urol 1972;107:273.

125. Nash PA, Bihrle R, Gleason PE, et al: Mohs' micrographic surgery and distal urethrectomy with immediate urethral reconstruction for glanular carcinoma in situ with significant urethral extension. Urology 1996;47:108.

126. Cook JL, Perone JB: A prospective evaluation of the incidence of complications associated with Mohs micrographic surgery. Arch Dermatol 2003;139:143.

127. Mohs FE, Snow SN, Larson PO: Mohs micrographic surgery for penile tumors. Urol Clin North Am 1992;19:291.

128. Wu JJ, Markus RF, Orengo IF: The increased competitiveness of Mohs micrographic surgery training. Dermatol Online J 2002;8:24.

129. Wawroschek F, Vogt H, Bachter D, et al: First experience with gamma probe guided sentinel lymph node surgery in penile cancer. Urol Res 2000;28:246.

130. Tanis PJ, Lont AP, Meinhardt W, et al: Dynamic sentinel node biopsy for penile cancer: Reliability of a staging technique. J Urol 2002;168:76.

131. Srinivas V, Joshi A, Agarwal B, et al: Penile cancer: The sentinel lymph node controversy. Urol Int 1991;47:108.

132. Fowler JE Jr: Sentinel lymph node biopsy for staging penile cancer. Urology 1984;23:352.

133. Akduman B, Fleshner NE, Ehrlich L, et al: Early experience in intermediate-risk penile cancer with sentinel node identification using the gamma probe. Urology 2001;58:65.

134. Fossa SD, Hall KS, Johannessen NB, et al: Cancer of the penis: Experience at the Norwegian Radium Hospital 1974-1985. Eur Urol 1987;13:372.

135. Horenblas S, van Tinteren H, Delemarre JF, et al: Squamous cell carcinoma of the penis, III: Treatment of regional lymph nodes. J Urol 1993;149:492.

136. Fraley EE, Zhang G, Manivel C, et al: The role of ilioinguinal lymphadenectomy and significance of histological differentiation in treatment of carcinoma of the penis. J Urol 1989;142:1478.

137. Ravi R, Chaturvedi HK, Sastry DV: Role of radiation therapy in the treatment of carcinoma of the penis. Br J Urol 1994;74:646.

138. Johnson DE, Lo RK: Management of regional lymph nodes in penile carcinoma: Five-year results following therapeutic groin dissections. Urology 1984;24:308.

139. Parra RO: Accurate staging of carcinoma of the penis in men with nonpalpable inguinal lymph nodes by modified inguinal lymphadenectomy. J Urol 1996;155:560.

140. Jacobellis U: Modified radical inguinal lymphadenectomy for carcinoma of the penis: Technique and results. J Urol 2003;169:1349.

141. Coblentz TR, Theodorescu D: Morbidity of modified prophylactic inguinal lymphadenectomy for squamous cell carcinoma of the penis. J Urol 2002;168:1386.

142. Catalona WJ: Modified inguinal lymphadenectomy for carcinoma of the penis with preservation of saphenous veins: Technique and preliminary results. J Urol 1988;140:306.

143. Bevan-Thomas R, Slaton JW, Pettaway CA: Contemporary morbidity from lymphadenectomy for penile squamous cell carcinoma: The M.D. Anderson Cancer Center Experience. J Urol 2002;167:1638.

144. Daseler E, Anson B, Reiman A: Radical excision of iliac and inguinal lymph glands: A study based on 450 anatomical dissections and supportive clinical observations. Surg Gynecol Obstet 1948;87:679.

145. Assimos DG, Jarow JP: Role of laparoscopic pelvic lymph node dissection in the management of patients with penile cancer and inguinal adenopathy. J Endourol 1994;8:365.

146. Ravi R: Prophylactic lymphadenectomy vs observation vs inguinal biopsy in node-negative patients with invasive carcinoma of the penis. Jpn J Clin Oncol 1993;23:53.

147. Srinivas V, Morse MJ, Herr HW, et al: Penile cancer: relation of extent of nodal metastasis to survival. J Urol 1987;137:880.

148. Ahmed T, Sklaroff R, Yagoda A: An appraisal of the efficacy of bleomycin in epidermoid carcinoma of the penis. Anticancer Res 1984;4:289.

149. Sklaroff RB, Yagoda A: Methotrexate in the treatment of penile carcinoma. Cancer 1980;45:214.

150. Ahmed T, Sklaroff R, Yagoda A: Sequential trials of methotrexate, cisplatin and bleomycin for penile cancer. J Urol 1984;132:465.

151. Gagliano RG, Blumenstein BA, Crawford ED, et al: cis-Diaminedichloroplatinum in the treatment of advanced epidermoid carcinoma of the penis: A Southwest Oncology Group Study. J Urol 1989;141:66.

152. Fisher H, Barada J, Horton J, et al: Neoadjuvant therapy with cisplatin and 5-fluorouracil for stage III squamous cell carcinoma of the penis. J Urol 1990;143(4 Suppl):352A.

153. Hussein AM, Benedetto P, Sridhar KS: Chemotherapy with cisplatin and 5-fluorouracil for penile and urethral squamous cell carcinomas. Cancer 1990;65:433.

154. Shammas FV, Ous S, Fossa SD: Cisplatin and 5-fluorouracil in advanced cancer of the penis. J Urol 1992;147:630.

155. Dexeus FH, Logothetis CJ, Sella A, et al: Combination chemotherapy with methotrexate, bleomycin and cisplatin for advanced squamous cell carcinoma of the male genital tract. J Urol 1991;146:1284.

156. Huang XY, Kubota Y, Nakada T, et al: Intra-arterial infusion chemotherapy for penile carcinoma with deep inguinal lymph node metastasis. Urol Int 1999;62:245.

157. Haas GP, Blumenstein BA, Gagliano RG, et al: Cisplatin, methotrexate and bleomycin for the treatment of carcinoma of the penis: A Southwest Oncology Group study. J Urol 1999;161:1823.

158. Pizzocaro G, Nicolai N, Piva L: Chemotherapy for cancer of the penis. In Raghavan D, Scher HI, Leibel, SA, Lange PH (eds): Principles and Practice of Genitourinary Oncology. Philadelphia, Lippincott-Raven, 1997, p 973.

159. Kattan J, Culine S, Droz JP, et al: Penile cancer chemotherapy: Twelve years' experience at Institut Gustave-Roussy. Urology 1993;42:559.

160. Mitropoulos D, Dimopoulos MA, Kiroudi-Voulgari A, et al: Neoadjuvant cisplatin and interferon-alpha 2B in the treatment and organ preservation of penile carcinoma. J Urol 1994;152:1124.

161. Pizzocaro G, Piva L: Adjuvant and neoadjuvant vincristine, bleomycin, and methotrexate for inguinal metastases from squamous cell carcinoma of the penis. Acta Oncol 1988;27:823.

162. Pizzocaro G, Piva L, Nicolai N: [Treatment of lymphatic metastasis of squamous cell carcinoma of the penis: Experience at the National Tumor Institute of Milan]. Arch Ital Urol Androl 1996;68:169.

163. Roth AD, Berney CR, Rohner S, et al: Intra-arterial chemotherapy in locally advanced or recurrent carcinomas of the penis and anal canal: An active treatment modality with curative potential. Br J Cancer 2000;83:1637.

164. Sarin R, Norman AR, Steel GG, et al: Treatment results and prognostic factors in 101 men treated for squamous carcinoma of the penis. Int J Radiat Oncol Biol Phys 1997;38:713.

165. Rozan R, Albuisson E, Giraud B, et al: Interstitial brachytherapy for penile carcinoma: A multicentric survey (259 patients). Radiother Oncol 1995;36:83.

III

166. Opjordsmoen S, Waehre H, Aass N, et al: Sexuality in patients treated for penile cancer: Patients' experience and doctors' judgement. Br J Urol 1994;73:554.

167. McLean M, Akl AM, Warde P, et al: The results of primary radiation therapy in the management of squamous cell carcinoma of the penis. Int J Radiat Oncol Biol Phys 1993;25:623.

168. Jackson SM: The treatment of carcinoma of the penis. Br J Surg 1966;53:33.

169. Hess F, Prignitz R, Walthers E: Treatment of penis carcinoma. Urol Int 1983;38:243.

170. Delannes M, Malavaud B, Douchez J, et al: Iridium-192 interstitial therapy for squamous cell carcinoma of the penis. Int J Radiat Oncol Biol Phys 1992;24:479.

171. Crook J, Grimard L, Tsihlias J, et al: Interstitial brachytherapy for penile cancer: An alternative to amputation. J Urol 2002;167:506.

172. Mazeron JJ, Langlois D, Lobo PA, et al: Interstitial radiation therapy for carcinoma of the penis using iridium 192 wires: The Henri Mondor experience (1970-1979). Int J Radiat Oncol Biol Phys 1984;10:1891.

173. Lutolf UM, Glanzmann C, Horst W: [Radiotherapy of penile carcinoma, indications and results]. Strahlentherapie 1976;152:333.

174. Gerbaulet A, Lambin P: Radiation therapy of cancer of the penis: Indications, advantages, and pitfalls. Urol Clin North Am 1992;19:325.

175. Krieg R, Hoffman R: Current management of unusual genitourinary cancers, Part 1: Penile cancer. Oncology (Huntingt) 1999;13:1347.

176. Modig H, Duchek M, Sjodin JG: Carcinoma of the penis: Treatment by surgery or combined bleomycin and radiation therapy. Acta Oncol 1993;32:653.

177. Palmieri G, Gridelli C, Vitale A, et al: Contemporary chemotherapy and radiotherapy for inguinal metastases of carcinoma of the penis: A case report. Tumori 1988;74:585.

178. Pedrick TJ, Wheeler W, Riemenschneider H: Combined modality therapy for locally advanced penile squamous cell carcinoma. Am J Clin Oncol 1993;16:501.

179. Edsmyr F, Andersson L, Esposti PL: Combined bleomycin and radiation therapy in carcinoma of the penis. Cancer 1985;56:1257.

180. Perez-Tamayot C, Winjnmaalen A, Pomp J, et al: Combined approach to squamous cell carcinoma of the penis (SCP). Proc Am Soc Clin Oncol 1987;6:109.

181. Fraley EE, Hutchens HC: Radical ilio-inguinal node dissection: The skin bridge technique: A new procedure. J Urol 1972;108:279.

182. Kuruvilla JT, Garlick FH, Mammen KE: Results of surgical treatment of carcinoma of the penis. Aust N Z J Surg 1941;41:157.

183. Whitmore WF Jr, Vagaiwala MR: A technique of ilioinguinal lymph node dissection for carcinoma of the penis. Surg Gynecol Obstet 1984;159:573.

184. Karakousis CP, Heiser MA, Moore RH: Lymphedema after groin dissection. Am J Surg 1983;145:205.

185. Dalbagni G, Zhang ZF, Lacombe L, et al: Female urethral carcinoma: An analysis of treatment outcome and a plea for a standardized management strategy. Br J Urol 1998;82:835.

186. Fair W, Yang C: Urethral carcinoma in males. In Kursh E (ed): Current Therapy in Genitourinary Surgery, 2nd ed. St. Louis, Mosby-Year Book, 1992, p 157.

187. Roberts TW, Melicow MM: Pathology and natural history of urethral tumors in females: Review of 65 cases. Urology 1977;10:583.

188. Kaplan GW, Bulkey GJ, Grayhack JT: Carcinoma of the male urethra. J Urol 1967;98:365.

189. Mevorach RA, Cos LR, di Sant'Agnese PA, et al: Human papillomavirus type 6 in grade I transitional cell carcinoma of the urethra. J Urol 1990;143:126.

190. Ray B, Canto AR, Whitmore WF Jr: Experience with primary carcinoma of the male urethra. J Urol 1977;117:591.

191. Severino LJ, Brockunier A Jr, Davidian, MM: Adenocarcinoma of the urethra during pregnancy: Report of a case. Obstet Gynecol 1977;50:22s.

192. Fagan G, Hertig A: Carcinoma of the female urethra: Review of literature. Obstet Gynecol 1955;6:1.

193. Marshall F, Uson A, Melicow M: Neoplasms and caruncles of the female urethra. Surg Gynecol Obstet 1960;110:723.

194. Monaco A, Murphy G, Dowling W: Primary cancer of the female urethra. Cancer 1958;11:1215.

195. Donat S, Cozzi P, Herr H: Surgery of penile and urethral carcinoma. In Wein A (ed): Campbell's Urology. 8th ed. Philadelphia, Saunders, 2002, pp 2983-2999.

196. Cupp MR, Malek RS, Goellner JR, et al: Detection of human papillomavirus DNA in primary squamous cell carcinoma of the male urethra. Urology 1996;48:551.

197. Wiener JS, Liu ET, Walther PJ: Oncogenic human papillomavirus type 16 is associated with squamous cell cancer of the male urethra. Cancer Res 1992;52:5018.

198. Grabstald H: Proceedings: Tumors of the urethra in men and women. Cancer 1973;32:1236.

199. Forman JD, Lichter AS: The role of radiation therapy in the management of carcinoma of the male and female urethra. Urol Clin North Am 1992;19:383.

200. Srinivas V, Khan SA: Male urethral cancer: A review. Int Urol Nephrol 1988;20:61.

201. Chitale SV, Szemere JC, Burgess NA, et al: Surgical technique for the conservative management of distal urethral melanoma. Br J Plast Surg 2001;54:361.

202. Vadmal MS, Steckel J, Teichberg S, et al: Primary neuroendocrine carcinoma of the penile urethra. J Urol 1997;157:956.

203. Sylora HO, Diamond HM, Kaufman, M, et al: Primary carcinoid tumor of the urethra. J Urol 1975;114:150.

204. Chen KT: Primary carcinoid tumor of the urethra. J Urol 2001; 166:1831.

205. Kobayashi T, Fukuzawa S, Oka H, et al: Isolated recurrence of prostatic adenocarcinoma to the anterior urethra after radical prostatectomy. J Urol 2000;164:780.

206. Fukata S, Inoue K, Moriki T, et al: A solitary metastasis of renal cell carcinoma to the urethra. J Urol 2000;163:1245.

207. Goldberg MG, Plaine L: Solitary metastasis of renal cell carcinoma to urethra. Urology 1990;35:351.

208. Lowe LH, Banks WJ, Allen TD: Urethral metastasis in Wilms' tumor. J Urol 1998;160:165.

209. Stanley K, Khoudary KP, Nasrallah PF: Urothelial extension of Wilms' tumor presenting as a prolapsing urethral mass. J Urol 1995;153:1981.

210. Weghaupt K, Gerstner GJ, Kucera H: Radiation therapy for primary carcinoma of the female urethra: A survey over 25 years. Gynecol Oncol 1984;17:58.

211. Srinivas V, Khan SA: Female urethral cancer: An overview. Int Urol Nephrol 1987;19:423.

212. Mostofi FK, Davis CJ Jr, Sesterhenn IA: Carcinoma of the male and female urethra. Urol Clin North Am 1992;19:347.

213. Fadl-Elmula I, Gorunova L, Mandahl N, et al: Chromosome abnormalities in squamous cell carcinoma of the urethra. Genes Chromosomes Cancer 1998;23:72.

214. Schellhammer PF, Whitmore WF Jr: Transitional cell carcinoma of the urethra in men having cystectomy for bladder cancer. J Urol 1976;115:56.

215. Suzuki K, Morita T, Tokue A: Primary signet ring cell carcinoma of female urethra. Int J Urol 2001;8:509.

216. Murphy DP, Pantuck AJ, Amenta PS, et al: Female urethral adenocarcinoma: Immunohistochemical evidence of more than 1 tissue of origin. J Urol 1999;161:1881.

217. Baldi A, Rossiello R, Di Marino M, et al: Colonic type adenocarcinoma of male urethra. In Vivo 2000;14:487.

218. Chan YM, Ka-Leung Cheng D, Nga-Yin Cheung A, et al: Female urethral adenocarcinoma arising from urethritis glandularis. Gynecol Oncol 2000;79:511.

219. Ogihara S, Kato H: Endocrine cell distribution and expression of tissue-associated antigens in human female paraurethral duct: possible clue to the origin of urethral diverticular cancer. Int J Urol 2000;7:10.

220. Maier U, Dorfinger K, Susani M: Clear cell adenocarcinoma of the female urethra. J Urol 1998;160:492.

221. Mai KT, Yazdi HM, Perkins DG, et al: Multicentric clear cell adenocarcinoma in the urinary bladder and the urethral diverticulum: Evidence of origin of clear cell adenocarcinoma of the female lower urinary tract from mullerian duct remnants. Histopathology 2000;36:380.

222. Seseke F, Zoller G, Kunze E: Clear cell adenocarcinoma of the male

urethra in association with so-called nephrogenic metaplasia. Urol Int 2001;67:104.

223. Collado A, Algaba F, Caparros J, et al: Clear cell adenocarcinoma in a female urethral diverticulum. Scand J Urol Nephrol 2000;34:136.

224. Grabstald H, Hilaris B, Henschke U, et al: Cancer of the female urethra. JAMA 1966;197:835.

225. Hettiarachchi JA, Johnson GB, Panageas E, et al: Malignant priapism associated with metastatic urethral carcinoma. Urol Int 2001;66:114.

226. Raghavaiah NV: Radiotherapy in the treatment of carcinoma of the male urethra. Cancer 1978;41:1313.

227. Bracken RB, Johnson DE, Miller LS, et al: Primary carcinoma of the female urethra. J Urol 1976;116:188.

228. Peterson DT, Dockerty MB, Utz DC, et al: The peril of primary carcinoma of the urethra in women. J Urol 1973;110:72.

229. Grigsby PW, Herr HW: Urethral Tumors. In Vogelzang NJ, Shipley WU, Scardino PT, Coffey DS, Miles BJ (eds): Comprehensive Textbook of Genitourinary Oncology. Philadelphia, Lippincott Williams & Wilkins, 2000, p 1133.

230. Lee KC: Carcinoma of the female urethra responsive to moderate dose chemoradiotherapy. J Urol 2000;163:905.

231. Hickey N, Murphy J, Herschorn S: Carcinoma in a urethral diverticulum: Magnetic resonance imaging and sonographic appearance. Urology 2000;55:588.

232. Kawada T, Hashimoto K, Tokunaga T, et al: Two cases of penile cancer: Magnetic resonance imaging in the evaluation of tumor extension. J Urol 1994;152:963.

233. Kageyama S, Ueda T, Kushima R, et al: Primary adenosquamous cell carcinoma of the male distal urethra: Magnetic resonance imaging using a circular surface coil. J Urol 1997;158:1913.

234. Hricak H, Marotti M, Gilbert TJ, et al: Normal penile anatomy and abnormal penile conditions: Evaluation with MR imaging. Radiology 1988;169:683.

235. Shiojima K, Akimoto T, Takahashi I, et al: Transvaginal ultrasonography of female urethral carcinoma treated with radiation therapy: Report of two cases. Radiat Med 1998;16:221.

236. Gheiler EL, Tefilli MV, Tiguert R, et al: Management of primary urethral cancer. Urology 1998;52:487.

237. Anderson KA, McAninch JW: Primary squamous cell carcinoma of anterior male urethra. Urology 1984;23:134.

238. Konnak JW: Conservative management of low grade neoplasms of the male urethra: A preliminary report. J Urol 1980;123:175.

239. Milosevic MF, Warde PR, Banerjee D, et al: Urethral carcinoma in women: Results of treatment with primary radiotherapy. Radiother Oncol 2000;56:29.

240. Kuettel MR, Parda DS, Harter KW, et al: Treatment of female urethral carcinoma in medically inoperable patients using external beam irradiation and high dose rate intracavitary brachytherapy. J Urol 1997;157:1669.

241. Dinney CP, Johnson DE, Swanson DA, et al: Therapy and prognosis for male anterior urethral carcinoma: An update. Urology 1994;43:506.

242. Johnson DW, Kessler JF, Ferrigni RG, et al: Low dose combined chemotherapy/radiotherapy in the management of locally advanced urethral squamous cell carcinoma. J Urol 1989;141:615.

243. Licht MR, Klein EA, Bukowski R, et al: Combination radiation and chemotherapy for the treatment of squamous cell carcinoma of the male and female urethra. J Urol 1995;153:1918.

244. Narayan P, Konety B: Surgical treatment of female urethral carcinoma. Urol Clin North Am 1992;19:373.

245. Dalbagni G, Donat SM, Eschwege P, et al: Results of high dose rate brachytherapy, anterior pelvic exenteration and external beam radiotherapy for carcinoma of the female urethra. J Urol 2001;166:1759.

246. Levinson AK, Johnson DE, Wishnow KI: Indications for urethrectomy in an era of continent urinary diversion. J Urol 1990;144:73.

247. Tobisu K, Tanaka Y, Mizutani T, et al: Transitional cell carcinoma of the urethra in men following cystectomy for bladder cancer: Multivariate analysis for risk factors. J Urol 1991;146:1551.

248. Sakai N, Yamada T, Asao T, et al: A case of urethral recurrence found 15 years after radical cystectomy. Int J Urol 1999;6:578.

249. Tongaonkar HB, Dalal AV, Kulkarni JN, et al: Urethral recurrences following radical cystectomy for invasive transitional cell carcinoma of the bladder. Br J Urol 1993;72:910.

250. Wolinska WH, Melamed MR, Schellhammer PF, et al: Urethral cytology following cystectomy for bladder carcinoma. Am J Surg Pathol 1977;1:225.

251. Kent D, Gee JR, Amato RJ, et al: Successful management of metastatic urethral cancer with organ preservation. J Urol 2001;166:2308.

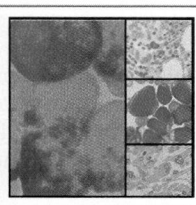

89

TESTICULAR CANCER

Eric J. Small

Jorge A. Garcia

Frank Torti

SUMMARY OF KEY POINTS

INCIDENCE
- Testicular cancer accounts for 1% of all male malignancies and 6000 to 8000 new cases a year in the United States.
- It is the most common malignancy among men aged 15 to 35.
- Seminoma represents 40% of all germ cell tumors.
- Nonseminoma accounts for 60% of all germ cell tumors, with embryonal elements most frequent.

DIFFERENTIAL DIAGNOSIS
- Exclude testicular torsion, hydrocele, varicocele, spermatocele, and epididymitis (these can coexist with germ cell tumors).
- Other malignancies to exclude are lymphoma and metastases from prostate cancer, lung cancer, or melanoma (generally in older age group).

DIAGNOSIS AND STAGING EVALUATION
- Complete history and physical examination.
- Bilateral testicular ultrasonography.
- Tumor serum markers: lactate dehydrogenase (LDH), β-human chorionic gonadotropin (βHCG), and α-fetoprotein (AFP).
- Hemogram, chemistry studies including renal function.

- Computed tomography (CT) of chest, abdomen, and pelvis.
- Additional imaging studies as appropriate (e.g., imaging of brain in patient with pure choriocarcinoma).
- Radical (inguinal) orchiectomy (transscrotal biopsy or orchiectomy should be avoided).

PRIMARY THERAPY
Seminoma
- Localized disease is curable with orchiectomy and low-dose adjuvant radiotherapy to lymph nodes in 98% of patients.
- Locally advanced disease (stage II) is curable with orchiectomy and radiotherapy to involved areas in 85 to 95% of patients with minimal to moderately bulky disease.
- Metastatic disease (stage III) or bulky locally advanced disease is curable in 90% of patients with combination chemotherapy.
- Postchemotherapy retroperitoneal lymphadenectomy can prevent subsequent relapse in selected patients.

Nonseminoma
- Clinically localized disease is curable with orchiectomy alone in 60% to 80% of patients.
- Risk of relapse is decreased with retroperitoneal lymphadenectomy, although in selected patients,

surveillance without surgery is an option.
- Adjuvant combination chemotherapy after lymphadenectomy might further decrease risk of relapse but does not affect survival rates.
- Nonbulky locally advanced (stage II) disease is cured with surgery alone in 40% to 60%.
- Moderate to bulky nodal disease requires combination chemotherapy.
- Metastatic disease (stage III) or bulky locally advanced disease is curable in 80% of patients with combination chemotherapy.
- Postchemotherapy retroperitoneal lymphadenectomy can prevent subsequent relapse in selected patients.

EFFECTIVE SECOND- AND THIRD-LINE THERAPIES
- Chemotherapy salvage rates are about 80% for patients who have failed surgical or radiation therapeutic treatments.
- Second-line chemotherapy for patients who have failed prior chemotherapy is curative in 20%.
- Subsequent high-dose therapy with autologous bone marrow transplant (ABMT) or peripheral stem cell transplant (PSCT) is possibly curative in 15% to 20% of those who have failed second-line therapy.

INTRODUCTION

Although testicular cancer accounts for only 1% of all male malignancies, the understanding and study of this disease are important for a variety of reasons. The evolution of therapy for germ cell tumors (GCTs) has been deliberate and thoughtful and has resulted in cure rates of 85%.[1] GCT therapy serves as a model for the treatment of curable cancers and is particularly notable because GCT occurs in young men who are entering their most productive

years. Nonetheless, challenges in the management of GCTs remain. Because of their young age, patients who have been cured are at risk of delayed, treatment-induced toxicity. Furthermore, an 85% cure rate also implies that 15% of patients with GCTs will not be cured and ultimately will succumb to their disease. An understanding of staging and risk assessment is crucial if patients with good risk features are not to be overtreated and exposed to undue toxic risks and if patients with poor risk features are to receive adequate (curative) therapy.

EPIDEMIOLOGY

Incidence

GCTs account for 1% of all male malignancies, and it is estimated that 7500 new cases were diagnosed in the United States in the year 2002.[2] Despite the overall curability of GCTs, approximately 400 men in the United States died in the year 2002 as a consequence of germ cell tumors. Although GCT is an uncommon malignancy, it is the most common malignancy among men aged 15 to 35. Seminoma accounts for 40% of all germ cell tumors, while nonseminoma germ cell tumors (NSGCTs) account for 60%.[3] Occasionally, GCT occurs in children (generally yolk sac tumors) and in men over 70 (generally spermatocytic seminoma), but by and large, it is a malignancy of early adulthood, with the incidence of seminoma peaking in the 25- to 45-year-old group. The highest incidence of nonseminoma occurs in a slightly younger group of men (15- to 30-year-old group).[3] Bilateral tumors occur in 2% to 4% of patients.[3,4]

Etiology

Although risk factors for the development of this disease are largely unknown, a history of cryptorchidism appears to be related to the development of GCT. The risk of developing GCT is 10- to 40-fold higher in cryptorchid testes, and it is anticipated that 12% of all GCTs arise in cryptorchid testes.[5] Conversely, from 1% to 5% of boys with a history of an undescended testicle will go on to develop GCT. The risk is highest (at approximately 5%) when a cryptorchid testis is retained intra-abdominally, falls to 1% if the testis is retained in the inguinal canal, and appears to fall further if the undescended testis is placed surgically in the scrotum (orchiopexy) before 6 years of age. One fourth of GCTs arising in patients with a history of cryptorchidism occur in the normal, descended testicle, however, suggesting that systemic sequelae of cryptorchidism (i.e., testicular atrophy) is of greater etiologic importance than local or anatomic abnormalities.[5]

In patients with testicular feminization syndrome and intra-abdominally retained gonads, a 40-fold increase of GCT is seen. In phenotypically female but genotypically male patients, this syndrome can be mistaken for ovarian cancer.[6]

Although the association between cryptorchidism and the development of GCT is indisputable, it is prudent to recall that a history of cryptorchidism is absent in nearly 90% of men with GCT. The contribution of orchitis, testicular trauma, or irradiation to the genesis of GCT is unknown, but it has been postulated that the final pathway common to all of these associations is testicular atrophy with increased follicle-stimulating hormone (FSH) drive.[7] There is growing support for the concept of transplacental damage to the fetal gonad by maternal estrogen levels as a contributing causative agent of germ cell cancer.[8]

Extragonadal GCTs appear to arise as a consequence of the malignant transformation of residual midline germinal elements, usually in the mediastinum or retroperitoneum, but occasionally in other locations such as the sacrococcygeal region and the pineal gland.[9] Whether these residual germinal elements are a consequence of abnormal germ cell migration is not known, and other factors that might contribute to the development of extragonadal GCT have not been identified.

MOLECULAR BIOLOGY

The cytogenetic and molecular biology of GCT has only recently begun to be understood. Most interest has focused on changes involving chromosome 12. The isochromosome of the short arm of chromosome 12, i(12p), has been reported in up to 90% of GCT patients.[10,11] Although it is occasionally found in gastric cancer, i(12p) is nearly a pathognomic feature of GCT of all histologic types, whether of gonadal or extragonadal origin. This cytogenetic abnormality has been reported in carcinoma in situ tissue, suggesting that it is an early marker, if not a cause, of germ cell tumorigenesis.[12] In patients with mediastinal GCT, in whom there is an increased incidence of hematologic malignancies (often acute myeloid leukemia), i(12p) can be found in both the mediastinal GCT tissue and in the leukemic cells, suggesting a common clonal origin for both.[13,14] The presence of i(12p) has been used diagnostically in patients with midline carcinomas of unknown origin, allowing, in one series, a definitive diagnosis of GCT in 28% of patients, and also serving as a marker of chemotherapy sensitivity (within the group of patients with midline malignancies of uncertain histogenesis).[15,16] The presence of three or more copies of i(12p) has been correlated with poor-prognosis GCT.[17] Other changes in chromosome 12 are seen in GCT. Deletions of the terminal portion of 12q have been observed in up to 44% of patients with GCT and in several GCT cell lines, suggesting the possibility of a tumor suppressor gene in this area.[18]

The gene or genes on i(12p) that could be involved in carcinogenesis have not been identified, although the oncogene c-Ki-ras-2, which is located on i(12p), has been implicated in GCT cell lines.[19] The Cyclin D2 gene has received much attention in both normal testicular development and the pathogenesis of GCT. It has an important role in cellular proliferation, and its expression is tightly regulated throughout the cell cycle. It facilitates passage of cells through the G1 cell-cycle checkpoint. The gene is located on the short arm of chromosome 12 and is overexpressed in nearly all GCTs. Cyclin D2 is therefore a candidate GCT oncogene.[20] Recently, activated mutations in the proto-oncogene c-kit have also been isolated from seminoma specimens.[21] c-kit encodes a transmembrane receptor tyrosine kinase that appears to have a role in normal spermatogenesis, and it is expressed in early fetal germ cells up to (but not beyond) 12 weeks of gestation. In addition, it has also been detected in carcinoma in situ (CIS) and seminoma cells, reflecting a possible role in GCT oncogenesis.[22,23] Epidermal growth factor receptor (EGFR) has also been found to be overexpressed in approximately 25% of the β-human

chorionic gonadotropin (HCG)-expressing component of mixed GCTs.[24] EGFR is a plasma glycoprotein which, after binding to its ligand, activates protein tyrosine kinase activity. This leads to activation of a cascade of biochemical and physiological responses that are involved in the mitogenic signal transduction of both normal and malignant cells.

HISTOLOGY AND NATURAL HISTORY

Overview of Histology

Most primary testicular cancers are of germinal origin and are felt by some to be the malignant counterparts of normal embryonic development. In this model, the normal embryonic development counterpart of seminoma is the spermatocyte, while pluripotential early cleavage-stage tissues are the counterparts of embryonal cell carcinoma. More differentiated malignancies find their normal tissue counterparts in tissues derived from the developing embryo, such as the embryo itself (teratoma), the yolk sac (yolk sac tumors), and the placenta (choriocarcinoma).

A commonly used histologic classification of testicular neoplasms is derived from the Armed Forces Institute of Pathology classification schema of Dixon and Moore,[25] which recognizes pure seminoma along with four other categories, each of which can occur with or without the following seminoma elements:

1. Embryonal carcinoma
2. Teratoma
3. Teratoma with foci of embryonal carcinoma and choriocarcinoma (also termed *teratocarcinoma*)
4. Choriocarcinoma with and without embryonal elements

The World Health Organization (WHO) international classification divides tumors into those of single histologic type (seminoma, spermatocytic seminoma, embryonal carcinoma, choriocarcinoma, teratoma, and yolk sac tumors) and those of more than one type, in which the listing and estimation of relative proportion of each type is required.[26] The major important differences between these two schemas is the recognition by the WHO schema of yolk sac tumors (endodermal sinus tumors) and spermatocytic seminoma as distinct categories (Table 89-1). Representative photomicrographs of various germ cell tumors can be seen in Figure 89-1.

Testicular cancers that are of nongerminal origin include specialized gonadal stromal neoplasms and sarcomas. These, in addition to adenocarcinoma (of the rete testis) and secondary (nonprimary) malignancies such as acute leukemia, lymphoma, carcinoma, and melanoma, comprise less than 5% of testicular neoplasms. The frequency and natural history of specific histologic subtypes are discussed in this chapter and are summarized in Table 89-2.

Overview of Natural History

The natural history of GCT is defined largely by lymphatic spread to the retroperitoneal lymph nodes early in the disease, with hematogenous dissemination developing later. Thus, virtually all GCTs with pulmonary or visceral metastases have concomitant retroperitoneal lymph node involvement. Pure choriocarcinoma is an exception, characterized by early hematogenous dissemination to the lungs, brain, and viscera.[27] The more aggressive biology of nonseminomatous GCT is evidenced by the 60% to 70% of patients with nonseminomatous GCT who will have nodal or other metastatic involvement at presentation, compared with 25% in patients with pure seminomas.[28-30] These figures are somewhat biased, as patients with clini-

TABLE 89-1

Histologic Classification of Testicular Tumors

DIXON AND MOORE	WHO
	Tumors of One Histologic Type
Seminoma	Seminoma
	Spermatocytic seminoma
Embryonal carcinoma	Embryonal carcinoma
	Polyembryoma
Teratoma, adult	Teratoma
	Mature
	Immature
	With malignant transformation
	Yolk sac tumor (embryonal carcinoma, juvenile type; endodermal sinus tumor)
Choriocarcinoma	Choriocarcinoma
	Tumors of More Than One Histologic Type
Teratoma with embryonal carcinoma ("teratocarcinoma")	Embryonal carcinoma with teratoma ("teratocarcinoma")
	Choriocarcinoma and any other types (specify)
	Other combinations (specify)

Adapted from Einhorn LH, Crawford ED, Shipley WU, et al: Cancer of the testes. In Devita VT (ed): Principles and Practice of Oncology, 3rd ed. Philadelphia, JB Lippincott, 1989, with permission.

TABLE 89-2

Frequency and Age Distribution of Germ Cell Tumors

	ALL GCT (%)	PEAK AGE
Histologic Subtype		
Seminoma	40	25–45
Classic and anaplastic	35	25–45
Spermatocytic	5	Average 65
Nonseminoma	60	15–35
Embryonal ± seminoma	24	20–30
Teratoma ± seminoma	5	
Teratoma + embryonal, choriocarcinoma, or both	25	
Choriocarcinoma (pure)	<1	
Yolk sac tumor (pure)	<1	
Site of Origin		
Gonadal	95–99	As above
Extragonadal	1–5	20–35

GCT, germ cell tumor.

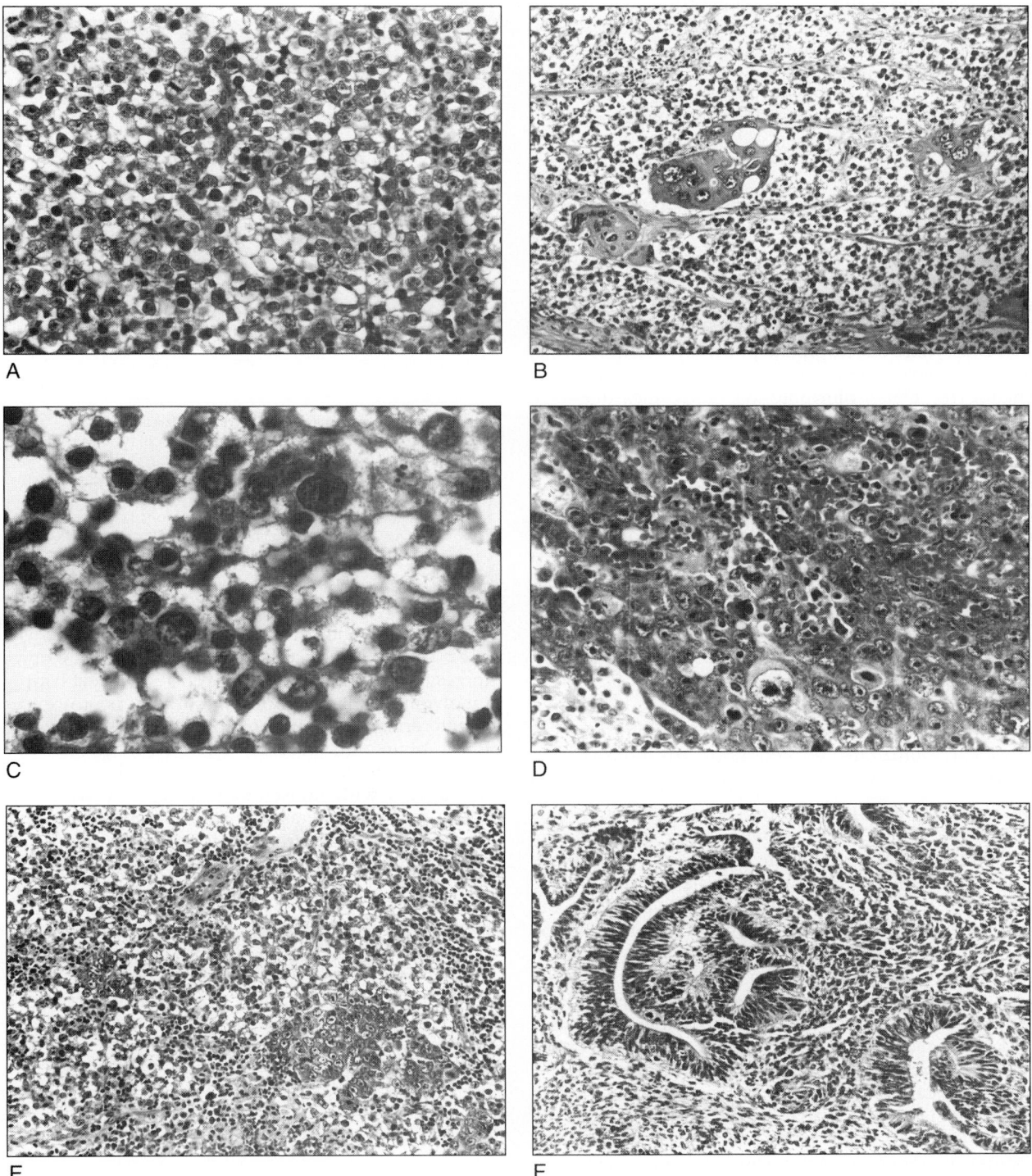

Figure 89-1. Representative histology of germ cell neoplasms. **A**, Classic seminoma. Note uniform cells with central, well-delineated nuclei. Occasional clear spaces represent areas of glycogen deposition. (H&E, ×50) **B**, Seminoma with giant syncytiotrophoblast cells. This histologic pattern may be seen in HCG-positive seminomas. Fibrovascular septae with a lymphoid infiltrate are a typical feature of seminoma. (H&E, ×25) **C**, Spermatocytic seminoma. Distinguished histologically from classic seminoma by relative lack of fibrovascular septae, lymphoid infiltrate, and marked variation of cell size (but not of cell shape). (H&E, ×100) **D**, Embryonal carcinoma. Compare with seminoma **(A)**, note cellular and nuclear pleomorphism and syncytial pattern (loss of cellular borders) (H&E, ×50) **E**, Mixed germ cell tumor, with seminoma and embryonal carcinoma elements. Note fibrovascular septae with lymphoid infiltrate characteristic of seminoma and islands of embryonal carcinoma. (H&E, ×25) **F**, Immature teratoma. Note primitive neural differentiation. (H&E, ×25)

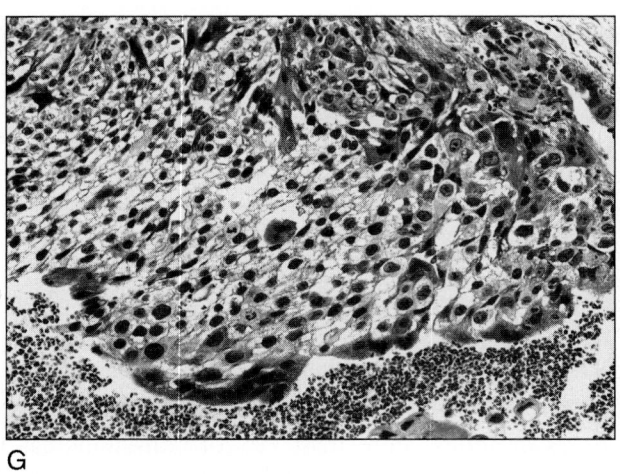

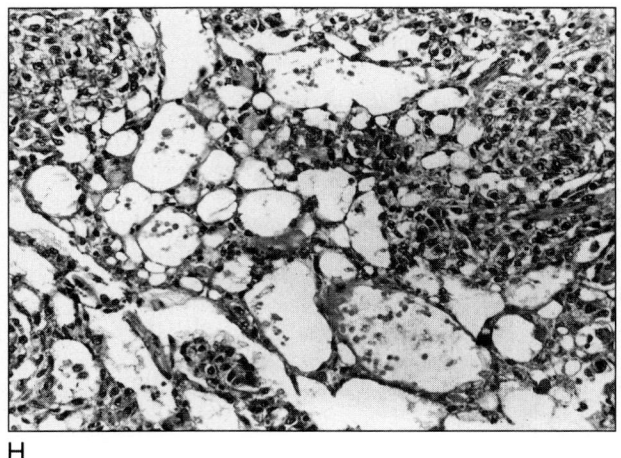

Figure 89-1, *cont'd.* Representative histology of germ cell neoplasms. **G,** Choriocarcinoma. The two cell types required for diagnosis are present. Syncytiotrophoblastic cells (giant cells with hyperchromatic nuclei and abundant eosinophilic cytoplasm) are seen in the upper right quadrant. Cytotrophoblasts (sheets of cells with single nuclei and abundant clear cytoplasm) comprise the midportion of this photomicrograph. Hemorrhagic infiltrate at the bottom of the photomicrograph is common in choriocarcinoma. (H&E, ×25). **H,** Yolk sac tumor, microcystic pattern. (H&E, ×25). (Courtesy of Dr. Noel Weidner, Department of Pathology, University of California, San Francisco.)

cal stage I seminoma (confined to testis) do not routinely undergo pathologic staging with a retroperitoneal lymph node dissection (RPLND), whereas pathologic staging is often undertaken in similar nonseminomatous patients.

Seminoma usually spreads to first-station para-aortic nodes, although (as with nonseminomatous GCT) pelvic nodes can be involved if the scrotal sac has been violated, either by the primary tumor or (in the case of transscrotal exploration) by inguinal surgery.[30-34] Although nodal involvement is less common in seminoma than in NSGCT, ureteral obstruction seems to occur more commonly than in nonseminomas because of either bulky disease or more diffuse, sheetlike spreading.[35] It is extremely unusual for seminomas to present with hepatic or pulmonary metastases; when they do, it is virtually always in the setting of retroperitoneal nodal involvement.

The distribution of retroperitoneal lymph node metastases in nonseminomatous GCT has been described by Ray and colleagues[36] and Donohue and coworkers,[37,38] and provides the basis for the specific surgical and

therapeutic approaches described in this chapter. Figure 89-2 diagrams the anatomy and distribution of retroperitoneal lymph node involvement in GCT. A right-sided testicular primary is most frequently found to have interaortocaval nodal metastases, followed (in order of decreasing frequency) by the precaval and preaortic nodes. Contralateral nodal involvement occurs in 15% of patients, but in virtually every case with contralateral involvement, ipsilateral nodes are involved also. Left testis tumors most frequently have nodal spread to the left para-aortic, preaortic, and interaortocaval nodes, in that order. Suprahilar nodal involvement does not occur in patients with microscopic or low-burden infrahilar disease (stage B1; see the discussion later in this chapter), whereas 25% of patients with gross infrahilar disease have been found to have positive suprahilar nodes.[36] Other nodal metastases are rare but can occur in the external iliac and obturator nodes if the primary tumor invades the epididymis or extends up the spermatic cord, or in inguinal lymph nodes if the tumor extends through the

Figure 89-2. Distribution of retroperitoneal nodal metastases in an early-stage nonseminoma germ cell tumor. **A,** Right; **B,** Left. (From Donohue JP, Sachary FM, Maynard BR: Distribution of nodal metastases in nonseminomatous testicular cancer. J Urol 1982;128:315.)

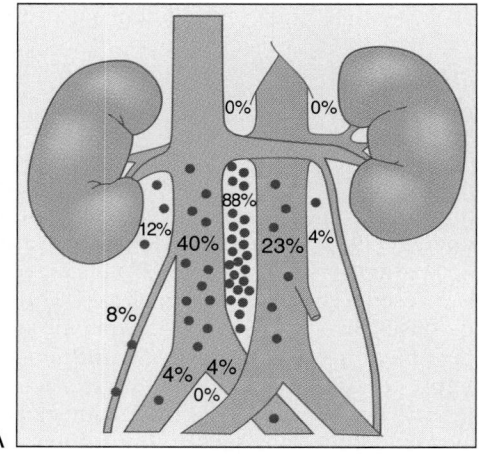

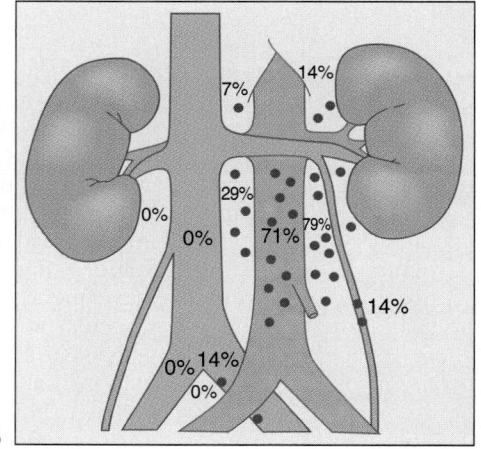

tunica vaginalis to involve the scrotum, or if transscrotal exploration has been used.[39-42]

Seminoma

Seminomas account for 40% of all GCTs. The three distinct histologic patterns that have been described historically are classic seminoma, anaplastic seminoma, and spermatocytic seminoma. A clinical distinction, however, can be made only between classic seminoma and spermatocytic seminoma, and the histologic definition of anaplastic seminoma (more than five mitotic figures per high-power field, cellular anaplasia, and tissue disruption) is of historic interest only, as neither response to therapy nor survival is affected adversely by the presence of anaplastic features.[43,44]

Classic seminoma usually presents in the fourth or fifth decade. It is localized to the testes (stage I) in approximately 70% of patients and is metastatic to lymph nodes (generally stage II) in 25%.[30] Metastases to lymph nodes occur in an orderly, sequential fashion along draining lymph node chains. Visceral metastases are present at presentation in less than 5% of patients, and in general they occur late in the course of the disease. Seminomas tend to appear homogeneous, with little necrosis or hemorrhage on gross inspection. Microscopically, they consist of sheets of uniform cells with large central hyperchromatic nuclei and clear or granular cytoplasm, which are divided by thin fibrous septations. Although lymphocytic infiltration and occasional giant cells may be seen, neoplasms in which any teratomatous or embryonal elements are seen are by definition not considered to be pure seminomas.[25]

Spermatocytic seminoma represents approximately 5% of all seminomas and warrants special consideration. It generally occurs in the sixth decade of life. Although it is more likely than typical seminoma to be bilateral (6% vs. 2%, respectively), it is nonetheless a fairly indolent malignancy in which metastatic events are distinctly uncommon.[45] Spermatocytic seminoma can be distinguished histologically from classic seminoma by the relative lack of compartmentalization of sheets of cells by fibrous septae, by the marked variation in cell size, and by the absence of lymphocytic infiltration.[12]

Embryonal Carcinoma

Pure embryonal carcinomas account for more than 60% of NSGCTs, although foci of embryonal elements can be found in a large majority of NSGCTs. Embryonal carcinoma occurs in 20- to 30-year-olds and is a highly malignant tumor characterized by rapid and bulky growth. In addition to lymphatic spread, these tumors are characterized by hematogenous spread of cancer cells, particularly to lung and liver. More than 60% of patients with embryonal carcinoma have metastases at presentation, and the likelihood of occult nodal metastases in clinical stage I (confined to testis) tumors is a function of the proportion of the tumor that is composed of embryonal carcinoma.[35,39,40,46-49] Furthermore, embryonal carcinoma has been reported to have the highest rate of

venous invasion, lymphatic invasion, and tunica (capsular) invasion in both stage I and II tumors.[48] Embryonal carcinomas exhibit focal necrosis and hemorrhage and are quite variable microscopically. Cellular features of embryonal carcinoma correlate with its more aggressive behavior and include anaplastic cells with embryoid features. Large pleomorphic nuclei, mitotic figures, and multinucleation are common also. Stroma varies from loose to thick and fibrous.[25]

Teratoma and Teratocarcinoma

Mature teratoma has elements of one or more of the three germinal layers that are fully differentiated. Pure teratoma is uncommon and makes up fewer than 5% of GCTs in adults. More than 75% of nonseminomas have been reported to have variable amounts of teratomatous elements, so that "pure" teratomas must be sampled carefully to exclude undifferentiated foci. The term *teratocarcinoma* refers to teratomas in combination with other elements, although some pathologists reserve the term for the combination of teratoma and embryonal carcinoma. When a teratoma has cellular and active stroma with mitotic figures, it is referred to as immature teratoma. Teratomas and teratocarcinomas are composed of solid and cystic spaces on cut surface, with areas of hemorrhage and necrosis. A histologic mix of fully differentiated cartilage, muscle, or epithelial tissue and malignant embryonal elements is seen. Predominant teratomatous features account for one third of teratocarcinomas, while approximately two thirds are mostly composed of nonteratomatous elements.[25] Mature teratoma is the least aggressive of the nonseminoma GCTs, although up to 30% of adult patients with clinical stage I teratoma treated with orchiectomy alone will subsequently relapse, suggesting that pure teratomas should not be exempted from the usual clinical and pathologic staging of GCT or from the usual subsequent therapeutic interventions.[49] The natural history of teratocarcinomas lies somewhere between that of mature teratoma and embryonal carcinoma, but for practical (diagnostic and therapeutic) purposes, teratocarcinomas can be grouped with embryonal cell carcinomas. The likelihood that residual or recurrent masses after treatment are composed of mature teratoma increases among patients with more extensive teratomatous elements at presentation and is discussed later in this chapter.

Choriocarcinoma

Choriocarcinoma is the most aggressive of the nonseminoma GCTs, with early hematogenous dissemination to lungs, liver, brain, and other visceral sites. Pure choriocarcinoma is a very rare disease and has a particularly poor prognosis because of its usual advanced stage at the time of diagnosis. Thus, if pure choriocarcinomas are excluded, the specific histologic subtype of NSGCT does not statistically influence survival. Pure choriocarcinoma is exceedingly rare, accounting for less than 0.5% of all testicular malignancies, but focal areas of choriocarcinoma are seen in approximately 12% of embryonal and terato-

carcinomas.[48] The microscopic diagnosis of choriocarcinoma requires the presence of two cell types—syncytiotrophoblastic cells (giant cells with multiple hyperchromatic nuclei and abundant eosinophilic cytoplasm) and cytotrophoblasts (sheets of cells with single nuclei, abundant clear cytoplasm, and well-defined borders)—arranged in papillary or pseudovillous patterns.[25]

Yolk Sac Tumors

Also known as endodermal sinus tumors, pure yolk sac tumors occur rarely, accounting for 1% of GCTs in adults. More commonly, yolk sac tumors in adults are found in combination with other tumor types, occurring in up to 70% of GCTs. In one series of 459 patients with stage I and II testicular cancer, the most common histology observed was a mixed one consisting of embryonal carcinoma plus yolk sac tumor and teratoma. Furthermore, the presence of teratoma and yolk sac tumor appeared to be associated with a large primary tumor size.[48] Although pure yolk sac tumors are considered conventionally to be more aggressive with early hematogenous distribution, recent histologic reviews have suggested that patients in whom yolk sac tumor elements are present are at lower risk of relapse than patients in whom they are absent.[47,48] The relatively high frequency with which yolk sac tumors and embryonal carcinoma are found together (50% of all tumors in some series) and the extremely rare occurrence of pure yolk sac tumors (1%) make this a difficult conclusion to substantiate.[47] Yolk sac tumors occur more commonly in children, in whom they appear to be a less aggressive histologic subtype.[50] The histology of yolk sac tumors, while characteristic, can be observed in several common patterns. These include a papillary pattern in which Schiller-Duval bodies (a fibrovascular core with a circle of cells around it, vaguely reminiscent of a glomerulus) can be seen, as well as microcystic, glanduloalveolar, and solid patterns.

Stromal Cell Tumors

Derived from the stromal and supporting cells surrounding germ cells, stromal cell tumors consist of Leydig cell tumors, Sertoli cell tumors, and granulosa cell tumors.[51-55] As a group, they account for 3% to 4% of primary testicular tumors but constitute nearly 20% of childhood testicular tumors. Although they are by and large benign, up to 10% can metastasize.[55] Histologic features appear to be useful in predicting the risk of disseminated disease, and management generally consists of orchiectomy and clinical staging with computed tomography (CT) scan, without use of RPLND. These tumors could be estradiol secreting; gynecomastia occurs in 30% of Sertoli cell tumors and in 15% of Leydig cell tumors.

Secondary (Metastatic) Neoplasms

Although the large majority of testicular neoplasms in young men are germ cell tumors, in men over 60 years of age, only 25% of malignancies are of germinal origin. Testicular malignancies in this age group are predominantly lymphomas, although metastases to the testicles—primarily from prostatic adenocarcinoma, lung carcinoma, and melanoma primary tumors—must also be considered.[56,57]

CLINICAL MANIFESTATIONS

The most common presentation of testicular cancer is testicular swelling (73% in one series of 450 patients).[48] A commonly held misconception is that testicular cancers are by and large painless and that painful testicular masses need not be evaluated for malignancy. In fact, testicular pain is a presenting feature of 18% to 46% of patients with GCT.[35,46,48] Acute pain can be associated with torsion of the neoplasm, infarction or bleeding in the tumor, or epididymitis. Signs and symptoms indistinguishable from acute epididymitis have been observed in up to one fourth of patients with testicular neoplasms. Less commonly presenting symptoms include gynecomastia in HCG-producing tumors such as choriocarcinoma (10%), back or flank pain from metastatic disease (10%), and infertility in fewer than 5% of tumors. Approximately 25% of patients with advanced disease have symptoms referable to their metastases, such as back pain.[46,58] This is frequently the presenting symptom in patients with primary retroperitoneal GCT. Pulmonary symptoms including shortness of breath, chest pain, and hemoptysis are rare but can occur in patients with advanced pulmonary disease or primary mediastinal GCT.

The physical examination of the testicles is performed by palpating fully all areas of the testicle between thumb and fingers. Testicular masses are firm to hard, and generally the scrotal sac is normal in appearance unless there is a large mass causing distension. The patient with a testicular mass must have a careful and complete physical exam, including examination for lymphadenopathy, intra-abdominal masses, hepatomegaly, bone tenderness, and pulmonary abnormalities.

The constellation of elicited symptoms and physical exam findings can offer a clue to the histology of a testicular mass. For example, it has been reported that pain more commonly occurrs in patients who have embryonal carcinoma elements in their tumors than in those without that histologic feature (56% vs. 37%; $P < 0.02$). The same study reported a significantly higher incidence of testicular swelling when the primary tumors contained teratoma or yolk sac tumor elements.[48] Primary tumors from patients with seminoma tend to be larger and more homogeneous, with diffuse involvement of the testicle, whereas embryonal and teratomatous elements tend to from smaller, discrete masses. Rapidly growing tumors, particularly those with extranodal dissemination, should raise the possibility of choriocarcinoma. These observations are, of course, no substitute for the appropriate clinical staging and histopathologic evaluation.

In addition to malignancy, the differential diagnosis of a testicular mass includes testicular torsion, hydrocele, varicocele, spermatocele, and epididymitis. Benign hydroceles tend to extend along the spermatic cord and

can be transilluminated. It is prudent to recall, however, that only a small percentage of testicular cancers is associated with hydroceles. Varicoceles occur in the venous pampiniform plexus of the spermatic cord and result in what has been described classically as a "bag of worms" on palpation. Spermatoceles are found in the posterior-superior portion of the scrotum and also transilluminate. As noted previously, testicular cancer is perhaps most often mistaken for epididymitis, which is marked by a swollen, extremely tender testicle with occasional fever and pyuria. Delays in treatment of testicular cancer of up to nine months have been observed as patients are treated for presumed epididymitis. Thus, the clinical diagnosis of epididymitis should prompt both a careful physical examination and ultrasonographic examination of the scrotum, particularly in those patients who fail to respond to a 10-day course of antibiotics.

EVALUATION OF THE PATIENT: DIAGNOSIS, CLINICAL STAGING, AND RISK ASSESSMENT

Diagnosis: Testicular Ultrasonography

The initial evaluation of a testicular mass is ultrasonographic evaluation. Testicular ultrasonography is a sensitive and specific test that can discriminate between a testicular neoplasm and nonmalignant processes included in the differential diagnosis, such as testicular torsion, hydrocele, varicocele, spermatocele, and epididymitis. Thus, the demonstration of hypoechoic or heterogeneous masses on ultrasonographic examination should prompt a thorough subsequent evaluation as will be described subsequently. Similarly, a negative ultrasonogram fairly reliably establishes the absence of intrascrotal GCT.[59-61] The obvious presence of a testicular mass on physical examination does not obviate the need for careful bilateral sonography, given the 2% to 4% incidence of bilateral lesions.[3,4] Extragonadal GCTs are a distinct clinical entity to be described shortly, constituting from 1% to 5% of all GCTs; in these patients, scrotal ultrasonography will be negative.[9]

Diagnosis: Orchiectomy

Any patient with a testicular mass or abnormal ultrasonography, or both, should have testicular carcinoma ruled out by a unilateral radical transinguinal orchiectomy. Orchiectomy is the definitive procedure for both pathologic diagnosis and local control of the primary tumor and in some cases could be a curative procedure.[28-30] Furthermore, important predictive factors that are crucial to risk assessment strategies used in the clinical management of these patients can be identified with routine histologic techniques.[28-30,47-49,62-65] The removal of suspicious testicles by inguinal orchiectomy should be undertaken even in patients in whom a diagnosis of disseminated GCT has been made by biopsy of a metastatic site, as the testes appear to be chemotherapy sanctuaries for cancer cells.[66]

Orchiectomy delay for up to two cycles of chemotherapy is occasionally indicated when control of metastatic disease must be obtained urgently. Although some debate remains, it appears that there exists a blood-testis barrier, so that viable GCTs can persist in the testis despite complete eradication of cancer from metastatic deposits by chemotherapy. Orchiectomy should therefore always be performed once control of metastatic disease is achieved.[67-69] Patients with a diagnosis of extragonadal GCT with normal testicular examinations and ultrasonograms need not undergo orchiectomy. Each testicle is evaluated and considered separately, so that in the 2% to 4% of patients with bilateral tumors, bilateral inguinal orchiectomies must be performed.[42] Transscrotal orchiectomies or needle biopsies are contraindicated absolutely, as they have been associated with up to 24% incidence of local recurrence or spread to inguinal lymph nodes.[42,70,71] Nonetheless, it is known that scrotal orchiectomy does not necessarily portend decreased survival if the patient is treated with aggressive local therapy (surgical resection of the inguinal portion of the spermatic cord in the event of a previous scrotal orchiectomy, and hemiscrotectomy or groin and scrotal irradiation for patients with NSGCT and seminoma, respectively, in whom a prior transscrotal biopsy has been undertaken) and careful follow-up. Patients who will be receiving chemotherapy do not require these local procedures, as chemotherapy protects against scrotal recurrence.[72,73]

Clinical Staging and Risk Assessment

The first step after the histologic confirmation of a GCT is to determine the extent of the disease (staging) so that appropriate therapy may be undertaken. An assessment of risk of metastases (in the case of local disease), or response to systemic therapy (in the case of advanced disease), utilizing the results of histopathologic, biochemical, and radiographic evaluations, should be an integral element of the staging process; such assessment is discussed in detail for each stage.

Tumor Markers

Tumor markers have become a fundamental component of the laboratory evaluation of patients with suspected testicular neoplasms, offering both diagnostic, staging, and prognostic information, as well as measuring disease progression and response to therapy.[74] Thus, along with the usual laboratory studies obtained for patients with suspected GCT, preorchiectomy levels of βHCG, AFP, and LDH are mandatory.

HCG is a glycoprotein of 45,000 MW. It consists of two covalently linked subunits, an α-subunit shared by luteinizing hormone (LH), follicle-stimulating hormone (FSH), and thyroid-stimulating hormone, and a unique β-subunit (β-HCG), which can be measured readily in serum. Although it normally is produced at high levels by the placenta, low levels are detectable in normal nonpregnant adults, including some men. HCG elevations are seen in neoplasms other than GCTs, including prostate, bladder,

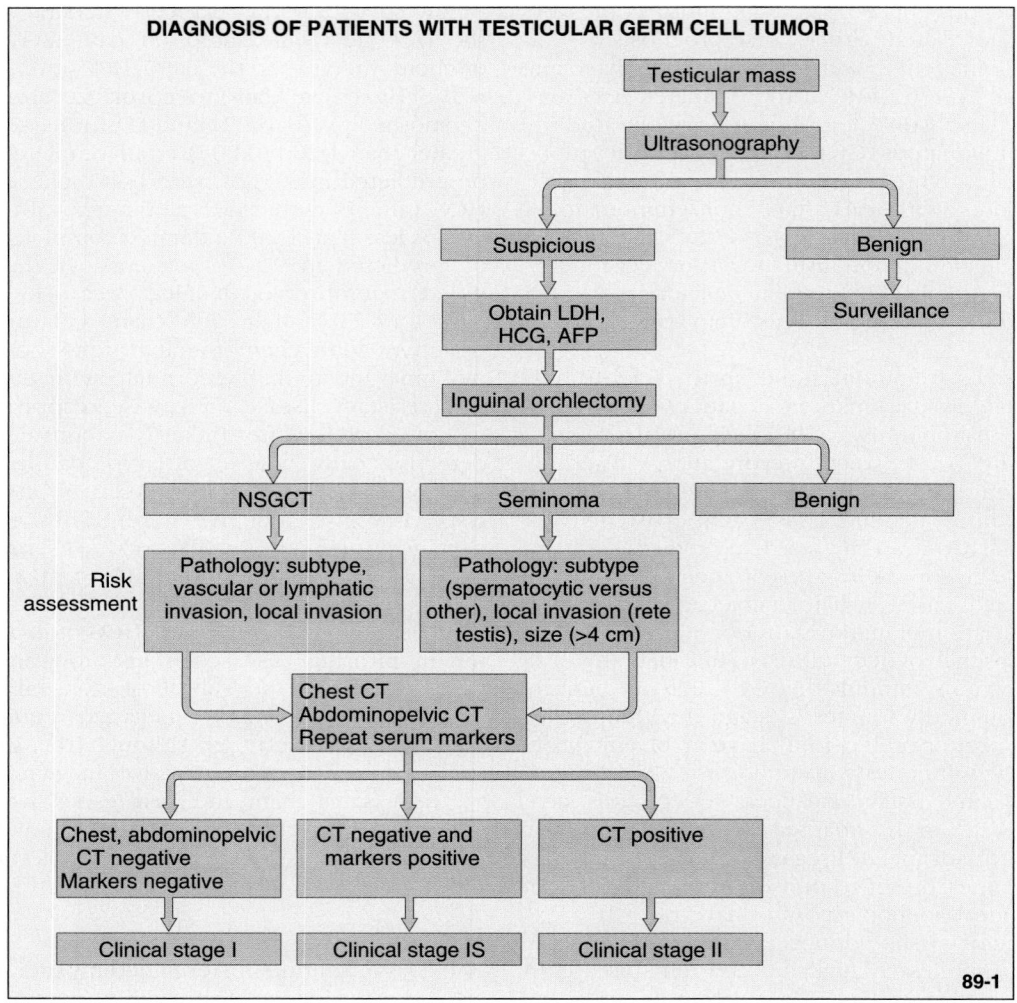

DIAGNOSIS OF PATIENTS WITH TESTICULAR GERM CELL TUMOR

89-1

ureteral, and renal cancers.[75-77] Spurious elevations have been noted in patients using marijuana.[78] Some patients who have undergone systemic therapy develop cisplatinum–induced testicular atrophy in the remaining testis, resulting in lower levels of testosterone, with a compensatory hypersecretion of LH to stimulate Leydig cell secretion of testosterone. Although HCG and LH are not immunologically cross-reactive, very high levels of LH might spuriously elevate measured HCG levels. When necessary, measurement of HCG levels 2 weeks after the administration of depotestosterone should rule out this possibility.[46] The biologic half-life of serum HCG is approximately 24 hours. In germ cell tumors, HCG is produced by syncytiotrophoblastic cells in embryonal carcinoma, choriocarcinoma, and seminoma. Extremely high levels of HCG are generally associated with choriocarcinoma. Although seminomas are generally felt to be marker negative, the incidence of HCG-positive seminoma varies from 5% to 40%. In general, these HCG elevations do not exceed a level of 100 mIU/mL and probably do not connote a worse prognosis.[79-86]

α-Fetoprotein (AFP) is a glycoprotein that is the major serum protein of the fetus. It is also an oncofetal protein, found not only in patients with nonseminomatous GCT but also in pregnant women (fetal hepatic production), in patients with hepatocellular carcinoma, and occasionally (at somewhat lower levels) in patients with cirrhotic livers demonstrating nodular regeneration or in patients with hepatitis. Its biologic half-life is 4 to 6 days. AFP elevations are most commonly seen in embryonal carcinoma and yolk sac tumors, with reports of up to 89% of tumors with yolk sac elements demonstrating elevated AFP.[48] Pure seminomas and pure choriocarcinomas do not produce AFP. Thus, in the absence of hepatitis or other causes of AFP, by definition the presence of an elevated AFP in a histologically pure seminoma identifies the presence of nonseminomatous elements and mandates that the management proceed accordingly.

Lactate dehydrogenase (LDH) is a nonspecific marker that appears to be related to tumor burden and that can serve as both an indicator of response to treatment and as a predictor of prognosis.[87] Interestingly, the gene for LDH isoenzyme 1 maps to chromosome 12, and the serum level of LDH isoenzyme 1 has been shown to correlate with the number of copies of i(12p) in the tumor, a fairly specific genetic marker of germ cell malignancies.[88]

Furthermore, the presence of three or more copies of i(12p) has been correlated with a worse prognosis.[17]

Overall, approximately 85% of nonseminomas have an elevation of either AFP or β-HCG; approximately 15% are marker negative.[76,89,90] AFP elevation alone is elevated in 40% of nonseminomatous GCTs, and β-HCG elevation alone is seen in 50% to 60%. It is important to note that up to 30% of patients with early-stage nonseminomatous GCTs have normal serum markers, so the absence of marker elevation should not influence the decision to perform an orchiectomy.[91] The incidence of serum marker elevation as a function of tumor histology is shown in Table 89-3.

Even though most seminomas and up to 15% of non-seminomatous GCTs are marker negative, AFP, LDH, and β-HCG levels should always be checked before and after orchiectomy. The correct interpretation of serum marker levels requires that the biologic half-life of AFP and HCG be taken into account. Thus, the persistence of elevated AFP or β-HCG levels higher than predicted by the half-lives of these glycoproteins after orchiectomy implies residual (occult) disease.[28,46] The converse, however, is not true: Normalization of markers after orchiectomy does not ensure the absence of occult disease. In fact, up to 60% of patients with nonseminomatous GCT felt on clinical grounds to be confined to the testis (stage I) with normal-ization of markers after orchiectomy have involvement of retroperitoneal lymph nodes with tumor.[28,29,47-49,62-65] The management of clinical stage I cancers reflects this fact and is discussed later in this chapter.

In patients with advanced disease, serum markers also can be used as a measure of response to therapy. Patients with retroperitoneal adenopathy who have been treated by lymphadenectomy should normalize their markers; failure to do so implies residual or recurrent disease.[28] The response of advanced GCT to chemotherapy can also be monitored by a fall in serum markers. In this situation, however—unlike the postorchiectomy or post-RPLND setting—tumor debulking is not instantaneous. Thus, the use of known half-lives to calculate the expected decay of levels of serum tumor markers is more difficult. A 10-fold decrease in the HCG level over a 3-week period has been observed empirically to be consistent with disease eradication.[46] Other investigators have shown that a durable complete response to chemotherapy could be predicted with a high degree of accuracy by the ratio of the HCG level measured on day 22 (after one cycle of chemotherapy) to the day 1 HCG level. In this schema, if the HCG level fails to normalize after one cycle of chemotherapy (day 22), and if the day-22/day-1 ratio is greater than 1:200 (0.005), an incomplete response could be predicted in 94% of patients. Conversely, if the day-22 HCG value is within normal range, or if the day-22/day-1 ratio is less than 1:200, a durable complete response could be predicted in 91% of patients.[92] Other reports have noted that observed half-life decays of greater than 7 days for AFP and greater than 4 days for HCG after treatment with chemotherapy are associated with poor outcome and probably correlate with the emergence of drug-resistant disease.[92] Likewise, reappearance of serum marker elevation after therapy is an invaluable method of detecting early relapse, often predating any radiologic evidence of relapse or recurrence.[46,93] On occasion, tumor lysis with chemotherapy will result in transient "flares" or rises in serum markers followed by a subsequent decline. The prognostic implications of such flares are not well understood.[94]

Measurements of AFP and β-HCG offer an excellent tool for monitoring disease progression and response to therapy so that the subset of nonseminomatous GCT patients who are marker negative requires particularly careful clinical scrutiny. Although the vast majority of seminomas are marker negative, in general their phenotype is less malignant, and their responsiveness to therapy is extremely high, making the usual absence of biochemical markers of disease less troublesome.

Radiologic Evaluation

The goal of routine postorchiectomy radiographic studies is to detect evidence of spread to the retroperitoneum and lungs. Accordingly, all patients with GCT should undergo CT of the chest, abdomen, and pelvis. Although some investigators have reported a 10% higher detection of metastatic disease by chest CT (compared with chest radiography), the value of the increased sensitivity of tomography has been disputed.[46] In one series of 120 patients staged with both chest radiograph and whole-lung tomograms, tomography led to a change in therapy in only one patient (0.8%).[95] Nonetheless, while interval

TABLE 89-3

Germ Cell Tumors and Serum Markers			
HISTOLOGY	MARKER NEGATIVE (%)	ELEVATED HCG ALONE (%)	ELEVATED AFP ALONE (%)
Seminoma	90	10 (usually <100 IU/mL)	0 (if +, by definition, NSGCT)
All NSGCT	15	50–60	40
Embryonal		0	10–40
Yolk sac tumors		Rare	80–90 (alone or with elevated HCG)
Choriocarcinoma (or syncytiotrophoblast elements)		>90 (level can be very high)	0

AFP, α-fetoprotein; HCG, human chorionic gonadotropin; NSGCT, nonseminoma germ cell tumor.

changes in the size of pulmonary nodules as a response to therapy can be monitored with a chest radiograph, many investigators recommend that the radiographic evaluation of pulmonary nodules for the purpose of initial staging, final documentation of response to therapy, and subsequent follow-up, should consist of a chest CT. Caution is warranted in the interpretation of chest CT scans of patients who have received bleomycin, as subclinical pulmonary fibrosis can have the appearance of metastatic nodules.[96,97] A comparison of chest CT scans before and after chemotherapy is usually all that is required for the distinction of progression of pulmonary nodules from bleomycin effects, obviating the need for biopsy.

No consensus exists as to the optimal method of staging retroperitoneal disease in GCTs. By and large, however, abdominal and pelvic CT has replaced the need for pedal lymphangiography (LAG), which produces considerably more morbidity and is also operator dependent.[46] Some radiation therapy centers require LAG for simulation and planning of fields (see the later discussion). In patients with nonseminomatous GCT, abdominopelvic CT understaging (false negatives) occurs in as high as 50% of patients, whereas overstaging (false positives) occurs in approximately 10% of patients.[28,29,47,48,62-65] Although LAG offers the advantage of demonstrating internal nodal architecture, a review of the literature found the sensitivity (about 72%) and the specificity (about 85%) to be the same with either LAG or CT in series in which histologic confirmation was obtained in all cases. A lower false-negative rate may be achieved with the combination of CT and LAG (sensitivity as high as 90%), although it appears to be at the expense of a higher false-positive rate (specificity as low as 63%) and is justified (but not required) only in the case of surveillance protocols for stage I NSGCT.[28] The sensitivity and specificity of abdominal CT for detecting lymph node metastases in patients with clinical stage I disease (testis-only disease) has been recently evaluated.[99] Using a cutoff of 10 mm or larger, a sensitivity of 37% and a specificity of 100% were observed, whereas if a 4-mm cutoff was used, sensitivity was greatly enhanced (93%) at the cost of decreased specificity (58%).

The exact incidence of occult retroperitoneal lymph node metastases in patients with seminoma who have normal CT or LAG evaluations (or both) is not known because these patients are typically treated with radiation therapy and do not undergo surgical exploration. Nonetheless, an estimated incidence of occult nodal metastases of 10% to 25% is generally accepted.[30,99,100]

More recently, FDG-PET [fluor-18-labeled deoxyglucose (FDG) positron emission tomography (PET)] has been used to identify viable cancer in residual postchemotherapy masses. Sensitivity and specificity of 88% and 95%, respectively, have been reported, along with high positive and negative predictive values (90% and 96%) in two multicenter trials.[101,102] Thus, FDG-PET could be a useful modality in evaluating postchemotherapy masses. By contrast, the utility of FDG-PET in the initial staging of GCT patients is less clear. Several reports including more than 110 patients evaluated the accuracy of FDG-PET compared with CT scan staging in patients with stage I and II GCTs. Sensitivity and specificity were reported as 73% to 94% and 40% to 78%, respectively. Moreover, FDG-PET was unable to detect either mature teratomas or lesions smaller than 5 mm in diameter.[103-105] Hence, FDG-PET is not used routinely or recommended as initial staging for stage I–II GCTs.

In summary, the major limitation of CT imaging is that although gross nodal disease can usually be detected, this is not the case for microscopic metastases. For this reason, an assessment of the risk of occult retroperitoneal nodal involvement based on histopathologic features is of importance and is described shortly.

Other imaging modalities, such as head CT and bone scan, are not undertaken routinely except as warranted by symptoms. One exception to this rule is for choriocarcinoma, in which an increased incidence of brain metastases mandates head CT.[27] Similarly, in patients with serum marker–positive GCT who have relapsed by serum markers but have a negative physical examination and a negative imaging evaluation consisting of an ultrasonogram of the contralateral testicle and abdominopelvic and chest CT, it is not unreasonable to complete the evaluation with a head CT and a bone scan.[99]

Staging

Several schemas are incorporated in the current staging of GCT. Lymphadenectomy is almost never undertaken as a primary therapeutic modality in seminoma, so it is staged clinically. Until recently, the standard treatment of nonseminomatous tumors has included a RPLND, so that most patients with nonseminomatous GCT were staged pathologically. Because up to 80% of patients with carefully staged clinical stage I nonseminomatous GCT tumors have been found to be free of retroperitoneal disease, some patients with clinical stage I nonseminomatous GCTs have been offered observation in lieu of lymphadenectomy (see later discussion). A clear distinction must be made in these patients (and in all patients with nonseminomatous GCTs) between clinical stage and pathologic stage. The development of an international consensus GCT risk classification schema has allowed the use of prognostic groupings as the basis of a revised staging classification. This revised (1997) TNM American Joint Committee on Cancer/Union Internationale Contre le Cancer (AJCC/UICC) classification (Table 89-4) continues to rely on anatomic disease extent and allows for the pathologic classification of lymph nodes, but for the first time, it also takes into account serum tumor markers. Patients who have only serologic marker evidence of disease are now classified as stage I-S.[106]

In general, stage I (or A) refers to tumors confined to the testis, with no evidence of nodal or pulmonary parenchymal involvement. Stage II (or B) denotes tumors with retroperitoneal lymph node metastases. Stage II patients are further subdivided by the relative tumor burden. In seminoma patients, burden is defined clinically by the size of nodal involvement detected by imaging studies, whereas in nonseminomatous GCT this is usually (but not always) a pathologic diagnosis. Stage IIA (or B1) implies minimal but definite nodal involvement, generally

TABLE 89-4

 TNM Classifications of Testis Tumors

Primary Tumor (pT)

The extent of primary tumor is classified after radical orchiectomy

pT	Primary tumor cannot be assessed (if no radical orchietomy has been performed TX is used)
pT0	No evidence of primary tumor (e.g., histologic scar in testis)
pTis	Intratubular germ cell neoplasia (carcinoma in situ)
pT1	Tumor limited to testis and epididymis without vascular/lymphatic invasion Tumor may invade into tunica albuginea but not tunica vaginalis
pT2	Tumor limited to testis and epididymis with vascular/lymphatic invasion, or tumor extending through tunica albuginea with involvement of tunica vaginalis
pT3	Tumor invades spermatic cord with or without vascular/lymphatic invasion
pT4	Tumor invades scrotum with or without vascular/lymphatic invasion

Regional Lymph Nodes (N)

Clinical

NX	Regional lymph nodes cannot be assessed
N0	No regional lymph node metastasis
N1	Metastasis with a lymph node mass 2 cm or less in greatest dimension; or multiple lymph nodes, none more than 2 cm in greatest dimension
N2	Metastasis with a lymph node mass more than 2 cm or less than 5 cm in greatest dimension; or multiple lymph nodes, any one mass more than 2 cm, but not more than 5 cm in greatest dimension
N3	Metastasis with a lymph node mass more than 5 cm in greatest dimension

Pathologic Classification of Regional Lymph Nodes (pN)

pNX	Regional lymph nodes cannot be assessed
pN0	No regional lymph node metastasis
pN1	Metastasis with a lymph node mass 2 cm or less in greatest dimension and 5 or fewer positive nodes, none more than 2 cm in greatest dimension
pN2	Metastasis with a lymph node mass, more than 2 cm but not more than 5 cm in greatest dimension; or more than 5 nodes positive, none more than 5 cm; or evidence of extranodal extension of tumor
pN3	Metastasis with a lymph node mass more than 5 cm in greatest dimension

Distant Metastasis (M)

MX	Distant metastasis cannot be assessed
M0	No distant metastasis
M1	Distant metastasis
M1a	Nonregional lymph node or pulmonary metastasis
M1b	Nonpulmonary visceral metastasis

Serum Tumor Markers (S)

SX	Marker studies not available or not performed
S0	Marker study levels within normal limits
S1	LDH <1.5 × normal and HCG (mIU/mL) <5000 and AFP (ng/mL) <1000
S2	LDH 1.5–10 × normal or HCG (mIU/mL) 5000–50,000 or AFP (ng/mL) 1000–10,000
S3	LDH >10 × normal or HCG (mIU/mL) >50,000 or AFP (ng/mL) >10,000

N indicates the upper limit of normal for the LDH assay

Staging Grouping

Stage 0	pTis	N0	M0	S0, SX
Stage I	pT1-4	N0	M0	SX
Stage IA	pT1	N0	M0	S0
Stage IB	pT2	N0	M0	S0
	pT3	N0	M0	S0
	pT4	N0	M0	S0
Stage IS	Any pT/Tx	N0	M0	S1–3
Stage II	Any pT/Tx	N1–3	M0	SX
Stage IIA	Any pT/Tx	N1	M0	S0
	Any pT/Tx	N1	M0	S1
Stage IIB	Any pT/Tx	N2	M0	S0
	Any pT/Tx	N2	M0	S1
Stage IIC	Any pT/Tx	N3	M0	S0
	Any pT/Tx	N3	M0	S1
Stage III	Any pT/Tx	Any N	M1, M1a	SX
Stage IIIA	Any pT/Tx	Any N	M1, M1a	S0
	Any pT/Tx	Any N	M1, M1a	S1
Stage IIIB	Any pT/Tx	N1–3	M0	S2
	Any pT/Tx	Any N	M1, M1a	S2
Stage IIIC	Any pT/Tx	N1–3	M0	S3
	Any pT/Tx	Any N	M1, M1a	S3
	Any pT/Tx	Any N	M1b	Any S

From American Joint Committee on Cancer: Manual for Staging of Cancer, 6th ed. New York, Springer-Verlag, 2002, with permission.

TABLE 89-5

Royal Marsden Clinical Staging Schema for Seminoma

STAGE	DEFINITION
I	Confined to testis
IIA	Abdominal nodal disease: <2 cm
IIB	Abdominal nodal disease: 2–5 cm
IIC	Abdominal nodal disease: >5 cm
III	Supradiaphragmatic nodal disease
IV	Extranodal disease

From American Joint Committee on Cancer: Manual for Staging of Cancer, 5th ed. Philadelphia, JB Lippincott, 1997, with permission.

of a microscopic nature; stage IIB (or B2) refers to macroscopic disease or a larger number of microscopic metastases, while stage IIC (or B3) indicates bulky retroperitoneal nodal disease. Stage III (or C) refers to disease that has spread beyond the retroperitoneum, usually to supradiaphragmatic lymph nodes, pulmonary parenchyma, or other sites including liver, bone, or brain. Some staging schemas, particularly those for seminoma, distinguish between stage III (supradiaphragmatic lymph nodes) and stage IV (any extranodal metastases, including pulmonary parenchyma, bone, and brain) (Table 89-5). The distinction of hepatic, central nervous system, and osseous metastases is not without merit, as patients with metastases to these regions clearly have a worsened prognosis.

MANAGEMENT OF LOW-STAGE DISEASE

The management of clinical stage I GCT is in part dependent on an assessment of the risk of occult nodal metastases. This assessment is in turn based on clinicopathologic features of the primary tumor, including serum marker elevation, size and extent of disease, and histologic features. Pure seminoma and NSGCT are considered separately.

Clinical Stage I Seminoma

Risk Assessment
A histologic diagnosis of pure seminoma implies an excellent prognosis. Pure seminoma is exquisitely sensitive to radiation therapy and can be sterilized readily by relatively low doses (25–35 Gy) of external-beam irradiation.[30] Consequently, prognostic factors are difficult to analyze in patients with early-stage seminoma, as the prognosis is so good that treatment failure is uncommon.

Prognostic factors that have been postulated as predictors of outcome include DNA ploidy status, mitotic rate, DNA S-phase percentage, presence of syncytiotrophoblasts, degree of lymphocytic infiltration of the primary tumor, and the expression of β-HCG and low-molecular-weight keratin on immunohistochemical analyses. None of these factors has been confirmed in prospective trials, however.[43,44,79-86] The utility of serum markers in seminoma patients is limited to the identification of nonseminomatous elements by an elevated AFP, even in the face of a histologic diagnosis of pure seminoma. Ten percent of pure seminoma patients will have an elevated β-HCG. By and large, this feature does not appear to connote a worse prognosis in stage I patients.[79-86]

For patients with stage I seminoma managed by surveillance (see the "Treatment" section), approximately 20% of patients will relapse. A pooled analysis of data from four surveillance series identified size of primary tumor (>4 cm) and rete testis invasion as independent predictors of relapse. Although previous studies suggested that patients under 30 years of age were at higher risk of relapse, this was not observed in this pooled analysis.[107] An increased incidence of pelvic nodal involvement is also seen in patients who have had previous inguinal surgery, or in whom the primary tumor has invaded scrotal skin. Scrotal skin involvement also predisposes to relapse in the hemiscrotum.[31-33] Finally, tumor invasion of the spermatic cord increases the risk of relapse in the inguinal orchiectomy scar.[34]

Treatment
Cancer confined to the testis is the most common presentation of seminoma, accounting for nearly 70% of all patients with this diagnosis.[28,30] For the last half century, the traditional management of these patients after an orchiectomy has consisted of radiation therapy to the para-aortic and pelvic (retroperitoneal) lymph nodes. Recent surveillance studies (to be described shortly) suggest that approximately 15% of clinical stage I seminoma patients in fact have occult retroperitoneal disease, indicating that the common practice of nodal irradiation is not unreasonable.

Conventional radiation fields for clinical stage I seminoma treat the para-aortic nodes from the diaphragm at the level of the T10 vertebral body down to the lower border of the L4 vertebral body, including the ipsilateral common iliac and external iliac nodes.[107] If pelvic nodes could be involved, the field is extended to include the ipsilateral inguinofemoral lymph nodes. Spermatic cord involvement necessitates a radiation field that covers the entire inguinal orchiectomy scar, while scrotal skin involvement mandates radiation to the hemiscrotum.[28,30-34]

The results of adjuvant radiation therapy in clinical stage I seminoma patients have been reviewed.[28,30] Most centers treat patients with 25 to 35 Gy to the retroperitoneal nodes in 15 to 20 fractions over a period of 3 to 4 weeks. In more than 2000 patients reported, the cause-specific 5-year survival is 97%. Most relapses occur within 2 years, and almost always within 5 years of treatment. Failures within the irradiated volume are extraordinarily uncommon; most relapses occur in the mediastinum, supraclavicular and cervical lymph nodes, or lung. Isolated recurrences might respond well to radiation therapy, although most radiation failures can be salvaged with systemic chemotherapy since the advent of cisplatinum-based chemotherapy. Prophylactic mediastinal and supraclavicular irradiation has been used as a means of reducing relapses in these regions, but has not been shown to confer a survival advantage.[108]

The side effects of the low doses of radiotherapy required for the treatment of stage I seminoma, discussed next, are mild and include mild nausea, possibly peptic ulcer disease, transient oligospermia, and a modest but measurable increase in the risk of subsequent (secondary) malignancies. The possibility of reducing both early and late radiation-associated toxicity, coupled with the availability of salvage therapy with excellent results, is the impetus behind the evaluation of lower doses of radiation as well as surveillance as a therapeutic option in clinical stage I seminoma. For example, the use of 26 Gy to the para-aortic region with the omission of iliac radiation results in a relapse rate of 3.7%, with only 0.8% isolated ipsilateral iliac responses and has been advocated by some to be appropriate therapy.[109]

Several large studies have evaluated the role of surveillance in patients with stage I seminoma, with similar results.[110-112] The risk of relapse within the first year is 5% to 10%, 10% to 15% in the second year, and 15% to 20% by the third year. As noted previously, two adverse prognostic factors can identify patients at high risk of relapse: tumor diameter greater than 4 cm and rete testis involvement. In a pooled analysis, the 5-year relapse-free survival for patients with 0 or 1 risk factors was 83% to 88%, whereas patients with two adverse factors had a 5-year relapse-free survival of 69%.[107] These data have allowed an estimation of the frequency of occult nodal metastases in clinical stage I seminoma. The most common site of relapse has been the para-aortic lymph nodes, with rare intrathoracic relapses. Despite these relapses, salvage therapy with either radiation or systemic therapy has been extremely successful, resulting in a cause-specific survival identical to historical experience with conventional radiotherapy (95%–100%).[110-113]

There is no consensus regarding the optimal follow-up protocol for seminoma surveillance. In general, patients are seen at 3- to 4-month intervals for 3 to 4 years, every 6 months for another 2 to 3 years, and then annually. At each visit, a clinical assessment, CT scan of the abdomen and pelvis, chest x-ray or chest CT, and serum markers are obtained.[112]

One or two cycles of single-agent carboplatin have also been explored as adjuvant therapy. An initial report by Oliver and colleagues[114] indicated that one cycle of adjuvant carboplatin appeared to be sufficient therapy. On the other hand, Dieckmann and coworkers[115] recently reported an 8.6% relapse rate in 93 patients treated with a single dose of carboplatin (400 mg/m²). By contrast, 32 patients who received two courses of carboplatin remain disease free after a 45-month follow-up period, suggesting that one cycle of carboplatin might not be sufficient when compared with adjuvant radiation therapy. A retrospective analysis of 107 stage I seminoma patients treated with two cycles of adjuvant carboplatin dosed at 400 mg/m² indicated no relapses with a median follow-up of 12 years (74 months, range 5–145 months).[116] No neurotoxicity, ototoxicity, or nephrotoxicity was observed, and hematologic toxicity was minimal (no grade 3 or 4 toxicity, with only 2% of patients experiencing grade 2 leukopenia). Although surveillance or adjuvant chemotherapy results are encouraging, these therapies still require large-scale

prospective randomized trials to assess their efficacy, as decades of experience have proven radiation therapy to be extremely efficacious and relatively nonmorbid, and no data exist comparing long-term risks of low-dose chemotherapy with those of radiation therapy.

Clinical Stage I Nonseminoma

Risk Assessment

Controversy over the optimal management of clinical stage I nonseminomatous GCT has prompted a search for prognostic factors that can be used to predict the risk of occult nodal involvement. Histologic subtype, local tumor extension, and vascular or lymphatic invasion have all been shown to correlate with occult nodal metastases (pathologic stage IIA) or a high risk of relapse (summarized in Table 89-6).

Several studies have identified histologic evidence of vascular or lymphatic invasion in the primary tumor as a predictor of either relapse or occult nodal involvement in clinical stage I patients who were followed after orchiectomy with surveillance or treated with RPLND. In patients with clinical stage I NSGCT, the Testicular Cancer Intergroup Study observed venous or lymphatic invasion in 23.6% and 9.2% of specimens, respectively, and in 55% and 45%, respectively, of specimens from patients with clinical stage II disease. Not only was vascular invasion more common in node-positive patients than in node-negative patients, but in node-negative patients treated with orchiectomy and RPLND alone, relapse was noted in 10 of 168 patients (6%) who demonstrated no vascular invasion, compared with 12 of 62 patients (19.4%) if vascular invasion were present.[48] Other studies have confirmed the significance of vascular or lymphatic invasion as a predictor of occult nodal metastases or relapse, either alone or in combination with other variables.[36,47,49,62,63,65] A British study of 259 clinical stage I nonseminomatous GCT patients identified invasion of veins or lymphatics, along with two histologic features (presence of embryonal carcinoma and absence of yolk sac tumor) as four factors most predictive of relapse. If three or four features were present, the likelihood of relapse or occult nodal involvement was 58%; patients with two positive risk factors had a 24% chance of relapse, whereas patients with zero or one risk factor relapsed only 9% of the time.[47] A Swedish/Norwegian study identified vascular invasion, absence of AFP before orchiec-

TABLE 89-6

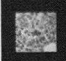 **Clinical Features Associated with High Risk of Occult Nodal Involvement in Clinical Stage I Nonseminomatous Germ Cell Tumors**

Vascular/lymphatic invasion
Embryonal carcinoma elements (>30%)
Absence of yolk sac elements
Absence of AFP preorchiectomy
Less than 50% teratoma
Local extension into paratesticular structures

See text for findings of individual studies.

tomy, or high T stage as predictive factors that identified high-risk patients with clinical stage I nonseminomatous GCT. For example, risk of relapse in AFP-negative patients was 77% if vascular invasion was present and 38% if no vascular invasion was noted.[62] In a Danish study, patients with vascular invasion had a risk of relapse of 36%, compared with patients with no vascular invasion, whose relapse rate was 13%.[63]

Another significant observation from the Testicular Cancer Intergroup Study was the confirmation that the presence of embryonal carcinoma clearly increased the risk of recurrence. Although this fact had been pointed out by other reports, the Testicular Cancer Intergroup Study demonstrated this relationship in 321 patients with either stage I or II nonseminomatous GCT who were treated with orchiectomy and lymphadenectomy only (Figure 89-3).[117] In general, the risk of relapse remained low until the percentage of embryonal carcinoma exceeded 30% to 40%. In this series, however, the percentage of embryonal carcinoma was not found to be a significant prognostic factor after adjustment for either vascular invasion or nodal stage.[48] Another large series of 292 patients with clinical stage I NSGCT suggested that embryonal carcinoma-predominant tumors were both more likely to have occult positive lymph nodes (32% vs. 15.6%) and were also considerably more likely to relapse after RPLND (21% vs. 3%).[118]

The absence of yolk sac elements is felt to be a marker of poor prognosis in patients with stage I NSGCT. The confirmation by the Testicular Cancer Intergroup Study that AFP production is linked to yolk sac histology suggests that the identification of AFP negativity as a marker of poor prognosis in stage I NSGCT is a reflection of the fact that yolk sac tumor histology appears to confer some benefit to these patients.[47,48,62] Fung and associates[41] have confirmed in their series of 60 nonseminomatous

GCTs the importance of vascular invasion as a negative prognostic marker but also have identified tumors with less than 50% teratoma as having a higher likelihood of relapse.

Local extension of tumor into paratesticular structures also appears to be predictive of higher relapse rates. Whereas some studies have noted higher relapse rates in patients with invasion of any structures outside the testis (rete testis, tunica albuginea, epididymis, or spermatic cord), others have noted that tumor involvement of only certain paratesticular structures carried an increased risk of relapse.[39,41] Thus, Sesterhenn and colleagues[48] report a 42% vs. 16% relapse rate after RPLND in stage I and II patients with and without tunica albuginea involvement. Other studies have suggested that involvement of the rete and epididymis (but not the tunica albuginea or spermatic cord) were associated with a higher risk of relapse.[40] Recent studies suggest that negative immunohistochemical staining with an antibody against the Ki-67 receptor, a marker of tumor proliferation, identifies a good risk population with a negative predictive value for occult nodal involvement of 88%, although this has not been confirmed by others.[118-120]

A variety of other factors have been shown to have no prognostic value. Increased levels of preorchiectomy β-HCG and AFP, the size of the primary tumor, or the side of the primary (right vs.left) do not appear to carry prognostic weight.[28,39-41]

Treatment

Clinical stage I NSGCTs account for approximately 50% of all NSGCTs.[121] Pathologic staging reduces this number to approximately 40%. The evolution of improved surgical technique, the increased capacity for judicious surveillance, and the advent of highly successful systemic chemotherapy all have served to make the management of clinical stage I NSGCT a controversial one.

Retroperitoneal Lymph Node Dissection. Before the advent of cisplatinum-based chemotherapy, it was recognized that radical RPLND offered the potential of cure, even to NSGCT patients with nodal metastases. This dissection is a full, bilateral procedure in which all lymphatic, neural, and connective tissue is removed from a field demarcated by the crus of the diaphragm superiorly to the bifurcation of the common iliacs inferiorly, and bordered laterally by the ureters.[122]

After RPLND, clinical stage I NSGCT patients are restaged as either pathologic stage I or pathologic stage IIA (microscopic nodal involvement). Survival data from clinical stage I NSGCT patients has been reviewed.[28] In the precisplatinum era, survival rates were 93% for patients with pathologic stage I tumors and 75% for patients with pathologic stage IIA tumors. Since the advent of cisplatinum-based chemotherapy, which is used in this setting as either salvage or adjunctive therapy, the long-term survival rate approaches 100% for patients with pathologic stage I tumors and 96% for patients with pathologic stage IIA tumors.[28,123]

A large prospective trial by the Testicular Cancer Intergroup Study enrolled 195 patients with pathologic

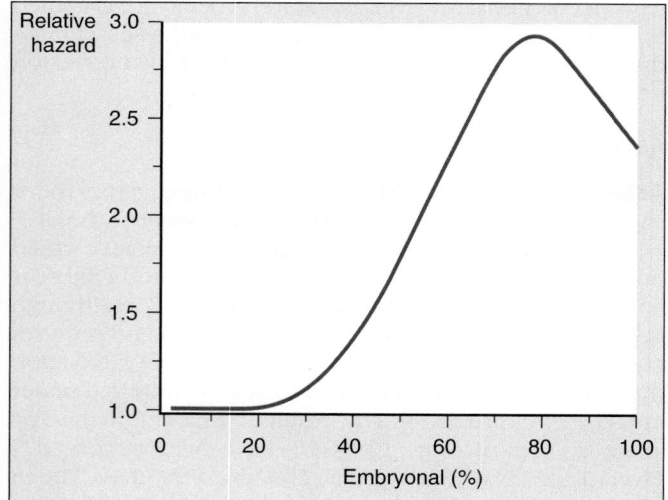

Figure 89-3. Relationship between percentage of embryonal carcinoma in the primary orchiectomy specimen and relative risk of recurrence. (From Sesterhenn IA, Weiss RB, Mostofi FK, et al: Prognosis and other clinical correlates of pathologic review in stage I and II testicular carcinoma: A report from the Testicular Cancer Intergroup study. J Clin Oncol 1992;10:69.)

stage II NSGCT (including 64 patients with pathologic stage IIA) who were randomized after RPLND to observation or immediate adjuvant chemotherapy.[123] For patients with pathologic stage I NSGCT, at a median follow-up of 45 months, 28 patients (10.5%) had recurrent disease and 6 had died, 2 of drug-resistant cancer. At the time of report, 98% of patients were alive and disease free. Other reports have corroborated these data.[122-124] One series reported 11 relapses (22%) in 50 NSGCT patients with low-volume nodal metastases who where managed expectantly after RPLND. Most relapses consisted of marker elevation. Five of the patients who suffered relapse had elevated markers before RPLND. The relative risk of relapse in patients with persistent marker elevation before RPLND was very high (8.0). These data indicate that patients with persistent marker elevation after orchiectomy should not undergo RPLND and should receive systemic therapy instead.[125]

By contrast, patients with pathologic stage IIA disease who are treated with orchiectomy and RPLND only will have a relapse rate as high as 30% to 40%, although some investigators have reported relapse rates in the 10% range in carefully selected patients with pathologic stage IIA disease.[122,123,126] Regardless of surgical cure rate, in the cisplatinum era, the overall survival of patients with pathologic stage IIA NSGCT treated initially with orchiectomy and RPLND is in the 96% to 99% range.[122,123,126] The integration of chemotherapy into treatment schemas for stage II NSGCT is discussed later in this chapter.

In experienced hands, a full RPLND is associated with low morbidity and mortality, but loss of ejaculatory function occurs in 65% to 100% of patients.[28,122,127] It has been stressed that disruption of these fibers results in retrograde ejaculation, but not in loss of potency, libido, or ability to have an orgasm.[122] The high incidence of ejaculatory dysfunction after full RPLND, coupled with an understanding of the pattern of nodal involvement in patients with low-volume disease, has led investigators to modify the traditional full RPLND. Extensive experience with full RPLND has allowed accurate mapping of nodal involvement in patients with low- and moderate-volume disease.[36-38] As described previously, this work has shown that suprahilar metastases are exceedingly rare in patients with low-volume retroperitoneal disease, and that patients with minimal-volume retroperitoneal disease almost always have unilateral retroperitoneal disease. Patients with left-sided primaries characteristically have nodal metastases to the upper left periaortic zone, while patients with right-sided primaries have involvement of the interaortocaval and precaval regions. These observations have led to modifications of the traditional full RPLND for patients with low-volume retroperitoneal disease, whereby a suprahilar dissection was eliminated and a limited dissection template was used, depending on the side of the primary. For right-sided lesions, dissection is limited on the left by the lateral margin of the aorta to the bifurcation, and for left-sided tumors, the right margin is the right renal hilum and the vena cava to the bifurcation.[122] The templates for right and left modified RPLND are illustrated in Figure 89-4. The benefits of a modified RPLND in this group of patients are shorter operative time, shorter postoperative ileus, and a significant reduction in ejaculatory dysfunction (30%–40% dysfunction after a right modified RPLND, and 60%–70% dysfunction after left modified RPLND). Furthermore, modification of the traditional full RPLND in patients with minimal retroperitoneal disease does not have an adverse effect on outcome, yielding surgical cure rates of approximately 90% in patients with pathologic stage I disease and 70% in patients with pathologic stage IIA disease and an overall long-term survival rate approaching 100%.[122]

The most recent modification in technique for RPLND in patients with low-stage NSGCT is the nerve sparing dissection described by Donohue and associates.[127,128] In this procedure, postganglionic sympathetic fibers from lumbar ganglia are identified prospectively and preserved before lymphadenectomy, with the intent to stage and treat in a standard fashion while preserving normal ejaculatory function. One hundred percent of 73 patients with clinical stage I disease who underwent a nerve-sparing lymphadenectomy at Indiana University had normal postoperative ejaculation. The distribution of pathologic stages and relapse pattern was no different from what has been described with full or modified RPLND. Of 73 clinical stage I patients, 14 (20%) were found to have occult nodal metastases. The relapse rate was 7% in the 61 patients with pathologic stage I disease and 28% in the 14 patients with pathologic stage IIA disease. All patients who suffered a relapse were salvaged with platinum-based chemotherapy.[122,127] (The characteristic relapse pattern after RPLND is discussed later and contrasted with the relapse pattern in similar patients who are not treated with an RPLND.) Thus, the nerve-sparing RPLND appears to be diagnostically and therapeutically as efficacious as more morbid full and modified retroperitoneal lymphadenectomies. Overall, approximately 30% of clinical stage I NSGCTs are found to have occult nodal involvement at RPLND and are classified as pathological stage IIA. The use of adjuvant chemotherapy in these patients is discussed later in the section on the treatment of stage II nonseminoma.

Alternatives to RPLND

Adjuvant Radiation Therapy. Some investigators have suggested that patients with clinical stage I NSGCT who are considered to be at high risk of relapse could potentially be treated with adjuvant chemotherapy or radiation therapy rather than with RPLND.[29,65] Although NSGCT is less radiosensitive than seminoma and requires considerably higher radiation doses (45–55 Gy), radiation therapy nonetheless could occasionally be required under unusual circumstances. The results of radiation therapy alone in clinical stage I NSGCT have been reviewed.[28] Overall survival rates from 70% to 90% have been reported; however, the advent of highly effective chemotherapy has largely obviated the role of radiation therapy in the treatment of clinical stage I NSGCT.

Adjuvant Chemotherapy. Up to 50% of patients with high-risk clinical stage I NSGCT are subsequently found to

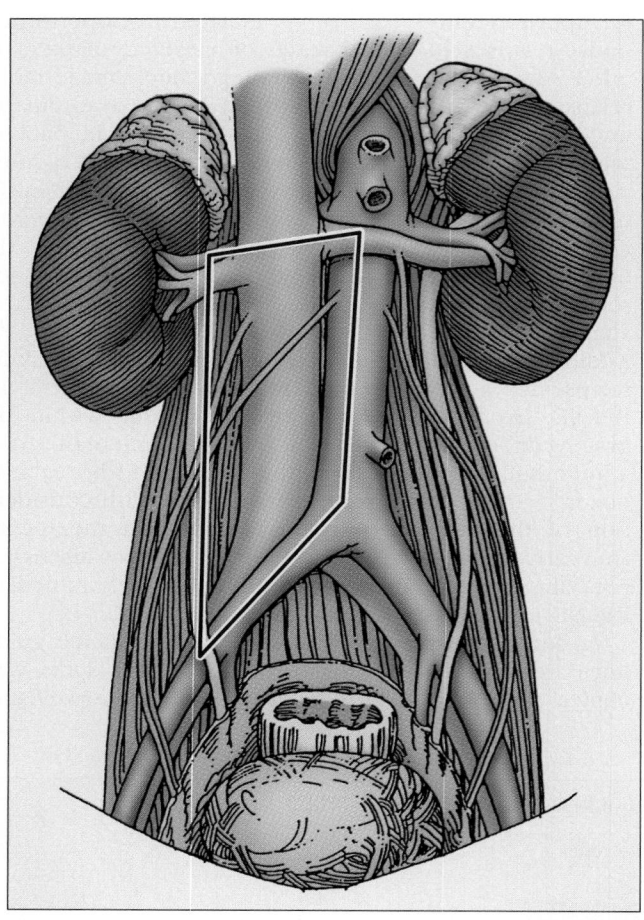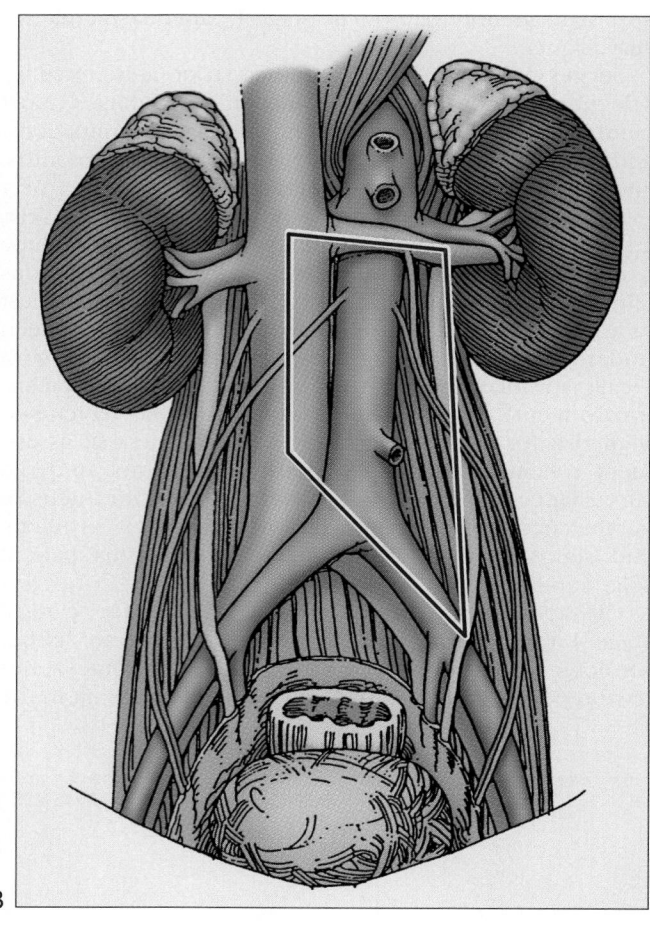

A   B

Figure 89-4. Templates for modified retroperitoneal lymphadenectomy. **A**, Right modified RPLND. **B**, Left modified RPLND. (From Foster RS, Donohue JP: Surgical treatment of clinical stage A nonseminomatous testis cancer. Semin Oncol 1992;19:166.)

have nodal involvement. As will be discussed later, some of these patients go on to receive chemotherapy after RPLND or in the salvage setting. It has therefore been suggested that chemotherapy might serve as effective primary adjunctive therapy after orchiectomy, thereby sparing patients an RPLND. Several investigators have used two cycles of cisplatin, etoposide, and bleomycin (PEB) in lieu of an RPLND and have reported very low relapse rates (generally <5%) in patients with median follow-ups as high as 4 to 6 years.[129-133] These results must be balanced with the concern that the use of primary chemotherapy exposes at least 50% of patients to unnecessary chemotherapy. Adjuvant chemotherapy for stage I NSGCT in lieu of an RPLND is generally not undertaken in the United States, in part due to these concerns, and in part due to the development of the nerve-sparing RPLND, which has reduced the risk of retrograde ejaculation (the major long-term complication of this procedure) to less than 1%. Adjuvant chemotherapy for stage I NSGCT is more commonly used in Europe.

Surveillance. The development of extraordinarily effective chemotherapy for disseminated NSGCT has also resulted in an effort to minimize "up-front" treatment for clinical stage I NSGCT. The strategy of surveillance after orchiectomy, followed by systemic therapy at the first sign of relapse, is based on the observation that only 20% to 40% of clinical stage I patients have occult nodal involvement, the belief that the majority of these patients can thus be spared the morbidity associated with RPLND, and confidence in chemotherapy as a curative "salvage" modality for those patients who do relapse.

Surveillance programs have been evaluated primarily in nonrandomized studies.[135] A summary of published results from nearly 600 patients who underwent surveillance after orchiectomy revealed a relapse rate of approximately 30% but an overall disease-free survival rate of more than 95%.[134] The Medical Research Council (UK) has reported on a prospective evaluation of surveillance in 373 patients with clinical stage I NSGCT. Although the 5-year rate of freedom from relapse was 73%, salvage surgical and chemotherapeutic interventions yielded an overall 5-year survival of 98%.[135] These data have been interpreted to suggest that the strategy of surveillance yields results equivalent to RPLND in carefully selected patients with clinical stage I NSGCT.[29,124] The selection of patients for surveillance might be enhanced by the use of a lymphangiogram and a CT scan, which, when negative,

appear to identify pathologic stage I patients suitable for surveillance.[136]

Successful surveillance requires strict adherence to selection criteria and surveillance methodologies. Most centers rely on serum markers, physical examinations, and chest radiographs obtained every 1 to 2 months, and on CT scan of the abdomen and pelvis every 3 or 4 months the first year, every 6 months the second year, and yearly thereafter.[29] Eligibility criteria must include a compliant and motivated patient in whom rigorous clinical staging (negative exam, serum markers, chest radiograph or CT, and abdominal/pelvic CT) has been undertaken. Most studies have excluded patients with locally advanced tumors (e.g., spermatic cord, scrotal sac involvement), and it has been suggested that patients at high risk for nodal metastases based on the risk assessment schemas outlined previously should not undergo surveillance alone.[29,65] Patient compliance with intensive surveillance programs remains a recognized problem, and successful surveillance mandates rigorous patient selection.[137-139]

Characteristically, relapses after RPLND for clinical stage I (pathologic stage I or IIA) NSGCT are either serologic or occur in the chest, although some series have reported from 4% to 6% of relapses occurring in the retroperitoneum.[28,122,123,125,127] Isolated retroperitoneal nodal relapses in the absence of elevated markers or other sites of relapse are exceedingly rare. Furthermore, relapses more than 2 years after RPLND are extraordinarily uncommon.[122,123] By contrast, most relapses in patients with clinical stage I disease who have elected orchiectomy alone followed with surveillance are identified by tumor markers and occur by and large in the retroperitoneum. Although some investigators have made the observation that the majority of these retroperitoneal relapses occur with bulky disease, there is no evidence to suggest that overall survival is affected.[28,134,135,138] Additionally, surveillance patients appear to be at risk for relapse for a longer period than patients treated with RPLND. Even though most relapses occur within the first year of instituting surveillance (median, 3 to 4 months), late relapses in the third to fifth years do occur.[111] These patterns of relapse, along with consideration of the morbidity involved with each therapeutic alternative, have formed the basis of a lively discussion regarding the relative merits of surveillance vs. immediate RPLND in patients with clinical stage I NSGCT.

As long as staging, treatment, and surveillance guidelines are observed strictly, nearly 100% of patients with clinical stage I NSGCT can be cured, whether surveillance

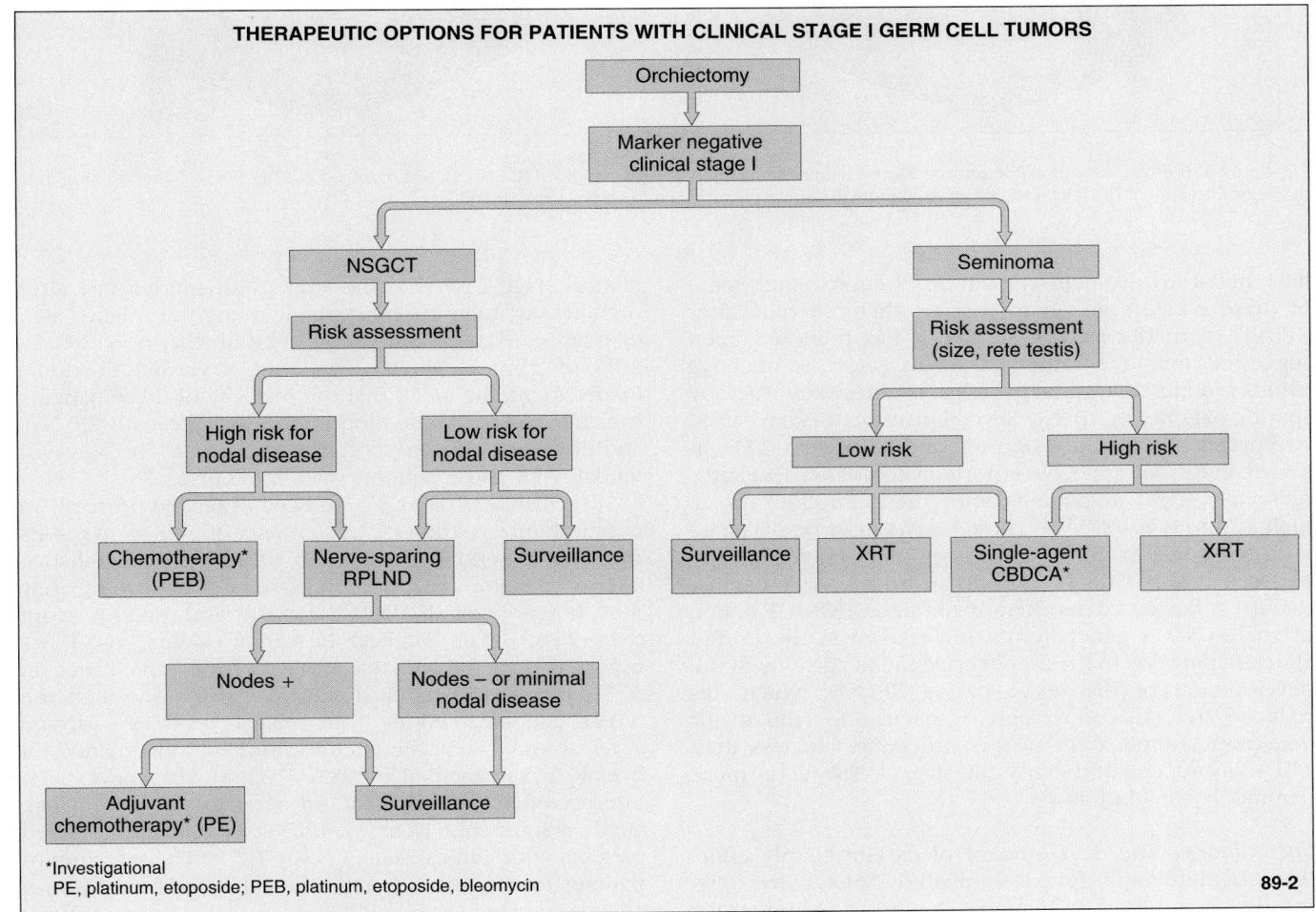

THERAPEUTIC OPTIONS FOR PATIENTS WITH CLINICAL STAGE I GERM CELL TUMORS

*Investigational
PE, platinum, etoposide; PEB, platinum, etoposide, bleomycin

or RPLND with or without adjuvant chemotherapy is used. Each patient with clinical stage I NSGCT must be informed of these alternatives and allowed to choose the methods of management most suited to his wishes and needs.

Stage II Seminoma: Treatment and Results

The Royal Marsden Hospital clinical staging system (see Table 89-5) divides stage II (abdominal) seminoma patients into subgroups on the basis of tumor bulk, as follows:

- Stage IIA, smaller than 2 cm;
- Stage IIB, from 2 cm to 5 cm; and
- Stage IIC, larger than 5 cm.

Historically, radiation therapy has been used for all stages of seminoma, allowing a retrospective analysis of failure rates and survival rates as a function of tumor mass. More recent series generally report better outcomes, perhaps because the era of CT scanning has allowed more precise definition of nodal margins and tumor volume.[140-146] Reviews of recent collected series have found recurrence rates of generally less than 5% in patients with masses less than 5 cm in size (stages IIA and IIB); 80% to 90% will be cured with standard abdominal radiation therapy alone. The use of salvage chemotherapy or radiation therapy (or both) in patients with masses smaller than 5 cm who relapse after initial radiotherapy results in a cause-specific survival of 95% to 100%.[30] Radiation therapy is therefore recommended for small-volume (<5 cm) retroperitoneal disease. The radiation field is generally limited to the infradiaphragmatic lymph nodes as in stage I disease. Relapses, when they occur, have largely been reported to occur outside the radiation ports.[46] Nonetheless, relapse in the mediastinum or supraclavicular nodes is a distinctly unusual event, and when it occurs, salvage with radiation therapy or chemotherapy is successful.[142,145] Thus, supradiaphragmatic radiotherapy is not warranted in these patients.

By contrast, failure rates of around 10% are reported in patients with masses between 5 cm and 10 cm in size, although some series have reported relapse rates as high as 40%.[147] The relapse rate after radiation therapy alone in patients with masses larger than 10 cm is unacceptably high, at approximately 35%.[30,140] Cure rates with radiation therapy alone for patients with IIC seminoma range from 30% to 60%, although an overall cause-specific survival of up to 90% can be expected with salvage chemotherapy.[147] Two major problems are associated with the use of radiotherapy alone for stage IIC seminoma. The first is a risk of mediastinal or supraclavicular relapse in up to 20% of patients.[142] In general, the degree of marrow compromise in patients receiving infra- and supradiaphragmatic radiation makes supradiaphragmatic radiation therapy an impractical solution to the problem. Second, it has been suggested that the radiation fields required for treating large masses, even if shrinking field techniques are used, make renal toxicity difficult to avoid.[109] In consequence, it is generally recommended that patients with stage IIC seminoma (masses >5 cm), and especially

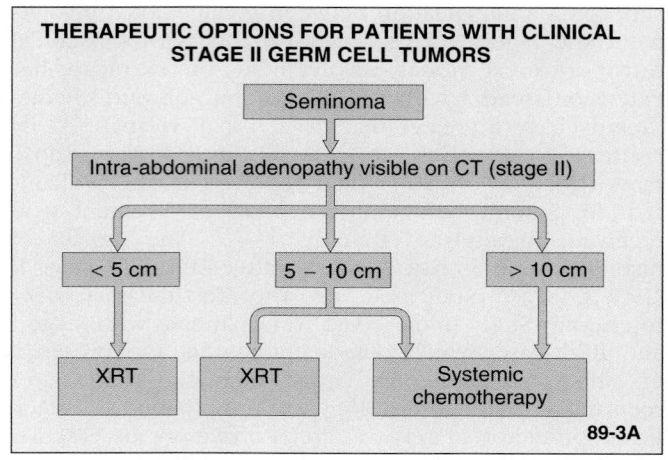

THERAPEUTIC OPTIONS FOR PATIENTS WITH CLINICAL STAGE II GERM CELL TUMORS

89-3A

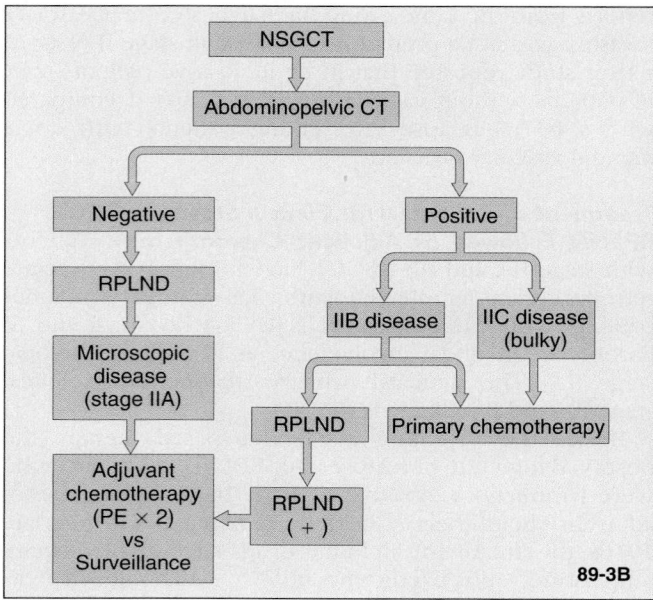

89-3B

patients with masses larger than 10 cm, be treated initially with chemotherapy. This approach is discussed shortly and results in cure rates from 85% to 95%.[30,109,147]

Stage II Nonseminoma

Risk Assessment

The identification of factors uniformly associated with a higher risk of relapse in patients with node-positive NSGCT after RPLND has not been possible. The Testicular Cancer Intergroup Study randomized 195 patients with completely resected retroperitoneal disease to observation or two cycles of adjuvant-based chemotherapy. Among the patients randomized to observation, approximately 50% subsequently relapsed.[123] Recurrence rates were higher among patients with advanced nodal stage: 40% for patients with microscopically positive nodes, 53% for nodes smaller than 2 cm, and 60% for nodes larger than 2 cm. Although these differences were not statistically significant, this study was likely underpowered to detect clinically significant differences. Other series have

supported an association between greater nodal involvement and higher relapse rates. Patients with substantial retroperitoneal nodal involvement or extracapsular extension treated with RPLND but no adjuvant chemotherapy have a greater than 50% risk of relapse.[28,62] By contrast, some series report significantly lower relapse rates (from 0% to 20%) than reported in the Williams trial, for patients with minimal nodal involvement who received no adjuvant therapy.[125,148,149] The impact of histologic type on risk of relapse after RPLND in stage II NSGCT was confirmed by the Testicular Cancer Intergroup Study pooled data from patients with stage I and II disease, which demonstrated that the presence of embryonal carcinoma clearly increased the risk of recurrence, although histology was not retained as a significant predictor of relapse after correction for vascular invasion or nodal involvement.[123] Although earlier reports from the same group had suggested that vascular invasion was not a predictor of relapse in stage II NSGCT, a later study reported that in node-positive patients, 24% of patients without vascular invasion relapsed, compared with a 63.5% relapse rate among patients with documented vascular invasion.[48,123]

Treatment of Patients with Clinical Stage II NSGCT

RPLND Followed by Adjuvant Chemotherapy. Patients with stage IIA and IIB NSGCT have minimal or moderate retroperitoneal lymphadenopathy. This category includes patients with clinical stage I NSGCT who are found to harbor occult nodal involvement at RPLND (pathologic stage IIA). The standard primary treatment for clinical stage IIA and B patients is RPLND.

Before the advent of cisplatinum-based therapy, the observed high rate of relapse after RPLND in patients who were lymph node positive was the basis for the use of adjuvant chemotherapy in these patients. Before the late 1970s, this treatment included drugs such as bleomycin, vinblastine, and dactinomycin.[150-152] Although it was acknowledged that more than 50% of patients would be treated unnecessarily, the poor prognosis of a relapse mandated this approach. Improvements in results of chemotherapy for systemic disease led to the use of platinum-based therapy in the adjuvant setting, although the utility of this approach had previously not been confirmed in a randomized prospective trial.[148] An international study by Williams and colleagues[123] was published in 1987; in this study, 195 patients with completely resected retroperitoneal disease (108 patients with pathologic stage II NSGCT) were randomized to either immediate adjuvant chemotherapy consisting of two cycles of cisplatinum, vinblastine, and bleomycin (PVB) or vinblastine, dactinomycin, bleomycin, cisplatinum, and cyclophosphamide (VAB-6), or no adjuvant therapy followed by chemotherapy at the time of relapse. With a median follow-up of 4 years, 49% of the patients in the observation arm relapsed, compared with 6% in the adjuvant therapy arm. Patients in the observation arm who relapsed were treated with salvage chemotherapy. Because of effective salvage therapy, the overall survival (97%) was the same in both arms. The authors concluded that the deferral of adjuvant treatment was appropriate

but also documented the effectiveness of a brief course of cisplatinum-based therapy in the prevention of relapse. Although this report included patients with a mixed group of stage II tumors, ranging from microscopic nodal involvement (N1) to grossly involved lymph nodes larger than 2 cm (N2b) and nodes with capsular penetration (N3b), no subgroup was identified in which adjuvant chemotherapy was mandatory. Nor was any subgroup identified with so favorable an outcome that adjuvant therapy was not necessary. Nevertheless, as noted, and despite the results of this study, nodal stage is felt by some to have value in predicting relapse.[125,148,149] For this reason, most centers recommend adjuvant chemotherapy over surveillance in patients with moderate retroperitoneal lymph node involvement (i.e., stage IIB disease), but an option for patients with minimal microscopic disease is surveillance after RPLND, as true pathologic stage IIA patients are at a very low risk of relapse (0%–10%).

Nonrandomized series have confirmed the high overall disease-free survival rate (98%–100%) observed with adjuvant chemotherapy administered after RPLND. Earlier studies used either PVB or one of the VAB regimens. Studies in the late 1980s, however, demonstrated that the substitution of etoposide for vinblastine produced equivalent survival with substantially less toxicity when used for patients with advanced disease.[153] Consequently, several centers have tested the substitution of etoposide for vinblastine in the adjuvant setting as well.[154-157] Bleomycin was omitted in two of these studies.[155,157] Survival in all of these series was 99% to 100%, with follow-up ranging from 30 to 72 months.

Taken together, these data demonstrate that excellent long-term survival can be achieved with RPLND followed by either observation (with salvage chemotherapy at relapse) or adjuvant chemotherapy. The disadvantage of adjuvant therapy is that it unnecessarily subjects approximately 50% of the patients (those who would have been cured with RPLND alone) to chemotherapy. Surveillance after RPLND avoids this problem, but it requires half the patients to endure the psychological trauma of recurrent disease. In addition, it requires patients to adhere to a frequent follow-up schedule, compliance with which is often difficult in this population of patients. In the Williams study,[123] for example, 25% of the patients made six or fewer follow-up visits. Finally, patients who do not receive adjuvant therapy will likely require more extensive chemotherapy for relapsed disease than had they been treated in the adjuvant setting. The excellent results of Motzer and colleagues[157] suggest that two cycles of etoposide and cisplatin might be adequate in the adjuvant setting, yet a chemotherapy-naive relapsed patient would probably receive either four cycles of etoposide and cisplatin or three cycles of PEB.

Primary Chemotherapy. Patients who have clinical stage IIC NSGCT have traditionally been grouped with those who have stage III disease when therapeutic options are being considered, and they are usually treated with systemic chemotherapy.[158] The rationale for this approach includes the excellent results of chemotherapy in "good-risk" disseminated disease, which includes patients with

clinical stage IIC NSGCT, along with the increased morbidity associated with RPLND for patients with bulky disease.[159,160]

The excellent response of advanced disease to systemic therapy on the one hand, and the possibility of cure without an RPLND in selected patients with clinical stage I disease on the other, are the basis for the experimental use of systemic chemotherapy without an RPLND in patients with clinical stage II NSGCT.[158,161-163] Two centers, the M.D.Anderson Cancer Center (MDA) and the Royal Marsden Hospital (RMH), have reported on the use of primary chemotherapy in patients with clinical stage II NSGCT.[158,163] Postchemotherapy RPLND was required in only 22% to 30% of these patients. Analysis of the clinical and histologic features of the 50 MDA patients suggested that patients with tumors larger than 5 cm had the highest frequency of postchemotherapy RPLND (33%), although this number did not reach statistical significance. At the RMH, 17% of 58 stage IIA patients (nodes <2 cm) required RPLND, compared with 39% of 64 stage IIB patients. In the MDA series, the most important predictor of the need for postchemotherapy RPLND was the presence of teratomatous elements in the primary tumor (36% incidence of need for RPLND in these patients, compared with only 8% of patients with embryonal with or without seminoma; $P = 0.014$). A 96% complete response rate with primary chemotherapy followed selectively by an RPLND was reported by MDA, while the 5-year actuarial survival probability for the RMH patients was 95%, with a median follow-up of 5.5 years. These series suggest that primary chemotherapy could be a therapeutic option for stage II NSGCT, obviating the need for surgery in 70% to 80% of patients. Patients particularly suited for this approach appear to be those with masses smaller than 2 cm in size, and with no teratomatous elements in their primary orchiectomy specimens. The risks of persistent disease or progression of residual teratoma for up to 10 years after apparent clinical eradication of stage II GCT (or both) have been cited as reasons for using this approach with caution.[164,165] The degree of retroperitoneal lymphadenopathy at which patients are directed toward primary chemotherapy rather than primary RPLND varies among institutions. Our approach at the University of California, San Francisco (UCSF) is to perform primary RPLND in all patients with clinical stage IIA and in most patients with stage IIB disease. For some patients with stage IIB disease who have more extensive and/or bilateral retroperitoneal disease (which would not be amenable to a modified or nerve-sparing RPLND, generally with masses >3–5 cm in size), we offer primary chemotherapy with a "good-risk" regimen such as PEB for three cycles or PE for four cycles. The role of adjunctive surgery after chemotherapy in disseminated disease is discussed later in this chapter.

MANAGEMENT OF ADVANCED DISEASE

The functional definition of advanced GCT includes those stages of tumor in which locally directed therapy (radiation therapy for seminoma, RPLND for NSGCT) offers unacceptably poor results. Thus, for NSGCT, lymph nodes larger than 2 cm define advanced disease for most investigators, whereas in seminoma, bulky IIC disease (generally masses >5 cm) is considered advanced disease. Stages III and IV are, of course, considered advanced.

The greatly improved prognosis for patients with disseminated GCT is largely attributable to a dramatic improvement in chemotherapy. The history of the development of chemotherapy for disseminated GCT has been described elsewhere, and only relatively recent developments pertinent to the clinical care of GCT patients are reviewed here.[46] Until the late 1970s, bleomycin and vinblastine were the chemotherapeutic gold standards for the care of disseminated GCT. The introduction of cisplatinum into combination chemotherapy regimens resulted in markedly superior response rates and long-term survival. Einhorn and coworkers[166-168] and the Southeastern Cancer Study Group (SECSG) demonstrated the utility of PVB and further refined their regimen by showing in randomized trials that lower dosage of vinblastine and the elimination of maintenance therapy did not affect response rates or long-term survival. Simultaneously, investigators at Memorial Sloan-Kettering Cancer Center (MSKCC) built upon the combination of vinblastine and bleomycin in their series of VAB protocols by first adding dactinomycin and then cisplatin.[169] Most recently, the discovery of etoposide as an active agent in advanced GCT led to the substitution of etoposide for vinblastine in the PVB regimen. A randomized trial comparing the etoposide-containing regimen (PEB) with PVB found that use of PEB resulted in an overall identical response rate, complete response rate, and 2-year survival rate, while significantly reducing the toxicity (primarily neuromuscular) associated with PVB, essentially making PVB obsolete (Table 89-7).[153]

Either PVB, PEB, or VAB-6 will result in approximately 80% of patients with advanced GCT achieving a complete response (CR) and 70% achieving long-term apparent cures. By the same token, however, 20% to 30% of patients still ultimately die from their disease. Studies of pretreatment clinical characteristics have sought to identify prognostic features that can prospectively be utilized to segregate this diverse group of advanced GCT patients into poor and good prognostic subsets. Proper identification of the subset of patients who are destined to relapse or fail to achieve a complete response to standard therapy is critical, to offer these "poor-risk" patients more aggressive investigational therapies aimed at improving response and cure rates. By contrast, "good-risk" patients are largely adequately treated with conventional therapy. Although the toxicities of these regimens are by and large manageable, they could account for considerable morbidity and on occasion even mortality. Thus, studies of pretreatment prognostic features have also sought to identify the "good-risk patient" cohort, for whom the investigation of less toxic but equally efficacious treatment is appropriate.

Risk Assessment

Several classification systems have been proposed as a means of distinguishing between "good-risk" and "poor-risk" patients with advanced GCT. In general, prognostic

Specific Malignancies

III

TABLE 89-7

Induction and Salvage Chemotherapy Regimens for Advanced Germ Cell Tumor

PEB (Every 21 Days) × 3–4

Indiana University
  CDDP 20 mg/m²/d, days 1–5
  VP-16 100 mg/m²/d, days 1–5
  Bleomycin 30 U, days 2, 9, and 16
Stanford University/Europe
  CDDP 100 mg/m²/d, day 1
  VP-16 150 mg/m²/d, days 1–3 (In Europe, days 1, 3, and 5)
  Bleomycin 15 U/m², days 1, 8, and 15

PE (Every 21 Days)

CDDP 20 mg/m²/d, days 1–5
VP-16 100 mg/m²/d, days 1–5 (In Europe, 150 mg/m2/, days 1, 3, and 5)

VAB-6 (Every 21–28 days)

Vinblastine 4 mg/m², day 1
Dactinomycin 1 mg/m², day 1
Bleomycin 30 mg, day 1
CDDP 120 mg/m², day 4
Cyclophosphamide 600 mg/m², day 1

VIP (Salvage) (Every 21 Days)

Vinblastine 0.11 mg/kg, days 1 and 2 or VP-16 75 mg/m²/d, days 1–5
Ifosfamide 1.2 g/m²/d, days 1–5 (with mesna)
CDDP 20 mg/m²/d, days 1–5

CDDP, *cis*-platinum; VP-16, etopside

factors are first identified by a retrospective statistical analysis of the relationship of the risk feature to outcome (generally complete response or survival). Although the specific clinical parameters used to define prognosis vary somewhat in these classification schemas, the pretreatment tumor burden has consistently been identified as an important predictive factor. Different researchers have defined tumor mass by size, number, and location of metastases. Other proposed pretreatment clinical features influencing prognosis in advanced GCT include histology (i.e., seminoma vs. nonseminoma), primary site, serum markers, and site of metastases.[47,170–174]

When these schemas were tested prospectively on independent data sets, they appeared to classify good-risk patients equally well but yielded markedly different complete response rates in the poor-prognosis groups.[175,176] To address this issue, a common classification system was developed by the International Germ Cell Cancer Collaborative Group (IGCCCG).[177] The IGCCCG database included 5202 patients with NSGCT and 660 patients with seminoma and was divided into a test set and a validation set. Prognostic factors for progression-free survival and survival were examined, and prognostic groups for seminoma and NSGCT were developed. The major independent prognostic factors for progression-free survival and overall survival were identified and used to establish prognostic groupings. For NSGCT, the independent high-risk factors identified were presence of mediastinal non-seminomatous primary tumor, presence of nonpulmonary visceral metastases (liver, bone, brain, etc.), and increased levels of tumor markers including β-HCG, AFP, and LDH

(Table 89-8). For seminoma patients, generally a group considered to carry a more favorable prognosis, the only significant prognostic factor was the presence of non-pulmonary visceral metastases.[30,147]

Although this system needs to be tested in a prospective fashion, it has been validated both on the IGCCCG validation set and on an independent data set.[178] In this system, good- and intermediate-prognosis patients have a testis or retroperitoneal primary, no nonpulmonary visceral metastases, and low serum tumor markers. Intermediate prognosis patients are the same as good-prognosis patients but have intermediate serum tumor markers. Poor-prognosis patients have a mediastinal primary, nonpulmonary visceral metastases, or high levels of serum tumor markers. Five-year overall survival for the good-, intermediate-, and poor-prognosis categories with current regimens is 92%, 80%, and 48%, respectively (see Table 89-8). By definition, seminomas are never poor prognosis. Seminomas are segregated into good-prognosis cases (any primary site, but with the presence of non-pulmonary visceral metastases), with a 72% 5-year survival.[177]

Several studies have confirmed the post-therapy rate of decline in marker concentration as a predictive marker of outcome in GCT patients. A recent study re-examined this issue in the context of the IGCCCG risk classification system. After adjusting for risk status, satisfactory marker decline (which was defined as a calculated half-life of 7 days or fewer for AFP and 3.5 days or fewer for HCG) predicted an improved CR proportion, 2-year event-free survival, and 2-year overall survival.[179]

Treatment of Good-Risk Advanced Germ Cell Tumors

All risk assessment schemas that were used before the development of the IGCCCG classification system were equally able to identify accurately a subgroup of good-prognosis testis cancer patients who had a high likelihood of obtaining a sustained complete response when treated with platinum-based therapy. In general, this group was made up of patients with marker elevation only or with small-volume infradiaphragmatic and/or supradiaphragmatic disease, and without visceral involvement.[175,180] Because it is not likely that the extraordinarily high cure rate for this group of patients can be improved upon, most efforts have been aimed at optimizing treatment with less toxic regimens that have equal efficacy.

Trials evaluating the elimination of bleomycin, a reduction in the number of chemotherapy cycles administered, or the substitution of carboplatin for cisplatin have been undertaken. In evaluating the results of these trials, several caveats hold. First, most of these trials have not used the new IGCCCG prognostic classification but rather have relied on different risk assessment schemas, making comparison between trials problematic. Second, most etoposide-containing regimens used in the United States (PEB, PE) administer a total of 500 mg/m² of etoposide (100 mg/m², days 1–5), whereas one European counterpart of these regimens administers 120 mg/m² on days 1 through 3, for a total of 360 mg/m². Finally, the inclusion

TABLE 89-8

International Consensus Advanced Germ Cell Tumor Prognostic Classification Schema

GOOD PROGNOSIS

Nonseminoma
56% of nonseminomas
5-year PFS, 89%
5-year survival, 92%
Testis or retroperitoneal primary
and
No nonpulmonary visceral metastases
and
Good markers (all of the following):
  AFP <1000 ng/mL
  HCG <5000 IU/L (1000 ng/mL)
  LDH <1.5 × upper limit of normal

Seminoma
90% of seminomas
5-year PFS, 82%
5-year survival, 86%
Any primary site
and
No nonpulmonary visceral metastases
and
Normal AFP, any HCG, any LDH

INTERMEDIATE PROGNOSIS

Nonseminoma
28% of nonseminomas
5-year PFS, 75%
5-year survival, 80%
Testis or retroperitoneal primary
and
No nonpulmonary visceral metastases
and
Intermediate markers (any of the following):
  AFP ≥1000 and ≤10,000 ng/mL
HCG ≥5000 IU/L and ≤50,000 IU/L
  or
LDH ≥1.5 × N and ≤10 × N

Seminoma
10% of seminomas
5-year PFS, 67%
5-year survival, 72%
Any primary site
and
Nonpulmonary visceral metastases
and
Normal AFP, any HCG, any LDH

POOR PROGNOSIS

Nonseminoma
16% of nonseminomas
5-year PFS, 41%
5-year survival, 48%
Mediastinal primary
  or
Nonpulmonary visceral metastases
  or
Poor markers (any of the following):
AFP >10,000 ng/ml
  or
HCG >50,000 IU/L (10,000 ng/mL)
  or
LDH >10 × upper limit of normal

Seminoma

No patients classified as poor prognosis

AFP, α-fetoprotein; HCG, human chorionic gonadotropin; LDH, lactate dehydrogenase; N, normal; PSF, progression-free survival.
Adapted from International Germ Cell Cancer Collaborative Group: International Germ Cell Consensus Classification: A prognostic factor-based staging system for metastatic germ cell cancers. J Clin Oncol 1997;15:594, with permission.

(or exclusion) of patients with advanced seminoma from good-risk trials has been inconsistent. IGCCCG data suggest that although seminoma is clearly a good-risk tumor, it should be evaluated in separate trials. In those series in which patients with advanced-stage seminoma were considered separately from NSGCT, platinum-containing regimens (including VIP, PEB, EP, and VAB-6) result in roughly comparable survival rates of around 90%.[30,177]

Results of Clinical Trials in Good-Prognosis Patients

As discussed previously, etoposide may be substituted for vinblastine in the PVB regimen, resulting in an improvement in the toxicity profile without loss of effectiveness. Using the Indiana University staging system, the SECSG reported on a randomized trial of four cycles of PVB vs. four cycles of PEB, with CR rates of 97% and 96%, respectively.[153] (Interestingly, the same study demonstrated PEB to be superior to PVB in the treatment of poor-prognosis advanced GCT patients.) A subsequent randomized trial by the SECSG demonstrated that in good-prognosis patients, three cycles of PEB are as efficacious as four cycles, with complete response rates of 97% and continuous complete remission rates of 92% in either regimen.[181] Moreover, the EORTC recently reported the results of a prospective randomized 2x2 factorial trial in IGCCC patients with good-prognosis GCT, which compared three vs. four cycles of therapy and PEB administered over 5 days (platinum 100 mg/m² daily for 5 days and etoposide 100 mg/m² daily for 5 days) or over 3 days,

but with the same total dose (platinum 20 mg/m^2 on day 1 and etoposide 100 mg/m^2 daily for 3 days).[182] Three cycles of PEB were therapeutically equivalent to four, and there was no difference in outcome between the 3- and 5-day schedules. By contrast, a multicenter phase III trial randomized patients to the "Indiana regimen" (platinum 20 mg/m^2 on days 1 through 5, etoposide 100 mg/m^2 on days 1 through 5, and bleomycin 30 units on days 1, 8, and 15 of each 21-day cycle) administered three times, vs. four cycles of a regimen used by the MRC/EOTRC (platinum 100 mg/m^2 on day 1, etoposide 120 mg/m^2 on days 1 through 3, and bleomycin 30 units on day 1 of each 21-day cycle). Although there was no statistically significant difference in response proportion between the two groups, overall survival was significantly better for those patients receiving the Indiana regimen, prompting the early termination of the study.[183] These studies have established three cycles of PEB using 100 mg/m^2 platinum and 500 mg/m^2 etoposide as a benchmark for other good-risk GCT trials.

The relatively high incidence of clinically apparent pulmonary toxicity from bleomycin, observed in up to 20% of patients, and a small but real bleomycin-related death rate of 2% to 4% (although data are largely from the era before routine monitoring of respiratory function), has been the impetus behind the evaluation of regimens for good-risk GCTs that delete bleomycin.[184]

MSKCC conducted a randomized comparison of their standard therapy for GCT (three cycles of VAB-6) and four cycles of a two-drug regimen of etoposide and cisplatinum (EP) in 170 good-risk patients as defined by the MSKCC risk criteria. Complete response rates of 92% and 95% (not statistically significant) were observed in the EP and VAB-6 arms, respectively. Although patients treated with EP had significantly less emesis, magnesium wasting, neutropenia, and thrombocytopenia, relapse-free and overall survival were similar in both arms.[185]

Although most investigators agree that three rather than four cycles of PEB are adequate in good-risk patients, the role of bleomycin remains hotly debated, in part due to the heterogeneity of the risk assessment schemas and regimens utilized.[180] Nevertheless, there now exist three published trials that suggest that bleomycin, while adding modest toxicity, appears to result in improved outcome in good-risk patients. One of these studies was an Australian study suggesting that PV was inferior to PVB.[186] (The fact that the introduction of PEB has made PVB largely obsolete makes this a study of historic interest only.) A second study conducted by the Eastern Cooperative Oncology Group (ECOG) compared three cycles of (U.S.) PE to the "benchmark" three cycles of (U.S.) PEB.[187] An interim analysis revealed an increased number of relapses, progressive disease, and higher likelihood of death for the two-drug combination (durable CR rate 86% for PEB vs. 70% for PE), resulting in early termination of the study. Finally, the EORTC randomized 450 patients to four cycles of (European) PE or four cycles of (European) PEB and found a significantly higher CR rate (95% vs. 87%) for patients on the three-drug combination.[188] In aggregate, these data suggest that the deletion of bleomycin from good-risk regimens is generally not appropriate. Whether four cycles of (U.S.) PE are adequate therapy is unknown, however—of the two trials using four cycles of PE as a comparator, the European Organization for Research and Treatment of Cancer (EORTC) trial noted previously used European PE, which contains less etoposide.[188] The second trial using PE was the MSKCC trial noted previously, in which PE was compared with a non-benchmark regimen, VAB-6.[185] At UCSF, our approach for good-risk patients has been to plan three cycles of (U.S.) PEB and to switch to four cycles of (U.S.) PE if pulmonary toxicity becomes apparent (see the later section on toxicity).

Carboplatin, a cisplatin analog with less nephrotoxicity and neurotoxicity than cisplatin, has also been evaluated in patients with good-risk GCT. The RMH reported on 76 patients with good prognosis by the MRC criteria who were treated in a one-arm study in which carboplatin was substituted for cisplatin in a PEB-like, three-drug regimen; four cycles of therapy were administered. The 2-year disease-free survival rate in this nonrandomized trial was comparable with historic controls reported with four cycles of PEB.[189] By contrast, the substitution of carboplatin for cisplatin in the two-drug regimen EP is inferior, as suggested by the results of a randomized trial of four cycles of EP given every 3 weeks vs. four cycles of EC (etoposide plus carboplatin) given every 4 weeks, in good-risk patients (MSKCC criteria). Although the CR rates were similar (88%–90%), unfavorable events (incomplete response or relapse) were more common in the EC arm (24% vs. 13%; $P = 0.04$), and EP patients had a superior event-free and relapse-free survival (87% vs. 76%).[190] Whether this difference was due to the difference in frequency of administration of each regimen (every 3 weeks for EP vs. every 4 weeks for EC) was addressed by an MRC/EORTC study, which randomized patients to receive either four cycles of European PEB (in which bleomycin was given on day 1 of each cycle only, as opposed to the usual three times per cycle) given every 3 weeks, or the same regimen (also given every 3 weeks) with the substitution of carboplatin for cisplatin. The carboplatin regimen was inferior with regard to the CR rate (87.3% vs. 94.4%) and with regard to 3-year survival (90% vs. 97%).[191] These studies have demonstrated fairly convincingly that there is no role for carboplatin in the treatment of good-risk GCTs.

In summary, although there has been a difference in the classification schemas used to identity good- vs. poor-prognosis patients with advanced GCT, all schemas are able to identify a good-prognosis subset of patients, in whom the likelihood of a complete response to chemotherapy is in the 90% to 95% range and in whom long-term survival can be expected in 85% to 90% of patients. Three cycles of PEB appears to be the standard, although some investigators believe that four cycles of PE are also acceptable. There is no role for substituting carboplatin for cisplatin.

Poor-Risk Advanced Germ Cell Tumors

The outlook for poor-risk patients is grim, with only 38% to 62% of patients achieving a complete response.

Thus, whereas the major concern in good-risk patients has been the reduction of toxicity, the major objective of clinical investigation in poor-risk patients has been to improve efficacy, with less concern for reducing toxicity. An equally important goal has been the accurate pretreatment identification of poor-risk patients, so that patients are not incorrectly classified as poor risk and thereby exposed unnecessarily to the toxicity of these regimens. The use of post-treatment variables—in particular, the rate of decline of the serum markers AFP and HCG—might also serve to identify the patient who is destined to fail standard induction chemotherapy.[192]

Results of Clinical Trials in Poor-Prognosis Patients

The results of clinical trials conducted in patients with poor-risk GCTs have been summarized.[193] Most trials have included only small numbers of patients in single-armed phase II trials, and a wide range of risk criteria has been utilized, making it difficult to compare these trials. The extraordinarily wide range of reported complete remission rates (38%–92%) is probably more a reflection of the diversity of the risk assessment schemas employed than of actual differences in efficacy of the regimens themselves.

Clinical trials in poor-prognosis patients have by and large relied on either or both of two approaches. The first has been to exploit agents that have been demonstrated to be efficacious in the salvage setting (e.g., etoposide, paclitaxel, and ifosfamide), whereas the second approach has evaluated the role of dose escalation.

Perhaps the earliest demonstration of a regimen providing poor-risk patients with an improved outcome was the SECSG study that randomized GCT patients to receive four cycles of either PVB or PEB. A subset analysis of poor-risk patients demonstrated that PEB resulted in a higher complete response proportion than PVB (68% and 38%, respectively, using the Indiana risk criteria).[153] This study established four cycles of PEB as a benchmark against which other high-risk GCT trials could be compared.

The appreciation of the activity of etoposide in the treatment of GCT (as in the PEB regimen) led to several trials in which etoposide was utilized in an induction regimen. The Southwest Oncology Group (SWOG) undertook a randomized comparison of standard PVB to a PVB regimen in which etoposide was substituted for bleomycin (termed *PEV*) in high-risk patients. This study demonstrated that the inclusion of etoposide did not improve the frequency of disease-free status (disease-free survival) (64.5% with PEV vs. 73% with PVB). Furthermore, some investigators have challenged the validity of the risk criteria used, given the high disease-free survival rate obtained with PVB.[194] The inclusion of etoposide in other nonrandomized trials does not appear to improve outcome.[193] The observation that the combination of ifosfamide, cisplatin, and etoposide (VIP) could salvage some patients who had failed induction therapy with PVB or PEB led to the use of the VIP regimen as primary induction therapy for high-risk GCT patients.[195,196] A randomized trial comparing standard induction therapy (PEB) with the VIP regimen normally used in the salvage setting (see Table 89-8) found no statistically significant difference in patients rendered disease free (51% vs. 57%), in relapse rate (17% vs. 14%), or in overall survival or progression-free survival (53% vs. 56%).[197] Furthermore, the VIP regimen was associated with increased (primarily hematologic) toxicity and thus cannot be recommended routinely as initial therapy for high-risk patients.

The apparent dose-response relationship for cisplatin in the 75 to 120 mg/m^2 range in GCT patients prompted several trials that tested the hypothesis that further dose escalation would result in improved efficacy in the high-risk subset.[198] A randomized comparison of a high-dose regimen (consisting of etoposide added to PVB with twice the standard dose of cisplatin) with standard PVB therapy for the therapy of high-risk patients with GCT was undertaken by the NCI.[199] Alhtough this trial demonstrated an apparent improvement in outcome (albeit with significant ototoxicity), a subsequent randomized trial conducted by the Southeastern Cancer Study Group and the SWOG comparing PEB with platinum dose-intense PEB in high-risk patients failed to demonstrate increased efficacy.[193]

Another approach tested in poor-risk patients with GCT has been the use of alternating non–cross-resistant therapy. The EORTC compared four cycles of PEB to four cycles of alternating cycles of PEB and PVB and could show no advantage to the alternating regimen.[200] A similar approach was developed by the MRC/EORTC and consisted of initial treatment with bleomycin, vincristine, and cisplatin (BOP) followed by a VIP-like regimen. Preliminary results from a randomized trial comparing PEB with BOP-VIP suggested no difference in outcome (CR rate, 59% and 58%, respectively; durable CR, 50% and 52%, respectively).[201] Several other alternating regimens have been studied, including POMB-ACE, which alternates platinum, vincristine, methotrexate, and bleomycin (POMB) with actinomycin, cyclophosphamide, and etoposide (ACE). This regimen has been reported to yield a survival rate higher than expected in IGCCCG-defined poor-risk patients (75% at 3 years vs. 50% expected) and in patients with primary mediastinal disease (73% 5-year survival vs. 40% expected).[202,203] A second regimen—BOP-CISCA-POMB-ACE, which alternates bleomycin, vincristine, and cisplatin (BOP); cisplatin, cyclophosphamide, and doxorubicin (CISCA); cisplatin, vincristine, methotrexate, and bleomycin (POMB); etoposide, dactinomycin, and cyclophosphamide (ACE)—has been reported to result in a 3-year PFS greater than expected in the IGCCCG-defined poor-risk patients (67% vs. 50%).[204] Although intriguing, testing in a randomized trial (e.g., vs. four cycles PEB) is essential before these regimens can be recommended.

The demonstration of the efficacy of high-dose chemotherapy (HDCT) with autologous hematopoietic stem cell support in the salvage treatment of relapsed and/or cisplatin-insensitive GCT formed the basis for treatment of selected high-risk patients with GCT using HDCT earlier in their courses, as part of their induction therapy rather than reserving it as salvage. During the same time period, carboplatin had been shown effective in the treatment of GCT, first as single-agent salvage therapy and then in

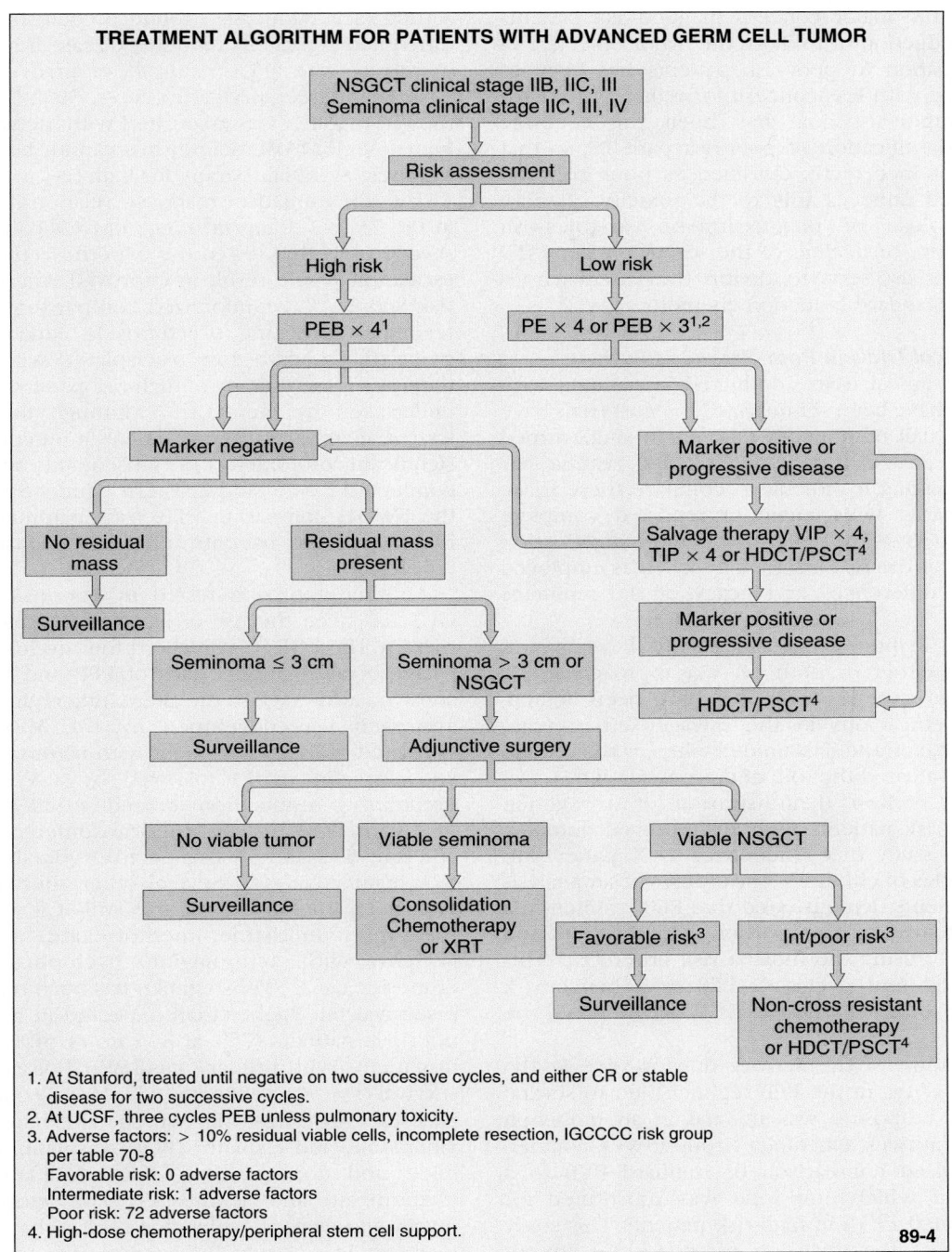

TREATMENT ALGORITHM FOR PATIENTS WITH ADVANCED GERM CELL TUMOR

1. At Stanford, treated until negative on two successive cycles, and either CR or stable disease for two successive cycles.
2. At UCSF, three cycles PEB unless pulmonary toxicity.
3. Adverse factors: > 10% residual viable cells, incomplete resection, IGCCCC risk group per table 70-8
   Favorable risk: 0 adverse factors
   Intermediate risk: 1 adverse factors
   Poor risk: 72 adverse factors
4. High-dose chemotherapy/peripheral stem cell support.

89-4

combination with etoposide and bleomycin as induction therapy for poor-risk NSGCT.[205,206] These observations, along with the potential for dose escalation with carboplatin, led to the use of HDCT in dose-intensity trials for high-risk tumors as well. In these trials, patients generally received one to two cycles of standard induction therapy followed by HDCT. Reasonable CR rates of 56% to 70% and durable CR rates of 46% to 64% have been described.[207–209]

With the availability of hematopoietic growth factors and peripheral-blood stem-cell transplantation, HDCT followed by peripheral stem-cell transplant (PSCT) has become an attractive option for poor-risk GCT patients. Several phase II trials have suggested that first-line HDCT is well tolerated and appears to confer a potential survival advantage in poor-risk patients, when compared with historical controls treated with standard therapy.[208,210] To compare front-line HDCT/PSCT with standard-dose chemotherapy in patients with poor-risk disease, a retrospective matched pair analysis was undertaken.[211] The results demonstrated a significant improvement in the 2-year PFS (75% vs. 59%) and OS (82% vs. 71%)

for patients receiving HDCT/PSCT. Although these data might support HDCT as first-line therapy in patients with poor-prognosis GCTs, clearly caution is warranted in their interpretation.[211] An intergroup study comparing two cycles of PEB followed by HDCT with four cycles of PEB alone as first-line therapy for patients with poor-prognosis GCT is ongoing and is expected to address this issue.

In summary, there is a lack of consensus regarding the optimal management of high-risk GCT. Off protocol, no particular regimen can be recommended over four cycles of PEB. Every effort should be made to enroll and treat patients with poor-prognosis GCT in clinical trials.

Unique, High-Risk Germ Cell Tumors: Brain Metastases and Extragonadal Disease

A mediastinal primary or the presence of nonpulmonary visceral metastasis in patients with NSGCT defines high-risk patients in the IGCCCG Consensus Risk Classification. This is corroborated by a review of nearly 800 patients by the MRC, which has reported 3-year survivals for 86 patients with liver, bone, or brain metastases of 52%, compared with a 3-year survival of 89% in 709 patients without metastases at one of these sites.[47] Two clinical scenarios that warrant special consideration are those involving extragonadal primary tumors and GCT brain metastases.

Extragonadal GCT

As discussed earlier, it is generally accepted that extragonadal GCTs are a consequence of malignant transformation of residual midline germinal elements, generally found in the retroperitoneum or mediastinum. From 1% to 5% of germ cell tumors are of extragonadal origin, and most but not all occur in men.[7] As noted previously, all patients with extragonadal GCT should undergo the standard evaluation for patients with GCTs, including bilateral testicular ultrasonography to rule out an unsuspected testicular primary.

Extragonadal GCT of nonseminomatous histology appears to be associated with Klinefelter's syndrome. In one series of 22 consecutive patients with nonseminomatous extragonadal GCT, 18% were found to have karyotypically defined Klinefelter's syndrome.[212] Hematologic malignancies have been observed to develop in approximately 10% of patients with the disease, usually within 2 years.[13] A common origin of the two malignancies is postulated based on a shared karyotypic abnormality [i(12p)].[14]

Seminomas account for approximately 30% to 40% of all these tumors. They appear to be somewhat slower growing than their nonseminomatous counterparts, and approximately 60% to 70% of patients with mediastinal seminoma have metastases at the time of diagnosis (compared with 85% to 90% in patients with nonseminomatous extragonadal GCT).[9] Although the lungs and intrathoracic structures are the most common sites of metastases, these tumors not uncommonly demonstrate

osseous metastases. Extragonadal seminoma, like its counterpart of gonadal origin, is exquisitely radiosensitive, and approximately 60% of patients can be cured with radiation therapy. Cisplatin-based chemotherapy, however, is generally considered to be the superior modality, with complete response rates of 67% to 89% reported.[9]

Nonseminomatous extragonadal GCTs constitute 60% to 70% of all extragonadal GCTs. In contrast to extragonadal seminoma, local treatment with radiation therapy has been unsuccessful, and chemotherapy is far less efficacious. A compilation of 158 cases of nonseminomatous extragonadal GCT noted an overall response to cisplatin-based therapy of 54% (range, 38%–68%) and a long-term disease-free survival rate of 42% (range, 22%–58%).[8] The optimal chemotherapy regimen is undefined; certainly these patients are in the poor-prognosis category and when possible should be enrolled in appropriate clinical trials. Unfortunately, patients with mediastinal NSGCT frequently demonstrate resistance not only to primary but also to salvage therapy. For example, a multivariate analysis of prognostic features in 283 heavily pretreated patients with GCT subsequently treated with HDC as salvage therapy demonstrated that a mediastinal site of origin clearly imparted an adverse prognosis.[213]

Brain Metastases

Brain metastases occur in less than 5% of patients with GCTs, most frequently in patients with choriocarcinoma or yolk sac elements.[46] The presence of brain metastases is a marker of a particularly poor prognosis. An MRC series of 795 patients included 16 patients with central nervous system (CNS) involvement, in whom the 3-year survival was 37%.[47] Similarly, Indiana University reported on 22 patients with brain metastases in whom the overall survival was 31.8%.[214] The Indiana experience, albeit before the advent of etoposide-based therapy, suggested that the brain was a sanctuary from PVB and that a subset of patients could be cured if aggressive multimodality therapy, employing surgery, radiation therapy, and chemotherapy, was utilized.[214] Other centers have advocated combined chemotherapy and radiotherapy with long-term disease-free intervals, or high-dose intravenous methotrexate along with intrathecal methotrexate.[215,216] It seems reasonable to conclude that unlike most malignancies, the presence of GCT CNS metastases should not preclude therapy with curative intent.

RISK ASSESSMENT OF RESIDUAL MASSES AFTER CHEMOTHERAPY: THE NEED FOR ADJUNCTIVE SURGERY

The advent of platinum-based chemotherapy has resulted in complete responses in a large percentage of patients with advanced GCT. Furthermore, a number of patients with partial responses can be converted surgically into complete responders. Surgery is unnecessary in some of these patients, however, as their postchemotherapy residual masses might not reveal any malignant cells on histologic review. Thus, the identification of patients likely to have residual malignancy is of importance.

Residual Masses in Seminoma

Residual masses after systemic therapy for advanced seminoma are observed in 60% to 85% of patients, while 15% to 45% of patients have normal radiographic evaluations after systemic therapy.[217-221] Residual masses after chemotherapy for advanced seminoma most typically result in obliteration of radiographic planes identified on CT. These findings usually represent a dense scirrhous response that merges with the great vessels and other retroperitoneal structures.[219] These "masses" are in fact usually not discreet or well-defined, generally are not easily resected, and occur in 40% to 60% of patients. Only 20% to 30% of patients have discreet residual masses, which are usually larger than 3 cm and are in fact resectable.[219-221] The morbidity associated with attempted resections of these masses—in particular, the schirrous, ill-defined type—has prompted an evaluation of features predictive of residual active seminoma.

Overall, it has been estimated that 20% to 25% of patients with residual masses after systemic therapy for advanced seminoma will have residual malignancy.[217,219-221] Motzer and coworkers[219] made the observation that nearly half (42%) of patients with residual abnormalities larger than 3 cm in size were found to have viable malignancy, whereas no patient with a normal imaging study or residual mass smaller than 3 cm who then underwent exploratory surgery was found to have viable tumor. The authors concluded that seminoma patients with residual abnormalities smaller than 3 cm should not undergo surgical exploration, whereas attempts to excise masses larger than 3 cm should be undertaken. More recently, FDG-PET (2-^{18}fluoro-2 deoxy-D glucose positron emission tomography) has been shown to be a useful predictor of viable tumor in postchemotherapy masses in patients with pure seminoma, correctly predicting 96% of residual masses 3 cm or smaller and 100% of masses larger than 3 cm. This study demonstrated a superior positive predictive value (100% vs. 50%) and negative predictive value (97% vs. 91%) compared with assessment of residual mass size ($\leq$ or $>$ 3 cm).[101] Other groups have recommended either radiation therapy or careful observation of patients with masses larger than 3 cm. Our practice at the University of California, San Francisco, has been to resect any masses larger than 3 cm. Patients who do not undergo surgical resection of residual masses can be imaged by FDG-PET, followed by careful surveillance with imaging studies every 2 to 3 months for the first year, and less frequently thereafter.

Residual Masses in Nonseminoma

Up to 60% to 70% of patients with advanced-stage NSGCT will be rendered clinically free of disease with platinum-based therapy, and an additional 10% to 20% of patients observed to have residual masses after systemic therapy can subsequently be rendered free of disease surgically. The role of adjunctive surgery in patients with NSGCT having postchemotherapy residual masses has been reviewed.[217] Most investigators agree that, except in rare circumstances, adjunctive surgery is not indicated in the presence of persistently elevated serum tumor markers. (The role of surgery in marker-positive patients is reviewed in the section on salvage therapy.) By contrast, the recommendations for adjunctive surgery in patients with postchemotherapy NSGCT in whom serum markers have normalized vary considerably.[217]

Viable malignant GCT cells are found in the surgical specimens of approximately 15% of patients who have residual masses after chemotherapy, although some series have reported residual malignancy in as few as 3% of patients.[222] Fibrosis/necrosis or teratoma are found in approximately 50% and 35% of patients with residual masses, respectively.[217,223-225] It is fairly clear that the histology of resected postchemotherapy masses carries significant prognostic implications. Patients with residual carcinoma in their specimens have an overall long-term survival of approximately 60% to 70%, whereas survival for patients with necrosis/fibrosis is in the 85%–90% range.[217,225-227] The presence of viable GCT cells in completely resected specimens has been termed a *surgical complete response*. A recent retrospective report from an international study group of 238 patients with viable GCT cells in resected postchemotherapy masses indicated 5-year progression-free survival and 5-year overall survival rates of 64% and 73%, respectively.[226] Three factors reportedly were associated with improved progression-free and overall survival: complete resection of residual masses, fewer than 10% malignant cells in the resected specimen, and initial IGCCC good-risk group classification. These data suggest that complete and aggressive resection of residual masses is warranted. Interestingly, for patients with residual cancer in their resected specimens in this nonrandomized retrospective analysis, an improved 5-year PFS (69% vs. 52%) was seen in patients who underwent postoperative chemotherapy compared with postoperative surveillance alone. Overall survival was not statistically different between the two groups, perhaps because those patients who underwent surveillance received adequate salvage therapy at the time of relapse.[226] Although teratoma in the residual mass could be histologically benign, the rationales for aggressive and complete early debulking of teratomas include the following:

1. The risk of local complications and of growth into unresectable lesions.
2. The risk of late recurrence.
3. The risk of malignant transformation into non–germ cell malignancies such as sarcomas and carcinomas.[167,219,228]

The association of teratoma and late relapse is discussed in the section on late consequences of therapy. Because the diagnosis of residual teratoma is usually made by excisional biopsy, it has not been possible to compare the outcome of patients with known teratoma that has not been resected with that of patients in whom the teratoma was excised. Nonetheless, most series have reported an overall survival of 85% or higher among patients who were found to have teratoma in their postchemotherapy resected specimens.[217,223-225,229]

Preoperative variables have been evaluated for their utility in predicting postoperative histologic diagnosis

(and potentially as a means of deriving guidelines for patients in whom postchemotherapy could be avoided).[217,225,228-231] Several series have identified the size of the residual retroperitoneal mass, the size of pre-chemotherapy mass, and/or the extent of shrinkage as predictive factors able to identify a group of patients at lower risk for postchemotherapy teratoma or malignancy. Some studies, but not all, have demonstrated that the presence of teratomatous elements in the prechemo-therapy biopsies is predictive of teratoma or malignancy in the postchemotherapy specimen.[228-231] Prechemo-therapy serum markers (high LDH, low AFP) also were identified by logistic regression as predictors of an increased likelihood of finding only necrotic debris.[229] Despite the predictive value of some of these variables, no single variable or group of variables appears to be consistently sufficiently predictive to allow the identifi-cation of patients in whom resection can be avoided. Thus, two separate studies have reported the risk of a false negative prediction (the likelihood of finding residual carcinoma or teratoma in patients predicted to have only necrosis/fibrosis) to be approximately 20%.[228,229] The identification of patients in whom postchemotherapy resection can be avoided remains controversial.[226] When postchemotherapy lymphadenectomy is undertaken, bilateral (non-nerve sparing) RPLND is recommended.[217]

Most investigators have recommended the resection of residual pulmonary nodules. From 10% to 30% of specimens have been reported as malignant, teratoma has been observed in 26% to 60%, and the fraction of specimens containing only necrosis or fibrosis has ranged from 14% to 64%.[227,229,232] In some series, up to one fifth of patients undergoing resection of pulmonary nodules required bilateral thoracotomies. In a series of 39 patients undergoing 47 procedures, the pathology at resection could not be correlated with prechemotherapy size of the nodule, with size of residual nodule, or with extent of shrinkage.[229] Similarly, in the same report, the pathology of residual mediastinal masses in 17 patients was not asso-ciated with prechemotherapy size or percent shrinkage, although the size of the residual mass appeared to be more strongly correlated with histology.[229] Furthermore, in patients who undergo resection of more than one tumor site, several studies have suggested that histology from the earlier procedure (e.g., RPLND) will be predictive of the histology from the later procedure (e.g., thoracotomy) only 53% to 65% of the time.[227,229,232,233] Thus, although as few as 10% of residual pulmonary nodules might harbor malignancy, the 25% to 60% incidence of teratoma, and the inability to predict which nodules will contain only fibrosis and necrosis, mandates surgical removal of all postchemotherapy residual masses.

SALVAGE THERAPY

Although 80% of patients with NSGCT can currently be cured with platinum-based therapy, 20% will ultimately die of their disease, either because they fail to achieve a complete response with induction therapy or because they relapse after becoming disease-free with primary therapy. Before the initiation of salvage therapy, the diagnosis of relapsed or primarily refractory GCT must be established clearly. In particular, false positive serologic data and the detection of falsely positive radiographic studies of the chest, as described previously, must be ruled out. Persistent or slowly growing masses, particularly in the absence of serologic progression, could represent benign teratoma.

Chemotherapy

Etoposide and ifosfamide are single agents with demonstrated activity in the salvage therapy of GCT, with response rates of 20% to 50% in patients previously treated with cisplatin, although currently they are rarely used as monotherapy agents.[234] Particularly intriguing is a report that oral etoposide has a response rate of 28% in patients with refractory GCT whose prior combination chemotherapy treatment included etoposide.[235]

Salvage combination chemotherapy regimens generally have included etoposide, ifosfamide, or both. Before the acceptance of etoposide as a standard agent in primary induction therapy, etoposide and platinum-containing regimens resulted in long-term disease-free survival of approximately 20%.[236] A salvage regimen utilizing etopo-side, dactinomycin, and methotrexate reported a conti-nuous complete remission (>5 years) in 29% of patients who had relapsed after PVB therapy.[237] The use of eto-poside combined with ifosfamide (as in the VIP regimen; see Table 89-7) resulted in a complete response rate of 33% (including surgical resection of residual masses) in patients previously treated with PVB.[194] Ifosfamide-containing salvage regimens for patients previously exposed to etoposide have either substituted vinblastine for etoposide (VeIP) but continued to utilize etoposide if the patient had been previously treated with vinblastine, or simply continued to use etoposide (VIP), regardless of prior etoposide treatment (see Table 89-7).[238] Either strategy has resulted in a 33% to 36% complete response rate (including surgically induced complete remissions), with 15% to 25% of patients remaining in durable com-plete responses.[194,195,238] Indiana University also reported on the results of salvage VeIP in 84 patients with refractory GCT, 77 of whom had been previously treated with etoposide-containing regimens. The overall complete response rate was 52%, and the authors reported a 33% long-term disease-free survival with a median follow-up of 17 months.[239] The MSKCC experience with salvage therapy consisting of the VAB-6 regimen, EP, or other cisplatin-based regimens suggested roughly equal complete response rates of 25% to 36%, regardless of regimen used, with an overall durable complete response rate of 23%.[240] Salvage therapy is considerably more successful in patients with recurrent seminoma. In this setting, VeIP results in an 83% CR rate, and 54% of patients remain alive and continuously disease-free.[241] For patients with relapsed or recurrent seminoma, this is clearly the most appropiate initial salvage therapy.

Paclitaxel has been substituted for vinblastine in the VeIP regimen on the basis of in vitro studies that showed synergy for the three drugs against resistant GCTs and the

single-agent activity of paclitaxel in phase II trials.[242,243] Overall, complete responses with the paclitaxel, ifosfamide, and cisplatin (TIP) regimen were seen in 23 of 30 patients. After a 2-year period, 85% of the patients were alive (median follow-up 33 months). These data suggest that selected patients who are not candidates for surgical salvage might benefit from this regimen.[244] There has been no comparison of TIP to VeIP, and randomized trials are required to identify the optimal salvage regimen in this group of patients.

High-Dose Chemotherapy

The use of HDCT with ABMT and/or autologous PSCT as salvage therapy for relapsed or refractory GCT has been fairly extensively explored and was reviewed recently.[213,245-260] The rationales for this approach include the following:

- GCTs are extremely chemosensitive and therefore potentially might demonstrate a dose-response relationship.
- GCT patients are generally young and otherwise healthy and can withstand the rigors of HDCT.
- Bone marrow involvement with metastatic GCT is distinctly uncommon.

Initial trials with HDCT used cyclophosphamide, etoposide, or thiotepa. Cisplatin, although certainly the most active single agent in the treatment of GCT, is poorly suited for dose intensification because of neurotoxicity, ototoxicity, and nephrotoxicity. Carboplatin, by contrast, is better suited for use in HDCT regimens, because its major toxicity is hematopoietic and because it is an active agent in the treatment of germ cell neoplasms. A high-dose carboplatinum and VP-16 regimen pioneered by Indiana University and Vanderbilt University resulted in an overall disease-free survival rate of 60% and has become a skeleton that other investigators have modified, often by the addition of an alkylating agent such as cyclophosphamide or ifosfamide.[245,261] These results compare favorably with those observed after standard-dose salvage chemotherapy with VeIP and suggested that early HDCT could be beneficial in patients with relapsed GCTs.

Several novel HDCT salvage regimens have been reported, including induction with TIP therapy followed by high-dose carboplatin, etoposide, and Thiotepa, as well as sequential dose-intensive paclitaxel, ifosfamide, carboplatin, and etoposide.[262-264] From 25% to 50% of patients appear to achieve durable remissions, so that the curative potential of HDC as salvage (and frequently third-line) therapy is fairly well established.[213] Preliminary reports from a randomized trial of four cycles of salvage VIP or VeIP vs. three cycles of VIP or VeIP followed by a single treatment of HDCT indicated no difference in response rates, however. Whether this will translate into survival differences, or whether more conventional double ("tandem") treatments with HDCT/PSCT are required, remains to be determined.[264] Treatment-related mortality of HDCT/PSCT has declined over the years to levels usually less than 5% to 10%. Nevertheless, HDCT in this setting remains imperfect. For example, very few patients with refractory mediastinal tumors will benefit from HDCT.

Surgery

In general, resection of residual masses after chemotherapy in patients with NSGCT should be reserved for individuals in whom serum tumor markers have normalized. Nonetheless, this approach has come under question recently. Several centers have reported on the results of surgical resection of solitary residual masses in highly selected patients with persistently elevated serum markers who were felt to be refractory to platinum (after either primary or salvage therapy).[265,266] In one series of 15 patients, nearly half (7) obtained lasting complete remissions. The clinical features associated with a likelihood of successful outcome included a retroperitoneal site and/or an elevated AFP only (all five patients with elevated preoperative HCG levels subsequently relapsed).[265] A second center reported on a series of 48 patients, of whom 10 (28%) achieved lasting remissions with salvage surgery alone, with a minimal follow-up of 23 months. In this series, preoperative factors that predicted for long-term remission were extent of disease at the time of surgery and recurrence more than 2 years after initial therapy.[267] A third report indicated a 37% "cure" rate in patients undergoing resection of residual masses in the setting of elevated serum markers.[266] Absolute conclusions regarding the role of salvage surgery cannot be drawn from such a small number of patients, and it must be borne in mind that this is a highly select group of patients. For example, the patients reported in one series accounted for only 4% of all patients who failed to achieve a complete response to induction therapy at that institution over a 10-year period.[265] Nonetheless, these data suggest that in very carefully selected chemorefractory patients, surgical resection of residual masses, despite the presence of positive serum markers, could be appropriate.

RISK ASSESSMENT IN PATIENTS WITH RELAPSED OR REFRACTORY GERM CELL TUMOR

An analysis of the clinical features of responding vs. nonresponding patients could serve to identify the subset of patients likely to benefit from each of the salvage modalities discussed previously and to identify those patients suited for novel therapeutic approaches.

Most clinical trials using standard-dose salvage chemotherapy have observed that survival or response (or both) are considerably lower in primarily refractory patients compared with patients who have had a prior response to chemotherapy.[195,238,240] MSKCC reported on 124 patients who were treated with salvage therapy. Patients who had relapsed after a prior complete response had a 2-year survival rate of 36%, compared with a 9% survival rate among patients with prior incomplete response to induction chemotherapy.[240] Similarly, the median survival for relapsed patients with GCT who were treated with VIP at Indiana University was 10.7 months if the previous best

response to chemotherapy had been either an incomplete response or a complete response of less than 2 months' duration, compared with 26 months among patients who had experienced previous complete responses lasting more than 2 months.[238] Other features observed to be predictive of improved survival or response (or both) in some but not all series include lower tumor burden.[195,238,240] Patients with extragonadal primary sites do poorly.[240] In a review of 203 patients treated with VIP or VeIP at three institutions, four independent prognostic factors have recently been identified:

1. Incomplete response at induction.
2. Extragonadal origin.
3. Presence of lung metastases.
4. Elevated serum marker level (HCG >10,000 mIU/mL, AFP >1000 ng/mL).

Patients with either marker elevation or extragonadal origin and at least one other poor prognostic feature had a complete response rate of 4%, with no long-term cures, whereas patients with testicular tumors and nonelevated markers were observed to have a complete response rate of 62% and a 3-year survival of 43%.[268]

HDCT appears to be able to overcome primary cisplatin resistance in some patients, although patients with refractory mediastinal germ cell tumors do not appear to benefit from this approach. In the series of 40 patients with recurrent or refractory germ cell cancer treated with HDCT and ABMT at Indiana University, 3 of 6 patients who obtained prolonged remissions were primarily refractory to cisplatin, whereas none of the 11 patients with extragonadal GCT obtained a complete remission.[239] Other centers have reported a complete response rate of approximately 15% in platinum-refractory patients.[249] A multivariate analysis of risk factors in 310 patients treated with HDC as salvage therapy at four centers in the United States and Europe reported that mediastinal NSGCT, primary platinum resistance, progressive disease before HDCT, and high HCG levels before HDC (>1000 IU/L) had independent (adverse) prognostic significance.[213] This risk assessment schema has held true in subsequent HDCT trials. In general, patients with more than two adverse features have a poor outcome, even with HDCT, with virtually no patients achieving continuous remissions and median survival less than 1 year.[262,264] Thus, it is probably reasonable to offer HDCT to patients whose disease has relapsed after platinum-based therapy. Additionally, high-risk patients, including those with extragonadal GCT, might best be served by induction therapy followed by consolidation with HDCT, as opposed to reserving HDCT for salvage, where it appears to be largely ineffective.

Patients who experience disease progression after HDCT or other second-line therapy do poorly. They often receive further chemotherapy and/or surgery. No single agent or combination has yet demonstrated significant activity in this subset of patients. Several studies have shown response rates of 11% to 26% for single-agent paclitaxel.[242,243] Some other agents (e.g., gemcitabine and oral etoposide) have also been reported to produce responses of 7% to 19%.[244,269] Chronic oral etoposide has also been used as maintenance treatment for patients at high risk of relapse or progression after salvage chemotherapy and as a palliative regimen for those patients with cisplatin-refractory disease.[270] The Eastern Cooperative Oncology Group evaluated the combination of paclitaxel and gemcitabine in patients whose disease had progressed after conventional salvage second-line therapy or during initial cisplatin-based therapy. A response rate of 21% was reported.[271] Despite response proportions of 10% to 20%, in general, complete responses are rare in these settings, and long-term survival is uncommon.[270] Regardless of regimen, integration of surgery as a component of therapy after HDCT therapy appears to be important.[271]

LATE CONSEQUENCES

Testicular cancer is a unique malignancy in terms of its curability. Long-term follow-up of patients treated with PVB or PEB suggests that the estimated probability of relapse-free survival for complete responders is in the 80% to 90% range.[272,273] Nonetheless, once a complete remission is obtained, patients remain at risk for two types of adverse late consequences: relapse (including contralateral primary testicular neoplasms) and toxicity from therapy.

Germ Cell Tumor Relapse

After obtaining complete remission, 8% to 15% of GCT patients relapse, usually within the first 2 years after treatment.[272,273] The timing of a relapse does not appear to be dependent on histology, extent of disease, or induction regimen utilized.[277]

Late recurrences, defined as relapses occurring more than 24 months after diagnosis, have been reported in 1.5% to 4% of patients achieving a complete response.[272,273-277] The majority of late relapses occur more than 5 years after initial diagnosis. One series of 83 patients reported that 60% of patients were symptomatic at late relapse, while 40% were not. Nearly 50% of relapses were retroperitoneal, and 35% were intrathoracic (including the mediastinum).[278] Proposed mechanisms for late relapses include the development of second primary lesions, growth of an occult contralateral testicle tumor that is not affected by chemotherapy because of the blood-testicular barrier, the "reactivation" of quiescent carcinoma, or malignant degeneration of mature teratoma. The latter argument is the most favored, as teratomatous elements are observed in either the orchiectomy or relapse specimens in most patients.[272,274] Teratomatous elements were present in the orchiectomy specimens of 66% of 21 NSGCT patients with a late relapse reported in three series.[272,274,275] Nonetheless, this theory accounts for neither the 33% of late relapse NSGCT patients who did not have teratoma described in their orchiectomy specimen (perhaps a microscopic focus was missed) nor the seven pure seminoma patients in these series who experienced a late relapse.

A late relapse should be treated aggressively as a de novo malignancy. Although the numbers are small, it

appears that 50% to 60% of late relapsing patients with NSGCT can be rendered free of disease with chemotherapy or surgery (or both), and approximately 70% of seminoma patients will achieve a no-evidence-of-disease (NED) status with chemotherapy or radiation therapy, or both.[274-276] A recent update on late relapse of GCTs suggests better outcomes with primary surgery as a single modality compared with primary chemotherapy as a single modality, although most of the patients who received chemotherapy had more advanced disease. Whether or not chemotherapy is used, aggressive surgical resection is warranted in this setting.[278]

Contralateral Testicular Cancer

Contralateral testicular cancer (CLTC), including synchronous neoplasms, has been reported to occur in 2% to 4% of patients.[3,4,278-281] A Dutch tumor registry study of 1909 men with testicular cancer, with a median follow up of 7.7 years, reported a 15-year actuarial risk of 2.4% for a CLTC.[278] The overall excess risk compared with the general population was 40-fold. This study also demonstrated that testicular cancer patients treated with chemotherapy (primarily PVB) had a significantly reduced risk of a contralateral tumor, compared with those patients treated with radiation therapy or surgery alone, and that this risk reduction lasted for a period of at least 5 years. These data appear to conflict with previous observations that preorchiectomy chemotherapy in clinical stage II patients failed to eradicate all of the intratesticular cancer and that cisplatin-based therapy failed, in one series, to prevent the recurrence of CLTC in 14 of 781 men.[66,163,282] Thus, despite the potential for the reduction of risk of CLTC by the use of chemotherapy, it must be assumed that all men with testicular cancer have a small but real risk of CLTC.

Early Detection of Recurrent GCT

The optimal schedule for follow-up of patients with GCTs in complete remission varies from center to center, but in general it consists of intensive follow-up during the first 12 months after completion of therapy (physical examinations, determination of serum marker levels, and chest radiograph every 4 to 6 weeks, with CT scans every 2 to 3 months) and a slightly diminished intensity of follow-up with scans every 4 months during the second year after therapy.[276] During the third through fifth years, this evaluation is generally undertaken every 6 months. After 5 years, guidelines are less well established, although most authors agree that the incidence of late recurrence mandates lifetime follow-up with at least an annual history, physical evaluation, tumor markers, and a chest x-ray.[272-276]

Toxicity

Although the acute toxicities of the various therapeutic modalities employed in the treatment of GCT are fairly self-apparent and well understood, only recently have the chronic toxic costs of treatment begun to be appreciated.

Just as we learned only in the 1990s of the toxic consequences of therapies used in the 1970s and 1980s, an understanding of the potential late consequences of today's therapeutic maneuvers must enter into risk-assessment strategies and accentuate the need for defining low-risk populations in whom less treatment is appropriate. The acute and chronic toxicities associated with surgery, radiation therapy, and chemotherapy have been reviewed and are summarized next.[122,184,283,284]

Acute Toxicities

The acute surgical morbidity of orchiectomy is minimal, similar to that seen with simple inguinal hernia repair. The surgical complications specific to retroperitoneal lymphadenectomy (apart from the usual general complications of major intra-abdominal surgery), which include retrograde ejaculation, have been described earlier in this chapter.[28,122,127,128] It is generally appreciated that RPLND after radiation therapy or combination therapy is more technically demanding and probably more morbid, as patients requiring RPLND have not only been debilitated by chemotherapy or radiation therapy but also are patients with bulkier tumors, greater invasion of normal tissue, and greater likelihood of fibrosis and/or necrosis of both residual malignant and surrounding nonmalignant tissue.[184]

The acute toxicities from radiation therapy are largely dose dependent and are less of an issue in seminoma patients, who usually are treated with 25 to 30 Gy. Nonetheless, acute gastrointestinal toxicity consisting of nausea, vomiting, and diarrhea has been described in up to 50% to 100% of patients.[284] Changes in total dosage, equipment used, and treatment planning have largely relegated radiation nephritis, pneumonitis, and bone marrow suppression to historical archives.

The acute toxicities associated with chemotherapy for GCT have been discussed extensively and largely represent the toxicities anticipated from the individual chemotherapeutic agents comprising these regimens. Advances in the development of antiemetic agents, the use of growth factors, and improvement of supportive measures have mitigated some of these toxicities. Nonetheless, specific acute toxicities that bear mention in context of the chemotherapy used for the treatment of GCT include myelosuppression, renal toxicity, pulmonary toxicity, and neuromuscular toxicity.

Myelosuppression is mild to moderate in patients treated with PVB, PEB, or EP and somewhat more severe with VAB-6. Considerably more myelosuppression occurs with VIP than with PEB.[196] The importance of timely administration of chemotherapy for patients with metastatic disease, even in the face of myelosuppression, has been demonstrated, although the wide availability of growth factors has largely made the issue moot.[285,286]

Nephrotoxicity associated with platinum-containing regimens is perhaps less severe in this group of young, generally otherwise healthy men than in an older group of oncologic patients. Nonetheless, the potential for chronic renal insufficiency (and for peripheral neurotoxicity and/or ototoxicity), the occasional incidence of urinary obstruction by tumor masses, and the need for platinum-

containing salvage regimens (VIP or high-dose carboplatinum) in up to 20% of patients mandates careful monitoring of renal function. As noted previously, in general, carboplatin should not be substituted for cisplatin unless mandated by impaired renal function.[190,191]

A recent review of the literature suggests that the incidence of thromboembolic events in GCT patients undergoing chemotherapy can be as high as 8%, with 83% of these being venous and 17% arterial.[287] Liver metastases and the administration of high doses of dexamethasone as antiemetic therapy were identified as risk factors for the development of thromboembolic complications.[287] Prophylactic anticoagulation is not routinely administered to patients with GCT receiving chemotherapy, however, given the relatively low risk of thromboembolic events.

The acute pulmonary toxicity of bleomycin is manifested as noninfectious pneumonitis. Up to 20% of GCT patients treated with bleomycin-containing regimens develop clinically apparent pneumonitis, and 3% to 4% of patients with GCT have died from pulmonary toxicity in some series. This is a dose-related complication, with a markedly increased incidence at cumulative doses greater than 400 U, although toxicity can occur at lower doses.[184] Although the single-breath-diffusing capacity for carbon monoxide (DLCO) is the most common test utilized to monitor for pulmonary toxicity of bleomycin, its utility remains controversial.[288-291] Despite this controversy, it seems reasonable to assess each patient's pulmonary function clinically before each bleomycin dose and with a DLCO before commencing each new cycle. Measured DLCO may be expressed as a percentage of the predicted DLCO. Bleomycin-stopping rules utilizing a greater than 10-point drop in this percentage have been recommended.

The neuromuscular toxicity associated with PVB has been attributed to cisplatin (peripheral sensory neuropathy, ototoxicity) and vinblastine (peripheral neuropathy, paralytic ileus, myalgias).[184] Peripheral sensory neuropathy and possibly autonomic dysfunction after cisplatin administration have been well described and will not be addressed further. A randomized comparison of PVB to PEB reported that 8% of patients receiving vinblastine (compared with 2% receiving etoposide) had severe abdominal cramping, and 14% of PVB-treated patients developed severe myalgias. Four percent of patients treated with PEB (as opposed to 11% of PVB-treated patients) developed severe paresthesias.[153] These data have resulted in the substitution of PEB for PVB as front-line therapy for advanced GCT. Nonetheless, because patients with GCT continue to receive cisplatin-based therapy, and because vinblastine is used in the salvage VeIP regimen, the potential for neuromuscular toxicity must be appreciated.

Chronic Toxicities of Radiation Therapy

The chronic toxicities associated with modern radiation therapy techniques for GCT are not known. Much of the available information regarding chronic toxicities is derived from late follow-up reports of patients treated on orthovoltage equipment, or using dated techniques, or both.[184] Nonetheless, it must be assumed that the potential for some of these toxicities persists even with modern techniques. Although only minimal late nephro-

toxicity and peripheral neurotoxicity have been described with radiation therapy, more common late toxicities include chronic peptic ulceration in 5% to 10% of patients, and of greatest concern, the development of delayed non–germ cell malignancies discussed shortly.[184,278,283,292,293] Several studies have suggested that testis cancer patients could be at an increased risk of developing a second, non–germ cell malignancy with long-term follow-up, although the relative impact of chemotherapy (vs. radiotherapy) is unknown.[186,278,283,292,293]

Chronic Toxicities of Chemotherapy

Renal, vascular, cardiac, neurologic, and reproductive toxicities and the risk of secondary malignancies comprise the major long-term toxicities of chemotherapy. The chronic renal toxicity associated with cisplatin administration has been reviewed.[184,294] Most studies suggest that the acute deterioration of renal function observed after cisplatin might be irreversible and might persist beyond 12 months, although overt renal failure is generally not observed. Presumed renovascular hypertension has been observed in up to 24% of men after cisplatin-based therapy, although it is not known whether this is a consequence of chemotherapy or of increased surveillance.

Chronic vascular toxicities associated with chemotherapy include Raynaud's phenomenon, vascular occlusive events, and potential alterations in cholesterol metabolism. The most common vascular toxicity in GCT patients treated with chemotherapy is Raynaud's phenomenon, occurring in 23% to 49% of patients, usually within a year of treatment.[184,294] Although the exact cause in this setting is unknown, it appears to occur after treatment with bleomycin alone and in combination with vinblastine, but the addition of cisplatin might double the incidence. Symptoms of Raynaud's phenomenon abate in approximately 50% of patients. The possibility of a relationship between platinum-based therapy and the less than 5% incidence of fatal major vascular occlusive events involving coronary, cerebral, or peripheral arterial circulation has been raised.[184,294]

The cardiovascular toxicities associated with chemotherapy agents are a cause of increased concern. Although previous follow-up studies of survivors of metastatic GCT have reported a prevalence of major cardiac events, ranging from 0% to 3%, recent studies with longer median follow-up times have observed a higher prevalence of major cardiac events of up to 6%, including myocardial infarction, angina pectoris, and myocardial ischema.[295] In part, this might be explained by the presence of an unfavorable cardiac risk profile (hypertension, obesity, and an elevated serum level of total cholesterol with a decrease of high-density lipoprotein [HDL] cholesterol level), which have been observed in patients who have received chemotherapy.[295] The mechanism explaining this increased cardiovascular risk profile is unknown.[296,297]

The chronic reproductive toxicities associated with chemotherapeutic treatment of GCT include oligo- and azoospermia and Leydig cell dysfunction.[184,294,298,308] The exact role of chemotherapy in this process is often unclear in the individual patient, as many men are hypofertile at the time of diagnosis of GCT, and up to 80%

are oligospermic after orchiectomy.[294,299] Many men also demonstrate Leydig cell dysfunction after orchiectomy, evidenced by elevated LH and FSH levels in the face of normal testosterone levels. In one series, only 11% of men treated with orchiectomy alone or orchiectomy plus radiation therapy had residual oligospermia or Leydig cell dysfunction.[298] By contrast, combination chemotherapy appears to have a profound impact on spermatogenesis and Leydig cell function. The same study reported azoospermia in 27% and Leydig cell dysfunction in 86% of patients after treatment with chemotherapy. Sperm counts generally increase in the second and third year after therapy and return to normal in about 50% of men. Approximately 25% of men are permanently azoospermic, and it appears that Leydig cell dysfunction could persist at 3 to 9 years after therapy.[184,293,298,300,301] These deleterious effects of chemotherapy on gonadal function appear to be similar for all regimens evaluated to date. The only exception might be short-course (two cycles) PEB, in which the gonadotoxic effects might be reversible in nearly all patients.[129] Nonetheless, oligospermic and even azoospermic patients have been able to father children, and approximately one third of men treated with chemotherapy are able to father healthy children.[294]

Secondary Malignancies

In a Danish tumor registry group of more than 6000 patients, in which it is likely that most were treated with radiation therapy, the relative risk of second solid malignancies is approximately 2, with a latency period of 10 or more years.[293] A Dutch tumor registry study of 1909 patients with testis cancer confirmed these results, reporting a lifetime relative risk of a secondary malignancy of 1.6 and of all gastrointestinal malignancies (the most common site of origin of secondary solid malignancies) of 2.9, with the greatest risk (relative risk [RR], 6.5) occurring more than 9 years after therapy. The 15-year actuarial risk of developing a second cancer was 9.8%.[278] Although it has been suggested that the risk of leukemia in patients treated with modern radiation therapy techniques does not appear to be elevated, the Dutch series suggests that the relative risk of leukemia after radiation therapy, although not as high as seen after chemotherapy, remains elevated at 5.2.[184,278] The latency period is shorter than with solid tumors, with the highest risk occurring at around 5 years after treatment. The combination of radiation therapy and chemotherapy resulted, in this study, in significantly higher risks of solid malignancies (RR, 9.5) and leukemia (RR, 66.7) than if either modality was used alone.[278] Kaldor and colleagues[302] summarized the incidence of second malignancies in 17,730 testis cancer patients identified from 11 population-based tumor registries. These authors found that survivors of testis cancer experienced 30% more tumors than expected for the general population, with a statistically significant increase in the likelihood of developing sarcoma (RR, 3.0), melanoma (RR, 1.8), non–Hodgkin's lymphoma (RR, 2.7), and leukemia (RR, 1.7). No information regarding the type of treatment delivered for the initial testis tumor was available in the study. Wanderas and colleagues[281] examined the risk of

subsequent non–germ cell tumors in 2006 Norwegian survivors of testis cancer who were followed for an average of 12.5 years after diagnosis of testis cancer. The relative risk for developing a second non–germ cell malignancy in this population was 1.65 when compared with the general population, and the cumulative risk of developing such a tumor was 7.8% after 15 years of follow-up. There was an increased risk of colorectal, gastric, hepatobiliary, lung, and bladder cancers, as well as melanoma and sarcoma. The highest relative risk for developing a second non–germ cell tumor was seen in patients treated with either radiation alone or with radiation plus chemotherapy. Bokemeyer and Schmoll[303] reported a cumulative incidence of 1.38% for the development of a secondary tumor in 1025 patients followed for an average of 61 months after treatment for testis cancer.

The risk of secondary leukemias after chemotherapy for the treatment of GCT is small but real. Alkylator-associated leukemias have occurred when these agents were used in the treatment of GCT.[184] More recent series suggest that acute leukemias are unlikely to occur after treatment with standard doses of PVB.[278] Although uncommon, etoposide-associated acute leukemias have been described, occurring in approximately 0.5% of patients. From a combined total of 881 patients with GCT treated on protocol at Indiana University and MSKCC, a total of four patients developed acute myeloid leukemia. All leukemias occurred in patients treated with high cumulative doses of etoposide (2 g/m^2 in all patients but one, who received 1.3 g/m^2) and were diagnosed from 2 to 4 years after treatment.[304,305] Two other centers have reported a total of six leukemias out of a total of 322 patients treated with etoposide (and none in a group of 318 men receiving platinum-based therapy without etoposide), with a somewhat higher cumulative risk (3.5%–4.7%) of developing leukemia at 5 years.[306,307] Bearing in mind that even the "easiest" adjuvant regimen consisting of two cycles of etoposide and cisplatin contain 1 g/m^2 of etoposide, careful and considered use of etoposide-containing regimens is warranted as further information accumulates.

Taken together, these data suggest that secondary malignancies are an expected late occurrence in patients with treated testicular cancer, with a relative risk of between 1.38 and 2.0. Radiation-containing treatment regimens could have a higher association with secondary solid tumors, whereas chemotherapy could be more likely to result in secondary leukemias. These risks, although quite small compared with the impact of not undergoing therapy, must nevertheless be considered in the therapeutic decision-making process and be discussed with each patient with GCT.

REFERENCES

1. Roth BJ, Nichols CR: Testicular cancer in the 90s: Victory—and a new call to arms. Semin Oncol 1992;19:117.
2. Jemal A, Thomas A, Murray T, et al: Cancer statistics, 2002. CA Cancer J Clin 2002;52:23–47.

3. Oliver RTD: A comparison of the biology and prognosis of seminoma and nonseminoma. In Horwich A (ed): Testicular Cancer—Clinical Investigation and Management. New York, Chapman & Hall Medical, 1991, p 95.

4. Dieckmann KP, Boeckmann W, Grosig W, et al: Bilateral testicular germ cell tumors: Report of nine cases and review of the literature. Cancer 1986;57:1254.

5. Gilbert JB, Hamilton JB: Incidence and nature of tumors in ectopic testes. Surg Gynecol Obstet 1940;71:731.

6. Rutgers JL, Scully RE: The androgen insensitivity syndrome (testicular feminization): A clinicopathologic study of 43 cases. Int J Gynecol Pathol 1991;10:126.

7. Carlsen E, Giwercman A, Keiding N, et al: Evidence for decreasing quality of semen during past 50 years. BMJ 192;305:609.

8. Swedlow AJ, De Stavola BL, Swanwick MA, Maconochie NE: Risks of breast and testicular cancers in young adult twins in England and Wales: Evidence on prenatal and genetic aetiology. Lancet 1997;350:1723.

9. Hainsworth JD, Greco A: Extragonadal germ cell tumors and unrecognized germ cell tumors. Semin Oncol 1992;19:119.

10. Kurie JM, Bosl GJ, Dmitrovsky E: Genetic and biologic aspects of treatment response and resistance in male germ cell cancer. Semin Oncol 1992;19:197.

11. Rodriguez E, Mathew S, Reuter V, et al: Cytogententic analysis of 124 prospectively ascertained male germ cell tumors. Cancer Res 1992;52:2285.

12. Vos A, Oosterhuis JW, deJong B, et al: Cytogenetics of carcinoma in situ of the testis. Cancer Genet Cytoget 1990;46:75.

13. Nichols CR, Roth B, Heerema N, et al: Hematologic neoplasia associated with primary mediastinal germ cell tumors—an update. N Engl J Med 1990;322:1425.

14. Ladanyi M, Samanieto F, Reuter VE, et al: Cytogenetic and immunohistochemical evidence for the germ cell origin of a subset of acute leukemias associated with mediastinal germ cell tumors. J Natl Cancer Inst 1990;82:221.

15. Motzer RJ, Rodriguez E, Reuter VE, et al: Genetic analysis as an aid in diagnosis of patients with midline carcinomas of uncertain histologies. J Natl Cancer Inst 1991;83:341.

16. Motzer RJ, Rodriguez E, Reuter VR, et al: Molecular and cytogenetic studies in the diagnosis of patients with poorly differentiated carcinomas of unknown primary site. J Clin Oncol 1995;13:274.

17. Bosl G, Dmitrovsky E, Reuter VE, et al: Isochrome of chromosome 12: Clinically useful marker for male germ cell tumors. J Natl Cancer Inst 1989;81:1874.

18. Saminiego F, Rodriguez E, Houldsworth J, et al: Cytogenentic and molecular analysis of human male germ cell tumors: Chromosome 12 abnormalities and gene amplification. Genes Chromosome Cancer 1990;1:289.

19. Wang LC, Vass W, Gao C, et al: Amplification and enhanced expression of the c-ki-ras2 proto-oncogene in human embryonal carcinoma. Cancer Res 1987;47:4192.

20. Houldsworth J, Reuter V, Bosl G, et al: Aberrant expression of cyclin D2 is an early event in male germ cell tumorigenesis. Cell Growth Differ 1997;8:293.

21. Chaganti RSK, Houldsworth J: Genetics and biology of adult human male germ cell tumors. Cancer Res 2000;60:1475–1482.

22. Madami A, Kemmer K, Sweeny C, et al: Expression of Kit and epidermal growth factor receptor (EGFR) in chemotherapy refractory non-seminomatous germ cell tumors [abstract]. Proc Am Soc Clin Oncol 2002;21:738.

23. Tian Q, Frierson H, Krystal G, et al: Activating c-kit gene mutations in human germ cell tumors. Am J Pathol 1999;154:1643–1647.

24. Moroni M, Veronese S, Sciavo R, et al: Epidermal growth factor receptor expression and activation in nonseminomatous germ cell tumors. Clin Cancer Res 2001;7:2770–2775.

25. Dixon RJ, Moore RA (eds): Atlas of Tumor Pathology, Fascicle 31B, Section 8. Washington, DC, Armed Forces Institute of Pathology, 1952.

26. Mostofi FK, Sobin LH: International Histological Classification of Tumors of Testis (No 16). Geneva, World Health Organization, 1977.

27. Mostofi FK, Price EB: Tumors of the male genital system. In Atlas of Tumor Pathology, 2nd series, Fascicle 8. Washington, DC, Armed Forces Institute of Pathology, 1973.

28. Fung CY, Garnick MB: Clinical stage I carcinoma of the testis: A review. J Clin Oncol 1988;6:734.

29. Rorth M: Therapeutic alternatives in clinical stage 1 nonseminomatous disease. Semin Oncol 1992;19:190.

30. Horwich A, Dearnaley DP: Treatment of seminoma. Semin Oncol 1992;19:171.

31. Zagars GK, Babaian RJ: Stage I testicular seminoma: Rationale for post-orchiectomy radiation therapy. Int J Radiat Oncol Biol Phys 1987;13:155.

32. Mason MD, Featherstone J, Olliff J, et al: Inguinal iliac lymph node involvement in germ cell tumours of the testis: Implications of radiological investigation and for therapy. Clin Oncol 1991;3:147.

33. Horwich A: Questions in the management of seminoma. Clin Oncol 1990;2:249.

34. Richie JP: Neoplasms of the testis. In Walsh PC, Retik AB, Stamey TA et al (eds): Campbell's Urology, vol 2, 6th ed. Philadelphia, WB Saunders, 1992.

35. Smith RB: Testicular carcinoma. In Haskell CM (ed): Cancer Treatment, 2nd ed. Philadelphia, WB Saunders, 1985.

36. Ray B, Hajdu SI, Whitmore WF: Distribution of retroperitoneal lymph node metastases in testicular germinal tumors. Cancer 1974;33:340.

37. Donohue JP, Sachary FM, Maynard BR: Distribution of modal metastases in nonseminomatous testic cancer. J Urol 1982;128:315.

38. Donohue JP: Transabdominal lymphadenectomy. In Donohue JP (ed): Testis Tumors. Baltimore, Williams & Wilkins, 1983.

39. Raghavan D, Peckham MJ, Heyderman E, et al: Prognostic factors in clinical stage I sonseminomatous germ cell tumours of the testis. Br J Cancer 1982;45:167.

40. Hoskin P, Dilly S, Easton D, et al: Prognostic factors in stage I nonseminomatous germ cell testicular tumors managed by orchiectomy and surveillance: Implications for adjuvant chemotherapy. J Clin Oncol 1986;4:1031.

41. Fung CY, Kalish LA, Brodsky G, et al: Stage I nonseminomatous testicular germ cell tumour: Prediction of metastatic potential by primary histopathology. J Clin Oncol 1988;6:1467.

42. Donohue JP: Surgical management of testicular cancer. In Einhorn LH (ed): Testicular Tumors, Managment and Treatment. New York, Masson, 1980.

43. Cockburn AG, Vugrin D, Batata M, et al: Poorly differentiated (anaplastic) seminoma of the testis. Cancer 1984;53:1991.

44. Percarpio B, Clements JC, McLeod DG, et al: Anaplastic seminoma: An analysis of 77 patients. Cancer 1979;43:2510.

45. Rosai U, Silber I, Khodadoust K: Spermatocytic seminoma. Clinicopathologic study of 6 cases and review of the literature. Cancer 1969;24:92.

46. Einhorn LH, Crawford ED, Shipley WU, et al: Cancer of the testes. In Devita VT (ed): Principles and Practice of Oncology, 3rd ed. Philadelphia, JB Lippincott, 1989.

47. Mead GM, Stennning SP, Parkinson MC, et al: The Second Medical Research Council study of prognostic factors in nonseminomatous germ cell tumors. J Clin Oncol 1992;10:85.

48. Sesterhenn IA, Weiss RB, Mostofi FK, et al: Prognosis and other clinical correlates of pathologic review in stage I and II testicular carcinoma: A report from the testicular cancer intergroup study. J Clin Oncol 1992;10:69.

49. Freedman LS, Parkinson MC, Jones WG, et al: Histopathology in the prediction of relapse of patients with stage I testicular teratoma treated by orchiectomy alone. Lancet 1987;2:294.

50. Drago JR, Nelson RP, Palmer JM: Childhood embryonal carcinoma of the testis. Urology 1978;12:499.

51. Mostofi FK, Theiss EA, Ashley DJB: Tumors of specialized gonadal stroma in human male patients: Androblastoma, Sertoli cell tumor, granulosa-theca cell tumor of the testis and gonadal stromal origin. Cancer 1959;12:944.

52. Holtz F, Abell MR: Testicular neoplasm in infants and children I: Tumors of non-germ cell origin. Cancer 1963;16:982.

53. Silverberg SG, Thompson JW, Higashi G, Baskin AM: Malignant interstitial cell tumor of the testis: Case report and review. J Urol 1966;96:356.

54. Hopkins GB: Interstitial cell tumor of the testis: Case report and review of the literature. J Urol 1970;103:449.

55. Unluer E, Ozcan D, Altin S: Malignant Leydig cell tumour of the

testis: A case report and review of the literature. Int Urol Nephrol 1990;22:455.

56. Doll DC, Weiss RB: Malignant lymphoma of the testis. Am J Med 1986;81:515.

57. Patel SR, Richardson RL, Kvols L: Metastatic cancer to the testes: A report of 20 cases and review of the literature. J Urol 1989;142:1003.

58. Bosl GJ, Vogelzang NJ, Goldman A, et al: Impact of delay in diagnosis on clinical stage of testicular cancer. Lancet 1981;2:970.

59. Feld R, Middleton WD: Recent advances in sonography of the testis and scrotum. Radiol Clin North Am 1992;30:1033.

60. Lerner RM, Mevorach RA, Hulbert WC, et al: Color Doppler US in the evaluation of acute scrotal disease. Radiology 1990;176:355.

61. Horstman WG, Melson GL, Middleton WD, et al: Testicular tumors: Findings with color Doppler US. Radiology 1992;167:631.

62. Klepp O, Olsson AM, Henrickson J, et al: Prognostic factors in clinical stage I nonseminomatous testicular germ cell tumors of the testis: Multivariate analysis of a prospective multicenter study. J Clin Oncol 1990;8:509.

63. Jacobsen GK, Rorth M, Osterlind K, et al: Histopathological features in stage I nonseminomatous testicular germ cell tumours correlated to relapse. APMIS 1990;98:377.

64. Stomper PC, Fung CY, Socinski MA, et al: Detection of retroperitoneal metastases in early-stage nonseminomatous testicular cancer: Analysis of different CT criteria. Am J Roentgenol 1987;149:1187.

65. Pont J, Holtl W, Kosak D, et al: Risk-adapted treatment choice in stage I nonseminomatous testicular germ cell cancer by regarding vascular invasion in the primary tumor: A prospective trial. J Clin Oncol 1990;8:16.

66. Chong C, Logthetis CJ, von Eschenbach A, et al: Orchiectomy in advanced germ cell cancer following intensive chemotherapy: A comparison of systemic to testicular response. J Urol 1986;136:1221.

67. Simmonds PD, Mead GM, Lee AHS, et al: Orchiectomy after chemotherapy in patients with metabolic testicular cancer: Is it indicated? Cancer 1995;75:1018.

68. Leibovitch I, Little JS Jr, Foster RS, et al: Delayed orchiectomy after chemotherapy for metabolic nonseminomatous germ cell tumors. J Urol 1996;155:952.

69. Dieckmann KP, Loy V: Intratesticular effects of cisplatin-based chemotherapy. Eur Urol 1995;28:25.

70. Markland C: Special problems in managing patients with testicular cancer. Urol Clin North Am 1977;4:427.

71. Gottesman JE: Radical inguinal orchiectomy. In Crawford ED, Das S (eds): Current Genitourinary Cancer Surgery. Philadelphia, Lea & Febiger, 1990.

72. Boileau MA, Steers WD: Testis tumors: The clinical significance of the tumor-contaminated scrotum. J Urol 1984;132:51.

73. Giquere JK, Stablein DM, Spaulding JT, et al: The clinical significance of unconventional orchiectomy approaches in testicular cancer: A report from the Testicular Cancer Intergroup Study. J Urol 1988;139:1225.

74. Klein EA: Tumor markers in testis cancer. Urol Clin North Am 1993;20:67.

75. Borkowski A, Muguardt C: Human chorionic gonadotropin in the plasma of normal, non-pregnant subjects. N Engl J Med 1979;301:298.

76. Braunstein GD, Vaitukaitis JL, Carbone PP, et al: Ectopic production of human chorionic gonadotropin by neoplasms. Ann Intern Med 1973;78:39.

77. Fukutani K, Libby JM, Panko WB, et al: Human chorionic gonadotropin detected in urinary concentrates from patients with malignant tumors of the testis, prostate, bladder, ureter, and kidney. J Urol 1983;129:74.

78. Garnick MB: Spurious rise in human chorionic gonadotropin induced by marijuana in patients with testicular cancer. N Engl J Med 1980;303:1177.

79. Javadpour N, McIntire KR, Waldmann TA, et al: The role of alpha fetoprotein and human chorionic gonadotropin in seminoma. J Urol 1978;120:687.

80. Mauch P, Weichselbaum R, Botnick L: The sign of positive chorionic gonadotropins in apparently pure seminoma of the testis. Int J Radiat Biol Phys 1979;5:887.

81. Swartz DA, Johnson DE, Hussey DH: Should an elevated human chorionic gonadotropin titer alter therapy for seminoma? J Urol 1984;131:63.

82. Mirimanoff RO, Shipley WU, Doseretz DE, et al: Pure seminoma of the testis: The results of radiation therapy in patients with elevated human chorionic gonadotropin titers. J Urol 1985;134:1124.

83. Loehrer PJ, Birch R, Williams SD, et al: Chemotherapy of metastatic seminoma: The Southeastern Cancer Study Group experience. J Clin Oncol 1987;5:1212.

84. Butcher DN, Gregory WM, Gunter PA, et al: The biological and clinical significance of HCG-containing cells in seminoma. Br J Cancer 1985;51:473.

85. Dieckmann KP, Due W, Bauer HW: Seminoma testis with elevated serum beta HCG-A category of germ cell cancer between seminoma and non-seminoma. Int J Urol Nephrol 1989;21:175.

86. Morgan DAL, Caillauld JM, Bellet D, et al: Gonadotrophin producing seminoma: A distinct category of germ cell neoplasm. Clin Radiol 1982;33:149.

87. Voneyben FE, Blaabjerg O, Madsen EL, et al: Serum lactate dehydrogenase isoenzyme-1 and tumor volume are indicators of response to treatment and predictors of prognosis in metastaic testicular germ cell tumours. Eur J Cancer 1992;28:410.

88. Voneyben FE, Degraaff WE, Marrink J, et al: Serum lactate dehydrogenase isoenzyme-1 activity in patients with testicular germ cell tumours correlates with the total number of copies of the short arm of chromosome 12 in the tumour. Mol Gen Genet 1991;235:140.

89. Kurman RJ, Scardino PT, Mcintire KR, et al: Cellular localization of alpha fetoprotein and human chorionic gonadotropin in germ cell tumors of the testis using an indirect immunoperoxidase technique: A new approach to classification utilizing tumor markers. Cancer 1977;40:2136.

90. Scardino PT, Cox DH, Waldman TA, et al: The value of serum tumor markers in the staging and prognoiss of germ cell tumors of the testis. J Urol 1977;118:994.

91. Picozzi VJ Jr, Freiha F, Hannigan JF, Torti FM: Prognostic significance of a decline in serum human chorionic gonadotropin levels after initial chemotherapy for advanced germ-cell carcinoma. Ann Intern Med 1984;100:183.

92. Lange PH, McIntire KR, Waldmann TA: Tumor markers in testicular tumor, current status and future prospects. In Einhorn LH (ed): Testicular Tumors: Managment and Treatment. New York, Masson, 1980.

93. Rathmell AJ, Brand IR, Carey BM, Jones WG: Early detection of relaspse after treatment for metastatic germ cell tumour of the testis: An excercise in medical audit. Clin Oncol 1993;5:34.

94. de Wit R, Sylvester R, Stoter G: Serum alpha-fetoprotein surges after the initiation of chemotherapy have a strong adverse prognostic significance in nonseminomatous testicular cancer. Proc Am Soc Clin Oncol 1997;16:318.

95. Jochelson MX, Garnick MB, Balikian JP, et al: The efficacy of routine whole lung tomography in germ cell tumors. Cancer 1984;54:1001.

96. Nachman JB, Baum ES, White H, et al: Bleomycin-induced pulmonary fibrosis mimicking recurrent metastatic disease in a patient with testicular cancer. Cancer 1981;47:236.

97. McCrea ES, Diaconis JN, Wade JC, et al: Bleomycin toxicity simulating metastatic nodules to the lungs. Cancer 1981;48:1096.

98. Hilton S, Herr HW, Teitcher JB, et al: CT detection of retroperitoneal lymph node metastases in patients with clinical stage I testicular nonseminomatous germ cell cancer. Am J Roentgenol 1997;169:521.

99. Heiken JP, Balfe DM, McClennan BC: Testicular tumors: Oncologic imaging and diagnosis. Int J Radiat Oncol Biol Phys 1984;10:275.

100. Maier JG, Sulak MH, Mittemeyer BT: Seminoma of the testis: Analysis of treatment success and failure. Am J Roentgenol 1968;102:596.

101. De Santis M, Bokemeyer C, Becherer A, et al: Predictive impact of 2-[18]fluoro-2-deoxy-d-glucose positron emission tomography for residual postchemotherapy masses in patients with bulky seminoma. J Clin Oncol 2001;19:3740–3744.

102. Bokemeyer C, Kollmannsberger C, Oechsle K, et al: Early prediction of treatment response to high-dose salvage

chemotherapy in patients with relapsed germ cell cancer using (^{18}F) FDG-PET. Br J Cancer 2002;86:506–511.

103. Hain SF, O'Doherty MJ, Timothy AR, et al: Fluorodeoxyclucose PET in the initial staging of germ cell tumours. Eur J Nuc Med 2000;27:590–594.

104. Cremerius U, Wilderberger J, Borchers H, et al: Does positron emission tomography using 18-fluoro-2-deoxyclucose improve clinical staging of testicular cancer? Results of a study in 50 patients. Urology 1999;54:900–904.

105. Albers P, Bender H, Yilmaz H, et al: Positron emission tomography in the clinical staging of patients with stage I and II testicular germ cell tumors. Urology 1999;53:808–811.

106. American Joint Committee on Cancer: Manual for Staging of Cancer, 6th ed. New York, Springer-Verlag, New York, Inc, 2002.

107. Warde P, Specht L, Horwich A, et al: Prognostic Factor for relapse in stage I seminoma managed by surveillance: A pooled analysis. J Clin Oncol 2002;20:4448–4452.

108. Hussey DH, Doornbos JF: Treatment, radiation therapy. In Johnson DE (ed): Testicular Tumors, 2nd ed. Flushing, NY, Medical Examination, 1976.

109. Bamberg M, Schmidberger H, Meisner C, et al: Radiotherapy for stages I and IIA/B testicular seminoma. Int J Cancer 1999;83: 823–827.

110. Horwich A, Alsanjari N, Ahern R, et al: Surveillance following orchidectomy for stage I testicular seminoma. Br J Cancer 1992;65:775.

111. Rabbani F, Sheinfeld J, Farivar-Mohseni H, et al: Low-volume nodal metastases detected at retroperitoneal lymphadenectomy for testicular cancer: Pattern and prognostic factors for relapse. J Clin Oncol 2001;19:2020–2025.

112. Thomas GM, Sturgeon JF, Alison M, et al: A study of post-orchidectomy surveillance in stage I testicular seminoma. J Urol 1989;142:313.

113. Oliver RTD, Ong J, Ostrowski J, Williams M: Radiotherapy, surveillance or platinum-based adjuvant chemotherapy for stage I germ cell tumors. Proc Am Soc Clin Oncol 1993;12:231.

114. Oliver TRD, Edmonds PM, Ong JYH, et al: Pilot studies of 2 and 1 course carboplatin as adjuvant for stage I seminoma: Should it be tested in a randomized trial against radiotherapy? Int J Radiat Oncol Biol Phys 1994;29:3.

115. Dieckmann KP, Bruggeboes B, Pichlmeier U, et al: Adjuvant treatment of clinical stage I seminoma: Is a single course of carboplatin sufficient? Urology 2000;55:102–106.

116. Reiter WJ, Brodowicz T, Alavi S, et al: Twelve-year experience with two courses of adjuvant single-agent carboplatin therapy for clinical stage I seminoma. J Clin Oncol 2001;19:101–104.

117. Moul JW, McCarthy WF, Fernandez EB, et al: Percentage of embryonal carcinoma and of vascular invasion predicts pathological stage in clinical stage I nonseminomatous testicular cancer. Cancer Res 1994;54:362.

118. Sweeney CJ, Hermans BP, Heilman DK, et al: Results and outcome of retroperitoneal lymph node dissection for clinical stage I embryonal carcinoma—predominant testis cancer. J Clin Oncol 2000;18:358.

119. Albers P, Bierhoff E, Neu D, et al: MIB-1 immunohistochemistry in clinical stage I nonseminomatous testicular germ cell tumors predicts patients at low risk for metastasis {see comments}. Cancer 1997;79:1710.

120. Heidenreich A, Schenkmann NS, Sesterhenn IA, et al: Immunohisto-chemical expression of Ki-67 to predict lymph node involvement in clinical stage I nonseminomatous germ cell tumors. J Urol 1997;158:620.

121. Schultz H: The Danish Testicular Carcinoma Study Group: Testicular carcinoma in Denmark 1976–1980. Stage and selected clinical parameters at presentation. Acta Radiol Oncol 1984; 23:249.

122. Foster RS, Donohue JP: Surgical treatment of clinical stage A nonseminomatous testis cancer. Semin Oncol 1992;19:166.

123. Williams SD, Stablein DM, Einhorn LH, et al: Immediate adjuvant chemotherapy versus observation with treatment at relapse in pathologic stage II testicular cancer. N Engl J Med 1987;317: 1433.

124. Foster RS, Roth BJ: Clinical stage I nonseminoma: Surgery versus surveillance. Semin Oncol 1998;25:145.

125. Rabbani F, Sheinfeld J, Farivar-Mohsenu H, et al: Low-volume nodal metastases detected at retroperitoneal lymphadenectomy for testicular cancer: Pattern and prognostic factors for relapse. J Clin Oncol 2001;19:2020–2025.

126. Richie JP, Kantoff PW: Is adjuvant chemotherapy necessary for patients with stage B1 testicular cancer? J Clin Oncol 1991;9:1393.

127. Donohue JP, Thornhill JA, Foster RS, et al: Primary retroperitoneal lymph node dissection in clinical stage A nonseminomatous germ cell testis cancer. Review of the Indiana University experience 1965–1989. Br J Urol 1993;71:326.

128. Donohue JP, Foster RS, Rowland RG, et al: Nerve sparing retroperitoneal lymphadenectomy. J Urol 1990;144:287.

129. Cullen MH, Stenning SP, Parkinson MC, et al: Short-course adjuvant chemotherapy in high-risk stage I nonseminomatous germ cell tumors of the testis: A Medical Research Council report. J Clin Oncol 1996;14:1106.

130. Oliver RT, Raja MA, Ong J, et al: Pilot study to evaluate impact of a policy of adjuvant chemotherapy for high risk stage I malignant teratoma on overall relapse rate of stage I cancer patients. J Urol 1992;148:1453.

131. Pont J, Albrecht W, Postner G, et al: Adjuvant chemotherapy for high-risk clinical stage I nonseminomatous testicular germ cell cancer: Long-term results of a prospective trial. J Clin Oncol 1996;14:441.

132. Studer UE, Fey MF, Calderoni A, et al: Adjuvant chemotherapy after orchiectomy in high-risk patients with clinical stage I nonseminomatous testicular cancer. Eur Urol 1993;23:444.

133. Bohlen D, Borner M, Sonntag R, et al: Long-term results following adjuvant chemotherapy in patients with clinical stage I testicular nonseminomatous malignant germ cell tumors with high risk factors. J Urol 1999;161:1148–1152.

134. Rorth M, Cullen MH, Horwich A, et al: Management of patients with nonseminomatous germ cell tumours stage I. In EORTC Gentiourinary Group Monograph 7: Prostate Cancer and Testicular Cancer. New York, Wiley-Liss, 1990.

135. Read G, Stenning SP, Cullen MH, et al: Medical Research Council prospective study of surveillance for stage I testicular teratoma. J Clin Oncol 1992;10:1762.

136. Freiha F, Torti FM: Orchiectomy only for clinical stage I nonseminomatous germ cell testis tumors: Comparison with pathologic stage I disease. Urology 1989;34:347.

137. Roeleveld TA, Horenblas S, Meinhardt W, et al: Surveillance can be the standard of care for stage I nonseminomatous testicular tumors and even high-risk patients. J Urol 2001;166:2177–2170.

138. Pizzocaro G, Zanoni F, Salvioni R, et al: Difficulties of a surveillance study omitt/ing retroperitoneal lymphadenectomy in clinical stage I nonseminomatous germ cell tumors of the testes. J Urol 1987;138:1393.

139. Young BJ, Bultz BD, Russell JA, et al: Compliance with follow-up of patients treated for nonseminomatous testicular cancer. Br J Cancer 1991;64:606.

140. Thomas G: Management of metastatic seminoma: role of radiotherapy. In Horwich A (ed): Testicular Cancer—Clinical Investigation and Management. New York, Chapman & Hall Medical, 1991.

141. Gregory C, Peckham MJ: Results of radiotherapy for stage II testicular seminoma. Radiother Oncol 1986;6:285.

142. Thomas GM, Rider WD, Dembo AJ, et al: Seminoma of the testis: Results of treatment and patterns of failure after radiation therapy. Int J Radiat Oncol Biol Phys 1982;8:165.

143. Evenson JF, Fossa SD, Kjellevold K, et al: Testicular seminoma: Analysis of treatment and failure for stage II disease. Radiother Oncol 1985;4:55.

144. Mason BR, Kearsley JH: Radiotherapy for stage II testicular seminoma: The prognostic influence of tumor bulk. J Clin Oncol 1988;6:1856.

145. Huben RP, Williams PD, Pontes JE, et al: Seminoma at Roswell Park, 1970 to 1979. An analysis of treatment failures. Cancer 1984;53:1451.

146. Kellokumpu-Lehtinen P, Halme A: Results of treatment in irradiated testicular seminoma patients. Radiother Oncol 1990;18:1.

147. Motzer RJ, Bosl GJ, Geller NL, et al: Advanced seminoma: The role of chemotherapy and adjunctive surgery. Ann Intern Med 1988;108:513.

148. Javadpour N, Young JD: Prognostic factors in non-seminomatious testicular cancer. J Urol 1986;135:497.

149. Pizzocaro G, Monfardini S: No adjuvant chemotherapy in selected patients with pathologic stage II nonseminomatous germ cell tumors of the testis. J Urol 1984;131:677.

150. Samuels ML, Johnson DE: Adjuvant therapy of testis cancer: The role of vinblastine and bleomycin. J Urol 1980;124:369.

151. Bredael JJ, Vugrin D, Whitmore WF: Selected experience with surgery and combination chemotherapy in the treatment of nonseminomatous germ cell tumors of the testis. J Urol 1984;131:677.

152. Vugrin D, Whitmore WF, Cvitkovic E, et al: Adjuvant chemotherapy combination of vinblastine, actinomycin D, bleomycin, and chlorambucil following retroperitoneal lymph node dissection for stage II testis cancer. Cancer 1981;47:840–844.

153. Williams SD, Birch R, Einhorn LH, et al: Treatment of disseminated germ cell tumors with cisplatin, bleomycin, and either vinblastine or etoposide. N Engl J Med 1987;316:1435.

154. Behnia M, Foster R, Roth B, et al: Adjuvant bleomycin, etoposide and cisplatin in fully resected stage B nonseminomatous testicular cancer. Proc Am Soc Clin Oncol 1996;15:249.

155. Culine S, Theodore C, Farhat F, et al: Cisplatin-based chemotherapy after retroperitoneal lymph node dissection in patients with pathological stage II nonseminomatous germ cell tumors. J Surg Oncol 1996;61:195.

156. Cushing B, Giller R, Marina N, et al: Results of surgery alone or surgery plus cisplatin, etoposide and bleomycin in children with localized gonadal malignant germ cell tumor: A pediatric intergroup report (POG9048/CCG8891). Proc Am Soc Clin Oncol 1997;16:511.

157. Motzer RJ, Sheinfeld J, Mazumdar M, et al: Etoposide and cisplatin adjuvant therapy for patients with pathologic stage II germ cell tumors. J Clin Oncol 1995;13:2700.

158. Horwich A, Dearnaley DP, Norman A, et al: Primary chemotherapy for stage II low volume non seminomatous germ cell tumours of the testis. Proc Am Soc Clin Oncol 1992;11:197.

159. Whitmore WF Jr: Surgical treatment of adult germinal testis tumors. Semin Oncol 1979;6:55.

160. Donohue JP, Rowland RG: The role of surgery in advanced testicular cancer. Cancer 1984;54:2716.

161. Vugrin D, Whitmore WF Jr: The role of chemotherapy and surgery in the treatment of retroperitoneal metastases in advanced nonseminomatous testis cancer. Cancer 1985;55:1874.

162. Oliver RTD, Freedman LS, Parkinson MC, Peckham MJ: Medical options in the managment of stages 1 and 2 testicular germ cell tumors. Urol Clin North Am 1987;14:721.

163. Logothetis CJ, Swanson DA, Dexeus F, et al: Primary chemotherapy for clinical stage II NSGCT of the testis: A follow-up of 50 patients. J Clin Oncol 1987;5:906.

164. Kamer M, Rowland RG, Einhorn LH, Donohue JP: Recurrent testis cancer: Seeding from retroperitoneal nodes after complete remission by chemotherapy. J Urol 1983;130:1196.

165. Ahmed T, Bosl GJ, Hajdu SI: Teratoma with malignant transformation in germ cell tumors in men. Cancer 1985;56:860.

166. Einhorn LH, Donohue JP: CDDP, vinblastine and bleomycin combination chemotherapy in disseminated testicular cancer. Ann Intern Med 1977;87:293.

167. Einhorn LH, Williams SD: Chemotherapy of disseminated testicular cancer. Cancer 1980;46:1339.

168. Einhorn LH, Williams SD, Troner M, et al: The role of maintenance therapy in disseminated testicular cancer. N Engl J Med 1981;305:727.

169. Bosl GJ, Gluckman R, Geller NL, et al: VAB-6: An effective chemotherapy regimen for patients with germ cell tumors. J Clin Oncol 1986;4:1493.

170. Bosl GJ, Geller NL, Cirrincione C, et al: Multivariate analysis of prognostic variables in patients with metastatic testicular cancer. Cancer Res 1983;43:3403.

171. Birch R, Williams S, Cone A, et al: Prognostic factors for favorable outcome in disseminated germ cell tumors. J Clin Oncol 1986;4:400.

172. Droz JP, Kramar A, Ghosn M, et al: Prognostic factors in advanced non seminomatous testicular cancer. A multivariate logistic regression analysis. Cancer 1988;62:564.

173. Stoter G, Sylvester R, Sleijfer D, et al: Multivariate analysis of prognostic factors in patients with disseminated non seminomatous testicular cancer: Results from a EORTC multi-institutional phase III study. Cancer Res 1987;47:2714.

174. Droz JP, Kramer A, Rey A: Prognostic factors in metastatic disease. Semin Oncol 1992;19:181.

175. Bajorin D, Katz A, Chan E: Comparison of criteria for assigning germ cell tumor patients to "good risk" and "poor risk" studies. J Clin Oncol 1988;6:786.

176. Bosl GJ, Geller NL, Bajorin D: Serum tumor markers and patient allocation to good risk and poor risk clinical trials in patients with germ cell tumors. Cancer 1991;67:1299.

177. International Germ Cell Cancer Collaborative Group: International Germ Cell Consensus Classification: A prognostic factor-based staging system for metastatic germ cell cancers. J Clin Oncol 1997;15:594.

178. Rodriguez P, Casanova L, Otero J, et al: Validation of International Classification (IGCCCG) for metastatic germ cell tumours treated with platinum-based chemotherapy. Proc Am Soc Clin Oncol 1997;16:341.

179. Mazumdar M, Bajorin DF, Bacick J, et al: Predicting outcome to chemotherapy in patients with germ cell tumors: The value of the rate of decline of human chorionic gonadotropin and alpha-fetoprotein during therapy. J Clin Oncol 2001;19:2534–2541.

180. Garrow GC, Johnson DH: Treatment of "good risk" metastatic testicular cancer. Semin Oncol 1992;19:159.

181. Einhorn LH, Williams SD, Loehrer PJ, et al: Evaluation of optimal duration of chemotherapy in favorable-prognosis disseminated germ cell tumors: A Southeastern Cancer Study Group protocol. J Clin Oncol 1989;7:387.

182. Horwich A, Oliver RTD, Wilkinson PM, et al: A medical research counsil randomized trial of single agent carboplatin versus etoposide and cisplatin for advanced metastatic seminoma. Br J Cancer 2000;12:1623–1629.

183. deWit R, Roberts JT, Wilkinson P, et al: Equivalence of three or four cycles of bleomycin, etoposide, and cisplatin chemotherapy and of a 3- or 5-day schedule in good prognosis germ cell cancer: A randomized study of the European Organization for Research and Treatment of Genitourinary Tract Cancer Cooperative Group and the Medical Research Council. J Clin Oncol 2001;6:1629–1640.

184. Boyer M, Raghavan D: Toxicity of treatment of germ cell tumors. Semin Oncol 1992;19:128.

185. Bosl GJ, Geller NL, Bajorin D, et al: A randomized trial of etoposide + cisplatin versus vinblastine + bleomycin + cisplatin + cyclophosphamide + dactinomycin in patients with good-prognosis germ cell tumors. J Clin Oncol 1988;6:1231.

186. Levi JA, Raghavan D, Harvey V, et al: The importance of bleomycin in combination chemotherapy for good-prognosis germ cell carcinoma. J Clin Oncol 1993;11:1300.

187. Loerher PJ, Elson P, Johnson DH, et al: A randomized trial of cisplatin plus etoposide with or without bleomycin in favorable-prognosis disseminated germ cell tumors: An ECOG study. Proc Am Soc Clin Oncol 1991;10:169.

188. deWit R, Storer G, Kaye SB, et al: Importance of bleomycin in combination chemotherapy for good-prognosis testicular non-seminoma: A randomized study of the European Organization for Research and Treatment of Cancer Genitourinary Tract Cancer Cooperative Group. J Clin Oncol 1997;15:1837.

189. Horwich A, Dearnaley DP, Nichols J, et al: Effectiveness of carboplatin, etoposide and bleomycin combination chemotherapy in good-prognosis metastatic testicular nonseminomatous germ cell tumors. J Clin Oncol 1991;9:62.

190. Bajorin DF, Sarosdy MF, Pfister DG, et al: Randomized trial of etoposide and cisplatin versus etoposide and carboplatin in patients with good-risk germ cell tumors: A multi-instutional study. J Clin Oncol 1993;11:598.

191. Horwich A, Sleijfer DT, Fossa SD, et al: Randomized trial of bleomycin, etoposide and cisplatin compared with bleomycin, etoposide and carboplatin in good-prognosis metastatic non-seminomatous germ cell cancer: A multi-institutional Medical

Research Council/European Organization for Research and Treatment of Cancer trial. J Clin Oncol 1997;15:1844.

192. Toner GJ, Geller NL, Tan C, et al: Serum tumor marker half-life during chemotherapy allows early prediction of complete response and survival in nonseminomatous germ cell tumors. Cancer Res 1990;50:5904.

193. Motzer RJ, Bajorin DF, Bosl GJ: Poor risk germ cell tumors: Current progress and future directions. Semin Oncol 1992;19:206.

194. Wozniak A, Samson M, Shah NT, et al: A randomized trial of cisplatin, vinblastine and bleomycin versus vinblastine, cisplatin, and etoposide in the treatment of advanced germ cell tumors of the testis: A Southwest Oncology Group study. J Clin Oncol 1991;9:70.

195. Loerher PJ, Einhorn LH, Williams SD: VP-16 plus ifosfamide plus cisplatin as salvage therapy in refractory germ cell cancer. J Clin Oncol 1986;4:528.

196. Harstrick A, Schmoll HJ, Wilke CH, et al: Cisplatin, etoposide, and ifosfamide salvage therapy for refractory or relapsing germ cell carcinoma. J Clin Oncol 1991;9:1549.

197. Nichols CR, Williams SD, Loehrer PJ, et al: Randomized study of cisplatin dose intensity in poor-risk germ cell tumors: A Southeastern Cancer Study Group and Southwest Oncology Group protocol. J Clin Oncol 191;9:1163.

198. Samson MK, Rivkin SE, Jones SE, et al: Dose-response and dose-survival advantage for high versus low-dose cisplatin combined with vinblastine and bleomycin in disseminated testicular cancer. Cancer 1984;53:1029.

199. Ozols RF, Ihde DC, Linehan M, et al: A randomized trial of standard chemotherapy versus a high-dose chemotherapy regimen in the treatment of poor prognosis nonseminomatous germ cell tumors. J Clin Oncol 1988;6:1031.

200. deWit R, Storer G, Sleijfer DT, et al: Four cycles of BEP versus an alternating regime of PVB and BEP in patients with poor-prognosis metastatic testicular non-seminoma: A randomised study of the EORTC Genitourinary Tract Cancer Cooperative Group. Br J Cancer 1995;71:1311.

201. Kaye SB, Mead GM, Fossa S, et al: An MRC/EORTC randomised trial in poor-prognosis metastatic teratoma, comparing BEP with BOP-VIP. Proc Am Soc Clin Oncol 1995;14:246.

202. Bower M, Newlands ES, Holden L, et al: Treatment of men with metastatic non-seminomatous germ cell tumours with cyclical POMB/ACE chemotherapy. Ann Oncol 1997;8:477.

203. Bower M, Brock C, Holden L, et al: POMB/ACE chemotherapy for mediastinal germ cell tumours. Eur J Cancer 1997;33:838.

204. Fizazi K, Prow DM, Do K-A, et al: Alternating dose-dense chemotherapy in patients with high volume disseminated non-seminomatous germ cell tumours. Br J Cancer 2002;86:1555–1560.

205. Motzer RJ, Bosl GJ, Tauer K, et al: Phase II trial of carboplatin in patients with advanced germ cell tumors refractory to cisplatin. Cancer Treat Rep 1987;71:197.

206. Motzer RJ, Cooper K, Geller NL, et al: Carboplatin, etoposide, and bleomycin for patients with poor-risk germ cell tumors. Cancer 1990;65:2465.

207. Chevreau C, Droz JP, Pico JL, et al: Early intensified chemotherapy with autologous bone marrow transplantation in first line treatment of poor risk non-seminomatous germ cell tumors. Preliminary results of a French randomized trial. Eur Urol 1993;23:213.

208. Motzer RJ, Mazumdar M, Gulati SC, et al: Phase II trial of high-dose carboplatin and etoposide with autologous bone marrow transplantation in first line therapy for patients with poor risk germ cell tumors. J Natl Cancer Inst 1993;85:1828.

209. Lotz JP, André T, Donsimone R, et al: High-dose chemotherapy with ifosfamide, carboplatin, and etoposide combined with autologous bone marrow transplantation for the treatment of poor prognosis germ cell tumors and metastatic trophoblastic disease in adults. Cancer 1995;75:874.

210. Motzer RJ, Mazumdar M, Bajorin DF, et al: High-dose carboplatin, etoposide and cyclophosphamide with autologous bone marrow transplantation in first-line therapy for patients with poor-risk germ cell tumors. J Clin Oncol 1997;15:2546–2552.

211. Bokemeyer C, Kollmannsberger C, Meisner A, et al: First-line high-dose chemotherapy compared with standard-dose PEB/VIP chemotherapy in patients with advanced germ cell tumors: A multivariate analysis and matched-pair analysis. J Clin Oncol 1999;11:3450–3456.

212. Nichols CR, Heerema NA, Palmer C, et al: Klinepelter's syndrome associated with primary mediastinal germ-cell tumors. J Clin Oncol 1987;5:1290.

213. Beyer J, Kramer A, Mandanas R, et al: High-dose chemotherapy as salvage treatment in germ cell tumors: A multivariate analysis of prognostic factors. J Clin Oncol 1996;14:2638.

214. Lester SG, Morphis JG, Hornback NB, et al: Brain metastases and testicular tumors: Need for aggressive therapy. J Clin Oncol 1984;2:1397.

215. Logothetis CJ, Samuels ML, Trindode A: The management of brain metastases in germ cell tumors. Cancer 1982;49:1278.

216. Rustin GJS, Newlands ES, Bagshawe KD, et al: Successful management of metastatic and primary germ cell tumors in the brain. Cancer 1986;57:2108.

217. Bajorin DF, Herr H, Motzer RJ, et al: Current perspectives on the role of adjunctive surgery in combined modality treatment for patients with germ cell tumors. Semin Oncol 1992;19:148.

218. Friedman EL, Garnick MB, Stomper PC, et al: Therapeutic guidelines and results in advanced seminoma. J Clin Oncol 1985;3:1325.

219. Motzer RJ, Bosl GJ, Heelan R, et al: Residual mass: An indication for further therapy in patients with advanced seminoma following systemic chemotherapy. J Clin Oncol 1987;5:1064.

220. Schultz S, Einhorn L, Concec D, et al: Management of postchemotherapy residual mass in patients with advanced seminoma: Indiana University experience. J Clin Oncol 1989;7:1497.

221. Fossa SD, Borge L, Gass N, et al: The treament of advanced metastatic seminoma: Experience in 55 cases. J Clin Oncol 1987;5:1071.

222. Freiha FS, Shortliffe D, Rose RV, et al: The extent of surgery after chemotherapy for advanced germ cell tumors. J Urol 1984;132:915.

223. Jansen RHL, Sylvestyer R, Sleyfer DT, et al: Long term follow-up of nonseminomatous testicular cancer patients with mature teratoma or carcinoma at post-chemotherapy surgery. Eur J Cancer 1991;27:695.

224. Geller NL, Bosl GJ, Chan EY: Prognostic factors for relapse after complete response in patients with metastatic germ cell tumors. Cancer 1989;63:440.

225. Nichols C, Gupta S, Loerher P, et al: Outcome in patients with residual germ cell cancer after post chemotherapy surgery. Proc Am Soc Clin Oncol 1987;6:100.

226. Fizazi K, Tjulandin S, Salvioni R, et al: Viable malignant cells after primary chemotherapy for disseminated nonseminomatous germ cell tumors: Prognostic factors and role of postsurgery chemotherapy: Results from an international study group. J Clin Oncol 2001;19:2647–2657.

227. Tiffany P, Morse MJ, Bosl G, et al: Sequential excision of residual thoracic and retroperitoneal masses after chemotherapy for stage III germ cell tumors. Cancer 1986;57:978.

228. Fossa SD, Ous S, Lien HH, et al: Post-chemotherapy lymph node histology in radiologically normal patients with metastatic nonseminomatous testicular cancer. J Urol 1989;141:557.

229. Toner GC, Panicek DM, Heelan RT, et al: Adjunctive surgery after chemotherapy for nonseminomatous germ cell tumors: Recommendations for patient selection. J Clin Oncol 1990;8:1683.

230. Donohue JP, Rowland RG, Kopecky K, et al: Correlation of computerized tomographic changes and histological findings in 80 patients having radical retroperitoneal lymph node dissection after chemotherapy for testis cancer. J Urol 1987;137:1176.

231. Levitt MD, Reynold PM, Sheiner HJ, et al: Nonseminomatous germ cell testicular tumors: Residual masses after chemotherapy. Br J Surg 1985;72:19.

232. Qvist HL, Fossa SD, Ous S: Post-chemotherapy tumor residuals in patients with advanced nonseminomatous testicular cancer. Is it necessary to resect all residual masses? J Urol 1991;145:300.

233. Brenner PC, Herr HW, Morse MJ, et al: Simultaneous retroperitoneal, thoracic and cervical resection of postchemotherapy residual masses in patients with metastatic

Specific Malignancies

III

nonseminomatous germ cell tumors of the testis. J Clin Oncol 1996;14:1765.

234. Saxman S: Salvage therapy in recurrent testicular cancer. Semin Oncol 1992;19:143.

235. Miller J, Einhorn LH: Phase II study of daily oral etoposide in refractory germ cell tumors. Semin Oncol 1990;17:36.

236. Hainsworth JD, Williams SD, Einhorn LH, et al: Successful treatment of resistant germinal neoplasms with VP-16-213 and cisplatin: Results of a Southeastern Cancer Study Group trial. J Clin Oncol 1985;3:666.

237. Levi JA, Thomson D, Harvey V, et al: Effective salvage chemotherapy with etoposide, dactinomycin, and methotrexate in refractory germ cell cancer. J Clin Oncol 1990;8:27.

238. Loerher PJ, Lauer R, Roth BJ, et al: Salvage therapy in recurrent germ cell cancer: Ifosfamide and cisplatin plus either vinblastine or etoposide. Ann Intern Med 1988;109:540.

239. McCaffrey JA, Mazumdar M, Bajorin DF, et al: Ifosfamide- and cisplatin-containing chemotherapy as first-line salvage therapy in germ cell tumors: Response and survival. J Clin Oncol 1997;15:2559.

240. Motzer RJ, Geller NL, Tan CCY, et al: Salvage chemotherapy for patients with germ cell tumors. Cancer 1991;67:1305.

241. Miller K, Loehrer P, Gonin R, et al: Salvage chemotherapy with vinblastine, ifosfamide and cisplatin in recurrent seminoma. J Clin Oncol 1997;15:1427.

242. Motzer RJ, Bajorin DF, Schwartz LH, et al: Phase II trial of paclitaxel shows antitumor activity in patients with previously treated germ cell tumors. J Clin Oncol 1994;12:2277–2283.

243. Bokemeyer C, Beyer J, Metzner B, et al: Phase II study of paclitaxel in patients with relapsed or cisplatin-refractory testicular cancer. Ann Oncol 1994;7:31–34.

244. Motzer R, Sheinfeld J, Mazumdar M, et al: Paclitaxel, ifosfamide and cisplatin second-line therapy for patients with relapsed testicular germ cell cancer. J Clin Oncol 2000;18:2413–2418.

245. Broun ER, Nichols CR, Kneebone P, et al: Long-term outcome of patients with relapsed and refractory germ cell tumors treated with high dose chemotherapy and autologous bone marrow rescue. Ann Intern Med 1992;117:124.

246. Nichols CR, Andersen J, Lazarus HM: High dose carboplatin and etoposide with autologous bone marrow transplantation in refractory germ cell cancer: An Eastern Cooperative Oncology Group protocol. J Clin Oncol 1992;10:558.

247. Droz JP, Pico JL, Kramar A: Role of autologous bone marrow transplantation in germ cell cancer. Urol Clin North Am 1993;5:270.

248. Barnett MJ, Coppin CML, Murray N, et al: Intensive therapy and autologous bone marrow transplantation for patients with poor prognosis nonseminomatous germ cell tumors. Proc Am Soc Clin Oncol 1991;10:165.

249. Elias A, Kantoff P, Ayash L, et al: High dose ifosfamide, carboplatin and etoposide (ICE) with autologous marrow support for germ cell carcinoma. Proc Am Soc Clin Oncol 1993;12:231.

250. Broun ER, Nichols CR, Turns M, et al: Early salvage therapy for germ cell cancer using high-dose chemotherapy with autologous bone marrow support. Cancer 1994;73:1716.

251. Broun ER, Nichols CR, Mandanas R, et al: Dose escalation study of high-dose carboplatin and etoposide with autologous bone marrow support in patients with recurrent and refractory germ cell tumors. Bone Marrow Transplant 1995;16:353.

252. Lampe H, Dearnaley DP, Price A, et al: High-dose carboplatin and etoposide for salvage chemotherapy of germ cell tumors. Eur J Cancer 1995;31A:717.

253. Rosti G, Albertazzi L, Salvioni R, et al: High-dose chemotherapy with autologous bone marrow transplantation in germ cell tumors: A phase II study. Ann Oncol 1992;3:809.

254. Siegert W, Beyer J, Strohscheer I, et al: High-dose treatment with carboplatin, etoposide, and ifosfamide followed by autologous stem-cell transplantation in relapsed or refractory germ cell cancer: A phase I/II study. J Clin Oncol 1994;12:1223.

255. Beyer J, Kingreen D, Krause M, et al: Long term survival of patients with recurrent or refractory germ cell tumors after high dose chemotherapy. Cancer 1997;79:161.

256. Margolin K, Doroshow JH, Ahn C, et al: Treatment of germ cell cancer with two cycles of high-dose ifosfamide, carboplatin, and etoposide with autologous stem-cell support. J Clin Oncol 1996;14:2631.

257. Rodenhuis S, van der Wall E, ten Bokkel Huinink WW, et al: Pilot study of a high-dose carboplatin-based salvage strategy for relapsing or refractory germ cell cancer. Cancer Invest 1995;13:355.

258. Motzer RJ, Mazumdar M, Bosl GJ, et al: High-dose carboplatin, etoposide, and cyclophosphamide for patients with refractory germ cell tumors: Treatment results and prognostic factors for survival and toxicity. J Clin Oncol 1996;14:1098.

259. Motzer RJ, Gulati SC, Crown JP, et al: High-dose chemotherapy and autologous bone marrow rescue for patients with refractory germ cell tumors: Early intervention is better tolerated. Cancer 1992;69:550.

260. Linkesch W, Greinix H, Kalhs P, et al: Long term results of phase I/II trial of CarboPEC with ABMT in refractory or relapsed NSGCT. Bone Marrow Transplant 1994;14(Suppl):S41

261. Bhatia S, Abonour R, Porcu P, et al: High-dose chemotherapy as initial salvage chemotherapy in patients with relapsed testicular cancer. J Clin Oncol 2000;18:3346–3351.

262. Rick O, Beyer J, Hartmann JT, et al: Salvage treatment with paclitaxel, ifosfamide, and cisplatin plus high-dose carboplatin, etoposide, and thiotepa followed by autologous stem-cell rescue in patients with relapsed or refractory germ cell cancer. J Clin Oncol 2001;19:81–88.

263. Motzer R, Mazumdar M, Sheinfeld J, et al: Sequential dose-intensive paclitaxel, ifosfamide, carboplatin, and etoposide salvage therapy for germ cell tumor patients. J Clin Oncol 2000;18:1173–1180.

264. Rosti G, Pico JL, Wandt H, et al: High-dose chemotherapy in the salvage treatment of patients failing first-line platinum chemotherapy for advanced germ cell tumor (GCT): First results of a prospective randomized trial of the European Group for Blood and Marrow Transplantation (EBMT): IT-94 [abstract]. Proc Am Soc Clin Oncol 2002;716:55.

265. Wood DP, Herr HW, Motzer RJ, et al: Surgical resection of solitary metastases after chemotherapy in patients with nonseminomatous germ cell tumors and elevated serum tumor markers. Cancer 1992;70:2354.

266. Eastham JA, Wilson TG, Russell C, et al: Surgical resection in patients with nonseminomatous germ cell tumor who fail to normalize serum tumor markers after chemotherapy. Urology 1994;43:74.

267. Murphy B, Breeden E, Donohue J, et al: Surgical salvage of chemorefractory germ cell tumors. Proc Am Soc Clin Oncol 1992;11:198.

268. Droz JP, Kramar A, Nichols C, et al: Second line chemotherapy with ifosfamide, cisplatin and either etoposide or vinblastine in recurrent germ cell cancer: Assignment of prognostic groups. Proc Am Soc Clin Oncol 1993;12:229.

269. Bokemeyer C, Gerl A, Schoffski P, et al: Gemcitabine in patients with relapsed or cisplatin-refractory testicular cancer. J Clin Oncol 1999;17:512–516.

270. Porcu P, Bhatia S, Sharma M, et al: Results of treatment after relpased from high-dose chemotherapy in germ cell tumors. J Clin Oncol 2000;18:1181–1186.

271. Hinton S, Catalano P, Einhorn L, et al: Phase II study of paclitaxel plus gemcitabine in refractory germ cell tumours (E9897): A trial of the Eastern Cooperative Oncology Group. J Clin Oncol 2002;20:1859–1863.

272. Roth BJ, Greist A, Kubilis PS, et al: Cisplatin-based combination chemotherapy for disseminated germ cell tumors: Long-term follow-up. J Clin Oncol 1988;6:1239.

273. Dearnaley DP, Horwich A, Hern R, et al: Combination chemotherapy with bleomycin, etoposide, and cisplatin (BEP) for metastatic testicular teratoma: Long-term follow-up. Eur J Cancer 1991;27:684.

274. Borge N, Fossa SD, Ous S, et al: Late recurrences of testicular cancer. J Clin Oncol 1988;6:1248.

275. DeLeo MJ, Greco FA, Hainsworth JD, Johnson DH: Late recurrence in long-term survivors of germ cell neoplasms. Cancer 1988;62:985.

276. Terebelo HR, Taylor HG, Brown A, et al: Late relapse of testicular cancer. J Clin Oncol 1983;1:566.

277. Baniel J, Foster RS, Gonin R, et al: Late relapse of testicular cancer. J Clin Oncol 1995;13:1170.

278. George DW, Foster RS, Hromas RA, et al: Update on late relpase of germ cell tumor: A clinical and molecular analysis. J Clin Oncol 2003;21:113–122.

279. van Leeuwen FE, Stiggelbout A, van den Belt-Dusebout RN, et al: Second cancer risk following testicular cancer: A follow-up study of 1,909 patients. J Clin Oncol 1993;11:415.

280. Vallis KA, Howard GC, Duncan W, et al: Radiotherapy for stages I and II testicular seminoma: Results and morbidity in 238 patients. Br J Radiol 1995;68:400.

281. Wanderas EH, Fossa SA, Tretli S: Risk of a second germ cell cancer after treatment of a primary germ cell cancer in 2201 Norwegian male patients. Eur J Cancer 1997;33:244.

282. Fossa SD, Aass N: Cisplatin-based chemotherapy does not eliminate the risk of a second testicular cancer. Br J Urol 1989;63:531.

283. Grossfeld GD, Small EJ: Long term side effects of treatment for testis cancer. Urol Clin North Am 1998;25:503.

284. Aass N, Fossa SD, Host H: Acute and subacute side effects due to infradiaphragmatic radiotherapy for testicular cancer: A prospective study. Int J Radiat Oncol Biol Phys 1992;22:1057.

285. Birch R, Loerher P, Williams S, et al: The effect of delay of therapy on response to cisplatin chemotherapy in disseminated germ cell tumor. Proc Am Soc Clin Oncol 1986;5:105.

286. Motzer RJ, Geller NL, Bosl GJ: The effect of a 7-day delay in chemotherapy cycles on complete response and event-free survival in good-risk disseminated germ cell tumor patients. Cancer 1990; 66:857.

287. Weijl NI, Rutten M, Zwinderman AH, et al: Thromboembolic events during chemotherapy for germ cell cancer: A cohort study and review of the literature. J Clin Oncol 2000;10:2169–2178.

288. Ginsberg SJ, Comis RL: The pulmonary toxicity of antineoplastic agents. Semin Oncol 1982;9:34.

289. Comis RL, Kuppinger MS, Ginsberg SJ, et al: Role of single breath diffusing capacity in monitoring the pulmonary effects of bleomycin in germ cell tumor patients. Cancer Res 1979; 39:5076.

290. Comis RL: Detecting bleomycin pulmonary toxicity: A continued conundrum. J Clin Oncol 1990;8:765.

291. McKeage MJ, Evans BD, Atkinson C, et al: Carbon monoxide diffusing capacity is a poor predictor of clinically significant bleomycin lung. J Clin Oncol 1990;8:779.

292. Aass N, Fossa SD, Aas M, et al: Renal function related to different treatment modalities for malignant germ cell tumors. Br J Cancer 1990;62:842.

293. Moeller H, Mellemgaard A, Jacobsen GK, et al: Incidence of second primary cancer following testicular cancer. Eur J Cancer 1993;29A:672.

294. Roth BJ, Einhorn LH, Greist A: Long-term complications of cisplatin-based chemotherapy for testis cancer. Semin Oncol 1988;15:345.

295. Meinardi MT, Gietema WTA, Van Der Graaf DJ, et al: Cardiovascular morbidity in long-term survivors of metastatic testicular cancer. J Clin Oncol 2000;18:1725–1732.

296. Raghavan D, Cox K, Childs A, et al: Hypercholesterolemia after chemotherapy for testis cancer. J Clin Oncol 1992;10:1386.

297. Ellis PA, Fitzharris BM, George PM, et al: Fasting plasma lipid measurements following cisplatin chemotherapy in patients with germ cell tumors. J Clin Oncol 1992;10:1609.

298. Hansen SW, Berthelsen JG, von der Maase H: Long term fertility and Leydig cell function in patients treated for germ cell cancer with cisplatin, vinblastine, and bleomycin versus surveillance. J Clin Oncol 1990;8:1695.

299. Foster RS, McNulty A, Rubin LR, et al: The fertility of patients with clinical stage I testis cancer managed by nerve sparing retroperitoneal lymph node dissection. J Urol 1994;152: 1139.

300. Brennemann W, Stoffel-Wagner B, Helmers A, et al: Gonadal function of patients treated with cisplatin based chemotherapy for germ cell cancer. J Urol 1997;158:844.

301. Stephenson WT, Poirier SM, Rubin L, et al: Evaluation of reproductive capacity in germ cell tumor patients following treatment with cisplatin, etoposide, and bleomycin. J Clin Oncol 1995;13:2278.

302. Kaldor JM, Day NE, Band P, et al: Second malignancies following testicular cancer, ovarian cancer and Hodgkin's disease: An international collaborative study among cancer registries. Int J Cancer 1987;39:571.

303. Bokemeyer C, Schmoll HJ: Secondary neoplasms following treatment of malignant germ cell tumors. J Clin Oncol 1993;11:1703.

304. Nichols CR, Breeden ES, Loehrer PJ, et al: Secondary leukemia associated with a conventional dose of etoposide: Review of serial germ cell tumor protocols. J Natl Cancer Inst 1993;85:36.

305. Bajorin DF, Motzer RJ, Rodriguez E, et al: Acute nonlymphocytic leukemia in germ cell tumor patients treated with etoposide-containing chemotherapy. J Natl Cancer Inst 1993;85:60.

306. Pedersen-Bjergaard J, Daugaard G, Hansen SW, et al: Increased risk of myelodysplasia and leukaemia after etoposide, cisplatin, and bleomycin for germ cell tumours. Lancet 1991;338:359.

307. Oliver RTD, Ong JYH, Raja MA, et al: Secondary leukaemia and etoposide. Lancet 1991;338:1269.

308. Li MC, Whitmore WF, Golbey R, et al: Effects of combined drug therapy on metastatic cancer of the testis. JAMA 1960;174:1271.

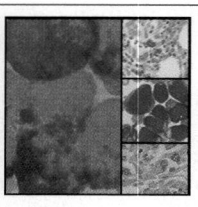

Anthony H. Russell

Michael V. Seiden

Linda R. Duska

Anne Kathryn Goodman

Susanna I. Lee

Subba R. Digumarthy

Arlan F. Fuller, Jr.

CANCERS OF THE CERVIX, VAGINA, AND VULVA

SUMMARY OF KEY POINTS

INCIDENCE

- An estimated 12,200 new cases of invasive cervical cancer are anticipated in 2003 in the United States, with 4100 deaths projected
- From 75% to 80% are squamous cell carcinomas
- Since the advent of cytologic screening in the 1940s, the incidence of cervical cancer has been decreasing; however, a steady increase in the incidence of preinvasive disease of the cervix has occurred

ETIOLOGY

Associated risk factors include race, early age at first coitus, multiple sexual partners, multiparity, lower socioeconomic standing, cigarette smoking, history of sexually transmitted diseases, immunosuppression, and oral contraceptive use

- Strong association with human papillomavirus (HPV)
- HPV serotypes 16, 18, 31, 33, 45, and 56 account for more than 80% of all invasive cervical cancers

EVALUATION AND STAGING

- Screening for cervical cancer has historically been done with the Papanicolaou (Pap) smear and pelvic examination
- Testing for DNA of high-risk oncogenic HPV may be used to triage atypical smears and to

reduce the frequency of cytologic screening
- Biopsies should be performed of gross lesions
- Patients without gross lesions but with abnormal cytology should undergo colposcopy with directed biopsies and endocervical curettage (ECC) or brushing
- Once a diagnosis of cancer is made, the patient requires a complete history and physical examination, including bimanual and rectovaginal examination, as well as supraclavicular and groin lymph node examination
- Cervical cancer is staged clinically, not surgically
- Assignment of stage of disease may be influenced by findings from chest and skeletal radiography, excretory urography (intravenous pyelogram; IVP), barium enema, cytoscopy, and proctoscopy
- Results of computed tomography (CT), magnetic resonance imaging (MRI), positron emission tomography (PET), or other imaging modalities do not influence assignment of International Federation of Obstetrics and Gynaecology (FIGO) stage, but may be important in directing therapy

PRIMARY THERAPY

High-grade dysplasia or carcinoma in situ may be treated with excisional cone biopsy (i.e., cervical conization

performed with loop electrosurgical excision procedure [LEEP], or cold-knife)
- Stage Ia1 (microinvasive cervical cancer 3 mm or less depth of invasion and 7 mm width or less) without lymph-vascular invasion is managed with conservative surgery (i.e., excisional conization or extrafascial hysterectomy)
- Stage Ia2 lesions (invasion of more than 3 mm depth, and lesion 7 mm width or less) or Ia1 lesions with lymph-vascular invasion are managed with modified radical hysterectomy
- Stage Ib lesions and stage IIa lesions may be managed with radical hysterectomy or radiation therapy with equivalent probability of cure but different morbidities. Selected surgical patients with adverse risk factors may benefit from adjuvant postoperative radiation or chemoradiation
- Patients with stage IIb to IVa are generally treated with radiation therapy with concurrent chemotherapy

THERAPY FOR RECURRENT DISEASE

- Disease that recurs centrally in the pelvis after radiation may be treated with radical exenterative surgery
- Locally recurrent disease after surgery is generally treated with radiation therapy or chemoradiation

INTRODUCTION

Cancers of the cervix, vulva, and vagina represent the major malignancies of the lower female genital tract. With the exception of the endocervix, this portion of the genital tract is available for physical examination, including direct visual inspection and palpation. Currently, cytologic screening and surveillance by Papanicolaou (Pap) smear, testing for the presence of oncogenic strains of the human papillomavirus (HPV), colposcopy, and a variety of confirmatory biopsy techniques, are capable of diagnosing preinvasive disease or very early stage invasive disease that can be treated with a high probability of cure.

Improvements in diagnostic imaging and assessment of disease extent before therapeutic intervention and more routine use of integrated, multimodality therapy together offer the opportunity for better outcomes for women with invasive local or regional disease.

Squamous cell carcinomas are the dominant histologic type in all three sites, with many tumors associated with oncogenic strains of HPV. In the last decade, improved understanding of HPV biology, the epidemiology and natural history of HPV infection, and early studies on HPV-directed vaccines offer hope that the incidence of invasive disease could decrease in the decades ahead. In the future, anticipated use of HPV-targeted vaccines in the pediatric population offers the potential to reduce dramatically worldwide morbidity and mortality associated with this group of diseases.

EPIDEMIOLOGY

For 2003, the American Cancer Society estimates that 12,200 cases of invasive cervical carcinoma and approximately 4100 cervical cancer deaths will occur in the United States, representing only 1.5% of the projected 270,600 annual cancer deaths in American women. A much larger population of American women (approximately fourfold) will be diagnosed with cervical dysplasia that will never develop invasive neoplasia.

Although cervical cancer is the third most common gynecologic malignancy in the United States, it ranks as the most common gynecologic malignancy worldwide and is the second most common cancer in women in the world, with an estimated 500,000 cases in 2003. Marked disparity in incidence exists between countries where routine gynecologic care and Pap smear screening are available, and countries in Latin America, the Caribbean, and Africa where cervical cancer is the most common cause of cancer-related death in women.[1]

It has long been appreciated that the incidence of invasive cervical carcinoma is related to sexual activity. Early age at first intercourse, multiple sexual partners, a history of venereal infection, and other parameters of sexual activity have long been recognized as factors associated with the development of invasive cervical cancer. Women from lower socioeconomic strata, black, and Hispanic populations have an increased frequency of disease. Incidence rates in the United States are estimated

at 8.1 new cases per 100,000 white women each year as compared with 11 per 100,000 in blacks and 14.4 per 100,000 in Hispanics.

Molecular epidemiologic studies have demonstrated that correlation of sexual activity with cervical carcinoma is related to transmission of the epithelial trophic and oncogenic HPV.[2-4] Most HPV infections are transient, resulting in no changes or low-grade intraepithelial lesions (cervical intraepithelial neoplasia; CIN 1) that will be spontaneously cleared in most young women.[5,6] Development of high-grade intraepithelial lesions will occur in a small minority of women, usually within 24 months.[7] High-grade lesions (CIN 2/3) may progress to invasive cervical cancer if not treated.[8,9]

Cases of CIN 2/3 that progress to invasive cancer will do so over a period of 8 to 12 years, which has been referred to as the detectable preclinical phase.[10-13] Thus the opportunities for early detection and intervention are abundant. However, an estimated half of the invasive cervical cancers diagnosed in the United States are found in women who have never been screened, and an additional 10% are diagnosed in women who have not been screened within the preceding 5 years.[14]

Based on a comprehensive review of available evidence, the American Cancer Society convened an expert panel in 2001 through 2002 to formulate detailed guidelines for the initiation of screening, screening intervals, discontinuation of screening, screening in the context of prior hysterectomy, and use of various screening tests.[15] A synopsis of their recommendations is found in Table 90-1.

HUMAN PAPILLOMAVIRUS BIOLOGY

The HPV is a double-stranded DNA virus in the Papovaviridae family (Fig. 90-1). This virus, constituted of approximately 8000 nucleotides, encodes seven early genes and two late genes, as well as having a small, untranslated region. Approximately 100 different serotypes with limited DNA homology have been identified. Although the identification of high-risk subtypes of HPV has been important in defining potential therapeutic targets for the prevention of cervical carcinoma, HPV infection has not adequately explained all of the biologic features of preinvasive disease and progression to invasive disease. Studies in sexually active college coeds demonstrated that infection with HPV is extremely common, occurring in up to 50% of women who become sexually active between the ages of 16 and 21 years, with the first abnormal Pap smear appearing in only a subset of women 1 year after infection. These infections are typically associated with low-grade dysplastic lesions and are usually transient. Persistent infection with associated high-grade dysplastic lesions is seen in only a small proportion of infected women (perhaps 1% or 2%). Biologic and/or immunologic cofactors that allow the persistence of HPV infection in a small subset of women remain unclear. Epidemiologic studies suggest that co-infection with herpes simplex virus type II (HSV), long-term oral contraceptive use, cigarette smoking, and high parity may increase the risk of persistent infection, carcinoma in situ

TABLE 90-I

American Cancer Society Guideline for Screening by Cytology for the Early Detection of Cervical Neoplasia and Cancer

- Cervical cancer screening should begin ~3 yr after the onset of vaginal intercourse and no later than age 21 yr*
- Women who are age 70 or older with an intact cervix and who have had 3 or more documented, consecutive, technically satisfactory normal/negative cervical cytology tests and no abnormal/positive cytology tests within the 10-yr period before age 70 may elect to cease cervical cancer screening†
- Screening with vaginal cytology tests after total hysterectomy (with removal of the cervix) for benign gynecologic disease is not indicated. The presence of CIN 2/3 is not considered benign. Women with a history of CIN 2/3 or without documentation of the absence of CIN 2/3 should be screened until three documented, consecutive, technically satisfactory normal/negative cervical cytology tests and no abnormal/positive cytology tests with a 10-year period are achieved†
- After initiation of screening, cervical screening should be performed annually with conventional cervical cytology smears or every 2 years using liquid-based cytology; at or after age 30, women who have had three consecutive, technically satisfactory normal/negative cytology results may be screened every 2–3 years‡

*Age 21 to initiate screening is a guideline for circumstances in which sexual history is not available because providers do not ask, or because patients are unable or unwilling to provide a history regarding consensual or non-consensual intercourse. It also is intended to protect victims of sexual abuse.
†Women who have a history of cervical cancer, in utero diethylstilbestrol exposure, or are immunocompromised [including human immunodeficiency virus positive (HIV⁺)] should continue screening absent severe comorbid or life-threatening illnesses.
‡More frequent screening may be advisable in women with in utero DES exposure, and women who are HIV⁺ or are immunocompromised by organ transplantation, chemotherapy, or prolonged corticosteroid treatment.

(CIS), and invasive disease.[16,17] Whereas long-term epidemiologic studies undertaken since appreciation of the role of HPV remain incomplete, it is known is that in the large majority of women, the period between HPV infection, dysplasia, and then invasive carcinoma is typically years to decades, offering the potential for screening and early intervention to change the natural history and morbidity associated with this disease.[18-22]

Molecular epidemiologic studies have divided HPV serotypes into high-risk, intermediate-risk, and low-risk subtypes for the development of cervical neoplasia.[23] Low-risk subtypes have been associated with venereal warts (condyloma acuminata) whereas intermediate- and high-risk subtypes have been associated with cervical dysplasia and invasive carcinoma. Recent worldwide review of HPV typing demonstrated that 87% of squamous cell carcinomas had identifiable HPV genome associated with the tumor as compared with 76.4% of adenocarcinomas. HPV-16 was the predominant type associated with between 46% and 63% of the squamous carcinomas, whereas HPV-18 was associated with 10% to 14% of squamous cell carcinomas. An additional 16 other HPV types were associated with the remaining 25% of cases, including HPV-45, -31, and -33. Most epidemiologic studies have demonstrated a higher incidence of HPV-18 (37% to 41%), followed by HPV-16 (26% to 36%) in women with adenocarcinoma of the cervix. Several authors have shown a positive association between the presence of certain HPV subtypes and prognosis. Barnes and colleagues[24] showed that, among invasive carcinomas, HPV-18 is associated with poorly differentiated histology and higher incidence of nodal metastases. Similarly,

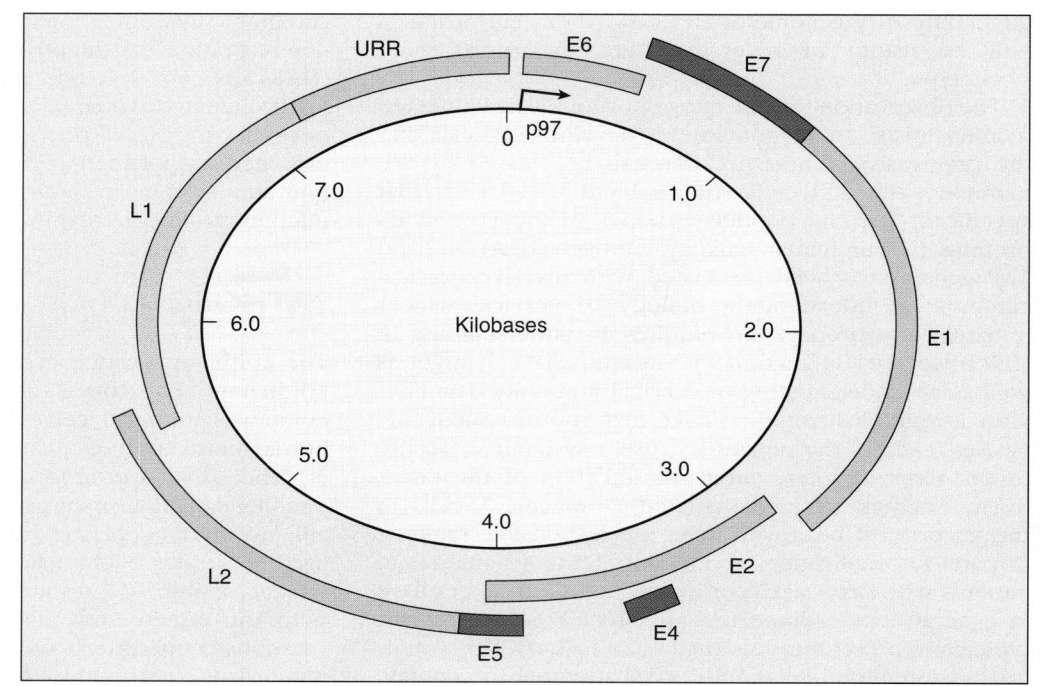

Figure 90-1. HPV Genome. The HPV virus is a double stranded DNA virus in the Papovaviridae family. This virus, constituted by approximately 8000 nucleotides, encodes seven early genes and two late genes, as well as having a small, untranslated region. Approximately 100 different serotypes with limited DNA homology have been identified. (From Basic biology and biochemistry of gynecologic cancer. In Hoskins WJ, Perez CA, Young RC (eds): Principles and Practice of Gynecologic Oncology, 2nd ed. Philadelphia, Lippincott-Raven, 1997, Fig. 3.6.)

Walker[25] reported that HPV-18–associated cancers were more likely to recur than were HPV-16–associated cancers. By contrast, HPV-16 was associated with large cell keratinizing tumors, and these tumors were less likely to recur.[26] Lombard[27] demonstrated HPV-18–associated tumors to have a relative risk of death 2.4 times greater than that observed for patients with HPV-16–associated tumors and 4.4 times greater than that for patients with a tumor associated with another HPV type.

The mechanism by which these epithelial trophic viruses cause neoplasia has been defined through an elaborate collection of experiments that have focused on the role of the E6 and E7 early genes. Virally encoded E6 binds to the p53 protein, leading to its ubiquination and targeting of this cellular checkpoint protein for proteosomal destruction. The E6 protein product also enters the nucleus and interacts with the other important nuclear proteins. The second virally encoded protein, E7, sequesters the retinoblastoma gene product (Rb) releasing the RB-associated E2F transcription factor, which results in the initiation of a number of nuclear events important in driving the cell through the cell cycle. Recent studies also suggested that p21 is sequestered and inactivated by the E7 protein. Elimination of the p53 and Rb checkpoint results in dysregulated cell growth and dysplasia. In addition, the E7/E6 proteins both independently lead to mitotic instability, with abnormality in chromosomal segregation during mitosis and increased chromosome instability. This may in part describe the long latency period between HPV infection and carcinoma. Loss-of-heterozygosity studies and other molecular events have defined chromosomal changes and changes in other oncogenic proteins that are neither primary nor secondary effects of HPV infection, but are due instead to co-infection or other non-HPV factors. Although data suggest that HPV infection may be critical in initiating the neoplastic transformation, it is not clear that therapy that targets the HPV genome or HPV-related protein products will be useful in reversing the fully transformed phenotype.

The observation that, in a large portion of HPV-infected women, invasive carcinoma never develops suggests that the preinvasive neoplastic cells can be cleared by the immune system. Recent studies identified T cells that specifically identify peptide epitopes of the E6 and E7 proteins. Certain human leukocyte antigen (HLA) DR2 and TAP genes have been associated with invasive cervical carcinoma. Understanding biology of cervical cancer initiation and propagation requires an understanding of HPV biology, its interaction with its epithelial cell target, as well as an understanding of cervical immunity. The HPV virus is epithelial trophic. Unlike that in other oncogenic viruses (such as the hepatitis viruses), systemic exposure to the virus is not required for infection of the target organ. Analysis has demonstrated E6-specific T cells in the majority of healthy women are responsible (at least in part) for eradication of infection. Tetramer analysis in patients with cervical CIS or invasive cervical cancer have in general demonstrated few HPV-16 E7-reactive T cells, typically representing less than 0.1% of the CD8+ T cells in the systemic circulation. Recent attempts to generate

productive and/or long-term HPV-16 infection have been accomplished by using an HPV-16 virus–like particle vaccine. In a recent randomized, placebo-controlled study, the delivery of three vaccinations at day 0, month 2, and month 6 reduced the risk of persistent new HPV-16 infection from 3.8 cases per 100 women-years at risk to 0 per 100 woman-years in the group that were vaccinated, for a 100% efficacy rate. In this study, involving 2392 young women between the ages of 16 and 23 years, nine cases of HPV-16–related CIN were noted, all in the placebo recipients.[28] Further study with this and other vaccines is ongoing.

Maiman, Fruchter, and associates[29-32] investigated the disease characteristics, recurrence risks, and survival rates of HIV-seropositive patients with CIN and invasive cervical cancer. HIV-infected women had significantly higher rates of recurrence of CIN after standard therapies than did seronegative women. HIV-infected women with cervical cancer had significantly more advanced disease than did those who were not infected. Only 3 (19%) of 16 HIV-seropositive patients were first seen with an early-stage disease (defined as stage Ia or nonbulky Ib) compared with 35 (52%) of 68 in the HIV-seronegative group. When upstaged based on surgicopathologic findings, only 1 (6%) HIV-infected patient had early-stage disease compared with 40% of uninfected patients. The response to therapy and prognosis were poorer among HIV-seropositive women, with higher recurrence and death rates. The majority of seropositive women had lymph node metastases and high-grade tumors. They were generally asymptomatic with respect to their HIV disease, but died of cervical cancer. The significant impact of immune status on disease progression was made evident by prolonged disease-free follow-up in seropositive patients with CD4 counts greater than 500/mm³, in contrast to those with CD4 counts less than 500/mm³. The observed marked increased risk of invasive cervical carcinoma in women infected with the HIV virus and the demonstration that highly effective antiretroviral therapy (HART) is capable of doubling the CIN regression rates in HIV-infected women, as compared with those women not receiving HART, provides suggestive, indirect clinical evidence supporting the critical importance of the intact immune system in limiting the progression of HPV infection to invasive cancer in healthier populations.

PATHOLOGY

The epithelium of the cervix is composed of squamous epithelium that covers the exocervix and glands and columnar epithelial cells that line the endocervix. The border between the squamous and columnar epithelium is called the *squamocolumnar junction*, the site of ongoing squamous metaplasia believed to be most vulnerable to viral neoplastic transformation. With increasing age, the squamocolumnar junction migrates from the exocervix into the distal endocervical canal (Fig. 90-2) with the region between the original and subsequent locations termed the *transformation zone*. The transformation zone is the most common location for detection

of early cervical cancers (Fig. 90-3) Tumors arising on the ectocervix are typically squamous cell carcinomas, whereas adenocarcinomas are more likely to have their epicenter in the endocervix.

A continuum appears to exist from CIN to frankly invasive squamous cell carcinoma (Fig. 90-4). The mean age of women with CIN is 15.6 years younger than that of women with invasive cancer, suggesting slow progression of CIN to invasive carcinoma.[18] The natural history of HPV infection and CIN in part reflects the host immune system response to the virus. Seventy-five percent of CIN 1 lesions will spontaneously regress or persist as CIN 1, without progression to invasive carcinoma.[18-21]

Miller[33] reported, in a 13-year observational study, that only 14% of CIN 3 lesions had progressed, whereas 61% persisted, and the remainder disappeared. Patients taking corticosteroids or other immunosuppressive drugs and patients with HIV infection are at higher risk of

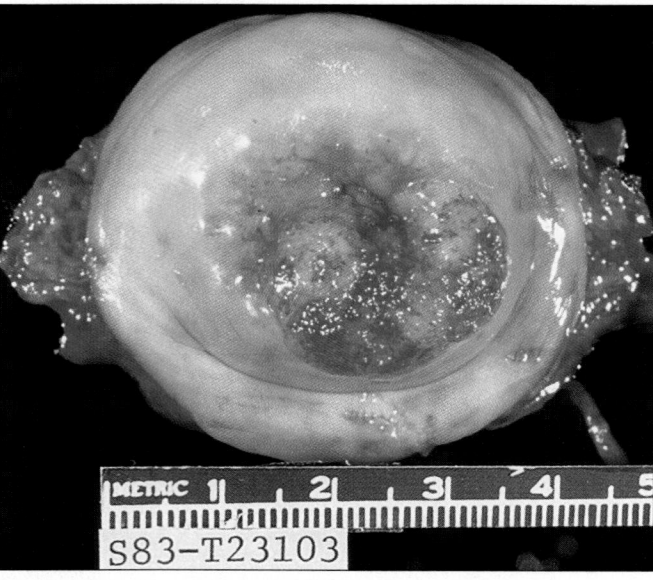

Figure 90-3. Invasive squamous cell carcinoma. A mass is present on the external OS. (Clement PB, Young RH: Atlas of Gynecologic Surgical Patholoy. Philadelphia, WB Saunders, 2000, p 103.)

progressing to invasive cancer and may have a shorter transit time for this progression.

Squamous Cell Carcinomas of the Cervix

Approximately 75% of invasive cervical carcinomas are squamous cell carcinomas. Tumor histology can range between well, moderately, or poorly differentiated tumors. Squamous carcinomas (Fig. 90-5) may be keratinizing (sometimes containing characteristic keratin pearls) or nonkeratinizing. Large cell and small cell variants exist. True verrucous cancers of the cervix are rare.

Cervical Adenocarcinomas

Adenocarcinomas comprise 15% to 25% of invasive cervical carcinomas. Typically arising in the endocervix, adenocarcinomas can be more difficult to detect on visual inspection of the cervix. These tumors may infiltrate deeply into the stroma of the cervix, sometimes with parametrial extension and nodal metastases without gross destruction of the exocervix. In addition to the classic endocervical type, histologic variants of adenocarcinoma include endometrioid carcinoma, villoglandular, mesonephric, serous, intestinal-type, and signet-ring morphologies.

Clinically important subtypes also include clear cell adenocarcinomas of the cervix associated with in utero diethylstilbestrol (DES) exposure, which tend to be diagnosed at a younger age than most other adenocarcinomas, and so-called "adeno malignum" or minimal deviation adenocarcinoma (Fig. 90-6), an entity associated with deceptively bland or benign-appearing cells, which may be cause for undertreatment of a true malignancy, with a significant likelihood of recurrence even when diagnosed at an early stage.[34,35]

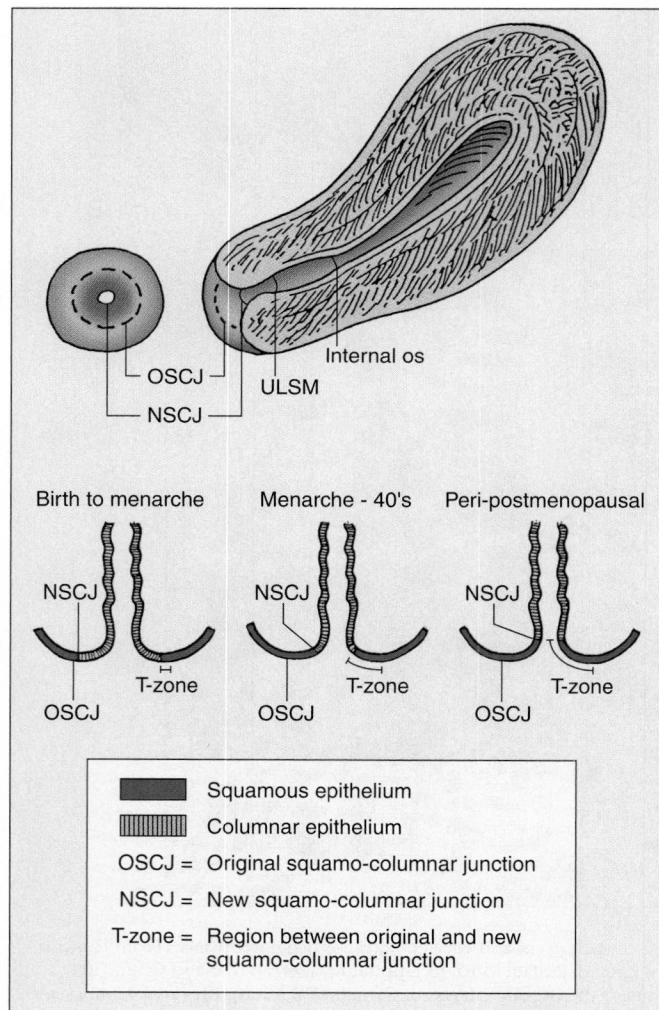

Figure 90-2. The transformation zone and squamocolumnar junction. (From Hoskins WJ, Perez CA, Young RC (eds): Principles and Practice of Gynecologic Oncology, 2nd ed. Philadelphia, Lippincott, 1997, p 678 and Berek JS, Hacker NF: Practical Gynecologic Oncology, 2nd ed. Baltimore, Williams & Wilkins, 1994.)

Specific Malignancies

III

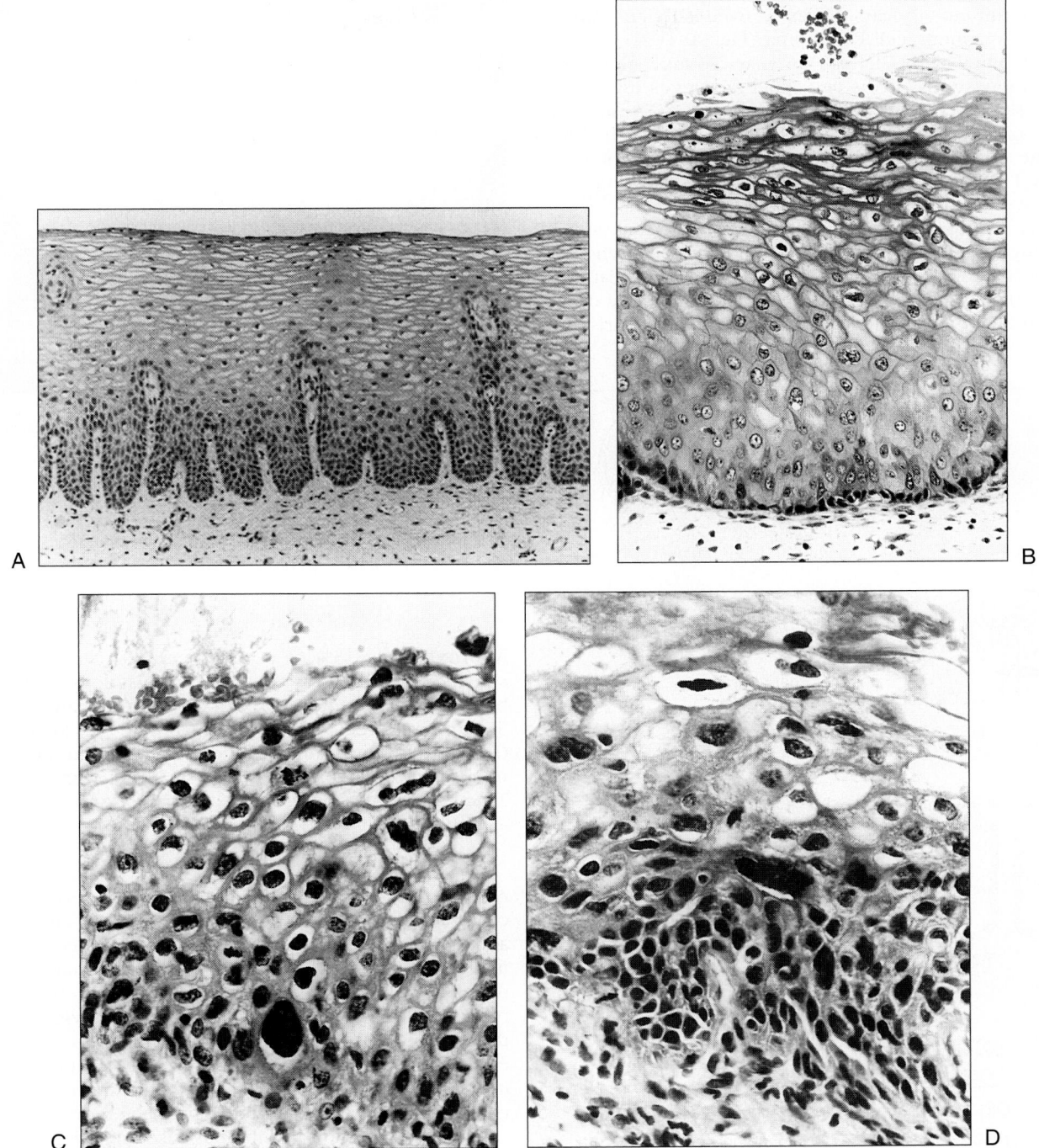

Figure 90-4. A–F, Histologic portraits of normal stratified squamous epithelium of the cervix and cervical intraepithelial neoplasia. (From Hoskins WJ, Perez CA, Young RC (eds): Principles and Practice of Gynecologic Oncology, 2nd ed. Philadelphia, JB Lippincott, 1997, p 678 and Crum CP: Papillomavirus-related changes and premalignant and malignant squamous lesions of the uterine cervix. In Clement PB, Young RH [eds]: Tumors and Tumorlike Lesions of the Uterine Corpus and Cervix. Contemporary Issues in Surgical Pathology, Vol 22. New York, Churchill Livingstone, 1993, p 91, with permission.)

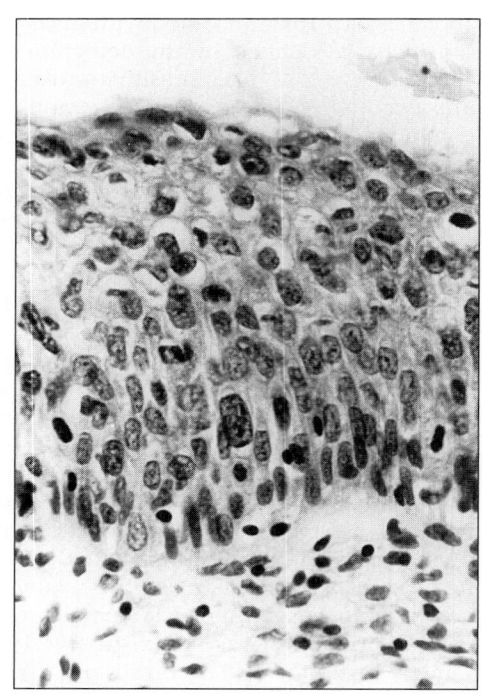
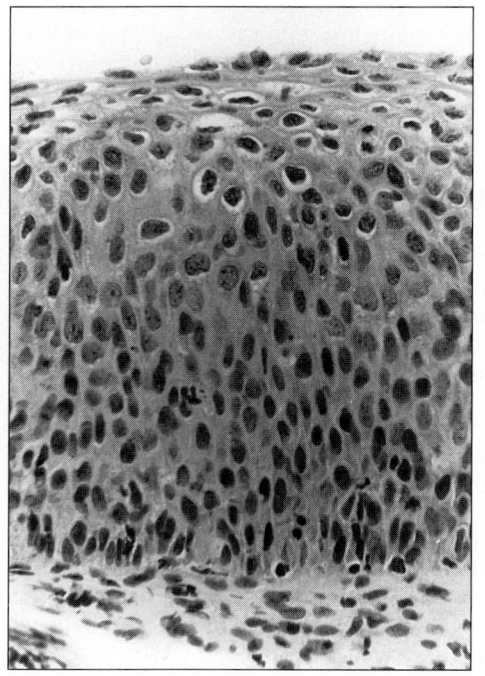

Figure 90-4, *cont'd.*

Adenosquamous Carcinomas

Adenosquamous carcinomas consist of a malignant glandular component and a malignant squamous component and comprise approximately one third of cervical carcinomas with glandular differentiation. Opinions vary regarding the prognosis of adenosquamous carcinoma compared with pure adenocarcinoma or pure squamous carcinoma when prognosis is adjusted for clinical stage at diagnosis. A clinically important variant of adeno-

squamous carcinoma is the so-called *glassy cell carcinoma,* thought to represent a very poorly differentiated adenosquamous carcinoma, the name of which derives from the ground-glass or granular appearance of the cytoplasm seen in many cases. Additional features may include an intense stromal inflammatory infiltrate composed predominantly of eosinophils and plasma cells. Some patients may have accompanying eosinophilia in their circulating blood, with elevated absolute eosinophil counts. This histologic type is associated with a rapid

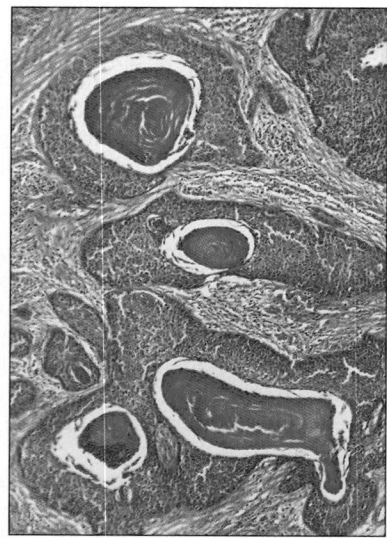

Figure 90-5. Invasive squamous cell carcinoma of the keratinizing type. (Clement PB, Young RH: Atlas of Gynecologic Surgical Pathology. Philadelphia, WB Saunders, 2000, p 103.)

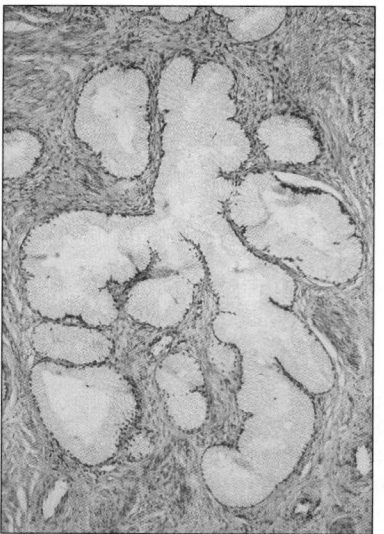

Figure 90-6. Adenoma malignum. A gland with a bizarre shape is lined by benign-appearing tumor cells. (Clement PB, Young RH: Atlas of Gynecologic Surgical Pathology. Philadelphia, WB Saunders, 2000, p 118.)

clinical rate of growth, proclivity for early regional dissemination, and increased risk of recurrence after surgical therapy or radiation therapy, even in the absence of other recognized adverse prognostic factors.[36-39]

NEUROENDOCRINE TUMORS OF THE CERVIX

Neuroendocrine tumors arising in the cervix include typical and atypical carcinoid tumors, and large cell and small cell neuroendocrine carcinomas. Both large cell and small cell neuroendocrine tumors resemble similar carcinomas arising in the lung and other aerodigestive sites and have a proclivity for early hematogenous dissemination.[40,41]

These tumors rarely may manifest clinical or biochemical evidence of ectopic hormone production. Treatment of neuroendocrine carcinomas of the cervix parallels the treatment of these histologic types at other primary sites, with an emphasis on systemic therapy soon after diagnosis, with surgery and/or radiation used as consolidative therapy for patients with clinically localized or only regional extent of disease.

Clinical Presentation

Preinvasive neoplastic disorders of the cervix are generally asymptomatic, hence the need for regular screening by cytologic evaluation of cells collected from the exocervix and endocervix. Early invasive cancers also may be asymptomatic, although some women will notice postcoital, intermenstrual, or postmenopausal spotting. Other symptoms may include malodorous vaginal discharge, dyspareunia, or cramping pelvic pain from uterine contractions caused by the accumulation of blood and uterine deciduas in menstruating patients with occlusion of the endocervical canal. Chronic blood loss may result in symptomatic anemia in some patients. Major hemorrhage is unusual except in locally advanced disease. Pelvic pain, lower extremity swelling (from occlusion of pelvic lymphatics or thrombosis of the external iliac vein), or problems with micturition or defecation indicate advanced regional disease and portend an ominous prognosis. Metastatic disease involving supraclavicular nodes, bones, or lungs can be the cause of presenting symptoms, but rarely in the absence of pelvic symptoms. Constitutional symptoms, including anorexia, dysgeusia, and weight loss, are most often seen in patients with very advanced disease.

Screening

Screening for cervical cancer and its precursors with the Pap smear and pelvic examination has resulted in dramatic reductions in cervical cancer mortality in every country where this has been widely used, and is arguably the most effective screening program in effect for any neoplastic disease, in male or female patients. Current screening guidelines of the American Cancer Society are outlined in Table 90-1. The false-negative rate of the Pap smear is about 10% to 15% in women with invasive cancer, but the sensitivity, as defined by the detection of biopsy-proven CIN, is 51%.[42-44] The sensitivity of the test may be improved by ensuring adequate sampling of the squamocolumnar junction and the endocervical canal. Smears without endocervical or metaplastic cells may be inadequate and should possibly be repeated.[45]

Factors contributing to abnormal cytologic smears include the presence of hemorrhage, necrosis, and intense inflammation. Thus gross symptomatic lesions should be sampled with biopsy rather than assessed with exfoliative cytology.

In the 1980s, cytology laboratories began reporting an increasing number of smears with changes of "squamous atypia" in response to concerns from clinicians over an unacceptably high false-negative cytology rate and increased recognition by cytopathologists of the cytologic changes associated with HPV infection. The use of multiple classification systems with inconsistently defined numeric grading conventions added further imprecision. In an attempt to eliminate confusion among clinicians and cytopathologists, a uniform system for reporting epithelial cell abnormalities was established in 1988 at a National Cancer Institute (NCI) workshop for reporting cervical and vaginal cytologic diagnoses.[46]

The Bethesda System has since been revised in 1991 and again in 2001 (Table 90-2)[47] to reflect laboratory and clinical experience gained since the original implementation, as well as the increased utilization of new technologies and results from interval research studies. An important contribution of the Bethesda System was the creation of a standardized format and nomenclature for cytology laboratory reports that includes both a descriptive diagnosis and an evaluation of specimen adequacy.

With the formulation of Bethesda 2001, a specimen is designated "satisfactory for evaluation" or "unsatisfactory for evaluation." The category "satisfactory but limited by..." has been eliminated as confusing. Minimal cellularity requirements for a specimen to qualify as satisfactory depend on specimen type, with an estimated 8000 to 12,000 well-visualized squamous cells for conventional smears and 5000 squamous cells for liquid-based preparations. Comments on partially obscuring inflammation or blood may be added to the "satisfactory" designation, with a specimen considered "partially obscured" when 50% to 75% of the epithelial cells cannot be visualized. When more than 75% of epithelial cells are obscured, a specimen is designated "unsatisfactory." A notation is made regarding the presence or absence of an endocervical/transformation zone component for specimens with adequate squamous cellularity, with the numeric criterion being at least 10 well-preserved endocervical or squamous metaplastic cells. Cell clusters are not required.

Squamous atypia is a mild cellular abnormality characterized by slight nuclear enlargement and minimal changes of the nuclear chromatin. Cellular changes that show morphologic features of papillomavirus infection or mild CIN (grade 1) are termed *low-grade squamous intraepithelial lesions* or LSILs. Cellular changes con-

TABLE 90-2

The 2001 Bethesda System

Specimen Adequacy

Satisfactory for evaluation (not presence of endocervical/transformation zone component)
Unsatisfactory for evaluation (specify reason)
Specimen rejected/not processed (specify reason)
Specimen processed and examined, but unsatisfactory for evaluation of epithelial abnormality because of (specify reason)

General Categorization (Optional)

Negative for intraepithelial lesion or malignancy
Epithelial cell abnormality
Other

Interpretation/Result

Negative for intraepithelial lesion or malignancy
  Organisms
    Trichomonas vaginalis
    Fungal organisms consistent with Candida sp.
    Shift in flora suggestive of bacterial vaginosis
    Bacteria morphologically consistent with Actinomyces sp.
    Cellular changes consistent with herpes simplex virus
  Other non-neoplastic findings (Optional. List not comprehensive)
    Reactive cellular changes associated with inflammation (includes typical repair)
      Radiation
      Intrauterine contraceptive device
    Glandular cells after hysterectomy
    Atrophy
Epithelial cell abnormalities
  Squamous cell
    Atypical squamous cells (ASC) of undetermined significance (ASC-US), cannot exclude HSIL (ASC-H)
    Low-grade squamous intraepithelial lesion (LSIL) encompassing human papillomavirus, mild dysplasia, cervical intraepithelial neoplasia (CIN) I
    High-grade squamous intraepithelial lesion (HSIL) encompassing moderate and severe dysplasia, carcinoma in situ; CIN 2 and CIN 3
    Squamous cell carcinoma
  Glandular cell
    Atypical glandular cells (AGCs) (specify endocervical, endometrial, or not otherwise specified)
    Atypical glandular cells, favor neoplastic (specify endocervical or not otherwise specified)
    Endocervical adenocarcinoma in situ (AIS)
    Adenocarcinoma
    Other (list not comprehensive)
      Endometrial cells in a woman 40 yr or older

Automated Review and Ancillary Testing

(Include as appropriate)

Educational Notes and Suggestions (Optional)

Adapted from Soloman D, Davey D, Kurman R, et al: The 2001 Bethesda System: Terminology for reporting results of cervical cytology. JAMA 2002;287:2114.

sistent with moderate (CIN 2) or severe (CIN 3) dysplasia are termed *high-grade squamous intraepithelial lesions* or HSILs. The division of SILs into high- and low-grade strata reflects accumulating evidence that LSIL is generally indicative of transient infection with HPV, particularly in young women, and does not routinely require colposcopy or treatment, whereas HSIL cytology detects precursor lesions that require further evaluation and treatment.

Important refinements in the 2001 Bethesda System relate to the reporting of equivocal results. Atypical squamous cells (ASCs) are now further qualified as "of undetermined significance" (ASC-US) or "cannot exclude HSIL" (ASC-H). The qualifier "undetermined significance" was retained, as some cases of ASC-US are associated with underlying CIN 2 or CIN 3. All ASCs are considered to be suggestive of SILs, and thus the category "ASCUS favor reactive" has been eliminated, with a portion of cases previously so designated being downgraded to "negative for intraepithelial lesion or malignancy." The new term ASC-H includes true HSIL and its mimics and is thought to have a positive predictive value for CIN 2 or CIN 3 intermediate between ASC-US and HSIL. The term *atypical glandular cells of undetermined significance* (AGUS) has been eliminated to avoid confusion with ASC-US. Glandular cell abnormalities are now classified as *atypical endocervical, endometrial,* or *glandular cells.* The term *atypical epithelial cells* may be used when a squamous versus glandular origin cannot be ascertained.

DIAGNOSIS

Management of the patient with an abnormal Pap smear with respect to further diagnostic assessments, therapeutic intervention, and subsequent surveillance follow-up is a complex arena in which guidelines continue to evolve. The American Society for Colposcopy and Cervical Pathology (ASCCP) has developed contemporary guidelines for management of cervical cytologic abnormalities and CIN based on current reporting terminology (Bethesda 2001), to which the reader is referred.[48,49] Techniques for further evaluation can include colposcopy, endocervical curettage or brushing, and cervical conization by cold knife or loop electrodiathermy excision procedure (LEEP).

Testing for high-risk, oncogenic HPV DNA[50-56] synchronously, or subsequent to cytologic screening, is proving to be a useful complementary tool in triage of patients with ASC-US smears and in determining the need for colposcopy and the intervals for repeated screening. It may be helpful in the follow-up of younger patients with LSIL smears, and a useful tool in identifying older women who can safely be screened at 3-year intervals instead of annually.

HPV triage of patients with an ASC-US smear is at least as sensitive as immediate colposcopy for ultimately detecting CIN 3 and results in referral of about half as many women to colposcopy. A follow-up strategy that uses repeated cytology is sensitive at an ASCUS referral threshold, but requires two follow-up visits and ultimately more colposcopic examinations than does HPV triage.[57]

Cytologic and HPV screening in women older than 30 years (after which most sexually active women have been exposed to HPV and have, or have not, spontaneously cleared the infection) may be a mechanism through which low-risk HPV-negative and cytologically negative patients can be identified for whom screening at 3-year intervals is prudent and appropriate.

Colposcopy

Patients with a gross lesion of the cervix should undergo cervical biopsy. For patients with an abnormal cytologic evaluation, without a gross lesion, a colposcopic examination with directed punch biopsies is required. Colposcopy allows the clinician to identify areas suggestive of dysplasia. A 3% acetic acid solution is applied to the cervix for 30 to 90 seconds, which causes a transient reaction with the envelope proteins of the papillomavirus, in addition to producing an osmotic dehydration of the dysplastic cells, thereby accentuating the optically dense chromatin to produce a whitish area. The skilled colposcopist can further distinguish between grades of dysplasia based on acetowhitening and types of vascular patterns (Fig. 90-7). An additional technique to help visualize abnormal areas is the application of quarter-strength Lugol's iodine after the initial inspection for acetowhitening. High-grade lesions turn mustard yellow.

Endocervical Curettage or Endocervical Brush

Study of the endocervical canal is required when no abnormalities are found on colposcopic examination, when the entire squamocolumnar junction cannot be visualized, or when atypical endocervical cells are present on Pap smear. Some experts advocate the use of endocervical curettage (ECC) as part of every colposcopic examination to safeguard against missing occult cancer within the endocervical canal. Others reserve ECC for patients with recurrent cytologic atypia after therapy. A sleeved endocervical brush is an alternative to ECC that is less uncomfortable for many patients. Recent, prospective comparison of ECC specimens with sleeved endocervical brush specimens (both obtained from the same patient sequentially after randomization with respect to the order of obtaining specimens) before cervical conization or hysterectomy revealed a higher rate of inadequate specimens from ECC, comparability of the two techniques with respect to sensitivity and specificity in unmatched analysis, and superior sensitivity of the sleeved endocervical brush in matched analysis. As the sleeved endocervical brush is at least isoeffective and possibly better than ECC but more comfortable for the patient, many clinicians prefer this maneuver, which may serve to increase patient compliance with subsequent surveillance follow-up and repeated assessment.[58]

Excisional Biopsy

Diagnostic cervical conization (cone biopsy) leads to an accurate diagnosis and decreases the incidence of inappropriate therapy in the following situations: (1)

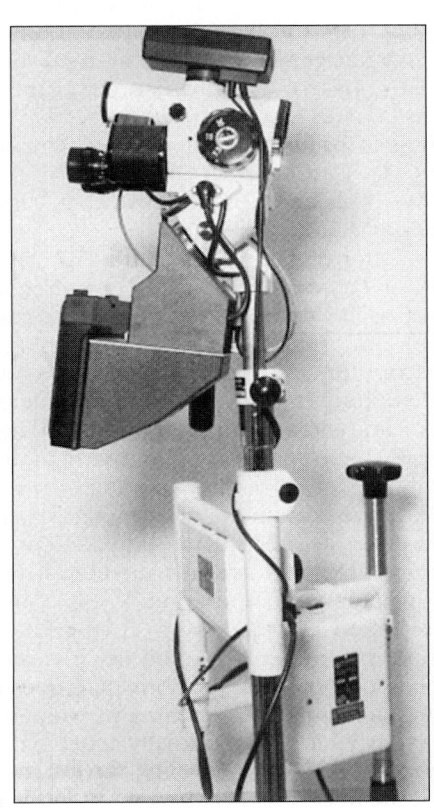
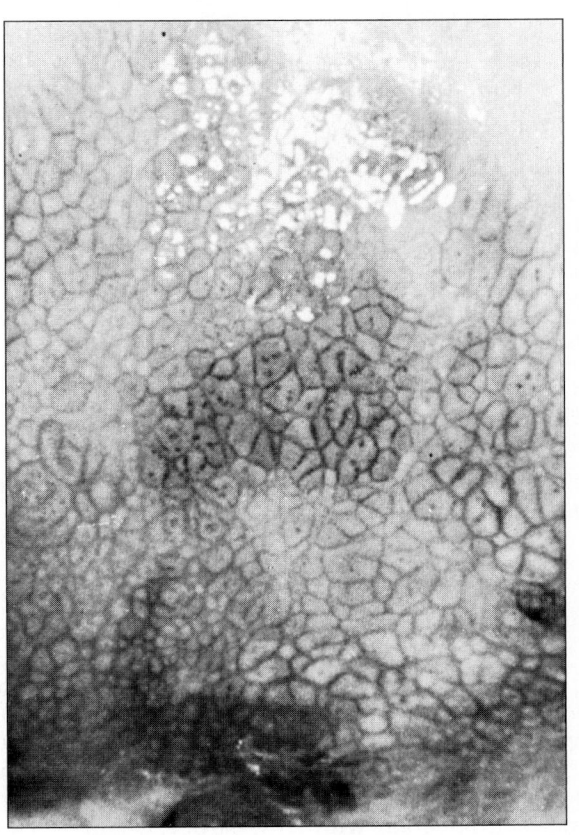

Figure 90-7. A, Colposcope. **B,** Colposcopic discovery of high-grade cervical dysplasia. (From Hoskins WJ, Perez CA, Young RC (eds): Principles and Practice of Gynecologic Oncology, 2nd ed. Philadelphia, Lippincott, 1997, p 678 and Morrow CP, Curtin JP: Synopsis of Gynecologic Oncology, 5th ed. San Francisco, Churchill Livingstone, 1998, p 107.)

the squamocolumnar junction is not visualized on colposcopy, (2) dysplastic epithelium extends into the endocervical canal, (3) cytology is suggestive of high-grade dysplasia or worse, (4) microinvasive carcinoma is found on directed biopsy, (5) sampling of the endocervical canal shows high-grade intraepithelial neoplasia, and (6) cytology is suggestive of adenocarcinoma in situ.

Loop Electrodiathermy Excision Procedure

LEEP uses wire-loop electrodes in conjunction with a radiofrequency alternating current to excise the entire transformation zone and distal canal under local anesthesia (Fig. 90-8). Compared with ablative procedures, LEEP has the major advantage of obtaining tissue for histologic evaluation. At many centers, LEEP has become the preferred treatment for CIN that can be adequately assessed with colposcopy.[59-71]

Complications include bleeding, with a reported incidence of 1% to 8%,[72,73] cervical stenosis (1%), and, rarely, pelvic cellulitis or adnexal abscess. In some cases, LEEP may not be an adequate alternative to formal excisional conization, such as in those patients in whom microinvasive or invasive cancer is suspected, or in

those with adenocarcinoma in situ, as it may inadequately treat disease within the cervical canal and complicate pathologic interpretation of the specimen. Appropriate application of this technique will yield tissue suitable for pathologic study and reliable diagnosis. Excess heat may result in thermal artifact that can compromise interpretation of margins and the therapeutic adequacy of the LEEP procedure.

Diagnostic or Therapeutic Excisional Conization (Cone Biopsy)

These operations must be performed under general or regional anesthesia. Complications include hemorrhage, sepsis, infertility, stenosis, and cervical incompetence, which occur in 2% to 12% of patients, depending on depth and geometry of excision.[74-76] Width and depth of the cone should be tailored to lesion topography, to produce the least amount of injury while providing clear surgical margins. Conization may be performed with a cold knife or with the carbon dioxide laser.

Patient Evaluation in Patients with Invasive Disease

A thorough history should be obtained before diagnostic assessments are initiated, because skilled questioning will elicit information that will serve to guide subsequent evaluation. A sexual history should be obtained from all patients, which may alert the physician to screen for human immunodeficiency virus and other sexually transmitted diseases. This also will serve to establish a baseline for sexual function and expectations that may be helpful in the post-treatment counseling and sexual rehabilitation of patients after completion of therapy. A complete history and systems review also should assess comorbid conditions (neurologic, cardiovascular, pulmonary, gastrointestinal, endocrine, etc.) that may affect the selection and implementation of treatment strategy.

A social assessment should be routinely obtained; this will assist in determining supportive interventions that may be necessary to facilitate patient compliance with complex diagnostic programs and multimodality treatment programs. In the United States, patients with advanced cervical cancer may be uninsured or underinsured, often will have cultural or language barriers to obtaining and complying with care, may have limited educational attainment and medical sophistication, and will have variable degrees of familial or other social support.

A general physical examination should be carried out with attention to accessible lymph node groups, including the supraclavicular nodes and the inguinal nodes. Physical examination also should assess the heart, lungs, and large vasculature (carotid, dorsalis pedis, posterior tibial, and femoral arteries; the aorta; and the veins of the lower extremities). Pelvic examination must include meticulous inspection of all potentially visible sites and palpation of the perineum, vulva, full length of the vaginal barrel, and the anorectum. Some patients will manifest areas of preinvasive disease at multiple separate sites along the

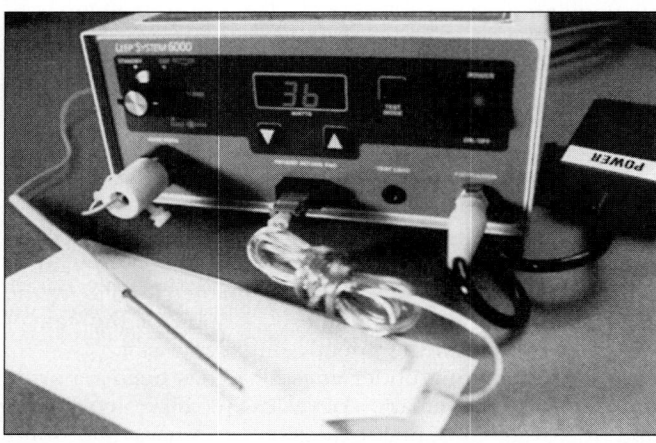

A

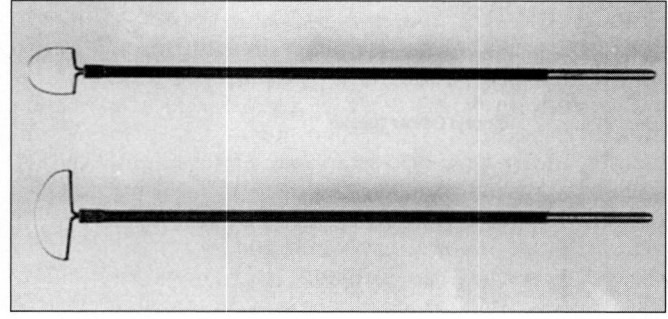

B

Figure 90-8. Equipment used for loop electrosurgical excision procedures (LEEP). **A,** Electrosurgical generator designed for LEEP. **B,** Large loop electrodes used for LEEP. (From Hoskins WJ, Perez CA, Young RC (eds): Principles and Practice of Gynecologic Oncology, 2nd ed. Philadelphia, Lippincott, 1997, p 678.)

Specific Malignancies

III

lower reproductive tract or synchronous invasive primary cancers of the lower reproductive tract and the anus representing "field cancerization" consequent to exposure to a common etiologic agent. Typically tumors arising from the ectocervix or transformation zone are easily visualized and sampled with biopsy. Occasionally tumors arising in the uterine corpus or lower uterine segment can invade the uterine cervix or protrude through the cervical os, causing confusion in the diagnosis. Often this can be sorted out by histopathology and by diagnostic imaging, with magnetic resonance imaging (MRI) being most useful in this context. Once the diagnosis of cervical carcinoma is established, staging includes careful clinical evaluation of the vagina, cervix, uterus, and parametria. The adnexal areas should be palpated as well, as some patients will harbor adnexal pathology (tubo-ovarian abscesses or, less commonly, adnexal metastases) that are optimally diagnosed and addressed before initiation of cancer treatment.

Conventionally, pelvic examinations in the setting of invasive cancer are performed under general or regional anesthesia (EUA) to assist in the most accurate possible physical evaluation of disease extent. Relaxation of the muscles of the pelvic floor and the opportunity to conduct vigorous and prolonged examination without inflicting discomfort or pain may identify disease extension that may be missed in an outpatient clinic examination. For example, EUA may be critical in very anxious, young, nulliparous women, as well as in elderly patients who may not be regularly sexually active and in whom the vagina may be stenotic. EUA also affords the opportunity to perform cystoscopy and proctosigmoidoscopy when indicated. However, in an era of cost containment and constrained health care resources, EUA may be omitted when a cooperative patient is amenable to satisfactory examination in the clinic or in rare circumstances in patients with locally extensive disease requiring rapid initiation of treatment.

Staging

The revised 1995 staging criteria (Table 90-3) of the International Federation of Obstetrics and Gynaecology (FIGO) are a mixture of histopathologic, clinical, and radiographic assessments that reflect the fact that invasive cervical cancer is most prevalent in less-developed portions of the globe where sophisticated and expensive imaging modalities may not be widely available. Cervical cancer is clinically staged and based primarily on inspection and palpation of the cervix, vagina, parametrium, and pelvic sidewalls. Only the subclassification of stage I (Ia1, Ia2) requires pathologic assessment. The FIGO staging system permits assessment through biopsy, physical examination, cystoscopy, proctoscopy, excretory urography (intravenous pyelography or IVP), and plain film radiography of the chest and skeletal system. Results of lymphangiography (LAG), computed tomography (CT), MRI, and positron emission tomography (PET) may be of great value in planning treatment, but do not influence assignment of clinical stage in the FIGO formalism. When findings are equivocal, by convention, a patient is assigned

to a lower stage. Once clinical stage has been assigned, it cannot be altered by subsequent events or findings. Findings from surgical evaluation (by laparoscopy or by surgical assessment of retroperitoneal lymph nodes via extraperitoneal or transperitoneal node dissection) will not alter assignment of clinical stage. However, these findings may profoundly influence subsequent treatment. Similarly, evidence of nodal or other spread discerned at the time of hysterectomy does not alter clinical stage.

A staging system based largely on findings from clinical pelvic examination is inherently imprecise and somewhat subjective, with overstaging and understaging of the parametria being the most problematic issue and the one most likely to alter management. However, FIGO stage does correlate with prognosis and does permit cautious interinstitutional and intrainstitutional comparisons of treatment outcomes.

Diagnostic Imaging Evaluation of Cervical Cancer

The goals of clinical staging in patients with invasive disease include determining the appropriateness and extent of initial surgical treatment, as opposed to initial treatment with combined radiation therapy and synchronous chemotherapy. Although not formally part of clinical staging, modern sophisticated diagnostic imaging can enhance clinical assessment of disease volume and extent in women with cervical carcinoma, thus refining both selection of treatment and technical implementation of treatment modalities.

The FIGO staging is based predominantly on clinical EUA, ultrasonography, intravenous urography, cystoscopy, proctoscopy, and chest radiography. Significant inaccuracies occur in this staging because of possible errors in gynecologic examination (24% to 39%).[77] The various imaging modalities have a complementary role in the accurate staging and complete evaluation of the cancer that have important therapeutic implications.

Endosonography under anesthesia has been reported to be of value in evaluation of vesical, rectal, vesicovaginal, and rectovaginal septal extension.[78] Transvaginal sonography has been shown to be accurate in the detection of bladder wall invasion.[79] However, ultrasound evaluation, although useful in addressing specific focused anatomic questions, is less useful for general evaluation of disease extent because it is subject to variables of patient habitus and operator variability. CT is a cross-sectional imaging modality useful in assessing advanced disease and identification of involved lymph nodes, distant metastases, and tumor recurrences (Fig. 90-9).[80] However, MRI provides better anatomic delineation and accurate estimation of the tumor size, volume, and local extent within the pelvis, which can influence the choice of therapy (Fig. 90-10). Involvement of the vagina, parametrium, pelvic wall muscles, ureter, bladder, and rectum can be better assessed for accurate staging (Fig. 90-11).[77] MRI before and after vaginal opacification with contrast medium can be used if imaging evaluation of the vaginal wall or fornices is required.[81] T_2-Weighted images obtained by using phased-array coil, fast-spin-echo or conventional

TABLE 90-3

American Joint Committee on Cancer and International Federation of Gynecology and Obstetrics Staging Systems for Cancer of the Uterine Cervix

AJCC TNM CATEGORIES	FIGO STAGES	
TX	–	Primary tumor cannot be assessed
T0	–	No evidence of primary tumor
Tis	0	Carcinoma in situ
T1	I	Cervical carcinoma confined to uterus (extension to corpus should be disregarded)
T1a	Ia	Invasive carcinoma diagnosed only by microscopy. All macroscopically visible lesions—even with superficial invasion—are T1b/Ib. Stromal invasion with a maximum depth of 5.0 mm measured from the base of the epithelium and a horizontal spread of 7.0 mm. Vascular space invasion, venous or lymphatic, does not affect classification
T1a1	Ia1	Measured stromal invasion ≤3.0 mm in depth and ≤7.0 mm in horizontal spread
T1a2	Ia2	Measured stromal invasion more than 3.0 mm and ≤5.0 mm with a horizontal spread ≤7.0 mm
T1b	Ib	Clinically visible lesion confined to the cervix or microscopic lesion greater than T1a2/Ia2
T1b1	Ib1	Clinically visible lesion ≤4.0 cm in greatest dimension
T1b2	Ib2	Clinically visible lesions >4.0 cm in greatest dimension
T2	II	Cervical carcinoma invades beyond uterus but not to pelvic wall or to the lower third of vagina
T2a	IIa	Tumor without parametrial invasion
T2b	IIb	Tumor with parametrial invasion
T3	III	Tumor extends to the pelvic wall, and/or involves the lower third of the vagina, and/or causes hydronephrosis or nonfunctioning kidney
T3a	IIIa	Tumor involves lower third of the vagina, no extension to pelvic wall
T3b	IIIb	Tumor extends to pelvic wall and/or causes hydronephrosis or nonfunctioning kidney
T4	IVa	Tumor invades mucosa of the bladder or rectum, and/or extends beyond true pelvis (Bullous edema is not sufficient to classify a tumor as T4)
M1	IVb	Distant metastasis

Regional Lymph Nodes (N)

NX	Regional lymph nodes cannot be assessed
N0	No regional lymph node metastasis
N1	Regional lymph node metastasis

Distant Metastasis (M)

MX	Distant metastasis cannot be assessed
M0	No distant metastasis
M1	Distant metastasis

Stage Grouping

Stage 0	Tis	N0	M0
Stage Ia1	T1a1	N0	M0
Stage Ia2	T1a2	N0	M0
Stage Ib1	T1b1	N0	M0
Stage Ib2	T1b2	N0	M0
Stage IIa	T2a	N0	M0
Stage IIb	T2b	N0	M0
Stage IIIa	T3a	N0	M0
Stage IIIb	T1	N1	M0
	T2	N1	M0
	T3a	N1	M0
	T3b	Any N	M0
Stage IVa	T4	Any N	M0
Stage IVb	Any T	Any N	M1

Notes about the Staging System

Stage 0 cases are those with full-thickness involvement of the epithelium with atypical cells but with no signs of invasion into the stroma. (Cases of stage 0 disease should not be included in any therapeutic statistics for invasive carcinoma.)

As a rule, it is impossible to estimate clinically whether a cancer of the cervix has extended to the corpus. Extension to the corpus should therefore be disregarded

A growth fixed to the pelvic wall by a short and indurated but not nodular parametrium should be assigned stage IIb. It is impossible at clinical examination to decide whether a smooth and indurated parametrium is truly cancerous or only inflammatory, and thus such cases should be classified as stage III only if the parametrium is nodular to the pelvic wall or if the growth itself extends to the pelvic wall

The presence of hydronephrosis or nonfunctioning kidney caused by stenosis of the ureter by cancer permits a case to be classified as stage III even if, according to the other findings, the case should be classified as stage I or stage II

The presence of bullous edema, as such, should not permit a case to be classified as stage IV. Ridges and furrows into the bladder wall should be interpreted as signs of submucous involvement of the bladder if they remain fixed to the growth at palposcopy (i.e., examination from the vagina or the rectum during cystoscopy). A finding of malignant cells in cytologic washings from the urinary bladder requires further examination and biopsy from the wall of the bladder

Specific Malignancies

TABLE 90-3

American Joint Committee on Cancer and International Federation of Gynecology and Obstetrics Staging Systems for Cancer of the Uterine Cervix—cont'd

Rules for Clinical Staging

The staging should be based on careful clinical examination and should be performed before any definitive therapy. Ideally, the examination should be performed under anesthesia by an experienced examiner

The clinical stage must under no circumstances be changed on the basis of subsequent findings

When doubt exists as to the assignment of stage, the case must be classified as the earlier stage. For staging purposes, the following examination methods are permitted: palpation, inspection, colposcopy, endocervical curettage, hysteroscopy, cystoscopy, proctoscopy, intravenous urography, and x-ray examination of the lungs and skeleton. Suspected bladder or rectal involvement should be confirmed by biopsy and histologic evidence

Findings on examinations such as lymphangiography, arteriography, venography, laparoscopy, and so forth are valuable for planning therapy, but because such studies are not yet generally available and because interpretation of the results is variable, the findings of such studies should not be the basis for changing the clinical staging

Infrequently, hysterectomy is performed in the presence of unsuspected extensive invasive cervical carcinoma. Such cases cannot be clinically staged or included in therapeutic statistics, but they should be reported separately

Only strict observance of the rules for clinical staging will allow meaningful comparison of results between clinics and modes of therapy

From Fleming I, Cooper JS, Henson DE, et al. (eds): AJCC Cancer Staging Manual. 5th ed. Philadelphia, Lippincott Williams & Wilkins, 1997, pp 189–194.

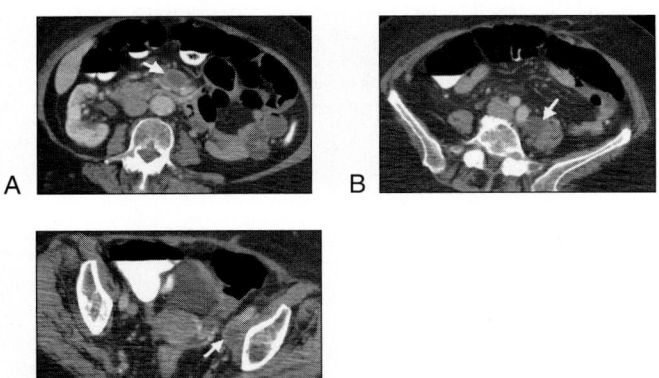

Figure 90-9. Pattern of nodal metastases (*arrows*) on CT. Necrosis is a frequent feature of squamous cell carcinoma **A,** Paraaortic node. **B,** Retroperitoneal node. **C,** External iliac node.

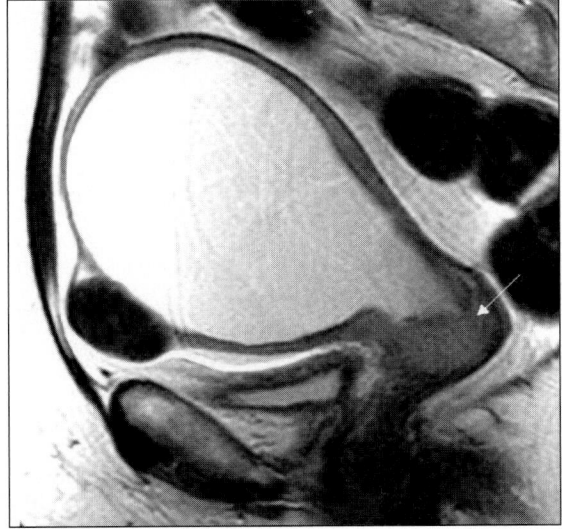

Figure 90-10. Cervical cancer MRI. T2-weighted sagittal image showing cervical mass (*arrow*) causing stenosis and fluid accumulation in uterus.

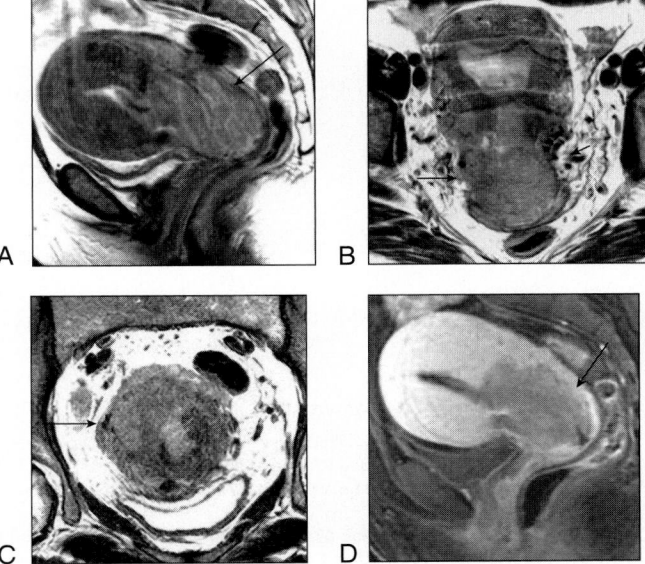

Figure 90-11. Cervical cancer MRI. **A,** Sagittal T2-weighted image showing heterogeneous isointense mass in cervix extending into posterior wall of uterine body. **B,** T2-weighted image sliced coronally through the cervix showing mass protruding into the uterine cavity (*arrow*). **C,** T2-weighted image sliced axially across the cervix showing bulky, eccentric cervical mass on the right side with spread beyond the T2 hypointense ring of the cervical stroma in to the parametrium. **D,** T1-weighted gadolinium-enhanced image revealing clear delineation of the mass relative to the adjacent uterus (*arrow*).

spin-echo techniques are accurate in local staging and lymph nodal assessment; the former technique is faster with increased resolution.[82] Dynamic contrast-enhanced T_1W images are helpful in identifying smaller tumors, fistulous tracts, and invasion into bladder and rectum.[77] Dynamic contrast-enhanced imaging is useful in differentiating areas composed predominantly of tumor cells (well-enhanced areas) from those of fibrous tissue with scattered cancer cells (poorly enhanced areas). This information can be helpful, as radiation therapy is more effective in well-enhancing tumors.[83]

MRI is very useful in the evaluation of tumor volume and enlarged lymph nodes, inherently important prognostic factors as well as determinants of the design of radiation treatment ports and selection of radiation dose. However, MRI cannot identify micrometastases to lymph nodes and differentiate malignant from nonmalignant enlargement. MRI with newer contrast agents like ultrasmall superparamagnetic iron oxide has been useful in distinguishing benign from malignant nodes.[84] The shape, volume, and direction of the growth of the tumor can be well assessed, and these are crucial for planning brachytherapy and external-beam radiotherapy.[77] MRI also is useful in the follow-up evaluation of the tumor, its response to treatment, and identification of recurrences. However, benign conditions like edema or inflammation sometimes cannot be differentiated from tumor. Dynamic contrast-enhanced MRI is useful in differentiating malignant lesions that usually have shorter and stronger enhancement than benign conditions in patients who have abnormalities after treatment for cervical cancer.[85]

Radical trachelectomy is an operation suitable for highly selected patients with small, generally exophytic squamous tumors involving mostly the exocervix, who desire conservation of reproductive capacity. The margin between the superior extent of the tumor and the uterine isthmus must be a minimum of 1.5 cm if uterine conservation is not to hazard unacceptable risk of cancer recurrence. MRI has been used preoperatively to assist in patient selection for this procedure by assessing proximal tumor extension with respect to the internal os.[86]

Functional imaging with PET using 2-fluorine 18-fluoro-2-deoxy-D-glucose (FDG) is more sensitive and specific than MRI in identifying malignant from nonmalignant involvement of lymph nodes and the extent of nodes involved. FDG-PET also is useful in evaluating locally recurrent lesions and differentiating them from scar tissue, and also has been used in whole-body screening for detecting recurrence. The main disadvantages of PET are high cost, low spatial resolution, and inability to determine the exact anatomic location and extent of the tumor.[87,88] The hybrid CT-PET scanner is likely to prove superior in spatial resolution and anatomic localization.

Laboratory Evaluation

Routine laboratory assessment should include complete blood counts with differential counts and red cell indices. Many patients with advanced disease will be anemic at the time of diagnosis, often reflecting chronic blood loss and iron deficiency. Anemic patients treated with radiation or chemoradiation have poorer outcomes than do patients with near-normal hemoglobin levels.[89-92] Anemia at diagnosis (before treatment) correlates significantly with reduced pelvic control and survival with univariate analysis, but not always when data are subjected to multivariate analysis. In contrast, multivariate analysis reveals that hemoglobin level during the course of radiation therapy or chemoradiation is a robust predictor of local outcome and survival.[89-92] Transfusion for anemic patients with maintenance of average weekly nadir hemoglobin levels at or above 11 to 12 g/dL through radiation therapy is associated with improvement in prognosis to that associated with patients with near-normal or normal hemoglobin levels at diagnosis.[89,91] This effect may be partially mediated through better tumor oxygenation and oxygen-enhanced radiation lethality to clonogenic cells as well as reduced angiogenesis in better-oxygenated tumors. With pelvic or extended-field radiation that will encompass a substantial percentage of adult bone marrow, hemoglobin may slowly decline, even when adequate iron stores are present and patients are supported with hematinics. Concurrent administration of cisplatin further aggravates this problem, and can result in clinically significant reduction in hemoglobin levels over the course of a 6- to 8-week program of chemoradiation, even in patients with normal hemoglobin levels at the time of diagnosis. Frequent monitoring of hemoglobin levels as well as white cell counts and platelets should be performed throughout a course of chemoradiation, and hemoglobin level should be supported, either by transfusion or through the use of recombinant erythropoietin. The minimal hemoglobin level required is uncertain, but it seems prudent to target a minimum of 12 g/dL.

Neutropenia may indicate supportive treatment with granulocyte–colony-stimulating factor (G-CSF) to avoid prolonged treatment interruptions that are known to adversely affect local tumor control in patients treated with radiation.[93,94] Absolute neutrophil counts should be monitored at least weekly in patients undergoing chemoradiation.

An elevated platelet count has been associated with advanced malignancy and is considered a consequence of increased platelet production.[95] Hernandez and associates[96] identified this effect in advanced cervical cancer, and Rodriguez and coworkers[97] identified the preoperative platelet count as an adverse prognostic factor, even for patients with stage Ib cervical carcinoma. The cumulative 5-year survival of women with a platelet count greater than 300,000 (85 women) was 65%, compared with 84% for the group with a normal value (134 women). At issue was the question of whether the value could have been elevated simply because of bleeding from the primary tumor, but no association was found with the preoperative hematocrit. This study of surgically treated patients with early disease also demonstrated that the effect was not a consequence of metastatic disease and did correlate with tumor volume, with nearly half of the patients with platelet counts in excess of 300,000 having "large" lesion size, in contrast to only 28% (32 of 114) patients with normal counts.[95] In a multivariate analysis, adjusting for age, race, tumor size, and presence of lymph node metastases, high platelet count was still associated with an adverse prognosis.

Additional laboratory tests should include a complete chemistry panel with serum electrolytes and measurements of renal and hepatic function. Electrolytes and renal function should be monitored repeatedly through a course of chemoradiation. Creatinine may be elevated secondary to hydroureter/hydronephrosis that may require ureteral stent placement or nephrostomies before radiation therapy, particularly if cisplatin chemotherapy is anticipated. Serum sodium and potassium may become abnormal during the course of chemoradiation, particularly in elderly patients, consequent to diarrhea with potassium loss, inadequate oral replenishment, and inadequate or inappropriate fluid intake.

TREATMENT OVERVIEW

The treatment of patients with cervical cancer is determined primarily by the stage and extent of disease. As a general rule, CIS and microinvasive cervical cancer with no greater than 3 mm of stromal invasion and no more than 7 mm breadth (FIGO stage Ia1) are managed with conservative surgery (excisional conization or extrafascial/simple hysterectomy). Microinvasive cervical cancer with 3 to 5 mm of stromal invasion and no more than 7 mm breadth (FIGO stage Ia2) may be managed with modified radical hysterectomy. Stages Ib1 and small-volume IIa may be managed with either radical surgery (generally radical hysterectomy or modified radical hysterectomy), radiation alone, or chemoradiation. Controversies surround the optimal management of patients with bulky stage Ib2 (>4 cm) cancer, who may be treated with triple-modality therapy in selected instances (surgery, radiation, chemotherapy in a variety of possible sequences).

After initial radical surgical therapy, patients with adverse histopathologic factors may be advised to undergo adjuvant pelvic radiation or adjuvant chemoradiation. Risk factors for recurrence include metastatic disease in regional nodes, positive surgical margins, parametrial extension, deep cervical stromal invasion, lymphovascular space invasion, and large tumor size.

Patients with large FIGO stage IIa or with stages IIb through IVa are conventionally managed with chemoradiation. Some patients with an incomplete response to chemoradiation may benefit from a combined approach using adjunctive hysterectomy to clear persistent central disease after chemoradiation. Patients with bulky Ib2 or IIa disease and rare patients with bulky central stage IIb lesions with minimal, medial parametrial invasion may be considered for this approach. For patients in whom disease recurs centrally in the pelvis after maximal chemoradiation, radical exenterative surgery can be performed, provided that no distant disease is present. Optimal candidates have mobile central disease without lymph node involvement.[98-100] Intraoperative radiation therapy (IORT) may be part of salvage surgery when lateral or posterior surgical margins will be predictably inadequate.[101,102] Recurrent disease after initial radical surgery has historically been treated with salvage radiation, but should currently be treated with chemoradiation.[103]

Superficial Ablative Therapy

A major deficiency of all ablative therapies is the absence of full histopathologic assessment of the lesion treated, and the hazard of undertreatment of an occult invasive lesion. For this reason, use of ablative techniques is appropriately declining. Three superficial ablative techniques used historically are electrocoagulation diathermy, cryosurgery, and CO_2 laser therapy.

Hysterectomy

Hysterectomy involves the removal of the uterus and varying amounts of surrounding tissue (Fig. 90-12). Because the risk of ovarian metastases is low (0.5%), ovarian preservation is generally recommended in premenopausal women, obviating the need for hormone replacement therapy.[104] An important exception is when nodal metastases from a primary cervical adenocarcinoma are detected intraoperatively, when the risk of ovarian metastasis escalates steeply, perhaps to as high as 25%.[105] Five types of hysterectomy have been described.[106]

Extrafascial or Simple Hysterectomy (Type I)
Extrafascial or simple hysterectomy involves the removal of the cervix, adjacent tissues, and a small cuff of the upper vagina in a plane outside the pubocervical fascia; it is appropriate treatment for stage Ia1 disease. Minimal disturbance occurs to the bladder and ureters, which decreases the risk of urinary complications.

Modified Radical Hysterectomy (Type II)
Modified radical or Wertheim's hysterectomy is less extensive than the radical hysterectomy and removes the cervix and proximal 1 to 2 cm of vagina, including the paracervical and parametrial tissues. The ureters are dissected to the point of entry to the bladder to allow safe removal of parametrial and paracervical tissue. The medial half of the cardinal ligaments and the uterosacral ligaments also are removed.

Radical Hysterectomy (Type III)
A radical (Meigs') hysterectomy includes removal of the uterus, cervix, and paracervical, parametrial, and paravaginal tissues to the pelvic sidewalls bilaterally in continuity, with as much of the uterosacral ligaments as possible. The uterine vessels are ligated at their origin, and the proximal one fourth to one third of the vagina and paracolpos is resected. Generally this operation will be performed in conjunction with bilateral therapeutic pelvic lymphadenectomies. Acute complications include blood loss (average, 800 mL), ureterovaginal fistula (1% to 2%), vesicovaginal fistula (<1%), pulmonary embolus (1% to 2%), small bowel obstruction (1%), and febrile morbidity (25% to 50%). Subacute complications include transient bladder dysfunction lasting 1 to 7 weeks (30%) and lymphocyst formation (<5%). Chronic complications include bladder hypotonia and atonia in about 3% of patients and, uncommonly, ureteral strictures. Rare patients may have transient or permanent lower extremity lymphedema.

Figure 90-12. Diagram of pelvic anatomy and types of hysterectomy. (From Berek JS, Hacker NF: Practical Gynecologic Oncology, 2nd ed. Baltimore, Williams & Wilkins, 1994.)

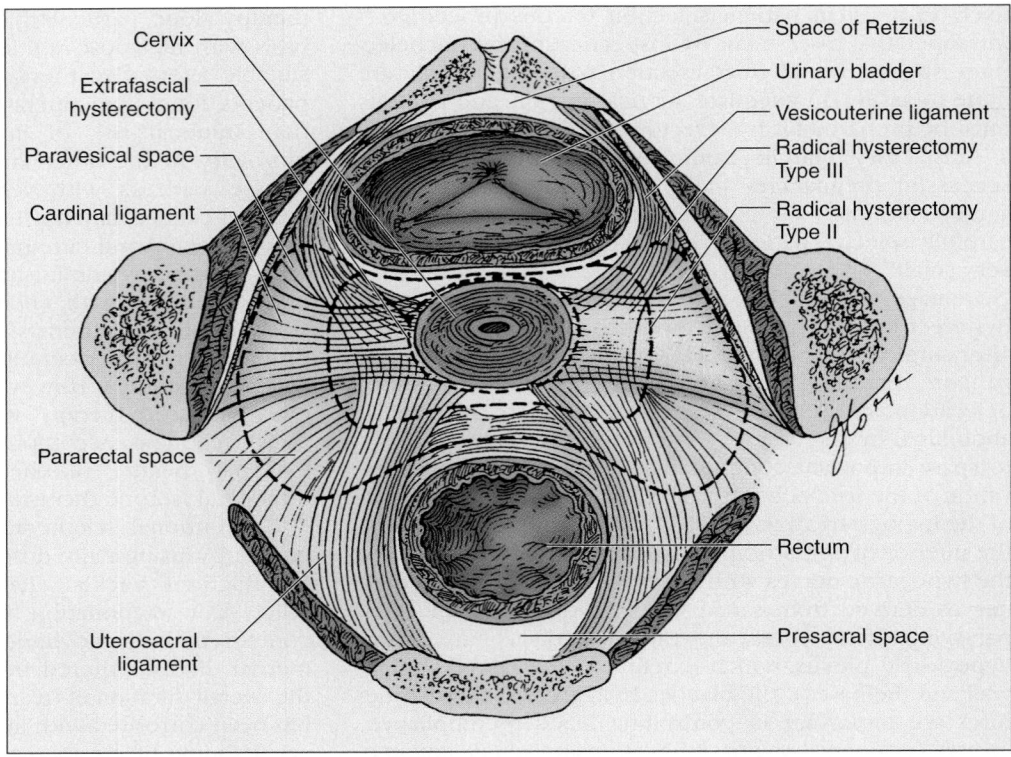

Extended Radical Hysterectomy (Type IV)

In addition to the tissue removed in the type III, extended radical surgery removes the periureteral tissue, the superior vesicle artery, and up to three fourths of the vagina. This procedure is rarely done, as patients with the anatomic extent of disease that would warrant such treatment should generally be treated with chemoradiation.

Partial Exenteration (Type V)

Partial exenteration is rarely performed, because radiation therapy should be reserved for patients with the extent of disease that would require surgery of this extent for gross anatomic clearance. Parts of the distal ureters and bladder are resected in this procedure. This may be appropriate initial surgery for patients with FIGO stage IVa cancer with large vesicovaginal fistulae and incontinence. However, vesicovaginal fistulae may scar closed in some patients after high-dose radiotherapy if the upper vagina is permitted to fuse shut, thus restoring urinary continence.

Surgical Alternatives to Conventional Radical Abdominal Hysterectomy

The late 1980s and the decade of the 1990s witnessed a proliferation of surgical techniques consequent to the availability of the sophisticated instruments and optical equipment required for laparoscopic surgery, a resurgence of interest in vaginal hysterectomy, and concerns about preserving reproductive potential in young women with early cervical cancer.

Radical vaginal hysterectomy carried out by the methods of Schauta-Stoeckel (less radical) or Schauta-Amreich (more radical) is a surgical alternative to radical or modified radical abdominal hysterectomy (types II and III) that may be associated with shorter hospital stays and more rapid recuperation. Laparoscopic radical hysterectomy is a technique that performs an operation comparable to a radical hysterectomy (type III hysterectomy) entirely through the laparoscope, including the vaginal closure.

Laparoscopy has been coordinated with vaginal hysterectomy, with varying amounts of surgery being carried out via the laparoscopic approach, ranging from pelvic and para-aortic lymphadenectomy, to lymphadenectomy plus important components of the radical hysterectomy.[107–109]

Radical trachelectomy is an operation suitable for selected patients with small, generally exophytic squamous tumors (usually <2 cm, although some patients with larger tumors have been treated in this fashion) involving primarily the exocervix who desire conservation of reproductive capacity. In this surgery, the main trunk of the uterine artery is preserved, although branches to the cervix and vaginal fornices are sacrificed before amputation of the cervix at a point approximately 5 mm caudal to the uterine isthmus. The uterus is suspended from the lateral stumps of the transected paracervical ligaments. Isthmic cerclage is performed in a fashion similar to that used as prophylaxis against miscarriage, and an anastomosis between the vaginal mucosa and the isthmic mucosa is performed. Variations on this surgery can be performed vaginally with laparoscopy, or abdominally. The margin between the superior extent of the tumor and the uterine isthmus must be a minimum of 1.5 cm, but preferably 2 cm. MRI can be used preopera-

tively to assist in patient selection for this procedure.[86] Intraoperative assessment by inspection of the trachelectomy specimen and frozen-section pathologic study are done to assure an adequate surgical margin, and patients must be prepared for hysterectomy in the eventuality that a satisfactory margin cannot be obtained. Numerous successful pregnancies have been reported after such surgery, although the risk of miscarriage is increased. In carefully selected patients, the risk of cancer recurrence is very small.[110-112]

Damage to the pelvic autonomic nerves during radical hysterectomy is responsible for much of the late morbidity after surgical treatment of FIGO stages Ia2 to IIa cervical cancer, including problems with bladder function, defecation, and sexual dysfunction. Nerve-sparing radical abdominal hysterectomy[113] is a procedure that endeavors to spare important components of the autonomic innervation of the true pelvis by identification and preservation of the hypogastric nerves, which carry sympathetic fibers; the inferior hypogastric plexus formed from the fusion of the hypogastic nerves with fibers of the pelvic splanchnic nerves derived from sacral roots S2 to S4, which carry parasympathetic fibers; and the most distal part of the hypogastric plexus, which extends to the lateral vaginal wall and the base of the bladder. In aggregate, these structures are important in controlling bladder compliance, urinary continence, vaginal lubrication and genital engorgement during sexual arousal, small muscle contractions with orgasm, and some rectal functions. This recent surgical innovation is intended not to compromise the efficacy of the cancer surgery, while preserving important components of quality of life in cancer survivors. Precise criteria for patient selection have not been defined.

Radiation Therapy

Radiation therapy for cervical cancer will generally consist of a combination of external radiation (teletherapy) and intracavitary or interstitial radioisotope therapy (brachytherapy). Roentgen discovered r-rays in 1895. Radium was discovered by the Curies in 1898. Biologic effects of so-called "Roentgen rays" on skin were soon appreciated after prolonged exposures. Serendipitous discovery of the acute biologic effect of exposure to radium was consequent to the discoverer of radioactivity, Becquerel, carrying a 200-mg sample in his vest pocket for 6 hours and subsequently experiencing an ulcerating burn. In 1901, roentgen rays were first applied to the cervix by using a transvaginal cone. Intracavitary brachytherapy for cervical cancer was first described with radium circa 1902. Interstitial brachytherapy with radium was first proposed by Alexander Graham Bell in 1903. In the past 100 years, the discipline of radiation oncology has evolved as a medical specialty because of continuous refinements in medical radiation dosimetry, increasing sophistication of equipment, and progress in understanding the biologic consequences of radiation exposure in both cancer and normal tissues and cell lines (radiobiology).

Patients with very small volume cervical tumors stages Ia1 to Ib1 (Ib1, <1 cm in diameter) can be successfully treated with intracavitary brachytherapy alone, with results that parallel the efficacy of surgery.[114] Brachy-

therapy alone, particularly if conducted on an outpatient basis with high-dose-rate technology (HDR) may serve as suitable alternative therapy for medically compromised patients for whom operative intervention implies more than minimal risk of intraoperative or perioperative morbidity. At the other end of the spectrum of invasive disease, patients with very extensive stage III or IVa cervical cancer may not have geometry compatible with brachytherapy, and cure may sometimes be accomplished with teletherapy administered alone (or more commonly in combination with chemotherapy) by using progressively smaller teletherapy treatment volumes carried to progressively higher cumulative radiation dose ("shrinking fields technique"). However, most patients treated with radiation-based therapy with curative intent will have their treatment accomplished with a combination of external beam (teletherapy) and intracavitary or interstitial isotope therapy (brachytherapy).

Conventional teletherapy is given in a fractionated course by using daily doses of 1.8 to 2 Gy per fraction, five fractions weekly. Selected patients may benefit from twice daily fractionation by using a "field within a field" concurrent boost to limited volumes of nodal or parametrial disease. Altered fractionation may serve to keep the overall duration of treatment as short as possible, which has been correlated with improved local control and survival. It should be emphasized that target volumes and teletherapy dose distributions are not standardized and should be based on pretreatment imaging studies that define disease extent rather than on FIGO stage. Depending on the presence or absence of nodal metastases and the anatomic level of nodal disease, teletherapy ports may encompass only nodes caudal to the bifurcations of the common iliac arteries (approximately at the interspace between the fifth lumbar vertebra and the first sacral segment), nodes to the level of the aortic bifurcation (approximately at the level of the third lumbar vertebra), or to a volume extending to encompass para-aortic nodes to the level of the cisterna chyli (approximately at the level of the twelfth thoracic vertebra). Treatment of such widely differing volumes, particularly when done with synchronous chemotherapy, implies substantial variability in acute symptomatic tolerance, hematologic tolerance, and potential delayed sequelae of treatment. Routine treatment of standard volumes is not a substitute for appropriate diagnostic assessment of disease extent and treatment tailored in consideration of both tumor and patient factors.

Conventionally, brachytherapy dose has been calculated and prescribed at points A and points B (Fig. 90-13). Doses to the bladder neck and anterior rectal wall (dose-limiting normal structures) are usually specified as well (Fig. 90-14).[115] Brachytherapy is generally accomplished by using one or two intracavitary or interstitial inpatient applications LDR (50 to 60 cGy/hr) technologies. Most applicators for intracavitary brachytherapy resemble the apparatus in Figure 90-15, and consist of an intrauterine tandem and paired colpostats or ovoids, which are placed in the lateral vaginal fornices, resulting in a classic pear-shaped isodose distribution. The customary strategy is intracavitary brachytherapy supplemented by tailored teletherapy treatment to boost volumes

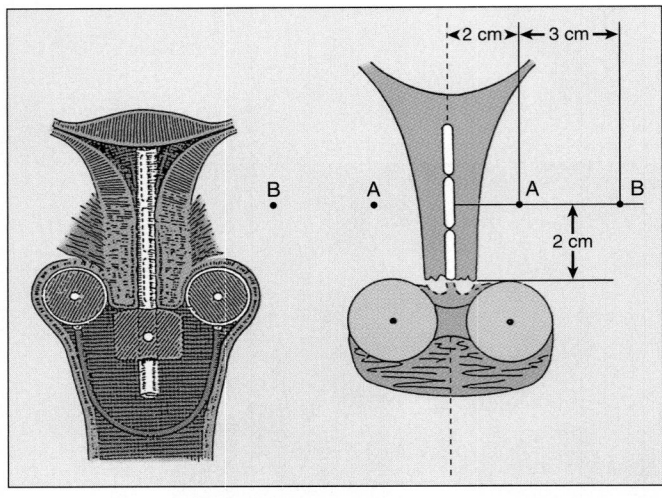

Figure 90-13. Points A and B for cervical radiation therapy. (From Hoskins WJ, Perez CA, Young RC (eds): Principles and Practice of Gynecologic Oncology, 2nd ed. Philadelphia, Lippincott, 1997, p 678.)

generally lateral and posterior to the cervix and medial parametria. In patients whose vaginal anatomy does not accommodate tandem and colpostat devices (a so-called "conical vagina" with flush or ablated fornices and a narrowed upper vagina) or patients with extensive, lateral parametrial invasion, interstitial implantation may provide more satisfactory dose distribution when gross tumor extends beyond the traditional pear-shaped dose envelope provided by intracavitary brachytherapy (Fig. 90-16). Both brachytherapy approaches have proponents and detractors. Both strategies are somewhat operator dependent. Such nonrandomized data as exist based on inter-institutional comparisons fail to demonstrate a clear superiority of one approach over the other, with respect to either long-term tumor control or normal tissue complications, among patients with stage III or IV disease. However, patients with stage II disease appeared to do somewhat better with intracavitary brachytherapy.[116]

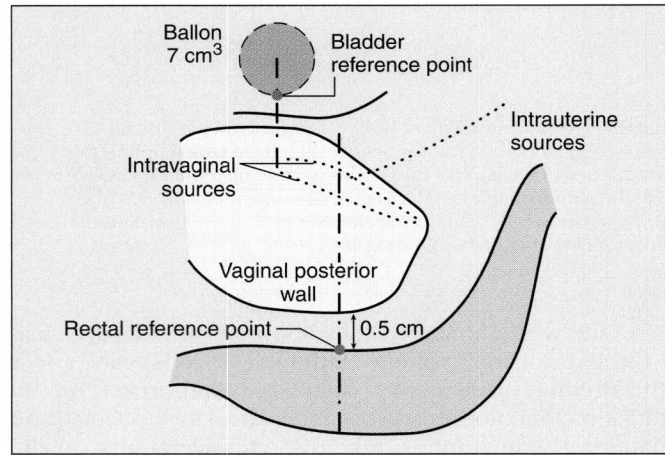

Figure 90-14. Rectal and bladder reference points according to the International Commission on Radiation Units and Measurements Report 38. (From Cox JD (ed): Radiation Oncology, 8th ed. St. Louis, Mosby, 2003, fig. 28-16.)

LDR brachytherapy procedures require insertion under anesthesia and hospitalization for radiation safety and patient immobilization. Alternatively, multiple outpatient intracavitary insertions may be performed by using HDR (100 cGy/min) remote afterloading technology. Commonly five intracavitary insertions are performed when HDR technology is used. Because of miniaturization of the high-activity source and the hardware used for treatment, these insertions may be accomplished under conscious sedation when cooperative patients with favorable vaginal anatomy are selected. Because of inherent biologic disadvantages associated with HDR brachytherapy, substitution of this technology for conventional LDR systems has been controversial. More tailored dose distributions can often be designed with the inherently more flexible HDR systems than with historically used LDR equipment using multiple sources with fixed physical dimensions and a limited spectrum of source strengths. Such comparative data as exist suggest that HDR and LDR technologies are approximately isoeffective for tumor control and roughly equivalent with respect to complications when appropriate dose-rate corrections have been applied.[117,118]

What seems increasingly clear is that either approach (LDR or HDR) in the hands of seasoned physicians with substantial brachytherapy experience is likely to be superior to the other approach in the hands of the inexperienced or the clinician who treats only a limited number of patients. It has often been said that brachytherapy is an art and not a science. The American Brachytherapy Society is involved in the commendable process of attempting to place brachytherapy on a more rational, scientific basis by developing guidelines grounded in established practice and data driven to replace what has often been based on subjective criteria and intuition coupled with the hard lessons of experience.[119,120] Improvements in diagnostic imaging (MRI, CT, PET, and combination, hybrid or fusion studies) are anticipated to facilitate these efforts by providing improved understanding of the spatial relations of brachytherapy sources and both cancer and dose-limiting normal tissues. This effort, however, remains a work in progress.

As partially art rather than pure science, brachytherapy is similar to surgery. Skills atrophy unless regularly used. Understanding that fact should stimulate consideration of referral of patients requiring brachytherapy to centers of excellence where annual volume provides greater assurance that the requisite skills and experience will be available.

The side effects of radiation therapy include both immediate and late effects. Acute reactions of radiation are seen in tissues with the most rapid cell-turnover rates such as skin, intestinal mucosa, urothelium, vaginal mucosa, and bone marrow. Acute side effects of pelvic irradiation include diarrhea, abdominal cramps, tenesmus, urinary frequency, urgency, and dysuria. Some women will experience vaginal bacterial overgrowth consequent to alterations in the integrity of the vaginal mucosa, causing symptoms of discharge and pruritis. Occasionally small-volume bleeding from the bladder or rectum may occur. Aggravation of hemorrhoidal disease is common. Older patients with extensive diverticular disease are vulnerable to development of diverticulitis under the influence of

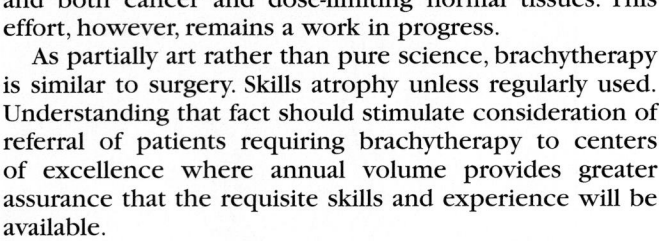
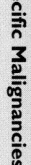

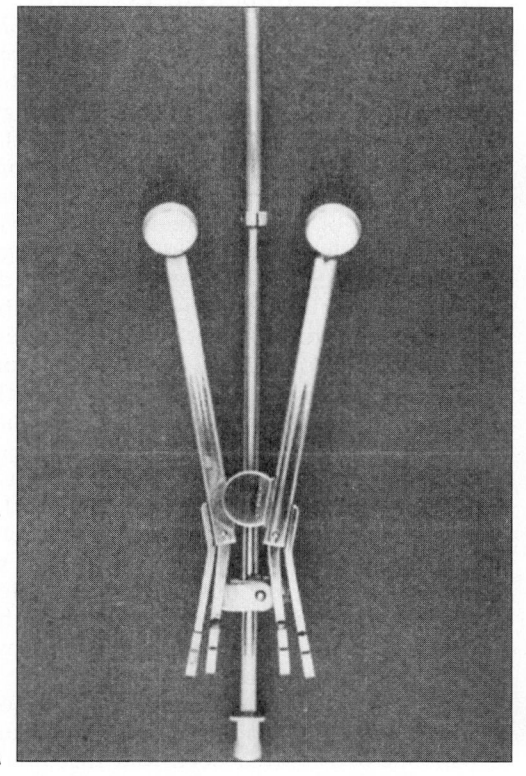

A

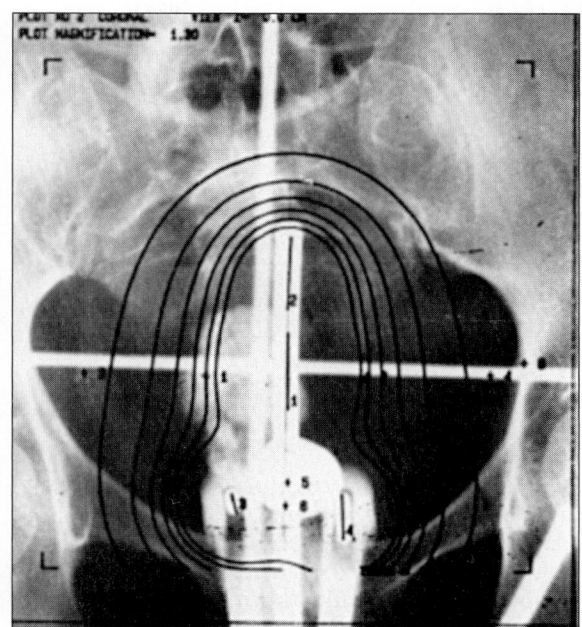

B

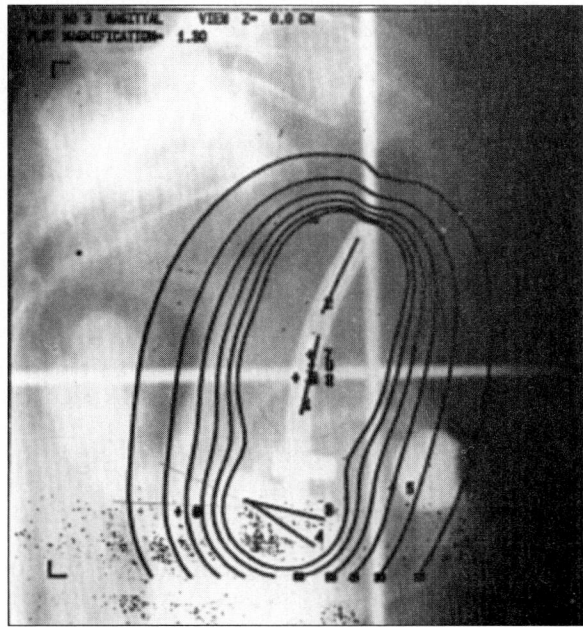

C

Figure 90-15. A, Intracavitary device for brachytherapy. **B** and **C,** Treatment plan for cervical carcinoma showing a radiograph of the intracavitary irradiation in situ with its isodose distribution in cGy/hr. (**B** and **C,** from Shingleton SM, Kim RY: Treatment of cancer of the cervix. In Gusberg SB, Shingleton HM, Neppe G [eds]: Female Genital Cancer. New York, Churchill Livingstone, 1988, p 297.)

pelvic radiotherapy, which may result in pain, bleeding, perforation, and significant delay in completion of treatment. Rare patients will experience bacterial overgrowth with *Clostridium difficile,* even in the absence antecedent antibiotic exposure. Severe, prolonged diarrhea poorly responsive to standard medications and dietary modification should arouse the clinician's suspicion. Not uncommonly, pelvic radiation will provoke a recrudescence of herpes simplex virus type II, usually manifest as focal,

discrete, well-marginated ulcerations on the labia caudal to the irradiated volume, although lesions may affect the urethra, bladder, and vagina. It is important for the radiation oncologist to recognize the labial lesions, the pattern of which tends to be discrete ulcerations, usually quite different from the more confluent, irregularly bordered, moist desquamative reaction seen with acute radiation dermatitis. Obviously, the treatment of these conditions will be quite different.

Figure 90-16. A, Device for interstitial brachytherapy. **B,** Diagrams of same device in coronal and sagittal planes. (From Hoskins WJ, Perez CA, Young RC (eds): Principles and Practice of Gynecologic Oncology, 2nd ed. Philadelphia, Lippincott, 1997, p 678.)

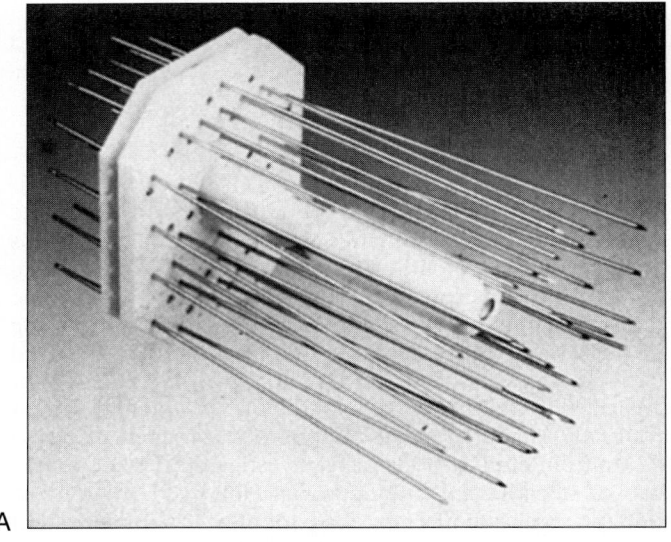

A

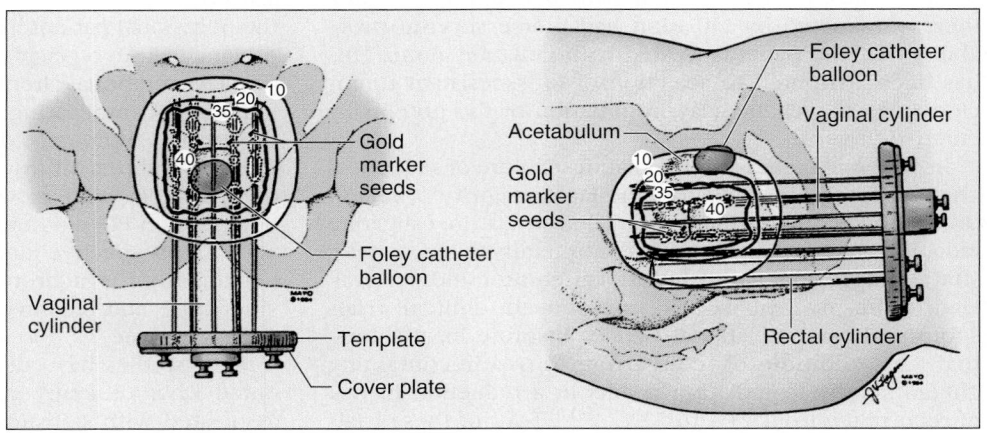

B

Late complications (onset months to years after radiotherapy) can be due to intimal proliferation in small arteries/arterioles with decreased blood supply and subsequent fibrosis or focal infarction. The larger the dose per treatment fraction, the greater the risk of late complications in normal tissues unavoidably included within the treatment volume. Late effects of pelvic irradiation may include chronic radiation cystitis with urothelial atrophy, irritative symptoms, and bleeding. In rare patients, vesicovaginal fistulae may develop, usually at the level of the bladder neck where brachytherapy dose is often highest. Vaginal stenosis with dyspareunia and compromised ability to perform surveillance follow-up is a somewhat avoidable consequence of radiation therapy if informed and compliant patients are provided with vaginal dilators and instructed in their use, as well as provided with vaginal estrogen cream. Chronic radiation proctitis or sigmoiditis with pain and small-volume bleeding can occur in some patients, with focal injury to the anterior rectal wall consequent to brachytherapy being the most common site for this late complication. Major hemorrhage is unlikely, except in patients with portal hypertension or therapeutic anticoagulation for medical comorbidities. Distressing bleeding can often be controlled through conservative, judicious laser ablation of bleeding telangiectatic vessels. Symptomatic large bowel stricture is uncommon, but may require fecal diversion in severe instances. Rectovaginal fistulae may be the consequence of severe injury to the rectovaginal septum and anterior rectal wall. Usually this complication will require permanent fecal diversion, but occasional patients can have segmental resection with re-establishment of intestinal continuity. Most intestinal injury is to small intestine, commonly manifested by obstructive symptoms. The usual site is in the terminal ileum, but focal jejunal injury may be seen, particularly in patients undergoing extended-field treatment to encompass para-aortic lymph nodes. If the ovaries are in the treatment field, ablation of both endocrine and reproductive function will be the inevitable consequence of pelvic radiotherapy administered in cancerocidal dose to premenopausal women. Symptoms of estrogen deprivation may take several months to develop after pelvic radiation, depending on the age of the patient and endogenous body stores of estrogen. Usually the endometrium is ablated consequent to high mucosal dose from intracavitary brachytherapy. Occasional patients will have remnants of functioning endometrium. With the almost inevitable occlusion of the endocervical canal after brachytherapy, painful hematometra may develop in such patients if

unopposed estrogen replacement therapy or cyclical hormone replacement is instituted. Generally, combined hormone replacement therapy will avoid this complication that may necessitate hysterectomy in severe cases.

Chemoradiation

Synchronous administration of radiation and cytotoxic chemotherapy will enhance acute radiation reactions within all tissues included in the treatment volume, resulting in more severe acute symptoms. Impact on chronic radiation injuries is less predictable. Anxiety regarding normal tissue tolerance, both immediate and late, delayed extrapolation of successful chemoradiation strategies for anal cancer to the larger volumes of vulnerable tissues routinely irradiated in the treatment of cervical cancer.

Multiple clinical trials have investigated the sequential use of neoadjuvant chemotherapy followed by conventional radical radiotherapy for patients.[121-124] In several of these studies, patients treated with neoadjuvant chemotherapy followed by radiation had worse survival probability than did patients treated with radiation alone. This has been attributed to selection of cross-resistant tumor clonogens as well as delay in initiation of the potentially curative therapy.

In dramatic contrast to the manifest failure of sequential chemotherapy and radiation, the large majority of recent prospective, randomized controlled trials investigating radiation and synchronous chemotherapy have demonstrated improvements in both local control and survival. Data from five phase III randomized clinical trials sponsored by the National Cancer Institute have shown that the addition of concurrent cisplatin-containing chemotherapy to radiation results in a reduction in risk of recurrence from 21% to 52%.[125-129] Four of these trials pertained to women with locally advanced cervical cancer, stages Ib2 to IVa. The fifth studied high-risk postoperative patients stages Ib to IIa with cancer extension to parametrium, surgical margins, or regional lymph nodes.

The optimal drug regimen is uncertain. Four of these trials had an experimental arm containing 5-fluorouracil (5-FU); however, the Gynecologic Oncology Group (GOG) prospectively compared weekly cisplatin with continuous-infusion 5-FU at 225 mg/m^2 for 5 days weekly (a lower daily dose than the 1000 mg/m^2/24 hr for 96 hours used in the previous positive studies) and terminated the study (GOG protocol 165) when it became clear that no possibility existed that the 5-FU arm might ultimately prove superior. Weekly cisplatin at a dose of 40 mg/m^2 for six doses has become the most commonly used regimen for concurrent chemotherapy with radiation for advanced cervical cancer.

However, the National Cancer Institute of Canada (NCIC) prospectively compared radiation alone with radiation plus weekly cisplatin in 259 patients with squamous cancers with bulky ($\geq$5 cm) stage Ib2 to IIa, or smaller tumors with positive nodes, and patients with stages IIb to IVa. The study was designed to have an 80% probability of detecting a 15% survival difference at 5 years. Although patients receiving the cisplatin regimen did marginally better, the study failed to find a statistically significant difference.[130]

The Radiation Therapy Oncology Group (RTOG) prospectively compared radiation alone administered to extended volumes (pelvis plus para-aortic nodes) with pelvic radiation with three synchronous cycles of 5-FU and CDDP, with one cycle administered synchronously with intracavitary brachytherapy. 5-FU was administered at 1000 mg/m^2/24 hr for 96 hours with each cycle, and cisplatin at 75 mg/m^2. The population of 403 patients composing the study population were identified and selected with entry criteria similar to those of the NCIC study (except that nonsquamous cancers were included). The relative risk of recurrence was 0.48 (90% confidence interval) in the chemoradiation arm compared with radiation alone.[127]

Ideally, a prospective study comparing weekly cisplatin at 40 mg/m^2 with the chemotherapy used in the RTOG study would resolve this controversy. It seems unlikely, however, that sufficient resources will be devoted to resolving this issue when the difference between the two arms of such a study could be expected to be modest. For the occasional patient in whom inadequate renal function precludes use of cisplatin, 5-FU by prolonged infusion provides a rational alternative.

Further complicating this issue are the three additional prospective, randomized studies that have found relapse-free survival benefit from the synchronous administration of epirubicin with radiation,[131] mitomycin-C with radiation,[132] or 5-FU plus mitomycin-C with radiation,[133] and a fourth prospective randomized trial that failed to detect benefit from synchronous administration of cisplatin, vincristine, and bleomycin with radiation compared with radiation alone.[134]

Most studies have demonstrated that the use of combined chemotherapy and radiation therapy has been associated with statistically significant increase in gastrointestinal and hematologic toxicity that, although significant, has been tolerable. Data suggest that synchronous administration of chemotherapy potentiates radiation effect in cycling, immediately responding cell systems, in both cancer and normal tissue. Thus both immediate normal tissue reactions and side effects are potentiated. Importantly, an increase in catastrophic late complications such as bowel obstruction, fistula formation, or second malignancies, has not been seen. Given the preponderance of evidence, which now suggests that synchronous radiation with radiopotentiating chemotherapy favorably affects probability of cancer-free survival, clinical research into the optimal drugs and schedule of administration is likely play a central role in clinical investigation for the foreseeable future.

TREATMENT OF LOCOREGIONAL DISEASE BY STAGE

Stage Ia1 and Ia2 (Microinvasion)

The purpose of defining microinvasion is to identify a group of patients not at risk for lymph node involvement and therefore treatable with conservative therapy. In the current staging classification, stage Ia1 is defined as a tumor with stromal invasion no greater than 3 mm in

depth beneath the basement membrane and no wider than 7 mm. Stage Ia2 is defined as a tumor with stromal invasion greater than 3 mm, no greater than 5 mm in depth, and no wider than 7 mm. Patients at highest risk for metastases or recurrence in this group appear to be those with evidence of tumor in the lymphovascular spaces.[135,136]

Patients with stage Ia1 disease can be adequately treated with therapeutic conization if conservation of reproductive capacity is desired, or extrafascial hysterectomy. The risk of pelvic lymph node metastases with 1 to 3 mm of stromal invasion is less than 1%.[137,138] For patients opting for therapeutic conization, the following histopathologic criteria should be met: (1) depth of stromal invasion 3 mm or less, (2) diameter of lesions less than 7 mm, (3) no lymphovascular invasion, and (4) clear margins. Patients treated with conization should be followed up closely with cytologic, colposcopic, and endocervical curettage evaluation every 3 months for the first year.[139] A vaginal or a type I abdominal hysterectomy (extrafascial) is appropriate treatment if future childbearing is not desired.

Microinvasive carcinoma with stromal invasion 3.1 to 5 mm is associated with a 5% risk of nodal metastases.[140] The preferred treatment for stage Ia2 is a modified radical (type II) hysterectomy with bilateral pelvic lymphadenectomy. Treatment with radiation also will have a high probability of success and may be preferable therapy in patients who are compromised surgical candidates based on age and comorbidities.

Stage Ib1, Ib2, and IIa

Stage Ib is defined as a clinically evident lesion confined to the cervix or preclinical lesions greater than those of Ia2. Patients with IIa disease have extension to the upper vagina without parametrial involvement. The incidence of pelvic nodal metastases is approximately 15% to 25% for patients with stage Ib disease.[140] Treatment must be directed toward the lymph nodes, cervix, parametrial tissue, paravaginal tissue, and upper vagina; therefore, a radical (type III) hysterectomy with bilateral pelvic lymphadenectomy and para-aortic lymph node evaluation has historically been the treatment of choice. Radiation therapy is as effective as surgery based on a prospective, randomized comparison conducted in Italy.[141] In that study, 337 analyzed patients (FIGO Ib1, Ib2, and IIa) were randomly assigned treatment with initial type III hysterectomy or with radiation therapy using a radiation dose (cumulative teletherapy and brachytherapy dose of 76 Gy at point A) which is substantially lower than the 85 to 90 Gy used in leading centers in the United States. Postoperative pelvic radiotherapy was administered to patients with positive nodes, positive margins, positive parametria, or less than 3 mm surgical margin. Forty-six (84%) of 55 patients with tumors larger than 4 cm in diameter received postoperative radiotherapy. Chemotherapy was not used. Five-year survival and disease-free survival were identical in both groups (83% and 74%, respectively). Serious complications were 28% in the group treated initially with surgery, and 12% in the radiotherapy group. Theoretically, results with chemoradiation might well be superior to those with surgery, but the

benefit for synchronous administration of chemotherapy has been documented only in patients with tumors larger than 4 cm (Ib2) or more advanced stages of disease.

Given that surgery and radiotherapy are approximately isoeffective with respect to cancer control, treatment is generally selected on the basis of physician and patient preference and differences in treatment-related morbidity. Surgery provides important prognostic information and offers premenopausal women the option of ovarian conservation, because the risk of ovarian metastases is only 0.5%.[104] Considerable debate concerns whether sexual function is more feasible or better after surgical treatment or radiotherapy. Both forms of treatment carry some risk of urologic injury or bowel injury. However, the nature of those complications, the ability to remedy those complications, and the impact of chronic complications on quality of life are both challenging to quantitate and vulnerable to quite subjective interpretation. Radiation carries a small but not trivial risk of late induction of second malignancies.

For patients with stage Ib1 who are young and free of major comorbid conditions, surgery tends to be the preferred option. In patients that are poor surgical risks or elderly, radiotherapy is more sensible. Radiotherapy is usually a combination of teletherapy intended to encompass the primary, microscopic regional extensions, and regional lymph nodes, supplemented by intracavitary brachytherapy intended selectively to carry gross disease to higher dose. When disease is very small (<1 cm in diameter), the risk of nodal metastases is low, and the treatment approach may be modified to intracavitary brachytherapy therapy alone with excellent results.[114]

The treatment of patients with stage Ib2 disease remains a source of continued controversy. With either surgery or radiotherapy, progressive decrements in survival probability are found as tumor size increases. In some centers, Ib2 patients continue to undergo initial surgery, recognizing that most will have indications for postoperative radiotherapy, but that surgery will clear gross central disease, which is the most likely site of pelvic failure in patients treated with radiation. Because the morbidity of combined therapy is clearly greater, some surgeons will limit the radicality of surgical extirpation in anticipation of postoperative radiotherapy in a sensible effort to limit morbidity.[142] Neoadjuvant chemotherapy with cisplatin, vincristine, and bleomycin for three cycles at 10-day intervals before attempted radical hysterectomy has been used with encouraging results in Ib2 cancers reported by Sardi and colleagues in Argentina.[143] Pathologic downstaging was observed in patients operated on after neoadjuvant chemotherapy compared with patients undergoing initial surgery. These results have not been reproduced in the context of a multi-institutional trial, when tested by the GOG.

Alternatively, radiation has been used as initial therapy supplemented by type I adjuvant hysterectomy to clear central disease. The GOG compared radical radiotherapy with attenuated preoperative radiotherapy supplemented by extrafascial hysterectomy.[144] A lower cumulative incidence of local relapse was noted in the radiotherapy plus hysterectomy group (at 5 years, 27% vs. 14%). No statistical differences were observed in outcomes

between regimens, except for the adjusted comparison of progression-free survival, although all indicated a slightly lower risk in the adjuvant hysterectomy regimen [unadjusted relative risk (URR) of progression, 0.77; $P = .07$; URR of death, $P = .26$; both one-tailed]. Because of preliminary analysis of this trial that suggested benefit from surgery in improved local control, the GOG carried out a successor trial in which all patients had attenuated preoperative radiotherapy, followed by extrafascial hysterectomy. Half of the patients were randomized to receive weekly cisplatin at 40 mg/m² during teletherapy. The rates of both progression-free survival ($P < .001$) and overall survival ($P = .008$) were significantly higher in the combined-therapy (chemoradiation) group at 4 years.[125]

Although interpretations of the outcomes of these studies vary, it has become less common to carry out adjunctive hysterectomy routinely in patients undergoing chemoradiation for Ib2 or bulky IIa disease. However, selected patients may benefit who have poor response to teletherapy and chemotherapy assessed at the time of intracavitary insertion, or who have poor vaginal anatomy, limiting the dose of brachytherapy that can be prudently prescribed.

Patients undergoing primary surgery for stage Ib and IIa cancer who are found to have adverse clinicopathologic prognostic factors may be advised to undergo adjuvant postoperative pelvic radiotherapy or adjuvant chemoradiation. Much effort has been expended in attempting to define clinicopathologic factors that reliably identify patients at high risk for failure after initial surgical therapy. Primary tumor size, depth of cervical invasion, and lymph-vascular space invasion (LVSI) are thought to be independent prognostic factors in node-negative patients with surgically treated Ib squamous carcinoma of the cervix.[145] Parametrial extension[146] and parametrial node metastasis,[147] independent of retroperitoneal lymph node status,[148] are predictive of an increased risk of recurrence in surgically treated patients. Positive or insecure margins including vaginal margins,[149] extension of cancer to the lower uterine segment,[150,151] and adverse histopathology[38] are additional parameters that may correlate with a more ominous outlook. Controversies persist concerning the relative importance of some of these factors in multivariant analysis. However, with consensus approaching unanimity, metastasis to pelvic lymph nodes is recognized as a dominant prognostic indicator.[152]

Two cooperative NCI-sponsored intergroup studies have been carried out prospectively evaluating adjuvant therapy for patients with adverse histopathologic features after radical hysterectomy. Sedlis[153] reported on 277 "intermediate risk" node-negative patients who were identified based on combinations of tumor size, depth of cervical stromal invasion, and lymphatic space invasion. Based on historic outcomes, these patients were estimated to have an approximate 25% to 27% probability of recurrence after surgery, with the pelvis being the most probable site of relapse. Patients were randomized to observation versus adjuvant pelvic teletherapy. Adjuvant radiation resulted in a 47% reduction in overall risk of recurrence from 28% to 15% ($P = .008$). In 18 of 137 irradiated patients, disease recurred with relapse within the pelvis compared with 30 of 140 observation patients

in whom recurrence had a pelvic component, suggesting that pelvic radiation prevented approximately 39% of the expected pelvic failures. This raises some concerns about the adequacy of the radiotherapy used, but also suggests that synchronous administration of chemotherapy may further improve outcome in this group of patients.

Peters[128] reported on 243 analyzable "high-risk" patients who had positive nodes, parametrial extension, or positive surgical margins. After radical hysterectomy, these patients were randomized to receive adjuvant pelvic radiotherapy, or the same adjuvant radiation regimen with two cycles of synchronous 5-FU and cisplatin followed by two further cycles of sequential 5-FU and cisplatin. Cisplatin was administered at 70 mg/m², and 5-FU was administered at 1000 mg/m²/24 hr for 96 hours with each cycle. The projected progression-free survival at 4 years was 80% for the patients in the radiation-plus-chemotherapy arm compared with 63% in patients receiving adjuvant radiation alone. Analysis of pattern of treatment failure at the time of initial recurrence reveals that 11 of 127 chemoradiation patients had a component of pelvic recurrence compared with 25 of 116 radiation patients, suggesting that the addition of chemotherapy resulted in a 60% reduction in the rate of pelvic failure. A component of distant metastatic spread was seen in 13 of 127 chemoradiation patients and 18 of 116 radiation patients, suggesting that the addition of chemotherapy resulted in a 34% reduction in distant spread. Paradoxically, the effect of the chemotherapy appears to have been greater on local disease than on distant dissemination, suggesting that the primary benefit may have been as a potentiator of local radiation effect.

In a small, randomized trial, Tattersall[154] reported that the addition of three cycles of cisplatin, vinblastine, and bleomycin before adjuvant pelvic radiation produced no benefit compared with immediate postoperative radiation therapy in Ib to IIa patients with pelvic node metastases. In a complementary, randomized trial in which all patients received adjuvant postoperative chemotherapy, Curtin[155] reported that the addition of delayed adjuvant radiation produced no benefit in either pelvic control or survival.

Stages IIb and III

In the United States, patients with advanced disease are treated with chemoradiation. Teletherapy with synchronous chemotherapy is supplemented with intracavitary brachytherapy whenever feasible. The Syed-Neblett or Martinez interstitial templates are alternative brachytherapy approaches that have the theoretic advantage of extending the brachytherapy isodoses laterally to treat pelvic side walls and parametrium.[156,157] However, it is unclear that this provides any advantage compared with conventional intracavitary brachytherapy supplemented by teletherapy boost treatments to limited volumes.

Stage IVa

Radiation therapy in combination with chemotherapy as a radiosensitizer rarely cures patients with these advanced

tumors. A primary pelvic exenteration may be considered for stage IVa disease with extension to the rectum or bladder, but survival is as high with radiation alone, with a lower urinary fistula rate of 3.8%.[140]

TREATMENT OF METASTATIC DISEASE AND SALVAGE CHEMOTHERAPY

Cervical cancer is not considered curable with chemotherapy. Chemotherapy has traditionally been reserved for patients with extrapelvic metastatic disease or recurrent disease who are not candidates for radiation therapy or exenterative surgery. In an important GOG study, Thigpen and colleagues[158] found that cisplatin has the greatest antitumor activity in advanced squamous carcinoma of the cervix, with a response rate of 20% to 25%. Unfortunately, in most series, responses to cisplatin are short-lived (3 to 6 months). The median duration of response for complete responders is 6 months, and the median survival is only 9 months.[159,160] Other agents reported to achieve partial responses (15% to 25%) include carboplatin, iphosphamide, 5-FU, doxorubicin, methotrexate, hexamethylmelamine, mitomycin-C, vinblastine, bleomycin, paclitaxel, topotecan, vinorelbine, and irinotecan. Little objective evidence suggests that combination chemotherapy is superior to single-agent cisplatin.

A small portion of patients will first be seen with advanced disease that is not amenable to radiation therapy with curative intent. In women in whom recurrent or persistent disease develops in the central pelvis after radical hysterectomy, on occasion, a cure may be achieved with radical salvage radiation or chemoradiation. A second small subset of patients with central pelvic recurrence after radiation therapy can be salvaged with aggressive surgical therapy, which often involves removal of the bladder or rectum or both. For patients with distant disease, the principle goal of therapy is palliation with an aim of reducing pain and suffering associated with metastatic lesions. No convincing data indicate that the delivery of systemic therapy in this clinical setting improves overall survival.

Numerous platinum combination–based regimens incorporating drugs such as doxorubicin, iphosphamide, bleomycin, and, most recently, paclitaxel, have demonstrated higher response rates (typically in the 20% to 40% range) with the combinations with greater toxicity. A limited number of reasonably well powered randomized trials comparing these doublets with either triplet regimens or singlet regimens have demonstrated that combination therapy leads to a slightly higher response rate and a longer progression-free survival that does not appear to affect overall survival.[161,162] Recently the GOG compared paclitaxel and cisplatinum with single-agent cisplatinum. In this study of 241 eligible women, the response rate to single-agent cisplatin was 19%. The response rate to the doublet was 36%. The median time to progression was prolonged from 2.8 months with cisplatin alone to 4.8 months for the doublet. Overall survival for the two arms was equivalent, with an 8.8-month median for cisplatin and a 9.7-month median for the doublet.[163]

The potential role of drugs such as epidermal growth factor–receptor inhibitors, angiogenesis inhibitors, and other molecularly targeted therapies, remains still largely unexplored in this disease. Preliminary evaluation of geftinib demonstrates only minimal activity in cervical cancer.

When interpreting clinical trials evaluating the efficacy of chemotherapy in cervical cancer, it is important to recall the patient population under study. Chemotherapy- and radiotherapy-naïve women receiving neoadjuvant therapy for bulky cervical tumors typically demonstrate response rates in excess of 50%. As discussed earlier, this response rate has not reproducibly translated into improved survival or cure. Response rates for recurrent disease outside of the radiation ports (such as pulmonary metastases or high para-aortic nodal recurrences) typically range between 10% and 20% for single-agent therapy and 20% and 45% for multiagent therapy. Finally, response rates for measurable tumors in the previously irradiated pelvis tend to be much lower, with complete responses rare, and response rates generally no higher than 10% to 15%. Evaluation is complicated in the irradiated pelvis, either with physical examination or radiologic studies, both of which are at times unable to distinguish postsurgical and postradiation changes from tumor recurrences, which are often infiltrating distorted tissue planes in the post-treatment pelvis.

Vulvar Cancer

SUMMARY OF KEY POINTS

EPIDEMIOLOGY

- The American Cancer Society estimates 4000 new cases of invasive vulvar cancer in the United States in 2003 with 800 deaths
- Vulvar cancers compose 4% of malignancies of the female genital tract
- Squamous cell carcinoma and its variants are the most prevalent histologies, comprising 90% of invasive lesions
- Vulvar melanoma, basal cell cancer, and rare sarcomas constitute most of the remaining tumors
- Adenocarcinoma and adenoidcystic carcinoma of the vestibular glands (Bartholin's gland) are less common than the squamous cancers arising from these structures
- Age-adjusted incidence increases steeply after age 70

ETIOLOGY

- An association is found with human papillomavirus (HPV) in approximately one third of cases, primarily in younger patients
- Vulvar cancer in older patients frequently arises in association with lichen sclerosis or squamous hyperplasia (hyperplastic dystrophy or lichen simplex chronicus), although these conditions are not clearly premalignant
- Chronic immunosuppression has been implicated in some cases

DIFFERENTIAL DIAGNOSIS

- Paget's disease of the vulva and vulvar intraepithelial neoplasia (VIN) are in the differential diagnosis of a vulvar lesion
- Giant condyloma may mimic vulvar neoplasia, and vulvar neoplasia may coexist with condyloma accuminata

EVALUATION

- Complete history and physical examination including a thorough pelvic examination and careful palpation of groin lymph nodes
- Diagnosis must be confirmed by vulvar biopsy

TREATMENT OF SQUAMOUS CELL CARCINOMA OF THE VULVA

- Treatment should individualized on the basis of disease volume and anatomic extent, histology, age, comorbidities, and patient preference
- Stage I lesions may be treated with radical local excision alone, or combined with inguinofemoral lymphadenectomy if depth of invasion exceeds 1 mm
- Surgery for stage II vulvar cancer usually consists of modified radical vulvectomy and inguinofemoral lymphadenectomy
- Locally extensive (T3,4) vulvar cancers, or cancers invading or encroaching on functionally important midline structures can be managed with synchronous preoperative chemotherapy and radiation (chemoradiation) followed by conservative excision of residual disease, or by radical chemoradiation alone
- Management of inguinofemoral nodes may consist of surgical dissection alone, or surgery coordinated with preoperative or postoperative radiation if nodes harbor metastatic deposits
- Surgery of the primary and the groin nodes may be conducted through separate incisions (triple incisions) to reduce both acute and late surgical morbidity
- Elective radiation or chemoradiation may be an alternative to surgical treatment of inguinofemoral nodes in selected patients with clinically and radiographically negative groin nodes
- Sentinel lymph node biopsy may be a useful discriminator to guide the selection and sequencing of modalities used to treat the groin nodes

EPIDEMIOLOGY

Vulvar cancer is predominantly a disease of postmenopausal women, most commonly observed in the seventh and eighth decades, and with a mean age at diagnosis of 65 years. Age-specific incidence rates in the United States increase steeply at age 70 and continue to increase beyond age 80 years.[164] The coincidence of vulvar intraepithelial neoplasia (VIN) or invasive squamous carcinoma of the vulva with in situ or invasive epidermoid carcinoma of the cervix has long been known, and synchronous or sequential (usually antecedent) cervical lesions may be present in as many as 20% of women with primary vulvar lesions. This observation suggests a common etiology in at least some patients.[165-171]

VIN, a precursor lesion, may often be multifocal. After conservative local excision of invasive vulvar cancer with preservation of clinically normal vulva, cancer may develop at anatomically distinct structures within conserved vulvar tissues. Rather than recurrence, this phenomenon may be a manifestation of the so-called "field change" model of oncogenesis, representing metachronous appearance of independent primaries.[172]

ETIOLOGY

Risk factors for the development of invasive vulvar cancer include a history of condyloma acuminatum, VIN, smoking, and chronic vulvar dystrophies including

lichen sclerosus and squamous hyperplasia (hyperplastic dystrophy).[173-176]

Vulvar carcinoma frequently coexists with vulvar dystrophy, particularly in older women, with dystrophic changes in adjacent skin in up to 50% of patients with invasive vulvar cancer.[177,178]

However, it is unknown whether lesions such as lichen sclerosus or squamous hyperplasia are true precursor lesions. Detection of human papillomavirus (HPV) in VIN or invasive disease is most common in young patients and less frequent in older patients.[179,180] These observations have led to the hypothesis that patients with vulvar cancer may be segregated into two broad groups: an older population with cancer arising in association with vulvar dystrophy and unassociated with HPV, and a younger population with HPV-associated tumors frequently adjacent to areas of VIN.[181,182]

An increasing incidence of VIN and reports of invasive vulvar cancer in young patients may be consequences of the sexual revolution and transmission of HPV. Invasive vulvar cancer has been reported in young patients with both naturally occurring and iatrogenic immune compromise.[183-188] Patients infected with the human immunodeficiency virus-1 (HIV-1) are much more likely to have HPV infection than are HIV-uninfected women and may be more vulnerable to development of VIN than are HIV-negative controls. VIN may be more difficult to clear in HIV-infected women and may progress to invasive disease with greater rapidity.[189,190]

Detection of the HIV in very young vulvar cancer patients raises the specter of increasing rates of vulvar as well as cervical cancer as the acquired immunodeficiency syndrome (AIDS) epidemic unfolds.[191]

NATURAL HISTORY

Vulvar Dystrophy

A patient with any degree of cellular atypia associated with vulvar dystrophy is at risk of invasive vulvar cancer. Patients with cellular atypia compose approximately 10% of those patients with histopathology-proven vulvar dystrophy, and in fewer than 5% of these patients will invasive vulvar cancer develop.[192] The International Society for the Study of Vulvar Disease (ISSVD) established a classification for vulvar dystrophies and atypias based on histopathology[193] (Table 90-4). The ISSVD now advises that "dystrophy" is no longer an acceptable term and recommends use of specific terminology (i.e., lichen sclerosus, lichen planus, lichen simplex chronicus, psoriasis), although these recommendations have not been uniformly adopted.[194-196]

Paget's Disease

Vulvar Paget's disease was first reported in 1901 by Dubreuilh.[197] The disease is seen predominantly in post-menopausal women, with common presenting symptoms of vulvar pruritus and soreness, sometimes accompanied by persistent oozing. Grossly, Paget's disease may have an

TABLE 90-4

Classification of Epithelial Disorders of the Vulva

Non-neoplastic epithelial disorders of the skin and mucosa
  Lichen sclerosus (lichen sclerosus et atrophicus)
  Squamous cell hyperplasia (formerly hyperplastic dystrophy)
  Other dermatoses
Classification of vulvar intraepithelial neoplasia

VIN 1	Mild dysplasia (formerly mild atypia)
VIN 2	Moderate dysplasia (formerly moderate atypia)
VIN 3	Severe dysplasia (formerly severe atypia)
CIS	Carcinoma in situ

From Ridley CM, Frankman O, Jones ISC, et al: New nomenclature for vulvar disease; report of the Committee on Terminology of the International Society for the Study of Vulvar Disease. J Reprod Med 1990;35:483.

eczematoid appearance. With extensive disease, it may appear raised and velvety. Under the light microscope, the presence of large, pale Paget's cells that are rich in mucopolysaccharide and that are periodic acid–Schiff (PAS)-positive, diastase resistant, are pathognomonic of this disorder (Fig. 90-17). Paget's cells stain for carcinoembryonic antigen (CEA), cytokeratin 7 (CK-7), and gross-cystic-disease fluid protein.[198,199] Paget's cells infrequently express CA-125, and testing for estrogen receptors is generally negative.[200,201] Many cases express c-erB2 (HER-2/neu), which is not believed to influence the risk of metastatic spread.[202,203] Nondiploid tumors are more likely to recur. Electron microscopic studies have demonstrated that Paget's cells are derived from the stratum germinativum of the epidermis.[204] Squamous keratinocytes, sweat gland cells, and hair follicles also are derived from this epidermal layer, possibly explaining the characteristic finding of more Paget's cells in juxtaposition to the basal layer of cells in the epidermis, as opposed to within higher strata.

In approximately one sixth of cases, Paget's disease involving the vulva has been associated with an underlying adenocarcinoma of the vulva, often arising in apocrine glands or within Bartholin's glands. Paget's disease also has been associated with a synchronous primary invasive cancer in another female genital tract site in approximately one fourth of patients.[205-207]

Wide local excision is recommended as treatment, with verification of surgical margins by frozen section.[208,209] Repeated excision is sometimes required for marginal recurrence.[210]

Intraepithelial Squamous Cell Neoplasia of the Vulva

The term *VIN* now replaces such terms as Bowen's disease, erythoplasia of Queyrat, carcinoma simplex, bowenoid papulosis, bowenoid dysplasia, hyperplastic dystrophy with atypia, and condylomatous dysplasia. The ISSVD recognizes squamous cell carcinoma in situ. The incidence of VIN has increased over the past 20-year period. Histopathologically, these lesions are characterized by varying degrees of cytoplasmic and nuclear maturation, giant cells with abnormal nuclei, and disruption of the

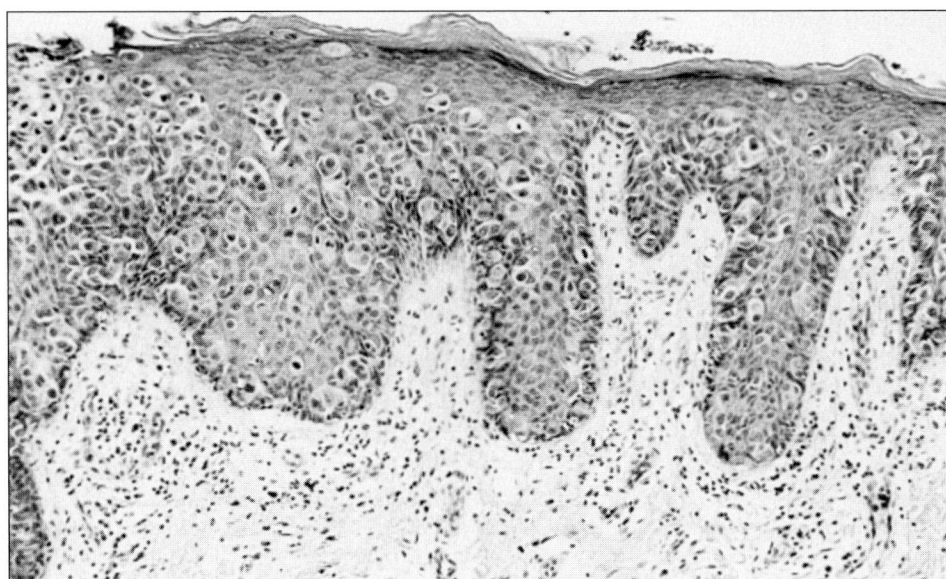

Figure 90-17. Histologic portrait of Paget's disease of the vulva. (From Quant E, Matin SA, Kraus CT: The vulva and vagina. In Silverberg SG [ed]: Principles and Practice of Surgical Pathology, 2nd ed. New York, Churchill Livingstone, 1990, p 1715.)

normal epithelial architecture (Fig. 90-18). On rare occasions, pearl formation at the base of the rete pegs can be seen, without significant abnormality in the overlying epithelium. Buscema and colleagues[211] reported that in approximately 4% of patients with VIN, invasive vulvar cancer developed. Fu and colleagues[212] observed that all intraepithelial lesions analyzed had an aneuploid DNA pattern when associated with HPV. The term *bowenoid papulosis* has historically been used as a synonym for multifocal intraepithelial neoplasia of the vulva. This lesion also is associated with HPV infection. The invasive potential of this entity appears to be very low. Therapy for VIN generally consists of surgical excision. Laser vaporization may be useful as an alternative when large areas would require excision or functionally important areas are involved, but carries a small risk of failure to detect areas of true invasion. The risk of occult invasion may be as high as 20% in patients with VIN 3.[213] Cavitational ultrasonic surgical aspiration (CUSA) provides another conservative surgical modality to treat VIN

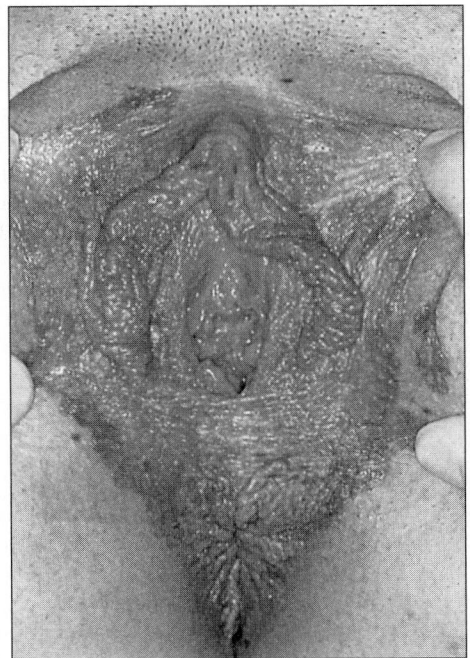
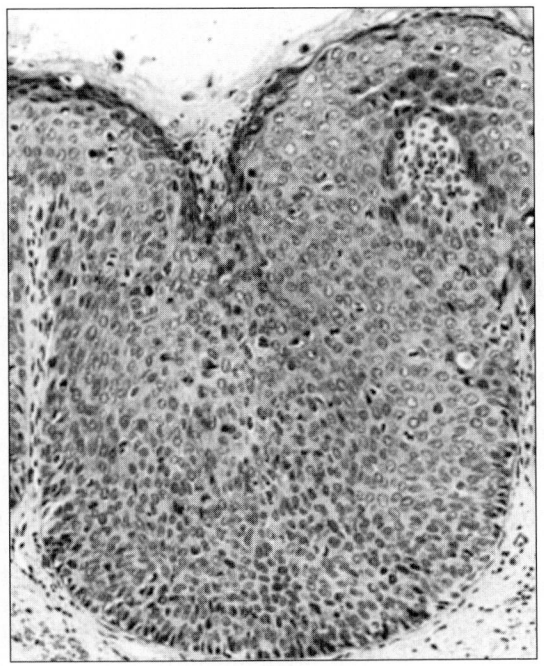

Figure 90-18. Characteristic gross (**A**) and histologic (**B**) features of vulvar intraepithelial neoplasia. (**A,** From Hoskins WJ, Perez CA, Young RC (eds): Principles and Practice of Gynecologic Oncology, 2nd ed. Philadelphia, Lippincott, 1997, p 678; **B,** From Deppe G, Lawrence WD: Vulvar dysplasia and neoplasia. In Gusberg SB, Shingleton HM, Neppe G [eds]: Female Genital Cancer. New York, Churchill Livingstone, 1988, p 223.)

with minimal loss of functionally important tissue and provision of tissue for histologic study.[214] Laser excision, by providing tissue for histologic evaluation, is less likely to miss a clinically occult area of invasion.[215]

Invasive Squamous Cell Carcinoma of the Vulva

Clinical Features

Histologically, squamous cell carcinoma accounts for more than 90% of cases of malignancy involving the vulva. Common presenting symptoms include chronic vulvar pruritus; a mass, lump, or sore; and small-volume bleeding. Most lesions involve the labia majora, whereas lesions originating on the labia minora and the clitoris occur less commonly. Lesions arising in the vestibular (Bartholin's) glands will first be seen as a swelling or mass, sometimes without invasion of overlying skin. Presentation with gross inguinal adenopathy is uncommon in the current era. In 10% of cases, the lesion will be too extensive to determine the site of origin, and in 5% of cases, the lesions are multifocal.[216]

Routes of Spread

Direct extension occurs to adjacent structures including the vagina, perineum, clitoris, and anus. The lymphatics of the vulva consist of a network that covers the entire labia minora, fourchette, prepuce, and distal vagina below the hymenal membrane. These coalesce anteriorly, forming larger trunks, which run laterally to the clitoris to the mons veneris, acquiring tributaries from the lymphatics of the labia majora, which run in a parallel fashion anteriorly from the perineal body. The vulvar lymphatics run through the vulva and do not cross the labiocrural fold. The lymphatics of the perineum, however, course lateral to the labiocrural fold through the superficial tissues of the upper medial thigh. In the treatment of patients with advanced vulvar cancer that extends beyond the vulva to the perineal skin, these more lateral channels must be taken into consideration. Similarly, direct proximal extension of an advanced vulvovaginal cancer along the vaginal cylinder may spread through vaginal lymphatics directly to pelvic nodes. At the mons veneris, the vulvar lymphatic trunks diverge laterally to the primary regional nodes, the ipsilateral or contralateral inguinal nodes. Study of the localization of dye or radiolabeled tracer in regional lymph nodes after focal injection of discrete sites in the vulva and on the perineum reveals that the lymphatic drainage of the perineum, clitoris, and anterior labia minora is bilateral, whereas the lymph flow from well-lateralized sites in the vulva is, predominantly, to the ipsilateral groin.[217,218] Discrete ($\leq$2 cm diameter), well-lateralized primary cancers limited to the vulva and not approaching midline structures rarely manifest spread to contralateral groin nodes in the absence of spread to ipsilateral nodes.[219-224]

From the superficial inguinal nodes, secondary lymphatic drainage is through the cribriform fascia to the femoral nodes (Fig. 90-19), with subsequent tertiary flow under the inguinal ligaments to the external iliac nodes. However, metastases have been reported to the femoral lymph nodes without involvement of the superficial inguinal lymph nodes, especially from carcinomas of the clitoris and Bartholin's gland.[225,226] A recent GOG study

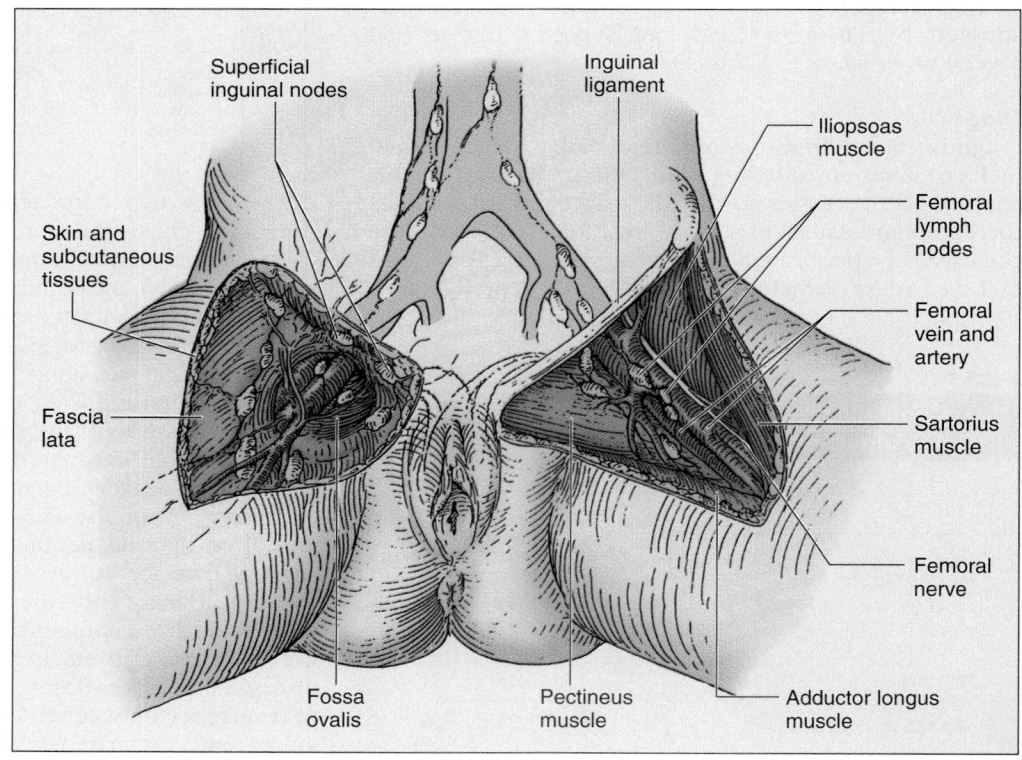

Figure 90-19. Regional lymph nodes in vulvar carcinoma: Inguinal and femoral. (From Berek JS, Hacker NF: Practical Gynecologic Oncology, 2nd ed. Baltimore, Williams & Wilkins, 1994.)

also found an unexpectedly high incidence of ipsilateral groin recurrences secondary to presumed involvement of lymph nodes deep to the cribriform fascia, despite having negative superficial nodes.[227] Levenback and colleagues[228] further supported these data by lymphatic mapping studies.

The frequency of lymph node metastases to the inguinofemoral nodes is related to the lesion size and depth of stromal invasion.[220,229] For lesions smaller than 1 cm in diameter, the incidence is approximately 5%. For lesions exceeding 4 cm, the rate of inguinofemoral lymph node metastases is 30% to 50%.[221,230] The overall incidence of metastases to the pelvic lymph nodes is 5% and is rare in the absence of three or more positive inguinofemoral lymph nodes. Hematogenous spread is rare in the absence of inguinofemoral lymph node involvement and usually occurs late in the course of the disease. However, in patients with three or more positive lymph nodes, the ultimate risk of hematogenous spread is 66%. By contrast, patients with fewer than three positive lymph nodes have only a 4% risk of hematogenous spread.[231,232] Sites of hematogenous spread include lung and bone.

Staging

Staging of invasive vulvar cancer is based on clinico-pathologic measurement and assessment of anatomic extent of the primary lesion; the presence, laterality, and extent of regional lymph node metastases; and the presence or absence of distant metastases including pelvic lymph nodes. Historically, staging evaluation of the inguinal lymph nodes was based on palpation and clinical impression. Because the clinical assessment of inguinal lymph nodes is associated with false-positive and false-negative rates of approximately 20%[233-238] (Table 90-5), a surgical staging system for vulvar cancer was initially adopted by FIGO in 1988 and subsequently revised several times since[239] (Table 90-6).

Diagnosis

Diagnosis of vulvar lesions requires a biopsy, which should include some surrounding skin and underlying dermis and connective tissue so that the pathologist can assess the depth and nature of stromal invasion. This procedure can usually be performed under local anesthesia. For lesions of 1 cm or less diameter, excisional biopsy is preferable.

TABLE 90-5

Clinical Assessment of Inguinofemoral Nodes by Palpation

	HISTOLOGICALLY (−)	HISTOLOGICALLY (+)
Clinically (−) (N = 451 patients)	363 (80.5%)	88 (19.5%)
Clinically (+) (N = 243 patients)	53 (21.8%)	190 (78.2%)

Pooled data, six institutions.[233-238]

TABLE 90-6

FIGO/AJCC/UICC 1997 TNM Classification and Stage Grouping

T	Primary tumor
TX	Primary tumor cannot be assessed
T0	No evidence of primary tumor
Tis	Carcinoma in situ (preinvasive carcinoma)
T1	Tumor confined to the vulva and perineum* ≤2 cm in greatest dimension
T1a	Tumor confined to the vulva or vulva and perineum, ≤2 cm in greatest dimension, and with stromal invasion ≤1 mm
T1b	Tumor confined to the vulva or vulva and perineum, ≤2 cm in greatest dimension, with stromal invasion >1 mm
T2	Tumor confined to the vulva and perineum >2 cm in greatest dimension
T3	Tumor of any size with adjacent spread to the lower urethra and/or vagina and/or anus
T4	Tumor of any size invading any of the following: the upper urethral mucosa, the bladder mucosa, the rectal mucosa, or tumor fixed to the bone
N	Regional lymph nodes†
N0	No nodal metastases
N1	Unilateral regional lymph node metastasis
N2	Bilateral regional lymph node metastasis
M	Distant metastasis
M0	No evidence of distant metastasis
M1	Any distant metastasis including pelvic lymph nodes

FIGO/AJCC/UICC Stage Grouping

0	TisN0M0
I	T1N0M0
II	T2N0M0
III	T3N0M0
	T1,2,3N1M0
IVa	T1,2,3N2M0
	T4NxM0
IVb	TxNxM1

(x denotes any T or N category)

AJCC, American Joint Commission on Cancer; FIGO, Federation Internationale de Gynecologie et d'Obstetrique; UICC, Union Internationale Contre le Cancer.
*The depth of invasion is defined as the measurement of the tumor from the epithelial-stromal junction of the adjacent most superficial dermal papilla to the deepest point of invasion.
†Note that assessment of inguinofemoral nodes is histologic.

The operative approach to the treatment of vulvar carcinoma, consisting of a radical en bloc resection of the vulva, was developed at the beginning of the 20th century in response to the combination of patients first seen with regionally advanced disease and the poor results (approximately 20% to 25% 5-year survival) achieved with limited surgical excision.[240]

Basset[241] first reported an en bloc operative removal of the vulva along with the regional lymph nodes, resulting in considerable improvement in 5-year survival (60% to 70%). Three decades later, Taussig[242] of the United States and Way[233,243] of the United Kingdom popularized this radical en bloc dissection that remained the standard of surgical care for vulvar cancer until the early 1980s. At that time, Hacker and others[244,245] introduced the concept of individualized and conservative surgery, proposing the use of separate groin incisions for women with stage I disease and demonstrating no difference in the incidence of recurrence between those women undergoing a radical vulvectomy compared with those undergoing a radical

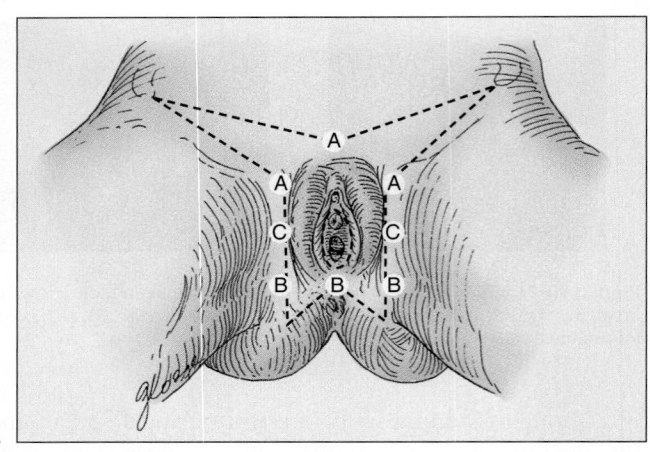
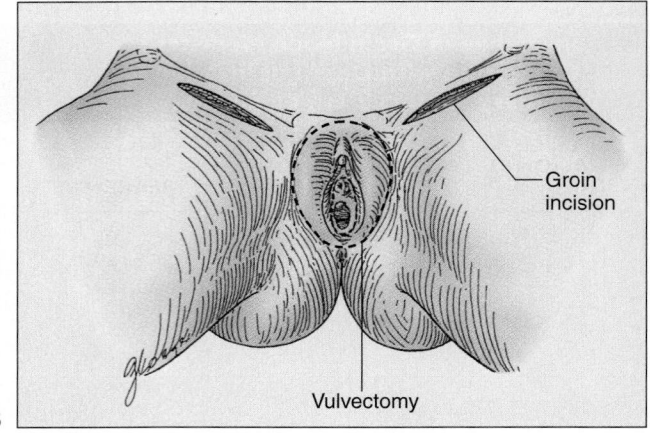

Figure 90-20. Comparison of incisions used for the en bloc vulvectomy and groin dissection (**A**) versus the modified radical vulvectomy with separate incisions for the groin dissection (**B**). (From Berek JS, Hacker NF: Practical Gynecologic Oncology, 2nd ed. Baltimore, Williams & Wilkins, 1994.)

local excision (modified radical vulvectomy). The trend over the past 20 years has been toward less radical surgery for early-stage vulvar cancer in an attempt to decrease the significant physical and psychologic morbidity associated with en bloc dissection (Fig. 90-20). Historically, exenterative procedures were undertaken to clear central disease in patients first seen with locally advanced disease.[246] Increasingly, treatment has evolved to include combinations of preoperative radiation or preoperative chemoradiation to reduce tumor volume sufficiently to permit clearance of central disease without sacrifice of functionally important midline structures.[244-248]

Surgical Techniques

Radical Local Excision. This technique involves a wide and deep excision of the lesion with the goal of clearing the lesion by 2 cm at all margins, except for posteriorly with perineal lesions in which the distance to the anus is limited. The incision should be carried down to the inferior fascia of the urogenital diaphragm, which is in a parallel plane to the fascia lata and the fascia over the symphysis pubis. The surgical defect is closed in two layers. Limitations to this conservative approach are encountered when cancer is in close proximity to functionally important midline structures (clitoris, urethra, anus). Eight millimeters or greater histopathologic margin (approximately equivalent to 1-cm clinical margin in tissue before fixation) serves as a useful discriminating boundary between patients who are likely to have excellent prospects for local control with surgery alone, as opposed to patients who have a substantial risk of local recurrence and who might require more extensive surgery initially or postoperative adjuvant radiotherapy[249-251] (Table 90-7).

Radical Vulvectomy. The radical vulvectomy may be performed through an incision separate from the groin dissection or in an en bloc fashion. The en bloc technique was based on the concern that leaving tissue between the primary tumor and the regional lymph nodes might leave microscopic foci tumor in the draining lymphatics.

However, squamous carcinoma most often spreads by embolization and not by permeation. Although rare instances of recurrence within the skin bridge have been reported, the experience with separate groin incisions has shown that very little chance of recurrence exists in the skin bridge without clinically suggestive groin nodes.[244] Wound seroma is the most common acute complication and occurs in approximately 15% of cases.[244,245] Other acute complications include urinary tract infection, wound cellulitis, temporary anterior thigh anesthesia from femoral nerve injury, thrombophlebitis, and rarely pulmonary embolus. The most common chronic complication now is leg edema. With the use of separate groin incisions, the incidence of this decreased from 31% to 14%.[244,245] Other chronic complications include genital prolapse, urinary stress incontinence (10%), temporary weakness of the quadriceps muscle, and introital stenosis. Rare late complications include pubic osteomyelitis, femoral hernia, and rectoperineal fistula. Farias-Eisner and associates[252] and Hacker and colleagues[220] observed a further reduction in acute and chronic morbidity when radical local excision of the primary lesion is used instead of radical vulvectomy.

Groin Lymph Node Dissection

The appropriate application of groin dissection is the single most important factor in decreasing the mortality

TABLE 90-7

Width of Surgical Margin and Risk of Local Recurrence		
AUTHOR	**MARGIN <8 MM**	**MARGIN ≥8 MM**
Heaps[249]	21/44 (48%)	0/91
Faul[250]	18/31 (58%)	NA
De Hullu[251]*	9/40 (23%)	0/39
NA, not applicable.		
*Surgical margin ≤8 mm vs. >8 mm.		

TABLE 90-8

■ Incidence of Groin Node Metastasis Correlated with Depth of Invasion for Primary Tumors 2 cm or Smaller			
DEPTH OF INVASION (MM)	**PATIENTS (NO.)**	**POSITIVE NODES (NO.)**	**PERCENTAGE**
≤1	120	0	0
1–2	121	8	6.6
1–3	97	8	8.2
1–4	50	11	22
1–5	40	10	25
>5	32	12	37.5

Pooled data, six series.[220,222,223,229,253,254]

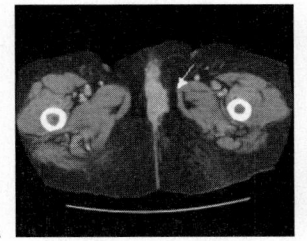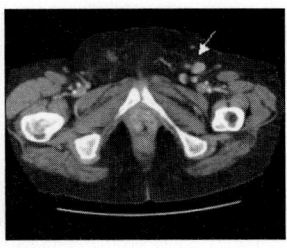

Figure 90-21. CT of vulvar cancer. **A,** Irregular thickening and growth involving the left vulva with distortion of contour (*arrow*). **B,** Enlarged left inguinal node (*arrow*).

of early vulvar cancer. The technique for groin dissection involves the removal of an ellipse of skin 1 cm below and parallel to the groin crease. The incision is carried down, with incising and dissecting, to the fascia lata and 2 cm above the inguinal ligament to remove the inguinal nodes. The saphenous vein is tied off, the fascia lata is then split, and the femoral nodes are dissected. Some surgeons will conserve the saphenous vein in an effort to decrease both acute and chronic morbidity. A suction drain is placed, and the wound closed in two layers.

Surgical specimens from patients with primary tumors 2 cm or smaller in diameter (T1) clearly show escalating risk of node metastasis with progressive depth of invasion (Table 90-8).[220,222,223,229,253,254] The probability of finding groin node metastasis is related to the size of the primary tumor, as shown in Table 90-9.[255,256] An infiltrative pattern of growth correlates with nodal spread,[257,258] and the presence of vascular or lymphatic space invasion substantially escalates the probability of finding metastases in dissected nodes.[255] The presence of metastatic spread to contralateral groin nodes in the absence of disease in ipsilateral nodes occurs in 15% or fewer of all patients with metastases to groin nodes,[259] generally in patients with larger lesions. Although described in two patients with lateralized T1 lesions,[169] the risk of contralateral nodal spread in the absence of ipsilateral metastasis is less than 1%.[170,230,234,235,259,260–264] When metastatic disease is present in multiple groin nodes, pelvic lymphadenectomy will detect disease in 15% to 25% of patients, but rarely when only one groin node is microscopically contaminated.[265,266]

TABLE 90-9

■ Primary Tumor Size and Risk of Groin Node Metastasis			
PRIMARY SIZE (CM)	**PATIENTS (NO.)**	**POSITIVE NODES (NO.)**	**PERCENTAGE**
≤2	75	5	6.7
2–4	78	19	24.4
>4	79	26	32.9

Pooled data, two series.[255,256]

A thoughtful appraisal of the risk of nodal spread and the anatomic level of potential contamination is an essential part of planning surgical therapy and determining target volume, dose, and technique for a course of radiation therapy. Diagnostic imaging may be helpful in the assessment of regional nodes in patients with vulvar cancer and tailoring the extent of surgery or radiation accordingly. Magnetic resonance imaging (MRI) is highly specific for the detection of inguinal nodal involvement (97% to 100%). Computed tomography (CT) also is useful in detecting nodal involvement (Fig. 90-21) that may be deeper in tissue than can be readily detected on physical examination. Fluorodeoxyglucose–positron emission tomography (FDG-PET) has a sensitivity of 67% to 80% in predicting lymph node metastasis. It also is more specific (90% to 95%) and is useful in planning radiation therapy and as an adjunct to lymphatic mapping and sentinel lymph node dissection.[267,268] Lymphoscintigraphy with technetium-99m (Tc-99m) sulfur colloid may be useful in the identification of sentinel nodes.[269]

Given the results of the Gynecologic Oncology Group (GOG) prospective randomized trial demonstrating better efficacy for adjuvant node radiation compared with pelvic node dissection, the indications for extending surgery proximal to the inguinal ligament are diminishing.[262]

RADIATION THERAPY

Radiotherapy is increasingly used in the curative management of vulvar cancer,[270–275] often in conjunction with synchronous administration of radiation potentiating chemotherapy (chemoradiation).[276–288]

Radiation salvages some patients with locoregional recurrence after radical vulvectomy and regional node dissection.[289] Postoperative radiation directed to the groins and pelvic nodes improves disease-free survival in patients with metastatic spread to two or more inguino-femoral nodes[262] and may further improve results if residual vulva and perineum (operative bed) are included within the irradiated volume.[290]

Preoperative radiation and chemoradiation have reduced the indications for exenterative surgery and may permit a substantial decrease in the volume of normal tissue that must be removed in patients with tumors invading or intimately approximating the anus, clitoris, urethra, and distal vagina.[270–274,282,283,288]

Postsurgical, central, limited-volume, local recurrence in the residual vulva, at the introital margin, or on the perineum will often be salvaged with secondary surgery, radiation, or combined-modality therapy.[289] A disease-free interval of 2 or more years and lack of involvement of regional nodes portend a favorable outcome with salvage therapy, although the majority of disease recurs within 2 years of initial surgery.[291,292] Under circumstances in which the anticipated surgical margin is less than that of the original surgery, when recurrence approaches or involves critical structures, or when the pattern of recurrence is multifocal, it is prudent to plan for delivery of radiation as at least a component of the salvage strategy. Regional relapse in the groin or in pelvic nodes is much less likely to be salvaged, regardless of the combination of modalities used.[289,292-294] Salvage radiation alone, in doses ranging from 63 Gy to 72 Gy with progressive volume reductions or partial treatment with brachytherapy, often controls small-volume recurrence. Preoperative radiation ranging in dose from 45 Gy to 54 Gy followed by local excision may be less injurious in terms of delayed normal tissue effects than a high radiation dose to a large perineal volume in the absence of surgery.[292]

Adjuvant Postoperative Radiotherapy

The GOG conducted a randomized trial comparing pelvic lymphadenectomy with radiotherapy directed to the bilateral groins and pelvic nodes (but not the tumor bed or perineum) in patients who were found to have groin node metastasis. A total of 114 eligible patients were randomized, of whom 40 had only one positive groin node. In 15 (28.3%) patients of 53 undergoing pelvic lymphadenectomy, disease had spread to pelvic nodes; 9 (60%) of these patients died of cancer within 1 year of study entry. The overall survival advantage for radiation at 2 years (68% for radiation, 54% for pelvic node dissection) was limited to patients with two or more involved groin nodes (63% for radiation, 37% for pelvic node dissection) and was attributable to a decrease in recurrence in the groin among the irradiated patients (5.1%) compared with those patients treated with surgery alone (23.6%). Lymphedema was reported in 19% of irradiated patients compared with 11% of patients treated with surgery alone. Of the 44 patients who had recurrence, only 11 patients failed with a component of "distant" disease (including three patients with relapse in the thigh, periaortic nodes, and abdominal skin), whereas 75% of relapsing patients failed with locoregional disease alone (vulvar area, groins, or pelvis). Eleven (25%) patients experienced recurrence in the unirradiated vulvar area; 10 of these had no other apparent sites of failure. As a consequence of this study, pelvic lymphadenectomy is less likely to be performed, and regional adjuvant radiation has become the standard of additional care for patients with metastasis to two or more regional nodes.[262] Areas of controversy in the postoperative adjuvant therapy of resected, node-positive vulvar cancer include whether patients with only one node contaminated should receive adjuvant therapy, whether patients with only unilateral groin node metastasis should have radiation delivered to the contralateral groin and pelvis, and whether synchronous administration of chemotherapy might further improve outcomes. Retrospective outcomes analysis of node-positive patients undergoing adjuvant groin and pelvic radiation suggests the wisdom of including the operative bed of the primary lesion within the treatment volume.[290]

Preoperative Chemoradiation

Under circumstances in which the extent of the primary disease suggests that postoperative radiation will be indicated, it is reasonable to consider preoperative radiation if it has the potential to reduce the scope of surgery and to conserve normal tissue structure and function or to convert the status of the patient from unresectable to operable.[270-274,282,283] An anticipated margin of 1 cm or less from structures that will not be surgically removed is a useful guide for selecting patients for preoperative radiation.[249-251] Tumors that encroach on the anal sphincter, abut the pubic arch, or involve more than the distal urethra should be considered for preoperative therapy. Patients with tumors that approach the clitoris or extend more than minimally past the vaginal introitus also should be considered for preoperative irradiation if conservation of sexual function is desired. Moderate-dose radiation (36 Gy to 54 Gy) has been given, followed by excision of residual palpable abnormalities that revealed no evidence of persistent cancer in 50% of cases (Table 90-10).

External-beam radiation is most commonly used, but interstitial or intracavitary brachytherapy may apply a higher dose to a discrete tissue volume where a surgical margin is anticipated to be inadequate.[270]

The GOG studied 73 patients with stage III to IV squamous cancers of the vulva who were judged not amenable to resection because of local disease extent beyond the conventional boundaries of radical vulvectomy. Preoperative chemoradiation, consisting of 47.6 Gy delivered in fractions of 1.7 Gy coordinated with two cycles of synchronous cisplatin and 5-fluorouracil (5-FU), converted 69 of 71 patients medically fit for surgery to having lesions considered amenable to resection. Ultimately, urinary and fecal continence was conserved in all but 3 patients. With the use of this approach, local tumor control has been excellent, with conservation of normal tissue

TABLE 90-10

Histologic Tumor Clearance by Preoperative Radiation

AUTHOR	PATIENTS	DOSE (GY)	NEGATIVE SPECIMEN	PERCENTAGE
Hacker[271]	8*	44–54	4	50
Acosta[272]	14	36–55	5	36
Jafari[273]	4	30–42	4	100
Total	26	30–55	13	50

Includes one patient who received additional 24 Gy by intravaginal mould.

Cycle #1	
Day	Mon. – Fri. Mon. – Fri. 1 2 3 4 5 6 7 8 9 10 11 12
Radiation 1.7 Gy/Fx	R R R R 0 0 R R R R R R R
5-FU 1,000 mg/M²/24 hrs Cisplatin 50 mg/M²	F F F F P 1½—2½ week planned rest

Cycle #2	
Day	Mon. – Fri. Mon. – Fri. 1 2 3 4 5 6 7 8 9 10 11 12
Radiation 1.7 Gy/Fx	R R R R 0 0 R R R R R R R
5-FU 1,000 mg/M²/24 hrs Cisplatin 50 mg/M²	F F F F P

*Patients who are judged to be unresectable following completion of 47.6 Gy preoperative chemoradiation receive additional 20 Gy in fractions of 1.7 Gy–2.0 Gy with reduced treatment volume encompassing gross residual disease, or may receive additional radiation dose via brachytherapy. A third cycle of chemotherapy is recommended if teletherapy is employed. The authors would suggest restricting the cumulative dose to 59.5 Gy/35 Fx in the interest of avoiding severe late skin effects.
R denotes a fraction of external radiation. A 4-hour minimum inter-treatment interval is mandatory, but 6 or more hours are suggested when practically feasible.
0 indicates a day without radiation treatment.
F signifies 5-fluorouracil by continuous intravenous infusion.
P indicates bolus cisplatin administration.

Figure 90-22. Time/Dose/Fractionation schedule: Phase II evaluation of preoperative chemoradiation for advanced vulvar cancer. GOG Protocol 101.[248]

integrity in many patients who would otherwise have required exenterative surgery for tumor clearance.[283] By using the identical regimen (Fig. 90-22) in 46 patients with extensive (matted, fixed, or ulcerated) and unresectable groin metastases, physicians of the GOG were ultimately able to resect groin nodes in 37 patients, of whom 15 had histologically negative groin specimens.[295] The observation of complete histologic clearance of malignancy after moderate-dose preoperative radiation (alone or coordinated with synchronous chemotherapy) serves to encourage efforts to control vulvar cancer with radiation-based therapy under circumstances in which surgery is either technically unfeasible or medically contraindicated.

Radical Radiation and Chemoradiation

Definitive radiation has been used to treat medically inoperable or technically unresectable patients. Historically, results have been poor, in terms of both tumor control and normal tissue sequelae, although the tumor-control probability for patients with disease of limited volume has approached that of surgery.[274,296,297] Results with radiation alone in recent years have improved with better technique and dosimetry.[275]

The favorable experience with chemotherapy and reduced-dose radiation in the treatment of cancers of the anal canal has prompted increasing utilization of this approach in the treatment of advanced vulvar cancer. Most published experiences used 5-FU, with or without cisplatin or mitomycin.[278-280,285-287,298-301] Retrospective comparison[301] suggests the superiority of chemoradiation compared with radiation alone, but prospective randomized data do not exist to validate the clinical impression of better results. Unquestionably, the administration of concurrent chemotherapy augments the acute reaction in normal tissues. Moist desquamation of the vulva necessitates treatment interruption in most patients. Hybrid dose/fractionation regimens have been developed to preserve dose intensity and to maximize potential synergistic effects. Twice-daily fractionation has become a popular strategy to exploit the radiation/drug interaction while minimizing the theoretical disadvantages of split-course radiation that is made mandatory by the enhanced effects in normal tissue.[248,286,287] Because of potential enhancement of late normal tissue effects, and because full radiation dose must be administered to some skin when treating what is fundamentally a skin cancer, it is advisable that total dose not exceed approximately 54 Gy in 30 fractions, 59.5 Gy in 35 fractions, or 64 Gy in 40 fractions to gross disease when chemoradiation is used, and that the volume receiving the full dose be as small as possible, while including all areas of initial measurable clinical involvement.

Elective Groin Radiation

A contributing factor to perioperative complications and chronic morbidity is the dissection of the inguinofemoral nodes.[302] In selected patients with limited primary tumors (T1a with ≤1 mm of invasion), omission of the node dissection is prudent. In others, limiting the groin dissection to superficial inguinal nodes (if histopathologically negative) has been an effective strategy for reducing acute and chronic morbidity. Preoperative identification of sentinel nodes may further enhance the safety of this approach. Elective irradiation of the clinically and radiographically negative groin nodes is an alternative strategy that has the theoretical advantage of treating all of the regional nodes rather than leaving some portion untreated. This approach also is applicable in patients with locally advanced primary tumors, in whom less than radical (superficial and deep) bilateral groin dissection would constitute less than adequate surgical treatment. Several series[303-306] have reported favorable results with elective or prophylactic groin irradiation (Table 90-11), but frequently in the setting in which groin nodes would be expected to be histologically uninvolved if treated surgically (T1 or T2 primary tumors of limited extent; Table 90-12).[307]

The GOG conducted a randomized trial comparing groin irradiation with groin dissection in otherwise

TABLE 90-11

Results of Elective Groin Radiation or Chemoradiation in Patients with Vulvar Cancer and Clinically Negative Inguinofemoral Lymph Nodes*

AUTHOR	PATIENTS	GROIN FAILURE	PERCENTAGE
Radiation Alone			
Frankendal[303]	12	0	0
Simonsen[304]	65	11	16.9
Boronow[270]	13	0	0
Perez[275]	39	2	5.1
Lee[305]	16	3	18.8
Petereit[306]	23	2	8.7
Stehman[308]	27	5	18.5
Total	195	23	11.8
Chemoradiation			
Leiserowitz[310]	19	0	0
Wahlen[311]	17	0	0
Total	36	0	0

*Patients with FIGO 1969 N0,1 negative groin nodes by clinical evaluation.

operable patients with resectable vulvar primaries.[308] The study was terminated early because of an unacceptable rate of groin relapse (5 of 27 patients, 18.5%) and subsequent death of cancer (all 5 patients) in the group of women randomized to radiation. Technical inadequacies in the radiation treatment that may have led to inadvertent underdosage of the nodes could have contributed to this outcome.[309]

At the Radiation Oncology Centers of Sacramento[310] and at Loma Linda University,[311] patients have undergone prophylactic chemoradiation to the groin nodes, generally as a component of preoperative or definitive chemoradiation for locally advanced primary cancers. Among 37

such patients treated, no groin relapses occurred (see Table 90-11). It remains unclear whether the better results reflect better radiation technique or the radiopotentiating effect of synchronous chemotherapy.

Radiation Techniques, Volumes, and Doses

No standard approach is found to the treatment of vulvar cancer with radiation. The circumstance of radiation (postoperative, preoperative, or as definitive treatment) will influence the designation of target volume, fractionation, and dose. Clinical and histopathologic characteristics of the primary and regional nodes may independently affect the selection of treatment parameters, which depends further on the scope of any coordinated surgery and whether chemotherapy is to be administered with radiation. Comorbidities in elderly patients may constrain the volume and intensity of treatment. Conservation of ovarian function and possible reproductive integrity in younger patients also may affect the technique of treatment.[312] No substitute can be found for comprehensive assessment of disease extent followed by tailored, individualized therapy that takes into account the intent of treatment (preoperative, definitive, adjuvant postoperative), patient comorbidities, and patient preference. A guideline for radiation doses and fractionation is found in Table 90-13.

Chemotherapy

Chemotherapy to potentiate the effectiveness of locoregional radiation is rapidly becoming the standard of care for patients receiving radiation as all or as a component of treatment for the vulvar primary and regional nodes. Prospective randomized data for chemoradiation versus radiation alone do not exist. However, it is the clinical impression of experienced clinicians that tumor control within the irradiated volume appears to be better

TABLE 90-12

Probability of Clinically Occult Metastasis to Inguinofemoral Lymph Nodes Correlated with Primary Tumor Category and Size

T STAGE (1997 FIGO)	N0* (1969 FIG0) N (%)	N1* (1969 FIGO) N (%)	TOTAL N (%)
T1	13/84 (15.5)	3/21 (14.3)	16/105 (15.2)
T2	17/56 (30.4)	4/14 (28.5)	21/70 (30)
T3	11/38 (28.9)	1/11 (9.1)	12/49 (24.4)
T4	0/1	0/0	0/1
Total	41/179 (22.9)	8/46 (17.4)	49/225 (21.7)
Clinical Tumor Size (cm)			
0–1.0	3/39 (7.7)	0/4	3/43 (7)
1.1–2.0	11/46 (23.9)	3/17 (17.6)	14/63 (22.2)
2.1–3.0	13/42 (31)	1/10 (10)	14/52 (26.9)
3.1–5.0	12/33 (36.4)	2/8 (25)	14/41 (34.1)
>5.0	1/10 (10)	2/5 (40)	3/15 (20)
Total†	40/170 (23.5)	8/44 (18.2)	48/214 (22.4)

*N0 denotes no palpable inguinal nodes; N1 denotes nodes palpable, nonsuggestive.
†Clinical tumor measurements not available for all patients.
Data from Gonzalez-Bosquet J, Kinney WK, Russell AH, et al: Risk of occult inguinofemoral lymph node metastasis from squamous carcinoma of the vulva. Int J Radiat Oncol Biol Phys 2003;57:419–424.

TABLE 90-13

Dose Guidelines

| | CANCER VOLUME | | | |
| | RADIATION ALONE | | CHEMORADIATION | |
TREATMENT INTENT	MICROSCOPIC	GROSS	MICROSCOPIC	GROSS
Preoperative	45–56	45–56	36–48	36–48
Postoperative	45–56	54–64 (+ margin)	36–48	45–56 (+ margin)
Radical	45–56	63–72	36–48	45–64

All doses expressed in Gray. Dose guidelines assume that treatment will be administered in fractions of 1.6 Gy to 1.8 Gy and that multiple daily fractions may be used for all or a part of the treatment. Higher total doses imply fraction size of 1.6 Gy, and lower total doses imply fraction size of 1.8 Gy. Dose guidelines should be interpreted in the contexts of tumor bulk, health of normal tissues unavoidably included within the treatment volume, tolerance, and response to treatment. Use of doses in the lower end of the range for gross disease is predicated on a biopsy at the completion of treatment confirming histologic clearance. Doses for gross disease should be applied with progressively shrinking volumes that confine high dose to not more, and possibly less, than the original volume of measurable disease.

than that historically achieved with radiation alone. Additionally, late radiation sequelae in normal tissues may be milder consequent to the use of lower total dose and lower dose per treatment fraction. Most chemoradiation has been done with 5-FU alone or in combination with cisplatin or mitomycin-C. Representative results of treatment are depicted in Table 90-14. Experience with radiation and concurrent bleomycin has been disappointing as both preoperative treatment[313] and treatment for extensive, inoperable disease,[314] with the majority of patients treated for locoregionally advanced disease manifesting persistent or recurrent disease within the irradiated volume.

Chemotherapy for Recurrent, Persistent, or Metastatic Vulvar Carcinoma

Recurrent or persistent vulvar carcinoma after surgical therapy is typically treated with surgical resection or radiation-based therapy or both. Vulvar carcinoma that recurs in a local or regional area of prior radiation is often considered for surgical resection. Tumors that are not controlled or amenable to surgical or radiotherapeutic approaches are difficult to manage because of a lack of active systemic agents; these tumors often are first seen in elderly patients with major comorbidities, and sometimes in individuals with altered immunity due to chronic

TABLE 90-14

Results of Radical Chemoradiation for Locoregional Advanced or Recurrent Cancers of the Vulva in Previously Untreated Patients

AUTHOR	PATIENTS STAGES (N)	DRUGS	RADIATION DOSE (GY)	COMPLETE RESPONSE	SUBSEQUENT LOCAL FAILURE	NED F/U (MO)
Thomas[284]	9 "Advanced"	F,M	40–64	6 (67%)	3 (50%)	NA
Berek[285]	12 III (8) IV (4)	F,P	44–54	8 (67%)	0	7–60
Russell[286]	18+ II (1) III (10) IV (6)	F,P M	46.8–56	16 (89%)	2 (13%)	2–52
Koh[287]	14+ III (4) IV (10)	F,P M	34–63.1	8 (57%)	1 (17%)	5–75
Eifel[298]	12 II (1) III, IV (11)	F,P	40–50	6 (50%)	1 (16%)	17–37
Cunningham[299]	14 III (9) IV (5)	F,P	50–65	9 (64%)	1 (11%)	7–81
Akl[300]	12 I (3) II (5) III (4)	F,M	30–36	12 (100%)	1 (8%)	8–125
Total	91			65 (71%)	9 (14%)	

F, 5-FU; M, mitomycin-C; NED, no evidence of disease; P, cisplatinum.

TABLE 90-15

Pattern of Recurrence* in 267 Patients for Whom Regional Therapy† Failed for Carcinoma of the Vulva

VULVA/PERINEUM N (%)	GROIN N (%)	PELVIS N (%)	DISTANT N (%)
162 (60.7)	62 (23.2)	42 (15.7)	51 (19.1)

*Because some patients manifested recurrence at more than one site, the total recurrences exceed 267, and the total of the percentages exceeds 100.
†The majority of patients underwent radical surgery. Adjunctive radiation was administered in some, and a small number were treated with radiation alone. Pooled data, seven series.[220,291–293,315–317]

immunosuppression. Because recurrent tumors are rare, no randomized phase III trials have evaluated systemic therapy. Very few phase II studies have been reported to guide clinicians in selecting treatment. The effectiveness of chemotherapy also is limited by the fact that many treatment failures are local, or locoregional,[220,291–293,315–317] and typically within a prior radiation field (Table 90-15). These radiation-resistant tumors are typically also resistant to chemotherapy. Responses to treatment may be difficult to evaluate because of extensive anatomic abnormalities associated with prior surgery and radiation. Only six agents have been evaluated as single agents, with trials including only 4 to 22 patients, with most of these trials done in the early 1980s. Doxorubicin (Adriamycin) and bleomycin have demonstrated some single-agent activity.[318–320] An anecdotal response has been reported with liposomal doxorubicin.[321] Unfortunately, the duration of response in most instances is disappointing and measured in months.

Combination chemotherapy regimens have been evaluated and have included bleomycin, along with a variety of agents (Table 90-16).[322–326] The largest experience is with the regimen of bleomycin, methotrexate,

and N-(2-chloroethyl)-N'-cyclohexyl-N-nitrosourea (CCNU) (BMC).[322,323] Activity has been seen in two separate phase II studies that included 53 patients and demonstrated 5 complete responses and 27 partial responses for an overall response rate of 60% in a group of patients with locally advanced squamous cell carcinoma of the vulva.

In vitro studies with squamous cell cancer lines of the vulva demonstrate high expression of the epidermal growth factor receptor and efficacy of ZD1839 in vitro either alone or in combination with chemotherapy.[327,328] The role of this targeted agent in the clinic awaits formal testing.

Other Histologic Types

Adenosquamous Carcinoma

The pathogenesis of adenosquamous carcinoma of the vulva remains controversial, as it has been since it was first described by Lever 45 years ago.[329] Initially, it was thought to arise from solar keratoses. However, this theory was later discounted, as cases were described in which vulvar sun exposure was not a factor.[329,330] A currently accepted theory is that the involved glandular elements produce mucin and have their origin from mucin-producing cells of the skin appendages.[331]

Adenosquamous cell carcinoma of the vulva appears to be a biologically distinct tumor. These lesions involving the vulva are highly aggressive, are first seen at a more advanced stage, and are associated with a higher incidence of lymph node metastases than are their corresponding squamous cell counterparts. Five-year survival rates reflect this trend: 5% and 62% for adenosquamous and squamous cell carcinomas, respectively.[332]

Melanoma

Malignant melanoma of the vulva is the second most common cancer of the vulva, accounting for approximately 10% of primary vulvar neoplasms and representing 0.05% to 0.5% of all malignancies of the female genital

TABLE 90-16

Combination Chemotherapy in Squamous Cell Carcinoma of the Vulva

REGIMEN	DOSE AND SCHEDULE	N	COMPLETE RESPONSES	PARTIAL RESPONSES	REFERENCES
Bleomycin, vincristine, mitomycin-C, cisplatin	15 mg/m² cont IV days 1–3 1.4 mg/m² IV day 3 10 mg/m² IV day 3 60 mg/m² IV day 3	23	3	4	325, 326
Bleomycin, methotrexate, CCNU	5 mg IM day 1–5 15 mg PO days 1 and 4 40 mg PO days 5–7	28	3	15	321
Bleomycin, methotrexate, CCNU	5 mg IM days 1–5, 8, 15, 22, 29, 36 15 mg PO days 1 and 4, 8, 15, 22, 29, 36 40 mg PO days 5–7	25	2	12	322
Bleomycin, methotrexate, cisplatin	15 mg IV days 1 and 8 300 mg/m² day 8 with rescue 100 mg/m² day 1	21	0	14	327

CCNU, N-(2-chloroethyl)-N-cyclohexyl-N-nitrosource.

tract. Even large, tertiary cancer referral centers will treat only one or two patients annually.[333-336]

Malignant melanoma occurs predominantly in postmenopausal white women, with a peak incidence between the 6th and 7th decades. These lesions may arise de novo or from preexisting junctional or compound nevi. Three basic histologic types exist: (1) superficial spreading melanoma is most common and tends to remain superficial in its early course; (2) lentigo malignant melanoma is a "flat freckle" that has a tendency to remain superficial; and (3) nodular melanoma is the most aggressive variety, carries the worst prognosis, and tends to invade deeply early.[334]

Amelanotic varieties of these lesions are very rare. These lesions tend to be asymptomatic and insidious. Any pigmented lesions on the vulva should be sampled with biopsy. Melanomas typically contain melanoma antigen and S-100 antigen and lack carcinoembryonic antigen (CEA). These immunohistochemical tests may be required to differentiate superficial spreading melanoma from Paget's disease.[337]

Staging. The prognosis for vulvar melanoma appears to correlate most closely with the level of skin involvement. Chung and colleagues[334] (Table 90-17) proposed a modified leveling system, retaining Clark's definitions[338] for levels I and V. Levels II, III, and IV are arbitrarily defined by using measurements in millimeters. Breslow's[339] measurements also may be used, but in the vestibule and perineum, because no keratin or granular layers exist, the system must be modified.

Treatment. For level I or II lesions (superficial), the risk of nodal spread is low, and wide local excision is adequate therapy. For deeper lesions, radical vulvectomy with en bloc bilateral inguinofemoral lymphadenectomy should be performed if the inguinofemoral nodes are positive. Estrogen receptors have been demonstrated in human melanomas, and a response to tamoxifen has been reported.[340] PET and sentinel-node groin biopsies may be tools to aid in selecting the extent of regional surgery. Systemic adjuvant therapies for vulvar melanoma parallel adjuvant strategies for cutaneous melanomas arising at other primary sites.

Prognosis. Melanomas of the vulva tend to spread earlier than squamous cell carcinoma and carry a worse prognosis overall. Chung and colleagues[334] reported corrected 5-year survival rates of 100%, 40%, and 20% for patients with level II, III or IV, and V lesions, respectively. The overall 5-year survival rate with negative and positive nodes is 38% and 13%, respectively.[341]

Basal Cell Carcinoma

Basal cell carcinomas represent approximately 2% of vulvar cancers. They usually affect postmenopausal white women and are locally aggressive, although nonmetastasizing. They are commonly seen on sun-exposed skin, but also can rarely be seen on the vulva. Their common appearance is a "rodent" ulcer with rolled edges and central ulceration. Wide local excision is the treatment of choice. Not unlike CIS and Paget's disease of the vulva, basal cell carcinomas are associated with a high incidence of antecedent or concomitant malignancy elsewhere in the body; a thorough search for other primary malignancies is always warranted.

Bartholin Gland Carcinoma

The Bartholin gland is situated inferior to the bulbocavernosus muscle and superior to the deep perineal muscles. The gland is composed of columnar epithelium and ducts are lined by stratified squamous epithelium and transitional cell epithelium. Therefore adenocarcinomas, squamous cell carcinomas, and rarely transitional cell carcinomas may arise from the Bartholin gland. Most primary adenocarcinomas of the vulva arise within these glands. The median age at diagnosis is 57 years. In 10% of patients, a history of preceding inflammation of the Bartholin gland is obtained. Malignancy arising from the Bartholin's gland constitutes approximately 4% to 7% of vulvar malignancy.

The criteria established by the Armed Forces Institute of Pathology for the diagnosis of Bartholin's gland carcinoma enjoy the broadest contemporary acceptance.[342] A primary Bartholin's cancer should show areas of apparent transition from normal elements to neoplastic ones on histologic study, should be histologically compatible with origin from Bartholin's gland, and should exist without evidence of primary cancer elsewhere. The Bartholin's complex comprises a duct that is lined by squamous epithelium as it enters the distal vagina. The more proximal portions of the ductal system are lined by transitional epithelium and may be lined by columnar epithelium before arborization into secretory glandular

TABLE 90-17

	Stages of Melanoma of the Vulva According to Three Different Systems of Criteria		
STAGE	**CLARK'S LEVELS**	**CHUNG**	**BRESLOW**
I	Intraepithelial	Intraepithelial	>0.76 mm
II	Into papillary dermis	≤1 mm from granular layer	0.76–1.50 mm
III	Filling dermal papillae	1.1–2 mm from granular layer	1.51–2.25 mm
IV	Into reticular dermis	>2 mm from granular layer	2.26–3.0 mm
V	Into subcutaneous fat	Into subcutaneous fat	>3 mm

From Berek JS, Hacker NF: Practical Gynecologic Oncology, 2nd ed. Baltimore, Williams & Wilkins, 1994.

elements. Squamous carcinoma constitutes approximately 35% to 50% of cases, with adenocarcinoma only slightly less common.[342-346] Adenosquamous carcinomas and transitional cell carcinomas make up a small minority of cases. Adenoid cystic carcinoma represents a distinct subset thought to be less likely to spread to regional nodes and associated with a long natural history and late recurrences, which may be either local or hematogenous.[347] Bartholin's gland carcinomas have been reported in younger women and in association with pregnancy,[342,343] although an etiologic relation is not apparent. Often first seen with a mass deep in the labia with intact overlying skin, Bartholin's gland carcinomas may be confused with a Bartholin's cyst or abscess, particularly if the patient is young. No persuasive evidence exists that squamous carcinomas of Bartholin's gland behave differently or should be managed differently from squamous cancers arising from other vulvar structures. However, it may be more difficult to accomplish conservative excision with adequate surgical margins in patients with Bartholin's gland cancers, and the majority of patients for whom surgical therapy fails have a component of locoregional recurrence.[345,346] The use of adjuvant postoperative radiation is common.[348,349] A retrospective review of 36 nonrandomized patients at M.D. Anderson Hospital and Tumor Institute revealed that in 6 (27%) of 22 patients treated with surgery alone local recurrence developed, whereas only 1 (7%) of 14 higher-risk patients selected to receive adjuvant radiation manifested local failure.[346]

Sarcoma

Vulvar sarcomas constitute 1% to 2% of vulvar malignancies and include leiomyosarcomas, rhabdomyosarcomas, angiosarcomas, neurofibrosarcomas, and epithelioid sarcomas. The prognosis appears to be dependent on three main determinants: lesion size, tumor contour, and mitotic activity. Lesions greater than 5 cm in diameter, with infiltrating margins, and demonstrating more than five mitotic figures per 10 high-power fields (HPFs) are most likely to recur. Wide local excision is the usual treatment.

Verrucous Carcinoma

Verrucous carcinoma of the vulva represents a variant of squamous cell carcinoma. These lesions were originally described as occurring in the oral cavity but also have been described involving the vagina, cervix, and vulva. The lesion grossly appears cauliflower-like in nature. Microscopically, the papillary fronds lack the connective tissue core that characterizes condyloma acuminata. These features are very similar to those of the giant condylomata Buschke-Loewenstein, possibly representing successive stages of the same pathologic process. Clinically, these tumors are very slow growing and carry a favorable prognosis. As metastasis to regional lymph nodes is rare, radical local excision is the standard treatment.[350-353] If suggestive groin nodes are present, fine-needle aspiration (FNA) or excisional biopsy should be carried out. Usually enlarged nodes will be caused by inflammatory hypertrophy, but if they do contain metastases, radical vulvectomy and bilateral groin lymph node dissections are indicated. Verrucous carcinoma has the reputation of being radioresistant, and reports of favorable outcomes after radiation are uncommon. Surgery remains the treatment of choice whenever feasible.

Cancer of the Vagina

SUMMARY OF KEY POINTS

EPIDEMIOLOGY
- For 2003, 2000 new cases of invasive vaginal cancer in the United States are estimated, with 800 deaths
- Primary vaginal cancer constitutes only 1% to 2% of malignancies of the female genital tract and 0.1% to 0.2% of all cancers
- The majority of vaginal malignancies (≤90%) are metastatic
- Squamous cell carcinomas compose approximately 80% of primary vaginal malignancies, whereas adenocarcinomas, melanomas, sarcomas, and lymphomas compose most of the remainder

ETIOLOGY
- Speculation occurs regarding the role of human papillomavirus (HPV) in vaginal carcinoma, but no conclusive etiologic link has been identified. Low socioeconomic status, a history of genital warts, a prior abnormal Papanicolaou (Pap) smear, early hysterectomy, and prior vaginal trauma may be associated risk factors
- The frequency with which vaginal intraepithelial neoplasia (VAIN) will progress to invasive malignancy is unknown, but the percentage is thought to be small

EVALUATION
- Up to 20% of patients are asymptomatic, with disease being diagnosed on routine pelvic examination and Pap smear
- Most patients initially have postcoital or postmenopausal painless bleeding or discharge
- Patients also may have symptoms related to the location of the tumor, such as urinary frequency or dysuria from anterior tumors, or constipation or tenesmus from posterior tumors
- Vaginal carcinoma may be identified by using colposcopy in the setting of an abnormal Pap smear
- Diagnosis is established by tissue biopsy of a gross or colposcopically detected lesion
- Vaginal cancer is staged clinically based on findings of physical examination, cystoscopy, proctoscopy, and chest radiography. Additional diagnostic assessments will not alter staging, but may be important in the design of a treatment program

TREATMENT
- Depending on location of cancer within the vagina, tumor size, and extent of invasion, surgery may be effective primary therapy in selected circumstances Patients with stage I disease that can be excised with negative surgical margins without compromising the function of the urinary bladder or rectum are appropriate candidates, as well as patients with stage IVa disease in whom urinary or fecal continence has already been destroyed by direct invasion of the cancer through the wall of adjacent viscera
- Radiation therapy is the treatment of choice for most other patients. Combined chemoradiation, similar to the approach used in anal, vulvar, and cervical cancers, has been reported in a limited numbers of patients, but has not been established as superior to radiation alone
- Patients with central recurrence after radiation may be candidates for surgical salvage, which usually will entail pelvic exenteration

EPIDEMIOLOGY

Primary vaginal cancers are rare, constituting only 1% to 2% of malignant neoplasms involving the female genital tract. By convention, with International Federation of Gynecology and Obstetrics (FIGO) criteria for classification and staging, any tumor that has extended to the cervix and has reached the external os should be classified as a cervical carcinoma. Similarly, any tumor extending to involve the vagina and vulva simultaneously is classified as vulvar carcinoma. In addition, if a patient has been previously treated for a cervical cancer, a subsequent vaginal cancer within 5 years (or 10 years, depending on the author) is considered a recurrence of the cervical cancer rather than a new primary cancer. Thus some tumors with their epicenters in the vagina will be classified as cervical or vulvar neoplasms by using the FIGO formalism, and other patients, who may have second primary vaginal malignancy as part of a "field cancerization" of the lower genital tract, will be classified as patients with recurrence of prior malignancy. These factors account for some of the rarity of primary vaginal cancer. Speculation occurs that the lack of a transformation zone and glandular tissue in the vagina (compared with the cervix) makes the vagina less likely to develop neoplasia.

The majority of cancers involving the vagina are metastatic. Vaginal involvement may occur by direct extension or by lymphatic or hematogenous spread. Primary tumors most commonly are the source of metastases involving the vagina include cancers of the endometrium, cervix, vulva, ovary, breast, colon and rectum, and kidney.[354-357]

Only 10% of vaginal cancers are primary in the vagina, and the majority of these are of squamous histology. Nonsquamous primary vaginal malignancies comprise a heterogeneous group of histologies as shown in Table 90-18.[358-367] Metastatic tumors are treated according to their primary site of origin, and not as vaginal cancers.

TABLE 90-18

Primary Vaginal Cancer: Reported Incidence of Histologic Types[358–367]

HISTOLOGY	NUMBER	PERCENTAGE
Squamous	627	83.4
Adenocarcinoma	70	9.3
Sarcoma	20	2.6
Melanoma	20	2.6
Undifferentiated	8	1.0
Small cell	5	0.7
Lymphoma	2	0.3
Carcinoid	1	0.1
Total	753	100

Modified from Berek JS, Hacker NF: Practical Gynecologic Oncology, 3rd ed. Lippincott Williams & Wilkins, 2000, p 598.

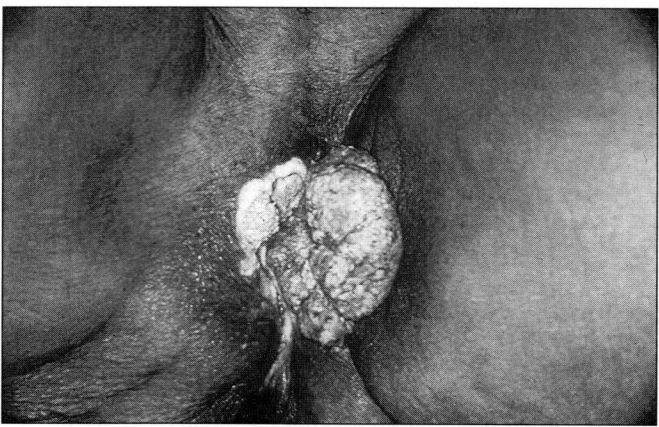

Figure 90-23. Locally recurrent verrucous cancer following radical vulvectomy. Warty, exophytic, cauliflower morphology is characteristic. This patient had persistent local disease, despite salvage chemoradiation consisting of 54 Gy in 30 fractions with twice daily fractionation over 7 weeks with three cycles of synchronous 5-fluorouracil and cisplatin. (Reproduced with permission from Russell AH: Vulva. In Leibel SA, Phillips TL (eds): Textbook of Radiation Oncology. Philadelphia, WB Saunders, 1998.)

Most women with vaginal squamous cancer are postmenopausal. More than 75% of patients are older than 50 years at diagnosis. Most single-institution series report average age in the fifth through seventh decades, with age ranges from the 20s to the 90s. A correlation is not found between age and stage of disease or survival. Squamous tumors may be nodular, ulcerative, indurative, or exophytic plaques of any size. Histologically, they are similar to squamous tumors from other sites. Approximately one third of these tumors are keratinizing, and more than one half are nonkeratinizing, moderately differentiated lesions. The degree of histologic differentiation of these tumors has not been shown to correlate with survival.[360,368–371]

Verrucous carcinoma is an uncommon variant of squamous cell carcinoma morphologically similar in the vagina to verrucous lesions of the vulva (Fig. 90-23). Grossly, it appears as a warty fungating mass. Histologically, it is composed of large papillary fronds covered by dense keratin. Its deep margin creates a pushing border of well-oriented rete ridges. This tumor rarely metastasizes but can extensively infiltrate into surrounding tissues, including the rectum and coccyx. This histologic variant of squamous cancer has a reputation of being resistant to control by conventional doses of radiation. Thus surgery is favored as a treatment modality when clinically feasible.

Adenocarcinomas occurring in the vagina include papillary, mucinous, adenosquamous, small cell, and clear cell variants. The best described of these are the clear cell malignancies, primarily because of their reported occurrence in young women who had been exposed to diethylstilbestrol (DES) in utero.[372,373] Clear cell carcinomas of the vagina are generally polypoid masses. Histologically, well-described patterns are noted: tubulocystic, solid, or papillary. They are generally diagnosed at an earlier clinical stage than is seen with squamous cell carcinomas; 74% of Registry patients were stage I, and 26% were stage II.

ETIOLOGY

The association of vaginal, vulvar, and cervical intraepithelial neoplasia (CIN) and human papillomavirus (HPV) has caused speculation as to the role of HPV in multifocal carcinoma of the lower female genital tract. Ikenberg and coworkers[374] were able to demonstrate the presence of HPV DNA in tumor tissue in 10 of 18 patients with vaginal cancer, suggesting a possible etiologic role for HPV in the development of vaginal neoplasia. Many women are first seen with multifocal disease of the genital tract, including dysplasias of vulva, vagina, and cervix. Unlike the cervix, where disease is usually present in the transformation zone, vaginal dysplasia can occur anywhere in the vaginal mucosa and is often multifocal. The natural history of vaginal intraepithelial neoplasia (VAIN) is not well understood, and the potential of VAIN to progress to invasive squamous malignancy is not known with precision. Aho and colleagues[375] identified 23 patients with VAIN followed up for at least 3 years without treatment. The mean age was 41 years. Half of the VAIN lesions were multifocal, and half were associated with either cervical intraepithelial neoplasia (CIN) or vulvar dysplasia. The spontaneous regression rate of VAIN was high (78%) including 4 of 5 VAIN 3 patients, but 2 cases (9%) progressed to invasive cancer. Studies by Benedet and Saunders[376] and by Lenehan and associates[377] have shown that only 3% to 5% of patients with VAIN treated with various methods actually progressed to having invasive vaginal carcinoma.

The clear cell variant of vaginal adenocarcinoma has been clearly linked to in utero exposure to DES. The Registry for Research on Hormonal Transplacental Carcinogenesis had accessioned more than 580 cases of clear cell carcinoma of the vagina and cervix. In utero exposure to synthetic estrogens accounted for only two thirds of reported cases. Work by Herbst and coworkers[378–380] suggests that the age distribution for clear cell adenocarcinoma of the vagina has two separate peaks. The first peak contained women with a mean age of 26 years, and the second peak contained women with a mean age of 71 years. The first peak contained all DES daughters, and

the second peak contained women born before 1950 and thus not exposed to DES. However, even when the DES daughters were excluded, a bimodal pattern was still observed. The authors suggested that this pattern might imply a genetic predisposition. The age range of DES-related clear cell adenocarcinoma is 7 to 42 years. The actual risk of clear cell adenocarcinoma developing in DES-exposed women is estimated at only 1 in 1000, with the highest risk in those women exposed before 12 weeks' gestation.[372] Although the risk of clear cell carcinoma of the vagina is small in DES-exposed women, 45% of these patients will have areas of vaginal adenosis, and 25% will have structural abnormalities of the uterus, cervix, or vagina. Thus it is recommended that women exposed to DES in utero be initially examined at menarche (approximately age 14 years) and that a careful examination of the cervix and the vagina be performed in addition to cytologic examinations. Colposcopy is unnecessary if the clinical and cytologic examinations are normal.

PATTERNS OF SPREAD

Vaginal cancer may spread by several routes:

1. Direct extension to adjacent soft-tissue structures such as the paracolpos/parametria, bladder, urethra, and rectum, with eventual involvement of the bony structures of the pelvis.
2. Lymphatic dissemination, the pattern of which will depend on the location of the primary tumor. The lymphatics of the upper vagina communicate with those of the cervix and drain into the pelvic nodes and then to the para-aortic nodes. The posterior vaginal wall drains into lymphatics that anastomose with the inferior gluteal, sacral, and deep pelvic nodes. The anterior wall is drained by lymphatics that drain to the lateral pelvic walls. The lymphatics of the distal one third of the vagina drain into the inguinofemoral nodes and then secondarily to the pelvic nodes.
3. Hematogenous dissemination to other organs, including the lungs, liver, and bone, is usually a late manifestation in the natural history of this disease.

SIGNS AND SYMPTOMS

Presenting symptoms commonly associated with this malignancy include painless spontaneous or postcoital vaginal bleeding or vaginal discharge. Because of the close proximity of the urethra to the vagina, anterior vaginal tumors may cause symptoms of urinary frequency or dysuria or both. Similarly, advanced posterior vaginal tumors may cause symptoms of tenesmus or constipation. Pelvic pain may be present when disease has extended beyond the vagina. Up to 20% of patients are asymptomatic, with disease detected on routine examination or Papanicolaou (Pap) smear. In a review of the literature by Plentl and Friedman[381] and colleagues in 1971, 51% of vaginal carcinomas arose in the upper vagina, 19% from the middle third, and 30% from the distal third. Fifty-seven percent of the tumors originated from the posterior wall, 27% from the anterior wall, and 16% from the lateral wall.[353] The most common site of occurrence of vaginal carcinoma is along the posterior wall in the upper one third of the vagina. Because the posterior blade of the speculum will often obscure this area, the speculum must be rotated to view the vaginal tube in its entirety.

DIAGNOSIS

The diagnosis of carcinoma of the vagina may be missed on initial examination, especially if the tumor is located anteriorly or posteriorly where the blades of a duckbill speculum may obscure a lesion. Thus the speculum must be rotated as it is withdrawn to allow circumferential visualization of all areas of the vaginal mucosa, and the speculum may require multiple insertions and withdrawals to accomplish this goal. If no lesion is detected in the setting of an abnormal Pap smear, use of Lugol's iodine to stain the vaginal mucosa and colposcopy may be helpful to direct biopsies. Diagnosis requires biopsy confirmation of a suspected lesion, as benign lesions such as vaginal warts (condyloma) may mimic the gross appearance of malignancy. An examination under anesthesia with directed biopsies may be necessary if the patient is elderly or has significant vaginal stenosis precluding a satisfactory office examination, or if cystoscopy or proctoscopy is indicated to evaluate the patient adequately because of the location and extent of the vaginal lesion.

STAGING

Vaginal cancers are staged according to criteria set forth by FIGO or by the American Joint Committee (Table 90-19). The staging of vaginal cancers is primarily clinical and is based on the findings on physical and pelvic examination, cystoscopy, proctoscopy, chest radiography, and skeletal radiography (if indicated for bone pain). Assignment of FIGO stage is necessary, but alone may be insufficient to direct therapy optimally. Rubin and colleagues[361] studied vaginal cancer patients spanning the years 1958 through 1980. In this study, 18% of patients had stage I tumors, and 46% had stage II tumors. Stock[382] reviewed patients spanning the years 1962 through 1992. In this study, 23% of patients had stage I disease, and 58% had stage II disease; the remaining patients had more advanced disease.

In addition to the standard staging investigation, an abdominopelvic computed tomography (CT) scan or pelvic magnetic resonance imaging (MRI) or both may be helpful to evaluate the extent of the primary tumor, confirm patency of the ureters, and screen for the possible presence of metastases to deep femoral, pelvic, and para-aortic lymph nodes.[383] Precise delineation of local disease extent may be helpful in planning intracavitary or interstitial brachytherapy. Positron emission tomography (PET) may be a clinically useful tool to assess for regional (lymphatic) and remote (hematogenous) dissemination,

TABLE 90-19

Vaginal Cancer: Staging Systems

TYPE	TNM	FIGO	DEFINITION
Primary tumor	TX		Primary tumor cannot be assessed
	T0		No evidence of primary tumor
	Tis	0	Carcinoma in situ
	T1	I	Tumor confined to the vagina
	T2	II	Tumor invades paravaginal tissues but not to the pelvic wall
	T3	III	Tumor extends to the pelvic wall
	T4	IVa	Tumor invades mucosa* of the bladder or rectum and/or extends beyond the true pelvis
		IVb	Distant metastasis
Regional lymph nodes	NX		Regional lymph nodes cannot be assessed
	N0		No regional lymph node metastasis
Upper 2/3 vagina	N1		Pelvic node metastasis
Lower 1/3 vagina	N1		Unilateral inguinal node metastasis
	N2		Bilateral inguinal node metastases
Distant metastasis	MX		Presence of distant metastasis cannot be assessed
	M0		No distant metastasis
	M1		Distant metastasis

*Presence of bullous edema is not sufficient evidence to classify as T4 or FIGO IVa.

but its value has not been prospectively evaluated in this context (Fig. 90-24).

A refinement of the AJCC/FIGO staging formalism has been proposed by Perez and colleagues[384] and is commonly used by radiation oncologists both in selection of radiation technique and in the reporting of outcomes after treatment. Patients with stage IIa have paravaginal extension only, whereas patients with stage IIb have extension to parametria. This distinction has both prognostic significance and a potential impact on the volume and technique of both teletherapy and brachytherapy (intracavitary vs. interstitial).

TREATMENT

Therapy for vaginal carcinoma must be highly individualized depending on tumor location, size, extent, and the functional status of both the vagina and adjacent organs. The close proximity of the bladder, urethra, and rectum limits the doses of radiation that can be given and restricts the surgical margins that can be obtained without performing an exenterative procedure. Up to 50% of patients with primary vaginal cancer may have had prior hysterectomy for malignant or benign indications.[382,385,386] In such patients, the presence of adhesions with fixed loops of small bowel or sigmoid colon above the vaginal apex also may affect selection of treatment modalities and techniques.

Additionally, psychosexual issues and attempting to maintain a patent and functional vagina in patients desirous of preserving the option of vaginal intercourse should be an important part of treatment planning.

Surgery

Surgery[359,387] in vaginal cancer is limited by the propensity of this cancer to spread to adjacent organs because of the lack of anatomic boundaries around the vagina. The use of surgery as a primary modality is limited to those cases in which negative margins can be achieved without significant loss of function of bladder and rectum. Surgery also can be used to salvage central pelvic recurrence after radiation.

Many authors in the past have considered radiation to be the primary treatment modality for vaginal cancer. Contributing to this recommendation has been the age of most patients with vaginal cancer and the complicating presence of multiple medical comorbidities. With improved anesthetic techniques and better postoperative care, surgery may be an option available to more women with vaginal cancer.

Surgery for vaginal cancer can be primary therapy or can be used as an adjunct to radiotherapy. Stage I vaginal cancer involving the upper vagina in a young woman can be treated with radical hysterectomy and radical upper vaginectomy with pelvic lymph node dissection. This approach in most cases allows preservation of both vaginal and ovarian function, particularly if no risk factors are found during surgery that would require postoperative radiotherapy.

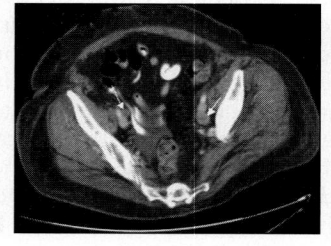
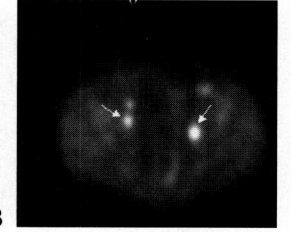

Figure 90-24. Vaginal cancer with lymphadenopathy. **A,** CT of pelvis showing mildly enlarged bilateral external iliac nodes suggestive of metastases (*arrows*). **B,** Axial FDG PET scan showing hypermetabolic nodes as hyperintense spots confirming metastases.

Specific Malignancies

III

Traditionally, later-stage vaginal cancers, particularly those in elderly women, have been treated primarily with radiation therapy. However, several recent series have suggested that judicious use of surgery may increase disease-free survival in carefully selected patients.

Tjama and associates[388] reported their experience treating 84 patients with primary invasive vaginal cancers in the Northern Gynecological Oncology Centre, where the policy tended toward operative management. In this series, the treatment was individualized based on patient age, medical status, size of tumor, location of lesion, and stage. Large lesions that did not permit negative margins were treated primarily with radiation, and adjuvant radiation was used postoperatively to treat patients who had positive retroperitoneal nodes or incomplete excision. Forty patients in this series were treated with surgery alone. Fifty-eight patients underwent exploratory laparotomy for either treatment or staging. Primary surgical treatment included radical vaginectomy, partial vaginectomy, wide local excision, and exenteration. This study demonstrated a significantly increased disease-free survival in patients who had surgery as part of their therapy or as their only therapy compared with patients who were treated with radiation alone. When stratified by stage, this difference was significantly different in those patients with stage II disease. In a multivariate analysis, surgical treatment and FIGO stage were the only significant predictors of improved disease-free survival. Unknown selection biases may have contributed substantially to these results, influencing treatment-modality choice and therefore outcomes.

The National Cancer Data Base study[389] reported surgery was used to treat 49% of patients with stage I disease, 28% of patients with stage II disease, and 25% of patients with advanced stage disease. Women with stage I disease treated with surgery only had a 5-year survival of 90% compared with 63% for women with stage I disease treated with radiotherapy only. Although this difference was statistically significant, differences among these patients with respect to age and medical comorbidities could not be assessed. Similar findings were demonstrated in stage II disease, in which surgery alone gave a 5-year survival rate of 70% compared with 57% for patients treated with radiotherapy alone. Nine women with advanced-stage disease had surgery, radiotherapy, and chemotherapy; remarkably, the 5-year survival for this group was 71%. These findings suggest that in selected cases, surgery may play a role in improving 5-year survival in all stages of disease.

Radiation Therapy

Radiation therapy using various combinations of teletherapy as well as interstitial and intracavitary therapy is generally considered the treatment of choice for most patients with more than small-volume stage I and II cancers of limited extent. The exact combinations of treatment again depend on the tumor location, volume and thickness, and depth of invasion beyond the vagina. Almost all patients with stage I lesions that are larger than 2 cm, and all patients with stage II to IV disease,

require initial treatment with external-beam therapy of approximately 45 to 50.4 Gy both to shrink the size of the primary tumor and to address potential sites of microscopic or clinically occult dissemination. Inclusion of pelvic or inguinofemoral lymph nodes or both in the field depends on the tumor location. Tumors extending to involve the distal third of the vagina should have inclusion of the inguinofemoral nodes as well as the pelvic nodes. Extended-field treatment to include the para-aortic lymph nodes is appropriate if these nodes have been found to contain metastatic disease by surgical excision or image-guided fine-needle aspiration. In physically vigorous patients absent major medical contraindications, elective extension of teletherapy treatment fields to encompass the common iliac or para-aortic node volumes may be appropriate when histologic proof of pelvic node metastasis has been established. External-beam therapy is generally followed by interstitial or intracavitary brachytherapy to a total tumor dose of approximately 75 to 85 Gy. For tumors involving the upper third of the vagina with intact uterus, intrauterine tandem and vaginal ovoids/colpostats may be used to obtain proper dose distributions encompassing the vaginal wall, paravaginal tissues, and parametria. For a patient in this category whose uterus has previously been surgically removed, a vaginal cylinder or colpostats may be used. Generally, the use of intracavitary vaginal brachytherapy is restricted to patients with tumor thickness of 5 mm or less because of the rapid fall-off of dose with distance from intracavitary isotope sources. For carcinomas with more than 5-mm thickness after teletherapy, the use of interstitial technique in addition to a vaginal cylinder will increase the depth of the radiation-dose distribution without delivering an excessive dose of radiation to the vaginal mucosa.[390] The treatment of small, superficial, stage I lesions may be satisfactory with brachytherapy alone, involving intracavitary cylinders with or without single-plane interstitial implants.[390,391]

The concomitant use of chemotherapeutic agents such as cisplatin and 5-fluorouracil (5-FU) as radiosensitizers for this malignancy has not been extensively studied. As the combination of radiation with synchronous chemotherapy (chemoradiation) has increasingly become the mainstay of therapy for locally advanced cervical cancer, anal cancer, and advanced vulvar cancer, extrapolation to squamous carcinoma of the vagina seems logical. The shared etiology suspected in many patients with primary squamous cancers of the anogenital area supports the notion that a successful treatment strategy used for one disease site also could be expected to be effective at adjacent disease sites. However, because of the rarity of patients with vaginal cancer, the use of chemoradiation in this context has not been prospectively evaluated in randomized cooperative group studies comparable to protocols that have been feasible in patients with cervical and anal cancers. Evans and coworkers[392] used 5-FU and mitomycin-C along with radiation to treat seven patients with vaginal cancer, including two patients with stage II disease, four patients with stage III disease, and one with stage IV disease. Four of seven were cancer free 19 to 39 months after treatment, including both patients with stage II disease.

Roberts and colleagues[393] reported on a series of 67 patients with advanced lower female genital tract carcinoma who were treated with chemoradiation. Included in this report were 7 patients with vaginal cancer, of whom 5 had stage III lesions, and 2 were recurrent cases. Three patients were treated with interstitial needles, and 2 with vaginal cylinder insertions in addition to teletherapy. Chemotherapy was reported to include cisplatin or 5-FU or both. In three patients, disease recurred locally, and one had a distant recurrence. In the series reported by Kirkbride and associates[394] from Toronto, 26 of 153 vaginal cancer patients were treated with combined-modality therapy with radiation and concurrent 5-FU with or without mitomycin-C. Of these patients, 20 of the 26 had stage III or IV disease, and the reported 5-year survival of 50% was significantly worse compared with surgery alone (87%) or radiation therapy alone (78%). Kirkbride and coworkers acknowledged probable selection bias in those patients advised to undergo chemoradiation based on advanced stage and extent of disease. A report from Sacramento, California, describes 14 patients with squamous carcinoma of the vagina who were treated with primary therapy consisting of synchronous radiation and chemotherapy.[395] Patients were judged not to be surgical candidates based on tumor size, location, and concerns related to urinary, bowel, or sexual function. Three patients were FIGO stage I; 10 patients, stage II (5 IIa and 5 IIb); and 1 patient, stage III. Radiation consisted of teletherapy alone (6 patients) or in combination with intravaginal brachytherapy (8 patients). Interstitial brachytherapy was not used. Total radiation dose ranged from 57 to 70.8 Gy (median, 63 Gy). Chemotherapy consisted of 5-FU alone (7 patients), or with cisplatin (6 patients) or mitomycin-C (1 patient). All patients received concomitant 5-FU during teletherapy. Seven patients also received either cisplatin (6 patients) or mitomycin-C (1 patient) as a second drug. 5-FU was administered as a 4-day continuous infusion with doses ranging from 750 to 1200 mg/m^2/24 hours. Cisplatin was administered at 100 mg/m^2 (usually on day 2 of each course of 5-FU), and mitomycin-C, at 10 mg/m^2. One patient received one cycle of chemotherapy, 8 patients received two cycles, and 5 patients received three cycles. Typically, chemotherapy was administered at 4-week intervals. In patients treated with three cycles of chemotherapy, radiation therapy was interrupted so that all chemotherapy could be administered concurrent with teletherapy. Only one patient's disease recurred locally at 7 months. Four patients died of intercurrent illness (46, 92, 104, and 109 months), and nine remained alive and cancer free 74 to 168 months after treatment (median, 100 months). Actuarial freedom from progression was 93% at 5 years. No vesicovaginal or enterovaginal fistulae were noted. Important in this report are the reduced total radiation doses used in the context of synchronous chemotherapy compared with customary radiation doses routinely given when radiation is used as monotherapy. This strategy parallels the use of chemoradiation with reduced radiation dose that has proven successful in increasing tumor-control rates while reducing late sequelae in patients treated for squamous or basaloid cancers of the anal canal.

Intervention by Stage

Stage I Disease

For disease involving the proximal vagina, if the uterus is still in situ, a radical hysterectomy, partial vaginectomy, and bilateral pelvic lymphadenectomy can be performed. In a patient with a prior hysterectomy, a radical upper vaginectomy and bilateral lymphadenectomies can be performed. For disease in proximity to the bladder neck or urethra in the anterior vagina, radiation will generally be preferable. Posterior tumors may be more amenable to a surgical approach. Lateral tumors in the middle or distal vagina with minimal invasion may be considered for wide local excision. Radiation therapy with brachytherapy alone may be considered for very small tumors less than 2 cm in largest diameter. Generally, radiation will consist of a combination of teletherapy and brachytherapy.

Stage II or III Disease

Before radiation, exploratory laparotomy may allow precise detailing of the areas of involvement, resection of bulky metastatic adenopathy, and ovarian transposition in premenopausal patients. Radiation therapy will consist of both teletherapy and brachytherapy in most patients, with treatment volume and techniques contingent on the location and extent of the primary, the presence and level of metastatic involvement of regional lymph nodes, and patient comorbidities. Some patients may be successfully treated with progressively shrinking teletherapy treatment volumes as an alternative to large-volume interstitial brachytherapy treatment.

Stage IVa Disease

For patients with a rectovaginal or vesicovaginal fistula or extensive bladder or rectal involvement who are in otherwise good medical condition, a pelvic exenterative procedure with vaginal reconstruction by using a gracilis myocutaneous flap or rectus abdominis myocutaneous flap may be the procedure of choice.[396,397] Rarely, in patients with fistulae who are not sexually active, the vagina may be allowed to fuse/scar shut after high-dose radiotherapy, thus effectively sealing the fistula and restoring continence. Treatment for most patients will involve radiotherapy, either as primary therapy or as adjuvant treatment after surgical clearance of central disease.

Patients with a Central Recurrence after Previous Surgery or Radiation Therapy

Radiation treatment will usually be the most appropriate intervention in patients previously treated with surgery. Surgery for local failure after radiation therapy will usually require anterior, posterior, or total pelvic exenteration. Repeated irradiation is rarely feasible.

Complications of Therapy

Complications from the use of radiation or surgery occur in 10% to 15% of patients. The close proximity of other organs to the vagina predisposes them to injury. These complications include rectovaginal or vesicovaginal

fistulae, radiation cystitis, radiation proctitis, rectal and vaginal strictures, and vaginal necrosis. To decrease the degree of vaginal stenosis after radiation therapy, patients should use a vaginal dilator, preferably on a daily basis. After radiation therapy, the vaginal mucosa may become thin and atrophic. Topical application of estrogen cream stimulates thickening of the vaginal mucosa after radiation and will decrease symptoms of vaginal mucosal atrophy that can include pruritus, discharge, and dyspareunia.[398,399]

PROGNOSIS

Because of the rarity of vaginal cancer, even large referral centers have only limited experience treating vaginal cancers, and thus data with respect to treatment and survival are scarce and based on retrospective series that may span multiple decades, during which both diagnostic assessments of treatment extent and treatment techniques have changed and evolved. Additionally, some published series have pooled patients with squamous cancers with patients with other histologic types. Others have included patients with noninvasive disease. Thus precision in assignment of prognosis remains elusive. Although the natural history and biologic behavior of vaginal squamous cancer mimics squamous cancer of the cervix,[354] the cure rates of vaginal neoplasms remain lower, and the morbidity associated with treatment may be higher because of the close proximity of functionally important organs, which limit the intensity of treatment and account for most of the late morbidity consequent to therapy.

The most important variable affecting prognosis is the clinical stage at presentation, which reflects the size and depth of tumor penetration.[391,400] Five-year survival estimates for all patients with this malignancy range from 42% to 56%. Rates of survival according to stage are as follows: stage I, 65% to 81%; stage II, 50% to 66%; stage III, 15% to 39%; and stage IV, 0 to 25%.

Adenocarcinoma

Fewer than 15% of primary vaginal neoplasms are adenocarcinomas. Adenocarcinomas occurring in the vagina include papillary, mucinous, adenosquamous, small cell, and clear cell variants. As glandular tissue is not normally present in the vagina, patients with adenocarcinoma must be carefully evaluated to exclude the probability that adenocarcinoma found in the vagina represents metastatic spread from another primary site. Potential primary sites are most likely to include endometrium, cervix, vulva (Bartholin's gland), ovary, breast, colon and rectum, and kidney.[354,357] The treatment for vaginal adenocarcinoma is similar to that for squamous cell carcinoma of the vagina. Because the majority of women afflicted with clear cell cancer of the vagina are young, efforts should be made to preserve vaginal and ovarian function. Surgical treatment of stage I and II disease has consisted of radical hysterectomy; vaginectomy, with formation of a split thickness of skin graft neovagina; and lymphadenectomy or local surgical excision followed by local irradiation to the tumor bed.[401] With use of local irradiation to a stage I lesion, consideration should be given to performing a pelvic lymphadenectomy, because 17% of stage I lesions have pelvic nodal metastases.[402] If treatment of larger or more advanced lesions with whole pelvic irradiation is to be undertaken, ovarian transposition before radiation should be considered. Prognosis with clear cell vaginal cancers is favorable. The overall actuarial 10-year survival rate is 79%. This improves to 90% for patients with stage I vaginal tumors. The best survival rates are associated with a tumor having a tubulocystic pattern. Persistent or recurrent disease has been noted in 25% of Registry patients. Most recurrences occur within 3 years of initial therapy; however, recurrences 20 years later have been reported.[402,403] One third of recurrences are detected at distant sites such as the lung or supraclavicular lymph nodes.

Sarcomas

Vaginal sarcomas make up 3% of primary vaginal carcinomas. Of the 68 cases of vaginal sarcoma reported by Peters and colleagues,[404] leiomyosarcomas accounted for 68% of the reported cases. Other reported sarcomas include endometrial stromal sarcoma, malignant mixed müllerian tumor, and rhabdomyosarcoma, among others.[405] Surgical resection is the treatment of choice. The benefit of chemotherapy or radiation therapy is unclear in the treatment of adult vaginal sarcomas. Embryonal rhabdomyosarcoma (sarcoma botryoides) is a highly malignant sarcoma that occurs in children aged 6 years or younger (mean age, 1.8 years). This sarcoma generally appears as soft nodules that fill and protrude from the vagina or as abnormal bleeding. The prognosis for patients with this malignancy has improved with the use of multimodality therapy including surgery, polyagent chemotherapy, and radiation.[406]

Endodermal Sinus Tumors

Endodermal sinus tumors are rare germ cell malignancies that occur primarily in the ovary but have been reported to occur at extragonadal sites including the vagina. This vaginal malignancy occurs in children younger than 2 years. It appears as abnormal bleeding or discharge in addition to the presence of a vaginal mass. As in its ovarian counterpart, α-fetoprotein can be detected in this malignancy and can be used as a serum tumor marker. Treatment consists of chemotherapy (vincristine, actinomycin D, and cyclophosphamide), as well as surgical excision, and occasionally radiation therapy.

Melanoma

Vaginal melanomas are rare but account for 2.7% of vaginal malignancies.[407-409] Three percent of malignant melanomas involve the female genital tract, with the vulva the most common site of occurrence. Melanomas arising in the vagina are thought to originate from in situ melanocytes in areas of melanosis or atypical melanocytic hyperplasia. These malignancies occur at a mean age of 55 years, with an age range of 22 to 83 years. Patients

typically are first seen with abnormal vaginal bleeding, discharge, or a mass. These tumors most frequently occur in the lower one third of the vagina on the anterior wall and appear as a blue-black or black-brown mass or plaque. They have a poor prognosis, with 5-year survival rates of 15% to 20%.[407-409] Management is surgical and, depending on the position of the lesion, may require exenterative procedures to obtain adequate margins. No established curative role is found for radiation, which is generally reserved for circumstances in which surgery either is not feasible or is refused. Local radiation may provide palliation and growth restraint in patients with proven metastatic deposits for whom exenterative surgery may not be appropriate. Adjuvant systemic therapy and treatment for disseminated melanoma parallels the treatment of melanoma arising at other sites.

CHEMOTHERAPY FOR PERSISTENT, RECURRENT, OR METASTATIC VAGINAL CANCER

Most cases of recurrent or persistent vaginal carcinoma occur in the vaginal vault, or pelvic, inguinal, and supra-clavicular nodes.[410] Dermal metastasis and lung and bone metastases also have been reported.[411,412] Very limited data exist on the treatment of vaginal cancer, with only few phase II studies describing single-agent experiences with squamous cell carcinoma of the vagina. Even fewer data are available for therapies for clear cell or adeno-carcinomas of the vagina. Responses have been reported to single-agent cisplatin and doxorubicin, and a single case reports a complete response to the combination of bleomycin, methotrexate, and cisplatin.[413-416]

REFERENCES

Cervix

1. National Institutes of Health Consensus Development Conference Statement: Cervical Cancer, April 13, 1996. J Natl Cancer Inst Monogr 1996;21:vii.
2. Bosch FX, Lorincz A, Munoz N, et al: The causal relation between human papillomavirus and cervical cancer. J Clin Pathol 2002;55:244–265.
3. Bosch FX, Manos MM, Munoz N, et al: Prevalence of human papillomavirus in cervical cancer: A worldwide perspective. International Biological Study on Cervical Cancer (IBSCC) Study Group. J Natl Cancer Inst 1995;87:796–802.
4. Walboomers JM, Jacobs MV, Manos MM, et al: Human papillomavirus is a necessary cause of invasive cervical cancer worldwide. J Pathol 1999;189:12–19.
5. Moscicki AB, Shiboski S, Broering J, et al: The natural history of human papillomavirus infection as measured by repeated DNA testing in adolescents and young women. J Pediatr 1998;132:277–284.
6. Ho GY, Bierman R, Beardsley L, et al: Natural history of cervicovaginal papillomavirus infection in young women. N Engl J Med 1998;338:423–428.
7. Koutsky LA, Holmes KK, Critchlow CW, et al: A cohort study of the risk of cervical intraepithelial neoplasia grade 2 or 3 in relation to papillomavirus infection. N Engl J Med 1992;327:1272–1278.
8. Park TW, Fujiwara H, Wright TC: Molecular biology of cervical cancer and its precursors. Cancer 1995;76:1902–1913.

9. Holloway P, Miller AB, Rohan T, et al: Natural history of dysplasia of the uterine cervix. J Natl Cancer Inst 1999;91:252–258.
10. Boyes DA, Worth AJ, Fidler HK: The results of treatment of 4389 cases of preclinical cervical squamous carcinoma. J Obstet Gynaecol Br Commonw 1970;77:769–780.
11. Eddy DM: The frequency of cervical cancer screening: comparison of a mathematical model with empirical data. Cancer 1987;60:1117–1122.
12. Celentano DD, de Lissovoy G: Assessment of cervical cancer screening and follow-up programs. Public Health Rev 1989;90;17:173–240.
13. Frame PS. Frame JS: Determinants of cancer screening frequency: The example of screening for cervical cancer. J Am Board Fam Pract 1998;11:87–95.
14. National Institutes of Health: Cervical cancer. NIH Consensus Statement, 1996 Apr 1–3;14–38.
15. Saslow D, Runowicz CD, Solomon D, et al: American Cancer Society guideline for the early detection of cervical neoplasia and cancer. CA Cancer J Clin 2002;52:342–362.
16. Smith JS, Herrero R, Bosetti C, et al: Herpes simplex virus-2 as a human papillomavirus cofactor in the etiology of invasive cervical cancer. J Natl Cancer Inst 2002;94:1604–1613.
17. Castellsague X, Bosch FX, Munoz N: Environmental co-factors in HPV carcinogenesis. Virus Res 2002; 89:191–199.
18. Schlecht NF, Platt RW, Duarte-Franco E, et al: Human papillomavirus infection and time to regression of cervical intraepithelial neoplasm. J Natl Cancer Inst 2003;95:1336.
19. Richart RM, Barron BA: A follow-up study of patients with cervical dysplasia. Am J Obstet Gynecol 1969;105:386.
20. Nasiell K, Nasiell M, Vaclavinkova V: Behavior of moderate cervical dysplasia during long-term follow-up. Obstet Gynecol 1984;61:451.
21. Green GH: The progression of preinvasive lesions of the cervix to invasion. N Z Med J 1974;80:279.
22. Miller AB: Control of carcinoma of the cervix by exfoliative cytology screening. In Coppleson M (ed): Gynecologic Oncology: Fundamental Principles and Clinical Practice. Edinburgh, Churchill Livingstone, 1981, p 381.
23. Clifford GM, Smith JS, Plummer M, Munoz N, Franceschi S: Human papillomavirus types in invasive cervical cancer worldwide: A meta-analysis. Br J Cancer 2003;88:63–73.
24. Barnes W, Delgado G, Kurman RJ, et al: Possible prognostic significance of human papillomavirus type in cervical cancer. Gynecol Oncol 1988;29:267.
25. Walker J, Bloss JD, Liao SY, et al: Human papillomavirus genotype as a prognostic indicator in carcinoma of the uterine cervix. Obstet Gynecol 1989;74:781–785.
26. Walton RJ: Cervical cancer screening programs: Epidemiology and natural history of carcinoma of the cervix. Can Med Assoc J 1982;114:1003.
27. Lombard I, Vincent-Salomon A, Validire P, et al: Human papillomavirus genotype as a major determinant of the course of cervical cancer. J Clin Oncol 1998;16:2613.
28. Koutsky LA, Ault KA, Wheeler CM, et al: A controlled trial of a human papillomavirus type 16 vaccine. N Engl J Med 2002;347:1645–1651.
29. Maiman M, Fruchter RG, Serur E, Remy JC, Feuer G, Boyce J: Human immunodeficiency virus infection and cervical neoplasia. Gynecol Oncol 1990;38:377–382.
30. Maiman M, Fruchter RG, Guy L, Cuthill S, Levine P, Serur E: Human immunodeficiency virus and invasive cervical carcinoma. Cancer 1993;71:402–406.
31. Fruchter RG, Maiman M, Sedlis A, et al: Multiple recurrences of cervical intraepithelial neoplasia in women with the immunodeficiency virus. Obstet Gynecol 1996;87:338–344.
32. Maiman M: Management of cervical neoplasia in human immunodeficiency virus-infected women. J Natl Cancer Inst Monogr 1998;23:43–49.
33. Miller AB: Control of carcinoma of the cervix by exfoliative cytology screening. In Coppleson M (ed): Gynecologic Oncology: Fundamental Principles and Clinical Practice. Edinburgh, Churchill Livingstone, 1981, p 381.
34. Gilks CB, Young RH, Aguirre P, et al: Adenoma malignum (minimal deviation adenocarcinoma) of the uterine cervix: A

clinicopathological and immunohistochemical analysis of 26 cases. Am J Surg Pathol 1989;13:717-729.

35. Kaminski PF, Norris HJ: Minimal deviation carcinoma (adenoma malignum) of the cervix. Int J Gynecol Pathol 1983;2:141-153.

36. Glucksman A, Cherry C: Incidence, histology and response to radiation of mixed carcinoma (adenoacanthoma) of the uterine cervix. Cancer 1956;9:971-9.

37. Littman P, Clement PB, Henriksen B, et al: Glassy cell carcinoma of the cervix. Cancer 1976;37:2238-2246.

38. Tamimi HK, Ek M, Hesla J, et al: Glassy cell carcinoma of the cervix redefined. Obstet Gynecol 1988;71:837-841.

39. Lotocki RJ, Krepart GV, Paraskevas M, et al: Glassy cell carcinoma of the cervix: A bimodal treatment strategy. Gynecol Oncol 1992;44:254-259.

40. Conner MG, Richter H, Moran CA, Hameed A, Albores-Saavedra J: Small cell carcinoma of the cervix: A clinicopathologic and immunohistochemical study of 23 cases. Ann Diagn Pathol 2002;6:345-348.

41. Chan JK, Loizzi V, Burger RA, Rutgers J, Monk BJ: Prognostic factors in neuroendocrine small cell cervical carcinoma: A multivariate analysis. Cancer 2003;97:568-574.

42. Walton RJ: Cervical cancer screening programs: Epidemiology and natural history of carcinoma of the cervix. Can Med Assoc J 1982;114:1003.

43. Nanda K, McCrory DC, Myers ER, et al: Accuracy of the Papanicolaou test in screening for and follow-up of cervical cytologic abnormalities: A systematic review. Ann Intern Med 2000;132:810-819.

44. Fahey MT, Irwig L, Macaskill P: Meta-analysis of Pap test accuracy. Am J Epidemiol 1995;141:680-689.

45. Kivlahan C, Ingram E: Papanicolaou smears without endocervical cells: Are they inadequate? Acta Cytol 1986;30:258.

46. The revised Bethesda system for reporting cervical/vaginal cytologic diagnoses: Report of the 1991 Bethesda workshop. Acta Cytol 1992;36:273

47. Solomon D, Davey D, Kurman R, et al: The 2001 Bethesda System: Terminology for reporting results of cervical cytology. JAMA 2002;287:2114.

48. Wright TC Jr, Cox JT, Massad LS, Twiggs LB, Wilkinson EJ: ASCCP-Sponsored Consensus Conference: 2001 consensus guidelines for the management of women with cervical cytologic abnormalities. JAMA 2002;85:642-647.

49. Wright TC Jr, Cox JT, Massad LS, Carlson J, Twiggs LB, Wilkinson EJ: American Society for Colposcopy and Cervical Pathology: 2001 consensus guidelines for the management of women with cervical intraepithelial neoplasia. Am J Obstet Gynecol 2003;189:295-304.

50. Clavel C, Masure M, Bory JP, et al: Hybrid Capture II-based human papillomavirus detection, a sensitive test to detect in routine high-grade cervical lesions: A preliminary study on 1518 women. Br J Cancer 1999;80:1306-1311.

51. Schiffman M, Herrero R, Hildesheim A, et al: HPV DNA testing in cervical cancer screening: Results from women in a high-risk province of Costa Rica. JAMA 2000;283:87-93.

52. Liaw KL, Glass AG, Manos MM, et al: Detection of human papillomavirus DNA in cytologically normal women and subsequent cervical squamous intraepithelial lesions. J Natl Cancer Inst 1999;91:954-960.

52. Remmink AJ, Walboomers JM, Helmerhorst TJ, et al: The presence of persistent high-risk HPV genotypes in dysplastic cervical lesions is associated with progressive disease: Natural history up to 36 months. Int J Cancer 1995;61:306-311.

54. Greenberg MD, Reid R, Schiffman M, et al: A prospective study of biopsy-confirmed cervical intraepithelial neoplasia grade 1: Colposcopic, cytological, and virological risk factors for progression. J Lower Genital Tract Dis 1999;3:104-110.

55. Nobbenhuis MA, Meijer CJ, van den Bule AJ, et al: Addition of high-risk HPV testing improves the current guidelines on follow-up after treatment for cervical intraepithelial neoplasia. Br J Cancer 2001;84:796-801.

56. Belinson J, Qiao YL, Pretorius R, et al: Shanxi province cervical cancer screening study: A cross sectional comparative trial of multiple techniques to detect cervical intraepithelial neoplasia. Gynecol Oncol 2001;83:439-444.

57. ASCUS-LSIL Triage Study (ALTS) Group: Results of a randomized trial on the management of cytology interpretations of atypical squamous cells of undetermined significance. Am J Obstet Gynecol 2003;188:1383-1392.

58. Boardman LA, Meinz H, Steinhoff MM, Heber WW, Blume J: A randomized trial of the sleeved cytobrush and the endocervical curette. Obstet Gynecol 2003;101:426-430

59. Phipps JM, Gunasekera PC, Lewis BV: Occult cervical carcinoma revealed by large loop diathermy. Lancet 1989;2:453.

60. Howe DT, Vincenti AC: Is large loop excision of the transformation zone (LLEZT) more accurate than colposcopically directed punch biopsy in the diagnosis of cervical intraepithelial neoplasia? Br J Obstet Gynaecol 1991;98:588.

61. Murdoch JB, Grimshaw RN, Monaghan JM: Loop diathermy excision of the abnormal cervical transformation zone. Int J Gynecol Cancer 1991;1:105.

62. Burger MPM, Hollema H: The reliability of the histologic diagnosis in colposcopically directed biopsies: A plea for LETZ. Int J Gynecol Cancer 1993;3:385.

63. Prendiville W, Cullimore J: Excision of the transformation zone using the low voltage diathermy (LVD) loop: A superior method of treatment. Colposc Gynaecol Laser Surg 1987;3:225.

64. Gunasekera PC, Phipps JM, Lewis BV: Large loop excision of the transformation zone (LLETZ) compared to carbon dioxide laser in the treatment of CIN: A superior mode of treatment. Br J Obstet Gynaecol 1990;97:995.

65. Prendiville W, Cullimore JM, Norman S: Large loop excision of the transformation zone (LLETZ): A new method of management for women with cervical intraepithelial neoplasia. Br J Obstet Gynaecol 1989;96:1054.

66. Bigrigg MA, Codling BW, Pearson P, et al: Colposcopic diagnosis and treatment of cervical dysplasia at a single clinic visit. Lancet 1990;2:336.

67. Luesley DM, Cullimore J, Redman CWE, et al: Loop diathermy excision of the cervical transformation zone in patients with abnormal cervical smears. BMJ 1990;300:1690.

68. Whiteley PF, Olah KS: Treatment of cervical intraepithelial neoplasia: Experience with low voltage diathermy loop. Am J Obstet Gynecol 1990;162:1272.

69. Murdoch JB, Grimshaw RN, Morgan PR, Monaghan JM: The impact of loop diathermy on the management of early invasive cervical cancer. Int J Gynecol Cancer 1992;2:129.

70. Mor-Yosef S, Lopes A, Pearson S, Monaghan JM: Loop diathermy cone biopsy. Obstet Gynecol 1990;75:884.

71. Wright TC, Richardt RM, Ferenczy A, Koulos J: Comparisons of specimens removed by CO_2 laser conization and the loop electrosurgical excision procedure. Obstet Gynecol 1992;79:147.

72. Luesley D, McCrum A, Terry PB, Wade-Evans T: Complications of cone biopsy related to the dimensions of the cone and the influence of prior colposcopic assessment. Br J Obstet Gynaecol 1985;92:158.

73. Larson G, Gullberg B, Grundell H: A comparison of laser and cold knife conization. Obstet Gynecol 1983;62:213.

74. Luesley D, McCrum A, Terry PB, Wade-Evans T: Complications of cone biopsy related to the dimensions of the cone and the influence of prior colposcopic assessment. Br J Obstet Gynaecol 1985;92:158.

75. Larson G, Gullberg B, Grundell H: A comparison of laser and cold knife conization. Obstet Gynecol 1983;62:213

76. Jordon JA: Symposium on cervical neoplasia, I: Excisional methods. Colposc Gynaecol Laser Surg 1984;1:271.

77. Nicolet V, Carignan L, Bourdon F, Prosmanne O: MR imaging of cervical carcinoma: A practical staging approach. Radiographics 2000;20:1539-1549.

78. Houvenaeghel G, Martino M, Resbeut M, et al: Pelvic staging of advanced and recurrent gynecologic cancers: Contribution of endosonography. Gynecol Oncol 1994;55:393-400.

79. Iwamoto K, Kigawa J, Minagawa Y, Miura H, Terakawa N: Transvaginal ultrasonographic diagnosis of bladder-wall invasion in patients with cervical cancer. Obstet Gynecol 1994;83:217-219.

80. Pannu HK, Corl FM, Fishman EK: CT evaluation of cervical cancer: Spectrum of disease. Radiographics 2001;21:1155-1168.

81. Lieven Van Hoe, Vanbeckevoort D, Oyen R, Itzlinger U, Vergote I: Cervical carcinoma: Optimized local staging with intravaginal contrast-enhanced MR imaging—preliminary results. Radiology 1999;213:608–611

82. KK Yu, Hricak H, Subak LL, Zaloudek CZ, Powell CB: Preoperative staging of cervical carcinoma: Phased array coil fast spin- echo versus body coil spin-echo T2-weighted MR imaging. Am J Roentgenol 1998;171:707–711.

83. Yamashita Y, Baba T, Baba Y, et al: Dynamic contrast-enhanced MR imaging of uterine cervical cancer: Pharmacokinetic analysis with histopathologic correlation and its importance in predicting the outcome of radiation therapy. Radiology 2000;216:803–809.

84. Harisinghani MG, Saini S, Weissleder R, et al: MR lymphangiography using ultrasmall superparamagnetic iron oxide in patients with primary abdominal and pelvic malignancies: radiographic-pathologic correlation. Am J Roentgenol 1999;172:1347–1351.

85. Hawighorst H, Knapstein G, Schaeffer U, et al: Pelvic lesions in patients with treated cervical carcinoma: Efficacy of pharmacokinetic analysis of dynamic MR images in distinguishing recurrent tumors from benign conditions. Am J Roentgenol 1996;166:401–408.

86. Peppercorn PD, Jeyarajah AR, Woolas R, et al: Role of MR imaging in the selection of patients with early cervical carcinoma for fertility-preserving surgery: Initial experience. Radiology 1999;212:395–399.

87. Reinhardt MJ, Ehritt-Braun C, Vogelgesang D, et al: Metastatic lymph nodes in patients with cervical cancer: Detection with MR imaging and FDG PET. Radiology 2001;218:776–782.

88. Park DH, Kim KH, Park SU, et al: Diagnosis of recurrent uterine cervical cancer: Computed tomography versus positron emission tomography. Korean J Radiol 2000;1:51–55.

89. Grogan M, Thomas GM, Melamed I, et al: The importance of hemoglobin levels during radiotherapy for carcinoma of the cervix. Cancer 1999;86:1528–1536.

90. Obermair A, Cheuk R, Horwood K, et al: Impact of hemoglobin levels before and during concurrent chemoradiotherapy on the response of treatment in patients with cervical carcinoma: Preliminary results. Cancer 2001;92:903–908.

91. Kapp KS, Poschauko J, Geyer E, et al: Evaluation of the effect of routine packed red blood cell transfusion in anemic cervix cancer patients treated with radical radiotherapy. Int J Radiat Oncol Biol Phys 2002;54:58–66.

92. Dunst J, Kuhnt T, Strauss HG, et al: Anemia in cervical cancers: impact on survival, patterns of relapse, and association with hypoxia and angiogenesis. Int J Radiat Oncol Biol Phys 2003;56:778–787.

93. Lanciano RM, Martz K, Coia LR, et al: Tumor and treatment factors improving outcome in stage III-B cervix cancer. Int J Radiat Oncol Biol Phys 1991;20:95–100.

94. Fyles A, Keane TJ, Barton M, et al: The effect of treatment duration in the local control of cervix cancer. Radiother Oncol 1992;25:273–279.

95. Tranum BL, Haut A: Thrombocytosis: Platelet kinetics in neoplasia. J Lab Clin Med 1974;84:615–619.

96. Hernandez E, Lavine M, Dunton CJ, Gracely E, Parker J: Poor prognosis associated with thrombocytosis in patients with cervical cancer. Cancer 1992;69:2975–2977.

97. Rodriguez GC, Clarke-Pearson DL, Soper JT, Berchuck A, Synan I, Dodge RK: The negative prognostic implications of thrombocytosis in women with stage IB cervical cancer. Obstet Gynecol 1994;83:445–448.

98. Shingleton HM, Soong SJ, Gelder MS, Hatch KD, Baker VV, Austin JM Jr: Clinical and histopathologic factors predicting recurrence and survival after pelvic exenteration for cancer of the cervix. Obstet Gynecol 1989;73:1027–1034.

99. Hatch KD, Shingleton HM, Soong SJ, Baker VV, Gelder MS: Anterior pelvic exenteration. Gynecol Oncol 1988;31:205–216.

100. Stanhope CR, Webb MJ, Podratz KC: Pelvic exenteration for recurrent cervical cancer. Clin Obstet Gynecol 1990;33:897–909.

101. Stelzer KJ, Koh WJ, Greer BE, et al: The use of intraoperative radiation therapy in radical salvage for recurrent cervical cancer: Outcome and toxicity. Am J Obstet Gynecol 1995;172:1881–1886.

102. Mahe MA, Gerard JP, Dubois JB, et al: Intraoperative radiation therapy in recurrent carcinoma of the uterine cervix: Report of the French intraoperative group on 70 patients. Int J Radiat Oncol Biol Phys 1996;34:21–26.

103. Thomas GM, Dembo AJ Black B, et al: Concurrent radiation and chemotherapy for carcinoma of the cervix recurrent after radical surgery. Gynecol Oncol 1987;27:254–260.

104. Tabata M, Ichinoe K, Sakuragi N, et al: Incidence of ovarian metastasis in patients with cancer of the uterine cervix. Gynecol Oncol 1987;28:255.

105. Natsume N, Aoki Y, Kase H, Kashima K, Sugaya S, Tanaka K: Ovarian metastasis in stage IB and II cervical adenocarcinoma. Gynecol Oncol 1999;74:255–258.

106. Piver MS, Rutledge F, Smith JP: Five classes of extended hysterectomy for women with cervical cancer. Obstet Gynecol 1974;44:265–272.

107. Nezhat CR, Burrell MO, Nezhat FR, Benigno BB, Welander CE: Laparoscopic radical hysterectomy with paraaortic and pelvic node dissection. Am J Obstet Gynecol 1992;166:864–865.

108. Nezhat CR, Nezhat FR, Burrell MO, et al: Laparoscopic radical hysterectomy and laparoscopically assisted vaginal radical hysterectomy with pelvic and paraaortic node dissection. J Gynecol Surg 1993;9:105–120.

109. Roy M, Plante M, Renaud MC, Tetu B: Vaginal radical hysterectomy versus abdominal radical hysterectomy in the treatment of early-stage cervical cancer. Gynecol Oncol 1996;62:336–339.

110. Dargent D, Martin X, Sacchetoni A, Mathevet P: Laparoscopic vaginal radical trachelectomy: A treatment to preserve the fertility of cervical carcinoma patients. Cancer 2000;88:1877–1882.

111. Roy M, Plante M: Pregnancies after radical vaginal trachelectomy for early-stage cervical cancer. Am J Obstet Gynecol 1998;179:1491–1496.

112. Covens A, Shaw P, Murphy J, et al: Is radical trachelectomy a safe alternative to radical hysterectomy for patients with stage IA-B carcinoma of the cervix? Cancer 1999;86:2273–2279.

113. Trimbos JB, Maas CP, Deruiter MC, Peters AA, Kenter GG: A nerve-sparing radical hysterectomy: Guidelines and feasibility in Western patients. Int J Gynecol Cancer 2001;11:180–186.

114. Hamberger AD, Fletcher GH, Wharton JT: Results of treatment of early stage I carcinoma of the uterine cervix with intracavitary radium alone. Cancer 1978;41:980–985.

115. International Commission on Radiation Units and Measurements. Dose and Volume Specification for Reporting Intracavitary Therapy in Gynecology. Bethesda, Md, International Commission on Radiation Units and Measurements, 1985.

116. Monk BJ, Tewari K, Burger RA, Johnson MT, Montz FJ, Berman ML: A comparison of intracavitary versus interstitial irradiation in the treatment of cervical cancer. Gynecol Oncol 1997;67:241–247.

117. Patel FD, Sharma SC, Negi PS, Ghoshal S, Gupta BD: Low dose rate vs. high dose rate. Int J Radiat Oncol Biol Phys 1994;28:335–341.

118. Shigematsu Y, Nishiyama K, Masaki N, et al: Treatment of carcinoma of the uterine cervix by remotely controlled afterloading intracavitary radiotherapy with high-dose rate: A comparative study with a low-dose rate system. Int J Radiat Oncol Biol Phys 1983;9:351–356.

119. Nag S, Chao C, Erickson B, et al, for the American Brachytherapy Society: The American Brachytherapy Society recommendations for low-dose-rate brachytherapy for carcinoma of the cervix. Int J Radiat Oncol Biol Phys 2002;52:33–48.

120. Nag S, Erickson B, Thomadsen B, Orton C, Demanes JD, Petereit D: The American Brachytherapy Society recommendations for high-dose-rate brachytherapy for carcinoma of the cervix. Int J Radiat Oncol Biol Phys 2000;48:201–211.

121. Souhami L, Gil R, Allan S, et al: A randomized trial of chemotherapy followed by pelvic radiation therapy in stage IIIB carcinoma of the cervix. J Clin Oncol 1991;9:970–977.

122. Tabata T, Takeshima N, Nishida H, Hirai Y, Hasumi K: A randomized study of primary bleomycin, vincristine, mitomycin and cisplatin (BOMP) chemotherapy followed by radiotherapy versus radiotherapy alone in stage IIIB and IVA squamous cell carcinoma of the cervix. Anticancer Res 2003;23:2885–2890.

123. Leborgne F, Leborgne JH, Doldan R, et al: Induction chemotherapy and radiotherapy of advanced cancer of the cervix: A pilot study

and phase III randomized trial. Int J Radiat Oncol Biol Phys 1997;37:343–350.

124. Chiara S, Bruzzone M, Merlini L, et al: Randomized study comparing chemotherapy plus radiotherapy versus radiotherapy alone in FIGO stage IIB-III cervical carcinoma. GONO (North-West Oncologic Cooperative Group). Am J Clin Oncol 1994;17:294–297.

125. Keys HM, Bundy BN, Stehman FB, et al: Cisplatin, radiation, and adjuvant hysterectomy compared with radiation and adjuvant hysterectomy for bulky stage IB cervical carcinoma. N Engl J Med 1999;340:1154–1161.

126. Rose PG, Bundy BN, Watkins EB, et al: Concurrent cisplatin-based radiotherapy and chemotherapy for locally advanced cervical cancer. N Engl J Med 1999;240:1144–1153.

127. Morris M, Eifel PJ, Lu J, et al: Pelvic radiation with concurrent chemotherapy compared with pelvic and para-aortic radiation for high risk cervical cancer. N Engl J Med 1999;340:1137–1143.

128. Peters WA III, Liu PY, Barrett RJ, et al: Cisplatin and 5-fluorouracil plus radiation therapy are superior to radiation therapy as adjunctive in high risk early stage carcinoma of the cervix after radical hysterectomy and pelvic lymphadenectomy: Report of a phase III inter-group study. J Clin Oncol 2000;18:1606–1613.

129. Whitney CW, Sause W, Bundy BN, et al: A randomized comparison of fluorouracil plus cisplatin versus hydroxyurea as an adjunct to radiation therapy in stages IIB-IVA carcinoma of the cervix with negative para-aortic lymph nodes. J Clin Oncol 1999;17:1339–1348.

130. Pearcey R, Brundage M, Drouin P, et al: Phase III trial comparing radical radiotherapy with and without cisplatin chemotherapy in patients with advanced squamous cell cancer of the cervix. J Clin Oncol 2002;20:966–972.

131. Wong LC, Ngan HY, Cheung AN, Cheng DK, Ng TY, Choy DT: Chemoradiation and adjuvant chemotherapy in cervical cancer. J Clin Oncol 1999;17:2055–2060.

132. Roberts KB, Urdaneta N, Vera R, et al: Interim results of a randomized trial of mitomycin-C as an adjunct to radical radiotherapy in the treatment of locally advanced squamous-cell carcinoma of the cervix. Int J Cancer 2000;90:206–223.

133. Lorvidhaya V, Chitapanarux I, Sangruchi S, et al: Concurrent mitomycin C, 5-fluorouracil, and radiotherapy in the treatment of locally advanced carcinoma of the cervix: A randomized trial. Int J Radiat Oncol Biol Phys 2003;55:1226–1232.

134. Tseng CJ, Chang CT, Lai CH, et al: A randomized trial of concurrent chemoradiotherapy versus radiotherapy in advanced carcinoma of the uterine cervix. Gynecol Oncol 1997;66:52–58.

135. Delgado G, Bundy B, Zaino R, et al: Prospective surgical-pathological study of disease-free interval in patients with stage IB squamous cell carcinoma of the cervix: A Gynecologic Oncology Group study. Gynecol Oncol 1990;38:353.

136. Bremer GL, Tiebosch ATMG, van der Putten HWHM, et al: Tumor angiogenesis: An independent prognostic parameter in cervical cancer. Am J Obstet Gynecol 1996;174:126.

137. Boyce J, Fruchter R, Nicastri A: Prognostic factors in stage I carcinoma of the cervix. Gynecol Oncol 1981;12:154.

138. Simon NL, Gore H, Shingleton HM, et al: Study of superficially invasive carcinoma of the cervix. Obstet Gynecol 1986;68:19.

139. Morrow CP, Curtin JP: Synopsis of Gynecologic Oncology. 5th ed. San Francisco, Churchill Livingstone, 1998, p 107.

140. Berek JS, Hacker NF: Practical Gynecologic Oncology, 2nd ed. Baltimore, Williams & Wilkins, 1994.

141. Landoni F, Maneo A, Colombo A, et al: Randomised study of radical surgery versus radiotherapy for stage Ib-IIa cervical cancer. Lancet 1997;350:535–540.

142. Boronow RC: The bulky 6-cm barrel-shaped lesion of the cervix: Primary surgery and postoperative chemoradiation. Gynecol Oncol 2000;78:313–317.

143. Sardi JE, Giaroli A, Sananes C, et al: Long-term follow-up of the first randomized trial using neoadjuvant chemotherapy in stage Ib squamous carcinoma of the cervix: The final results. Gynecol Oncol 1997;67:61–69.

144. Keys HM, Bundy BN, Stehman FB, et al: Gynecologic Oncology Group: Radiation therapy with and without extrafascial hysterectomy for bulky stage IB cervical carcinoma: A randomized trial of the Gynecologic Oncology Group. Gynecol Oncol 2003;89:343–353.

145. Delgado G, Bundy B, Zaino R, Sevin BU, Creasman WT, Major F: Prospective surgical-pathological study of disease-free interval in patients with stage IB squamous cell carcinoma of the cervix: A Gynecologic Oncology Group study. Gynecol Oncol 1990;38:352–357.

146. Inoue T, Okumura M: Prognostic significance of parametrial extension in patients with cervical carcinoma stages IB, IIA, and IIB: A study of 628 cases treated by radical hysterectomy and lymphadenectomy with or without postoperative irradiation. Cancer 1984;54:1714–1719.

147. Burghardt E, Haas J, Girardi F: The significance of the parametrium in the operative treatment of cervical cancer. Baillieres Clin Obstet Gynaecol 1988;2:879–888.

148. Zreik TG, Chambers JT, Chambers SK: Parametrial involvement, regardless of nodal status: A poor prognostic factor for cervical cancer. Obstet Gynecol 1996;87:741–746.

149. Estape RE, Angioli R, Madrigal M, et al: Close vaginal margins as a prognostic factor after radical hysterectomy. Gynecol Oncol 1998;68:229–232.

150. Noguchi H, Shiozawa K, Tsukamoto T, Tsukahara Y, Iwai S, Fukuta T: The postoperative classification for uterine cervical cancer and its clinical evaluation. Gynecol Oncol 1983;16:219–231.

151. Gonzalez D, Ketting BW, van Bunningen B, van Dijk JD: Carcinoma of the uterine cervix stage IB and IIA: Results of postoperative irradiation in patients with microscopic infiltration in the parametrium and/or lymph node metastasis. Int J Radiat Oncol Biol Phys 1989;16:389–395.

152. Fuller AF Jr, Elliott N, Kosloff C, Hoskins WJ, Lewis JL Jr: Determinants of increased risk for recurrence in patients undergoing radical hysterectomy for stage IB and IIA carcinoma of the cervix. Gynecol Oncol 1989;33:34–39.

153. Sedlis A, Bundy BN, Rotman MZ, Lentz SS, Muderspach LI, Zaino RJA: Randomized trial of pelvic radiation therapy versus no further therapy in selected patients with stage IB carcinoma of the cervix after radical hysterectomy and pelvic lymphadenectomy: A Gynecologic Oncology Group study. Gynecol Oncol 1999;73:177–183.

154. Tattersall MH, Ramirez C, Coppleson M: A randomized trial of adjuvant chemotherapy after radical hysterectomy in stage Ib-IIa cervical cancer patients with pelvic lymph node metastases. Gynecol Oncol 1992;46:176–181.

155. Curtin JP, Hoskins WJ, Venkatraman ES, et al: Adjuvant chemotherapy versus chemotherapy plus pelvic irradiation for high-risk cervical cancer patients after radical hysterectomy and pelvic lymphadenectomy (RH-PLND): A randomized phase III trial. Gynecol Oncol 1996;61:3–10.

156. Syed AM, Puthawala AA, Abdelaziz NN, et al: Long-term results of low-dose rate interstitial-intracavitary brachytherapy in the treament of carcinoma of the cervix. Int J Rad Oncol Biol Phys 2002;54:67–78.

157. Martinez A, Cox RS, Edmundson GK: A multiple-site perineal applicator (MUPIT) for treatment of prostatic, anorectal and gynecologic malignancies. Int J Radiat Oncol Biol Phys 1984;10:297.

158. Thigpen T, Shingleton H, Homesley H, et al: Cis-platinum in treatment of advanced or recurrent squamous cell carcinoma of the cervix: A phase II study of the Gynecologic Oncology Group. Cancer 1981;48:889.

159. Bonomi P, Blessing JA, Stehman FB, et al: Randomized trial of three cisplatin dose schedules in squamous cell carcinoma of the cervix: A Gynecologic Oncology Group study. J Clin Oncol 1985;3:1079.

160. Thigpen JT: Chemotherapy of gynecologic cancer. In Perry MC (ed): The Chemotherapy Source Book, 2nd ed. Baltimore, Williams & Wilkins, 1996, p 1253.

161. Omura GA, Blessing JA, Vaccarello L, et al: Randomized trial of cisplatin versus cisplatin plus mitolactol versus cisplatin plus ifosfamide in advanced squamous carcinoma of the cervix: A Gynecologic Oncology Group study. J Clin Oncol 1997;15:165–171.

162. Bloss JD, Blessing JA, Behrens BC, et al: Randomized trial of cisplatin and ifosfamide with or without bleomycin in squamous carcinoma of the cervix: A Gynecologic Oncology Group study. J Clin Oncol 2002;20:1832–1837.

163. Moore DH, Blessing JA, McQuellon RP, et al: Phase III study of cisplatin with or without paclitaxel in stage IVB, recurrent or persistent squamous cell carcinoma of the cervix: A Gynecologic Oncology Group Study. J Clin Oncol (in press).

Vulva

164. Henson D, Tarone R: An epidemiologic study of cancer of the cervix, vagina, and vulva based on the Third National Cancer Survey in the United States. Am J Obstet Gynecol 1977;129:525.

165. Marcus SL: Multiple squamous cell carcinomas involving the cervix, vagina, and vulva: The theory of multicentric origin. Am J Obstet Gynecol 1960;80:802.

166. Stern BD, Kaplan L: Multicentric foci of carcinomas arising in structures of cloacal origin. Am J Obstet Gynecol 1969;104:255.

167. Jimerson GK, Merrill JA: Multicentric squamous malignancy involving both the cervix and vulva. Cancer 1970;26:150.

168. Franklin EW, Rutledge FD: Epidemiology of epidermoid carcinoma of the vulva. Obstet Gynecol 1972;39:165.

169. Figge DC, Gaudenz R: Invasive carcinoma of the vulva. Am J Obstet Gynecol 1974;119:382.

170. Choo YC, Morley GW: Double primary epidermoid carcinoma of the vulva and cervix. Gynecol Oncol 1980;9:324.

171. Sherman KJ, Daling JR, Chu J, et al: Multiple primary tumours in women with vulvar neoplasms: A case-control study. Br J Cancer 1988;57:423.

172. ISSVD Task Force: Microinvasive cancer of the vulva: Report of the ISSVD Task Force. J Reprod Med 1984;29:454.

173. Daling JR, Chu J, Weiss NS, et al: The association of condylomata acuminata and squamous carcinoma of the vulva. Br J Cancer 1984;50:533.

174. Newcomb PA, Weiss NS, Daling JR: Incidence of vulvar carcinoma in relation to menstrual, reproductive, and medical factors. J Natl Cancer Inst 1984;73:391.

175. Mabuchi K, Bross DS, Kessler II: Epidemiology of cancer of the vulva: A case-control study. Cancer 1985;55:1843.

176. Brinton LA, Nasca PC, Mallin K, et al: Case-control study of cancer of the vulva. Obstet Gynecol 1990;75:859.

177. Buscema J, Stern J, Woodruff JD: The significance of the histologic alterations adjacent to invasive vulvar carcinoma. Am J Obstet Gynecol 1980;137:902.

178. Zaino RJ, Husseinzadeh N, Nahhas W, et al: Epithelial alterations in proximity to invasive squamous carcinoma of the vulva. Int J Gynecol Pathol 1982;1:73.

179. Crum CP: Carcinoma of the vulva: Epidemiology and pathogenesis. Obstet Gynecol 1992;79:448.

180. Ansink AC, Heintz APM: Epidemiology and etiology of squamous cell carcinoma of the vulva. Eur J Obstet Gynecol Reprod Biol 1993;48:111.

181. Brinton LA, Nasca PC, Mallin K, et al: Case-control study of cancer of the vulva. Obstet Gynecol 1990;75:859.

182. Neill SM, Lessana-Leibowitch M, Pelisse M, et al: Lichen sclerosus, invasive squamous cell carcinoma and human papillomavirus. Am J Obstet Gynecol 1990;162:1633.

183. Porreco R, Penn I, Droegmuller W, et al: Gynecologic malignancies in immunosuppressed organ homograft recipients. Obstet Gynecol 1975;45:359.

184. Caterson RJ, Furber J, Murray J, et al: Carcinoma of the vulva in two young renal allograft patients. Transplant Proc 1984;16:559.

185. Halpert R, Fruchter RG, Sedlis A, et al: Human papillomavirus and lower genital neoplasia in renal transplant patients. Obstet Gynecol 1986;68:251.

186. Giaquinto C, Del Mistro A, De Rossi A, et al: Vulvar carcinoma in a 12-year old girl with vertically acquired human immunodeficiency virus infection. Pediatrics 2000;106:E57.

187. Wright TC, Koulos JP, Liu P, et al: Invasive vulvar carcinoma in two women infected with the human immunodeficiency virus. Gynecol Oncol 1996;60:500.

188. Al-Ghamdi Freedman A, Miller D, Poh D, Rosin C, Zhang M, Gilks CB: Vulvar squamous cell carcinoma in young women: A clinicopathologic study of 21 cases. Gynecol Oncol 2002;84:94-101.

189. Korn AP, Abercrombie PD, Foster A: Vulvar intraepithelial neoplasia in women infected with human immunodeficiency virus-1. Gynecol Oncol 1996;61:384.

190. Kuhn L, Sun XW, Wright TC Jr: Human Immunodeficiency virus infection and female lower genital tract malignancy. Curr Opin Obstet Gynecol 1999;11:35.

191. Abercrombie PD, Korn AP: Vulvar intraepithelial neoplasia in women with HIV. AIDS Patient Care STDS 1998;12:251.

192. Hording U, Junge J, Puolsen H, et al: Vulvar intraepithelial neoplasia. Obstet Gynecol 1995;56:276.

193. Ridley CM, Frankman O, Jones ISC, et al: New nomenclature for vulvar disease: Report of the Committee on Terminology of the International Society for the Study of Vulvar Disease. J Reprod Med 1990;35:483.

194. Ridley CM: ISSVD new nomenclature for vulvar disease. Am J Obstet Gynecol 1989;160:769-770.

195. Wilkinson EJ: Normal histology and nomenclature of the vulva, and malignant neoplasms, including VIN. Dermatol Clin 1992;10:283-329.

196. Wilkinson EJ: Vulvar intraepithelial neoplasia and squamous cell carcinoma with emphasis on new nomenclature. Prog Reprod Urinary Tract Pathol 1990;2:1-20.

197. Dubreuilh W: Pigmentation of the skin due to *Demodex folliculorum*. Br J Dermatol 1901;13:403.

198. Nadji M, Ganji P: The application of immunoperoxidase techniques in the evaluation of vulvar and vaginal disease. In Wilkinson EJ (ed): Contemporary Issues in Surgical Pathology, Vol. 9. New York, Churchill Livingstone, 1987, p 239.

199. Chan TY, Alt SZ, Mandavilli SR, Carun RW, Sherman ME: Immuno-histochemical analysis of Paget's disease of the vulva: Implications for histogenetics and diagnosis. Mod Pathol 1999;12:114A.

200. Ford LC, Berek JS, Lagasse LD, Hacker NF, Heins YL, DeLange RJ: Estrogen and progesterone receptor sites in malignancies of the uterine cervix, vagina, and vulva. Gynecol Oncol 1983;15:27-31.

201. Crawford D, Nimmo M, Clement PB, et al: Prognostic factors in Paget's disease of the vulva: A study of 21 cases. Int J Gynecol Pathol 1999;18:351-359.

202. Chen CH, Ji H, Suh KW, et al: Control of HPV-associated malignancies grown in liver with DNA vaccine. Mod Pathol 1999;12:114A.

203. Scheistroen M, Trope C, Kaern J, et al: DNA ploidy and expression of p53 and c-erb-2 in extramammary Paget's disease of the vulva. Gynecol Oncol 1997;64:88-92.

204. Koss LG, Brockunier A Jr: Ultrastructural aspects of Paget's disease of the vulva. Arch Pathol 1969;87:592.

205. Creasman WT, Gallagher S, Rutledge F: Paget's disease of the vulva. Gynecol Oncol 1975;3:133.

206. Hart WR, Millman RB: Progression of intraepithelial Paget's disease of the vulva to invasive carcinoma. Cancer 1977;40:2333.

207. Parmley TH, Woodruff JD, Julian CG: Invasive vulvar Paget's disease. Obstet Gynecol 1975;46:341.

208. Kodama S, Kaneko T, Saito M, et al: A clinicopathologic study of 30 patients with Paget's disease of the vulva. Gynecol Oncol 1995;56:63.

209. Stacy D, Burrell MO, Franklin EW III: Extramammary Paget's disease of the vulva and anus: Use of intraoperative frozen section margins. Am J Obstet Gynecol 1986;155:519.

210. Bergan S, DiSaia PJ, Liao SY, Berman ML: Conservative management of extramammary Paget's disease of the vulva. Gynecol Oncol 1989;33:151.

211. Buscema J, Woodruff JD, Parmley TH, et al: Carcinoma in situ of the vulva. Obstet Gynecol 1980;55:225.

212. Fu YS, Reagan JW, Townsend DE, Kaufman RH, et al: Nuclear DNA study of vulvar intraepithelial and invasive squamous neoplasms. Obstet Gynecol 1981;57:643.

213. Husseinzadeh N, Recinto C. Frequency of invasive cancer in surgically excised vulvar lesions with intraepithelial neoplasia (VIN 3). Gynecol Oncol 1999;73:119-120.

214. Miller BE. Vulvar intraepithelial neoplasia treated with cavitational ultrasonic surgical aspiration. Gynecol Oncol 2002;85:114-118 Gynecol Oncol 1999;75:277-281.

215. Sideri M, Spinaci L, Spolti N, Schettino F: Evaluation of CO(2) laser excision or vaporization for the treatment of vulvar intraepithelial neoplasia. Gynecol Oncol 2002;85:114-118.

216. Zacur H, Genandry R, Woodruff JD: The patient-at-risk for development of vulvar cancer. Gynecol Oncol 1980;9:199.

217. Parry-Jones E: Lymphatics of the vulva. J Obstet Gynecol Br Empire 1963;70:751.

218. Iversen T, Aas M: Lymph drainage from the vulva. Gynecol Oncol 1983;16:179.

219. Iversen T, Abeler V, Aalders J: Individualized treatment of stage I carcinoma of the vulva. Obstet Gynecol 1981;57:85.

220. Hacker NF, Berek JS, Lagasse LD, et al: Individualization of treatment for stage I squamous cell vulvar carcinoma. Obstet Gynecol 1984;63:155.

221. Wharton JT, Gallagher S, Rutledge FN: Microinvasive carcinoma of the vulva. Obstet Gynecol 1974;118:159.

222. Parker RT, Duncan I, Rampone J, et al: Operative management of early invasive epidermoid carcinoma of the vulva. Am J Obstet Gynecol 1975;123:349.

223. Magrina JF, Webb MJ, Gaffey TA, et al: Stage I squamous cell cancer of the vulva. Am J Obstet Gynecol 1979;134:453.

224. Buscema J, Stern JL, Woodruff JD: Early invasive carcinoma of the vulva. Am J Obstet Gynecol 1981;140:563.

225. Chu J, Tamimi HK, Figge DC: Femoral node metastases with negative superficial inguinal nodes in early vulvar cancer. Am J Obstet Gynecol 61:408, 1983

226. Burke TW, Levenback C, Coleman TL, et al: Surgical therapy of T1 and T2 vulvar carcinoma: Further experience with radical wide excision and selective inguinal lymphadenectomy. Gynecol Oncol 1995;57:215.

227. Stehman FB, Bundy BN, Dvoretsky PM, Creasman WT: Early stage I carcinoma of the vulva treated with ipsilateral superficial inguinal lymphadenectomy and modified radical hemivulvectomy: A prospective study of the Gynecologic Oncology Group. Obstet Gynecol 1992;79:490.

228. Levenback C, Burke TW, Morris M, et al: Potential applications of intraoperative lymphatic mapping in vulvar cancer. Gynecol Oncol 1995;59:216.

229. Hoffman JS, Kumar NB, Morley GW: Microinvasive squamous carcinoma of the vulva: Search for a definition. Obstet Gynecol 1983;61:615.

230. Boyce J, Fruchter RG, Kasambilides E, et al: Prognostic factors in carcinoma of the vulva. Gynecol Oncol 1985;20:364.

231. Homesley HD, Bundy BN, Sedlis A, et al: Assessment of current International Federation of Gynecology and Obstetrics staging of vulvar carcinoma relative to prognostic factors for survival: A Gynecologic Oncology Group study. Am J Obstet Gynecol 1991;164:997.

232. Hacker NF: Current treatment of small vulvar cancers. Oncology 1980;4:21.

233. Way S: Carcinoma of the vulva. Am J Obstet Gynecol 1960;79:692–697.

234. Morley GW. Infiltrative carcinoma of the vulva: results of surgical treatment. Am J Obstet Gynecol 1976;124:874–888.

235. Iversen T, Aalders JG, Christensen A, Kolstad P: Squamous cell carcinoma of the vulva: A review of 424 patients, 1956–1974. Gynecol Oncol 1980;9:271–279.

236. Rutledge F, Smith JP, Franklin EW: Carcinoma of the vulva. Am J Obstet Gynecol 1970;106:1117–1130.

237. Morris JM: A formula for selective lymphadenectomy: Its application to cancer of the vulva. Obstet Gynecol 1977;50:152–158.

238. Goplerud DR, Keettel WC. Carcinoma of the vulva: A review of 156 cases from the University of Iowa hospitals. Am J Obstet Gynecol 1968;100:550–553.

239. Fleming I, Cooper JS, Henson DE, et al (eds): AJCC Cancer Staging Manual, 5th ed. Philadelphia, Lippincott Williams & Wilkins, 1997, pp 181–184.

240. Blair-Bell W, Datnow MM: Primary malignant diseases of the vulva, with special reference to treatment by operation. J Obstet Gynaecol Br Commonw 1938;43:755.

241. Basset A: Traitement chirurgical operatoire de l'epithelioma primitif du clitoris. Rev Chir 1912;46:546.

242. Taussig FJ: Cancer of the vulva: An analysis of 155 cases. Am J Obstet Gynecol 1940;40:764.

243. Way S: The anatomy of the lymphatic drainage of the vulva and its influence on the radical operation for carcinoma. Ann R Coll Surg Engl 1948;3:187.

244. Hacker NF, Leuchter RS, Berek JS, et al: Radical vulvectomy and bilateral inguinal lymphadenectomy through separate groin incisions. Obstet Gynecol 1981;58:574.

245. Magrina JF, Gonzalez-Bosquet J, Weaver AL, et al: Primary squamous cell cancer of the vulva: Radical versus modified radical vulvar surgery. Gynecol Oncol 1988;71:116.

246. Cavanagh D, Shepherd JH: The place of pelvic exenteration in the primary management of advanced carcinoma of the vulva. Gynecol Oncol 1982;13:318.

247. Boronow RC, Hickman BT, Reagan MT, et al: Combined therapy as an alternative to exenteration for locally advanced vulvovaginal cancer. Am J Clin Oncol 1987;10:171.

248. Moore DH, Thomas GM, Montana GS, et al: Preoperative chemoradiation for advanced vulvar cancer: A phase II study of the Gynecologic Oncology Group. Int J Radiat Oncol Biol Phys 1998;42:79.

249. Heaps JM, Fu YS, et al: Surgical-pathologic variables predictive of local recurrence in squamous cell carcinoma of the vulva. Gynecol Oncol 1990;38:309–314.

250. Faul CM, Mirmow D, Huang Q, et al: Adjuvant radiation for vulvar carcinoma: Improved local control. Int J Radiat Oncol Biol Phys 1997;38:381–389.

251. De Hullu JA, Hollema H, et al: Vulvar carcinoma: The price of less radical surgery. Cancer 2002;95:2331–2338.

252. Farias-Eisner R, Cirisano FD, Grouse D, et al: Conservative and individualized surgery for early squamous carcinoma of the vulva: the treatment of choice for stage I and II (T1-2N0-1M0) disease. Gynecol Oncol 1994;53:55.

253. Wilkinson EJ, Rico MJ, Pierson KK: Microinvasive carcinoma of the vulva. Int J Gynecol Pathol 1982;1:29.

254. Kneale BLG, Elliott PM, McDonald IA: Microinvasive carcinoma of the vulva: Clinical features and management. In Coppleson M (ed): Gynecologic Oncology. Edinburgh, Churchill Livingstone, 1981, p 320.

255. Franklin EW, Rutledge FN: Prognostic factors in epidermoid carcinoma of the vulva. Obstet Gynecol 1971;37:892.

256. Krupp PJ, Lee FYL, Bohm JW: Prognostic parameters and clinical staging criteria in epidermoid carcinoma of the vulva. Obstet Gynecol 1975;46:84.

257. Hacker NF, Nieberg RK, Berek JS, et al: Superficially invasive vulvar cancer with nodal metastases. Gynecol Oncol 1983;15:65.

258. Crissman JD, Azoury RS: Microinvasive carcinoma of the vulva: A report of two cases with regional lymph node metastasis. Diag Gynecol Obstet 1981;3:75.

259. Krupp PJ, Bohm JW: Lymph gland metastases in invasive squamous cell carcinoma of the vulva. Am J Obstet Gynecol 1978;130:943.

260. DiSaia PJ, Creasman WT, Rich WM: An alternative approach to early cancer of the vulva. Am J Obstet Gynecol 1979;133:825.

261. Green TH Jr: Carcinoma of the vulva: A reassessment. Obstet Gynecol 1978;52:462.

262. Homesley HD, Bundy BN, Sedlis A, et al: Radiation therapy versus pelvic node resection for carcinoma of the vulva with positive groin nodes. Obstet Gynecol 1986;68:733.

263. Dean RE, Taylor ES, Weisbrod DM, et al: The treatment of premalignant and malignant lesions of the vulva. Am J Obstet Gynecol 1974;119:59.

264. Benedet JL, Turko M, Fairey RN, et al: Squamous carcinoma of the vulva: Results of treatment, 1938–1976. Am J Obstet Gynecol 1979;134:201.

265. Curry SL, Wharton JT, Rutledge F: Positive lymph nodes in vulvar squamous carcinoma. Gynecol Oncol 1980;9:63.

266. Hacker NF, Berek JS, Lagasse LD, et al: Management of regional lymph nodes and their prognostic influence in vulvar cancer. Obstet Gynecol 1983;61:408.

267. Aslam Sohaib SA, Richards PS, Ind T, et al: MR imaging of carcinoma of the vulva. Am J Roentgenol 2002;178:373–377.

268. Cohn DE, Dehdashti F, Gibb RK, et al: Prospective evaluation of positron emission tomography for the detection of groin node metastases from vulvar cancer. Gynecol Oncol 2002;85:179–184.

269. Moore RG, DePasquale SE, Steinhoff MM, et al: Sentinel node identification and the ability to detect metastatic tumor to inguinal lymph nodes in squamous cell cancer of the vulva. Gynecol Oncol 2003;89:475–479.

270. Boronow RC, Hickman BT, Reagan MT, et al: Combined therapy as an alternative to exenteration for locally advanced vulvovaginal cancer. Am J Clin Oncol 1987;10:171.

271. Hacker NF, Berek JS, Juillard GJF, et al: Preoperative radiation therapy for locally advanced vulvar cancer. Cancer 1984;54:2056.

272. Acosta AA, Given FT, Frazier AB, et al: Preoperative radiation therapy in the management of squamous cell carcinoma of the vulva: Preliminary report. Am J Obstet Gynecol 1978;132:198.

273. Jafari K, Magalotti M: Radiation therapy in carcinoma of the vulva. Cancer 1981;47:686.

274. Fairey RN, MacKay PA, Benedet JL, et al: Radiation treatment of carcinoma of the vulva, 1950–1980. Am J Obstet Gynecol 1985;151:591.

275. Perez CA, Grigsby PW, Galakatos A, et al: Radiation therapy in management of carcinoma of the vulva with emphasis on conservation therapy. Cancer 1993;71:3707.

276. Kalra JK, Grossman AM, Krumholz BA, et al: Preoperative chemoradiotherapy for carcinoma of the vulva. Gynecol Oncol 1981;12:256.

277. Levin W, Goldberg G, Altaras M, et al: The use of concomitant chemotherapy and radiotherapy prior to surgery in advanced stage carcinoma of the vulva. Gynecol Oncol 1986;25:20.

278. Whitaker SJ, Kirkbride P, Arnott SJ, et al: A pilot study of chemo-radiotherapy in advanced carcinoma of the vulva. Br J Obstet Gynaecol 1990;97:436.

279. Evans LS, Kersh CR, Constable WC, et al: Concomitant 5-fluorouracil, mitomycin-C, and radiotherapy for advanced gynecologic malignancies. Int J Radiat Oncol Biol Phys 1988;15:901.

280. Carson LF, Twiggs LB, Adcock LL, et al: Multimodality therapy for advanced and recurrent vulvar squamous cell carcinoma. J Reprod Med 1990;35:1029.

281. Roberts WS, Hoffman MS, Kavanagh JJ, et al: Further experience with radiation therapy and concomitant intravenous chemo-therapy in advanced carcinoma of the lower female genital tract. Gynecol Oncol 1991;43:233.

282. Landoni F, Maneo A, Zanetta G, et al: Concurrent preoperative chemotherapy with 5-fluorouracil and mitomycin C and radiotherapy (FUMIR) followed by limited surgery in locally advanced and recurrent vulvar carcinoma. Gynecol Oncol 1996;61:321.

283. Moore DH, Thomas GM, Montana GS, et al: Preoperative chemoradiation for advanced vulvar cancer: A phase II study of the Gynecologic Oncology Group. Int J Radiat Oncol Biol Phys 1998;42:79.

284. Thomas G, Dembo A, DePetrillo A, et al: Concurrent radiation and chemotherapy in vulvar carcinoma. Gynecol Oncol 1989;34:263.

285. Berek JS, Heaps JM, Fu YS, et al: Concurrent cisplatin and 5-flourouracil chemotherapy and radiation therapy for advanced-stage squamous carcinoma of the vulva. Gynecol Oncol 1991;42:197.

286. Russell AH, Mesic JB, Scudder SA, et al: Synchronous radiation and cytotoxic chemotherapy for locally advanced or recurrent squamous cancer of the vulva. Gynecol Oncol 1992;47:14.

287. Koh WJ, Wallace JH 3rd, Greer BE: Combined radiotherapy and chemotherapy in the management of local-regionally advanced vulvar cancer. Int J Radiat Oncol Biol Phys 1993;26:809.

288. Lupi G, Raspagliesi F, Zucali R, et al: Combined preoperative chemoradiotherapy followed by radical surgery in locally advanced vulvar carcinoma: A pilot study. Cancer 1996;77:1472–1478.

289. Prempree T, Amornmarn R: Radiation treatment of recurrent carcinoma of the vulva. Cancer 1984;54:1943.

290. Dusenbery KE, Carlson JW, LaPorte JJ, et al: Radical vulvectomy with postoperative nodal radiotherapy: A reappraisal of the vulvar central block. Int J Radiat Oncol Biol Phys 1994;29:989–998.

291. Podratz KC, Symmonds RE, Taylor WF: Carcinoma of the vulva: Analysis of treatment failures. Am J Obstet Gynecol 1982;143:340.

292. Tilmans AS, Sutton GP, Look KY, et al: Recurrent squamous carcinoma of the vulva. Am J Obstet Gynecol 1992;167:1383.

293. Piura B, Masotina A, Murdoch J, et al: Recurrent squamous cell carcinoma of the vulva: A study of 73 cases. Gynecol Oncol 1993;48:189.

294. Buchler DA, Kline JC, Tunca JC, et al: Treatment of recurrent carcinoma of the vulva. Gynecol Oncol 1979;8:180.

295. Montana GS, Thomas GM, Moore DH, et al: Preoperative chemo-radiation for carcinoma of the vulva with N2/N3 nodes: A Gynecologic Oncology Group study. Int J Radiat Oncol Biol Phys 2000;48:1007.

296. Frischbier HJ, Thomsen K: Treatment of cancer of the vulva with high energy electrons. Am J Obstet Gynecol 1971;111:431.

297. Pirtoli L, Rottoli ML: Results of radiation therapy for vulvar carcinoma. Acta Radiol Oncol 1982;21:45.

298. Eifel PJ, Morris M, Burke TW, et al: Prolonged continuous infusion cisplatin and 5-fluorouracil with radiation for locally advanced cancer of the vulva. Gynecol Oncol 1995;59:51.

299. Cunningham MJ, Goyer RP, Gibbons SK, et al: Primary radiation, cisplatin, and 5-fluorouracil for advanced squamous carcinoma of the vulva. Gynecol Oncol 1997;66:258.

300. Akl A, Akl M, Boike G, et al: Preliminary results of chemoradiation as a primary treatment for vulvar carcinoma. Int J Radiat Oncol Biol Phys 2000;48:415.

301. Han SC, Kim DH, Higgins SA, et al: Chemoradiation as primary or adjuvant treatment for locally advanced carcinoma of the vulva. Int J Radiat Oncol Biol Phys 2000;47:1235.

302. Gould N, Kamelle S, Tillmanns T, et al: Predictors of complications after inguinal lymphadenectomy. Gynecol Oncol 2001;82:329.

303. Frankendal B, Larsson L-G, Westling P: Carcinoma of the vulva: Results of an individualized treatment schedule. Acta Radiol Ther Phys Biol 1973;12:165.

304. Simonsen E, Nordberg U-B, Johnsson J-E, et al: Radiation therapy and surgery in the treatment of regional lymph nodes in squamous cell carcinoma of the vulva. Acta Radiol Oncol 1984;23:433.

305. Lee WR, McCollough WM, Mendenhall WM, et al: Elective inguinal lymph node irradiation for pelvic carcinomas. Cancer 1993;72:2058.

306. Petereit DG, Mehta MP, Buchler DA, et al: Inguinofemoral radiation of N0,N1 vulvar cancer may be equivalent to lymphadenectomy if proper radiation technique is used. Int J Radiat Oncol Biol Phys 1993;27:963.

307. Gonzalez-Bosquet J, Kinney WK, Russell AH, et al: Risk of occult inguinofemoral lymph node metastasis from squamous carcinoma of the vulva. Int J Radiat Oncol Biol Phys 2003;57:419–424.

308. Stehman FB, Bundy B, Thomas G, et al: Groin dissection versus groin radiation in carcinoma of the vulva: A Gynecologic Oncology Group study. Int J Radiat Oncol Biol Phys 1992;24:389–396.

309. Koh WJ, Chiu M, Stelzer KJ, et al: Femoral vessel depth and the implications for groin node radiation. Int J Radiat Oncol Biol Phys 1993;27:969.

310. Leiserowitz GS, Russell AH, Kinney WK, et al: Prophylactic chemoradiation of inguino-femoral lymph nodes in patients with locally advanced vulvar cancer. Gynecol Oncol 1994;54:112.

311. Wahlen SA, Slater JD, Wagner RJ, et al: Concurrent radiation therapy and chemotherapy in the treatment of primary squamous cell carcinoma of the vulva. Cancer 1995;75:2289.

312. Serkjes K, Wysocka B, Emerich J, et al: Salvage hemipelvis radiotherapy with fertility preservation in an adolescent with recurrent vulvar carcinoma. Gynecol Oncol 2002;85:381.

313. Scheistroen M, Trope C: Combined bleomycin and irradiation in preoperative treatment of advanced squamous cell carcinoma of the vulva. Acta Oncol 1992;32:657.

314. Iversen T: Irradiation and bleomycin in the treatment of inoperable vulval carcinoma. Acta Obstet Gynecol Scand 1982;61:195–197.

315. Bryson SCP, Dembo AJ, Colgan TJ, et al: Invasive squamous cell carcinoma of the vulva: Defining low and high risk groups for recurrence. Int J Gynecol Cancer 1991;1:25.

316. Malfetano J, Piver MS, Tsukada Y, et al: Stage III and IV squamous cell carcinoma of the vulva. Gynecol Oncol 1986;23:192–198.

317. Cavanagh D, Fiorica JV, Hoffman MS, et al: Invasive carcinoma of the vulva: Changing trends in surgical management. Am J Obstet Gynecol 1990;163:1007.

318. Deppe G, Cohen CJ, Bruckner HW: Chemotherapy of squamous cell carcinoma of the vulva: A review. Gynecol Oncol 1979; 7:345–348.

319. Deppe G, Bruckner HW, Cohen CJ: Adriamycin treatment of advanced vulvar carcinoma. Obstet Gynecol 1977;50:13s–14s.

320. Srivannaboon S, Boonyanit S, Vatananusara C, Sophak P: A clinical trial of bleomycin on carcinoma of the vulva: A preliminary report. J Med Assoc Thai 1973;56:101–108.

321. Huang GS, Juretzka M, Ciaravino G, Kohler S, Teng NN: Liposomal doxorubicin for treatment of metastatic chemorefractory vulvar adenocarcinoma. Gynecol Oncol 2002;87:313–318.

322. Durrant KR, Mangioni C, Lacave AJ, et al: Bleomycin, methotrexate, and CCNU in advanced inoperable squamous cell carcinoma of the vulva: A phase II study of the EORTC Gynaecological Cancer Cooperative Group (GCCG). Gynecol Oncol 1990;37:359–362.

323. Wagenaar HC, Colombo N, Vergote I, et al: Bleomycin, methotrexate, and CCNU in locally advanced or recurrent, inoperable, squamous-cell carcinoma of the vulva: EORTC Gynaecological Cancer Cooperative Group Study: European Organization for Research and Treatment of Cancer. Gynecol Oncol 2001;81:348–354.

324. Belinson JL, Stewart JA, Richards AL, McClure M: Bleomycin, vincristine, mitomycin-C, and cisplatin in the management of gynecological squamous cell carcinomas. Gynecol Oncol 1985;20:387–393.

325. Shimizu Y, Hasumi K, Masubuchi K. Effective chemotherapy consisting of bleomycin, vincristine, mitomycin C, and cisplatin (BOMP) for a patient with inoperable vulvar cancer. Gynecol Oncol 1990;36:423–427.

326. Benedetti-Panici P, Greggi S, Scambia G, Salerno G, Mancuso S: Cisplatin (P), bleomycin (B), and methotrexate (M) preoperative chemotherapy in locally advanced vulvar carcinoma. Gynecol Oncol 1993;50:49–53.

327. Sirotnak FM, Zakowski MF, Miller VA, Scher HI, Kris MG: Efficacy of cytotoxic agents against human tumor xenografts is markedly enhanced by coadministration of ZD1839 (Iressa), an inhibitor of EGFR tyrosine kinase. Clin Cancer Res 2000;6:4885–4892.

328. Mamot C, Drummond DC, Greiser U, et al: Epidermal growth factor receptor (EGFR)-targeted immunoliposomes mediate specific and efficient drug delivery to EGFR- and EGFRvIII-overexpressing tumor cells. Cancer Res 2003;63:3154–3161.

329. Lever WF: Adenoacanthoma of the sweat glands: Carcinoma of the sweat glands with glandular and epidermal elements: Report of four cases. Arch Dermatol Syphilol 1947;56:157.

330. Johnson WC, Helwig EB: Adenoid squamous cell carcinoma (adenoacanthoma): A clinicopathologic study of 155 patients. Cancer 1966;19:1939.

331. Underwood JW, Adcodk LL, Okagaki T: Adenosquamous carcinoma of skin appendages of the vulva. Cancer 1978;42:1851

332. Berek JS, Hacker NF: Practical Gynecologic Oncology, 3rd ed. Baltimore, Lippincott Williams & Wilkins, 2000.

333. Podratz KC, Gaffey TA, Symmonds RE, et al: Melanoma of the vulva: An update. Gynecol Oncol 1983;16:153.

334. Chung AF, Woodruff JM, Lewis JL Jr: Malignant melanoma of the vulva: A report of 44 cases. Obstet Gynecol 1975;45:638.

335. Verschraegen CF, Benjabipal M, Supakarapongkul W, et al: Vulvar melanoma at the M.D. Anderson Cancer Center: 25 years later. Int J Gynecol Cancer 2001;11:359.

336. Morrow CP, Rutledge FN: Melanoma of the vulva. Obstet Gynecol 1972;39:745.

337. Shah KD, Tabibzadch SS, Gerber MA: Immunohistochemical distinction of Paget's disease from Bowen's disease and superficial spreading melanoma with the use of monoclonal cytokeratin antibodies. Am J Clin Pathol 1987;88:689.

338. Clark WH, From L, Bernardino EA Mihm MC: The histogenesis and biologic behavior of primary malignant melanomas of the skin. Cancer Res 1969;29:705–711.

339. Breslow A: Thickness, cross-sectional area and depth of invasion in the prognosis of cutaneous melanoma. Ann Surg 1970;172:902–908.

340. Masiel A, Buttrick P, Bitran J: Tamoxifen in the treatment of malignant melanoma. Cancer Treat Rep 1981;65:531.

341. Phillips GL, Bundy BN, Twiggs LB, Okagaki T, Kucera PR, Stehman FB: Malignant melanoma of the vulva treated by radical hemivulvectomy. Cancer 1994;73:2626–2632.

342. Chamlian DK, Taylor HB: Primary carcinoma of Bartholin's gland: A report of 24 patients. Obstet Gynecol 1972;39:489:143.

343. Barclay DL, Collins CG, Macey HB: Cancer of the Bartholin gland: A review and report of 8 cases. Obstet Gynecol 1964;24:329.

344. Leuchter RS, Hacker NF, Voet RL, et al: Primary carcinoma of the Bartholin gland: A report of 14 cases and review of the literature. Obstet Gynecol 1982;60:361.

345. Wheelock JB, Goplerud DR, Dunn LJ, et al: Primary carcinoma of the Bartholin gland: A report of ten cases. Obstet Gynecol 1984;63:820.

346. Copeland LJ, Sneige N, Gershenson DM, et al: Bartholin gland carcinoma. Obstet Gynecol 1986;67:794.

347. Copeland LJ, Sneige N, Gershenson DM, et al: Adenoid cystic carcinoma of Bartholin gland. Obstet Gynecol 1986;67:115.

348. Cardosi RJ, Speights A, Fiorica JV, et al: Bartholin's gland carcinoma: A 15-year experience. Gynecol Oncol 2001;82:247.

349. Balat O, Edwards CL, Delclos L, et al: Advanced primary carcinoma of the Bartholin gland: Report of 18 patients. Eur J Gynaecol Oncol 2001;22:46.

350. Gallousis S: Verrucous carcinoma: Report of three vulvar cases and review of the literature. Obstet Gynecol 1972;40:502.

351. Japaze H, Dinh TV, Woodruff JD: Verrucous carcinoma of the vulva: Study of 24 cases. Obstet Gynecol 1982;60:462.

352. Foye G, Marsh MR, Minkowitz S: Verrucous carcinoma of the vulva. Obstet Gynecol 1969;34:484.

353. Lucas WE, Benirschke K, Lebherz TB: Verrucous carcinoma of the female genital tract. Am J Obstet Gynecol 1974;119:435.

Vagina

354. Dunn LJ, Napier JG: Primary carcinoma of the vagina. Am J Obstet Gynecol 1966;96:1112.

355. Way S: Vaginal metastases of carcinoma of the body of the uterus. Br J Obstet Gynaecol 1951;58:558.

356. Bergman F: Carcinoma of the ovary: A clinicopathologic study of 86 autopsied cases with special reference to mode of spread. Acta Obstet Gynecol Scand 1966;45:211.

357. Nergrum TA: Vaginal metastases of hypernephroma. Acta Obstet Gynecol Scand 1966;45:515.

358. Peters WA III, Kumar NB, Morley GW: Carcinoma of the vagina. Cancer 1985;55:892.

359. Ball HG, Berman ML: Management of primary vaginal carcinoma. Gynecol Oncol 1982;14:154.

360. Perez CA, Arneson AN, Dehner LP, Galakatos A: Radiation therapy in carcinoma of the vagina. Obstet Gynecol 1974;44:862.

361. Rubin SC, Young J, Mikuta JJ: Squamous carcinoma of the vagina: Treatment complications and long-term followup. Gynecol Oncol 1985;20:346.

362. Pride GL, Buchler DA: Carcinoma of vagina 10 or more years following pelvic irradiation therapy. Am J Obstet Gynecol 1977;127:513–518.

363. Houghton CRS, Iversen T: Squamous cell carcinoma of the vagina: A clinical study of the location of the tumor. Gynecol Oncol 982;13:365–372.

364. Benedet JL, Murphy KJ, Fairey RN, Boyes DA: Primary invasive carcinoma of the vagina. Obstet Gynecol 1983;62:715–719.

365. Sulak P, Barnhill D, Heller P, et al: Nonsquamous cancer of the vagina. Gynecol Oncol 1988;29:309–320.

366. Eddy GL, Marks RD, Miller MC III, Underwood PB Jr: Primary invasive vaginal carcinoma. Am J Obstet Gynecol 1991;165:292–298.

367. Ali MM, Huang DT, Gopelrud DR, et al: Radiation alone for carcinoma of the vagina: Variation in response related to the location of the primary tumor. Cancer 1996;77:1934–1939.

368. Gallup DG, Talledo E, Shah KJ, Hayes C: Invasive squamous cell carcinoma of the vagina: A 14-year study. Obstet Gynecol 1987;69:782.

369. Underwood RB, Smith RT: Carcinoma of the vagina. JAMA 1971;217:46.

370. Pride GL, Schultz AE, Chuprevich TW, et al: Primary invasive squamous carcinoma of the vagina. Obstet Gynecol 1979;53:218.

371. Rutledge F: Cancer of the vagina. Am J Obstet Gynecol 1967;97:635.

372. Herbst AL, Scully RE: Adenocarcinoma of the vagina in adolescence: A report of 7 cases including 6 clear-cell carcinomas (so-called mesonephromas). Cancer 1970;25:745.

373. Melnick S, Cole P, Anderson D, Herbst A: Rates and risks of diethylstilbestrol-related clear-cell adenocarcinoma of the vagina and cervix: An update. N Engl J Med 1987;316:514.

374. Ikenberg H, Runge M, Goppinger A, Pfleiderer A: Human papillomavirus DNA in invasive carcinoma of the vagina. Obstet Gynecol 1990;76:432-438.

375. Aho M, Vesterinen E, Meyer B, Purola E, Paavonen J: Natural history of vaginal intraepithelial neoplasia. Cancer 1991;68: 195-197.

376. Benedet JL, Saunders BH: Carcinoma in situ of the vagina. Am J Obstet Gynecol 1984;148:695.

377. Lenehan PM, Meffe F, Lickrish GM: Vaginal epithelial neoplasia: Biologic aspects and management. Obstet Gynecol 1986;68:333.

378. Herbst AL, Ulfelder H, Poskanzer DC: Adenocarcinoma of the vagina: Association of maternal stilbestrol therapy with tumor appearance in young women. N Engl J Med 1971;284:878-881.

379. Herbst AL: Diethylstilbestrol and adenocarcinoma of the vagina. Am J Obstet Gynecol 1999;181:1576-1579.

380. Herbst AL: Adult sequelae of fetal exposure to diethylstilbestrol (DES): Diagnosis, monitoring, fertility management, health outcomes. In Mishell DR Jr, Stencheuer MA, Droegemueller W, Herbst AL (eds): Comprehensive Gynecology, 3rd ed. St. Louis, Mosby-Yearbook, 1997, pp 389-402.

381. Plentl AA, Friedman EA: Lymphatic System of the Female Genitalia: The Morphologic Basis of Diagnosis and Therapy. Philadelphia, WB Saunders, 1971.

382. Stock RG, Chen ASJ, Seski J: A 30-year experience in the management of primary carcinoma of the vagina: Analysis of prognostic factors and treatment modalities. Gynecol Oncol 1995;56:45-52.

383. Chang YC, Hricak H, Thurnher S, Lacey CG: Vagina: Evaluation with MR imaging, Part II: Neoplasms. Radiology 188;169:175-179.

384. Perez CA, Arneson AN, Galakatos A, et al: Malignant tumors of the vagina. Cancer 1973;31:36-44.

385. Choo YC, Anderson DG: Neoplasms of the vagina following cervical carcinoma. Gynecol Oncol 1982;14:125-132.

386. Kanbour AI, Klionsky B, Murphy AI: Carcinoma of the vagina following cervical cancer. Cancer 1974;34:1838-1841.

387. Davis KP, Stanhope CR, Gaton, et al: Invasive vaginal carcinoma: Analysis of early-stage disease. Gynecol Oncol 1991;42:131.

388. Tjama WAA, Monaghan JM, deBarros Lopes A, Naik R, Nordin AJ, Weyler JJ: The role of surgery in invasive squamous carcinoma of the vagina. Gynecol Oncol 2001;81:360-365.

389. Creasman WT, Phillips JL, Menck HR: The National Cancer Data Base Report on cancer of the vagina. Cancer 1998;83:1033-1040.

390. Stock RG, Mychalczak B, Armstrong JG, et al: The importance of brachytherapy technique in the management of primary carcinoma of the vagina. Int J Radiat Oncol Biol Phys 1992;24:747.

391. Chyle V, Zagars GK, Wheeler JA, et al: Definitive radiotherapy for carcinoma of the vagina: Outcome and prognostic factors. Int J Radiat Oncol Biol Phys 1996;35:891.

392. Evans LS, Kersh CR, Constable WC, et al: Concomitant 5-fluorouracil, mitomycin-C, and radiotherapy for advanced gynecologic malignancies. Int J Radiat Oncol Biol Phys 1988;15:901-906.

393. Roberts WS, Hoffman MS, Kavanagh JJ, et al: Further experience with radiation therapy and concomitant intravenous chemotherapy in advanced carcinoma of the lower female genital tract. Gynecol Oncol 1991;43:233-236.

394. Kirkbride P, Fyles A, Rawlings GA, et al: Carcinoma of the vagina: Experience at the Princess Margaret Hospital (1974-1989). Gynecol Oncol 1995;56:435-443.

395. Dalrymple JL, Russell AH, Lee SW, et al: Chemoradiation for primary invasive squamous carcinoma of the vagina. Int J Gynecol Cancer 2004;14:110-117.

396. Berek JS, Hacker NF, Lagasse LD: Vaginal reconstruction performed simultaneously with pelvic exenteration. Obstet Gynecol 1984;63:318.

397. Benson C, Soisson AP, Carlson J, et al: Neovaginal reconstruction with a rectus abdominis myocutaneous flap. Obstet Gynecol 1993;81:871.

398. Abitol MM, Davenport JH: The irradiated vagina. Obstet Gynecol 1974;44:249-256.

399. Pitkin RM, Van Voorhis LW. Postirradiation vaginitis: An evaluation of prophylaxis with topical estrogen. Radiology 1971;99:417-421.

400. Perez CA, Bedwinek JM, Breaux SR: Patterns of failure after treatment of gynecologic tumors. Cancer Treat Symp 1983;2:217.

401. Senekjian EK, Frey KW, Anderson D, Herbst AL: Local therapy in stage I clear cell adenocarcinoma of the vagina. Cancer 1987;60: 1319.

402. Robboy SJ, Herbst AL, Scully RE: Clear-cell adenocarcinoma of the vagina and cervix in young females: Analysis of 37 tumors that persisted or recurred after primary therapy. Cancer 1974;34:606.

403. Fishman DA, William S, Small W Jr, et al: Late recurrences of vaginal clear cell adenocarcinoma. Gynecol Oncol 1996;62:128.

404. Peters WA, Kumar NB, Andersen WA, Morley GW: Primary sarcoma of the adult vagina: A clinicopathologic study. Obstet Gynecol 1985;65:699.

405. Curtin JP, Saigo P, Slucher B, et al: Soft-tissue sarcoma of the vagina and vulva: A clinicopathologic study. Obstet Gynecol 1995;86:269.

406. Andrassy RJ, Hays DM, Raney RB, et al: Conservative surgical management of vaginal and vulvar pediatric rhabdomyosarcoma: A report from the Intergroup Rhabdomyosarcoma Study III. J Pediatr Surg 1995;30:1034.

407. Curtin JP, Morrow CP: Melanoma of the female genital tract. In Coppleson M (ed): Gynecologic Oncology: Fundamental Principles and Clinical Practice. London, Churchill Livingstone, 1992, p 1059.

408. Weinstock MA: Malignant melanoma of the vulva and vagina in the United States: Patterns of incidence and population-based estimates of survival. Am J Obstet Gynecol 1994;171:1225.

409. Lee RB, Buttoni L, Dhru K, Tamimi H: Malignant melanoma of the vagina: A case report of progression from preexisting melanosis. Gynecol Oncol 1984;19:238.

410. Tarraza MH Jr, Muntz H, Decain M, Granai OC, Fuller A Jr: Patterns of recurrence of primary carcinoma of the vagina. Eur J Gynaecol Oncol 1991;12:89-92.

411. Koenigs KP, Campbell DR, Magrina J, Ruth WE: Pulmonary lymphangitic carcinomatosis from vaginal carcinoma presenting as congestive heart failure. Obstet Gynecol 1983;61:760-763.

412. Corey JP, Nelson E, Crawford M, Riester JW, Geiss R: Metastatic vaginal carcinoma to the temporal bone. Am J Otol 1991;12:128-131.

413. Thigpen JT, Blessing JA, Homesley HD, Berek JS, Creasman WT: Phase II trial of cisplatin in advanced or recurrent cancer of the vagina: A Gynecologic Oncology Group Study. Gynecol Oncol 1986;23:101-104.

414. Piver MS, Barlow JJ, Xynos FP: Adriamycin alone or in combination in 100 patients with carcinoma of the cervix or vagina. Am J Obstet Gynecol 1978;131:311-313.

415. Holleboom CA, Kock HC, Nijs AM, Leers WH: cis-Diamminechloroplatinum in the treatment of advanced primary squamous cell carcinoma of the vaginal wall: A case report. Gynecol Oncol 1987;27:110-115.

416. Katib S, Kuten A, Steiner M, Yudelev M, Robinson E: The effectiveness of multidrug treatment by bleomycin, methotrexate, and cis-platinum in advanced vaginal carcinoma. Gynecol Oncol 1985;21:101-102.

Specific Malignancies

III

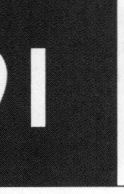
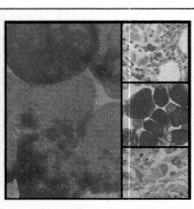

91 CANCER OF THE UTERUS

Eleanor E. R. Harris

S. Jack Wei

Christina Chu

Geza Acs

SUMMARY OF KEY POINTS

INCIDENCE
- Each year, there are an estimated 40,100 new cases of endometrial cancer and 6800 related deaths in the United States.
- Endometrial adenocarcinomas account for 95% these cases, and 5% are uterine sarcomas.

ETIOLOGY AND EPIDEMIOLOGY
- The median age of onset for endometrial cancer is 65.8 years; most cases occur after menopause.
- Hormonally dependent subtypes arise in hypertrophic endometrium.
- Lifetime estrogen exposure contributes to the risk of disease.
- Hormonally independent types occur at an older age and arise in atrophic endometrium.
- Other risk factors include family history, certain systemic diseases, and tamoxifen use.

PATHOLOGY AND BIOLOGY
- Atypical hyperplasia confers a 25% risk of invasive cancer.
- Aggressive subtypes include uterine serous, clear cell, and sarcomas.
- Estrogen and progesterone receptor expression influence biologic behavior.
- Uterine serous pathogenesis is p53-mediated.

CLINICAL FINDINGS
- Abnormal uterine bleeding and discharge are present in 90% of cases.
- Biopsy or dilation and curettage is required for diagnosis.

DIFFERENTIAL DIAGNOSIS AND STAGING
- Other causes of uterine bleeding include atrophy, infection, medications, coagulopathy, polyps and fibroids, and nongynecologic malignancies.
- Staging is surgical and is based on whether disease is confined to the uterus.
- Clinical staging is used for patients with inoperable disease.

PRIMARY THERAPY
- Surgery, including hysterectomy, bilateral salpingo-oophorectomy, lymph node sampling, and pelvic washings, is performed in all patients with operable disease; lymph node sampling may be omitted in patients with grade 2 tumors limited to the endometrium or grade 1 tumors with less than 50% invasion.
- Adjuvant radiation to the pelvis is indicated for patients with high-risk factors, including high-grade lesions, deep myometrial invasion, and spread to the lymph nodes.
- Systemic treatment with doxorubicin, cisplatin, and cyclophosphamide is used for metastatic disease.
- Radiation alone is used for patients with inoperable disease and for palliation.

SALVAGE THERAPY
- Pelvic recurrence after surgery alone is treated with radiation therapy.
- Salvage after surgery and radiation therapy is seldom successful, although systemic therapy may be used.

COMPLICATIONS
- Surgical and radiation complications include bladder or bowel dysfunction.

PROGNOSIS
- Survival is strongly correlated with stage and extent of disease as defined by depth of invasion, adnexal spread, and peritoneal cytology.
- Survival is worse when the tumor is of high grade or has aggressive histologic features.

INCIDENCE

Endometrial cancer is the fourth most common cancer among women, ranking after breast, lung, and colon cancer, and is the most common gynecologic cancer in the United States. According to Cancer Statistics for 2003, there were 40,100 estimated new cases of endometrial cancer in the United States and 6800 deaths attributable to this disease.[1] The probability of endometrial cancer is highest at 60 to 79 years of age, when the relative risk reaches 1.59, compared with 0.73 from 40 to 59 years of age and 0.05 for age younger than 39 years.

The overall 5-year survival rate for all women diagnosed with endometrial cancer from 1992 to 1998 was 86%, which has increased compared with the previous two decades. Most endometrial cancers are stage I (confined to the uterus) at diagnosis.

According to the Surveillance, Epidemiology, and End Results (SEER) Program of the National Cancer Institute, localized disease represented 73% of all cases diagnosed from 1992 to 1999, regional disease represented 15% of cases, and distant disease represented only 8% of cases, with 4% of cases unstaged.[2] In this survey, the overall survival rate for all stages of endometrial cancer diagnosed from 1992 to 1999 was 84%; for localized disease, it was

96%. The overall survival rate for regional disease was 65%; for distant disease, it was only 26%.

The most common pathologic subtype is endometrioid adenocarcinoma, which arises from the endometrium and accounts for approximately 80% of malignant endometrial neoplasms. Aggressive variants of adenocarcinomas, including uterine serous and clear cell histologies, have a much poorer prognosis. Less common are uterine sarcomas, which arise from the myometrium or other mesenchymal elements of the uterine wall and account for only 2% to 5% of uterine malignancies.[3] Of uterine sarcomas, carcinosarcoma (or mixed malignant mullerian tumors [MMMTs]) is the most common (8.2 per million women per year), followed by leiomyosarcoma (LMS; [6.4 per million]), both of which are somewhat more common in African American women than in white women. The incidence of MMMT increases with age, whereas the incidence of LMS peaks in middle age and then declines. The next most common type is endometrial stromal sarcoma (ESS; [1.8 per million]). The final group is known as unclassified (0.7 per million), and includes rhabdomyosarcoma, angiosarcoma, fibrosarcoma, chondrosarcoma, and liposarcoma.

ANATOMY

Anatomically, the uterus is contiguous with the cervix, and the two structures are separated at a narrowing known as the isthmus, at which point the epithelium begins to transition from endometrial glands to mucus-secreting columnar epithelium.[4] The body, or corpus, of the uterus is typically 7 to 8 cm long, 5 to 7 cm wide, and 2 to 3 cm thick. The corpus is located superior to the bladder, from which it separated by the vesicouterine pouch, and normally projects anteriorly, but in some women, may be retroverted.

Posteriorly, it is separated from the sigmoid colon by peritoneum and from the rectum by the rectouterine pouch (pouch of Douglas). The fallopian tubes extend laterally from the cornu of the fundus, the superiormost portion of the corpus, and open into the peritoneal cavity adjacent to the ovaries. The corpus and adnexa are enclosed in the broad ligaments, which are folds of the peritoneum that hold the uterus in position, although it is mobile enough to move with filling and emptying of the adjacent bladder. The round and uterosacral ligaments also extend from the uterine wall to the pelvic wall through the broad ligaments. The round ligaments course toward the deep inguinal ring, and the uterosacral ligaments course posteriorly toward the sacrum.

The main blood supply to the uterus is via the uterine arteries, branches of the internal iliac arteries. They enter the broad ligaments near the lateral vaginal fornices and cross the ureters superiorly, adjacent to the uterine cervix. The uterine fundus is also supplied by the ovarian arteries, which are branches of the aorta. These vessels form a vascular plexus and anastomose with each other. The uterine venous plexus drains to the uterine veins. The lymphatics follow the vascular structures. The lymphatics that supply the fundus drain to the aortic lymph nodes, and those that supply the lower portions of the uterus drain to the internal and external iliac nodes. Lymphatics may also run along the round ligaments toward the superficial inguinal nodes. The uterus is innervated by the inferior hypogastric plexus.

EPIDEMIOLOGY

The median age at diagnosis of endometrial cancer is 65.8 years, and most patients diagnosed with endometrial cancer are postmenopausal.[5] Table 91-1 shows the distribution of endometrial cancer by age as reported by the SEER program. Endometrial adenocarcinomas appear to have two distinct mechanisms of pathogenesis.[6] Most adenocarcinomas (type I) arise in normal or hypertrophic endometrium, are associated with hyperplasia, are well differentiated and express steroid hormone receptors, and are hormonally responsive. Others (type II) arise in atrophic endometrium, are associated with endometrial intraepithelial carcinoma without high levels of steroid receptor expression, and do not appear to be related to hormonal exposure. Type I tumors have a better prognosis overall than type II tumors. Pathologic comparison between cancers that occur in women who did or did not use estrogen replacement shows that in nonusers, cancers are more likely to be of lower grade, whereas those in users are more likely to be clear cell or adenosquamous.[7]

Endometrial cancer is uncommon in young women. A family history of endometrial cancer in a first-degree relative or a family history of hereditary nonpolyposis colorectal cancer syndrome (HNPCC) is a risk factor for endometrial cancer in the premenopausal years. Carriers of the HNPCC mutation have a 50% to 60% lifetime risk of endometrial cancer, with a median age of younger than 50 years.[8] Other risk factors for younger women include the use of hormone-replacement therapy, nulliparity, and other reproductive factors similar to those seen in older women.[9]

Compared with older women, young women have a similar stage distribution at diagnosis, with most cancers

TABLE 91-1

Incidence by Age, 1996–2000

AGE (YR)	INCIDENCE PER 100,000 FEMALES
25–29	1.3
30–34	2.8
35–39	6.1
40–44	12.5
45–49	24.0
50–54	47.9
55–59	68.4
60–64	86.5
65–69	94.4
70–74	101.9
75–79	99.0
80–84	95.2
85+	71.3

SEER Incidence Data, Cancer Statistic Review, 1975–2000.

diagnosed as stage I. Younger women are more likely to have lower-grade, less deeply invasive cancers, and they have an overall survival rate similar to that of older women.[10,11] In contrast, elderly patients (older than 75 years of age) have a higher incidence of poorly differentiated cancers, aggressive histology, and lack of steroid receptor expression, consistent with nonendometrioid patterns of tumorigenesis.[12] When outcomes are examined by race, African American women have a somewhat lower incidence of endometrial cancer, but a worse overall survival rate compared with white women.[13] African American women are diagnosed more often with aggressive histologies, with higher-grade tumors, and at later stages.

The etiology of uterine sarcomas is not well understood. One factor is previous exposure to pelvic irradiation. Secondary uterine sarcomas and carcinomas have been reported after irradiation for cervical and rectal cancers,[14,15] with a median latency period of 17 years and an absolute risk of 0.03% to 0.8%.[16] A study of endometrial sarcomas and reproductive factors showed that LMS is associated with early menarche, induced abortions, and breast-feeding, and both LMS and ESS are associated with later menopause.[17]

ETIOLOGY AND PATHOGENESIS

For cancers arising in hypertrophic or active endometrium, risk factors are related to lifetime estrogen exposure, known as the unopposed estrogen effect. According to this hypothesis, exposure to unopposed estrogen leads to increased proliferative activity of the endometrial cells, resulting in increased DNA replication errors and somatic mutations. Table 91-2 lists known risk factors for endometrial adenocarcinomas. Higher endogenous estrogen exposure associated with nulliparity, lower gravidity, early menarche, late menopause, estrogen-producing ovarian tumors, or obesity is associated with an increased risk of endometrial cancer.[18–20] High circulating blood levels of androstenedione, estrone, and estradiol are associated with a threefold to fourfold increased risk.[21] Exogenous estrogen sources, such as hormone-replacement therapy without progestins, also increase risk. The use of unopposed estrogens for 3 or more years is associated with a fivefold increased risk of invasive endometrial cancer.[22] The use of progesterones in a hormone-replacement regimen may actually decrease the risk of cancer through downregulation of hormone receptors.[23] Cancers occurring in women who used combined estrogen and progestin hormone-replacement therapy tend to be tumors of low stage and grade.[24] A family history of endometrial cancer in a first-degree relative is associated with a relative risk of 1.5, although only approximately 1% of endometrial cancers are attributable to genetic factors.[25] Family history appears to be a more significant risk factor in young women (younger than 50 years of age at diagnosis).[26] For the uterine serous subtype, women are at increased risk for concurrent or subsequent breast cancer.[27] Breast cancers are diagnosed in 25% of women with uterine serous carcinoma (USC), compared with 3% of those with endometrioid carcinoma, implicating a genetic or biologic link. Endometrial cancer is part of the spectrum of cancer predisposition in families with HNPCC syndrome, which results from mutations in DNA mismatch repair genes. Women with HNPCC have a 50% to 60% lifetime risk of endometrial cancer.

Other systemic diseases and lifestyle factors affect the risk of endometrial cancer. Obesity, diabetes, and hypertension all increase the risk. Hypertension and diabetes may be associated with increased risk, mainly in women who are also obese, however. Overall, nearly 40% of the risk of endometrial cancer can be attributed to obesity.[28] Obesity from an early age, substantial weight gain over time, and marked obesity all confer higher risks than moderate obesity.[29] When examined by degree of obesity as measured by body mass index (BMI), in comparison with lean women, women who are overweight (BMI 28 to 29.9) have a relative risk of 1.5 compared with women with a lower BMI. Women who are obese (BMI 30 to 33.9) have a 2.9 relative risk, and women who are markedly obese (BMI ≥ 34) have a relative risk of 6.3.[30] Some studies show an association between endometrial cancer and dietary intake of fat, suggesting that a healthier diet and reduction of dietary fat may reduce the risk.[31,32] Diabetes confers a relative risk of approximately 4,[33] and the risk is highest for women who are both obese and diabetic.[34,35] There may be a link between ovarian hyperandrogenism, leading to progesterone deficiency, lifetime weight gain, and chronic hyperinsulinism, all of which are associated with an increased risk of endometrial cancer.

A potential causal link between treatment of breast cancer with the antiestrogen drug tamoxifen and the development of endometrial cancer was first suggested in 1985.[36] This was later confirmed by the results of large series from the Netherlands Cancer Institute and the National Surgical Adjuvant Breast Project (NSABP). The Netherlands Cancer Institute identified 98 patients who had endometrial cancer after treatment for breast cancer, and performed a matched case–control study among women who did not have endometrial cancer.[37] Among patients with endometrial cancer, 24% had taken tamoxifen compared with 20% of control subjects. The

TABLE 91-2

Risk Factors for Endometrial Adenocarcinoma

RISK FACTOR	RELATIVE RISK
Nulliparity[19]	1.4
Endogenous estrogen levels[32]	2.0–3.8
Estrogen use[22]	5
Obesity[29]	
High body mass index	3.2
Substantial weight gain	3.5
Diabetes[33]	4.1
Obesity + diabetes[34,35]	3–8.0
Hypertension[33]	1.6
Tamoxifen[38]	2.2
Oral contraceptives[8]	0.5

Specific Malignancies

III

risk of endometrial cancer increased with the duration of tamoxifen use. Those treated for 5 years or longer had a 3.0 relative risk of endometrial cancer compared with control subjects. The NSABP analyzed data from the B-14 study, in which 2834 women with node-negative, estrogen receptor–positive breast cancers were randomized to receive placebo or tamoxifen 20 mg daily.[38] Twenty-three of 24 cases of endometrial cancer occurring in women entering this trial occurred in the tamoxifen arm. These were mostly favorable cancers: 88% were stage I at diagnosis, and 78% were low or intermediate grade. The authors calculated an annual hazard rate of endometrial cancer development in women taking tamoxifen as 1.6 per 1000 patient-years and 0.2 per 1000 patient-years in the placebo group. However, the use of tamoxifen resulted in a 38% improvement in disease-free survival for breast cancer, which far outweighed the risk of endometrial cancer. Only four deaths caused by endometrial cancer were observed

Known protective factors against endometrial cancer include full-term pregnancy, multiparity or incomplete pregnancies, older age at menarche, older age at first birth, and oral contraceptive use. The use of oral contraceptives for 1 to 5 years is associated with a relative risk of 0.2, and use for at least 1 year reduces the risk of endometrial cancer by approximately 45%.[8] Increasing physical activity decreases the risk of endometrial cancer independently of weight and parity.[39] Interestingly, cigarette smoking decreases the risk of endometrial cancer, but this effect may be limited to postmenopausal women or those taking hormone-replacement therapy.[40] It has been postulated that components of cigarette smoke may suppress endogenous estrogens or may be associated with lower body weight as a potential mechanism for the protective effect. Clearly, the risks of smoking greatly outweigh any potential benefit with respect to endometrial cancer.

PATHOLOGY

Hyperplasia

Proliferative diseases of the endometrium represent a broad continuum of morphologic and cellular changes, ranging from simple hyperplasia to invasive carcinoma. Hyperplasia is an abnormal proliferation of the endometrial glands, and in some cases, it precedes endometrial cancer as a premalignant phase. According to the World Health Organization (WHO) and International Federation of Gynecologic Oncologists (FIGO), hyperplasia is classified as simple or complex, with or without atypia.

Simple hyperplasia is the most common type. It is a benign change that causes thickening of the endometrium, with dilation and an increased number of endometrial glands, but minimal crowding or glandular complexity. Such changes are rarely associated with malignant progression. Complex hyperplasia is characterized by increased endometrial thickness caused by crowding of the glands, which have irregularity, including uterine processes and diminished stromal spaces.

TABLE 91-3

Progression in Endometrial Hyperplasia

TYPE OF HYPERPLASIA	PROGRESSION TO CANCER (%)[41]
Simple, no atypia	1
Complex, no atypia	3
Simple with atypia	8
Complex with atypia	29

Epithelial pseudostratification in two to four layers can occur with a variable amount of mitotic activity. These lesions are associated with a 3% rate of malignant progression.[41] Most of both types of lesions without atypia regress.

Atypical hyperplasia is characterized by an increased number of atypical cells, regardless of whether the gland appears morphologically simple or complex; however, affected glands usually appear complex. Cellular features may include an increased nuclear-to-cytoplasmic ratio, enlargement, nuclear hyperchromatism, and irregular enlargement with prominent nucleoli. If atypia is present in a biopsy or endometrial curettage, the reported risk of finding adenocarcinoma after hysterectomy is 14% to 57%, with an average risk of approximately 25%.[42] Among such cancers, myometrial invasion is common, and up to 20% are grade 2 or 3. Although Pap smear is not a reliable screening test for endometrial cancer, findings on Pap smears known as atypical glandular cells of undetermined significance (AGUS) may be of endometrial origin. Among patients undergoing biopsy for a finding of AGUS on Pap smear, 13% have endometrial cancers, 11% have endometrial hyperplasia, and 7% have squamous lesions; therefore, one-third of women with this finding on Pap smear have a significant endometrial lesion.[43] Table 91-3 lists the risk of progression to malignancy based on the type of hyperplasia seen.

Endometrioid Adenocarcinoma

Adenocarcinomas arising from hypertrophic endometrium or associated with atypical hyperplasia are typically of the endometrioid type (Fig. 91-1). For all of these subtypes, the median age at diagnosis is approximately 65 years. Table 91-4 lists the various types of endometrial carcinomas classified by the International Society of Gynecologic Pathologists (ISGP). Endometrioid adenocarcinomas are the most common type, arising from the endometrium and representing approximately 75% of cases.[44] Villoglandular carcinomas make up approximately 7% of adenocarcinomas. They tend to be of lower grade and lack the anaplasia associated with USC. They otherwise have a similar median age, depth of invasion, and frequency of nodal spread compared with the endometrioid type.[45] Secretory carcinomas are found in only 2% of cases, and tend to be of low grade and well differentiated, with a favorable outcome. Progesterone administration may cause a secretory appearance of atypical

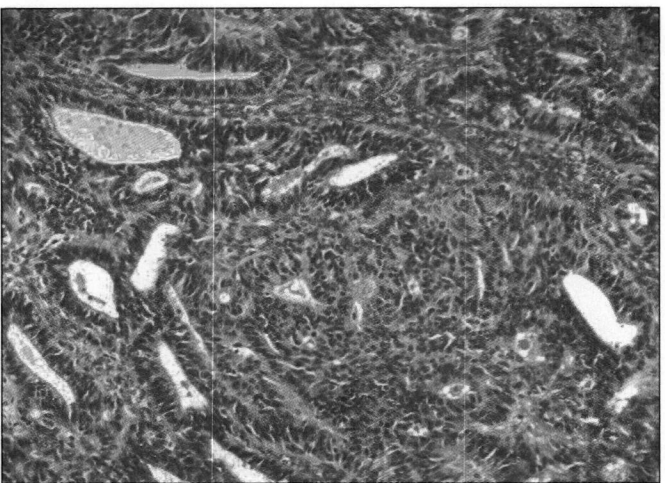

Figure 91-1. Endometrial adenocarcinoma. International Federation of Gynecology and Obstetrics grade 1.

hyperplasia or low-grade adenocarcinoma. Ciliated cell carcinomas are composed primarily of ciliated cells that are typically confined to benign endometrial proliferations, but occasionally form cancers that invade the myometrium.[46] Approximately 25% of endometrial adenocarcinomas show focal squamous differentiation. In the late 1960s, a distinction was made between tumors in which the squamous component appeared well differentiated (adenoacanthoma) and those in which it appeared poorly differentiated (adenosquamous carcinoma). Numerous studies confirmed the significantly better

TABLE 91-4

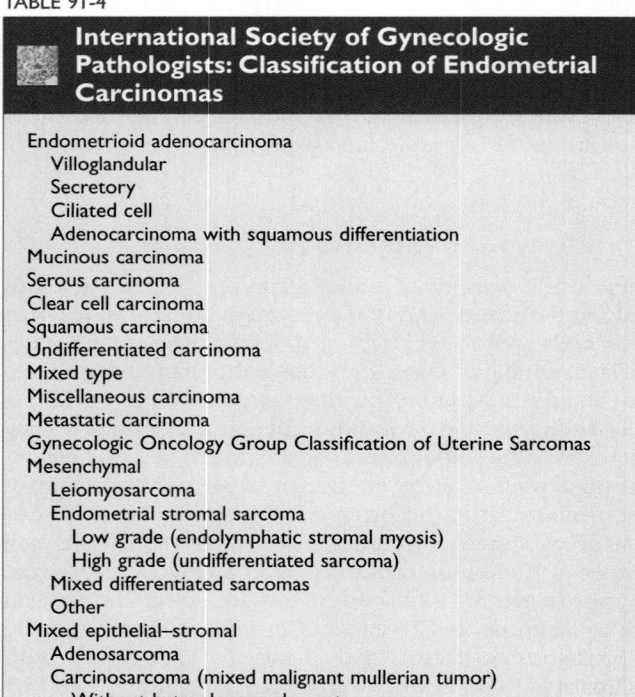

International Society of Gynecologic Pathologists: Classification of Endometrial Carcinomas

Endometrioid adenocarcinoma
  Villoglandular
  Secretory
  Ciliated cell
  Adenocarcinoma with squamous differentiation
Mucinous carcinoma
Serous carcinoma
Clear cell carcinoma
Squamous carcinoma
Undifferentiated carcinoma
Mixed type
Miscellaneous carcinoma
Metastatic carcinoma
Gynecologic Oncology Group Classification of Uterine Sarcomas
Mesenchymal
  Leiomyosarcoma
  Endometrial stromal sarcoma
    Low grade (endolymphatic stromal myosis)
    High grade (undifferentiated sarcoma)
  Mixed differentiated sarcomas
  Other
Mixed epithelial–stromal
  Adenosarcoma
  Carcinosarcoma (mixed malignant mullerian tumor)
    Without heterologous elements
    With heterologous elements

prognosis associated with adenoacanthoma compared with adenosquamous carcinoma. However, in large studies in which the glandular and squamous components were graded separately, differentiation of the squamous component closely paralleled that of the endometrial component. Thus, the prognosis can be predicted by the grade of the glandular component alone. Accordingly, the ISGP and WHO recommend the use of the term *adenocarcinoma with squamous differentiation* to describe these tumors, and grading is based solely on the glandular component.

Adenocarcinomas are further characterized by grade and depth of invasion. Grade 1, or low-grade, lesions are well differentiated; grade 2 lesions are moderately differentiated; and grade 3, or high-grade, lesions are poorly differentiated. Histologic grading according to FIGO uses either architectural patterns or nuclear features. Grade 1 tumors are composed of cells and glands that closely resemble those of normal endometrium and show well-preserved glandular growth patterns, with 5% or less solid growth; grade 2 contains 6% to 50% solid growth; and grade 3 tumors have more than 50% nonsquamous solid growth.[47] Although this system relies predominantly on the architectural pattern of the glands, FIGO recommends that in cases where there is severe nuclear atypia that is inappropriate for the architectural grade, the overall grade of the tumor should be raised by one level. In addition, in cases of serous and clear cell carcinomas, nuclear grading takes precedence. In the nuclear grading system, grade 1 has uniform oval nuclei, with evenly distributed chromatin; grade 3 has large pleomorphic nuclei, with prominent nucleoli and clumped chromatin; and grade 2 is intermediate between these features.[48] Higher grade is associated with myometrial invasion, lymph node metastasis, and a poorer overall prognosis. The Gynecologic Oncology Group (GOG) found that high-grade tumors made up 42% of those with deep myometrial invasion, compared with 7% of tumors with no myometrial invasion.[49] Depth of invasion is determined by measuring the extension of cancer into the myometrium divided by the total width of the myometrium. The depth of myometrial invasion has been categorized by both thirds and halves. For staging purposes, FIGO classifies the depth of invasion as limited to the endometrium, less than one half of the myometrium, or more than one half of the myometrium. Deeper invasion is associated with a higher risk of nodal metastasis.

Serous Carcinoma

USC represents 5% to 10% of endometrial carcinomas (Figs. 91-2 and 91-3). The median age at diagnosis is 63 years.[50] This subtype arises in atrophic endometrium from a putative precursor lesion known as endometrial intraepithelial carcinoma. It is not hormonally mediated. It typically has a uterine growth pattern, with severe nuclear atypia and a high nuclear-to-cytoplasmic ratio. These cancers are considered high grade, and the depth of invasion may not always be great. Morphologic features include marked nuclear pleomorphism, multinucleated

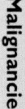

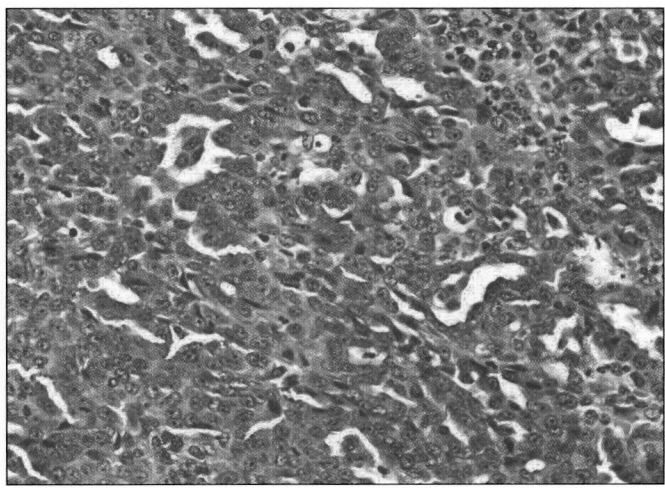

Figure 91-2. Serous carcinoma grade 3, low power.

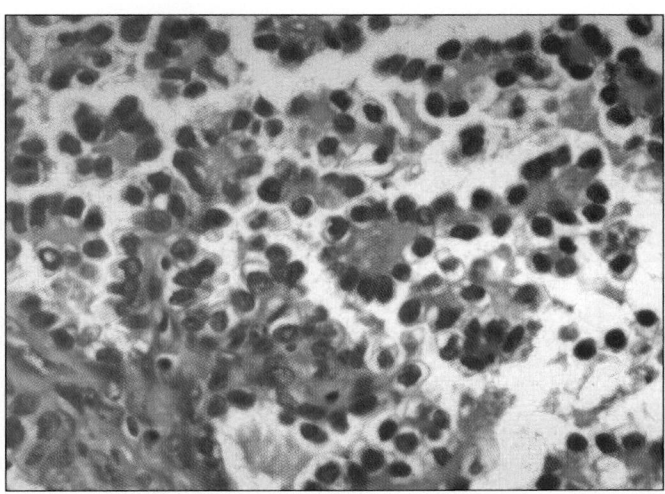

Figure 91-4. Clear cell carcinoma.

cells, hobnail cells, psammoma bodies, uneven uterine borders, and inflammation.[51] Most have lymphovascular invasion, and lymph node metastases are present in 36% of women with no myometrial invasion, 50% with invasion of the inner half, and 40% with invasion of the outer half.[52] These cancers have a high rate of intra-abdominal spread and distant metastases.[53] Because of these features, uterine serous cancers are upstaged postoperatively from clinical stage I/II to stage III/IV in nearly 50% of patients. Survival rates are only 30% to 50%, even for tumors confined to the uterus, and median survival is significantly shorter than for endometrioid carcinoma.

Clear Cell Carcinoma

Carcinomas with clear cell features arise in the uterus, ovary, vagina, and cervix, and have been associated with in utero exposure to the synthetic estrogen diethylstilbestrol (DES), which was prescribed to women during pregnancy

for certain complications between 1940 and 1971. In daughters of women who took this agent, the overall risk of clear cell carcinoma of the gynecologic tract is estimated at 0.1%.[54] Clear cell endometrial cancers account for approximately 5% of adenocarcinomas (Fig. 91-4). The median age at diagnosis is 66 years.[55] Cells form cystic, solid, or tubular cellular patterns, and the cytoplasm appears clear or light pink on staining with hematoxylin and eosin. This cytoplasmic material is glycogen-positive. Nucleic size varies, but a high mitotic count is often present and the cells are generally considered high grade. Although pelvic failures occur in approximately one third of patients postoperatively without adjuvant radiation, unlike serous carcinoma, this subtype has only a 15% rate of intra-abdominal failure. Relapse in the lung, liver, and bone occurs in 25% of patients. The 5-year disease-free survival rate is approximately 40%.[56] The survival rate is 72% for stage I disease and 60% for stage II disease; these rates are more favorable than for serous cancers.[57]

Other Carcinomas (Mucinous, Squamous, Undifferentiated, Mixed, Metastatic)

There are a variety of other relatively rare subtypes of endometrial cancer. Mucinous cancers contain more than 50% cells with periodic acid-Schiff–positive diastase-resistant mucin.[58] These cells have abundant cytoplasmic mucin, and the tumors produce large amounts of mucopolysaccharides. Morphologically similar tumors may occur in other abdominal organs, such as the gastrointestinal tract or ovary, so metastasis should be excluded. For primary cases, the prognosis appears to be similar to that of endometrioid carcinoma. Primary squamous cell cancer of the endometrium is exceedingly rare, reported in approximately 100 cases in the literature. The median age at diagnosis is 67 years.[59] Chronic pyometra may be a predisposing factor, and these are associated with nulliparity. If the cervix is involved, the tumor should be considered a primary cervical cancer; therefore, no stage II squamous carcinomas of the endometrium can be

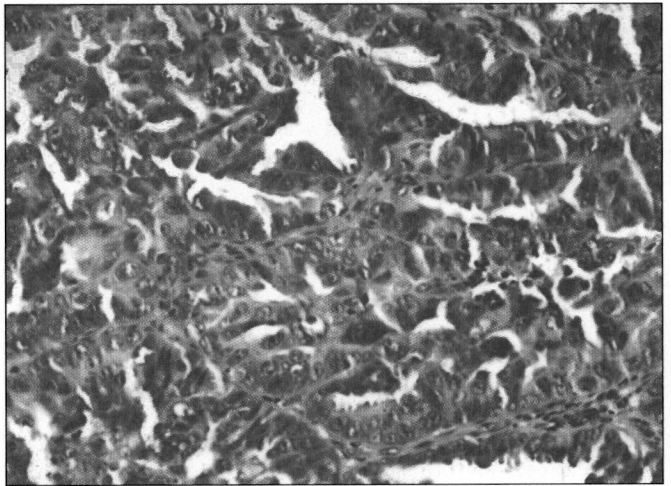

Figure 91-3. Serous carcinoma grade 3, high power.

reported. Survival appears to be similar to that of adeno-carcinoma (80% for stage I disease at 3 years). Undifferentiated carcinomas show no clear glandular or squamous differentiation, and some may be small cell carcinomas. They may stain for epithelial or neurosecretory antigens. Mixed-cell carcinomas are composed of at least 30% each of two or more pure cell types. If serous or undifferentiated components are present, the prognosis is worse than for pure high-grade endometrioid cancers.[60] Other extragenital cancers may metastasize to the endometrium or myometrium. One study found that primary tumors originated in the breast (43%), colon (18%), stomach (11%), pancreas (11%), gallbladder (5%), lung (5%), urinary bladder (3%), or thyroid (2%), or as cutaneous melanoma (3%).[61] Among those, metastatic disease in the uterus was the first indicator of the primary cancer in 25% of cases.

Uterine Sarcoma

Uterine sarcomas arise primarily from the mesenchymal or muscle elements of the uterus. They may be comprised of pure mesenchymal elements or of mixed mesenchymal and epithelial elements. The proposed GOG classification is shown in Table 91-3. The most common types are MMMT, carcinosarcoma, LMS, and ESS. All of the subtypes combined occur rarely, with uterine sarcomas accounting for only 5% of all malignant uterine neoplasms.

Leiomyosarcoma

LMS accounts for approximately 25% of uterine sarcomas, or 1% of malignant uterine neoplasms (Fig. 91-5). The median age at diagnosis is 52 years. Benign leiomyomas occur commonly in the uterus; however, LMS is believed to arise independently, and malignant transformation of a leiomyoma is considered exceedingly rare. LMS is typically a solitary lesion that irregularly permeates the adjacent myometrium, and may show areas of hemorrhage and necrosis. The tumor arises from the myometrium and may be located deep in the uterine wall. Histologically, the tumors are densely cellular and are composed of bundles

of spindle cells. The degree of smooth muscle differentiation is variable. Nuclear and cellular pleomorphism, nuclear hyperchromasia, and multinucleate giant cells are common. To differentiate LMS from benign leiomyoma, the following factors should be considered: patient age, tumor size, gross appearance of the tumor, invasiveness of the tumor margins, vascular invasion, cytologic atypia, tumor cell necrosis, and mitotic activity. In approximately 27% of cases, LMS metastasizes to the lymph nodes, and 50% of cases recur, with lung the most common site.[62]

Endometrial Stromal Sarcoma

Endometrial stromal tumors are usually defined as neoplasms composed of stromal cells similar to those of normal proliferative-phase endometrium. Classically, endometrial stromal tumors have been divided into two categories: benign stromal nodule, if the margins are smooth, and ESS, if the margins are infiltrating (Fig. 91-6). Sarcomas are further subdivided into those with fewer than 10 mitoses per 10 high-power fields (low grade) and those with 10 or more mitoses per 10 high-power fields (high grade).[63] The tumors formerly regarded as high-grade stromal sarcomas are a heterogeneous group, composed partly of tumors made up of endometrial stromal cells, but also of anaplastic tumors composed of tumor cells that show marked cytologic atypia. The latter tumors occur at an older age and are associated with a much worse prognosis. Histologically, they more closely resemble the sarcomatous components of a carcinosarcoma rather than an endometrial stromal tumor. Based on these features, endometrial stromal tumors have been recently reclassified as endometrial stromal nodule, ESS, and undifferentiated uterine sarcoma.[64,65]

ESS is a malignant tumor with infiltrative margins. These tumors are composed of cells similar to those of endometrial stroma. Histologically, the tumor cells are uniform, with scant cytoplasm. A striking feature of many ESS lesions, and the origin of their older name, "endolymphatic stromal myosis," is the serpentine processes of the tumor that infiltrate between muscle fibers and into lymphatic

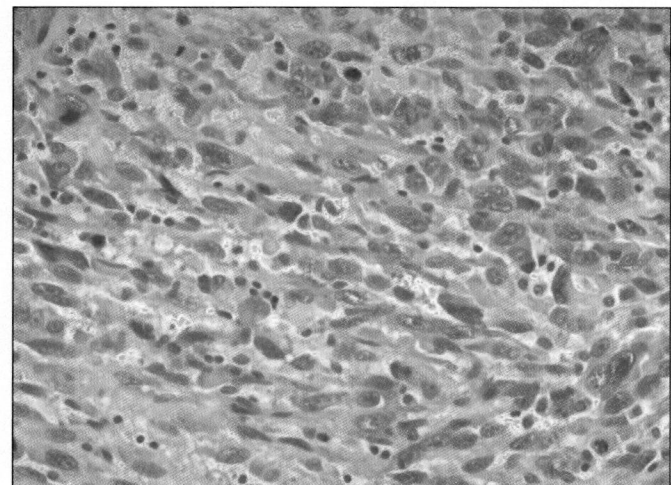

Figure 91-5. Leiomyosarcoma.

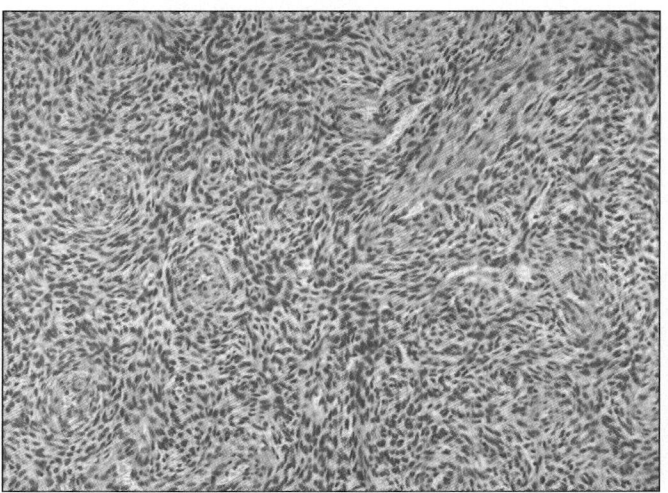

Figure 91-6. Endometrial stromal sarcoma.

spaces. Nuclear atypia is typically mild, and mitotic activity is usually less than 10 per 10 high-power fields. Mitotic count is not a criterion for diagnosis, however. These tumors generally express estrogen and progesterone receptors and are responsive to progesterone therapy.[66] The clinical course is indolent and characterized by long disease-free intervals, although 36% of patients, even with stage I disease, relapse, and 10% die of disease.

Undifferentiated uterine sarcoma is a rare malignant tumor composed of pleomorphic mesenchymal cells that have a high mitotic index and do not resemble the cells of the endometrial stroma. These tumors are found in older women (median age, 58 to 61 years).[67] These tumors behave aggressively, with 55% of patients with disease confined to the uterus having recurrent disease at a median of 5 months, in both the pelvis and the abdomen.[68]

Malignant Mixed Mullerian Tumor (Carcinosarcoma)

MMMT represents approximately 50% of all uterine sarcomas, or 3% of all uterine neoplasms. They occur at a median age of 66 years.[69] These tumors contain mixed epithelial and mesenchymal elements (Fig. 91-7). Adenosarcoma is a tumor with malignant mesenchymal stroma and benign epithelial elements. Carcinosarcomas contain both malignant mesenchymal and epithelial elements, typically adenocarcinoma. The stromal component is usually high grade. The mesenchymal component is classified as either homologous (composed of cell types that are normally found in the uterus, such as ESS, fibrosarcoma, LMS, and undifferentiated sarcoma) or heterologous (composed of cell types that are not normally found in the uterus). Each type accounts for approximately half of cases of MMMT. The heterologous elements are found in association with fully differentiated sarcoma, and include rhabdomyosarcoma, chondrosarcoma, and osteosarcoma, in order of decreasing frequency. Although these tumors are heterogeneous, in general, stage and depth of invasion correlate with prognosis. Other prognostic factors may include extensive tumor, lympho-

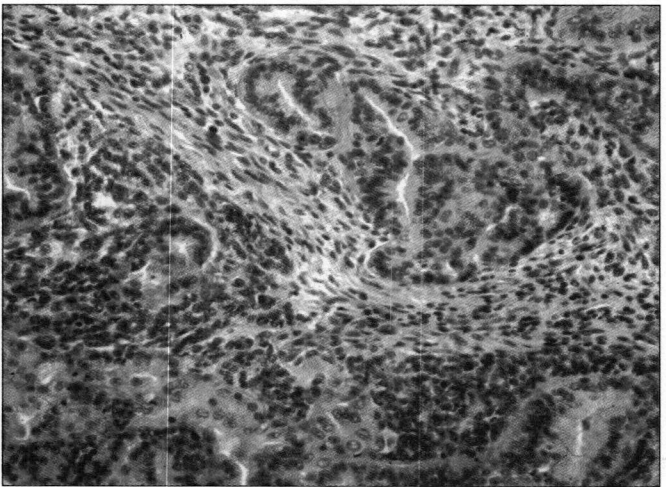

Figure 91-7. Malignant mixed mullerian tumor.

vascular invasion, extrauterine disease, and heterologous elements.[70] Nodal metastases are seen in approximately 35% of cases, and tend to arise from the epithelial component. However, recurrences are often secondary to sarcomatous elements. The overall 5-year survival rate is 40% to 50%.[71]

MOLECULAR PATHOLOGY AND BIOLOGY

Endometrioid Adenocarcinoma

Approximately 57% of endometrial adenocarcinomas express estrogen receptors (ER) and progesterone receptors (PR), whereas 24% are negative for either receptor.[72] Expression correlates with tumor differentiation and stage. Both ER and PR are expressed by approximately 80% of grade 1 cancers and 60% to 70% of grade 2 cancers. For grade 3 cancers, ER is expressed in 46% and PR is expressed in 59%.[73] Expression also differs among histologic types, with much lower levels found in higher-grade histologic types, such as uterine serous compared with endometrioid carcinomas. In patients whose tumors are ER-positive and PR-positive or ER-negative and PR-positive, survival is significantly better than in patients with tumors that are either ER-negative and PR-negative or ER-positive and PR-negative.[74] Some studies also found ER status to be prognostic.[75,76] When tumors metastasize, loss of PR expression is more common than loss of ER expression.[77] In vitro studies show that the PR isoform PRB is downregulated in more poorly differentiated cancers that do not respond to progesterone therapy.[78] For ER isoforms, a higher ratio of ER-beta expression correlates significantly with deeper myometrial invasion and more advanced disease.[79] Genetic analysis of DNA from human endometrial cancers has shown that certain polymorphisms on the ER-alpha gene are present at different frequencies, suggesting that inherited alterations in the ER gene may either predispose to or protect against endometrial cancer.[80] More information about the role of specific steroid-receptor isoforms in uterine tissues and how they are expressed at different stages of disease may lead to the development of selective receptor modulators, potentially improving treatment outcomes.

The endometrial hormonal pathways interact with other molecular pathways, further explicating potential mechanisms for tumorigenesis and progression. The proto-oncogene transmembrane receptor Her2/neu (c-erbB2) is a member of the epidermal growth factor family of receptor tyrosine kinases and is overexpressed in approximately one third of breast cancers. A monoclonal antibody therapy that targets the gene expression has been developed. Her2 is overexpressed in approximately 10% to 20% of endometrial cancers, correlating with higher grade, advanced disease, and loss of ER expression.[81-83] Her2 overexpression is seen in 27% of patients with metastatic disease compared with only 4% with early-stage disease. One study showed that Her2 overexpression correlates with a poorer overall survival and that the use of radiation therapy or chemotherapy in these patients is associated with improved survival.[84] Overexpression of the oncogene p53, found in approximately 15% of endometrial cancers, may also correlate with worse prognosis and predict for recurrence.[85] The finding that p53 is almost never overexpressed in endometrial hyperplasia suggests that this particular mutation occurs late in the course of tumorigenesis.[86]

Serous and Clear Cell Carcinomas

USC and clear cell carcinoma (CCC) have often been studied together, for both clinical outcomes and biologic parameters. Unlike the endometrioid subtype, both subtypes are associated with lack of hormonal dependence and an increase in atrophic endometrium.

Immunohistochemical profiles comparing the endometrioid and USC subtypes for ER, PR, and the expression of p53 and HER2/neu show that USC cancers are usually negative for ER and PR, whereas 80% overexpress p53 and 45% overexpress Her2/neu.[87] Another study found that 80% of USC cancers highly express Her2, and that USC cancer cell lines express Her2 at higher levels than do either breast or ovarian cells.[88] These cell lines are resistant to chemotherapy, but exposure to trastuzumab (Herceptin), the monoclonal antibody that targets Her2, is cytotoxic, suggesting that Herceptin may be a useful therapy for USC cancers.

Overexpression of the p53 oncogene appears to play an important role in the biology of USC cancers, which show significantly higher expression of p53 than do endometrioid subtypes (75% to 85%).[89,90] Unlike the endometrioid subtypes, p53 mutations occur early in USC tumorigenesis. USC cancers and their putative precursor, endometrial intraepithelial carcinoma, both commonly have abnormal p53 overexpression.[91] A p53 mutation is associated with loss of ER and PR expression, and even among USC cancers, confers poorer overall survival.[92]

CCC has a distinctive molecular profile. Similar to USC, it shows low expression of ER and PR, but its immunoreactivity for p53 is significantly lower than that for USC.[93] CCC without serous features is associated with hyperplastic endometrium in 40% of cases. These findings suggest that CCC is a distinct biologic subtype from both USC and endometrioid cancers.

Other molecular markers have been studied for both endometrioid and USC/CCC cancer types. Overexpression of the epidermal growth factor receptor, which occurs in 50% of endometrial cancers, strongly correlates with squamous differentiation,[94] nonendometrial subtypes, and metastasis (76%), and also predicts a poorer survival in patients with endometrioid subtypes.[95] DNA aneuploidy is associated with higher pathologic stage, higher grade, and more frequent lymph node involvement, and is found in most cases of USC and CCC.[96] Metallothioneins are low-molecular-weight proteins that have metastatic potential and are expressed in endometrial carcinomas. They are associated with higher grade, higher stage, and uterine serous subtypes.[97] High levels of cathepsin D protease, another metastatic marker, correlate with high-grade tumors, the USC subtype, positive nodal status, and deep myometrial invasion.[98] Microsatellite instability has

been found in approximately one third of endometrioid carcinomas, but does not correlate well with other prognostic factors.[99] Early use of gene microarrays identified 24 transcripts that distinguish USC from endometrioid cancers, promising to expand the base of knowledge about molecular differences that may lead to targeted therapies.[100] The prognostic or therapeutic usefulness of these markers remains to be determined.

Sarcoma

Little is known about the biology of uterine mesenchymal tumors because of their rarity and heterogeneity. Most studies have combined the different types of sarcomas. Histologic grade is a prognostic factor. Mitotic count also predicts for outcome in some sarcomas.[101] Sarcomas express ER and PR less frequently than carcinomas, with overall ER positivity of 48% and PR positivity of 30%.[102] Most sarcomas do not respond to hormonal therapy. Aneuploidy, which is found in approximately half of sarcomas, and mean S-phase fraction occur more often in higher-stage, more poorly differentiated sarcomas that have a higher mitotic index.[103] The histologic features do not clearly correlate with outcome, and survival rates are similar among the three main subtypes, LMS, MMMT, and ESS.

CLINICAL PRESENTATION AND PATIENT EVALUATION

Most patients (80%) with both carcinomas and sarcomas have abnormal postmenopausal uterine bleeding. Endometrial cancer may also cause menorrhagia or other abnormal bleeding patterns in premenopausal women. Profuse serous or serosanguinous discharge is a presenting symptom in 10% of cases. Sarcomas may cause a rapidly enlarging uterine mass, or may be associated with symptomatic fibroids. The differential diagnosis includes other types of gynecologic cancers, such as cervical or vaginal tumors, and gastrointestinal and bladder cancers.[104] Nonmalignant causes of bleeding or discharge include atrophy, infection, or pyometra; traumatic lesions or foreign bodies; polyps or fibroids (leiomyomas); adenomyosis; and endometriosis. Iatrogenic causes include the use of hormonal medications, hypothalamic depressants, digitalis, phenytoin, and anticoagulants. Systemic diseases that may cause abnormal bleeding include liver disease and coagulation disorders.

These symptoms should be evaluated routinely with pelvic examination and office endometrial biopsy or dilation and curettage. Although Pap smear is not an effective screening or diagnostic test for endometrial cancer, it should be performed to assess cervical pathology. Biopsies are subject to sampling error. If biopsy findings are negative for cancer, but symptoms persist, fractional dilation and curettage should be performed. A biopsy finding of atypical hyperplasia also needs further sampling, because 15% to 25% of patients with this finding have carcinoma.[105] Samples should be taken separately from the cervix and uterus so that an endocervical lesion may be differentiated from a lesion in the lower uterine segment. Biopsy specimens should be obtained from any suspicious masses that are visible in the uterine cavity at the time of the procedure. Sarcomas, especially LMS, may be located submucosally.

Less commonly, patients present with more advanced disease in the absence of uterine bleeding. In this case, symptoms are related to a large tumor mass, and may include pelvic pain, hematuria or hematochezia, rectal obstruction, renal failure as a result of hydronephrosis, and abdominal discomfort and distension. Patients with advanced cases have a pelvic mass on examination. Metastatic disease commonly occurs in the lungs, and there may be associated pulmonary symptoms.

Screening for endometrial cancer should be considered in special populations. Women who take tamoxifen for the treatment for breast cancer have twice the risk of endometrial cancer as the general population. Analysis of NSABP data shows that the average annual hazard rate for endometrial cancer within 5 years of follow-up is 1.2 per 1000 patient-years, with a cumulative hazard rate of 6.3 per 1000 patient-years.[38]

In a randomized study of ultrasonography or office hysteroscopy for endometrial assessment in asymptomatic women using tamoxifen, the sensitivity and specificity of transvaginal ultrasonography for cancer detection were 85% and 100%, respectively. For office hysteroscopy, they were 77% and 92%, respectively.[106] Transvaginal ultrasound detects a high percentage of cases of endometrial thickening. Women who take tamoxifen have a significantly thicker endometrium than those who do not, and this correlates with duration of exposure.[107] However, nearly half of women who have undergone follow-up hysteroscopy and sampling have either a benign or an atrophic endometrium, resulting in a high false-positive rate, even with up to 10 mm of endometrial thickening.[108] Despite concerns about cost-effectiveness, it is reasonable to perform annual pelvic examination and transvaginal ultrasound in women taking tamoxifen, because the benefit of early cancer detection is significant. Hysteroscopy and biopsy may be performed as indicated, based on the findings of these examinations. Women with HNPCC have a 50% lifetime risk of endometrial cancer, which is the most common noncolonic cancer in these families. Although optimal screening protocols in this population have not been established, routine annual screening with pelvic examination and transvaginal ultrasound is recommended.[109] Prophylactic hysterectomy may be considered after childbearing is completed.

LABORATORY AND IMAGING STUDIES

After the pathologic diagnosis is established, a thorough history should be obtained and physical examination should be performed to document signs of local or metastatic disease and to determine risk factors for cancer as well as comorbidities that may affect the patient's ability to tolerate surgery or other therapy. An examination performed under anesthesia may be indicated for patients with apparent locally advanced disease, and at this time, cystoscopy and proctoscopy may be performed to document invasion of the bladder or rectosigmoid colon.

Further evaluation of the gastrointestinal tract, including colonoscopy and upper endoscopy, is indicated for mucinous tumors, which may be of gastrointestinal origin, or those with symptoms related to the upper bowel. Because the lung is a common site of metastasis, a chest x-ray is part of the initial evaluation. Abnormalities seen on chest x-ray should be further evaluated by computed tomography (CT) scan of the chest with contrast. A mammogram should be performed if a screening study has not been performed in the last year. Imaging of the brain is performed only if indicated by history or examination. Patients undergoing surgery also need cardiac evaluation, including an electrocardiogram, and further studies as indicated for surgical clearance.

Routine blood work, including urinalysis, blood counts, liver function tests, electrolyte levels, renal function tests, and bleeding times are obtained for workup and pre-surgical clearance. The tumor marker CA-125 is elevated preoperatively in the serum of approximately 20% of patients with endometrial carcinomas, and is correlated with stage.[110] Elevated CA-125 levels predict for occult extrauterine or metastatic disease.[111]

To assist with preoperative staging and management decisions, imaging of the urogenital tract may include intravenous pyelogram or CT scan of the abdomen and pelvis with contrast. Because endometrial cancer is a surgically staged disease, routine preoperative CT scan is often omitted. In cancers with grade 2 to 3 or high-risk histologic features on biopsy, surgical staging, including nodal sampling, is performed. Therefore, CT scan is not needed to assess the lymph nodes. However, in patients with medically inoperable disease or when more advanced or metastatic disease is suspected, CT scan may be useful to evaluate the extent of abdominopelvic and nodal disease. Magnetic resonance imaging scans improve on the evaluation of myometrial and cervical invasion and may be warranted in patients with medically inoperable disease and in other specific situations.[112] Transvaginal ultrasound is also useful for assessing myometrial invasion and tumor size. Accurate prediction of myometrial invasion by ultrasound compared with pathologic assessment is 70% to 100%.[113,114]

STAGING

In 1988, FIGO instituted a surgical staging system for endometrial cancer. Before this system was introduced, FIGO used a clinical staging system based on the extent of disease within the uterus that could be assessed primarily by physical examination (Table 91-5). The surgical staging system should be used for all patients who undergo hysterectomy for the treatment of endometrial cancer. Because this system requires specific assessment of the adnexa, lymph nodes, and peritoneal cytology, appropriate surgery for endometrial cancer includes total abdominal hysterectomy, bilateral salpingo-oophorectomy, pelvic and para-aortic lymph node sampling, and pelvic washings.

TABLE 91-5

STAGE	DESCRIPTION
International Federation of Gynecology and Obstetrics Staging Systems for Endometrial Cancer	
FIGO 1988 Staging of Carcinoma of the Corpus Uteri	
IA G123	Tumor limited to the endometrium
IB G123	Invasion to less than one half of the myometrium
IC G123	Invasion to more than one half of the myometrium
IIA G123	Endocervical glandular involvement only
IIB G123	Cervical stromal invasion
IIIA G123	Tumor invades serosa and/or adnexa, and/or positive peritoneal cytology
IIIB G123	Vaginal metastases
IIIC G123	Metastases of pelvic and/or para-aortic lymph nodes
IVA G123	Tumor invasion of the bladder and/or bowel mucosa
IVB	Distant metastases, including intra-abdominal and/or inguinal lymph nodes
FIGO 1971 Staging of Corpus Cancer	
I	Confined to the corpus
Ia	Length of the uterine cavity ≤8 cm
Ib	Length of the uterine cavity >8 cm
II	Carcinoma involves the corpus and cervix
III	Carcinoma extends outside the corpus, but not outside the true pelvis (may involve the vaginal wall or parametrium but not the bladder or rectum)
IV	Carcinoma involves the bladder or rectum or extends outside the true pelvis

FIGO, International Federation of Gynecology and Obstetrics.

Biopsy specimens of suspicious nodules in the abdomen or pelvis should be obtained. However, for superficial grade 1 or noninvasive grade 2 cancers, the risk of lymph node involvement is sufficiently low that nodal sampling is sometimes omitted. Surgery may be significantly modified in patients with known metastatic disease, when surgery is used for debulking or palliation of symptomatic disease, in which case thorough staging is not indicated. Generally, the pelvic and para-aortic nodes should be sampled, regardless of whether they appear grossly suspicious. Only 10% of patients with clinical stage I cancer have palpably enlarged pelvic lymph nodes, whereas the risk of pelvic nodal metastasis ranges from 3% to 34%, depending on the grade and depth of invasion.[49] Adequate nodal sampling of the obturator, external iliac, and para-aortic regions suffices. Pathologic assessments included in the staging system are grade, depth of myometrial invasion, peritoneal cytology, cervical invasion, serosal or adnexal involvement, vaginal invasion, and lymph node metastases. The FIGO 1971 clinical staging system is used for patients who are not surgical candidates. Whether the staging is based on surgical or clinical staging systems should be clearly documented. These staging systems may also be used for uterine sarcoma, for which there is no specific system.

In the GOG study of the patterns of spread in surgically staged patients, lymph node involvement strongly correlated with grade and depth of invasion.[49] The risk of pelvic nodal metastasis in patients with clinical stage I disease is less than 10% in all tumors with superficial invasion or invasion of up to two thirds of the myometrium only, regardless of the grade (range 0% to 9%). Tumors invading more than two thirds of the myometrial

depth have a higher risk of pelvic node metastases, depending on the grade. For grade 1, the risk is 11%; for grade 2, it is 19%; and for grade 3, it is 34%.

Furthermore, the grade and depth of invasion are strongly correlated; 58% of grade 3 tumors show deep invasion. Para-aortic nodal metastases are present in 14% of grade 2 deeply invasive tumors and in 23% of grade 3 deeply invasive tumors. Approximately 20% of patients with clinical stage I disease have occult extrauterine disease in the nodes or washings. Downstaging is uncommon. Surgical staging more accurately predicts for survival than clinical staging. In one study, survival for patients with clinical stage I, II, and IV disease were 83%, 64%, and 8%, respectively; survival rates for patients with surgical stage I, II, III, and IV disease were 89%, 100%, 58%, and 24%, respectively.[115]

PROGNOSIS

The most important prognostic factors in endometrial carcinoma are the stage or extent of disease, grade, depth of invasion, and histologic subtype. The prognosis for uterine-confined, stage I disease is excellent, and survival is highly correlated with extrauterine disease. These factors affect the risk of extrauterine spread and recurrence and therefore affect survival.

Stage

The staging system for endometrial cancer reflects the extent of disease, in which stage I disease is confined to the uterus. Stage II disease has extension to the cervix only, is relatively uncommon, and is often reported to occur with stage I. In stage III and IV disease, there is extension beyond the uterus or pelvis. Overall survival rates are approximately 90% for stage I/II disease, 60% for stage III disease, and 25% for stage IV disease.

Histologic Subtype

The most common histologic type, as well as one of the most favorable, is endometrioid adenocarcinoma. Other adenocarcinomas, including uterine serous and CCC, have a much higher propensity for both nodal and extrauterine spread; therefore, their prognosis is much poorer. Squamous carcinomas and undifferentiated subtypes also behave aggressively. Overall survival among patients with endometrioid adenocarcinoma is more than 90%, compared with only 33% for all unfavorable histologies combined.[116] High-grade sarcomas also have a poorer prognosis than endometrioid adenocarcinoma.

Depth of Invasion

Depth of invasion of the myometrium is the most important pathologic feature with respect to lymph node metastasis. Pelvic node metastases are found in 1% of superficial tumors, 5% of tumors with invasion of the inner third of the myometrium, 6% with invasion of the middle third, and 25% with deep invasion of the outer third.[49] Para-aortic nodal metastases are seen in 1%, 3%, 1%, and 17%, respectively. Depth of invasion correlates with grade, and more than half of grade 3 cancers have deep invasion. Although the depth of invasion is commonly recorded by thirds, the FIGO surgical staging system defines invasion as endometrium only, inner half of the myometrium, or outer half of the myometrium.

Grade

Histologic grade is one of the primary predictors of extra-uterine spread. Higher grade is associated with both deeper myometrial invasion and lymph node metastasis. Grade 1 cancers have a 3% risk of pelvic lymph node spread, compared with 9% for grade 2 and 18% for grade 3.[49] Para-aortic nodes are involved in 2% of grade 1 tumors, 5% of grade 2 tumors, and 11% of grade 3 tumors. The presence of both high histologic grade and deep myometrial invasion conveys the highest risk of nodal spread: 34% to the pelvic nodes and 23% to the para-aortic nodes. The correlation is not absolute, however, and 10% of grade 1 tumors show deep invasion, whereas 3% of grade 3 tumors are superficial.

Adnexal Involvement

Only 5% to 6% of surgically staged patients with clinical stage I disease have isolated adnexal involvement.[49] This pathologic finding is associated with a 32% risk of pelvic lymph node metastases, and 23% have para-aortic lymph node spread, compared with only 8% and 5% risk of pelvic or para-aortic nodal spread, respectively, without adnexal involvement.

Positive Peritoneal Cytology

Positive peritoneal washings are often a marker for other extrauterine spread. More than half of patients with positive pelvic washings have adnexal or other areas of pelvic spread of disease. Approximately 10% of patients with FIGO stage I endometrial cancer have positive peritoneal washings. This finding is associated with depth of invasion, high grade, and positive nodes, appearing to place these patients at high risk for recurrence.[117]

In a series of 270 patients with stage I disease, 5% had positive washings, correlating with tumor grade and depth of invasion.[118] Peritoneal cytology was found to predict for survival; however, peritoneal cytology may not identify additional patients whose prognosis is not apparent from grade and depth of invasion.

Lymphovascular Invasion

Lymphovascular invasion is present in 15% of endometrial cancers, conferring a 27% risk of pelvic nodal spread and a 19% risk of para-aortic nodal spread, compared with 7% and 9%, respectively, if the feature is absent.[49] Capillary space invasion correlates with poorer disease-free survival.[119]

Age

Older age is associated with a worse prognosis.[120] Age is also associated with an increased risk of high-risk histology, such as uterine serous type, higher grade, deep invasion, and higher stage, possibly reflecting more aggressive biologic behavior of hormone-independent cancers that occur at a higher median age. However, when endometrial cancers with similar pathologic features are compared, survival rates are not significantly different by age. In patients younger than 60 years of age, the rate is 74%; at 60 to 69 years of age, it is 70%; and at 70 years of age or older, it is 60%.[121]

TREATMENT OF EARLY-STAGE ENDOMETRIAL CANCER

FIGO stage I and II endometrial carcinoma includes tumors that are confined to the uterus or extend to the uterine cervix only. The overall survival rate for these patients is quite good. Five-year overall survival rates of 76% to 100% and 46% to 85% for patients with stage I and II disease, respectively, have been reported (Tables 91-6 and 91-7). Treatment mainly consists of surgical resection, with adjuvant radiation therapy reserved for patients who have risk factors for recurrence. If recurrences occur after early-stage endometrial cancer, they are predominantly local, and the addition of radiation therapy to the management of early-stage endometrial carcinoma has been shown to decrease the rate of local recurrence. Definitive radiation therapy is largely reserved for patients whose disease is medically inoperable or who refuse surgical resection.

TABLE 91-6

Results of Postoperative External Beam Radiation Therapy for Stage I Endometrial Cancer

STUDY	NO. OF PATIENTS	STAGE	RADIATION TECHNIQUE	5-YR LOCAL CONTROL (%)	5-YR OVERALL SURVIVAL RATE (%)
Aalders et al.[135]	263	I	EBRT + ICRT	91	89
Roberts et al.[156]	190	IB, IC, II	EBRT	96 (2-year)	96 (3-year)
Creutzberg et al.[157]	354	I	EBRT	96	81
Sainz de la Cuesta et al.[158]	28	IB	EBRT or ICRT	97	NR
Grigsby et al.[159]	142	I	EBRT, ICRT, or EBRT + ICRT	IA: 92 IB: 86	NR
Irwin et al.[160]	322	I	EBRT, ICRT, or EBRT + ICRT	77 (DFS)	81
Podczaski et al.[161]	148	I/II (occult)	EBRT	95	NR
Weiss et al.[162]	61	IC	EBRT	100	98
Stryker et al.[186]	79	I	EBRT ± ICRT	98	NR
Algan et al.[187]	75	I	EBRT + ICRT	89	83

DFS, disease-free survival; EBRT, external beam radiation therapy; ICRT, Intracavitary radiation therapy; NR, not reported.

Surgery

Surgical Technique

Surgery should be performed with an incision that allows for adequate examination of the abdomen and pelvis as well as retroperitoneal lymph node sampling if indicated. On entry into the abdominal cavity, pelvic washings should be obtained for cytologic analysis. Next, a thorough inspection of all peritoneal surfaces should be performed, and biopsy should be performed on any suspicious lesions. Before the uterus is removed, the fallopian tubes should be clamped or occluded with clips to prevent retrograde spillage of tumor. Extrafascial hysterectomy with bilateral salpingo-oophorectomy may then be completed. The specimen may be bivalved in the operating room, away from the surgical field, and examined to determine the depth of myometrial invasion of tumor, or in the pathology department as part of frozen-section evaluation. In cases of deep myometrial invasion, grade 2 or 3 disease, or obvious extrauterine tumor, pelvic and para-aortic lymph nodes should be sampled.

For selected patients who are at high risk for perioperative complications and whose tumors appear clinically confined to the uterus, vaginal hysterectomy may be an alternative.[122] Although this approach may offer reduced surgical morbidity, it has several disadvantages. A vaginal approach may make removal of the ovaries difficult. In addition, peritoneal cytology, thorough abdominal exploration, and lymphadenectomy are not feasible. To overcome these obstacles, some advocate laparoscopically assisted vaginal hysterectomy combined with laparoscopic lymphadenectomy.[123] The laparoscopic surgery consists of initial laparoscopic examination of the abdominal cavity followed by sampling of the para-aortic and pelvic lymph nodes through the same incisions. The hysterectomy may be performed vaginally, with laparoscopic assistance, to ensure ovarian removal. The procedure is converted to an open laparotomy if the laparoscopy proves to be too difficult or inadequate, or if excessive blood loss occurs. Approximately 80% to 90% of laparoscopic resections are successful and do not require conversion.[124] Although laparoscopy increases the total time of operation, the postsurgical hospital stay is shorter.[125] Although rates of complications, lymph node counts, recurrence, and survival rates are reportedly equivalent compared with traditional total abdominal hysterectomy, the technique has yet to be validated.[126-129] Some have reported increased need for blood transfusion

TABLE 91-7

Results of Postoperative External Beam Radiation Therapy for Stage II Endometrial Cancer

STUDY	NO. OF PATIENTS	STAGE	RADIATION TECHNIQUE	5-YR LOCAL CONTROL (%)	5-YR OVERALL SURVIVAL RATE (%)
Greven et al.[119]	26	II	EBRT ± ICRT	88	72
Lanciano et al.[165]	70	II	EBRT ± ICRT	87	70
Eltabbakh et al.[166]	48	II	EBRT ± ICRT	94	92
Sartori et al.[167]	133	II	EBRT	89	80
Onsrud et al.[229]	40	II	EBRT + ICRT	82	85
Grigsby et al.[159]	90	II	ICRT ± EBRT	91	78
Greven et al.[164]	24	II	EBRT	94	NR

DFS, disease-free survival; EBRT, external beam radiation therapy; ICRT, Intracavitary radiation therapy; NR, not reported.

ADJUVANT RADIATION THERAPY FOR EARLY-STAGE ENDOMETRIAL CANCER

One of the most controversial aspects of clinical management of endometrial cancer involves the use of adjuvant postoperative radiation therapy for stage I disease, particularly determining who benefits from it and who may safely avoid it. The recommendations for adjuvant radiation therapy are influenced by the risk of nodal metastases and the rate of vaginal recurrence. According to a Gynecologic Oncology Group (GOG) pathologic study, patients with deep myometrial invasion and grade 2 or 3 tumors have a 19% to 34% risk of pelvic lymph node metastasis.[49] The risk is increased by positive peritoneal cytology, location in the lower uterine segment or cervix, adnexal involvement, and capillary space invasion. The risk of vaginal recurrence after surgery alone is greater with grade 2 or 3 histology, deep myometrial invasion, lymphovascular space invasion, large tumor size, location in the lower uterine segment or cervix, and close or positive margins. Adjuvant radiation is extremely effective at preventing pelvic and vaginal recurrence, but is associated with an increased risk of late side effects. It can also be argued that radiation therapy for isolated vaginal recurrence is relatively effective salvage treatment and thus may be reserved for tumors that recur.

Although three randomized trials have addressed the question of postoperative radiation in early-stage disease, all have been criticized. All three trials entered patients that were predominantly at low or intermediate risk for recurrence. The Post-Operative Radiation Therapy in Endometrial Cancer (PORTEC) study excluded high-risk patients from eligibility, including those with high-grade or deeply invasive tumors.[157] In the Norwegian Radium Hospital (NRH) trial, 50% of the patients entered had stage IB grade 1 or 2 adenocarcinomas, and only 18% had stage IC grade 3 tumors.[155] In GOG 99, only 18% of patients entered had grade 3 disease, and 20% had deep myometrial invasion (outer one third).[156] Two trials (NRH and PORTEC) did not include surgical lymph node staging. Although GOG 99 did require surgical staging, the median number of lymph nodes recovered was reportedly relatively low. The therapeutic benefit of nodal sampling and its role in reducing pelvic recurrence is controversial. Therefore, all three randomized trials addressing the role of adjuvant radiation in early stage endometrial cancer included a preponderance of intermediate risk patients, diluting the ability to detect a benefit in the patients at highest risk for pelvic recurrence, those with high grade and deep myometrial invasion. In addition, none of these trials has adequately assessed the benefit of adjuvant radiation after comprehensive surgical staging. Not surprisingly, no overall survival benefit for adjuvant radiation has been reported in these trials. GOG 99 showed a significantly improved 2-year progression-free interval in the adjuvant radiation arm ($P = 0.004$), and a 3-year overall survival of 96% in the radiation arm versus 89% in the observation arm ($P = 0.09$).

What is not controversial is that adjuvant radiation has been consistently shown to significantly reduce the pelvic and vaginal recurrence rates in stage I endometrial cancer patients. In the NRH trial (in which all patients received vaginal brachytherapy and were randomized to pelvic radiation or no further treatment), the vaginal and pelvic recurrence rate in the observation arm was 6.9% compared with 1.9% in the radiation arm ($P = 0.01$). The PORTEC trial reported locoregional recurrences rates of 14% in the observation arm compared to 4% in the radiation arm ($P < 0.001$). GOG 99 reported a crude vaginal and pelvic recurrence rate 8.5% in the observation arm and 1.5% in the radiation arm (three patients, two of whom refused radiation after randomization). When risk factors for recurrence were examined in the NRH trials, the greatest benefit of adjuvant radiation was for patients with high-grade and deeply invasive tumors.

Complications are increased by the use of both surgery and pelvic radiation. The NRH reported a crude grade 3 or 4 complication rate of 0.7% after postoperative vaginal brachytherapy alone (one fistula and one urethral stricture), and 0.7% after postoperative pelvic radiation and brachytherapy (including one death due to postoperative infection after a bowel obstruction, and one bladder necrosis). The PORTEC trial included no vaginal brachytherapy, and reported treatment related complications (grade 1 to 4) of 25% in the radiation arm compared to 6% in the observation arm, of which 68% overall were grade 1 toxicities. Grade 3 toxicity occurred in seven patients (0.09%), six of whom received radiation therapy. Grade 4 toxicity occurred in one patient from the radiation arm who had Crohn's disease, therefore should not have been offered adjuvant irradiation.

Based on the patterns of nodal metastases and patterns of recurrence, a management algorithm has been developed for the use of postoperative radiation therapy stage I and II endometrial cancer patients. A multidisciplinary approach is recommended, involving gynecologic oncologists and radiation oncologists in the patients' care. Low risk patients have a sufficiently small risk of nodal or vaginal recurrence that they require no adjuvant therapy, including stage IA grade 1 to 2 and stage IB grade 1. The recurrence pattern in intermediate-risk patients is predominantly vaginal. These patients may be offered observation vs. vaginal brachytherapy alone after a discussion of the risks and benefits of both approaches and the salvage rates after recurrence. This category includes stage IA, grade 3, stage IB grade 2 or 3, and stage IC, grade 1 or 2. The recurrence pattern for high-risk patients includes both vaginal and pelvic relapses; therefore they should be offered pelvic radiation with or without vaginal brachytherapy. This category includes stage IC, grade 3 and stage II. Vaginal brachytherapy in addition to pelvic radiation is considered for stage II patients (those with extension to the cervix) unless they have undergone a radical hysterectomy and margins are widely negative, and for some stage IC grade 3 patients, including those with large tumors (>4 cm) in the lower uterine segment or extensive lymphovascular invasion. The daily fraction size for vaginal brachytherapy when given in combination with external beam pelvic irradiation should not exceed 500 cGy. Any patient with very close or positive margins postoperatively should be offered vaginal brachytherapy at a minimum. Patients who have not undergone an adequate pelvic lymph node sampling (several nodes from each side of the pelvis) should be offered pelvic irradiation, even if they have only intermediate risk features.

LAPAROSCOPIC SURGERY FOR ENDOMETRIAL CANCER

Total abdominal hysterectomy and bilateral salpingo-oophorectomy, with lymph node sampling in selected patients, is the standard surgical approach for management of early endometrial cancer. While vaginal hysterectomy has been utilized in women at high risk for perioperative morbidity, the technique does not allow for adequate peritoneal exploration, or for lymphadenectomy. However, laparoscopically assisted vaginal hysterectomy may be combined with laparoscopic lymph node sampling to provide a means of adequate staging, as well as to potentially decrease postoperative stay. While laparoscopic-assisted vaginal hysterectomy may be a technically feasible option for surgical management, long-term data on recurrence and survival have yet to be characterized by randomized controlled clinical trials.

and increased operative times for the laparoscopic approach as well as a small number of deaths directly related to complications associated with laparoscopy. Vaginal cuff recurrence associated with laparoscopically assisted vaginal hysterectomy has also been reported.[130] A GOG study is currently accruing patients to a large prospective randomized trial to compare the abdominal and laparoscopic approaches for the management of endometrial cancer.

For patients with disease spread outside of the uterus, more aggressive surgical options exist. Radical hysterectomy, with removal of the uterus, cervix, parametria, and upper vagina, may be an option for those with disease involving the cervix.[131] Fewer than 10% of patients have stage IV disease.[132] Although overall survival for these patients is less than 10%, aggressive surgical cytoreduction may improve survival.[133-135]

Surgical removal of the uterus provides a therapeutic benefit and is important for accurate staging. Surgical staging can result in upstaging in 12% of patients with stage I disease and 27% with stage II disease as well as downstaging in 59% of patients with stage II disease, compared with preoperative clinical staging.[136] In addition, surgical staging allows for full evaluation of histologic grade. Histologic grade based on the biopsy specimen differs from the histologic grade based on the surgical specimen after hysterectomy in more than 20% of cases.[137,138] Surgical staging is also vital for assessing the depth of myometrial invasion and determining the presence of lymphovascular invasion, all of which are critical in guiding adjuvant therapy.

Surgical Staging of Lymph Nodes

Extended surgical staging, including sampling of the pelvic and para-aortic lymph nodes, may be performed at the time of the surgery. When the tumor is limited to the uterine corpus, occult metastases to the lymph nodes most frequently occur to the external iliac and obturator lymph node chains.[139] Spread to the common iliac lymph nodes is more common when there is cervical extension of the primary disease. Isolated involvement of the para-aortic lymph nodes can occur, although it is uncommon without pelvic lymph node spread. Lymph node metastases can significantly alter the treatment plan, and removal of the lymph nodes has a strong role in improving staging.[140] However, lymphadenectomy has not been shown to improve survival, other than in small retrospective studies.[139,141] A review of more than 9000 women with endometrial cancer who were registered into the National Cancer Institute SEER database showed that the 5-year relative survival of 2831 women with stage I endometrial cancer who underwent sampling of the pelvic lymph nodes was nearly identical to that of 6363 women with stage I disease who did not undergo lymph node sampling.[142]

Risk factors for metastases to clinically uninvolved lymph nodes include myometrial invasion to the outer third of the myometrium, involvement of the lymphovascular space, involvement of the cervix, and high-grade histology. Patients with stage I carcinomas without these adverse risk factors have histologically involved lymph nodes less than 10% of the time, and lymph node sampling may be omitted in these cases.[143,144] In a nonrandomized prospective trial of 332 patients with endometrial carcinoma who did not have significant risk factors for lymph node metastases, treatment with hysterectomy and adjuvant postoperative vaginal brachytherapy alone without lymphadenectomy resulted in a 30-year disease-free survival rate of 96.7%.[145] The presence of any of these risk factors can increase the risk of pelvic or para-aortic lymph node involvement to 14% to 31%, and sampling of the pelvic and para-aortic lymph nodes to allow for complete pathologic staging is indicated.[146,147] To identify patients who are at high risk for lymph node involvement, frozen-section examination of the uterine specimen may be performed at the time of surgery to determine the grade, depth of invasion, and presence of lymphovascular invasion.

Surgery as a Single Modality

Several series examined the outcomes of patients with stage I/II endometrial cancer who underwent hysterectomy without adjuvant treatment, listed in Table 91-8. Berchuck and associates[148] reviewed a series of 354 patients with stage I/II endometrial adenocarcinoma from Duke University who underwent postsurgical surveillance.

Twelve percent of patients had recurrent disease. Of the patients with recurrence, 27% had isolated vaginal recurrences, 27% had pelvic recurrences with vaginal or abdominal involvement, 29% had pelvic recurrences with other distant sites, 10% had isolated lung recurrences, and 7% had recurrences at other distant sites. Another study from the University of Alabama–Birmingham reviewed 613 patients with stage I endometrial carcinoma who underwent primary surgery.[149] The 5-year overall survival rate was 98%, and the 5-year disease-free survival rate was 93%. For patients with stage IB disease, 99% did not receive adjuvant treatment and only 5% of those patients had recurrent disease. All patients who had a recurrence within the pelvis or vagina underwent successful salvage treatment with radiation therapy. For patients with stage IC disease, 69% did not receive adjuvant therapy.

TABLE 91-8

Results of Surgery Alone for Early-Stage Endometrial Carcinoma

STUDY	NO. OF PATIENTS	STAGE	5-YR LOCAL CONTROL (%)	5-YR OVERALL SURVIVAL RATE (%)
Kilgore et al.[141]	74	IA-IC	NR	98
Berchuck et al.[148]	354	I/II	93	NR
Straughn et al.[149]	374	IB/IC	93	98
Chen[150]	18	I	100	100
Larson et al.[151]	199	I–II	97	92
Orr et al.[263]	61	IA	100	100
Roberts et al.[156]	200	IB, IC, II	88 (2-year PFS)	89 (3-year)
Creutzberg et al.[157]	361	I	86 (DFS)	85
Sainz de la Cuesta et al.[158]	58	IB	95	NR
Irwin et al.[160]	228	I	93	90
Podczaski et al.[161]	152	I/II	93	NR
Sartori et al.[167]	70	II	81	76

DFS, disease free survival; NR, not reported; PFS, progression-free survival.

Recurrence was seen in only 8% of those patients. A small prospective series of 33 patients with stage I endometrial carcinoma who had poor prognostic features, including deep myometrial invasion or histologic grade 3 tumors, had surgery alone as primary treatment for endometrial cancer.[150] All 18 patients who had disease confined to the uterus were without evidence of disease at their latest follow-up. However, 73.3% of patients (11 of 15) with spread beyond the uterus had a recurrence. Larson and associates[151] reviewed 207 women with uterine-confined endometrial carcinoma who underwent surgery without adjuvant radiation therapy. Forty-five percent were considered to be in a low-risk group, with grade 1 tumors and invasion through less than 50% of the myometrium. The 5-year recurrence-free survival rate was 95% in these patients. In 47% of patients with additional risk factors, but histologically confirmed negative nodes, the 5-year recurrence-free survival rate was 89%.

A factor that favors the use of surgery only in these patients is the high rate of salvage for recurrences. Patients who have a recurrence after surgery alone often undergo successful salvage treatment, with external beam radiation therapy to the pelvis, vaginal brachytherapy, or most commonly, a combination of both. The 5-year disease-free survival rate after salvage radiation therapy is 62% to 92% for these patients.[152,153] The long-term complication rate is 15% after salvage radiation therapy in patients with grade 2 or 3 disease.[154]

External Beam Radiation Therapy

Endometrial carcinoma is a radiosensitive tumor, and the addition of radiation can result in very high rates of locoregional control. Adverse risk factors, such as extension beyond the corpus to the uterine cervix, deep myometrial invasion, or high-grade histology, significantly increase the risk of locoregional recurrence after surgery alone. In these patients, adjuvant radiation therapy has been used successfully to significantly reduce the risk of local recurrence. In addition, radiation has been used with some success as primary treatment of patients who are poor surgical candidates, those with medically inoperable disease, and those who refuse surgical removal of the uterus.

Postoperative External Beam Radiation Therapy for Stage I Disease

Several randomized studies have explored the benefit of adjuvant external beam radiation therapy (see Table 91-6). A study by Aalders and associates[155] randomized 540 patients with stage I endometrial adenocarcinoma who underwent hysterectomy and received 60 Gy postoperative radiation delivered via intravaginal radium implants to receive either no further treatment or an additional 40 Gy to the pelvis via external beam radiation therapy. The results showed a significant reduction in the 5-year local recurrence rate in the group receiving pelvic radiation (1.9% vs. 6.9%, P < 0.01); however, no survival advantage was seen because of an increase in the rate of distant metastases in the group receiving additional radiation therapy. Subgroup analysis showed that patients who had the greatest reduction in local recurrence rates were those with grade 3 tumors as well as those with more than 50% myometrial invasion.

GOG protocol 99 randomized 390 patients with stage IB or IC or occult stage IIA or IIB endometrial cancer to treatment with surgery alone vs. surgery with 50.4 Gy postoperative external beam radiation therapy.[156] Most patients had stage IB (60%) and grade 1 or 2 disease (80%). Median follow-up was 56 months. The results showed a 2-year progression-free interval rate of 96% in the irradiated patients compared with 88% for patients in the observation arm (P = 0.004). Importantly, all patients in this study were required to undergo surgical lymph node staging, and the benefit in progression-free survival was seen, even in patients who had pathologically uninvolved lymph nodes. In addition, although 17 patients in the observation arm had failure in the pelvis or vagina, only 3 patients in the radiation arm had locoregional failure and 2 of those 3 did not actually receive radiation treatment.

Although preliminary 3-year overall survival was higher in the radiation arm compared with the observation arm (96% vs. 89%), this difference was not statistically significant ($P = 0.09$), largely because of the high rate of salvage in patients who had a recurrence.

Another prospective randomized trial supporting the use of adjuvant radiation for early-stage endometrial cancer was conducted by the Post-Operative Radiation Therapy in Endometrial Cancer (PORTEC) Study Group in the Netherlands.[157] Only patients with intermediate-risk stage I endometrial carcinoma were enrolled. Patients who were eligible had grade 1 tumors with 50% or more myometrial invasion, grade 2 tumors with any depth of invasion, or grade 3 tumors with less than 50% myometrial invasion. Treatment consisted of total abdominal hysterectomy and bilateral salpingo-oophorectomy (TAH-BSO), with or without external beam radiation (46 Gy given as 2 Gy daily) delivered to the whole pelvis after surgery. Overall, 715 patients were randomized to receive postoperative radiation therapy vs. no further treatment. Patients were followed for a median of 52 months. The 5-year local and regional recurrence rate was 4% in the group receiving postoperative radiation therapy compared with 14% in the group undergoing no further treatment ($P < 0.001$). The overall incidence of distant metastasis was similar in both groups (8% vs. 7% for the radiation and observations arms, respectively). Despite this improvement in locoregional control, there was no difference in overall survival, again largely due to the high rate of salvage for patients who had a recurrence. The 5-year overall survival rate was 81% in the radiation therapy group compared with 85% in the observation group ($P = 0.31$). The rate of death of endometrial cancer was also similar between the two groups (9% vs. 6% for the radiation therapy group and the observation group, respectively; $P = 0.37$). On multivariate analysis, the only factors predicting for locoregional recurrence were patient age and the postoperative radiation therapy. Histologic grade and depth of myometrial invasion both showed a trend toward predicting recurrence; however, neither reached statistical significance. In terms of patterns of failure, 75% (30 of 40) of patients who had a local recurrence had that recurrence within the vaginal vault. An increase in late toxicity was associated with radiation treatment. Twenty-five percent of patients receiving radiation therapy had grade 1 to 4 late toxicity compared with 6% of the observation group ($P < 0.001$). However, only 7 patients had grade 3 toxicity, and 1 patient who had Crohn's disease had grade 4 gastro-intestinal toxicity.

Many retrospective series examined the efficacy of postoperative radiation therapy in stage I endometrial cancer. In one series, 124 patients with stage IB endometrial carcinoma were reviewed at Massachusetts General Hospital.[158] All patients underwent hysterectomy, and 62 patients did not receive any adjuvant therapy. Only 3% (4 of 124) of the patients had a recurrence. One of the four patients who had a relapse had received adjuvant therapy, and that patient had a grade 3 tumor. In another retrospective series from Washington University, 858 patients with clinical stage I endometrial cancer were treated with TAH-BSO and radiation therapy.[159] The study included a wide variety of radiation techniques, including external beam radiation therapy and intracavitary brachytherapy as well as both preoperative and postoperative radiation, and included patients treated over a long period. The 5-year progression-free survival rate was 92% for patients with stage IA disease and 86% for patients with stage IB disease.

A series from Princess Margaret Hospital compared 228 patients who underwent surgery alone for stage I endometrial carcinoma with 217 patients who received adjuvant external beam radiation therapy with intracavitary boost and 97 patients who received adjuvant external beam radiation therapy only.[160] Overall, local control was the same among the three groups (93% to 95%). However, patients receiving radiation were more likely to have more than 50% myometrial invasion and grade 3 tumors. Another series reviewed 300 patients with endometrial cancer confined to the uterus who underwent hysterectomy.[161] Patients with high-risk features for local recurrence received adjuvant radiation therapy. Treatment with radiation resulted in a pelvic control rate of 95%, and recurrences were more likely to be distant than local. The use of radiation therapy correlated with patient prognosis. A smaller series from the University of Chicago reviewed the outcomes of women with stage IC endometrial carcinoma who were treated with external beam radiation therapy to the whole pelvis without the addition of intracavitary brachytherapy.[162] No patient had local recurrence, and the 5-year disease-free and overall survival rates were 87% and 98%, respectively.

For patients who are good candidates for postoperative radiation, the interval between the completion of surgery and the initiation of radiation appears to significantly affect local control. In a retrospective study by Ahmad and colleagues,[163] patients with endometrial cancer who were treated with postoperative radiation had a significantly decreased 5-year disease-specific survival from 89% to 81% ($P < 0.005$ with multivariate analysis) when the interval between surgery and radiation was longer than 6 weeks compared to less than 6 weeks. In addition, an increased surgery-to-radiation interval showed a trend toward worsened local control (88% for interval < 6 weeks vs. 84% for interval > 6 weeks; $P = 0.06$ with multivariate analysis).

Postoperative Radiation Therapy for Stage II Disease

Cervical invasion in endometrial cancer results in an increased risk of local recurrence, particularly at the vaginal cuff. In the setting of known cervical extension, wider resection, such as a radical hysterectomy, is often performed at the time of surgery. Often, occult cervical involvement is seen only on pathologic examination of the surgical specimen. In either case, postoperative radiation therapy is usually indicated to reduce the risk of local recurrence.

Aside from the inclusion of patients with occult stage IIA or IIB disease in the GOG 99 trial, there are no randomized trials that specifically address the role of adjuvant radiation therapy in patients with stage II endometrial carcinoma. Nevertheless, several retrospective series support its use in these patients (see Table 91-7). Greven and Olds[164] reported a 5-year overall survival rate of 86% for patients with stage II disease treated with surgery and adjuvant radiation. Lanciano and associates[165] reviewed 184 patients with stage II carcinoma of the endometrium who received a variety of treatments, including TAH-BSO with preoperative radiation therapy, postoperative radiation therapy, or both, or who received radiation therapy alone or radical hysterectomy alone. The overall 5-year disease-free survival and overall survival rates were 79% and 70%, respectively. The only predictors of recurrence on multivariate analysis were histologic subtype and grade. There was no difference in disease-free survival on subgroup analysis with respect to the timing of radiation to surgery. In a series at the University of Vermont, 48 women with stage II endometrial carcinoma were treated with TAH followed by pelvic external beam radiation therapy, vaginal cuff radiation, or radical hysterectomy alone.[166] The 5-year overall survival rate was 92%, and the 5-year disease-free survival rate was 90%. None of the 31 patients treated with both external beam radiation therapy and vaginal cuff boost or with radical hysterectomy had a recurrence. Seventeen percent of patients who received total abdominal hysterectomy with only pelvic radiation or vaginal cuff radiation had a local recurrence. The authors concluded that the use of both pelvic external beam radiation therapy and vaginal cuff radiation was warranted in this group of patients. Sartori and associates[167] reviewed 203 patients with stage IIA and IIB endometrial carcinoma, among whom 66% underwent simple hysterectomy and 34% underwent radical hysterectomy. Adjuvant radiation was delivered to 59% of patients with stage IIA disease and 73% of patients with stage IIB disease. Overall survival was better in patients undergoing radical hysterectomy (10-year overall survival 74% vs. 94%; $P < 0.05$) compared with simple hysterectomy. Overall survival did not differ between the two treatment groups (10-year overall survival 73% vs. 75% for irradiated patients and observation patients, respectively). However, the overall recurrence rate was lower in patients receiving adjuvant radiation (11.3% vs. 18.6%).

Preoperative Radiation

An alternative approach to postoperative radiation therapy for early-stage carcinoma is the administration of radiation therapy before surgical resection of the uterus, via external beam radiation therapy, brachytherapy, or a combination. Preoperative radiation has the potential advantages of sterilizing the tumor before surgery and increasing the ease of resection by decreasing tumor bulk, particularly in patients with extensive involvement of the uterine cervix. There are no randomized studies comparing the relative efficacy of preoperative radiation therapy with postoperative radiation; however, several retrospective studies indicate that preoperative radiation is a reasonable option for patients with early-stage endometrial cancer (Table 91-9). One retrospective study of patients with stage I endometrial carcinoma compared treatment with hysterectomy alone with hysterectomy and preoperative radiation with cesium implants.[168] The 5-year disease-free survival rates were similar in the two groups (94% vs. 91%); however, the treatment groups were unbalanced. Patients receiving preoperative radiation were more likely to have adverse prognostic features that placed them at higher risk for local recurrence. A study from the Mallinckrodt Institute of Radiology reviewed the results of 90 patients with stage II endometrial cancer, most of whom were treated with a combination of preoperative external beam radiation therapy and intracavitary low-dose-rate brachytherapy.[169] The 5- and 10-year disease-free survival rates for these patients were 78% and 75%, respectively. Bruckman and colleagues[170] reported the results of 40 patients with stage II endometrial cancer treated with 40 Gy external beam radiation therapy with an additional 40 mgh Ra Eq radiation delivered via intracavitary brachytherapy followed by surgery. In these patients, the 5-year relapse-free survival rate was 78% and the 5-year overall survival rate was 80%. Overall, for stage I or II disease, the addition of preoperative radiation resulted in a 5-year disease-free survival rate of 80% to 88% and a 5-year overall survival rate of 82% to 95%.[171-173]

Grigsby and colleagues[159] reported a decrease in progression-free survival with doses of less than 3500 mgh Ra Eq delivered via intracavitary cesium implants. This decrease was greatest for high-grade tumors, although doses greater than 3500 mgh Ra Eq resulted in equivalent results (5-year progression-free survival rate of 87%) for all grades. The results of these retrospective studies of preoperative radiation therapy are similar to historical results for patients with early-stage endometrial cancer

TABLE 91-9

Results of Preoperative Radiation Therapy for Early-Stage Endometrial Cancer

STUDY	NO. OF PATIENTS	STAGE	RADIATION TECHNIQUES	5-YR DISEASE-FREE SURVIVAL RATE (%)	5-YR OVERALL SURVIVAL RATE (%)
Grigsby et al.[159]	685	I	ICRT ± postop EBRT	96	88
Sause et al.[168]	112	I	ICRT	94	NR
Bruckman et al.[170]	40	II	ICRT ± EBRT	100 (LC)	80
Ritcher et al.[284]	161	I	EBRT	NR	95
Reisinger et al.[285]	30	II	EBRT ± ICRT	97 (LC)	69
Higgins et al.[171]	74	II	EBRT ± ICRT	88	NR
Baram et al.[172]	109	IB	EBRT	91	72

EBRT, external beam radiation therapy; ICRT, intracavitary radiation therapy; LC, local control; NR, not reported.

treated with hysterectomy followed by adjuvant radiation. Preoperative radiation is a viable option for the treatment of patients with stage I/II disease; however, care must be taken to deliver adequate doses, particularly in patients with risk factors for recurrence, such as high-grade disease or deep myometrial invasion.

Postoperative Radiation Therapy for High-Risk Histology

Several histologic subtypes of endometrial carcinoma have a significantly higher risk of extrauterine spread and a greater propensity for local recurrence, most notably, USC and CCC. These histologic subtypes have shown a propensity for distant spread, and when compared with other stage-matched endometrial carcinomas, they have significantly worse outcomes. The propensity of USC to spread can be seen even without definitive evidence of local invasion. Lymph node metastases can be seen in more than 35% of patients with USC who do not have evidence of myometrial invasion on pathologic examination. Patients with stage I/II USC have a recurrence rate of 38% compared with 22% for CCC and 20% for grade 3 adenocarcinoma.[173] Survival is also worse for these variant histologies, with an estimated 5-year overall survival rate of 32% to 44% for patients with USC and a 5-year overall survival rate of 59% to 72% for those with CCC.[174]

Because of the probability of intraperitoneal spread with USC and CCC, the use of whole-abdominal irradiation has been explored in several studies. At Stanford University, eight patients with stage I or II USC or CCC were treated with adjuvant whole-abdominopelvic irradiation.[175] The 3-year disease-free and overall survival rates were both 87%. Another study reviewed the results of 78 patients with stage I/IIIA (positive washings only) endometrial cancer who had USC.[176] Fifty-eight patients received whole-abdominal radiation therapy and had a significantly better 5-year disease-specific survival rate than those who received either less extensive radiation therapy or no adjuvant therapy (75% vs. 41%). These studies show that the use of whole-abdominal radiation therapy can improve disease control in patients with these aggressive histologies and should be considered as part of treatment for all patients with these variant histologies, even those with early-stage disease. Alternative approaches to the treatment of these high-risk histologies include the use of chemotherapy.

Brachytherapy

Intravaginal brachytherapy has been used, both alone, as the primary means of radiation treatment, or in conjunction with external beam radiation therapy. For early-stage disease, brachytherapy offers the advantage of delivering a high dose of radiation locally while minimizing the volume of surrounding normal structures receiving a high dose of radiation. Previously, brachytherapy consisted mainly of low-dose-rate intracavitary insertions; however, this requires inpatient hospitalization and lengthy insertion times that increase the risk of radiation exposure to medical personnel. Increasingly, high-dose-rate techniques with remote afterloading of the radiation source have been used, eliminating the need for hospitalization and minimizing radiation exposure to medical personnel. In appropriately selected patients, brachytherapy offers results similar to those of external beam radiation therapy, and high-dose rate brachytherapy appears to offer similar rates of control to low-dose-rate techniques.

Low-Dose-Rate Brachytherapy

In addition to the preoperative use of low-dose-rate brachytherapy, with or without external beam radiation that was described previously, low-dose-rate brachytherapy has been used postoperatively to decrease the risk of local recurrence at the vaginal cuff (Table 91-10). In the randomized trial by Aalders,[155] all patients were treated postoperatively with 60 Gy intracavitary radium and randomized to receive either an additional 40 Gy external beam radiation therapy to the pelvis or no further therapy.[166] Although the addition of external beam radiation therapy resulted in improved vaginal and pelvic control, the patients benefiting the most from pelvic irradiation were those with high-grade lesions and deep myometrial invasion. Patients without these features who were treated with brachytherapy only had excellent rates of local control without the addition of external beam radiation. For patients who had less than 50% myometrial invasion and received only intracavitary radiation, the vaginal and pelvic recurrence rate was 4.3%. In addition, patients receiving brachytherapy only who had grade 1 tumors had a vaginal and pelvic recurrence rate of 3.6%, whereas those with grade 2 tumors had a local recurrence rate of 3.2%. High rates of local control with postoperative

TABLE 91-10

Results of Postoperative Low-Dose-Rate Brachytherapy After Hysterectomy

STUDY	NO. OF PATIENTS	STAGE	RADIATION TECHNIQUES	5-YR LOCAL CONTROL (%)	5-YR SURVIVAL RATE (%)
Aalders et al.[135]	277	I	ICRT	96	91
Marchetti et al.[177]	68	I	ICRT	100	97
Irwin et al.[178]	217	I	ICRT + EBRT	95	82
Greven et al.[179]	41	I/II	ICRT + EBRT	93	NR
Randall et al.[180]	102	I	ICRT + EBRT	94	NR

EBRT, external beam radiation therapy; ICRT, intracavitary radiation therapy; NR, not reported.

low-dose-rate brachytherapy alone in appropriately selected patients also have been seen retrospectively. In one study, 68 patients with grade 1 or 2 tumors and less than 50% myometrial invasion were treated with postoperative intracavitary radium only. At a median follow-up of 4.8 years, none of the patients had a vaginal recurrence.[177] For patients without significant risk factors for nodal dissemination, postoperative low-dose-rate brachytherapy alone provides excellent local control.

The role of adding a brachytherapy boost to external beam radiation in patients who are at risk for nodal dissemination, but at low risk for local recurrence, is less clear. A retrospective study from Princess Margaret Hospital described 550 patients with stage I endometrial carcinoma who were treated with surgery alone, surgery followed by external beam radiation, or surgery with external beam radiation and intracavitary brachytherapy.[178] Local control rates were similar among the three groups (93% vs. 94% vs. 95%). Grade 3 or 4 toxicity was higher in the patients receiving both external beam radiation and intracavitary brachytherapy. The rate of grade 3 or 4 bowel toxicity was 9.7% when patients received both compared with 5% when they received external beam radiation as their only postoperative adjuvant therapy. Vaginal stenosis was also worse for patients receiving external beam radiation therapy and brachytherapy (21% having grade 3 or worse) compared with those receiving postoperative external beam radiation only (3%).

Although the authors concluded that the addition of neither external beam radiation nor brachytherapy improved local control, patients receiving external beam radiation therapy were more likely to have more than 50% myometrial invasion than patients undergoing surgery alone. In addition, most patients receiving brachytherapy had involvement of the lower uterine segment, increasing the risk of local recurrence. Greven and colleagues[179] retrospectively reviewed the outcomes of 270 patients with stage I or II endometrial carcinoma who received either external beam radiation therapy alone or external beam radiation therapy with the addition of a brachytherapy boost. Of the 97 patients receiving a brachytherapy

boost, low-dose-rate therapy was used in 41 patients. The 5-year pelvic control rates were similar in those who received a brachytherapy boost and those who did not (96% vs. 94%). Pelvic control rates remained similar when patients were analyzed separately by stage. In addition, a non–statistically significant increase in grade 3 and 4 small bowel complications was seen in the group receiving brachytherapy. Other retrospective studies also did not show improved local control, but showed increased complication rates from adding intracavitary radiation to external beam radiation for patients with low risk of nodal spread.[180] Currently, it appears that for patients who are at risk for nodal spread, external beam radiation therapy alone provides adequate regional and local control. For patients who are at low risk for nodal spread, but have risk factors for vaginal recurrence, such as involvement of the lower uterine segment, the addition of postoperative brachytherapy alone provides excellent local control.

High-Dose-Rate Brachytherapy

Although there are no prospective randomized data on high-dose-rate brachytherapy, a number of retrospective and institutional studies indicate that high-dose-rate brachytherapy is an effective means of providing local control for selected patients, with an acceptable level of toxicity (Table 91-11). A series from Memorial Sloan-Kettering Cancer Center examined 233 patients with stage IB, grade 1 or 2 endometrial carcinoma who were treated with simple hysterectomy followed by postoperative high-dose-rate intravaginal brachytherapy consisting of 21 Gy in 7-Gy fractions given at 2-week intervals.[181] The 5-year vaginal and pelvic control rate was 96%, and the 5-year overall survival rate was 94%. The actuarial rate of complications of grade 3 or higher at 5 years was 2%. Noyes and associates[182] performed a phase II trial on 63 patients with stage IA and grade 3 or stage IB and grade 1/2 disease, all of whom received high-dose-rate brachytherapy alone postoperatively. Most received a total dose of 32.4 Gy in two fractions delivered to the surface of the vaginal ovoids. With a median follow-up of 1.6 years, no patient had a vaginal cuff recurrence. Anderson and colleagues[183] reviewed 102 patients with stage IB and IC

TABLE 91-11

Results of Postoperative High-Dose-Rate Brachytherapy Alone After Hysterectomy

STUDY	NO. OF PATIENTS	STAGES	5-YR LOCAL CONTROL (%)	5-YR OVERALL SURVIVAL RATE (%)
Noyes et al.[182]	63	I, IIA	98	NR
Alektiar et al.[181]	233	IB2–3	96	94
MacLeod et al.[286]	141	I–II	99	91
Fanning et al.[44]	66	IG3, IC, II	100	84
Horowitz et al.[287]	164	IB, IC, II	98	87
Petereit et al.[188]	191	I	100	95
Anderson et al.[183]	102	IB, IC	97	84
Mandell et al.[184]	330	I/II	97	I: 92
				II: 82
Nori et al.[185]	173	I/II	96	91

NR, not reported.

endometrial carcinoma who were treated postoperatively with a relatively lower dose of high-dose-rate brachytherapy, using 15 Gy in three fractions of 5 Gy after hysterectomy. The 5-year locoregional control rate was 97%, with only one patient experiencing a failure at the vaginal cuff, comparable to the rate with higher doses. A number of other institutional series showed similar excellent local control with postoperative high-dose-rate brachytherapy only in appropriately selected patients. These results are similar to historical results seen with low-dose-rate brachytherapy.

The use of high-dose-rate brachytherapy after external beam radiation has been described in a number of nonrandomized series. Several studies included both patients receiving postoperative external beam radiation alone and those receiving postoperative external beam radiation with a high-dose-rate intracavitary brachytherapy boost. However, direct comparisons between these two groups is difficult in these retrospective studies because patients receiving both modes of radiation therapy often have independent risk factors for local recurrence. Mandell and associates[184] reviewed 330 patients with either high-risk stage I or stage II endometrial carcinoma who were treated with a combination of 40 Gy external beam radiation therapy and a vaginal vault boost of 21 Gy. The overall pelvic and vaginal recurrence rate was 3.7%. Nori and associates[185] reviewed 300 patients with stage I or II endometrial carcinoma who were treated with hysterectomy and high-dose-rate brachytherapy. External beam radiation therapy was given to patients with high-risk features. With a median follow-up of 12 years, actuarial progression-free survival was 96.6%.

Importantly, at long-term follow-up, no grade 3 or 4 toxicities were seen in any patient. Another retrospective study examined the results of 86 patients with stage I and occult stage II endometrial cancer who were treated with surgery followed by external beam radiation in one of three different fractionation schedules, with or without intracavitary brachytherapy.[186] No difference was seen in rates of local recurrence, and on multivariate analysis, the addition of brachytherapy did not affect survival. A retrospective series from Fox Chase Cancer Center looked at 98 patients with pathologic stage I/II endometrial cancer.[187] Most patients received postoperative external beam radiation with a high-dose-rate brachytherapy boost; however, 17 patients received postoperative brachytherapy only. At 5 years, 89% of the entire population was free from pelvic recurrence.

As with low-dose-rate brachytherapy, it is unclear whether the addition of high-dose-rate brachytherapy to external beam radiation improves local control. In addition, intravaginal brachytherapy may lead to an increased incidence of complications, such as vaginal stenosis, particularly when combined with external beam radiation. The long-term incidence may be decreased with physical adhesiolysis, either with a dilator, by stent, or through sexual intercourse. These patients require close, appropriate follow-up. Overall, these series indicate that the addition of high-dose-rate brachytherapy alone after hysterectomy results in high rates of local control in patients who are at low risk for nodal spread. Rates of acute toxicity may be somewhat higher with the use of high-dose-rate brachytherapy.[188] The dose received by the surrounding normal tissue is critically dependent on positioning of the applicator. In one study, it resulted in a change in the distance from the rectal wall to the applicator of a median of 10.5 mm between two consecutive placements of the applicator.[189] The treatment must be planned appropriately, and the position of the applicator for each treatment must be verified to minimize radiation dose to the surrounding normal tissues.

TREATMENT OF PATIENTS WITH MEDICALLY INOPERABLE DISEASE

Patients who refuse surgery or have medically inoperable disease may be treated with primary radiation therapy alone. External beam radiation, with or without vaginal brachytherapy, is often used; however, in patients who are at low risk for spread beyond the uterus, vaginal brachytherapy alone may be used. Table 91-12 reviews results with radiation alone. In Patanaphan and colleagues,[190] the 5-year overall survival rate was 46% for

TABLE 91-12

Results of Treatment with Radiation Only

STUDY	NO. OF PATIENTS	STAGES	5-YR LOCAL CONTROL (%)	5-YR OVERALL SURVIVAL RATE (%)
Patanaphan et al.[190]	54	I	NR	75 (OS)
Langren et al.[191]	124	I, II	I: 78 II: 82	I: 77 (OS) II: 65 (OS)
Kupelian et al.[192]	137	I, II	86	I: 87 (DSS) II: 88 (DSS)
Chao et al.[193]	101	I	IA: 100 IB: 88	IA: 80 (DFS) IB: 84 (DFS)
Fishman et al.[194]	54	I, II	NR	I: 80 (CSS) II: 85 (CSS)

CSS, cancer specific survival; DFS, disease free survival; DSS, disease specific survival; NR, not reported; OS, overall survival.

all patients receiving radiation alone, and the 5-year overall survival for patients with stage I, grade I disease was only 75%. Langren and associates[191] retrospectively reviewed 124 patients with stage I and II endometrial cancer who were treated with radiation alone. Although the 5-year overall survival rate was low because of the medical comorbidities of this patient population (stage I, 77%; stage II, 65%), radiation alone achieved acceptable rates of local control. At 5 years, 78% of patients with stage I disease and 82% of patients with stage II disease were free from pelvic recurrence. Several institutional series showed the effectiveness of radiation alone for stage I and II endometrial carcinoma. Kupelian and colleagues reviewed 152 patients who were treated with radiation therapy alone.[192] Most patients (116 of 152) were treated with brachytherapy alone. Patients with stage I disease and those with stage II disease had 5-year disease-specific survival rates of 87% and 88%, respectively. Intrauterine recurrence was seen in 14% of patients with stage I or II disease, and extrauterine recurrence was seen in 3%. Chao and colleagues[193] reviewed 101 patients treated with primary radiation therapy at Washington University. All patients had either stage IA (18 patients) or IB disease (83 patients). Most patients were treated with both whole-pelvic irradiation and intracavitary boost, although a wide range of techniques was used. Pelvic control was achieved in 100% of patients with stage IA and 88% of patients with stage IB disease. The 5-year disease-free survival rate was 80% for stage IA and 84% for stage IB.

In another series from Yale University, 54 patients with medically inoperable stage I or II endometrial adeno-carcinoma were treated with radiation alone.[194] These patients were matched 2:1 by age, stage, and grade with patients who underwent surgical treatment for endo-metrial cancer. The cancer-specific survival rate was some-what worse for patients undergoing primary radiation treatment. For patients with stage I disease, the 5-year actuarial cancer-specific survival rate was 80% for patients treated with radiation alone compared with a 5-year cancer-specific survival rate of 98% for those undergoing surgery. For patients with stage II disease, the 5-year actuarial cancer-specific survival rate was 85% and 100% for patients with inoperable and operable disease, respectively. A significant difference in 5-year overall survival was seen between inoperable and operable disease (30% and 24% for stage I and II inoperable disease vs. 88% and 85% for stage I and II operable disease). However, for patients receiving radiation only who did not die of intercurrent illness, there was no significant difference in median survival between patients with inoperable vs. operable disease.

For patients who are not good candidates for surgical removal of the uterus because of coexisting medical conditions and who are at low risk for nodal spread, brachytherapy alone may be used as the primary therapy for endometrial cancer. Although low-dose-rate brachy-therapy may require anesthesia, it can also be performed with epidural anesthesia in some patients. It is less invasive than hysterectomy and is generally well tolerated, with a low procedural complication rate.[195] Grigsby and colleagues[169] reviewed the outcomes of 26 patients with

stage II disease who were treated with low-dose-rate intracavitary brachytherapy alone.[176] The 5-year disease-free survival rate was 53% in this group, with a high major complication rate of 19%. In another retrospective study, the 5-year disease-free survival rate for stage IA, IB, and II disease treated with high-dose-rate brachytherapy alone was 85%, 73%, and 69%, respectively.[196] Another study reported a 3-year disease-free survival rate of 85% in patients with stage I, medically inoperable endometrial cancer treated with high-dose-rate brachytherapy alone; however, complication rates were again high, at 21%.[197] Overall survival is low in these patients because of their medical comorbidities, and complication rates are higher than in medically operable patients. The results with brachytherapy alone are worse than those with treatment that includes surgical resection, even for very early-stage disease; however, brachytherapy offers a reasonable option for treatment in patients who are poor surgical candidates.

No randomized studies have been conducted directly comparing radiation alone and surgery alone for early-stage endometrial cancer. Surgery remains the treatment of choice for patients who are medically fit; however, for patients who are medically inoperable, radiation therapy alone offers a viable alternative for treatment and provides good rates of local control.

TREATMENT OF ADVANCED ENDOMETRIAL CANCER

Although most patients are diagnosed with endometrial cancer at an early stage of disease, 10% to 15% have advanced disease at presentation. This group includes patients with positive pelvic and para-aortic lymph nodes, local invasion into other pelvic organs, pelvic recurrence at the vaginal cuff or in the pelvic lymph nodes, and distant metastases. Patients may be categorized according to pathologic stage or clinical stage III and IV disease. Hysterectomy remains the primary treatment for operable advanced-stage cancers. Radiation therapy is often used postoperatively to reduce the risk of local recurrence, treat areas of residual disease, or palliate symptoms of recurrent cancer. It may also be used preoperatively in patients with technically inoperable disease or even as primary therapy in patients with medically inoperable disease. Although radiation therapy has not improved overall survival in these cases, it is very effective for both locoregional control and palliation. Adjuvant radiation has a particularly important role in endometrial cancer, given the relatively low rates of response to chemotherapeutic agents.

GOG protocol 122 randomized patients with stage III and IV disease and maximal postoperative residual disease of 2 cm to receive either whole-abdominal irradiation or seven cycles of systemic chemotherapy with cisplatin and doxorubicin.[198] The radiation arm included a pelvic boost and the para-aortic fields in the case of positive para-aortic nodes. Progression-free survival at 24 months for cisplatin and doxorubicin is 59% vs. 46% for whole-abdominal irradiation. Overall survival at 24 months is 70% in patients who received cisplatin and doxorubicin and 59% in patients who received whole-abdominal irradiation. This is at the cost of increased incidence of adverse affects in the cisplatin and doxorubicin arm, including sustained peripheral neuropathy, compared with limited fatigue and gastrointestinal problems, which had essentially resolved 6 months after treatment in the radiation arm.[199] The ongoing GOG trial (protocol 184) includes a similar patient cohort, all of whom receive pelvic radiation, with or without para-aortic fields, and then are randomized to receive cisplatin and doxorubicin, with or without paclitaxel.

Pathologic Stage III Disease

The results of therapy for stage III disease depend on whether patients have pathologic stage III diagnosed after surgical staging or whether they have clinical stage III disease. When staged surgically, stage III disease includes stage IIIA disease diagnosed by positive washings alone or by microscopic extension to the serosa or adnexa and stage IIIC disease diagnosed by microscopic lymph node involvement. Clinical stage III disease involves gross extra-uterine extension, pelvic adenopathy that is detectable on preoperative scans, and clinically evident vaginal extension. Thus clinical stage III disease comprises bulkier tumors by definition, and often includes patients requiring radical surgery, such as an exenteration, or those with technically inoperable disease. Inevitably, outcomes are poorer for these patients. For patients with pathologic stage III disease treated with hysterectomy and postoperative radiation, 5-year disease-free survival rates of 64% and pelvic recurrence rates of 21% have been reported.[200] Predictors of survival include grade, depth of invasion, number of extrauterine sites of disease, and USC or CCC. Grade is the strongest predictor of pelvic recurrence; histologic features and the number of extrauterine sites are predictors of abdominal recurrence.

Pathologic Stage IIIA Disease

The most favorable outcome is among the subgroup of patients with stage III disease who have positive peritoneal washings as the sole criterion of advanced disease (approximately 5% of patients). The selection of adjuvant treatment for these patients is controversial, and the prognostic significance of this finding remains uncertain. Approximately 10% of patients with FIGO stage I endometrial cancer have positive peritoneal washings. More than half of patients with positive pelvic washings also have adnexal or other areas of pelvic spread of disease. This finding is associated with depth of invasion, high-grade histology with positive nodes, and positive cytology, is predictive of survival.[201,202] Table 91-13 shows the results of series examining the effect of positive cytology, with recurrence rates of 0% to 46% and disease-free survival rates of 17% to 100%, highlighting the difficulty in interpreting positive cytology as a prognostic marker. Overall, peritoneal cytology may not identify additional patients who are candidates for postoperative therapy, but are not identified by grade and depth of invasion.

Despite data suggesting a poorer prognosis for these patients, only a few series have reported exclusively on outcomes in patients with pathologic stage IIIA disease. In a series by Creasman and associates,[203] 26 patients with stage I disease and positive peritoneal washings had a 34% recurrence rate compared with 9% among women with

TABLE 91-13

Results of Stage IIIA Cancer with Positive Peritoneal Washings Only

STUDY	NO. OF PATIENTS	ADJUVANT TREATMENT	RECURRENCE RATE (%)	DISEASE-FREE SURVIVAL (%)
Turner et al.[288]	28	None	32	84 (5-yr OS)
Yazigi et al.[289]	10	None	10	87 (5-yr OS)
Zuna et al.[290]	8	None	—	17
Morrow et al.[143]	14	None	7	76 (5-yr RFI)
	18	Pelvic RT	28	(all patients)
Creasman et al.[203]	13	None	46	—
	23	IP P-32	13	—
Soper et al.[204]	43	IP P-32 (all) Pelvic RT-3; ICRT	8	89
Lurain et al.[291]	30	Pelvic RT; ICRT; CT or hormones	17	—
Konski et al.[96]	11	Pelvic RT	9	100
	8	WART	25	75
Martinez et al.[292]	18	WART	11	73
Mazurka et al.[207]	16	Hormones or CT (N = 13)	25	—
Piver et al.[208]	25	Progestins	0	100
Kennedy et al.[118]	14	Various (CT, P-32, hormone)	—	67
Harouny et al.[293]	41	Various (pre-op RT, pelvic RT, CT, hormone)	29	71

CT, chemotherapy; ICRT, intracavitary radiation therapy; IP, intraperitoneal; OS, overall survival; RFI, recurrence free interval; RT, radiation therapy; WART, whole abdominal radiation therapy.

negative washings. Of 13 patients with no extrauterine disease and positive cytology, 46% died of disseminated intraperitoneal recurrence. The investigators subsequently treated 23 patients with malignant washings with intra-abdominal P-32 colloid postoperatively and concluded that P-32 therapy was efficacious because none of these patients had pelvic or abdominal recurrence, although distant disease developed in three.

In a report by Soper and associates,[204] 65 women with clinical stage I to III endometrial cancer and malignant cytologic findings were treated with intraperitoneal radioactive P-32 suspension. The authors reported an 8% intraperitoneal recurrence rate, with most patients having simultaneous extraperitoneal metastases. Chronic bowel symptoms were not seen in patients receiving P-32 alone, but occurred in 29% of women who also received external irradiation to the pelvis. Two of these patients died. Potish[205] described a 5-year relapse-free survival rate of 77% in women with microscopic peritoneal spread treated with whole-abdominal radiation, and an overall 4% rate of bowel obstructions. The use of adjuvant radiation in patients with positive cytology as the only evidence of extrauterine spread remains controversial, although it is frequently offered. Whether to offer pelvic or whole-abdominal radiation remains unclear.

Hormonal therapy with progestins or systemic chemotherapy has also been used as an adjuvant in small groups of patients with isolated positive washings. These small series reported relapse rates of 0% to 25% and disease-free survival rates of 67%, compared with 85%.[206,207] Piver[208] conducted a pilot study of 25 patients with surgical stage I disease and malignant pelvic washings who were treated with progesterone. Twenty-two patients underwent second-look laparoscopy, and 95% had no evidence of disease, with negative washings. One patient with persistent positive washings was treated with an additional year of progestin therapy and remained free of disease. Although these data are intriguing, too few patients were treated exclusively with hormonal therapy to permit an assessment of the efficacy of this therapy compared with adjuvant radiation, although either treatment appears superior to no adjuvant therapy. Most patients have other risk factors for pelvic or distant recurrence that guide treatment decisions, including grade, depth of invasion, and invasion of the lymphovascular space.

Patients with pathologic stage III disease as a result of isolated adnexal involvement also comprise a more favorable subset among patients with stage III disease. Direct transtubal invasion or lymphatic spread may occur. Because some of these patients may have concurrent early-stage ovarian cancers, careful pathologic assessment is warranted. A GOG study reported that 5% of surgically staged patients with clinical stage I disease had adnexal involvement.[49] This pathologic finding is associated with a 32% risk of pelvic lymph node metastasis, and 23% of patients have para-aortic lymph node spread. In the largest reported subgroup of 42 patients with isolated adnexal involvement, Greven noted a 5-year survival rate of 60%, compared with 54% for the entire group of patients with pathologic stage III disease.[200] The grade and depth of myometrial invasion further defined the prognosis for

these patients, in whom high-grade disease reduced the survival rate to 40% and invasion through more than one third of the myometrium resulted in a 47% survival rate. Most patients had received postoperative pelvic irradiation, with or without a boost. Isolated abdominal failure in this series was uncommon, at 7%. Nori and colleagues[209] analyzed a group of patients treated with surgery and either preoperative or postoperative pelvic irradiation with an intravaginal boost, including 21 patients with microscopic involvement of the adnexa and 12 patients with gross adnexal involvement. The 5-year survival rate was better for those with microscopic invasion (80%) than for those with gross invasion of the adnexa (40%), even though this was the only extrauterine disease.

Several other smaller series that analyzed this subset of patients reported 5-year relapse-free survival rates of 60% to 90% in patients treated postoperatively with either pelvic[210,211] or whole-abdominopelvic radiation.[212,213] Overall, the small numbers of patients in these reports preclude any conclusion about the relative efficacy of pelvic vs. whole-abdominal radiation in this subset of patients. Adjuvant pelvic therapy is usually offered to patients without significant comorbidity.

Pathologic Stage IIIC Disease

Patients at highest risk for recurrence are those with positive pelvic or para-aortic lymph nodes. A GOG study examined pathologic factors in patients with clinical stage I/II endometrial cancer.[49] In a series of 1180 women, 13% overall had positive pelvic nodes (3% grossly positive), and approximately one third of patients with positive pelvic nodes also had para-aortic nodal metastases. Lymph nodes were involved in 51% of women with extrauterine disease, 32% with adnexal invasion, and 25% with deep myometrial invasion. Patients with positive pelvic nodes who were treated with postoperative pelvic irradiation had a 5-year disease-free survival rate of 72%. The presence of positive pelvic lymph nodes only was more favorable than involvement of the para-aortic nodes as well. The recurrence rate was 28% for those with positive pelvic nodes compared with 40% for those with positive aortic nodes. Of patients with positive para-aortic nodes, 77% received postoperative radiation, with a 5-year disease-free survival rate of 36%. In a small study of 17 patients with nodal spread confined to the pelvic nodes, in which all of the patients received postoperative radiation, the 5-year overall survival rate was 72%.[214] Better survival rates have been reported for patients with microscopically positive lymph nodes vs. grossly involved nodes. One series reported a mean survival rate of more than 60 months if nodes were microscopically involved compared with 35 months for grossly involved nodes.[215]

Outcomes with adjuvant radiation (with or without systemic therapy) have been retrospectively reviewed, although treatment techniques have varied significantly. Table 91-14 shows the results of various series. In a recent study of 47 patients with stage IIIC disease, 36% had whole-abdominal radiation, 19% had extended pelvic and para-aortic nodal irradiation, and 17% had pelvic irradiation alone.[216] In addition, 17% were treated with chemo-

TABLE 91-14

Results for Stage IIIC Patients with Positive Pelvic or Para-aortic Lymph Nodes				
STUDY	**NO. OF PATIENTS**	**TREATMENT**	**RELAPSE RATE (%)**	**5-YR SURVIVAL RATE (%)**
Nelson et al.[214]	17 (+ pelvic LNs only)	PRT or WART	PA LNs: 12 DM: 12	72
McMeekin et al.[216]	47	WART; EFRT; PRT; ± CT or progestins	Pelvic: 9 DM: 21	65
Martinez et al.[292]	8	WART, PA + pelvic boost	NS	70 (RFS)
Mundt et al.[121]	30	PRT or EFRT	Pelvic: 23 DM: 40 PA LNs: 13 Abdomen:13	34 (DFS)
Rose et al.[220]	17	EFRT + Megace	DM: 29	53
Onda et al.[221]	20	CT + EFRT	NS	75 (+PA LNs) 100 (+ pelvic LNs only)

CT, chemotherapy; DFS, disease free survival; DM, distant metastases; EFRT, extended field radiation therapy; LN, lymph node; NS, not stated; PA, para-aortic; PRT, pelvic radiation therapy; RFS, relapse free survival; WART, whole abdominal radiation therapy.

therapy and 11% with progestins. The 5-year overall survival rate was 65%, with distant metastases seen in 21% and pelvic recurrence in 9%. Predictors of treatment failure included depth of invasion and positive cytologic findings or adnexal involvement. The role of the various adjuvant treatments used, however, could not be clearly defined. Patients in whom nodal disease is confined to the pelvic lymph nodes and whose para-aortic lymph nodes are negative are still at risk for para-aortic recurrence. Mundt and colleagues[217] reported 30 patients with stage IIIC disease, all of whom had positive pelvic nodes. Of these patients, 54% had positive para-aortic lymph nodes all were treated with TAH-BSO followed by pelvic or extended-field radiation.[217] They noted a 5-year disease-free survival rate of 34%, with 23% of patients experiencing pelvic failure (including four vaginal failures), 13% having abdominal failure, and 13% having para-aortic failure. Distant metastases occurred in 40%. No patient who was treated with extended-field irradiation had a para-aortic nodal recurrence, although 8 of 10 had positive para-aortic nodes at surgery. Treatment was well tolerated, with only two late sequelae occurring, one case of chronic enteritis and one bowel obstruction.

For patients with positive para-aortic nodes and no other abdominal disease, the optimal radiation field remains uncertain. Potish and colleagues[218] reported 48 women treated with extended para-aortic fields, half of whom had abnormal lymphangiograms and half of whom had pathologically documented nodal metastases. They found that 88% of recurrences were outside the radiation fields, including 44% of first failures in the abdomen. In this series, survival was better in clinically staged than in surgically staged patients (57% vs. 47%), suggesting uncertainty about clinical staging of nodal disease.

Corn and associates[219] examined outcomes in 50 women, 26 with pathologically staged para-aortic nodal involvement and 24 diagnosed with lymphangiography, treated preoperatively and postoperatively or primarily with extended-field radiation. Para-aortic lymph node dissection significantly decreased the rate of para-aortic failure, and the authors reported only three abdominal failures. Two other series examined the effect of extended-field irradiation in patients with pathologically documented para-aortic nodal spread. In one group of 26 patients, 17 received extended-field radiation treatment, most with adjuvant megestrol (Megace). The remaining nine patients received Megace or chemotherapy alone.[220] The overall survival rate was significantly improved in the irradiated group (53% vs. 22%). In the second series, 20 patients with para-aortic metastases received three cycles of postoperative chemotherapy followed by extended-field irradiation.[221] The 5-year survival rate was 75% for those with positive para-aortic nodes, compared with 100% if only the pelvic nodes were positive. Reported series of patients treated with whole-abdominal radiation represented heterogeneous stage and histologic groups, and generally included small numbers of patients with para-aortic metastases as the primary reason for the use of whole-abdominal radiation fields.

Clinical Stage III and IV Disease

The 1971 FIGO staging system is based on findings on clinical examination.[222] In that era, fewer patients were treated with surgery, and primary irradiation was often used. Clinical stage III endometrial cancer was defined as carcinoma extending outside the uterus, but not outside the true pelvis. Stage IV disease included invasion of the bladder or rectum, or disease beyond the true pelvis.

Clinical Stage III Disease

Treatment of clinical stage III endometrial cancer has included radiation alone or surgery and radiation. Grigsby and associates[223] reported a series including 27 patients with clinical stage III disease treated with total hysterectomy and salpingo-oophorectomy combined with preoperative or postoperative irradiation. The 5-year disease-free survival rate was 33%, with a distant metastatic rate of 48%

and a pelvic recurrence rate of 33%. Aalders and colleagues[224] compared outcomes in 108 patients who had clinical stage III disease with 67 patients who had pathologic stage III disease. Radical surgery was possible in 70% of patients with pathologic stage III disease compared with only 13% of those with clinical stage III disease. Therefore, 66 patients were treated with radiation alone. Surgical debulking was an important prognostic factor. The 5-year overall survival rate was 16% vs. 40% for those with clinical vs. pathologic stage III disease, respectively. In a series by Greven and colleagues,[200] 52 patients had clinical stage III disease, 20 of whom had radiation alone after biopsy. The overall survival rate for patients with this stage of disease was 36%, with a median survival of 9 months for patients treated with radiation alone compared with 60 months for patients treated with surgery and radiation. The group treated with radiation only also showed very poor pelvic control, with 89% having pelvic failure. In the patients who received combined treatment, the 5-year survival rate was 48%, with 40% having pelvic failure. Isolated abdominal failure was much less common, at 6%, but 38% overall had a component of abdominal failure and 16% had distant metastases alone. Thus, although a combined treatment approach of surgery and adjuvant irradiation results in superior outcomes to radiation alone for patients with clinical stage III disease, these patients still have a high rate of pelvic and abdominal failure.

In some patients with locally advanced disease, surgery may only be able to achieve debulking. Bulky residual disease has been defined as greater than 2 cm residual tumor after primary surgery. This may include pelvic implants, residual nodal disease, or intraperitoneal deposits. There appears to be a benefit with respect to recurrence and survival if tumor is optimally debulked. Surgery is followed by adjuvant irradiation to the pelvis, para-aortic nodes, or whole abdomen, as indicated by the location of residual disease. In a study of surgical cytoreduction in 65 patients with stage IVB disease, optimal debulking to less than 1 cm residual disease was accomplished in 55%.[225] Those patients had a significantly improved median survival of 34 months vs. 11 months for those with bulkier residual disease. Among those with optimal cytoreduction, adjuvant chemotherapy or radiation was associated with improved survival. In another series of patients with stage IV disease, including 24 patients who had optimal debulking to less than 2 cm residual disease and 31 patients with bulkier residual or unresectable peritoneal carcinomatosis, median survivals were 31, 12, and 3 months, respectively.[226]

Whole-abdominal radiation for bulky residual disease appears to be inadequate, and patients with greater than 2 cm residual disease seldom achieve adequate control.[213] This may be related to the lower radiation doses that are achievable with whole-abdominal radiation because of limitations of dose tolerance for the small bowel, liver, and kidneys. Limited-field boosts to areas of bulky residual disease should be considered, particularly for the para-aortic nodes, which can be treated at higher doses without exposing the liver or kidneys to excessive radiation. For patients with bulky disease confined to the pelvis, preoperative radiation may be considered to improve the likelihood of optimal surgical resection.

Clinical Stage IV Disease

Patients with stage IVA disease, presenting with invasion of the bladder or rectum, with or without lymph node metastases, should be treated similarly to those with stage III disease, with combined surgery and radiation, with or without systemic therapy. Preoperative radiation may be considered in patients with marginally operable or inoperable disease confined to the pelvis. Although few data exist on the use of this approach in endometrial cancer, it has been used successfully in a variety of other pelvic malignancies. Patients with stage IVB disease are rare, and are most often treated palliatively. Residual or progressive pelvic disease can be a major source of symptoms in these patients. The 5-year survival rate is approximately 0% to 10%.[227,228] Surgical debulking may be of benefit, or may be considered for palliation of symptoms.

For patients with advanced inoperable disease, palliative radiation therapy should be considered. Patients with stage IV disease are also candidates for systemic chemotherapy or hormonal therapy. Bulky disease requires high-dose irradiation, even for palliation. Unfortunately, because of poor tolerance of the bowel to high dose fractions of radiation, palliative treatment may require several weeks of daily therapy. Conventional doses of 45 to 55 Gy external irradiation may be followed by low-dose-rate or high-dose-rate brachytherapy, depending on the location and extent of disease. Palliation of bleeding may also be accomplished with brachytherapy alone. This approach is useful for debilitated patients. One group of 27 patients with endometrial cancer who were not considered surgical candidates, usually because of age or comorbidities, received 1 to 3 doses of 10-Gy fractions to the pelvis.[229] Bleeding resolved in 90% of cases, malodorous discharge was reduced in 38%, and 22% had a complete tumor response, with a median survival of 9 months. Only three patients had significant bowel effects. The Radiation Therapy Oncology Group (RTOG) reported a phase II trial in patients with advanced pelvic malignancies treated with accelerated split-course irradiation, consisting of three courses over 6 days in 12 fractions, with 2- or 4-week breaks between each course.[230] Patients who completed all three courses had a 42% response rate, and therapy was well tolerated.

For patients with distant metastases or distant relapses after primary therapy, chemotherapy or hormonal therapy is the mainstay of initial treatment. The most common sites of distant metastases are lung (35%), liver (29%), omentum or peritoneum (25%), gastrointestinal tract (21%), and bone (15%), with rare instances of adrenal (10%) or brain (6%) involvement.[231] Radiation is rarely used for visceral disease; however, palliative irradiation is indicated in specific cases, including patients with painful bony metastases, symptomatic brain metastases, spinal cord compression, and airway obstruction. Short courses of hypofractionated radiation are most commonly used over 1 to 2 weeks. Therapy is delivered to the whole brain or to the painful portion of involved bone.

SYSTEMIC THERAPY FOR ENDOMETRIAL CANCER

The role of chemotherapy in early-stage endometrial cancer is limited. The primary pattern of failure in these patients is locoregional; therefore, the benefit of adding systemic therapy is mainly reserved for patients with more advanced disease. However, for certain high-risk, early-stage tumors, particularly CCC and USC, systemic dissemination remains a substantial risk. The use of chemotherapy has been examined in these patients. At M.D. Anderson Cancer Center, 62 patients with high-risk stage I or clinically occult stage II endometrial cancer, including grade 3 tumors, deep myometrial invasion, and high-risk histologic types (CCC or USC), were prospectively treated with postoperative cisplatin, doxorubicin, and cyclophosphamide chemotherapy.[232] The addition of chemotherapy did not appear to decrease the rate of distant failure in women who had extrauterine disease; however, in patients with uterine-confined disease, the recurrence rate was 24%, with an observed progression-free interval of more than 36 months. In a small prospective study from Sweden, 31 patients with stage I, grade 3, or USC were treated with hysterectomy, postoperative radiation, and chemotherapy consisting of cisplatin and epirubicin.[233] At median follow-up of 32 months, none of the patients had recurrent disease.

A GOG study addressed the issue of chemotherapy after surgery and postoperative radiation therapy in patients with high-risk, early-stage endometrial cancer. However, the study included patients with nodal metastases as well as adnexal metastases. In addition, there were many protocol violations and patients who were lost to follow-up, making a more definitive analysis of outcome difficult. Although the results of these small trials are promising, chemotherapy is rarely used in patients with early-stage disease because of the risk of increased toxicity with chemotherapy and the lack of definitive data documenting a benefit. In general, chemotherapy is reserved for patients with more advanced or metastatic endometrial cancer.

Adjuvant chemotherapy for women with recurrent or advanced endometrial cancer did not prolong survival over more traditional treatment with radiation. Only one large randomized trial studied the effect of adjuvant chemotherapy. In 1990, Morrow and associates[234] treated 181 patients who had poor prognostic factors with postoperative radiation therapy. Patients were then randomized to receive either observation only or treatment with intravenous doxorubicin to a total dose of 500 mg/m^2. No significant difference in recurrence rates was noted between the two groups.

A variety of single agents for the treatment of metastatic or recurrent disease have been studied in phase II trials. Drugs with a reported response rate of more than 20% include 5-fluorouracil, cyclophosphamide, ifosfamide, doxorubicin, platinum, and paclitaxel. In particular, paclitaxel has a response rate of 27% to 38% when used as first- or second-line therapy.[235-237]

Several multiple-agent combinations have also been tested. A GOG study randomized patients to receive either doxorubicin or cisplatin plus doxorubicin.[238] A significant improvement was noted in both response rate (45% vs. 27%) and progression-free survival (13 months vs. 8 months) for the combination. A smaller study conducted by the European Organization of Research and Treatment of Cancer (EORTC) Gynecological Cancer Group showed similar results, although no significant difference in overall survival was noted.[239] The combination of paclitaxel and carboplatin has also been investigated, with reported response rates of 50% to 78%.[240,241]

Patient accrual was recently completed for two GOG trials of combination therapy for patients with advanced or recurrent endometrial cancer; the results should be forthcoming. These trials include a study comparing 24-hour administration of paclitaxel, doxorubicin, and granulocyte-colony-stimulating factor (G-CSF) with a combination of cisplatin and doxorubicin, and another study comparing 3-hour administration of paclitaxel, doxorubicin, cisplatin, and G-CSF with doxorubicin and paclitaxel.

HORMONAL THERAPY FOR ENDOMETRIAL CANCER

The mainstay of hormonal therapy for endometrial cancer is treatment with progestins, either megestrol acetate or medroxyprogesterone acetate. These agents yield overall response rates of 15% to 25%. Dose does not appear to be related to response. Thigpen and associates[242] randomized 299 women with advanced or recurrent endometrial cancer to receive medroxyprogesterone acetate either 200 or 1000 mg daily. The overall response rate was 25% in women receiving the low-dose regimen compared with 15% in those receiving the high-dose regimen. Median progression-free survival for both groups was approximately 2 to 3 months. Lentz and associates[243] administered high-dose megestrol acetate 800 mg daily to women with advanced or recurrent endometrial cancer and noted a 24% overall response rate, similar to the rate reported with lower-dose regimens.

Tamoxifen is the most widely studied nonprogestational hormonal agent for the treatment of endometrial cancer. In a review of eight studies, Moore and colleagues[244] reported a pooled response rate of 22%. Other agents, such as goserelin acetate and danazol, have shown limited activity.[245,246] Although the results have not yet been published, accrual to a GOG crossover trial was recently completed. This trial is evaluating doxorubicin, cisplatin, paclitaxel, and G-CSF and tamoxifen and megestrol acetate in patients with advanced or recurrent endometrial cancer.

SYSTEMIC THERAPY FOR UTERINE SARCOMA

Uterine sarcomas have a high rate of recurrence, even in the setting of stage I disease, and tend to recur at distant sites, making the need for effective systemic chemotherapy a pressing issue. Chemotherapy has no proven role in the adjuvant treatment of completely resected stage I disease. Omura and colleagues[247] randomized 156 patients with stage I and II uterine sarcomas to receive either observation or adjuvant doxorubicin. No statistical difference was seen in recurrence rate, progression-free interval, or overall survival rate.

A current phase III GOG study is comparing accelerated hyperfractionated whole-abdominal radiation therapy with combination chemotherapy with ifosfamide-mesna and cisplatin for optimally debulked stage I to IV carcinosarcoma. For single-agent treatment of patients with advanced or recurrent disease, ifosfamide (30% response rate for chemotherapy-naïve patients[248]) and cisplatin (18% to 19% response[249,250]) showed the most activity against carcinosarcoma. A recent study of paclitaxel showed moderate activity, with an 18% response rate.[251]

Combination therapy with cisplatin and ifosfamide may offer a small improvement in progression-free interval over single-agent therapy, although no improvement in overall survival was noted.[252] Currently, a GOG study is comparing the combination of ifosfamide and paclitaxel with ifosfamide alone. For patients with LMS, doxorubicin has shown to be the most effective single agent (25% response rate), although ifosfamide has also demonstrated some antitumor activity.[253,254]

COMPLICATIONS OF TREATMENT

Overall, surgery, including staging of lymph nodes, is well tolerated; however, the addition of lymphadenectomy to TAH-BSO increases the risk of vascular injuries, hematomas, and lymphocysts.[255] In addition, approximately 10% to 20% of patients undergoing lymphadenectomy have lower-extremity lymphedema.[256] The addition of lymphadenectomy to adjuvant radiation therapy also increases postoperative hospitalization rates and results in a higher rate of severe complications.[257,258] The risk of complications from lymphadenectomy is related to the number of lymph nodes removed at surgery.[259] Despite these increased risks, the importance of accurate staging of the lymph nodes cannot be overstated, and surgical staging of lymph nodes should be performed in appropriately selected patients.

Although pelvic radiation is generally well tolerated, the acute and long-term effects of this treatment have been well documented. Long-term follow-up from the PORTEC trial showed that the 5-year actuarial rate of late complications of grade 1 to 4 disease was 26% in patients who received radiation compared with 4% in those who did not ($P < 0.0001$).[157] Although 63% of the patients had some degree of acute toxicity, most of these patients had symptoms that resolved without further complications and only 2% discontinued treatment because of their symptoms. However, the most important predictor of long-term toxicity was acute symptoms. These rates of complications are similar to those reported in other series in which whole-pelvic irradiation was delivered, either preoperatively or postoperatively.[260] In an attempt to

decrease the radiation dose received by the surrounding normal tissues, several recent studies examined the dosimetric advantages of using intensity-modulated radiation therapy in the treatment of endometrial carcinoma. The results of these studies suggest that the volume of normal tissue, namely bladder, rectum, and small bowel, receiving high doses of radiation can be significantly reduced while adequate coverage of the postoperative planning target volume is delivered.[261,262] The potential advantages of intensity-modulated radiation therapy in decreasing normal tissue toxicity must be weighed against the potential risk of decreased margin on the target volume and increased volume of normal tissue receiving low doses of radiation. This increases the need for proper patient positioning and adequate immobilization to minimize treatment-to-treatment variations in patient position. Because of its potential to deliver a highly conformal radiation dose, intensity-modulated radiation therapy holds promise in improving the toxicity profile of pelvic irradiation. However, further studies are needed to assess the long-term outcome in patients treated with this therapy.

When extended-field or whole-abdominal irradiation is given, the treatment technique must minimize exposure to normal tissues, in particular, small bowel, liver, and kidneys. The most common acute effects of large abdominopelvic radiation fields are acute gastrointestinal symptoms, including nausea, vomiting, diarrhea, and cramping. Loss of fluid and electrolytes through vomiting and diarrhea may lead to acute dehydration, so antiemetics and antidiarrheals should be prescribed early in therapy and patients must be monitored closely. Myelosuppression through exposure of the bone marrow may also occur; therefore, blood counts should be monitored and supportive therapy given accordingly. Four-field pelvic arrangements, including anterior, posterior, and lateral fields, often allow for blocking of anterior segments of the small bowel. When the para-aortic nodes or whole abdomen is treated, larger volumes of small bowel are inevitably included, leading to a greater likelihood of acute enteritis. Typically, the whole-abdomen dose is limited to 25 to 30 Gy, keeping exposure of the kidneys to less than 20 Gy and exposure of the whole liver to less than 22 to 25 Gy. Doses of greater than 45 to 50 Gy to large volumes of small bowel significantly increase the risk of late complications. Series using these dose parameters and techniques report late bowel complications, primarily small bowel obstruction, in 3% to 12% of patients with extended-field irradiation[217,221] and in 0% to 9% of patients with whole-abdominal irradiation.[205,263,264,292]

TREATMENT OF RECURRENT DISEASE

Incidence of Pelvic Recurrence

Recurrence in the pelvis after hysterectomy is common in patients with endometrial cancer. Most locoregional recurrences are diagnosed in the first 2 to 3 years after initial treatment. For patients with pathologic stage I/II disease, the main risk factors for pelvic recurrence are high-grade histologic features and myometrial invasion of more than one third to one half of the myometrial width. With no postoperative adjuvant therapy, the risk of pelvic recurrence in these patients has been reported to be 10% to 40%. This risk is reduced to less than 5% with adjuvant pelvic irradiation, with or without a vaginal brachytherapy boost.[155,265,266] The distant metastatic rate and overall survival rate are not altered by the addition of adjuvant pelvic irradiation. Most series reported failures as total pelvic recurrences, including the vaginal cuff, pelvic lymph nodes, or other limited pelvic sites. High-risk patients with stage I disease, such as those with high-grade disease or deep invasion, appear to have a 15% risk of vaginal recurrence at 10 years when treated with initial surgery alone.[267] A randomized GOG study compared surgery alone with surgery and postoperative pelvic irradiation for "intermediate-risk" patients, including those with stage IB, IC, and occult stage II disease (GOG 99).[156] Early results showed a 2-year progression-free rate of 88% for surgery alone and a rate of 96% for surgery with postoperative irradiation ($P = 0.004$). When patterns of recurrence were examined, 13 vaginal recurrences were noted among 202 women who were randomized to undergo surgery alone (6%), compared with 3 vaginal recurrences in 190 women who were randomized to receive adjuvant irradiation (1.6%). Four pelvic and vaginal recurrences occurred in the surgery-only arm, compared with none in the adjuvant radiation arm. Patients with extrauterine disease have a higher risk of pelvic recurrence, depending on the type and number of extrauterine sites of disease.

A group of Dutch institutions conducted the PORTEC randomized trial of surgery alone (without lymphadenectomy) vs. surgery and postoperative pelvic radiation for selected patients with stage I disease (grade 1 disease and > 50% myometrial invasion, grade 2 disease and any level of invasion, and grade 3 disease and < 50% invasion).[157] Cancer-related deaths at 5 years occurred in 6% in the surgery-only arm and in 9% in the adjuvant radiation arm. However, locoregional recurrences were significantly reduced in the adjuvant radiation arm. Locoregional relapses were seen in 14% after surgery alone and in 4% after adjuvant radiation at 5 years. In 73% of cases, relapse was confined to the vagina. Adjuvant pelvic radiation reduced recurrences in both the vaginal vault and pelvis compared with surgery alone. This study also found that salvage treatment for vaginal relapse was associated with a 3-year survival rate of 69%, compared with 13% after pelvic or distant relapse. This salvage rate was better in the surgery arm, presumably because high-dose radiation could be delivered more readily for salvage therapy when none was given postoperatively.

Treatment of Pelvic Recurrence

Exenteration

Surgical treatment of pelvic relapse often requires partial or total exenteration. Barakat and associates[264] reported 44 patients treated with exenteration for recurrent endometrial cancer in the pelvis (location not otherwise described), 77% of whom had received previous irradiation. The median interval to recurrence in this series was 28 months, and half of the patients required total exenteration. The median survival after salvage surgery was 10 months, with nine patients (20%) alive at more than 5 years. However, 80% had major postoperative complications.

Radical Radiation

Radical irradiation is usually the treatment of choice for patients initially treated with surgery alone. High-dose pelvic radiation with intravaginal brachytherapy is effective salvage therapy. Isolated vaginal recurrences are more successfully treated than recurrences of the pelvic side wall or pelvic lymph nodes, but pelvic lymph node recurrences may still require high-dose palliation. Factors associated with treatment outcome for recurrence include tumor size, grade, location in the vagina (distal vs. apical), and disease-free interval.[268]

Outcome

Prognostic factors and outcomes in patients with pelvic recurrences have been examined. Methods of salvage therapy have varied, depending on the presentation and extent of recurrent disease and the type of previous therapy. A series of 42 women with recurrent endometrial cancer after surgery alone were treated at Princess Margaret Hospital, all with combined external beam and intracavitary therapy to a median total dose of 81.5 Gy.[269] The median time to recurrence postoperatively was 1.3 years. The 5- and 10-year survival rates after salvage treatment were 53% and 41%, respectively. The rate of local control was 65%, and was affected by vaginal stage and the size of the recurrence. The authors also noted that the rate of local control differed by vaginal location (66% for apex and 100% for distal) compared with central pelvic sites (44%). Although local control was better with a total dose of greater than 80 Gy (72% vs. 54% for < 80 Gy), this was not statistically significant. Sears and associates[270] reported 45 patients who had not received postoperative pelvic radiation therapy and then had vaginal (85%) or pelvic (15%) recurrence of endometrial cancer. Recurrences were analyzed by the corresponding change in the grade of vaginal cancer. The median time to recurrence was 12 months, and long-term median follow-up had elapsed. Salvage treatment consisted of external beam radiation alone in 40%, external beam radiation and brachytherapy in 56%, and brachytherapy alone in 4%, with a median dose of 50 Gy. The 5-year disease-specific survival rate was 51%, the overall survival rate was 44%, and the locoregional control rate was 54%. Factors associated with local control were vaginal stage of recurrent disease, tumor size, technique of radiation boost, time to recurrence, and age. The disease-specific survival rate was influenced by local control (74% for local control vs. 23% without local control).

An Austrian series of 56 patients with pelvic relapse after hysterectomy included 41% who had received adjuvant irradiation, and 71% of recurrences were vaginal.[271] A reirradiation dose of approximately two thirds of the initial dose was used in previously irradiated patients (30 to 40 Gy,), and was increased as the interval

Specific Malignancies

from the previous radiation therapy increased. Nearly half of the patients were treated with pelvic radiation and brachytherapy, 25% had brachytherapy alone, and 16% had external irradiation only, whereas 12% had no radiation therapy. Better 3-year survival rates were seen in patients who had no previous irradiation (59% vs. 25%), low-grade disease (48% vs. 22%), a relapse-free interval of more than 2 years (55% vs. 35%), and recurrence only in the vagina (54% vs. 19%). A series of 26 patients treated with external radiation therapy or brachytherapy for locoregional recurrence of endometrial cancer reported a 5-year overall survival rate of 44%.[272] These authors also noted that the size of recurrent disease affected the success of salvage therapy. Locoregional control was achieved in 100% of patients with recurrent tumors smaller than 2 cm, 83% of patients with tumors 2 to 4 cm, and 67% of those with tumors larger than 4 cm. Also, the use of combined external irradiation and brachytherapy resulted in 100% locoregional control, whereas the use of either treatment mode alone resulted in a second relapse in 4 of 10 patients.

Other series had less promising results, possibly because of the extent of pelvic recurrence. Kuten and associates[273] reviewed a group of patients with recurrent disease, only 33% of whom had isolated vaginal recurrence, whereas another third had simultaneous pelvic and distant recurrence. For the entire group, the rate of locoregional control was only 35%, and the 5-year survival rate was 18%. The overall vaginal control rate was 82%, and patients with isolated vaginal recurrence had a 5-year progression-free survival rate of 40%. No patients with pelvic recurrence were alive beyond 1.5 years. In a study of 73 women undergoing salvage radiation therapy for

pelvic recurrence after surgery alone, 60% received combined external radiation and brachytherapy, 23% received brachytherapy alone, and 17% received external radiation alone, to a mean physical dose of 76 Gy.[274] Most patients in this study had vaginal stage II (60%) or III (34%) disease. The 5-year survival rate was 25%, and the response rate was 73%, with 67% experiencing progressive disease, slightly more than half of whom had local progression.

Isolated Vaginal Recurrence

Salvage therapy for isolated vaginal recurrence may include treatment with external beam irradiation plus a vaginal brachytherapy boost, or intravaginal brachytherapy alone. Several series examined the prognosis and outcomes for this selected group of patients, and these studies are summarized in Table 91-15. Overall survival rates after salvage therapy for vaginal recurrence range from 25% to 69%. In the largest retrospective series from M.D. Anderson Cancer Center, 91 patients with isolated vaginal recurrence received pelvic radiation alone (31%), brachytherapy alone (12%), or a combination of both modalities (57%).[275] At a median follow-up of 58 months, the 5-year local control rate was 75% and the overall survival rate was 43%. Predictors of better local control included combined-modality irradiation and dose greater than 80 Gy. Curran and associates[276] reported 55 women with isolated vaginal recurrence after hysterectomy. Nearly half received pelvic radiation and vaginal brachytherapy, 30% had external radiation alone, and 7% had brachytherapy alone, to a median dose of 60 Gy. The 5-year survival rate was 31% and the 5-year pelvic control rate was 42%. The outcome was highly dependent on the radiation dose, with a 68% pelvic control rate at 5 years if

TABLE 91-15

Results for Treatment of Isolated Vaginal Recurrence

STUDY	NO. OF PATIENTS	TREATMENT	PELVIC CONTROL*	5-YR SURVIVAL RATE
Curran [276]	55	Pelvic RT and/or Brachy	Stage* I: 100	85
			Stage IIA: 53	59
			Stage IIB: 35	26
Wylie [269]	46	Pelvic RT ± ICRT	Stage I: 94	71
			Stage IIA: 65	61
			Stage IIB: 45	27
Sears [270]	39	Pelvic RT and/or Brachy	Stage I: 77	44
			Stage II: 51 (entire group)	
Greven [277]	18	Pelvic RT and ICRT	44	33
Kuten [273]	17	Pelvic RT and/or Brachy	82 (vaginal control)	40 (PFS)
Colombo [279]	35	ICRT (LDR)	86	57
Morgan [278]	34	Pelvic RT and/or Brachy	85	68
Tewari [281]	30	Interstitial (LDR) ± Pelvic RT	83	65
Charra [283]	37	Interstitial (LDR) ± Pelvic RT	70	56
Nag [154]	10	Interstitial (LDR)	64	42
	5	Pelvic RT + Interstitial (LDR)	100	
Pai [280]	20	IC RT (HDR) ± Pelvic RT	74 (10 year)	71 (CSS)
Jhingran [275]	91	Pelvic RT and/or Brachy (LDR)	75	43

Brachy, brachytherapy (various); CSS, cause specific survival; HDR, high dose rate; ICRT, intracavitary radiation therapy; LDR, low dose rate; PFS, progression-free survival; RT, radiation therapy.
*Stage refers to the extent of recurrent vaginal disease.

60 Gy or more was delivered, compared with 10% for those receiving less than 60 Gy (including some patients who received no radiation). The 5-year survival rate was also worse for patients receiving reirradiation, 16% at 5 years vs. 48% for those receiving a first course of radiation therapy. Using the vaginal carcinoma staging criteria to describe the extent of disease, this study found that survival rates diminished as the "stage" of recurrent disease increased. In addition, better pelvic control rates were seen in recurrences located in the vaginal apex than in the suburethral area (56% vs. 20%).

Greven and Olds[277] treated 18 patients with isolated vaginal recurrence with a combination of external pelvis radiation and intravaginal ovoids. They achieved a 3-year local control rate of 44% and an overall survival rate of 33% at a follow-up of 3 to 10 years. Morgan and colleagues[278] used pelvic fields and either intracavitary or interstitial brachytherapy in 34 patients with isolated vaginal recurrence, resulting in a pelvic control rate of 85%, a 5-year survival rate of 68%, and a disease-free survival rate of 60%. Better control rates were seen in patients with disease of less than 2 cm and in those treated with radiation doses greater than 60 Gy. A group of patients from the University of Milan who had isolated vaginal recurrence after surgery alone were treated with low-dose-rate intravaginal ovoids or cylinders to a dose of 60 to 70 Gy at the vaginal surface.[279] The median time to relapse was 14 months. Vaginal recurrences were located in the upper third of the vagina in 69%, in the middle third in 9%, in the lower third in 11%, and diffusely in 11%. All patients had a complete response to therapy, and 12% subsequently had treatment failure, for an overall local control rate of 86%.

Low-dose-rate brachytherapy, as described in the previous studies, is believed to provide equivalent tumor control rates compared with high-dose-rate therapy. Both methods have been widely used in the adjuvant postoperative setting to deliver a vaginal cuff boost, with or without external pelvic irradiation. Pai and associates[280] reported the use of high-dose-rate intracavitary brachytherapy for isolated vaginal recurrence. Thirteen of 20 patients received external pelvic radiation (44 Gy) and a high-dose-rate vaginal boost (24 Gy). The others were treated with high-dose-rate intracavitary therapy alone (35 Gy). Complete response was noted in 90%, with second local relapses occurring within 30 months in 22%, for a 10-year local control rate of 74%. The 10-year disease-free survival rate was 46% and the complication rate was 15%, with no grade 3 or 4 late complications. This study suggests that high-dose-rate intravaginal therapy is also an effective treatment for vaginal recurrence and is well tolerated.

Interstitial brachytherapy has also been used for the treatment of vaginal wall recurrences. Tewari and associates[281] reported 30 patients who had isolated vaginal relapse after initial surgery alone (18 patients), who were treated with external irradiation followed by an interstitial implant, or with implant alone for previously irradiated patients (12 patients). The method used was the Syed-Neblett vaginal template, placed transperineally, for a cumulative dose of 86 Gy in the patients with post-operative relapse and 98.5 Gy in the reirradiation group. All of the recurrent tumors were larger than 2 cm, with a median time to relapse of 29 months from initial diagnosis. Complete clinical responses were noted in 93%, with 18% second local relapses at a median interval of 16 months. The median survival after recurrence was 60 months, with a 5-year survival rate of 65%. Only five patients had major morbidity, including fistula (n = 2), stricture (n = 1), and proctitis (n = 2). Nag and colleagues[282] also used a perineal interstitial template for vaginal recurrences, combining external beam radiation with a 30-Gy boost for postoperative relapses and using 50 to 55 Gy interstitial therapy alone for previously irradiated patients.[282] They reported an overall local control rate of 66% and a 5-year survival rate of 42%. A French group used an intravaginal template with embedded needles to treat recurrences in the vaginal vault, and achieved a 70% rate of local control and an overall survival rate of 56%.[283] Thus interstitial brachytherapy provides a reasonable chance of local control, and may be used to treat more extensive tumors that are not amenable to simple intravaginal brachytherapy.

FUTURE ISSUES

Endometrial cancer largely presents at an early stage, when surgery is possible and often curative. However, a number of high-risk features require patients to undergo adjuvant radiation therapy postoperatively. Current screening methods are relatively insensitive, and new imaging modalities, such as magnetic resonance imaging and ultrasound, may be combined with molecular markers to identify patients at even earlier stages of disease.

One of the biggest areas of controversy in early-stage endometrial cancer involves which patients benefit from adjuvant therapy and whether this should include pelvic irradiation, with or without a vaginal brachytherapy boost. Because bimodality therapy is associated with an increased risk of both acute and long-term sequelae, better criteria for adjuvant therapy in the various subsets of patients with stage I disease may allow fewer patients to be exposed to the risks of combined surgery and radiation. In addition, the use of less invasive and less extensive laparoscopic surgical approaches for both primary surgery and staging procedures may further reduce the risk of side effects. In patients destined to be long-term survivors, the focus must now turn to reducing treatment sequelae and addressing quality-of-life issues. The outcomes for patients with high-risk histologic features remain poor, necessitating the study of more effective systemic agents.

In advanced endometrial cancer, both local control and distant metastases are important challenges. Unfortunately, active systemic chemotherapy and hormonal regimens have not been well defined. Thus trials examining new systemic agents are warranted. Newer biologic agents may be useful in certain subsets of patients. The participation of willing patients in collaborative group trials should be strongly encouraged so that these questions and others can be answered. Current protocols are looking at the use of adjuvant chemotherapy for early-stage disease and at multiagent chemotherapy regimens for advanced or recurrent disease. Future protocols may involve newer biologic agents, such as COX-2 inhibitors, and newer hormonal agents, such as fulvestrant, an ER downregulator. Finally, these studies will use molecular analyses to identify biomarkers for prognosis.

REFERENCES

1. Jemal A, Murray T, Samuels A, et al: Cancer Statistics, 2003. CA Cancer J Clin 2003;53:5-26.
2. Ries LAG, Eisner MP, Kosary CL, et al: SEER Cancer Statistics Review, 1975-2000. National Cancer Institute, 2003.
3. Harlow BL, Weiss NS, Lofton S: The epidemiology of sarcomas of the uterus. J Natl Cancer Inst 1986;76:399-402.
4. Moore KL: The perineum and pelvis. In Gardner JM (ed): Clinically Oriented Anatomy, 2nd ed. Baltimore, Williams & Wilkins, 1985, pp 373-380.
5. Partridge EE, Shingleton HM, Menck HR: The National Cancer Data Base report on endometrial cancer. J Sur Oncol 1996;61:111-123.
6. Bokhman JV: Two pathogenetic types of endometrial carcinoma. Gynecol Oncol 1983;15:10-17.
7. Nyholm HC, Nielsen AL, Norup P: Endometrial cancer in postmenopausal women with and without previous estrogen replacement treatment: Comparison of clinical and histopathological characteristics. Gynecol Oncol 1993;49:229-235.
8. Berends MJ, Kleibeuker JH, de Vries EG, et al: The importance of family history in young patients with endometrial cancer. Eur J Obstet Gynecol Reprod Biol 1999;82:139-141.
9. Parslov M, Lidegaard O, Klintorp S, et al: Risk factors among young women with endometrial cancer: A Danish case-control study. Am J Obstet Gynecol 2000;182:23-29.
10. Evans-Metcalf ER, Brooks SE, Reale FR, Baker SP: Profile of women 45 years of age and younger with endometrial cancer. Obstet Gynecol 1998;91:349-354.
11. Patsner B: Endometrial cancer in women 45 years of age or younger. Eur J Gynaecol Oncol 2000;21:249-250.
12. Deligdisch L, Kase NG, Bleiweiss IJ: Endometrial cancer in elderly women: A histologic and steroid receptor study. Gerontology 2000;46:17-21.
13. Hicks ML, Phillips JL, Parham G, et al: The National Cancer Data Base report on endometrial carcinoma in African-American women. Cancer 1998;83:2629-2637.
14. Hoffman M, Roberts WS, Cavanagh D: Second pelvic malignancies following radiation therapy for cervical cancer. Obstet Gynecol Surv 1985;40:611-617.
15. Norris HJ, Taylor HB: Postirradiation sarcomas of the uterus. Obstet Gynecol 1965;26:689-694.
16. Mark RJ, Poen J, Tran LM, et al: Postirradiation sarcoma of the gynecologic tract: A report of 13 cases and a discussion of the risk of radiation-induced gynecologic malignancies. Am J Clin Oncol 1996;19:59-64.
17. Schwartz SM, Weiss NS, Daling JR, et al: Incidence of histologic types of uterine sarcoma in relation to menstrual and reproductive history. Int J Cancer 1991;49:362-367.
18. McPherson CP, Sellers TA, Potter JD, et al: Reproductive factors and risk of endometrial cancer: The Iowa Women's Health Study. Am J Epidemiol 1996;143:1195-1202.
19. Lambe M, Wuu J, Weiderpass E, Hsieh CC: Childbearing at older age and endometrial cancer risk (Sweden). Cancer Causes Control 1999;10:43-49.
20. Parazzini F, Negri E, La Vecchia C, et al: Role of reproductive factors on the risk of endometrial cancer. Int J Cancer 1998;76:784-786.
21. Potischman N, Hoover RN, Brinton LA, et al: Case-control study of endogenous steroid hormones and endometrial cancer. J Natl Cancer Inst 1996;88:1127-1135.
22. Shapiro JA, Weiss NS, Beresford SA, Voigt LF: Menopausal hormone use and endometrial cancer, by tumor grade and invasion. Epidemiology 1998;9:99-101.
23. Dai D, Wolf DM, Litman ES, et al: Progesterone inhibits human endometrial cancer cell growth and invasiveness: Downregulation of cellular adhesion molecules through progesterone B receptors. Cancer Res 2000;62:881-886.
24. McGonigle KF, Karlan BY, Barbuto DA, et al: Development of endometrial cancer in women on estrogen and progestin hormone replacement therapy. Gynecol Oncol 1994;55:126-132.
25. Parazzini F, La Vecchia C, Moroni S, Chatenoud L, Ricci E: Family history and the risk of endometrial cancer. Int J Cancer 1994;59:460-462.
26. Gruber SB, Thompson WD: A population-based study of endometrial cancer and familial risk in younger women: Cancer and Steroid Hormone Study Group. Cancer Epidemiol Biomarkers Prev 1996;5:411-417.
27. Geisler JP, Sorosky JI, Duong HL, et al: Papillary serous carcinoma of the uterus: Increased risk of subsequent or concurrent development of breast carcinoma. Gynecol Oncol 2001;83:501-503.
28. Kaaks R, Lukanova A, Kurzer MS: Obesity, endogenous hormones, and endometrial cancer risk: A synthetic review. Cancer Epidemiol Biomarkers Prev 2002;11:1531-1543.
29. Olson SH, Trevisan M, Marshall JR: Body mass index, weight gain, and risk of endometrial cancer. Nutr Cancer 1995;23:141-149.
30. Weiderpass E, Persson I, Adami HO: Body size in different periods of life, diabetes mellitus, hypertension, and risk of postmenopausal endometrial cancer (Sweden). Cancer Causes Control 2000;11:185-192.
31. Goodman MT, Hankin JH, Wilkens LR: Diet, body size, physical activity, and the risk of endometrial cancer. Cancer Res 1997;57:5077-5085.
32. Potischman N, Swanson CA, Brinton LA: Dietary associations in a case-control study of endometrial cancer. Cancer Causes Control 1993;4:239-250.
33. Maatela J, Aromaa A, Salmi T, et al: The risk of endometrial cancer in diabetic and hypertensive patients: A nationwide record-linkage study in Finland. Ann Chir Gynaecol Suppl 1994;208:20-24.
34. Salazar-Martinez E, Lazcano-Ponce EC, Lira-Lira GG, et al: Case-control study of diabetes, obesity, physical activity and risk of endometrial cancer among Mexican women. Cancer Causes Control 2000;11:707-711.
35. Shoff SM, Newcomb PA: Diabetes, body size, and risk of endometrial cancer. Am J Epidemiol 1998;148:234-240.
36. Killackey MA, Hakes TB, Pierce VK: Endometrial adenocarcinoma in breast cancer patients receiving antiestrogens. Cancer Treat Rep 1985;69:237-238.
37. van Leeuwen FE, Benraadt J, Coebergh JW, et al: Risk of endometrial cancer after tamoxifen treatment of breast cancer. Lancet 1994;343:448-452.
38. Fisher B, Costantino JP, Redmond CK, et al: Endometrial cancer in tamoxifen-treated breast cancer patients: Findings from the National Surgical Adjuvant Breast and Bowel Project (NSABP) B-14. J Natl Cancer Inst 1994;86:527-537.
39. Terry P, Baron JA, Weiderpass E, et al: Lifestyle and endometrial cancer risk: A cohort study from the Swedish Twin Registry. Int J Cancer 1999;82:38-42.
40. Terry PD, Rohan TE, Franceschi S, Weiderpass E: Cigarette smoking and the risk of endometrial cancer. Lancet Oncol 2002;3: 470-480.
41. Kurman RJ, Kaminski PF, Norris HJ: The behavior of endometrial hyperplasia: A long-term study of "untreated" hyperplasia in 170 patients. Cancer 1985;56:403-412.
42. Janicek MF, Rosenshein NB: Invasive endometrial cancer in uteri resected for atypical endometrial hyperplasia. Gynecol Oncol 1994;52:373-378.
43. Chhieng DC, Elgert P, Cohen JM, Cangiarella JF: Clinical implications of atypical glandular cells of undetermined significance, favor endometrial origin. Cancer 2001;93:351-356.
44. Fanning J, Evans MC, Peters AJ, et al: Endometrial adenocarcinoma histologic subtypes: Clinical and pathologic profile. Gynecol Oncol 1989;32:288-291.
45. Zaino RJ, Kurman RJ, Brunetto VL, et al: Villoglandular adenocarcinoma of the endometrium: A clinicopathologic study of 61 cases. A Gynecologic Oncology Group Study. Am J Surg Pathol 1998;22:1379-1385.

46. Hendrickson MR, Kempson RL: Ciliated carcinoma: A variant of endometrial adenocarcinoma. A report of 10 cases. Int J Gynecol Pathol 1983;2:1–12.

47. Shepherd JH: Revised FIGO staging for gynaecological cancer. Br J Obstet Gynaecol 1989;96:889–892.

48. Connelly PJ, Alberhasky RC, Christopherson WM: Carcinoma of the endometrium: III. Analysis of 865 cases of adenocarcinoma and adenoacanthoma. Obstet Gynecol 1982;59:569–575.

49. Creasman WT, Morrow CP, Bundy BN, et al: Surgical pathologic spread patterns of endometrial cancer: A Gynecologic Oncology Group Study. Cancer 1987;60(Suppl 8):2035–2041.

50. Christopherson WM, Alberhasky RC, Connelly PJ: Carcinoma of the endometrium: II. Papillary adenocarcinoma. A clinical pathological study: 46 cases. Am J Clin Pathol 1982;77:534–540.

51. Demopoulos RI, Genega E, Vamvakas E, et al: Papillary carcinoma of the endometrium: Morphometric predictors of survival. Int J Gynecol Pathol 1996;15:110–118.

52. Goff BA, Kato D, Schmidt RA, et al: Uterine papillary serous carcinoma: Patterns of metastatic spread. Gynecol Oncol 1994;54:264–268.

53. Cirisano FD Jr, Robboy SJ, Dodge RK, et al: Epidemiologic and surgicopathologic findings of papillary serous and clear cell endometrial cancers when compared to endometrioid carcinoma. Gynecol Oncol 1999;74:385–394.

54. Kaufman RH, Adam E: Findings in female offspring of women exposed in utero to diethylstilbestrol. Obstet Gynecol 2002;99:197–200.

55. Abeler VM, Vergote IB, Kjorstad KE, Trope CG: Clear cell carcinoma of the endometrium: Prognosis and metastatic pattern. Cancer 1996;78:1740–1747.

56. Murphy KT, Rotmensch J, Yamada SD, Mundt AJ: Outcome and patterns of failure in pathologic stages I-IV clear-cell carcinoma of the endometrium: Implications for adjuvant radiation therapy. Int J Radiat Oncol Biol Phys 2003;55:1272–1276.

57. Carcangiu ML, Chambers JT: Early pathologic stage clear cell carcinoma and uterine papillary serous carcinoma of the endometrium: Comparison of clinicopathologic features and survival. Int J Gynecol Pathol 1995;14:30–38.

58. Tiltman AJ: Mucinous carcinoma of the endometrium. Obstet Gynecol 1980;55:244–247.

59. Goodman A, Zukerberg LR, Rice LW, et al: Squamous cell carcinoma of the endometrium: A report of eight cases and a review of the literature. Oncology 1996;61:54–60.

60. Tornos C, Silva EG, Khorana SM, Burke TW: High-stage endometrioid carcinoma of the ovar: Prognostic significance of pure versus mixed histologic types. Am J Surg Pathol 1994;18:687–693.

61. Kumar NB, Hart WR: Metastases to the uterine corpus from extragenital cancers: A clinicopathologic study of 63 cases. Cancer 1982;50:2163–2169.

62. Goff A, Rice LW, Fleischhacker D, et al: Uterine leiomyosarcoma and endometrial stromal sarcoma: Lymph node metastases and sites of recurrence. Gynecol Oncol 1993;50:105–109.

63. Norris HJ, Taylor HB: Mesenchymal tumors of the uterus: I. A clinical and pathological study of 53 endometrial stromal tumors. Cancer 1966;19:755–766.

64. Chang KL, Crabtree GS, Lim-Tan SK, et al: Primary uterine endometrial stromal neoplasms: A clinicopathologic study of 117 cases. Am J Surg Pathol 1990;14:415–438.

65. Roth LM (ed): Contemporary Issues in Surgical Pathology. New York, Churchill Livingstone, 1993, pp 265–328.

66. Tosi P, Sforza V, Santopietro R: Estrogen receptor content, immunohistochemically determined by monoclonal antibodies, in endometrial stromal sarcoma. Obstet Gynecol 1989;73:75–78.

67. DeFusco PA, Gaffey TA, Malkasian GD Jr, et al: Endometrial stromal sarcoma: Review of Mayo Clinic experience, 1945–1980. Gynecol Oncol 1989;35:8–14.

68. Gadducci A, Sartori E, Landoni F, et al: Endometrial stromal sarcoma: Analysis of treatment failures and survival. Gynecol Oncol 1996;63:247–253.

69. Gallup DG, Gable DS, Talledo OE, Otken LB Jr: A clinical-pathologic study of mixed mullerian tumors of the uterus over a 16-year period: The Medical College of Georgia experience. Am J Obstet Gynecol 1989;161:533–538; discussion 538–539.

70. Macasaet MA, Waxman M, Fruchter RG, et al: Prognostic factors in malignant mesodermal (mullerian) mixed tumors of the uterus. Gynecol Oncol 1985;20:32–42.

71. Spanos WJ Jr, Wharton JT, Gomez L, et al: Malignant mixed mullerian tumors of the uterus. Cancer 1984;53:311–316.

72. Kleine W, Maier T, Geyer H, Pfleiderer A: Estrogen and progesterone receptors in endometrial cancer and their prognostic relevance. Gynecol Oncol 1990;38:59–65.

73. Creasman WT, Soper JT, McCarty KS Jr, et al: Influence of cytoplasmic steroid receptor content on prognosis of early stage endometrial carcinoma. Am J Obstet Gynecol 1985;151:922–932.

74. Sutton GP, Geisler HE, Stehman FB, et al: Features associated with survival and disease-free survival in early endometrial cancer. Am J Obstet Gynecol 1989;160:1385–1391; discussion 1391–1393.

75. Chambers JT, MacLusky N, Eisenfield A, et al: Estrogen and progestin receptor levels as prognosticators for survival in endometrial cancer. Gynecol Oncol 1988; 31:65–81.

76. Martin JD, Hahnel R, McCartney AJ, Woodings TL: The effect of estrogen receptor status on survival in patients with endometrial cancer. Am J Obstet Gynecol 1983;147:322–324.

77. Runowicz CD, Nuchtern LM, Braunstein JD, Jones JG: Heterogeneity in hormone receptor status in primary and metastatic endometrial cancer. Gynecol Oncol 1990;38:437–441.

78. Kumar NS, Richer J, Owen G, et al: Selective down-regulation of progesterone receptor isoform B in poorly differentiated human endometrial cancer cells: Implications for unopposed estrogen action. Cancer Res 1998;58:1860–1065.

79. Takama F, Kanuma T, Wang D, et al: Oestrogen receptor beta expression and depth of myometrial invasion in human endometrial cancer. Br J Cancer 2001;84:545–549.

80. Sasaki M, Tanaka Y, Kaneuchi M, et al: Polymorphisms of estrogen receptor alpha gene in endometrial cancer. Biochem Biophys Res Commun 2002;297:558–564.

81. Berchuck A, Rodriguez G, Kinney RB, et al: Overexpression of HER-2/neu in endometrial cancer is associated with advanced stage disease. Am J Obstet Gynecol 1991;164:15–21.

82. Rolitsky CD, Theil KS, McGaughy VR, et al: HER-2/neu amplification and overexpression in endometrial carcinoma. In J Gynecol Pathol 1999;18:138–143.

83. Niederacher D, An HX, Cho YJ, et al: Mutations and amplification of oncogenes in endometrial cancer. Oncology 1999;56:59–65.

84. Saffari B, Jones LA, el-Naggar A, et al: Amplification and overexpression of HER-2/neu (c-erbB2) in endometrial cancers: Correlation with overall survival. Cancer Res 1995;55:5693–5698.

85. Coronado PJ, Vidart JA, Lopez-Asenjo JA, et al: P53 overexpression predicts endometrial carcinoma recurrence better than HER-2/neu overexpression. Eur J Obstet Gynecol Reprod Biol 2001;98:103–108.

86. Eissa S, Abu Saada M, el-Sharkawy T: Flow cytometric cell cycle kinetics and quantitative measurement of c-erbB-2 and mutant p53 proteins in normal, hyperplastic, and malignant endometrial biopsies. Clin Biochem 1997;30:209–214.

87. Halperin R, Zehavi S, Habler L, et al: Comparative immunohistochemical study of endometrioid and serous papillary carcinoma of endometrium. Eur J Gynaecol Oncol 2001;22:122–126.

88. Santin AD, Bellone S, Gokden M, et al: Overexpression of HER-2/neu in uterine serous papillary cancer. Clin Cancer Res 2002;8:1271–1279.

89. Kounelis S, Kapranos N, Kouri E, et al: Immunohistochemical profile of endometrial adenocarcinoma: A study of 61 cases and review of the literature. Mod Pathol 2000;13:379–388.

90. Moll UM, Chalas E, Auguste M, et al: Uterine papillary serous carcinoma evolves via a p53-driven pathway. Hum Pathol 1996;27:1295–300.

91. Kovalev S, Marchenko ND, Gugliotta BG, et al: Loss of p53 function in uterine papillary serous carcinoma. Hum Pathol 1998;29:613–619.

92. Bancher-Todesca D, Gitsch G, Williams KE, et al: p53 protein overexpression: A strong prognostic factor in uterine papillary serous carcinoma. Gynecol Oncol 1998;71:59–63.

93. Lax SF, Pizer ES, Ronnett BM, Kurman RJ: Clear cell carcinoma of the endometrium is characterized by a distinctive profile of p53, Ki-67, estrogen, and progesterone receptor expression. Hum Pathol 1998;29:551–558.

Specific Malignancies

III

94. Jasonni VM, Santini D, Amadori A, et al: Epidermal growth factor receptor expression and endometrial cancer histotypes. Ann N Y Acad Sci 1994;30:298–305.

95. Khalifa MA, Mannel RS, Haraway SD, et al: Expression of EGFR, HER-2/neu, P53, and PCNA in endometrioid, serous papillary, and clear cell endometrial adenocarcinomas. Gynecol Oncol 1994;53: 84–92.

96. Konski AA, Domenico D, Irving D, et al: Clinicopathologic correlation of DNA flow cytometric content analysis (DFCA), surgical staging, and estrogen/progesterone receptor status in endometrial adenocarcinoma. Am J Clin Oncol 1996;19:164–168.

97. McCluggage WG, Maxwell P, Hamilton PW, Jasani B: High metallothionein expression is associated with features predictive of aggressive behaviour in endometrial carcinoma. Histopathology 1999;34:51–55.

98. Nazeer T, Church K, Amato C, et al: Comparative quantitative immunohistochemical and immunoradiometric determinations of cathepsin D in endometrial adenocarcinoma: Predictors of tumor aggressiveness. Mod Pathol 1994;7:469–474.

99. Catasus L, Machin P, Matias-Guiu X, Prat J: Microsatellite instability in endometrial carcinomas: Clinicopathologic correlations in a series of 42 cases. Hum Pathol 1996;29:1160–1164.

100. Risinger JI, Maxwell GL, Chandramouli GV, et al: Microarray analysis reveals distinct gene expression profiles among different histologic types of endometrial cancer. Cancer Res 2003;63:6–11.

101. Pautier P, Genestie C, Rey A, et al: Analysis of clinicopathologic prognostic factors for 157 uterine sarcomas and evaluation of a grading score validated for soft tissue sarcoma. Cancer 2000;88: 1425–1431.

102. Wade K, Quinn MA, Hammond I, et al: Uterine sarcoma: Steroid receptors and response to hormonal therapy. Gynecol Oncol 1994;39:364–367.

103. Malmstrom H, Schmidt H, Persson PG, et al: Flow cytometric analysis of uterine sarcoma: Ploidy and S-phase rate as prognostic indicators. Gynecol Oncol 1992;44:172–177.

104. Brenner PF: Differential diagnosis of abnormal uterine bleeding. Am J Obstet Gynecol 1996;175:766–769.

105. Tavassoli F, Kraus FT: Endometrial lesions in uteri resected for atypical endometrial hyperplasia. Am J Clin Pathol 1978;70: 770–779.

106. Timmerman D, Deprest J, Bourne T, et al: A randomized trial on the use of ultrasonography or office hysteroscopy for endometrial assessment in postmenopausal patients with breast cancer who were treated with tamoxifen. Am J Obstet Gynecol 1998;179:62–70.

107. Love CD, Muir BB, Scrimgeour JB, et al: Investigation of endometrial abnormalities in asymptomatic women treated with tamoxifen and an evaluation of the role of endometrial screening. J Clin Oncol 1999;17:2050–2054.

108. Gerber B, Krause A, Muller H, et al: Effects of adjuvant tamoxifen on the endometrium in postmenopausal women with breast cancer: A prospective long-term study using transvaginal ultrasound. J Clin Oncol 2000;18:3464–3470.

109. Burke W, Petersen G, Lynch P, et al: Recommendations for follow-up care of individuals with an inherited predisposition to cancer: I. Hereditary nonpolyposis colon cancer. Cancer Genetics Studies Consortium. JAMA 1997;277:915–919.

110. Ginath S, Menczer J, Fintsi Y, et al: Tissue and serum CA125 expression in endometrial cancer. Int J Gynecol Cancer 2002;12:372–375.

111. Patsner B, Mann WJ, Cohen H, Loesch M: Predictive value of preoperative serum CA 125 levels in clinically localized and advanced endometrial carcinoma. Am J Obstet Gynecol 1988;158:399–402.

112. Belloni C, Vigano R, del Maschio A, et al: Magnetic resonance imaging in endometrial carcinoma staging. Gynecol Oncol 1990;37:172–177.

113. Rullo S, Piccioni MG, Framarino dei Malatesta ML, et al: Sonographic, hysteroscopic, histological correlation in the early diagnosis of endometrial carcinoma. Eur J Gynaecol Oncol 1991;12:463–446.

114. Shipley CF, Smith ST, Dennis EJ, Nelson GH: Evaluation of pretreatment transvaginal ultrasonography in the management of patients with endometrial carcinoma. Am J Obstet Gynecol 1992;167:406–441.

115. Vardi JR, Tadros GH, Anselmo MT, Rafla SD: The value of exploratory laparotomy in patients with endometrial carcinoma according to the new International Federation of Gynecology and Obstetrics staging. Obstet Gynecol 1992;80:204–208.

116. Wilson TO, Podratz KC, Gaffey TA, et al: Evaluation of unfavorable histologic subtypes in endometrial adenocarcinoma. Am J Obstet Gynecol 1990;162:418–423.

117. McLellan R, Dillon MB, Currie JL, Rosenshein NB: Peritoneal cytology in endometrial cancer: A review. Obstet Gynecol Surv 1989;44:711–719.

118. Kennedy AW, Webster KD, Nunez C, Bauer LJ: Pelvic washings for cytologic analysis in endometrial adenocarcinoma. J Reprod Med 1993;38:637–642.

119. Greven KM, Corn BW, Case D, et al: Which prognostic factors influence the outcome of patients with surgically staged endometrial cancer treated with adjuvant radiation? Int J Radiat Oncol Biol Phys 1997;39:413–418.

120. Kosary CL: FIGO stage, histology, histologic grade, age and race as prognostic factors in determining survival for cancers of the female gynecological system: An analysis of 1973-87 SEER cases of cancers of the endometrium, cervix, ovary, vulva, and vagina. Semin Surg Oncol 1994;10:31–46.

121. Mundt AJ, Waggoner S, Yamada D, et al: Age as a prognostic factor for recurrence in patients with endometrial carcinoma. Gynecol Oncol 2000;79:79–85.

122. Bloss JD, Berman ML, Bloss LP, Buller RE: Use of vaginal hysterectomy for the management of stage endometrial cancer in the medically compromised patient. Gynecol Oncol 1991;40:74–77.

123. Childers JM, Surwit EA: Combined laparoscopic and vaginal surgery for the management of two case of stage I endometrial cancer. Gynecol Oncol 1992;45:46–51.

124. Eltabbakh GH, Shamonki MI, Moody JM, Garafano LL: Hysterectomy for obese women with endometrial cancer: Laparoscopy or laparotomy? Gynecol Oncol 2000;78:329–335.

125. Fram KM: Laparoscopically assisted vaginal hysterectomy versus abdominal hysterectomy in stage I endometrial cancer. Int J Gynecol Cancer 2002;12:57–61.

126. Gemignani ML, Curtin JP, Zelmanovich J, et al: Laparoscopic-assisted vaginal hysterectomy for endometrial cancer: Clinical outcomes and hospital charges. Gynecol Oncol 1999;73:5–11.

127. Malur S, Possover M, Michels W, Schneider A: Laparoscopic-assisted vaginal versus abdominal surgery in patients with endometrial cancer: A prospective randomized trial. Gynecol Oncol 2001;80:239–244.

128. Scribner DR Jr, Walker JL, Johnson GA, et al: Surgical management of early-stage endometrial cancer in the elderly: Is laparoscopy feasible? Gynecol Oncol 2001;83:563–868.

129. Eltabbakh GH, Shamonki MI, Moody JM, Garafano LL: Laparoscopy as the primary modality for the treatment of women with endometrial carcinoma. Cancer 2001;91:378–387.

130. Chu CS, Randall TC, Bandera CA, Rubin SC: Vaginal cuff recurrence of endometrial cancer treated by laparoscopic-assisted vaginal hysterectomy. Gynecol Oncol 2003;88:62–65.

131. Rutledge F: The role of radical hysterectomy in adenocarcinoma of the endometrium. Gynecol Oncol 1974;2:331–347.

132. Wolfson AH, Sightler SE, Markoe AM, et al: The prognostic significance of surgical staging for carcinoma of the endometrium. Gynecol Oncol 1992;45:142–146.

133. Mohan DS, Samuels MA, Selim MA, et al: Long-term outcomes of therapeutic pelvic lymphadenectomy for stage I endometrial adenocarcinoma. Gynecol Oncol 1998;70:165–171.

134. Goff BA, Goodman A, Muntz HG, et al: Surgical stage IV endometrial carcinoma: A study of 47 cases. Gynecol Oncol 1994;52:237–240.

135. Aalders JG, Abeler V, Kolstad P: Stage IV endometrial carcinoma: A clinical and histopathological study of 83 patients. Gynecol Oncol 1984;17:75–84.

136. Wolfson AH, Sightler SE, Markoe AM, et al: The prognostic significance of surgical staging for carcinoma of the endometrium. Gynecol Oncol 192;45:142–146.

137. Oakley G, Nahhas WA: Endometrial adenocarcinoma: Therapeutic

impact of preoperative histopathologic examination of endometrial tissue. Eur J Gynaecol Oncol 1989;10:55-260.

138. DuBeshter B, Deuel C, Gillis S, et al: Endometrial cancer: The potential role of cervical cytology in current surgical staging. Obstet Gynecol 2003;101:445-450.

139. Mariani A, Webb MJ, Keeney GL, Podratz KC: Routes of lymphatic spread: A study of 112 consecutive patients with endometrial cancer. Gynecol Oncol 2001;81:100-104.

140. Chuang L, Burke TW, Tornos C, Marino BD, et al: Staging laparotomy for endometrial carcinoma: Assessment of retroperitoneal lymph nodes. Gynecol Oncol 1995;58:189-193.

141. Kilgore LC, Partridge EE, Alvarez RD, et al: Adenocarcinoma of the endometrium: Survival comparisons of patients with and without pelvic lymph node sampling. Gynecol Oncol 1995;56:29-33.

142. Trimble EL, Kosary C, Park RC: Lymph node sampling and survival in endometrial cancer. Gynecol Oncol 1998;71:340-343.

143. Morrow CP, Bundy BN, Kurman RJ, et al: Relationship between surgical-pathological risk factors and outcome in clinical stage I and II carcinoma of the endometrium: A Gynecologic Oncology Group study. Gynecol Oncol 1991;40:55-65.

144. Mariani A, Webb MJ, Keeney GL, et al: Predictors of lymphatic failure in endometrial cancer. Gynecol Oncol 2002;84:437-442.

145. Eltabbakh GH, Piver MS, Hempling RE, Shin KH: Excellent long-term survival and absence of vaginal recurrences in 332 patients with low-risk stage I endometrial adenocarcinoma treated with hysterectomy and vaginal brachytherapy without formal staging lymph node sampling: Report of a prospective trial. Int J Radiat Oncol Biol Phys 1997;38:73-380.

146. Mariani A, Webb MJ, Keeney GL, et al: Predictors of lymphatic failure in endometrial cancer. Gynecol Oncol 2002;84:437-442.

147. Lampe B, Kurzl R, Hantschmann P: Prognostic factors that predict pelvic lymph node metastasis from endometrial carcinoma. Cancer 1994;74:2502-2508.

148. Berchuck A, Anspach C, Evans AC, et al: Postsurgical surveillance of patients with FIGO stage I/II endometrial adenocarcinoma. Gynecol Oncol 1995;59:20-24.

149. Straughn JM Jr, Huh WK, Kelly FJ, et al: Conservative management of stage I endometrial carcinoma after surgical staging. Gynecol Oncol 2002;84:194-200.

150. Chen SS: Operative treatment in stage I endometrial carcinoma with deep myometrial invasion and/or grade 3 tumor surgically limited to the corpus uteri: No recurrence with only primary surgery. Cancer 1989;63:1843-1845.

151. Larson DM, Broste SK, Krawisz BR: Surgery without radiotherapy for primary treatment of endometrial cancer. Obstet Gynecol 1998;91:355-359.

152. Jereczek-Fossa B, Badzio A, Jassem J: Recurrence endometrial cancer after surgery alone: Results of salvage radiotherapy. Int J Radiat Oncol Biol Phys 2000;48:405-413.

153. Hasbini A, Haie-Meder C, Morice P, et al: Outcome after salvage radiotherapy (brachytherapy +/- external) in patients with vaginal recurrence from endometrial carcinomas. Radiother Oncol 2002;65:23-28.

154. Nag S, Yacoub S, Copeland LJ, Fowler JM: Interstitial brachytherapy for salvage treatment of vaginal recurrences in previously unirradiated endometrial cancer patients. Int J Radiat Oncol Biol Phys 2002;54:1153-1159.

155. Aalders J, Abeler V, Kolstad P, Onsrud M: Postoperative external irradiation and prognostic parameters in stage I endometrial carcinoma: Clinical and histopathologic study of 540 patients. Obstet Gynecol 1980;56:419-427.

156. Roberts JA, Brunetto VL, Keyes HM, et al: A phase II randomized study of surgery vs. surgery plus adjuvant radiation therapy in intermediate risk endometrial cancer. Gynecol Oncol 1998;68:135.

157. Creutzberg CL, van Putten WL, Koper PC, et al: Surgery and postoperative radiotherapy versus surgery alone for patients with stage-1 endometrial carcinoma: Multicentre randomized trial. Lancet 2000;355:1404-1411.

158. Sainz de la Cuesta R, Goff BA, et al: Postoperative management of patients with stage Ib endometrial carcinoma. Eur J Gynaecol Oncol 1996;17:338-341.

159. Grigsby PW, Perez CA, Kuten A, et al: Clinical stage I endometrial cancer: Results of adjuvant irradiation and patterns of failure. Int J Radiat Oncol Biol Phys 1991;21:379-385.

160. Irwin C, Levin W, Fyles A, et al: The role of adjuvant radiotherapy in carcinoma of the endometrium. Results in 550 patients with pathologic stage I disease. Gynecol Oncol 1998;70:247-254.

161. Podczaski E, Kaminski P, Gurski K, et al: Detection and patterns of treatment failure in 300 consecutive cases of "early" endometrial cancer after primary surgery. Gynecol Oncol 1992;47:323-327.

162. Weiss MF, Connell PP, Waggoner S, et al: External pelvic radiation therapy in stage IC endometrial carcinoma. Obstet Gynecol 1999;93:599-602.

163. Ahmad NR, Lanciano RM, Corn BW, Schultheiss T: Postoperative radiation therapy for surgically staged endometrial cancer: Impact of time factors (overall treatment time and surgery-to-radiation interval) on outcome. Int J Radiat Oncol Biol Phys 1995;33:837-842.

164. Greven K, Olds W: Radiotherapy in the management of endometrial carcinoma with cervical involvement. Cancer 1987;60:1737-1740.

165. Lanciano RM, Curran WJ Jr, Greven KM, et al: Influence of grade, histologic subtype, and timing of radiotherapy on outcome among patients with stage II carcinoma of the endometrium. Gynecol Oncol 1990;39:368-373.

166. Eltabbakh GH, Moore AD: Survival of women with surgical stage II endometrial cancer. Gynecol Oncol 1999;74:80-85.

167. Sartori E, Gadducci A, Landoni F, et al: Clinical behavior of 203 stage II endometrial cancer cases: The impact of primary surgical approach and adjuvant radiation therapy. Int J Gynecol Cancer 2001;11:430-437.

168. Sause WT, Fuller DB, Smith WG, et al: Analysis of preoperative intracavitary cesium application versus postoperative external beam radiation in stage I endometrial carcinoma. Int J Radiat Oncol Biol Phys 1990;18:1011-1017.

169. Grigsby PW, Perez CA, Camel HM, et al: Stage II carcinoma of the endometrium: Results of therapy and prognostic factors. Int J Oncol Biol Phys 1985;11:1915-1923.

170. Bruckman JE, Goodman RL, Murthy A, Marck A: Combined irradiation and surgery in the treatment of stage II carcinoma of the endometrium 1978;42:1146-1151.

171. Higgins RV, van Nagell JR Jr, Horn EJ, et al: Preoperative radiation therapy followed by extrafascial hysterectomy in patients with stage II endometrial carcinoma. Cancer 1991;68:1261-1264.

172. Baram A, Figer A, Inbar M, et al: Endometrial carcinoma stage I: Comparison of two different treatment regimes. Evaluation of risk factors and its influence on prognosis, suggested step by step treatment protocol. Gynecol Oncol 1985;22:294-301.

173. Cirisana FD Jr, Robboy SJ, Dodge RK, et al: The outcome of stage I-II clinically and surgically staged papillary serous and clear cell endometrial cancers when compared with endometrioid carcinoma. Gynecol Oncol 2000;77:55-65.

174. Carcangiu ML, Chambers JT: Early pathologic stage clear cell carcinoma and uterine papillary serous carcinoma of the endometrium: Comparison of clinicopathologic features and survival. Int J Gynecol Pathol 1995;14:30-38.

175. Smith RS, Kapp DS, Chen Q, Teng NN: Treatment of high-risk uterine cancer with whole abdominopelvic radiation therapy. Int J Radiat Oncol Biol Phys 2000;48:767-778.

176. Lim P, Al Kushi A, Gilks B, et al: Early stage uterine papillary serous carcinoma of the endometrium: Effect of adjuvant whole abdominal radiotherapy and pathologic parameters on outcome. Cancer 2001;91:752-757.

177. Marchetti DL, Piver MS, Tsukada Y, Reese P: Prevention of vaginal recurrence of stage I endometrial adenocarcinoma with postoperative vaginal radiation. Obstet Gynecol 1986;67:399-402.

178. Irwin C, Levin W, Fyles A, et al: The role of adjuvant radiotherapy in carcinoma of the endometrium: Results in 550 patients with pathologic stage I disease. Gynecol Oncol 1998;70:247-254.

179. Greven KM, D'Agostino RB Jr, Lanciano RM, Corn BW: Is there a role for a brachytherapy vaginal cuff boost in the adjuvant management of patients with uterine-confined endometrial cancer? Int J Radiat Oncol Biol Phys 1998;42:101-104.

180. Randall ME, Wilder J, Greven K, Raben M: Role of intracavitary cuff boost after adjuvant external beam irradiation in early endometrial carcinoma. Int J Radiat Oncol Biol Phys 1990;19:49-54.

181. Alektiar KM, McKee A, Venkatraman E, et al: Intravaginal high-dose-rate brachytherapy for stage IB (FIGO Grade 1,2) endometrial cancer. Int J Radiat Oncol Biol Phys 2002;53:707–713.

182. Noyes WR, Bastin K, Edwards SA, et al: Postoperative vaginal cuff irradiation using high dose rate remote afterloading: A phase II clinical protocol. Int J Radiat Oncol Biol Phys 1995;32:1439–1443.

183. Anderson JM, Stea B, Hallum AV, et al: High-dose rate postoperative vaginal cuff irradiation alone for stage IB and IC endometrial cancer. Int J Radiat Oncol Biol Phys 2000;46:417–425.

184. Mandell L, Nori D, Anderson L, Hilaris B: Postoperative vaginal radiation in endometrial cancer using a remote afterloading technique. Int J Radiat Oncol Biol Phys 1985;11:473–478.

185. Nori D, Merimsky O, Batata M, Caputo T: Postoperative high dose-rate intravaginal brachytherapy combined with external irradiation for early stage endometrial cancer: A long-term follow-up. Int J Radiat Oncol Biol Phys 1994;30:831–837.

186. Stryker JA, Podczaski E, Kaminski P, Velkley D: Adjuvant external beam therapy for pathologic stage I and occult stage II endometrial carcinoma. Cancer 1991;67:2872–2879.

187. Algan O, Tabesh T, Hanlon A, et al: Improved outcome in patients treated with postoperative radiation therapy for pathologic stage I/II endometrial cancer. Int J Radiat Oncol Biol Phys 1996;35:925–933.

188. Petereit DG, Sarkaria JN, Chappell RJ: Perioperative morbidity and mortality of high-dose-rate gynecologic brachytherapy. Int J Radiat Oncol Biol Phys 1998;42:1025–1031.

189. Hoskin PJ, Cook M, Bouscale D, Cansdale J: Changes in applicator position with fractionated high dose rate gynaecological brachytherapy. Radiother Oncol 1996;40:59–62.

190. Patanaphan V, Salazar OM, Chougule P: What can be expected when radiation therapy becomes the only curative alternative for endometrial cancer? Cancer 1985;55:1462–1467.

191. Langren RC, Fletcher GH, Delclos I, Wharton JT: Irradiation of endometrial cancer in patients with medical contraindications to surgery or with unresectable lesions. Am J Roentgenol 1976;126:148–154.

192. Kupelian PA, Eifel PJ, Tornos C, et al: Treatment of endometrial carcinoma with radiation therapy alone. Int J Radiat Oncol Biol Phys 1993;27:817–824.

193. Chao CK, Grigsby PW, Perez CA, et al: Medically inoperable stage I endometrial carcinoma: A few dilemmas in radiotherapeutic management. Int J Radiat Oncol Biol Phys 1996;34:27–31.

194. Fishman DA, Roberts KB, Chambers JT, et al: Radiation therapy as exclusive treatment for medically inoperable patients with stage I and II endometrioid carcinoma with endometrium. Gynecol Oncol 1996;61:189–196.

195. Chao CK, Grigsby PW, Perez CA, et al: Brachytherapy-related complications for medically inoperable stage I endometrial carcinoma. Int J Radiat Oncol Biol Phys 1995;31:37–42.

196. Knocke TH, Kucera H, Weidinger B, et al: Primary treatment of endometrial carcinoma with high-dose-rate brachytherapy: Results of 12 years of experience with 280 patients. Int J Radiat Oncol Biol Phys 1997;37:359–365.

197. Nguyen TV, Petereit DG: High-dose-rate brachytherapy for medically inoperable stage I endometrial cancer. Gynecol Oncol 1998;71:196–203.

198. Randall ME, Brunetto G, Muss H, et al: Whole abdominal radiation versus combination doxorubicin-cisplatin chemotherapy in advanced endometrial carcinoma: A randomized phase III trial of the Gynecologic Oncology Group. Proc ASCO 2003;22:2.

199. Watkins-Bruner D, Barsevik A, Tian C, et al: Quality of life trade-off to incremental gain in survival on Gynecologic Oncology Group (GOG) Protocol 122: Whole abdominal radiation vs. doxorubicin-platinum (AP) chemotherapy in advanced endometrial cancer. Proc ASCO 2003;22:449.

200. Greven KM, Lanciano RM, Corn B, et al: Pathologic stage III endometrial carcinoma: Prognostic factors and patterns of recurrence. Cancer 1993;71:3697–3702.

201. McLellan R, Dillon MB, Currie JL, Rosenshein NB: Peritoneal cytology in endometrial cancer: A review. Obstet Gynecol Surv 1989;44:711–719.

202. Kennedy AW, Webster KD, Nunez C, Bauer LJ: Pelvic washings for cytologic analysis in endometrial adenocarcinoma. J Reprod Med 1993;38:637–642.

203. Creasman WT, DiSaia PJ, Blessing J, et al: Prognostic significance of peritoneal cytology in patients with endometrial cancer and preliminary data concerning therapy with intraperitoneal radiopharmaceuticals. Am J Obstet Gynecol 1981;141:921–929.

204. Soper JT, Creasman WT, Clarke-Pearson DL, et al: Intraperitoneal chromic phosphate P 32 suspension therapy of malignant peritoneal cytology in endometrial carcinoma. Am J Obstet Gynecol 1985;153:191–196.

205. Potish RA: Abdominal radiotherapy for cancer of the uterine cervix and endometrium. Int J Radiat Oncol Biol Phys 1989;16:1453–1458.

206. Kennedy AW, Webster KD, Nunez C, Bauer LJ: Pelvic washings for cytologic analysis in endometrial adenocarcinoma. J Reprod Med 1993;38:637–642.

207. Mazurka JL, Krepart GV, Lotocki RJ: Prognostic significance of positive peritoneal cytology in endometrial carcinoma. Am J Obstet Gynecol 1988;158:303–306.

208. Piver MS: Progesterone therapy for malignant peritoneal cytology surgical stage I endometrial adenocarcinoma. Semin Oncol 1988;15:50–52.

209. Nori D, Hilaris BS, Tome M, et al: Combined surgery and radiation in endometrial carcinoma: An analysis of prognostic factors. Int J Radiat Oncol Biol Phys 1987;13:489–497.

210. Bruckman JE, Bloomer WD, Marck A, et al: Stage III adenocarcinoma of the endometrium: Two prognostic groups. Gynecol Oncol 1980;9:12–17.

211. Antoniades J, Brady LW, Lewis GC: The management of stage III carcinoma of the endometrium. Cancer 1976;38:1838–1842.

212. Potish RA, Twiggs LB, Adcock LL, Prem KA: Role of whole abdominal radiation therapy in the management of endometrial cancer: Prognostic importance of factors indicating peritoneal metastases. Gynecol Oncol 1985;21:80–86.

213. Greer BE, Hamberger AD: Treatment of intraperitoneal metastatic adenocarcinoma of the endometrium by the whole-abdomen moving-strip technique and pelvic boost irradiation. Gynecol Oncol 1983;16:365–373.

214. Nelson G, Randall M, Sutton G, et al: FIGO stage IIIC endometrial carcinoma with metastases confined to pelvic lymph nodes: Analysis of treatment outcomes, prognostic variables, and failure patterns following adjuvant radiation therapy. Gynecol Oncol 1999;75:211–214.

215. Katz LA, Andrews SJ, Fanning J: Survival after multimodality treatment for stage IIIC endometrial cancer. Am J Obstet Gynecol 2001;184:1071–1073.

216. McMeekin DS, Lashbrook D, Gold M, et al: Analysis of FIGO stage IIIc endometrial cancer patients. Gynecol Oncol 2001;81:273–278.

217. Mundt AJ, Murphy KT, Rotmensch J, et al: Surgery and postoperative radiation therapy in FIGO stage IIIC endometrial carcinoma. Int J Radiat Oncol Biol Phys 2001;50:1154–1160.

218. Potish RA, Twiggs LB, Adcock LL, et al: Paraaortic lymph node radiotherapy in cancer of the uterine corpus. Obstet Gynecol 1985;65:251–256.

219. Corn BW, Lanciano RM, Greven KM, et al: Endometrial cancer with para-aortic adenopathy: Patterns of failure and opportunities for cure. Int J Radiat Oncol Biol Phys 1992;24:223–227.

220. Rose PG, Cha SD, Tak WK, et al: Radiation therapy for surgically proven para-aortic node metastasis in endometrial carcinoma. Int J Radiat Oncol Biol Phys 1992;24:229–233.

221. Onda T, Yoshikawa H, Mizutani K, et al: Treatment of node-positive endometrial cancer with complete node dissection, chemotherapy and radiation therapy. Br J Cancer 1997;75:1836–1841.

222. International Federation of Gynecology and Obstetrics: Classification and staging of malignant tumors in the female pelvis. Int J Gynaecol Obstet 1971;9:172.

223. Grigsby PW, Perez CA, Kuske RR, et al: Results of therapy, analysis of failures, and prognostic factors for clinical and pathologic stage III adenocarcinoma of the endometrium. Gynecol Oncol 1987;27:44–57.

224. Aalders JG, Abeler V, Kolstad P: Clinical (stage III) as compared to subclinical intrapelvic extrauterine tumor spread in endometrial

carcinoma: A clinical and histopathological study of 175 patients. Gynecol Oncol 1984;17:64–74.

225. Bristow RE, Zerbe MJ, Rosenshein NB, et al: Stage IVB endometrial carcinoma: The role of cytoreductive surgery and determinants of survival. Gynecol Oncol 2000;78:85–91.

226. Chi DS, Welshinger M, Venkatraman ES, Barakat RR: The role of surgical cytoreduction in stage IV endometrial carcinoma. Gynecol Oncol 1997;67:56–60.

227. Pliskow S, Penalver M, Averette HE: Stage III and stage IV endometrial carcinoma: A review of 41 cases. Gynecol Oncol 1990;38:210–215.

228. Burke TW, Heller PB, Woodward JE, et al: Treatment failure in endometrial carcinoma. Obstet Gynecol 1990;75:96–101.

229. Onsrud M, Hagen B, Strickert T: 10-Gy single-fraction pelvic irradiation for palliation and life prolongation in patients with cancer of the cervix and corpus uteri. Gynecol Oncol 2001;82:167–171.

230. Spanos WJ Jr, Perez CA, Marcus S, et al: Effect of rest interval on tumor and normal tissue response: A report of phase III study of accelerated split course palliative radiation for advanced pelvic malignancies (RTOG-8502). Int J Radiat Oncol Biol Phys 1993;25:399–403.

231. Salazar OM, Feldstein ML, DePapp EW, et al: Endometrial carcinoma: Analysis of failures with special emphasis on the use of initial preoperative external pelvic radiation. Int J Radiat Oncol Biol Phys 1977;2:1101–1107.

232. Burke TW, Gershenson DM, Morris M, et al: Postoperative adjuvant cisplatin, doxorubicin, and cyclophosphamide (PAC) chemotherapy in women with high-risk endometrial cancer. Gynecol Oncol 1994;55:47–50.

233. Rosenberg P, Boeryd B, Simonsen E: A new aggressive treatment approach to high-grade endometrial cancer of possible benefit to patients with stage I uterine papillary cancer. Gynecol Oncol 1993;48:32–37.

234. Morrow CP, Bundy BN, Homesley HD, et al: Doxorubicin as an adjuvant following surgery and radiation therapy in patients with high-risk endometrial carcinoma, stage I and occult stage II: A Gynecologic Oncology Group Study. Gynecol Oncol 1990;36:166–171.

235. Lissoni A, Zanetta G, Losa G, et al: Phase II study of paclitaxel as salvage treatment in advanced endometrial cancer. Ann Oncol 1996;7:861–863.

236. Woo HL, Swenerton KD, Hoskins PJ: Taxol is active in platinum-resistant endometrial adenocarcinoma. Am J Clin Oncol 1996;19:290–291.

237. Lincoln S, Blessing JA, Lee RB, Rocereto TF: Activity of paclitaxel as second-line chemotherapy in endometrial carcinoma: A Gynecologic Oncology Group study. Gynecol Oncol 2003;88:277–281.

238. Thigpen JT, Blessing JA, DiSaia PJ, et al: A randomized comparison of doxorubicin alone versus doxorubicin plus cyclophosphamide in the management of advanced or recurrent endometrial carcinoma: A Gynecologic Oncology Group study. J Clin Oncol 1994;12:1408–1414.

239. Aapro MS, Van Wijk FH, Bolis G, et al: Doxorubicin versus doxorubicin and cisplatin in endometrial carcinoma: Definitive results of a randomised study (55872) by the EORTC Gynaecological Cancer Group. Ann Oncol 2003;14:441–448.

240. Hoskins PJ, Swenerton KD, Pike JA, et al: Paclitaxel and carboplatin, alone or with irradiation, in advanced or recurrent endometrial cancer: A phase II study. J Clin Oncol 2001;19:4048–4053.

241. Price FV, Edwards RP, Kelley JL, et al: A trial of outpatient paclitaxel and carboplatin for advanced, recurrent, and histologic high-risk endometrial carcinoma: Preliminary report. Semin Oncol 1997;24:S15-78–S15-82.

242. Thigpen JT, Brady MF, Alvarez RD, et al: Oral medroxyprogesterone acetate in the treatment of advanced or recurrent endometrial carcinoma: A dose-response study by the Gynecologic Oncology Group. J Clin Oncol 1999;17:1736–1744.

243. Lentz SS, Brady MF, Major FJ, et al: High-dose megestrol acetate in advanced or recurrent endometrial carcinoma: A Gynecologic Oncology Group Study. J Clin Oncol 1996;14:357–361.

244. Moore TD, Phillips PH, Nerenstone SR, Cheson BD: Systemic treat-ment of advanced and recurrent endometrial carcinoma: Current status and future directions. J Clin Oncol 1991;9:1071–1088.

245. Asbury RF, Brunetto VL, Lee RB, et al: Goserelin acetate as treatment for recurrent endometrial carcinoma: A Gynecologic Oncology Group study. Am J Clin Oncol 2002;25:557–560.

246. Covens A, Brunetto VL, Markman M, et al: Phase II trial of danazol in advanced, recurrent, or persistent endometrial cancer: A Gynecologic Oncology Group study. Gynecol Oncol 2003;89:470–474.

247. Omura GA, Blessing JA, Major F, et al: A randomized clinical trial of adjuvant Adriamycin in uterine sarcomas: A Gynecologic Oncology Group Study. J Clin Oncol 1985;3:1240–1245.

248. Sutton GP, Blessing JA, Rosenshein N, et al: Phase II trial of ifosfamide and mesna in mixed mesodermal tumors of the uterus: A Gynecologic Oncology Group study. Am J Obstet Gynecol 1989;161:309–312.

249. Thigpen JT, Blessing JA, Beecham J, et al: Phase II trial of cisplatin as first-line chemotherapy in patients with advanced or recurrent uterine sarcomas: A Gynecologic Oncology Group study. J Clin Oncol 1991;9:1962–1966.

250. Thigpen JT, Blessing JA, Orr JW Jr, DiSaia PJ: Phase II trial of cisplatin in the treatment of patients with advanced or recurrent mixed mesodermal sarcomas of the uterus: A Gynecologic Oncology Group Study. Cancer Treat Rep 1986;70:271–274.

251. Curtin JP, Blessing JA, Soper JT, DeGeest K: Paclitaxel in the treatment of carcinosarcoma of the uterus: A gynecologic oncology group study. Gynecol Oncol 2001;83:268–270.

252. Sutton G, Brunetto VL, Kilgore L, et al: A phase III trial of ifosfamide with or without cisplatin in carcinosarcoma of the uterus: A Gynecologic Oncology Group Study. Gynecol Oncol 2000;79:147–153.

253. Omura GA, Major FJ, Blessing JA, et al: A randomized study of Adriamycin with and without dimethyl triazenoimidazole carboxamide in advanced uterine sarcomas. Cancer 1983;52:626–632.

254. Sutton GP, Blessing JA, Barrett RJ, McGehee R: Phase II trial of ifosfamide and mesna in leiomyosarcoma of the uterus: A Gynecologic Oncology Group study. Am J Obstet Gynecol 1992;166:556–559.

255. Moore DH, Fowler WC Jr, Walton LA, Droegemueller W: Morbidity of lymph node sampling in cancers of the uterine corpus and cervix. Obstet Gynecol 1989;74:180–184.

256. Nunns D, Williamson K, Swaney L, Davy M: The morbidity of surgery and adjuvant radiotherapy in the management of endometrial carcinoma. Int J Gynecol Cancer 2000;10:233–238.

257. Lewandowski G, Torrisi J, Potkul RK, et al: Hysterectomy with extended surgical staging and radiotherapy versus hysterectomy alone and radiotherapy in stage I endometrial cancer: A comparison of complication rates. Gynecol Oncol 1990;36:401–404.

258. Corn BW, Lanciano RM, Greven KM, et al: Impact of improved irradiation technique, age, and lymph node sampling on the severe complication rate of surgically staged endometrial cancer patients: A multivariate analysis. J Clin Oncol 1994;12:510–515.

259. Franchi M, Ghezzi F, Riva C, et al: Postoperative complications after pelvic lymphadenectomy for the surgical staging of endometrial cancer. J Surg Oncol 2001;78:232–237.

260. Greven KM, Lanciano RM, Herbert SH, Hogan PE: Analysis of complications in patients with endometrial cancer receiving adjuvant irradiation. Int J Radiat Oncol Biol Phys 1991;21:919–923.

261. Roeske JC, Lujan A, Rotmensch J, Waggoner SE, Yamada D, Mundt AJ: Intensity-modulated whole pelvic radiation therapy in patients with gynecologic malignancies. Int J Radiat Oncol Biol Phys 2000;48:1613–1621.

262. Mundt AJ, Lujan AE, Rotmensch J, et al: Intensity-modulated whole pelvic radiation therapy in patients with gynecologic malignancies. Int J Radiat Oncol Biol Phys 2002;52:1330–1337.

263. Orr JW Jr, Holiman JL, Orr PF: Stage I corpus cancer: Is teletherapy necessary? Am J Obstet Gynecol 1997;176:777–788.

264. Barakat RR, Goldman NA, Patel DA, et al: Pelvic exenteration for recurrent endometrial cancer. Gynecol Oncol 1999;75:99–102.

265. Kadar N, Malfetano JH, Homesley HD: Determinants of survival of surgically staged patients with endometrial carcinoma histologically confined to the uterus: Implications for therapy. Obstet Gynecol 1992;80:655–659.

266. Carey MS, O'Connell GJ, Johanson CR, et al: Good outcome associated with a standardized treatment protocol using selective postoperative radiation in patients with clinical stage I adenocarcinoma of the endometrium. Gynecol Oncol 1995;57:138-144.

267. Elliott P, Green D, Coates A, et al: The efficacy of postoperative vaginal irradiation in preventing vaginal recurrence in endometrial cancer. Cancer 1994;4:84-89.

268. Ingersoll FM: Vaginal recurrence of carcinoma of the corpus: Management and prevention. Am J Surg 1971;121:473-477.

269. Wylie J, Irwin C, Pintilie M, et al: Results of radical radiotherapy for recurrent endometrial cancer. Gynecol Oncol 2000;77:66-72.

270. Sears JD, Greven KM, Hoen HM, Randall ME: Prognostic factors and treatment outcome for patients with locally recurrent endometrial cancer. Cancer 1994;74:1303-1308.

271. Vavra N, Denison U, Kucera H, et al: Prognostic factors related to recurrent endometrial carcinoma following initial surgery. Acta Obstet Gynecol Scand 1993;72:205-209.

272. Hoekstra CJ, Koper PC, van Putten WL: Recurrent endometrial adenocarcinoma after surgery alone: Prognostic factors and treatment. Radiother Oncol 1993;27:164-166.

273. Kuten A, Grigsby PW, Perez CA, et al: Results of radiotherapy in recurrent endometrial carcinoma: A retrospective analysis of 51 patients. Int J Radiat Oncol Biol Phys 1989;17:29-34.

274. Jereczek-Fossa B, Badzio A, Jassem J: Recurrent endometrial cancer after surgery alone: Results of salvage radiotherapy. Int J Radiat Oncol Biol Phys 2000;48:405-413.

275. Jhingran A, Burke TW, Eifel PJ: Definitive radiotherapy for patients with isolated vaginal recurrence of endometrial carcinoma after hysterectomy. Int J Radiat Oncol Biol Phys 2003;56:1366-1372.

276. Curran WJ Jr, Whittington R, Peters AJ, Fanning J: Vaginal recurrences of endometrial carcinoma: The prognostic value of staging by a primary vaginal carcinoma system. Int J Radiat Oncol Biol Phys 1988;15:803-808.

277. Greven K, Olds W: Isolated recurrences of endometrial adenocarcinoma and their management. Cancer 1987;60:419-421.

278. Morgan JD, Reddy S, Sarin P, et al: Isolated vaginal recurrences of endometrial cancer. Radiology 1993;189:609-613.

279. Colombo A, Cormio G, Placa F, et al: Brachytherapy for isolated vaginal recurrences from endometrial carcinoma. Tumori 1998;84:649-651.

280. Pai HH, Souhami L, Clark BG, Roman T: Isolated vaginal recurrences in endometrial carcinoma: Treatment results using high-dose-rate intracavitary brachytherapy and external beam radiotherapy. Gynecol Oncol 1997;66:300-307.

281. Tewari K, Cappuccini F, Syed AM, et al: Interstitial brachytherapy in the treatment of advanced and recurrent vulvar cancer. Am J Obstet Gynecol 1999;181:91-98.

282. Nag S, Martinez-Monge R, Copeland LJ, et al: Perineal template interstitial brachytherapy salvage for recurrent endometrial adenocarcinoma metastatic to the vagina. Gynecol Oncol 1997;66:16-19.

283. Charra C, Roy P, Coquard R, et al: Outcome of treatment of upper third vaginal recurrences of cervical and endometrial carcinomas with interstitial brachytherapy. Int J Radiat Oncol Biol Phys 1998;40:421-426.

284. Ritcher N, Lucas WE, Yon JL Jr, Sanford FG: Preoperative whole pelvic external irradiation in stage I endometrial cancer. Cancer 1981;48:59-62.

285. Reisinger SA, Staros EB, Feld R, Mohiuddin M, Lewis GC: Preoperative radiation therapy in clinical stage II endometrial carcinoma. Gynecol Oncol 1992;45:174-178.

286. MacLeod C, Fowler A, Duval P, et al: High-dose-rate brachytherapy alone post-hysterectomy for endometrial cancer. Int J Radiat Oncol Biol Phys 1998;42:1033-1039.

287. Horowitz NS, Peters WA III, Smith MR, Dresher CW, Atwood M, Mate TP: Adjuvant high dose rate vaginal brachytherapy as treatment of stage I and II endometrial carcinoma. Obstet Gynecol 2002;99:235-240.

288. Turner DA, Gershenson DM, Atkinson N, Sneige N, Wharton AT: The prognostic significance of peritoneal cytology for stage I endometrial cancer. Obstet Gynecol 1989;74:775-780.

289. Yazigi R, Piver MS, Blumenson L: Malignant peritoneal cytology as prognostic indicator in stage I endometrial cancer. Obstet Gynecol 1983;62:359-362.

290. Zuna RE, Behrens A: Peritoneal washing cytology in gynecologic cancers: Long-term follow-up of 355 patients. J Natl Cancer Inst 1996;88:980-987.

291. Lurain JR, Rumsey NK, Schink JC, Wallemark CB, Chmiel JS: Prognostic significance of positive peritoneal cytology in clinical stage I adenocarcinoma of the endometrium. Obstet Gynecol 1989;74:175-179.

292. Martinez A, Podratz K, Schray M, Malkasian G: Results of whole abdominopelvic irradiation with nodal boost for patients with endometrial cancer at high risk of failure in the peritoneal cavity: A prospective clinical trial at the Mayo Clinic. Hematol Oncol Clin North Am 1988;2:431-446.

293. Harouny VR, Sutton GP, Clark SA, Geisler HE, Stehman FB, Ehrlich CE: The importance of peritoneal cytology in endometrial carcinoma. Obstet Gynecol 1988;72(3 Pt 1):394-398.

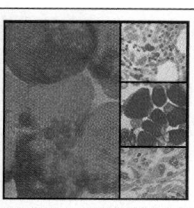

OVARIES AND FALLOPIAN TUBES

James Tate Thigpen

92

SUMMARY OF KEY POINTS

CELOMIC EPITHELIAL CARCINOMA

Basic Characteristics
- Ninety percent of the 23,300 new cases and 13,900 deaths annually in the United States
- Derived from celomic epithelium lining the peritoneal cavity, most commonly from that which invests the ovary
- Most common route of spread: dissemination throughout peritoneal cavity
- Significant prognostic factors: age, histologic type and grade, extent of disease at diagnosis

Screening and Prophylaxis
- High-risk individuals: those with one or more first-order relatives with ovarian carcinoma
- No proven effective screening tests available, although transvaginal sonography and serial CA-125 and proteomic serum patterns under evaluation
- Prophylactic oophorectomy still of no proven value

Initial Evaluation and Management
- Emphasis in initial evaluation placed on the peritoneal cavity, an emphasis requiring exploratory laparotomy in those not clearly stage IV
- Minimum requirements for appropriate laparotomy: surgery through an incision adequate to inspect the entire peritoneal surface, multiple peritoneal biopsies in the absence of gross extrapelvic disease, and a maximal attempt at surgical cytoreduction, including total abdominal hysterectomy, bilateral salpingo-oophorectomy, and omentectomy

Management of Advanced (Stage III–IV) Disease
- After surgery, systemic therapy to include at least a platinum compound

- Combination chemotherapy favored by the weight of evidence with preferred combination, paclitaxel-carboplatin: paclitaxel (175 mg/m^2 IV over 3 hours) followed by carboplatin [area under the curve (AUC), 6 to 7.5 IV] repeated every 3 weeks for six cycles
- Controversial issues: the roles of new agents; the role of dose-intense therapy supported by marrow reconstitution; the role of intraperitoneal therapy; and the role of maintenance paclitaxel

Management of Limited (Stage I–II) Disease
- After careful exploratory laparotomy, patients divided into low-risk and high-risk groups based on the presence of one or more high-risk features: poorly differentiated neoplasm, extracystic tumor, positive peritoneal washings, ascites, or extraovarian disease
- Those at low risk of recurrence (no high-risk features): total abdominal hysterectomy, bilateral salpingo-oophorectomy, and omentectomy followed by observation
- Those at high risk of recurrence (one or more high-risk features): the same surgery as in those at low risk followed by adjuvant platinum-based chemotherapy (paclitaxel/carboplatin for three cycles)

Salvage Therapy for Recurrent Disease
- Patients divided into platinum-sensitive and platinum-resistant groups
- Platinum-sensitive patients (responded to initial platinum-based therapy and experienced at least a 6-month platinum-free interval before relapse): retreatment with taxane/platinum combination
- Platinum-resistant patients (progressed on platinum-based therapy, best response to platinum-based therapy stable disease, or

relapsed during or within 6 months of platinum-based therapy): treatment with drugs producing responses (weekly paclitaxel, docetaxel, pegylated liposomal doxorubicin, oral etoposide, topotecan, tamoxifen, gemcitabine, navelbine, ifosfamide)
- Offering no proven advantage over intravenous therapy at standard doses to these patients: intraperitoneal therapy, high-dose therapy with marrow reconstitution, radiation therapy, and biologic agents

GERM CELL CANCERS

Basic Characteristics
- Germ cell cancers comprise 5% of all cancers of the ovary in the United States
- Histologies: dysgerminomas and nondysgerminomas (endodermal sinus tumors, mixed cell tumors, immature teratomas, embryonal carcinomas, and choriocarcinomas)
- Tumor markers are an important means of detecting early recurrence and monitoring the progress of therapy: α-fetoprotein and human chorionic gonadotropin
- For management purposes, two major groups of patients (1) stages I to III completely resected and (2) incompletely resected stage III to IV disease

Stages I to III Completely Resected
- Initial management: complete resection of disease
- Adjuvant therapy: combination chemotherapy (either bleomycin/etoposide/cisplatin or vincristine/actinomycin/cyclophosphamide)

Stages III to IV Incompletely Resected
Systemic therapy:
bleomycin/etoposide/cisplatin

All
Close follow-up after chemotherapy, including monthly assessments of

SUMMARY OF KEY POINTS—cont'd

tumor markers, physical examination, and chest radiography

RARE MALIGNANT OVARIAN TUMORS
- Less than 5% of ovarian cancer: granulosa cell tumors, thecoma-fibroma tumors, Sertoli-Leydig cell tumors, gynandroblastomas, and steroid cell tumors
- Treatment of choice: surgical resection with little known about the use of radiation or systemic

therapy as either adjuvant treatment or management for advanced or recurrent disease

CANCER OF THE FALLOPIAN TUBE
- Rare (300 cases annually in the United States), with more than 90% of all cases papillary serous adenocarcinomas
- Pattern of spread similar to that of celomic epithelial carcinoma of the ovary

- Surgical resection the mainstay for most patients with disease confined to the fallopian tube
- Radiation or chemotherapy reserved for cases with penetration to or beyond the serosa, with evidence favoring management similar to that used for advanced ovarian carcinoma

INTRODUCTION

Cancers of the ovary and fallopian tube together account for most deaths resulting from cancer of the female genital tract. This relates primarily to the fact that, unlike other common malignant gynecologic neoplasms (cancers of the endometrium and cervix), cancers of the ovary and fallopian tube are first seen at relatively advanced stages of disease because of the lack of an effective early diagnostic test. Ovarian cancers are far more common than tubal malignancies and provide most of the data on which the management of both malignancies is based. This chapter first addresses cancers of the ovary extensively, followed by a discussion of cancers of the fallopian tube.

CANCER OF THE OVARY

Cancer of the ovary will be newly diagnosed in more than 23,300 women in the United States each year and will cause the death of more than 13,900 American women annually.[1] The lifetime likelihood that ovarian cancer will develop in a woman is estimated to be between 1 in 60 and 1 in 70, with a higher frequency associated with certain familial syndromes.[2-5] This group of cancers includes three major types: celomic epithelial carcinoma of the ovary, germ cell neoplasms, and stromal tumors. Each of these groups is discussed separately.

Celomic Epithelial Carcinoma

Almost 90% of cancers of the ovary are celomic epithelial carcinoma, which is one of the three most common gynecologic cancers. Management of these lesions evolves from an understanding of certain basic aspects of the disease process.

Basic Characteristics

Clinically Relevant Disease Features. Celomic epithelial carcinomas may arise in any part of the peritoneal cavity,

although most appear to arise from the celomic epithelium that invests the ovary during embryonic development. The reasons for the preference for ovarian celomic epithelium are not entirely clear. It has been speculated that repeated rupture and repair of this portion of the celomic epithelium with the process of ovulation affords a greater opportunity for mutations that lead to malignancy. Such speculation is supported by observations that associate multiple pregnancies and the use of birth control pills, which suppress ovulation, with a decreased risk for ovarian carcinoma.[6]

Furthermore, most of these lesions arise in invaginated epithelium in areas of repair after ovulation, developing as though within a cyst. The process eventually penetrates the capsule of the ovary, forms tumor excrescences on the surface of the ovary, and then disseminates primarily by direct spread throughout the peritoneal cavity. Subsequent spread via lymphatic and hematogenous dissemination also occurs. This pattern of evolution of the disease is reflected in the International Federation of Gynecology and Obstetrics (FIGO) staging system[7] (Table 92-1), in which the most common stage at presentation is stage III, characterized by spread outside the pelvis to involve the peritoneal cavity. Because the process is an intra-abdominal disease that produces few symptoms before intraperitoneal dissemination and is not amenable to early diagnosis by currently available screening techniques, essentially 70% to 75% of patients are first seen with advanced (stage III or IV) rather than limited (stage I or II) disease.

Several characteristics of celomic epithelial carcinomas distinguish their clinical management from that of the other two common gynecologic cancers: endometrial and cervical cancer. First, the primary route of spread, dissemination throughout the peritoneal cavity, opens the possibility for therapy directed toward the peritoneal cavity. Second, unlike the other two common gynecologic cancers, these lesions usually are first seen at a relatively advanced stage (stage III or IV), which necessitates a larger role for systemic therapy in the management of these cases. Finally, volume of residual disease at initiation of systemic therapy influences subsequent response to

TABLE 92-1

FIGO Staging System for Ovarian Carcinoma

STAGE	DESCRIPTION
I	Growth limited to the ovaries
IA	One ovary; no ascites; capsule intact; no tumor on external surface
IB	Two ovaries; no ascites; capsule intact; no tumor on external surface
IC	One or both ovaries with either surface tumor; ruptured capsule; or ascites or peritoneal washings with malignant cells
II	Pelvic extension
IIA	Involvement of uterus and/or tubes
IIB	Involvement of other pelvic tissues
IIC	Stage IIA or IIB with factors as in stage IC
III	Peritoneal implants outside pelvis and/or positive retroperitoneal or inguinal nodes
IIIA	Grossly limited to true pelvis; negative nodes; microscopic seeding of abdominal peritoneum
IIIB	Implants of abdominal peritoneum ≤2 cm; nodes negative
IIIC	Abdominal implants >2 cm and/or positive retroperitoneal or inguinal nodes
IV	Distant metastases

FIGO, International Federation of Gynecology and Obstetrics.
Data from the New FIGO stage grouping[7].

chemotherapy and survival. The smaller the largest residual nodule, the more likely the disease will regress with drug therapy[8-11] (Table 92-2) and the more likely the patient will live longer[12-14] (Table 92-3).

Other disease characteristics have been observed to influence outcome (Table 92-4). Shortened survival is associated with older age[15] and more poorly differentiated disease. These factors do not, however, affect therapeutic decisions, except for the role of histologic grade in limited disease, a role discussed later. Histologic subtype also affects survival: patients who have clear cell or mucinous carcinomas have shorter survival, whereas those with tumors of low malignant potential ("borderline carcinomas") have a markedly better survival. These subtypes constitute less than 10% of all celomic epithelial tumors. Because no alternative therapeutic choice offers greater benefit for mucinous or clear cell carcinomas, these

TABLE 92-3

Impact of Volume of Residual Disease on Survival in Patients with Advanced Ovarian Carcinoma

REGIMEN	MINIMAL (MO)	BULKY (MO)
PAC (GOG)[8,9]	42	19
L-PAM (GOG)[13,14]	33	13

L-PAM, melphalan; PAC, cisplatin + doxorubicin + cyclophosphamide.

histologic types do not currently influence therapeutic decisions. Conversely, tumors of low malignant potential do influence therapeutic choices, as will be discussed.

Tumors of Low Malignant Potential. Celomic epithelial tumors of low malignant potential account for approximately 15% of ovarian carcinomas.[16] Patients with these lesions tend to be younger than those with invasive ovarian carcinoma (average age at onset, 49 years).[17] The sine qua non of the diagnosis is the absence of invasion of the stroma.[18] The vast majority of cases display serous or mucinous histology with bilaterality in roughly one third of serous tumors.

Recognition of these tumors is important because both prognosis and management differ greatly, as opposed to standard management of invasive ovarian carcinomas.[19-21] In general, management should begin with an exploratory laparotomy and resection of as much disease as possible. Pathology should be reviewed carefully to ensure that no areas of invasive carcinoma are present.[22] After surgery, patients should be observed until such time as the disease begins to behave in a more aggressive fashion. At that point, chemotherapy may be used, although its efficacy in this setting is not clear.

Extraovarian Peritoneal Serous Papillary Carcinoma. It has long been recognized that celomic epithelial carcinomas can arise in portions of the peritoneal cavity other than the surface of the ovaries. The Gynecologic Oncology Group (GOG) undertook a study of these extra-

TABLE 92-2

Impact of Volume of Residual Disease on Pathologic Complete Response to Combination Chemotherapy in Patients with Advanced Ovarian Carcinoma

REGIMEN	MINIMAL	BULKY
PAC (GOG)[8,9]	45/137 (33%)	13/107 (12%)
PAC (Ehrlich)[10]	5/17 (30%)	5/39 (13%)
HCAP (Greco)[11]	18/21 (86%)	3/29 (10%)
CHEX-UP (Young)[12]	5/14 (36%)	5/37 (14%)

CHEX-UP, cyclophosphamide + hexamethylmelamine + 5-fluorouracil + cisplatin; HCAP, hexamethylmelamine + cyclophosphamide + doxorubicin + cisplatin; PAC, cisplatin + doxorubicin + cyclophosphamide.

TABLE 92-4

Prognostic Factors in Ovarian Carcinoma

FACTOR	DESCRIPTION
Age	Older patients have poorer survival
Grade	Poorly differentiated lesions are associated with poorer survival
Histologic type	Clear cell and mucinous histologies are associated with poorer survival. Tumors of low malignant potential imply a much better survival
Stage	More-extensive disease, as reflected in the FIGO staging system, produces poorer survival
Volume of disease	In patients with stage III disease, larger volume of residual disease leads to poorer survival

ovarian peritoneal papillary serous carcinomas to determine whether they responded in a similar fashion to standard treatment for celomic epithelial carcinomas of the ovary.[23] The study of 47 women with these extraovarian celomic epithelial carcinomas showed that, when the data are compared with results of treatment of ovarian carcinomas with the same chemotherapy, similar response rates, surgical complete response rates, and survivals are observed. This is the basis on which these lesions are now included in trials of chemotherapy for ovarian carcinoma.

FIGO Stage. The factor that most influences management is the extent of disease at diagnosis (stage). This discussion is organized accordingly: A general approach to initial evaluation and surgical management is followed by a discussion of the role of chemotherapy both in previously untreated patients with advanced disease and in patients with recurrent or persistent disease. The management of patients with limited lesions is then considered.

Initial Evaluation and Management

Patients with celomic epithelial carcinomas generally are first seen with complaints of a full or heavy sensation in the pelvis or with increasing abdominal girth. Unfortunately, these symptoms usually reflect the presence of advanced disease. Efforts directed to earlier diagnosis have largely been unsuccessful, with the possible exception of the application of certain tools to patient populations at high risk for the development of ovarian carcinoma.

High-Risk Patients, Screening, and Genetic Testing.

Within the past decade, interest in using family history to identify patients at high risk of the development of ovarian carcinoma has escalated.[2,24-26] Data now suggest that women with one first-order relative with ovarian carcinoma have a 3.6-fold higher risk than that of the general population. For those who have two or more relatives with ovarian carcinoma, at least one of whom is a first-order relative, risk is considerably higher, with estimates as great as 50% or better reported, but not necessarily substantiated.

Certain hereditary syndromes have been described.[3,25] These include hereditary breast/ovarian cancer syndromes associated with changes at chromosome 17q (*BRCA1*) and at chromosome 13q (*BRCA2*) and hereditary nonpolyposis colon cancer syndromes (Lynch syndrome II with an association with colon and endometrial cancers as well), which exhibit *hMLH1*, *hMSH2*, and *hPMS2* mutations. These familial ovarian cancers typically appear at a younger age than does sporadic ovarian carcinoma and, despite pathologic factors that should portend a poor survival, predict a significantly better survival than that associated with sporadic ovarian cancer of the same stage.[4,5,25-29] Both hereditary breast/ovarian syndrome and hereditary nonpolyposis colon cancer syndromes appear to be vertically transmitted by an autosomal dominant mode, with incomplete penetrance. Familial ovarian cancer registries have now identified a number of women who either fit one of these syndromes or have at least one first-order relative with ovarian cancer.

These observations raise at least four significant questions with regard to management. First, should prophylactic oophorectomy be recommended to women at high risk? The largest experience with prophylactic oophorectomy comes from the Gilda Radner Familial Ovarian Cancer Registry. To date, 324 women with at least one first-order relative with ovarian cancer have undergone prophylactic oophorectomy. The relatively short follow-up evaluation of most of these women shows that in six, celomic epithelial carcinomas of the peritoneal cavity have developed, for an overall rate of 1.8%.[30] Although this rate is low, it already exceeds the rate of ovarian carcinoma in the general population. Other reports have documented the occurrence of primary peritoneal neoplasms in women who have previously undergone oophorectomy.[31] This raises questions about the value of prophylactic oophorectomy in preventing the development of celomic epithelial carcinomas. No prospective trials have been conducted to examine this question. The weight of evidence suggests that the procedure should not be routinely recommended until further follow-up is available to determine whether a further significant increase in the incidence of peritoneal malignancies will occur. The exception to this may be those women who have a true hereditary syndrome with a very high risk of developing ovarian carcinoma, although no clinical trial documents the value of prophylactic oophorectomy even in this population.[32,33]

Second, how should patients at high risk be monitored; or, more simply put, do we have valid screening tests? Family history clearly identifies a high-risk population. Logic dictates that screening leading to early diagnosis would result in a higher cure rate. The problem is the lack of evidence that any monitoring technique yields early diagnosis at a reasonable rate. Both CA-125 and transvaginal sonography have been recommended for screening. Evidence is lacking that CA-125 leads to early diagnosis.[4] By contrast, transvaginal sonography has proved capable of identifying ovarian carcinoma at a limited stage in two series.[5,30] The drawback for the technique is that 15 to 40 laparotomies have to be done to diagnose one case of limited ovarian carcinoma. At least for the present, neither approach can be recommended for routine screening, although selected high-risk patients, with a clear understanding of the attendant difficulties, can be screened with transvaginal sonography.[34,35]

More recently, new technology has offered some hope of an effective approach to screening for ovarian carcinoma. Investigators at the United States National Cancer Institute reported the use of proteomic patterns in serum to identify patients with ovarian cancer.[36] In a population of 50 patients with ovarian cancer and 66 patients with nonmalignant disease, the test reportedly had a sensitivity of 100%, a specificity of 95%, and a positive predictive value of 94% for correctly identifying those with or without ovarian cancer. Unfortunately, the calculation of the positive predictive value did not take into account the prevalence of the disease in the target population. When this deficiency is corrected, the true positive predictive value is 1%, not 94%. This is less than the positive predictive value reported for the use of CA-125 alone.[37] Before proteomic patterns can be recommended to screen for ovarian carcinoma, further retrospective and prospective studies are required.

Third, should patients with positive family histories be offered genetic testing? Approximately 10% of ovarian carcinoma is associated with inheritance of an autosomal dominant genetic mutation and a resultant strong family history of ovarian carcinoma and certain other associated cancers such as breast cancer.[38] These cases fall into two broad categories. The first is commonly called the breast and ovarian cancer syndrome and is associated with mutations at two loci: *BRCA1* on chromosome 17q21 (75% to 90% of breast and ovarian cancer syndrome) and *BRCA2* on chromosome 13q12 (10% to 25% of breast and ovarian cancer syndrome). In published series, these mutations account for approximately 7% of ovarian carcinoma. The second is commonly called the HNPCC (hereditary nonpolyposis colorectal carcinoma) syndrome and is associated with mutations that include three known genes: *hMSH1* (45% to 50% of cases of HNPCC syndrome), *hMLH1* (45% to 50% of cases of HNPCC syndrome), and *hPMS2* (<5% of cases of HNPCC syndrome). These lesions account for approximately 3% of ovarian carcinoma.

Although the risk of inheriting a mutation from a parent carrier is 50%, the actual risk of developing a cancer varies from as high as 80% to 85% to as low as 16% for different mutations.[38] This variability of risk and the previously discussed controversy about the efficacy of prophylactic oophorectomy raise questions about the role of genetic testing in individuals with family histories of ovarian carcinoma. The American Society of Clinical Oncology (ASCO) recently issued an updated policy statement about genetic testing and cited three criteria for determining when genetic testing should be offered (Table 92-5).[39] Such testing should only be done if counseling before and after the test is available to discuss such issues as the risks and benefits of genetic testing as well as the efficacy, or lack thereof, of interventions prompted by the tests.

Fourth, might interventions other than prophylactic oophorectomy be efficacious in high-risk women? Oral contraceptives have been reported to reduce the risk of ovarian carcinoma by as much as 50% after prolonged (>10 years) use.[40-42] At least some reports suggest that the effects of such oral contraceptive use on cancer incidence may differ between those with positive family histories and those with a true hereditary syndrome associated with *BRCA1* or *BRCA2*,[43,44] with an actual increase in breast cancer risk among those *BRCA1* or *BRCA2* women taking tamoxifen for chemoprevention.[45] Although this implies a need for caution, at least one study reports that prolonged oral contraceptive use reduces the risk of ovarian cancer in women with pathogenic mutations in the *BRCA1* or *BRCA2* gene,[46] whereas another shows no impact, negative or positive, of oral contraceptives on ovarian cancer risk.[47] In the absence of clear-cut evidence for a benefit, the role of oral contraceptives to prevent ovarian cancer is not established; hence they should not be used for such a purpose at present.

Other hormone use also has been evaluated. At least some reports show a direct correlation between postmenopausal estrogen-replacement therapy and risk for development of ovarian carcinoma that ranges from a relative risk of 1.59 to 2.81.[48-50] This correlation appears to hold only for those patients taking estrogen only and not for those taking a combined estrogen/progesterone regimen. Other studies have failed to find such a correlation.[51] In women who are ovarian cancer survivors, no evidence is found that estrogen use increases the likelihood of relapse or shortens survival.[52]

Finally, one report assessed the relation between raloxifene and risk for ovarian carcinoma.[53] This study was actually a meta-analysis of seven randomized placebo-controlled trials of raloxifene involving a total of 9837 women. The relative risk associated with the use of raloxifene was 0.50. This suggests no adverse effect, but it does not prove a beneficial effect.

In summary, no scientifically proven screening approach exists for ovarian carcinoma. In addition, no clear role is seen for the use of interventions in the high-risk patient, although the ovarian consensus statement recommends the use of screening with transvaginal sonography and prophylactic oophorectomy in women with true hereditary syndromes. The basis for this recommendation is expert opinion and not appropriate definitive trials.

Initial Evaluation. The initial evaluation of patients with suspected ovarian carcinoma, after the usual history, physical examination, laboratory testing, and CA-125, should be directed toward a detailed assessment of the abdominal cavity. Although a variety of imaging techniques for the abdominal cavity are now available, including sonography, computed tomography (CT), magnetic resonance imaging (MRI), and special isotopic scanning techniques, none provides the level of detailed study necessary for accurate staging of ovarian carcinoma. At the very least, CT scanning of the abdominal cavity, chest radiography, and bone scanning should be done.

Unless this evaluation demonstrates evidence of disease outside the abdominal cavity, exploratory laparotomy is an essential part of the initial evaluation of the patient. The laparotomy should be done through an incision adequate to evaluate the entire peritoneal surface, including the undersurface of the diaphragm and the right

TABLE 92-5

Criteria* for Offering Genetic Testing[39]

- Individual has personal or family history features suggestive of a genetic cancer susceptibility condition
- Test can be adequately interpreted
- Results will aid in diagnosis or influence the medical or surgical management of the patient or family members at hereditary risk of cancer

*Genetic testing must include pre- and post-test counseling, which should include a discussion of the risks and benefits of testing and the interventions prompted by the testing.

Specific Malignancies

III

paracolic gutter, as well as the para-aortic lymph nodes. If no evidence of gross disease is found outside the pelvis, multiple biopsies of the peritoneal surface should be obtained. Many patients with the disease apparently confined to the pelvis will have evidence of microscopic seeding of the abdominal peritoneum in one or more biopsies. At the conclusion of this procedure, accurate staging of the disease will have been accomplished and will serve to direct further management.

Therapeutic Role of Surgery

Volume of residual disease is related both to response to chemotherapy and to survival. As a result, the standard of care of patients with ovarian carcinoma with disease confined to the abdominal cavity is to resect as much disease as possible at initial laparotomy. This approach applies to patients with limited disease that can be completely removed, as well as to those with advanced disease that can be only partially resected. Data on which this approach has been based are retrospective analyses showing that patients who initiate chemotherapy with small-volume disease (no nodule larger than 2 cm in diameter remaining in the abdominal cavity) have both a higher frequency of pathologic complete response and a superior survival with chemotherapy[8,10-14,117] (see Tables 92-2 and 92-3).

Several major questions have been raised about the value of cytoreductive surgery in patients with advanced disease not amenable to a "curative" resection. First and foremost, detractors have pointed out that approximately one half of the population of patients with small-volume disease consists of those patients with stage IIIA or IIIB disease—patients who already have small-volume disease at the time the abdomen was opened without any surgical cytoreduction. According to this line of reasoning, the improved results in small-volume disease relate entirely to this portion of the patients who presumably have biologically less aggressive disease. A retrospective analysis of a GOG database of patients with small-volume disease provided some support for this view.[14] Operative notes on the population in the database were reviewed to separate the patients into two groups: those who had stage IIIA or IIIB disease, and those who had stage IIIC disease that was successfully surgically cytoreduced to small-volume residual disease. Patients who required surgical cytoreduction had an inferior survival as compared with those who already had small-volume disease at the time the abdomen was opened. Whereas this investigation shows a difference between these two patient groups, however, it does not prove that surgical cytoreduction has no value, in the absence of a population for comparison in which chemotherapy was started with large-volume disease.

The only way to address the question of the value of cytoreductive surgery is to conduct a randomized trial in which all patients are randomized to surgical cytoreduction or no surgical cytoreduction and then analyzed by intent to treat. No such study assessing initial surgical cytoreduction has been successfully completed. Two prospective randomized phase III trials, however, have evaluated the role of interval cytoreduction[54,55] (Table 92-6).

TABLE 92-6

Results of Two Studies of Interval Surgical Cytoreduction

PARAMETER	ALL	IDS	NO IDS
EORTC Study[54]			
Patients	408	150	149
Response after 3 cycles			
Complete response	17%		
Partial response	55%		
Progression-free survival		15 mo	12.5 mo
Survival		27 mo	19 mo
GOG Study[55]			
Patients	425	216	209
Progression-free survival		10.5 mo	10.8 mo
Survival		32 mo	33 mo

IDS, interval debulking surgery.

In a European trial by the European Organization for Research and Treatment of Cancer (EORTC),[54] patients with advanced disease received three courses of cisplatin plus cyclophosphamide and were then randomized to receive either three more courses of the same chemotherapy or interval cytoreductive surgery, followed by three more cycles of cisplatin plus cyclophosphamide. The group receiving interval cytoreductive surgery demonstrated a statistically significantly superior progression-free and overall survival.

A GOG study[55] took patients with stage IIIC disease who had undergone an aggressive attempt at initial surgical cytoreduction and still had large-volume disease remaining and randomized them to either six cycles of paclitaxel plus cisplatin or three cycles of paclitaxel plus cisplatin followed by interval surgical cytoreduction and then three more cycles of paclitaxel plus cisplatin. This trial showed no difference between the two study arms.

The most rational interpretation of these two studies rests on an understanding of the differences in study execution. In the European trial, initial surgery was performed by surgeons with a varied training background and, in many instances, probably did not represent a true aggressive attempt at surgical cytoreduction. In the GOG study, conversely, virtually every patient underwent an initial attempt at aggressive surgical cytoreduction by a trained gynecologic oncologist. What the two trials show is that patients with a less than optimal initial attempt at surgical cytoreduction benefit from interval bulk reduction, whereas those who undergo an aggressive initial surgery and still have large-volume disease do not benefit from interval surgery.

Based on the weight of current evidence, patients, except for those with obvious stage IV disease, should undergo an initial laparotomy with intent to carry out maximal surgical cytoreduction. This should improve response to chemotherapy as well as survival. Those who have a less aggressive initial operation should be considered for interval surgical cytoreduction.

Management of Advanced Disease

Patients with stage III or IV disease, on completion of initial surgery, should receive systemic therapy for control of disease. Fortunately, celomic epithelial carcinoma is a chemosensitive disease—hence the significant therapeutic options for patients with advanced disease.

Active Agents. A number of cytotoxic agents as well as biologic and hormonal agents have activity against celomic epithelial neoplasms[6-8,10-15,24-26,117] (Table 92-7). Response rates reported for each of the active agents vary as a result of several factors: (1) volume of residual disease in the patient population at the initiation of therapy; (2) dose and schedule of the agent under study; and (3) whether the patient population has received prior cytotoxic therapy to which the neoplasm has become clinically resistant, as evidenced by clinical progression during therapy. With the reservation that these factors cannot be sorted out in many of the single-agent studies reported, it is possible to point to certain active cytotoxic drugs of major interest: the platinum compounds, the taxanes, the mustard-type alkylating agents, the anthra-cyclines (including pegylated liposomal encapsulated doxorubicin), the topoisomerase I inhibitors, oral etoposide, gemcitabine, vinorelbine, and hexamethylmelamine. In addition, among hormonal and biologic agents, interferon alpha and gamma and tamoxifen display activity. Among these, the platinum compounds and paclitaxel deserve specific comment because of their current major relevance to front-line therapy for newly diagnosed disease.

Platinum Analogues. The platinum analogues are the most systematically evaluated and active cytotoxic drugs. Cisplatin demonstrates clear-cut activity in patients with no prior chemotherapy, as well as in those refractory to prior alkylating agents.[56,60-63] Carboplatin produces less neurotoxicity and nephrotoxicity than cisplatin, in exchange for thrombocytopenia as the dose-limiting adverse effect, and exhibits activity similar to that seen with cisplatin.[63]

Taxanes. Paclitaxel, a diterpenoid extracted from the bark of *Taxus brevifolia* (the Western yew tree), acts to enhance tubulin polymerization and microtubule stability and hence to produce microtubule bundling throughout the cell.[116] This stability leads to inhibition of the dynamic reorganization of the microtubular structure of the cell before cell division. This unique mechanism of action accounts for the apparent lack of cross-resistance between this drug and the platinum analogues.

Paclitaxel demonstrated significant activity in four phase II trials in patients who had received prior platinum-based combination chemotherapy[65-68] (Table 92-8). In two of the four trials, responses were documented in both platinum-sensitive and platinum-resistant patients. Adverse effects, including myelosuppression, hypersensitivity reactions, and significant arrhythmias requiring continuous cardiac monitoring during therapy, were frequent and severe but manageable and resulted in no deaths attributable to toxicity. The occurrence of significant anaphylactic episodes in the initial experience with the drug led to the use of premedication with steroids and H_1 and H_2 blockers in the phase II trials, with the resultant virtual elimination of significant hypersensitivity reactions. The dose-limiting toxicity is myelo-

TABLE 92-7

Active Single Agents in Celomic Epithelial Carcinoma of the Ovary*[48-107]

	PATIENTS	
DRUG	N	PERCENT†
Alkylating agents[56]	1,371	33
Ifosfamide[56-59]	98	15
Cisplatin[56,60,61]	190	32
Carboplatin[56,62,63]	82	24
Oxaliplatin[64]	45	16
Paclitaxel[65-68]	157	35
Docetaxel[69-73]	423	29
Doxorubicin[56]	102	33
5-Fluorouracil[56]	126	29
Methotrexate[56]	34	18
Mitomycin[56]	49	16
Hexamethylmelamine[74-81]	296	23
Topotecan[82-86]	352	17
Irinotecan[87]	29	17
Pegylated liposomal doxorubicin[88-93]	557	18
Oral etoposide[94-98]	193	28
Gemcitabine[99-101]	109	16
Vinorelbine[102-106]	156	22
Dihydroxybusulfan[56]	26	27
Galactitol[56]	39	15
5-Fluorouracil/leucovorin[107]	44	14
Mitoxantrone[108]	33	15
Treosulfan[109]	80	19
Oral trofosfamide[110]	31	16
Progestins[56]	176	12
Tamoxifen[111-113]	141	14
Prednimustine[56]	36	28
Mifepristone[114]	34	26
Interferon-α[56]	21	19
Interferon-γ[56]	14	29
Trastuzumab[115]	41	7

*Response rate, >15%.
†Response rate percentage.

TABLE 92-8

Phase II Trials of Taxol as Salvage Therapy in Patients with Ovarian Carcinoma

INVESTIGATORS	NO. OF PATIENTS	RESPONSE (%)
McGuire et al.[67]	40	30
Sensitive	15	40
Resistant	25	24
GOG (Thigpen et al.)[65]	43	35
Sensitive	16	44
Resistant	27	30
Einzig et al.[66]	30	20
Kohn et al.[68]	44	48

suppression, which, with 24-hour infusions, is severe but brief.

The other taxane, docetaxel, has been less extensively evaluated.[69-73] Activity appears to be similar to that of paclitaxel. Whether toxicity differs significantly awaits publication of randomized trials that have evaluated this, but docetaxel may be less neurotoxic but more myelosuppressive on the basis of data available to date.

In summary, a variety of drugs have activity against ovarian carcinoma. The most important of these are the platinum compounds and the taxanes. Other agents of particular interest exhibit the ability to obtain responses in patients who have progressed on paclitaxel-platinum front-line therapy and include: oral etoposide, topotecan, tamoxifen, gemcitabine, navelbine, ifosfamide, and possibly doxil.

Combination Chemotherapy. An extensive series of questions had to be addressed to evolve effective regimens for the treatment of advanced ovarian carcinoma after surgical cytoreduction. Over the last two decades, the major themes that have keyed the development of current therapy include the evolution of platinum-based combination chemotherapy, assessment of the value of dose intensity, the defining of the role of paclitaxel, the determination of which platinum compound to use, and the ascertainment of the role, if any, of maintenance or consolidation therapy for those who respond to front-line therapy. Each of these issues is discussed, and a brief look at other significant issues follows.

Evolution of Platinum-based Combination Chemotherapy. A multitude of trials have made a firm case for the value of combination chemotherapy compared with treatment with single agents. The most significant of these studies were three large, randomized trials.[8,9,117] The conclusions from these three GOG studies, supported by other trials of systemic therapy, formed the basis for practice at the end of the 1980s.[118]

The first two GOG trials were successive studies in patients with bulky advanced disease[8,117] (Table 92-9). The first of these (GOG Protocol 22) compared melphalan alone with either melphalan plus hexamethylmelamine or doxorubicin plus cyclophosphamide.[117] The only statistically significant difference observed was a greater clinical complete response rate in those patients treated with doxorubicin plus cyclophosphamide, as compared with those receiving melphalan alone. This was the basis for selection of the two-drug combination as the control arm of the second trial (GOG Protocol 47), which compared doxorubicin plus cyclophosphamide with the same two drugs plus cisplatin.[8] Results showed a statistically significant improvement in clinical complete response rate, overall response rate, progression-free interval, and survival in those patients treated with the three-drug cisplatin-based combination.

The third critical study (GOG Protocol 52), in patients with minimal residual disease (defined as those with stage III disease and no nodules larger than 1 cm in diameter), compared the three-drug combination with cisplatin

plus cyclophosphamide[9] (Table 92-10). The pathologic complete response rates, as documented at second-look laparotomy, were not significantly different, nor were any differences noted in progression-free interval or survival.

These three trials make a strong case for the combination of cisplatin plus cyclophosphamide as the standard chemotherapy for advanced or recurrent ovarian carcinoma by the late 1980s. Four other studies focusing on the substitution of carboplatin for cisplatin expanded somewhat the meaning of standard chemotherapy.[119-122] These studies compared the relative efficacy of cisplatin-based versus carboplatin-based regimens (Table 92-11). The trial of the Southwest Oncology Group compared cyclophosphamide (600 mg/m^2) plus either cisplatin (100 mg/m^2) or carboplatin (300 mg/m^2) in patients with bulky stage III or IV disease.[119] The study showed no significant differences between the two regimens with regard to response rate, progression-free interval, or survival. The toxicity of the two regimens was different, with the cisplatin regimen producing greater adverse effects. The National Cancer Institute of Canada trial compared essentially the same regimens, except for a

TABLE 92-9

Results of Two GOG Studies of Combination Chemotherapy in Large-Volume Advanced Ovarian Carcinoma[8,117]

PARAMETER	GOG PROTOCOL 22		GOG PROTOCOL 47	
	L-PAM	AC	AC	PAC
Patients	64	72	120	107
CR	20%	32%	26%	51%
Total response (CR + PR)	37%	49%	48%	76%
CR			4/23	13/39
PCR/total			3%	12%
Duration	8 mo	10 mo	9 mo	15 mo
Median survival	12 mo	14 mo	16 mo	20 mo

AC, doxorubicin (50 mg/m^2) plus cyclophosphamide (500 mg/m^2), both IV, every 3 weeks, for eight courses; CR, complete response; L-PAM, melphalan (0.2 mg/kg/d PO), for 5 days every 4 to 6 weeks, for 10 courses or 18 months; PAC, cisplatin (50 mg/m^2) plus doxorubicin and cyclophosphamide as in AC, all IV, every 3 weeks, for eight courses; PCR, pathologic complete response; PR, partial response.

TABLE 92-10

Results of a GOG Study of Minimal Residual Stage III Ovarian Carcinoma[9]

PARAMETER	PAC	PC
Patients	173	176
Early recurrence	19	30
Refused second look	36	37
Residual disease	73	67
Pathologic complete response (%)	45 (26%)	42 (24%)

PAC, cisplatin (50 mg/m^2) plus doxorubicin (50 mg/m^2) plus cyclophosphamide (500 mg/m^2), all IV every 3 weeks, for eight cycles; PC, cisplatin (50 mg/m^2) plus cyclophosphamide (1000 mg/m^2), both IV, every 3 weeks, for eight cycles.

TABLE 92-11

Randomized Trials Comparing Cisplatin-based with Carboplatin-based Combination Chemotherapy in Advanced, Predominantly Large-Volume Ovarian Carcinoma[119-122]

STUDY AND REGIMEN	RESPONSE	SURVIVAL
Alberts et al.[119] (342 patients)		
Carboplatin (300 mg/m^2), q4wk	cCR, 34%	20 mo
Cyclophosphamide (600 mg/m^2), q4wk	pCR, 12%	
Cisplatin (100 mg/m^2), q4wk	cCR, 27%	17 mo
Cyclophosphamide (600 mg/m^2), q4wk	pCR, 7%	
ten Bokkel et al.[120] (339 patients)		
Cyclophosphamide (100 mg/m^2 PO), d14–28	cCR, 24%	107 wk
Hexamethylmelamine (150 mg/m^2 PO), d14–28		
Doxorubicin (35 mg/m^2 IV), d1		
Carboplatin 350 mg/m^2 IV), d1		
Cyclophosphamide (100 mg/m^2 PO), d14–28	cCR, 23%	108 wk
Hexamethylmelamine (150 mg/m^2 PO), d14–28		
Doxorubicin (35 mg/m^2 IV), d1		
Cisplatin (20 mg/m^2 IV), d1–5		
Pater et al.[121] (447 patients)		
Carboplatin (300 mg/m^2), q4wk	pCR, 13%	24 mo
Cyclophosphamide (600 mg/m^2), q4wk		
Cisplatin (75 mg/m^2), q4wk	pCR, 18%	23 mo
Cyclophosphamide (600 mg/m^2), q4wk		
Edmondson et al.[122] (103 patients)		
Carboplatin (150 mg/m^2), q4wk		20 mo
Cyclophosphamide (1000 mg/m^2), q4wk		
Cisplatin (60 mg/m^2), q4wk		27 mo
Cyclophosphamide (1000 mg/m^2), q4wk		

cCR, clinical complete response; pCR, pathologic complete response.

slightly lower cisplatin dose of 75 mg/m^2, with similar results.[121]

The study conducted by the Gynaecological Cancer Cooperative Group for the EORTC compared two four-drug combinations consisting of cyclophosphamide, doxorubicin, and hexamethylmelamine with either cisplatin or carboplatin.[120] No significant differences were noted with regard to response rate, progression-free interval, or survival.

The trial conducted by investigators at the Mayo Clinic is flawed by a major design problem.[122] The dose intensity of carboplatin is well below that of cisplatin in the other arm, making it difficult to determine whether the differences in progression-free interval and survival favoring the cisplatin regimen were related to a different platinum compound or to a lower dose intensity of the carboplatin. This study has two other distinguishing features from the other three trials. The number of patients in the trial is considerably smaller and included 65% with small-volume disease.

In summary, these seven randomized trials[8,9,117,119-122] defined four major concepts about standard chemotherapy for advanced ovarian carcinoma as of 1990. First, combination chemotherapy is superior to single-agent therapy. Second, platinum-based combination chemotherapy offers significant advantages over non–platinum-based regimens. Third, carboplatin offers certain advantages over cisplatin in terms of altered and more tolerable toxicity with no diminution in efficacy. Finally, two-drug combinations of a platinum compound and an alkylating agent offer benefits equivalent to those

achieved with more complex regimens. Three major themes dominated clinical research in the 1990s in attempts to improve further on systemic therapy for advanced disease: dose intensity, the development of combinations of a platinum compound and paclitaxel, and the choice of platinum compound.

Dose Intensity. Although debated to some extent, the concept of the importance of dose intensity to the success of chemotherapy in the management of celomic epithelial carcinomas of the ovary has been generally well accepted among oncologists. In vitro data support the efficacy of increasing drug levels in enhancing cell kill in cultures of ovarian cancer cells.[123] In patients who have experienced recurrence after prior platinum-based chemotherapy for ovarian carcinoma, responses to higher doses of the same platinum compound[124] or to greater exposure as a result of intraperitoneal administration[125] have been cited as evidence that enhanced dose can result in response when lower doses have failed. The use of hypertonic saline to permit escalation of cisplatin dose to 200 mg/m^2 per course in combination with cyclophosphamide has been reported to yield high response rates superior to those achieved with lower-dose regimens.[126] Finally, meta-analyses have been reported to show a correlation between dose intensity of platinum and response.[127,128] These kinds of evidence have provided strong support for the value of dose intensity in the treatment of ovarian carcinoma.

At first glance, the case for dose intensity would appear to be very solid. However, several significant questions remain. First, with regard to reported responses of "refractory" ovarian carcinoma to higher doses of drug, it is becoming increasingly apparent that such responses do not occur in patients whose disease progresses with the lower-dose therapy, but rather in patients in whom recurrent disease develops some time after completing prior therapy. For example, Ozols and colleagues[129] reported a series of 30 patients with "refractory" ovarian carcinoma who were treated with high-dose carboplatin (800 mg/m^2/35 d). Although eight responses were observed, Ozols and colleagues also noted that "no responses were observed from high-dose carboplatin in [9] patients who had progressive disease during prior therapy with a cisplatin-based regimen." Similar observations emerge from second-line phase II studies of intraperitoneal chemotherapy. In other words, patients whose tumors are clinically resistant to platinum-based chemotherapy do not benefit from treatment with higher doses of the same or similar drugs.

Second, the reported improvement in response rate seen with high-dose cisplatin regimens has been reappraised in light of the significant neurotoxicity that emerged from these studies.[126] Although not a randomized comparison, it is instructive to compare the results of GOG studies with regimens using 50 mg/m^2 of cisplatin in the combination regimen with results of using high-dose cisplatin. In patients with minimal residual stage III disease (no nodule >2 cm remaining), the high-dose regimen (cisplatin, 200 mg/m^2, plus cyclophosphamide, 1000 mg/m^2 repeated every 4 weeks) yielded a pathologic complete response rate of 38%,[126] whereas the GOG regimen (cisplatin, 50 mg/m^2, plus cyclophosphamide, 1000 mg/m^2 every 3 weeks) yielded a pathologic complete response rate of 30%.[9] In patients with bulky stage III or stage IV disease, the high-dose regimen (same as noted earlier) yielded a pathologic complete response rate of 12%,[126] whereas the GOG regimen (cisplatin, 50 mg/m^2, plus doxorubicin, 50 mg/m^2, plus cyclophosphamide, 500 mg/m^2, repeated every 3 weeks) yielded a pathologic complete response rate of 11%.[8] Thus no evidence exists that the high-dose cisplatin regimen yielded a superior result, even though the dose intensity of the platinum compound as a function of dose and time was 3 times as high.

Third, although a dose-intensity meta-analysis conducted by Levin and Hryniuk[127] indeed documented a dose-response relation for cisplatin, this relation held only over the range of 0.4 to 0.8. For purposes of this meta-analysis, the "standard" regimen used a cisplatin dose equivalent to 15 mg/m^2 per week. The dose-response relation for cisplatin thus held over a range of 6 mg/m^2 per week to 12 mg/m^2 per week. This equates to a highest dose of 36 mg/m^2 every 3 weeks. This meta-analysis thus supplied no support for the use of doses higher than those used by the GOG in their relatively low-dose cisplatin regimens.

An extended meta-analysis by the same investigators[128] included more studies in the higher dose range. This study demonstrated the superiority of combination chemotherapy over single agents and also noted a correlation between response and cisplatin dose up to a level of 25 mg/m^2/week (or 75 mg/m^2 every 3 weeks). In this analysis, the investigators also suggested that total dose delivered might be as important as dose intensity. Neither meta-analysis, however, offered any evidence supporting the importance of total dose or of a correlation between response and dose intensity for any drug other than cisplatin; and neither was able to support the importance of cisplatin dose intensity beyond 25 mg/m^2/week.

These considerations raise serious questions about the value of dose-intense regimens in the treatment of ovarian carcinoma. Addressing these issues appropriately requires randomized prospective trials. Eight such studies have been reported (Table 92-12).[130-137]

Studies Showing No Advantage from Dose Intensity. GOG Protocol 97[130] randomized patients with large-volume disease defined as having nodules larger than 1 cm or stage IV disease to receive either eight cycles of cisplatin (50 mg/m^2) plus cyclophosphamide (500 mg/m^2) every 3 weeks or four cycles of cisplatin (100 mg/m^2) plus cyclophosphamide (1000 mg/m^2) every 3 weeks. A total of 458 eligible patients was randomized, of whom 130 had measurable disease. Prognostic features were evenly distributed between the two treatment arms. If the prescribed low dose is assigned a dose intensity of 1.0, the actual received dose intensity for the low-dose regimen was 0.95, and for the high-dose regimen, 1.90. A twofold difference in dose intensity was thus achieved. No difference in total dose received was noted between the two arms as planned.

With regard to response, of 60 patients assigned to the high-dose arm, 19 (32%) achieved a clinical complete response; 16 (27%), a partial response; 18 (30%), stable disease; and 7 (12%), increasing disease. The overall response rate for the high-dose arm was thus 59%. Of 70 patients assigned to the low-dose arm, 27 (39%) achieved a clinical complete response; 18 (26%), a partial response; 24 (34%), stable disease; and 1 (1%), increasing disease. The overall response rate for the low-dose arm was thus 65%. No statistically significant differences were noted between the two arms with regard to response.

With regard to progression-free interval and survival, all 458 patients were included in the analysis. Median progression-free intervals for the low-dose and high-dose regimens, respectively, were 12 and 13 months, whereas median survivals were 24 and 21 months, respectively. No significant differences were observed in either parameter.

The high-dose regimen was associated with more severe or life-threatening (grade 3 or 4) toxicity, which included more leukopenia (82% vs. 40%), more thrombocytopenia (22% vs. 1%), more anemia (9% vs. 2%), more nausea and vomiting (16% vs. 3%), and more nephrotoxicity (5% vs. 1%). Very few cases of grade 3 or 4 neurotoxicity were seen.

This GOG study was designed as a pure dose-intensity study only in patients with large-volume disease. No evidence exists that a twofold increase in dose intensity yields any greater patient benefit over the range of doses used in this trial for patients with large-volume disease, but it is clear that the higher-dose regimen was more toxic.

TABLE 92-12

TRIAL	PLATINUM DI	RESPONSE	SURVIVAL
Showing No Difference			
GOG[122]	Cisplatin, 16.7 mg/m^2/wk	65%	21 mo
	Cisplatin, 33.3 mg/m^2/wk	59%	24 mo
GICOG[124]	Cisplatin, 25 mg/m^2/wk	61%	33 mo
	Cisplatin, 50 mg/m^2/wk	66%	36 mo
GONO[125]	Cisplatin, 12.5 mg/m^2/wk	61%	24 mo
	Cisplatin, 25 mg/m^2/wk	58%	29 mo
London[126]	Carboplatin, AUC 6	57%	HR 0.91
	Carboplatin, AUC 12	63%	
Danish[127]	Carboplatin, AUC 8		33% 3 yr
	Carboplatin, AUC 4		30% 3 yr
Austrian[128]	Cisplatin, 25 mg/m^2/wk	42%	38 mo
	Cis, 25 mg/m^2 + Carbo 75 mg/m^2/wk	39%	42 mo
Showing a Difference			
Scottish[123]	Cisplatin, 16.7 mg/m^2/wk	34%	27% 4 yr
	Cisplatin, 33.3 mg/m^2/wk	61%	32% 4 yr
Hong Kong[129]	Cisplatin, 15–20 mg/m^2/wk	30%	30% 3 yr
	Cisplatin, 30–40 mg/m^2/wk	55%	60% 3 yr

Seven Randomized Trials of Platinum Dose Intensity in Advanced Ovarian Carcinoma[130–137]

DI, dose intensity.

A GICOG trial[132] randomized 306 patients with advanced disease to either cisplatin, 75 mg/m^2 every 3 weeks for six cycles, or cisplatin, 50 mg/m^2 weekly for 9 weeks. The actual received dose intensity of the high-dose regimen was twice that of the low-dose regimen, and no differences existed in the total dose delivered in either arm of the trial. In contrast to the GOG study, 45% of the patients in this study had small-volume advanced disease. No significant differences were observed between the arms with regard to pathologic complete response (24% high-dose vs. 28% low-dose), progression-free interval (21 vs. 18 months), and survival (36 vs. 33 months). Like the GOG study, this was a trial of pure dose intensity, because each regimen delivered the same total dose of drug. Also like the GOG trial, this study provides no support for the importance of dose intensity over the range of cisplatin dose intensity from 25 mg/m^2/week to 50 mg/m^2/week.

A GONO trial[133] randomized 145 patients with large-volume advanced disease to receive cyclophosphamide, 600 mg/m^2, plus epirubicin, 60 mg/m^2, plus either cisplatin, 50 mg/m^2, or cisplatin, 100 mg/m^2, every 4 weeks for six cycles. In contrast to the GOG and GICOG trials, this study called for the delivery of twice as much total dose of cisplatin in the high-dose regimen. Actual received dose intensity achieved a 2:1 ratio between the high-dose and low-dose regimens and evaluated the range of cisplatin dose intensity from 12.5 mg/m^2/week to 25 mg/m^2/week. No significant differences were noted with regard to clinical response (57.5% high-dose vs. 61.1% low-dose), pathologic complete response (9.6% high-dose vs. 18.1% low-dose), progression-free interval (18 months high-dose vs. 13 months low-dose), and survival (29 months high-dose vs. 24 months low-dose). The high-dose regimen was clearly more toxic. The trial

provides no support for the importance of either dose intensity or total dose over the range of cisplatin dose intensity tested (12.5 mg/m^2/week to 25 mg/m^2/week).

A London GOG trial[134] randomized 241 patients with either small-volume or large-volume advanced disease to single-agent carboplatin dosed to an area under the curve (AUC) of either 6 for six courses or 12 for four courses at 4-week intervals. In the high-dose arm, dose intensity was doubled, and total dose increased by 22%. No significant differences were noted with respect to response (63% high-dose vs. 57% low-dose), progression-free interval (hazard ratio, 0.98), and survival (hazard ratio, 0.91). This trial also provides no support for the importance of dose intensity or total dose over the range tested.

In a DACOVA trial,[135] Danish investigators randomized 222 patients with advanced ovarian carcinoma to carboplatin dosed to an AUC of either 4 or 8, every 4 weeks for six cycles. No differences were observed with respect to pathologic complete response or survival.

An Austrian trial[136] approached the problem of platinum dose intensity by combining cisplatin and carboplatin. A total of 253 patients with stages IC to IV disease were randomized either to cisplatin, 100 mg/m^2, plus carboplatin, 300 mg/m^2, or to cisplatin, 100 mg/m^2, plus cyclophosphamide, 600 mg/m^2 monthly, for six cycles. Actual received dose intensity for platinum was 1.6-fold greater with the cisplatin/carboplatin regimen. The platinum-intensified regimen produced more myelo-suppression, ototoxicity, and gastrointestinal toxicity. The cisplatin/carboplatin regimen produced a response rate of 39%, a complete response rate of 26%, a progression-free median survival of 22 months, and an overall median survival of 42 months. These results were not significantly different from those seen with the cisplatin/cyclophosphamide regimen: 42% response rate, 26% complete response rate, 25-month median progression-free survival, and 38-month median overall survival. This trial thus failed to confirm an advantage for a 1.6-fold increase in platinum dose intensity.

These observation contradict the dogma that higher-dose schedules yield better results. Several possible explanations may be found. First, total dose instead of dose intensity may be important. At least four of the six studies, however, used differences in both dose intensity and total dose and showed no advantage. Second, dose intensity may be relatively ineffective in large-volume disease and still yield better results in patients with small-volume disease. All but the GOG trial, however, included patients with small-volume disease, with no advantage noted in the small-volume subset. Third, a twofold increase in dose intensity may be too small to permit observation of differences. Finally, and perhaps most devastatingly, once a certain threshold is reached, further escalation in dose intensity may yield no further benefit.

Studies Showing an Advantage for Dose Intensity. A Scottish trial,[131] a study from the Scottish Gynaecology Cancer Trials Group, randomized 159 patients with stages IC to IV disease to cyclophosphamide, 750 mg/m², plus either cisplatin, 50 mg/m², or cisplatin, 100 mg/m², every three weeks. Actual received dose intensity for the higher-dose versus the lower-dose regimen was 1.8 to 1. The lower-dose regimen produced significantly less neurotoxicity. At 4 years of follow-up, 32% of those receiving the higher dose regimen were alive as compared to 27% of those on the lower-dose regimen. The ratio of deaths among those receiving the higher-dose regimen versus that of those receiving the lower-dose regimen was 0.52 at 2 years and 0.68 at 4.75 years. These results suggest that, in contrast to results in the previous five studies, an advantage that diminished with time occurred for the higher-dose regimen. The investigators' conclusion was that the optimal dose of cisplatin would be 75 mg/m² every 3 weeks.

This trial has major problems. First, 49 (31%) of the 159 patients had stage IC or II disease. The heterogeneous patient population resulting from the inclusion of these limited-disease patients makes interpretation of results very difficult, especially when one considers the relatively small total number of patients in the study. Second, the actual difference in 4-year survival of less than 6% is not impressive; and the relative death rate of the higher-dose versus the lower-dose regimen after the first 2 years is 1.30. The overall advantage for the higher-dose regimen is significant only at *P* = .061. Finally, the choice of 75 mg/m² every 3 weeks as the optimal dose of cisplatin does not follow from the results of the study, which did not deal with the recommended dose.

A Hong Kong trial[137] is the smallest of the randomized studies, with only 50 patients entered. The patient population is not well characterized. Cisplatin doses on the two regimens were 60 mg/m² and 120 mg/m², respectively. The higher-dose regimen yielded a response rate of 55% and a 3-year survival of 60% as compared with lower-dose results of a response rate of 30% and 3-year survival

of 30%. Even though these results suggest that the higher-dose regimen offered an advantage, the size of the trial and the poor characterization of the patient population make the conclusions less convincing.

Conclusions Regarding Dose Intensity. In conclusion, the case for the use of regimens with greater dose intensity, especially greater dose intensity of the platinum compound, is unclear at best. To understand the apparent contradiction between in vitro data and clinical results, one must look to certain basic principles on which the concept of the value of dose intensity is based. By using a somatic mutation theory for drug resistance, Coldman and Goldie[138] postulated that the failure to cure a patient of malignancy results from either the failure to eradicate all drug-sensitive cells because of insufficient drug dose intensity or the emergence of cells resistant to the drug regimen. Enhanced dose intensity functions in two ways to improve the likelihood of cure: (1) eradicating all sensitive cells, and (2) eliminating cells likely to mutate to resistance before such mutations take place. No evidence exists that drug resistance can be overcome in vivo by enhancement of dose intensity over the range that can be clinically achieved.

If these considerations are translated into simple terms, increasing dose intensity yields increasing clinical response rates up to the point at which all sensitive cells have been eradicated. Further increase in dose intensity cannot be expected to yield further improvement in results over the currently achievable range. The only basis on which an increased cure rate can be expected from dose escalation is that the drugs are started before the emergence of resistant cells, an unlikely circumstance in patients with advanced disease.

Role of Paclitaxel

A new agent with a unique mechanism of action, paclitaxel has significant activity in ovarian carcinoma as second-line therapy with a response rate in excess of 20% in patients, regardless of prior response to platinum-based chemotherapy. These results marked paclitaxel as probably non–cross-resistant with the platinum compounds and alkylating agents and suggested a major role for the drug in first-line treatment of ovarian carcinoma. These data prompted four major randomized trials testing paclitaxel in front-line combination chemotherapy.

GOG Protocol 111[139] randomized 386 newly diagnosed patients with large-volume advanced ovarian carcinoma to six cycles of cisplatin, 75 mg/m², plus either cyclophosphamide, 750 mg/m², or paclitaxel, 135 mg/m², over a 24-hour period preceding the cisplatin. The paclitaxel-based regimen proved superior in regard to overall response rate (73% vs. 60%; *P* = .01), clinical complete response rate (51% vs. 31%; *P* = .01), percentage grossly disease free at second-look laparotomy (40% vs. 24%; *P* = .001), progression-free survival (median, 18 vs. 13 months; *P* < .001), and overall survival (median, 38 vs. 24 months; *P* < .001) (Table 92-13). Analysis of comparative risk demonstrated a 33% reduction in morbidity and mortality with the addition of paclitaxel to first-line

TABLE 92-13

Results of GOG Protocol 111 and EORTC/NCIC OV 10: Cisplatin plus Either Cyclophosphamide or Taxol[139,140]

| | GOG 111* | | OV 10† | |
	TP	CP	TP	CP
Clinical response rate	73%	60%	59%	45%
Clinical complete response rate	51%	31%	41%	27%
Grossly disease-free second look	40%	24%	—	—
Pathologic complete response	26%	20%	—	—
Progression-free survival	18 mo	13 mo	15.5 mo	11.5 mo
Overall survival	38 mo	24 mo	35.6 mo	25.8 mo

*TP, paclitaxel, 135 mg/m²/24h, plus cisplatin, 75 mg/m² q3w; CP, cyclophosphamide, 750 mg/m² plus cisplatin, 75 mg/m² q3w. Each regimen given for six cycles; all differences statistically significant except pathologic complete response, for which $P = .08$.
†TP, paclitaxel, 175 mg/m²/3h, plus cisplatin, 75 mg/m² q3w; CP, cyclophosphamide, 750 mg/m², plus cisplatin, 75 mg/m² q3w. Each regimen given for up to nine cycles; all differences statistically significant.

chemotherapy. Although increased myelosuppression, cardiac problems, and alopecia were found with the paclitaxel-based regimen, no major clinical consequences occurred. In particular, the frequency of grade 3 or 4 neurotoxicity was the same with the two regimens. The conclusion of the GOG is that paclitaxel plus cisplatin is the new standard of care for ovarian carcinoma.

In OV-10,[140] a Canadian/European consortium randomized patients with advanced disease to either cyclophosphamide, 750 mg/m², plus cisplatin, 75 mg/m², every 3 weeks for six to nine cycles, or paclitaxel, 175 mg/m² over a 3-hour period, followed by cisplatin, 75 mg/m² every 3 weeks for six to nine cycles. This trial shows superiority for the paclitaxel/cisplatin regimen with regard to response (59% vs. 45%), clinical complete response (41% vs. 27%), progression-free survival (15.5 months vs. 11.5 months), and overall survival (35.6 months vs. 25.8 months). This study confirms GOG 111 and conclusively establishes paclitaxel plus a platinum compound as the standard of care.

GOG Protocol 132[141] was completed before availability of the final analysis of GOG Protocol 111. This trial randomized 613 newly diagnosed patients with large-volume advanced disease to six cycles of either cisplatin, 100 mg/m² every 3 weeks, paclitaxel, 200 mg/m² over a

24-hour period every 3 weeks, or paclitaxel plus cisplatin, as in GOG Protocol 111 (Table 92-14). No differences were observed among the three arms with respect to survival. The paclitaxel regimen arm was inferior with respect to response and progression-free survival. It is important to note, however, that this trial did not serve as a confirmatory trial for GOG Protocol 111 for a very important reason. At the time of accrual to GOG Protocol 111, paclitaxel was not commercially available in the United States; whereas it was commercially available at the time of accrual to GOG Protocol 132. Very few of the patients on the nonpaclitaxel regimen in GOG Protocol 111 received paclitaxel at the time of first relapse. Conversely, vast majority of patients on the single-agent regimens of GOG Protocol 132 received the other drug before progression of disease. This pattern of second-line therapy blunts differences among the three regimens.

International Collaborative Ovarian Neoplasm (ICON3)[142] (Table 92-15) is the most recently completed of the four trials and the largest (2074 patients). Several features of this trial distinguish it from the other three and dictate how this study should be evaluated. First, the study included patients with all stages of disease, I to IV. Patients with stage I to II disease represent 20% of the patients; hence the patient population is very heterogeneous. Second, the regimens are not so well defined as those in the other three trials. A choice was made

TABLE 92-14

Results of GOG Protocol 132: Comparison of Cisplatin versus Paclitaxel versus Cisplatin plus Paclitaxel[141]

	P	T	TP
Clinical response rate	67%	42%	66%
Clinical complete response rate	42%	21%	43%
Progression-free survival	16.4 m	10.8 m	14.1 m
Overall survival	30.2 m	25.9 m	26.3 m

P, cisplatin, 100 mg/m² q3wk; T, paclitaxel, 200 mg/m²/24hr q3wk; TP, paclitaxel, 135 mg/m²/24hr, plus cisplatin, 75 mg/m² q3wk. Each regimen given for six cycles. Only statistically significant differences are in failure rates: paclitaxel alone is inferior to the other two.

TABLE 92-15

Results of ICON3: Comparison of Carboplatin or CAP versus Paclitaxel versus Carboplatin plus Paclitaxel[142]

	CONTROL*	TP†
Progression-free survival	16.1 mo	17.3 mo
Overall survival	36.1 mo	35.4 mo

*Control regimens included carboplatin or CAP q3wk: carboplatin, AUC minimum 5, CAP, cyclophosphamide, 500 mg/m², doxorubicin, 50 mg/m², cisplatin, 50 mg/m².
†TP, paclitaxel, 175 mg/m²/3hr, carboplatin, AUC minimum 5, every 3 weeks. Each regimen given for six cycles.

between two regimens for the control arm, and those arms involving carboplatin allowed a range of AUC doses so long as a minimum was met. That a choice of control regimens was made is perhaps not so much a problem as it might have been, because the results of a randomized trial comparing the two has since been reported as showing no differences.[143] Third, the randomization was 2:1 favoring the control arm, so that twice as many patients were assigned to the control regimens as to paclitaxel plus carboplatin. Fourth, quality control was not so tight as in the other three trials. No pathology review is planned. Surgical requirements were nonexistent. No audit of data is planned. These factors detract from the credibility of this trial as compared with the other three.

The trial shows no significant differences between the control regimens and the experimental regimen in terms of progression-free and overall survival. This contradicts the results of GOG 111 and OV 10. The deficiencies of the study, however, are such that this trial should not detract from the results of the earlier studies.

Conclusions from these four studies should be based not only on the study results but also on the quality of the study design and execution. Two trials (GOG 111 and OV 10) show a clear advantage for a taxane/platinum combination. One trial (GOG 132) shows no difference, but crossover before progression in all likelihood means that the study actually evaluated concurrent versus sequential use of the two agents. Even in this setting, the concurrent arm was judged to be the treatment of choice because the overall toxicity was less with the concurrent regimen. The last trial (ICON3) has a number of design problems and lack of data audits; hence its contrary result should be regarded circumspectly. On the basis of these considerations, the current standard of care should be a combination of paclitaxel plus a platinum compound.

Choice of Platinum Compound

Initial studies of paclitaxel in front-line therapy involved regimens with cisplatin. Interest in substitution of carboplatin for cisplatin results from the ease of administration and decreased nonhematologic toxicity associated with carboplatin. Concerns about the use of carboplatin with paclitaxel focused on an interaction between the two agents.[144] This interaction decreases the amount of thrombocytopenia observed with carboplatin such that suppression is less severe, and recovery is usually complete by 3 weeks instead of 4, as is seen with carboplatin alone. The mechanism for this interaction is not yet clear; hence it is not clear whether the same mechanism might also result in tumor protection. This would result in less efficacy than is observed with paclitaxel/cisplatin. This concern led to three phase III trials comparing paclitaxel plus cisplatin with paclitaxel plus carboplatin.[145-147]

The Dutch trial[145] randomized 208 advanced-disease patients to paclitaxel, 175 mg/m^2/3 hr, plus either cisplatin, 75 mg/m^2, or carboplatin, AUC 5 every 3 weeks for at least six cycles. No differences in efficacy were observed, and the carboplatin-based regimen had a better toxicity profile. The study, however, was too small to permit definite conclusions to be drawn about therapeutic equivalence between the two regimens.

The AGO trial[146] randomized 798 advanced-disease patients to paclitaxel, 185 mg/m^2/3 hr, plus either cisplatin, 75 mg/m^2, or carboplatin, AUC 6 every 3 weeks for six cycles. No differences were observed between the two regimens with regard to progression-free or overall survival, with small trends favoring the cisplatin regimen. The cisplatin-based regimen was more toxic and produced a significantly inferior quality of life.

GOG Protocol 158[147] randomized 798 patients with small-volume residual advanced disease to either paclitaxel, 135 mg/m^2/24 hr, plus cisplatin, 75 mg/m^2, or paclitaxel, 175 mg/m^2/3 hr, plus carboplatin, AUC 7.5. This study differs from the other two in several important ways. First, the use of the 24-hour infusion of paclitaxel with cisplatin served to decrease the amount of neurotoxicity seen with the cisplatin-based regimen. Second, as a result of the 24-hour infusion, the dose of paclitaxel was different in the two regimens. Third, and most important, the dose of carboplatin was substantially higher in this trial. The study showed no difference in progression-free and overall survival between the two regimens, but a strong trend favored the carboplatin-based regimen, with a hazard ratio for survival of 0.86. As a result of the escalated dose of carboplatin, the toxicity of the carboplatin-based regimen was substantially greater than reported in the other two trials and did not differ greatly from that seen with the cisplatin-based regimen.

Conclusions from these three trials point to no major differences in efficacy between paclitaxel/cisplatin and paclitaxel/carboplatin. The observed trends, however, raise serious questions about the optimal dose of carboplatin in combination with paclitaxel. At the very least, when combining carboplatin with paclitaxel, an AUC of 6 of carboplatin should be used; and serious consideration should be given to the higher AUC of 7.5.

Consolidation or Maintenance Therapy

For patients with advanced ovarian carcinoma, response rates now approach 90%, clinical complete response rates reach 75%, and median survivals range from 26 months for patients with bulky residual disease to more than 60 months for patients with small-volume residual disease. Despite these excellent results, almost 75% of those who achieve a clinical complete response will relapse eventually and die of their disease.

In addition to the continuing effort to improve further the clinical complete response rate, investigators have conducted studies of ways to consolidate or maintain these responses. Over the last 20 years, none of these studies had produced a positive result.[148] The most recent reports focused on consolidation after six initial cycles of paclitaxel plus carboplatin with four cycles of topotecan.[149,150] Neither study showed any advantage for the consolidation therapy. No evidence now supports a role for consolidation therapy.

The one exception to the plethora of negative studies is a recent phase III randomized trial of extended-duration paclitaxel as maintenance therapy.[151] This study differs from prior trials in two significant respects. First, only those who responded to front-line therapy with a clinical complete response were eligible. Second, evidence

TABLE 92-16

Results of SWOG/GOG Intergroup Study of Maintenance Therapy*

	3 CYCLES	12 CYCLES
Patients	107	115
Recurrences	34	20
Progression-free survival[†]	28 mo	21 mo

*Comparison of 3 versus 12 cycles of monthly paclitaxel in those with clinical complete response to front-line paclitaxel plus cisplatin[151]
[†]The difference in progression-free survival was statistically significant (P = .0023).

suggests that extension of the duration of paclitaxel therapy may be beneficial. This includes anecdotal reports of responses to paclitaxel that did not develop until as late as the twelfth cycle of therapy and preclinical observations of an antiangiogenic effect of paclitaxel over a prolonged period of treatment.[152]

Originally designed to accrue 450 patients with clinical complete responses to paclitaxel/platinum and to randomize these patient to either 12 or 3 additional monthly cycles of paclitaxel, 175 mg/m^2/3 hr, the study was closed early because of extreme differences in progression-free survival favoring the 12 additional cycles (Table 92-16). Because of patient choice to cross over to the 12-cycle regimen after study closure, survival is not assessable. Toxicity was obviously greater in the 12-cycle regimen, but only 13 patients in the entire study dropped out because of toxicity. Although one study requires confirmation, the trial should certainly prompt discussion of this issue with each patient; and the evidence poses a convincing case for using 12 additional cycles of paclitaxel monthly as maintenance therapy. Whether 12 cycles is enough could be questioned because of the observation of an increase in recurrence rate after cessation of the paclitaxel on each arm.

Current Standard of Care

Based on the series of studies cited over the last two decades, a solid case points to the combination of paclitaxel, 175 mg/m^2/3 hr, plus carboplatin, AUC 6 to 7.5 every 3 weeks, for six cycles as the current standard of care. With this approach, an overall response rate of 95%, a clinical complete response rate of 75%, a pathological complete response rate of 50%, a progression-free survival of 15 to 24 months, and an overall survival of 26 to more than 60 months should result. These results will vary according to the volume of residual disease, with those patients with small-volume residual disease (no nodule left >2 cm diameter) experiencing better outcome.

After this, the issue of maintenance therapy with 12 cycles of paclitaxel should be discussed with the patient. Patient preference will play a large role in determining whether an individual patient will receive maintenance therapy.

Controversies and Issues

Studies of patients with advanced disease address a number of additional issues: optimal paclitaxel schedule,

intraperitoneal chemotherapy, high-dose chemotherapy with stem cell support, integration of new agents (both cytotoxic and biologic) into front-line therapy, the role of second-look laparotomy, and the role of CA-125 in assessing response and progression.

Paclitaxel Schedule. Paclitaxel was initially studied in a number of different schedules from weekly to every-3-week schedules and from 1-hour to 120-hour infusion durations. By 1990, investigators were exclusively using a 24-hour infusion given every 3 weeks because of the higher incidence of hypersensitivity reactions with shorter infusions. Since then, shorter and longer infusions as well as weekly schedules have been studied.

A great deal of interest focused on the potential for shorter infusions because of the inconvenience of 24-hour infusions. A landmark phase III trial of 3-hour versus 24-hour infusions of paclitaxel as a single agent in relapsed ovarian cancer established the feasibility of short infusions preceded by premedication to prevent hypersensitivity reactions.[153] The study dispelled the myth that the 24-hour infusion had superior efficacy by showing no difference in response rate, progression-free survival, and overall survival. In terms of toxicity, the 3-hour infusion produced significantly less myelosuppression in exchange for increased neurotoxicity and other nonhematologic toxicities.

The theoretical advantages of even longer infusions also have been examined. Two studies of 96-hour infusions, prompted by suggestions in breast cancer that this length of infusion produced responses in some patients for whom shorter infusions had failed, defined no role for this approach. Markman and colleagues[154] treated 30 patients, for whom either a 3-hour or a 24-hour infusion had failed, with a 96-hour infusion of a total dose of 140 mg/m^2, to be repeated every 3 weeks. No objective responses were observed, although the regimen was well tolerated. Subsequently the GOG randomized patients with newly diagnosed advanced ovarian carcinoma to either paclitaxel, 135 mg/m^2/24 hr, plus cisplatin, 75 mg/m^2 every 3 weeks for six cycles, or paclitaxel, 120 mg/m^2/96 hr, plus cisplatin, 75 mg/m^2, every 3 weeks for six cycles.[155] No differences in efficacy were observed. Therefore no reason exists to use a 96-hour infusion in the treatment of ovarian carcinoma.

Of potentially greater interest is a weekly schedule of paclitaxel. An initial phase I study of 40 to 100 mg/m^2/1 hr of paclitaxel weekly demonstrated that this approach was feasible and also suggested potential activity (four responses among 13 patients).[156] This study also suggested that these weekly infusions produced fewer adverse effects. Subsequently a phase II trial treated 53 patients with paclitaxel, 80 mg/m^2/1 hr weekly, and reported 13 (25%) responses.[157] A randomized phase III trial of weekly versus every-3-week paclitaxel (67 mg/m^2/3 hr weekly versus 200 mg/m^2/3 hr every 3 weeks), however, showed no difference in efficacy and a small advantage for the weekly regimen in terms of toxicity.[158] It should be pointed out that the dose of the every-3-week schedule is higher than is generally used in ovarian carcinoma, and this may account for the greater toxicity seen with that schedule.

In summary, these data on schedule taken together provide the following points that should be considered in the application of paclitaxel to the treatment of ovarian carcinoma. First, efficacy does not appear to be affected by schedule. Second, toxicity does vary with schedule. Longer infusions produce more myelosuppression, whereas shorter infusions produce more nonhematologic toxicity, such as neurotoxicity. With appropriate premedication, hypersensitivity does not appear to be a major problem regardless of infusion duration. Finally, although the weekly schedule is certainly efficacious and feasible, it appears to offer insufficient advantage in general to justify the greater inconvenience of weekly treatments.

Intraperitoneal Chemotherapy

In an effort directed at achieving ever greater dose intensity, three randomized trials involving intraperitoneal therapy have been reported. The first of these studies, an Intergroup study of the Southwest Oncology Group (SWOG) and the GOG, randomized 654 patients with small-volume residual disease to cyclophosphamide, 600 mg/m^2 intravenously, plus cisplatin, 100 mg/m^2, either intravenously or intraperitoneally.[159] Results show a statistically significant small survival advantage and less tinnitus, clinical hearing loss, and neurotoxicity for those patients on the intraperitoneal regimen. The study has a flaw in execution (extension of the accrual goal to increase the size of a subset and then an analysis using all patients, an approach which introduces statistical bias) but does suggest an advantage for intraperitoneal chemotherapy. Somewhat counterintuitively, the study shows that the treatment advantage exists only in those with somewhat larger nodules (0.5 to 2.0 cm) rather than the expected 0- to 0.5-cm subgroup.

GOG Protocol 114,[160] a second Intergroup trial involving intraperitoneal therapy, randomized small-volume patients to either paclitaxel plus cisplatin as given in GOG Protocol 111 or two cycles of carboplatin dosed to an AUC of 9 at 4-week intervals followed by six cycles of paclitaxel, 135 mg/m^2 intravenously over 24 hours, followed by intraperitoneal cisplatin, 100 mg/m^2 every 3 weeks. The 523 patients with no nodule larger than 1-cm diameter were randomized to study. The intraperitoneal regimen was superior with regard to progression-free survival (median, 27.6 vs. 22.5 months; $P = .02$), but only a marginal difference in overall survival was observed (median, 52.9 vs. 47.6 months; $P = .056$).[160] The gain in efficacy, similar to that seen in the prior intraperitoneal study,[159] came at the expense of significantly more toxicity of all types on the intraperitoneal regimen.

The third intraperitoneal study, GOG Protocol 172,[161] randomized 417 small-volume (<1.0-cm nodules) patients to either paclitaxel plus cisplatin, as given in GOG Protocol 111, or six cycles of paclitaxel, 135 mg/m^2 intravenously over 24 hours on day 1, intraperitoneal cisplatin, 100 mg/m^2 on day 2, and intraperitoneal paclitaxel, 80 mg/m^2 on day 8, with the regimen repeated every 3 weeks. Toxicity was dramatically greater on the intraperitoneal regimen to the extent that a substantial portion

of the patients were unable to complete six cycles of therapy. Analysis of survival awaits sufficient deaths. Progression-free survival, however, is superior on the intraperitoneal regimen, with a hazard ratio of 0.73.

These three trials make the case that intraperitoneal chemotherapy yields a superior survival compared with standard intravenous chemotherapy in patients with small-volume residual advanced ovarian carcinoma. This benefit is bought at the expense of significantly more toxicity, to the extent that a substantial portion of the patients cannot complete six cycles of therapy. At least at the present, the toxicity of the intraperitoneal regimens tested precludes their routine clinical use. Current efforts are directed at the development of less toxic intraperitoneal regimens that preserve the apparent survival benefit of the approach.

Stem Cell–Supported High-Dose Chemotherapy. The alternative to intraperitoneal chemotherapy for the achievement of higher dose intensity is the use of stem cell–supported high-dose chemotherapy. As with the use of this approach in other cancers, most studies are small and uncontrolled and show high response rates but short response durations and short survivals.[162] The largest study to date reports on the use of stem cell–supported high-dose chemotherapy in 421 patients for whom prior chemotherapy failed.[163] The population had an average age of 48 years, and 59% were platinum sensitive. The reported response rate was 70% (47% complete response and 23% partial response). Two-year progression-free survival was 12%, and 2-year overall survival was 35%. Although these numbers appear promising, patients with similar demographic and disease features fare considerably better with either intraperitoneal chemotherapy or standard intravenous chemotherapy.

To settle the issue of the role of high-dose chemotherapy with stem-cell support, a randomized phase III trial should be conducted. Two attempts, one in Europe and one in the United States, have failed to accrue sufficient patients. Until such a trial demonstrates the value of this approach, high-dose therapy should be reserved for clinical trials, preferably phase III clinical trials.

Integration of New Cytotoxic and Biologic Agents into Front-Line Therapy. The last 10 years saw a veritable explosion of discovery of new agents, both cytotoxic and biologic, with activity in ovarian carcinoma. Many of these agents are active in patients with disease that is still platinum sensitive, but activity in platinum-resistant disease is minimal or nonexistent. Of particular interest for incorporation into front-line therapy are those agents with activity in patients who have progressed on or shortly after completion of a paclitaxel/platinum front-line regimen. Such agents may be considered at least partially clinically non–cross-resistant with the taxanes and platinum compounds and thus may add additional benefit to front-line regimens.

At least four cytotoxic agents have activity in patients with "paclitaxel/platinum-resistant" disease: oral etoposide,[94] pegylated liposomal doxorubicin,[88,89] topotecan,[84,86] and gemcitabine.[99-101] These four agents have been the focus of efforts by an international consortium to integrate one or more into front-line therapy. Oral etoposide was dropped from further efforts because of the occurrence of three cases of acute myeloid leukemia among 52 patients in the study of paclitaxel plus carboplatin plus escalating duration of prolonged oral etoposide.[164] The other three agents are being evaluated in an ongoing GOG/ Gynecologic Cancer Intergroup trial (Table 92-17), which assesses the impact of a third agent added either as a component of a triplet or as part of a sequential doublet.

Biologic agents of interest as part of front-line therapy now include tyrosine kinase inhibitors (Iressa); monoclonal antibodies that target either epidermal growth factor receptor (EGFR; C-225), HER2-neu (trastuzumab), or vascular endothelial growth factor (VEGF; bevacizumab); agents that reverse resistance (cyclosporine and valspodar); and gamma interferon. Of these, data are available on trastuzumab, cyclosporine, valspodar, and gamma interferon.

The GOG studied trastuzumab in a population of patients with recurrent or refractory ovarian carcinoma.[115] Of a total of 837 patients screened; 95 overexpressed HER2-neu ($2^+/3^+$ by immunohistochemistry). Of these 95, 41 were eligible and assessable and agreed to participate in the trial. Among the 41 treated with trastuzumab, one complete and two partial responses resulted. Investigators concluded that HER2-neu overexpression occurred less frequently than previously reported (12% instead of 25%) and that treatment with trastuzumab had at best modest activity (7%).

The GOG also evaluated cyclosporine (cyclosporin A) for potential ability to reverse resistance to cisplatin.[165] Preclinical data had suggested that cyclosporin A could inhibit P-glycoprotein and reverse *MDR*-mediated resistance to cisplatin. Among 26 patients with platinum-resistant disease, only three responses to cisplatin plus cyclosporin A occurred. These data were considered insufficient justification for further study. A related compound (cyclosporine D analogue), valspodar, subsequently underwent a phase II and a phase III study of its ability to reverse MDR-mediated resistance to paclitaxel. The GOG phase II study[166] administered the combination to

58 patients with clinical resistance to paclitaxel. Five responses resulted and prompted the performance of a phase III trial by an international consortium.[167] This phase III study in patients with newly diagnosed ovarian carcinoma sought to determine whether the concurrent administration of valspodar with paclitaxel/ carboplatin produced results superior to that of chemotherapy alone. The study report showed no significant differences in efficacy or toxicity. All trends in both efficacy and toxicity favored the chemotherapy-alone regimen. These three trials suggest that these two compounds have no significant role in the management of ovarian carcinoma.

Studies of gamma interferon report significant activity against ovarian carcinoma by either intraperitoneal or intravenous routes.[168] These results prompted a phase III trial of cyclophosphamide/cisplatin with or without gamma interferon administered by the subcutaneous route.[169] Although this study had to be stopped prematurely because of the emergence of paclitaxel/carboplatin as the new standard of care, the trial did show a statistically significant difference in progression-free survival favoring the gamma interferon regimen. As a result, gamma interferon is being evaluated in an ongoing phase III trial of paclitaxel/carboplatin with or without gamma interferon.

Among other biologic agents, agents directed against VEGF attract the greatest interest because of studies suggesting that high levels of VEGF in tumor specimens are associated with a poorer prognosis.[170] At this point, however, no data define a clear role for any biologic agent.

Role of CA-125. CA-125, a mucin-like glycoprotein, increases in response to disturbances of the celomic epithelium. The marker is most closely associated with the assessment of patients with ovarian carcinoma. As discussed earlier, the marker has no defined role in the early detection of ovarian carcinoma. The major clinical role is the assessment of disease status in patients receiving treatment for advanced disease.[171] Because of the difficulty in accurately assessing tumor response in a neoplasm often confined to the peritoneal cavity, interest has developed in defining ways to use CA-125 levels to determine response.[172] Current proposals focus on definitions based on a 50% or 75% decrease of CA-125 levels during the course of therapy and are currently under review by a committee of the Gynecologic Cancer Intergroup.[173]

Until standard definitions are developed, the marker should be confined to allowing a rough idea of whether disease is responding and should not be used as a response criterion. Decreasing CA-125 levels suggest a favorable response of tumor to therapy, whereas increasing levels suggest progression of disease. Certain principles should guide such a use. First, no single CA-125 value should dictate management decisions; a series of increasing or decreasing values (usually three or more) should be required. Second, changes in the CA-125 should not result in action until the changes are corroborated by other objective evidence.

Second-Look Laparotomy. Second-look laparotomy is an exploratory laparotomy performed at the conclusion of

TABLE 92-17

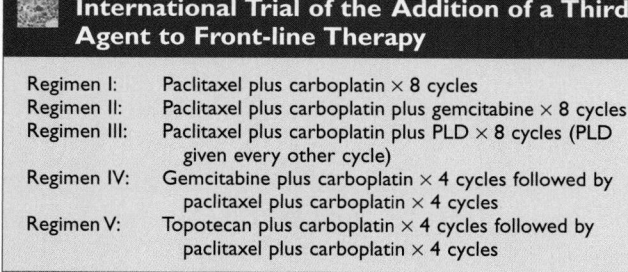

Schema for GOG Protocol 182, an International Trial of the Addition of a Third Agent to Front-line Therapy

Regimen I:	Paclitaxel plus carboplatin × 8 cycles
Regimen II:	Paclitaxel plus carboplatin plus gemcitabine × 8 cycles
Regimen III:	Paclitaxel plus carboplatin plus PLD × 8 cycles (PLD given every other cycle)
Regimen IV:	Gemcitabine plus carboplatin × 4 cycles followed by paclitaxel plus carboplatin × 4 cycles
Regimen V:	Topotecan plus carboplatin × 4 cycles followed by paclitaxel plus carboplatin × 4 cycles

PLD, pegylated liposomal doxorubicin.
Accrual goal, 4000 patients.

front-line chemotherapy. The purpose of the procedure is to determine disease status accurately so that decisions regarding further management can be made.[174] Patients selected as candidates for second-look laparotomy usually are in one of two categories: those with a clinical complete response to front-line therapy and those who are potential candidates for secondary surgical cyto-reduction. Among patients undergoing second-look laparotomy, 40% will have no pathologic evidence of disease; yet half of those with a pathologic complete response will relapse.[175,176]

After widespread use in the 1980s, second-look laparotomies are now performed less frequently. Reasons cited for decrease in use of the procedure usually focus on the failure of studies to show that patients who undergo second-look laparotomy have an improved survival as a result. The most recent and largest study evaluating second-look laparotomy[147,177] came from data collected in a study of paclitaxel/carboplatin versus paclitaxel/cisplatin in patients with small-volume residual stage III ovarian carcinoma (GOG Protocol 158). Institutions were required to specify whether women with clinical complete responses on the study would undergo second-look laparotomy at the conclusion of the protocol-assigned therapy. Roughly half of the patients entered in the study did undergo the procedure. GOG investigators compared the outcome for those patients who did or did not have a second look. No differences were observed; hence the investigators concluded that second-look laparotomy was of no value.

The problem with the study is the same flaw seen in other reported studies. The potential value of second-look laparotomy lies in the information gleaned from the procedure. What determines whether that value is realized is the value of the management decision made on the basis of the information. The proper study should specify the management choice to be made for each finding at second look so that the study evaluates the package of second-look plus a specified management versus no second look. In conclusion, second-look laparotomy is currently not recommended for routine clinical use.

Summary of Management of Advanced Disease

Patients with advanced ovarian carcinoma should undergo an initial attempt at surgical cytoreduction followed by chemotherapy. The best evidence shows that paclitaxel combined with carboplatin is the regimen of choice. On completion of initial chemotherapy, the use of an additional 12 cycles of paclitaxel monthly as maintenance therapy should be discussed with the patient. Dose-intense regimens, intraperitoneal therapy, and the addition of a third agent to front-line therapy offer no established advantage and hence should be reserved for clinical trials.

Management of Limited Disease

Patients with stage I or II disease compose approximately 25% of all patients with celomic epithelial carcinoma of the ovary. Only a small proportion of these are ever entered onto clinical trials, however; hence until recently, it was difficult to provide definitive guidelines for the

---

THERAPEUTIC DECISIONS IN NEWLY DIAGNOSED CELOMIC EPITHELIAL CARCINOMA

Newly diagnosed patients with celomic epithelial carcinoma of the ovary must be carefully staged so that appropriate treatment decisions can be made. This necessitates an exploratory laparotomy in all but those who have obvious stage IV disease. At laparotomy, as much disease as possible should be resected. Decisions are then governed by the surgical stage of the disease.

For patients with stage I or II disease, total abdominal hysterectomy and bilateral salpingo-oophorectomy should be done. This should be followed by adjuvant therapy if any of the following are present: poorly differentiated disease (grade 3), tumor excrescences on the surface of the ovary, ascites, positive peritoneal cytology, or extraovarian disease. The adjuvant therapy of choice at our institution is platinum-based chemotherapy: carboplatin (AUC, 7.5 IV) after paclitaxel (175 mg/m^2/3hr IV) every 3 weeks for three cycles. At the conclusion of treatment, close observation will suffice.

For patients with stage III or IV disease, an aggressive attempt at surgical cytoreduction should be followed by platinum-based combination chemotherapy for six cycles. The optimal regimen is the combination of paclitaxel, 175 mg/m^2 over a 3-hour period, plus carboplatin, AUC 6 to 7.5, every 3 weeks for six cycles. At the conclusion of initial chemotherapy, the physician should discuss the issue of maintenance paclitaxel, 175 mg/m^2 over a 3-hour period, monthly for 12 cycles.

---

management of these patients. Recent randomized trials form the basis of current management principles.

General Considerations. Certain characteristics of the primary lesion are important in determining the prognosis of the patient with limited disease: histologic grade, location of the primary tumor, ascites, peritoneal cytology, and, to a lesser extent, histologic type. These characteristics permit separation of the patient population into those at low risk of recurrence and those at high risk[178] (Table 92-18). Patients at low risk of recurrence exhibit all the following characteristics: one or both ovaries involved, grade 1 or 2 (well or moderately differentiated), intracystic (no tumor on the external surface of the ovary), no ascites, negative peritoneal cytology, and no extraovarian disease. Patients at high risk have any one of the following characteristics: grade 3 (poorly differentiated), extracystic (tumor on the surface of the ovary), ascites, positive peritoneal cytology, or extraovarian (stage II) disease. Patients at low risk of recurrence have a 5-year survival that exceeds 90%, whereas those at high risk have a substantially lower survival.[179]

The assignment of a patient to a risk category should be based on a careful exploratory laparotomy performed through an incision that permits the exploration of the entire abdominal contents. Ascites should be noted, and samples for cytology taken. In the absence of ascites, peritoneal washings for cytology should be obtained.

TABLE 92-18

Risk Groups for Limited Ovarian Carcinoma

GROUP	CHARACTERISTICS
Low risk	Grade 1 or 2 disease
	Intact capsule
	No tumor on external surface
	Negative peritoneal cytology
	No ascites
	Growth confined to ovaries
High risk	Grade 3 disease
	Ruptured capsule
	Tumor on external surface
	Positive peritoneal cytology
	Ascites
	Growth outside ovaries

If any high-risk factors are present, the patient is considered high risk.
Data from Young et al.[179]

The capsule of the tumor should be inspected for excrescences, dense adherence, or rupture. The peritoneal surface should be carefully examined for implants of tumor. Areas requiring particular attention include the undersurface of the diaphragm, the paracolic gutters, and the omentum. Biopsies should be obtained of any suggestive lesion and, in the absence of suggestive areas, of multiple sites. The para-aortic nodes should be examined and sampled. Finally, after inspection of the entire peritoneal surface, a total abdominal hysterectomy, bilateral salpingo-oophorectomy, and omentectomy should be carried out.

Because selection of therapy will be based on risk category, a detailed staging procedure is mandatory. In a series of 100 patients referred after initial laparotomy-based diagnosis of stage I or II ovarian carcinoma and then re-explored, 31 were found to have more advanced disease than noted at initial laparotomy. Such upstaging may have a significant impact on choice of therapy.

Management. The initial approach to patients with limited disease should be surgical resection of disease.

This should be combined with a careful staging laparotomy that defines in detail the anatomic extent of disease. Controversy, however, characterizes recommendations for the use of adjuvant therapy after surgical resection. At least three different approaches have been used in uncontrolled trials: abdominopelvic radiation therapy, intraperitoneal radioactive chromic phosphate (^{32}P), and chemotherapy.

Radiation Therapy. The use of radiation therapy in the management of ovarian carcinoma fell into disfavor because of two flawed approaches to its use: pelvic radiation therapy as an adjuvant to surgical resection of stage I disease[180,181] and abdominopelvic radiation therapy in patients with gross disease. The first approach failed because a significant proportion of the patients treated with pelvic fields already had at least microscopic disease outside the pelvis. The second approach attempted the

eradication of disease too bulky to handle with the doses achievable to a whole abdominal field. Results with abdominopelvic radiation therapy as an adjuvant treatment in patients with stage I through III disease and no gross residual suggest that the potential role of radiation therapy should be reconsidered.

Investigators at the Princess Margaret Hospital in Toronto, Ontario, Canada, randomized patients with stage I, stage II, and minimal residual stage III disease to either abdominopelvic radiation to a total of 22.5 cGy by a moving-strip technique or pelvic radiation with or without chlorambucil. Patients with stage III disease were not randomized to pelvic radiation alone. The study demonstrated clear superiority for abdominopelvic radiation.[182] A follow-up trial that compared abdominopelvic radiation by a moving strip and open field technique showed no difference.[183]

A subsequent analysis of patients receiving abdominopelvic radiation in these two studies looked at the results in patients at intermediate or high risk of recurrence on the basis of histologic type, grade, and stage.[184] Of 211 patients at intermediate risk, only 60 were assigned to stage I; 5-year survival was 75%. Of 88 patients at high risk of recurrence, there were 72 stage III and 16 stage II patients; 5-year survival was 32%. Two groups of patients did not benefit from abdominopelvic radiation: those with stage I grade I and those with large-volume disease (nodules >2 cm).

An important problem with these studies is the lack of careful surgical staging, as evidenced by the large number (155 of 325) assigned to stage II, an uncommon stage in appropriately evaluated patients. This is a major inconsistency in a patient population that purports to serve as the basis for determining prognostic features that can identify low-risk, intermediate-risk, and high-risk patient subsets.

Despite the questionable nature of the surgical staging, the Princess Margaret Hospital experience makes a strong case for a role for abdominopelvic radiation in the management of patients with limited disease at significant risk for recurrence. The comparisons with pelvic radiation with or without chlorambucil do not permit conclusions as to the relative merits of abdominopelvic radiation versus chemotherapy, because the chemotherapy used consisted of suboptimal doses of a single alkylating agent.

Supporting these observations are a number of uncontrolled reports in the literature.[185,186] These experiences confirm that patients with gross disease, particularly those with nodules greater than 2 cm in diameter, do not benefit significantly from radiation.

In contrast to these experiences is one earlier M.D. Anderson Hospital trial of 149 patients with stage I, II, or minimal residual stage III disease randomized to either abdominopelvic radiation by the moving-strip technique or oral melphalan. Ten-year follow-up evaluation showed no difference in survival.[187] The study has been criticized for imbalances in prognostic factors favoring the chemotherapy regimen and for problems with the radiation technique used.

Based on present evidence, abdominopelvic radiation cannot be recommended as adjuvant therapy in limited disease. Studies suggesting efficacy have critical flaws. Further study, however, is indicated on the basis of the Princess Margaret Hospital experience.

Radioactive Isotopes. The intraperitoneal administration of radioactive isotopes to treat limited-stage ovarian cancer after surgical resection has been proposed as a promising approach.[188-194] Early studies were characterized by: small numbers of patients accrued over many years, lack of control groups, and inadequate surgical staging. Despite these limitations, reported survival rates were sufficiently high to include this modality as one treatment regimen in three major randomized trials described.[179,195,196]

This approach is based on the facts that ovarian carcinoma spreads initially primarily by intraperitoneal seeding and that ^{32}P is an emitter of beta-radiation, which has a maximum tissue penetration of 3 to 4 mm, with an effective penetration of probably no more than 2 mm. Whereas ^{32}P could not be expected to be effective in patients with visible disease, it may well be an effective agent in patients with microscopic or no documentable residual disease after surgical resection. Uncontrolled trials in limited disease as well as reports of efficacy in patients who have achieved a pathologic complete response of more advanced disease with initial chemotherapy supported the possible efficacy of this approach.[186] A subsequent randomized trial (GOG Protocol 95) comparing intraperitoneal ^{32}P with cyclophosphamide/cisplatin showed a superior progression-free survival with chemotherapy and also highlighted distribution problems and bowel toxicities associated with ^{32}P. The GOG investigators concluded that chemotherapy was the preferred treatment for high-risk limited ovarian carcinoma and essentially laid to rest any role of ^{32}P.[197]

Single Alkylating Agents. Single alkylating agents, most commonly melphalan, appear to offer benefit in uncontrolled trials.[187,197] One series compared melphalan with abdominopelvic radiation and showed similar survival between the two regimens and an advantage for melphalan because of less toxicity.[187] The other study retrospectively evaluated 50 patients with limited disease accrued over a 13-year period and treated with single-agent melphalan.[197] Survival at 2 years was 98%, and at 4 years, 94%. Consistency of surgical staging techniques was not documented in the report. To draw definite conclusions about the efficacy of melphalan from these reports is impossible, but survival figures suggest that melphalan may be an effective adjuvant therapy.

Randomized Trials. Superseding the previously described uncontrolled trials are nine major randomized trials comparing modalities as adjuvant therapy in patients with limited disease: GOG Protocol 1, a National Cancer Institute of Canada Clinical Trials Group study, two critically important trials from the combined efforts of the Ovarian Cancer Study Group and the GOG, two European trials, two additional studies of the GOG, and the combined analysis of two European trials (ICON1/ACTION).

GOG Protocol 1. GOG Protocol 1, conducted during 1970 to 1976, was a phase III trial of patients with stage I ovarian carcinoma.[181] Although all patients underwent exploratory laparotomy, routine exploration of the diaphragm, lymph node sampling, peritoneal cytology, and omentectomy were not required because the importance of these procedures as a part of careful staging was not fully understood. After surgical resection of disease, patients were randomized to either no further therapy, pelvic radiation to 50 cGy, or chemotherapy consisting of melphalan (0.2 mg/kg/d PO) for 5 days every 4 weeks. Of the 168 patients entered into the study, only 86 were both eligible and evaluable, a major problem.

An analysis of prognostic factors showed an even distribution of prognostic factors, except that the control arm contained a greater percentage of favorable histology and stage IA. Among 29 patients randomized to no further therapy, five (17%) recurrences were found; among 23 given pelvic radiation, seven (30%) had a recurrence; and among 34 receiving melphalan, only two (6%) had recurrence. The difference between melphalan and pelvic radiation was significant ($P < .05$).

This trial suggests that patients with limited disease benefit from the use of adjuvant melphalan, but flaws in study execution and the relatively small number of evaluable patients prevent definitive conclusions. The results do indict pelvic radiation as an inadequate approach. The analysis of prognostic factors also points to the importance of grade, histologic type, and extracystic tumor in determining patient outcome.

National Cancer Institute of Canada Clinical Trials Group Study. This investigation of patients with stage I or IIA high risk (defined by rupture of a malignant ovarian cyst, poorly differentiated disease, extracystic excrescences of tumor, or positive peritoneal cytology), stage IIB, or stage III with disease confined to the pelvis[195] randomized subjects to pelvic radiation to 45 cGy plus either abdominal radiation to 22.5 cGy, radioactive chromic phosphate 15 mCi IP, or melphalan (8 mg/m^2/d PO) for 4 days every 4 weeks for 18 months. Of 257 eligible and evaluable patients, 107 were randomized to abdominopelvic radiation, 106 to pelvic radiation plus melphalan, and 44 to pelvic radiation plus IP ^{32}P. The arm including IP chromic phosphate was closed early because of an unacceptably high incidence of delayed toxicity. No differences in disease-free or overall survival or in recurrence rate were noted among the three arms. The investigators concluded that the survival results of all three arms point to the need for further improvement in adjuvant therapy.

Ovarian Cancer Study Group and GOG Studies. These studies were conducted from 1976 to 1986.[179] The first study, OCSG/GOG Protocol 7601, randomized 81 patients with stage I disease at low risk of recurrence (defined as those patients with well- or moderately well-differentiated intracystic lesions associated with no extraovarian neoplasm, no ascites, and negative peritoneal cytology after a careful and detailed exploratory laparotomy) to either no further therapy (38 patients) or melphalan

TABLE 92-19

Results of OCSG/GOG Protocol 7601*,179

	OBSERVATION	MELPHALAN
Patients	38	43
Recurrences	4	1
Deaths	4	2
Disease-free 5-yr survival	91%	98%
Overall 5-yr survival	94%	98%

*Randomized trial of patients at low risk of recurrence.

TABLE 92-20

Results of OCSG/GOG Protocol 7602*,179

	IP ^{32}P	MELPHALAN
Patients	73	68
Recurrences	14	13
Deaths	16	15
Disease-free 5-yr survival	80%	80%
Overall 5-yr survival	78%	81%

IP, intraperitoneal.
*Randomized trial of patients at high risk of recurrence.

(0.2 mg/kg/d PO) for 5 days every 4 weeks for up to 12 cycles (43 patients). At a median follow-up in excess of 6 years, only six deaths have been observed—four in the control arm and two in the melphalan arm. Five recurrences have been observed, four in the control arm and one in the melphalan arm. No significant differences in recurrence rate, disease-free survival, and survival were noted between the two arms (Table 92-19).

The second trial, OCSG/GOG Protocol 7602, involving 141 patients with stage I high-risk disease [defined as having one or more high-risk feature (i.e., poorly differentiated disease, extracystic tumor, ascites, positive peritoneal cytology, or extraovarian lesions) or stage II disease completely resected] randomized subjects to either intraperitoneal radioactive chromic phosphate, 15 mCi (73 patients), or melphalan (0.2 mg/kg/d PO) for 5 days every 4 weeks for up to 12 cycles (68 patients). At a median follow-up of more than 6 years, 34 (24%) recurrences were seen, 16 (22%) of 73 in the ^{32}P arm and 18 (26%) of 68 in the melphalan arm. Over the same period, 31 (22%) deaths occurred, 16 (22%) of 73 in the ^{32}P arm and 15 (22%) of 68 in the melphalan arm. The 5-year disease-free survival for both arms is 80%. No significant differences between arms are present in regard to recurrence rate, disease-free survival, or overall survival (Table 92-20).

Italian Trial. An Italian trial,[198] reported in 1992, grouped patients with limited disease into three categories: a low-risk group including stage IA G1 and IB G1 with no extracystic involvement (93 patients); an intermediate-risk group including stage IAG2-3 and stage IBG2-3 with no extracystic involvement (91 patients); and a high-risk group including stage I patients with extracystic involvement (185 patients) (Table 92-21). Patients in the low-risk group were followed up on no active treatment after surgical resection and demonstrated a 5-year disease-free survival of 90% with five relapses and three disease-related deaths.

Patients in the intermediate-risk group were randomized to either cisplatin, 50 mg/m^2 every 4 weeks for six cycles, or no further treatment after surgical resection. The 5-year disease-free survival in the cisplatin arm was 76%, whereas it was 58% in the control arm. Eighteen relapses and nine disease-related deaths were observed. The difference in disease-free survival was significant ($P < .05$), in favor of the cisplatin arm.

Patients in the high-risk group were randomized to either cisplatin (50 mg/m^2) every 4 weeks for six cycles or chromic phosphate (15 mCi IP). The 5-year disease-free survival in the cisplatin arm was 84% versus 61% in the ^{32}P arm, a difference that was statistically significant ($P < .01$) in favor of the cisplatin arm. Forty relapses and 25 disease-specific deaths were observed.

Norwegian Study. A Norwegian study[199] reported in 1992 randomized 265 patients with stage I limited disease to either cisplatin or intraperitoneal ^{32}P, as in the Italian trial. The trial is difficult to interpret on the basis of the only report to date because of the inclusion of patients with borderline lesions (low malignant potential) and because of a failure to separate patients into low-risk and high-risk groups.

GOG Protocol 95. The GOG randomized 205 patients with high-risk limited disease after complete surgical resection to adjuvant therapy consisting of either intraperitoneal ^{32}P or three cycles of cyclophosphamide, 1000 mg/m^2, plus cisplatin, 100 mg/m^2.[200] The percentage recurrence free at 5 years was 77% on the chemotherapy regimen versus 66% with ^{32}P. The estimated relative risk is 0.693, favoring

TABLE 92-21

Results of a Randomized Trial Involving 369 Patients with Stage I Ovarian Carcinoma

TREATMENT	RELAPSES	DEATHS	5-YR DFS (%)
Group A: IAiG1 and IBiG1 (n = 93)	5	3	
No further therapy			90
Group B: IAiG2-3 and IBiG2-3 (n = 91)	18	9	
No further therapy			58
Cisplatin			76
Group C: IAii, IBii, and IC (n = 185)	40	25	
^{32}P			61
Cisplatin			84

DFS, disease-free survival; i, no extracystic tumor; ii, extracystic tumor.
In group B, DFS is significantly different ($P < .05$) in favor of cisplatin. In group C, DFS is significantly different ($P < .01$) in favor of cisplatin.
Data from Bolis et al.[198]

Specific Malignancies

III

TABLE 92-22

Results of GOG Protocol 95*

	IP ^{32}P	CP†	RR
Patients	98	107	
Recurrence free at 5 yr	66%	77%	0.693†
Alive at 5 yr	76%	84%	

IP, intraperitoneal; RR, relative risk.
*Randomized trial of patients at high risk of recurrence.[200]
†Cyclophosphamide, 1000 mg/m^2, plus cisplatin, 100 mg/m^2. Repeat every 3 wk times 3.
‡P = .075.

TABLE 92-23

Results of ICON1/ACTION*,[201]

	OBSERVATION	CHEMOTHERAPY	RR
Patients	460	465	
Recurrence free at 5 yr	65%	76%	0.64†
Alive at 5 yr	74%	82%	0.67‡

RR, relative risk.
*Randomized trial of patients at high risk of recurrence.
†P = .001.
‡P = .008.

the chemotherapy regimen (P = .075). Survival at 5 years was 84% for the chemotherapy and 76% for the ^{32}P group. Patients receiving the intraperitoneal ^{32}P experienced problems with distribution of the compound in the abdominal cavity and also with bowel toxicities. The GOG concluded from these data that chemotherapy represented the preferred treatment (Table 92-22).

ICON1/ACTION. The combined efforts of the ICON and the EORTC produced a combined analysis of two randomized studies of adjuvant chemotherapy in patients with limited disease.[201] Both groups required that patients have stage I to IIA disease and that patients be randomized after surgical resection to either no further therapy or adjuvant chemotherapy containing a platinum compound. Of 925 patients were randomized to the two studies, at a median follow-up of 4 years, 245 patients had either died or disease had recurred. Recurrence-free survival at 5 years was 76% in the chemotherapy arm and 65% in the observation arm [relative risk (RR) = 0.64; P = .001]. Overall survival at 5 years was 82% in the chemotherapy arm and 74% in the observation arm (RR = 0.67; P = .008). This study marks the first report of an improved overall survival with chemotherapy and establishes chemotherapy as the standard of care after surgery in patients with high-risk limited disease (Table 92-23).

GOG Protocol 157. The GOG randomized 457 patients with high-risk limited ovarian carcinoma after complete surgical resection to paclitaxel, 175 mg/m^2/3 hr, plus carboplatin, AUC 7.5, every 3 weeks for either three or six cycles.[202] The basis for this trial included the prior studies that showed an advantage for chemotherapy in high-risk limited disease[200,201] and the randomized trials that established paclitaxel/carboplatin as the standard of care for advanced disease.[139,140,146,147] The chemotherapy regimen adopted was that used in GOG Protocol 158.[147] A large proportion of the patients failed to meet the surgical requirements of the trial (107 of 457 or 23%), so the study was analyzed both with and without these patients. Both analyses showed a reduction in recurrence rate that did not reach statistical significance (RR, 0.69 without the surgical exclusions and 0.77 with the exclusions, neither statistically significant). Both also showed no significant difference in survival at 5 years (73 to 24) (Table 92-24).

Conclusions. The results of the nine randomized trials provide guidelines for the management of patients with limited disease. First, the trials demonstrate the importance of careful surgical staging to establish patient risk of recurrence. Second, patients at low risk of recurrence have a 5-year survival exceeding 90% with or without adjuvant therapy. Additional treatment after surgical resection does not appear to be indicated. Third, patients at high risk of recurrence appear to benefit from adjuvant therapy. The weight of evidence supports the use of cisplatin-based chemotherapy as the adjuvant therapy of choice. Although definitive statements about regimen and duration are difficult, it would seem reasonable to use paclitaxel/carboplatin, as in GOG Protocol 157, for at least three cycles of therapy.

Management of Recurrent, Persistent, or Progressive Disease

Although debate continues about the optimal choice of drugs, dose schedule, and route of administration, platinum-based combination chemotherapy yields the following results in patients with advanced disease:[139,140,146,147] overall response rate of 95%, clinical complete response rate of 75%, pathologic complete response rate of 40% to 50%, a 10-year survival rate of 15% to 40%, and a recurrence rate after clinical complete response of 75% and after pathologic complete response of 40% to 60%. Patients who initiate front-line therapy with small-volume residual disease will fare better than those who start chemotherapy with large-volume residual disease. The fact remains, however, that a majority (60% to 75%) of patients with ovarian carcinoma will require

TABLE 92-24

Results of GOG Protocol 157*,[202]

	TP × 3*	TP × 6†	RR
Patients	213	216	
Recurrence free at 5 yr	75%	81%	0.77‡
Alive at 5 yr	79%	84%	

*Randomized trial of patients at high risk of recurrence.
†Paclitaxel, 175 mg/m^2/3hr plus carboplatin, AUC 7.5. Repeat every 3 wk.
‡P = .109.

THERAPEUTIC CHOICES IN RECURRENT, PERSISTENT, OR PROGRESSIVE CELOMIC EPITHELIAL CARCINOMA

Choices of therapy for progressive, persistent, or recurrent celomic epithelial carcinoma of the ovary hinges on the patient's response to front-line therapy. Those patients who respond to initial chemotherapy, who become disease free, and who experience a treatment-free interval of 6 months or longer are highly likely, at recurrence, to be responsive to platinum-based salvage therapy. These platinum-sensitive patients should be retreated with a platinum-based combination regimen. The currently preferred regimen is carboplatin (AUC, 6 to 7.5 IV) after paclitaxel (175 mg/m²/3 hr IV) every 3 weeks. Those who fail to respond should be deemed platinum resistant and treated accordingly. Those who respond and become disease free with a treatment-free interval of at least 6 months should once again receive platinum-based therapy.

Those patients whose disease progresses while receiving initial therapy, who have persistent disease at the conclusion of initial treatment, or whose tumor recurs within 6 months of initial therapy should be regarded as platinum resistant. These patients should be treated with regimens that induce responses in platinum-resistant disease. Repeated platinum-based therapy is not indicated. Single agents that achieve responses in resistant patients include weekly paclitaxel, docetaxel, pegylated liposomal doxorubicin, oral etoposide, topotecan, tamoxifen, gemcitabine, navelbine, and ifosfamide. No evidence supports the use of combinations in resistant patients. Therapy should be continued until disease progression or achievement of complete response.

Approaches that should be reserved for clinical trials only include high-dose therapy with autologous bone marrow transplantation (ABMT) or peripheral stem-cell support, intraperitoneal therapy, and biologic agents.

further therapy for recurrent, persistent, or progressive disease. The factors that affect the choice of that therapy and the specific options available are now considered.

Recurrent Disease Population. Long-term follow-up evaluation of 726 women treated for ovarian carcinoma on GOG protocols[203,204] identified a number of characteristics associated with increased likelihood of recurrence: clear cell or mucinous histology, non–platinum-based treatment, poor performance status, older age, higher stage, clinically measurable disease, larger residual tumor volume, and ascites. In addition, an analysis of those factors that predict recurrence after pathologic complete response[205] shows that histologic grade is an important determinant of relapse rate, with grade 1, 22%; grade 2, 39%; and grade 3, 56%.

None of these factors provides guidance in the selection of appropriate subsequent therapy. An additional factor that does appear, however, to provide a basis for choosing salvage therapy is the result of immediately preceding therapy. Patients who respond to previous platinum-based therapy and who demonstrate a signi-

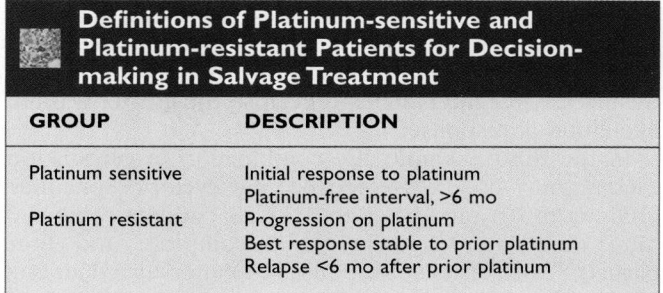

TABLE 92-25

Definitions of Platinum-sensitive and Platinum-resistant Patients for Decision-making in Salvage Treatment	
GROUP	**DESCRIPTION**
Platinum sensitive	Initial response to platinum Platinum-free interval, >6 mo
Platinum resistant	Progression on platinum Best response stable to prior platinum Relapse <6 mo after prior platinum

ficant treatment-free interval have a high probability of responding again to platinum-based treatment.[206-211] Patients who progressed during or shortly after completion of platinum-based therapy are unlikely to respond to further treatment with a platinum compound and should be considered for therapy with non–cross-resistant agents.[65-115] Discussion of salvage therapy is based on this division of patients into "sensitive" and "resistant" populations based on responsiveness to initial platinum-based treatment (Table 92-25).

Management of Platinum-Sensitive Patients

Importance of Treatment-Free Interval. Until recently, most studies of patients who have recurrent, persistent, or progressive disease after initial chemotherapy focused on the identification of the activity of new drugs or approaches as a basis for the subsequent testing of these active regimens in phase III studies of front-line therapy. As a result, determination of optimal therapy for this setting was extrapolated from data collected for other purposes. These efforts have led to the conclusion that the most important determinant of the likelihood of a response in the setting of progressive, persistent, or recurrent disease is the treatment-free interval.

Succinctly stated, the duration of the interval from the conclusion of preceding therapy to the need for further therapy influences the likelihood of the patient's responding to the chosen further therapy. The longer the interval, the greater the likelihood of a response.[210] To illustrate this principle, four among many studies are examined.

In the first example, IV cisplatin-based therapy as salvage treatment was evaluated retrospectively in 72 patients with measurable disease who had received at least two cisplatin- or carboplatin-based regimens and had demonstrated a platinum-free interval of at least 4 months between the completion of the first regimen and initiation of the second.[210] The overall response rate was 43% (31 of 72 with 10 pathologic complete responses). Response rate increased as the platinum-free interval increased. In those with an interval of 5 to 12 months, the response rate was 27% (5% pathologic complete responses); 13 to 24 months, 33% (11% pathologic complete responses); and more than 24 months, 59% (pathologic complete responses, 22%).

In the second example, a salvage regimen of weekly cisplatin combined with either epirubicin or etoposide[211] yielded a 60% response rate (25% complete response) with a median duration of response of 7 months and a median survival of 13.5 months in 40 patients who had responded to initial platinum-based therapy. The longer the disease-free interval before relapse, the greater was the likelihood of response.

In the third example, the combination of carboplatin (300 mg/m^2) on day 8 preceded by cyclophosphamide (100 mg/m^2/d) on days 1 to 7 in 28 patients produced nine objective responses (five complete and four partial).[208] Six of these responses (46%) occurred among 13 patients who were initial responders and hence platinum sensitive. Only three responses (20%) were observed among the 15 platinum-resistant patients. The relatively high response rate among the platinum-resistant group may be accounted for by the response definitions, because the platinum-resistant group included patients with platinum-free intervals of up to 12 months' duration.

The fourth example evaluated the platinum analogue iproplatin at an initial dose of 270 mg/m^2 in patients with recurrent disease after prior cisplatin or carboplatin treatment.[209] Among 78 resistant patients, nine responses (three complete and six partial, 12%) were observed. Among the 19 sensitive patients, five responses (two complete and three partial, 26%) were observed.

These four examples demonstrate that patients who respond to platinum-based therapy initially and relapse after a significant platinum-free interval have a high likelihood of responding again to IV platinum-based treatment. The correct definition of a significant platinum-free interval is unclear, although the data suggest that the longer the interval, the more likely the response. Most studies use the interval of 6 months as the point that defines platinum sensitivity.

Choice of Regimen. The principle of the treatment-free interval appears to apply regardless of the drug or regimen chosen.[90] Virtually all active drugs tested to date appear to fare better in the platinum-sensitive group than in the platinum-resistant group. The frequency of response, however, does appear to depend on the drug chosen. For any given point along the plot of treatment-free interval, the frequency of response to platinum-based therapy is 1.5 to 2.0 times greater than that reported with nonplatinum agents or regimens.[85,86,90,208-211] In addition, the duration of response and survival is better with platinum-based regimens than with alternative, non–platinum-containing regimens.[212]

Debate has focused on whether a platinum compound as a single agent offered a less-toxic and equally efficacious alternative to combination chemotherapy in the setting of platinum-sensitive disease. A phase III trial has directly addressed this question. ICON4 randomized patients with platinum-sensitive disease, defined as a treatment-free interval from prior therapy of at least 6 months, to a platinum-containing regimen with or without a taxane.[213] The vast majority of patients received either single-agent carboplatin or a combination of paclitaxel/carboplatin. The analysis showed that the patients receiving the taxane/platinum regimen had a superior response rate

TABLE 92-26

	Results of ICON4/OVAR 2.2[*,113]		
	PLATINUM	**TAXANE/ PLATINUM**	**RR**
Patients	410	392	
Response	54%	66%	
Progression free at 1 yr	40%	50%	0.76[†]
Alive at 2 yr	50%	57%	0.82[‡]

RR, relative risk.
*Randomized trial of patients with platinum-sensitive recurrent disease
[†]$P < .001$.
[‡]$P = .023$.

(66% vs. 54%; $P = .06$), a superior progression-free survival (50% progression-free vs. 40% at 1 year, HR = 0.76; $P < .001$), and a superior overall survival (57% alive vs. 50% at 2 years, HR = 0.82; $P = .023$) (Table 92-26). This is the first study in the second-line setting to show a survival advantage for combination chemotherapy over a single agent and establishes a taxane/platinum combination as the preferred treatment for patients with platinum-sensitive disease (a confirmatory trial will be required to make this the standard of care).

Dose-Intense Second-Line Chemotherapy. Studies of dose-intense approaches to salvage chemotherapy for ovarian carcinoma[163,214-216] purport to show an advantage for such approaches based on the observation of responses in the recurrent-disease situation. The problem with the interpretation of many of these reports is the lack of information on prior response to platinum-based treatment. Without such data, one cannot determine whether the observed responses occurred only in platinum-sensitive patients at a rate expected with standard IV platinum therapy or whether platinum-resistant patients are responding to the higher-dose schedules.

Two reports[206,207] do provide this critical information. The first of these is a study of high-dose carboplatin (800 mg/m^2 IV) every 5 weeks in 30 patients previously treated with cisplatin.[206] Eight objective responses (27%) were observed, none in patients with progressive disease during platinum-based therapy.

The second report examined retrospectively two phase II trials of salvage cisplatin-based intraperitoneal therapy.[207] Among 89 patients, 52 were considered platinum sensitive, and 37 platinum resistant. Among the sensitive patients, 29 (56%) developed an objective response; 17 were pathologic complete responses. Among the resistant patients, only four responded (11%), all partial.

These two reports suggest that the increase in dose intensity achievable by dose escalation or intraperitoneal administration of drug cannot overcome true clinical resistance. Although this does not rule out the ability of an even greater dose intensity to overcome resistance, the fact that intraperitoneal drug administration with a fairly significant enhancement of drug exposure to cells did not yield a significant response rate in resistant patients certainly argues against the likelihood that other dose-intense programs will succeed. Conversely, the activity of these approaches in sensitive patients is on the same order as that reported with standard intravenous doses of platinum-based regimens.[162] Little evidence so far support the routine clinical use of such dose-intense approaches in the salvage setting.

Conclusions. Evidence supports the use of platinum-based therapy to treat patients with recurrent disease who responded to prior platinum-based therapy and experienced at least a 6-month treatment-free interval before recurrence. In such a setting, platinum-based therapy is far more likely to produce a response than any other alternative. Furthermore, recent evidence supports the use of a taxane/platinum-based combination regimen. The goal of therapy in this setting should be both improvement in survival and palliation. Dose-intense approaches do not appear to offer any advantage over standard intravenous doses.

Management of Platinum-Resistant Patients. Successful management of platinum-resistant patients (<6-month treatment-free interval after a preceding platinum-based regimen) depends on the identification of agents that are non–cross-resistant with the platinum compounds. Until 1989, essentially no such agents had been identified. Now a number of agents have been shown to produce objective responses in patients who have failed to respond to platinum-based initial therapy. Among these are: paclitaxel,[56,65-68] docetaxel,[69-73] pegylated liposomal doxorubicin,[88-93] oral etoposide,[94-98] topotecan,[82-86] tamoxifen,[111-113] gemcitabine,[99-101] vinorelbine,[102-106] and ifosfamide.[56-59] Although each of these agents appears to be more active in platinum-sensitive patients, major interest has been generated primarily by their activity in resistant patients.

In platinum-resistant patients, paclitaxel achieves responses in 24% to 30% of patients in phase II trials.[65-68] This agent is clearly the treatment of choice in patients whose disease has failed to achieve an objective response to initial platinum-based regimens. Because paclitaxel is now a part of standard front-line therapy, current focus is on those agents with activity in patients who have disease resistant to both the platinum compounds and paclitaxel. Six agents have demonstrated such activity: docetaxel, weekly paclitaxel, pegylated liposomal doxorubicin, topotecan, oral etoposide, and gemcitabine.

To date, no evidence suggests an advantage for combination chemotherapy over single-agent therapy in the platinum-resistant setting; hence platinum-resistant patients should be treated with single-agent therapy consisting of one of the six agents with demonstrated activity against resistant disease. The goal in this setting is palliative because no evidence indicates that therapy in this setting prolongs survival.

Other potential options for treatment of resistant ovarian carcinoma include more dose-intense therapy, biologic agents, and hormones. The lack of evidence supporting the value of more dose-intense approaches has been described. Insufficient data are available to establish the value of biologic agents in resistant disease.

Conclusions Regarding Salvage Therapy. The current management of patients with ovarian carcinoma who have recurred after initial platinum-based chemotherapy rests on consideration of the results of the initial chemotherapy. Patients who respond to the initial platinum-based therapy and relapse after a platinum-free interval should be considered clinically sensitive to further platinum-based treatment. Recent evidence suggests that combination chemotherapy with a taxane/platinum combination produces a superior response rate and progression-free and overall survival. Such therapy will yield response rates as high as 60% with up to 25% of patients achieving a complete response and also median survivals that exceed 2 years. No evidence indicates that more dose-intense approaches yield better results in these patients than results with standard intravenous schedules.

Patients who fail to respond to initial platinum-based therapy or who relapse shortly after completion of initial therapy should be regarded as clinically resistant to further platinum-based treatment. These patients should be treated with drugs that have been shown to have activity against resistant disease: weekly paclitaxel, docetaxel, pegylated liposomal doxorubicin, oral etoposide, topotecan, tamoxifen, gemcitabine, navelbine, and ifosfamide. No evidence exists that combinations of these drugs are more effective than single-agent therapy.

Controversial Issues. Two specific situations in the management of patients with recurrent, persistent, or progressive disease deserve further comment: patients with a rising CA-125 as the only evidence of recurrence or progression and potential candidates for secondary surgical cytoreduction.

Patients with Increasing CA-125 Only. With the advent of the widespread use of CA-125 to monitor patients with ovarian carcinoma, an increasingly common situation to confront the physician is that of the patient who develops an increasing CA-125 but is otherwise free of any evidence, objective or otherwise, of recurrence and is asymptomatic. Because of the high level of awareness of CA-125, patients naturally obsess about their CA-125 values and often demand that the physician intervene with therapy in such a situation. Unanswered as yet is the question as to what is the best choice for these patients: treatment or observation until the development of other objective evidence of disease or of symptoms.

Until recently, all treatment in the second-line setting was regarded as purely palliative. In such circumstances, the rationale for waiting until the patient developed either symptoms or other objective evidence of recurrence, which was almost always followed shortly thereafter by symptoms, was obvious. Except for those patients who demanded treatment, the general recommendation was that treatment should await the onset of symptoms or the appearance of other objective evidence of disease.

With the report of the results of ICON4/OVAR 2.2[213] and the demonstration that survival could be improved by treatment in the platinum-sensitive setting, the question of immediate treatment should be revisited. As of this writing, no such study is under way; hence treatment decisions must be made in the absence of definitive evidence. The best recommendation is to discuss the issue with the patient. In the absence of a preference on the patient's part, a policy of watchful waiting until the development of symptoms would seem to be most prudent.

Potential Candidates for Secondary Surgical Cytoreduction. Secondary surgical cytoreduction is debulking performed in the patient with recurrent, persistent, or progressive disease before the use of second-line chemotherapy.[217] Mixed results have been reported with secondary debulking.[218,219] Benefit appears to depend on careful selection of candidates for the procedure. Patients whose disease can be surgically cytoreduced to the point that no gross disease remains appear to be the patients who benefit from the procedure.[220] The procedure should therefore probably be reserved for those patients in whom the surgeon feels that complete resection of all gross disease can be achieved. To some extent, the benefit observed also depends on the availability of chemotherapy that will follow the procedure and to which the patient is likely to be sensitive.

Special Situations

The natural history and spread patterns of celomic epithelial carcinomas of the ovary create at least two special circumstances with which the clinician must deal: intestinal obstruction and malignant effusions.

Intestinal Obstruction. Up to one half of patients with ovarian carcinoma develop symptoms of gastrointestinal (GI) obstruction (nausea, vomiting, abdominal pain, and obstipation), most commonly related to progressive cancer rather than adhesions.[221,222] Small bowel and, to a lesser extent, colonic and gastric outlet obstruction can occur. Nonoperative management with intravenous hydration, intestinal intubation, and parenteral hyperalimentation is acceptable initial management, but only 10% to 30% of cases of true obstruction will be relieved by such an approach, with the majority of those so relieved developing recurrent obstruction within 1 month.[223,224]

Surgical management of intestinal obstruction is the remaining option if no relief is obtained with noninvasive measures. If they are used indiscriminately, median survival after such an approach is uniformly less than 8 months and not dramatically different from that seen in patients managed without surgery. The selection of those patients to be considered for surgery will depend on several features: performance status, contraindications to general anesthesia, and availability of effective postoperative chemotherapy. Particularly in those patients who are still potentially sensitive to chemotherapy, surgical relief of the obstruction is warranted.[225]

Malignant Effusions. Although malignant effusions associated with ovarian carcinoma can involve any one of three cavities (peritoneal, pleural, or pericardial), only the first two are sufficiently common to warrant detailed consideration. With regard to the first of these, ascites is by far the most common of the effusions. At initial diagnosis, ascites is frequent but seldom severe enough to require specific intervention and usually responds to systemic chemotherapy with resolution after one to two cycles of treatment.[226] For cases resistant to systemic chemotherapy and productive of significant problems, paracentesis provides symptomatic relief. Intraperitoneal bleomycin[227,228] and peritoneovenous shunts[229,230] have been used in particularly troublesome cases, but success is temporary and most often related to concomitant chemotherapy the patient received.

Pleural effusions occur in 25% to 30% of patients and are cytologically positive for malignant cells in 75% of cases.[231] When symptomatic, these effusions should be approached with thoracentesis. For patients receiving first-line chemotherapy, the pleural effusion usually responds and does not become a recurring problem; whereas patients with recurrent disease and associated pleural effusion, particularly those with platinum-resistant disease, can experience major problems with rapid reaccumulation of fluid after thoracentesis. In such cases, drainage of the fluid with a thoracostomy tube can provide complete resolution of the problem in 36% to 55% of patients.[232,233] Instillation of sclerosing agents such as tetracycline, talc, or bleomycin can significantly improve the rate at which complete resolution is observed.[234] Those with persistent problems after all these measures can be considered for pleurectomy or thoracoscopic pleurodesis.[235,236]

Germ Cell Cancers

Approximately 5% of ovarian cancer consists of germ cell carcinomas, which are classified into two broad groups: dysgerminomas and nondysgerminomas[237] (Table 92-27). The same staging system as that used for celomic epithelial carcinomas is used for these tumors. Management begins with exploratory laparotomy to determine extent of disease and to permit surgical resection, if

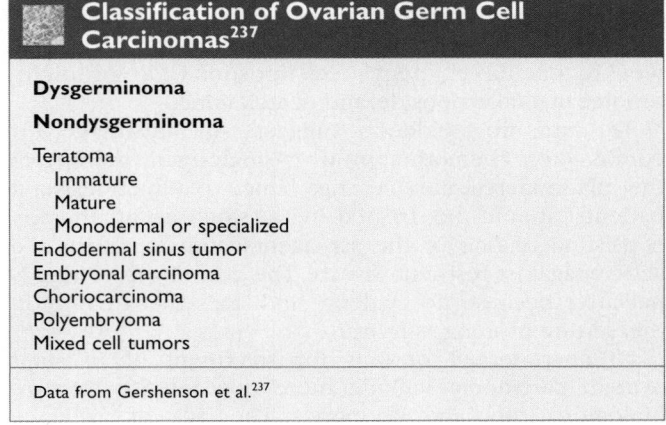

TABLE 92-27

Classification of Ovarian Germ Cell Carcinomas[237]

Dysgerminoma

Nondysgerminoma

Teratoma
  Immature
  Mature
  Monodermal or specialized
Endodermal sinus tumor
Embryonal carcinoma
Choriocarcinoma
Polyembryoma
Mixed cell tumors

Data from Gershenson et al.[237]

possible. Subsequent treatment depends on histology and findings at laparotomy that place patients into one of two groups: those with stage I to III disease completely resected and those with incompletely resected stage III and IV disease. Therapeutic decisions, however, are based on comparisons with historic controls, because these lesions are sufficiently uncommon that randomized trials are not feasible.

Tumor Markers

Ovarian germ cell tumors produce markers in most cases. α-Fetoprotein elevations have been noted in patients with endodermal sinus tumors, immature teratomas, mixed germ cell tumors, embryonal carcinomas, and polyembryomas. Elevations of human chorionic gonadotropin have been observed with choriocarcinomas, embryonal carcinomas, polyembryomas, mixed cell tumors, and less commonly, dysgerminomas. These markers are useful in assessing response to chemotherapy and in monitoring patients in complete remission for evidence of recurrence.

Stage I to III Completely Resected

In patients with completely resected stage I, II, or III endodermal sinus tumors, mixed cell tumors, embryonal carcinomas, choriocarcinomas, and immature teratoma, the recurrence rate is sufficiently high to warrant adjuvant therapy. The largest experience with adjuvant chemotherapy is that of the GOG in studies evaluating adjuvant VAC (vincristine, actinomycin D, and cyclophosphamide) and adjuvant BEP (bleomycin, etoposide, and cisplatin).[238-240]

The relative value of these regimens is best established by comparison with historic data on no adjuvant therapy (Table 92-28), which shows a steady increase in the percentage of patients remaining disease free at 16 months of follow-up, as treatment progresses from no adjuvant through VAC to BEP. On the basis of these data, adjuvant BEP is the treatment of choice for patients with completely resected stage I to III disease and specific histologies: immature teratoma grade 2 and 3, endodermal

TABLE 92-28

GOG Trials of Adjuvant Chemotherapy for Ovarian Germ Cell Carcinoma

THERAPY	EST AND MCT	IMMATURE TERATOMA
No adjuvant	34/165 (21%)[‡]	36/56 (64%)
VAC*	53/82 (65%)	59/70 (84%)
BEP[†]	30/31 (97%)	18/19 (95%)

EST, endodermal sinus tumor; MCT, mixed cell tumor.
*VAC, vincristine (1.5 mg/m² IV, max 2 mg), q2wk, × 12, actinomycin D (350 μg/m²/d IV) × 5 days q4wk × 6, and cyclophosphamide (150 mg/m²/d IV) × 5 days q4wk × 6.
[†]BEP, bleomycin (20 U/m² IV, max 30 units) per week × 9, etoposide (100 mg/m²/d IV, × 5 q3wk × 3, and cisplatin, (20 mg/m²/d IV, × 5 q3wk × 3.
[‡]Percentage of patients remaining disease free at a median follow-up of 16 months after completion of therapy.
Data from Slayton et al.[238] and Williams et al.[239]

sinus tumor, mixed cell tumor, embryonal carcinoma, and choriocarcinoma. For other histologic types, data are insufficient to permit definitive conclusions.

Stage III Incompletely Resected and Stage IV Disease

At least two chemotherapy regimens are active in patients with advanced or recurrent disease: VAC and PVB (cisplatin, vinblastine, and bleomycin)[240] (Table 92-29). The cisplatin-based combination yields higher response rates and a greater percentage of patients who remain disease free for extended periods. The current study of the GOG evaluates a combination of bleomycin, etoposide, and cisplatin.

Rare Malignant Ovarian Tumors

Accounting for less than 5% of all malignant ovarian tumors are a variety of rare ovarian neoplasms, including granulosa cell tumors, thecoma-fibroma tumors, Sertoli-Leydig cell tumors, gynandroblastomas, and steroid cell tumors. Such lesions are best treated with surgical resection if only limited disease is present. Appropriate management of more-advanced disease is unclear.

THERAPEUTIC DECISION IN NEWLY DIAGNOSED GERM CELL CARCINOMAS

Patients with germ cell carcinomas should be divided into two groups: those with stage I to III disease that has been completely resected and those with incompletely resected stage III and IV disease. After complete resection, patients with endodermal sinus tumor, mixed cell tumor, embryonal carcinoma, choriocarcinoma, or immature teratomas, grade 2 or 3, should receive adjuvant therapy consisting of VP-16 (100 mg/m²/d IV) plus cisplatin (20 mg/m²/d IV) for 5 days every 3 weeks for three cycles, and bleomycin (30 units IV) weekly for the 9 weeks of the three cycles. Second-look laparotomy at the conclusion of therapy is unnecessary if all clinical evidence of disease has disappeared and if both α-fetoprotein and human chorionic gonadotropin levels are normal.

Patients with incompletely resected stage III and IV disease, regardless of histologic type, should be treated with four cycles of the combination described earlier. Those with complete remission, including normalization of α-fetoprotein and human chorionic gonadotropin, can be followed with no further treatment. Those with persistent disease will require further therapy with other active agents, but the precise nature of this therapy has not been defined. Other active drugs include actinomycin D, ifosfamide, and other alkylating agents, anthracyclines, methotrexate, and the vinca alkaloids.

Because most tumors produce either α-fetoprotein or human chorionic gonadotropin, or both, therapy should be monitored with the appropriate markers. Subsequent follow-up management of complete responders also should include the marker(s) that were positive.

TABLE 92-29

GOG Trials of Two Three-Drug Combinations in Incompletely Resected Stage III and IV Germ Cell Carcinomas of the Ovary[240]

HISTOLOGY AND THERAPY	CR	PR	DISEASE FREE
Immature teratoma			
VAC*	—	—	4/8 (50%)
PVB†	2/9 (22%)	2/9 (22%)	12/24 (50%)
Endodermal sinus tumor and mixed cell tumor			
VAC	—	—	3/14 (21%)
PVB	13/24 (54%)	8/24 (33%)	31/58 (53%)
Dysgerminoma			
PVB	3/4 (75%)	1/4 (25%)	7/8 (88%)
Choriocarcinoma			
PVB	2/3 (67%)	1/3 (33%)	2/3 (67%)

CR, complete response; PR, partial response.
*VAC, vincristine (1.5 mg/m^2 IV, max 2 mg), q2wk × 12, actinomycin D (350 µg/m^2/d IV), × 5 days q4wk × 6, and cyclophosphamide (150 mg/m^2/d IV), × 5 days q4wk × 6.
†PVB, vinblastine (12 mg/m^2 IV) q3wk × 4, bleomycin (20 U/m^2 IV, max 30 units) per week, and 12 cisplatin (20 mg/m^2/d IV), × 5 q3wk × 3–4.
Data from Williams et al.[240]

Although both radiation therapy and chemotherapy have been used in the management of advanced disease and as adjuvant therapy for limited disease, evidence is largely anecdotal. It is thus not possible to make definitive recommendations for the management of more advanced cases.

CANCER OF THE FALLOPIAN TUBE

The fallopian tube is the least common site of origin in the female genital tract for cancer. The most common histologic type of cancer, accounting for 90% of all malignancies of the tube, is papillary serous adenocarcinoma, but even this type is rare, with only 300 cases reported annually in the United States. The pattern of spread is similar to that seen with celomic epithelial lesions of the ovary, with dissemination throughout the peritoneal cavity perhaps the most important route of spread; hence it is often difficult to distinguish between ovarian and fallopian tube primary tumors. Criteria have been set for lesions designated to be of fallopian tube origin[241,242]: the main tumor arises from the endosalpinx and is in the tube, the histologic pattern shows a papillary pattern, a transition zone between benign and malignant epithelium must be demonstrable if the wall is involved, and the ovaries and endometrium must be either normal or less involved than the tube.

As a reflection of the propensity of tubal cancer to spread by intraperitoneal dissemination, 5-year survival rates correlate well with the degree to which the primary lesion penetrates the wall of the tube: 91% for intramucosal lesions, 53% for those with mucosal wall invasion, and 25% or less for lesions that penetrate the tubal serosa.[243] The actual staging system used, however, is a modification of the FIGO staging system for ovarian cancer (see Table 92-1).

In contradistinction to ovarian cancer, fallopian tube cancers tend to be first seen at an earlier stage of development, with roughly 33% as stage I, 33% as stage II, and 33% as more-advanced disease. The mainstay of therapy for patients with limited disease is surgical resection. Whether postoperative radiation therapy is of value as an adjuvant treatment in patients whose tumors have been completely resected is unclear in the absence of a randomized trial. If radiation therapy does have a role, it would seem to be in patients who have no gross disease. Studies of chemotherapy in fallopian tube carcinoma are anecdotal. Agents noted to produce responses are the same noted to be active in celomic epithelial carcinoma of the ovary. It would seem reasonable to base the choice of systemic therapy in advanced or recurrent disease on extrapolation from data in ovarian carcinoma.

THERAPEUTIC DECISIONS IN FALLOPIAN TUBE CARCINOMAS

Firm recommendations on the management of fallopian tube carcinomas are difficult because of the lack of extensive clinical studies. With the best evidence available, four basic groups of patients are found.

INTRAMUCOSAL LESIONS ONLY
For patients with intramucosal lesions only, cure is excellent with surgical resection. Patients should undergo total abdominal hysterectomy and bilateral salpingo-oophorectomy and be monitored closely with no further therapy.

MUCOSAL WALL INVASION
For patients with mucosal wall invasion, the recurrence rate is approximately 50%. These patients are candidates for adjuvant therapy, but no data support the use of such treatment. If adjuvant therapy is to be used, choices similar to those for high-risk ovarian carcinoma seem reasonable. If radiation therapy is to be used, it would seem appropriate to treat the entire abdominal cavity. A preferable approach would be the use of platinum-based chemotherapy, on the assumption that this disease responds similar to celomic epithelial carcinoma.

PENETRATION OF THE SEROSA
For patients with penetration of the serosa but no gross spread, recurrence rate exceeds 75%. An even stronger case for the use of adjuvant therapy can be made. The choices are similar to those noted earlier.

For patients with obvious spread of disease to locoregional and distant sites, platinum-based chemotherapy is a reasonable choice. The overall strategy should be similar to that used for patients with advanced or recurrent celomic epithelial carcinoma of the ovary.

FUTURE DIRECTIONS

The development of additional information about the nature and management of germ cell cancers and rarer malignant tumors of the ovary as well as fallopian tube cancer will continue to be restricted by the low frequency of these lesions. With regard to celomic epithelial carcinomas of the ovary, however, progress should continue to be rapid. Current and future investigational efforts focus on several distinct areas: biology of ovarian carcinoma, screening and early detection, the proper role of surgery, new agents and their role in systemic therapy, and the role of dose-intense approaches.

First, with regard to the biology of ovarian carcinoma, specific studies are seeking (1) to characterize factors associated with ovarian carcinoma and its outcome such as specific genetic defects associated with hereditary ovarian carcinoma, various oncogenes, and DNA ploidy; (2) to identify features predictive of the likelihood of developing ovarian carcinoma; and (3) to ascertain the biologic reasons for the observation that more-aggressive disease is associated with older patients. As these and other investigations expand the understanding of the basic nature of ovarian carcinoma, the development of better and more specific methods for early detection and treatment of the disease should be possible. Where this line of work will ultimately lead is speculative but exciting.

Second, the evolution of effective techniques for screening for and early detection of ovarian carcinoma has a high priority in ovarian carcinoma, the only one of the major gynecologic cancers for which early detection is not the rule. Most interest centers on the potential for transvaginal sonography, especially when enhanced by color-flow Doppler, to permit earlier detection of disease. The recent report of potential value for proteomic patterns in the serum for early detection of ovarian carcinoma has focused on the biologic front as well. Confirmation of the value of such approaches must await larger trials.

Third, although the efficacy of initial surgical cytoreduction in patients with stage III disease has been accepted on the basis of retrospective analyses, prospective trials are needed to address several important questions. Two trials of interval surgical cytoreduction at the midpoint of a series of chemotherapy courses suggest a role for this procedure in patients with a less than optimal initial surgical effort. Prospective randomized trials of initial or secondary surgical cytoreduction have not been performed. Investigations of the relative merits of each of these approaches versus no surgery are needed, as well as trials evaluating which of these points in the therapy represents the optimal time to introduce surgical resection into the management of advanced disease. Such studies are difficult to conduct because of the widespread acceptance of the role of surgical cytoreduction in ovarian carcinoma.

Fourth, efforts continue to investigate the role of new agents in the management of ovarian carcinoma. Current interest continues to center on further delineation of the role of a number of promising new cytotoxic and biologic agents. The plethora of new agents with activity in patients who are clinically resistant to the platinum compounds and paclitaxel opens the possibility for the addition of clinically non–cross-resistant drugs to front-line paclitaxel/platinum therapy. Defining the role of these new agents is of paramount importance.

Finally, dose intensity continues to command significant interest. Three basic ways to enhance the dose intensity have been proffered: escalation of dose within the range that can be achieved without marrow reconstitution, high-dose chemotherapy with support of autologous bone marrow transplant or peripheral stem cell transfusion, and, in the case of ovarian carcinoma, intraperitoneal administration of drug. Eight randomized trials of dose escalation over a standard range of doses have been completed. Six show no advantage to a doubling of dose intensity, and the other two have major design problems. Further exploration of this approach seems unwarranted.

Although uncontrolled studies and anecdotal reports of high-dose chemotherapy with marrow reconstitution appear promising, the highly selected nature of the patients and the expense of the procedures mandate that randomized, comparative trials demonstrate the superiority of this approach over standard therapy before it can be considered a valid part of the therapeutic armamentarium.

Intraperitoneal administration of drug, although under study for more than a decade, still has no defined role in management. In the salvage setting, it appears to have no advantage over intravenous therapy. In the setting of first-line treatment, three large randomized trials in patients with small-volume disease show small advantages at the expense of markedly enhanced toxicity. The final determination of the role, if any, for intraperitoneal therapy awaits the development of less-toxic regimens. If a role for intraperitoneal therapy exists, data show that it will be in only those patients with extremely small-volume disease or perhaps no residual disease; hence its role will be a very narrow one.

In conclusion, the future holds the promise of continuing advances in the management of patients with celomic epithelial carcinoma of the ovary. Although the explosion of knowledge of the basic nature of the disease holds the greatest potential for improvement, the identification of an effective screening technique, the clarification of the role of surgery in advanced disease, and the introduction of exciting new biologic and cytotoxic agents offer the promise of better treatment in the immediate future. The great promise of dose-intense regimens, still worthy of further investigation, suffers from a growing body of evidence that no advantage is obtained at least over the clinically achievable range of doses unsupported by marrow reconstitution.

REFERENCES

1. Jemal A, Thomas A, Murray T, Thun M: Cancer statistics, 2002. CA Cancer J Clin 2002;52:23–47.
2. Lynch HT, Watson P, Lynch JF, et al: Hereditary ovarian cancer: Heterogeneity in age at onset. Cancer 1993;71:573–581.

3. Lynch HT, Casey MJ, Shaw TG, Lynch JF: Hereditary factors in gynecologic cancer. Oncologist 1998;3:319–338.

4. Rubin SC, Benjamin I, Behbakht K, et al: Clinical and pathological features of ovarian cancer in women with germ-line mutations of BRCA1. N Engl J Med 1996;335:1413–1416.

5. Buller RE, Anderson B, Connor JP, et al: Familial ovarian cancer. Gynecol Oncol 1993;51:160–166.

6. WHO Collaborative Study of Neoplasia and Steroid Contraceptives: Epithelial ovarian cancer and combined oral contraceptives. Int J Epidemiol 1989;18:538.

7. The new FIGO stage grouping for primary carcinoma of the ovary (1985). Gynecol Oncol 1986;25:383.

8. Omura G, Blessing J, Ehrlich C, et al: A randomized trial of cyclophosphamide and doxorubicin with or without cisplatin in advanced ovarian carcinoma. Cancer 1986;57:1725–1730.

9. Omura G, Bundy B, Berek J, et al: Randomized trial of cyclophosphamide plus cisplatin with or without doxorubicin in ovarian carcinoma: A Gynecologic Oncology Group study. J Clin Oncol 1989;7:457–465.

10. Ehrlich C, Einhorn L, Williams S, et al: Chemotherapy for stage III-IV epithelial ovarian cancer with cis-dichlorodiammine-platinum, II: Adriamycin, and cyclophosphamide: a preliminary report. Cancer Treat Rep 1979;63:281–288.

11. Greco F, Julian C, Richardson R, et al: Advanced ovarian cancer: Brief intensive combination chemotherapy and second-look operation. Obstet Gynecol 1981;58:199–205.

12. Young R, Howser D, Myers C, et al: Combination chemotherapy (CHex-UP) with intraperitoneal maintenance in advanced ovarian adenocarcinoma. Proc ASCO 1981;22:465.

13. Gall S, Bundy B, Beecham J, et al: Therapy of stage III (optimal) epithelial carcinoma of the ovary with melphalan or melphalan plus Corynebacterium parvum (a Gynecologic Oncology Group study). Gynecol Oncol 1986;25:26–36.

14. Hoskins W, Bundy B, Thigpen T, Omura G: The influence of cytoreductive surgery on recurrence-free interval and survival in small-volume stage III epithelial ovarian cancer: A Gynecologic Oncology Group study. Gynecol Oncol 1992;47:159–166.

15. Thigpen T, Brady M, Omura G, et al: Age as a prognostic factor in ovarian carcinoma: The Gynecologic Oncology Group experience. Cancer 1993;71:606–614.

16. Colgan T, Norris H: Ovarian epithelial tumors of low malignant potential: A review. Int J Gynecol Pathol 1983;1:367–382.

17. Pecorelli S, Odicino F, Maisonneuve P, et al: Carcinoma of the ovary. J Epidemiol Biostat 1998;3:75–102.

18. Russell P: Surface epithelial-stromal tumors of the ovary. In Kurman R (ed): Blaustein's Pathology of the Female Genital Tract. New York, Springer-Verlag, 1994, pp 705–782.

19. Menzin A: Update on low malignant potential ovarian tumors. Oncology 2000;14:897–906.

20. Burger C, Prinssen H, Baak J, et al: The management of borderline epithelial tumors of the ovary. Int J Gynecol Cancer 2000;10:181–197.

21. Sykes P, Quinn M, Rome R: Ovarian tumors of low malignant potential: A retrospective study of 234 patients. Int J Gynecol Cancer 1997;7:218–226.

22. Sengupta P, Shanks J, Buckley C, et al: Requirement for expert histopathological assessment of ovarian cancer and borderline tumours. Br J Cancer 2000;82:760–762.

23. Bloss J, Brady M, Liao S, et al: Extraovarian peritoneal serous papillary carcinoma: A phase II trial of cisplatin and cyclophosphamide with comparison to a cohort with papillary serous ovarian carcinoma: A Gynecologic Oncology Group study. Gynecol Oncol 2003;89:148–154.

24. Piver MS, Baker TR, Jishi MF, et al: Familial ovarian cancer: a report of 658 families from the Gilda Radner Familial Ovarian Cancer Registry (1981-1991). Cancer 1993;71:582–588.

25. Srivastava A, McKinnon W, Wood M: Risk of breast and ovarian cancer in women with strong family histories. Oncology 2001;15:889–902.

26. Watson P, Butzow R, Lynch H, et al: The clinical features of ovarian cancer in hereditary nonpolyposis colorectal cancer. Gynecol Oncol 2001;82:223–228.

27. Boyd J, Sonoda Y, Federici M, et al: Clinicopathologic features of BRCA-linked and sporadic ovarian cancer. JAMA 2000;283:2260–2265.

28. Ben David Y, Chetrit A, Hirsh-Yechezkel G, et al: Effect of BRCA mutations on the length of survival in epithelial ovarian tumors. J Clin Oncol 2002;20:463–466.

29. Cass I, Baldwin R, Varkey T, et al: Improved survival in women with BRCA-associated ovarian carcinoma. Cancer 2003;97:2187–2195.

30. Piver MS, Jishi MF, Tsukada Y, et al: Primary peritoneal carcinoma after oophorectomy in women with a family history of ovarian cancer. Cancer 1993;71:2751–2755.

31. Eisen A, Rebbeck T, Wood W, Weber B: Prophylactic surgery in women with a hereditary predisposition to breast and ovarian cancer. J Clin Oncol 2000;18:1980–1995.

32. Kerlikowske K, Brown J, Grady D: Should women with familial ovarian cancer undergo prophylactic oophorectomy? Obstet Gynecol 1992;80:700–707.

33. Scheuer L, Kauff N, Robson M, et al: Outcome of preventive surgery and screening for breast and ovarian cancer in BRCA mutation carriers. J Clin Oncol 2002;20:1260–1268.

34. ACOG Committee on Gynecologic Practice: The role of the generalist obstetrician-gynecologist in the early detection of ovarian cancer. Gynecol Oncol 2002;87:237–239.

35. NIH Consensus Development Panel on Ovarian Cancer: Ovarian cancer: Screening, treatment, and follow-up. JAMA 1995;273:491–497.

36. Petricoin E, Ardekani A, Hitt B, et al: Use of proteomic patterns in serum to identify ovarian cancer. Lancet 2002;359:572–577.

37. Jacobs I, Davies A, Bridges J, et al: Prevalence screening for ovarian cancer in postmenopausal women by CA-125 measurement and ultrasonography. Br Med J 1993;306:1030–1034.

38. Boyd J: Molecular genetics of hereditary ovarian cancer. Oncology 1998;12:399–406.

39. ASCO Working Group on Genetic Testing for Cancer Susceptibility: American Society of Clinical Oncology policy statement update: Genetic testing for cancer susceptibility. J Clin Oncol 2003;21:2397–2406.

40. Gwinn M, Lee N, Rhodes P, et al: Pregnancy, breast feeding, and oral contraceptives and the risk of epithelial ovarian cancer. J Clin Epidemiol 1990;43:559–568.

41. Weiss N, Lyon J, Liff J, et al: Incidence of ovarian cancer in relation to the use of oral contraceptives. Int J Cancer 1981;28:669–671.

42. Parazzini F, La Vecchia C, Negri E, et al: Oral contraceptive use and the risk of ovarian cancer: An Italian case control study. Eur J Cancer 1991;27:594–598.

43. Grabrick D, Hartmann L, Cerhan J, et al: Risk of breast cancer with oral contraceptive use in women with a family history of breast cancer. JAMA 2000;284:1791–1798.

44. Ursin G, Henderson B, Haile R, et al: Does oral contraceptive use increase the risk of breast cancer in women with BRCA1/BRCA2 mutations more than in other women? Cancer Res 1997;57:3678–3681.

45. Eeles R, Powles T, Ashley S, et al: BRCA1, BRCA2 mutation and pedigree analysis to determine genetic risk in the UK Royal Marsden Hospital Tamoxifen Prevention Trial. Br J Cancer 2000;83(Suppl 1):25(abstr).

46. Narod S, Risch H, Moslehi R, et al: Oral contraceptives and the risk of hereditary ovarian cancer. N Engl J Med 1998;339:424–428.

47. Modan B, Hartge P, Hirsh-Yechezkel G, et al: Parity, oral contraceptives, and the risk of ovarian cancer among carriers and noncarriers of a BRCA1 or BRCA2 mutation. N Engl J Med 2001;345:235–240.

48. Risch H: Estrogen replacement therapy and risk of epithelial ovarian cancer. Gynecol Oncol 1996;63:254–257.

49. Rodriguez C, Patel A, Calle E, et al: Estrogen replacement therapy and ovarian cancer mortality in a large prospective study of US women. JAMA 2001;285:1460–1465.

50. Lacey J, Mink P, Lubin J, et al: Menopausal hormone replacement therapy and risk of ovarian cancer. JAMA 2002;288:334–341.

51. Sit A, Modugno F, Weissfeld J, et al: Hormone replacement formulations and risk of ovarian carcinoma. Gynecol Oncol 2002;86:118–123.

52. Guidozzi F, Daponte A: Estrogen replacement therapy for ovarian carcinoma survivors. Cancer 1999;86:1013–1018.

53. Neven P, Goldstein S, Ciaccia A, et al: The effect of raloxifene on the incidence of ovarian cancer in postmenopausal women. Gynecol Oncol 2002;85:388–390.

54. van der Burg MEL, van Lent M, Buyse M, et al: The effect of debulking surgery after induction chemotherapy on the prognosis in advanced epithelial ovarian cancer. N Engl J Med 1995;332:629.

55. Rose P, Nerenstone S, Brady M, et al: A phase III randomized study of interval secondary cytoreduction in patients with advanced stage ovarian carcinoma with suboptimal residual disease: A Gynecologic Oncology Group study. Proc ASCO 2002;21:201a(abstr).

56. Thigpen JT: Single agent chemotherapy in the management of ovarian carcinoma. In Alberts DS, Surwit EA (eds): Ovarian Carcinoma. Boston, Martinus Nijhoff, 1985, pp 115–146.

57. Sutton GP, Blessing JA, Photopoulos G, et al: Gynecologic Oncology Group experience with ifosfamide. Semin Oncol 1990;17(Suppl 4):6–10.

58. Markman M, Hakes T, Reichman B, et al: Ifosfamide and mesna in previously treated advanced epithelial ovarian cancer: Activity in platinum-resistant disease. J Clin Oncol 1992;10:243–248.

59. Markman M, Kennedy A, Sutton G, et al: Phase 2 trial of single agent ifosfamide/mesna in patient with platinum/paclitaxel refractory ovarian cancer who have not previously been treated with an alkylating agent. Gynecol Oncol 1998;70:272–274.

60. Wiltshaw E, Kroner T: Phase II trial of cis-dichlorodiammineplatinum (II) (NSC-119875) in advanced adenocarcinoma of the ovary. Cancer Treat Rep 1976;60:55–60.

61. Thigpen T, Lagasse L, Homesley H, et al: Cisplatinum in the treatment of advanced or recurrent adenocarcinoma of the ovary: A phase II study of the Gynecologic Oncology Group. Am J Clin Oncol 1983;6:431–435.

62. Kjorstad K, Bertelsen K, Slevin M, et al: Phase II trial of carboplatin in ovarian cancer. Proc ASCO 1986;5:116.

63. Pecorelli S, Bolis G, Vassena L, et al: Randomized comparison of cisplatin and carboplatin in advanced ovarian cancer. Proc ASCO 1988;7:136.

64. Piccart M, Green J, Lacave A, et al: Oxaliplatin or paclitaxel in patients with platinum-pretreated advanced ovarian cancer: A randomized phase II study of the European Organization for research and Treatment of Cancer Gynecology Group. J Clin Oncol 2000;18:1193–1202.

65. Thigpen T, Blessing J, Ball H, et al: Phase II trial of taxol as second-line therapy for ovarian carcinoma: A Gynecologic Oncology Group study. J Clin Oncol 1994;12:1748–1753.

66. Einzig A, Wiernik P, Sasloff J, et al: Phase II study and long-term follow-up of patients treated with taxol for advanced ovarian adenocarcinoma. J Clin Oncol 1992;10:1748–1756.

67. McGuire W, Rowinsky E, Rosenshein N, et al: Taxol: A unique antineoplastic agent with significant activity in advanced ovarian epithelial neoplasms. Ann Intern Med 1989;111:273–279.

68. Kohn E, Sarosy G, Bicher A, et al: Dose-intense taxol: High response rate in patients with platinum-resistant recurrent ovarian cancer. J Natl Cancer Inst 1994;86:18–24.

69. Verschraegen C, Sittisomwong T, Kudelka A, et al: Docetaxel for patients with paclitaxel-resistant mullerian carcinoma. J Clin Oncol 2000;18:2733–2739.

70. Francis P, Schneider J, Hann L, et al: Phase II trial of docetaxel in patients with platinum-refractory advanced ovarian cancer. J Clin Oncol 1994;12:2301–2308.

71. Kaye S, Piccart M, Aapro M, et al: Phase II trials of docetaxel (Taxotere) in advanced ovarian cancer: An updated review. Eur J Cancer 1997;33:2167–2170.

72. Rose P, Blessing J, Ball H, et al: A phase II study of docetaxel in paclitaxel-resistant ovarian and peritoneal carcinoma: A Gynecologic Oncology Group study. Gynecol Oncol 2003;88:130–135.

73. Piccart M, Gore M, Ten Bokkel Huinink W, et al: Docetaxel: An active new drug for treatment of advanced epithelial ovarian cancer. J Natl Cancer Inst 1995;87:676–681.

74. Manetta A, Tewari K, Podczaski E: Hexamethylmelamine as a single second-line agent in ovarian cancer: Follow-up report and review of the literature. Gynecol Oncol 1997;66:20–26.

75. Vergote I, Himmelmann A, Frankendal B, et al: Hexamethyl-melamine as second-line therapy in platin-resistant ovarian cancer. Gynecol Oncol 1992;47:282–286.

76. Markman M, Blessing J, Moore D, et al: Altretamine in platinum-resistant and platinum-refractory ovarian cancer: A Gynecologic Oncology Group phase II trial. Gynecol Oncol 1998;69:226–229.

77. Moore D, Valea F, Crumpler L, et al: Hexamethylmelamine/altretamine as second-line therapy for epithelial ovarian carcinoma. Gynecol Oncol 19932;51:109–112.

78. Rustin G, Nelstrop A, Crawford M, et al: Phase II trial of oral altretamine for relapsed ovarian carcinoma: Evaluation of defining response by serum CA125. J Clin Oncol 1997;15:172–176.

79. Keldsen N, Havsteen H, Vergote I, et al: Altretamine in the treatment of platinum-resistant ovarian cancer: A phase II study. Gynecol Oncol 2003;88:118–122.

80. Malik I: Altretamine is an effective palliative therapy of patients with recurrent epithelial ovarian cancer. Jpn J Clin Oncol 2001;31:69–73.

81. Rosen G, Lurain J, Newton M: Hexamethylmelamine in ovarian cancer after failure of cisplatin-based multiple-agent chemotherapy. Gynecol Oncol 1987;27:173–179.

82. Kudelka A, Tresukosol D, Edwards C, et al: Phase II study of intravenous topotecan as a 5-day infusion for refractory epithelial ovarian carcinoma. J Clin Oncol 1996;14:1552–1557.

83. Creemers G, Bolis G, Gore M, et al: Topotecan, an active drug in the second-line treatment of epithelial ovarian cancer: Results of a large European phase II study. J Clin Oncol 1996;14:3056–3061.

84. Ten Bokkel Huinink W, Gore M, Carmichael J, et al: Topotecan versus paclitaxel for the treatment of recurrent epithelial ovarian cancer. J Clin Oncol 1997;15:2183–2193.

85. McGuire W, Blessing J, Bookman M, et al: Topotecan has substantial antitumor activity as first-line salvage therapy in platinum-sensitive epithelial ovarian carcinoma: A Gynecologic Oncology Group study. J Clin Oncol 2000;18:1062–1067.

86. Bookman M, Malmstrom H, Bolis G, et al: Topotecan for the treatment of advanced epithelial ovarian cancer: An open-label phase II study in patients treated after prior chemotherapy that contained cisplatin or carboplatin and paclitaxel. J Clin Oncol 1998;16:3345–3352.

87. Bodurka D, Levenback C, Wolf J, et al: Phase II trial of irinotecan in patients with metastatic epithelial ovarian cancer or peritoneal cancer. J Clin Oncol 2003;21:291–297.

88. Muggia F, Hainsworth J, Jeffers S, et al: Phase II study of liposomal doxorubicin in refractory ovarian cancer: Antitumor activity and toxicity modification by liposomal encapsulation. J Clin Oncol 1997;15:987–993.

89. Gordon A, Granai C, Rose P, et al: Phase II study of liposomal doxorubicin in platinum- and paclitaxel-refractory epithelial ovarian cancer. J Clin Oncol 2000;18:3093–3100.

90. Gordon A, Fleagle J, Guthrie D, et al: Recurrent epithelial ovarian carcinoma: A randomized phase III study of pegylated liposomal doxorubicin versus topotecan. J Clin Oncol 2001;19:3312–3322.

91. Markman M, Kennedy A, Webster K, et al: Phase 2 of liposomal doxorubicin (40 mg/m^2) in platinum/paclitaxel-refractory ovarian and fallopian tube cancers and primary carcinoma of the peritoneum. Gynecol Oncol 2000;78:369–372.

92. Rose P, Maxson J, Fusco N, et al: Liposomal doxorubicin in ovarian, peritoneal, and tubal carcinoma: A retrospective comparative study of single-agent dosages. Gynecol Oncol 2001;82:323–328.

93. Campos S, Penson R, Mays A, et al: The clinical utility of liposomal doxorubicin in recurrent ovarian cancer. Gynecol Oncol 2001;81:206–212.

94. Rose P, Blessing J, Mayer A, Homesley H: Prolonged oral etoposide as second-line therapy for platinum-resistant and platinum-sensitive ovarian carcinoma: A Gynecologic Oncology Group study. J Clin Oncol 1998;16:405–410.

95. Hoskins P, Swenerton K: Oral etoposide is active against platinum-resistant epithelial ovarian cancer. J Clin Oncol 1994;12:60–63.

96. Seymour M, Mansi J, Gallagher C, et al: Protracted oral etoposide in epithelial ovarian cancer: A phase II study in patients with relapsed or platinum-resistant disease. Br J Cancer 1994;69:191–195.

97. Markman M, Hakes T, Reichman B, et al: Phase 2 trial of chronic low-dose oral etoposide as salvage therapy of platinum-refractory ovarian cancer. J Cancer Res Clin Oncol 1992;119:55-57.

98. Tuxen M, Lund B, Hansen O, et al: Oral etoposide in elderly previously untreated ovarian cancer patients with residual disease. Int J Gynecol Cancer 1997;7:213-217.

99. Friedlander M, Millward M, Bell D, et al: A phase II study of gemcitabine in platinum pre-treated patients with advanced epithelial ovarian cancer. Ann Oncol 1998;9:1343-1345.

100. Shapiro J, Millward M, Rischin D, et al: Activity of gemcitabine in patients with advanced ovarian cancer: Responses seen following platinum and paclitaxel. Gynecol Oncol 1996;63:89-93.

101. Lund B, Hansen O, Theilade K, et al: Phase II study of gemcitabine in previously treated ovarian cancer patients. J Natl Cancer Inst 1994;86:1530-1533.

102. George M, Heron J, Kerbrat P, et al: Navelbine in advanced ovarian epithelial cancer: A study of the French Oncology Centers. Semin Oncol 1989;(Suppl 4):30-32.

103. Sorensen P, Hoyer M, Jakobsen A, et al: Phase II study of vinorelbine in the treatment of platinum-resistant ovarian carcinoma. Gynecol Oncol 2001;81:58-62.

104. Burger R, DiSaia P, Roberts J, et al: Phase II trial of vinorelbine in recurrent and progressive epithelial ovarian cancer. Gynecol Oncol 1999;72:148-153.

105. Gershenson D, Burke T, Morris M, et al: A phase I study of daily ×3 schedule of intravenous vinorelbine for refractory epithelial ovarian cancer. Gynecol Oncol 1998;70:404-409.

106. Bajetta E, Leo A, Biganzoli L, et al: Phase II study of vinorelbine in patients with pretreated advanced ovarian cancer: Activity in platinum-resistant disease. J Clin Oncol 1996;14:2546-2551.

107. Look K, Muss H, Blessing J, Morris M: A phase II trial of 5-fluorouracil and high-dose leucovorin in recurrent epithelial ovarian carcinoma: A Gynecologic Oncology Group study. Am J Clin Oncol 1995;18:19-22.

108. Markman M, Lichtman S, Homesley H, et al: Phase 2 trial of moderately high dose single agent mitoxantrone in platinum and paclitaxel-refractory ovarian cancer. Gynecol Oncol 1998;70:123-126.

109. Gropp M, Meier W, Hepp H: Treosulfan as an effective second-line therapy in ovarian cancer. Gynecol Oncol 1998;71:94-98.

110. Gunsilius E, Gierlich T, Mross K, et al: Palliative chemotherapy in pretreated patients with advanced cancer: Oral trofosfamide is effective in ovarian carcinoma. Cancer Invest 2001;19:808-811

111. Hatch K, Beecham J, Blessing J, Creasman W: Responsiveness of patients with advanced ovarian carcinoma to tamoxifen. Cancer 1991;68:269-271.

112. Shirey D, Kavanagh J, Gershenson D, et al: Tamoxifen therapy of epithelial ovarian cancer. Obstet Gynecol 1985;66:575-578.

113. Schwartz P, Keating G, MacLusky N, et al: Tamoxifen therapy for advanced ovarian cancer. Obstet Gynecol 1982;59:583-588.

114. Rocereto T, Saul H, Aikins J, Paulson J: Phase II study of mifepristone in refractory ovarian cancer. Gynecol Oncol 2000;77:429-432.

115. Bookman M, Darcy K, Clarke-Pearson D, et al: Evaluation of monoclonal humanized anti-HER2 antibody, trastuzumab, in patients with recurrent or refractory ovarian or primary peritoneal carcinoma with overexpression of HER2: A phase II trial of the Gynecologic Oncology Group. J Clin Oncol 2003;21:283-290.

116. Rowinsky EK, Donehower RC, Jones RJ, Tucker RW: Microtubule changes and cytotoxicity in leukemic cell lines treated with taxol. Cancer Res 1988;48:4093-4100.

117. Omura G, Morrow P, Blessing J, et al: A randomized comparison of melphalan versus melphalan plus hexamethylmelamine versus Adriamycin plus cyclophosphamide in ovarian carcinoma. Cancer 1983;51:783-789.

118. Thigpen T, Vance R, Lambuth B, et al: Chemotherapy for advanced or recurrent gynecologic cancer. Cancer 1987;60:2104-2116.

119. Alberts DS, Green SJ, Hannigan EV, et al: Improved efficacy of carboplatin plus cyclophosphamide versus cisplatin plus cyclophosphamide: Preliminary report by the Southwest Oncology Group of a phase III randomized trial in stages III and IV suboptimal ovarian cancer, abstracted. Proc ASCO 1989;8:151.

120. ten Bokkel Huinink WW, van der Burg MEL, van Oosterom AT, et al: Carboplatin in combination therapy for ovarian cancer. Cancer Treat Rev 1988;15(Suppl B):9-15.

121. Pater J: Cyclophosphamide/cisplatin versus cyclophosphamide/carboplatin in macroscopic residual ovarian cancer: Initial results of a National Cancer Institute of Canada Clinical Trials Group trial, abstracted. Proc ASCO 1990;9:155.

122. Edmondson JH, McCormack GM, Wieand HS, et al: Cyclophosphamide-cisplatin versus cyclophosphamide-carboplatin in stage III-IV ovarian carcinoma: A comparison of equally myelosuppressive regimens. J Natl Cancer Inst 1989;81:1500-1504.

123. Alberts DS, Young L, Mason NL, et al: In vitro evaluation of anticancer drugs against ovarian cancer at concentrations achievable by intraperitoneal administration. Semin Oncol 1985;12:38-42.

124. Ozols R, Corden B, Jacob J, et al: High-dose cisplatinum in hypertonic saline. Ann Intern Med 1984;100:19-24.

125. Howell S, Zimm S, Markman M, et al: Long-term survival of advanced refractory ovarian carcinoma patients with small-volume disease treated with intraperitoneal chemotherapy. J Clin Oncol 1987;5:1607-1612.

126. Ozols R: High dose therapy with cisplatin and its analogs in ovarian cancer: Current status and future studies. ASCO Educ Book 1987, pp 69-70.

127. Levin L, Hryniuk WM: Dose intensity analysis of chemotherapy regimens in ovarian carcinoma. J Clin Oncol 1987;5:756-767.

128. Levin L, Simon R, Hryniuk W: Importance of multiagent chemotherapy regimens in ovarian carcinoma: Dose intensity analysis. J Natl Cancer Inst 1993;85:1732-1742.

129. Ozols RF, Ostchega Y, Curt G, Young RC: High-dose carboplatin in refractory ovarian cancer patients. J Clin Oncol 1987;5:197-201.

130. McGuire WP, Hoskins WJ, Brady MF, et al: Assessment of dose-intensive therapy in suboptimally debulked ovarian cancer: A Gynecologic Oncology Group study. J Clin Oncol 1995;13:1589-1599.

131. Kaye S, Lewis C, Paul J, et al: Randomized study of two doses of cisplatin and cyclophosphamide in epithelial ovarian cancer. Lancet 1992;340:329-333.

132. Colombo N, Pittelli M, Parma G, et al: Cisplatin dose intensity in advanced ovarian cancer: A randomized study of conventional dose versus dose-intense cisplatin monochemotherapy. Proc ASCO 1993;12:255(abstr).

133. Conte P, Bruzzone M, Carnino F, et al: High-dose versus low-dose cisplatin in combination with cyclophosphamide and epidoxorubicin in suboptimal ovarian cancer: A randomized study of the Gruppo Oncologico Nord-Ouest. J Clin Oncol 1996;14:351-356.

134. Gore M, Mainwaring P, Macfarlane V, et al: Randomized trial of dose-intensity with single agent carboplatin in patients with epithelial ovarian cancer. J Clin Oncol 1998;16:2426-2434.

135. Jakobsen A, Bertelsen K, Andersen JE, et al: Dose-effect study of carboplatin in ovarian cancer: A Danish Ovarian Cancer Group Study. J Clin Oncol 1997;15:193-8.

136. Dittrich C, Obermair A, Kurz C, et al: Prospective randomized trial of cisplatin/carboplatin versus conventional cisplatin/cyclophosphamide in epithelial ovarian cancer: First results of the impact of platinum dose intensity on patient outcome. Proc Am Soc Clin Oncol 1996;15:279(abstr).

137. Ngan H, Choo Y, Cheung M, et al: A randomized study of high-dose versus low-dose cisplatin combined with cyclophosphamide in the treatment of advanced ovarian cancer. Chemotherapy 1989;35:221-227.

138. Coldman A, Goldie J: Impact of dose-intense chemotherapy on the development of permanent drug resistance. Semin Oncol 1987;14:29-33.

139. McGuire WP, Hoskins WJ, Brady MF, et al: Cyclophosphamide and cisplatin compared with paclitaxel and cisplatin in patients with stage III and stage IV ovarian cancer. N Engl J Med 1996;334:1-6.

140. Piccart MJ, Bertelsen K, James K, et al: Randomized Intergroup trial of cisplatin-paclitaxel versus cisplatin-cyclophosphamide in women with advanced epithelial ovarian cancer: Three-year results. J Natl Cancer Inst 2000;92:699-708.

141. Muggia FM, Braly PS, Brady MF, et al: Phase III randomized study of

cisplatin versus paclitaxel versus cisplatin and paclitaxel in patients with suboptimal stage III or IV ovarian cancer: A Gynecologic Oncology Group study. J Clin Oncol 2000;18:106–115.

142. The International Collaborative Ovarian Neoplasm (ICON) Group: Paclitaxel plus carboplatin versus standard chemotherapy with either single-agent carboplatin or cyclophosphamide, doxorubicin, and cisplatin in women with ovarian cancer: the ICON3 randomised trial. Lancet 2002;360:505–515.

143. The International Collaborative Ovarian Neoplasm (ICON) Group: ICON2: randomised trial of single-agent carboplatin against three-drug combination of CAP (cyclophosphamide, doxorubicin, and cisplatin) in women with ovarian cancer. Lancet 1988;352:1571–1576.

144. Pertussini E, Ratajczak J, Majka M, et al: Investigating the platelet-sparing mechanism of paclitaxel/carboplatin combination chemotherapy. Blood 2001;97:638–644.

145. Neijt J, Engelholm S, Tuxen M, et al: Exploratory phase III study of paclitaxel and cisplatin versus paclitaxel and carboplatin in advanced ovarian cancer. J Clin Oncol 2000;18:3084–3092.

146. DuBois A, Lueck H, Meier W, et al: Cisplatin/paclitaxel vs carboplatin/paclitaxel in ovarian cancer: Update of an Arbeitsgemeinschaft Gynaekolgische Onkologie study group trial. Proc ASCO 1999;18:356a(abstr).

147. Ozols R, Bundy B, Fowler J, et al: Randomized phase III study of cisplatin/paclitaxel versus carboplatin/paclitaxel in optimal stage III epithelial ovarian cancer: A Gynecologic Oncology Group trial. Proc ASCO 1999;18:356a(abstr).

148. Ozols R: Maintenance therapy in advanced ovarian cancer: Progression-free survival and clinical benefit. J Clin Oncol 2003;21:2451–2453.

149. Pignata S, Deplacido S, Scambia G, et al: Topotecan vs nihil after response to carboplatin and paclitaxel in advanced ovarian cancer: Early results of the MITO-1 study. Proc ASCO 2003;22:446(abstr).

150. Pfisterer J, Lotholary A, Kimmig R, et al: Paclitaxel/carboplatin vs. paclitaxel/carboplatin followed by topotecan in first-line treatment of ovarian cancer FIGO stages IIB-IV: Interim results of a gynecologic cancer Intergroup phase III trial of the AGO Ovarian Cancer Study Group and GINECO. Proc ASCO 2003;22:446(abstr).

151. Markman M, Liu P, Wilczynski S, et al: Phase III randomized trial of 12 versus 3 months of maintenance paclitaxel in patients with advanced ovarian cancer after complete response to platinum and paclitaxel-based chemotherapy: A Southwest Oncology Group and Gynecologic Oncology Group trial. J Clin Oncol 2003;21:2460–2465.

152. Browder T, Butterfield C, Kraling B, et al: Antiangiogenic scheduling of chemotherapy improves efficacy against experimental drug-resistant cancer. Cancer Res 2001;60:1878–1886.

153. Eisenhauer E, ten Bokkel Huinink W, Swenerton K, et al: European-Canadian randomized trial of paclitaxel in relapsed ovarian cancer: High-dose versus low-dose and long versus short infusion. J Clin Oncol 1994;12:2654–2666.

154. Markman M, Rose P, Jones E, et al: Ninety-six-hour infusional paclitaxel as salvage therapy of ovarian cancer patients previously failing treatment with 3-hour or 24-hour paclitaxel infusion regimens. J Clin Oncol 1998;16:1849–1851.

155. Hurteau J: Personal communication on behalf of the GOG.

156. Fennelly D, Aghajanian C, Shapiro F, et al: Phase I and pharmacologic study of paclitaxel administered weekly in patients with relapsed ovarian cancer. J Clin Oncol 1997;15:187–192.

157. Markman M, Hall J, Spitz D, et al: Phase II trial of weekly single-agent paclitaxel in platinum/paclitaxel-refractory ovarian cancer. J Clin Oncol 2002;20:2365–2369.

158. Andersson H, Boman K, Ridderheim M, et al: An updated analysis of a randomized study of single agent paclitaxel given weekly vs every 3 weeks to patients with ovarian cancer treated with prior platinum therapy. Proc ASCO 2000;19:380a.

159. Alberts DS, Liu PY, Hannigan EV, et al: Intraperitoneal cisplatin plus intravenous cyclophosphamide versus intravenous cisplatin plus intravenous cyclophosphamide for stage III ovarian cancer. N Engl J Med 1996;335:1950–1955.

160. Markman M, Bundy B, Alberts D, et al: Phase III trial of standard-dose intravenous cisplatin plus paclitaxel versus moderately high-dose carboplatin followed by intravenous paclitaxel and intraperitoneal cisplatin in small-volume stage III ovarian carcinoma: An Intergroup study of the Gynecologic Oncology Group, Southwestern Oncology Group, and Eastern Cooperative Oncology Group. J Clin Oncol 2001;19:1001–1007.

161. Armstrong D, Bundy B, Baergen R, et al: Randomized phase III study of intravenous paclitaxel and cisplatin versus intravenous paclitaxel, intraperitoneal cisplatin and intraperitoneal paclitaxel in optimal stage III epithelial ovarian cancer: A Gynecologic Oncology Group trial (GOG 172). Proc ASCO 2002;21:201a.

162. Thigpen T: Dose-intensity in ovarian carcinoma: Hold, enough? J Clin Oncol 1997;15:1291–1293.

163. Stiff P, Veum-Stone J, Lasarus H, et al: High-dose chemotherapy and autologous stem-cell transplantation for ovarian cancer: An autologous blood and marrow transplant registry report. Ann Intern Med 2000;133:504–515.

164. Rose P, Rodriguez M, Waggoner S, et al: Phase I study of paclitaxel, carboplatin, and increasing days of prolonged oral etoposide in ovarian, peritoneal, and tubal carcinoma: A Gynecologic Oncology Group study. J Clin Oncol 2000;18:2957–2962.

165. Manetta A, Blessing J, Hurteau J: Evaluation of cisplatin and cyclosporin A in recurrent platinum-resistant ovarian cancer: A phase II study of the Gynecologic Oncology Group. Gynecol Oncol 1998;68:45–46.

166. Fracasso P, Brady M, Moore D, et al: Phase II study of paclitaxel and valspodar in refractory ovarian carcinoma: A Gynecologic Oncology Group study. J Clin Oncol 2001;19:2975–2982.

167. Joly F, Mangioni C, Nicolleto M, et al: A phase 3 study of PSC 833 in combination with paclitaxel and carboplatin versus paclitaxel and carboplatin alone in patients with stage IV or suboptimally debulked stage III epithelial ovarian cancer or primary cancer of the peritoneum. Proc ASCO 2002;21:202a(abstr).

168. Pujade-Lauraine E, Guastalla J, Colombo N, et al: Intraperitoneal recombinant interferon gamma in ovarian cancer patients with residual disease at second-look laparotomy. J Clin Oncol 1996;14:343–350.

169. Windbichler G, Hausmaninger H, Stummvoll W, et al: Interferon-gamma in the first-line therapy of ovarian cancer: A randomized phase III trial. Br J Cancer 2000;82:1138–1144.

170. Paley P, Staskus K, Gebhard K, et al: Vascular endothelial growth factor expression in early stage ovarian carcinoma. Cancer 1997;80:98–106.

171. Markman M: The role of CA-125 in the management of ovarian cancer. Oncologist 1997;2:6–9.

172. Bridgewater J, Nelstrop A, Rustin G, et al: Comparison of standard and CA-125 response criteria in patients with epithelial ovarian cancer treated with platinum or paclitaxel. J Clin Oncol 1999;17:501–508.

173. Rustin G, Nelstrop A, Bentzen S, et al: Selection of active drugs for ovarian cancer based on CA-125 and standard response rates in phase II trials. J Clin Oncol 2000;18:1733–1739.

174. Berek J, Hacker N, Lagasse L, et al: Second look laparotomy in stage III epithelial ovarian cancer: Clinical variables associated with disease status. Obstet Gynecol 1984;64:207–212.

175. Potter M, Hatch K, Soong S, et al: Second look laparotomy and salvage therapy: A research modality only? Gynecol Oncol 1992;44:3–9.

176. Podratz K, Kinney W: Second-look operation in ovarian cancer. Cancer 1993;71:1551–1558.

177. Greer B, Bundy B, Ozols R, et al: Implications of second-look laparotomy in the context of Gynecologic Oncology Group Protocol 158: A non-randomized comparison using an explanatory analysis. Gynecol Oncol 2003;88:156(abstr).

178. Day TG, Smith JP: Diagnosis and staging of ovarian carcinoma. Semin Oncol 1975;2:217.

179. Young RC, Walton L, Ellenberg SS, et al: Adjuvant therapy in stage I and stage II epithelial ovarian cancer: Results of two prospective randomized trials. N Engl J Med 1990;322:1021–1027.

180. Bush RS, Allt WEC, Beale FA, et al: Treatment of epithelial carcinoma of the ovary: operation, irradiation and chemotherapy. Am J Obstet Gynecol 1977;127:692–704.

181. Hreshchyshyn MM, Park RC, Blessing JA, et al: The role of adjuvant therapy in stage I ovarian cancer. Am J Obstet Gynecol 1980;138:139–145.

182. Dembo AJ, Bush R, Beale F et al: The Princess Margaret study of ovarian cancer: Stages I, II and asymptomatic III presentation. Cancer Treat Rep 1979;63:249–254.

183. Dembo AJ, Bush R, Beale F, et al: A randomized clinical trial of moving strip versus open field whole abdominal irradiation in patients with invasive epithelial cancer of ovary. Int J Radiat Oncol Biol Phys Suppl 1983;9:97.

184. Dembo AJ: Abdominopelvic radiotherapy in ovarian cancer: A 10-year experience. Cancer 1985;55:2285–2290.

185. Martinez A, Schray M, Howes A, Bagshaw M: Postoperative radiation therapy for epithelial ovarian cancer: The curative role based on a 24-year experience. J Clin Oncol 1985;3:901–911.

186. Haas J, Mansfield C, Hartman G, et al: Results of radiation therapy in the treatment of epithelial carcinoma of the ovary. Cancer 1980;46:1950–1956.

187. Smith J, Rutledge F, Delclos L: Postoperative treatment of early cancer of the ovary: A random trial between postoperative irradiation and chemotherapy. Natl Cancer Inst Monogr 1975;42:149–153.

188. Allen C: Adjunctive irradiation treatment for ovarian carcinoma. Northwest Med 1967;66:1040–1044.

189. Aure J, Hoeg K, Kolstad P: Radioactive colloidal gold in the treatment of ovarian carcinoma. Acta Radiat Ther Phys Biol 1871;10:399–407.

190. Buchsbaum H, Keetel W, Latourette H: The use of radioisotopes as adjunct therapy of localized ovarian cancer. Semin Oncol 1975;2:247–251.

191. Decker D, Webb M, Holbrook M: Radiocolloid treatment of epithelial cancer of the ovary: late results. Am J Obstet Gynecol 1973;115:751–758.

192. Hilaris B, Clark D: The value of postoperative intraperitoneal injection of radiocolloids in early cancer of the ovary. Am J Roentgenol 1971;112:749–754.

193. Pezner R, Stevens K, Tong D, et al: Limited epithelial carcinoma of the ovary treated with curative intent by the intraperitoneal installation of radiocolloids. Cancer 1987;42:2563–2571.

194. Piver S, Lele S, Bakshi S, et al: Five and ten year estimated survival and disease-free rates after intraperitoneal chromic phosphate: Stage I ovarian adenocarcinoma. Am J Clin Oncol 1988;11:515–519.

195. Klaassen D, Shelley W, Starreveld A, et al: Early stage ovarian cancer: A randomized clinical trial comparing whole abdominal radiotherapy, melphalan, and intraperitoneal chromic phosphate: A National Cancer Institute of Canada Clinical Trials Group report. J Clin Oncol 1988;6:1254–1263.

196. Spencer R, Marks R, Fenn J, et al: Intraperitoneal P-32 after negative second-look laparotomy in ovarian carcinoma. Cancer 1989;63:2434–2437.

197. Gallion H, Van Nagell J, Donaldson E, et al: Adjuvant oral alkylating chemotherapy in patients with stage I epithelial ovarian cancer. Cancer 1989;63:1070–1073.

198. Bolis G, Colombo N, Favalli G, et al: Randomized multicenter clinical trials in stage I epithelial ovarian cancer. Proc ASCO 1992;11:225.

199. Vergote I, Kaern J, Trope C: Adjuvant treatment of stage I ovarian cancer: How can we prevent overtreatment? Proc ASCO 1992;11:225.

200. Young R, Brady M, Nieberg R, et al: Randomized clinical trial of adjuvant treatment of women with early (FIGO I-IIA high risk) ovarian cancer. Proc ASCO 1999;18:357a.

201. Vergote I, Trimbos B, Guthrie D, et al: Results of a randomized trial in 923 patients with high-risk early ovarian cancer, comparing adjuvant chemotherapy with no further treatment following surgery. Proc ASCO 2001;20:201a(abstr).

202. Bell J, Brady M, Lage J, et al: A randomized phase III trial of three versus six cycles of carboplatin and paclitaxel as adjuvant treatment in early stage ovarian epithelial carcinoma: A Gynecologic Oncology Group study. Gynecol Oncol 2003;88:156(abstr).

203. Neijt JP, ten Bokkel Huinink WW, van der Burg ME, et al: Long-term survival in ovarian cancer: Mature data from The Netherlands Joint Study Group for Ovarian Cancer. Eur J Cancer 1991;27:1367–1372.

204. Omura GA, Brady MF, Homesley HD, et al: Long-term follow-up and prognostic factor analysis in advanced ovarian carcinoma: The Gynecologic Oncology Group experience. J Clin Oncol 1991;9:1138–1150.

205. Rubin SC, Hoskins WJ, Saigo PE, et al: Prognostic factors for recurrence following negative second-look laparotomy in ovarian cancer patients treated with platinum-based chemotherapy. Gynecol Oncol 1991;42:137–141.

206. Ozols RF, Ostchega Y, Curt G, Young RC: High-dose carboplatin in refractory ovarian cancer patients. J Clin Oncol 1987;5:197–201.

207. Markman M, Reichman B, Hakes T, et al: Responses to second-line cisplatin-based intraperitoneal therapy in ovarian cancer: Influence of a prior response to intravenous cisplatin. J Clin Oncol 1991;9:1801–1805.

208. van der Burg ME, Hoff AM, van Lent M, et al: Carboplatin and cyclophosphamide salvage therapy for ovarian cancer patients relapsing after cisplatin combination chemotherapy. Eur J Cancer 1991;27:248–250.

209. Weiss G, Green S, Alberts DS, et al: Second-line treatment of advanced measurable ovarian cancer with iproplatin: A Southwest Oncology Group Study. Eur J Cancer 1991;27:135–138.

210. Markman M, Rothman R, Hakes T et al: Second-line platinum therapy in patients with ovarian cancer previously treated with cisplatin. J Clin Oncol 1991;9:389–393.

211. Zanaboni F, Scarfone G, Presti M, et al: Salvage chemotherapy for ovarian cancer recurrence: Weekly cisplatin in combination with epirubicin or etoposide. Gynecol Oncol 1991;43:24–28.

212. Cantu M, Buda A, Parma G, et al: Randomized controlled trial of single-agent paclitaxel versus cyclophosphamide, doxorubicin, and cisplatin in patients with recurrent ovarian cancer who responded to first-line platinum-based regimens. J Clin Oncol 2002;20:1232–1237.

213. Ledermann J on behalf of ICON and AGO collaborators: Randomised trial of paclitaxel in combination with platinum chemotherapy versus platinum-based chemotherapy in the treatment of relapsed ovarian cancer (ICON4/OVAR 2.2). Proc ASCO 2003;22:446.

214. Ozols RF, Ostchega Y, Myers CE, et al: Cisplatin in hypertonic saline in refractory ovarian cancer. J Clin Oncol 1985;3:1246–1250.

215. Markman M: Intraperitoneal chemotherapy. Semin Oncol 1991;18:248–254.

216. McGuire WP, Rowinsky EK: Old drugs revisited, new drugs, and experimental approaches in ovarian cancer therapy. Semin Oncol 1991;18:255–269.

217. Berek J, Hacker N, Lagasse L, et al: Survival of patients following secondary cytoreductive surgery in ovarian cancer. Obstet Gynecol 1983;61:189.

218. Morris M, Gershenson D, Wharten T, et al: Secondary cytoreductive surgery for recurrent epithelial ovarian cancer. Gynecol Oncol 1989;34:334–338.

219. Janicke F, Holscher M, Kuhn W, et al: Radical surgery procedure improves survival time in patients with recurrent ovarian cancer. Cancer 1992;70:2129–2136.

220. Vaccarello L, Rubin S, Vlamis V, et al: Cytoreductive surgery in ovarian carcinoma patients with a documented previously complete surgical response. Gynecol Oncol 1995;57:61–65.

221. Lund B, Hansen M, Lundvall F, et al: Intestinal obstruction in patients with advanced carcinoma of the ovaries treated with combination chemotherapy. Surg Gynecol Obstet 1989;169:213–218.

222. Krebs H, Helmkamp F: Management of intestinal obstruction in ovarian cancer. Oncology 1989;3:25–36.

223. Helmkamp B, Kimmel J: Conservative management of small bowel obstruction. Am J Obstet Gynecol 1985;152:677–679.

224. Krebs H, Goplerud D: The role of intestinal intubation in obstruction of the small intestine due to carcinoma of the ovary. Surg Gynecol Obstet 1984;158:467–471.

225. Piver S, Barlow J, Lele S, Frank A: Survival after ovarian cancer induced intestinal obstruction. Gynecol Oncol 1982;13:44–49.

226. Ozols R, Rubin S, Thomas G, et al: Epithelial ovarian cancer. In Hoskins W, Perez C, Young R (eds): Principles and Practice of

Gynecologic Oncology, 3rd ed. Philadelphia, JB Lippincott, 2000, pp 981–1058.

227. Paladine W, Cunningham T, Sponzo R, et al: Intracavitary bleomycin in the management of malignant effusions. Cancer 1976;38:1903–1908.

228. Ostrowski M: An assessment of the long-term results of controlling the reaccumulation of malignant effusions using intracavity bleomycin. Cancer 1986;57:721–727.

229. Souter R, Wells C, Tarin D, Kettlewell M: Surgical and pathologic complications associated with peritoneovenous shunts in management of malignant ascites. Cancer 1985;55:1973–1975.

230. Edney J, Hill A, Armstrong D: Peritoneovenous shunts palliate malignant ascites. Am J Surg 1989;158:598–601.

231. Kerr V, Cadman E: Pulmonary metastases in ovarian cancer. Cancer 1985;56:1209–1213.

232. Johnston N: The malignant pleural effusion: A review of the cytopathologic diagnosis of 584 specimens from 472 consecutive patients. Cancer 1985;56:905–910.

233. O'Neill W, Spurr C, Muss H, et al: A prospective study of chest tube drainage and tetracycline sclerosis versus chest tube drainage in treatment of malignant pleural effusion. Proc ASCO 1980;21:349.

234. Austin E, Flye M: The treatment of recurrent malignant pleural effusion. Ann Thorac Surg 1979;28:190–203.

235. Martini N, Bains M, Beattie E: Indications for pleurectomy in malignant effusion. Cancer 1975;35:734–738.

236. Boutin C, Viallat C, Cargnino P, Farisse P: Thoracoscopy in malignant pleural effusions. Am Rev Respir Dis 1981;124:588–592.

237. Gershenson DM, Malone JM Jr: Chemotherapy for malignant germ cell tumors of the ovary. In Deppe G (ed): Chemotherapy of Gynecologic Cancer, 2nd ed. New York, Wiley-Liss, 1990, pp 217–239.

238. Slayton RE, Park RC, Silverberg SG, et al: Vincristine, dactinomycin and cyclophosphamide in the treatment of malignant germ cell tumors of the ovary: A Gynecologic Oncology Group study, a final report. Cancer 1985;56:243–248.

239. Williams S, Blessing J, Liao S, et al: Adjuvant therapy of ovarian germ cell tumors with cisplatin, etoposide, and bleomycin: A trial of the Gynecologic Oncology Group. J Clin Oncol 1994;12:701.

240. Williams SD, Blessing JA, Moore DH, et al: Cisplatin, vinblastine, and bleomycin in recurrent ovarian germ cell tumors: A trial of the Gynecologic Oncology Group. Ann Intern Med 1989;3:22–27.

241. Sedlis A: Primary carcinoma of the fallopian tube. Obstet Gynecol Surv 1961;16:209.

242. Yoonessi M: Carcinoma of the fallopian tube. Obstet Gynecol Surv 1979;34:257.

243. Schiller HM, Silverberg SG: Staging and prognosis in primary carcinoma of the fallopian tube. Cancer 1971;28:389.

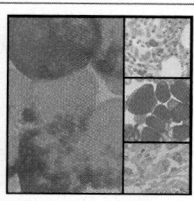

GESTATIONAL TROPHOBLASTIC DISEASE

Donald Peter Goldstein

Ross Stuart Berkowitz

SUMMARY OF KEY POINTS

INCIDENCE

- The incidence of complete hydatidiform mole is approximately 1 in 1500 pregnancies in the United States.
- The incidence of partial hydatidiform mole is approximately 1 in 750.
- Repeat moles occur in 1 in 100 pregnancies, and third moles occur in 1 in 25 pregnancies.

ETIOLOGY/EPIDEMIOLOGY

- Complete hydatidiform mole is usually due to an androgenetic diploid conception, in which a haploid sperm fertilizes an egg lacking female chromosomes.
- A partial hydatidiform mole develops when dispermy occurs and the resulting conceptus is triploidy.

PATHOLOGY/BIOLOGY

- Earlier diagnosis of complete hydatidiform mole due to improved ultrasound and human chorionic gonadotropin assays has made the pathologic diagnosis of complete hydatidiform mole more difficult because of its resemblance to partial hydatidiform mole and nonmolar abortions.
- Hydatidiform mole is characterized by hydropic villi with trophoblastic hyperplasia.
- Invasive mole is characterized by invasion of myometrium by hydropic villi surrounded by hyperplastic trophoblasts.
- Choriocarcinoma is characterized by sheets of neoplastic cyto- and syncytiotrophoblasts invading tissue

and is associated with necrosis and hemorrhage. Hematogenous spread occurs early.
- Placental site trophoblastic tumor is a rare form of choriocarcinoma made up of mononuclear cells from the implantation site that invade myometrium. Placental site trophoblastic tumor metastasizes late and is relatively resistant to chemotherapy.

CLINICAL FINDINGS

- Hydatidiform mole presents in the first trimester with vaginal bleeding.
- Complete hydatidiform mole is usually diagnosed by ultrasound because of the abnormal appearance of the placenta and the absence of a fetus.
- Partial hydatidiform mole could be difficult to diagnose by ultrasound and is usually confirmed pathologically.
- Persistent gestational trophoblastic disease after molar pregnancy is usually nonmetastatic and is characterized by a rising hCG level and persistent bleeding.
- Metastatic gestational trophoblastic disease after hydatidiform mole usually involves the lungs, and more rarely, brain, liver, and other sites.
- The diagnosis of gestational trophoblastic disease after a miscarriage or term pregnancy can be delayed and can present with significant disease.

STAGING/CLASSIFICATION

The 2002 International Federation of Gynecologists and Obstetricians

Staging System combines an anatomic description of the disease (i.e., stages I, II, III, IV) with a prognostic scoring system.

PRIMARY THERAPY

- Single-agent therapy is usually curative in patients with stage I, II, and III disease who have low prognostic scores.
- Patients with stage II, III, and IV disease who have high-risk scores require combination chemotherapy for optimal outcome.
- Survival rates are 100% in patients with stage I, II, and III disease and 80% in patients with stage IV disease.
- Response to therapy and remission is determined by hCG levels, which should be tested weekly during chemotherapy.
- Patients with high-risk disease should be treated with three to four consolidation courses after the hCG titre normalizes.

COMPLICATIONS

- Toxicity from the chemotherapeutic agents is the most common complication.
- Other complications relate to the extent of disease and usually are due to internal bleeding.

PROGNOSIS

- Most women survive their disease and are able to achieve subsequent pregnancy.
- The vast majority of patients are cured and are able to return to normal soon after attaining a normal hCG titre.

INTRODUCTION

Terminology

Gestational trophoblastic disease (GTD) is a biologically unique disease for several reasons:

- It elaborates the tumor marker, human chorionic gonadotropin (hCG).
- It is exquisitely sensitive to chemotherapy.
- It has a unique immunobiological relationship with its host.

GTD is one of the rare human malignancies that can be cured predictably even in the presence of widespread metastases. GTD originates from placental tissue and is made up of a group of interrelated tumors that are classified histologically as complete hydatifiform mole (CHM) and partial hydatidiform mole (PHM), invasive mole (IM), choriocarcinoma (CCA), and placental site trophoblastic tumor (PSTT). The term *gestational trophoblastic neoplasm* (GTN) is used interchangeably because treatment is frequently undertaken without knowledge of the precise histology. We will use this term throughout this chapter when describing those patients who require treatment after any antecedent pregnancy.

It is well recognized that these conditions have varying propensities for local invasion and metastases. When persistent GTN develops after evacuation of an hydatidiform mole (HM), the resulting tumor, histologically speaking, is either an invasive mole, choriocarcinoma, or, on rare occasion, placental site trophoblastic tumor. The tumor that develops after a term pregnancy or miscarriage histologically is choriocarcinoma or placental site trophoblastic tumor, as there is no molar disease in these gestations. When GTN develops after an ectopic pregnancy, it can present histologically as hydatidiform mole, choriocarcinoma, or placental site trophoblastic tumor.

Incidence

The reported incidence of GTD varies significantly in different regions of the world. The frequency of molar pregnancy in Asian countries is seven to ten times greater than the reported incidence in Europe or North America.[1] Japan has a reported incidence of 2 in 1000 pregnancies, which is two- to threefold higher than the incidence in Europe or North America. The incidence of hydatidiform mole in Taiwan is 1 in 125 pregnancies. In Ireland, the incidence of complete and partial moles has been determined to be 1 in 1945 and 1 in 695 pregnancies, respectively.[2] In the United States, hydatidiform moles are observed in 1 in 600 therapeutic abortions and in 1 in 1000 to 1 in 1200 pregnancies.

The overall incidence of invasive mole has been estimated at 1 in 15,000 pregnancies. Approximately 15% to 29% of hydatidiform moles will result in invasive mole. Choriocarcinoma is reported to occur in 1 in 40,000 pregnancies. Approximately 3% to 5% of hydatidiform moles progress to choriocarcinoma, which accounts for almost 50% of cases. Twenty-five percent of choriocarcinoma cases follow abortion or tubal pregnancy (1 in 15,000), and 25% are associated with term pregnancies (1 in 50,000).

Relevant Historical Issues

GTD has an ancient and interesting history going back to Hippocrates, who in 400 B.C. described the passage of hydropic villi from the uterus as "uterine dropsy." The first recorded description of molar pregnancy appeared in *Uterus Hydropii* by Aetius of Amida (483–565 B.C.), who observed that "when the menses have been suppressed for some time and the patient has not become pregnant, the uterus becomes filled with tumor and small bladder-like objects are developed in the fluid." In 1565, Von Grafenburg first described the clinical condition of what we now call a "classical mole." In 1827, Velpeau and Boivin correctly observed that hydatids represented cystic dilatation of chorionic villi. In 1895, Marchand reasoned that choriocarcinoma is an epithelial tumor from the trophoblast.

An important milestone in the history of GTD occurred in 1928, when Ascheim and Zondek first described a reliable pregnancy test, which became the basis for the early measurements of hCG. In 1963, MacVicor and Donald first used ultrasound in the diagnosis of molar pregnancy. Kajii and Ohama[3] in 1977 elucidated the androgenetic origin of hydatidiform moles. Finally, in 1978, Szulman and Surti[4] described the genetic basis for partial mole as a triploid gestation.

Prior to the introduction of chemotherapy, survival with GTN remained limited and precarious, as the only form of treatment consisted of hysterectomy or local excision of metastatic sites where possible. In 1959, Brewer[5] reviewed survival with choriocarcinoma at the Albert Mathieu Chorioepithelioma Registry at Northwestern University. Only 6 of 103 patients with metastatic CCA were free of disease at 5 years after their diagnosis. Their group also analyzed the 5-year survival rates in patients with nonmetastatic CCA treated by hysterectomy. Only 29 of 70 patients (41%) with presumably localized tumor survived despite prompt hysterectomy. The remaining patients developed metastases after the operative procedure and died from widely disseminated disease.

A new era in the management of GTN was inaugurated in 1956, when Li and colleagues[6] reported the complete regression of metastatic CCA in three women treated with methotrexate. In 1961, Hertz and coworkers[7] reported the initial 5-year experience with chemotherapy for metastatic GTN from the National Cancer Institute. Complete remission was achieved with methotrexate in 28 of 63 patients (47%) with metastatic disease. After obtaining dramatic results with chemotherapy in disseminated disease, Hertz and associates[8] successfully employed chemotherapy for nonmetastatic tumors. During the 1960s, it became apparent that certain patients with metastatic GTN were relatively resistant to single-agent chemotherapy and experienced a high mortality rate. In 1965, Ross and colleagues[9] reported that patients with prolonged delay in diagnosis, high hCG levels, and liver and/or brain metastases were resistant to treatment with single-agent therapy. The use subsequent use of intensive combination chemotherapy for so-called high-risk metastatic disease has resulted in substantial improvement in survival.

During the past three decades, the management of GTN has been guided by the results from various regional centers. Virtually all patients with nonmetastatic and low-risk metastatic GTN now can expect to achieve cure with chemotherapy, with preservation of reproductive function in the vast majority of cases. Patients with widespread disease also can anticipate a 70% to 80% survival rate. GTN represents one of the most dramatic successes of chemotherapy in the treatment of human malignancy.

EPIDEMIOLOGY

Although much of the geographic variation in the incidence of molar disease could in fact be due to differences in reporting rather than to true differences in incidence, the high incidence of molar pregnancy in some populations has been attributed to nutritional and socio-economic factors. Acosta-Sisson and Espaniola[10] carefully studied cases of molar pregnancy that were managed at the Philippine General Hospital. Hydatidiform mole was detected infrequently among wealthy Filipino patients. Although molar pregnancy was diagnosed in 1 in 200 pregnancies in indigent patients, molar gestation occurred in only 1 in 2000 pregnancies in the affluent population. In Korea, the incidence of molar pregnancy has shown a considerable and continuing decrease over the past four decades, presumably due in part to changing social conditions, including completion of childbearing at an earlier age and improved nutrition.[11]

Low levels of carotene (vitamin A precursor) and animal fat intake might explain some of the global differences in the incidence of complete mole. We have observed in a case-controlled study that the risk of complete molar pregnancy is associated with low levels of consumption of these nutrients.[12] Parazzini and colleagues[13] also reported from Italy that low carotene consumption was associated with molar pregnancy. Geographic areas with a high incidence of vitamin A deficiency correspond to regions with a high incidence of molar pregnancy.

The risk of having a complete molar pregnancy also increases with increasing maternal age.[1] Women older than age 40 have a 5- to 10-fold greater risk of having a complete molar gestation. Ova from older women could be more susceptible to faulty fertilization and abnormal embryonic development. There does not appear to be any significant association with gravidity or the age of the male consort. The risk for both complete and partial molar pregnancy is increased in women with histories of prior spontaneous abortion and infertility.[14]

Certain epidemiologic features of complete and partial mole differ markedly. Parazzini and coworkers[14] reported that the risk for partial mole was not associated with maternal age. Additionally, the risk for partial mole has been reported to be associated with the use of oral contraceptives and a history of irregular menstruation, but not with dietary factors.[15] Therefore, the risk of partial mole appears to be associated with reproductive history rather than dietary factors.

ETIOLOGY AND PATHOGENESIS

Our perspectives on the etiology and pathogenesis of hydatidiform mole and GTN have become focused significantly over the past few years. The etiology of HM appears to be due to abnormal gametogenesis and fertilization. Recent studies have defined two different forms of HM: partial and complete. They are distinct cytogenetic processes with characteristic clinical and histopathologic findings and do not represent a transition from normal to molar gestation.

Partial hydatidiform moles usually have a triploid karyotype (69 chromosomes) derived from two paternal and one maternal haploid sets of chromosomes. Most have a 69,XXX or 69,XXY genotype derived from a haploid ovum with dispermic fertilization. Lawler and coworkers[16] and Lage and associates[17] reported that 93% and 90%, respectively, of partial moles were triploid. More recent data from our institution presents convincing evidence that all partial moles are triploid. Genest and colleagues[18] reviewed 19 presumed nontriploid partial moles using standardized histologic diagnostic criteria and repeat flow cytometry; on re-evaluation, none of these cases was convincingly a nontriploid partial mole. This finding suggests that nontriploid partial moles might not exist. When a fetus is present in conjunction with a partial mole, it generally exhibits the stigmata of triploidy, including growth retardation and multiple congenital anomalies such as syndactyly, hydrocephaly, omphalocoele, and hare lip (Fig. 93-1).

Complete hydatidiform mole, in contrast, usually has a chromosomal complement totally derived from the paternal genome, while the maternal chromosomes are either inactivated or absent. The 46,XX genotype is most common, representing in most cases reduplication of the haploid genome of one sperm. A smaller portion of complete moles have 46,XY karyotype, consistent with dispermic fertilization. It appears that molar disease, both

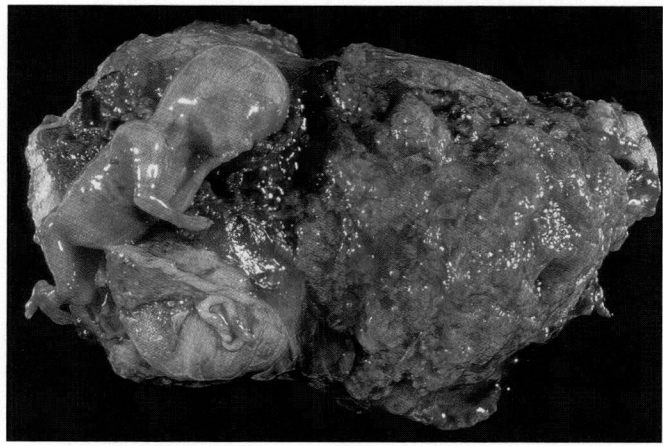

Figure 93-1. Fetus of partial molar pregnancy showing characteristic malformations, including omphalocele, syndactyly, and hare lip deformity.

partial and complete, is associated with excess male genetic composition due to an abnormality of the egg, which is either devoid of maternal chromosomal material or allows for dispermy.

Several growth factors and oncogenes have been studied in molar tissues and CCA.[19] Increased expression of p53 and c-fms has been observed in CHM, and increased ras and c-myc RNAS have been measured in CCA.[20,21] Fulop and associates[22] have investigated the expression of various growth factors and oncogenes in normal placenta, complete and partial mole, and CCA. CHM and CCA were characterized by overexpression of c-myc, c-erb B-2, and bcl-2, and these oncoproteins could be important in the pathogenesis of GTN. Expression of c-fms protein did not differ between normal placenta and GTN. CHM and CCA were also characterized by increased expression of p53, p21, Rb, and MdM2. The p53 gene was studied to detect any mutation in 22 complete moles and 11 choriocarcinomas that had increased expression of p53. Because only one nonsense mutation in p53 was detected by polymerase chain-reaction analysis, it is likely that the overexpressed p53 protein was the wild type. Although studies have identified increased expression of several growth factors in GTN, the precise molecular pathogenesis has not been determined. It was observed that the level of expression of epidermal growth factor receptor (EGFR) in CCA and the syncytio- and cyto-trophoblast of complete mole was significantly greater than the expression of EGFR in syncytio- and cytotrophoblast of placenta and partial mole.[23] This observation was consistent in both immunohistochemic and in situ hybridization studies. In complete mole, strong expression of EGFR and c-erbB-3 in the extravillous trophoblasts was significantly associated with the development of postmolar tumor. The EGFR-related family of oncogenes might be important in the pathogenesis of GTN.

Extracellular proteinases such as matrix metallo-proteinases (MMPs) are thought to be important in modulating both cell-matrix interactions and the degradation of the basement membrane necessary for invasion and metastases. CCA exhibits significantly stronger expression of MMP-1 and MMP-2 and decreased expression of tissue inhibitor of MMP-1 (TIMP-1) than the syncytiotrophoblast of complete and partial mole and normal placenta.[24] The increased expression of MMP-1 and MMP-2 and decreased expression of TIMP-1 in CCA could contribute to the invasiveness of CCA cells.

Certain genes are expressed normally on either the maternal or paternal allele, and this occurrence is described as parental imprinting. Modification of parental imprinting has been associated with tumor formation; both complete moles and CCA have relaxation of parental imprinting.[25] Relaxation of parental imprinting could be important in the pathogenesis of GTN.

PATHOLOGY

Hydatidiform moles may be categorized as either complete or partial based on gross morphology, histopathology, and karyotype (Table 93-1).

TABLE 93-1

Features of Complete and Partial Moles

FEATURE	COMPLETE MOLE	PARTIAL MOLE
Fetal or embryonic tissue	Absent	Present
Hydropic villi	Diffuse	Focal
Trophoblast hyperplasia	Diffuse	Focal
Scalloping of chorionic villi	Absent	Present
Trophoblastic stromal inclusions	Absent	Present
Karyotype	46,XX; 46,XY	69,XXY;69,XYY

Complete Hydatidiform Mole

Complete hydatidiforme mole (CHM) is a pregnancy characterized by vesicular swelling of placental villi and the absence of an intact fetus. Microscopically, there is proliferation of the trophoblast (both cyto- and syncytio-trophoblast) with varying degrees of hyperplasia and dysplasia (Fig. 93-2). The chorionic villi are fluid-filled and distended, and blood vessels are absent or scant. Complete mole undergoes early and total hydatidiform enlargement of the villi in the absence of a fetus or embryo, and the trophoblastic cells are hyperplastic.

The pathologic features of complete molar pregnancy have changed significantly over the past two decades due to earlier diagnosis and uterine evacuation.[26] Whereas cavitation and circumferential trophoblastic proliferation were present in three quarters of complete moles in the past, these findings are now present in fewer than half the cases. Mosher and coworkers[27] compared pathologic findings of 23 current complete moles (1994 through 1997; mean gestational age, 8.5 weeks) with 20 past complete moles (1969 through 1975; mean gestational age, 17 weeks). Histologically, complete moles now encountered have smaller mean maximal villous diameter (5.7 mm vs. 8.2 mm), less circumferential trophoblastic hyperplasia (39% vs. 75%), more primitive villous stroma (70% vs. 10%), and less global necrosis (22% vs. 54%). Keep

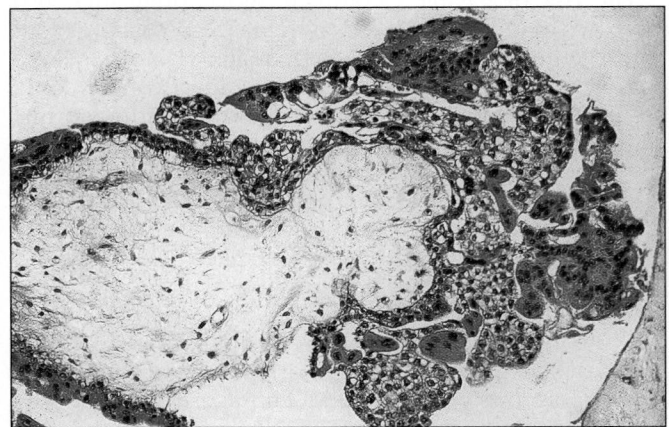

Figure 93-2. Photomicrograph of complete hydatidiform mole showing diffusely hydropic chorionic villi and diffuse trophoblastic hyperplasia. Embryonic tissue is not present.

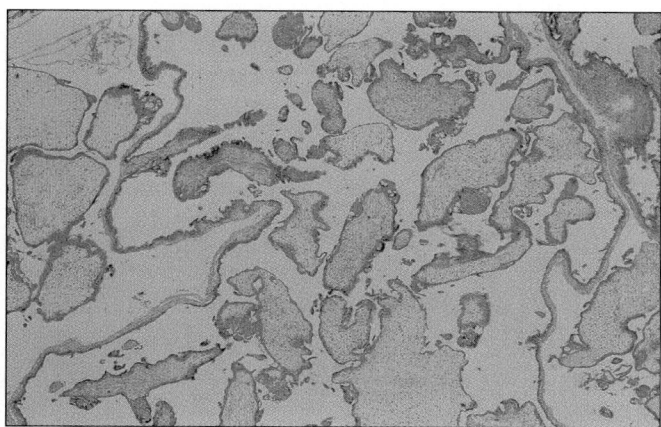

Figure 93-3. Photomicrograph of partial hydatidifrom mole showing varying-sized chorionic villi with focal trophoblastic hyperplasia, stromal trophoblastic inclusions, and villous scalloping. Fetal tissue is present.

and coworkers[28] observed that early complete moles were characterized by focal trophoblastic hyperplasia, minimal villous cavitation, and hypercellular primitive stroma. Complete moles are now often characterized by subtle morphologic alterations that could result in their misclassification as partial moles or nonmolar hydropic abortions. DNA ploidy studies or karyotyping are useful adjuncts in these circumstances.[18]

Partial Hydatidiform Mole

Partial hydatidiform mole (PHM) is characterized by the following pathologic features:

- Varying-sized chorionic villi with focal swelling and focal trophoblastic hyperplasia.
- Focal, mild atypia of implantation-site trophoblast.
- Marked villous scalloping and prominent stromal trophoblastic inclusions.
- Identifiable fetal or embryonic tissues (Fig. 93-3).

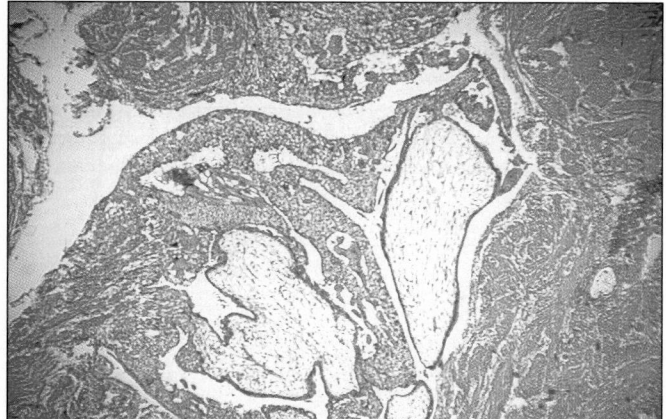

Figure 93-4. Invasive mole with hydropic villous and hyperplastic trophoblast invading myometrium.

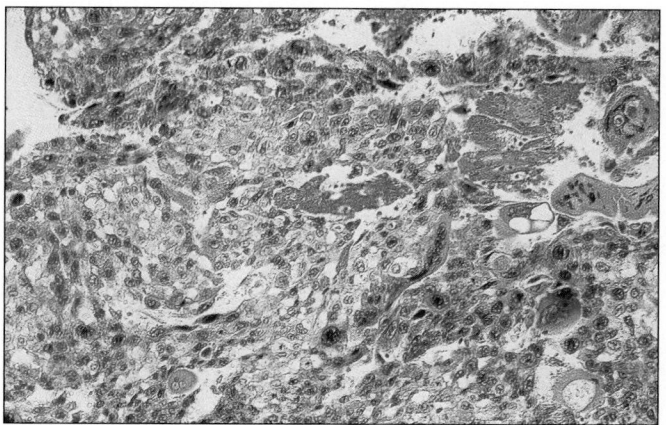

Figure 93-5. Photmicrograph of choriocarcinoma showing sheets of anaplastic cyto- and syncytiotrophoblasts.

Invasive Mole

Invasive mole is a tumor arising from a hydatidiform mole that invades the myometrium by direct extension or by venous channels. It also metastasizes to distant sites in about 15% of cases, most commonly to the lungs and vagina. The tumor is characterized by swollen placental villi and accompanying hyperplastic trophoblast, which is usually dysplastic when located in sites outside the uterine cavity (Fig. 93-4).

Choriocarcinoma

Choriocarinoma is a highly malignant tumor characterized by abnormal trophoblastic hyperplasia and anaplasia, absence of chorionic villi, hemorrhage, and necrosis (Fig. 93-5). It can invade the uterine wall directly or metastasize by vascular channels to the myometrium and distant sites, most commonly to the lungs, vagina, brain, liver, spleen, kidneys, and intestines.

Placental Site Trophoblastic Tumor

Placental site trophoblastic tumor (PSTT) is an extremely rare tumor that arises from the placental implantation site and is monocellular. Tumor cells infiltrate the myometrium and grow between smooth muscle cells with vascular invasion (Fig. 93-6). PSTT differs from CCA primarily in the absence of an alternating pattern of cyto- and syncytiotrophoblast, in that the cells are morphologically of one population (intermediate trophoblast), and in that hemorrhage and necrosis are less evident. There are no placental villi. Human placental lactogen is present in the tumor cells, whereas immunoperoxidase staining for hCG is positive in only scattered cells. Serum hCG levels are relatively low compared with those seen in CCA. There appears to be a direct correlation between the mitotic activity of the tumor and the prognosis.[29]

IMMUNOBIOLOGY

The remarkable curability of GTN might be attributable partly to a host immunologic response to paternal

Specific Malignancies

III

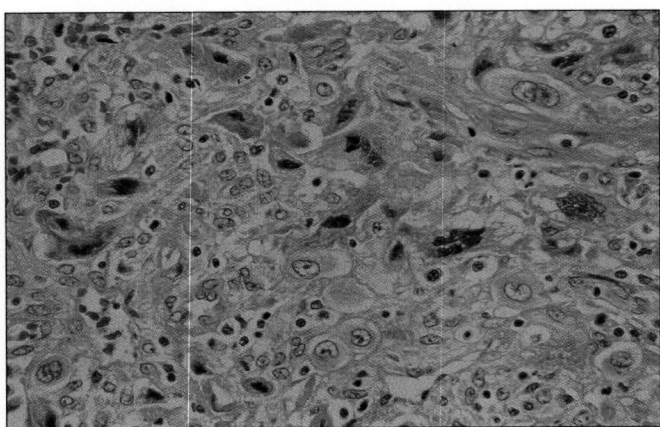

Figure 93-6. Photomicrograph of placental site trophoblastic tumor composed almost entirely of mononuclear cells of the intermediate trophoblast.

antigens expressed on trophoblastic cells.[30] The prognosis of patients with gestational CCA has been related to the intensity of lymphocytic and monocytic infiltration at the tumor-host interface.[31] Because the lymphocytes and macrophages that infiltrate gestational CCA are probably exposed to paternal antigens and oncoproteins, the immune cells could become activated. Immunologically active cells might promote the regression of GTN through their release of cytokines. Cytokines have been reported to inhibit the proliferation of CCA cells in vitro and to increase the HLA expression of CCA cells in vitro, thereby increasing immunogenicity.[32]

It has been theorized that the development and progression of GTN could be favored by histocompatibility between the patient and her partner. If the patient and her partner are histocompatible, the trophoblastic tumor that bears paternal antigens might not be immunogenic in the maternal host. The intensity of the host's immunologic response might depend on the immunogenicity of the trophoblastic tumor. On the other hand, histocompatibility between the patient and her partner does not appear to be a prerequisite for the development of persistent GTN.[33] HLA systems could, however, influence the clinical course of rapidly progressive and fatal GTN. Tomoda and colleagues[34] reported that drug-resistant CCA was associated with increased histocompatibility between the patient and her partner. Similarly, Morgenson and coworkers[35] observed that histocompatibility between patients and partners was associated with a greater risk of metastatic disease. Because all chromosomes in a CHM are paternal in origin, a CHM is a complete allograft and could stimulate a vigorous immune response by the maternal host. There is evidence for both a cellular and a humoral response to CHM. When compared with normal placentas, molar implantation sites have fivefold increase infiltration by helper T cells.[36] Circulating immune complexes have also been measured in patients with CHM and have been noted to increase as the patient entered remission.[37]

Circulating immune complexes in patients with CHM have been demonstrated to contain paternal HLA

antigens.[38] The maternal host with a CHM is therefore sensitized to paternal HLA antigens. The distribution of HLA antigens in molar chorionic villi has been determined by immunofluorescent assays.[39] HLA A, B, C antigens were detected on the stromal cells of molar chorionic villi but not on the villous trophoblast; however, the molar villous fluid that bathes the stromal cells does not contain soluble HLA antigen.[32] The maternal host could therefore be sensitized to paternal HLA antigen when the villous trophoblastic layer is disrupted and HLA-positive villous stromal cells are released into the circulation.

CLINICAL PRESENTATION

Complete Molar Pregnancy

The clinical presentation of CHM has changed dramatically over the past two decades in the wake of the widespread use of ultrasound and the availability of improved methods for hCG testing. Whereas CHM was usually diagnosed in the second trimester prior to 1980, the diagnosis of CHM is now usually made in the first trimester, before the classic clinical signs and symptoms appear. Table 93-2 summarizes the signs and symptoms of classical CHM and PHM. When patients with CHM present with these classical signs and symptoms, they are at high risk for developing GTN. Soto-Wright and associates[26] compared the clinical presentation and outcome of patients with CHM at the New England Trophoblastic Disease Center (NETDC) between 1988 and 1993 with those of patients between 1965 and 1975. Despite the change in presentation, there was no change in the incidence of GTN disease requiring treatment.

Vaginal Bleeding

Vaginal bleeding was the most common presenting symptom in patients with CHM, occurring in 89% to 97% of cases. Bleeding varied from bright red to dark and from heavy to light flow. Molar chorionic villi may separate from the decidua and disrupt vessels, leading to the distension of the endometrial cavity by large volumes of retained blood. Retained blood can undergo oxidation and lead to the prune juice–like fluid that is pathognomonic of this condition. The amount of blood loss can be

TABLE 93-2

Presenting Signs and Symptoms of Classical Complete and Partial Hydatidiform Moles		
SIGN	**COMPLETE MOLE**	**PARTIAL MOLE**
	N=306 (%)	**N=81 (%)**
Vaginal bleeding	97	73
Excessive uterine size	51	4
Theca lutein cysts >6 cm	50	0
Pre-eclampsia	27	3
Hyperemesis	26	0
Hyperthyroidism	7	0
Trophoblastic emboli	2	0

considerable, resulting in anemia (hemoglobin <10 g/100 mL). Vaginal bleeding continues to be the most common presenting symptom, occurring in 84% of our current patients; however, anemia is seen in only 5% of our current patients.

Theca Lutein Cysts

The reported frequency of theca lutein cysts (TLC) depends on the method of diagnosis. Ultrasonically, TLC greater than 5 cm in diameter were detected in 46% of 50 patients with CHM, whereas clinical examination detected TLC in only 26%.[40,41] Although TLC are generally 6 to 12 cm in diameter, they can enlarge considerably to more than 20 cm in size after molar evacuation and can cause significant symptoms, including abdominal pain, swelling, and respiratory difficulties. They are usually multicystic and bilateral and contain serosanguinous or amber-colored fluid (Fig. 93-7). TLC usually develop in patients with very high serum hCG levels and result from hyperstimulation of the ovaries.

Other signs of ovarian hyperstimulation may also be encountered, including ascites and pleural effusion. TLC generally resolve slowly over an interval of 8 to 12 weeks in concert with regressing hCG levels.

The most common complications of TLC are torsion or rupture. Kohorn[42] reported that 3 of 127 patients with CHM developed torsion. Similarly, Montz and coworkers[41] noted that only 2 of 102 patients with TLC developed torsion or rupture. If patients develop severe symptoms of pelvic or abdominal pressure, pain, or respiratory compromise, TLC may be decompressed by ultrasound-guided or laparoscopic aspiration. Similarly, ovarian rupture or torsion may also be managed by laparoscopy. TLC are encountered rarely today because of earlier diagnosis and lower hCG levels.

Excessive Uterine Size

In the classic mole, uterine size was excessively enlarged in 35% to 50% of patients. Uterine size is related to the amount of retained blood and the extent of trophoblastic

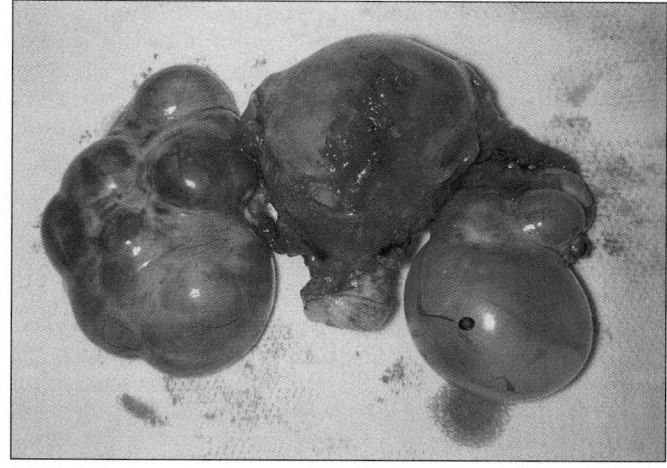

Figure 93-7. Theca lutein cysts associated with complete hydatidiform mole with high hCG levels.

proliferation. Excessive uterine enlargement is usually associated with serum hCG levels in excess of 100,000 mIU/mL. Currently, because of earlier diagnosis, excessive uterine size is seen at the NETDC in only 28% of patients.

High Serum hCG Levels

Serum hCG levels greater than 100,000 mIU/mL are usually encountered when the uterus is larger than dates. It is important to remember that levels of hCG of this magnitude can also occur in normal pregnancy at 10 to 12 weeks and in multiple gestation.

Hyperemesis Gravidarum

Hyperemesis requiring antiemetic therapy was formerly seen in 20% to 26% of patients with CHM. This symptom was usually associated with excessive uterine enlargement and high hCG levels. It is generally believed that high estrogen levels are the main cause. Only 8% of our current patients present with hyperemesis.

Pre-eclampsia

Pre-eclampsia was a complication of CHM in 12% to 27% of patients. It developed almost exclusively in patients with excessive uterine size and high hCG levels. When pre-eclampsia developed in the second trimester, it was considered to be pathognomonic of complete molar gestation. It is interesting that eclamptic convulsions were rarely observed. In contrast, between 1988 and 1993, only 1 of 74 patients with CHM presented at the NETDC with pre-eclampsia.

Hyperthyroidism

Patients with CHM whose hCG levels are greater than 100,000 mIU/mL are more likely to be hyperthyroid. There is conflicting data as to the cause of the hyperthyroid state, but it is now generally believed that that hCG has intrinsic thyrotropin activity.[43] Patients with poorly controlled or untreated hyperthyroidism may develop thyroid storm at the time of anesthesia induction and evacuation. Thyroid storm is characterized by hyperthermia, delirium, coma, atrial fibrillation, and eventual cardiovascular collapse. As a precautionary measure, it is recommended that beta-blocking agents be administered before evacuation in patients whose hCG levels exceed 100,000 mIU/mL or where there is chemical evidence of elevated total T_4 and T_3. Hyperthyroidism is rarely encountered in our current patients.

Respiratory Insufficiency

Acute respiratory insufficiency was encountered in 2% of patients with CHM in the earlier series. This complication occurred almost exclusively in patients with high hCG levels and excessive uterine size, the same group of patients who are at risk of developing pre-eclampsia and hyperthyroidism. This complication is virtually never encountered currently due to earlier diagnosis.

Respiratory insufficiency presents with anxiety, dyspnea, tachynea, hemoptysis, and tachycardia, in most cases immediately after molar evacuation. Pulmonary insufficiency can be due to many causes, including trophoblastic embolization, cardiovascular complications of

Specific Malignancies

III

thyroid storm, pre-eclampsia, and massive fluid replacement. Chest x-rays generally show bilateral pulmonary infiltrates that typically clear spontaneously, usually in 72 to 96 hours. Auscultation of the chest reveals diffuse rales. Arterial blood gases usually show hypoxia and respiratory alkalosis. Because this condition is self-limiting, treatment is supportive and consists of appropriate cardiovascular and respiratory measures. On rare occasions, it could be necessary to place patients on mechanical ventilation in anticipation of recovery.

Partial Molar Pregnancy

Patients with partial molar pregnancy typically present with symptoms indistinguishable from those of a threatened or spontaneous miscarriage (rather than with the classical symptoms of CHM), unless diagnosis is delayed until the second trimester. Eighty-one patients with PHM were studied at the NETDC between 1979 and 1984.[44] Vaginal bleeding tends to be less intense than in CHM, and anemia is rare. Excessive uterine size and pre-eclampsia were detected in only three and two patients, respectively. Szulman and Surti[45] and Czernobilsky and coworkers[46] reported that only 11% of 81 and 8% of 25 patients with PHM, respectively, had excessive uterine enlargement. Pre-eclampsia occurred in only 4% in both studies. Furthermore, none of our patients exhibited prominent theca lutein cyst, hyperthyroidism, or hyperemesis. The diagnosis of PHM is usually suggested by ultrasonography and confirmed by pathologic review of curettage material. hCG levels in patients with PHM are usually not as elevated as in those with CHM. When PHM progresses into the second trimester, the ultrasound diagnosis becomes more accurate because of the obvious fetal malformations associated with triploidy and the extent of vesicular change of the placenta. These patients with PHM whose diagnosis is delayed until the second trimester will, in many instances, recapitulate the classical signs and symptoms associated with CHM with regard to the incidence of pre-eclampsia, hyperthyroidism, trophoblastic embolization, and other complications.

Gestational Trophoblastic Neoplasm

Gestational trophoblastic neoplasm is the term used when there is clinical, radiologic, pathologic, and/or hormonal evidence of persistent gestational trophoblastic disease, which can follow any type of antecedent pregnancy. Rarely, the antecedent pregnancy cannot be determined. Postmolar GTN is diagnosed by a plateau in the level of hCG over at least 3 consecutive weeks, a 10% or greater rise in hCG for three or more values over at least 2 weeks, persistence of hCG 6 months after molar evacuation, or histologic evidence of invasive mole, CCA, or PSTT. GTN comprises two distinct disease entities—nonmetastatic or metastatic—based on whether there is evidence of disease beyond the uterus.

Nonmetastatic GTN

Nonmetastatic or locally invasive GTN develops in about 15% of patients after molar evacuation and infrequently

---

MOLAR PREGNANCY

The advent of transvaginal ultrasound and sensitive hCG assays has made it possible for clinicians to diagnose molar pregnancy at an earlier gestational age. This has led to a significant decrease in the incidence of associated medical complications. Despite earlier diagnosis, however, the incidence of persistent gestational trophoblastic neoplasm after complete hydatidiform mole has not changed. Therefore, careful hCG monitoring after molar evacuation is essential for the early detection and successful management of persistent gestational trophoblastic neoplasm.

PERSISTENT GESTATIONAL TROPHOBLASTIC NEOPLASM
The diagnosis of persistent gestational trophoblastic neoplasm is made by detecting an inappropriate level of hCG after any type of antecedent pregnancy. Prompt intervention is the key to reduced morbidity and mortality. Appropriate metastatic work-up should be undertaken, and appropriate stage and prognostic scores should be assigned to the patient so that optimal therapy can be initiated with well-established treatment protocols. Patients with unusual presentation or high-risk factors should either be referred to or be treated in collaboration with a referral center.

FUTURE REPRODUCTIVE FUNCTION
Patients with either a molar pregnancy or gestational trophoblastic neoplasm can be reassured that their reproductive function can be preserved despite the use of potent chemotherapeutic agents. Although the risk of subsequent molar gestation is increased, other abnormalities of pregnancy do not seem to be a problem. After a later pregnancy, hCG testing after a delivery or miscarriage is advised to detect the rare case of choriocarcinoma.

---

following other pregnancies. These patients usually present with irregular vaginal bleeding, theca lutein cyst, uterine subinvolution or asymmetrical enlargement, and elevated hCG levels. The tumor can erode into uterine vessels causing vaginal bleeding, or it can perforate through the myometrium producing intraperitoneal hemorrhage. The presence of bulky necrotic tumors that is characteristic of CCA can serve as a nidus for sepsis, particularly *Clostridium welchii*. The presence of deep myometrial invasion can be confirmed by curettage, laparoscopy, or imaging studies such as ultrasound, magnetic resonance imaging (MRI), or angiography.

Metastatic GTN
Metastatic GTN occurs in approximately 5% of patients after molar evacuation and infrequently after other gestations. Although invasive mole can metastasize to distant sites, most metastatic GTN is generally associated with CCA, which has the propensity for early vascular invasion and widespread dissemination. Because trophoblastic tumors are highly vascular, metastatic lesions often present with signs and symptoms of spontaneous bleeding. The most common metastatic sites are the lung (80%), vagina (30%), brain (10%), and liver (10%). As a general rule, cerebral and hepatic metastases are un-

common unless there is concurrent involvement of the lungs and/or vagina.

Pulmonary Metastases. The pulmonary parenchyma is the most common site of metastasis. Eighty percent of patients with metastatic disease have lung involvement. Patients with pulmonary involvement can present with cough, chest pain, hemoptysis, and/or dyspnea or an asymptomatic lesion on chest x-ray. Respiratory symptoms can have an acute onset or be chronic. Pulmonary involvement produces four principle radiologic patterns:

1. Discrete rounded densities.
2. "Snowstorm" or alveolar pattern.
3. Embolic pattern resulting from pulmonary artery occlusion.
4. Pleural effusion.

Patients can develop pulmonary hypertension in the absence of substantial parenchymal involvement. Because the respiratory symptoms and radiographic findings can be striking, the patients may be thought to have a primary pulmonary disease. Unfortunately, the diagnosis of GTN might be made only after thoracotomy is performed. Therefore, it is important to obtain an hCG level in all women of reproductive age who have unexplained respiratory symptoms or a lesion on chest x-ray. Gynecologic symptoms could be minimal or absent in patients with extensive pulmonary involvement. In fact, the reproductive organs could be free of trophoblastic tumor in patients with widespread metastases. Early respiratory failure requiring mechanical ventilation can develop in patients with extensive pulmonary involvement. Kelly and associates[47] and Bakri and colleagues[48] reported 100% mortality in 11 and 8 patients, respectively, with early respiratory failure. Vaccarello and coworkers,[49] however, reported one patient who was cured after mechanical ventilation for respiratory failure. Risk factors for early respiratory failure within 1 month of presentation include greater than 50% lung opacification, dyspnea, anemia, cyanosis, and pulmonary hypertension. With chemotherapy, patients could develop bleeding into metastatic sites and potentially worsen pulmonary symptoms and radiologic findings. Kelly and associates[47] observed that reducing the initial dose of chemotherapy did not protect against early respiratory failure and recommended administering intensive chemotherapy at the outset.

Vaginal Metastases. Thirty percent of patients with metastatic disease have vaginal involvement. Vaginal metastases occur most commonly suburethrally or in the fornices and cause purulent discharge or irregular bleeding (Fig. 93-8). Vaginal lesions are highly vascular and can bleed vigorously if biopsied. Surgical excision of a vaginal metastasis should be avoided, except in unusual circumstances, due to the risk of hemorrhage that could be difficult to control. We have observed that after instituting chemotherapy when some tumor shrinkage has occurred, the vaginal lesion can be excised with less risk.

Hepatic Metastases. Choriocarcinoma involves the liver in 10% of patients who develop disseminated disease.

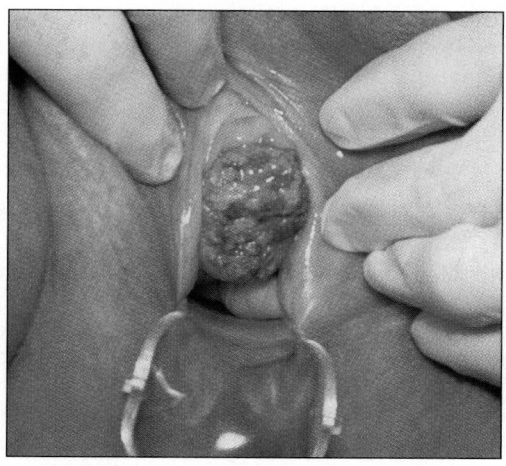

Figure 93-8. Vaginal metastasis of choriocarcinoma.

Hepatic metastases are encountered almost exclusively in patients who have extensive tumor burdens and prolonged delays in diagnosis. Hepatic lesions can cause liver rupture with exsanguinating intraperitoneal hemorrhage; however, patients with liver metastases usually do not present with symptoms that are related to hepatic involvement. Bakri and colleagues[50] noted that only 5 of 19 patients (26%) presented with jaundice, intra-abdominal bleeding, or epigastric pain.

Brain Metastases. Cerebral lesions also occur in approximately 10% of patients with metastatic GTN. Cerebral involvement is usually seen in patients with advanced disease and histologically is almost always related to CCA. The main presenting symptoms of brain metastases are headache, vomiting, seizures, and focal neurologic signs such as slurred speech, hemiparesis, or visual disturbances.

Neurologic symptoms usually result from increased intracranial pressure or intracerebral bleeding. Bakri and associates[51] and Athanassiou and colleagues[52] reported that 20 of 23 patients (87%) and 66 of 69 patients (96%), respectively, with brain involvement had neurologic complaints. Furthermore, Liu and coworkers[53] reported that all 34 patients with brain metastases presented with neurologic symptoms.

Cerebral lesions are associated with elevated levels of hCG in the cerebrospinal fluid (CSF). Bagshawe and Harland[54] reported that the plasma-to-CSF hCG ratio was less than 60 in patients with cerebral involvement; however, a single plasma-to-CSF hCG ratio can be misleading because rapid changes in the hCG levels in the serum might not be reflected promptly in the CSF.[55] With earlier diagnosis of GTN and the advent of improved imaging techniques (particularly MRI), occult brain metastases are now frequently being detected before patients present with neurologic symptoms.

Other Metastatic Sites. Gastrointestinal, renal, and splenic metastases are seen only in patients with advanced disease, most commonly in patients with post-term CCA, where there has been a delay in diagnosis. Abdominal computed tomography (CT) scanning is useful for the early detection of metastases to these sites. Testing for hematochezia should also be part of the work-up in any patient who presents with metastatic GTN.

LABORATORY AND IMAGING STUDIES

The optimal management of GTN requires a thorough evaluation of the extent of the disease prior to treatment. All patients with persistent disease should undergo a thorough pretreatment evaluation, to include a complete history and physical examination, baseline levels of peripheral blood and platelet counts, hCG titer, hepatic, thyroid and renal function tests, and stool guiac tests. A pelvic sonogram is helpful in detecting adnexal involvement, the presence of residual tissue in the uterine cavity, or the presence of deep myometrial invasion. A baseline chest x-ray should be performed in all patients at the time of molar evacuation to identify pre-existing pulmonary disease that might be misinterpreted if the patient were to develop postmolar GTN. Asymptomatic patients with a normal pelvic examination or sonogram and chest x-ray are very unlikely to have liver or brain metastases. Patients with vaginal or lung metastases and/or an histologic diagnosis of CCA, however, should undergo CT scans of the chest and abdomen and MRI scanning of the brain because they are more likely to have distant metastases.

hCG Measurement

A reliable assay for total hCG is central to the management of patients with trophoblastic disease. The assay must measure all portions of the hCG molecule, particularly free beta subunit, nicked hCG, and hyperglycosylated hCG.[56] Several commercial assays do not measure free beta subunit or nicked hCG and do not differentially recognize hyperglycosylated hCG. Practically speaking, however, the available clinical assays for β-hCG are adequate in the vast majority of patients for diagnosis, monitoring therapy, and follow-up to ensure that the patient remains in complete gonadotropin remission. Physicians treating patients with GTN, however, must recognize the limitations of the assay they are using and base clinical decisions on the clinical, morphologic, and radiologic findings, as well as on hormonal results.

Patients with CHM commonly have markedly elevated pre-evacuation hCG levels. Genest and coworkers[57] noted that 46% of 153 patients with CHM managed at the NETDC between 1980 and 1990 had pre-evacuation hCG levels above 100,000 mIU/mL. Patients with PHM less commonly present with markedly elevated hCG values. Czernobilsky and associates[46] reported that only 1 of 17 patients with PHM presented with urinary hCG levels above 300,000 mIU/mL. Review of our own data at the NETDC noted that only 2 of 30 patients with PHM presented with levels greater than 100,000 mIU/mL.[44]

Complete and partial moles also differ in their levels of free beta and alpha subunits of hCG. Whereas complete moles have higher percentages of free beta hCG, partial moles have higher levels of free alpha hCG.[58] The mean ratios of percentage free beta to percentage free alpha hCG in complete and partial mole are 20.9 and 2.4, respectively.

Ultrasonography

Sonographic examination of the first-trimester uterus, particularly when combined with transvaginal color Doppler flow, has made possible the detection of abnormalities of early pregnancy. The diagnosis of molar pregnancy is nearly always made by sonography except in very early pregnancy. The indications for ultrasound in pregnant patients when molar disease or GTN is suspected include the following:

- First-trimester bleeding
- The appearance of signs and symptoms of molar pregnancy
- Unusually high hCG levels

The ultrasonographic appearance of CHM does not vary considerably between the first and second trimester. At either stage, complex, echogenic masses with multiple small cystic spaces are visible within the uterus, and no fetus is identifiable (Fig. 93-9).

Two sonographic features have been described that are significantly associated with PHM: focal cystic changes in the placenta and a ratio of the transverse-to-anteroposterior dimension of the gestational sac greater than 1.5.[59] Changes in the shape of the gestational sac could be part of the embryopathy of triploidy. On rare occasions, particularly when PHM has progressed into the late first or early second trimester, the sonogram will show the presence of a fetus with multiple congenital abnormalities associated with a focally hydropic placenta, oligohydramnios, and abnormal placental Doppler flow pattern. These changes might not be visible in the first trimester.

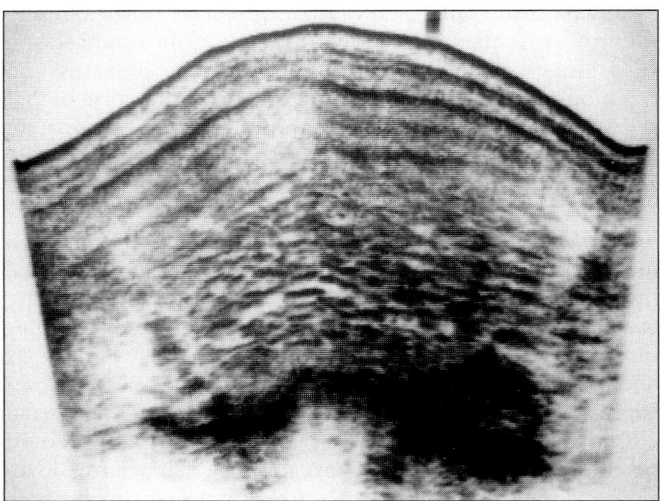

Figure 93-9. Ultrasound of complete hydatidiform mole characterized by absence of fetus and amniotic sac and presence of "Swiss cheese" pattern representing hydropic villi surrounded by blood and hyperplastic trophoblast.

Ultrasound is also used after molar evacuation when there is abnormal bleeding or a rising hCG level, to determine whether there is sufficient residual tissue in the uterine cavity to justify another evacuation or whether there is evidence of invasive disease or adnexal involvement. Ultrasonography can help the clinician select patients who will benefit from hysterectomy because it can detect accurately the presence of extensive uterine trophoblastic tumor.

Ultrasonography is also useful in monitoring the progress of theca lutein cyst regression and aids in decompression when the cysts cause symptoms such as pain and difficult respiration.

Computed Tomography and Magnetic Resonance Imaging

When a patient develops persistent GTN, the current standard of care is to obtain a CT scan of the chest rather than a plain radiographic film to look for metastatic lesions, particularly for those patients who are thought to have nonmetastatic disease and who are likely candidates for primary surgical treatment. The findings of occult metastatic disease on chest CT scan would mandate that chemotherapy be included in the treatment protocol. Because it is unusual for metastatic sites other than the vagina or pelvis to be involved in the absence of pulmonary metastases, a full metastatic work-up is usually not indicated unless lung involvement is observed. When a chest CT is positive, metastatic work-up should consist of an abdominal CT scan to detect liver, renal, splenic, and gastrointestinal involvement, and a CT or MRI scan of the head. These new radiologic techniques for brain imaging have greatly enhanced our ability to diagnose asymptomatic cerebral lesions, which allows for earlier intervention before irreversible neurologic changes occur.

STAGING/CLASSIFICATION

Three staging/classification systems are in use for evaluating patients with persistent GTN. Classification helps clinicians estimate prognosis and select optimal therapy, and it can be used as a basis for comparison of results among multiple treatment centers.

National Institutes of Health Clinical Classification

The National Institutes of Health (NIH) Clinical Classification separates patients with nonmetastatic disease from those with metastases because virtually all patients with nonmetastatic disease can be cured with single-agent chemotherapy or hysterectomy (Table 93-3).[60] Patients with metastatic disease are further subdivided into low-risk and high-risk disease categories based on five risk factors. "Risk" in this context refers to the likelihood that the patient will develop drug resistance and ultimately die of her disease. Patients are classified as being at "high risk" based on the presence of one or more of the following:

TABLE 93-3

NIH Clinical Classification of GTN

Nonmetastatic

Metastatic

Good prognosis
  Duration of disease <4 months from antecedent pregnancy or onset of symptoms
  Pretreatment serum hCG level <40,000 mIU/mL
  No prior chemotherapy
  No evidence of brain and/or liver metastases
  Antecedent pregnancy not term
Poor prognosis
  Duration of disease >4 months from antecedent pregnancy or onset of symptoms
  Pretreatment serum hCG level >40,000 mIU/mL
  Prior chemotherapeutic failure
  Evidence of brain and/or liver metastases
  Antecedent pregnancy term

- Pretreatment serum hCG level in excess of 40,000 mIU/mL.
- Duration of disease longer than 4 months from the antecedent pregnancy event, or from onset of symptoms to treatment if the antecedent pregnancy is not known.
- Metastases to sites other than the lungs or vagina.
- Antecedent term pregnancy.
- Prior unsuccessful chemotherapy.

International Federation of Gynecologists and Obstetricians Staging

The first anatomic staging system for GTN, adopted by the Cancer Committee of the International Federation of Gynecologists and Obstetricians (FIGO) in 1982 and modified in 1992, was based on material presented by Dr. H.C. Sung at a meeting of the International Society for the Study of Trophoblastic Disease (ISSTD) in Beijing in 1979. The FIGO system delineates stages as follows:

- **Stage I** includes all patients with persistently elevated hCG levels and tumor confined to the uterus.
- **Stage II** includes all patients with disease outside the uterus but localized to the vagina and/or pelvic structures.
- **Stage III** encompasses all patients with pulmonary metastases with or without uterine, vaginal, or pelvic lesions. Precise histologic diagnosis is not easily obtained in this group of patients without biopsy or available tissue from another source. Nonetheless, we do not advocate performing thoracotomy or other invasive procedures merely to obtain information regarding the histologic pattern of the metastatic site, as treatment is based on staging rather than pathology.
- **Stage IV** includes patients with far advanced disease with involvement of one or more of the following organs: brain, liver, kidney, spleen, or gastrointestinal tract. Patients with stage IV disease are more likely to become drug resistant and are, therefore, in the highest risk category. Patients with stage IV disease invariably

have histologic evidence of CCA, which is more likely to follow a nonmolar pregnancy.

World Health Organization Prognostic Score

In addition to anatomic staging, other variables are needed to predict the likelihood that a patient will develop drug resistance and to serve as a guide to the selection of an appropriate chemotherapy regimen. In 1983, the World Health Organization (WHO) adopted a modification of the Bagshawe prognostic scoring system, which was based on a number of clinical, radiologic, hormonal, and demographic factors, each of which was considered an independent variable and assumed to be additive.[61] Patients with prognostic scores of 7 or lower are considered to be at low risk of developing drug resistance and are ideal candidates for single-agent chemotherapy. When the prognostic score is greater than 7, the patient is considered to be at high risk for developing drug resistance and requires combination therapy to obtain optimal treatment outcomes. In general, patients with stage I tumors have low risk scores and patients with stage IV tumors have high risk scores. Therefore, the prognostic scoring system is most useful when it applies to stages II and III in that it helps to identify patients who require more intensive therapy for best results.

The variables that are included in the prognostic score include tumor volume (hCG measurement, size, and number of metastases), site of involvement, prior chemotherapy exposure, and duration of disease. Ross and co-workers[9] reported in 1965 that patients with high hCG levels, prolonged delays in diagnosis, and brain or liver metastases were relatively resistant to single-agent chemotherapy. Hammond and colleagues[60] observed further in 1973 that patients with prior chemotherapy exposure or antecedent term pregnancy were also relatively unresponsive to single-agent therapy. The importance and reliability of these prognostic factors have been confirmed by other investigators.

CCA after term pregnancy has been noted to be a poor prognostic factor and to have distinctive clinical features. We reviewed the experience with post-term CCA at the NETDC from 1964 to 1996.[62] Seven of 44 patients (16%) presented with clinical evidence of maternal-fetal bleeding that resulted in severe fetal anemia and non-immune hydrops or third trimester bleeding. Although none of the infants had evidence of metastatic CCA, rare cases of fetal involvement by CCA have been reported and are usually associated with either fetal or neonatal death. The time interval from delivery to diagnosis, sites of metastases, and pretreatment hCG level were all significant risk factors in predicting outcome. All 31 of our patients with a WHO score less than or equal to 8 survived, whereas 6 of 13 patients (46%) with a WHO score greater than 8 succumbed to their disease.

During the past 5 years, the ISSTD, the International Gynecologic Cancer Society, and FIGO have moved to modify the staging systems for trophoblastic disease by combining the basic FIGO stages with the WHO Prognostic Score (Table 93-4).

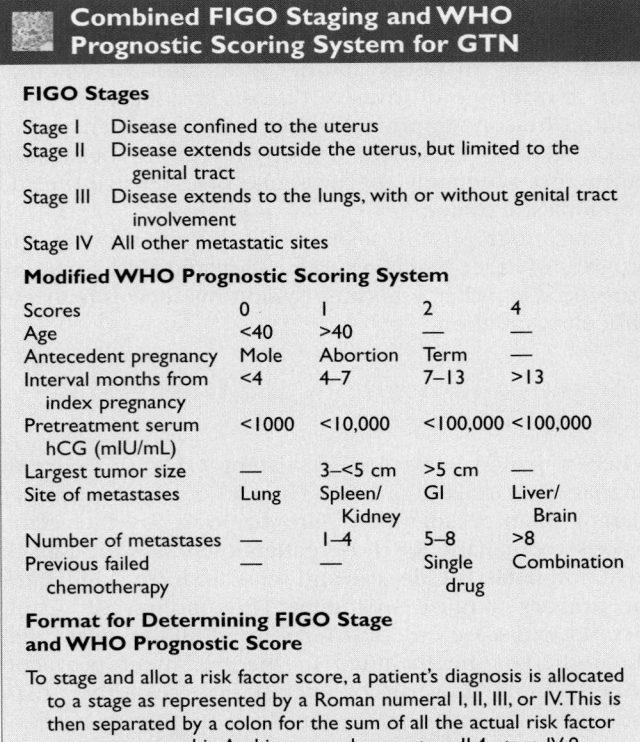

TABLE 93-4

Combined FIGO Staging and WHO Prognostic Scoring System for GTN

FIGO Stages

Stage I	Disease confined to the uterus
Stage II	Disease extends outside the uterus, but limited to the genital tract
Stage III	Disease extends to the lungs, with or without genital tract involvement
Stage IV	All other metastatic sites

Modified WHO Prognostic Scoring System

Scores	0	1	2	4
Age	<40	>40	—	—
Antecedent pregnancy	Mole	Abortion	Term	—
Interval months from index pregnancy	<4	4–7	7–13	>13
Pretreatment serum hCG (mIU/mL)	<1000	<10,000	<100,000	<100,000
Largest tumor size	—	3–<5 cm	>5 cm	—
Site of metastases	Lung	Spleen/ Kidney	GI	Liver/ Brain
Number of metastases	—	1–4	5–8	>8
Previous failed chemotherapy	—	—	Single drug	Combination

Format for Determining FIGO Stage and WHO Prognostic Score

To stage and allot a risk factor score, a patient's diagnosis is allocated to a stage as represented by a Roman numeral I, II, III, or IV. This is then separated by a colon for the sum of all the actual risk factor scores expressed in Arabic numerals, e.g., stage II:4, stage IV:9.

PRIMARY TREATMENT

Molar Pregnancy

The primary management of molar pregnancy is surgical evacuation. Before proceeding with surgery, however, the patient should be thoroughly evaluated to identify the presence of medical complications such as pre-eclampsia, electrolyte imbalance due to hyperemesis, hyperthyroidism, and anemia, which might complicate the surgical procedure. After evacuation, the clinician must be committed to conscientious hCG follow-up to screen for persistent GTN and to counseling regarding the management of future pregnancies.

Surgical Management
Once the patient's medical condition has stabilized, a decision must be made regarding the most appropriate surgical treatment. If the patient no longer desires to preserve fertility, hysterectomy should be considered. At the time of hysterectomy, prominent theca lutein cyst can be decompressed. The advantage of removing the uterus is that it eliminates the possibility that the patient will develop nonmetastatic disease. Although hysterectomy eliminates the risk of local invasion, however, it does not obviate the need for chemotherapy if metastases pre-exist or subsequently appear.

Suction curettage is the preferred method of evacuation, regardless of uterine size, in patients who desire to preserve fertility. At the time of evacuation, if the uterus is larger than 12 weeks' size, it is advisable to administer oxytocin at the onset of cervical dilatation to facilitate uterine involution. In larger uteri, as the cervix is being dilated, the surgeon might encounter brisk bleeding due to the release of retained blood. Shortly after commencing suction evacuation, uterine bleeding is generally well controlled, and the uterus involutes rapidly. If the uterus is larger than 14 weeks' size, it is helpful for the surgeon to massage the uterine fundus to stimulate uterine contraction. When suction evacuation is thought to be complete, a gentle sharp curettage should be performed to remove any residual chorionic tissue. It is important to avoid too vigorous curettement because of the risk of inducing uterine synechiae (Asherman's syndrome). Patients who are Rh negative should receive Rh immune globulin at the time of evacuation because RH D factor is expressed on trophoblast.

Some authors have proposed using cervical ripening agents to facilitate cervical dilatation and prevent trauma. In general, we have not found this to be necessary. The size of the curette to be used is determined by the uterine size. Generally, a 10-mm or 12-mm suction curette suffices, and greater dilatation of the cervix is not necessary. Patients with large-for-dates uteri and high hCG levels should be observed for signs and symptoms of acute respiratory insufficiency postoperatively, which could indicate that massive trophoblastic embolization has occurred.

Role of Prophylactic Chemotherapy

Patients with complete mole with high pre-evacuation hCG levels (>100,000 mIU/mL) and signs of marked trophoblastic growth (excessive uterine size) are at increased risk (40%) of developing persistent GTN (Table 93-5).[63] In these patients, the use of chemotherapy prophylactically at the time of evacuation has been shown to reduce the incidence of persistent GTN.[64,65] The administration of Mtx or actinomycin D (Act D) reduced the incidence of postmolar tumor from 47% to 14% and from 50% to 14%, respectively. None of the patients in either series developed metastatic disease.

Prophylaxis should also be considered in situations in which hCG follow-up is either unavailable or unreliable. An earlier diagnosis of molar pregnancy has been associated with a decrease in the number of patients who present clinically with high-risk moles. Despite earlier

TABLE 93-5

	NO. OF PATIENTS (%)	
OUTCOME	**LOW-RISK**	**HIGH-RISK**
Normal involution	486/506 (96)	212/352 (60)
Persistent GTN		
Nonmetastatic	17/506 (3.4)	109/352 (31)
Metastatic	3/506 (0.6)	31/352 (8.8)
Totals	506/858 (59)	352/858 (41)

Sequelae* of Low- and High-Risk Complete Hydatidiform Mole

*All patients managed by evacuation without prophylactic chemotherapy.

diagnosis, however, the incidence of persistent GTN remains unchanged, suggesting that the development of persistent GTN is inherent in the malignant potential of the molar pregnancy itself rather than being due to other factors such as duration of gestation or completeness of the evacuation.

Persistent GTN

Persistent GTN can occur after any antecedent pregnancy. The clinical presentation is more important in determining prognosis than the precise histologic diagnosis, which might not be available. Infrequently, the diagnosis is made solely on the basis of a rising or plateaued hCG level in the absence of a documented pregnancy or of any clinical, radiologic, or pathologic evidence of trophoblastic tissue. When this occurs, it is important to make certain that the hCG being measured by the assay is true rather than a false-positive test (the so-called Phantom hCG).[66] Postmolar GTN is diagnosed on the basis of a rising (increase of 10%) or plateauing (<10% for at least 3 weeks, or four values over 14 days) hCG value. Abnormal vaginal bleeding, subinvolution of the uterus, and cystic ovaries can be present. Women with GTN after nonmolar pregnancies can present with subtle signs and symptoms, making diagnosis difficult. Abnormal bleeding after any pregnancy should be evaluated promptly with an hCG test. Because metastases from CCA have been reported in virtually every anatomic site, a diagnosis of persistent GTN should be considered in any woman of reproductive age who presents with metastatic disease from an unknown primary site.

Chemotherapeutic Agents

Single-Agent Chemotherapy. Single-agent chemotherapy with either methotrexate or actinomycin D has induced comparable and excellent remission rates in both nonmetastatic and metastatic GTN.[67]

An optimal regimen should maximize the cure rate while minimizing toxicity. Table 93-6 summarizes the various protocols that are in use for the primary treatment of both nonmetastatic and low-risk metastatic GTN. Several regimens of methotrexate and actinomycin D have induced complete remission in 70% to 100% of patients with nonmetastatic GTN and in 50% to 70% of patients with low-risk metastatic GTN. Fortunately, if a patient develops resistance to the single agent utilized initially, she usually can achieve remission with the alternative drug. Bagshawe and Wilde[68] first reported in 1964 on administering methotrexate with folinic acid to reduce chemotherapeutic toxicity.

Methotrexate plus folinic acid has remained the primary treatment of nonmetastatic and low-risk metastatic GTN at the Charing Cross Hospital. Although methotrexate plus folinic acid is highly effective, a 20% rate of resistance and 6% toxicity were observed.

Methotrexate plus folinic acid has also been the preferred single-agent regimen at the NETDC for the treatment of GTN since 1974.[69] Between September 1974 and September 1984, 185 patients with GTN were treated

TABLE 93-6

Single-Agent Regimens for Low-Risk GTN	
METHOTREXATE REGIMENS	**REMISSIONS (%)**
5-day MTX	93.0
Mtx 0.5 mg/kg IV or IM daily for 5 days	
Pulse MTX	81.0
Mtx 50 mg/m² IM weekly	
MTX/FA	90.2
Mtx 1 mg/kg IM or IV on days 1, 3, 5, 7	
FA 0.1 mg/kg PO on days 2, 4, 6, 8	
High-dose MTX/FA	61
Mtx 100 mg/m² IV bolus	
Mtx 200 mg/m² 12 hr infusion	
FA 15 mg q 12 hrs × 4 doses IM or PO	
beginning 24 hours after starting Mtx	
Actinomycin D Regimens	
5-day Act D	94.0
Act D 12 µg/kg IV push daily for 5 days	
Pulse Act D	94.0
Act D 1.25 mg/m² IV push q 2 wks	

with primary methotrexate/folinic acid at the NETDC. Complete gonadotropin remission was achieved in 147 of 163 patients (90%) with Stage I GTN and in 15 of 22 patients (68%) with low-risk stage II and III GTN. Among the 23 patients resistant to methotrexate/folinic acid, 14 (61%) subsequently achieved remission with actinomycin D, and 9 required combination chemotherapy. Thrombocytopenia, granulocytopenia, and hepatotoxicity occurred in only 11 (6%), 3 (2%), and 26 (14%) patients, respectively. One patient required platelet transfusion and developed sepsis due to myelosuppression. No patient developed alopecia. The effectiveness of this methotrexate/folinic acid protocol could be due partly to the prolonged exposure to methotrexate. When methotrexate is administered at a higher dose (300 mg/m² over 12 hours and 30 minutes), the remission rate declines to 69% in patients with nonmetatastic GTN. Although methotrexate and actinomycin D are the two most commonly used single agents in GTN in the United States and abroad, 5-fluorouracil (5-FU) has been the preferred single-agent chemotherapy in China. Sung and associates[70] reported that 5-FU induced complete remission in 93% of patients with stage I GTN and in 86% of patients with stage II disease.

Etoposide administered orally has also been shown to be highly effective in the treatment of nonmetastatic and metastatic GTN by the Hong Kong group, who reported complete sustained remission in 56 of 60 patients (93%).[71]

Combination Regimens. Triple chemotherapy with methotrexate/folinic acid, actinomycin D, and cyclophosphamide (MAC) had been the preferred combination drug

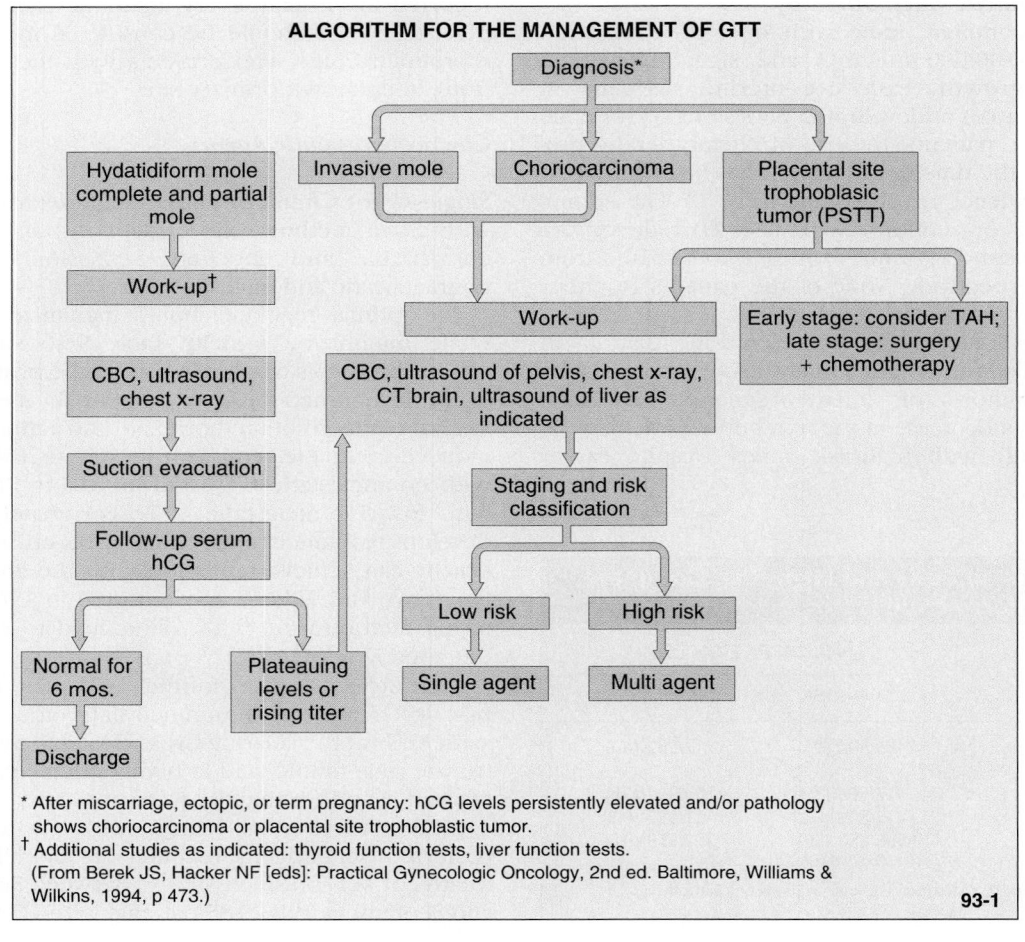

ALGORITHM FOR THE MANAGEMENT OF GTT

* After miscarriage, ectopic, or term pregnancy: hCG levels persistently elevated and/or pathology
   shows choriocarcinoma or placental site trophoblastic tumor.
† Additional studies as indicated: thyroid function tests, liver function tests.
(From Berek JS, Hacker NF [eds]: Practical Gynecologic Oncology, 2nd ed. Baltimore, Williams & Wilkins, 1994, p 473.)

93-1

TABLE 93-7

Protocol for MAC Regimen

DAY	DRUG	DOSE
1	Mtx	1.0 mg.kg IM or IV
	Act D	12 μg/kg IV push
	Cyclophosphamide	3 mg/kg IV bolus
2	FA	0.1 mg/kg IM or PO
	Act D	12 μg/kg IV push
	Cyclophosphamide	3 mg/kg IV bolus
3	Mtx	1.0 mg.kg IM or IV
	Act D	12 μg/kg IV push
	Cyclophosphamide	3 mg/kg IV bolus
4	FA	0.1 mg/kg IM or PO
	Act D	12 μg/kg IV push
	Cyclophosphamide	3 mg/kg IV bolus
5	Mtx	1.0 mg.kg IM or IV
	Act D	12 μg/kg IV push
	Cyclophosphamide	3 mg/kg IV bolus
6	FA	0.1 mg/kg IM or PO
7	Mtx	1.0 mg.kg IM or IV
8	FA	0.1 mg/kg IM or IV

regimen at the NETDC in patients with high-risk GTN (Table 93-7). This regimen, however, has been shown to be associated with a low success rate in patients with high-risk GTN who have prognostic scores greater than 7. Summarizing the data from six centers, triple therapy induced complete remission in 47 of 92 patients (51%) with metastatic GTN and high-risk WHO scores.

Bagshawe[72] reported an 83% remission rate in patients with metastatic GTN and high-risk WHO scores, using a special combination regimen. This regimen, which includes etoposide, methotrexate/folinic acid, actinomycin D, cyclophosphamide, and vincristine (EMA-CO), is currently the preferred treatment for patients with metastatic GTN who have high-risk WHO scores (Table 93-8). If patients prove resistant to EMA-CO, they might then successfully be treated with a modification of this regimen by substituting etoposide and cisplatin on day 8 (EMA-CE) (Table 93-9). Bower and colleagues[73] reported that EMA-

TABLE 93-8

Protocol for EMA-CO Regimen

DAY	DRUG	DOSE
1	Etoposide	100 mg/m² by infusion in 200 mL saline over 30 min
	Act D	0.5 mg IV push
	Mtx	100 mg/m² IV push
		200 mg/m² by infusion over 12 hr
2	Etoposide	100 mg/m² by infusion in 200 mL saline over 30 min
	Act D	0.5 mg IV push
	FA	15 mg q12 hours × 4 doses IM or PO beginning 24 hours after starting Mtx
8	Cyclophosphamide	600 mg/m² by infusion in saline over 30 min
	Oncovin (vincristine)	1.0 mg/m² IV push

TABLE 93-9

Protocol for EMA-CE Regimen

DAY	DRUG	DOSE
1	Etoposide	100 mg/m² by infusion in 200 mL saline over 30 min
	Act D	0.5 mg IV push
	Mtx	100 mg/m² IV push
		1000 mg/m² by infusion over 12 hr
2	Etoposide	100 mg/m² by infusion in 200 mL saline over 30 min
	Act D	0.5 mg IV push
	FA	30 mg q12 hours × 6 doses IM or PO beginning 32 hours after starting Mtx
8	Cisplatin	60 mg/m² with prehydration
	Etoposide	100 mg/m² by infusion in 200 mL saline over 30 min

CE induced remission either alone or in conjunction with surgery in 16 of 21 patients (76%) resistant to EMA-CO. Unfortunately, the use of etoposide in GTN has been reported to increase the risk of later secondary tumors—including myeloid leukemia, melanoma, colon cancer, and breast cancer. The increased risk for breast cancer did not become apparent until after 25 years. Among all patients who were treated with etoposide, 1.5% subsequently developed leukemia. Etoposide, therefore, should be used only in patients who require it to achieve remission, most commonly patients with metastatic disease and high-risk WHO scores. When patients with nonmetastatic and low-risk metastatic disease prove resistant to single-agent therapy, we now administer triple therapy (MAC) at our center before using regimens that contain etoposide.

Second-line therapy with cisplatin, vinblastine, and bleomycin (VBP) could also be effective in patients with drug-resistant GTN. This regimen has been shown to induce complete remission in 18%, 57%, and 63% of patients with drug resistant GTN.[75]

The potential role of autologous bone marrow transplantation or stem cell rescue in GTN has yet to be defined. Individual cases have been reported in which high-dose chemotherapy with autologous bone marrow techniques have been successful in inducing remission in patients refractory to the usual regimens.

Efforts continue to identify new agents that are effective in treating patients with GTN. Although ifosfamide and taxol are both active, further studies are needed to better define their roles as primary and second-line therapy in the treatment of this disease.

Patients who require combination chemotherapy must be treated intensively to attain remission. We administer combination chemotherapy as frequently as toxicity permits (usually at 2- to 3-week intervals) until the patient attains three consecutive undetectable hCG values. After the patient achieves normal β-hCG levels, three to four additional courses of chemotherapy are administered to reduce the risk of relapse. Relapse can be attributed to the fact that residual disease is present, producing hCG below the threshold of assay systems currently in use.

Stage I (Nonmetastatic Disease)

The protocols for the management of stage I disease at the NETDC are shown in the nearby box. The treatment of stage I GTN is either surgical or medical, depending on the patient's desire to preserve fertility. Hysterectomy is advisable as initial treatment in patients with stage I nonmetastatic disease GTN who no longer wish to preserve fertility. The use of hysterectomy to treat nonmetastatic disease results in a reduced number of courses of chemotherapy and in a shorter duration and lower dose of chemotherapy required to achieve remission.[76] Adjuvant chemotherapy administered at the time of surgery is indicated to eradicate any occult metastases and to reduce the likelihood of tumor dissemination at the time of surgery. Adjuvant chemotherapy administered at the time of surgery has not been associated with increased postoperative morbidity. Nonmetastatic PSTT should be treated with hysterectomy because of this tumor's poor response to chemotherapy. Once PSTT metastasizes, the survival rate is extremely low despite multimodal therapy.[77] Thirty-one patients treated by primary hysterectomy and adjuvant chemotherapy all achieved complete remission with no additional therapy.

Results of Treatment. Between July 1965 and May 2002, 528 patients with stage I disease were treated at the NETDC (Table 93-10). Complete sustained remission was achieved in 446 patients (92%) with single-agent therapy. The remaining 43 patients resistant to single-agent chemotherapy subsequently attained remission either with further chemotherapy or surgical intervention. If a patient no longer wishes to preserve fertility, hysterectomy with adjuvant single-agent chemotherapy may be performed as primary treatment. Thirty-one patients were treated with this approach at the NETDC, and all achieved complete, sustained remission with no further therapy. The use of chemotherapy at the time of hysterectomy has not been associated with an increased risk of postoperative morbidity.

TREATMENT PROTOCOL FOR STAGE I GTN

INITIAL
Sequential Mtx/Act D or hysterectomy with adjuvant chemotherapy

RESISTANT TO BOTH SINGLE AGENTS
Combination chemotherapy
Hysterectomy with adjuvant chemotherapy
Local uterine resection
Pelvic intrarterial infusion

FOLLOW-UP HCG
Weekly until normal for 3 weeks, then monthly until normal for 1 year

CONTRACEPTION
12 consecutive months of normal hCG tests

TABLE 93-10

Results of Treatment in Stage I GTN (1965–2002)

REMISSION THERAPY	NO. OF PATIENTS (%)	NO. OF REMISSIONS (%)
Initial	**485 (92)**	
Sequential Mtx/Act D		446 (92)
Hysterectomy		31 (6.4)
MAC		3 (0.6)
EMA		5 (1.0)
Resistant	**43 (8.1)**	
MAC		16 (37.2%)
EMA		20 (46.5)
EITP*		1 (2.3)
Hysterectomy		3 (7.0)
Local resection		2 (4.7)
Pelvic infusion		1 (2.3)
Total	**528**	**528 (100)**

*E, etoposide; I, ifosfamide; P, platinum; T, taxol.

Method of Administration. At the NETDC, β-hCG levels are measured weekly after each course of chemotherapy and serve as the primary basis for determining the need for additional treatment in patients with stage I GTN. After the first treatment, further chemotherapy is withheld as long as the hCG level falls progressively. A second course of the same agent is administered under the following conditions:

- β-hCG level plateaus for more than 2 consecutive weeks or re-elevates, or
- β-hCG levels do not decline by one log (10-fold) within 18 days after completing the first treatment.

If a second course of methotrexate/folinic acid is necessary, the dosage of methotrexate remains unaltered if the patient's response to the first treatment has been adequate. An adequate response is defined as a fall in the β-hCG level by one log (10-fold) after a course of chemotherapy. When the response to the first treatment is inadequate, the dose of methotrexate is increased by 50%. If the response is inadequate to two consecutive courses of methotrexate/folinic acid, the patient is considered to be resistant to methotrexate, and actinomycin D is instituted promptly. If a patient fails to respond to sequential methotrexate/actinomycin D, then combination chemotherapy using methotrexate, actinomycin D, and cytoxan (MAC) is administered at 3-week intervals or as frequently as toxicity permits until the patient's β-hCG level becomes undetectable. Patients who require combination chemotherapy should be treated intensively to attain remission. To prevent relapse, at least two additional courses of chemotherapy should be administered after the patient achieves undetectable hCG levels.

Stages II and III

The NETDC protocol for the management of stages II and III GTN is outlined in the nearby box. Although low-risk patients (WHO score of 7 or lower) are treated with

---

TREATMENT PROTOCOL FOR STAGES II AND III GTN

LOW RISK

Initial	Sequential Mtx/Act D
Resistant to both single agents	Combination chemotherapy or local resection with adjunctive CT

HIGH RISK

Initial	Combination chemotherapy
Resistant	Second-line combination chemotherapy or local resection with adjunctive CT
Follow-up hCG	Weekly until normal for 3 weeks, then monthly until normal for 12 months
Contraception	12 consecutive months of normal hCG tests

---

primary single-agent chemotherapy with methotrexate or actinomycin D, patients with high-risk scores (WHO score greater than 7) require primary combination chemotherapy to achieve optimal outcomes. Patients resistant to single-agent chemotherapy are then treated with combination chemotherapy, either MAC or EMA-CO. Patients resistant to MAC should then receive EMA-CO, and those resistant to EMA-CO may be treated with a modification of that regimen by substituting cisplatin and etoposide on day 8 and escalating the dose of methotrexate infusion to 1 g/m^2 (EMA-CE).

Management of Vaginal Metastases. Because trophoblastic tissue is highly vascular, vaginal metastases can bleed profusely. When bleeding is a problem, it could be necessary to pack the lesion or to perform a wide local excision. The administration of one or two courses of chemotherapy could result in the development of avascular planes around the vaginal tumor, making excision less bloody.

Angiographic embolization of the hypogastric artery or of the specific vessels feeding the tumor could be required to control hemorrhage from a vaginal metastasis. Extension of tumor to the adnexa should be monitored by ultrasound when asymptomatic. These tumor deposits usually resolve once chemotherapy is administered; however, surgical intervention could be required if signs of intra-abdominal bleeding appear.

Management of Lung Metastases. Thoracotomy has a limited role in the management of stage III GTN. Thoracotomy should be performed initially if there is the possibility that the lesion is an hCG-producing primary lung tumor. Pulmonary resection is also indicated if a patient has a persistent viable nodule despite intensive chemotherapy. Before undertaking thoracotomy, however, a metastatic work-up should be carried out to exclude the presence of other metastatic sites. Excision of persistent nodules in the face of complete gonadotropin remission is

not indicated, because treated pulmonary nodules can fibrose and remain indefinitely on chest x-ray. If there is any question regarding the viability of a pulmonary lesion, a scan with radioisotope-labeled antibody to hCG or a positron emission tomography (PET) scan could be helpful. These scans might also be useful in identifying occult sites of viable tumor. Tomoda and colleagues[78] reviewed their experience with pulmonary resection in 19 patients with chemotherapy-resistant GTN and proposed the following criteria for successful resection:

- Good surgical candidate.
- Primary malignancy is controlled.
- No evidence of other metastatic sites.
- Pulmonary metastasis localized to one lung.
- hCG level below 1000 mIU/mL.

In Tomoda's series, complete remission was achieved in 14 of 15 patients who met all five criteria, but in none of the 4 patients who had one or more unfavorable clinical features. Similarly, Jones and coworkers[79] reported that six of nine carefully selected patients with drug-resistant pulmonary GTN attained complete remission after lung resection. Several investigators have reported that the achievement of nondetectable hCG levels within 1 to 2 weeks after resection of a solitary pulmonary nodule is highly predictive of a favorable outcome. Survival after salvage surgery is also influenced by other factors, such as the number of preoperative chemotherapy regimens, the number of disease sites, and the patient's WHO score.

Results of Treatment. Between July 1965 and May 2002, all 28 patients with stage II disease treated at the NETDC achieved remission. Single-agent chemotherapy induced complete remission in 16 of 20 (80%) low-risk patients. In contrast, only two of eight high-risk patients achieved remission with single-agent treatment. Between July 1965 and May 2002, 152 out of 153 patients (99%) with stage III GTN attained complete remission. Single-agent chemotherapy induced complete remission in 85 of 104 patients (82%) with low-risk disease and in 13 of 49 patients (27%) with high-risk disease. All patients who were resistant to single-agent treatment later achieved remission with combination chemotherapy.

Stage IV
The protocol for the management of patients with stage IV GTN at the NETDC is summarized in the nearby box. All patients are managed with primary combination chemotherapy with EMA-CO. In the presence of cerebral metastases, the methotrexate dosage in the infusion is increased to 1 g/m^2, and whole-head irradiation is administered immediately. Patients with disease resistant to EMA-CO may then be treated with EMA-CE. When cerebral metastases are detected, whole-brain irradiation should be instituted promptly. Brain irradiation is both hemostatic and tumoricidal. The concurrent use of combination chemotherapy and brain irradiation appears to reduce the risk of spontaneous bleeding in cerebral metastases. Yordan and associates[80] reported that deaths

---

**TREATMENT PROTOCOL
FOR STAGE IV GTN**

INITIAL
Combination chemotherapy
With brain metastases—whole head irradiation (3000
  cGy), craniotomy as indicated
With liver metastases—resection to manage complications

RESISTANT
Second-line chemotherapy
Local resection as indicated
Hepatic artery infusion as indicated

FOLLOW-UP hCG
Weekly until normal for 3 weeks, then monthly for 24
  consecutive months

CONTRACEPTION
24 consecutive months of normal hCG values

---

due to central nervous system involvement occurred in 11 of 25 patients (44%) treated with chemotherapy alone but in none of 18 patients treated with both brain irradiation and chemotherapy. Newland and colleagues,[81] on the other hand, have reported excellent remission rates in patients with cerebral metastases treated with chemotherapy alone. Thirty of 35 patients (86%) with cerebral lesions achieved sustained remission with intensive combination chemotherapy that included high-dose intravenous and intrathecal methotrexate.

Management of Cerebral Metastases. Craniotomy should be reserved for patients who develop progressive neurologic deterioration, indicating the need for acute decompression or for control of bleeding. In rare instances, cerebral metastases that are resistant to chemotherapy could be amenable to local resection, particularly if they are localized in the periphery. Evans and co-workers[82] reported complete remission in three of four patients who underwent craniotomy to relieve intracranial pressure and in two of three patients undergoing craniotomy for resection of chemotherapy-resistant tumor. Athanassiou and colleagues[52] similarly reported that four of five patients undergoing craniotomy for acute intracranial complications were ultimately cured. Most patients with cerebral metastases who achieve remission have little or no residual neurologic deficits, unless there has been an acute hemorrhagic episode.

Management of Hepatic Metastases. The management of liver metastases is particularly difficult and problematic. If a patient is resistant to chemotherapy, hepatic arterial infusion might induce remission in selected cases. Hepatic resection might also be necessary to control acute hepatic bleeding or to remove localized areas of resistant tumor. Grumbine and associates[83] reported the use of selective occlusion of the hepatic arteries and concurrent combination chemotherapy in a patient with bleeding liver

metastases who ultimately attained remission. Wong and colleagues[84] also noted that 9 out of 10 patients with hepatic involvement achieved complete remission with primary intensive combination chemotherapy without hepatic irradiation. Bakri and colleagues[50] similarly reported that five of eight patients (63%) with liver metastases who were treated with combination chemotherapy alone attained remission. Liver metastases could cause capsular rupture with profuse intraabdominal hemorrhage.

Role of Hysterectomy. Hysterectomy may be performed in patients with metastatic GTN to control uterine bleeding or sepsis. Furthermore, in patients with bulky tumor growth in the uterus, hysterectomy could substantially reduce tumor burden and thereby reduce the amount of chemotherapy required to induce remission. Hammond and coworkers[76] reported that patients who underwent hysterectomy had a shorter duration of hospitalization and chemotherapy.

Results of Treatment. Prior to 1975, only 6 of 20 patients (30%) with stage IV disease achieved remission. After 1975, 16 (79%) of 19 patients attained remission. This dramatic improvement in survival resulted both from the introduction of multimodal therapy early in the course of treatment and from the availability of supportive treatments that help control life-threatening drug-induced toxicity.

FOLLOW-UP

After Evacuation of a Molar Pregnancy

Complete Mole
Patients with CHM should be followed with weekly β-hCG tests after evacuation until the β-hCG levels are undetectable for 3 consecutive weeks. Tests should then continue monthly for 6 months.

Partial Mole
After evacuation of a PHM, we recommend that patients be followed weekly until β-hCG levels are undetectable for 3 weeks, and then monthly for 3 months if the β-hCG level normalizes by 7 weeks. Patients should be followed monthly for 6 months if the β-hCG level takes longer than 7 weeks to become undetectable.

Postevacuation Contraception
Patients should be counseled to use effective contraception during the entire interval of β-hCG follow-up. We do not encourage the insertion of intrauterine devices until the patient achieves undetectable β-hCG levels because of the risk of infection or perforation if residual tumor is present. If the patient does not desire surgical sterilization, her options are, therefore, either hormonal or barrier methods. The incidence of postmolar tumor has been reported to be increased in patients who start oral contraceptives before the β-hCG level becomes undetect-

able.[85] Data from the NETDC, the Gynecologic Oncology Group, and the Brewer Center, however, indicate that oral contraceptives do not appear to increase the risk of postmolar GTN.[86]

Another important reason to place patients on oral contraceptives during follow-up is to prevent cross-reactivity with luteinizing hormone. After multiple courses of chemotherapy, ovarian steroidal function could be damaged, particularly in patients in their late 30s and 40s. When ovarian function is damaged, luteinizing hormone levels can rise, and due to cross-reactivity, the patients could be thought falsely to have persistent low levels of β-hCG.

After completion of the prescribed follow-up period, pregnancy may be undertaken. Patients should be counseled that they are at increased risk of another molar pregnancy in any subsequent gestation. For that reason, we highly recommend that a pelvic ultrasound be performed at 10 weeks of gestation. There is also evidence that patients who have been treated for GTN have a higher incidence of another trophoblastic event after any subsequent pregnancy. Therefore, all patients with a history of molar pregnancy or GTN should undergo β-hCG testing at the 6-week postpartum or postabortal visit.

After Treatment for GTN

Stages I–III
All patients with stages I, II, and III GTN should be followed with weekly β-hCG values until they become undetectable for 3 consecutive weeks; testing then should continue monthly for 12 months. During the entire period of gonadotropin monitoring, patients must be encouraged to use effective contraception. When patients have completed the prescribed period of follow-up, they are free to try for pregnancy. Patients may be reassured that subsequent pregnancies are associated with no increased risk of spontaneous abortions, congenital malformations, prematurity, or other major obstetrical complications.

Stage IV
Patients with Stage IV disease should be followed with weekly β-hCG values until they are normal for 3 consecutive weeks and should then be followed monthly for 24 months. A more prolonged follow-up is required for patients with stage IV disease because of the increased risk of late recurrence.

Management of Primary Treatment Failure

When patients become resistant to or relapse after treatment with primary and secondary chemotherapy as manifested either by a plateau in or a re-elevation of the β-hCG level, it is necessary to re-evaluate her status, looking for occult metastases that might be protected from the effects of drug therapy. Mutch and colleagues[87] reported recurrences after initial remission in 2% of patients with nonmetastatic GTN, in 4% of patients with good-prognosis metastatic disease, and in 13% of patients with poor-prognosis disease. Relapses developed within

3 and 18 months in 50% and 85% of patients, respectively. We have observed relapses after initial remission in 3% of patients with stage I, 8% with stage II, 4% with stage III, and 9% with stage IV disease.[88] The mean time to recurrence from the last undetectable hCG level was 6 months, and this rate did not differ among the four FIGO stages. All patients with stage I, II, and III GTN who relapsed were subsequently cured, whereas both stage IV patients with recurrent disease succumbed. Patients with uncomplicated molar pregnancy who spontaneously resolve their β-hCG levels rarely recur after 3 weeks of undetectable tests.

Role of Surgery
In contrast to its limited role in primary therapy, surgery can play an important role in the treatment of patients who prove resistant to first- and second-line therapy. Surgical removal of resistant disease of the uterus, lung, brain, liver, spleen, and gastrointestinal tract should be undertaken to reduce tumor burden and prevent bleeding when it is apparent that these metastatic sites no longer respond to either primary or salvage therapy.

Salvage Chemotherapy
Resistance to primary and secondary chemotherapy regimens requires the use of salvage regimens in addition to surgery and radiation therapy. A number of well-recognized protocols have been used with some success in this situation, including VBP and EMA-CE.

Phantom Choriocarcinoma
Some patients can have a false-positive elevation in serum β-hCG measurement due to the presence of circulating heterophile antibody.[66] These patients with so-called phantom choriocarcinoma often have no clear antecedent pregnancy and no progressive rise in their β-hCG levels. The possibility of false-positive hCG measurement should be considered and evaluated by sending both serum and urine samples to an hCG reference laboratory. Patients with phantom hCG generally have no measurable hCG in a parallel urine sample, and their titers do not dilute on the hCG assay.

Subsequent Pregnancy

Pregnancy after Complete Hydatidiform Mole
Patients with molar pregnancies can anticipate normal reproduction in the future. Patients with CHM treated at the NETDC had 1278 later pregnancies between June 1965 and November 2001 (Table 93-11). These pregnancies resulted in 877 (69%) normal, full-term live births, 95 (7%) premature deliveries, 11 ectopic pregnancies, and 7 still births. First-trimester spontaneous abortions occurred in 221 pregnancies (17%). Major and minor congenital malformations were detected in only 40 infants. Primary cesarean section was consistent with the normal population at 19%.

Pregnancy after Partial Hydatidiform Mole
Between June 1965 and November 2001, patients with PHM at the NETDC had 251 subsequent gestations, which

TABLE 93-11

Subsequent Pregnancy Outcome in CHM (1965–2002)

OUTCOME	NUMBER (%)
Total pregnancies	1254
Total deliveries	962
Term live	862 (68.7)
Preterm	93 (7.4)
Stillbirth	7 (0.6)
Congenital anomalies	38 (3.0)
C/S (1979–2000)	67 (18.8)
Spontaneous abortions	223 (17.8)
Therapeutic abortions	40 (3.2)
Ectopic pregnancy	11 (0.9)
Repeat molar pregnancy	18 (1.4)

TABLE 93-13

Subsequent Pregnancy Outcome in Patients Treated for GTN

OUTCOME	NUMBER (%)
Total pregnancies	537
Total deliveries	404
Term live	365 (67.8)
Preterm	32 (0.6)
Stillbirth	8 (1.5)
Congenital anomalies	10 (1.9)
C/S (1979–2000)	58 (19.2)
Spontaneous abortions	91 (16.8)
Therapeutic abortions	27 (5.0)
Ectopic pregnancy	7 (1.3)
Repeat molar pregnancy	6 (1.1)

resulted in 189 (75%) term live births, 1 still birth, 1 ectopic pregnancy, and 4 premature deliveries (Table 93-12). First-trimester spontaneous abortions occurred in 38 (15%) pregnancies, and major and minor congenital anomalies were detected in only 3 infants.

After a patient has had a molar pregnancy, she has an increased risk of developing another molar pregnancy at a later conception.[89] Thirty-four (1 in 150) of our patients had at least two molar gestations between June 1965 and November 2001. Patients can have an initial CHM or PHM and then, in a later pregnancy, they can develop the other type of molar disease. Following two molar pregnancies, 34 patients had 35 later conceptions resulting in 20 (57%) full-term normal deliveries, 7 (20%) molar pregnancies (6 complete, 1 partial), 3 spontaneous abortions, 1 ectopic pregnancy, 1 intrauterine death, and 3 therapeutic abortions. Bagshawe and colleagues[90] also reported that the risk of a third molar disease after two episodes of molar pregnancy was 15%. In six of our cases, we have documented that the patient had different partners at the time of conception of different molar pregnancies.

Pregnancy after GTN

Patients treated successfully with chemotherapy can also generally experience normal reproductive function. Table 93-13 summarizes the experience at the NETDC in

TABLE 93-12

Subsequent Pregnancy Outcome in PHM (1975–2002)

OUTCOME	NUMBER (%)
Total pregnancies	218
Total deliveries	167
Term live	162 (74.3)
Preterm	4 (1.8)
Stillbirth	1 (0.5)
Congenital anomalies	3 (1.4)
C/S (1979–2000)	23 (13.8)
Spontaneous abortions	35 (16.1)
Therapeutic abortions	11 (5.0)
Ectopic pregnancy	1 (0.5)
Repeat molar pregnancy	4 (1.8)

581 pregnancies that occurred between June 1965 and November 2001. These later pregnancies resulted in 393 (68%) full-term live births, 35 premature deliveries, 7 ectopic pregnancies, and 9 still births. First-trimester spontaneous abortions occurred in 16%, and major and minor abnormalities were detected in only 10 infants. It is reassuring that the frequency of congenital anomalies is not increased despite the use of chemotherapeutic agents, which are both teratogenic and mutagenic.

Our experience is in general agreement with that of other centers regarding the pregnancy outcome after chemotherapy for GTN. A total of 2038 subsequent pregnancies have been reported, which resulted in 77% full-term live births, 5% premature deliveries, 1% stillbirths, and 14% spontaneous miscarriages. Although the frequency of still births appears somewhat increased, congenital anomalies were noted in only 1.8% of patients, which is consistent with the general population. Woolas and associates[91] noted that there were no differences in either conception rate or pregnancy outcome between women treated with single agents and those treated with combination chemotherapy. Furthermore, only 7% of women who wished to become pregnant after GTN failed to conceive.

Psychosocial Consequences of GTN

Women who develop GTN can experience significant mood disturbance, marital and sexual problems, and concerns over future fertility.[92] Because GTN is a consequence of pregnancy, patients and their partners must confront the loss of a pregnancy at the same time they face concerns regarding malignancy. Patients can experience clinically significant levels of anxiety, fatigue, anger, confusion, sexual problems, and concern for future pregnancy that last for protracted periods of time. Patients with metastatic disease and active disease are particularly at risk of serious psychological disturbances.

Psychosocial assessments and interventions should be provided to patients with GTN and their partners and should be targeted particularly to patients in the metatastic and active disease groups. The psychological and social stresses related to persistent GTN can last for many years beyond achieving remission.

ISSUES FOR THE FUTURE

Survival in GTN has improved dramatically over the past three decades because of the introduction of sensitive and specific hCG assays for diagnosis, treatment, and follow-up and because of the introduction of effective chemotherapy regimens based on patients' risk profiles. Further advances in the treatment of GTN can be achieved through earlier detection and intervention and through the introduction of effective chemotherapeutic protocols for resistant disease.

It is well recognized that the treatment of patients, particularly those with high-risk GTN, by physicians experienced in the management of this disease achieves optimal results. Therefore, prompt referral to or consultation with treatment centers is always in the best interest of the patient.

REFERENCES

1. Bracken MB: Incidence and aetiology of hydatidiform mole: An epidemiologic review. Br J Obstet Gynecol 1987;94:1123.
2. Jeffers MD, O'Dwyer P, Curran B, et al: Partial hydatitiform mole: A common but undiagnosed condition. Int J Gynecol Pathol 1993;12:315.
3. Kajii T, Ohama K: Androgenetic origin of hydatidiform mole. Nature 1977;268:633.
4. Szulman AE, Surti U: The syndromes of hydatidiform mole: I. Cytogenetic and morphologic correlations. Am J Obstet Gynecol 1978;131:665.
5. Brewer JI: The Albert F. Mathieu Chorionepithelioma Registry. Ann NY Acad Med 1959;80:140.
6. Li MC, Hertz R, Spencer DB: Effect of methotrexate therapy on chorcorcinoma and chorioadenoma. Proc Sci Exp Biol Med 1956;93:361.
7. Hertz R, Lewis JL Jr, Lipsett MB: Five years' experience with chemotherapy of metastatic choriocarcinoma and related trophoblastic tumors in women. Am J Obstet Gynecol 1961;82:631.
8. Hertz R, Ross GT, Lipsett MB: Primary chemotherapy of nonmetastatic trophoblastic disease in women. Am J Obstet Gynecol 1963;86:808.
9. Ross GT, Goldstein DP, Hertz R, et al: Sequential use of methotrexate and actinomycin D in the treatment of metastatic choriocarcinom and related trophoblastic diseases in women. Am J Obstet Gynecol 1965;93:223.
10. Acosta-Sisson H, Espaniola N: Clinicopathologic study from thirty-two cases of chorionepithelioma. Am J Obstet Gynecol 1941;42:878.
11. Martin BH, Kim JM: Changes in gestational trophoblastic tumors over four decades: A Korean experience. J Reprod Med 1998;43:60.
12. Berkowitz RS, Cramer DW, Bernstein MR, et al: Risk factors for complete molar pregnancy from a case-control study. Am J Obstet Gynecol 1985;152:1016.
13. Parazzini F, Mangili G, LaVecchia C, et al: Dietary factors and risk of trophoblastic disease. Am J Obstet Gynecol 1988;158:93.
14. Parazzini F, Mangili G, LaVecchia C, et al: Risk factors for gestational trophoblastic disease: A separate analysis of complete and partial hydatidiform moles. Obstet Gynecol 1991;78:1039.
15. Berkowitz RS, Bernstein MR, Harlow BL: Case-control study of risk factors for partial molar pregnancy. Am J Obstet Gynecol 1995;173:788.
16. Lawler SD, Fisher RA, Dent J: A prospective genetic study of complete and partial hydatidiform moles. Am J Obstet Gynecol 1991;164:1270.
17. Lage JM, Mark SD, Roberts D, et al: A flow cytometric study of 137 fresh hydropic placentas: Correlation between types of hydatidiform moles and DNA ploidy. Obstet Gynecol 1992;79:403.
18. Genest DR, Ruiz RE, Weremowicz S, et al: Do non triploid partial hydatidiform moles exist? A histologic and flow cytometric reevaluation of nontriploid specimens. J Reprod Med 2002;47:363.
19. Fulop V, Mok SC, Gati I, et al: Recent advances in molecular biology of gestational trophoblastic diseases: A review. J Reprod Med 2002;47:369.
20. Cheung ANY, Srivastava G, Pittaluga S, et al: Expression of c-myc and c-fms oncogenes in hydatidiform mole and human normal placenta. J Clin Pathol 1994;46:204.
21. Cheung ANY, Srivastava G, Chung LP, et al: Expression of the p53 gene in trophoblastic cells in hydatidiform mole and normal human placenta. J Reprod Med 1994;39:223.
22. Fulop V, Mok SC, Genest DR, et al: p53, p21, Rb, and MdM2 oncoproteins: Expression in normal placenta, partial and complete mole and choriocarcinoma. J Reprod Med 1998;43:119.
23. Fulop V, Mok SC, Genest DR, et al: c-myc, c-erbB-2, c-fms, and bcl-2 oncoproteins: Expression in normal placenta, partial and complete mole and choriocarcinoma. J Reprod Med 1998;43:101.
24. Vegh GL, Tuncer ZS, Fulop V, et al: Matrix metalloproteinases and their inhibitors in gestational trophoblastic diseases and normal placenta. Gynecol Oncol 1999;75:248.
25. Mutter GL, Stewart CL, Chaponot ML, et al: Oppositely imprinted genes H19 and insulin-like growth factor 2 are co-expressed in human androgenetic trophoblast. Am J Hum Genet 1993;53:1096.
26. Soto-Wright V, Bernstein MR, Goldstein DP, et al: The changing clinical presentation of complete molar pregnancy. Obstet Gynecol 1995;86:775.
27. Mosher R, Goldstein DP, Berkowitz RS, et al: Complete hydatidiform mole—comparison of clinicopathologic features, current and past. J Reprod Med 1998;43:21.
28. Keep D, Zaragoza MV, Hasold T, et al: Very early complete hydatidiform mole. Hum Pathol 1996;27:708.
29. Feltmate CM, Genest DR, Wise L, et al: Placental site trophoblastic tumor. A 17-year experience at the New England Trophoblastic Disease Center. Gynecol Oncol 2001;82:415.
30. Berkowitz TRS, Goldstein DP, Anderson DJ: Recent advances in understanding the immunology of gestational trophobolastic disease—a review. Trophoblast Res 1987;2:123.
31. Ito H, Sekine T, Komuro N, et al: Histologic stromal reaction of the host with gestational choriocarcinoma and its relation to clinical stages, classification and prognosis. Am J Obstet Gynecol 1981;140:781.
32. Berkowitz RS, Hill JA, Kurtz CB, et al: Effects of products of activated leukocytes (lymphokines and monokines) jn the growth of malignant trophoblast cells in vitro. Am J Obstet Gynecol 1988;158:199.
33. Berkowitz RS, Hornig-Rohan J, Martin-Alosco S, et al: HLA antigen frequency distribution in patients with gestational chorio-carcinoma and their husbands. Placenta Suppl 1981;3:263.
34. Tomoda Y, Fuma M, Saiki N, et al: Immunological studies in patients with trophoblastic neoplasia. Am J Obstet Gynecol 1976;126:6561.
35. Morgenson B, Kissmeyer-Nielson F, Hauge M: Histocompatibility antigens on the HL-A locus in gestational choriocarcinoma. Transplant Proc 1969;1:76.
36. Berkowitz RS, Mostoufizadeh M, Kabawat SE, et al: Immuno-pathologic study of the implantation site in molar pregnancy. Am J Obstet Gynecol 1982;144:925.
37. Berkowitz RS, Lahey SJ, Rodrick ML, et al: Circulating immune complex levels in patients with molar pregnancy. Obstet Gynecol 1983;61:165.
38. Lahey SJ, Steele G Jr, Berkowitz RS, et al: Identification of maternal with placental HLA antigen immunoreactivity from purported circulating immune complexes inpatients with gestational trophoblastic neoplasms. J Natl Cancer Inst 1984;72:983.
39. Berkowitz RS, Anderson DJ, Hunter NJ, et al: Distribution of major histocompatibility (HLA) antigens in chorionic villi of molar pregnancy. Am J Obstet Gynecol 1983;146:221.
40. Santos-Ramos R, Forney JP, Schwartz BE: Sonographic findings and clinical correlations in molar pregnancy. Obstet Gynecol 1980;56:186.
41. Montz FJ, Schlaerth JB, Morrow CP: The natural history of theca lutein cysts. Obstet Gynecol 1988;72:247.
42. Kohorn EI: Molar pregnancy: Presentation and diagnosis. Clin Obstet Gynecol 1984;27:181.

Specific Malignancies

III

43. Nisula BC, Taliadouros GS: Thyroid function in gestational trophoblastic neoplasia: Evidence that the thyrotropic activity of chorionic gonadotropin mediates the thyrotoxicosis of choriocarcinoma. Am J Obstet Gynecol 1980;138:77.

44. Berkowitz RS, Goldstein DP, Bernstein MR: Natural history of partial molar pregnancy. Obstet Gynecol 1986;66:677.

45. Szulman AE, Surti U: The clinicopathologic profile of partial hydatidiform mole. Obstet Gynecol 1982;59:597.

46. Czernobilsky B, Barash A, Lancet M: Partial mole: A clinicopathologic study of 25 cases. Obstet Gynecol 1982; 59:75.

47. Kelly MP, Rustin GJS, Ivory C, et al: Respiratory failure due to choriocarcinoma: A study of 103 dyspneic patients. Gynecol Oncol 1990;38:149.

48. Bakri YN, Berkowitz RS, Khan J, et al: Pulmonary metastases of gestational trophoblastic tumor: Risk factors for early respiratory failure. J Reprod Med 1994;39:174.

49. Vaccarello L, Apte SM, Diaz P, et al: Respiratory failure from metastatic choriocarcinoma: A survivor of mechanical ventilation. Gynecol Oncol 1997;67:111.

50. Bakri YN, Sughi J, Amer M, et al: Liver metastases of gestational trophoblastic tumor. Gynecol Oncol 1993;l48:110.

51. Bakri YN, Berkowitz RS, Goldstein DP, et al: Brain metastases of gestational trophoblastic tumor. J Reprod Med 1994;39:179.

52. Athanassiou A, Begent RHJ, Newlands ES, et al: Central nervous system metastases of choriocarcinoma: 23 years' experience at Charing Cross Hospital. Cancer 1983;52:1728.

53. Liu TL, Deppe G, Chang QT, et al: Cerebral metastatic chorio-carcinoma in the People's Republic of China. Gynecol Oncol 1983;15:166.

54. Bagshawe KD, Harland S: Immunodiagnosis and monitoring of gonadotropin-producing metastases in the central nervous system. Cancer 1976;38:112.

55. Berkowitz RS, Osathanondh R, Goldstein DP, et al: Cerebraospinal fluid human chorionic gonadotropin levels in normal pregnancy and choriocarcinoma. Surg Obstet Gynecol 1981;153:687.

56. Cole LA: New perspectives in measuring human chorionic gonadotropin levels for measuring and monitoring trophoblastic disease. J Reprod Med 1994;39:193.

57. Genest DR, Laborde O, Berkowitz RS, et al: A clinocpathologic study of 153 cases of complete hydatidiform mole (1980-1990): Histologic grade lacks prognostic significance. Obstet Gynecol 1991;78:402.

58. Berkowitz RS, Ozturk M, Goldstein DP, et al: Human chorionic gonadotropin and free subunits' serum levels in patients with partial and complete hydatidiform moles. Obstet Gynecol 1989;74:212.

59. Fine C, Bundy AL, Berkowitz RS, et al: Sonographic diagnosis of partial hydatidiform mole. Obstet Gynecol 1989;73:414.

60. Hammond CB, Borchert LG, Tyrey L, et al: Treatment of metastatic trophoblastic disease: Good and poor prognosis. Am J Obstet Gynecol 1973;115:451.

61. Bagshawe KD: Risks and prognostic factors in trophoblastic neoplasia. Cancer 1976;38:1373.

62. Rodabaugh KJ, Bernstein MR, Goldstein DP, et al: Natural history of post-term choriocarcinoma. J Reprod Med 1998;43:76.

63. Goldstein DP, Berkowitz RS: Prophylactic chemotherapy of complete molar pregnancy. Semin Oncol 1995;22:157.

64. Kim DS, Moon H, Kim KT, et al: Effects of prophylactic chemotherapy for persistent trophoblastic disease in patients with complete hydatidiform mole. Obstet Gynecol 1986;67:690.

65. Limpongsanurak S: Prophylactic actinomycin D for high-risk complete hydatidiform mole. J Reprod Med 2001;46:110.

66. Cole LA, Butler S: Detection of hCG in trophoblastic disease—the USA hCG Reference Service Experience. J Reprod Med 2002;47:4333.

67. Holmesley HD: Single-agent therapy for non-metastatic and low-risk, metastatic gestational trophoblastic disease. J Reprod Med 1998;43:69.

68. Bagshawe KD, Wilde CE: Infusion therapy for pelvic trophoblastic tumors. J Obstet Gynaecol Br Commonw 1964;71:565.

69. Berkowitz RS, Goldstein DP, Bernstein MR: Ten years' experience with methotrexate and folinic acid as primary therapy for gestational trophoblastic disease. Gynec Oncol 1986;23:111.

70. Sung HC, Wu PC, Yang HY: Re-evaluation of 5-fluorouracil as a single therapeutic agent for gestational trophoblastic neoplasms. Am J Obstet Gynecol 1984;150:69.

71. Wong LC, Choo YC, Ma HK: Primary oral etoposide therapy in gestational trophoblastic disease: An update. Cancer 1986;58:14.

72. Bagshawe KD: Treatment of high risk choriocarcinoma. J Reprod Med 1984;29:813.

73. Bower M, Newlands ES, Holden L, et al: EMA/CO for high risk gestational trophoblastic tumors: Results from a cohort of 272 patients. J Clin Oncol 1997;15:2636.

74. Rustin GJS, Newlands ES, Lutz JM, et al: Combination but not single-agent methotrexate chemotherapy for gestational trophoblastic tumors increases the incidence of second tumors. J Clin Oncol 1996;14:L2767.

75. DuBeshter B, Berkowitz RS, Goldstein DP, et al: Vinblastine, cisplatin and bleomycin as salvage therapy for refractory high-risk metastatic gestational trophoblastic disease. J Reprod Med 1989;34:189.

76. Hammond CB, Weed JC, Currie JL: The role of operation in the current therapy of gestational trophoblastic disease. Am J Obstet Gynecol 1980;136:844.

77. Papadopoulos AJ, Foskett M, Sekl MJ, et al: Twenty-five years' clinical experience with placental site trophoblastic tumors. J Reprod Med 2002;47:460.

78. Tomoda Y, Arii Y, Kaseki S, et al: Surgical indications for resection in pulmonary metastases of choriocarcinoma. Cancer 1980;46:2723.

79. Jones WB, Romain K, Erlandson RA, et al: Thoracotomy in the management of gestational choriocarcinoma: A clinicopathologic study. Cancer 1993;72:2175.

80. Yordan EL Jr, Schlaerth J, Gaddis O, et al: Radiation therapy in the management of gestational choriocarcinoma metastatic to the central nervous system. Obstet Gynecol 1987;69:627.

81. Newland ES, Holdlen L, Seckl MJ, et al: Management of brain metastases in patient with high risk gestational trophoblastic tumors. J Reprod Med 2002;47:465.

82. Evans AC Jr, Soper JT, Clarke-Pearson DL, et al: Gestational trophoblastic disease metastatic to the central nervous system. Gynecol Oncol 1995;59:226.

83. Grumbine FC, Rosenshein NB, Brereton HD, et al: Management of liver metastases from gestational trophoblastic neoplasia. Am J Obstet Gynecol 1980;137:959.

84. Wong LC, Choo YC, Ma HK: Hepatic metastases in gestational trophoblastic disease. Obstet Gynecol 1986;67:107.

85. Stone M, Dent J, Kardana A, et al: Relationship of oral contraception to development of trophoblastic tumour following evacuation of an hydatidiform mole. Br J Obstet Gynecol 1976;83:913.

86. Berkowitz RS, Goldstein DP, Marean AR, et al: Oral contraceptives and postmolar trophoblastic disease. Obstet Gynecol 1981;58:474.

87. Mutch DG, Soper JT, Babcock CJ, et al: Recurrent gestational trophoblastic disease. Experience of the Southeastern Regional Trophoblastic Disease Center. Cancer 1990;66:978.

88. Goldstein DP, Zanten-Przybysz I, Bernstein MR, et al: Revised FIGO staging system for gestational trophoblastic tumors: Recommendations regarding therapy. J Reprod Med 1998;43:37.

89. Lurain JR, Sand PK, Carson SA, et al: Pregnancy outcome subsequent to consecutive hydatidiform moles. Am J Obstet Gyecol 1982;142:1060.

90. Bagshawe KD, Dent J, Webb J: Hydatidiform mole in England and Wales 1973–1983. Lancet 1986;2:673.

91. Woolas RP, Bower M, Newlands ES, et al: Influence of chemotherapy for gestational trophoblastic disease on subsequent pregnancy outcome. Br J Obstet Gynaecol 1998;105:1032.

92. Wenzel LB, Berkowitz RS, Robinson S, et al: Psychological, social, and sexual effects of gestational trophoblastic disease on patients and partners. J Reprod Med 1994;39:163.

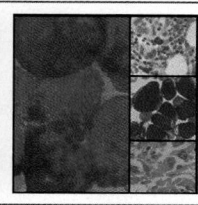

CANCER OF THE BREAST

Martin D. Abeloff

Antonio C. Wolff

William C. Wood

Beryl McCormick

Barbara L. Weber

SUMMARY OF KEY POINTS

INCIDENCE AND EPIDEMIOLOGY

- Breast cancer is the most frequently diagnosed cancer in women in the United States, accounting for an estimated 276,000 new cases (217,000 invasive cancers and 59,000 in situ carcinomas) and more than 40,000 deaths in 2001
- In the United States, the age-specific incidence of breast cancer increases with age, to a lifetime risk of breast cancer of 1 in 8 (to 110 years of age); by age 40, approximately 1 in 250 women will have been diagnosed with breast cancer annually; at 60 years of age, the figure is 1 in 35 women
- Incidence rates rose 21% from 1973 to 1990, but then began to decline; mortality rates have stayed relatively constant until recently, when annual decreases have been seen
- Age, family history, and both endogenous and exogenous ovarian hormone exposure have an important effect on risk and have been incorporated into models that predict individual risk of breast cancer; diet, alcohol use, and other factors play a smaller role
- Inherited mutations in *BRCA1*, *BRCA2*, and *CHEK2* play a role in the development of breast cancer and can be directly tested in individuals

BIOLOGY AND ESTIMATION OF RISK

- The expression of nuclear estrogen and progesterone receptors plays an important role in the differentiation and growth of normal breast epithelium and the response of breast cancer cells to hormonal therapeutics
- ERBB2 (HER2) is a growth-signaling molecule on the surface of normal breast cells that is overexpressed in approximately one third of breast cancer cells, contributing to growth autonomy and genomic instability

- *TP53* is a tumor-suppressor gene that is mutated in 30% to 50% of breast cancers; loss of normal TP53 function is associated with a poor prognosis and reduced likelihood of treatment response, possibly because of decreased response to apoptotic signaling, increased genome instability, and angiogenesis
- *BRCA1* and *BRCA2* are tumor-suppressor genes that play a critical role in the cellular response to DNA damage; inherited mutations in these genes are associated with an increased risk of breast cancer
- Regardless of the criteria used by an individual physician and patient to define high risk, four possible actions may be taken, some of which can be used simultaneously: (1) enhanced surveillance, (2) behavioral modification, (3) chemopreventive strategies, and (4) prophylactic mastectomy or oophorectomy

SCREENING AND DIAGNOSIS

- Despite recent challenges to the benefits of mammographic screening, the United States Preventive Service Task Force and many other organizations recommend screening mammography, with or without clinical breast examination, every 1 to 2 years for women 40 years of age and older
- Microcalcification and soft tissue density are the major indications for biopsy in mammographic screening; the mammographic abnormality with the highest rate of malignancy is a mass density with associated calcification
- Computer-assisted digitized mammographic imaging, magnetic resonance imaging, positron emission tomography, and radionuclide scanning are under intense investigation as emerging techniques for breast imaging

- For patients with breast symptoms or palpable abnormalities, mammography characterizes the suspicious area, evaluates the remainder of the breast for occult lesions, and assesses the contralateral breast
- Malignant breast masses classically are nontender and firm, with irregular borders
- Diagnostic methods include fine-needle aspiration cytology, needle core biopsy with ultrasound or stereotactic guidance, and excisional biopsy, with or without wire or tack localization

MANAGEMENT OF NONINVASIVE DISEASE

- Lobular carcinoma in situ (LCIS) is a nonpalpable lesion that is usually discovered with another indicator for biopsy; it is more common in premenopausal women and accounts for 30% to 50% of cases of carcinoma in situ
- LCIS has a propensity for multicentricity and bilaterality; it is an indicator of risk of subsequent invasive breast cancer
- Management of LCIS had shifted toward observation after biopsy rather than mastectomy; increasing evidence shows that tamoxifen should be considered as a preventive approach; the multifocal nature of LCIS makes margin clearance an unrealistic and unnecessary goal
- Unlike LCIS, ductal carcinoma in situ (DCIS), is almost always first identified by mammography; the peak incidence is between 51 and 59 years of age, and it accounts for most of the increasing number of carcinoma in situ lesions diagnosed
- DCIS is more likely to be localized to one area of the breast; thus, most patients are candidates for breast conservation; tamoxifen should also be considered

MANAGEMENT OF EARLY INVASIVE DISEASE (STAGES I AND II)

- Patients should undergo a complete history and physical examination
- Hemogram and renal and hepatic function tests as well as serum alkaline phosphatase evaluation should be performed in all patients
- Bilateral mammography is indicated for all patients; other imaging studies are recommended only to evaluate specific signs or symptoms or in patients with locally advanced disease
- Prognostic factors include pathologic tumor size, hormone receptors, axillary nodal status, histologic subtype, tumor grade, and perhaps age; new biologic prognosticators require further study before routine application
- Overexpression of HER2 identifies patients with metastatic disease who might benefit from trastuzumab therapy, but its utility as a prognostic factor in early-stage disease is still under evaluation
- Promising results have been shown with microarray-based expression profiling as a potential means of gauging prognosis or predicting response to therapy
- The revised American Joint Committee on Cancer TNM staging system takes into account the increasing use of novel imaging and pathology techniques, such as sentinel node biopsy and immunochemistry; it also considers the number of involved nodes a strong prognostic factor
- Axillary dissection of level I and II nodes remains a valuable staging procedure; however, sentinel lymph node mapping is being used in lieu of axillary dissection for patients with clinically negative axillae. Large prospective, controlled, and randomized trials are comparing these two axillary staging techniques
- For patients with stage I and II disease, breast conservation and modified radical mastectomy are the therapeutic options; for most patients, breast conservation is an acceptable approach
- Factors that affect local control in breast conservation include pathologic margin evaluation, extensive intraductal component, age, and the presence of multiple tumors
- Adjuvant therapy with cytotoxic drugs or endocrine treatment, or both, is recommended for patients with node-positive disease
- Pathologic tumor size, hormone-receptor status, histologic subtype, and nuclear grade are used to select patients with node-negative disease for adjuvant therapy
- The results of the meta-analysis performed by the Early Breast Cancer Trialists' Collaborative Group (EBCTCG) show that the survival benefits of adjuvant chemotherapy and endocrine therapy persist after 15 years of follow-up
- Challenges that require resolution include identification of biologic parameters that more precisely predict the natural history of disease and the response to systemic therapy; more effective treatments are clearly needed

MANAGEMENT OF LOCALLY ADVANCED DISEASE

- Patients with locally advanced disease (stage III) are a heterogeneous group, including those with T3N1, T0–3N2–3, and T4N0–3 disease
- Multimodality therapy is recommended for virtually all patients with locally advanced disease; the sequence of chemotherapy, surgery, and radiation is largely dependent on the operability of the primary disease
- For women with inoperable or inflammatory breast cancer (or both), preoperative chemotherapy is recommended, followed by surgery, radiation, and endocrine therapy, if appropriate. Preoperative endocrine therapy for patients with receptor-positive disease is also a reasonable option

MANAGEMENT OF LOCALLY RECURRENT DISEASE

- Local recurrence is an indicator of systemic relapse in most cases; an exception may be local relapse in a breast that has undergone conservation therapy
- Selection of the treatment modality is largely dependent on the extent of local and regional failure and the presence of distant metastases
- Surgical removal alone may be sufficient in some cases, but it is frequently combined with locoregional radiation and/or systemic therapy

MANAGEMENT OF METASTATIC DISEASE

- Although a small percentage of patients with metastatic breast cancer achieve long-term disease-free survival, this stage of disease essentially is not curable and therapy is largely palliative
- A wide range of systemic, local, and supportive therapies are available for the palliation of metastatic breast cancer
- The selection of endocrine, cytotoxic, or biologic therapy is usually based on disease-free interval, receptor status, HER2 status, site of metastasis, performance status, age, and previous exposure to systemic therapy

INTRODUCTION

Breast cancer is the most common cancer in women in the United States and the second leading cause of death from malignancy in women. The effect of breast cancer on U.S. society, however, exceeds even those impressive numbers in that this disease has had dramatic social, psychological, cultural, and even political consequences. Recent cancer statistics show the good news that in the 1990s death rates from breast cancer have been decreasing in the United States and the United Kingdom, despite the increasing incidence of breast cancer during this period. However, the magnitude of the decrease in death rates in African Americans and other minority groups has not been as great. The most likely cause is lack of access to early-detection programs and treatment services, although biologic differences have not been excluded.

Certain key factors led to changes in the management of breast cancer and ultimately improvement in death rates. These factors include incremental improvements in the screening and early diagnosis of breast cancer throughout the last century as well as improvements, refinements, and innovations in surgery and radiation therapy. Other factors include new adjuvant endocrine therapies, cytotoxic drugs, biologic therapies, and combinations of these treatments, as well as a vigorous patient advocacy movement that not only has facilitated and accelerated research efforts, but also has made therapy more accessible to the U.S. population. The marked increase in the understanding of the molecular and cellular biology of breast cancer is also beginning to yield new molecularly targeted diagnostic and therapeutic approaches, and progress in prevention is also being made. This chapter reviews the epidemiologic and biologic basis of the current understanding of breast cancer, and emphasizes the collaborative, multidisciplinary, preventive, diagnostic, treatment, and supportive care approaches that are required to continue making significant progress against this disease.

TABLE 94-1

Risk of Breast Cancer in U.S. Women

AGE RANGE	BREAST CANCER RISK
30–40 yr	1:252
40–50 yr	1:68
50–60 yr	1:35
60–70 yr	1:27
Lifetime (to age 110 yr)	1:8

www.cancer.gov

INCIDENCE AND EPIDEMIOLOGY

In the United States, breast cancer is the most frequently diagnosed cancer in women, with 217,000 new cases of invasive disease, 59,000 new cases of in situ disease, and more than 40,000 deaths estimated in 2004 (American Cancer Society, www.cancer.org). Breast cancer accounts for 30% of all cancers diagnosed and 16% of all cancer deaths in U.S. women.[1] Worldwide, particularly in developed countries, breast cancer is a major public health problem, with 1 million new cases diagnosed annually.[2]

In the United States, the lifetime risk of female breast cancer is estimated at 1 in 8.[1] However, more than half of this risk is incurred after 60 years of age, and the risk of 1 in 8 is not reached until 110 years of age[3] (Table 94-1 and Fig. 94-1). In addition, risk is very heterogenous in the population. Therefore, individual risk assessment is considerably more useful than population risk in the development of clinical management strategies. Means of estimating individual risk are discussed later in this chapter.

Breast cancer incidence rates vary markedly between populations, with the highest rates in Western countries (>100 cases/100,000 women) and the lowest rates in Asian countries (10 to 15 cases/100,000 women).[2] However, incidence rates have increased rapidly in countries

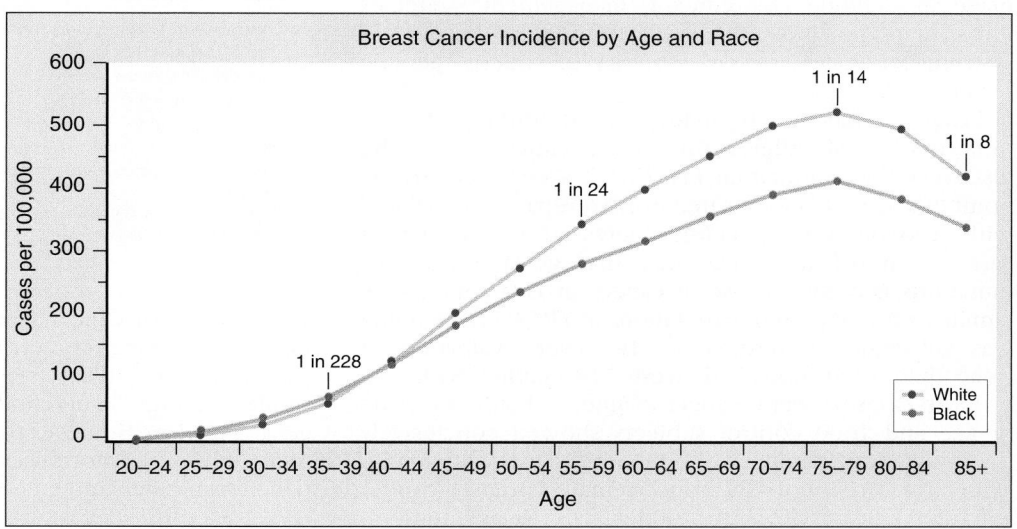

Figure 94-1. Incidence of breast cancer by age and race. The increased incidence in black women before 45 years of age is seen. After 45 years of age, incidence rates in white women are higher but mortality rates are lower than in black women. Risk figures are shown above the curve. The commonly cited 1 in 8 lifetime risk of breast cancer in U.S. women is not reached until 85 years of age or older. (Surveillance, Epidemiology, and End Results [SEER], 2003, http://seer.cancer. gov/.)

Specific Malignancies

such as Japan, where major lifestyle changes have occurred in the last 50 years. When women from Asia or other low-risk areas migrate to an area of high risk, they gradually assume the risk of the high-risk population.[4] Interestingly, the difference in breast cancer incidence between Asian and Western populations is primarily the result of much lower incidence rates of postmenopausal breast cancer in Asian countries, because premenopausal breast cancer rates are similar in Asian and Western countries. These data suggest that underlying genetic factors that contribute primarily to breast cancer in young women are similar in both populations, but hormone exposure and lifestyle factors that vary widely between continents may play an important role in defining postmenopausal breast cancer risk.[5]

EPIDEMIOLOGY AND RISK FACTORS

Risk factors associated with the development of breast cancer are summarized in Table 94-2 and are discussed briefly in the next section.

Family History and Inherited Risk Factors

Many studies show that the risk of breast cancer in an individual increases with the number of affected relatives. A particularly strong effect is seen in women who have relatives diagnosed with premenopausal breast cancer. Between 10% and 20% of women with breast cancer have an affected first- or second-degree relative, and 50% report at least one affected relative of any type.[6] Approximately 5% of women with breast cancer have a family history that suggests a single high-risk susceptibility gene mutation.[7,8] Two such genes have been isolated, BRCA1[9] and BRCA2.[10] However, these genes account for only 30% to 40% of cases of breast cancer that appears in families as an autosomal dominant trait, leaving the cause in a substantial number of high-risk families unexplained.[11,12] Several large international consortia have been assembled to isolate additional high-risk breast cancer susceptibility genes, so far, to no avail. However, substantial progress has been made in defining risk-reducing management strategies for women with BRCA1 and BRCA2 mutations, providing a strong rationale for women at risk to undergo genetic testing.[13-15]

Progress has been made in identifying lower-penetrance risk alleles for breast cancer, with the discovery that a mutation in CHEK2, a cell-cycle checkpoint kinase that is implicated in DNA repair, is associated with a twofold to threefold increased risk of breast cancer.[16] Initial data suggested that germline CHEK2 mutations may be a cause of cancer in Li-Fraumeni–like families without germline mutations in TP53[17]; this finding was subsequently refuted.[16,18] However, evaluation of more than 1000 individuals from 718 families with two or more cases of breast cancer diagnosed before 60 years of age and 1600 control subjects showed conclusively that the CHEK2 mutation 1100delC is associated with a relative risk of 2.2 for female breast cancer ($P < 0.0000001$). CHEK2 1100delC also was found in

TABLE 94-2

Risk Factors for Breast Cancer

RISK FACTOR	RISK	REFS
Family History		
First-Degree Relative		134–136
Premenopausal diagnosis	OR 3.0	
Bilateral disease	OR 5.0	
Premenopausal diagnosis and bilateral disease	OR 9.0	
Postmenopausal diagnosis	OR 1.5	
Second-Degree Relative		137
Premenopausal diagnosis	OR 1.2	
Postmenopausal diagnosis	No increased risk	
Germline Mutations		
BRCA1/BRCA2	60%–80% lifetime risk	138–140
TP53	30%–40% lifetime risk	141
CHEK2	OR 2.2	16
Dietary Fat Intake	No consistent association	20, 142
Alcohol		22, 23
3–9 drinks/wk	OR 1.3	
≥10 drinks/wk	OR 1.6	
Oral Contraceptives		25
Current Users	OR 1.2	
1–4 yr after stopping	OR 1.16	
5–9 yr after stopping	OR 1.07	
>10 yr after stopping	OR 1.0	
Hormone Replacement Therapy*	OR 1.1–1.4	26, 27
Reproductive Factors		32
Menarche before 16 yr	OR 1.2	
Menopause after 50 yr	OR 1.5	
Nulliparity	OR 2.0	
Breast-feeding	4.3% decreased risk/yr	39
Benign Breast Disease		40
Fibrocystic disease	No increased risk	
Ductal hyperplasia	OR 1.3	
Atypical ductal hyperplasia	OR 4.3	
Atypical ductal hyperplasia and family history	OR 11.0	41
Breast Irradiation†		
Contralateral breast irradiation	No increased risk	49, 50
Mantle radiation for Hodgkin's disease	OR 39.0	47
Atomic bomb survivors	OR 13.0	45

OR, odds ratio.
*Combined estrogen and progestin therapy for at least 5 years after natural menopause.[27]
†Adolescent or premenopausal exposure. No increased risk reported for postmenopausal exposure.

13.5% of breast cancer families with at least one case of male breast cancer, conferring a relative risk of 10 for male breast cancer.[16] A large Finnish study recently reported similar findings.[16] The clinical utility of testing for such a gene is unclear. However, these low-penetrance genes may ultimately prove more useful as part of a risk assessment panel than as an independent predictor of risk, such as BRCA1 and BRCA2.

Diet

Dietary ingestion of fat has been associated with increased levels of plasma estrogen. Marked reduction in fat intake can be associated with reductions in plasma estradiol levels within a few weeks of dietary alteration.[19] However, although many studies have been performed, conclusive evidence separating fat intake from a number of other factors that could affect breast cancer risk has been difficult to produce. One meta-analysis of 12 studies that included more than 10,000 subjects found a positive correlation between fat intake and breast cancer in postmenopausal women.[20] However, a pooled analysis of cohort studies showed no evidence of a link between dietary fat intake and breast cancer.[21] The Women's Health Initiative, a large epidemiologic study sponsored by the National Cancer Institute (NCI), will randomize women to low-fat or standard diets to determine whether reducing dietary fat intake decreases the risk of breast cancer.

Alcohol Consumption

Alcohol consumption was associated with the risk of breast cancer in a number of studies, including two large prospective cohort studies.[22,23] Odds ratios range from 1.2 to 1.6, with the highest risk seen in women who consume more than the equivalent of three glasses of wine daily. It is unclear why even modest alcohol consumption should affect the incidence of breast cancer, and many researchers regard the association of alcohol and breast cancer with skepticism. Recent studies show that ethanol ingestion can increase the levels of sex steroid hormones in nonalcoholic premenopausal women, but the mechanism remains unknown.[24]

Oral Contraceptives

Oral contraceptive use is associated with a very slight increase in breast cancer risk (relative risk = 1.2) for current users vs. never-users. However, breast cancer risk associated with the use of oral contraceptives disappears with time when use is discontinued. One to 4 years after discontinuation the relative risk is 1.16, at 5 to 9 years after use the risk is 1.07, and by 10 years from last use, breast cancer risk of ever-users is not different from never-users.[25]

Hormone Replacement Therapy

Results of the many studies of hormone replacement therapy (HRT) and the risk of breast cancer have been mixed, with some detecting no measurable risk and others estimating a relative risk of 1.1 to 1.4.[26] As with oral contraceptives, this risk dissipates after estrogen use is discontinued. Recent data from the Women's Health Initiative randomized trial of estrogen and progesterone in healthy postmenopausal women found a 26% increase in the risk of breast cancer over a mean follow-up of 5.2 years.[27] This effect varied over time, and no increase in breast cancer risk was seen until after the first 4 years of therapy. This trial confirmed the benefit of HRT in prevention of osteoporotic fractures (relative risk = 0.66), but did not show a benefit in prevention of coronary heart disease (relative risk = 1.29). Thus, routine use of postmenopausal HRT for prevention of coronary heart disease is no longer recommended for all women, irrespective of breast cancer risk.[28-30] Short-term use of postmenopausal HRT (<5 years) for relief of postmenopausal symptoms remains a reasonable option for some women. Longer use for prevention of osteoporosis may be beneficial for women at high risk for osteoporotic fracture and at relatively low risk for breast cancer[28-30] and must be considered in the context of effective nonhormonal interventions for the management of osteoporosis.

Menstrual and Reproductive Factors

Breast cancer risk has been consistently linked to age at menarche and age at menopause, surrogates for the lifetime number of ovarian cycles. Each earlier year at menarche and later year at menopause (using ages 16 and 50 years as benchmarks, respectively) is associated with a 4% to 5% increase in the risk of breast cancer.[31,32] Other well-established hormonal risk factors are age at first live birth and parity. First live birth before 20 years of age is associated with a breast cancer risk that is 50% lower than that associated with first live birth after 35 years of age.[33] In addition, women with three or more live births have a significantly lower risk of breast cancer than nulliparous women.[31,34,35] Some studies suggest that abortions are associated with an increased risk of breast cancer[36,37]; however, the largest, most methodologically sound study using population-based data from a national health registry found no such association.[38] A recent working group of epidemiologists and other scientists constituted by the NCI also concluded that there was no association between induced or spontaneous abortion and the risk of breast cancer. Finally, breast-feeding appears to have a small protective effect against breast cancer, possibly by allowing a final cellular differentiation step in breast epithelium to take place.[39]

Benign Breast Disease

Benign breast lesions, such as papillomas, fibroadenomas, and those commonly referred to as fibrocystic change, are not premalignant lesions and are not associated with an increased risk of breast cancer. However, proliferative changes, primarily ductal or lobular hyperplasia, confer a relative risk of 1.5 to 2, and atypical hyperplasia is associated with a substantially increased relative risk of 3 to 5.[40] In women with a family history of breast cancer, atypical proliferative changes were associated with a relative risk of 11 in one study.[41] These data are important considerations in patient management and also suggest a recognizable process of malignant transformation from normal to hyperplastic to atypical epithelium, followed by progression to ductal carcinoma in situ (DCIS) and ultimately to invasive breast cancer.

Ionizing Radiation

Low-dose radiation exposure to the breast is clearly carcinogenic,[42-44] with the risk of breast cancer increasing with exposure dose.[43,45–47] This risk is also age-dependent, with women exposed during adolescence having the greatest risk and women exposed after 50 years of age having virtually no added risk. There has been concern about whether radiation scatter to the contralateral breast during the treatment of primary breast cancer (100 to 200 cGy[48]) increases the risk of contralateral breast cancer. However, several studies show this not to be the case.[49,50] The latent period between exposure and the diagnosis of breast cancer is 10 to 15 years or longer. Previously, the population at greatest risk for radiation-induced breast cancer was Japanese women who survived the atomic attacks at Hiroshima and Nagasaki.[45,46] Now it is young women who receive radiation therapy for Hodgkin's disease (relative risk = 39).[47] In the future, it may be women exposed in nuclear accidents, such as the Chernobyl nuclear disaster in 1986.

MODELS TO ESTIMATE THE RISK OF BREAST CANCER

One widely used means of assessing individual risk, commonly called the Gail model,[51] was derived from a prospective analysis of women undergoing regular mammographic screening. This model incorporates family history of breast cancer, previous breast biopsy (including atypical ductal hyperplasia), age at menarche, and first live birth as risk factors, and accounts for racial differences in breast cancer incidence. The Gail model was used to determine eligibility for the National Surgical Adjuvant Breast and Bowel Project (NSABP) breast cancer chemoprevention trial of tamoxifen vs. placebo. It is now commonly used to identify women who may benefit from tamoxifen as a chemopreventive agent and is available for use on the NCI Web site (http://bcra.nci.nih.gov/brc/q1.htm).

The Claus model, another commonly used tool for predicting breast cancer risk, was derived from data collected in the Cancer and Steroid Hormone (CASH) study.[52] Estimates derived from the Claus model are based solely on family history, and include age at which affected relatives were diagnosed as an important component of risk. These estimates are provided as a series of tables that list individual risk estimates at 10-year intervals from 20 to 80 years of age. One limitation of the Gail model is the inclusion of only first-degree relatives, thus underestimating risk in the 50% of families with cancer in the paternal lineage. The Claus model incorporates maternal and paternal breast cancer history, first- and second-degree relatives, and age at diagnosis of breast cancer. Concordance of the Gail and Claus models is only fair, with the greatest discrepancies seen with nulliparous women, those with multiple benign breast biopsy findings, and those with a strong paternal family history, because paternal relatives are not included in the Gail model (reviewed by Domchek and associates[53]).

BIOLOGY

A clear understanding of the underlying genetic and biologic differences between normal and malignant breast epithelium and a system of classifying breast cancers based on the specific molecular differences found in individual breast cancers form the basis for developing effective targeted therapies and ultimately for curing breast cancer. Several genes are very well studied in breast cancer, including the estrogen receptors (ERs) and progesterone receptors (PRs) ERBB2, TP53, BRCA1, and BRCA2. The biologic function of these genes and their relevance to breast cancer are discussed later. In addition, high-throughput, whole-genome technologies have been applied in recent years in an attempt to identify additional genes that are important in the genesis of breast cancer and to link clinical outcome to molecular profiles. Data from these studies are also summarized.

Estrogen Receptors (ER-α and ER-β)

Both normal breast epithelium and many malignant breast tumors are dependent on estrogen for growth and cell survival. This effect is mediated by ER, a nuclear transcription factor that binds estrogen as ligand, induces ER homodimer formation, and activates the promoter of several genes (including PR) that induce cell proliferation and confer resistance to apoptosis (reviewed by Osborne and associates[54]). DNA binding by ER homodimers is mediated by a specific sequence motif (estrogen-responsive elements) found in the promoter of estrogen-responsive genes.[55] Breast cancers that express high levels of ER are, at least initially, responsive to hormonal therapies, such as tamoxifen and aromatase inhibitors.

ER was long believed to be a single molecule, but it was recently discovered that two distinct molecules exist, ER-α and ER-β. ER-β is transcribed from a distinct gene on a different chromosome, with different affinities for ligand and responses to antagonists.[56] ER-α is believed to be the predominant form in breast cancer, but ER-β has important physiologic effects as well.[57] The combined function of the two different estrogen receptors may explain in part the differing tissue-specific effects of antiestrogens.

Approximately 15% of normal breast epithelial cells express ER, are evenly distributed throughout the breast, and do not proliferate. Proliferative cells are even less prevalent, but are often adjacent to ER-positive cells, leading to the hypothesis that breast epithelium proliferates through the paracrine effects of factors secreted from ER-positive cells that act locally on ER-negative cells.[58] ER-positive and ER-negative cells are not distinguishable histologically, and nothing is known about interconversion between the cell types. It is a common misconception that ER-positive cells are the proliferative component of mammary epithelium. ER expression and BrdU staining of proliferating cells are almost completely mutually exclusive in normal breast epithelium. However, ER and BrdU are commonly coexpressed in breast cancer cells. Interestingly, in normal breast, coexpression of ER and Ki-67, another marker of proliferation, increases with age, correlating with the risk of breast cancer as determined by other measures.[59] Because proliferative mammary epithelial cells are almost uniformly ER-negative and tumor progenitors require proliferation for clonal expansion, it has been hypothesized that most breast cancers arise from ER-negative cells that acquire ER expression. Thus, altered regulation of this tightly controlled system, allowing proliferation of ER-positive cells, may be a cause of altered proliferative control in cancer rather than a marker for the cell of origin. Changes in ER expression also occur with tumor progression, with studies showing ER expression in approximately 30% of cases of DCIS and in nearly 60% of metastases,[60] providing support for the theory that cells transition from ER-negative to ER-positive as they become malignant, not the more widely assumed converse.

Progesterone Receptor (PGR)

Progesterone has complex growth effects in hormone-responsive tissues. It is generally agreed that progesterone blocks estrogen-stimulated endometrial proliferation. Most in vitro studies of normal and malignant breast cell cultures similarly suggest that progestins reduce the mitogenic effect of estrogen.[61] However, in vivo studies suggest the opposite, with the primary effect of progesterone on breast epithelium being proliferative and progesterone antagonists blocking estrogen-stimulated breast epithelial proliferation (reviewed by Klijn and associates[62]). Recent epidemiologic evidence also suggests that progesterone, used in hormone replacement regimens to balance the growth-stimulating effect of unopposed estrogen on endometrium, is associated with an increased risk of breast cancer.[27] Both estrogen and progesterone are necessary for normal breast development. Mouse models in which PGR has been "knocked out" suggest that estradiol stimulates ductal elongation and progesterone induces lobuloalveolar development.[63]

PGR is an estrogen-regulated gene with an active estrogen-responsive element in its promoter. Therefore, almost all breast cancers that are ER-positive are also PGR-positive. PGR uses separate promoters and translational start sites to produce two isoforms, PRA and PRB, which are identical except for an additional 165 amino acids that are present only in the amino terminus of PRB. Although PRA and PRB share several structural domains, they are distinct transcription factors that mediate different response genes to distinct physiologic effect with little overlap.[64] PRB functions as a transcriptional activator in most cells, whereas PRA is transcriptionally inactive for the most part and functions as a ligand-dependent repressor of steroid hormone-receptor transcriptional activity, explaining the discordant growth effects in various tissues. The N-terminus of PGR mediates a progestin-dependent interaction of PR with various cytoplasmic signaling molecules, including SRC tyrosine kinases inducing potent activation of these kinases and downstream MAP kinase signaling playing an important role in progestin-related growth effects in breast epithelial cells.[65]

TP53

TP53 is an important tumor-suppressor gene for many tissues, including the breast. Between 30% and 50% of breast cancers have somatic TP53 mutations,[66] and many women with germline mutations in TP53 (Li-Fraumeni syndrome) who survive childhood cancers later have breast cancer.[67] Interestingly, 50% to 70% of breast cancers in women with germline BRCA1 mutations also have TP53 mutations, suggesting an interaction between these genes in the development of breast cancer.[68] TP53 is believed to function as a critical component of the cellular response to DNA damage, signaling through p21 for cell-cycle arrest to allow adequate time for high-fidelity repair, or through BAX for apoptosis in the setting of more extensive damage (reviewed by Ryan and associates[69]; Fig. 94-2). Several mouse models have been instructive in defining the role of TP53 in the development of breast cancer. In most cases, the absence of normal TP53 in the mammary gland is not associated with a higher incidence of tumors. However, mammary gland–specific loss of TP53 function reduces the latency of mammary tumor development when these mice are crossed with transgenic animals overexpressing MYC, ERBB2, IGF1, or WNT1. These data suggest that TP53 promotes mammary tumor development, but may not be an initiating event.[70]

Initial studies evaluating a potential association between tumor TP53 mutations and breast cancer outcome with immunohistochemical staining for TP53 as a surrogate marker of TP53 mutations produced ambiguous results, presumably because of the variability in this assay. However, more recent studies using direct mutation detection show a strong association between TP53 mutations and poor prognosis. TP53 mutations are among the most promising prognostic indicators in breast cancer.[71-74]

Although the biologic explanation underlying the association between TP53 mutations and poor prognosis is not known, TP53-mutant tumors may have reduced sensitivity to conditions that induce apoptosis, marked genomic instability,[75,76] increased proliferative capacity,[77] or enhanced angiogenesis.[78,79]

TP53 mutations are linked to drug resistance in breast cancer as well,[80] and are a strong predictor of treatment failure.[72,81] TP53 mutations are associated with resistance to tamoxifen,[73,82] radiation therapy,[83,84] and doxorubicin[74] in most studies, although some studies found no correlation.[84,85] Mutations in genes regulated by the TP53 pathway also correlate with drug resistance. Low levels of expression of BAX, a proapoptotic protein regulated by wild-type TP53, are associated with resistance to drugs and radiation therapy in breast cancer.[86-89]

ERBB2

The proto-oncogene ERBB2 (HER-2/neu) encodes a transmembrane tyrosine kinase receptor, a family of related growth factor receptors that includes EGFR, ERBB3 (HER3), and ERBB4 (HER4).[90] The ligands for these receptors, known as heregulins, are a family of growth factors that bind to ERBB3 and ERBB4, inducing heterodimerization with ERBB2 and subsequent transduction of downstream signals (Fig. 94-3).[91-93] Amplification of ERBB2 or protein overexpression is found in 20% to 30% of breast cancers,[94] and is associated with a more aggressive clinical course and decreased survival time

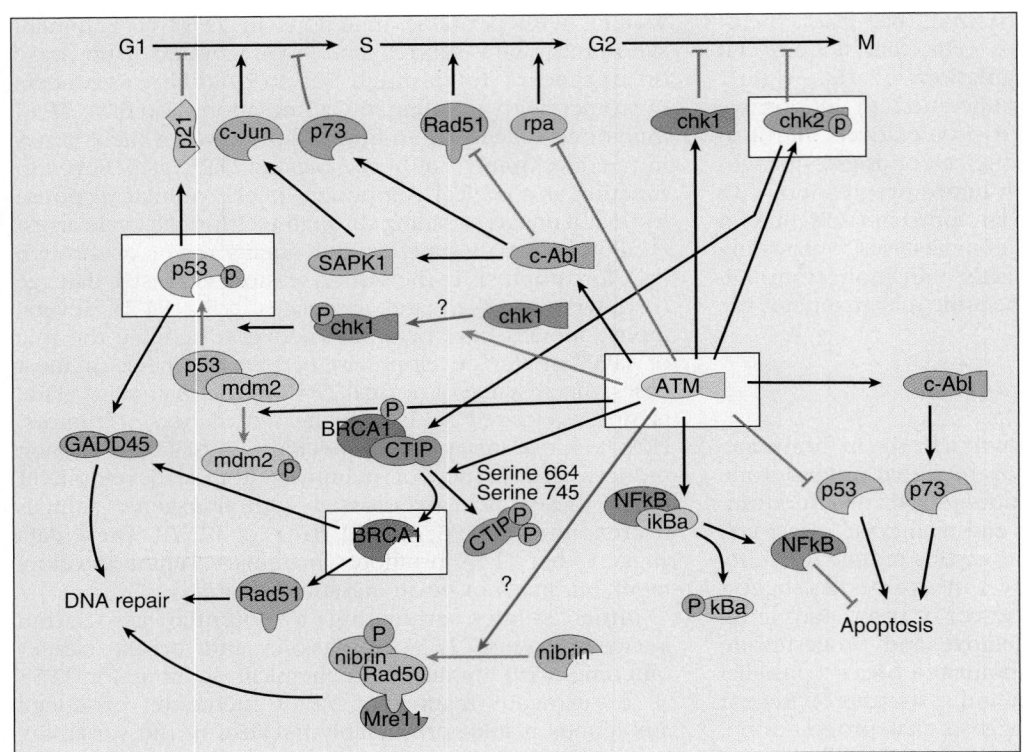

Figure 94-2. DNA damage response pathways and breast cancer. These pathways show the primary cellular responses to double-stranded DNA breaks in human cells. These pathways and a number of their molecular components are important in maintaining genome stability. This function is believed to play a central role in breast cancer tumor suppression. Inherited mutations in the four pathway members outlined by white boxes—BRCA1, TP53 (p53), chk2, and ATM—cause increased susceptibility to breast cancer in the women who carry them. In addition, TP53 mutations are among the most common mutations that occur in sporadic breast cancers. (Modified from Biocarta http://www.biocarta.com/index.asp.)

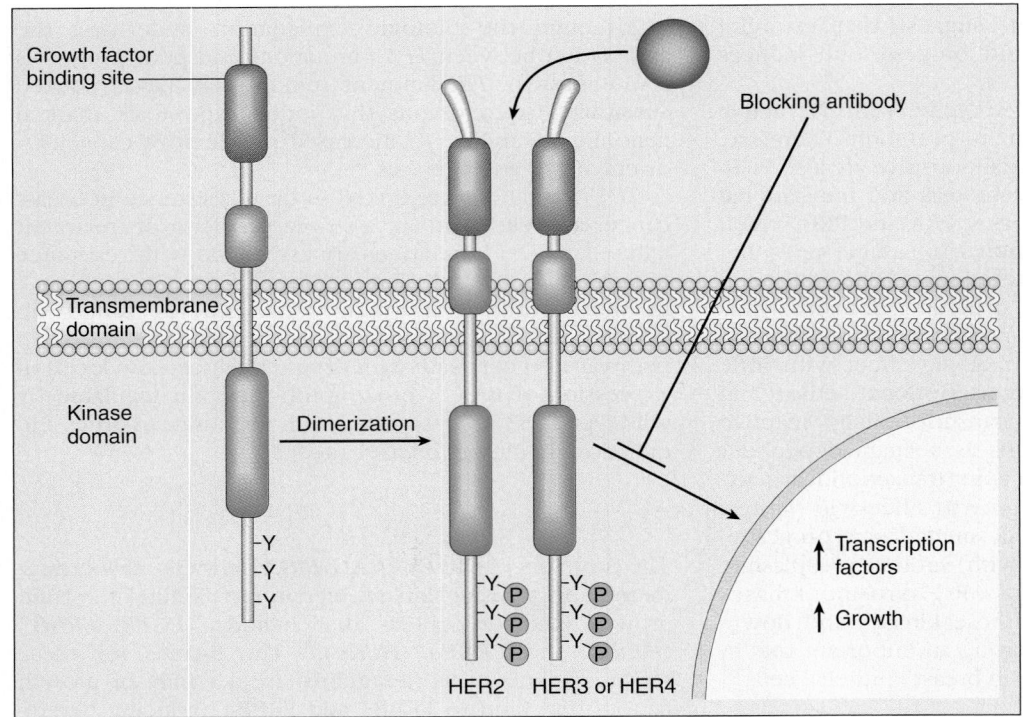

Figure 94-3. ERRB2 (HER2/neu) growth signaling and inhibition. ERBB2, a member of the epidermal growth factor receptor family, is overexpressed in more than 30% of breast cancers and is associated with an aggressive clinical course. ERBB2 receptors exist on the cell surface in the inactive monomeric form until ligand binding results in autophosphorylation and activation. In the activated state, these receptors initiate a signaling cascade that results in upregulation of genes that control cell growth and oncogenesis. Blocking antibodies have been developed that inhibit this process and are effective in the treatment of some breast cancers with ERBB2 overexpression.

compared with tumors with normal levels of ERBB2.[95,96] Several cellular pathways are altered by increased *ERBB2* expression that could explain this clinical behavior. Most directly, overexpression of tyrosine kinase receptors is a well-studied means of producing growth signal autonomy in cancers. It has been particularly well studied in breast cancer, and, as a result, a humanized monoclonal antibody (trastuzumab) that blocks ERBB2 signaling has been approved for breast cancer treatment.

Recent data suggest that overexpression of *ERBB3* also contributes to the malignant phenotype by enhancing cell motility, possibly enhancing metastatic potential, and by transducing antiapoptotic signals, prolonging cell survival, contributing to genome instability, and inducing drug resistance (reviewed by Skorski[97]). With regard to metastatic behavior, heregulin is a potent migratory factor for breast cancer cells, inducing formation of motile actin cytoskeleton structures.[98] Heregulin, which signals through ERBB2 after dimerization with ERBB3, stimulates actin reorganization, the development of motile structures, such as filopodia and lamellipodia, and induces motility in breast cancer cell lines in vitro. Heregulin also stimulates p21-activated kinase (PAK1), a kinase involved in promoting cell migration. Clinically, this may have relevance to the development of metastatic disease, which as noted earlier, is associated with breast cancers that overexpress *ERBB2*.

In addition to enhancing cell motility, overexpression of receptor tyrosine kinases appears to confer drug resistance by enhancing repair of the double-strand breaks induced in DNA by active agents, such as doxorubicin,[99] prolonging activation of cell-cycle checkpoints that allow repair to occur, and upregulating antiapoptotic members of the *BCL2* family. This enhanced repair capability is directly related to receptor tyrosine kinase catalytic activity.[100] Dissociation of cell-cycle checkpoints and the DNA damage response also is an important component of DNA damage tolerance. Finally, *ERBB2* expression results in downregulation of *BAX* and upregulation of *BCL2* and *BCL-X_L*, reducing apoptotic signaling, enhancing genome instability, and further enhancing resistance to chemotherapeutic agents.[101-103] These effects result in resistance to chemotherapeutic agents that induce DNA damage by enhancing repair of these lesions and increasing cell tolerance of spontaneous and drug-induced genomic instability, further contributing to malignant progression.

BRCA1

It has been more than 8 years since the tumor-suppressor gene *BRCA1* was first identified,[9,10,104] enabling studies of its function and its role in breast tumorigenesis. It is now believed that BRCA1 is a multifunctional protein involved in maintaining genomic stability and the cellular response to DNA damage (reviewed by Venkitaraman[105]; Fig. 94-4). However, it remains unknown why, given the universal requirement for BRCA1 function, breast cancer is the predominant lesion in women with inherited *BRCA1* mutations and why *BRCA1* mutations have not been reported in sporadic breast tumors.

BRCA1 is required for the cellular response to DNA.[106,107] BRCA1 acts as a coactivator of TP53-responsive genes, and is central to modulating cellular response to DNA damage, suggesting that regulating expression of genes that mediate apoptosis and cell cycling is part of this process.[108-110] BRCA1 also binds Rad51,[111] which concatamerizes around the DNA helix during repair and replication, suggesting a direct role in maintenance and repair of chromosome structure. As might be expected based on this observation, *BRCA1*-associated cancers are often aneuploid, high-grade lesions.[112] Finally, it was recently discovered that ATM, the protein kinase mutated

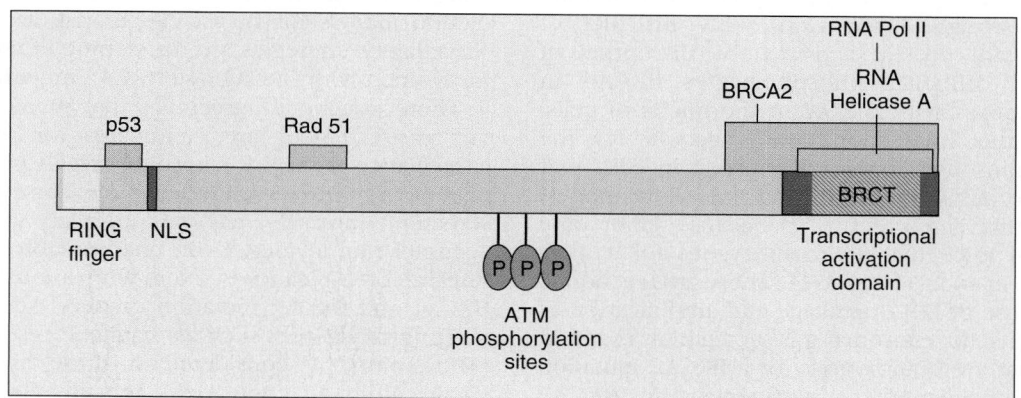

Figure 94-4. BRCA1 binding partners of known function. An important means of identifying the biologic function of uncharacterized genes is by defining what proteins their product binds to. In the case of BRCA1, which was identified by positional cloning, the first hint that it was important in the cellular response to DNA damage came from the discovery that it binds to TP53,[109] known to be an important component of this pathway. The discovery that BRCA1 and BRCA2 bind to each other places them in the same pathways.[123] The subsequent discovery that they both bind to Rad51,[111] also a key component of DNA damage response, provided a mechanism for their action. Interaction with RNA polymerase II shows that another important function of BRCA1 is regulating the expression of other genes.[946] Most recently, BRCA1 was shown to interact with SWI/SNF complexes that alter transcription through chromatin remodeling,[947] and with XIST, the small noncoding RNA that is essential for X inactivation.[948] The meaning of the BRCA1–XIST interaction is unclear, but given the dramatically higher risk in female carriers of BRCA1 mutations compared with male carriers, it is intriguing to speculate that BRCA1 regulation of sex chromosome inactivation may be important in breast cancer tumor suppression. BRCT, BRCA1 carboxyl terminus; NLS, nuclear localization signal.

in ataxia telangiectasia, phosphorylates BRCA1 after DNA damage occurs by ionizing radiation.[113] There is some, albeit controversial, evidence that ATM heterozygotes are at increased risk for breast cancer.[114-117] Once it is phosphorylated by ATM, BRCA1 associates with the hRad50-hMre11-p95 complex,[118] a group of proteins that directly bind damaged DNA.[119] These findings and other studies that identified BRCA1 binding partners were recently integrated by evidence of a "super complex" consisting of 40 BRCA1-associated proteins.[120] Nine of these proteins have known functions in the recognition of abnormal or damaged DNA, suggesting that BRCA1 may function as a coordinator of many cellular processes involved in the maintenance of genomic stability. These data suggest a model in which ATM senses DNA damage and phosphorylates a number of proteins that are important in protecting the cell from the effect of that damage, including BRCA1 and TP53. These genes then cooperate in initiating further amplification of DNA damage response signals by upregulating a number of other genes, and in the case of BRCA1, directly binding to protein complexes that are involved in DNA repair.

BRCA2

BRCA2 was discovered approximately 1 year after *BRCA1*, and has a similar clinical signature, with breast cancer as the predominant cancer in families with germline mutations and mutations in sporadic breast cancers being very rare (reviewed by Welsch and King[121]). BRCA2 also is linked to the cellular response to DNA damage, and it was found to bind to RAD51, a protein involved in recombination-mediated DNAl repair.[122] Finally, BRCA2 is believed to bind to BRCA1, providing additional evidence that BRCA2 is a critical component of DNA damage response and that this pathway is central to protecting women from breast cancer.[123]

BRCA2 also participates in the regulation of mitotic checkpoints through interaction with hBUBR1, a mitotic checkpoint protein activated by disruption of microtubules.[124] hBUBR1 phosphorylates BRCA2 in vitro and colocalizes with BRCA2 in the nuclei of cells. Disruption of this interaction could account for the extensive chromosomal abnormalities seen in cells that lack normal *BRCA2*. A murine BRCA2 "knockout model" suggests that this is correct,[125,126] because embryonic fibroblasts from mice that are homozygous for a truncating mutation in exon 11 of *BRCA2* show gross genomic instability because of DNA breakage and amplification of centrosomes. This chromosomal mis-segregation found in murine cells that are homozygous for a BRCA2 mutation suggests a mechanism for tumorigenesis in *BRCA2* mutation carriers.

It was recently shown that homozygous germline BRCA2 mutations are responsible for Fanconi anemia (FA) subtypes B and D1.[127] FA is a rare autosomal recessive cancer susceptibility disorder characterized by cellular hypersensitivity to mitomycin C. There are believed to be eight complementation groups. Six of the eight FA genes were previously identified, but the genes responsible for FA subtypes B and D1 remained unidentified. Patients with FA-B and FA-D1 have mutations in both copies of *BRCA2*, and express only truncated BRCA2 protein. Functional complementation of FA-D1 fibroblasts with wild-type *BRCA2* complementary DNA restores mitomycin C resistance, linking the six cloned FA genes with *BRCA1* and *BRCA2* in a common pathway involved in response to DNA damage.[127]

MANAGEMENT OF PATIENTS AT HIGH RISK FOR BREAST CANCER

Once an individual patient's risk has been estimated, it is a matter of personal opinion as to what constitutes high risk. For many women, a relative risk of 1, with a lifetime probability of 1 in 8 of being diagnosed with breast cancer, is already high. For others, a relative risk of 2 or more would be considered high risk. Whatever criteria an individual physician and patient use to define high risk, four possible actions may be taken, some of which can be used simultaneously. These actions include the following: (1) enhanced surveillance, (2) behavioral modification, (3) chemopreventive strategies, and (4) prophylactic mastectomy or oophorectomy.

Increased Surveillance

As discussed in the section on mammographic screening, the United States Preventive Task Force recommends screening mammography, with or without clinical breast examination, every 1 to 2 years for women 40 years of age and older. Although this task force recommended mammographic screening only as a category B intervention on the grounds that the quality of evidence was fair and the net gain moderate, and although controversy remains about the utility of routine screening before 50 years of age, ample evidence supports increased surveillance in women at high risk for breast cancer. A number of prediction models for breast cancer risk are available, and surveillance strategies are developing rapidly, particularly for women with BRCA1 and BRCA2 mutation carriers.[128]

There is general agreement that women at high risk for breast cancer are candidates for mammographic surveillance in their 40s. In some cases, earlier initiation of mammographic screening may be appropriate. Shorter screening intervals may be necessary because of the accumulating evidence of unacceptably high rates of interval breast cancers, even with annual screening, in BRCA1 and BRCA2 mutation carriers. Additionally, other imaging modalities, such as magnetic resonance imaging (MRI), must be considered in these high-risk groups. Finally, although controversy remains about the role of breast self-examination in the general population, experts in the surveillance of high-risk women still recommend monthly breast self-examination for women with BRCA1 and BRCA2 mutations.[129]

Behavior Modification

Multidisciplinary centers that provide counseling for women who are at substantial risk for breast cancer are well established throughout the United States. These multidisciplinary consultations provide recommendations for a range of surveillance and interventional approaches. In addition to the available surgical and medical preventive strategies, modification of lifestyle factors, such as obesity, high-fat diet, alcohol consumption, and lack of exercise, should be discussed. It will probably be many years before it is possible to say conclusively whether lifestyle modification changes a woman's risk. In the meantime, patients and their physicians must choose whether and how to modify lifestyle factors.

Chemoprevention

Tamoxifen was studied as a chemopreventive agent for breast cancer in four randomized prospective clinical trials. A significant reduction in breast cancer risk with tamoxifen was seen in the NSABP P-1 study[130] and the International Breast Cancer Intervention Study (IBIS-I).[131] Futher analysis of the patients in the NSABP P-1 study showed that tamoxifen reduced the incidence of breast cancer among BRCA2 carriers by 62%, but not among BRCA1 carriers.[132] However, two European chemoprevention studies performed at the Royal Marsden Hospital[133] and by the Italian Tamoxifen Prevention Study Group,[134] respectively, did not show a decrease in the incidence of breast cancer in women using tamoxifen.

Based in large part on compelling evidence from the NSABP study, which showed a 49% reduction in overall risk of invasive breast cancer with the use of tamoxifen, a number of review groups, including the American Society of Clinical Oncology Technology Assessment Working Group, recommended that tamoxifen should at least be considered to reduce the risk of breast cancer in women with a defined 5-year projected risk of 1.66 or greater. However, this group of studies had considerable methodologic differences, and further studies are needed to better define the role of chemoprevention in high-risk women. Furthermore, the NSABP study was not designed to show a difference in death rate from breast cancer as a primary endpoint.

Two selective estrogen-receptor modulators (SERMs), tamoxifen and raloxifene, are being compared in the NSABP STAR trial. This chemoprevention trial has accrued well, and it is anticipated that outcomes will be first reported in 2007. Another International Breast Cancer Intervention Study (IBIS-II) is randomizing high-risk postmenopausal women to receive the aromatase inhibitor anastrozole or placebo.

It is not known whether SERMs reduce the incidence of breast cancer by preventing the formation of cancer or by a treatment effect on small, clinically occult cancers. The use of these agents outside of a clinical trial requires an in-depth assessment of the risks and benefits of using the specific drug in an individual patient.

Prophylactic Mastectomy or Oophorectomy

Prophylactic mastectomy and oophorectomy are highly controversial preventive approaches to breast cancer.

In recent years, considerable new data has been obtained on the use of these prophylactic surgical procedures in patients with hereditary breast or ovarian cancer syndrome. Current data show that prophylactic mastectomy is effective in preventing breast cancer in patients with either a strong family history of breast and/or ovarian cancer[135] or a genetic predisposition to breast cancer.[15] Additional data show that prophylactic contralateral mastectomy can reduce the risk of breast cancer in patients with a previous diagnosis of unilateral disease.[136] A high prevalence of premalignant lesions is seen in prophylactically removed breasts from women who are at hereditary risk for breast cancer.[137]

Oophorectomy was first performed as a therapeutic procedure for advanced breast cancer more than 100 years ago and as hormonal adjuvant treatment of primary breast cancer more than 50 years ago. Uncertainty remains about the appropriate use of oophorectomy in adjuvant treatment, so it should not be surprising that preventive oophorectomy in high-risk women remains controversial. Again, the identification of women with BRCA1 or BRCA2 mutations has provided an opportunity to study this prophylactic procedure. Initial results show that bilateral prophylactic oophorectomy reduces the risk of breast cancer and epithelial ovarian cancer in this population.[13]

DETECTION OF BREAST CANCER

Despite a lifetime probability currently estimated as 1 in 8 (in women who live to be 110 years of age) for breast cancer, only 30% of all women have one or more identifiable risk factors.[51,138,139] Although these risk factors affect the parameters for breast cancer screening, current screening and education programs must include all women. The goal of breast cancer screening is early detection of malignancy at a stage that will lead to a reduction in mortality and morbidity. For breast cancer, the ideal screening program is sensitive enough to detect occult cancer with a minimum of false-positive findings. In addition, a screening program for breast cancer should be safe, relatively easy to provide to the public, acceptable to both patients and physicians, and cost-effective.

During the last 40 years, an intense effort has been mounted to evaluate the efficacy of mammography, clinical breast examination, and patient self-examination as tools for breast cancer screening. These efforts have included a number of case-control and cohort clinical trials as well as eight major randomized, prospectively controlled studies (Table 94-3). More than 650,000 women have participated in the randomized trials alone.[140-167]

Film-screen mammography remains the best available screening tool for breast cancer.[140,156,159,161,162] Randomized comparisons with the new generation of digital mammography units suggest that they are now capable of an equivalent level of detection. Computer-aided diagnosis allows a digital reading of the mammogram to identify areas that meet a computer pattern of discrimination. This allows a technique in addition to that of the radiologist's eye to discriminate abnormal-appearing areas. Some newer applications "learn" from the radiologist's

TABLE 94-3

Clinical Trials Testing the Efficacy of Screening

LOCATION	START OF STUDY	AGE RANGE (YR)	SCREENED GROUP	CONTROL GROUP	GROUPS	INTERVAL BETWEEN SCREENINGS (MO)	BREAST CANCER MORTALITY RELATIVE RISK*	P
United States	1963	40–64	31,131	31,565	PE + M vs. control	12 (3 times)	0.71 at 10 yr	<0.05
Malmö, Sweden	1976	45–69	21,088	21,195	M vs. control	18–24	0.96 at 9 yr	NS
Two counties in Sweden	1977	40–74	77,000	56,000	M vs. control	24 (for those 40–49 yr) 33 (for those 50–74 yr)	0.70 at 11 yr	<0.05
United Kingdom	1979	45–64	45,841 (group 1) 63,636 (group 2)	127,117 (group 3)	PE + M (group 1) BSE (group 2) Control (group 3)	12 (for PE) 24 (for M)	0.80 at 7 yr	NS
Edinburgh	1979	45–64	23,226	21,904	PE + M vs. control	12 (for PE) 24 (for M)	0.83 at 7 yr	NS
Stockholm	1981	40–64	40,000	20,000	M vs. control	28	0.76 at 7 yr	NS
Canada	1980	40–49	25,000	25,000	PE vs. M vs. one PE	12	NA	NA
		50–59	20,000	20,000	PE + M vs. PE	12	NA	NA

BSE, breast self-examination; M, mammography; NA, not available; NS, not significant (P = 0.05); PE, physical examination.
*Relative risk of death among the women who were screened compared with control subjects.
Adapted from Harris JR, Lippman ME, Veronesi U, Willett W: Breast cancer (three parts), N Engl J Med 327:319, 390, 473, 1992. Copyright Massachusetts Medical Society, 1992.

over-read of their identification points. The degree of benefit offered by these computer-aided programs is still under study, but appears promising.[168-170] An effective search for occult breast cancer requires aggressive interpretation of radiographs (i.e., a high index of suspicion) and an aggressive approach to biopsy. It is necessary to accept much less test specificity to avoid or minimize the incidence of interval breast cancers. In other words, the goal for optimizing breast cancer screening must be a higher rate of false-positive findings so that the risk of false-negative findings may be virtually eliminated.[171] In breast cancer screening, the discovery of smaller tumors has the added benefit of increasing the number of patients who can be treated by breast-conserving approaches.[172]

While mammography is the best screening tool, it detects only 85% to 90% of biopsy-proven cancers.[173] As a result, mammography is not a substitute for tissue sampling and histologic evaluation of any palpable abnormality, nor is it a substitute for careful physical examination.[174-176] The results of prospective trials to evaluate screening tools for occult breast tumor confirmed the importance of combining mammography and physical examination.[140,156,159,161,162,166] Although the efficacy of breast cancer screening has been challenged repeatedly, it is considered to have established benefit for women older than 50 years of age. Three considerations remain under investigation: (1) the efficacy of screening in women 40 to 49 years of age, (2) the value of screening in women in the 9th and 10th decades of life, and (3) the optimal interval for screening.

Screening

The efficacy of screening for occult cancer is heavily dependent on the following factors: (1) tumor growth rate, (2) the sensitivity of the test related to tumor volume, and (3) interval between screens. Growth rates of breast cancer vary, and some younger women have more rapidly growing tumors.[177] Moskowitz[178] reported a mean detection lead time gained by screening of 2 ± 0.5 years in younger women and of 4 ± 0.5 years in women older than 50 years of age.

Despite this knowledge, the many recent trials designed to test the efficacy of screening are based on widely varying screening methods, with the expected result of a confusing set of published recommendations. Some investigators claim efficacy only for women older than 50 years of age.[179-181] Some recommend cessation of screening beyond 69 years of age. However, clinical trial data for women in their 70s and 80s are inadequate for developing such a policy.[171] Some studies used only mammography without physical examination, others performed screens at biennial or triennial intervals, and some used only single lateral views of the breast.

In determining the efficacy of screening, four biases must be considered: lead-time bias, length bias, selection bias, and overdiagnosis bias. Lead-time bias is the interval that the diagnosis has been advanced by screening. Length bias concerns the timing of detection. When screening is infrequent, fast-growing tumors are not detected as early in their natural history as more slowly growing tumors. Thus, the outcome of cancers detected by screening is better than that for interval cancers. Selection bias is an obvious factor. For example, women who participate in breast cancer screening may be more health conscious; it is likely that their outcomes would be better, even in the absence of screening. Overdiagnosis has always been a concern in screening for cancer. Detection of breast lesions of questionable malignancy affects mortality data because these lesions would not be diagnosed without screening. It is not known how many of these very early in situ cancers would progress to become invasive malignancies.

These biases complicate the design and evaluation of screening trials. Randomized controlled trials, with the mortality rate of the the study population as the end point, are the only means of effectively eliminating these biases. In evaluating the results of screening trials, several points must be remembered. First, the survival and case fatality rates of patients with breast cancer are not adequate endpoints for determining results. Second, the closest end-point for studying the mortality rate in a population is an observed reduction in the incidence of advanced disease. Finally, if screening detected an excessive number of cancers that were not destined to be lethal, then the death rate among the screened women would not be altered and no benefit would be observed.

Before 1977, no formal guidelines existed for screening women for occult breast cancer. The publication of the Health Insurance Plan (HIP) of Greater New York Screening Project, conducted in the 1960s, led the NCI and the American Cancer Society to support a nationwide breast cancer screening project to evaluate further the efficacy of screening by mammography and physical examination. The Breast Cancer Detection Demonstration Project (BCDDP) took place in 29 centers, and 280,222 women were screened over a period of 5 years.[182] The basis for the development of the BCDDP was the observations of the HIP study.

Although the study is well documented, it is important to review the design and findings of the HIP landmark clinical trial. The HIP study invited women 40 to 69 years of age who were enrolled in the HIP of Greater New York to be screened for breast cancer.[183,184] The HIP project was the first randomized controlled trial and included annual clinical examinations and mammography for 4 years. Using pairwise allocation, 62,000 women were randomized to the study group or the control group. Of the total population, 45% were 40 to 49 years of age at study entry. Of the 31,000 women in the study group, 65% attended one or more screening sessions. Because it was not possible to identify within the control group women who would decline screening, the outcome of the control group was evaluated in relation to the total study group.

A surprising aspect of the initial evaluation of the results was the striking difference in the effectiveness of screening at different ages. At 5 years, the HIP study found a 50% decrease in mortality rate in women older than 50 years of age, but only a 5% decrease in mortality rate in women younger than 50 years of age.[183] However, after further follow-up, this difference in effectiveness began to change. With follow-up, the mortality rate in women younger than 50 years of age showed a 23.5% decrease, and it became statistically significant at year 18 of follow-up.[182] In women older than 50 years of age, the reduction in mortality became evident at approximately the fourth year of follow-up. Significantly, a reduction in mortality rate in younger women took longer than a decade to manifest.[185] Women who refused screening or who had interval cancers had no reduction in mortality rate.

For the first time, the results of the HIP study provided strong evidence that early detection of breast cancer increased the duration of survival. The trial was not designed to test for a differential effect of age on screening, and the difference observed could be the result of chance[143,185] or poorer survival of patients with stage I disease in the control group rather than the benefit that mammography and physical examinations provided the test group.[182,185]

In preparation for launching of the BCDDP, screening guidelines were set forth by a consensus development meeting on breast cancer screening held at the NCI in 1977. The 1977 guidelines recommended annual mammograms for all women older than 50 years of age; mammograms for women 40 to 49 years of age if they, their mother, or their sister had breast cancer; and mammograms for women 35 to 39 years of age if they had a history of breast cancer.

The 5-year results from the BCDDP, first reported in 1982, indicated that approximately one third of the breast cancers found were in women 35 to 49 years of age.[140] As a result of early data from the BCDDP clinical trial, the American Cancer Society published criteria for tests suitable for inclusion in a cancer-related health workup.[186,187] These criteria led to several modifications of the guidelines for breast cancer screening. The major unanswered question was the efficacy of mammography in younger women. These guidelines considered ongoing technical improvements in mammography (significantly improved resolution using very fine-grain x-ray film, intensifying screens, and breast compression). In addition, switching from tungsten as the x-ray tube target to molybdenum targets produced lower-energy x-rays that were more appropriate for imaging breast soft tissue. Changes in the design of the x-ray tube also permitted better cooling of the tube, enabling the use of smaller focal spots on the tube target, and as a result, greater image resolution and fine detail.

In addition to the HIP trial and the BCDDP study, five randomized clinical trials have been performed in Sweden. These include the Swedish two-county trial (two trials), the Malmö trial, the Stockholm trial, and the Gothenburg trial.[166] Other randomized controlled trials took place in Edinburgh (the Edinburgh Trial) and Canada (the National Breast Screening Study). In the Swedish two-county trial, which began in 1977 in Kopperberg, 38,562 women 40 to 74 years of age were assigned to screening and 18,478 were assigned to a control group. Randomization was not performed on an individual basis, but rather by power to detect reductions in the mortality rate of 30% or less. Only the HIP trial and the Kopperberg trial reached statistical significance for a decrease in mortality rate.[181] Excluding the National Breast Screening Study, which cannot be compared because of marked differences in design, a meta-analysis of the results of the other studies showed statistical significance, for a decrease of 25% to 30% in mortality rate.

By 1987, enough data had accumulated about mammography screening to lead the American College of Radiology to develop a consensus for new, universally acceptable screening guidelines. Twelve national organizations participated. Again, controversy focused on the value of screening women younger than 50 years of age and the appropriateness of a baseline study in women 35 to 39 years of age. Most of the participants agreed that the HIP and BCDDP data could not be ignored. The HIP trial, after 18 years of follow-up and with two separate analyses, showed decreases in mortality rates of 24% and 25%, respectively, in younger women.[141,143,188]

After months of debate, the 12 participating organizations adopted the following guidelines[189]:

1. Clinical examination and film-screen mammography are complementary, and both are required to maximize detection rates.
2. The screening process should begin at 40 years of age, and should consist of physical examination and mammography performed at 1- to 2-year intervals.
3. Beginning at 50 years of age, both clinical examination and mammography should be performed annually.
4. The recommendations apply only to women without signs or symptoms of breast cancer.

The participants agreed that no new evidence supported either the efficacy of regular breast self-examination or previous recommendations for a baseline mammogram at 35 years of age.

In October 1991, a workshop was held to determine whether new information warranted further modification of these guidelines.[190] Cost-effectiveness, legislative effects, and barriers to implementation were discussed at length, and it was concluded that no evidence indicated a change. The committee also concluded that no known factors existed to mitigate against screening elderly women (older than 65 years of age) as long as life expectancy was sufficient to realize a benefit for detection of early breast cancer.

In February 1993, the NCI held an International Workshop on Screening for Breast Cancer to conduct a thorough and objective review of the most recent data from clinical trials on breast cancer screening. Investigators representing the eight randomized controlled trials in women 40 to 74 years of age presented published and unpublished data. The findings of the workshop were published in a special article in the *Journal of the National Cancer Institute*.[191] The following conclusions were reported: randomized controlled trials of breast cancer screening did not show a survival benefit at 5 to 7 years for women 40 to 49 years of age; benefit was uncertain at 10 to 12 years, and if present, was marginal; in women 50 to 69 years of age, the mortality rate decreased by 33%; and there are no data on the efficacy of screening in women older than 70 years of age.

Four years later, in January 1997, the NCI conducted a consensus conference in an effort to establish guidelines for screening. The panel concluded that there were not enough data to support the recommendation of screening for all women in their 40s.[192] This announcement produced a significant professional and public outcry, and in March 1997, the NCI National Advisory Board voted to change the NCI guidelines to include a mammogram every 1 to 2 years for women 40 to 49 years of age and at average risk.[193]

In 2000, doubts about the validity of five of the randomized trials were raised by Gotzsche and Olsen,[194,195] and their conclusions engendered vigorous debate. In response, the Swedish workers conducted an overview of four of their trials and published their conclusions in *The Lancet*. They indicated that the benefit of breast screening was associated with a reduction in the breast cancer mortality rate of 21%, persisting for a median of 15.8 years. Three additional working groups met in response to these critiques. A working group of the International Agency for Cancer Research met in Lyon in March 2002, and concluded that many criticisms raised by Gotzsche and Olsen were unsubstantiated. The United States Preventive Service Task Force (USPSTF) that was charged to produce evidence-based reviews of preventive interactions concluded that mammographic screening could be recommended as a category B intervention, on the grounds that the quality of evidence was fair and the net gain moderate. The reduction in the breast cancer mortality rate in women who were invited to undergo screening was approximately 23%. Their conclusion was, "The USPSTF recommends screening mammography with or without clinical breast examination every one to two years for women aged 40 and older. The USPSTF concludes that the evidence is insufficient to recommend for or against routine clinical breast examination alone. The USPSTF concludes that the evidence is insufficient to recommend for or against teaching or performing routine breast self examination." In 2002, a global summit on mammographic screening was organized at the European Institute of Oncology in Milan. Recent results from the seven randomized trials were presented and discussed in detail in light of the criticism of Gotzsche and Olsen. The considerations that were raised did not detract from the conclusion that screening mammography reduced the mortality rate from breast cancer in women invited to be screened in well-organized clinical trials. Women who actually obtained mammograms had a greater benefit.

This controversy about the efficacy of screening for women 40 to 49 years of age is ongoing because breast cancer is less frequent in this age group, and there is a greater likelihood that mammographic abnormalities will prove benign on biopsy. Data showing that tumors grow more rapidly in this decade suggest that a more aggressive screening program is indicated (i.e., annually rather than every 24 months).[192] Even the best screening tends to detect breast cancer at a fairly late stage of growth, usually when the tumor is 0.5 cm in diameter. At this volume, the breast cancer has been present for 1 to 6 years, has been through many cell divisions, and if invasive, has had the opportunity to metastasize.

A recent report indicated that the ongoing screening program involving a significant proportion of women in Sweden has been associated with a decline in mortality from breast cancer in participating counties.[196] Evidence is overwhelming that screening for breast cancer with mammography and clinical examination can significantly decrease the number of women who die of this cancer. A significant number of incident cases occur in the fourth decade of life and may include a subset with a more rapid growth rate and more aggressive biologic characteristics.

These data argue for at least the individualization of screening recommendations for women 40 to 49 years of age, with particular attention to women with significant risk factors.[196-198]

Patient Compliance

As discussed earlier, the primary objective of breast cancer screening is the discovery of occult tumors at an early stage, which will result in a decreased mortality rate and an increased number of patients who are candidates for conservative breast therapy. Over the last decade, aggressive public education programs conducted by the American Cancer Society, the NCI, and public interest groups led to a dramatic increase in mammographic screening in the United States. A particular concern was marked underuse by women of minority groups. Over the last decade, the use of mammography has increased dramatically and the racial gap has virtually disappeared. Between 60% and 70% of white and African American women in the United States had a mammogram within the last year.[199,200] Several studies suggested that the most important intervention ultimately is one-to-one counseling by the health care provider to the woman.[201,202] Despite these achievements and extensive publicity about the effect breast cancer screening has had on lowering the mortality rate from this cancer, there is a significant need to improve compliance with breast cancer screening guidelines.

Various studies show that feelings of susceptibility were an important factor in determining the usefulness of screening.[203] Studies also show a significant lack of knowledge about the benefits of mammography and about breast cancer screening guidelines.[204,205] Other studies found that fear of radiation, embarrassment, pain associated with compression, and anxiety about what might be discovered are significant barriers to participation in screening.[205]

Several studies have been performed to determine methods of intervention that can increase the use of screening. These studies clearly show the importance of providing women with information as well as the value of the health care provider in communicating this knowledge and urging compliance.[206-209] In a study conducted in two rural southern Minnesota counties, vouchers for free mammography significantly improved compliance rates.[202] Champion[201] presented a theoretical model for mammographic use (Fig. 94-5). The results of the study showed the importance of providing information about mammography together with individually tailored "belief" counseling. Media intervention in any format has little effect on compliance and limited long-range benefit. Perhaps the real message in these investigations is the need for a greater emphasis on intervention at the health care provider level. Educational programs targeted at primary care physicians should become a priority.[202]

Sensitivity of Mammography

Mammography is more effective in detecting occult malignancy as patients age and breast tissue becomes

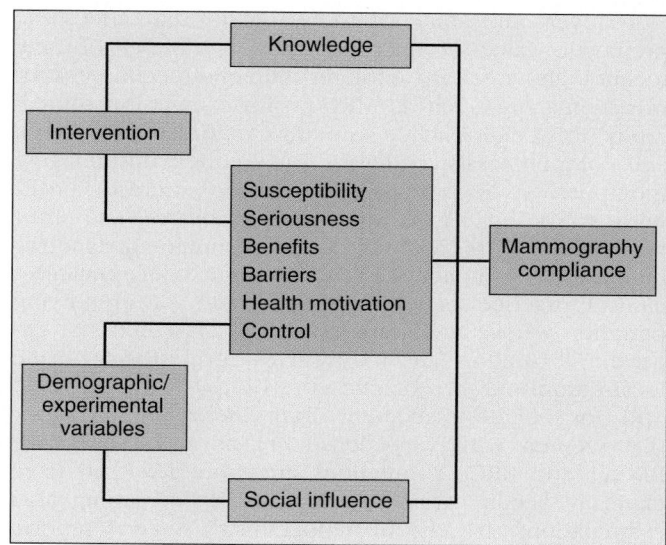

Figure 94-5. Theoretical model for mammography use. (Adapted from Champion VL: Strategies to increase mammography utilization. Med Care 1994;32:118.)

replaced with fat.[210] The density of the breast on film-screen mammography most directly affects the risk of false-negative and false-positive interpretation.[211] Several factors affect breast density. Age is the most significant factor, with more premenopausal women, especially those 40 to 49 years of age, having breasts that are more glandular and thus more dense. HRT in postmenopausal women may increase breast density.[211] For premenopausal women, mammographic sensitivity may be increased by scheduling evaluation during the first 2 weeks of the menstrual cycle, corresponding with the follicular phase.[212,213]

The sensitivity, or accuracy, of film-screen mammography is also affected by the experience of the radiologist, as shown in a study in which 150 mammograms were randomly selected from a pool of previously interpreted studies. Ten radiologists with varying levels of mammography experience then read the films. In a multivariate analysis, the rate at which the radiologist obtained regular feedback and the total lifetime number of mammograms read were independently associated with the number of times that immediate workup was recommended in patients with cancer. The most experienced radiologist had the highest sensitivity in diagnosing breast cancer.[214]

Another study evaluated 492 occult mammographically detected lesions that had been surgically excised.[215] Each mammographically detected lesion was classified as to risk according to the Breast Imaging Reporting and Data System (BI-RADS) for determining indications for biopsy. Features with the highest positive predictive value for carcinoma were spiculated margins (81%), irregular shape (73%), linear calcification (81%), and segmented (74%) or linear calcification distribution (68%). These category 5 features had an 81% positive predictive value compared with a positive predictive value of 34% for category 4 lesions.

To overcome some of the variables that affect the predictive value of mammography, a number of new technologies are being explored. Emerging techniques for breast imaging, such as MRI, positron emission tomography (PET), radionuclide scanning (scintimammography), and computer-assisted digitized mammographic imaging (computed radiography), are receiving interest.[215] MRI with spin-echo T1-weighted images before and after IV injection of 0.15 mmol/kg gadolinium-diethylenetriamine penta-acetic acid (DTPA) has gained acceptance in clinical practice as a useful technique for identifying patients whose mammograms are classified as uncertain.[216] Studies are in progress to perform needle localization and stereotactic core biopsy using real-time MRI for needle placement. Data increasingly suggest that women with very dense breasts and those with BRCA1 and BRCA2 mutations are more likely to have clinically occult carcinoma detected by screening MRI examinations than by mammograms.[217] Several reports indicate that PET scanning is useful for localizing occult carcinoma of the breast and identifying occult tumor in axillary lymph nodes.[218,219]

Just as exciting are the studies of scintimammography using specific antibodies or pharmaceuticals that localize to tumors. In a study of 84 patients using ^{99m}Tc tetrofosmin, sensitivity was 90%, specificity was 80%, the positive predictive value was 71%, and the negative predictive value was 93% for planar images. These values were 93%, 76%, 68%, and 95%, respectively, for single-photon emission computed tomography (SPECT).[220]

The Elderly Patient

The life expectancy for women in the United States increased from 79.0 years in 1996 to 79.8 years in 2001. Biologic parameters suggest a higher prevalence of more aggressive tumors in younger women, with less aggressive tumors occurring in older women. Clinical observations supporting this hypothesis showed that poorly differentiated tumors are less frequently seen and that hormone-receptor-rich tumors are more often seen in the elderly population.[221,222] Tabar and colleagues[223] showed that for a given tumor size, the likelihood of nodal involvement is lower in older women than in younger women. These data suggest that it may be appropriate to increase the screening interval to 2 years in older women. However, there is no age at which sufficient data suggest that screening can be abandoned. At 80 years of age, the average life expectancy for women is longer than 9 years. At 90 years of age, the average life expectancy is nearly 5 years. Clearly, individuals may be more or less likely to experience this life expectancy, depending on comorbid conditions and functional status.

In a survey of 576 primary care physicians, 90% were aware of the importance of screening mammography and believed that it could detect early cancer in women 65 years of age and older.[224,225] Even so, evidence clearly shows that fewer elderly women are being screened annually, even those with a history of breast cancer. Mandelblatt and colleagues[226] reported that in each age group (65 to 69 years of age, 70 to 74 years of age, 75 to 79 years of age, 80 to 84 years of age, and older than 85 years of age) breast cancer screening saves lives. These benefits were found in all age groups, and even in patients with comorbid disease. The magnitude of the benefit, as expected, decreased with age and with the severity of comorbid disease. A cost-benefit analysis of annual screening showed a value of $13,200 to $34,600 for each year of life saved. This can be compared with the cost of treating mild to moderate hypertension, which is $16,000 to $72,000 per year of life saved.[226]

Wilson and colleagues[227] attempted to determine the differences in stage of breast cancer in elderly women based on whether the tumor was discovered by physical examination or by mammography only. They found that 17 cancers detected by annual screening differed significantly from 45 cancers in patients who did not undergo screening. Tumor diameter was 1.1 cm vs. 2.1 cm. Of the 17 screen-detected cancers, 14 were classified as minimal, whereas only 15 of 45 tumors detected otherwise were so classified. These results were obtained with a positive breast biopsy rate of 70%, and led to treatment of significantly more patients with more conservative surgery. The detection of a greater number of minimal cancers, permitting less surgery, is an important factor in the efficacy of therapeutic interventions for the elderly.

Quality of Life and Harms Associated with Screening

Although most women are willing to accept false-positive test results, abnormal screening test results affect well-being, anxiety, and health care costs. The anxiety and psychosocial distress associated with false-positive readings may be trenchant, and their severity is inversely related to the interval between the abnormal finding and identification of the tumor as benign. However, concern about false-positive mammographic results and the possibility of needle biopsy is a source of anxiety that leads some women to avoid screening.[228-231] Some studies show that physicians overestimate concerns about screening and do not refer older women for mammography based on anticipated patient refusal.[232,233]

Screening Women at Increased Risk

Women who meet the criteria for hereditary breast cancer, as defined by a careful, three-generation family history, should be considered for additional screening. Options include the following: (1) initiation of screening 10 years before the onset of a first-degree relative's breast cancer, or at 30 years of age; (2) the addition of MRI screening; (3) shorter screening intervals (e.g., every 6 months); and (4) the addition of ultrasound screening. A woman with *BRCA1* or *BRCA2* mutations may have a risk as high as 20% with certain mutations by 40 years of age. MRI appears to be the most sensitive technique for screening these very young women.[234,235] The role of clinical examination and breast self-examination in high-risk women seems particularly limited.[236,237] Shorter screening intervals have been based on modeling data, and no prospective data have validated this recommendation. Although MRI shows improved sensitivity, it has lower specificity than mammography and may lead to additional fine-needle aspiration (FNA) or core biopsy in these young women at high risk.

Ductal lavage is promoted as a screening technique in asymptomatic women who are considered at increased risk. The goal of this technique was to provide stratification for women at increased risk in terms of intervention (e.g., tamoxifen). Although numerous research studies are underway, no data recommend the use of ductal lavage, alone or in combination with other screening techniques, and the technique remains investigational.

MAMMOGRAPHIC ABNORMALITIES

The value of mammography is heavily dependent on the technical expertise available in obtaining the study as well as on the experience of the radiologist interpreting the study.[238] Vigorous compression is essential to even out the breast tissue over the film to provide more uniform exposure and less scattered radiation. Compression decreases the possibility that glandular areas will obscure masses or calcification. It also avoids motion, which causes loss of fine resolution. Additional views may be required to image all of the breast tissue, especially tissue adjacent to the chest wall. Magnification films are valuable for evaluating areas of architectural distortion and fine calcification.

Many studies show the importance of significant experience in administering mammograms (radiographs) and interpreting the results.[214] Distinct advantages for the patient occur when mammography is provided by a dedicated mammography unit with a full-time technical team and an experienced radiologist. When more than one radiologist specializing in breast radiology reviews films, the accuracy of interpretation is further increased.

Masses

Benign masses are typically well defined, with sharp margins, and have little effect on the surrounding breast architecture. Fibroadenomas, papillomas, intramammary lymph nodes, and cysts are the most common causes of benign mammographic density (Fig. 94-6). Malignant breast densities classically have irregular borders that blend into the surrounding tissue. Often they appear to infiltrate the breast background tissue and have a stellate appearance. Usually, there is some distortion of adjacent breast stroma. The following questions remain to be answered:

1. Is this really a mass? (It must be identified in more than one view, and special views may be required.)
2. Where is it located?
3. Are there associated calcifications?
4. Is the mass solid or cystic? (This usually requires ultrasonography.)
5. Is the mass new?

The mammographic abnormality that has the highest rate of malignancy is a mass density shown on radiograph with associated calcification (Figs. 94-7, 94-8, and 94-9). Associated calcification increases the rate of positivity for malignancy from 13% with density alone to 29% for density containing microcalcifications.[239]

Calcifications

Malignant calcifications are typically linear, small (<1 mm) in diameter, nonuniform in size, and clustered. Between 20% and 25% of clustered microcalcifications are positive for cancer on biopsy. Benign calcifications are usually larger and coarser, and are often round, with smooth

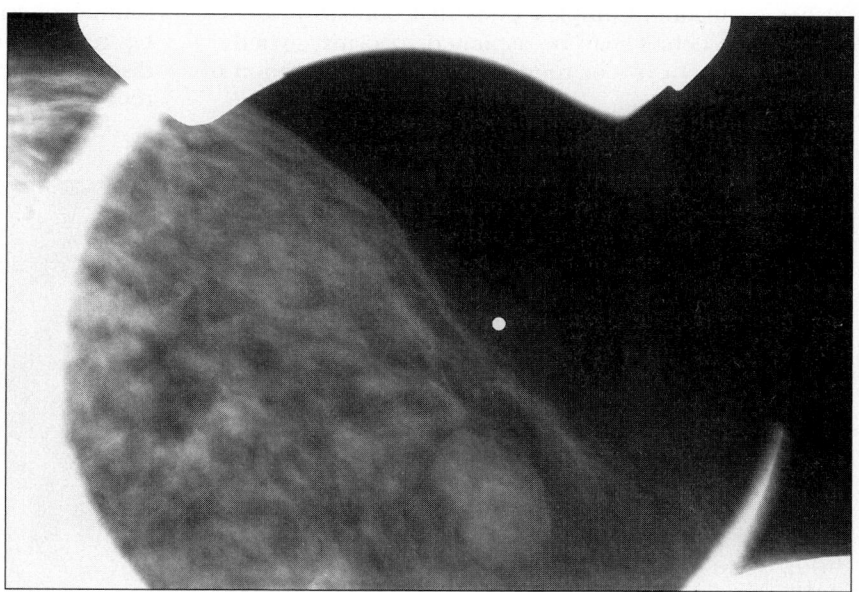

Figure 94-6. Magnified view showing that a palpable lump is uniform in density, lacks microcalcifications, and has sharp, clear borders. Biopsy established the lump to be fibroadenoma.

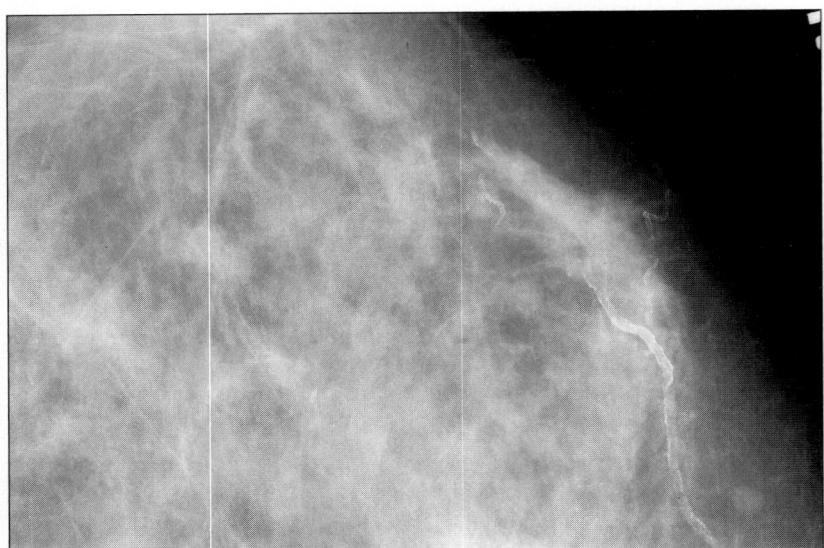

Figure 94-7. Mammogram showing arterial calcifications in an otherwise normal examination.

margins. Table 94-4 lists various types and distributions of calcifications. Benign causes of microcalcification include involuting fibroadenoma, arteriosclerosis, sclerosing adenosis, fat necrosis, and previous mastitis with ductal calcium deposits.

Ultrasonography

Diagnostic ultrasonography has not proved useful in showing malignancy of the breast when tumors are less than 1 cm in diameter. This modality is of greatest use when the mammographic findings are equivocal and when examination shows multiple areas of abnormality (Fig. 94-10).[240-242] Ultrasonography is very accurate (>95%) in the diagnosis of breast cysts. Cysts have well-demarcated, smooth margins and an echo-free center (Fig. 94-11). They are usually rounded and thin-walled, and produce distal shadowing.[243] Clear cysts require no further evaluation. Complex cysts that contain evidence of tissue or debris may be aspirated to clarify whether they are simply cysts or represent cystic degeneration of a tumor.

Ultrasonic image texture analysis is an effective way to distinguish benign from malignant breast lesions. This technique is a simple way to reduce the number of biopsies performed on benign lesions without missing additional cancers.[244] Doppler flow analysis may provide additional information about solid lesions. Malignant tumors show increased blood flow compared with benign tumors, resulting in a characteristic blood flow signal. Also, Doppler flow imaging is helpful in evaluating the response of breast cancers to primary medical therapy.[245]

APPROACH TO THE PATIENT

The surgeon is the physician most often involved in evaluating the patient who has symptoms of breast disease. The basis for referral to the surgeon may include a palpable lump discovered on self-examination or during routine physical examination. Alternatively, patients may be referred because of a mammographic abnormality discovered on routine screening mammogram. Most reports indicate that between 15% and 30% of biopsy

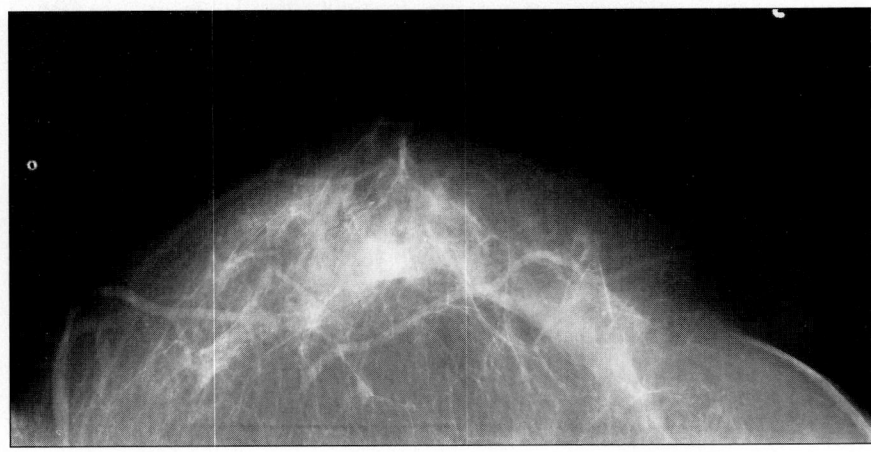

Figure 94-8. Pleomorphic calcifications in an area of extensive ductal carcinoma in situ.

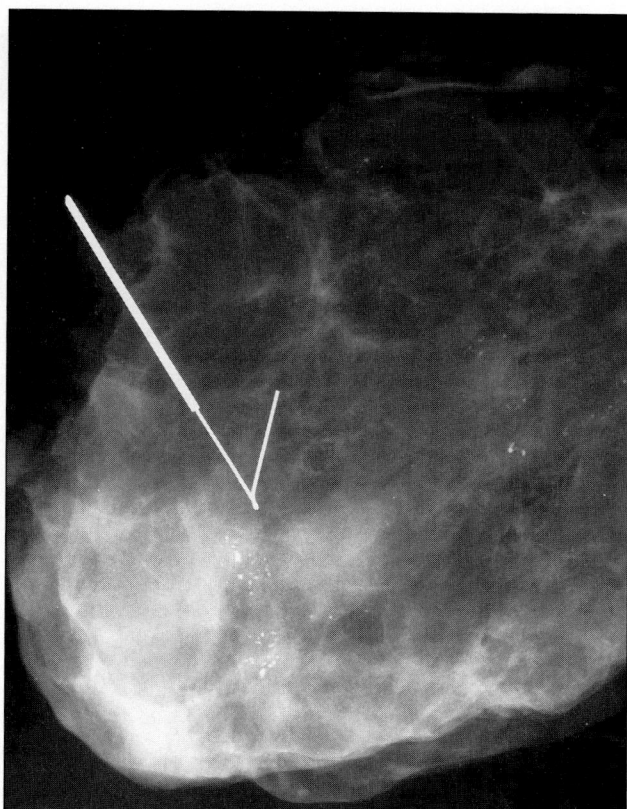

Figure 94-9. Specimen radiograph confirming removal of the clustered microcalcifications. Histopathologic examination showed ductal carcinoma in situ.

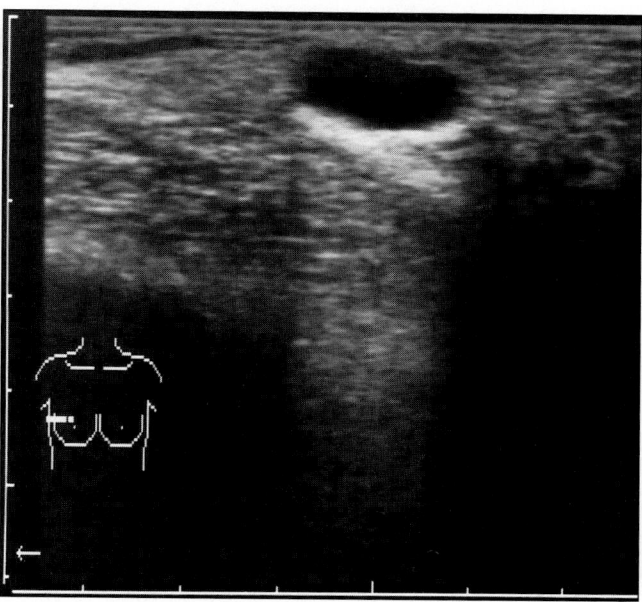

Figure 94-11. Ultrasonography of the breast showing the palpable lump to be cystic. Cystic lesions have a characteristic hypoechoic pattern, with prominent acoustic shadowing.

specimens obtained for mammogram abnormalities are positive for carcinoma. In 45% of cases, microcalcification is the indication for biopsy, and in 43% of patients, the indication is soft tissue density.[246] Biopsy specimens of clustered microcalcifications were positive for cancer in only 11.5% of patients, and highly suspicious breast densities were positive in 74% of cases. When densities appeared only moderately suspicious, the incidence of cancer was only 5.4%.[247]

Management of the Palpable Mass

A number of patients are self-referred because they discovered a change in their breast tissue during regular self-examination or because they accidentally discovered a lump. Others are referred because of a lump detected during examination by a health care provider. The determination of whether a palpable abnormality is a significant breast mass (i.e., malignant) can be difficult, especially in premenopausal women. In general, if a palpable mass is determined to be solid, histologic diagnosis is required.

An area of abnormal thickening in the breast that is not dominant and discrete (asymmetrical thickening compared with the same area in the opposite breast) usually suggests a benign change. Such areas of thickening may be safely observed for one or two menstrual cycles. Patients with a palpable mass or a new breast symptom should have mammography. Ultrasonography may also be useful; often it is the only test needed to evaluate adolescents and young women 20 to 30 years of age.

The goals of mammography for patients with breast symptoms or positive findings on examination are different from the goals of screening. For the patient with a breast lump, the goals of mammography are to

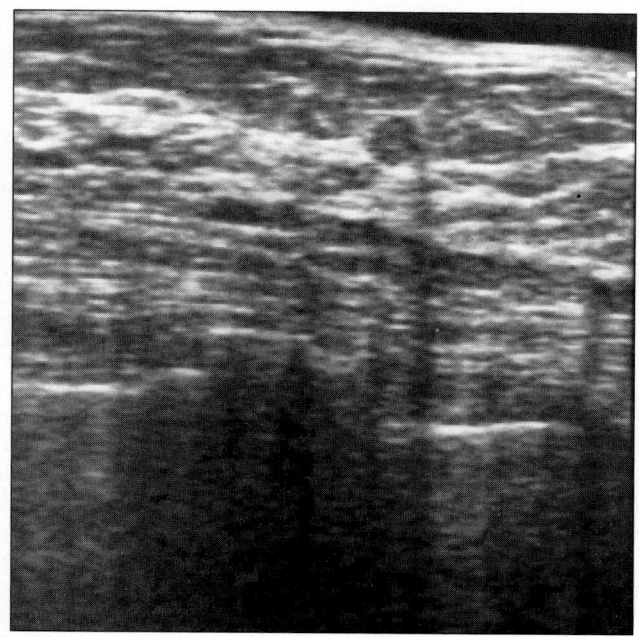

Figure 94-10. Ultrasonography confirms the presence of a solid mass.

TABLE 94-4

Types and Distributions of Calcifications

TYPE OF CALCIFICATION	DESCRIPTION
Typical Benign	
Skin (dermal)	Typical lucent-centered deposits that are pathognomonic. Atypical forms may be confirmed by tangenital views to be in the skin.
Vascular	Parallel track or linear tubular calcifications that are clearly associated with blood vessels.
Coarse or popcorn-like	The classic calcifications produced by an involuting fibroadenoma.
Large rod-like	Benign calcifications forming continuous rods that may occasionally be branching. They are usually more than 1 mm in diameter, and may have lucent centers, if calcium surrounds rather than fills an ectatic duct. These are the kinds of calcifications found in secretory disease, "plasma cell mastitis," and duct ectasia.
Round	When multiple, they may vary in size. They are usually considered benign, and when small (<1 mm), they frequently are formed in the acini of lobules. When <0.5 mm, the term "punctate" can be used.
Lucent-centered	Benign calcifications ranging from <1 mm to ≥1 cm. These deposits have a smooth surface, are round or oval, and have a lucent center. The "wall" that is created is thicker than the "rim" or "eggshell" type of calcifications. Included are areas of fat necrosis, calcified debris in ducts, and occasional fibroadenomas.
Eggshell or rim	Very thin, benign calcifications that appear as calcium deposited on the surface of a sphere. These deposits are usually <1 mm thick when viewed on edge. Although fat necrosis can produce these thin deposits, calcifications in the walls of cysts are the most common "rim" calcifications.
Milk of calcium	Consistent with sedimented calcifications in cysts. On the craniocaudal image, they are often less evident and appear as fuzzy, round, amorphous deposits; on the 90-degree lateral view, they are sharply defined, similunar, crescent-shaped, curvilinear, or linear, defining the dependent portions of cysts.
Suture	Calcium deposited on suture material. They are relatively common in the postirradiated breast. They are typically linear or tubular in appearance, and knots are frequently visible.
Dystrophic	Calcifications that usually form in the irradiated breast or in the breast after trauma. Although irregular in shape, they are usually >0.5 mm in size. They often have lucent centers.
Punctate	Round or oval, >0.5 mm, with well-defined margins.
Intermediate Concern	
Amorphous or indistinct	Often round or flake-shaped calcifications that are so small or hazy that a more specific morphologic classification cannot be determined
Higher Probability of Malignancy	
Pleomorphic or heterogeneous (granular)	Usually more conspicuous than the amorphic forms. They are neither typically benign nor typically malignant irregular calcifications. They vary in size and shape and are usually <0.5 mm in diameter.
Fine linear, or fine linear branching (casting)	Thin, irregular calcifications that appear linear, but are discontinuous and <0.5 mm wide. Their appearance suggest filling of the lumen of a duct involved irregularly by breast cancer.
Distribution Modifiers	Used as modifiers of the basic morphologic description. These terms describe the arrangement of the calcification. Multiple similar groups may be indicated when there is more than one group of calcifications that are similar in morphology and distribution.
Grouped or clustered	Although historically the term "clustered" has connoted suspicion, the term is now used as a neutral distribution modifier and may reflect benign or malignant processes. It is used when multiple calcifications occupy a small volume (<2 mL) of tissue.
Linear	Calcifications are arrayed in a line that may have branch points.
Segmental	Worrisome in that their distribution suggests deposits in a duct and its branches, raising the possibility of multifocal breast cancer in a lobe or segment of the breast. Although benign causes of segmental calcifications exist (e.g., secretory disease), this distribution is of greater concern when the morphology of the calcifications is not specifically benign.
Regional	Calcifications scattered in a large volume of breast tissue and not necessarily conforming to a duct distribution. They are likely benign, but are not everywhere in the breast, and do not fit the other, more suspicious categories.
Diffuse/scattered	Calcifications that are distributed randomly throughout the breast.

Adapted from Breast Imaging Reporting and Data System: American College of Radiology, 1998, p 27.

provide an image and therefore to characterize the area of palpable abnormality, to evaluate the remaining breast for signs of additional occult lesions, and to evaluate the contralateral breast.

Whether a mammogram is obtained in women younger than 35 years of age depends on the character of the palpable abnormality (e.g., the level of concern about potential malignancy on examination). Ultrasonography is simple to perform and may distinguish a solid mass from a cystic mass; a cyst can usually be aspirated. Cytologic examination of aspirated fluid is not indicated because cysts are rarely positive for carcinoma. Follow-up of these patients in 3 to 4 months is generally indicated, and most breast surgeons excise a chronically recurring cyst or a cyst with bloody fluid.

A solid mass, as confirmed by mammography, ultrasonography, or needle aspiration, requires histologic confirmation of its character. If the cytologic findings indicate cancer, then definitive therapy is planned. If they do not, then cytologic or core biopsy diagnosis must be consistent with the findings that led to the biopsy. If the lesion is highly suspicious, negative findings on FNA or core biopsy will not completely remove suspicion unless they show a histologic explanation of the findings. When cytologic findings are nondiagnostic, excision of the lesion offers both patient and surgeon peace of mind. The finding of proliferative epithelium, or atypia, affects the risk of subsequent breast cancer. Atypical hyperplasia is found in 4% to 10% of benign biopsy specimens. Associated risk relates strongly to family history. Table 94-5 shows the relative associated risks for patients with benign histologic findings.

FNA has many advantages in evaluating a solid breast mass. The finding of a benign explanation for the density may be reassuring. It also allows a sufficient diagnosis to indicate the margin of excision, should primary excision be required for a malignant tumor. Having a preoperative diagnosis also allows sentinel lymph node biopsy to be combined with excision of the tumor. Both false-negative and false-positive rates of FNA are extremely dependent on the expertise of the cytologist. If physical examination and mammograms both suggest a benign lesion and FNA cytologic findings are consistent, the likelihood of a

TABLE 94-5

American Board of Pathology Histologic Classification of Benign Disease

HISTOPATHOLOGY	APPROXIMATE RELATIVE RISK
Nonproliferative	No added risk
Cysts	
Duct ectasia	
Calcification	
Fibroadenoma	
Milk ductal epithelial hyperplasia	
Sclerosing adenosis	No added risk
Papillomatosis	Slight added risk
Radial scars	
Complex sclerosing lesions	?
Moderate florid hyperplasia	1.5:1 to 2:1
Atypical hyperplasia (ductal and lobular)	4:1
Extensive ductal involvement of atypical hyperplasia	7:1
Lobular carcinoma in situ	10:1
Ductal carcinoma in situ	10:1

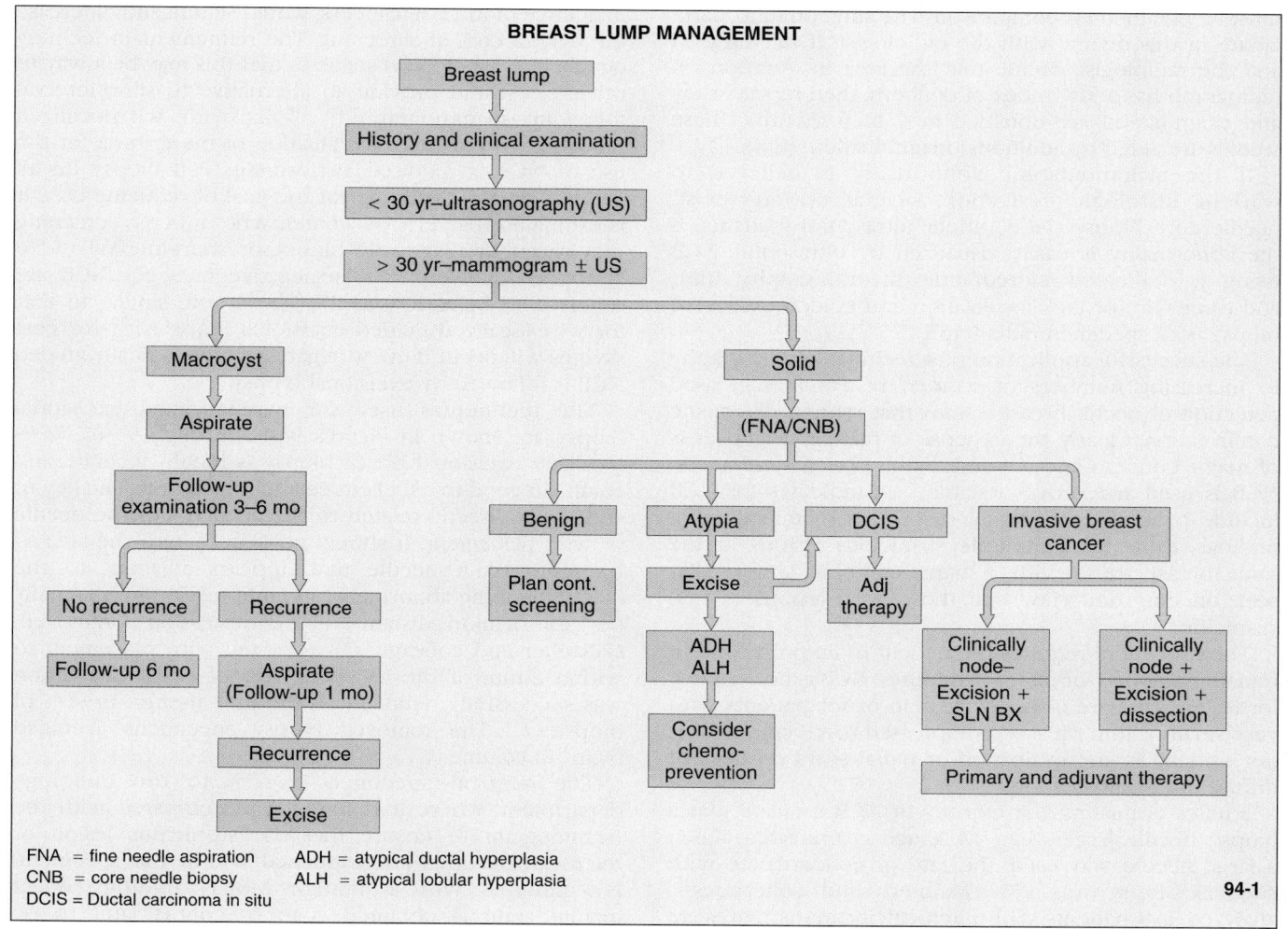

BREAST LUMP MANAGEMENT

FNA = fine needle aspiration
CNB = core needle biopsy
DCIS = Ductal carcinoma in situ
ADH = atypical ductal hyperplasia
ALH = atypical lobular hyperplasia

94-1

Specific Malignancies

III

missed breast cancer is less than 1%.[248,249] If the findings of any of the three tests are suspicious, a more aggressive biopsy to prevent progression of breast cancer is strongly recommended.

Management of the Nonpalpable Mammogram Abnormality

The surgeon is commonly faced with a patient who is asymptomatic and has a normal breast examination, but has an abnormal mammogram. The mammographic criteria for biopsy are fairly well accepted as the following: (1) a localized soft tissue density that was not previously seen; (2) a localized soft tissue density that has changed on successive studies; (3) a localized soft tissue density with ill-defined borders or stellate distortion of the stroma (or both); and (4) a focus of suspicious microcalcification, with or without soft tissue density (see Table 94-4).

If these findings are seen on screening mammograms, diagnostic mammograms, including magnification views, are required to confirm the abnormality. Often mammographic changes are not as clear as those listed in Table 94-4. The mammography report may state "cannot exclude an early breast cancer" or "clinical correlation is recommended." In these situations, all previous mammograms must be obtained for comparison. The surgeon must participate in this review with the radiologist. If the surgeon and the radiologist decide that the area in question on radiograph has a low index of concern, then repeat study and examination are obtained in 4 to 6 months. These studies are aided by additional magnification views.

If the mammographic abnormality is believed to warrant histologic evaluation, several options exist: needle core biopsy (NCB) under ultrasound guidance if the abnormality is easily visualized by ultrasound; NCB using a dedicated stereotactic mammography unit; and three-wire or tack localization and guided excisional biopsy with specimen radiography.[249-252]

The successful application of screening mammography to increasing numbers of women results in increased detection of occult breast lesions that require diagnostic confirmation. Clearly, the expense of further diagnoses is of major concern and is considerably less if stereotactic NCB is used and proves reliable.[253] Candidates for NCB include patients with highly suspicious mammographic findings, those with multiple suspicious lesions in the same breast, those with a mammographic abnormality seen on only one view, and those with lesions of low suspicion.

The procedure requires the patient to lie prone and to remain immobile for 30 to 45 minutes. NCB is not suitable for lesions that are close to the skin or for patients with very small or thin breasts (compressed to <3 cm). NCB is not optimal in the evaluation of radial scars or areas of diffuse microcalcification.

Studies evaluating the efficacy of NCB indicate that a biopsy needle larger than 14 gauge is preferred. When a large needle was used, the rate of concordance with surgical biopsy was 97%. Mainiero and colleagues[254] analyzed 118 patients with microcalcifications that were stereotactically sampled with a mean of seven cores. They found microcalcifications in 86% of patients and determined a diagnosis in 52%. Much more important is the finding that 60% of patients who were diagnosed by stereotactic cores as having DCIS were found to have invasive cancer at biopsy. Similarly, studies show that when core biopsy shows typical ductal hyperplasia, open surgical biopsy shows DCIS in 30% to 50% of cases. This is similar to finding atypical ductal hyperplasia in 50% of patients whose biopsy showed carcinoma.[255,256] Thus, excisional biopsy is indicated in the following situations: (1) for a nondiagnostic core biopsy, (2) when atypical ductal hyperplasia is found, (3) when DCIS is present, (4) when the patient has a radial scar, and (4) when calcifications cannot be sampled. All patients with benign histologic features should have a 6-month follow-up two-view mammogram, and a system must be in place to ensure compliance.

As discussed earlier, a goal in screening for occult breast cancer has been a low positive predictive value for mammographic findings leading to biopsy. On biopsy, approximately two benign tumors are found for each cancer that is discovered, but some authors argue that biopsy should be performed when the chance of finding cancer reaches 10%. Driving the rate of positive biopsy findings even lower, with the goal of decreasing the incidence of interval cancers, would significantly increase the overall cost of screening. The refinement in technology for the use of NCB suggests that this may be a way to reduce cost and provide an alternative to short-interval follow-up mammography.[257,258] As with wire-localized biopsy, however, careful evaluation of the criteria for the use of NCB is required. Performing NCB biopsy on all patients would clearly defeat the goal of reducing cost. It is estimated that 11% of women who undergo screening require either diagnostic biopsy or short-interval (4- to 6-month) follow-up.[259] False-negative rates for NCB are reported to be as low as 2%,[249,259] a rate similar to that for wire-localized guided excisional biopsies.[252] No cost savings will occur if every negative stereotactically guided NCB is followed by excisional biopsy.

The techniques used for wire-localized excisional biopsy are shown in Figures 94-12 through 94-16. Wire-localized excisional breast biopsy is highly accurate and results in good to excellent cosmetic outcome. The key to success is directly related to the accuracy of the needle or wire placement. It should go directly into the area to be removed. A needle that appears adjacent to the mammographic abnormality in compression may actually be 1 cm or more distant when compression is removed. Gallagher and colleagues[251] reported wire placement to within 2 mm of the lesion in 96% of cases. The lesion was successfully removed on the first attempt in 96% of biopsies.[251] The removed biopsy specimens averaged 6 cm^3 in volume.

The surgical specimen is sent to the radiology department, where it is filmed and compared with the mammogram to ensure that the suspicious lesion or microcalcifications are contained within the specimen. For patients with a benign biopsy finding, repeat mammogram is obtained 4 to 6 months later to re-

Figure 94-12. Excision of nonpalpable mammographic abnormalities. **A,** Kopans hook wire and localizing needle (Kopans, Bloomington, IL). **B,** The incision is placed near or directly over the spot where the tip of the wire and the radiographic lesion are located. In this case, a circumareolar incision was ideal. The skin welt that is seen is the result of infiltration with local anesthetic (1% lidocaine with 1:200,000 epinephrine). (From Baker RR, Niederhuber J: The Operative Management of Breast Disease. Philadelphia, WB Saunders, 1994.)

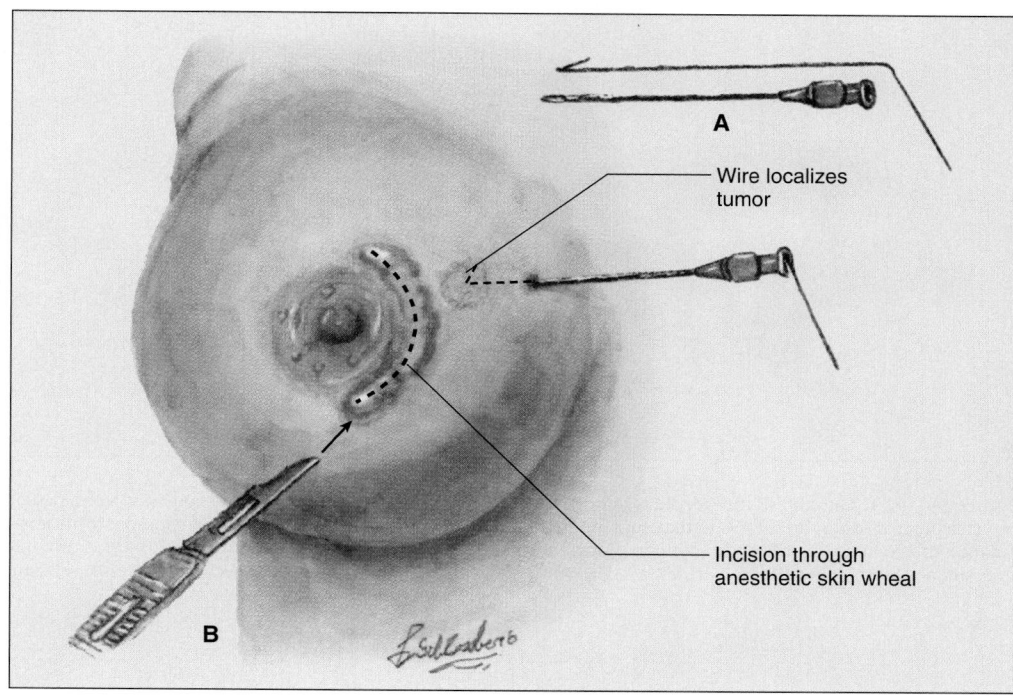

establish a baseline and confirm clearing of the suspicious abnormality.

STAGING AND PROGNOSTIC EVALUATION

Once the pathologic diagnosis of breast cancer is established, the clinician should promptly obtain the staging information necessary to make therapeutic recommendations and decisions. Completing the staging evaluation in a timely fashion is important for both medical and psychological reasons. Obtaining essential information and avoiding unnecessary tests are important for medical, psychological, and economic reasons.

The primary goal of staging evaluation is to assess whether the patient is potentially curable by surgery, with or without radiation therapy, or whether she has advanced disease beyond reasonable expectation of cure with surgery or radiation therapy. If the patient has

Figure 94-13. Skin hooks are retracted as the surgeon raises a flap toward the point of entrance of the localizing needle. An Allis clamp is used to grasp the breast tissue as the area surrounding the end of the hook wire is dissected. (From Baker RR, Niederhuber J: The Operative Management of Breast Disease. Philadelphia, WB Saunders, 1994.)

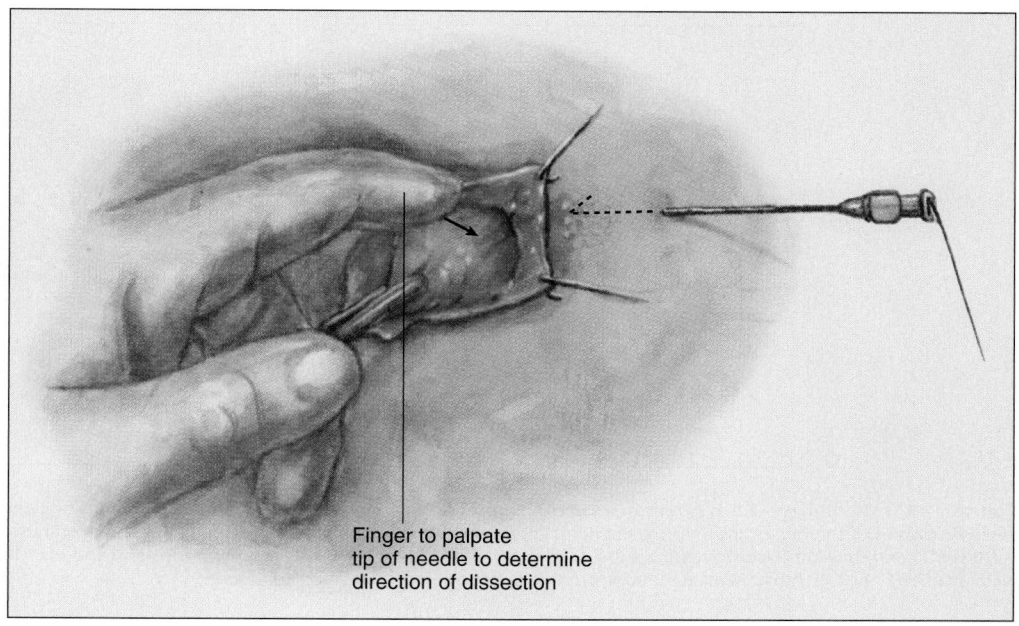

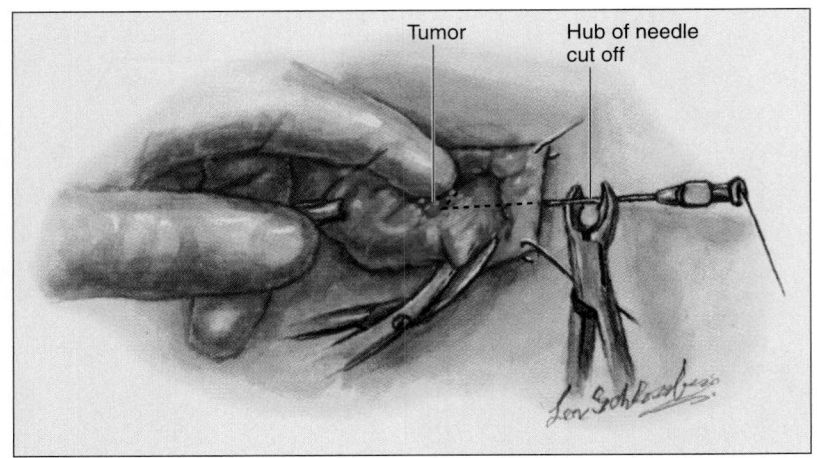
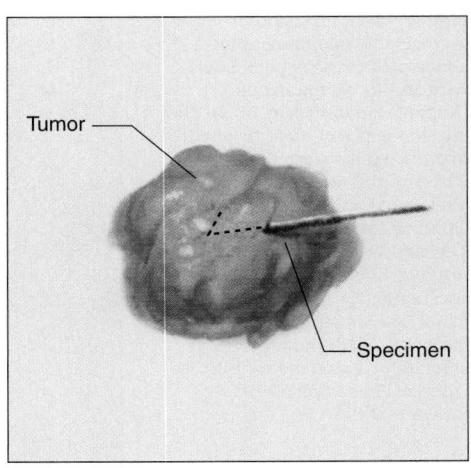

Figure 94-14. A, The hub of the needle is cut off with a wire cutter, allowing the needle and wire to be passed through the skin flap. The surgeon can sharply excise the breast tissue that surrounds the tip of the hook wire, including the mammographic abnormality. **B,** After a specimen radiograph is taken to confirm the radiographic abnormality, the specimen containing the hook wire is oriented and marked for histopathologic assessment. (From Baker RR, Neiderhuber J: The Operative Management of Breast Disease. Philadelphia, WB Saunders, 1994.)

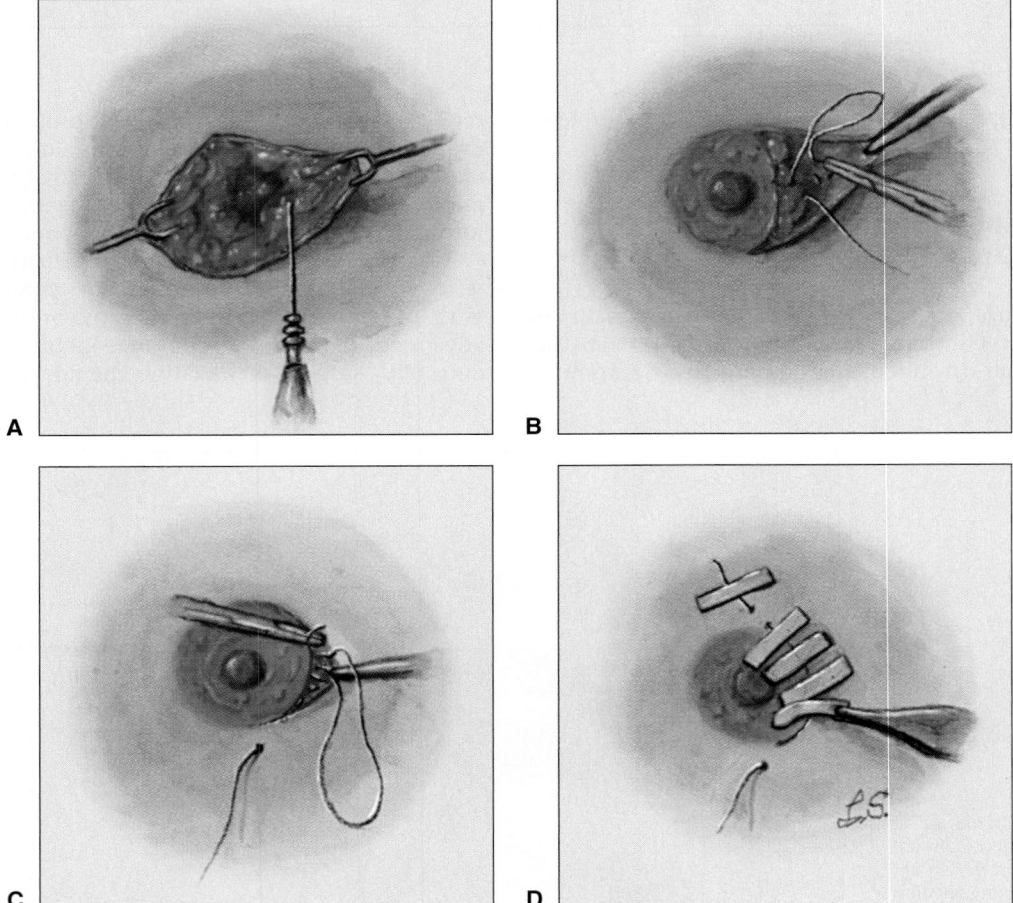

Figure 94-15. After the specimen is removed, careful hemostasis is obtained with electrocautery **(A).** The deep tissues are never reapproximated to avoid distortion of the breast and poor cosmetic result if subsequent irradiation is required **(B).** The deep dermis is closed with 3-0 absorbable sutures **(C),** and the skin is closed with a subcuticular pull-out suture of 5-0 Prolene. Steristrips **(D)** and dressings are applied. (From Baker RR, Neiderhuber J: The Operative Management of Breast Disease. Philadelphia, WB Saunders, 1994.)

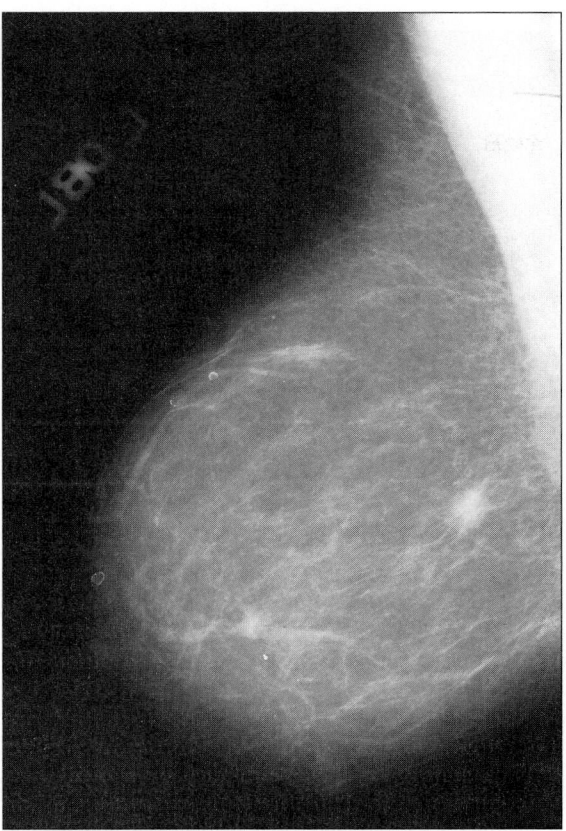

Figure 94-16. Lateral oblique view showing a nonpalpable speculated density with ill-defined borders. Wire localization biopsy confirmed the presence of an invasive ductal cancer.

curable disease, staging data can be further used to predict the natural history of the breast cancer, make a decision about the need for systemic adjuvant therapy, and aid in the selection of specific adjuvant treatment. Ideally, the staging parameters (particularly biologic factors) predict the response to adjuvant therapy and serve as measurable markers of otherwise clinically occult, micrometastatic disease. Unfortunately, these goals cannot be met with available prognosticators.

2003 Update of the TNM Staging System

In January 2003, the American Joint Committee on Cancer (AJCC) [www.cancerstaging.org; last accessed April 22, 2003] released the sixth edition of the Cancer Staging Manual with a revision of the TNM staging system for breast cancer (Table 94-6).[260,261] This revision considers the increasing use of novel imaging and pathology techniques, such as sentinel node biopsy and immunohistochemistry. It also considers the number of involved lymph nodes (a strong prognostic factor) in staging allocation. The main changes in the TNM staging system include the following: (1) the distinction beween micrometastases and isolated tumor cells on the basis of size and histologic evidence of malignant activity; (2) identifiers to indicate the use of sentinel lymph

node dissection and immunohistochemical or molecular pathology techniques; (3) indication of the number of malignant lymph nodes as shown by routine hematoxylin and eosin staining (preferred method) or by immunohisto-chemistry staining (i.e., pN1 for 1 to 3 involved lymph nodes, pN2 for 4 to 9 involved lymph nodes, and pN3 for 10 or more lymph nodes); (4) reassignment of metastasis to the infraclavicular nodes as N3 disease and down-staging of ipsilateral supraclavicular node involvement from M1 to N3; and (5) staging of internal mammary lymph nodes based on detection by sentinel node biopsy (N1 disease), radiologic or clinical examination (N2 disease), or concomitant axillary nodal involvement (N3 disease).

Undoubtedly, the TNM staging system for breast cancer has become more complex, although the allocation of specific TNM combinations to different stage groupings remains the same. A major exception is the creation of a new stage IIIc to include patients with exclusively TanyN3M0 disease. This revised staging system acknowl-edges the heterogeneity of breast cancer and facilitates the collection of uniform data from international databases. These changes make the breast cancer staging system more consistent with existing clinical consensus about diagnostic and treatment standards and allow researchers to better assess the long-term outcome of specific patient subgroups and the effect of novel imaging and pathologic techniques.[261]

Pathologic Factors

Increasing pathologic size of the primary tumor is inversely related to disease-free survival and overall survival rates (Table 94-7). Although concern has been expressed about the variability in correlation between tumor size and outcome in node-negative patients, recent analyses show that tumor size is a powerful predictor of recurrence in node-negative (T1N0M0 and T2N0M0) breast cancer.[262]

The increasing use of systemic adjuvant therapy in patients with tumors with a maximal diameter greater than 1 cm or other unfavorable histologic and biologic parameters challenged the utility of lymph node dis-section for staging purposes. Histologic status of the axillary lymph nodes remains the single most important prognostic factor for operable breast cancer (Table 94-8). Axillary staging is an essential procedure because of the power of axillary lymph node status as a prognostic factor, the importance of informing patients about their prognosis, and the potential to modify adjuvant therapeutic options for patients with involved vs. uninvolved axilla.[263] Sentinel node biopsy in experienced hands is gaining widespread acceptance as the preferred staging procedure.

Many pathologic factors, including histologic subtype, nuclear and histologic grade, and lymphatic or vascular invasion, have been evaluated as prognosticators of clinical course or response to therapy. Although each of these histologic parameters can be a useful predictor in expert hands, histologic subclassification has the greatest applicability. Most invasive breast cancers are epithelial

TABLE 94-6

 American Joint Committee on Cancer TNM Staging System for Breast Cancer

TNM STAGING

Primary Tumor (T)

Definitions for classifying the primary tumor (T) are the same for clinical and for pathologic classification. If the measurement is made by the physical examination, the examiner uses the major headings (T1, T2, or T3). If other measurements, such as mammographic or pathologic measurements, are used, the subsets of T1 can be used. Tumors should be measured to the nearest 0.1-cm increment.

TX	Primary tumor cannot be assessed
T0	No evidence of primary tumor
Tis	Carcinoma in situ
Tis (DCIS)	Ductal carcinoma in situ
Tis (LCIS)	Lobular carcinoma in situ
Tis (Paget's)	Paget's disease of the nipple with no tumor

Note: Paget's disease associated with a tumor is classified according to the size of the tumor.

T1	Tumor 2 cm or less in greatest dimension
T1mic	Microinvasion 0.1 cm or less in greatest dimension
T1a	Tumor more than 0.1 cm but not more than 0.5 cm in greatest dimension
T1b	Tumor more than 0.5 cm but not more than 1 cm in greatest dimension
T1c	Tumor more than 1 cm but not more 2 cm in greatest dimension
T2	Tumor more than 2 cm but not more than 5 cm in greatest dimension
T3	Tumor more than 5 cm in greatest dimension
T4	Tumor of any size with direct extension to (a) chest wall or (b) skin, only as described below
T4a	Extension to chest wall, not including pectoralis muscle
T4b	Edema (including peau d'orange) or ulceration of the skin of the breast or satellite skin nodules confined to the same breast
T4c	Both T4a and T4b
T4d	Inflammatory carcinoma

Regional Lymph Nodes (N)

Clinical

NX	Regional lymph nodes cannot be assessed (e.g., previously removed)
N0	No regional lymph node metastasis
N1	Metastasis to movable ipsilateral axillary lymph node(s)
N2	Metastases in ipsilateral axillary lymph nodes fixed to one another (matted) or in clinically apparent* ipsilateral internal mammary nodes in the absence of clinically evident axillary lymph node metastasis
N2a	Metastases in ipsilateral axillary lymph nodes fixed to one another (matted) or to other structures
N2b	Metastases only in clinically apparent ipsilateral internal mammary nodes and in the absence of clinically evident axillary lymph node metastasis
N3	Metastasis in ipsilateral infraclavicular lymph node(s), with or without axillary lymph node involvement, or in clinically apparent ipsilateral internal mammary lymph node(s) and in the presence of clinically evident axillary lymph node metastasis; or metastasis in ipsilateral supraclavicular lymph node(s), with or without axillary or internal mammary lymph node involvement
N3a	Metastasis in ipsilateral infraclavicular lymph node(s)
N3b	Metastasis in ipsilateral internal mammary lymph node(s) and axillary lymph node(s)
N3c	Metastasis in ipsilateral supraclavicular lymph node(s)

Pathologic (pN)[†]

PNX	Regional lymph nodes cannot be assessed (e.g., previously removed or not removed for pathologic study)
PN0	No regional lymph node metastasis histologically and no additional examination for isolated tumor cells (ITCs)

Note: ITCs are defined as single tumor cells or small cell clusters not greater than 0.2 mm that are usually detected only by immunohistochemical (IHC) or molecular methods, but may be verified on hematoxylin and eosin stains. ITCs do not usually show evidence of malignant activity (e.g., proliferation or stromal reaction).

pN0(i−)	No regional lymph node metastasis histologically, negative IHC
pN0(i+)	No regional lymph node metastasis histologically, positive IHC, no IHC cluster greater than 0.2 mm
pN0(mol−)	No regional lymph node metastasis histologically, negative molecular findings (RT-PCR)
pN0(mol+)	No regional lymph node metastasis histologically, positive molecular findings (RT-PCR)
pN1	Metastasis in 1 to 3 axillary lymph nodes, or in internal mammary nodes with microscopic disease detected by sentinel lymph node dissection, but not clinically apparent[‡]
pN1mi	Micrometastasis (greater than 0.2 mm, none greater than 2.0 mm)
pN1a	Metastasis in 1 to 3 axillary lymph nodes
pN1b	Metastasis in internal mammary nodes with microscopic disease detected by sentinel lymph node dissection, but not clinically apparent
pN1c	Metastasis in 1 to 3 axillary lymph nodes and in internal mammary nodes with microscopic disease detected by sentinel lymph node dissection, but not clinically apparent. (If associated with greater than 3 positive axillary lymph nodes, the internal mammary nodes are classified as pN3b to reflect increased tumor burden)
pN2	Metastasis in 4 to 9 axillary lymph nodes or in clinically apparent internal mammary lymph nodes in the absence of of axillary lymph node metastasis
pN2a	Metastasis in 4 to 9 axillary lymph nodes (at least one tumor deposit greater than 2.0 mm)
pN2b	Metastasis in clinically apparent internal mammary lymph nodes in the absence of axillary lymph node metastasis

TABLE 94-6

American Joint Committee on Cancer TNM Staging System for Breast Cancer—*cont'd*

pN3	Metastasis in 10 or more axillary lymph nodes, in infraclavicular lymph nodes, or in clinically apparent ipsilateral internal mammary lymph nodes in the presence of 1 or more positive axillary lymph nodes; or in more than 3 axillary lymph nodes with clinically negative microscopic metastasis in internal mammary lymph nodes; or in ipsilateral supraclavicular lymph nodes
pN3a	Metastasis in 10 or more axillary lymph nodes (at least one tumor deposit greater than 2.0 mm), or metastasis to the infraclavicular lymph nodes
pN3b	Metastasis in clinically apparent ipsilateral internal mammary lymph nodes in the presence of 1 or more positive axillary lymph nodes; or in more than 3 axillary lymph nodes and in internal mammary lymph nodes with microscopic disease detected by sentinel lymph node dissection, but not clinically apparent
pN3c	Metastasis in ipsilateral supraclavicular lymph nodes

Distant Metastasis (M)

MX	Distant metastasis cannot be assessed
M0	No distant metastasis
M1	Distant metastasis

STAGE GROUPING

Stage 0	Tis	N0	M0
Stage I	T1§	N0	M0
Stage IIA	T0	N1	M0
	T1§	N1	M0
	T2	N0	M0
Stage IIB	T2	N1	M0
	T3	N0	M0
Stage IIIA	T0	N2	M0
	T1§	N2	M0
	T2	N2	M0
	T3	N1	M0
	T3	N2	M0
Stage IIIB	T4	N0	M0
	T4	N1	M0
	T4	N2	M0
Stage IIIC	Any T	N3	M0
Stage IV	Any T	Any N	M1

Note: Stage designation may be changed if postsurgical imaging studies show distant metastases, provided that the studies are carried out within 4 months of diagnosis in the absence of disease progression and provided that the patient has not received neoadjuvant therapy.

HISTOPATHOLOGIC TYPE

The histopathologic types are the following:

In situ Carcinomas

NOS (not otherwise specified)
Intraductal
Paget's disease and intraductal

Invasive Carcinomas

NOS
Ductal
Inflammatory
Medullary, NOS
Medullary with lymphoid stroma
Mucinous
Papillary (predominantly micropapillary pattern)
Tubular
Lobular
Paget's disease and infiltrating
Undifferentiated
Squamous cell
Adenoid cystic
Secretory

HISTOPATHOLOGIC GRADE (G)

All invasive breast carcinomas except medullary carcinoma should be graded. The Nottingham combined histologic grade (Elston-Ellis modification of the Scarff-Bloom-Richardson grading system) is recommended.[1,2] The tumor grade is determined by assessing the morphologic features (tubule formation, nuclear pleomorphism, and mitotic count), assigning a value of 1 (favorable) to 3 (unfavorable) to each feature, and adding the scores for the three categories. A combined score of 3 to 5 points is grade 1, a combined score of 6 to 7 points is grade 2 and a combined score of 8 to 9 points is grade 3.

Continued

TABLE 94-6

American Joint Committee on Cancer TNM Staging System for Breast Cancer—cont'd

1. Elston CW, Ellis IO: Pathological prognostic factors in breast cancer. I. The value of histologic grade in breast cancer experience from a large study with long-term follow-up. Histopathology 1991;19:403–410.
2. Fitzgibbons PL, Page DL, Weaver D, et al: Prognostic factors in breast cancer. College of American Pathologists consensus statement 1999. Arch Pathol Lab Med 2000;124:966–978.

Histologic Grade (Nottingham Combined Histologic Grade Is Recommended)

GX   Grade cannot be assessed
G1   Low combined histologic grade (favorable)
G2   Intermediate combined histologic grade (moderately favorable)
G3   High combined histologic grade (unfavorable)

NOS, not otherwise specified; RT-PCR, reverse transcriptase polymerase chain reaction.
*Clinically apparent is defined as detected by imaging studies (excluding lymphoscintigraphy) or by clinical examination or grossly visible pathologically.
†Classification is based on axillary lymph node dissection with or without sentinel lymph node dissection. Classification based solely on sentinel lymph node dissection without subsequent axillary node dissection is designated (sn) for "sentinel node" (e.g., pN0[i+] [sn]).
‡Not clinically apparent is defined as not detected by imaging studies (excluding lymphoscintigraphy) or by clinical examination.
§T1 includes T1mic.
National Comprehensive Cancer Network, Inc., version 1, 2003;10/29/02 © 2003.
Used with the permission of the American Joint Committee on Cancer (AJCC), Chicago, Illinois. The original and primary source for this information is the AJCC Cancer Staging Manual, 6th ed. (2002) published by Springer-Verlag New York. (For more information, visit www.cancerstaging.net.) Any citation or quotation of this material must be credited to the AJCC as its primary source. The inclusion of this information herein does not authorize any reuse or further distribution without the expressed, written permission of Springer-Verlag New York, Inc., on behalf of the AJCC.

TABLE 94-7

Tumor Size and Outcome in Operable Breast Cancer

| | TOTAL NO. OF PATIENTS | SURVIVAL (%) RELATED TO TUMOR SIZE | | | | | |
| | | 2 CM | | 2–5 CM | | >5 CM | |
AUTHORS		5 YR	10 YR	5 YR	10 YR	5 YR	10 YR
Carter et al.	24,740	91		80		63	
Schottenfeld et al.	304	92	79	71	57	55	40
Nemoto et al.	13,384	[62]		[49]		[34]	

[ ], disease-free survival.
Adapted from Yeh I, Fowble B, Viglione MJ, et al: Pathologic assessment and pathologic prognostic factors in operable breast cancer. In Fowble B, Goodman RL, Glick JH, Rosato EF (eds): Breast Cancer Treatment: A Comprehensive Guide to Treatment. St. Louis, Mosby-Year Book, 1991, p 171.

TABLE 94-8

Axillary Node Status and Outcome in Operable Breast Cancer

| | SURVIVAL (%) RELATED TO NODES | | | | | |
| | NEGATIVE NODES | | 1–3 POSITIVE NODES | | 4 POSITIVE NODES | |
AUTHORS	5 YR	10 YR	5 YR	10 YR	5 YR	10 YR
Moon et al.						
Milan	89 [81]	–	68 [53]	–	48 [31]	–
Royal Marsden	66 [69]	–	70 [51]	–	42 [32]	–
M.D. Anderson	–	–	91 [69]	–	53 [43]	–
Carter et al.	92	–	81	–	57	–
Valagussa et al.	88 [79]	83 [74]	69 [46]	54 [33]	42 [26]	26 [15]
Ariel	81	63	66	53	48	23
Fisher et al.	78	65	62	38	32	13

Adapted from Yeh I, Fowble B, Viglione MJ, et al: Pathologic assessment and pathologic prognostic factors in operable breast cancer. In Fowble B, Goodman RI, Glick JH, Rosato EF (eds): Breast Cancer Treatment: A Comprehensive Guide to Treatment. St. Louis, Mosby-Year Book, 1991, p 171.

TABLE 94-9

Histologic Classification and Incidence of Invasive Breast Cancer

HISTOLOGIC TYPE	INCIDENCE (%)
Invasive ductal carcinoma	85
Invasive lobular carcinoma	4–10
Mucinous carcinoma	
Medullary carcinoma	
Papillary carcinoma	3–6
Tubular carcinoma	
Adenoid cystic carcinoma	
Secretory (juvenile) carcinoma	
Apocrine carcinoma	
Carcinoma with metaplasia	

Adapted from Azzopardi JG, Chepick OF, Hartman WH, et al: The World Health Organization histological typing of breast tumors, 2nd ed. Am J Clin Pathol 1982;78:806. Copyright © 1982, American Society of Clinical Pathologists.

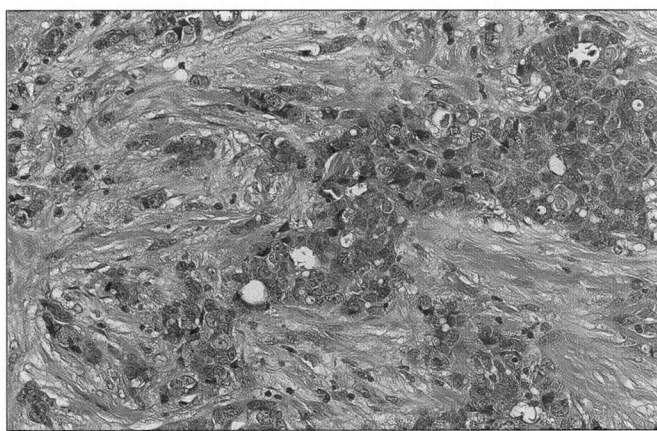

Figure 94-18. Invasive lobular carcinoma. The tumor cells are small, and form linear, single files.

neoplasms. The rarer sarcomas, lymphomas, and non-epithelial tumors are discussed elsewhere. Infiltrating breast cancers are histologically heterogeneous, but most of them are adenocarcinomas arising from the terminal ducts. Invasive ductal carcinoma, which accounts for approximately 85% of breast cancers (Table 94-9),[264] has no specific histologic features (Fig. 94-17). Invasive lobular carcinoma accounts for 5% to 10% of breast cancers. Its overall prognosis is similar to that of the invasive ductal subtype. Microscopically, lobular carcinoma is characterized by single-filing ("Indian file") of small, regular epithelial cells that tend to grow around ducts and lobules (Fig. 94-18).

Many special types of breast carcinoma are less common than the invasive ductal and lobular kinds, and they usually have a more favorable prognosis. These include mucinous, papillary, tubular, and adenoid cystic carcinoma. The better prognoses associated with these special histologic subtypes have been most clearly defined in node-negative patients. Rosen and colleagues[262] found that patients with node-negative disease with special

tumor types that were 3 cm or smaller had a good prognosis, equivalent to that of patients with infiltrating ductal or lobular carcinoma 1 cm or less in diameter. The clinical and biologic features of 444 patients with tubular carcinoma and 1221 patients with mucinous carcinoma were compared with those of 43,587 patients with infiltrating ductal carcinoma, not otherwise specified.[265] Because of the favorable characteristics and excellent prognoses of these types of breast carcinoma, the investigators concluded that axillary node dissection may not be beneficial in tubular carcinoma, regardless of size, or in mucinous carcinoma 1 cm or smaller. The response of these special histologic types to systemic adjuvant therapy has not been adequately studied, but in most cases, this therapy is not required. Mucinous (colloid) carcinoma is characterized microscopically by abundant accumulation of extracellular mucin around tumor cells (Fig. 94-19).

The histopathologic features that define medullary carcinoma include a well-circumscribed border, intense reaction with lymphocytes and plasma cells, poorly

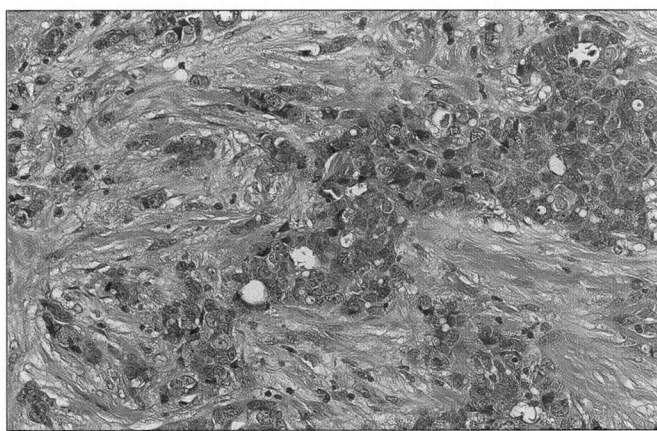

Figure 94-17. Typical infiltrating ductal carcinoma. Irregularly dispersed glands and cords of tumor cells are set in a desmoplastic stroma.

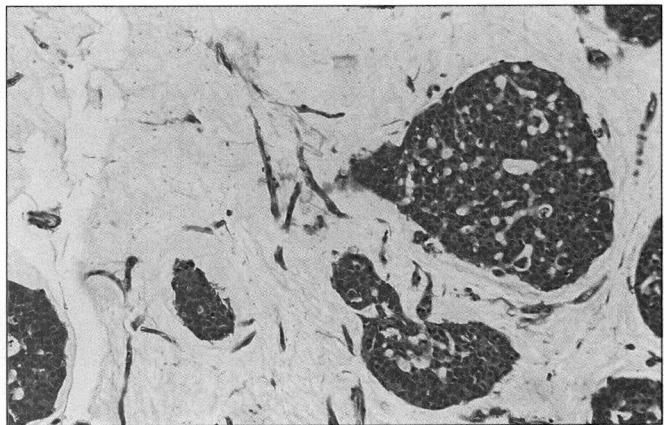

Figure 94-19. Invasive mucinous (colloid) carcinoma. Bland nests of tumor cells float in abundant extracellular mucin.

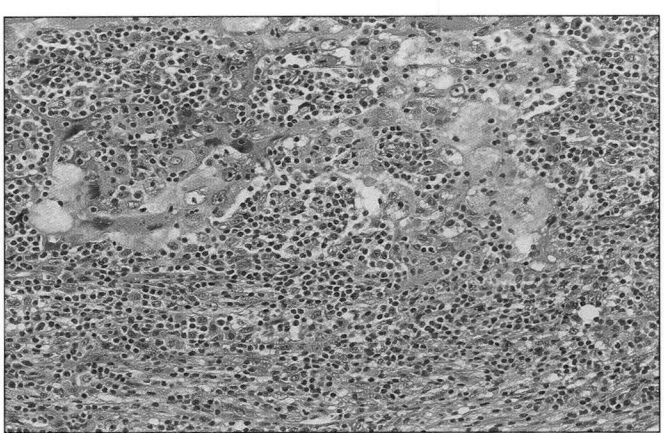

Figure 94-20. Medullary carcinoma characterized by a well-defined border, an intense lymphoplasmacytic reaction, and pleomorphic tumor cells with vesicular chromatin.

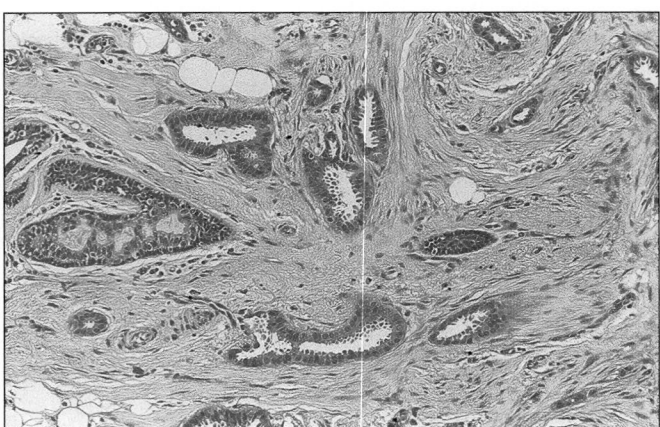

Figure 94-22. Infiltrating tubular carcinoma. The invasive glands are irregularly dispersed, lack a second myoepithelial cell layer, and are set in a desmoplastic stroma. Tubular carcinoma resembles normal breast ducts. Two normal ducts, seen in the center, appear darker than the tubular carcinoma and have two cell layers.

differentiated nuclei, a syncytial growth pattern, and little or no intraductal carcinoma (Fig. 94-20). The more favorable prognosis requires the presence of all of these characteristics. Thus, atypical medullary tumors do not have the same excellent outcome. Furthermore, the risk of incorrectly labeling an aggressive, poorly differentiated carcinoma as medullary carcinoma led some to exclude the latter from the special types of breast cancer with favorable prognoses. A frond-forming growth pattern characterizes papillary carcinoma (Fig. 94-21). Tubular carcinoma is distinguished by the proliferation of small glands that resemble normal mammary ducts (Fig. 94-22).

Studies of the prognostic value of other pathologic factors, such as histologic grade, vascular-lymphatic invasion, inflammatory response, and tumor necrosis,

showed considerable variation. However, some studies showed that nuclear grade, as determined by expert breast pathologists, had predictive power equivalent to that of newer biologic parameters.[266] The major criticism of nuclear grade is the lack of observer consistency in making this subjective classification. New quantitative techniques for computerized image analysis may help to overcome the obstacles to routine application of nuclear grade as a prognostic factor.

Various prognostic indices incorporating several parameters have been intensively studied. The Nottingham Prognostic Index,[267] which is derived from tumor size, nodal status, and tumor grade, was validated by the German Breast Cancer Study Group[268] in a series of 600 patients with node-negative breast cancer.

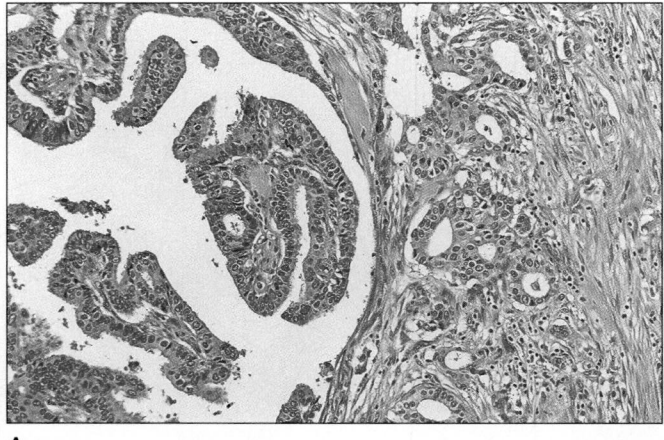

A

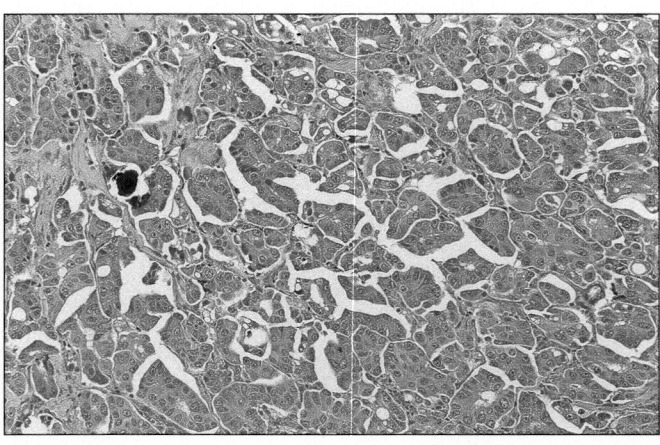

B

Figure 94-21. A, Invasive carcinoma arising in papillary ductal carcinoma in situ (invasive papillary carcinoma). The in situ component seen on the right has a frond-like appearance, and the invasive carcinoma component on the left consists of irregularly shaped small glands. **B,** Invasive micropapillary carcinoma of the breast. The tumor resembles ovarian serous carcinoma, and small clusters of invasive tumor cells are separated from the stroma by spaces. A psammoma body is seen.

TABLE 94-10

Criteria for Evaluating Clinically Useful Tumor Markers

Identification of a Potential Marker

What is the distribution of the marker in normal and abnormal tissues?

What is the prevalence of the marker in the patient population of interest?

What is the source of specimens examined? Institutional or cooperative group tissue or serum banks?

Does the marker appear to predict outcome (prognostic factor) or response to therapy (predictive factor)?

Development and Validation of a Clinical Assay

Has the assay target that best correlates with the intended marker objective been identified (e.g., gene amplification, protein expression)?

Has the optimal specimen source for the assay been identified (e.g., paraffin block, fresh tumor tissue, peripheral blood, urine)?

Have the conditions of the assay been optimized and standardized? Has its reproducibility in other labs been tested?

Has standardized and cross-validated scoring system been developed?

Have the sensitivity and specificity of the assay been validated against a gold standard?

Validation of the Clinical Usefulness of the Marker

Has this marker been validated in a patient population different than the one used to develop the predictive and prognostic model?

Does the presence of the marker discriminate between patient subsets according to the outcome of interest?

Is the prognostic or predictive information provided by the marker independent of other established markers?

Has a prospective randomized trial using the proposed marker been performed using the information provided by the assay to stratify patients according to risk or to select planned therapy?

Predictive and Prognostic Factors

Although it is easy to describe the risk of recurrence in a population of patients, this exercise is difficult in an individual patient, and physicians rely heavily on prognostic factors. A pure prognostic factor should reflect the biologic features of the tumor and predict patient outcome in the absence of therapy.[269-271] A pure predictive factor should assess the responsiveness of an individual patient's cancer to a particular type of therapy. Most factors have mixed characteristics, with variable strength, and few have been properly validated (Table 94-10). TNM staging (i.e., tumor size and axillary node status) remains the most important prognostic factor.

Other accepted factors include tumor grade, lymphatic or vascular invasion, and tumor type (e.g., small mucinous and tubular cancers).[272,273] Although ER and PR are strong predictive factors for benefit from endocrine therapy, they are only weak prognostic factors for favorable outcome (Table 94-11). The potential role of factors such as bone marrow micrometastases and circulating epithelial cells remains uncertain.

HER2 (ERBB2) and ER are examples of weak prognostic factors with a strong predictive component for response to specific therapies that can help to individualize treatment recommendations for women at high risk for recurrence. Women whose tumors overexpress or amplify the HER2 receptor may be less likely to respond to endocrine manipulations. These women may consider the addition of adjuvant chemotherapy, even if their tumors do not exceed 1 cm and carry ER or PR.[274] *HER2* overexpression also identifies patients with metastatic disease who might benefit from trastuzumab therapy.[275] Many other individual prognostic or predictive factors are under investigation. Levels of urokinase-type plasminogen activator and its inhibitor PAI-1 had strong prognostic value in a group of 118 women with node-negative breast cancer who did not receive adjuvant systemic therapy and had more than 10 years of follow-up.[276] In addition to individual factors, powerful emerging technologies, such as proteomics or gene arrays, hold the potential to identify patterns of expression of genes or proteins at baseline or in response to therapy that may have prognostic or predictive value, and to assist in treatment decision-making for individual women.[277-280]

Initial studies with array-based expression profiling (Fig. 94-23) to classify breast carcinomas showed the ability of the technology to classify correctly ER-negative and ER-positive tumors[281,282] and to differentiate *BRCA1*-related tumors from *BRCA2*-related and sporadic tumors.[277,283] The ER-positive group was characterized by high expression of many genes expressed by breast luminal cells, and the ER-negative group showed gene expression characteristic of basal epithelial cells. However, a third group showed genes related to *HER2* overexpression,[281] suggesting that this molecular characteristic may have equal or greater weight than ER expression in subclassifying breast cancers. Finally, a small group of breast cancers cluster with normal breast epithelium and are referred to as normal breast-like.

TABLE 94-11

Relationship of Estrogen Receptor (ER) to Disease-Free and Overall Survival at 5 Years

TRIAL	DISEASE-FREE SURVIVAL (%)			OVERALL SURVIVAL (%)		
	ER+	ER–	P	ER+	ER–	P
NSABP	74	66	<0.001	92	82	<0.0001
San Antonio	76	67	<0.001	84	75	<0.0001

NSABP, National Surgical Adjuvant Breast and Bowel Project.
Adapted from McGuire WL, Tandon AK, Allred DC, et al: Treatment decisions in axillary node–negative breast cancer patients. J Natl Cancer Inst Monogr 1992;11:173.

Specific Malignancies

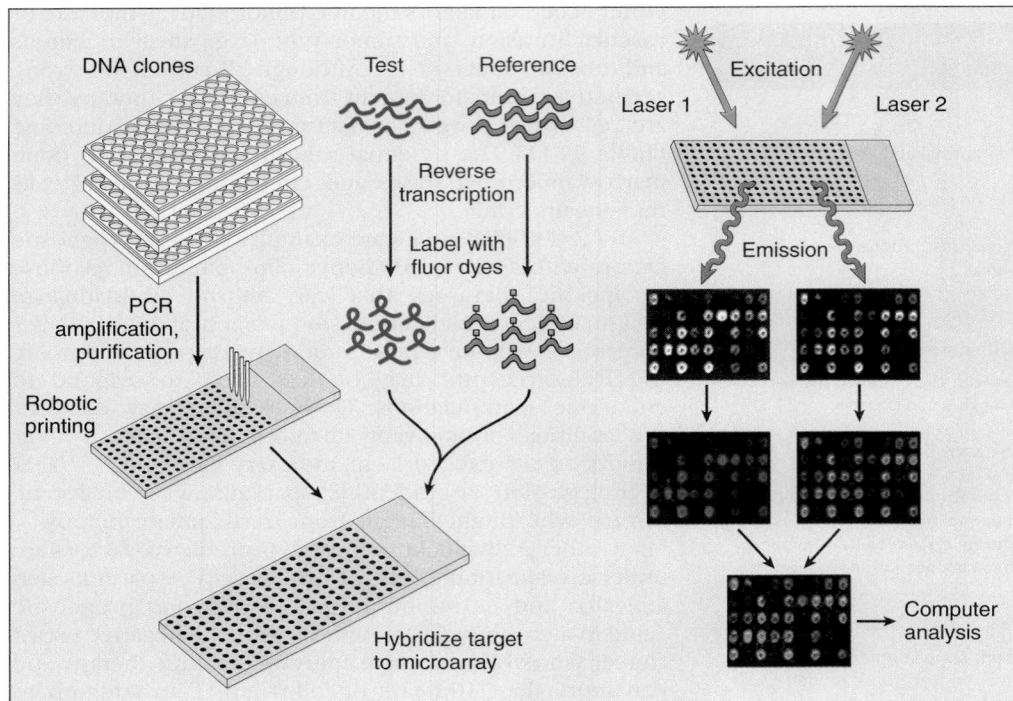

Figure 94-23. Microarray analysis. Microarrays are made by spotting small amounts of DNA onto a glass slide or other solid support with a specially designed robot. Either DNA, for comparative genomic hybridization (CGH) [array CGH], or reverse-transcribed RNA, for expression profiling, is labeled with fluorescent dye and hybridized to the slides. The signal is read by a laser scan and fed into a computer for analysis. Array CGH provides a genome-wide view of deletions and amplifications, and expression profiling provides a comprehensive analysis of transcript (messenger RNA) levels for every gene represented on the microarray. More than 30,000 spots can be stamped onto a standard microscope slide, allowing analysis of most of the genes in the human genome simultaneously. PCR, polymerase chain reaction.

Initial efforts to classify breast tumors by molecular profiling lacked direct clinical correlation. Prognostic information that can identify those who will do well without chemotherapy, those who will clearly benefit from chemotherapy, and those who may do poorly despite chemotherapy is key to the advancement of breast cancer treatment. Several reports show a link between microarray-based tumor expression profiles and clinical outcome.[277,284,285]

The first such study used expression profiling of FNA in women undergoing preoperative chemotherapy for breast cancer in an attempt to define gene expression profiles associated with clinical response.[285] Expression profiles were analyzed before and after treatment using an array containing 4800 genes. An algorithm based on expression patterns of 37 genes correctly predicted clinical response in all 10 patients studied. Genes associated with response to chemotherapy included *KIT* (a growth factor receptor), *ERG* (a transcription factor), *CD44,* and others.

In a subsequent study, 78 breast cancers were examined using expression profiling in an attempt to predict clinical outcome.[284] From a set of 8100 genes, 456 were identified that optimally characterized these tumors. Hierarchical clustering using this gene set showed the previously described subgroups: ER-positive or luminal tumors, ER-negative or basal tumors, tumors expressing *HER2*, and normal-breast-like tumors.[281] The ER-positive or luminal group could be divided into three subgroups. Group A had the highest expression of ER, whereas groups B and C had comparatively lower expression of luminal-specific genes, including ER. Group C also had increased expression of a panel of genes representing several signaling pathways. These groups were analyzed for correlation with disease-free and overall survival rates. ER-negative or basal tumors and those overexpressing *HER2* fared worst, whereas group A ER-positive or luminal tumors had the best overall and disease-free survival rates. Group B and C ER-positive or luminal tumors and normal-breast-like tumors had intermediate outcomes, suggesting that this technology will allow prognostically important segregation of subgroups of ER-positive breast cancers with different disease outcomes.[284]

In the most extensive and informative study performed to date, expression profiles of 117 primary breast tumors were compared with known prognostic markers.[277] Expression profiling with 25,000 genes provided intitally separated the tumors into two groups. In one group, only 34% of patients had distant metastasis at 5 years; in the second group, 70% of patients had metastatic disease. The second group contained 34 of the 39 clinically ER-negative tumors in the sample as well as 16 of the 18 *BRCA1*-related tumors.[277]

Next, 231 genes were selected that had a correlation coefficient that was significantly associated with disease outcome. From these, 70 genes were identified for optimal accuracy in predicting recurrent disease. Using this classification, the outcome of 83% of patients was predicted correctly.[277] Finally, the data were reanalyzed using an optimal threshold so that 10% or fewer of patients in the poor-prognosis group would be misclassified. Genes with increased expression in the poor-prognosis group compared with the good-prognosis group included cyclin E2 (a cell-cycle regulator), *MMP9* (a metalloproteinase), *FLT1* (a growth factor receptor), and others. However, this group did not include several genes that were previously considered important, such as cyclin D1 (a cell-cycle

Figure 94-24. Annual age-adjusted incidence rates of invasive breast cancer, ductal carcinoma in situ, and lobular carcinoma in situ per 100,000 women in Los Angeles County, CA, from 1972 through 1998. Rates include women of all racial and ethnic groups. Rates are standardized to the 1970 U.S. population. (From Bernstein L: The epidemiology of breast cancer in situ. In Silverstein M: Ductal Carcinomas in Situ of the Breast, 2nd ed. Philadelphia, Lippincott Williams & Wilkins, 2002, pp 22–34.)

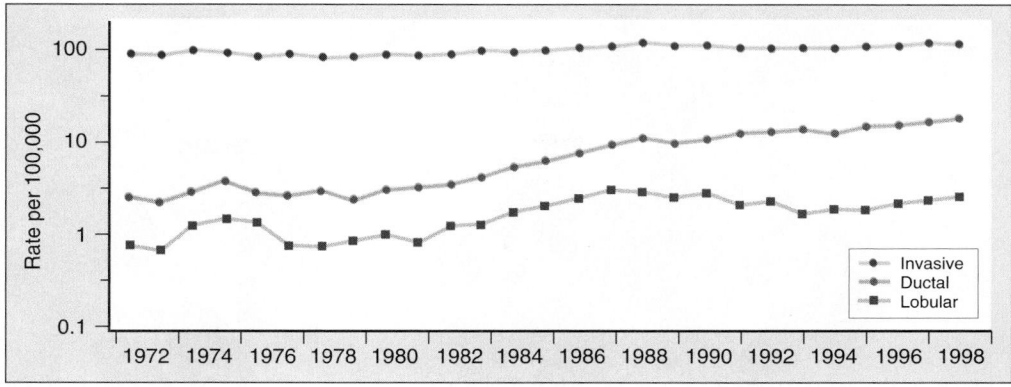

regulator), *ERα, PAI* (a serine protease inhibitor), *ERBB2* (a growth factor receptor), and *MYCC*.[277] After cross-validation was performed, the poor-prognosis profile was associated with an odds ratio of 15 for an interval of 5 years or longer to the development of metastases. A multivariate analysis was performed with currently available prognostic factors (grade, tumor size >2 cm, angioinvasion, age <40 years, and ER-negative status). This analysis showed that the poor-prognosis microarray profile was an independent predictor of clinical outcome, with an odds ratio of 18 (95% confidence interval [CI], 3 to 94). The findings suggested that expression profiling of breast cancer may result in better prediction of which patients will benefit from chemotherapy, sparing many women unnecessary toxicity.[277] These data also provide stunning evidence that the genetic program of a cancer cell at diagnosis defines its biologic behavior many years later. This finding refutes a competing hypothesis suggesting that additional genetic changes are acquired in residual cells after treatment and lead to the development of metastatic disease.

MANAGEMENT OF NONINVASIVE BREAST CANCER

Much evidence supports the view that the development of malignancy is a multistep process and that invasive breast cancer has a preinvasive phase. During the carcinoma in situ (CIS) phase, normal epithelial cells undergo enough genetic alterations to result in malignant transformation.[286] Transformed epithelial cells proliferate and pile up within lobules or ducts, but lack the additional required genetic alteration that enables cells to penetrate the investing basement membrane.

As discussed later, nowhere in cancer therapy has more controversy existed than in the appropriate management of in situ breast cancer. Because of the increasing acceptance of breast cancer screening in the United States, CIS accounts for an increasing proportion of all new breast cancers. Between 1975 and 1978, surveys suggested an incidence of pure in situ lesions of 1.4% to 5.1%.[287] In 2001, nearly 20% of all new breast cancers in the United States were DCIS; the denominator does not include cases of lobular carcinoma in situ (LCIS;

Fig. 94-24). Thus, debate continues about the natural history of CIS. Which CIS is preinvasive cancer and which is simply a marker of unstable epithelium that represents an increased risk of subsequent invasive cancer? In the future, these answers may become obvious through genomic research, but traditional methods of estimating risk are still in use.

Lobular Carcinoma in Situ

Although breast CIS was first reported in 1932 by Broders,[286] in 1941, Foote and Steward[288] first described a noninvasive malignancy confined to the lobules and terminal ducts, and referred to this entity as LCIS. The authors described this lesion as rare and reported it as the sole finding in 2 of the 300 mastectomy specimens reviewed. In another 12 patients, it was associated with conventional infiltrating lobular cancer, leading the authors to conclude that the in situ form and the invasive lesion constituted a single malignant process.[288]

Anatomy and Pathology

The original description of LCIS characterized the lesion as a lobular unit with its cluster of ductules or acini filled, distorted, and distended by proliferating epithelial cells (Fig. 94-25). Anderson and Vindelboe[289] described the cells as having a fairly uniform pattern of clear cytoplasm containing rounded, bland nuclei. Intercellular spaces are preserved, and clear vacuoles within the cytoplasm may displace the nucleus. This type is often called "classical" LCIS. Lesser forms of lobular unit involvement are known as lobular hyperplasia, although a consensus definition of these two pathologic entities has not been reached. Some investigators argue that the word *carcinoma* should not be included in the term and that it is better to refer to atypical lobular hyperplasia and LCIS as "lobular neoplasia."[290] However, LCIS is a well-established entity and should remain as the descriptive label, because it is a recognized risk factor for the development of invasive breast cancer.

LCIS is a microscopic diagnosis, not a gross abnormality. The diagnosis is not associated with a mammographic abnormality. It is believed to account for 17% to 20% of all diagnosed cases of CIS.[291-293] Its incidence is discussed in the next section. If LCIS is discovered after needle-

Specific Malignancies

III

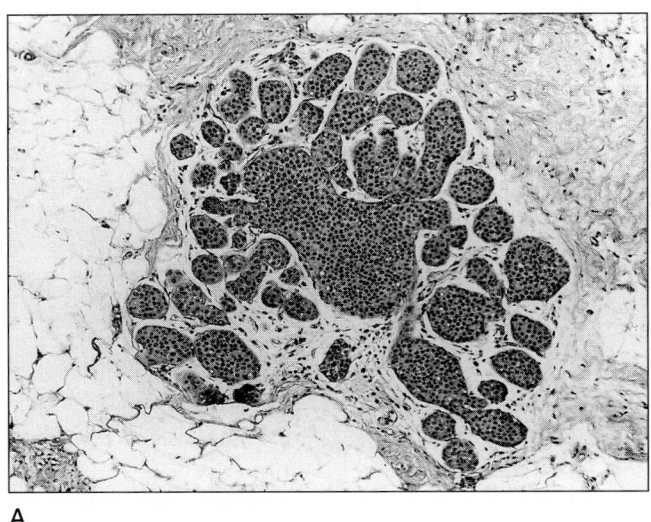

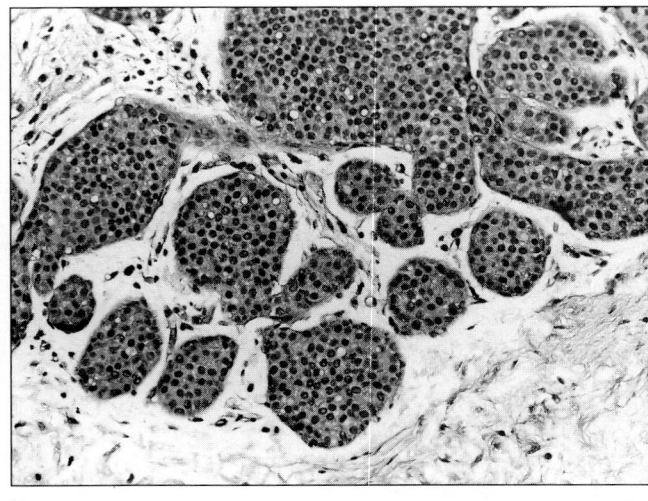

A   B

Figure 94-25. A, Lobular carcinoma in situ. The lobular unit (see Fig. 94-27) is distended and distorted by proliferating cells. The cells are uniform and round, with bland nuclei. **B,** The same example seen at a higher power.

localization biopsy of suspicious microcalcifications, the calcification is almost always outside the LCIS.[291,294-296] The only exception is the rare fibroadenoma that contains a focus of LCIS within the mass.[297]

Incidence

LCIS is usually discovered in association with another indicator for biopsy, such as a cyst or a fibroadenoma. It is a disease of younger women. In a report by Haagensen and colleagues,[290] 90% of the 211 patients with LCIS were premenopausal. LCIS is rare before 35 years of age and even rarer in women older than 75 years of age.[298-304] Figures 94-24 and 94-26 show the incidence of LCIS and DCIS in Los Angeles County, both over time since 1972 and by patient age.

Because LCIS is most often an incidental finding on a biopsy performed for other reasons, several pathology series retrospectively reviewed "benign" breast biopsy specimens to establish the true incidence of LCIS. Reports range from from 0.5% to 3.6%.[305-308] A greater use of mammography and a tendency to perform a more

thorough histologic evaluation of biopsy tissue appear to have contributed to an increase in the diagnosis of LCIS.[298,301] LCIS is more common in premenopausal women, but no evidence shows a hormonal etiology and no association has been noted with the use of exogenous estrogen.

Multicentricity and Bilaterality

LCIS is often multicentric and has an increased incidence of bilaterality.[291,302] The incidence of multicentricity was reported by Benfield and colleagues[303] as 86%, by Carter and Smith[304] as 63%, by Dall'Olmo and associates[306] as 56%, by Ringberg and associates[307] as 65%, by Schwartz and colleagues[308] as 67%, and by Rosen and associates[309] as 48%. The incidence of bilaterality was reported by Farrow[310] as 18%, by Carter and Smith[304] as 37%, by Urban[311] as 35%, by Rosen and colleagues[312] as 35%, and by Ringberg and associates[307] as 69%. This extensive literature was summarized by Nielsen and associates,[313] who reported multicentricity in 42% to 86% of cases and bilaterality in 9% to 69% of cases. However, it is possible

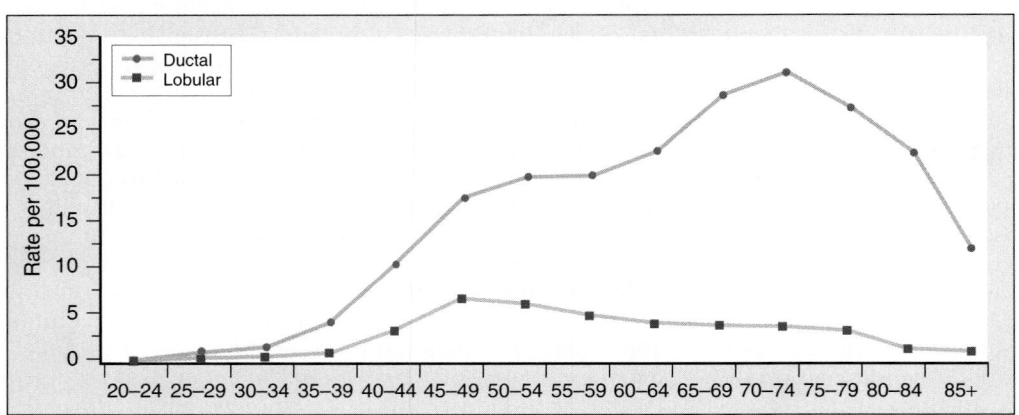

Figure 94-26. Average annual age-specific incidence rates of ductal carcinoma in situ and lobular carcinoma in situ per 100,000 women in Los Angeles County, CA, from 1972 to 1998. Rates include women of all racial and ethnic groups. (From Bernstein L: The epidemiology of breast cancer in situ. In Silverstein M: Ductal Carcinomas in Situ of the Breast, 2nd ed. Philadelphia, Lippincott Williams & Wilkins, 2002, pp 22-34.)

that the presence of bilateral and multicentric LCIS could approach 100% if the histopathologic search and extent of resection were comprehensive. The real importance of these observations is not the frequency of multicentric LCIS, but the correlation of this finding with the increased risk of subsequent invasive cancer and therefore increased mortality.

Incidence of Coexisting Invasive Cancer

In the premammography era, Carter and Smith[304] found that 3 of 49 patients with LCIS had invasive cancer in a subsequent mastectomy specimen. Benfield and colleagues[303] and Dall'Olmo and associates[306] did not find invasive cancer in their patients with LCIS. Ringberg and associates[307] found two invasive cancers associated with 16 LCIS tumors. Rosen and associates[309] reported two invasive cancers in 50 patients with LCIS. Rosen and colleagues[312] also looked at the risk of an occult contralateral invasive cancer and found six invasive cancers in 63 patients undergoing random biopsy of the contralateral breast. Although they are not perfect statistical models, these reviews suggest that the risk of a concurrent occult ipsilateral invasive cancer is low (<13%) and that the risk of an occult contralateral invasive cancer is even lower.

LCIS as a Marker for Invasive Cancer

Finding LCIS in breast biopsy specimens has its real value as an indicator of risk for the subsequent development of invasive breast cancer. This conclusion originated in retrospective studies by Haagensen and associates,[290,314] Rosen and colleagues,[309,315] and Page and associates.[305] The work of Rosen and associates, reported in 1978 and 1979, is perhaps the best known. Rosen and colleagues[309,315] reviewed 8607 "benign" biopsy specimens at Memorial Sloan-Kettering Cancer Center. They identified 99 women with LCIS who received no further surgical intervention. Of these, 84 had available follow-up data at a mean time of 24 years. Of the 29 subsequent cases of invasive breast carcinoma that were diagnosed, 12 were in the same breast, 9 were in the contralateral breast,

7 were bilateral, and 1 was at an unknown site.[315] The incidence of cancer was nine times greater than in the normal population, an overall risk similar to that reported by Page and associates.[305] However, in the Page study, of 44 women with LCIS who were followed for longer than 18 years, the risk was highest in the first 15 years. In contrast, in the Rosen study, the risk was observed through the 24-year study period.

The real significance of LCIS is as a predictor of risk for subsequent invasive cancer. These and other reports suggest that this risk is 7 to 12 times that in the general population (Table 94-12).

Treatment

Many studies have debated the appropriate management of LCIS. Over the years, the approach has included ipsilateral mastectomy with contralateral (mirror image) biopsy, bilateral mastectomy, and, more recently, biopsy with observation.[291,314-320] Because the risk of subsequent invasive breast cancer is fairly evenly divided between the index breast and the contralateral breast, similar management for both breasts is appropriate. DCIS may accompany LCIS. In such situations, therapy is dictated by the histologic pattern and risks of the DCIS component.

Management decisions in LCIS must take into account the patient's desires, anxiety level, and associated risk factors. It is reasonable to consider LCIS a marker of risk for subsequent invasive breast cancer in either breast and to follow these patients closely. Importantly, women who had LCIS were eligible for the NSABP P-1 tamoxifen prevention study, and a decrease in the risk of subsequent invasive breast cancer was seen in subjects receiving tamoxifen. Based on this result, the U.S. Food and Drug Administration approved this hormone as a risk-reduction agent, and it is another management option for women who have biopsy-proven LCIS. In the STAR trial, the NSABP is currently testing raloxifene against tamoxifen in a similar group of women who are at increased risk for breast cancer. More years of follow-up are required to fully evaluate these studies, to determine how long such chemoprevention is required, and to

TABLE 94-12

Risk of Subsequent Invasive Breast Cancer in Patients with Lobular Carcinoma in Situ: Follow-up Studies

STUDY	NO. OF PATIENTS	FOLLOW-UP (YR)	INVASIVE CANCER (%)	RELATIVE RISK
Salvadori et al.	80	5	6.3	10.3
Ottesen et al.	69	5	11.6	11.0
Fisher et al.	182	5	3.3	—
Andersen	47	15	26.4*	12.0
Haagensen et al	287	16.3	18	6.9
Wheeler et al.	32	17.5	12.5	—
Page et al.	44	18	23	9.0
Bodian et al.	236	18	26†	5.4
Rosen et al.	99	24	34.5‡	9.0

*Includes two patients with bilateral tumors counted separately.
†Includes ductal carcinoma in situ and invasive carcinoma.
‡Percentage calculated for 84 patients with follow-up.
From Schnitt S, Morrow M: Lobular carcinoma in situ: Current concepts and controversies. Semin Diagn Pathol 1999;16:210.

identify the risk-benefit ratio with tamoxifen and related therapies.[130]

Ductal Carcinoma in Situ

Noninvasive ductal carcinoma, or DCIS, is defined as "a proliferation of malignant cells confined within the basement membrane of the ducts of the breast."[321] Before the widespread use of mammography, DCIS was not commonly diagnosed and usually presented as a palpable mass or bloody nipple discharge. The increasing use of screening mammography resulted in a significant increase in the number of patients diagnosed with DCIS. Most of these cases are clinically occult.

Anatomic Histology

The terminal ductal lobular unit has been proposed as the site of origin of most breast cancer,[322,323] including DCIS (Fig. 94-27). In contrast to LCIS, which tends to be multicentric, DCIS is likely to be confined to one branching ductal system in the breast. As this disease becomes better understood, a picture of the spectrum of histologic subtypes of DCIS is emerging.

In the past, the pathologic classification of DCIS was based on the architectural patterns of DCIS as seen microscopically. These patterns included a solid pattern of growth filling the duct, a cribriform pattern characterized by well-defined holes seen within the growth pattern in the duct (Fig. 94-28), a comedo pattern with necrosis seen in the center of the duct (Fig. 94-29), and both micropapillary (Fig. 94-30) and papillary (Fig. 94-31) variants, characterized by frond-like projections of tumor cells into the lumen of the duct. Pathology reports commonly describe two or even three subtypes of DCIS in the same specimen, when using this system. A number of other classification systems have been proposed in the United States and Europe.

To clarify these pathology classification schemas and, more importantly, to identify subtypes of DCIS that may predict patient prognosis or response of the DCIS to

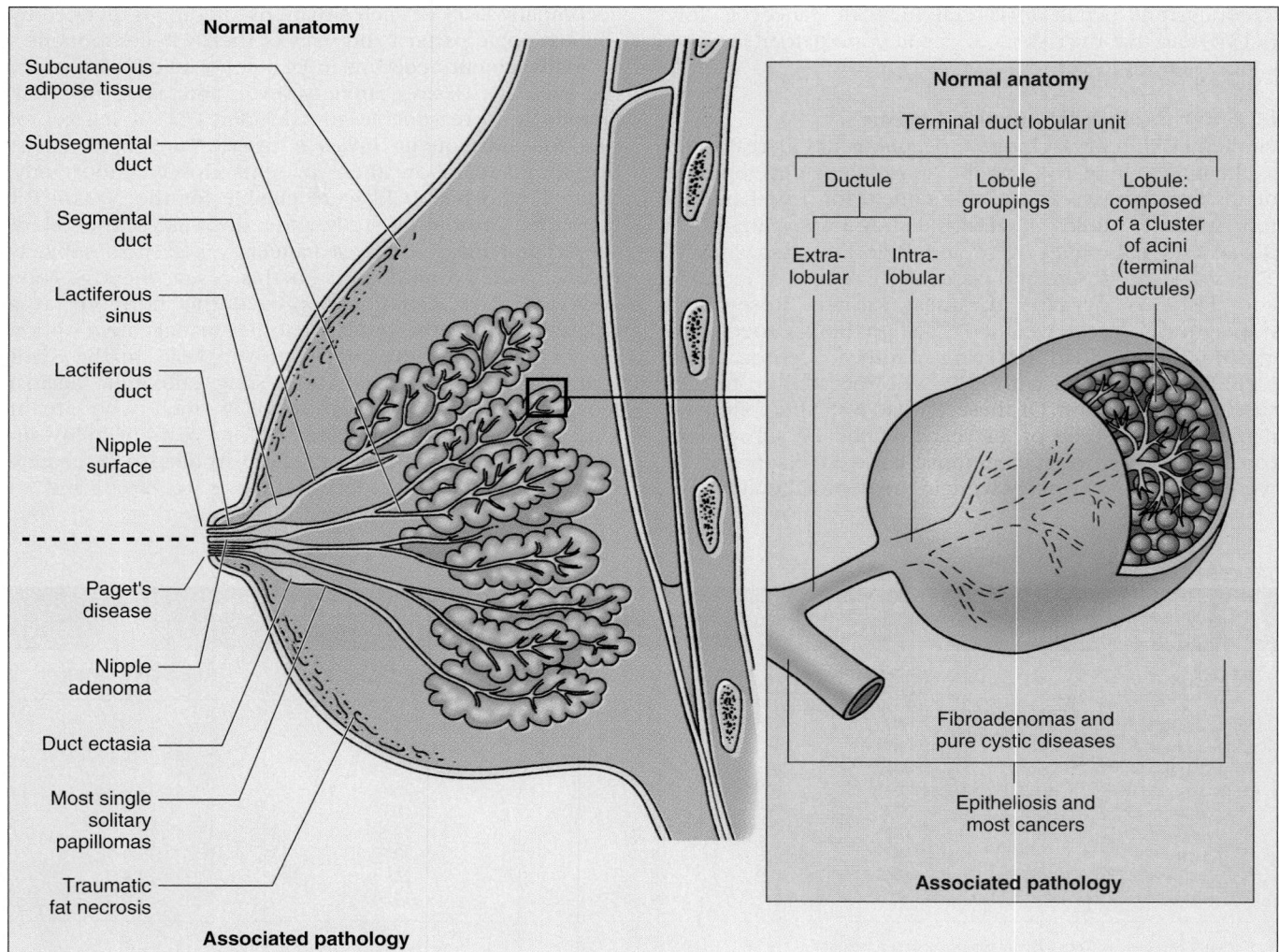

Figure 94-27. Anatomy of the breast, showing the organization of the elements of the terminal duct lobular unit and their relationship to specific pathologic abnormalities. (From Hayes D: Breast cancer. In Skarin AT [ed]: Atlas of Diagnostic Oncology. Philadelphia, JB Lippincott, 1991, p 64.)

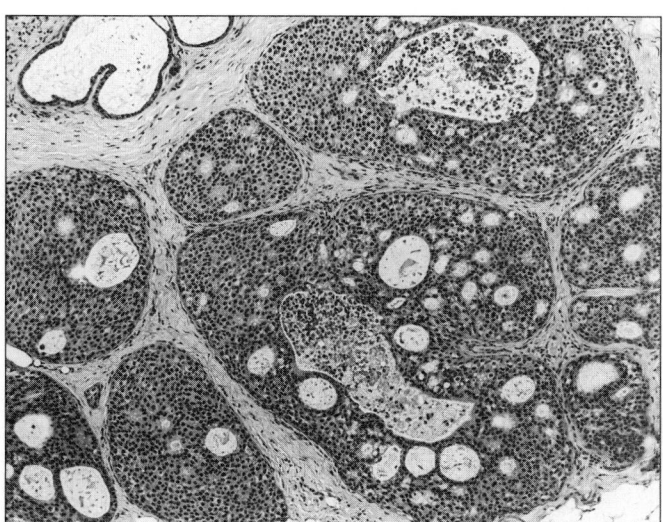

Figure 94-28. Cribriform ductal carcinoma in situ, which accounts for most of the ductal carcinoma in situ detected. It is characterized by interconnecting strands of hyperchromatic cells. Few necrotic cells are seen, and arches of connecting strands appear rigid.

various clinical interventions, a consensus conference was held in 1997. This conference included 19 breast pathologists from the United States and Europe as well as experts in breast imaging, surgery, and radiation oncology. The conference reached a consensus on issues such as pathologic classification, methods of determining the size and extent of the DCIS, methods of determining margin width, and most importantly, the procedure for processing the specimen in the pathology laboratory to ensure that all pertinent information can be obtained from the tissue.[321]

Significant recommendations of the report on the classification of DCIS included noting the nuclear grade of the cancer cells, the proportion of involved ducts showing necrosis, the polarization of the cells around the intercellular spaces, and the architectural pattern. Nuclear grade was determined to be the most important feature, and low-grade and high-grade lesions were described. Low-grade lesions had monotonous nuclei, measuring 1.5 to 2 times the size of a normal red blood cell, with finely dispersed chromatin and only occasional nucleoli and mitotic figures. High-grade lesions had markedly pleomorphic nuclei, measuring more than 2.5 times the size of a normal red blood cell, with irregular chromatin distribution and prominent nucleoli with conspicuous mitoses. Intermediate-grade nuclei were defined as those not meeting the criteria for high-grade or low-grade lesions.[321]

Necrosis was also defined as the presence of ghost cells and karyorrhectic debris. It was further quantified as "comedo," with central-zone necrosis, or "punctate," with nonzonal necrosis and without a linear pattern within the ducts. The traditional architectural patterns were also noted as appropriate to mention in the pathology report, independently of the other pathologic features.[321]

Tissue processing in the pathology laboratory was also described, because it is key in determining such information as lesion size and margin width. Important steps to follow included orientation of the specimen by the surgeon; radiograph of the specimen when feasible; inking of the surface of the specimen for margin information, unless the surgeon sends separate margin specimens; and, most importantly, processing the specimen in sequence in separate cassettes.

The size of the lesions can be determined in several ways. If DCIS is closely associated with linear or branching-type calcifications, the mammogram size can

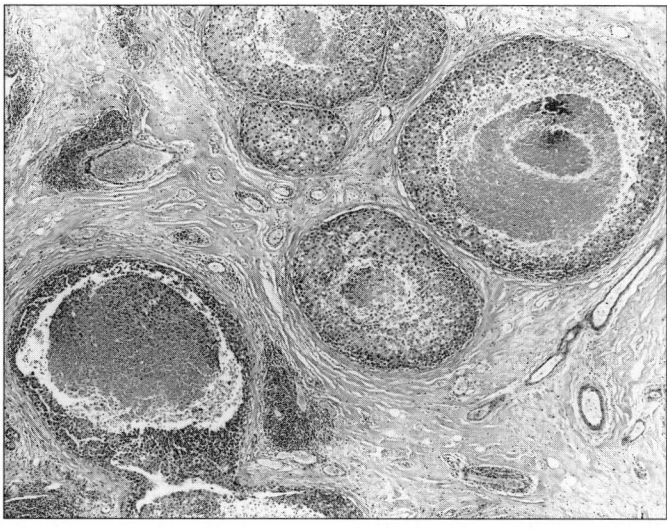

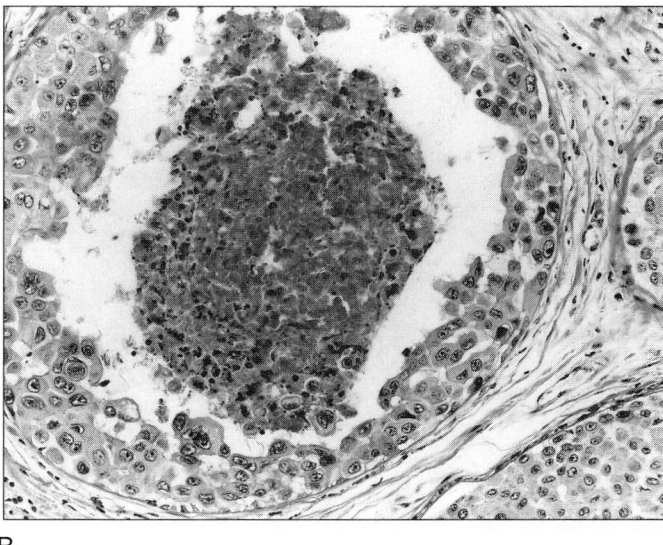

A   B

Figure 94-29. A, Comedo ductal carcinoma in situ (DCIS). The ducts are expanded by sheets of proliferating cells with areas of central necrosis. The sheets of cells show more pleomorphism than is common with other histologic types of DCIS. A higher incidence of microinvasion is also seen with comedo DCIS. **B,** The same example seen at a higher power.

Specific Malignancies

III

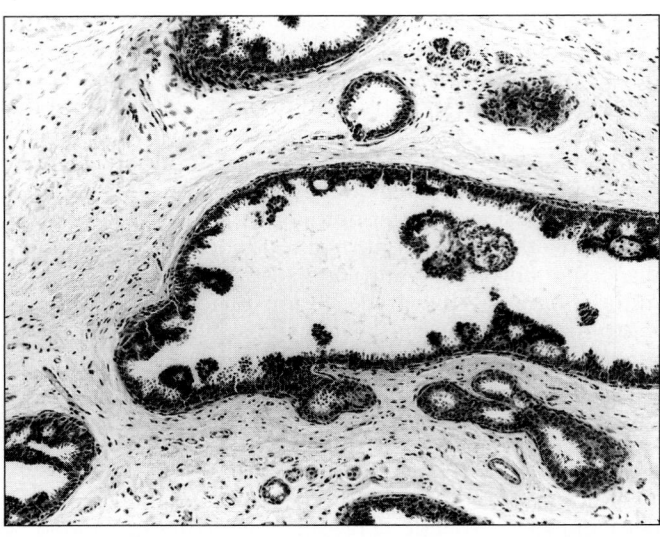

A

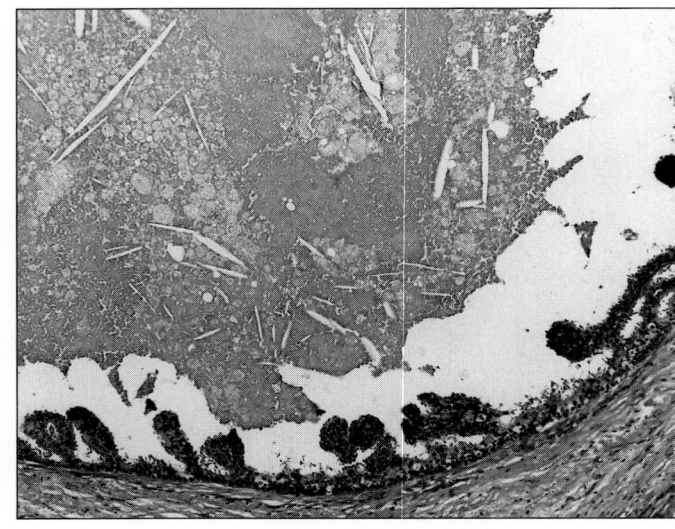

B

Figure 94-30. A, Micropapillary ductal carcinoma in situ is characterized by small papillary projections of neoplastic cells. The papillary projections are frond-like, with a narrow base, and arise from the intersurface of ductal spaces. They are several cells thick. **B,** The same example seen at a higher power.

provide minimum size information. If DCIS is seen microscopically on only one slide, measurement across this slide is also a meaningful estimate of size. When DCIS is present on multiple slides, the pathologist should note the number of sequential slides or segments that show DCIS. Margin information is usually described in terms of the width of the closest margin, using the distance from the inked margin to the nearest involved duct.[321] Like size, this measurement is an estimate, because the pathologist can view only a finite number of representative sections. In the unsampled tissue, the margin may actually be closer than the distance recorded in the sampled slides.

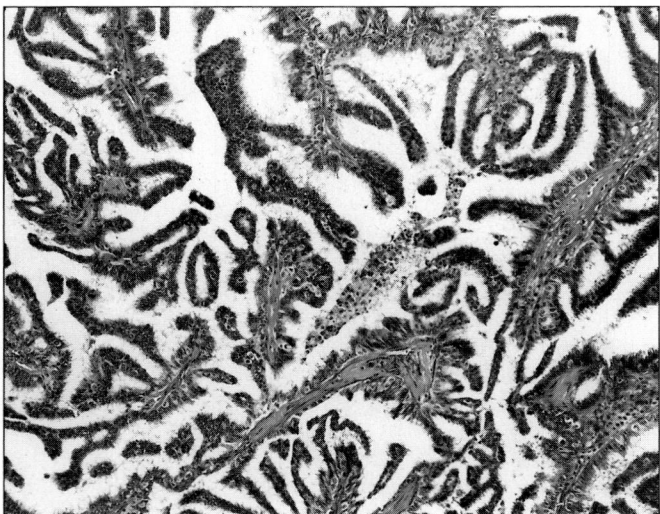

Figure 94-31. Papillary ductal carcinoma in situ. In contrast to the micropapillary form, fibrovascular fronds are seen, similar to a duct papilloma. The fibrovascular fronds are covered by multiple layers of neoplastic cells with hyperchromatic nuclei.

Incidence and Multicentricity

Mammographic screening and an aggressive approach to histologic confirmation of suspicious radiographic abnormalities contributed to an increased incidence of CIS, especially DCIS. Autopsy series suggest that as many as 16% of asymptomatic women have occult DCIS lesions.[313,324] Frykberg and associates[325] collected a series of 18 recent reports suggesting (when pooled) that DCIS was present in 7% of 6287 breast biopsy specimens of nonpalpable mammographic abnormalities. DCIS was also identified in 30% of 1455 nonpalpable carcinomas.

Figure 94-24 shows the incidence of DCIS, from 1974 through 1992, based on Surveillance, Epidemiology, and End Results data. In Figure 94-26, trends in incidence by age show a marked increase in women older than 50 years of age.[326]

The reports on the multicentricity of DCIS often present less than convincing data. As a result, the literature contains a wide range of data on the incidence of multicentricity. McDivitt[327] characterized multicentric DCIS as two or more separate foci of carcinoma within the breast that are believed to have developed independently from the same carcinogenic stimulus. Lagios and associates[328] suggested defining multicentricity as a second separate focus of DCIS at least 5 cm distant from the primary site. With complete sectioning of the breast after mastectomy, this group found an incidence of multicentricity with this definition of 14% when primary lesions were less than 2.5 cm in diameter and of 54% when the primary lesion was larger than 2.5 cm.

Multifocality and residual DCIS within the same breast duct segment, which does not always correspond to the index "quadrant," should not be confused with true multicentricity. Holland wrote extensively on this topic, proposing that most DCIS is distributed along a duct segment. When several foci of calcifications were seen on the mammogram, he found that these areas are often "connected" at the light microscopy level. In a careful study that correlated whole-organ sectioning after mastectomy, using light microscopy and x-rays of each section, Holland and Faverly[329] measured the distance, or gaps, between areas of DCIS, and defined this as "discontinuous" DCIS. In a study of 60 women treated with mastectomy for DCIS, they found this discontinuous pattern of growth in 30 cases. However, only 8% of the patients had a gap distance of greater that 10 mm. In the remaining cases, the gap was less than 5 mm in 19 women and less than 10 mm in 25 cases.

Clinical Diagnosis

Unlike LCIS, DCIS is almost always diagnosed by mammography. Even when palpable DCIS is present, the mammographic findings are quite characteristic, with a diffuse, often linear, and extensive pattern of pleomorphic calcifications.[330-332] However, the screening mammogram is usually the first indication of DCIS. Several patterns of calcifications raise the suspicion of the diagnostic radiologist. These include linear or casting-type calcifications, fine or "powdery" calcifications, and irregularly shaped calcifications described by Tabar and colleagues as "crushed stone."[333] Although any pathologic grade of DCIS can be diagnosed with any type of calcification, the most common associations are high-nuclear-grade lesions with the linear pattern and low- to intermediate-nuclear-grade lesions with a fine or powdery pattern.[333] Less likely mammographic findings include architectural distortion or a mass.

Bloody nipple discharge can also be a symptom of DCIS. A galactogram is indicated in this situation and may show a filling defect. Paget's disease of the breast, another form of DCIS, commonly causes a crusty, eczema-like change in the skin of the nipple, and bleeding may be noted. Approximately half of these women have a palpable mass as well. In those who do not, a recent series found a negative mammogram in 63% of women with nipple changes only.[333]

Clinical research on MRI for DCIS is ongoing in many centers equipped with a dedicated breast coil. Although some technical problems must be overcome in imaging DCIS with MRI, it has proven useful in evaluating the extent of residual disease in women requiring re-excision after initial biopsy.[334,335]

FNA is not ideal for evaluating DCIS. For years, when mammographic abnormalities suggested DCIS, needle-localization-directed open biopsy with specimen radiography was the standard approach. Recently, with the availability of large-gauge, image-guided automated core biopsy devices, this technique has become accepted in appropriate cases.[336]

Biology

DCIS by definition has intact basement membrane on light microscopy.[337] Defective basement membranes, however, have been found when DCIS lesions are stained with periodic acid-Schiff reagent and examined by electron microscopy.[337] Unlike pure DCIS, when micro-invasion is present, type IV collagen and lamina are lost from the basement membrane in association with loss of membrane continuity.[338] Such observations lend weight to the argument that DCIS is a precursor of invasive ductal cancer.

Not all cases of DCIS progress to invasive cancer. Identifying the predictors of this process is a major challenge in understanding the biology of this disease. Traditional ways of classifying pathology subtypes of DCIS have not provided these data. A recent subset analysis by histologic type of the 1010 women in the European Organization for Research on the Treatment of Cancer (EORTC) 10853 trial concluded that histologic type was not related to the risk of invasive recurrence. However, patients with poorly differentiated or high-grade DCIS who had a recurrence with invasive carcinoma had a significantly higher risk of metastatic disease than those with well-differentiated DCIS who had an invasive recurrence.[339]

An understanding of DCIS at the genetic level is the goal of many ongoing studies. However, to quote D. Craig Allred on this subject, "Unfortunately, very little is known about this biology. Certain alterations appear to play particularly important roles, such as over-expression and perhaps mutation of ER, amplification and overexpression of erbB2 and mutation of p53. Other studies assessing allelic imbalance emphasize that many other important genetic defects are yet to be discovered."[340]

Treatment

Today, most DCIS is diagnosed by mammography. Approximately 72% of cases are detected by calcification alone, 12% by calcification and a soft tissue density, and 10% by a soft tissue abnormality.[332,341] The surgeon, when offering the patient a breast-conserving approach, must be confident that the remaining breast is free of suspicious mammographic abnormalities. Other clusters of micro-calcification within the breast take on greater significance after a diagnosis of DCIS is established, and biopsy of these may be appropriate. Coordination between the pathologist and the breast-imager is very important in documenting the relationship between calcium observed on film and in the specimen. When a patient has extensive areas of suspicious calcification, the entire area must be cleared surgically to ensure the success of breast conservation.[342,343] When this is not possible, simple mastectomy with reconstruction, if the patient desires, is appropriate local treatment.

Schnitt and colleagues[344,345] and Lagios and associates[346,347] proposed a number of important guidelines for managing patients with DCIS who are candidates for breast conservation. Guidelines for DCIS therapy have been significantly influenced by a number of retrospective reports on follow-up of patients treated with excision only[311,346-361] or with excision plus irradiation.[356,362-365] More importantly, these retrospective study results have been used to design large, prospective phase III trials.

The need for radiation after wide excision was first tested prospectively by the NSABP group in a randomized trial.[366] This study randomized 818 women with DCIS to receive lumpectomy, with or without radiation. Patients were stratified by method of detection (i.e., mammogram

GUIDELINES FOR EVALUATION AND TREATMENT OF NONPALPABLE DUCTAL CARCINOMA IN SITU (DCIS)

1. Careful multiview mammography with or without ultrasonography and including magnification views
     Document extent of disease
     Identify other areas of microcalcification
2. Suspicious microcalcifications and densities cleared with needle localization biopsy
3. Specimen radiography with magnification techniques
4. Radiograph-directed histopathologic evaluation with:
     Orientation of specimen by surgeon
     Multicolored inked margins
5. Complete pathologic description to include:
     Type of DCIS and size of tumor
     Relationship to microcalcifications
     Distance of lesion from inked margins
     Presence of multifocality
     Presence or risk of microinvasion
6. Repeat mammography with magnification to confirm successful clearing of suspicious areas
7. Repeat breast excision if:
     Residual microcalcifications are found
     Margins are unacceptable

only or palpable mass) as well as by age. Negative tumor margins were required, and were defined as no DCIS seen at the inked margin. After a median of 12 years of follow-up, the local failure rate in the index breast was 17% in women randomized to receive radiation, compared with 39.7% in the observed group. However, similar to the findings of studies of invasive cancer, this significant difference in local control did not translate to any difference in survival for the women in this trial.

A similar large phase III trial comparing radiation with observation after wide local excision for women with DCIS was undertaken by the EORTC group. This study randomized 1010 women to the same two local treatment arms of lumpectomy and radiation vs. lumpectomy only. This study is less mature than the B-17 study, but it showed a similar rate of local control to the NSABP B-17 study at the same point in follow-up. With a median follow-up of 4.25 years, the 4-year local control rate was 84% in the excision-only group, compared with 91% in women randomized to radiation.[367] As the retrospective collaborative DCIS study has shown at 15 years of follow-up, these studies suggest that over time, the in-breast failure rate continues to increase slowly. Again, survival in patients with DCIS was the same in both treatment arms.

Several breast surgeons published individual series of patients with DCIS treated with wide excision only. Patient selection clearly plays a role in this kind of reporting. Nonetheless, local control rates in these retrospective studies are quite good, and the results generated another series of cooperative group trials. Factors believed to predict a favorable outcome[368–374] include small size, low pathology grade, older patient age, and wide surgical margins. Several U.S. trials are ongoing to test these

hypotheses. The Eastern Cooperative Oncology Group (ECOG) recently closed an observation-only registry trial, and the Radiation Therapy Oncology Group (RTOG) has an ongoing open phase III trial, randomizing selected low-risk patients with DCIS to wide excision, with or without radiation.

In general, a woman's risk of local failure in the index breast after wide excision appears to be reduced by a factor of approximately one half by the addition of whole-breast radiation to a dose of 50 Gy. Because survival remains excellent, whatever local treatment is selected, involving the patient in a decision, based on her assessed risk and the relative benefits and risks of radiation, appears appropriate for women in lower-risk groups. These groups are defined as age older than 50 years[370] as well as by tumor grade, size, and margin width, and likely by other factors yet to be described.

The NSABP B-24 study tested the role of tamoxifen, in addition to lumpectomy and radiation therapy, in a prospective trial of 1804 women. With a median follow-up of 74 months, with the addition of tamoxifen to 50 Gy radiation, the risk of ipsilateral invasive recurrence was reduced by approximately 50%. No significant reduction in noninvasive recurrence was seen. Predictably, the addition of tamoxifen decreased the risk of a contralateral breast event by approximately 1.5%.[342] A similar trial in the United Kingdom showed no effect of tamoxifen over that achieved by radiation, with a median follow-up of 3 years.[375] Maturity of these and other trials exploring the role of antiestrogen therapy in the management of women with DCIS will be needed before any firm treatment decisions can be reached.

With the availability of sentinel lymph node mapping, some surgical groups advocate this procedure in selected women with DCIS. In general, this procedure is considered in women in whom microinvasion cannot be excluded based on the findings of core biopsy or in those who opt to undergo simple mastectomy. The rationale is to avoid a situation in which invasive carcinoma is discovered after definitive local surgery and the opportunity to perform a sentinel node procedure has been lost, committing the patient to formal node dissection.[375]

Male breast cancer accounts for only approximately 1% of all cases of breast cancer. Men with DCIS are estimated to be only 7% of that already small group, so aside from case reports, little information exists on the management of this unusual entity.[376]

MANAGEMENT OF EARLY INVASIVE DISEASE (STAGES I AND II)

The management of early invasive breast cancer is multidisciplinary. Patients should be evaluated by a team of breast cancer specialists representing the subspecialties of breast imaging, surgical oncology, radiation oncology, and medical oncology. Approximately 75% of patients with newly diagnosed breast cancer have tumors less than 5 cm in diameter. The vast majority of tumors are 2 cm or less. Of these patients, 75% have node-negative disease.

Patients with stage I and II disease usually have two options: breast conservation and mastectomy with or without reconstruction. Careful histologic assessment of the resected tumor, with particular attention to size, histologic margins, and histologic features, is important for the decision. Other important factors include the extent of the intraductal component, the histology of the intraductal component if present, and prognostic information obtained from a study of specific tumor markers. It is important to determine carefully the patient's needs, expectations, and understanding of available therapeutic options.

The goal of breast conservation is an acceptable cosmetic outcome without sacrificing disease-free survival and overall survival. Most patients with stage I or II breast cancer can be managed well with breast conservation. If the size or location of the tumor relative to the size of the breast suggests that resection of the tumor would cause significant distortion of the breast, induction (preoperative chemotherapy) accomplishes two goals. Eighty percent of breast cancers are reduced in diameter by more than 50% after induction chemotherapy. This reduction may allow a considerably improved cosmetic result. An additional benefit is the identification of patients who do not respond to the induction protocol. This allows consideration of other systemic regimens as adjuvant therapy. The best management of nonresponding breast cancers is the subject of ongoing clinical trials. A large NSABP clinical trial randomized more than 1500 women with breast cancer to doxorubicin and cyclophosphamide (AC) for four cycles followed by primary therapy or primary therapy followed by four cycles of adjuvant AC. More women who received induction chemotherapy were able to have breast conservation. Because the great majority of women with breast cancer, whether node-negative or node-positive, receive adjuvant chemotherapy, moving its use to the preoperative period appears to offer the advantage of increasing the feasibility of breast conservation. However, a survival advantage has not been seen for preoperative therapy.

Increased understanding of the biologic behavior and the patterns of spread of breast cancer, advances in cytotoxic chemotherapy and endocrine therapy, and studies of these principles in animal tumor models provided an excellent scientific basis for investigation of adjuvant therapy in humans. These clinical trials were carried out under the rationales that breast cancer is no longer curable once clinically detectable distant metastasis occurs and that treatment of micrometastatic disease could either cure or at a minimum prolong disease-free survival.

Assessment of the indication for adjuvant therapy in an individual patient should be based on the risk of recurrence and death of breast cancer in the specific patient, the anticipated net benefits of therapy, and other relevant medical and psychosocial factors. Many decisions about adjuvant therapy must be based on data that are subject to a wide range of interpretation. Patients must be well informed and educated about the advantages and disadvantages of such therapy, and should play an active role in the decision-making process.[377]

Breast-Conservation Therapy with Surgery and Radiation

Fortunately, for most patients with stage I and II disease, breast conservation is an acceptable therapy. The appropriateness of breast conservation is one of the most studied treatment decisions in modern medicine. In the 1920s and 1930s, pioneering investigators (e.g., Keynes[378] in England, Peters[379] in Canada, Baclesse[380] in France, and Mustakallio[381] in Finland) began to treat groups of women with breast-conserving partial mastectomy followed by irradiation to the intact breast, challenging the need for total mastectomy. Results from these early studies were promising. Keynes[378] and Peters[379] compared their breast-conserving results with those of similarly staged patients who were treated contemporaneously with radical surgery. The results showed no differences in survival for patients who elected a breast-sparing approach. Baclesse[380] showed that local control could be obtained in a substantial majority of patients treated with radiation as a sole therapy, even those with locally advanced tumors.

Many single institutions began to use nonmastectomy therapy, including excision plus radiation therapy, for their patients with breast cancer, first in European and Canadian centers and later in the United States. In the early 1970s, several European reports created worldwide interest in nonmastectomy treatment, because of the excellent results seen in series of several hundred patients.[382,383] The first small series in the United States was published in 1975 by Prosnitz and Goldenberg[384] from Yale University. Soon thereafter, the Joint Center for Radiation Therapy in Boston, led by Weber and Hellman,[385] began to publish their results, which were also encouraging. Dozens of single-institution experiences have been reported in the literature. Selected series are shown in Table 94-13. They have consistently shown that crude local recurrence rates range from 5% to 10% and that survival is equivalent to the expected survival of a group of similar patients treated with mastectomy.

If only single-institution studies made up the mainstay of evidence showing the efficacy of breast-sparing therapy, some doubt might remain about the equivalence of this technique compared with mastectomy. Selection bias in single-institution studies could place more favorable patients into the lumpectomy group, creating a false impression of the success of this treatment. The only scientifically valid test of a new treatment is a randomized comparison with standard therapy. Six randomized prospective trials comparing lumpectomy plus radiation with mastectomy have been performed and published in the literature.[386-388] Details of these trials are presented in Table 94-14. Nearly 4000 women have been randomized between the two therapies. The outcome at 5, 10, 15, and now 20 years shows that survival in the two groups is identical as an overview and in each individual trial. It is inconceivable that these survival curves will separate, and thus women who choose breast-sparing therapy do not pay a survival price compared with those having a mastectomy. The data are so convincing that in 1990, the NCI held a consensus development conference

TABLE 94-13

Single-Institution Experience with Excision Plus Radiation in the Treatment of Primary Breast Cancer

AUTHOR	NO. OF PATIENTS	DATES	10-YR BREAST RECURRENCE RATE (%)
Ayme et al.*	1775	1960–1982	13
Heimann et al†	869	1984–1994	3††
Kini et al.‡	400	1980–1987	10
Grosse et al§	3072	1972–1995	10
Mansfield et al.‖	1070	1982–1994	14
Gage et al.#	1628	1968–1986	13
Pierce et al.¶	429	1984–1995	11
Haffty et al.**	973	1970–1989	16

*Ayme Y, Amalric R, Kurtz JM, Spitalier JM: Long-term results of conservation treatment of operable breast cancer. Ann N Y Acad Sci 1993;698:259.
†Heimann R, Powers C, Halpem HJ, et al: Breast preservation in stage I and II carcinoma of the breast: The University of Chicago experience. Cancer 1996;78:1722.
‡Kini VR, White JR, Horwitz EM, et al: Long term results with breast-conserving therapy for patients with early stage breast carcinoma in a community hospital setting. Cancer 1998;82:127.
§Grosse A, Schreer I, Frischbier HJ, et al: Results of breast conserving therapy for early breast cancer and the role of mammographic follow-up. Int J Radiat Oncol Biol Phys 1997;38:761.
‖Mansfield CM, Komarnicky LT, Schwartz GF, et al: Ten year results in 1070 patients with stages I and II breast cancer treated by conservative surgery and radiation therapy. Cancer 1995;75:2328.
#Gage I, Recht A, Gelman R, et al: Long-term outcome following breast-conserving surgery and radiation therapy. Int J Radiat Oncol Biol Phy 1995;33:245.
¶Pierce I, Strawderman MH, Douglas KR, Lichter AS: Conservative surgery and radiotherapy for early-stage breast cancer using a lung density correction: The University of Michigan experience. Int J Radiat Oncol Biol Phys 1998;39:921.
**Haffty BG, Reiss M, Beinfeld M, et al: Ipsilateral breast tumor recurrence as a predictor of distant disease: Implications for systemic therapy at the time of local relapse. J Clin Oncol 1996;14:52.
††Five-year rate.

of the previous biopsy site to ensure complete clearing of the tumor. The first step is to determine whether re-excision is indicated. The goal of re-excision is to achieve absolutely clear margins. Evidence suggests that even microscopically positive margins are associated with a higher risk of local failure after radiation therapy.

Even with positive surgical margins, only approximately 50% of re-excision specimens show residual tumor.[390,391] Thus, it is difficult to predict whether a woman will be a candidate for breast-sparing therapy based on the findings of initial biopsy. Even in women who appear to have widespread disease with many areas of margin positivity, little or no residual disease may be seen on re-excision.

The risk of local failure is related to the amount of breast resected. A tumorectomy that achieves negative margins for invasive cancer is sufficient. There is no need to have 1- or 2-cm margins beyond the invasive component. Where there is an extensive intraductal component (>25% of the volume of the lesion is DCIS) there must be a clear margin beyond the DCIS. Although the margin beyond an invasive component of a few cells may be sufficient, several millimeters (3 to 10 mm) of normal breast duct must be excised to ensure that all of the DCIS component of the lesion has been removed. This resection can be a tumorectomy with an effort to obtain approximately 2-cm margins around the tumor, or it may be more radical, such as segmental or quadrant resection. Although the risk of local recurrence decreases in direct proportion to the extent of resection, as expected, the cosmetic result also declines with more aggressive resection.

The ideal approach is re-excision of the previous biopsy site, unless the tumor is small and careful analysis of the initial biopsy material confirms the appropriate margins. For re-excision, sharp dissection is preferred. Electrocautery should be avoided until the specimen is removed. This technique avoids cautery artifacts that might obscure a positive margin.

Patients must be thoroughly informed about the indications for re-excision and the possibility, although fortunately rare, that the histologic features of the specimen will dictate a change in therapy. For example, a re-excision specimen sometimes contains extensive or multifocal intraductal cancer. Some of these patients have intraductal cancer that is not marked by calcification that

on the treatment of early breast cancer, and declared that breast-sparing therapy was not only equivalent to mastectomy, but was actually the "preferable" treatment, because it preserved the breast, with all of the attendant psychological and body image advantages associated with a lesser surgical procedure.[389]

Resection of the Primary Lesion

In some cases, breast conservation involves re-excision

TABLE 94-14

Randomized Trials Comparing Lumpectomy Plus Radiation to Mastectomy

TRIAL	NO. OF PATIENTS	MAXIMUM TUMOR SIZE	FOLLOW-UP (YR)	SURVIVAL (%) MASTECTOMY	SURVIVAL (%) LUMPECTOMY
NSABP	1217	4	12	60	62
Institut Gustave-Roussy	179	2	14.5	65	73
Milan	701	2	16	71	72
EORTC	874	5	8	73	71
Danish	618	5	6	82	79
NCI	237	5	10	75	77

extends into unknown areas of the breast. If all apparent intraductal cancer cannot be removed surgically, the risk of local failure can become unacceptably high and dictates planning for mastectomy and reconstruction.

Once the tumor has been removed, sutures or numbered tags are placed on the specimen so that it can be oriented, and the entire specimen has its surface inked in some fashion to allow evaluation of the histologic margins.[392-396] Different colored inks may be used to represent different surfaces. The specimen is then cut and histologic sections prepared. Extra attention is paid to areas near the surgical margin wherever tumor is seen to encroach grossly. A thorough histopathologic evaluation can be done in a reproducible fashion, and a template for reporting surgical pathology in patients who undergo lumpectomy can be used to ensure that no important details are neglected.[397]

A few additional points about the surgical technique are warranted. Although the primary goal is to avoid recurrence, the secondary goal is to avoid any evidence of the disease or its treatment. Consequently, whenever possible, a circumareolar incision provides optimal cosmetic results. In tumors located in the upper inner quadrant of the breast, where incisions are most visible, particular effort should be made to use a circumareolar incision, if feasible. Clearly, the primary consideration is clearance of the tumor, not cosmesis. Some surgeons always make the incision directly over the tumor mass, in an effort to provide better tumor control. However, there is no evidence that this is the case. Several small surgical clips placed in the tumorectomy wall guide the radiation oncologist for precise placement of a radiation boost when indicated (Fig. 94-32). Reapproximation of breast

tissue is associated with greater distortion of breast shape than occurs when complete hemostasis is achieved and this cavity is filled with a small seroma. As that heals, the cavity constricts and usually provides optimal cosmesis. No drain should be used. Any axillary incision should be separate from the breast excision. If the cavities or incisions are connected, the cosmetic result suffers.

Although most women today can have breast-conserving surgery, there are several contraindications. These are based on the premise that all invasive or pre-invasive cancer should be removed surgically and that breast conservation depends on radiation to the breast.

1. Patients with previous chest wall radiation require evaluation by a radiation oncologist to determine the feasibility of breast conservation.
2. Other contraindications to breast or chest wall radiation include scleroderma, cutaneous lupus, and other active collagen disease of these tissues.
3. Diffuse suspicious calcifications make definition of preinvasive cancer impossible.
4. Multiple or diffuse cancers or extensive DCIS may preclude breast conservation.
5. Residual disease after induction therapy may make it difficult to achieve acceptable cosmesis with breast conservation. This is a highly personal decision that the patient must make in conjunction with her physician.

Axillary Staging

The second aspect of breast-conservation therapy involves staging the axilla (Fig. 94-33). Although many studies suggested that a panel of prognostic indicators and molecular markers of the primary tumor might eventually be a better predictor of outcome than the number of involved lymph nodes, no combination of such parameters has been validated.

When suspicious axillary lymph nodes are present, axillary dissection should take place. Originally, axillary lymph nodes, including level III nodes medial to the medial border of the pectoralis minor muscle, were carefully removed. These dissections were associated with a higher incidence of lymphedema of the arm than limiting dissection to levels I and II. No oncologic detriment from leaving the level III nodes in place has been shown. Level I and II dissection is now the standard for axillary clearance. This type of axillary dissection is associated with the lowest risk of regional failure.

When axillary dissection is performed, care is taken to preserve the lateral and medial pectoral nerves, the long thoracic nerve, and the thoracodorsal nerve. It is usually possible to preserve the upper branches of the inner costobrachial sensory nerve to the inner posterior arm, avoiding the troublesome dysphoric sensations associated with dense numbness in the distribution of this nerve. Carefully sparing the brachial lymphatics that lie anterior to the axillary vein and brachial plexus minimizes the risk of lymphedema. Lymphedema is associated with body habitus, and people with obesity are at risk, despite optimal surgical technique.

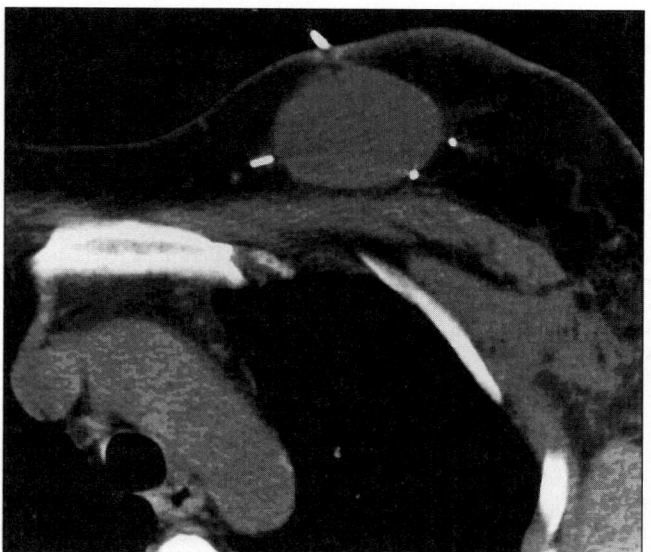

Figure 94-32. Computed tomography scan showing metallic clips left by the surgeon in the tumor bed. These clips greatly facilitate performance of boost therapy to the tumor bed with radiation.

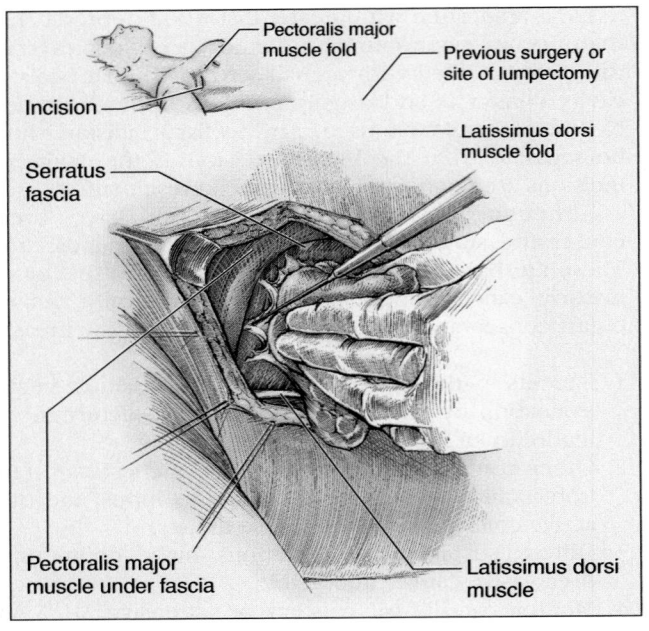

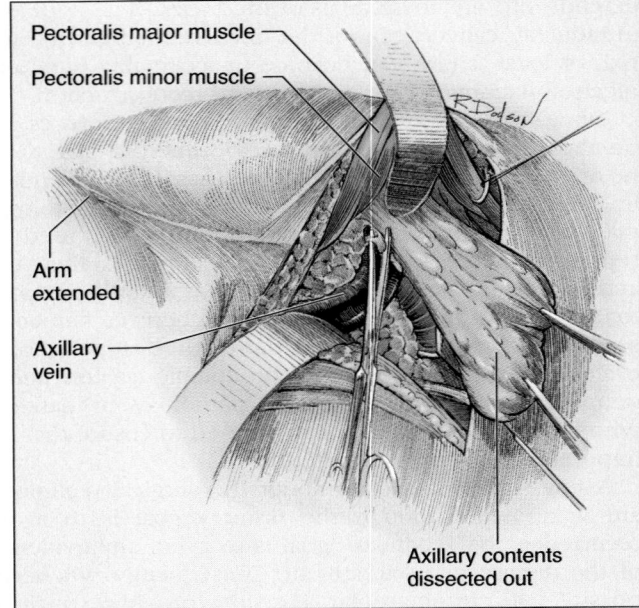

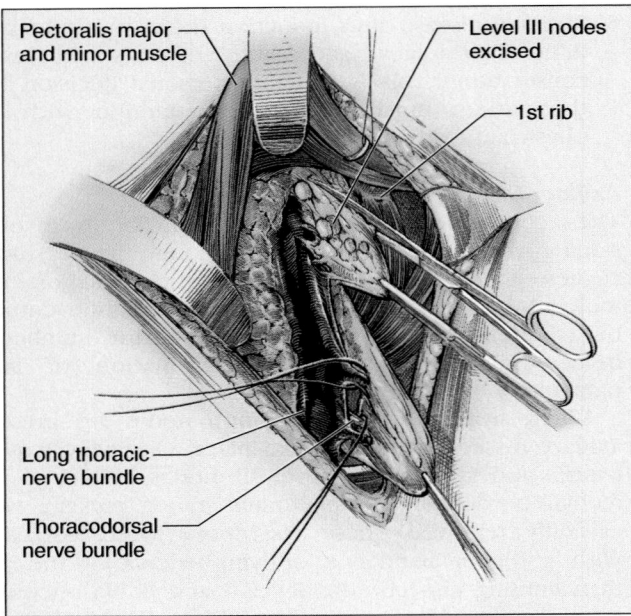

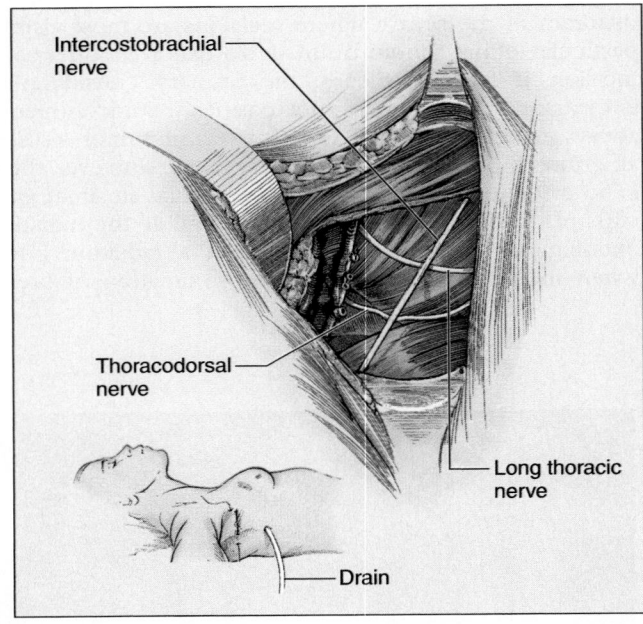

Figure 94-33. A, The incision for axillary node dissection is placed at the inferior aspect of the axillary hairline, and extends from the lateral border of the pectoralis major muscle to the anterior border of the latissimus dorsi muscle. Nylon traction sutures are placed in the dermis. Flaps are raised superiorly and inferiorly. **B,** The pectoralis major and minor muscles are retracted to facilitate dissection of the lymph node–bearing fatty tissue from beneath the muscles and away from the axillary vein and chest wall. **C,** Excision of level III lymph nodes (highest level near the entrance of the axillary vein into the chest) is easily accomplished, even through the small axillary incision, with the arm rotated upward. **D,** The completed dissection, showing the isolated nerves to the serratus muscles, the latissimus dorsi muscle, the pectoral muscles, and the sensory nerve to the inner aspect of the upper arm.

Sentinel Lymph Node Mapping

Sentinel lymph node mapping (SLN) has largely replaced axillary dissection for patients with clinically negative axillae.

Many believe that SLN will soon replace axillary dissection for the majority of patients. However, others strongly believe that axillary lymphadenectomy provides excellent local control of the disease, providing a modest improvement in survival. When performed by an experienced surgeon, it is rarely associated with long-term morbidity.[398-402]

The movement toward SLN is influenced significantly by the trend toward mammographically detected occult breast cancers and the resultant increase in negative axillary dissections.[401,402] With T1a, b, and c tumors, the incidence of axillary metastasis is 10% to 15%, 15%, and approximately 30%, respectively.[403] Sentinel lymph node procedures can be performed on an outpatient basis, theoretically decreasing the costs associated with management of early-stage breast cancer.

The concept of the sentinel lymph node originated in 1977, when Cabanas[404] described mapping the first lymph node draining penile carcinoma. In 1992, Morton and colleagues[403] at the John Wayne Cancer Center in Los Angeles reported the identification of a sentinel "blue"node in patients with cutaneous melanoma. The sentinel lymph node procedure correctly determined regional node status in 99% of the 82% of patients in whom the node could be identified and in 95% of all patients with positive findings on regional node dissection.

In 1993, Krag and colleagues[405] first reported SLN in breast cancer using radioisotope localization. Their report was followed by a study by Guiliano and associates[406] of the John Wayne Cancer Center using the blue dye techniques established for melanoma. In these reports, the radioisotope technique correctly identified the sentinel lymph node in 82% of 22 patients, with 100% accuracy. The blue dye method identified the sentinel lymph node in 65% of 173 patients studied, with a 96% accuracy rate. As recently reviewed, 14 published reports validated the sentinel lymph nodes by concurrent axillary dissection.[407,408]

Guiliano and colleagues[409] showed that, with experience, the blue dye technique identified the sentinel lymph node in 93% of patients. Those reporting the use of isotope and blue dye simultaneously appear to shorten the learning curve and result in slightly better identification of sentinel lymph nodes.[410,411] The combined approach appears best, although some surgeons specializing in breast cancer use dye alone. When a single lymph node is identified, the risk of a false-negative result is increased over that associated with two or three sentinel lymph nodes. Consequently, the effort needed to identify a second sentinel lymph node seems well spent.

Identification of sentinel lymph nodes has also focused attention on methods of enhancing the accuracy of pathologic assessment. Serial sectioning and immuno-histochemical staining using antibodies to cytokeratin are the most practical means of searching for micro-metastases. Turner and colleagues[412] reported the results of a careful assessment by serial sectioning and immuno-histochemistry of 60 patients with a negative sentinel lymph node who had axillary dissection with similar examination of the remaining nodes. Only 1 of 1087 non-sentinel nodes was positive for metastases (0.1%). Reverse transcriptase polymerase chain reaction can enhance the detection of even a few cancer cells in a sentinel lymph node. However, there is no protein unique to breast cancer, such as tyrosinase in melanoma. Reverse transcriptase polymerase chain reaction would also require an investigation as to the meaning of positivity in terms of, for example, the decision to perform complete axillary dissection. There is considerable controversy about the staging of patients whose sentinel lymph nodes appear negative by standard hematoxylin and eosin examination, but who have a micrometastasis found by immunohisto-chemistry or reverse transcriptase polymerase chain reaction evidence of a few cancer cells. The latest TNM staging manual suggests classifying these patients as node-negative, with a subscript to indicate these additional findings. Some European centers consider these patients node-positive.

Contraindications to sentinel lymph node biopsy include clinically suspicious axillary lymph nodes and a tumor arising from the axillary tail of the breast. If no sentinel lymph node can be identified, or if it contains tumor cells, axillary dissection should be performed. Some prefer to perform SLN and biopsy before induction chemotherapy, but data from NSABP B-27 study indicate that sentinel node biopsy is a reliable procedure following preoperative chemotherapy (Mamounas, ASCO 2002). Studies show that it can be performed after induction chemotherapy, although current data suggest a higher false-negative rate than is usually associated with this technique. Some authors recommend sentinel lymph node biopsy for patients with DCIS when high grade or when microinvasion is present. No data suggest that micrometastases found in this case represent more than the debris of core biopsy being cleared by the lymphatic system. When a very large area of DCIS is present and mastectomy is required, axillary dissection can be eliminated when the sentinel lymph node is negative.

Several prospective randomized trials are in progress, and physicians are encouraged to provide prospective patients with information about these options. These studies should provide important data about the ability of SLN alone to provide long-term regional control. Clearly, SLN requires a team approach, involving a surgeon, a nuclear medicine physician, and a dedicated breast pathologist. A significant learning phase is required for a surgeon wishing to use SLN. Lymph node dissection should be performed during this learning phase to avoid understaging women who then might not receive adequate adjuvant therapy.

SENTINEL LYMPH NODE MAPPING

RADIOISOTOPE
Europe: ^{99m}Tc colloidal albumin (unfiltered) [ideal particle size 10 to 200 nm] 0.1 to 0.6 mCi/4 mL normal saline injected subdermally or into the breast.

United States: ^{99m}Tc sulfur colloid 0.3 to 1.0 mCi in 4 mL normal saline is injected subdermally or into the breast 1 to 4 hours before surgery; a handheld gamma probe is used.

BLUE DYE
Between 4 and 5 mL isosulfan blue dye is injected subdermally beneath the areola or into the breast parenchyma on the axillary side or at the tumor site. Breast is massaged for 5 minutes before the low axilla is explored.

TABLE 94-15

				LOCAL RECURRENCE	
TRIAL	**NO. OF PATIENTS**	**LARGEST TUMOR SIZE (CM)**	**SURGICAL PROCEDURE**	**EXCISION**	**E + XRT**
Milan	567	2.5	Quadrantectomy	12%*	2%*
NSABP	1262	4	Wide excision	35%	10%
Ontario	837	4	Wide excision	35%	11%
Sweden	381	2	Sector resection	18%	2%
Scottish	585	4	Wide excision	25%	6%
British	418	5	Wide excision	35%	13%

*Total recurrence rate.
NSABP, National Surgical Adjuvant Breast and Bowel Project.

Irradiation of the Intact Breast

Before considering how to irradiate the breast, the physician should determine whether the postexcision breast requires radiation. Several single-institution studies showed a 25% to 40% risk of breast recurrence after lumpectomy alone without radiation.[413–416] Six prospective randomized studies reported on lumpectomy, with or without radiation (Table 94-15).[417] All six studies showed a statistically significant reduction in local recurrence of breast cancer in the irradiated group. No subsets of women have been identified who do as well without radiation as they do with it, although such subsets of patients have been aggressively sought.[418] Current recommendations are to irradiate the breast after lumpectomy to achieve the lowest possible recurrence rate.

Nevertheless, as tumors get smaller, the success of lumpectomy alone increases. More and more very small invasive cancers are being diagnosed through mammography screening. Should these women receive radiation? Thus far, clinical trials have not identified a subgroup of these patients in which radiation therapy should routinely not be employed. Alternative treatments such as partial breast irradiation may reduce the cost and morbidity of treatment and are especially important in countries in which radiation therapy equipment is a scarce resource,[419] but these modalities remain investigational.

When radiation therapy is elected, the whole breast is treated through a pair of tangentially directed fields to a dose of 4500 to 5000 cGy over 5 to 12 weeks.[420,421] The fields are designed to skim along the chest wall and irradiate the smallest amount of underlying lung. In left-sided primary lesions, the fields should result in the lowest possible exposure of the heart (Fig. 94-34). At the conclusion of whole-breast treatment, it is customary to apply a boost dose to the tumor bed to bring the total dose to at least 6000 cGy. Lower total doses are associated with a higher breast failure rate.[422] However, the need for a breast boost in all patients is controversial. For example, in the NSABP lumpectomy trial, no boost to the tumor bed was given and a recurrence rate of 10% was noted.[423]

This recurrence rate is comparable to that reported in most single-institution series in which a radiation boost was applied. However, the NSABP trial required that negative surgical margins be obtained at the first attempt at excision. Patients with a positive surgical margin were removed from the study and treated with mastectomy. Thus, the relevance of the NSABP experience is unclear when re-excisions are frequently performed and patients with positive focal margins are at times treated. A randomized trial performed in Lyon, France, showed a 25% reduction in the recurrence rate when a boost was used.[424] However, the patients in that study had favorable features (small tumors and free margins) and the absolute recurrence risk was reduced from 4.5% to 3.6% at 5 years. A randomized prospective EORTC trial is also evaluating the need for a boost in patients undergoing lumpectomy.[425] Most institutions currently recommend a boost for all patients who are treated with lumpectomy and irradiation,[426] and 80% to 90% of patients receive boost treatment.[427] The boost is accomplished quickly and easily

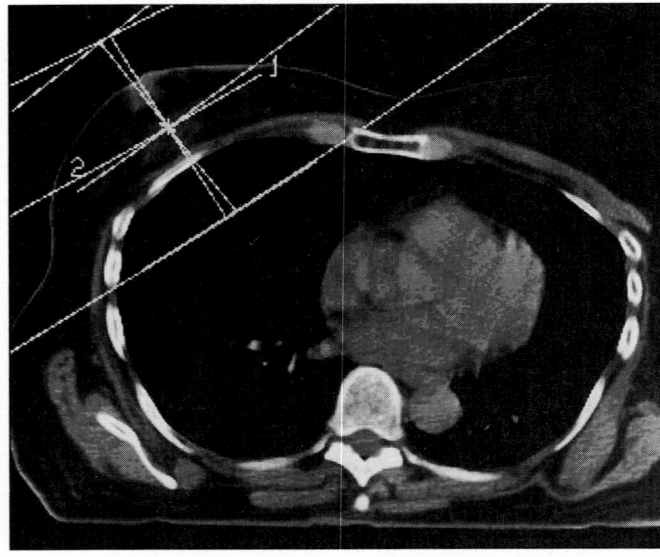

Figure 94-34. The standard field configuration for breast cancer. Two tangentially directed fields encompass the breast with a minimal amount of underlying lung tissue. The contralateral breast and all of the critical structures are spaced.

on a linear accelerator equipped with electron-beam capability, and requires six to eight additional treatments.[421] Localizing the target within the breast for boost purposes can be accomplished by computed tomography,[428-430] by ultrasound,[431] or by clips left in the tumor bed.[432] Morbidity associated with a boost is virtually nil.

No radiation to the axilla itself is indicated once surgical excision of the axillary lymph nodes has been performed.[433-435] Much clinical experience indicates that the axilla is the site of first breast cancer failure in fewer than 1% of patients who have had an axillary dissection.[436,437] Axillary recurrences occur in approximately 2% of patients with negative nodes or one to three positive nodes and in patients with axillary dissection who received irradiation to the breast only after lumpectomy.[426] Widespread extracapsular extension and gross tumor left behind in the axilla are the only indications for specifically irradiating the dissected axilla. Microscopic extracapsular nodal extension appears to have little effect on the local control rate in the axilla after surgery alone, and can safely be ignored.[438,439] A clinically negative axilla that is undissected is well controlled by axillary irradiation of 45 to 50 cGy.[440] In patients who are at low risk for axillary involvement, a pair of tangential breast fields appears adequate to control the axilla in most cases, because the low axilla is included in such fields.[441] In patients with positive axillary nodes found on axillary dissection, most investigators use a small field that irradiates the supraclavicular nodes and the apex of the axilla (level III nodes).[442-444] Some institutions prefer to use this field only in patients with four or more positive nodes, whereas other institutions apply it to all axillary-positive patients. However, some investigators perform no nodal irradiation, even when axillary nodes are positive. For example, all NSABP trials prohibit irradiation of the axillary apex and supraclavicular fossa, and the recurrence rate in regional nodal sites in their hands has been acceptably low.[423,443]

Complications of Treatment

Complications after breast conservation occur in a minority of treated patients. More than 90% of patients report an excellent cosmetic result. As noted, the more extensive the breast resection, the more likely that deformity of the breast and a less-than-acceptable result will occur.

Table 94-16 summarizes the complications of lumpectomy and radiation. Approximately 5% to 20% of patients

TABLE 94-16

Complications of Therapy	
COMPLICATION	**FREQUENCY (%)**
Arm edema	5–20
Rib fractures	5
Radiation pneumonitis	1
Brachial plexus damage	<1
Second nonbreast malignancy	<0.1
Poor cosmetic outcome	5

have measurable arm edema. Factors associated with edema include the extent of axillary dissection, postoperative wound complications, and the use of direct axillary radiation.[445-447] In the NCI series, the rate of arm edema in the lumpectomy group was identical to the rate after mastectomy.[421] This implies that the axillary dissection performed in both sets of patients, rather than the specific treatment to the breast, is likely responsible for the arm edema.

Rib fractures are seen in approximately 2% to 5% of patients treated with radiation.[448,449] In this setting, most rib fractures are asymptomatic and are detected on a bone scan or chest x-ray that is performed for other reasons. Rib fracture should always be included in the differential diagnosis of a previously irradiated patient with breast cancer who has chest wall or rib tenderness and whose bone scan shows an area of tracer uptake in the ribs of the treated chest wall. No specific therapy is indicated for these rib fractures, and they heal spontaneously.

Approximately 1% or fewer of patients treated with radiation have symptomatic radiation pneumonitis.[450,451] This complication is more frequent in patients who have received chemotherapy and radiation that included a field to the supraclavicular lymph nodes.[450] In almost all patients, pneumonitis resolves either spontaneously or with a short course of steroid therapy, and no long-term sequelae occur. In some patients, radiation causes scarring in the small rim of lung treated in the tangential fields. This scarring can appear as a density in the lung field underlying the treated breast on routine chest radiograph. The diagnosis of radiation-induced scarring can be made with a computed tomography scan that shows lung changes confined to the area of high-dose irradiation just underneath the anterior chest wall.[452] These patients usually need no specific therapy, and lung biopsy is not needed.

Rarely, breast irradiation leads to late cardiac damage.[453,454] Much of this information comes from treatment of the postmastectomy chest wall, especially when radiation was directed specifically at the internal mammary nodes. Recent studies suggest that few patients have sufficient cardiac volume within the radiation port to place them at risk for later damage and that these patients can be recognized in advance. With sophisticated treatment planning, these complications can be avoided.[455-458] A supraclavicular portal sometimes results in brachial plexus injury,[459] greatly increasing in frequency if large daily dose fractions are used.[460] In rare cases, years later, radiation results in a soft tissue sarcoma within the radiation portal.[461-463] The incidence of this extremely serious complication is approximately 0.1%.

Follow-up

After radiation is completed, patients are typically seen at 3- to 4-month intervals for the first 2 years, at 6-month intervals for up to 5 years after treatment, and yearly thereafter. The first post-treatment mammogram is obtained 4 to 5 months after radiation therapy, after resolution of the acute radiation edema. Subsequent mammograms are ordered yearly thereafter. In this setting, mammographically detected local recurrences are smaller and more often noninvasive compared with recurrences detected by physical examination, attesting to the importance of mammographic follow-up.[464] Other follow-up studies, such as blood tests and radiographic examinations, are performed as indicated in the general follow-up of patients with breast cancer. They are not routinely recommended for screening in an otherwise asymptomatic patient.

In most centers, local in-breast failure is managed with mastectomy. Although there are reports of successful treatment either by excision alone, especially for late recurrences,[465] or by excision plus additional local radiation, these techniques are not considered part of standard care. Patients who have a local failure have a 5-year survival rate of 60% to 80%.[466-468] However, they are two to four times more likely to have a distant failure than those who do not have an in-breast failure.[469,470] Some investigators have used this knowledge to suggest that patients with in-breast failure, especially those with early recurrences, should be treated with adjuvant therapy in an effort to reduce metastatic risk. The adjuvant therapies used in this patient group at the time of initial diagnosis vary greatly, affecting the choice of possible systemic therapy at recurrence. In addition, variations occur in clinical recurrence patterns. For these reasons, designing a clinical trial to address this question is not likely.

FACTORS THAT AFFECT OUTCOME

Patient Age

It is widely acknowledged that younger patients (<35 years of age) have a higher rate of lumpectomy failure than do older patients. Virtually every series that addressed this question confirmed this fact (Table 94-17). Young women have a higher rate of chest wall failure after mastectomy than do older patients. This effect has been known for many decades,[471] but was confirmed in modern series, including a detailed analysis from M.D. Anderson Cancer Center.[472]

Why this should be the case is not entirely clear. It is well established that tumors in younger women are histopathologically more aggressive than those in older women. They have a higher incidence of extensive intraductal carcinoma (EIC), high nuclear grade, lymphatic space invasion, and tumor necrosis.[473,474] It is likely that the recurrence patterns seen in these young women are related to a combination of these adverse histologic features.

Tumor Size

When lumpectomy and the use of radiation are examined as a function of tumor size, there is a dramatic fall-off in the application of breast-sparing therapy for T2 tumors in comparison with smaller T1 tumors. In general, patients with T2 tumors receive breast-sparing treatment less than half as frequently as patients with T1 tumors, partly because of the appearance of larger 4- and 5-cm tumors in small-breasted patients, in whom tumor-clearing lumpectomy would result in substantial cosmetic distortion. The important factor in the decision should not be tumor size, but cosmetic results, as well as the other histologic factors that are described later.

Women whose primary tumor size makes it difficult to perform a cosmetically acceptable excision can have their tumor reduced with preoperative chemotherapy and can then have breast-conserving therapy. The NSABP B-18 trial

TABLE 94-17

	Age as a Factor in Local Breast Recurrence**			
AUTHOR	**DEFINITION OF "YOUNG" AGE (YR)**	**NO. OF YOUNG/NO. OF RECURRENCES (%)**	**NO. OF OLDER/NO. OF RECURRENCES (%)**
Boyages et al.*	≤34	61/15 (25)	722/76 (11)
Delouche et al.†	≤40	71/14 (20)	339/26 (8)
Forquet et al.‡	≤32	35/12 (34)	383/44 (11)
Haffty et al.§	≤50	135/24 (18)	248/26 (10)
Kurtz‖	≤39	210/41 (20)	1172/106 (9)
Ryoo et al.#	≤40	51/8 (16)	346/18 (5)
Solin et al.¶	≤35	88/12 (14)	808/42 (5)
Total		651/126 (19)	4014/338 (8)

*Boyages J, Recht A, Connolly I, et al: Factors associated with local recurrence as a first site of failure following the conservative treatment of early breast cancer. Recent Results Cancer Res 1989;115:92.
†Delouche G, Bachelot F, Premont M, Kurtz JM: Conservation treatment of early breast cancer: Long term results and complications. Int J Radiat Oncol Biol Phy 1987;13:29.
‡Fourquet A, Campana F, Zafrani, et al: Prognostic factors of breast recurrence in the conservative management of early breast cancer: A 25-year follow-up. Int J Radiat Oncol Biol Phys 1989;17:719.
§Haffty BG, Fischer D, Rose M, et al: Prognostic factors for local recurrence in the conservatively treated breast cancer patient: A cautious interpretation of the data. J Clin Oncol 1991;9:997.
‖Kurtz JM, Jacquemier J, Amalric R, et al: Why are local recurrences after breast-conserving therapy more frequent in younger patients? J Clin Oncol 1990;8:591.
#Ryoo MC, Kagan AR, Wollin M, et al: Prognostic factor for recurrence and cosmesis in 393 patients after radiation therapy for early mammary carcinoma. Radiology 1989;172:555.
¶Solin LJ, Fowble B, Schultz DJ, Goodman RL: Age as a prognostic factor for patients treated with definitive irradiation for early stage breast cancer. Int J Radiat Oncol Biol Phys 1989;16:373.
**Any locoregional failure.

randomized more than 1500 women with localized breast cancer to receive systemic chemotherapy for four cycles, either before or after local therapy. Overall, 67.8% of women in the preoperative arm vs. 59.8% in the postoperative arm underwent breast-conservation therapy. No difference in survival was noted between the two groups, confirming the safety of preoperative chemotherapy.[475,476] Thus, tumor size alone should no longer be a deterrent for women who desire breast-sparing therapy.

Histology

Schnitt and colleagues[477] in Boston noted that the histologic pattern within a breast tumor was a strong predictor for subsequent in-breast failure. They noted that a breast cancer lesion could contain intraductal carcinoma in four specific patterns: (1) entirely absent; (2) present admixed within the invasive component, but not adjacent to the invasive tumor; (3) present adjacent to the invasive tumor, but not within the invasive cancer; and (4) present both within and adjacent to the invasive breast cancer lesion (Fig. 94-35). They defined the fourth category (intraductal carcinoma within and adjacent to the invasive cancer) as an extensive intraductal component (EIC). More specifically, they observed that DCIS had to be a prominent feature of the invasive cancer, at least 25% of the tumor area. No specific amount of DCIS adjacent to the tumor was required. Tumors that were predominantly DCIS with small areas of minimal invasion were classified as EIC-positive tumors (pattern 5).

When these investigators plotted the risk of local breast failure as a function of EIC, the results were dramatic. The 5-year actuarial recurrence rate for 103 patients with EIC-positive tumors was 24% vs. less than 6% for 280 women with EIC-negative tumors.[478] Furthermore, the pattern of recurrence was different in these two groups, with 88% of EIC-positive patients vs. 55% of EIC-negative patients having a true recurrence. This suggested that there might be a greater tumor burden inadvertently left behind at the site of the primary excision in patients with EIC-positive disease.

MAKING LUMPECTOMY AND RADIATION AVAILABLE TO PATIENTS WITH BREAST CANCER

Data show that a relatively small percentage of U.S. women are being treated with breast-sparing techniques, even though such techniques are known to be equal to mastectomy. Also, in the words of the NCI Consensus Conference on the Treatment of Early Breast Cancer, these techniques represent the "preferred" therapy.[479] Data from the American College of Surgeons show that in 1995, 58% of stage I and 36% of stage II cancers were treated with breast-sparing techniques.[480] Overall, twice as many patients received breast-sparing treatment in 1995 compared with 1985. The most recent international adjuvant therapy hormonal trial, the Anastrozole or Tamoxifen Alone or in Combination (ATAC) trial, noted

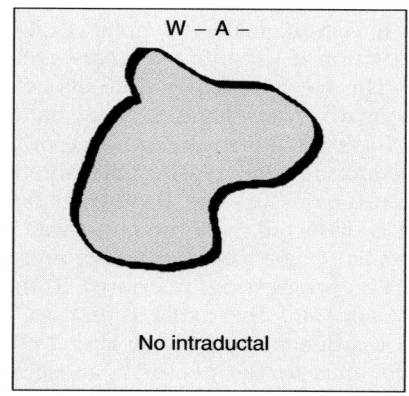

1.

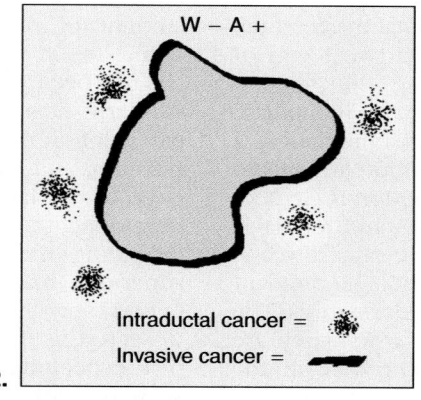

2.

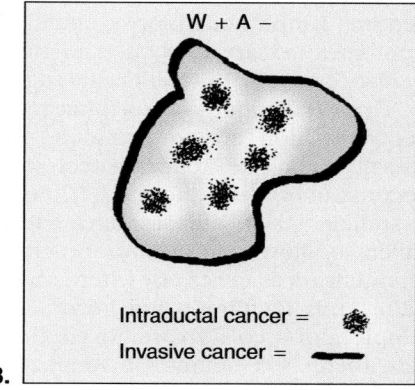

3.

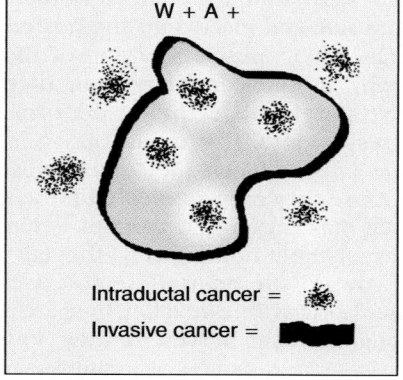

4.

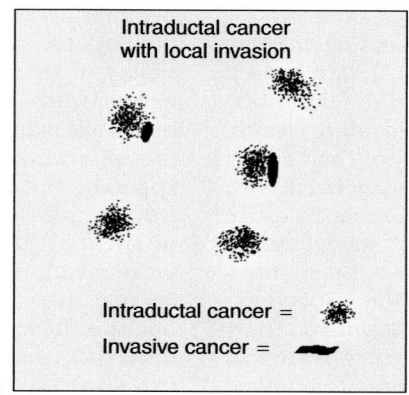

5.

Figure 94-35. Patterns of invasive and intraductal cancer. A, intraductal cancer adjacent to the primary tumor; W, intraductal cancer within the primary tumor.

that breast-conservation therapy for early-stage tumors appears to be more common in Europe, Australia, and New Zealand than in the United States. This suggests that the continued reduction in the percentage of mastectomies is plateauing. This is surprising, particularly in view of the demonstrated effects of induction chemotherapy to shrink tumors that would otherwise make breast-conserving therapy problematic.

There is still a marked geographic variation in the United States in the use of nonmastectomy techniques.[481-484] Why lumpectomy rates are so low in some areas and vary so much by geographic locale is not entirely known. However, some physicians in active practice still believe that mastectomy is the "best" treatment for breast cancer, despite overwhelming evidence of the equivalence of nonmastectomy therapy. However, no data support these prejudices. Over time, the use of nonmastectomy techniques should continue to increase.

MASTECTOMY

For several decades, modified radical mastectomy has supplanted the previous generally applied surgical management of primary breast cancer, which is radical mastectomy. Sentinel lymph node biopsy has made axillary dissection for staging unnecessary in women with no suspicious palpable lymphadenopathy and negative findings on sentinel lymph node biopsy. Total mastectomy has supplanted modified radical mastectomy for this group of node-negative patients who require mastectomy. When axillary dissection is indicated by the finding of suspicious axillary lymph nodes or metastatic disease on sentinel lymph node biopsy, modified radical mastectomy combines axillary dissection of the lower two levels of axillary nodes with total mastectomy.

Three techniques for total mastectomy with immediate reconstruction are in common use. In some cases, a fourth technique, total mastectomy without immediate reconstruction, is performed. When this option is elected, a sufficient skin ellipse about the nipple and areola is taken to allow skin closure to achieve the same level of skin tension as exists elsewhere on the thorax. Redundant skin tends to fibrose and become pachydermatous. The nipple and areola are removed, because when they are left, there is a definite incidence of recurrence in the ducts of the nipple and subareolar tissue. Options for mastectomy include the following: (1) total mastectomy, (2) skin-sparing mastectomy, (3) areolar-sparing mastectomy, and (4) nipple-sparing mastectomy. The last option is the same operation that was previously described as "subcutaneous mastectomy." This procedure leaves sufficient subareolar tissue to allow the nipple and areola to retain their shape. It is consequently associated with recurrence of tumor in the nipple and areola. Because much has been written about the risks of subcutaneous mastectomy, the term *nipple-sparing* has been introduced in an apparent attempt to revive this procedure. Areola-sparing mastectomy is a skin-sparing mastectomy in which the nipple is excised and later reconstructed, but the areola is spared. This has been more often talked about than attempted, and there is no series of areola-sparing mastectomy with significant follow-up to evaluate its safety or cosmetic advantage. Skin-sparing mastectomy is performed through a circumareolar incision that removes the nipple and areola, but spares the entire skin envelope and inframammary fold. This is an extremely advantageous approach when immediate reconstruction is performed. Retention of the normal skin envelope enables the breast to mimic the other breast exactly, and tailoring procedures on the contralateral breast are rarely required. In these immediate reconstructions, nipple reconstruction and tattooing of the neoareola are performed weeks to months later.

When surgery is performed through incisions other than circumareolar incisions, the incision is placed so that the scar will not be visible in a bathing suit or low-cut dress. When elliptical or transverse incisions are used for a total mastectomy, it is ideal to excise any previous biopsy scar as well as the nipple–areolar complex.

Skin flaps are carefully developed with a combination of scalpel and electrocautery dissection. The flaps are sufficiently thin to remove all apparent breast tissue, but need not remove the subcutaneous tissue of the flaps. This tissue carries the blood vessels to the skin and is of cosmetic importance. Depending on the body habitus of the patient, the flaps may contain from 1 to 8 mm of subcutaneous fat. In a standard modified radical or total mastectomy, the inferior flap extends inferiorly below the inframammary crease for approximately 2 cm onto the interior fascia of the rectus muscle. If immediate reconstruction is to be performed, the dissection usually ends at the inframammary crease. Sparing the inframammary crease is associated with leaving a minuscule amount of residual breast. It makes a great deal of difference in reconstruction if the inframammary crease has not been ablated. The superior flap is then dissected similarly, just to beneath the clavicle. The medial extension of the skin flaps reaches the lateral edge of the sternum, and the lateral extension reaches the anterior edge of the latissimus dorsi. When the flaps have been developed, the breast is dissected from the chest wall by dissecting the pectoralis major fascia off the muscle superiorly and medially, progressing inferiorly. If total mastectomy is performed and the axilla is not to be dissected, as the breast is dissected from the lateral edge of the pectoralis major muscle, the pectoralis muscle is seen beneath it. The surgeon should spare the medial pectoral nerves, which wrap around the lateral border of the pectoralis minor muscle and insert into the posterior aspect of the pectoralis major muscle. Division of these nerves leads to atrophy in the central portion of the pectoralis major muscle. If total mastectomy is performed, the dissection progresses into the axilla above any apparent breast tissue and includes the lower axillary lymph nodes, only because they are admixed with the tail of Spence. During total mastectomy, no attempt is made to remove the axillary lymph nodes. Only the tail of Spence that extends toward the axilla is removed. The breast is then swept inferiorly, with care taken to spare the thoracodorsal and long thoracic nerves in their lower extent as the breast tissue is removed. If a skin-sparing procedure is performed, a suture is used to identify a margin of the specimen so that the pathology department can orient it properly for assessing marginal clearance.

If the axilla is to be dissected, either in continuity or as a separate axillary dissection as part of breast-conserving surgery, the axilla is best entered from within the fascia of the pectoralis major muscle posteriorly. Coming down two fingerbreadths from the uppermost extent of the pectoralis major fascia posteriorly, a transverse incision is made. This incision goes through the pectoralis major fascia and 1 mm beneath it, through the claypectoral fascia. Fat from the axilla then pops through this division of the clavipectoral fascia. The inferior border of the axillary vein is two fingerbreadths below the highest extent of the pectoralis major fascia. This is important because the lymphatics of the arm pass anterior to the axillary vein. Staying below the axillary vein minimizes the risk of subsequent lymphedema of the arm. A single dose of perioperative antibiotics further minimizes occult cellulitis that could scar axillary lymphatics in healing.

The landmark for the axillary anatomy is the thoracodorsal vein, which is one fingerbreadth out from the chest, 2 cm lateral to the chest wall, and passing dorsally into the dorsal inferior aspect of the axillary vein. When it is identified, the thoracodorsal nerve is seen to emerge from behind the axillary vein, just medial to the thoracodorsal vessels. It joins these vessels, continuing onto the anterior surface of the thoracodorsal vein. Between 1 and 2 cm below the axillary vein, the highest branch of the intercostobrachial nerve is seen coming from the chest wall and going to the arm. It is important, and usually possible, to spare and clear this nerve branch. This avoids the dysesthesias associated with its division and total numbness of the inner posterior arm. These technical steps minimize the sensory complications and lymphedema associated with axillary dissection. When the thoracodorsal nerve has been identified, sweeping the axillary fat downward off of the chest wall moves the level II axillary nodes out from behind the pectoralis minor muscle and clears the long thoracic nerve safely. The long thoracic nerve is always found in the same anterior-posterior plane as the thoracodorsal nerve, but is immediately applied to the chest wall. At this point, the three major midaxillary nerves have been identified. If the medial pectoral nerves were not previously identified by sweeping the fatty tissue off of the lateral border of the pectoralis minor muscle, the medial pectoral nerves will not be seen coming around the lateral border of the pectoralis minor and entering the posterior aspect of the pectoralis major. The axillary contents can now be cleared inferiorly, with all of the important nerves and vessels in view. When axillary dissection is complete, the remainder of the breast flap division allows the specimen to be handed off. If this was done through a circumareolar incision, the specimen may be too large to be delivered and a tennis racket incision 1 to 2 cm lateral to the circumareolar incision will allow the specimen to be retracted. When hemostasis is complete, the plastic surgeon can reconstruct the breast according to the patient's body habitus. For a very small-breasted woman, an expander can be placed beneath the pectoralis major and partially expanded to allow the skin anterior to the muscle to achieve normal tension. For a fuller breast, the latissimus dorsi can be freed, swung around anteriorly, and joined to the lateral border of the pectoralis major muscle with a prosthesis lying deep to the muscle. This muscle cover provides the reconstructed breast with a very natural feel. For a larger-breasted woman, optimal reconstruction may involve a transverse rectus abdominis myocutaneous (TRAM) flap, either free or pedicled, using the fatty tissue of the lower abdomen supported on its muscular vessels.

ADJUVANT IRRADIATION

At one point, irradiation of the chest wall after mastectomy was almost universally applied in the treatment of breast cancer, largely because of the more advanced nature of breast cancer in the early decades of the 20th century, with an attendant high rate of local chest wall failure. As surgical techniques improved and as clinicians began to take a more rigorous scientific look at breast cancer therapy, the need for postoperative chest wall irradiation began to be questioned. Possibly the first randomized prospective clinical trial testing one form of cancer therapy against another was the first Manchester, England, trial of immediate vs. delayed chest wall irradiation in postmastectomy patients, begun in 1948. Since that time, more than 30 randomized trials of postmastectomy irradiation have been performed. Although chest wall radiation dramatically reduced the risk of subsequent chest wall recurrence and decreased the chance of dying of breast cancer, the overall survival rate in irradiated women was not significantly increased.

However, in the era of aggressive systemic chemotherapy for node-positive patients, postmastectomy chest wall irradiation is being re-examined.[485,486] Two modern randomized trials of chest wall radiation show a survival advantage for this therapy in premenopausal women with positive nodes, all receiving CMF chemotherapy (oral cyclophosphamide 100 mg/m^2 on days 1 to 14, methotrexate 40 mg/m^2 on days 1 and 8, and 5-fluorouracil 600 mg/m^2 on days 1 and 8, administered every 28 days). These trials are summarized in Table 94-18 and show that obtaining maximum initial local control of breast cancer is important in achieving the best survival results.[487] Similar survival benefits were shown in a nonrandomized review of patients with 10 or more positive lymph nodes who were treated with chemotherapy, with or without radiation.[488] Additional attention must be paid to the use of postmastectomy chest wall irradiation, not only for its ability to reduce the risk of local failure, but also for its potential to enhance survival.[489]

ADJUVANT SYSTEMIC THERAPY

Decisions about whether to offer an individual patient adjuvant systemic therapy (e.g., endocrine manipulation, chemotherapy, or both) should balance the risk of relapse, the potential absolute benefit of therapy, and existing

INDICATIONS FOR POSTMASTECTOMY RADIATION

Tumor >5 cm
T4 tumor
Involvement of 4 or more axillary lymph nodes
Gross extracapsular nodal disease
Residual disease after mastectomy

ADDITIONAL CONSIDERATIONS

Involvement of 1 to 3 axillary lymph nodes
Gross multifocality
Extension into the nipple or skin

comorbidities. In general, women who have early breast cancer with a moderate to high risk of relapse are offered adjuvant systemic therapy, and there has been a steady decrease in the threshold to offer therapy. More than 50% of newly diagnosed breast cancers express the ER or PR, and these patients are candidates for endocrine therapy. Treatment with tamoxifen or other therapies that modulate estrogen exposure to the tumor cells is generally well tolerated, and most women with hormone-receptor-positive invasive breast cancer benefit from this treatment if contraindications do not exist.[490] Combination chemotherapy is associated with a proportional reduction in the annual odds of recurrence of up to 33%.[491] Many clinicians offer adjuvant chemotherapy to otherwise healthy women if the absolute reduction in the risk of recurrence is 3% or greater at 5 years.[492] However, given similar odds, individual women may make very different decisions about treatment.[493]

TABLE 94-18

Trials of Postmastectomy Radiation Therapy

FEATURE	BRITISH COLUMBIA	DBCG
Years of accrual	1978–1986	1982–1989
No. of patients randomized	318	1708
Surgery	MRM	TM + AXD
Chemotherapy	CMF	CMF
Radiation therapy dose	37.5 Gy	48–50 Gy
Locoregional failure		
With radiation therapy	13%	9%
Without radiation therapy	33%	32%
	$P = 0.003$	$P < 0.001$
Disease-free survival		
With radiation therapy	50%	48%
Without radiation therapy	33%	34%
	$P = 0.007$	$P < 0.001$
Overall survival		
With radiation therapy	54%	54%
Without radiation therapy	46%	45%
	$P = 0.07$	$P = <0.001$
Follow-up (yr)	15	10

AXD, axillary node dissection; CMF, cyclophosphamide, methotrexate, and 5-fluorouracil; DBCG, Danish Breast Cancer Cooperative Group; MRM, modified radical mastectomy; TM, total mastectomy.

Evidence indicates that patients with breast cancer overestimate the value of systemic therapy, do not recall receiving quantitative estimates of the potential benefit of adjuvant treatment, and are willing to accept remarkably low incremental benefits.[494] Therefore, quantitative tools to help patients and health care providers estimate the potential benefit from adjuvant systemic therapy have been developed, such as the online programs *Adjuvant!*[495] and *Numeracy*[496] (www.adjuvantonline.com and www.mhs.mayo.edu/adjuvant; last accessed June 13, 2003). Useful clinical practice guidelines also include the U.S. NCI Network (annual updates),[497] the St. Gallen International Consensus Meeting (updated every 2 years),[498,499] the Cancer Care Ontario Practice Guidelines Initiative on lymph node–negative disease (last updated February 2002),[500] and ad hoc panels such as the November 2000 U.S. National Institutes of Health (NIH) Conference.[501]

Large databases indicate that the 5-year survival rate in women with small endocrine-responsive tumors is not likely to be affected by their disease, and chemotherapy offers minimal potential benefit.[502,503] However, the NSABP evaluated the long-term outcomes of 1259 patients with node-negative breast cancer whose tumors were 1 cm or smaller (19% ER-negative). Significant improvement was seen with chemotherapy in recurrence-free survival and overall survival for both ER-positive and ER-negative women.[504] Alternatively, only 6 to 7 of 100 women with tumors 1 cm or smaller may benefit from chemotherapy, and more than 90% do not require or do not benefit from the therapy, highlighting the need for sufficiently strong prognostic factors to separate those who are at risk for recurrence from those who are not at risk. However, strong evidence supports the use of tamoxifen in women with small (<1.0 cm) endocrine-responsive tumors treated with lumpectomy and radiation therapy. NSABP B-21 showed a 63% reduction in the hazard rate of ipsilateral recurrence and a 55% reduction in the risk of contralateral breast cancer when tamoxifen was added to breast-conservation therapy (lumpectomy plus radiation therapy).[505] Although prospective randomized controlled trials of adjuvant systemic therapy were first initiated approximately 40 years ago, until recently, considerable controversy continued about the lasting benefits of such treatment. These uncertainties were largely a result of the modest treatment benefits obtained with available systemic therapies as well as the considerable heterogeneity in the clinical course of early breast cancer. Decisions about breast cancer care are mostly based on large data sets from prospective randomized clinical trials comparing adjuvant systemic regimens with other regimens or placebo. These trials vary by type of agent investigated, treatment duration, and number of agents. To minimize the inherent biases of varied designs and the small power of individual trials to identify therapeutic differences, groups of investigators have successfully performed systematic reviews of multiple studies that examined similar questions.

Thus, the small to modest therapeutic effects noted in individual clinical studies could be of great value if applied to the large population of women with breast cancer. To detect whether a specific treatment modality used for patients with operable breast cancer had an effect on overall survival and to determine the magnitude of this effect, since 1985, the Early Breast Cancer Trialists' Collaborative Group (EBCTCG, or the Oxford Overview) has performed at intervals of 5 years an ongoing combined analysis, or meta-analysis, of all available randomized trials. This remarkable worldwide collaboration resulted in reports at regular intervals on the utility of polychemotherapy, tamoxifen, and ovarian ablation in early breast cancer.[490,491,506] Preliminary results of the most recent systematic review were released in 2000.[507]

As a result of the Oxford Overview and information gained from individual trials, general conclusions can be reasonably drawn about the effectiveness of adjuvant systemic therapy. A significant survival advantage after polychemotherapy was unequivocally shown in all adequately studied age categories. However, the magnitude of benefit appears to be less in older women. Likewise, chemotherapy has been effective in patients with node-negative or node-positive disease. Polychemotherapy is superior to monochemotherapy, and chemotherapy administered for 12 months or longer has not been associated with greater benefit than shorter duration of treatment (e.g., 6 months). Increasing evidence indicates additional benefit of combining chemotherapy and tamoxifen in receptor-positive patients. Although controversy remains, anthracycline-containing regimens appear to have greater effects on recurrence and survival than standard CMF regimens.

The Oxford Overview also shows that adjuvant tamoxifen improves survival. These survival benefits are irrespective of age or menopausal status. The hormone-receptor status of the primary tumor is the strongest predictor of the magnitude of the treatment benefit of tamoxifen. In contrast to chemotherapy, more prolonged administration of tamoxifen (i.e., 5 years) provides greater benefit than a single year of administration. Some studies show no additional benefit when tamoxifen is continued beyond 5 years, but this question has not been resolved.

A provocative and significant observation in the initial Oxford Overview was the finding that ovarian ablation resulted in a reduction in mortality rate in women younger than 50 years of age that was comparable to the effects of polychemotherapy. Many questions remain about the appropriate role of adjuvant ovarian ablation in premenopausal patients. Large international clinical trials led by the International Breast Cancer Study Group (IBCSG) began in 2003.

A stated goal of the Oxford Overview is to bring the results closer to the patient and thus to provide an understandable quantitative estimate of the degree of benefit of a specific therapy. Estimate of this benefit is based on the concept that the absolute increase in the 10-year overall survival rate depends on both the reduction in relative risk and the baseline prognosis of the treated cohort. Table 94-19 provides critical information for decision making by patients and physicians. For example, a woman with "good-prognosis" stage I disease has a 10% to 20% baseline risk of death from breast cancer and can expect an absolute benefit of approximately 4% (reduction of 4 deaths per 100 women treated) from treatment that persistently reduces the annual odds of death by 30%. For a woman with stage II disease and a significantly worse 10-year risk of death of 40% to 80%, the absolute benefit from the same treatment would be 12%. For a therapy that is 50% less effective (i.e., reduction of annual odds of death by 15%), the absolute benefit would be proportionally reduced by approximately half. In discussing these findings with patients, it is important for clinicians to recall that the overview results provide information about predicted outcomes for populations, but do not provide insight into the distribution of benefit among individual patients. One common interpretation is that the treatment benefit is shared among patients, with most having some benefit. When discussing the potential benefits of adjuvant systemic therapy, it is important to consider the estimated individual risk, comorbidity, and personal patient preferences.

TABLE 94-19

Correlation Between Absolute Reduction in Mortality Rate and Baseline Prognosis and Reduction in Odds of Death*			
		APPROXIMATE ABSOLUTE BENEFIT: DIFFERENCE IN NUMBER ALIVE SEVERAL YEARS LATER IF 100 WOMEN HAVE A PERSISTENT REDUCTION IN ANNUAL ODDS OF DEATH OF	
10-YR RISK OF DEATH FROM BREAST CANCER (%)	**EXAMPLE OF PATIENTS WITH EARLY BREAST CANCER AT SUCH RISK**	**30%**	**15%**
10–20	Stage I, good prognosis	4	2
20–40	Stage I, poor prognosis	8	4
40–80	Stage II, any prognosis	12[†]	6[†]

*These eventual absolute benefits apply chiefly to survival, where annual risk reductions may well be persistent. Elsewhere, they may be less if (as will be seen for many analyses of recurrence-free survival) the reduction in annual risk is substantial for only the first few years.
[†]For stage II, once approximately half of the untreated women have died, the absolute benefit from a persistent odds reduction may not depend much on prognosis or on duration of follow-up.
Adapted from Early Breast Cancer Trialists' Collaborative Group: Systemic treatment of early breast cancer by hormonal, cytotoxic, or immune therapy: 3 randomized trials involving 31,000 recurrences and 24,000 death among 75,000 women. Lancet 1992;339:1.

Adjuvant Chemotherapy

The 1995 Oxford Overview on polychemotherapy analyzed data from 17,723 study participants in 47 of 53 identified clinical trials that addressed questions of adjuvant chemotherapy versus none, duration of chemotherapy, and type of regimen (containing vs. not containing anthracycline).[491] This systematic review showed that administration of polychemotherapy for several months was associated with a significant reduction in annual odds of recurrence (23.5%; standard deviation [SD], 2.1; 2 P < 0.00001) and mortality rate (15.3%; SD, 2.4; 2 P < 0.00001). The benefit was greater in younger women. Women with node-negative and those with node-positive disease benefited equally from adjuvant chemotherapy. The 2000 update of the Oxford Overview showed persistent benefits extending to 15 years (Fig. 94-36).[501]

Data from three important large clinical trials that randomized patients with breast cancer to receive chemotherapy vs. no chemotherapy were reported after the 1995 Oxford Overview. These trials include Southwest Oncology Group (SWOG) 8814 in patients with node-positive disease and NSABP B-20 and IBCSG trial IX in patients with node-negative disease. In SWOG 8814 (Intergroup 0100), 1477 postmenopausal women with node-positive, receptor-positive breast cancer were randomized to receive tamoxifen alone or chemotherapy with cyclophosphamide, doxorubicin, and fluorouracil (CAF) with concurrent or sequential tamoxifen (CAFT). With 8-year follow-up, chemoendocrine therapy was associated with improved disease-free survival and overall survival rates (5-year disease-free survival rate 76% vs. 67% for CAFT and tamoxifen, respectively [hazard ratio T:CAFT, 1.43; 95% CI, 1.18 to 1.72]; 5-year overall survival 84% vs. 79% for CAFT and tamoxifen, respectively,).[508] NSABP B-20 randomly assigned 2306 patients with axillary-node-negative, ER-positive breast cancer to receive tamoxifen alone, six cycles of classic CMF plus tamoxifen, or methotrexate and 5-fluorouracil plus tamoxifen. Disease-free survival and overall survival rates were improved in women who received combination chemotherapy and tamoxifen compared with tamoxifen alone. The NSABP investigators concluded that women of all ages with node-negative, ER-positive disease benefited from the addition of CMF-based chemotherapy to tamoxifen.[509] Finally, in IBCSG trial IX 1669, postmenopausal women with node-negative disease received three cycles of classic CMF and tamoxifen or tamoxifen alone. Nearly two thirds of the study participants had ER-positive disease. With a 71-month follow-up, the addition of chemotherapy improved disease-free survival and overall survival rates in women with ER-negative disease (5-year disease-free survival rate, 84% with CMF plus tamoxifen vs. 69% with tamoxifen [risk ratio, 0.52; 95% CI, 0.34 to 0.79]; 5-year overall survival rate, 89% with CMF plus tamoxifen vs. 81% with tamoxifen [risk ratio, 0.51; 95% CI, 0.30 to 0.87]).[510] These recent data on node-negative patients are important for two reasons. First, despite the use of what might be considered suboptimal chemotherapy (i.e., three instead of six cycles of CMF), a statistically significant survival advantage in long-term outcome was seen in ER-negative

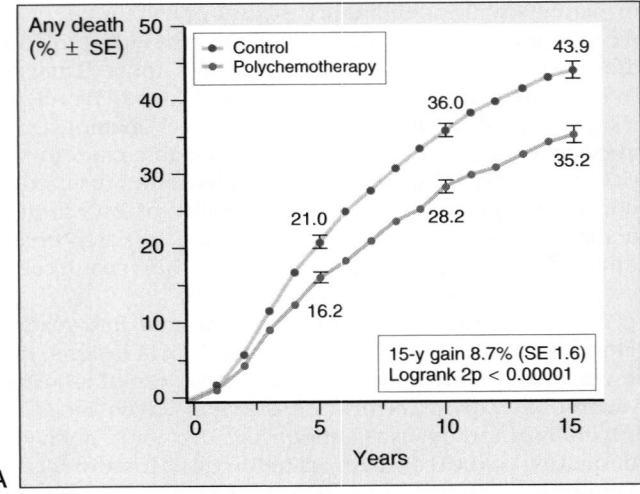

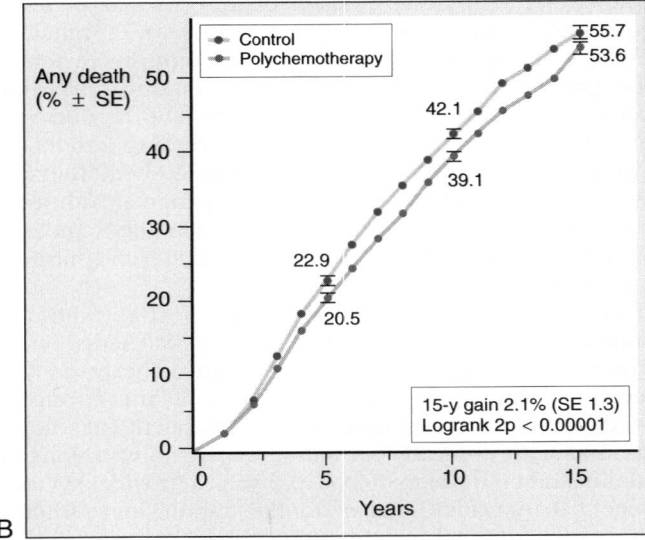

Figure 94-36. Comparison of death from any cause in patients receiving polychemotherapy vs. those not receiving polychemotherapy. **A,** Life-table curve: 6901 women younger than 50 years of age, 35% node-positive. **B,** 18,629 women 50 to 69 years of age, 70% node-positive. SE, standard error. (From the 2000 Early Breast Cancer Trialists' Collaborative Group.)

women. The long-term outcome of patients with ER-negative disease who were treated with chemotherapy was similar to that of women with ER-positive cancer who were treated with tamoxifen, with or without chemotherapy. These results led to speculation that longer duration of CMF chemotherapy or the use of anthracycline-based therapy could be associated with further improvement in outcomes in both the ER-negative and ER-positive groups. Second, little data were available on the use of adjuvant chemotherapy in truly postmenopausal women, and IBCSG trial IX showed no benefit from the addition of chemotherapy to tamoxifen in women with ER-positive disease. This is the largest chemotherapy trial in postmenopausal patients with node-negative breast cancer. After these data were released, the NSABP performed a retrospective analysis of its trials involving patients with breast cancer who had negative axillary nodes (including B-20). Patients older than 50 years of age were divided into two retrospective subgroups (50 to 59 years of age vs. older than 59 years of age).[511] These data continue to show a trend for benefit with the addition of chemotherapy in patients 50 to 59 years of age. However, no benefit was seen for women older than 59 years of age. These results emphasize the need for further investigation of the role of chemotherapy in older women with high-risk primary breast cancer, especially those with endocrine-responsive disease. They also seem to confirm observations that endocrine-unresponsive tumors may be more sensitive to chemotherapy.[512-514]

HER2 Status

The 2000 update of the American Society of Clinical Oncology Clinical Practice Guidelines on the use of tumor markers in breast cancer states that *HER2* "overexpression should be evaluated on every primary breast cancer either at the time of diagnosis or at the time of recurrence."[515] An emerging pattern suggests a potential role as a prognostic factor for worse outcome[516] and as a predictive factor for benefit from adjuvant anthracycline,[517-519] but not for lack of benefit from adjuvant CMF[520] or tamoxifen.[521] This topic is controversial because of the retrospective nature, small sample size, and inadequate design of these studies. At the same time, determination of HER2 status in primary tumors appears justified, especially if it helps to identify patients who are candidates for adjuvant trials with trastuzumab. In this case, inadequate standardization of HER2 assays used in clinical practice outside high-volume central facilities increases the risk of false-positive HER2 results, which can expose patients to unnecessary toxicity and decrease the statistical power of ongoing adjuvant trials of trastuzumab.[522,523]

Choice and Duration of Anthracycline Regimens

The Oxford Overview on polychemotherapy showed that anthracycline-containing regimens provided a significant proportional reduction in recurrence and mortality rates compared with CMF-based regimens (Fig. 94-37). However, NSABP studies comparing just four cycles of AC vs. six cycles of classic CMF showed both regimens to offer a similar survival benefit.[524,525] At the same time, studies comparing six cycles of CAF[526] or six cycles of CEF (with epirubicin)[527,528] with CMF showed a survival benefit favoring an anthracycline-based regimen. French Adjuvant Study Group trial 01 also showed a disease-free survival and overall survival advantage favoring six vs. three cycles of FEC 50 (epirubicin 50 mg/m^2 every 21 days). Ongoing trials in North America are directly comparing shorter vs. longer duration of anthracycline therapy in an attempt to resolve the duration issue.

Doxorubicin is the anthracycline that is most commonly used in the United States. Epirubicin, the 4'-epimer of doxorubicin, is more commonly used in Europe and Canada. Epirubicin has an improved safety profile compared with doxorubicin and thus dose can be escalated further, but direct comparison trials are lacking. The National Cancer Institute of Canada (NCI-C) MA-5 trial used CEF 120 (cyclophosphamide 75 mg/m^2 orally

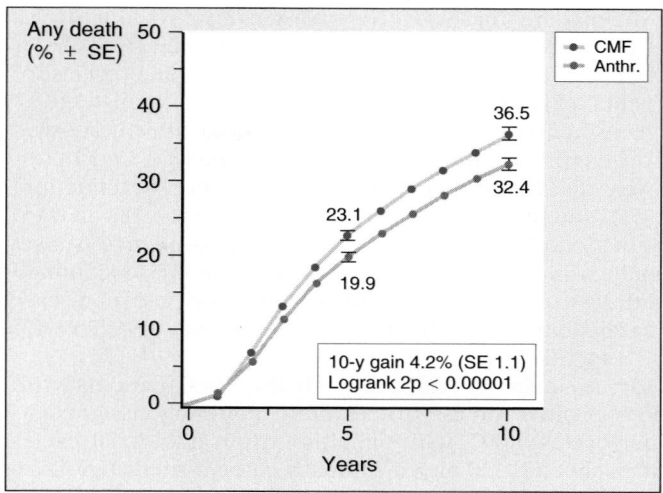

Figure 94-37. Comparison of death from any cause in patients receiving anthracycline-based regimens vs. CMF (oral cyclophosphamide 100 mg/m^2 on days 1 to 14, methotrexate 40 mg/m^2 on days 1 and 8, and 5-fluorouracil 600 mg/m^2 on days 1 and 8, administered every 28 days). Ten-year life-table curve: 13,552 women, 62% node-positive, 65% entry at younger than 50 years of age. SE, standard error. (From the 2000 Early Breast Cancer Trialists' Collaborative Group.)

on days 1 to 14, epirubicin 60 mg/m^2 on days 1 and 8, and 5-fluorouracil 500 mg/m^2 on days 1 and 8, with cotrimoxazole two tablets twice daily for the duration of chemotherapy) in patients with node-positive disease. Results showed better 5- and 10-year relapse-free survival and overall survival rates compared with classic CMF in premenopausal, node-positive patients.[526,527] CEF was associated with a small risk of congestive heart failure (4 cases, 1.1% vs. 1 case, 0.3%; $P = 0.047$), but no greater risk of acute leukemia. However, a study of 777 premenopausal and postmenopausal patients younger than 70 years of age who had node-positive breast cancer showed no advantage with a different schedule of epirubicin given as epirubicin and cyclophosphamide (60 or 100 mg/m^2 every 21 days) compared with classic CMF, although an overall survival advantage favored patients who received a higher vs. a lower dose of epirubicin.[529] An epirubicin dose-response relationship was also seen in disease-free and overall survival rates in the French Adjuvant Study Group trial using FEC100 vs. FEC50 (epirubicin 100 mg/m^2 vs. 50 mg/m^2 every 21 days) in node-positive patients.[530] Although epirubicin has a higher threshold than doxorubicin for the clinical development of congestive heart failure (mg/mg basis), indirect evidence of myocardial damage (e.g., decreased left ventricular ejection fraction, elevated plasma markers of myocardial injury) is also seen, even after just a few cycles of adjuvant epirubicin.[531]

Role of Taxanes

The observed activity of taxanes in advanced disease led to several prospective clinical trials examining their role in the adjuvant setting. Cancer and Leukemia Group B (CALGB) trial 9344 (Intergroup 0148) randomized 3170 women with node-positive breast cancer to four cycles of AC with three dose levels of doxorubicin (60, 75, or 90 mg/m^2), with or without four additional cycles of paclitaxel 175 mg/m^2. All cycles were administered 3 weeks apart. Escalating the dose of doxorubicin showed no benefit, but the addition of paclitaxel offered better 5-year disease-free survival (65% vs. 70%; hazard reduction, 17%) and overall survival rates (77% vs. 80%; hazard reduction, 18%).[532] An unplanned retrospective subset analysis indicates that benefit from taxane was confined almost exclusively to women with ER-negative disease (hazard ratio 0.72; 95% CI, 0.59 to 0.86 vs. 0.91; 95% CI, 0.78 to 1.07).[533]

In a similar NSABP study (B-28), 3060 patients with node-positive breast cancer were randomly assigned to four cycles of AC, with or without four additional cycles of paclitaxel 225 mg/m^2. Initially, after a median follow-up of 34 months, disease-free survival and overall survival rates were similar in both groups (disease-free survival rate approximately 81% in both arms; overall survival rates 90% and 92% for AC and AC followed by paclitaxel, respectively).[533] However, a significant 17% ($P < 0.008$) improvement in disease-free survival rate was seen after a median follow-up of 64 months.[534] The benefit from paclitaxel began to emerge at approximately 3 years, and an overall survival benefit might be seen with longer follow-up. Subset analysis showed that this benefit was not affected by hormone-receptor status. One important difference between the CALGB and NSABP trials is the timing of tamoxifen administration. In the CALGB study, tamoxifen was recommended to all receptor-positive women for 5 years after the completion of chemotherapy. In the NSABP study, tamoxifen was initiated at the start of chemotherapy for all women who were older than 50 years of age and for those younger than 50 years of age with hormone-receptor-positive disease. Patients in the NSABP trial also had smaller tumors, with fewer lymph nodes involved. Overall, these data seem to confirm the clinical utility of paclitaxel after AC in the adjuvant treatment of patients with node-positive breast cancer, regardless of hormone-receptor status.

In a third, smaller study at the M.D. Anderson Cancer Center, 524 women with primary operable breast cancer received eight cycles of 5-fluorouracil, doxorubicin, and cyclophosphamide (FAC) or four cycles of paclitaxel 175 mg/m^2 followed by four cycles of FAC. With a median follow-up of 48 months, both groups had similar relapse-free survival and overall survival rates.[535]

Breast Cancer International Research Group (BCIRG) study 001 evaluated 1491 node-positive patients treated in the adjuvant setting with TAC (docetaxel 75 mg/m^2, doxorubicin 50 mg/m^2, and cyclophosphamide 500 mg/m^2) vs. a standard FAC regimen. At 33-month median follow-up, TAC offered better disease-free survival (82% and 74%; relative risk, 0.64; $P = 0.0002$) and overall survival rates (relative risk, 0.71; $P = 0.049$). However, greater toxicity was seen with TAC (febrile neutropenia, 24% vs. 2%; grade 3 to 4 infection, 2.8% vs. 1.3%; and congestive heart failure, 1.2% vs. 0.1%).[536] Recent studies in high-risk, node-negative or node-positive disease will provide additional information. Among these studies are

ECOG 2197 (Intergroup trial), comparing AC vs. AT (doxorubicin 60 mg/m^2 and docetaxel 60 mg/m^2); ECOG 1199 (Intergroup trial), comparing AC followed by paclitaxel or docetaxel, weekly or every 3 weeks (four arms); NSABP B-30, comparing 6 months of AC followed by docetaxel vs. either 3 months of AT or TAC; and BCIRG trial 005, comparing six cycles of TAC vs. four cycles of AC followed by four cycles of docetaxel.

Dose Intensity

Dose intensity is the total dose of a specific agent that is administered over a set time. The dose of each course or cycle is increased (i.e., increased total dose), and many of these regimens require colony-stimulating factor support. CALGB 8541 examined three variations of CAF in patients with node-positive breast cancer. Variations included the following: low-dose treatment (four cycles of cyclophosphamide 300 mg/m^2, doxorubicin 30 mg/m^2, and fluorouracil 300 mg/m^2); intermediate-dose treatment (six cycles of cyclophosphamide 400 mg/m^2, doxorubicin 40 mg/m^2, and fluorouracil 400 mg/m^2); and high-dose treatment (four cycles of cyclophosphamide 600 mg/m^2, doxorubicin 60 mg/m^2, and fluorouracil 600 mg/m^2).[537] Subgroups of patients in this trial appear to have benefited from dose intensification (e.g., women whose tumors overexpress *HER2*), but these data await further validation. Nine-year median follow-up shows a disease-free survival and overall survival advantage favoring the intermediate-dose and high-dose groups compared with the low-dose group. French Adjuvant Study Group trial 01 in node-positive patients showed significant improvement in disease-free survival and overall survival outcomes with six cycles of FEC 50 (epirubicin 50 mg/m^2) compared with three cycles of FEC 75 or FEC 50.[538] French Adjuvant Study Group trial 05 in patients with node-positive disease showed a relapse-free survival (65% vs. 52%) and overall survival advantage (76% vs. 65%) of FEC 100 compared with FEC 50.[529] However, escalation of doses of doxorubicin in CALGB 9344[532] and cyclophosphamide in NSABP B22 and B25[539,540] beyond standard doses of AC (doxorubicin 60 mg/m^2 and cyclophosphamide 600 mg/m^2 every 21 days for four cycles) showed no benefit from dose intensification. These data do not allow direct comparison between doxorubicin and epirubicin. However, they suggest a minimum threshold for individual-agent dosing, with no advantage from further dose escalation.

Dose Density

Dose density is the administration of a higher dose of an agent per unit of time (i.e., mg/m^2 per week). Thus, the dose of each course may be increased, decreased, or equivalent to the standard dose, but the interval between two courses is shortened. The Goldie-Coldman hypothesis suggested that the use of several non-cross-resistant agents simultaneously would provide the best chance of a cure in cancer therapy by preventing spontaneous mutations of tumor cells that account for drug resistance and treatment failure.[541] However, Norton and Simon[542] suggested in another mathematical model that crossover intensification might result in greater regression of small-volume tumors.

They also suggested that sequential single-agent therapy may be a better way to deliver chemotherapy because each drug can be delivered at its maximum tolerated dose, without compromise as a result of combination with other agents. The Milan group showed a survival advantage of sequential therapy (four cycles of doxorubicin followed by eight cycles of CMF) vs. alternating therapy.[543] The Memorial Sloan-Kettering group piloted a sequential dose-dense approach with doxorubicin, paclitaxel, and cyclophosphamide[544] that served as the basis for CALGB 9741 (Intergroup trial) in patients with node-positive breast cancer. These patients were randomly assigned using a 2×2 factorial model to one of four regimens: four cycles of single-agent sequential doxorubicin, paclitaxel, and cyclophosphamide, administered every 3 weeks or every 2 weeks, or four cycles of AC followed by four cycles of paclitaxel, administered every 3 weeks or every 2 weeks. Patients who received the dose-dense regimens also received granulocyte colony-stimulating factor. Results indicate better 3-year disease-free survival (85% vs. 81%) and overall survival rates (92% vs. 90%), favoring every-2-week (dose-dense) vs. conventional every-3-week schedules, but similar outcomes in the combined vs. sequential regimens.[545] Other than an increased risk of anemia and the need for blood transfusion with dose-dense AC followed by paclitaxel, toxicity was not increased in the dose-dense regimens, and fewer cases of neutropenia were reported with concomitant use of granulocyte colony-stimulating factor.

Myeloablative Regimens

Although adjuvant chemotherapy improved both disease-free survival and overall survival rates, many women still have recurrences and die of breast cancer. A logical extension of preclinical and clinical data was that dose intensification with high-dose chemotherapy and autologous marrow support might improve outcome. Based on preclinical experiments and encouraging responses in women with heavily pretreated advanced breast cancer, several early-phase clinical trials were performed in women with nonmetastatic, high-risk breast cancer.[546,547] Unfortunately, the promise of high-dose chemotherapy has not been fulfilled, and data show a marginal clinical benefit.[548,549] Evidence suggests that patient selection was largely responsible for the promising results of uncontrolled phase II trials. Because of the high toxicity profile of myeloablative chemotherapy, entry criteria for these studies were very strict. As a result, there may be a patient selection bias in the enrollment to high-risk and metastatic disease trials.[550,551] Several recent adjuvant trials await data maturity, but newer therapies and targeted approaches may improve the outcome of standard therapies, superseding the question of high-dose therapy.

Adjuvant Endocrine Therapy

Breast cancer is often an estrogen-dependent disease, and endocrine therapy offers the most favorable risk-benefit ratio among existing systemic therapy options. Surgical hormonal manipulation[552] (e.g., oophorectomy, adrenalec-tomy, and hypophysectomy) in metastatic disease is considered the first example of targeted antitumor therapy, which has been largely supplanted by targeted pharmacologic approaches (e.g., SERMs, aromatase inhibitors, and pure antiestrogens). Tamoxifen is the standard agent for premenopausal women in the adjuvant setting.[553] However, recent data suggest an increasing role for aromatase inhibitors in postmenopausal women.[554,555] Ovarian ablation appears to offer similar benefit to CMF-based chemotherapy, but ongoing studies are investigating its role vis-à-vis chemotherapy in premenopausal women with endocrine responsive disease.

Adjuvant Tamoxifen

SERMs may function as estrogen-receptor agonists, antagonists, or mixed agonist-antagonists, depending on the target tissue. Major examples include triphenylethylene derivatives (e.g., tamoxifen), nonsteroidal antiestrogens (e.g., the benzothiophene raloxifene), and steroidal antiestrogens (e.g., ICI 182,780, or fulvestrant). Tamoxifen is the SERM with the longest track record in breast cancer and is approved in the United States for risk reduction in high-risk women, for reduction in the risk of invasive breast cancer after breast conservation in women with DCIS, in the adjuvant treatment of both node-negative and node-positive hormone-receptor-positive disease, and in the management of advanced disease. Because of the potentially undesirable effects in the uterus, vagina, and central nervous system, other SERMs have been evaluated in the laboratory and in the clinic, aiming for greater efficacy and lower toxicity,[556] but they have not been approved in the adjuvant setting.

Tamoxifen is associated with an increase in bone mineral density in the axial skeleton and with stabilization in the appendicular skeleton in postmenopausal women.[557,558] Despite an observed bone mineral loss in the lumbar spine and hip in premenopausal women,[559] the NSABP P-01 prevention study showed a reduction (relative risk, 0.81; 95% CI, 0.63 to 1.05) in fractures of the hip, radius, and spine in all age groups, especially among those 50 years of age and older.[560] Tamoxifen is associated with a reduction in low-density-lipoprotein cholesterol.[561] Initial evidence suggested that it might reduce the risk of coronary heart disease.[562-566] However, this was not confirmed by the Oxford Overview.[490]

EBCTCG Systematic Review on Tamoxifen

The 1995 Oxford Overview on adjuvant tamoxifen confirmed its role as the mainstay of endocrine therapy for all women with ER-positive disease, regardless of patient age or menopausal status. Its database of 37,000 women treated in 55 trials of adjuvant tamoxifen vs. no tamoxifen, started before 1990, contains 87% of the worldwide evidence.[490] No meaningful benefit was seen in nearly 8000 women with low or no ER protein detected in their primary tumor. The proportional reduction in the risk of recurrence observed in trials of 1, 2, and approximately 5 years of tamoxifen administration among 30,000 patients with ER-positive (n = 18,000) or ER-unknown disease (n = 12,000) after approximately 10 years of follow-up were significant (21%, SD, 3; 29%, SD, 2;

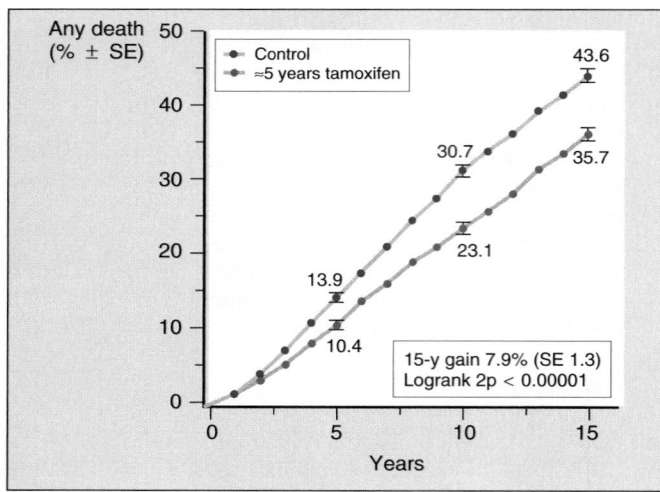

Figure 94-38. Comparison of death from any cause in patients receiving 5 years of tamoxifen vs. those not receiving 5 years of tamoxifen. (Life-table curve: 10,386 women, all ages 80% estrogen-receptor-positive, 30% node-positive.) SE, standard error. (From the 2000 Early Breast Cancer Trialists' Collaborative Group.)

and 47%, SD, 3, respectively), with a highly significant trend toward greater effect with longer duration of treatment. A significant proportional reduction in the risk of death was similarly observed with increased duration of therapy (12%, SD, 3; 17%, SD, 3; and 26%, SD, 4, respectively). The relative improvement in survival increased throughout the first 10 years and was equal in patients with node-positive and node-negative disease. A 46% reduction (SD, 9) in new contralateral breast cancer was seen, similar to that observed in NSABP prevention trial P-01.[560] The 2000 update of the Oxford Overview showed persistent survival benefits extending to 15 years (Fig. 94-38).[501]

Duration of Adjuvant Tamoxifen Treatment
The 1995 Oxford Overview does not address the use of tamoxifen beyond 5 years.[490] In the largest available trial (NSABP B-14), 2818 patients were initially randomized to receive 5 years of tamoxifen or placebo.[567,568] Of these, 643 patients who remained disease-free after 5 years of tamoxifen were subsequently randomized to receive an additional 5 years of tamoxifen or placebo.[569] In another group of 1211 registered patients who were eligible for NSABP B-14, 510 patients who were disease-free after 5 years of tamoxifen were also randomly assigned to receive 5 more years of tamoxifen or placebo.[570] Results showed better disease-free survival (92% vs. 86%; $P = 0.003$) and distant disease-free survival rates (96% vs. 90%; $P = 0.01$) in the patients who discontinued tamoxifen at 5 years (median follow-up of 5.6 years after randomization), with similar survival rates (96% vs. 94%; $P = 0.08$), now updated to 7 years since rerandomization.[570] Two other studies addressed this issue. The Scottish trial in 1327 patients with node-negative disease showed similar results in 342 of the 667 original patients who were initially randomized to tamoxifen and underwent a second randomization,[571,572] with 15 years of median follow-up.[573] A smaller

study of 194 patients with node-positive disease showed a small favorable trend for longer duration of tamoxifen therapy.[574] Two large, ongoing international trials enrolling approximately 20,000 patients (Adjuvant Tamoxifen Long vs. Short [ATLAS] and Adjuvant Tamoxifen Treatment, Offer More? [aTTom]) may help to answer this question. However, most ongoing studies of adjuvant endocrine therapy in postmenopausal patients are examining the role of aromatase inhibitors.[575]

Ovarian Ablation
The ovary is the primary site of estrogen production in premenopausal women. In 1896, Sir George Beatson[552] first reported the benefits of oophorectomy as palliative therapy for several young women with metastatic breast cancer. Randomized trials of ovarian ablation as an adjuvant strategy to suppress or ablate ovarian function began in 1948,[576] but interest in ovarian ablation decreased with the advent of adjuvant chemotherapy and tamoxifen. Recently, there has been renewed interest in this approach because of the recognition of its beneficial adjuvant effects, the availability of medical forms of ovarian suppression, and the use of steroid receptors to identify targeted populations. Permanent ovarian ablation can be effected by surgical oophorectomy, which has faster onset and uses a laparoscopic approach, or radiation therapy, which has slower onset and is sometimes partially effective. Temporary ovarian suppression results from long-term administration of luteinizing hormone–releasing hormone (LHRH) agonists. Ovarian suppression or ablation is a potential indirect result of adjuvant chemotherapy. The risk of chemotherapy-related amenorrhea increases with age, duration of adjuvant chemotherapy, and the use of certain cytotoxic agents, such as cyclophosphamide. The benefit of adjuvant chemotherapy may be due in part to ovarian suppression.[577]

Over the last 20 years, ovarian suppression with long-term administration of LHRH analogs (e.g., goserelin, leuprolide, and triptorelin) has emerged as a treatment strategy by decreasing ovarian production of estrogen by acting on the hypothalamic-pituitary axis (downregulation of pituitary LHRH receptors, suppression of gonadotropin secretion by the pituitary, and loss of ovarian steroid production). This simple, reversible intervention allows fertility to be preserved, and its short-term use (2 to 5 years) minimizes the side effects associated with prolonged estrogen deficiency. The optimal duration of therapy is unknown.[578]

The most informative data set on ovarian ablation as adjuvant therapy for premenopausal breast cancer comes from the Oxford Overview.[506] This review includes the results of 12 randomized trials of surgical or radiation-induced ovarian ablation that were started before 1980 (2102 women <50 years of age and 1354 women ≥50 years of age). These data show that ovarian ablation as a single treatment in women younger than 50 years of age led to a 25% reduction (SD, 7%) in the annual odds of recurrence and a 24% reduction (SD, 7%) in the annual odds of death, regardless of nodal status.[501] The 2000 update of the Oxford Overview showed persistent benefits extending to 15 years (Fig. 94-39).

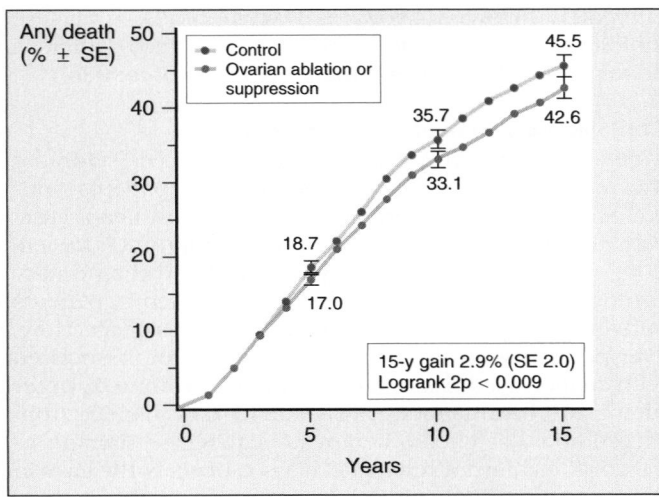

Figure 94-39. Comparison of death from any cause in patients undergoing ovarian ablation or suppression vs. those not undergoing the treatment. (Life-table curve: 7601 women, 53% estrogen-receptor-positive, 61% node-positive.) SE, standard error. (From the 2000 Early Breast Cancer Trialists' Collaborative Group.)

Ovarian ablation appeared to be more effective in women with ER-positive tumors than in those with ER-negative tumors. These data are limited and showed a reduced effect in women also treated with chemotherapy. This is likely caused by a lack of benefit in women with chemotherapy-induced menopause. The Oxford Overview did not detect any benefit from ovarian ablation in women 50 years of age and older.

A number of studies compared the efficacy of combination chemotherapy with ovarian ablation or suppression, with or without tamoxifen, in premenopausal women. In aggregate, these studies suggest that the two forms of therapy are similar in effectiveness.[579-582] However, the studies have several limitations. For instance, eligibility was not always limited to patients with hormone-receptor-positive breast cancer; tamoxifen was not administered to women in the chemotherapy arms, based on a previous belief that it was ineffective in premenopausal women; most of the trials used non-anthracycline-containing chemotherapy regimens; and finally, most of the studies had small sample sizes and lacked statistical power. Studies also examined whether ovarian suppression in addition to adjuvant chemotherapy improves outcome for premenopausal women with early-stage breast cancer.[583-587] Similar limitations apply to their conclusions.

Two expert panels reviewed the international database on adjuvant ovarian ablation or suppression. The 2000 NIH Consensus Conference concluded that adjuvant chemotherapy should be recommended to most premenopausal women with early breast cancer and that adjuvant hormonal therapy with tamoxifen should be offered to most women with steroid-receptor-positive invasive breast cancer.[501] Ovarian ablation or suppression was believed to be an acceptable alternative to 5 years of treatment with tamoxifen in selected women. However, available data were not believed to support the addition of ovarian ablation or suppression to adjuvant chemotherapy followed by tamoxifen. The most recent St. Gallen conferences on adjuvant therapy for primary breast cancer reported that endocrine therapy (including ovarian suppression or ablation and tamoxifen) is equivalent to adjuvant chemotherapy for premenopausal women with endocrine-responsive breast cancer.[498,499] Several important questions remain, such as the role of ovarian ablation or suppression in the subgroup of premenopausal women with hormone-receptor-positive breast cancer who do not become postmenopausal with chemotherapy (the value of chemotherapy followed by ovarian ablation or suppression); the optimal duration of therapy; the utility of combined endocrine therapy; the identification of predictive factors other than steroid-receptor status; and long-term side effects.

Aromatase Inhibitors

The conversion of androgen to estrogen in peripheral tissues is the primary source of estrogen in postmenopausal women, and the aromatase enzyme is present in a number of tissues (e.g., muscle, fat, skin, neural tissues, and breast). Levels of estrogen and aromatase are elevated in malignant breast tissue, and aromatase inhibitors can block the action of the enzyme and reduce estrogen production. Available drugs include type 1 steroidal non-reversible inhibitors (e.g., exemestane and formestane) and type 2 nonsteroidal reversible inhibitors (e.g., letrozole, and anastrozole).[588] First-generation inhibitors (e.g., aminoglutethimide) were associated with significant toxicity in the adjuvant setting because of the nonspecific effects that occur at several steps in the steroid biosynthetic pathway.[589] A marginal benefit was seen compared with tamoxifen.[590] The more specific (and less toxic) third-generation aromatase inhibitors supported the initiation of several adjuvant trials in postmenopausal women.

The first such trial reported is the ATAC trial,[591] a double-blind, placebo-controlled trial including 9366 postmenopausal women with operable breast cancer of any steroid-receptor status who completed local therapy with or without chemotherapy. Patients were randomized to receive tamoxifen (20 mg orally daily), anastrozole (1 mg orally daily), or the combination for 5 years. Their median age was 64 years, 84% had hormone-receptor-positive disease, 61% had node-negative disease, and 21% received adjuvant chemotherapy before trial entry. At a median follow-up of 33 months, the 3-year disease-free survival rate was 89.4% for anastrozole, 87.4% for tamoxifen, and 87.2% for the combination, a significant difference favoring anastrozole. Subset analysis showed that the advantage of anastrozole was seen only in women with hormone-receptor-positive breast cancer. There was also a significant difference in contralateral invasive breast cancer (30 cases in the tamoxifen arm vs. 9 cases in the anastrozole arm), but no difference in mortality rate. Anastrozole was associated with fewer hot flashes, less vaginal bleeding, and fewer thromboembolic, ischemic, and cerebrovascular events. However, it was associated with more spine and wrist fractures and musculoskeletal symptoms. These short-term results favor the use of anastrozole and argue against additional value for combination therapy. An update at 47 months comparing anastrozole vs. tamoxifen continues to favor the aromatase inhibitor (4-year disease-free survival rate, 86.9% vs. 84.5%).[592] These data led to the approval of anastrozole by the U.S. Food and Drug Administration as a form of adjuvant endocrine therapy for postmenopausal patients with endocrine-responsive breast cancer.

While acknowledging that data from several large trials were still not available, an expert panel from the American Society of Clinical Oncology urged caution and recommended tamoxifen as the standard initial adjuvant endocrine therapy in these patients.[555] Anastrozole can be considered for women who have a contraindication to tamoxifen or who have breast cancer while receiving raloxifene or tamoxifen. Aromatase inhibitors should not be used as monotherapy in premenopausal women or those with endocrine-unresponsive disease. Ongoing clinical trials are examining the role of other aromatase inhibitors and the optimal sequence of endocrine therapy.

Perhaps of greater significance are the results of the NCI-C MA17 intergroup trial, published in the *New England Journal of Medicine* in 2003, that randomized postmenopausal patients who were disease-free after an average of 5 years of adjuvant tamoxifen to an additional 5 years of letrozole or placebo. The primary endpoint was disease-free survival (including new contralateral breast cancer), and after a median follow-up of 2.4 months there were 75 local or metastatic recurrences of breast cancer or new primary cancers in the contralateral breast in the letrozole group compared to 132 in the placebo group. The estimated 4-year disease-free survival rates were 93% and 87%, respectively ($P \leq 0.001$), and these data for the first time support the continuation of endocrine therapy past 5 years of tamoxifen. The recommendation of the trial's data safety and monitoring committee to unblind the study and offer letrozole to the patients on placebo generated much controversy, but this decision was supported by other groups such as NSABP, whose ongoing trial B-33, comparing exemestane versus placebo following 5 years of tamoxifen, has since been suspended.

Low levels of toxicities such as low-grade hot flashes, arthritis, arthralgia, and myalgia were observed in patients treated with letrozole in MA17, but so was a lesser frequency of vaginal bleeding. The rate of osteoporosis (a major complication seen with upfront use of anastrozole in the ATAC trial) was somewhat increased (5.8% in the letrozole group vs. 4.5% in the placebo group, $P = 0.07$), but fracture rates were not increased, possibly due to the prior use of tamoxifen. These data from MA17 are of great interest to postmenopausal patients with ER-positive breast cancer. However, several questions remain unanswered, such as the optimal duration of letrozole therapy after 5 years of tamoxifen, the role of longer aromatase inhibitor therapy in patients who received initial endocrine therapy with 5 years of anastrozole or sequential tamoxifen-anastrozole, and the role of bisphosphonates to reduce the risk of osteoporosis and related complications associated with the adjuvant use of aromatase inhibitors. More recent data (published by Coombes and colleagues in the *New England Journal of Medicine* in March 2004) indicate that 2 to 3 years of

tamoxifen followed by 2 to 3 years of an aromatase inhibitor (5 years total of endocrine therapy) offers a better disease-free survival than 5 years of tamoxifen.

Combined Chemoendocrine Therapy

Adjuvant endocrine therapy has a more favorable therapeutic index than chemotherapy in patients with endocrine-responsive breast cancer. In postmenopausal women, tamoxifen is a more efficacious adjuvant intervention,[593] and endocrine therapy is considered the primary component of any adjuvant systemic regimen in patients with endocrine-responsive disease, regardless of age. However, patients who also have prognostic factors associated with an increased risk of recurrence and death (e.g., larger tumors or lymph node involvement) may benefit from the addition of chemotherapy to endocrine therapy as part of the adjuvant regimen. This is especially the case in premenopausal women, in part because of the ovarian suppression caused by chemotherapy.

In the 1995 Oxford Overview on polychemotherapy,[491] chemotherapy in women younger than 50 years of age reduced the proportional risk of recurrence and death compared with no therapy (37%, SD, 4; and 28%, SD, 5, respectively) or when added to tamoxifen compared with tamoxifen alone (21%, SD, 13; and 25%, SD, 14, respectively). These figures are imprecise because very few women younger than 50 years of age (<650) participated in trials of tamoxifen, with or without chemotherapy. Chemotherapy was still beneficial in women 50 to 69 years of age in similar scenarios, although to a lesser degree with regard to both recurrence and death, compared with no therapy (22%, SD, 4; and 12%, SD, 4, respectively) or compared with tamoxifen alone (19%, SD, 3; and 11%, SD, 4, respectively). These data suggest that chemotherapy offers risk reduction benefit to all subgroups, although the Oxford Overview data suggested a lesser beneficial effect of chemotherapy in endocrine-responsive disease and in older women.[491] The role of adding chemotherapy in low-risk, older patients, such as those with node-negative, endocrine-responsive disease who will be treated with 5 years of adjuvant tamoxifen, is unclear. Few data are available on polychemotherapy in women 70 years of age and older.[491]

The 1995 Oxford Overview on polychemotherapy was limited by the absence of mature data on three of the largest trials ever conducted on the role of chemotherapy when added to tamoxifen. These studies included IBCSG IX (1669 postmenopausal patients)[594] and NSABP B-20 (2306 premenopausal and postmenopausal patients) in patients with node-negative disease,[509,568] and SWOG 8814 (Intergroup 0100 [1477 postmenopausal patients]) in those with node-positive disease.[508] These studies were discussed earlier in this chapter. These results confirm the survival benefit from even a short course (three cycles) of CMF in older women with node-negative, endocrine-unresponsive disease. At the same time, they reinforce the cautionary tone that permeates recent clinical practice guidelines and consensus statements about the use of chemotherapy in postmenopausal women with endocrine-responsive disease who will receive 5 years of adjuvant tamoxifen.[497,498,499,501] These data on combined systemic therapy address whether additional benefit is associated with adding chemotherapy to tamoxifen. Approximately 20% of patients in the ATAC trial (usually node-positive patients) received chemotherapy in addition to endocrine therapy,[591] but it is not known whether these findings on combined chemoendocrine therapy are applicable to the aromatase inhibitors.

SWOG 8814 (Intergroup 0100) also addressed the important issue of timing when combining chemotherapy and endocrine therapy, and indicated a survival advantage associated with sequential vs. concurrent administration of chemotherapy and tamoxifen.[595] A smaller Spanish trial (GEICAM 9401) comparing epirubicin and cyclophosphamide with sequential vs. concurrent tamoxifen showed a trend favoring a sequential approach.[596]

Preoperative Systemic Therapy

Chemotherapy in early breast cancer has traditionally been administered after definitive breast surgery. Prognostic information (e.g., tumor size and nodal status) is used to help to identify patients with a high-risk profile who might derive benefit from systemic therapy. Adjuvant systemic therapy after surgery has been the gold standard for examining the effect of new treatment strategies on disease-free survival and overall survival rates in the adjuvant setting. These endpoints require large sample sizes and long-term follow-up to achieve the number of events required to assess the effect of the investigational arm on the end point of interest. This problem is compounded by the increasing number of patients diagnosed with earlier stages of disease. Preoperative systemic therapy has been traditionally reserved for women with locally advanced breast cancer (LABC) to enhance the likelihood of negative surgical margins or even breast preservation.[597,598] Preclinical data suggest that the administration of systemic therapy before surgery may be associated with early eradication of micrometastases and improved long-term outcomes by decreasing the risk of drug resistance and leading to more favorable growth kinetics.[599,600] Preoperative systemic therapy offers a small increase in the rate of breast conservation over the same therapy given after surgery, although it offers no survival advantage.[601,602]

However, pathologic complete response after preoperative systemic therapy appears to correlate with long-term disease-free survival or overall survival.[514,603,604] In addition, the initial response to preoperative systemic therapy offers the potential of in vivo assessment of sensitivity or resistance to treatment (clinical or tissue samples).[605-607] There are concerns that preoperative therapy might lead to the loss of baseline parameters (e.g., tumor size and lymph node involvement) that are generally used to guide recommendations for adjuvant therapy. Perhaps more importantly, the identification of intermediate (surrogate) markers (tissue and blood) that correlate with outcome after preoperative systemic therapy might allow a greater number of trials with smaller sample sizes to test new adjuvant treatment modalities. In patients treated with preoperative systemic therapy, it is advisable to request immunohistochemistry studies in the initial biopsy specimen, in case no residual disease is identified at surgery after therapy.

Preoperative systemic endocrine therapy is also an attractive alternative to chemotherapy. Letrozole appears to be as active as tamoxifen as induction therapy in patients with locally advanced ER-positive disease. An exploratory analysis of this concept in a small study shows a better response with letrozole in patients with HER2-positive disease.[608]

Secondary Effects of Adjuvant Systemic Therapy

Complications of Chemotherapy

As more patients with earlier stages of disease are offered adjuvant systemic therapy, its short- and long-term effects on quality of life must be carefully weighed. Chemotherapy commonly administered to patients with breast cancer (e.g., CMF, FAC, FEC, AC, or taxane-based regimens) is generally well tolerated. Acute life-threatening toxicity in patients receiving the therapy is quite rare. Common short-term effects include alopecia, myelosuppression, gastrointestinal symptoms, and febrile neutropenia or neutropenic infection. Peripheral neuropathy, arthralgia, and myalgia are also seen with taxanes. The effect of anemia on quality of life and cognitive function is the subject of ongoing investigation.[609] Although many women accept these short-term toxicities, increasingly, attention is being placed on late effects from systemic therapy as the number of patients who will become long-term survivors is increasing. For some, the actual absolute reduction in risk of recurrence and death is relatively small compared with the potential risk of late toxicity.

Anthracycline-related cardiac toxicity is a potential concern. Long-term follow-up data indicate an 8% increased risk of systolic dysfunction 10 years after therapy with a median dose of doxorubicin of 294 mg/m^2.[610] Cardioprotective drugs, such as dexrazoxane, are approved only for use in patients with advanced disease.[611,612] The risk of clinical congestive heart failure associated with conventional doses of anthracyclines is quite small ($\leq 1\%$), and ongoing studies are examining the value of markers of myocardial injury (e.g., troponin) and dysfunction (e.g., brain natriuretic peptide) to prospectively identify patients at risk for late onset of myocardial dysfunction.[613,614] Nuclear medicine scans have no proven value as predictors for anthracycline-related cardiac dysfunction.[615]

Secondary acute myeloid leukemia and myelodysplastic syndrome are rare events. They occur early on, usually after therapy with alkylating agents (e.g., cyclophosphamide), topoisomerase II inhibitors (e.g., anthracyclines), and antimetabolites (e.g., methotrexate).[540,616,617] Thus far, taxanes have not been associated with this complication.[531] The incidence of acute myeloid leukemia or myelodysplastic syndrome after four cycles with conventional doses of AC (60 and 600 mg/m^2) at 5 years is 0.21%, compared with 1.01% in patients treated with two to four cycles of AC with a fourfold increase in the cyclophosphamide dose per cycle.[618]

Young women are at risk for premature menopause after adjuvant chemotherapy.[577] This risk increases with age and duration of treatment, and CMF-based chemotherapy is associated with a 70% risk of ovarian failure in women older than 40 years of age.[619] Preliminary data from BCIRG trial 001 also suggest an increased risk of amenorrhea with a docetaxel-based regimen, such as TAC, compared with a standard anthracycline regimen, such as FAC.[535] Although ovarian suppression as a result of chemotherapy may further decrease the odds of recurrence and death in premenopausal women with endocrine-responsive disease, premature menopause can have a significant effect on quality of life because of severe hot flashes and vaginal dryness. Hot flashes resulting from discontinuation of HRT or induction of menopause are a common symptom after chemotherapy, with only partial remedies.[619-622]

For women who retain fertility, pregnancy does not appear to increase the risk of another breast cancer event.[623] Women who have chemotherapy-induced ovarian failure after adjuvant chemotherapy are at risk for rapid bone loss and complications from osteoporosis.[624] Preliminary evidence suggests that bisphosphonates help to mitigate this potentially serious complication.[625]

Symptoms of fatigue, weight gain, and cognitive dysfunction are reported with some frequency after the completion of therapy. Weight gain is a common symptom associated with induction of menopause,[626,627] and it may be related to factors such as changes in food consumption, decreased physical activity, or reduced basal metabolic rate.[628] Cognitive dysfunction may cause short-term memory loss in patients receiving treatment. Long-term effects include poor memory, impaired concentration, and language deficits.[629-631] The association with chemotherapy is confounded by factors such as onset of menopause, discontinuation of menopausal replacement therapy, and use of endocrine therapy with antiestrogens. However, although long-term survivors report more frequent physical and menopausal symptoms than healthy women, their health-related quality of life and sexual functioning are comparable to those reported in healthy, age-matched control subjects,[632] with no evidence of global or permanent impairment.[633]

Complications of Tamoxifen

Although tamoxifen is associated with an increase in bone mineral density in the axial skeleton[557,558] and the NSABP P-01 prevention study showed a reduction (relative risk, 0.81; 95% CI, 0.63 to 1.05) in fractures of the hip, radius, and spine in all age groups (especially those 50 years of age and older),[560] bone mineral loss is observed in the lumbar spine and hip in premenopausal women receiving tamoxifen.[559] Tamoxifen is associated with a reduction in low-density-lipoprotein cholesterol,[561] and individual studies suggested that tamoxifen might reduce the risk of coronary heart disease.[562-566] However, the Oxford Overview did not show any statistically significant effect of cardiac or vascular events on overall survival.[490]

Similar to its antiestrogen effects in breast tissue, the toxicity profile of tamoxifen is also related to its tissue-specific SERM. The 1995 Oxford Overview showed a higher incidence of uterine malignancies (ratio of incidence rates, 2.58; SD, 0.35).[490] Similar findings were observed in the three largest trials of 5 years of tamoxifen therapy (NSABP B-14,[570,634] Scottish study,[573] and

Stockholm B study).[635] The absolute excess in deaths is 1 or 2 per 1000 after 10 years (0.2 per 1000 woman-years), which is half of the absolute decrease seen in contralateral breast cancer.[490] Although uterine cancer is likely to be diagnosed at an early stage and cured with surgery alone, longer duration of tamoxifen therapy is associated with worse histology and higher grade,[636] with a 15% risk of death.[637] It is now believed that 2% to 5% of all cases represent uterine sarcoma.[638] The NSABP database, with nearly 18,000 patients in six separate studies, showed an incidence of adenocarcinoma of the uterus of 2.2 per 1000 woman-years in the tamoxifen arms compared with 0.71 in the nontamoxifen arms. Perhaps more important for daily practice, tamoxifen is expected to cause endometrial thickness, and neither transvaginal ultrasound[639] nor endometrial biopsy[640] is a useful screening tool in asymptomatic patients. Instead, women who are taking tamoxifen should simply continue their otherwise routine gynecologic evaluation and notify their physicians of abnormal vaginal spotting or bleeding. The Oxford Overview did not show an increase in the incidence of other tumors.[490]

Fewer than 1% of patients taking tamoxifen have thromboembolic complications,[560,567] but this is most marked with concomitant tamoxifen and IV administration of CMF.[641] Tamoxifen is associated with increased rates of hot flashes, vaginal discharge, and night sweats, but without a statistically significant effect on quality of life.[642] Hot flashes are a common and vexing symptom.[643] Selective serotonin reuptake inhibitors (e.g., paroxetine,[644] fluoxetine,[622] and venlafaxine[645]) appear to be the most effective agents, but other pharmacologic interventions have been investigated, such as clonidine,[646] vitamin E, gabapentin, soy phytoestrogens, and progestational agents, with intense debate about the safety of the latter two drugs.[647] Some other popular remedies, such as black cohosh,[621] offer little benefit.

Weight gain is commonly observed in patients with breast cancer,[619] and tamoxifen is associated with a small risk of inducing menopause, especially in patients older than 45 years of age.[619] Sarcopenic obesity is a simultaneous increase in fat mass and decrease in lean body mass that occurs in association with a number of medical conditions, including long-term corticosteroid use, prolonged physical inactivity, aging, and menopause.[622,623] The large NASBP prevention trial P-01 showed no detrimental effects on quality of life, mood, or sexual function in the tamoxifen-treated group.[648] Sexual dysfunction is rare and is more commonly associated with chemotherapy.[649] Ocular toxicities (e.g., corneal changes, tamoxifen retinopathy, and posterior subcapsular opacities) are rare,[650,651] but the NSABP recommends at least a baseline ophthalmologic evaluation.

Other Late Complications

As more women with early-stage breast cancer become long-term survivors, concerns about cancer recurrence are expected to decrease, and it is sometimes difficult for patients and their physicians to separate age-related symptoms from those that might be related to long-term effects of therapy. Data on the safety of menopausal

ADJUVANT SYSTEMIC TREATMENT FOR PATIENTS WITH OPERABLE BREAST CANCER

TREATMENT ACCORDING TO RESPONSIVENESS TO ENDOCRINE THERAPY

RISK GROUP	Endocrine-Responsive Disease		Endocrine-Nonresponsive Disease	
	Premenopausal	Postmenopausal	Premenopausal	Postmenopausal
Node-negative disease, minimal risk	Tamoxifen or none	Tamoxifen or none	Not applicable	Not applicable
Node-negative disease, average risk	Tamoxifen (± ovarian ablation),[*,†] or tamoxifen (± ovarian ablation) preceded by chemotherapy	Tamoxifen or tamoxifen preceded by chemotherapy	Chemotherapy	Chemotherapy
Node-positive disease	Tamoxifen (± ovarian ablation)[*,†] preceded by chemotherapy, or tamoxifen (± ovarian ablation)[*,†]	Tamoxifen preceded by chemotherapy or tamoxifen	Chemotherapy	Chemotherapy

*Some advocate the addition of ovarian ablation to tamoxifen in all women <35 yr.
†The addition of ovarian ablation to tamoxifen in women who do not receive chemotherapy or who remain premenopausal after chemotherapy is being evaluated by the Suppression of Ovarian Function Total (SOFT) International Breast Cancer Study Group trial 24-02. Evidence suggests that a few years of treatment with ovarian ablation alone offers similar survival outcome to chemotherapy; Most of these trials did not use anthracycline regimens or tamoxifen.
‡Tamoxifen and anastrozole are appropriate options for initial endocrine therapy in postmenopausal patients. Choice of drug should take into consideration toxicity profile and individual patient factors.
§Postmenopausal women who remain free of recurrence after 5 years of tamoxifen should consider up to 5 years of the aromatase inhibitor letrozole.
Adapted from Goldhirsch A, Wood WC, Geller RD, et al: Meeting highlights: Updated International Expert Consensus on the primary therapy of early breast cancer. J Clin Oncol 2003;21:3357–3365.

hormone replacement therapy in breast cancer survivors are limited, and are mostly derived from cohort and case-control studies.[652-654] Prospective randomized trials are lacking.[655] The use of complementary and alternative medications is a common and unreported practice among patients,[656] but few prospective controlled studies have been conducted.[657] Fatigue is another common symptom, especially in patients with higher levels of depression, pain, and sleep disturbance. Increasing evidence also shows that adjuvant chemotherapy may have long-term effects on cognitive function.[631]

Sexual disturbances are also common. A study in premenopausal women treated with goserelin vs. tamoxifen vs. the combination vs. no adjuvant endocrine therapy, with or without chemotherapy, found temporary disturbances in women treated with goserelin alone, no disturbances with tamoxifen alone, and lasting effects from a short course of adjuvant chemotherapy.[658] The investigators concluded that menopause induction might be a factor. Concerns about preserving fertility may play a role in the decision of young women considering ovarian ablation instead of chemotherapy in the adjuvant setting. Anecdotal reports suggest the possible use of LHRH analogs to prevent chemotherapy-induced amenorrhea among young women, but data on the effectiveness of this strategy to preserve fertility are lacking.[659]

DEFINITION OF RISK CATEGORIES FOR PATIENTS WITH NODE-NEGATIVE BREAST CANCER

RISK	ENDOCRINE-RESPONSIVE DISEASE	ENDOCRINE-NONRESPONSIVE DISEASE
Minimal	ER, PR, or both, expressed, and all of the following features: $pT \leq 2$ cm, Grade 1, Age ≥ 35 yr	Not applicable
Average	ER, PR, or both, expressed, and at least one of the following features: $pT > 2$ cm, Grade 2–3, Age < 35 yr	ER and PR absent

ER, estrogen receptor; PR, progesterone receptor; pT, pathologic tumor size.
Adapted from Goldhirsch A, Wood WC, Geller RD, et al: Meeting highlights: Updated International Expert Consensus on the primary therapy of early breast cancer. J Clin Oncol 2003;3357–3365.

Treatment Recommendations

Guidelines have been developed to help to identify patients who might benefit from adjuvant systemic therapy. These include the annual update of the U.S. National Comprehensive Cancer Network (NCCN) guidelines,[497] the biennial St. Gallen International Consensus Meeting,[499] the Cancer Care Ontario Practice Guidelines Initiative on node-negative disease,[500] and ad hoc panels, such as the November 2000 U.S. NIH Consensus Development Conference on adjuvant therapy for breast cancer.[501]

Endocrine therapy should be considered in all patients who have endocrine-responsive invasive disease because it reduces the annual odds of recurrence and death in all age and risk groups. In patients with very small tumors or small tumors with a favorable prognosis (e.g., pure lobular or pure tubular cancers), the risk may be low enough that no therapy is an option. This group may include patients who are at risk for significant complications (e.g., tamoxifen and thromboembolic disease; aromatase inhibitors and osteoporosis and bone fracture). Women with low levels of ER or PR by immunohistochemistry should not be erroneously labeled as having endocrine-unresponsive disease (false-negative result), because they may benefit from adjuvant endocrine therapy.[660]

The NIH Consensus panel made the following recommendations for endocrine therapy:

1. The decision to recommend adjuvant hormonal therapy should be based on ER and PR status as determined by immunohistochemical staining. If the specimen is insufficient, positivity is assumed, especially in postmenopausal women.
2. There is insufficient evidence to support the use of *HER2* expression to influence the choice of endocrine therapy.
3. Tamoxifen should not be offered to women with endocrine-unresponsive (ER-negative, PR-negative) disease.
4. Five years of adjuvant tamoxifen therapy should be recommended for all women with endocrine-responsive (ER- or PR-positive) disease, regardless of age, menopausal status, axillary lymph node status, tumor size, or use of adjuvant chemotherapy. Possible exceptions include women with small (<1 cm), node-negative tumors who wish to avoid the side effects of tamoxifen.
5. Ovarian ablation or suppression may be considered an alternative to chemotherapy in premenopausal women.[501]

These recommendations emphasize that the benefit from adjuvant tamoxifen far outweighs most risks (e.g., endometrial cancer and venous thromboembolism), and that screening tests such as transvaginal ultrasonography and endometrial biopsy are not recommended in asymptomatic women receiving tamoxifen. No data support the use of other SERMs (e.g., raloxifene and toremifene) in the adjuvant setting. However, preliminary results from the ATAC trial support the use of the aromatase inhibitor anastrozole instead of tamoxifen in postmenopausal women.[555,591] As previously noted in this chapter, postmenopausal women who have completed 5 years of tamoxifen can also benefit from an additional 5 years of letrozole.

Administration of polychemotherapy for several months appears to provide optimal benefit in reducing the risk of recurrence and death. Anthracycline-containing regimens offer a small but statistically significant improvement in survival compared with nonanthracycline regimens. No meaningful improvement in survival is observed with more dose-intensive treatment regimens, such as high-dose chemotherapy with peripheral stem cell support.[545,546] Recent updates on the role of paclitaxel after AC as adjuvant therapy for node-positive disease confirmed a survival benefit. It is difficult to identify specific groups of patients who may not require adjuvant chemotherapy. Women with node-negative cancers smaller than 1 cm in diameter and those with favorable histologic subtypes without lymph node involvement may do well without chemotherapy. The benefit from chemotherapy in women 70 years of age and older is controversial. A sequential approach, with combined chemotherapy followed by tamoxifen, is preferred over their concomitant use.[595] Efficacy data favor the use of the classic CMF regimen with oral cyclophosphamide over CMF variants, especially if combined with sequential tamoxifen.[661]

The chemotherapy benefit seen in premenopausal women appears to be due in part to ovarian suppression, even if temporary. Ongoing studies with contemporary chemotherapy regimens will help to determine whether a few years of ovarian ablation plus tamoxifen or an aromatase inhibitor adds to or eliminates the need for cytotoxic chemotherapy. A growing consensus indicates that adjuvant chemotherapy in truly postmenopausal women with node-negative, endocrine-responsive disease offers little additional benefit to women who are committed to 5 years of treatment with tamoxifen.[511,593,594]

Follow-up

There is significant interest in identifying post-treatment surveillance strategies for early detection of breast cancer recurrence. These strategies must take into account the effect on several outcomes of interest, such as survival, quality of life, reduction in toxicity, and cost-effectiveness. Clinical practice guidelines issued by the American Society of Clinical Oncology concluded that sufficient data exist to recommend monthly breast self-examination, annual mammography, and a clinical evaluation every 3 to 6 months for 3 years, then every 6 to 12 months for 2 years, and then annually.[662] Data were insufficient to recommend imaging studies (e.g., bone scan, chest x-ray, ultrasound, and computed tomography scans) other than the annual screening mammogram. Although preliminary evidence suggests a potential role for screening for the MUC-1 gene product (CA 27.29 antigen),[663] its effect on the endpoints of interest is unknown. Tumor markers are not recommended for post-treatment surveillance because few data show their usefulness in improving survival and quality of life.[662] Patients should continue their routine health maintenance evaluation, including other cancer screening, and report any new symptom of concern, such as new pain, dyspnea, or weight loss, to their physicians.

New Strategies in Adjuvant Treatment

Greater understanding of the molecular pathophysiology of breast cancer should help with the identification and integration of novel and more selective therapies into daily practice. The identification of patients who are at risk for recurrence (prognostic markers) and are most likely to benefit from a specific intervention (predictive markers) remains a challenge. A further challenge is the selection of those who are most likely to benefit and least likely to be harmed by systemic therapies with a narrow therapeutic index. There is significant interest in developing more effective diagnostic, prognostic, and predictive markers. Promising technologies include gene expression profiles using microarray techniques.[277,278] Proteomics to identify serum biomarkers with predictive or prognostic value[279,280] hold the potential for large-scale tumor profiling.

HER2 overexpression in breast cancer tissue is the most recent example of targeted therapy. Based on clinical evidence of activity as a single agent[664,665] and the survival advantage when added to chemotherapy in patients with metastatic disease,[666] ongoing randomized trials of the recombinant monoclonal anti-HER2 antibody trastuzumab are examining its role in patients with early-stage, node-positive disease. The potential risk of cardiac dysfunction seen in randomized trials of trastuzumab in metastatic disease (especially if combined with anthracyclines) poses a significant challenge in its development in the adjuvant setting.[667,668]

Significant bone mineral loss is seen in premenopausal women who have chemotherapy-induced ovarian failure after adjuvant therapy.[669] Bisphosphonates have a potential role in minimizing this bone loss,[625] but their use must be confirmed in larger efficacy trials. Postmenopausal women who discontinue menopausal replacement therapy have more significant bone loss than non-HRT users. This effect is not ameliorated by therapy with tamoxifen (or toremifene), with or without clodronate.[670] Bisphosphonates reduce the risk of bone-related complications in patients with metastatic disease.[671-673] However, data from small trials on the use of adjuvant bisphosphonates to reduce the risk of bone or visceral recurrence are conflicting.[674-676] Larger studies are ongoing.

New cytotoxic drugs, such as the oral fluoropyrimidine capecitabine, are being tested in the adjuvant setting, both in combination and in single-agent regimens. Preoperative systemic therapy offers the opportunity for early in vivo assessment of response at surgery.[606] Ongoing studies will confirm whether pathologic response after preoperative systemic therapy can serve as an early surrogate prognostic and/or predictive marker.

MANAGEMENT OF LOCALLY ADVANCED BREAST CANCER

Locally advanced breast cancer (LABC) has always included a heterogeneous group of presentations. With the 2002 changes to the AJCC staging system, LABC can technically include a patient with a clinically apparent internal mammary or paraclavicular node as well as the more commonly accepted presentations, including a primary breast cancer larger than 5 cm, disease fixed to the chest wall or involving the skin, or bulky palpable disease in the axilla. Inflammatory breast cancer is sometimes included in the category of LABC, but is discussed separately in this chapter.

With such a broad spectrum of presentations, survival rates for LABC vary significantly among series, reflecting institutional differences in therapeutic policies and patient selection bias. Although some series report 5-year survival rates of greater than 70%,[677,678] these series exclude patients with inflammatory disease, the most aggressive form of nonmetastatic breast cancer. Comparison of treatment results among institutions requires critical review to assess the comparability of patient groups.

The philosophy toward the management of LABC has changed significantly through the years. Historically, surgery and radiation therapy were the only treatments available. However, with the advent of chemotherapy, multimodality approaches that emphasize systemic therapy have become the standard of treatment.

Surgery or Radiation Therapy Alone

In 1943, Haagensen and Stout[679] observed clinical signs of advanced-stage breast cancer and correlated these clinical findings with operative results and overall survival rates. From their observations, they established the first criteria of inoperability. These criteria represented clinical findings associated with such a poor survival rate that aggressive surgery was not warranted, and included extensive edema of the skin of the breast, satellite tumor nodules in the skin, inflammatory cancer, involvement of supraclavicular or internal mammary nodes, and preoperative arm edema as a result of massive axillary node involvement. Five additional factors, the "Grave signs," were also identified with advanced-stage disease. They included edema limited to one third of the skin over the breast, skin ulceration, fixation of tumor to the chest wall, axillary nodes measuring at least 2.5 cm, and axillary nodes fixed to either the skin or structures in the axilla. Although local recurrence rates after mastectomy were increased in the presence of one Grave sign compared with early-stage disease, continued use of mastectomy was justified (Table 94-20). Combinations of any two or more Grave signs increased the rate of local recurrence and decreased the 5-year survival rate even further. These patients were considered clinically inoperable and usually were referred for palliative radiation therapy.

Because many patients with categorically inoperable breast cancer were referred for radiation, data were soon collected evaluating the ability of radiation therapy to achieve locoregional control in LABC. The doses administered to the breast in earlier studies were limited by acute skin reactions from the available orthovoltage treatment units. To reduce acute skin toxicity, Baclesse[680] developed a protracted radiation fractionation to deliver high doses to the breast and regional nodes over a long interval. With doses of up to 9000 R over a minimum of

TABLE 94-20

Radical Mastectomy Results Among Patients with Grave Signs

CLINICAL SIGN	NO. OF CASES	LOCAL RECURRENCE (%)	5-YR DISEASE-FREE SURVIVAL (%)
Limited skin edema	75	32	23
Skin ulceration	14	14	36
Fixation to the chest wall	20	40	5
Axillary nodes ≥2.5 cm	24	13	38
Fixed axillary nodes	8	13	13

From Haagensen CD, Stout AP: Carcinoma of the breast, criteria of operability. Ann Surg 1943;118:859.

3 months, durable locoregional control was achieved in 58% of patients with T3 and T4 disease. Fletcher and Montague[681] achieved a 68% rate of locoregional control using similar fractionation. Their study included some patients with inflammatory disease.

Using standard fractionation, a review of the literature suggests a dose–response relationship for locally advanced disease (Table 94-21). Bruckman and colleagues[682] found significant improvement in local control in patients receiving a total dose of 60 Gy or greater vs. less than 60 Gy, with 5-year control rates of 78% vs. 39%, respectively. Researchers at the Princess Margaret Hospital and the Institute Gustave-Roussy reviewed the outcome of 463 patients with breast cancer treated by radiation therapy alone. They generated a model predicting local control using tumor size, tumor fixation, and nodal fixation.[683] Although both tumor dose and tumor size were independent predictors for local control, dose was the most significant factor predicting for recurrence, with dose increases of 15 Gy resulting in twofold differences in rates of local control. Complications, however, were also increased. Spanos and associates[684] reported an increased rate of fibrosis and necrosis of the chest wall with doses greater than 81 Gy. These complications continued to occur at a similar rate among survivors living more than 10 years from treatment. Bedwinek and colleagues[685] found that 19% of patients treated with high-dose radiation had moderate to severe breast fibrosis. Other complications included breast edema, arm edema, brachial plexus injury, and shoulder stiffness.

Radiation therapy has been administered as an adjuvant to mastectomy for LABC, both preoperatively and postoperatively. Postoperative therapy is usually delivered to patients with operable disease. Preoperative radiation therapy has been used to convert unresectable or marginally resectable cancers into technically resectable disease. From series in which radiation therapy was delivered preoperatively, pathologic review of mastectomy specimens yields information about the ability of radiation therapy to sterilize disease. Despite delivery of 60 to 70 Gy to the breast and regional nodes, Zucali and associates[686] found 75% of mastectomy specimens to

TABLE 94-21

Radiation Therapy Alone in Locally Advanced Breast Cancer

REFERENCE	YEARS OF TREATMENT	NO. OF PATIENTS	INFLAMMATORY CARCINOMA	RADIATION DOSE (GY)	5-YR SURVIVAL (%)	LOCO-REGIONAL CONTROL (%)	NOTES
Fletcher et al.*	1948–1962	273	47 (17)	80–100	Inflammatory 12 Noninflammatory 28	68	Protracted therapy over 10–11 weeks
Bruckman et al.†	1968–1976	116	18 (15)	40–85	25	64	Therapy over 6.5 weeks; 41 patients received adjuvant therapy
Treurniet-Donker et al.‡	1965–1974	129	25 (19)	46–70	17	60 with MeV 30 with orthovoltage	Local control evaluated at 40 months among responders
Almaric et al.§	1960–1974	341	0	75–80	37**	59	
Bedwinek et al.‖	1960–1975	83	29 (35)	40–70		Inflammatory 48 Noninflammatory 39	
Chu et al.#	1958–1978	147	0	60–70	24	49	63 patients received adjuvant therapy
Alderman et al.¶		18		100		100	

*Fletcher GH, Montague ED: Radical irradiation of advanced breast cancer. Am J Roentgenol Radium Ther Nucl Med 1965;93:573.
†Bruckman JE, Harris JR, Levene MB, et al: Results of treating stage III carcinoma of the breast by primary radiation therapy. Cancer 1979;43:985.
‡Treurniet-Donker A, Hop W, Hold-Sijtseona S: Radiation treatment of stage III mammary carcinoma: A review of 129 patients. Int J Radiat Oncol Biol Phys 1980;6:1477.
§Almaric R, Santamaria F, Robert F, et al: Radiation therapy with or without primary limited surgery for operable breast cancer. Cancer 1982;49:30.
‖Bedwinek J, Rao DV, Perez C, et al: Stage III and localized stage IV breast cancer: irradiation alone vs. irradiation plus surgery. Int J Radiat Oncol Biol Phys 1982;8:31.
#Chu AM, Cope O, Doucette J, et al: Non-metastatic locally advanced cancer of the breast treated with radiation. Int J Radiat Oncol Biol Phys 1984;10:2299.
¶Alderman S: Combination teletherapy and iridium implantation in the treatment of locally advanced breast cancer. Cancer 1976;38:1936.
**Disease-free survival.

contain residual tumor in patients with a complete clinical response. This and other series using preoperative radiation therapy confirmed the need to deliver high-dose radiation therapy for durable local control if patients were treated with radiation therapy only.

The combination of mastectomy and lower-dose radiation therapy has increased the overall rate of locoregional control. In a series from M.D. Anderson, 376 women with noninflammatory LABD were treated with mastectomy followed by external beam radiation therapy.[687] The chest wall and nodes received a minimum of 50 Gy over 5 weeks, followed by a 10- to 20-Gy boost limited to the scar. With median follow-up of 17.7 years, the rate of locoregional control was 88% for stage IIIA disease and 74% for stage IIIB disease. Thus, with only 50 Gy delivered after mastectomy, locoregional control rates were improved relative to historical controls treated with radiation therapy only. Bedwinek and colleagues[685] compared the complications seen in patients treated with radiation therapy with and without mastectomy. The fibrosis, shoulder stiffness, and brachial plexus injury seen with high doses of external beam radiation therapy alone were not apparent with surgery and postoperative radiation therapy. Arm edema, however, was increased compared with patients treated with radiation therapy only.

Retrospective comparisons between radiation therapy alone and surgery with preoperative or postoperative radiation therapy showed a significant benefit in locoregional control and overall survival for combined locoregional therapy.[678,685,686,688] These results, however, reflect significant bias in patient selection. Patients with resectable or borderline resectable lesions tended to be treated with combined local therapy, whereas those with categorically inoperable disease usually received radiation therapy only. Because no large prospective trials randomized patients to radiation therapy alone vs. mastectomy and postoperative radiation therapy, local control and survival with radiation therapy with and without surgery cannot be directly compared.

Systemic Therapy

Rationale
Despite improvements in locoregional control with surgery and radiation therapy, the predominant pattern of failure in LABD remained distant metastatic disease.[679,686,689] The probability of distant dissemination is strongly associated with the rate of axillary node involvement, and nodal involvement is, by definition, frequent in these patients.[678,679,687,690,691] With the development of systemic therapies to address micrometastatic disease, chemotherapy has become as important as locoregional treatment of LABD. In some studies, chemotherapy was delivered after the completion of locoregional therapy (i.e., adjuvant chemotherapy). This approach has the theoretical advantage of delivering chemotherapy when the tumor burden is minimal, decreasing the risk of chemoresistant cells. In other series of operable and inoperable cases, chemotherapy was administered initially (preoperative therapy), followed by local therapy and additional adjuvant chemotherapy.

The rationale for this approach includes delivery of systemic therapy early in treatment to attempt to reduce subclinical micrometastatic disease, reduce local and regional tumor bulk, and increase the likelihood of successful surgical resection. In addition, the appropriateness of the systemic agents chosen can be assessed by following the patient's locoregional clinical response.

Pilot studies also showed the ability of induction chemotherapy to sterilize tumor, now recognized as a prognostic factor for women with LABC. Feldman and associates[692] reported results of a study in which patients received FAC (5-fluorouracil, doxorubicin, and cyclophosphamide) followed by mastectomy and radiation therapy. Seventeen percent of patients had no gross residual disease at surgery. Of these women, 40% had no microscopic residual disease in their mastectomy specimens, and the overall pathologic complete response was 7%. A study from Johns Hopkins reported a 17% pathologic complete response using an intensive doxorubicin- and antimetabolite-based regimen.[693] Both series included patients with inflammatory disease.

With the introduction of colony-stimulating factors, dose escalation in this group of women has been possible. This dose escalation, coupled with novel combinations of chemotherapy, has continued to result in increasing response rate to systemic treatment.

Retrospective Trials
Multiple retrospective studies showed a survival benefit with the addition of chemotherapy to local therapy, when compared with historical control subjects treated with local therapy only. In some series, chemotherapy was administered after surgery, but most recent series combined preoperative and postsurgical therapy. Other endpoints for comparison of these studies include local control rates, clinical tumor response, and pathologic tumor response when patients undergo mastectomy. In some cases, the clinical response has been judged significant, and a significant proportion of women were able to undergo less invasive procedures than mastectomy.

This approach is shown in a report of 372 patients with LABC who were treated with FAC at M.D. Anderson between 1989 and 1996. After preoperative chemotherapy, these women underwent either segmental mastectomy and axillary node dissection (29%) or modified radical mastectomy (71%). The decision about the type of surgery was based on the clinical response of the tumor and initial prechemotherapy disease bulk. In this series, 31% of primary tumors were smaller than 5 cm, and 20% of women had no clinically detectable axillary adenopathy at diagnosis. After the surgical procedure, all of the women had more chemotherapy and then locoregional radiation therapy. With a median follow-up of 58 months, patients were analyzed by complete pathologic response vs. incomplete pathologic response at the time of surgery. Twelve percent of patients achieved complete pathologic response, and that subset of women had 5-year overall and disease-free survival rates of 89% and 87%, respectively. In comparison, the subset of women who had less than complete pathologic response had an overall survival rate of 64% and a disease-free survival rate of 58% at 5 years. In the subset of patients undergoing segmental mastectomy, the 5-year survival rate was 82%, compared with 66% for those who needed mastectomy after chemotherapy.[694]

Many chemotherapy combinations have been used for this group of patients, with similar results. Each series had different entry criteria, however, reflecting the heterogeneity of LABC.

Randomized Trials
Trials Evaluating Systemic Therapy Plus Local Radiation with Radiation Only.
EORTC Breast Cancer Cooperative trial 10792, the largest randomized trial completed in patients with LABC, was reanalyzed 8 years after trial closure. Specifically, 410 patients with LABC, including 48 women with inflammatory disease, were randomized to receive radiation therapy alone, radiation therapy with chemotherapy, radiation therapy with hormonal therapy, or radiation therapy with both chemotherapy and hormonal therapy. Patients who were randomized to receive chemotherapy received 12 cycles of CMF. Premenopausal women who were randomized to receive hormonal therapy received ovarian irradiation, whereas postmenopausal women who were randomized to receive hormonal therapy received tamoxifen. With a median follow-up of 8 years, both hormonal therapy and chemotherapy reduced the risk of locoregional failure from approximately 60% to 47%. Hormonal therapy significantly improved survival, with a 25% reduction in the death hazards ratio. Unlike an interim analysis that showed a significant improvement in survival in the chemotherapy arm, this benefit did not remain statistically significant with further follow-up. In the most recent analysis, however, the greatest survival benefit was observed in women who received both hormonal therapy and chemotherapy with radiation, with a 35% reduction in the death hazards risk.[695]

Trials Comparing Multimodality Therapy.
Randomized trials showed suboptimal local control with either mastectomy or radiation therapy after primary chemotherapy (Table 94-22). Perloff and associates[696] from CALGB reported locoregional failure rates of 19% and 27% after preoperative chemotherapy with mastectomy vs. radiation therapy, respectively, with only 3-year follow-up. Similar findings were reported by DeLena and associates in Milan, with locoregional failure rates of 30% and 31% reported with mastectomy and radiation therapy, respectively, after primary therapy with doxorubicin and vincristine at 3 years of follow-up.[697]

Based on these results, other studies evaluated mastectomy, with or without postoperative radiation therapy, in conjunction with chemotherapy.[677,697] In an ECOG study, patients randomized to receive radiation therapy after mastectomy and adjuvant chemotherapy had a 15% rate of local failure as first failure, compared with a local failure rate of 24% in the absence of radiation therapy.[697] In the Helsinki trial reported by Klefstrom and associates,[677] crude rates of local failure as first failure exceeded 50% for patients receiving adjuvant chemotherapy without radiation therapy compared with 20% for those receiving adjuvant radiation therapy and 13% for those receiving the combination of radiation therapy and adjuvant chemotherapy after mastectomy. It appears that maximal locoregional control in LABC is achieved with the combination of surgery, radiation therapy, and chemotherapy, although large-scale trials have not been performed

TABLE 94-22

Locoregional Control in Randomized Trials in Locally Advanced Breast Cancer

REFERENCE	NO. OF PATIENTS	SCHEMA	LOCOREGIONAL CONTROL (%)	FOLLOW-UP (YR)
DeLena et al.*	132	AV { RM → AV	70	3
		RT → AV	69	
Perloff et al.†	133	CAFVP { M → CAFVP	81	3
		RT → CAFVP	73	
Klefstrom et al.‡	120	M { RT	80	
		VAC ± levamisole	43	5
		RT + VAC	87	
Olson et al.§	312	M + CAFTH { RT	85	
		Observation	76	9
Papaioannou et al.‖	105	VACMF + M + Oophor { RT + VACMF	92	2
		Observation	89	

AV, doxorubicin, vincristine; CAFVP, cyclophosphamide, doxorubicin, 5-fluorouracil, vincristine, prednisone; M, mastectomy; Oophor, oophorectomy; RM, radical mastectomy; RT, radiation therapy; VAC, vincristine, doxorubicin, cyclophosphamide; VACMF, vincristine, doxorubicin, cyclophosphamide, methotrexate, 5-fluorouracil.

*DeLena M, Varini M, Zucali R, et al: Multi-modal treatment for locally advanced breast cancer: Results of chemotherapy-radiotherapy versus chemotherapy-surgery. Cancer Clin Trials 1981;4:229.

†Perloff M, Lesnick GJ, Korzun A, et al: Combination chemotherapy with mastectomy or radiotherapy for stage III breast carcinoma: A Cancer and Leukemia Group B study. J Clin Oncol 1988;6:261.

‡Klefstrom P, Grohn P, Heinonen E, et al: Adjuvant postoperative radiotherapy, chemotherapy and immunotherapy in stage III breast cancer. Cancer 1987;60:936.

§Olson JE, Neuberg D, Pandya KJ, et al: The role of radiotherapy in the management of operable locally advanced breast cancer. Cancer 1997;79:1138.

‖Papaioannou A, Lissaios B, Vasilaros S, et al: Pre- and postoperative chemoendocrine treatment with or without postoperative radiotherapy for locally advanced breast cancer. Cancer 1983;51:1284.

comparing locoregional outcomes after contemporary chemotherapy and radiation therapy with or without mastectomy. However, given the success shown with postmastectomy radiation therapy, the combined use of mastectomy and radiation therapy (with chemotherapy) is the most common locoregional treatment approach in LABC.

Breast-Conservation Therapy

As described earlier, induction chemotherapy has the ability to cytoreduce locoregional disease. Some patients receiving primary chemotherapy achieve complete clinical response. Attention has been directed toward the identification of patients with an excellent response to preoperative therapy who are possible candidates for breast conservation. The goals of this approach are the same as for women with early-stage disease who are candidates for breast conservation (i.e., optimal locoregional control with acceptable cosmesis of the treated breast).

To study the feasibility of breast preservation in advanced disease, mastectomy specimens from 143 patients with stage IIB and III breast cancer who were treated at M.D. Anderson Cancer Center were retrospectively analyzed after preoperative chemotherapy.[698] Using the criteria for breast preservation in early-stage disease, 23% of these women would have been good candidates for breast conservation after receiving preoperative chemotherapy. Based on this experience, breast conser-

vation is now offered to appropriate candidates with LABC using similar criteria as in early-stage disease, as discussed earlier. Investigators at the NCI and the University of Michigan reported their results with breast conservation using a selection process based on biopsy-proven pathologic criteria.[699,700] Investigators at both institutions prospectively administered primary chemotherapy and performed a biopsy at the primary site, either after maximal clinical response (NCI study) or after a fixed number of cycles (Michigan study). For patients with a complete pathologic response, definitive locoregional radiation therapy was delivered. The more conventional mastectomy with postoperative radiation therapy was administered to patients with residual disease at biopsy. With a median follow-up of 5.3 years, the 5-year actuarial locoregional failure rate as first site of first failure was 23% with breast conservation in the NCI series.[699] Similarly, with a median follow-up of 4.5 years, the 5-year actuarial estimate of locoregional failure as isolated first failure was 18% in the Michigan series.[700]

Representative trials using breast preservation in LABC are shown in Table 94-23. Breast conservation in locally advanced disease is under study in many centers in conjunction with aggressive induction chemotherapy. Although in general, local control is maximally achieved with mastectomy and postoperative radiation therapy, in selected subgroups of patients who respond to preoperative chemotherapy, breast-conserving therapy

TABLE 94-23

Breast Preservation Studies in Stage III Disease

REFERENCE	NO. OF PATIENTS	% INFLAMMATORY	CHEMOTHERAPY	RADIATION DOSE (GY)	LOCOREGIONAL CONTROL (%)
Pierce et al.*	107	43	CAMFPT	60	77
Hery et al.†	25	0	CAVF	60–75	76
Lamb et al.‡	65	100	CA/CMF‡‡	60–73	54
Borger et al.§	209	0	CMF ± AV§§	65	45–47
Baillet et al.‖	134	5	VTMFA	65–75	80
Touboul et al.#	97	0	CAVF	65–75	80 with RT alone
					77 with lumpectomy
Ahern et al.**	67	0	AC/CMF or NC/CMF	80	86 for tumors <10 cm
					50 for tumors >10 cm
Merajver et al.††		40	CAMFPT	64	82

AC, doxorubicin, cyclophosphamide; AV, doxorubicin, vincristine; CA, cyclophosphamide, doxorubicin; CAMFPT, cyclophosphamide, doxorubicin, methotrexate, 5-fluorouracil, prednisone, tamoxifen; CAVF, cyclophosphamide, doxorubicin, vincristine, 5-fluorouracil; CMF, cyclophosphamide, methotrexate, 5-fluorouracil; NC, Novantrone, cyclophosphamide; RT, radiation therapy; VTMFA, vinblastine, thiotepa, methotrexate, 5-fluorouracil, doxorubicin.
*Pierce L, Lippman M, Ben-Baruch N, et al: The effect of systemic therapy on local-regional control in locally advanced breast cancer. Int J Radiat Oncol Biol Phys 1992;23:949.
†Hery M, Namer M, Moro M, et al: Conservative treatment of locally advanced breast cancer. Cancer 1986;57:1744.
‡Lamb C, Eberlein T, Parker L, et al: Results of radical radiotherapy for inflammatory breast cancer. Am J Surg 1991;162:236.
§Borger J, van Tienhover G, Passchier D, et al: Primary radiotherapy of breast cancer: treatment results in locally advanced breast cancer and in operable patients selected by positive axillary apex biopsy. Radiother Oncol 1992;25:1.
‖Baillet F, Rozec C, Ucla L, et al: Tratment of locally advanced breast cancer without mastectomy: 5- and 10-yr results of 135 tumors larger than 5 cm treated by external beam therapy, brachytherapy and neoadjuvant chemotherapy [abstract]. In Pisa Symposia in Oncology. Breast Cancer from Biology to Therapy, 1992, p 22.
#Touboul E, Lefranc J-P, Blondon J, et al: Primary chemotherapy and preoperative irradiation for patients with stage II larger than 3 cm or locally advanced non-inflammatory breast cancer. Radiother Oncol 1997;42:219.
**Ahern V, Barraclough B, Bosch C, et al: Locally advanced breast cancer: Defining an optimum treatment regimen. Int J Radiat Oncol Biol Phys 1994;28:867.
††Merajver SD, Weber BL, Cody r, et al: Breast conservation and prolonged chemotherapy for locally advanced breast cancer: the University of Michigan Experience. J Clin Oncol 1997;15:2873.
‡‡Administered to 72% of patients.
§§Administered to 30% of patients.

appears to yield local control rates similar to those attainable with mastectomy and radiation therapy.

Strategies for Improved Response and Outcome

Because most series show superior survival in patients with a complete pathologic response to preoperative therapy, strategies have been designed with this goal in mind. Efforts to improve response to chemotherapy include attempts to synchronize tumor cells with hormonal agents. Conte and associates[701] used estrogenic recruitment in conjunction with cytotoxic chemotherapy and achieved a 15% clinical complete response rate. The 3-year rate of progression-free survival was 54%. A subsequent randomized trial with FAC chemotherapy, with or without diethylstilbestrol,[702] showed higher response and disease-free survival rates for patients receiving estrogenic recruitment. Survival rates did not improve with estrogenic stimulation, with 4-year survival rates of 74% and 77%, respectively, with and without diethylstilbestrol. Others also found higher objective response rates with hormonal manipulation, without improvements in overall survival rates.[699,700,703] Pierce and associates[699] and Lippman and colleagues[704] at the NCI also used a strategy for hormonal synchronization with both estrogens and antiestrogens in their approach to locally advanced disease. Despite complete clinical response rates of 50% with stage IIIA disease and 57% with inflammatory disease, the 5-year survival rates did not significantly differ from survival results in other series that did not use hormonal synchronization.

Another strategy for improved response is the use of non-cross-resistant therapies. Clinical trials show a trend toward improved disease-free and overall survival rates among patients receiving both methotrexate- and doxorubicin-based regimens. In a prospective trial from the North Central Treatment Group in conjunction with the Mayo Clinic, objective responses were achieved in 65% of women after alternating preoperative chemotherapy, with 5-year relapse-free and overall survival rates of 42% and 57%, respectively.[703] Given the excellent response rates to taxanes in metastatic breast cancer and the significant disease-free and overall survival benefit shown by the addition of paclitaxel in stage II disease,[705] taxanes are used extensively as non-cross-resistant agents with doxorubicin in stage III breast cancer.

The use of ablative chemotherapy with bone marrow or stem cell[706,707] rescue is also under study. Mulder and colleagues[708] described 19 patients with locally advanced disease who had a complete response to induction chemotherapy and underwent autologous transplant. After a median observation time of 48 months, 58% of patients were disease-free. It is difficult to attribute this outcome to a specific part of this regimen, because some patients survived disease-free for longer than 36 months without intensification and transplant. Ayash and colleagues[707] from the Dana Farber Cancer Institute and Wake Forest University reported their results in women with stage IIIB disease. With a patient population consisting primarily of women with stage IIIB disease, the 30-month disease-free survival rate was 64%. For patients with complete pathologic response or microscopic or gross residual disease after induction chemotherapy and intensification, 30-month disease-free survival rates were 100%, 70%, and 38%, respectively. Although these results compare favorably with published results of women treated with conventional therapy, follow-up is much too short to allow comparisons between series. A small randomized trial of conventional therapy vs. transplant from the Netherlands was reported for stage II and III disease and showed no difference in disease-free and overall survival rates with high-dose therapy.[709] Thus, the potential benefit of aggressive therapy with bone marrow transplant compared with results achieved with induction and maintenance therapy await the outcome of large randomized trials.

Advances in breast imaging are also emerging as tools to select patients for further therapy after preoperative chemotherapy. ^{99m}Tc sestamibi scans performed before and after chemotherapy showed an ability to assess response, when correlated with later pathology findings at surgery.[710,711] A recent study using PET imaging with ^{18}fluorodeoxyglucose (FDG) was similarly successful in predicting response to preoperative treatment. Histopathologic response was predicted in this small study of 22 women, with an accuracy of 88%.[712]

Biologic markers, as discussed elsewhere in this chapter, will likely play a significant role in tailoring multimodality treatments in this complex group of tumors. Similarly, initial studies with sentinel lymph node mapping after preoperative chemotherapy showed that a sentinel node was identified in 82% of cases. The sentinel node was predictive of the final pathology of the full dissection that followed in each case.[713] Results from NSABP B-27 also confirm the feasibility of performing sentinel lymph node biopsy after preoperative chemotherapy.[714]

INFLAMMATORY DISEASE

Inflammatory breast cancer is the most aggressive form of nonmetastatic breast cancer. Although it accounts for only 1% to 4% of breast cancers in the United States, it has a striking presentation.[715,716] Characteristics essential to the clinical diagnosis include rapid enlargement and generalized induration of the breast, often without an associated mass. Haagensen and Stout[679] described erythema of the skin affecting more than one third of the breast as the most distinctive clinical feature of the disease. Flattening and retraction of the nipple, with diffuse breast warmth and peau d'orange, are common in inflammatory disease, and most patients have palpable axillary adenopathy. Approximately 35% of patients with inflammatory carcinoma have obvious metastases at diagnosis.[717] A history of treatment with systemic antibiotics for presumed mastitis is common with this carcinoma before a biopsy establishes the true diagnosis.

Pathologic Findings

Pathologically, inflammatory cancer is not a distinct histologic entity. However, dermal lymphatic involvement is the pathologic hallmark of the disease. Since the first description by Bryant[718] in 1887, many studies have associated the clinical findings with carcinoma in the lymphatics of the skin. Thorough examination of mastectomy specimens confirms dermal lymphatic involvement in as many as 70% of women with clinical signs of inflammatory carcinoma.[719,720]

Dispute exists in the literature about the criteria necessary to diagnose inflammatory breast cancer. Although some believe that clinical findings alone are adequate to make the diagnosis, others argue that a skin biopsy confirming dermal lymphatic involvement is essential. A review from the Mallinckrodt Institute examining prognostic factors in inflammatory cancer found no difference in outcome among patients diagnosed based on either clinical findings or dermal lymphatic involvement.[709]

It is unclear whether patients with either clinical or pathologic criteria alone have comparable clinical outcomes. Such determination would require a prospective trial. Critical review of the literature is required if these subsets are to be compared, because different series include patients diagnosed on the basis of clinical or pathologic criteria, or both.

Multimodality Therapy

Combined-modality therapy with chemotherapy and locoregional treatment has become the standard approach to the treatment of inflammatory breast cancer, similar to the evolution of treatment for other types of LABC. Survival comparisons between historical control subjects treated with local therapy only and patients receiving systemic therapy in addition to local therapy showed marked improvements in survival with the addition of chemotherapy.[721] Although patients with inflammatory cancer were included in the Netherlands Cancer Institute[722] and EORTC trials,[723] which randomized women to receive chemotherapy or hormonal therapy, separate survival analyses were not performed for the subset of patients with inflammatory disease.

However, retrospective data are convincing for a survival benefit and support the routine use of systemic therapy in this disease (Table 94-24). Depending on the choice of chemotherapeutic and locoregional treatment, disease-free survival rates at 5 years generally exceeded 25% to 30%, with 5-year survival rates approaching 40%.

In many trials, response to chemotherapy was an important predictor of survival.[721,724,725] One hundred seventy-eight women with this disease were treated in four successive protocols at M.D. Anderson between 1974 and 1993.[724] In each trial, either FAC or FAC plus vincristine and prednisone (FACVP) was administered as primary therapy, followed by either radiation therapy alone or surgery and radiation therapy with adjuvant chemotherapy. Seventy-two percent of patients achieved at least a partial response, and 12% achieved a complete clinical response. The median disease-free and overall

TABLE 94-24

STUDY	TREATMENT PROGRAM	NO. OF PATIENTS	PATIENTS RENDERED DISEASE-FREE (%)	MEDIAN SURVIVAL TIME (MO)	5-YR SURVIVAL RATE (%)
DeLena et al.	CT + RT ± CT	36	73	25	NA
Chu et al.	RT + H	14	NA	15	NA
	RT + CT	16	NA	>26	NA
Pouillart et al.	CT + RT + CT	77	51	34	NA
Zylberberg et al.	CT + S + CT ± RT	15	100	>50	70
Pawlicki et al.	CT ± S + RT	72	NA	NA	NA
Loprinzi et al.	S + CT + RT + CT	9	100	>25	55
Keiling et al.	CT + S + CT	41	100	NR	63
Jacquillat et al.	CT + RT + CT + H	66	100	NR	66
Alberto et al.	CT + S + CT + RT	22	95	26	10
Ferriere et al.	CT + RT ± S + CT	75	93	NR	54
Pourny et al.	CT + S ± RT + CT	33	82	70	60
Chevallier et al.	CT + RT ± CT ± S	178	83	37	32
Rouesse et al.	CT + RT + CT + H	91	41	36	40
Israel et al.	CT + S + CT	25	96	NR	62
Krutchik et al.	CT + RT + CT	32	NA	24	NA
Brun et al.	CT + RT + S + CT	26	NA	31	NA
Thoms et al.	CT + S + CT + RT	61	NA	61	35
Swain et al.	CT + RT + S + CT + H	45	NA	36	NR
Fields et al.	CT + S + RT + CT	37	NA	49	44
Maloisel et al.	CT + S + CT + RT + H	43	NA	46	75
Koh et al.	CT + RT + CT	40	NA	39	37
	CT + S + CT + RT	23	NA	38	30
	CT + S + CT + RT	43	NA	31	40

CT, chemotherapy; H, hormone therapy; NA, not available; NR, not reached; RT, radiation therapy; S, surgery.
Adapted from Hortobagyi G, Singletary S, Strom E: Treatment of locally advanced and inflammatory breast cancer. In Harris J, Lippman M, Morrow M, Osborne CK (eds): Diseases of the Breast, 2nd ed. Philadelphia, Lippincott Williams & Wilkins, 2000, p 651.

survival rates for the entire group were 21 months and 40 months, respectively. When both disease-free and overall survival rates were analyzed by response to chemotherapy, both outcomes significantly differed. Disease-free survival rates at 120 months were approximately 48%, 28%, and 10% for those with complete response, partial response, and less than partial response, respectively. Overall survival rates were approximately 42%, 30%, and 8%, respectively. Maloisel and colleagues[726] reported similar results in a series of 43 patients with inflammatory disease. The most significant prognostic factor was residual tumor after primary chemotherapy, with an 80% predicted 5-year disease-free survival rate in patients responding vs. 30% for patients not responding.

Although most series correlated response with outcome, more than 50% of women with inflammatory breast cancer die within 5 years after receiving optimal therapy. Locoregional control appears to be optimized in most series with the combination of surgery and radiation therapy in conjunction with systemic therapy.[727-729] Retrospective data from Mallinckrodt showed a significant improvement in local control and disease-free survival rates with surgery.[728] Only 19% of patients who underwent mastectomy in addition to radiation therapy had locoregional failure compared with 70% who had radiation therapy alone. Chemotherapy was also associated with improved local control. In a large French series of patients with inflammatory disease, mastectomy was an important component in optimizing locoregional control and disease-free survival in patients who achieved an objective response to primary chemotherapy.[727] In contrast, Buzdar and colleagues[724] reviewed multiple trials of inflammatory cancer from M.D. Anderson that collectively did not show a benefit in local control with the addition of surgery to radiation therapy. With the addition of surgery, however, a lower dose of radiation therapy was used, decreasing the number of late complications. Therefore, for decreased radiation-induced sequelae, and in most series, improved locoregional control, both mastectomy and radiation therapy are generally incorporated into most therapeutic strategies.

The M.D. Anderson group reported a series of women treated with FACVP. This treatment was followed by mastectomy in patients showing a complete clinical response and by more chemotherapy and then mastectomy in the remaining patients. Postoperatively, additional chemotherapy was delivered, followed by an escalating dose of radiation using a novel, twice-daily fraction. Doses as high as 66 Gy were delivered, and significant improvement was noted with the highest doses, compared with internal control subjects who were treated at lower doses. At 5 years, the local control rate was 84% with the highest doses, compared with 57% with lower doses of radiation, with some doses delivered twice daily. Respective disease-free and overall survival rates were 38% and 46% for the highest doses, compared with 26% and 35% for lower doses. Radiation complications were comparable in both groups.[730]

Breast conservation has been attempted in women with inflammatory disease, based on clinical and pathologic response to primary chemotherapy. In a series by Brun and colleagues,[731] all patients received two cycles of primary chemotherapy followed by locoregional radiation. Patients with clinically residual disease underwent extended simple mastectomy, and chemotherapy was resumed for six additional cycles. Despite persistent disease in patients receiving mastectomy, local control was improved with surgery vs. radiation alone; 2% of patients treated with mastectomy had a locoregional recurrence compared with 44% who had a complete response after treatment with radiation therapy. Pierce and colleagues[699] from the NCI also found improvement in locoregional control using mastectomy and postoperative radiation therapy in patients who had a pathologic partial response with T4 lesions, compared with radiation therapy only among those who had a pathologic complete response. Patients with inflammatory disease who were treated with breast conservation had inferior cosmesis compared with that in women with early-stage disease who were treated with breast-conserving therapy as a result of technical factors necessary to achieve the full dose to the skin. Therefore, despite reports of the successful use of breast conservation in the treatment of inflammatory disease, inferior rates of local control compared with mastectomy plus radiation therapy in most series and technical factors associated with treatment support further study of the feasibility of breast conservation for the treatment of inflammatory cancer in a protocol setting before this technique is routinely accepted.

MANAGEMENT OF LOCALLY RECURRENT DISEASE

Locoregional recurrence is often the first sign of treatment failure. After mastectomy, locoregional failure rates of 5% to greater than 30% have been reported. This risk is related to the extent of axillary node involvement and tumor size at initial diagnosis.[679,732-751] In an ECOG study, Recht and colleagues[752] calculated the incidence of locoregional failure for more than 2000 women who received four randomized protocols after primary treatment with modified radical mastectomy. Table 94-25 lists the risk of isolated locoregional failure and locoregional failure with distant failure for this group of women by primary tumor size and number of pathologically involved lymph nodes. The site of locoregional failure is also noted. Chest wall and supraclavicular and infraclavicular failures were most common. Internal mammary node failures were least common, with only two noted, explaining their absence from the table.

Thorough axillary dissection, although primarily of prognostic value, results in major reduction in the risk of axillary and intrapectoral recurrence.[753] Patients who did not have axillary dissection as part of their initial resection have a 16% to 23% incidence of nodal failure.[754,755] As discussed elsewhere in this chapter, adjuvant locoregional radiation also decreases the risk of locoregional failure after mastectomy.

Most local recurrences are discovered early, with a median time of onset of less than 2 years from the original

TABLE 94-25

Ten-Year Cumulative Incidence of Isolated LRF, LRF with or without Simultaneous DF, DF Only, and Specific Sites of LRF in Relation to Conventional Groupings of Tumor Size and Number of Involved Nodes

TUMOR SIZE, NO. OF NODES	NO. OF PATIENTS	ISOLATED LRF		LRF ± DF		DF ONLY		LOCAL		SUPRACLAVICULAR–INFRACLAVICULAR		AXILLARY	
		%	SE	%	SE	%	SE	%	SE	%	SE	%	SE
T1, 1–3	407	9.1	1.5	12.4	1.7	23.2	2.2	8.5	1.4	3.9	1.0	2.0	0.7
T2, 1–3	576	7.0	1.1	12.1	1.4	28.0	1.9	7.5	1.1	4.1	0.8	1.1	0.4
T3, 1–3	35	22.9	7.2	31.4	8.0	37.4	8.5	25.7	7.5	2.9	2.9	2.9	2.9
T1, 4–7	180	11.1	2.4	19.9	3.1	34.0	3.6	12.3	2.5	7.7	2.1	2.4	1.2
T2, 4–7	349	16.9	2.1	26.7	2.5	34.1	2.7	15.0	2.0	9.5	1.6	6.8	1.4
T3, 4–7	33	28.7	8.3	44.8	9.2	29.0	8.4	25.7	8.1	15.9	6.7	6.2	4.4
T1, ≥8	110	19.6	3.9	32.7	4.6	39.3	4.8	15.9	3.6	14.9	3.5	11.3	3.1
T2, ≥8	297	19.6	2.4	32.7	2.8	45.8	3.0	15.9	2.2	15.7	2.2	6.8	1.5
T3, ≥8	29	7.3	5.1	33.2	9.5	46.8	10.0	18.5	7.9	18.2	7.7	4.0	4.1

DF, distant failure; LRF, locoregional failure; SE, standard error.
Adapted from Recht A, Gray R, Davidson N, et al: Locoregional failure 10 years after mastectomy and adjuvant chemotherapy with or without tamoxifen without irradiation: Experience of the Eastern Cooperative Group. J Clin Oncol 1999;17:1693.

diagnosis.[744,750,751,756-761] Even so, it is not uncommon to see local failure many years after initial therapy. Once local failure occurred, the mean time until distant disease manifested was 14.6 months in one study.[748] Patients with more advanced disease at diagnosis, as expected, had a shorter interval between the diagnosis of locoregional disease and the development of distant metastases.[744] In addition, the shorter the time from primary treatment to local failure, the shorter the time from local failure to detectable distant disease. In a group of 90 patients with local failure, Aberizk and colleagues[755] found that each year 20% of the patients had systemic failure.

Information about recurrence in the breast after breast conservation is available from many single-institution studies (see Table 94-13) and randomized trials (see Table 94-15). Overall, approximately 5% to 15% of patients treated with lumpectomy and radiation have some type of recurrence during the follow-up period.

Failure in the irradiated breast can take two distinct forms. The first is a true recurrence of the original tumor. These true recurrences, by definition, occur at or near the site of the tumor bed, which is defined as being within the same quadrant as the original primary lesion.[762] They are most common during the first 5 years of follow-up. In large series with follow-up far beyond 5 years, a second pattern of local failure is seen. These patients have a tumor elsewhere in the breast, separate from the location of the index tumor, and likely a new primary tumor that developed since the original diagnosis and treatment. In a recent report from the Milan group that had 20-year follow-up, Veronesi and associates[763] noted a total of 30 women with recurrent tumor in the radiated breast after quadrantectomy. Of these, 10 appeared in the location of the scar and 20 appeared in other breast quadrants. Bartelink,[764] reporting for the EORTC trial of mastectomy vs. breast-conserving surgery and radiation, noted that only 47% of recurrences were located in the primary tumor region after more than 5 years of follow-up.

Detection and Treatment

The benefit of mammography in follow-up of the chest after mastectomy, especially in patients with reconstruction, has not been well studied. Fajardo and colleagues[765] obtained mediolateral oblique films and when possible craniocaudal mammograms on the treated chests of 865 patients who underwent mastectomy. The incidence of recurrence was 4.5%, and the mean time to diagnosis was 3.5 years. However, abnormal findings on physical examination were the primary diagnostic criteria in these patients. In this study, mammograms were not positive in any patients who had negative findings on physical examination.

When local chest wall recurrence is discovered after mastectomy, a variety of treatments have been used. Selection of the treatment modality depends greatly on the type and extent of local and regional failure, the previous local and systemic therapies used at the time of diagnosis, the extent of other distant disease, and the patient's overall condition. Because so many variables exist, designing a prospective study to identify optimal treatment is not feasible.

Surgical removal alone may be sufficient in some cases. For example, if the recurrence is a small, isolated lesion in the scar or skin flap, simple excision alone sometimes offers long-term local control.[766-768] Generally, a 2- or 3-cm margin and primary closure are appropriate. Some patients may have an isolated axillary or interpectoral nodal recurrence. Surgical excision of these nodal recurrences is the initial treatment of choice. If the original axillary dissection appears to have been incomplete, it is advisable to convert the axilla to an anatomically thorough dissection. In 1992, Salvadori and colleagues[767] described the use of surgery in a series of 39 patients. With a mean follow-up of 48 months, 32 patients were free of local recurrence and 21 were alive and disease-free. These patients appeared to have had thick flaps and inadequate

Specific Malignancies

III

axillary dissections at the time of original mastectomy. Of these patients, 21 received additional chemotherapy with six cycles of CMF.

In 1993, Dahlstrom and colleagues[769] reported their experience in Denmark. Between 1983 and 1987, they treated 98 women with locally recurrent breast cancer with wide surgical excision. Twenty-nine of the 98 patients had radiation to the local recurrence first, without complete remission, and subsequently underwent surgery. Of the 98 patients, 45% had another local failure. The median duration of local control was 21 months.

Radiation therapy is used more often than surgery when locoregional disease is detected. If recurrences are surgically excised, radiation often follows.[755,770-775] With radiation alone, complete response rates of 60% to 70% are reported, with 5-year survival rates of 20% to 40%. When radiation is used, the entire chest wall and supraclavicular nodal region are usually treated. Small fields of radiation have a high rate of failure, and failure to treat the supraclavicular nodal region resulted in a 16% recurrence rate after radiation compared with a rate of 6% when these nodes were included in the field.[773]

Systemic chemotherapy successfully controlled local recurrence in only approximately 50% of patients.[751,776] As a result, multidrug chemotherapy is rarely used without some type of local treatment. Although it is impossible to cite good prospective data to guide treatment planning for locoregional failure, it appears that as chest wall disease becomes more extensive (increase in the number and size of lesions), treatment must be more aggressive to achieve control. For patients with more advanced or diffuse locoregional disease, a multidisciplinary approach to therapy is warranted.

RECURRENCE AFTER BREAST-CONSERVATION THERAPY

In contrast to locoregional recurrence after total mastectomy, recurrence in the breast after breast-conservation therapy does not necessarily signal great risk of systemic disease. It may represent actual recurrence at or near the site of the original primary lesion, or it may be a new primary lesion, especially when located in a different quadrant of the breast.

The incidence of breast recurrence in patients treated with adequate local lumpectomy and breast radiation is 10% to 20% at 10 years (see Table 94-13).[777] The treatment of choice for patients who have a failure in the conserved breast is salvage mastectomy, with reconstruction if desired. Other approaches, such as tumorectomy and multidrug chemotherapy, are experimental.

Fowble and colleagues[778] at the University of Pennsylvania report a 5-year actuarial survival of 84% in 52 patients treated by mastectomy at the time of recurrence. Kurtz and associates[747] reported a 5-year survival rate of 69% and a 10-year survival rate of 57%.[747] Other series report survival rates of 60% to 75% at 5 years from the time of salvage surgery. This number does not apply to all women in a given series who have local failure in the breast, but rather to those who are able to undergo mastectomy.

In the surgical management of these women, it is important to consider the decreased blood supply and decreased skin elasticity from the previous radiation. Skin closure should be accomplished at salvage mastectomy, keeping the possibility of delayed healing in mind. For some of the same reasons, reconstruction with a tissue expander often results in increased incidence of necrosis, infection, and capsular contracture. Reconstruction with autologous tissue is preferred.[779]

The decision to use additional multidrug chemotherapy or hormone therapy is based on the nature of the breast recurrence as well as on whether the patient previously received adjuvant chemotherapy. As with local recurrence after mastectomy, prospective studies do not appear feasible, but each case must be considered by an experienced multidisciplinary breast team.

Special Problems

Patients who undergo unsuccessful radiation therapy, chemotherapy, or a combination of the two in an attempt to control locoregional disease present a special challenge for the surgeon. Surgery should be attempted in these patients because failure to control local disease results in a considerable decrease in quality of life. These patients often have painful, ulcerating, bleeding, and chronically infected local tumors. Surgery should be aggressive, frequently including the ribs and intercostal muscles. As emphasized, the extent of locoregional recurrence is a major influence on the design of a treatment plan. Therapy decisions are also significantly affected by the recognition that such disease is a marker for distant disease. For these reasons, a multimodality approach appears to have the best chance of providing real patient benefit.

MANAGEMENT OF METASTATIC DISEASE

The primary goal of therapy in patients with metastatic breast cancer is palliation and prolongation of life with quality, because many if not most patients with metastatic (advanced) breast cancer ultimately die of their disease.[780] Institutional databases show an improvement in the survival of patients with metastatic disease over the last quarter century.[781] This effect is likely a combined result of more effective therapies and diagnosis at earlier phases of metastatic disease (stage migration). The median survival of patients treated with modern chemotherapy regimens is approximately 2 years.[782] At the same time, there is increasing recognition that some patients may become long-term survivors. A very small cohort of patients with "oligometastatic" disease may benefit from aggressive therapy, such as surgical resection of an isolated visceral metastasis with curative intent.[783]

Approximately 75% of metastases occur within the first 5 years after the diagnosis of early-stage disease. Unfortunately, a smaller risk of recurrence persists and metastases have been documented as late as 20 to 30 years after the initial diagnosis. Although most patients with metastatic disease are likely to have disease progression soon, certain clinical and tumor characteristics are useful in predicting prognosis. Patients with a long interval since initial diagnosis, excellent performance status, endocrine-responsive disease, bone or soft tissue disease, and few sites of visceral involvement are likely to have a better long-term prognosis. These factors clearly reflect the biology of the disease affecting an individual patient.[784-786] Available locoregional systemic and supportive care treatments can result in significant regression of disease, relief of symptoms, and in some cases prolongation of survival. Although the goal of treatment of metastatic breast cancer is seldom cure, palliation with improved quality of life can be achieved in many patients.

Preliminary evidence indicates a role for combined multimodality therapy in patients with small-volume (preferably isolated) metastatic disease.[787,788] However, combined-modality therapy in patients with oligo-metastatic disease must be properly tested in randomized trials specifically designed to answer this question.[783] If confirmed, this could also have significant implications and force re-examination of the current recommendations for no surveillance in the absence of specific symptoms. Also, more effective surveillance tools would be required.

Previous exposure to adjuvant therapy predicts a lower response to first-line chemotherapy in patients with metastatic breast cancer.[789] However, retrospective data suggest that patients who have a recurrence long after completing adjuvant therapy may respond to similar regimens.[790] IBCSG data suggest that quality-of-life scores may correlate with outcome in metastatic breast cancer, but not in early-stage disease.[791] Improvement in symptoms such as pain, shortness of breath, and abnormal mood may correlate with greater response to therapy.[792]

Evaluation of Suspected Metastases

Many patients who have metastatic disease after adjuvant systemic therapy have nonspecific symptoms, such as new pain, weight loss, or dyspnea. When recurrence is suspected, biopsy confirmation of an accessible lesion is considered whenever possible. The diagnosis of recurrence must be confirmed in patients with a single isolated suspected site of disease and in cases in which a tissue specimen may be required for determination of endocrine-receptor or HER2 status. Clinicians should be wary of solitary lesions seen on bone scintigraphy or computed tomography scan because they may not represent metastatic breast cancer. In the appropriate clinical setting, imaging studies without tissue confirmation may be acceptable evidence of metastatic disease, such as multiple areas of osseous lytic or blastic metastases or multiple sites with visceral involvement. Baseline imaging studies, including bone scintigraphy, computed tomography, and plain x-rays, will provide a baseline for the evaluation of response to the planned treatment modality.

Prompt initiation of supportive measures and specific anticancer therapy in patients with significant symptoms or life-threatening complications (e.g., spinal cord compression, destructive bone lesions in weight-bearing areas, hypercalcemia, and symptomatic pleural or pericardial effusions and ascites) can offer significant palliation of symptoms. The role of PET with the glucose analog FDG as an adjunct to the evaluation of patients with metastatic disease remains investigational.[793] Recent reports suggest a possible increase in the prevalence of central nervous system involvement.[794] This may result from the increased use of more effective systemic therapy, but with little central nervous system penetration.[795,796]

Endocrine Therapy

The primary goals in the treatment of systemic recurrence are improved quality of life and prolonged survival. Effective therapies with minimal toxicity, such as endocrine therapy, are highly desirable and should be considered a primary option over cytotoxic chemotherapy. Beatson[552] introduced the first endocrine treatment and the first systemic and targeted therapy for breast cancer in the late 19th century, when he used surgical oophorectomy in the treatment of patients with metastatic disease. Surgical ablative procedures remained the dominant form of endocrine therapy until the second half of the 20th century, when a number of hormonal agents were effective in advanced disease.

Although the clinical factors discussed earlier are important in the selection of systemic therapy, routine measurement of ER and PR expression to identify patients who may respond to endocrine therapy may be the single most important initial test. Endocrine therapy offers the highest therapeutic yield to patients with endocrine-responsive metastatic disease. It is considered the standard approach in patients who have endocrine-responsive disease and few symptoms.

SERMs

Tamoxifen 20 mg daily is the most commonly used SERM. Toremifene is now available for use in this patient population, but has a similar profile and is cross-resistant with tamoxifen.[797] PET with either FDG or the estrogen analog 16α-[18]fluoroestradiol-17β before and after treatment with tamoxifen can assess the functional status of the ER in vivo (metabolic flare) and may predict response to tamoxifen in patients with ER-positive disease.[798] Raloxifene has only modest activity, and is not approved for the treatment of metastatic breast cancer.[799] Acquired resistance to tamoxifen may be explained by a variety of mechanisms, such as mutations in the ER, changes in tamoxifen metabolism, levels of intracellular tamoxifen, and differential expression of steroid-receptor transcriptional coactivators and corepressors.[800-805]

Aromatase Inhibitors

In postmenopausal women with no or distant previous exposure to antiestrogen agents, the nonsteroidal aromatase inhibitors anastrozole[806,807] and letrozole[808] show similar or modestly superior efficacy compared with tamoxifen. In patients who were recently exposed to tamoxifen, the use of a selective, third-generation aromatase inhibitor may be the preferred initial approach.[588] These drugs appear to be ineffective in premenopausal women, and may induce virilization in young women. Nonsteroidal

Specific Malignancies

aromatase inhibitors (e.g., anastrozole and letrozole) are more active and less toxic than megestrol acetate as second-line therapy[809,810] and than the first-generation drug aminoglutethimide.[811] Anastrozole has similar activity to tamoxifen as first-line therapy.[812] The steroidal aromatase inactivator exemestane is active after administration of tamoxifen,[813] megestrol acetate,[814] or a nonsteroidal aromatase inhibitor.[815]

Letrozole appears to be a more potent suppressor of total-body aromatization and plasma estrogen levels than anastrozole in patients with breast cancer.[816] However, direct comparison as second-line therapy in metastatic breast cancer did not show convincing clinical advantage of one drug over the other,[817] and either drug may be considered a first-line option in these patients.[808,818,819] Circulating levels of estrone and estradiol decrease similarly in both responders and nonresponders after therapy with an aromatase inhibitor, suggesting that intratumoral aromatase activity could play a more significant role in differentiating these two groups of patients.[820] Few data suggest that the sequence of therapy matters (i.e., a SERM followed by an aromatase inhibitor, or vice versa). Although steroidal inactivators and nonsteroidal inhibitors differ in pharmacokinetics, selectivity, and potency,[821] it is unclear whether there is a true clinical difference between steroidal and nonsteroidal agents.

Ovarian Ablation

In premenopausal women with endocrine-responsive disease and recent exposure to tamoxifen, the preferred endocrine therapy is ovarian ablation with surgical or medical techniques (LHRH agonist). Although the former induces a postmenopausal state more rapidly, the latter is reversible. Radiation ablation is less reliable and technically more challenging, and the results are not as immediate.[822,823] Adrenalectomy and hypophysectomy induce greater toxicity and are no longer recommended. Data show both an overall survival advantage and a progression-free survival advantage with the addition of tamoxifen to an LHRH agonist,[824,825] but no data are available on the use of ovarian ablation plus an aromatase inhibitor.

Other Antiestrogens

The nonsteroidal pure antiestrogen fulvestrant (ICI 182780) specifically downregulates the ER and has none of the agonistic activity of tamoxifen.[826] Preclinical studies indicate growth inhibition of the breast and endometrium, neutral behavior regarding bones and lipids, and no crossing of the blood-brain barrier.[827] It is as effective as anastrozole in patients whose disease progressed during previous endocrine therapy,[828-830] and it is well tolerated in monthly deep intramuscular gluteal injections. Ongoing studies are comparing it with tamoxifen as first-line therapy. Less frequently used endocrine therapies include progestins (megestrol acetate), androgens (fluoxymesterone), and high-dose estrogen (ethynil estradiol). After first- or second-line therapy, few efficacy data are available to aid in selection of the optimal sequence and decisions are frequently made based on the toxicity profile of individual drugs.

Chemotherapy

Patients with symptomatic visceral disease, ER- and PR-negative disease, or disease that is resistant to endocrine therapy should receive chemotherapy. Given the palliative goal and the toxicities of cytotoxic therapy, the challenge for the oncologist is in deciding when to initiate chemotherapy. Many appropriate chemotherapy regimens are available, and little evidence recommends combination therapy over sequential single-agent chemotherapy (Table 94-26).

There is often a fine line between premature use of chemotherapy in the asymptomatic patient without disease-related complications vs. delaying therapy until deterioration of performance status significantly decreases the likelihood of response. There is considerable interest in identifying biologic parameters that may predict the success of specific chemotherapy regimens. Although expression of the multidrug-resistance phenotype and overexpression of the *HER2* gene correlated with poor response to chemotherapy in some adjuvant studies, evidence is insufficient to justify the routine use of such biologic factors in clinical decision-making in metastatic disease other than for identification of patients with *HER2*-positive diseases that could be offered trastuzumab. Patients with disease that does not express hormone receptors are more likely to respond to chemotherapy.[513] The organ distribution of metastases and the patient's symptoms, history of exposure to chemotherapy, and general medical condition are helpful considerations when determining the time of initiation of chemotherapy. In patients without significant organ dysfunction, increased age alone does not preclude chemotherapy.

Single-Agent Chemotherapy

Commonly used single-agent chemotherapy drugs in patients with advanced disease include anthracyclines, taxanes, vinorelbine, and capecitabine. If no data suggest a markedly strong benefit of one class of drugs over another, decisions should be made based on patient convenience and toxicity profile. Other active agents include gemcitabine, platinum compounds, etoposide, vinblastine, and continuous-infusion 5-fluorouracil.

The activity of taxanes in patients with anthracycline-resistant disease is well documented,[831,832] and docetaxel is active in a small number of patients with paclitaxel-resistant disease.[833] Doses higher than paclitaxel 175 mg/m² and docetaxel 100 mg/m² as single agents are associated with increased toxicity without further clinical benefit.[834-836] Taxanes appear to have a better toxicity profile compared with either doxorubicin[837,838] or a CMF-based regimen.[839] Weekly taxane regimens appear less toxic and may be more active and better tolerated,[840,841] including in elderly patients.[842] Results from studies comparing weekly vs. every-3-week regimens are not yet available. Capecitabine is active in patients who showed disease progression after previous taxane regimens.[843]

Combination Chemotherapy

Commonly used combination chemotherapy regimens include FAC/CAF (5-fluorouracil, doxorubicin, and cyclo-

TABLE 94-26

Preferred Chemotherapy Regimens for Recurrent or Metastatic Breast Cancer

PREFERRED DRUGS*	PREFERRED COMBINATIONS*	OTHER ACTIVE DRUGS
Anthracyclines	AC (doxorubicin and cyclophosphamide)	Continuous infusion 5-fluorouracil
Capecitabine	AT (doxorubicin and docetaxel, doxorubicin and paclitaxel)	Oral etoposide
Taxanes	CAF/FAC (cyclophosphamide, doxorubicin, and 5-fluorouracil)	Platinoids (platin-based)
Vinorelbine	CMF (cyclophosphamide, methotrexate, and 5-fluorouracil)	Vinblastine
	EC (epirubicin and cyclophosphamide)	Gemcitabine
	FEC (5-fluorouracil, epirubicin, and cyclophosphamide)	
	XT (capecitabine and docetaxel)	

*Drugs and regimens listed in alphabetical order. Despite higher initial response rates, there is no compelling evidence that combination chemotherapy offers improved survival compared with sequential single-agent therapy.
Adapted from NCCN Practice Guidelines for Breast Cancer, Version 1.20 (www.nccn.org), National Comprehensive Cancer Network, 2003.

phosphamide), FEC (with epirubicin), AC, epirubicin and cyclophosphamide, AT (doxorubicin plus docetaxel or paclitaxel), and CMF. A survival advantage was seen in randomized trials of first-line therapy in metastatic breast cancer (paclitaxel vs. CMFP[839]) and in trials in patients previously exposed to anthracycline-containing regimens (docetaxel vs. mitomycin and vinblastine[844]).

However, such survival advantage correlates with whether or not patients who showed disease progression while receiving the nontaxane regimen were subsequently crossed over to a taxane drug.[839,844] Similar findings were seen in a study of docetaxel with or without capecitabine in patients with metastatic breast cancer who were previously treated with an anthracycline.[845] In this study, only a small fraction of patients who were initially treated with docetaxel alone subsequently crossed over to capecitabine at progression. This combination is promising and is being evaluated in the adjuvant setting.

Because anthracyclines and taxanes are among the most active drugs in advanced disease, combination regimens were explored in early research studies.[846] Data suggest a higher response rate in many trials comparing combination vs. sequential single agents[782] or vs. a standard AC combination.[847-849] However, none showed a survival advantage in the anthracycline and taxane arm, possibly because many patients in the control arm ultimately received a taxane drug at the time of disease progression. A Milan trial combining doxorubicin and paclitaxel showed pharmacokinetic interference of paclitaxel on doxorubicin elimination, resulting in a lower threshold for cardiac toxicity.[846] This risk appears to be minimized if the cumulative dose of doxorubicin is limited to 360 mg/m². In patients treated with FAC, the combined use of dexrazoxane appears to be cardioprotective.[612] However, its use is restricted to patients who received a cumulative dose of doxorubicin of greater than 300 mg/m² because of concerns about its possible cancer-protective effect.[611] Despite many years of investigation involving thousands of patients, most of whom unfortunately were enrolled in small, single-arm studies, no evidence supports the standard use of high-dose myelo-

ablative therapy with autologous stem cell rescue in patients with metastatic breast cancer.[850]

HER2-Targeted Therapy

Anti-HER2 therapy with the recombinant monoclonal antibody trastuzumab is a more recent example of targeted therapy. Its potential benefits are restricted to women whose tumors overexpress *HER2*, and evidence does not support its use against HER2-negative disease. Although data do not show a survival advantage with combined cytotoxic therapy in metastatic disease, this benefit was seen when trastuzumab was added to anthracycline and cyclophosphamide or paclitaxel.[666] Excessive cardiac toxicity limits the ability to combine anthracyclines with trastuzumab.[667]

Many consider trastuzumab the mainstay of therapy in HER2-positive disease. However, the sequential approach of trastuzumab followed by chemotherapy (or the combination) vs. upfront combined therapy has not been tested. No data are available on combining endocrine therapy with trastuzumab vs. either treatment alone. Single-agent therapy with trastuzumab is an active option, with minimal toxicity seen in both first-[665] and second-line[664] settings, and it is considered a reasonable option for front-line therapy. Although most clinical trial data used a weekly intravenous schedule, pharmacokinetic data suggest its possible use once every 3 weeks.[851]

Despite concerns about potential cardiac toxicity from trastuzumab, especially in patients previously treated with an anthracycline, there are no accepted standards for monitoring cardiac function during therapy.[668] Identification of patients who may be candidates for trastuzumab therapy is limited by the inadequacy of nonstandardized HER2 assays used in clinical practice,[522,523,852] perhaps not unlike early experience with hormone-receptor testing. Until these issues are resolved, most ongoing clinical trials now require HER2 testing in higher-volume, central laboratory facilities.

Trastuzumab has been safely combined with taxanes,[853,854] vinorelbine,[855] and other drugs in small phase II studies. Despite promising preclinical data and

SELECTION OF SYSTEMIC THERAPY FOR PATIENTS WITH METASTATIC BREAST CANCER

PATIENT GROUP	PREVIOUS ADJUVANT THERAPY	SUGGESTED INITIAL THERAPY	SUBSEQUENT THERAPY (IF INITIAL RESPONSE OR LONG DISEASE STABILIZATION)
ER+, PR+ disease, including bone or soft tissue or asymptomatic visceral disease	Endocrine therapy previous 12 mo (e.g., SERM or AI)	Premenopausal: Switch to ovarian ablation ± AI Postmenopausal: Switch to AI, SERM, or fulvestrant	Attempt remaining endocrine options Note: If disease is refractory to endocrine therapy, switch to chemotherapy alone if HER2 is not overexpressed or to trastuzumab ± chemotherapy if HER2 is overexpressed
	No previous endocrine therapy or >12 months ago	Premenopausal: Tamoxifen ± ovarian ablation Postmenopausal: AI or SERM	
ER−, PR disease ER+, PR+ disease refractory to endocrine therapy or symptomatic visceral disease		Trastuzumab ± chemotherapy* or chemotherapy alone[†]	Secondline chemotherapy[†,‡,§]

AI, aromatase inhibitor; SERM, selective estrogen-receptor modulator (tamoxifen or toremifene).
*Randomized data showed a survival benefit of paclitaxel plus trastuzumab vs. paclitaxel alone. Single-arm trials have shown the safety and activity of combinations with docetaxel, vinorelbine, and platinum compounds.
[†]Sequential single-agent chemotherapy is the preferred approach. Combination chemotherapy may be useful in symptomatic patients because of the greater likelihood of response. However, combination chemotherapy does not show evidence of a survival benefit over sequential single-agent therapy.
[‡]Consider discontinuation of cytotoxic therapy if no response is seen after three sequential regimens or in patients with poor performance status (Eastern Cooperative Oncology Group performance status ≥3).
[§]The continuation of trastuzumab on progression while on combination trastuzumab with chemotherapy remains investigational.

widespread adoption in clinical practice, however, no clinical evidence supports the continuation of trastuzumab in patients with disease progression, and any such studies are limited by the long half-life of trastuzumab.

Bisphosphonates

Bone is the most common site of metastatic disease and ultimately is affected in most patients.[856] Monthly injections of bisphosphonates for up to 2 years can reduce the risk of skeletal events in patients who have lytic bone metastases and are receiving systemic therapy.[857,858] Pamidronate therapy administered for longer than 2 years appears safe,[859] but the optimal duration of therapy is unknown and costs can be substantial.[860] Zoledronate is an effective alternative to pamidronate because of its shorter infusion time.[861]

New Approaches

The marked increase in understanding of the cellular and molecular biology of breast cancer led to a striking increase in novel therapies for breast cancer and a significant shift away from the high-dose-chemotherapy hypothesis that "more is better," to a more rational, targeted approach first attempted with endocrine therapy. Targeted anti-HER2 therapy with trastuzumab is now being tested in the adjuvant setting. Other examples in patients with advanced disease include therapies targeting the epidermal growth factor family of receptors,[862,863] matrix metalloproteinases,[864] vascular endothelial growth factor receptors and other angiogenesis targets,[865,866] the AKT/PI3K pathway,[867] and farnesyl transferases.[868] The redundancy of many of these pathways suggests the potential need for a combination of drugs targeting multiple steps or more promiscuous drugs that interact with multiple targets.[869] These studies include combinations of existing hormonal and cytotoxic drugs, and the design of these studies is challenging. Patients must have access to high-quality, well-conducted studies to ensure that useful data are generated, are properly interpreted, and lead to improved cancer care. An important challenge in the treatment of patients with breast cancer is how best to identify those who are most likely to benefit from specific interventions while avoiding unnecessary toxic exposure in those who are unlikely to benefit.

UNUSUAL PROBLEMS ENCOUNTERED IN BREAST CANCER

Male Breast Cancer

Male breast cancer is rare, accounting for 0.2% of male cancers and fewer than 1% of new breast cancers.[870] A higher incidence is reported in Jewish men, men with a history of mumps orchitis after 20 years of age, and men with Klinefelter's syndrome.[871,872] Mutations in the BRCA2 gene predispose men to breast cancer and may account for up to 40% of all cases.[873,874] The vast majority (87%) of male breast cancers are infiltrating ductal carcinoma.[872] More often, it has a pure infiltrating histology, without an intraductal component. Lobular carcinomas are extremely unusual, and most tumors are unilateral, firm, painless masses. Nipple discharge should be taken seriously and is an indication for FNA or core or excisional biopsy. When no mass is palpable, a ductogram with contrast injected into the affected duct may help to localize the abnormal area. Mammography and ultrasound may be of help, but the former is difficult to obtain, especially in thin men. A negative finding on FNA or core biopsy requires an excision procedure, and cytologic findings that show gynecomastia require close follow-up. Most breast cancers in men are ER- and PR-positive, and a third overexpress *HER2*, p53, and EGFR.[870,875]

The standard treatment of male breast cancer was extrapolated from the treatment of female disease. Modified radical mastectomy is the most common surgical approach, often followed by radiation therapy in high-risk patients. The current trend in early-stage disease is a multidisciplinary approach that often includes surgery (including axillary lymph node staging), radiation therapy, and adjuvant systemic therapy with chemotherapy or endocrine therapy (usually tamoxifen). Because most patients have endocrine-responsive disease, orchiectomy is often used in patients with advanced disease.[876] Endocrine therapies that induce responses include androgens (75%), antiandrogens (57%), steroids (50%), estrogens (32%), progestins (50%), and tamoxifen (49%).[877] The LHRH agonist buserelin, in combination with the antiestrogen cyproterone acetate, is also effective.[878] Aromatase inhibitors are of potential interest in men with metastatic disease. However, approximately 80% of circulating estrogens are derived from the aromatization of precursor androgens. The remaining estrogens come from direct testicular secretion. This may explain the apparent lower response rate observed with the first-generation aromatase inhibitor aminoglutethimide compared with tamoxifen[879] and the low levels of activity seen with anastrozole.[880] These observations suggest that orchiectomy and tamoxifen remain the endocrine therapies of choice in men with breast cancer.

Breast Cancer and Pregnancy

Breast Cancer during Pregnancy

Carcinoma of the breast is associated with pregnancy in approximately 1 to 3 patients in 10,000 deliveries.[881]

It is the most common malignancy associated with pregnancy.[882] Although this number is relatively low, it is expected to increase because of a number of factors. For example, the risk of breast cancer increases with age. The average age at first full-term pregnancy, another known risk factor, has risen dramatically in the last two decades. Statistics show a 60% increase in the rate of first full-term pregnancy in women older than 30 years of age since 1975.[883] In addition, women who delayed pregnancy for educational or professional reasons, or both, may have other risk factors, such as being white, college-educated, and socioeconomically privileged.[884]

The advanced level of disease and the poor prognosis associated with gestational breast cancer is linked to a delay in diagnosis. Little evidence supports the theory that endocrine changes during pregnancy may be a risk factor for mammary cancers.[883] For this reason, the obstetrician must pursue early signs of breast cancer actively via a thorough breast examination. Thorough examination of the breast should take place during the first obstetric visit, before the breast becomes engorged or hypertrophic. In an older female population planning pregnancy, it is worth considering mammography before planned conception. Diagnosis and staging are far more difficult in pregnant women because of physiologic changes in the mother and radiation risk to the fetus. Mammograms are not routinely performed, because little information can be gained as a result of increased breast density. Ultrasonography may be used safely to differentiate cysts from solid masses. MRI is particularly useful for the diagnosis of bone, liver, or brain metastasis. Routine bone scintigraphy is contraindicated in pregnant patients.[884,885]

Biopsy of a mass during pregnancy is difficult and must be undertaken with extreme care to avoid infection and milk fistulas in the lactating breast. FNA and stereotactic NCB are the initial procedures used in evaluating a breast mass.[886] Some surgeons prefer to suppress lactation preoperatively with bromocriptine. Biopsy can almost always be performed under local anesthesia; however, no evidence shows that general anesthesia poses significant risk to either the mother or the fetus if proper precautions are taken.[887] Modified radical mastectomy is the treatment of choice for breast cancer during pregnancy. Depending on the extent of disease and the predicted delivery date, breast conservation may be considered. Tumor excision and axillary dissection are performed during pregnancy, followed by breast irradiation after delivery.[887] Survival is not improved by therapeutic abortion, and pregnancy-associated breast cancer should be treated using the same decision tree that would be appropriate for a nonpregnant patient.[886,888]

In most cases, chemotherapeutic agents are not recommended in the pregnant patient because of concerns about teratogenesis. The effect on the fetus is also related to drug dosage, gestational age, and tolerance of the individual patient. Cytotoxic chemotherapy, however, has been administered, mostly after the first trimester, without identifiable damage to the fetus. Data from the M.D. Anderson Cancer Center described 24 pregnant patients with primary or recurrent cancer of the breast. These patients were treated over an 8-year period with outpatient chemotherapy, surgery, or surgery plus radiation therapy, as clinically indicated.[889] These patients received a median of four cycles of combination chemotherapy with 5-fluorouracil, doxorubicin, and cyclophosphamide during the second and third trimesters. Mean gestational age at delivery was 38 weeks, and no antepartum complications temporally attributable to systemic therapy were noted. In the immediate postpartum period, all of the infants appeared well. The authors concluded that breast cancer can be treated with chemotherapy during the second and third trimesters of pregnancy with minimal complications of labor and delivery. However, the small potential for complications must not be disregarded.[884,890] Early in pregnancy, therapeutic abortion greatly simplifies the treatment of early-stage breast cancer but does not improve treatment outcome.[881] No reports show that breast cancer is harmful to the fetus, because these cells cannot traverse the placenta, as in some cases of melanoma, lymphosarcoma, or leukemia.[881] Therefore, each patient and family must make an informed decision on an individual basis.

A rare condition known as gestational squamous cell carcinoma has been reported, and appears to have an aggressive course.[891] It appears to have a worse prognosis than the nongestational squamous cell carcinoma detected in postmenopausal women.

Pregnancy after Breast Cancer

Many women now emerge from treatment for breast cancer with fertility intact, and 5% to 8% of these women will become pregnant.[883] The literature suggests that patients who have a subsequent pregnancy after breast cancer have a higher survival rate than control subjects. However, these statistics may not be accurate for a number of reasons. First, not all pregnancies are reported. Second, those with a better prognosis are more likely to pursue pregnancy. Finally, most clinicians recalled a number of reported cases from memory, and it is natural to remember the patients who have done well.[892]

Kroman and colleagues[893] analyzed 5725 women with primary breast cancer who were 45 years of age or younger at the time of diagnosis and treatment. Of these women, 173 subsequently became pregnant, and those who had a full-term pregnancy had a nonsignificantly reduced risk of death (relative risk, 0.55; 95% CI, 0.28 to 1.06) compared with those who had no full-term pregnancy. The IBCSG identified in their clinical trial database 94 patients who became pregnant after a diagnosis of breast cancer, including 8 who had a relapse during pregnancy. The investigators compared the outcome of these patients with the outcome of 188 matched, controlled patients from the same database, and showed no adverse effect from pregnancy on survival.[623] A similar pattern was seen in 47 patients younger than 35 years of age who were treated with adjuvant chemotherapy at M.D. Anderson and subsequently became pregnant.[894] Thus, there is no evidence that pregnancy after breast cancer treatment increases the risk of a worse outcome.

Axillary Metastases with Occult Breast Cancer

A woman who has enlarged axillary lymph nodes despite normal findings on breast examination and mammogram requires careful evaluation for possible breast cancer.[895-897] Further evaluation of the patient with a normal mammogram includes gadolinium-enhanced breast MRI and PET scans.[898,899] The first step is to exclude infection. Although most enlarged axillary nodes are caused by infection, the most common malignant cause in women is lymphoma. However, in the absence of other adenopathy or physical findings, the diagnosis of breast cancer must be pursued. Unknown primary cancers of the gastrointestinal tract, lung, and thyroid are occasionally the cause.[900-902] The initial workup after mammography includes chest radiograph and computed tomography of the chest, abdomen, and pelvis to look for possible primary cancers. FNA or CNB of the axillary mass is usually the first invasive procedure.

It is mandatory to determine whether the specimen contains ER or PR. Patients whose histopathologic features are consistent with an occult primary breast lesion are typically offered modified radical mastectomy, but breast conservation is now considered in the absence of positive findings on physical examination or mammography. Occult cancer is found in approximately 71% of mastectomy specimens. The 5- and 10-year survival rates are essentially the same as for T1N1 and T2N1 tumors. Even patients in whom a primary breast cancer is not identified are treated in the same way as patients with N1 breast cancer, with appropriate adjuvant therapy.[903] Some reports suggest that these patients can be successfully treated with irradiation of the breast without mastectomy. This treatment may be an alternative for women who want to preserve their breast.[904-907]

Paget's Disease of the Breast

Paget's disease of the breast is a cutaneous manifestation of underlying breast malignancy. This eczematoid lesion (often weeping, red, and crusting in late presentation) occurs in approximately 1% to 4% of patients with breast cancer. Reports vary as to the proportion of patients who have an associated mass. Kister and Haagensen[908] found a palpable tumor in 58% of 159 patients. A study of patients from the Portuguese Institute of Oncology (Lisbon) noted a palpable mass in only 28% of 109 patients.[909] Ashikari and associates[910] described an associated mass in 55% of 214 patients. In most patients with Paget's disease of the breast, a carcinoma can be pathologically identified in the underlying breast with the aid of immunohistochemistry.[911,912] Paget's disease is a carcinoma of glandular origin, and Paget's cells are spread through the epidermis as a result of motility induced by a chemotactic factor released by epidermal cells.[913]

The greatest prevalence of Paget's disease of the breast occurs in the sixth decade of life. The infrequency of early diagnosis is associated with a delay in recognition of early symptoms. Although an early sign of Paget's disease is severe itching accompanied by erosive nipple changes, the median delay between first symptom and diagnosis is approximately 6 months, and may be as long as several years.[914] Paget's disease associated with a palpable underlying tumor can be treated with breast conservation with removal of the nipple–areolar complex. This procedure usually leaves an acceptable breast mound for subsequent reconstruction of the nipple–areolar complex. Sentinel node biopsy is an appropriate method for evaluating axillary status.

This disease shows the importance of physical examination and physician-patient education. Early-stage Paget's disease of the breast is almost universally associated with prolonged disease-free survival. It is unfortunate that the average patient with this disease must wait so long for the diagnosis to be recognized. To maximize survival, Paget's disease of the breast must be detected before it progresses from nipple erosion to an underlying palpable mass. Several conditions mimic Paget's disease of the breast secondary to underlying breast cancer, including erosive adenomatosis of the nipple and pemphigus vulgaris of the nipple.[915,916]

Cystosarcoma Phyllodes and Sarcomas

Sarcomas of the breast are rare, representing fewer than 1% of malignant breast tumors.[917–920] Included in this group are benign and malignant forms of cystosarcoma phyllodes (CSP) [approximately 0.5%], carcinosarcoma, and sarcoma.[921,922] CSP was first described in 1838 by Johannes Müller,[923] who believed the tumors to be benign. CSP tumors are classified as either benign or malignant. In reported reviews, 20% to 50% were classified as malignant.[922–930] These tumors have a characteristic leaf-like architecture, with clefts lined by epithelial cells, and are often (approximately 25%) associated with fibroadenomas.[922] Some authors refer to benign CSP as giant fibroadenomata, reserving the term CSP for the malignant lesion. The average age at presentation is the mid-40s.

In treating CSP, it is important to differentiate benign from malignant lesions. Several histologic characteristics are considered indicators of malignant CSP, including increased cellularity, subepithelial stromal overgrowth, and stromal anaplasia.[931] Norris and Taylor[932] and Lester and Stout[933] reviewed the correlation between histologic features and malignant potential. Norris and Taylor[932] concluded that important criteria for malignant potential included tumor size, contour, degree of cellular atypia, and mitotic activity. For example, in their series of 94 patients, no deaths occurred in patients whose tumors had fewer than three mitotic figures per high-power field. They also determined that if microscopic evaluation of the widely excised CSP tumor found the tumor to be fixed to adjacent breast tissue, malignancy should be suspected.

Hawkins and colleagues[934] retrospectively studied 33 patients with CSP, 8 of whom had metastases. The most reliable predictor of metastases was stromal overgrowth. Degree of mitotic activity, nuclear pleomorphism, and infiltrating margins were also important markers for malignancy, as were necrosis and tumor size. Initial evaluation of suspected fibroadenoma or CSP of the breast should include FNA or CNB. The biopsy findings can provide the information needed to plan the surgical excision.

Rajan and colleagues[935] at Memorial Sloan-Kettering Cancer Center reviewed the pathologic features and clinical course of 45 adolescent girls and young women 10 to 24 years of age who had CSP. Of these patients, 34 had benign CSP and 11 had malignant CSP. Follow-up was obtained in 36 patients. Six patients (16%) had local recurrence, and all of these had microscopically positive margins. Mitotic activity was the most important factor in determining malignancy.

CSP tumors are treated with wide local excision to include a sufficient margin of normal breast tissue from the tumor bed. Even benign tumors have a high incidence of local recurrence if they are simply shelled out of the breast tissue. In reported series, the incidence of local recurrence after excision of benign CSP is between 11% and 20%.[922,924,926,928,929,936,937] Meticulous effort is required to obtain an adequate tissue margin. This may result in cosmetic deformity, which can be addressed after a careful histopathologic study is completed and the magnitude of deformity is established by completion of the healing process. Recurrences of benign CSP may be re-excised, again with wide margins. Some cases are better managed by mastectomy and reconstruction. If a diagnosis of malignant CSP is established or strongly suspected after thorough pathologic review, then total mastectomy is performed. Advanced disease is treated in the same way as metastasis from extremity or truncal sarcoma.

In addition to malignant CSP, sarcomas of the breast include a wide range of histologic types, such as carcinosarcoma, osteosarcoma, liposarcoma, angiosarcoma, malignant histiocytoma, leiomyosarcoma, stromal sarcoma, and mixed types.[938–940] Carcinosarcoma is different in that it is composed of a combination of malignant epithelial cells, as would be found in breast adenocarcinoma, in addition to malignant stromal cells characteristic of sarcoma. These tumors may behave somewhat differently from pure sarcomas. For example, they can extend to the axillary lymph nodes. Treatment of carcinosarcoma usually includes mastectomy with adequate tissue margins, including muscle and skin if necessary and complete axillary dissection. If axillary extension is found, adjuvant chemotherapy with a doxorubicin-containing regimen should be considered. The role of chest wall irradiation is affected by tumor size, location, and margins.

The M.D. Anderson study of 60 patients reported a mean age for occurrence of breast sarcoma of 48 years and a mean tumor size of 6.49 cm.[939] The disease-free survival rate was 33% at 5 years and 31% at 10 years. The overall survival rate was 50% at 5 years and 41% at 10 years. This study showed that patients with tumors less than 5 cm had a much better prognosis.

North and colleagues[940] at the Roswell Park Cancer Institute reviewed 25 patients treated for breast sarcoma between 1964 and 1995. Of these patients, 24 were female and only 1 was male. The median age at diagnosis was 55 years. Ten of the tumors were angiosarcomas. Twenty-one of the 25 patients were treated by mastectomy. The overall survival rate was 61% at 5 years and 36% at 10 years. Because breast sarcomas tend to be mobile, well-demarcated, painless masses, they are difficult to differentiate from benign fibroadenomas.[941] For these reasons, PET scanning with FDG may be useful in determining that a benign-appearing mass is a breast sarcoma. It also may be useful in defining the extent of spread of the sarcoma.[942]

For sarcomas of the breast, surgical therapy is determined by tumor size. Because these tumors do not spread directly to lymph nodes, dissection of the nodes is not indicated. An exception may be liposarcoma, which may have a 10% incidence of nodal involvement. Tumor spread to the lymph nodes is part of the hematogenous systemic spread of the tumor. Wide local excision is adequate primary surgical treatment for most lesions, with attention given to obtaining wide margins, including deep muscle, if indicated. Depending on their location, tumors larger than 5 cm and high-grade tumors may require mastectomy, possibly with chest wall resection. The surgeon must approach these tumors according to the established guidelines for sarcoma surgery. Adjuvant radiation therapy is used in almost all cases, but prospective data are not available to support this decision. Local failures are best treated with repeat surgical excision. If radiation was not used at the time of treatment of the primary tumor, then it is used after re-excision. Little information is available about preoperative or adjuvant polychemotherapy for breast sarcomas.[943,944] Regimens used to downstage other sarcomas, such as extremity sarcomas, are occasionally considered in patients with large, bulky tumors.[945]

The rarity of breast sarcomas limits the rigorous evaluation of therapeutic options. Even so, it seems appropriate to approach sarcomas of the breast using therapeutic methods that have evolved from treating soft tissue sarcomas of the extremities and trunk.

REFERENCES

1. Cancer Facts and Figures. Atlanta, GA: American Cancer Society, 1999.
2. Key TJ, Verkasalo PK, Banks E: Epidemiology of breast cancer. Lancet Oncol 2001;2:133–140.
3. Breast Cancer Statistics, 2002. National Cancer Institute. www.cancer.gov.
4. Ziegler RG, Hoover RN, Pike MC, et al: Migration patterns and breast cancer risk in Asian-American women. J Natl Cancer Inst 1993;85:1819–1827.
5. King SE, Schottenfeld D: The "epidemic" of breast cancer in the US: Determining the factors. Oncology 1996;10:453–62; discussion 462, 464, 470–472.
6. Newman B, Moorman PG, Millikan R, et al: The Carolina Breast Cancer Study: Integrating population-based epidemiology and molecular biology. Breast Cancer Res Treat 1995;35:51–60.
7. Slattery ML, Kerber RA: A comprehensive evaluation of family history and breast cancer risk: The Utah Population Database (see comments). JAMA 1993;270:1563–1568.
8. Colditz GA, Willett WC, Hunter DJ, et al: Family history, age, and risk of breast cancer: Prospective data from the Nurses' Health Study (published erratum appears in JAMA 1993;270:1548) [see comments]. JAMA 1993;270:338–343.
9. Miki Y, Swensen J, Shattuck-Eidens D, et al: A strong candidate for the breast and ovarian cancer susceptibility gene BRCA1. Science 1994;266:66–71.
10. Wooster R, Bignell G, Lancaster J, et al: Identification of the breast cancer susceptibility gene BRCA2 (see comments) [published erratum appears in Nature 1996;379:749]. Nature 1995;378:789–792.
11. Couch FJ, DeShano ML, Blackwood MA, et al: BRCA1 mutations in women attending clinics that evaluate the risk of breast cancer (see comments). N Engl J Med 1997;336:1409–1415.
12. Peto J, Collins N, Barfoot R, et al: Prevalence of BRCA1 and BRCA2 gene mutations in patients with early-onset breast cancer (see comments). J Natl Cancer Inst 1999;91:943–949.
13. Rebbeck TR, Lynch HT, Neuhausen SL, et al: Prophylactic oophorectomy in carriers of BRCA1 or BRCA2 mutations. N Engl J Med 2002;346:1616–1622.
14. Rebbeck TR, Levin AM, Eisen A, et al: Breast cancer risk after bilateral prophylactic oophorectomy in BRCA1 mutation carriers (see comments). J Natl Cancer Inst 1999;91:1475–1479.
15. Meijers-Heijboer H, van Geel B, van Putten WL, et al: Breast cancer after prophylactic bilateral mastectomy in women with a BRCA1 or BRCA2 mutation. N Engl J Med 2001;345:159–164.
16. Meijers-Heijboer H, van den Ouweland A, Klijn J, et al: Low-penetrance susceptibility to breast cancer due to CHEK2(*)1100delC in noncarriers of BRCA1 or BRCA2 mutations. Nat Genet 2002;31:55–59.
17. Bell DW, Varley JM, Szydlo TE, et al: Heterozygous germ line hCHK2 mutations in Li-Fraumeni syndrome. Science 1999;286:2528–2531.
18. Sodha N, Williams R, Mangion J, Bullock SL, Yuille MR, Eeles RA: Screening hCHK2 for mutations. Science 2000;289:359.
19. Freedman LS, Clifford C, Messina M: Analysis of dietary fat, calories, body weight, and the development of mammary tumors in rats and mice: A review. Cancer Res 1990;50:5710–5719.
20. Howe GR, Hirohata T, Hislop TG, et al: Dietary factors and risk of breast cancer: Combined analysis of 12 case-control studies. J Natl Cancer Inst 1990;82:561–569.
21. Boyd NF, Greenberg C, Lockwood G, et al: Effects at two years of a low-fat, high-carbohydrate diet on radiologic features of the breast: Results from a randomized trial. Canadian Diet and Breast Cancer Prevention Study Group. J Natl Cancer Inst 1997;89:488–496.
22. Harvey EB, Schairer C, Brinton LA, Hoover RN, Fraumeni JF Jr: Alcohol consumption and breast cancer. J Natl Cancer Inst 1987;78:657–661.
23. Willett WC, Stampfer MJ, Colditz GA, Rosner BA, Hennekens CH, Speizer FE: Moderate alcohol consumption and the risk of breast cancer. N Engl J Med 1987;316:1174–1180.
24. Reichman ME, Judd JT, Longcope C, et al: Effects of alcohol consumption on plasma and urinary hormone concentrations in premenopausal women. J Natl Cancer Inst 1993;85:722–727.
25. Breast cancer and hormonal contraceptives: Collaborative reanalysis of individual data on 53,297 women with breast cancer and 100,239 women without breast cancer from 54 epidemiological studies. Collaborative Group on Hormonal Factors in Breast Cancer. Lancet 1996;347:1713–1727.
26. Breast cancer and hormone replacement therapy: Collaborative reanalysis of data from 51 epidemiological studies of 52,705 women with breast cancer and 108,411 women without breast cancer. Collaborative Group on Hormonal Factors in Breast Cancer. Lancet 1997;350:1047–1059.
27. Rossouw JE, Anderson GL, Prentice RL, et al: Risks and benefits of estrogen plus progestin in healthy postmenopausal women: Principal results from the Women's Health Initiative randomized controlled trial. JAMA 2002;288:321–333.
28. Postmenopausal hormone replacement therapy for primary prevention of chronic conditions: Recommendations and rationale. Ann Intern Med 2002;137:834–839.
29. Mosca L, Collins P, Herrington DM, et al: Hormone replacement therapy and cardiovascular disease: A statement for healthcare professionals from the American Heart Association. Circulation 2001;104:499–503.
30. Nelson HD: Assessing benefits and harms of hormone replacement therapy: Clinical applications. JAMA 2002;288:882–884.
31. Kvale G, Heuch I: Menstrual factors and breast cancer risk. Cancer 1988;62:1625–1631.
32. Kvale G: Reproductive factors in breast cancer epidemiology. Acta Oncol 1992;31:187–194.

33. Leon DA: A prospective study of the independent effects of parity and age at first birth on breast cancer incidence in England and Wales. Int J Cancer 1989;43:986–991.

34. Layde PM, Webster LA, Baughman AL, Wingo PA, Rubin GL, Ory HW: The independent associations of parity, age at first full term pregnancy, and duration of breastfeeding with the risk of breast cancer: Cancer and Steroid Hormone Study Group. J Clin Epidemiol 1989;42:963–973.

35. Albrektsen G, Heuch I, Kvale G: The short-term and long-term effect of a pregnancy on breast cancer risk: A prospective study of 802,457 parous Norwegian women. Br J Cancer 1995;72:480–484.

36. Pike MC, Henderson BE, Casagrande JT, Rosario I, Gray GE: Oral contraceptive use and early abortion as risk factors for breast cancer in young women. Br J Cancer 1981;43:72–76.

37. Brind J, Chinchilli VM, Severs WB, Summy-Long J: Induced abortion as an independent risk factor for breast cancer: A comprehensive review and meta-analysis. J Epidemiol Community Health 1996;50:481–496.

38. Melbye M, Wohlfahrt J, Olsen JH, et al: Induced abortion and the risk of breast cancer. N Engl J Med 1997;336:81–85.

39. Breast cancer and breastfeeding: Collaborative reanalysis of individual data from 47 epidemiological studies in 30 countries, including 50302 women with breast cancer and 96973 women without the disease. Lancet 2002;360:187–195.

40. Dupont WD, Parl FF, Hartmann WH, et al: Breast cancer risk associated with proliferative breast disease and atypical hyperplasia. Cancer 1993;71:1258–1265.

41. Dupont WD, Page DL: Risk factors for breast cancer in women with proliferative breast disease. N Engl J Med 1985;312:146–151.

42. Baral E, Larsson LE, Mattsson B: Breast cancer following irradiation of the breast. Cancer 1977;40:2905–2910.

43. Howe GR, McLaughlin J: Breast cancer mortality between 1950 and 1987 after exposure to fractionated moderate-dose-rate ionizing radiation in the Canadian fluoroscopy cohort study and a comparison with breast cancer mortality in the atomic bomb survivors study. Radiat Res 1996;145:694–707.

44. Preston DL, Mattsson A, Holmberg E, Shore R, Hildreth NG, Boice JD Jr: Radiation effects on breast cancer risk: A pooled analysis of eight cohorts. Radiat Res 2002;158:220–235.

45. Tokunaga M, Land CE, Tokuoka S, Nishimori I, Soda M, Akiba S: Incidence of female breast cancer among atomic bomb survivors, 1950-1985. Radiat Res 1994;138:209–223.

46. Land CE, Hayakawa N, Machado SG, et al: A case-control interview study of breast cancer among Japanese A-bomb survivors: I. Main effects. Cancer Causes Control 1994;5:157–165.

47. Bhatia S, Meadows AT, Robison LL: Second cancers after pediatric Hodgkin's disease (letter; comment). J Clin Oncol 1998;16:2570–2572.

48. Fraass BA, Roberson PL, Lichter AS: Dose to the contralateral breast due to primary breast irradiation. Int J Radiat Oncol Biol Phys 1985;11:485–497.

49. Boice JD, Harvey EB, Blettner M, Stovall M, Flannery JT: Cancer in the contralateral breast after radiotherapy for breast cancer. 1992;326:781–785.

50. Horn PL, Thompson WD: Risk of contralateral breast cancer: Associations with histologic, clinical, and therapeutic factors. Cancer 1988;62:412–424.

51. Gail MH, Brinton LA, Byar DP, et al: Projecting individualized probabilities of developing breast cancer for white females who are being examined annually (see comments). J Natl Cancer Inst 1989;81:1879–1886.

52. Claus EB, Risch N, Thompson WD: Autosomal dominant inheritance of early-onset breast cancer: Implications for risk prevention. Cancer 1994;73:643–651.

53. Domchek SD, Eisen A, Calzone K, Stopfer J, Blackwood A, Weber BL: Application of breast cancer risk prediction models in clinical practice. J Clin Oncol 2003;21:593–601.

54. Osborne MP, Bradlow HL, Wong GY, Telang NT: Upregulation of estradiol C16 alpha-hydroxylation in human breast tissue: A potential biomarker of breast cancer risk (see comments). J Natl Cancer Inst 1993;85:1917–1920.

55. Klinge CM: Estrogen receptor interaction with estrogen response elements. Nucleic Acids Res 2001;29:2905–2919.

56. Mosselman S, Polman J, Dijkema R: ER beta: Identification and characterization of a novel human estrogen receptor. FEBS Lett 1996;392:49–53.

57. Katzenellenbogen BS, Katzenellenbogen JA: Estrogen receptor transcription and transactivation: Estrogen receptor alpha and estrogen receptor beta. Regulation by selective estrogen receptor modulators and importance in breast cancer. Breast Cancer Res 2000;2:335–344.

58. Clarke RB, Howell A, Potten CS, Anderson E: Dissociation between steroid receptor expression and cell proliferation in the human breast. Cancer Res 1997;57:4987–4991.

59. Shoker BS, Jarvis C, Sibson DR, Walker C, Sloane JP: Oestrogen receptor expression in the normal and pre-cancerous breast. J Pathol 1999;188:237–244.

60. Nass SJ, Herman JG, Gabrielson E, et al: Aberrant methylation of the estrogen receptor and E-cadherin 5′ CpG islands increases with malignant progression in human breast cancer. Cancer Res 2000;60:4346–4348.

61. Soderqvist G: Effects of sex steroids on proliferation in normal mammary tissue. Ann Med 1998;30:511–524.

62. Klijn JG, Setyono-Han B, Foekens JA: Progesterone antagonists and progesterone receptor modulators in the treatment of breast cancer. Steroids 2000;65:825–830.

63. Humphreys RC, Lydon J, O'Malley BW, Rosen JM: Mammary gland development is mediated by both stromal and epithelial progesterone receptors. Mol Endocrinol 1997;11:801–811.

64. Horwitz KB: The structure and function of progesterone receptors in breast cancer. J Steroid Biochem 1987;27:447–457.

65. Boonyaratanakornkit V, Scott MP, Ribon V, et al: Progesterone receptor contains a proline-rich motif that directly interacts with SH3 domains and activates c-Src family tyrosine kinases. Mol Cell 2001;8:269–280.

66. Coles C, Condie A, Chetty U, Steel CM, Evans HJ, Prosser J: p53 mutations in breast cancer. Cancer Res 1992;52:5291–5298.

67. Nichols KE, Malkin D, Garber JE, Fraumeni JF Jr, Li FP: Germ-line p53 mutations predispose to a wide spectrum of early-onset cancers. Cancer Epidemiol Biomarkers Prev 2001;10:83–87.

68. Bertwistle D, Ashworth A: Functions of the BRCA1 and BRCA2 genes. Curr Opin Genet Dev 1998;8:14–20.

69. Ryan KM, Phillips AC, Vousden KH: Regulation and function of the p53 tumor suppressor protein. Curr Opin Cell Biol 2001;13:332–337.

70. Blackburn AC, Jerry DJ: Knockout and transgenic mice of Trp53: What have we learned about p53 in breast cancer? Breast Cancer Res 2002;4:101–111.

71. Thorlacius S, Borresen AL, Eyfjord JE: Somatic p53 mutations in human breast carcinomas in an Icelandic population: A prognostic factor. 1993;53:1637–1641.

72. Kovach JS, Hartmann A, Blaszyk H, Cunningham J, Schaid D, Sommer SS: Mutation detection by highly sensitive methods indicates that p53 gene mutations in breast cancer can have important prognostic value. Proc Natl Acad Sci USA 1996;93:1093–1096.

73. Bergh J, Norberg T, Sjogren S, Lindgren A, Holmberg L: Complete sequencing of the p53 gene provides prognostic information in breast cancer patients, particularly in relation to adjuvant systemic therapy and radiotherapy. Nature Med 1995;1:1029–1034.

74. Aas T, Borresen AL, Geisler S, et al: Specific P53 mutations are associated with de novo resistance to doxorubicin in breast cancer patients. Nature Med 1996;2:811–814.

75. Bardeesy N, Beckwith JB, Pelletier J: Clonal expansion and attenuated apoptosis in Wilms' tumors are associated with p53 gene mutations. Cancer Res 1995;55:215–219.

76. Moll UM, Ostermeyer AG, Ahomadegbe JC, Mathieu MC, Riou G: p53 mediated tumor cell response to chemotherapeutic DNA damage: A preliminary study in matched pairs of breast cancer biopsies. Hum Pathol 1995;26:1293–1301.

77. Tada M, Iggo RD, Ishii N, et al: Clonality and stability of the p53 gene in human astrocytic tumor cells: Quantitative analysis of p53 gene mutations by yeast functional assay. Int J Cancer 1996;67:447–450.

78. Fontanini G, Vignati S, Lucchi M, et al: Neoangiogenesis and p53 protein in lung cancer: Their prognostic role and their relation

with vascular endothelial growth factor (VEGF) expression. Br J Cancer 1997;75:1295–1301.

79. Takahashi Y, Bucana CD, Cleary KR, Ellis LM: p53, vessel count, and vascular endothelial growth factor expression in human colon cancer. Int J Cancer 1998;79:34–38.

80. Lowe SW, Bodis S, McClatchey A, et al: p53 status and the efficacy of cancer therapy in vivo. Science 1994;266:807–810.

81. Clahsen PC, van de Velde CJ, Duval C, et al: p53 protein accumulation and response to adjuvant chemotherapy in premenopausal women with node-negative early breast cancer. J Clin Oncol 1998;16:470–479.

82. Berns EM, Klijn JG, van Putten WL, et al: p53 protein accumulation predicts poor response to tamoxifen therapy of patients with recurrent breast cancer. J Clin Oncol 1998;16:121–127.

83. Formenti SC, Dunnington G, Uzieli B, et al: Original p53 status predicts for pathological response in locally advanced breast cancer patients treated preoperatively with continuous infusion 5-fluorouracil and radiation therapy. Int J Radiat Oncol Biol Phys 1997;39:1059–1068.

84. Degeorges A, de Roquancourt A, Extra JM, et al: Is p53 a protein that predicts the response to chemotherapy in node negative breast cancer? Breast Cancer Res Treat 1998;47:47–55.

85. Rozan S, Vincent-Salomon A, Zafrani B, et al: No significant predictive value of c-erbB-2 or p53 expression regarding sensitivity to primary chemotherapy or radiotherapy in breast cancer. Int J Cancer 1998;79:27–33.

86. Veronese S, Mauri FA, Caffo O, et al: Bax immunohistochemical expression in breast carcinoma: A study with long term follow-up. Int J Cancer 1998;79:13–18.

87. Krajewski S, Blomqvist C, Franssila K, et al: Reduced expression of proapoptotic gene BAX is associated with poor response rates to combination chemotherapy and shorter survival in women with metastatic breast adenocarcinoma. Cancer Res 1995;55:4471–4478.

88. Kapranos N, Karaiosifidi H, Valavanis C, Kouri E, Vasilaros S: Prognostic significance of apoptosis related proteins Bcl-2 and Bax in node-negative breast cancer patients. Anticancer Res 1997;17:2499–2505.

89. Bargou RC, Daniel PT, Mapara MY, et al: Expression of the bcl-2 gene family in normal and malignant breast tissue: Low bax-alpha expression in tumor cells correlates with resistance towards apoptosis. Int J Cancer 1995;60:854–859.

90. Lupu R, Cardillo M, Harris L, Hijazi M, Rosenberg K: Interaction between erbB-receptors and heregulin in breast cancer tumor progression and drug resistance. Semin Cancer Biol 1995;6:135–145.

91. Plowman GD, Green JM, Culouscou JM, Carlton GW, Rothwell VM, Buckley S: Heregulin induces tyrosine phosphorylation of HER4/p180erbB4. Nature 1993;366:473–475.

92. Sliwkowski MX, Schaefer G, Akita RW, et al: Coexpression of erbB2 and erbB3 proteins reconstitutes a high affinity receptor for heregulin. J Biol Chem 1994;269:14661–14665.

93. King CR, Borrello I, Bellot F, Comoglio P, Schlessinger J: EGf binding to its receptor triggers a rapid tyrosine phosphorylation of the erbB-2 protein in the mammary tumor cell line SK-BR-3. EMBO J 1988;7:1647–1651.

94. Ross JS, Fletcher JA: The HER-2/neu oncogene in breast cancer: Prognostic factor, predictive factor, and target for therapy. Stem Cells 1998;16:413–428.

95. Slamon DJ, Godolphin W, Jones LA, et al: Studies of the HER-2/neu proto-oncogene in human breast and ovarian cancer. Science 1989;244:707–712.

96. Muss HB, Thor AD, Berry DA, et al: c-erbB-2 expression and response to adjuvant therapy in women with node-positive early breast cancer (see comments) [published erratum appears in N Engl J Med 1994;331:211]. N Engl J Med 1994;330:1260–1266.

97. Skorski T: Oncogenic tyrosine kinases and the DNA-damage response. Nat Rev Cancer 2002;2:351–360.

98. Adam L, Vadlamudi R, Kondapaka SB, Chernoff J, Mendelsohn J, Kumar R: Heregulin regulates cytoskeletal reorganization and cell migration through the p21-activated kinase-1 via phosphatidylinositol-3 kinase. J Biol Chem 1998; 273:28238–28246.

99. Raderschall E, Stout K, Freier S, Suckow V, Schweiger S, Haaf T: Elevated levels of Rad51 recombination protein in tumor cells. Cancer Res 2002;62:219–225.

100. Pietras RJ, Fendly BM, Chazin VR, Pegram MD, Howell SB, Slamon DJ: Antibody to HER-2/neu receptor blocks DNA repair after cisplatin in human breast and ovarian cancer cells. Oncogene 1994;9:1829–1838.

101. Kumar R, Mandal M, Lipton A, Harvey H, Thompson CB: Over-expression of HER2 modulates bcl-2, bcl-XL, and tamoxifen-induced apoptosis in human MCF-7 breast cancer cells. Clin Cancer Res 1996;2:1215–1219.

102. Amarante-Mendes GP, Naekyung Kim C, Liu L, et al: Bcr-Abl exerts its antiapoptotic effect against diverse apoptotic stimuli through blockage of mitochondrial release of cytochrome C and activation of caspase-3. Blood 1998;91:1700–1705.

103. Li Y, Upadhyay S, Bhuiyan M, Sarkar FH: Induction of apoptosis in breast cancer cells MDA-MB-231 by genistein. Oncogene 1999;18:3166–3172.

104. Hall JM, Lee MK, Newman B, et al: Linkage of early-onset familial breast cancer to chromosome 17q21. Science 1990;250:1684–1689.

105. Venkitaraman AR: Cancer susceptibility and the functions of BRCA1 and BRCA2. Cell 2002;108:171–182.

106. Moynahan ME, Chiu JW, Koller BH, Jasin M: BRCA1 controls homology-directed DNA repair. Mol Cell 1999;4:511–518.

107. Scully R, Chen J, Ochs RL, et al: Dynamic changes of BRCA1 subnuclear location and phosphorylation state are initiated by DNA damage. Cell 1997;90:425–435.

108. Somasundaram K, Zhang H, Zeng YX, et al: Arrest of the cell cycle by the tumour-suppressor BRCA1 requires the CDK-inhibitor p21WAF1/CiP1. Nature 1997;389:187–190.

109. Zhang H, Somasundaram K, Peng Y, et al: BRCA1 physically associates with p53 and stimulates its transcriptional activity. Oncogene 1998;16:1713–1721.

110. Harkin DP, Bean JM, Miklos D, et al: Induction of GADD45 and JNK/SAPK-dependent apoptosis following inducible expression of BRCA1. Cell 1999;97:575–586.

111. Scully R, Chen J, Plug A, et al: Association of BRCA1 with Rad51 in mitotic and meiotic cells. 1997;88:265–275.

112. Anonymous: Pathology of familial breast cancer: Differences between breast cancers in carriers of BRCA1 or BRCA2 mutations and sporadic cases. Breast Cancer Linkage Consortium (see comments). Lancet 1997;349:1505–1510.

113. Cortez D, Wang Y, Qin J, Elledge SJ: Requirement of ATM-dependent phosphorylation of BRCA1 in the DNA damage response to double-strand breaks (see comments). Science 1999;286:1162–1166.

114. Athma P, Rappaport R, Swift M: Molecular genotyping shows that ataxia-telangiectasia heterozygotes are predisposed to breast cancer. Cancer Genet Cytogenet 1996;92:130–134.

115. Easton DF: Cancer risks in A-T heterozygotes. Int J Radiat Biol 1994;66:S177–S182.

116. Janin N, Andrieu N, Ossian K, et al: Breast cancer risk in ataxia telangiectasia (AT) heterozygotes: Haplotype study in French AT families. Br J Cancer 1999;80:1042–1045.

117. FitzGerald MG, Bean JM, Hegde SR, et al: Heterozygous ATM mutations do not contribute to early onset of breast cancer (see comments). Nat Genet 1997;15:307–310.

118. Zhong Q, Chen CF, Li S, et al: Association of BRCA1 with the hRad50-hMre11-p95 complex and the DNA damage response. Science 1999;285:747–750.

119. Haber JE: The many interfaces of Mre11. Cell 1998;95:583–586.

120. Wang Y, Cortez D, Yazdi P, Neff N, Elledge S, Qin J: BASC, a super complex of BRCA1-associated proteins involved in the recognition and repair of aberrant DNA structures. Genes Dev 2000;14:927–939.

121. Welsch PL, King MC: BRCA1 and BRCA2 and the genetics of breast and ovarian cancer. Hum Mol Genet 2001;10:705–713.

122. Yuan SS, Lee SY, Chen G, Song M, Tomlinson GE, Lee EY: BRCA2 is required for ionizing radiation-induced assembly of RAD51 complex in vivo. Cancer Res 1999;59:3547–3551.

123. Chen J, Silver DP, Walpita D, et al: Stable interaction between the products of the BRCA1 and BRCA2 tumor-suppressor genes in mitotic and meiotic cells. Mol Cell 1998;2:317–328.

124. Futamura M, Arakawa H, Matsuda K, et al: Potential role of BRCA2 in a mitotic checkpoint after phosphorylation by hBUBR1. Cancer Res 2000;60:1531–1535.

125. Tutt A, Gabriel A, Bertwistle D, et al: Absence of BRCA2 causes genome instability by chromosome breakage and loss associated with centrosome amplification. Curr Biol 1999;9:1107–1110.

126. Patel KJ, Vu VP, Lee H, et al: Involvement of BRCA2 in DNA repair. Mol Cell 1998;1:347–357.

127. Howlett NG, Taniguchi T, Olson S, et al: Biallelic inactivation of BRCA2 in Fanconi anemia. Science 2002;297:606–609.

128. Domchek SM, Eisen A, Calzone K, et al: Application of breast cancer risk prediction models in clinical practice. J Clin Oncol 2003;21:593.

129. DeMichele A, Weber BL: Risk management in BRCA1 and BRCA2 mutation carrier: Lessons learned, challenges posed. J Clin Oncol 2002;20:1164.

130. Fisher B, Costantino JP, Wickerham DL, et al: Tamoxifen for prevention of breast cancer: Report of the National Surgical Adjuvant Breast and Bowel Project P-1 study. J Natl Cancer Inst 1998;90:1371.

131. Cuzick J, Forbes J, Edwards R, et al: First results from the International Breast Cancer Intervention Study (IBIS-I): A randomized prevention trial. Lancet 2002;360:817.

132. King M-C, Wieand S, Hale K, et al: Tamoxifen and breast cancer incidence among women with inherited mutations in BRCA1 and BRCA2. JAMA 2001;286:2251.

133. Powles TJ: The Royal Marsden Hospital (RMH) trial: Key points and remaining questions. Ann N Y Acad Sci 2001;949:109.

134. Veronesi V, Maisonneuve P, Costa A, et al: Prevention of breast cancer with tamoxifen: Preliminary findings from the Italian randomized trial among hysterectomised women. Lancet 1998;352:93.

135. Hartmann LC, Schaid DJ, Woods JE, et al: Efficacy of bilateral prophylactic mastectomy in women with a family history of breast cancer. N Engl J Med 1999;340:77.

136. McDonnell SK, Schaid DJ, Myers JL, et al: Efficacy of contralateral prophylactic mastectomy in women with a personal and family history of breast cancer. J Clin Oncol 2001;19:3938.

137. Hoogerbrugge N, Bult P, de Widt-Leveit LM, et al: High prevalence of premalignant lesions in prophylactically removed breasts from women at hereditary risk for breast cancer. J Clin Oncol 2003;21:41.

138. Cancer Statistics Review: 1973–1994. NIH Pub. No. 97-2789. Bethesda, National Cancer Institute, 1997.

139. Miller BA, Ries LA, Hankey BF, et al: Cancer Statistics Review 1973–1989. DHEW Publ. No. (NIH) 92-2789. Bethesda, National Cancer Institute, 1992.

140. Baker LH: Breast Cancer Demonstration Project: Five-year summary report. Cancer 1982;33:194.

141. Shapiro S: Periodic screening for breast cancer: The Health Insurance Plan Project and its sequelae, 1963–1989. Baltimore, Johns Hopkins University Press, 1988.

142. Shapiro S, Venet W, Strax P, et al: Ten- to fourteen-year effect of screening on breast cancer mortality. J Natl Cancer Inst 1982;69:349.

143. Chu KC, Smart CR, Tarone RE: Analysis of breast cancer mortality and stage distribution by age for the Health Insurance Plan clinical trial. J Natl Cancer Inst 1988;80:1125.

144. Tabar L, Fagerberg CJ, Gad A, et al: Reduction in mortality from breast cancer after mass screening with mammography: Randomized trial from the Breast Cancer Screening Working Group for the Swedish National Board of Health and Welfare. Lancet 1985;1:829.

145. Holmberg LH, Tabar L, Adami HO, et al: Survival in breast cancer diagnosed between mammographic screening examinations. Lancet 1983;2:27.

146. Tabar L, Fagerberg G, Duffy SW, et al: The Swedish two county trial for mammographic screening for breast cancer: Recent results and calculation of benefit. J Epidemiol Community Health 1989;43:107.

147. Tabar L, Fagerberg G, Duffy SW, et al: Update of the Swedish two-county program of mammographic screening for breast cancer. Radiol Clin North Am 1992;30:187.

148. Tabar L, Fagerberg CG, South MC, et al: The Swedish two-county trial of mammographic screening for breast cancer: Recent results on mortality and tumor characteristics. In Miller AB Jr, Chamberlain J, Day NE, et al (eds): Cancer Screening. Cambridge, Cambridge University Press, 1991, p 23.

149. Andersson K, Aspegren K, Janzon L, et al: Mammographic screening and mortality from breast cancer: The Malmö mammographic screening trial. BMJ 1988;297:943.

150. Janzon L, Andersson I: Malmö mammographic screening trial. In Miller AB Jr, Chamberlain J, Day NE, et al (eds): Cancer Screening. Cambridge, Cambridge University Press, 1991, p 637.

151. Frisell J, Eklund G, Hellstrom L, et al: Analysis of interval breast carcinomas in a randomized screening trial in Stockholm. In Breast Cancer Research and Treatment, vol 9. Boston, Martinus-Nijhoff, 1987, p 219.

152. Frisell J, Eklund G, Hellstrom L, et al: The Stockholm breast cancer screening trial: 5-year results and stage at discovery. Breast Cancer Res Treat 1989;13:79.

153. Frisell J, Eklund G, Hellstrom L, et al: Randomized study of mammography screening: Preliminary report on mortality in the Stockholm trial. Breast Cancer Res Treat 1991;18:49.

154. Frisell J, Glas U, Hellstrom L, et al: Randomized mammographic screening for breast cancer in Stockholm Breast Cancer Research and Treatment, vol 8. Boston, Martinus-Nijhoff, 1986, p 45.

155. Rutgvist LE, Miller AB, Anderson I, et al: Reduced breast cancer mortality with mammography screening: An assessment of currently available data. Int J Cancer Suppl 1990;5:76.

156. von Rosen A, Frisell J, Glas U, et al: Non-palpable invasive carcinomas from the Stockholm screening project. Acta Oncol 1989;28:23.

157. Baines CJ, McFarlane DV, Miller AB: Sensitivity and specificity of first screen mammography in 15 NBSS centers. Can Assoc Radiol J 1988;39:273.

158. Baines CJ, Miller AB, Bassett AA: Physical examination: Its role as a single screening modality in the Canadian National Breast Screening Study. Cancer 1989;63:1816.

159. Miller AB, Baines CJ, To T, et al: Canadian National Breast Screening Study: 1. Breast cancer detection and death rates among women ages 40 to 49 years. Can Med Assoc J 1992;147:1459.

160. Miller AB, Baines CJ, To T, et al: Canadian National Breast Screening Study: 2. Breast cancer detection and death rates among women 50 to 59 years. Can Med Assoc J 1992;1457:1477.

161. Roberts MM, Alexander FE, Anderson TJ, et al: Edinburgh trial of screening for breast cancer: Mortality at seven years. Lancet 1990;335:241.

162. Roberts MM, Alexander FE, Anderson TH, et al: The Edinburgh randomized trial of screening for breast cancer: Description of method. Br J Cancer 1984;50:1.

163. Chamberlain J, Coleman D, Ellman R, et al: Sensitivity and specificity of screening in the UK trial for early detection of breast cancer. In Miller AB Jr, Chamberlain J, Day NE, et al (eds): Cancer Screening. Cambridge, Cambridge University Press, 1991, p 3.

164. Trial of early detection of breast cancer: Description of method. Br J Cancer 1981;44:618.

165. UK Trial of Early Detection of Breast Cancer Group: First results on mortality reduction in the UK Trial of Early Detection of Breast Cancer Group. Lancet 1988;2:411.

166. Nyström L, Rutqvist LE, Wall S, et al: Breast cancer screening with mammography: An overview of the Swedish randomized trials. Lancet 1993;341:973.

167. Elwood JM, Cox B, Richardson AK: The effectiveness of breast cancer screening by mammography in younger women. Online J Curr Clin Trials 1993.

168. Huo Z, Giger ML, Vyborny CJ, Metz CE: Breast cancer: Effectiveness of computer-aided diagnosis observer study with independent database of mammograms. Radiology 2002;224:560–568.

169. Vyborny CJ, Giger ML, Nishikawa RM: Computer-aided detection and diagnosis of breast cancer. Radiol Clin North Am 2000;38:725–740.

170. Huo Z, Giger ML, Olopade OI, et al: Computerized analysis of digitized mammograms of BRCA1 and BRCA2 gene mutation carriers. Radiology 2002;225:519–526.

171. Solin LJ, Legorreta A, Schultz DJ, et al: The importance of mammary screening relative to the treatment of women with carcinoma of the breast. Arch Intern Med 1994;154:745.

172. Gayler BW, Brem RF: Mammography. In Niederhuber JE (ed): Current Therapy in Oncology. St. Louis, Mosby-Year Book, 1993, p 86.

173. Kopans DB: Detecting breast cancer not visible by mammography. J Natl Cancer Inst 1992;84:745.

174. McKenna RJ, Green P, Winchester DP, et al: Breast self-examination and breast physical examination. Cancer 1992;69:2003.

175. Senie RT, Lesser M, Kinne DW, Rosen PP: Method of tumor detection influences disease-free survival of women with breast carcinoma. Cancer 1994;73:1666.

176. Kusama S, Spratt JS, Donega WL, et al: The gross rates of growth of mammary carcinoma. Cancer 1972;30:594.

177. Day NE, Chamberlain J, Hakama M, et al: UICC project on screening for cancer: Report on the workshop on screening for breast cancer. Int J Cancer 1986;38:303.

178. Moskowitz M: Guidelines for screening for breast cancer: Is a revision in order? Radiol Clin North Am 1992;30:221.

179. US Preventive Services Task Force: Guide to clinical preventive services. Washington, DC, U.S. Department of Health and Human Services, 1989, p 26.

180. Shapiro S: Screening: Assessment of current studies. Cancer 1994;74:231.

181. Shapiro S, Strax P, Venet L, et al: Changes in 5-year breast cancer mortality in a breast cancer screening program. In Seventh National Cancer Conference Proceedings. American Cancer Society, 1974, p 663.

182. Beaker O, Shapiro S, Smart C: Report of the Working Group to review the National Cancer Institute American Cancer Society Breast Cancer Detection Demonstration Projects. J Natl Cancer Inst 1972;62:639.

183. Shapiro S, Venet W, Strax P, Venet L: Periodic screening for breast cancer: The Health Insurance Plan Project and its sequelae, 1963–1986. Baltimore, Johns Hopkins University Press, 1988.

184. Chu KC, Connor RJ: Analysis of the temporal patterns of benefits in the Health Insurance Plan of Greater New York trial by stage and age. Am J Epidemiol 1991;13:1039.

185. Breslow L, Thomas LB, Upton AC: Final reports of the National Cancer Institute Ad Hoc Working Groups on Mammography in Screening for Breast Cancer and summary report of their joint findings and recommendations. J Natl Cancer Inst 1977;59:467.

186. American Cancer Society Mammographic Guidelines 1983: Background, statement and update of cancer related check-up guidelines for breast cancer detection in asymptomatic women ages 40 to 49. CA Cancer J Clin 1983;33:254.

187. The Workshop Group: Reducing deaths from breast cancer in Canada. Can Med Assoc J 1989;141:199.

188. Shapiro S, Venet W, Strax P, Venet L: Current results of the breast cancer screening randomized trial: The Heath Insurance Plan (HIP) of Greater New York study. In Day NE, Miller AB (eds): Screening for Breast Cancer. Toronto, Hans Huber, 1988, p 3.

189. American Cancer Society Workshop on Guidelines and Screening for Breast Cancer: October 11–13, 1991 Proceedings. Cancer Suppl 1992;69:1885.

190. Screening recommendations of the forum panel. J Gerontol 1992;47.

191. Fletcher SW, Black W, Harris R, et al: Results of the International Workshop on Screening for Breast Cancer. J Natl Cancer Inst 1993;85:1644.

192. Fletcher SW: Whither scientific deliberation in health policy recommendations? Alice in Wonderland of breast cancer screening. N Engl J Med 1997;336:1180.

193. Eastman P: NCI adopts new mammography screening guidelines for women. J Natl Cancer Inst 1997;89:538.

194. Gotzsche PC, Olsen O: Is screening for breast cancer with mammography justifiable? Lancet 2000;355:129–134.

195. Olsen O, Gotzsche PC: Cochrane review on screening for breast cancer with mammography. Lancet 2001; 358:1340–1342.

196. Duffy S, Tabar L, Chen HH, et al: The impact of organized mammographic service screening on breast cancer mortality in seven Swedish counties. Cancer 2002;95:458–469.

197. Harris R: Breast cancer among women in their forties: Toward a reasonable research agenda. J Natl Cancer Inst 1994;86:410.

198. Champion VL: The relationship of selected variables to breast cancer detection behaviors in women 35 and older. Oncol Nurs Forum 1991;18:733.

199. Breen N, Wagener D, Brown ML, et al: Progress in cancer screening over a decade: Results of cancer screening from the 1987, 1992, and 1998 NHIS. National Health Interview Surveys. J Natl Cancer Inst 2001;93:1704–1713.

200. Lannin DR, Mathews HF, Mitchell J, Swanson MS: Impacting cultural attitudes in African-American women to decrease breast cancer mortality. Am J Surg 2002;184:418–423.

201. Champion VL: Strategies to increase mammography utilization. Med Care 1994;32:118.

202. Stoner TJ, Dowd B, Carr WP, et al: Do vouchers improve breast cancer screening rates? Results from a randomized trial. Health Services Res 1998;33:11.

203. Schechter C, Vanchieri C, Crofton C: Evaluating women's beliefs and perceptions in developing mammography promotion messages. Public Health Rep 1990;105:253.

204. Slenker SE, Grant MC: Attitudes, beliefs, and knowledge about mammography among women over forty years of age. J Cancer Educ 1989;4:61.

205. Eley JW, Hill HA, Chen VW, et al: Racial differences in survival from breast cancer: Results of the National Cancer Institute Black/White Cancer Survival Study. JAMA 1994;272:947.

206. Simon MS, Gimotty PA, Coombs J, et al: Factors affecting participation in a mammography screening program among members of an urban Detroit health maintenance organization. Cancer Detect Prevent 1998;22:30.

207. Kerlikowske K: Timeliness of follow-up after abnormal screening mammography. Br Cancer Res Treat 1996;40:53.

208. Rimer B, King E: Why aren't older women getting mammograms and clinical breast exam? Women's Health Issues 1992;2:94.

209. Fox S, Stein J: The effect of physician patient communication on mammography utilization by different ethnic groups. Med Care 1991;29:1065.

210. Kerlikowske K: Effect of age, breast density, and family history on the sensitivity of first screen mammography. JAMA 1996;276:33.

211. Laya MB: Effect of estrogen replacement therapy on the specificity and sensitivity of screening mammography. J Natl Cancer Inst 1996;88:643.

212. Baines CJ, Vidmar M, McKeown-Eyssen G, Tibshirani R: Impact of menstrual phase on false-negative mammograms in the Canadian National Breast Screening Study. Cancer 1997;80:720.

213. White E, Velentgas P, Mandelson MT, et al: Variation in mammographic breast density by time in menstrual cycle among women aged 40 to 49 years. J Natl Cancer Inst 1998;90:906.

214. Liberman L, Abramson AF, Squires FB, et al: The breast imaging reporting and data system: Positive predictive value of mammographic features and final assessment categories. Am J Roentgenol 1998;171:35.

215. Salvatore M, Del Vecchio S: Dynamic imaging: Scintimammography (review). Eur J Radiol 1998;27(S2):259.

216. Sardanelli F, Melani E, Ottonello C, et al: Magnetic resonance imaging of the breast in characterizing positive or uncertain mammographic findings. Cancer Detect Prev 1998;22:39.

217. Tilanus-Linthorst M, Verhoog L, Obdeijn IM, et al: A BRCA1/2 mutation, high breast density and prominent pushing margins of a tumor independently contribute to a frequent false-negative mammography. Int J Cancer 2002;102:91–95.

218. Block EF, Meyer MA: Positron emission tomography in diagnosis of occult adenocarcinoma of the breast. Am Surg 1998;64:906.

219. Smith IC, Ogston KN, Whitford P, et al: Staging of the axilla in breast cancer: Accurate in vivo assessment using positron emission tomography with 2-(fluorine-18)-fluro-2-deoxy-D-glucose. Ann Surg 1998;228:220.

220. Lind P, Umschaden HW, Forsthuber E, et al: Scintimammography using Tc-99m tetrofosmin. Acta Med Aust 1997;24:50.

221. Nixon AJ, Neuberg D, Hayes DF, et al : Relationship of patient age to pathologic features of the tumor and prognosis for patients with stage I or II breast cancer. J Clin Oncol 1994;12:888–894.

222. Balducci L, Schapira DV, Cox CE, Greenberg HM, Lyman GH: Breast cancer of the older woman: An annotated review. J Am Geriatr Soc 1991;39:1113–1123.

223. Tabar L, Vitak B, Chen HH, et al: The Swedish Two-County Trial twenty years later: Updated mortality results and new insights from long-term follow-up. Radiol Clin North Am 2000;38: 625–651.

224. Weinberger M, Saunders A, Samsa G, et al: Breast cancer screening in older women: Practices and barriers reports by primary care physicians. J Am Geriatr Soc 1991;39:22.

225. Morrow M: Breast disease in elderly women. Surg Clin North Am 1994;74:145.

226. Mandelblatt J, Wheat M, Monane M, et al: Breast cancer screening for elderly women with and without co-morbid conditions. Ann Intern Med 1992;116:722.

227. Wilson TE, Helvie MA, August DA: Breast cancer in the elderly patient: Early detection with mammography. Radiology 1994;190:203.

228. Fentiman IS: Psychological sequelae of screening women with a family history of breast cancer. Eur J Cancer 1998;34: 1991–1992.

229. Gilbert FJ, Cordiner CM, Affleck IR, Hood DB, Mathieson D, Walker LG: Breast screening: The psychological sequelae of false-positive recall in women with and without a family history of breast cancer. Eur J Cancer 1998;34:2010–2014.

230. Lowe JB, Balanda KP, Del Mar C, Hawes E: Psychologic distress in women with abnormal finds in mass mammography screening. Cancer 1999;85:1114–1118.

231. Lampic C, Thurfjell E, Bergh J, Sjoden PO: Short- and long-term anxiety and depression in women recalled after breast cancer screening. Eur J Cancer 2001;37:463–469.

232. Weinberger M, Saunders AF, Samsa GP, et al: Breast cancer screening in older women: Practices and barriers reported by primary care physicians. J Am Geriatr Soc 1991;39:22–29.

233. Fox SA, Roetzheim RG, Kington RS: Barriers to cancer prevention in the older person. Clin Geriatr Med 1997;13:79–95.

234. Kuhl KC, Schmutzler RK, Luetner CC, et al: Breast MR imaging screening in 192 women proved or suspected to be carriers of a breast cancer susceptibility gene: Preliminary results. Radiology 2000;215:267–279.

235. Tilanus-Linthorst MM, Obdeijn IM, Bartels KC, de Konig HJ, Oudkerk M: First experiences in screening women at high risk for breast cancer with MR imaging. Breast Cancer Res Treat 2000;63: 53–60.

236. Scheuer L, Kauff N, Robson M, et al: Outcome of preventive surgery and screening for breast and ovarian cancer in BRCA mutation carriers. J Clin Oncol 2002;20:1260–1268.

237. DeMichele A, Weber BL: Risk management in BRCA1 and BRCA2 mutation carriers: Lesions learned, challenges posed. J Clin Oncol 2002;20:1164–1166.

238. Baines CJ, Miller AB, Kopans DB: Canadian national breast screening study: Assessment of technical quality by external review. Am J Radiol 1990;155:743.

239. Sailors DM, Crabtree JD, Land RL, et al: Needle localization for nonpalpable breast lesions. Am Surg 1994;60:186.

240. Kopans DB, Meyer JF, Lindfors KK: Whole breast ultrasound imaging: Four year follow-up. Radiology 1985;157:505.

241. Egan R, Egan KL: Detection of breast cancer: Comparison of water-bath whole breast sonography, mammography and physical examination. Am J Roentgenol 1985;145:1.

242. Skoone P, Engeldal K, Skjennald A: Interobserver variation in the interpretation of breast imaging: Comparison of mammography, ultrasonography, and both combined in the interpretation of palpable noncalcified breast masses. Acta Radiol 1997;38:497.

243. Sickles EA, Filley RA, Callen PW: Benign breast lesions: Ultrasound detection and diagnosis. Radiology 1984;151:467.

244. Garra BS, Krasner BH, Horii SC, et al: Improving the distinction between benign and malignant breast lesions: The value of sonographic texture analysis. Ultrason Imaging 1993;15:267.

245. Kedar RP, Cosgrove DO, Smith IE, et al: Breast carcinoma: Measurement of tumor response to primary medical therapy with color Doppler flow imaging. Radiology 1994;190:825.

246. Morrow M: Management of nonpalpable breast lesions. PPO Updates 1990;4:1.

247. Moskowitz M: The predictive value of certain mammographic signs in screening for breast cancer. Cancer 1983;51:1007.

248. Azavedo E, Auer G, Svane G: Sterotactic fine needle biopsy in mammographically detected nonpalpable lesions. Lancet 1989;1:1033.

249. Parker SH, Lovin JD, Jobe WE, et al: Nonpalpable breast lesions: Sterotactic automated large-core biopsies. Radiology 1991;180:403.

250. Parker SH, Lovin JD, Jobe WE, et al: Stereotactic breast biopsy with a biopsy gun. Radiology 1990;176:741.

251. Gallagher W, Cardenosa G, Rubens J: Minimal volume excision of nonpalpable breast lesions. Am J Radiol 1989;153:947.

252. Homer MJ, Smith TJ, Safari H: Prebiopsy needle localization: Methods, problems and expected results. Radiol Clin North Am 1992;30:139.

253. Schmidt RA: Stereotactic breast biopsy. CA Cancer J Clin 1994;44:172.

254. Mainiero MB, Philpotts LE, Lee CH, et al: Stereotaxic core needle biopsy of breast microcalcifications: Correlation of target accuracy and diagnosis with lesion size. Radiology 1996;198:665.

255. Jackman RJ, Nowels KW, Shepard MJ, et al: Stereotaxic large-core needle biopsy of 450 nonpalpable breast lesions with surgical correlation in lesions with cancer or atypical hyperplasia. Radiology 1994;193:91.

256. Liberman L, Cohen MA, Dershaw DD, et al: Atypical ductal hyperplasia diagnosed a stereotaxic core biopsy of breast lesions: An indication for surgical biopsy. Am J Roentgenol 1995;164: 1111.

257. Sullivan DC: Needle core biopsy of mammographic lesions. Am J Roentgenol 1994;162:601.

258. Meyer JE: Value of large core biopsy of occult breast lesions. Am J Roentgenol 1992;185:991.

259. Lindfors KK, Rosenquist CJ: Needle core biopsy guided with mammography: A study of cost effectiveness. Radiology 1994;190:217.

260. Greene FL, Page DL, Fleming ID, et al: AJCC Cancer Staging Manual, 6th ed. New York, Springer-Verlag, 2002.

261. Singletary SE, Allred C, Ashley P, et al: Revision of the American Joint Committee on Cancer Staging System for Breast Cancer. J Clin Oncol 20:3628–3636, 2002 (early release www.jco.org July 9, 2002).

262. Rosen PP, Groshen S, Kinne DW, Norton L: Factors influencing prognosis in node negative breast carcinoma: Analysis of 767 T1N0M0/T2N0M0 patients with long term follow-up. J Clin Oncol 1993;11:2090.

263. Lin PP, Allison DC, Wainstock J, et al: Impact of axillary lymph node dissection on the therapy of breast cancer patients. J Clin Oncol 1993;11:1536.

264. Azzopardi JG, Chepick OF, Hartman WH, et al: The World Health Organization histological typing of breast tumors, 2nd ed. Am J Clin Pathol 1982;78:806.

265. Diab SG, Clark GM, Osborne CK, et al: Tumor characteristics and clinical outcome of tubular and mucinous breast carcinomas. J Clin Oncol 1999;17:1442.

266. Fisher ER, Redmond C, Fisher B, Bass G: Pathologic findings from the National Surgical Adjuvant Breast and Bowel Projects (NSABP): Prognostic discriminants for 8-year survival. Cancer 1990;65:2121.

267. Todd JH, Williams MR: Confirmation of prognostic index in primary breast cancer. Br J Cancer 1987;56:489.

268. Sauerbrei W, Hubner K, Schmoor, et al: German Breast Cancer Study group: Validation of existing and development of new prognostic classifications schemes in node negative breast cancer. Breast Cancer Res Treat 1997;42:149.

269. McGuire WL, Clark GM: Prognostic factors and treatment decisions in axillary-node-negative breast cancer. N Engl J Med 1992;326:1756–1761.

270. Gasparini G: Prognostic variables in node-negative and node-positive breast cancer. Breast Cancer Res Treat 1998;52:321–331.

271. Hayes DF, Trock B, Harris AL: Assessing the clinical impact of prognostic factors: When is "statistically significant" clinically useful? Breast Cancer Res Treat 1998;52:305–319.

272. Isaacs C, Stearns V, Hayes DF: New prognostic factors for breast cancer recurrence. Semin Oncol 2001;28:53–67.

273. Clark GM: Interpreting and integrating risk factors for patients with primary breast cancer. J Natl Cancer Inst Monogr 2001;17–21.

274. Yamauchi H, Stearns V, Hayes DF: The role of c-erbB-2 as a predictive factor in breast cancer. Breast Cancer 2001;8:171–183.

275. Mass R: The role of HER-2 expression in predicting response to therapy in breast cancer. Semin Oncol 27:46–52; discussion 2000;92–100.

276. Zemzoum I, Kates RE, Ross JS, et al: Invasion factors uPA/PAI-1 and HER2 status provide independent and complementary information on patient outcome in node-negative breast cancer. J Clin Oncol 2003;21:1022–1028.

277. van't Veer LJ, Dai H, van de Vijver MJ, et al: Gene expression profiling predicts clinical outcome of breast cancer. Nature 2002;415:530–536.

278. van de Vijver MJ, He YD, van't Veer LJ, et al: A gene-expression signature as a predictor of survival in breast cancer. N Engl J Med 2002;347:1999–2009.

279. Rai AJ, Zhang Z, Rosenzweig J, et al: Proteomic approaches to tumor marker discovery. Arch Pathol Lab Med 2002;126:1518–1526.

280. Li J, Zhang Z, Rosenzweig J, et al: Proteomics and bioinformatics approaches for identification of serum biomarkers to detect breast cancer. Clin Chem 2002;48:1296–304.

281. Perou CM, Sorlie T, Eisen MB, et al: Molecular portraits of human breast tumours. Nature 2000;406:747–752.

282. West M, Blanchette C, Dressman H, et al: Predicting the clinical status of human breast cancer by using gene expression profiles. Proc Natl Acad Sci USA 2001;98:11462–11467.

283. Hedenfalk I, Duggan D, Chen Y, et al: Gene-expression profiles in hereditary breast cancer. N Engl J Med 2001;344:539–548.

284. Sorlie T, Perou CM, Tibshirani R, et al: Gene expression patterns of breast carcinomas distinguish tumor subclasses with clinical implications. Proc Natl Acad Sci USA 2001;98:10869–10874.

285. Sotiriou C, Powles TJ, Dowsett M, et al: Gene expression profiles derived from fine needle aspiration correlate with response to systemic chemotherapy in breast cancer. Breast Cancer Res 2002;4:R3.

286. Broders AC: Carcinoma in-situ contracted with benign penetrating epithelium. JAMA 1932;99:1670.

287. Rosner D, Bedwani RN, Vana J, et al: Noninvasive breast carcinoma: Results of a national survey by the American College of Surgeons. Ann Surg 1980;192:139.

288. Foote FW, Steward FW: Lobular carcinoma in-situ: A rare form of mammary cancer. Am J Pathol 1941;17:491.

289. Anderson JA, Vendelboe ML: Cytoplastic mucous globules in lobular carcinoma in situ. Am J Surg Pathol 1981;5:251.

290. Haagensen CD, Lane N, Lattes R, et al: Lobular neoplasia (so-called lobular carcinoma in situ) of the breast. Cancer 1978;42:737.

291. Kinne DW: Lobular carcinoma in situ. In Gump FF (ed): Breast Cancer in High-Risk Patients. Surg Oncol Clin North Am 1993;2:65.

292. Landercasper J, Gundersen SB, Gundersen AL, et al: Needle localization and biopsy of nonpalpable lesions of the breast. Surg Gynecol Obstet 1987;164:399.

293. Tinnemans GM, Wobbes T, Holland R, et al: Mammographic and histopathologic correlation of nonpalpable lesions of the breast and the reliability of frozen section diagnosis. Surg Gynecol Obstet 1987;165:523.

294. Poole GV Jr, Choplin RH, Sterchi MJ, et al: Occult lesions of the breast. Surg Gynecol Obstet 1986;163:107.

295. Pole TL Jr, Fechner RE, Wilhelm MC, et al: Lobular carcinoma in situ of the breast: Mammographic features. Radiology 1988;168:63.

296. Sonnefeld MR, Frenna TH, Weidnes N, et al: Lobular carcinoma in situ: Mammographic-pathologic correlation of needle-directed biopsy. Radiology 1991;181:363.

297. Nguyen J, McMullen K, Sardi A: Lobular carcinoma in situ within a fibroadenoma. J La State Med Soc 1991;143:33.

298. Page DL, Jopaze H: Non infiltrating (in situ) carcinoma. In Bland KI, Copeland EM (eds): The Breast, Comprehensive Management of Benign and Malignant Diseases. Philadelphia, WB Saunders, 1991, p 169.

299. Frykberg ER, Santiago F, Betsill WL Jr, O'Brien PH: Lobular carcinoma in situ of the breast. Surg Gynecol Obstet 1987;164:285.

300. Newman W: Lobular carcinoma of the female breast: Report of 73 cases. Ann Surg 1966;164:305.

301. Giordano JM, Klopp CT: Lobular carcinoma in situ: Incidence and treatment. Cancer 1973;31:105.

302. Swain SM: Non-invasive breast cancer: Lobular carcinoma in situ. Incidence, presentation, guidelines to treatment. Oncology 1989;3:35.

303. Benfield JR, Jacobson M, Warner NE: In situ lobular carcinoma of the breast. Arch Surg 1965;91:130.

304. Carter D, Smith RRL: Carcinoma in situ of the breast. Cancer 1977;40:1189.

305. Page DL, Kidd TE, DuPont WD, et al: Lobular neoplasia of the breast: Higher risk for subsequent invasive cancer predicted by more extensive disease. Hum Pathol 1991;22:1232.

306. Dall'Olmo CA, Ponka JL, Horn RC, Rui R: Lobular carcinoma of the breast in situ: Are we too radical in its treatment? Arch Surg 1975;110:537.

307. Ringberg A, Palmer B, Linell F: The contralateral breast at reconstructive surgery after breast operation: A histopathological study. Breast Cancer Res Treat 1982;2:151.

308. Schwartz GF, Feig SA, Potefsky AS: Significance and staging of nonpalpable carcinomas of the breast. Surg Gynecol Obstet 1988;166:6.

309. Rosen PP, Senie R, Schottenfeld D, Askihri R: Non-invasive breast carcinoma: Frequency of unsuspected invasion and implications for treatment. Ann Surg 1979;189:377.

310. Farrow JH: The James Ewing Lecture: Current concepts in the detection and treatment of the earliest of the early breast cancers. Cancer 1979;25:468.

311. Urban JA: Biopsy of the "normal" breast in treating breast cancer. Surg Clin North Am 1969;49:291.

312. Rosen PP, Braun DW, Lyngholm B, et al: Lobular carcinoma in situ of the breast: Preliminary results of treatment by ipsilateral mastectomy and contralateral breast biopsy. Cancer 1981;47:813.

313. Nielsen M, Jensen J, Andersen J: Precancerous and cancerous breast lesions during lifetime and at autopsy. Cancer 1984;54:612.

314. Haagensen CD, Bodian C, Haagensen DE Jr: Breast Carcinoma Risk and Detection. Philadelphia, WB Saunders, 1981, p 238.

315. Rosen PP, Lieberman PH, Braun DW, et al: Lobular carcinoma in situ of the breast. Am J Surg Pathol 1978;2:225.

316. Ottesen GL, Graversen HP, Blichert-Toft M, et al: Lobular carcinoma in situ of the female breast: Short-term results of a prospective nationwide study. Am J Surg Pathol 1993;17:14.

317. Sunshine JA, Moseley HS, Fletcher WS, et al: Breast carcinoma in situ: A retrospective review of 112 cases with a minimum 10 year follow-up. Am J Surg 1985;150:44.

318. Kinne DW, Petrek JA, Osborne MP, et al: Breast carcinoma in situ. Arch Surg 1989;124:33.

319. Rosen PP, Brown DW, Kinne DW: The clinical significance of pre-invasive carcinoma. Cancer 1980;46:919.

320. Walt AJ, Simon M, Swanson GM: The continuing dilemma of lobular carcinoma in situ. Arch Surg 1992;127:904.

321. The Consensus Conference Committee: Consensus Conference on the Classification of Ductal Carcinoma in Situ. Cancer 1997;80:1798–1802.

322. Wellings SR, Jensen HM: On the origin and progression of ductal carcinoma in the human breast. J Natl Cancer Inst 1973;50:1111.

323. Alpers CH, Wellings SR: The prevalence of carcinoma in situ in normal and cancer-associated breasts. Hum Pathol 1985;16:796.

324. Nielsen M, Thomsen JL, Primdahl S, et al: Breast cancer and atypia among young and middle-aged women: A study of 110 medico-legal autopsies. Br J Cancer 1987;56:814.

325. Frykberg ER, Masood S, Copeland EM, Bland KI: Ductal carcinoma in situ of the breast: Collective review. Surg Gynecol Obstet 1993;177:425.

326. Bernstein L: The epidemiology of breast cancer. In Silverstein M (ed): Ductal Carcinoma in Situ of the Breast, 2nd ed. Philadelphia, Lippincott Williams & Wilkins, 2002, p 23.

327. McDivitt RW: Breast cancer multicentricity. In McDivitt RW, Oberman HA, Ozello L (eds): The Breast. Baltimore, Williams & Wilkins, 1984.

328. Lagios MD, Westdahl PR, Margohn FR, et al: Duct carcinoma in situ: Relationship of extent of noninvasive disease to the frequency of occult invasion, multicentricity, lymph node

metastases, and short-term treatment failures. Cancer 1982;50:1309.

329. Holland R, Faverly D: The local distribution of ductal carcinoma in situ of the breast: Whole-organ studies. In Silverstein M (ed): Ductal Carcinoma in Situ of the Breast, 2nd ed. Philadelphia, Lippincott Williams & Wilkins, 2002, pp 240–248.

330. Ikeda DM, Anderson I: Ductal carcinoma in situ: Atypical mammographic appearances. Radiology 1989;172:661.

331. Dershaw DD, Abramson A, Kinne DW: Ductal carcinoma in situ: Mammographic findings and clinical implications. Radiology 1989;170:411.

332. Stomper PC, Mergolin FR: Ductal carcinoma in situ: The mammographic perspective. Am J Radiol 1994;162:585.

333. Tabar L, Gad A, Parsons W, Neeland D: Mammographic appearances of in situ carcinomas. In Silverstein M (ed): Ductal Carcinoma in Situ of the Breast, 1997, Philadelphia, Lippincott Williams & Wilkins, pp 95–117.

334. Orel S, Reynolds C, Schnall M, et al: Breast carcinoma: MR imaging before re-excisional biopsy. Radiology 1997;205:429–436.

335. Soderstrom C, Harms S, Farrell R, et al: Detection with MR imaging of residual tumor in the breast soon after surgery. Am J Roentgenol 1997;168:485–488.

336. Berg W: Imaging the local extent of disease. Semin Breast Dis 2001;4:153–173.

337. Ozzello L: Intraepithelial carcinoma of the breast. In Hollman KH, Verley JM (eds): New Frontiers in Mammary Pathology. New York, Plenum Press, 1983.

338. Barsky SH, Siegal GP, Jannetta F, et al: Loss of basement membrane components by invasive tumors but not by their benign counterparts. Lab Invest 1983;49:140.

339. Bijker N: Analysis of EORTC trial 10853. Fifth EORTC/EUSOMA DCIS Consensus Conference, Leyden, The Netherlands, May 2002.

340. Allred DC: Biologic characteristics of ductal carcinoma in situ. In Silverstein M (ed): Ductal Carcinoma in Situ of the Breast, 2nd ed. Philadelphia, Lippincott Williams & Wilkins, 2002, pp 37–48.

341. Stomper PC, Connolly JL, Meyer JE, Haris JR: Clinically occult ductal carcinoma in situ detected with mammography: Analysis of 100 cases with radiologic pathologic correlation. Radiology 1989;172:225.

342. Fisher B, Digman J, Wolmark N, et al: Tamoxifen in treatment of intraductal breast cancer: National Surgical Adjuvant Breast and Bowel Project B-24 randomised controlled trial. Lancet 1999;353: 1993–2000.

343. McCormick B, Rosen P, Kinne, D et al: Duct carcinoma in situ of the breast: An analysis of local control after conservation surgery and radiotherapy. Int J Radiat Oncol Biol Phys 1991;21:289–292.

344. Schnitt SJ, Harris JR: Ductal carcinoma in situ (intraductal carcinoma) of the breast. PPO Updates 1988;2:1.

345. Schnitt SJ, Silen W, Sadowsky NL, et al: Ductal carcinoma in situ (intraductal carcinoma) of the breast. N Engl J Med 1988;31:898.

346. Lagios MD, Margolin FR, Westdahl PR, et al: Mammographically detected duct carcinoma in situ: Frequency of local recurrence following tylectomy and prognostic effect of nuclear grade on local recurrence. Cancer 1989;63:618.

347. Lagios M: Duct carcinoma in situ: Pathology and treatment. Surg Clin North Am 1990;70:853.

348. Bedwani R, Vana J, Rosner D, et al: Management and survival of female patients with "minimal" breast cancer: As observed in the long-term and short-term surveys of the American College of Surgeons. Cancer 1981;47:2769.

349. Fisher ER, Leeming R, Anderson S, et al: Conservative management of intraductal carcinoma (DCIS) of the breast. J Surg Oncol 1991;47:139.

350. Baird RM, Worth A, Hislop G: Recurrence after lumpectomy for comedo-type intraductal carcinoma of the breast. Am J Surg 1990;159:479.

351. Millis RR, Thynne GSJ: In situ intraductal carcinoma of the breast: A long term follow-up study. Br J Surg 1975;62:957.

352. von Reuden DG, Wilson RE: Intraductal carcinoma of the breast. Surg Gynecol Obstet 1984;158:105.

353. Ashikari R, Hajdu SI, Robbins GF: Intraductal carcinoma of the breast (1960–1969). Cancer 1971;28:1182.

354. Arnessen L-G, Fagerberg G, Gronroft O: Is sector resection sufficient for cure of in situ ductal cancer of the breast? Fourth EORTC Breast Cancer Working Conference, London, July 1987.

355. Price P, Sinnett HD, Gusterson B, et al: Duct carcinoma in situ: Predictors of local recurrence and progression in patients treated by surgery alone. Br J Cancer 1990;61:869.

356. Fisher ER, Sass R, Fisher B, et al: Pathologic findings from the National Surgical Adjuvant Breast Project (Protocol 6) I: Intraductal carcinoma (DCIS). Cancer 1986;57:197.

357. Salvadori D: Ductal carcinoma in situ: Retrospective analysis of 50 patients including 19 treated with breast conservation (abstracted). Castlemarquet, The Netherlands, EORTC in Situ Breast Cancer Workshop, 1988.

358. Gallagher WJ, Koerner RD, Wood WC: Treatment of intraductal carcinoma with limited surgery: Long-term followup. J Clin Oncol 1989;7:376.

359. Carpenter R, Boulter PS, Cooke T, et al: Management of screen-detected ductal carcinoma in situ of the female breast. Br J Surg 1989;76:564.

360. Page DL, Dupont WD, Rogers LW, Nandenberg M: Intraductal carcinoma of the breast: Follow-up after biopsy only. Cancer 1982;49:751.

361. Fowble BL: Intraductal non-invasive breast cancer: A comparison of local treatments. Oncology 1989;3:51.

362. Stotter AT, McNeese M, Oswald MJ, et al: The role of limited surgery with radiation and primary treatment of ductal in situ breast cancer. Int J Radiat Oncol Biol Phys 1990;18:283.

363. Solin LJ, Fowble B, Martz KL, et al: Definitive radiation for early stage breast cancer: The University of Pennsylvania experience. Int J Radiat Oncol Biol Phys 1988;14:235.

364. Silverstein MJ, Rosser R, Gierson E, et al: Intraductal breast carcinoma (DCIS): A therapeutic dilemma. Proc Am Soc Clin Oncol 1988;7:25.

365. Bornstein B, Recht A, Connolly JL, et al: Results of treating ductal carcinoma in situ of the breast with conservative surgery and radiation therapy. Cancer 1991;67:7.

366. Fisher E, Dignam J, Tan-Chiu E, et al: Pathologic findings from the National Surgical Adjuvant Breast Project (NSABP): Eight-year update of protocol B-17. Cancer 1999;86:429–438.

367. Julien J, Bijker N, Fentiman I, et al: Radiotherapy in breast-conserving treatment for ductal carcinoma in situ: First results of the EORTC randomized phase III trial 10853. Lancet 2000;355:528–533.

368. Vicini F, Recht A: Age at diagnosis and outcome for women with ductal carcinoma in situ of the breast: A critical review of the literature. J Clin Oncol 2002;20:2736–2744.

369. Van Zee K, Liberman L, Samli B, et al: Long term follow-up of women with ductal carcinoma in situ treated with breast-conserving surgery: The effect of age. Cancer 1999;86: 1757–1767.

370. Solin L, Fourquet A, Vicini F, et al: Mammographically detected ductal carcinoma in situ of the breast treated with breast-conserving surgery and definitive breast radiation: Long-term outcome and prognostic significance of patient age and margin status. Int J Radiat Oncol Biol Phys 2001;50:991–1002.

371. Solin L, Yeh I, Kurtz J, et al: Ductal carcinoma in situ (intraductal carcinoma) of the breast treated with breast-conserving surgery and definitive irradiation. Cancer 1993;71:2532–2542.

372. Kestin L, Goldstein N, Lacerna M, et al: Factors associated with local recurrence of mammographically detected ductal carcinoma in situ in patients given breast-conserving therapy. Cancer 2000;88:596–607.

373. Cutuli B, Cohen-Solal-Le C, LaFontan B, et al: Breast conservation therapy for ductal carcinoma in situ of the breast: The French cancer centers' experience. Int J Radiat Oncol Biol Phys 2002;53:868–879.

374. Sposto R, Epstein M, Silverstein M: Predicting local recurrence in patients with ductal carcinoma in situ. In Silverstein M (ed): Ductal Carcinoma of the Breast, 2nd ed. Philadelphia, Lippincott Williams & Wilkins, 2002, pp 255–263.

375. Houghton J, George WD: Radiotherapy and tamoxifen after complete excision of ductal carcinoma in situ of the breast. In Silverstein M (ed): Ductal Carcinoma of the Breast, 2nd ed. Philadelphia, Lippincott Williams & Wilkins, 2002, pp 453–455.

376. Camus M, Joshi M, Mackarem G, et al: Ductal carcinoma in situ of the male breast. Cancer 1994;74:1289–1293.

377. Levine MN, Jafni A, Markham B, MacFarlane D: A bedside decision instrument to elicit a patient's preference concerning adjuvant chemotherapy for breast cancer. Ann Intern Med 1992;117:53.

378. Keynes G: Conservative treatment of cancer of the breast. BMJ 1937;2:643.

379. Peters MV: Wedge resection with or without radiation in early breast cancer. Int J Radiat Oncol Biol Phys 1977;2:1151.

380. Baclesse F: Roentgen therapy as the sole method of treatment of cancer of the breast. Am J Roentgenol 1949;62:311.

381. Mustakallio S: Conservative treatment of breast carcinoma review of 25 years follow up. Clin Radiol 1972;23:110.

382. Pierquin B, Baillet F, Wilson JF: Radiation therapy in the management of primary breast cancer. Am J Roentgenol 1976;127: 645.

383. Calle R, Pilleron JP, Schlienger P, Vilcoq JR: Conservative management of operable breast cancer: Ten years experience at the Foundation Curie. Cancer 1978;42:2045.

384. Prosnitz LR, Goldenberg IS: Radiation therapy as primary treatment for early stage carcinoma of the breast. Cancer 1975;35:1587.

385. Weber E, Hellman S: Radiation as primary treatment for local control of breast carcinoma: A progress report. JAMA 1975;234:608.

386. Morrow M. Rational local therapy for breast cancer (editorial). N Engl J Med 2002;347:1270–1271.

387. Veronesi U, Cascinelli N, Mariani L, et al: Twenty-year follow-up of a randomized study comparing breast-conserving surgery with radical mastectomy for early breast cancer. N Engl J Med 2002; 347:1227–1231.

388. Fisher B, Anderson S, Bryant J, et al: Twenty-year follow-up of a randomized trial comparing total mastectomy, lumpectomy, and lumpectomy plus irradiation for the treatment of invasive breast cancer. N Engl J Med 2002;345:1233–1240.

389. NIH Consensus Conference: Treatment of early-stage breast cancer. JAMA 1991;265:391.

390. Solin LJ, Fowble B, Martz K, et al: Results of re-excisional biopsy of the primary tumor in preparation for definitive irradiation of patients with early stage breast cancer. Int J Radiat Oncol Biol Phys 1986;12:721.

391. McCormick B, Kinne D, Petrek J, et al: Limited resection for breast cancer: A study of inked specimen margins before radiotherapy. Int J Radiat Oncol Biol Phys 1987;13:1667.

392. Margolese R, Poisson R, Shibata H, et al: The technique of segmental mastectomy (lumpectomy) and axillary dissection: A syllabus from the National Surgical Adjuvant Breast Project workshops. Surgery 1987;102:828.

393. Gould EW, Robinson PG: The pathologist's examination of the "lumpectomy": The pathologists' view of surgical margins. Semin Surg Oncol 1992;8:129.

394. Rosen PP: Pathological assessment of nonpalpable breast lesions. Semin Surg Oncol 1991;7:257.

395. Connolly JL, Schnitt SJ: Evaluation of breast biopsy specimens in patients considered for treatment by conservative surgery and radiation therapy for early breast cancer. Pathol Annu 1988;1:1.

396. Denham JW, Sillar RW, Clarke D: Boost dosage to the excision site following conservative surgery for breast cancer: It's easy to miss! Clin Oncol (R Coll Radiol) 1991;3:257.

397. Recommendations for the reporting of breast carcinoma: Association of Directors of Anatomic and Surgical Pathology. Am J Clin Pathol 1995;104:614.

398. Petrek JA, Blackwood MM: Axillary dissection: Current practice and technique. Curr Probl Surg 1995;33:259.

399. Roses DF, Brooks AD, Harris MN, et al: Complications of level I and II axillary dissection in the treatment of carcinoma of the breast. Ann Surg 1999;230:194.

400. Rosen PP, Groshen S: Factors influencing survival and prognosis in early breast carcinoma (TINOMO-TINIMO): Assessment of 644 patients with a mean follow-up of 18 years. Surg Clin North Am 1990;70:937.

401. Miller BA, Feuer EJ, Hankey BF: Recent incidence trends for breast cancer in women and the relevance of early detection: An update. CA Cancer J Clin 1993;43:27.

402. Cady B, Stone M, Schuller JG, et al: The new era in breast cancer: Invasion, size and nodal involvement dramatically decreasing as a result of mammographic screening. Arch Surg 1996;131:301.

403. Morton DL, Wen DR, Wong JH, et al: Technical details of intraoperative lymphatic mapping for early stage melanoma. Arch Surg 1992;127:392.

404. Cabanas R: An approach for the treatment of penile carcinoma. Cancer 1977;39:456.

405. Krag ND, Weaver DL, Alex JC, et al: Surgical resection and radiolocalization of the sentinel lymph node in breast cancer using a gamma probe. Surg Oncol 1993;2:335.

406. Guiliano AE, Kirgan DM, Guenther JM, et al: Lymphatic mapping and sentinel lymphadenectomy for breast cancer. Ann Surg 1994;220:391.

407. Brady MS, Coit DG: Sentinel lymph node evaluation in melanoma. Arch Dermatol 1997;133:1014.

408. Cody HS: Sentinel lymph node mapping in breast cancer. Oncology 1999;13:25 (a review with discussions of the article by Crag D, 13:35; Kimme W, 13:36; and Hiagh PI, Guiliano AE, 13:39).

409. Guiliano AE, Jones RC, Brennan M, et al: Sentinel lymphadenectomy in breast cancer. J Clin Oncol 1997;15:2345.

410. O'Hea BJ, Hill ADK, El-Shirbing A, et al: Sentinel lymph node biopsy in breast cancer: Initial experience at Memorial Sloan-Kettering Cancer Center. J Am Coll Surg 1998;186:423.

411. Barnwell JM, Arredondo MA, Kollmorgen D, et al: Sentinel node biopsy in breast cancer. Ann Surg Oncol 1998;5:126.

412. Turner RR, Ollela DW, Drasne WL, et al: Histologic validation of the sentinel lymph node hypothesis for breast carcinoma. Ann Surg 1997;226:271.

413. Kantorowitz DA, Poulter CA, Rubin P, et al: Treatment of breast cancer with segmental mastectomy alone or segmental mastectomy plus radiation. Radiother Oncol 1989;15:141.

414. Freeman CR, Belliveau NJ, Kim TH, Boivin JF: Limited surgery with or without radiotherapy for early breast carcinoma. J Can Assoc Radiol 1981;32:125.

415. Greening WP, Montgomery AC, Growing NF: Report on pilot study of treatment of breast cancer by quadratic excision with axillary dissection and no other therapy. J R Soc Med 1978;71:261.

416. Tagart RE: Partial mastectomy for breast cancer. BMJ 1978;2: 1268.

417. Liljegren G, Holmberg L, Adami G, et al: Sector resection with or without postoperative radiotherapy for stage I breast cancer: Five year results of a randomized trial. J Natl Cancer Inst 1994;86:717.

418. Schnitt SJ, Hayman J, Gelman R, et al: A prospective study of conservative surgery alone in the treatment of selected patients with stage I breast cancer. Cancer 1996;77:1094.

419. Lichter AS: Conservative treatment of breast cancer: How much is required? J Natl Cancer Inst 1992;84:659.

420. Winchester DP, Cox JD: Standards for diagnosis and management of invasive breast cancer. CA Cancer J Clin 1998;48:83.

421. Lichter AS, Fraass BA, Yanke B: Treatment techniques in the conservative management of breast cancer. Semin Radiat Oncol 1992;2:94.

422. Harris JR, Connolly JL, Schnitt SJ, et al: Clinical-pathologic study of early breast cancer treated by primary radiation therapy. J Clin Oncol 1983;1:184.

423. Fisher B, Anderson S, Redmond CK, et al: Reanalysis and results after 12 years of follow-up in a randomized clinical trial comparing total mastectomy with lumpectomy with or without irradiation in the treatment of breast cancer. N Engl J Med 1995;333:1456.

424. Romestaing P, Lehingue Y, Carrie C, et al: Role of a 10-Gy boost in the conservative treatment of early breast cancer: Results of a randomized clinical trial in Lyon, France. J Clin Oncol 1997;15:963.

425. van Tienhoven G, van Bree BJ Mijnheer, Bartelink H: Quality assurance of the EORTC trial 22881/10882: Assessment of the role of the booster dose in breast conserving therapy: An overview. Strahlenther Onkol 1997;173:201–207.

426. Recht A, Harris JR: To boost or not to boost, and how to do it. Int J Radiat Oncol Biol Phys 1991;20:177.

427. Kutcher GL, Smith AR, Fowble BL, et al: Treatment planning for primary cancer: A pattern of care study. Int J Radiat Oncol Biol Phys 1996;36:731.

428. Solin LJ, Danoff BF, Schwartz GF, et al: A practical technique for the localization of the tumor volume in definitive irradiation of the breast. Int J Radiat Oncol Biol Phys 1985;11:1215.

429. Regine WF, Ayyangar KM, Komarnicky LT, et al: Computer-CT planning of the electron boost in definitive breast irradiation (see comments). Int J Radiat Oncol Biol Phys 1991;20:121.

430. Messer PM, Kirikuta IC, Bratengeiger K, Flentje M: CT planning of boost irradiation in radiotherapy of breast cancer after conservative surgery. Radiother Oncol 1997;42:239.

431. DeBiose DA, Horwitz EM, Martinez AA, et al: The use of ultrasonography in the localization of the lumpectomy cavity for interstitial brachytherapy of the breast. Int J Radiat Oncol Biol Phys 1997;38:755.

432. Solin LJ, Chu JCH, Larsen R, et al: Determination of depth for electron breast boosts. Int J Radiat Oncol Biol Phys 1987;13:1915.

433. Hoskin PJ, Rajan B, Ebbs S, et al: Selective avoidance of lymphatic radiotherapy in the conservative management of early breast cancer. Radiother Oncol 1992;25:83.

434. Solin LJ: Radiation treatment volumes and doses for patients with early-stage carcinoma of the breast treated with breast-conserving surgery and definitive irradiation. Semin Radiat Oncol 1992;2:82.

435. Dewar JA, Sarrazin D, Benhamou E, et al: Management of the axilla in conservatively treated breast cancer: 592 patients treated at Institut Gustave-Roussy. Int J Radiat Oncol Biol Phys 1987;13:475.

436. Halverson KJ, Taylor ME, Perez CA, et al: Regional nodal management and patterns of failure following conservative surgery and radiation therapy for stage I and II breast cancer. Int J Radiat Oncol Biol Phys 1993;26:593.

437. Recht A, Houlihan MJ: Axillary lymph nodes and breast cancer: A review. Cancer 1995;76:1491.

438. Donegan WL, Stine SB, Samter TG: Implications of extracapsular nodal metastases for treatment and prognosis of breast cancer. Cancer 1993;72:778.

439. Pierce LJ, Oberman HA, Strawderman MH, Lichter AS: Microscopic extracapsular extension in the axilla: Is this an indication for axillary radiotherapy? Int J Radiat Oncol Biol Phys 1995;33:253.

440. Haffty BG, Fischer D, Fischer JJ: Regional nodal irradiation in the conservative treatment of breast cancer. Int J Radiat Oncol Biol Phys 1990;19:859.

441. Wong JS, Recht A, Beard CJ, et al: Treatment outcome after tangential radiation therapy without axillary dissection in patients with early-stage breast cancer and clinically negative axillary nodes. Int J Radiat Oncol Biol Phys 1997;39:915.

442. Solin LJ, Fowble BL, Martz KL, et al: Results of the 1983 patterns of care process survey for definitive breast irradiation. Int J Radiat Oncol Biol Phys 1991;20:105.

443. Recht A: Nodal treatment for patients with early stage breast cancer: Guilty or innocent? Radiother Oncol 1992;25:79.

444. Vicini FA, Horwitz EM, Lacerna MD, et al: The role of regional nodal irradiation in the management of patients with early-stage breast cancer treated with breast-conserving therapy. Int J Radiat Oncol Biol Phys 1997;39:1069.

445. Larson D, Weinstein M, Goldberg I, et al: Edema of the arm as a function of the extent of axillary surgery in patients with stage I–II carcinoma of the breast treated with primary radiotherapy. Int J Radiat Oncol Biol Phys 1986;12:1575.

446. Pezner RD, Patterson MP, Hill LR, et al: Arm lymphedema in patients treated conservatively for breast cancer: Relationship to patient age and axillary node dissection technique. Int J Radiat Oncol Biol Phys 1986;12:2079.

447. Liljegen G, Holmberg L: Arm morbidity after sector resection and axillary dissection with or without postoperative radiotherapy in breast cancer stage I: Results from a randomised trial. Uppsala-Orebro Breast Cancer Study Group. Eur J Cancer 1997;33:193.

448. Pierce SM, Recht A, Lingos TI, et al: Long-term radiation complications following conservative surgery (CS) and radiation therapy (RT) in patients with early stage breast cancer. Int J Radiat Oncol Biol Phys 1993;23:915.

449. Markiewicz DA, Schultz DJ, Haas J, et al: The effect of sequence and type of chemotherapy and radiation therapy on cosmesis and complications after breast conservation therapy. Int J Radiat Oncol Biol Phys 1996;35:661.

450. Lingos TI, Recht A, Vicini F, et al: Radiation pneumonitis in breast cancer patients treated with conservative surgery and radiation therapy. Int J Radiat Oncol Biol Phys 1991;21:355.

451. Graves TA, Bland KI: Surgery for early and minimally invasive breast cancer. Curr Opin Oncol 1996;8:468.

452. Srinivasan G, Kurtz DW, Lichter AS: Pleural-based changes on chest x ray after irradiation for primary breast cancer: Correlation with findings on computerized tomography. Int J Radiat Oncol Biol Phys 1983;9:1567.

453. Rutqvist LE, Lax I, Fornander T, Johansson H: Cardiovascular mortality in a randomized trial of adjuvant radiation therapy versus surgery alone in primary breast cancer. Int J Radiat Oncol Biol Phys 1992;22:887.

454. Paszat LF, Mackillop WJ, Groome PA, et al: Mortality from myocardial infarction after adjuvant radiotherapy for breast cancer in the surveillance, epidemiology, and end-results cancer registries. J Clin Oncol 1998;16:2625.

455. Rutqvist LE, Liedberg A, Hammar N, Dalberg K: Myocardial infarction among women with early-stage breast cancer treated with conservative surgery and breast irradiation. Int J Radiat Oncol Biol Phys 1998;40:359.

456. Nixon AJ, Manola J, Gelman R, et al: No long-term increase in cardiac-related mortality after breast-conserving surgery and radiation therapy using modern techniques. J Clin Oncol 1998;16:1374.

457. Gyenes G, Gagliardi G, Lax I, et al: Evaluation of irradiated heart volumes in stage I breast cancer patients treated with postoperative adjuvant radiotherapy. J Clin Oncol 1997;15:1348.

458. Gagliardi G, Lax I, Soderstrom S, et al: Prediction of excess risk of long-term cardiac mortality after radiotherapy of stage I breast cancer. Radiother Oncol 1998;46:63.

459. Salner AL, Botnick LE, Herzog AG, et al: Reversible brachial plexopathy following primary radiation therapy for breast cancer. Cancer Treat Rep 1981;65:797.

460. Olsen NK, Pfeiffer P, Mondrup K, Rose C: Radiation-induced brachial plexus neuropathy in breast cancer patients. Acta Oncol 1990;29:885.

461. Wijnmaalen A, Van OB, Van GB, et al: Angiosarcoma of the breast following lumpectomy, axillary lymph node dissection, and radiotherapy for primary breast cancer: Three case reports and a review of the literature. Int J Radiat Oncol Biol Phys 1993;26:135.

462. Strobbe LJ, Peterse HL, van Tinteren H, et al: Angiosarcoma of the breast after conservation therapy for invasive cancer, the incidence and outcome: An unforseen sequela. Breast Cancer Res Treat 1998;47:101.

463. Karlsson P, Holmberg E, Johansson KA, et al: Soft tissue sarcoma after treatment for breast cancer. Radiother Oncol 1996;38:25.

464. Orel SG, Fowble BL, Solin LJ, et al: Breast cancer recurrence after lumpectomy and radiation therapy for early-stage disease: Prognostic significance of detection method. Radiology 1993;188:189.

465. Kurtz JM, Jacquemier J, Amalric R, et al: Is breast conservation after local recurrence feasible? Eur J Cancer 1991;27:240.

466. Mulleen EE, Deutsch M, Bloomer WD: Salvage radiotherapy for local failures of lumpectomy and breast irradiation. Radiother Oncol 1997;42:25.

467. Abner AL, Recht A, Eberlein T, et al: Prognosis following salvage mastectomy for recurrence in the breast after conservative surgery and radiation therapy for early-stage breast cancer. J Clin Oncol 1993;11:44.

468. Stotter A, Atkinson EN, Fairston BA, et al: Survival following locoregional recurrence after breast conservation therapy for cancer. Ann Surg 1990;212:166.

469. Salvadori B: Local recurrences after breast-conserving treatment: An open problem. Semin Surg Oncol 1996;12:46.

470. Fisher B, Anderson S, Fisher ER, et al: Significance of ipsilateral breast tumor recurrence after lumpectomy. Lancet 1991;338:327.

471. Lewis D, Rinehoff WF: A study of the operations for the cure of carcinoma of the breast performed at Johns Hopkins Hospital from 1889–1931. Ann Surg 1932;95:336.

472. Matthews RH, McNeese MD, Montague ED, Oswald MJ: Prognostic implications of age in breast cancer patients treated with tumorectomy and irradiation or with mastectomy. Int J Radiat Oncol Biol Phys 1988;14:659.

473. Nixon AJ, Schnitt S, Connolly JL, et al: Relationship of patient age to pathologic features of the tumor and the risk of local recurrence for patients with stage I and II breast cancer treated with conservative surgery and radiation therapy. Int J Radiat Oncol Biol Phys 1992;24:221.

474. Kurtz JM, Jacquemier J, Amalric R, et al: Why are local recurrences after breast-conserving therapy more frequent in younger patients? J Clin Oncol 1990;8:591.

475. Fisher B, Brown A, Mamounces E, et al: Effect of preoperative chemotherapy on local-regional disease in women with operable breast cancer: Findings from NSABP B-18. J Clin Oncol 1997;15:2483.

476. Fisher B, Bryant J, Wolmark N, et al: Effect of preoperative chemotherapy on the outcome of women with operable breast cancer. J Clin Oncol 1998;16:2672.

477. Schnitt SJ, Connolly JL, Harris JR, et al: Pathologic predictors of early local recurrence in stage I and II breast cancer treated by primary radiation therapy. Cancer 1984;53:1049.

478. Boyages J, Recht A, Connolly JL, et al: Early breast cancer: Predictors of breast recurrence for patients treated with conservative surgery and radiation therapy. Radiother Oncol 1990;19:29.

479. Lazovich DA, White E, Thomas DB, Moe RE: Underutilization of breast-conserving surgery and radiation therapy among women with stage I or II breast cancer. JAMA 1991;266:3433.

480. Osteen RT, Steele GJ, Menck HR, Winchester DP: Regional differences in surgical management of breast cancer. CA Cancer J Clin 1992;42:39.

481. Bland KI, Menck HR, Scott-Conner CE, et al: The National Cancer Base 10-year survey of breast carcinoma treatment at hospitals in the United States. Cancer 1998;83:1262.

482. Nattinger AB, Gottlieb MS, Veum J, et al: Geographic variation in the use of breast-conserving treatment for breast cancer. N Engl J Med 1992;326:1102.

483. Farrow DC, Hunt WC, Samet JM: Geographic variation in the treatment of localized breast cancer (see comments). N Engl J Med 1992;326:1097.

484. Albain KS, Green SR, Lichter AS, et al: Influence of patient characteristics, socioeconomic factors, geography, and systemic risk on the use of breast-sparing treatment in women enrolled in adjuvant breast studies: An analysis of two intergroup trials. J Clin Oncol 1996;14:3009.

485. Fowble B: Postmastectomy radiation: Then and now. Oncology (Huntingt) 1997;11:213,

486. Pierce LJ, Lichter AS: Defining the role of post-mastectomy radiotherapy: The new evidence. Oncology (Huntingt) 1996;10:991.

487. Recht A, Bartelink H, Fourquet A, et al: Postmastectomy radiotherapy: Questions for the twenty-first century. J Clin Oncol 1998;16:2886.

488. Diab SG, Hilsenbeck SG, de Moor C, et al: Radiation therapy and survival in breast cancer patients with 10 or more positive axillary lymph nodes treated with mastectomy. J Clin Oncol 1998;16:1655.

489. Hellman S: Stopping metastases at its source. N Engl J Med 1997;337:996.

490. Tamoxifen for early breast cancer: An overview of the randomised trials. Early Breast Cancer Trialists' Collaborative Group (see comments)]. Lancet 1998;351:1451–1467.

491. Polychemotherapy for early breast cancer: An overview of the randomised trials. Early Breast Cancer Trialists' Collaborative Group. Lancet 1998;352:930–942.

492. Lippman ME, Hayes DF: Adjuvant therapy for all patients with breast cancer? J Natl Cancer Inst 2001;93:80–82.

493. Simes RJ, Coates AS: Patient preferences for adjuvant chemotherapy of early breast cancer: How much benefit is needed? J Natl Cancer Inst Monogr 2001;30:146–152.

494. Ravdin PM, Siminoff IA, Harvey JA: Survey of breast cancer patients concerning their knowledge and expectations of adjuvant therapy. J Clin Oncol 1998;16:515–521.

495. Ravdin PM, Siminoff LA, Davis GJ, et al: Computer program to assist in making decisions about adjuvant therapy for women with early breast cancer. J Clin Oncol 2001;19:980–991.

496. Loprinzi CL, Thome SD: Understanding the utility of adjuvant systemic therapy for primary breast cancer. J Clin Oncol 2001;19:972–979.

497. NCCN practice guidelines for breast cancer, version 1.2003 (www.nccn.org, last accessed April 24, 2003), National Comprehensive Cancer Network, 2003.

498. Goldhirsch A, Glick JH, Gelber RD, et al: Meeting highlights: International Consensus Panel on the Treatment of Primary Breast Cancer. Seventh International Conference on Adjuvant Therapy of Primary Breast Cancer. J Clin Oncol 2001;19:3817–3827.

499. Goldhirsch A, Wood WC, Geller RD, et al: Meeting highlights: Updated International Expert Consensus on the primary therapy of early breast cancer. J Clin Oncol 2003;21:3357–3365.

500. The Cancer Care Ontario Practice Guidelines Initiative Breast Cancer Disease Site Group: Adjuvant systemic therapy for node-negative breast cancer (www.ccopebc.ca/guidelines/bre/cpg1_8.html, last accessed January 26, 2003), 2002.

501. National Institutes of Health Consensus Development Panel: National Institutes of Health Consensus Development Conference statement. Adjuvant therapy for breast cancer, November 1–3, 2000. J Natl Cancer Inst 2001;93:979–989.

502. Morrow M, Krontiras H: Who should not receive chemotherapy? Data from American databases and trials. J Natl Cancer Inst Monogr 2001;30:109–113.

503. Bergh J, Holmquist M: Who should not receive adjuvant chemotherapy? International databases. J Natl Cancer Inst Monogr 2001;30:103–108.

504. Fisher B, Dignam J, Tan-Chiu E, et al: Prognosis and treatment of patients with breast tumors of one centimeter or less and negative axillary lymph nodes. J Natl Cancer Inst 2001;93:112–120.

505. Fisher B, Bryant J, Dignam JJ, et al: Tamoxifen, radiation therapy, or both for prevention of ipsilateral breast tumor recurrence after lumpectomy in women with invasive breast cancers of one centimeter or less. J Clin Oncol 2002;20:4141–4149.

506. Ovarian ablation in early breast cancer: Overview of the randomised trials. Early Breast Cancer Trialists' Collaborative Group (see comments). Lancet 1996;348:1189–1196.

507. Eifel P, Axelson JA, Costa J, et al: National Institutes of Health Consensus Development Conference Statement: Adjuvant therapy for breast cancer, November 1–3, 2000. J Natl Cancer Inst 2001;93:979–989.

508. Albain K, Green S, Ravdin P, et al: Overall survival after cyclophosphamide, Adriamycin, 5-FU, and tamoxifen (CAFT) is superior to T alone in postmenopausal, receptor(+), node(+) breast cancer: New findings from phase III Southwest Oncology Group Intergroup trial S8814 (INT-0100) [abstract 94]. Proc Am Soc Clin Oncol 2001;20:24a.

509. Fisher B, Dignam J, Wolmark N, et al: Tamoxifen and chemotherapy for lymph node-negative, estrogen receptor-positive breast cancer (see comments). J Natl Cancer Inst 1997;89:1673–1682.

510. International Breast Cancer Study Group (IBCSG): Endocrine responsiveness and tailoring adjuvant therapy for postmenopausal lymph node-negative breast cancer: A randomized trial. J Natl Cancer Inst 2002;94:1054–1065.

511. Fisher B, Jeong JH, Bryant J, et al: Findings from two decades of National Surgical Adjuvant Breast and Bowel Project clinical trials involving breast cancer patients with negative axillary nodes (abstract 16). Breast Cancer Res Treat 2002;76(Suppl 1):S32.

512. Colleoni M, Minchella I, Mazzarol G, et al: Response to primary chemotherapy in breast cancer patients with tumors not expressing estrogen and progesterone receptors. Ann Oncol 2000;11:1057–1059.

513. Lippman ME, Allegra JC, Thompson EB, et al: The relation between estrogen receptors and response rate to cytotoxic chemotherapy in metastatic breast cancer. N Engl J Med 1978;298:1223–1228.

514. Kuerer HM, Newman LA, Smith TL, et al: Clinical course of breast cancer patients with complete pathologic primary tumor and axillary lymph node response to doxorubicin-based neoadjuvant chemotherapy. J Clin Oncol 1999;17:460–469.

515. Bast RC Jr, Ravdin P, Hayes DF, et al: 2000 update of recommendations for the use of tumor markers in breast and colorectal cancer: Clinical practice guidelines of the American Society of Clinical Oncology. J Clin Oncol 2001;19:1865–1878.

516. Andrulis IL, Bull SB, Blackstein ME, et al: neu/erbB-2 amplification identifies a poor-prognosis group of women with node-negative breast cancer: Toronto Breast Cancer Study Group. J Clin Oncol 1998;16:1340–1349.

517. Budman DR, Berry DA, Cirrincione CT, et al: Dose and dose intensity as determinants of outcome in the adjuvant treatment of breast cancer: The Cancer and Leukemia Group B. J Natl Cancer Inst 1998;90:1205–1211.

518. Paik S, Bryant J, Park C, et al: erbB-2 and response to doxorubicin in patients with axillary lymph node-positive, hormone receptor-negative breast cancer (see comments). J Natl Cancer Inst 1998;90:1361–1370.

519. Thor AD, Berry DA, Budman DR, et al: erbB-2, p53, and efficacy of adjuvant therapy in lymph node-positive breast cancer (see comments). J Natl Cancer Inst 1998;90:1346–1360.

520. Menard S, Valagussa P, Pilotti S, et al: Response to cyclophosphamide, methotrexate, and fluorouracil in lymph node-positive breast cancer according to HER2 overexpression and other tumor biologic variables. J Clin Oncol 2001;19:329–335.

521. Pritchard KI: Endocrine therapy of advanced disease: Analysis and implications of the existing data. Clin Cancer Res 2003;9:460S–467S.

522. Paik S, Bryant J, Tan-Chiu E, et al: Real-world performance of HER2 testing: National Surgical Adjuvant Breast and Bowel Project experience. J Natl Cancer Inst 2002;94:852–854.

523. Roche PC, Suman VJ, Jenkins RB, et al: Concordance between local and central laboratory HER2 testing in the breast intergroup trial N9831. J Natl Cancer Inst 2002;94:855–857.

524. Fisher B, Brown AM, Dimitrov NV, et al: Two months of doxorubicin-cyclophosphamide with and without interval reinduction therapy compared with 6 months of cyclophosphamide, methotrexate, and fluorouracil in positive-node breast cancer patients with tamoxifen-nonresponsive tumors: Results from the National Surgical Adjuvant Breast and Bowel Project B-15. J Clin Oncol 1990;8:1483–1496.

525. Fisher B, Anderson S, Tan-Chiu E, et al: Tamoxifen and chemotherapy for axillary node-negative, estrogen receptor-negative breast cancer: Findings from National Surgical Adjuvant Breast and Bowel Project B-23. J Clin Oncol 2001;19:931–942.

526. Hutchins L, Green S, Ravdin P, et al: CMF with and without tamoxifen in high-risk node-negative breast cancer patients and a natural history follow-up study in low-risk-node-negative patients (abstract 2). Proc Am Soc Clin Oncol 1998;17:1a.

527. Levine MN, Bramwell VH, Pritchard KI, et al: Randomized trial of intensive cyclophosphamide, epirubicin, and fluorouracil chemotherapy compared with cyclophosphamide, methotrexate, and fluorouracil in premenopausal women with node-positive breast cancer. National Cancer Institute of Canada Trials Group. J Clin Oncol 1998;16:2651–2658.

528. Pritchard K, Levine M, Bramwell V, et al: A randomized trial comparing CEF to CMF in premenopausal women with node positive breast cancer: Update of NCIC CTG MA.5 (abstract 17). Breast Cancer Res Treat 2002;76(Suppl 1).

529. Piccart MJ, DiLeo A, Beauduin M, et al: Phase III trial comparing two dose levels of epirubicin combined with cyclophosphamide with cyclophosphamide, methotrexate, and fluorouracil in node-positive breast cancer. J Clin Oncol 2001;19:3103–3110.

530. French Adjuvant Study Group: Benefit of a high-dose epirubicin regimen in adjuvant chemotherapy for node-positive breast cancer patients with poor prognostic factors: 5-year follow-up results of French Adjuvant Study Group 05 randomized trial. J Clin Oncol 2001;19:602–611.

531. Meinardi MT, van Veldhuisen DJ, Gietema JA, et al: Prospective evaluation of early cardiac damage induced by epirubicin-containing adjuvant chemotherapy and locoregional radiotherapy in breast cancer patients. J Clin Oncol 2001;19:2746–2753.

532. Henderson IC, Berry DA, Demetri GD, et al: Improved outcomes from adding sequential paclitaxel but not from escalating doxorubicin dose in an adjuvant chemotherapy regimen for patients with node-positive primary breast cancer. J Clin Oncol 2003;21:976–983.

533. Piccart MJ, Lohrisch C, Duchateau L, et al: Taxanes in the adjuvant treatment of breast cancer: Why not yet? J Natl Cancer Inst Monogr 2001;30:88–95.

534. Mamounas EP, Bryant J, Lembersky BC et al: Paclitaxel (T) following doxorubicin/cyclophosphamide (AC) as adjuvant chemotherapy for node-positive breast cancer: Results from NSABP B-28 (abstract 12). Proc Am Soc Clin Oncol 2003;22:4.

535. Buzdar AU, Singletary SE, Valero V, et al: Evaluation of paclitaxel in adjuvant chemotherapy for patients with operable breast cancer: Preliminary data of a prospective randomized trial. Clin Cancer Res 2002;8:1073–1079.

536. Nabholtz J-M, Pienkowski T, Mackey J, et al: Phase III trial comparing TAC (docetaxel, doxorubicin, cyclophosphamide) with FAC (5-fluorouracil, doxorubicin, cyclophosphamide) in the adjuvant treatment of node positive breast cancer (BC) patients: Interim analysis of the BCIRG 001 study (abstract 141). Proc Am Soc Clin Oncol 2002;21:36a.

537. Wood WC, Budman DR, Korzun AH, et al: Dose and dose intensity of adjuvant chemotherapy for stage II, node-positive breast carcinoma. N Engl J Med 1994;330:1253–1259.

538. Fumoleau P, Kerbrat P, Romestaing P, et al: Randomized trial comparing six versus three cycles of epirubicin-based adjuvant chemotherapy in premenopausal, node-positive breast cancer patients: 10-year follow-up results of the French Adjuvant Study Group 01 trial. J Clin Oncol 2003;21:298–305.

539. Fisher B, Anderson S, Wickerham DL, et al: Increased intensification and total dose of cyclophosphamide in a doxorubicin-cyclophosphamide regimen for the treatment of primary breast cancer: Findings from National Surgical Adjuvant Breast and Bowel Project B-22. J Clin Oncol 1997;15:1858–1869.

540. Fisher B, Anderson S, DeCillis A, et al: Further evaluation of intensified and increased total dose of cyclophosphamide for the treatment of primary breast cancer: Findings from National Surgical Adjuvant Breast and Bowel Project B-25. J Clin Oncol 1999;17:3374–3388.

541. Goldie JH, Coldman AJ: A mathematic model for relating the drug sensitivity of tumors to their spontaneous mutation rate. Cancer Treat Rep 1979;63:1727–1733.

542. Norton L, Simon R: The Norton-Simon hypothesis revisited. Cancer Treat Rep 1986;70:163–169.

543. Bonadonna G, Zambetti M, Valagussa P: Sequential or alternating doxorubicin and CMF regimens in breast cancer with more than three positive nodes: Ten-year results. JAMA 1995;273:542–547.

544. Hudis C, Seidman A, Baselga J, et al: Sequential dose-dense doxorubicin, paclitaxel, and cyclophosphamide for resectable high-risk breast cancer: Feasibility and efficacy. J Clin Oncol 1999;17:93–100.

545. Citron ML, Berry DA, Cirrincione C, et al: A randomized trial of dose dense vs. conventionally scheduled and sequential vs. concurrent combination chemotherapy as post-operative adjuvant treatment of node-positive primary breast cancer: First report of Intergroup C9741-CALGB 9741. J Clin Oncol 2003;21:1431–1439.

546. Hortobagyi GN: High-dose chemotherapy for primary breast cancer: Facts versus anecdotes. J Clin Oncol 1999;17:25–29.

547. Antman KH: Overview of the six available randomized trials of high-dose chemotherapy with blood or marrow transplant in breast cancer. J Natl Cancer Inst Monogr 2001;30:114–116.

548. Tallman MS, Gray R, Robert NJ, et al: Conventional adjuvant chemotherapy with or without high dose chemotherapy and autologous stem cell transplantation in high risk breast cancer. N Engl J Med 2003;349:17–26.

549. Rodenhuis S, Bontenbal M, Beex LV et al: High dose chemotherapy with hematopoietic stem cell rescue for high risk breast cancer. N Engl J Med 2003;349:7–16.

550. Garcia-Carbonero R, Hidalgo M, Paz-Ares L, et al: Patient selection in high-dose chemotherapy trials: Relevance in high-risk breast cancer. J Clin Oncol 1997;15:3178–3184.

551. Rahman ZU, Frye DK, Buzdar AU, et al: Impact of selection process on response rate and long-term survival of potential high-dose chemotherapy candidates treated with standard-dose doxorubicin-containing chemotherapy in patients with metastatic breast cancer (see comments). J Clin Oncol 1997;15:3171–3177.

552. Beatson G: On the treatment of inoperable cases of carcinoma of the mamma: Suggestions for a new method of treatment with illustrative cases. Lancet 1896;2:104–107.

553. Osborne CK: Tamoxifen in the treatment of breast cancer. N Engl J Med 1998;339:1609–1618.

554. Ravdin P: Aromatase inhibitors for the endocrine adjuvant treatment of breast cancer. Lancet 2002;359:2126–2127.

Specific Malignancies

555. Winer EP, Hudis C, Burstein HJ, et al: American Society of Clinical Oncology technology assessment on the use of aromatase inhibitors as adjuvant therapy for women with hormone receptor-positive breast cancer: Status report 2002. J Clin Oncol 2002;20:3313–3327 (early release www.jco.org July 1, 2002).

556. Osborne CK, Zhao H, Fuqua SA: Selective estrogen receptor modulators: Structure, function, and clinical use. J Clin Oncol 2000;18:3172–3186.

557. Love RR, Mazess RB, Barden HS, et al: Effects of tamoxifen on bone mineral density in postmenopausal women with breast cancer. N Engl J Med 1992;326:852–856.

558. Kristensen B, Ejlertsen B, Dalgaard P, et al: Tamoxifen and bone metabolism in postmenopausal low-risk breast cancer patients: A randomized study. J Clin Oncol 1994;12:992–997.

559. Powles TJ, Hickish T, Kanis JA, et al: Effect of tamoxifen on bone mineral density measured by dual-energy x-ray absorptiometry in healthy premenopausal and postmenopausal women. J Clin Oncol 1996;14:78–84.

560. Fisher B, Costantino JP, Wickerham DL, et al: Tamoxifen for prevention of breast cancer: Report of the National Surgical Adjuvant Breast and Bowel Project P-1 study. J Natl Cancer Inst 1998;90:1371–1388.

561. Love RR, Newcomb PA, Wiebe DA, et al: Effects of tamoxifen therapy on lipid and lipoprotein levels in postmenopausal patients with node-negative breast cancer. J Natl Cancer Inst 1990;82:1327–1332.

562. Adjuvant tamoxifen in the management of operable breast cancer: The Scottish Trial. Report from the Breast Cancer Trials Committee, Scottish Cancer Trials Office (MRC), Edinburgh. Lancet 1987;2:171–175.

563. Love RR, Wiebe DA, Newcomb PA, et al: Effects of tamoxifen on cardiovascular risk factors in postmenopausal women. Ann Intern Med 1991;115:860–864.

564. McDonald CC, Stewart HJ: Fatal myocardial infarction in the Scottish adjuvant tamoxifen trial: The Scottish Breast Cancer Committee. BMJ 1991;303:435–437.

565. Rutqvist LE, Mattsson A: Cardiac and thromboembolic morbidity among postmenopausal women with early-stage breast cancer in a randomized trial of adjuvant tamoxifen: The Stockholm Breast Cancer Study Group. J Natl Cancer Inst 1993;85:1398–1406.

566. Costantino JP, Kuller LH, Ives DG, et al: Coronary heart disease mortality and adjuvant tamoxifen therapy. J Natl Cancer Inst 1997;89:776–782.

567. Fisher B, Costantino J, Redmond C, et al: A randomized clinical trial evaluating tamoxifen in the treatment of patients with node-negative breast cancer who have estrogen-receptor-positive tumors. N Engl J Med 1989;320:479–484.

568. Fisher B, Jeong JH, Dignam J, et al: Findings from recent national surgical adjuvant breast and bowel project adjuvant studies in stage I breast cancer. J Natl Cancer Inst Monogr 2001;30:62–66.

569. Fisher B, Dignam J, Bryant J, et al: Five versus more than five years of tamoxifen therapy for breast cancer patients with negative lymph nodes and estrogen receptor-positive tumors. J Natl Cancer Inst 1996;88:1529–1542.

570. Fisher B, Dignam J, Bryant J, et al: Five versus more than five years of tamoxifen for lymph node-negative breast cancer: Updated findings from the National Surgical Adjuvant Breast and Bowel Project B-14 randomized trial. J Natl Cancer Inst 2001;93:684–690.

571. Stewart HJ: The Scottish trial of adjuvant tamoxifen in node-negative breast cancer: Scottish Cancer Trials Breast Group. J Natl Cancer Inst Monogr 1992;311:117–120.

572. Stewart HJ, Forrest AP, Everington D, et al: Randomised comparison of 5 years of adjuvant tamoxifen with continuous therapy for operable breast cancer: The Scottish Cancer Trials Breast Group. Br J Cancer 1996;74:297–299.

573. Stewart HJ, Prescott RJ, Forrest APM: Scottish adjuvant tamoxifen trial: A randomized study updated to 15 years. J Natl Cancer Inst 2001;93:456–462.

574. Tormey DC, Gray R, Falkson HC: Postchemotherapy adjuvant tamoxifen therapy beyond five years in patients with lymph node-positive breast cancer: Eastern Cooperative Oncology Group (see comments). J Natl Cancer Inst 1996;88:1828–1833.

575. Abrams JS: Tamoxifen: Five versus ten years. Is the end in sight? J Natl Cancer Inst 2001;93:662–664.

576. Clarke MJ: Ovarian ablation in breast cancer, 1896 to 1998: Milestones along hierarchy of evidence from case report to Cochrane review. BMJ 1998;317:1246–1248.

577. Bines J, Oleske DM, Cobleigh MA: Ovarian function in premenopausal women treated with adjuvant chemotherapy for breast cancer. J Clin Oncol 1996;14:1718–1729.

578. Emens LA, Davidson NE: Adjuvant hormonal therapy for premenopausal women with breast cancer. Clin Cancer Res 2003;9:486S–494S.

579. Adjuvant ovarian ablation versus CMF chemotherapy in premenopausal women with pathological stage II breast carcinoma: The Scottish trial. Scottish Cancer Trials Breast Group and ICRF Breast Unit, Guy's Hospital, London (see comments). Lancet 1993;341:1293–1298.

580. Thomson CS, Twelves CJ, Mallon EA, et al: Adjuvant ovarian ablation vs CMF chemotherapy in premenopausal breast cancer patients: Trial update and impact of immunohistochemical assessment of ER status. Breast 2002;11:419–429.

581. Ejlertsen B, Dombernowsky P, Mouridsen HT, et al: Comparable effect of ovarian ablation (OA) and CMF chemotherapy in premenopausal hormone receptor positive breast cancer patients (PRP) [abstract 248]. Proc Am Soc Clin Oncol 1999;18:66a.

582. Jonat W, Kaufmann M, Sauerbrei W, et al: Goserelin versus cyclophosphamide, methotrexate, and fluorouracil as adjuvant therapy in premenopausal patients with node-positive breast cancer: The Zoladex Early Breast Cancer Research Association Study. J Clin Oncol 2002;20:4628–4635.

583. Davidson N, O'Neill A, Vukov A, et al: Effect of chemohormonal therapy in premenopausal, node (+), receptor (+) breast cancer: An Eastern Cooperative Oncology Group phase III intergroup trial (E5188, INT-0101) [abstract 249]. Proc Am Soc Clin Oncol 1999;18:67a.

584. Baum M: Adjuvant treatment of premenopausal breast cancer with Zoladex and tamoxifen. Breast Cancer Res Treat 1999;57:30.

585. Rutqvist LE: Zoladex® and tamoxifen as adjuvant therapy in premenopausal breast cancer: A randomised trial by the Cancer Research Campaign (CRC) Breast Cancer Trials Group, the Stockholm Breast Cancer Study Group, The South-East Sweden Breast Cancer Group & the Gruppo Interdisciplinare Valutazione Interventi in Oncologia (GIVIO) [abstract 251]. Proc Am Soc Clin Oncol 1999;18:67a.

586. The International Breast Cancer Study Group: Randomized controlled trial of ovarian function suppression plus tamoxifen versus the same endocrine therapy plus chemotherapy: Is chemotherapy necessary for premenopausal women with node-positive, endocrine-responsive breast cancer? First results of International Breast Cancer Study Group 11-93. Breast 2001;10:130–138.

587. Castiglione-Gertsch M, O'Neill A, Gelber RD, et al: Is the addition of adjuvant chemotherapy always necessary in node negative (N-) pre/perimenopausal breast cancer patients (pts) who receive goserelin? First results of IBCSG trial VIII (abstract 149). Proc Am Soc Clin Oncol 2002;21:38a.

588. Goss PE, Strasser K: Aromatase inhibitors in the treatment and prevention of breast cancer. J Clin Oncol 2001;19:881–894.

589. Jones AL, Powles TJ, Law M, et al: Adjuvant aminoglutethimide for postmenopausal patients with primary breast cancer: Analysis at 8 years. J Clin Oncol 1992;10:1547–1552.

590. Boccardo F, Rubagotti A, Amoroso D, et al: Sequential tamoxifen and aminoglutethimide versus tamoxifen alone in the adjuvant treatment of postmenopausal breast cancer patients: Results of an Italian cooperative study. J Clin Oncol 2001;19:4209–4215.

591. Anastrozole alone or in combination with tamoxifen versus tamoxifen alone for adjuvant treatment of postmenopausal women with early breast cancer: First results of the ATAC randomised trial. Lancet 2002;359:2131–2139.

592. Baum M, Buzdar A, Cuzick J, et al: Anastrozole alone or in combination with tamoxifen versus tamoxifen alone for adjuvant treatment of postmenopausal women with early-stage breast cancer: Results of the ATAC (Arimidex, Tamoxifen Alone or in Combination) trial efficacy and safety update analyses. Cancer 2003;98:1802–1810.

593. Wolff AC, Abeloff MD: Adjuvant chemotherapy for postmenopausal lymph node-negative breast cancer: It ain't necessarily so. J Natl Cancer Inst 2002;94:1041–1043.

594. Endocrine responsiveness and tailoring adjuvant therapy for postmenopausal lymph node-negative breast cancer: A randomized trial. J Natl Cancer Inst 2002;94:1054–1065.

595. Albain KS, Green SJ, Ravdin PM, et al: Adjuvant chemohormonal therapy for primary breast cancer should be sequential instead of concurrent: Initial results from intergroup trial 0100 (SWOG-8814) [abstract 143]. Proc Am Soc Clin Oncol 2002;21:37a.

596. Pico C, Martin M, Jara C, et al: Epirubicin-cyclophosphamide (EC) chemotherapy plus tamoxifen (T) administered concurrent (Con) versus sequential (Sec): Randomized phase III trial in postmenopausal node-positive breast cancer (BC) patients. GEICAM 9401 study (abstract 144). Proc Am Soc Clin Oncol 2002;21:37a.

597. Esteva FJ, Hortobagyi GN: Locally advanced breast cancer. Hematol Oncol Clin North Am 1999;13:457–472, vii.

598. Swain SM: Locally advanced noninflammatory breast cancer. Cancer Invest 1999;17:211–219.

599. Fisher B, Gunduz N, Saffer EA: Influence of the interval between primary tumor removal and chemotherapy on kinetics and growth of metastases. Cancer Res 1983;43:1488–1492.

600. Fisher B, Saffer E, Rudock C, et al: Effect of local or systemic treatment prior to primary tumor removal on the production and response to a serum growth-stimulating factor in mice. Cancer Res 1989;49:2002–2004.

601. Powles TJ, Hickish TF, Makris A, et al: Randomized trial of chemoendocrine therapy started before or after surgery for treatment of primary breast cancer. J Clin Oncol 1995;13:547–552.

602. Fisher B, Brown A, Mamounas E, et al: Effect of preoperative chemotherapy on local-regional disease in women with operable breast cancer: Findings from National Surgical Adjuvant Breast and Bowel Project B-18 (see comments). J Clin Oncol 1997;15:2483–2493.

603. Fisher B, Bryant J, Wolmark N, et al: Effect of preoperative chemotherapy on the outcome of women with operable breast cancer. J Clin Oncol 1998;16:2672–2685.

604. Meric F, Mirza NQ, Buzdar AU, et al: Prognostic implications of pathological lymph node status after preoperative chemotherapy for operable T3N0M0 breast cancer. Ann Surg Oncol 2000;7:435–440.

605. Fisher B, Mamounas EP: Preoperative chemotherapy: A model for studying the biology and therapy of primary breast cancer. J Clin Oncol 1995;13:537–540.

606. Wolff AC, Davidson NE: Primary systemic therapy in operable breast cancer. J Clin Oncol 2000;18:1558–1569.

607. Cleator S, Parton M, Dowsett M: The biology of neoadjuvant chemotherapy for breast cancer. Endocr Relat Cancer 2002;9:183–195.

608. Ellis MJ, Coop A, Singh B, et al: Letrozole is more effective neoadjuvant endocrine therapy than tamoxifen for ErbB-1- and/or ErbB-2-positive, estrogen receptor-positive primary breast cancer: Evidence from a phase III randomized trial. J Clin Oncol 2001;19:3808–3816.

609. Demetri GD, Gabrilove JL, Blasi MV, et al: Benefits of epoetin alfa in anemic breast cancer patients receiving chemotherapy. Clin Breast Cancer 2002;3:45–51.

610. Zambetti M, Moliterni A, Materazzo C, et al: Long-term cardiac sequelae in operable breast cancer patients given adjuvant chemotherapy with or without doxorubicin and breast irradiation. J Clin Oncol 2001;19:37–43.

611. Swain SM, Whaley FS, Gerber MC, et al: Delayed administration of dexrazoxane provides cardioprotection for patients with advanced breast cancer treated with doxorubicin-containing therapy (see comments). J Clin Oncol 1997;15:1333–1340.

612. Swain SM, Whaley FS, Gerber MC, et al: Cardioprotection with dexrazoxane for doxorubicin-containing therapy in advanced breast cancer. J Clin Oncol 1997;15:1318–1332.

613. Suter TM, Meier B: Detection of anthracycline-induced cardiotoxicity: Is there light at the end of the tunnel? Ann Oncol 2002;13:647–649.

614. Cardinale D, Sandri MT, Martinoni A, et al: Myocardial injury revealed by plasma troponin I in breast cancer treated with high-dose chemotherapy. Ann Oncol 2002;13:710–715.

615. Sabel MS, Levine EG, Hurd T, et al: Is MUGA scan necessary in patients with low-risk breast cancer before doxorubicin-based adjuvant therapy? Multiple gated acquisition. Am J Clin Oncol 2001;24:425–428.

616. Ghalie RG, Goodkin DE: Secondary leukemia after adjuvant chemotherapy for breast cancer. J Clin Oncol 2001;19:1231–1233.

617. Pagano L, Pulsoni A, Mele L, et al: Acute myeloid leukemia in patients previously diagnosed with breast cancer: Experience of the GIMEMA group. Ann Oncol 2001;12:203–207.

618. Smith RE, Bryant J, DeCillis A, et al: Acute myeloid leukemia and myelodysplastic syndrome after doxorubicin-cyclophosphamide adjuvant therapy for operable breast cancer: The national surgical adjuvant breast and bowel project experience. J Clin Oncol 2003;21:1195–1204.

619. Goodwin PJ, Ennis M, Pritchard KI, et al: Risk of menopause during the first year after breast cancer diagnosis. J Clin Oncol 1999;17:2365–2370.

620. Van Patten CL, Olivotto IA, Chambers GK, et al: Effect of soy phytoestrogens on hot flashes in postmenopausal women with breast cancer: A randomized, controlled clinical trial. J Clin Oncol 2002;20:1449–1455.

621. Jacobson JS, Troxel AB, Evans J, et al: Randomized trial of black cohosh for the treatment of hot flashes among women with a history of breast cancer. J Clin Oncol 2001;19:2739–2745.

622. Loprinzi CL, Sloan JA, Perez EA, et al: Phase III evaluation of fluoxetine for treatment of hot flashes. J Clin Oncol 2002;20:1578–1583.

623. Gelber S, Coates AS, Goldhirsch A, et al: Effect of pregnancy on overall survival after the diagnosis of early-stage breast cancer. J Clin Oncol 2001;19:1671–1675.

624. Shapiro CL, Manola J, Leboff M: Ovarian failure after adjuvant chemotherapy is associated with rapid bone loss in women with early-stage breast cancer. J Clin Oncol 2001;19:3306–3311.

625. Vehmanen L, Saarto T, Elomaa I, et al: Long-term impact of chemotherapy-induced ovarian failure on bone mineral density (BMD) in premenopausal breast cancer patients: The effect of adjuvant clodronate treatment. Eur J Cancer 2001;37:2373–2378.

626. Goodwin PJ, Ennis M, Pritchard KI, et al: Adjuvant treatment and onset of menopause predict weight gain after breast cancer diagnosis. J Clin Oncol 1999;17:120–129.

627. Demark-Wahnefried W, Peterson BL, Winer EP, et al: Changes in weight, body composition, and factors influencing energy balance among premenopausal breast cancer patients receiving adjuvant chemotherapy. J Clin Oncol 2001;19:2381–2389.

628. Goodwin PJ: Weight gain in early-stage breast cancer: Where do we go from here? J Clin Oncol 2001;19:2367–2369.

629. Schagen SB, van Dam FS, Muller MJ, et al: Cognitive deficits after postoperative adjuvant chemotherapy for breast carcinoma. Cancer 1999;85:640–650.

630. van Dam FS, Schagen SB, Muller MJ, et al: Impairment of cognitive function in women receiving adjuvant treatment for high-risk breast cancer: High-dose versus standard-dose chemotherapy. J Natl Cancer Inst 1998;90:210–218.

631. Brezden CB, Phillips KA, Abdolell M, et al: Cognitive function in breast cancer patients receiving adjuvant chemotherapy. J Clin Oncol 2000;18:2695–2701.

632. Ganz PA, Rowland JH, Desmond K, et al: Life after breast cancer: Understanding women's health-related quality of life and sexual functioning. J Clin Oncol 1998;16:501–514.

633. Dorval M, Maunsell E, Deschenes L, et al: Long-term quality of life after breast cancer: Comparison of 8-year survivors with population controls. J Clin Oncol 1998;16:487–494.

634. Fisher B, Costantino JP, Redmond CK, et al: Endometrial cancer in tamoxifen-treated breast cancer patients: Findings from the National Surgical Adjuvant Breast and Bowel Project (NSABP) B-14. J Natl Cancer Inst 1994;86:527–537.

635. Rutqvist L, Johansson H, Signomklao T, et al: Adjuvant tamoxifen therapy for early stage breast cancer and second primary malignancies. Stockholm Breast Cancer Study Group. J Natl Cancer Inst 1995;87:645–651.

636. Bergman L, Beelen ML, Gallee MP, et al: Risk and prognosis of endometrial cancer after tamoxifen for breast cancer: Comprehensive Cancer Centres' ALERT Group. Assessment of liver and endometrial cancer risk following tamoxifen. Lancet 2000;356:881–887.

637. Barakat RR: Screening for endometrial cancer in the patient receiving tamoxifen for breast cancer (editorial; comment). J Clin Oncol 1999;17:1967–1968.

638. Wysowski DK, Honig SF, Beitz J: Uterine sarcoma associated with tamoxifen use. N Engl J Med 2002;346:1832–1833.

639. Love CDB, Muir BB, Scrimgeour JB, et al: Investigation of endometrial abnormalities in asymptomatic women treated with tamoxifen and an evaluation of the role of endometrial screening. J Clin Oncol 1999;17:2050.

640. Barakat RR, Gilewski TA, Almadrones L, et al: Effect of adjuvant tamoxifen on the endometrium in women with breast cancer: A prospective study using office endometrial biopsy. J Clin Oncol 2000;18:3459–3463.

641. Pritchard KI, Paterson AH, Paul NA, et al: Increased thromboembolic complications with concurrent tamoxifen and chemotherapy in a randomized trial of adjuvant therapy for women with breast cancer: National Cancer Institute of Canada Clinical Trials Group Breast Cancer Site Group. J Clin Oncol 1996;14:2731–2737.

642. Ganz PA: Impact of tamoxifen adjuvant therapy on symptoms, functioning, and quality of life. J Natl Cancer Inst Monogr 2001;30:130–134.

643. Stearns V, Hayes DF: Cooling off hot flashes. J Clin Oncol 2002;20:1436–1438.

644. Stearns V, Isaacs C, Rowland J, et al: A pilot trial assessing the efficacy of paroxetine hydrochloride (Paxil) in controlling hot flashes in breast cancer survivors. Ann Oncol 2000;11:17–22.

645. Loprinzi CL, Kugler JW, Sloan J, et al: Venlafaxine alleviates hot flashes: An NCCTG trial (abstract 4). Proc Am Soc Clin Oncol 2000;19:2a.

646. Pandya KJ, Raubertas RF, Flynn PJ, et al: Oral clonidine in postmenopausal patients with breast cancer experiencing tamoxifen-induced hot flashes: A University of Rochester Cancer Center Community Clinical Oncology Program study. Ann Intern Med 2000;132:788–793.

647. Loprinzi CL, Barton DL, Rhodes D: Management of hot flashes in breast-cancer survivors. Lancet Oncol 2001;2:199–204.

648. Day R, Ganz PA, Costantino JP, et al: Health-related quality of life and tamoxifen in breast cancer prevention: A report from the National Surgical Adjuvant Breast and Bowel Project P-1 Study. J Clin Oncol 1999;17:2659–2669.

649. Ganz PA, Desmond KA, Belin TR, et al: Predictors of sexual health in women after a breast cancer diagnosis. J Clin Oncol 1999;17:2371–2380.

650. Nayfield S, Gorin M: Tamoxifen-associated eye disease: A review. J Clin Oncol 1996;14:1018–1026.

651. Gorin MB, Day R, Costantino JP, et al: Long-term tamoxifen citrate use and potential ocular toxicity. Am J Ophthalmol 1998;125:493–501.

652. DiSaia PJ, Brewster WR, Ziogas A, et al: Breast cancer survival and hormone replacement therapy: A cohort analysis. Am J Clin Oncol 2000;23:541–545.

653. Col NF, Hirota LK, Orr RK, et al: Hormone replacement therapy after breast cancer: A systematic review and quantitative assessment of risk. J Clin Oncol 2001;19:2357–2363.

654. O'Meara ES, Rossing MA, Daling JR, et al: Hormone replacement therapy after a diagnosis of breast cancer in relation to recurrence and mortality. J Natl Cancer Inst 2001;93:754–761.

655. Cuzick J: Is hormone replacement therapy safe for breast cancer patients? J Natl Cancer Inst 2001;93:733.

656. Boon H, Stewart M, Kennard MA, et al: Use of complementary/alternative medicine by breast cancer survivors in Ontario: Prevalence and perceptions (see comments). J Clin Oncol 2000;18:2515–2521.

657. Jacobson JS, Workman SB, Kronenberg F: Research on complementary/alternative medicine for patients with breast cancer: A review of the biomedical literature. J Clin Oncol 2000;18:668–683.

658. Berglund G, Nystedt M, Bolund C, et al: Effect of endocrine treatment on sexuality in premenopausal breast cancer patients: A prospective randomized study. J Clin Oncol 2001;19:2788–2796.

659. Fox KR, Ball JE, Mick R, et al: Preventing chemotherapy-associated amenorrhea (CRA) with leuprolide in young women with early-stage breast cancer (abstract 98). Proc Am Soc Clin Oncol 2001;20:25a.

660. Harvey JM, Clark GM, Osborne CK, et al: Estrogen receptor status by immunohistochemistry is superior to the ligand-binding assay for predicting response to adjuvant endocrine therapy in breast cancer. J Clin Oncol 1999;17:1474–1481.

661. Goldhirsch A, Coates AS, Colleoni M, et al: Adjuvant chemoendocrine therapy in postmenopausal breast cancer: Cyclophosphamide, methotrexate, and fluorouracil dose and schedule may make a difference. International Breast Cancer Study Group. J Clin Oncol 1998;16:1358–1362.

662. Smith TJ, Davidson NE, Schapira DV, et al: American Society of Clinical Oncology 1998 update of recommended breast cancer surveillance guidelines. J Clin Oncol 1999;17:1080–1082.

663. Chan DW, Beveridge RA, Muss H, et al: Use of Truquant BR radioimmunoassay for early detection of breast cancer recurrence in patients with stage II and stage III disease. J Clin Oncol 1997;15:2322–2328.

664. Cobleigh MA, Vogel CL, Tripathy D, et al: Multinational study of the efficacy and safety of humanized anti-HER2 monoclonal antibody in women who have HER2-overexpressing metastatic breast cancer that has progressed after chemotherapy for metastatic disease. J Clin Oncol 1999;17:2639–2648.

665. Vogel CL, Cobleigh MA, Tripathy D, et al: Efficacy and safety of trastuzumab as a single agent in first-line treatment of HER2-overexpressing metastatic breast cancer. J Clin Oncol 2002;20:719–726.

666. Slamon DJ, Leyland-Jones B, Shak S, et al: Use of chemotherapy plus a monoclonal antibody against HER2 for metastatic breast cancer that overexpresses HER2. N Engl J Med 2001;344:783–792.

667. Seidman A, Hudis C, Pierri MK, et al: Cardiac dysfunction in the trastuzumab clinical trials experience. J Clin Oncol 2002;20:1215–1221.

668. Speyer J: Cardiac dysfunction in the trastuzumab clinical experience. J Clin Oncol 2002;20:1156–1157.

669. Ganz PA, Greendale GA: Menopause and breast cancer: Addressing the secondary health effects of adjuvant chemotherapy. J Clin Oncol 2001;19:3303–3305.

670. Saarto T, Vehmanen L, Elomaa I, et al: The effect of clodronate and antioestrogens on bone loss associated with oestrogen withdrawal in postmenopausal women with breast cancer. Br J Cancer 2001;84:1047–1051.

671. Hillner BE, Ingle JN, Berenson JR, et al: American Society of Clinical Oncology guideline on the role of bisphosphonates in breast cancer: American Society of Clinical Oncology Bisphosphonates Expert Panel. J Clin Oncol 2000;18:1378–1391.

672. Ali SM, Esteva FJ, Hortobagyi G, et al: Safety and efficacy of bisphosphonates beyond 24 months in cancer patients. J Clin Oncol 2001;19:3434–3437.

673. Diel IJ, Solomayer E-F, Gollan C, et al: Bisphosphonates in the reduction of metastases in breast cancer: Results of the extended follow-up of the first study population (abstract 314). Proc Am Soc Clin Oncol 2000;19:82a.

674. Diel IJ, Solomayer EF, Costa SD, et al: Reduction in new metastases in breast cancer with adjuvant clodronate treatment (see comments). N Engl J Med 1998;339:357–363.

675. Powles TJ, McCloskey E, Paterson AH, et al: Oral clodronate and reduction in loss of bone mineral density in women with operable primary breast cancer. J Natl Cancer Inst 1998;90:704–708.

676. Saarto T, Blomqvist C, Virkkunen P, et al: Adjuvant clodronate treatment does not reduce the frequency of skeletal metastases in node-positive breast cancer patients: 5-year results of a randomized controlled trial. J Clin Oncol 2001;19:10–17.

677. Klefstrom P, Grohn P, Heinonen E, et al: Adjuvant postoperative radiotherapy, chemotherapy, and immunotherapy in stage III breast cancer. Cancer 1987;60:936.

678. Toonkel L, Fix I, Jacobson L, et al: Locally advanced breast carcinoma: Results with combined regional therapy. Int J Radiat Oncol Biol Phys 1986;12:1583.

679. Haagensen CD, Stout AP: Carcinoma of the breast, criteria of operability. Ann Surg 1943;118:859, 1032.

680. Baclesse F: Roentgen therapy as the sole method of treatment on cancer of the breast. Am J Roentgenol 1949;62:311.

681. Fletcher GH, Montague ED: Radical irradiation of advanced breast cancer. Am J Roentgenol Radium Ther Nucl Med 1965;93:573.

682. Bruckman JE, Harris JR, Levene MB, et al: Results of treating stage III carcinoma of the breast by primary radiation therapy. Cancer 1979;43:985.

683. Arriagada R, Mouriesse H, Sarrazin D, et al: Radiotherapy alone in the Gustave-Roussy Institute and the Princess Margaret Hospital. Int J Radiat Oncol Biol Phys 1985;11:1751.

684. Spanos WJ, Montague ED, Fletcher GH: Late complications of radiation only for advanced breast cancer. Int J Radiat Oncol Biol Phys 1980;6:1473.

685. Bedwinek J, Rao DV, Perez C, et al: Stage III and localized stage IV breast cancer: Irradiation alone vs. irradiation plus surgery. Int J Radiat Oncol Biol Phys 1982;8:31.

686. Zucali R, Uslenghi C, Kenda R, et al: Natural history and survival of inoperable breast cancer treated with radiotherapy and radiotherapy followed by radical mastectomy. Cancer 1976;37:1422.

687. Strom EA, McNeese MD, Fletcher GH, et al: Results of mastectomy and postoperative irradiation in the management of locoregionally advanced carcinoma of the breast. Int J Radiat Oncol Biol Phys 1991;21:319.

688. Graham MV, Perez CA, Kuske RR, et al: Locally advanced (noninflammatory) carcinoma of the breast: Results and comparison of various treatment modalities. Int J Radiat Oncol Biol Phys 1991;21:311.

689. Pearlman N, Fracchia A: Primary inoperable cancer of the breast. Surg Gynecol Obstet 1976;143:909.

690. Fracchia AA, Evans JF, Eisenberg BL: Stage III carcinoma of the breast. Ann Surg 1989;192:705.

691. Vilcoq J, Fourquet A, Jullien D, et al: Prognostic significance of clinical nodal involvement in patients treated by radical radiotherapy for a locally advanced breast cancer. Am J Clin Oncol 1984;7:625.

692. Feldman L, Hortobagyi G, Buzdar A, et al: Pathological assessment of response to induction chemotherapy in breast cancer. Cancer Res 1986;46:2578.

693. Armstrong D, Beveridge R, Donehower R, et al: Sixteen-week dose-intense chemotherapy for inoperable, locally advanced breast cancer (abstract). Breast Cancer Res Treat 1991;19:160.

694. Kuere H, Newman L, Smith T, et al: Clinical course of breast cancer patients with complete pathologic primary tumor and axillary lymph node response to doxorubicin-based neoadjuvant chemotherapy. J Clin Oncol 1999;17:460–469.

695. Bartelink H, Rubens RD, et al: Hormonal therapy prolongs survival in irradiated locally advanced breast cancer: A European Organization for Research and Treatment of Cancer Randomized Phase III Trial. J Clin Oncol 1997;15:207.

696. Perloff M, Lesnick GJ, Korzun A, et al: Combination chemotherapy with mastectomy or radiotherapy for stage III breast carcinoma: A Cancer and Leukemia Group B study. J Clin Oncol 1988;6:261.

697. Olson JE, Neuberg D, Pandya KJ, et al: The role of radiotherapy in the management of operable locally advanced breast cancer. Cancer 1997;79:1138.

698. Singletary S, McNeese M, Hortobagyi G: Feasibility of breast conservation surgery after induction chemotherapy for locally advanced breast carcinoma. Cancer 1991;69:2849.

699. Pierce L, Lippman M, Ben-Baruch N, et al: The effect of systemic therapy on local-regional control in locally advanced breast cancer. Int J Radiat Oncol Biol Phys 1992;23:949.

700. Merajver SD, Weber BL, Cody R, et al: Breast conservation and prolonged chemotherapy for locally advanced breast cancer: The University of Michigan Experience. J Clin Oncol 1997;15:2873.

701. Conte PF, Alama A, Bertelli G, et al: Chemotherapy with estrogenic recruitment and surgery in locally advanced breast cancer: Clinical and cytokinetic results. Int J Cancer 1987;40:490.

702. Chu AM, Cope O, Doucette J, et al: Non-metastatic locally advanced cancer of the breast treated with radiation. Int J Radiat Oncol Biol Phys 1984;10:2299.

703. Pisansky TM, Loprinzi CL, Cha SS, et al: A pilot evaluation of alternating preoperative chemotherapy in the management of patients with locoregionally advanced breast carcinoma. Cancer 1996;77:2520.

704. Lippman ME, Cassidy J, Wesley M, et al: A randomized attempt to increase the efficacy of cytotoxic chemotherapy in metastatic breast cancer by hormonal synchronization. J Clin Oncol 1984;2:28.

705. Henderson IC, Berry D, Demetri G, et al: Improved disease-free and overall survival from the addition of sequential paclitaxel but not from escalation of doxorubicin dose level in adjuvant chemotherapy of patients with node positive primary breast cancer. Proc Annu Meet Am Soc Clin Oncol 1998;17:A390A.

706. Blumenschein GR, Decker P, DiStefano A, et al: CAVe/XRT/McCFUD as an alternative to high dose chemotherapy (HDC) and autologous bone marrow support (ABMS) for patients (pts) with advanced primary breast cancer (meeting abstract). Proc Annu Meet Am Soc Clin Oncol 1996;15:A243.

707. Ayash L, Elias A, Ibrahim J, et al: High-dose multimodality therapy with autologous stem-cell support for stage IIIB breast carcinoma. J Clin Oncol 1998;16:1000.

708. Mulder N, Mulder P, Sleijfer D, et al: Induction chemotherapy and intensification with autologous bone marrow reinfusion in patients with locally advanced and disseminated breast cancer. Eur J Cancer 1993;29A:668.

709. Rutgers E, Richel DJ, Baars JW, et al: A randomized phase II study of adjuvant high-dose chemotherapy in high risk breast cancer (abstract no. 26). 51st Annual Cancer Symposium, jointly sponsored by the Society of Surgical Oncology & World Federation of Surgical Oncology Societies, March 26–29, 1998, San Diego, CA, 1998, p 13.

710. Sciuto R, Pasqualoni R, Bergomi S, et al: Prognostic value of (99m) Tc-sestamibi washout in predicting response of locally advanced breast cancer to neoadjuvant chemotherapy. J Nucl Med 2002;43:745–751.

711. Mankoff D, Dunnwald L, Gralow J, et al: Monitoring the response of patients with locally advanced breast carcinoma to neoadjuvant chemotherapy using [technetium 99m]-sestamibi scintimammography. Cancer 1999;11:2410–2423.

712. Schelling M, Avril N, Nahrig J, et al: Positron emission tomography using [(18)F] flourodeoxyglucose for monitoring primary chemotherapy in breast cancer. J Clin Oncol 2000;18:1689–1695.

713. Cohen L, Breslin T, Kuerer H, et al: Identification and evaluation of axillary sentinel lymph nodes in patients with breast carcinoma treated with neoadjuvant chemotherapy. Am J Surg Pathol 2000;24:1266–1272.

714. Mamounas EP, Brown A, et al: Accuracy of sentinel node biopsy after neoadjuvant chemotherapy in breast cancer: Updated results from NSABP B-27 (abstract 140). Proc Am Soc Clin Oncol 2002;21:36a.

715. Lee B, Tannenbaum N: Inflammatory carcinoma of the breast: A report of 28 cases from the breast clinic of Memorial Hospital. Surg Gynecol Obstet 1924;39:580.

716. Taylor G, Meltzer A: Inflammatory carcinoma of the breast. Am J Cancer 1938;33:33.

717. Delarue J, May-Levin F, Mouriesse H, et al: Estrogen and progesterone cytosolic receptors in clinically inflammatory tumors of the human breast. Br J Cancer 1981;44:911.

718. Bryant J: Diseases of the Breast. London, England, Cassell, 1887, p 171.

719. Drolias C, Sewell C, McSweeney M: Inflammatory carcinoma of the breast. Ann Surg 1976;184:217.

720. Camp ED: Inflammatory cancer of the breast. Am J Surg 1976;131:583.

721. Rouesse S, Sarrazin D, Mouriesse H, et al: Primary chemotherapy in the treatment of inflammatory breast carcinoma: A study of 230 cases from the Institute Gustave-Roussy. J Clin Oncol 1986;4:1765.

722. Koning C, Hart G: Long-term follow-up of a randomized trial on adjuvant chemotherapy and hormonal therapy in locally advanced breast cancer. Int J Radiat Oncol Biol Phys 1998;41:397.

723. Bartelink H, Rubens RD, et al: Hormonal therapy prolongs survival in irradiated locally advanced breast cancer: A European Organization for Research and Treatment of Cancer randomized phase III trial. J Clin Oncol 1997;15:207.

724. Buzdar AU, Singletary SE, Booser DJ, et al: Combined modality treatment of stage III and inflammatory breast cancer. Surg Oncol Clin North Am 1995;4:715.

Specific Malignancies

III

725. Israel L, Brew J, Morere J: Two years of high dose cyclophospha-mide and 5-fluorouracil followed by surgery after 3 months for acute inflammatory breast carcinomas: A phase II study of 25 cases with a median follow-up of 35 months. Cancer 1986; 57:24.

726. Maloisel F, Dufour P, Bergerat J, et al: Results of initial doxorubicin, 5-fluorouracil, and cyclophosphamide combination chemotherapy for inflammatory carcinoma of the breast. Cancer 1990;65:851.

727. Chevallier B, Bastit P, Graic Y, et al: The Centre H. Becquerel studies in inflammatory non metastatic breast cancer: Combined modality approach in 178 patients. Br J Cancer 1993;67:594.

728. Fields JN, Perez CA, Kuske RR, et al: Inflammatory carcinoma of the breast: Treatment results on 107 patients. Int J Radiat Oncol Biol Phys 1989;17:249.

729. Stephens FO: Intraarterial induction chemotherapy in locally advanced stage III breast cancer. Cancer 1990;66:645.

730. Liao Z, Strom E, Buzdar A, et al: Locoregional irradiation for inflammatory breast cancer: Effectiveness of dose escalation in decreasing recurrence. Int J Radiat Oncol Biol Phys 2000;47: 1191–1200.

731. Brun B, Otmezguine Y, Feuilhade F, et al: Treatment of inflamma-tory breast cancer with combination chemotherapy and mastec-tomy versus breast conservation. Cancer 1988;61:1096.

732. Valagussa P, Bonadonna G, Veronesi U: Patterns of relapse and survival following radical mastectomy: Analysis of 716 consecutive patients. Cancer 1978;14:1170.

733. Stotter AT, McNeese MD, Ames FC, et al: Predicting the rate of locoregional failure after breast conservation therapy for early breast cancer. Cancer 1989;64:2217.

734. Warrens S, Tompkins VN: Significance of the extent of axillary metastases in carcinoma of the female breast. Surg Gynecol Obstet 1943;76:327.

735. Conway H, Neuman CG: Evaluation of skin grafting in technique of radical mastectomy in relation of local recurrence of carcin-oma. Surg Gynecol Obstet 1949;88:45.

736. Hickey RC, Kerr HD, Tidrick RT, et al: Cancer of the breast, 1661 patients: I. Considerations in future therapy. Arch Surg 1956;73:654.

737. Auchincloss H: The nature of local recurrence following radical mastectomy. Cancer 1958;11:611.

738. Zimmerman KW, Montague ED, Fletcher GH: Frequency, anatomical distribution and management of local recurrences after definitive therapy for breast cancer. Cancer 1966;19:67.

739. Spratt JS: Locally recurrent cancer after radical mastectomy. Cancer 1967;20:1051.

740. Deck KB, Kern WH: Local recurrence of breast cancer. Arch Surg 1976;111:323.

741. DiPietro S, Bertario L, Cant G, Re A: An analysis of 800 breast cancer patients relapsed after radical mastectomy. Tumori 1976;62:99.

742. Clark RM, Wilkinson RH, Mahoney IJ, et al: Breast cancer: A 21 year experience with conservative surgery and radiation. Int J Radiat Oncol Biol Phys 1982;8:967.

743. Kurtz JM, Spilalier J-M, Amalric R: Late recurrence after lumpectomy and irradiation. Int J Radiat Oncol Biol Phys 1983;9:1191.

744. Gilliland MD, Barton R, Copeland EM: The implications of local recurrence of breast cancer as the first site of therapeutic failure. Ann Surg 1983;197:284.

745. Recht A, Silver B, Schnitt S, et al: Breast relapse following primary radiation therapy for early breast cancer: I. Classification, frequency and salvage. Int J Radiat Oncol Biol Phys 1985;11:1271.

746. Donegan WL, Perez-Mesa CM, Watson FR: A biostatistical study of locally recurrent breast carcinoma. Surg Gynecol Obstet 1966;122:529.

747. Kurtz J, Spitalier J-M, Amalric R, et al: Mammary recurrences in young women younger than forty. Int J Radiat Oncol Biol Phys 1988;15:271.

748. Stotter A, Atkinson EN, Fairston BA, et al: Survival following locoregional recurrence after breast conservation therapy for cancer. Ann Surg 1990;212:166.

749. Recht A, Hayes DF: Local recurrence following mastectomy. In Harris JR, Hellman S, Hendersen K, Kinne DW (eds): Breast Diseases, 2nd ed. Philadelphia, JB Lippincott, 1991, p 529.

750. Greco M, Cascinelli N, Galluzzo D, et al: Locally recurrent breast cancer after radical surgery. Eur J Surg Oncol 1992;18:209.

751. Kennedy MJ, Abeloff MD: Management of locally recurrent breast cancer. Cancer 1993;71:2395.

752. Recht A, Gray R, Davidson N, et al: Locoregional failure 10 years after mastectomy and adjuvant chemotherapy with or without tamoxifen without irradiation: Experience of the Eastern Cooperative Oncology Group. J Clin Oncol 1999;17:1689–1700.

753. Tough ICK: The significance of recurrence in breast cancer. Br J Surg 1966;53:897.

754. Hietanen P: Relapse pattern and follow-up of breast cancer. Ann Clin Res 1986;18:134.

755. Aberizk WJ, Silver B, Hendersen IC, et al: The use of radiotherapy in treatment of isolated locoregional recurrence of breast carcinoma after mastectomy. Cancer 1986;58:1214.

756. Dao TL, Nemoto N: The clinical significance of skin recurrence after radical mastectomy in women with cancer of the breast. Surg Gynecol Obstet 1963;117:447.

757. Karabali-Dalamaga S, Souhami RL, O'Higgins NJ, et al: Natural history and prognosis of recurrent breast cancer. BMJ 1978; 2:730.

758. Matsumoto K: Prognostic analysis of recurrent breast cancer. Jpn J Clin Oncol 1985;15:595.

759. Rosenman J, Bernard S, Kober C, et al: Local recurrences in patients with breast cancer at the North Carolina Memorial Hospital (1970–1982). Cancer 1986;57:1421.

760. Crile G: Low incidence of local recurrence after conservative operations for cancer of the breast. Ann Surg 1972;175:249.

761. Fentiman IS, Matthews PN, Davison OW, et al: Survival following local skin recurrence after mastectomy. Br J Surg 1985;72:14.

762. Recht A, Silen W, Schnitt S, et al: Time course of local recurrence following conservative surgery and radiotherapy for early stage breast cancer. Int J Radiat Oncol Biol Phys 1988;15:255–261.

763. Veronesi U, Cascinelli N, Mariani L, et al: Twenty-year follow-up of a randomized study comparing breast-conservation surgery with radical mastectomy for early breast cancer. N Engl J Med 2002;347:1227–1231.

764. Bartelink H: Editorial comment. Eur J Cancer 2001;37:2143–2146.

765. Fajardo LL, Roberts CC, Hunt KR: Mammographic surveillance of breast cancer patients: Should the mastectomy site be imaged? Am J Radiol 1993;161:953.

766. Donegan W: Local and regional recurrence. In Donegan W, Spratt D (eds): Cancer of the Breast. Philadelphia, WB Saunders, 1979.

767. Salvadori B, Rovini D, Squicciarini P, et al: Surgery for local recurrences following deficient radical mastectomy for breast cancer: A selected series of 39 cases. Eur J Surg Oncol 1992;18:438.

768. Humphrey LJ, Moore DL, Lytle GH: Postmastectomy locally recurrent breast cancer. J Surg Oncol 1990;43:88.

769. Dahlstrom KK, Anderson AP, Andersen M, Krag C: Wide local excision of recurrent breast cancer in the thoracic wall. Cancer 1993;72:774.

770. Chu F, Lin F-J, Kim JH, et al: Locally recurrent carcinoma of the breast: Results of radiation therapy. Cancer 1976;37:2677.

771. Beck TM, Hart NE, Woodward DA, Smith C: Local or regional recurrent carcinoma of the breast: Results of therapy in 121 patients. J Clin Oncol 1983;1:400.

772. Deutsch M, Parsons JA, Mittal BB: Radiation therapy for locally regional recurrent breast cancer. Int J Radiat Oncol Biol Phys 1986;12:2061.

773. Hulverson KJ, Perez CA, Kucke RR, et al: Isolated local-regional recurrence of breast cancer following mastectomy: Radiotherapeutic management. Int J Radiat Oncol Biol Phys 1990;19:851.

774. Chen KK-Y, Montague E, Oswald MJ: Results of irradiation in the treatment of loco-regional breast cancer recurrence. Cancer 1985;56:1269.

775. Fowble B: The role of radiotherapy in the treatment and prevention of local-regional recurrence following mastectomy for operable breast cancer. Int J Radiat Oncol Biol Phys 1986;12: 2209.

776. Janjan NA, McNeese MD, Buzdar AU, Montague ED: Management of loco-regional recurrent breast cancer. Cancer 1986;58:1552.

777. Recht A, Silen W, Schnitt SJ, et al: Time course of local recurrence following conservation surgery and radiotherapy for early stage breast cancer. Int J Radiat Oncol Biol Phys 1988;15:255.

778. Fowble B, Solin LJ, Schultz DJ, et al: Breast recurrence following conservative surgery and radiation: Pattern of failure, prognosis and pathologic findings from mastectomy specimens with implications for treatment. Int J Radiat Oncol Biol Phys 1990;19:833.

779. Disa J, Petrek J: Surgical management after local failure in the irradiated breast. Semin Breast Dis 1999;2:252–257.

780. Clark GM, Sledge GW Jr, Osborne CK, et al: Survival from first recurrence: Relative importance of prognostic factors in 1,015 breast cancer patients. J Clin Oncol 1987;5:55–61.

781. Giordano SH, Buzdar AU, Kau S-WC, et al: Improvement in breast cancer survival: results from M.D. Anderson Cancer Center protocols from 1975–2000 (abstract 212). Proc Am Soc Clin Oncol 2002;21:54a.

782. Sledge GW, Neuberg D, Bernardo P, et al: Phase III trial of doxorubicin, paclitaxel, and the combination of doxorubicin and paclitaxel as front-line chemotherapy for metastatic breast cancer: An intergroup trial (E1193). J Clin Oncol 2003;21:588–592.

783. Hortobagyi G: Can we cure limited metastatic breast cancer? J Clin Oncol 2002;20:620–623.

784. Tomiak E, Piccart M, Mignolet F, et al: Characterisation of complete responders to combination chemotherapy for advanced breast cancer: A retrospective EORTC Breast Group study. Eur J Cancer 1996;32A:1876–1887.

785. Greenberg PA, Hortobagyi GN, Smith TL, et al: Long-term follow-up of patients with complete remission following combination chemotherapy for metastatic breast cancer. J Clin Oncol 1996;14:2197–2205.

786. Falkson G, Holcroft C, Gelman RS, et al: Ten-year follow-up study of premenopausal women with metastatic breast cancer: An Eastern Cooperative Oncology Group study. J Clin Oncol 1995;13:1453–1458.

787. Holmes F, Buzdar A, Kau S, et al: Combined-modality approach for patients with isolated recurrences of breast cancer (IV-NED): The M.D. Anderson experience. Breast Dis 1994;7:7–20.

788. Rivera E, Holmes FA, Buzdar AU, et al: Fluorouracil, doxorubicin, and cyclophosphamide followed by tamoxifen as adjuvant treatment for patients with stage IV breast cancer with no evidence of disease. Breast J 2002;8:2–9.

789. Pierga JY, Asselain B, Jouve M, et al: Effect of adjuvant chemotherapy on outcome in patients with metastatic breast carcinoma treated with first-line doxorubicin-containing chemotherapy. Cancer 2001;91:1079–1089.

790. Cara S, Tannock IF: Retreatment of patients with the same chemotherapy: Implications for clinical mechanisms of drug resistance. Ann Oncol 2001;12:23–27.

791. Coates AS, Hurny C, Peterson HF, et al: Quality-of-life scores predict outcome in metastatic but not early breast cancer: International Breast Cancer Study Group. J Clin Oncol 2000;18:3768–3774.

792. Geels P, Eisenhauer E, Bezjak A, et al: Palliative effect of chemotherapy: Objective tumor response is associated with symptom improvement in patients with metastatic Breast Cancer. J Clin Oncol 2000;18:2395–2405.

793. Cook GJ, Houston S, Rubens R, et al: Detection of bone metastases in breast cancer by 18FDG PET: Differing metabolic activity in osteoblastic and osteolytic lesions. J Clin Oncol 1998;16:3375–3379.

794. Miller KD, Weathers T, Haney LG, et al: Occult central nervous system (CNS) involvement in patients (pts) with metastatic breast cancer: Prevalence, predictive factors and impact on overall survival (abstract 214). Breast Cancer Res Treat 2001;69:240.

795. Crivellari D, Pagani O, Veronesi A, et al: High incidence of central nervous system involvement in patients with metastatic or locally advanced breast cancer treated with epirubicin and docetaxel. Ann Oncol 2001;12:353–356.

796. Chock JY, Domchek S, Burstein HJ, et al: Central nervous system (CNS) metastases in women who receive trastuzumab for metastatic breast cancer (MBC) [abstract 218]. Proc Am Soc Clin Oncol 2002;21:55a.

797. Buzdar AU, Hortobagyi GN: Tamoxifen and toremifene in breast cancer: Comparison of safety and efficacy (see comments). J Clin Oncol 1998;16:348–353.

798. Mortimer JE, Dehdashti F, Siegel BA, et al: Metabolic flare: Indicator of hormone responsiveness in advanced breast cancer. J Clin Oncol 2001;19:2797–2803.

799. Gradishar W, Glusman J, Lu Y, et al: Effects of high dose raloxifene in selected patients with advanced breast carcinoma. Cancer 2000;88:2047–2053.

800. Jiang SY, Langan-Fahey SM, Stella AL, et al: Point mutation of estrogen receptor (ER) in the ligand-binding domain changes the pharmacology of antiestrogens in ER-negative breast cancer cells stably expressing complementary DNAs for ER. Mol Endocrinol 1992;6:2167–2174.

801. Crewe HK, Notley LM, Wunsch RM, et al: Metabolism of tamoxifen by recombinant human cytochrome P450 enzymes: Formation of the 4-hydroxy, 4′-hydroxy and N-desmethyl metabolites and isomerization of trans-4-hydroxytamoxifen. Drug Metab Dispos 2002;30:869–874.

802. Osborne CK, Wiebe VJ, McGuire WL, et al: Tamoxifen and the isomers of 4-hydroxytamoxifen in tamoxifen-resistant tumors from breast cancer patients. J Clin Oncol 1992;10:304–310.

803. Osborne CK, Coronado E, Allred DC, et al: Acquired tamoxifen resistance: Correlation with reduced breast tumor levels of tamoxifen and isomerization of trans-4-hydroxytamoxifen. J Natl Cancer Inst 1991;83:1477–1482.

804. Wiebe VJ, Osborne CK, McGuire WL, et al: Identification of estrogenic tamoxifen metabolite(s) in tamoxifen-resistant human breast tumors. J Clin Oncol 1992;10:990–994.

805. Girault I, Lerebours F, Amarir S, et al: Expression analysis of estrogen receptor alpha coregulators in breast carcinoma: Evidence that NCOR1 expression is predictive of the response to tamoxifen. Clin Cancer Res 2003;9:1259–1266.

806. Nabholtz JM, Buzdar A, Pollak M, et al: Anastrozole is superior to tamoxifen as first-line therapy for advanced breast cancer in postmenopausal women: Results of a North American multicenter randomized trial. J Clin Oncol 2000;18:3758–3767.

807. Bonneterre J, Thurlimann B, Robertson JF, et al: Anastrozole versus tamoxifen as first-line therapy for advanced breast cancer in 668 postmenopausal women: Results of the tamoxifen or arimidex randomized group efficacy and tolerability study. J Clin Oncol 2000;18:3748–3757.

808. Mouridsen H, Gershanovich M, Sun Y, et al: Superior efficacy of letrozole versus tamoxifen as first-line therapy for postmeno-pausal women with advanced breast cancer: Results of a phase III study of the International Letrozole Breast Cancer Group. J Clin Oncol 2001;19:2596–2606.

809. Buzdar A, Douma J, Davidson N, et al: Phase III, multicenter, double-blind, randomized study of letrozole, an aromatase inhibitor, for advanced breast cancer versus megestrol acetate. J Clin Oncol 2001;19:3357–3366.

810. Dombernowsky P, Smith I, Falkson G, et al: Letrozole, a new oral aromatase inhibitor for advanced breast cancer: Double-blind randomized trial showing a dose effect and improved efficacy and tolerability compared with megestrol acetate (see comments). J Clin Oncol 1998;16:453–461.

811. Gershanovich M, Chaudri HA, Campos D, et al: Letrozole, a new oral aromatase inhibitor: Randomised trial comparing 2.5 mg daily, 0.5 mg daily and aminoglutethimide in postmenopausal women with advanced breast cancer. Letrozole International Trial Group (AR/BC3). Ann Oncol 1998;9:639–645.

812. Buzdar A, Nabholtz JM, Robertson JF, et al: Anastrozole (Arimidex) versus tamoxifen as first-line therapy for advanced breast cancer (ABC) in postmenopausal (PM) women? Combined analysis from two identically designed multicenter trials (abstract 609D). Proc Am Soc Clin Oncol 2000;19:154a.

813. Jones S, Vogel C, Arkhipov A, et al: Multicenter, phase II trial of exemestane as third-line hormonal therapy of postmenopausal women with metastatic breast cancer: Aromasin Study Group. J Clin Oncol 1999;17:3418–3425.

814. Kaufmann M, Bajetta E, Dirix LY, et al: Exemestane is superior to megestrol acetate after tamoxifen failure in postmenopausal women with advanced breast cancer: Results of a phase III randomized double-blind trial. The Exemestane Study Group. J Clin Oncol 2000;18:1399–1411.

Specific Malignancies

III

815. Lønning PE, Bajetta E, Murray R, et al: Activity of exemestane in metastatic breast cancer after failure of nonsteroidal aromatase inhibitors: A phase II trial. J Clin Oncol 2000;18:2234–2244.

816. Geisler J, Haynes B, Anker G, et al: Influence of letrozole and anastrozole on total body aromatization and plasma estrogen levels in postmenopausal breast cancer patients evaluated in a randomized, cross-over study. J Clin Oncol 2002;20:751–757.

817. Rose C, Vtoraya O, Pluzanska A, et al: Letrozole (Femara) vs. anastrozole (Arimidex): Second-line treatment in postmenopausal women with advanced breast cancer (abstract 131). Proc Am Soc Clin Oncol 2002;21:34a.

818. Bonneterre J, Buzdar A, Nabholtz JM, et al: Anastrozole is superior to tamoxifen as first-line therapy in hormone receptor positive advanced breast carcinoma. Cancer 2001;92:2247–2258.

819. Buzdar AU: Superior efficacy of letrozole versus tamoxifen as first-line therapy. J Clin Oncol 2002;20:876–878.

820. Bajetta E, Zilembo N, Bichisao E, et al: Tumor response and estrogen suppression in breast cancer patients treated with aromatase inhibitors. Ann Oncol 2000;11:1017–1022.

821. Johnson PE, Buzdar A: Are differences in the available aromatase inhibitors and inactivators significant? Clin Cancer Res 2001;7:4360s–4368s; discussion 4411s–4412s.

822. Dees EC, Davidson NE: Ovarian ablation as adjuvant therapy for breast cancer. Semin Oncol 2001;28:322–331.

823. Counsell R, Bain G, Williams MV, et al: Artificial radiation menopause: Where are the ovaries? Clin Oncol (R Coll Radiol) 1996;8:250–253.

824. Klijn JG, Blamey RW, Boccardo F, et al: Combined tamoxifen and luteinizing hormone-releasing hormone (LHRH) agonist versus LHRH agonist alone in premenopausal advanced breast cancer: A meta-analysis of four randomized trials. J Clin Oncol 2001;19:343–353.

825. Klijn JGM, Beex LVAM, Mauriac L, et al: Combined treatment with buserelin and tamoxifen in premenopausal metastatic breast cancer: A randomized study. J Natl Cancer Inst 2000;92:903–911.

826. Howell A, Osborne CK, Morris C, et al: ICI 182,780 (Faslodex): Development of a novel, "pure" antiestrogen. Cancer 2000;89:817–825.

827. Howell A: Preliminary experience with pure antiestrogens. Clin Cancer Res 2001;7:4369s–4375s; discussion 4411s–4412s.

828. Henderson IC: A rose is no longer a rose. J Clin Oncol 2002;20:3365–3368 (early release www.jco.org July 9, 2002).

829. Osborne CK, Pippen J, Jones SE, et al: Double-blind, randomized trial comparing the efficacy and tolerability of fulvestrant versus anastrozole in postmenopausal women with advanced breast cancer progressing on prior endocrine therapy: Results of a North American trial. J Clin Oncol 2002;20:3386–3395 (early release www.jco.org July 1, 2002).

830. Howell A, Robertson JFR, Albano JQ, et al: Fulvestrant, formerly ICI 182,780, is as effective as anastrozole in postmenopausal women with advanced breast cancer progressing after prior endocrine treatment. J Clin Oncol 2002;20:3396–3403 (early release www.jco.org July 1, 2002).

831. Valero V, Holmes FA, Walters RS, et al: Phase II trial of docetaxel: A new, highly effective antineoplastic agent in the management of patients with anthracycline-resistant metastatic breast cancer. J Clin Oncol 1995;13:2886–2894.

832. Rivera E, Holmes FA, Frye D, et al: Phase II study of paclitaxel in patients with metastatic breast carcinoma refractory to standard chemotherapy. Cancer 2000;89:2195–2201.

833. Valero V, Jones SE, Von Hoff DD, et al: A phase II study of docetaxel in patients with paclitaxel-resistant metastatic breast cancer. J Clin Oncol 1998;16:3362–3368.

834. Winer E, Berry D, Duggan D, et al: Failure of higher dose paclitaxel to improve outcome in patients with metastatic breast cancer: Results from CALGB 9342 (abstract 388). Proc Am Soc Clin Oncol 1998;17:101a.

835. Smith RE, Brown AM, Mamounas EP, et al: Randomized trial of 3-hour versus 24-hour infusion of high-dose paclitaxel in patients with metastatic or locally advanced breast cancer: National Surgical Adjuvant Breast and Bowel Project Protocol B-26. J Clin Oncol 1999;17:3403–3411.

836. Salminen E, Bergman M, Huhtala S, et al: Docetaxel: Standard recommended dose of 100 mg/m(2) is effective but not feasible for some metastatic breast cancer patients heavily pretreated with chemotherapy. A phase II single-center study. J Clin Oncol 1999;17:1127.

837. Chan S, Friedrichs K, Noel D, et al: Prospective randomized trial of docetaxel versus doxorubicin in patients with metastatic breast cancer: The 303 Study Group. J Clin Oncol 1999;17:2341–2354.

838. Paridaens R, Biganzoli L, Bruning P, et al: Paclitaxel versus doxorubicin as first-line single-agent chemotherapy for metastatic breast cancer: A European organization for research and treatment of cancer randomized study with cross-over. J Clin Oncol 2000;18:724.

839. Bishop JF, Dewar J, Toner GC, et al: Initial paclitaxel improves outcome compared with CMFP combination chemotherapy as front-line therapy in untreated metastatic breast cancer. J Clin Oncol 1999;17:2355–2364.

840. Burstein HJ, Manola J, Younger J, et al: Docetaxel administered on a weekly basis for metastatic breast cancer. J Clin Oncol 2000;18:1212–1219.

841. Perez EA, Vogel CL, Irwin DH, et al: Multicenter phase II trial of weekly paclitaxel in women with metastatic breast cancer. J Clin Oncol 2001;19:4216–4223.

842. Hainsworth JD, Burris HA III, Yardley DA, et al: Weekly docetaxel in the treatment of elderly patients with advanced breast cancer: A Minnie Pearl Cancer Research Network phase II trial. J Clin Oncol 2001;19:3500–3505.

843. Blum JL, Dieras V, LoRusso PM, et al: Multicenter, phase II study of capecitabine in taxane-pretreated metastatic breast carcinoma patients. Cancer 2001;92:1759–1768.

844. Nabholtz JM, Senn HJ, Bezwoda WR, et al: Prospective randomized trial of docetaxel versus mitomycin plus vinblastine in patients with metastatic breast cancer progressing despite previous anthracycline-containing chemotherapy: 304 Study Group. J Clin Oncol 1999;17:1413–1424.

845. O'Shaughnessy J, Miles D, Vukelja S, et al: Superior survival with capecitabine plus docetaxel combination therapy in anthracycline-pretreated patients with advanced breast cancer: Phase III trial results. J Clin Oncol 2002;20:2812–2823.

846. Gianni L, Munzone E, Capri G, et al: Paclitaxel by 3-hour infusion in combination with bolus doxorubicin in women with untreated metastatic breast cancer: High antitumor efficacy and cardiac effects in a dose-finding and sequence-finding study (see comments). J Clin Oncol 1995;13:2688–2699.

847. Biganzoli L, Cufer T, Bruning P, et al: Doxorubicin and paclitaxel versus doxorubicin and cyclophosphamide as first-line chemotherapy in metastatic breast cancer: The European Organization for Research and Treatment of Cancer 10961 Multicenter Phase III Trial. J Clin Oncol 2002;20:3114–3121.

848. Luck HJ, Thomssen C, Untch M, et al: Multicentric phase III study in first line treatment of advanced metastatic breast cancer (ABC): Epirubicin/paclitaxel (ET) vs epirubicin/cyclophosphamide (EC). A study of the AGO Breast Cancer Group (abstract 280). Proc Am Soc Clin Oncol 2000;19:73a.

849. Nabholtz JM, Falkson C, Campos D, et al: Docetaxel and doxorubicin compared with doxorubicin and cyclophosphamide as first-line chemotherapy for metastatic breast cancer: Results of a randomized, multicenter, phase III trial. J Clin Oncol 2003;21:968–975.

850. Stadtmauer EA, O'Neill A, Goldstein LJ, et al: Conventional-dose chemotherapy compared with high-dose chemotherapy plus autologous hematopoietic stem-cell transplantation for metastatic breast cancer. N Engl J Med 2000;342:1069–1076.

851. Leyland-Jones B, Arnold A, Gelmon K, et al: Pharmacologic insights into the future of trastuzumab. Ann Oncol 2001;12(Suppl 1):S43–S47.

852. Zujewski JA: "Build quality in": HER2 testing in the real world. J Natl Cancer Inst 2002;94:788–789.

853. Seidman AD, Fornier M, Esteva F, et al: Final report: Weekly (W) herceptin (H) and taxol (T) for metastatic breast cancer (MBC). Analysis of efficacy by HER2 immunophenotype [immunohistochemistry (IHC)] and gene amplification [fluorescent in-situ hybridization (FISH)] (abstract 319). Proc Am Soc Clin Oncol 2000;19:83a.

854. Kuzur ME, Albain KS, Huntington MO, et al: A phase II trial of docetaxel and herceptin in metastatic breast cancer patients

overexpressing HER-2 (abstract 512). Proc Am Soc Clin Oncol 2000;19:131a.

855. Burstein HJ, Kuter I, Campos SM, et al: Clinical activity of trastuzumab and vinorelbine in women with HER2-overexpressing metastatic breast cancer. J Clin Oncol 2001;19:2722-2730.

856. Solomayer EF, Diel IJ, Meyberg GC, et al: Metastatic breast cancer: Clinical course, prognosis and therapy related to the first site of metastasis. Breast Cancer Res Treat 2000;59:271-278.

857. Hortobagyi GN, Theriault RL, Lipton A, et al: Long-term prevention of skeletal complications of metastatic breast cancer with pamidronate: Protocol 19 Aredia Breast Cancer Study Group. J Clin Oncol 1998;16:2038-2044.

858. Theriault RL, Lipton A, Hortobagyi GN, et al: Pamidronate reduces skeletal morbidity in women with advanced breast cancer and lytic bone lesions: A randomized, placebo-controlled trial. J Clin Oncol 1999;17:846-854.

859. Lipton A, Theriault RL, Hortobagyi GN, et al: Pamidronate prevents skeletal complications and is effective palliative treatment in women with breast carcinoma and osteolytic bone metastases: Long term follow-up of two randomized, placebo-controlled trials. Cancer 2000;88:1082-1090.

860. Hillner BE, Weeks JC, Desch CE, et al: Pamidronate in prevention of bone complications in metastatic breast cancer: A cost-effectiveness analysis. J Clin Oncol 2000;18:72-79.

861. Berenson JR, Rosen LS, Howell A, et al: Zoledronic acid reduces skeletal-related events in patients with osteolytic metastases. Cancer 2001;91:1191-1200.

862. Moulder SL, Yakes FM, Muthuswamy SK, et al: Epidermal growth factor receptor (HER1) tyrosine kinase inhibitor ZD1839 (Iressa) inhibits HER2/neu (erbB2)-overexpressing breast cancer cells in vitro and in vivo. Cancer Res 2001;61:8887-8895.

863. Hidalgo M, Siu LL, Nemunaitis J, et al: Phase I and pharmacologic study of OSI-774, an epidermal growth factor receptor tyrosine kinase inhibitor, in patients with advanced solid malignancies. J Clin Oncol 2001;19:3267-3279.

864. Hidalgo M, Eckhardt SG: Development of matrix metalloproteinase inhibitors in cancer therapy. J Natl Cancer Inst 2001;93:178-193.

865. Sledge GW Jr: Vascular endothelial growth factor in breast cancer: Biologic and therapeutic aspects. Semin Oncol 2002;29:104-110.

866. Miller KD, Sweeney CJ, Sledge GW Jr: Redefining the target: Chemotherapeutics as antiangiogenics. J Clin Oncol 2001;19:1195-1206.

867. Hidalgo M, Rowinsky EK: The rapamycin-sensitive signal transduction pathway as a target for cancer therapy. Oncogene 2000;19:6680-6686.

868. Johnston SR: Farnesyl transferase inhibitors: A novel targeted therapy for cancer. Lancet Oncol 2001;2:18-26.

869. Arteaga CL: Molecular therapeutics: Is one promiscuous drug against multiple targets better than combinations of molecule-specific drugs? Clin Cancer Res 2003;9:1231-1232.

870. Giordano SH, Buzdar AU, Hortobagyi GN: Breast cancer in men. Ann Intern Med 2002;137:678-687.

871. Evans DB, Crichlow RW: Carcinoma of the male breast and Klinefelter's syndrome: Is there an association? CA Cancer J Clin 1987;37:246-251.

872. Donegan WL, Redlich PN, Lang PJ, et al: Carcinoma of the breast in males: A multiinstitutional survey. Cancer 1998;83:498-509.

873. Couch FJ, Farid LM, DeShano ML, et al: BRCA2 germline mutations in male breast cancer cases and breast cancer families. Nat Genet 1996;13:123-125.

874. Thorlacius S, Olafsdottir G, Tryggvadottir L, et al: A single BRCA2 mutation in male and female breast cancer families from Iceland with varied cancer phenotypes. Nat Genet 1996;13:117-119.

875. Rayson D, Erlichman C, Suman VJ, et al: Molecular markers in male breast carcinoma. Cancer 1998;83:1947-1955.

876. Kraybill WG, Kaufman R, Kinne D: Treatment of advanced male breast cancer. Cancer 1981;47:2185-2189.

877. Jaiyesimi IA, Buzdar AU, Sahin AA, et al: Carcinoma of the male breast. Ann Intern Med 1992;117:771-777.

878. Lopez M, Natali M, DiLauro L, et al: Combined treatment with buserelin and cyproterone acetate in metastatic male breast cancer. Cancer 1993;72:502-505.

879. Harris AL, Dowsett M, Stuart-Harris R, et al: Role of aminoglutethimide in male breast cancer. Br J Cancer 1986;54:657-660.

880. Giordano SH, Valero V, Buzdar AU, et al: Efficacy of anastrozole in male breast cancer. Am J Clin Oncol 2002;25:235-237.

881. van der Vange N, van Dongen JA: Breast cancer and pregnancy. Eur J Surg Oncol 1991;17:1.

882. Kuerer HM, Cunningham JD, Brower ST, Tartter PI: Breast carcinoma associated with pregnancy and lactation. Surg Oncol G: 1997;6:93-98.

883. Titcomb CL: Breast cancer and pregnancy. Hawaii Med J 1990;49:18.

884. Petrek JA: Breast cancer during pregnancy. Cancer 1994;74(Suppl):518.

885. Samuels TH, Liu FF, Yaffe M, Haider M: Gestational breast cancer. Can Assoc Radiol J 1998;49:172.

886. Sorosk JI, Scott-Conner CE: Breast disease complicating pregnancy. Obstet Gynecol Clin North Am 1998;25:353.

887. Hoover HC: Breast cancer during pregnancy and lactation. Surg Clin North Am 1990;70:1151.

888. Espie M, Cuvier C: Treating breast cancer during pregnancy: What can be taken safely? Drug Safety 1998;18:135.

889. Berry DL, Theriault RL, Holmes FA, et al: Management of breast cancer during pregnancy using a standardized protocol. J Clin Oncol 1999;17:855-861.

890. Ebert U, Loffler H, Kirch W: Cytotoxic therapy and pregnancy. Pharmacol Ther 1997;74:207.

891. Zanconati F, Zanella M, Falconieri G, Di Bonito L: Gestational squamous cell carcinoma of the breast: An unusual mammary tumor associated with aggressive clinical course. Pathol Res Pract 1997;193:783.

892. Petrek JA: Pregnancy safety after breast cancer. Cancer 1994;74(Suppl):528.

893. Kroman N, Jensen MD, Melbye M, et al: Should women be advised against pregnancy after breast-cancer treatment? Lancet 1997;350:319.

894. Lozada JA, Shullaih SA, Hoy E, et al: Effects of pregnancy following treatment for breast cancer on survival and risk of recurrence (abstract 145). Proc Am Soc Clin Oncol 2001;20:37a.

895. Owen HW, Dockery MB, Gray HK: Occult carcinoma of the breast. Surg Gynecol Obstet 1954;58:302.

896. Westbrook KC, Gallagher HS: Breast carcinoma presenting as an axillary mass. Am J Surg 1971;122:607.

897. Ashikari R, Rosen PP, Urban JA, et al: Breast cancer presenting as an axillary mass. Ann Surg 1976;183:415.

898. Block EF, Meyer MA: Positron emission tomography in diagnosis of occult adenocarcinoma of the breast. Am Surg 1998;64:906.

899. Tilanus-Linthorst MM, Obdeijn AI, Bontenbal Mand Oudkerk M: MRI in patients with axillary metastases of occult breast carcinoma. Breast Cancer Res Treat 1997;44:179.

900. Iglehart JD, Ferguson BJ, Shingleton WW, et al: An ultrastructural analysis of breast carcinoma presenting as isolated axillary adenopathy. Ann Surg 1982;196:8.

901. Kemeny MM, Rivera DE, Terz JJ, et al: Occult primary adenocarcinoma with axillary metastases. Am J Surg 1986;152:43.

902. Baron PL, Moore MP, Kinne DW, et al: Occult breast cancer presenting with axillary metastases. Arch Surg 1990;125:210.

903. Knapper WH: Management of occult breast cancer presenting as an axillary metastasis. Semin Surg Oncol 1991;17:311.

904. Merson M, Andreola S, Galimberti V, et al: Breast carcinoma presenting as axillary metastases without evidence of a primary tumor. Cancer 1992;70:504.

905. Vilcoq JR, Calle R, Ferme F, Veith F: Conservative treatment of axillary adenopathy due to probable subclinical breast cancer. Arch Surg 1982;117:1136.

906. Baron PL, Moore MP, Kinne DW, et al: Occult breast cancer presenting with axillary metastases: Updated management. Arch Surg 1990;125:210.

907. Campana F, Fourquet M, Ashby A, et al: Presentation of axillary lymphadenopathy without detectable breast primary (T_0N_{1b} breast cancer): Experience at Institut Curie. Radiother Oncol 1989;15:321.

908. Kister SJ, Haagensen CD: Paget's disease of the breast. Am J Surg 1970;119:606.

909. Ascensao AC, Marques MSJ, Capitao-Mor M: Paget's disease of the nipple. Dermatologica 1985;170:170.
910. Ashikari P, Vanuytsel L, Rihinders A, et al: Breast conserving treatment of Paget's disease. Radiother Oncol 1990;17:305.
911. Vielh P, Validire P, Kheirallah S, et al: Paget's disease of the nipple without clinically and radiologically detectable breast tumor: Histochemical and immunohistochemical study of 44 cases. Pathol Res Pract 1993;189:150.
912. Yim HJ, Wick MR, Relpott GW, et al: Underlying pathology in mammary Paget's disease. Ann Surg Oncol 1997;4:287.
913. Potter CR, Eeckout I, Schelfhout AM, et al: Keratinocyte induced chemotaxis in the pathogenesis of Paget's disease of the breast. Histopathology 1994;24:349.
914. Schwartz GF, Carter WB, Finkel GC: Paget's carcinoma of the breast. Surg Oncol Clin North Am 1993;2:93.
915. Miller L, Tyler W, Maroon M, Miller OF: Erosive adenomatosis of the nipple: A benign imitator of malignant breast disease. Cutis 1997;59:91.
916. Kobayoshi TK, Ueda M, Nishimno T, et al: Scrape cytology of pemphigus vulgaris of the nipple, a mimicker of Paget's disease. Diagn Cytopathol 1997;16:156.
917. Barnes L, Pietruszka M: Sarcomas of the breast: A clinicopathological analysis of ten cases. Cancer 1977;40:1577.
918. Callery CD, Rosen PP, Kinne DW: Sarcoma of the breast: Study of 32 patients with reappraisal of classification and therapy. Ann Surg 1985;201:527.
919. Khanna S, Gupta S, Khanna NM: Sarcomas of the breast: Homogenous or heterogenous? J Surg Oncol 1981;18:119.
920. May DS, Stroup NE: The incidence of sarcomas of the breast among women in the U.S. 19731986. Plast Reconstruct Surg 1991;87:193.
921. Reynolds J, Mies C, Daly JM: Mesenchymal infiltrating tumors. In Bland KI, Copeland EM (eds): The Breast: Comprehensive Management of Benign and Malignant Diseases. Philadelphia, WB Saunders, 1991, p 210.
922. Schnabel FR: Cystosarcoma phyllodes. In Gump FE, Cady B (eds): Breast Cancer in High Risk Patients. Surg Oncol Clin North Am 1993;2:107.
923. Müller J: Uber den feineren Bau und die Formen der Krankhaften art Geschwulste. Berlin, Reimer, 1838, p 54.
924. Treves N, Sunderland DA: Cystosarcoma phyllodes of the breast: A malignant and benign tumor. Cancer 1951;4:1286.
925. Halverson JD, Hori-Rubaina JM: Cystosarcoma phyllodes of the breast. Am Surg 1974;40;295.
926. Pietruszka M, Barnes L: Cystosarcoma phyllodes: A clinicopathologic analysis of 42 cases. Cancer 1978;41:1974.
927. Al-Jurf A, Hawk WA, Crile G: Cystosarcoma phyllodes. Surg Gynecol Obstet 1978;146:358.
928. Contarini O, Urdaneta LF, Hagen W, et al: Cystosarcoma phyllodes of the breast: A new therapeutic proposal. Am Surg 1982;48:157.
929. Hines JR, Murad TM, Beal JM: Prognostic indicators in cystosarcoma phyllodes. Am J Surg 1987;153:276.
930. Murad TM, Hines JR, Beal J, et al: Histopathological and clinical correlations of cystosarcoma phyllodes. Arch Pathol Lab Med 1988;112:752.
931. Azzopardi JG: Problems in breast pathology. In Bennington J (ed): Major Progress in Pathology. Philadelphia, WB Saunders, 1979, p 346.
932. Norris JH, Taylor HB: Relationship of histologic features to behavior of cystosarcoma phyllodes. Cancer 1967;20:2090.
933. Lester J, Stout AP: Cystosarcoma phyllodes. Cancer 1954;7:335.
934. Hawkins RE, Schofield JB, Fisher C, et al: The clinical and histologic criteria that predict metastases from cystosarcoma phyllodes. Cancer 1992;69:141.
935. Rajan PB, Cranor ML, Rosen PP: Cytosarcoma phyllodes in adolescent girls and young women: A study of 45 patients. Am J Surg Pathol 1998;22:64.
936. Hajdu SI, Espinosa MH, Robbins GF: Recurrent cystosarcoma phyllodes: A clinicopathologic study of 32 cases. Cancer 1976;138:1402.
937. McGregor GI, Knowling MA, Este FA: Sarcoma and cystosarcoma phyllodes tumors of the breast: A retrospective review of 58 cases. Am J Surg 1994;167:477.
938. Ciatto S, Bonardi R, Cataliotti L, Cardona G: Sarcomas of the breast: A multi-center series of 70 cases. Neoplasma 1992; 39:375.
939. Gutman H, Pollock RE, Ross MI, et al: Sarcoma of the breast: Implication for extent of therapy. Surgery 1994;116:505.
940. North JH, McPhee M, Arredondo M, Edge SB: Sarcoma of the breast: Implications of the extent of local therapy. Am Surg 1998;64:1059.
941. Moore MP, Kinne DW: Breast sarcoma. Surg Clin North Am 1996;76:383.
942. Bakheet SM, Powe J, Ezzat A, et al: F-18 FDG whole-body positron emission tomography scan in primary breast sarcoma. Clin Nucl Med 1998;23:604.
943. Pezzi CM, Pollock RE, Evans HL, et al: Preoperative chemotherapy for soft-tissue sarcomas of the extremities. Ann Surg 1990; 211:476.
944. Glenn J, Kinsella T, Glatstein E, Tepper J: A randomized prospective trial of adjuvant chemotherapy in adults with soft tissue sarcomas of the head and neck, breast and trunk. Cancer 1985;55: 1206.
945. Bramwell V, Rousse J, Steward W: European experience of adjuvant chemotherapy for soft tissue sarcomas: Interim report of a randomized trial of CYVADIC versus control. In Ryan JR, Baker LO (eds): Recent Concepts in Sarcoma Treatment: Proceedings of the International Symposium on Sarcomas. Boston, Kluwer Academic, 1988.

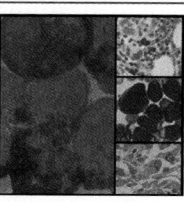

95

SARCOMAS OF BONE

James R. Neff

SUMMARY OF KEY POINTS

INCIDENCE AND EPIDEMIOLOGY
- More than 2400 new cases are diagnosed annually in the United States.
- No specific etiologic agents are identified in the majority of cases.
- Secondary neoplasms are related to known oncogenic factors (e.g., ionizing radiation, alkylating chemotherapy agents, combinations of both).
- Hereditary cancer syndromes (tumor suppressor genes) are responsible for some cases.

DIAGNOSIS AND RADIOGRAPHIC STAGING
- Needle or open biopsy (most tumors are not homogenous) is the most important staging method.
- Pathology review: immunohistochemistry and cytogenetics are important.
- Electron microscopic (EM) tissue occasionally is required and may be discarded if not used.
- Magnetic resonance imaging (MRI) scan of primary tumor is the superior imaging method for both low- and high-grade tumor.
- Chest x-ray is appropriate for low-grade tumor; computed tomography (CT) scan of the chest is better for high-grade tumor.
- Thallium-201 (^{201}Tl) and positron emission tomography (PET) scans can be used to monitor chemotherapy-related tumor necrosis.
- Rapid whole-body STIR MRI complements technetium-99m (^{99m}Tc) bone scan as a survey tool.

PROGNOSTIC FACTORS
- Multiagent neoadjuvant chemotherapy administration
- Tumor response to neoadjuvant chemotherapy
- Surgical margins of resection (minimum of a "wide" margin)
- Adjuvant chemotherapy administration
- Greater than 10-cm-diameter high-grade tumor: poor prognosis

STAGING SYSTEM
- American Joint Committee on Cancer (AJCC) now monitors location, grade (high and low grade), depth, and size (8 cm), designates "skip" lesions (T_3), and separates metastasis to bone from other sites (MIa, MIb).
- Musculoskeletal Tumor Society monitors location (intra- and extracompartmental), grade (high- and low-grade), and metastasis ("skip" lesions, nodal, bone, and lung are all lumped together in M).

PRIMARY THERAPY
- Limb-sparing procedures are appropriate for 70% to 90% of patients with localized extremity disease, without increasing the risk of developing local recurrence and/or metastatic disease.
- Local recurrence rates for limb-sparing procedures approach 5% or less.
- Reconstruction methods can be tailored to patient needs, expectations, acceptance, and functionality.
- New and improved biocompatible implant materials and improved designs are available.
- Improvements have been made in quality control of tissue bank (e.g., procurement of materials, testing).

FUTURE TRENDS
- The search continues for new drugs, drug schedules, potentiating agents, and improved dose intensity.
- Identification of risk factors (e.g., cytogenetic, molecular genetic, and signal transduction abnormalities) will improve to identify new methods of potential treatment.
- Imaging techniques will be refined further to indirectly predict good and poor response to chemotherapy in surgically inaccessible tumors.
- Continue to refine treatment methods to maximize therapy and minimize toxicity, improve quality control and delivery of radiotherapy techniques (i.e., intensity modulated radiation therapy), and decrease treatment-related and late effects of treatment.

STAGING AND BIOPSY

Approximately 2400 new malignant tumors of bone (excluding multiple myeloma) and 8300 new connective tissue tumors are diagnosed each year in the United States. More of these arise in and around the buttock, proximal thigh, and knee than at any other anatomic site. For children under the age of 15, the 5-year relative survival rate with management of primary tumors of bone has improved from 54% in 1976 to 73% in 1998 ($P < 0.05$).[1] The management of these patients, from initial evaluation and biopsy through surgical therapy and long-term follow-up, is labor intensive and technically demanding. With improved imaging technology and the varied multidisciplinary modes of therapy, the subspecialty of musculoskeletal oncology has evolved to provide the depth of knowledge required for optimum management of these patients.

Compartmental Surgical Concepts

In 1958, Bowden and Booher[2] described the concepts of compartmental confinement of soft-tissue tumors in the extremity. Independently, using stereoscopic biplanar angiography, Stener[3,4] was able to define the involved muscle compartment by correlating the image with the longitudinal axis of the tumor. After removal of the tumor, a procedure then referred to as myectomy, the lesion and margins were pathologically evaluated, confirming that the tumor often was confined within the anatomic fascial compartment.

Simon and Enneking,[5] in a study of 54 patients with soft-tissue sarcoma of the extremity, correlated the clinicopathologic findings with subsequent outcome and correlated local control with the surgical margins actually achieved. The authors were able to define appropriate bone and soft-tissue compartmental margins necessary for local primary tumor control without the use of neoadjuvant or adjuvant therapy.

Surgical theory regarding management of musculoskeletal neoplasms requires acceptance of a fundamental hypothesis: Solid tumors grow centrifugally from a central point and spread along predictable anatomic paths. They begin in mesenchymal tissue or bone and enlarge within that anatomic structure, growing along routes of least resistance. Only when large will a tumor violate major bone or fascial boundaries and invade another compartment. This compartment theory applies to skeletal and soft-tissue neoplasms. Determining the extent of compartment growth is critical for obtaining surgical control of local tumor; it is not a substitute for recognizing and treating systemic disease.

Surgical Staging System

The development of a useful and credible staging system requires the systematic collection and correlation of clinicopathologic data with extensive pathologic support and long-term patient management and follow-up. Enneking and associates[6] combined the concepts of a simplified pathologic grade (benign, low-grade, and high-grade) and clinical stage (compartmental vs. extracompartmental) and correlated these parameters with documented pathologic margins to define the surgical margins required for adequate local control. These correlative data were linked to a staging system common to both bone and soft-tissue lesions and were used for management of patients with tumors of the trunk, spine, and extremities.

Currently, the staging system adopted by the Musculoskeletal Tumor Society (MSTS) in 1980 and modified in 1986 is accepted by most musculoskeletal oncologists.[7,8] The system conveniently integrates tumor grade and patient stage with easily definable surgical margins derived from histopathologic observations. The knowledge of invasive tumor growth and local spread of bone and soft-tissue malignancies aids in management.

Characteristically, sarcomas grow at the expense of normal tissues by invasion, expansion, and flattening of normal tissues. The flattened area, called the zone of compression, is surrounded by condensed, atrophic, and edematous vascular tissue usually best defined by magnetic resonance imaging (MRI) and usually containing the neovascularity seen on conventional and digital angiography. This region is designated as the reactive zone. The combination of the zone of compression and the reactive zone pathologically comprises the pseudocapsule.

The compartmental fascia surrounding the lesion provides a rigid anatomic barrier to tumor growth. Infiltrative growth seen in tumors that develop in muscle usually occurs longitudinally in the planes of least resistance between muscle fibers and along the surrounding fascia. The proximal and distal extent of the tumor is often less well defined both radiographically and pathologically. Wide resections should include generous proximal and distal margins whenever possible.

In an effort to consolidate tumor grade classifications, tumors are separated into three grades: benign (G0), low-grade malignant (G1), and high-grade malignant (G2). Low-grade malignant lesions (G1), comprising Broder's I and II lesions, have a low probability of metastasis (25%). The majority of these tumors can be managed by relatively conservative surgical procedures. High-grade lesions (G2), Broder's III and IV tumors, have a significantly higher incidence of local persistence and metastases, requiring more radical surgical procedures and possibly neoadjuvant and/or adjuvant multidisciplinary therapy. Table 95-1

TABLE 95-1

Surgical Grade (G)

LOW (G1)	HIGH (G2)
Parosteal osteosarcoma	Classic osteosarcoma
Periosteal osteosarcoma	High-grade surface
Low-grade central osteosarcoma	Paget's sarcoma of bone
Intraosseous osteosarcoma	Radiation sarcoma
Secondary chondrosarcoma	Primary chondrosarcoma
	Dedifferentiated chondrosarcoma
	Mesenchymal chondrosarcoma
Clear cell chondrosarcoma	
Fibrosarcoma, Kaposi's sarcoma	Fibrosarcoma
Atypical malignant fibrous histiocytoma	Malignant fibrous histiocytoma (MFH)
	MFH of bone
	Undifferentiated primary sarcoma
Giant cell tumor, bone	Giant cell sarcoma, bone
Hemangioendothelioma	Angiosarcoma
Hemangiopericytoma	Hemangiopericytoma
Myxoid liposarcoma	Pleomorphic liposarcoma
	Neurofibrosarcoma (schwannoma)
Clear cell sarcoma	Rhabdomyosarcoma
Epithelioid sarcoma	Synovial sarcoma
Chordoma	Ewing's sarcoma of bone
Adamantinoma	PNET (primitive neuroepithelial tumor)
Alveolar cell sarcoma	Askin's tumor
Other and Undifferentiated	Alveolar cell sarcoma
	Other and undifferentiated

Modified from Enneking WF, Spanier SS, Goodman MA: A system for the surgical staging of musculoskeletal sarcoma. Clin Orthop 1980;153:106.

TABLE 95-2

Surgical Sites (T)

INTRACOMPARTMENTAL (T1)	EXTRACOMPARTMENTAL (T2)
Intraosseous	Soft tissue extension
Intra-articular	Soft tissue extension
Superficial to deep fascia	Deep fascial extension
Parosseous	Intraosseous or extrafascial
Intrafascial compartments	Extrafascial planes or spaces
Ray of hand or foot	Mid- and hindfoot
Anterolateral leg	Popliteal "space"
Posterior leg	Groin-femoral triangle
Middle thigh	Intrapelvic (retroperitoneal)
Posterior thigh	Midhand
Buttocks	Antecubital fossa
Dorsal forearm	Axilla
Volar forearm	Periclavicular
Anterior arm	Paraspinal
Posterior arm	Head and neck
Periscapular	

Adapted from Enneking WF, Spanier SS, Goodman MA: A system for the surgical staging of musculoskeletal sarcoma. Clin Orthop 1980;153:106.

is a representative grouping of both low- and high-grade malignant tumors of bone and soft-tissue origin.

The anatomic setting or topography (T) in which the tumor arises can be used to define surgical margins and procedures intended to leave the patient locally tumor free. Known anatomic fascial compartments are listed in Table 95-2. These compartments, as well as each individual bone, are known to serve as anatomic barriers to infiltrative tumor growth.

Metastatic spread is designated as M. Patients without evidence of metastatic disease after radiographic staging are designated M0. In general, metastatic disease evident in the lung, the lymph nodes, or as an intramedullary "skip" lesion has poor prognostic significance and is designated M1.

The surgical staging system classifies bone and soft-tissue tumors by a combination of grade (G0, G1, and G2), anatomic setting (T1 or T2), and the absence or presence of metastases (M0 or M1). The surgical stage combines tumor grade and metastatic status (designated by I, low-grade; II, high-grade; and III, metastasis). The stage is subdivided according to the compartmental anatomic

status of the tumor (e.g., A, intracompartmental; B, extra-compartmental). To illustrate, a low-grade intracompartmental tumor without distant metastases would be designated as stage IA, whereas a high-grade extracompartmental tumor without recognizable metastases would be defined as stage IIB. Patients with metastatic disease are classified as stage III.

Surgical procedures are defined by the relationship of the circumferential surgical plane of dissection and the pseudocapsule. Surgical margins are defined as intra-lesional, marginal, wide, and radical (Table 95-3). Examples of intralesional margins include curettage of a presumed benign tumor or cytoreductive debulking procedures. Marginal margins, achieved when the plane of dissection passes through the reactive zone of the pseudocapsule, are suitable for management of the majority of benign tumors. Such margins are accomplished when the surgeon "shells out" a neoplasm, cleaving the tissue between the reactive zone and the zone of compression. This technique leaves behind viable tumor satellites at the periphery of the lesion; thus, marginal margins are not sufficient for local control of malignant or benign "aggressive" lesions.

Wide margins are curative for benign tumors and most malignant low-grade lesions that are less infiltrative. Margins are defined as wide when the plane of dissection passes through absolutely normal nonreactive tissue well removed from the pseudocapsule. The intent is to remove as much length of the muscle from origin to insertion as possible so that any longitudinal infiltrative tumor growth is included. Wide margins are often sufficient for control of high-grade intracompartmental malignant lesions, but only after the patient has demonstrated a good or excellent response to neoadjuvant chemotherapy or preoperative radiotherapy.

Radical margins are achieved when the plane of dissection passes entirely outside the limiting fascia of the involved anatomic compartment from origin to insertion. Radical margins generally provide adequate local control for most high-grade malignant neoplasms, either with or without other adjuvant modalities.[9]

The surgical staging system defined here has been tested clinically and found useful as assessed by the clinical and functional results. Criticisms of the system include concern for its apparent lack of sensitivity to some patient populations (e.g., 95% of all conventional osteosarcomas are stage IIB). Pressures are mounting to

TABLE 95-3

Surgical Margins

MARGIN	PLANE OF DISSECTION	POTENTIAL RESULT
Intralesional	Cytoreductive surgery (i.e., curettage)	Retained macroscopic disease
Marginal	"Shelled out"—plane through reactive zone of pseudocapsule	Leaves satellite microscopic disease
Wide	Intracompartmental en bloc with cuff of absolutely normal tissue	May leave satellite lesions
Radical	Extracompartmental en bloc from origin to insertion	No residual local tumor

Adapted from Enneking WE, Spanier SS, Goodman MA: A system for the surgical staging of musculoskeletal sarcoma. Clin Orthop 1980;153:106.

TABLE 95-4

Definition of TNM

Primary Tumor (T)

TX	Primary tumor cannot be assessed
T0	No evidence of primary tumor
T1	Tumor ≤8 cm in greatest dimension
T2	Tumor >8 cm in greatest dimension
T3	Discontinuous tumors in the primary bone site

Adapted from Greene FL, Page DL, Fleming ID, et al (eds): AJCC Cancer Staging Manual, 6th ed. New York, Springer Verlag, 2002.

TABLE 95-6

Stage Grouping

Stage IA	T1	N0	M0	G1,2 low grade
Stage IB	T2	N0	M0	G1,2 low grade
Stage IIA	T1	N0	M0	G3,4 high grade
Stage IIB	T2	N0	M0	G3,4 high grade
Stage III	T3	N0	M0	Any G
Stage IVA	Any T	N0	M1a	Any G
Stage IVB	Any T	N1	Any M	Any G
	Any T	Any N	M1b	Any G

Adapted from Greene FL, Page DL, Fleming ID, et al (eds): AJCC Cancer Staging Manual, 6th ed. New York, Springer Verlag, 2002.

modify the surgical staging system to include dimensions of the lesion, as does the American Joint Commission Staging System.[10-16]

The American Joint Committee on Cancer (6th edition) has made significant progress in adapting the TNM staging system to bone. The topography (T) of the primary tumor now includes size based on relevant published reviews, in which the greatest dimension (8 cm for Ewing tumor and 9 cm for conventional osteosarcoma) has replaced the compartment concept. Also, T3 has now been assigned to those patients developing "skip" metastases (Table 95-4).

The problem of defining histopathologic grade (G) has been addressed and now essentially consists of low- and high-grade lesions (Table 95-5). G1 and G2 have been combined into low-grade and G3 and G4 into high-grade histopathology. Currently, all Ewing tumors are classified as G4 or high grade. This grouping is now identical to the G1 and G2 of the MSTS staging system.

The stage groupings are shown in Table 95-6. Here, the committee has appropriately addressed the difference in prognosis of those patients sustaining metastases to lung (M1a) and to other sites, including bone (M1b). A summary of notable changes is reviewed in Table 95-7. Overall, the new classification system more closely approaches the MSTS staging system.

In many institutions, physicians are required to use and stage patients using the AJCC system. These new changes will enhance significantly the ability of orthopaedic oncologists to combine both systems for classification and staging responsibilities. As cytogenetic and molecular diagnostics continue to identify potential prognostic indicators, these dynamic staging systems must continue to adapt and expand.[16]

Radiographic Staging

Conventional bone radiography remains the single most useful initial study for bone tumor evaluation. The study consists of anteroposterior (AP) and lateral projections of the lesion obtained by a technique sufficient to evaluate cancerous trabeculation in normal bone. Benign bone lesions often result in expansion of the cortex (a time-dependent process) and can be recognized by a thin rim of reactive vertically oriented spicules of new bone completely circumscribing the lesion and described as "well marginated." This reactive bone margin is the soft-tissue analog of a true capsule. In contrast, malignant neoplasms and acute and subacute infectious processes result in ill-defined or "poorly marginated" radiographic margins with little or no reactive bone, loss of medullary trabeculation, and endosteal cortical erosion, suggesting an active but destructive process at the tumor/host bone interface. The pathologic process biologically overwhelms the normal time-dependent reactive processes of bone formation. Therefore, the radiographic presence or absence of a reactive rim of bone is often useful in predicting the biologic aggressiveness of the pathologic process (Table 95-8).

The use of ^{99m}Tc bone scintigraphy remains the standard for surveying the skeleton for multiple osseous

TABLE 95-5

Histologic Grade (G)

GX	Grade cannot be assessed
G1	Well differentiated – low grade
G2	Moderately differentiated –low grade
G3	Poorly differentiated – high grade
G4*	Undifferentiated – high grade

*Ewing's sarcoma is classified as G4.
Adapted from Greene FL, Page DL, Fleming ID, et al (eds): AJCC Cancer Staging Manual, 6th ed. New York, Springer Verlag, 2002.

TABLE 95-7

Summary of Changes

- T1 has changed from "Tumor confined within the cortex" to "Tumor ≤8 cm in greatest dimension."
- T2 has changed from "Tumor invades beyond the cortex" to "Tumor >8 cm in greatest dimension."
- T3 designation of skip metastasis is defined as "Discontinuous tumors in the primary bone site." By defining skip metastases as two or more discontinuous lesions occurring within a single bone, the AJCC system eliminates appropriately 5% of transarticular skip lesion, as demonstrated in Figure 95-1. This designation is a stage III tumor that was not previously defined.
- M1 lesions have been divided into M1a and M1b.
- M1a is lung-only metastases.
- M1b is metastases to other distant sites, including lymph nodes.
- In the stage grouping, stage IVA is M1a, and stage IVB is M1b.

Adapted from Greene FL, Page DL, Fleming ID, et al (eds): AJCC Cancer Staging Manual, 6th ed. New York, Springer Verlag, 2002.

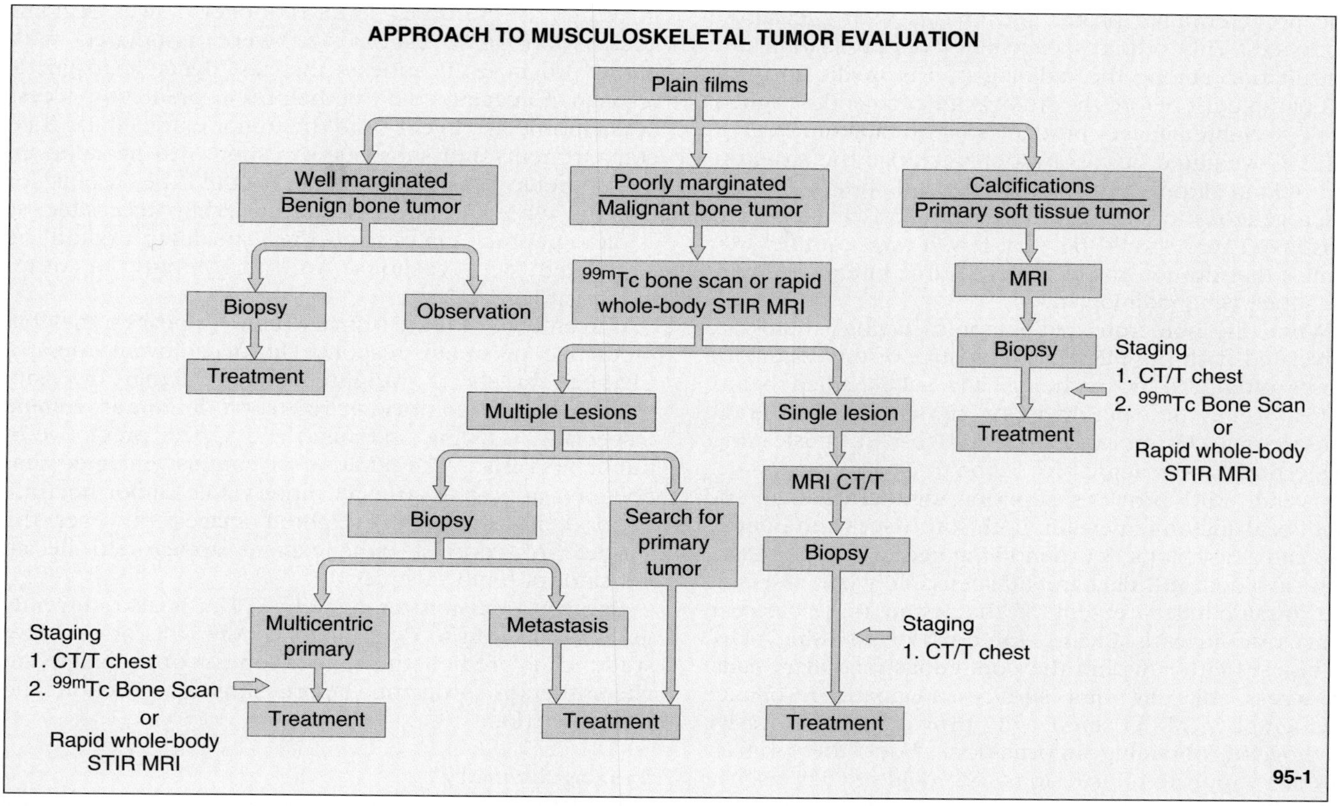

APPROACH TO MUSCULOSKELETAL TUMOR EVALUATION

Plain films

Well marginated
Benign bone tumor

Poorly marginated
Malignant bone tumor

Calcifications
Primary soft tissue tumor

Biopsy

Observation

^{99m}Tc bone scan or rapid
whole-body STIR MRI

MRI

Treatment

Biopsy

Staging
1. CT/T chest
2. ^{99m}Tc Bone Scan
or
Rapid whole-body
STIR MRI

Multiple Lesions

Single lesion

Treatment

Biopsy

Search for
primary
tumor

MRI CT/T

Biopsy

Multicentric
primary

Metastasis

Staging
1. CT/T chest

Staging
1. CT/T chest
2. ^{99m}Tc Bone Scan
or
Rapid whole-body
STIR MRI

Treatment

Treatment

Treatment

95-1

lesions. The test can be administered as a single delayed static study or can be displayed in multiple timed phases to evaluate the vascularity of the lesion. The initial study (blood pool) can be followed by the delayed static total body AP and posteroanterior (PA) scan, and possibly by single photon emission computed tomography (SPECT) imaging. The latter study serves to better localize and separate lesions too close in proximity to be distinguished by conventional two-plane imaging. A "cold" scan correlating with a poorly marginated lesion could be helpful in developing a differential diagnosis that must include

multiple myeloma, chordoma, and histiocytic lesions in bone.

More recently, the use of ^{201}Tl scans to monitor histologic response of the tumor to therapy or possible local recurrence has been demonstrated to be a useful adjunct for bone and soft-tissue scintigraphy.[17]

Conventional polytomography and computed tomography (CT) are useful to evaluate the bone margins of the lesion (margination) and are superior to MRI in demonstrating mineralization of tumor matrix (osteosarcoma) or punctate calcification (e.g., hemangiomas, cartilaginous lesions, necrosis). Computed tomography is also useful in identifying and localizing homogeneous, low-density soft-tissue masses, such as intramuscular lipomas and pseudotumors that are not isodense with muscle or the surrounding tissue.

Computed tomography also remains the standard for evaluation of the chest for occult metastases. The cross-sectional display usually provides sufficient resolution (<0.5 cm) to demonstrate subpleural metastases long before they become evident on plain chest films. Before definitive therapy or local management of a potentially malignant lesion, a staging CT evaluation of the chest and mediastinum should be performed.[18]

MRI has diminished the need for invasive angiography in many instances.[19-22] The introduction of contrast enhancement and gaiting has broadened the scope of this application.

The majority of bone and soft-tissue lesions, however, are best evaluated by a single well-planned MRI using spe-

TABLE 95-8

Radiographic Techniques Available

1. Plain films—loss of trabeculation, matrix identification, calcification, etc.
2. Polytomes—evaluate margination, matrix identification, calcification, etc.
3. Bone scan—three phases to evaluate vascularity, static skeletal survey
4. Rapid whole body STIR MRI—excellent survey study with cooperative patients and in institutions using these techniques
5. CT—margination, matrix identification, calcification, cortical disruption, axial localization of lesion
6. MRI—excellent soft tissue contrast, sometimes nearly diagnostic; T_1 best for anatomy, contrast enhancement, MRA capability, best overall single study when properly monitored by a physician
7. PET—adds metabolic parameter used to monitor effectiveness of neoadjuvant chemotherapy
8. Other— ^{201}Tl scan, gallium scan, PET scan

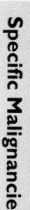

Specific Malignancies

III

cific predetermined planes and images with specialized sequences. This requires excellent communication and consultation among the radiologist, orthopedic surgeon, and pathologist before the study is initiated and designed. The T_1-weighted images produce superior anatomic detail, while T_2-weighted images best characterize the structure and composition of the lesion (solid, homogeneous, heterogeneous, cystic, or combinations of these characteristics). There should be very few, if any, "routine" MRI studies that do not involve considerable interaction with the supervising radiologist.

When the numerous radiographic staging studies are correlated with the MRI characteristics of the lesion, the tumor often can be pathologically subclassified before biopsy (e.g., hemangiomas or lipoma vs. low-grade liposarcoma). On occasion, the MRI can be misleading, suggesting a more aggressive lesion.[23]

Overall, MRI provides superior sagittal, coronal, and multiaxial anatomic detail in both soft tissues and bone. It also can assist biopsy by identifying necrotic tumor tissue to be avoided. MRI data are indispensable when assessing the intramedullary extent of the lesion (e.g., osteosarcoma, osteomyelitis, Ewing's sarcoma) or assessing "skip" metastases either within the contiguous medullary canal or across adjacent joint surfaces. Magnetic resonance angiography (MRA) soon will provide a noninvasive method of obtaining information about the primary vascular supply to bone lesions and could predict vascular anomalies in the affected limbs.[24] Conventional angiography might still be required in instances in which the vascular supply to the tumor and the integrity of the limb must be determined preoperatively. Selective embolization can be useful in some instances to diminish tumor vascularity preoperatively.

Considerable interest currently exists in developing an in vivo noninvasive study to evaluate the efficacy of chemotherapeutic agents on tumor tissues. Patients undergoing primary or neoadjuvant chemotherapy for either Ewing's sarcoma or osteosarcoma would benefit if the effectiveness of the neoadjuvant chemotherapy agents could be ascertained without obtaining additional biopsy material. Adjustments in drug dose or scheduling or alternative chemotherapeutic agents could be introduced before anticipated limb-preserving surgery.

Reddick and associates[24] evaluated the kinetic parameters of a two-compartment pharmokinetic model of a low-molecular-weight contrast agent between the vasculature and the tumor extracellular fluid. It was hypothesized that the transfer rate of the contrast (which does not cross the cellular membrane) would provide a surrogate measure of drug access to the tumor (regional access) transported across the vessel wall, governed by the surface area of exchange, transvascular concentration of the drug, and pressure gradient. Thirty-one patients who had high-grade osteosarcoma with resectable nonmetastatic primary lesions were assessed. Results demonstrated that correlation with histologic grade of response was not a statistically significant prognostic factor in the patients ($P = 0.884$); however, regional contrast access after preoperative chemotherapy was significantly predictive of disease-free survival ($P = 0.035$)

in a Cox proportional hazards model. Lower regional access and small tumor size were associated with better prognosis. It appears that fast dynamic magnetic resonance imaging could be helpful in predicting access of chemotherapy agents into the tumor extracellular fluid compartments and subsequent response to neoadjuvant chemotherapy. This information would be useful for patients whose lesions are not surgically accessible, as a radiographic analysis of the "specimen" could be correlated with response to radiotherapy or other treatment modalities.

Currently, MRI of the primary tumor appears somewhat predictive of tumor response to neoadjuvant therapy. Changes in the T_2-weighted image signal intensity correlate with an obvious reduction in tumor volume (especially in Ewing's sarcoma) and appear predictive of tumor necrosis.[25] The addition of contrast enhancement does not appear to provide more viable tumor/necrotic tumor contrast than T_2-weighted images; however, the absence of contrast enhancement appears to be an indicator of tumor necrosis.[24-27]

Positron emission tomography (PET) is also currently under evaluation to determine whether this noninvasive study can predict the effectiveness of neoadjuvant chemotherapy programs before surgical resection and reconstruction.

Imaging Summary

Early detection of occult metastases to bone remains a priority among both medical and surgical oncologists. Metastases to bone become detectable with conventional plain film technology only after 50% of the bone mineral content has been lost.[28,29] Cortical destruction often can be detected with computed tomography (CT) by imaging of contiguous tomographic planes. Bone scintigraphy, however, is more sensitive than either plain x-ray or CT when ^{99m}Tc-methylene diphosphonate is used. Bone scintigraphy allows for a total body imaging assessment, thereby providing valuable noninvasive staging data.[30] Although scintigraphy is very sensitive, it lacks diagnostic specificity. Numerous studies comparing scintigraphy with regional MRI have demonstrated both the superior sensitivity and the specificity of MRI.[31-37]

With the development of rapid or turbosequences and with declining imaging costs, there is renewed interest in developing and using MRI (TurboSTIR MRI) as a whole-body screening technology for metastatic disease.[38-43]

Eustace and coauthors[44] studied 25 patients with known or suspected skeletal metastases, comparing whole-body turbo short inversion recovery MRI with ^{99m}Tc-methylene diphosphonate planar scintigraphy. In each patient, 16 coronal slices were acquired using a maximum of four overlapping coronal images. Their results revealed metastases at 57 of 175 possible sites with a sensitivity of 96.5%, a specificity of 100%, and a positive predictive value of 100%. MRI has known improved spacial and contrast resolution, improved anatomic detail, and direct visualization of the bone marrow and tumor. Scintigraphy, on the other hand, demonstrated metastases at 43 of 175 possible sites, with a sensitivity of 72%, a specificity of 98%, and a positive predictive value of 95%.

Exact correlation between both techniques was demonstrated in 19 of the 25 patients (76%). A discrepancy was observed between both techniques in six patients (24%). Unsuspected visceral metastases were detected in six patients, and one unsuspected cerebral metastasis was also detected. Whole-body respiratory-gaited MRI was completed in a mean time of 40 minutes and was dictated by the respiratory rate. They concluded that whole-body TurboSTIR MRI is a reliable and effective method, with a unique potential of screening for skeletal metastases and with better sensitivity than conventional planar bone scintigraphy.[44]

Staging Biopsy

Often considered a simple procedure, the staging biopsy might well be the most important procedure performed in the patient's management. The placement, length, and orientation of the biopsy scar and the anatomic compartments contaminated during the biopsy procedure dictate which tissues and how many surgical compartments will require removal for local tumor management and limb-sparing surgery. A thorough knowledge of the soft-tissue anatomic planes and muscle compartments is mandatory before proceeding with bone or soft-tissue biopsy. Consideration should be given to the location and type of biopsy to be used, whether fine-needle aspiration (FNA), open biopsy, or both if sufficient tissue for diagnosis is not obtained with aspiration.

OSTEOSARCOMA

Osteosarcoma, the most common primary sarcoma of bone, is a complex and heterogeneous set of neoplasms. It is characterized by a bimodal age distribution, with the first peak in the second and third decades of life and the second much later, in the sixth and seventh decades. Osteosarcoma is associated with other underlying disease processes.

INCISIONAL BIOPSY*

1. Planning—plan most appropriate biopsy tract, avoid transverse incisions
2. Use pneumatic tourniquet after gravity exsangunation
3. Avoid contamination of joint
4. Avoid exposure of neurovascular structures
5. Monitor biopsy with frozen sections
6. Microbiologic culture if question
7. Maintain integrity of deep tumor/host margin—could extend necessary surgical margin
8. Absolute hemostasis—thrombogenic agents (thrombin, Oxycel, Avitene, etc.)
9. Hemostatic closure of pseudocapsule
10. Subcuticular closure and adhesive strips

*Soft tissue lesions 2.5–3.0 cm.

GUIDELINES FOR EXCISIONAL BIOPSY: SOFT TISSUE LESIONS LESS THAN 2.5 TO 3.0 CM

1. Planning—must provide potentially curative margins
2. Superficial lesions—must include contiguous deep fascia as deep margin
3. Deep lesions—myectomy where possible
4. Obtain appropriate sterile specimens prior to contamination of specimen (e.g., cytogenetics,)
5. Absolute hemostasis
6. Avoid drain—when necessary place drain tract in-line and 1 cm from incision to facilitate re-excision if necessary
7. Subcuticular closure and supportive skin adhesive strips

Epidemiology

Conventional, or classic, osteosarcoma comprises the majority of all osteosarcomas. It occurs primarily in the metaphyses of adolescents with open physes or in young adults. Most patients with classic osteosarcoma are under the age of 30 years, and many have no apparent predisposing factors.[51] The lesion most often arises in the larger, more active epiphyses (e.g., distal femur, proximal tibia, proximal humerus) but also can arise in the flat bones of the pelvis, skull, scapula, and ribs and in the spine. Overall, the majority of the lesions develop in the extremities and pelvis.[52]

An epidemiologic study conducted in Sweden between 1971 and 1984 investigated possible changes in the typical features of 227 conventional osteosarcomas. The mean annual incidence was 2.1 per million. The male/female ratio of 1.6:1.0 remained unchanged over the study period, as did the location and distribution of the tumors. The only clear change over the study period was an increase in the age of patients, beyond the classical peak age range of 10 to 29 years.[53]

Ten percent of patients develop osteosarcoma after the age of 60. This group comprises the second peak of the bimodal age distribution curve. In these older patients, the anatomic region of presentation differs substantially from the sites of classic osteosarcoma. Whereas more than 50% of patients with classic osteosarcoma develop lesions in the region of the knee (the largest and most active epiphyses), only 15% of the older patients develop osteosarcoma at that site. Moreover, osteosarcomas in the older population characteristically present in regions that have had previous radiotherapy, underlying Paget's disease of bone, fibrous dysplasia, or some other pathologic abnormality. In many ways, the older group can be thought of as having "secondary" osteosarcoma.[54]

An estimated 2000 malignant bone tumors are diagnosed in the United States each year. Approximately 750 of these patients have classic or conventional osteosarcomas. Males are affected slightly more often than females. Females develop classic osteosarcoma slightly earlier than males, and there appears to be no race predi-

Specific Malignancies

III

lection.[55] Although the common histologic presentation of malignant cells producing osteoid would suggest a homogenous group of tumors, the morphologic appearance can vary considerably, ranging from classic osteosarcoma (45% of cases) through fibroblastic (9%), chondroblastic (27%), anaplastic (17%), telangiectatic, low-grade central, and other osteosarcomas (2%).[56]

A separate group of osteosarcoma variants, including high-grade surface, extraskeletal, pagetoid, intracortical, low-grade central osteosarcoma, parosteal and periosteal osteosarcomas, small-cell osteosarcoma, secondary tumors, and therapy-related tumors will be discussed in a later section of this chapter.

Histology

Proposed histologic grading systems for osteosarcoma appear to be of little value. Attempting to grade an osteosarcoma presents many difficulties that limit the usefulness of any grading system. For example, many tumors are heterogeneous, and tissues sampled from separate areas of the same tumor may give different impressions. The number of mitoses, the degree of cellularity, and cellular anaplasia or pleomorphism can differ from site to site within the same tumor. For this reason, it is impractical to grade a small biopsy. Moreover, tumors of identical histologic appearance often differ in their clinical behavior based on differences in location. All "classic" or conventional osteosarcomas are considered high grade.

Telangiectatic osteosarcoma, a predominantly lytic, destructive osteosarcoma variant, becomes fatal rapidly. Histologically, it is composed of single or multiple dilated spaces containing blood or degenerated tumor cells and lined by anaplastic, mitotically active sarcoma cells.[57] Telangiectatic osteosarcoma must be differentiated from aneurysmal bone cyst, to which it can be similar in appearance both radiographically and histologically.

A review of 124 patients with telangiectatic osteosarcoma spanning the years 1921–1979 suggested no differences in survival compared with patients with conventional osteosarcoma. Further analysis demonstrated that the favorable outcome in 17 of the patients with telangiectatic osteosarcoma was related to their being treated with multiagent chemotherapy. Twenty-five patients had received this therapy, and 17 were free of disease at 5.5 years, demonstrating the response to chemotherapy in this highly vascular tumor.[58]

Cytogenetic Findings

A small subset of osteosarcomas is hereditary.[59] Osteosarcoma in siblings occurs in fewer than 1 in 1000 to 1 in 3000 osteosarcoma patients.[60,61] Observation of two or more affected siblings in a family indicates an underlying genetic predisposition.[61-68] When siblings in multiple generations are affected, an autosomal dominant disorder is most likely responsible. One example would be the hereditary form of retinoblastoma. Individuals with hereditary retinoblastoma (germline retinoblastoma gene mutation) have a 2000-fold risk of developing osteosarcoma in the second decade of life when compared with the general population.[69-74]

The gene for retinoblastoma (RB) has been localized to the long arm of chromosome 13 (13q14). The RB gene is recognized as the prototype of a tumor suppressor gene and has been implicated in the pathogenesis of a number of human neoplasms.[74,75] A tumor suppressor gene normally functions by restraining cell (tumor) growth, so loss of function or inactivation of a tumor suppressor gene results in tumor growth. Loss of 13q14 (the RB gene) is thought to be responsible for the development of retinoblastoma.[75-79] A two-hit kinetic model for this class of genes was proposed by Knudson.[80] For hereditary retinoblastoma, the primary mutation in one RB locus occurs in germinal cells; for sporadically occurring retinoblastoma, the primary mutation exists in somatic cells. The second step, responsible for malignant transformation, is the loss of function of the remaining normal homologue in somatic cells by some chromosomal rearrangement or mutation identified as loss of heterozygosity for markers in or around the RB gene.[69,71-83] Molecular analyses of both sporadic osteosarcomas and osteosarcomas from patients with retinoblastoma have revealed homozygous loss of RB gene function in a high percentage of cases.[69,70,76-88] Assessment of loss of heterogosity (LOH) at the RB gene in a study by Feugeas and colleagues[89] revealed that RB gene locus LOH could be an early predictive feature for osteosarcomas with a potentially unfavorable outcome. Osteosarcoma develops in 12% of patients with bilateral retinoblastoma, yet as many as 70% of osteosarcomas have a dysfunctional RB gene product.[57,90-95] Thus other oncogenes are likely implicated in the oncogenesis of osteosarcoma.

Several investigators have demonstrated that the mutational profiles of the RB gene in osteosarcoma are basically the same as for retinoblastoma and that mutation of the RB gene plays an essential role in the development of osteosarcoma.[76,84] Besides loss of gene function at the locus on chromosome 13, however, loss of heterozygosity for other chromosomal loci such as 3q, 17p, and 18q has been implicated.[84,96-101]

Adjuvant Chemotherapy and Early Surgical Recommendations

A review reporting data on 1337 patients with osteogenic sarcoma undergoing adequate surgery (primarily amputations) between 1946 and 1971 revealed survival rates of 19.7% at 5 years and 16% at 10 years. Virtually all of the metastases occurred within 2 years from the time of surgery. It was concluded that because the majority of patients had amputations or disarticulations for management of their primary tumor, 80% must have had microscopic, subclinical pulmonary metastases at the time of surgery, as measured by full-lung tomography and plain films.[102]

Reasoning that chemotherapy should be most effective for patients with microscopic disease, investigators initiated numerous nonrandomized adjuvant (postoperative) clinical trials in the early 1970s.[103-112] The role of adjuvant chemotherapy in the treatment of osteosarcoma became better defined. The single-agent, high-dose methotrexate (HDMTX) with leucovorin rescue was used to manage 12 patients with classic nonmetastatic osteosarcoma.[113] The disease-free survival rate at 12 years was 42%. The adjuvant use of doxorubicin (also as a single agent) produced similar results, with approximately 40% of patients remaining free of disease at 5 years. These and other studies demonstrated the efficacy of single agents as adjuvants in the treatment of osteosarcoma when compared with historical controls.[114]

These studies did not have randomized designs, and there was increasing concern whether chemotherapy was truly controlling disease. Such concerns were voiced by Taylor and coworkers,[115] who reported a retrospective review demonstrating no difference in relapse-free survival between patients receiving vincristine plus high-dose methotrexate and control subjects. A later small pilot study randomizing 38 patients seemed to support the conclusion of no difference between patients receiving vincristine with high-dose methotrexate and control subjects.[116]

To better assess the role of adjuvant chemotherapy in osteosarcoma of the extremity, a multi-institutional osteosarcoma study was conducted between June 1982 and August 1984. After surgical management of the primary tumor, 113 patients were eligible for random assignment either to treatment by adjuvant chemotherapy or to observation. Thirty-six patients were randomized, 18 to adjuvant multiagent chemotherapy and 18 to observation. Of the 18 patients in the observation group, only 2 remained disease-free, compared with 11 of the 18 patients who received adjuvant chemotherapy.

Seventy-seven patients refused randomization; of these, 59 elected adjuvant chemotherapy and 18 chose observation. Of the 18 electing observation, 15 (83%) have relapsed. Of the 59 evaluable patients electing adjuvant chemotherapy, 23 (39%) have relapsed. The projected 6-year event-free survival was 11% for the untreated group and 61% for the adjuvant chemotherapy group ($P < 0.001$). Adjuvant chemotherapy clearly had a significant impact on the disease-free survival for patients with nonmetastatic osteosarcoma of the extremities.[117,118]

Early Surgical Management

Originally, disarticulation or resection of the entire involved bone was recommended for surgical management of osteosarcoma.[119] This was due in part to the intramedullary origin of the tumor with proximal intramedullary growth and the reported 25% incidence of intramedullary "skip" metastases.[120] Later studies reviewing the local recurrence rates for patients whose primary management was transmedullary amputation alone revealed local recurrences in approximately 5% to 10%, suggesting that the incidence of "skip" or intraosseous metastasis was probably lower than originally believed. The general standard of surgical management of patients with extremity osteosarcoma in 1980 included transmedullary amputation approximately 5 to 7 cm proximal to the intramedullary extent of the tumor.[121]

Neoadjuvant Chemotherapy and Development of Limb-Sparing Rationale

Successful treatment of metastatic osteosarcoma to the lung provided clinical and histopathologic evidence that HDMTX and doxorubicin given before thoracotomy could diminish demonstrable pulmonary disease and produce significant tumor necrosis. The histopathologic response of pulmonary metastases to chemotherapy before thoracotomy became a prognostic factor.[122]

The use of preoperative chemotherapy was extended to selected patients in an attempt to contain growth of the primary tumor while awaiting construction of a custom prosthesis (usually 12–16 weeks).[122-124] The sequence of several courses of primary chemotherapy and subsequent surgery afforded the opportunity to examine and histopathologically grade the tumor tissue response to multiple chemotherapy agents. Patients with greater than 90% tumor necrosis (good) were shown to have a better disease-free survival than those with a poor (<90%) response to chemotherapy.[125]

In 1983, a review of the 8-year experience from Memorial Sloan-Kettering Cancer Center (MSKCC) reported the results of 185 protocol-treated patients with primary osteosarcoma. Surgical treatment consisted of 99 patients having had amputations, while 86 had limb-preserving resections and reconstruction. Even though the reviewers reported a 92% continuously disease-free group of 73 T10-treated patients, there were 14 therapy-related deaths, with 10 lethal complications related to surgery (8 died of distant disease after local recurrence). Four deep surgical infections had resulted in amputation, and one patient died of infection in this group of immunocompromised patients.[126,127]

A multidisciplinary consensus conference held in 1985 at the National Institutes of Health evaluated the role of limb-sparing procedures in more than 2000 patients with primary bone and soft-tissue sarcomas. The conference recognized and established the safety and efficacy of limb-preservation procedures, providing an alternative to amputation in appropriately selected patients.[128]

All current nonmetastatic osteosarcoma protocols provide for primary or neoadjuvant chemotherapy followed by radiographic reassessment to establish or measure a radiographic response to neoadjuvant chemotherapy and to stage the patient surgically in preparation for a limb-sparing procedure. A variety of surgical reconstruction techniques have been used in limb-sparing surgery, including the use of deep-frozen or irradiated allografts, custom tumor or modular prostheses, arthrodesis, or rotationplasty.

Radiographic Staging Studies

The ^{99m}Tc bone scan has been considered superior to other imaging studies for surveying the skeleton for metastatic or multiple lesions and for later detecting the development of skeletal metastases.[129] Before the common use of MRI, CT was the standard by which the primary lesion and contiguous bone were evaluated radiographically. The imaging qualities of CT in osteosarcoma could demonstrate some "skip" lesions, but each study was time-consuming and costly. Less well-mineralized lesions were often isodense with adjacent soft tissue, making interpretation difficult.[130-132] Retrospective review of CT data demonstrated that the degree of intramedullary extension of the tumor predicted the subsequent development of pulmonary metastases.[133]

MRI is the single most useful study in evaluating the intraosseous and extraosseous extent of the primary tumor and in detecting intramedullary or transarticular "skip" metastases. It has been well demonstrated that MRI better identifies the edema (high water content) in and around the reactive zone of the pseudocapsule illuminating the potential surgical margin. MRI has also been shown to be superior to CT in displaying the medullary canal extent of the tumor, suspected "skip" lesions, soft-tissue extension, and overall anatomic location of an extremity tumor.[134] MRI with or without MRA is also the single most valuable tool for planning limb-sparing surgical procedures.[135-137] Radiologic staging and presurgical planning have been improved significantly by the use of MRI.[138,139] Serial MRI is less reliable, however, in evaluating tumor response to primary chemotherapy and are more predictive of a poor rather than a good response. By demonstrating an increase in size of the tumor, more bone destruction, and soft-tissue invasion on serial studies, MRI is more accurate as a measure of a poor chemotherapy response.[25,140,141]

Metastases to bone and/or lung are usually assessed by a whole-body ^{99m}Tc bone scan and a complete CT of the chest and mediastinum. Regional lymph node involvement is unusual unless the tumor directly involves the skin or regional lymphatic structures.

MRI can also be used as a survey study using a rapid whole-body STIR technique.[44] Mazumdar and colleagues[142] assessed whole-body fast inversion recovery MR imaging of small cell neoplasms in seven pediatric patients as a method of distant imaging for metastatic disease, using turbo STIR and turbo spin-echo T_1-weighted sequences from cranial vertex through both feet in a coronal plane. The fast MR imaging was performed in conjunction with routine MR imaging of the primary tumor. The researchers identified 24 skeletal lesions using turbo STIR sequences and 20 lesions using T_1-weighted spin-echo imaging. The marrow lesions were measurable at sizes as small as 6 to 9 mm. They concluded that whole-body turbo STIR MR imaging is equivalent to bone scintigraphy for detecting metastases in patients with small round cell tumors.

Daldrup-Link and coworkers[143] compared whole-body MR using a conventional T_1-weighted spin-echo sequence, skeletal scintigraphy, and positron emission tomography (PET) for diagnostic accuracy to detect bone metastases. The study included 39 patients, many of whom eventually preferred only T_1-weighted images because of the faster acquisition time. The researchers concluded that whole-body MR imaging had a higher sensitivity than skeletal scintigraphy but a lower sensitivity than PET for the assessment of bone marrow metastases. Sensitivities for the detection of bone metastases were 90% for PET, 82%

for whole-body MR imaging (T_1-weighted sequences), and 71% for bone scintigraphy (p < 0.05).

O'Connell and associates[144] have added the technical innovation of a moving tabletop to reduce requirements for the operator to reposition the patient, thus eliminating additional localizing scans and decreasing total exam and room time (Fig. 95-1).

PET scans have been used in an attempt to stage and separate high-grade from low-grade tumors.[145] Brenner and associates[146] summarized the current usefulness of ^{18}F-FDG PET in patients with osteosarcoma. High-

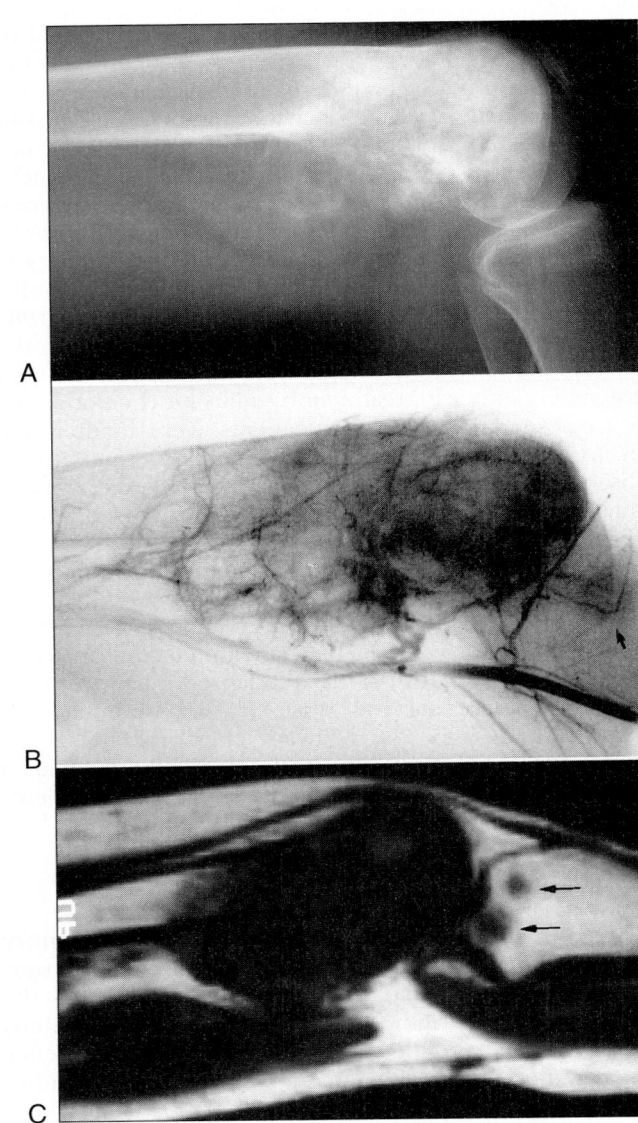

Figure 95-1. Images obtained while evaluating a biopsy-proved osteosarcoma of the distal femur in a 21-year-old woman. **A,** Lateral x-ray demonstrates the lesion in the distal femur with a posterior mass. There is no suggestion of a "skip" lesion in the proximal tibia. **B,** Preoperative angiogram demonstrates the posterior soft tissue mass, and one "skip lesion (*arrow*) can be identified. **C,** Sagittal T_1-weighted MR of the distal femur clearly demonstrates two "skip" lesions (*arrows*)—one that was recognized in the angiogram and one that was not previously evident. The serial images further demonstrate the improved sensitivity and specificity of MRI as a staging tool.

resolution CT has been shown to be superior to ^{18}F-FDG PET for detecting pulmonary metastases and is not recommended to detect bone metastases except when a suspected "skip" lesion has been identified on MRI.

Because the overall ^{18}F-FDG uptake values differ between different tumor grades, PET does not make it possible to differentiate between high- and low-grade osteosarcoma. It could be useful, however, in determining the appropriate area to biopsy to identify viable representative tumor tissue and also in distinguishing benign aggressive lesions from other lesions where local recurrence is likely.

^{18}F-FDG PET could be most useful in determining the response to neoadjuvant chemotherapy and in demonstrating a region of viable tumor remixing. The timing between the initiation of preoperative chemotherapy and the point at which ^{18}F-FDG PET becomes predictive remains uncertain. The response to soft-tissue postchemotherapy inflammation and healing surrounding the tumor must be characterized before this technique becomes predictive of preoperative response to chemotherapy.

Patient follow-up differentiating postoperative tissue changes and possible tumor recurrence also remains promising. Orthopaedic implants often hamper assessment by CT or MRI, and sequential ^{18}F-FDG PET scans could differentiate between recurrent tumors and the normal healing process. Also, because ^{18}F-FDG PET provides scanning of the entire patient, it could be useful when combined with CT of the chest to detect first evidence of pulmonary metastasis. New PET agents are being developed to assess hypoxia (18F-misonidazole) and DNA synthesis and cell proliferation (11C-thymidine).

In summary, PET has potential usefulness in osteosarcoma for

- Predicting outcome as well as tumor response to chemotherapy
- Differentiating postoperative changes from residual tumor
- Imaging the whole body for detecting hematogenous metastases
- Possibly differentiating benign from metastatic bone and lung lesions

On the other hand, PET is not useful in osteosarcoma for

- Primary staging evaluation
- Tumor grading

PET scans also add a physiologic and biochemical parameter to the tumor best shown by MRI.[147]

Serial ^{201}Tl scans are currently recommended to replace gallium-67 (^{67}Ga) scans as a method of assessing preoperative tumor response to chemotherapy.[140] A pretreatment limited ^{201}Tl scan of the involved extremity is recommended for comparison with a similar scan after completion of primary chemotherapy to assess the tumor response. Thallium chloride is actively transported intracellularly and has been shown to have an affinity for a variety of osteosarcomas and soft-tissue sarcomas. Nine of 10 patients with a high-grade sarcoma of bone or soft tissue who demonstrated reduced thallium uptake after primary chemotherapy later were shown to have at least 95% tumor necrosis after histopathologic review of the surgical specimen.[17,148-150]

Current Chemotherapy Treatment and Surgical Management

A number of single- and multi-institutional studies have reported the results of treatment protocols, including multiagent neoadjuvant chemotherapy, limb-sparing surgery, and adjuvant chemotherapy. Surgical resection of the primary tumor usually followed in 10 to 13 weeks. Limb preservation was elected if the tumor had responded favorably; clinically, evidence of favorable response included diminished local pain and improved flexion contracture, and radiographically, evidence consisted of mineralization of the previously unmineralized soft-tissue portion of the tumor on CT and/or MRI and retention of a normal fatty tissue plane between vascular and neural structures and the tumor. If, however, the lesion enlarged and the vessels became involved secondarily (poor response), ablative surgery was recommended. Once the operative wounds had healed (usually within 3 weeks), adjuvant chemotherapy was initiated and maintained for approximately 40 weeks, depending on the particular study.[151-168]

Wilkins and colleagues[169] described their results at two institutions with a dose-intensified neoadjuvant protocol using intravenous doxorubicin and intra-arterial cisplatin administered until a maximum angiographic response was observed (usually four courses). The 417 patients with primary high-grade osteosarcoma of a limb were evaluated, with 43 completing a limb-sparing procedure and 41 of those having greater than 90% tumor necrosis. During an average follow-up of 92 months (range 20–178 months), 39 patients were continuously free of disease, 3 died of disease, 1 died from other causes, and 4 had no evidence of disease 11 to 51 months after pulmonary relapse. There were no local recurrences, and 10-year survival and event-free survival were projected at 92% and 84%, respectively. This protocol, although similar to others previously reported, requires extraordinary resources, making it unlikely that a similar study could be carried out in an extensive cooperative manner.[170,171]

Long-term outcomes were studied by Bacci and coauthors,[172] who reported the results of treatment of 164 patients with nonmetastatic extremity osteosarcoma followed for a minimum of 10 years. Preoperative chemotherapy consisted of high-dose methotrexate, cisplatin, and adriamycin. Postoperatively, good responders ($\geq$ 90% tumor necrosis) received the same three drugs, while poor responders (<90% tumor necrosis) received ifosfamide and etoposide in addition to the three-drug chemotherapy regimen. Follow-up showed that 101 patients (61%) remained continuously free of disease, 61 had relapsed, and 2 had died of adriamycin-related cardiotoxicity. There were no differences in outcome between good and poor responders.

Limb-preserving surgery was performed in 136 of the patients (82%) in the Bacci study, and 117 (71%) had a good histologic response. Despite the large percentage of patients with limb-sparing procedures, only four local recurrences developed (2.4%). The complications of chemotherapy included adriamycin-induced cardiotoxicity (six patients) and secondary malignancies (seven patients) at a median followup of 11.5 years.

In 1997, Bramwell[173] reviewed original articles published from 1991 through 1996 that reported studies meeting the following criteria:

- Availability of at least 15 patients for analysis
- Minimum follow-up of 12 months or median follow-up of at least 24 months
- All patients with histologically confirmed extremity osteosarcoma and no metastatic disease at diagnosis
- All patients having definitive surgery as an option
- All patients receiving some form of adjuvant systemic chemotherapy

The review sought to provide answers to important questions about the role of chemotherapy in the management of patients with nonmetastatic osteosarcoma of the extremities, and recent studies have allowed the expansion of the original list of nine questions. The illustration of the "Approach to the Treatment of Osteosarcoma" identifies some of the regions of the treatment strategy reviewed by Bramwell.

1. Does Adjuvant Chemotherapy Improve Survival?

Yes. The study by Link and coworkers[118] clearly demonstrated the role of adjuvant chemotherapy in the treatment of patients with conventional osteosarcoma. The role of adjuvant chemotherapy was also confirmed by another study that provided additional objective evidence for the efficacy of multiagent chemotherapy in preventing and/or delaying relapse.[174]

2. Are the Results of the Rosen T10 Protocol Reproducible at Different Institutions and in Different Settings?

Yes. The five studies reviewed by Bramwell[118,175–178] approached the results of Rosen and associates;[126] three were multicenter studies, and two were reports from a single institution. Bramwell concluded that, although the Rosen T10 regimen is complex and toxic, it can be given in a multicenter setting without apparent major compromise in efficacy.

3. Is Chemotherapy with Two of the Most Active Drugs (Doxorubicin and Cisplatin) an Effective Adjuvant Treatment, Comparable to Other Multiagent Regimens?

Yes. Bramwell concluded that reports of outcomes were similar for the doxorubicin/cisplatin regimen used in two consecutive European Osteosarcoma Intergroup protocols when compared with results from multicenter studies using the T10 regimen.[178,179]

4. Does Histopathologic Response to Neoadjuvant Chemotherapy Correlate with Reduced Local Recurrence and/or Improved Survival?

Probably. The reports by Picci and colleagues[180] (Bologna, 355 patients), Kempf-Bielack and coworkers[181] (COSS, 504 patients), and Delépine and associates[182] (Paris, 112 patients) all demonstrated that a good response to neoadjuvant chemotherapy was an independent

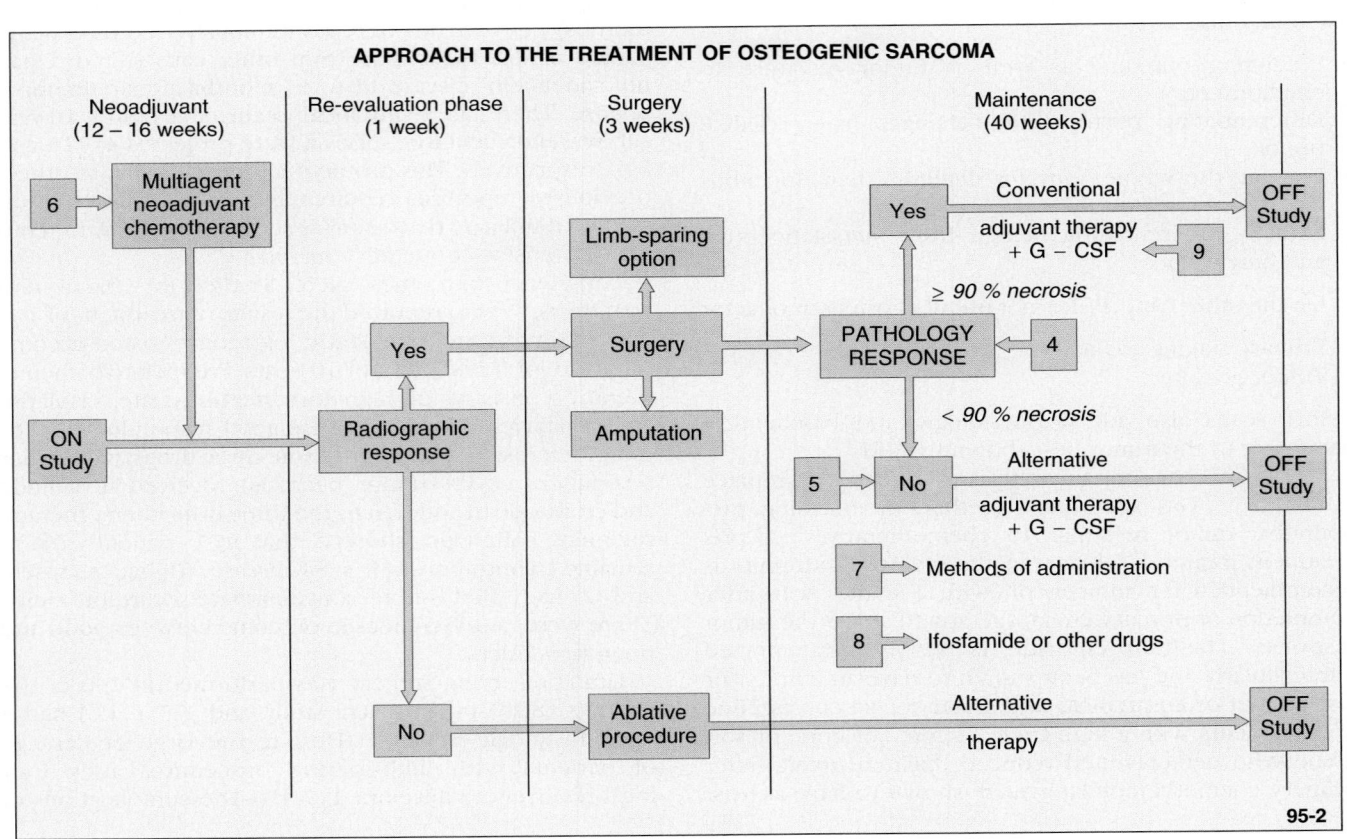

APPROACH TO THE TREATMENT OF OSTEOGENIC SARCOMA

95-2

prognostic factor. Meyers and colleagues[183] reported the relationship between duration of preoperative chemotherapy and histopathologic response. In univariate analysis, the duration of preoperative chemotherapy did not correlate with relapse-free survival. With longer preoperative treatment, a greater proportion of patients had a favorable histopathologic response to therapy, but the correlation of the response with outcome decreased. Bramwell[173] postulated that with prolonged preoperative chemotherapy, a good response to chemotherapy might lose its prognostic significance. The recent CCG-782 study published by Provisor and coworkers[184] involving 268 patients with nonmetastatic osteosarcoma of the extremity used the resected tumor histologic response to neoadjuvant chemotherapy to determine postoperative chemotherapy. In 206 patients, the tumor was morphometrically assessed for residual viable tumor; 28% displayed a good (<5% viable tumor) histologic response, while the remaining patients were judged to have a poor histologic response (>5% residual viable tumor). Those patients having a good response had an 8-year postoperative event-free survival of 81% and a survival rate of 81%. Patients with a poor histologic response had an 8-year postoperative event-free survival of 46% and an overall survival rate of 52%. The researchers concluded that event-free and overall survival appeared to be related directly to histologic response to neoadjuvant chemotherapy.

5. Does a Change to Alternative Adjuvant Postoperative Chemotherapy for Patients Whose Tumors Show a Poor Histopathologic Response to Neoadjuvant Chemotherapy Improve Survival?

Not Proven. The data are conflicting regarding the efficacy of salvage chemotherapy. A retrospective study reported by Benjamin and associates[185] compared outcomes from three consecutive cohorts of patients receiving intra-arterial cisplatin and intravenous doxorubicin between 1980 and 1992. In cohort 1 (37 patients), the postoperative chemotherapy was the same. In cohort 2 (59 patients), the postoperative chemotherapy for poor responders consisted of high-dose methotrexate, bleomycin, cyclophosphamide, and dactinomycin alternating between doxorubicin and dacarbazine. In cohort 3 (28 patients between 1988 and 1992), poor responders were managed with three alternating regimens of high-dose methotrexate, ifosfamide, and doxorubicin/dacarbazine. The significant 5-year relapse-free survival for poor responders for the three cohorts was 13%, 34%, and 67%. Bramwell believes that, although the results appear significant, they could also be explained on the basis of small sample size, increasing dose intensity, total dose, and increased duration of preoperative chemotherapy.[186]

6. Does Primary or Neoadjuvant Chemotherapy Improve Survival?

Not Proven. The role of neoadjuvant chemotherapy in facilitating limb preservation appears to be well established.[180,187] Investigators from the Rizzoli Institute in Bologna have shown by multivariate analysis that the incidence of local recurrence in 355 patients was related closely to surgical margins ($P < 0.0001$) and response to preoperative chemotherapy ($P < 0.0001$). There were 28

patients who experienced local recurrence (7%), and 3 of those patients survived (11%). Six of 10 patients not receiving preoperative chemotherapy developed local recurrence.

Preliminary results addressing this question were reported in an abstract summarizing the data from 106 patients admitted to the Pediatric Oncology Group Study 8651 and randomized to immediate surgery or to preoperative chemotherapy with high-dose methotrexate, doxorubicin, and cisplatin for two cycles (10 weeks). Except for timing, the chemotherapy was identical for both groups. The preliminary 2-year results for relapse-free survival were 70% for the neoadjuvant group (45 patients evaluable) and 73% for the postoperative chemotherapy group (56 patients evaluable). The study remains plagued by slow accrual.[188]

Goorin and associates[189] attempted to resolve the issue of presurgical chemotherapy vs. immediate surgery in their report of the results of treatment of 100 patients with nonmetastatic osteosarcoma of the extremity. Fifty-five patients were assigned randomly to immediate surgery and 45 were assigned to immediate chemotherapy followed 10 weeks later with surgical therapy. There was little difference in event-free survival between both groups, and the number of limb-preserving procedures was nearly equal in both groups (55% with immediate surgery and 50% with presurgical chemotherapy). Although the percentages of patients in the two groups are similar, the overall percentage of patients receiving limb-sparing procedures was much lower than the usual 60% to 90% limb-preserving procedures reported. In the Goorin study, there was no advantage in event-free survival for patients given presurgical chemotherapy. Only one local recurrence was reported among all 100 patients.

7. Are Specific Drugs or Their Methods of Administration Important in Determining Outcomes?

Yes. Following are studies related to specific drugs.

Methotrexate. Delépine and colleagues[190] published a meta-analysis of the relationship of total dose and dose intensity of methotrexate (MTX) from nine single-institution and nine multi-institution randomized trials. They concluded that both methotrexate dose and dose intensity had major prognostic value.

Cisplatin. Intravenous administration appears to be as effective as the intra-arterial route of administration.[191]

Doxorubicin. A meta-analysis of 16 regimens published by a group from the National Cancer Institute found that dose intensity was the most important determinant of a favorable outcome, defined as a good histopathologic response to neoadjuvant chemotherapy.[192] Other studies likewise support the importance of doxorubicin treatment in patients with osteosarcoma.[193,194]

8. Do New Agents Incorporated into Intensive Multiagent Regimens Improve Pathologic Response and/or Survival?

Yes. Preliminary trials incorporating ifosfamide into multiagent chemotherapy appear promising.[195-199]

9. Can Dose Intensity of Treatment be Increased with Granulocyte Colony Stimulating Factor (G-CSF)?

Yes. In a pilot study, the European Osteosarcoma Intergroup demonstrated the use of G-CSF–supported increased dose intensity, making chemotherapy every two weeks feasible.[200] Thrombocytopenia remained dose limiting, and whether attainable dose intensification improves survival remains uncertain.

10. Does the Histologic Subtype of High-grade Osteosarcoma Correlate with the Histologic Response to Chemotherapy?

Yes. Bacci and colleagues[201] at the Rizzoli Institute in Bologna correlated the histopathologic response to preoperative chemotherapy in 1058 patients with conventional osteosarcoma of the extremity. They classified the tumors as osteoblastic (70%), chondroblastic (13%), fibroblastic (9%), and telangiectatic (6%). At diagnosis, 911 patients had localized disease, and 147 had resectable pulmonary metastases. The response to preoperative chemotherapy was good (90% or more tumor necrosis) in 59% of patients and poor (<90% tumor necrosis) in 41%. Notably, the rate of good responders was significantly higher (P = 0.0001) in patients with fibroblasts (83%) and telangiectatic tumors (80%) than in those with osteoblastic (62%) and chondroblastic (60%) tumors. In all subtypes (excepting the chondroblastic), the 5-year overall survival rate was significantly higher (P = 0.0001) in good responders (68%) than in poor responders (52%).

These data correlate well with the report by Hauben and coworkers[202] of 570 patients from two consecutive trials of the European Osteosarcomas Intergroup. Using similar histopathologic characteristics and response to chemotherapy criteria, 71% had osteoblasts, 10% had chondroblastic tumors, and 9% had fibroblastic tumors. Response to neoadjuvant chemotherapy was also similar, with 71% of fibroblastic tumors having a good response and only 50% of chondroblasts having a good response. It appears that the subtype classification is important and reliable in predicting the response to preoperative chemotherapy and (possibly) prognosis.

11. Can Chemotherapy for Nonmetastatic Extremity Osteosarcoma in Highly Selected Patients with Small Favorable Lesions Be Curative and Abrogate Surgery?

In General, No. Jaffe and colleagues[203] in the Department of Pediatrics at the University of Texas M.D. Anderson Cancer Center attempted the cure of 31 patients with nonmetastatic osteosarcoma. Their protocol for selection included initial treatment with chemotherapy comprised of high-dose methotrexate and leucovorin rescue (MTX-LF) in three patients and intra-arterial cisplatin in 28 patients. After response at 3 months, entry into the study was permitted, and chemotherapy treatment was maintained for a total of 18 to 21 months with a combination of MTX-LF, intra-arterial cisplatin, and doxorubicin. Only 3 of 31 patients (10%) were cured exclusively with chemotherapy. Four additional patients requested surgical extirpation of the tumor after the cessation of chemotherapy. Histopathologic examination revealed no evidence of viable tumor. Adding these patients to the three mentioned earlier yields a total of seven patients (23%) having a cure from chemotherapy alone. As the expected cure rate with conventional strategies is 50% to 65%, the authors concluded that their results do not justify the option of current forms of chemotherapy as exclusive treatments for osteosarcoma.

12. Does Local Recurrence During the Treatment Phase of Nonmetastatic Osteosarcoma Have an Effect on Long-term Survival?

Apparently So. Two recent studies indicate that local recurrence within 18 to 24 months of surgery has a substantial negative influence on long-term survival.

Ferrari and colleagues[204] at three Italian institutions reviewed the data on patients treated for nonmetastatic osteosarcoma of the extremities between October 1986 and June 1995, finding 162 patients with recurrence or relapse. The main prognostic factors for postrelapse survival were the relapse-free interval, site of metastasis, and number of pulmonary nodules. Complete surgical resection of the recurrence was found to be pivotal in the strategy of treatment. When the risk factors were combined, patients with a relapse-free interval longer than 24 months and with only one or two pulmonary nodules had a postrelapse survival of 72%. Patients with a short relapse-free interval and three or more lung pulmonary nodules had a poor postrelapse survival of 5%. Patients with unresectable recurrence did receive benefit from second-line chemotherapy, but the authors' data did not support the generalized use of chemotherapy after complete surgical resection of the first recurrence.

Weeden and colleagues[205] reported the effect of local recurrence on survival of 559 patients entered into two randomized controlled trials of the European Osteosarcoma Intergroup using preoperative chemotherapy, but without a survival benefit between chemotherapy arms. Data on histological response were included, with a good histopathologic response defined as 90% or greater necrosis. A "landmark" method of statistical analysis proved most beneficial in the analysis, with a consensus time point chosen at 18 months from surgery. Forty-two patients (8%) were considered to have had a local recurrence as determined by direct contact with the treating physician.

The landmark analysis allowed assessment of 440 patients at 18 months, and 22 patients (5%) had experienced a local recurrence. Patients with a local recurrence had a fourfold greater risk of death during the 18 months after surgery. To investigate whether the choice of the time point had an effect on the conclusion, similar analyses were conducted with landmark time points at 1 and 2 years. In general, the proportion of the patients and recurrences varied; the proportion of the recurrence remained fairly steady.

Using a multivariate proportional hazards model, 368 patients were assessed to investigate the relative prognostic importance of histological response and local recurrence. It appears clear that histologic response to chemotherapy and local recurrence had a significant effect on survival.

Analysis of the Resected Specimen

DNA analysis of osteosarcomas after preoperative chemotherapy appears prognostically informative. Conversion from an aneuploid to a diploid state in osteosarcoma correlates with a good histopathologic response (necrosis) to the chemotherapy.[206,207] It has been suggested that an altered ploidy pattern, by indicating changes in the tumor cell population that are more subtle than the estimation of necrosis as an indicator of drug-induced cytotoxicity, allows a better identification of poor responders for alternative chemotherapy protocols.

Morphometric analysis of pathologic specimens was instituted after it was recognized that chemotherapy-induced necrosis correlated with clinical outcome. Picci and coauthors[208] described their methodology in 50 patients. Necrosis was divided into three categories: good (100%–80% necrosis), fair (80%–50% necrosis), and poor (<50% necrosis). Depending on the system used, tumor necrosis ranging from 60% to 95% is common. The information gained has prognostic significance. Winkler and associates[209] were early to report that patients with unfavorable pathologic responses to preoperative chemotherapy experienced a poorer (49%) disease-free survival than patients with a favorable pathologic response (87%) (P = 0.005). Glasser and coworkers[210] later reviewed 279 consecutive patients with stage II osteosarcoma of the appendicular skeleton treated between 1976 and 1986. Continuous disease-free survival for the overall group was 70% at 5 years and 69% at 10 years. The only independent predictor of a favorable outcome was found to be the histopathologic response to chemotherapy as defined by pathologic review of the surgical specimen.

A current literature review by Davis and colleagues[211] attempted to identify prognostic factors that could influence survival in patients with nonmetastatic high-grade osteosarcoma of the extremities. Eight previously reported large series of patients included sufficient data to evaluate the numerous identified variables. Only two variables proved significant to univariate analysis: tumor size and chemotherapy-induced tumor necrosis after primary chemotherapy. Only tumor necrosis remained significant after multivariate analysis, however. Other large series have demonstrated similar prognostic responses to neoadjuvant chemotherapy.[122,125,128,152–168,183,184,210]

Risk of Developing Metastatic Disease While Awaiting Limb-Sparing Surgery

To identify the potential risks of awaiting limb-sparing surgery vs. immediate amputation, the results of data on 279 patients treated at Memorial Sloan-Kettering between 1975 and 1984 were reviewed retrospectively. Sixty-three patients completing primary surgery and adjuvant chemotherapy were compared with patients having primary chemotherapy followed by surgery and adjuvant chemotherapy. Univariate analysis showed no difference in outcome between patients having limb-sparing procedures and those having amputations (P = 0.34).[183]

A multi-institutional retrospective study evaluating patients with nonmetastatic osteosarcoma of the distal femur reported treatment results for 227 patients managed by limb-sparing procedures, above-knee amputation, and hip disarticulation between July 1975 and June 1980. The Kaplan-Meier estimates for the three surgical groups revealed no significant difference in continuous disease-free and ultimate survival for each group (Mantel-Cox test, P = 0.8) after a median follow-up of 5.5 years. The continuously disease-free survival rate for the entire group was 42%, with an overall survival of 55% at five years. The researchers concluded that limb-sparing procedures for osteosarcoma of the distal end of the femur did not compromise either disease-free or overall survival. Outcome results showed that one third of patients with limb-sparing procedures required at least one additional surgical procedure, and one fourth eventually required amputation.[212]

A follow-up of the aforementioned study 8 years later reviewed the original 227 patients. Two hundred thirteen patients had been classified as having stage IIB osteosarcomas. Seventy-three patients had had limb-preserving procedures, 115 had had above-knee amputations, and 39 had had hip disarticulations. Eighty-four percent of patients were followed for a minimum of 10 years. The Kaplan-Meier estimate of disease-free survival for all patients at 10 years was 41%. Fourteen of the original 17 patients experiencing a local recurrence in the first study did so within the first 2 years after the index procedure, and only one of the original 17 patients survived. There were nine local recurrences after above-knee amputations and eight after limb-sparing procedures. No patient having a hip disarticulation (radical margin) developed a local recurrence. Although the function of patients with limb-sparing procedures was superior to that of both the amputation and the disarticulation groups, no differences could be identified regarding patient acceptance or psychosocial outcome (quality of life) among the three operative groups.[213]

Table 95-9 summarizes recent data regarding treatments for nonmetastatic osteosarcoma reported by 10 internationally recognized institutions. The table suggests that results have improved due to management by multiagent neoadjuvant chemotherapy combined with adequate local surgery performed by experienced musculoskeletal surgeons. Several conclusions can be drawn from these studies:

1. Patients requesting limb-sparing operations do not appear to be at greater risk for development of local or distant relapse than patients having transmedullary amputations.
2. The administration of sequential multiagent adjuvant chemotherapy has significantly improved the disease-free survival for patients without metastasis.
3. The risk of local recurrence appears to be no greater in patients completing limb-preserving procedures than for those having an amputation.[156,158–161,163–167,183]

Relationship of Surgical Margins, Neoadjuvant Chemotherapy, and Local Recurrence

Four of the institutions reporting data shown in Table 95-9 also provided data on the pathologic margins

TABLE 95-9

Summary of Recent Studies of Patients Treated for Nonmetastatic Osteosarcoma

INSTITUTION	NO. NON METASTATIC EXT. TOTAL*	RESECTION*	ROTATION-PLASTY*	AMPUTATION*	LOCAL CONTROL*	DISEASE-FREE SURVIVAL
M.D. Anderson	60	31	—	28	4 (7%)	74% (TIOS-III)
Dana Farber	74	36	—	38	1 (1%)	87%
Memorial Sloan-Kettering	271	159	9	103	18 (7%)	77%
Vienna University Clinic	73	41	22	10	2 (3%)	76.7%
Birmingham Service	99	74	—	15	4 (4%)	48%
French Study	100	79	3	18	1 (1%)	82%
Brazil Group	92	34	—	58	6 (7%)	41.1%
Mie Japan	52	25	—	27	2 (4%)	58.9%
COSS 86	159	65	39	44	3 (2%)	84%
Rizzoli Institute	125	106	9	10	1 (0.08%)	87%

*Number of patients.

achieved at surgery and correlated the surgical margins with locally recurrent disease. Of the 271 margins reported by Memorial Sloan-Kettering, 266 were adequate (261 wide and 5 radical) and 5 were inadequate (3 marginal and 2 intralesional). Of the 18 locally persistent tumors, however, all developed in patients thought to have wide margins. There were no locally recurrent tumors from the five known inadequate surgical margins.[163] The University of Vienna group reported 61 margins as wide, with 12 inadequate (nine marginal and three intralesional) margins. Only two local recurrences developed, one in a patient having an intralesional amputation and the other with a marginal resection and reconstruction.[162]

A similar review from Birmingham, England, revealed 23 marginal and 15 intralesional margins in 99 patients, with a 4.5% recurrence rate.[163] The French study reported 100 patients with nonmetastatic osteosarcoma managed by neoadjuvant chemotherapy and surgery with "numerous" marginal margins but no intralesional margins. They reported one local recurrence.[164] The Rizzoli Institute study, reporting 125 patients retrospectively, identified 15 patients with inadequate margins. Only one patient has developed a local recurrence.[158]

To better illustrate the relationship between surgical margins and local recurrence, Picci and colleagues[180] reported on a single-institution study retrospectively reviewing 355 patients with nonmetastatic high-grade osteosarcoma of the pelvis and extremities. The surgical margins, percentage of tumor necrosis, and local control were correlated with clinical outcome. The average length of follow-up was 65 months for surviving patients.

Pathologic review demonstrated less than wide margins in 65 of the 355 patients. The most common anatomic site for inadequate margins was the popliteal region near the vascular and neural structures, where 20 of 140 patients were found to have inadequate margins (either marginal or intralesional). Only 7 of the 20 patients developed local recurrence, however. Only 3 of 15 patients with inadequate margins associated with lesions

around major joints developed locally persistent disease. The intramedullary canal was the site of inadequate margins in 20 of 237 patients, and 6 developed local recurrence. It is of interest that 7 of the 11 patients with intralesional surgical margins and 16 of 21 with contaminated margins did not develop local recurrence. These findings could not be explained on the basis of poor survival or early death. The observation is believed to be related to the effectiveness of preoperative chemotherapy at producing tumor necrosis and the development of a "mature" capsule surrounding the tumor where satellite tumor nodule formation had been suppressed.[214]

An analysis of the most recent group, 164 patients with nonmetastatic osteosarcoma of the extremities, also came from the Rizzoli Institute. Limb-sparing procedures were performed in 136 patients (83%), 18 patients (11%) had amputation, and 10 (5%) had rotationplasty. Seven of the 136 patients had resections of the proximal fibula and did not require reconstruction, while 79 of the remaining patients underwent prosthetic reconstructions, 32 allograft reconstructions, 10 arthrodeses, 6 autogenous reconstructions including a vascularized fibula, and 2 autogenous bone graft reconstructions.

The surgical margins were reviewed. In amputations, 18 margins were wide or greater; in rotationplasty, nine were wide and one was intralesional. In the other limb-salvage procedures, 110 patients had wide margins, 12 were marginal, 7 had intralesional margins, and 7 had wide contaminated margins. Although 27 patients had inadequate margins, only 3 developed local recurrence, all within the first 2 years after diagnosis.

Complications of surgery included 18 nerve palsies, 12 graft fractures, 2 cases of prosthetic loosening, and 1 subluxation of the prosthesis. Ninety-seven of the 102 complications occurred in limb-preserving procedures. One patient underwent a late amputation for control of infection. No complications were observed in patients having an amputation, whereas three of nine patients having rotationplasty developed major complications.[168]

Surgical Therapy

Limb-preserving procedures are currently performed in approximately 60% to 90% of osteosarcoma patients with nonmetastatic extremity tumors, in contrast to the previously reported high amputation rates. Limb-sparing procedures are now encouraged. Advances in chemotherapy, imaging technology, implant design and materials, and subspecialization in orthopedic oncology have reversed the trends of previous decades. Limb preservation, however, has not altered disease-free survival rates when compared with ablative procedures.[212,213,215] Local recurrence after neoadjuvant chemotherapy and resection/amputation has improved significantly (0.8 to 7%) (see Table 95-9).

Problems associated with limb sparing and improved function include an increased early complication rate of 25% to 35%.[158,161,168,216] Many reconstruction alternatives are available, and the method chosen depends on such variables as patient age and employability, tumor location and size, and the potential of the elected procedure to provide curative margins. Of paramount importance are recognition of the patient's desires and discussion of realistic expectations.

Lindner and associates[217] from the University of Muenster reported their results of a study with 133 patients who had high-grade osteosarcoma of the extremities treated with intravenous neoadjuvant chemotherapy and surgery between 1978 and 1994. Seventy-nine patients had limb-preserving procedures, including 32 with endoprosthesis, 39 with allograft replacement, 6 with autograft reconstruction, and 2 with shortening procedures. Twenty-one patients had rotationplasty, while 33 patients elected amputation. Using the MSTS (1993) functional evaluation scale, major complications were experienced after all procedures, with 20 of 32 patients with endoprosthetic procedures experiencing a major complication and 6 of the 20 requiring removal of the prosthesis. Twenty of the 39 patients with allografts developed a major complication, and 6 of those required removal as well. Ten of the 21 patients with rotationplasty also developed major complications, but none required revision to amputation. Eight of the 33 patients treated by transmedullar amputation developed a major complication, with 3 of the 8 requiring a more proximal reamputation. The researchers concluded that the extent of preoperative primary tumor necrosis, surgical margins, and tumor volume were the most important oncologic prognostic factors, and that functional outcome after rotationplasty was superior to that of amputation and other limb-preserving techniques.

Intra-articular Resections

Intra-articular resections are amenable to custom tumor prostheses, autoclaved autograft/prosthesis composites, and allograft/total joint replacement composites.[218-240] Early function is excellent; however, the implant has a finite lifespan requiring later revision surgery. Osteoarticular allografts perform better and are more frequently used in upper-extremity reconstructions. These options result in mobile joints.

Extra-articular Resections

Extra-articular resections frequently result in arthrodesis. Resection-arthrodesis is employed exclusively by some surgeons for lesions around the knee in skeletally mature patients. Others choose arthrodesis only when the primary lesion produces an extraosseous mass projecting into and destroying the quadriceps mechanism (stage IIB) adjacent to the knee joint. Usually, resection of such a lesion is done by an extra-articular resection that includes the quadriceps mechanism with the transmedullary margin from 3 cm to 5 cm distant from the closest extent of the lesion and a subadventitial dissection of the vessels. Reconstruction of the surgical defect is generally performed in one of two ways:

1. A large turn-around coronally fashioned graft of either the proximal tibia (tibial turn-back) or the distal femur (femoral turn-down)
2. A structural allograft[241-247]

For the rare intraosseous lesion (stage IIA) or situations with the primary lesion projecting laterally, some surgeons prefer to reconstruct the extremity using a custom articulated prosthesis, where impact loading of the prosthesis can be protected with a functioning quadriceps mechanism.

Lesions arising in the proximal humeral metaphysis and the scapula can be managed by prosthetic replacement, osteoarticular allograft replacement, arthrodesis, resection of the body of the scapula, or a Tikhoff-Linbergtype procedure.[248] The experience of the Mayo Clinic was reviewed recently by O'Connor, Sim, and Chao,[248] who described the treatment of 53 patients with malignant bone tumors of the shoulder girdle with an average follow-up of 5.3 years (median, 4.6 years). A variety of surgical procedures and reconstruction methods were used to achieve wide margins in 40 of 53 patients, with 13 patients having marginal resection margins. Four patients (two after wide resection, two after marginal resection) experienced locally recurrent disease. The functional results, including some of the just-reported patients from the Mayo Clinic, are the subject of another report.[249]

Rotationplasty

Rotationplasty is a third alternative. A minimum of a "wide" margin must be achieved for adequate local control of high-grade primary sarcomas of bone (e.g., conventional osteosarcoma, high-grade surface osteosarcoma, malignant fibrous histiocytoma of bone, Ewing's sarcoma). If there is neural involvement from lesions arising around the knee, then the equivalent of a wide amputation must be performed. If the nerve is spared, then consideration should be given to limb-sparing resection. For skeletally immature patients, tibial rotationplasty should be considered. A similar procedure of hip rotationplasty has been described and used by others for proximal femoral tumors.[250]

Tibial rotationplasty was first described by Borggreve in 1930 for management of a limb markedly shortened by tuberculosis involvement of the knee.[251] In 1950, Van Nes[252] and others extended the use of the procedure to treat congenital femoral focal limb deficiencies.[253-255] The first tibial rotationplasty used for reconstruction after a radical resection of the distal femur for osteosarcoma was performed by Dr. Martin Salzer and coworkers in Vienna in 1974 and reported in 1981.[256]

The largest collective experience, reported in 1991, involved 70 patients with sarcoma of bone managed with rotationplasty.[257] Forty-seven patients had stage IIB osteosarcoma; other conditions included malignant fibrous histiocytoma of bone (six patients), parosteal osteosarcoma (three patients), chondrosarcoma (three patients), Ewing's sarcoma (three patients), giant cell tumor of bone (three patients), periosteal osteosarcoma (one patient), and undifferentiated sarcoma of bone (two patients). Sixty-two of the lesions originated in the distal femur, six involved the diaphysis, and two originated in the tibia. The follow-up ranged from 2 years to 12.8 years, with a mean follow-up of 4.3 years. Kaplan-Meier analysis revealed a 70% probability of survival and a 58% probability of disease-free survival with a minimum of 2 years' follow-up.[258]

The surgical oncology principles of tibial rotationplasty yield surgical margins comparable to those of a transmedullary amputation.[257,258] In patient selection, the only absolute requirement is the absence of tumor involvement of the sciatic nerve and a previously untraumatized, essentially normal functioning foot and ankle. The procedure as described is applicable for lesions involving the distal one half of the femur and the proximal one third of the tibia that spare both the peroneal and tibial divisions of the nerve. Large, locally invasive lesions of the distal femur, even with knee joint involvement, are often amenable to tibial rotationplasty.

The procedure ideally is used in young, skeletally immature patients in whom the anticipated adult limb length inequality (associated with the loss of the distal femoral and proximal tibial epiphyses) can be compensated for by reconstructing the limb somewhat longer at the time of surgery. The desired final effect is to have the axis of rotation of the rotated ankle joint slightly proximal to the axis of rotation of the normal knee at skeletal maturity. In general, it is better to have the operated limb slightly shorter rather than longer at skeletal maturity (Fig. 95-2).

In adults, the limb must be reconstructed to the appropriate length initially, making primary skin closure critical. Commonly, entire muscle groups not required for function (e.g., portions of the hamstrings or quadriceps group) may be compartmentally resected to provide sufficient space for the rotated limb within the soft-tissue skin envelope for primary wound closure.

Resection and Distraction Osteogenesis

The results of treating patients having a local resection for tumor of bone and treatment using bone transport (10 patients), shortening-distraction (3 patients), and distraction osteogenesis (6 patients) have been reported.[259] Ten complications in 19 patients were treated successfully; however, the usefulness of this technique remains doubtful for patients requiring prolonged adjuvant chemotherapy.

Although distraction osteogenesis has been considered unpredictable in managing surgical defects in patients requiring concomitant chemotherapy, Tsuchiya and colleagues[260] recently reported the results of treatment of

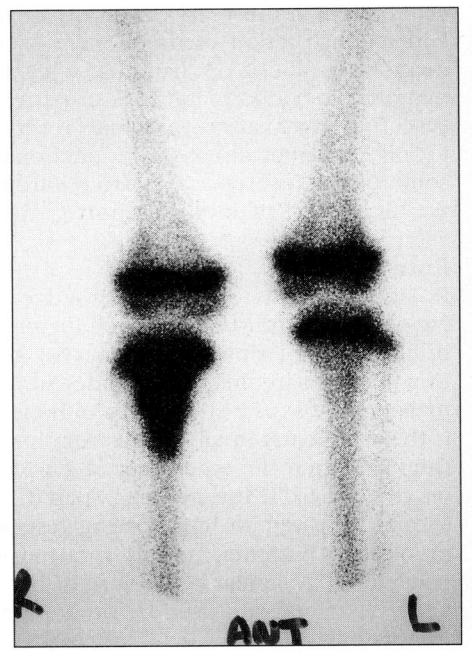
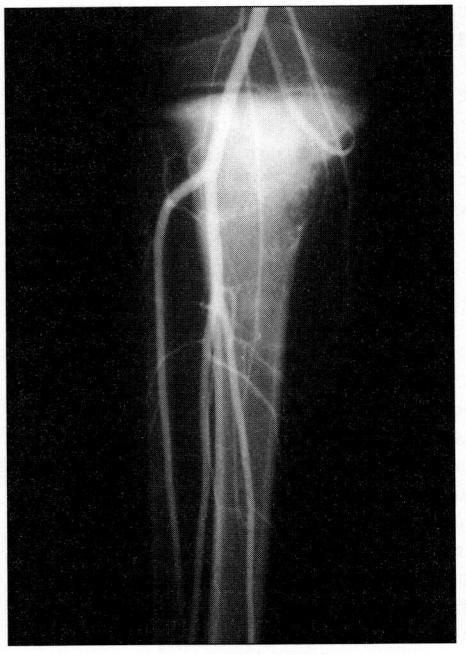

Figure 95-2. A, This ^{99m}Tc bone scan demonstrates an area of increased uptake in the right proximal tibial metaphysis of a 10-year-old male who developed a painful mass in the region 3 months prior to examination. An open biopsy demonstrated high-grade osteoblastic osteosarcoma. The patient was otherwise free of disease. **B,** An arteriogram was performed to demonstrate appropriate vascular anatomy and response to chemotherapy after completing 12 weeks of intensive neoadjuvant multiagent chemotherapy. Because of the patient's age and the anticipated limb length inequality at skeletal maturity, the parents elected to pursue tibial rotationplasty.

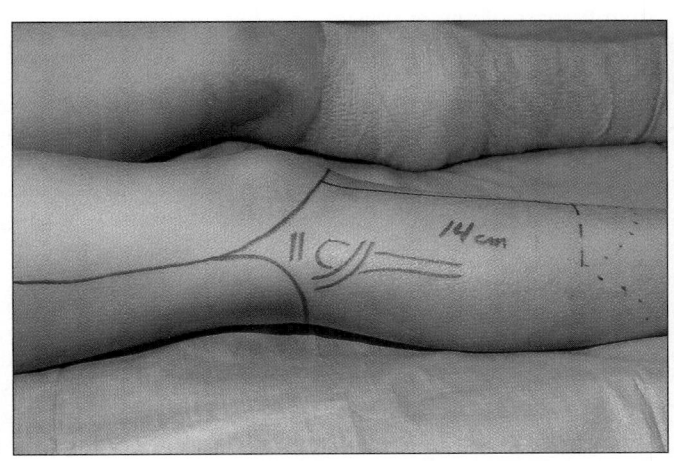
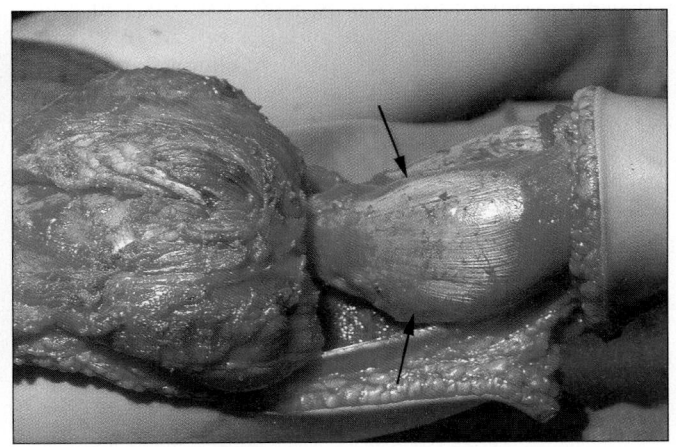
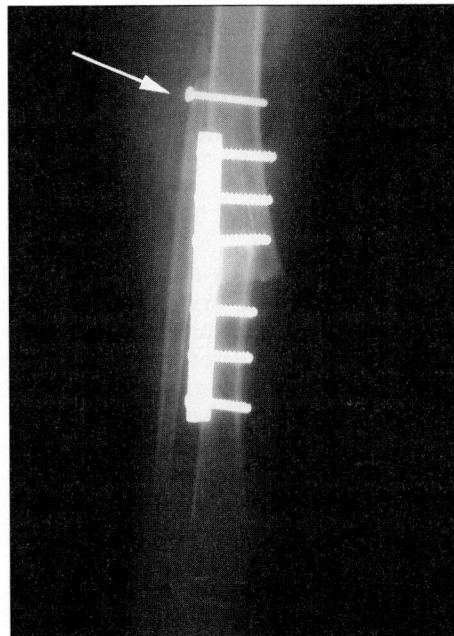
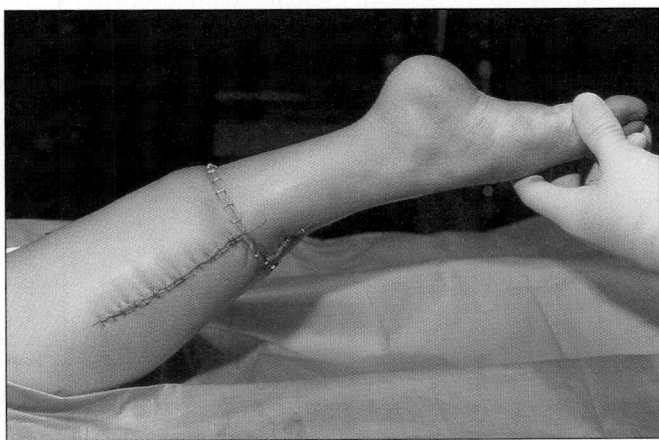
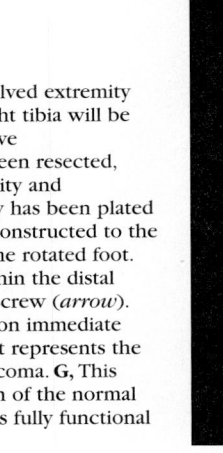
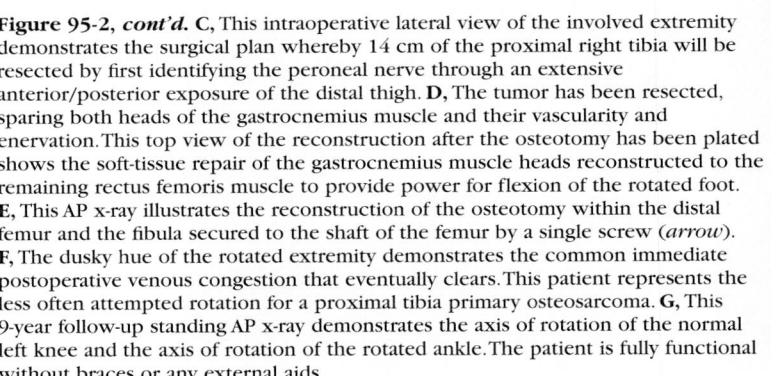

Figure 95-2, *cont'd.* C, This intraoperative lateral view of the involved extremity demonstrates the surgical plan whereby 14 cm of the proximal right tibia will be resected by first identifying the peroneal nerve through an extensive anterior/posterior exposure of the distal thigh. **D,** The tumor has been resected, sparing both heads of the gastrocnemius muscle and their vascularity and enervation. This top view of the reconstruction after the osteotomy has been plated shows the soft-tissue repair of the gastrocnemius muscle heads reconstructed to the remaining rectus femoris muscle to provide power for flexion of the rotated foot. **E,** This AP x-ray illustrates the reconstruction of the osteotomy within the distal femur and the fibula secured to the shaft of the femur by a single screw (*arrow*). **F,** The dusky hue of the rotated extremity demonstrates the common immediate postoperative venous congestion that eventually clears. This patient represents the less often attempted rotation for a proximal tibia primary osteosarcoma. **G,** This 9-year follow-up standing AP x-ray demonstrates the axis of rotation of the normal left knee and the axis of rotation of the rotated ankle. The patient is fully functional without braces or any external aids.

Specific Malignancies

11 patients with juxta-articular osteosarcoma around the knee. The five males and six females had six distal femoral and five proximal tibial lesions. Eight patients had high-grade lesions requiring pre- and postoperative chemotherapy. The response to preoperative chemotherapy was judged to be complete in seven patients (100% necrosis) and partial (90% necrosis) in one patient.

The authors included patients in whom at least 1 cm of epiphysis could be preserved after achieving a wide margin. Three methods of bone transport were used:

1. Intramedullary nailing, used after transport to allow for removal of the fixator
2. Distraction, initiated at one to two weeks after the index procedure and proceeding at 1 mm per day
3. Weightbearing allowed with crutches and active range of motion encouraged

Chemotherapy was continued during the postoperative period using intravenous cisplatin, caffeine with doxorubicin, and HD-MTX with citrovorum factor and vincristine for three courses.

Results revealed no tumor contamination of the operative site. The duration of external fixation was 297 days (± 131.7 days) with a mean length gained at 9.7 cm (± 3.7 cm). Ten patients had a full range of knee motion, and one had 50% of normal motion. Two patients died, one from distant relapse at 13 months and the other from fulminant hepatitis 49 months after surgery. The success of this modest series appears to establish distraction osteogenesis as another potential method of reconstruction after tumor ablation about the knee while preserving the articular surface and intra-articular ligamentous structures.

Ablation or primary amputation may be considered for patients with pathologic fracture and patients younger than 9 years of age in whom lower-extremity limb length inequality would be considerable.[241,242] Also, stage IIB lesions arising below the knee and below the elbow are best treated by primary amputation. It should be recognized, however, that selected patients with favorable lesions arising below the knee and elbow might also be candidates for limb-sparing procedures. Also, some pathologic fractures have been shown to heal during intensive neoadjuvant chemotherapy.[261]

Physeal-Sparing Technique

Canadell and colleagues[262] have described an innovative physeal-sparing procedure in skeletally immature patients in whom the primary tumor was limited to the metaphysis. During the neoadjuvant chemotherapy phase, distraction forces were applied to the epiphysis, "pulling" the tumor away from the epiphysis and providing new, widened uninvolved metaphyseal bone for a margin of resection without sacrificing the adjacent joint. The procedure was used in 20 patients with a mean follow-up of 54 months without evidence of local recurrence (Fig. 95-3).

An Expandable Prosthesis

The Phenix (Phenix Medical, Paris, France) is an ingenious custom-designed prosthetic system that can be used in the upper and lower extremities. The lower-extremity distal femoral design is an offset hinge coupled by an axle to a titanium tube that is secured within the medullary

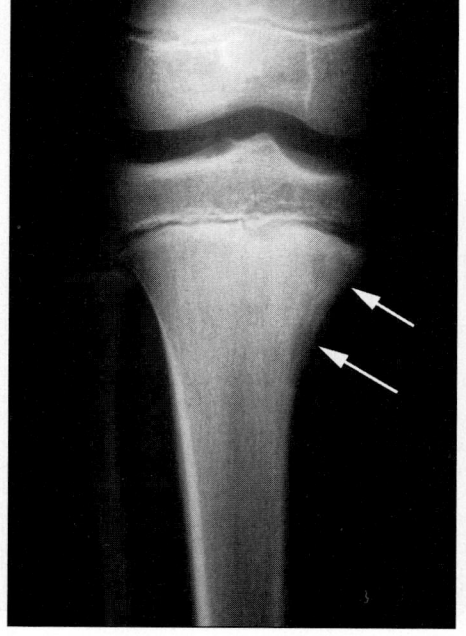
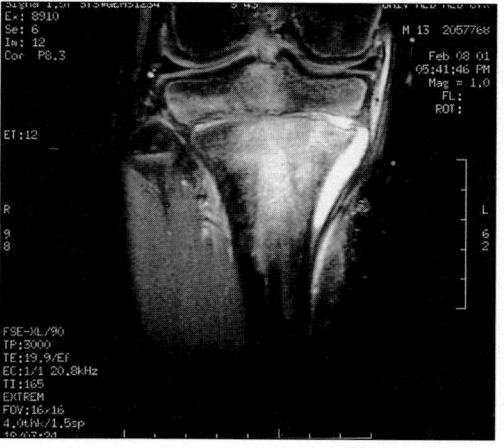

Figure 95-3. A, This AP x-ray of a male, age 12 years and 6 months, shows increased density over the medial tibial metaphysis (*arrows*). **B,** This pretreatment AP fat suppression MR image illustrates the extra-osseous extension of the tumor and sparing of the medial proximal tibial epiphysis.

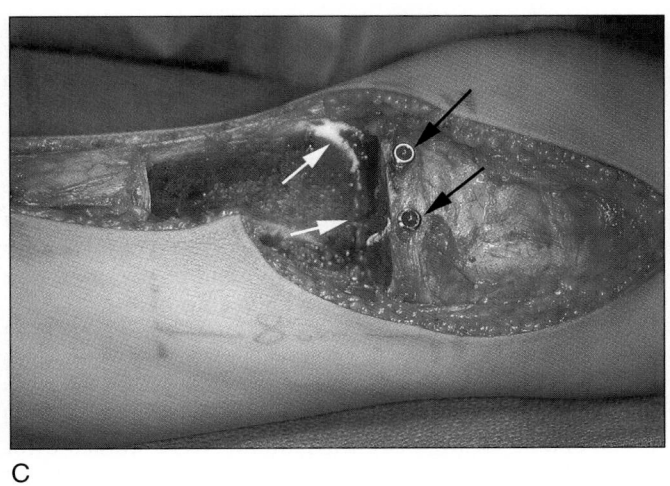

C

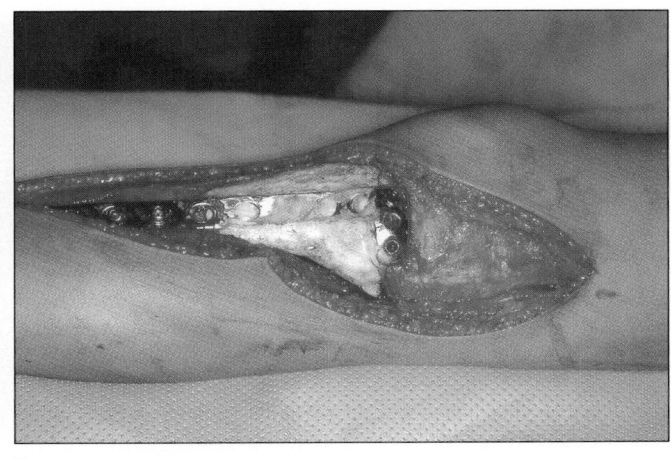

D

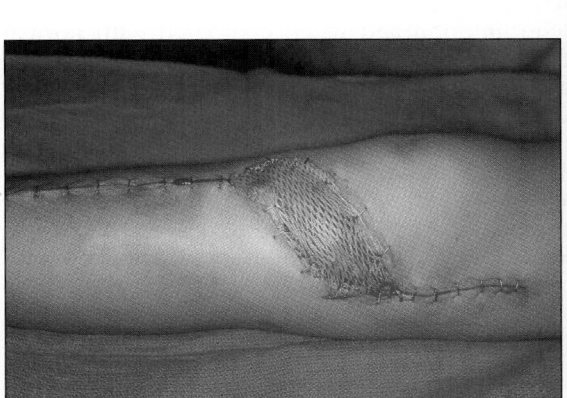

E

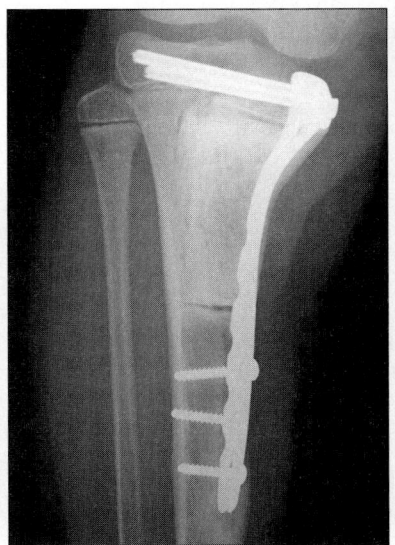

F

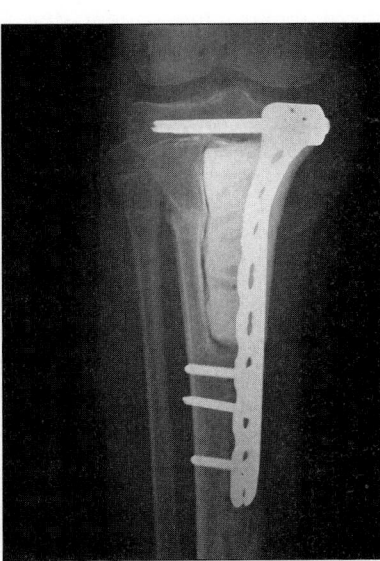

H

Figure 95-3, *cont'd.* **C,** The response to preoperative chemotherapy was excellent, and at 12 weeks the patient was essentially asymptomatic. A follow-up MR scan demonstrated only minimal residual medial metaphyseal disease. The family refused rotationplasty, expandable prosthetic replacement, or amputation and requested a partial physeal-sparing procedure, sparing the articular surface medially and the growth plate and tibial apophysis laterally, followed by periodic operative procedures to correct the anticipated varus deformity associated with continued lateral tibial physeal growth. This photo demonstrates the heads of screws in the epiphysis (*black arrows*) with the tumor resected, sparing the tibial apophysis and lateral tibial epiphysis (*white arrows*). **D,** A plate has been attached to the tibial plateau and secured to the tibial shaft. The defect was filled with chilled methyl methacrylate, to be removed at a later date for periodic correction of the anticipated varus deformity. **E,** A medial gastrocnemius flap was rotated with a meshed split thickness skin graft for closure and to use the underlying gastrocnemius fascia of the medial head to reconstruct the medial collateral ligament that had been resected. **F,** This x-ray demonstrates the normal lateral tibial growth, resulting in a 15-degree varus deformity at 18 months. **G,** The patient was returned to the operating room, where the plate and methyl methacrylate were removed. A chevron osteotomy of the lateral aspect of the tibia metaphysis allowed correction of the deformity. **H,** This x-ray represents the end result 6 months after the first correction (total 24 months post therapy). It is anticipated that at least one or perhaps two additional corrections will be required before skeletal maturity is attained.

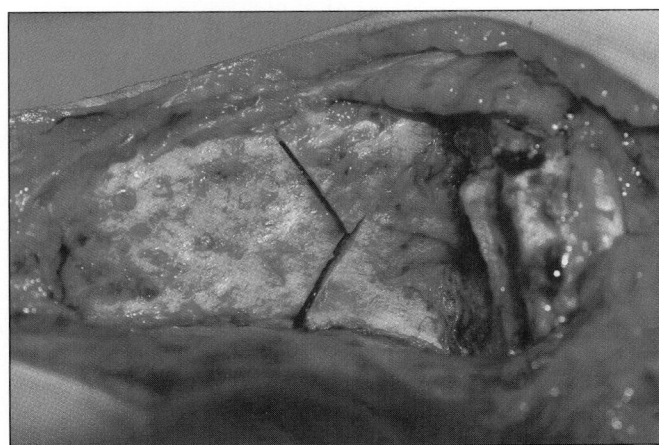

G

canal of the resected shaft of the femur. The tube-within-a-tube design allows for expansion while controlling rotation and bending loads. The distal femoral body is composed of a poly-ether-ether ketone. The expansions module placed within the sliding tube consists of a compressed spring embedded in a heat-sensitive polyethylene material which, when heated by an external induction coil, softens to allow expansion of the compressed spring, resulting in elongation of the prosthetic interlocking screws. Removal of the induction coil results in hardening of the material once again, preserving the kinetic energy in the spring for further use at another limb-lengthening session.

Wilkins and Soubeiran[263] reported their results of treatment with seven Phenix implants in six patients who had successful resections for osteosarcoma, with one in the humerus, one in the proximal tibia, and five in the distal femur. One patient developed an infection after revision for a post-traumatic failure of the first Phenix prosthesis. The average age of the patients was 15 years (range 8 to 31 years).

Twenty-one expansions were required in six patients, and the mean lengthening was 8 mm. No acute or immediate complications were reported.

Other Considerations

The potential deleterious effect of concomitant pregnancy and osteosarcoma was reviewed by Huvos and associates.[264] They reviewed the clinical outcomes of 18 pregnant females with osteosarcoma and found that the overall prognosis was no worse than for age- and sex-matched controls. The two clinical states appeared to be independent of each other. They advised against therapeutic abortion during the last two trimesters of pregnancy but suggested that consideration be given to an elective abortion during the first trimester.

Functional Results of Surgical Therapy

The functional outcome of surgical therapy should be considered by the surgeon when assessing the physical demands and needs of the patient. Upper-extremity reconstructive procedures should attempt to maximize function as much as possible, as the extremity does not need to be reconstructed to weight-bearing tolerance. Lower extremity and pelvic reconstructive procedures require greater attention to stability, durability, and mobility.

Renard and colleagues[265] from the Netherlands reported retrospective results in 77 patients treated between 1975 and 1995 for sarcomas in the lower extremity. They compared functional results using the MSTS (1993) criteria and the quality of life for groups of 52 patients having limb-sparing surgery and 25 having ablative treatment. Follow-up extended for a minimum of 97 months for the limb-sparing group and 112 months for the ablative group. Ten of the 25 patients in the ablative group had amputation as a method of treatment for complications associated with limb-sparing procedures. Treatment of tumors involving the pelvis to distal femur and proximal tibia were included. When all anatomic groups of limb-preserving procedures were combined and these patients were compared with patients managed by amputation, the functional score of the limb-sparing group was significantly better (P = 0.0001) than for those having an ablative procedure after a mean duration of 97 months follow-up.

Oxygen consumption studies of gait suggest that patients with rotationplasty compare favorably with patients having a below-knee amputation and function better than most with an above-knee amputation.[266-269]

Harris and coauthors[242] studied the function of 22 patients who had surgical management for malignant neoplasms around the knee. Seven had an above-knee amputation, nine had resection/arthrodesis, and six had replacement arthroplasty. All patients were available for physical examination and measurement of consumption of oxygen, and all answered questionnaires on function and psychological effects.

All patients walked at similar speeds that were significantly slower than normal matched subjects. All patients walked with comparable efficiency at three velocities (free walking, 25% faster, and 50% faster), as measured by oxygen consumption and when compared with normal controls. For patients who had had an arthroplasty, efficiency tended to improve slightly at greater velocities. The times required to climb a flight of stairs and to step up and down a curb were similar for those with an arthroplasty and those with an arthrodesis, and both groups accomplished the tasks faster than those who had had an amputation. The times taken to descend the steps, stand from a supine position, and stand from a sitting position were similar for all three groups.

Other findings with regard to function for the different treatment groups are summarized next.

Physical Capacity
Amputation. Patients who underwent amputation experienced difficulty walking up and down steep inclines, on slippery surfaces, and on uneven ground. They also had difficulty squatting (prosthetic ankles do not dorsiflex) and ran with a skip-hop pattern. They had little to moderate phantom limb pain, but skin irritation was frequent, and they required crutches to get into and out of a tub or shower. Overall, however, this group of patients worried least about damaging the prosthesis or injuring the involved limb.

Arthrodesis. This group of patients had the most stable affected limbs when walking on uneven ground and on slippery surfaces or down hills. They ran with a skip-hop pattern and easily kept up with their peers. They could squat or kneel with the involved limb projecting either in the front or back, with enough stability to have both hands free for work, and they could climb ladders and jump from short heights. As a group, these patients performed more physically demanding work than the other groups.

Arthroplasty. Patients who had undergone arthroplasty walked better in crowds and on snow, sat easily and could rise from a chair with ease, and could drive automobiles normally. Half of the patients required a hand rail while descending steps one at a time. More could flex the limb sufficiently to squat on the opposite (normal) knee. They often refrained from kneeling because of pressure on the prosthesis. These patients were the most protective of all, limiting their recreational activity, and were the most sedentary of any of the groups.[242]

Rotationplasty. Most of the rotationplasty patients very active, with general disregard for the well-being of the limb or prosthesis. All of them shared problems associated with patients with a below-knee amputation (e.g., difficulty walking on steep slopes or uneven ground, inability to squat with ease). Oxygen consumption studies of gait suggest that patients with rotationplasty compare favorably with patients having a below-knee amputation, functioning better than most with an above-knee amputation and as well as those who have had endoprosthetic replacement.[266-269]

Activities and Quality of Life After Rotationplasty

At least two studies have examined general activities and quality of life for persons who have undergone rotationplasty. Hillman and associates[270] compared functional results in 34 patients treated with endoprostheses and 33 patients treated with rotationplasty. The rotationplasty patients were under the age of 24 years and had a minimum follow-up of 2 years. Results were evaluated using the 1993 version of the MSTS functional scoring system and the core quality of life questionnaire of the European Organization for Research and Treatment of Cancer (EORTC). Patients treated by rotationplasty had better scores related to role functioning that included hobbies and work, had better ability to function without external aids, and were less inhibited when performing daily and sporting tasks. Most were less concerned than their counterparts about restrictions of activities involving sporting activities and work. Patients treated by endoprosthetic replacement had slightly more complaints of discomfort, and more (6 of 34 patients) used external aids than did those with rotationplasty (1 of 33 patients). Neither group was unhappy; however, some patients with rotationplasty appeared more self-conscious.

Veenstra and colleagues[271] from the Netherlands assessed the quality of life and psychosocial functioning of 33 of 34 patients with a minimum age of 16 years who had large malignancies of the distal femur treated by rotationplasty between 1981 and 1994. The mean follow-up period was 6.3 years (range, 1 to 11 years). The general quality of life (QOL) was assessed with the EORTC QLQ-C30 cancer-specific QOL questionnaire. When compared with healthy counterparts, patients with rotationplasty had significantly poorer performance functionally but were superior psychosocially. Nine of 33 patients reported a negative effect on social contact, while 17 of 30 reported that the operation exerted no influences on social contacts. Seventeen did not feel limited in initiating intimate relationships, while 13 felt slightly to moderately limited, and 1 felt very limited. There was no apparent difference between males and females regarding the effect of surgery. Twenty-one of 33 patients reported that they were sexually active during the months before surgery. Eleven patients reported no sexuality problems, while 10 reported a small to moderate degree of inhibition. Physical function and prosthetic use assessment revealed that 21 of 33 patients did not use extended aids, and 8 of 33 used a single crutch periodically. No patient was confined to a wheelchair; 12 patients used a normal bicycle regularly, and 15 required a shortened crank. Thirty-two of 33 patients reported wearing their prostheses from early morning to late at night, and all but 2 reported no difficulty sitting. The researchers concluded that rotationplasty was an excellent operative procedure for managing large tumors of the distal femur. Although the patients' level of physical functioning was below that of their normal peers, patients treated with rotationplasty experienced an overall QOL similar to that of their normal peers and functioned comparably in a psychosocial context.

Validation of a Functional Evaluation System

Lee and coworkers[272] evaluated the Musculoskeletal Tumor Society functional evaluation system using the Nottingham Health Profile, the Short Form-36, and the EuroQOL protocol to measure the quality of life of patients with malignant musculoskeletal tumors. Forty-nine patients were assessed, and osteosarcoma about the knee was the most common condition. Prosthetic reconstructions had been completed in 55.1% of patients.

All of the items of the lower extremity were related to the same function—walking ability. The Musculoskeletal Tumor Society system had a strong correlation with other QOL measures in the construct validity and reliability, but the sociologic domains of the system were so comprehensive that it could not represent the quality of life properly. The preoperative and postoperative status of the patients could not be compared using this system. The overall validity and reliability of the Musculoskeletal Tumor Society system appeared appropriate; however, the system could require the additional development of domains for evaluating the quality of life in patients with musculoskeletal tumors.

Endoprosthetic Longevity, Complications, and Outcome

The longevity and survivorship of endoprostheses used to reconstruct surgical resection defects in bone are specific to both design and site. Prosthetic reconstruction, especially involving the proximal femur, distal femur and proximal tibia, and shoulder remains a favorite method of reconstruction for many musculoskeletal oncologists.

Proximal Humerus

Wittig and coauthors[273] described the single-surgeon experience of 23 patients with osteosarcoma of the proximal humerus that included 1 stage IIA lesion, 18 stage IIB lesions, and 4 stage III lesions. Twenty-two of the 23 patients were treated surgically with an extra-articular resection that included the deltoid muscle and the rotator cuff, while 1 patient was treated with a transarticular resection sparing the shoulder abductors.

The patients ranged in age from 10 to 77 years, and there were 12 males and 11 females. The overall follow-up spanned 6 to 234 months (median, 76 months). All survivors were followed for a minimum of 2 years or until death. Eighteen of the 23 patients received induction chemotherapy. Five patients did not have induction chemotherapy because they were participants in a protocol randomizing patients to either induction chemotherapy or surgery plus adjuvant chemotherapy or immediate surgery followed by adjuvant chemotherapy. All patients received postoperative adjuvant chemotherapy according to standard protocol administration.

Before 1988, 10 patients received custom proximal humeral replacements, and after 1988, 13 modular segmental prosthetic replacements permitting intra-operative sizing were used. Three-mm Dacron tapes and dynamic muscle transfers were used for suspension of the prosthesis to the clavicle and scapula. There were no local recurrences in any of the 23 patients. Prosthetic survival for the 15 survivors was 100% at a median follow-up of 120 months (range, 24 to 234 months). No prosthesis required revision. There was one instance of aseptic loosening. Complications included transient nerve palsies (two anterior intra-osseous nerve palsies; two radial nerve palsies; four combined radial and ulnar nerve palsies). All nerve palsies resolved within 6 to 12 months after surgery. There were two instances of minor skin necrosis that healed with conservative measures. One patient developed a periprosthetic fracture 15 years after surgery and secondary to local trauma. The fracture healed without consequence.

Functional outcome as recorded by the Musculoskeletal Tumor Society Extremity Functional Scores ranged from 24 to 27 (80%–90%). All shoulders were stable, and all patients could perform the activities of daily living with the involved extremity.

Pelvis

Recent studies have examined reconstruction and other considerations related to surgical therapy for pelvic primaries. Schwameis and associates[274] described the results of the Austrian experience of reconstruction of the pelvis in children and adolescents. Thirty patients, ages 19 years or younger, managed with malignant tumors of bone of the pelvis were treated between 1970 and 1998. Ten pelvic defects were reconstructed using an endo-prosthesis, and in 20 patients, reconstruction was completed using autologous grafts (7 patients), allograft/prosthetic composites (2 patients), methyl methacrylate reconstruction (1 patient), iliosacral arthrodesis (1 patient), modified girdle stone procedure (3 patients), or resection/arthroplasty (6 patients).

After a mean follow-up of 52 months (range, 2 to 241 months), 15 patients were continuously free of disease, 2 were alive with disease, and 13 had died of their disease. Musculoskeletal Tumor Society ratings revealed an 81% functional status after autograft, 73% functional status after allograft, and 60% functional status after endoprosthetic reconstruction.

Reoperations were significant in that those patients receiving allograft reconstruction required an average of 3.5 reoperations, while those receiving endoprosthetic reconstruction required an average of 2.5 reoperations. Only 0.8 reoperations per patient were necessary after the other described methods of reconstruction.

Satcher and coworkers[275] described the results of patients undergoing reconstruction for pelvic deficits associated with tumor resection in and about the acetabulum in a slightly older population. The review was limited to peri-acetabular resections and included patients with primary malignancies and metastatic disease. The authors described a reconstruction technique utilizing numerous Steinman pins placed within the residual and remaining bone to reconstruct the acetabular structures with methyl methacrylate and (occasionally) autoclaved autograft bone in combination with total hip arthroplasty. Their study included 15 patients from two institutions between 1985 and 2000.

The surgical method using Steinman pins with methyl methacrylate incorporated a constrained polyethylene acetabular component cemented into a bed interdigitating with the Steinman pins. Fifteen of 24 patients identified were available for the study. Indications for the reconstruction included the ability to achieve a wide margin and spare the superior and inferior gluteal nerves. The average age was 48 years (range, 8 to 70 years), and there were seven females and 8 males. The average follow-up was 56 months (range, 12 to 164 months). Seven patients were continuously free of disease, two were alive with disease, and six were dead as a consequence of their disease. The five-year survival rate for patients with chondrosarcoma (12 of 15 patients) was 60%.

The surgical technique included an extended iliofemoral approach. After tumor resection, the pelvis was reconstructed using autoclaved autograft or the cement and Steinman technique. The criterion for use of the autoclaved autograft was at least two thirds of the acetabular surface remaining in the resected specimen after stripping all of the soft tissue and tumor from the specimen. The autoclaved bone was then replaced in the surgical defect and used as a bulk "allograft." Steinman pins and cement were used in areas where there were major deficiencies.

Functional results were graded overall excellent or good for 87% of the patients. Of note was the time required to return to independent gait for those with acetabulum restoration. Their recovery time in general approximated those patients with routine total hip arthroplasty.

Ozaki and associates[276] described a single institution's experience evaluating the incidence and characteristics of sacral infiltration in pelvic sarcoma. Fifty-one patients with pelvic sarcoma (chondrosarcoma, 15 patients; Ewing's sarcoma, 23 patients; osteosarcoma, 13 patients) adjacent to the sacroiliac joint had surgical therapy. Tumor infiltration into the sacrum was suspected based on the preoperative imaging in 18 patients; 15 of 18 had histologic tumor invasion. There was a significant difference of median volume of sarcomas with and without infiltration. One of 23 Ewing's sarcomas, 7 of 15 chondrosarcomas, and 7 of 13 osteosarcomas penetrated the sacroiliac joint in the sacrum. Diagnosis appeared to be the most important factor influencing sacral infiltration. Risk factors included elderly age status, large tumors, and the diagnosis of osteosarcoma and chondrosarcoma. The authors concluded that elderly patients having lesions abutting the sacroiliac joint with known invasive characteristics could require an extended medial margin into the ala of the sacrum to provide a "wide" margin.

Proximal Femur

Two types of proximal femoral reconstruction are available for comparison:

1. Megaprosthesis: large metallic prosthesis, often modular in design, used to replace the entire proximal femur and occasionally the acetabulum. Reattachment of ligamentous structures to the prosthesis is facilitated by holes or rings designed into the prosthesis, to which the ligaments can be sutured securely. There is very little evidence to suggest secure long-term reattachment other than to the scar enveloping the prosthesis.
2. Allograft/prosthetic composite, consisting of a long-stemmed proximal femoral prosthesis placed within a proximal femoral allograft, securely cemented into the allograft and remaining shaft of the host bone. Advantages over megaprostheses include the ability to repair host ligaments to the retained ligaments on the allograft. There is histologic evidence that the host and allograft ligamentous structures do unite by scar formation, with less than normal tensile strength.

Survival of prostheses replacing the proximal femur is generally reported as between 88% and 100% at 5 years.[277-279] A direct comparison of megaprostheses and allograft/prosthetic composites used to reconstruct the proximal femur has demonstrated a survival advantage for composites.[280] Stability of the hip remains a concern, with dislocation rates reported at between 2% and 14%, while aseptic loosening remains low for proximal femoral reconstruction.[277-279,281-284]

Distal Femoral Prosthetic Replacement

Two prosthetic designs are available for the review:

1. The simple hinged-knee prosthetic does not allow for rotation but only for flexion and extension.
2. The kinematic rotation hinge knee prosthetic allows for rotation, flexion, and extension through an offset hinge that provides stability in full extension.

The most important cause of failure for distal femoral prosthetic replacement remains aseptic loosening, found in 0% to 11% of patients.[279,285,286] In 218 reconstructions, the overall survival for patients with the simple hinge design was 80% at 5 years, 65% at 10 years, and 53% at 20 years.[285] The rotating kinematic hinge design has a better record, with 5- and 10-year survival rates of 90% and 80%, respectively.[278] It is suggested that the rotation of the normal knee simulated by the improved design diminishes impact torsional loading of the cement/bone interface, which often is responsible for loosening.

At present, several modular tumor prosthetic systems are available for reconstruction of tumor resection about the knee. Also, some physicians continue to prefer custom design prostheses that have a standard modular rotating hinge implant combined with a custom design for the stem, providing better fit and fill. Results with one modular tumor system used in large numbers by two separate groups have recently been published. Mittermayer and associates[287] recently reported on the University of Vienna's treatment of 100 patients with primary lower extremity uncemented reconstruction using the Kotz Modular Femur Tibia Reconstruction System between 1982 and 1989. Forty-one patients were followed for a mean of 138 months (51 patients had died and 8 were lost to follow-up). Nine patients required revision for aseptic loosening, and two required two such revisions. Four patients developed deep infections. Fourteen patients required reoperation for early failure of the polyethylene bushings.

A large multicenter Canadian study reported by Malo and colleagues[288] addressed the question of stem fixation and fixed vs. rotation hinge design of the knee in the Kotz design prosthesis. Thirty-one patients with Kotz fixed hinge and uncemented stem constructs were compared with 25 patients with the KMRS cemented stem and rotating hinge design using the MSTS (1987 and 1993) functional assessment, the Toronto Extremity Salvage Score (TESS), and the Short Form-36 Physical Component Score for a follow-up period of at least 1 year. Results in the two groups of implants were comparable, except that the uncemented group had an average of 2 cm greater length of resection. The outcomes of the MSTS (1993) ($P = 0.006$) and the TESS ($P = 0.03$) assessment suggest that cemented stem fixation and a less constrained knee design was preferable, even though the study was designed to assess functional issues from the patient's perspective.

Virolainen and coworkers[289] reported the experimental results of healing and extracortical fixation in six mongrel dogs treated by bilateral femoral diaphyseal resections and reconstruction using a porous-coated segmental implant. One side was left without autologous graft, while the experimental side was reconstructed with eight strips of corticocancellous bone placed evenly about the implant/bone junctions. Cancellous graft was placed under and between the corticocancellous grafts. At 12 weeks, the contact area and volume of callus was greater on the experimental side ($P < 0.05$). Mechanical stiffness was 18-fold greater ($P < 0.007$), and torque to failure of extracortical bridging was fivefold greater ($P < 0.05$) on the experimental side. The authors concluded that extra-cortical bridging could be accomplished with autologous corticocancellous bone graft significantly enhancing implant fixation.

Proximal Tibial Prosthetic Replacement

Two factors play a role in rather poor performance of implants used to reconstruct the proximal tibia:

1. Difficulty in obtaining good soft-tissue coverage.
2. Poor reconstructive options for extensor mechanism reconstitution.

Specific Malignancies

III

Allograft/prosthetic composites appear to have improved survivorship and function compared with megaprostheses and remain a favorite method of reconstruction because the composites provide the ability to reconstruct the host patellar tendon with the remaining allograft patellar tendon. The routine use of the rotation of a medial gastrocnemius flap either with or without skin has improved coverage of the prosthesis and local nutrition. Infection, however, remains an inordinately high risk, up to 31% (Fig. 95-4).[277]

Allografts

The experience using large-bone allografts for reconstruction in high-grade osteosarcoma at the Rizzoli Institute in Bologna was recently reviewed by Donati and colleagues.[290] Between 1986 and 1994, 112 large-bone allograft reconstructions were performed. Forty-one were used for arthrodesis of the knee and three in the ankle. Thirty-nine were used as intercalary grafts (Fig. 95-5) and 22 as osteoarticular allografts (3 humeral, 6 in the distal femur, and 13 in the proximal tibia). Seven

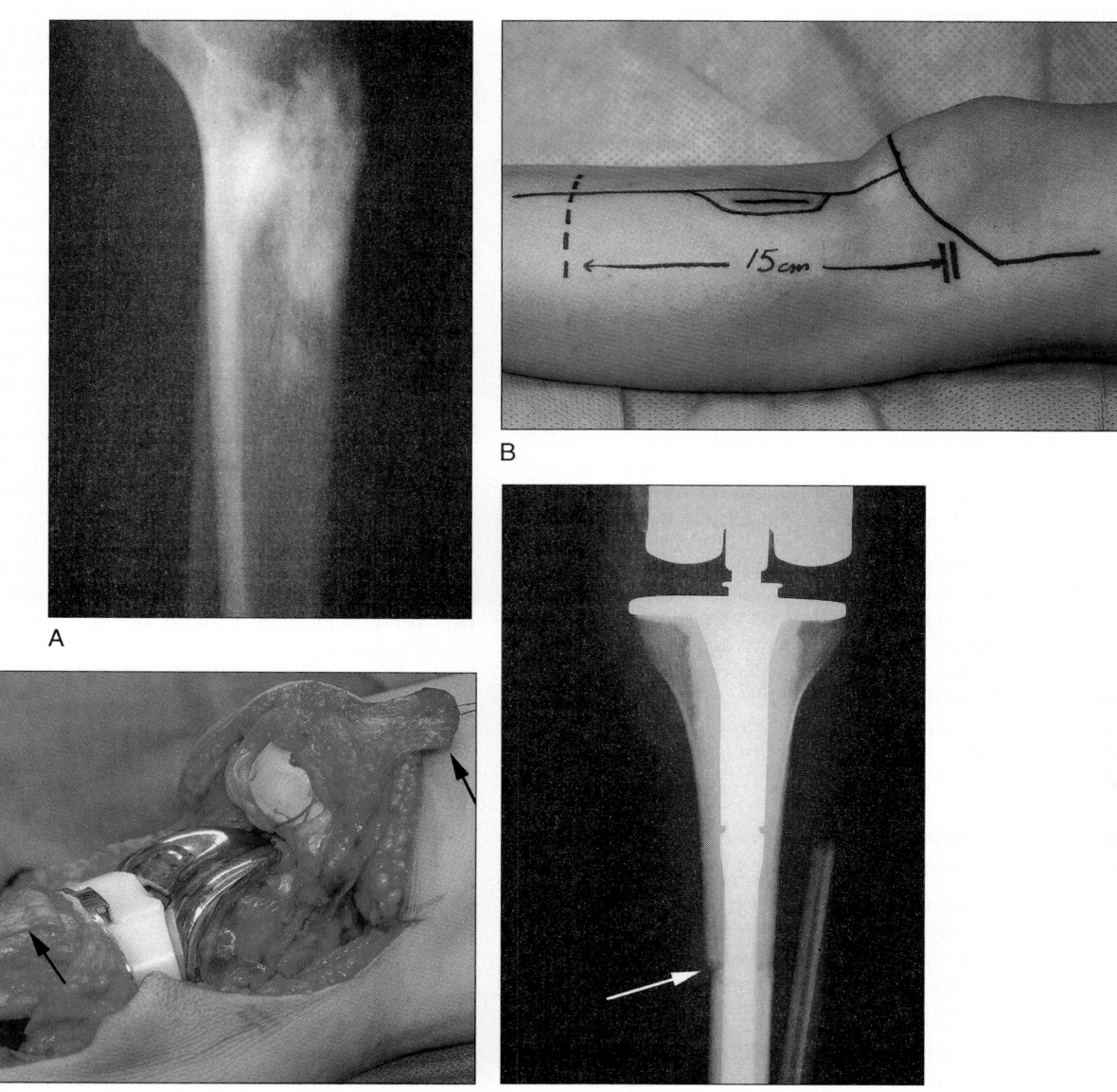

Figure 95-4. A, A 27-year-old female developed a painful mass in the left proximal tibia approximately 3 weeks prior to medical evaluation. This lateral x-ray of the tibia demonstrates a dense, bone-producing lesion in the metaphysis associated with a soft-tissue mass in the anterior compartment. **B,** An open biopsy confirmed osteoblastic osteosarcoma, and all staging studies suggested that the patient was otherwise free of disease. After 12 weeks of standard preoperative multiagent chemotherapy, the patient was taken to the operating room to resect 15 cm of the proximal tibia and adjuvant soft tissue to include the patellar tendon and the proximal fibula while sparing the peroneal nerve. **C,** This intraoperative photo after the tumor was resected demonstrates the reconstruction using a deep frozen allograft with the retained allograft patellar tendon (*double arrows*). The prosthesis has been secured, and the host patellar tendon (*single arrow*) will be woven and sutured to the allograft tendon to restore the resected extensor mechanism. **D,** This AP x-ray taken 3 months postoperatively demonstrates the composite allograft/prosthetic hybrid secured with methyl methacrylate and shows that the host/grft juncture (*white arrow*) with supplemental bone graft is healing with evidence of callus.

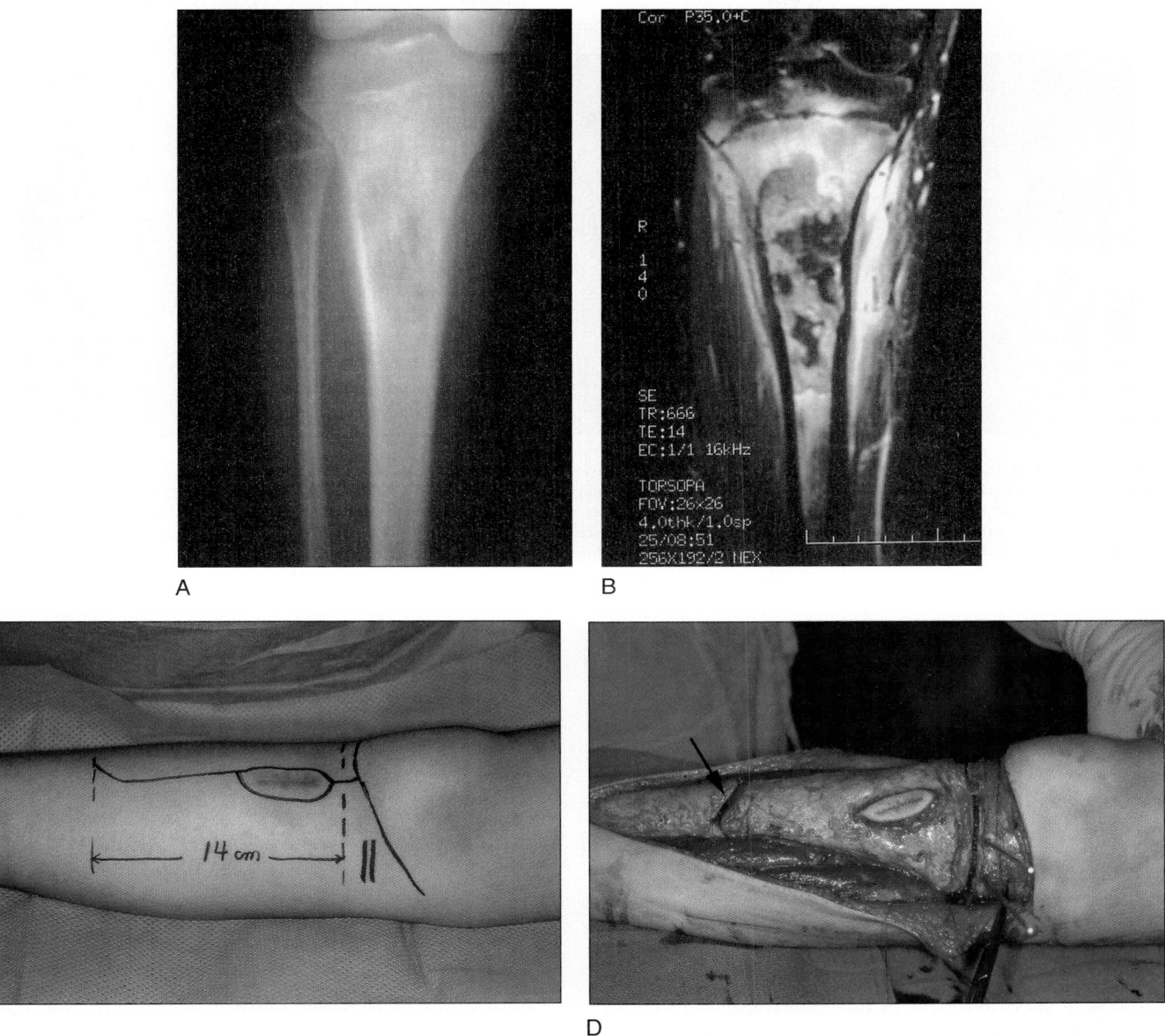

A

B

C

D

Figure 95-5. A, This 16-year-old skeletally mature male athlete developed pain and tenderness in the right proximal tibia while practicing for a winter sport 6 weeks before medical evaluation. There was no history of trauma, fever, or chills. **B,** This STIR image of the right proximal tibia demonstrates intramedullary destruction and a medial metaphyseal soft tissue mass. The physis and physeal plate, although edematous, appear to be spared. **C,** The preoperative chemotherapy response proved to be excellent, with the clinical absence of pain, mass, and knee stiffness. The preoperative MR also demonstrated loss of edema and consolidation of the small medial soft-tissue mass, with resolution of all signal adjacent to the closing proximal tibial epiphysis. The patient requested a joint-sparing procedure if at all possible. **D,** This intraoperative photo demonstrates the resection margin just proximal to the tibial physis, including the tibial tubercle and patellar tendon. A distal chevron osteotomy was performed 14 cm distal to the proximal osteotomy. The specimen was cut immediately on the back table to be certain that the proximal and distal margins were free of disease.

Continued

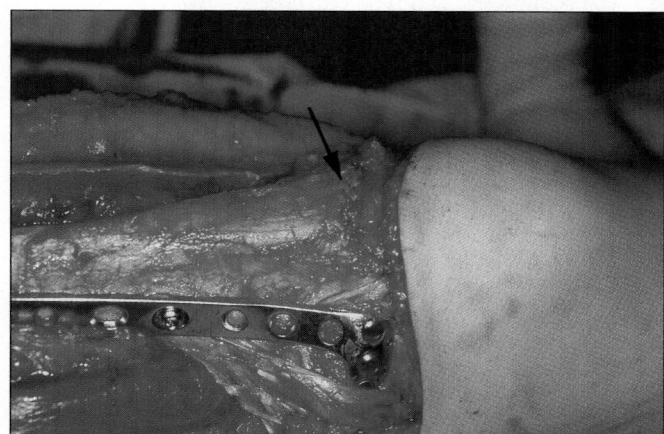

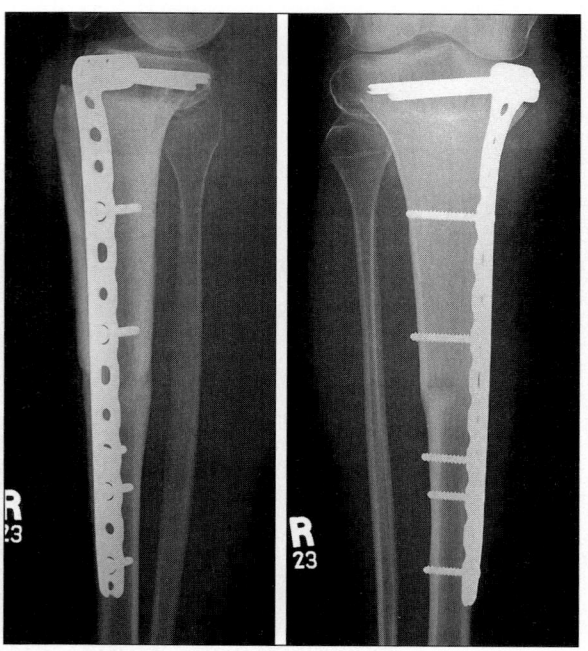

Figure 95-5, *cont'd*. E, A deep frozen allograft with ligaments attached was matched to the bone size and used to fill the defect anatomically while providing an allograft patellar tendon for reconstruction. The arrow demonstrates the suture line used to reconstruct the allograft/host patellar tendon while retaining the host tibial plateau and intra-articular ligaments. A medial gastrocnemius flap and meshed split thickness skin graft was used to cover the construct. **F,** This composite AP and lateral x-ray represents the 18-month follow-up with complete proximal and distal host/allograft incorporation. The patient has returned to competitive swimming without external aids or a brace.

composite constructs were reported, with two in the proximal and distal humerus, one in the proximal femur, and four in the proximal tibia. Complications included delayed union (greater than 1 year without radiographic union) in 49% and fracture in 30%. There were no deep infections. Using the modification of the Mankin scale by Gebhardt and coworkers,[291] good to excellent functional results were reported in 74% of the 92 patients available for review (Fig. 95-6).

There has been increasing interest in identifying osteotrophic growth factors that enhance the ability to heal bone defects and improve osteointegration of bone/implant and host bone/allograft junctures. Seven bone morphogenic proteins have been identified.[292] Cook and associates[293] reported the rapid healing (8 weeks) of a 1.5-cm skeletal defect in the rabbit with 6.25 mg of osteogenic protein-1 and demineralized bone matrix. Extending their work on osteogenic protein-1 to assess enhancement of healing of cortical allograft strut grafts to the femur of adult dogs, Cook and associates[294] found incorporation of the struts in four weeks, compared with eight weeks for the control site.

Alternative Methods of Cementless Implant Fixation

Recently, Bini and colleagues[295] reported their results of treating five patients requiring intra-articular resection of the distal femur and custom prosthetic reconstruction using compliant prestress, cementless fixation. Based on extensive animal studies, their methods were used to secure the femoral implant using Belleville spring washers and multiple transverse femoral pins to maintain a bone/implant interforce pressure of 1200 N. Four of the five surviving patients were followed for greater than 3 years with excellent radiographic and clinical results.

Cost Effectiveness of Limb Preservation

Over the past 30 years, both surgical techniques and prosthetic designs have evolved to the point that limb-preserving procedures for extremity bone sarcomas have become commonplace.[125] The use of multiagent neoadjuvant chemotherapy in conjunction with intensive adjuvant chemotherapy regimens has resulted in 60% to 65% event-free survival.[118] Approximately 80% to 85% of patients are now offered limb-sparing procedures.[296]

Procedures to preserve limbs and limb function have also been refined to offer reconstruction opportunities, ranging from joint-sparing amputation to the insertion of custom design prostheses. Functional outcome studies have assessed quality of life of matched groups and have failed to demonstrate a clear difference.[297-299]

Tumor prostheses have been available for many years, and considerable experience has accumulated in their use and design.[300-302] Limb-sparing procedures by experienced subspecialty-trained orthopedic surgeons do not compromise patient survival when compared with amputation.[213]

Grimer and associates[303] have derived a formula to calculate the ongoing costs of limb preservation based on actual costs and the use of historical data to demonstrate the likelihood of additional surgery or revision. The

Figure 95-6. A, This AP x-ray demonstrates the third failure of a distal femoral osteoarticular allograft in a 36-year-old male (*white arrow*) used to reconstruct the skeletal defect for treatment of an osteosarcoma of the distal right femur 18 years previously. **B,** The patient requested a more permanent type of reconstruction involving the use of a custom prosthesis. The modularity of this implant can be observed using a conical couple for assembly and disassembly if repair is required at a later date. **C,** This lateral intraoperative photo demonstrates the entire construct, with intramedullary fixation proximally and a kinematic rotating hinge-like design for the joint. This prosthesis will allow for flexion/extension and rotation to stimulate near-normal knee function.

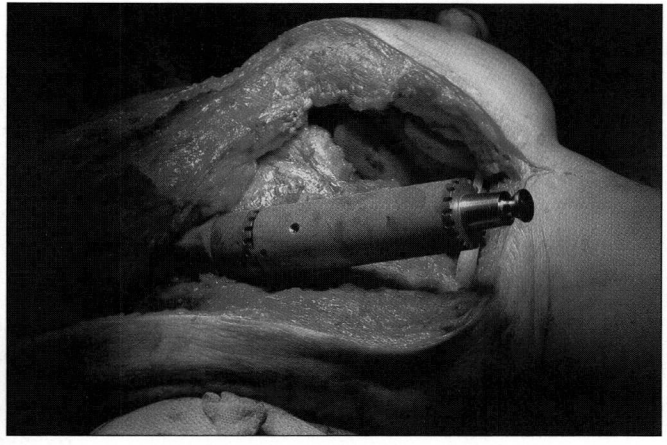

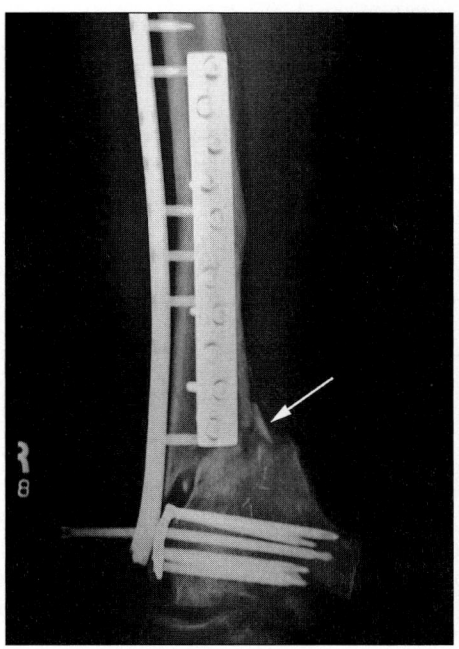

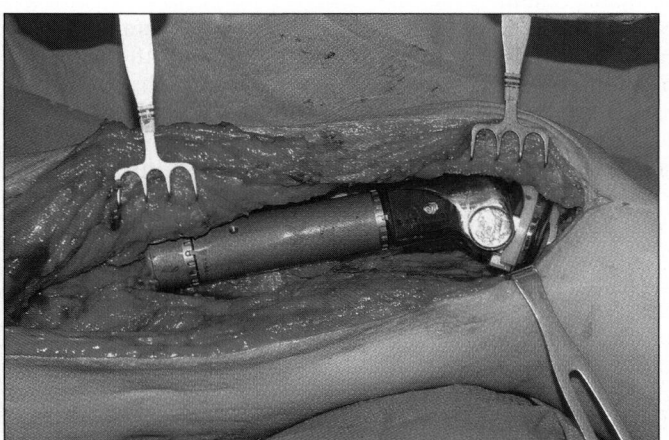

published failure rate for aseptic loosening in a large series of endoprostheses around the knee was 50% at 20 years' follow-up, for an average revision rate of 2.5% per year. Infection was calculated at 1.5% per year, and all risk factors were assumed to be constant over time. The authors concluded that the average cost saving for custom prosthetic reconstruction over amputation surgery during a 20-year period was approximately 70,000 British pounds at 1997 prices.

Management of Patients with High-Grade Osteosarcoma and Pathologic Fractures

The incidence of the development of pathologic fracture of the extremity in patients with high-grade osteosarcoma varies from 10% to 13%.[304,305] The fracture could be a consequence of the naturally destructive nature of the tumor and thinned cortex or of the biopsy defect violating the thinned cortex and adding to the stress riser already present (see "Biopsy"). The development of a pathologic fracture before biopsy has traditionally been thought to be associated with a poor prognosis, often leading to treatment that includes an immediate amputation followed by adjuvant multiagent chemotherapy.[211]

The development of a pathologic fracture is multifactorial and often depends on the following factors:

1. The histopathologic subtype of the lesion—the more destructive lesions, such as telangiectatic osteosarcoma, result in a thinned expanded cortex subject to fracture, while others might produce malignant mineralized osteoid with less destruction but markedly reduced strength.
2. Location of lesion (e.g., lesion involves a weight-bearing bone, such as the proximal femur).
3. The general athletic activity of the patient.
4. The degree or severity of the trauma required to produce the fracture.

Before the advent of neoadjuvant chemotherapy, the majority of patients developing pathologic fractures were treated by amputation.[306,307] Jaffe and colleagues,[304] however, observed that some pathologic fractures would heal while under the influence of systemic chemotherapy. They observed "reduction of the associated soft-tissue mass, repair of periosteum, and deposition of new mineral in the tumor and about the fracture." These observations made the closed management of some selected pathologic fractures feasible during treatment with neoadjuvant

Specific Malignancies

III

chemotherapy and in preparation for a limb-preserving procedure.

The subsequent healing of the fracture is also a function of the response of the tumor to neoadjuvant chemotherapy. Patients with healing fractures in general would be expected to have better overall outcomes than those without a favorable histopathologic healing response to primary chemotherapy.

Current recommendations for treatment of patients developing pathologic fractures from tumors potentially sensitive to chemotherapy include the following:

1. The patient must have the ability to tolerate conventional intensive chemotherapy.
2. The fracture must be treatable by closed means—either immobilization (usually upper extremity fractures) or use of external fixators well removed from the tumor margins, fracture braces, or traction for lower extremity fracture management.
3. The fracture should be monitored by physical examination (e.g., decreased motion and pain) and the demonstration of a radiographically favorable response (e.g., increased maturation of the tumor, increased mineral deposition, subperiosteal new bone). If no evidence of improvement or favorable tumor response can be demonstrated after each chemotherapy course, then consideration must be given to immediate limb-preserving surgery or amputation.
4. Patients with stage III disease may elect to consider amputation to concentrate all efforts on intensive treatment of metastatic disease and subsequent pulmonary or metastatic resection.
5. Proceed with an ablative procedure when there are no good limb-sparing alternatives available (e.g., pathologic fracture in a bone with multiple "skip" lesions).

Experience is limited in patients who develop pathologic fractures and are treated with multiagent preoperative chemotherapy followed by a limb-preserving procedure. Consequently, it is not certain whether waiting creates additional risks of a poor outcome. Current small retrospective reviews suggest that patients with pathologic fracture who can tolerate both the proposed method of fracture treatment and intensive multiagent chemotherapy do not appear to have a greater risk of an unfavorable outcome, unless the fracture demonstrates poor healing and unfavorable clinical response to treatment.[305,308,309]

Metachronous Osteosarcoma

Aung and colleagues[310] described a single-institution assessment of patients developing metachronous skeletal osteosarcoma between 1973 and May 2000. A retrospective review of records from 426 patients with nonmetastatic high-grade and primary osteosarcoma showed 23 patients, with a median age of 18.7 years, who developed metachronous osteosarcoma. Initial therapy included combination chemotherapy and surgery. Treatment of the metachronous relapse consisted of chemotherapy or radiation alone, or surgery with or without additional individualized chemotherapy.

The median time to the diagnosis of a metachronous lesion was 1.4 years, with a range of 0.2 to 11.3 years. Patients who developed late metachronous osteosarcoma experienced significantly longer postmetachronous osteosarcoma survival compared with those whose metachronous disease developed early. For the former group, the 2- and 5-year postmetachronous osteosarcoma survival rates were 72.7% and 61%, respectively. In contrast, all five patients who developed metachronous disease between 12 and 24 months died within 1.5 years of follow-up. Among patients developing late metachronous disease, further analysis based on type of therapy suggested that those treated with combined modality (including surgery and aggressive chemotherapy) for their metachronous disease fared better than those who received monotherapy. The authors also concluded that local therapy with surgery directed at the bulky primary tumor is the only effective method for local control.

Rodriguez and associates[311] described the treatment of five patients in whom primary osteosarcoma had been treated effectively with chemotherapy and resection of the primary tumor, and in whom another osteosarcoma developed at another site but without pulmonary metastases. The interval between management of the primary tumor and the subsequent development of another, apparently unrelated metachronous osteosarcoma ranged from 99 to 150 months. All patients remained otherwise free of disease 24 to 96 months after treatment of the metachronous lesion, except for one patient who developed acute myelogenous leukemia, most likely as a late effect from chemotherapy. Fitzgerald and colleagues[312] reported that among 800 patients, 12 developed metachronous osteosarcoma and none developed pulmonary metastases, a response quite different from patients reported with primary metastatic osteosarcoma.

Metastatic Disease

Primary osteosarcoma can arise in many tissues other than bone (e.g., kidney, liver, and cervix), but metastases in these other tissues are far more common. Metastatic disease is principally the result of hematogenous spread to the lungs and bone, followed by secondary involvement of kidney, liver, and brain. Regional lymph nodes are involved in fewer than 10% of cases. Metastatic disease at diagnosis does not preclude long-term disease-free survival when the disease is sensitive to chemotherapy and managed appropriately.[313-315]

Aggressive surgical treatment of pulmonary metastases (often requiring more than one procedure) can yield disease-free survivals from 17% to as high as 40%.[316-318] Generally favorable prognostic indicators include metastasis later than one year from original diagnosis, unilateral disease, presence of fewer than five nodules, and completeness of resection. Early pulmonary metastases; unresectable bilateral disease, and hilar, nodal, or pleural-based lesions have a poor prognosis.[319-321]

Bacci and coauthors[322] from the Rizzoli Institute reported their results of treatment of 44 patients with osteosarcoma of the extremity with detectable pulmonary metastases between January 1993 and June 1995. Of these patients, 12 were ineligible; 4 also had metastases to bone, 3 had metastases to lung and bone, 3 were over 50 years of age, and the remaining 2 had been treated at another institution. Thirty-six patients were eligible for the study. Ten patients thought to have pulmonary metastases, however, later were proven to have benign conditions at thoracotomy. Twenty-three patients were evaluable, having completed primary chemotherapy consisting of methotrexate, cisplatin, doxorubicin, and ifosfamide as defined by their protocol OS/N5.

After primary chemotherapy, lung metastases disappeared in 3 of the 23 evaluable patients, whereas in four the pulmonary disease was assessed as unresectable. All seven patients received surgical therapy for the primary tumor only. In the remaining 16 patients, simultaneous resection of the primary tumor and of the pulmonary metastases was performed. Remission was complete in 15 of the 16 patients and incomplete in 1. Ten patients (55.5%) remained continuously free of disease at a mean follow-up of 30 months.

Kaste and coworkers[323] reported the experience of St. Jude Children's Research Hospital in evaluating 215 patients with extremity osteosarcoma, of whom 32 (15%) had evidence of metastatic disease. Thirty-one patients demonstrated evidence of pulmonary metastases, and only one demonstrated metastases to bone. The histologic subtype most commonly associated with metastases was the osteoblastic subtype (n = 17). Original imaging was available for 28 of the 32 patients. One of 32 had solitary bone metastases without evidence of lung involvement. Four (14%) had calcifications within the pulmonary nodules, and both the number of nodules and the number of lobes involved were found to be significant predictors of survival (P = 0.0009; P = 0.04, respectively); multiple nodes were bilateral in 61% of patients. In the nonmetastatic cohort, the 5-year survival rate plus or minus standard error was 69% plus or minus 4%, and the 5-year event-free survival plus or minus standard error was 52% plus or minus 4%. This is in contrast to the results of the metastatic group (n = 32), in which the 5-year survival plus or minus standard error was 29% plus or minus 8%, and the 5-year event-free rate was 14% plus or minus 7%. Notably, the risk of death increased 1.4-fold for each additional lobe involved with pulmonary metastases (95% confidence interval [CI]: 1.018). The authors found a 2-year event-free survival rate similar to those previously reported, in spite of the inclusion of cases accrued over a 20-year span. Bacci[322] has reported a 2-year survival estimate of 45% for patients with resected pulmonary metastases. The 2-year survival estimated for their cohort was 52%. Meyers and colleagues[319] reported a 5-year survival estimate of 11% compared with the reported cohort estimate of 14% of patients presenting with metastases. They concluded that not only the number of pulmonary metastases but also their distribution among pulmonary lobes affected survival.

The Cooperative German-Austrian-Swiss Osteosarcoma Study Group recently reported their findings with patients with proven high-grade osteosarcoma of the extremities or trunk registered between 1979 and December 1998.[324]

Of the total 1765 patients, 202 (11.4%) had clinically detected metastatic osteosarcoma. In univariate analysis, survival of the patients with metastases was correlated significantly with patient age, site of primary tumor, number and location of metastases, number of involved organ systems, histological response of the primary tumor to preoperative chemotherapy, and completeness and time point of surgical resection of all tumor sites. After Cox multivariate regression analysis, however, only multiple metastases at diagnosis and macroscopically incomplete surgical resection remained significantly associated with poor outcomes. At a median follow-up of 1.9 years, 60 patients were alive, and 37 of the original 202 were in complete and continuous surgical remission. Overall actuarial survival at 5 years was 29% and at 10 years, 24%. The researchers concluded that the number of metastases and the completeness of surgical resection of all clinically detected tumor sites are of independent prognostic value in patients with proven primary metastatic osteosarcoma.

Stem cell transplantation was used by Fagioli and colleagues[325] in treating a 12-year-old male with a grade IV fibroblastic osteosarcoma of the distal femur. After neo-adjuvant chemotherapy, a local resection was performed, and the femur was reconstructed with a Katz prosthesis. Histopathologic review of the resected specimen revealed no visible cells. At 44 months, the patient underwent left lung metastectomy, and at 52 months he developed multiple osseous metastases. Allogeneic stem cell transplantation was performed using cells from an HLA-identical brother, and full donor chimerism was achieved. Complete remission was achieved on day 116. On day 210, the patient relapsed with a scapular metastasis.

Late Effects of Therapy

Psychosocial Outcomes

Nagarajan and associates[326] from the University of Minnesota described psychosocial outcomes (education, employment, health insurance, and marriage) for survivors of pediatric lower-extremity bone tumors. The long-term Childhood Cancer Survivor Study is a multi-institutional cohort study comprising 14,054 individuals who have survived 5 or more years after treatment for cancer diagnosed during childhood or adolescence. The 694 survivors who had osteosarcoma or Ewing's sarcoma of the lower extremity or pelvis were classified by amputation status and age at diagnosis. The median age at diagnosis was 14 years, and median follow-up since diagnosis was 16 years.

Amputation status and age at diagnosis had no significant influence on any of the measured psychosocial outcomes. Education was a significant positive predictor of employment, having health insurance, and being currently in a first marriage. Male gender predicted having been employed, and female gender predicted having health insurance and marriage. Compared with siblings, amputees had significant deficits in education, employment, and health insurance. The authors concluded, however, that overall, no differences were found between amputees and nonamputees. Gender and education played a prominent role. When compared with siblings, amputees in this cohort could have benefitted from additional support.

Survivors were grouped into one of two categories according to the type of surgically controlled procedure—those treated with and without amputation. Survivors of lower-extremity bone tumors had high rates of employment (97%), graduation (high school, 93%; college, 50%), and marriage (67%). Thirty percent reported health insurance problems, and 87% had health insurance. The study reported a higher percentage of amputees than would normally be observed in current studies, but this is thought to be a reflection of the indications for limb-sparing and amputation surgery at the time the patients were under treatment.

Second Malignant Neoplasms

Aung and associates[327] retrospectively reviewed the experience of the Memorial Sloan-Kettering Cancer Center with long-term survivors of osteosarcoma and the subsequent development of secondary malignancies. The patients were treated between February 1973 and March 2000, and all had received chemotherapy and/or surgery. Chemotherapy consisted of a combination of agents that included high-dose methotrexate, doxorubicin, bleomycin, cyclophosphamide, dactinomycin, vincristine, cisplatin, and ifosfamide. Of 509 patients, 14 were identified as having developed secondary malignant neoplasms. The time interval from diagnosis of the primary osteosarcoma to the development of the secondary malignant neoplasm ranged from 1.3 years to 13.1 years (median 5.5 years). The second neoplasms occurred in the central nervous system in four patients. There were two cases of acute myeloid leukemia and one case each of myelodysplasic syndrome, non-Hodgkin lymphoma, high-grade pleomorphic sarcoma, leiomyosarcoma, fibrosarcoma, carcinoma of the breast, and mucoepidermoid carcinoma. The standard incidence was 4.6% when patients with a history of retinoblastoma or Rothmund-Thompson syndrome were excluded.

Osteosarcoma After Allogeneic Bone Marrow Transplantation

Bielack and coworkers[328] reported on four patients who were identified by searching the database for the Cooperative Osteosarcoma Study Group (COSS) for patients whose osteosarcoma arose after hematopoietic stem cell transplantation (HSCT). Transplant indications in the patients affected had been acute lymphoblastic leukemia (three patients) and sickle cell disease (one patient). A stem cell source was bone marrow in all cases (three allogeneic, one syngenic). All four patients had received allocating agents as part of their conditioning regimen and/or first-line therapy. The conditioning regimen included total-body irradiation in three patients. Two lesions occurred in the distal femur and two in the proximal tibia. In one patient with a proximal tibial lesion, another lesion was discovered in the pubis of the pelvis. One patient refused surgery and received radiotherapy, subsequently developing a myelodysplastic syndrome

requiring reconditioning and an additional peripheral blood stem cell transplant from the same donor. The patient with two lesions underwent resection of both lesions of the proximal tibia and pubis and was alive with stable disease at 4.5 years. The third and fourth patients both underwent limb-sparing surgery; one remained alive without evidence of disease three years after surgical resection, and the other completed the adjuvant portion of chemotherapy. The authors concluded that osteosarcoma should be included as a potential late effect from bone marrow transplantation.

OSTEOSARCOMA VARIANTS

This section discusses variants of classic osteosarcoma. Some of these subtypes are low grade and well differentiated, have low metastatic potential, and usually do not require adjuvant therapy.[329] The more common high-grade variants will also be reviewed. Although osteogenic lesions arising in the jaw are more common than the recognized variants of osteosarcoma, this subtype will not be addressed in this chapter.

High-Grade Variants

High-Grade Surface Osteosarcoma

Epidemiology. Of the more aggressive surface osteosarcoma variants, the least common is high-grade surface osteosarcoma. It is most frequently reported in the second and third decades of life and, unlike classic osteosarcoma, is four times more frequent in males than females. The femur appears to be the most frequent site of involvement; these tumors are rarely observed in the flat bones.[330]

Radiographic Features. No roentgenographic features reliably distinguish high-grade surface osteosarcoma from other surface osteosarcomas. Some lesions appear radiographically destructive, while others tend to mineralize more heavily. Some may even present with a sunburst appearance. The only common denominator known is that high-grade surface osteosarcomas usually arise from the surface of long bones and tend to be slightly more diaphyseal in location. The tumors generally demonstrate intense uptake on ^{99m}Tc bone scintigraphy. CT best demonstrates the site of peripheral surface origin, while MRI shows possible marrow involvement and the anatomic features of the lesion on T_1-weighted images.[331]

Differential Diagnosis. In some instances, high-grade surface osteosarcoma can be radiographically indistinguishable from low-grade parosteal osteosarcoma and periosteal osteosarcoma. Occasionally, myositis ossificans can be confused with the lesion, but it is usually associated with trauma and the subsequent onset of tenderness.[332]

Histopathology. The histopathologic appearance is best characterized by cartilage intermixed with high-grade anaplastic osteoid-producing cells. Often, histopathology is the only reliable method to differentiate these radiographically similar tumors of bone from one another.

Chemotherapy. Wold and colleagues[333] reported on nine patients with high-grade surface osteosarcoma. Seven of the nine died as a result of their disease. Currently, the majority of musculoskeletal oncologists would recommend conventional multiagent neoadjuvant chemotherapy as presently recommended for conventional osteosarcoma, followed by limb-sparing surgery and adjuvant chemotherapy for treatment.

Surgical Therapy. Surgical management of the tumor requires a minimum of a wide surgical margin after primary chemotherapy, with an intramedullary margin of 3 cm to 5 cm as calculated from the preoperative MRI. Pulmonary metastases should be pursued aggressively with surgical removal and adjuvant chemotherapy.

Prognosis. The number of patients treated and reported with high-grade surface osteosarcomas is too small to analyze. It is likely, however, that the disease-free survival rate is similar to that for patients with conventional osteosarcoma.

Extraskeletal Osteosarcoma

Extraskeletal osteosarcoma is an uncommon variant of high-grade osteosarcoma, characterized histopathologically by the production of malignant osteoid and bone arising in soft tissue. Although primary osteosarcoma in rare instances arises in other organs, the majority of these lesions are found in soft tissues of the lower extremity and buttock, upper extremity, and retroperitoneum.[334-340]

Epidemiology. Extraskeletal osteosarcoma differs from conventional or "classic" osteosarcoma in that the majority of patients are older than 50 years of age. The tumors most often arise beneath the deep fascia, and 10% to 15% of patients have a history of antecedent trauma.[340]

The etiology of extraskeletal osteosarcoma remains unknown except for patients who have had external-beam radiotherapy (postradiation sarcoma) for other reasons. The subsequent development of extraskeletal osteosarcoma within the radiation therapy field after a latent period remains a well-known risk. Of the 88 patients reported by Chung and Enzinger[342] with extraskeletal osteosarcoma, 5 had previously undergone radiotherapy.

Radiographic Features. The majority of lesions can be palpated and identified with plain x-rays of the extremity using soft-tissue techniques. Although the mass is commonly ill defined, matrix mineralization can often be identified as a "fluffy" density. If abundant cartilage is present, punctate calcifications can be evident.

As expected in conventional osteosarcoma, extraskeletal osteogenic lesions are often well demonstrated by intense uptake on ^{99m}Tc bone scan. Pulmonary metastases and local lymph node involvement can occasionally be demonstrated by bone scintigraphy. To assess potential metastatic disease, a ^{99m}Tc three-phase bone scan or a rapid whole-body STIR MRI and CT of the chest should be completed for appropriate radiographic staging.

CT of the lesion with both bone and soft-tissue techniques will often identify the mineralized tumor matrix or cartilagenous calcification. MRI offers no specific benefit over CT in evaluating this lesion, as medullary canal involvement is not an issue. The cross-sectional display and compartmental anatomy demonstrated by CT generally identify both the axial location of the tumor and the anatomic compartment involved. The regional, retroperitoneal, and mediastinal lymph nodes should also be evaluated.

Radiographically, both myositis and extraskeletal osteosarcoma demonstrate bone production, and differentiation can be difficult. Myositis characteristically arises adjacent to bone and demonstrates a lucent zone between the lesion and the underlying cortex. Also, maturation of myositis often exhibits mature, well-marginated bone at the periphery of the lesion. Extraskeletal osteosarcoma, on the other hand, displays tumor bone more centrally with an indistinct, poorly marginated peripheral margin in the region of the frequently loculated advancing invasive tumor growth. Parosteal osteosarcoma pathologically and radiographically also demonstrates central maturation with peripheral immature tissue similar to extraskeletal osteosarcoma, but it arises immediately adjacent to bone.

Clinical Manifestations. Extraosseous osteosarcoma must be distinguished from myositis ossificans, with which it is commonly confused. Patients with myositis usually have a distinct history of trauma, either acute or chronic, followed by pain and local tenderness. Extraskeletal osteosarcoma usually grows more slowly, remains mobile in the adjacent soft tissues, and is nontender until late in clinical stages of the disease. Myositis, on the other hand, usually appears rapidly, is tender and edematous, and can be fixed to deep osseous structures.

Differential Diagnosis. The most common ossifying lesion presenting in soft tissue is myositis ossificans. Parosteal osteosarcoma characteristically arises from the posterior aspect of the distal femoral metaphysis in young adults (third and fourth decade). The characteristic thin rim of mature reactive bone often demonstrated best on CT usually separates myositis from parosteal and extraskeletal sarcomas, which tend to be more mature centrally. The invasive, more immature peripheries of malignant tumors are often isodense and blend into the surrounding soft tissues. MRI probably provides better information than CT to differentiate between myositis ossificans, intramuscular hemangioma, parosteal osteosarcoma, high-grade surface osteosarcoma, and pseudotumors of the thigh.

Surgical Therapy. Clinically, the lesion appears indurated when palpating the relaxed surrounding muscle. Pathologically, lobulation is common and must be taken into account when planning surgical therapy and the biopsy tract. The preoperative staging CT and/or MRI should be reviewed carefully so as to avoid contamination of uninvolved anatomic compartments. Representative tissue must be obtained through a judiciously placed longitudinal skin biopsy incision. Experienced pathologists are often reluctant to interpret needle biopsies from this rare and unusual tumor.

The literature clearly illustrates that most surgeons do not appreciate the invasive and lobulated growth potential of this primary malignant tumor. In two large retrospective representative studies, the local recurrence rates were 50% (13 of 26 patients) and 43% (38 of 88 patients).[341,342]

Chemotherapy. Extraskeletal osteosarcoma is considered a high-grade tumor producing metastases to lung, bone, and (occasionally) regional lymph nodes. For patients who can medically tolerate intensive neoadjuvant chemotherapy, three cycles of multiagent chemotherapy would usually be used before a limb-sparing procedure. With intensive primary chemotherapy tailored specifically to sarcomas of bone and soft tissue, the majority of lesions can be removed surgically, with wide margins for appropriate local control. Adjuvant chemotherapy should be initiated after wound healing. Radiotherapy is not used commonly as a therapeutic modality except for palliation in patients with systemic disease.

Pagetoid Osteosarcoma

Sarcoma originating as a complication of Paget's disease of bone was first recognized by Paget himself in 1877. The patient he described subsequently developed fibrosarcoma of the involved radius and died. Of his 23 reported patients, 5 similarly developed sarcoma within the involved bone and died.

Epidemiology. Approximately 5% of the osteosarcomas reported in large series are complications of Paget's disease of bone. Pagetoid osteosarcoma is twice as common in males as in females. The exact frequency of sarcomatous change in patients with uncomplicated Paget's disease is unknown; reports range from 1% to 12%. Sarcoma tends to develop in patients with polyostotic bone involvement (90%) and is distinctly unusual in patients with monostotic disease (10%). The lesion develops in bone showing the characteristic radiographic accentuated trabeculations of Paget's disease, not in otherwise normal bone.[343] Schmorl,[344] in an autopsy study, reported a 3% incidence of Paget's disease in humans over the age of 40 years. The distribution of involved areas in uncomplicated Paget's disease revealed involvement of the pelvis and sacrum to be most common (56%), followed by the spine (50%), right femur (31%), and cranium (25%). Sites less commonly involved were the sternum, pelvis, left femur, clavicle, tibia, ribs, and humerus. In contrast, the distribution of sarcoma arising in Paget's disease is most common in the pelvis (ilium, 34%), humerus (22%), and femur (19%) and is distinctly uncommon in the spine.[345] Lesions arising in the vertebral bodies are usually associated with previous irradiation. The reason for the common sarcomatous involvement of the humerus and the rarity of involvement of the spine is unknown.[346]

Radiographic Features. The classic conventional radiographic change observed with malignant degeneration in pagetic bone is loss or destruction of the usually distinct but accentuated trabeculation. A recent observation by Colarinha and colleagues[347] using ^{201}Tl to differentiate between benign and malignant polyostotic lesions might be helpful.

Scintigraphy using ^{99m}Tc MDP and ^{201}Tl was performed in a patient with polyostotic Paget's disease and sarcomatous degeneration in the right ilium. The ^{99m}Tc MDP imaging revealed abnormal uptake in both types of lesions, while the ^{201}Tl imaging showed increased uptake in the sarcomatous lesion only. These new findings, in conjunction with the observation of a soft-tissue mass in and around the suspected lesion on MRI, could assist in earlier diagnosis and treatment.

Pathologic Features. The histopathologic subtypes differ among pathologists. Huvos and coauthors[348] reported a fibrohistiocytomatous histology to be the most common (26%), while others have reported osteosarcoma (59%) as the most frequently observed subtype.[343] Histopathologic interpretation appears to account for these differences.

Prognosis. The overall prognosis for patients with sarcoma of Paget's disease is worse than for patients with classic osteosarcoma. The disease is usually fatal with or without adjuvant chemotherapy. The majority of patients are best managed surgically by a "wide" amputation for local control and relief of pain. The majority of patients die within three years.

Postradiation Osteosarcoma of Bone

Epidemiology. Postirradiation sarcoma occurs after 3 to 10 years and arises within the radiation therapy portal of treatment for an osseous or extraosseous benign or malignant tumor; it occurs twice as commonly in females. Secondary osteosarcoma or malignant fibrous histiocytoma arises mainly in two groups of patients:

1. Those treated for childhood tumors such as retinoblastoma, who could be genetically predisposed to secondary tumors developing both inside and outside the field of irradiation; and
2. Those treated for adult tumors such as Hodgkin's lymphoma, who have little evidence of genetic disposition toward secondary malignancies but develop the secondary tumor within the radiation field.[349-352]

In general, induction of the tumor appears to be related to dosage, type and site of radiation, age of the patient, and concomitant use of chemotherapeutic agents. The interval between exposure and the development of the tumor ranges from 2.75 years to 41 years, with an average of 13.4 years. Secondary solid tumors have a longer latency period than leukemia when they are related to chemotherapy and radiotherapy.[353,354] Histopathologic subtypes reported for radiation-induced sarcomas include osteosarcoma (50%), fibrosarcoma (40%), and less commonly, chondrosarcoma (4%).[355]

Clinical Manifestations. The development of increasing pain and swelling within a previously irradiated portal should alert the physician to the possibility of malignant change. In contrast to conventional osteosarcoma, the most commonly involved osseous sites are the ilium, proximal femur, and proximal humerus.[349] Whether the underlying bone was normal or abnormal at the time of initiation of treatment appears to make little difference in the latent period.

Pathologic Findings. In the Huvos series,[349] fibrohistiocytomatous lesions were most common (38%), followed by osteoblastic (18%) and chondroblastic (12%) lesions. The 5-year survival rate was 17%. The poor prognosis is thought to be related to the secondary neoplasm arising in the central marrow-bearing anatomic regions involved by the index disease process (e.g., sternum, spine, pelvis). (See the section on round cell tumor for information about treatment-related sarcomas.)

Radiographic Features. The most common radiographic feature of malignant change is destruction of the underlying bone within the radiation portal. Serial ^{99m}Tc bone scans might show evidence of increased uptake in the anatomic region in question when compared with earlier studies. CT often demonstrates destruction and an associated soft-tissue mass. The presence or absence of demonstrable calcification or tumor matrix mineralization is dependent on the differentiation of the tumor.

Using the criteria described by Arlen and colleagues,[356] Sheppard and Libshitz[357] identified 63 patients with postradiation sarcomas. There were 43 females and 20 males, with a mean age of 52.8 years. The mean radiation dose delivered was 50.1 Gy, with a mean latency period for the development of the sarcoma of 15.5 years. The most common primary diagnoses were carcinoma of the breast, lymphoma, and head and neck cancer. The most common histopathologies included osteosarcoma and malignant fibrous histiocytoma. The most common imaging findings were bone destruction with an associated soft-tissue mass. The authors concluded that postradiation sarcomas, although uncommon, are not rare. They could demonstrate no pathognomonic radiographic findings other than appreciation of the expected latency and knowledge of the anatomic site of the previous radiation porthole.

Differential Diagnosis. The development of pain in a previously irradiated anatomic region must be evaluated clinically. The differentiation between radiation necrosis and pathologic or insufficiency fracture could be very difficult. A helpful feature is the clinicoradiologic course of radiation necrosis, resulting in bone resolution that often is associated with multiple pathologic fractures (e.g., multiple ribs) and that occurs over a larger area of the therapy field.

Surgical Therapy. Because of the usual overlying leatherlike skin and soft-tissue changes, limb-sparing procedures rarely are offered as surgical therapy for adult secondary irradiation sarcomas. When they occur as a complication

of treatment of childhood tumors, however, radical procedures such as rotationplasty of the proximal or distal femur or proximal tibia occasionally can be offered for patients in whom the tumor and associated soft-tissue changes can be resected, leaving nonirradiated tissues for reconstruction. The majority of adult and elderly patients are offered an ablative procedure well above and proximal to the affected anatomic part.[358]

Small Cell Osteosarcoma

Small cell osteosarcoma, once thought to be a variant of another tumor type, now appears to be a recognized variant of osteosarcoma.

A recent and detailed report by Nakajima and coworkers[359] reviewed 72 cases of small cell osteosarcoma (22 from the Mayo Clinic files and 50 from their consultation files) and described the clinicopathologic features of this unusual entity.

Clinical Features. The patients reviewed included 39 males (63.8%) and 33 females (45.8%) ranging in age from five to 71 years (mean, 24.8 years; median, 20 years). More than half the patients were in the second or third decade of life.

Forty-four tumors (63.8%) involved the long bones, and 22 tumors (31.9%) occurred in femurs, with 6 developing proximally, 4 in the midshaft, and 11 in the distal one third. Twelve tumors arose in the humerus, including eight proximally, three in the midshaft, and one in the distal one third. Three patients presented with multiple lesions, and two presented with pulmonary metastases.

Pain and swelling were the most common symptom and sign. One patient with a vertebral lesion developed sudden paraplegia. The duration of symptoms and signs varied from 4 days to 10 years (average, 15.4 months; median, 6 months).

Radiographic Features. Imaging studies were available for 35 patients. The lesions were generally characterized as destructive and had the appearance of an aggressive process, with 20 of the 35 clearly suggestive of conventional osteosarcoma arising in the metaphysis. The remaining studies displayed primarily a destructive and osteolytic process, with no mineralization of the adjacent soft-tissue mass.

Differential Diagnosis. The differential diagnosis includes Ewing's sarcoma, malignant lymphoma, and metastatic and small cell carcinoma of the lung.

Pathological Findings. Osteoid production was identified in all tumors. Nakajima identified a round cell type and a short, spindle cell type, with the round cell variety subdivided into three additional groups based on size: very small (25 tumors), small (27 tumors), and medium size (16 tumors). Four tumors were identified as being of the short, spindle cell type.

Chemotherapy. The data suggest that the chemotherapy regimen should be based on and similar to treatment of conventional osteosarcoma.

Surgical Therapy. Although early reports suggested that amputation or disarticulation was required for local control, median survival time for patients who had surgery with additional chemotherapy was 13.4 years. Current recommendations for treatment include multiagent neoadjuvant chemotherapy, surgical resection, and limb-sparing surgery with a minimum of wide margins, followed by adjuvant chemotherapy. Patients reviewed who had had marginal or contaminated margins had poor prognoses.[360-366]

Osteosarcoma over the Age of 40

A recent monumental review by the European Musculo-skeletal Oncology Society has made a significant contribution to knowledge of osteosarcoma in patients over the age of 40 years.[367] Using the retrospective experience of 12 centers, they studied outcomes of treatment in 481 patients with osteosarcoma, including 272 males, 206 females, and 3 unclassified, all over the age of 40.

Forty-two patients (28 males, 14 females) with Pagetoid osteosarcoma had a mean age of 71 years (range, 47–88 years). The most commonly involved bones were the pelvis (12 patients) and the femur (12 patients). Only 14 of the 42 patients underwent surgery, and five procedures resulted in local recurrence (four of nine limb-preserving procedures and one of five amputations). Although the median survival was 9 months, one patient with an osteosarcoma of the tibia who was treated with an amputation lived for 8 years. Only two patients had chemotherapy.

Forty-one patients (29 females, 12 males) with a mean age of 58 years (range, 40–82 years) developed radiation-induced osteosarcoma. The majority of the tumors developed in the axial skeleton and were related to radiation treatment for ovarian or cervical carcinoma (pelvis, 12 patients) and breast cancer (scapula, 11 patients). Only 12 of the 41 patients had no axial tumors. Twenty-nine patients had surgery, including 19 patients with limb-preserving procedures and 8 with primary amputations. Eleven patients developed local recurrence, with two occurring in the amputee group and six in the limb-preserving group. Patients with axial tumors did worse (5-year survival 28%) than those with primary tumor of the limb (5-year survival 55%).

Twenty-six patients had low-grade osteosarcoma (parosteal and low-grade central osteosarcoma), including 14 tumors in the femur. Only two of these patients had chemotherapy. Twenty-five had local limb-sparing procedures, and one had an amputation. Four developed local recurrence, and only one subsequently died as a result of local recurrence. The 5-year survival for the group was 88%.

The review covered 220 patients for whom follow-up data were available and who had high-grade nonmetastatic osteosarcoma not related to Paget's disease or radiation, and not involving the pelvis, skull, or spine. Thirteen patients had intracompartmental disease (stage IIA), and 151 had extracompartmental disease (stage IIB), with 104 cases involving the distal femur, 48 the tibia, 34 the proximal femur, 19 the proximal humerus, and 8 the fibula. Eighty-six patients had an amputation, and 126 had a limb-sparing procedure (23 excision alone, 7 allograft reconstruction, and 78 endoprosthesis). One hundred twenty-nine patients had a minimum of a "wide" surgical margin, and 37 were believed to have marginal or intralesional margins. Local recurrence occurred in 25 patients (5% amputees, 13% with limb-preserving procedures, and 24% of those with excision alone). Eleven of 129 patients (9%) with what were believed to be "wide" or radial margins experienced local recurrence. Overall, survival was 46% at 5 years and 33% at 10 years. Of the 154 patients able to receive chemotherapy (i.e., doxorubicin, cisplatin, ifosfamide, and methotrexate), 29% were over the age of 60 years, and 80% were under 60 years of age. Overall, improved outcomes were related to the ability to receive chemotherapy (age <60 years) and location of the lesion (lower limb). These data suggest that patients over the age of 40 years who have conventional high-grade osteosarcoma and are capable of withstanding cytotoxic chemotherapy might do as well with comprehensive multimodal treatment as younger patients under 40.

Low-Grade Variants

Low-Grade Central Osteosarcoma

Epidemiology. This well-differentiated osteosarcoma variant can be characterized by its presentation primarily in young adults and its intraosseous location. The original series described by Unni and colleagues[368] included 27 patients with pain and swelling as the most common presenting complaints; the onset of their symptoms occurred from one to 20 years before medical evaluation. The ages ranged from 10 to 65 years. A more recent review (from the same institution) of 80 patients with low-grade central osteosarcoma involved 41 males and 39 females, with a mean age of 28.2 years. Skeletal distribution of the tumors was similar to that seen with conventional osteosarcoma.[369]

Radiographic Features. A review of 74 patients with histopathologically proven low-grade central lesions revealed 64 tumors involving the medullary canal and ten of cortical origin.[369] Forty-three of the 64 long-bone lesions had a metaphyseal location, 11 were diaphyseal/metaphyseal, and 10 were diaphyseal. Eleven patients were skeletally immature at the time of diagnosis, and no tumor was observed to have violated or crossed the epiphysis. Larger lesions readily crossed the physeal scar after adult epiphyseal closure. Occasionally, the tumor penetrated and destroyed the cortex. Poor margination was observed radiographically in 50 of 74 patient x-rays reviewed, and 51 patients (69%) showed x-ray evidence of tumor matrix mineralization.

Histopathology. Many tumors appeared well differentiated, and some appeared strikingly similar to fibrous dysplasia. The tissue was composed primarily of spindle cells with scarce mitotic figures with minimal atypia. Osteoid content was variable.[370-372]

Differential Diagnosis. As mentioned, differentiation of low-grade central osteosarcoma from benign bone tumors can be difficult. Low-grade central osteosarcoma appears histopathologically similar to fibrous dysplasia and to benign spindle cell lesions, such as desmoplastic fibroma and low-grade fibrosarcoma.

Surgical Therapy. Wide excision is the treatment of choice. Intralesional or marginal margins resulted in 11 patients, with 11 tumors reoccurring within a mean time of 3.9 years after suboptimal surgical therapy. Two of the 11 patients died as a result of their disease between 2 and 48 years after diagnosis.[369]

Chemotherapy. Chemotherapy is probably not useful in the initial treatment of this disease; however, 15% of patients experience tissue transformation from low-grade to high-grade osteosarcoma. Those patients with high-grade tumors might benefit from conventional multiagent chemotherapy.

Intracortical Osteosarcoma
Epidemiology. In 1960, Jaffe[373] published the original description of intracortical osteosarcoma observed in two patients. The low-grade lesion often presents in diaphyseal cortical bone of either the tibia (most common) or the femur. Unlike periosteal osteosarcoma, the intracortical lesion arises within diaphyseal cortical bone and rarely penetrates into or invades the medullary canal.[374]

Differential Diagnosis. In some instances, intracortical osteosarcoma can mimic the radiographic appearance of osteoid osteoma or osteoblastoma, but the lesion should not be assumed to be benign. It also can resemble adamantinoma radiographically. The lesion can demonstrate cortical destruction on plain film or CT evaluation.

Surgical Therapy. With either CT or MRI as a guide, the lesion should be excised, along with the adjacent biopsy tract and contiguous soft-tissue. If the lesion does not penetrate the endosteal surface of bone and the MRI marrow signal is otherwise normal, then a hemisection of the shaft with normal uninvolved margins (wide) could be sufficient for surgical treatment, if supplemented with bone graft and possibly internal fixation. If there is a suggestion of marrow involvement, either by biopsy contamination or by direct tumor extension, then the entire shaft should be included circumferentially. With improved imaging techniques and appropriate preoperative planning, past errors that resulted in marginal resections should now be minimized if not eliminated.

Hermann and coworkers[375] described a delay in diagnosis of an 11-year-old male's anterior tibia lesion, which was later proven to be intracortical osteosarcoma. The differential diagnosis included osteoid osteoma or

Brodie's abscess. Clinical history did not support the radiographic suspicion of osteoid osteoma because of the absence of pain relieved by nonsteroidal anti-inflammatory medications. Only later did pain become an issue. Because the outcome for this tumor is so favorable, the delay in diagnosis played no part in the overall favorable outcome. Griffith and associates,[376] reviewing the available literature on the least common osteosarcoma variant, found that five patients were free of disease 3 to 10 years after primary surgery. Death has been described as a consequence of this disease after a 26-year follow-up, however.[377]

The use of neoadjuvant or adjuvant chemotherapy should be individualized, based on the size of the lesion, histopathologic interpretation, duration of symptoms, and the margins obtained at the time of wide excision.[378]

Periosteal Osteosarcoma
In 1955, Lichtenstein[379] described an unusual periosteal lesion of the humerus and another in the femur that produced cartilage as well as malignant osteoid. Cooper[378] later reported a recurrent lesion previously managed by local resection of the ulna, which he described as juxta-cortical chondrosarcoma. Schajowicz[381,382] brought attention to three brothers with juxtacortical chondrosarcoma.

The publication by Unni and colleagues[383] in 1976 clarified the issue and focused on the osteoid component seen in the lesion. They described the entity currently recognized as periosteal osteogenic sarcoma.

Epidemiology. Periosteal osteosarcoma is an uncommon low-grade osteosarcoma variant arising primarily in the cortical shaft of the tibia and femur. Radiographically, the lesion arises from the surface of the bone, contiguous with the cortex, producing a "scalloped" appearance. A soft-tissue mass within the scalloped lesion can be seen on CT or MRI. Magnetic resonance imaging frequently predicts the absence of marrow involvement beyond the scalloped margins.

Pathologic Features. Histologically, the lesion consists of intermediate-grade malignant chondroblastic tissue, anaplastic spindle cells, and malignant osteoid. Metastatic disease occurs in approximately 15% of patients.[383]

Surgical Therapy. Treatment consists of en bloc excision with a wide margin and reconstruction, sparing the limb in the majority of cases. When the lesion arises in the femur, the tumor could circumferentially involve the cortex, requiring an intercallary resection of the shaft and reconstruction. Neoadjuvant chemotherapy could be useful in some patients with large lesions; however, adjuvant chemotherapy is generally not indicated in the routine treatment of this disease unless pulmonary metastases are evident or develop postoperatively.

Parosteal Osteosarcoma
Epidemiology. Parosteal osteosarcoma comprises approximately 4% of all osteosarcomas and is slightly more common in adult females during the third decade

of life. The most common site of presentation is the posterior aspect of the distal femoral metaphysis (72%), followed by the proximal humeral metaphysis and the proximal tibia.[384] The lesion consistently presents as a fixed, painless hard mass.[383]

Radiographic Features. Radiographically, the lesion consists of a dense lobulated bone and soft-tissue mass arising from the posterior aspect of the distal femoral metaphysis. Usually, there is an ill-defined separation or lucent zone between the lesion and the cortex (best demonstrated by polytomography or CT). The peripheral margin of the lesion (zone of maturation) is poorly marginated radiographically and less mature pathologically. The lesion is often demonstrated by intense uptake on ^{99m}Tc bone scan. Untreated lesions usually do not involve the medullary canal, which can best be evaluated with MRI.

Pathologic Features. Histopathologically, the tumor consists of fibroblastic, cartilaginous, and osseous components, all of which are evaluated individually and graded according to the highest-grade malignancy. The most mature and well-differentiated elements are often seen centrally. The outer zone of the tumor is composed of less mature hypercellular elements.

A system of grading has been applied to parosteal osteosarcoma (grades I, II, and III). Patients with lesions containing foci of high-grade malignancy (grade III) have survival rates similar to patients with conventional osteosarcoma.[383,385] These patients are potential candidates for neoadjuvant and/or adjuvant chemotherapy.

Surgical Therapy. After radiographic staging, treatment for lesions without intramedullary involvement requires local excision with wide margins, most often resulting in a limb-sparing procedure (Fig. 95-7). Vascular displace-

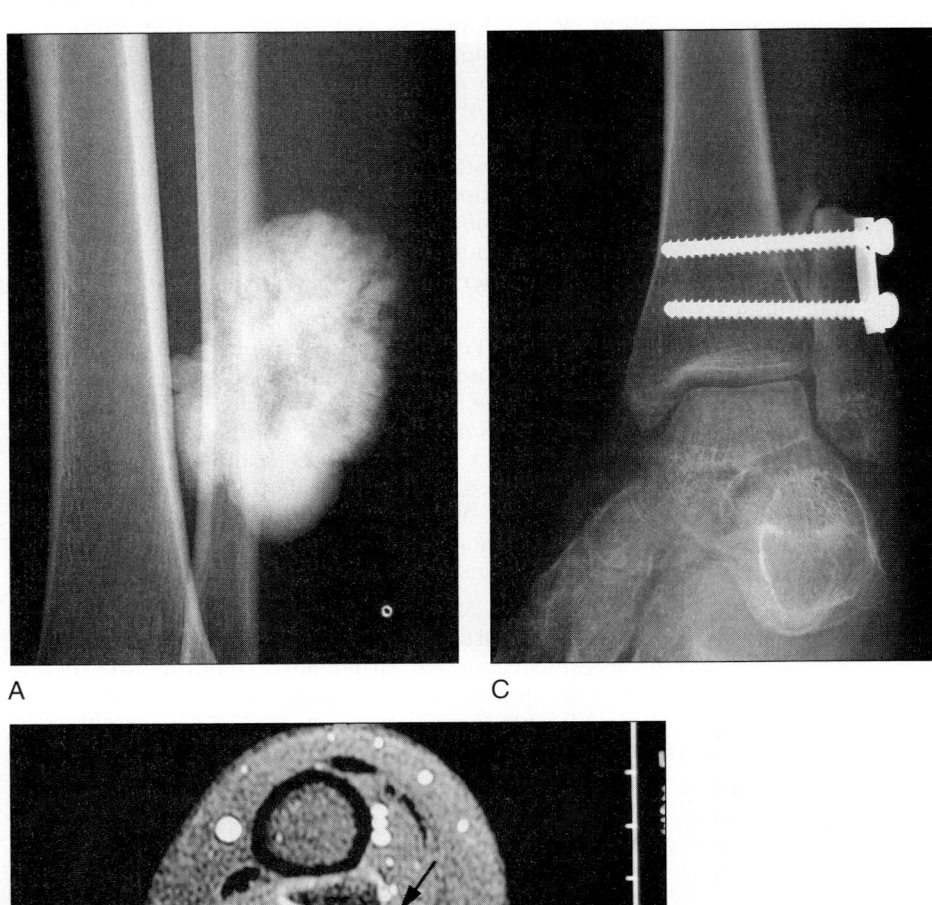

A

C

B

Figure 95-7. A, This 31-year-old female had noted a painless mass posterior to the left fibula 24 months before medical evaluation. The patient denied any local trauma. **B,** The axial fat suppression MR with contrast demonstrates the mineralized central position (*black areas*) with the typical bright circumferential ring of enhancement typical for parosteal osteosarcoma. Also note the normal fatty marrow signal (*arrow*) without the suggestion of tumor involvement. **C,** This AP postoperative x-ray demonstrates the resection margin of the distal fibula and the operative synostosis to stabilize the lateral malleolus.

ment is usually not a contraindication for local resection and limb preservation. If the MRI demonstrates evidence of intramedullary involvement, the entire circumference of the involved bone and the contiguous overlying soft tissues must be resected. Patients with intramedullary involvement either primarily or secondarily from local recurrence do not necessarily have a worse prognosis.[386]

CHONDROSARCOMA

Chondrosarcoma is second only to osteosarcoma in frequency as a primary malignant bone tumor. Chondrosarcoma characteristically produces cartilage matrix from neoplastic tissue devoid of osteoid. Ossification, calcification, and myxoid changes can occur.

Epidemiology

Chondrosarcoma comprises approximately 20% of all malignant bone tumors. The tumor arises predominantly in individuals in the third decade of life or beyond, with nearly equal distribution among males and females. Pain (often ill defined) and a mass are the most common presenting complaints. The majority of lesions in adults arise in regions of the skeleton preformed from cartilage, with the pelvis most commonly affected (approximately 30%). Other locations frequently involved include the proximal and distal femoral diaphysis, ribs, and proximal humerus.[387-391] Chondrosarcoma rarely occurs in the spine.[392-396]

When a potentially malignant cartilage tumor is considered, age and location are important factors.[397,398] In adults of middle to advanced age, central lesions are more likely to be malignant than lesions in peripheral locations (hands and feet).[399-401] The craniofacial region is the site in 13% of patients under the age of 21 years, compared with 3.5% in older patients.[402-405] The younger group has fewer malignancies of the ribs and sternum (4%) than do the older patients (10%).[387,406-410]

Etiology and Pathogenesis

Chondrosarcoma can conveniently be divided into primary and secondary lesions. Primary or central chondrosarcoma arises de novo from previously normal-appearing bone preformed from cartilage. Secondary or peripheral tumors arise or develop from preexisting benign cartilage lesions, such as the cartilaginous portion of an osteochondroma or a benign enchondroma.[411] Both tend to appear at least 15 to 20 years after skeletal maturity and usually demonstrate radiographic enlargement (osteochondroma) or endosteal erosions (enchondroma).[412] Pain is the most common initial symptom. The anatomic location (T) and histopathologic grade (G) are important factors in determining whether the lesions are categorized as central (primary) or peripheral (secondary).

Primary or central chondrosarcomas comprise approximately two thirds of reported chondrosarcomas and usually represent high-grade neoplasms capable of producing metastases and of infiltrating and invading the surrounding soft tissues (Fig. 95-8). Extraskeletal chondro-

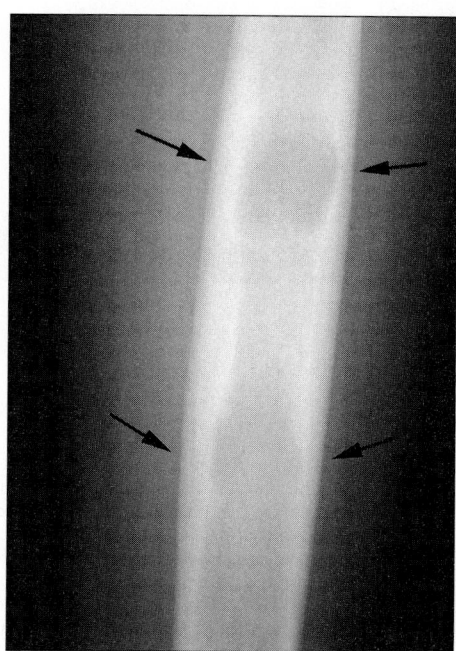
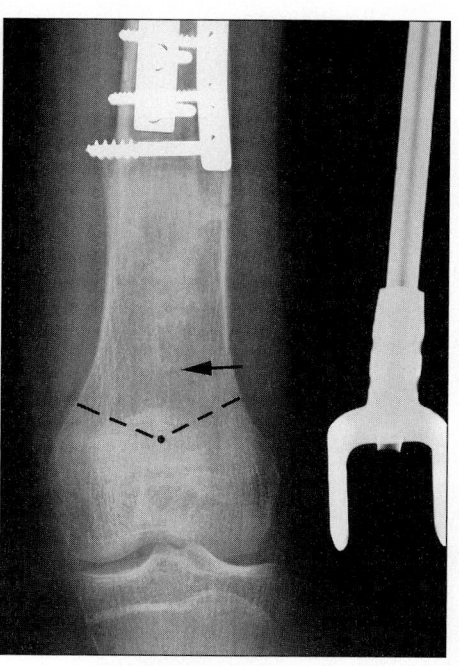

Figure 95-8. A, This x-ray, taken 6 years previously, demonstrates a lobulated intramedullary lesion (*arrows*) with expansion of the cortex, later proven to be primary low-grade chondrosarcoma. The lesion was resected and reconstructed using an intercallary deep frozen allograft at age 8 years. **B,** Five years later and approaching skeletal maturity at age 14 years, the patient developed discomfort in the distal left femur, where this AP x-ray demonstrates a likely distal marginal recurrence (*arrow*). The plate fixing the more proximal allograft can be seen. Open biopsy confirmed low-grade chondrosarcoma. A joint-sparing procedure was designed around a distal chevron osteotomy (*dashed line*), leaving a 2-cm distal margin. A custom tong-like implant can be seen laterally in the measurement film with the intramedullary nail to aid preoperative planning.

Continued

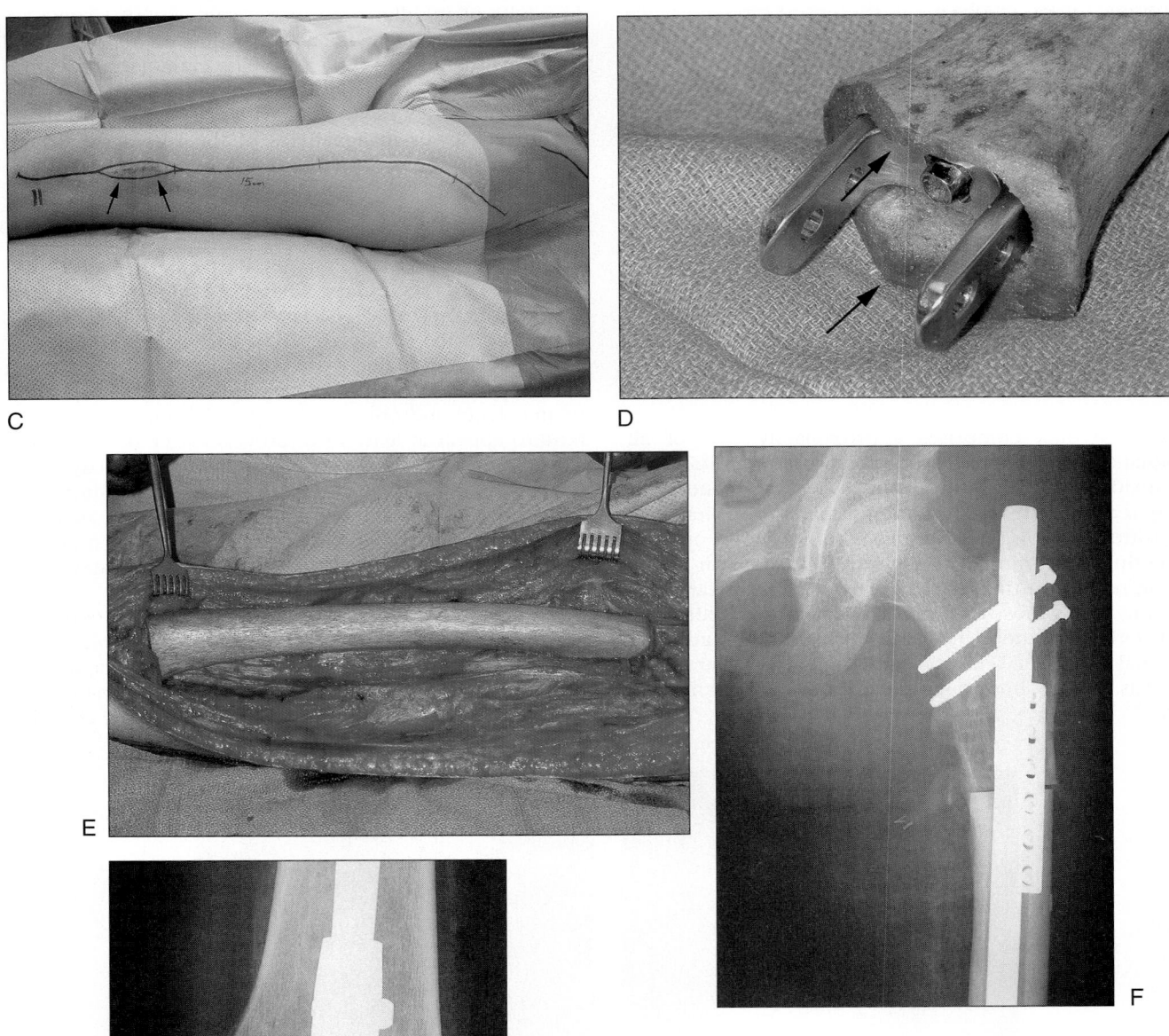

Figure 95-8, *cont'd*. C, This intraoperative photo demonstrates the recent biopsy scar (*arrows*) and the intended operative exposure, leaving the biopsy tract intact with the resection specimen. **D,** This photo shows the transepiphyseal tong-like terminal device on the end of the IM nail within the intramedullary canal of a deep frozen allograft. The distal osteotomy was fashioned with a complementary interlocking chevron osteotomy (*arrows*) to interlock with the host distal femoral osteotomy. **E,** The terminal device has been seated and secured distally, and proximal interlocking screws have been inserted through the intramedullary rod. This lateral view of the femur shows the complete construct. **F,** The AP x-ray of the proximal femur demonstrates the host/allograft juncture secured with an ancillary plate anteriorly, with the interlocking screws securing the proximal fixation. **G,** This AP x-ray of the distal femur illustrates the distal joint-sparing construct interlocking the inherently stable chevron allograft/host osteotomy.

sarcoma usually represents fewer than 5% of lesions.[413-415] Dedifferentiated chondrosarcoma is the most aggressive and malignant expression of chondroid tumors.[416,417] All of these lesions are considered high-grade.

The peripheral or secondary tumors are usually low grade, except for lesions arising in patients with Ollier's disease or Maffucci's syndrome, in which dedifferentiation is known to occur.[418-420] Approximately one third of chondrosarcomas reported are either secondary or peripheral in location.

Secondary chondrosarcoma is rare, comprising approximately 1% of all malignant bone tumors. Secondary chondrosarcoma can arise in solitary osteochondroma (Fig. 95-9), multiple osteochondroma, Ollier's disease, Maffucci's syndrome, synovial chondromatous fibrous dysplasia, and as a complication of radiation therapy. Large single-institution studies of secondary chondrosarcoma as a consequence of either single or multiple osteochondroma are helpful in better defining the appropriate method of management.

Ahmed and associates[421] described the Mayo Clinic experience with 107 patients developing secondary chondrosarcoma (61 with solitary and 46 with multiple lesions). They observed that the average age of onset was approximately 1 to 2 decades younger than patients who developed primary chondrosarcoma. The incidence of sarcomatous degeneration was 7.6% for the 802 patients with single osteochondroma and 36.3% for the 120 patients with multiple osteochondroma. Among patients with multiple osteochondroma, 28 patients had hereditary tendencies, while 14 did not.

In both groups, the flat bones were the most common site for malignant degeneration (ilium 19.7%, pubis 19.7%), with the proximal femur and distal femur as the second and third most common sites. Males were more commonly affected than females (ratio in solitary osteochondroma, 1.2:1; in multiple osteochondroma, 1.9:1). Multiplanar imaging, such as CT scanning or MRI, provided the most useful information in defining the relationship of the lesion to the underlying bone, matrix mineralization, presence of soft-tissue mass, and cortical destruction. Overall, MRI was found to be superior to CT scanning.

Cartilaginous cap thickness was available from 39 tumors, with a mean thickness of 3.9 cm (range, 0.5-15.0 cm), and dimensions were available on 77 tumors with a mean size of $9.5 \times 9.5 \times 9.5$ cm (range, 1.5 $\times 1.5 \times 1.5$ cm to $24 \times 24 \times 15$ cm). Permeation, manifested as nodules of cartilage separated from the main tumor and present in the secondary soft tissue, was present in 61 patients (39 in solitary osteochondroma and 22 in multiple osteochondroma). Ninety-seven tumors (60 solitary and 37 multiple) were considered grade I/II, while 10 (1 solitary and 9 multiple) were grade II/III. No grade III tumors were identified.

Radiographic Features

Primary or central chondrosarcomas arising from cartilaginous preformed bone can demonstrate cortical destruction and loss of normal medullary bone trabeculations. Evidence of punctate calcifications and destruction

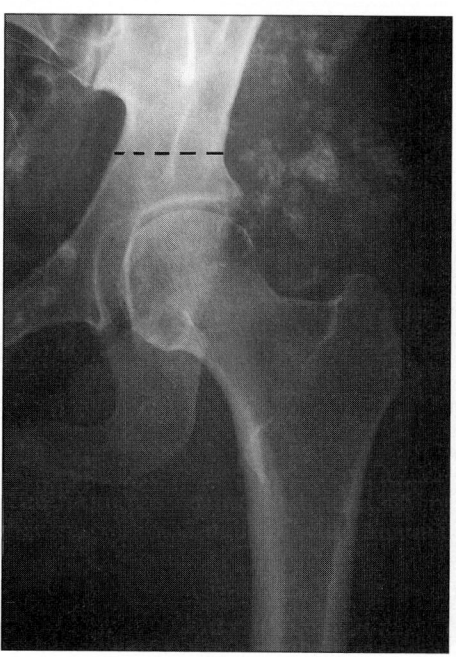
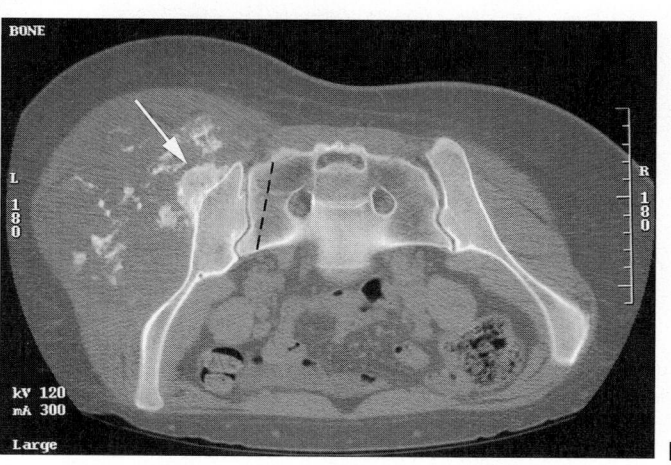

Figure 95-9. A, This AP x-ray of the left hip of a 33-year-old female reveals evidence of matrix calcification in the left buttock, thought to be responsible for pain and mass effect. The dashed lines illustrate the intended line of bone resection later used for resection. **B,** A CT scan was performed illustrating calcifications within the lesion believed to have grown as a secondary chondrosarcoma from the small osteochondroma (*white arrow*) from the outer table of the left ilium. The dashed line also illustrates the intended osteotomy through the left ala of the sacrum, used later to accomplish the resection of the ilium.

Continued

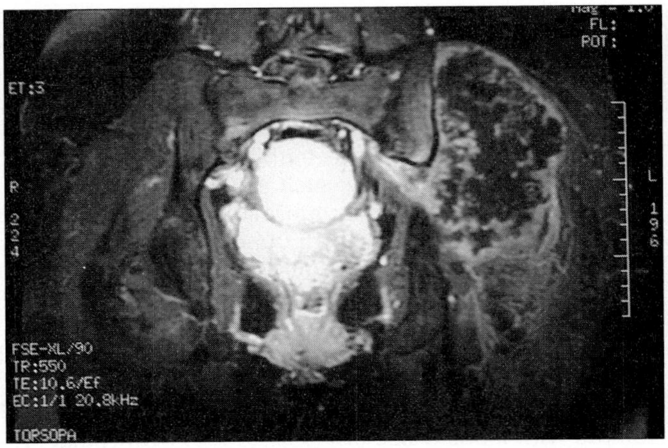

C

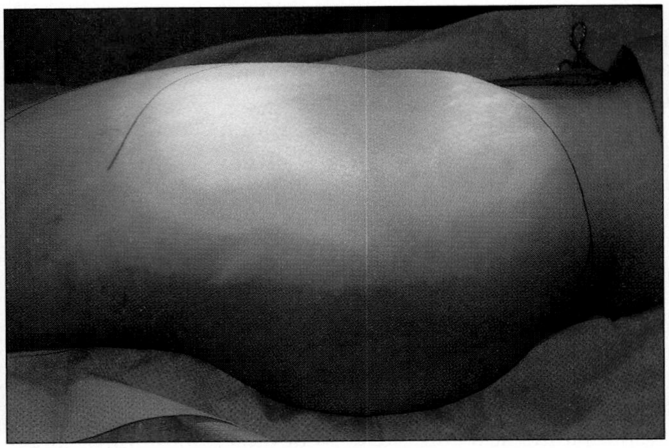

D

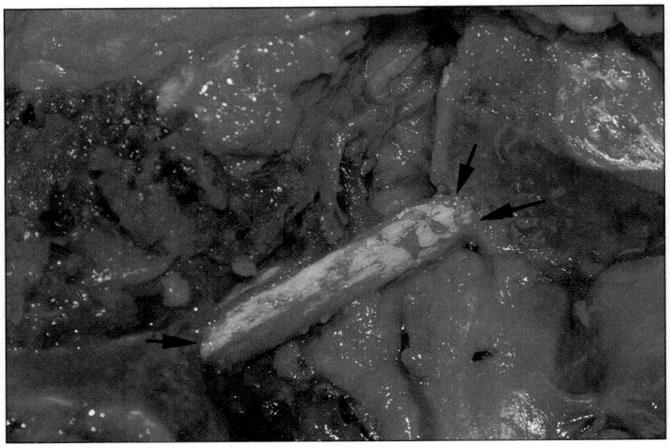

E

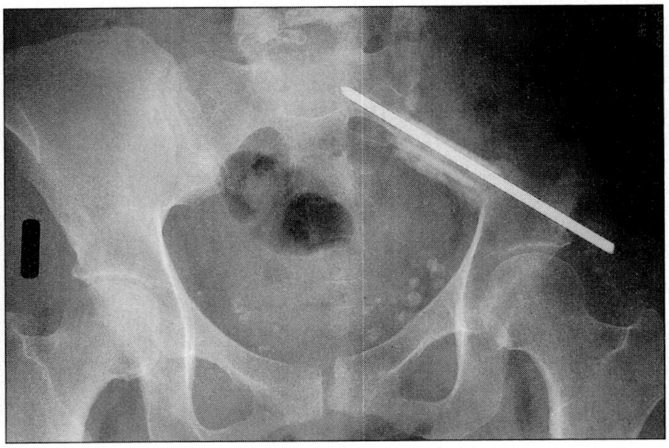

F

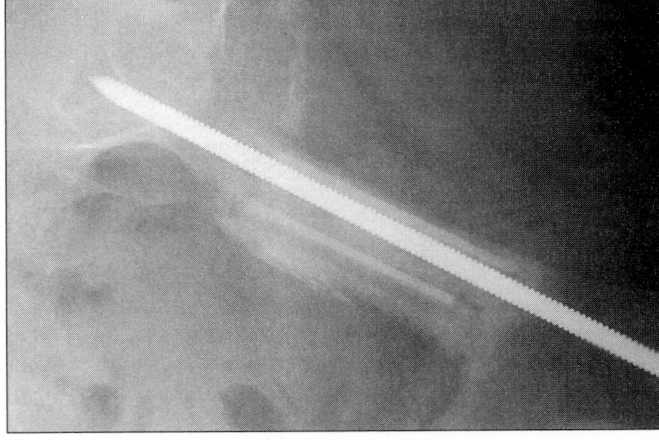

G

Figure 95-9, *cont'd.* C, The fat suppression MR demonstrates the lesion abutting the left sacro-iliac joint and extending into the soft tissues. A radical iliectomy was designed preoperatively with the bone resection margin through the supra-acetabulum region of the left hip and through the left ala of the sacrum. **D,** This intraoperative photo demonstrates the comprehensive exposure required for resection of the lesion sparing the superior gluteal vessel and nerve. **E,** This photo demonstrates the free fibular graft obtained from the left leg, spanning the defect between the dome of the acetabulum (*left, single arrow*) and the remaining left ala of the sacrum (*right, two arrows*). **F,** An AP of the pelvis 3 months after surgery demonstrates the secure free fibular graft stabilized with a Steinmann pin. The overall symmetry of the pelvis appears excellent. **G,** This close-up x-ray of the fibular graft demonstrates new bone about the underside and periphery of the fibular pelvic-stabilizing grafts at 6 months.

is commonly seen in chondrosarcoma. Lesions arising in the pelvis might not be recognized until late. Plain films of the pelvis are not sufficiently sensitive to identify small tumors.[99m]Tc bone scintigraphy is one of the most useful radiographic screening exams for chondrosarcoma. Magnetic resonance imaging most often demonstrates both the intramedullary extent of the tumor and the extraosseous extension and is necessary for appropriate preoperative planning.

Secondary or peripheral chondrosarcoma arises from preexisting lesions.[412] The slow increase in size of a previously recognized osteochondroma or increasing low-grade pain associated with an intramedullary lesion with punctate calcifications usually alerts the patient and physician to possible pathologic change. Computed tomography or MRI typically shows the remains of an osteochondroma with a thicker, less distinct cartilage cap. Central lesions might demonstrate endosteal erosion, destruction of calcifications, and associated cortical thickening.[422] Both lesions are usually identified on bone scintigraphy. If a previous bone scan is available, comparison with later scans usually shows evidence of increasing uptake, suggesting pathologic change. It is recommended that patients with Maffucci's or Ollier's disease have bone scans every 3 to 5 years after recognition of their disease to monitor potential malignant transformation.[418]

Geirnaerdt and colleagues[423] evaluated 37 patients with benign and malignant cartilaginous tumors using fast contrast-enhanced MRI in an effort to distinguish between malignant and benign lesions. Start of enhancement was considered early within 10 seconds, delayed between 10 seconds and 2 minutes, and late after 5 minutes on spin-echo images. The findings were correlated with surgical specimens in 27 cases, curettage material in 3, and biopsy material in 7.

Early enhancement was seen in chondrosarcoma but not in enchondroma and was observed in osteochondromata only after cessation of skeletal growth. The sensitivity was 89%, specificity 84%, positive predictive value 84%, and negative predictive value 89%. Differentiation of malignancy from benignity on the basis of early and exponential enhancement revealed a sensitivity of 61%, a specificity of 95%, a positive predictive value of 92%, and a negative predictive value of 72%. The start of enhancement and the combination of start and progression of enhancement correlated significantly (P < .001) with benign and malignant tumors.

Clear Cell Chondrosarcoma

Clear cell chondrosarcomas are expansile and osteolytic lesions most commonly arising in the epiphyseal regions of long bones (proximal femur and humerus). They are often described as cystic. They typically originate in the mature secondary ossification center, expanding and invading the surrounding soft tissues. The male-to-female ratio is 3:1, and the condition most often occurs after the first decade of life, with a rather even distribution up to the seventh decade.

Dedifferentiated Chondrosarcoma

Dedifferentiated chondrosarcomas also arise from pre-existing lesions that become dedifferentiated to a far more aggressive and malignant neoplasm, such as high-grade malignant fibrous histiocytoma of bone. The foci of dedifferentiated tissue usually destroy the underlying chondroid matrix and calcifications, leaving an area devoid of calcification and often producing a contiguous soft-tissue mass.

Pathologic Features

Many benign cartilaginous lesions mimic low-grade malignant lesions and must be distinguished histopathologically for appropriate treatment.[424,425] The clinical, radiographic, and histopathologic features must be correlated for an accurate diagnosis.[426,427]

Pain and an enlarging lesion in an adult are the most significant clinical factors in establishing a diagnosis of a low-grade malignant cartilage lesion. Lichtenstein and Jaffe[428] established the histopathologic criteria for malignancy, which include an increased number of binucleate cartilage cells, often associated with giant multinucleated cartilage cells. Multiple fields must be evaluated to observe focal areas of increased cellular activity. Most secondary chondrosarcomas will be found to be low grade.

Primary or central chondrosarcomas are more cellular, producing less chondroid tissue and more often, lobules of tumor tissue in the surrounding pseudocapsule. Radiographically, the majority demonstrate cortical disruption, loss of normal medullary trabeculations, and bone destruction. Occasionally, myxoid and cystic changes occur, and ossification can still be identified. Other, more aggressive lesions demonstrate spindle tumor cells growing in sheets. Cartilaginous tumors are not homogenous, and multiple fields must be evaluated to grade these tumors accurately.[429]

Clear cell chondrosarcoma is often diagnosed radiographically and confirmed histopathologically. Benign giant cells can be identified among the fine line of calcification between proliferating binucleated tumor cells. The tumor cells have a characteristic clear cytoplasm with distinct cytoplasmic borders. Lobulation is less prominent.[430-432]

Surgical Therapy

Surgical therapy varies from intralesion curettage for the very-low-grade lesions to radical amputations for the more aggressive high-grade chondrosarcomas and the dedifferentiated variety.[226,387,389-392,433] Secondary, very low-grade lesions arising from osteochondromatas or enchondromas with only minimal histopathologic suggestion of malignancy can be controlled by excision, with a cuff of normal tissue encompassing the cartilaginous cap, or by vigorous curettage. Secondary lesions arising from enchondromas with a more typical histopathology of binucleate and giant chondroid-producing cells should be treated with wide intramedullary and surrounding soft-tissue margins.

A study at the Mayo Clinic involved 107 patients with secondary chondrosarcoma (61 with solitary and 46 with multiple).[421] Overall, no patient with a wide resection developed locally recurrent disease; however, 45 patients did experience local recurrence (20 solitary chondrosarcomas and 25 multiple osteochondromas). The number of local recurrences ranged from 1 to 11, with 52 recurrences in 20 patients with solitary chondrosarcoma and 72 recurrences in patients with multiple osteochondromas. The average interval between surgery and the first local recurrence was 44.6 months for patients with solitary lesions and 24 months for patients with multiple lesions. Thirty patients in this series died, including 18 dying as a consequence of tumor. Patients with grade II tumor, tumors of the trunk, and multiple lesions were most likely to succumb to their disease. The majority of local recurrences developed within the first 5 years, and clinical follow-up should continue for at least 10 and preferably 15 years.

High-grade primary lesions should be managed with a minimum of a wide margin (surgical plane passing through absolutely normal nonreactive tissue) or an amputation or disarticulation with wide margins. Because tumor growth occurs by expansion of the tumor mass and by lobulation, generous soft-tissue margins must be provided to include all tumor tissue.[393,434,435] Cartilagenous tumor cells can survive in even the most hostile environments and can easily be implanted in the soft-tissues.

Clear cell chondrosarcoma also requires a wide margin for local control. Most often, the difficulty arises in making the appropriate diagnosis. Cystic formation within the lesion, along with the presence of giant cells, often leads to an incorrect diagnosis, such as aneurysmal bone cyst (Fig. 95-10). Intralesional curettage is not sufficient to manage this distinct but rare entity.[430,431]

Dedifferentiated chondrosarcoma is managed surgically with wide to radical margins. The majority of patients who develop high-grade tumors benefit from neoadjuvant and/or adjuvant chemotherapy and radical surgery. Often, patients require compartmental margins because of the location, local tumor invasion, and infiltrative nature of the dedifferentiated element of the tumor. Few patients survive this disease.[391,416,417,432]

Extraskeletal chondrosarcoma is also considered high grade and is managed surgically by either wide or compartmental margins. Unfortunately, the majority of high-grade chondrosarcomas respond only to surgical therapy. Radiotherapy and multiagent chemotherapy may be used for palliation.

EWING'S SARCOMA

The pathologic process currently known as Ewing's sarcoma was described as early as 1866 by Lücke.[436] It became widely known in 1921, as James Ewing described the condition as endothelial myeloma, a lesion he believed to be of perivascular endothelial origin. In 1939, Ewing reclassified the tumor as a neoplasm separate from osteosarcoma.[437]

A number of cell types have been proposed as the cell of origin. In addition to pericytic cells, these include mesenchymal, myeloid, reticular, neuroepithelial, and primitive multipotential cells.[436-444] Ewing's sarcoma is one of the recognized small round cell tumor variants. Commonly, sophisticated immunochemistry, electron microscopy, and cytogenetic and molecular genetic techniques are required to distinguish Ewing's sarcoma from other small round cell neoplasms. These entities include neuroblastoma, embryonal rhabdomyosarcoma, osteomyelitis, small cell osteosarcoma, and non-Hodgkin's lymphoma.[438]

Epidemiology

Ewing's sarcoma is the third most common primary sarcoma of bone, comprising approximately 10% of all primary bone tumors.[439] As with many pediatric solid tumors, males are slightly more affected than females. The peak incidence in males is between 10 and 14 years of age, while in females it is 5 to 9 years (range, 1 year to 80 years). Ewing's sarcoma is distinctly rare in blacks and uncommon in Chinese.[440,441] The majority of patients present for medical treatment between 5 and 30 years of age.

Etiology and Pathogenesis

Evidence of cytogenetic and molecular genetic abnormalities shared with the more differentiated peripheral neuroectodermal tumor (PNET) suggests that Ewing's sarcoma is a tumor of parasympathetic nerve origin.[445] Identification of primitive neuroectodermal tumor of bone, however, is reserved for those tumors that show some evidence of neurosecretory-type granules on electron microscopy and that demonstrate positive immunoreactive markers for neuron-specific enolase (NSE) and neurofilaments. Cell membrane neural antigens and acetylcholinesterase production have also been demonstrated.[446-448]

Clinical Manifestations

Ewing's sarcoma arises from within the medullary canal of bone. Distant metastases are most common to the lung and bone. The tumor often produces a painful soft-tissue mass overlying and surrounding the involved bone. Ewing's sarcoma of the extremities primarily affects the long tubular bones, such as the femur, tibia, proximal fibula, and humerus. Approximately 20% to 40% of lesions arise in the pelvis and flat bones and often produce bizarre and unusual symptoms that result in delays in diagnosis.

Tumors arising in the pelvis are often large (>10 cm in diameter) at the time of diagnosis, and many patients have demonstrable distant disease at diagnosis. Primary tumors arising in the spine most often present with pain and can exhibit a rapidly progressive neurologic deficit. This symptom complex frequently precipitates an emergent decompressive laminectomy, at which time the diagnosis is often made.

Patients often appear systemically ill. Clinical manifestations include rapid growth, local pain, and low-grade fever. Pathologically, hemorrhage and necrosis are common. Unfortunately, patients' use of aspirin products in an attempt to control discomfort and fever can result in even greater intralesional hemorrhages, leading to further swelling and pain.

Radiographic Features

Ewing's sarcoma characteristically produces a permeative destructive pattern in bone often associated with a soft-tissue mass. In tubular bones, the lesions most often arise in the diaphysis or the metaphyseal/diaphyseal region and can demonstrate both an extrinsic pressure phenomenon and bone hypertrophy. As mentioned, plain films of the pelvis can be deceptively normal, while a ^{99m}Tc bone scan, CT or MRI, and other investigative measures might demonstrate both the destructive process and the extent of marrow involvement. Consequently, plain films of the

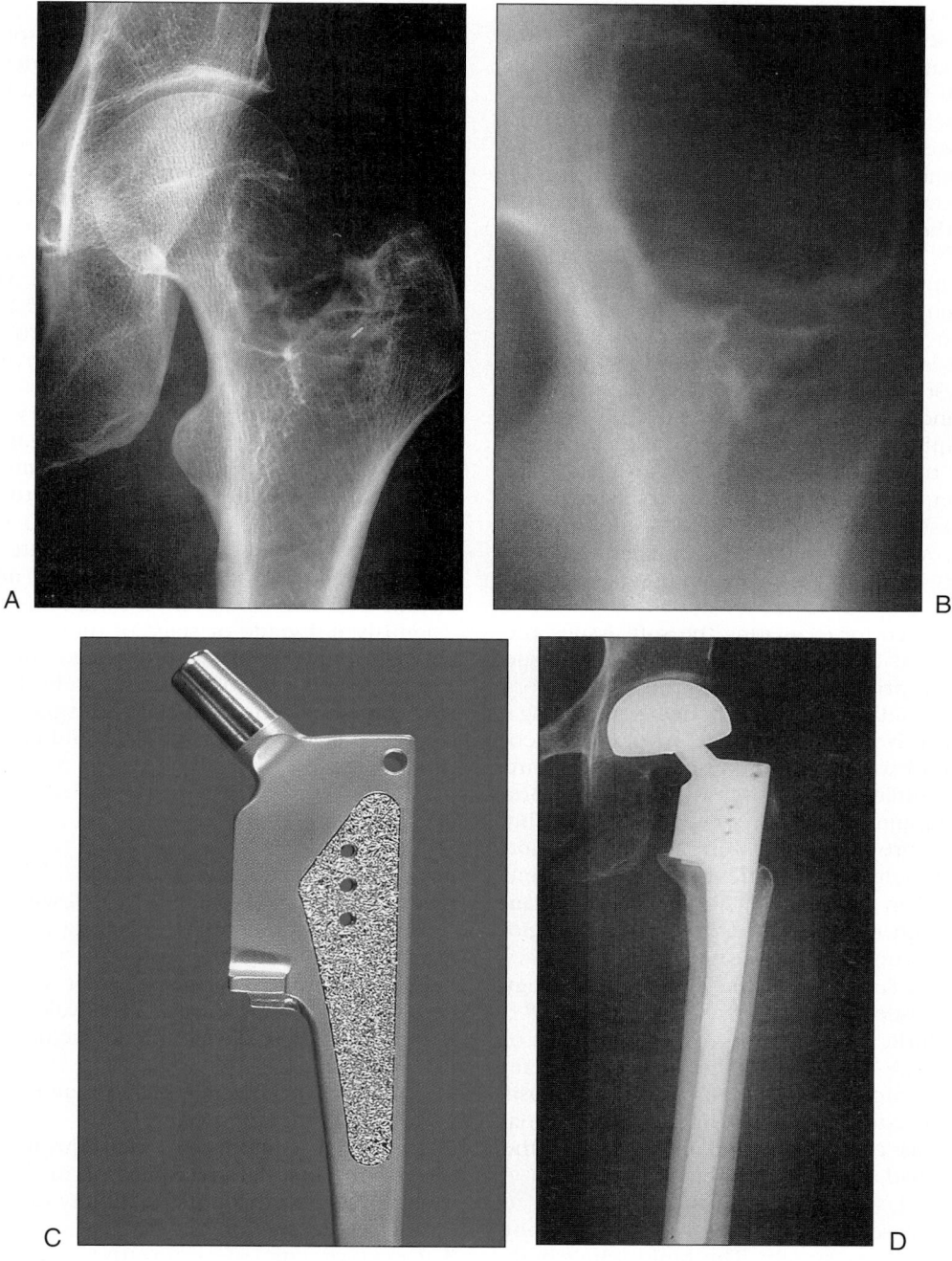

Figure 95-10. A, After 6 months of pain and discomfort involving the left anterior thigh and groin, an AP radiograph of the proximal femur revealed a relatively well-marginated lesion involving the lateral neck and greater trochanter of the proximal femur in a 38-year-old male. **B,** Conventional AP polytomes of the lesion confirmed a relatively well-marginated lesion of the proximal femur and trochanter. No radiographically identifiable matrix could be identified within the lesion. Open biopsy was performed, revealing a cellular cartilaginous neoplasm composed of large cells with clear cytoplasm. The combination of the location of the lesion, its radiographic "soap bubble appearance, and the histopathology confirmed the diagnosis of clear cell chondrosarcoma. **C,** This photo illustrates a press-fit custom titanium calcar-replacing prosthesis with titanium mesh for bone ingrowth used for reconstruction. **D,** Radiograph demonstrating the AP projection of the custom titanium press-fit (cementless) proximal femoral prosthesis.

pelvis or other deep structures should not be used alone as a screening method, but only in conjunction with other studies.

Bone scintigraphy often aids in identifying the bone or bones involved and to some extent the degree of intramedullary involvement. The conventional ^{99m}Tc bone scan is ideal to screen for metastatic disease.[36] To gain additional information regarding the extent and location of involvement of the primary lesion, occasionally SPECT is required. [67]Ga scintigraphy can often assist in identifying the soft-tissue extent of disease. Comparative serial ^{201}Tl scans of the primary tumor are reported as helpful in assessing the effectiveness of neoadjuvant chemotherapy before and after the completion of the neoadjuvant multi-agent regimen. [201]Tl and ^{99m}Tc scintigraphy in primary bone tumors are most effective when used in conjunction with other imaging modalities, such as CT and MRI.[148] [67]Ga and ^{99m}Tc phosphate compounds alone are inadequate to assess the tumor's response to therapy.[449]

CT of the chest to assess the presence of pulmonary metastases is mandatory to stage a patient with Ewing's sarcoma radiographically. The use of CT in the evaluation of the primary tumor can be valuable in illustrating bone destruction, but it might not demonstrate the associated soft-tissue mass, which is often isodense with the surrounding soft tissues. The CT information can be supplementary to the superior imaging data obtained from MRI.

MRI is ideally suited for evaluating the soft tissues, the intramedullary extent of disease, and adjacent soft-tissue involvement of the primary lesion. Currently, for tumors arising in the medullary canal of bone (e.g., Ewing's sarcoma, histiocytic lymphoma of bone, myeloma, osteosarcoma, and chrondrosarcoma), MRI remains the standard by which other studies are compared for staging, preoperative planning, and patient follow-up.[22] MRI probably has contributed more to the appropriate surgical and radiotherapy management of patients with bone and soft-tissue lesions than any other technology. A physician-monitored MRI often eliminates the need for CT, angiography, and conventional tomography of the primary tumor. An excellent summary of the diagnostic strategy for bone and soft-tissue tumors is available for review.[18]

PET alone has little application in the management of patients with Ewing's sarcoma but has provided useful data regarding chemotherapy-induced tumor necrosis before and after neoadjuvant chemotherapy. Sequential PET and ^{201}Tl scans could be useful in predicting the effectiveness of neoadjuvant chemotherapy regimens.

The use of rapid whole-body or turboSTIR MRI to detect occult metastases complements bone scintigraphy for total-body skeletal assessment. The rapid whole-body STIR MRI has the added advantage of detecting soft-tissue and unrecognized central nervous system (CNS) metastases.[44] With continued development, this study could become commonplace in future staging studies.

Differential Diagnosis

The histopathologic similarity of Ewing's sarcoma to other small round cell tumors results in a diagnostic challenge for the surgical pathologist. The lesion must be distinguished from lymphoma of bone, rhabdomyosarcoma, metastatic neuroblastoma, small cell osteosarcoma, osteomyelitis, metastatic small cell carcinoma of the lung, mesenchymal chondrosarcoma, and occasionally, metastatic hemangiopericytoma. The responsible surgeon must obtain viable tissue for routine histopathology, touch preparations, sterile tissue for cytogenetics, a small sample for electron microscopy, and tissue and fluid for culture and sensitivity.

The challenges of diagnosis were illustrated by Wurtz and associates[450] in a retrospective review of a single institution with 68 patients who had primary bone sarcoma of the pelvic girdle. They found that the average duration of symptoms before accurate diagnosis was 10 months (range, 1 month to 4 years). Common symptoms included buttock pain (35%), presence of a mass (30%), sciatica (29%), groin pain (26%), and low back pain (21%). Inaccurate diagnoses were made in 44% of patients (e.g., herniated disc, spinal stenosis, spondylolisthesis, bursitis, stress fracture, urinary retention, etc.). Inappropriate treatment for these diagnoses included seven operative procedures (two laminectomies, two débridements, one hip arthrotomy, one total knee replacement, and one inguinal herniorrhaphy). On the average, 7 months elapsed before an accurate diagnosis was made. Review of the clinical data did not find an association between duration of symptoms before accurate diagnosis and grade or stage of tumors or an association between duration of symptoms and survival (P = 0.54). The grade and stage of the tumor were strongly associated with outcome, however, with low-grade tumor proving to be a favorable prognostic indicator for survival (P = 0.006).

Surgical Therapy

Radiotherapy, with few exceptions, has been the treatment of choice for patients with Ewing's sarcoma until recently. Developments in surviving patients have led to a reassessment of the role of surgery in providing management of the primary tumor with sustained local control and minimal risk of developing a secondary malignancy. These developments include:

1. A local recurrence rate higher than initially appreciated with radiotherapy alone.[451,452]
2. Improved combination neoadjuvant chemotherapy, resulting in a marked reduction in the soft-tissue mass and thus improving the feasibility of surgical resection and reconstruction.
3. Development of innovative surgical techniques combined with the use of soft-tissue flaps for improved wound coverage and limb function.
4. Advances in modular tumor prosthesis design, using improved materials that are resistant to fatigue and early failure.
5. Realization of the oncogenic potentiation of combined chemotherapy and radiotherapy for development of late secondary malignancies within the radiation portal and tumor bed of surviving patients.

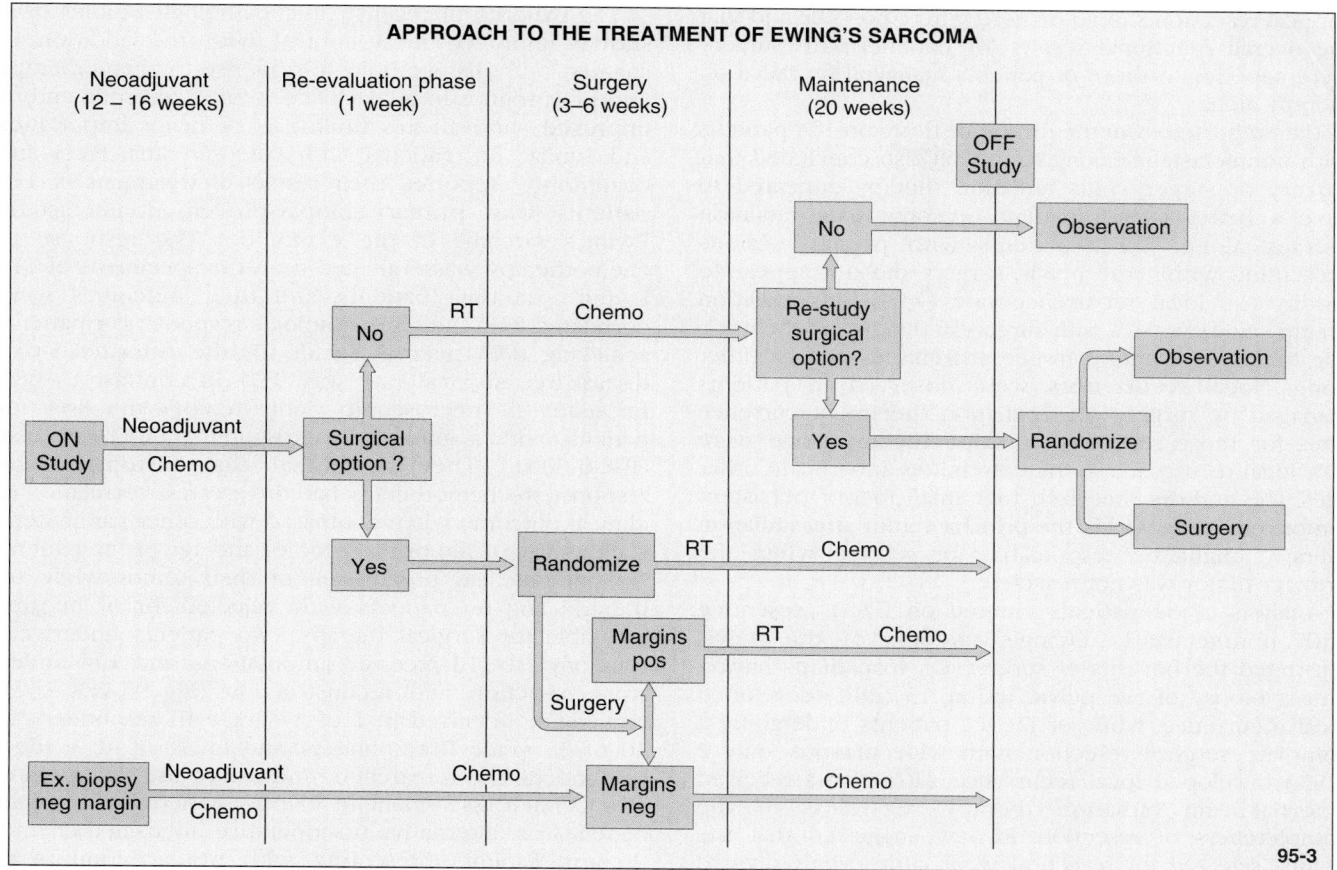

APPROACH TO THE TREATMENT OF EWING'S SARCOMA

95-3

The role of surgical therapy as an adjunct in the treatment of patients with Ewing's sarcoma of bone is now well established. Since Ewing's original description of the use of a radium pack in treating a patient with Ewing's sarcoma of the ulna, surgery (primarily amputation, etc.) has been reserved primarily for the management of bulky destructive lesions, pathologic fractures, or local failures of radiation therapy. It was well recognized that radiation therapy could control the primary tumor until the majority of patients developed systemic disease and died, usually within 2 years.

The development of aggressive multiagent adjuvant chemotherapy in the 1970s was an attempt to control the late development of systemic disease. It soon became apparent that aggressive induction chemotherapy before local therapy often resulted in tumor regression.[453] As more patients survived their disease, the issue of local control became more important.

Current Considerations in Surgical Therapy

In 1975, Pritchard and coworkers[454] reported a retrospective review of 194 patients with nonmetastatic Ewing's sarcoma treated between 1912 and 1968. They concluded that survival improved when the primary tumor presented in the extremities rather than in other sites. For patients with primary extremity lesions who had had surgical treatment, 44.7% survived for 5 years, whereas patients managed by nonsurgical means experienced a 13.1% survival. The most common method of surgical management was amputation. The 5- and 10-year survival rates for all patients who had surgery was approximately 30%; in patients treated by nonsurgical methods, the survival rate was 10%.

These retrospective data could be compared with the IESS-I prospective data involving 334 patients with Ewing's sarcoma. Fifty-seven patients had either a partial or complete surgical resection even though the protocol did not request surgical therapy. None of the primary tumors appeared to be favorable for resection. A statistically significant advantage in prognosis was suggested in both time to relapse ($P = 0.03$) and survival ($P = 0.01$) for patients receiving surgery over patients receiving radiation therapy alone.[455] A later IESS-I review of patients with primary rib lesions, however, suggested that the apparent prognostic advantage of patients undergoing surgical excision of the ribs could have been explained by patient selection.[456]

In 1981, Rosen and coworkers[457] published their 10-year experience of 67 consecutive patients with nonmetastatic Ewing's sarcoma. Of the 34 patients receiving radiation therapy as the only mode of local therapy, 7 (21%) developed local recurrence. No local relapses were reported among the 13 patients who had amputation alone (primarily distal lesions) or among the 20 who had surgery plus radiation therapy. The authors concluded that surgical resection should be used where possible and that the overall functional results for patients with surgery were superior to those of patients managed by radiation therapy alone.

Data reported from the Rizzoli Institute on 124 patients with nonmetastatic Ewing's sarcoma also concluded that surgery or surgery plus radiation therapy appeared to have a better overall patient outcome than radiation therapy alone.[458] For patients with primary lesions presenting within the pelvis, surgery did not appear to modify the local recurrence rate (43% with radiation therapy alone vs. 33% with surgery and radiation therapy). For tumors presenting in the extremities and/or other bones, local recurrences were observed in patients managed by surgery plus radiation therapy. Recurrence rates for those receiving radiation therapy alone were 30% local recurrence in the extremities and 18% in other sites. The authors theorized that small foci of persistent tumor remaining within the primary tumor after radiation therapy might be responsible for relapse when the primary tumor was not resected.

Analysis of 62 patients entered on IESS-I presenting with nonmetastatic Ewing's sarcoma of the pelvis illustrated the benefits of surgery. Of 46 patients having only a biopsy of the pelvic lesion, 13 (28%) developed local recurrence, while of the 11 patients undergoing a complete surgical resection with wide margins, only 2 (18%) developed local recurrence. All patients received external-beam radiation therapy regardless of the completeness of resection. Review suggested that the lesions selected for resection were fairly evenly divided among primary tumors of the ilium, pubis, and sacrum. Of the 29 patients with tumors of the ilium, 8 (28%) developed local recurrence after biopsy alone, while no patient undergoing a complete surgical resection developed local recurrence.[459] Other reports demonstrating improved local control in surgically treated patients include those by Wilkins and colleagues[460] from the Mayo Clinic, Juergens and coworkers[461] from Germany, and Sailer and associates[462] from Boston.

To better determine the effects of size of the tumor and local failure for patients treated with radiotherapy alone, Göbel and associates[463] concluded that the improved prognosis enjoyed by patients managed by surgery was due in part to a biased distribution of smaller tumor volumes. It appeared that more patients with smaller tumors were being managed by surgical therapy.

Toni and others[464] reviewed 131 patients from 1972 to 1987 with primary nonmetastatic Ewing's sarcoma limited to the extremities. Local treatment of the primary tumor included amputation, resection with or without radiotherapy, or radiotherapy alone. All patients were analyzed for prognostic significance along with time to relapse at both local and distant sites. The surgical specimens were sectioned, and all surgical margins were classified according to the previously described Musculoskeletal Surgical Staging System. Sixty-nine of 131 patients (53%) had either an amputation or surgical resection. Thirty-eight patients (29%) had wide margins and no adjuvant radiotherapy. The local recurrence rate for patients managed by surgery alone was 5%.

The majority of recent clinicopathologic studies have shown improved local control with the addition of surgery.[465,466] Histopathologic response to chemotherapy appears prognostic for reduced local recurrence and/or improved survival; this finding is of major importance and similar for patients with osteosarcoma. Picci and coauthors[467] reported their results of treatment of 118 patients with primary biopsy-proven, nonmetastatic Ewing's sarcoma of the extremities. The response to chemotherapy was evaluated from the specimens of 118 Ewing's sarcoma patients, and their outcomes were correlated with the histopathologic response. For patients achieving 100% necrosis (grade III), the estimated 5-year disease-free survival rate was 95%, in contrast to 68% for grade II (microscopic viable tumor) and 34% for patients with a grade I (macroscopic tumor) response (P < 0.0001). They concluded that histopathologic response to chemotherapy had the greatest correlation to clinical outcome when compared with other parameters, such as size of the primary tumor and age of the patient. No patients had progression of their tumor while on therapy, and no patients were rejected for or became ineligible for surgical therapy. Two patients underwent rotationplasty, 12 received amputations, and 104 underwent resection and reconstruction (Fig. 95-11). Local recurrence occurred in 2 of 37 grade III responders, in 10 of 35 grade II responders, and in 31 of 46 grade I responders. The researchers propose to use this method of specimen assessment to identify patients who might benefit from alternative postoperative intensified chemotherapy. Patients presenting with primary tumors of sacrum, pelvis, and spine, however, have a poor prognosis. The overall impact of operative treatment on outcome or survival of patients with Ewing's sarcoma of the pelvis or sacrum has recently been questioned.[468]

Paulussen and colleagues[469] described the final results of the CESS 86 study aimed at improving event-free survival in patients with high-risk, localized Ewing's tumor of bone. Between January 1986 and July 1991, 470 patients with localized Ewing's tumor of bone were enrolled in CESS 86. Of the 301 patients meeting the inclusion criteria, 180 were male (60%). The median age at diagnosis was 15 years (range, 8.5 months to 47 years). The patients were treated in 92 institutions in Germany, Austria, the Netherlands, and Switzerland. Open biopsies were performed in all patients. Metastases were excluded by chest CT scan, bone marrow aspirates from two or more distant sites, and whole-body technetium bone scan. Tumor volumes were calculated using plain radiograph and computed-tomography scans.

Tumor volume was used to allocate the patients to risk groups. The median tumor volume was 145 mL (range, 2 mL to 2069 mL). Exact tumor volumes were available in 228 patients: 86 patients (38%) had tumor volumes of less than 100 mL; 57 patients (26%) had tumor volumes of 100 mL to 200 mL; and 85 patients (37%) had tumor volumes greater than 200 mL. Patients were allocated into two risk groups and treated accordingly. Patients with small (<100 mL) extremity tumors were classified as "standard risk" patients (n = 52), and patients with tumor volumes of greater than 100 mL (n = 177) and/or central-axis tumors

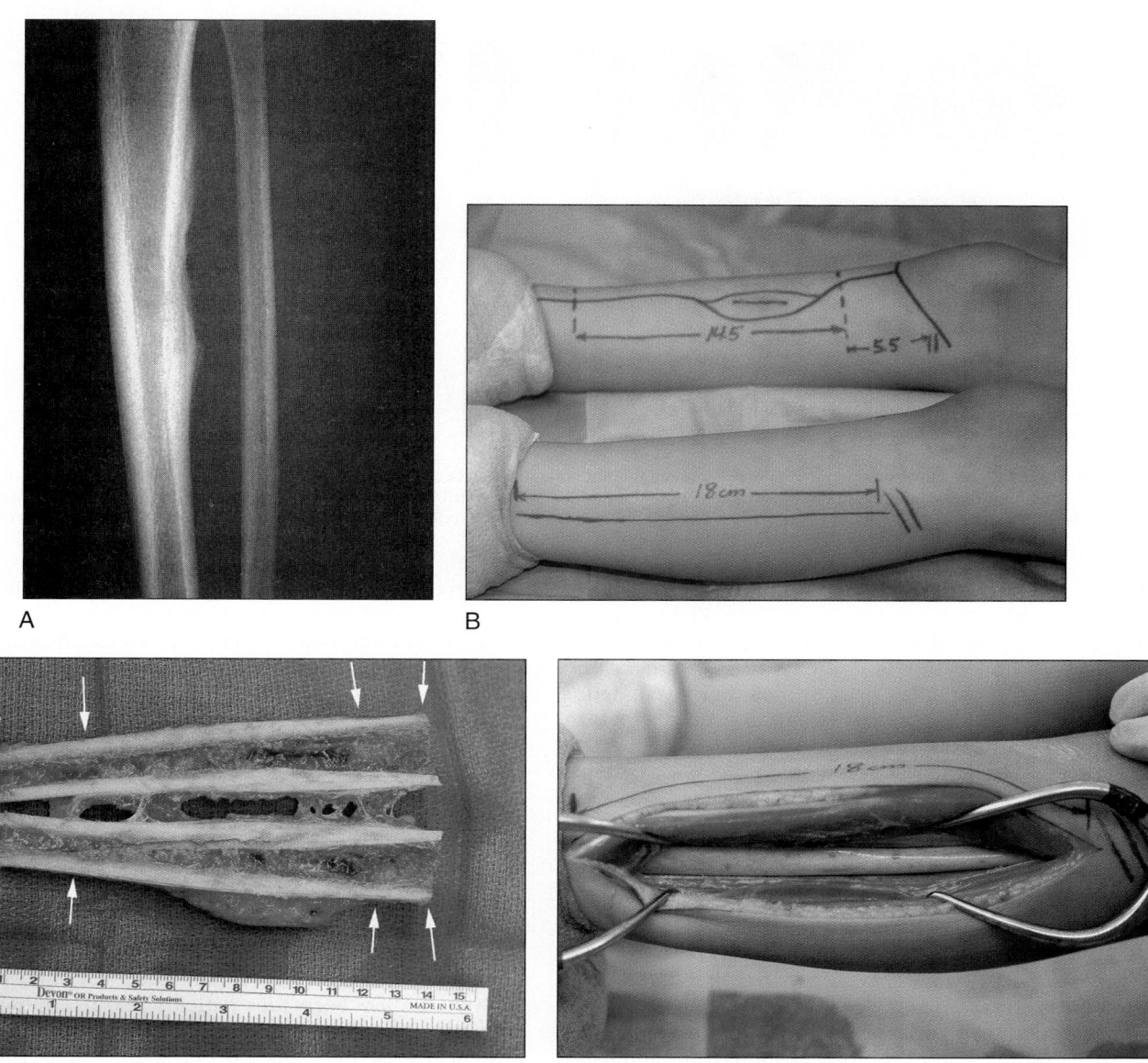

A

B

C

D

Figure 95-11. A, This lateral x-ray of the right leg of a 7-year-old white male demonstrates a destructive lesion in the diaphysis, later proven to be Ewing's sarcoma. The patient was found to be otherwise free of disease. **B,** After completing 12 weeks of standard preoperative multiagent chemotherapy, a restaging MR suggested an excellent response, with evidence of a normal marrow signal both proximal and distally to the diaphyseal tumor. It was elected to proceed with a resection of 14.5 cm of the midshaft of the right tibia, sparing 5.5 cm of proximal tibia and reconstructing the surgical defect with an 18-cm left free fibular graft. **C,** The surgical resection specimen was taken to the back table and split to be certain that the proximal (*right arrows*) and distal intramedullary margin (*left arrows*) were appropriate. **D,** Using separate gowns, gloves, and instruments, a free avascular fibular graft was obtained from the left midshaft fibula with iliac crest graft as well.

Continued

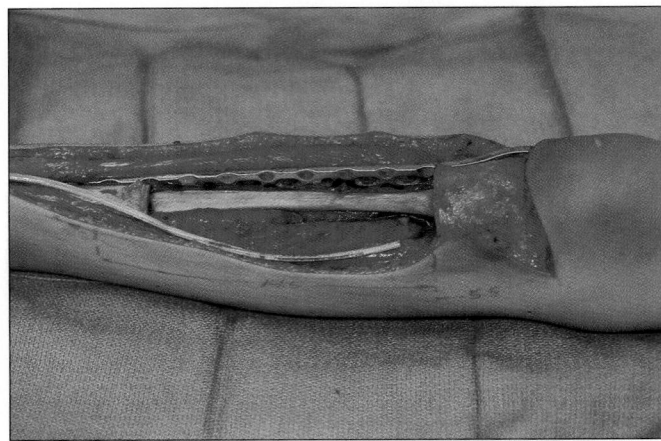

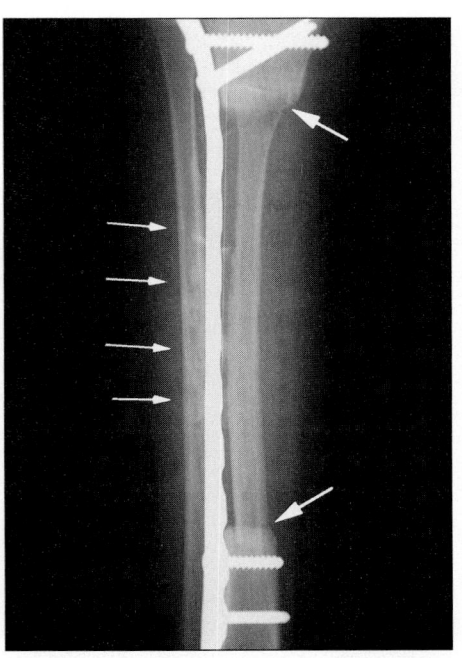

E

F

Figure 95-11, *cont'd.* **E,** This intraoperative photo illustrates the fibular graft in place and secured with a bone plate. Iliac crest autologous graft was used to augment the proximal and distal host/graft bone juncture. **F,** This 6-month postoperative x-ray demonstrates the developing synostosis between the fibula and free fibular graft (*small white arrows*) and healing of the proximal and distal host-graft bone junctures (*single arrows*).

(skull, shoulder, chest, spine, pelvic bones; n = 164) were classified as high-risk patients (n = 241). Eight patients could not be classified on the basis of these criteria. Local therapy was surgery for 68 patients (23%), surgery and radiation for 146 patients (49%), or radiotherapy alone for 82 patients (28%). Local therapy was delivered at a median of 12 weeks after diagnosis, and five had local therapy after the end of chemotherapy. Eighty percent of patients received local therapy between 9 and 20 weeks.

In CESS 86, larger tumors were observed more frequently than expected from the results of CESS 81. This resulted in changing the prognostic threshold of volume to 200 mL rather than 100 mL. The 10-year event-free survival rate was 52%. The event-free survival did not differ between the high-risk and standard-risk therapy groups. Tumor volume of greater than 200 mL and poor histologic response had a negative impact on event-free survival. In multivariant analyses, small tumor volumes of less than 200 mL, good histologic response, and intensive chemotherapy argued for a fair outcome.

Bacci and coworkers[470] retrospectively reviewed 91 consecutive patients treated for Ewing's sarcoma of the femur in an attempt to eliminate selection bias toward those treated with surgery with or without radiotherapy and those treated by radiotherapy alone at other locations. Chemotherapy consisted of four different protocols of neoadjuvant and adjuvant management. The primary tumor was treated by surgery alone in 54 patients, by surgery plus radiotherapy in 13, and by radiotherapy alone in 23 patients. One patient was treated by chemotherapy alone.

At a median follow-up of 10 years, 48 patients (53%) remained free of disease, 39 (43%) developed relapse,

and two died of chemotherapy toxicity; two developed a radiation-induced second tumor. The probability of survival without local recurrence was significantly higher (P = 0.01) for patients who were treated by surgery with or without radiotherapy (88%) than for patients who received radiotherapy alone (59%). The 5- and 10-year overall survival rates were 64% and 57%, respectively. The authors concluded that patients with Ewing's sarcoma of the femur achieved better local control with surgery alone or surgery plus radiotherapy than by radiotherapy alone.

Sluga and associates[471] analyzed the impact of wide surgical margins of resection of the primary tumor in the treatment of Ewing's sarcoma. They reviewed 86 patients who had systemic chemotherapy and surgery (biopsy in 6 patients and tumor resection in 80 patients) between 1980 and 1984. Forty-four patients also had radiotherapy as part of local control therapy (Fig. 95-12). The 5-year overall disease-free survival rate was 59.4%. The 5-year disease-free survival rate for patients having radical or wide surgical margins was 58.2%, while the rate for patients with marginal or intralesional resection margins was 40.1%. Two patients with inadequate resection margins developed local recurrences. The authors also noted that patients having a good histologic response to neoadjuvant chemotherapy had a 5-year overall survival rate of 80.2%, vs. 41.7% for those with a poor response. They concluded that adequate surgical margins (either radical or wide) significantly affected the outcome of patients with Ewing's sarcoma.

Surgical treatment of patients with Ewing's sarcoma arising in pelvic bones has improved, principally because of improved imaging techniques, improved neoadjuvant

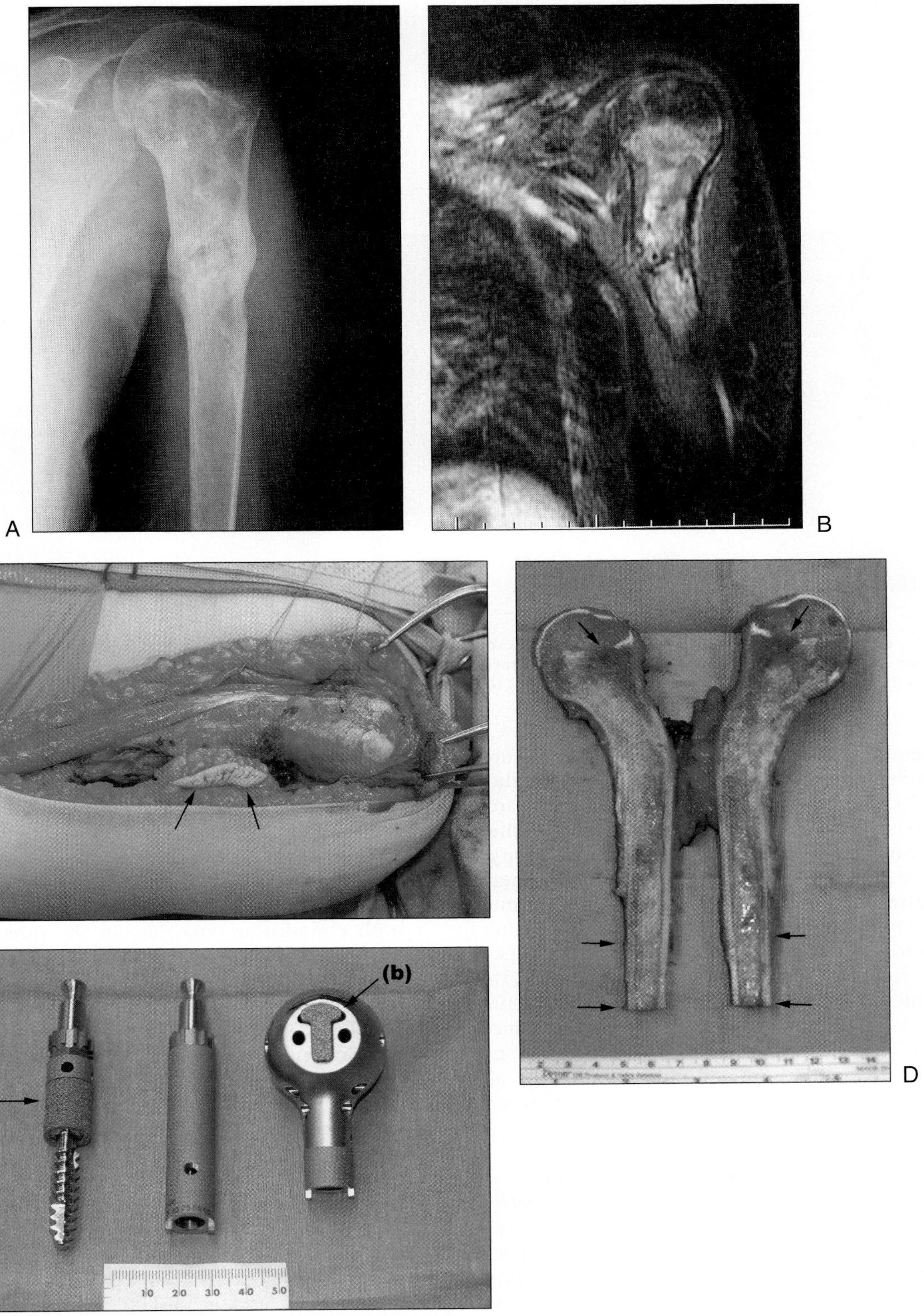

Figure 95-12. A, This internal rotation AP x-ray demonstrates an attempt at healing of a pathological fracture through a previously irradiated Ewing's sarcoma of the left nondominant humerus of a 12-year-old female after completing chemotherapy. **B,** The coronal MR better demonstrates a nonunion and angulation. There was a clinical concern regarding persistent tumor in the proximal humerus. After a prolonged period of conservative care, it was elected to proceed with resection and reconstruction using a custom modular titanium prosthesis. **C,** This intraoperative view demonstrates the circumferential anterior exposure of the proximal two thirds of the humerus, sparing the rotator cuff and radial nerve. The arrows identify the contiguous previous biopsy incision and the humerus to provide an en bloc "wide" resection. **D,** Once removed, the specimen is split to confirm appropriate margins distally (2.5 cm; *arrows*). Note the closure of the epiphysis in the humeral head after external beam radiotherapy (*arrow* in humeral head). **E,** A custom modular titanium prosthesis was designed and constructed using tantalum trabecular metal to allow bone ingrowth, promote extracortical fixation of the implant/host juncture, and allow for soft-tissue reattachment to the humeral head.

Continued

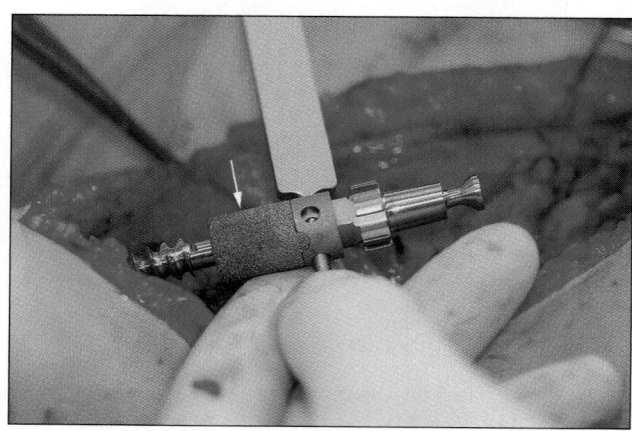

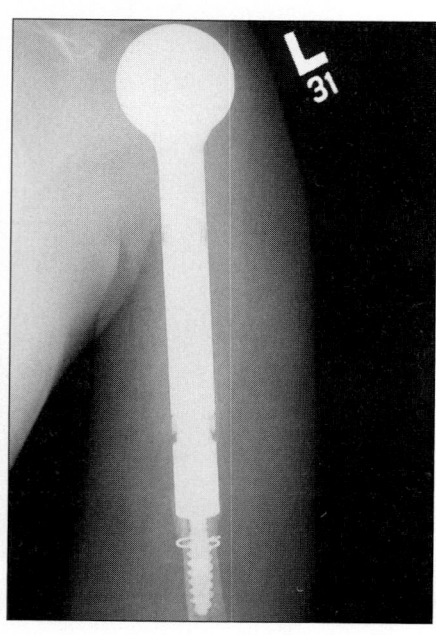

Figure 95-12, *cont'd.* **F,** This intraoperative view demonstrates securing of the implant to bone using a screw design to bring the tantalum trabecular metal (*arrow*) in juxtaposition to the shaft of the resection margin to promote extracortical bone bridging. **G,** This postoperative x-ray demonstrates the construct after reconstructing the rotator cuff to the implant and closure.

chemotherapy regimens, and an improved surgical understanding of the disease. Frassica and coauthors[472] reviewed 21 patients with nonmetastatic Ewing's sarcoma of the pelvis. Thirteen of the 21 received chemotherapy and radiation therapy, and 8 received chemotherapy and local operative resection with or without postoperative radiotherapy. The actuarial 5-year overall survival rate for patients having chemotherapy and radiation therapy without surgical resection was 25%, while patients with a surgical resection had a 75% survival rate (P < 0.005, log-rank method). The actuarial overall 5-year survival was 45% for patients presenting without evidence of metastases. The rate of local failure was 44% for the group managed by chemotherapy and radiation therapy alone, compared with 13% for patients with a local resection (P > 0.25, log-rank method).

Surgical Therapy for Pelvic and Axial Primaries

Although patients with Ewing's sarcoma of the pelvis are not recommended as candidates for surgical resection, some institutions have elected to resect pelvic primary lesions, regardless of their location, that have responded well to neoadjuvant chemotherapy as an alternative to radiation therapy. Reconstruction techniques are limited to arthrodesis, soft-tissue interpositional arthroplasty, custom prosthetic implants, and allograft reconstruction. Ozaki and colleagues[473] from Münster, Germany, reported their results of pelvic allograft reconstruction, comparing patients with 7 chondrosarcomas, 14 Ewing's sarcomas, and 1 osteosarcoma. Patients with Ewing's sarcoma and osteosarcoma had neoadjuvant chemotherapy, while the seven patients with chondrosarcoma did not. All pelvic allografts were procured, prepared, and stored as

recommended by the European Association for Musculo-skeletal Transplantation, using cobalt γ radiation for sterilization. All patients received perioperative antibiotics, and all drains were removed within ten days.

Eight allografts became infected between 2 weeks and 15 months, with two other patients sustaining fractures. Early infections were observed more often in patients with chondrosarcoma than in the others, who had had chemotherapy. Three patients were converted to saddle prostheses, three patients had no further reconstructive surgery, and two had hemipelvectomies. The authors concluded that risk factors for infection were large tumors and prolonged operating time.

Carrie and coworkers,[474] in a report by the French Society of Pediatric Oncology, described the results of treatment of nonmetastatic pelvic Ewing's sarcoma since January of 1984. Records of 59 children were reviewed retrospectively, and 53 patients were eligible for review of their local control. Local treatment included surgery alone in 17 patients, radiation therapy in 27 patients, and a combination of surgery plus radiation therapy in nine patients. Six patients relapsed locally only. Eight relapsed both locally and at distant sites, and nine developed distant metastases only. Overall survival rate appeared less favorable for patients receiving radiotherapy alone compared with patients receiving surgery or combined modality treatment (44% vs. 72%, P = 0.043). The authors emphasized the importance of surgery wherever possible as one of the modalities of therapy. They concluded that surgery or a combination of surgery and radiation therapy is the best method of local treatment in cases in which surgery is an option. Radiotherapy alone should be reserved for patients with inoperable lesions.

Shamberger and colleagues[475] reported the results of treatment of 98 of 869 patients (11.3%) who had primary tumors of the chest wall. The median follow-up was 3.47 years, and the 5-year event-free survival rate was 56% for chest wall lesions. Ten of 20 (50%) initial resections resulted in negative margins, compared with 41 of 53 (70%) negative margins with delayed resections after chemotherapy (P = .043). The event-free survival rate did not differ by timing of surgery (P = .69) or type of local control (P = .17). Initial chemotherapy decreased the percentage of patients needing radiotherapy. Seventeen of 24 (70.8%) with initial surgery received radiotherapy, compared with 34 of 71 patients (47.8%) who started with chemotherapy (P = .061). In cases of delayed operation—excluding those patients who received only radiation therapy for local control—only 25 of 62 patients needed radiotherapy (40.3%; P = .016). The authors concluded that complete tumor resection with a negative microscopic margin and consequent avoidance of external beam radiation and its potential complications are increased with neoadjuvant chemotherapy and delayed resection of chest wall Ewing's sarcoma/PNET.

Survival After Recurrence of Ewing's Tumor

Although the outcome is generally poor for patients experiencing recurrent Ewing's sarcoma, certain patient subgroups could differ appreciably in their likelihood of survival, as shown in studies in the United States and Europe.

A review of the St. Jude Children's Research Hospital experience between 1979 and 1999 included consecutive institutional protocols (ES-79, ES-87, and EW-92).[476] A retrospective medical chart and database review was performed to identify patients and disease characteristics at the time of diagnosis of Ewing's tumor and at the time of recurrence, and to record the treatment received and the outcome after recurrence. Seventy-one patients were identified, with 34 (47.9%) having distant recurrence, 25 (35.2%) having local recurrence, and 12 (16.9%) having both distant and local recurrence, all at a median of 1.7 years after diagnosis. The probability of a 5-year postrecurrence survival was 17.7% plus or minus 4.5%. Interestingly, however, recurrence 2 years or more after diagnosis predicted a significantly better outcome (5-year postrecurrence survival 34.9% ± 8.5%) compared with earlier recurrence (5.0% ± 2.8%; P < 0.001). Patients who had both local and distant recurrences fared more poorly, with a 5-year postrecurrence survival rate of 12.5% plus or minus 8.3%, compared with patients who had local recurrence alone (21.7% ± 7.8%) or distant recurrence alone (17.6% ± 6.1%). Among patients with local recurrence alone, those who underwent salvage procedures with radical surgery had a significantly higher five-year postrecurrence survival estimates (31.4% ± 11.6%) compared with the other patients (9.1% ± 6.1%; P = 0.023). Pulmonary radiation also significantly improved the outcome of patients with isolated pulmonary recurrence (5-year postrecurrence survival estimate 30.3% ± 12.5% vs. 16.7% ± 10.8%, respectively; P = 0.018). The authors concluded that favorable out-comes are most likely among patients who experience recurrence two years or more after diagnosis and among patients who have local recurrence that can be treated with radical surgery and intensive chemotherapy.

Similarly, Catterill and coauthors,[477] in an analysis of 975 patients from the European Intergroup Cooperative Ewing's Sarcoma Study group, documented a relationship between survival and length of time before recurrence. Patients who relapsed within two years of diagnosis had a less favorable prognosis than those who relapsed later (5-year survival after relapse, 4% vs. 23%, respectively; P < .0001), findings similar to those observed in osteosarcoma patients.

Current Guidelines for Surgical Therapy

All active multimodality Ewing's sarcoma protocols have provisions and recommendations for limited surgery in an effort to avoid the late effects of therapy where possible. Most surgical procedures have been limited to resection of expendable bones after a favorable neoadjuvant chemotherapy response. These include the rays of the hands and feet, the proximal four fifths of the fibula, the pubis and ilium of the pelvis, ribs, distal four fifths of the clavicle (Fig. 95-13), the body of the scapula, and other small, well-localized lesions. The majority of these procedures should not require reconstruction because of the occasional need for adjuvant radiation therapy to the surgical bed and prolonged intensive adjuvant chemotherapy.[478] As neoadjuvant chemotherapy becomes more effective in reducing tumor bulk and as more sophisticated and accurate noninvasive imaging techniques become available, local resections with clear margins (4 cm–5 cm) followed by reconstructive techniques are becoming commonplace.

Surgical resection should be considered after induction chemotherapy in patients presenting with small primary lesions of the metacarpals or metatarsals, when a ray amputation with a minimum of a wide margin could render the patient free of disease. In general, the hand and the foot do not tolerate radiotherapy well. Small midtarsal lesions and lesions arising in the os calcis can sometimes be treated with radiation therapy in the mature skeleton, but the majority of larger lesions in skeletally immature patients are better managed by Syme's amputation or distal tibiotalar disarticulation. Lesions of the tibia should not be considered for resection except in instances in which satisfactory tumor margins can be ensured (4 cm–5 cm) and in which postoperative radiation therapy is unlikely to be required. The majority of non-prosthetic reconstructive procedures will not tolerate the addition of radiotherapy.

Commonly, the proximal four fifths of the fibula can be resected with satisfactory margins, leaving at least 6 cm distally for satisfactory ankle function with little or no morbidity. A tibiofibular synostosis should be performed in skeletally immature patients to prevent proximal migration of the lateral malleolus. A recent report of five children with nonmetastatic Ewing's sarcoma of the distal fibula suggests that distal fibulectomy yielded near normal functional results, with a mean follow-up of 8 years.[479]

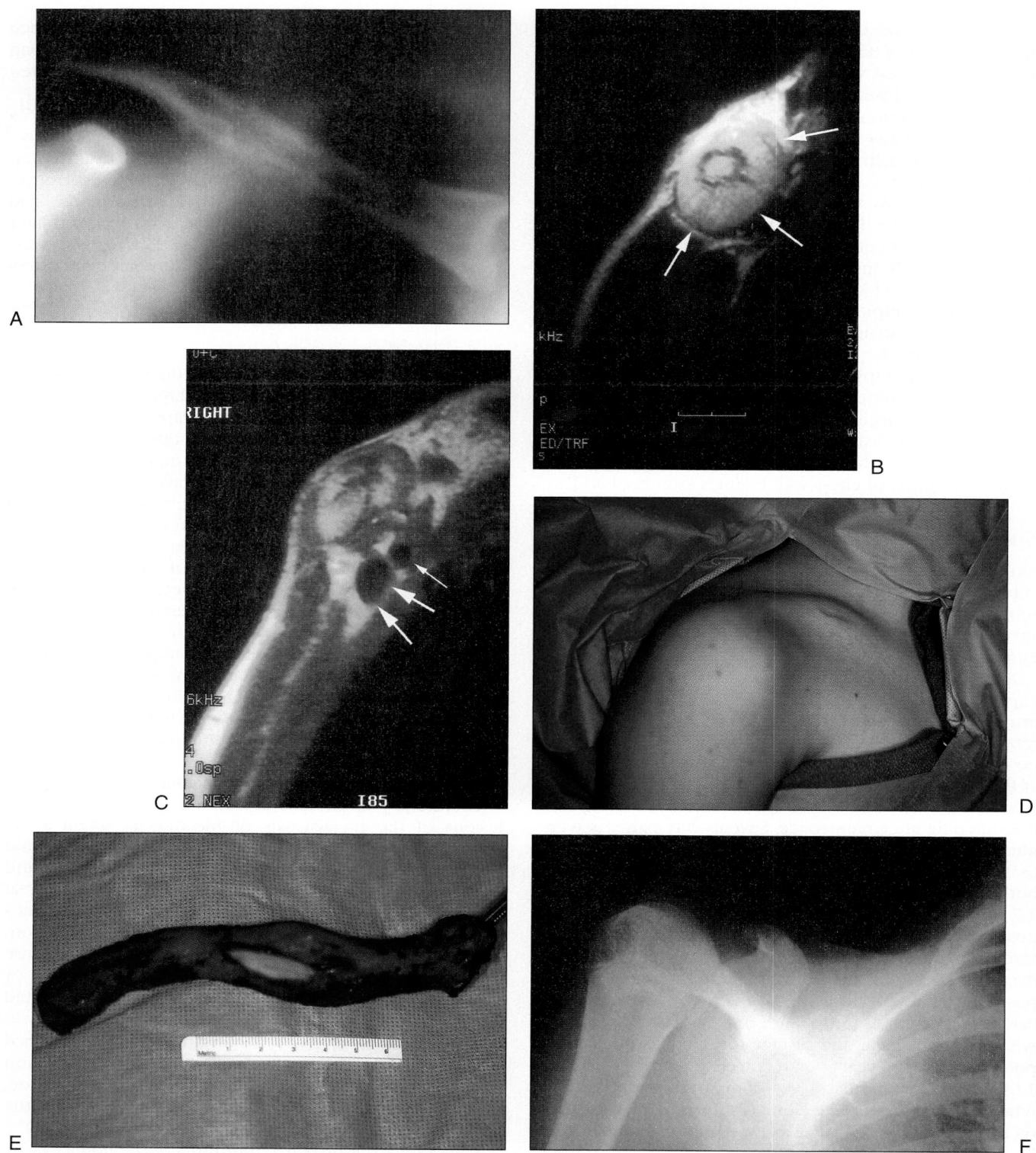

Figure 95-13. A, This 14-year-old, right-hand-dominant female was evaluated for increasing pain and development of a mass involving the right clavicle over the past 2 years. This AP tomogram demonstrated local bone destruction and loss of trabeculation along the entire length of the right clavicle. **B,** The initial axial MR view of the clavicle demonstrates the extraosseous tumor component (*arrows*) of the later biopsy, proven, to be Ewing's tumor of bone. **C,** After completion of 12 weeks of standard preoperative multiagent chemotherapy, a preoperative comparison MR scan demonstrates the radiographic response to therapy and the adjacent major vessels (*arrows*). **D,** This intraoperative photo demonstrates the biopsy tract inline with the clavicle in the proximal one third of the clavicle. **E,** This photo of the resected specimen demonstrates the extraperiosteal resection of an expendable bone with wide curative margins by disarticulating the sternoclavicular and acromioclavicular joints and sparing the major vessels to the dominant arm. **F,** This off treatment x-ray of the right shoulder reveals the total absence of the right clavicle.

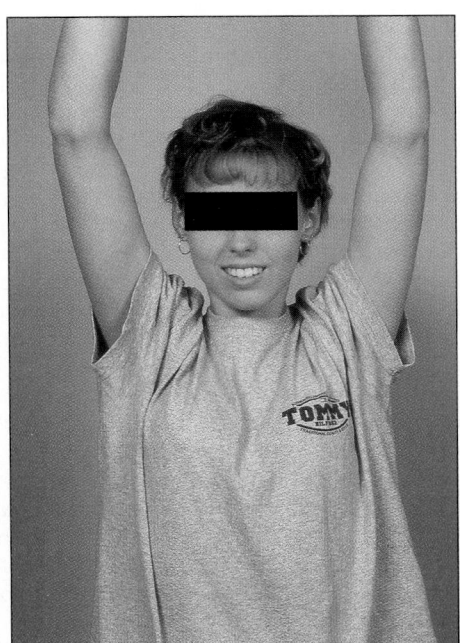

G

Figure 95-13, *cont'd*. G, This 2-year follow-up photo demonstrates the complete function and normal range of motion of the right shoulder.

Neoplasms about the knee could be amenable to local resection and prosthetic replacement in cases in which considerable destruction of bone by the tumor would likely lead to pathologic fracture and probably late amputation. This decision should be made before radiotherapy. Allograft or prosthetic ingrowth materials can also be used to reconstruct the shaft of the femur as an alternative to amputation; however, the majority of the primary lesions will be managed by external-beam radiation therapy.

Destructive lesions about the proximal femur and acetabulum can sometimes be managed by resection and reconstruction in cases in which pathologic fractures and poor joint function could be anticipated. Modular titanium prostheses or allograft/prosthetic composites can be used to reconstruct the hip and proximal femur in patients for whom abduction function can be retained reliably.

Well-localized lesions presenting in the pelvis that are responsive to neoadjuvant chemotherapy—primarily those confined to the ilium and the pubis—are often resectable. Also, tumors arising in the lower portion of the sacrum and coccyx are amenable to sacral amputation with minimal neurologic sequelae. Before undertaking these technically demanding procedures, however, the surgeon should carefully consider the anticipated difficulty of resection and the resultant physical deficit. (See the later discussion on sacral chordoma.)

All of the procedures just discussed are predicated on a satisfactory tumor response characterized by the following:

- A significant decrease in pain
- A nearly complete regression in size of the lesion, as shown by MRI

- Possible healing of an underlying pathologic fracture
- Improved range of near-painless motion of nearby joints

Rib primaries are best managed by excisional biopsy at the time of diagnosis in an effort to prevent contamination of the pleural cavity. Incisional biopsy should be reserved for larger lesions, with the wide resection of the recommended entire rib and surrounding soft tissue completed after induction chemotherapy.

Primary tumors presenting in the body of the scapula that preserve the glenoid structures and the chest wall can be resected without significant functional deficit. Lesions presenting in the region of the glenoid are managed by radiation therapy or by resection/arthroplasty. Small lesions in the acromion and in the spine of the scapula might also be amenable to excision.

The outer four fifths of the clavicle can be resected without significant physical impairment; however, tumors in the proximal one fifth of the clavicle and the sternum are best managed by primary radiation therapy.

Resection of the proximal humerus and reconstruction are often associated with loss of active abduction and therefore should be reserved for patients with extensive destruction. Resection and allograft (osteoarticular or composite) reconstruction yields satisfactory results. In general, functional deficits and limb length inequalities are better tolerated in the upper extremity than in the lower extremity.

Amputation

Although the role of amputation in the surgical management of Ewing's sarcoma remains controversial, primary amputation or disarticulation might offer a clinical option that is superior to the prolonged morbidity associated with pathologic fracture or severe limb length inequality, which can result in late or delayed amputation. Large destructive lesions in males under the age of ten years and in females under the age of 8 years may be managed by primary amputation or a primary limb-sparing option (rotationplasty, etc.). Amputation should be considered when epiphysiodesis of the opposite limb does not provide a reasonable treatment option to approach equalization of lower limb lengths at skeletal maturity.[480]

Prognosis

Location

Clearly, location of the primary lesion in patients with nonmetastatic disease has a profound relationship to long-term survival. Patients with lesions arising below the elbow and below the mid-calf who are treated appropriately have five-year survival rates approaching 80%. Large bulky lesions presenting in the pelvis in nonresectable sites yield 5-year survival rates of less than 25%.[472]

Histopathologic Response to Chemotherapy

Location and size of the primary lesion, however, are not the only determinants of survival. The histopathologic response of the tumor to neoadjuvant chemotherapy has

Specific Malignancies

been shown to be important in predicting outcome.[481] Patients completing systemic neoadjuvant chemotherapy and managed by surgical resection and reconstruction were evaluated using a pathologic grading system independent of change in tumor volume. The resection specimens were sectioned and mapped for review to determine the extent of tumor necrosis. Patients whose specimens displayed complete tumor necrosis with no identifiable foci of tumor tissue (grade III) were projected to have a 90% continuous disease-free survival. Those with lesser degrees of necrosis (grades II and I) were projected to have 53% and 32% 5-year disease-free survival rates.

Wunder and coworkers[482] reviewed the histopathological response to preoperative chemotherapy of 74 patients with an operative resection specimen, correlating the response as a predictor of the overall outcome of multimodality therapy. The minimum duration of follow-up was 5 years. The operative specimens were reviewed, and the histopathological response to chemotherapy was graded semiquantitatively. Grade I represented 50% or less necrosis; grade II, 50% to 90%; grade III, 90% to 99%; and grade IV, 100% necrosis. Of the 74 specimens, 44 (59%) were either grade IV or grade III, while 14 (19%) were grade I and 16 (22%) were grade II. The two most important predictors of event-free survival were histological response to preoperative chemotherapy ($P = 0.0001$), followed by size of the primary tumor ($P = 0.001$). At 5 years, the event-free survival for grade I patients was zero. Grade II responders experienced a 6/16 event-free survival, and for grades III and IV, 37 of 44 patients (84%) experienced a 5-year event-free survival. The risk of local recurrence was also strongly associated with the quality of the operative margins. There were four local recurrences (6%) after 67 resections thought to have negative margins. The authors concluded that histopathological response to preoperative chemotherapy and size of the primary tumor were the most important clinical predictors of outcome of operative treatment for nonmetastatic Ewing's sarcoma.

In the CESS 81 study by Sauer and colleagues[483] for the German Society of Paediatric Oncology, a subset of patients (n = 29) were treated with low-dose radiotherapy (36 Gy). At 18 weeks, having completed the neoadjuvant chemotherapy, the patients underwent either surgery alone, radiation therapy alone, or combined surgery and radiotherapy. Patients treated with wide margins received no further local therapy. The overall survival at 4 years was 62%, and the local failure rate was 3% (1/31). The patients managed with radiotherapy alone had a local failure rate of 46%, and patients treated with combined surgery (incomplete resection) and radiotherapy (36 Gy) had an overall survival of 66% at 4 years, with a local failure rate of 17% (5/29).

Merchant and colleagues[484] reported the results of a retrospective review of treatment of 25 patients at the Memorial Sloan-Kettering Cancer Center for whom treatment was initiated between 1979 and 1996. At the time of diagnosis, 21 of the 25 patients had prognostically unfavorable tumors, including the presence of metastatic disease (n = 12) and axial primary (n = 17) and a tumor measuring greater than 8 cm (n = 18). The primary tumor was completely resected (wide local excision) in 13 patients, with marginal excision in 7 patients, and biopsy only in the remaining 5 patients. The median dose of irradiation to the primary site was 30 Gy. At a median follow-up time of 67 months, 28% of the surviving patients had failed distantly, and an additional 28% were found to have progression of previously established metastatic disease. No patient failed locally. The median overall survival time was 43 months. The authors concluded that limited surgery with postoperative radiation is one strategy that promises to achieve local control while diminishing late effects.

Bacci and associates[485] described their results of treatment of 44 patients with nonmetastatic PNET of bone treated with neoadjuvant chemotherapy. A six-drug regimen of chemotherapy (vincristine, doxorubicin, dactinomycin, cyclophosphamide, ifosfamide, and etoposide) was administered to all patients. Local treatment consisted of surgery in 20 patients, surgery followed by radiotherapy in 13 patients, and radiotherapy in 11 patients. The 5-year event-free survival and overall survival were 54.2% and 62.7%, respectively. The prognostic significance of neural differentiation was assessed by comparison with 138 concomitant patients with typical Ewing's sarcoma. These patients were treated with the same protocol, and 103 (75%) remained continuously event-free, 34 (24%) relapsed, and one patient died of chemotherapy-related toxicity. The authors concluded that the PNET patients treated with this chemotherapy regimen had a significantly worse prognosis than those patients with typical Ewing's sarcoma (5-year event-free survival 54.2% vs. 70.6%, $P < .012$; 5-year overall survival, 62.7% vs. 78.3%, $P < .002$). The authors also concluded that studies of new adjuvant therapies for Ewing's sarcoma should consider neural differentiation as a potential risk factor.

Of all the variables assessed, only grade of tumor necrosis was associated with disease-free survival ($P = 0.004$). There was, however, a trend for tumor volume to be associated with disease-free survival ($P = 0.06$).[481]

Future improvement in the clinical outcome of Ewing's sarcoma and closely related tumors will depend on the introduction of new and more effective chemotherapeutic agents and improved dose intensity. Ifosfamide, first synthesized in the 1950s and used in combination with MESNA as a uroprotective agent, appears to offer encouraging results when combined with granulocyte colony growth factors.

De Alava and colleagues[486] performed a clinical and pathological analysis of 99 patients with Ewing's sarcoma in whom EWS-FWI1 fusion transcripts were identified by reserve-transcriptase polymerase chain reaction (RT-PCR) and for whom adequate follow-up data were available. Median follow-up for the 99 patients was 26 months (range, 1 to 140 months). Tumors in 64 patients contained the type 1 fusion, and 35 contained the less common fusion types. They hypothesized that the type 1 EWS-FLI1 fusion could result in a tumor intrinsically less aggressive or more chemosensitive than other fusion types. It appears that recognition of a type 1 EWS-FLI1 fusion transcript could be an indicator of favorable prognosis.

Increasing the dose intensity of chemotherapy was the focus of a study by Hawkins and colleagues,[487] who reviewed the results of treatment of 23 children and adolescents with metastatic sarcomas treated with intensive chemotherapy supported by G-CSF and peripheral blood stem cells. Seventeen patients (74%) achieved a complete response, with an event-free survival of 39% at 2 years. It was concluded that the peripheral blood stem cell-supported multicycle chemotherapy is a feasible method of increasing chemotherapy dose intensity in patients with metastatic sarcomas.

The reliability of custom modular prosthetic implants continues to improve, further expanding the chemotherapy/surgery envelope.

Late Effects of Treatment

Functional Results

The long-term functional outcome of patients with primary tumors treated with chemotherapy and radiation therapy alone appears to be multifactorial. Studies regarding the effects of irradiation on bone and growth cartilage were first described by Perthes in 1903, when he observed abnormalities of growth and deformity.[488] Later, chondrogenesis was arrested experimentally in the growth plate by Rubin and associates.[489] Hinkle and colleagues[490] demonstrated a minimum threshold dose required to produce deformity and found that the minimum dose increased with age. Currently, it is generally accepted that the pathologic and biomechanical changes associated with high-dose irradiation of bone include decreased vascularity, cellularity, and bone metabolism, with increased porosity and loss of mechanical strength, impaired fracture healing, and periosteal fibrosis.[491]

The soft-tissue and skeletal effects of irradiation are related to the following factors:

- Skeletal maturity of the patient
- The volume of tissue treated
- The total dose and dose rate
- The energy and delivery system of the beam
- Concomitant chemotherapy treatment
- Inclusion of major joints or growth centers

The first clinical reports of patients surviving Wilms' tumor showed that 11 of 12 who received radiation therapy developed hypoplasia of the ilium.[492] Lewis and coauthors[493] reported functional effects in 55 patients with Ewing's sarcoma treated with radiation therapy. They noted, as others did, that limb length and functional deficits of the upper extremities were much better tolerated than similar deficits developing in the lower extremities. They recommended primary amputation for some distal destructive lesions in young patients. Ten of 31 reported patients were judged to have nonfunctional extremities secondary to radiation therapy.

Robertson and coauthors[494] reported limb length inequalities in 12 of 67 patients surviving childhood cancer who had received radiotherapy. All the children survived to skeletal maturity. Seven of the 12 patients reported symptoms. The development of limb length inequality was shown to be uniformly related to long bone physeal radiation of 45 Gy or greater.

Additional comorbidities include soft-tissue atrophy and fibrosis, joint stiffness, and pathologic fracture of the previously treated bone. Jentzsch and colleagues[495] reported that 9 of 40 patients who completed treatment sustained a pathologic fracture with Ewing's sarcoma of the lower extremity. They found slow and delayed fracture healing, with two patients sustaining re-fracture. All eventually healed by closed means. Later, Springfield and Pagliarulo[494] reported the results of a retrospective analysis of patients receiving chemotherapy and radiotherapy for primary Ewing's sarcoma of the extremities. Twenty-eight patients were followed for a minimum of 2 years or until their deaths. Seventeen patients had primary lesions presenting in the humerus or femur. All 17 received chemotherapy and radiation therapy, with doses ranging from 50 to 60 Gy administered by a shrinking field technique. Two of the eight patients with humeral primaries and five of nine patients with femoral primaries sustained pathologic fractures without significant trauma. Of the five femoral fractures, four were in the subtrochanteric region, and all had a cortical window removed at the time of biopsy. Only two patients developed pathologic fractures through the cortical defect. Springfield and Pagliarulo[496] strongly recommend rebiopsy to assess possible persistent disease, followed by internal fixation and the addition of autogenous bone graft.

Secondary Malignancies

In 1979, Chan and coauthors[497] reported that among 24 patients with primary Ewing's sarcoma of the pelvis who had survived for 5 years, 4 developed secondary malignancies within the irradiated fields and died. Three of the four patients also had received intensive chemotherapy. Also, Strong and associates[498] reported an increased hazard of developing secondary malignancy in patients treated with radiation therapy, with a cumulative cancer risk of 35% over 10 years. The administration of intensive chemotherapy in five or more courses appeared to exert an enhancing effect, increasing the rate of development of new tumors. Li[499] also reported a 12% risk of developing a new cancer in 15 of 410 patients who survived childhood cancers.

Most recently, Tucker and coworkers[500] estimated the subsequent risk of development of bone cancer in 9170 patients surviving 2 or more years. Data on treatment were evaluated on 64 patients in whom bone cancer developed after childhood cancer. Patients who had received radiation therapy had a 2.7-fold risk of developing a secondary malignancy. The dose response appeared to reach a 40-fold risk after doses to bone of more than 60 Gy. Similar numbers of patients were treated with orthovoltage and megavoltage, and the patterns of risk among categories of doses did not differ according to the type of voltage. Also, after adjusting for radiation therapy, treatment with alkylating agents also appeared to increase the subsequent risk of bone cancer.

Coleman[501,502] reported that an average latent period for development of treatment-induced solid tumors was 10 to 15 years, with a 10% actuarial risk at 10 years for pediatric patients. The Late Effects Study Group confirmed the risk in 1985.[531] Smith and associates,[504] summarizing the treatment of 25 long-term survivors of Ewing's sarcoma, reported that one patient developed acute myelogenous leukemia at 15 months and one patient developed osteosarcoma 3 years after treatment. The actuarial risk of developing a second malignancy at 5 years was 8%, with a 4% risk of developing a secondary bone sarcoma.

Future Directions

With evolving and intensified induction and maintenance chemotherapy and improved imaging and patient selection techniques (e.g., MRI, PET, rapid whole-body STIR MRI), many patients not previously suitable for limb-sparing procedures could become candidates for local resection and reconstruction. As mentioned previously, resection of expendable bones usually does not require reconstruction. If the margins are not adequate for local control, postoperative radiation therapy can be administered without significantly altering the result in constructs not requiring bone graft healing and incorporation.

The radiotherapy data from the Pediatric Oncology Group 8346 Study determined that patients who had appropriate radiotherapy after induction chemotherapy with no deviations of radiation therapy had a 5-year local control rate of 80%.[505] Those patients discovered to have minor deviations from appropriate radiotherapy had a 5-year local control rate of 48%, and those with major deviations had a 16% 5-year local control rate. The local control rate for those 21 patients having a surgical resection with wide margins and an additional 16 patients (total 26%) requiring postoperative radiation therapy with inadequate margins was also approximately 80%.

Donaldson and colleagues[505] reviewed the end results of POG #8346, evaluating 178 eligible patients, of whom 141 (79%) had only local disease and 37 (21%) metastatic disease. Thirty-seven patients with localized disease underwent local resection, and 16 (43%) of those required postoperative radiotherapy. The 5-year event-free survival for the surgical patients was 80%. The remaining 104 patients with local disease were eligible for randomization or assignment to receive radiotherapy. The 5-year event-free survival for these patients was 41%. The 5-year local control rate for the surgical patients, either with or without postoperative radiotherapy, was 88%, while the rate for the patients undergoing radiotherapy alone was 65%. The quality of the radiotherapy correlated with outcome. Patients who had appropriate radiotherapy (treatment of appropriate volumes) had a 5-year local control rate of 80%, while those with minor deviations had a 5-year local control rate of 48%, and those with major deviations had a local control rate of only 16%. The local failure was within an irradiated volume in 62% of patients and outside the irradiated volume in 24% of cases. It was clear that adequate involved field radiotherapy requires treatment to appropriate volumes, as defined by high-quality MRI images, and full radiation doses.

The use of brachytherapy or intraoperative radiation therapy (IORT) at the time of local resection could also extend the reconstruction techniques to include the use of autogeneic tissues. If radiation therapy is required for treatment of contaminated surgical margins after resection, therapy can often be tailored individually to the margins requiring treatment, thereby protecting other normal tissues and structures. Also, muscle pedicle flaps protected at the time of irradiation can be rotated into the operative field to provide additional blood supply and coverage to free or vascularized graft materials. Experience with these techniques suggests that the grafts do unite and revascularize, but at a slightly slower rate than in patients not receiving radiation therapy.[506]

The increasing role of surgical therapy in the local management of patients with Ewing's sarcoma appears to be beneficial with respect to overall disease-free survival and reduction of treatment-related late effects. It should be the common goal of all oncologists to optimize therapy wherever possible to provide the patient with the best overall clinical and functional results.

MALIGNANT FIBROUS HISTIOCYTOMA OF BONE

Malignant fibrous histiocytoma (MFH) of bone is a rare tumor of histiocytic origin first described in 1972.[507] Excluding dedifferentiated chondrosarcoma, MFH of bone is classified into primary and secondary categories, which are related to the absence or presence of a known predisposing and underlying pathologic entity such as bone infarction, fibrous dysplasia, or Paget's disease of bone. Some tumors also appear to be associated with orthopedic implants and could be metal induced.[508] The literature previously referred to MFH as pleomorphic spindle cell sarcoma, poorly differentiated fibrosarcoma of bone, and other titles until its identity as a separate neoplasm was established.[509,510]

Epidemiology

Approximately 70% of malignant fibrous histiocytomas of bone are primary tumors, and 30% are secondary.[511] There is a slight male predominance. The primary variety tends to affect younger patients, while the secondary neoplasms are seen predominantly in the sixth and seventh decades of life. A painful fixed mass adjacent to a major joint is the most common presentation.

Radiographic Features

Pronounced loss of normal trabeculation associated with permeative cortical destruction is the characteristic radiographic appearance. Invasion into adjacent soft tissue with the development of a large soft-tissue mass is not uncommon. The proximal tibia and distal femoral metaphyses are most frequently affected, followed by the pelvis, proximal humeral metaphysis, and scapula. A little more than one half of the tumors originate in the lower extremity.[512]

Large, destructive lesions originating in weight-bearing bones are often painful and, if unrecognized and untreated, can lead to pathologic fracture. Periosteal new bone formation and endosteal scalloping are rarely seen in malignant fibrous histiocytoma of bone. Computed tomography is useful in defining the extent of bone destruction; however, MRI with contrast enhancement of the extremity is the single study of choice to provide maximum data.[22,513]

Secondary MFH of bone is by definition associated with an underlying or preexisting condition. There appears to be a clear association with bone infarction as a preexisting condition. Radiographically, the remaining punctate calcifications can be seen about the periphery of the lesion, with destruction and loss of radiographic detail evident within the lesion. Also, a contiguous soft-tissue mass is commonly present.

Patients with known Paget's disease of bone, hereditary dysplasias of bone, or prior treatment with radiotherapy are at risk to develop secondary malignant fibrous histiocytomas of bone. These patients are often older than those developing the primary subtype.

Pathologic Features

Regardless of the primary or secondary classification, the overwhelming majority of these lesions are high-grade malignancies. Only 10% or fewer are low grade. Histologically, the tumor is composed of fibroblasts in a storiform (whorling or cartwheel) pattern with multinucleated giant cells, inflammatory cells, and histiocytes with numerous foamy mononuclear or multinucleated giant cells (xanthomatous variant). Mitotic figures are frequent, with considerable pleomorphism.

Other lesions that must be considered in the differential diagnosis of malignant fibrous histiocytoma of bone include fibrosarcoma, malignant schwannoma, leiomyosarcoma, malignant giant cell tumor of bone, spindle-cell osteosarcoma, and dedifferentiated chondrosarcoma (with prominent spindle-cell component).[514-518] Malignant fibrous histiocytoma of bone demonstrates immunoreactivity for vimentin, glycoprotein, α_1-antitrypsin, α_1-antichymotrypsin, and the bacteriolytic enzyme, lysozyme.[519] These tumors are commonly S-100 negative. Ultrastructurally, the lesions seem to derive from a primitive mesenchysmal stem cell that might be shared with the common progenitor cell of osteosarcoma.[519]

Surgical Therapy

Spanier and coworkers[509] reviewed more than 400 primary bone tumors in 1975 to identify 11 primary bone tumors with the histopathologic features of primary malignant fibrous histiocytoma of bone. Radiographically, the lesions reported developed in the long bones and were metaphyseal and destructive, often producing pathologic fracture. Nine of the 11 patients developed pulmonary metastases, and three developed regional lymph node involvement less than 2 years after diagnosis. The average survival for six of the nine patients was 12 months. Six patients who developed metastases had no

further treatment. The remaining three received additional treatment; two patients received systemic chemotherapy, and one had additional radiotherapy. All demonstrated a partial response.[509]

Mirra and associates,[520,521] Dorfman and colleagues,[522] and Michael and Dorfman[523] drew attention to the association of MFH with underlying bone infarcts. Two cases of fibrosarcoma arising at sites of bone infarction had also been reported by Furey and coauthors.[524] McCarthy and associates[525] reported a clinicopathologic analysis of 35 patients and described four with multicentric distribution at the time of diagnosis. The authors recommended amputation as the surgical procedure of choice.

Ghandur-Mnaymneh and colleagues[526] described 6 new patients and reviewed the literature, reporting on a total of 74 patients followed for at least 5 years. Analysis of data showed a 36.5% 5-year survival rate. Thirteen of 74 patients (17.6%) survived from 5 to 38 years, demonstrating certain similarities to osteosarcoma.

Capanna and associates[527] reported on the largest series of 90 patients with MFH of bone, with 68 patients undergoing surgical therapy and 20 of 60 receiving chemotherapy. The overall survival rate was 34% at 5 years and 28% at 10 years. With adequate surgery (a wide margin) and chemotherapy, however, the 5-year survival rate improved to 57%.

The chemotherapy regimen for MFH of bone is evolving. A regimen of vincristine, high-dose methotrexate with citrovorum rescue, and doxorubicin has been reported as successful in preventing distant disease at 42 to 48 months.[528] At present, combination chemotherapy that includes doxorubicin, ifosfamide, and dacarbazine (DTIC) with mesna uroprotection (MAID) is another alternative being evaluated (Fig. 95-14).

The value of high-dose methotrexate-based neoadjuvant chemotherapy in the treatment of MFH of bone has recently been reported by Ham and colleagues.[529] They compared the outcomes of 17 patients diagnosed since 1977 with MFH of bone. Ten patients (59%) completed treatment with four courses of neoadjuvant chemotherapy with HD-MTX, vincristine, doxorubicin, cyclophosphamide, bleomycin, and dactinomycin, or with HD-MTX, epidoxorubicin, and carboplatin. Three patients completed tumor resection, two had curettage with cryotherapy, two had an amputation, and three had a local resection with endoprosthetic reconstruction.

Neoadjuvant MTX-containing chemotherapy was contraindicated in five patients (29%) due to age, cardiac insufficiency, or a mental disorder. Five of the six patients who received no HD-MTX-based neoadjuvant chemotherapy developed metastatic disease (83%), with a median time to metastatic disease of 17 months (range, 3–44 months). In contrast, in the 10 patients who completed treatment with HD-MTX-based neoadjuvant chemotherapy, at a mean follow-up of 9.8 years (range, 2.3–15.7 years) after diagnosis, no local recurrence or distant metastases were diagnosed (P < .005). The authors concluded that neoadjuvant HD-MTX-containing chemotherapy, when combined with appropriate surgery, dramatically improved the prognosis of patients with MFH of bone.

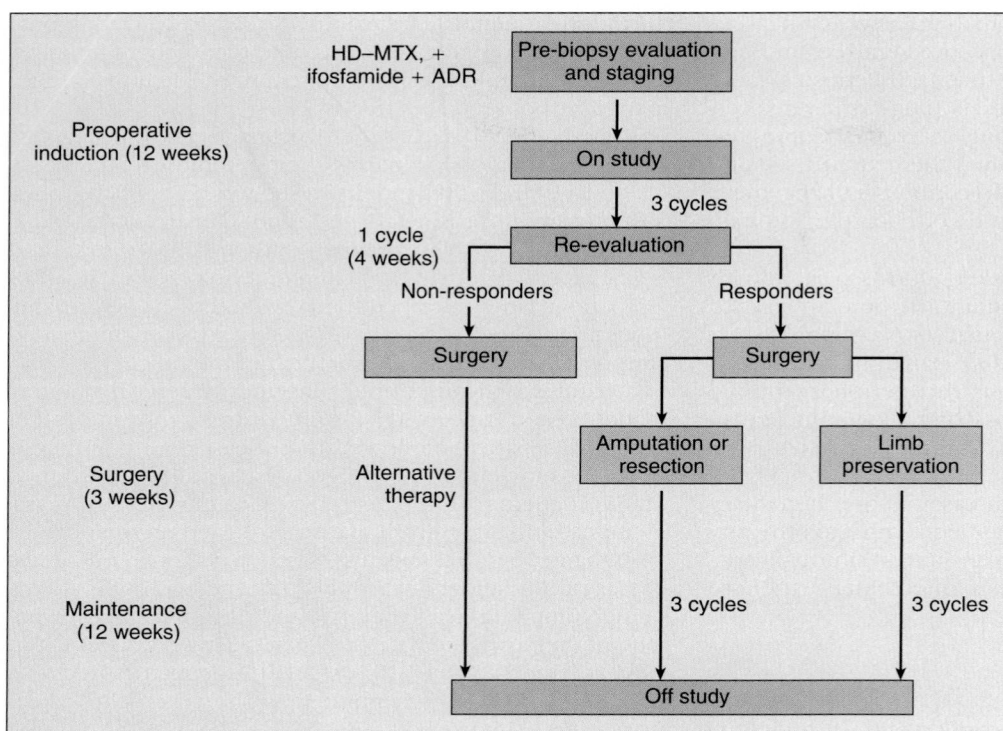

Figure 95-14. Malignant fibrous histiocytoma of bone commonly responds to intensive multidrug chemotherapy regimens similar to the soft-tissue counterpart. This schema is under investigation for management of adult patients with biopsy-proved nonmetastatic nonosteogenic primary sarcomas of bone presenting in anatomic regions where limb-preserving procedures could be used. This particular schema uses three cycles of primary chemotherapy. If the patient experiences pain relief, decreased size of the lesion, and MRI evidence demonstrating increased tumor necrosis on re-evaluation, the patient is said to be a responder. Once the decision has been made as to response, the patient is managed either by a limb-sparing procedure or by amputation. If pathologic review of the specimen suggests a satisfactory or excellent response, the patient may continue on the same chemotherapy combination. If the pathologic analysis suggests a poor response, an alternative chemotherapy can be used.

Nonmetastatic primary malignant fibrous histiocytoma of bone is best managed in a manner similar to primary osteosarcoma of adolescents and young adults (Fig. 95-15). After diagnostic biopsy, neoadjuvant chemotherapy can be administered and the primary tumor response monitored by clinical and radiographic parameters. The majority of tumors respond clinically with relief of pain, resolution of the associated joint contracture, diminished local edema, and reduction in the size of the soft-tissue component. Radiographic response to neoadjuvant chemotherapy is best confirmed by a reduction in size of the soft-tissue component and diminished or absent contrast enhancement on follow-up MRI evaluation.

The surgical planning and the construction of a custom implant can be completed during the neoadjuvant treatment schedule. A three-week "window" in the protocol has been developed after completion of the third or fourth three-week course of chemotherapy (Table 95-10). If the patient is a limb-sparing candidate, a surgical procedure with a minimum of a wide margin can usually be performed following the determinants of limb-sparing surgery. Should the lesion prove to be unresectable, an ablative procedure with a minimum of a wide to compartmental margin should be performed. When a limb-sparing option is available, most musculoskeletal oncologists would utilize either a custom implant arthroplasty, a resection/arthrodesis, an allograft, an allograft/prosthetic implant composite, or rotationplasty. Treatment of patients with primary nonmetastatic malignant fibrous histiocytoma of bone essentially parallels that of patients with nonmetastatic osteosarcoma.

Adamantinoma of Bone

Although similar in name, adamantinoma of bone is not related to ameloblastoma of the mandible derived from Rathke's pouch. First described by Dockerty and Myerding and later refined by Cohn and colleagues[531] from the Mayo Clinic in 1962, this rare, low-grade malignant lesion arises predominantly in the tibia (90%), with the next most common site the fibula.[531-534] When adamantinoma involves trabecular bones of the upper extremity, the ulna predominates. There appears to be no definite sex predominance, and the majority of tumors appear in the second and third decades of life.

The most common symptom is the onset of pain and later, a "swelling," most often in the midshaft of the tibia (70%). Radiographically, the lesion is well marginated and appears to begin within the medullary cavity, eventually expanding the medullary cavity and resulting in thinning of the cortex, which can lead to bowing of the tibia or pathological fracture (Fig. 95-16). Other less common lesions, according to Czerniak and colleagues,[532] appear to

TABLE 95-10

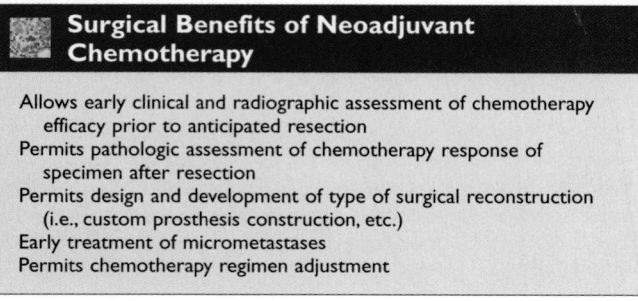

Surgical Benefits of Neoadjuvant Chemotherapy

Allows early clinical and radiographic assessment of chemotherapy efficacy prior to anticipated resection
Permits pathologic assessment of chemotherapy response of specimen after resection
Permits design and development of type of surgical reconstruction (i.e., custom prosthesis construction, etc.)
Early treatment of micrometastases
Permits chemotherapy regimen adjustment

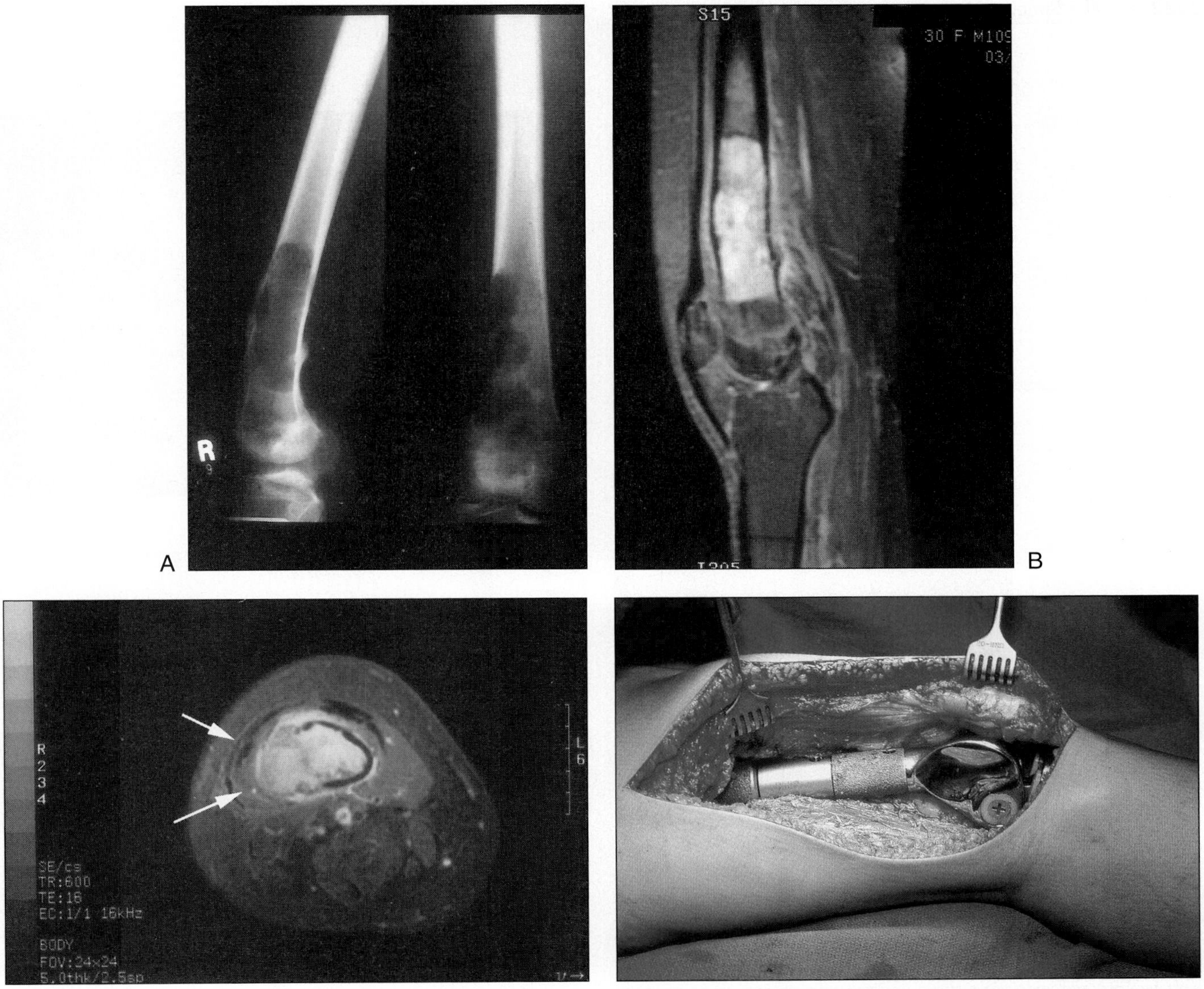

Figure 95-15. A, This 30-year-old female sustained a fall in the snow resulting in pain in the right distal thigh. The AP and lateral x-ray demonstrate a destructive expansible lesion in the metaphysis of the femur without radiographic evidence of matrix calcifications or mineralization. **B,** The sagittal fat suppression MR scan of the thigh demonstrates the extent of disease and surrounding edema. Examination revealed a lateral soft-tissue mass. **C,** The axial view of the same MR sequence demonstrates penetration of the lateral cortex and the extent of the adjacent soft-tissue mass (*white arrows*). An open biopsy proved malignant fibrous histiocytoma of bone. The patient completed three courses of multiagent systemic chemotherapy before consideration of surgical resection. **D,** The patient remained otherwise free of disease, with a good MR contrast-assessed histopathologic response to preoperative chemotherapy. The lesion was resected with a minimum of a 2-cm proximal bone margin and was reconstructed using a modular distal femoral prosthesis. **E,** This AP and lateral composite x-ray demonstrates the postoperative results. In general, this tumor is managed in a fashion similar to conventional osteosarcoma of bone.

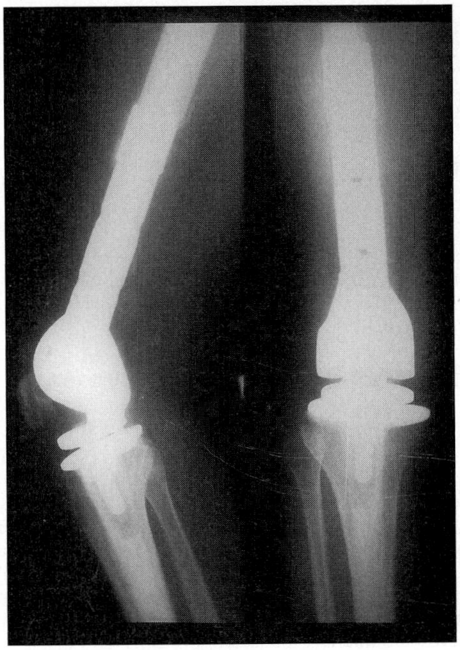

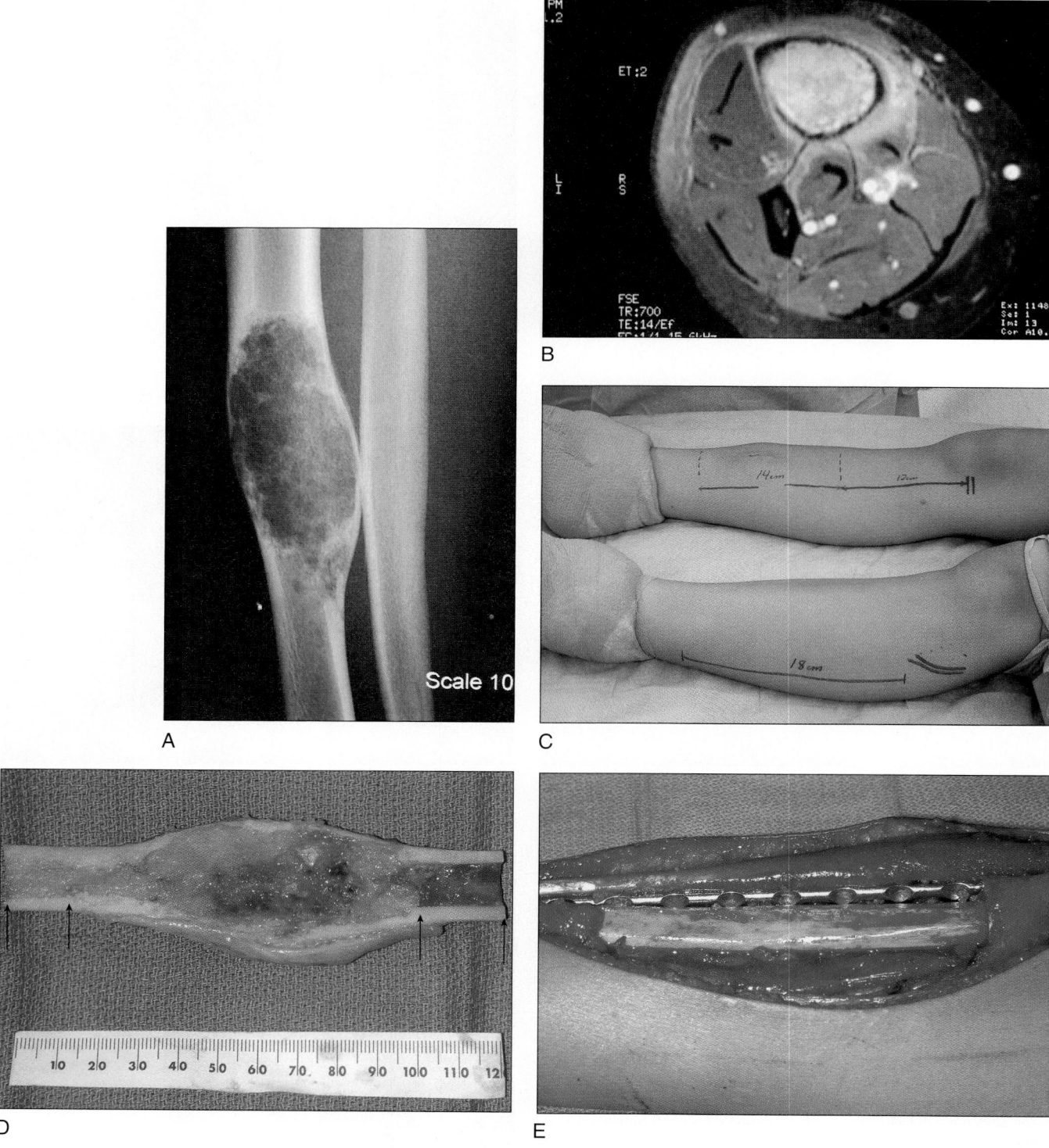

Figure 95-16. A, This 16-year-old skeletally mature female was seen for increasing right leg pain made worse by weight bearing. The lateral digital film demonstrates an expansile intramedullary midshaft tibia mass with cortical thinning and destruction. A total body STIR MR revealed no other detectable lesions. Physical examination revealed no café-au-lait cutaneous pigmentation. **B,** This axial MR view demonstrates expansion and thinning of the cortex, destruction of the medullary bone and inner cortex without tumor necrosis, and surrounding soft-tissue edema. **C,** An open biopsy revealed adamantinoma of bone. This intra-operative view demonstrates the intended surgical procedure, resecting 14 cm of the diaphysis of the tibia and reconstructing the skeletal defect with a free avascular left fibula graft supplemented with autologous iliac crest bone graft. **D,** After resection, the lesion was taken to the back table and split to confirm appropriate proximal (*right arrows*) and distal (*left arrows*) intramedullary margins. **E,** A continuous strength locking screw plate was used to maintain reduction and to secure the fibular graft, having been shaped to fit within the proximal and distal medullary canal. The proximal and distal host/graft osteotomy sites were supplemented with autologous iliac crest bone graft.

arise from the cortex, much like osteofibrous dysplasia and dedifferentiated to adamantinoma.[535,536] Radiographically, the lesions appear to arise within the cortex and then later involve the medullary cavity. They also can be multicentric, involving several apparently separate areas of the cortex rather than the center of the "classic" variety, which appears to arise from a single region. Clinically, some osteofibrous varieties with multiple focal epithelial elements tend to pursue a course similar to osteofibrous dysplasia, while the classic variety pursues a slowly progressive course.

The Association of Orthopaedic Implants and Malignancy

The concern regarding the use of metallic implants in humans and late development of malignancies is well known.[508,537-543] McDougall[544] first reported a high-grade vascular lesion in association with plate and screw fixation in 1956. Since then, 38 cases have been reported and well summarized by McDonald and coauthors[543] in a review of the literature. Their review suggests that the latency period is longer for nonarthroplasty malignancies (mean 19.4 years) than for malignancies associated with arthroplasty (mean 6.0 years). Implant infection does not appear to be a factor.

Malignancy associated with arthroplasty also appears to lack a cause-and-effect relationship.[537,543] McDonald[543] also reviewed 25 reported cases of malignancies associated with arthroplasty and could find no correlation with metal-on-metal implants, loosening and infection, or the metallurgy (including CoCr alloys to near-pure titanium). It was clear, however, that the outcomes of treatment for malignancy overall were poor for both nonarthroplasty and arthroplasty groups. It is suspected that numerous cases have not been reported.

PRIMARY TUMORS OF THE SPINE

It is estimated that less than 10% of all primary bone tumors—approximately one per million per year—arise in the spine.[545] Metastatic disease to the spine that results in spinal cord compression, on the other hand, approximates 8.5 per 100,000 per year.[546] The vertebral column remains the most common site of developing skeletal metastases, resulting in approximately 20,000 patients per year

---

CRITERIA FOR METAL-ASSOCIATED NEOPLASIA

1. Tumor must arise within the direct vicinity of the metallic implant
2. Minimum latency of 2 years
3. No obvious predisposing factors for development of secondary malignancies (e.g., prior radiation, chronic infection, bone infarction)
4. Histology must reflect nonmetastatic histogenesis (e.g., sarcomas, not carcinomas)

---

requiring treatment.[547] Autopsy studies of patients dying of disseminated cancer demonstrated vertebral metastases in 14% to 41%, intradural/extramedullary metastases in 5% to 8%, and intramedullary metastases to the cord in 1%.[548-552] Therefore, metastatic disease must be considered and excluded during evaluation of a patient suspected of having a primary bone tumor of the spine.

It is also important to recognize that unusual entities such as tophaceous gout, pigmented villonodular synovitis, brown tumor of hyperparathyroidism, Rosai-Dorfman disease, and Hodgkin's disease can affect the spine as well.[553-558]

General Considerations

Symptoms
Pain is the most common presenting symptom in more than 80% of patients and is often associated with considerable delay in diagnosis.[559,560] The symptoms are often vague, ill-defined, and slow to localize to a more specific region of the anatomy. Unilateral radiculopathy may be ascribed to disc disease; however, bilateral involvement must be recognized as unusual and requires radiographic and medical evaluation. Less commonly, some patients present with the onset of spinal cord compression without any antecedent history of pain.

Age
The age of the patient is important when evaluating a patient with a suspected lesion involving the vertebral column. Patients under the age of 18 years are 80% more likely to have a benign lesion than those over 18 years of age, even though single metastatic vertebral lesions are far more common than primary malignant spinal neoplasms.[561-563] The incidence of spinal cord compression among children undergoing treatment for sarcoma is approximately 5%.[564] The childhood tumors that more commonly produce spinal cord compression arising either as a primary tumor of the spine or as the result of metastatic disease include Ewing's sarcoma, metastatic neuroblastoma, osteosarcoma, lymphoma, and others.

Benign primary tumors of bone arising in the vertebral column also can produce spinal cord compression, either by direct pressure or as a result of pathologic fracture and collapse. They are more common in the first two decades of life. Because of the occasional similarity of the radiographic appearance of benign and malignant primary neoplasms of the spine, it is important to understand the pathologies and the most common radiographic sites and locations of primary benign and malignant bone tumors that arise in the spine. Table 95-11 lists the more common benign and malignant primary tumors of the spine, together with their most common sites of location.

Staging and Biopsy of Primary Tumors of the Spine

Surgical Staging Systems
The surgical staging system proposed by Enneking[8] is more difficult to apply to primary tumors arising in the spine. As noted by others, extraosseous extension could

TABLE 95-11

Anatomic Distribution of Vertebral Lesions		
ANTERIOR ELEMENTS OF THE SPINE	**POSTERIOR ELEMENTS OF THE SPINE**	**BOTH ANTERIOR AND POSTERIOR ELEMENTS OF THE SPINE**
Multiple myeloma	Osteoid osteoma	Metastasis (spares disk end plates)
Hemangioma	Osteoblastoma	Infection (involves disk end plates)
Paget's disease of bone	Aneurysmal bone cyst	Classic osteosarcoma
Histiocytosis × (vertebra plana)		Postradiation sarcoma
Giant cell tumor of bone		Malignant histiocytoid variety
Reparative granuloma		Osteosarcoma
Ewing's sarcoma (PNET)		Osteochondroma
Lymphoma of bone		Primary chondrosarcoma
Malignant fibrous histiocytoma		Secondary chondrosarcoma
Chordoma		

represent extension into the surrounding paravertebral soft tissues or, more problematically, extension into the epidural or intradural tissues. Tomita and colleagues[565] reported a system for surgical staging of vertebral tumors in which stage I represents intracompartmental involvement, stage II represents extraosseous extension, and stage III is reserved for tumors invading and extending into adjacent vertebrae. Each vertebral body is considered as one compartment. Unfortunately, no method was proposed to differentiate lesions specifically involving the extradural region and/or paraspinous tissues. The surgical implications of these seemingly similar events, however, differ considerably from one another.

A separate surgical staging system has been proposed by Boriani and coworkers[566] (WBB) to recognize the apparent inadequacies of the MSTS-adopted system. Using a clock-face 12-sector staging system as viewed from cephalad to caudad, in which 1 and 12 represent the left and right sides of the spinous process, respectively, these authors distinguish five separate centrifugal surrounding tissue layers (A, B, C, D, and E), beginning with intradural involvement (A) and extending out to paraspinous muscle involvement (E) (Fig. 95-17).

To test the adequacy of the staging systems, the three participating institutions jointly staged 36 patients with benign giant cell tumors of the spine using the WBB and MSTS systems. Only patients with three-dimensional imaging and who had completed their definitive surgical therapy at one of three cooperating institutions between 1974 and 1991 were included. The 36 patients described all met the criteria, with 42% of the lesions in the lumbar spine, while 36% and 22% were evaluated in the thoracic and cervical spines, respectively. Ten patients (28%) presented with pathologic fractures. No tumors were identified that involved only the posterior elements.

Twenty-eight patients had no prior treatment before referral. Five of the 28 having no prior treatment subsequently developed local recurrence (18%), while 5 of 6 patients managed before referral (83%) experienced recurrence. The authors state that these relatively pathologically homogenous lesions tended to recur locally more often if there was radiographic evidence of tumor extension into the spinal canal and/or into the paraspinous

musculature. Given so few cases, the classification system, when applied to this particular study, did not appear to be predictive of local recurrence or poor outcome.

Benign "aggressive" and low-grade malignant tumors will require clean contaminated or "wide" potentially curative surgical margins, regardless of the classification system. The WBB method does not address the biology or

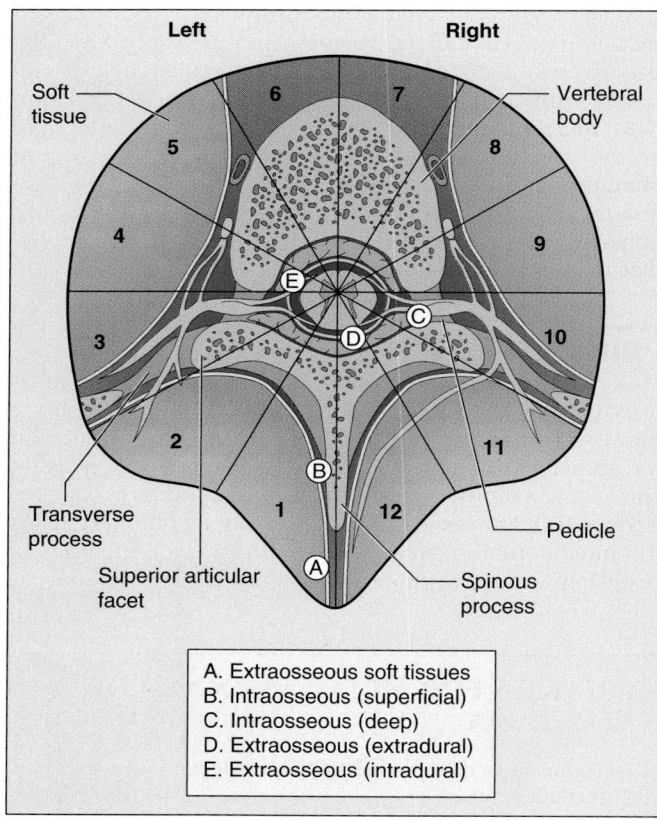

Figure 95-17. Representation of the current staging scheme proposed by Weinstein-Boriani-Biagini, with 12 radically distributed zones beginning at the spinous process and five separate tissue layers designed to distinguish intramedullary and extradural involvement from bone and soft-tissue paravertebral extension. The system does not recognize grade (G) or longitudinal compartmental margins (T).

grade of the lesion (G) nor the ill-defined, longitudinal anatomic paraspinous compartmental margins (T). The WBB system does provide a more accurate description than the MSTS system of the axial distribution of tumor involvement. It was recognized by Weinstein and McLain[562] that 76% of all primary malignant tumors arise in the vertebral body, whereas only 36% of lesions occurring in the posterior elements were malignant. Perhaps in time, both systems could be integrated to provide a more comprehensive method of staging that might lead to better surgical management and possibly predict a superior approach to surgical therapy.

Radiographic Staging

Conventional x-rays of the spine do not necessarily identify the region of skeletal involvement.[568] Bone scintigraphy is also less reliable than previously believed.[569] Kori and associates[29] demonstrated that at least 50% of the bone must be destroyed before a lesion can be identified clearly with conventional x-ray techniques. If there is sufficient clinical concern regarding the presence of an occult pathologic process, either a spiral CT or an MRI of the area in question could be required to appreciate the underlying pathologic process.[31,570] Once a lesion is detected, more specific imaging techniques can be used to better assess the vascularity of the lesion (via contrast enhancement), or myelographic techniques can be used to identify intradural or cord involvement.[571] The current radiographic standard for accurate staging of primary tumors of the spine is MRI, possibly supplemented by other studies.[572]

Biopsy

Most often, a pathologic diagnosis will be required before surgical therapy, whether it is obtained as a frozen section followed by definitive surgical management or as a separate procedure that allows for additional preoperative planning and/or the use of neoadjuvant chemotherapy or preoperative radiotherapy. In many instances, preoperative imaging can provide sufficient information that the frozen section or a squash-smear preparation will provide diagnostic confirmatory evidence to proceed with definitive therapy in one procedure.

The appropriate diagnosis of a malignant primary tumor of the spine often requires more tissue.[573,574] The technique of fine needle aspiration could require several passes through the same skin puncture wound, but using a starburst pattern to assess several areas within a potentially nonhomogenous lesion. More complex lesions often provide only nonspecific radiographic information while identifying the anatomic location and extent.

Some surgeons prefer a semi-open transpedicular fluoroscopic controlled biopsy from a limited posterior surgical approach (Fig. 95-18).[575] As in the management of all sarcomas of bone or soft tissue, the biopsy track must be considered contaminated and be included in the carefully planned en bloc resection.[576-578]

Hadjipavlou and colleagues[579] described the results of 71 percutaneous transpedicular biopsy specimens taken from 68 patients with cervical, thoracic, lumbar, and sacral vertebral lesions. Sixty-one procedures were performed using fluoroscopic guidance, and seven procedures used computed tomography; local anesthesia was administered

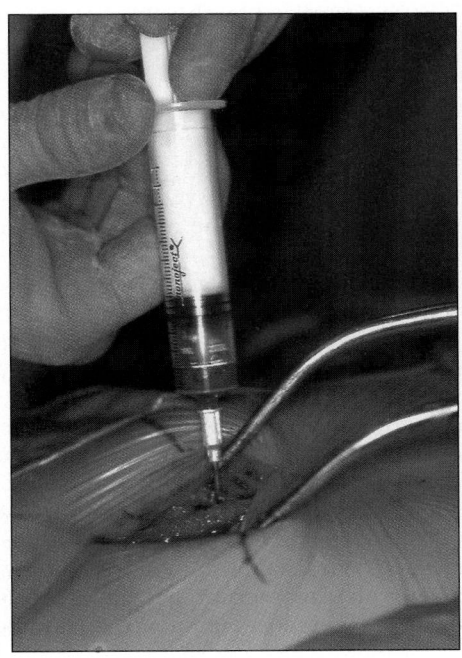
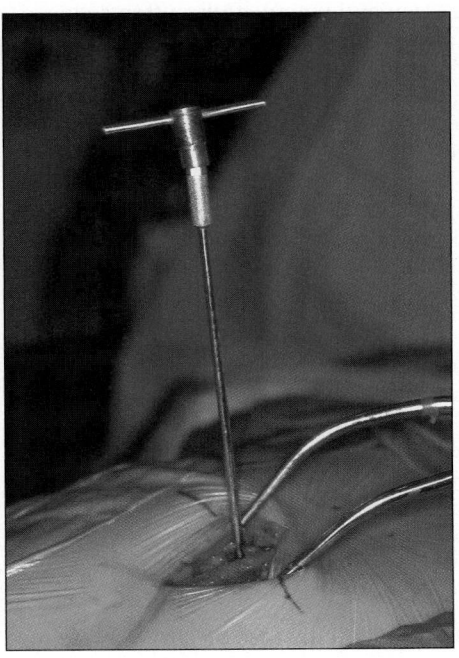

Figure 95-18. A, Intraoperative photo demonstrating the use of a Craig needle to obtain a left transpedicular fluoroscopically controlled biopsy from a thoracic vertebral body using a limited posterior exposure. When the pathologic process is limited to the body without producing an extraosseous paravertebral mass, anterior contamination can be eliminated using this technique. **B,** During the same or a different procedure, and when the tumor produces sufficient bone destruction, a much smaller needle can be passed down through the pedicle to obtain fluid and small bits of material for cytology and/or culture and sensitivity using fluoroscopic control.

for all patients. Twenty-one patients were diagnosed with infectious spondylodiscitis, three with tuberculosis, two with coccidiomycosis, two with brucellosis, and one with blastomycosis. Six had primary neoplasms, 14 had metastatic neoplasms, and 5 had osseous repair from insufficiency fractures. There were seven patients with osteoporotic fractures and one with Paget's disease of bone. In the four remaining patients, the biopsy was initially negative but was later proven to be a false negative because of faulty technique. The authors concluded that percutaneous transpedicular biopsy of lesions within the vertebral body is cost effective and efficacious, and false negatives can be controlled by strict adherence to technical details outlined in the procedure.

With the introduction of video-assisted thoracoscopic surgery, some authors have introduced this technology as an adjunct to biopsy techniques to evaluate thoracic tumors of the spine.[580] To assess a potentially malignant pathologic process confined to the vertebral body, the authors prefer a posterior transpedicular biopsy to minimize contamination of other tissues. For those lesions that do produce a soft-tissue mass, a well-monitored CT-guided biopsy will most often provide tissue sufficient for diagnosis. In the authors' opinion, techniques that potentially contaminate the pleural cavity often render the tumor inoperable and should be avoided if at all possible.

Benign Tumors of the Spine

Osteoid Osteoma of the Spine
Clinical Presentation. Approximately 10% of all osteoid osteomas occur in the spine, and most present in the posterior elements. Painful scoliosis and unexplained vertebral pain in children and young adults, often relieved with nonsteroidal anti-inflammatory drugs (NSAIDs) or aspirin, commonly is associated with this small lesion that is difficult to find and identify. The facet inflammatory synovitis, painful motion, and muscle spasm commonly result in the development of functional scoliosis.[581,582] The intense pain experienced by patients with these tumors is thought to be associated with excessive prostaglandin E2 production by the tumor, resulting in the surrounding inflammatory effect.[583,584] The pain is characteristically worse at night.

Radiographic Features. Osteoid osteoma is usually less than 1.5 cm in diameter and characteristically arises in the posterior elements of the spine. The lesion is encased in dense reactive bone in response to prostaglandin E2 production surrounding the nidus. Plain x-rays are notoriously normal and can be confused with sclerosing osteomyelitis of Garrés. The majority of lesions are discovered after bone scintigraphy or CT.

Histopathology. The nidus consists of an interlacing network of immature bone trabeculae, usually measuring less than 1 cm in diameter and distributed in a background of vascular connective tissue. Prominent benign-appearing osteoblasts rim the osteoid trabeculae. Numerous multinucleated giant cells are present in the

---

> ## OSTEOID OSTEOMA
>
> ### INCIDENCE AND CLINICAL FINDINGS
> 1. Majority of patients <20 years of age
> 2. Male predilection 2:1
> 3. Age range between 5 and 30 years
> 4. 10% occur in spine (posterior elements)
>
> ### RADIOGRAPHIC FINDINGS
> 1. Nidus—osteolytic region <1.5 cm (diaphyseal/metaphyseal)
> 2. Within nidus—may have small central irregular bony opacity
> 3. Nidus surrounded by dense "halo" of reactive bone

---

background. Clinical management consists of either medical or surgical therapy. When surgically accessible, or when prolonged NSAID use is contraindicated, the lesion can be excised surgically with wide margins and the skeletal defect grafted when necessary. When the lesion is located in surgically inaccessible regions, such as the vertebral column or immediately adjacent to an open physis, medical management using NSAIDs may be advised (Fig. 95-19). The risks of medical therapy are basically those associated with the prolonged use of NSAIDs.[585]

Osteoblastoma of the Spine
Osteoblastoma is a progressively enlarging osteoid-containing lesion most often presenting in the posterior elements of the spine and, in contrast to osteoid osteoma, it is characterized by the absence of intense pain and by the dense surrounding reactive bone.

Clinical Presentation. The average age at onset is 17 years (range, 3–78 years). Ninety percent of cases occur before age 30 years.[586,587] The majority of lesions arise in the spinous and transverse processes of the posterior neural arch of the spine. Multifocal lesions have also been reported.[588]

The clinical presentation is usually associated with dull, aching pain, unlike the intense night pain described in patients with osteoid osteoma. Also, the pain is usually not relieved by aspirin or NSAIDs. Tumors presenting in the spinous processes often enlarge to become tender to palpation, while others expand and project into the neural canal, producing symptoms of spinal cord compression. Lesions expanding in the region of the pedicle or transverse process can produce unilateral radicular and peripheral nerve compression symptoms when restricting an adjacent neural foramen. Primary osteoblastomas arising in the sacrum generally involve the posterior elements and most commonly expand posteriorly.

Radiographic Features. Osteoblastoma is characteristically larger than 1.5 cm in diameter, expansile, and well marginated, with a thin rim of reactive bone formation. The central portion of the tumor demonstrates an intra-

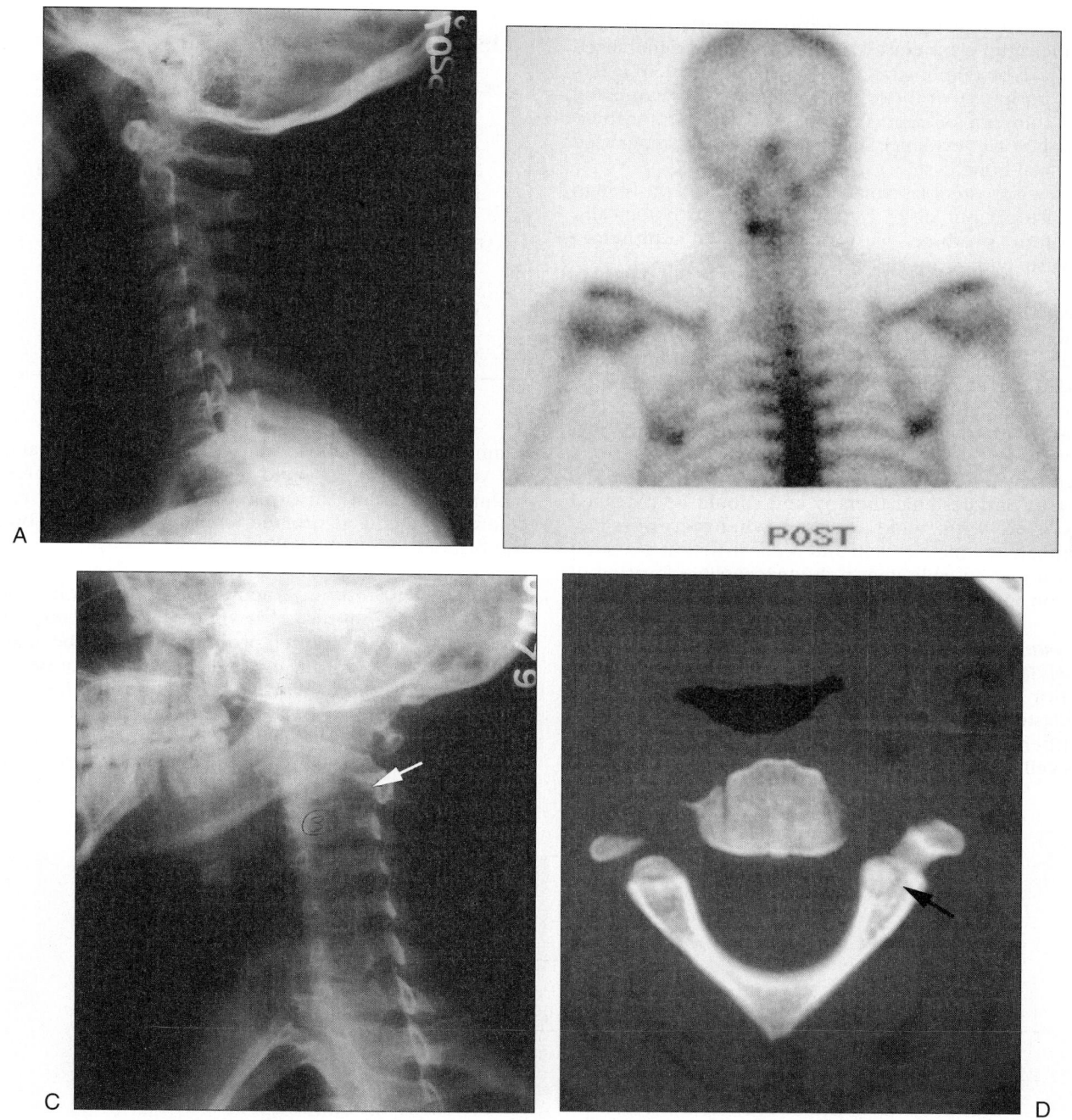

Figure 95-19. A, An 18-year-old female collegiate varsity swimmer developed increased pain in the left midcervical region over 3 months. This lateral cervical spine x-ray was interpreted as normal. **B,** The PA view of the ^{99m}Tc bone scan revealed an area of intense uptake in the left facet of C2. **C,** The right posterior oblique film was also originally interpreted as normal until a bone scan was performed and a lesion was discovered in the region of the left C2 facet (*arrow*). **D,** A targeted CT was performed that demonstrated nidus of ab osteoid osteoma (<1.0 cm diameter) with the characteristic surrounding "halo" in the left facet of C2 (*arrow*). The patient was offered medical or surgical therapy with fusion. The patient elected medical therapy with NSAIDs. The patient is nearly symptom free after 6 months of therapy.

lesional granular appearance related to the punctate mineralization of the osteoid. Localization of the lesion is facilitated by increased focal uptake with bone scintigraphy, with a targeted CT/T or MRI.

"Aggressive" osteoblastoma, considered a separate pathologic entity, represents a borderline malignant lesion between benign osteoblastoma and osteosarcoma. They are characteristically even larger (>3 cm in diameter) and tend to occur in a slightly older population. The tumor can have an aneurysmal or expanded radiographic appearance.

Histopathology. This tumor is also characterized as having a "nidus," with a network of immature bone trabeculae rimmed with benign-appearing osteoblasts and multinucleated giant cells. Varying degrees of mineralized osteoid can be demonstrated. In contrast to osteoid osteoma, the periphery of the lesion is usually well marginated with a thin rim of reactive bone and can demonstrate histopathologic evidence of a secondary or engrafted aneurysmal bone cyst.

Aggressive osteoblastomas appear similar to a benign osteoblastoma but differ by being larger; pathologically, they often produce or form sheets of epitheloid osteoblasts within the lesion.[589,590]

Surgical Therapy. There is currently no medical management for osteoblastoma, and radiotherapy is to be avoided if at all possible. Intralesional excision, resulting in an extended currettage that includes the entire surrounding reactive bone and followed by autogeneic bone grafting, is most often curative for large benign osteoblastoma (Fig. 95-20).

Aggressive osteoblastoma, on the other hand, often can recur after intralesional therapy and should be managed by excision with wide margins whenever possible. Unfortunately, wide excision and reconstruction are often technically impossible due to the inaccessible location of the lesion and adjacent critical, nonexpendable structures.

Aneurysmal Bone Cyst of the Spine

Clinical Presentation. This lesion also presents in the posterior elements, similar to osteoid osteoma and osteoblastoma and in contrast to giant cell tumor, which most often involves the anterior vertebral elements. Pain and swelling with palpable tenderness are the most

---

OSTEOBLASTOMA

INCIDENCE AND CLINICAL FINDINGS
1. Most common between 10 and 20 years of age
2. Dull pain most common (slow growing)
3. 30%–40% originate in the posterior elements of the spine and may present with a neurologic functional deficit while the remainder occur at other sites

RADIOGRAPHIC FINDINGS
1. Mixed osteolytic and blastic response
2. Often >1.5 cm in diameter
3. Well-defined radiographic margins with punctate calcifications present within
4. May expand the cortex

---

common presenting symptoms. The majority of patients are younger than 30 years of age. Lesions that present within the sacrum can expand to enormous proportions before producing neurologic compromise of the bowel and bladder.

Radiographic Features. Aneurysmal bone cyst is characterized radiographically as having a ballooned-out, soap-bubble appearance. It often produces loss of trabeculation and local destruction of the underlying bone. The remaining thin rim of reactive bone about the lesion can usually be identified on CT/T, and layering of complex fluid levels within can likewise be identified. Magnetic resonance imaging with contrast enhancement usually

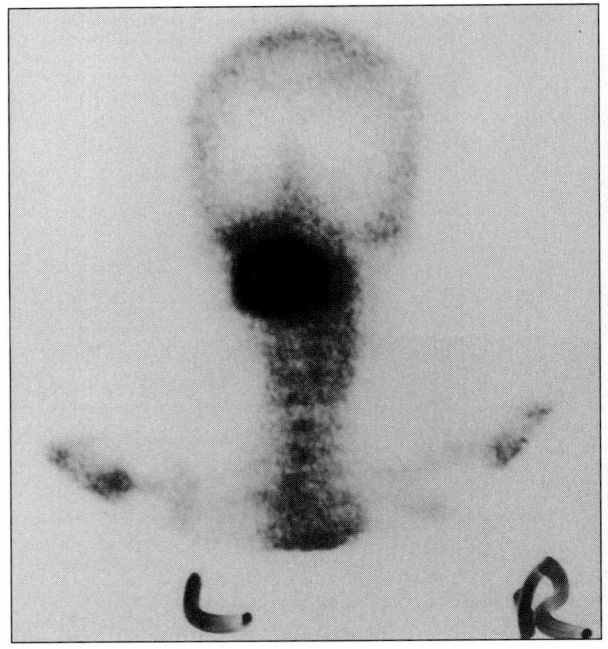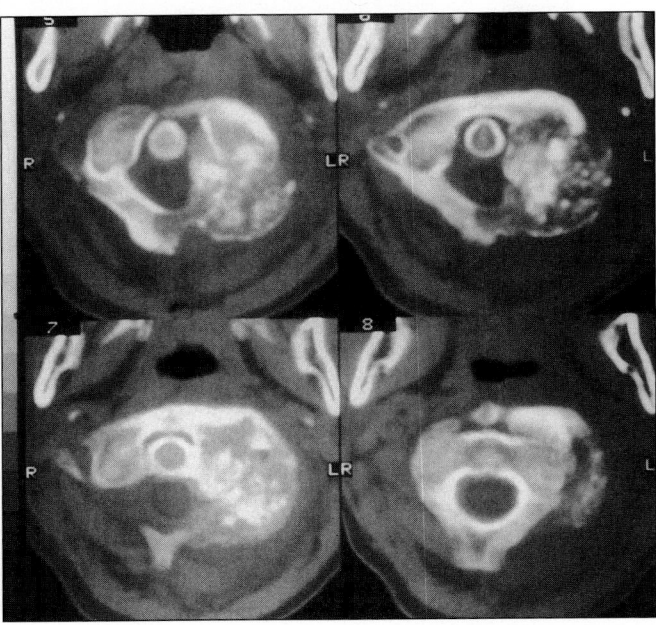

Figure 95-20. A, This PA ^{99m}Tc bone scan demonstrates intense uptake in the left suboccipital region of a 10-year-old male who was symptomatic with local pain 6 to 8 months before medical evaluation. No neurologic deficits could be identified on physical examination. **B,** Multiple images of a targeted CT through the region of C1–2 demonstrates an expansile lesion involving the left posterior elements of C1 with mineralization of the tumor matrix. The course of the right vertebral artery can be evaluated only on the right side.

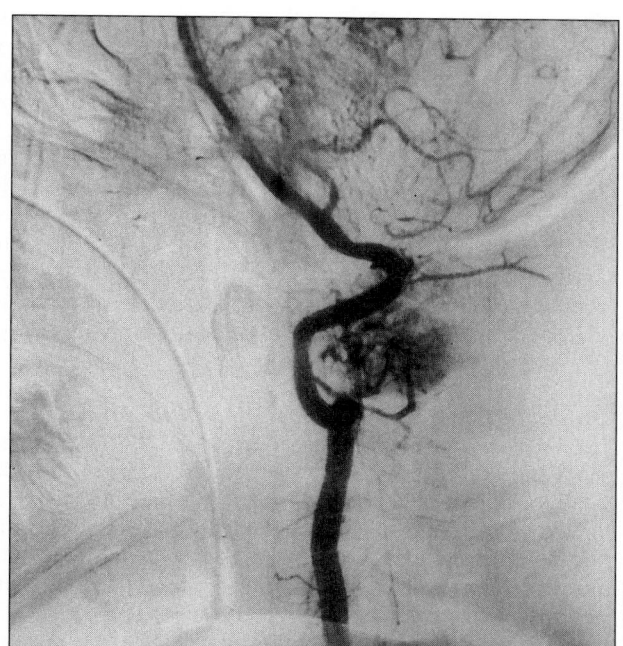

C

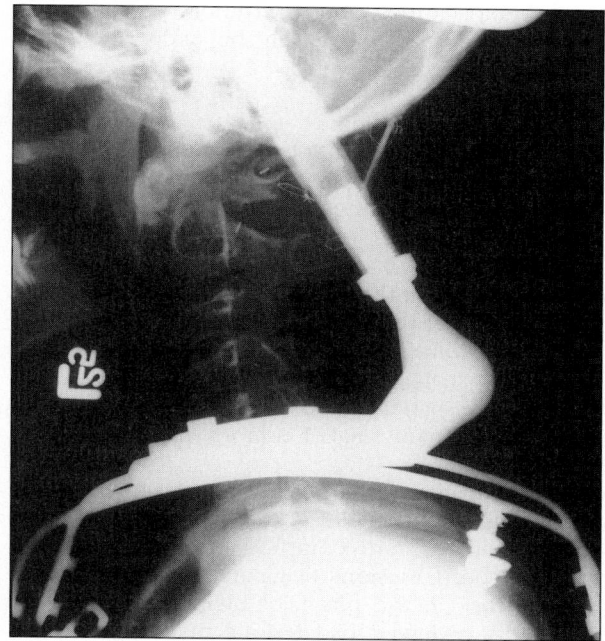

D

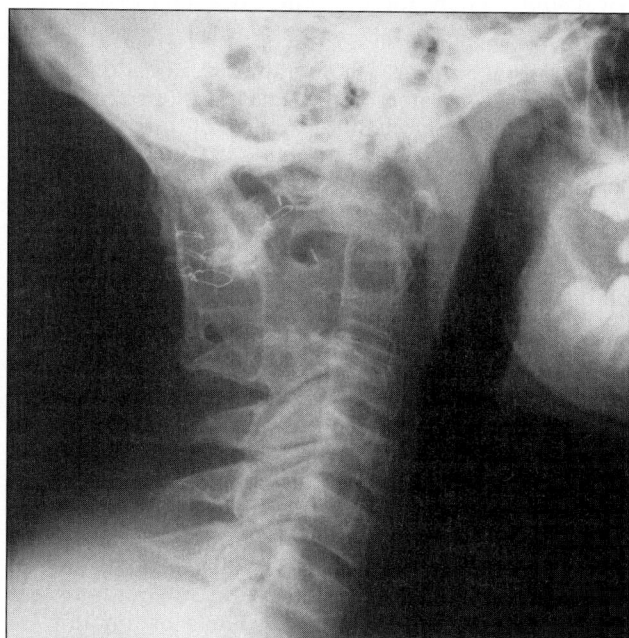

E

Figure 95-20, *cont'd.* **C,** A lateral view of a selective left carotid angiogram demonstrates the anterior position of the vertebral artery and the associated tumor blush. **D,** With the patient prone and the head rigidly immobilized, a left posterior cervical approach was performed in which the lesion was removed piecemeal with subsequent clean contaminated margins. The resection was reconstructed using autogeneic full-thickness iliac crest bone graft wired to the outer table of the skull and the posterior elements of C2. The patient was immobilized in a halo-vest jacket for 6 months. **E,** This lateral C-spine film demonstrates the 5-year follow-up without evidence of persistent disease. The patient lacks 10 degrees of full flexion and 20 degrees of right and left lateral gaze.

demonstrates the bone contour and local anatomy best on T_1-weighted images, while characterizing the enhancing cyst wall on T_2-weighted images. The differential diagnosis includes telangiectatic osteosarcoma, secondary aneurysmal bone cyst associated with underlying chondroblastoma or osteoblastoma, and the posterior extension of a giant cell tumor of bone.

Histopathology. The primary cyst typically demonstrates large, cavernous blood-filled spaces lined by a thin pseudoendothelial cyst wall. Hemosiderin-laden macro-

phages are numerous, with multinucleated giant cells present and in juxtaposition to the cyst lining embedded in a fibrovascular meshwork of benign-appearing tissue.

Surgical Therapy. Because these cysts commonly communicate with interanastomosing vascular channels and the systemic vascular system, injection of sclerosing agents or crystalline steroid compounds is to be avoided. Surgical curettage of the cyst wall, including mechanical debridement of the surrounding reactive bone with a high-speed bur followed by the addition of autogeneic

Specific Malignancies

III

bone graft, is most often curative. Tumors presenting in the transverse process can usually be excised without reconstruction.

Osteochondroma of the Spine
Clinical Presentation. This indolent, slow-growing tumor of the spine can present as a mass with no pain; with pain and no neurologic involvement; or with any combination of a mass, pain, and the presence of a neurologic deficit.[591] In patients with known hereditary multiple exostoses, the diagnosis may be inferred. For lesions to present as a mass with or without pain, in general, they must protrude away from the neurologic elements. Lesions producing radicular pain usually involve an adjacent peripheral nerve root. Those patients presenting with spinal cord compression often have smaller tumors that project into the neural canal.

Kak and colleagues[592] reported on 3 patients and reviewed 10 others with solitary osteochondroma of the spine causing spinal cord compression. Among the 13 patients reviewed, 10 lesions originated in the vertebral body, and 5 arose in the posterior elements. Also, 9 of the 13 patients reviewed had lesions that involved the cervical spine, where there is little extradural "space."

Radiographic Features. Radiographic evaluation often identifies the associated bone stalk that remains contiguous with the intramedullary canal of the associated bone. On occasion, only the punctate calcifications of the cartilaginous cap are evident on plain films or, if not, a CT scan most often identifies the stalk and the punctate calcifications present within the cartilaginous cap.[593] If a neurologic deficit is evident, contrast-enhanced CT of the spine or MRI is recommended.

Surgical Therapy. Surgical therapy consists of excision to include the cartilaginous cap and overlying perichondrium and bursa. Obviously, location and the ability to protect the surrounding neurologic structures dictate whether the lesion can be removed without morselization. The important surgical principle for complete removal is to include the stalk if present and all of the surrounding cartilage tissue and adjacent soft tissue that could have embedded cartilage in it. The complete removal of all cartilage-bearing tissues is paramount for local control.

Primary Malignant Tumors of the Spine

Osteogenic Sarcoma of the Spine
Epidemiology. Osteosarcoma of the spine is fortunately rare, with approximately 1% of reported cases presenting in the spine.[594-596] A clinicopathologic review of 10 patients identified by a retrospective review of more than 1000 patients demonstrated ages ranging from 3 to 64 years, with a mean age of 35 years. Six patients were believed to have conventional osteosarcomas, and four had secondary osteosarcomas (three females with tumors secondary to Paget's disease, and one patient with a postradiation osteosarcoma).

Clinical Presentation. All patients presented with complaints of pain, except for a 3-year-old child who presented with a mass. Three tumors presented in the thoracic spine, seven presented in the lumbar spine, and only one presented with a compression fracture. The overall prognosis was poor, with seven patients dying within 1 year of diagnosis and only one patient living longer than 1 year. Treatment was inconsistent, with seven patients undergoing decompression laminectomy and an attempt at local tumor excision. Nine patients received radiotherapy, with five of the nine also receiving chemotherapy. There were no instances of a complete histologic response to chemotherapy.[597]

Radiographic Features and Differential Diagnosis. The radiographic appearance of patients with osteogenic sarcoma of the spine can vary greatly. The tumor produces malignant osteoid that is often visible on plain films of excellent quality or on CT scans. Bone scintigraphy is usually successful in identifying the involved bone and/or multicentric lesions. Occasionally, telangiectatic osteosarcoma can present as a "cold" bone scan.

CT is valuable in identifying the extent of the soft-tissue mass by detecting mineralization within the soft-tissue extension. CT remains the standard of care for evaluating the lungs for possible metastatic disease. MRI, however, remains the single most useful study. Angiography has virtually been replaced by MRI except to identify the small segmented vessels that supply the spinal cord.

The differential diagnosis of primary tumors arising in the spine includes osteoblastoma, aneurysmal bone cyst, giant cell tumor of bone, osteoid osteoma, eosinophilic granuloma, malignant degeneration of preexisting bone lesion (e.g., Ollier's disease), and metastasis. Osteoblastoma characteristically arises in the posterior elements (including the transverse processes), while giant cell tumor most commonly arises in the vertebral body. Postradiation sarcoma of bone must be considered for patients who have had radiotherapy for treatment of other diseases, and especially for those patients treated concomitantly with alkylating chemotherapeutic agents (associated with promoting development of a secondary malignancy).

ANEURYSMAL BONE CYST

INCIDENCE AND CLINICAL FINDINGS
1. 75% observed prior to age 20
2. Pain and swelling most common sign
3. 20% originate in the posterior elements of the spine
4. Spine lesions commonly present with increasing neurologic findings

RADIOGRAPHIC FINDINGS
1. 50% suggest subperiosteal origin
2. Metaphyseal/diaphyseal location
3. Involves primarily posterior elements of spine
4. Fusiform expansile lesion could involve adjacent vertebra

Surgical Therapy. The appropriate treatment of patients with osteosarcoma of the spine is becoming increasingly clear.[597-599] In 1989, Ogihara and associates[600] reported on a 15-year-old patient managed by posterior decompressive laminectomy of T4 and a COMPADRI-III chemotherapy regimen, in which doxorubicin was the primary agent. The patient remained disease free for 6 years.

A report on 24 patients with osteosarcoma of the spine better illustrates the combined role of surgery, chemotherapy, and radiotherapy. Thirteen of these patients had conventional osteosarcoma, and 11 had secondary tumors. Thirteen patients treated between 1949 and 1977 with limited surgery and radiotherapy were compared with 11 patients treated between 1978 and 1984 with more aggressive surgery, combination chemotherapy, and radiotherapy. Five patients from the second group were long-term survivors. Complete surgical resection was used when anatomically possible, after several cycles of neoadjuvant chemotherapy. Radiation therapy was added when complete excision was not possible.[601]

With improvements in both imaging capabilities and spinal instrumentation, more aggressive procedures (spondylectomies) are possible with a resultant mechanically stable spine. After diagnosis—usually requiring a decompressive laminectomy—multiagent neoadjuvant chemotherapy followed by staged radical surgery and spine stabilization could offer superior results.

Cohen and coauthors[602] have described a two-staged technique for total spondylectomy for lesions involving the cervical spine. Preoperative chemotherapy consisted of high-dose methotrexate with leucovorin rescue, cisplatin, and doxorubicin. After achieving a near-complete response, the lesion at C6 was re-evaluated, with the tumor involving both pedicles of C6. Posterior extension was visible dorsal to the lamina, and only mild cord compression was evident.

The authors described the first posterior stage, requiring the resection of the posterior elements and a transpedicular C6 vertebrectomy with the placement of a temporary vertebrectomy defect spacer. Posterior instrumentation was achieved between C3 and T3. This consisted of lateral mass screws and thoracic pedicle screws, rods, and cross-links. The posterior elements of C3–C4 and T1–T3 were decorticated, and allograft chips were then placed in an attempt for autofusion.

The anterior approach was then staged 1 week later and performed in the supine position. An anterior exposure was achieved, and the vertebral bodies between C5 and C7 were resected as a single block. The temporary cage at C6 was removed. A Synmesh cage was filled with allograft and Grafton to span the C5–C7 vertebrectomy defect.

Surgical "wide" margins are not possible in the cervical spine because of the need to preserve both the cervical nerve roots and the vertebral arteries. After systemic multiagent chemotherapy, however, it might be possible to achieve a near-complete 100% necrosis, in which a clean contaminated type of margin might result in prolonged survival and possibly cure. With the evolution of ever more sophisticated spinal implants and their flexibility of application, there has been renewed interest in managing patients with nonmetastatic primary bone tumors of the spinal column after completion of a neoadjuvant course of chemotherapy.

Adjuvant chemotherapy and possibly radiotherapy could be used to prolong survival. Long-term survival appears dependent on the dose intensity and duration of the chemotherapeutic agents used and on the overall chemosensitivity of the primary tumor (responders vs. nonresponders).

Malignant Fibrous Histiocytoma of the Spine

Although they are extraordinarily rare as a primary tumor of the spine, single skeletal metastases to the vertebral column from an otherwise well-managed primary malignant fibrous histiocytoma of bone or soft tissue occasionally can present several years after initial therapy.[603-605] Regardless of the origin of the tumor, malignant fibrous histiocytoma of bone is treated identically to osteosarcoma, with multiagent neoadjuvant chemotherapy followed by surgical resection with wide margins and adjuvant chemotherapy.[606,607] The only difference in the local treatment is the frequent addition of radiation therapy if wide margins are not achieved. Malignant fibrous histiocytoma also can arise as a secondary malignancy from previous treatment of disease.[608-616]

Chondrosarcoma of the Spine

Epidemiology. Primary and/or secondary chondrosarcoma arising in the vertebrae is uncommon and represents approximately 7% to 10% of patients reported in a large series. It remains the most common primary tumor of bone in the middle to late decades of life, however, with the exception of multiple myeloma.

Embryologically, growth centers are present at three separate centers during development from immature cartilage (Fig. 95-21). Therefore, it is not surprising that cartilagenous tumors appear to arise from both the anterior and posterior elements.

Shives and colleagues[393] reported their results of treatment of patients with 20 stage IB (low-grade, extracompartmental) chondrosarcomas of the spine managed at the Mayo Clinic. All but two patients presented with pain, and eight also had an associated mass. One additional patient noted only a mass, while another presented with paresis without local symptoms. Nine of 20 patients presented with neurologic symptoms, 2 with weakness, and 2 with sensory loss only, and the remaining 5 had both motor and sensory loss. There were 16 males and 4 females, with a mean age of 45 years.

The distribution of primary tumors from several larger series of patients reported is demonstrated in Table 95-12 (excluding the sacrum). There appears to be a slight predilection of tumors in the cervical spine, with fewer lesions presenting in the lumbar spine. In the Mayo Clinic review, eight tumors arose in the posterior elements and three in the body alone, while nine tumors involved both anterior and posterior elements. Four tumors arose in preexisting osteochondromas. Overall outcomes were not included due to the number of years spanned by the paper and the advent of superior imaging and

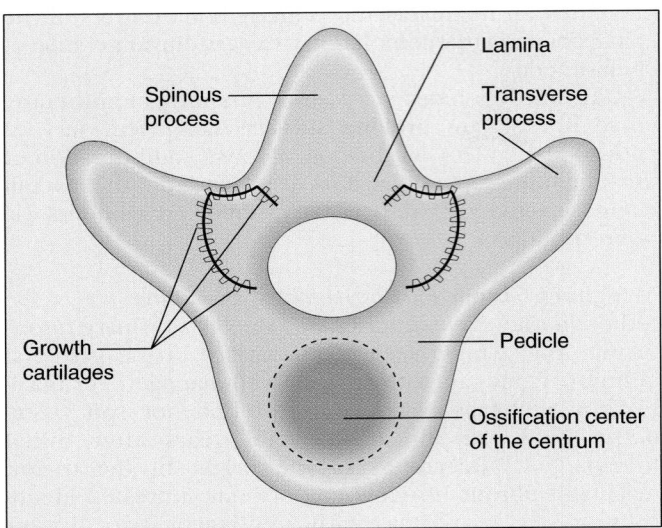

Figure 95-21. The developing vertebral body contains one ossification center, while three growth cartridges develop bilaterally to form the neural arch, with one for the pedicle, lamina, and transverse process. Union of the growth centers does not occur until the sixth to seventh year of life.

reconstruction techniques. Only the paper by Shives and colleagues[393] attempted to control for the change of imaging techniques over time. Only 1 of 20 patients was considered inoperable compared with other reports.

Radiographic Features. Characteristically, malignant cartilaginous neoplasms are radiographically poorly marginated. Ten of 20 patients reported by Shives and colleagues[393] had radiographs available to review. Tumors in all 10 patients were poorly marginated, without evidence of rimming reactive bone, supporting their later histopathologic findings of malignancy. Characteristic matrix calcification was present in 7 of 10 tumors. Extension into adjacent soft tissues was present in nine tumors, and cortical destruction was radiographically demonstrable in all 10.

Histopathology. Chondrosarcoma arising in the spine had histopathologic features identical to those presenting at other sites. Hypercellularity, myxoid changes, and double-nucleated cells represent the predominant features

of a chondrosarcoma. In general, the tumor behaves biologically by pushing the adjacent soft tissues aside and by lobulation rather than by invading adjacent tissues. Of the four chondrosarcomas of the spine reported by Eriksson and coauthors,[615] two were low grade (grade I), and two were high grade (grade II). Among the 20 patients reported by Shives and colleagues,[391] 15 tumors were low grade (grade I), and 5 were high grade (grade II). Of those earlier tumors reported by others as inoperable (see Table 95-12), the majority were larger lesions in which wide surgical margins were impossible to achieve.

Surgical Therapy. Chondrosarcoma is one of the more operable tumors of the spine, often originating asymmetrically and producing a lobulated mass that pushes aside structures with minimal soft-tissue invasion. Chondrosarcomas usually can be well demonstrated by CT or illuminated radiographically with contrast-enhanced MRI, making surgical planning easier and more predictable. Also, because chondrosarcoma tends to be less invasive than other tumor types, resection of smaller amounts of surrounding normal tissue is required to achieve a wide surgical margin.

Tumors can invade the neural canal, encroaching on the dura, and can produce spinal cord compression above the vertebra of L1 or peripheral nerve root involvement below the level of the conus. As with all malignant tumors of the spine, the tumor and biopsy tract must be removed en bloc with the primary tumor, with a minimum of a wide bone and soft-tissue margin for adequate local control (Fig. 95-22). When dura is involved, the dura must be resected en bloc with the lesion to maintain a wide margin. Of the 20 patients described by Shives and coworkers,[393] 11 had intralesion margins (e.g., piecemeal removal, curettage) and all 11 patients experienced persistent progressive disease. Six patients had clean contaminated margins (i.e., intralesional margins converted to wide margins by excising the pseudocapsule and surrounding reactive tissue). Three developed progressive disease and died, while the other three remain free of local recurrence after more than 5 years. Similarly, Wuisman and colleagues[618] compared treatment of four patients with secondary chondrosarcoma of the spine with 45 patients having nonspinal secondary chondrosarcomas of the spine managed by surgery. One patient, having had a wide en bloc resection, remains free of

TABLE 95-12

			LOCATION			
STUDY	**NO. OF PATIENTS**	**NO. REPORTED**	**C-SPINE**	**T-SPINE**	**L-SPINE**	**CONSIDERED INOPERABLE**
Scandinavica (1957)	9	9	4	4	1	Not reported
Memorial (1978)	14	14	6	5	3	Not reported
MGH (1980)	4/43	4/43	Distribution not reported			4/4
Rizzoli Inst. (1981)	7/125	7/125	0	4	3	6/7
Mayo Clinic (1989)	37/553	20/553	4	11	5	1/20

Incidence of Anatomic Location of Primary Spine Tumors (Excluding Sacrum)

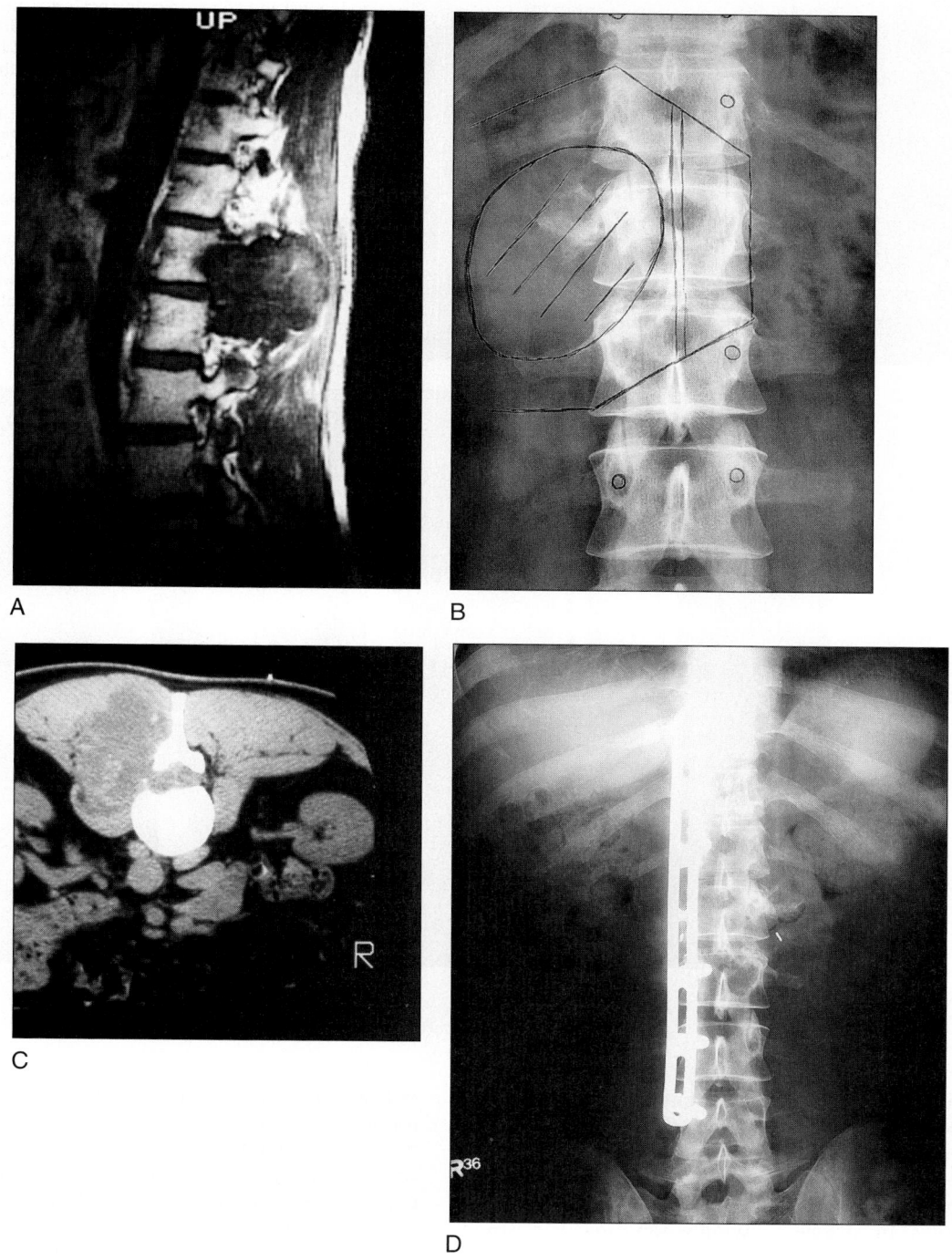

Figure 95-22. A, 30-year-old male was seen and evaluated 18 months after developing increasing left midlumbar spine pain. Plain films demonstrated the absence of the left transverse process of L1. The T_1-weighted MRI of the spine demonstrated an irregular infiltrative asymmetric lesion involving the left paraspinous musculature and lateral elements of L1 and part of T12 and L2. An open biopsy revealed grade II chondrosarcoma. **B,** This PA radiograph of the thoracolumbar junction demonstrates the region of the tumor (*cross-hatching*) with the area outlined, demonstrating the structures that would require removal to obtain a wide surgical margin. A myelogram demonstrated tumor invading the canal through the left foramen of L1. A two-stage procedure was planned, whereby a right hemilaminectomy of L1 and transverse-oblique laminotomies of T12 and L2 would be performed from the right side posteriorly, followed by instrumentation of the right pedicles of T10, T11, T12, L2, and L3 with VSP instrumentation. **C,** The CT scan demonstrates the encroachment of the left L1 foramen and neural canal by tumor displacing the dura to the right. A fat plane can be identified between the tumor and the dura. These findings require the resection of the potentially involved dura with the specimen to complete an en bloc resection with wide margins. **D,** This AP x-ray demonstrates the completion of the first stage of a two-stage procedure. The plate was applied to the right pedicles of T10, T11, T12 and L2, L3, and L4. Hemilaminectomies were performed on the right, as well as oblique laminectomies illustrated in **(B).**

Continued

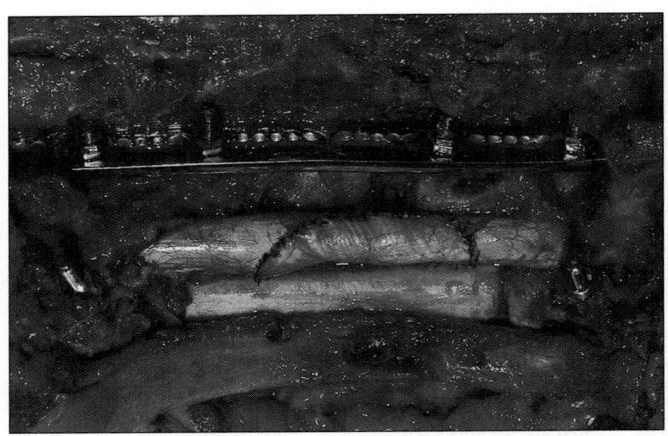

E

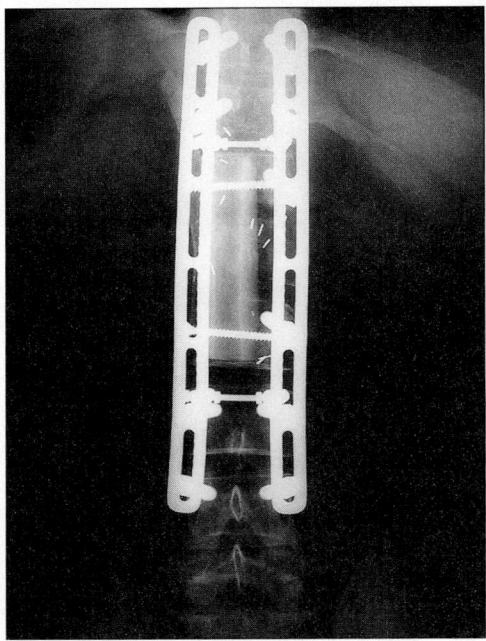

F

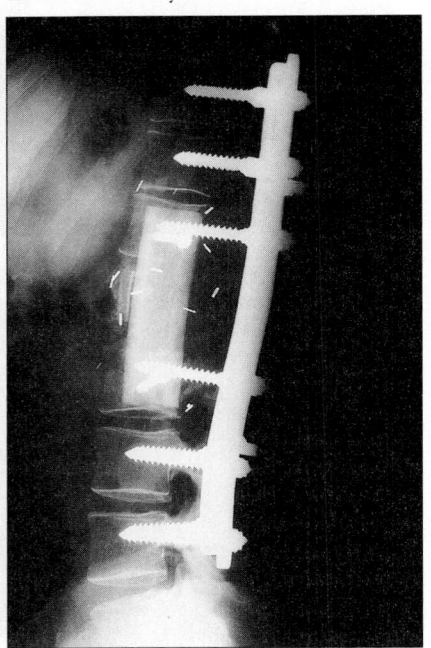

G

Figure 95-22, *cont'd.* E, Two weeks later, through a thoracoabdominal and communicating posterior midline exposure, the lesion was removed successfully en bloc with wide margins to include the lower oblique one-half of T12, L1, and the upper oblique one-half of L2 and in continuity with the involved dura of L1. A dural patch was required for repair. This intraoperative photo demonstrates the previously applied first-stage plate at the top with the dural repair beneath. A cylindric full-thickness segment of femoral allograft was used to restore the continuity of the anterior column (below the dura). A vascularized rib graft can be seen below, curving up to about the allograft. **F,** This AP x-ray demonstrates the postoperative completed construct with four cross-connectors. The patient was immobilized in a TLSO jacket for 1 year and has consistently used an abdominal/lumbar support since his procedure. This AP x-ray was taken at the patient's 10-year re-evaluation. **G,** This lateral x-ray also demonstrates a stable construct at 10 years without hardware failure or allograft resorption. The patient remains continuously disease free at 12 years.

disease, while the other three patients with intralesional margins experienced local recurrence and have died of their disease.

Primary Ewing's Sarcoma of the Spine

Epidemiology. In primary Ewing's sarcoma, the spine remains an unusual site for the development of primary disease. Whitehause and Griffiths[619] reviewed the literature and found a 3.5% incidence of spine as a primary site in 1020 cases. Pilepich and associates[620] described the early results of treatment of IESS-1 and found 22 of 271 registered patients with primary involvement of the spine. As mentioned previously, the disease is rarely if ever seen in the black population.

Clinical Manifestations. Approximately 75% of patients with Ewing's sarcoma present before the age of 20 years and 90% before the age of 30 years.[621,622] Kaspers and colleagues[623] reviewed 15 cases from the literature and found that 100% of patients presented with either back or radicular pain, and 83% presented with paresis with or without sensory disturbances of one or both lower extremities, and with bowel and bladder symptoms. The mean age at diagnosis was 17.5 years (range, 4 to 47 years), and the mean diagnostic delay was 5.8 months.

Radiographic Features. The tumor is classically destructive, producing loss of trabeculation with permeative changes and cortical destruction of bone. Plain films used to evaluate the spine are frequently inadequate. The study of choice remains a contrast-enhanced, physician-monitored MRI of the involved area with multiplanar reconstruction of the region in question. Some lesions in contrast result in a solitary ivory apparence or in vertebra plana that often mimics eosinophilic granuloma.[624-626]

Skeletal assessment or staging is best performed using bone scintigraphy or rapid whole-body STIR MRI. Computed tomography remains the standard by which to assess the lungs for pulmonary metastases.

Differential Diagnosis. Primary Ewing's sarcoma of the spine does not produce any radiographically identifiable matrix and results in a nonspecific and varied radiographic appearance. Metastases, infection, eosinophile granuloma, and primary hematologic processes of the spine can often be confused with Ewing's sarcoma.

Treatment. Because of the difficulty in achieving a complete resection with wide margins, the majority of patients initially have a decompressive laminectomy for immediate relief of neurologic symptoms and to obtain biopsy material. Grubb and coauthors[627] reported their results of 36 patients diagnosed and managed at the Mayo Clinic between 1951 and 1988. The mean age of patients at diagnosis was 17 years (range, 5 to 40 years). Neurologic symptoms were recorded in 58% of patients. Forty-seven percent had a decompressive laminectomy for early treatment and a biopsy. Three of the four patients with thoracic or thoracolumbar tumors treated by laminectomy without a stabilizing procedure developed progressive kyphosis.

Sixteen of 36 patients were registered in the Intergroup Ewing's Sarcoma Study (IESS). Intensive chemotherapy was administered to 32 patients, and all patients received radiotherapy. The 5-year survival rate was 33%, with nine patients free of disease at 6 to 184 months and a mean survival time of 2.9 years. No significant correlation could be identified between location of the tumor in the spine, length of disease-free survival, overall survival, or incidence of metastatic disease. Those patients enrolled in the IESS, however, had significantly better rates of disease-free survival and overall survival.[627]

In most instances, the tumor is sensitive to neoadjuvant chemotherapy and radiotherapy. If radiotherapy is used, it can often be delayed until the treatment window at 12 to 13 weeks usually reserved for surgery (see the earlier discussion on treatment of Ewing's sarcoma). If acute cord compression is an issue, however, radiotherapy can be used initially to relieve compression of the dura and the surrounding neural elements.

Stability of the Spine. Because Ewing's sarcoma is usually very destructive and the tumor characteristically involves the anterior spinal elements, many of the patients subsequently develop significant kyphosis after induction chemotherapy, radiotherapy and vertebral collapse, or decompressive laminectomy alone. If there is clear radiographic suggestion that the anterior spine elements will collapse with therapy, consideration must be given to stabilizing the spine—posteriorly initially, and possibly anteriorly after completion of therapy.

Surgical Therapy. Ideally, if there is concern about destabilizing the spine either by therapy or decompressive laminectomy, the spine should be stabilized initially with posterior pedicle fixation to include (in most cases) two motion segments above and two motion segments below the lesion. By placing all the bone screws in the pedicles before decompression or biopsy, subsequent surgical contamination of the wound after biopsy usually does not result in seeding the other vertebral bodies. The wound can be managed initially by copious irrigation and drained closure, followed by chemotherapy and possibly radiotherapy, if required.

Fessler and coauthors[628] described a posterior lateral parascapular extrapleural approach to the upper thoracic vertebrae and the results of treatment in four patients. The parascapular musculature is reflected off the spinous processes (trapezius, levator scapulae, and rhomboid muscles) and retracted laterally to expose the underlying ribs. With a double-lumen endotracheal tube in place, the involved ribs are removed, retracting the paraspinal muscle mass dorsally and medially. The lung is deflated, and the thoracic cage is opened dorsally. The intercostal nerve, artery, and veins are ligated, and the suture is used later to act as a guide for the decompression or as a guide to the thecal sac. The resected rib serves as bone graft for reconstruction.

If the patient responds well to treatment after decompression and posterior pedicle instrumentation zand remains otherwise free of distant disease, the authors prefer to defer any secondary surgical procedures until the entire chemotherapy program has been completed (i.e., the upper limb of the approach to the treatment of Ewing's sarcoma). The surgical procedures for spondylectomy to achieve either wide or clean contaminated margins after radiotherapy and chemotherapy are usually complex, requiring combined anterior and posterior surgical exposures. These frequently are associated with numerous complications that could require more than the three weeks normally allowed within the treatment protocol. By delaying surgical therapy until the completion of chemotherapy, it is much easier to provide superior care, to devote full time and effort to achieve wide surgical margins, and to treat any complications appropriately without fear of interrupting the chemotherapy schedule.

Late Effects of Radiation Therapy for Treatment of Malignant Childhood Tumors. Skeletal complications and late effects from irradiation of bone are well documented and include scoliosis, kyphosis, chest and rib deformities, limb-length discrepancy, hypoplasia of the ilium, exostoses, and secondary postradiation sarcomas.[629,630] As more and more children managed by multimodal therapy survive their disease, the late and lasting therapy-related effects become more evident.

Butler and colleagues[635] published their retrospective review of 143 patients who received radiotherapy for childhood tumors and survived to skeletal maturity. Fifty (35%) developed scoliosis. Patients with Wilms' tumor and neuroblastoma developed curves in 63% and 83% of cases, respectively. The mean dose for treatment of neuroblastoma was 1960 cGy, and a mean of 2825 cGy was given for treatment of Wilms' tumor. Although the spine was treated symmetrically, the soft tissues treated were very asymmetric compared with those patients treated for Hodgkin's disease. Even though the mean dose of 3460 cGy was higher for patients with Hodgkin's disease, the treatment fields were symmetric; consequently, the scoliosis curves in 17 patients (39%) were all less than 20 degrees.

Chest and rib deformities were seen in 36% of patients after treatment, with 35% of females also having breast asymmetry.

Kidney Autotransplantation. If the primary tumor is located adjacent to the renal fossa where external-beam radiotherapy might result in a significant loss of renal function, consideration must be given to autotransplantation of the kidney. This well-tolerated procedure must be planned for before radiotherapy to protect the kidneys, allowing for well-planned, uncompromised radiotherapy treatment.[636]

Giant Cell Tumors of the Spine

Epidemiology. Giant cell tumor of the vertebral column is uncommon above the sacrum. Shankman and coauthors[637] reviewed 1277 cases of giant cell tumor and found only 34 (2.7%) reported in the spine. A report from the Rizzoli Instituto in Bologna reviewed 314 patients with giant cell tumor and nine patients (2.9%) who presented with spinal primary tumors.[638] It appears that lesions in the vertebral column above the sacrum are more or less equally distributed in the cervical, thoracic, and lumbar spine. In general, the overall incidence of giant cell tumor presenting in the spine is approximately 3.2%.[639-643]

Clinical Manifestations. There appears to be a predilection for female patients with giant cell tumor of the spine. Dahlin[644] reported 23 female and 8 male patients with primary giant cell tumor of the spine. Savini and associates[638] reported 7 of 9 females, and Sanjay and colleagues[645] reviewed 17 females and 7 males with giant cell tumor affecting the spine. The majority of patients were diagnosed in the second and third decades of life, with age ranging between 6 and 66 years. The most common presenting symptom was pain, followed by neurologic symptoms and then deformity.[638,644,646]

Radiographic Features. The preoperative x-rays were available for 18 of 24 patients reviewed from the Mayo Clinic, and all demonstrated an osteolytic but relatively well-marginated lesion devoid of matrix mineralization. More than half of the lesions demonstrated expansion of the existing cortex. Two large tumors involved the subchondral bone and disc extending into the adjacent vertebrae. Pathologic fracture and soft-tissue extension were relatively common. Two patients developed asynchronous multicentric lesions, with one in the spine and one developing in an extremity.[645]

Differential Diagnosis. In contrast to aneurysmal bone cyst (ABC), osteoblastoma, and osteoid osteoma, giant-cell tumors of the spine develop primarily in the anterior vertebral elements and, less commonly, involve the neural arch. Of these comparable entities, ABC is the most similar in appearance and can often be excluded by the absence of a cavernous blood-filled septated cyst, most often diagnostic of ABC. Benign osteoblastoma most often demonstrates both osteogenesis and prominent osteoid trabeculae formed throughout the tumor.[644]

Surgical Therapy. The consensus among musculoskeletal oncologists is to excise the lesion, then to perform reconstruction using autogeneic bone and/or allograft. Larsson and coauthors[646] reported four nonsacral lesions treated using various methods. One skeletally immature male was treated with external-beam radiotherapy using 3100 cGy for a relatively undisplaced tumor of C5. The tumor primarily had involved the body, one pedicle, and one lamina. The pain was relieved in 14 days. Spinal deformity resulted in partial collapse; however, a 14-year follow-up did demonstrate fusion developing between the fourth, fifth, and sixth cervical vertebrae with a 20-degree gibbus deformity.

One other patient with a primary tumor of the body of T12 was treated with radiotherapy (5000 cGy) after intralesional surgical treatment, demonstrating nearly complete destruction of the body. Although the patient originally was paraplegic, the spinal cord function returned to the point at which the patient could work full-time walking with a cane.[646]

Two other patients with lesions in the bodies of T12 and L1 both had partial or subtotal excision and no instrumentation. Neither patient experienced local recurrence.[646]

Savini and associates[638] reported the results of treatment of nine patients, one treated with radiotherapy alone without success. The patient died as a consequence of the disease 30 months later. Two other patients had intralesional excision followed by radiotherapy. One patient died of pulmonary metastases 30 months later, and the other developed recurrence 6 years later that required radiotherapy.

Their best results were reported for patients having clean contaminated excision followed by reconstruction, made possible by better and improved surgical technique and spinal instrumentation. In all three patients, no local recurrence occurred, and all constructs appeared to be stable and healed.

Surgical therapy for 24 patients described by Sanjay and coauthors[645] from the Mayo Clinic was reported as requiring one- or two-stage procedures and was somewhat site dependent. Ideally, a wide margin should be achieved; however, spondylectomy for a benign tumor has associated risks.[647,648]

Fourteen patients had a one-stage procedure, eight by an anterior approach and six by a posterior approach. Ten patients had a two-stage procedure, or both an anterior and a posterior approach. Tumors involving the arch were usually treated by a laminectomy, including removal of the tumor with clean contaminated margins and posterior fusion. Tumors confined to the body anteriorly were treated by a one-stage anterior procedure with stabilization and bone grafting. Seven cases involved the vertebral body only, and three involved both the body and the posterior arch, managed by a two-stage procedure that included excision of the tumor with anterior and posterior stabilization.

Complications included two perioperative problems, involving a dural leak and a hematoma that required reoperation. Two patients experienced late complications, one each with an anterior and posterior nonunion and both requiring reinstrumentation and autogeneic bone grafting. Both patients ultimately achieved solid fusions with excellent functional results.

Local control after the index procedure was achieved in 14 patients. Ten patients developed local recurrence. Of the 10 patients with locally persistent disease, all patients had attempts at re-excision, with 6 patients requiring additional radiotherapy in cases in which the quality of the margins could not be ensured.

At the time of the report, two deaths appeared to be tumor related. One patient had developed a radiation-induced secondary sarcoma, and one patient died from a deep infection. The use of radiotherapy in patients with giant cell tumor remains controversial.[644,649-651] Rock and coauthors[652] reported a 10% incidence of subsequent development of a radiation-induced sarcoma from treatment of benign giant cell tumor of bone.

Neoplastic Epidural Spinal Cord Compression

Pathophysiology. The pathophysiology of epidural spinal cord compression is important to understand. The slowly enlarging extradural mass results in early obstruction of the epidural venous plexus and enhances vasogenic edema. Dysfunction of the normal specialized spinal cord/blood barrier results in increased permeability, with extravasation of protein-bound and water-soluble materials into the normally restricted extracellular space of the neural tissues. As a result, the neural tissue becomes edematous. In the late stages of development, there is a rapid decrease in spinal cord blood flow at the site of compression, resulting in irreversible loss of function.[653-665]

Treatment

High-Dose Dexamethasone Therapy. The use of high-dose steroids in the treatment of spinal cord compression is well accepted and is supported by numerous animal model studies.[653,654,656,659] It is presumed that the effects observed are related to the anti-inflammatory properties induced by the steroid therapy. Vecht and coauthors[666] reported their results of a randomized prospective study designed to evaluate either initial high-dose dexamethasone (100 mg) and conventional (10-mg intravenous bolus) treatment of patients with spinal cord compression followed by a 16-mg daily oral dose. No dose effect was observed on neurologic function or outcome; however, the authors did report substantial pain relief. Steroid-related improvement is most often related to the oncolytic effect, as in leukemias and lymphoma.[667] Nonlymphoproliferative neoplasms, such as metastases and primary sarcomas of bone, rarely if ever respond as dramatically to high-dose steroid therapy.

It is important to use systemic steroid therapy carefully, however. It has been shown that both duration and total dose predicted subsequent patient complications (e.g., gastric intestinal bleeding, rectosigmoid perforation). Because major complications can occur in patients receiving steroids, they should be tapered to a lower dose or discontinued as soon as clinically possible.[671]

Surgical Therapy for Tumors of the Spine. The vascularity of the spinal cord depends primarily on three longitudinal arterial vessels: the anterior median longitudinal trunk, and a pair of posterolateral trunks that ramify between the emerging posterior nerve roots. Medullary feeders or radicular arteries reinforce the longitudinal vessels at various levels. The artery of Adamkiewicz, also a radicular vessel, occurs on the left side between T7 and L4 in 80% of patients, and most occur from T9 to T11. Even though the artery of Adamkiewicz is preserved surgically, it does not ensure normal function of the cord, as the anterior medial longitudinal vessel is probably the most important vessel supplying the cord.[672]

The first reported spondylectomy was performed by Lievre and colleagues,[673] with piecemeal removal of a giant cell tumor in the fourth lumbar vertebra. Stener,[392] in 1971, described a one-stage posterior total spondylectomy for chondrosarcoma arising asymmetrically in the seventh vertebral body. Reconstruction involved posterior internal fixation and anterior autogeneic structural graft material. His techniques were refined in 1984 and summarized in 1989.[674-676] The advent of improved anterior and posterior spinal instrumentation, together with multimodal chemotherapy and/or radiotherapy, have made some previously inoperable tumors now amenable to surgery.[677-687]

The overall goal of surgical therapy is to achieve a wide pathologically confirmed margin. Morselization and piecemeal removal of a primary spinal bone tumor should be considered only after a "good" preoperative chemotherapy response has been achieved or after the completion of preoperative radiotherapy in which clean contaminated margins can be ensured. A recent review of treatment of spinal tumors by Bell[688] outlines many of the current methods and recommendations for treatment of patients with tumors of the spine.

Currently, the majority of surgeons use either a single- or two-stage procedure for surgical treatment. By first stabilizing the spine posteriorly with pedicle fixation, the appropriate laminotomies and required exposure posteriorly are completed before closure and completion of the first stage. The second-stage resection is completed 10 to 14 days later through a combined sufficient thoracoabdominal and posterior spine incision to obtain anterior and posterior exposure and to ensure an exposure large enough to obtain a wide, potentially curative margin.[689,690]

CHORDOMA

Cervical and Sacrococcygeal Chordoma

Embryology

The notochord is a unique tissue that reaches maturity in the 11-mm embryo. In the second gestational month, the

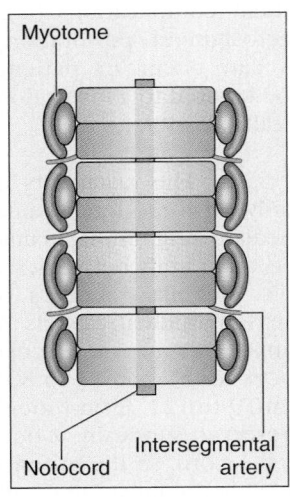
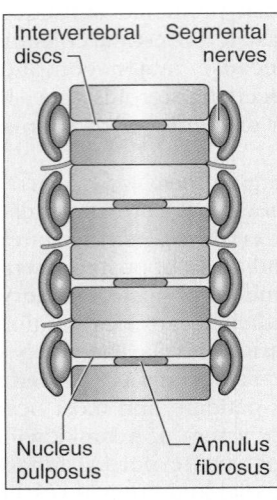

Figure 95-23. A, The formation of less dense cephalic and more dense caudal sclerotoma surrounding the notochord at four weeks. **B,** At 11 weeks' gestation, the precartilaginous vertebral bodies have formed by the upper and lower halves of two successive sclerotomas, while the notochord has degenerated except in the region of the intervertebral disk.

notochordal tissue is essentially obliterated (Fig. 95-23). As the developing vertebrae emerge, notochordal tissue nests are displaced peripherally and caudally, leaving behind microscopic foci of notochord tissue adjacent to the vertebral bodies and distally in the body of the sacrum and coccyx. It is from these aberrant tissue nests in the sphenooccipital and sacrococcygeal regions that the malignant neoplasm chordoma arises.[691]

Incidence and Distribution

Chordoma is a rare tumor arising anteriorly in the body of the vertebrae: Fewer than 1500 cases have been reported. The overall incidence is not well established because many chordomas are not reported. Two independent Scandinavian studies, however, estimated an annual incidence of approximately 0.5 per million population.[694-695]

The distribution of chordoma in 80 patients, as reported by the Memorial Sloan-Kettering Institute, included 53 cases (66%) located in the sacrum, 24 (30%) in vertebral bodies, and 3 (4%) in the spheno-occipital region.[696] Reviews of the literature, however, suggest that an average of 50% arise in the sacrum, 35% in the spheno-occipital region, and the remaining 15% in the vertebrae.[692,697-700] This distribution of vertebral lesions suggests that the tumor arises most often in the cervical spine, less often in the thoracic spine, and least often in the lumbar spine. The spheno-occipital variety usually occurs in individuals between the ages of 10 and 40 years, while those developing sacrococcygeal lesions are generally over the age of 40. The mean age of patients with sacrococcygeal lesions has been reported as 56 years and of those with vertebral lesions, 47 years. The male-to-female ratio is 2:1.[701]

Interestingly, a case of intradural chordoma without bone involvement was reported recently by Steenberghs and colleagues.[702] They described a 50-year-old patient with a 28-year history of chronic low back pain who later was proven to have a disseminated intradural chordoma involving the thoracolumbosacral spinal cord and eventually extending into the paraspinal muscles. This would appear to be the first case described in an intradural location.

Pathologic Features

In general, few pathologic entities are likely to be confused with chordomas. Crapanzano and coworkers[703] reviewed transcutaneous FNA biopsies to diagnose chordoma accurately using cytologic material for ThinPrep, cytologic smears, and cell blocks from 12 patients with chordoma. They concluded that the cytomorphologic features of chordoma allow accurate diagnosis by FNA biopsy. They also noted that features associated with dedifferentiation include increased pleomorphism of the physaliphorous cells and could include nuclear inclusions, bi- or multinucleation, and rarely, mitotic figures. Transrectal FNA should be avoided.

Chordomas are of basically three overlapping histopathologic types: conventional, chondroid, and those with a malignant spindle cell component. Microscopically, the conventional subtype (the most common) consists of polyhedral cells with distinct cytoplasmic membranes and intracytoplasmic vacuoles. These "physaliferous" cells can be extraordinarily large.[704] Other tumors demonstrate chondroid and fibrous differentiation. Occasionally, an association with secondary malignant fibrous histiocytoma has been reported.[705-709]

Chordomas are immunoreactive with cytokeratin, epithelial membrane antigen, S-100 protein, vimentin, and neurofilaments.[710-714] These characteristics are helpful in distinguishing chordoma from chondrosarcoma, malignant fibrous histiocytoma of bone, and metastatic mucin-producing adenocarcinoma.

Vertebral Chordoma

Clinical and Radiographic Manifestations

The clinical features and management of vertebral and sacral chordomas are sufficiently different that each will be described separately. Vertebral lesions are most often associated with ill-defined symptoms, usually occurring in younger middle-aged patients. The pain and discomfort is characteristically associated with either radicular pain or a disturbance of balance or gait. It is not uncommon for symptoms to be present for more than 1 year.[689] Thoracic and cervical vertebral involvement can be associated with the onset of a cough or dysphagia.[715] Because the tumors project anteriorly, they are rarely if ever palpable. Local tenderness could be elicited by percussion of cervical or lumbar lesions, while bilateral rib compression might identify the thoracic region of interest.

Radiographically, chordoma can often be seen originating in the vertebral body as a destructive, well-marginated lesion. Characteristically, smaller lesions radiographically preserve the adjacent discs, while larger lesions involving more than one vertebral body can destroy the intervening disks.[716] The often-associated soft-tissue mass projects anteriorly, elevating the anterior

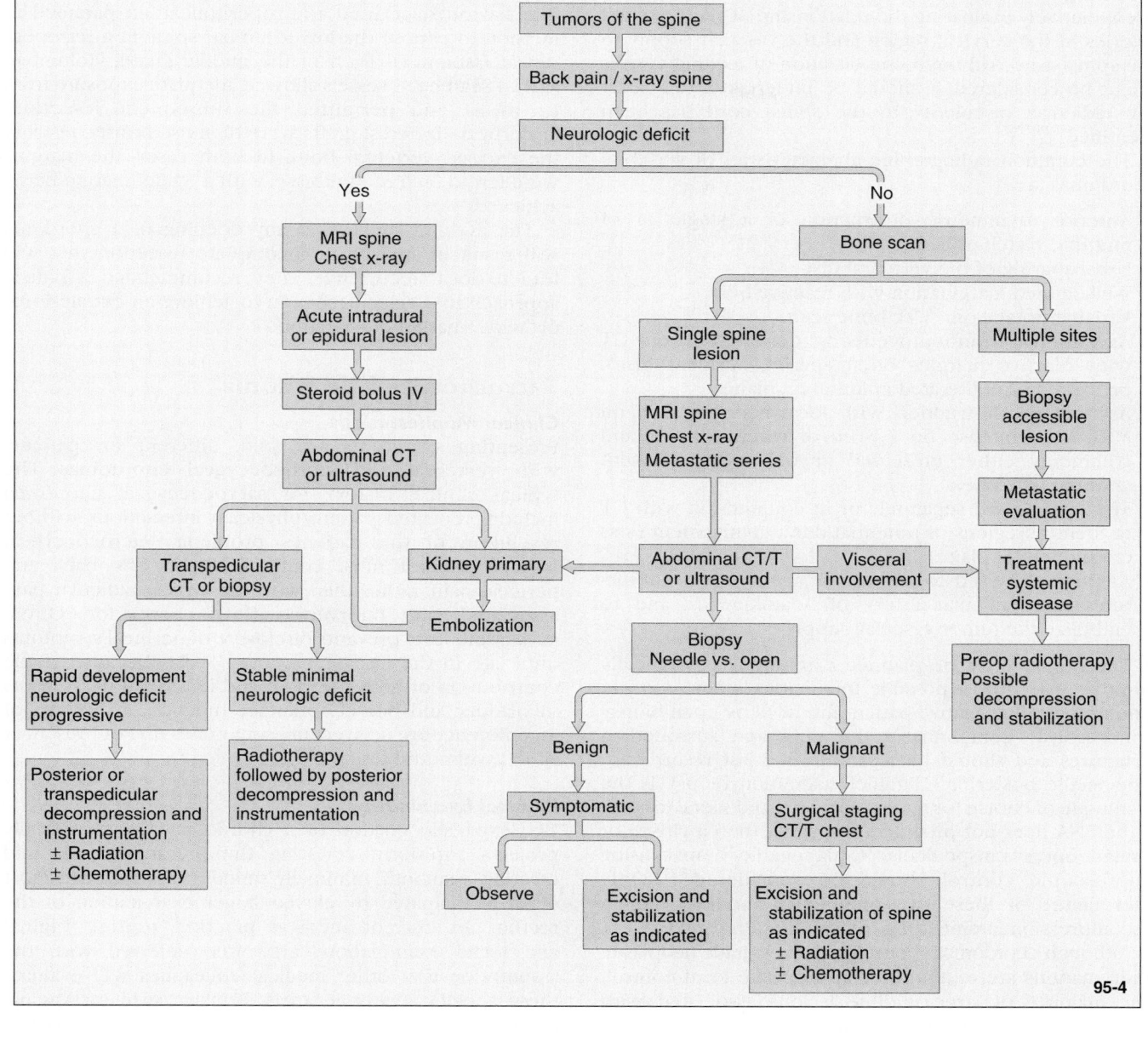

Flowchart: Tumors of the spine

Tumors of the spine → Back pain / x-ray spine → Neurologic deficit

Yes branch:
- MRI spine / Chest x-ray
- Acute intradural or epidural lesion
- Steroid bolus IV
- Abdominal CT or ultrasound
  - Transpedicular CT or biopsy
    - Rapid development neurologic deficit progressive → Posterior or transpedicular decompression and instrumentation ± Radiation ± Chemotherapy
    - Stable minimal neurologic deficit → Radiotherapy followed by posterior decompression and instrumentation
  - Kidney primary → Embolization

No branch:
- Bone scan
  - Single spine lesion
    - MRI spine / Chest x-ray / Metastatic series
    - Abdominal CT/T or ultrasound ← (Kidney primary) / → Visceral involvement
    - Biopsy Needle vs. open
      - Benign → Symptomatic → Observe / Excision and stabilization as indicated
      - Malignant → Surgical staging CT/T chest → Excision and stabilization of spine as indicated ± Radiation ± Chemotherapy
  - Multiple sites
    - Biopsy accessible lesion
    - Metastatic evaluation
    - Treatment systemic disease
    - Preop radiotherapy Possible decompression and stabilization

95-4

longitudinal ligament. When originating in the thoracic vertebrae, chordoma can present asymptomatically as a posterior mediastinal tumor.[717,718]

The ^{99m}Tc bone scan can be utilized to define a chordoma; however, on occasion the lesions may appear scintigraphically photopenic.[719,720] This would appear to be a radioscintigraphy characteristic of vertebral and sacral chordoma.

CT of vertebral chordoma is superior to plain films. The CT finding for 19 patients with axial chordoma was reviewed by Krol and associates.[721] These authors emphasized areas of low attenuation producing a heterogeneous scan associated with a disproportionately large soft-tissue component. The neoplasm can present asymmetrically within the body of the vertebrae. Epidural

tumor extension was demonstrated in all spinal cases. Contrast enhancement was also occasionally useful.[722-724]

Myelography continues to be helpful in demonstrating extradural involvement of a chordoma. Epidural tumor can extend well beyond the area of osseous destruction. Myelography can be combined with CT to better define the extent of the lesion within the neural canal and involvement of adjacent soft-tissue structures.[724]

MRI with and without contrast appears to be the single most valuable study when correlated with the initial plain films. Sze and associates[725] reported a comparative study of 20 intracranial and cervical chordomas studied with CT and MRI. The two methods were comparable in detecting the neoplasm, but MRI was considerably better in delineating the full epidural and soft-tissue extent of the tumor.

Specific Malignancies

III

Angiography of vertebral chordomas can be helpful in preoperatively evaluating the relationship of the vertebral arteries in the cervical region and the vascular supply to the spinal cord. Although embolization of feeding vessels might be considered, it should be undertaken only after the radicular vascularity to the spinal cord has been identified.[724,726]

The common radiographic characteristics of vertebral chordomas are:

- Anterior asymmetric destruction of a single or of multiple vertebral bodies.
- Usual sparing of the vertebral disc.
- Well-defined margination with reactive bone.
- Variable uptake on ^{99m}Tc bone scan.
- Asymmetric nonhomogeneous destruction on CT with reactive margins often sparing adjacent discs; preserved or obliterated epidural fat plane.
- Asymmetric destruction with focal necrosis seen on MRI. Hyperintense on T_2, rim of reactive bone, and commonly, either preserved or obliterated adjacent epidural fat plane.
- Myelogram used separately or in conjunction with CT to identify regions of potential dural involvement (loss of epidural fat plane).
- Angiography used to identify adjacent vascular structures and radicular artery of Adamkiewicz, and to embolize the tumor vascular supply.

The biopsy must be planned carefully if a potentially curative procedure is possible. Injudicious laminectomy in a neurologically negative patient followed by open biopsy unnecessarily contaminates the dura and surrounding structures and should be reserved as a last resort only. Fine-needle posterior CT-guided aspiration biopsy is the technique of choice for almost all spinal and sacral lesions. If the FNA does not provide a diagnosis, then a closed or limited open transpedicular Craig needle biopsy using fluoroscopic control should be considered.[727] Only after failure of these two techniques should an open decompression laminectomy/biopsy be performed.

Although chordoma is considered a low-grade neoplasm, wide margins are required for appropriate local control. The majority of large midline lesions associated with epidural involvement are not likely to maintain normal neurologic function with en bloc wide resections. The majority of patients managed surgically require a one-stage posterior approach that includes laminectomy followed by subtotal intralesional therapy.[701,711,713,717,718,728-730] Many staged well-planned procedures result in wide, clean contaminated margins with the potential for local recurrence.[689,731,732] Only small lesions located eccentrically lend themselves to complete single or staged resection with potentially curative wide margins.

Bosma and coworkers[733] described the technique they used in two cases for removal of primary lumbar vertebral body chordomas. They employed a two-stage procedure, with the first stage using a posterior approach and a midline exposure with pedicle instrumentation and fixation. The pedicles were transected posteriorly adjacent to the dura, and the nerve roots were protected. The lamina and the pedicles were removed in one piece, with

the transverse processes disconnected and left behind. The second stage used a retroperitoneal left paramedian incision to expose the lower lumbar spine in a retroperitoneal fashion. Division of the middle sacral, iliolumbar, and L4 segmental vessels allowed adequate exposure from L4 to S1 and permitted the subsequent resection. Tricortical iliac crest grafts were then used to reconstruct the excised vertebral body. In both cases, the margins were felt to be free of disease, with a "wide" margin being achieved.

The authors stated that any opening of a chordoma will result in spillage or incomplete resection that will lead to local recurrence. They recommended a radical approach to surgical resection to achieve an extralesional or "wide" margin of resection.

Sacrococcygeal Chordoma

Clinical Manifestations

Presenting symptoms are quite different for patients with vertebral and sacrococcygeal chordomas. The typical clinical history for sacrococcygeal chordoma includes repeated patient/physician interactions without resolution of the patient's problems. Sacrococcygeal lesions manifest most commonly with low back and perineal pain, rather than with the typical radicular pain associated with intervertebral disc herniation. Often, patient modesty prevents disclosure of perineal symptoms until late in the disease process.[734] Also, because of the contribution of both the right and left sacral nerve roots to bladder and bowel sphincter function, symptoms of incontinence are delayed and sometimes do not present at all in asymmetric lesions.[735]

Physical Examination

The expansile portion of a chordoma characteristically projects anteriorly, deviating the presacral fascia and creating a smooth, minimally tender mass that can most often be palpated by gloved finger examination of the rectum. In current medical practice, routine vaginal and rectal examinations are often deferred with the assumption that other medical colleagues will evaluate these specific anatomic areas. Females seen for vaginal examinations are evaluated with respect to the pelvic contents, but little attention is directed to the lower sacrum or coccyx. Rectal examinations for males with prostatic enlargement usually do not make reference to the coccyx or sacrum. The majority of sacrococcygeal chordomas can be palpated by vaginal and rectal examinations.

Radiographic Evaluation

If a lesion in the pelvis or lower sacrococcygeal region is suspected but cannot be palpated physically, the radiographic evaluation is crucial to define the extent and location of the lesion, along with the relationship of adjacent and potentially involved vital structures.[736] The most common plain-film radiographic finding is loss of normal bone trabeculations and possible cortical destruction. A lateral projection of the sacrum might reveal an associated asymmetric soft-tissue mass projecting anteriorly and deviating the normal rectal gas shadow. These findings are often retrospective, however. It is generally recognized that a plain AP film of the pelvis is not sufficiently sensitive to detect small underlying lesions of the coccyx, sacrum, or pelvis and should not be used as a screening method.[737] In assessment of a neoplastic process in the pelvis, sacrum, or coccyx, a minimal evaluation must also include a ^{99m}Tc bone scan.

Differential Diagnosis (Radiographs)

Besides chordoma, the radiographic differential diagnosis includes:

1. Metastatic disease (most common neoplastic deposit in the sacrum)
2. Benign disease
   a. Aneurysmal bone cyst
   b. Giant cell tumor of bone
   c. Arachnoid cyst
   d. Epithelioma
   e. Neurofibroma
   f. Early phase (destructive) of Paget's disease of bone
   g. Teratoma of the sacrum
3. Malignant primary and "benign aggressive" lesions
   a. Desmoplastic fibroma
   b. "Aggressive" giant cell tumor of bone
   c. Ewing's sarcoma
   d. Malignant schwannoma

The ^{99m}Tc bone scan often detects skeletal lesions arising in the sacrococcygeal region and the pelvis. To evaluate the pelvis, however, the urinary bladder contents must be evacuated and the perineum cleaned before examination. Multiple views of the pelvis are beneficial in localizing the area of the abnormality. An improved evaluation of the sacrum can be achieved with an additional static sequence, a Chassard Lapine ("squat shot") view performed by directly viewing the cleansed perineum from below, distinguishing anterior from posterior structures. As mentioned previously, chordoma might not be well visualized using conventional ^{99m}Tc scintigraphy.[738]

Once a lesion has been recognized, the next most appropriate study should provide maximum information and resolution of the anatomic structures involved. The cross-sectional display of CT and the multiaxial display of MRI provide superior three-dimensional information to localize and characterize the lesion.[739,740] These data may also be used to assist and facilitate biopsy and subsequent surgical resection. A physician-monitored MRI of the sacrococcygeal region, sciatic notch contents, sacroiliac joints, and adjacent ilium provides superior anatomic detail with predetermined sequences and image planes to appropriately evaluate the vertebrae, sacrum, and pelvic contents.[741,742]

The common radiographic characteristics of sacrococcygeal chordoma are:

- Symmetric or asymmetric destruction anteriorly in the body of the sacrum or coccyx (Fig. 95-24).
- Variable uptake in a single lesion on ^{99m}Tc bone scan, possibly requiring a Chassard Lapine ("squat shot") view.

- CT—nonhomogeneous lesion originating in the body of the sacrum and projecting anteriorly, with evidence of reactive bone and preserved presacral fascia and associated presacral fat plane.
- MRI—single most valuable study demonstrating either a symmetric or asymmetric, well-marginated, nonhomogeneous destructive lesion originating in the body of the sacrum or coccyx and projecting anteriorly and/or laterally with preserved presacral fascia, perineural fat, and presacral fat plane (see Fig. 95-24).
- Myelogram—infrequently required to demonstrate region of epidural involvement; could be necessary for planning dural transection level if not well seen on MRI.
- Angiography—used to identify major contributing vessels followed by embolization where appropriate. Could be of major importance when using a one-stage posterior approach for resection.

Surgical Therapy for Sacrococcygeal Chordoma

Biopsy. Posterior midline needle or open biopsies should be used exclusively for biopsy purposes. Needle biopsies with either sonographic or CT guidance to avoid areas of necrosis should be reserved for centers where pathologists are experienced in obtaining and interpreting small tissue samples. The presacral fascia with the adjacent fat plane between the rectum and sacrum is the only anterior surgical margin and should be preserved at all costs. Transrectal biopsy is absolutely contraindicated to evaluate lesions in the retrorectal area and sacrum.

Open biopsy techniques uniformly provide sufficient tissue for diagnosis. The sacral incision should be oriented longitudinally in the midline, with the deeper surgical planes angling appropriately to avoid contamination of the dura and to gain access to the lesion. The characteristically gelatinous chordoma tissue can be obtained atraumatically by use of a suction trap or curette. The previously outlined principles of tissue collection and open biopsy technique should be followed.

Subtotal and Total Sacral Amputation. Surgical amputation with a minimum of wide margins is generally accepted as the best treatment to produce cure. Radiotherapy should be reserved for management of patients with surgically inaccessible lesions and for patients with positive surgical margins or recurrent disease after attempted curative sacral amputation.

Three types of procedures are used for the surgical management of sacral chordomas:

1. A single posterior midline exposure with the patient in the prone position.
2. A combined anteroposterior approach with the patient in the lateral decubitus position.
3. A two-stage anterior and posterior approach, turning the patient from the supine to the prone position.

All of the procedures have merit, and each has specific indications.

Most authors agree that small tumors (involving the sacrum below S3) can be excised through a transperineal

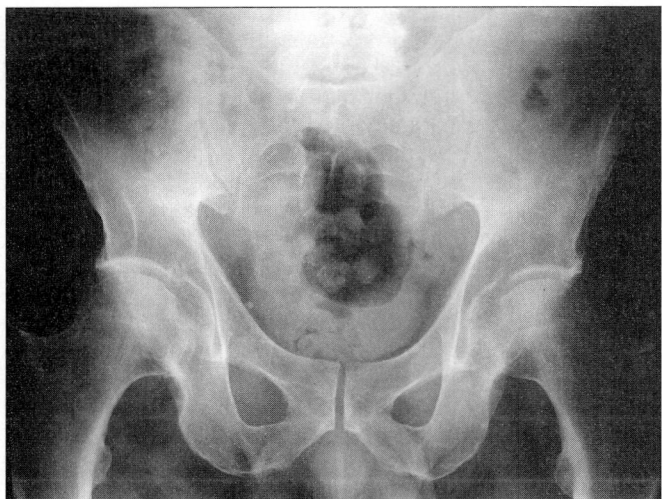

A

Figure 95-24. A, AP radiograph of the pelvis of a 56-year-old male with a 3-year history of ill-defined low back and buttock pain. No rectal examination was reported done until the patient was evaluated for bowel complaints. **B,** MRI of the pelvis demonstrated a mass projecting from the anterior lower (S3 and below) sacral elements. This axial view of the biopsy-proven chordoma demonstrates the preserved fat plane between the tumor and rectum (*arrows*). **C,** Sagittal T_1-weighted image clearly demonstrates the region of anterior sacral involvement and the preserved fat plane between the tumor and rectum (*small arrows*). The large arrow indicates the location of the sacral amputation (S3) used to potentially cure this patient, who is currently 2 years free of disease.

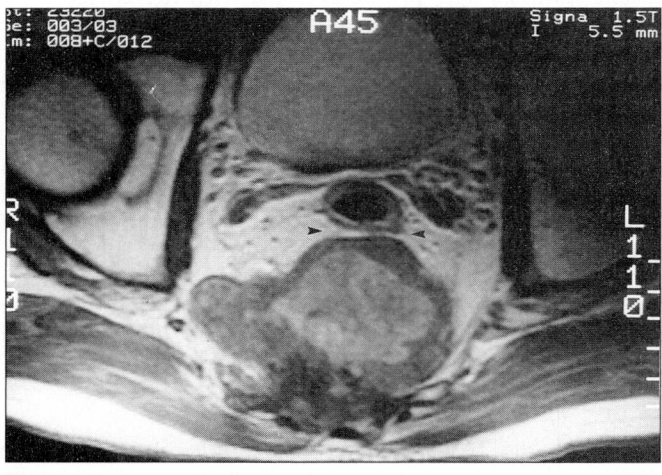

B

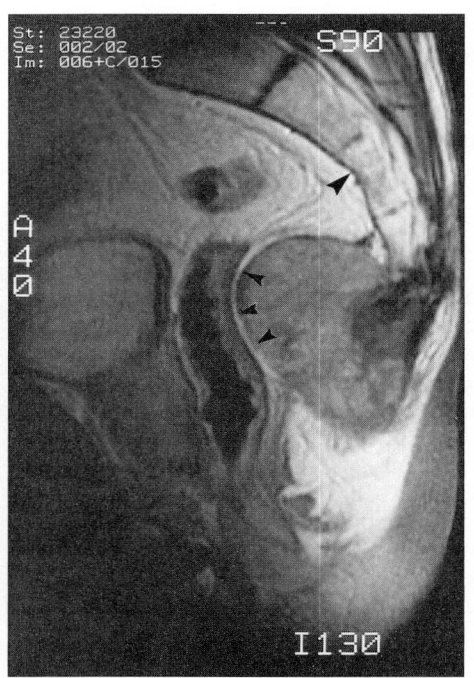

C

Kraske approach. Of the 63 patients reported by Uhlig and Johnson,[741] the majority were managed by a single posterior approach.

MacCarty and coauthors[744] used the Kraske or posterior approach exclusively for lesions of all sizes, with some lesions reportedly extending to S1. Of the 18 patients originally described, however, only 7 were locally free of disease from 1 to 12 years later. The follow-up report also revealed an operative mortality of 1 in 18 patients.[745]

Sampson and coauthors[746] described 21 patients with sacrococcygeal chordoma, all managed by the posterior approach. Four patients required a resection margin at the S1-sparing level, while seven required S2-sparing procedures. Ten patients had wide excisions, and one additional patient had a wide contaminated margin. Three patients had a marginal excision, with the remaining

seven having intralesional therapy. Four of 21 patients experienced a local recurrence.

Thirteen patients received preoperative radiotherapy, and five completed the course postoperatively. Three patients had postoperative radiotherapy after intralesional surgical therapy. The authors recommended preoperative radiotherapy for large lesions that might be entered inadvertently at the time of resection.

Other surgeons advocate either a combined abdomino-sacral single-stage approach or an anteroposterior two-stage procedure. Localio and colleagues[747] described a combined abdominosacral approach for amputation of sacrococcygeal chordoma in 1967. In their procedure, the patient was placed in the right lateral decubitus position and could be rolled to nearly a prone position once the drapes were applied. A left paramedian incision was used from symphysis to umbilicus, and a left retroperitoneal approach was made to expose and mobilize the rectum from the lesion through the presacral fat plane. The middle and lateral sacral vessels were dissected and ligated, and the upper and lower extents of the lesion were identified.

With the rectum mobilized, attention was directed posteriorly, where the proximal sacral amputation level could be ascertained from the abdominal exposure. Huth and coauthors[748] and Karakousis,[749] using a similar one-stage anteroposterior approach, have reported apparent success.

Bowers[750] described the management of a patient with a large vascular giant cell tumor of the sacrum, in which an attempt was made to excise the lesion from posteriorly. The procedure was abandoned due to uncontrolled bleeding after apparent hemostatic control of the middle and lateral sacral vessels. Two weeks later, the lesion was first visualized anteriorly through a left rectus incision, and visible pulsatile flow through the lesion could be controlled by ligation of the internal iliac vessels. The wound was closed temporarily and the patient was turned prone, and then the sacrum was amputated safety through the S2 foramen. These observations, in addition to the need to better identify the anterior extent of large tumors, led to the development of a two-stage anterior/posterior procedure described in detail by Stener and Gunterberg.[751]

Two-Stage Anteroposterior Procedure Preserving the Rectum.

The two-stage anteroposterior procedure is initiated in the supine position, with a comprehensive "smile" incision that allows a retroperitoneal approach to both lateral borders and the promontory of the sacrum. The rectum can be mobilized from the tumor through the fibrofatty tissue plane anterior to the presacral fascia. Once the full extent of the tumor has been evaluated, the tumor is devascularized by ligating the middle and lateral sacral vessels. Both ureters are identified. The internal iliac vessels can be divided surgically or controlled with vascular tapes during the remainder of the procedure. The anterior osteotomy site is selected, and the appropriate uninvolved sacral nerves and neural foramen are identified.

The presacral fascia and periosteum are incised well about the lesion near the sacral promontory and then dissected subperiosteally distally to create an anatomic plane between normal bone and the tumor. In this instance, the plane of dissection would be through the inferior endplate of S1, potentially preserving the S1 and S2 nerve roots. Once the flap of tissue has been created, the anterior one half of the transverse sacral osteotomy is completed as shown in Figure 95-25. Figure 95-25E demonstrates an osteotomy through the anterior one half of the body of S2, preserving the second sacral nerve root. Figure 95-25F illustrates preservation of the S1 nerve roots, while Figure 95-25G demonstrates an extensive amputation that includes the nerve roots of S1 but preserves sufficient pelvic strength for unassisted ambulation.[752] Figure 95-25E demonstrates why many

authors believe that the single-stage posterior approach is appropriate for lesions involving the body of S3 and below. The surgeon's finger can be introduced through the sciatic notch anteriorly to palpate the upper extent of the lesion and direct the appropriate level of amputation laterally and posteriorly.

Hemostasis is secured, a moist counted lap pack is positioned between the rectum, vascular structures, and the lesion, and the wound is closed permanently. The patient is now turned to the prone position, where the rectum is surgically sutured closed and isolated from the prepared posterior surgical field. The previous midline biopsy incision is included in the posterior incision, shown to the right in Figure 95-25A. Proximal and lateral extensions of the incision can be made to gain additional lateral exposure. Figure 95-25H demonstrates the posterior exposure after a total laminectomy at L5 and S1, tracing the nerve roots into their respective foramen. The dural sac has been amputated and suture ligated. The remaining musculature is dissected from the lateral border of the sacrum, incising the sacrotuberous ligament near its attachment along with the sacrospinous ligament and coccygeus muscle. The pyriformis muscle is transected as far laterally as possible, protecting the sciatic nerve. The surgeon's finger can now be introduced through the sciatic notch to palpate the level of the previous transverse anterior osteotomy and thereby direct the posterior cut to interconnect with the anterior osteotomy. The involved sacral nerve roots are incised, sparing those that are not involved, and the lesion is removed. The vascular tapes about the internal iliac vessels are removed, and hemostasis is controlled. Drains are inserted, and the wound is closed permanently.

Two-stage Anteroposterior Procedure Including the Rectum.

If the rectum is to be included in the specimen, the bowel must be prepared mechanically and chemically. Some surgeons choose a midline abdominal incision for anterior exposure in the lithotomy position. The peritoneal cavity must be entered. After division of the superior rectal vessels, the bowel is divided at the rectosigmoid junction, and dissection is directed distally and anteriorly to the rectum to communicate with a skin incision around the previously sutured and closed rectum. The middle rectal vessels are divided and cut, further mobilizing the rectum. The procedure proceeds as previously described, except that the rectum is included with the specimen. A formal colostomy is performed once the mobilization and amputation procedures have been completed, requiring that the patient be turned one more time to the supine position.

High sacral amputations through the body of S1 remain anatomically stable.[753] Total sacrectomy has been reported both without and with pelvic stabilization.[728,752,754] Anorectal function, associated neurologic deficits, and sexual function after major sacral resections and amputations have been investigated extensively.[755-757] The detailed myoelectric studies by Gunterberg and colleagues[755-757] demonstrated that bilateral loss of S2–S5 resulted in severe sexual and anorectal dysfunction. When

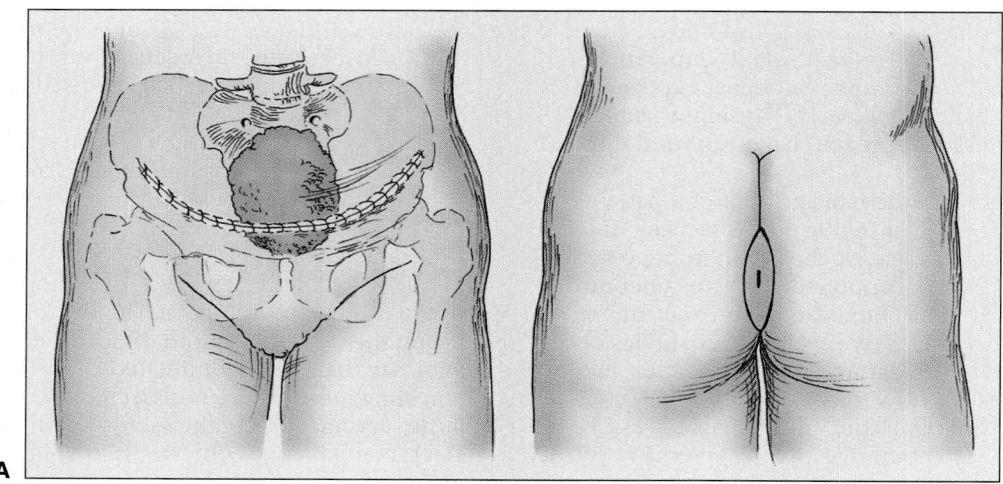

A

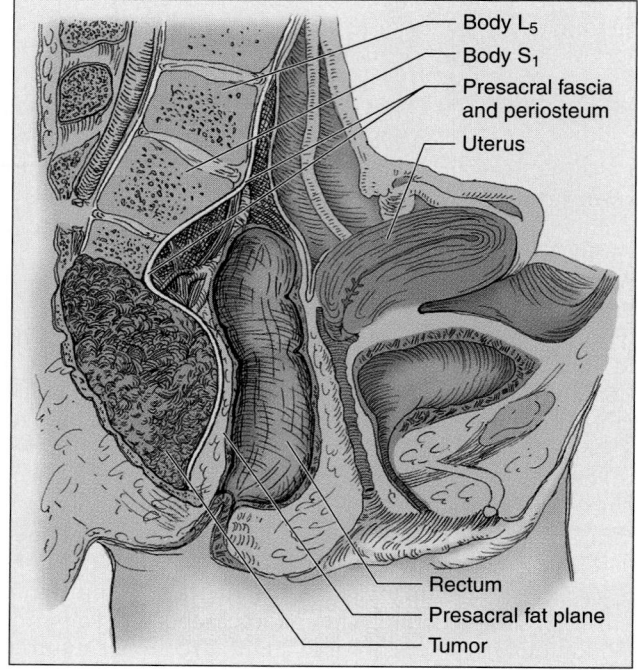

B

Body L$_5$
Body S$_1$
Presacral fascia
and periosteum
Uterus

Rectum
Presacral fat plane
Tumor

Figure 95-25. A, The anterior "smile" incision used for the retroperitoneal exposure when perserving the rectum (*left*). A midline transperitoneal incision is advised when resection of the rectum and the sacrum is required. The midline posterior incision encompassing a midline longitudinal biopsy incision (*right*). For larger resections, proximal lateral extensions of the incision could be required. **B,** Sagittal midline illustration demonstrating the relationship of the female viscera with the lesion and the critical planes of dissection. The presacral fascia and vertebral periosteum act as an anatomic barrier to tumor growth and must remain intact. The importance of the fat plane between the rectum and sacrum is demonstrated.

Continued

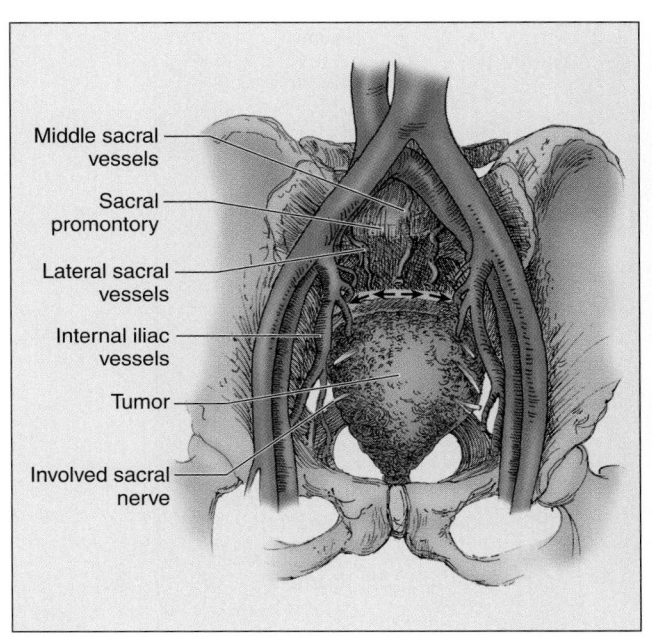

Middle sacral vessels

Sacral promontory

Lateral sacral vessels

Internal iliac vessels

Tumor

Involved sacral nerve

C

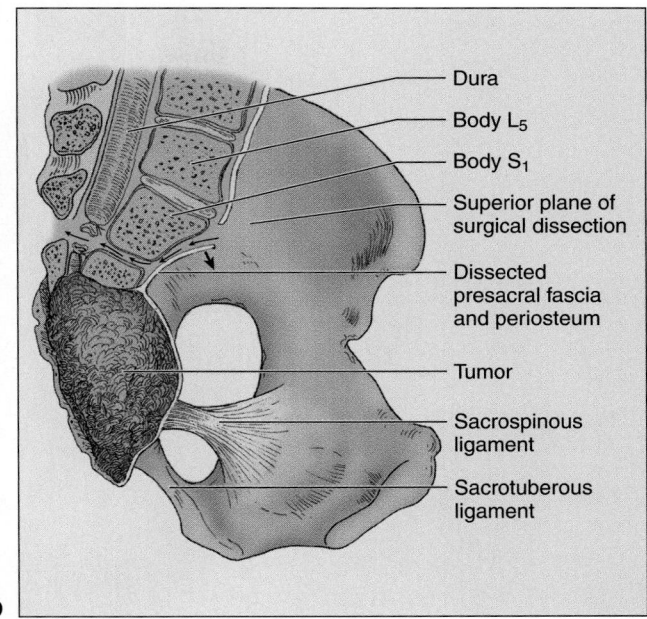

Dura

Body L₅

Body S₁

Superior plane of surgical dissection

Dissected presacral fascia and periosteum

Tumor

Sacrospinous ligament

Sacrotuberous ligament

D

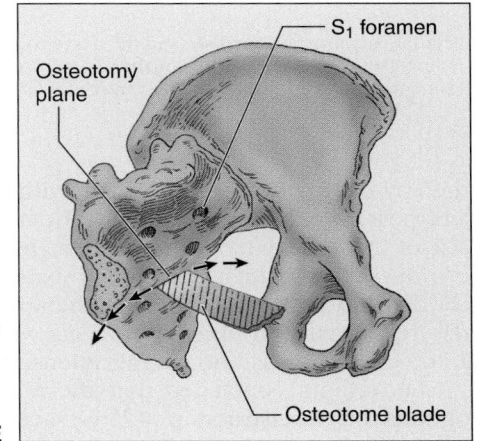

S₁ foramen

Osteotomy plane

Osteotome blade

E

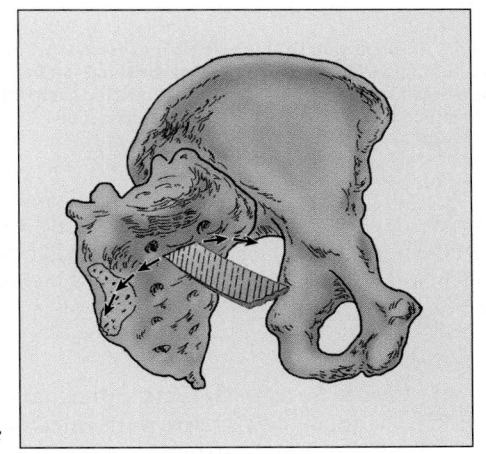

F

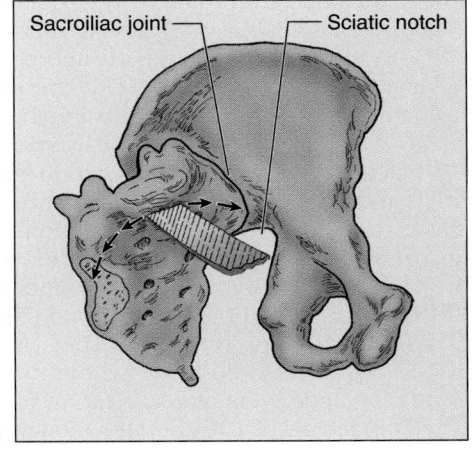

Sacroiliac joint

Sciatic notch

G

Figure 95-25, *cont'd*. C, Anterior mobilization of the rectum and exposure for vascular control. The middle and lateral sacral vessels are ligated, and vascular control is gained of both internal iliac vessels. Both gutters on either side of the tumor mass are devascularized and dissected as far distally as possible before anterior wound closure. A counted lap pack is placed in the region of dissection, to be removed later from the posterior approach. **D,** Similar sagittal illustration, but with the viscera removed, demonstrates the mobilization of the rectum from the tumor anteriorly and the sacral promontory presacral facia/periosteal incision with subperiosteal dissection of the preplanned transverse sacral osteotomy. **E–G,** Anterior sacral osteotomies performed to preserve S2 (E), S1 (F), and L5 (G). The osteotomy cuts are made only through the anterior cotex (arrows) and most are to the region of the sciatic notch superior to the tumor margin. The osteotomy is completed from the posterior approach when the surgeon's gloved finger can be placed in the sciatic notch to palpate the appropriate anterior level of the osteotomy cut.

Continued

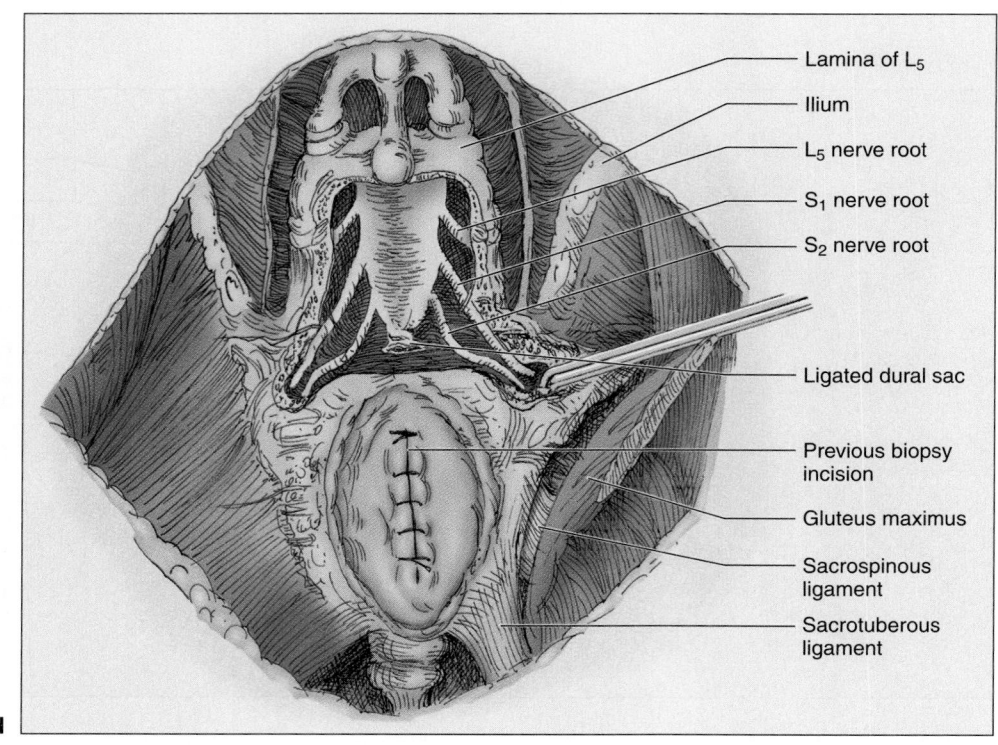

Lamina of L₅
Ilium
L₅ nerve root
S₁ nerve root
S₂ nerve root

Ligated dural sac

Previous biopsy incision

Gluteus maximus

Sacrospinous ligament

Sacrotuberous ligament

H

Figure 95-25, cont'd. H, Salient points of the posterior dissection. Total laminectomy exposes the dural sac and the nerve roots. The roots to be preserved are traced to their respective foramen and the dural sac transected below. The posterior sacrum is further exposed, taking down the gluteus maximus muscle and transecting the sacrouberous and sacrospinous ligamenta along with the pyriformis muscle as far laterally as possible. The amputation is completed, sparing the appropriate nerve roots.

S3 was retained, sexual and bladder dysfunction were only partially impaired. On the other hand, unilateral loss of S1–S2 resulted in little or no abnormality. Every effort should be made to spare uninvolved sacral roots whenever possible.[758]

Reconstruction of Large Sacral Defects. Miles and coauthors[759] reviewed a total of 27 flaps performed in 25 patients for sacral defect reconstruction after total sacrectomy. Diagnoses included chordoma (n = 13), giant cell carcinoma (n = 2), sarcoma (n = 5), rectal adenocarcinoma (n = 4), and radiation-induced necrosis (n = 1). The size ranged from 18 cm² to 450 cm² (mean, 189.8 cm²). Ten patients, including five who had preoperative radiation, underwent transpelvic vertical rectus abdominis myocutaneous flap reconstruction for sacral defects with a mean size of 203.3 cm². Of these, five patients had complications (four had minor wound dehiscences, and one had seroma). Eight patients, including one who had preoperative radiotherapy, underwent bilateral gluteal advancement flap reconstruction for sacral defects with a mean size of 198.0 cm². They had no complications. Two patients, both of whom had preoperative radiotherapy, underwent gluteal rotation flap reconstruction for sacral defects of 120 cm² and 144 cm². Both had complications (one partial flap loss and one nonhealing wound requiring a free flap). Three patients, including one who had had preoperative radiation

therapy, underwent reconstruction with combined gluteal and posterior thigh flaps for sacral defects with a mean size of 246 cm²; two of these patients had partial necrosis of the posterior thigh flaps. Three patients, all of whom had had postoperative radiation therapy, underwent free flap reconstruction for sacral defects with a mean size of 144.3 cm². They had no complications.

The authors concluded that there are three reliable options for reconstruction of large sacral wound defects: bilateral gluteal advancement flaps, transpelvic rectus myocutaneous flaps, and free flaps. In patients with no preoperative radiation therapy and intact gluteal vessels, the use of bilateral gluteal advancement flaps should be considered. In patients with a history of radiation to the sacral area and in patients whose gluteal vessels have been damaged, the use of a transpelvic rectus abdominis myocutaneous flap should be considered. If the transpelvic rectus abdominis flap can not be used because of previous abdominal surgery, a free flap should be considered as a last option.

Prognosis. Local recurrence is directly related to the adequacy of the initial surgery requiring a minimum of a wide margin. Ishii and associates[760] reported on four patients with sacral chordoma managed by local en bloc resection who experienced local recurrence. All four had an en bloc resection through the S2–S3 region for sacral chordomas located below S3. The primary recurrences were noted to be along the lateral margin of the remaining sacrum in all patients. The authors were concerned that the preoperative MRI had not appropriately identified the lateral projection in the region of origin of the gluteus maximus or piriformis muscle, resulting in tumor perhaps being left behind and leading to local recurrence. They therefore recommended that the S2–S3 sacrectomy be performed to include a portion of the sacroiliac joint together with portions of the origin of the gluteus maximus and the piriformis muscles.

The surgical principles outlined and developed by Stener and Gunterberg, when used appropriately and by skilled surgeons, result reliably in a wide amputation. These procedures are technically demanding and should not be undertaken by the unprepared. Even in the best of hands, however, 5% to 40% of patients will develop distant disease.

The single-institution experience from the Musculoskeletal Tumor Center at the Sahlgrenska University Hospital in Göteborg, Sweden, has been updated regarding the prognosis of patients with chordoma of the sacrum and the mobile spine.[761] The results of treatment and follow-up of 30 patients with sacral and 9 patients with mobile spine chordomas (size range, 3–20 cm; mean size, 8 cm) occurring in 22 women and 17 men with a median age of 55 years were analyzed. The preferred method of diagnosis was spine needle aspiration.

The final surgical margins were wide in 23 patients and marginal or intralesional in 16. The mean follow-up was 8.1 years (range, 0.1–23 years). Seventeen patients (44%) developed local recurrence, and 11 patients (28%) developed metastases. The estimated 5–10–15–20–year survival rates were 84%, 64%, 52%, and 52%, respectively. Local recurrences were significantly associated with increased risks of metastases and tumor-related death (P <0.001). The authors recognized that large tumor size, performance of an invasive morphologic diagnostic procedure outside of the tumor's center, inadequate surgical margins, microscopic tumor necrosis, and local recurrence were significant risk factors.[761]

The average time to distant failure is 3 years. The lung, liver, bone, lymph nodes, skin, and subcutaneous tissues are only a few of the regions of reported metastases.[762-766] Because metastasis can occur up to 10 years later, long-term follow-up is required.

Data reported by Sundaresan[767] suggest that survival rates are similar for patients treated by surgery alone or by surgery plus radiotherapy. Median survival with both forms of treatment is 6 years, and 66% of the patients with sacrococcygeal lesions survive for 5 years. The 10-year survival for that group is 40%, with a constant risk of dying from disease.[768]

SUMMARY

The sarcomas of bone and chordoma represent a heterogeneous group of tumors arising in somewhat predictable locations throughout the entire skeleton. The diagnosis and surgical planning have improved significantly with the addition of physician-monitored MRI and the other associated multiaxial display imaging techniques. Also, the addition of sophisticated immunohistochemistry and cytogenetic techniques has made differentiation of similar-appearing lesions easier. The increasing complexity of the management of these patients, including primary chemotherapy and limb- and function-preserving surgery, requires a dedicated team of nurses, technicians, and physicians working to provide and implement the therapeutic modalities necessary to cure previously incurable diseases.

REFERENCES

Staging and Biopsy

1. Landis S, Murray T, Bolden S, Wingo P: Cancer statistics, 1999. CA Cancer J Clin 1999;49:31.
2. Bowden L, Booher R: Principles and technique of resection of soft parts for sarcoma. Surgery 1958;44:963.
3. Stener B, Stener I: Malignant tumors of the soft tissues of the thigh. Acta Chir Scand 1958;115:457.
4. Stener B: The management of soft tissue tumors. Int Orthop (SICOT) 1978;1:289.
5. Simon M, Enneking W: The management of soft tissue sarcomas of the extremities. J Bone Joint Surg 1976;58A:317.
6. Enneking W, Spanier S, Goodman M: A system for the surgical staging of musculoskeletal sarcoma. Clin Orthop 1980;153:106.
7. Enneking W, Spanier S, Goodman M: Current concepts review. The surgical staging of musculoskeletal sarcoma. J Bone Surg 1980;62A:1027.
8. Enneking W: A system of staging musculoskeletal neoplasms. Clin Orthop 1986;204:9.
9. Enneking W, Spanier S, Malawer M: The effect of the anatomic setting on the results of surgical procedures for soft parts sarcoma of the thigh. Cancer 1981;47:1005.
10. Hadju S: Pathology of Soft Tissue Tumors. Philadelphia, Lea & Febiger, 1979.
11. Rydholm A, Rööser B: Surgical margins for soft-tissue sarcoma. J Bone Joint Surg 1987;69A:1074.
12. Suit H, Mankin H, Schiller A, et al: Staging systems for sarcoma of soft tissue and sarcoma of bone. Cancer Treat Symp 1985;3:29.
13. Beahrs O, Henson D, Hutter R, Myers M: Manual for Staging of Cancer, 3rd ed. Philadelphia, JB Lippincott, 1988.
14. Olson P, Everson L, Griffiths H: Staging of musculoskeletal tumors. Radiol Clin North Am 1994;32:151.
15. Spanier S, Shuster J, Vander Griend R: The effect of local extent of the tumor on prognosis in osteosarcoma. J Bone Joint Surg 1990;72A:643.
16. Greene FL, Page DL, Fleming ID, et al (eds.) AJCC Cancer Staging Manual, 6th ed. New York, Springer Verlag, 2002.
17. Menendez L, Fideler B, Mirra J: Thallium-201 scanning for the evaluation of osteosarcoma and soft-tissue sarcoma. J Bone Joint Surg 1993;75A:526
18. Simon M, Finn H: Diagnostic strategy for bone and soft-tissue tumors. J Bone Joint Surg 1993;75A:622
19. Turner D: Nuclear magnetic resonance in oncology. Semin Nucl Med 1985;25:210.
20. Dalinka M, Zlatkin M, Chao P, et al: The use of magnetic resonance imaging in the evaluation of bone and soft tissue tumors. Radiol Clin North Am 1990;28:461.
21. Exner G, von Hochstetter A, Augustiny N, von Schulthess G: Magnetic resonance imaging in malignant bone tumours. Int Orthop 1990;14:49.
22. Sundaram M, McLeod R: MR imaging of tumor and tumorlike lesions of bone and soft tissue. Am J Roentgenol 1990;155:817.
23. Hayes C, Conway W, Sundaram M: Misleading aggressive MR imaging appearance of some benign musculoskeletal lesions. Radiographics 1992;12:1119.
24. Reddick WE, Wang S, Xiong X, Glass JO, Wu S, Kaste SC, et al: Dynamic magnetic resonance imaging of regional contrast access

as an additional prognostic factor in pediatric osteosarcoma. Cancer 2001;91:2230–2237.

25. Swan J, Weber D, Korosec F, et al: Technical note. Combined MRI and MRA for limb salvage planning. J Comput Assist Tomogr 1993;17:339.

26. Holscher H, Bloem J, Nooy M, et al: The value of MR imaging in monitoring the effect of chemotherapy on bone sarcomas. Am J Roentgenol 1990;154:763.

27. Fletcher B: Response of osteosarcoma and Ewing sarcoma to chemotherapy: Imaging evaluation. Am J Roentgenol 1991;157:825.

28. Gold R, Seeger L, Bassett L, Steckel R: An integrated approach to the evaluation of metastatic bone disease. Radiol Clin North Am 1990;28:471.

29. Kori S, Krol G, Foley K: Computed tomographic evaluation of bone and soft tissue metastases. In Weiss GH (ed): Bone Metastases. Boston, GK Hall, 1983, p 245.

30. Gosfield E, Alavi A, Kneeland B: Comparison of radionuclide bone scans and magnetic resonance imaging in detecting spinal metastases. J Nucl Med 1993;34:2191.

31. Avrahami E, Tadmor R, Dally O, Hadar H: Early MR demonstration of spinal metastases in patients with normal radiographs and CT and radionuclide bone scans. J Comput Assist Tomogr 1989; 13:598.

32. Delbeke D, Powers T, Sandler M: Negative scintigraphy with positive magnetic resonance imaging in bone metastases. Skeletal Radiol 1990;19:113.

33. Algra P, Bloem J, Tissing H, et al: Detection of vertebral metastases: Comparison between MR imaging and bone scintigraphy. Radiographics 1991;11:219.

34. Mehta R, Wilson M, Perlman S: False negative bone scan in extensive metastatic disease: CT and MR findings. J Comput Assist Tomogr 1989;13:717.

35. Kattapuram S, Khurana J, Scott J, El Khoury G: Negative scintigraphy with positive magnetic resonance imaging in bone metastasis. Skeletal Radiol 1990;19:204.

36. Frank J, Ling A, Patronas N, et al: Detection of malignant bone tumors: MR imaging vs scintigraphy. Am J Radiol 1990;155:1043.

37. Aitchison F, Poon F, Hadley M, et al: Vertebral metastases and equivocal bone scan: Value of magnetic resonance imaging. Nucl Med Commun 1992;13:429.

38. Johnson K, Leavitt G, Kayser H: Total body MR imaging in as little as 18 seconds. Radiology 1997;202:262.

39. Dwyer A, Frank J, Sank V, et al: Short T-1 inversion recovery pulse sequence: Analysis and initial experience in cancer imaging. Radiology 1988;168:827.

40. Jones K, Unger E, Granstrom P, et al: Bone marrow imaging using STIR at 0.5 Tesla and 1.5 Tesla. Magn Reson Imaging 1992;10:169.

41. Constable R, Smith R, Gore J: Signal to noise and contrast in fast spine echo (FSE) and inversion recovery FSE imaging. J Comput Assist Tomogr 1992;16:41.

42. Jones K, Mulkern R, Mantello M: Brain hemorrhage: Evaluation with fast spin echo and conventional dual spin echo images. Radiology 1992;182:53.

43. Hennig J, Naurth A, Friedburg H: RARE imaging: A fast imaging method for clinical MR. Magn Reson Imaging 1986;3:823.

44. Eustace S, Tello R, DeCarvalho V, et al: A comparison of whole-body turboSTIR MR imaging and planar 99m-Tc-methylene diphosphonate scintigraphy in the examination of patients with suspected skeletal metastases. Am J Radiol 1997;169:1655

45. Koss L, Woyke S, Wlodzimierz O: Aspiration Biopsy: Cytologic Interpretation and Histologic Bases. New York, Igaku-Shoin, 1984.

46. Wakely P, Kardos T, Frable W: Application of fine needle aspiration biopsy to pediatrics. Hum Pathol 1988;19:1383.

47. Bommer K, Ramzy I, Mody D: Fine-needle aspiration biopsy in the diagnosis and management of bone lesions: A study of 450 cases. Cancer 1997;81:148.

48. Taylor S, Nunez C: Fine needle aspiration biopsy in a pediatric population. Cancer 1984;54:1449.

49. McGahey BE, Moriarty AT, Nelson WA, Hull MT: Fine-needle aspiration biopsy of small round blue cell tumors of childhood. Cancer 1992;69:1067.

50. Davies N, Livesley P, Cannon S: Recurrence of an osteosarcoma in a needle biopsy tract. J Bone Joint Surg 1993;75B:977.

Osteosarcoma

51. Huvos A: Bone Tumors, Diagnosis, Treatment and Prognosis. Philadelphia, WB Saunders, 1991, p 98.

52. Dahlin D: Bone Tumors: General Aspects and Data on 6,221 Cases. Springfield, IL, Charles C Thomas, 1978, p 269.

53. Stark A, Kreicbergs A, Nilsonne U, Silfverswärd C: The age of osteosarcoma patients is increasing. An epidemiological study of osteosarcoma in Sweden 1971 to 1984. J Bone Joint Surg 1990;72B:89.

54. Huvos A: Osteogenic sarcoma of bones and soft tissues in older persons. A clinicopathologic analysis of 117 patients older than 60 years. Cancer 1986;57:1442.

55. Dix D, McDonald M, Cohen P: Adolescent bone cancer: is the growth spurt implicated? [letter]. Eur J Cancer Clin Oncol 1983;19:859.

56. Huvos A: Bone Tumors, Diagnosis, Treatment and Prognosis, 2nd ed. Philadelphia, WB Saunders, 1991.

57. Matsuno T, Unni K, McLeod R, Dahlin D: Telangiectatic osteogenic sarcoma. Cancer 1976;38:2538.

58. Huvos A, Rosen G, Bretsky S, Butler A: Telangiectatic osteogenic sarcoma: A clinicopathological study of 124 patients. Cancer 1982;49:1679.

59. Hansen M: Molecular genetic considerations in osteosarcoma. Clin Orthop 1991;270:237.

60. Coley B: Neoplasms of Bone, 2nd ed. New York, Paul B Hoebner, 1980.

61. Schimke R, Lowman J, Cowan G: Retinoblastoma and osteogenic sarcoma in siblings. Cancer 1974;34:2077.

62. Swaney J: Familial osteogenic sarcoma. Clin Orthop 1973;97:64.

63. Mulvihill J, Gralnick J, Whang-Peng J, Leventhal B: Multiple childhood osteosarcomas in an American Indian family with erythroid macrocytosis and skeletal anomalies. Cancer 1977;40:3115.

64. Smith J, Ali K, Caces J, et al: Familial cancer: the occurrence of bone cancer in male members of a family in multiple generations. Clin Res 1980;28:869A.

65. Miller C, McLaughlin R: Osteosarcoma in siblings. Report of two cases. J Bone Joint Surg 1977;59A:261.

66. Colyer R: Osteogenic sarcoma in siblings. Johns Hopkins Med J 1979;145:131.

67. Olsen J: Osteogenic sarcoma in siblings. Ugeskr Laeger 1983;145:1065.

68. Schey W, Pinsky S, Post M: Bone tumors in identical twins. Clin Nucl Med 1977;2:82.

69. Hansen M, Koufos A, Gallie B, et al: Osteosarcoma and retinoblastoma: A shared chromosomal mechanism revealing recessive predisposition. Proc Natl Acad Sci USA 1985;82:6216.

70. Dryja T, Rapaport J, Epstein J, et al: Chromosome 13 homozygosity in osteosarcoma without retinoblastoma. Am J Hum Genet 1986;38:59.

71. Jensen R, Miller R: Retinoblastoma-epidemiologic characteristics. N Engl J Med 1971;285:307.

72. Matsunaga E: Hereditary retinoblastoma: Host resistance and second primary tumors. J Natl Cancer Inst 1980;65:47.

73. Der Kinderen D, Koten J, Wolterbeck R, et al: Non-ocular cancer in hereditary retinoblastoma survivors and relatives. Ophthal Paediatr Genet 1987;8:23.

74. Gallie B: Retinoblastoma gene mutations in human cancer. N Engl J Med 1994;330:786.

75. Cryns V, Thor A, Xu H-J, et al: Loss of the retinoblastoma tumor-suppressor gene in parathyroid carcinoma. N Engl J Med 1994;330:757.

76. Friend S, Bernards R, Rogelj S, et al: A human DNA segment with properties of the gene that predisposes to retinoblastoma and osteosarcoma. Nature 1986;323:643.

77. Lee W-H, Bookstein R, Hong F, et al: Human retinoblastoma susceptibility gene: Cloning, identification and sequence. Science 1987;235:1394.

78. Fung Y-K, Murphree A, T'ang A, et al: Structural evidence for the authenticity of the human retinoblastoma gene. Science 1987;236:1657.

79. Araki N, Uchida A, Kimura T, et al: Involvement of the retinoblastoma gene in primary osteosarcomas and other bone and soft-tissue tumors. Clin Orthop 1991;270:271.

80. Knudson A Jr: Mutation and cancer: Statistical study of retinoblastoma. Proc Natl Acad Sci USA 1971;68:820.

81. Cavenee W, Dryja T, Phillips R, et al: Expression of recessive alleles by chromosomal mechanisms in retinoblastoma. Nature 1983; 305:779.

82. Dryja R, Cavanee W, White R, et al: Homozygosity of chromosome 13 in retinoblastoma. N Engl J Med 1984;310:510.

83. Stanbridge E: Functional evidence for human tumor suppressor genes: Chromosome and molecular genetic studies. Cancer Surv 1992;12:5.

84. Toguchida J, Ishizaki K, Sasaki M, et al: Chromosomal reorganization for the expression of recessive mutation of retinoblastoma susceptibility gene in the development of osteosarcoma. Cancer Res 19988;48:3939.

85. Scheffer H, Haandrikman A, Oosterhuis J, et al: Loss of heterozygosity of chromosome 13 in osteosarcoma. Pediatr Res 1986;20:1045.

86. Friend S, Horowitz J, Gerber M, et al: Deletions of a DNA sequence in retinoblastomas and mesenchymal tumors: Organization of the sequence and its encoded protein. Proc Natl Acad Sci USA 1987; 84:9059.

87. Weichselbaum R, Beckett M, Diamond A: Some retinoblastomas, osteosarcomas, and soft tissue sarcomas may share a common etiology. Proc Natl Acad Sci USA 1988;85:2106.

88. Reissmann P, Simon J, Lee W, Slamon D: Studies of the retinoblastoma gene in human sarcomas. Oncogene 1989;4:839.

89. Feugeas O, Guriec N, Babin-Boilletor A, et al: Loss of heterozygosity of the RB gene is a poor prognostic factor in patients with osteosarcoma. J Clin Oncol 1996;14:467.

90. Scheffer H, Kruize Y, Osinga J, et al: Complete association of loss of heterozygosity of chromosomes 13 and 17 in osteosarcoma. Cancer Genet Cytogenet 1991;53:45.

91. Abramson D, Ronner H, Ellsworth R: Second tumors in non-irradiated bilateral retinoblastoma. Am J Ophthalmol 1979;87:624.

92. Strong L, Knudson A: Second cancers in retinoblastoma. Lancet 1973;2:1086.

93. Chen P, Scully P, Shew J, et al: Phosphorylation of the retinoblastoma gene product is modulated during the cell cycle and cellular differentiation. Cell 1989;58:1193.

94. Fung U, Murphree A, T'Ang A, et al: Structural evidence for the authenticity of the human retinoblastoma gene. Science 1987;236:1657.

95. Goddard A, Balakier H, Canton M, et al: Infrequent genomic rearrangement and normal expression of the putative RB1 gene in retinoblastoma tumors. Mol Cell Biol 1988;8:2082.

96. Masuda H, Miller C, Koeffler H, et al: Rearrangement of the p53 gene in human osteogenic sarcomas. Proc Natl Acad Sci USA 1987;84:7716.

97. Mulligan L, Matlashewski G, Scrable H, Cavenee W: Mechanisms of p53 loss in human sarcomas. Proc Natl Acad Sci USA 1990;87: 5863.

98. Yamaguchi T, Toguchida J, Yamamuro T, et al: Allelotype analysis in osteosarcomas: Frequent allele loss on 3q, 13q, 17p, and 18q. Cancer Res 1992;52:2419.

99. Toguchida J, Yamaguchi T, Tirchie B, et al: Mutation spectrum of the p53 gene in bone and soft tissue sarcomas. Cancer Res 1992;52:6194.

100. Oliner J, Kinzler K, Meltzer P, et al: Amplification of a gene encoding a p53-associated protein in human sarcomas. Nature 1992;358:80.

101. Ladanyi M, Cha C, Lewis R, et al: MDM2 gene amplification in metastatic osteosarcoma. Cancer Res 1993;53:16.

102. Carter S: The dilemma of adjuvant chemotherapy for osteosarcoma. Cancer Clin Trials 1980;3:29.

103. Breur K, Cohen P, Schweisguth O, Hart A: Irradiation of the lungs as an adjuvant therapy in the treatment of osteosarcoma of the limbs: An EORTC randomized study. Eur J Cancer 1978;14:461.

104. Carter S: Adriamycin—a review. J Natl Cancer Inst 1975;55:1265.

105. Cortes E, Holland J, Wang J, et al: Amputation and adriamycin in primary osteogenic sarcoma. N Engl J Med 1974;291:998.

106. Cortes E, Holland H, Wang J, et al: Adriamycin and amputation in primary osteogenic sarcoma. Proc Am Soc Clin Oncol 1974;15:170.

107. Cortes E, Holland J, Glidewell O: Amputation and adriamycin in primary osteosarcoma: A 5-year report. Cancer Treat Rep 1978;62:271.

108. Djerassi I, Rominger C, Kim J, et al: Phase I study of high doses of methotrexate with citrovorum factor in patients with lung cancer. Cancer 1972;30:22.

109. Eilber F, Grant T, Morton D: Adjuvant therapy for osteosarcoma: Preoperative and postoperative treatment. Cancer Treat Rep 1978;62:213.

110. Etcubanas E, Wilbur J: Adjuvant chemotherapy for osteogenic sarcoma. Cancer Treat Rep 1978;62:283.

111. Fossati-Bellani F, Gasparini M, Gennari L: Adjuvant treatment with adriamycin in primary operable osteosarcoma. Cancer Treat Rep 1978;62:279.

112. Gottlieb J, Baker L, Quagliana J, et al: Chemotherapy of sarcomas with a combination of adriamycin and dimethyltriazno imidazole carboxamide. Cancer 1972;30:1632.

113. Jaffe N, Frei E III, Traggis D, Bishop Y: Adjuvant methotrexate and citrovorum-factor treatment of osteogenic sarcoma. N Engl J Med 1974;291:994.

114. Goorin A, Abelson H, Frei E: Osteosarcoma: Fifteen years later. N Engl J Med 1985;313:1637.

115. Taylor W, Ivins J, Dahlin D: Trends and variability in survival from osteosarcoma. Mayo Clin Proc 1978;53:695.

116. Edmonson J, Green S, Ivins J, et al: A controlled pilot study of high dose methotrexate as post-surgical adjuvant chemotherapy for primary osteosarcoma. J Clin Oncol 1984;2:152.

117. Link M, Goorin A, Miser A, et al: The effect of adjuvant chemotherapy on relapse-free survival in patients with osteosarcoma of the extremity. N Engl J Med 1986;314:1600.

118. Link M, Goorin A, Horowitz M, et al: Adjuvant chemotherapy of high-grade osteosarcoma of the extremity. Updated results of the multi-institutional osteosarcoma study. Clin Orthop 1991;270:8.

119. Malawer M, Dunham W: Skip metastases in osteosarcoma: Recent experiences. J Surg Oncol 1983;22:236.

120. Enneking W, Kagan A: "Skip" metastases in osteosarcoma. Cancer 1975;46:2192.

121. Companacci M, Laus M: Local recurrences after amputation for osteosarcoma. J Bone Joint Surg 1980;62B:201.

122. Rosen G, Marcove R, Caparros B: Primary osteogenic sarcoma. The rationale for preoperative chemotherapy and delayed surgery. Cancer 1979;43:2163.

123. Marcove R: En bloc resection for osteogenic sarcoma. Can J Surg 1978;20:521.

124. Watts H: Introduction to resection of musculoskeletal sarcomas. Clin Orthop 1980;153:31.

125. Rosen G, Murphy M, Huvos A, et al: Chemotherapy, en bloc resection and prosthetic bone replacement in the treatment of osteogenic sarcoma. Cancer 1976;37:1.

126. Rosen G, Marcove R, Huvos A., et al: Primary osteogenic sarcoma: Eight-year experience with adjuvant chemotherapy. J Cancer Res Clin Oncol 1983;106(Suppl):55.

127. Rosen G, Caparros B, Huvos A, et al: Preoperative chemotherapy for osteogenic sarcoma: selection of postoperative adjuvant chemotherapy based on the response of the primary tumor to preoperative chemotherapy. Cancer 1982;49:1221.

128. Conference NIOHC: Limb-sparing treatment of adult soft-tissue sarcomas and osteosarcomas. JAMA 1985;25413:1791.

129. McKillop J, Etcubanas E, Goris M: The indications for and limitations of bone scintigraphy in osteogenic sarcoma: A review of 55 patients. Cancer 1981;59:1133.

130. de Santos L, Bernardino M, Murray J: Computed tomography in the evaluation of osteosarcoma: Experience with 25 cases. Am J Roentgenol 1979;132:535.

131. Destouet J, Gilula L, Murphy W: Computed tomography of long-bone osteosarcoma. Radiology 1979;131:439.

132. Schreiman J, Crass J, Wick M, et al: Osteosarcoma: Role of CT in limb-sparing treatment. Radiology 1986;161:485.

133. Hermann G, Leviton M, Mendelson D, et al: Osteosarcoma: Relationship between extent of marrow infiltration on CT and frequency of lung metastases. Am J Roentgenol 1986;149:1203.

134. Zimmer W, Berquist T, McLeod R, et al: Bone tumors: Magnetic resonance imaging versus computed tomography. Radiology 1985;155:709.

135. Powers J: Magnetic resonance imaging in marrow diseases. Clin Orthop 1986;206:79.

136. Sundaram M, McGuire M, Herbold D, et al: Magnetic resonance imaging in planning limb-salvage surgery for primary malignant tumors of bone. J Bone Joint Surg 1986;68A:809.

137. Swan J, Weber D, Korosec F, et al: Combined MRI and MRA for limb salvage planning. J Comput Assist Tomogr 1993;17:339.

138. Gillespy T III, Manfrini M, Ruggieri P, et al: Staging of intraosseous extent of osteosarcoma: Correlation of preoperative CT and MR imaging with pathologic macroslides. Radiology 1988;167:765.

139. Bloem J, Taminiau A, Eulderink F, et al: Radiologic staging of primary bone sarcoma: MR imaging, scintigraphy, angiography, and CT correlation with pathologic examination. Radiology 1988; 169:805.

140. Fletcher B: Response of osteosarcoma and Ewing sarcoma to chemotherapy: Imaging evaluation. Am J Roentgenol 1991;157:825.

141. Lawrence J, Babyn P, Chan H, et al: Extremity osteosarcoma in childhood: Prognostic value of radiologic imaging. Radiology 1993;189:43.

142. Mazumdar A, Siegel MJ, Narra V, Luchtman-Jones L: Whole-body fast inversion recovery MR imaging of small cell neoplasms in pediatric patients: A pilot study. Am J Roentgenol 2002;179: 1261-1266.

143. Daldrup-Link HE, Franzius C, Link TM et al: Whole-body MR imaging for detection of bone metastases in children and young adults: Comparison with skeletal scintigraphy and FDG PET. Am J Roentgenol 2001;177:229-236.

144. O'Connell MJ, Hargaden G, Powell T, Eustace SJ: Whole-body turbo short Tau inversion recovery MR imaging using a moving tabletop. Am J Roentgenol 2002;179:866-868.

145. Adler L, Blair H, Makley J, et al: Noninvasive grading of musculoskeletal tumors using PET. J Nucl Med 1991;32:1508.

146. Brenner W, Kohuslavizki KH, Eary JF: PET imaging of osteosarcoma. J Nucl Med 2003;44(6):930-942.

147. Seeger L, Gold R, Chandnani B: Diagnostic imaging of osteosarcoma. Clin Orthop 1991;270:254.

148. Ramanna L, Waxman A, Binney G, et al: Thallium-201 scintigraphy in bone sarcoma: Comparison with gallium-67 and technetium-MDP in the evaluation of chemotherapeutic response. J Nucl Med 1990;31:567.

150. Rosen G, Loren G, Brien D, et al: Serial thallium-201 scintigraphy in osteosarcoma: Correlation with tumor necrosis after preoperative chemotherapy. Clin Orthop 1993;293:302.

151. Ohtomo K, Terui S, Yokoyama R, et al: Thallium-201 scintigraphy to assess effect of chemotherapy in osteosarcoma. J Nucl Med 1996;37:1444.

152. Ettinger L, Douglass H Jr, Mindell E, et al: Adjuvant adriamycin and cisplatin in newly diagnosed, nonmetastatic osteosarcoma of the extremity. J Clin Oncol 1986;4:353.

153. Krailo M, Ertel I, Makley J, et al: A randomized study comparing high dose methotrexate with moderate dose methotrexate as components of adjuvant chemotherapy in childhood nonmetastatic osteosarcoma: A report from the Children's Cancer Study Group. Med Pediatr Oncol 1987;15:69.

154. Sweetnam R: Malignant bone tumor management, thirty years of achievement. Clin Orthop 1989;247:67.

155. Tomita K, Tsuchiya H: Intermediate results and functional evaluation of limb-salvage surgery for osteosarcoma: An intergroup study in Japan. J Surg Oncol 1989;41:71.

156. Winkler K, Bielack S, Delling G, et al: Effect of intraarterial versus intravenous cisplatin in addition to systemic doxorubicin, high-dose methotrexate, and ifosfamide on histologic tumor response in osteosarcoma (Study COSS-86). Cancer 1990;66:1702.

157. Bacci G, Picci P, Ruggieri P, et al: Primary chemotherapy and delayed surgery (neoadjuvant chemotherapy) for osteosarcoma of the extremities. Cancer 1990;65:2539.

158. Bacci G, Picci P, Pignatti G, et al: Neoadjuvant chemotherapy for nonmetastatic osteosarcoma of the extremities. Clin Orthop 1991;l270:87.

159. Goorin A, Andersen J: Experience with multiagent chemotherapy for osteosarcoma. Improved outcome. Clin Orthop 1991;270:22.

160. Jaffe N, Smith D, Jaffe J, et al: Intraarterial cisplatin in the management of stage IIB osteosarcoma in the pediatric and adolescent age group. Clin Orthop 1991;270:15.

161. Glasser D, Lane J: Stage IIB osteogenic sarcoma. Clin Orthop 1991;270:29.

162. Kropej D, Schiller C, Ritschl P, et al: The management of IIB osteosarcoma: Experience from 1976 to 1985. Clin Orthop 1991;270:40.

163. Carter S, Grimer R, Sneath R: A review of 13-years experience of osteosarcoma. Clin Orthop 1991;270:45.

164. Dubousset J, Missenard G, Kalifa C: Management of osteogenic sarcoma in children and adolescents. Clin Orthop 1991; 270:52.

165. Petrilli S, Penna V, Lopes A, et al: IIB osteosarcoma: Current management, local control, and survival statistics Sao Paulo, Brazil. Clin Orthop 1991;270:60.

166. Ogihara Y, Sudo A, Gujinami S: Current management, local management, and survival statistics of high grade osteosarcoma: Experience in Japan. Clin Orthop 1991;270:72.

167. Winkler K, Bieling P, Bielack S, et al: Local control and survival from the cooperative osteosarcoma study group studies of the German Society of Pediatric Oncology and the Vienna Bone Tumors Registry. Clin Orthop 1991;270:79.

168. Bacci G, Picci P, Ferrari S, et al: Primary chemotherapy and delayed surgery for non-metastatic osteosarcoma of the extremities. Results of 144 preoperatively treated with high-dose methotrexate (IV) followed by cisplatinum (IV) and Adriamycin (IV). Cancer 1993;72:3227.

169. Wilkins RM, Cullen JW, Odom L, et al: Superior survival in treatment of primary nonmetastatic pediatric osteosarcoma of the extremity. Ann Surg Onc 2003;10(5):498-507.

170. Souhami RL, Craft AW, van der Eijken JW, et al: Randomized trial of two regimens of chemotherapy in operable osteosarcoma: A study of the European Osteosarcoma Intergroup. Lancet 1997; 350:911-917.

171. Uchida A, Myoui A, Araki N, Yoshikawa et al: Neoadjuvant chemotherapy for pediatric osteosarcoma patients. Cancer 1997;79:411-415.

172. Bacci G, Ferrari S, Bertoni F, Ruggieri P, et al: Long-term outcome for patients with nonmetastatic osteosarcoma of the extremity treated at the Instituto Ortopedico Rizzoli according to the Instituto Ortopedico Rizzoli/Osteosarcoma-2 Protocol: An updated report. J Clin Oncol 2000;18(24):4016-4027.

173. Bramwell V: The role of chemotherapy in the management of non-metastatic operable extremity osteosarcoma. Semin Oncol 1997;24:561.

174. Eilber F, Giuliano A, Eckardt J, et al: Adjuvant chemotherapy for osteosarcoma: A randomized prospective trial. J Clin Oncol 1987;5:21.

175. Miser J, Krailo M: The Childrens Cancer Group (CCG) studies. In Humphrey G (ed): Osteosarcoma in Adolescents and Young Adults. Boston, Kluwer Academic, 1993, p 287.

176. Saeter G, Alvegrd T, Elomaa I, et al: Treatment of osteosarcoma of the extremities with the T-10 protocol, with emphasis on the effects of preoperative chemotherapy with single-agent high-dose methotrexate: A Scandinavian Sarcoma Group study. J Clin Oncol 1996;9:1766.

177. Kalifa C, Razafindrakoto H, Vassal G, et al: The experience of the pediatric department of the Gustave Roussy Institute. In Humphrey G (ed): Osteosarcoma in Adolescents and Young Adults. Boston, Kluwer Academic, 1993, p 347.

178. Ekert H, Tiedemann K: Osteosarcoma: experience with the Rosen T1-protocol at RCH, Melbourne. In Humphrey G (ed): Osteosarcoma in Adolescents and Young Adults. Boston, Kluwer Academic, 1993, p 355.

179. Bramwell V, Burgers M, Sneath R, et al: A comparison of two short intensive adjuvant chemotherapy regimens in operable osteosarcoma of limbs in children and young adults: The first study of the European Osteosarcoma Intergroup. J Clin Oncol 1992;10:1579.

180. Picci P, Sangiorgi L, Rougraff B, et al: The relationship of chemotherapy-induced necrosis and surgical margins to local recurrence in osteosarcoma. J Clin Oncol 1994;12:2699.

181. Kempf-Bielack B, Bielack S, Bieling P, et al: Local failure (LF) of osteosarcoma (OS): risk factors and prognosis. Results of the Co-operative OS Study group (COSS) [abstract]. Proc Am Soc Clin Oncol 1996;15:520.

182. Delépine N, Delépine G, Alkallaf S, et al: Local relapses following limb sparing salvage surgery for osteosarcoma: Prognostic factors and influence of chemotherapy [abstract]. Proc Am Soc Clin Oncol 196;15:526.

183. Meyers P, Heller G, Healey J, et al: Chemotherapy for non-metastatic osteogenic sarcoma: The Memorial Sloan-Kettering Experience. J Clin Oncol 1992;10:5.

184. Provisor AJ, Ettinger LJ, Nachman JB, et al: Treatment of nonmetastatic osteosarcoma of the extremity with preoperative and postoperative chemotherapy: A report from the Children's Cancer Group. J Clin Oncol 1997;15:76.

185. Benjamin R, Patel S, Armen T, et al: The value of ifosfamide in postoperative neoadjuvant chemotherapy of osteosarcoma [abstract]. Proc Am Soc Clin Oncol 1995;14:516.

186. Jaffe N, Patel S, Benjamin R: Chemotherapy in osteosarcoma. Hematol Oncol Clin North Am 1995;9:825.

187. Gherlinzoni F, Picci P, Bacci G, Campanacci D: Limb sparing versus amputation in osteosarcoma. Correlation between local control, surgical margins and tumor necrosis: Istituto Rizzoli experience. Ann Oncol 1992;3(Suppl):S23.

188. Goorin A, Baker A, Gieser P, et al: No evidence for improved event free survival (EFS) with presurgical chemotherapy (PRE) for non-metastatic extremity osteogenic sarcoma (OGS): Preliminary results of randomized Pediatric Oncology Group (POG) Trial 8651 [abstract]. Proc Am Soc Clin Oncol 1995;14:444.

189. Goorin AM, Schwartzentruber DJ, Devidas M, et al: Presurgical chemotherapy compared with immediate surgery and adjuvant chemotherapy for nonmetastatic osteosarcoma: Pediatric Oncology Group Study POG-8561 J Clin Oncol 2003;21(8):1574–1580.

190. Delépine N, Cornille H, Delépine G, Desbois J: Prognostic value of total dose and dose intensity of methotrexate in multidrug treatment of osteosarcoma [abstract]. Proc Am Soc Clin Oncol 1994;13:413.

191. Bacci G, Picci P, Avella M, et al: Effect of intra-arterial versus intravenous cisplatin in addition to systemic Adriamycin and high-dose methotrexate on histologic tumor response of osteosarcoma of the extremities. J Chemother 1992;4:189.

192. Smith M, Ungerleider R, Horowitz M, Simon R: Influence of doxorubicin dose intensity on response and outcome for patients with ostegenic sarcoma and Ewing's sarcoma. J Natl Cancer Inst 1991;83:1460.

193. Bacci G, Picci P, Ferrari S, et al: Influence of adriamycin dose in the outcome of patients with osteosarcoma treated with multidrug neoadjuvant chemotherapy: Results of two sequential studies. J Chemother 1993;5:237.

194. Winkler K, Beron G, Delling G, et al: Neoadjuvant chemotherapy of osteosarcoma: Results of a randomized cooperative trial (COSS-82) with salvage chemotherapy based on histological tumor response. J Clin Oncol 1988;6:329.

195. Miser J, Arndt C, Smithson W, et al: Treatment of high-grade osteosarcoma (OGS) with ifosfamide (IFOS), mesna (MES), adriamycin (ADR), high-dose methotrexate (HDMTX) with or without cisplatin (CDDP). Results of two pilot trials [meeting abstract]. Proc Am Soc Clin Oncol 1994;13:41.

196. Bacci G, Picci P, Ferrari S, et al: Neoadjuvant chemotherapy for the treatment of osteosarcoma of the extremities: Excellent response of the primary tumor to preoperative treatment with methotrexate, cisplatin, adriamycin, and ifosfamide. Preliminary results. Chir Organi Mov 1995;LXXX:1.

197. Epelman S, Siebel N, Melaragno R, et al: Treatment of newly diagnosed high grade osteosarcoma (OS) with ifosfamide (IFOS), adriamycin (ADR) and cisplatin (CDP) without high dose methotrexate [abstract]. Proc Am Soc Clin Oncol 1995;14:439.

198. Biron P, Blay J, Belouineau F, et al: Pilot study of the HELP regimen in osteosarcoma [abstract]. Proc Am Soc Clin Oncol 1993;12:471.

199. Meyer W, Pratt C, Harper J, et al: Ifosfamide (IFOS) and carboplatin (CARBO) window therapy in previously untreated osteosarcoma (OS) [abstract]. Proc Am Soc Clin Oncol 1995;14:442.

200. Ornadel D, Souhami R, Whelan J, et al: Doxorubicin and cisplatin with granulocyte colony-stimulating factor as adjuvant chemotherapy for osteosarcoma: Phase II trial of the European Osteosarcoma Intergroup. J Clin Oncol 1994;12:1842.

201. Bacci G, Bertoni F, Longhi A, et al: Neoadjuvant chemotherapy for high-grade central osteosarcoma of the extremity. Histologic response to preoperative chemotherapy correlates with histologic subtype of the tumor. Cancer 2003;97:3068–3075.

202. Hauben EI, Weeden S, Pringle J, et al: Does the histological subtype of high grade-central osteosarcoma influence the response to treatment with chemotherapy and does it affect overall survival? A study of 570 patients of two consecutive trials of the European Osteosarcoma Intergroup. Eur J Cancer 2002;38:1218–1225.

203. Jaffe N, Carrasco H, Raymond K, et al: Can cure in patients with osteosarcoma be achieved exclusively with chemotherapy and abrogation of surgery? Cancer 2002;95:2202–2210.

204. Ferrari S, Briccoli A, Mercuri M, et al: Postrelapse survival in osteosarcoma of the extremities: Prognostic factors for long-term survival. J Clin Oncol 2003;21:710–715.

205. Weeden S, Grimer RJ, Cannon SR, Taminiau AHM, Uscinska BM: The effect of local recurrence on survival in resected osteosarcoma. Eur J Canc 2001;37:39–46.

206. Bosing T, Toessner A, Hiddemann W, et al: Cytostatic effects in osteosarcoma as detected by flow cytometric DNA analysis after preoperative chemotherapy according to the COSS 80/82 protocol. J Cancer Res 1987;113:369.

207. Baldini N, Gebhardt M, Springfield D, et al: Effect of preoperative chemotherapy on nuclear DNA content in osteosarcoma. Chir Organi Mov 1990;75:22.

208. Picci P, Bacci G, Campanacci M, et al: Histologic evaluation of necrosis in osteosarcoma induced by chemotherapy. Cancer 1985;56:1515.

209. Winkler K, Beron G, Kotz R, et al: Neoadjuvant chemotherapy for osteogenic sarcoma: Results of a cooperative German/Austrian study. J Clin Oncol 1984;2:617.

210. Glasser D, Lane J, Huvos A, et al: Survival, prognosis, and therapeutic response in osteogenic sarcoma. Cancer 1992;69:698.

211. Davis A, Bell R, Goodwin P: Prognostic factors in osteosarcoma: A critical review. J Clin Oncol 194;12:423.

212. Simon M, Aschliman M, Thomas N, Mankin H: Limb-salvage treatment versus amputation for osteosarcoma of the distal end of the femur. J Bone Joint Surg 1986;68A:1331.

213. Rougraff B, Simon M, Kneisl J, et al: Limb-salvage compared with amputation for osteosarcoma of the distal end of the femur. J Bone Joint Surg 1994;76A:649.

214. Malawer M, Bush R, Reaman G, et al: Impact of two cycles of preoperative chemotherapy with intraarterial cisplatin and intravenous doxorubicin on the choice of surgical procedure for high-grade bone sarcoma of the extremities. Clin Orthop 1991;270:214.

215. Springfield D, Schmidt R, Graham-Pole J, et al: Surgical treatment of osteosarcoma. J Bone Joint Surg 1988;70A:1124.

216. Simon M: Limb salvage for osteosarcoma current concepts review. J Bone Joint Surg 1988;70A:307.

217. Lindner NJ, Ramm O, Hillmann A, et al: Limb salvage and outcome of osteosarcoma. Clin Orthop 1999;358:83.

218. Otis J, Lane J, Kroll M: Energy cost during gait in osteosarcoma patients after resection and knee replacement and after above the knee amputation. J Bone Joint Surg 1985;67A:606.

219. Sim F, Beauchamp C, Chao E: Reconstruction of musculoskeletal defects about the knee for tumors. Clin Orthop 1987;221:188.

220. Ritschl P, Braun O, Pongracz N, et al: Modular reconstruction system for the lower extremity. In Enneking W (ed): Limb Salvage in Musculoskeletal Oncology. New York, Churchill Livingstone, 1987, p 237.

221. Malawer M, McHale K: Limb-sparing surgery for high-grade malignant tumors of the proximal tibia. Surgical technique and a method of extensor mechanism reconstruction. Clin Orthop 1989;239:231.

222. Horowitz S, Lane J, Otis J, Healey J: Prosthetic arthroplasty of the knee after resection of a sarcoma in the proximal end of the tibia. J Bone Joint Surg 1991;73A:286.

223. Eckhardt J, Eilber F, Rosen G, et al: Endoprosthetic replacement for stage IIB osteosarcoma. Clin Orthop 1991;270:202.

224. Mercuri M, Capanna R, Manfrini M, et al: The management of malignant bone tumors in children and adolescents. Clin Orthop 1991;264:156.

225. Thompson V, Steggall C: Chondrosarcoma of the proximal portion of the femur treated by resection and bone replacement. A six-year result. J Bone Joint Surg 1956;33A:357.

226. Smith W, Simon M: Segmental resection for chondrosarcoma. J Bone Joint Surg 1975;57A:1097.

227. Johnston J, Harries T, Alexander C, Alexander AH: Limb salvage procedure for neoplasms about the knee by spherocentric total knee arthroplasty and autogenous autoclaved bone grafting. Clin Orthop 1983;181:137.

228. Ku J, Smith P, Goldstein S, Matthews L: An experimental investigation of the fate of autogenous autoclaved bone grafts. Orthop Trans 1985;9:340.

229. Smith W, Struhl S: Replantation of an autoclaved autogenous segment of bone for treatment of chondrosarcoma. J Bone Joint Surg 1988;70A:70.

230. Freiberg A, Saltzman C, Smith W: Replantation of an autoclaved, autogenous humerus in a patient who had chondrosarcoma. J Bone Joint Surg 1992;74A:438.

231. Mankin H, Fogelson F, Thrasher A, Jaffer F: Massive resection and allograft transplantation in the treatment of malignant bone tumors. N Engl J Med 1976;294:1247.

232. Mankin H, Doppelt S, Sullivan T, Tomford W: Osteoarticular and intercalary allograft transplantation in the management of malignant tumors of bone. Cancer 1982;50:613.

233. Mankin H, Doppelt S, Tomford W: Clinical experience with allograft implantation. The first ten years. Clin Orthop 1983;174:69.

234. Sim F, Chao E: Segmental prosthetic replacement of the knee after tumor resection. In Enneking W (ed): Limb salvage in musculoskeletal oncology. New York, Churchill Livingstone, 1987, p 379.

235. Lord C, Gebhardt M, Tomford W, Mankin H: Infection in bone allografts. Incidence, nature, and treatment. J Bone Joint Surg 1988;70A:369–376.

236. Gitelis S, Heligman D, Quill G, Piasecki P: The use of large allografts for tumor reconstruction and salvage of the failed total hip arthroplasty. Clin Orthop 1988;231:62.

237. Gebhardt M, Mankin H: The use of proximal tibial allografts in the reconstruction of tumors and other defects. In Yamamuro T (ed): New Developments for Limb Salvage in Musculoskeletal Tumors. New York, Springer Verlag, 1989, p 573.

238. Gebhardt M, Flugstad D, Springfield D, Mankin H: The use of bone allografts for limb salvage in high-grade extremity osteosarcoma. Clin Orthop 1991;270:181.

239. Gitelis S, Piasecki P: Allograft prosthetic composite arthroplasty for osteosarcoma and other aggressive bone tumors. Clin Orthop 1991;270:197.

240. Vander Griend R: The effect of internal fixation on the healing of large allografts. J Bone Joint Surg 1994;76A:657.

241. Waters R, Perry J, Antonelli D, Hislop H: Energy cost of walking of amputees: The influence of level of amputation. J Bone Joint Surg 1976;58A:42.

242. Harris I, Leff A, Gitelis S, Simon M: Function after amputation, arthrodesis, or arthroplasty for tumors about the knee. J Bone Joint Surg 1990;72A:1477.

243. D'Aubigné R, Dejouany H: Diaphyso-epiphyseal resection for bone tumour at the knee. With reports of nine cases. J Bone Joint Surg 1958;40B:385.

244. Enneking W, Shirley P: Resection-arthrodesis for malignant and potentially malignant lesions about the knee using an intramedullary rod and local bone grafts. J Bone Joint Surg 1977;59A:223.

245. Campanacci M, Costa P: Total resection of the distal femur or proximal tibia for bone tumours: Autogenous bone grafts and arthrodesis in twenty-six cases. J Bone Joint Surg 1979;61B:455.

246. Enneking W, Eady J, Burchardt H: Autogenous cortical bone grafts in the reconstruction of segmental skeletal defects. J Bone Joint Surg 1980;62A:1039.

247. Neff J: Experience in the use of a custom modular titanium intramedullary rod in resection/arthrodesis of the knee. In Yamamuro T (ed): New Developments for Limb Salvage in Musculoskeletal Tumors. Tokyo, Springer-Verlag, 1989, p 263.

248. O'Connor MI, Sim FH, Chao EY: Limb salvage for neoplasms of the shoulder girdle. Intermediate reconstructive and functional results. J Bone Joint Surg 1996;78A:1872.

249. Damron TA, Rock MG, O'Connor MI, et al: Functional laboratory assessment after oncologic shoulder joint resections. Clin Orthop 1998;348:124.

250. Winkelmann W: Hip rotationplasty for malignant tumors of the proximal part of the femur. J Bone Joint Surg 1986;68A:362.

251. Borggreve J: Kniegelenksersatz durch das in der Beinlangsachse um 180 degree gedrehte Fussgelenk. Arch Orthop Unfall Chir 1930;28:175.

252. Van Nes C: Rotation-plasty for congenital defects of the femur. Making use of the ankle of the shortened limb to control the knee joint of a prosthesis. J Bone Joint Surg 1950;32B:12.

253. Kostiuk J, Gillespie R, Hall J, Hubbard S: Van Nes rotational osteotomy for treatment of proximal femoral focal deficiency and congenital short femur. J Bone Joint Surg 1975;57A:1039.

254. Kritter A: Tibial rotation-plasty for proximal femoral focal deficiency. J Bone Joint Surg 1977;59A:927.

255. Torode I, Gillespie R: Rotationplasty of the lower limb for congenital defects of the femur. J Bone Joint Surg 1983;65B:569.

256. Salzer M, Knahr K, Kotz R, Kristen H: Treatment of osteosarcomata of the distal femur by rotation-plasty. Arch Orthop Trauma Surg 1981;99:131.

257. Gottsauner-Wolf F, Kotz R, Knahr K, et al: Rotationplasty for limb salvage in the treatment of malignant tumors at the knee. J Bone Joint Surg 1991;73A:1365.

258. Kotz R, Salzer M: Rotation-plasty for childhood osteosarcoma of the distal part of the femur. J Bone Joint Surg 1982;64A:959.

259. Tsuchiya H, Tomita K, Minematsu K, et al: Limb salvage using distraction osteogenesis. A classification of the technique. J Bone Joint Surg 1997;79B:403.

260. Tsuchiya H, Abdel-Wanis ME, Sakurakichi K, et al: Osteosarcoma around the knee. J Bone Joint Surg (Br) 2002;84B:1162–1166.

261. Jaffe N, Knapp J, Chuang V, et al: Osteosarcoma: Intra-arterial treatment of the primary tumor with cis-diammine-dichloroplatinum II (CDP). Angiographic, pathologic, and pharmacologic studies. Cancer 1983;51:402.

262. Canadell J, Forriol F, Cava JA: Removal of metaphyseal tumours with preservation of the epiphysis. Physeal distraction before excision. J Bone Joint Surg (Br) 1994;76B:127–132.

263. Wilkins RM, Soubeiran A: The Phenix expandable prosthesis. Clin Orthop 2001;382:51–58.

264. Huvos A, Butler A, Bretsky S: Osteogenic sarcoma in pregnant women. Prognosis, therapeutic implications and literature review. Cancer 1985;56:2326.

265. Renard AJ, Veth RP, Schreuder HW, et al: Function and complications after ablative and limb-salvage therapy in lower extremity sarcoma of bone. J Surg Oncol 2000;73(4):198.

266. Knahr K, Kotz R, Kristen H, et al: Clinical evaluation of patients with rotationplasty. In Enneking W (ed): Limb salvage in musculoskeletal oncology. Bristol-Myers/Zimmer Orthopaedic Symposium. New York, Churchill Livingstone, 1987, p 429.

267. Knahr K, Kristen H, Ritschl P, et al: Prosthetic management and functional evaluation of patients with resection of the distal femur and rotationplasty. Orthopedics 1987;10:1241.

268. McClenaghan B, Krajbich J, Pirone A, et al: Comparative assessment of gait after limb-salvage procedures. J Bone Joint Surg 1989;71A:1178.

269. Cammisa F Jr, Glasser D, Otis J, et al: The Van Nes tibial rotationplasty. A functionally viable reconstructive procedure in children who have a tumor of the distal end of the femur. J Bone Joint Surg 1990;72A:1541.

270. Hillmann A, Hoffmann C, Gosheger G, et al: Malignant tumor of the distal part of the femur or the proximal part of the tibia: Endoprosthetic replacement or rotationplasty. J Bone Joint Surg 1999;81A:4;462.

271. Veenstra KM, Sprangers MA, van der Eijken JW, Taminiau AH: Quality of life in Survivors with a Van Ness-Borggreve rotationplasty after bone tumour resection. J Surg Oncol 2000;73:192.

272. Lee SH, Kim DJ, Oh JH, et al: Validation of a functional evaluation system in patients with musculoskeletal tumors. Clin Orthop 2003;411:217–226.

273. Wittig JC, Bickels J, Kellar-Graney KL, Kim FH, Malawer MM: Osteosarcoma of the proximal humerus: Long-term results with limb-sparing surgery. Clin Orthop 2002;397:156–176.

274. Schwameis E, Dominkus M, Krepler P, et al: Reconstruction of the pelvis after tumor resection in children and adolescents. Clin Orthop 2002;402:220–235.

275. Satcher Jr RL, O'Donnell RJ, Johnston JO: Reconstruction of the pelvis after resection of tumors about the acetabulum. Clin Orthop 2003;409:209–217.

276. Ozaki T, Rodl R, Gosheger G, et al: Sacral infiltration in pelvic sarcomas. Clin Orthop 2003;407:152–158.

277. Horowitz S, Glasser D, Lane J, Healey J: Prosthetic and extremity survivorship after limb salvage for sarcoma. How long do the reconstructions last? Clin Orthop 1993;293:280.

278. Malawer M, Chou L: Prosthetic survival and clinical results with use of large-segment replacements in the treatment of high-grade bone sarcomas. J Bone Joint Surg 1995;77A:1154.

279. Zwart H, Taminiau A, Schimmel J, van Horn J: Kotz modular femur and tibial replacement. 28 tumor cases followed for 3 (1–8) years. Acta Orthop Scand 1994;65:315.

280. Zehr R, Enneking W, Scarborough M: Allograft-prosthesis composite vs. megaprosthesis in proximal femoral reconstruction. In Campanacci M, Capanna R (eds): Eighth International Symposium on Limb Salvage: 1995 May 10–12; Florence, Italy. Florence, 1995, p 58.

281. Capana R, Leonessa C, Bettelli G, et al: Modular Kotz prosthesis. The Rizzoli experience. In Yamamuro T (ed): New Developments for Limb Salvage in Musculoskeletal Tumors. New York, Springer Verlag, 1989, p 37.

282. Eckhardt J, Pignatti G, Eilber F, et al: Management of failed endoprosthetic implants: The UCLA experience. In Langlais F, Tomeno B (eds): Limb Salvage: Major Reconstruction in Oncologic and Nontumoral Conditions. New York, Springer Verlag, 1990, p 479.

283. Khong K, Chao E, Sim F: Long-term performance of custom prosthetic replacement for neoplastic disease of the proximal femur. In Yamamuro T (ed): New Developments for Limb Salvage in Musculoskeletal Tumors. New York, Springer Verlag, 1990, p 403.

284. Unwin P, Walker P, Briggs T, et al: Aseptic loosening in 1001 cases of cemented custom-made bone tumour replacements of the lower limb. In Campanacci M, Capanna R (eds): Eighth International Symposium on Limb Salvage; 1995 May 10–12; Florence, Italy. Florence, 1995, p 47.

285. Unwin P, Cobb H, Walker P: Distal femoral arthroplasty using custom-made prostheses. The first 218 cases. J Arthroplasty 1993;8:259.

286. Shih L, Sim F, Pritchard D, et al: Segmental total knee arthroplasty after distal femoral resection for tumor. Clin Orthop 1993; 292:269.

287. Mittermayer F, Krepler P, Dominkus M, Schwameis E, Sluga M, Heinzl H, Kotz R: Long-term followup of uncemented tumor endoprostheses for the lower extremity. Clin Orthop 2001;388:167.

288. Malo M, Davis AM, Wunder J, Masri BA, Bell RS, Isler MH, Turcott RE: Functional evaluation in distal femoral endoprosthetic replacement for bone sarcoma. Clin Orthop 2001;389:173.

289. Virolainen P, Inque N, Nagao M, et al: Autogenous only grafting for enhancement of extracortical tissue formation over porous-coated segmental replacement prostheses. J Bone J Surg 1999;81A(4): 493–499.

290. Donati D, Di Liddo M, Zavatta M, Manfrini et al: Massive bone allograft reconstruction in high-grade osteosarcoma. Clin Orthop 2000;377:186.

291. Gebhardt MC, Flugstad DI, Springfield DS, Mankin HJ: The use of bone allografts for limb salvage in high-grade extremity osteosarcoma. Clin Orthop 1991;270:181–196.

292. Wozney JM, Rosen V, Celeste AJ, et al: Novel regulators of bone formation: Molecular clones and activities. Science 1988;242: 1528–1534.

293. Cook SD, Baffes GC, Wolfe MW et al: The effect of recombinant human osteogenic protein-1 on healing of large bone defects in rats. J Bone Joint Surg (Am) 1994;76A:827–838.

294. Cook SD, Barrack RL, Santman M, et al: Strut allograft healing to the femur with recombinant human osteogenic protein-1. Clin Orthop 2000;381:47–57.

295. Bini S, Johnson J, Martin D: Compliant Pre Stress Fixation in Distal Femur: Three Year Follow-up Data. Abstract Book. Combined Meeting of the American and European Musculoskeletal Tumor Societies. Washington, DC, 1998, p 164.

296. Picci P, Capanna R, Bacci G, et al: Margins, necrosis and local recurrence after conservative surgery in osteosarcoma. Chir Organi Mov 1990;75(Suppl):82.

297. Weddington WJ, Segraves K, Simon M: Psychological outcome of extremity sarcoma survivors undergoing amputation or limb salvage. J Clin Oncol 1985;3:1393.

298. Postma A, Kingma A, De Ruiter J, et al: Quality of life in bone tumour patients comparing limb salvage and amputation of the lower extremity. J Surg Oncol 1992;51:47.

299. Harrish J, Leff A, Gitelis S, Simon M: Function after amputation, arthrodesis or arthroplasty for tumours about the knee. J Bone Joint Surg 1990;72A:1477.

300. Dobbs H, Scales J, Wilson J, et al: Endoprosthetic replacement of the proximal femur and acetabulum: A survival analysis. J Bone Joint Surg 1981;63B:219.

301. Roberts P, Chan D, Grimer R, et al: Prosthetic replacement of the distal femur for primary bone tumors. J Bone Joint Surg 1991;73B:762.

302. Ross A, Wilson J, Scales J: Endoprosthetic replacement of the proximal humerus. J Bone Joint Surg 1987;69B:656.

303. Grimer RJ, Carter SR, Pynsent PB: The cost-effectiveness of limb salvage for bone tumours. J Bone Joint Surg 1997;79B:558.

304. Jaffe N, Spears R, Eftekhari F, et al: Pathologic fracture in osteosarcoma. Impact of chemotherapy on primary tumor and survival. Cancer 1987;59:701.

305. Scully S, Temple H, O'Keefe R, et al: The surgical treatment of patients with osteosarcoma who sustain pathologic fractures. Clin Orthop 1996;324:227.

306. Coley B, Sharp G: Pathologic fractures in primary bone tumors of the extremities. Am J Surg 1930;9:251.

307. Coley B, Pool J: Factors influencing prognosis in osteogenic sarcoma. Ann Surg 1940;122:1114.

308. Wurtz D, Peabody T, Simon M: Oncologic outcomes of patients who have pathologic fractures of high-grade conventional osteosarcomas. Clin Orthop 1998.

309. Abudu A, Sferopoulos N, Tillman R, et al: The surgical treatment and outcome of pathological fractures in localized osteosarcoma. J Bone Joint Surg 1996;78B:694.

310. Aung L, Gorlick R, Healey JH, et al: Metachronous skeletal osteosarcoma in patients treated with adjuvant and neoadjuvant chemotherapy for nonmetastatic osteosarcoma. J Clin Oncol 2003;21:342–348.

311. Rodriguez EK, Hornicek FJ, Gebhardt MC, Mankin HJ: Metachronous osteosarcoma: A report of five cases. Clin Orthop 2003;411:227–235.

312. Fitzgerald RH, Dohlin DC, Sim FH: Multiple metachronous osteogenic sarcoma. J Bone Joint Surg 1973;55A:595–605.

313. Marina N, Pratt C, Rao B, et al: Improved prognosis of children with osteosarcoma metastatic to the lung(s) at the time of diagnosis. Cancer 1992;70:2722.

314. Meyers P, Heller G, Healey J, et al: Osteogenic sarcoma with clinically detectable metastasis at initial presentation. J Clin Oncol 1993;11:449.

315. Harris M, Gieser P, Link M, et al: Treatment of metastatic osteosarcoma at diagnosis: A Pediatric Oncology Group study. Proc Am Soc Clin Oncol 1995;14:445.

316. Belli L, Scholl S, Livartowski A, et al: Resection of pulmonary metastases in osteosarcoma: A retrospective analysis of 44 patients. Cancer 1989;63:2546.

317. Huth J, Eilber F: Patterns of recurrence after resection of osteosarcoma of the extremity. Arch Surg 1989;124:122.

318. Carter S, Grimer R, Sneath R, Matthews H: Results of thoracotomy in osteogenic sarcoma with pulmonary metastases. Thorax 1991;46:727.

319. Meyer W, Schell M, Kumar M, et al: Thoracotomy for pulmonary metastatic osteosarcoma: An analysis of prognostic indicators of survival. Cancer 1987;59:374.

320. Snyder C, Saltzman D, Ferrell K, et al: A new approach to the resection of pulmonary osteosarcoma metastases. Clin Orthop 1991;270:247.

Specific Malignancies

III

321. Burk C, Belasco J, O'Neill J Jr, Lange B: Pulmonary metastases and bone sarcomas. Surgical removal of lesions appearing after adjuvant chemotherapy. Clin Orthop 1991;262:88.

322. Bacci G, Mercuri M, Briccoli A, et al: Osteogenic sarcoma of the extremity with detectable lung metastases at presentation. Results of treatment of 23 patients with chemotherapy followed by simultaneous resection of primary and metastatic lesions. Cancer 1997;79:245.

323. Kaste SC, Pratt CB, Cain AM, et al: Metastases detected at the time of diagnosis of primary pediatric extremity osteosarcoma at diagnosis. Imaging Features. Cancer 1999;86:1602-1608.

324. Kager L, Zoubek A, Potschger U, et al: Primary metastatic osteosarcoma: Presentation and outcome of patients treated on neoadjuvant cooperative osteosarcoma study group protocols. J Clin Oncol 2003;21:2011-2018.

325. Fagioli F, Berger M, del Prever AB, et al: Regression of metastatic osteosarcoma following non-myeloablative stem cell transplantation. A case report. Haematologica 2003;88(5):ECR16.

326. Nagarajan R, Neglia JP, Clohisy DR, et al: Education, employment, insurance, and marital status among 694 survivors of pediatric lower extremity bone tumors. A report from the Childhood Cancer Survivor Study. Cancer 2003;97:2554-2564.

327. Aung L, Gorlick RG, Shi W, et al: Second malignant neoplasms in long-term survivors of osteosarcoma. Cancer 2002;95:1728-1734.

328. Bielack SS, Rerin JS, Dickerhoff R, et al: Osteosarcoma after allogeneic bone marrow transplantation. A report of four cases from the Cooperative Osteosarcoma Study Group. Bone Marrow Transplant 2003;31:353-359.

Osteosarcoma Variants

329. Dahlin D, Unni K: Osteosarcoma of bone and its important recognizable varieties. Am J Surg Pathol 1977;1:61.

330. Schajowicz F, McGuire M, Araujo S, et al: Osteosarcomas arising on the surface of long bones. J Bone Joint Surg 1988;76A:555.

331. Raymond A: Surface osteosarcoma. Clin Orthop 1991;270:140.

332. Sonneland P, Unni K: High-grade "surface" osteosarcoma arising from femoral shaft. Skeletal Radiol 1984;11:77.

333. Wold L, Unni K, Beabout J, Pritchard D: High-grade surface osteosarcoma. Am J Surg Pathol 1984;8:181.

334. Present D, Bertoni F, Laus M, et al: Case Report 565. Skeletal Radiol 1989;18:471.

335. Greenspan A, Steiner G, Norman A, et al: Case Report 436. Skeletal Radiol 1987;18:489.

336. Tarr R, Kerner T, McCook B, et al: Primary extraosseous osteogenic sarcoma of the mediastinum: Clinical, pathologic and radiologic correlation. South Med 1988;J81:1317.

337. Young R, Rosenberg A: Osteosarcoma of the urinary bladder. Report of a case and review of the literature. Cancer 1987;59:174.

338. von Hochstetter A, Hättenschwiler J, Vogt M: Primary osteosarcoma of the liver. Cancer 1987;60:2312.

339. Bloch T, Roth L, Stehman FB, et al: Osteosarcoma of the uterine cervix associated with hyperplastic and atypical mesonephric rests. Cancer 1988;62:1594.

340. Reznik M, Lenelle J: Primary intracerebral osteosarcoma. Cancer 1991;68:793.

341. Bane B, Evans H, Ro JY, et al: Extraskeletal osteosarcoma. A clinicopathologic review of 26 cases. Cancer 1990;65:2762.

342. Chung E, Enzinger F: Extraskeletal osteosarcoma. Cancer 1987;60:1132.

343. Schajowicz F, Araujo E, Berenstein M: Sarcoma complicating Paget's disease of bone. J Bone Joint Surg 1983;65B:299.

344. Schmorl G: Uber Osteitis deformans Paget. Virchows Arch (Pathol Anat) 1932;283:694.

345. Healey J, Buss D: Radiation and Pagetic osteogenic sarcomas. Clin Orthop 1991;270:128.

346. Schajowicz F: Tumors and Tumorlike Lesions of Bones and Joints. New York, Springer Verlag, 1981.

347. Colarinha P, Fonseca A, Salgado L, Vieira M: Diagnosis of malignant change in Paget's disease by T1-201. Clin Nucl Med 1996;21:299.

348. Huvos A, Butler A, Bretsky S: Osteogenic sarcoma associated with Paget's disease. Cancer 1983;52:1489.

349. Huvos A, Woodard H, Cahan S, et al: Postradiation osteosarcoma and bone and soft tissues. Cancer 1985;55:1244.

350. Meadows A, Strong L, Li F, et al: Bone sarcoma as a second malignant neoplasm in children: Influence of radiation and genetic predisposition. Cancer 1980;46:2603.

351. Abramson D, Ellsworth R, Kitchin F, Tung G: Second nonocular tumors in retinoblastoma survivors. Are they radiation induced? Opthalmology 1984;91:1351.

352. Coleman M, Bell C, Fraser P: Second primary malignancy after Hodgkin's disease, ovarian cancer, and cancer of the testes: A population based cohort study. Br J Cancer 1987;56:349.

353. Tucker M, Coleman C, Cox R, et al: Risk of second cancers after treatment for Hodgkin's disease. N Engl J Med 1988;318:76.

354. Nadeem S, Feun L, Bruce-Gregorios J, Green B: Post radiation sarcoma (malignant fibrous histiocytoma) of the cervical spine following ependymoma (a case report). J Neuro-oncol 1991;11:263.

355. Schajowicz F: Tumors and Tumorlike Lesions of Bone and Joints. New York, Springer Verlag, 1981.

356. Arlen M, Higinbotham N, Huvos A, et al: Radiation-induced sarcoma of bone. Cancer 1971;28:1087.

357. Sheppard DG, Libshitz HI: Post-radiation sarcomas: A review of the clinical and imaging features in 63 cases. Clin Radiol 2001;56: 22-29.

358. Frassica F, Sim F, Frassica D, Wold L: Survival and management considerations in post-irradiation osteosarcoma and Paget's osteosarcoma. Clin Orthop 1991;270:120.

359. Nakajima H, Sim FH, Bond JR, Unni KK: Small cell osteosarcoma of bone. Review of 72 cases. Cancer 1997;79:2095.

360. Sim F, Unni K, Beabout J, Dahlin D: Osteosarcoma with small cells simulating Ewing's tumor. J Bone Joint Surg 1979;61A:207.

361. Ayala A, Ro J, Raymond A, et al: Small cell osteosarcoma: A clinicopathologic study of 27 cases. Cancer 1989;64:2162.

362. Bertoni F, Present D, Bacchini P, et al: The Instituto Rizzoli experience with small cell osteosarcoma. Cancer 1989;64:2591.

363. Dickersin G, Rosenberg A: The ultrastructure of small-cell osteosarcoma, with a review of the light microscopy and differential diagnosis. Hum Pathol 1991;22:267.

364. Martin S, Dwyer A, Kissane J, Costa J: Small-cell osteosarcoma. Cancer 1982;50:990.

365. Sanjay B, Ray G, Vishwakarma G: A small-cell osteosarcoma with multiple skeletal metastases. Arch Orthop Trauma Surg 1988;107:58.

366. Hartman K, Triche T, Kinsella T, Miser J: Prognostic value of histopathology in Ewing's sarcoma: Long-term follow-up of distal extremity primary tumors. Cancer 1991;67:163.

367. Grimer RJ, Cannon SR, Taminiau AM, et al: Osteosarcoma over the age of forty. Euro J Cancer 2003;39:157.

368. Unni K, Dahlin D, McLeod R, Pritchard D: Interosseous well- differentiated osteosarcoma. Cancer 1977;40:1337.

369. Kurt A, Unni K, McLeod R, Pritchard D: Low-grade intraosseous osteosarcoma. Cancer 1990;65:1418.

370. Sundaram M, Herbold D, McGuire M: Case report 370. Skeletal Radiol 1986;15:338.

371. Sim F, Kurt A, McLeod R, Unni K: Case Report 628. Skeletal Radiol 1990;19:457.

372. Campanacci M, Bertoni F, Capanna R, Cervellati C: Central osteosarcoma of low-grade malignancy. Ital J Orthop Traumatol 1981;7:71.

373. Jaffe H: Intracortical osteogenic sarcoma. Bull Hosp Jt Dis 1960;21:189.

374. Kyriakos M: Intracortical osteosarcoma. Cancer 1980;46:2525.

375. Hermann G, Klein MJ, Springfield D, et al: Intracortical osteosarcoma; two-year delay in diagnosis. Skeletal Radiol 2002;31:592-596.

376. Griffith JF, Kumta SM, Chow LTC, et al: Intracortical osteosarcoma. Skeletal Radiol 1998;27:228-232.

377. Scranton PEJ, DeCicco FA, Totten RS, et al: Prognostic factors in osteosarcoma. A review of 20 years experience at the University of Pittsburgh Health Center Hospital. Cancer 1975;36:2179-2191.

378. Vigorita VJ, Ghelman B, Jones JK, Marcove RC: Intracortical osteosarcoma. Am J Surg Pathol 1984;8:65.

379. Lichtenstein L: Tumors of periosteal origin. Cancer 1955;8:1060.

380. Cooper R: Juxtacortical chondrosarcoma. J Bone Joint Surg 1965;47A:524.

381. Schajowicz F, Bessone J: Chondrosarcoma in three brothers. J Bone Joint Surg 1967;49A:129.
382. Schajowicz F: Juxtacortical chondrosarcoma. J Bone Joint Surg 1977;59B:473.
383. Unni K, Dahlin D, Beabout S, Ivins J: Parosteal osteogenic sarcoma. Cancer 1976;37:2466.
384. Ahuja S, Villacin A, Smith J, et al: Juxtacortical (parosteal) osteogenic sarcoma. J Bone Joint Surg 1977;59:532.
385. Campanacci M, Picci P, Gherlinzoni F, et al: Parosteal osteosarcoma. J Bone Joint Surg 1984;66B:313.
386. Okada K, Frassica F, Sim F, et al: Parosteal osteosarcoma. J Bone Joint Surg 1994;76A:366.

Chondrosarcoma

387. Marcove R: Chondrosarcoma: Diagnosis and treatment. Orthop Clin North Am 1977;8:811.
388. Pritchard D, Lunke R, Taylor W, et al: Chondrosarcoma: A clinicopathologic and statistical analysis. Cancer 1980;45:149.
389. Gitelis S, Bertoni F, Picci P, Campanacci M: Chondrosarcoma of bone: the experience at the Instituto Ortopedico Rizzoli. J Bone Joint Surg 1981;63A:1248.
390. Huvos A, Rosen G, Dabska M, Marcove R: Mesenchymal chondrosarcoma. A clinicopathologic analysis of 35 patients with emphasis on treatment. Cancer 1983;51:1230.
391. Healey J, Lane J: Chondrosarcoma. Clin Orthop 1986;204:119.
392. Stener B: Total spondylectomy in chondrosarcoma arising from the seventh thoracic vertebra. J Bone Joint Surg 1971;53B:288.
393. Shives T, McLeod R, Unni K, Schray M: Chondrosarcoma of the spine. J Bone Joint Surg 1989;71A:1158.
394. Lee S-T, Lui T-N, Tsai M-D: Primary intraspinal dura mesenchymal chondrosarcoma. Surg Neurol 1989;31:54.
395. Kretzschmar H, Eggert H: Mesenchymal chondrosarcoma of the craniocervical junction. Clin Neurol Neurosurg 1990;92:343.
396. Venderhooft J, Conrad E, Anderson P, et al: Intradural recurrence with chondrosarcoma of the spine. Clin Orthop 1993;294:90.
397. Aprin H, Riseborough E, Hall J: Chondrosarcoma in children and adolescents. Clin Orthop 1982;166:226.
398. Young C, Sim F, Unni K, McLeod R: Chondrosarcoma of bone in children. Cancer 1990;66:1641.
399. Dahlin D, Salvador A: Chondrosarcomas of bones of the hands and feet: A study of 30 cases. Cancer 1974;34:755.
400. Roberts R, Price C: Chondrosarcoma of the bones of the hand. J Bone Joint Surg 1977;59B:213.
401. Nelson D, Abdul-Karim F, Carter J, Makley J: Chondrosarcoma of small bones of the hand arising from enchondroma. J Hand Surg 1990;15A:655.
402. Arlen M, Tollefsen H, Huvos A, Marcove R: Chondrosarcoma of the head and neck. Am J Surg 1970;120:456.
403. Lacovara J, Patterson K, Reaman G: Primary nasal chondrosarcoma. The pediatric experience. Am J Pediatr Hematol Oncol 1992;14:158.
404. Mark R, Tran L, Sercarz J, et al: Chondrosarcoma of the head and neck. The UCLA experience 1955–1988. Am J Clin Oncol 1993;16:232.
405. Stapleton S, Wilkins P, Archer D, Uttley D: Chondrosarcoma of the skull base: A series of eight cases. Neurosurgery 1993;32:348.
406. Ahmed H: A case of chondrosarcoma of rib involving the right upper lobe. Br J Surg 1964;51:390.
407. Kadokura M, Takaba T, Yamamoto N, et al: A case of chondrosarcoma of rib origin with intrathoracic extension. Kyobu Geka 1984;37:804.
408. Marcove R, Huvos A: Cartilaginous tumors of the ribs. Cancer 1971;27:794.
409. Pandolfo I, Gaeta M, Balandino A, et al: Costal chondrosarcoma with pleural seeding: CT findings. J Comput Assist Tomogr 1985;9:408.
410. Arnold P, Pairolero P: Chondrosarcoma of the manubrium. Resection and reconstruction with pectoralis major muscle. Mayo Clin Proc 1978;53:54.
411. Garrison R, Unni K, McLeod R, et al: Chondrosarcoma arising in osteochondroma. Cancer 1982;49:1890.
412. Norman A, Sissons H: Radiographic hallmarks of peripheral chondrosarcoma. Radiology 1984;151:589.

413. Wu K, Collon D, Guise E: Extra-osseous chondrosarcoma. Report of five cases and review of the literature. J Bone Joint Surg 1980;62A:189.
414. Hachitanda Y, Tsuneyoshi M, Daimaru Y, et al: Extraskeletal myxoid chondrosarcoma in young children. Cancer 1988;61:2521.
415. Chetty R: Extraskeletal mesenchymal chondrosarcoma of the mediastinum. Histopathology 1990;17:261.
416. Sissons H, Matlen J, Lewis M: Dedifferentiated chondrosarcoma. Report of an unusual case. J Bone Joint Surg 1991;73A:294.
417. Potts M, Rose G, Milroy C, Wright J: Dedifferentiated chondrosarcoma arising in the orbit. Br J Ophthalmol 1992;76:49.
418. Voutsinas S, Wynne-Davies R: The infrequency of malignant disease in diaphyseal oclasis and neurofibromatosis. J Med Genet 1983;20:345.
419. Harris W: Chondrosarcoma complicating total hip arthroplasty in Maffucci's syndrome. Clin Orthop 1990;260:212.
420. Bushe K, Naumann M, Warmuth-Metz M, et al: Maffucci's syndrome with bilateral cartilaginous tumors of the cerebellopontine angle. Neurosurgery 1990;25:625.
421. Ahmed AR, Tan T, Unni KK, et al: Secondary chondrosarcoma in osteochondroma: Report of 107 patients. Clin Orthop 2003;411:193–206.
422. Hudson T, Springfield D, Spanier S, et al: Benign exostoses and exostotic chondrosarcomas: Evaluation of cartilage thickness by CT. Radiology 1984;152:595.
423. Geirnaerdt MJA, Hogendoorn PCW, Bloem JL, Taminiau AHM, van der Woude HJ: Cartilaginous tumors: Fast contrast-enhanced MR imaging. Radiology 2000;214:539–546.
424. Sanerkin N: The diagnosis and grading of chondrosarcoma of bone. A combined cytologic and histologic approach. Cancer 1980;45:582.
425. Rosenthal D, Schiller A, Mankin H: Chondrosarcoma: correlation of radiological and histological grade. Radiology 1984;150:21.
426. Mankin H, Cantley K, Lippiello L, et al: The biology of human chondrosarcoma. I. Description of the cases, grading, and biochemical analyses. J Bone Joint Surg 1980;62A:160.
427. Mankin H, Cantley K, Schiller A, Lippiello L: The biology of human chondrosarcoma. II. Variation in chemical composition among types and subtypes of benign and malignant cartilage tumors. J Bone Joint Surg 1980;62A:176.
428. Lichtenstein L, Jaffe H: Chondrosarcoma of bone. Am J Pathol 1943;19:553.
429. Alho A, Connor J, Mankin H, et al: Assessment of malignancy of cartilage tumors using flow cytometry. A preliminary report. J Bone Joint Surg 1983;65A:779.
430. Unni K, Dahlin D, Beabout J, Sim J: Chondrosarcoma: Clear-cell variant, a report of sixteen cases. J Bone Joint Surg 1976;58A:676.
431. Charpentier Y, Forest M, Postel M, et al: Clear-cell chondrosarcoma. A report of five cases including ultrastructural study. Cancer 1979;44:622.
432. McCarthy E, Dorfman H: Chondrosarcoma of bone with dedifferentiation: A study of eighteen cases. Hum Pathol 1982;13:36.
433. Marcove R, Mike V, Hutter R, et al: Chondrosarcoma of the pelvis and upper end of the femur. An analysis of factors influencing survival time in one hundred and thirteen cases. J Bone Joint Surg 1972;54A:561.
434. Marcove R, Stovell P, Huvos A, Bullough P: The use of cryosurgery in the treatment of low and medium grade chondrosarcoma. A preliminary report. Clin Orthop 1977;122:147.
435. Marcove R: A 17-year review of cryosurgery in the treatment of bone tumors. Clin Orthop 1982;163:231.

Ewing's Sarcoma

436. Lücke A: Beitrage zur Geschwulstlehre. Virchows Arch (Path Anat) 1866;35:524.
437. Ewing J: A review of the classification of bone tumors. Surg Gynecol Obstet 1939;68:971.
438. Huvos A: Bone Tumors: Diagnosis, Treatment and Prognosis. Philadelphia, WB Saunders, 1979.
439. Larsson S, Lorentzon R: The geographic variation and incidence of malignant primary bone tumors in Sweden. J Bone Joint Surg 1974;56A:592.

440. Glass A, Fraumeni J: Epidemiology of bone cancer in children. J Natl Cancer Inst 1970;44:187.

441. Li F, Tu J, Liu F, Shiang E: Rarity of Ewing's sarcoma in China. Lancet 1980;1:1255.

442. Aurias A, Rimbaud C, Buffe D, et al: Chromosomal translocations in Ewing's sarcoma. N Engl J Med 1983;309:496.

443. Turc-Carel C, Philip I, Berger M-P, et al: Chromosomal translocations in Ewing's sarcoma. N Engl J Med 1983;309:497.

444. Turc-Carel C, Aurias A, Mugneret F, et al: Chromosomes in Ewing's sarcoma. I. An evaluation of 85 cases and remarkable consistency of 5(11;22)(Q24;q12). Cancer Genet Cytogenet 1988;32:229.

445. Cavazzana A, Miser J, Jefferson J, Triche T: Experimental evidence for a neural origin of Ewing's sarcoma of bone. Am J Pathol 1987;127:507.

446. Horowitz M: Ewing's sarcoma: Current status of diagnosis and treatment. Oncology 1989;3:101.

447. Lipinski M, Braham K, Philip I, et al: Neuroectodermal-associated antigens on Ewing's sarcoma cell lines. Cancer Res 1987;47:183.

448. McKeon C, Thiele C, Ross R, et al: Indistinguishable patterns of proto-oncogene expression in two distinct but closely related tumors: Ewing's sarcoma and neuroepithelioma. Cancer Res 1988;48:4307.

449. Caner B, Kitapci M, Aras T, et al: Increased accumulation of Hexakis (2-methoxyosysobutyl-isonitrile) technetium in osteosarcoma and its metastatic lymph nodes. J Nucl Med 1991;32:1977.

450. Wurtz LD, Peabody TD, Simon MA: Delay in the diagnosis and treatment of primary bone sarcoma of the pelvis. J Bone J Surg 1999;81A(3):317-325.

451. Bader J, Horowitz M, Dewan R, et al: Intensive combined modality therapy of small round cell and undifferentiated sarcomas in children and young adults: Local control and patterns of failure. Radiother Oncol 1989;16:189.

452. Hayes F, Thompson E, Meyer W, et al: Therapy for localized Ewing's sarcoma of bone. J Clin Oncol 1989;7:208.

453. Hayes F, Thompson E, Hustu H, et al: The response of Ewing's sarcoma to sequential cyclophosphamide and adriamycin induction therapy. J Clin Oncol 1983;1:45.

454. Pritchard D, Dahlin D, Dauphine R, et al: Ewing's sarcoma: A clinicopathological and statistical analysis of patients surviving five years or longer. J Bone Joint Surg 1975;57A:10.

455. Pritchard D: Surgical experience in the management of Ewing's sarcoma of bone. Natl Cancer Inst Monogr 1981;56:169.

456. Thomas P, Perez C, Neff J, et al: The management of Ewing's sarcoma: Role of radiotherapy in local tumor control. Can Treat Rep 1984;68:703.

457. Rosen G, Caparros B, Nirenberg A, et al: Ewing's sarcoma: Ten-year experience with adjuvant chemotherapy. Cancer 1981;47:2204.

458. Bacci G, Picci P, Gherlinzoni F, et al: Localized Ewing's sarcoma of bone: Ten years' experience at the Instituto Ortopedico Rizzoli in 124 cases treated with multimodality therapy. Eur J Can Clin Oncol 1985;21:163.

459. Evans R, Newbit M, Askin F, et al: Local recurrence, rate and sites of metastases, and time to relapse as a function of treatment regimen, size of primary and surgical history in 62 patients presenting with nonmetastatic Ewing's sarcoma of the pelvic bones. Int J Radiat Oncol Biol Phys 1985;11:129.

460. Wilkins R, Pritchard D, Burgert E Jr, Unni K: Ewing's sarcoma of bone: experience with 140 patients. Cancer 1986;58:2551.

461. Jürgens H, Exner U, Gadner H, et al: Multidisciplinary treatment of primary Ewing's sarcoma of bone. A 6 year experience of a European cooperative trial. Cancer 1988;61:23.

462. Sailer S, Harmon D, Mankin H, et al: Ewing's sarcoma: Surgical resection as a prognostic factor. Int J Radiol Oncol Biol Phys 1988;15:43.

463. Göbel V, Jürgens H, Etspuler G, et al: Prognostic significance of tumor volume in localized Ewing's sarcoma of bone in children and adolescents. J Cancer Res Clin Oncol 1987;113:187.

464. Toni A, Neff J, Sudanese A, et al: The role of surgical therapy in patients with nonmetastatic Ewing's sarcoma of the limbs. Clin Orthop 1993;286:225.

465. Bacci G, Toni A, Avella M, et al: Long-term results in 144 localized Ewing's sarcoma patients treatment with combined therapy. Cancer 1989;63:1477.

466. Nesbit M Jr, Gehan E, Burgert E Jr, et al: Multimodal therapy for the management of primary, nonmetastatic Ewing's sarcoma of bone. A long-term follow-up of the First Intergroup Study. J Clin Oncol 1990;8:1664.

467. Picci P, Böhling T, Bacci G, et al: Chemotherapy-induced tumor necrosis as a prognostic factor in localized Ewing's sarcoma of the extremities. J Clin Oncol 1997;15:1553.

468. Evans R, Nesbit M, Gehan E, et al: Multimodal therapy for the management of localized Ewing's sarcoma of pelvic and sacral bones. A report from the Second Intergroup Study. J Clin Oncol 1991;9:1173.

469. Paulussen M, Ahrens S, Dunst J, et al: Localized Ewing tumor of bone: Final result of the cooperative Ewing's sarcoma study CESS 86. J Clin Oncol 2001;19(6):1818-1829.

470. Bacci G, Ferrari S, Longhi A, Versari, et al: Local and systemic control in Ewing's sarcoma of the femur treated with chemotherapy, and locally by radiotherapy and/or surgery. J Bone Joint Surg (Br) 2003;85B:107-114.

471. Sluga M, Windhager R, Lang S, et al: The role of surgery and resection margins in the treatment of Ewing's sarcoma. Clin Orthop 2001;392:394-399.

472. Frassica F, Frassica D, Pritchard D, et al: Ewing sarcoma of the pelvis. J Bone Joint Surg 1993;75A:1457.

473. Ozaki T, Hillmann A, Bettin D, et al: High complication rates with pelvic allografts. Experience of 22 sarcoma resections. Acta Orthop Scand 1996;67:333.

474. Carrie C, Mascard E, Gomez F, et al: Nonmetastatic pelvic Ewing sarcoma: Report of the French Society of Pediatric Oncology. Med Pediatr Oncol 1999;33:444-449.

475. Shamberger RC, Gebhardt MC, Neff JR, Tarbell NJ, Marcus KC, Sailer SL, et al: Ewing sarcoma/primitive neuroectodermal tumor of the chest wall: The impact of initial versus delayed resection on tumor margins, survival, and use of radiation therapy. Ann Surg 2003, in press.

476. Rodriguez-Galindo C, Billups CA, Kun LE, Rao BN, Pratt CB, Merchant TE, et al: Survival after recurrence of Ewing tumors. The St. Jude Children's Research Hospital Experience, 1979-1999. Cancer 2002;94:561-569.

477. Catterill SJ, Ahrens S, Paulussen M, Jürgens HF, Voûte PA, Gadner H, et al: Prognostic factors in Ewing's tumor of bone: Analysis of 975 patients from the European Intergroup Cooperative Ewing's Sarcoma Study Group. J Clin Oncol 2000;18:3108-3114.

478. Neff J: Nonmetastatic Ewing's sarcoma of bone: The role of surgical therapy. Clin Orthop 1986;204:111.

479. Norman-Taylor F, Sweetnam D, Dixsen J: Distal fibulectomy for Ewing's sarcoma. J Bone Joint Surg 1994;76B:559.

480. Horowitz M, Neff J, Kun L: Ewing's sarcoma. Radiotherapy versus surgery for local control. Pediatr Clin North Am 1991;38:365.

481. Picci P, Rougraff B, Bacci G, et al: Prognostic significance of histopathologic response to chemotherapy in nonmetastatic Ewing's sarcoma of the extremities. J Clin Oncol 1993;11:1763.

482. Wunder JS, Paulian G, Huvos AG, et al: The histological response to chemotherapy as a predictor of the oncological outcome of operative treatment of Ewing sarcoma. J Bone Joint Surg 1998;80:1020-1033.

483. Sauer R, Jürgens H, Burgers, JMV, et al: Prognostic factors in the treatment of Ewing's sarcoma. The Ewing's sarcoma study group of the German Society of Paediatric Oncology CESS 81. Radiother Oncol 1987;10:101-110.

484. Merchant TE, Kushner BH, Sheldon JM, LaQuaglia M, Healey JH: Effect of low-dose radiation therapy when combined with surgical resection for Ewing sarcoma. Med Pediatr Oncol 1999;33:65-70.

485. Bacci G, Ferrari S, Bertoni F, Donati Det al: Neoadjuvant chemotherapy for peripheral malignant neuroectodermal tumor of bone: Recent experience at the Instituto Rizzoli. J Clin Oncol 2000;18(4):885.

486. De Alava E, Kawai A, Healey JH, et al: EWS-FLI1 fusion transcript structure is an independent determinant of prognosis in Ewing's sarcoma. J Clin Onol 1998;16:1248-1255.

487. Hawkins DS, Felgenhauer J, Park J, Kreissman S, Thompson B, Douglas J, et al: Peripheral blood stem cell support reduces the toxicity of intensive chemotherapy for children and adolescents with metastatic sarcomas. Cancer 2002;95:1354-1365.

488. Perthes G: Uber den einfluss der rontgenstralen auf epitheliale gewebe, inbessondere auf das carcinom. Arch Klin Chir 1903;79:955.

489. Rubin P, Andrews J, Swarm R, Gump H: Radiation induced dysplasias of bone. Am J Roentgenol 1959;82:206.

490. Hinkle C, Parker B, Kaplan H: The effects of roentgen rays upon the long bones of albino rats. II. Histopathological changes involving endochondral growth centers. Am J Roentgenol 1943;49:321.

491. Sugimoto M, Takahashi S, Toguchida J, et al: Changes in bone after high-dose irradiation: Biomechanics and histomorphology. J Bone Joint Surg 1991;73B:492.

492. Vaeth J, Levitt S, Jones M, Holtfreter C: Effects of radiation therapy in survivors of Wilms' tumors. Radiology 1962;79:560.

493. Lewis R, Marcove R, Rosen G: Ewing's sarcoma: Functional effects of radiation therapy. J Bone Joint Surg 1987;59A:325.

494. Robertson W Jr, Butler M, D'Angio G, Rate W: Leg length discrepancy following irradiation for childhood tumors. J Pediatr Orthop 1991;11:284.

495. Jentzsch K, Binder H, Cramer H, et al: Leg function after radiotherapy for Ewing's sarcoma. Cancer 1981;47:1267.

496. Springfield D, Pagliarulo C: Fractures of long bones previously treated for Ewing's sarcoma. J Bone Joint Surg 1985;67A:477.

497. Chan R, Sutow W, Lindberg R, et al: Management and results of localized Ewing's sarcoma. Cancer 1979;43:1001.

498. Strong L, Herson J, Osborne B, Sutow W: Risk of radiation- related subsequent malignant tumors in survivors of Ewing's sarcoma. J Natl Cancer Inst 1979;62:1401.

499. Li F: Second malignant tumors after cancer in childhood. Cancer 1977;40:1899.

500. Tucker M, D'Angio G, Boice J Jr, et al: Bone sarcomas linked to radiotherapy and chemotherapy in children. N Engl J Med 1987;317:588.

501. Coleman C: Secondary neoplasma in patients treated for cancer: Etiology and perspective. Radiat Res 1982;92:188.

502. Coleman C: Editorial: secondary malignancy after treatment of Hodgkin's disease: An evolving picture. J Clin Oncol 1986;4:821.

503. Meadows A, Baum E, Fossati-Bellani F, et al: Second malignant neoplasms in children: An update from the late effects study group. J Clin Oncol 1985;3:532.

504. Smith L, Cox R, Donaldson S: Second cancers in long-term survivors of Ewing's sarcoma. Clin Orthop 1992;274:275.

505. Donaldson SS, Torrey M, Link MP, et al: A multidisciplinary study investigating radiotherapy in Ewing's sarcoma: End results of POG #8346. Int J Radiat Oncol Biol Phys 1998;42:125.

506. Metaizeau H, Olive D, Bey P, et al: Resection followed by vascularized bone autograft in patients with possible recurrence of malignant bone tumors after conservative treatment. J Pediatr Surg 1984;19:116.

Malignant Fibrous Histiocytoma of Bone

507. Feldman F, Norman D: Intra- and extraosseous malignant fibrous histiocytoma (malignant fibrous xanthome). Radiology 1972;104:497.

508. Ward J, Thorbury D, Lemons H, Dunham W: Metal induced sarcoma: A case report and literature review. Clin Orthop 1990;252:299.

509. Spanier S, Enneking W, Enriquez P: Primary malignant fibrous histiocytoma of bone. Cancer 1975;36:2084.

510. Huvos A: Primary malignant fibrous histiocytoma of bone: Clinicopathologic study of 18 patients. NY State J Med 1976;76:552.

511. Huvos A: Bone Tumors: Diagnosis, Treatment and Prognosis, 2nd ed. Philadelphia, WB Saunders, 1991.

512. Huvos A, Heilweil M, Bretsky S: The pathology of malignant fibrous histiocytoma of bone. A study of 130 patients. Am J Surg Pathol 1985;9:853.

513. Paling M, Hyams D: Computed tomography in malignant fibrous histiocytoma. J Comput Assist Tomogr 1982;6:785.

514. Taconis W, van Rijssel T: Fibrosarcoma of long bones. A study of the significance of areas of MFH. J Bone Joint Surg 1985;67B:111.

515. Jacobs R, Fox T: Neurilemmoma of bone. A case report with a review of the literature. Clin Orthop 1972;87:248.

516. von Hochstetter A, Eberle H, Ruttner J: Primary leiomyosarcoma of extragnathic bones. Case report and review of the literature. Cancer 1984;53:2194.

517. Roessner A, Hobik H, Grundmann E: Malignant fibrous histiocytoma of bone and osteosarcoma. A comparative light and electron microscopic study. Pathol Res Pract 1979;164:385.

518. Dahlin D, Beabout J: Dedifferentiation of low-grade chondrosarcomas. Cancer 1971;28:461.

519. Katenkamp D, Stiller D: Malignant fibrous histiocytoma of bone. Light microscopic and electron microscopic examination of four cases. Virchows Arch (Pathol Anat) 1981;391:323.

520. Mirra J, Bullough P, Marcove R, et al: Malignant fibrous histiocytoma and osteosarcoma in association with bone infarcts: Report of four cases, two in caisson workers. J Bone Joint Surg 1974;56A:932.

521. Mirra J, Gold R, Marafiote R: Malignant (fibrous) histiocytoma arising in association with a bone infarct in sickle-cell disease: Coincidence or cause-and-effect? Cancer 1977;39:186.

522. Dorfman H, Norman A, Wolff H: Fibrosarcoma complicating bone infarction in a caisson worker. J Bone Joint Surg 1966;48A:528.

523. Michael R, Dorfman H: Malignant fibrous histiocytoma associated with bone infarcts. Clin Orthop 1976;118:180.

524. Furey J, Ferrer-Torells M, Reagan J: Fibrosarcoma arising at the site of bone infarcts. A report of two cases. J Bone Joint Surg 1960;42A:802.

525. McCarthy E, Matsuno T, Dorfman H: Malignant fibrous histiocytoma of bone: A study of 35 cases. Hum Pathol 1979;10:57.

526. Ghandur-Mnaymneh L, Zych G, Mnaymneh W: Primary malignant fibrous histiocytoma of bone: Report of six cases with ultrastructural study and analysis of the literature. Cancer 1982;49:698.

527. Capanna R, Bertoni F, Bacchini P, et al: Malignant fibrous histiocytoma of bone. The experience at the Rizzoli Institute: Report of 90 cases. Cancer 1984;54:177.

528. Weiner M, Sedlis M, Johnston A, et al: Adjuvant chemotherapy of malignant fibrous histiocytoma of bone. Cancer 1983;51:25.

529. Ham SJ, Hoekstra JH, van der Graaf WT, et al: The value of high-dose methotrexate-based neoadjuvant chemotherapy in malignant fibrous histiocytoma of bone. J Clin Oncol 1996;14:490–496.

530. Kanamori M, Antonescu CR, Scott M, et al: Extra copies of chromosomes 7,8,12,19, and 21 are recurrent in adamantinoma. J Mol Diagn 2001;3(1):16–21.

531. Cohn BT, Brahms MA, Froimson AI: Metastasis of adamantinoma sixteen years after knee articulation: Report of a case. J Bone Joint Surg 1986;68:772–776.

532. Czerniak B, Rojas-Corona RR, Dorfman HD: Morphologic diversity of long bone adamantinoma. The concept of differentiated (regressing) adamantinoma and its relationship to osteofibrous dysplasia. Cancer 1989;64:2319–2334.

533. Kenney GL, Unni KK, Beabout JW, Pritchard DJ: Adamantinoma of lone bones: A clinicopathologic study of 85 cases. Cancer 1989;64:730–737.

534. Park YK, Unni KK, McLeod RA, Pritchard DJ: Osteofibrous dysplasia: Clinicopathologic study of 80 cases. Hum Pathol 1993;24:1339–1347.

535. Bridge JA, Deminski A, DeBoer J, Travis J, Neff JR: Clonal chromosomal abnormalities in osteofibrous dysplasia: Implications for histopathogenesis and its relationship with adamantinoma. Cancer 1994;73:1746–1752.

536. Weiss SW, Dorfman HD: Adamantinoma of long bone: An analysis of nine new cases with emphasis on metastasizing lesions and fibrous dysplasia-like changes. Hum Pathol 1977;8:141–153.

537. Tharani R, Dorey FJ, Schmalzried TP: The risk of cancer following total hip or knee arthroplasty. JBJS 2001;83-A:5,774.

538. Matsuno T, Kaneda K, Takeda N: Development of angiosarcoma at the site of a bone infarct. Clin Orthop 1996;327:259.

539. Gillespie WJ, Henry DA, O'Connell DL, et al: Development of hematopoietic cancers after implantation of total joint replacement. Clin Orthop 1996;329(Suppl):S290–S296.

540. Lewis CG, Sunderman FW: Metal carcinogenesis in total joint arthroplasty—animal models. Clin Orthop 1996;329S:S264.

541. Visuri T, Pukkala E, Paavolainen P, Pulkkinen P, Riska E: Cancer risk after metal on metal and polyethylene on metal total hip arthroplasty. Clin Orthop 1996;329S:S280.

542. Billings S, Wurtz D, Tejada E, Henley JD: Occult sarcoma of the femoral head in patients undergoing total hip arthroplasty. J Bone Joint Surg 2000;82-A:1536.

543. McDonald DJ, Enneking WF, Sundaram M: Metal-associated angiosarcoma of bone: Report of two cases and review of the literature. Clin Orthop 2002;396:206.

544. McDougall A: Malignant tumour at site of bone plating. J Bone Joint Surg 1956;38B:709.

Primary Tumors of the Spine

545. Companacci M: Bone and Soft Tissue tumors. Bologna, Aulo Gagy Editore, 1990.

546. Murray P: Functional outcome and survival in spinal cord injury secondary to neoplasia. Cancer 1985;55:197.

547. Schaberg J, Gainor B: A profile of metastatic carcinoma of the spine. Spine 1985;10:19.

548. Abrams H, Spiro R, Goldstein N: Metastases in carcinoma. Analysis of 1000 autopsied cases. Cancer 1950;3:74.

549. Young J, Funk F: Incidence of tumor metastasis to the lumbar spine: A comparative study of roentgenographic changes and gross lesions. J Bone Joint Surg 1953;35A:55.

550. Gonzalez J, Garcia-Bunuel R: Meningeal carcinomatosis. Cancer 1976;37:2906.

551. Patchell R, Posner J: Neurologic complications of systemic cancer. Neurol Clin 1985;3:729.

552. Chason J, Walker F, Landers J: Metastatic carcinoma in the central nervous system and dorsal root ganglia. Cancer 1963;16:781.

553. Ishida T, Dorfman H, Bullough P: Tophaceous pseudogout (tumoral calcium pryophosphate dihydrate crystal deposition disease). Hum Pathol 1995;26:587.

554. Clark L, McCormick P, Domenico D, Savory L: Pigmented villonodular synovitis of the spine. Case report. J Neurosurg 1993;79:456.

555. Chan K, Chow YY, Ghadially F, et al: Rosai-Dorfman disease presenting as spinal tumor. J Bone Joint Surg 1985;67A:1425.

556. Moridaira K, Handa H, Murakami H, et al: Primary Hodgkin's disease of the bone presenting with an extradural tumor. Acta Haematol 1994;92:148.

557. Yokota N, Kuribayashi T, Nagamine M, et al: Paraplegia caused by brown tumor in primary hyperparathyroidism. J Neurosurg 1989;71:446.

558. Motateanu N, Déruaz J, Fankauser H: Spinal tumour due to primary hyperparathyroidism causing sciatica: Case report. Neuroradiology 1994;36:134.

559. Janin Y, Epstein J, Carras R, Khan A: Osteoid osteomas and osteoblastomas of the spine. Neurosurgery 1981;8:31.

560. Dreghorn C, Newman R, Hardy G, Dickson R: Primary tumors of the axial skeleton: Experience of the Leeds Regional Bone Tumor Registry. Spine 1990;15:137.

561. Delamarter R, Sachs B, Thompson G, et al: Primary neoplasms of the thoraco and lumbar spine: An analysis of 29 consecutive cases. Clinical Orthop 1990;256:87.

562. Weinstein J, McLain R: Primary tumors of the spine. Spine 1987;12:843.

563. Paillas J-E, Alliez B, Pellet W: Primary and secondary tumors of the spine. In Vinken PJ, Bruyn GW (eds): Handbook of Clinical Neurology, vol. 20. Amsterdam, North-Holland Publishing, 1976, p 19.

564. Klein S, Sanford R, Muhlbauer M: Pediatric spinal epidural metastases. J Neurosurg 1991;74:70.

565. Tomita K, Tsuchiya H, Kawahara N: New proposal on surgical staging of vertebral tumour (VTS) for spine salvage surgery. Limb salvage: Current trends. Proceedings of the 7th International Symposium for ISOLS, Singapore, 1993, p 548.

566. Boriani S, Weinstein J, Biagini R: Spine update. Primary bone tumors of the spine, terminology and surgical staging. Spine 1997;22:1036.

567. Hart R, Boriani S, Currier B, Weinstein J: A system for surgical staging and management of spine tumors. Spine 1997;22:1773.

568. Edelstyn G, Gillespie P, Greggell F: The radiological demonstration of skeletal metastases. Clin Radiol 1967;18:158.

569. Galasko CS: The significance of occult skeletal metastases detected by skeletal scintigraphy in patients with otherwise apparently early mammary carcinoma. Br J Surg 1975;62:694.

570. Kamholtz R, Sze G: Current imaging in spinal metastatic disease. Semin Oncol 1991;18:158.

571. Kramer E, Rafto S, Packer R, Zimmerman R: Comparison of myelography with CT follow-up versus gadolinium MRI for subarachnoid metastatic disease in children. Neurology 1991;41:46.

572. Yuh W, Zachar C, Barloon T, et al: Vertebral compression fractures: Distinction between benign and malignant causes with MR imaging. Radiology 1989;172:215.

573. Dollahite H, Tatum L, Moinuddin S, Carnesale P: Aspiration biopsy of primary neoplasms of bone. J Bone Joint Surg 1989;71A:1166.

574. Herkowitz H, Wesolowski D: Percutaneous biopsy of the spine: Techniques, results and complications. In Garvin S (ed): Complications of Spine Surgery. Baltimore, Williams & Wilkins, 1989, p 342.

575. Mondal A, Misra D: CT-guided needle aspiration cytology (FNAC) of 112 vertebral lesions. Indian J Pathol Microbiol 1994;37:255.

576. Mankin H, Lange T, Spanier S: The hazards of biopsy in patients with malignant primary bone and soft-tissue tumors. J Bone Joint Surg 1982;64A:1121.

577. Springfield D, Enneking W, Neff J, Makley J: Principles of tumor management. In Murray J (ed): Instructional Course Lectures, vol 33. St. Louis, Mo, Mosby, 1984, p1.

578. Simon M, Biermann J: Biopsy of bone and soft-tissue lesions. J Bone Joint Surg 1993;75A:616.

579. Hadjipavlou AG, Kontakis GM, Gaitanis JN, Katonis PG, Lander P, Crow WN: Effectiveness and pitfalls of percutaneous transpedicle biopsy of the spine. Clin Orthop 2003;411:54-60.

580. Huang T, Hsu R, Liu H, et al: Technique of video-assisted thoracoscopic surgery for the spine: New approach. World J Surg 1997;21:358.

581. Kiers L, Shield L, Cole W: Neurological manifestation of osteoid osteoma. Arch Dis Child 1990;65:851.

582. Wold L, Pritchard D, Beabout JW, Wilson D: Prostaglandin synthesis by osteoid osteoma and osteoblastoma. Mod Pathol 1988;1:129.

583. Makeley J, Dunn M: Prostaglandins: A mechanism for pain mediation in osteoid osteoma. Orthop Trans 1982;6:72.

584. Greco F, Tamburrelli F, Crabattoni G: Prostaglandins in osteoid osteoma. Int Orthop 1991;15:35.

585. Kneisl J, Simon M: Medical management compared with operative treatment for osteoid osteoma. J Bone Joint Surg 1992;74:179.

586. McLeod R, Dahlin D, Beabout J: The spectrum of osteoblastoma. AJR Am J Roentgenol 1976;126:321.

587. Byers P: Solitary benign osteoblastic lesions of bone. Osteoid osteoma and benign osteoblastoma. Cancer 1968;22:43.

588. Schajowicz F, Lemos C: Osteoid osteoma and osteoblastoma. Closely related entities of osteoblastic derivation. Acta Orthop Scan 1970;41:272.

589. Dorfman H: Case records of the Massachusetts General Hospital, case #40. N Engl J Med 1980;303:866.

590. Roessner A, Metze K, Heymer B: Aggressive osteoblastoma. Pathol Res Pract 1985;179:433.

591. Loftus CM, Rozario RA, Prager R, Scott RM: Solitary osteo-chondroma of T4 with thoracic cord compression. Surg Neurol 1979;13:355.

592. Kak VK, Prabhakar S, Khosla V, Banerjee A: Solitary osteochondroma of spine causing spinal cord compression. Clin Neurol Neurosurg 1985;87:135.

593. Malat J, Virapongse C, Levine A: Solitary osteochondroma of the spine. Spine 1986;11:625.

594. Marsh H, Choi C-B: Primary osteogenic sarcoma of the cervical spine originally mistaken for benign osteoblastoma. J Bone Joint Surg 1970;52A:1467.

595. Fielding J, Fietti VJ, Hughes J, Gabrielian J-C: Primary osteogenic sarcoma of the cervical spine. J Bone Joint Surg 1976; 58A:892.

596. Mnaymneh W, Brown M, Tejada F, Morrison G: Primary osteogenic sarcoma of the second cervical vertebra. Case report. J Bone Joint Surg 1979;61A:460.

597. Barwick K, Huvos A, Smith J: Primary osteogenic sarcoma of the vertebral column. A clinicopathologic correlation of ten patients. Cancer 1980;46:595.

598. Gandolfi A, Bordi C: Primary osteosarcoma of the cervical spine causing neurological symptoms. Surg Neurol 1984;21:441.

599. Patel D, Hammer R, Levin B, Fisher M: Primary osteogenic sarcoma of the spine. Skeletal Radiol 1984;12:276.

600. Ogihara Y, Sekiguchi K, Tsuruta T: Osteogenic sarcoma of the fourth thoracic vertebra. Long-term survival by chemotherapy only. Cancer 1984;53:2615.

601. Sundaresan N, Rosen G, Huvos A, Krol G: Combined treatment of osteosarcoma of the spine. Neurosurgery 1988;23:714.

602. Cohen ZR, Fourney DR, Marco RX, et al: Total cervical spondylectomy for primary osteogenic sarcoma. Case report and description of operative technique. J Neurosurg (Spine 3) 2002;97:386–392.

603. Maillefert J, Guy F, Coudert B, et al: Multifocal malignant fibrous histiocytoma of the spine. Rev Rheum Engl Ed Fr 1997;64:274.

604. Nishida J, Sim F, Wenger D, Unni K: Malignant fibrous histiocytoma of bone. A clinicopathologic study of 81 patients. Cancer 1997;79:482.

605. Sturm P, Abramovitz J, Wagner D, et al: Malignant fibrous histiocytoma of the spine. A case report and review of the literature. Spine 1992;17:975.

606. Bernini J, Fort D, Pritchard M, et al: Adjuvant chemotherapy for treatment of unresectable and metastatic angiomatoid malignant fibrous histiocytoma. Cancer 1994;74:962.

607. Bacci G, Mercuri M, Ruggieri M, et al: Neoadjuvant chemotherapy for malignant fibrous histiocytoma of bone and for osteosarcoma of the limbs: A comparison between the results obtained for 21 and 144 patients, respectively, treated during the same period with the same chemotherapy protocol. Chir Organi Mov 1996;81:139.

608. Ortiz-Cruz E, Quinn R, Fanburg J, et al: Late development of a malignant fibrous histiocytoma at the site of a giant cell tumor. Clin Orthop 1995;318:199.

609. Theegarten D, Sardisong F, Philippou S: Malignant fibrous histiocytoma in the area of a total endoprosthesis of the hip joint. Chirurg 1995;66:158.

610. Aboulafia A, Littelton K, Shmookler B, Malawer M: Malignant fibrous histiocytoma at the site of hip replacement in association with chronic infection. Orthop Rev 1994;23:427.

611. Mainetti C, Masouye I, Salomon D, et al: L-tryptophan-induced eosinophilia-myalgia syndrome associated with primary cutaneous malignant fibrous histiocytoma and extraabdominal desmoid tumor. Cancer 1993;72:2712.

612. Helio H, Kivioja A, Karaharju E, et al: Malignant fibrous histiocytoma arising in a previous site of fracture and osteomyelitis. Eur J Surg Oncol 1993;19:479.

613. Cossetto D, Nade S, Blackwell J: Malignant fibrous histiocytoma in Paget's disease of bone. A report of 7 cases. Aust NZ J Surg 1992;62:52.

614. Lindeman G, McKay M, Taubman K, Bilous A: Malignant fibrous histiocytoma developing in bone 44 years after shrapnel trauma. Cancer 1990;66:2229.

615. Kennedy C, Stoker D: Malignant fibrous histiocytoma complicating chronic osteomyelitis. Clin Radiol 1990;41:435.

616. Spirtos G, Qadri A, Phillips A: Malignant fibrous histiocytoma (MFH) arising within a cholecystectomy incision: A cause-and-effect relationship is possible between previous surgery and the development of a malignant fibrous histiocytoma within the operative site. J Surg Oncol 1988;38:267.

617. Eriksson AI, Schiller A, Mankin HJ: The management of chondrosarcoma of bone. Clin Orthop 1980;153:44.

618. Wuisman PIJM, Jutte PC, Ozaki T: Secondary chondrosarcoma in osteochondromas. Medullary extension in 15 of 45 cases. Acta Orthop Scand 1997;68:396.

619. Whitehause G, Griffiths G: Roentgenologic aspects of spinal involvement by primary and metastatic Ewing's tumor. J Can Assoc Radiol 1976;27:290.

620. Pilepich MV, Vietti TJ, Nesbit ME, et al: Ewing's sarcoma of the vertebral column. Int J Radiat Oncol Biol Phys 1981;7:27.

621. Mirra J: Bone Tumors: Diagnosis and Treatment. Philadelphia, JB Lippincott, 1980.

622. Dahlin D, Coventry M, Scanlon P: Ewing's sarcoma. J Bone Joint Surg 1961;43A:185.

623. Kaspers G, Kamphorst W, van de Graaff M, et al: Primary spinal epidural extraosseous Ewing's sarcoma. Cancer 1991;68:648.

624. Mohan V, Sabri T, Gupta R, Das D: Solitary ivory vertebra due to primary Ewing's sarcoma. Pediatr Radiol 1992;22:388.

625. Poulsen J, Jensen J, Thommesen P: Ewing's sarcoma simulating vertebra plana. Acta Orthop Scand 1975;46:211.

626. O'Donnell J, Brown L, Herkowitz H: Vertebra plana-like lesions in children: Case report with special emphasis on the differential diagnosis and indications for biopsy. J Spinal Disord 1991;4:480.

627. Grubb M, Currier B, Pritchard D, Ebersold M: Primary Ewing's sarcoma of the spine. Spine 1994;19:309.

628. Fessler RG, Dietze DD, MacMillan M, Peace D: Lateral parascapular extrapleural approach to the upper thoracic spine. J Neurosurg 1991;75:349–355.

629. Katzman W, Waugh T, Berdon W: Skeletal changes following irradiation of childhood tumors. J Bone Joint Surg 1969;51A:825.

630. Littman P, D'Angio G: Growth considerations in the radiation therapy of children with cancer. Annu Rev Med 1979;30:405.

631. Mayfield J, Riseborough E, Jaffe N, Nehme M: Spinal deformity in the children treated for neuroblastoma. J Bone Joint Surg 1981;63A:183.

632. Neuhauser E, Wittenborg M, Berman L, Cohen J: Irradiation effects of roentgen therapy on the growing spine. Radiology 1952;57:637.

633. Riseborough E, Grabias S, Burton R, Jaffe N: Skeletal alterations following irradiation for Wilms' tumor. J Bone Joint Surg 1976;58A:526.

634. Rutherford H, Dodd G: Complications of radiation therapy: growing bone. Semin Roentgenol 1974;9:15.

635. Butler MS, Robertson WW Jr, Rate W, et al: Skeletal sequelae of radiation therapy for malignant childhood tumors. Clin Orthop 1990;251:235.

636. Hitchcock R, Kohler J, Duffy P, Malone P: Renal autotransplantational kidney saving procedure before spinal radiotherapy. Pediatr Hematol Oncol 1993;10:333.

637. Shankman S, Greenspan A, Klein M, Lewis M: Giant cell tumor of the ischium: A report of two cases and review of the literature. Skeletal Radiol 1988;17:46.

638. Savini R, Gherlinzoni F, Morandi M, et al: Surgical treatment of giant-cell tumor of the spine: The experience at the Istituto Ortopedico Rizzoli. J Bone Joint Surg 1983;65A:1283.

639. Rockwell M, Small C: Giant-cell tumors of bone in South India. J Bone Joint Surg 1961;43A:1035.

640. Reddy C, Rao P, Rajakumari K: Giant-cell tumors of bone in South India. J Bone Joint Surg 1974;56A:617.

641. Tuli S, Varma B, Srivastava T: Giant-cell tumour of bone: A study of natural course. Int Orthop 1978;2:207.

642. Sung H, Kuo D, Shu W, et al: Giant-cell tumor of bone: Analysis of two hundred and eight cases in Chinese patients. J Bone Joint Surg 1982;64A:755.

643. Larsson S-E, Lorentzon R, Boquist L: Giant-cell tumor of bone: A demographic, clinical and histopathological study of all cases recorded in the Swedish Cancer registry for the years 1958 through 1968. J Bone Joint Surg 1975;57A:167.

644. Dahlin D: Giant-cell tumor of vertebrae above the sacrum: A review of 31 cases. Cancer 1977;39:1350.

645. Sanjay BK, Sim FH, Unni KK, et al: Giant-cell tumours of the spine. J Bone Joint Surg 1993;75B:148.

646. Larsson S-E, Lorentzon R, Boquist L: Giant-cell tumors of the spine and sacrum causing neurological symptoms. Clin Orthop 1975;111:201.

647. Lièvre J-A, Darcy M, Pradat P, et al: Tumeur à Cellules Géantes du Rachis Lombaire, Spondylectomie Totale en Deux Temps. Rev Rheum 1968;35:125.

648. Stener B, Johnsen O: Complete removal of three vertebrae for giant-cell tumour. J Bone Joint Surg 1971;53B:278.

649. Cahan W, Woodard H, Higinbotham N, et al: Sarcoma arising in irradiated bone. Cancer 1948;1:3.

650. Keplinger J, Bucy P: Giant-cell tumors of the spine. Ann Surg 1961;154:648.

651. Goldenberg R, Campbell C, Bonfiglio M: Giant-cell tumor of bone: An analysis of two hundred and eighteen cases. J Bone Joint Surg 1970;52A:619.

652. Rock M, Pritchard D, Unni K: Metastases from histologically benign giant-cell tumor of bone. J Bone Joint Surg 1984;66A:269.

653. Ushio Y, Posner R, Posner J, Shapiro W: Experimental spinal cord compression by epidural neoplasms. Neurology 1977;27:422.

654. Ikeda H, Ushio Y, Hayakawa T, Mogami H: Edema and circulatory disturbance in the spinal cord compressed by epidural neoplasms. J Neurosurg 1980;52:203.

655. Kato M, Ushio Y, Hayakawa T, et al: Circulatory disturbance of the spinal cord with epidural neoplasm in rats. J Neurosurg 1985; 63:260.

656. Delattre J, Arbit E, Thaler H, et al: A dose-response study of dexamethasone in a model of spinal cord compression caused by epidural tumor. J Neurosurg 1989;70:920.

657. Siegal T, Siegal T, Sandbank U, et al: Experimental neoplastic spinal cord compression: Evoked potentials, edema, prostaglandins, and light and electron microscopy. Spine 1987;12:440.

658. Siegal T, Siegal T, Shapira Y, et al: Indomethacin and dexamethasone in experimental neoplastic spinal cord compression: part I. Effect on water content and specific gravity. Neurosurgery 1988;22:328.

659. Siegal T, Shohami E, Shapira Y, Siegal T: Indomethacin and dexamethasone in experimental neoplastic spinal cord compression: Part II. Effect on edema and prostaglandin synthesis. Neurosurgery 1988;22:334.

660. Siegal T, Siegal T, Shohami E, Shapira Y: Comparison of soluble dexamethasone sodium phosphate with free dexamethasone and indomethacin in the treatment of experimental neoplastic spinal cord compression. Spine 1988;13:1171.

661. Siegal T, Siegal T, Shapira Y, et al: The early effect of steroidal and non-steroidal anti-inflammatory agents on neoplastic epidural cord compression. Ann N Y Acad Sci 1989;559:488.

662. Siegal T, Siegal T, Shohami E, Lossos F: Experimental neoplastic spinal cord compression: Effect of ketamine and MK-801 on edema and prostaglandins. Neurosurgery 1990;26:963.

663. Siegal T, Siegal T: Experimental neoplastic spinal cord compression: Effect of anti-inflammatory agents and glutamate receptor antagonists on vascular permeability. Neurosurgery 1990;26:967.

664. Siegal T, Siegal T: Participation of serotonergic mechanisms in the pathophysiology of experimental neoplastic spinal cord compression. Neurology 1991;41:574.

665. Siegal T, Siegal T: Serotonergic manipulations in experimental neoplastic spinal cord compression. J Neurosurg 1993;78:929.

666. Vecht C, Haaxma-Reiche H, van Putten W, et al: Initial bolus of conventional versus high-dose dexamethasone in metastatic spinal cord compression. Neurology 1989;39:1255.

667. Posner J, Howieson J, Cvitkovic E: "Disappearing" spinal cord compression: Oncolytic effects of glucocorticoids (and other chemotherapeutic agents) on epidural metastases. Ann Neurol 1977;2:409.

668. Fadul C, Lemann W, Thaler H, et al: Perforation of the gastrointestinal tract in patients receiving steroids for neurologic disease. Neurology 1988;38:348.

669. Weissman D: Glucocorticoid treatment for brain metastases and epidural cord compression: A review. J Clin Oncol 1988;6:543.

670. Martenson J, Evans R Jr, Lie M, et al: Treatment outcome and complications in patients treated for malignant epidural spinal cord compression. J Neuro-oncol 1985;3:77.

671. Findlay G: Adverse effects of the management of malignant spinal cord compression. J Neurol Neurosurg Psychiatry 1984;47:761.

672. Dommisse G: The blood supply of the spinal cord. A critical vascular zone in spinal surgery. J Bone Joint Surg 1974;56B:225.

673. Lievre J, Darcy M, Pradat P, et al: Tumeur a cellues geantes du rachis lombaire, spondylectomie totale en deux temps. Rev Rheum 1968;35:125.

674. Stener B: Total spondylectomy for removal of a giant cell tumor in the eleventh thoracic vertebra. Spine 1977;2:197.

675. Stener B: Surgical Treatment of Giant Cell Tumors, Chondrosarcomas, and Chordomas of the Spine. Berlin, Heidelberg, Springer Verlag, 1984.

676. Stener B: Complete removal of vertebrae for extirpation of tumors. Clin Orthop 1989;245:72.

677. Luque ER: The anatomic basis and development of segmental spinal instrumentation. Spine 1982;7:256.

678. Luque E: Treatment of scoliosis without arthrodesis or external support. Orthop Trans 1977;1:37.

679. Steffee AD, Biscup RS, Sitkowski DJ: Segmental spine plates with pedicle screw fixation. A new internal fixation device for disorders of the lumbar and thoracolumbar spine. Clin Orthop 1986;203:45.

680. Boucher H: A method of spinal fusion. J Bone Joint Surg 1959;41B:248.

681. Harrington P, Dickson J: Spinal instrumentation in the treatment of severe progressive spondylolisthesis. Clin Orthop 1976;117:157.

682. Pennel G, McDonald G, Dale G: A method of spinal fusion using internal fixation. Clin Orthop 1964;35:86.

683. Roy-Camille R: Personal communication, 1984.

684. Hall DJ, Webb JK: Anterior plate fixation in spine tumor surgery. Indications, technique, and results. Spine 1991;16:580.

685. Black R, Eng P, Gardner V, et al: A contoured anterior spinal fixation plate. Clin Orthop 1988;227:135.

686. Kaneda K, Abumi K, Fujiya M: Burst fractures with neurologic deficits of the thoraco-lumbar spine: Results of anterior decompression and stabilization with anterior instrumentation. Spine 1984;9:788.

687. Siegal T, Siegal T: Vertebral body resection for epidural compression by malignant tumours. J Bone Joint Surg 1985;67A:375.

688. Bell G: Surgical treatment of spinal tumors. Clin Orthop 1997;335:54.

689. Sundaresan N, DiGiacinto G, Krol G, Hughes J: Spondylectomy for malignant tumor of the spine. J Clin Oncol 1989;7:1485.

690. Tomita K, Kawahara N, Toribatake Y, et al: Total en bloc spondylectomy for malignant vertebral tumourinnovative surgical technique of spine salvage. Spine 1997;22:324.

Chordoma

691. Horwitz T: Chordal ectopia and its possible relation to chordoma. Arch Pathol 1941;31:354.

692. Mabrey R: Chordoma: A study of 150 cases. Am J Cancer 1935;25:501.

693. Rich T, Schiller A, Suit H, Mankin H: Clinical and pathologic review of 48 cases of chordoma. Cancer 1985;56:182.

694. Bjornsson J, Wold L, Ebersold M, Laws E: Chordoma of the mobile spine. A clinicopathologic analysis of 40 patients. Cancer 1993;71:735.

695. Poavolainen P, Teppo L: Chordoma in Finland. Acta Orthop Scand 1976;47:46.

696. Higinbotham N, Phillips R, Farr H, Huster H: Chordoma. Thirty-five year study at Memorial Hospital. Cancer 1967;20:1841.

697. Dahlin D, MacCarty C: Chordoma. A study of fifty-nine cases. Cancer 1952;5:1170.

698. Wellinger C: Rachicial chordoma. I. Review of the literature since 1960. Rev Rheum Mal Osteoartic 1975;42:109.

699. Wellinger C: Rachicial chordoma. II. Review of the literature since 1960. Rev Rheum Mal Osteoartic 1975;42:195.

700. Wellinger C: Rachicial chordoma. III. Review of the literature since 1960. Rev Rheum Mal Osteoartic 1975;42:287.

701. Sundaresan N, Galicich J, Chu F, Huvos A: Spinal chordomas. J Neurosurg 1979;50:312.

702. Steenberghs J, Kiekens C, Menten J, Monstrey J: Intradural chordoma without bone involvement. Case report and review of the literature. J Neurosurg (Spine 1) 202;97:94–97.

703. Crapanzano JP, Ali SZ, Ginsberg MS, Zakowski MF: Chordoma. A cytologic study with histologic and radiologic correlation. Cancer (Cancer Cytopathol) 2001;93:40–51.

704. Hruban R, Traganos F, Reuter V, Huvos A: Chordomas with spindle cell components. A DNA flow cytometric and immunohistochemical study with histogenetic implications. Am J Surg Pathol 1990;137:435.

705. Huvos A: Bone Tumors: Diagnosis, Treatment and Prognosis, 2nd ed. Philadelphia, WB Saunders, 1991.

706. Chu R: Chondroid chordoma of the sacrococcygeal region. Arch Pathol Lab Med 1987;111:861.

707. Makek M, Leu H: Malignant fibrous histiocytoma arising in a recurrent chordoma. Case report and electron microscopic findings. Virchows Arch (Pathol Anat) 1982;397:241.

708. Halpern J, Kopolovic J, Carane R: Malignant fibrous histiocytoma developing in irradiated sacral chordoma. Cancer 1984;53:2661.

709. Belza M, Urich H: Chordoma and malignant fibrous histiocytoma: Evidence of transformation. Cancer 1986;58:1082.

710. Meis J, Raymond A, Evans H, et al: Dedifferentiated chordoma. A clinicopathologic and immunohistochemical study of three cases. Am J Surg Pathol 1987;11:516.

711. Nakamura Y, Becker L, Marks A: S-100 protein in human chordoma and human and rabbit notochord. Arch Pathol Lab Med 1983;107:118.

712. Salisbury J, Isaacson P: Demonstration of cytokeratins and an epithelial membrane antigen in chordomas and human fetal notochord. Am J Surg Pathol 1985;9:791.

713. Uhrenholt L, Stimpel H: Histochemistry of sacrococcygeal chordoma. Acta Pathol Microbiol Scand 1985;93:203.

714. Abenoza P, Sibley R: Chordoma: An immunohistologic study. Hum Pathol 1986;17:744.

715. Cotler H, Cotler J, Cohn H, et al: Intrathoracic chordoma presenting as a posterior superior mediastinal tumor. Spine 1983;8:781.

716. Firooznia H, Pinto R, Lin H: Chordoma: Radiologic evaluation of 20 cases. Am J Roentgenol 1976;127:797.

717. Crowe G, Muldoon P: Thoracic chordoma. Thorax 1951;6:403.

718. Castellano G, Johnston H: Intrathoracic chordoma presenting as a posterior mediastinal tumor. South Med J 1975;68:109.

719. Rossleigh M, Smith J, Yeh S: Scintigraphic features of primary sacral tumors. J Nucl Med 1986;27:627.

720. Brooks M, Kleefield J, O'Reilly F, et al: Thoracic chordoma with unusual radiographic features. Comput Radiol 1987;11:85.

721. Krol G, Sundaresan N, Deck M: Computed tomography of axial chordomas. J Comput Assist Tomogr 1983;7:286.

722. Firooznia H, Golimbu C, Rafii M, et al: Computed tomography of spinal chordomas. J Comput Tomogr 1986;10:45.

723. Meyer J, Lipke R, Lindfors K, et al: Chordomas: Their CT appearance in the cervical, thoracic and lumbar spine. Radiology 1984;153:693.

724. Pinto R, Lin H, Firooznia H, Lefleur R: The osseous and angiographic features of vertebral chordomas. Neuroradiology 1975;9:230.

725. Sze G, Uichanco L III, Brant-Zawadzki M, et al: Chordomas: MR Imaging. Radiology 1988;166:187.

726. Dommisse G: The blood supply of the spinal cord. A critical vascular zone in spinal surgery. J Bone Joint Surg 1974;56B:225.

727. Renfrew D, Whitten C, Wiese J, et al: CT-guided percutaneous transpedicular biopsy of the spine. Radiology 1991;180:574.

728. Edwards C: Spinal Reconstruction in Tumor Management. Berlin, Heidelberg, Springer Verlag, 1984.

729. Bridge J, Pickering D, Neff J: Cytogenetic and molecular cytogenetic analysis of sacral chordoma. Cancer Genet Cytogenet 1994;75:23.

730. Sandberg A, Bridge J: The Cytogenetics of Bone and Soft Tissue Tumors. Austin, Tx, RG Landes, 1994.

731. Gregorius F, Batzdorf U: Removal of thoracic chordoma by staged laminectomy and thoractomy: Case report. Am J Surg 1979;45:535.

732. Sundaresan N, Huvos A, Krol G, et al: Surgical treatment of spinal chordomas. Arch Surg 1987;122:1479.

733. Bosma JJ, Pigott JD, Pennie BH, Jaffray DC: En bloc removal of the lower lumbar vertebral body for chordoma. Report of two cases. J Neurosurg (Spine 2) 2001;94:284-291.

734. Drukker B, Lee C, Kim T: Sacral chordoma. A rare cause of chronic pelvic and low back pain. Obstet Gynecol 49(Suppl)1977;64.

735. Sundaresan N: Spinal chordomas. Clin Orthop 1986;204:135.

736. Stephens G, Schwartz H: Lumbosacral chordoma resection: Image integration and surgical planning. J Surg Oncol 1993;54:226.

737. Smith J, Ludwig R, Marcove R: Sacrococcygeal chordoma. A clinicoradiological study of 60 patients. Skeletal Radiol 1987;16:37.

738. Shih W, Reba R, Huang T: Scintigraphic photopenia in sacrococcygeal chordoma. Eur J Nucl Med 1983;8:279.

739. Levine E, Batnitzky S: Computed tomography of sacral and presacral lesions. Crit Rev Diagn Imaging 1984;21:307.

740. Wetzel L, Levine E: MR imaging of sacral and presacral lesions. Am J Radiol 1990;154:771.

741. Yuh W, Flickinger F, Barloon T, Montgomery W: MR imaging of unusual chordomas. J Comput Assist Tomogr 1988;12:30.

742. Rosenthal D, Scott J, Mankin H, et al: Sacrococcygeal chordoma: Magnetic resonance imaging and computed tomography. Am J Radiol 1985;145:143.

743. Uhlig B, Johnson R: Presacral tumors and cysts in adults. Dis Colon Rectum 1975;18:581.

744. MacCarty C, Waugh J, Mayo C, Coventry M: The surgical treatment of presacral tumors: A combined problem. Proc Staff Meetings Mayo Clin 1952;27:73.

745. MacCarty C, Waugh J, Coventry M, O'Sullivan D: Sacrococcygeal chordomas. Surg Gynecol Obstet 1961;113:551.

746. Samson I, Springfield D, Suit H, Mankin H: Operative treatment of sacrococcygeal chordoma. J Bone Joint Surg 1993;75A:1476.

747. Localio S, Francis K, Rossano P: Abdominosacral resection of sacrococcygeal chordoma. Ann Surg 1967;166:394.

748. Huth J, Dawson E, Eilber F: Abdominosacral resection for malignant tumors of the sacrum. Am J Surg 1984;148:157.

749. Karakousis C: Sacral resection with preservation of continence. Surg Gynecol Obstet 1986;163:270.

750. Bowers R: Giant cell tumor of the sacrum: A case report. Ann Surg 1948;128:1164.

751. Stener B, Gunterberg B: High amputation of the sacrum for extirpation of tumors. Spine 1978;3:351.

752. Shikata J, Yamamuro T, Kotoura Y, et al: Total sacrectomy and reconstruction for primary tumors. J Bone Joint Surg 1988;70A:122.

753. Gunterberg B, Romanus B, Stener B: Pelvic strength after major amputation of the sacrum. Acta Orthop Scand 1976;47:635.

754. Tomita K, Tsuchiya H: Total sacrectomy and reconstruction for huge sacral tumors. Spine 1990;15:1223.

755. Gunterberg B, Norlén L, Stener B, Sundin T: Neurologic evaluation after resection of the sacrum. Invest Urol 1975;13:183.

756. Gunterberg G, Kewenter J, Petersén I, Stener B: Anorectal function after major resections of the sacrum with bilateral or unilateral sacrifice of sacral nerves. Br J Surg 1976;63:546.

757. Gunterberg B, Petersén I: Sexual function after major resections of the sacrum with bilateral or unilateral sacrifice of sacral nerves. Fertil Steril 1976;27:1146.

758. Neff J: Technique of Subtotal and Total Sacral Amputation for Neoplasm. New York, Thieme Medical, 1994.

759. Miles WK, Chang DW, Kroll SS, et al: Reconstruction of large sacral defects following total sacrectomy. Plast Reconstr Surg 2000;105:2387-2394.

760. Ishii K, Kazuhiro C, Watanabe M, Yabe H, Fujimura Y, Toyama Y: Local recurrence after S2-3 sacrectomy in sacral chordoma. Report of four cases. J Neurosurg (Spine 1) 2002;97:98-101.

761. Bergh P, Kindblom LG, Gunterberg B, et al: Prognostic factors in chordoma of the sacrum and mobile spine. A study of 39 patients. Cancer 2000;88:2122-2134.

762. Whitaker R, Cast I: Prolonged survival in a case of sacrococcygeal chordoma with metastases. Br J Surg 1969;56:392.

763. Graf L: Sacrococcygeal chordoma with metastases. Arch Pathol 1944;37:136.

764. Chambers P, Schwinn C: Chordoma. A clinicopathologic study of metastasis. Am J Clin Pathol 1979;72:765.

765. Markwalder T, Markwalder R, Robert J, Krneta A: Metastatic chordoma. Surg Neurol 1979;12:473.

766. Chalmers J, Coulson W: A metastasising chordoma. J Bone Joint Surg 1960;42B:556.

767. Sundaresan N: Chordomas. Clin Orthop 1986;204:135.

768. Mindell E: Current concepts review. Chordoma. J Bone Joint Surg 1981;63A:501.

SUGGESTED READINGS

Cytogenetics

Sandberg AA, Bridge JA: Updates on the cytogenetics and molecular genetics of bone and soft tissue tumors: Dermatofibrosarcoma protuberans and giant cell fibroblastoma. Cancer Genet Cytogenet 2003; 140:1-12.

Sandberg AA, Bridge JA: Updates on the cytogenetics and molecular genetics of bone and soft tissue tumors: Osteosarcoma and related tumors. Cancer Genet Cytogenet 2003;145:1-30.

Specific Malignancies

III

Sandberg AA, Bridge JA: Updates on the cytogenetics and molecular genetics of bone and soft tissue tumors: Alveolar soft part sarcoma. Cancer Genet Cytogenet 2002;136:1-9.

Sandberg AA, Bridge JA: Updates on the cytogenetics and molecular genetics of bone and soft tissue tumors: Chondrosarcoma and other cartilaginous neoplasms. Cancer Genet Cytogenet 2002;143:1-31.

Sandberg AA, Bridge JA: Updates on the cytogenetics and molecular genetics of bone and soft tissue tumors: congenital (infantile) fibrosarcoma and mesoblastic nephroma. Cancer Genet Cytogenet 2002;132:1-13.

Sandberg AA, Bridge JA: Updates on the cytogenetics and molecular genetics of bone and soft tissue tumors: Desmoplastic small round-cell tumors. Cancer Genet Cytogenet 2002; 138:1-10.

Sandberg AA, Bridge JA: Updates on the cytogenetics and molecular genetics of bone and soft tissue tumors: Gastrointestinal stromal tumors. Cancer Genet Cytogenet 2002;135:1-22.

Sandberg AA, Bridge JA: Updates on the cytogenetics and molecular genetics of bone and soft tissue tumors: Synovial sarcoma. Cancer Genet Cytogenet 2002;133:1-23.

Sandberg AA, Bridge JA: Updates on the cytogenetics and molecular genetics of bone and soft tissue tumors: Clear cell sarcoma (malignant melanoma of soft parts). Cancer Genet Cytogenet 2001;130:1-7.

Sandberg AA, Bridge JA: Updates on the cytogenetics and molecular genetics of bone and soft tissue tumors: Mesothelioma. Cancer Genet Cytogenet 2001;127:93-110.

Sandberg AA, Bridge JA: Updates on cytogenetics and molecular genetics of bone and soft tissue tumors: Ewing sarcoma and peripheral primitive neuroectodermal tumors. Cancer Genet Cytogenet 2000;123:1-26.

Surgical Technique

Abe E, Sato K, Tazawa H, Murai H, Okada K, Shimada Y, Morita H: Total spondylectomy for primary tumor of the thoracolumbar spine. Spinal Cord 2000;38:146-152.

Ariel I, Shah H: The conservative hemipelvectomy. Surg Gynecol Obstet 1977; 144:407.

Bailey R, Stevens DB: Radical exarticulation of the extremities for the curative and palliative treatment of malignant neoplasms. J Bone Joint Surg 1961;43A:845.

Banks S, coleman S: Hemipelvectomy: Surgical techniques. J Bone Joint Surg 1956;384:1147.

Beck N, Bickel W: Interinnomino-abdominal amputations. Report of twelve cases. J Bone Joint Surg 1948;30A:201.

Bowden L, Booher R: Surgical considerations in the treatment of sarcoma of the buttock. Cancer 1953;6:89.

Boyd J: Anatomic disarticulation of the hip. Surg Gynecol Obstet 1947;84:346.

Burwell H: Resection of the shoulder with humeral suspension for sarcoma involving the scapula. J Bone Joint Surg 1965;47B:300.

Cammisa FJ, Glasser D, Otis J, et al: The Van Ness tibial rotationplasty. A functionally viable reconstructive procedure in children who have a tumor of the distal end of the femur. J Bone Joint Surg 1990;72A:1541.

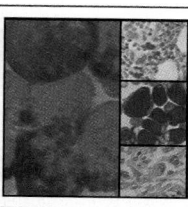

SARCOMAS OF SOFT TISSUE

Peter W. T. Pisters

Vivien H.C. Bramwell

Brian P. Rubin

Brian O'Sullivan

SUMMARY OF KEY POINTS

INCIDENCE AND EPIDEMIOLOGY

- 8300 new cases annually in the United States
- No specific etiologic agent identifiable in the majority of cases
- Occasional cases related to previous radiation, chemical exposure, alkylating chemotherapeutic agents, or chronic lymphedema
- Genetic conditions related to soft tissue sarcoma include neurofibromatosis, tuberous sclerosis, basal cell nevus syndrome, Gardner's syndrome, and Li-Fraumeni syndrome

DIAGNOSIS AND EVALUATION OF EXTENT OF DISEASE

- Core-needle biopsy (large lesions) or excisional biopsy (small lesions)
- Pathologic review of histologic subtype, grade, and assessment of margins (excisional biopsies)
- MRI or CT of primary site
- Chest x-ray for low-grade tumors and high-grade T1 lesions, chest CT for high-grade T2 tumors

PROGNOSTIC FACTORS

- High-grade histology, deep location, and T2 tumor size are independent adverse prognostic factors for distant metastasis and survival
- Presentation with recurrent disease or positive surgical margin (gross or microscopic) are independent adverse prognostic factors for local recurrence
- Individual patient prognosis can be predicted from handheld computer-based nomogram

STAGING SYSTEMS

AJCC (UICC) system employs criteria that include grade, size, and location relative to the investing muscular fascia, nodal status, and distant metastases

PRIMARY THERAPY

- Surgical resection with an adequate margin of normal tissue; for extremity lesions, a limb-sparing approach is possible in more than 90% of patients and offers survival comparable to amputation without the associated morbidity
- For most patients, local control is improved with preoperative or postoperative radiotherapy

RECURRENT DISEASE

- Local recurrence rates vary depending on the anatomic site of the primary and the adequacy of local therapy; for extremity lesions, approximately 20% of patients develop locally recurrent disease
- Chemotherapy with selective use of metastasectomy is the mainstay of therapy for patients with metastatic disease
- For the small subset of patients who develop isolated (solitary) pulmonary metastases, 20% to 50% 3-year survival rates have been reported with pulmonary metastasectomy

INTRODUCTION

Soft tissue sarcomas comprise a group of relatively rare, anatomically and histologically diverse neoplasms. These tumors share a common embryologic origin, arising primarily from tissues derived from the mesoderm. The notable exceptions are neurosarcomas, primitive neuro-ectodermal tumors, and possibly Ewing's sarcomas, which are believed to arise from tissues of ectodermal origin. Despite the fact that the somatic soft tissues account for as much as 75% of total body weight, neoplasms of the soft tissues are comparatively rare, accounting for 1% of adult malignancies and 15% of pediatric malignancies. The annual incidence of soft tissue sarcomas in the United States is about 8300 new cases, comparable to the incidence of testicular cancer.[1] However, an estimated 3900 patients die annually of soft tissue sarcoma—a rate nearly 10-fold greater than is seen with testicular cancer—emphasizing the comparatively high overall mortality rate seen with this tumor.

The first portion of this chapter reviews the available literature on the evaluation and treatment of extremity sarcoma (which account for 50% of all lesions). Other specific anatomic sites are reviewed at the end of the chapter.

ETIOLOGY AND EPIDEMIOLOGY

Environmental Factors

No specific etiologic agent is identified in the majority of patients with soft tissue sarcoma (STS). There are a number of recognized associations between environmental factors and the subsequent development of sarcoma; these are summarized in Table 96-1. The development of sarcoma has been reported after the use of ionizing

TABLE 96-1

Soft Tissue Sarcoma: Predisposing Environmental Factors

FACTOR	AGENT	PATIENT POPULATION	COMMENT
Radiotherapy	Ortho- and megavoltage radiation	Therapeutic radiation patients	Most commonly osteosarcoma; dose-response relationship
Chemotherapy	Alkylating agents: cyclophosphamide, melphalan, procarbazine, nitrosourea, and chlorambucil	Pediatric cancer patients	Relative risk of bone sarcoma increased with cumulative drug exposure
Chemical exposure	Phenoxyacetic acids: 2,4-dichlorophenoxyacetic acid (2,4-D); 2,4,5 trichlorophenoxy acetic acid (2,4,5-T); 2 methyl-4 chlorophenoxyacetic acid (MCPA)	Forestry and agricultural workers	Phenoxy herbicide and defoliant exposure
	2,3,7,8-tetrachlorodibenzo-p-dioxin (TCDD); dioxin	Vietnam veterans	No clear link demonstrable for dioxin (Agent Orange)
	Chlorophenols	Sawmill workers	
	Thorotrast	Diagnostic x-ray patients	Hepatic angiosarcoma
	Vinyl chloride	Vinyl chloride workers	Hepatic angiosarcoma
	Arsenic	Vineyard workers	Hepatic angiosarcoma after exposure to arsenical herbicides
Chronic lymphedema		Postsurgery patients Postradiation patients Patients with congenital Lymphadema or filariasis	Stewart-Treves syndrome (lymphangiosarcoma)

radiation for the treatment of lymphoma[2]; solid tumors of the head and neck,[3] breast,[4,5] gynecologic organs, and skin; benign conditions including endometriosis, tuberculous arthritis,[6] and benign thymic enlargement. The vast majority of radiation-associated sarcomas are high grade lesions (87%), and the predominant histology is osteosarcoma[7,8]—a historical observation before the era of megavoltage radiation possibly linked to the greater absorption of orthovoltage radiation by bone as compared to soft tissue. Malignant fibrous histiocytoma, angiosarcoma, and other mesenchymal subtypes have also been reported after therapeutic radiation.[7-9] By criteria described initially by Cahan and colleagues,[10] radiation-induced sarcomas arise no sooner than 4 years after the therapeutic radiation[11,12] and often arise decades later. More recently, however, a shorter 2-year period after diagnosis has been utilized to define radiation-related disease. Contrary to early theories, recent studies have suggested that both orthovoltage and megavoltage treatments are sarcomagenic[8,13] at doses of 8.8 to 70 Gy. In a carefully conducted case-control analysis, the Late Effects Study Group found 64 cases of osteosarcoma in 9170 patients who had survived more than 2 years after the diagnosis of a variety of cancers. A clear dose-response relationship was found between the radiation dose and the subsequent development of osteosarcoma, with a relative risk ranging from 0.6 in patients who received less than 10 Gy to 38.3 in those who received more than 60 Gy.[14] A complete understanding of underlying biology of radiation-induced malignancy remains elusive. Host-related factors (especially young age) and treatment (especially its intensity) seem to both play a role in a complex relationship.[15] Underlying genetic susceptibility is also important and is governed by factors such as deletion or mutation of tumor suppresser gene and DNA repair genes, which likely means that subgroups of the populations have vastly enhanced risk than had previously been anticipated while others are at lower risk than was appreciated in the past. In addition it is highly probably that the greater intensity of multimodality treatments for cancer that have been introduced over recent years with the goal of improving cancer control and survival are going to result in an increase in the rate of radiation-induced malignancies. Of the latter, the overwhelming tumor is sarcoma at risk especially if one considers its baseline incidence rates.[15]

Sarcomas have also been associated with exposure to various chemical agents. A number of conflicting reports have emerged suggesting a relationship between occupational exposure to phenoxyacetic acids (found in some herbicides) and chlorophenols (found in some wood preservatives). Several studies from Sweden have established a link between phenoxy herbicide exposure in forestry workers and the subsequent development of sarcoma.[16-19] However, additional investigations from the United States, New Zealand, and Finland have not confirmed this relationship.[20-22] Similarly, there has been no demonstrable increase in the risk of sarcoma in Vietnam veterans exposed to Agent Orange (dioxin or TCDD [2,3,7,8-tetrachlorodibenzo-p-dioxin]).[23] Hepatic angiosarcomas have been associated with exposure to a number of compounds including Thorotrast (a colloidal suspension of thorium dioxide formerly used as an intravenous contrast agent in radiologic imaging procedures),[24-26] vinyl chloride,[27-29] and arsenic.[30,31]

Recent studies have suggested a relationship between exposure to alkylating chemotherapeutic agents and the subsequent development of sarcomas. Osteosarcomas have been reported after cyclophosphamide treatment for pediatric acute lymphoblastic leukemia.[32,33] In the recent report from the Late Effects Study Group, prior chemotherapy, particularly with melphalan, procarbazine, nitrosoureas, or chlorambucil, was found to be an independent risk factor for the development of sarcoma.[14] The relative risk of sarcoma increased with cumulative drug exposure.

Chronic lymphedema can be a factor in the development of lymphangiosarcoma. These neoplasms have been noted to arise in the chronically lymphedematous arms of women treated for breast cancer with radical mastectomy (Stewart-Treves syndrome).[34,35] Lower extremity lymphangiosarcomas have also been observed in patients with congenital lymphedema or filariasis complicated by chronic lymphedema.[36]

A recent history of trauma is often elicited from sarcoma patients, particularly those with extremity sarcoma. Usually, the interval between the traumatic event and the diagnosis of sarcoma is short, making a causal relationship unlikely. Some reports have suggested, however, that chronic inflammatory processes may be a risk factor for sarcoma. Shrapnel, bullets, intramuscular iron injections, and foreign body implants have been implicated.[37]

Genetic Predisposition

Germline mutations may play an important role in the development of soft tissue sarcomas (Table 96-2). These genetic changes are identified or similar to the genetic changes seen in corresponding sporadic sarcomas (Table 96-3). Mechanistically, the proteins encoded by the altered genes are involved in maintenance of the genome through DNA repair and the cell cycle.

The epidemiologic relationship between the development of soft tissue sarcoma and inherited syndromes associated with a predisposition to neoplasia (e.g., neurofibromatosis and Li-Fraumeni syndrome) has been appreciated for more than 2 decades.[38,39] For example, patients with neurofibromatosis have a 7% to 10% lifetime risk of developing a malignant peripheral nerve sheath tumor (MPNST).[40] A sudden increase in the size of any neurofibroma suggests malignant transformation.[41,42] The mechanisms underlying the transformation from a benign neurofibroma to MPNST are not completely understood.

However, loss-of-function mutations in the NF1 gene, which are found in patients with neurofibromatosis, result in activation of the RAS signaling pathway, a well-known mechanism identified in a variety of cancers.[43] It has been observed that secondary MPNSTs (arising from a prior neurofibroma) have deletions and mutations of 17p (particularly 17p12-17p13.1) at the region of the TP53 tumor suppressor gene.[44-46] Thus, it has been postulated that an initial alteration in the NF1 gene contributes to the formation of a benign neurofibroma through activation of the RAS pathway and that secondary mutations in the TP53 gene allow the transformation into MPNST. Since mutations in TP53 lead to an inability to control DNA damage via the cell cycle, they also enable rapid accumulation of other mutations, which encode mutant proteins that undoubtedly play an important role in sarcomagenesis.

The Li-Fraumeni syndrome was identified when relatives of pediatric soft tissue sarcoma patients were noted to have an increased frequency of diverse and often multiple primary cancers.[38,47] The neoplasms noted in relatives included some soft tissue sarcomas, premenopausal breast cancers, brain tumors, adrenocortical carcinomas, leukemias, and sometimes germ cell tumors.[48] Follow-up of Li-Fraumeni kindreds over 2 decades has revealed that the majority of individuals develop cancer at young ages, with 79% of those affected younger than 45 years at the time of diagnosis of malignancy.[49] The observed cancer distribution in families is believed to fit a rare autosomal dominant mode of genetic transmission with high penetrance.[50] Recent molecular genetic studies have identified germline TP53 mutations in the majority of patients with Li-Fraumeni syndrome.[51] Germline mutations in CHK2, another component of the cell cycle checkpoint machinery encoded by a gene located on 22q11, are responsible for another subgroup of patients with Li-Fraumeni syndrome.[52]

Pediatric patients with familial retinoblastoma have a 13q chromosomal deletion[53] and an increased incidence of osteosarcoma and other neoplasms, including soft tissue sarcoma.[14,54,55] The retinoblastoma (Rb1) protein is expressed ubiquitously in normal cells and is a well-

TABLE 96-2

Germline Mutations Associated with Soft Tissue Sarcomas

SYNDROME	INHERITANCE PATTERN	LOCUS	GENE	ASSOCIATED SOFT TISSUE SARCOMAS
Familial gastrointestinal stromal tumor syndrome	AD	4q12	KIT	Gastrointestinal stromal tumor
Familial infiltrative fibromatosis	AD	5q21	APC	Desmoid fibromatosis
Li-Fraumeni syndrome	AD	17p13	TP53	Multiple types
		22q11	CHK2	
Neurofibromatosis type 1 (von Recklinghausen's disease)	AD	17q11	NF1	Malignant peripheral nerve sheath tumors
Retinoblastoma	AD	13q14	RB1	Multiple types
Rhabdoid predisposition syndrome	AD	22q11	SNF5/INI1	Malignant rhabdoid tumors
Werner's syndrome	AR	8p11-12	WRN	Multiple types

AD, autosomal dominant; AR, autosomal recessive.

Specific Malignancies

III

TABLE 96-3

Molecular Alterations Identified in Sarcoma

TUMOR TYPE	CHARACTERISTIC CYTOGENETIC EVENTS	MOLECULAR EVENTS	FREQUENCY	DIAGNOSTIC UTILITY?
Alveolar soft part sarcoma	t(X;17)(p11;q25)	ASPL-TFE3 fusion	>90%	Yes
Extraskeletal myxoid chrondrosarcoma	t(9;22)(q22;q12)	EWS-NR4A3 fusion	>75%	Yes
	t(9;17)(q22;q11)	TAF2N-NR4A3 fusion	<10%	Yes
	t(9;15)(q22;q21)	TCF12-NR4A3 fusion	<10%	Yes
Clear cell sarcoma	t(12;22)(q13;q12)	EWS-ATF1 fusion	>75%	Yes
Desmoplastic small round cell tumor	t(11;22)(q13;q12)	EWS-WT1 fusion	>75%	Yes
Dermatofibrosarcoma protuberans	Ring form of chromosomes 17 and 22	COL1A1-PDGFB fusion	>75%	Yes
	t(17;22)(q21;q13)	COL1A1-PDGFB fusion	10%	Yes
Ewing's sarcoma/peripheral primitive neuroectodermal tumor	t(11;22)(q24;q12)	EWS-FLI1 fusion	>80%	Yes
	t(21;22)(q12;q12)	EWS-ERG fusion	5–10%	Yes
	t(2;22)(q33;q12)	EWS-FEV fusion	<5%	Yes
	t(7;22)(p22;q12)	EWS-ETV1 fusion	<5%	Yes
	t(17;22)(q12;q12)	EWS-E1AF fusion	<5%	Yes
	inv(22)(q12;q12)	EWS-ZSG fusion	<5%	Yes
Fibrosarcoma, infantile	t(12;15)(q13;q26)	ETV6-NTRK3 fusion	>75%	Yes
	Trisomies 8, 11, 17 and 20		>75%	Yes
Gastrointestinal stromal tumor	Monosomies 14 and 22		>75%	Yes
	Deletion of 1p		>25%	No
		KIT mutation	>90%	Yes
Inflammatory myofibroblastic tumor	2p23 rearrangement	ALK fusion genes	50%	Yes
Leiomyosarcoma	Deletion of 1p		>50%	No
Liposarcoma				
Well-differentiated	Ring form of chromosome 12		>75%	Yes
Myxoid/round cell	t(12;16)(q13;p11)	TLS-CHOP fusion	>75%	Yes
Pleomorphic	Complex	EWS-CHOP fusion	<5%	Yes
Malignant fibrous histiocytoma	Complex		>90%	No
Malignant peripheral nerve sheath tumor	Complex		>90%	No
Myxofibrosarcoma (myxoid malignant fibrous histiocytoma)	Ring form of chromosome 12		?	?
Neuroblastoma				
Good prognosis	Hyperdiploid, no 1p deletion		90%	Yes
Poor prognosis	1p deletion		90%	Yes
	Double minute chromosomes	N-myc amplification	>25%	Yes
Rhabdoid tumor	Deletion of 22q	INI1 inactivation	>90%	Yes
Rhabdomyosarcoma				
Alveolar	t(2;13)(q35;q14)	PAX3-FKHR fusion	>75%	Yes
	T(1;13)(p36;q14), double minutes	PAX7-FKHR fusion	10–20%	Yes
Embryonal	Trisomies 2q, 8, and 20		>75%	Yes
		Loss of heterozygosity at 11p15	>75%	Yes
Synovial sarcoma				
Monophasic	t(X;18)(p11;q11)	SYT-SSX1 or SYT-SSX2 fusion	>90%	Yes
Biphasic	t(X;18)(p11;q11)	SYT-SSX1 fusion	>90%	Yes

known tumor suppressor, involved in maintaining the integrity of the genome through control of the cell cycle. Interestingly, not only is the Rb1 gene mutated in osteosarcomas associated with retinoblastoma, but abnormality or absence of the Rb1 gene product has also been observed in multiple other malignancies, including sporadic osteosarcomas, breast cancer,[56] small cell lung cancer,[57] and soft tissue sarcomas.[58]

Familial infiltrative fibromatosis, also known as hereditary desmoid disease, is caused by germline mutations in the APC gene.[59-61] Patients with this syndrome develop desmoid fibromatosis at a younger age than do patients with sporadic desmoids. Patients with familial adenomatous polyposis also harbor germline mutations in the APC gene; this helps to explain Gardner's syndrome, which is characterized by the development of desmoid tumors as well as polyposis.[62] The APC gene is involved in the WNT or wingless cell-signaling pathway. One of the normal functions of the APC protein, is to bind β-catenin.[63] Thus loss-of-function mutations of APC result in the activation of transcription of oncogenes by β-catenin. Mutations in APC and β-catenin are also identified in sporadic desmoid fibromatosis.[64-66]

Rhabdoid predisposition syndrome is due to inactivating germline mutations in the INI1 gene.[67] Patients with this syndrome develop one or more extrarenal and/or renal rhabdoid tumors. INI1 is a member of the SWI/SNF protein complex, which controls gene expression globally through its ability to alter chromatin structure.[68] Thus loss of INI1 gene expression results in other changes in gene expression, specifically activation of oncogenes. Rhabdoid tumors have loss of function mutations in both copies of the INI1 gene.[69]

Werner's syndrome is a rare genetic instability syndrome caused by mutations in the WRN gene.[70,71] Affected patients age prematurely and are at greatly increased risk for a variety of cancers including soft tissue sarcomas. The WRN gene encodes a protein believed to be involved in DNA repair, and loss of WRN protein function leads to genetic instability, accumulation of genetic mutations, and ultimately predisposition to rapid aging and cancer.

Germline mutations in the KIT oncogene are found in patients with familial gastrointestinal stromal tumor syndrome.[72,73] Activating KIT mutations are also identified in approximately 90% of sporadic gastrointestinal stromal tumors (GISTs).[74] Patients with the familial syndrome develop, to varying degrees, skin hyperpigmentation, urticaria pigmentosa, and cutaneous mast cell disease in addition to one or more GISTs.[75] Activating KIT mutations have been shown to lead to ligand-independent activation of the KIT receptor tyrosine kinase pathway, which results in dysregulated cell growth, and are thought to be the first step in the pathogenesis of GISTs.[72] Interestingly, the identification of the important role of KIT in the pathogenesis of GISTs has led to treatment with imatinib mesylate.[76] A small-molecule drug specifically inhibits the KIT pathway (see sections on Prognostic Factors as Therapeutic Targets and GISTs).

Chromosomal Rearrangements

A large number of sarcomas have been found to have consistent chromosomal abnormalities (see Table 96-3).[77] These chromosomal rearrangements are important diagnostically, may be important prognostically (see section on "Potential Molecular Prognostic Factors"), have shed light on the pathogenesis of sarcomas, and may provide targets for pharmacologic therapy (see section on treatment of GISTs). Benign soft tissue neoplasms also harbor chromosomal rearrangements.

Chromosomal translocations are the most common cytogenetic abnormality in soft tissue neoplasms and are likely responsible for the initiation of tumorigenesis in most cases.[77] Deletions and trisomies have also been reported and are thought to represent secondary changes involved in tumor progression. Deletions tend to represent loss of tumor suppressor genes, whereas trisomies indicate the presence of an oncogene. Although we know a lot about the primary tumorigenic events in many sarcomas, defining the secondary changes has been much more problematic and is an area of intense study.

Cloning and molecular analysis of the various genetic aberrations that characterize different sarcomas have revealed the different pathogenetic mechanisms that underlie these tumors. Translocations typically create chimeric transcription factors or growth factors that result in deregulation of transcription or growth control. A typical example of a chimeric transcription factor is the PAX3-FKHR fusion protein, which has been shown to activate a complex myogenic transcriptional program when the protein is expressed in a fibroblast cell line.[78]

Infantile fibrosarcoma is characterized by a translocation involving chromosomes 12 and 15 that encodes a chimeric ETV6-NTRK3 constitutively activated growth factor receptor.[79] Other oncogenic proteins appear to act by a mechanism that remodels chromatin structure, which is known to have a profound influence on gene expression (e.g. INI1 mutations in rhabdoid tumors).[69]

Specific chromosomal rearrangements are very useful in the diagnosis of soft tissue sarcomas. Beyond the obvious benefit of providing further objective proof of a diagnosis in morphologically typical cases, the detection of chromosomal aberrations may facilitate the diagnosis of lesions that are difficult to characterize by standard histopathologic, ultrastructural, and immunohistochemical techniques.[80,81] For example, the presence of the translocation t(X;18)(p11;q11) has been used to confirm the diagnosis of synovial sarcoma in poorly differentiated cases that were diagnostically very challenging.[82-84] Similarly, the finding of the characteristic translocation t(11;22)(q24;q12) in a small round blue cell tumor supports the diagnosis of Ewing's sarcoma/PNET (primitive neuroectodermal tumor).[85]

Translocations can be identified by cytogenetic analysis, fluorescence in situ hybridization (FISH), or reverse transcriptase polymerase chain reaction (RT-PCR). A detailed description of these techniques is beyond the scope of this chapter, but each technique has its advantages and disadvantages. Cytogenetic analysis requires fresh (living) tissue since the cells need to be cultured before karyotypic analysis. This technique is becoming more widely available than before, owing to the availability of overnight transport of biologic specimens and "for profit" core facilities. FISH is a technologically sophisticated technique that does not require fresh or frozen tissue. FISH is easier to perform on cytogenetic cultures or frozen tissue, however, so these are still preferable to paraffin-embedded material. RT-PCR is an extremely sensitive technique that can be performed on fresh, frozen, or paraffin-embedded tissues. The major drawback of RT-PCR is the relatively high false-positive rate, which results from its sensitiveness. Meticulous care is required to prevent problems from contamination.

Although RT-PCR can be performed on paraffin-embedded tissue, it is preferable to perform the analysis on fresh or frozen tissue. Since all of these techniques either require or are easier to perform on fresh or frozen tissue, it is advisable to freeze and store a portion of any suspected sarcoma or poorly differentiated neoplasm for potential molecular analysis.

Many sarcomas are characterized by several different translocations, some of which are mutually exclusive (see Table 96-3). For instance, alveolar rhabdomyosarcoma is characterized by a translocation involving chromosomes 2 and 13, which results in fusion of the PAX3 and FKHR genes, or by a translocation involving chromosomes 1 and 13, which results in fusion of the PAX7 and FKHR genes.[86-89] Sarcomas within a subtype may also have differences in the specific exons involved in each of these different translocations. It has been proposed that this heterogeneity may result in differences in prognosis (see "Potential Molecular Prognostic Factors"). For example,

Ewing's sarcoma/PNET and synovial sarcoma possess genetic variations that have been suggested to have prognostic significance.[90-93] Future research may establish whether cytogenetic and molecular factors can be used as a basis for therapeutic decisions and the prediction and evaluation of response to treatment.

The identification of genetic alterations with high specificity for different sarcomas will also identify specific therapeutic targets. This has already resulted in the successful treatment of two different sarcomas, GISTs and dermatofibrosarcoma protuberans (DFSP).[76,94] About 90% of GISTs harbor activating mutations in the KIT oncogene, which result in ligand-independent activation of the KIT receptor tyrosine kinase pathway.[74] Imatinib mesylate, a small-molecule drug that is administered orally and inhibits the KIT pathway, has been shown to be very efficacious in the treatment of GIST (see the section on investigational new drugs in the chemotherapy section). DFSP is characterized by translocations involving the COL1A1 and PDGFβ genes, which result in activation of the platelet-derived growth factor-β PDGFβ pathway. Imatinib mesylate is also active against the PDGFβ pathway and has been shown to be effective in the treatment of a small number of DFSPs.

PATHOLOGY

Soft tissue sarcomas have been described at virtually all anatomic sites. The anatomic sites and site-specific histologic subtypes of 4207 sarcomas treated at a single referral institution are outlined in Figure 96-1. Approximately half of all soft tissue sarcomas occur in the extremities (lower, 34%; upper, 14%), where the most common histopathologic subtypes are well-differentiated, myxoid, and round cell liposarcoma (28%) and malignant fibrous histiocytoma (pleomorphic undifferentiated sarcoma) (24%). Retroperitoneal sarcomas comprise 15% of all soft tissue

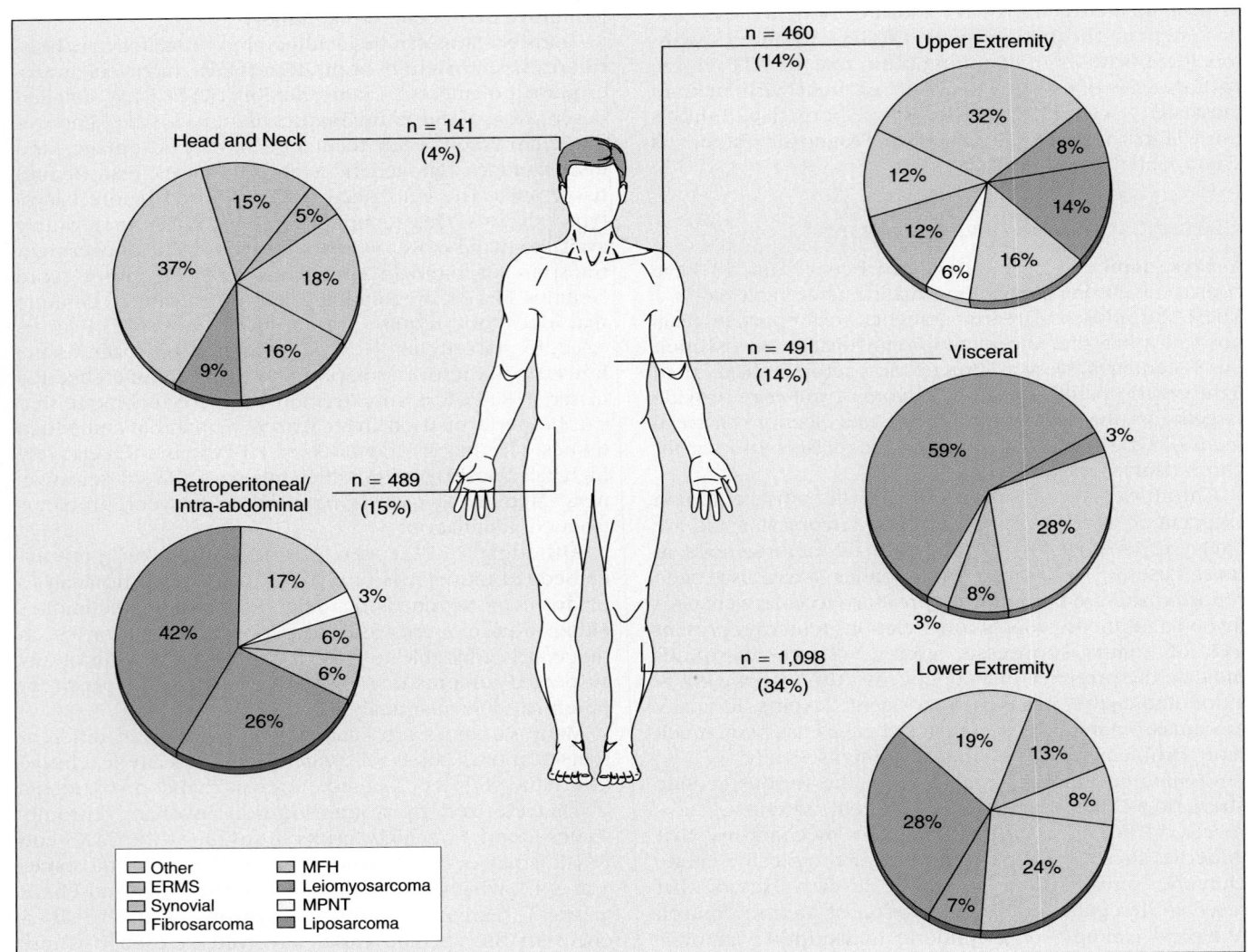

Figure 96-1. Anatomic distribution and site-specific histiotypes of 4207 adult patients with soft tissue sarcomas seen at the University of Texas M.D. Anderson Cancer Center, 1996–2003.

sarcomas, with well-differentiated or dedifferentiated lipo-sarcoma being the predominant histologic subtype (42%). The visceral sarcomas make up an additional 14%, while the head and neck sarcomas comprise approximately 4%.

Classification

In broad terms, sarcomas can be classified into neoplasms arising in bone and those arising from the soft tissues. Sarcomas of the soft tissues can be further grouped into those that arise from viscera (gastrointestinal, genito-urinary, and gynecologic organs) and those that arise from nonvisceral soft tissues (muscle, tendon, adipose, pleura, and connective tissue).

An alternative way to index soft tissue sarcomas is by their differentiation; tumors can be grouped broadly into adipocytic tumors, fibroblastic/myofibroblastic tumors, so-called fibrohistiocytic tumors, smooth muscle tumors, pericytic (perivascular) tumors, primitive neuroecto-dermal tumors (PNETs), skeletal muscle tumors, vascular tumors, osseous tumors, and tumors of uncertain differen-tiation (Table 96-4).[95] Classification is based on clinical, histologic, ultrastructural, immunohistochemical, and genetic features. Electron microscopic evidence of cellular substructures, neurofibrils, microfilaments, actin-myosin complexes, dense bodies, etc., often helps to clarify the tissue of origin.[96] However, the widespread availability of commercial antibodies for immunohistochemical has diminished the need for electron microscopic examina-tion in many cases. Immunohistochemical staining for proteins characteristic of smooth muscle (smooth muscle actin and desmin), skeletal muscle (muscle-specific actin, desmin, and myogenin), blood vessels (factor VIII, CD34, and CD31), and epithelial tissue (epithelial membrane antigen and cytokeratins) often facilitates reliable classification.[97,98]

The tissue of origin classification scheme is the most commonly used scheme and is the basis for the recent World Health Organization (WHO) classification system for sarcomas.[95,99] The WHO classification system is repro-ducible for most sarcomas. As the degree of histologic differentiation declines, however, the determination of tissue of origin becomes increasingly difficult. In parti-cular, despite advanced immunohistochemical techniques, electron microscopy, and molecular analysis, determining the tissue of origin for some soft tissue tumors is difficult, occasionally arbitrary, and sometimes impossible. This leads to significant disparities in diagnoses among pathol-ogists. Discrepancies between the original histologic diag-nosis and the subsequent diagnosis by an expert reviewer have been noted in as many as 25% of cases.[100,101] Review of tissue specimens by an expert at a regional sarcoma center is therefore imperative, as the degree of expertise in correctly diagnosing rare and unusual sarcomas is directly related to the number of sarcomas that a pathologist has seen.

It is important to classify soft tissue sarcomas as precisely as possible because of major differences in their clinical behavior and in their susceptibility to different therapies. For example, a few soft tissue sarcomas, including epithelioid sarcoma, clear cell sarcoma, angio-

---

TABLE 96-4

Histologic Classification of STS

Adipocytic Sarcomas

Atypical lipomatous tumor/well-differentiated liposarcoma
Dedifferentiated liposarcoma
Myxoid liposarcoma
Pleomorphic liposarcoma

Fibroblastic/Myofibroblastic Sarcomas

Malignant solitary fibrous tumor
Inflammatory myofibroblastic tumor
Myxoinflammatory fibroblastic sarcoma
Infantile fibrosarcoma
Adult fibrosarcoma
Myxofibrosarcoma (myxoid malignant fibrous histiocytoma)
Low-grade fibromyxoid sarcoma
Sclerosing epithelioid fibrosarcoma

So-called Fibrohistiocytic Sarcomas

Pleomorphic malignant fibrous histiocytoma/undifferentiated
    high-grade pleomorphic sarcoma
Giant cell malignant fibrous histiocytoma/undifferentiated
    pleomorphic sarcoma with giant cells
Inflammatory malignant fibrous histiocytoma/undifferentiated
    pleomorphic sarcoma with prominent inflammation

Smooth Muscle Sarcomas

Leiomyosarcoma

Skeletal Muscle Sarcomas

Embryonal rhabdomyosarcoma
Alveolar rhabdomyosarcoma
Pleomorphic rhabdomyosarcoma

Vascular Sarcomas

Epithelioid hemangioendothelioma
Angiosarcoma

Osseous Sarcomas

Extraskeletal osteosarcoma

Sarcomas of Uncertain Differentiation

Synovial sarcoma
Epithelioid sarcoma
Alveolar soft part sarcoma
Clear cell sarcoma of soft tissue
Extraskeletal myxoid chondrosarcoma
Desmoplastic small round cell tumor
Extrarenal rhabdoid tumor
Intimal sarcoma

---

sarcoma, and rhabdomyosarcoma, have a greater risk of regional lymph node metastasis.[102,103] In one single-institution study, the overall rate of nodal metastasis at the time of sarcoma presentation was only 2.7%; however, the rate was much higher for angiosarcoma (13.5%), embryonal rhabdomyosarcoma (13.6%), and epithelioid sarcoma (16.7%).[102]

Patterns of distant metastases also differ for subtypes of sarcoma. For example, myxoid liposarcoma tends to metas-tasize to soft tissue sites including the retroperitoneum,[104] and patients with myxoid liposarcoma often present with metastatic disease. Therefore if a myxoid liposarcoma is identified in the abdomen, the thighs should be examined for an occult primary tumor. The vast majority of so-called primary myxoid liposarcomas of the abdomen/retroperitoneum are actually metastatic myxoid liposarcomas or misdiagnosed dedifferentiated liposarcomas, which often mimic myxoid liposarcoma.[105]

Patterns of local spread also differ dramatically among subtypes of sarcoma. For example, DFSP has a propensity to infiltrate subcutaneous adipose tissue in a manner that is very difficult to detect; and thus wide surgical excision of DFSP is essential. When planning a surgery for DFSP, the surgeon should regard the grossly observable lesion as "the tip of the iceberg." Angiosarcoma also spreads very diffusely and is difficult to define grossly.

Histologic Grading

Histologic classification alone does not always provide enough information to predict the clinical behavior of soft tissue sarcomas. For many sarcomas, histologic grading provides additional information that can aid in predicting biologic behavior and planning treatment. The spectrum of grades varies among specific histologic subtypes (Fig. 96-2). For example, leiomyosarcomas exhibit wide variations in grade and should always be graded, while Ewing's sarcomas/PNETs are always high-grade and therefore do not require grading. In careful comparative multivariate analyses, histologic grade has been the most important prognostic factor in assessing the risk for distant metastasis and tumor-related mortality.[106-108]

Several grading systems have been proposed, but there is no consensus regarding the specific morphologic criteria that should be employed in the grading of soft tissue sarcomas. The two most important criteria appear to be the mitotic index and extent of tumor necrosis.

Two of the most commonly employed grading systems are the U.S. National Cancer Institute (NCI) system developed by Costa and colleagues[109] and the FNCLCC system (Federation Nationale des Centres de Lutte Contre le Cancer) developed by the French Federation of Cancer Centers Sarcoma Group.[110] The NCI system is based on the tumor's histologic subtype and amount of tumor necrosis, but cellularity, nuclear pleomorphism, and mitotic index are considered for certain subtypes. The FNCLCC system employs a score generated by evaluation of three parameters: tumor differentiation, mitotic rate, and amount of tumor necrosis. The prognostic values of these two grading systems were retrospectively compared in a population of 410 adult patients with nonmetastatic soft tissue sarcoma.[111] Significant discrepancies were observed in one third of cases. An increased number of grade III tumors, reduced number of grade II tumors, and better correlation with overall and metastasis-free survival were observed in favor of the FNCLCC system.[111] Thus in the absence of other comparative data, the FNCLCC system may be the best presently available grading system.

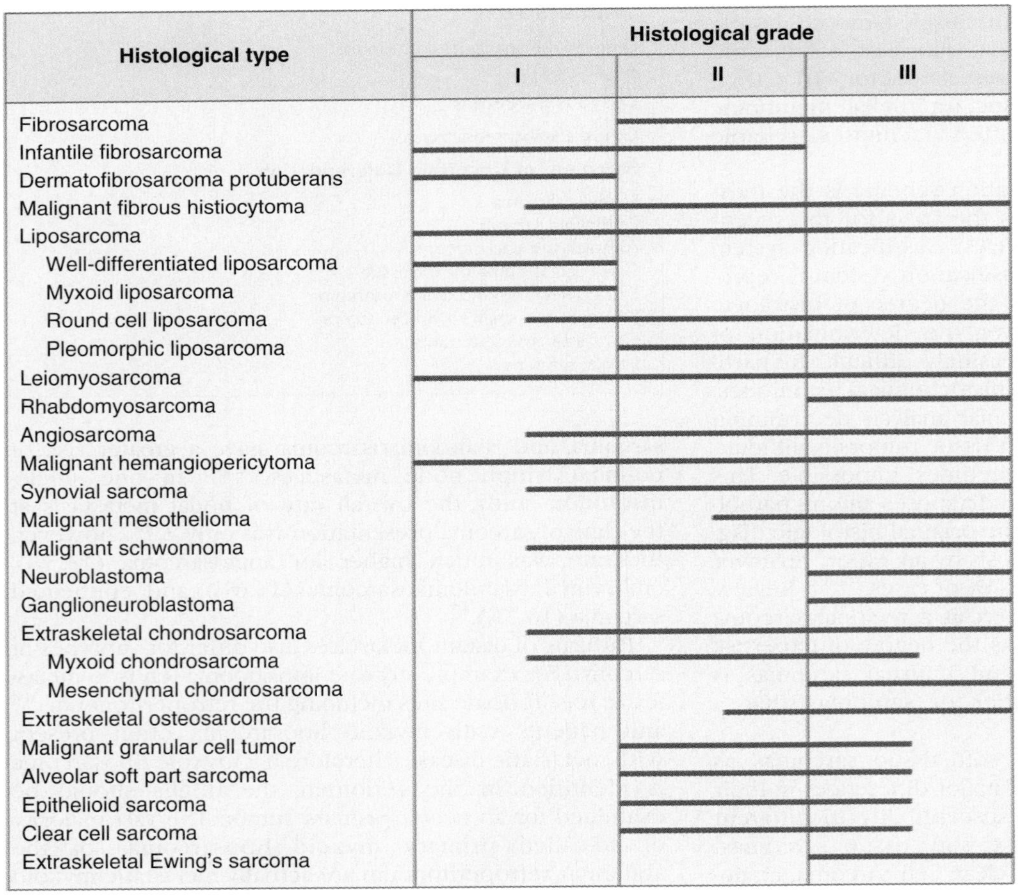

Histological type	Histological grade		
	I	II	III
Fibrosarcoma		────────	────────
Infantile fibrosarcoma	────────	────────	
Dermatofibrosarcoma protuberans	────────	────────	
Malignant fibrous histiocytoma	────	────────	────────
Liposarcoma			
Well-differentiated liposarcoma	────────	────────	
Myxoid liposarcoma	────────	────────	
Round cell liposarcoma		────────	────────
Pleomorphic liposarcoma		────────	────────
Leiomyosarcoma	────────	────────	────────
Rhabdomyosarcoma			────────
Angiosarcoma	────────	────────	────────
Malignant hemangiopericytoma	────────	────────	────────
Synovial sarcoma	────	────────	────────
Malignant mesothelioma		────	────────
Malignant schwannoma	────	────────	────────
Neuroblastoma			────────
Ganglioneuroblastoma			────────
Extraskeletal chondrosarcoma			
Myxoid chondrosarcoma	────	────────	
Mesenchymal chondrosarcoma			────────
Extraskeletal osteosarcoma			────────
Malignant granular cell tumor		────────	────────
Alveolar soft part sarcoma		────────	────────
Epithelioid sarcoma		────────	────────
Clear cell sarcoma		────────	────────
Extraskeletal Ewing's sarcoma			────────

Figure 96-2. The spectrum of grades observed among histologic subtypes of soft tissue sarcoma. (Reprinted with permission from Enzinger FM, Weiss SW: Malignant tumors of uncertain type. In Enzinger FM, Weiss SW [eds]: Soft Tissue Tumors, 3rd ed. St. Louis, Mosby, 1995, p 1067.)

CLINICAL PRESENTATION AND DIAGNOSIS

The majority of patients present with a painless mass, although pain is noted at presentation in up to a third of cases.[112] Delay in diagnosis of sarcomas is common, with the most common incorrect diagnosis for extremity and trunk lesions being lipoma or hematoma.

Physical examination should include an assessment of the size and mobility of the mass. Its relationship to the fascia (superficial versus deep) and nearby neurovascular and bony structures should be noted. A site-specific neurovascular examination and assessment of regional lymph nodes should also be performed.

Biopsy

Biopsy of the primary tumor is essential for most patients presenting with soft tissue masses. In general, any soft tissue mass in an adult that is asymptomatic or enlarging, is larger than 5 cm, or persists beyond 4 to 6 weeks should be biopsied. The preferred biopsy approach is generally the least invasive technique required to allow a definitive histologic diagnosis and assessment of grade. In most centers, core-needle biopsy provides satisfactory tissue for diagnosis[113-115] and has been demonstrated to result in substantial cost savings compared to open biopsy.[115] Direct palpation can be used to guide needle biopsy of most superficial lesions, but less accessible sarcomas often require an image-guided biopsy to sample safely the most heterogeneous component of the mass. Needle tract tumor recurrences after closed biopsy are rare but have been reported,[116] leading some surgeons to advocate tattooing the biopsy site for subsequent excision or for inclusion in radiotherapy treatment volumes (Fig. 96-3). In some centers, fine-needle aspiration may be an acceptable biopsy technique for primary soft tissue masses provided that an experienced sarcoma cytopathologist is available.[117-119] Due to the frequent difficulty in accurately diagnosing these lesions even when adequate tissue is available, however, the major utility of fine-needle aspiration in most centers is in the diagnosis of suspected recurrent sarcoma.

Incisional or excisional biopsy is rarely required but may be performed when a definitive diagnosis cannot be achieved by less invasive means. Several technical points merit comment. Relatively small, superficial masses that can easily be removed should be biopsied by complete excision with microscopic assessment of surgical margins. Incisional and excisional biopsies should be performed with the incision oriented longitudinally (for extremity lesions) to facilitate subsequent wide local excision. The incision should be centered over the mass at its most superficial point. Care should be taken not to raise tissue flaps. Meticulous hemostasis should be ensured to prevent dissemination of tumor cells into adjacent tissue planes by hematoma. All excisional biopsy specimens should be sent fresh, sterile, and anatomically oriented for pathologic analysis. At definitive resection of a previously biopsied sarcoma, the previous surgical biopsy scar should be excised en bloc with the tumor.

Imaging

Optimal imaging of the primary tumor is dependent on the anatomic site. For soft tissue masses of the extremities, magnetic resonance imaging (MRI) has been regarded as the imaging modality of choice (Fig. 96-4). This is because MRI enhances the contrast between tumor and muscle and between tumor and adjacent blood vessels and provides multiplanar definition of the lesion.[120,121] However, a study by the Radiation Diagnostic Oncology Group that compared MRI and computed tomography (CT) in patients with malignant bone (n = 183) and soft tissue (n = 133) tumors showed no specific advantage of MRI over CT from a diagnostic standpoint.[122] For pelvic lesions, the multiplanar capability of MRI may provide superior single-modality imaging (Fig. 96-5A and B, p. 2583). The multiplanar capability is also helpful for visualization disease in noncoplanar ways when employing conformal radiotherapy technique and is an especially helpful adjunct when using image fusion techniques or to visualize peritumoral edema that may harbor sarcoma cells. In the retroperitoneum and abdomen, CT usually provides satisfactory anatomic definition of the lesion (Fig. 96-6, p. 2584). Occasionally, MRI with gradient sequence imaging can better delineate the relationship of the tumor to midline vascular structures, particularly the inferior vena cava and aorta. More invasive studies such as angiography or cavography are almost never required for the evaluation of soft tissue sarcomas.

The utility of 18F-fluorodeoxyglucose positron emission tomography (FDG PET) in the evaluation and treatment of STS has been a subject of recent studies and has been reviewed in detail elsewhere. The technique utilizes radio-labeled glucose analogues,[19] which are taken up at increased rates by malignant tumors. Pilot studies of PET in soft tissue sarcoma suggest that by evaluating tumor metabolic activity, PET scans may allow for noninvasive

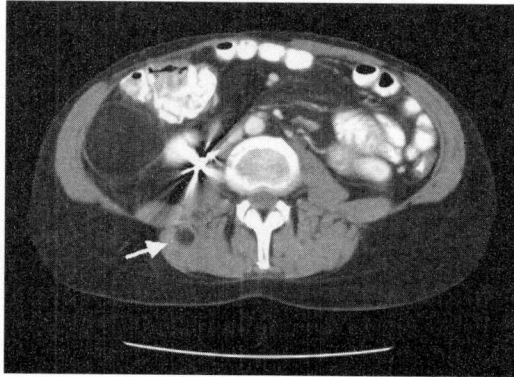

Figure 96-3. Axial CT image of a recurrent well-differentiated low-grade liposarcoma of the retroperitoneum. Note the tumor nodule *(arrow)* representing a tumor implant within muscle from a previous needle biopsy that was obtained through the posterior abdominal wall. It is beneficial to consider the location of biopsy tracts so that subsequent surgery or radiotherapy includes the area of the biopsy (see text).

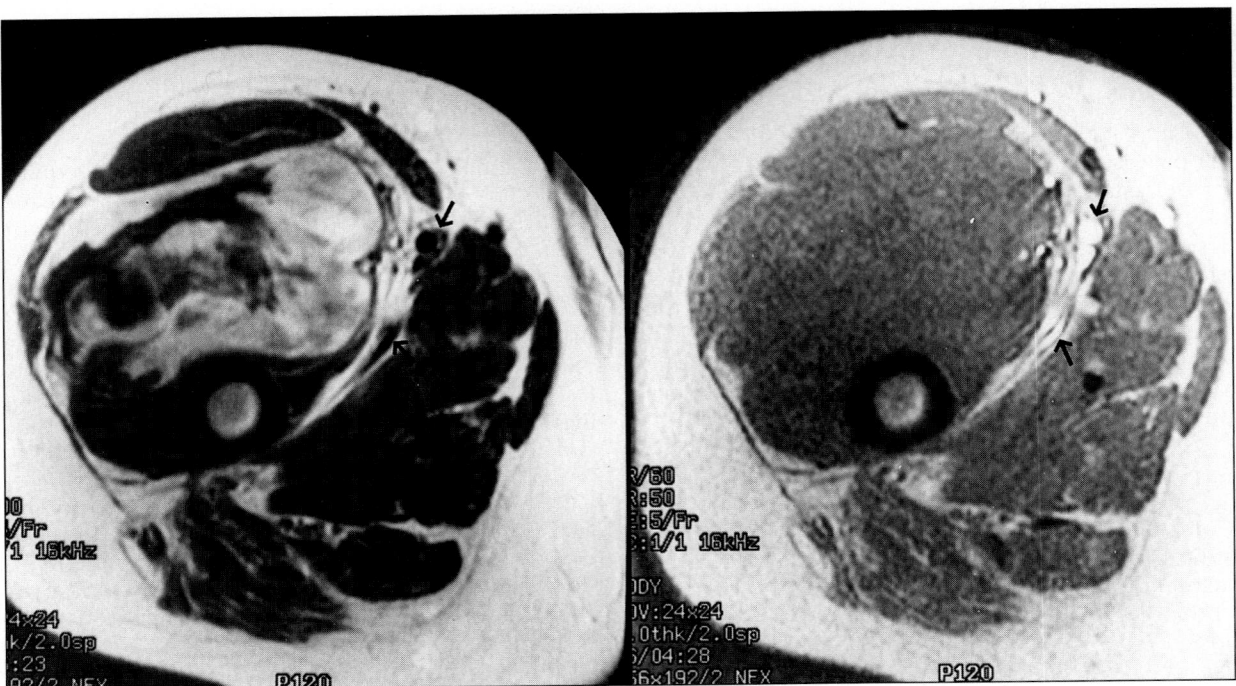

Figure 96-4. 47-year-old male with malignant fibrous histiocytoma of the left thigh. Axial contrast enhanced T1-weighted *(left)* and flow sensitive gradient *(right)* images reveal a large mass in the vastus intermedius muscle. A plane is identified between the mass and the profunda femoris and superficial femoral vessels *(arrows)*.

assessment of tumor grade.[123] Recent preliminary studies have demonstrated that PET may be helpful in the assessment of locally recurrent soft tissue sarcoma[124] and in the evaluation of response to therapy.[125,126] The role and cost-effectiveness of PET in the staging of soft tissue sarcoma remain incompletely defined, and thus further studies will be required to define fully the role for FDG PET in the diagnosis, evaluation, and treatment of STS.

STAGING

The relative rarity of soft tissue sarcomas, the anatomic heterogeneity of these lesions, and the presence of more than 30 recognized histologic subtypes of variable grade have made it difficult to establish a functional system that can accurately stage all forms of this disease. The recently revised staging system (sixth edition) of the American Joint Committee on Cancer (AJCC) and the International Union Against Cancer (UICC) is the most widely employed staging system for soft tissue sarcomas.[127] This staging system is a revision of the original AJCC system, which was first published in 1977; it incorporates histologic grade into the conventional TNM system (Table 96-5). The 2002 sixth edition classification has identical T and N categories as the 1997 fifth edition TNM, but has some modifications to the stage groupings. For the detailed background to these changes the reader is referred to a more complete discussion. All soft tissue sarcoma subtypes are included except dermatofibrosarcoma protuberans, a condition considered to have only borderline malignant potential.

Four distinct histologic grades are recognized, ranging from well-differentiated to undifferentiated. Histologic grade and tumor size are the primary determinants of clinical stage (see Table 96-5). Tumor size is further substaged as "a" (a superficial tumor that arises outside the investing fascia) or "b" (a deep tumor that arises beneath the fascia or invades the fascia). The system is designed to

TABLE 96-5

AJCC/UICC Staging System for Soft Tissue Sarcomas

T1		=5 cm		
T1a		Superficial to muscular fascia		
T1b		Deep to muscular fascia		
T2		>5 cm		
T2a		Superficial to muscular fascia		
T2b		Deep to muscular fascia		
N1		Regional nodal involvement		
G1		Well-differentiated		
G2		Moderately differentiated		
G3		Poorly differentiated		
G4		Undifferentiated		
Stage IA	G1, 2	T1a, b	N0	M0
Stage IB	G2, 2	T2a, b	N0	M0
Stage IIA	G3, 4	T1a, b	N0	M0
Stage IIB	G3, 4	T2a	N0	M0
Stage III	G3, 4	T2b	N0	M0
Stage IV	Any G	Any T	N1	M0
	Any G	Any T	Any N	M1

Modified from Greene FL et al (eds.): UICC TNM Classification of Malignant Tumors, 6th ed. [LOC.], Springer Verlag, 2002.

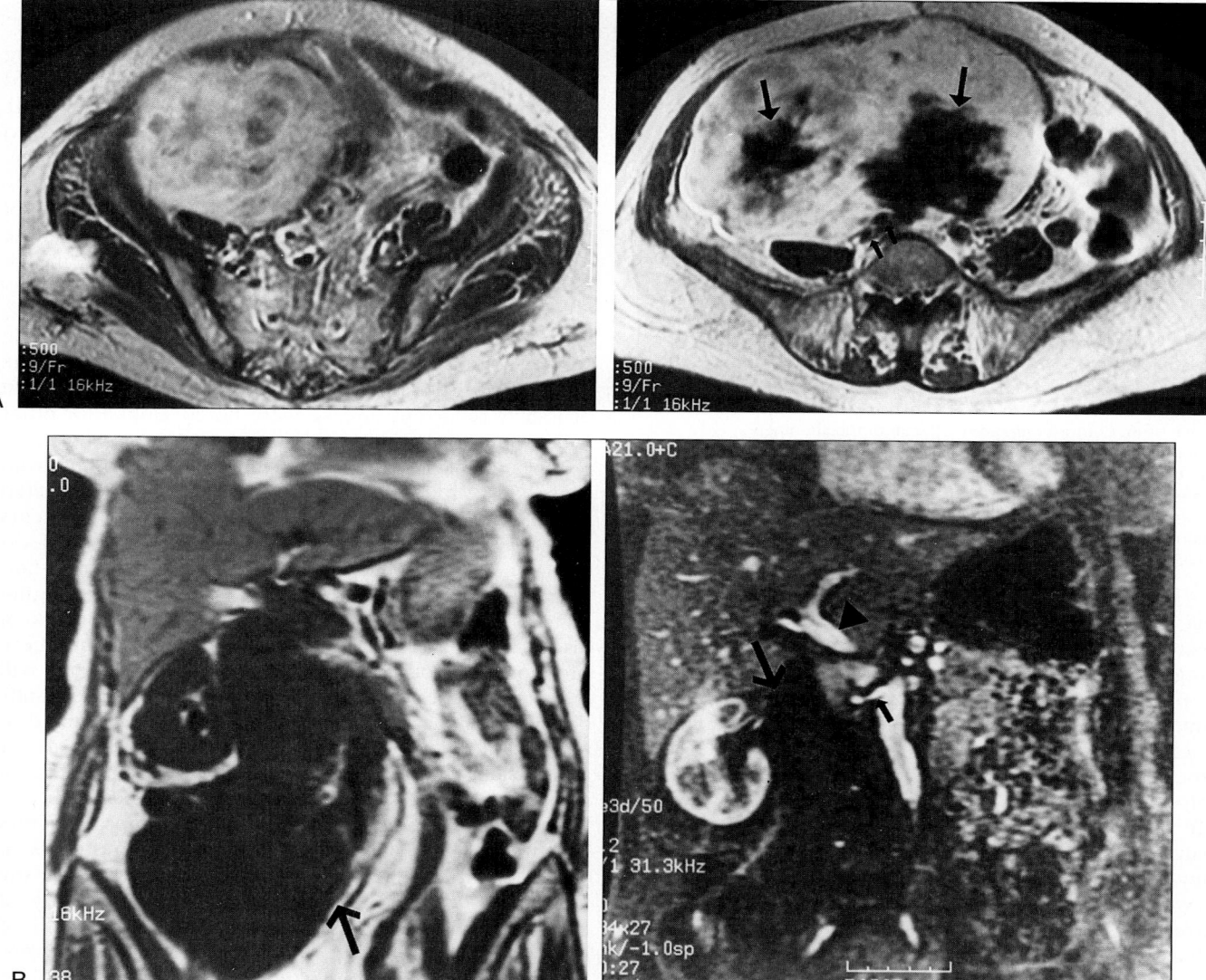

Figure 96-5. A, 74-year-old female with retroperitoneal malignant fibrous histiocytoma extending into the upper pelvis. Axial contrast enhanced T1-weighted images reveal a large heterogenous mass with foci of necrosis *(large arrows).* Note relationship to common iliac vessels *(small arrows).* **B,** Same patient as in **(A).** Coronal T1-weighted *(left)* and source MR images *(right)* from contrast enhanced 3D MR angiogram reveal large abdominal mass *(large arrows)* closely abutting the right renal capsule. Note relationship to aorta. The right renal artery is visualized *(small arrow)* as is the portal vein *(arrowhead).*

optimally stage extremity tumors but is also applicable to torso, head and neck, and retroperitoneal lesions; it should not be used for sarcomas of the gastrointestinal tract. This staging system has been validated based on analysis of 1146 patients presenting with primary extremity soft tissue sarcoma at the Memorial Sloan-Kettering Cancer Center. Stage-specific survival plots are outlined in Figure 96-7.

A major limitation of the present staging system is that it does not take into account the anatomic site of soft tissue sarcomas. Anatomic site, however, is an important determinant of outcome. Patients with retroperitoneal and visceral sarcomas have a worse overall prognosis than do patients with extremity tumors. Although site is not

incorporated as a specific component of any present staging system, outcome data should be reported on a site-specific basis.

PROGNOSTIC FACTORS

Conventional Clinicopathologic Factors

Thorough understanding of the clinicopathologic factors known to impact outcome is essential in formulating a treatment plan for the patient with soft tissue sarcoma. Over the past decade, many multivariate analyses of prognostic factors for patients with localized sarcoma

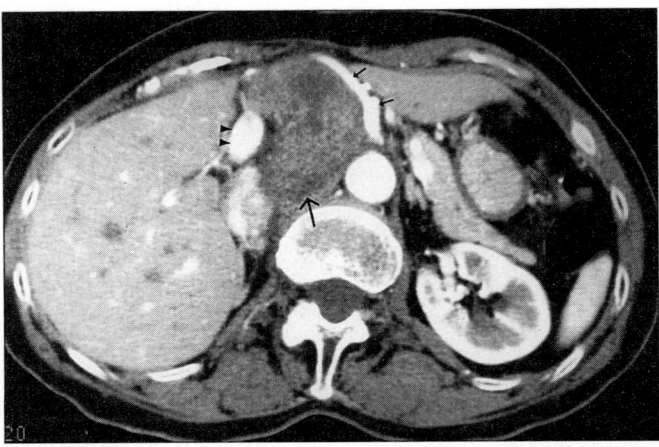

Figure 96-6. Contrast enhanced CT scan of the abdomen demonstrating a retroperitoneal malignant fibrous histiocytoma. Note large mass *(large arrow)* between aorta and inferior vena cava with abutment and displacement of celiac axis and hepatic artery *(small arrows)*. The portal vein *(arrowheads)* is well visualized and low attenuation foci in the liver, which are unopacified hepatic veins, are incidentally visualized.

have been reported. With few exceptions,[106,107,128,129] most studies have analyzed fewer than 300 patients (range, 82 to 297 patients). At least three detailed analyses of prognostic factors in soft tissue sarcoma merit comment.[106,107,128] The initial study of prognostic factors in extremity sarcoma from Memorial Sloan-Kettering Cancer Center evaluated clinicopathologic prognostic factors in a series of 423 patients with localized extremity soft tissue sarcoma seen from 1968 to 1978.[128] This analysis, among the first to discriminate between specific clinical end points, clearly established the clinical profile of what is now accepted as the high-risk patient with extremity soft tissue sarcoma: the patient with a large (>5 cm), high-grade, deep lesion. The adverse prognostic significance of a high tumor grade, deep tumor location, and tumor size greater than 5 cm was also noted in the recent report of the French Federation of Cancer Centers

study of 546 patients with sarcomas of the extremities, head and neck, trunk wall, retroperitoneum, and pelvis.[107]

A follow-up report from Memorial Sloan-Kettering evaluated clinicopathologic prognostic factors that had been documented prospectively in a population of 1041 patients with extremity soft tissue sarcoma.[106] The end points for the multivariate analyses were local recurrence, distant recurrence (metastasis), and disease-specific survival. Results of the regression analyses for each of these end points are summarized in Table 96-6. These results, using prospectively acquired data, confirm the initial observations made at that institution using an independent data set.[128] In addition the previously unappreciated prognostic significance of specific histologic subtypes and the increased risk for adverse outcome associated with a microscopically positive surgical margin or locally recurrent disease were noted. Unlike for other solid tumors, the adverse prognostic factors for local recurrence of a soft tissue sarcoma are different from those that predict distant metastasis and tumor-related mortality (see Table 96-6).[106] In other words, patients with a constellation of adverse prognostic factors for local recurrence are not necessarily at increased risk for distant metastasis or tumor-related death. Therefore staging systems that are designed to stratify patients for risk of distant metastasis and tumor-related mortality using these prognostic factors (such as the AJCC/UICC system) will not stratify patients for risk of local recurrence. The results of these multivariate analyses should be incorporated in the design of new staging systems and clinical trials for soft tissue sarcoma, and the identification of individual patients at high risk for distant recurrence and death.

It should be emphasized that the prognostic factors identified have been derived primarily from studies of patients with localized extremity sarcomas. Despite the fact that extremity sarcomas make up the majority of sarcomas, these results may not be optimally generalized to the greater population of soft tissue sarcoma patients. Separate reviews of prognostic factors for sarcomas of the retroperitoneum,[130,131] head and neck,[132-135] gastrointestinal tract,[136,137] colon and rectum,[138] uterus,[139] synovial

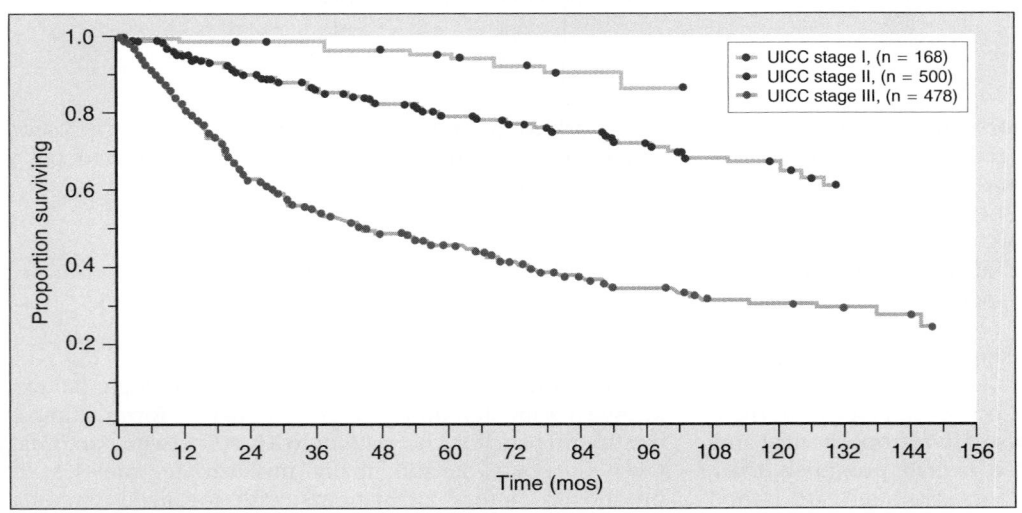

Figure 96-7. Overall survival by AJCC stage in a population of 1146 patients with primary extremity sarcoma treated at the Memorial Sloan-Kettering Cancer Center.

TABLE 96-6

Multivariate Analysis of Prognostic Factors in Patients with Extremity Soft Tissue Sarcoma

ENDPOINT	ADVERSE PROGNOSTIC FACTOR	RELATIVE RISK
Local recurrence	Age >50 years	1.6
	Local recurrence at presentation	2.0
	Microscopically positive margin	1.8
	Fibrosarcoma	2.5
	Malignant peripheral nerve tumor	1.8
Distant recurrence	Size 5.0–10.0 cm	1.9
	Size > 10.0 cm	1.5
	High-grade	4.3
	Deep location	2.5
	Local recurrence	1.5
	Leiomyosarcoma	1.7
	Other nonliposarcoma histology	1.6
Disease-specific survival	Size > 10.0 cm	2.1
	Deep location	2.8
	Local recurrence at presentation	1.5
	Leiomyosarcoma	1.9
	Malignant peripheral nerve tumor	1.9
	Microscopically positive margin	1.7
	Lower extremity site	1.6

Adverse prognostic factors identified are independent by Cox regression analysis.
Modified from Pisters PWT, Leung DHY, Woodruff JM, et al: Analysis of prognostic factors in 1041 patients with localized soft tissue sarcomas of the extremities. J Clin Concol 1996;14:1679.

sarcomas,[140,141] malignant fibrous histiocytoma,[142-144] and Ewing's sarcoma[145-148] have been reported.

Potential Molecular Prognostic Factors

Attention has recently been focused on the evaluation of molecular pathologic prognostic factors. Specific molecular parameters evaluated for prognostic significance have included p53,[149] mdm2,[149] Ki-67,[149] altered expression of the retinoblastoma gene product (pRb)[58,150] in high-grade sarcomas, and the presence of the SYT-SSX fusion transcripts in synovial sarcoma[92] or EWS-FL11 fusion transcripts in Ewing's sarcoma.[90,91]

A preliminary report evaluating the prognostic role of pRb expression in 44 primary and 12 metastatic high-grade human sarcomas by immunohistochemical methods and western blotting demonstrated that alterations in pRb are more commonly associated with high-grade tumors, metastatic lesions, and decreased survival.[58] However, a subsequent report from the same group in an expanded population of 174 adult patients with soft tissue sarcoma revealed that pRb alterations were frequently observed in both low- and high-grade lesions and that altered pRb expression did not correlate with known predictors of survival and was not an independent predictor of long-term outcome.[150] These studies and the now well-documented phenomenon of late (>5 years post-treatment) recurrence of soft tissue sarcoma[151] underscore the importance of long-term follow-up and relatively large sample size in these types of analyses.

p53 is a tumor suppressor gene located on chromosome 17. Somatic p53 mutations have been reported in 4% to 65% of patients with soft tissue sarcoma.[152-156] Detection of p53 has also been correlated with reduced overall survival in immunohistochemical studies of paraffin-embedded soft tissue sarcomas. Data on the underlying prognostic significance of p53 status are conflicting, with some investigators reporting no independent adverse prognostic significance by regression analysis[149,157] and others reporting a highly significant correlation between p53/mdm2 status and outcome.[158]

Ki-67, an antigen expressed throughout the majority of the cell cycle, is utilized as a measure of dividing cells.[159] Preliminary reports of series of heterogeneous sarcomas in adults suggested that proliferative index as measured by Ki-67 nuclear staining correlated with histologic grade, but was not of independent prognostic significance when histologic grade was taken into account.[157,160] However, additional studies in larger numbers of patients have demonstrated that Ki-67 status is an independent prognostic factor.[149,161,162] An initial immunohistochemical analysis of a cohort of 65 soft tissue sarcomas and a subsequent analysis of 132 soft tissue sarcomas from the French Federation of Cancer Centers Sarcoma Group demonstrated the adverse prognostic significance of increased Ki-67 activity.[161,162]

Heslin and colleagues evaluated the potential prognostic significance of pRb, p53, mdm2, and Ki-67 by immunohistochemical techniques in a population of 121 patients with primary, high-grade extremity sarcomas and compared these factors to conventional clinicopathologic prognostic factors (median follow-up, 64 months).[149] Clinicopathologic and molecular factors found to be statistically significant adverse prognostic factors in both univariate and multivariate analyses for the separate end points of distant metastasis and tumor-related mortality included tumor size greater than 5 cm, microscopically positive surgical margin, and a Ki-67 score of greater than 20 (>20% nuclear staining). Overexpression of p53 or mdm2 or deletion of pRb did not correlate with an increased risk of distant metastasis or tumor-related mortality.

Synovial sarcoma is characterized by a specific chromosomal translocation, t(X;18)(p11;q11), which is seen in more than 90% of these tumors.[82,84] This had led to studies evaluating the potential prognostic significance of SYT-SSX fusion transcripts, which arise from this translocation.[92] The t(X;18)(p11;q11) translocation fuses the SYT gene from chromosome 18 to either of two homologous genes at Xp11, SSX1, or SSX2. The fusion transcripts SYT-SSX1 and SYT-SSX2 are believed to function as aberrant transcriptional regulators. The prognostic significance of these alternative forms of the SYT-SSX fusion gene and the relationship of these fusion transcripts and synovial sarcoma tumor morphology (monophasic versus biphasic subtype) were examined in 45 patients with synovial sarcoma.[92] There was a significant correlation ($P = 0.003$) between histologic subtype and fusion transcript type; all 12 biphasic synovial sarcomas had an SYT-SSX1 fusion transcript, whereas 17 (52%) of 33 monophasic tumors were positive for SYT-SSX1. Moreover the presence of the SYT-SSX1 transcript was an independent adverse prognostic factor for metastasis-free survival. Thus

SYT-SSX fusion transcripts may be used as a diagnostic marker for synovial sarcoma, and transcript subtype should be confirmed as an independent prognostic factor.

Ewing's sarcomas are characterized by a translocation involving chromosomes 22 and 11: t(11;22)(q24;q12).[85] Recent studies have evaluated the prognostic significance of transcripts produced by the fusion of the EWS and FL11 genes from chromosomes 22 and 11. The most common EWS-FL11 fusion, designated as type 1, is found in 65% of Ewing's sarcomas.[163,164] Two groups have demonstrated that type 1 EWS-FL11 fusion transcripts are associated with a more favorable prognosis.[90,91] De Alava and colleagues[91] have demonstrated that the prognostic significance of type 1 EWS-FL11 fusion transcripts is independent of tumor site, stage, and size. However, these observations were made with a short follow-up (median 26 months; range, 1 to 140 months), and thus additional studies and longer follow-up are needed to further substantiate these interesting observations. The biologic basis for these observations is unknown. Additional studies that examine the relationship between EWS-FL11 transcript subtype and proliferative rate, apoptosis, and response to treatment are warranted.

Although specific cellular and molecular parameters have been identified as having independent prognostic significance, there is presently no consensus on how specific molecular prognostic factors should be utilized in clinical practice. Until more data are available, molecular prognostic factors proven to be of prognostic significance (e.g., Ki-67) should be considered for inclusion as stratification criteria in clinical trials.

Prognostic Factors as Therapeutic Targets

The prognosis of gastrointestinal stromal tumors (GISTs) is poor,[165] and these tumors rarely respond to conventional systemic chemotherapy. One of the more exciting discoveries in GIST research in recent years is targeted molecular therapy, which will be discussed later in the chapter. The proto-oncogene c-Kit is the cellular homologue of the oncogene v-Kit (a feline sarcoma virus). c-Kit encodes a transmembrane tyrosine kinase receptor that is structurally similar to platelet-derived growth factor and provides selective targets of key aberrations in the molecular signaling implicated in the pathogenesis of GISTs and other tumors (e.g., dermatofibrosarcoma protuberans or DFSP). An interesting additional feature of c-Kit expression in GIST is that different types and locations of mutations in c-Kit appear independently significant for predicting disease-free survival irrespective of treatment with kinase receptor inhibitors.[166] CD117 expression was uniformly evident in a recent study of nonimatinib-treated GIST cases.[74,166] Of interest, c-Kit was highly phosphorylated in all cases, even in those few that lacked demonstrable sequence mutations.[74] The c-Kit mutations that were seen were located in exon 11 (juxtamembrane domain, seen in 71% of tumors), exon 9 (the extracellular region, 13%), exon 13 (first lobe of the split-kinase domain, 4%), and exon 17 (phosphotransferase domain, 4%). The subset of patients with exon 11 mutations resulting in point single amino acid substitutions

(i.e., missense codon mutations) fared much better than did patients with deletion/insertion mutations of exon 11 (5-year recurrence free survival rate of 89% ± 11% versus 37% ± 10%, respectively). A potential explanation for this finding is that exon 11 missense mutations are detected in lower-grade, favorable outcome GISTs.[166] While it is conceivable that the type of mutation is a surrogate for the behavior of a GIST, however, it is also plausible that the type of mutation represents the initial pathogenetic mechanism, making it a true prognostic marker and target. Finally, in vitro studies suggest that GISTs with regulatory-region KIT mutations are more likely to respond to imatinib than are GISTs with enzymatic-region mutations.[167]

Predicting Individual Prognosis

Kattan and colleagues have recently observed that information that is appropriate for researchers is not as helpful for patients with cancer who must plan in a different way for the future.[168] Patients' main preoccupation is to obtain a predicted probability of individual (i.e., personal) survival unencumbered by specific knowledge of prognostic factors, relative risk, or the risk group in which he/she may belong. Kattan and colleagues have constructed and validated a nomogram to predict the probability of 12-year sarcoma-specific death based on a prospective series of patients (Fig. 96-8).[168] This tool is useful for individual patient counseling, follow-up scheduling, and clinical trial eligibility assessment and is further facilitated by being also available for personal handheld computer devices. This sarcoma-specific computer application is available at www.nomograms.org.

TREATMENT OF LOCALIZED PRIMARY SOFT TISSUE SARCOMA

Surgery

Limb-Sparing Surgery versus Amputation

Surgical resection remains the cornerstone of therapy for localized soft tissue sarcoma, and the prototypical situations concern the management of lesions arising in the extremity, the most common anatomic site. Over the past 20 years, there has been a marked decline in the rate of amputation as the primary therapy for extremity soft tissue sarcoma. With the widespread application of multimodality treatment strategies, less than 10% of patients presently undergo amputation.[169,170] The current use of limb-sparing multimodality treatment approaches for patients with extremity sarcoma is largely based on a randomized prospective study from the U.S. NCI in which patients with extremity sarcomas amenable to limb-sparing surgery were randomized to receive amputation or limb-sparing surgery with postoperative radiotherapy.[171,172] Both arms of this trial included postoperative chemotherapy with doxorubicin, cyclophosphamide, and methotrexate. With more than 9 years of follow-up evaluation, 5 (19%) of 27 patients randomly assigned to receive limb-sparing surgery and postopera-

Figure 96-8. Postoperative nomogram for 12-year sarcoma-specific death risk. Fibro, fibrosarcoma; GR, grade; Leiomyo, leiomyosarcoma; Lipo, liposarcoma; MFH, malignant fibrous histiocytoma; MPNT, malignant peripheral nerve sheath tumor; SSD, sarcoma-specific death. (Reproduced with permission from Kattan M: Statistical prediction models, artificial neural networks, and the sophism "I am a patient, not a statistic." J Clin Oncol 2002;20:885.)

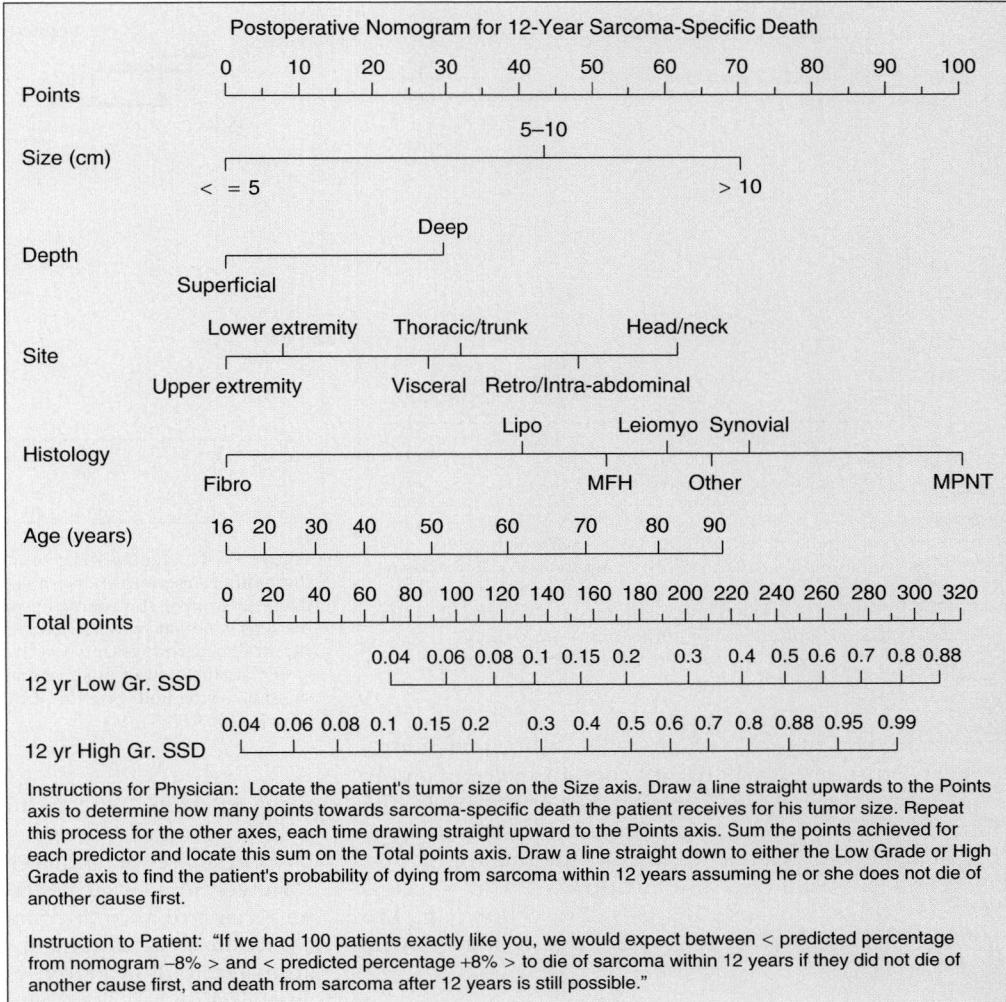

tive radiation with chemotherapy had local recurrences, as compared to 1 (6%) of 17 patients in the amputation plus chemotherapy arm ($P = 0.22$) (Fig. 96-9).[172] The disease-free survival rate was 63% for limb-sparing surgery versus 71% for amputation ($P = 0.52$) (Fig. 96-10), and the overall survival rate was 70% for limb-sparing surgery versus 71% for amputation ($P = 0.97$). This study established that for patients for whom limb-sparing surgery is an option, a multimodality approach employing limb-sparing surgery combined with postoperative radiotherapy yields disease-related survival rates comparable to those for amputation while simultaneously preserving a functional extremity.

Currently, at least 90% of patients with localized extremity sarcomas can undergo limb-sparing procedures.[169,173] Most surgeons consider definite major vascular, bony, or nerve involvement as relative indications for amputation. Complex en bloc bone, vascular, and nerve resections with interposition grafting can be undertaken, but the associated morbidity is high. Therefore for a few patients with critical involvement of major bony or neurovascular structures, amputation remains the only surgical option but offers the prospect of prompt rehabilitation with excellent local control and survival.[172]

Completeness of Resection
Satisfactory local resection involves resection of the primary tumor with a margin of normal tissue around the lesion. The width of the margin should differ depending upon whether adjuvant radiotherapy is used or not. It is clear that dissection along the tumor pseudocapsule (enucleation) is associated with local recurrence rates ranging between 33% and 63%.[174-176] Wide local excision with a margin of normal tissue around the lesion is associated with local recurrence rates in the range of 10% to 31% as noted in the control arms (surgery alone) of the randomized trials evaluating postoperative radiotherapy.[177,178] Unlike for malignant melanoma, a disease for which there are randomized data to address adequate margin size, there are no comparable data available to define what constitutes a satisfactory gross resection margin for a sarcoma. In general every effort should be made to achieve a wide margin (2 cm is a frequently cited arbitrary choice) around the tumor mass, except in the

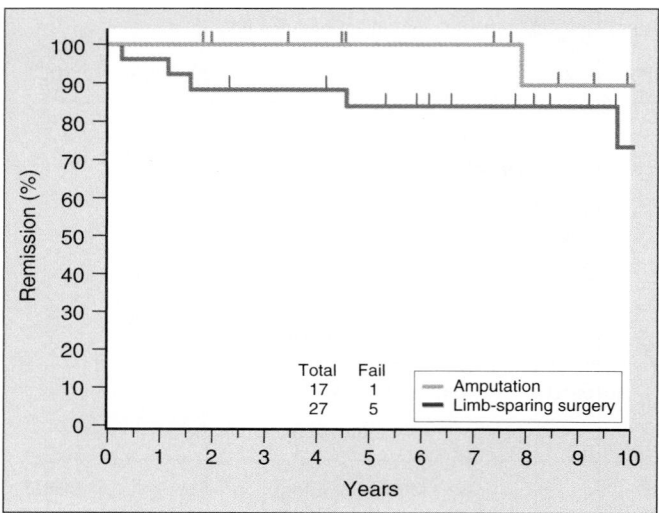

Figure 96-9. Local recurrence rates in patients with high-grade extremity sarcomas randomized to receive amputation or limb-sparing surgery. All patients were treated with adjuvant chemotherapy using doxorubicin, cyclophosphamide, and methotrexate. Median follow-up > 9 years; P = 0.22. (Reprinted with permission from Yang JC, Rosenberg SA: Surgery for adult patients with soft tissue sarcomas. Semin Oncol 1989;16:289.)

immediate vicinity of functionally important neurovascular structures, where, in the absence of frank neoplastic involvement, dissection is performed in the immediate perineural or perivascular tissue planes. The 2-cm choice is unnecessary if radiotherapy is also used since substantial modification of the surgical approach with much closer margins of resection (e.g., 1 to 2 mm) is made possible, and even large lesions can be

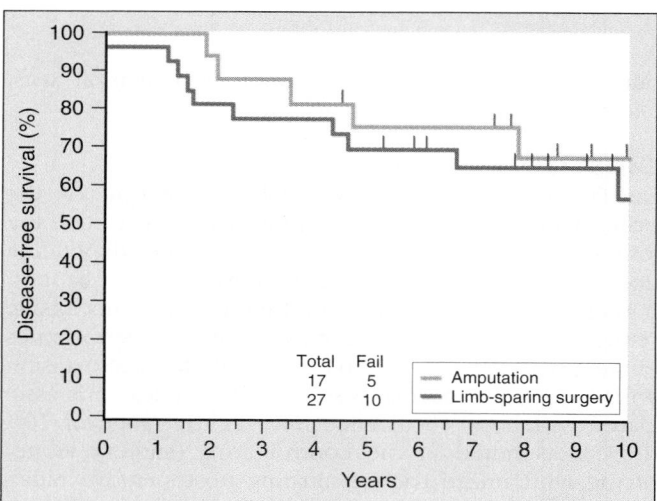

Figure 96-10. Disease-free survival rates for patients with high-grade extremity sarcomas randomized to receive amputation or limb-sparing surgery. All patients were treated with adjuvant chemotherapy using doxorubicin, cyclophosphamide, and methotrexate. Median follow-up > 9 years; P = 0.52. (Reprinted with permission from Yang JC, Rosenberg SA: Surgery for adult patients with soft tissue sarcomas. Semin Oncol 1989;16:289.)

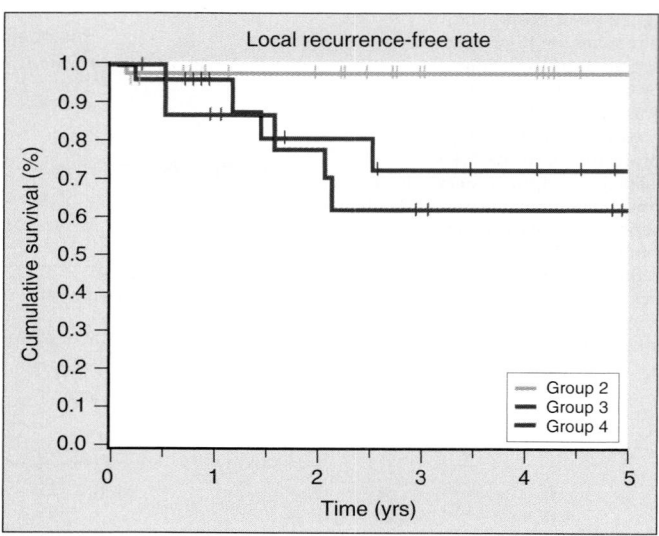

Figure 96-11. Kaplan-Meier estimate for local recurrence-free rate for three different groups of positive margin categories (see text for details). Group 1 (low-grade liposarcoma with positive resection margins is not shown). Tick marks represent censored cases. (Reproduced with permission from Gerrand CH, Wunder JS, Kandel RA, et al: Classification of positive margins after resection of soft-tissue sarcoma of the limb predicts the risk of local recurrence. J Bone Joint Surg Br 2001;83:1149.)

managed conservatively in that setting. Technical details of the surgical approach to extremity sarcomas are beyond the scope of this chapter but are comprehensively reviewed in a surgical atlas.[179] At the same time it is also important to bear in mind that involved (i.e., positive) resection margins remain an adverse finding even when adjuvant radiotherapy is used, notwithstanding the amelioration of risk that radiation treatment provides. Data from Memorial Sloan-Kettering Hospital, Princess Margaret Hospital, and Massachusetts General Hospital suggest an additional absolute reduction of local control of approximately 10% to 15% for patients with positive margins compared to those with microscopically negative surgical margins.[179-182]

In considering the existing outcome data, it is important to bear in mind that these data consider the rubric "positive margins" in a uniform way, although in reality this is unlikely to be the case. In fact, positive resection margins have different causes. One is oncologically inadequate surgery where positive resection margins may have been avoidable in another surgeon's hands. When this is the case, microscopically positive surgical margins can be considered a technical failure. Alternatively, positive resection margins may arise in anatomically adverse presentations where locally advanced disease challenges the goals of conservative resection from the outset. In another study from the Princess Margaret Hospital, Gerrand and colleagues evaluated the type of microscopically positive margin as a prognostic factor and defined four groups in this setting.[183] Patients with low-grade liposarcomas and microscopically positive surgical margins (group 1) have a low risk of local failure (4.2%), as do those in whom a positive margin is anticipated before surgery in order to preserve critical structures and radiotherapy is given to sterilize the minimal residual disease (group 2). However, two categories of positive margins are associated with a higher risk of local recurrence: (1) patients who present after prereferral unplanned excision and who have a positive margin on subsequent reexcision (group 3); and (2) those with unanticipated positive margins occurring during primary sarcoma resection (group 4) (Fig. 96-11). For group 3, an "unplanned excision" is defined as an excisional biopsy or resection carried out without adequate preoperative staging or consideration of the need to remove normal tissue around tumor, an adverse feature reported by the same authors previously.[184] These data appear to support the premise that, provided adjuvant radiotherapy is administered, a very small amount of residual disease resulting from a "planned" positive margin at the site of a critical anatomic structure (group 2, local recurrence rate of 3.6% and 95% confidence interval 0 to 10.4) is not associated with the same deleterious risk that occurs with a positive margin that follows major contamination due to "shell out" intralesional surgery (group 3, local recurrence rate of 31.6% and 95% confidence intervals 10.7 to 52.5) or inadvertent contamination of the wound (group 4, local recurrence rate of 37.5% and 95% confidence interval 13.8 to 61.2).[183] These data seem particularly relevant to anatomic sites where achievement of adequate resection margins is a perennial problem, such as the head and neck, as evidenced by recent results from a prospective series where the outcome approaches that of extremity and body wall sarcomas.[185] We would caution, however, that such results are probably not attainable without a defined management protocol and joint multidisciplinary assessment before treatment is undertaken since there exist issues that merit discussion at the individual case level (e.g., the complex relationship between tissues to be resected and reconstructed, and the radiotherapy volumes and doses, all of which can influence each other in the decision algorithm).

Lymph Node Dissection

Given the low (2% to 3%) prevalence of lymph node metastasis in adults with sarcomas,[102,103] there is no role for routine regional lymph node dissection. Patients with angiosarcoma, embryonal rhabdomyosarcoma, and epithelioid histiotypes have an increased incidence of lymph node metastasis and should be carefully examined for adenopathy. Therapeutic lymph node dissection (curative) results in a 34% actuarial survival rate,[102] and thus the rare patients with regional nodal involvement who have no evidence of extranodal disease should undergo therapeutic lymphadenectomy. Patients with adverse features at the time of dissection (i.e., extracapsular extension beyond the lymph nodes into perinodal fat, or positive or doubtful margins on the neurovascular bundle) or where treatment into the next grossly uninvolved lymph node echelon is not feasible with surgery should also be considered for additional adjuvant nodal irradiation. The principles underlying this approach have recently been outlined.[186]

Surgery Alone

Although the majority of patients with extremity soft tissue sarcoma should be treated with preoperative or postoperative radiotherapy, recent reports suggest that concomitant radiotherapy may not be required for selected patients with completely resected, small, primary soft tissue sarcomas (Table 96-7).[187-190] Rydholm and colleagues have reported their experience with 70 patients with subcutaneous or intramuscular extremity sarcomas treated with wide surgical resection and microscopic assessment of surgical margins.[189] Negative histologic margins were obtained for 32 of 40 subcutaneous and 24 of 30 intramuscular tumors. The 56 patients with microscopically negative margins received no postoperative radiotherapy, yet only 4 (7%) developed local recurrence. A study from Brigham and Women's Hospital reported similar results for a selected group of 74 patients with primary extremity STS treated by surgery without radiotherapy.[190] The 10-year actuarial local control rate was 93% plus or minus 4%. The absolute gross margin was a significant predictor of local recurrence; patients with a close gross margin of less than 1 cm had a 10-year local control rate of 87% plus or minus 6% compared to 100% for patients with a closest gross margin of 1 cm or greater ($P = 0.04$). The generally favorable local control rates with surgery alone reported by these and other[187,191]

TABLE 96-7

Results of Surgery Alone for Selected Patients with Soft Tissue Sarcoma

FIRST AUTHOR	INSTITUTION	NO. OF PATIENTS	SELECTION CRITERIA	ADJUVANT RADIATION (NO.)	LOCAL RECURRENCE (%)	DISTANT RECURRENCE (%)
Geer[188]	MSKCC	174	T1 size, primary tumor	117	10	5
Rydholm[189]	Lund, Sweden	56	G/M margin negative	0	7	NR
Baldini[190]	BWH	74	T1 size, G/M margin negative	0	7	12
Karakousis[187]	RPCI	116	2 cm G margin	0	10	NR
Fabrizio*	Mayo	34	Not stated	0	15	12

BWH, Brigham and Women's Hospital; G/M, gross/microscopic; Mayo, Mayo Clinic; MSKCC, Memorial Sloan-Kettering Cancer Center; NR, not reported; RPCI, Roswell Park Cancer Institute.
*Fabrizio PL, Stafford SL, Pritchard DJ: Extremity soft-tissue sarcomas selectively treated with surgery alone. Int S Radiat Oncol Biol Phys 2000;48:227.

investigators in these series of highly selected patients are comparable to local recurrence rates observed for more heterogeneous patient populations treated with conventional multimodality therapy incorporating preoperative or postoperative radiotherapy (Table 96-8).[66,177,192-198] These data support the hypothesis that selected patients with small, primary soft tissue sarcomas can be treated with surgical resection alone without preoperative or postoperative radiotherapy.

It is difficult to define the precise selection criteria that should be used to identify patients with primary sarcoma who can safely undergo treatment by surgery without radiotherapy. Most investigators have limited this approach to patients with carefully selected T1 tumors that can be resected with clear margins (see Table 96-7). In contrast, Karakousis and colleagues did not consider absolute tumor size but instead utilized surgical resection alone for all patients in whom a minimum intracompartmental margin of 2 cm could be maintained circumferentially, irrespective of tumor size.[187] Karakousis and colleagues recently updated the results for high-grade STS of the policy of limiting the use of postoperative radiation treatment for tumors resected with positive or "narrow" (less than 2 cm) resection margins.[199] This approach has yielded useful data because the consistent application of this treatment approach resulted in a local recurrence rate of 19% with "wide" margin surgery alone compared to 24% after "narrow" margin surgery and adjuvant radiotherapy.[199] Although the results provide some clarity about the 2 cm or greater margin benchmark, it would be useful to also have similar data from other groups for a variety of margin widths to draw conclusions about when it is safe to withhold radiotherapy. Moreover the authors acknowledge the potential to treat a greater proportion of cases with radiotherapy and lower the 19% local recurrence rate in some of those "favorable cases" currently treated with surgery alone by widening the indication for adjuvant radiotherapy in a proportion of these patients.[199] This view would certainly be consistent with contemporary observations such as the local

recurrence rate of 7% in cases undergoing combined modality treatment such as those in the recent Canadian randomized trial (see section "Preoperative or Postoperative Radiotherapy").[200]

Factors other than anatomic location, tumor size, and the feasibility of achieving an R0 resection (macroscopically and microscopically complete) should be considered when selecting patients for treatment by surgery alone. For example, the issue of whether the patient has had a prior "unplanned" excision (referred to earlier) is important. At the Princess Margaret Hospital, a significantly higher rate of local recurrence was apparent in patients who were treated after unplanned excision on the outside compared to patients who received their treatment at their institution (22% versus 7%, $P = 0.03$).[184] It is important to remember that unplanned excision is very common in the community setting when small soft tissue lesions are often excised without image guidance under the presumption that they are benign. Therefore while it is reasonable to attempt a reexcision if considered feasible, patients who have undergone unplanned excision should also be strongly considered for adjuvant radiation.

Preoperative or Postoperative Radiotherapy

Conservative (limb-sparing) surgery and radiotherapy have been combined to optimize local control for patients with localized soft tissue sarcoma. Radiotherapy can be administered preoperatively,[192-194,201,202] postoperatively,[196,203,204] or by interstitial techniques (brachytherapy).[66,195,205-209]

Local Control
Data from two randomized controlled trials (RCTs)[71,177] have confirmed earlier retrospective reports suggesting that surgery combined with radiotherapy results in superior local control compared to surgery alone.[193,196,198] Yang and colleagues from the NCI recently reported on a RCT of postoperative external-beam radiotherapy

TABLE 96-8

Local Control with Surgery and Radiotherapy for Localized Soft Tissue Sarcoma

RADIOTHERAPY APPROACH	FIRST AUTHOR	RADIATION DOSE (GY)	STUDY DESIGN	NO. OF PATIENTS	LOCAL FAILURE (%)	SUBSET
Preoperative EBRT	Suit[192]	50–56	Retrospective	89	17	
	Barkley[193]	50	Retrospective	110	10	
	Brant[194]	50.4	Retrospective	58	9	
	O'Sullivan[200]	50	RCT	94	7	
Brachytherapy	Pisters[182]	42–45	RCT	119	9	(high-grade)
				45	23	(low-grade)
Postoperative EBRT	Lindberg[196]	60–75	Retrospective	300	22	
	Karakousis[197]	45–60	Retrospective	53	14	
	Suit[192]	60–68	Retrospective	131	12	
	Yang[177]	45+18	RCT	91	0	(high-grade)
				50	5	(low-grade)
	O'Sullivan[200]		RCT	96	7	

EBRT, external beam radiotherapy; RCT, randomized controlled trial.
Randomized controlled trials and selected nonrandomized retrospective series.

(EBRT).[177] One hundred forty-one patients with localized extremity soft tissue sarcomas amenable to limb-sparing resection were randomly assigned to receive post-operative EBRT or no radiotherapy. All patients with high-grade lesions received postoperative chemotherapy. In the subset of 91 patients with high-grade lesions, there have been no local recurrences noted in the 44 patients who received postoperative radiotherapy (with chemotherapy) versus 9 local recurrences (19%) in the 47 patients who received postoperative chemotherapy alone ($P = 0.0003$). In the 50 patients with low-grade sarcomas, 1 (4%) of 26 patients who received adjuvant radiotherapy has had a local recurrence versus 8 (33%) of 24 patients treated by surgical resection alone ($P = 0.016$). However, there was no improvement in survival noted with adjuvant radiotherapy in the entire cohort of patients or in any subgroup.

The second RCT of postoperative radiotherapy was conducted at Memorial Sloan-Kettering Cancer Center, where investigators studied adjuvant brachytherapy for patients with extremity and superficial trunk soft tissue sarcomas.[182] One hundred sixty-four patients with extremity or superficial trunk soft tissue sarcomas were randomly assigned to receive adjuvant brachytherapy (42 to 45 Gy with an iridium-192 implant) or no postoperative radiotherapy after complete resection of their sarcomas. Randomization took place in the operating room after gross total resection thereby limiting the potential bias that might influence the extent of surgical resection in a comparative trial. Sixty-eight of 119 patients with high-grade tumors also received chemotherapy. With a median follow-up of 76 months, 5-year actuarial local control rates were significantly better in the group treated with adjuvant brachytherapy (82%) than in those who received surgery alone (69%). Subset analysis demonstrated that the local control advantage of brachytherapy was confined to patients with high-grade lesions, for whom the 5-year local control rate was 89% (versus 66% in the surgery-only group) (Fig. 96-12). Patients with low-grade soft tissue sarcomas did not appear to experience the same local control benefit with adjuvant brachytherapy.[182,209] As

noted in the NCI RCT,[177] the improvement in local control did not translate into any detectable survival difference between the brachytherapy and no-brachytherapy arms of the trial.

Local failure rates with combined-modality regimens incorporating surgery and radiotherapy are generally less than 15% (see Table 96-8). Despite theoretical advantages that may favor preoperative radiation, brachytherapy, or postoperative radiation, there does not appear to be a major difference in local control rates among these radiation techniques, although at present data comparing the approaches are sparse.

Relationship Between Local Control and Survival
Whether local control impacts overall survival for patients with soft tissue sarcoma remains unclear and highly controversial.[210-214] Only an adequately powered prospective randomized trial can assess the precise nature of any relationship between local control and overall survival. Three RCTs have evaluated local control and survival in the context of defining treatment approaches for soft tissue sarcoma. In a randomized trial of amputation versus conservative surgery plus radiation from the NCI, local recurrence rates were 19% in the limb-sparing arm versus 6% in the amputation arm ($P = 0.022$).[171,172] Despite this, overall survival rates were equivalent at 70% for limb-sparing surgery and 71% for amputation ($P = 0.97$). In the randomized trials of postoperative radiotherapy,[177,182] the improvement in local control noted in patients treated with surgery plus radiotherapy did not translate into any detectable survival advantage. Thus none of the currently available data from prospective RCTs support the hypothesis that better local control enhances survival in patients with sarcoma. Methodologically, the available trials are problematic for this issue because the outcome of interest (i.e., a difference in survival consequent on a differential in local control) would require a prohibitively large sample size. Thus it is most improbable for these trials to be capable of demonstrating an effect with their modest sample sizes intended for evaluation of different outcomes. Indeed it is most unlikely if even a meta-analysis

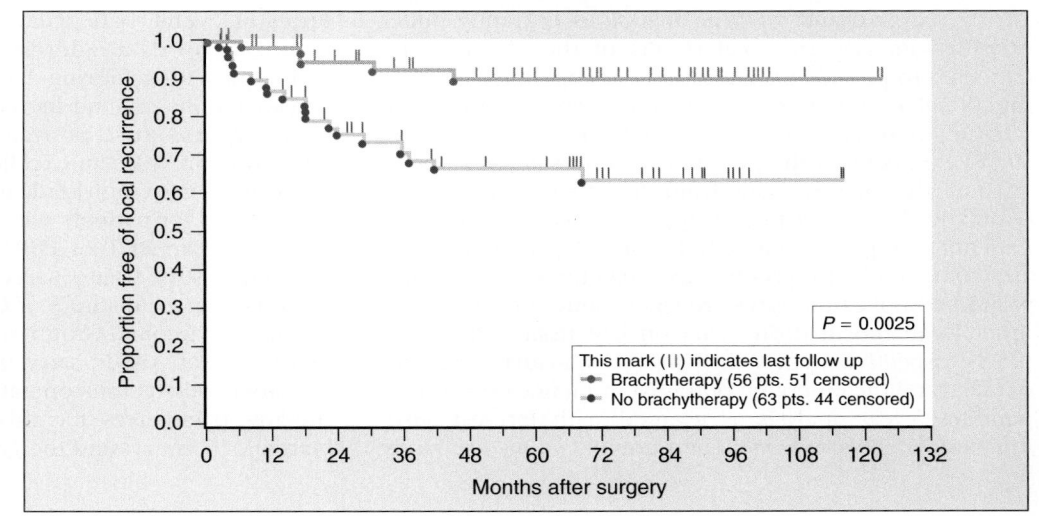

Figure 96-12. Local recurrence-free survival in patients with high-grade sarcoma treated in the Memorial Sloan-Kettering Cancer Center randomized trial of postoperative brachytherapy versus surgery alone. A statistically significant difference was noted in local recurrence-free survival with brachytherapy. $P = 0.0025$. (Reprinted with permission from Pisters PW, Harrison LB, Leung DH, et al: Long-term results of a prospective randomized trial of adjuvant brachytherapy in soft tissue sarcoma. J Clin Oncol 1996;14:859.)

of the trials could demonstrate this. Furthermore data from nonrandomized studies support the concept that there is little, if any, relationship between local control and survival. In a recent series from Sweden, the outcome of patients who were treated with an inadequate excision was compared with that of patients who had an adequate operation.[213] Local recurrence was 3.5 times more common after inadequate excision, but there was no difference in the incidence or timing of distant metastases. The power of the RCTs reported so far to detect a difference in survival is relatively small, and a large number of patients may be required to demonstrate that prevention of local recurrence impacts survival.[211] Stotter and colleagues have argued that local recurrence is a time-dependent variable and should be considered as such in multivariate studies.[210] Analysis in this fashion of the data from a nonrandomized study demonstrates a statistically significant relationship between local control and survival. Other retrospective analyses have yielded similar conclusions.[215,216]

For a more detailed description of the methodological problems associated with time-dependent variables and the use of surrogate end points that emerge after the initial sarcoma treatment, the reader is referred elsewhere.[217] In this context, it is clearly important to distinguish between the well-defined adverse prognostic impact of subsequent local recurrence on survival[106,214,218] and the unproven positive effect of improved local control (i.e., prevention of local recurrence with improved local therapy) on survival. The former phenomenon may be a manifestation of more aggressive tumor biology, that is, biologically more aggressive lesions may recur locally and metastasize more frequently.

Treatment Sequencing: Preoperative versus Postoperative Treatment

Of further interest, an improvement in overall survival (crude rate of 85% versus 72% in favor of postoperative radiotherapy, $P = 0.0481$) has emerged and was only partially explained by increased deaths in the postoperative arm unrelated to sarcoma (Fig. 96-13).[200] This observation is of obvious oncologic interest. Longer follow-up is clearly required and a 5-year analysis is currently under way. In summary, the final results of the SR2 trial are expected to provide insight into the comparative efficacy, functional outcome, economic costs, and complication rates of these two options for EBRT, and potentially on survival outcome if the preliminary results are sustained.

Until the mature data from the Canadian Sarcoma Group RCT are available, it appears reasonable to treat patients with postoperative EBRT since local control rates are comparable to preoperative techniques but major wound complication rates are significantly lower. On the other hand the maturing data on late tissue effects for these respective approaches in the Canadian trial are salutary, and the emerging potential influence on survival, pending 5-year analysis, is awaited with interest. Also, in anatomic sites where wound complications are rarely

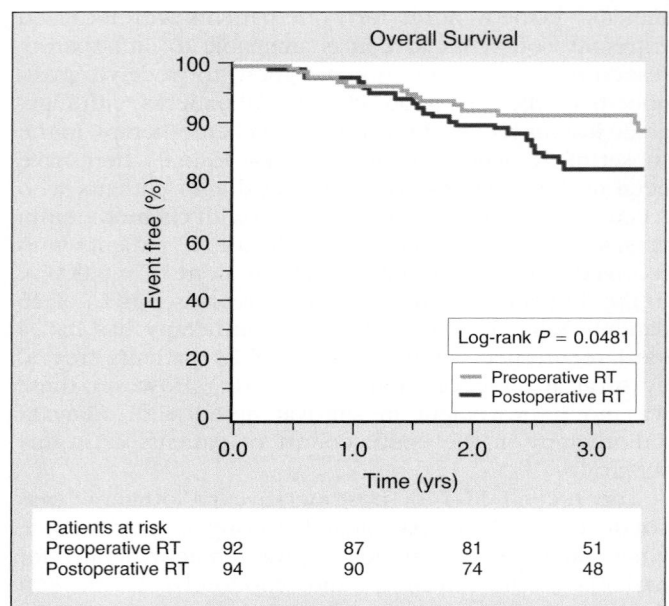

Figure 96-13. Actuarial probability of overall survival for preoperative versus postoperative radiotherapy in extremity soft tissue sarcoma. (Reproduced with permission from O'Sullivan B, Davis AM, Turcotte R, et al: Preoperative versus postoperative radiotherapy in soft-tissue sarcoma of the limbs: A randomised trial. Lancet 2002;359:2235.)

seen (i.e., the upper extremity) the rationale for wound complication avoidance as a reason to favor the use of postoperative radiotherapy is not as sound. In particular the obvious advantage to preoperative radiotherapy in the proximal arms and shoulder is apparent where avoidance of large volume and higher dose irradiation that may treat the lung or brachial plexus can be achieved. These principles are also reasonable in the head and neck based on the recent Princess Margaret Hospital data.[185]

On the other hand, with brachytherapy, the patient's entire local treatment (surgery plus radiation) can be completed in 10 to 14 days. This has significant cost advantages[219] and also has significant implications in terms of overall patient convenience. In the absence of comparative data addressing the efficacy of these techniques in achieving local control, these additional considerations assume increased importance. Where the necessary expertise is available for brachytherapy, this technique provides an excellent, cost-effective alternative for patients with high-grade lesions. Brachytherapy should not be used for patients with low-grade sarcomas.[209]

Recently, an RCT of EBRT for patients with localized extremity soft tissue sarcoma was reported by the National Cancer Institute of Canada Clinical Trials Group/Canadian Sarcoma Group in which 190 patients with extremity soft tissue sarcoma were randomized to preoperative versus postoperative radiation.[200] The radiotherapy parameters for this protocol required a field margin of 5 cm around the gross tumor volume (GTV) for the initial phase of treatment (i.e., treatment to 50 Gy in 25 fractions) and this generally included any peritumoral edema seen on MRI, irrespective of grade or size of the tumor. Subsequently, a reduced volume field was treated to a total combined dose of 66 Gy in all postoperative cases and in those preoperative patients where the resection margins were involved.

The results of this trial are complex because the primary end point that powered the trial, and hence its sample size, was the cumulative incidence of acute wound complications 120 days after protocol surgery in both arms of the study. Nevertheless the local control rates after 3.3 years of median follow-up are identical in both arms of the study (7%).

Wound Complication Rates and Post-treatment Function

The results of the Canadian RCT may provide insight into the comparative efficacy, functional outcome, economic costs, and complication rates of pre- and postoperative treatment sequencing for EBRT. In the absence of a clear local control advantage to any specific radiation technique, clinicians have considered other factors in formulating standards of care. Such factors have included wound complication rates, financial costs, patient convenience, health-related quality of life and physical function, radiotherapy toxicity, and perhaps even overall survival.

It is clear that while field size and radiation dose may be minimized with preoperative radiotherapy,[220] major wound complications after preoperative radiotherapy and surgery have been reported to be in the 20% to 35% range.[221,222] In the Canadian Sarcoma Group RCT, wound complications were defined as secondary wound surgery, hospital admission for wound care, deep packing, or prolonged dressings within 120 days after tumor resection. By these criteria, preoperative radiation had a significantly higher rate (35% versus 17%, $P = 0.01$) of wound complications than did postoperative EBRT. Of note, the risk was confined to the lower extremity.[200]

Taken in isolation, the wound complication fact alone can be expected to cause some groups to continue to favor postoperative radiotherapy though this may change as data has now emerged from the Canadian RCT that late tissue outcomes strongly favor the preoperative approach and a putative survival advantage needs to await mature follow-up.[223] Thus the radiotherapy toxicity rates after 2 years differed between the arms of the study. The rates of grade 2 or greater fibrosis and edema were significantly higher in the postoperative arm compared to preoperative radiotherapy, and were independently associated with the larger irradiation volumes and doses used in postoperative radiotherapy.[223] Short-term functional outcome in the SR2 trial has also been reported and continues to be collected prospectively.[224] Two validated instruments—the Toronto Extremity Salvage Score (TESS) and the Short Form-36 quality of life instrument (SF-36)—were applied, as was the observer-based Musculoskeletal Tumor Society Rating Scale (MSTS).[224] Patients treated with postoperative radiotherapy had better function with higher MSTS, TESS, and SF-36 bodily pain scores at 6 weeks after surgery than did those treated with preoperative radiation, but there were no differences at later time points up to 1 year. Thus, the timing of radiotherapy has minimal impact on the function of STS patients in the first year after surgery, but thereafter significant factors likely come into play. These include the apparently deteriorating late tissue sequelae caused by larger doses and volumes. Of interest, patients who experience wound complications appear to continue to suffer some impaired function. Further follow-up will be required to assess the ongoing evolution of these competing risks.

Conformal Radiotherapy and Intensity-Modulated Radiotherapy

Soft tissue sarcoma present in virtually any anatomic site and the capacity for unusual presentation is almost limitless. This may result in circumstances in which conventionally delivered radiotherapy is impossible due the magnitude of the volume to be treated, uncertainty in defining the target for radiotherapy, or more usually because of the proximity of normal tissues to the intended target volume. While some presentations are extremely problematic (e.g., uncertain targets due to organ mobility or imprecise anatomic issues resulting from poor definition of tumor location related to imaging limitations or inadequate surgical and/or pathological description), others can be addressed by novel methods of radiotherapy delivery. Leading the advances in this field is intensity-modulated radiotherapy (IMRT). IMRT is an advanced form of three-dimensional conformal radiotherapy in which radiation beams are not only shaped at their perimeters, but also include variable intensity across the profiles of the beams. This permits the creation of exquisite conformation of dose to targets of irregular shape while generating high dose gradients between tumor and normal tissues. A full discussion of the potential uses of IMRT in soft tissue sarcoma is beyond the scope of this chapter but is discussed in detail elsewhere.[225] It may be administered preoperatively, postoperatively, or as a sole modality with specific indications. Some applications include its use in lesions adjacent to the spine or critical anatomical structures of the head and neck, and in the retroperitoneum to permit liver avoidance (as well as to permit spinal cord, kidney, and intestinal dose limitation) especially in lesions involving the right upper abdominal quadrant. Avoidance of late toxicity to anatomic structures such as weight-bearing bone at risk for fracture after treatment of extremity sarcomas seems also to be feasible.[226] Although these approaches are promising, their precise contribution and role need to be evaluated.[227]

Conventional Radiotherapy Without Surgery

Radiotherapy alone has been employed as primary therapy for patients with locally advanced, inoperable soft tissue sarcoma and patients who present with stage IV disease. Efforts to use radiation as the primary treatment have demonstrated that high doses (more than 65 Gy) are required to achieve local control rates between 30% and 60%[228,229] and that there appears to be an inverse relationship between tumor size and local control rates. In a series of 35 patients treated with high-dose (>65 Gy) primary radiotherapy, for tumor sizes less than 5 cm, 5 to 10 cm, and larger than 10 cm, the local control rates were 88%, 53%, and 33%, respectively.[230] In general, local control rates with radiation alone are inferior to those after surgery, and thus primary radiation should be reserved for patients who are medically unfit for surgery, have technically unresectable tumors, or refuse surgery as initial therapy. However, some caution is necessary in interpreting such results in a scientifically valid manner. Encumbered with such adverse selection factors, radiotherapy outcome would never be comparable to surgery. Moreover, surgery has the added advantage over radiotherapy alone because its use for locally advanced cases is ordinarily also combined with adjuvant radiotherapy.

Neutron Radiotherapy

Neutron radiotherapy has been emphasized by certain groups because of the lower oxygen enhancement ratio (OER) compared to x-rays and the consequent attractive possibility of overcoming the biological phenomenon that hypoxic cells generally limit the curability of malignancy with x-rays. Additional differences from x-rays are the reduced repair of sublethal and potentially lethal damage. These neutron effects are less vulnerable to the differential radiosensitivities associated with different phases of the cell cycle. It should be apparent that some of these repair phenomena also impact negatively on the tolerance of normal tissues. Neutrons have been employed in a number of pilot studies, primarily in patients with locally advanced disease, with 60 to 70% local control rates.[231-233]

In a recent large series, 220 patients with locally advanced sarcomas were treated with neutron radiotherapy. Ninety-four patients with gross residual disease after resection were treated with neutron therapy alone; among these patients, 27% had major morbidity, 26% had 5-year survival, and 56% had local control. One hundred four patients with microscopically positive margins of resection received a neutron boost dose; they had 7% morbidity, 65% 5-year survival, and 78% local control rates. These results suggest that for patients with gross residual disease, neutron beam radiation may provide improved local control compared to conventional external-beam treatment, but this data should continue to be interpreted with caution when one considers the late tissue sequelae that appear to result from neurton beam radiation use. Comparative studies are needed to define the precise role of neutron beam therapy in the treatment of soft tissue sarcoma. Apart from unresectable disease, it seems unclear where the benefit of neutron therapy may accrue when one considers the exceptionally favorable results of conventional x-ray treatment combined with surgery and the more adverse normal tissue tolerance to neutron therapy.

Adjuvant Chemotherapy

In the past 30 years, improvements in surgical and radiotherapy techniques have led to impressive rates of local control, particularly in extremity STS, with concomitant sparing of normal tissues and preservation of limb and/or organ function. Regrettably, in the same period, much less progress has been made in finding ways to eradicate the micrometastases that are the ultimate cause of death in many individuals presenting with apparently localized soft tissue sarcoma. The discovery that doxorubicin had significant antitumor activity against adult STS prompted the initiation of multiple RCTs during the period 1973 to 1990 to evaluate the benefit of doxorubicin alone or in combination with other agents after the completion of local treatment. However, most of these trials were too small to detect moderate treatment effects reliably.

The statistical technique of meta-analysis may overcome the problem of inadequate power of small RCTs,

TABLE 96-9

Adjuvant Doxorubicin-Based Chemotherapy for Localized STS: Sarcoma Meta-Analysis Collaboration Results

SURVIVAL OUTCOME	NO. OF TRIALS	NO. OF PATIENTS	HAZARD RATIO (95% CI)	P VALUE	10-YEAR SURVIVAL BENEFIT (%)
Overall, All patients	14	1544	0.89 (0.76–1.03)	0.12	4
Overall, Extremity only	12	886	0.80 (NA)	0.029	7
Recurrence-free	14	1366	0.75 (0.64–0.87)	0.0001	10
Local recurrence-free	13	1315	0.73 (0.56–0.94)	0.016	6
Metastasis-free	13	1315	0.70 (0.57–0.85)	0.0003	10

Adapted from Tierney JF: Adjuvant chemotherapy for localised resectable soft-tissue sarcoma of adults: Meta-analysis of individual data. Lancet 1997;350:1647.

TABLE 96-10

	Post 1992 Randomized Controlled Trials of Adjuvant Chemotherapy versus Observation in STS						
						SURVIVAL	
STUDY	**CHEMOTHERAPY REGIMEN**	**NO. OF PATIENTS**	**DISEASE SITES**	**FOLLOW-UP**		**RFS**	**OS**
Italian Cooperative*[237]	Epirubicin + Ifosfamide + G-GSF (×5)	53	Limb (grade III > 5 cm)	59 mos (median)		48 mos	75 mos
	Control	51				16 mos	46 mos
						p=0.04	p=0.03
Australian Cooperative[†238]	Ifosfamide + Doxorubicin + Dacarbazine (IFADIC) + G-CSF ×6	31	Limb 47, Trunk 12 (grade II/III)	41 mos (mean)		77%	NR
	Control	28				57%	NR
						p=0.1	p=0.4

G-CSF, granulocyte colony stimulating factor; mos, months; NR, not reported at defined follow-up time; OS, overall survival; RFS, recurrence-free survival.
*Median recurrence-free plus overall survival
[†](1) comparison % recurrence-free plus overall survival after mean observation period 41 (8–84) mos. (2) overall survival plotted but actuarial results not reported at defined follow-up time(s).
Outcome data provided in original papers.

and meta-analyses based on individual patient data (IPDMA) can minimize other potential biases (e.g., exclusion of unpublished trials, variable follow-up, postrandomization exclusions, and differing definition of end points) inherent in analyses limited to published results. In 1997, the Sarcoma Meta-Analysis Collaboration (SMAC) published an IPDMA of outcomes for 1568 soft tissue sarcoma patients included in 14 RCTs that completed accrual by December 1992.[234] As outlined in Table 96-9, significant improvements were found in local and distant relapse-free intervals and recurrence-free survival, but these improvements did not translate into a significant overall survival benefit, except in the subgroup of patients with limb extremity sarcomas.

When interpreting the SMAC results, it is instructive to compare them with the IPDMAs that have provided conclusive evidence of the benefits of adjuvant chemotherapy and hormone therapy in early breast cancer.[235,236] In contrast with the approximately 1500 patients included in the SMAC IPDMA, the Early Breast Cancer Collaborative Trials Group identified 47 trials that recruited 18,000 patients for comparisons of adjuvant chemotherapy versus no adjuvant chemotherapy. The power of large numbers, even in the setting of meta-analysis, is self-evident. Compounding the problem of small numbers of soft tissue sarcoma cases, STSs as a group show marked heterogeneity in pathology and site of origin; this is much less evident in breast cancer. For example, it has been suggested that in the SMAC meta-analysis, chemotherapy benefits for extremity (57% of total) and high-grade STSs were obscured by inclusion of sarcomas at other locations (head, neck, trunk, and uterus) and those of low (5%) or unknown grade (28%). Another point of contrast with breast cancer is the relative paucity of drugs active against soft tissue sarcoma. Only two agents (doxorubicin and ifosfamide) have reproducibly produced overall response rates exceeding 20% in patients with advanced disease. This provides limited opportunity to exploit the potential

advantages of combination chemotherapy. Of the 14 trials included in the SMAC meta-analysis, 6 used doxorubicin alone, and the remaining 8 were trials of combination chemotherapy. Only one unpublished soft tissue sarcoma trial (29 patients) examined the combination of doxorubicin with ifosfamide. Not surprisingly, the SMAC analysis was not able to demonstrate that combination chemotherapy had a superior effect on treatment outcomes.

Since the SMAC meta-analysis, full reports have been published on two additional RCTs (Table 96-10) examining high-dose anthracycline and ifosfamide-based regimens supported by granulocyte colony-stimulating factor (G-CSF). In the Italian Cooperative Group study,[237] accrual was terminated, based on an early stopping rule, after half the planned number of patients had been recruited. The median recurrence-free survival and overall survival (see Table 96-10) were significantly better for the chemotherapy group, but a high cumulative incidence of late distant relapses was noted (2 year: 28% versus 45%, $P = 0.08$; 4 year: 44% versus 45%, $P = 0.94$ for chemotherapy versus control groups, respectively), although 4-year overall survival remained better for the chemotherapy group (69% versus 50%, $P = 0.04$). Longer follow-up is needed to document whether there will be a persistent survival advantage in this trial. With high-grade STS, most distant relapses will occur within 5 years. Improved treatments and supportive care may extend survival for patients with metastasis, and there may be more salvage options for patients who have not already received chemotherapy; thus patients may die at different rates in the two arms of clinical trials that compare local treatment plus chemotherapy to local treatment alone.

The authors of the second study, a prospective randomized feasibility trial, concluded that a regimen of six cycles of ifosfamide, doxorubicin, and dacarbazine given concurrently with postoperative hyperfractionated radiotherapy (during cycles 3 and 4 when doxorubicin was omitted from the regimen) was manageable and tolerable but did not translate into significant benefits in recurrence-free survival ($P = 0.1$ versus control arm), time to local failure ($P = 0.09$), or overall survival ($P = 0.4$).[238] A third RCT, from another Italian center, has been published in abstract form.[239] Only 19 of 41 patients in the chemotherapy arm received an intensive epirubicin/ifosfamide combination (the remainder received single-agent epirubicin), and the study was underpowered for efficacy end points.

So can any definite recommendations be made regarding the use of adjuvant chemotherapy in adult soft tissue sarcoma? Since 1995, the European Organization for the Research and Treatment of Cancer (EORTC) has been recruiting patients into an RCT (protocol 62931) of high-dose doxorubicin and ifosfamide versus control, which should be completed within the next 1 to 2 years, and outcome data will provide additional data to address this question. In an editorial[240] that accompanied the report of the Italian Cooperative Group Trial,[237] Bramwell concluded that a specific standard of care was not yet clear and that the situation would take some time to change. A Canadian practice guideline[241] on this topic has suggested, "It is reasonable to consider anthracycline-based adjuvant chemotherapy in patients who have had removal of a sarcoma with features predicting a high likelihood of relapse (deep location, size > 5 cms, high histological grade)." With the current state of knowledge, we believe this is a reasonable approach. One of the high-dose anthracycline and ifosfamide regimens used in recent RCTs seems a logical choice for adjuvant treatment but may not be suitable for the substantial minority of patients who are older than 70 years (this group has been excluded from RCTs evaluating these regimens). Ultimately, the decision of whether to administer adjuvant chemotherapy and the regimen chosen will depend on a number of considerations, including risk of relapse, physician preferences (which may also depend on patient age and comorbid conditions), referral practices, and available resources.

Neoadjuvant Chemotherapy

Given that the role of postoperative adjuvant chemotherapy for patients with adult soft tissue sarcoma remains controversial, it is hardly surprising that the advantages of chemotherapy given before surgery (neoadjuvant therapy) are even less clear, particularly as there have been no adequately powered RCTs addressing this issue. Neoadjuvant chemotherapy has theoretical benefits that include:

1. Destruction of the primary tumor may reduce the risk of contamination at surgery and permit closer margins with less tissue loss and functional disability but improved local control.
2. Extensive delays in initiating chemotherapy resulting from complex surgery and/or radiotherapy are avoided; for rapidly growing tumors, this earlier elimination of micrometastases may improve survival, although this has not been proven.

Numerous neoadjuvant treatment approaches and preoperative drug regimens have been explored. Intra-arterial (IA) administration of drugs such as doxorubicin or cisplatin has been evaluated, in some cases in conjunction with radiotherapy, isolated limb perfusion, and/or hyperthermia. The IA route delivers drugs more directly to the tumor but is more complex, expensive, and prone to complications compared with the intravenous (IV) route. In the one small RCT on route of administration, there were no differences in rates of local control or overall failure between neoadjuvant chemotherapy given IA or IV.[242,243] In a series of nonrandomized studies reflecting the evolution of neoadjuvant treatment at their center over a 20-year period, the University of California, Los Angeles (UCLA) group treated a total of 498 patients with neoadjuvant chemotherapy.[244] The combination of chemotherapy and 28-Gy radiotherapy before surgery provided the best local control with the lowest complication rate. Based on results of the RCT described earlier, IA doxorubicin was replaced by IV doxorubicin, and cisplatin and ifosfamide were added to the most recent protocol.[244] In the whole group of 498 patients, the overall local recurrence rates were 11% at 5 years and 15% at 10 years, and corresponding overall survival rates were 71% and 66%. The local recurrence rate was lower and overall survival rate higher for patients who had no residual tumor (38%) or greater than 95% necrosis (14%) after neoadjuvant chemotherapy, compared with those who had less than 95% necrosis. In a multivariate analysis, pathologic necrosis was an independent predictor of local recurrence and overall survival. The percentage of patients with 95% or greater necrosis increased to 48% with the addition of ifosfamide, as compared to 13% for patients in all other protocols combined.

Pisters and colleagues have reviewed the long-term results of neoadjuvant chemotherapy given at the University of Texas M.D. Anderson Cancer Center for stage IIIB extremity sarcomas between 1986 and 1990.[245] All patients received doxorubicin-based regimens; at that time, ifosfamide was rarely used (3 patients). In 75 patients, the overall clinical objective response rate (complete response plus partial response) was 27%. At a median follow-up of 85 months, the 5-year actuarial local recurrence-free survival, overall recurrence-free survival and overall survival were 83%, 52%, and 59%, respectively. In contrast with the UCLA group's results[244] for pathologic response, there were no differences in any outcomes between responding and nonresponding patients. In the M.D. Anderson expe-rience, complete pathologic response was an infrequent event, occurring in only 8% of patients treated between 1984 and 1992.[246] Five of these patients were long-term survivors after a median follow-up of 76 months.

In a separate analysis at M.D. Anderson, 65 patients (42 extremity and 23 retroperitoneal sarcomas) were treated at the same center between 1991 and 1996 with doxorubicin or ifosfamide-based neoadjuvant chemotherapy; 34% achieved a radiographic partial response and 9% a minor response.[247] Patients having partial response had higher rates of negative-margin resections, local recurrence-free survival, and overall survival than did non-responders. Postoperative morbidity was also evaluated in a larger cohort of 105 patients (71 extremity and 34 retroperitoneal STS) treated at M.D. Anderson during the same period, of whom 50 received ifosfamide as well as doxorubicin.[248] The authors found no evidence that preoperative chemotherapy increased surgical complications (e.g., wound infections and other wound problems), length of hospital stay, rate of readmission, or rate of reoperation.

A number of other institutions have recently reported, mostly in abstract form, their experience with neoadjuvant chemotherapy using doxorubicin and ifosfamide-based regimens that in many cases included cisplatin.[249-252] In most of these studies, radiotherapy followed chemotherapy and was given preoperatively or postoperatively.

The EORTC has performed the only RCT assessing preoperative chemotherapy for soft tissue sarcoma (three cycles of doxorubicin and ifosfamide plus G-CSF) versus no preoperative chemotherapy (control).[253] A total of 150 patients with high-risk STS (≥8 cm any grade, or grade II/III tumors < 8 cm, or grade II/III local recurrence tumors/inadequate surgery) were randomized, of whom 134 were considered eligible for outcome assessment. Radiotherapy was indicated for tumors excised with close or microscopically positive margins and was given in 46% of patients in the chemotherapy arm and 54% of patients in the control arms. Limb salvage was possible in 89% of patients, and chemotherapy did not affect postoperative wound healing. Grade 4 toxicities were rare, although there was one death due to neutropenic fever. At a median follow-up of 7.3 years, the 5-year recurrence-free survival and overall survival rates were 56% versus 52% ($P = 0.36$) and 65% versus 64% ($P = 0.22$) for the chemotherapy and control arms, respectively. Although originally planned as a phase III trial with adequate numbers to detect a 15% difference in 5-year overall survival, the study was closed after completion of the phase II section because of slow accrual. Most groups have concluded that for large high-grade tumors, preoperative chemotherapy is feasible, does not increase postoperative morbidity, increases the rate of operability, and may enhance local control. The beneficial effects on distant metastases and overall survival, if any, are less clear.

It is impossible to determine from the results of the phase II retrospective or prospective series whether preoperative neoadjuvant chemotherapy reduces distant metastases and improves survival, and the EORTC RCT was too small to illuminate this issue. Preoperative chemotherapy, particularly in combination with preoperative radiotherapy, can induce substantial rates of pathological necrosis, may increase operability in large high-grade tumors, and leads to impressive rates of local control. It is not clear, however, that these results are better than would be achieved with preoperative radiotherapy alone, particularly if radiation is delivered using modern intensity-modulated techniques; and most neoadjuvant chemotherapy regimens are associated with substantial toxicity. The contribution of drugs such as cisplatin and dacarbazine (agents with poor activity in metastatic soft tissue sarcoma) other than increasing toxicity can be questioned. There is a clear need for an RCT comparing neoadjuvant chemoradiotherapy with preoperative radiotherapy alone in patients with large high-grade soft tissue sarcoma. As this will require international collaboration and opinions regarding the value of chemotherapy are often entrenched, this may never occur. Preoperative chemoradiotherapy should be delivered only in centers experienced in these techniques, providing further rationale for referral of the majority of patients with soft tissue sarcomas to centers that can provide multidisciplinary assessment and treatment. Alternative techniques to achieve local control in large high-grade extremity soft tissue sarcoma are discussed in the next section.

Combined Preoperative Chemotherapy and Radiotherapy

With the advances made with combined-modality treatment of other solid tumors, there has been interest in combined-modality preoperative treatment (concurrent or sequential chemotherapy and radiation) for patients with localized soft tissue sarcomas. Concurrent doxorubicin-based chemoradiation has been employed extensively by Eilber and colleagues at the University of California, Los Angeles.[256,257] This treatment protocol involved intra-arterial doxorubicin with unusually high-dose per fraction radiotherapy (35 Gy of external-beam radiotherapy delivered in 10 daily fractions, which was reduced to 17.5 Gy in 5 daily fractions to minimize local toxicity). A subsequent prospective randomized trial compared preoperative IA doxorubicin to IV doxorubicin, both followed by 28 Gy of radiation delivered over 8 days followed by surgical resection.[258] No differences in local recurrence or survival were noted.

The combination of regional chemotherapy and concurrent radiotherapy originally pioneered by Eilber and colleagues has been modified and utilized by other groups.[259-261] Investigators from the University of Illinois treated 55 patients with a 10-day preoperative regimen of intra-arterial doxorubicin (10 mg/m^2/day) with concomitant radiotherapy (25 Gy; 2.5 Gy/fraction × 10 fractions).[261] With a mean follow-up of 94 months, local control was 85%. Complications related to the therapy occurred in 26% of patients and required further operative management in 7% of patients. Temple and colleagues treated a group of 42 patients with a similar regimen of 60 to 90 mg of doxorubicin infused IA or IV over a 3-day period followed by sequential radiotherapy (30 Gy; 3 Gy/fraction × 10 fractions).[260] Resection of the residual post-treatment mass was performed 4 to 6 weeks later. At a median follow-up of 6 years, local control was achieved in 39 of 40 patients, although two patients were excluded from this analysis because clear margins were not obtained at the time of surgery. Intra-arterial infusion-related complications occurred in 4 (11%) of 35 patients. Objective radiographic and pathologic response rates were not reported, and thus the efficacy of concurrent chemoradiation therapy in achieving cytoreduction to an extent sufficient to convert lesions resectable by amputation only to lesions

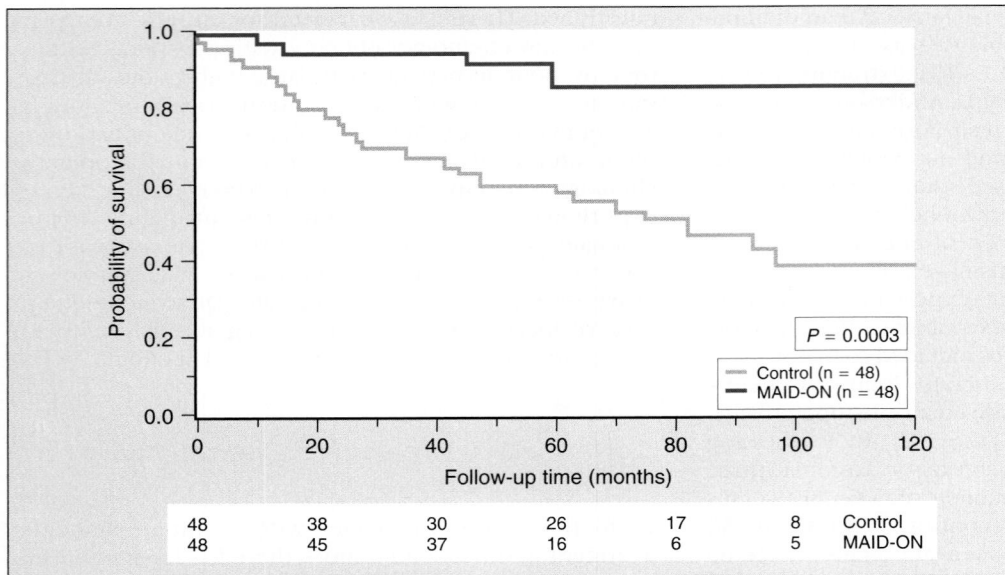

Figure 96-14. Actuarial probability of overall survival for MAID-chemoradiotherapy and surgery versus control patients. The significant difference between both groups with respect to cause of death was distant metastasis (see text for details). (Reproduced with permission from Delaney TF, Spiro IJ, Suit HD, et al: Neoadjuvant chemotherapy and radiotherapy for large extremity soft-tissue sarcomas. Int J Radiat Oncol Biol Phys 2003;56:1117.)

amenable to a limb-sparing approach remains largely anecdotal. Moreover whether preoperative chemoradiation approaches offer local control advantages over conventional treatment approaches employing surgery with preoperative or postoperative radiotherapy is also not apparent. In fact, with current local control rates exceeding 90%, it is difficult to appreciate how this may be further improved using preoperative chemotherapy, unless the strategy involved a radiotherapy dose reduction to ameliorate normal tissue toxicity.

Alternative chemoradiation sequencing has been employed by investigators from Massachusetts General Hospital, who have recently reported mature data from a sequential chemoradiation strategy in the treatment of patients with large (>8 cm) localized, high-grade extremity soft tissue sarcomas.[254] This treatment protocol involved interdigitating courses of chemotherapy and radiotherapy: three courses of doxorubicin, ifosfamide, mesna, and dacarbazine; and two 22-Gy courses of radiation (11 fractions each) for a total preoperative radiation dose that is lower than is usually used (44 Gy). This was followed by surgical resection with microscopic assessment of surgical margins. An additional 16-Gy (8-fractions) boost dose was delivered for microscopically positive surgical margins. The strategy therefore usefully addresses the dual problems of local control and metastatic risk. The outcomes of 48 patients treated with this regimen between June 1989 and March 1999 have been compared to those of a matched series of historic controls (treated between January 1988 and March 1997).[254] The 5-year actuarial local control, distant metastasis–free survival, and overall survival rates (%) for the sequential chemoradiation group are 92, 75, and 87, respectively. For the matched historic controls, these rates (%) are 86, 47, and 58, respectively. The protocol was toxic with 29% experiencing confluent moist skin desquamation, 25% requiring hospitalization at some time for febrile neutropenia, and G-CSF needed in 81%. Wound-healing complications evaluated using recently described criteria[200] were apparent in 29% of cases and confined to the lower extremities as was also observed in the Canadian Sarcoma Group treatment sequencing RCT.[200] One patient died from late marrow dysfunction attributed to chemotherapy. Although the results are encouraging from a tumor standpoint (Fig. 96-14), they will require prospective comparative studies for confirmation and especially because of the local and systemic toxicity associated with this approach.[262] An ongoing Radiation Therapy Oncology Group protocol (RTOG-95-14) has also investigated this treatment approach (see section on preoperative chemotherapy).[255] While the RTOG phase II results are similar in terms of tumor outcome to the data of DeLaney and colleagues, they too are characterized by concerning features of significant toxicity including marrow dysplasia and treatment-related death.

Hyperthermic Isolated Limb Perfusion and Whole Body Hyperthermia with Chemotherapy

Hyperthermic isolated limb perfusion (HILP) and whole-body hyperthermia are two investigational techniques that continue to receive considerable attention, particularly in Europe. HILP (with tumor necrosis factor α [TNFα], interferon α [IFNα], and melphalan) has been used as an neoadjuvant therapy to render tumors resectable and as a primary therapy to avoid amputation for nonresectable extremity soft tissue sarcoma.[263-265] Overall response rates in three series, which recruited 55, 35, and 41 patients, respectively, ranged from 72% to 91%, and limb salvage surgery was possible in 84% to 91% of cases. Small numbers of patients experienced subsequent local recurrence, and some of these patients needed later amputations. Not surprisingly, many patients ultimately developed and died of distant metastases. HILP has also been advocated to facilitate palliative limb salvage in patients with regional and/or distant metastases from unresectable stage IVA or IVB soft tissue sarcoma.[266]

Various techniques of regional or whole-body hyperthermia have been combined with a variety of chemotherapy regimens.[267-272] A group from Munich has evaluated preoperative chemotherapy (four cycles of doxorubicin, ifosfamide, and etoposide) combined with regional hyperthermia (RHT) followed by surgery and adjuvant treatment (same chemotherapy ± radiation). Median follow-up times were 58 months for the RHT-91 protocol (59 patients) and 30 months for the RHT-95 protocol.[271] All patients had grade II/III tumors 5 cm or larger with extracompartmental extension. Clinical response rates were 42% and 33% for the two protocols, with respective local progression-free survival rates of 58% and 57%. Corresponding overall survival rates were 42% and 48%, respectively. These results are now being evaluated in a phase III RCT (EORTC 62961/ESHO RHT-95). The assumption has been made that preoperative chemotherapy with doxorubicin, ifosfamide, and etoposide is effective for patients with high-risk localized disease in this setting, and patients are being randomized to receive preoperative etoposide, ifosfamide, and doxorubicin (EIA, four cycles) plus RHT (two fractions) versus EIA chemotherapy alone.

TREATMENT OF SARCOMA PATIENTS AT SPECIALTY CENTERS

Recent data on other tumor types have demonstrated improved outcomes for patients who required complex treatment and are treated at specialty centers.[273] The most comprehensive data addressing this issue in soft tissue sarcoma come from Sweden, where Gustafson and colleagues analyzed the quality of treatment in a population-based series of 375 patients with primary soft tissue sarcomas arising in the extremities ($n = 329$) or the trunk ($n = 46$).[274] Comparisons were made between patients referred to a specialty soft tissue tumor center before surgery ($n = 195$), those referred after surgery ($n = 102$), and those not referred for treatment of the primary tumor ($n = 78$). The total number of operations for the primary tumor was 1.4 times higher in the patients not referred and 1.7 times higher in the patients referred after surgery than in patients referred before surgery. Of greatest significance, however, was the finding that the local recurrence rate was 2.4 times higher in the patients not referred and 1.3 times higher in the patients referred after surgery than in patients referred to a specialty soft tissue tumor center before any manipulation of their tumor. These findings support the principle of centralizing treatment of these rare tumors, which frequently require complex multimodality therapy.

TREATMENT OF LOCALLY RECURRENT SOFT TISSUE SARCOMA

Incidence of Local Recurrence

Despite optimal multimodality therapy, at least 20% to 30% of soft tissue sarcoma patients will develop recurrent disease, with a median disease-free interval of 18 months.[106,275] Not surprisingly, local recurrence rates are a function of the primary tumor site and are highest for retroperitoneal and head and neck sarcomas. This is due in part to the fact that adequate surgical margins are technically more difficult to attain in these locations. Indeed, while acknowledging our earlier discussion relating the type of positive margin,[183] by multivariate analysis, an unqualified positive surgical margin is an adverse prognostic factor associated with local recurrence operation for recurrent disease.[106,107] In addition, employment of conventional standard-dose postoperative radiotherapy (60 to 65 Gy) is often limited in the retroperitoneum and head and neck by the relative radiosensitivity of surrounding structures. These factors result in local recurrence rates of 38% for high-grade retroperitoneal sarcomas[130] and 48% for high-grade head and neck sarcomas,[276] compared to 5% to 25% for extremity lesions (see Table 96-8). It should also be acknowledged, however, that the rarity of nonextremity lesions probably results in a more varied approach to management, which may influence the ultimate outcome and may have also influenced the ability to design and execute clinical trials in the past. It would seem that properly applied principles of local management can achieve similar results even in sites with traditionally poor results such as the head and neck where disease access is limited by proximity to critical local anatomy.[185]

Surgery and Radiotherapy

Locally recurrent soft tissue sarcoma generally presents as a nodular mass or series of nodules arising in the surgical scar or radiation port. Patients with retroperitoneal recurrences usually present with nonspecific symptoms, often after the recurrence has reached substantial size.

Treatment approaches for patients with locally recurrent soft tissue sarcoma need to be individualized, based on local anatomic constraints and the limitations on present treatment options imposed by prior therapies. In general all such patients should be evaluated for re-resection of their local recurrence. The results of such "salvage surgery" are good, with two thirds of patients surviving long-term.[277,278]

If no prior radiotherapy was employed, adjuvant radiation should be utilized after surgery for locally recurrent disease. Occasionally, subtherapeutic or low-dose radiation was previously employed, and such patients may be candidates for additional adjuvant radiation by external-beam or brachytherapy approaches. Patients who have had a full course of prior radiation should be managed on an individual basis.

In a recent series of 40 patients with recurrent extremity sarcoma, limb salvage was possible by combining limb-sparing re-resection with adjuvant brachytherapy.[279] A median dose of 45 Gy was possible with this technique despite the fact that most patients had received prior external-beam radiation. The 5-year actuarial local control rate was 68%, with satisfactory limb preservation. However, brachytherapy should be used with caution in patients with locally recurrent low-grade sarcomas since it appears to be ineffective against low-grade sarcomas.[182,209]

Catton and colleagues from the Princess Margaret Hospital also employed conservative surgery and reirradiation (external-beam or brachytherapy) for treatment of local recurrences arising in a previous radiation field in a subset of 10 extremity sarcoma patients.[280] With a relatively short median follow-up of 24 months for the entire cohort, local control in the patients treated with further surgery and reirradiation was 100%.[280] Similarly, Nori and colleagues at Memorial Sloan-Kettering Cancer Center and Pearlstone and colleagues at the M.D. Anderson Cancer Center reported a local control rate of 82.5% (33/40) and 65% (17/26), respectively, when using conservative surgery and reirradiation with brachytherapy.[279,281] However, despite these encouraging findings, amputation or protocol-based HILP may be the only options for local control in some patients who were previously treated with radiation and have recurrent extremity sarcoma.

TREATMENT OF METASTATIC SOFT TISSUE SARCOMA

The most common site of metastasis from soft tissue sarcoma of the extremity is the lung. Indeed, the lungs are the only site of recurrence in approximately 20% of all patients with primary extremity and trunk soft tissue sarcomas.[275,282] Primary visceral and gastrointestinal sarcomas also commonly metastasize to the liver. Extrapulmonary metastases are uncommon forms of first metastasis and usually occur as a late manifestation of widely disseminated disease.[275] An obvious exception is in myxoid liposarcoma where unpredictable and aberrant recurrences are a hallmark of disease behavior.[104,283] Evidence strongly suggests that apparently isolated soft tissue masses that manifest in this disease are metastases, sharing the same molecular lineage with the original primary tumor.[284] For sarcomas in general, the median survival from the time of development of metastatic disease is 8 to 12 months. Optimal treatment of patients with metastatic soft tissue sarcoma requires an understanding of the natural history of the disease and individualized selection of treatment options based on specific patient factors, disease factors, and limitations imposed by prior treatment.

Surgical Resection

The current surgical approach for pulmonary metastases from soft tissue sarcoma is based on an extrapolation of the observations of Martini, Marcove, and colleagues in a series of patients with osteosarcoma treated at Memorial Sloan-Kettering Cancer Center in the 1960s. It had been observed that in a series of 184 patients undergoing amputation for osteosarcoma, 75% developed metastatic disease to the lungs within 18 months of amputation; and there were no 5-year survivors among this group.[285] In the absence of any effective systemic therapy for this disease, efforts were made to resect such metastatic lesions in later patients. Martini and colleagues reported successful complete resection in 22 of 28 patients, with a substantial 5-year overall disease-free survival rate of 32%.[286]

Multiple investigators have since reported their experience with pulmonary metastasectomy for metastatic soft tissue sarcoma in adults.[287-298] Three-year overall disease-free survival rates after thoracotomy for pulmonary metastasectomy have ranged from 23% to 54%, as outlined in the selected series summarized in Table 96-11.[287-291,298,299] With the exception of a study that evaluated the development and treatment of pulmonary metastases in patients with extremity sarcomas using a prospective sarcoma database (3-year survival rate of 23% after complete resection),[291] most studies have been retrospective analyses of the results of pulmonary resection in populations of carefully selected patients with metastatic sarcoma from heterogeneous primary sites. This may account for some of the variability in the reported survival rates.

Many investigators believe that repeated thoracotomies to render patients free of disease from pulmonary soft tissue sarcoma metastases are justified in the absence of effective systemic therapy. Several series of reoperative pulmonary metastasectomy have been published.[300,301] In

TABLE 96-11

	NO. OF PATIENTS					
FIRST AUTHOR/ INSTITUTION	**TOTAL**	**PULMONARY METASTASES**	**SURGICAL TREATMENT**	**COMPLETE RESECTION (%)**	**MEDIAN SURVIVAL (MO)**	**3-YEAR SURVIVAL (%)**
Creagan/Mayo[287]	112	112	112	64 (57%)	18	29
Putnam/NCI[288]	487	93	68	51 (75%)	23	32
Jablons/NCI[289]	74	57	57	49 (86%)	27	35
Casson/MDACC[290]	68	68	68	58 (85%)	25	42
Verazin/Roswell[307]	78	78	78	61 (78%)	21	21.5, (5 yr)
Gadd/MSKCC[291]	716	135	78	65 (83%)	19	23
Van Geel/EORTC[298]	255	255	255	255 (100%)	NR	54

Survival Following Complete Resection of Pulmonary Metastases from Soft Tissue Sarcoma in Adults

EORTC, European Organization for Research and Treatment of Cancer; Mayo, Mayo Clinic; MDACC, University of Texas M.D. Anderson Cancer Center; MSKCC, Memorial Sloan-Kettering Cancer Center; NCI, U.S. National Cancer Institute; Roswell, Roswell Park Cancer Institute.

an NCI series, 72% of 43 patients could be rendered free of disease at the second thoracotomy, with a median survival duration from the time of the second thoracotomy of 25 months.[300] In a report from the M.D. Anderson Cancer Center of a series of 34 patients undergoing reoperation for a second pulmonary metastasis after successful initial metastasectomy, factors predicting long-term survival included the presence of a solitary metastasis and the ability to perform a complete resection.[301] This study also illustrated the significant survival duration many of these patients enjoy: The median survival in the 19 patients who had unifocal recurrent metastatic disease was 65 months as compared to 14 months in the 15 patients with complete resection of two or more sites of recurrent disease.

It remains difficult to predict which patients will benefit from pulmonary resection. A number of different clinical criteria have been evaluated by univariate analysis, including the disease-free interval,[287,288,299,302] number of metastatic nodules,[299,302-305] and tumor doubling time.[299,305,306] Multivariate analyses from both the NCI and Roswell Park Cancer Institute confirm that a short disease-free interval (as a surrogate end point of adverse behavior) and incomplete pulmonary resection are adverse prognostic factors for survival of patients with pulmonary metastases.[289,307] A multivariate analysis from the M.D. Anderson Cancer Center suggested that, in addition, the presence of more than three metastatic pulmonary nodules on preoperative chest CT is an adverse prognostic sign.[290]

The ability to completely resect all pulmonary disease is perhaps the most important prognostic factor impacting survival after pulmonary metastasectomy; patients with residual pulmonary disease have a median survival of 9 months versus 27 months ($p_2 < 0.0001$) for patients rendered completely free of disease at thoracotomy.[289,291] In a series of 65 patients with metastatic pulmonary lesions from extremity sarcoma from the Memorial Sloan-Kettering Cancer Center, the median survival after complete resection was 19 months versus 10 months for patients who had incomplete resections and 8 months for patients who did not undergo surgery ($P = 0.005$).[291] The 3-year overall survival rate after complete resection was 23% compared to 2% in those treated nonsurgically ($P < 0.001$). The clinical criteria of disease-free interval, tumor doubling time, and number of nodules can serve as general prognostic indicators in patients being considered for pulmonary metastasectomy, but no single criterion should be used to exclude patients from surgery.

The ability to achieve complete resection and the number of pulmonary nodules present appear to best define the prognosis for patients postoperatively. Although carefully selected patients may benefit from surgical resection of pulmonary metastases, however, this treatment approach is feasible in only a small fraction of patients who develop pulmonary metastases. This is best illustrated by data from Memorial Sloan-Kettering, where a population of 716 patients with primary extremity sarcoma were followed for the subsequent development and treatment of pulmonary metastases (Fig. 96-15). Of the initial cohort, 148 patients (21%) developed pulmo-

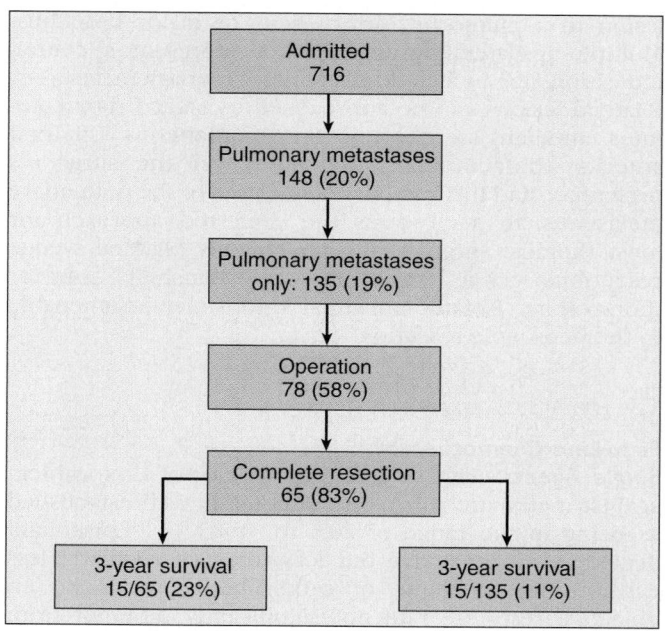

Figure 96-15. Risk for and subsequent management of pulmonary metastases in 716 patients with primary or locally recurrent extremity soft tissue sarcoma. (Reprinted with permission from Brennan MF: The surgeon as a leader in cancer care: Lessons learned from the study of soft tissue sarcoma. J Am Coll Surg 1996;182:520.)

nary metastases. Isolated pulmonary metastases occurred in 135 (91%) of these 148 patients. Of the 135 patients with pulmonary-only metastases, 78 (58%) were considered to have operable disease, and 65 (83%) of those taken to thoracotomy were able to undergo complete resection of all their pulmonary metastatic disease. This group represents only 44% of patients with pulmonary metastases. Median survival from the time of complete resection was 19 months, and the 3-year overall survival rate was 23%. All patients who did not undergo thoracotomy died within 3 years. For the entire cohort of 135 patients developing pulmonary-only metastases, the 3-year overall survival rate was only 11% (see Fig. 96-15).

The rather disappointing overall results of treatment for pulmonary metastases underscore the importance of careful patient selection for resection of pulmonary metastases. The following criteria are generally agreed upon: (1) the primary tumor is controlled or is controllable; (2) there is no extrathoracic disease; (3) the patient is a medical candidate for thoracotomy and pulmonary resection; and (4) complete resection of all disease appears possible.[308] With careful patient selection, the morbidity of thoracotomy can be limited to the subset of patients who are most likely to benefit from this aggressive treatment approach.

Wedge excision with negative margins is the procedure of choice for patients who undergo surgery for isolated pulmonary metastases. Formal segmentectomy, lobectomy, and mediastinal lymph node dissection are not necessary and do not contribute to improved local control. Occasionally, lobectomy or even pneumonectomy is required because of the proximity of the metastatic lesion to a pulmonary artery, vein, or major bronchus. Multiple ipsilateral lesions do not represent a contra-indication, nor, in fact, do bilateral pulmonary metastases. Bilateral lesions can be approached by staged thoracotomies, median sternotomy, or simultaneous bilateral anterior thoracotomies, depending on the surgeon's preference and the number and location of the pulmonary metastases. In such cases the preferred approach for most thoracic surgeons is simultaneous bilateral wedge resections via a sternotomy or "clamshell" anterior thoracotomy. Isolated unilateral lesions may be amenable to thoracoscopic resection.

Chemotherapy

First-Line Chemotherapy

Single Agents. The single-agent activity of doxorubicin against metastatic soft tissue sarcoma is well established as being in the range of 20% to 30%.[309-311] Epirubicin, developed as an active but less toxic (particularly less cardiotoxic) analogue of doxorubicin, produced an objective response rate not significantly different from that of doxorubicin (18% versus 25%, $P = 0.33$) in an EORTC RCT of 167 patients receiving equimolar doses (75 mg/m^2) of the drugs.[312] There is some evidence of a dose-response relationship with epirubicin; a dose-escalation study showed response rates of 17%, 44%, and 100% for 140 mg/m^2, 160 mg/m^2, and 180 mg/m^2 of epirubicin, respectively.[313] Only three patients were entered at the maximum tolerated dose of 180 mg/m^2, and 160 mg/m^2 was recommended for routine clinical use. However, the EORTC group, in a three-arm RCT of 334 patients, was unable to demonstrate any benefit from either of two schedules of epirubicin (150 mg/m^2) compared with doxorubicin (75 mg/m^2); all regimens produced response rates of 14% to 15%.[314] Furthermore there was considerably more myelosuppression in the two epirubicin arms, with two toxic deaths. Nevertheless, particularly in Europe, epirubicin has commonly been substituted for doxorubicin in high-dose regimens, based on its better toxicity profile.

A number of studies of liposomal anthracyclines have suggested these agents have lower rates of cardiotoxicity but variable activity.[315-319] An EORTC phase II RCT [320] demonstrated low activity for both doxorubicin and liposomal doxorubicin (Doxil)—9% versus 10%—but different spectrums of toxicity, with less myelosuppression and with palmer-plantar erythrodysthesia (grade 3, 20%) as the dose-limiting toxicity in the Doxil arm. The EORTC is further exploring Doxil in combination with ifosfamide.

Lack of response rather than cardiotoxicity is the main limiting factor for anthracycline use in palliative chemotherapy of STS. Nonetheless, strategies to reduce anthracycline toxicity are of particular importance in the adjuvant setting.[321] Dexrazoxane is undoubtedly cardioprotective when given with doxorubicin.[322] Concerns about the possibility of tumor protection point to a need for further RCTs in STS.

After the reports of several randomized studies documenting activity ranging from 24% to 67%,[323-325] Bramwell and colleagues performed an RCT comparing ifosfamide (5 g/m^2 by 24-hour infusion) with cyclophosphamide (1.5 g/m^2).[326] Respective response rates were 18% and 8%, but the difference was not statistically significant ($P = 0.13$).

Indirect data from several RCTs in which ifosfamide and/or cyclophosphamide were added to doxorubicin have provided additional evidence that ifosfamide is a more active analogue than cyclophosphamide.[309] Questions about the optimal scheduling of ifosfamide (multiple daily bolus doses versus continuous infusion) have never been satisfactorily resolved and are confounded by dose differences in many studies. Two consecutive phase II studies by investigators at M.D. Anderson evaluated ifosfamide (14 g/m^2), given as a 72-hour continuous infusion or a 2-hour infusion for 3 consecutive days. Respective response rates were 19% and 42%.[327] In an EORTC RCT comparing 5 g/m^2 ifosfamide over 24 hours with 3 g/m^2 ifosfamide over 4 hours on days 1 to 3, response rates were 3% and 17.5%. However, a subsequent EORTC study showed no difference in response rates for 9 g/m^2 ifosfamide by CIV or intermittent bolus injection[328] (see "High-Dose Ifosfamide").

Combination Chemotherapy. In the 1970s and early 1980s before the widespread availability of ifosfamide, most combination chemotherapy regimens were based on doxorubicin and dacarbazine. The addition of cyclophosphamide and vincristine which are active against childhood sarcomas, created a regimen called CyVADIC, for which the Southwest Oncology Group reported response rates as high as 59% in patients with metastatic disease.[329] Later investigators were unable to reproduce such high response rates with the same regimen, however, and summary data on variants of the CyVADIC regimen revealed an overall response rate of 35% in 2092 patients.[330]

Most regimens now used for first-line chemotherapy are based on the combination of doxorubicin and ifosfamide. A recent systematic search of the literature[331] found 3 phase III RCTs and 16 phase II trials (excluding phase I studies and those recruiting less than 25 patients) in adult STS that used combination regimens including an anthracycline and ifosfamide. Although the response rate varied widely from 25% to 56% in the phase II studies, they were at the lower end of this range in the three RCTs.[332-334] In the Eastern Cooperative Oncology Group (ECOG) study[332] of 178 patients, the response rate was significantly higher for doxorubicin/ifosfamide than for doxorubicin alone (34% versus 20%, $P = 0.03$) although median survivals were similar. In an EORTC study of 471 patients, however, there were no significant differences in response rate (28% versus 23%) or median survival for doxorubicin/ifosfamide versus doxorubicin alone.[333] In an intergroup trial of 340 patients, the ifosfamide-containing regimen MAID was shown to produce a significantly higher response rate (32% versus 17%, p < 0.002) than doxorubicin/dacarbazine, but with no overall survival benefit.[334]

Bramwell and colleagues performed a meta-analysis of eight RCTs, that compared doxorubicin-based combinations with single-agent doxorubicin.[310] In these eight studies with a total of 2281 patients, 10 combination regimens were evaluated; five included ifosfamide (two) or dacarbazine (three) and the remaining five used other drugs with low known single-agent activity. There were no significant benefits in terms of response rate (OR [odds ratio] = 0.79, P = 0.10) or overall survival (OR 0.84, P = 0.13) for combination chemotherapy. Inclusion of a small RCT (106 patients)[335] that compared epirubicin (180 mg/m^2) with epirubicin (180 mg/m^2) plus cisplatin (120 mg/m^2) and reported respective response rates of 29% and 54% (P = 0.025) did not significantly alter the meta-analysis results. Based on single-agent doxorubicin's lower overall toxicity than that of combination regimens, Bramwell and colleagues suggested that, for chemotherapy given with palliative intent, doxorubicin alone was a reasonable first-line option,[310] a conclusion also reached in a commentary by Santoro.[336] This leaves open the possibility of further second-line chemotherapy with ifosfamide in fit patients progressing on or relapsing after a response to doxorubicin therapy. Whether patients with advanced sarcomas should be treated with chemotherapy at all is also a topic of debate.[337]

One reason for the lack of convincing evidence that standard-dose combination chemotherapy improves outcomes compared with single-agent doxorubicin for metastatic STS may be that dose of the drugs in combination regimens are often reduced below optimum levels to limit toxicity. In STS, dose-response relationships have been suggested for both doxorubicin and ifosfamide, but myelosuppression, particularly neutropenia, limits the doses that can be safely delivered. Use of hematopoietic growth factors or autologous stem cell transplantation permits substantial dose escalation of these agents. In a systematic review, Verma and Bramwell identified seven phase I trials, five phase II trials, and two RCTs exploring dose-escalated regimens of doxorubicin and ifosfamide, with and without other agents for metastatic STS.[331] Most regimens included the growth factors G-CSF or GM-CSF, but in two trials autologous stem cell transplantation was used. In the phase I studies, the maximum tolerated doses were in the range of a 2-fold increase of the doxorubicin or epirubicin dose (over a standard dose of 75 mg/m^2) and a 2.4 to 2.8-fold increase of the ifosfamide dose (over a standard dose of 5 g/m^2). Significant toxicities included anemia, thrombocytopenia, nephrotoxicity, and neurotoxicity; severe neutropenia and febrile neutropenia were also seen at the higher doses. In a recently reported study,[338] De Pas and colleagues reported no nephrotoxicity or neurotoxicity with ifosfamide infused over 12 days at 15 g/m^2 (given with doxorubicin, 75 mg/m^2), although myelosuppression was dose limiting. Although not the primary objective, response rates were reported for all these phase I studies and were in the range of 28% to 58%. Additionally, for the five phase II studies of dose-escalated doxorubicin and ifosfamide (only studies with more than 20 evaluable patients were included), response rates were 31% to 65%. In a phase II study that was not included in the review, a response rate of 40% in 70 patients was documented.[339]

In contrast with these promising results in phase I/II studies, response data in the RCTs have been disappoint-ing. In an EORTC trial in 314 patients with metastatic STS, standard-dose doxorubicin (50 mg/m^2) plus ifosfamide (5 g/m^2) was compared with higher-dose doxorubicin (75 mg/m^2) with the same dose of ifosfamide plus GM-CSF.[340] Respective response rates were 21% and 23%, with similar median overall survivals (56 versus 55 weeks); but median progression-free survival was significantly longer in the high-dose arm (19 versus 29 weeks, P = 0.03). In the other RCT included in Verma and Bramwell's review, as yet reported only in abstract form,[341] 162 patients were randomized to receive standard-dose MAID or MAID with doses escalated 25% plus G-CSF support. Respective response rates were 37% versus 43% (P not significant), but no survival data were reported. There were five toxicity-related deaths, however, all in the dose-escalated MAID arm. In a third RCT, 180 mg/m^2 epirubicin and 150 mg/m^2 epirubicin, each combined with cisplatin but with no growth factor support, were compared in 151 patients.[335] There was a higher response rate (51% versus 28%, P = 0.004) and a marginal effect on overall survival (P = 0.06) with the higher-dose regimen. As all three RCTs were quite limited tests of dose escalation, more RCTs are needed before it can be concluded that such regimens are a more effective option than conventional-dose chemotherapy.

Omission of dacarbazine may reduce the toxicity of high-dose doxorubicin/ifosfamide regimens. A trial comparing standard-dose ifosfamide (6 g/m^2) with high-dose ifosfamide (12 g/m^2), both combined with doxorubicin (60 mg/m^2) and supported by G-CSF, is in progress. To date, only preliminary data on toxicity in 63 patients[342] have been reported.

Possible reasons for the lack of a clear benefit of dose-escalated therapy in the RCTs are discussed by Verma and Bramwell[331] and include tumor heterogeneity, difficulties in eradicating large tumor burdens, and the appropriate-ness of the drugs, doses, and schedules used.

Second-Line Chemotherapy

High-Dose Ifosfamide. Although ifosfamide is often used as a first-line agent, it is clearly active as second-line therapy in patients progressing or relapsing after doxorubicin-based regimens. Early studies of ifosfamide suggested there was a dose-response relationship,[343] and several groups have documented responses to high-dose ifosfamide in patients not responding to lower doses of the drug.[344-347] Nevertheless dose-escalation studies of ifosfamide have produced conflicting results. Doses of 12 g/m^2 without and 14 to 18 g/m^2 with growth factor support seem achievable and have produced response rates of 33% to 45%, but nephrotoxicity and neurotoxicity are considerable.[327,341,347] Frustaci and colleagues found high-dose ifosfamide to be well tolerated when infused at 1 g/m^2/day over 21 days.[348] In 36 patients, they were able to administer up to three cycles of median duration 15 days, producing a response rate of 24%. Myelosuppression was dose limiting, but there was no significant nephro-toxicity or neurotoxicity. Pharmacokinetic data, reported by Cerny and colleagues demonstrated that ifosfamide doses greater than 14 to 16 g/m^2 given over 5 days resulted in a relative decrease of the active metabolite phosphoramide mustard, suggesting dose-dependent saturation or inhibition of ifosfamide metabolism.[349]

Despite encouraging phase II trial results, the advantages of increasing the dose of ifosfamide are far from clear, based on recent EORTC studies. The response rate rates for 9 g/m^2 (3 g/m^2 over 4 hours, days 1 to 3) and 5 g/m^2 (24-hour continuous IV) were 3% and 17.5%, respectively, in an RCT of 101 patients.[350] Escalation to 12 g/m^2 as a 3-day continuous IV infusion produced a response rate of 16% in a phase II study of 124 patients.[351] In the most recent EORTC RCT of first-line chemotherapy, the response rates were 11%, 6.5%, and 9.4% for 75 mg/m^2 doxorubicin, 3 g/m^2 ifosfamide over 4 hours on days 1 to 3, and 9 g/m^2 ifosfamide 24-hour continuous infusion, respectively. In addition to these disappointingly low and similar response rates, there were no differences in progression-free survival between the three arms.[328]

Other Marketed Drugs Alone or in Combination. Collected response rate data for many drugs studied in phase II trials for metastatic STS have been published in a number of reviews.[309,352,353] Dacarbazine has been used most extensively, either as a first-line agent in combination with doxorubicin and ifosfamide (MAID) or as a second-line salvage treatment. Demetri and colleagues found an overall 16% response rate for dacarbazine in 109 patients from collected phase II studies.[309] Although dacarbazine is commonly given in divided doses over 3 to 5 days, Buesa showed that doses of 1.2 g/m^2 over 20 minutes are feasible and active, as well as more convenient.[354] The current availability of portable infusion pumps means prolonged infusions are also feasible. Although Rosen and colleagues reported a response rate of 27% lasting 2 to 18 months or longer, Reichardt and colleagues were not able to confirm this high rate of activity when they gave 12- to 14-day infusions of 200 to 225 mg/m^2/day dacarbazine, observing only disease stabilization in 8 of 25 heavily pretreated patients.[355]

There is conflicting evidence on the activity of cisplatin and carboplatin against metastatic STS, although most reviews have reported response rates of less than 15%.[309,352,353] Low response rates are also seen for etoposide given as a single agent.[309,326,356] Promising early data on docetaxel[357] could not be reproduced in later studies,[336,358-361] and paclitaxel similarly has little activity.[362-364] Objective response rates have also been very low (3% to 5%) in 3 phase II studies of gemcitabine,[365-367] although the M.D. Anderson group described a response rate of 18% in 39 patients, if GISTs were excluded.[362]

Despite poor levels of activity as single agents, some of the preceding drugs have been incorporated into nonanthracycline-based salvage regimens. Based on encouraging data in pediatric sarcomas, etoposide has been combined with ifosfamide, although with variable results.[361,368-371] All but one such study produced response rate in the range of 38% to 46%; because ifosfamide given alone has produced up to 67% in phase II studies, however, these results are difficult to interpret. Combinations of paclitaxel or docetaxel with gemcitabine are being evaluated, with preliminary reports of encouraging synergistic activity.[372-374] Temozolomide,[375-377] raltitrexed,[378]

irinotecan,[379] sargramostim,[380] topotecan,[381,382] and vinorelbine[383] seem to have minimal activity in STS, despite their proven value in other tumor types.

Investigational New Drugs. The identification of a specific molecular target (the tyrosine kinase receptor KIT) in a rare type of soft tissue sarcoma (GIST) and successful treatment with a drug (imatinib) that inhibits that target provide a model for future drug development in soft tissue sarcoma. Although it is unlikely that the pathogenesis of most soft tissue sarcoma will prove to be driven by a single genetic mutation, better molecular differentiation of STSs into categories with similar molecular characteristics may facilitate future studies of highly targeted drugs. At an NCI sponsored "State of the Science" meeting on soft tissue sarcoma, Demetri pointed out that the ideal target would meet four conditions: (1) a single validated molecule critical to STS pathogenesis in humans; (2) expressed and active; (3) a target for which there are no alternative pathways to bypass the blockade; and (4) necessary and sufficient for sarcoma survival.[227] Other potential targets are discussed elsewhere in this chapter.

Complex sarcomas with diverse karyotypes and/or drug-resistance mutations are likely to require drugs used in combination to block multiple targets. Recent reviews have described signal transduction pathways in sarcoma as therapeutic targets,[384] the potential use of antiangiogenesis agents,[385] and new approaches to immunotherapy.[386] Early reports of antiangiogenesis therapies have shown limited benefit in STS,[387,388] but many agents remain to be evaluated.

Of drugs currently in phase II development, ET743 (ecteinascidin 743), a DNA guanine-specific minor groove-binding agent, seems to have the most potential across the spectrum of sarcomas. Hints of activity in bone and STSs were observed in phase I trials[389,390] and appeared to be confirmed in phase II trials of this agent. Demetri and colleagues reported a response rate of 18% in 34 chemonaive sarcoma patients and 9% in 34 who had received prior chemotherapy. George and colleagues reported a lower progression rate (5%) but a substantial proportion (19%) of patients with minor responses or stable disease.[391] Two European trials described response rates of 11% to 12% in previously treated sarcoma patients.[392,393] Occasional severe toxicities, sometimes lethal, seemed to be related to elevated baseline liver function tests.

Although the majority of patients with metastatic soft tissue sarcoma will not have access to phase II studies of investigational agents, where these are available trial entry should be encouraged. Use of an investigational agent as a first- or second-line therapy for metastatic disease should also be considered. Investigational agents given as third- or fourth-line treatments may be doomed to failure because of acquired drug resistance, whereas both doxorubicin and ifosfamide have already been shown to have activity in the salvage therapy setting and thus remain options if investigational agents fail.

Unique Routes of Delivery. Some experimental studies have evaluated intraperitoneal delivery of cytotoxic agents, usually doxorubicin and cisplatin sometimes with hyperthermia, in sarcomas confined to the peritoneal cavity after resection of all visible abdominal disease.[352,394,395] Evaluation of any benefit is a major challenge in these studies, however, and this technique may be less suitable for sarcomas than for epithelial cancers.

Another novel approach is isolated lung perfusion with doxorubicin after resection of pulmonary metastases, in general a more common situation in soft tissue sarcomas. To date, studies of isolated pulmonary perfusion have focused on feasibility rather than outcomes.[396]

SPECIAL SITES AND SUBTYPES OF SARCOMA

Retroperitoneal Sarcomas

Retroperitoneal sarcomas are relatively uncommon, accounting for approximately 15% of all sarcomas (see Fig. 96-1). The most common histologic subtypes are liposarcoma and leiomyosarcoma, found in 42% and 26% of cases, respectively (see Fig. 96-1). Nearly 80% of patients present with an abdominal mass, and 50% of patients report pain at the time of presentation.[178] Patients commonly describe nonspecific gastrointestinal symptoms. Other commonly noted symptoms include neurologic symptoms (primarily sensory) in 27% and weight loss in 7%.[178,397] These tumors often grow to substantial size before a patient's nonspecific complaints are evaluated or an abdominal mass is noted on physical examination.

CT and MRI are the primary methods used to image retroperitoneal tumors (see Figs. 96-3, 96-5, and 96-6).[398–400] These modalities allow assessment of the consistency of the mass (cystic or solid components, associated necrosis), the mass's precise anatomic location, and the extent of any regional disease and confirm function of the contralateral kidney. CT of the abdomen and pelvis usually provides images satisfactory for treatment planning. Occasionally, MRI with gradient sequence imaging may be helpful in defining long segment vascular anatomy for surgical planning. For patients with an abnormal chest radiograph, chest CT should be performed to exclude the possibility of metastatic disease.

The differential diagnosis for a retroperitoneal mass is relatively limited. Physical examination should include a testicular examination in men to evaluate the possibility of a primary testicular neoplasm. Laboratory tests should include the common serum markers for germ cell tumors, beta-human chorionic gonadotropin, and alpha-fetoprotein. If physical examination is suggestive of malignancy or biochemical markers are elevated, testicular ultrasonography should be performed. This may obviate laparotomy for patients with metastatic testicular tumors and allow identification of primary retroperitoneal germ cell tumors.

In general, preoperative biopsy is not necessary when surgical resection is planned for a resectable primary retroperitoneal mass. For clearly unresectable lesions or in cases in which physical examination or laboratory studies suggest a lymphoma or germ cell tumor, a needle biopsy may facilitate diagnosis. Percutaneous core- or fine-needle biopsy may also be helpful if preoperative chemotherapy and/or radiotherapy are planned.

Surgical resection with negative margins remains the standard primary treatment for patients with localized retroperitoneal sarcoma. Because en bloc multiorgan resection may be required to achieve negative margins, all patients should have preoperative bowel preparation and assessment of bilateral renal function by CT. Resectability rates in recent series combining patients with primary and recurrent lesions have ranged from 25% to 96% (Table 96-12).[178,397,401–406] Resectability rates at different institutions are difficult to compare and interpret because these rates are a function of the referral pattern, the criteria used to determine which patients will undergo surgical exploration, and the skill and experience of the surgeons.[405,407,408] For patients with primary lesions, grossly complete resection is possible in up to 78% of cases.[130,405] The most common reasons for unresectability are the presence of major vascular involvement (aorta or vena cava), peritoneal implants, or distant metastases.[178] Resection of adjacent retroperitoneal or intra-abdominal organs, frequently the kidney, colon, or pancreas, is required in 50% to 80% of cases to permit complete resection.[178,403,409] Partial resections or debulking procedures have been performed, but there is no evidence that partial resection improves survival (Fig. 96-16).[178,409] In general until effective adjuvant therapy is available for gross

TABLE 96-12

Resectability Rates for Retroperitoneal Sarcomas in Selected Series

FIRST AUTHOR	INSTITUTION	ACCRUAL PERIOD (YRS)	TOTAL NO. OF PATIENTS	NO. COMPLETELY RESECTED	RESTABILITY RATE (%)
Glenn[401]	NCI	19	50	37	74
Karakousis[402]	Roswell Park	24	68	27	40
Dalton[403]	Mayo Clinic	19	116	63	54
Jaques[178]	MSKCC	5	114	67	59
Alvarenga[397]	Royal Marsden	20	110	28	25
Karakousis[405]	Roswell Park	17	87	83	95
Kilkenny[406]	University of Florida	25	63	49	78

MSKCC, Memorial Sloan-Kettering Cancer Center; NCI, U.S. National Cancer Institute.

Specific Malignancies

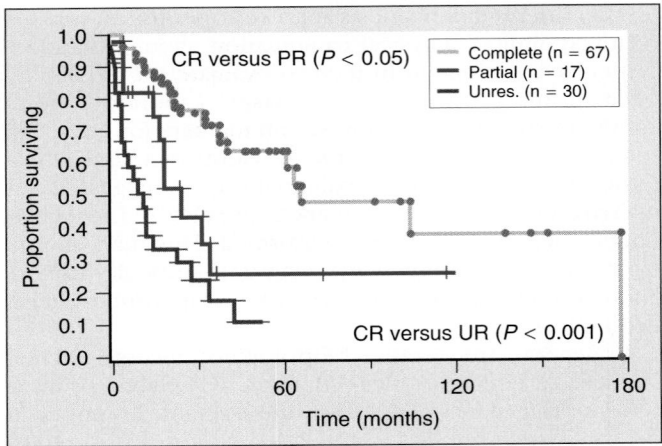

Figure 96-16. Proportion of patients with retroperitoneal sarcoma surviving from the date of first operation at Memorial Sloan-Kettering Cancer Center for patients undergoing complete (gross negative margin), incomplete (gross positive margin), or no resection. (Reprinted with permission from Jaques DP, Coit DG, Hajdu SI, et al: Management of primary and recurrent soft-tissue sarcoma of the retroperitoneum. Ann Surg 1990;212:51.)

residual disease, deliberate partial resection outside the confines of a clinical trial should be reserved for relief of bowel obstruction or palliation of other critical manifestations of advanced disease.

Results from published series demonstrate 5-year overall survival rates in the range of 54% to 64% for patients with completely resected retroperitoneal sarcoma.[130,178,403,405,406] Overall survival rates for patients with incompletely resected disease range from 10% to 36%. Adequate margins are often difficult to obtain in retroperitoneal sarcoma surgery because of the proximity of critical organs, vascular structures, and the spine. Consequently, recurrent disease remains a significant problem, with recurrence developing alone or with systemic relapse in 46% to 59% of patients with completely resected tumors.[131,178,403,405,410]

A number of recent studies have evaluated prognostic factors for retroperitoneal sarcomas by univariate and multivariate analysis.[130,131,397,403,410] For patients presenting without metastatic disease, complete surgical resection and histologic grade were the primary determinants of survival in several multivariate analyses.[130,397,403,406,410] Some investigators have also found that large tumor size (>10 cm) and fixation to adjacent retroperitoneal structures other than neurovascular bundles or bone were significant adverse factors for survival by multivariate analysis.[403] Patients undergoing a grossly complete resection have a 60% 5-year overall survival rate and a median survival of 64 months (see Fig. 96-16). This is significantly better than those of patients who have an incomplete resection (grossly positive margins) or unresectable disease. For patients with low-grade lesions, the median survival (80 months versus 20 months) and 5-year overall survival rate (70% versus 25%) are significantly better than for with patients with high-grade lesions.[178]

The unfavorable results of outcome for retroperitoneal sarcoma logically points to the need to investigate adjuvant approaches. The obvious candidates include preoperative and postoperative radiotherapy. Detailed discussions of the pertinent issues in these approaches are available[411,412] and are summarized in the following section.

Surgery Plus Radiation Treatment

Postoperative EBRT has been shown to reduce local recurrence rates for extremity and superficial trunk sarcomas. However, gastrointestinal toxicities or neurotoxicities often limit the delivery of sufficient radiation doses to the retroperitoneum. Several retrospective studies have suggested that postoperative EBRT may improve local control after grossly complete resection[178,208,402,410,413–417] while other small retrospective reports have not suggested any improvement in local control with postoperative radiotherapy.[178,208,402]

However, these series have included small numbers of patients (<30 to 40), no standard treatment protocol, and variable details on histopathology, extent of resection, and margin status. The largest study addressing this issue was reported by the French Cancer Federation Sarcoma Group with the suggestion that postoperative radiotherapy was associated with significantly reduced local recurrence compared to surgery alone.[418] In this report, 145 patients presented with localized nonmetastatic retroperitoneal sarcoma. As is typical for this disease, the tumors were large (median size 15 cm, range 2 to 70 cm) and only a minority (6%) were T1 lesions. As in others series, liposarcoma was unusually well represented (30%). Their patients may differ from those in other reports in that only 27 cases (19%) had grade 1 lesions. A significant number of patients (31%) had neurovascular or bone involvement. Complete resection took place in 94 of the 145 patients (65%), and 60 of these patients received radiotherapy to a median dose of 50 Gy. Of the 94 patients that underwent complete resection, the 5-year actuarial local recurrence–free interval was 60% for those treated with radiotherapy compared to 23% for those who did not receive postoperative radiotherapy ($P = 0.0021$). Clearly, the likely possibility of selection bias must be considered in interpreting these results since patients with large and more complex (i.e., unusually located or infiltrating) lesions and patients who experienced postoperative morbidity are less likely to have been treated with radiotherapy.

Preoperative EBRT for retroperitoneal sarcoma offers certain theoretical and practical advantages: (1) high-dose treatment may minimize the risk of tumor implantation in the peritoneal cavity after a marginal resection by sterilizing a large number of tumor cells; (2) partial tumor regression may facilitate grossly complete resection; (3) anatomic issues, including the tumor displacement of critical radiosensitive organs (bowel predominantly) away from the preoperative radiation field, thereby reducing toxicity and improving tolerance; and (4) an intact peritoneum offers a mechanical barrier to tumor seeding during the time radiotherapy is being administered before resection and division of these membranes. Moreover postoperative radiotherapy is problematic if bowel is tethered in the radiotherapy target area, making it impossible to treat some patients, at least without unnecessary risk of complications.

Two recent series, the first from the Princess Margaret Hospital (PMH) and the other from the University of Texas M.D. Anderson Cancer Center (MDACC) are informative because acute toxicity resulting from preoperative radiotherapy was differentiated prospectively from the effects of other treatments.[419,420] In the PMH series, the median preoperative dose of radiotherapy comprised 45 Gy in 25 fractions. Although the median radiation volume exceeded 7L, preoperative external-beam radiation therapy was associated with European Organization for the Research and Treatment of Cancer/Radiation Therapy Oncology Group (EORTC/RTOG) acute toxicity scores of less than or equal to two in all patients who underwent resection. Furthermore no patient was hospitalized for acute toxicity, and there were no treatment interruptions or requirements for cessation of treatment because of acute toxicity. The remarkably low toxicity of the preoperative course with enormous radiotherapy volumes in the study has been attributed to the displacement of bowel outside the target volume. At the same time brachytherapy used postoperatively in selected cases did appear to be associated with toxicity, and also does not appear to have contributed to enhanced tumour outcome. Late toxicity resulted in death in 4.3% (2 of 46) and with life-threatening illness in 2.2% (1 of 46) of patients, all of whom had been treated with brachytherapy to the upper abdomen. The 2-year overall survival and disease-free survival for resected retroperitoneal sarcoma were 88% and 80%, respectively. Significantly better 2-year disease-free survival was achieved in patients with primary (as opposed to recurrent) disease and in those with low-grade tumors (93% and 95%, respectively).[419] Similarly, in the MDACC phase I trial (*n* = 35) the tolerance of preoperative radiotherapy is also reported. The MDACC trial differed from the PMH study in that it also evaluated outcome after preoperative doxorubicin in addition to concurrent allocation to 1 of 6 sequential 1.8-Gy-per-fraction escalating radiotherapy protocols (from 18 to 50.4 Gy), and used intraoperative electron-beam as the boost technique in localized retroperitoneal tissue sarcoma.[420] At the highest radiation dose of 50.4 Gy, 2 (18%) of 11 patients had grade 3 or 4 nausea. Twenty-nine patients (83%) underwent laparotomy; six patients had interval disease progression and did not undergo surgery. Grossly complete resection (R0 or R1) was performed in 26 (90%) of 29 patients who had surgery. Intraoperative electron-beam was feasible and successfully administered to 22 patients who had R0 or R1 resections. This trial demonstrates that preoperative external-beam radiation can be safely administered to a total dose of 50.4 Gy with continuous-infusion doxorubicin.

The three papers with sufficient follow-up that describe the use of preoperative radiotherapy with a brachytherapy or electron boost reported improved outcomes compared to most other series, especially for primary (as opposed to recurrent) presentation cases,[419,421,422] and presumably the MDACC trial will demonstrate similar findings with maturation of the data.[420] However, again we caution against overinterpretation of results that could be explained by surgical technique at major referral sarcoma centers or by case selection; of note, none of the four studies provides a comparison control group from which to infer efficacy. Similarly, it remains unclear what contribution is being provided by the use of brachytherapy or intraoperative radiotherapy (as opposed to the preoperative external-beam radiotherapy, common to all four studies), which should probably remain protocol-based in expert hands or be reserved for individual nonstandard clinical use.

Intraoperative Radiation Treatment

Intraoperative radiotherapy (IORT) offers the advantage of a direct boost dose to the tumor bed, thereby allowing a reduction in the dose of relatively more toxic concomitant EBRT. However, critical evaluation of its role is especially problematic because of treatment selection factors (both medical and technical) along with the fact that any observations of efficacy are confounded by the frequent use of additional fractionated external-beam radiotherapy in the "adjuvant package." Therefore a clear demonstration of the effectiveness of intraoperative radiotherapy is lacking, although its potential value should continue to be evaluated in appropriate investigational protocols. The same situation applies to the use of adjuvant brachytherapy approaches to dose augmentation in the retroperitoneum.

The efficacy of combined adjuvant IORT and EBRT has been evaluated in two recent series, one from Massachusetts General Hospital and the second from the Mayo Clinic,[421-423] and in a previous report from the U.S. National Cancer Institute (NCI).[424] The latter was a prospective trial in which 30 patients with completely resected retroperitoneal sarcomas were randomly assigned to receive IORT (11 to 15 MeV electron beam to a dose of 20 Gy) with low-dose postoperative EBRT (35 to 40 Gy) or to receive high-dose postoperative EBRT (50 to 55 Gy) alone.[424] IORT with low-dose EBRT was associated with a significantly lower rate of gastrointestinal toxicity (7% versus 60%), but no differences were noted in local control, disease-free survival, or overall survival. The rates of 5-year disease-free (20%) and overall survival (40%) seen in this study were comparable to those observed with surgery alone.[208,403] The reports from Massachusetts General Hospital and the Mayo Clinic described preoperative high-dose EBRT (40 to 50 Gy), instead of postoperative administration, with IORT (using electron beam to a dose of 8.75 to 30 Gy, depending on the series).[421,422] Both papers report on overall toxicity without differentiation between the influence of preoperative external beam and the boost after resection. This likely arose because of retrospective toxicity data collection in the two studies, which is further confounded by the frequent use of IORT in each.[421,422] The inference from our analysis of the results of both studies is that much of the toxicity seems related to use of IORT and is not from preoperative external-beam radiotherapy.

In summary, in the management of retroperitoneal sarcoma, complete surgical resection remains the standard of care. In selected patients with advanced disease, some disabling symptoms may be palliated by low to moderate dose EBRT. As for extremity sarcomas, there are no presently available data to support the use of routine adjuvant chemotherapy for these patients. Given the relatively high complication rates of high-dose external-beam radiation to the retroperitoneum, and the lack of clear demonstrable clinical benefit, routine preoperative or postoperative EBRT is not recommended outside the setting of a clinical trial and clinicians should be encouraged to enter patients in ongoing trials at referral centers.[411,425,426]

Chemotherapy

Retrospective studies have not demonstrated any benefit for preoperative[427] or postoperative[130,178,402] doxorubicin-based chemotherapy for retroperitoneal sarcomas. In fact, in one small RCT, there appeared to be an adverse effect of chemotherapy.[428] In another study, six complete responses were seen in 23 patients who received high-dose doxorubicin/ifosfamide/DDP (cisplatin) with concurrent radiotherapy.[242] Neoadjuvant chemotherapy has been combined with hyperthermia[429] and preoperative radiotherapy[420] without excessive toxicity. Idoxuridine was used as a radiosensitizer in a small pilot study.[430] These techniques remain experimental, however, and need further assessment, eventually in RCTs, to evaluate their place in the management of retroperitoneal sarcomas.

Gastrointestinal Stromal Tumors (GISTs)

Gastrointestinal stromal tumors (GISTs) arise from the gastrointestinal tract. This group of soft tissue tumors has become increasingly recognized as a separate subtype of sarcoma defined pathologically by expression of the growth factor receptor c-Kit (CD117). The management of these tumors has undergone significant recent change with the development and availability of imatinib mesylate, an agent with significant clinical benefit for patients with advanced GISTs. Details of the molecular pathology of GISTs are addressed in the sections "Potential Molecular Prognostic Factors" and "Prognostic Factors as Therapeutic Targets."

This section of the chapter will cover the evaluation and treatment of patients with GISTs. Consideration of these issues is often aided by subclassification by clinical staging into patients with localized, nonmetastatic (resectable) disease and patients with metastatic GIST.

Localized (Surgically Resectable) GISTs

Patients with localized GISTs are best treated with surgical resection of the primary tumor. Surgical resection generally requires segmental resection of the involved section of the gastrointestinal tract without local or regional lymphadenectomy. Since GISTs were only recently pathologically defined, there are few reports outlining the natural history of localized GISTs (excluding other forms of mural gastrointestinal neoplasms). Moreover the natural history of patients with localized disease stratified by c-Kit mutation subclassification is not well characterized at this time.

Details of the natural history of patients with surgically treated gastrointestinal leiomyosarcoma, the vast majority of whom may have what we currently would classify as GISTs, are outlined in prior reports.[138,431,432] These reports emphasize the importance of macroscopically and microscopically complete surgical resection and the adverse prognostic significance of large tumor size and high tumor grade (as assessed by light microscopic criteria). Although surgical resection has been the mainstay of therapy for patients with localized GISTs, a recently published analysis of 200 patients by DeMatteo and colleagues noted only a 54% disease-specific survival rate for patients in whom a grossly complete resection of their primary GIST had been achieved and the median survival in patients with metastatic disease was only 20 months.[433]

The role for imatinib mesylate in the preoperative and postoperative treatment of patients with localized GISTs is unknown. Two important trials of the American College of Surgeons Oncology Group (ACSOG; www.ACOSOG.org) will clarify the potential role for adjuvant imatinib mesylate. The first, ACOSOG Z9000, is a phase II trial of adjuvant imatinib mesylate, 400 mg daily in patients with complete resected high-risk (tumor size >10cm, tumor rupture at surgery, or multifocal [<5] tumors) GISTs. This trial is designed to determine whether these patients have prolonged survival compared to historical controls. ACOSOG Z9000 was closed to accrual in the summer of 2003 having accrued 89 eligible patients. The second trial, ACOSOG Z9001, is a randomized placebo controlled trial of imatinib mesylate in the management of patients with localized, completely resected GISTs. Three hundred eighty eligible patients will be randomized to receive postoperative imatinib mesylate (400 mg daily) or placebo for 1 year after the complete resection of localized GISTs. Accrual to this intergroup trial has been excellent to date. Results of this study will clarify the potential role for adjuvant imatinib mesylate in this disease.

Metastatic GISTs

The primary sites of failure for most patients with recurrent GIST are liver, peritoneum, or sometimes both sites. At this point, there is no standard algorithm for the management of patients with metastatic GISTs. In general, classification of such patients into those with radiographically resectable and unresectable disease is helpful in considering therapeutic options.

Metastasectomy. Patients with recurrent GISTs should be evaluated for metastasectomy. Results of surgical series of patients with metastatic leiomyosarcoma (many of whom likely had the relatively newly described entity GIST) suggest that complete resection of isolated hepatic or peritoneal metastases may improve survival and should be attempted if feasible in good risk patients.[431,434,435]

The role for pre- or postmetastasectomy imatinib mesylate is not defined at this writing. In general, consideration of imatinib mesylate for treatment of clinically occult micrometastatic disease is reasonable when one takes into account the considerable risk of having occult residual disease after metastasectomy and the belief that many systemic agents may be optimally administered when the volume of residual disease is low. For these reasons, further studies will need to explore the optimal ways to combine imatinib mesylate and metastasectomy.

Chemotherapy: Imatinib Mesylate.
GISTs are resistant to conventional cytotoxic chemotherapy agents with response rates that are typically in the single digit range. In the era of imatinib mesylate, there is no defined role for conventional chemotherapy agents in this disease.

The identification of mutations of c-Kit, which cause constitutive activation of the KIT tyrosine kinase receptor pathway in GIST, prompted treatment in 1996 of a Finnish patient with imatinib,[436] a tyrosine kinase inhbitor that is highly effective against chronic myeloid leukemia. An impressive response led to rapid initiation of phase I[437] and randomized phase II studies of imatinib for GISTs.[438] In an EORTC study, 40 patients, of whom 36 had GISTs, were treated at dose levels ranging from 400 mg/day to 1000 mg/day orally. There were 19 patients that had partial responses (54%) and 13 with stable disease (37%). Four of five of non-GIST patients progressed. The most common side effects of imatinib were nausea, vomiting, edema, and rash. In a multicenter phase II study, 147 patients were randomly assigned to receive 400 mg or 600 mg of imatinib daily. Although no patient had a complete response during treatment, 79 (54%) had a PR and 41 (28%) had stable disease. The median duration of response had not been reached at a median follow-up of 24 weeks from the onset of response.[76] There were no significant differences in response rate or toxicities between the two doses, with edema, diarrhea, and fatigue being the most common side effects. Gastrointestinal hemorrhage occurred in approximately 5% of patients.

Two RCTs of imatinib have been completed in North America[439] and Europe,[440] accruing 746 and 946 patients, respectively, with locally advanced or metastatic GIST. They compared 400 mg and 800 mg of imatinib and assessed overall survival, progression-free survival (PFS), and toxicity. Preliminary data on PFS do not indicate superiority of the higher dose level, which is more toxic. For patients with GISTs refractory to imatinib there is interest in a compound SU 11248 targeting multiple tyrosine kinases (KIT, PDGF-R, FLT3, and VEGF-R) that induced disease regression or stability in 11 (61%) of 18 patients in a phase I study.[441]

Singer and colleagues reported that c-Kit mutation type affects outcome.[166] They found a 5-year recurrence-free survival rate of 89% for patients with GISTs expressing missense exon 11 mutations compared with 40% ($P = 0.03$) for GISTs with other mutation types. The same group reported a higher PR rate to imatinib (72% versus 32%, $P = 0.0033$) for patients with exon 11 versus exon 9 mutations.[442]

Other soft tissue tumors that express activated tyrosine kinase receptors include desmoids and dermatofibrosarcoma protuberans (DFSP [PDGFß]) and desmoplastic round cell tumor (KIT). Case reports of patients with DFSP have documented responses to imatinib.[94,443,444] Not unexpectedly, in an EORTC study, Judson and colleagues demonstrated that most STSs, which do not generally express activated tyrosine kinase receptors, do not respond to imatinib.[445]

Head and Neck Sarcomas

Head and neck sarcomas are uncommon, accounting for only 4% of all sarcomas and less than 1% of head and neck malignancies in adults. (A detailed discussion of the current state of knowledge for adult and pediatric head and neck sarcoma is also available elsewhere.[446]) The most common histologic subtypes in adults are fibrosarcoma (18%), malignant fibrous histiocytoma (16%), and rhabdomyosarcoma (15%).[276,447] In recent large series of 176,[276] 188,[448] and 254[449] patients with head and neck sarcomas, the most common anatomic sites were the neck (23% to 38%) and paranasal sinuses (14% to 30%).

In the pediatric population, 40% of all soft tissue sarcomas occur in the head and neck, where the most common histologies are neuroblastoma and embryonal rhabdomyosarcoma. The treatment of these lesions in the pediatric population is beyond the scope of this chapter and is reviewed in the chapter on pediatric tumors.

Methods of diagnosis, imaging, and biopsy for head and neck sarcomas do not differ substantially from those for other head and neck tumors. Wide surgical excision with negative margins is the therapeutic mainstay for head and neck sarcomas. Regional lymph node metastases are rare, occurring in only 4% to 6% of patients in large series.[448,449] Thus, in the absence of clinically positive lymph nodes, regional lymphadenectomy is not routinely required.

Recent series have identified prognostic factors for head and neck sarcomas.[132-135,276,448,449] Multivariate analyses of patients with head and neck sarcomas identified high histologic grade and positive surgical margins as independent adverse prognostic factors for survival.[134,135] Age greater than 60 years at diagnosis was also found to be an independent adverse prognostic factor in one multivariate analysis.[135] Additional data from the Mayo Clinic confirm that the presence of metastases is associated with a poor (25%) 5-year overall survival rate and that certain histologic subtypes (angiosarcoma and nonorbital rhabdomyosarcoma) may have an adverse prognosis.[449]

Patterns of failure for head and neck sarcomas reflect the difficulty in obtaining adequate surgical margins in the head and neck region. Local recurrence remains a significant problem, with overall rates of local recurrence ranging from 14% to 48%,[276,448,450] making it important to consider appropriately applied principles of sarcoma management with combined modality approaches where appropriate. As with sarcomas elsewhere in the body, biologic behavior is a function of histologic grade, with local recurrence rates ranging from 22% for low-grade head and neck sarcomas to 48% for high-grade lesions.[276] Systemic recurrence develops in 12% to 31% of patients despite complete resection.[276,450] Overall 5-year survival rates are 45% to 68%.[276,448,449,451]

Radiation Treatment
Based on experience gained in treating extremity sarcomas, adjuvant radiotherapy should be considered whenever there is doubt as to the adequacy of surgical margins or the location of the tumor precludes complete excision. Evidence for the benefit of adjuvant radiotherapy is less plentiful than in extremity lesions and probably

relates to the rarity of these lesions and the absence of randomized trials addressing the specific issues for these lesions. However, Tran and colleagues from the University of California, Los Angeles have shown that local control was 52% with surgery alone versus 90% in head and neck patients treated with combined radiotherapy and surgery.[132] Additional evidence from the Princess Margaret Hospital reveals that head and neck STS patients with clear surgical margins or microscopic residuum had similar local failure rates (26% and 30% failure, respectively), provided radiotherapy was administered.[452] Indeed these outcomes for radiotherapy after R0/R1 resections approach those achieved in extremity sarcoma.

One strategy to improve outcome in head and neck sarcomas is through the use of preoperative radiotherapy. This approach may have particular advantages in this site because of the smaller volumes of radiotherapy and the lower doses that can be used compared to the postoperative treatment in difficult surgical access locations, especially in the base of skull. Obvious advantages provided relate to the ability to spare critical anatomy such as the optic structures (globes, optic nerves, and the optic chiasm), as well as the brain stem and spinal cord. If for no other reason, the preoperative approach promotes collaboration between the surgical and radiation oncologist, facilitates a complete management plan to be fashioned before any surgical intervention, and maximizes the opportunity to achieve control even when disease may be resected with a small but planned positive margin against critical unexpendable anatomy, as discussed earlier.[183]

In a prospective series of 40 patients (excluding rhabdomyosarcoma) with adverse selection criteria managed with preoperative radiotherapy between 1989 and 1999 at the Princess Margaret Hospital, 7 local relapses manifested (overall control rate of 82.5%).[185] This population of head and neck patients included five patients with intracranial extension, one with spinal cord compression, more than half were greater than 5 cm in size (a formidable problem for lesions in this anatomical location), and 85% were deep to the investing fascia. The series also contained four angiosarcoma patients, a group of patients with sinister local control probability (see vascular tumors later). In fact three of the seven local failures occurred in the angiosarcoma patients. If the series is confined to more usual soft tissue sarcoma, the local control rate is 33 out of 36 (92%). The metastatic relapse-free rate also exceeded 80% in this series, potentially related in part to the smaller overall dimension of sarcomas in this location compared to sarcomas elsewhere. Also the improved local control compared to a previous series of patients treated at the same institution may have contributed to this amelioration because the local control rate in the earlier series was substantially lower and death from concurrent local and metastatic disease was evident.[452]

Wound complications, assessed by the Canadian trial criteria,[200] were also seen with less frequency in this prospective study of head neck lesions (overall rate of 8 of 40 or 20%)[185] than were noted earlier with preoperative radiotherapy in extremity lesions. This may relate to the greater use of flaps for head and neck reconstruction.

At present, useful guidelines for using preoperative radiotherapy in the head and neck are: (1) the need to maximally restrict radiotherapy volumes in some anatomic sites (e.g., close to critical anatomy); (2) the desire to minimize radiation dose in some situations (e.g., where critical neurological tissues are in close proximity, as in the optic structures); and (3) a desire not to irradiate new tissues, especially vascular reconstructions vulnerable to the effects of high-dose postoperative radiotherapy.

Genitourinary Sarcomas

Although soft tissue sarcomas of the genitourinary tract are uncommon in adults, they account for up to 8% of all malignant disease in children younger than 15 years.[453] The management of genitourinary sarcomas in children has been more successful than in adults and is discussed in detail elsewhere in this book. In the Memorial Sloan-Kettering Cancer Center adult sarcoma database, only 43 sarcomas (2.7%) were of genitourinary origin. The paratesticular region (33%) and prostate/seminal vesicles (28%) are the most frequent sites of genitorurinary sarcomas, followed by the bladder (23%) and kidneys (16%). The most common histologic subtypes in adults are leiomyosarcoma (44%) and rhabdomyosarcoma (33%), although a spectrum of other histologic subtypes has been reported.[454]

A feature of genitourinary sarcomas that distinguishes them from other sarcomas is the fact that the vast majority of these lesions are of high histologic grade. In a recent report from the Memorial Sloan-Kettering Cancer Center, fully 86% of genitourinary sarcomas were high grade and 56% were larger than 5 cm.[454] Similar findings have been recently reported from the M.D. Anderson Cancer Center, where 15 (88%) of 17 primary sarcomas of the kidney met pathologic criteria for high-grade classification and tumor size ranged from 5.5 to 23 cm.[455] These findings have obvious prognostic implications, and recent series report relatively poor 5-year overall survival rates for patients with high-grade histology (48% versus 100% for low-grade lesions) or large tumor size (30% for lesions ≥ 5cm versus 83% for lesions < 5 cm).

The primary treatment for genitourinary sarcomas, as with sarcomas elsewhere in the body, is complete resection with histologically negative margins. There are no comparative trials specifically evaluating adjuvant therapy in this subgroup of sarcomas, but most investigators have extrapolated from the lessons learned with extremity soft tissue sarcoma and employ adjuvant therapy for patients with high-risk lesions, including those with high histologic grade, large tumor size, microscopically positive margins, gross residual disease, or unfavorable anatomic site (prostate or kidney). Using preoperative chemoradiation and surgery for patients with nonbulky sarcomas of the bladder and prostate and postoperative chemoradiation after radical surgery for patients with bulky disease, investigators at UCLA and at the City of Hope have reported encouraging results, with 9 of 11 patients with leiomyosarcomas alive with no evidence of disease at a mean follow-up of 61 months.[456] These promising results are similar to those reported from the

Mayo Clinic for a subset of seven patients with bladder sarcomas treated with preoperative radiotherapy and cystectomy[457] and are superior to those observed in a small series of patients treated with surgery alone.[458]

Paratesticular and spermatic cord sarcomas, if managed appropriately, can provide satisfactory outcome as reported in recent small series from the Princess Margaret Hospital (PMH)[459] and the M.D. Anderson Cancer Center.[460] Simple excision proved to be inadequate treatment for sarcomas in the spermatic cord and paratesticular region. In the PMH report wide repeat excision revealed microscopic residual disease in 27% of completely excised cases. These series suggest that adjuvant radiation should be considered for these patients as well as those with narrow repeat resection margins. Definitive conclusions on multimodality therapy for genitourinary sarcomas await further experience in larger numbers of patients.

The comparative infrequency of these lesions and the lack of a uniform staging system lead to difficulties in comparison of series and identification of prognostic factors. Prognostic factors for survival were analyzed in the series from the Memorial Sloan-Kettering Cancer Center and, by univariate analysis, favorable prognostic variables included tumor diameter less than 5 cm, low histologic grade, paratesticular or bladder (versus kidney or prostate) tumor site, and complete surgical resection.[454] No significant differences in survival were noted based on patient age, sex, or histologic subtype. A poor prognosis for patients with primary renal sarcomas has also been observed at M.D. Anderson with 13 of 15 evaluable patients dead of disease after a mean of 23 months.[455] Complete tumor resection was possible in 72% of patients in the series of 43 adult genitourinary sarcomas from Memorial Sloan-Kettering. The 5-year overall survival rate was 64% for this group of patients. No patient with an incomplete resection survived 5 years.

Unfortunately, as with head and neck rhabdomyosarcomas, the favorable results observed in pediatric patients with genitourinary rhabdomyosarcoma treated with a multimodality approach (58% to 74% 5-year overall survival)[461,462] have not been observed in adults in one study, only 5 (36%) of 14 adults were alive at the time of analysis (median follow-up, 32 months) despite aggressive multimodality therapy.[454]

Uterine Sarcomas

Uterine sarcomas are uncommon neoplasms that comprise between 2% and 4% of uterine malignancies.[463,464] The three main histologic subtypes in a recent series of 66 uterine sarcomas were as follows: mixed mesodermal (mullerian) tumors, 48%; leiomyosarcomas, 36%; and endometrial stromal tumors, 15%.[465] As with patients who have adenocarcinomas of the uterus, most patients with uterine sarcomas present with vaginal bleeding (77% to 99%) or pelvic pain (30%).[466-469] A palpable pelvic mass is present in 20% to 50% of patients.[469,470] The diagnostic workup is similar to that for the common uterine neoplasms and involves an outpatient biopsy or fractional dilatation and curettage. Imaging studies including CT and

MRI are employed preoperatively in patients with positive preoperative biopsy findings or those with clinically apparent masses on examination.

The standard treatment approach for patients with localized disease is total abdominal hysterectomy with bilateral salpingo-oophorectomy. Complete abdominal exploration is important from the standpoint of prognosis, but since there are virtually no survivors among patients in whom extrauterine disease is found at the time of exploration, therapeutic extrapelvic dissection has no role. In a review of 423 patients from the West Midlands Cancer Registry, 5-year survival rates for patients with stage I, II, III, and IV (International Federation of Gynecology and Obstetrics staging system) uterine sarcomas were 51%, 13%, 10%, and 3%, respectively.[139]

Adjuvant radiation has been evaluated by a number of investigators. To date, no completed RCT has evaluated the impact of adjuvant radiotherapy on disease-free survival or local recurrence using surgery alone as a control. A Gynecologic Oncology Group (GOG) trial evaluating the role of postoperative radiotherapy closed because of poor patient accrual. Retrospective comparison of treatment results obtained with surgery alone versus surgery and postoperative radiotherapy has not demonstrated any significant difference in overall survival or disease-free survival rates.[465,471-476] Multiple retrospective evaluations have suggested, however, that patients treated with adjuvant radiotherapy have significantly improved local control with significantly improved freedom from local (pelvic) recurrence compared to patients treated with surgery alone.[465,472-475] These results parallel the findings noted for patients with extremity sarcomas—demonstrable improvement in local control with adjuvant radiation but no impact on survival, although the same concerns exist pertaining to the small sample size to detect an effect of this kind.[177,182]

Several investigators have recently identified prognostic factors for survival in uterine sarcoma.[139,477] Multivariate analysis of 423 cases of uterine sarcoma demonstrated that advanced tumor stage, poor histologic grade, increased age, and leiomyosarcoma histologic subtype (versus mixed mullerian tumors) are characteristics that adversely affect survival.[139] A similar multivariate analysis by the GOG of prognostic factors in 453 patients with uterine sarcomas demonstrated that factors related to progression-free interval were histologic grade, histologic type (homologous versus heterologous mixed mullerian tumors), adnexal spread, and lymph node metastasis.[477] These prognostic factors are of importance for selecting adjuvant therapy for individual patients and in designing future clinical trials in uterine sarcoma.

Chemotherapy

There is some evidence that mixed mullerian sarcomas (MMS) respond well to DDP chemotherapy alone[478] or in combination with other drugs.[479] Ifosfamide also seems to be active in MMS,[479] but doxorubicin may be of more limited value.[480] In a GOG study[481] in which 76 patients with completely resected MMS were given three cycles of adjuvant ifosfamide/DDP, 2-year recurrence-free survival (63%) and overall survival (74%) rates were better than for historical controls, but clearly an RCT is needed to establish any true benefit for this regimen.

Paclitaxel combined with topotecan produced a 29% response rate in 45 patients with MMS,[482] and a retrospective analysis of MMS of the ovary found a very high response rate (72%) for a combination of paclitaxel and DDP.[483] Further exploration of agents active in epithelial ovarian cancer may be justified in MMS.

In contrast, uterine leiomyosarcoma, which often metastasizes to the lung rather than the liver, responds reasonably well to doxorubicin.[480] With respect to adjuvant chemotherapy, no significant differences in recurrence, progression-free survival, or overall survival rates were evident in a GOG RCT of 156 patients comparing doxorubicin (60 mg/m^2) with no adjuvant chemotherapy after resection of stage I uterine sarcomas.[471] This trial was underpowered to detect small differences in outcome, however.

Desmoid Tumors (Aggressive Fibromatoses)

Desmoid tumor is an uncommon malignancy. It is estimated that approximately 700 to 900 new cases (3 to 4 cases per million) occur annually in the United States.[481,484] The tumor arises principally from the connective tissue of muscle and the overlying fascia or muscular aponeurosis. Clinically, the tumor presents as a poorly circumscribed, painless mass and is commonly located in the muscles of the shoulder and pelvic girdle and frequently in the thigh. It is most common in patients between the ages of 20 and 40 years with a peak incidence of 25 to 35 years. Aggressive fibromatosis, extra-abdominal desmoid, well-differentiated nonmetastasizing fibrosarcoma, and grade I fibrosarcoma are terms that have also been used to describe this lesion.

Surgery and Radiation

Surgical resection remains the mainstay of therapy for desmoid tumors. Wide local resection with negative microscopic margins (R0) is the optimal surgical therapy. When resection is performed with positive microscopic surgical margins, local recurrence rates are substantially higher. Unfortunately, there are relatively few large series that outline actuarial local recurrence-free survival rates

stratified by microscopic margin status for patients treated by surgery alone. Series from the M.D. Anderson Cancer Center (MDACC), Massachusetts General Hospital (MGH), and Memorial Sloan-Kettering Cancer Center (MSKCC) with margin-specific local recurrence rates are summarized in Table 96-13.[485–487] The experience of these institutions suggests that the local control rates for patients treated by surgery alone is on the order of 50% when microscopic surgical margins are positive (R1 resection), compared to approximately 75% when microscopic surgical margins are negative (R0 resection). As a consequence of the propensity for local recurrence, many groups have utilized postoperative external-beam radiotherapy for patients undergoing local excision (R0 or R1).[485,486] Postoperative external-beam radiotherapy is usually given to patients who are thought to be at higher risk for local recurrence. However, some groups employ external-beam radiation for patients who have undergone an R0 resection (because of the generally high local recurrence rates associated with surgical treatment alone) and also for most patients who have undergone an R1 resection. The criteria for selecting patients for postoperative radiation vary widely and are often subjective.

Interpretation of the limited literature on the use of external-beam radiotherapy in the management of localized desmoid tumors is hampered by the rarity of the lesion and the absence of margin-specific actuarial local recurrence rates for large series of consecutively treated patients. Retrospective comparisons stratified by margin status suggest that local recurrence rates may be reduced for patients treated with combined-modality therapy. The data substantiating this are all retrospective, nonrandomized, single-institution experiences and thus there is no clearly defined consensus on the role of radiation therapy in the management of patients with desmoid tumors.

Chemotherapy

Patients with desmoid tumors usually present to a medical oncologist only if they have progressed after surgery and radiotherapy and are considered inoperable or are located at sites not amenable to full-dose radiotherapy. These tumors are rarely life threatening, although some tumors, especially the intra-abdominal desmoids seen in Gardner's syndrome, may become so due to pressure on or invasion

TABLE 96-13

Local Recurrence-Free Rates Following Surgery for Patients with Desmoid Tumors

INSTITUTION	NO. OF PATIENTS	FOLLOW-UP (MO)	OVERALL (%)	LOCAL RECURRENCE-FREE SURVIVAL	
				R0 (%)	R1 (%)
MGH[485]	51	12–59	69	77	56*
MDACC[486]	122	113	62	73†	46†
MSKCC[487]	128	88	71	86*	49*

MDACC, University of Texas M.D. Anderson Cancer Center; MGH, Massachusetts General Hospital; MSKCC: Memorial Sloan-Kettering Cancer Center; R0, microscopically negative surgical margins; R1, microscopically positive surgical margins.
*Using 5-year actuarial analysis.
†Using 10-year actuarial analysis.

of vital organs. Rare responses have been reported to non-steroidal anti-inflammatory drugs or anti-estrogens.[488-490] Weiss and Lackman were the first to report responses of desmoids to low-dose chemotherapy with methotrexate (50 mg/week) and vinblastine (10 mg/week).[490] Regressions are often slow, and toxicity usually requires dosing to be extended to 2-week intervals. Several groups have since confirmed the activity of this combination.[491-493] A much more aggressive regimen of continuous infusion doxorubicin and dacarbazine[494,495] has produced substantial regressions in desmoids secondary to Gardner's syndrome. This regimen produces substantial toxicity, however, and should be reserved for those with aggressive symptomatic disease. A case report documented a response of a desmoid to single-agent doxorubicin,[496] and this may be a less toxic alternative.

Breast Sarcomas

Primary sarcomas of the breast account for less than 1% of all primary breast neoplasms.[497] They should be distinguished from cystosarcoma phyllodes, sarcomatoid carcinoma, and carcinosarcoma of the breast, which are all distinct clinical conditions. The most common histologic subtypes of breast sarcomas are malignant fibrous histiocytoma, liposarcoma, and fibrosarcoma.[498,499] A disproportionate number of angiosarcomas appear to arise in the breast either de novo[500] or after breast-conservation surgery with adjuvant radiation.[501-503] In general, however, the etiology of most breast sarcomas is unknown. An association between augmentation mammoplasty with silicone prostheses and development of breast sarcoma had been postulated, but analysis of the NCI's Surveillance, Epidemiology and End Results (SEER) Program database failed to demonstrate any relationship.[504]

On physical examination, breast sarcomas are usually well circumscribed, firm, mobile, and painless. Mammography frequently demonstrates a well-circumscribed lesion, in contrast to the irregular, stellate appearance of most mammary carcinomas. With the advent of fine-needle aspiration biopsy, an increasing number of these lesions are diagnosed preoperatively. This is of importance in planning an operative approach for these patients. As breast sarcomas rarely spread to regional lymph nodes,[505-507] axillary lymph node dissection is not indicated for patients with a clinically negative axilla. The treatment of choice for breast sarcomas is wide local excision with histologically negative margins. Depending on the relative proportions of the tumor and the breast, this sometimes necessitates total mastectomy.

Adverse prognostic factors for survival include high histologic grade and an infiltrative histologic pattern.[499,505,507,508] A recent retrospective review of 83 patients with primary breast sarcomas treated predominantly with surgery and selective use of adjuvant chemotherapy and/or radiation revealed 10-year overall and disease-free survival rates of 62% and 50%, respectively.[499] On the basis of this report and early reports,[505-507] it appears that patients with primary breast sarcomas have a similar natural history, prognostic factors, and outcome after combined-modality treatment to patients with extremity sarcomas.

There is no clearly defined role for adjuvant radiotherapy in this disease, although it would appear prudent to offer radiation to patients at high risk for local recurrence (microscopically positive margins or presentation with recurrent breast sarcoma). In addition, in a report of a mixed group of breast sarcomas and phylloides tumors at the Princess Margaret Hospital, breast conservation seemed to be attainable using conservative margin-negative excision and adjuvant radiotherapy in an organ-preserving approach consistent with the contemporary management for both breast cancer and soft tissue sarcoma.[509]

Vascular Sarcomas

The collective term "vascular sarcomas" includes the histologic subtypes of angiosarcoma, hemangiosarcoma, lymphangiosarcoma, and malignant hemangiopericytoma. Together these lesions account for approximately 4% of all soft tissue sarcomas.[510] A minority of these lesions are associated with well-known environmental factors, as noted in Table 96-1. In a national review of 99 Japanese patients with angiosarcoma, angiosarcoma was most commonly located on the head or face (29 patients) and was found to be associated with several predisposing conditions, including chronic pyothorax (6), use of Thorotrast in the liver (5), previous radiotherapy (4), and chronic lymphedema (1).[511] Virtually all of the literature on these rare neoplasms focuses on individual histologic and site-specific subtypes and includes pediatric patients. These facts, and the relative infrequency of these lesions, make general estimates of survival difficult for adult patients with vascular soft tissue sarcomas.

In a review of 69 patients with vascular sarcomas from Memorial Sloan-Kettering Cancer Center, 35 patients (51%) had angiosarcoma, 28 (41%) had malignant hemangiopericytoma, and 6 (9%) had lymphangiosarcoma.[510] No anatomic site was spared from involvement. The most common sites of involvement for angiosarcomas and malignant hemangiopericytomas were similar: visceral, retroperitoneum, head and neck, and extremities. The six lymphangiosarcomas in this series all occurred in an edematous extremity.

Cutaneous angiosarcoma is a variant of angiosarcoma that often arises in the head and neck and frequently diffusely infiltrates the dermis of the scalp or tissues of the face.[512] In the head and neck, cutaneous angiosarcoma may be difficult to treat by surgery alone because of the infiltrating nature of the disease and the anatomic constraints of the head and neck that make wide surgical margins difficult to achieve. Patients may be optimally treated by surgery to remove all macroscopic disease and subsequent radiotherapy to address the high risk of microscopic residual disease.[512]

Overall survival rates for patients with localized disease who undergo curative resection are similar for angiosarcomas and malignant hemangiopericytomas (68% to 72%). A clear survival advantage for patients with low-grade lesions was not demonstrable in this study, although other investigators have reported such a relationship for cutaneous angiosarcomas.[513] Several investigators have suggested that tumor size may be an important prognostic factor for survival in patients with malignant hemangiopericytomas[514,515] and angiosarcomas of the face and scalp,[516,517] although no relationship was noted in the study from Memorial Sloan-Kettering.

Surgery

By definition, these lesions are vascular and this should be borne in mind when planning preoperative biopsy and surgery. In the study from Memorial Sloan-Kettering, perioperative bleeding was noted in 33% of patients, with 18 of 69 patients experiencing extensive blood loss (>1000 cc) and two deaths related to hemorrhage.[510] Frozen section control of microscopic surgical margins is advisable given the locally infiltrative nature of many angiosarcomas, particularly those arising on the scalp.

Adjuvant Therapy

There is no clearly defined role for adjuvant radiation or chemotherapy for vascular sarcomas, although it seems reasonable to extrapolate from data derived from extremity lesions and offer adjuvant radiotherapy for patients with high-risk lesions. Unfortunately, aggressive surgical approaches may prove disappointing due the unusual capability of this disease to exhibit edge recurrence and manifest disease relatively remote from the initial site of presentation (Fig. 96-17A and B). Alternative radiotherapy techniques such as modulated electron radiotherapy (MERT) are promising and may be applied in the future to the treatment of wide field areas requiring only superficial penetration at depth, as is the case in craniofacial angiosarcoma. Considering the proximity of the brain and eyes in these lesions, limiting the depth of penetration and consequent reduction in dose to tissues deeper to tumor is the attractive aspect of this technology.[518]

There have been anecdotal reports that paclitaxel may be specifically active in angiosarcomas.[364,519] Interferon-α is active against benign capillary hemangiomas of infancy and malignant vascular lesions such as HIV-related Kaposi's sarcoma. Burgess and colleagues reported sporadic responses in a variety of angiomatous tumors to a combination of interferon-α and 13-cis-retinoic acid.[520] These intriguing reports need to be validated in larger studies.

Chemotherapy Considerations for Specific Histologic Subtypes

Synovial Sarcomas

Rosen and colleagues[521] were the first to suggest that synovial sarcomas were particularly responsive to ifosfamide. They documented 3 complete responses and 9 partial responses in 13 patients (9 of whom had received prior doxorubicin-based chemotherapy) with metastatic synovial sarcomas. These investigators also reported on 14 patients with localized synovial sarcomas who received adjuvant doxorubicin/ifosfamide/DDP chemotherapy.[522] There was one patient with local recurrence, but the remaining 13 patients (93%) remained disease free at a median follow-up period of 37 (6 to 85) months. In a large EORTC phase II trial of 124 patients with advanced STS receiving ifosfamide (12 g/m^2), the overall response rate rate for all histological subtypes was 16%,[351] but 8 (44%) of 18 patients with synovial sarcoma responded. Edmonson and colleagues described a higher response

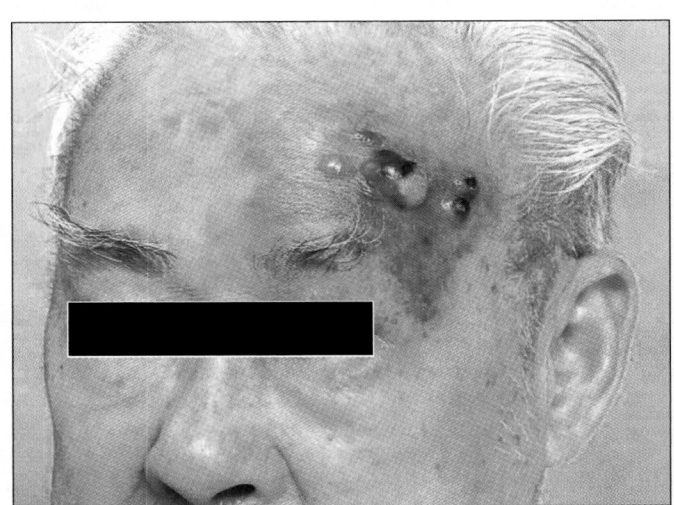
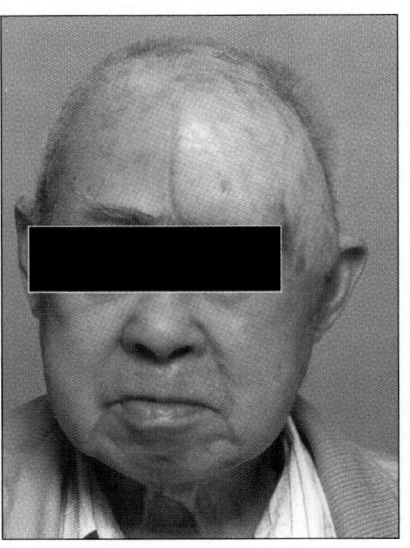

Figure 96-17. **A,** Angiosarcoma of the scalp and facial areas in an older male. Note the infiltrative and multinodular nature of this process characterized by mottled discoloration and ecchymosis in the upper eyelid and facial tissues adjacent to the lesion. These lesions pose a formidable challenge in achieving local control due to their propensity to manifest out-of-field recurrences after wide field surgical and radiotherapy interventions **(B)**, as well as a high predilection to fail in regional lymph nodes and distant sites. **B,** The same patient as in **(A)** showing the irradiated skin and the flap and reconstructed tissues at the site of wide field radiotherapy and surgery to the scalp for angiosarcoma. Unfortunately, this patient continued to manifest disease in other areas of the scalp remote from the treated areas that were managed with small field radiotherapy fields. This pattern of disease, including the ability to control disease locally but with relentless failure beyond the surgical and radiotherapy fields, is characteristic of angiosarcoma.

rate in synovial sarcomas for doxorubicin/ifosfamide than for doxorubicin alone (88% versus 20%, P = 0.02) in the setting of an RCT of multiple histologic subtypes of STS.[332] A subsequent ECOG phase II study of doxorubicin/ ifosfamide in synovial sarcomas showed 5 partial responses (42%) in 12 patients; however, the median survival for the whole group was only 11 months, and the trial was closed because of poor accrual.[523] In many studies evaluating ifosfamide, including some of the RCTs, the question of response by histologic subtype has not been addressed, and most of the data on histologic variations in response are anecdotal. As many of these patients are young and fit, inclusion of ifosfamide in first-line chemotherapy for metastatic disease seems reasonable. If the circumstances merit adjuvant chemotherapy, an anthracycline/ifosfamide combination would be a logical choice.

Liposarcomas

Activation of the PPARγ nuclear receptor stimulates terminal differentiation in preadipocytes. Troglitazone, used in the treatment of diabetes mellitus, is an activating ligand for PPARγ. Biopsies pre- and post-troglitazone therapy were obtained in 34 of 49 patients with different types of liposarcomas entering a phase II trial.[524] Five of seven (71%) evaluable patients with myxoid/round cell disease exhibited histologic evidence of lineage-appropriate differentiation of liposarcoma cells, whereas only one of three (33%) patients with high-grade pleomorphic disease showed such changes.[525] Although this study provides proof-of-concept data, the clinical significance is uncertain as responses to troglitazone were not documented.

Pediatric Sarcomas in Adults

Embryonal rhabdomyosarcomas and the PNETs (primitive neuroectodermal tumors), including extraskeletal Ewing's sarcoma, all seem to be chemosensitive when they occur in the adult age group. Adult patients with these tumors should receive aggressive combination chemotherapy similar to that offered to children with the same disease.[526,527] Nevertheless the outcome is likely to be poorer for adults with "pediatric sarcomas" than for pediatric sarcoma patients.

REFERENCES

1. Jemal A, Murray T, Samuels A, et al: Cancer Statistics, 2003. CA Cancer J Clin 2003;53:5.
2. Smith J: Postradiation sarcoma of bone in Hodgkin disease. Skeletal Radiol 1987;16:524.
3. Coia LR, Fazekas JT, Kramer S: Postirradiation sarcoma of the head and neck: A report of three late sarcomas following therapeutic irradiation for primary malignancies of the paranasal sinus, nasal cavity, and larynx. Cancer 1980;46:1982.
4. Arbabi L, Warhol MJ: Pleomorphic liposarcoma following radiotherapy for breast carcinoma. Cancer 1982;49:878.
5. Hatfield PM, Schulz MD: Postirradiation sarcoma: Including five cases after x-ray therapy of breast carcinoma. Radiology 1970;96:593.
6. Becker AJ: Zur Frage des Rontgensarkomas, zugleich ein Beitrag zur Pathogenese des Sarkomas. Muench Med Wochenschr 1922;69:623.
7. Brady MS, Gaynor JJ, Brennan MF: Radiation-associated sarcoma of bone and soft tissue. Arch Surg 1992;127:1379.
8. Robinson E, Neugut AI, Wylie P: Clinical aspects of postirradiation sarcomas. J Natl Cancer Inst 1988;80:233.
9. Pitcher ME, Davidson TI, Fisher C, et al: Post irradiation sarcoma of soft tissue and bone. Eur J Surg Oncol 1994;20:53.
10. Cahan WG, Woodward HQ, Higinbotham NL, et al: Sarcoma arising in irradiated bone: Report of 11 cases. Cancer 1948;1:3.
11. Arlen M, Higinbotham NL, Huvos AG, et al: Radiation-induced sarcoma of bone. Cancer 1971;28:1087.
12. Feigen M: Should cancer survivors fear radiation-induced sarcomas? Sarcoma 1997;1:5.
13. Davidson TI, Westbury G, Harmer CL: Radiation-induced soft-tissue sarcoma. Br J Surg 1986;73:308.
14. Tucker MA, D'Angio GJ, Boice JD Jr, et al: Bone sarcomas linked to radiotherapy and chemotherapy in children. N Engl J Med 1987;317:588.
15. Spiro IJ, Suit HD: Radiation-induced bone and soft tissue sarcomas: Clinical aspects and molecular biology. Cancer Treat Res 1997; 91:143.
16. Hardell L: Malignant mesenchymal tumors and exposure to phenoxy acids: A clinical observation. Lakartidningen 1977;74:2753.
17. Hardell L, Sandstrom A: Case-control study: Soft-tissue sarcomas and exposure to phenoxyacetic acids or chlorophenols. Br J Cancer 1979;39:711.
18. Eriksson M, Hardell L, Ber NO, et al: Soft-tissue sarcomas and exposure to chemical substances: A case-referent study. Br J Ind Med 1981;38:27.
19. Hardell L, Eriksson M: The association between soft tissue sarcomas and exposure to phenoxyacetic acids: A new case-referent study. Cancer 1988;62:652.
20. Hoar SK, Blair A, Holmes FF, et al: Agricultural herbicide use and risk of lymphoma and soft-tissue sarcoma. JAMA 1986;256:1141.
21. Smith AH, Pearce NE, Fisher DO, et al: Soft tissue sarcoma and exposure to phenoxyherbicides and chlorophenols in New Zealand. J Natl Cancer Inst 1984;73:1111.
22. Riihimaki V, Asp S, Hernberg S: Mortality of 2,4-dichlorophenoxyacetic acid and 2,4,5-trichlorophenoxyacetic acid herbicide applicators in Finland: First report of an ongoing prospective cohort study. Scand J Work Environ Health 1982;8:37.
23. Kang H, Enzinger FM, Breslin P, et al: Soft tissue sarcoma and military service in Vietnam: A case-control study. J Natl Cancer Inst 1987;79:693.
24. MacMahon HE, Murphy AS, Bates MI: Endothelial cell sarcoma of liver following Thorotrast injections. Am J Pathol 1947;23:585.
25. DaSilva-Horta J: Late lesions in man caused by colloidal thorium dioxide (Thorotrast). Arch Pathol 1956;62:403.
26. DaSilva-Horta J, Abbatt JD, DaMotta LC: Malignancy and other effects following the administration of Thorotrast. Lancet 1965;2:201.
27. Creech JL Jr, Makk L: Liver disease among polyvinyl chloride production workers. Ann N Y Acad Sci 1975;246:88.
28. Creech JL Jr, Johnson MN: Angiosarcoma of liver in the manufacture of polyvinyl chloride. J Occup Med 1974;16:150.
29. Lloyd JW: Angiosarcoma of the liver in vinyl chloride/polyvinyl chloride workers. J Occup Med 1975;17:333.
30. Roth F: Arsen-Lieber Tumoren (Hemangioendothelioma). Krebsforschung 1957;61:468.
31. Roth F: The sequelae of chronic arsenic poisoning in Moselle vintners. German Med Monthly 1957;2:172.
32. Gohokar D, Borges A, Shetty P: Osteogenic sarcoma developing after successful therapy of acute lymphocytic leukemia. Am J Pediatr Hematol Oncol 1986;8:259.
33. Shaw PJ, Bergin M, Stevens M: Osteogenic sarcoma following acute lymphoblastic leukemia. Am J Pediatr Hematol Oncol 1988;10:81.
34. Stewart FW, Treves N: Lymphangiosarcoma in post mastectomy lymphedema: A report of six cases of elephantiasis chirurgica. Cancer 1948;1:64.
35. Woodward AH, Ivins JC, Soule EH: Lymphangiosarcoma arising in chronic lymphedematous extremities. Cancer 1972;30:562.
36. Muller R, Hajdu SI, Brennan MF: Lymphangiosarcoma associated with chronic filarial lymphedema. Cancer 1987;59:179.
37. Brand KG: Foreign body induced sarcomas. In Becker FF (ed): Cancer. New York, Plenum, 1975, p 485.

38. Li FP, Fraumeni JF Jr: Soft-tissue sarcomas, breast cancer, and other neoplasms: A familial syndrome? Ann Intern Med 1969;71:747.

39. Knight WA III, Murphy WK, Gottlieb JA: Neurofibromatosis associated with malignant neurofibromas. Arch Dermatol 1973;107:747.

40. Sorensen SA, Mulvihill JJ, Nielsen A: Long-term follow-up of von Recklinghausen neurofibromatosis: Survival and malignant neoplasms. N Eng J Med 1986;314:1010.

41. Barker D, Wright E, Nguyen K, et al: Gene for von Recklinghausen neurofibromatosis is in the pericentromeric region of chromosome 17. Science 1987;236:1100.

42. Fountain JW, Wallace MR, Bruce MA, et al: Physical mapping of a translocation breakpoint in neurofibromatosis. Science 1989;244:1085.

43. Legius E, Marchuk DA, Collins FS, et al: Somatic deletion of the neurofibromatosis type 1 gene in a neurofibrosarcoma supports a tumour suppressor gene hypothesis. Nat Genet 1993;3:122.

44. Menon AG, Anderson KM, Riccardi VM, et al: Chromosome 17p deletions and p53 gene mutations associated with the formation of malignant neurofibrosarcomas in von Recklinghausen neurofibromatosis. Proc Natl Acad Sci USA 1990;87:5435.

45. Legius E, Dierick H, Wu R, et al: TP53 mutations are frequent in malignant NF1 tumors. Genes Chromosomes Cancer 1994;10:250.

46. Lothe RA, Slettan A, Saeter G, et al: Alterations at chromosome 17 loci in peripheral nerve sheath tumors. J Neuropathol Exp Neurol 1995;54:65.

47. Li FP, Fraumeni JF Jr: Rhabdomyosarcoma in children: Epidemiologic study and identification of a familial cancer syndrome. J Natl Cancer Inst 1969;43:1365.

48. Hartley AL, Birch JM, Kelsey AM, et al: Are germ cell tumors part of the Li-Fraumeni cancer family syndrome? Cancer Genet Cytogenet 1989;42:221.

49. Li FP, Fraumeni JF Jr, Mulvihill JJ, et al: A cancer family syndrome in 24 kindreds. Cancer Res 1988;48:5358.

50. Strong LC, Stine M, Norsted TL: Cancer in survivors of childhood soft tissue sarcoma and their relatives. J Natl Cancer Inst 1987;79:1213.

51. Malkin D, Li FP, Strong LC, et al: Germ line p53 mutations in a familial syndrome of breast cancer, sarcomas, and other neoplasms. Science 1990;s250:123.

52. Bell DW, Varley JM, Szydlo TE, et al: Heterozygous germ line hCHK2 mutations in Li-Fraumeni syndrome. Science 1999;286:2528.

53. Cavenee WK, Hansen MF, Nordenskjold M, et al: Genetic orgin of mutations predisposing to retinoblastoma. Science 1985;228:1.

54. Hansen MF, Koufos A, Gallie BL, et al: Osteosarcoma and retinoblastoma: A shared chromosomal mechanism revealing recessive predisposition. Proc Natl Acad Sci USA 1985;82:6216.

55. Draper GJ, Sanders BM, Kingston JE: Second primary neoplasms in patients with retinoblastoma. Br J Cancer 1986;53:661.

56. Lee EY, To H, Shew JY, et al: Inactivation of the retinoblastoma susceptibility gene in human breast cancers. Science 1988;241:218.

57. Harbour JW, Lai SL, Whang-Peng J, et al: Abnormalities in structure and expression of the human retinoblastoma gene in SCLC. Science 1988;241:353.

58. Cance WG, Brennan MF, Dudas ME, et al: Altered expression of the retinoblastoma gene product in human sarcomas. N Eng J Med 1990;323:1457.

59. Maher ER, Morson B, Beach R, et al: Phenotypic variation in hereditary nonpolyposis colon cancer syndrome: Association with infiltrative fibromatosis (desmoid tumor). Cancer 1992;69:2049.

60. Scott RJ, Froggatt NJ, Trembath RC, et al: Familial infiltrative fibromatosis (desmoid tumours) (MIM135290) caused by a recurrent 3'APC gene mutation. Hum Mol Genet 1996;5:1921.

61. Eccles DM, van der LR, Breukel C, et al: Hereditary desmoid disease due to a frameshift mutation at codon 1924 of the APC gene. Am J Hum Genet 1996;59:1193.

62. Gardner E: Cancer of the lower digestive tract in one family group. Am J Hum Genet 1950;2:41.

63. Korinek V, Barker N, Morin PJ, et al: Constitutive transcriptional activation by a beta-catenin-Tcf complex in APC-/- colon carcinoma. Science 1997;275:1784.

64. Okamoto M, Sato C, Kohno Y, et al: Molecular nature of chromosome 5q loss in colorectal tumors and desmoids from patients with familial adenomatous polyposis. Hum Genet 1990;85:595.

65. Alman BA, Li C, Pajerski ME, et al: Increased beta-catenin protein and somatic APC mutations in sporadic aggressive fibromatoses (desmoid tumors). Am J Pathol 1997;151:329.

66. Shitoh K, Konishi F, Iijima T, et al: A novel case of a sporadic desmoid tumour with mutation of the beta catenin gene. J Clin Pathol 1999;52:695.

67. Biegel JA, Zhou JY, Rorke LB, et al: Germline and acquired mutations of INI1 in atypical teratoid and rhabdoid tumors. Cancer Res 1999;59:74.

68. Biegel JA, Kalpana G, Knudsen ES, et al: The role of INI1 and the SWI/SNF complex in the development of rhabdoid tumors: Meeting summary from the workshop on childhood atypical teratoid/rhabdoid tumors. Cancer Res 2002;62:323.

69. Versteege I, Sevenet N, Lange J, et al: Truncating mutations of hSNF5/INI1 in aggressive paediatric cancer. Nature 1998;394:203.

70. Schellenberg G, et al: Werner syndrome. In Scriver CR, Beaudet AL, Sly WS, Valle D (eds): The Metabolic and Molecular Basis of Inherited Disease. New York, McGraw-Hill, 2001, p 785.

71. Yu CE, Oshima J, Fu YH, et al: Positional cloning of the Werner's syndrome gene. Science 1996;272:258.

72. Hirota S, Isozaki K, Moriyama Y, et al: Gain-of-function mutations of c-kit in human gastrointestinal stromal tumors. Science 1998;279:577.

73. Nishida T, Hirota S, Taniguchi M, et al: Familial gastrointestinal stromal tumours with germline mutation of the KIT gene. Nat Genet 1998;19:323.

74. Rubin BP, Singer S, Tsao C, et al: KIT activation is a ubiquitous feature of gastrointestinal stromal tumors. Cancer Res 2001;61:8118.

75. Rubin BP, Fletcher JA, Fletcher CD: Molecular Insights into the histogenesis and pathogenesis of gastrointestinal stromal tumors. Int J Surg Pathol 2000;8:5.

76. Demetri GD: Targeting the molecular pathophysiology of gastrointestinal stromal tumors with imatinib: Mechanisms, successes, and challenges to rational drug development. Hematol Oncol Clin North Am 2002;16:1115.

77. Rubin BP, Fetcher JA: Basic concepts in molecular cytogenetics of soft tissue tumors for the clinician. Semin Musculoskelet Radiol 1999;3:173.

78. Khan J, Simon R, Bittner M, et al: Gene expression profiling of alveolar rhabdomyosarcoma with cDNA microarrays. Cancer Res 1998;58:5009.

79. Knezevich SR, McFadden DE, Tao W, et al: A novel ETV6-NTRK3 gene fusion in congenital fibrosarcoma. Nat Genet 1998;18:184.

80. Fletcher JA, Kozakewich HP, Hoffer FA, et al: Diagnostic relevance of clonal cytogenetic aberrations in malignant soft-tissue tumors. N Eng J Med 1991;324:436.

81. Kushner BH, LaQuaglia MP, Cheung NK, et al: Clinically critical impact of molecular genetic studies in pediatric solid tumors. Med Pediatr Oncol 1999;33:530.

82. Sreekantaiah C, Ladanyi M, Rodriguez E, et al: Chromosomal aberrations in soft tissue tumors: Relevance to diagnosis, classification, and molecular mechanisms. Am J Pathol 1994;144:1121.

83. Karakousis CP, Dal Cin P, Turc-Carel C, et al: Chromosomal changes in soft-tissue sarcomas: A new diagnostic parameter. Arch Surg 1987;122:1257.

84. Limon J, Mrozek K, Mandahl N, et al: Cytogenetics of synovial sarcoma: Presentation of ten new cases and review of the literature. Genes Chromosomes Cancer 1991;3:338.

85. Turc-Carel C, Aurias A, Mugneret F, et al: Chromosomes in Ewing's sarcoma: An evaluation of 85 cases of remarkable consistency of t(11; 22)(q24; q12). Cancer Genet Cytogenet 1988;32:229.

86. Barr FG: Molecular genetics and pathogenesis of rhabdomyosarcoma. J Pediatr Hematol Oncol 1997;19:483.

87. Barr FG, Galili N, Holick J, et al: Rearrangement of the PAX3 paired box gene in the paediatric solid tumour alveolar rhabdomyosarcoma. Nat Genet 1993;3:113.

88. Davis RJ, D'Cruz CM, Lovell MA, et al: Fusion of PAX7 to FKHR by the variant t(1;13)(p36;q14) translocation in alveolar rhabdomyosarcoma. Cancer Res 1994;54:2869.

89. Galili N, Davis RJ, Fredericks WJ, et al: Fusion of a fork head

domain gene to PAX3 in the solid tumour alveolar rhabdomyo-sarcoma. Nat Genet 1993;5:230.

90. Zoubek A, Dockhorn-Dworniczak B, Delattre O, et al: Does expression of different EWS chimeric transcripts define clinically distinct risk groups of Ewing tumor patients? J Clin Oncol 1996;14:1245.

91. De Alava E, Kawai A, Healey JH, et al: EWS-FLII fusion transcript structure is an independent determinant of prognosis in Ewing's sarcoma. J Clin Oncol 1998;16:1248.

92. Kawai A, Woodruff JM, Healey JH, et al: SYT-SSX gene fusion as a determinant of morphology and prognosis in synovial sarcoma. N Eng J Med 1998;338:153.

93. Ladanyi M, Antonescu CR, Leung DH, et al: Impact of SYT-SSX fusion type on the clinical behavior of synovial sarcoma: A multi-institutional retrospective study of 243 patients. Cancer Res 2002;62:135.

94. Rubin BP, Schuetze SM, Eary JF, et al: Molecular targeting of platelet-derived growth factor B by imatinib mesylate in a patient with metastatic dermatofibrosarcoma protuberans. J Clin Oncol 2002;20:3586.

95. Fletcher CDM, Unni KK, Mertens F (eds): Pathology and Genetics of Tumours of Soft Tissue and Bone. Lyon, France, IARC Press, International Agency for Research on Cancer, p 2002.

96. Van Haelst UJGM: Electron microscopy in the study of soft tissue tumors: Diagnosis/differential diagnosis and histogenesis. In Van Oosterom AT, van Unnik JAM (eds): Management of Soft Tissue and Bone Sarcomas. New York, Raven, 1986, p 77.

97. Brooks JJ: Immunochemistry in sarcomas. In Ryan JR, Baker LO (eds): Recent Concepts in Sarcoma Treatment. Boston, Kluwer Academic, 1988, p 48.

98. Fletcher CDM: The use of immunohistochemistry in the diagnosis of soft tissue tumours. Histopathology 1986;10:771.

99. Weiss SW, Sobin LH: Histologic typing of soft tissue tumors. In Weiss SW (eds): Soft Tissue Sarcoma 2nd ed. Berlin, Springer-Verlag, 1994, p 7.

100. Presant CA, Russell WO, Alexander RW, et al: Soft-tissue and bone sarcoma histopathology peer review: The frequency of disagreement in diagnosis and the need for second pathology opinions. The Southeastern Cancer Study Group experience. J Clin Oncol 1986;4:1658.

101. Shiraki MJ, Enterline HT, Brooks JJ, et al: Pathologic analysis of advanced adult soft tissue sarcomas, bone sarcomas, and mesotheliomas. The Eastern Cooperative Oncology Group (ECOG) experience. Cancer 1989;64:484.

102. Fong Y, Coit DG, Woodruff JM, et al: Lymph node metastasis from soft tissue sarcoma in adults: Analysis of data from a prospective database of 1772 sarcoma patients. Ann Surg 1993;217:72.

103. Weingrad DN, Rosenberg SA: Early lymphatic spread of osteogenic and soft-tissue sarcomas. Surgery 1978;84:231.

104. Estourgie SH, Nielsen GP, Ott MJ: Metastatic patterns of extremity myxoid liposarcoma and their outcome. J Surg Oncol 2002; 80:89.

105. Hasegawa T, Seki K, Hasegawa F, et al: Dedifferentiated liposarcoma of retroperitoneum and mesentery: Varied growth patterns and histological grades—a clinicopathologic study of 32 cases. Hum Pathol 2000;31:717.

106. Pisters PWT, Leung DHY, Woodruff JM, et al: Analysis of prognostic factors in 1041 patients with localized soft tissue sarcomas of the extremities. J Clin Oncol 1996;14:1679.

107. Coindre JM, Terrier P, Bui NB, et al: Prognostic factors in adult patients with locally controlled soft tissue sarcoma: A study of 546 patients from the French Federation of Cancer Centers Sarcoma Group. J Clin Oncol 1996;14:869.

108. Coindre JM, Terrier P, Guillou L, et al: Predictive value of grade for metastasis development in the main histologic types of adult soft tissue sarcomas: A study of 1240 patients from the French Federation of Cancer Centers Sarcoma Group. Cancer 2001;91:1914.

109. Costa J, Wesley RA, Glatstein EJ, et al: The grading of soft tissue sarcomas: Results of a clinicohistopathologic correlation in a series of 163 cases. Cancer 1984;53:530.

110. Trojani M, Contesso G, Coindre JM, et al: Soft-tissue sarcomas of adults: Study of pathological prognostic variables and definition of a histopathological grading system. Int J Cancer 1984;33:37.

111. Guillou L, Coindre JM, Bonichon F, et al: Comparative study of the National Cancer Institute and French Federation of Cancer Centers Sarcoma Group grading systems in a population of 410 adult patients with soft tissue sarcoma. J Clin Oncol 1997;15:350.

112. Lawrence WJ, Donegan WL, Natarajan N, et al: Adult soft tissue sarcomas: A pattern of care survey of the American College of Surgeons. Ann Surg 1987;205:349.

113. Heslin MJ, Lewis JJ, Woodruff JM, et al: Core needle biopsy for diagnosis of extremity soft tissue sarcoma. Ann Surg Oncol 1997;4:425.

114. Ball AB, Fisher C, Pittam M, et al: Diagnosis of soft tissue tumours by Tru-Cut biopsy. Br J Surg 1990;77:756.

115. Skrzynski MC, Biermann JS, Montag AG, et al: Diagnostic accuracy and charge-savings of outpatient core needle biopsy compared with open biopsy of musculoskeletal tumors. J Bone Joint Surg Am 1996;78:644.

116. Schwartz HS, Spengler DM: Needle tract recurrences after closed biopsy for sarcoma: Three cases and review of the literature. Ann Surg Oncol 1997;4:228.

117. Akerman M, Idvall I, Rydholm A: Cytodiagnosis of soft tissue tumors and tumor-like conditions by means of fine needle aspiration biopsy. Arch Orthop Trauma Surg 1980;96:61.

118. Kissin MW, Fisher C, Webb AJ, et al: Value of fine needle aspiration cytology in the diagnosis of soft tissue tumours: A preliminary study on the excised specimen. Br J Surg 1987;74:479.

119. Layfield LJ, Anders KH, Glasgow BJ, et al: Fine-needle aspiration of primary soft-tissue lesions. Arch Pathol Lab Med 1986;110:420.

120. Chang AE, Matory YL, Dwyer AJ, et al: Magnetic resonance imaging versus computed tomography in the evaluation of soft tissue tumors of the extremities. Ann Surg 1987;205:340.

121. Hanna SL, Fletcher BD: MR imaging of malignant soft-tissue tumors. Magn Reson Imaging Clin N Am 1995;3:629.

122. Panicek DM, Gatsonis C, Rosenthal DI, et al: CT and MR imaging in the local staging of primary malignant musculoskeletal neoplasms: report of the Radiology Diagnostic Oncology Group. Radiology 1997;202:237.

123. Ioannidis JP, Lau J: 18F-FDG PET for the diagnosis and grading of soft-tissue sarcoma: A meta-analysis. J Nucl Med 2003;44:717.

124. Kole AC, Nieweg OE, van Ginkel RJ, et al: Detection of local recurrence of soft-tissue sarcoma with positron emission tomography using [18F]fluorodeoxyglucose. Ann Surg Oncol 1997;4:57.

125. Schuetze SM, Conrad C, Bruckner J, et al: FDG PET response to neoadjuvant chemotherapy predicts survival in patients with soft tissue sarcoma. Proc Am Soc Clin Oncol 2001;20:348a.

126. Bredella MA, Caputo GR, Steinbach LS: Value of FDG positron emission tomography in conjunction with MR imaging for evaluating therapy response in patients with musculoskeletal sarcomas. AJR Am J Roentgenol 2002;179:1145.

127. Greene FL et al: Soft tissue sarcoma. In AJCC Cancer Staging Manual. New York, Springer-Verlag, 2002, p 193.

128. Gaynor JJ, Tan CC, Casper ES, et al: Refinement of clinicopathologic staging for localized soft tissue sarcoma of the extremity: A study of 423 adults. J Clin Oncol 1992;10:1317.

129. Collin CF, Godbold J, Hajdu SI, et al: Localized extremity soft tissue sarcoma: An analysis of factors affecting survival. J Clin Oncol 1987;5:601.

130. Bevilacqua RG, Rogatko A, Hajdu SI, et al: Prognostic factors in primary retroperitoneal soft-tissue sarcomas. Arch Surg 1991;126:328.

131. Heslin MJ, Lewis JJ, Nadler E, et al: Prognostic factors associated with long-term survival for retroperitoneal sarcoma: implications for management. J Clin Oncol 1997;15:2832.

132. Tran LM, Mark R, Meier R, et al: Sarcomas of the head and neck: Prognostic factors and treatment strategies. Cancer 1992; 70:169.

133. Kowalski LP, San CI: Prognostic factors in head and neck soft tissue sarcomas: analysis of 128 cases. J Surg Oncol 1994;56:83.

134. Kraus DH, Dubner S, Harrison LB, et al: Prognostic factors for recurrence and survival in head and neck soft tissue sarcomas. Cancer 1994;74:697.

135. Le QT, Fu KK, Kroll SS, et al: Prognostic factors in adult soft-tissue sarcomas of the head and neck. Int J Radiat Oncol Biol Phys 1997;37:975.

Specific Malignancies

III

136. McGrath PC, Neifeld JP, Lawrence W Jr., et al: Gastrointestinal sarcomas: Analysis of prognostic factors. Ann Surg 1987;206:706.

137. Ng EH, Pollock RE, Romsdahl MM: Prognostic implications of patterns of failure for gastrointestinal leiomyosarcomas. Cancer 1992;69:1334.

138. Meijer S, Peretz T, Gaynor JJ, et al: Primary colorectal sarcoma: A retrospective review and prognostic factor study of 50 consecutive patients. Arch Surg 1990;125:1163.

139. Olah KS, Dunn JA, Gee H: Leiomyosarcomas have a poorer prognosis than mixed mesodermal tumours when adjusting for known prognostic factors: The result of a retrospective study of 423 cases of uterine sarcoma. Br J Obstet Gynaecol 1992; 99:590.

140. Rooser B, Willen H, Hugoson A, et al: Prognostic factors in synovial sarcoma. Cancer 1989;63:2182.

141. Singer S, Baldini EH, Demetri GD, et al: Synovial sarcoma: Prognostic significance of tumor size, margin of resection, and mitotic activity for survival. J Clin Oncol 1996;14:1201.

142. Le Doussal V, Coindre JM, Leroux A, et al: Prognostic factors for patients with localized primary malignant fibrous histiocytoma: A multicenter study of 216 patients with multivariate analysis. Cancer 1996;77:1823.

143. Pezzi CM, Rawlings MS Jr., Esgro JJ, et al: Prognostic factors in 227 patients with malignant fibrous histiocytoma. Cancer 1992;69: 2098.

144. Rooser B, Willen H, Gustafson P, et al: Malignant fibrous histiocytoma of soft tissue. A population-based epidemiologic and prognostic study of 137 patients. Cancer 1991;67:499.

145. O'Connor MI, Pritchard DJ: Ewing's sarcoma. Prognostic factors, disease control, and the reemerging role of surgical treatment. Clin Orthop 1991;262:78.

146. Sauer R, Jurgens H, Burgers JM, et al: Prognostic factors in the treatment of Ewing's sarcoma. The Ewing's Sarcoma Study Group of the German Society of Paediatric Oncology CESS 81. Radiother Oncol 1987;10:101.

147. Daugaard S, Sunde LM, Kamby C, et al: Ewing's sarcoma: A retrospective study of prognostic factors and treatment results. Acta Oncol 1987;26:281.

148. Aparicio J, Munarriz B, Pastor M, et al: Long-term follow-up and prognostic factors in Ewing's sarcoma: A multivariate analysis of 116 patients from a single institution. Oncology 1998;55:20.

149. Heslin MJ, Cordon-Cardo C, Lewis JJ, et al: Ki-67 detected by MIB-1 predicts distant metastasis and tumor mortality in primary, high grade extremity soft tissue sarcoma. Cancer 1998;83:490.

150. Karpeh MS, Brennan MF, Cance WG, et al: Altered patterns of retinoblastoma gene product expression in adult soft-tissue sarcomas. Br J Cancer 1995;72:986.

151. Lewis JJ, Leung DHY, Casper ES, et al: Multifactorial analysis of long-term follow-up (more than 5 years) of primary extremity sarcoma. Arch Surg 1999;134:199.

152. Toguchida J, Yamaguchi T, Dayton SH, et al: Prevalence and spectrum of germline mutations of the p53 gene among patients with sarcoma. N Eng J Med 1992;326:1301.

153. Toguchida J, Yamaguchi T, Ritchie B, et al: Mutation spectrum of the p53 gene in bone and soft tissue sarcomas. Cancer Res 1992;52:6194.

154. Wadayama B, Toguchida J, Yamaguchi T, et al: p53 expression and its relationship to DNA alterations in bone and soft tissue sarcomas. Br J Cancer 1993;68:1134.

155. Andreassen A, Oyjord T, Hovig E, et al: p53 abnormalities in different subtypes of human sarcomas. Cancer Res 1993; 53:468.

156. Stratton MR, Moss S, Warren W, et al: Mutation of the p53 gene in human soft tissue sarcomas: Association with abnormalities of the RB1 gene. Oncogene 1990;5:1297.

157. Yang P, Hirose T, Hasegawa T, et al: Prognostic implication of the p53 protein and Ki-67 antigen immunohistochemistry in malignant fibrous histiocytoma. Cancer 1995;76:618.

158. Wurl P, Meye A, Schmidt H, et al: High prognostic significance of Mdm2/p53 co-overexpression in soft tissue sarcoma of the extremities. Oncogene 1998;16:1183.

159. Gerdes J: Ki-67 and other proliferation markers useful for immunohistological diagnostic and prognostic evaluations in human malignancies. Semin Cancer Biol 1990;1:199.

160. Drobnjak M, Latres E, Pollack D, et al: Prognostic implications of p53 nuclear overexpression and high proliferation index of Ki-67 in adult soft-tissue sarcomas. J Natl Cancer Inst 1994;86:549.

161. Levine EA, Holzmayer T, Bacus S, et al: Evaluation of newer prognostic markers for adult soft tissue sarcomas. J Clin Oncol 1997;15:3249.

162. Rudolph P, Kellner U, Chassevent A, et al: Prognostic relevance of a novel proliferation marker, ki-s11, for soft tissue sarcoma: A multivariate study. Am J Pathol 1997;150:1997.

163. Zucman J, Melot T, Desmaze C, et al: Combinatorial generation of variable fusion proteins in the Ewing family of tumours. EMBO J 1993;12:4481.

164. Delattre O, Zucman J, Melot T, et al: The Ewing family of tumors— a subgroup of small round-cell tumors defined by specific chimeric transcripts. N Eng J Med 1994;331:294.

165. Di Matteo G, Pescarmona E, Peparini N, et al: Histopathological features and clinical course of the gastrointestinal stromal tumors. Hepatogastroenterology 2002;49:1013.

166. Singer S, Rubin BP, Lux ML, et al: Prognostic value of KIT mutation type, mitotic activity, and histologic subtype in gastrointestinal stromal tumors. J Clin Oncol 2002;20:3898.

167. Heinrich MC, Rubin BP, Longley BJ, et al: Biology and genetic aspects of gastrointestinal stromal tumors: KIT activation and cytogenetic alterations. Hum Pathol 2002;33:484.

168. Kattan MW, Leung DH, Brennan MF: Postoperative nomogram for 12-year sarcoma-specific death. J Clin Oncol 2002;20:791.

169. Williard WC, Collin CF, Casper ES, et al: The changing role of amputation for soft tissue sarcoma of the extremity in adults. Surg Gynecol Obstet 1992;175:389.

170. Williard WC, Hajdu SI, Casper ES, et al: Comparison of amputation with limb-sparing operations for adult soft tissue sarcoma of the extremity. Ann Surg 1992;215:269.

171. Rosenberg SA, Tepper JE, Glatstein EJ, et al: The treatment of soft-tissue sarcomas of the extremities: Prospective randomized evaluations of (1) limb-sparing surgery plus radiation therapy compared with amputation and (2) the role of adjuvant chemotherapy. Ann Surg 1982;196:305.

172. Yang JC, Rosenberg SA: Surgery for adult patients with soft tissue sarcomas. Semin Oncol 1989;16:289.

173. Brennan MF, Casper ES, Harrison LB, et al: The role of multimodality therapy in soft-tissue sarcoma. Ann Surg 1991;214:328.

174. Bowden L, Booher RJ: The principles and techniques of resection of soft parts for sarcomas. Surgery 1958;44:963.

175. Cantin J, McNeer GP, Chu FC, et al: The problem of local recurrence after treatment of soft tissue sarcoma. Ann Surg 1968;168:47.

176. Gerner RE, Moore GE, Pickren JW: Soft tissue sarcomas. Ann Surg 1975;181:803.

177. Yang JC, Chang AE, Baker AR, et al: A randomized prospective study of the benefit of adjuvant radiation therapy in the treatment of soft tissue sarcomas of the extremity. J Clin Oncol 1998;16:197.

178. Jaques DP, Coit DG, Hajdu SI, et al: Management of primary and recurrent soft-tissue sarcoma of the retroperitoneum. Ann Surg 1990;212:51.

179. Karakousis CP: Surgery for soft tissue sarcomas. In Bland KI, Karakousis CP, Copeland EM (eds): Atlas of Surgical Oncology. Philadelphia, WB Saunders, 1995, p 283.

180. LeVay J, O'Sullivan B, Catton C, et al: Outcome and prognostic factors in soft tissue sarcoma in the adult. Int J Radiat Oncol Biol Phys 1993;27:1091.

181. Sadoski C, Suit HD, Rosenberg AE, et al: Preoperative radiation, surgical margins, and local control of extremity sarcomas of soft tissues. J Surg Oncol 1993;52:223.

182. Pisters PW, Harrison LB, Leung DH, et al: Long-term results of a prospective randomized trial of adjuvant brachytherapy in soft tissue sarcoma. J Clin Oncol 1996;14:859.

183. Gerrand CH, Wunder JS, Kandel RA, et al: Classification of positive margins after resection of soft-tissue sarcoma of the limb predicts the risk of local recurrence. J Bone Joint Surg Br 2001; 83:1149.

184. Noria S, Davis A, Kandel R, et al: Residual disease following unplanned excision of soft-tissue sarcoma of an extremity. J Bone Joint Surg Am 1996;78:650.

185. O'Sullivan B, Gullane P, Irish J, et al: Preoperative radiotherapy for adult head and neck soft tissue sarcoma (STS): Assessment of wound complication rates and cancer outcome in a prospective series. World J Surg 2003;27:875–883.

186. O'Sullivan B, Wunder J, Pisters PWT: Target description for radiotherapy of soft tissue sarcoma. In Gregoire V, Scalliet P, Ang KK (eds): Clinical Target Volumes in Conformal Radiotherapy and Intensity Modulated Radiotherapy. Heidelberg, Germany, Springer-Verlag, 2003, p 205.

187. Karakousis CP, Proimakis C, Walsh DL: Primary soft tissue sarcoma of the extremities in adults. Br J Surg 1995;82:1208.

188. Geer RJ, Woodruff JM, Casper ES, et al: Management of small soft-tissue sarcoma of the extremity in adults. Arch Surg 1992;127: 1285.

189. Rydholm A, Gustafson P, Rooser B, et al: Limb-sparing surgery without radiotherapy based on anatomic location of soft tissue sarcoma. J Clin Oncol 1991;9:1757.

190. Baldini EH, Goldberg J, Jenner C, et al: Long-term outcomes after function-sparing surgery without radiotherapy for soft tissue sarcoma of the extremities and trunk. J Clin Oncol 1999; 17:3252.

191. Alektiar KM, Leung D, Zelefsky MJ, et al: Adjuvant radiation for stage II-B soft tissue sarcoma of the extremity. J Clin Oncol 2002;20:1643.

192. Suit HD, Mankin HJ, Schiller AL: Results of treatment of sarcoma of soft tissue by radiation and surgery at Massachusetts General Hospital. Cancer Treat Symp 1985;3:33.

193. Barkley HT Jr, Martin RG, Romsdahl MM, et al: Treatment of soft issue sarcomas by preoperative irradiation and conservative surgical resection. Int J Radiat Oncol Biol Phys 1988;14:693.

194. Brant TA, Parsons JT, Marcus RB Jr, et al: Preoperative irradiation for soft tissue sarcomas of the trunk and extremities in adults. Int J Radiat Oncol Biol Phys 1990;19:899.

195. Harrison LB, Franzese F, Gaynor JJ, et al: Long term results of a prospective trial of adjuvant brachytherapy in the management of completely resected soft tissue sarcomas of the extremity and superficial trunk. Int J Radiat Oncol Biol Phys 1993;27:259.

196. Lindberg RD, Martin RG, Romsdahl MM, et al: Conservative surgery and postoperative radiotherapy in 300 adults with soft-tissue sarcomas. Cancer 1981;47:2391.

197. Karakousis CP, Emrich LJ, Rao UN, et al: Feasibility of limb salvage and survival in soft tissue sarcomas. Cancer 1986;57:484.

198. Suit HD, Mankin HJ, Wood WC, et al: Treatment of the patient with stage M0 soft tissue sarcoma. J Clin Oncol 1988;6:854.

199. Karakousis CP, Zografos GC: Radiation therapy for high grade soft tissue sarcomas of the extremities treated with limb-preserving surgery. Eur J Surg Oncol 2002;28:431.

200. O'Sullivan B, Davis AM, Turcotte R, et al: Preoperative versus postoperative radiotherapy in soft-tissue sarcoma of the limbs: a randomised trial. Lancet 2002;359:2235.

201. Lindberg RD: Treatment of localized soft tissue sarcomas in adults at M. D. Anderson Hospital and Tumor Institute (1960–1981). Cancer Treat Symp 1985;3:59.

202. Enneking WF, McAuliffe JA: Adjunctive preoperative radiation therapy in treatment of soft tissue sarcomas: A preliminary report. Cancer Treat Symp 1985;3:37.

203. Leibel SA, Tranbaugh RF, Wara WM, et al: Soft tissue sarcomas of the extremities: Survival and patterns of failure with conservative surgery and postoperative irradiation compared to surgery alone. Cancer 1982;50:1076.

204. Suit HD, Mankin HJ, Wood W, et al: Preoperative, intraoperative, and postoperative radiation in the treatment of primary soft tissue sarcoma. Cancer 1985;55:2659.

205. Shiu MH, Hilaris BS, Harrison LB, et al: Brachytherapy and function-saving resection of soft tissue sarcoma arising in the limb. Int J Radiat Oncol Biol Phys 1991;21:1485.

206. Willett CG, Suit HD: Limited surgery and external beam irradiation in soft tissue sarcoma. Adv Oncol 1989;5:26.

207. Habrand JL, Gerbaulet A, Pejovic MH, et al: Twenty years experience of interstitial iridium brachytherapy in the management of soft tissue sarcomas. Int J Radiat Oncol Biol Phys 1991;20:405.

208. Brennan MF, Hilaris BS, Shiu MH, et al: Local recurrence in adult soft-tissue sarcoma: A randomized trial of brachytherapy. Arch Surg 1987;122:1289.

209. Pisters PWT, Harrison LB, Woodruff JM, et al: A prospective randomized trial of adjuvant brachytherapy in the management of low grade soft tissue sarcomas of the extremity and superficial trunk. J Clin Oncol 1994;12:1150.

210. Stotter AT, A'Hern RP, Fisher C, et al: The influence of local recurrence of extremity soft tissue sarcoma on metastasis and survival. Cancer 1990;65:1119.

211. Barr LC, Stotter AT, A'Hern RP: Influence of local recurrence on survival: A controversy reviewed from the perspective of soft tissue sarcoma. Br J Surg 1991;78:648.

212. Rooser B, Gustafson P, Rydholm A: Is there no influence of local control on the rate of metastases in high-grade soft tissue sarcoma? Cancer 1990;65:1727.

213. Gustafson P, Rooser B, Rydholm A: Is local recurrence of minor importance for metastases in soft tissue sarcoma? Cancer 1991;67:2083.

214. Lewis JJ, Leung DHY, Heslin MJ, et al: Association of local recurrence with subsequent survival in extremity soft tissue sarcoma. J Clin Oncol 1997;15:646.

215. Rooser B, Attewell R, Berg NO, et al: Survival in soft tissue sarcoma: Prognostic variables identified by multivariate analysis. Acta Orthop Scand 1987;58:516.

216. Emrich LJ, Ruka W, Driscoll DL, et al: The effect of local recurrence on survival time in adult high-grade soft tissue sarcomas. J Clin Epidemiol 1989;42:105.

217. O'Sullivan B, Pisters PWT: Staging and prognostic factor evaluation in soft tissue sarcoma. In Pollock RE (ed): Emerging Perspectives in Soft Tissue Sarcoma. Philadelphia, WB Saunders, 2003, p 333.

218. Eilber FC, Rosen G, Nelson SD, et al: High-grade extremity soft tissue sarcomas: Factors predictive of local recurrence and its effect on morbidity and mortality. Ann Surg 2003;237:218.

219. Janjan NA, Yasko AW, Reece GP, et al: Comparison of charges related to radiotherapy for soft tissue sarcomas treated by preoperative external beam irradiation versus interstitial implantation. Ann Surg Oncol 1994;1:415.

220. Nielsen OS, Cummings B, O'Sullivan B, et al: Preoperative and postoperative irradiation of soft tissue sarcomas: effect of radiation field size. Int J Radiat Oncol Biol Phys 1991;21:1595.

221. Bujko K, Suit HD, Springfield DS, et al: Wound healing after preoperative radiation for sarcoma of soft tissues. Surg Gynecol Obstet 1993;176:124.

222. Peat BG, Bell RS, Davis A, et al: Wound-healing complications after soft-tissue sarcoma surgery. Plast Reconstr Surg 1994;93:980.

223. O'Sullivan B, Davis A: A randomized phase III trial of preoperative compared to postoperative radiotherapy in extremity soft tissue sarcoma. Proc ASTRO 2001;51:151.

224. Davis AM, O'Sullivan B, Bell RS, et al: Function and health status outcomes in a randomized trial comparing preoperative and postoperative radiotherapy in extremity soft tissue sarcoma. J Clin Oncol 2002;20:4472.

225. O'Sullivan B, Ward I, Haycocks T, et al: Techniques to modulate radiotherapy toxicity and outcome in soft tissue sarcoma. Curr Opin Oncol 2003;4:453–464.

226. Chan MF, Chui CS, Schupak K, et al: The treatment of large extraskeletal chondrosarcoma of the leg: Comparison of IMRT and conformal radiotherapy techniques. J Appl Clin Med Phys 2001;2:3.

227. Borden EC, Baker LH, Bell RS, et al: Soft tissue sarcomas of adults: State of the translational science. Clin Cancer Res 2003;9:1941.

228. Lindberg RD: Soft tissue sarcoma. In Fletcher CDM (ed): Textbook of Radiotherapy. Philadelphia, Lea and Febiger, 1980, p 922.

229. Suit HD: Sarcomas of the soft tissue. In Third Annual Current Approaches to Radiation Oncology, Biology, and Physic. San Francisco, University of California, 1983, p 138.

230. Tepper JE, Suit HD: Radiation therapy alone for sarcoma of soft tissue. Cancer 1985;56:475.

231. Salinas R, Hussey DH, Fletcher GH, et al: Experience with neutron therapy for locally advanced sarcomas. Int J Radiat Oncol Biol Phys 1980;6:267.

232. Laramore GE, Griffith JT, Boespflug M, et al: Fast neutron radiotherapy for sarcomas of soft tissue, bone, and cartilage. Am J Clin Oncol 1989;12:320.

233. Pelton JG, DelRowe JD, Bolen JW, et al: Fast neutron radiotherapy

for soft tissue sarcomas. University of Washington experience and review of world's literature. Am J Clin Oncol 1986;9:397.

234. Tierney JF: Adjuvant chemotherapy for localised resectable soft-tissue sarcoma of adults: Meta-analysis of individual data. Lancet 1997;350:1647.

235. Tamoxifen for early breast cancer: An overview of the randomized trials. Early Breast Cancer Trialists' Collaborative Group. Lancet 1998;351:1451.

236. Polychemotherapy for early breast cancer: An overview of the randomized trials. Early Breast Cancer Trialists' Collaborative Group. Lancet 1998;352:930.

237. Frustaci S, Gherlinzoni F, De Paoli A, et al: Adjuvant chemotherapy for adult soft tissue sarcomas of the extremities and girdles: Results of the Italian randomized cooperative trial. J Clin Oncol 2001;19:1238.

238. Brodowicz T, Schwameis E, Widder J, et al: Intensified adjuvant IFADIC chemotherapy for adult soft tissue sarcoma: A prospective randomized feasibility trial. Sarcoma 2000;4:151.

239. Petrioli R, Frediani B, Manganelli A, et al: Comparison between a cisplatin-containing regimen and a carboplatin-containing regimen for recurrent or metastatic bladder cancer patients: A randomized phase II study. Cancer 1996;77:344.

240. Bramwell VH: Adjuvant chemotherapy for adult soft tissue sarcoma: Is there a standard of care? J Clin Oncol 2001;19:1235.

241. Figueredo A, Bramwell VHC, Bell R, et al: Adjuvant chemotherapy following complete resection of soft tissue sarcoma in adults: A clinical practice guideline. Sarcoma 2002;6:5.

242. Eilber FR, Eckardt J, Rosen G, et al: Preoperative therapy for soft tissue sarcoma. Hematol Oncol Clin North Am 1995;9:817.

243. Eilber FR, Eckardt J: Surgical management of soft tissue sarcomas. Semin Oncol 1997;24:526.

244. Eilber FC, Rosen G, Eckardt J, et al: Treatment-induced pathologic necrosis: A predictor of local recurrence and survival in patients receiving neoadjuvant therapy for high-grade extremity soft tissue sarcomas. J Clin Oncol 2001;19:3203.

245. Pisters PWT, Patel SR, Varma DGK, et al: Preoperative chemotherapy for stage IIIB extremity soft tissue sarcoma: long-term results from a single institution. J Clin Oncol 1997;15:3481.

246. Pisters PWT, Patel SR, Varma DGK, et al: Pathologic complete response (pCR) following preoperative multimodality therapy for stage IIIB extremity soft tissue sarcoma (STS): Implications for the design of multimodality trials. Proc Am Soc Clin Oncol 1997;16:499a.

247. Meric F, Hess K, Varma DG, et al: Radiographic response to neoadjuvant chemotherapy is a predictor of local control and survival in soft tissue sarcomas. Cancer 2002;95:1120.

248. Meric F, Milas M, Hunt K, et al: Impact of neoadjuvant chemotherapy on postoperative morbidity in soft tissue sarcomas. Proc Am Soc Clin Oncol 1999;18:546a.

249. Saghatchian M, Bonvalot S, Terrier P, et al: Intensive induction chemotherapy in adult patients with advanced soft tissue sarcoma (ASTS): Clinical and histological response, surgical impact and follow-up after resection. Proc Am Soc Clin Oncol 2000;19:562a.

250. De Paoli A, Gherlinzoni F, Buonadonna A, et al: Feasibility of pre- or postoperative (Op) combined chemotherapy (CT) and radiation therapy (RT) in adult soft tissue sarcomas of extremities or girdles (STS): A pilot study. Proc Am Soc Clin Oncol 2001;20:290b.

251. Wodajo F, Wittig J, Kumar D, et al: Successful treatment of high-grade soft tissue sarcoma with induction chemotherapy: Clinicopathologic analysis of thick capsule formation allowing less extensive "Marginal" surgical resection. Proc Am Soc Clin Oncol 2001;20:290b.

252. Edmonson JH, Petersen IA, Shives TC, et al: Chemotherapy, irradiation, and surgery for function-preserving therapy of primary extremity soft tissue sarcomas: Initial treatment with ifosfamide, mitomycin, doxorubicin, and cisplatin plus granulocyte macrophage-colony-stimulating factor. Cancer 2002;94:786.

253. Gortzak E, Azzarelli A, Buesa J, et al: A randomized phase II study on neoadjuvant chemotherapy for 'high-risk' adult soft-tissue sarcoma. Eur J Cancer 2001;37:1096.

254. Delaney TF, Spiro IJ, Suit HD, et al: Neoadjuvant chemotherapy and radiotherapy for large extremity soft-tissue sarcomas. Int J Radiat Oncol Biol Phys 2003;6:1117.

255. Kraybill WG, Spiro IJ, Harris JA, et al: Radiation Therapy Oncology Group (RTOG) 95-14: A phase II study of neoadjuvant chemotherapy (CT) and radiation therapy (RT) in the management of high risk (HR), high grade, soft tissue sarcomas (STS) of the extremities and body wall. Proc Am Soc Clin Oncol 2003;20:815.

256. Eilber FR et al: Neoadjuvant chemotherapy, radiation, and limited surgery for high grade soft tissue sarcoma of the extremity. In Ryan JR, Baker, LO (eds): Recent Concepts in Sarcoma Treatment. Dordrecht, The Netherlands, Kluwer Academic, 1988, p 115.

257. Eilber FR, et al: Postoperative adjuvant chemotherapy (Adriamycin) in high grade extremity soft tissue sarcoma: A randomized prospective trial. In Salmon SE (ed): Adjuvant Therapy of Cancer, 5th ed. New York: Grune and Stratton, 1987, p 719.

258. Eilber FR, Giuliano AE, Huth JF, et al: Intravenous (IV) vs. intraarterial (IA) Adriamycin, 2800 radiation and surgical excision for extremity soft tissue sarcomas: A randomized prospective trial. Proc Am Soc Clin Oncol 1990;9:309.

259. Wanebo HJ, Temple WJ, Popp MB, et al: Preoperative regional therapy for extremity sarcoma: A tricenter update. Cancer 1995;75:2299.

260. Temple WJ, Temple CLF, Arthur K, et al: Prospective cohort study of neoadjuvant treatment in conservative surgery of soft tissue sarcomas. Ann Surg Oncol 1997;4:586.

261. Levine EA, Trippon M, DasGupta TK: Preoperative multimodality treatment for soft tissue sarcomas. Cancer 1993;71:3685.

262. O'Sullivan B, Bell RS: Has "MAID" made it in the management of high-risk soft-tissue sarcoma? Int J Radiat Oncol Biol Phys 2003;56:915.

263. Eggermont AMM, Shraffordt Koops H, Lienard D, et al: Isolated limb perfusion with high-dose tumor necrosis factor-α in combination with interferon-α and melphalan for nonresectable extremity soft tissue sarcomas: A multicenter trial. J Clin Oncol 1996;14:2653.

264. Gutman M, Inbar M, Lev-Shlush D, et al: High dose tumor necrosis factor-alpha and melphalan administered via isolated limb perfusion for advanced limb soft tissue sarcoma results in a >90% response rate and limb preservation. Cancer 1997;79:1129.

265. Hohenberger P, Kettelhack C, Schlag PM: Follow-up results after hyperthermic isolated limb perfusion (ILP) with rhTNFα followed by radical surgery for soft tissue sarcoma. Proc Am Soc Clin Oncol 1998;17:510a.

266. Plaat BE, Hoekstra HJ, Koops HS, et al: Hyperthermic isolated limb perfusion (HILP) with TNFalpha-melphalan induces apoptosis and inhibits proliferation in soft tissue sarcomas. Proc Am Soc Clin Oncol 1997;16:500a.

267. Rossi CR, Vecchiato A, Foletto M, et al: Phase II study on neoadjuvant hyperthermic-antiblastic perfusion with doxorubicin in patients with intermediate or high grade limb sarcomas. Cancer 1994;73:2140.

268. Rossi CR, Foletto M, Di Filippo F, et al: Soft tissue limb sarcomas: Italian clinical trials with hyperthermic antiblastic perfusion. Cancer 1999;86:1742.

269. Wiedemann GJ, Katschinski DM, Westerman A, et al: A systemic hyperthermia Oncologic Working Group Trial: Ifosfamide (IFO)000, carboplatin (CBDCA) and etoposide (VP-10) combined with aquatherm induced 41.8C whole body hyperthermia (WBH) for refractory sarcoma. Proc Am Soc Clin Oncol 2000;19:562a.

270. Issels RD, Abdel-Rahman S, Wendtner C, et al: Neoadjuvant chemotherapy combined with regional hyperthermia (RHT) for locally advanced primary or recurrent high-risk adult soft-tissue sarcomas (STS) of adults: Long-term results of a phase II study. Eur J Cancer 2001;37:1599.

271. Wendtner C, Abdel-Rahman S, Falk MH, et al: Treatment of 113 high risk soft tissue sarcomas (HR-STS) of adults: Two consecutive phase II studies (RHT-91 and RHT-95) of neoadjuvant chemotherapy (XT) combined with regional hyperthermia (RHT). Proc Am Soc Clin Oncol 2000;19:557a.

272. Wendtner C, Abdel-Rahman S, Baumert J, et al: Response to neoadjuvant thermochemotherapy as significant prognosticator for long-term survival of patients with retroperitoneal or visceral high-risk soft-tissue sarcomas. Proc Am Soc Clin Oncol 2001;20:348a.

273. Birkmeyer JD, Siewers AE, Finlayson EV, et al: Hospital volume and surgical mortality in the United States. N Engl J Med 2002;346:1128.

274. Gustafson P, Dreinhofer KE, Rydholm A: Soft tissue sarcoma should be treated at a tumor center: A comparison of quality of surgery in 375 patients. Acta Orthop Scand 1994;65:47.

275. Potter DA, Glenn J, Kinsella TJ, et al: Patterns of recurrence in patients with high-grade soft-tissue sarcomas. J Clin Oncol 1985;3:353.

276. Farhood AI, Hajdu SI, Shiu MH, et al: Soft tissue sarcomas of the head and neck in adults. Am J Surg 1990;160:365.

277. Singer S, Antman KH, Corson JM, et al: Long-term salvageability for patients with locally recurrent soft-tissue sarcomas. Arch Surg 1992;127:548.

278. Midis GP, Pollock RE, Chen NP, et al: Locally recurrent soft tissue sarcoma of the extremities. Surgery 1998;123:666.

279. Nori D, Schupak K, Shiu MH, et al: Role of brachytherapy in recurrent extremity sarcoma in patients treated with prior surgery and irradiation. Int J Radiat Oncol Biol Phys 1991;20:1229.

280. Catton CN, Davis A, Bell RS, et al: Soft tissue sarcoma of the extremity: Limb salvage after failure of combined conservative therapy. Radiother Oncol 1996;41:209.

281. Pearlstone D, Janjan NA, Feig BW, et al: Re-resection with brachytherapy for locally recurrent soft tissue sarcoma arising in a previously radiated field. Cancer J Sci Am 1999;5:26.

282. Brennan MF: The surgeon as a leader in cancer care: lessons learned from the study of soft tissue sarcoma. J Am Coll Surg 1996;182:520.

283. Pearlstone DB, Pisters PW, Bold RJ, et al: Patterns of recurrence in extremity liposarcoma: Implications for staging and follow-up. Cancer 1999;85:85.

284. Antonescu CR, Elahi A, Healey JH, et al: Monoclonality of multifocal myxoid liposarcoma: Confirmation by analysis of TLS-CHOP or EWS-CHOP rearrangements. Clin Cancer Res 2000;6:2788.

285. Marcove RC, Mike V, Hajek JV, et al: Osteogenic sarcoma in childhood. N Y State J Med 1971;71:855.

286. Martini N, Huvos AG, Mike V, et al: Multiple pulmonary resections in the treatment of osteogenic sarcoma. Ann Thorac Surg 1971;12:271.

287. Creagan ET, Fleming TR, Edmonson JH, et al: Pulmonary resection for metastatic nonosteogenic sarcoma. Cancer 1979;44:1908.

288. Putnam JB Jr, Roth JA, Wesley MN, et al: Analysis of prognostic factors in patients undergoing resection of pulmonary metastases from soft tissue sarcomas. J Thorac Cardiovasc Surg 1984;87:260.

289. Jablons D, Steinberg SM, Roth JA, et al: Metastasectomy for soft tissue sarcoma: Further evidence for efficacy and prognostic indicators. J Thorac Cardiovasc Surg 1989;97:695.

290. Casson AG, Putnam JB Jr, Natarajan G, et al: Five-year survival after pulmonary metastasectomy for adult soft tissue sarcoma. Cancer 1992;69:662.

291. Gadd MA, Casper ES, Woodruff JM, et al: Development and treatment of pulmonary metastases in adult patients with extremity soft-tissue sarcoma. Ann Surg 1993;218:705.

292. Huth JF, Holmes EC, Vernon SE, et al: Pulmonary resection for metastatic sarcoma. Am J Surg 1980;140:9.

293. McCormack PM, Martini N: The changing role of surgery for pulmonary metastases. Ann Thorac Surg 1979;28:139.

294. Morrow CE, Vassilopoulos PP, Grage TB: Surgical resection for metastatic neoplasms of the lung. Experience at the University of Minnesota Hospitals. Cancer 1980;45:2981.

295. Mountain CF, McMurtrey MJ, Hermes KE: Surgery for pulmonary metastasis: a 20-year experience. Ann Thorac Surg 1984;38:323.

296. Pastorino U, Valente M, Gasparini M, et al: Lung resection for metastatic sarcomas: Total survival from primary treatment. J Surg Oncol 1989;4:275.

297. Rizzoni WE, Pass HI, Wesley MN, et al: Resection of recurrent pulmonary metastases in patients with soft-tissue sarcomas. Arch Surg 1986;121:1248.

298. Van Geel AN, Pastorino U, Jauch KW, et al: Surgical treatment of lung metastases: The European Organization for Research and Treatment of Cancer Soft Tissue and Bone Sarcoma Group study of 255 patients. Cancer 1996;77:675.

299. Roth JA, Putnam JB Jr, Wesley MN, et al: Differing determinants of prognosis following resection of pulmonary metastases from osteogenic and soft tissue sarcoma patients. Cancer 1985;55:1361.

300. Pogrebniak HW, Roth JA, Steinberg SM, et al: Reoperative pulmonary resection in patients with metastatic soft tissue sarcoma. Ann Thorac Surg 1991;52:197.

301. Casson AG, Putnam JB Jr, Natarajan G, et al: Efficacy of pulmonary metastasectomy for recurrent soft tissue sarcoma. J Surg Oncol 1991;47:1.

302. Takita H, Edgerton F, Karakousis CP, et al: Surgical management of metastases to the lung. Surg Gynecol Obstet 1981;152:191.

303. Putnam JB Jr, Roth JA, Wesley MN, et al: Survival following aggressive resection of pulmonary metastases from osteogenic sarcoma: analysis of prognostic factors. Ann Thorac Surg 1983; 36:516.

304. Regnard JF, Cerrina J, Silbert D: Curative surgical treatment of pulmonary metastases. In Third European Conference on Clinical Oncology. Stockholm, Sweden, 1985, p 58.

305. Ramming KP: Surgery for pulmonary metastases. Surg Clin North Am 1980;60:815.

306. Joseph WL, Morton DL, Adkins PC: Prognostic significance of tumor doubling time in evaluating operability in pulmonary metastatic disease. J Thorac Cardiovasc 1971;Surg 61:23.

307. Verazin GT, Warneke JA, Driscoll DL, et al: Resection of lung metastases from soft-tissue sarcomas: A multivariate analysis. Arch Surg 1992;127:1407.

308. McCormack PM: Surgical resection of pulmonary metastases. Semin Surg Oncol 1990;6:297.

309. Demetri GD, Elias AD: Results of single-agent and combination chemotherapy for advanced soft tissue sarcomas: Implications for decision making in the clinic. Hematol Oncol Clin North Am 1995;9:765.

310. Bramwell VH, Anderson D, Charette ML: Doxorubicin-based chemotherapy for the palliative treatment of adult patients with locally advanced or metastatic soft-tissue sarcoma: A meta-analysis and clinical practice guideline. Sarcoma 2000;4:103.

311. Van Glabbeke M, van Oosterom AT, Oosterhuis JW, et al: Prognostic factors for the outcome of chemotherapy in advanced soft tissue sarcoma: An analysis of 2,185 patients treated with anthracycline-containing first-line regimens: A European Organization for Research and Treatment of Cancer Soft Tissue and Bone Sarcoma Group study. J Clin Oncol 1999;17:150.

312. Mouridsen HT, Bastholt L, Somers R, et al: Adriamycin versus epirubicin in advanced soft tissue sarcomas: A randomized phase II/phase III study of the EORTC Soft Tissue and Bone Sarcoma Group. Eur J Cancer Clin Oncol 1987;23:1477.

313. Lopez M, Vici P, Lauro L, et al: Increasing single epirubicin doses in advanced soft tissue sarcomas. J Clin Oncol 2002;20:1329.

314. Nielsen OS, Dombernowsky P, Mouridsen H, et al: High-dose epirubicin is not an alternative to standard-dose doxorubicin in the treatment of advanced soft tissue sarcomas: A study of the EORTC Soft Tissue and Bone Sarcoma Group. Br J Cancer 1998;78:1634.

315. Casper ES, Schwartz GK, Sugarman A, et al: Phase I trial of dose-intense liposome-encapsulated doxorubicin in patients with advanced sarcoma. J Clin Oncol 1997;15:2111.

316. Garcia A, Kempf R, Rogers M, et al: A phase II study of Doxil (liposomal doxorubicin): Lack of activity in poor prognosis soft tissue sarcomas. Ann Oncol 1998;10:1131.

317. Toma S, Tucci A, Villani G, et al: Liposomal doxorubicin (Caelyx) in advanced pretreated soft tissue sarcomas: A phase II study of the Italian Sarcoma Group (ISG). Anticancer Res 2000; 20:485.

318. Skubitz KM: Early results of pegylated liposomal doxorubicin (Doxil) in refractory sarcoma. Proc Am Soc Clin Oncol 1998;17:524a.

319. Chidiac T, Budd GT, Pelley R, et al: Phase II trial of liposomal doxorubicin (Doxil) in advanced soft tissue sarcomas. Invest New Drugs 2000;18:253.

320. Judson I, Radford JA, Harris M, et al: Randomised phase II trial of pegylated liposomal doxorubicin (DOXIL/CAELYX) versus doxorubicin in the treatment of advanced or metastatic soft tissue sarcoma: A study by the EORTC Soft Tissue and Bone Sarcoma Group. Eur J Cancer 2001;37:870.

321. Casper ES, Gaynor JJ, Hajdu SI, et al: A prospective randomized trial of adjuvant chemotherapy with bolus versus continuous infusion of doxorubicin in patients with high-grade extremity soft

tissue sarcoma and an analysis of prognostic factors. Cancer 1991;68:1221.

322. Seymour L, Bramwell V, Moran LA: Use of dexrazoxane as a cardioprotectant in patients receiving doxorubicin or epirubicin chemotherapy for the treatment of cancer. The Provincial Systemic Treatment Disease Site Group. Cancer Prev Control 1999;3:145.

323. Antman KH, Montella D, Rosenbaum C, et al: Phase II trial of ifosfamide with mesna in previously treated metastatic sarcoma. Cancer Treat Rep 1985;69:499.

324. Stuart-Harris R, Harper PG, Kaye SB, et al: High-dose ifosfamide by infusion with mesna in advanced soft tissue sarcoma. Cancer Treat Rev 1983;Suppl A:163.

325. Bramwell VH, Mouridsen HT, Santoro A, et al: Cyclophosphamide versus ifosfamide: Final report of a randomized phase II trial in adult soft tissue sarcomas. Eur J Cancer Clin Oncol 1987; 23:311.

326. Bramwell VHC, Mouridsen HT, Santoro A, et al: Cyclophosphamide versus ifosfamide: final report of a randomized phase II trial in adult soft tissue sarcomas. Eur J Cancer Clin Oncol 1987;23:311.

327. Patel SR, Vadhan-Raj S, Papadopoulos NJ, et al: High-dose ifosfamide in bone and soft tissue sarcomas: Results of phase II and pilot studies—dose-response and schedule dependence. J Clin Oncol 1997;15:2378.

328. Lorigan P, Verweij J, Papai Z, et al: Randomized phase III trial of two investigational schedules of ifosfamide versus standard dose doxorubicin in patients with advanced or metastatic soft tissue sarcoma. (ASTS). Proc Am Soc Clin Oncol 2002;21:405a.

329. Gottlieb JA, Baker LH, O'Bryan RM, et al: Adriamycin (NSC-123127) used alone and in combination for soft tissue and bony sarcoma. Cancer Chemother Rep 1975;6:271.

330. Crawford SM, Jerwood D: An assessment of the relative importance of the components of CYVADIC in the treatment of soft-tissue sarcomas using regression meta-analysis. Med Inform (Lond) 1994;19:311.

331. Verma S, Bramwell V: Dose-intensive chemotherapy in advanced adult soft tissue sarcoma. Expert Rev Anticancer Ther 2002;2:201.

332. Edmonson JH, Ryan LM, Blum RH, et al: Randomized comparison of doxorubicin alone versus ifosfamide plus doxorubicin or mitomycin, doxorubicin, and cisplatin against advanced soft tissue sarcomas. J Clin Oncol 1993;11:1269.

333. Santoro A, Tursz T, Mouridsen HT, et al: Doxorubicin versus CYVADIC versus doxorubicin plus ifosfamide in first-line treatment of advanced soft tissue sarcomas: A randomized study of the European Organization for Research and Treatment of Cancer Soft Tissue and Bone Sarcoma Group. J Clin Oncol 1995;13:1537.

334. Antman KH, Crowley J, Balcerzak SP, et al: An Intergroup phase III randomized study of doxorubicin and dacarbazine with or without ifosfamide and mesna in advanced soft tissue and bone sarcomas. J Clin Oncol 1993;11:1276.

335. Jelic S, Kovcin V, Milanovic N, et al: Randomised study of high-dose epirubicin versus high-dose epirubicin-cisplatin chemotherapy for advanced soft tissue sarcoma. Eur J Cancer 1997;33:220.

336. Santoro A: Advanced soft tissue sarcoma: how many more trials with anthracyclines and ifosfamide? Ann Oncol 1999;10:151.

337. Benjamin RS, Rouesse J, Bourgeois H, et al: Should patients with advanced sarcomas be treated with chemotherapy? Eur J Cancer 1998;34:958.

338. De Pas T, Curigliano G, Masci G, et al: Phase I study of 12-day prolonged infusion of high-dose ifosfamide and doxorubicin as first-line chemotherapy in adult patients with advanced soft tissue sarcomas. Ann Oncol 2002;13:161.

339. Lopez-Pousa A, Buesa J, Montalar J, et al: First-line doxorubicin and scalated high-dose ifosfamide in advanced soft tissue sarcoma (STS) patients: A phase II study of the Spanish Group for Research on Sarcomas (GEIS). Proc Am Soc Clin Oncol 2000;19:564a.

340. Le Cesne A, Judson I, Crowther D, et al: Randomized phase III study comparing conventional-dose doxorubicin plus ifosfamide versus high-dose doxorubicin plus ifosfamide plus recombinant human granulocyte-macrophage colony-stimulating factor in advanced soft tissue sarcomas: A trial of the European Organization for Research and Treatment of Cancer Soft Tissue and Bone Sarcoma Group. J Clin Oncol 2000;18:2676.

341. Bui NB, Demaille M, Chevreau C, et al: qMAID vs MAID + 25% with G-CSF in adults with advanced soft tissue sarcoma (STS). First results of a randomized study of the FNCLCC Sarcoma Group. Proc Am Soc Clin Oncol 1998;17:517a.

342. Biermann JS, Taylor J, Cook T, et al: Toxicity data from a randomized phase II evaluation of 6 g/m2 of ifosfamide (standard dose-IFOS) plus doxorubicin (DOX) versus 12 g/m2 of ifosfamide (high-dose-IFOS) plus doxorubicin in patients with high-grade soft tissue sarcomas (HGSTS). Proc Am Soc Clin Oncol 2002;21:405a.

343. Benjamin RS, Legha SS, Patel SR, et al: Single-agent ifosfamide studies in sarcomas of soft tissue and bone: The M. D. Anderson experience. Cancer Chemother Pharmacol 1993;31 Suppl 2:S174–S179.

344. Elias AD, Eder JP, Shea T, et al: High-dose ifosfamide with mesna uroprotection: A phase I study. J Clin Oncol 1990;8:170.

345. Cinat G, Mickiewicz E, Cabalar M, et al: High dose ifosfamide (HDIFO): A regimen that deserves to be taken into account in previously treated sarcoma bearing patients (Pts). Proc Am Soc Clin Oncol 2000;19:576a.

346. Deligny N, Demaille M, Bui NB, et al: Phase II trial of high dose of ifosfamide (HDI) in adult patients with advanced soft tissue sarcomas (ASTS). Proc Am Soc Clin Oncol 2001;20:292b.

347. Le Cesne A, Antoine E, Spielmann M, et al: High-dose ifosfamide: Circumvention of resistance to standard-dose ifosfamide in advanced soft tissue sarcomas. J Clin Oncol 1995;13:1600.

348. Frustaci S, Comandone A, Bearz A, et al: Efficacy and tolerability of an ifosfamide continuous infusion (IFO-c.i.) soft tissue sarcoma (STS) patients (pts). Proc Am Soc Clin Oncol 1998;17:518a.

349. Cerny T, Leyvraz S, von Briel T, et al: Saturable metabolism of continuous high-dose ifosfamide with mesna and GM-CSF: A pharmacokinetic study in advanced sarcoma patients. Swiss Group for Clinical Cancer Research (SAKK). Ann Oncol 1999v;10:1087.

350. Van Oosterom A, Krzemienlecki K, Nielsen OS, et al: Randomized phase II study of the EORTC Soft Tissue and Bone Sarcoma (STSBS) Group comparing two different ifosfamide (IF) regimens in chemotherapy untreated advanced soft tissue sarcomas (STS) patients (pts). Proc Am Soc Clin Oncol 1997;16:496a.

351. Nielsen OS, Judson I, van Hoesel Q, et al: Effect of high-dose ifosfamide in advanced soft tissue sarcomas. A multicentre phase II study of the EORTC Soft Tissue and Bone Sarcoma Group. Eur J Cancer 2000;36:61.

352. Keohan ML, Taub RN: Chemotherapy for advanced sarcoma: Therapeutic decisions and modalities. Semin Oncol 1997;24:572.

353. Mertens WC, Bramwell VHC: Adjuvant chemotherapy for soft tissue sarcomas. Cancer Treat Res 1991;56:93.

354. Buesa JM, Mouridsen HT, van Oosterom AT, et al: High-dose DTIC in advanced soft-tissue sarcomas in the adult. A phase II study of the EORTC Soft Tissue and Bone Sarcoma Group. Ann Oncol 1991;2:307.

355. Reichardt P, Tilgner J, Mrozek A, et al: Continuous infusion of Dtic in heavily pretreated patients (Pts.) with metastatic soft tissue sarcoma (STS). Proc Am Soc Clin Oncol 2000;19:564a.

356. Keizer HJ, Crowther D, Nielsen OS, et al: EORTC Group phase II study of oral etoposide for pretreated soft tissue sarcomas. Sarcoma 1997;1:99.

357. Van Hoesel QG, Verweij J, Catimel G, et al: Phase II study with docetaxel (Taxotere) in advanced soft tissue sarcomas of the adult. EORTC Soft Tissue and Bone Sarcoma Group. Ann Oncol 1994;5:539.

358. Amodio A, Carpano S, Vici P, et al: Phase II trial of docetaxel in anthracycline-refractory patients with advanced soft tissue sarcomas. Proc Am Soc Clin Oncol 1998;17:518a.

359. Verweij J, Lee SM, Ruka W, et al: Randomized phase II study of docetaxel versus doxorubicin in first- and second-line chemotherapy for locally advanced or metastatic soft tissue sarcomas in adults: A study of the european organization for research and treatment of cancer soft tissue and bone sarcoma group. J Clin Oncol 2000;18:2081.

360. Kostler WJ, Brodowicz T, Attems Y, et al: Docetaxel as rescue medication in anthracycline- and ifosfamide-resistant locally advanced or metastatic soft tissue sarcoma: Results of a phase II trial. Ann Oncol 2001;12:1281.

361. Edmonson JH, Ebbert LP, Nascimento AG, et al: Phase II study of docetaxel in advanced soft tissue sarcomas. Am J Clin Oncol 1996;19:574.

362. Patel SR, Gandhi V, Jenkins J, et al: Phase II clinical investigation of gemcitabine in advanced soft tissue sarcomas and window evaluation of dose rate on gemcitabine triphosphate accumulation. J Clin Oncol 2001;19:3483.

363. Gian VG, Johnson TJ, Marsh RW, et al: A phase II trial of paclitaxel in the treatment of recurrent or metastatic soft tissue sarcomas or bone sarcomas. J Exp Ther Oncol 1996:186.

364. Casper ES, Waltzman RJ, Schwartz GK, et al: Phase II trial of paclitaxel in patients with soft-tissue sarcoma. Cancer Invest 1998;16:442.

365. Merimsky O, Meller I, Flusser G, et al: Gemcitabine in soft tissue or bone sarcoma resistant to standard chemotherapy: A phase II study. Cancer Chemother Pharmacol 2000;45:177.

366. Svancarova L, Blay JY, Judson IR, et al: Gemcitabine in advanced adult soft-tissue sarcomas. A phase II study of the EORTC Soft Tissue and Bone Sarcoma Group. Eur J Cancer 2002;38:556.

367. Okuno S, Ryan LM, Edmonson JH, et al: Phase II trial of gemcitabine in patients with advanced sarcomas (E1797): A trial of the Eastern Cooperative Oncology Group. Cancer 2003;97:1969.

368. Skubitz KM, Hamdan H, Thompson RC Jr: Ambulatory continuous infusion ifosfamide with oral etoposide in advanced sarcomas. Cancer 1993;72:2963.

369. Yalcin S, Gullu I, Barista I, et al: Treatment of advanced refractory sarcomas with ifosfamide and etoposide combination chemotherapy. Cancer Invest 1998;16:297.

370. Saeter G, Alvegard TA, Monge OR, et al: Ifosfamide and continuous infusion etoposide in advanced adult soft tissue sarcoma. A Scandinavian Sarcoma Group Phase II Study. Eur J Cancer 1997;33:1551.

371. Papai Z, Bodoky G, Szanto J, et al: The efficacy of a combination of etoposide, ifosfamide, and cisplatin in the treatment of patients with soft tissue sarcoma. Cancer 2000;89:177.

372. Colterelli T, Germino J, Shanabrook L, et al: A phase II trial of gemcitabine, paclitaxel and carboplatin in stage IVB soft tissue sarcoma. Proc Am Soc Clin Oncol 2001;20:295b.

373. Hensley ML, Maki R, Venkatraman E, et al: Gemcitabine and docetaxel in patients with unresectable leiomyosarcoma: results of a phase II trial. J Clin Oncol 2002;20:2824.

374. Leu K, Zalupski M, Sondak VK, et al: Gemcitabine and docetaxel in sarcoma. Sarcoma 2002;27.

375. Taub RN, Keohan ML, Plitsas M, et al: Phase II study of temozolomide in advanced sarcomas. Proc Am Soc Clin Oncol 2000;19:555a.

376. Woll PJ, Judson I, Lee SM, et al: Temozolomide in adult patients with advanced soft tissue sarcoma: A phase II study of the EORTC Soft Tissue and Bone Sarcoma Group. Eur J Cancer 1999;35:410.

377. Garcia del Muro X, Lopez-Pousa A, Buesa J, et al: Temozolomide as a 6-week oral schedule in advanced soft tissue sarcoma (STS): A phase II trial of the Spanish Group for Research on Sarcomas (GEIS). Proc Am Soc Clin Oncol 2001;20:354a.

378. Blay JY, Judson I, Rodenhuis S, et al: Phase II study of raltitrexed (Tomudex) for patients with advanced soft tissue sarcomas refractory to doxorubicin-containing regimens. Anticancer Drugs 1999;10:873.

379. De Angelo D, Naujoks R, Manola JB, et al: Phase II study of irinotecan (CPT-11) in relapsed or refractory soft tissue sarcoma (STS). Proc Am Soc Clin Oncol 2000;19:555a.

380. Carson E, Zalupski M, Redman B, et al: Phase II trial of sargramostim (yeast-derived recombinant human GM-CSF) as monotherapy for advanced sarcomas. Proc Am Soc Clin Oncol 2000;19:563a.

381. Bramwell VH, Eisenhauer EA, Blackstein M, et al: Phase II study of topotecan (NSC 609 699) in patients with recurrent or metastatic soft tissue sarcoma. Ann Oncol 1995;6:847.

382. Budd GT, Rankin C, Hutchins LF, et al: Phase II trial of topotecan by continuous infusion in patients with advanced soft tissue sarcomas, a SWOG study. Southwest Oncology Group. Invest New Drugs 2002;20:129.

383. Fidias P, Demetri GD, Harmon DC: Navelbine shows activity in previously treated sarcoma patients: Phase II results from MGH/ Dana-Farber/Partners Cancer Care Study. Proc Am Soc Clin Oncol 1998;17:1977.

384. Tuveson DA, Fletcher JA: Signal transduction pathways in sarcoma as targets for therapeutic intervention. Curr Opin Oncol 2001;13:249.

385. Heymach JV: Angiogenesis and antiangiogenic approaches to sarcomas. Curr Opin Oncol 2001;13:261.

386. Maki RG: Immunity against soft-tissue sarcomas. Curr Oncol Rep 2003;5:282.

387. Patel SR, Jenkins J, Papadopolous N, et al: Pilot study of vitaxin: An angiogenesis inhibitor in patients with advanced leiomyosarcomas. Cancer 2001;92:1347.

388. Masci G, Casati G, Crescenzi V: Synthesis and LC characterization of clenbuterol molecularly imprinted polymers. J Pharm Biomed Anal 2001;25:211.

389. Delaloge S, Yovine A, Taamma A, et al: Ecteinascidin-743: A marine-derived compound in advanced, pretreated sarcoma patients—preliminary evidence of activity. J Clin Oncol 2001;19:1248.

390. Taamma A, Riofrio M, Cvitkovic E, et al: Ecteinascidin-743 (ET-743) 24 hours continuous infusion (CI): Clinical and pharmacokinetic phase I study in solid tumor patients (Pts.). Proc Am Soc Clin Oncol 1998;17:232a.

391. George S, Maki RG, Harmon DC, et al: Phase II study of ecteinascidin-743 (ET-743) given by 3-hour IV infusion in patients (pts) with soft tissue sarcomas (STS) failing prior chemotherapies. Proc Am Soc Clin Oncol 2002;21:408a.

392. LeCesne A, Blay J-Y, Judson I, et al: ET-743 is an active drug in adult soft-tissue sarcoma (STS): A STBSG-EORTC phase II trial. Proc Am Soc Clin Oncol 2001;20:353a.

393. Dileo P, Casali P, Bacci G, et al: Phase II evaluation of 3-hour infusion ET-743 in patients with recurrent sarcomas. Proc Am Soc Clin Oncol 2002;21:408a.

394. Eilber FC, Rosen G, Forscher C, et al: Surgical resection and intraperitoneal chemotherapy for recurrent abdominal sarcomas. Ann Surg Oncol 1999;6:645.

395. Rossi CR, Foletto M, Mocellin S, et al: Hyperthermic intraoperative intraperitoneal chemotherapy with cisplatin and doxorubicin in patients who undergo cytoreductive surgery for peritoneal carcinomatosis and sarcomatosis: phase I study. Cancer 2002;94:492.

396. Putnam JB Jr, Madden T, Tran H, et al: Isolated single lung perfusion (ISLP) with adriamycin for unresectable sarcomatous metastases. Proc Am Soc Clin Oncol 1997;16:500a.

397. Alvarenga JC, Ball AB, Fisher C, et al: Limitations of surgery in the treatment of retroperitoneal sarcoma. Br J Surg 1991;78:912.

398. Neifeld JP, Walsh JW, Lawrence W Jr: Computed tomography in the management of soft tissue tumors. Surg Gynecol Obstet 1982;155:535.

399. Sundaram M, McLeod RA: MR imaging of tumor and tumor like lesions of bone and soft tissue. Am J Roentgenol 1990;155:817.

400. Manaser BJ, Ensign MF: Imaging of musculoskeletal tumors. Semin Oncol 1991;18:140.

401. Glenn J, Sindelar WF, Kinsella TJ, et al: Results of multimodality therapy of resectable soft-tissue sarcomas of the retroperitoneum. Surgery 1985;97:316.

402. Karakousis CP, Velez AF, Emrich LJ: Management of retroperitoneal sarcomas and patient survival. Am J Surg 1985;150:376.

403. Dalton RR, Donohue JH, Mucha PJ, et al: Management of retroperitoneal sarcomas. Surgery 1989;106:725.

404. Storm FK, Mahvi DM: Diagnosis and management of retroperitoneal soft-tissue sarcoma. Ann Surg 1991;214:2.

405. Karakousis CP, Velez AF, Gerstenbluth R, et al: Resectability and survival in retroperitoneal sarcomas. Ann Surg Oncol 1996;3:150.

406. Kilkenny JW, Bland KI, Copeland EM: Retroperitoneal sarcoma: The University of Florida experience. J Am Coll Surg 1996;182:329.

407. Karakousis CP, Kontzoglou K, Driscoll DL: Resectability of retroperitoneal sarcomas: A matter of surgical technique? Eur J Surg Oncol 1995;21:617.

408. Karakousis CP, Gerstenbluth R, Kontzoglou K, et al: Retroperitoneal sarcomas and their management. Arch Surg 1995;130:1104.

409. McGrath PC, Neifeld JP, Lawrence W Jr., et al: Improved survival following complete excision of retroperitoneal sarcomas. Ann Surg 1984;200:200–204.

410. Catton CN, O'Sullivan B, Kotwall C, et al: Outcome and prognosis in retroperitoneal soft tissue sarcoma. Int J Radiat Oncol Biol Phys 1994;29:1005.

411. Nielsen OS, O'Sullivan B: Retroperitoneal soft tissue sarcomas: A treatment challenge and a call for randomized trials. Radiother Oncol 2002;65:133.

412. Pisters PWT, O'Sullivan B: Retroperitoneal sarcomas: Combined-modality treatment approaches. Curr Opin Oncol 2002;14:400.

413. Bose B: Primary malignant retroperitoneal tumours: analysis of 30 cases. Can J Surg 1979;22:215.

414. Cody HSI, Turnbull AD, Fortner JG, et al: The continuing challenge of retroperitoneal sarcomas. Cancer 1981;47:2147.

415. Harrison LB, Gutierrez E, Fischer JJ: Retroperitoneal sarcomas: the Yale experience and a review of the literature. J Surg Oncol 1986;32:159.

416. Wist E, Solheim OP, Jacobsen AB, et al: Primary retroperitoneal sarcomas: A review of 36 cases. Acta Radiol Oncol 1985;24:305.

417. Tepper JE, Suit HD, Wood WC, et al: Radiation therapy of retroperitoneal soft tissue sarcomas. Int J Radiat Oncol Biol Phys 1984;10:825.

418. Stoeckle E, Coindre JM, Bonvalot S, et al: Prognostic factors in retroperitoneal sarcoma: A multivariate analysis of a series of 165 patients of the French Cancer Center Federation Sarcoma Group. Cancer 2001;92:359.

419. Jones JJ, Catton CN, O'Sullivan B, et al: Initial results of a trial of preoperative external-beam radiation therapy and postoperative brachytherapy for retroperitoneal sarcoma. Ann Surg Oncol 2002;9:346.

420. Pisters PW, Ballo MT, Fenstermacher MJ, et al: Phase I trial of preoperative concurrent doxorubicin and radiation therapy, surgical resection, and intraoperative electron-beam radiation therapy for patients with localized retroperitoneal sarcoma. J Clin Oncol 2003;21:3092.

421. Gieschen HL, Spiro IJ, Suit HD, et al: Long-term results of intraoperative electron beam radiotherapy for primary and recurrent retroperitoneal soft tissue sarcoma. Int J Radiat Oncol Biol Phys 2001;50:127.

422. Petersen IA, Haddock MG, Donahue JH, et al: Use of intraoperative electron beam radiotherapy in the management of retroperitoneal soft tissue sarcomas. Int J Radiat Oncol Biol Phys 2002;52:469.

423. Willett CG, Suit HD, Tepper JE, et al: Intraoperative electron beam radiation therapy for retroperitoneal soft tissue sarcoma. Cancer 1991, 1991;68:278.

424. Kinsella TJ, Sindelar WF, Lack EE, et al: Preliminary results of a randomized study of adjuvant radiation therapy in resectable adult retroperitoneal soft tissue sarcomas. J Clin Oncol 1988;6:18.

425. Brennan MF: Retroperitoneal sarcoma: time for a national trial? Ann Surg Oncol 2002;9:324.

426. Pisters PW, O'Sullivan B: Retroperitoneal sarcomas: Combined modality treatment approaches. Curr Opin Oncol 2002;14:400.

427. Storm FK, Eilber FR, Mirra JJ, et al: Retroperitoneal sarcomas: A reappraisal of treatment. J Surg Oncol 1981;17:1.

428. Glenn J, Kinsella TJ, Glatstein EJ, et al: A randomized, prospective trial of adjuvant chemotherapy in adults with soft tissue sarcomas of the head and neck, breast, and trunk. Cancer 1985;55:1206.

429. Wendtner CM, Abdel-Rahman S, Krych M, et al: Response to neoadjuvant chemotherapy combined with regional hyperthermia predicts long-term survival for adult patients with retroperitoneal and visceral high-risk soft tissue sarcomas. J Clin Oncol 2002;20:3156.

430. Robertson JM, Sondak VK, Weiss SA, et al: Preoperative radiation therapy and iododeoxyuridine for large retroperitoneal sarcomas. Int J Radiat Oncol Biol Phys 1995;31:87.

431. Ng EH, Pollock RE, Munsell MF, et al: Prognostic factors influencing survival in gastrointestinal leiomyosarcomas. Implications for surgical management and staging. Ann Surg 1992;215:68.

432. Conlon KC, Casper ES, Brennan MF: Gastrointestinal sarcomas: analysis of prognostic variables. Ann Surg Oncol 1995;2:26.

433. DeMatteo RP, Lewis JJ, Leung D, et al: Two hundred gastrointestinal stromal tumors: Recurrence patterns and prognostic factors for survival. Ann Surg 2000;231:51.

434. Demers ML, Roh MS, Ellis LM: Liver resection improves survival for metastatic sarcoma. Proc Soc Surg Onc 1993;181.

435. Jaques DP, Coit DG, Casper ES, et al: Hepatic metastases from soft-tissue sarcoma. Ann Surg 1995;221:392.

436. Joensuu H, Roberts PJ, Sarlomo-Rikala M, et al: Effect of the tyrosine kinase inhibitor STI571 in a patient with a metastatic gastrointestinal stromal tumor. N Engl J Med 2001;344:1052.

437. Van Oosterom AT, Judson IR, Verweij J, et al: Update of phase I study of imatinib (STI571) in advanced soft tissue sarcomas and gastrointestinal stromal tumors: A report of the EORTC Soft Tissue and Bone Sarcoma Group. Eur J Cancer 2002;38 Suppl 5:S83–S87.

438. Demetri GD, von Mehren M, Blanke CD, et al: Efficacy and safety of imatinib mesylate in advanced gastrointestinal stromal tumors. N Engl J Med 2002;347:472.

439. Benjamin RS, Rankin C, Fletcher CD, et al: Phase III dose-randomized study of imatinib mesylate (STI571) for GIST: Intergroup S0033 early results. Proc Am Soc Clin Oncol 2003;22:814.

440. Verweij J, Casali P, Zalcberg J, et al: Early efficacy comparison of two doses of imatinib for the treatment of advanced gastrointestinal stromal tumors (GIST): Interim results of randomized phase III trial from the EORTC-STBSG, ISG and AGITG. Proc Am Soc Clin Oncol 2003;22:814.

441. Demetri GD, George S, Heinrich M, et al: Clinical activity and tolerability of the multi-targeted tyrosine kinase inhibitor SU11248 in patients (pts) with metastatic gastrointestinal stromal tumor (GIST) refractory to imatinib mesylate. Proc Am Soc Clin Oncol 2003;22:814.

442. Heinrich M, Corless C, Blanke CD, et al: KIT mutational status predicts clinical response to STI571 in patients with metastatic gastrointestinal stroma tumors (GISTs). Proc Am Soc Clin Oncol 2002;21:2a.

443. Awan R, Dixon R, Antonescu CR, et al: Patients with metastatic sarcoma arising from dermatofibrosarcoma protruberans (DFSP) may respond to imatinib (ST1571, Gleevec). Proc Am Soc Clin Oncol 2002;21:410a.

444. Mace J, Sybil BJ, Sondak V, et al: Response of extraabdominal desmoid tumors to therapy with imatinib mesylate. Cancer 2002;95:2373.

445. Judson I, Verweij J, van Oosterom A, et al: Imatinib (Gleevec), an active agent for gastrointestinal stromal tumors (GIST), but not for other soft tissue sarcoma (STS) subtypes not characterized for KIT and PDGF-R expression: Results of EORTC phase II studies. Proc Am Soc Clin Oncol 2002;21:403a.

446. O'Sullivan B et al: Soft tissue and bone sarcomas of the head and neck. In Harrison LB, Sessions RB, and Hong WK (eds): Head and Neck Cancer: A Multidisciplinary Approach. Philadelphia: Lippincott, p 2003 (in press).

447. Shah JP: Soft-tissue sarcomas. Problems Gen Surg 1988;5:58.

448. Weber RS, Benjamin RS, Peters LJ, et al: Soft tissue sarcomas of the head and neck in adolescents and adults. Am J Surg 1986;152:386.

449. Freedman AM, Reiman HM, Woods JE: Soft-tissue sarcomas of the head and neck. Am J Surg 1989;158:367.

450. McKenna WG, Barnes MM, Kinsella TJ, et al: Combined modality treatment of adult soft tissue sarcomas of the head and neck. Int J Radiat Oncol Biol Phys 1987;13:1127.

451. Figueiredo MT, Marques LA, Campos Filho N: Soft-tissue sarcomas of the head and neck in adults and children: Experience at a single institution with a review of literature. Int J Cancer 1988;41:198.

452. Le Vay J, O'Sullivan B, Catton C, et al: An assessment of prognostic factors in soft-tissue sarcoma of the head and neck. Arch Otolaryngol Head Neck Surg 1994;120:981.

453. Maurer HM, Ragab AH: Rhabdomyosarcoma. In Sutow WW, Fernbach DJ, Vietti TJ (eds): Clinical Pediatric Oncology. St. Louis, Mosby, 1984, p 622.

454. Russo DP, Brady MS, Conlon KC, et al: Adult urological sarcoma. J Urol 1992;147:1032.

455. Grignon DJ, Ayala AG, Ro JY, et al: Primary sarcomas of the kidney: A clinicopathologic and DNA flow cytometric study of 17 cases. Cancer 1990;65:1611.

456. Ahlering TE, Weintraub P, Skinner DG: Management of adult sarcomas of the bladder and prostate. J Urol 1988;140:1397.

457. Sen SE, Malek RS, Farrow GM, et al: Sarcoma and carcinosarcoma of the bladder in adults. J Urol 1985;133:29.

458. Swartz DA, Johnson DE, Ayala AG, et al: Bladder leiomyosarcoma: A review of 10 cases with 5 year follow-up. J Urol 1985;133:200.

459. Catton C, Jewett M, O'Sullivan B, et al: Paratesticular sarcoma: Failure patterns after definitive local therapy. J Urol 1999;161:1844.

460. Ballo MT, Zagars GK, Pisters PW, et al: Spermatic cord sarcoma: Outcome, patterns of failure and management. J Urol 2001;166:1306.

461. Loughlin KR, Retik AB, Weinstein HJ, et al: Genitourinary rhabdomyosarcoma in children. Cancer 1989;63:1600.

462. Crist WM, Garnsey L, Beltangady MS, et al: Prognosis in children with rhabdomyosarcoma: A report of the Intergroup Rhabdomyosarcoma Studies I and II. Intergroup Rhabdomyosarcoma Committee. J Clin Oncol 1990;8:443.

463. Curtin JP, et al: Corpus: Mesenchymal tumors. In Hoskins WJ, Perez CA, Young RC (eds): Principles and Practice of Gynecologic Oncology, 2d ed. Philadelphia, Lippincott, 1997, p 897.

464. Levenback CF, Tortolero-Luna G, Pandey DK, et al: Uterine sarcoma. Obstet Gynecol Clin North Am 1996;23:457.

465. Echt G, Jepson J, Steel J, et al: Treatment of uterine sarcomas. Cancer 1990;66:35.

466. Kahanpaa KV, Wahlstrom T, Grohn P, et al: Sarcomas of the uterus: A clinicopathologic study of 119 patients. Obstet Gynecol 1986;67:417.

467. De Fusco PA, Gaffey TA, Malkasian GD Jr, et al: Endometrial stromal sarcoma: Review of Mayo Clinic experience, 1945–1980. Gynecol Oncol 1989;35:8.

468. Dreisler A, Lykkesfeldt G: [Sarcoma of the uterus. A retrospective clinical study of 56 cases.] Ugeskr Laeger 1985;147:3698.

469. Geraci P, Maggio S, Adragna F, et al: Uterine sarcomas: A retrospective study of 17 cases. Eur J Gynaecol Oncol 1988;9:497.

470. Larson B, Silfversward C, Nilsson B, et al: Mixed mullerian tumours of the uterus-prognostic factors: A clinical and histopathologic study of 147 cases. Radiother Oncol 1990;17:12.

471. Omura GA, Blessing JA, Major FJ, et al: A randomized clinical trial of adjuvant adriamycin in uterine sarcomas: A Gynecologic Oncology Group study. J Clin Oncol 1985;3:1240.

472. Badib AO, Vongtama V, Kurohara SS, et al: Radiotherapy in the treatment of sarcomas of the corpus uteri. Cancer 1969;24:724.

473. DiSaia PJ, Castro JR, Rutledge FN: Mixed mesodermal sarcoma of the uterus. Am J Roentgenol Radium Ther Nucl Md 1973;117:632.

474. Salazar OM, Bonfiglio TA, Patten SF, et al: Uterine sarcomas: Natural history, treatment and prognosis. Cancer 1978;42:1152.

475. Vongtama V, Karlen JR, Piver SM, et al: Treatment, result and prognostic factors in stage I and II sarcomas of the corpus uteri. AJR Am J Roentgenol 1976;126:139.

476. Wen BC, Tewfik FA, Tewfik HH, et al: Uterine sarcoma: A retrospective study. J Surg Oncol 1987;34:104.

477. Major FJ, Blessing JA, Silverberg SG, et al: Prognostic factors in early-stage uterine sarcoma: A Gynecologic Oncology Group study. Cancer 1993;71:1702.

478. Thigpen T, Vance R, Lambuth B, et al: Chemotherapy for advanced or recurrent gynecologic cancer. Cancer 1987;60:2104.

479. Sutton G, Brunetto VL, Kilgore L, et al: A phase III trial of ifosfamide with or without cisplatin in carcinosarcoma of the uterus: A Gynecologic Oncology Group Study. Gynecol Oncol 2000;79:147.

480. Omura GA, Major FJ, Blessing JA, et al: A randomized study of Adriamycin with and without dimethyl triazenoimidazole carboxamide in advanced uterine sarcomas. Cancer 1983;52:626.

481. Sutton G, Blessing J, Carson L, et al: Adjuvant ifosfamide, mesna, and cisplatin in patients with completely resected stage I or II carcinosarcoma of the uterus: A study of the Gynecologic Oncology Group. Proc Am Soc Clin Oncol 1997;16:362a.

482. Fuller AF, Penson R, Supko JG, et al: A phase I/II and pharmacokinetic study of 96-hour infusional topotecan and paclitaxel chemotherapy for recurrent müllerian tumors. Proc Am Soc Clin Oncol 2000;19:292a.

483. Duska LR, Garrett A, Eltabbakh GH, et al: Paclitaxel and platinum chemotherapy for malignant mixed mullerian tumors of the ovary. Gynecol Oncol 2002;85:459.

484. Enzinger FM, Weiss SW: Malignant tumors of uncertain type. In Enzinger FM, Weiss SW (eds): Soft Tissue Tumors, 3d ed. St. Louis: Mosby, 1995, p 1067.

485. Spear MA, Jennings LC, Mankin HJ, et al: Individualizing management of aggressive fibromatoses. Int J Radiat Oncol Biol Phys 1998;40:637.

486. Ballo MT, Zagars GK, Pollack A, et al: Desmoid tumor: Prognostic factors and outcome after surgery, radiation therapy, or combined surgery and radiation therapy. J Clin Oncol 1999;17:158.

487. Posner MC, Shiu MH, Newsome JL, et al: The desmoid tumor: Not a benign disease. Arch Surg 1989;124:191.

488. Klein WA, Miller HH, Anderson M, et al: The use of indomethacin, sulindac, and tamoxifen for the treatment of desmoid tumors associated with familial polyposis. Cancer 1987;60:2863.

489. Procter H, Singh L, Baum M, et al: Response of multicentric desmoid tumours to tamoxifen. Br J Surg 1987;74:401.

490. Weiss AJ, Lackman RD: Low-dose chemotherapy of desmoid tumors. Cancer 1989;64:1192.

491. Azzarelli A, Gronchi A, Bertulli R, et al: Low-dose chemotherapy with methotrexate and vinblastine for patients with advanced aggressive fibromatosis. Cancer 2001;92:1259.

492. Skapek SX, Hawk BJ, Hoffer FA, et al: Combination chemotherapy using vinblastine and methotrexate for the treatment of progressive desmoid tumor in children. J Clin Oncol 1998;16:3021.

493. Reich S, Overberg-Schmidt US, Buhrer C, et al: Low-dose chemotherapy with vinblastine and methotrexate in childhood desmoid tumors. J Clin Oncol 1999;17:1086.

494. Patel SR, Evans HL, Benjamin RS: Combination chemotherapy in adult desmoid tumors. Cancer 1993;72:3244.

495. Hamilton L, Blackstein M, Berk T, et al: Chemotherapy for desmoid tumours in association with familial adenomatous polyposis: A report of three cases. Can J Surg 1996;39:247.

496. Seiter K, Kemeny N: Successful treatment of a desmoid tumor with doxorubicin. Cancer 1993;71:2242.

497. Petrek JA: Other cancer of the breast. In Harris JA, Hellman S, Henderson IC, Kinne DW (eds): Breast Diseases. Philadelphia: Lippincott, 1991, p 804.

498. Pollard SG, Marks PV, Temple LN, et al: Breast sarcoma: A clinicopathologic review of 25 cases. Cancer 1990;66:941.

499. Zelek L, Llombart-Cussac A, Terrier P, et al: Prognostic factors in primary breast sarcomas: A series of patients with long-term follow-up. J Clin Oncol 2003;21:2583.

500. Rosen PP, Kimmel M, Ernsberger D: Mammary angiosarcoma: The prognostic significance of tumor differentiation. Cancer 1988;62:2145.

501. Taghian A, de Vathaire F, Terrier P, et al: Long-term risk of sarcoma following radiation treatment for breast cancer. Int J Radiat Oncol Biol Phys 1991;21:361.

502. Stokkel MP, Peterse HL: Angiosarcoma of the breast after lumpectomy and radiation therapy for adenocarcinoma. Cancer 1992;69:2965.

503. Edeiken S, Russo DP, Knecht J, et al: Angiosarcoma after tylectomy and radiation therapy for carcinoma of the breast. Cancer 1992;70:644.

504. Engel A, Lamm SH, Lai SH: Human breast sarcoma and human breast implantation: A time trend analysis based on SEER data (1973–1990). J Clin Epidemiol 1995;48:539.

505. Christensen L, Schiodt T, Blichert TM, et al: Sarcomas of the breast: A clinico-pathological study of 67 patients with long term follow-up. Eur J Surg Oncol 1988;14:241.

506. Callery CD, Rosen PP, Kinne DW: Sarcoma of the breast: A study of 32 patients with reappraisal of classification and therapy. Ann Surg 1985;201:527.

507. Gutman H, Pollock RE, Ross MI, et al: Sarcoma of the breast: implications for extent of therapy. The M. D. Anderson experience. Surgery 1994;116:505.

508. Terrier P, Terrier Lacombe MJ, Mouriesse H, et al: Primary breast sarcoma: A review of 33 cases with immunohistochemistry and prognostic factors. Breast Cancer Res Treat 1989;13:39.

509. McGowan TS, Cummings BJ, O'Sullivan B, et al: An analysis of 78 breast sarcoma patients without distant metastases at presentation. Int J Radiat Oncol Biol Phys 2000;46:383.

510. Karpeh MS, Caldwell C, Gaynor JJ, et al: Vascular soft-tissue sarcomas: An analysis of tumor-related mortality. Arch Surg 1991;126:1474.

511. Naka N, Ohsawa M, Tomita Y, et al: Angiosarcoma in Japan: A review of 99 cases. Cancer 1995;75:989.

512. Morrison WH, Byers RM, Garden AS, et al: Cutaneous angiosarcoma of the head and neck. Cancer 1995;76:319.

513. Girard C, Johnson WC, Graham JH: Cutaneous angiosarcoma. Cancer 1970;26:868.

514. Auguste LJ, Razack MS, Sako K: Hemangiopericytoma. J Surg Oncol 1982;20:260.

515. Enzinger FM, Smith BH: Hemangiopericytoma. An analysis of 106 cases. Hum Pathol 1976;7:61.

516. Maddox J, Evans HL: Angiosarcoma of skin and soft tissue: A study of 44 cases. Cancer 1981;48:1907.

517. Holden CA, Spittle MF, Jones EW: Angiosarcoma of the face and scalp, prognosis and treatment. Cancer 1987;59:1046.

518. Ma CM, Pawlicki T, Lee MC, et al: Energy- and intensity-modulated electron beams for radiotherapy. Phys Med Biol 2000;45:2293.

519. Fata F, O'Reilly E, Ilson D, et al: Paclitaxel in the treatment of patients with angiosarcoma of the scalp or face. Cancer 1999;86:2034.

520. Burgess MA, Patel SR, Plager C, et al: A preliminary evaluation of a combination of interferon alpha and dis-retinoic acid in patients with certain vascular tumors—malignant and benign. Proc Am Soc Clin Oncol 1996;15:525.

521. Rosen G, Forscher C, Lowenbraun S, et al: Synovial Sarcoma: Uniform response of metastases to high dose ifosfamide. Cancer 1994;73:2506.

522. Kampe CE, Rosen G, Eilber F, et al: Synovial sarcoma: A study of intensive chemotherapy in 14 patients with localized disease. Cancer 1993;72:2161.

523. Edmonson JH, Ryan L, Blum RH: Phase II study of ifosfamide plus doxorubicin in patients with advanced synovial sarcomas: An ECOG Study. Proc Am Soc Clin Oncol 2001;20:293b.

524. Demetri GD, Spiegelman BM, Fletcher CDM, et al: Differentiation of liposarcomas in patients treated with the PPAR-g Ligand Troglitazone: Documentation of biologic activity in myxoid/round cell and pleomorphic subtypes. Proc Am Soc Clin Oncol 1999;18:535a.

525. Demetri GD, Fletcher CD, Mueller E, et al: Induction of solid tumor differentiation by the peroxisome proliferator-activated receptor-gamma ligand troglitazone in patients with liposarcoma. Proc Natl Acad Sci USA 1999;96:3951.

526. Ferrari A, Dileo P, Casanova M, et al: Rhabdomyosarcoma in adults: A retrospective analysis of 171 patients treated at a single institution. Cancer 2003;98:571.

527. Little DJ, Ballo MT, Zagars GK, et al: Adult rhabdomyosarcoma: Outcome following multimodality treatment. Cancer 2002;95:377.

528. Kattan M: Statistical prediction models, artificial neural networks, and the sophism "I am a patient, not a statistic." J Clin Oncol 2002;20:885.

529. Fabrizio PL, Stafford SL, Pritchard DJ: Extremity soft-tissue sarcomas selectively treated with surgery alone. Int J Radiat Oncol Biol Phys 2000;48:227.

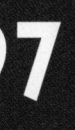
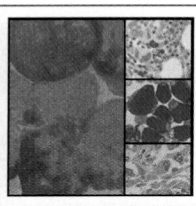

UNKNOWN PRIMARY CANCER

Katrina Y. Glover

Gauri R. Varadhachary

Renato Lenzi

Martin N. Raber

James L. Abbruzzese

SUMMARY OF KEY POINTS

INCIDENCE
- The incidence of unknown primary carcinoma ranges from 0.5 to 9% of all patients diagnosed with cancer.
- At M.D. Anderson Hospital from January 1987 to June 1995, unknown primary carcinoma accounted for 1.5% of all cancer referrals.

EVALUATION
- Controversy exists over the extent of evaluation needed to exclude a definable primary cancer.
- Biopsy of a metastatic site is recommended early to establish the diagnosis and help direct further workup.
- Basic evaluation includes the following:
  - History and physical examination (including breast and pelvic examinations in women and testis and prostate examinations in men)
  - SMA-12, complete blood cell count, prostate-specific antigen test in men, chest radiography, abdominal and pelvic computed tomographic scan, and mammography in women
- Testing for immunohistochemical markers (including CK7, CK20, TTF-1)
- The diagnostic utility of positron emission tomography (PET) and

its cost effectiveness are controversial and currently being studied.
- The role of DNA microarray and gene profiling in this subset is evolving.

DIFFERENTIAL DIAGNOSIS
- Diagnosis is made in patients with a biopsy-proved malignancy, when the site of origin is not obvious after preceding evaluation.
- Careful consultation with a pathologist is critical to exclude highly treatable malignancies (e.g., lymphoma, breast cancer, germ cell cancers).
- Newer diagnostic tools, including new immunohistochemical stains, and molecular markers promise the ability to identify the site of origin in a greater proportion of cases.

PRIMARY THERAPY
- It is important to identify specific patients who may have clinical/pathologic features of six highly treatable unknown primary carcinoma subsets (minority of patients):
  - Women with axillary adenopathy (adenocarcinoma or carcinoma)
  - Women with peritoneal carcinomatosis
  - Patients with poorly differentiated or undifferentiated carcinoma

- Males with the extragonadal germ cell syndrome
- Patients with neuroendocrine carcinoma
- Patients with high cervical adenopathy (squamous carcinoma)
- For the majority of patients, who belong to no identifiable subset, primary therapy consists of the following:
  - Systemic therapy: adeno-carcinoma: paclitaxel/carboplatin ± etoposide; CDDP/5-fluorouracil/leucovorin
  - Carcinoma: paclitaxel/carboplatin ± etoposide; CDDP/etoposide
  - Squamous carcinoma: CDDP/5-fluorouracil/leucovorin
  - Local therapy: resection ± radiation therapy; observation with best supportive care

SECOND- OR THIRD-LINE THERAPY
- No highly effective salvage systemic regimens are in use.
- Gemcitabine has produced low objective response rates and symptomatic improvement as single-agent therapy in the second-line setting.
- The role of newer agents such as irinotecan is unknown; patients should be encouraged to participate in clinical trials for novel agents.

INTRODUCTION

Despite the increasing array of sophisticated diagnostic tools available to establish the diagnosis of human neoplasia, oncologists have struggled to understand a subset of patients with metastatic cancer in whom detailed investigations fail to identify a primary anatomic site. The reported incidence of unknown primary carcinoma (UPC) varies with the practice setting and the definition used, but averages 0.5% to 9% of all patients who are diagnosed with cancer.[1] Identification of the primary lesion largely forms the basis for predicting the expected behavior and

assigning appropriate therapy of malignant diseases; thus the absence of a primary carcinoma poses a major challenge. The inability to identify a primary carcinoma also generates anxiety for the patient who may feel that the physician's evaluation has been inadequate or that the prognosis would be improved if a primary site could be established.

As suggested by the foregoing variable incidence statistics, the definition of UPC has not been standardized, varying in published reports mainly with regard to the extent of evaluation required to accept this diagnosis. For the purpose of this chapter we will define patients with UPC as having a biopsy-proved malignancy for which the anatomic origin remains unidentified after history and physical examination (including breast palpation and pelvic examination in women and testicular and prostate examination in men), laboratory studies including liver and renal function tests, hemogram, chest x-ray, computed tomography of abdomen and pelvis, mammography in women, and measurement of prostate-specific antigen in men. All positive findings on this initial evaluation are then investigated in detail.[2] Depending on the clinical situation, additional studies might include sputum cytologic test, computed tomography of the chest, breast ultrasonography, or gastrointestinal endoscopy. To further define the patient population most investigators have excluded from analysis rare instances in which soft tissue sarcoma or melanoma present without a definite primary site,[2] concentrating clinical research efforts on the vast majority of patients with common epithelial histologies such as adenocarcinoma, carcinoma, squamous carcinoma, and neuroendocrine carcinoma.

The approach to patients with UPC is based on the generally held belief that this group of patients is heterogeneous; they may have any one of numerous underlying primary cancers that remain occult during the lifetime of the patient. This concept is supported by studies showing that a detailed postmortem anatomic investigation will establish a primary cancer in many, if not the majority, of these patients.[3,4] However, clinically these small primary tumors usually remain undiagnosed during the course of the patient's disease. Although heterogeneous in their origins, detailed clinical and biochemical study of unknown primary carcinoma cells may represent a valuable resource with which to dissect the metastatic phenotype.[5,6] More recent approaches involve simultaneous determination of a large number of molecular markers with tools such as DNA microarrays and RT-PCR (reverse transcriptase–polymerase chain reaction). Such approaches promise to identify the site of origin in a larger proportion of UPCs,[7,8] although poorly differentiated tumors may still elude accurate classification.[9] Also, the heterogeneity of this population may make them the natural population to evaluate experimental approaches such as immunotherapy and antiangiogenesis. As is the case for the specific well-defined primary neoplasms discussed elsewhere in this text, it is the phenomenon of metastasis, as purely exemplified by the UPC patient, that causes the vast majority of cancer deaths.

ETIOLOGY AND EPIDEMIOLOGY

Whether there are specific etiologic factors relevant to UPC is not known. Although a history of cigarette smoking can be frequently elicited (Table 97-1), the heterogeneity of UPC makes it unlikely that specific etiologic agents will be associated with this disease. The fact that numerous occult anatomic sites can give rise to carcinomas that present with only metastatic disease supports the possibility that specific interactions of genetic and environmental insults could give rise to genomic and biochemical changes which lead to the early development of the metastatic phenotype without the associated

TABLE 97-1

Characteristics of 1109 Patients with Unknown Primary Carcinoma		
	UNKNOWN PRIMARY CARCINOMA (N = 1109)	**ALL PATIENTS REFERRED TO M.D. ANDERSON***
CHARACTERISTIC	**NO. OF PATIENTS (%)**	**NO. OF PATIENTS (%)**
Age		
0–39	108 (9.7)	9674 (17.6)
40–49	175 (15.8)	9706 (17.7)
50–59	283 (25.5)	12,158 (22.1)
60–69	346 (31.2)	14,112 (25.7)
>70	197 (17.8)	9289 (16.9)
Sex		
Female	537 (48.4)	26,970 (49.1)
Male	572 (51.6)	27,969 (50.9)
Ethnicity		
White	962 (86.8)	43,788 (79.7)
Hispanic	78 (7.0)	6267 (11.4)
Black	48 (4.3)	3909 (7.1)
Other	21 (1.9)	975 (1.8)
Smoking History		
Smokers	608 (54.8)	N/A
Nonsmokers/unknown	501 (45.2)	N/A

N/A, not available.
*Total number of patients referred with diagnosis of malignancy recorded from 1/1/87 to 6/30/95: 54,939 patients.

changes supporting local growth in the organ of origin. Although this concept must be considered highly speculative, it is a hypothesis that can be tested through analysis of available biomarkers such as oncogenes and tumor suppressor genes that have been characterized for cancers with known anatomic origins such as lung, pancreatic, breast, and colorectal carcinomas. Either the absence of genetic changes typical for malignancies with established primary cancers or the presence of unusual variants of known genetic alterations would support this hypothesis. It is likely that as the genomic and proteomic characterization of malignancies is refined, fewer and fewer malignancies may be assigned to the UPC designation.

The epidemiologic characteristics of 1109 consecutive UPC patients referred to the M.D. Anderson Cancer Center from January 1987 to June 1995 are presented in Table 97-1. These data are juxtaposed with the overall referral population during the same time period. Although the family history frequently identifies additional cancers with established origins in other family members, no clearly familial instances of UPC have been identified or reported.

HISTOLOGIC PRESENTATIONS

The frequency of specific histologic diagnoses established in UPC depends to some extent on the patient population

TABLE 97-2

Histologic Types Identified in 1109 Consecutive Patients with Unknown Primary Carcinoma

HISTOLOGIC TYPE	M.D. ANDERSON		HAINSWORTH ET AL[13]	
	NO. OF PATIENTS*	PERCENTAGE TOTAL	NO. OF PATIENTS†	PERCENTAGE TOTAL
Adenocarcinoma	646	58.3	—	31.8
Well differentiated	14			
Moderately differentiated	45		—	
Poorly differentiated	220		70	
Mucinous	46		—	
No descriptor/other	321		—	
Carcinoma	317	28.6		44.1
Poorly differentiated	161		97	
Undifferentiated	21		—	
Large cell	9		—	
Small cell	14		—	
No descriptor/other	112		—	
Squamous	68	6.1	5	2.3
Neuroendocrine	48	4.3	25	11.4
Adenosquamous	7	0.6	0	0
Pathology not Available for Review/Other	23	2.1	23	10.4

*Total number of patients, 1109.
†Total number of patients, 220.

chosen for study. For example, most recent investigators have excluded the well-characterized group of patients with metastatic squamous carcinomas to cervical lymph nodes.[10-12] The specific histologic diagnoses identified in a series of 1109 consecutive patients with UPC are outlined in Table 97-2 and are contrasted with another reported series.[13] The low frequency of squamous carcinoma reflects the direct referral of patients with squamous cell carcinoma involving high or mid-cervical lymph nodes to head and neck oncologists for management.

BIOLOGIC CHARACTERISTICS

The biology of UPC has been partially characterized through the evaluation of patient subsets using as primary end points responsiveness to therapy and survival. When all patients are considered, UPC is a highly aggressive neoplasm with an overall median survival time of 3 to 4 months in older series.[14] More recent studies have documented median survival times of 9 to 12 months.[15-18] In our series of 1109 consecutive patients the median survival period was 11 months. The survival curve for these patients is presented in Figure 97-1.

The survival times for the four most frequently encountered pathologic subtypes are presented in Figure 97-2. The median survival for patients with squamous carcinoma (exclusive of patients with mid-high cervical adenopathy) was 24 months, adenocarcinoma was 9 months, carcinoma was 12 months, and neuroendocrine carcinoma was 33 months. The state of differentiation or mucin production did not appear to significantly influ-

ence the poor survival of patients with adenocarcinoma (Fig. 97-3). Using univariate and multivariate analyses, various groups have assessed the influence of other clinical-pathologic features of UPC on survival. These data are summarized in Table 97-3. Culine and associates[19] also developed and validated a prognostic model to predict the length of survival in patients with UPCs. Univariate and multivariate prognostic factor analyses were conducted in a population of 150 unselected

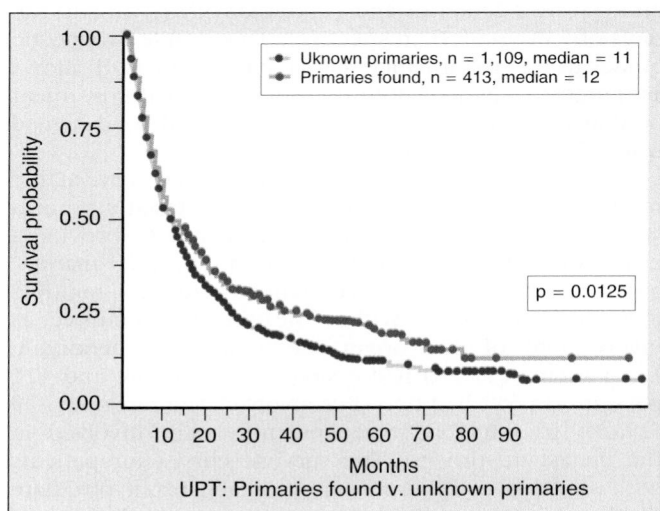

Figure 97-1. Survival curves for 1109 patients with unknown primary carcinoma (UPC) versus 413 patients referred with UPC in whom the primary cancer site was found.

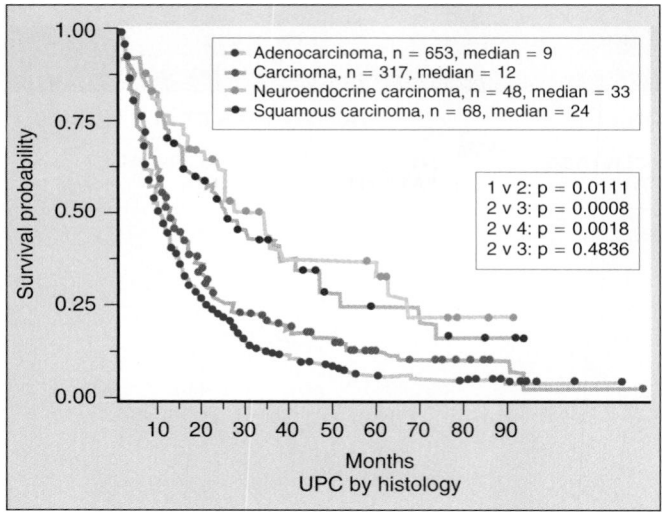

Figure 97-2. Survival curves of the major histologic subtypes of unknown primary carcinoma.

patients and led to the construction of two successive classification schemes. When studying the clinical variables only, poor performance status and presence of liver metastases were retained in the multivariate analysis. The first classification scheme consisted of three groups of patients with median survival times of 10.8, 6.0, and 2.4 months, according to the number of adverse prognostic factors. When serum lactate dehydrogenase (LDH) was introduced in a further step, liver metastases were no longer of significance. The second classification scheme therefore included performance status and elevated serum LDH. Good-risk and poor-risk patients were identified with median survival times of 11.7 months and 3.9 months and 1-year survival rates of 45% and 11%, respectively. Validation of the second classification was obtained using an external data set; and the median survival times of patients assigned to the good-risk group and poor-risk group were 12 months and 7 months with 1-year survival rates of 53% and 23%, respectively. This simple prognostic model using performance status and serum LDH allows assignment of patients into two subgroups with divergent outcomes. Additional prospective trials will be designed using this prognostic model.

To assess the impact of disease extent on survival, the number of organ sites involved in the metastatic process was assessed at presentation in our series to provide a crude quantitation of tumor burden. For this analysis, involvement of an organ, even when there were multiple individual metastases within the site, was counted as involvement of one organ site. Using this definition, 133 patients (37.5%) had a single involved site and 122 patients (34.5%) had two sites involved. The remaining 99 (28.0%) patients had three or more sites involved in the metastatic process. The survival curves for patients with one, two, and three or more organ sites involved are displayed in Figure 97-4. The median survival time for patients with one site of involvement was 10 months, with two sites of involvement 8.0 months, and with three or more sites of involvement 6.0 months. These survival

curves are statistically different by the Cox-Mantel log-rank test ($P = 0.028$). Other studies have documented similar results.[18]

The question of whether the biology of UPC is fundamentally different from known primary carcinoma with systemic metastases remains controversial.[20] Nystrom and associates have argued that the distribution of metastatic sites in patients with UPC where the primary cancer is subsequently found is sufficiently different from known primary carcinoma to support the hypothesis that UPC is biologically unique.[21] However, analysis of our series shows few significant differences in the pattern of metastases (Table 97-4) or in overall survival for true UPC versus patients in whom the primary lesion was found (see Fig. 97-1). Continued study of UPC will be necessary to resolve this controversy.

The reason the primary organ site cannot be diagnosed remains unknown. Previous investigators have speculated that the tumor may remain below the limits of clinical or radiographic detection or that it spontaneously regressed.[22] Another possibility would be that a clinically detectable primary cancer never develops due to the development of specific genetic changes that support metastatic but not local growth. Continued investigation has resulted in greater understanding of the biologic features of unknown primary carcinomas characterized by aneuploidy, chromosomal abnormalities, oncogenes, tumor suppressor genes, and microvessel density.

Aneuploidy is a well-recognized phenomenon occurring in 70% to 90% of solid tumors[23–25] and is defined as a chromosome complement that is not a simple multiple of the haploid set. Increasing evidence indicates that for many carcinomas, such as breast, prostate, and colorectal cancers, a diploid DNA content is associated with a more favorable prognosis.[26] Hedley and associates[27] measured the cellular DNA content of tumor biopsy specimens of 152 patients with metastatic adenocarcinoma or undifferentiated carcinoma of unknown primary site in order to determine favorable subgroups. Aneuploidy was found in the specimens of 70% of the patients. There were no significant differences between men and women, and there was no obvious relationship to the various patterns of metastatic involvement. The median survival of patients with diploid tumors was 4.2 months versus 4.8 months for patients with aneuploid tumors. Of the 46 patients with diploid tumors, 9 (18%) survived for more than 2 years, compared with 10 (9%) of 106 patients with aneuploid tumors. These results indicate that the incidence of aneuploidy in this heterogeneous group of patients is similar to that reported for carcinomas with known primary tumors. However, in contrast to many of these tumor types, in this single study conducted by Hedley and associates, metastatic adenocarcinomas of unknown primary origin that are diploid are not associated with a more favorable prognosis than are those of known primary origin.[27]

Chromosome Abnormalities

Evaluation of chromosomal abnormalities in UPC is an emerging area of investigation, and as such, relatively few

Figure 97-3. A, Influence of cellular differentiation on the survival of patients with unknown primary adenocarcinoma. **B,** Influence of cellular differentiation on the survival of patients with unknown primary carcinoma.

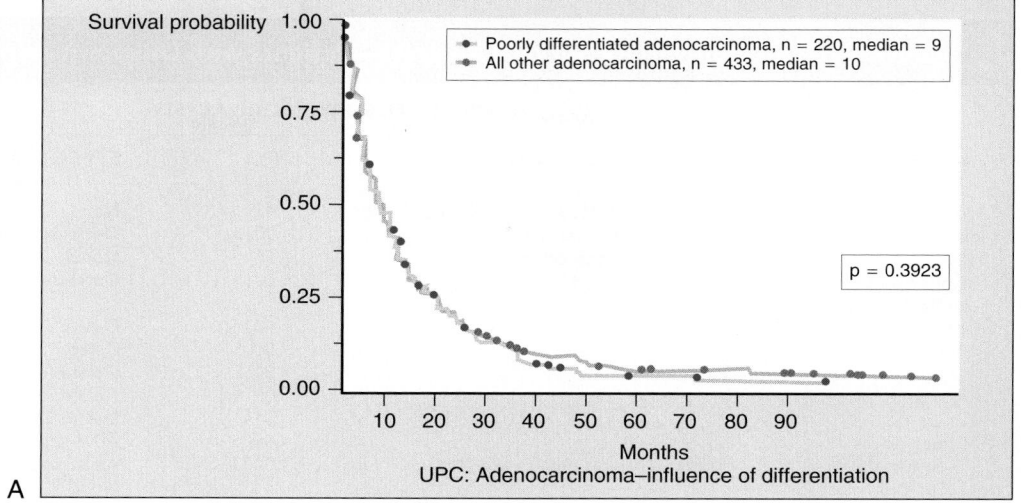

A

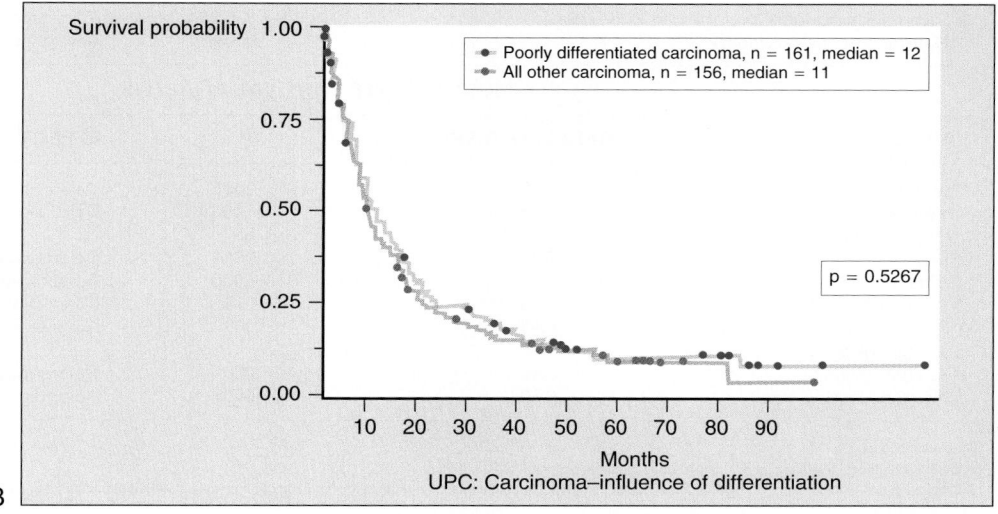

B

studies have been performed. Abbruzzese[5] and Bell[28] developed a research program aimed at identifying common karyotypic changes in UPC. The karyotypes of 13 of 20 UPC patients were determined and in 12 of the analyzed cell lines abnormalities were identified in the short arm of chromosome 1. The abnormalities detected included deletion of 1p, translocations, isochromosome 1q, and gene amplification. These findings were consistent with earlier descriptions of chromosome 1p abnormalities in advanced malignancy as described by Atkin[29] and Mertens and associates.[30]

Motzer and associates[31,32] used karyotyping to determine the frequency of specific abnormalities of chromosome 12 in patients with UPC. It was hypothesized that patients with undifferentiated carcinoma of unknown primary origin responding to cisplatin-based chemotherapy had unrecognized germ cell tumors and that isochromosome 12p, i(12p), a specific chromosomal marker

characterizing germ cell tumors, could be used to identify such patients. Thirty percent of patients had an increased 12p copy number or deletion of the long arm of chromosome 12, which proved predictive of response thereby validating the hypothesis. Complete response to cisplatin-based therapy was achieved in patients with specific chromosomal aberrations associated with germ cell tumors, and objective responses were achieved in 75% of these patients, compared with 17% of patients without these aberrations. Summersgill and associates[33] and Ilson and associates[34] found similar associations for UPC patients with undifferentiated carcinoma. Thus, for patients with undifferentiated carcinoma, i(12p) correlated with a good response to platin-based chemotherapy, though lack of i(12p) may not exclude a small percentage of responses; i(12p) occurs in over 80% of the germ cell tumors and only sparsely in a few other lesions (acute leukemia, embryonal rhabdomyosarcoma, and neuroepi-

Specific Malignancies

III

TABLE 97-3

Univariate and Multivariate Survival Analyses—Patients with Unknown Primary Carcinoma

UNIVARIATE SURVIVAL ANALYSIS

VARIABLE	GROUPING	P*	EFFECT ON SURVIVAL
Age, years	20–39, 40–49, 50–59, 60–69, 70+	.43	None
Sex	Male, female	.0018	Decreased survival for men
Race	White, other	.86	None
No. of organ sites	1, 2, 3+	.0018	Decreased survival with more organ sites
Involved organ sites			
Lung	—	.0014	Deleterious
Bone	—	.0005	Deleterious
Liver	—	.0050	Deleterious
Pleura	—	.0019	Deleterious
Brain	—	.014	Deleterious
Lymph nodes	—	<.0001	Advantageous
Axillary	—	.0003	Advantageous
Supraclavicular	—	.44	None
Peritoneum	—	.59	None
Skin	—	.69	None
Histologic type			
Adenocarcinoma	—	<.0001	Deleterious
Carcinoma	—	.0058	Advantageous
Squamous carcinoma	—	.058	Advantageous
Neuroendocrine carcinoma	—	.0009	Advantageous

MULTIVARIATE SURVIVAL ANALYSIS

VARIABLE	RELATIVE RISK†	P*	EFFECT ON SURVIVAL
Male sex	1.39	.0007	Deleterious
Increasing no. of organ sites	1.23	<.0001	Deleterious
Involved organ sites			
Liver	1.33	.0064	Deleterious
Lymph nodes (all sites)	.46	<.0001	Advantageous
Supraclavicular	1.56	.013	Deleterious
Peritoneum	0.59	.0099	Advantageous
Histologic type			
Adenocarcinoma	1.46	.0001	Deleterious
Neuroendocrine carcinoma	0.30	.0005	Advantageous

*Log rank test.
†Calculated from the Cox proportional hazards regression.
Adapted from Abbruzzese JL, Abbruzzese MC, Lenzi R, et al: Analysis of a diagnostic strategy for patients with suspected tumors of unknown origin. J Clin Oncol 1995;13:2094.

thelioma), and therefore, determination of the presence or absence of i(12p) can help diagnose extragonadal germ cell tumors in patients with UPC.[35]

Oncogenes

The oncogenes *ras*, *c-myc*, *bcl-2*, and *her-2/neu* are overexpressed in a variety of solid tumors. The levels of these genes are thought to be useful prognostic factors, though reports on *c-myc* and *bcl-2* are often conflicting. Pavlidis and associates[36] found a high rate of overexpression of *c-myc* (96%), *ras* (92%), and *c-erbB₂* (65%). Investigators found that the overexpression did not have a further relationship with histologic or clinical parameters or a diagnostic or prognostic value.

Briasoulis and associates[37] studied levels of *bcl-2* expression in 40 patients with UPC (8% squamous, 36% adenocarcinoma, and 55.5% poorly differentiated carci-

noma). Staining was evaluated based on intensity (+1 to +3) and the percentage of positive cells (1% to 100%). *Bcl-2* was expressed in almost half of the tumors. This finding was not expected because in most studies, *bcl-2* had been found to be upregulated in premalignant lesions rather than advanced malignancies and had also been associated with a less aggressive phenotype.[38,39] In this study, the level of *bcl-2* expression, by itself, had no prognostic value. When combined with a high level of expression of p53, high expression of *bcl-2* showed a trend toward a higher response to platinum-based chemotherapy.

Hainsworth and associates[40] stained 100 tumor specimens of poorly differentiated adenocarcinoma (PDA) or poorly differentiated carcinoma (PDC) of unknown primary site for Her-2 protein. The samples of 10 patients (11%) overexpressed Her-2. These investigators did not observe any major difference in the overall response rate

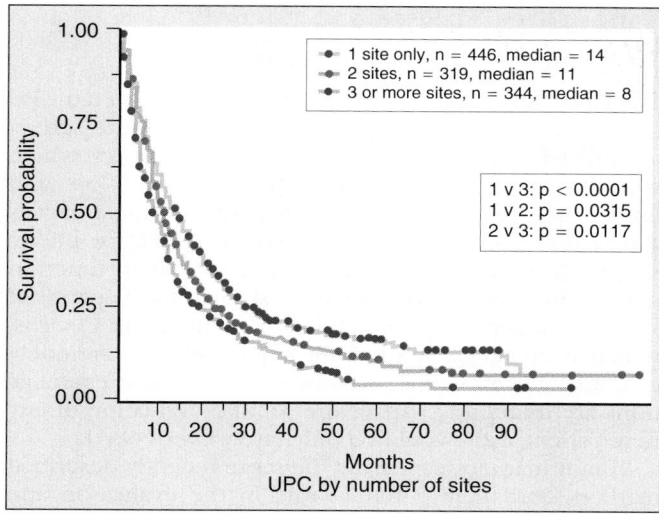

Figure 97-4. Survival of unknown primary carcinoma patients versus number of involved organ sites.

to chemotherapy between the patients whose cancer overexpressed Her-2 and those who did not. Evaluation of the efficacy of trastuzumab in selected UPC patients with Her-2 overexpression is warranted.

Tumor Suppressor Genes

It is now known that a large number of gene deletions or allelic inactivation occur in most human cancers. Many of these genetic alterations result in the activation of oncogenes or in the loss of tumor suppressor genes and have been localized to specific chromosomes. To date, p53 is the best-known and most widely studied tumor suppressor gene. p53 can control tumor development by arresting cell cycle or initiating apoptosis of damaged cells. p53 mutations are common and occur in about 55% of all human cancers.[41-43]

Briasoulis and associates[37] evaluated p53 expression using immunohistochemistry in 47 cases of UPC (4 squamous carcinoma, 17 adenocarcinoma, 26 PDC). Staining was evaluated based on intensity (+1 to +3) and percentage of positive cells (1% to 100%). More than 70% of the tumors expressed p53; 53% expressed a high level and 47% expressed a low level of immunohistochemical staining. In this study, p53 expression alone had no prognostic value.

Bar-eli and associates[44] also investigated the frequency of p53 mutations in a series of 15 UPC biopsies and 8 cell lines established from UPCs. Mutations in the conserved regions of p53 gene were analyzed by single-strand conformation polymorphism analysis of exons 5 to 9 and were verified by direct DNA sequencing of PCR products. The p53 gene was mutated in 6 of 23 (26%) patients with UPC. Therefore, despite the fact that UPCs represent bad prognostic tumors that are often aneuploid, the frequency of p53 mutation was relatively low in this study. This finding suggests that p53 mutations may not play a major role in the development and progression of UPC. The discrepancy between the results of these two studies may be due to discordance between the results of immunohistochemical and genetic molecular methods in detecting the p53 abnormalities, which may occur in 25% of tumors.

No research is available on metastasis-suppressor genes in UPC, which seems to play an important role in regulating the growth of disseminated cancer cells at secondary sites.

Microvessel Density

Compelling evidence indicates that angiogenesis, as measured by microvessel density (MVD), correlates with the incidence of metastases in several solid tumors. Hillen and associates aimed to identify a specific biologic role for angiogenesis in the metastatic phenotype of the UPC by comparing MVD in liver metastasis of UPC with MVD in liver metastasis of colon and breast tumors.[45] No

TABLE 97-4

Comparison of Metastatic Involvement of Common Sites with Known Primary Carcinomas versus Unknown Primary Carcinomas

	METASTATIC ORGAN SITE INVOLVEMENT (%)†					
	BONE		**LUNG**		**LIVER**	
PRIMARY SITE	**KNOWN**	**UPC-PRIMARY***	**KNOWN**	**UPC-PRIMARY***	**KNOWN**	**UPC-PRIMARY***
Lung	38	40	28	N/A	15	19
Breast	49	34	27	19	34	19
Pancreas	4	14	14	3	82	76
Prostate	88	50	6	50	4	0
Colorectal	3	4	21	20	77	92

N/A, data not available.
*Patients presenting with unknown primary carcinoma in whom the primary site was subsequently discovered.
†Known primaries, N = 2287; UPC in whom primary site discovered, N = 413.
Hess KC, Abruzzese JL, unpublished data.

Specific Malignancies

III

difference was found between MVD in liver metastasis of UPC and known primary tumors. In UPC, as in other solid tumors, high MVD correlated with short survival in univariate and multivariate analyses.

EVALUATION OF THE PATIENT

Considerable controversy surrounds the optimal evaluation of patients with UPC. It is clear that this diagnosis creates a serious dilemma for the clinician because treatment planning is based on both the anatomic origin and histologic type of the malignancy. Often there is the perception that the physician's efforts to locate a primary cancer have been somehow inadequate and that the prognosis and treatment of the malignancy would be radically altered if the primary tumor could be found.

An effective strategy would take into account the projected natural history and duration of survival and provide a reasonable probability of locating the primary anatomic site without compromising quality of life with difficult and time-consuming diagnostic studies. The overall goal is to rapidly identify the treatable patient subsets or occult primary lesions through a rational, calculated approach.

History and Physical Examination

This aspect of the evaluation of the patient with suspected UPC is one of the most important and is often overlooked. The history is critical because it can define areas of concern, which will require more detailed evaluation, such as the respiratory system in a smoker who presents with a supraclavicular node, cough, and hemoptysis. A detailed review of systems is mandatory, for it may elicit symptoms that were not immediately brought to the physician's attention. Attention also should be paid to history of previous biopsies, removed lesions, as well as spontaneously regressing lesions. The family history occasionally can be helpful, especially if the patient belongs to a specific ethnic group that is known to be at high risk for malignancies at specific sites (e.g., gastric cancer in Japanese populations or hepatocellular carcinoma or nasopharyngeal carcinoma in the Chinese) or belongs to a family that is known to be genetically predisposed to malignancies at specific sites (e.g., families with hereditary nonpolyposis colon cancer or hereditary breast malignancies).

The physical examination should be rigorous and should in all cases include careful palpation of the thyroid, breasts, lymph nodes, liver, and prostate. All patients should have a digital rectal examination with stool tested for occult blood. Genital examination, including a pelvic examination in women and careful palpation of the testes in men, is mandatory. Although these recommendations are routine, in our experience these aspects of the evaluation of the patient with UPC are frequently overlooked. When carefully performed, these examinations sometimes provide the probable diagnosis or at a minimum allow the clinician to formulate a directed laboratory and radiographic evaluation.

Laboratory Studies and Serum Tumor Markers

The laboratory evaluation of patients with suspected UPC should begin with a complete blood cell count to screen for anemia (particularly to look for iron deficiency, which would suggest chronic gastrointestinal blood loss and immediately focus attention on the gastrointestinal tract as a potential primary site), urinalysis (to check for microscopic hematuria or proteinuria), and liver function studies, in some cases including studies for hepatitis B surface antigen or prior exposure to hepatitis C virus, which would suggest a risk for hepatocellular carcinoma or cholangiocarcinoma. Because many of these examinations are frequently part of the routine evaluation of any new patient, they would be only rarely overlooked.

Tumor markers, especially the more recently described markers, and their potential role in the evaluation and management of patients with UPC have been reviewed.[46] As part of the routine evaluation of UPC patients five markers deserve special recognition. The beta subunit of human chorionic gonadotropin (β-hCG) has been classically associated with nonseminomatous germ cell tumors, and is useful both for diagnosis and during follow-up, often confirming the adequacy of therapy.[47] Alpha-fetoprotein (AFP) is also useful for the evaluation of nonseminomatous germ cell tumors as well as hepatocellular carcinoma.[47] Although many previous publications suggested that the presence of elevated β-hCG or AFP identified patients with marked chemotherapy responsiveness and good survival (see following section on Poorly Differentiated and Undifferentiated Carcinoma), in one study the presence of abnormal plasma levels of AFP or β-hCG did not identify patients with better overall survival.[48] In fact, for the subset of patients diagnosed with poorly differentiated carcinoma or poorly differentiated adenocarcinoma for whom both markers were available, those with AFP levels below 2.8 ng/mL or β-hCG levels below 3.4 mIU/mL survived longer. Thus, reliance on the use of these tumor markers to identify treatment-responsive patients with UPC does not appear to be justified.

Measurement of prostate-specific antigen (PSA) is very useful in men with adenocarcinoma and predominantly skeletal metastases. Elevation of PSA can provide a confirmation of metastatic prostate cancer, but the physician should be wary of the occasional coexistence of early prostate cancer with a more aggressive synchronous neoplasm. Serum measurements of PSA should frequently be coupled with immunohistochemical staining for PSA in tumor tissue because rare patients have been reported with metastatic cancer and clinical features atypical for metastatic prostate cancer.[49,50]

The extensively used tumor marker carcinoembryonic antigen (CEA) also has been argued to have a role in the evaluation of patients with UPC. The diagnostic utility of CEA was analyzed in a group of 32 patients initially diagnosed with UPC with the adenocarcinoma histologic type.[51] In this study 10 patients had a CEA of greater than 10 ng/mL and of these patients the anatomic site of primary tumor was established as lung (5), pancreas (2), ovary (2), and bile duct (1). However, although the CEA appeared to be useful in this study, in our analysis of 147 patients with UPC who had a panel of tumor markers analyzed, 41 had a value over 10 ng/mL, and this finding did not appear to significantly impact on the probability of establishing a primary tumor site (Abbruzzese and associates; unpublished data).

Another marker, which is frequently ordered during the evaluation and management of patients with UPC, is CA125. This marker was initially derived from a human ovarian carcinoma cell line, and its elevation in women with UPC is frequently suggested as a marker for chemotherapy sensitivity to agents that are used in the management of ovarian cancer. However, preliminary studies failed to validate this hypothesis, suggesting that the clinical presentation and histology were more predictive.[52] The exact role of other tumor markers such as CA19-9 and CA15-3 remains unclear, but they appear to be limited in their ability to establish a specific primary site or identify patients who respond to chemotherapy.

Pathologic Evaluation

General Considerations

An accurate pathologic assessment of biopsy material is essential in the initial evaluation of the patient with suspected UPC. In this context the pathologist is usually able to confirm that the lesion is neoplastic and frequently able to judge if the lesion is primary or metastatic.[2] However, in some situations it may be impossible to determine if the tumor has arisen from the biopsied organ site. This problem often complicates the cytologic evaluation of fine needle aspirate specimens and emphasizes the need for close communication between the clinician and pathologist. Frequently, exchange of available clinical information may lead to additional tissue procurement for analysis using one or more of the more detailed diagnostic studies that follow. Typically, the pathologist puts the tissue specimen through one to four different steps, depending on the need. These studies include light microscopy, immunohistochemical stains, electron microscopy, and chromosomal studies including cytogenetics.

Light Microscopy

The initial pathologic assessment of the biopsy specimen is light microscopic examination of paraffin sections stained with hematoxylin and eosin. Based on established cytologic criteria the pathologist can usually classify the tumor into broad groups such as carcinoma, sarcoma, or lymphoma.[53] Additionally, many carcinomas will be immediately recognized as manifesting at least some glandular differentiation (adenocarcinoma). When glandular differentiation is absent patients with UPC will be frequently diagnosed with poorly differentiated carcinoma or undifferentiated carcinoma. Other specimens will lack any cytologic distinguishing features, in which case a diagnosis of an undifferentiated malignancy is reported. In those groups with poorly differentiated carcinoma, undifferentiated carcinoma, or undifferentiated malignancy, additional pathologic studies, including histochemistry, immunohistochemistry, and electron microscopy, are most frequently and productively employed.[54] On light microscopy about 60% of the cases are reported as adenocarcinoma and 5% as squamous carcinoma; in 35% of cases light microscopy is not very helpful, and poorly differentiated adenocarcinoma, poorly differentiated carcinoma, or poorly differentiated neoplasm is then reported.

Immunohistochemistry

Immunohistochemical markers play a significant role in the diagnosis and workup of UPC. They help define tumor lineage by using peroxidase-labeled antibody against specific tumor antigens. Direct discussions between the pathologist and clinician are critical to ensure the most accurate pathologic characterization possible. Random use of large numbers of tissue markers is rarely helpful for establishing a diagnosis or planning therapy. The role of antibodies against AFP, β-hCG, PSA, and some other markers is well established (Table 97-5). More recently, cytokeratins and thyroid transcription factor (TTF-1) are gaining more importance as markers for the identification of the origin of the carcinoma.[55-60]

Cytokeratin 20 (CK20) is a low-molecular-weight cytokeratin, which is expressed in the normal glands

TABLE 97-5

Tumors Markers Useful in the Diagnosis of Unknown Primary Carcinoma		
HISTOLOGIC DIAGNOSIS APPLICATION	**TISSUE MARKER**	**DIAGNOSTIC**
Poorly Differentiated Carcinoma or Undifferentiated Carcinoma	1. Leukocyte common antigen (LCA)	Lymphoma
	2. Ki 1 (CD30)	Ki 1 lymphoma
	3. Human chorionic gonadotropin (β-hCG)	Germ cell neoplasm
	4. Alpha-fetoprotein (AFP)	Germ cell neoplasm
	5. Chromogranin	Neuroendocrine carcinoma
	6. S-100	Melanoma
	7. HMB-45	Melanoma
Adenocarcinoma	1. Estrogen receptor (ER)	Breast cancer
	2. Progesterone receptor (PR)	Breast cancer
	3. Prostate-specific antigen (PSA)	Prostate cancer
	4. Alpha-fetoprotein (AFP)	Hepatoma
	5. Thyroglobulin	Thyroid cancer

Specific Malignancies

III

as well as the tumors of the gastrointestinal epithelium, urothelium, and Merkel cell.[55-57] Cytokeratin 7 (CK7) is found in tumors of the lung, ovary, endometrium, and breast but not in the gastrointestinal tract. TTF-1 is a 38-kDa homeodomain-containing nuclear protein that plays a role in the transcriptional activation during embryogenesis in the thyroid, diencephalon, and respiratory epithelium.[55-57] TTF-1 staining is typically positive for lung and thyroid cancers. In 2002, Roh and associates[55] described the utility of TTF-1 and CK20 in identifying the origin of metastatic carcinomas of cervical lymph nodes. They stained 68 specimens with TTF-1 and CK20. The primary sites were lung (29 cases), stomach (13 cases), colorectum (3 cases), and other sites (23 cases). TTF-1 expression was detected in 69% of metastatic lung carcinomas and in none of the gastrointestinal carcinomas. CK20 expression was detected in 68.8% of gastrointestinal tumors and in none of the metastatic lung carcinomas. Jang and associates[56] looked at the utility of these markers in identifying the origin of malignant effusions. The primary sites of the tumors examined were lung (16), ovary (15), stomach (9), colon (8), and breast (8). The lung adenocarcinomas showed TTF-1 positivity in 81% of the cases (13 of 16) but all the nonpulmonary adenocarcinomas lacked TTF-1 staining. The CK7–/CK20+ immunophenotype was seen in 63% of colonic adeno-carcinomas and in none of the lung, breast, or ovary tumors. The CK7+/CK20– staining was seen in 100% of

lung, 88% of breast, and 87% of cancers that originated from the ovary. They concluded that TTF-1 immunostaining was useful in differentiating between pulmonary and nonpulmonary origin of adenocarcinoma in malignant effusions. The combination of CK7–/CK20+ staining is useful in identifying colon adenocarcinoma. In 2000, Rubin and associates[57] looked at the role of CK7 and CK20 in determining the origin of metastatic carcinoma of unknown primary site. Some data suggest the role of cytokeratin 5/6 as a marker for squamous cell carcinoma in poorly differentiated tumors if mesothelioma is ruled out.[58-60] Based on Rubin's data[57] and other studies with these recent markers, we describe a simple algorithm for providing clinicians some guidance on using these immunohistochemical markers to identify the site of origin provided that gastric, pancreatic and hepatobiliary cancers are ruled out (not always possible).

Electron Microscopy

Electron microscopy offers the option of looking at the ultrastructural features of a given cell. Patients with adenocarcinoma will typically show microvilli and mucin, neuroendocrine tumors may show secretory granules, and a melanoma will usually show premelanosomes. Electron microscopy is used infrequently today because of the improvement in immunohistochemical markers. Also, it requires pathologists who are experienced in the technique; it can be time-consuming and rarely offers

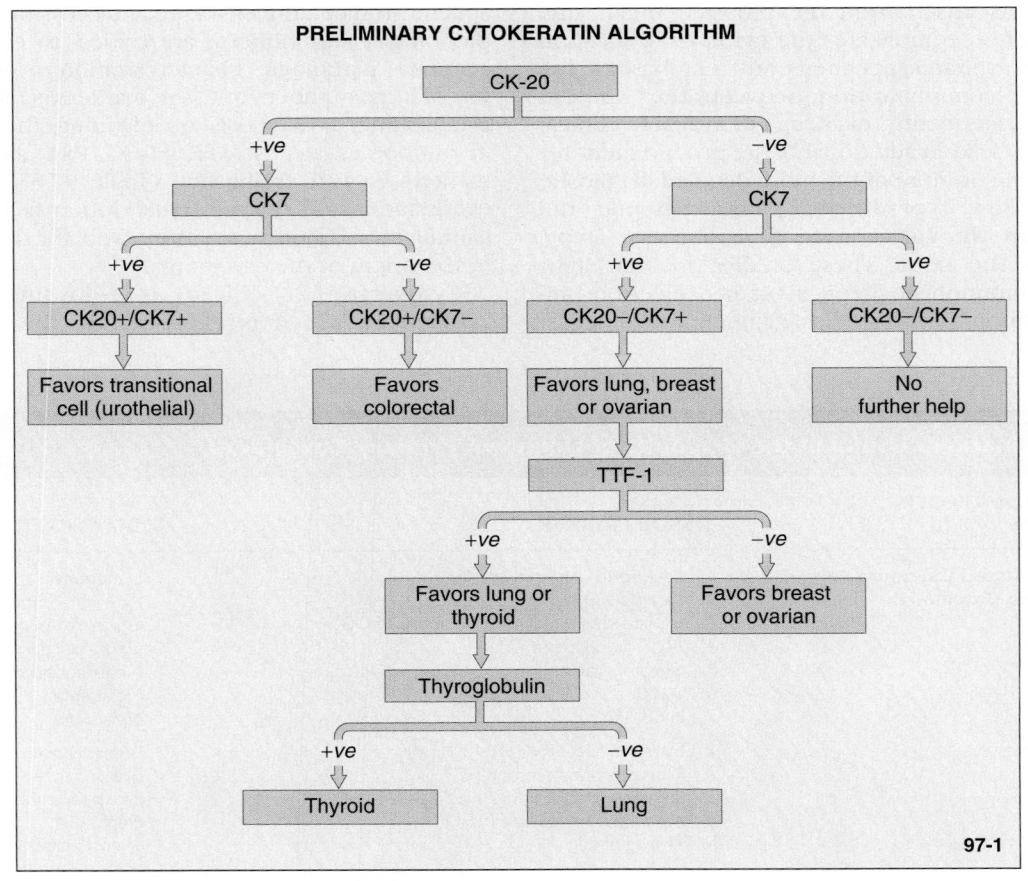

PRELIMINARY CYTOKERATIN ALGORITHM

97-1

information that changes the overall management. It may, however, be useful in some cases of poorly differentiated neoplasm.

Chromosomal Studies
Chromosomal aberrations in UPC and the significance of isochromosome (12p) have been discussed earlier (see Biologic Characteristics).

Radiographic Studies

Chest Radiographs and Plain Films
The chest x-ray is essential in the evaluation of patients with UPC. Given the large numbers of patients with UPC who will eventually be diagnosed with lung cancer, the chest radiograph should be part of the routine evaluation of these patients irrespective of whether there are respiratory symptoms. However, in this setting, Nystrom and associates have pointed out that the chest x-ray must be interpreted with caution.[3] This study demonstrated that the chest x-ray often could not conclusively distinguish primary lung cancer from metastatic disease to the lungs. This problem is further complicated by the fact that some malignancies (notably breast, renal, and colorectal cancers) can metastasize to endobronchial sites and thus mimic primary bronchogenic carcinoma. In this situation a bronchoscopic biopsy with detailed histologic or cytologic analysis of the neoplastic tissue will sometimes clarify the situation.

Other routine radiographic films are generally reserved for evaluation of symptomatic sites, such as painful bone lesions. Interpretation of these films must also be handled with caution because the degree of bony destruction needed to visualize an abnormality may not be present initially.[61] Radionuclide bone scan will often resolve this issue.

Contrast Radiographic Studies
Contrast radiographic studies (e.g., upper GI series, barium enema, intravenous pyelogram) have a low diagnostic yield and should generally be reserved for patients with symptoms or signs referable to the organ system in question. Two studies have looked at the diagnostic accuracy of these examinations.[3,62] In over 200 examinations only 7.4%, 11%, and 8% of upper GI, barium enemas, or intravenous pyelograms, respectively, were positive. In addition, biopsy confirmation of the abnormalities identified radiographically was made in only half of the cases. Thus the false positive rates from these studies were significant and could easily lead to inappropriate management based on faulty information.

Radionuclide Imaging
With the advent of computed tomography, radionuclide imaging of the liver is performed very infrequently in the evaluation of patients with UPC. Bone scanning, however, remains a useful diagnostic adjunct to stage patients with UPC (especially those complaining of bone pain) but is unlikely to provide information as to the site of the primary lesion. Using this modality in conjunction with routine x-rays, sites of significant destruction in major weight-bearing bones can be anticipated before devastating pathologic fractures develop. Radionuclide thyroid scanning is often performed for the evaluation of patients who present with papillary adenocarcinomas in cervical nodes, but is infrequently positive.[63] Thus, at this time radionuclide imaging cannot be recommended as a routine diagnostic study in patients with UPC, but can be helpful with assessment of disease extent.

Mammography
Bilateral mammography should be a part of the routine evaluation of all women with UPC.[2] Despite the relatively low numbers of occult breast cancer accounting for UPC (4% to 8%), at least one study documented a 7.5% rate of positive examinations.[64] Even with the apparent low yield from this evaluation, the good response of breast cancer to local and systemic therapy justifies the procedure in this patient population.

Computed Tomography
The role of computed tomography (CT) of the chest in the evaluation of patients with UPC is currently unclear. Although chest CT can accurately document mediastinal adenopathy,[65] it frequently overestimates the amount of metastatic parenchymal pulmonary involvement. The additional lesions visualized by chest CT (as compared to chest x-ray and whole lung tomography) are in many cases not malignant.[66,67] Until more evidence is available, routine use of the chest CT cannot be recommended. However, this study should be obtained to follow up an abnormal but nondiagnostic chest x-ray or positive sputum cytologic test.

The role for CT of the abdomen is much better defined and appears particularly useful in the detection of occult pancreatic primaries. Two relatively recent studies have addressed this issue. In one study, CT of the abdomen detected the primary site in 16 of 46 patients.[68] The primary sites documented included pancreas (6), ovary (2), hepatoma (2), kidney (2), lung (1), adrenal gland (1), gallbladder (1), and stomach (1). The second series, from the Mayo Clinic, identified the primary site in one third (31 of 98) of patients with clinically occult tumor.[68] In addition, this study pointed out that tissue confirmation could be obtained from the suspected primary site through the use of CT-directed needle aspiration biopsies. Thus, although it appears that CT of the abdomen should be considered a standard procedure in the evaluation of patients with UPC, the primary cancers identified are frequently difficult to treat, causing at least one group to question the cost-to-benefit relationship in this patient population.[2]

In the pelvis a combination of CT and pelvic ultrasound may be justified. In one prospective study of 24 patients with pelvic masses palpable by gynecologic examination, additional clinical information was provided by ultrasound in 71% and by CT scan in 63% of these patients.[69] However, in three patients both modalities failed to detect tumor recurrence. More problematic, however, is the usefulness of pelvic ultrasound or pelvic CT for patients without palpable abnormalities by gynecologic examination. There is no prospective study analyzing these diagnostic examinations in this group of patients. The most efficient evaluation includes pelvic CT, which is performed with CT of the abdomen.[2]

Magnetic Resonance Imaging

Enthusiasm for magnetic resonance imaging (MRI) is high. As the technical capabilities of this diagnostic modality evolve it may be increasingly indicated in the diagnosis and management of patients with UPC. Currently, however, few prospective or retrospective studies are available to suggest a broad role for MRI in evaluating UPC. One application that appears promising is in the evaluation of female patients with isolated axillary lymph node metastases and suspected occult primary breast carcinoma. In a recently reported series of 12 female patients presenting with isolated axillary lymphadenopathy pathologically confirmed to contain metastatic adenocarcinoma, 9 had a primary malignancy localized to the breast identified by MRI.[70] Thus at this time MRI should be limited to clinical situations in which it appears that the additional information to be gained will significantly alter the therapeutic approach recommended to an individual patient.

Positron Emission Tomography Imaging

Positron emission tomography with ^{18}F-fluoro-2-deoxy-D-glucose ($[^{18}F]$-FDG-PET) is a noninvasive nuclear imaging technique that has been proved to be a valuable diagnostic tool in identifying primary malignant tumors, assessing the extent of metastatic disease, and localizing carcinoma of unknown primary origin. Several studies have been conducted to determine the value of FDG-PET imaging in detecting occult primary tumors after unsuccessful conventional diagnostic evaluation in patients with metastatic disease from an unknown primary cancer. The majority of studies consist of a small number of evaluable patients[71-74] and focus primarily on patients with cervical or supraclavicular lymphadenopathy. In 1998, Kole and associates[71] evaluated the role of PET imaging in 29 patients with various histologic types of metastasis from a UPC after unsuccessful conventional diagnostic workup. PET imaging identified the primary tumor in 7 patients (24%), but survival was not altered by discovery of the primary tumor. In 1999, Lassen and associates prospectively studied 20 patients who underwent a PET scan after standard evaluation and the PET results were verified either histologically or by the clinical course of the disease.[72] All the metastatic lesions were visible with PET. In 13 patients, PET suggested the site for primary tumor, and this site was verified in 9 (45%) either histologically or by the clinical course of the disease. Eight of these patients had primary lung cancer and one had carcinoma of the base of the tongue. In most patients PET had no treatment-related implications. In 2000, Jungehulsing and associates[73] evaluated the use of PET imaging in 27 patients with head and neck lymphadenopathy and presumed UPC after unsuccessful conventional diagnostic evaluation failed to reveal the primary tumor. PET imaging revealed a primary tumor in 7 patients (24%). In 2002 Johansen and associates[74] evaluated 42 patients with squamous cell or undiffer-

entiated metastatic disease from a UPC. Potential focal pathologic uptake indicated a primary tumor in 20 of 42 cases (48%). After PET imaging, additional investigations confirmed the primary tumor in 10 patients (24%). In general, PET consistently visualized known metastatic lesions and resulted in the identification rates of a primary tumor ranging from 8% to 53%.

Although PET appears to be a promising diagnostic modality, its high cost, limited availability, elevated false-positive rate of up to 20%, and lack of improved survival rates after identification of the primary tumor preclude its routine use in the standard evaluation of patients with UPC. The combination of functional and anatomic imaging (PET/CT) is currently being evaluated and will very likely reduce the false-positive rate associated with PET imaging as a single diagnostic modality. The most practical approach would be to utilize PET imaging after conventional diagnostic evaluation has failed to locate a primary cancer, but before other advanced diagnostic tests are performed. The cost effectiveness of the use of PET scan in cancer of unknown primary site is not yet determined.

Molecular Markers by Gene Expression

Although few individual markers can identify a tumor's site of origin with a high degree of confidence (PSA and Mammoglobin are possible exceptions), metastatic tumors do appear to have distinguishable patterns of gene expression when a large number of markers are examined with tools such as DNA microarrays or RT-PCR (reverse transcriptase–polymerase chain reaction) assay.

Ramaswamy and associates[9] subjected 218 tumor tissues spanning 14 common tumor types (representing ~80% of the new cancer diagnoses in the United States) and 90 normal tissue samples to oligonucleotide microarray gene expression analysis. They used the relative levels of expression of 16,063 genes and expressed sequence tags to evolve a predictive support vector machine (SVM) algorithm. The algorithm was then tested on an independent group of 54 tumors, yielding an overall prediction accuracy of 78%. Although greatest accuracy required using all 16,063 genes, accuracy was still above 70% with fewer than 50 genes. Of the 54 independent tumors tested, 8 were metastatic tumors, of which 6 were accurately identified, suggesting that the cancers retain the markers of their tissue of origin throughout metastatic evolution, and that gene expression–based approaches to the diagnosis of UPCs may be feasible. Most of the tumor types that could not be accurately classified were moderately or poorly differentiated (high-grade) carcinomas. It can be difficult to classify such tumors with traditional methods because they often lack the characteristic morphologic hallmarks of the organ from which they arise. It has been assumed that these tumors are nonetheless fundamentally molecularly similar to their better-differentiated counterparts, apart from a few differences that might account for their clinically aggressive nature. However, Ramaswamy and associates[9] suggest that poorly differentiated tumors may not simply lack a few key markers of differentiation, but rather may have fundamentally distinct gene expression patterns, having a significant implication for the management of patients with these cancers.

Su and associates[75] used a set of 100 primary carcinomas from 10 common tumor types (prostate, breast, lung, ovary, colorectum, kidney, liver, pancreas, bladder/ureter, and gastroesophagus), which collectively account for 70% of all cancer-related deaths in the United States. They extracted mRNA from the tumors, and then used an Affymetrix oligonucleotide microarray to identify genes that were differentially expressed. A predictive algorithm was developed using 110 genes of the 9198 genes that were minimally expressed in these tumors. The algorithm was then tested against an additional 75 blinded samples and accurately predicted the tumor of origin in over 90% of the cases.

Dennis and associates[76] used a different approach to identify predictive markers, starting with published data on differential gene expression by tumor type. They identified 61 candidate tumor markers whose expression pattern was predicted to be characteristic of the site of origin and tested 11 of them against adenocarcinoma samples (breast, ovary, stomach, pancreas, lung). The actual expression patterns were consistent with those predicted in seven cases (64%), with three agreeing exactly. By extending this approach, it may be possible to identify a smaller subset (10 to 20 genes) of highly predictive markers that could be applicable to more commonly used laboratory techniques such as immunohistochemistry.

The foregoing work holds out the promise that in a large proportion of UPCs, the site of origin can be identified using arrays of molecular markers, though with one caveat. The underlying assumption is that UPCs are no different from other metastatic lesions, and retain the molecular markers associated with their tissue of origin identity, an assumption that needs to be tested.

CLINICAL MANIFESTATIONS AND MANAGEMENT

The clinical presentations of UPC are extremely varied. Historically, patients have frequently been characterized as to whether they have disease above or below the diaphragm.[77] However, given the heterogeneity and widespread metastases that characterize this disease, this arbitrary division is of doubtful value. Other investigators have effectively used other approaches to subclassify patients based largely on clinicopathologic criteria of histologic type, involved organ sites, and responsiveness to therapy. This approach has led to the definition of clinically defined patient subsets, which will be discussed subsequently. Despite these efforts at subclassification, the majority of patients present with solitary or multiple areas of involvement in a variety of visceral sites. Thus, in most cases the presenting symptoms and physical signs simply reflect the neoplastic involvement of these organ sites. The most common organ sites encountered are listed in Table 97-6, with lung, bone, lymph nodes, and liver the most frequently encountered. Table 97-6 also shows the histologic spectrum of disease associated

---

THE M.D. ANDERSON APPROACH TO THE PATIENT WITH NEWLY DIAGNOSED CARCINOMA OF UNKNOWN PRIMARY SITE

Patients with physical or radiographic evidence of metastatic cancer should undergo biopsy early in their evaluation. This approach confirms the diagnosis and provides histologic or cytologic information that will help in the planning of additional evaluation and treatment.

The essential diagnostic evaluation includes history, physical examination, CB count, SMA-12, PSA in men, chest radiography, CT of abdomen and pelvis, and mammography in women. Further investigations are performed only on the basis of positive findings from these screening studies. Patients are then readily classified and treated as outlined here.

IMPORTANT TREATABLE SUBSETS (MINORITY OF PATIENTS) AND THEIR MANAGEMENT

Clinic Subset	Management
Women with adenopathy (adenocarcinoma and carcinoma)	Same as for stage II breast cancer
Women with peritoneal carcinomatosis (papillary adenocarcinoma)	Same as for stage III ovarian cancer
Poorly differentiated and undifferentiated carcinoma (controversial subset)	Platin-based combination chemotherapy (carboplatin/paclitaxel ± etoposide or cisplatin/etoposide)
Extragonadal germ cell syndrome	Same as for nonseminomatous germ cell tumor
Neuroendocrine carcinoma	Same as for carcinoid/pancreatic islet cell carcinoma; cisplatin-based chemotherapy for poorly differentiated neuroendocrine tumors
High- and mid-cervical adenopathy (squamous cell carcinoma)	Surgical resection of palpable disease + curative radiation therapy to the neck

---

with each site as well as the other frequently involved metastatic sites encountered. Of the sites listed, only isolated involvement of lymph nodes was associated with significantly superior survival relative to the UPC population as a whole.[78]

The treatment of UPC continues to evolve. While the majority of patients are treated with systemic chemotherapy, the careful integration of surgery, radiation therapy, and even periods of observation are important in the overall management of these patients.[79-81] Observation is particularly important for patients with single sites of disease who have received adequate local therapy.

The most common problem is treatment of the patient with progressive metastatic adenocarcinoma involving two or more organ sites. Treatment of these patients

TABLE 97-6

Clinical Characteristics of Common Subsets of Unknown Primary Carcinomas

INVOLVED SITE (NO. OF PATIENTS)	NO. OF PATIENTS WITH ONE SITE ONLY	NO. OF PATIENTS WITH MULTIPLE SITES	HISTOLOGIC TYPE (SITE ONLY/SITE + OTHER)				
			ADENOCARCINOMA	CARCINOMA	SQUAMOUS	NEUROENDOCRINE	OTHER
Bone (318)	73	245	45/139	21/80	2/13	2/10	3/3
Lung (296)	21	275	13/175	5/72	0/13	0/10	1/5
Lymph nodes (479)	138	341	56/202	55/96	25/26	2/12	0/5
Liver (365)	139	226	93/129	24/72	2/6	18/15	2/4
Pleura (122)	31	91	25/71	6/17	0/0	0/0	0/3
Brain (79)	18	61	9/35	5/12	0/9	0/1	4/4
Skin (38)	9	29	2/15	6/7	0/4	1/3	0/0

METASTATIC INVOLVED SITE	ADDITIONAL INVOLVED SITES							MEDIAN SURVIVAL (MOS)	
	BONE	LUNG	LIVER	PLEURA	SKIN	NODES	BRAIN	SITE ONLY	SITE + OTHER
Bone	—	96	84	29	14	97	24	9	8
Lung	96	—	81	41	11	139	33	20	8
Lymph nodes	97	139	105	37	17	—	32	29	12
Liver	84	81	—	13	3	105	9	9	7
Pleura	29	41	13	—	0	37	3	9	8
Brain	24	33	9	3	2	32	—	16	8
Skin	14	11	3	0	—	17	2	*	8

*Median not yet reached.

remains suboptimal and probably awaits discovery of novel strategies applicable to other highly resistant adenocarcinomas such as those originating in the lung or gastrointestinal tract. This situation is contrasted with the management of the favorable subsets described next. These favorable patients have been grouped together primarily on the basis of their responsiveness to therapy. The numbers of patients who fall into these favorable groups are small, but they are important to recognize because specific treatment may significantly extend survival.

Favorable Clinical Subsets

Squamous Carcinoma Involving Mid-High Cervical Lymph Nodes

High cervical adenopathy with squamous cell carcinoma has been mentioned previously because of its well-defined natural history, high frequency of identification of the primary site, and responsiveness to therapy.[10-12] With appropriate evaluation, including direct visualization of the hypopharynx, nasopharynx, larynx, and upper esophagus, an occult primary lesion will frequently be identified. When no primary site is found, aggressive local therapy is applied to the involved neck.[12,81] From 30% to 50% 5-year survival rates have been reported with radical neck surgery, high-dose radiotherapy, or a combination of both modalities. A potential advantage of radiation therapy is that the suspected primary anatomic sites (nasopharynx, oropharynx, and hypopharynx) can be included in the radiation port.[81] The role of chemotherapy in these patients is unclear. However, one randomized

study suggested that chemotherapy with cisplatin and 5-fluorouracil improved the response rate and median survival when compared to radiation alone.[82]

Adenocarcinoma involving mid-high cervical nodes and lower cervical or supraclavicular adenopathy of all histologic types carry a much poorer prognosis.[83] These patients are managed with local measures (usually radiation therapy), or they may be candidates for systemic chemotherapy protocols.

Women with Isolated Axillary Adenopathy

Isolated axillary adenopathy secondary to metastatic adenocarcinoma usually occurs in women and has unique clinical features. Many of these women have occult primary breast cancers that can be identified in 40% to 70% of these patients who undergo mastectomy.[84,85] In this setting repeat biopsy of involved axillary nodes for estrogen and progesterone levels should be considered in view of the influence of this information on diagnosis and management. Management is based on the treatment of stage II breast cancer and should include both local and systemic therapies. Prognosis following treatment is comparable to women with stage II breast cancer. Older series have advocated modified radical mastectomy and axillary dissection for primary treatment.[84-86] However, a reported series of 42 patients suggested that survival was superior in patients receiving systemic chemotherapy, and local control was improved by irradiating the breast and axilla.[64] The actuarial disease-free survival rate in this study was 71% at 5 years and 65% at 10 years. This nonoperative approach has been outlined in a study by Lenzi and colleagues.[87]

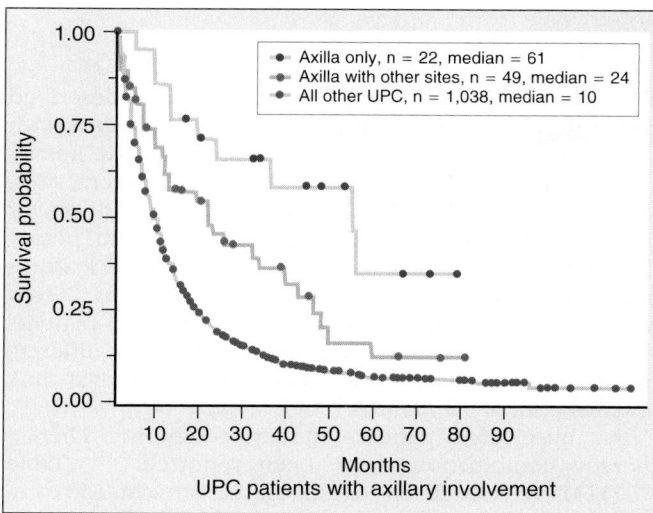

Figure 97-5. Survival of unknown primary carcinoma (UPC) patients with isolated axillary adenopathy versus those with axillary adenopathy with other metastatic sites versus UPC patients without axillary nodal involvement.

Patients with axillary adenopathy and involvement of additional sites (usually liver or bone) or with nonadenocarcinoma histologic type compose a much more heterogeneous group comprising equal numbers of men and women as well as a broader histologic spectrum with poorly differentiated carcinoma and neuroendocrine carcinomas represented in addition to adenocarcinoma.[88] Despite this heterogeneity, the survival of patients with axillary adenopathy and other involved organ sites is intermediate between that of the overall UPC population and women with isolated axillary adenopathy (Fig. 97-5).

The management of patients with involvement of the axilla as well as other sites or nonadenocarcinoma histology is less certain. These patients are generally approached using a combination of local and systemic modalities and may again be good candidates for novel systemic chemotherapy protocols.

Women with Peritoneal Carcinomatosis
Women with diffuse peritoneal carcinomatosis with adenocarcinoma compose another recognized subset. These patients form a distinctive subset because of their clinical similarities to patients with ovarian carcinoma. Often papillary histologic type and elevations in CA125 will be found but exploratory laparotomy fails to document a primary.[89,90] Other workers have also recognized this patient subset, terming this syndrome *peritoneal papillary serous carcinoma* or *multifocal extraovarian serous carcinoma*. These patients frequently respond to platinum-based chemotherapy.[90-92] Many patients in these series also underwent exploratory laparotomy with surgical debulking followed by chemotherapy. Median survival times are reported to be 16 months to 2 years.

The natural histories of males with isolated peritoneal carcinomatosis or patients with histologic features inconsistent with ovarian carcinoma or additional meta-static sites are much more poorly characterized, but overall survival, even with therapy, is poor.[93]

Poorly Differentiated and Undifferentiated Carcinoma
Approximately one third of patients with UPC will be defined as having this histologic picture of poorly differentiated or undifferentiated carcinoma. In this subset detailed histochemical or immunohistochemical studies are most likely to identify highly treatment-responsive patients with lymphoma (leukocyte common antigen), germ cell (β-hCG, AFP), or neuroendocrine (neuron-specific enolase, chromogranin) neoplasms (see Table 97-6). Additionally, Greco and Hainsworth have identified a group of patients with poorly differentiated carcinoma or poorly differentiated adenocarcinoma that are responsive to platinum-based chemotherapy.[1] Most of these patients had clinical features (young age, mediastinal/retroperitoneal involvement, and rapid growth) of the extragonadal germ cell syndrome.[94] Many of these patients will be male and have elevated β-hCG or AFP. Recently, Motzer and coworkers identified abnormalities in chromosome 12 specific for germ cell neoplasms in a group of male patients with poorly differentiated carcinoma involving midline structures, confirming the germ cell origin of these tumors.[31]

Combination chemotherapy regimens specific for germ cell carcinoma of testicular origin have usually been employed in the treatment of these patients.[15,47,94-96] In selected patients, these regimens have produced documented complete responses and an actual 10-year disease-free survival rate of 16%.[13]

Despite these favorable results, one analysis of this "favorable" subset failed to confirm that UPC patients with poorly differentiated carcinoma (PDC) or poorly differentiated adenocarcinoma (PDA) enjoyed prolonged survival.[48] The exact reasons for the failure of this newer study to confirm the earlier studies is unknown. However, insight into this question can be achieved by analyzing the patients reported in this analysis. From the population of 1400 patients referred with suspected UPCs a primary tumor[2] was established in 365 patients. The most frequent primary tumors diagnosed included 70 patients considered to have highly treatable tumors: 28 patients with breast cancer, 20 patients with lymphoma, 11 patients with ovarian cancer, 6 patients with germ cell tumors, and 5 patients with other hematologic malignancies. This study also clearly showed that the survival of UPC patients with squamous or neuroendocrine features have survival times that are superior to those for patients with PDC or PDA. Thus, the PDC and PDA populations analyzed in this study reflect the biology of these patients' malignancies after patients with slower-growing tumors (e.g., neuroendocrine cancers) or chemotherapy-responsive tumors (e.g., lymphomas, other hematologic malignancies, germ cell tumors, breast cancer, ovarian cancer) had been excluded.

Increasingly frequent use of special pathologic studies, including immunohistochemistry, is likely to be responsible for the ease with which patients with lymphoma, neuroendocrine, germ cell, and other malignancies can be excluded from the PDC or PDA groups. Many of these patients were often included in earlier series of PDC and PDA patients, which potentially confounded data on chemotherapy responsiveness and survival.

Poorly Differentiated Neuroendocrine Carcinoma

Poorly differentiated neuroendocrine carcinoma is an emerging clinicopathologic entity recognized primarily for its responsiveness to therapy. There is probably considerable overlap with extrapulmonary small cell carcinomas, anaplastic carcinoid, anaplastic islet cell tumors, Merkel cell tumors, and paragangliomas. Histologically these tumors are very poorly differentiated, but histochemical stains are positive for chromogranin or neuron-specific enolase. These patients often present with diffuse hepatic or bone metastases but do not have the indolent histologic or clinical features of typical carcinoid tumors, islet cell tumors, or paragangliomas, and thus observation may not be appropriate. These tumors are also frequently responsive to cisplatin-based chemotherapy.[97,98]

Unknown Primary Carcinoma in Unselected Patients

The optimistic results for the favorable patients described earlier do not apply to the vast majority of patients with UPC. Two thirds of UPC patents have metastatic adenocarcinoma with involvement of two or more visceral sites, usually some combination of liver, lung, lymph nodes, or bone. In addition, many men and women with poorly differentiated carcinoma have none of the clinical features outlined previously and respond poorly to therapy.[48] Even in series showing optimistic results for selected patients with poorly differentiated carcinoma or poorly differentiated adenocarcinoma, the overall median survival time remains poor at 12 months.[13]

For unselected patients numerous empiric chemotherapy combinations have been reported[99-116] (Table 97-7). Many have been based on Adriamycin (doxorubicin), 5-fluorouracil, or cisplatin. Little information is

TABLE 97-7

Chemotherapeutic Trials in Unknown Primary Carcinoma

AUTHOR	REFERENCE	HISTOLOGIC TYPE	REGIMEN	NO. OF PATIENTS	RESPONSE (%)	MEDIAN SURVIVAL (MOS)
Moertel et al	99	Adeno	5-FU	88	16	NS*
Moertel et al	99	Adeno	Mitomycin-C	9	22	NS
Moertel et al	99	Adeno	5-FU/Mito-C	7	0	NS
Moertel et al	99	Adeno	5-FU/BCNU	11	18	NS
McKeen et al	100	Adeno	5-FU/Adria/Mito-C	28	22	NS
Rodnick et al	101	Adeno	5-FU/Adria/Mito-C	14	7	+3
Woods et al	102	Adeno/UC	Adria/Mito-C	25	36	4.5
Valentine et al	103	Adeno/UC	Cytoxan/Adria/5-FU	14	14	7+
Bedikian et al	104	Adeno/UC	Cytoxan/MTX/5-FU	22	5	2
Bedikian et al	104	Adeno/UC	Tegafur/Cytoxan/Adria/Cisplatin	21	29	4.5
Pasterz et al	18	Adeno/UC	5-FU/Adria/Cytoxan/Cisplatin	44	28	NS
Greco et al	15	PDC/PDA	CDDP/vinblastine bleo ± doxorubicin	68	56% (22% CR)	18*
Goldberg et al	105	Adeno	5-FU/Adria Mito-C	45	30% (9% CR)	>10
Walach	106	Adeno	CTX/VNCR MTX/5-FU	21	48% (29% CR)	NS*
Shildt et al	107	Adeno	5-FU vs 5-FU/Adria/Cytoxan	36	0	3
Anderson et al	108	Carcinoma	VNCR/Adria/CTX	20	50% (20% CR)	NS
Raber et al	109	Adeno/UC	CDDP/VP-16/5-FU	16	17%	NS
LeChevalier et al	110	Adeno	MTX-FAM	19	37%	6+
Lenzi et al	111	Adeno/PDC	CDDP/5-FU/folinic	31	30	18
Hainsworth et al	112	PDC	CDDP/etoposide	32	60 (32% CR)	NS
Hainsworth et al	118	Adeno/PDC/PDA	Paclitaxel/carboplatin etoposide	55	47	13.4
Greco et al	115	PDA/PDC/ Neuroendocrine/ Small cell	Docetaxel + cisplatin	26	26	8
			Docetaxel + carboplatin	47	22	12
			Carboplatin + paclitaxel	77	47.8	13
Briasoulis et al	116	carcinoma PDA, PDC			68.4	15
					15.1	10

Adeno, adenocarcinoma; Adria, Adriamycin; bleo, bleomycin; CDDP, cis-diamminedichloroplatinum; CR, complete response; CTX, cyclophosphamide; 5-FU, 5-fluorouracil; Mito, mitomycin C; MTX, methotrexate; NS, not stated; PDA, poorly differentiated adenocarcinoma; PDC, poorly differentiated carcinoma; UC, undifferentiated carcinoma; VNCR, vincristine; VP-16, etoposide.
*Calculated from data presented.

available on the use of biologic agents alone or with chemotherapy. Response rates generally range from 20% to 30%, but most responses are partial and brief, resulting in little or no impact on median survival. The recent availability of new antineoplastic agents with broad-spectrum activity and potential efficacy in the treatment of UPC renewed interest in empiric chemotherapy for these patients. The taxanes, gemcitabine, and the topoisomerase I inhibitors represent such agents with potential efficacy in the treatment of UPC.

Taxane-based regimens evaluated in phase II clinical trials have included the following combinations: (1) paclitaxel/carboplatin/etoposide; (2) paclitaxel/carboplatin; (3) docetaxel/platinum; and (4) paclitaxel/carboplatin/gemcitabine.[115-117] Overall response rates with taxane-based regimens have ranged between 24% and 47%. Longer median survival times have also been observed with taxane-based regimens, ranging from 9 to 11 months as compared to a range of 5 to 8 months utilizing older gastrointestinal and breast cancer chemotherapy regimens. One report using carboplatin, paclitaxel, and etoposide reported that 47% (25 of 53 patients) had objective responses.[118] In this series seven patients (13%) experienced complete responses. However, the actuarial median survival time for the entire group was 13.4 months. The disappointing aspect of this survival statistic is that it is not substantially different from the 11-month median survival time reported in large consecutive series of UPC patients.[74,119]

Gemcitabine is a pyrimidine analog antimetabolite with single-agent activity in several solid tumors, and has also been found to be useful as secondary therapy for some patients with UPC. Hainsworth and associates[120] conducted a phase II trial evaluating single-agent gemcitabine in the second-line therapy of patients with UPC. Thirty-five patients (90%) had previously received treatment with chemotherapy containing both a platinum agent and a taxane. This study showed an 8% (3 of 36 evaluable patients) partial response rate, and 25% (9 patients) had minor responses or stable disease with reduced symptoms. The median time to progression was 5 months. These results show that as a second-line treatment for UPC, gemcitabine has a relatively low level of clinical activity in a refractory patient population, although a portion of patients experienced symptomatic improvement.

Because of the previously demonstrated activity of gemcitabine against a variety of advanced adenocarcinomas gemcitabine was evaluated with combination chemotherapy as a front-line agent. Greco and associates[121] evaluated the efficacy and toxicity of gemcitabine, carboplatin, and paclitaxel in previously untreated patients with UPC. Twenty-eight (25%) of 113 assessable patients had a major objective response. The median progression-free survival time was 6 months with a median survival time for the entire group of 9 months. Actuarial survival at 1 and 2 years was 42% and 23%, respectively. This study showed that combination chemotherapy with gemcitabine, carboplatin, and paclitaxel followed by weekly paclitaxel was well tolerated. However, the survival seen in this poor prognosis group of patients is notable and

similar to that seen in other taxane-based regimens for these patients. Newer regimens continue to be tested, and some evidence suggests that even poor prognosis patients may benefit.

FUTURE DIRECTIONS

Near-term research in UPC will continue to focus on the identification and treatment of patient subsets. This approach has been very successful in dealing with the inherent heterogeneity of UPC. Sophisticated data collection and computer–based analysis will foster these studies. The role of DNA microarray in this subset is evolving, as discussed earlier. Patients who do not fit a treatable subtype, as discussed in this chapter, should be encouraged to get involved in clinical trials for novel therapies. From a more distant perspective, research into the metastatic phenotype through an analysis of UPC cells may identify specific molecular and biochemical targets, which could be therapeutically exploitable for patients with UPC. These targets may be applicable to other metastatic malignancies as well. We would anticipate that the molecular characterization of UPC will not only improve our understanding of metastases but through comparison with known primary carcinomas eventually will resolve the question of anatomic origin.

REFERENCES

1. Greco FA, Hainsworth JD: Cancer of unknown primary site. In De Vita VT Jr, Hellman S, Rosenberg SA (eds): Cancer: Principles and Practice of Oncology, 5th ed. Philadelphia, Lippincott, 1997, pp 2423–2443.
2. Abbruzzese JL, Abbruzzese MC, Lenzi R, Hess KR, Raber MN: Analysis of a diagnostic strategy for patients with suspected tumors of unknown origin. J Clin Oncol 1995;13:2094.
3. Nystrom JB, Weiner JM, Wolf RM, et al: Identifying the primary site in metastatic cancer of unknown origin: Inadequacy of roentgenographic procedures. JAMA 1979;241:381.
4. Le Cesne A, Le Chevalier T, Caille P, et al: Metastases from cancers of unknown primary site: Data from 302 autopsies. Presse Med 1991;20:1369.
5. Abbruzzese JL, Lenzi R, Raber MN, Pathak S, Frost P: The biology of unknown primary tumors. Semin Oncol 1993;20:238.
6. van de Wouw AJ, Jansen RL, Speel EJ, Hillen HF: The unknown biology of the unknown primary tumour: A literature review. Ann Oncol 2003;14:191.
7. Dennis JL, Vass JK, et al: Identification from public data of molecular markers of adenocarcinoma characteristic of the site of origin. Cancer Res 2002;62:5999.
8. Su AI, Welsh JB, et al: Cancer research. molecular classification of human carcinomas by use of gene expression signatures. Cancer Res 2001;61:7388.
9. Ramaswamy S, Tamayo P, et al: Multiclass cancer diagnosis using tumor gene expression signatures. PNAS 2001;98(26):15149.
10. Jesse RH, Perez CA, Fletcher GH: Cervical lymph node metastases: Unknown primary cancer. Cancer 1973;31:854.
11. Wang RC, Geopfert H, Barber AE, Wolf P: Unknown primary squamous cell carcinoma metastatic to the neck. Arch Otolaryngol Head Neck Surg 1990;116:1388.
12. Marcial-Vega VA, Cardenes H, Perez CA, et al: Cervical metastases from unknown primaries: Radiotherapeutic management and appearance of subsequent primaries. J Radiat Oncol Biol Phys 1990;19:919.
13. Hainsworth JD, Johnson DH, Greco FA: Cisplatin-based combination chemotherapy in the treatment of poorly

differentiated carcinoma and poorly differentiated adenocarcinoma of unknown primary site: Results of a 12-year experience. J Clin Oncol 1992;10:912.

14. Newman KH, Nystrom JS: Metastatic cancer of unknown origin: Non-squamous cell type. Semin Oncol 1982;9:427.

15. Greco FA, Vaughn WK, Hainsworth JD: Advanced poorly differentiated carcinoma of unknown primary site: Recognition of a treatable syndrome. Ann Intern Med 1986;104:547.

16. Sporn JR, Greenberg BR: Empiric chemotherapy in patients with carcinoma of unknown primary site. Am J Med 1990;88:49.

17. Kambhu SA, Kelsen D, Fiore J, et al: Metastatic adenocarcinomas of unknown primary site. Am J Clin Oncol 1990;13:55.

18. Pasterz R, Savaraj N, Burgess M: Prognostic factors in metastatic carcinoma of unknown primary. J Clin Oncol 1986;4:1652.

19. Culine S, et al: Development and validation of a prognostic model to predict the length of survival in patients with carcinomas of an unknown primary site. J Clin Oncol 2002;20(24):4679.

20. Frost P, Raber M, Abbruzzese J: Unknown primary tumors—Are they a unique subgroup of neoplastic disease? Cancer Bull 1987;39:216.

21. Nystrom JS, Weiner JM, Heffelfinger-Juttner J, Irwin LE: Metastatic and histologic presentations in unknown primary cancer. Semin Oncol 1977;4:53.

22. Holmes FF, Fouts TL: Metastatic cancer of unknown primary site. Cancer 1970;26:816.

23. Barlogie B, et al: Flow cytometry in clinical cancer research. Cancer Res 1983;43(9):3982.

24. Jallepalli PV, Lengauer C: Chromosome segregation and cancer: Cutting through the mystery. Nat Rev Cancer 2001;1(2):109.

25. Shackney SE, Shankey TV: Common patterns of genetic evolution in human solid tumors. Cytometry 1997;29(1):1.

26. Williams NN, Daly JM: Flow cytometry and prognostic implications in patients with solid tumors. Surg Gynecol Obstet 1990;171(3):257.

27. Hedley DW, Leary JA, Kirsten F: Metastatic adenocarcinoma of unknown primary site: Abnormalities of cellular DNA content and survival. Eur J Cancer Clin Oncol 1985;21(2):185.

28. Bell CW, Pathak S, Frost P: Unknown primary tumors: Establishment of cell lines, identification of chromosomal abnormalities, and implications for a second type of tumor progression. Cancer Res 1989;49(15):4311.

29. Atkin NB: Chromosome 1 aberrations in cancer. Cancer Genet Cytogenet 1986;21(4):279.

30. Mertens F, et al: Chromosomal imbalance maps of malignant solid tumors: A cytogenetic survey of 3185 neoplasms. Cancer Res 1997;57(13):2765.

31. Motzer RJ, Rodriguez E, Reuter VE, et al: Genetic analysis as an aid in diagnosis for patients with midline carcinomas of uncertain histologies. J Natl Cancer Inst 1991;83:341.

32. Motzer RJ, et al: Molecular and cytogenetic studies in the diagnosis of patients with poorly differentiated carcinomas of unknown primary site. J Clin Oncol 1995;13(1):274.

33. Summersgill B, et al: Establishing germ cell origin of undifferentiated tumors by identifying gain of 12p material using comparative genomic hybridization analysis of paraffin-embedded samples. Diagn Molec Pathol 1998;7(5):260.

34. Ilson DH, et al: Genetic analysis in the diagnosis of neoplasms of unknown primary tumor site. Semin Oncol 1993;20(3):229.

35. Sandberg AA, Meloni AM, Suijkerbuijk RF: Reviews of chromosome studies in urological tumors. III. Cytogenetics and genes in testicular tumors. J Urol 1996;155(5):1531.

36. Pavlidis N, et al: Overexpression of C-myc, Ras and C-erbB-2 oncoproteins in carcinoma of unknown primary origin. Anticancer Res 1995;15(6B):2563.

37. Briasoulis E, et al: Bcl2 and p53 protein expression in metastatic carcinoma of unknown primary origin: Biological and clinical implications. A Hellenic Co-operative Oncology Group study. Anticancer Res 1998;18(3B):1907.

38. Kaklamanis L, et al: Early expression of bcl-2 protein in the adenoma-carcinoma sequence of colorectal neoplasia. J Pathol 1996;179(1):10.

39. Pezzella F, et al: bcl-2 protein in non-small-cell lung carcinoma [comment]. N Engl J Med 1993;329(10):690.

40. Hainsworth JD, Lennington WJ, Greco FA: Overexpression of Her-2 in patients with poorly differentiated carcinoma or poorly differentiated adenocarcinoma of unknown primary site. J Clin Oncol 2000;18(3):632.

41. Hollstein M, et al: p53 mutations in human cancers. Science 1991;253(5015):49.

42. Soong R, et al: Concordance between p53 protein overexpression and gene mutation in a large series of common human carcinomas. Hum Pathol 1996;27(10):1050.

43. Vousden KH, Woude GF: The ins and outs of p53 [comment]. Nat Cell Biol 2000;2(10):E178.

44. Bar-Eli M, et al: p53 gene mutation spectrum in human unknown primary tumors. Anticancer Res 1993;13(5A):1619.

45. Hillen HF, et al: Microvessel density in unknown primary tumors. Int J Cancer 1997;74(1):81.

46. Shahangian S, Fritsche HA: Serum tumor markers as diagnostic aids in patients with unknown primary tumors. Cancer Bull 1989;41:152.

47. Jones A, Farrow G, Richardson FL: The extragonadal germ cell cancer syndrome: The Mayo Clinic experience. In Fer MF, Greco FA, Oldham RK (eds): Poorly Differentiated Neoplasms and Tumors of Unknown Origin. Orlando, Grune & Stratton, 1986, p 203.

48. Lenzi R, Hess KR, Abbruzzese MC, Raber MN, Ordoñez N, Abbruzzese JL: Poorly differentiated carcinoma and poorly differentiated adenocarcinoma of unknown origin: Favorable subsets of patients with unknown primary carcinoma? J Clin Oncol 1997;15:2056.

49. Gentile PS, Carloss HW, Huang TY, et al: Disseminated prostate carcinoma simulating primary lung cancer. Cancer 1988;62:711.

50. Tell DT, Khoury JM, Taylor HG, et al: Atypical metastasis from prostate cancer: Clinical utility of the immunoperoxidase technique for prostate specific antigen. JAMA 1985;253:3574.

51. Koch M, McPherson TA: Carcinoembryonic antigen levels as an indicator of the primary site in metastatic disease of unknown origin. Cancer 1981;48:1242.

52. Abbruzzese J, Raber M, Frost P: The role of CA-125 in patients with unknown primary tumors. Proc Am Soc Clin Oncol 1990;9:118.

53. Mackay B, Ordoñez NG: The role of the pathologist in the evaluation of poorly differentiated tumors and metastatic tumors of unknown origin. In Fer MF, Greco AF, Oldham RK (eds): Poorly Differentiated Neoplasms and Tumors of Unknown Origin. Orlando, Grune & Stratton, 1986, p 3.

54. Hainsworth JD, Wright EP, Johnson DH, et al: Poorly differentiated carcinoma of the unknown primary site: Clinical usefulness of immunoperoxidase staining. J Clin Oncol 1991;9:1931.

55. Roh MS, Hong SH: Utility of thyroid transcription factor-1 and cytokeratin 20 in identifying the origin of metastatic carcinomas of cervical lymph nodes. J Korean Med Sci 2002;4:512.

56. Jang KY, Kang MJ, Lee DG, Chung MJ: Utility of thyroid transcription factor-1 and cytokeratin 7 and 20 immunostaining in the identification of origin in malignant effusions. Anal Quant Cytol Histol 2001;6:400.

57. Rubin BP, Skarin AT, et al: Use of cytokeratin 7 and 20 in determining the origin of metastatic carcinoma of unknown primary, with special emphasis on lung cancer. Eur J Cancer Prevention 2001;10:77.

58. Chu PG, Weiss LM: Expression of cytokeratin 5/6 in epithelial neoplasms: An immunohistochemical study of 509 cases. Mod Pathol 2002;15(1):6.

59. Ordonez NG: Value of cytokeratin 5/6 immunostaining in distinguishing epithelial mesothelioma of the pleura from lung adenocarcinoma. Am J Surg Pathol 1998;22(10):1215.

60. Kaufmann O, Fietze E, et al: Value of p63 and cytokeratin 5/6 as immunohistochemical markers for the differential diagnosis of poorly differentiated and undifferentiated carcinomas. Am J Clin Pathol 2001;116 (6):823.

61. Cirtrin DL, Bessent RG, Greig WR: A comparison of the sensitivity and accuracy of the ^{99m}Tc-phosphate bone scan and skeletal radiograph in the diagnosis of bone metastases. Clin Radiol 1977;28:107.

62. Stewart JF, Tattersall MHN, Woods RL, et al: Unknown primary adenocarcinoma: Incidence of over investigation and natural history. BMJ 1979;1:1530.

63. Didolkar MS, Fanous N, Elias EG, et al: Metastatic carcinoma from occult primary tumors: A study of 254 patients. Ann Surg 1977;186:625.

64. Ellerbrook N, Holmes F, Singletary E, et al: Treatment of patients with isolated axillary nodal metastases from an occult primary carcinoma consistent with breast origin. Cancer 1990;66:1461.

65. Heitzman ER, Bernardino ME, Wallace S, et al: Computed tomography of the thorax. Am J Roentgenol 1981;136:2.

66. Muhm JR, Brown LR, Crowe, et al: Comparison of whole lung tomography and computed tomography for detecting pulmonary nodules. Am J Roentgenol 1978;131:981.

67. Schaner EG, Chang AE, Doppman JL, et al: Comparison of computed and conventional whole lung tomography in detecting pulmonary nodules: A prospective radiologic-pathologic study. Am J Roentgenol 1978;131:51.

68. Karsell PR, Sheedy PF II, O'Connell MJ: Computed tomography in search of cancer of unknown origin. JAMA 1982;248:340.

69. Walsh JW, Rosenfield AT, Jaffe CC, et al: Prospective comparison of ultrasound and computed tomography in the evaluation of gynecologic pelvic masses. Am J Roentgenol 1978;131:995.

70. Morris EA, Schwartz LH, Dershaw DD, et al: MR imaging of the breast in patients with occult primary breast carcinoma. Radiology 1997;205:437.

71. Kole AC, et al: Detection of unknown occult primary tumors using positron emission tomography. Cancer 1998;82(6):1160.

72. Lassen U, et al: ^{18}F-FDG whole body positron emission tomography (PET) in patients with unknown primary tumours (UPT). Eur J Cancer 1999;35(7):1076.

73. Jungehulsing M, et al: 2[F]-fluoro-2-deoxy-D-glucose positron emission tomography is a sensitive tool for the detection of occult primary cancer (carcinoma of unknown primary syndrome) with head and neck lymph node manifestation. Otolaryngol Head Neck Surg 2000;123(3):294.

74. Johansen J, et al: Implication of ^{18}F-fluoro-2-deoxy-D-glucose positron emission tomography on management of carcinoma of unknown primary in the head and neck: A Danish cohort study. Laryngoscope 2002;112(11):2009.

75. Su AI, Welsh JB, et al: Molecular classification of human carcinomas by use of gene expression signatures. Cancer Res 2001;61:7388.

76. Dennis JL, et al: Identification from public data of molecular markers of adenocarcinoma characteristic of the site of origin. Cancer Res 2002;62(21):5999.

77. Ultmann JE, Philips TL: Cancer of unknown primary site. In DeVita VT Jr, Hellman S, Rosenberg SA (eds): Cancer: Principles and Practice of Oncology, 4th ed. Philadelphia, JB Lippincott, 1989.

78. Abbruzzese JL, Abbruzzese MC, Hess KR, Raber MN, Lenzi R, Frost P: Unknown Primary Carcinoma: Natural history and prognostic factors in 657 consecutive patients. J Clin Oncol 1994;12:1272.

79. Raber MN, Abbruzzese JL, Frost P: Unknown primary tumors. Curr Opin Oncol 1992;4:3.

80. Abbruzzese JL: Carcinoma of Unknown Primary. In Kirkwood JM, Lotze MT, Yasko JM (eds): Current Cancer Therapeutics, 3rd ed. New York, Churchill Livingstone, 1998, pp 309–316.

81. Carlson LS, Fletcher GH, Oswald MJ: Guidelines for the radiotherapeutic techniques for cervical metastases from an unknown primary. Int J Radiat Oncol Biol Phys 1986;12:2101.

82. De Braud F, Heilbrun LK, Ahmed K, et al: Metastatic squamous cell carcinoma of an unknown primary localized to the neck. Advantages of an aggressive treatment. Cancer 1989;64:510.

83. Lee NK, Byers RM, Abbruzzese JL, Wolf P: Metastatic adenocarcinoma to the neck from an unknown primary. Am J Surg 1991;162:306.

84. Patel J, Nemoto T, Rosner D, et al: Axillary lymph node metastasis from an occult breast cancer. Cancer 1981;47:2923.

85. Ashikari R, Rosen PP, Urban JA, Senoo T: Breast cancer presenting as an axillary mass. Ann Surg 1976;183:415.

86. Rosen PP: Axillary lymph node metastases in patients with occult noninvasive breast carcinoma. Cancer 1980;46:1298.

87. Lenzi R, Kim EE, Raber MN, Abbruzzese JL: Detection of primary breast cancer presenting as metastatic carcinoma of unknown primary origin by ^{111}In-pentetreotide scan. Ann Oncol 1998;9:213.

88. Lenzi R, Abbruzzese MC, Raber MN, Abbruzzese JL: Clinical outcomes of patients with metastatic carcinomas of unknown

89. August CZ, Murad TM, Newton M: Multiple focal extraovarian serous carcinoma. Int J Gynecol Pathol 1985;4:11.

90. Dalrymple JC, Bannatyne P, Russell P, et al: Extraovarian peritonaeal serous papillary carcinoma. A clinicopathologic study of 31 cases. Cancer 1989;64:110.

91. Strnad CM, Grosh WN, Baxter J, et al: Peritoneal carcinomatosis of unknown primary site in women. Ann Intern Med 1989;111:213.

92. Ransom DT, Patel SR, Keeney GL, et al: Papillary serous carcinoma of the peritoneum. A review of 33 cases treated with platin-based chemotherapy. Cancer 1990;66:1091.

93. Lenzi R, Abbruzzese MC, Raber MN, Abbruzzese JL: Clinical outcomes of patients with metastatic carcinomas of unknown primary presenting with peritoneal carcinomatosis. Proc Am Soc Clin Ocol 1997;16:295 (abstract).

94. van der Gaast A, Verweij J, Henzen-Logmans SC, et al: Carcinoma of unknown primary: Identification of a treatable subset? Ann Oncol 1990;1:119.

95. Richardson RL, Shoumacher RA, Fer MF, et al: The unrecognized extragonadal germ cell cancer syndrome. Ann Intern Med 1981;94:181.

96. Fox RM, Woods RL, Tattersall MHN: Undifferentiated carcinoma in young men: The atypical teratoma syndrome. Lancet 1979;1:1316.

97. Hainsworth JD, Johnson DH, Greco FA: Poorly differentiated neuroendocrine carcinoma of unknown primary site. A newly recognized clinicopathologic entity. Ann Intern Med 1988;109:364.

98. Moertel CG, Kvols LK, O'Connell MJ, Rubin J: Treatment of neuroendocrine carcinomas with combined etoposide and cisplatin. Evidence of major therapeutic activity in the anaplastic variants of these neoplasms. Cancer 1991;68:227.

99. Moertel CG, Reitmeier RJ, Schutt AJ, et al: Treatment of the patient with adenocarcinomas of unknown origin. Cancer 1972;30:1469.

100. McKeen E, Smith F, et al: Fluorouracil (F), Adriamycin (A), and mitomycin (M), FAM for adenocarcinoma of unknown origin. Proc AACR ASCO 1980;21:358.

101. Rodnick S, Tremont S, et al: Evaluation and therapy of adenocarcinoma of unknown primary (ACUP). Proc AACR ASCO 1981;22:379.

102. Woods RL, Fox RM, et al: Metastatic adenocarcinomas of unknown primary site. N Engl J Med 1980;303:87.

103. Valentine J, Rosenthal S, et al: Combination chemotherapy of adenocarcinoma of unknown primary origin. Cancer Clin Trials 1979;2:265.

104. Bedikian AY, Bodey GP, et al: Sequential chemotherapy for adenocarcinoma of unknown primary. Am J Clin Oncol 1983;6:219.

105. Goldberg R, Smith F, et al: Treatment of adenocarcinoma of unknown primary with fluorouracil, adriamycin, and mitomycin-C (FAM). Proc ASCO 1986;5:129.

106. Walach N: Treatment of adenocarcinoma of unknown origin with cyclophoshamide (C), oncovin (O), methotrexate (M), and 5-fluorouracil (F), (COMF). Proc ASCO 1986;5:125.

107. Shildt RA, Kennedy PS, et al: Management of patients with metastatic adenocarcinoma of unknown origin: A Southwest Oncology Group Study. Cancer Treat Rep 1983;67:77.

108. Anderson H, Thatcher N, et al: VAC (vincristine, Adriamycin, cyclophosphamide) chemotherapy for metastatic carcinoma from an unknown primary site. Eur J Cancer Clin Oncol 1983;19:49.

109. Raber MN, Faintuch J, Abbruzzese JL, et al: Continuous infusion 5-fluorouracil, etoposide and cis-diamminedichloroplatinum in patients with metastatic carcinoma of unknown primary origin. Ann Oncol 1991;2:519.

110. LeChevalier T, Tremblay J, et al: Phase II trial of methotrexate-FAM in adenocarcinoma of unknown primary. Proc ASCO 1987;6:130.

111. Lenzi R, Abbruzzese J, Amato R, et al: Cisplatin, 5FU and folinic acid for the treatment of carcinomas of unknown primary: A phase II study. Proc Am Soc Clin Oncol 1991;10:301.

112. Hainsworth JD, Johnson DH, Greco FA: The role of etoposide in the treatment of poorly differentiated carcinoma of unknown primary site. Cancer 1991;67:310.

113. Abbruzzese JL, Raber M, Vrijhof W, et al: A phase I trial of laboratory derived synergistic chemotherapeutic combination:

2'deoxy-5-azacytidine (DAC) and cisplatin (CDDP). Proc Am Assn Cancer Res 1991;32:304.

114. Kelsen D, Martin DS, Coloriore J, et al: A Phase II trial of biochemical modulation using *N*-phosphonacetyl-L-aspartate, high-dose methotrexate, high-dose 5-flourouracil, and leucovorin in patients with adenocarcinoma of unknown primary site. Cancer 1992;70:1988.

115. Greco FA, et al: Carcinoma of unknown primary site: Phase II trials with docetaxel plus cisplatin or carboplatin. Ann Oncol 2000;11(2):211.

116. Briasoulis E, et al: Carboplatin plus paclitaxel in unknown primary carcinoma: A phase II Hellenic Cooperative Oncology Group Study. J Clin Oncol 2000;18(17):3101.

117. Greco FA, et al: Taxane-based chemotherapy for patients with carcinoma of unknown primary site. Cancer J 2001;7(3):203.

118. Hainsworth JD, Erland JB, Kalman LA, et al: Carcinoma of unknown primary site: Treatment with 1-hour paclitaxel, carboplatin, and extended-schedule etoposide. J Clin Oncol 1997;15:2385.

119. Hess K, Abbruzzese MC, Lenzi R, et al: Classification and regression tree analysis of 1000 consecutive patients with unknown primary carcinoma. Proc Am Soc Clin Oncol 1996;15:452 (abstract).

120. Hainsworth JD, et al: Gemcitabine in the second-line therapy of patients with carcinoma of unknown primary site: A phase II trial of the Minnie Pearl Cancer Research Network. Cancer Invest 2001;19(4):335.

121. Ayoub JP, Hess KR, Abbruzzese MC, Lenzi R, Raber MN, Abbruzzese JL: Unknown primary tumors metastatic to liver. J Clin Oncol 1998;16:2105.

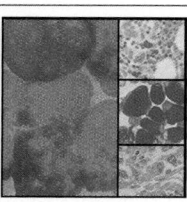

HIV-ASSOCIATED MALIGNANCIES

Richard F. Ambinder

98

SUMMARY OF KEY POINTS

INCIDENCE
- Non-Hodgkin's lymphoma, Hodgkin's disease, and Kaposi's sarcoma (KS) all occur with increased incidence in HIV-infected patients.
- Kaposi's sarcoma occurs in HIV patients also infected with KS herpesvirus (KSHV). Outside of Africa and some Mediterranean populations, Kaposi's sarcoma occurs mainly in men who have sex with men.
- Lymphoma occurs across all HIV risk groups and is most commonly aggressive with diffuse histologic features.

ETIOLOGY AND PATHOGENESIS
- Kaposi's sarcoma is always associated with KSHV; immunocompromise, inflammatory cytokines, and perhaps the HIV TAT protein contribute to pathogenesis.
- Lymphoma in HIV patients is associated with Epstein-Barr virus (EBV) approximately half of the time; immunocompromise, chronic antigen stimulation, and perhaps inflammatory cytokines contribute to pathogenesis.

EVALUATION OF KAPOSI'S SARCOMA
Evaluation of KS patients involves:
- Determination of CD4+ T-cell count and HIV load

- Biopsy to confirm diagnosis
- Computed tomographic scan of chest and abdomen
- Gastrointestinal endoscopy if clinically indicated

TREATMENT OF KAPOSI'S SARCOMA
- Institution of highly active antiretroviral therapy and treatment of opportunistic infections constitute an important step in the treatment of KS.
- If disease is symptomatic, rapidly progressive, or there is visceral involvement, institute systemic therapy with liposomal anthracycline or paclitaxel; all patients should be receiving *Pneumocystis* prophylaxis, and many patients will require hematopoietic growth factors.
- If disease is indolent and highly active antiretroviral therapy has just been initiated or major changes have been made, consider observation, interferon, thalidomide, or experimental therapy.
- For a few lesions, consider topical therapy, injection of lesions, or radiation therapy.

EVALUATION OF LYMPHOMA
- Determination of CD4+ T-cell count and HIV load.
- Assessment for signs of tumor lysis.

- Extranodal presentations of lymphoma are common, as are constitutional symptoms.
- Staging for systemic lymphoma should include testing lactate dehydrogenase levels; imaging of chest, abdomen, and brain; bone marrow biopsy; and lumbar puncture.

TREATMENT OF LYMPHOMA
- Allopurinol and hydration constitute the first step in treatment, even before staging is complete.
- Chemotherapy (CHOP, CDE, EPOCH regimens) with *Pneumocystis* prophylaxis and hematopoietic growth factors.
- Intrathecal prophylaxis is appropriate for patients with Burkitt's or Burkitt-like lymphoma or with EBV-associated non-Hodgkin's lymphoma.
- Antiretroviral therapy should be initiated in conjunction with cytotoxic chemotherapy or shortly thereafter, except possibly in association with continuous infusion regimens when it may be appropriate to delay or interrupt antiretroviral therapy until the conclusion of cytotoxic chemotherapy.

INTRODUCTION

In 1981 the first cases of *Pneumocystis carinii* pneumonia in gay men were reported.[1] Fatal opportunistic infections and other complications of immunodeficiency were consecutively confirmed in homosexual men, persons who injected drugs, their sexual partners, and men with hemophilia. In 1983 human immunodeficiency virus (HIV-1) was cultured from the lymph node of a patient.[2] The origins of the HIV/AIDS (acquired immunodeficiency syndrome) epidemic remain obscure, but by 2003, more than 42 million people worldwide were infected with HIV and approximately 3 million had died from AIDS in the previous year.[3] HIV infection has now become the fourth leading cause of death worldwide. In the United States, approximately 1 million people are infected and almost half a million have died with HIV infection. AIDS-related mortality rate has dramatically declined among patients with access to antiretroviral therapy. From the beginning of the epidemic, an increased incidence of Kaposi's sarcoma (KS) and lymphoma were recognized in association with AIDS. This chapter reviews aspects of HIV infection and AIDS and presents the management of KS and lymphoma in HIV-infected patients.

HIV INFECTION

The virus is transmitted sexually, parenterally, and vertically.[3,4] Worldwide, heterosexual transmission is most common. The highest risk of sexual transmission is associated with receptive anal intercourse. In the United States, men who have sex with men are the largest HIV risk group. Injection drug use is also a major contributor to the epidemic. Health care workers are at risk, but barrier precautions, safer needle devices, attention to safe practices, and related technical innovations have reduced exposure.[5]

HIV is associated with a spectrum of disease from asymptomatic to profoundly immunocompromised. HIV RNA levels are important predictors of the rate of progression, while CD4+ T-cell counts are markers of immunologic status. In untreated patients, the plasma HIV load reaches a fairly constant level within about 6 months of primary infection. The host cytotoxic T-cell response may be an important determinant of this "set point." Some diseases are specifically associated with low CD4+ T-cell counts. For example, *Pneumocystis* pneumonia typically occurs in patients with less than 200 cells/μL, and primary brain lymphoma typically occurs in patients with less than 50 cells/μL.[6]

A variety of constitutional signs and symptoms are common in HIV-infected patients, even in the absence of opportunistic infection and malignancy, and include anorexia, nausea, vomiting, and weight loss. Persistent fever is not uncommon, but always requires a search for opportunistic infections. Typically this investigation involves a chest radiograph, sinus computed tomographic (CT) scan, blood cultures for bacteria and atypical mycobacteria, and serum cryptococcal antigen test. Neurologic problems include AIDS dementia complex, HIV myelopathy, and various peripheral neuropathies.

Opportunistic infections that commonly occur in HIV-infected patients include *Pneumocystis carinii* pneumonia, chronic sinusitis, oral and esophageal candidiasis, herpes simplex infections, shingles, cytomegalovirus retinitis, and enterocolitis associated with *Campylobacter*, *Salmonella*, *Shigella*, adenovirus, cytomegalovirus, or various protozoans (*Cryptosporidium*, *Entamoeba histolytica*, *Giardia,* and others). A variety of infections manifest in the central nervous system, including toxoplasmosis, progressive multifocal leukoencephalopathy, and cryptococcal meningitis. Skin infections with molluscum contagiosum and dermatophytic fungi are also common. Several of these infections can be prevented with appropriate prophylaxis (Table 98-1).[7]

Antiretroviral therapy is generally recommended for all patients with acute HIV infection or within the first 6 months after seroconversion.[8-10] In addition, antiretroviral therapy is recommended for all patients with symptomatic AIDS, thrush, or unexplained fever and patients with CD4+ T-cell counts below 200/mm³. For asymptomatic patients with CD4+ T-cell counts above 200/mm³ many would initiate therapy only for patients with higher viral loads. Drugs approved for the suppression of viral replication include nucleoside analog reverse transcriptase

TABLE 98-1

Prophylaxis of Opportunistic Infections

CD4+ T-CELL COUNT	PROPHYLACTIC REGIMEN
CD4+ <200/mm³	*Pneumocystis carinii* pneumonia (PCP) prophylaxis with trimethoprim-sulfamethoxazole (TMP-SMX), dapsone, or aerosolized pentamidine
CD4+ <100/mm³	Toxoplasmosis prophylaxis in patients who are seropositive for *Toxoplasma gondii.* TMP-SMX administered as PCP prophylaxis also protects against toxoplasmosis. A variety of other agents are available for patients not receiving TMP-SMX.
CD4+ <50/mm³	*Mycobacterium avium* complex (MAC). Clarithromycin (daily) or azithromycin (weekly) are the drugs of choice.

inhibitors, non-nucleoside reverse transcriptase inhibitors, protease inhibitors, and, most recently, an inhibitor of fusion of the viral envelope with CD4+ T cells.[11,12] In parallel to the treatment of chemotherapy-responsive malignancies, combination antiretroviral therapy with two or more agents appears to be the most effective way to suppress viral replication and reduce the emergence of resistant virus. Non-nucleoside reverse transcriptase inhibitors are associated with the most rapid mutations to high-level resistance and should never be used alone. Protease inhibitors are sometimes associated with lipodystrophy, a disorder associated with fat redistribution. The only envelope fusion inhibitor that is approved, enfuvirtide, is available only parenterally, and is approved only for resistant virus.[11] A convenient guide to the medical management of HIV infection, which is updated regularly, can be found at http://www.hopkins-aids.edu/publications/abbrevgd/abbrevgd.html.

KAPOSI'S SARCOMA

Epidemiology

Before AIDS, KS was a rare disease recognized in older men of Eastern European or Mediterranean descent, in parts of Africa where it often occurred in children, and in organ transplant recipients.[13] Among AIDS patients, KS is the most common cancer. The risk of an HIV-infected patient developing KS in the era before highly active antiretroviral therapy was estimated to be greater than 1000 times the risk in the HIV-uninfected population.[14] With antiretroviral therapy the incidence has diminished substantially.[15,16] The risk of KS is not evenly distributed among HIV risk groups. The KS herpesvirus (KSHV), also referred to as HHV-8, is a required cofactor.[13] In contrast to most human herpesviruses, which are ubiquitous, KSHV infection is uncommon in most populations worldwide. Rates of infection are higher in central and southern Africa and intermediate in Mediterranean and Eastern European countries.

Men who have sex with men are at especially high risk for KSHV infection.[17] Sexual transmission may be inferred from several studies, but the precise mode of transmission remains poorly understood. In contrast, patients who acquire HIV infection through nonsexual blood-borne exposure (intravenous drug use, transfusion of blood or blood products) are at considerably lower risk for KSHV infection and for the development of KS. Among individuals who are seropositive for KSHV and HIV, the sequence of exposure is an important risk factor for the development of KS.[18] When KSHV seroconversion follows HIV seroconversion, the risk of developing KS is higher. Presumably this reflects the impact of HIV on establishing an effective primary immune response to KSHV.

Pathogenesis

KS lesions are composed of spindle-shaped cells between collagen bundles, neovascular slit-like spaces, extravasated erythrocytes, hemosiderin-laden macrophages, and a variable infiltrate of plasma cells, lymphocytes, and other inflammatory cells.[19] Spindle cells show nuclear pleomorphism in the later stages. Lesions begin in the dermis and progress from macular to plaque to tumor stage. In the early macular stage, spindle cells form irregular slits and clefts. A sparse infiltrate is composed of lymphocytes and plasma cells in the perivascular spaces. Nuclear atypia and mitoses are absent. In the plaque stage, the entire dermis is involved, and extravasated erythrocytes and hemosiderin-laden macrophages appear. With progression to the tumor stage, spindle cells come to predominate. Nuclear atypia and mitoses are present.

Spindle cells express endothelial and macrophage markers and are thought to originate from circulating peripheral blood hematopoietic precursor cells.[20-22] At least in organ transplant recipients, tumor cells may be of donor origin.[23] These cells often do not express factor VIII but do express CD34. In many instances KS lesions are clonal.[24,25] KS may possibly begin as a polyclonal inflammatory lesion and only sometimes progress to oligoclonal or monoclonal neoplasia. Immunohistochemistry and in situ hybridization show that KSHV is present in spindle cells, some epithelial cells, and some of the cells of the inflammatory infiltrate.[26,27]

KSHV is invariably present in KS lesions.[28] Electron microscopy shows evidence of viral production in some cells in KS lesions (Fig. 98-1), but spindle cells are generally latently infected (Fig. 98-2). Several viral genes are implicated in aspects of regulation of cellular growth, apoptosis, immune regulation, and angiogenesis.[29] Curiously, many of the genes that have functional properties that suggest they might play a role in transformation are lytic cycle genes and are not expressed in most of the spindle cells of KS lesions. These include the viral interferon regulatory factors (v-IRFs), an antiapoptotic protein viral BCL-2 (v-BCL-2), viral interleukin 6 (v-IL-6), a G-protein-coupled receptor (GPCR), and K1, a transmembrane glycoprotein with transforming properties. The viral proteins that are expressed in latently infected spindle cells are LANA, a nuclear protein required for maintenance of the viral episome; v-CYC, a cyclin-D

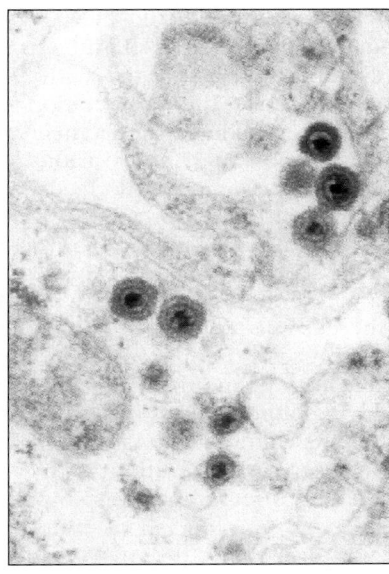

Figure 98-1. Electron micrograph showing herpesvirus particles budding from spindle cells in a Kaposi's sarcoma (KS) lesion. (Courtesy of Jan Orenstein.)

homolog that may disrupt usual pathways of cell cycle inhibition; and v-FLIP, an antiapoptotic protein that blocks death signals and may induce survival signals. The molecular biology of the virus and its role in transformation are discussed further in Chapter 12.

The immune system seems to play a determining role in the pathogenesis of KS. In organ transplant recipients, reduction or withdrawal of immunosuppression is often associated with tumor regression.[17] The virus itself expresses a number of genes that modify immune function. Viral genes modulate the actions of interferon and downregulate the display of major histocompatibility complex (MHC) class I and natural killer (NK) cell receptor ligands.[30-33] Cytotoxic T-cell responses to viral

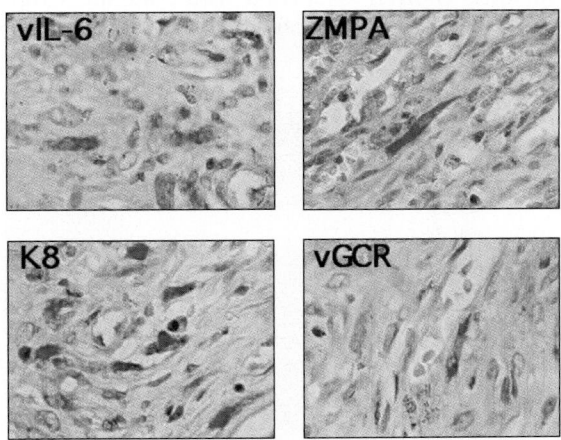

Figure 98-2. Kaposi's sarcoma herpesvirus (KSHV) antigens in spindle cells of a nodular KS lesion. Immunohistochemistry showing punctate nuclear LANA (brown spots) in many cells with v-GCR expression (red cytoplasm) in a few scattered lytic cells with nuclei that are devoid of LANA.

lytic antigens are readily detected in KSHV-seropositive individuals, but are diminished in HIV-infected individuals.

Cytokine dysregulation associated with HIV infection may specifically enhance the proliferation of this neoplasm. In vitro interleukin-6, tumor necrosis factor-α, interleukin-1-β, interleukin-8, and various chemokines will stimulate proliferation of KS-derived cells. The HIV TAT protein may directly upregulate KSHV genes.[34] Epidemiologic evidence also supports a direct role for HIV in the pathogenesis of KS insofar as KS is less common in areas of Africa where there is infection with HIV-2 than in areas where there is infection with HIV-1.[35] Opportunistic infections often precede the presentation or an exacerbation of KS. While both phenomena may reflect a deterioration of underlying immune status, several investigators have suggested that altered cytokine and inflammatory mediator production in association with opportunistic infection may have a direct impact on KS pathogenesis.[36]

Clinical Aspects

KS lesions typically arise on the skin or mucous membranes as flat deep purple plaques (Fig. 98-3). These plaques may progress to form nodules. Many parts of the body may be involved, and the clinical problems associated with KS vary as a function of location. Lesions are generally not pruritic or painful (except occasionally when they involve the plantar surface of the feet). The most frequent sites of disease are the skin, mucous membranes, lymph nodes, and gastrointestinal tract. Skin lesions most often appear on the legs and face (especially nose and ears) and are often symmetrically distributed. The oral hard palate is also commonly involved. KS virtually never involves brain parenchyma.

KS lesions have a distinctive appearance that is highly suggestive with regard to diagnosis. However, other entities occasionally are confused with KS. Prominent among them is bacillary angiomatosis, a benign disease associated with a slow-growing, fastidious, gram-negative bacillus and treated with antibiotic therapy.[37] Bacillary angiomatosis is often associated with systemic symptoms such as fever, chills, and headache. Therefore, a biopsy is

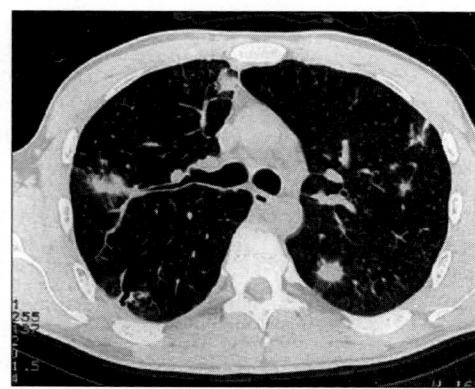

Figure 98-4. Computed tomographic scan of the chest shows a nodular lesion with characteristic flame-like appearance adjacent to right upper bronchus. (Courtesy of Elliot Fishman.)

generally indicated in order to confirm the diagnosis. This is most commonly a punch biopsy of a skin lesion, but at times lymph node biopsy, transbronchial or other endoscopic biopsy, or pleural biopsy is required. Once a diagnosis has been established, visualization of a characteristic lesion by bronchoscopy without biopsy or characteristic CT findings (flame-shaped hemorrhages) are generally regarded as adequate to diagnose pulmonary KS (Fig. 98-4). Gallium scan may be useful in differentiating pulmonary KS from *Pneumocystis* pneumonia as the inflammatory infiltrates in *Pneumocystis* pneumonia are gallium-avid and KS lesions are not. On the other hand, KS lesions are usually thallium-avid.

Lesion location is an important determinant of symptoms. Facial lesions are particularly likely to be cosmetically disturbing. Lesions of the lower extremities often lead to lymphatic obstruction with painful edema. Pulmonary lesions are often associated with dyspnea (but rarely hemoptysis). Gastrointestinal lesions may be associated with pain, cramping, diarrhea, and bleeding or may be entirely asymptomatic.

Staging and Prognosis

Standard tumor-node-metastases (TNM) staging has not proved particularly useful for KS, partly because KS is a multicentric disease and partly because the status of HIV disease is of overriding importance. The AIDS Clinical Trials Study Group (ACTG) developed a staging system specifically for KS occurring in HIV-infected individuals.[38] Devised in the era before the introduction of highly active antiretroviral therapy, this system classified patients as good risk or poor risk based on the extent of tumor (confined to skin or minimal disease vs. edema, ulcers, and extensive oral, visceral, or gastrointestinal invasion), immune status as measured by CD4+ T-cell count (at 200/mm^3, below 200/mm^3), and evidence of HIV-associated systemic symptoms; it proved to be a reasonable predictor of survival.

A relationship between the response to highly active antiretroviral therapy as reflected by measurements of HIV load and clinical regression of KS has been reported.[39]

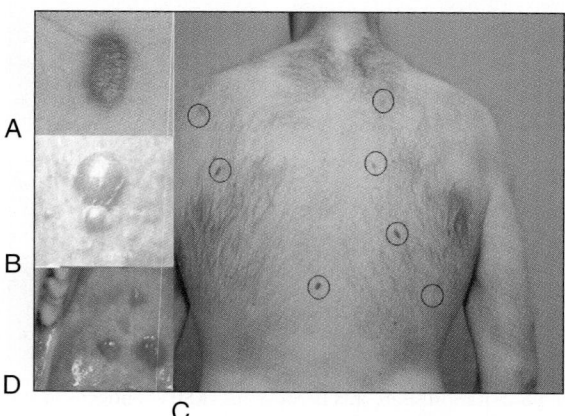

Figure 98-3. KS lesions. **A,** Plaque lesion. **B,** Nodular lesions. **C,** Near symmetric distribution of lesions on the trunk. Lesions are circled. **D,** Lesions on the hard palate.

Specific Malignancies

III

> ## TREATMENT OF KAPOSI'S SARCOMA
>
> Treatment with liposomal anthracycline: Liposomal doxorubicin is administered at a dose of 20 mg/m^2 intravenously every 2 to 3 weeks. Granulocyte colony-stimulating factor (G-CSF) is used as needed. Once a maximum response is attained, treatment is discontinued.
>
> Treatment with paclitaxel: Paclitaxel is administered at 100 mg/m^2 infused over 3 hours every 2 weeks. G-CSF is routinely used. Once a maximum response is attained, treatment is discontinued.
>
> Treatment with interferon-α: Therapy begins at 1 million units per day and then escalates as tolerated up to 9 MU per day over a period of 2 months. Interferon is associated with flu-like symptoms of fevers, chills, myalgias, and fatigue. These symptoms typically diminish, and tolerance improves with time. Treatment at night and the use of acetaminophen and nonsteroidal anti-inflammatory medications improve the tolerability of the regimen. Patients who respond or have stable disease are continued on treatment until disease progression.

The value of quantitative measurement of KSHV copy number in blood (plasma, serum, peripheral blood mononuclear cells) as a prognostic factor is under investigation. The presence of KSHV in peripheral blood mononuclear cells is more common in KSHV-seropositive patients with KS lesions than in KS-seropositive patients without lesions.[40] Furthermore, among men with KS, viral DNA is most likely to be detected in patients with new lesions. KSHV load in peripheral blood mononuclear cells may be a better predictor of clinical progression of KS than either CD4+ T-cell count or HIV viral load.[40] Antiretroviral therapy is sometimes associated with disappearance of measurable KSHV in plasma.[39] However, KSHV copy number does not correlate well with clinical response in patients treated with liposomal doxorubicin.[41] Thus, the utility and biologic importance of such measurements have yet to be defined.

Therapy

Management of HIV and Opportunistic Infection

Highly active antiretroviral therapy has profoundly altered the survival of patients with KS. The Multicenter AIDS Cohort Study showed an 81% reduced risk of death for patients with KS who were treated with highly active antiretroviral therapy.[42] The only form of KS clearly implicated in directly causing the death of patients is pulmonary KS. In the era before highly active antiretroviral therapy, KS was associated with a 90% mortality rate attributable to disease progression. In patients treated with highly active antiretroviral therapy, KS is associated with a 47% mortality rate.[43] The impact of antiviral therapy may be multifaceted. Restoration of immune function must be of major importance, but antiviral therapy may also reduce exposure to HIV proteins such as TAT and a variety of inflammatory cytokines associated with opportunistic infections also thought to play a role in KS progression. Some protease inhibitors also have direct antiangiogenic

and antineoplastic effects.[44,45] Thus, therapy begins with ensuring that the antiretroviral regimen has been optimized and opportunistic infections treated. In the absence of rapidly progressing disease (more than 10 new lesions in the past month), lymphedema, or symptomatic visceral or cosmetically disfiguring disease, it is often appropriate to wait several months to assess the full impact of the initiation of antiretroviral therapy before embarking on systemic therapies.

Systemic Therapy

Interferon-α is active in a subset of patients.[46] The mechanism of action may involve antiviral, immune modulatory, antiproliferative, or antiangiogenic properties. Uncertainties with regard to mechanism notwithstanding, interferon-α has activity in the treatment of KS. Early investigations showed that response rates to treatment were correlated with CD4+ T-cell lymphocyte counts.[47,48] In patients with CD4+ T-cell counts above 400/mm^3, the response rate was approximately 40%, whereas in patients with CD4+ T-cell counts below 200/mm^3 response rates were less than 10%. High doses (36 MU/day or 30 MU/m^2 three times weekly) were required to achieve these response rates. In combination with zidovudine, interferon-α showed activity against KS even in patients with CD4 lymphocyte counts below 200/mm^3 as well as evidence of HIV suppression. However, the combination was associated with myelosuppression and hepatotoxicity. In combination with nonmyelosuppressive antiretroviral regimens, interferon appears to be effective in lower doses (1 million units per day) than when used alone.[46] Time to interferon response of 8 to 12 weeks precludes its use in patients with very symptomatic or aggressive disease. On the other hand, responses are often long-lasting, particularly complete responses. This period is longer than the response duration typically associated with cytotoxic chemotherapy. Furthermore, even patients with widespread disseminated disease can have complete clinical responses.

Although a variety of single agents and combinations of agents have been studied in the past, single-agent therapy with a liposomal anthracycline or with paclitaxel is now the standard of care. Liposomal formulation of anthracyclines leads to altered pharmacokinetic profiles. Thus, liposomal doxorubicin has both a prolonged plasma half-life, increased concentration in tumor tissues, and decreased concentration in normal tissues.[49] In phase III trials, liposomal doxorubicin and liposomal daunorubicin have been shown to be at least as effective and less toxic than combination regimens including nonliposomal anthracyclines.[50,51] Liposomal anthracyclines are generally well tolerated, with myelosuppression as the major limiting toxicity. A "hand-foot" syndrome is occasionally seen and often responds to steroids.[52] Alopecia is rare, and cardiotoxicity is very rare.

Paclitaxel is an active agent for treatment of refractory KS.[53-55] In an initial trial, patients with advanced KS were treated with 135 mg/m^2 escalated to 175 mg/m^2 every 3 weeks. The response rate was 71.4%. Responses were seen in all four assessable patients who had previously received anthracycline therapy for KS and in patients with pulmonary KS. In a subsequent study, patients who had failed one or more chemotherapy regimens including combination chemotherapy and chemotherapy with liposomal daunorubicin were treated with paclitaxel 100 mg/m² every 2 weeks.[55] Among these poor prognosis patients with a median CD4+ T-cell count of 5/mm³, 53% responded. The same regimen in naive patients yielded an overall response rate of 70%. Alopecia, nausea, vomiting, myalgias, and myelotoxicity often requiring growth factor support are common toxicities.

Thalidomide also shows activity against KS.[56,57] Regimens studied include daily doses of 100 mg for 8 weeks, dose escalation beginning at 200 mg daily to tolerance, and treatment with 200 mg to 600 mg daily.[58,59] Sedation, depression, fever, rash, and neurologic toxicity have all been reported. The antineoplastic activity of thalidomide is poorly understood. Thalidomide inhibits tumor necrosis factor (TNF) production, alters T-cell response, and modulates T_H1 cytokine production. Although only a minority of patients respond, its oral availability and toxicity profile make it an attractive alternative for patients who do not require immediate responses and in patients who cannot tolerate myelosuppressive regimens.

Local Therapies

Local therapies are appropriate for patients with a few lesions and slowly progressive disease. For example, a patient with maximally suppressed HIV-1 and indolent but cosmetically disturbing facial lesions may benefit from local treatment. Local therapy avoids immunosuppression associated with cytotoxic chemotherapy but does nothing to interrupt or slow systemic progression and the appearance of new lesions. Alitretinoin (9-cis-retinoic acid) is administered as a topical gel applied twice daily initially and increasing up to four times daily as tolerated.[60] Four to 8 weeks of therapy are typically required before responses are seen. Responses occur even in patients with low CD4+ T-cell counts. Irritation at the site of gel application is common. Intralesional injections with vinblastine, interferon, or sodium tetradecyl sulfate all have a high response rate, but regrowth is common.[61,62] Similarly, liquid nitrogen is effective for the treatment of small lesions, particularly on the face.[63]

Radiation therapy is an effective and widely used local treatment.[63-66] Response rates are generally 80% to 90%. A variety of dosing schedules have been used. In a randomized study, three radiation prescriptions were compared: 8 Gy in one fraction, 20 Gy in 10 fractions, and 40 Gy in 20 fractions. Each treatment scheme led to flattening of lesions. However, as might be expected, the highest dose was associated with the greatest chance for complete clearing of lesions and the longest duration of benefit. Thus, single fractions are most appropriate for patients with very short life expectancies and to provide symptomatic rather than cosmetic relief. The conjunctiva, oral pharynx, and other sensitive tissues require different doses and fractionation schemes than most cutaneous lesions.

Antiherpesvirus Agents

Some retrospective evidence suggests that antiviral agents that block lytic KSHV infection may inhibit the development of KS. In vitro ganciclovir and foscarnet are active in inhibiting lytic KSHV replication. Acyclovir is not. Three studies have demonstrated a decreased incidence of KS in patients with HIV treated with either ganciclovir or foscarnet regimens but not acyclovir.[67-69] Thus, there is interest in the possibility that agents with similar in vitro activity might block the development of KS. In contrast, these agents appear to have no activity in the treatment of established KS. Presumably the resistance of established KS to such treatments reflects the predominantly latent state of the viral genome in tumors.

LYMPHOMA

Epidemiology

Both non-Hodgkin's and Hodgkin's lymphomas are increased in incidence in patients with HIV infection, although the increase in the non-Hodgkin's lymphomas is much greater, and only aggressive B-cell non-Hodgkin's lymphomas have been formally recognized as AIDS-defining illnesses. In contrast to the situation with KS, lymphomas occur in all HIV populations and show no marked predilection for men who have sex with men or other particular risk groups. Early data from cancer and AIDS registries in the United States showed that the relative risk of non-Hodgkin's lymphoma within 3.5 years of another AIDS diagnosis was 165-fold compared to persons without AIDS.[70] Particular types of lymphoma showed a much more dramatic increase in incidence. Thus, brain lymphoma was increased 3600-fold in comparison with the general population.[71] The risks for high-grade diffuse immunoblastic and Burkitt's lymphomas were increased 652-fold and 261-fold, respectively. The risk for Hodgkin's lymphoma in HIV-infected persons is increased 5- to 9-fold.[72-74]

With highly active antiretroviral therapy, the overall incidence of lymphoma is decreasing, with the most marked decrease occurring in primary brain lymphoma.[75-78] The length of time with HIV infection prior to diagnosis of lymphoma is increasing, as is the CD4+ T-cell count at the time of diagnosis.

Histology and Pathogenesis

The spectrum of lymphomas in the general population includes indolent and aggressive, follicular and diffuse, B- and T-cell tumors, and Hodgkin's and non-Hodgkin's histologic types. In patients with HIV infection, the increased incidence of lymphomas is mainly an increase in aggressive B-cell tumors with diffuse architecture and in Hodgkin's lymphoma.[76,79] Diffuse immunoblastic, Burkitt's (and Burkitt-like), and diffuse large B-cell lymphomas each account for approximately one third of the total of non-Hodgkin's lymphomas. Recently, polymorphic lymphoproliferative disorders such as those seen in transplant recipients have also been described.[80] Surface markers characteristic of B cells (CD19, CD20, CD22) are generally expressed, with the notable exception of primary effusion lymphomas. The latter often exhibit an indeterminate phenotype with expression of lymphoid activation markers.[79] Mixed cellularity is the most common Hodgkin's lymphoma subtype in the HIV-infected population, whereas lymphocyte-predominant Hodgkin's lymphoma is quite rare.[74,81-83]

Epstein-Barr virus (EBV) is presumed to play a key role in the pathogenesis of lymphomas that carry the viral genome.[84] This type describes approximately half of the lymphomas that arise in HIV-infected patients. In contrast to KSHV, EBV is a ubiquitous virus. EBV has a tropism for B lymphocytes and mediates growth transformation of primary B cells into long-term proliferating lymphoblastoid cell lines. It is associated with lymphoma across the spectrum of immunocompromised patients including patients with congenital immunodeficiency and transplant recipients. The molecular biology of the virus and its role in transformation are discussed further in Chapter 12.

Particular anatomic sites and particular histologic types are especially likely to be EBV-associated. Primary brain lymphomas and lymphomas with central nervous system involvement in AIDS patients are virtually always EBV-positive (Fig. 98-5).[85-89] Lymphomas with immunoblastic features, primary effusion lymphomas, plasmablastic oral lymphomas, and Hodgkin's disease are also usually EBV-associated.[79,82] Curiously, although EBV was discovered in African Burkitt's lymphoma and nearly 100% of endemic Burkitt's lymphoma is EBV-associated, AIDS-associated Burkitt's or Burkitt-like lymphoma is the histologic type least frequently associated with EBV (20% to 30%).[79]

Burkitt's lymphomas occur earlier in the course of HIV disease than diffuse immunoblastic or diffuse large cell lymphomas.[76] In one series, the median CD4+ T-cell count in patients with Burkitt's lymphoma was 270/mm[3] whereas it was 99/mm[3] for diffuse immunoblastic and diffuse large cell lymphomas.[90] Among patients with lymphoma as an AIDS-defining event, Burkitt's lymphoma accounted for 47% of lymphomas occurring as the first manifestation of AIDS, whereas it accounted for only 13% of non-Hodgkin's lymphoma that developed after another AIDS-related event. Isolated extranodal lymphomas were histologically diffuse immunoblastic or large cell types (97%) and were associated with a median CD4+ T-cell count of 70/mm[3]. Primary central nervous system lymphomas represent the extreme end of this spectrum and are associated with a particularly low CD4+ T-cell count.[88] It has been suggested that highly active antiretroviral therapy has changed the character of lymphomas occurring in HIV patients with a shift away from lymphomas of postgerminal center origin.[91]

Clinical Aspects

Advanced stage, extranodal disease, and constitutional symptoms are frequently seen in patients with HIV and lymphoma.[92-95] Approximately 90% have some extranodal involvement, and in 30% all disease is extranodal. The gastrointestinal tract is a particularly frequent site of extranodal involvement. Sites not generally involved by lymphoma arising in other settings such as heart, common bile duct, and rectum are seen in AIDS patients. Similarly, brain and skin may be involved by Hodgkin's lymphoma at presentation in HIV patients. Pleural, pericardial, or peritoneal cavities may harbor lymphomatous effusions in the absence of any "solid" tumor mass.

Constitutional symptoms are much more common in association with lymphoma in HIV patients than in other hosts. As in patients with KS, the presence of such symptoms in patients with lymphoma should prompt a search for opportunistic infections. However, in contrast to the KS situation, even after opportunistic infections are excluded, constitutional symptoms are common.

Biopsy is required for the diagnosis of lymphoma with the possible exception of primary central nervous system lymphoma, as discussed later.[84] Computed tomography or magnetic resonance imaging of the chest and abdomen is often useful in identifying lesions likely to yield diagnostic material. Gastrointestinal tract lesions will occasionally be detected only by endoscopy. Persistent generalized lymphadenopathy is common in patients with HIV infection, but asymmetrically enlarged nodes should always be biopsied. Biopsy of a node that shows benign hyperplasia does not exclude the possibility of lymphoma elsewhere, and several biopsies may be required to establish a diagnosis. Even in the absence of cytopenias, bone marrow biopsy will sometimes yield a diagnosis (Fig. 98-6). Bone marrow–only presentations of Hodgkin's lymphoma are not uncommon.

The location of the pathologic lesion is important in determining the type of biopsy to be performed. Lesions in the brain or other organs devoid of lymphoid tissue are adequately assessed by needle biopsy. Lymph nodes are best assessed by excisional biopsy, which allows assessment of architecture. Failure to identify a clonal population by flow cytometry or other molecular diagnostics does not exclude lymphoma. Whether technical artifact or distinctive pathogenesis, clonality could not be

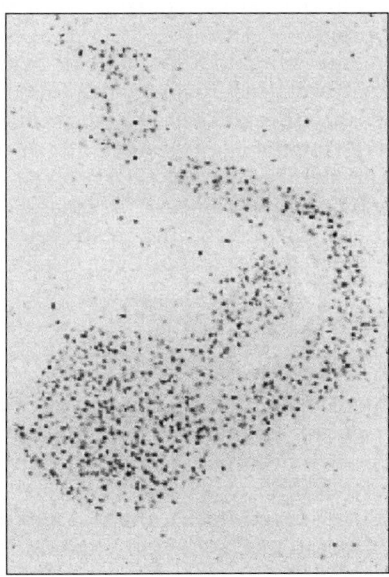

Figure 98-5. In situ hybridization demonstrating the presence of Epstein-Barr virus (EBV) RNA in brain lymphoma. Tumor cells are clustered around a vessel.

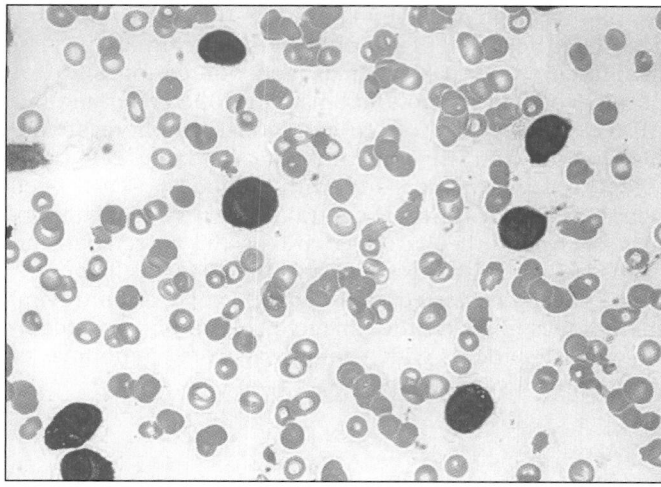

A

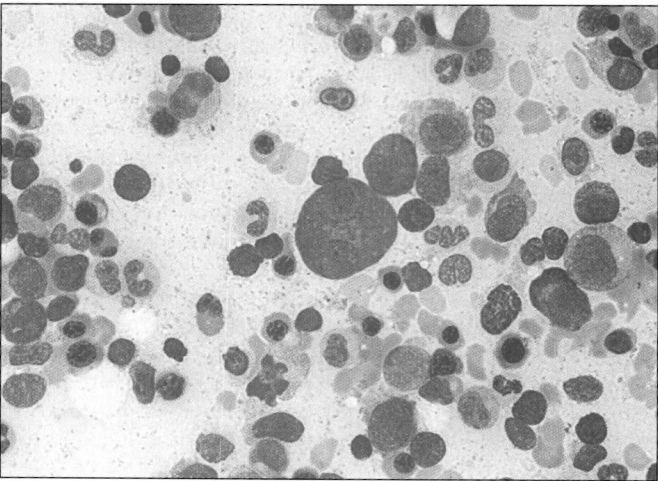

B

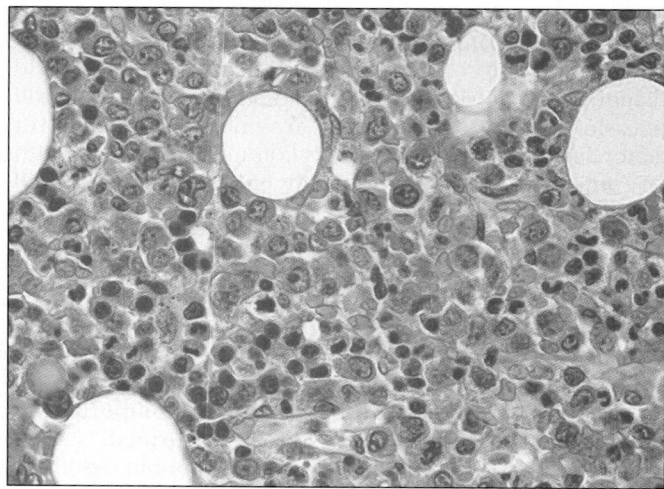

C

Figure 98-6. Plasma cell leukemia in an HIV patient. **A,** Peripheral blood smear. **B,** Aspirate. **C,** Bone marrow biopsy.

demonstrated in a sizable percentage of lymphomatous lesions in a San Francisco series.[96]

Staging of non-Hodgkin's lymphomas in AIDS patients requires that the brain be imaged, by magnetic resonance or computed tomography. In addition, in patients with EBV-positive tumors and in patients with Burkitt's, Burkitt-like, or immunoblastic lymphomas, a diagnostic lumbar puncture is indicated. An initial dose of prophylactic intrathecal chemotherapy (cytosine arabinoside or methotrexate) is often administered at the time of the diagnostic lumbar puncture.

Although brain lymphomas are common in patients with HIV, toxoplasmosis is the most common intracranial mass lesion.[97] Ring-enhancing unifocal or multifocal lesions are common in both diseases. Yet biopsy is sometimes associated with morbidity and even fatality, particularly in patients with lymphoma.[98] Thus, rather than prompt biopsy of suspicious lesions, empiric treatment for presumed toxoplasmosis is standard in seropositive patients. Biopsy is pursued only if a patient fails to respond to toxoplasmosis therapy or if there is evidence of progression over a 2-week therapeutic trial.

A variety of approaches to differentiate neoplastic and non-neoplastic lesions have been explored.[99-102] Positron emission tomography (PET) with ^{18}F-fluoro-2-deoxyglucose (FDG) has been able to accurately differentiate between lymphoma and infectious intracranial lesions in three studies.[103] Single-photon emission computed tomography (SPECT) with thallium-201 has generally identified patients with primary central lymphoma but has also occasionally mislabeled patients with infectious lesions.[104-106]

A nonradiographic approach to diagnosis of primary brain lymphoma involves the polymerase chain reaction (PCR) for EBV DNA in cerebrospinal fluid.[107,108] Although PCR will occasionally detect EBV DNA in cerebrospinal fluid, in other settings, such as acute infectious mononucleosis with neurologic manifestations, viral DNA is rarely detected in the cerebrospinal fluid of HIV patients without lymphoma.

Poor prognostic indicators for patients with AIDS and non-Hodgkin's lymphoma include absolute CD4+ T-cell count below 100/mL, age over 35 years, injection drug use, poor performance status, stage III or IV disease, elevated lactate dehydrogenase (LDH) level, and history of a previous AIDS-defining illness.[109,110] In the era of highly active antiretroviral therapy, the response to antiviral therapy has emerged as the most important prognostic factor.[78]

Therapy

Patients with HIV often have very aggressive, rapidly proliferating tumors. Attention to the possibility of tumor lysis syndrome with prompt assessment of renal function, serum electrolytes, and hyperuricemia is critical. Patients should always be started on allopurinol and aggressively hydrated, even before the staging evaluation is complete. Rapid assessment and treatment can be critically important in patients with aggressive lymphomas.

Before *Pneumocystis* prophylaxis and hematopoietic growth factors, lymphoma regimens in AIDS patients

TREATMENT OF NON-HODGKIN'S LYMPHOMA

Treatment is with standard dose CHOP: cyclophosphamide (750 mg/m^2), doxorubicin (75 mg/m^2), vincristine (1.5 mg/m^2), prednisone (100 mg/day for 5 days); repeated every 3 weeks. A maximum of six cycles is given. G-CSF is routinely prescribed. Dose adjustments are made for toxicity.

Patients with EBV-associated lymphoma, except Hodgkin's lymphoma, or with Burkitt's or Burkitt-like lymphoma receive intrathecal prophylaxis with 12 mg of methotrexate and 100 mg hydrocortisone administered five times during the first two cycles of systemic chemotherapy.

Patients with evidence of lymphomatous meningitis receive whole-brain radiation and intrathecal chemotherapy (three times per week until clear; the interval of treatments is then tapered to once a week for a month, then once a month for a total of 6 months).

were associated with a high treatment-related mortality rate.[111] A randomized trial of standard versus reduced dose therapies showed that reduced dose therapies did not compromise overall or disease-free survival but were associated with a decrease in the percentage of patients developing severe toxicities.[112] In profoundly immunocompromised patients, the antitumor effects of cytotoxic chemotherapy had to be balanced against associated myelosuppressive and immunosuppressive effects. With the advent of improved prophylaxis of opportunistic infections, highly effective antiretroviral therapy, and perhaps some change in the character of the tumors emerging in patients, the landscape has changed.

A first question addressed in the era of highly active antiretroviral therapy was the safety of the combination of antiretroviral therapy and cytotoxic chemotherapy. Data from retrospective series and from trials combining cytotoxic chemotherapy regimens with antiretroviral regimens have been published.[113,114] Although some interactions have been reported with altered clearance rates or serum concentrations of cyclophosphamide, doxorubicin, and indinavir, adverse interactions have been modest or negligible with the exception of regimens that include zidovudine. It is worth noting, however, that some of the protease inhibitors (e.g., ritonavir) are potent inhibitors of the P450 system and have not been carefully studied in combination with cytotoxic chemotherapeutic agents.

Infusional regimens have attracted a great deal of interest. Cyclophosphamide, doxorubicin, and etoposide (CDE) administered as a 96-hour infusion has yielded impressive results in single-institution and in multi-institution studies with and without highly active antiretroviral therapy.[113,115] A follow-up multi-institutional study investigated the use of infusional therapy in 107 patients. Patients treated with the infusional therapy and highly active antiretroviral therapy had a median overall survival time of almost 18 months, and those treated with the same therapy and only a single antiretroviral agent

(didanosine) had a median survival time of approximately 8 months. Combination of the regimen with rituximab yielded a complete response rate of 76% and a significant increase in overall survival (70% at 2 years).[116] A different continuous infusion regimen used in a single institution study also yielded impressive results.[91] Cyclophosphamide, doxorubicin, etoposide, vincristine, and prednisone (EPOCH) given by continuous infusion yielded a 92% disease-free survival time of 53 months. These survival outcomes represent a dramatic improvement over what was reported in cooperative group trials from before the highly active antiretroviral therapy era. Whether the improved survival reflects changing pathogenesis of lymphoma in HIV-infected patients, the importance of improved antiretroviral therapy following lymphoma therapy, the use of continuous infusion, or the particular choice of agents is not clear.

One of the complexities of infusional chemotherapy relates to possible metabolic interactions with antiretroviral agents. The possibility of important, possibly adverse, interactions led the investigators studying one of the infusional therapies to not initiate antiretroviral therapy until the conclusion of cytotoxic chemotherapy.[91] Viral load increased modestly during therapy. It plateaued between cycle 4 and cycle 6. At 3 months after starting or restarting antiretroviral therapy, viral loads declined to below baseline. There was no evidence that therapy led to the emergence of antiviral resistance. To the contrary, resistance mutations became transiently undetectable during therapy. CD4+ T cells decreased but recovered to baseline within 6 to 12 months. *Pneumocystis* prophylaxis should probably be administered to all patients undergoing intensive chemotherapy regardless of CD4+ T-cell count, whereas *Mycobacterium avium* complex prophylaxis is administered only to patients with CD4+ T-cell counts below 50/mm^3.[93]

Most patients with HIV infection and Hodgkin's lymphoma present with advanced-stage disease. Thus, combination chemotherapy is virtually always the mainstay of therapy. Doxorubicin (Adriamycin), bleomycin, vinblastine, and dacarbazine (ABVD) was studied by the AIDS Clinical Trials Group in the era before highly active antiretroviral therapy.[73]

A variety of salvage therapies have been evaluated, often with disappointing results.[94] ESHAP (etoposide, methylprednisolone, cisplatin, and high-dose cytarabine) chemotherapy is a commonly used regimen.[117] Increasingly, high-dose therapy with autologous peripheral stem cell transplantation is being used as consolidation.[118,119] Time to engraftment, infectious complications in the post-transplant period, and conditioning regimen complications are similar to those seen in patients without HIV infection. High-dose therapy with peripheral stem cell transplant is rapidly becoming established as the appropriate salvage for patients with chemotherapy-responsive relapse of either Hodgkin's or non-Hodgkin's lymphoma.

What should be regarded as "standard therapy" for AIDS lymphoma? Except in the most immunocompromised patients, standard dose lymphoma therapy including doxorubicin is appropriate. Among the choices that might

APPROACH TO AIDS PATIENTS WITH BRAIN LYMPHOMA

In the presence of characteristic lesion(s) on magnetic resonance imaging and thallium or PET studies, we accept detection of EBV DNA by PCR in spinal fluid as diagnostic of brain lymphoma. In instances in which lumbar puncture is contraindicated, brain biopsy is required for diagnosis. Patients are treated with radiation therapy.

be considered as standards are CHOP chemotherapy, CDE (cyclophosphamide, doxorubicin, etoposide) chemotherapy, and EPOCH chemotherapy. The benefits of rituximab in the treatment of AIDS-associated B-cell lymphomas have yet to be documented. A recent report from the AIDS Malignancy Consortium has suggested that there is reason for caution in this regard. The optimal integration of antiretroviral therapy with chemotherapy remains uncertain but long-term lymphoma-free survival can be achieved with concomitant or delayed antiretroviral therapy. Patients who relapse and are in good condition are appropriate candidates for salvage and may benefit from high-dose therapy with stem cell rescue or other aggressive interventions.

Radiation therapy has been the mainstay of treatment for brain lymphomas.[120] Retrospective studies show tumor responses, improvement in quality of life, and longer survival with treatment, but long-term survival is rare. Small series with high-dose methotrexate or ganciclovir and zidovudine have been reported.[121-123]

Other Malignancies in Patients with HIV Infection

With highly active antiretroviral therapy, the spectrum of malignancies in HIV-infected patients has been changing.[124] Non-AIDS-defining cancers have been reported with increased incidence, including those most common in the general population (lung cancer, colon cancer, skin cancers) as well as multiple myeloma and related plasma cell disorders, anal cancer, and cervical cancer. Lung and colon cancers may be indistinguishable from those appearing in the general population. Plasma cell dyscrasias in this population are quite distinctive, however. They are EBV-associated and often present with visceral or leukemic involvement.[125] Although cervical cancer has been recognized by the Centers for Disease Control as an AIDS-defining illness, an excess of cervical cancer attributable to HIV remains to be conclusively demonstrated.[92,126] However, some evidence suggests that HIV-infected women with cervical cancer are more likely to have advanced disease at presentation and to have a higher recurrence rate than non-HIV-infected women. Furthermore, cervical intraepithelial neoplasia occurs more frequently in women with HIV infection. Anal cancer occurs with a 40- to 80-fold excess in people with AIDS compared to the general population. Receptive anal intercourse is also a well-established risk factor for this cancer, and the relative contributions of HIV infection and

behavior have not been fully defined. Leiomyosarcomas in visceral organs occur with dramatically increased frequency in patients with HIV infection, particularly pediatric patients, but remain rare. The approach to treatment of these disorders does not differ from that in the non-HIV-infected population or has yet to be defined, although, clearly, cognizance of the special risks associated with chemotherapy is important.

THE EMERGING IMPORTANCE OF AIDS ONCOLOGY

With an improved prognosis for patients with HIV infection as a result of advances in supportive care and antiretroviral therapy, the neoplastic complications of HIV infection grow in importance. In the early days of the epidemic, the treatment of malignancies with curative intent might have been regarded as only marginally important in patients who were otherwise doomed to a short survival by virtue of their retroviral infection. However, for an increasing number of patients, HIV infection is most appropriately viewed as a chronic disease that requires a collaborative and multidisciplinary effort on the part of primary care and subspecialty providers, and the nihilism of the past should be replaced by a cautious optimism. It is now clear that durable remissions will translate into long-term survival in patients whose HIV load can be suppressed to very low or undetectable levels. The challenge that remains is to further develop specific therapies for HIV-associated malignancies and to integrate these approaches with the growing armamentarium of antiretroviral therapies.

REFERENCES

1. Gottlieb MS, Schroff R, Schanker HM, et al: *Pneumocystis carinii* pneumonia and mucosal candidiasis in previously healthy homosexual men: Evidence of a new acquired cellular immunodeficiency. N Engl J Med 1981;305:1425–1431.
2. Barre-Sinoussi F, Chermann JC, Rey F, et al: Isolation of a T-lymphotropic retrovirus from a patient at risk for acquired immune deficiency syndrome (AIDS). Science 1983;220:868–871.
3. UNAIDS/WHO: AIDS epidemic update 2002.
4. Sepkowitz KA: AIDS—The first 20 years. N Engl J Med 2001;344:1764–1772.
5. Gerberding JL: Clinical practice. Occupational exposure to HIV in health care settings. N Engl J Med 2003;348:826–833.
6. Bartlett J: The Johns Hopkins Hospital 2002 Guide to Medical Care of Patients with HIV Infection, 10th ed. Philadelphia, Lippincott Williams & Wilkins, 2001.
7. Kaplan JE, Masur H, Holmes KK: Guidelines for preventing opportunistic infections among HIV-infected persons—2002. Recommendations of the U.S. Public Health Service and the Infectious Diseases Society of America. MMWR Recomm Rep 2002;51:1–52.
8. Thorner A, Rosenberg E: Early versus delayed antiretroviral therapy in patients with HIV infection: A review of the current guidelines from an immunological perspective. Drugs 2003;63:1325–1337.
9. Trotta MP, Ammassari A, Melzi S, et al: Treatment-related factors and highly active antiretroviral therapy adherence. J Acquir Immune Defic Syndr 2002;31(Suppl 3):S128–S131.
10. Dybul M, Fauci AS, Bartlett JG, et al: Guidelines for using antiretroviral agents among HIV-infected adults and adolescents. Ann Intern Med 2002;137:381–433.

11. Steinbrook R: HIV infection—A new drug and new costs. N Engl J Med 2002;348:2171–2172.

12. Tashima KT, Carpenter CC: Fusion inhibition—A major but costly step forward in the treatment of HIV-1. N Engl J Med 2003;348: 2249–2250.

13. Moore PS: The emergence of Kaposi's sarcoma-associated herpesvirus (human herpesvirus 8). N Engl J Med 2000;343: 1411–1413.

14. Dal Maso L, Serraino D, Franceschi S: Epidemiology of AIDS-related tumours in developed and developing countries. Eur J Cancer 2001;37:1188–1201.

15. Grulich AE, Li Y, McDonald AM, et al: Decreasing rates of Kaposi's sarcoma and non-Hodgkin's lymphoma in the era of potent combination anti-retroviral therapy. AIDS 2001;15:629–633.

16. Carrieri MP, Pradier C, Piselli P, et al: Reduced incidence of Kaposi's sarcoma and of systemic non-Hodgkin's lymphoma in HIV-infected individuals treated with highly active antiretroviral therapy. Int J Cancer 2003;103:142–144.

17. Moore PS: Transplanting cancer: Donor-cell transmission of Kaposi sarcoma. Nat Med 2003;9:506–508.

18. Jacobson LP, Jenkins FJ, Springer G, et al: Interaction of human immunodeficiency virus type 1 and human herpesvirus type 8 infections on the incidence of Kaposi's sarcoma. J Infect Dis 2000;181:1940–1949.

19. Safai B: Kaposi's sarcoma and acquired immunodeficiency syndrome. In DeVita Jr VT, Hellman S, Rosenberg SA (eds): AIDS: Etiology, Diagnosis, Treatment and Prevention. Philadelphia, Lippincott-Raven, 1997, p 295.

20. Dupin N, Fisher C, Kellam P, et al: Distribution of human herpesvirus-8 latently infected cells in Kaposi's sarcoma, multicentric Castleman's disease, and primary effusion lymphoma. Proc Natl Acad Sci USA 1999;96:4546–4551.

21. Antman K, Chang Y: Kaposi's sarcoma. N Engl J Med 2000;342:1027–1038.

22. Kahn HJ, Bailey D, Marks A: Monoclonal antibody D2-40, a new marker of lymphatic endothelium, reacts with Kaposi's sarcoma and a subset of angiosarcomas. Mod Pathol 2002;15: 434–440.

23. Barozzi P, Luppi M, Facchetti F, et al: Post-transplant Kaposi sarcoma originates from the seeding of donor-derived progenitors. Nat Med 2003;9:554–561.

24. Rabkin CS, Janz S, Lash A, et al: Monoclonal origin of multicentric Kaposi's sarcoma lesions. N Engl J Med 1997;336:988–993.

25. Gill PS, Tsai YC, Rao AP, et al: Evidence for multiclonality in multicentric Kaposi's sarcoma. Proc Natl Acad Sci USA 1998;95: 8257–8261.

26. Hayward GS: Human herpesvirus 8 latent-state gene expression and apoptosis in Kaposi's sarcoma lesions. J Natl Cancer Inst 1999;91:1705–1707.

27. Cannon JS, Nicholas J, Orenstein JM, et al: Heterogeneity of viral IL-6 expression in HHV-8-associated diseases. J Infect Dis 1999;180:824–828.

28. Moore PS, Chang Y: Molecular virology of Kaposi's sarcoma-associated herpesvirus. Philos Trans R Soc Lond B Biol Sci 2001;356:499–516.

29. Masood R, Cesarman E, Smith DL, et al: Human herpesvirus-8-transformed endothelial cells have functionally activated vascular endothelial growth factor/vascular endothelial growth factor receptor. Am J Pathol 2002;160:23–29.

30. Chatterjee M, Osborne J, Bestetti G, et al: Viral IL-6-induced cell proliferation and immune evasion of interferon activity. Science 2002;298:1432–1435.

31. Means RE, Ishido S, Alvarez X, et al: Multiple endocytic trafficking pathways of MHC class I molecules induced by a herpesvirus protein. Embo J 2002;21:1638–1649.

32. Paulson E, Tran C, Collins K, et al: KSHV-K5 inhibits phosphorylation of the major histocompatibility complex class I cytoplasmic tail. Virology 2002;288:369–378.

33. Ishido S, Choi JK, Lee BS, et al: Inhibition of natural killer cell-mediated cytotoxicity by Kaposi's sarcoma-associated herpesvirus K5 protein. Immunity 2000;13:365–374.

34. Mortreux F, Gabet AS, Wattel E: Molecular and cellular aspects of HTLV-1 associated leukemogenesis in vivo. Leukemia 2003;17:26–38.

35. Ariyoshi K, Schim van der Loeff M, Cook P, et al: Kaposi's sarcoma in the Gambia, West Africa is less frequent in human immunodeficiency virus type 2 than in human immunodeficiency virus type 1 infection despite a high prevalence of human herpesvirus 8. J Hum Virol 1998;1:193–199.

36. Krown SE: Clinical overview: Issues in Kaposi's sarcoma therapeutics. J Natl Cancer Inst Monogr 1998;23:59–63.

37. Koehler JE: Bartonella-associated infections in HIV-infected patients. AIDS Clin Care 1995;7:97–102.

38. Krown SE, Testa MA, Huang J: AIDS-related Kaposi's sarcoma: Prospective validation of the AIDS Clinical Trials Group staging classification. AIDS Clinical Trials Group Oncology Committee. J Clin Oncol 1997;15:3085–3092.

39. Gill J, Bourboulia D, Wilkinson J, et al: Prospective study of the effects of antiretroviral therapy on Kaposi sarcoma–associated herpesvirus infection in patients with and without Kaposi sarcoma. J Acquir Immune Defic Syndr 2002;31:384–390.

40. Cannon MJ, Dollard SC, Black JB, et al: Risk factors for Kaposi's sarcoma in men seropositive for both human herpesvirus 8 and human immunodeficiency virus. AIDS 2003;17:215–222.

41. Nunez M, Saballs P, Valencia ME, et al: Response to liposomal doxorubicin and clinical outcome of HIV-1-infected patients with Kaposi's sarcoma receiving highly active antiretroviral therapy. HIV Clin Trials 2001;2:429–437.

42. Tam HK, Zhang ZF, Jacobson LP, et al: Effect of highly active antiretroviral therapy on survival among HIV-infected men with Kaposi sarcoma or non-Hodgkin lymphoma. Int J Cancer 2002;98:916–922.

43. Holkova B, Takeshita K, Cheng DM, et al: Effect of highly active antiretroviral therapy on survival in patients with AIDS-associated pulmonary Kaposi's sarcoma treated with chemotherapy. J Clin Oncol 2001;19:3848–3851.

44. Pati S, Pelser CB, Dufraine J, et al: Antitumorigenic effects of HIV protease inhibitor ritonavir: Inhibition of Kaposi sarcoma. Blood 2002;99:3771–3779.

45. Sgadari C, Barillari G, Toschi E, et al: HIV protease inhibitors are potent anti-angiogenic molecules and promote regression of Kaposi sarcoma. Nat Med 2002;8:225–232.

46. Krown SE, Li P, Von Roenn JH, et al: Efficacy of low-dose interferon with antiretroviral therapy in Kaposi's sarcoma: A randomized phase II AIDS clinical trials group study. J Interferon Cytokine Res 2002;22:295–303.

47. Krown SE: Interferon and other biologic agents for the treatment of Kaposi's sarcoma. Hematol Oncol Clin North Am 1991;5: 311–322.

48. Krown SE, Gold JW, Niedzwiecki D, et al: Interferon-alpha with zidovudine: Safety, tolerance, and clinical and virologic effects in patients with Kaposi sarcoma associated with the acquired immunodeficiency syndrome (AIDS). Ann Intern Med 1990;112:812–821.

49. Sharpe M, Easthope SE, Keating GM, et al: Polyethylene glycol-liposomal doxorubicin: A review of its use in the management of solid and haematological malignancies and AIDS-related Kaposi's sarcoma. Drugs 2002;62:2089–2126.

50. Northfelt DW, Dezube BJ, Thommes JA, et al: Pegylated-liposomal doxorubicin versus doxorubicin, bleomycin, and vincristine in the treatment of AIDS-related Kaposi's sarcoma: Results of a randomized phase III clinical trial. J Clin Oncol 1998;16: 2445–2451.

51. Stewart S, Jablonowski H, Goebel FD, et al: Randomized comparative trial of pegylated liposomal doxorubicin versus bleomycin and vincristine in the treatment of AIDS-related Kaposi's sarcoma. International Pegylated Liposomal Doxorubicin Study Group. J Clin Oncol 1998;16:683–691.

52. Gordon KB, Tajuddin A, Guitart J, et al: Hand-foot syndrome associated with liposome-encapsulated doxorubicin therapy. Cancer 1995;75:2169–2173.

53. Welles L, Saville MW, Lietzau J, et al: Phase II trial with dose titration of paclitaxel for the therapy of human immunodeficiency virus-associated Kaposi's sarcoma. J Clin Oncol 1998;16: 1112–1121.

54. Saville MW, Lietzau J, Pluda JM, et al: Treatment of HIV-associated Kaposi's sarcoma with paclitaxel. Lancet 1995;346:26–28.

55. Tulpule A, Groopman J, Saville MW, et al: Multicenter trial of low-dose paclitaxel in patients with advanced AIDS-related Kaposi sarcoma. Cancer 2002;95:147–154.

56. Krown SE: Management of Kaposi sarcoma: The role of interferon and thalidomide. Curr Opin Oncol 2001;13:374–381.

57. Levine AM, Tulpule A: Clinical aspects and management of AIDS-related Kaposi's sarcoma. Eur J Cancer 2001;37:1288–1295.

58. Fife K, Howard MR, Gracie F, et al: Activity of thalidomide in AIDS-related Kaposi's sarcoma and correlation with HHV8 titre. Int J STD AIDS 1998;9:751–755.

59. Little RF, Wyvill KM, Pluda JM, et al: Activity of thalidomide in AIDS-related Kaposi's sarcoma. J Clin Oncol 2000;18:2593–2602.

60. Miles SA, Dezube BJ, Lee JY, et al: Antitumor activity of oral 9-cis-retinoic acid in HIV-associated Kaposi's sarcoma. AIDS 2002;16:421–429.

61. Flaitz CM, Nichols CM, Hicks MJ: Role of intralesional vinblastine administration in treatment of intraoral Kaposi's sarcoma in AIDS. Eur J Cancer B Oral Oncol 1995;31B:280–285.

62. Ramirez-Amador V, Esquivel-Pedraza L, Lozada-Nur F, et al: Intralesional vinblastine vs. 3% sodium tetradecyl sulfate for the treatment of oral Kaposi's sarcoma. A double blind, randomized clinical trial. Oral Oncol 2002;38:460–467.

63. Webster GF: Local therapy for mucocutaneous Kaposi's sarcoma in patients with acquired immunodeficiency syndrome. Dermatol Surg 1995;21:205–208.

64. Kirova YM, Belembaogo E, Frikha H, et al: Radiotherapy in the management of epidemic Kaposi's sarcoma: A retrospective study of 643 cases. Radiother Oncol 1998;46:19–22.

65. Meyer JL: Whole-lung irradiation for Kaposi's sarcoma. Am J Clin Oncol 1993;16:372–376.

66. Stelzer KJ, Griffin TW: A randomized prospective trial of radiation therapy for AIDS-associated Kaposi's sarcoma. Int J Radiat Oncol Biol Phys 1993;27:1057–1061.

67. Mocroft A, Youle M, Gazzard B, et al: Anti-herpesvirus treatment and risk of Kaposi's sarcoma in HIV infection. Royal Free/Chelsea and Westminster Hospitals Collaborative Group. AIDS 1996;10:1101–1105.

68. Glesby MJ, Hoover DR, Weng S, et al: Use of antiherpes drugs and the risk of Kaposi's sarcoma: Data from the Multicenter AIDS Cohort Study. J Infect Dis 1996;173:1477–1480.

69. Jones JL, Hanson DL, Chu SY, et al: AIDS-associated Kaposi's sarcoma. Science 1995;267:1078–1079.

70. Cote TR, Biggar RJ, Rosenberg PS, et al: Non-Hodgkin's lymphoma among people with AIDS: Incidence, presentation and public health burden. AIDS/Cancer Study Group. Int J Cancer 1997;73:645–650.

71. Cote TR, Manns A, Hardy CR, et al: Epidemiology of brain lymphoma among people with or without acquired immunodeficiency syndrome. AIDS/Cancer Study Group. J Natl Cancer Inst 1996;88:675–679.

72. Goedert JJ, Cote TR, Virgo P, et al: Spectrum of AIDS-associated malignant disorders. Lancet 1998;351:1833–1839.

73. Levine AM, Li P, Cheung T, et al: Chemotherapy consisting of doxorubicin, bleomycin, vinblastine, and dacarbazine with granulocyte-colony-stimulating factor in HIV-infected patients with newly diagnosed Hodgkin's disease: A prospective, multi-institutional AIDS clinical trials group study (ACTG 149). J Acquir Immune Defic Syndr 2000;24:444–450.

74. Levine AM: Hodgkin's disease in the setting of human immunodeficiency virus infection. J Natl Cancer Inst Monogr 1998;95:37–42.

75. Sparano JA, Anand K, Desai J, et al: Effect of highly active antiretroviral therapy on the incidence of HIV-associated malignancies at an urban medical center. J Acquir Immune Defic Syndr 1999;21(Suppl 1):S18–S22.

76. Besson C, Goubar A, Gabarre J, et al: Changes in AIDS-related lymphoma since the era of highly active antiretroviral therapy. Blood 2001;98:2339–2344.

77. Kirk O, Pedersen C, Cozzi-Lepri A, et al: Non-Hodgkin's lymphoma in HIV-infected patients in the era of highly active antiretroviral therapy. Blood 2001;98:3406–3412.

78. Hoffmann C, Wolf E, Fatkenheuer G, et al: Response to highly active antiretroviral therapy strongly predicts outcome in patients with AIDS-related lymphoma. AIDS 2003;17:1521–1529.

79. Knowles DM, Pirog EC: Pathology of AIDS-related lymphomas and other AIDS-defining neoplasms. Eur J Cancer 2001;37:1236–1250.

80. Nador RG, Chadburn A, Gundappa G, et al: Human immunodeficiency virus (HIV)-associated polymorphic lymphoproliferative disorders. Am J Surg Pathol 2003;27:293–302.

81. Spina M, Vaccher E, Nasti G, et al: Human immunodeficiency virus-associated Hodgkin's disease. Semin Oncol 2000;27:480–488.

82. Siebert JD, Ambinder RF, Napoli VM, et al: Human immunodeficiency virus-associated Hodgkin's disease contains latent, not replicative, Epstein-Barr virus. Hum Pathol 1995;26:1191–1195.

83. Tirelli U, Errante D, Dolcetti R, et al: Hodgkin's disease and human immunodeficiency virus infection: Clinicopathologic and virologic features of 114 patients from the Italian Cooperative Group on AIDS and Tumors. J Clin Oncol 1995;13:1758–1767.

84. Ambinder RF: Epstein-Barr virus associated lymphoproliferations in the AIDS setting. Eur J Cancer 2001;37:1209–1216.

85. MacMahon EM, Glass JD, Hayward SD, et al: Epstein-Barr virus in AIDS-related primary central nervous system lymphoma. Lancet 1991;338:969–973.

86. Carbone A: AIDS-related non-Hodgkin's lymphomas: From pathology and molecular pathogenesis to treatment. Hum Pathol 2002;33:392–404.

87. Anthony IC, Crawford DH, Bell JE: B lymphocytes in the normal brain: Contrasts with HIV-associated lymphoid infiltrates and lymphomas. Brain 2003;126:1058–1067.

88. Camilleri-Broet S, Davi F, Feuillard J, et al: AIDS-related primary brain lymphomas: Histopathologic and immunohistochemical study of 51 cases. The French Study Group for HIV-Associated Tumors. Hum Pathol 1997;28:367–374.

89. Cingolani A, Gastaldi R, Fassone L, et al: Epstein-Barr virus infection is predictive of CNS involvement in systemic AIDS-related non-Hodgkin's lymphomas. J Clin Oncol 2000;18:3325–3330.

90. Roithmann S, Toledano M, Tourani JM, et al: HIV-associated non-Hodgkin's lymphomas: Clinical characteristics and outcome. The experience of the French Registry of HIV-associated tumors. Ann Oncol 1991;2:289–295.

91. Little RF, Pittaluga S, Grant N, et al: Highly effective treatment of acquired immunodeficiency syndrome-related lymphoma with dose-adjusted EPOCH: impact of antiretroviral therapy suspension and tumor biology. Blood 2003;101:4653–4659.

92. Gates AE, Kaplan LD: AIDS malignancies in the era of highly active antiretroviral therapy. Oncology (Huntingt) 2002;16:441–451, 456, 459.

93. Gates AE, Kaplan LD: AIDS malignancies in the era of highly active antiretroviral therapy. Oncology (Huntingt) 2002;16:657–665; discussion 665, 668–670.

94. Levine AM, Scadden DT, Zaia JA, et al: Hematologic aspects of HIV/AIDS. Hematology (Am Soc Hematol Educ Program) 2001;463–478.

95. Sparano JA: Clinical aspects and management of AIDS-related lymphoma. Eur J Cancer 2001;37:1296–1305.

96. Kaplan LD, Shiramizu B, Herndier B, et al: Influence of molecular characteristics on clinical outcome in human immunodeficiency virus-associated non-Hodgkin's lymphoma: Identification of a subgroup with favorable clinical outcome. Blood 1995;85:1727–1735.

97. Sacktor N, Lyles RH, Skolasky R, et al: HIV-associated neurologic disease incidence changes: Multicenter AIDS Cohort Study, 1990–1998. Neurology 2001;56:257–260.

98. Skolasky RL, Dal Pan GJ, Olivi A, et al: HIV-associated primary CNS lymphoma: Morbidity and utility of brain biopsy. J Neurol Sci 1999;163:32–38.

99. Pomper MG, Constantinides CD, Barker PB, et al: Quantitative MR spectroscopic imaging of brain lesions in patients with AIDS: Correlation with [11C-methyl]thymidine PET and thallium-201 SPECT. Acad Radiol 2002;9:398–409.

100. Heald AE, Hoffman JM, Bartlett JA, et al: Differentiation of central nervous system lesions in AIDS patients using positron emission tomography (PET). Int J STD AIDS 1996;7:337–346.

101. Lorberboym M, Estok L, Machac J, et al: Rapid differential diagnosis of cerebral toxoplasmosis and primary central nervous system lymphoma by thallium-201 SPECT. J Nucl Med 1996;37:1150–1154.

102. Gianotti N, Marenzi R, Messa C, et al: Thallium-201 single photon emission computed tomography in the management of contrast-enhancing brain lesions in a patient with AIDS. Clin Infect Dis 1996;23:185–186.

103. Miller RF, Hall-Craggs MA, Costa DC, et al: Magnetic resonance imaging, thallium-201 SPET scanning, and laboratory analyses for discrimination of cerebral lymphoma and toxoplasmosis in AIDS. Sex Transmit Infect 1998;74:258–264.

104. Licho R, Litofsky NS, Senitko M, et al: Inaccuracy of Tl-201 brain SPECT in distinguishing cerebral infections from lymphoma in patients with AIDS. Clin Nucl Med 2002;27:81–86.

105. Skiest DJ, Erdman W, Chang WE, et al: SPECT thallium-201 combined with *Toxoplasma* serology for the presumptive diagnosis of focal central nervous system mass lesions in patients with AIDS. J Infect 2000;40:274–281.

106. Berger JR: Mass Lesions of the Brain in AIDS: The Dilemmas of Distinguishing Toxoplasmosis from Primary CNS Lymphoma. Am J Neuroradiol 2003;24:554–555.

107. Bossolasco S, Cinque P, Ponzoni M, et al: Epstein-Barr virus DNA load in cerebrospinal fluid and plasma of patients with AIDS-related lymphoma. J Neurovirol 2002;8:432–438.

108. Cingolani A, De Luca A, Larocca LM, et al: Minimally invasive diagnosis of acquired immunodeficiency syndrome-related primary central nervous system lymphoma. J Natl Cancer Inst 1998;90:364–369.

109. Gisselbrecht C, Oksenhendler E, Tirelli U, et al: Human immunodeficiency virus–related lymphoma treatment with intensive combination chemotherapy. French-Italian Cooperative Group. Am J Med 1993;95:188–196.

110. Vaccher E, Tirelli U, Spina M, et al: Age and serum lactate dehydrogenase level are independent prognostic factors in human immunodeficiency virus–related non-Hodgkin's lymphomas: A single-institute study of 96 patients. J Clin Oncol 1996;14:2217–2223.

111. Gill PS, Levine AM, Krailo M, et al: AIDS-related malignant lymphoma: Results of prospective treatment trials. J Clin Oncol 1987;5:1322–1328.

112. Kaplan LD, Straus DJ, Testa MA, et al: Low-dose compared with standard-dose m-BACOD chemotherapy for non-Hodgkin's lymphoma associated with human immunodeficiency virus infection. National Institute of Allergy and Infectious Diseases AIDS Clinical Trials Group. N Engl J Med 1997;336:1641–1648.

113. Sparano JA, Wiernik PH, Hu X, et al: Pilot trial of infusional cyclophosphamide, doxorubicin, and etoposide plus didanosine and filgrastim in patients with human immunodeficiency virus–associated non-Hodgkin's lymphoma. J Clin Oncol 1996;14: 3026–3035.

114. Ratner L, Lee J, Tang S, et al: Chemotherapy for human immunodeficiency virus–associated non-Hodgkin's lymphoma in combination with highly active antiretroviral therapy. J Clin Oncol 2001;19:2171–2178.

115. Sparano JA, Wiernik PH, Strack M, et al: Infusional cyclophosphamide, doxorubicin, and etoposide in human immunodeficiency virus and human T-cell leukemia virus type I-related non-Hodgkin's lymphoma: A highly active regimen. Blood 1993;81:2810–2815.

116. Spina M, Sparano JA, Jaeger U, et al: Rituximab and chemotherapy is highly effective in patients with CD20-positive non-Hodgkin's lymphoma and HIV infection. AIDS 2003;17:137–138.

117. Bi J, Espina BM, Tulpule A, et al: High-dose cytosine-arabinoside and cisplatin regimens as salvage therapy for refractory or relapsed AIDS-related non-Hodgkin's lymphoma. J Acquir Immune Defic Syndr 2001;28:416–421.

118. Krishnan A, Zaia J, Molina A: Stem cell transplantation and gene therapy for HIV-related lymphomas. J Hematother Stem Cell Res 2002;11:765–775.

119. Krishnan A, Molina A, Zaia J, et al: Autologous stem cell transplantation for HIV-associated lymphoma. Blood 2001;98: 3857–3859.

120. Donahue BR, Sullivan JW, Cooper JS: Additional experience with empiric radiotherapy for presumed human immunodeficiency virus–associated primary central nervous system lymphoma. Cancer 1995;76:328–332.

121. Raez L, Cabral L, Cai JP, et al: Treatment of AIDS-related primary central nervous system lymphoma with zidovudine, ganciclovir, and interleukin 2. AIDS Res Hum Retroviruses 1999;15:713–719.

122. Alfandari S, Bourez JM, Senneville E, et al: Methotrexate for suspected cerebral lymphoma in AIDS. AIDS 1998;12:1246–1247.

123. Jacomet C, Girard PM, Lebrette MG, et al: Intravenous methotrexate for primary central nervous system non-Hodgkin's lymphoma in AIDS. AIDS 1997;11:1725–1730.

124. Grulich AE, Li Y, McDonald A, et al: Rates of non-AIDS-defining cancers in people with HIV infection before and after AIDS diagnosis. AIDS 2002;16:1155–1161.

125. Carraway H, Ambinder RF: Plasma cell dyscrasia, Hodgkin lymphoma, HIV, and Kaposi sarcoma–associated herpesvirus. Curr Opin Oncol 2002;14:543–545.

126. Frisch M, Smith E, Grulich A, et al: Cancer in a population-based cohort of men and women in registered homosexual partnerships. Am J Epidemiol 2003;157:966–972.

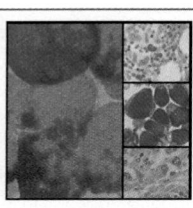

PEDIATRIC SOLID TUMORS

Jeffrey S. Dome

Carlos Rodriguez–Galindo

Sheri L. Spunt

Victor M. Santana

SUMMARY OF KEY POINTS

OSTEOSARCOMA

Incidence
- Four new cases per 1 million persons per year among children younger than 15 years.
- Most common bone tumor in children and adolescents.

Differential Diagnosis
- Other lytic bone lesions, including eosinophilic granuloma and giant cell tumor, must be excluded.
- At pathologic examination, tumors must be differentiated from fibrosarcoma and chondrosarcoma.

Staging Evaluation
Staging always should include complete history and physical examination, complete blood cell count (CBC), serum chemical analysis (including alkaline phosphatase), and imaging studies of the primary tumor and chest.

Primary Therapy
- The primary tumor is managed surgically with a limb-sparing operation or amputation.
- Adjuvant chemotherapy incorporating high-dose methotrexate is used preoperatively to manage presumed micrometastatic disease and to guide further therapy.
- Methotrexate responders have a more than an 80% chance of cure.
- Primary pulmonary metastatic disease is managed surgically, although adjuvant chemotherapy may reduce the extent of resection.

Effective Second-Line Therapy
- Pulmonary metastatic disease is managed surgically.
- Post-thoracotomy adjuvant chemotherapy is of unproven benefit.
- Local recurrence is managed surgically.
- Further adjuvant chemotherapy with non–cross-resistant agents is of uncertain benefit.

EWING'S SARCOMA FAMILY TUMORS

Incidence
- The incidence of Ewing's sarcoma family tumors is 2.8 new cases per 1 million persons per year among children younger than 15 years.
- Ewing's sarcoma is the second most common bone tumor among children and adolescents.

Differential Diagnosis
- Rule out osteomyelitis, especially when the patient has a fever.
- Lesions to be excluded include benign tumors of bone that manifest as lytic lesions (e.g., eosinophilic granuloma and giant cell tumor), malignant tumors (e.g., osteosarcoma, primary lymphoma of bone), and metastatic lesions from a nonosseous tumor (e.g., neuroblastoma).

Staging Evaluation
Staging always should include a complete history and physical examination, CBC, serum chemical analysis (including lactate dehydrogenase), bone marrow biopsy, and imaging studies of the primary tumor, bones, and chest.

Primary Therapy
- Always use multimodal therapy consisting of chemotherapy, radiation therapy, surgery, or a combination of these treatments.
- Specific local treatment depends on the primary site. Consider surgical extirpation in expendable bones (proximal part of the fibula, rib, clavicle, iliac wing).
- Unresectable tumors generally necessitate a combined approach of chemotherapy, radiation therapy, and surgery.
- Localized disease is curable with combined therapy in more than 70% of cases. Metastatic disease is curable in 30% to 40% of cases.

Effective Second-Line Therapy
- Effective second-line therapy has not been established.
- Local recurrence may be amenable to surgical extirpation.

NEUROBLASTOMA

Incidence
- Among white children younger than 15 years, 10.5 new cases occur per 1 million persons per year. Among black children the incidence is 8.8 new cases per 1 million persons per year.
- Neuroblastoma is the most common extracranial solid tumor in children.

Differential Diagnosis
- Disseminated bone disease can resemble systemic infection, inflammatory disease, osteomyelitis, or rheumatoid arthritis.
- Paraneoplastic syndromes associated with neuroblastoma (vasoactive intestinal peptide syndrome, opsoclonus-myoclonus-ataxia syndrome) must be differentiated from primary inflammatory bowel disease and neurologic disease.
- Neuroblastoma must be differentiated from other small round blue cell neoplasms of childhood (e.g., Ewing's sarcoma, primitive neuroectodermal tumor, non-Hodgkin's lymphoma, and undifferentiated soft-tissue sarcoma).
- In as many as 10% of tumors, catecholamines are not produced. In 1%, the absence of an obvious primary lesion confounds the diagnosis.

Staging Evaluation
Staging always should include a complete history and physical examination, CBC, serum chemical analysis (e.g., lactate dehydrogenase), quantitative urine catecholamines, bone marrow examination, skeletal

scintigraphy, and imaging studies of the primary tumor and chest.

Primary Therapy
- Specific treatment depends on stage, age, and biologic features of the tumor.
- With few exceptions (completely resected primary tumor, infants with stable stage 4S disease), multiple-agent chemotherapy is the backbone of multimodality treatment.
- Survival depends on stage and biologic features (e.g., tumor histopathology and *MYCN* gene amplification).
- The overall survival rate for stage I tumors is 90%; for stage 2A tumors, the survival rate is greater than 80%.
- Overall survival among patients with advanced-stage disease is poor. Sixty percent of children with stages 2B and 3 tumors live, and fewer than 15% with metastatic disease are long-term survivors.

Effective Second-Line Therapy
No second-line therapy has proved beneficial.

WILMS' TUMOR

Incidence
Eight cases per 1 million persons per year among children younger than 15 years

Etiology/Epidemiology
- Mean age at diagnosis is 44 months for unilateral tumors and 31 months for bilateral tumors.
- Familial cases account for 1.5% of cases of Wilms' tumor.
- Associated with Wilms' tumor are aniridia, genitourinary anomaly, mental retardation (WAGR syndrome), Denys-Drash syndrome, and Beckwith-Wiedemann syndrome.
- No firmly established environmental factors have been identified.

Pathology/Biology
- The main histologic subtypes are favorable and anaplastic.
- Implicated genes and loci include WT1 (11p13), WT2 (11p15), FWT1 (17q12-q21), FWT2 (19p13), and chromosomes 1p, 16q, and 7p.

- Mutations of the p53 gene are associated with anaplastic tumors.

Clinical Findings
An asymptomatic abdominal mass is found in most patients, as are abdominal pain, hematuria, hypertension, congenital anomalies (genitourinary malformations, aniridia, and hemihypertrophy).

Differential Diagnosis
- Neuroblastoma.
- Renal neoplasms (clear cell sarcoma, rhabdoid tumor, congenital mesoblastic nephroma, renal cell carcinoma).
- Benign renal processes (nephrogenic rests, multicystic or polycystic kidneys, hydronephrosis, renal carbuncles, hemorrhage).

Staging Evaluation
- Complete history and physical examination with careful attention to blood pressure and associated congenital anomalies.
- CBC, serum chemical analysis, urinalysis, abdominal ultrasonography or computed tomography (CT), chest radiography with or without chest CT.

Primary Therapy
- Surgery: Surgical resection of tumor, usually before chemotherapy in North America.
- Chemotherapy: Stages I and II favorable histology—vincristine and actinomycin D; stages III and IV favorable histology, stage I anaplastic histology—vincristine, doxorubicin, actinomycin D; stages II through IV anaplastic histology—vincristine, cyclophosphamide, doxorubicin, carboplatin, etoposide.
- Radiation therapy: Stages III and IV favorable histology and stages I through IV anaplastic histology.

Salvage Therapy
- Recurrent disease is effectively managed with radiation therapy and chemotherapeutic agents not administered during initial treatment.
- Patients initially treated aggressively may respond to ifosfamide, carboplatin, and etoposide-based regimens.

Complications
Renal failure (<1%), congestive heart failure in patients who receive doxorubicin (4.4%), pregnancy-related complications in girls who receive flank irradiation, and second malignant neoplasm (1.6%)

Prognosis
- Favorable histology: 85% 4-year relapse-free survival, 90% 4-year overall survival rate.
- Anaplastic histology: 50% 4-year relapse-free survival, 50% 4-year overall survival rate.

RENAL CELL CARCINOMA

Incidence
- Four cases per 10 million persons per year among children younger than 20 years of age.
- Median age at diagnosis is 9 years.

Differential Diagnosis
Typical presentation includes an abdominal mass, hematuria, pain, and rarely polycythemia.

Staging Evaluation
Complete history and physical examination; complete blood cell count; serum chemical analysis; imaging studies of abdomen, pelvis, and chest.

Primary Therapy
- Nephrectomy of the involved kidney.
- For metastatic disease, interleukin-2 or interferon-alpha–based therapy is recommended.

RHABDOMYOSARCOMA

Incidence
- Among children younger than 20 years, 4.3 new cases occur per 1 million persons per year.
- Rhabdomyosarcoma is the most common soft-tissue sarcoma among children and adolescents.

Differential Diagnosis
- Other benign and malignant soft-tissue tumors must be excluded.
- At pathologic examination rhabdomyosarcoma must be differentiated from the other small round blue cell tumors of childhood (e.g., Ewing's sarcoma, neuroblastoma, non-Hodgkin's lymphoma).

Staging Evaluation
Staging always should include a thorough history and physical examination; CBC; serum chemical analysis; imaging studies of the primary tumor, regional lymph nodes, and lungs; bone scintigraphy; and bone marrow examination.

Primary Therapy
- Primary therapy is chemotherapy with surgery, radiation therapy, or both. Specific treatment depends on age, primary site, histologic subtype, and extent of disease.
- Mutilating surgery must be avoided because the tumor is sensitive to both chemotherapy and radiation therapy.
- Overall survival exceeds 70% but depends on extent of disease. More than 90% of patients with localized, resectable tumors survive, but fewer than 20% of patients with metastatic disease survive.

Effective Second-Line Therapy
Cure rarely is possible except for patients with local recurrence of an embryonal or botryoid tumor amenable to surgical extirpation.

NONRHABDOMYOSARCOMA SOFT-TISSUE SARCOMA

Incidence
- Among persons younger than 20 years, 6.2 new cases occur per 1 million persons per year.
- Peaks in incidence occur among infants and among children older than 10 years.

Differential Diagnosis
Benign soft-tissue tumors, rhabdomyosarcoma, extraosseous Ewing's sarcoma

Staging Evaluation
- Staging always should include a thorough history and physical examination and imaging studies of the primary tumor and lungs.
- Imaging of regional lymph nodes, liver, and bones is indicated in some clinical settings.

Primary Therapy
- Surgical excision with or without radiation therapy for patients with resectable tumors.

- Chemotherapy may provide some benefit for patients with high-grade tumors larger than 5 cm in diameter and for those with unresectable or metastatic tumors.
- Survival depends on the size and grade of the tumor and extent of disease. Patients with localized tumors 5 cm or smaller or localized low-grade tumors larger than 5 cm in diameter have a survival rate exceeding 85%. Approximately 50% of patients with high-grade tumors larger than 5 cm or with unresectable disease survive. The survival rate is less than 10% among patients with metastatic disease.

Effective Second-Line Therapy
Cure generally is possible only for patients with local recurrence amenable to surgical extirpation and for those with surgically resectable distant recurrence of low-grade tumor.

RETINOBLASTOMA

Incidence and Clinical Forms
- Among children younger than 5 years, 11 new cases occur per 1 million persons per year.
- The two clinical forms are as follows:
  1. Hereditary, bilateral, or multifocal (40% of cases)—characterized by germline mutations of *RB1*. Inherited from an affected survivor or a silent carrier parent or the result of a new germline mutation.
  2. Nonhereditary, unilateral or unifocal (60% of cases)—15% of unilateral cases represent germline mutations.

Clinical Manifestations and Differential Diagnosis
- Clinical manifestations: Leukocoria in more than 50% of cases, strabismus in 20% to 25%.
- Differential diagnosis: Coats' disease, retinopathy of prematurity, persistent hyperplastic primary vitreous, *Toxocara* uveitis, toxoplasmosis.

Staging Evaluation
- Management depends on tumor size and on the presence of intraocular and extraocular extension.

- Indirect ophthalmoscopic examination of both eyes under general anesthesia always is required.
- Imaging studies are helpful in staging—ultrasonography, orbital and cerebral CT, and magnetic resonance imaging (MRI).
- Bone marrow and cerebrospinal fluid examinations are reserved for patients with extraocular disease, optic nerve involvement, or choroid invasion.

Treatment
- Treatment must be individualized and depends on laterality, potential for vision, and tumor extent.
- Enucleation is reserved for cases in which there is no potential for useful vision. Cryotherapy and photocoagulation are useful for small primary or recurrent tumors.
- Radiation therapy is the treatment of choice for controlling local disease and preserving vision for larger tumors.
- Chemotherapy is restricted to patients with advanced intraocular disease or with extraocular disease.

HEPATOBLASTOMA

Incidence
Among children younger than 15 years, 1.5 new cases occur per 1 million persons per year.

Etiology/Epidemiology
- Median age at diagnosis is 18 months.
- The tumor is associated with familial adenomatous polyposis and Beckwith-Wiedemann syndrome.
- Association with low birth weight has been found.

Pathology/Biology
- The major histologic subtypes are fetal, embryonal, macrotrabecular, and small cell (anaplastic).
- The tumor is associated with mutations of the *APC* and β-catenin genes and loss of heterozygosity at 11p15, the site of the *IGF2* gene.

Clinical Findings
- An asymptomatic abdominal mass is present in most patients.
- Other findings are anorexia, weight loss, vomiting, and precocious puberty (2% of cases).

SUMMARY OF KEY POINTS—*cont'd*

Differential Diagnosis
Other malignant (hepatocellular carcinoma, embryonal sarcoma, rhabdomyosarcoma, angiosarcoma, teratoma) and benign (hemangioma, hemangioendothelioma, hamartoma, adenoma) tumors.

Staging Evaluation
- Staging includes a complete history and physical examination with attention to congenital abnormalities or signs of precocious puberty.
- Laboratory tests (e.g., CBC, serum chemical analysis, α-fetoprotein, β human chorionic gonadotropin).
- Diagnostic imaging (CT or MRI of the abdomen, chest CT).

Primary Therapy
- Cure is possible only when complete surgical excision is performed. If complete excision is not feasible, liver transplantation should be considered.
- Adjuvant chemotherapy (cisplatin based, in conjunction with doxorubicin or 5-fluorouracil) is useful preoperatively for achieving resectability and postoperatively for preventing distant metastasis.

- Radiation therapy has a limited and ill-defined role.

Salvage Therapy
Recurrent disease confers a poor prognosis, but repeated resection of local and metastatic recurrences has lengthened the survival period.

Complications
Hearing loss and nephrotoxicity (related to cisplatin), cardiac toxicity (related to doxorubicin), second malignant neoplasms.

Prognosis
- Localized disease: 60% to 70% 5-year relapse-free survival rate, 70% to 80% 5-year overall survival rate.
- Metastatic disease: 25% to 30% 5-year relapse-free survival rate, 50% to 60% 5-year overall survival rate.

ADRENOCORTICAL CARCINOMA

Incidence
- Two to three new cases per 10 million persons per year in the United States.

- Ten- to fifteenfold increase in incidence in Southern Brazil.

Etiology/Epidemiology
Associated with germline P53 mutations and Li-Fraumeni syndrome.

Differential Diagnosis
Other androgen- or cortisol-producing conditions such as Cushing's syndrome or ovarian or testicular tumors.

Staging Evaluation
Imaging studies of the abdomen, pelvis, and chest; skeletal scintigraphy; and measurement of blood and urine concentrations of adrenocortical hormones.

Primary Therapy
- Complete surgical removal of the tumor.
- Mitotane-based therapy or chemotherapy with cisplatin.

Effective Second-Line Therapy
Recurrent disease can be managed with further surgery or experimental agents.

INTRODUCTION

Solid tumors account for 60% of all pediatric malignant neoplasms, approximately 3700 cases being newly diagnosed each year in the United States. The spectrum of tumor types that occur in children is much different from that observed in adults. Included among the diverse group of pediatric neoplasms are brain tumors of the central nervous system (35%); neuroblastoma (15%); soft-tissue sarcoma, including rhabdomyosarcoma (10%); bone tumors, including osteosarcoma and Ewing's sarcoma (8%); retinoblastoma (5%); and miscellaneous tumors, including hepatoblastoma, germ cell tumors, and melanoma (17%). Enormous progress has been made in the diagnosis and management of these tumors since the original demonstration of the chemosensitivity of Wilms' tumor to actinomycin D in 1966. Cure rates for most childhood solid tumors have increased as much as 50% since the mid 1970s. The increase is largely attributable to improved understanding of prognostically important biologic features, improvement in the precision of clinical staging systems, and development of more effective treatment, often incorporating a combination of chemotherapy, surgery, and radiation therapy.[1,2]

OSTEOSARCOMA

Epidemiology

Osteosarcoma, a malignant neoplasm derived from primitive mesenchymal cells and characterized by the presence of osteoid-producing spindle cell stroma is the most common malignant bone tumor in the pediatric age group.[3] Osteosarcoma ranks tenth among all newly reported pediatric cancers in the United States, accounting for 2.6% of all neoplasms in children. The estimated annual incidence is 3.9 cases per million white children and 4.5 per million African American children.[4] Most osteosarcomas occur during the first two decades of life, a period characterized by rapid skeletal growth. Boys are affected more commonly than girls. Several observations support the association between skeletal growth velocity and osteosarcoma. First, patients with osteosarcoma tend to be taller than their counterparts without this disease. Second, in female patients osteosarcoma develops at an earlier age than in male patients, perhaps because of differences in the timing of onset of puberty and the growth spurt.[5]

Biology

Unlike osteosarcoma in adults, in whom more than 25% of tumors arise in preexisting pathologic osseous conditions such as Paget's disease or fibrous dysplasia, most pediatric osteosarcomas arise spontaneously in areas of bone without any abnormality.[3] Irradiation is the best-characterized etiologic factor contributing to the development of secondary osteosarcoma. In a study involving 91 patients with second malignant bone sarcomas, osteosarcoma accounted for 72 cases, 52 (72%) of these cases occurring within previously irradiated fields.[6] The median time for development of the secondary tumor was 9.6 years.

Children with hereditary retinoblastoma are at increased risk of development of secondary nonocular tumors irrespective of previous radiation to the primary site.[7,8] The estimated 50-year cumulative incidence of secondary neoplasms in children with retinoblastoma is 51% in hereditary cases and 5% in nonhereditary cases. Osteosarcoma is the most common second neoplasm in these children, accounting for as many as 44% of cases.[8]

Alterations in components of the cell cycle control system appear to characterize the ontogeny of osteosarcoma. Studies of the retinoblastoma gene (*RB1*) have shown that alterations affect the *RB1* gene in as many as 80% of cases[9] and that other events, such as *CDK4* alterations, also may result in *RB1* inactivation.[10] In experimental models, introduction of the *RB1* gene into *RB1*-deleted osteosarcoma cell lines suppressed the tumorigenic potential of these cells.[11] However, the ontogeny of osteosarcoma is complex and likely involves several genetic alterations other than loss of *RB1* function. Other genetic abnormalities have been reported, including allelic loss at chromosome 17p, 25% to 50% of osteosarcomas having structural alterations at 17p13 of the p53 tumor suppressor gene.[12,13] Additional genetic abnormalities associated with osteosarcoma include amplification of the *MDM-2* gene, whose protein product is important in regulation of p53 function. Tumors with *MDM-2* amplification appear to display clinically aggressive behavior characterized by either local or distant metastasis.[14] Allelic loss at other chromosomal loci, including chromosomes 3q, 13q, and 18q, have been observed in as many as 75% of osteosarcomas karyotypically analyzed. This finding suggests the presence of at least two other potential tumor suppressor genes involved in the multistep process of tumor development and progression in osteosarcoma.[15,16]

The peak incidence of osteosarcoma coincides with the adolescent growth spurt. This finding has led to the hypothesis that the altered hormonal milieu of adolescents may play a role in development of osteosarcoma. It is therefore possible that the insulin-like growth factor I (IGF-I)–insulin-like growth factor I receptor (IGF-IR) axis may be involved in the unregulated proliferation of osteoblasts that occurs in osteosarcoma. IGF-I functions as a mitogen in human and mouse osteosarcoma cells, and osteosarcoma cell lines depend on IGF-I for in vitro growth.[17] Although the levels of IGF-I and its binding protein (IGFBP-3) are not elevated in patients with osteosarcoma, other components of the IGF-I signaling pathway may be involved in the development and progression of osteosarcoma.[18]

Pathology

Osteosarcoma is characterized by the presence of spindle cell stroma that produces osteoid. Conventional osteosarcoma can be subdivided histologically into three major groups depending on the predominant cell type. Approximately 50% of tumors are categorized as osteoblastic, because the predominant extracellular element is osteoid. Twenty-five percent of tumors are chondroblastic with a prominent cartilaginous component. Approximately 25% have a herringbone pattern similar to that observed in fibrosarcoma and are therefore called *fibroblastic*. No significant differences in overall outcome are apparent among these three histologic subtypes.[3] A distinctive histologic subtype of osteosarcoma is telangiectatic osteosarcoma, which accounts for approximately 5% to 10% of cases. This tumor is characterized radiographically by a purely lytic bone lesion. However, not all lytic osteosarcomas are telangiectatic. Telangiectatic osteosarcoma is characterized by the presence of single or multiple cystic cavities containing blood or necrotic tissue divided by septa composed of anaplastic sarcoma cells. Osteoid production is minimal.[3] Prognosis with current therapy is similar to that of the other histologic groups.[19]

Other descriptive classification schemes for osteosarcoma are based on the location of the primary tumor. Periosteal osteosarcoma is an extremely rare variant. It typically involves the diaphysis of the femur or tibia and is always located in the superficial cortex of the bone. Radiographically the tumor is limited to the periphery of the cortex, and the medullary portion of the bone is spared. Local recurrence is common, and wide surgical excision is the treatment of choice.[20] Parosteal osteosarcoma occurs more commonly in women and affects patients in the second to fourth decades of life. Most of these tumors are located in the posterior aspect of the femoral shaft; they are seen radiographically as a large, lobulated mass attached to the cortex by a broad base. Most of these tumors are low grade and often are cured by radical resection alone.[21] However, high-grade transformation can occur either as a primary event or after several local recurrences.[22]

Approximately 5% of all osteosarcomas are multifocal, involving two or more bones at the time of diagnosis. Multifocal osteosarcoma has a more aggressive clinical behavior, which leads to a high incidence of pulmonary metastasis and a very poor prognosis.[23]

Clinical Manifestations

Pain is the most common symptom in children and adolescents with osteosarcoma.[3] The pain often is insidious and usually involves the area affected by tumor. The appearance of sudden and severe pain is commonly associated with pathologic fracture. Swelling around the affected bone is the second most common clinical finding. The tumor may be easily palpable when located in areas

Specific Malignancies

III

such as the anterior surface of the femur but may manifest only as leg edema when occurring in difficult-to-appreciate areas such as the popliteal fossa. A painful limp that increases with weight bearing is the third most common symptom. Systemic symptoms such as fever and weight loss are uncommon.

Osteosarcoma most commonly involves the long bones, most tumors occurring around the knee. The most frequent sites of involvement are the distal part of the femur, the proximal portion of the tibia, and the proximal part of the humerus. The axial skeleton, including the pelvis, is rarely affected in children (fewer than 10% of cases) but is more frequently involved in patients older than 60 years.[3,24] Overt macroscopic metastatic disease occurs in 20% of cases and carries a grave prognosis.[24-26]

Laboratory and Radiologic Evaluation

Laboratory evaluation often is unrevealing. Elevations of serum lactate dehydrogenase (LDH) and alkaline phosphatase levels are the most common laboratory abnormalities. The latter appears to correlate with osteoblastic activity and has therefore proved useful in monitoring response to therapy.[27]

Radiologic evaluation of a patient with osteosarcoma must include assessment of the primary site as well as a search for distant metastatic lesions. Plain radiography is the most effective method of detection of bone tumors.[28,29] The main limitation of plain radiography is accurate delineation of local tumor extent. Characteristic radiologic findings in osteosarcoma commonly include a metaphyseal permeative lesion with periosteal new bone formation and destruction of preexisting cortical bone. A soft-tissue mass is present in more than 90% of cases. Other radiologic signs commonly associated with osteosarcoma include cumulus cloud–like density and the presence of Codman's triangle (Fig. 99-1A). A baseline chest radiograph should be obtained to search for distant metastatic lesions. Angiography usually is reserved for patients who receive intra-arterial chemotherapy or for those who need optimal vessel visualization before limb salvage.[29]

Computed tomography (CT) of the primary tumor is accurate in assessment of degree of tumor calcification and ossification, which are important in assessment of response to therapy.[29] Chest CT always should be performed at the time of diagnosis for documentation of metastatic disease. Findings at magnetic resonance imaging (MRI) offer the best estimate of intramedullary tumor extension, joint and vascular involvement, detection of skip metastatic lesions, and delineation of the soft-tissue component (Fig. 99-1B). The blood supply and vascularity of the tumor can be better appreciated with administration of gadopentetate dimeglumine (Gd-DTPA), a paramagnetic contrast material. MRI is helpful in assessing response to chemotherapy, as evidenced by changes in signal intensity on T_2-weighted images and alterations in the enhancement of tumor tissue after administration of Gd-DTPA (Fig. 99-2).[29] Dynamic contrast-enhanced MRI (DEMRI) is a valuable method for assessing microcirculation in osteosarcoma.[30] DEMRI can be used

to evaluate changes in regional contrast access during chemotherapy. The findings appear to correlate accurately with histologic response and outcome, allowing early identification of patients at risk of recurrence.[31] Radionuclide bone scans with ^{99m}Tc-labeled bone-seeking phosphate compounds are particularly useful in detection of metastatic bone lesions.[29] Thallium bone scintigraphy also is useful in the diagnosis of osteosarcoma; its primary role may be in assessing response to chemotherapy.[32]

Biopsy of the primary tumor should be carefully done, preferably by the surgeon who will ultimately perform the definitive operation. In performance of biopsy of a suspected bone tumor, the following basic principles should be observed: (1) avoidance of transverse incisions, which can make subsequent surgery difficult; (2) avoidance of contamination of multiple compartments and hematoma formation, because successful limb-sparing procedures can be jeopardized; and (3) if feasible, biopsy of the soft-tissue component only.

Prognostic Factors

The most important adverse prognostic factor in patients with osteosarcoma is the presence of metastatic disease.[24] In addition, primary tumor location is associated with outcome. Children with primary tumors of the tibia and distal femur appear to have a more favorable prognosis than those with axial primary tumors. This finding highlights the importance of complete surgical resection in the management of this malignant disease.[24,33] For patients with localized disease, factors associated with poor prognosis include measures of tumor burden, such as tumor size, and levels of alkaline phosphatase and LDH,[24,27,34] as well as more biologic measures, such as poor histologic response to preoperative chemotherapy,[33] hyperdiploidy,[35] and increased expression of P-glycoprotein[36] or Ki-67.[37] The percentage of tumor necrosis following preoperative chemotherapy is the most consistent and important factor associated with outcome in children and adolescents with localized osteosarcoma. A favorable response (more than 90% tumor necrosis) correlates with excellent overall survival. Patients who have less than 90% tumor necrosis are considered poor responders and usually have a poor prognosis.[24,33,38] Because of this strong correlation between degree of histologic response to preoperative chemotherapy and outcome, noninvasive methods, such as DEMRI, used for monitoring tumor response can be used to evaluate changes in regional contrast access during chemotherapy.[31]

Treatment

Optimal management of osteosarcoma consists of multiple-agent chemotherapy and local control measures, including amputation or limb-sparing surgical procedures. Before the development of limb-sparing procedures, amputation was the standard surgical method used to treat and cure patients with osteosarcoma. Amputation is now generally reserved for patients with primary tumors deemed unresectable. Limb function following below-the-knee amputation usually is excellent. Over the

Figure 99-1. A, Plain radiograph shows osteosarcoma involving right distal femur. A poorly defined, permeative destructive pattern; periosteal reaction; formation of Codman's triangle; and an associated soft-tissue mass are apparent. **B,** Sagittal T_2-weighted magnetic resonance image of the same patient shows abnormally dark signal intensity from the intramedullary space consistent with tumor involvement by osteosarcoma. The associated posterior soft-tissue mass is evident. Areas of bright focal signal enhancement represent intramedullary hemorrhage.

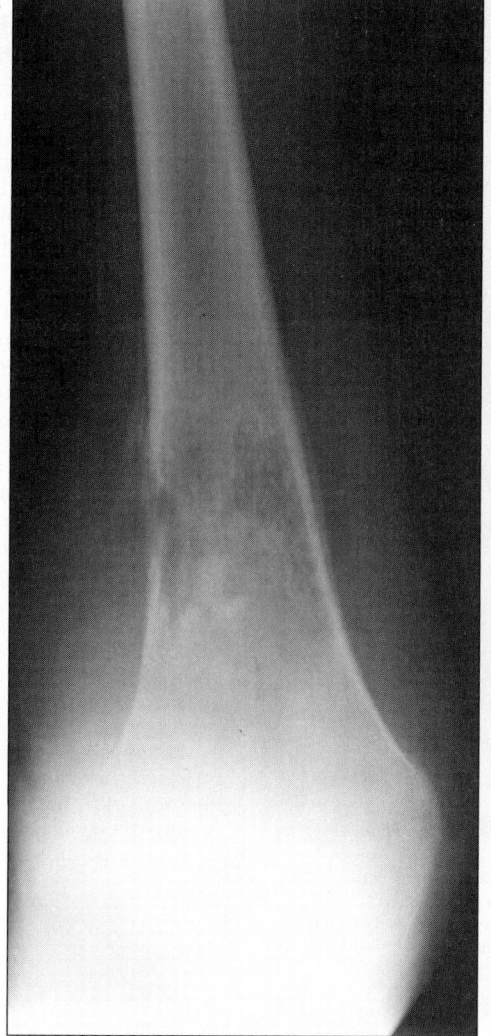

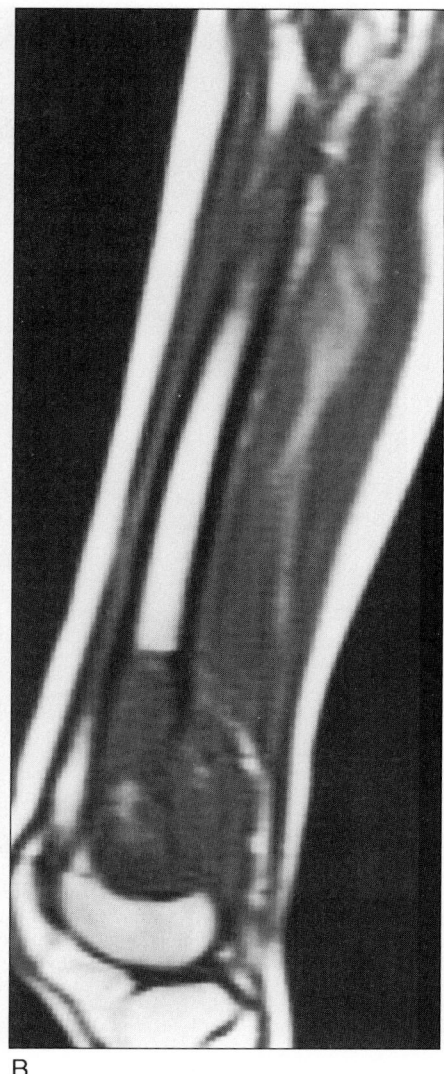

A

B

past several years, the role of limb-sparing procedures has increased dramatically. As a result of refinements in neoadjuvant chemotherapy, bioengineering, and imaging techniques, it is estimated that as many as 80% of patients with osteosarcoma will eventually be candidates for limb-sparing procedures.[39] The criteria for limb-sparing procedures include (1) absence of major neurovascular involvement by tumor, (2) feasibility of wide surgical excision to include a normal muscle cuff in all directions and en bloc removal of all biopsy sites, (3) resection of the adjacent joint and capsule, (4) adequate motor reconstruction with regional muscle transfer, and (5) adequate soft-tissue coverage.[40] In the past, immature skeletal age and primary tumor of the humerus were relative contraindications; however, new expandable prosthetic devices may help overcome this problem.[39,41] More recent improvements have been concentrated on achieving noninvasive extension of prostheses. One of such methods is the Phenix technology (Repiphysis). The basic principle involves storage of energy in a spring maintained

compressed by an original locking system. Prosthetic lengthening is performed through exposure to an external electromagnetic field that pilots the locking system and allows controlled release of the spring energy (Fig. 99-3). Prosthetic expansion of several millimeters can be achieved with each procedure, and the total duration of the procedure is less than 30 seconds[42] (Fig. 99-4). Thus limb-sparing procedures are considered feasible in the care of most children and adolescents with osteosarcoma. When these procedures are appropriately performed, the risk of local recurrence is low (less than 5%).[43] However, long-term functional outcome must be carefully compared with that obtained with amputation alone. Complications of limb-sparing surgery include infection, nonunion, fracture, and unstable joints.

Before the introduction of adjuvant chemotherapy, more than 80% of patients with osteosarcoma had metastatic disease and died of the disease.[44] Trials of single-agent chemotherapy began in the 1960s and early 1970s and established, in a nonrandomized manner, a

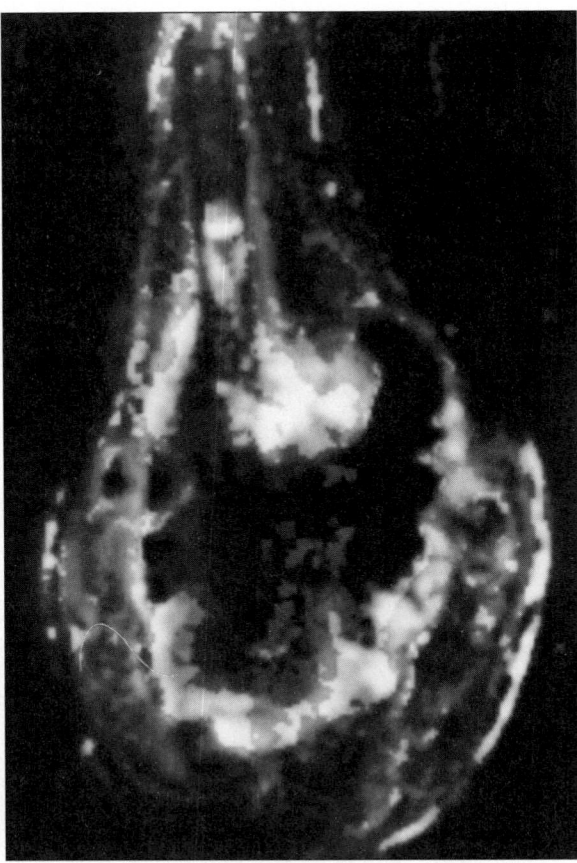

Figure 99-2. Dynamic, paramagnetic, contrast-enhanced magnetic resonance image of a patient with right distal osteosarcoma. At subsequent pathologic examination, the focal areas of increased signal intensity were found to represent nests of viable tumor.

ST. JUDE CHILDREN'S RESEARCH HOSPITAL APPROACH TO THE MANAGEMENT OF OSTEOSARCOMA

The standard approach in the management of osteosarcoma is the use of a platinum-based chemotherapy regimen followed by resection of the primary tumor. For patients with nonmetastatic disease, we have substituted carboplatin for cisplatin in a combination regimen that also includes high-dose methotrexate, doxorubicin, and ifosfamide. Local control is performed after three courses of chemotherapy, and postoperative chemotherapy is not modified on the basis of histologic response unless we document progression of the disease. Most patients with extremity osteosarcoma are candidates for limb salvage surgery. Amputation is performed only in selected cases. For patients with immature skeleton and growth potential, we use the Phenix (Repiphysis) device, which allows noninvasive lengthening.

In patients with metastatic and unresectable disease at diagnosis, we continue to use cisplatin in combination with high-dose methotrexate, ifosfamide, and doxorubicin. We perform aggressive resection of the primary site and all sites of metastasis. For patients with unresectable disease, we use radiation therapy, although the outcome for this group of patients is very poor.

The few patients with local recurrence after a limb-sparing procedure undergo amputation. Recurrent disease to the lungs is managed with aggressive surgery, and repeated thoracotomy usually is needed. Systemic chemotherapy with second-line regimens is added in cases of early recurrence or unresectable disease.

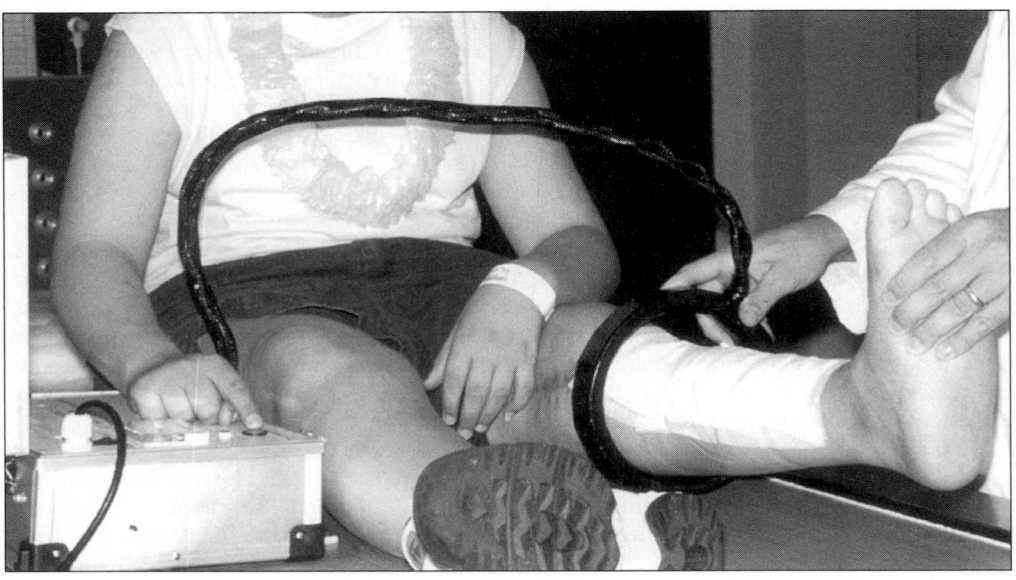

Figure 99-3. Activation of Phenix (Repiphysis) device expansion in treatment of a 13-year-old boy. Activating device is on the left. The electromagnetic coil is being held over the annular protuberance within the implant.

Figure 99-4. Radiographs show expandable portion of the Phenix (Repiphysis) device. The titanium tubular portion expands out of the polymeric tube. The increased distance between barrel and stem indicates the amount of expansion that occurred (*arrows*).

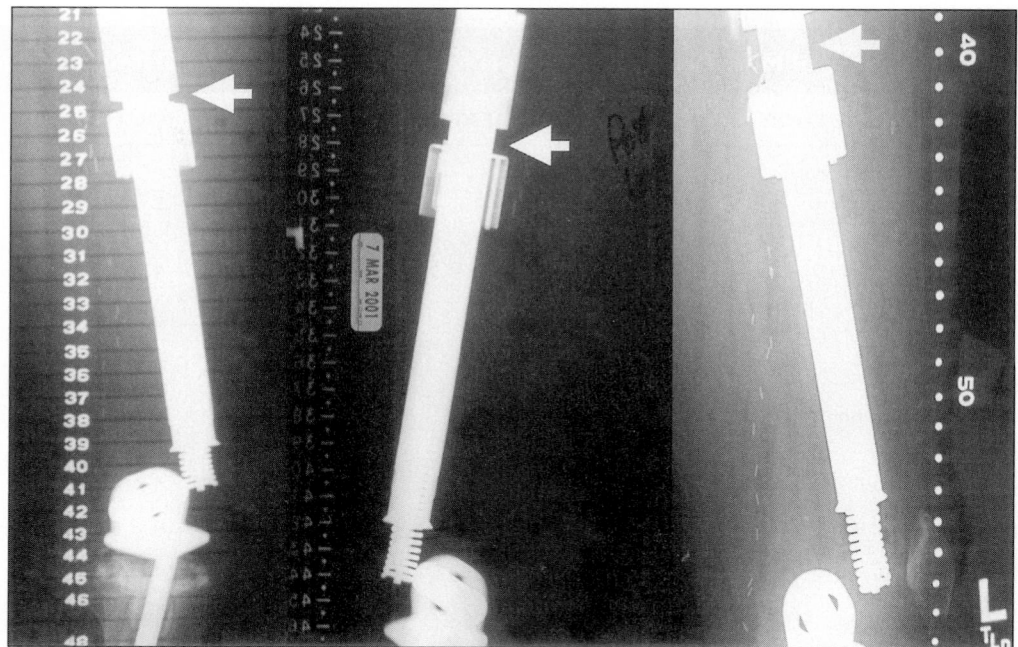

role for the use of chemotherapy in the management of osteosarcoma. Responses with single-agent high-dose methotrexate or doxorubicin occurred in 20% to 40% of patients with metastatic disease.[44,45] Since then, different combinations of platinum compounds, doxorubicin, and high-dose methotrexate have formed the basis of standard chemotherapy regimens that lead to cure in 50% to 75% of patients with nonmetastatic disease (Table 99-1).

For more than two decades, therapy for nonmetastatic osteosarcoma has followed the basic guidelines of the T-10 protocol,[46] and most of the current treatment strategies have evolved from lessons learned with it. The T-10 protocol and its variants consist of a multiple-agent regimen of high-dose methotrexate, doxorubicin, cisplatin, and a combination of bleomycin, cyclophosphamide, and dactinomycin. When the T-10 protocol guidelines are used, the 5-year actuarial event-free survival (EFS) rate may approach 70%.[33,34] However, these results are not always reproducible, and multi-institutional U.S. and European studies conducted according to similar guidelines have shown lower EFS rates, usually of 50% to 60%.[47-51] The lack of reproducibility of the results of the original study may be attributed in part to the complexity of the treatment. In a study performed by the European Osteosarcoma Intergroup, patients were randomized to receive the T-10 protocol or a much simpler treatment of six courses of a combination of cisplatin and doxorubicin.[47] Only one half of the patients randomized to the T-10–like arm completed all scheduled therapy, whereas 94% of the patients in the short-treatment group received the six courses of chemotherapy. The results for both treatment groups were identical, suggesting that a simple, two-drug regimen of cisplatin and doxorubicin can cure more than one half of patients with nonmetastatic osteosarcoma.[52]

One of the major contributions of the T-10 protocol and its predecessor T-7 is that the histologic response to neoadjuvant chemotherapy is the most important prognostic factor in the care of patients with nonmetastatic disease.[33] However, intensification of postoperative[33,48,49] or preoperative[34] chemotherapy with cisplatin and doxorubicin has not improved outcome. To increase the proportion of good histologic responders, some authors have investigated intra-arterial administration of cisplatin. However, in the context of an aggressive, multiple-agent treatment, intra-arterial infusion of cisplatin does not offer any significant advantages.[53] In recent years, ifosfamide has been incorporated into therapeutic regimens for osteosarcoma. After early reports showed that ifosfamide as a single agent achieved response rates of 10% to 60% in patients with advanced or refractory osteosarcoma,[54-56] some investigators began to use the agent in salvage therapy regimens for poor responders.[51,57] More recently, ifosfamide has been incorporated into front-line therapy in many regimens.[53,57-60] Whether incorporating the agent into standard treatment will improve the cure rate is unknown.[60] The Children's Oncology Group is investigating the role of ifosfamide in a randomized study. Because studies have shown that administering an alkylating agent with etoposide produces a synergistic antitumor effect,[61] several investigators have administered ifosfamide and etoposide together on a fractionated dosing schedule over 3 to 5 days. In patients with refractory osteosarcoma, some of whom had previously been treated with ifosfamide, the combination of ifosfamide and etoposide achieved response rates of 15% to 48%.[62-65] Thus this combination is being used increasingly to manage osteosarcoma.[57,66] More recently, investigators in the Pediatric Oncology Group have reported response rates of 59% in patients with untreated metastatic osteo-

TABLE 99-1

Summary of Most Relevant Protocols for the Management of Osteosarcoma

PROTOCOL/AUTHOR	N	TREATMENT		OUTCOME	COMMENTS
		Preoperative	Postoperative		
T-10/Meyers et al[34]	31	MTX-BCD	GR: + DOX PR: + CDDP/DOX	5-yr EFS: 73%	No advantage of intensified postoperative treatment of PR
T-12/Meyers et al[34] MIOS/Link et al[50]	36	MTX-BCD-DOX-CDDP	Same	5-yr EFS: 78%	No advantage of intensified neoadjuvant treatment
	77	None	MTX-BCD-DOX-CDDP	2-yr DFS: 66%	Randomized study demonstrating need for chemotherapy
	36	Surgery alone		2-yr DFS: 17%	
CCG-782/Provisor et al[49]	268	MTX-BCD	GR: + DOX PR: + DOX-CDDP	8-yr EFS: 53% GR: 81% PR: 46%	No advantage of intensified postoperative treatment of PR
COSS-82 arm A/Winkler et al[51]	59	MTX-BCD	GR: Same PR: + CDDP/DOX	4-yr EFS: 49%	
COSS-82 arm B	66	MTX-DOX-CDDP	GR: Same PR: + IFO	4-yr EFS: 68%	IFO for PR not advantageous
COSS-86 low risk Fuchs et al[53]	41	MTX-DOX-CDDP	Same	10-yr EFS: 66%	No difference IA vs IV administration of CDDP
COSS-86 high risk	128	MTX-DOX-CDDP-IFO	Same	10-yr EFS: 67%	Use of IFO for high-risk patients
EOI-1/Bramwell et al[52]	142	CDDP-DOX × 3	CDDP-DOX × 3	5-yr DFS: 57%	
	140	CDDP-DOX-MTX × 2	CDDP-DOX-MTX × 2	5-yr DFS: 41%	Value of a two-drug short regimen with CDDP-DOX
EOI-2/Souhami et al[47]	192	MTX-DOX	+ BCD-CDDP	5-yr PFS: 44%	Two-drug short regimen may be better than longer, more complex protocols
	199	CDDP-DOX	Same	5-yr PFS: 44%	
IOR-1/Ferrari et al[48]	127	MTX-CDDP	GR: + DOX-BCD PR: MTX-DOX-BCD	12-yr DFS: 46%	HD MTX better than MD MTX
IOR-2/Bacci et al[75]	164	MTX-CDDP-DOX	GR: Same PR: + IFO/ETO	5-yr DFS: 63% GR: 67% PR: 56%	Importance of dose intensity IFO/ETO good salvage for PR
IOR-3/Bacci et al[57]	139	MTX-CDDP-DOX	GR: Same PR: + IFO	3-yr DFS: 60%	No benefit of IFO for PR
IOR-4/Bacci et al[69]	133	MTX-CDDP-DOX-IFO	Same	5-yr EFS: 56%	No benefit of intensified therapy with IFO
SJ-OS91/Meyer et al[59]	47	CBP-IFO	Same + DOX-MTX	3-yr EFS: 72%	CBP is a good alternative to CDDP for nonmetastatic disease

BCD, bleomycin-cyclophosphamide-dactinomycin; CBP, carboplatin; CCG, Children's Cancer Group; CDDP, cisplatin; COSS, Cooperative Osteosarcoma Study; DFS, disease-free survival; DOX, doxorubicin; EFS, event-free survival; EOI, European Osteosarcoma Intergroup; ETO, etoposide; GR, good histologic responders; HD, high-dose; IA, intra-arterial; IFO, ifosfamide; IOR, Istituto Ortopedico Rizzoli; IV, intravenous; MD, moderate dose; MIOS, Multi-Institutional Osteosarcoma Study; MTX, methotrexate; PFS, progression-free survival; PR, poor histologic responders; SJ-OS, St. Jude Osteosarcoma.

sarcoma receiving this combination.[67] The combination of ifosfamide and etoposide appears more effective than ifosfamide alone in untreated patients with metastatic osteosarcoma.[56,67] These results support performance of additional studies of this combination in the treatment of patients with nonmetastatic disease.

Cisplatin is one of the most active agents against osteosarcoma. However, the toxicity of this agent is substantial: hearing loss and renal impairment can be permanent for some patients. Substitution of carboplatin for cisplatin was investigated at St. Jude Children's Research Hospital. In the context of a multiple-agent chemotherapeutic approach with high-dose methotrexate, ifosfamide, and doxorubicin, use of carboplatin resulted in a 3-year EFS rate of 72%, an outcome comparable with that of cisplatin-based therapy but with less long-term toxicity.[59] However,

incorporation of carboplatin in future osteosarcoma trials needs further evaluation, because there are reports that in the treatment of patients with metastatic disease, carboplatin as a single agent has poor antitumor effect.[68]

Approximately 20% of patients with osteosarcoma have clinically detectable metastatic disease at diagnosis, and their outcome usually is very poor.[25,26] Treatment of these patients must combine a very aggressive multimodal approach that entails intensive preoperative and postoperative chemotherapy and resection of both the primary tumor and metastatic lesions. When these guidelines are followed, contemporary protocols that incorporate ifosfamide or the combination of ifosfamide and etoposide along with high-dose methotrexate, doxorubicin, and cisplatin result in 2- to 5-year progression-free survival rates of 25% to 45%.[56,67,69]

Lung metastasis develops in most patients in whom therapy fails. The ability to control pulmonary micrometastatic disease after completion of therapy would certainly result in a significant improvement in outcome. In an animal model, administration of liposome-encapsulated muramyl tripeptide phosphatidylethanolamine (L-MTP-PE) resulted in activation of pulmonary macrophages and eradication of pulmonary micrometastatic lesions.[70] Use of L-MTP-PE is an attractive strategy that deserves further clinical investigation.

Some authors have reported overexpression of *HER2/erbB-2* (measured by immunohistochemistry) in approximately 40% of osteosarcoma tumor samples and correlation of this overexpression with more aggressive behavior and adverse outcome.[71] If this correlation holds true, the use of anti-*HER2* monoclonal antibodies may be an attractive therapeutic strategy for this group of high-risk patients. However, studies using either immunofluorescence[72] or fluorescence in situ hybridization[73] have not shown amplification of the *HER-2/neu* gene in patients with osteosarcoma.

Finally, administration of high doses of the bone-seeking radiopharmaceutical samarium-153 ethylene diamine tetramethylene phosphonate ([153]Sm-EDTMP) may provide good pain palliation with minimal nonhematologic toxicity for patients with local recurrences or bone metastasis of osteosarcoma, and its role may be expanding.[74]

EWING'S SARCOMA FAMILY TUMORS

Epidemiology

The term *Ewing's sarcoma family tumors* (ESFT) defines a group of small round cell neoplasms of neuroectodermal origin that manifest as a continuum of neurogenic differentiation. On this continuum Ewing's sarcoma of bone represents the least differentiated and primitive neuroectodermal tumors, and peripheral neuroepithelioma represents the most differentiated forms. Ewing's sarcoma is the second most common malignant bone tumor in children and adolescents. The estimated incidence among white children younger than 15 years is 2.8 cases per 1 million persons.[4] The tumor is rare in the nonwhite population, and boys are predominantly affected in most series. Most cases occur during the second decade of life.[76] The location of the tumor varies. Although most Ewing's sarcomas arise in bone, a significant proportion arise in soft tissue.[77] The most common locations are the chest wall, pelvis, and extremities, but any bone can be involved.[76,78]

Biology

The histogenesis of Ewing's sarcoma has been a source of controversy since its first description in 1921. Various hypotheses have been proposed in an attempt to identify the possible cell of origin in Ewing's sarcoma. Among these, cells of endothelial, pericytic, myeloid, mesenchymal, and neuroectodermal origin have been suggested.[79] The existence of either a mesenchymal stem cell or an early primitive neuroectodermal cell that has retained its ability for multilineage differentiation is the currently accepted hypothesis. It is now well accepted that ESFT constitute a single group of neurally derived neoplasms that share unique immunocytochemical, cytogenetic, and molecular markers.[79,80]

Nearly all ESFT have a reciprocal translocation that involves the *EWS* gene in chromosome 22q12.[81] The t(11;22) is the most commonly observed translocation (85% to 95% of cases) and juxtaposes the DNA-binding domain of the human homologue of the murine *Fli1* gene in chromosome 11 with the 5' end of *EWS* in chromosome 22 (Fig. 99-5). The most common fusions occur between exon 7 of *EWS* and exon 6 of *FLI1* (type 1; 55%–60% of cases) and between exon 7 of *EWS* and exon 5 of *FLI1* (type 2; 25% of cases).[81] The type of fusion transcript appears to be prognostically relevant, because type 1 fusion appears to be associated with a lower proliferative rate.[82] The t(11;22) appears to play a pivotal role in development of ESFT, because the *EWS-FLI1* fusion transcript can transform NIH 3T3 cells.[83] As many as 10% of ESFT contain an alternative translocation between chromosomes 21 and 22. This translocation fuses the *ERG* gene on chromosome 21 and the *EWS* gene on chromosome 22, producing an *ERG-EWS* fusion transcript.[81] Finally, rare cases of ESFT contain a t(7;22)(p22;q12) that fuses the *ETV1* and *EWS* genes.[84] The mechanism by which these fusion transcripts become tumorigenic is poorly understood, although it has been postulated that this chimeric transcript can transcriptionally deregulate members of the manic fringe family of genes, which are instrumental in somatic development.[85] The IGF-I/IGF-IR pathway is actively involved in the cell transformation and inhibition of apoptosis induced by *EWS-FLI1*.[86-88]

Pathology

Microscopic examination shows Ewing's sarcoma is the prototypic small round blue cell tumor of childhood. The ultrastructural and immunocytochemical characteristics of this and other small round cell tumors of childhood are shown in Table 99-2. Ewing's sarcoma is characterized by the presence of a dimorphic pattern of densely packed cells with variable amounts of large clear cytoplasm. Individual cells have an ellipsoid nucleus without distinct cytoplasmic outlines. The cells are primitive, show a paucity of organelles, and often contain large amounts of intracellular glycogen. Various microscopic patterns, including the diffuse, lobular, organoid, and filigree patterns, have been described.[89] Immunocytochemical analysis shows vimentin and HBA-71 reactivity. The latter monoclonal antibody specifically recognizes the cell-surface antigen [p30/p32]MIC-2, which is normally expressed as a component of the T-cell receptor complex.[89,90] When overt neural differentiation is present, the term *peripheral neuroectodermal tumor* or *peripheral neuroepithelioma* is used (Table 99-2). In these cases, the cells are round with more abundant cytoplasm but do not show mature neural elements, such as nerve bundles and mats of neuropile.[89] The term *extraosseous Ewing's sarcoma* has been reserved for neoplasms that cannot be differentiated

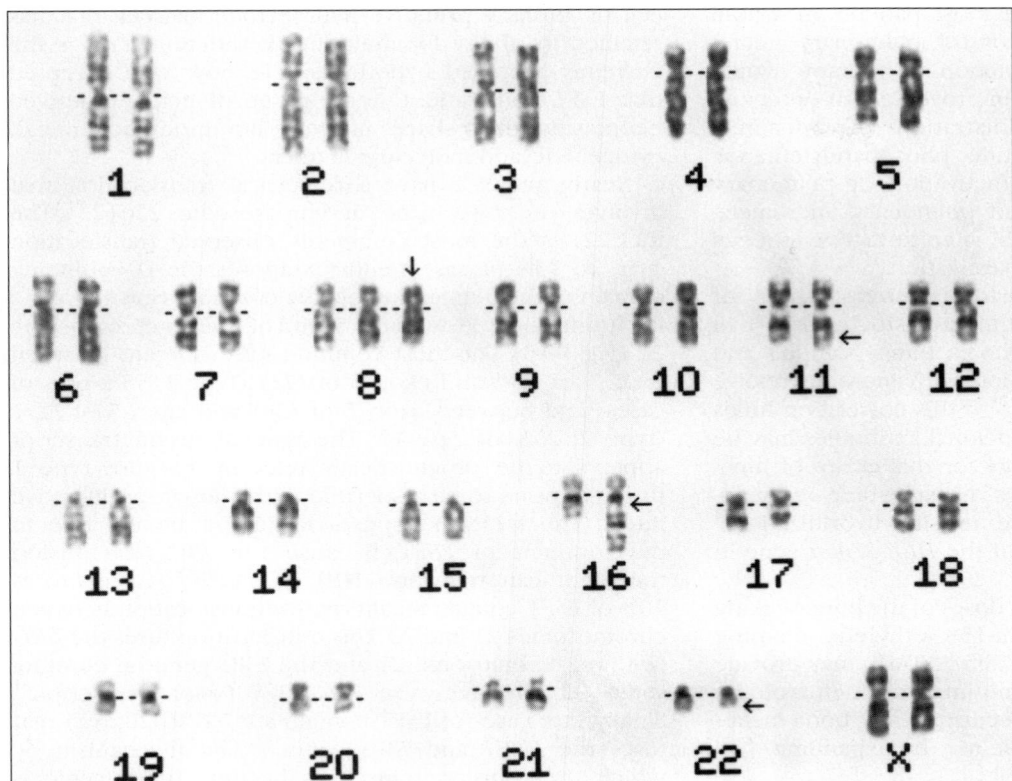

from Ewing's sarcoma at light microscopic examination but arise exclusively in soft tissue.[79,89] Patients with this histologic variety accounted for 5% of all subjects in the Intergroup Rhabdomyosarcoma Study,[77] although extraosseous tumors are now managed in the same manner as classic Ewing's sarcoma of bone. Despite these histologic distinctions, Ewing's sarcoma of bone, extraosseous Ewing's sarcoma, primitive neuroectodermal tumors, and peripheral neuroepithelioma are unified by the presence of the same oncogenic events and should therefore be considered the same neoplasm and thus managed in a similar manner. The advent of molecular diagnostic techniques has allowed development of sensitive tests, such as reverse transcriptase polymerase chain reaction (RT-PCR), which is accurate in detection of *EWS-FLI1* and *EWS-ERG* fusion transcripts at levels well below those commonly found with routine cytogenetic studies.[91] RT-PCR is a useful adjunct in the diagnosis of Ewing's sarcoma, particularly in differential diagnosis from other soft-tissue small round cell tumors, such as rhabdomyosarcoma.

Clinical Manifestations

Ewing's sarcoma commonly manifests during the second decade of life (median age, 13 years) with localized pain and a visible palpable mass.[76,92] Fewer than 3% of cases occur in children younger than 3 years.[93] Boys are more commonly affected than girls. Pathologic fractures may be present in as many as 15% of children and adolescents before diagnosis.[94] Back pain, extremity weakness, or altered sensation should raise suspicion of the presence of primary or metastatic disease. Systemic manifestations such as fever are more frequent than in osteosarcoma. Almost one half of patients have symptoms referable to the primary tumor for more than 3 months before the diagnosis is made. Ewing's sarcoma has a tendency to involve the shaft of long tubular bones, pelvis, and ribs, but almost every bone can be affected. Chest wall Ewing's sarcoma is known as *Askin's tumor* (Fig. 99-6). Approximately 20% to 25% of patients have metastatic disease when they arrive for evaluation. The most common sites of metastatic disease are the lungs, followed by the bones and bone marrow.

Laboratory and Radiologic Evaluation

Patients with suspected Ewing's sarcoma should be thoroughly evaluated to define the extent of local disease and the presence of metastatic lesions. Initial laboratory studies include complete blood cell count and erythrocyte sedimentation rate, serum electrolytes, LDH, renal and liver function tests, alkaline phosphatase, calcium, phosphorus, magnesium, and coagulation profile. In Ewing's sarcoma, elevation of erythrocyte sedimentation rate and serum LDH is not uncommon. Bone marrow aspiration and biopsy should be performed, and evaluation with molecular techniques such as RT-PCR is recom-

TABLE 99-2

Differential Diagnosis of Small Blue Round Cell Tumors with Electron Microscopy, Immunocytochemistry, and Molecular Cytogenetics

MODALITY	TUMOR TYPE				
	EWING'S SARCOMA	PNET	NEUROBLASTOMA	HEMATOLYMPHOID NEOPLASMS	RHABDOMYOSARCOMA
Electron microscopy					
Cell processes	Inconspicuous	Present	Prominent	Inconspicuous	Inconspicuous
External lamina	Absent	Absent	Absent	Absent	Present
Intracellular junctions	Primitive	Synaptic	Desmosomes, synaptic junctions	Absent	Inconspicuous
Filaments	Absent	Variable	Neurofilaments 8–12 nm in diameter	Absent	Present: dense Z-line-like structures Mixture of thin and thick filaments or myosin-ribosome complexes
Microtubules	Inconspicuous	Variable	Prominent, 24–30 nm in diameter	Absent	Inconspicuous
Granules	Absent neurosecretory granules (NSG)	Sporadic NSG	NSG 90–240 nm in diameter	Lysosomes only	Lysosomes only
Glycogen	Prominent	Variable	Inconspicuous	Inconspicuous	Prominent
Organelles	Sparse	Variable	Variable	Sparse	Variable
Immunocytochemistry					
Vimentin	+	+	−	±	+
HBA-71	+	+	−	±	±
NSE	±	+	+	−	±
Leu 7 (CD 57)	±	+	+	−	−
Cytokeratin	±	±	−	−	±
Neurofilaments	−	±	±	−	±
S-100	−	±	±	−	−
Muscle-specific actin	−	±	−	−	+
Desmin	−	±	−	−	+
MyoD1	−	−	−	−	+
LCA	−	−	−	+	−
Chromogranin	−	−	+	−	−
Synaptophysin	−	±	+	−	−
β₂-Microglobulin	+	+	−	+	+
Cytogenetics					
t(11;22), t(21;22), t(7;22)	+	+	−	−	−
t(2;13), t(1;13)	−	−	−	−	+
t(1;14), t(2;5), t(14;14), 14q11 abnormalities, t(8;14), t(2;8), t(8;22)	−	−	−	+	−
Loss of 1p36	±	−	+	−	−
Gene(s) involved					
EWS, FL1, ERG, ETV1	+	+	−	−	−
C-myc, TAI, HOX 11, LYL-1, etc.	−	−	−	+	−
PAX3, FKHR, PAX7	−	−	−	−	+
N-myc	−	−	+	−	−

+, present; −, absent; ±, present or absent; PNET, primitive neuroectodermal tumor.

mended. Important imaging studies are chest radiography, plain radiography of primary and metastatic sites, bone scintigraphy, CT of the chest , and MRI of the primary site with T_1- and T_2-weighted sequences as well as DEMRI.[29,95]

In Ewing's sarcoma plain radiographs typically show a diaphyseal destructive lesion with a laminated periosteal reaction and large soft-tissue mass (Fig. 99-7A). We favor MRI over CT for defining the intramedullary component of the primary tumor and the extent of soft-tissue mass (Fig. 99-7B). In contrast to the situation in osteosarcoma, DEMRI findings are not a reliable prognostic indicator.[96] However, newer techniques such as positron emission tomography appear useful in noninvasive evaluation of response to chemotherapy.[97]

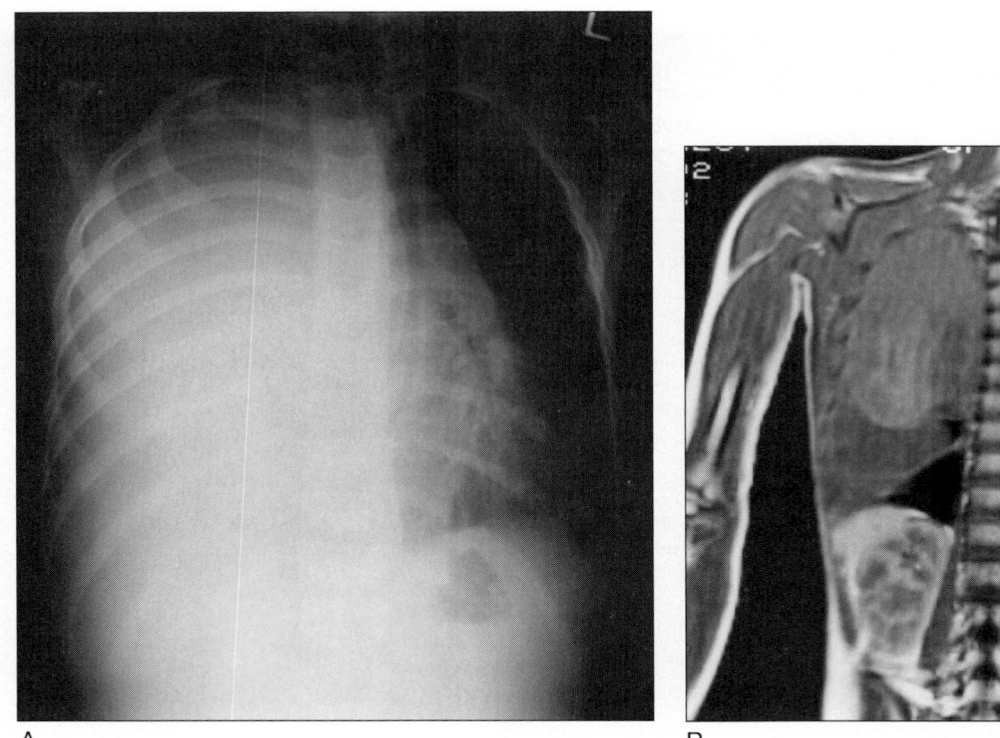

A   B

Figure 99-6. A, Plain radiograph of a primitive neuroectodermal tumor involving the chest wall shows complete opacification of the right hemithorax, marked mediastinal shift, and slight tracheal narrowing. **B,** Coronal T_1-weighted magnetic resonance image shows a large right intrathoracic mass with subjacent pleural effusion and small localized area of normal aerated lung parenchyma.

Prognostic Factors

A variety of initial clinical features have been correlated with outcome of therapy for Ewing's sarcoma. Two major European retrospective studies analyzed factors that are prognostically important in Ewing's sarcoma.[76,78] Both studies included patients treated in different European protocols over a 25-year period. The results confirmed the classic clinical features associated with poor prognosis, such as metastatic disease, older age, large tumors, and trunk and pelvic primary sites. However, both studies also showed that with refinement in the multidisciplinary approach to this disease that entails newer and more intensive chemotherapeutic regimens and superior local control measures, some of these classic prognostic factors are being redefined. Although large tumors have classically been associated with worse prognosis, this feature may be less important with more aggressive treatment. For example, in the early St. Jude studies, tumors larger than 8 cm in diameter were associated with worse prognosis.[98] However, tumor size disappeared as a prognostic factor in the more intensive St. Jude EW92 protocol.[99] In the Cooperative Ewing's Sarcoma Studies (CESS81), tumors larger than 100 cm^3 were associated with worse outcome.[100] With treatment improvements, the tumor size associated with worse prognosis has increased to 200 cm^3.[101] Tumor location also seems to be losing its prognostic significance with newer treatments. Although

pelvic and axial tumors classically were associated with worse outcome in the early studies,[98,102,103] differences in outcome were minimal in subsequent studies.[99,104,105] The first Pediatric Oncology Group–Children's Cancer Group Ewing trial (POG-8850/CCG-7881), an investigation of the effect of addition of ifosfamide and etoposide to the standard VACD regimen (vincristine, actinomycin D, cyclophosphamide, and doxorubicin) showed that addition of the drug pair abrogated the negative prognostic implications of large tumor size (>8 cm) and pelvic location. However, the benefit of addition of ifosfamide and etoposide was not seen in patients older than 18 years.

A newer prognostic factor is degree of histologic response to chemotherapy.[106,107] European studies consistently have shown the prognostic value of histologic response, the significance of which stands across protocols and appears to be independent of the drugs used. Patients with good histologic responses had a significantly better outcome than those with poor responses in the consecutive REN-1, -2, and -3 trials in Italy[78,107] and in the CESS-81[100] and CESS-86[108] trials in Germany. Thus degree of histologic response appears to be one of the most relevant prognostic factors. Type of fusion transcript also seems to influence the clinical behavior of ESFT. Although the biologic behavior of tumors with fusion *EWS-FLI1* does not differ from the behavior of tumors with *EWS-ERG* fusion,[109] the type of *EWS-FLI1* fusion may

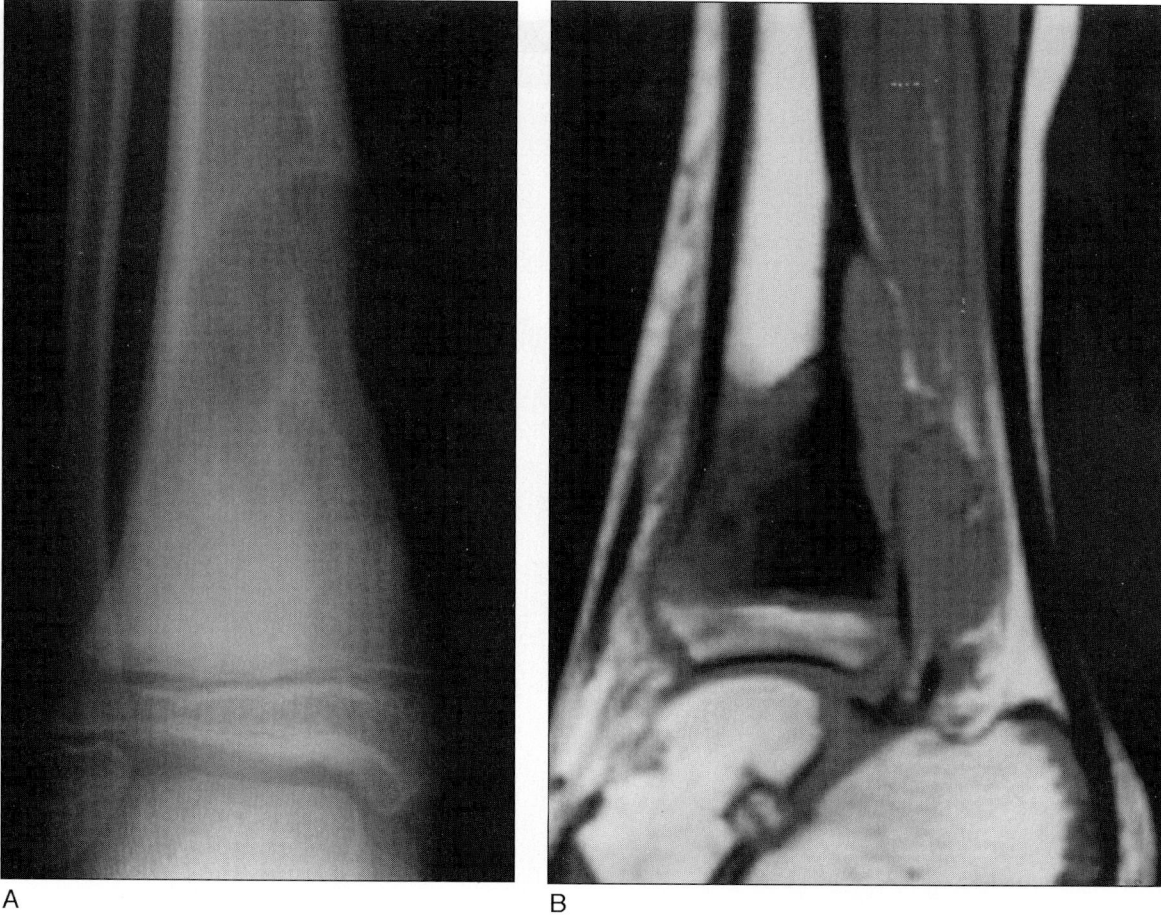

Figure 99-7. A, Plain radiograph of Ewing's sarcoma of the right distal tibia shows a poorly marginated destructive lesion with associated periosteal reaction. **B,** Sagittal T$_1$-weighted magnetic resonance image of the same lesion shows well-demarcated dark signal intensity defining the intramedullary extent of the tumor contrasted against the bright signal intensity derived from intramedullary fat. The soft-tissue component of the tumor is evident in the posterior aspect.

significantly affect prognosis. The hybrid transcripts resulting from fusion of exons 7 and 6 of the *EWS* and *FLI1* genes, respectively (type 1 fusion), seem to result in sarcoma of a less aggressive behavior than other fusion types.[110,111] Because ESFT manifest a continuum of neuroectodermal differentiation, the histologic diversity may reflect different biologic behaviors. However, there is no evidence to suggest the degree of neuroectodermal differentiation in ESFT correlates with prognosis.[112] The most important prognostic factor is the presence of metastatic disease at diagnosis.[76] Advances in management of ESFT have resulted in only very modest improvement in outcome among patients with metastatic lesions.[76,99,113] However, even among patients with metastatic disease, there is heterogeneity. With an appropriately intensive treatment that includes bilateral lung radiation, the European Intergroup Cooperative Ewing's Sarcoma Studies (EICESS) have shown that patients with isolated metastatic lesions in the lung may have a better prognosis, albeit still inferior to that of patients with localized disease. Patients with extrapulmonary metastasis have a worse prognosis.[114,115]

With the use of molecular techniques in the staging of ESFT, it is evident that a significant proportion of patients with localized disease (20%–30%) have micrometastatic disease in the bone marrow detected by PCR.[116-118] In patients with lung metastasis and those with bone metastasis, this proportion is 40% and 90%, respectively.[117] The prognostic significance of this microstaging for patients with localized disease is still unclear. Although the presence of tumor cells in peripheral blood may lack significance, detection of tumor cells in bone marrow by molecular techniques may be predictive of unfavorable outcome.[117,118]

Treatment

Before the introduction of systemic chemotherapy, fewer than 20% of children with Ewing's sarcoma treated with either surgery or radiation therapy alone were expected to be long-term survivors.[119] In the last three decades, major advances have been made in the management of Ewing's sarcoma. These advances derive largely from cooperative trials (Table 99-3). The first

TABLE 99-3

Management of Nonmetastatic Ewing's Sarcoma Family of Tumors

STUDY	NO. OF PATIENTS	REGIMEN	RESULTS 5-YR DFS	COMMENTS
IESS Studies				
IESS-I[120] (1973–1978)	342	VAC	24%	Value doxorubicin
		VAC + WLI	44%	Worse results for pelvic ESFT
		VACD	60%	Benefit of WLI?
IESS-II[104] (1978–1982)	214	VACD-HD	73%	Value of aggressive cytoreduction
		VACD-MD	56%	
First POG-CCG[127] (1988–1993)	NA	VACD	53%	Value of combination IE
		VACD + IE	68%	
Second POG-CCG[133] (1995–1998)	492	VCD+IE 48 weeks	75%	No differences between standard and dose-intensified therapy
		VCD+IE 30 weeks	76%	
St. Jude Studies				
ES-79[98] (1978–1986)	52	VACD	82% <8 cm	Tumor size as prognostic factor
			64% ≥ 8 cm	
EW-87[126] (1987–1991)	26	Therapeutic window with IE	Clinical responses in 96%	Combination IE is very effective in ESFT
EW-92[99] (1992–1996)	34	VCDIE × 3 VCD/IE intensification	78%	Tumor size (</≥8 cm) is not a prognostic factor with intensive treatment
CESS Studies				
CESS-81[100] (1981–1985)	93	VACD	Tumor size: 80% <100 mL 31% >100 mL Viable tumor: 79% <10% 31% >10%	Tumor size (</>100 mL) and histologic response are prognostic factors
CESS-86[108] (1986–1991)	301	SR:VACD	52%	Intensive treatment with ifosfamide for high-risk patients.
		HR:VAID	51% (10 yr)	Tumor volume >200 mL suggests poor prognosis
UKCCSG/MRC Studies				
ET-1[103] (1978–1986)	120	VACD	36% Extr. 52% Axial 38% Pelvic 13%	Tumor site is most important prognostic factor
ET-2[105] (1987–1993)	201	VAID	62% Extr. 73% Axial 55% Pelvic 41%	Importance of administration of high-dose alkylating agents
EICESS Studies				
EICESS-92 (1992–1999)[129]	470	SR:VAID/VACD	79%/71%	Volume (>200 mL) and histologic response as prognostic factor
		HR:VAID/EVAID	54%/62%	

CESS, Cooperative Ewing's Sarcoma Studies; DFS, disease-free survival; EICESS, European Intergroup Cooperative Ewing's Sarcoma Studies; ESFT, Ewing's sarcoma family of tumors; EVAID, etoposide, vincristine, actinomycin D, ifosfamide, doxorubicin; HD, high-dose; HR, high risk; IE, ifosfamide and etoposide; IESS, Intergroup Ewing Sarcoma Study; MD, moderate-dose; NA, not available; POG-CCG, Pediatric Oncology Group–Children's Cancer Group; SR, standard risk; UKCCSG/MRC, United Kingdom Children's Cancer Study Group and Medical Research Council; VAC, vincristine, actinomycin D, cyclophosphamide; VACD, VAC plus doxorubicin; VCD, vincristine, cyclophosphamide, doxorubicin; WLI, whole-lung irradiation.

studies conducted by the Intergroup Ewing Sarcoma Study (IESS) showed the importance of adjuvant chemotherapy that included a combination of alkylating agents and anthracyclines (IESS-I and II).[104,120] Thereafter conventional management of Ewing's sarcoma included local control measures in combination with administration of VACD.[98,100,103] More recently, incorporation of ifosfamide (VAID) has resulted in modest benefit for patients with high-risk features.[105,108] Preclinical and clinical evidence indicates that combined administration of etoposide and alkylators has a synergistic antitumor effect[61-63,121] and that the efficacy of both agents improves with fractionated administration.[122-125] Combined admin-

istration of ifosfamide and etoposide (IE) has been shown to be very active in untreated patients with Ewing's sarcoma.[126] Two randomized studies were conducted to investigate the effect of adding etoposide to VACD/VAID regimens.[127,128] In EICESS-92, patients with localized high-risk disease (>200 cm^3) receiving VAID did not seem to benefit from the addition of etoposide.[128] The first POG-CCG Ewing's sarcoma trial (POG-8850/CCG-7881) was an investigation of incorporation of the IE combination in front-line management of ESFT. Patients were randomized to receive VACD with or without IE.[127] Patients receiving IEVACD appeared to have a more favorable outcome.[127,129]

ST. JUDE CHILDREN'S RESEARCH HOSPITAL APPROACH TO THE MANAGEMENT OF EWING'S SARCOMA FAMILY TUMORS

For patients with nonmetastatic disease, regardless of the size and site of the tumor, we use intensive multiple-agent chemotherapy with alternating courses of vincristine, cyclophosphamide, and doxorubicin with ifosfamide and etoposide. Local control is undertaken after approximately four courses of induction chemotherapy. If the disease is considered resectable, surgery is the treatment of choice for local control, and it is always performed with curative intent. Radiation therapy is used for unresectable disease and for close or microscopic surgical margins. The same approach is followed for patients with metastatic disease to the lungs only with addition of radiation therapy to the lungs.

For patients with bone or bone marrow metastasis we continue to evaluate the role of intensive chemotherapy and consolidation with high-dose chemotherapy and autologous hematopoietic stem cell rescue. In these patients, aggressive local control of the primary tumor and bone metastasis is performed.

All patients with recurrent disease receive second-line systemic therapy. Patients with local recurrence undergo aggressive surgery when possible, and patients with metastasis to the lungs receive whole-lung radiation.

Incorporation of granulocyte colony-stimulating factor into treatment regimens for many types of cancer has allowed modest dose intensification of multiple-agent chemotherapy by increasing the total dose per cycle[99,130,131] or shortening the time between treatments.[132] For ESFT, this strategy is based on using high cumulative doses of alkylating agents and topoisomerase-II inhibitors.[99,130]

When these general treatment guidelines are followed, the disease-free survival rate for patients with localized, low-risk disease approaches 70% to 75%, whereas the overall survival rate for this group of patients may be greater than 80%.[99]

The importance of dose intensification in the management of ESFT was evaluated in the second POG-CCG Ewing's sarcoma trial (POG-9354/CCG-7942). In that trial, patients were randomized to receive alternating courses of vincristine, doxorubicin, and cyclophosphamide with ifosfamide and etoposide over either 48 or 30 weeks. The early results of that randomized trial demonstrated no difference in outcome between the standard and the dose-intensified arms.[133]

Despite improvement, the prognosis for patients with metastatic disease continues to be very poor, and only 20% to 25% survive (Table 99-4).[113,114,134] Several institutions have used treatment intensification, by which very high doses of different agents are administered in a short time. In the case of ESFT, this is a very attractive alternative, because ESFT are highly sensitive to alkylating agents, which have a steep dose-response curve. Although most patients treated in this manner may have good clinical and histologic responses, the final results are not better than those obtained with conventional therapy.[130,135,136]

Other protocols have been used to investigate the possibility of maintaining intensive treatments for more extended periods in an attempt to improve outcome for all patients with Ewing's sarcoma. At St. Jude Children's Research Hospital, the EW92 protocol was used to evaluate the feasibility of aggressive early induction with vincristine, cyclophosphamide, doxorubicin, ifosfamide, and etoposide (VCDIE), followed by prolonged maintenance therapy with intensification of alkylating agents

TABLE 99-4

Management of Metastatic Ewing's Sarcoma Family of Tumors without Hematopoietic Stem Cell Transplantation

STUDY	NO. OF PATIENTS	REGIMEN	RESULTS (5-YR DFS)	COMMENTS
IESS Studies				
IESS I–II[134] (1975–1985)	122	VACD	30%	
First POG-CCG[135] (1988–1993)	121	Reg. A: VACD	19%	Addition of IE does not improve results
		Reg. B: VACD+IE		
European Studies				
ET-1[103] (1978–1986)	22	VACD	9%	
ET-2[105]	42	VAID	23%	
EICESS[114] (1990–1995)	171	VAID±etoposide	27%	Pulmonary metastasis managed with RT: 40%
			Lungs: 34%	
			Bone/bone marrow: 28%	
			Combined: 14%	
Intensification Protocols				
First POG-CCG[135] (1988–1993)	60	Reg. C: VACD+IE	26%	Intensification does not improve results Incidence t-AML: 22.7%
EW-92[99]	19	VCDIE × 3 VCD/IE	27%	Intensification does not improve results High toxicity Incidence t-AML: 8%

±, with or without; DFS, disease-free survival; EICESS, European Intergroup Cooperative Ewing's Sarcoma Studies; IE, ifosfamide and etoposide; IESS, Intergroup Ewing Sarcoma Study; POG-CCG, Pediatric Oncology Group–Children's Cancer Group; RT, radiation therapy; t-AML, therapy-related acute myeloid leukemia; VACD, vincristine, actinomycin D, cyclophosphamide, and doxorubicin; VCD, vincristine, cyclophosphamide, doxorubicin.

and etoposide.[99] The results were not better than less aggressive regimens for patients with localized disease, and no significant benefit was obtained for patients with metastatic disease. Important findings were that only 66% of patients completed therapy and that intensification was feasible in only 25% of the patients.

Use of protocols that include intensification of alkylators and topoisomerase-II inhibitors has resulted in a significant increase in the incidence of treatment-related leukemia and myelodysplastic syndrome (t-AML/MDS). This therapeutic strategy appears to be strongly leukemogenic, and patients are at increased risk of development of both alkylator-related and etoposide-related t-AML/MDS.[135,137,138] With current therapies, the cumulative incidence of t-AML/MDS 5 years after treatment appears to be 8% to 10%. This increased risk of t-AML/MDS appears to be related to both the increase in the total cumulative doses and dose intensification. The role of hematopoietic growth factors in this complication is unknown.

New drugs and new drug combinations continue to be investigated in the care of patients with Ewing's sarcoma. Topotecan appears to be the most promising of the newest generation of anticancer drugs for this population. In a phase II study of topotecan as single agent at a dose of 2 mg/m^2 per day for 5 consecutive days, responses were observed in 10% of patients with refractory cases of ESFT.[139] A phase II study of topotecan (0.75 mg/m^2 per day for 5 days) and cyclophosphamide (250 mg/m^2 per day for 5 days) in patients with refractory solid tumors showed responses in 36% of patients with ESFT.[140] The results provided a firm basis for further evaluation of the combination of topotecan and cyclophosphamide in this population.

Advances in management of ESFT have resulted in only modest improvement in outcome among patients with metastatic disease.[76,99,113] However, with appropriately intensive treatment that includes bilateral lung radiation, patients with isolated lung metastasis may have a better prognosis than patients with extrapulmonary metastasis.[114,115] It is therefore for patients with bone and bone marrow metastasis that more intense therapies may have a role. ESFT are very sensitive to alkylators, a group of agents with a very steep dose-response curve, which provides the basis for the use of consolidation with myeloablative therapy and autologous hematopoietic stem cell transplantation (HSCT). The results of treatment with megatherapy and HSCT for patients with high-risk ESFT must be analyzed with caution given the lack of randomized studies and the heterogeneity of patients and treatments. Results of most retrospective European and American studies do not seem to support the use of this approach.[114,141-143] However, in more recent results reported by the European Bone Marrow Transplant Registry there appears to be an advantage to conditioning regimens that incorporate high doses of alkylating agents, generally busulfan and melphalan.[144,145] Administration of total-body irradiation does not seem to provide any additional benefit and only adds toxicity.[143,144] The European cooperative group is conducting a randomized study to evaluate the role of HSCT in the care of patients with metastatic Ewing's sarcoma.

Improvement in outcome among patients with ESFT also must be attributed to improvement in local control, which is largely related to advances in planning radiation therapy[100,101] and better surgical approaches. Advances in systemic therapy by means of incorporation of new drugs and treatment intensification also appear to contribute to better local control.[105,146-148] With current multimodal intensive protocols, rates of local recurrence have decreased significantly, and there appears to be little difference in efficacy between surgery and radiation therapy for local control.[99,146,147,149] Surgery continues to offer slightly better results, but this observation is biased by the fact that small lesions are more likely to be managed surgically.[103,150-152] For unresectable tumors or in case of gross residual disease, recommended doses are 55 to 60 Gy. Doses of 40 to 45 Gy are used for microscopic disease. The risk of secondary sarcoma after radiation therapy is not negligible.[153] This risk is dose dependent, but attempts at using lower doses of radiation therapy have been associated with higher local recurrence rates.[154]

NEUROBLASTOMA

Epidemiology

Neuroblastoma is the most common extracranial solid tumor of childhood, accounting for 8% to 10% of all pediatric cancers.[155] In the United States, the annual incidence is approximately 8 new cases per 1 million children per year with 550 newly diagnosed cases. The median age at diagnosis is 2 years. Most (85%) of the cases are diagnosed by 5 years of age. Neuroblastoma is extremely rare in children older than 10 years. Familial cases occur. Neuroblastoma also has been found in patients with neurofibromatosis, Hirschsprung's disease, Beckwith-Wiedemann syndrome, and fetal hydantoin syndrome.[156-160] Microscopic neuroblast nodules are found in the adrenal glands of 2% to 3% of infants who die of nonmalignant causes before 3 months of age.[161,162] It is uncertain whether these nodules represent spontaneous regression of congenital neuroblastoma or maturation of the tumor into asymptomatic benign tumors.

Mass screening programs for detection of neuroblastoma in early infancy with assays for urinary catecholamine metabolites have been conducted in Japan, Germany, and the United States.[163-166] In general, patients with disease detected in these programs have early-stage disease and otherwise excellent outcome.[167,168] However, mass screening has not resulted in a reduction in mortality from neuroblastoma. In addition, early detection has not changed outcome among patients with tumors that have biologic features associated with a poor prognosis.[169]

Biology

Neuroblastoma originates in neural crest cells of the sympathetic nervous system and, not unexpectedly, secretes a variety of neurogenically derived substances, including catecholamines, neuron-specific enolase (NSE), and ferritin.[170-175] Urinary excretion of abnormally high levels of catecholamine metabolites occurs in 75% to 90% of patients and is related to the degree of tumor differentiation. The metabolites most often measured in evaluation of suspected neuroblastoma are urinary vanillylmandelic acid and homovanillic acid. Levels of these catecholamines are sensitive indicators of disease status. At diagnosis other biologic markers, such as NSE, serum ferritin, and ganglioside G_{D2}, are present in high concentration in the serum of most patients with neuroblastoma.[176-181] None of these biologic markers is specific, but their presence at diagnosis may be associated with extent of disease.

Cytogenetic studies of neuroblastoma have demonstrated chromosomal abnormalities in most cases. The most common cytogenetic abnormalities in neuroblastoma are double-minute chromatin bodies (DM), homogeneously staining regions (HSRs), and nonrandom deletion or loss of heterozygosity of the short arm of chromosome 1.[169,182-187] DMs and HSRs both represent cytogenetic manifestations of amplified sequences of the *MYCN* cellular oncogene.[188,189] Amplified *MYCN* (more than 10 copies/cell) is present in approximately 30% of neuroblastomas. It is associated with the presence of advanced disease at diagnosis and poor outcome, even in

patients who have early-stage disease or who come to medical attention in infancy.[190-192] The DNA content of the tumor (ploidy) has been shown to correlate with therapeutic outcome and survival among infants with this tumor. Infants with hyperdiploid tumors (DNA index greater than 1.0) have a more favorable outcome than those with diploid tumors (DNA index, 1.0).[193-196] Results suggest that the presence of either *MYCN* amplification or diploid cellular DNA tumor content identifies whether an infant has a poor prognosis with current therapeutic regimens, independent of stage.[194,197,198] However, for children older than 24 months with disseminated disease, the DNA content of the tumor does not appear to have prognostic importance.[193,195]

Pathology

Neuroblastoma is one of the small round blue cell tumors of childhood. It originates from neural crest cells from within the sympathetic nervous system. Neuroblastoma can be classified pathologically into three broad histologic subgroups: neuroblastoma, ganglioneuroblastoma, and ganglioneuroma[199-201] (Fig. 99-8). These subgroups appear

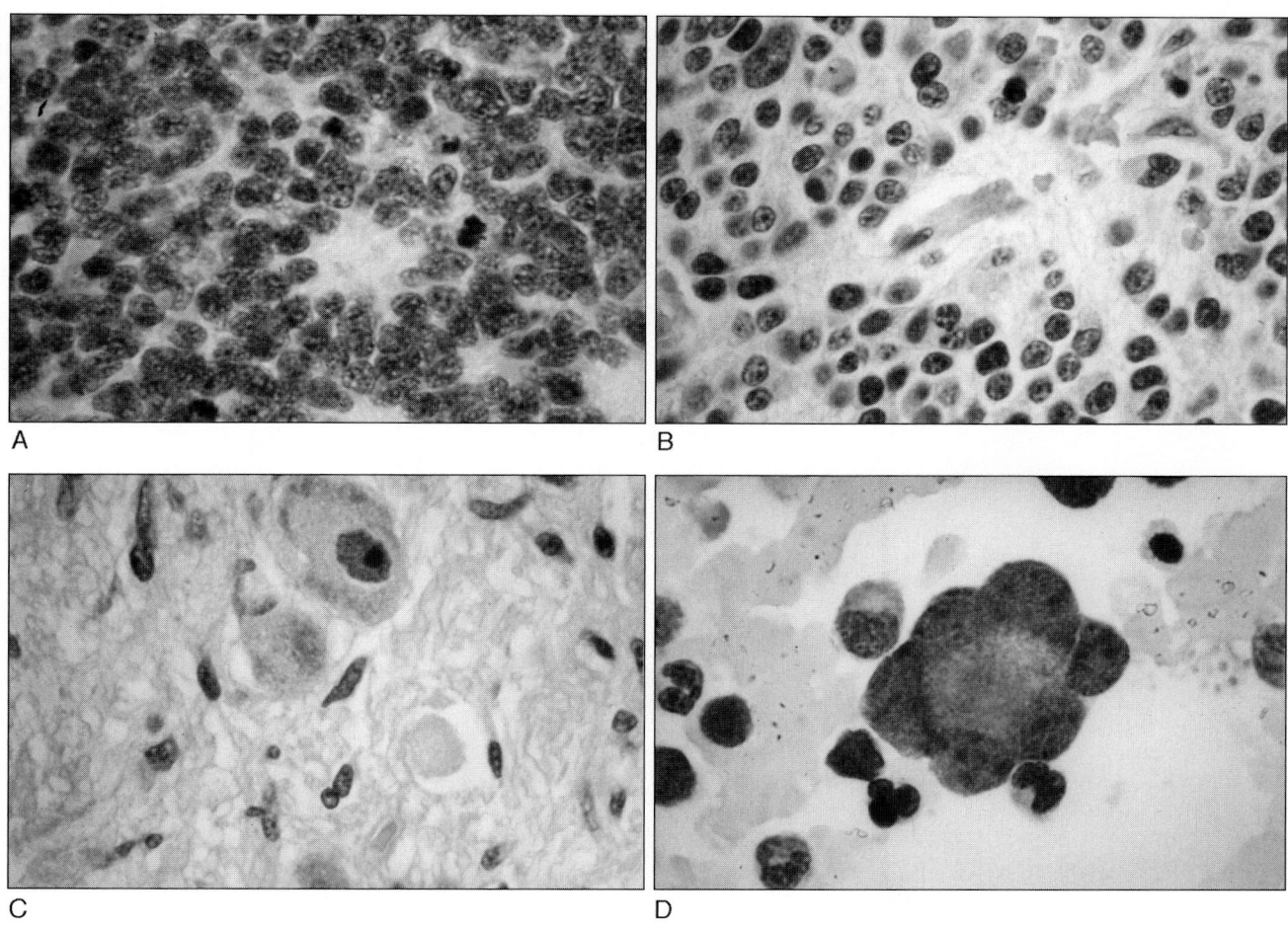

Figure 99-8. A, Neuroblastoma with nest of dense primitive cells surrounding a fibrillar center. **B,** Ganglioneuroblastoma consisting of primitive cells but with increased amounts of fibrillar material. **C,** Ganglioneuroma with well-differentiated ganglion cells, Schwann cells, and nerve bundles. **D,** Bone marrow involvement with metastatic neuroblastoma forming a pseudorosette.

Specific Malignancies

III

to recapitulate stages in the normal differentiation of neural crest stem cells. For example, neuroblastoma is the most primitive entity and is characterized by diffuse growth of undifferentiated neuroblastic cell nests irregularly separated by thin fibrovascular septa[202,203] (Fig. 99-8A). By contrast, benign ganglioneuroma consists of mature ganglion cells embedded in bulky stroma composed of Schwann cell sheets enveloping neuritic processes and perineural and endoneural elements (Fig. 99-8C). Between these two extremes is the transitional form known as *ganglioneuroblastoma* (Fig. 99-8B). These transitional forms have been subclassified into intermixed and nodular diffuse ganglioneuroblastoma. Composite (nodular) tumor is a ganglioneuroma that contains one or more discrete nodules of pure neuroblastoma. Intermixed (diffuse) tumor contains a mixture of primitive and differentiating neuroblasts with bizarre, immature, and mature ganglion cells. Patients frequently have tumors with mixtures of these cell types, and evidence supports the clinical observation that neuroblastoma can sometimes mature into benign ganglioneuroma. Spontaneous regression and therapy-induced maturation can occur.[204]

In 1999, the International Neuroblastoma Pathology Classification was established to standarize the terminology and criteria for the prognostic evaluation of the morphologic features of neuroblastic tumors in an age-linked framework.[202]

Clinical Manifestations

The clinical manifestations of neuroblastoma are varied. Nonspecific constitutional symptoms, such as fever, general malaise, and pain, are frequent initial features. The most common sites of primary tumors are the abdomen (adrenal gland or paraspinal ganglia) or the thorax (usually the posterior mediastinum). In infants, the distribution is slightly different in that a higher proportion of primary tumors occur in the thoracic cavity than is the case in older children. Common manifestations include a hard, painless mass in the neck, a localized intrathoracic mass found incidentally on a chest radiograph, or a palpable abdominal mass. A palpable abdominal mass can result from an enlarging primary adrenal or retroperitoneal tumor or from hepatomegaly secondary to tumor metastasis. Children may appear chronically ill and irritable and have periorbital ecchymosis, scalp nodules, and bone pain from widespread metastasis to the bone marrow or bone (Figs. 99-8D and 99-9). Lower limb paresis secondary to epidural extension of a primary paraspinal tumor growing through the intervertebral foramen can cause signs of spinal cord compression. Intermittent abdominal pain, malaise, failure to gain weight, and recurrent, unexplained fever may be present for prolonged periods before neuroblastoma is diagnosed.

Seventy-five percent of patients with neuroblastoma have metastatic disease at the time of diagnosis. The most common sites of metastasis are lymph nodes (local or distant), bone marrow, liver, skin, orbit, and bone (facial bones, skull, appendicular skeleton). Nearly one half of patients have widespread skeletal metastasis at diagnosis.[205,206] The bones of the skull and orbit are frequently affected, so proptosis, ecchymosis, and masses beneath the scalp are frequent findings (see Fig. 99-9). Lung metastatic lesions are extremely uncommon when the patient is first examined.[207] Horner's syndrome (ipsilateral miosis, ptosis, and anhydrosis) may be present in patients with lesions originating in the cervical or upper thoracic sympathetic ganglia. Less frequent is the syndrome of opsomyoclonus. Patients with this syndrome

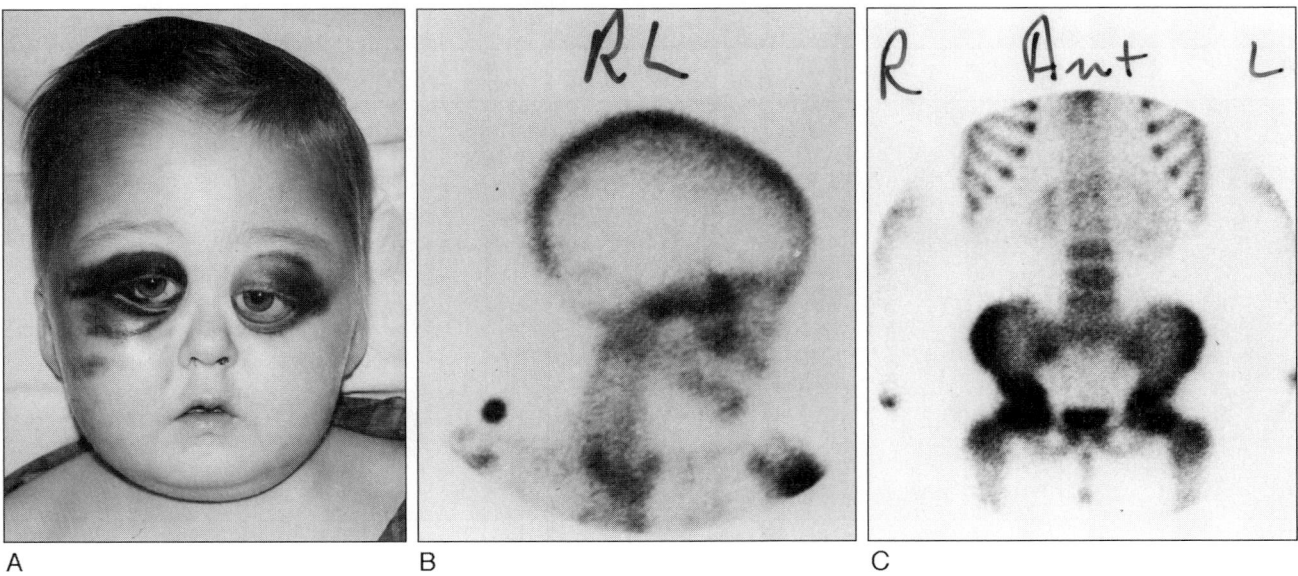

A   B   C

Figure 99-9. A, Periorbital ecchymosis secondary to metastatic orbital neuroblastoma. **B,** Radionuclide bone scan shows orbital and calvarial metastatic disease. **C,** Bone scan shows diffuse pelvic bone involvement with metastatic neuroblastoma.

have acute cerebellar encephalopathy, truncal ataxia, and rapid and random eye movements (so-called dancing eyes, dancing feet).[208] The pathophysiologic mechanism of this syndrome is unknown, but metabolic and immunologic causes have been invoked. A syndrome of chronic watery diarrhea may occur in patients with neuroblastoma. Increased serum levels of vasoactive intestinal peptide, which lead to increased intestinal motility and secretions, have been found in some cases.

Laboratory and Radiologic Evaluation

When neuroblastoma is suspected, evaluation should be performed to establish the diagnosis, determine the extent of disease, and obtain tumor material for molecular and genetic analyses. The physical examination should include special attention to blood pressure, asymmetric pupil size, facial sweating, lower limb weakness and other signs of spinal cord compression, and evidence of increased intracranial pressure. In addition, during the clinical examination, one should carefully document the size of palpable masses, enlarged lymph nodes, cutaneous lesions, and the liver.

Laboratory studies include complete blood cell count, renal and liver function studies, coagulation screen, urinalysis, and urine catecholamine assay. Serum often is obtained for NSE, ferritin, and ganglioside G_{D2} determinations, because the results may be helpful in prognosis.[173,178,209-211]

Staging of neuroblastoma requires radiologic studies and marrow aspiration and biopsy to determine the extent of local disease and distant spread. The minimal evaluation for metastatic disease includes skeletal scintigraphy and bone marrow aspiration. CT has generally replaced intravenous pyelography, arteriography, and inferior vena cavography (Fig. 99-10). Ultrasonographic studies of the abdomen and pelvis may be useful in evaluation of mass lesions and the degree of compression of vital structures

causing secondary complications. MRI may further improve the accuracy of determination of the anatomic extent of disease, especially in evaluation of tumors impinging on the spinal cord and evaluation for the presence of hepatic metastasis.[212] CT- or MRI-based myelography is necessary in evaluation of all patients with neurologic evidence of cord involvement.[213] Scans performed with radionuclides, such as [131]I-*m*-iodobenzylguanidine (MIBG) may be more accurate and sensitive for detection of nonosseous as well as osseous disease.[214-218] Newer modalities such as neural cell–specific monoclonal antibody conjugated to ^{131}I or ^{123}I are currently investigational. When tumor material is obtained, it should be submitted for determination of DNA content (tumor cell ploidy), presence of *MYCN* genomic amplification, and cytogenetic analysis.

The differential diagnosis suggested by the early manifestations of the tumor is broad because the initial symptoms can be so vague. The presence of an abdominal mass may suggest Wilms' tumor, hydronephrotic kidney, enlarged spleen or liver, lymphoma, germ cell tumor, and mesenteric cyst. Compression of vital structures in the neck and mediastinum can cause superior vena cava syndrome indistinguishable from that caused by other tumors.[219] Persistent diarrhea suggests the presence of a malabsorptive state. Arterial hypertension may be attributed to intrinsic renal disease or pheochromocytoma.[220] Bone pain can simulate rheumatic fever, rheumatoid arthritis, osteomyelitis, and acute leukemia. When initial signs are attributable to widespread lymphatic metastasis, a broad range of differential diagnoses, including primary tumor of the lymphoreticular system, storage disease, acute infection, and primary hematologic disorder, must be considered.

The diagnosis of neuroblastoma is established by pathologic evaluation of tumor tissue obtained at biopsy or by documentation of bone marrow involvement at bone marrow trephine biopsy or aspiration with the

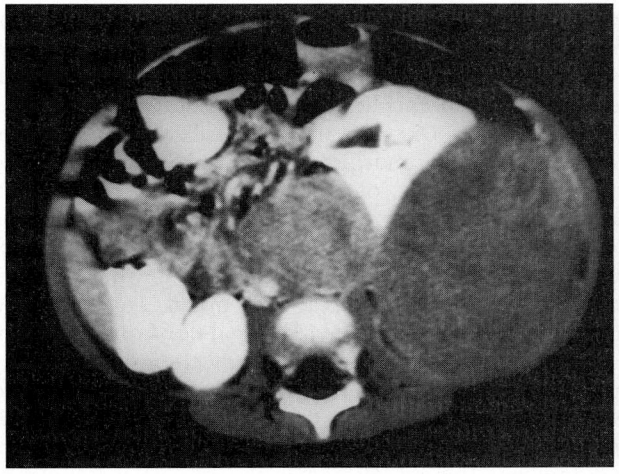
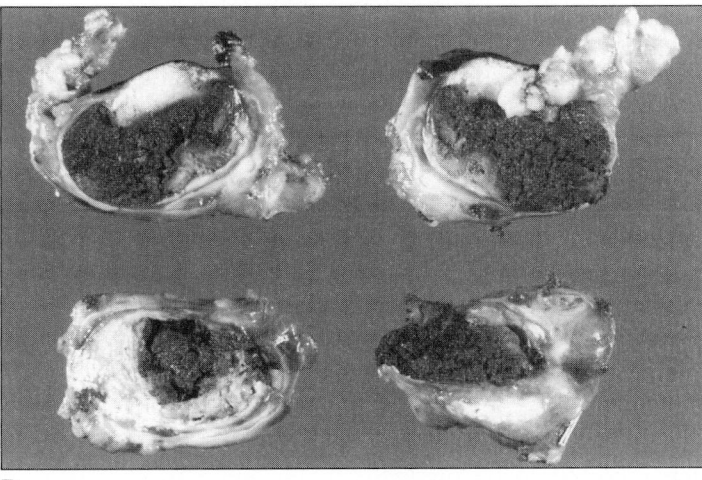

A   B

Figure 99-10. A, Computed tomographic scan shows adrenal neuroblastoma at diagnosis. **B,** Serial sections through adrenal neuroblastoma show tumor with large areas of diffuse hemorrhage and calcification.

TABLE 99-5

International Staging System for Neuroblastoma

STAGE	DESCRIPTION
I	Localized tumor confined to area of origin; complete gross excision with or without microscopic residual disease; identifiable ipsilateral and contralateral lymph nodes microscopically negative
2A	Unilateral tumor with incomplete gross excision; identifiable ipsilateral and contralateral lymph nodes microscopically negative
2B	Unilateral tumor with complete or incomplete gross excision; positive ipsilateral lymph nodes; identifiable contralateral lymph nodes microscopically negative
3	Unresectable unilateral tumor infiltrating across the midline with or without regional lymph node involvement; or unilateral tumor with contralateral lymph node involvement; or midline tumor with bilateral lymph node involvement
4	Metastatic tumor involvement to distant lymph nodes, bone, bone marrow, liver, or other organs (except as defined in stage 4S)
4S	Localized primary tumors as defined in stage I or 2 with dissemination limited to liver, skin, or bone marrow involvement <10% (but not bone); limited to infants younger than I year

presence of characteristic clumps or syncytia of tumor cells together with increased urine or serum levels of catecholamines or metabolites.[221] If the histologic diagnosis is equivocal, genetic features characteristic of neuroblastoma, such as deletion of chromosome 1p or *MYCN* genomic amplification, support the diagnosis. Several staging systems have been used to classify disease extent. The Evans and Pediatric Oncology Group staging systems were historically the most widely used in the United States. To facilitate comparison of clinical studies, the International Neuroblastoma Staging System (INSS) (Table 99-5), which is based on clinical, radiographic, and surgical evaluation, was developed by consensus of major pediatric oncology groups in the United States, Europe, and Japan.[222-227] The INSS uses the most important components of the Evans (e.g., midline extension) and the Pediatric Oncology Group (e.g., histologically positive or negative lymph nodes) systems. The main differences between these systems relate to surgical-pathologic staging and definitions distinguishing grossly unresected localized tumors from regional disease.[226]

Prognostic Factors

Although many factors have been investigated and purported to have prognostic significance in neuroblastoma, the most significant in prediction of cure are age and stage at diagnosis.[172,228,229] Children with low-stage disease have a good prognosis, regardless of age. In general, extent of disease at diagnosis is inversely related to cure. In infants, the DNA content of tumor cells has been reported to be predictive of response to chemotherapy and ultimate outcome. Infants with hyperdiploid tumors fare better than those with diploid tumors.[195] In children with metastatic disease, the most significant

prognostic variable is age at diagnosis. Children younger than 12 months at diagnosis have a significantly greater chance of cure.[230,231] In older children with disseminated disease, the prognosis is dismal, although improvements in response and survival have been reported with modern treatment modalities.

A variety of biologic markers of neuroblastoma have been used to identify whether a patient is at prognostically low, intermediate, or high risk. These markers include tumor markers, such as urinary catecholamine excretion, serum levels of ferritin, NSE, LDH, and ganglioside G_{D2}. Histologic subclassification based on degree of differentiation or presence or absence of stroma, mitoses, or karyorrhexis also has been used as a prognostic indicator (Shimada histopathologic classification). However, identification of various biologic and genetic features, such as the karyotype, DNA index determined by flow cytometry, *MYCN* copy number, deletion of regions of chromosome 1p, P-glycoprotein expression, and expression of the nerve growth receptor TRK-A, has defined subsets of patients with different outcomes of therapy.[183,197,198,232,233] For example, *MYCN* amplification can be used as a marker of poor outcome independent of age, whereas TRK-A appears to be a marker of favorable outcome.[234,235] Clinical studies are being conducted in an attempt to correlate the most informative combination of biologic markers, age, and stage to develop appropriate risk-directed therapeutic groups[236] (Table 99-6).

Treatment

A complete pathologic evaluation in conjunction with assessment of clinical features is important, because management of neuroblastoma is based on extent of disease. Accurate staging of the tumor at diagnosis is essential. Staging includes diagnostic imaging, pathologic assessment of lymph node involvement in locoregional disease, liver biopsy in the case of primary abdominal disease in infants, and determination of the presence of hematogenous dissemination (usually to bone or to bone marrow).[237] Patients with tumors localized to one side of the midline or that cross the midline without encasement of major blood vessels are candidates for primary surgical resection.[238-241] With local disease, complete gross surgical resection gives an excellent chance of cure without additional therapy. If the patient has localized unresectable disease, potentially morbid surgical procedures should be avoided because of the excellent outcome with chemotherapy in this setting. If the tumor cannot be excised because it encases major blood vessels, surgery is performed for diagnostic purposes or for palliation if the tumor is compressing a vital organ. This situation includes dumbbell tumors with spinal cord compression, in which rapid response to chemotherapy generally obviates laminectomy.[242] In patients with disseminated disease when they come to medical attention, initial aggressive surgical approaches have been shown to be of no significant benefit. However, the potential benefit of resection of bulky primary tumors after reductive chemotherapy in disseminated disease (delayed or second-look resection) is currently under investigation.

TABLE 99-6

Risk Categorization of Neuroblastoma on the Basis of Clinical and Biologic Features

INSS STAGE	AGE	MYCN STATUS	SHIMADA FEATURES	DNA PLOIDY*	RISK GROUP
1	0–21 yr	Any	Any	Any	Low
2A/2B	<365 d	Any	Any	Any	Low
	≥365 d–21 yr	Nonamplified	Any	—	Low
	≥365 d–21 yr	Amplified	Favorable	—	Low
	≥365 d–21 yr	Amplified	Unfavorable	—	High
3	<365 d	Nonamplified	Any	Any	Intermediate
	<365 d	Amplified	Any	Any	High
	≥365 d–21 yr	Nonamplified	Favorable	—	Intermediate
	≥365 d–21 yr	Nonamplified	Unfavorable	—	High
	≥365 d–21 yr	Amplified	Any	—	High
4	<365 d	Nonamplified	Any	Any	Intermediate
	<365 d	Amplified	Any	Any	High
	≥365 d–21 yr	Any	Any	—	High
4S	<365 d	Nonamplified	Favorable	>1	Low
	<365 d	Nonamplified	Any	1	Intermediate
	<365 d	Nonamplified	Unfavorable	Any	Intermediate
	<365 d	Amplified	Any	Any	High

INSS, International Neuroblastoma Staging System.
*DNA ploidy: DNA index (DI) >1 or 1. Hypodiploid tumors (DI <1, considered favorable ploidy) are treated as tumors with DI >1.

ST. JUDE CHILDREN'S RESEARCH HOSPITAL APPROACH TO THE MANAGEMENT OF NEUROBLASTOMA

We use a risk-categorization algorithm in which therapy for neuroblastoma is prescribed on the basis of clinical and biologic features. For patients with completely resected tumors independent of age or tumor biology, we recommend no further treatment after surgery and close monitoring and follow-up evaluation. In the event of disease recurrence, further surgical treatment with or without chemotherapy is instituted. Similarly, patients younger than 1 year with incomplete resection or limited nodal metastasis (in the absence of unfavorable biologic features) undergo no further therapy after surgery. Patients younger than 1 year with unresectable tumors (i.e., stage 3) and absence of the MYCN gene amplification receive a shortened course of chemotherapy comprising cyclophosphamide, doxorubicin, etoposide, and carboplatin. We administer chemotherapy to patients with epidural tumor in an attempt to avoid laminectomy. All patients older than 1 year with metastatic disease or unfavorable biologic features (e.g., MYCN gene amplification) or unfavorable histologic findings are treated in research studies that incorporate an induction phase with alkylating agents (e.g., cyclophosphamide), cisplatin, doxorubicin, and etoposide followed by surgery for removal of the primary lesion and a consolidation phase with high-dose chemotherapy with or without radiation and autologous hematopoietic stem cell transplantation followed by 6 months of oral retinoic acid. Pilot studies incorporating new agents, such as topotecan and irinotecan, also are under investigation. When primary treatment fails, experimental therapies with biologic agents (anti-GD$_2$ antibodies), MIBG therapy, or new cytotoxics usually are recommended.

Radiation therapy often is used for management of neuroblastoma and is particularly useful in treating patients with tumors that are localized but unresectable, even after initial chemotherapy and second-look surgery. Because of the high frequency of metastatic disease, radiation therapy has a relatively limited role in initial overall treatment of a child with neuroblastoma. Indications for radiation therapy include control of local tumors unresponsive or resistant to chemotherapy and not amenable to surgical extirpation, palliative management of unresectable or metastatic disease, and management of 4S neuroblastoma (in selected cases). The last indication is based on the observation that infants with bona fide stage 4S disease sometimes respond to subtherapeutic doses of radiation (400–800 cGy) delivered to ports that do not encompass all known sites of disease.

Chemotherapy is the primary modality of treatment of most children with neuroblastoma, because the disease is frequently widespread at diagnosis.[243-246] A variety of single agents (cyclophosphamide, melphalan, doxorubicin, cisplatin, epipodophyllotoxin, vincristine) produce responses in patients with neuroblastoma, but significant and durable responses have been achieved only with combination chemotherapy.[247-250] In general, pairs of these drugs, such as cyclophosphamide and doxorubicin or cisplatin and etoposide, delivered in a cytokinetically rational manner are more effective in producing responses than are single agents. Although improvement in survival of infants with advanced-stage disease and children with locally unresectable disease has resulted from implementation of various chemotherapeutic regimens, the outlook for older children with advanced disease has not changed dramatically. Only 20% to 25% of these patients survive 5 years from diagnosis.[243] These studies have shown, however, that among older children the complete response rate and disease-free interval have increased with more intensive combination chemotherapy, encouraging further development and refinement of this therapy.

Some current therapeutic regimens for neuroblastoma are so intensive that myelosuppression can be the dose-limiting toxicity. This problem can be overcome with hematopoietic stem cell transplantation. High-dose chemotherapy with bone marrow transplantation may be useful in the care of patients with a poor long-term prognosis who have achieved complete remission or at least substantial partial remission with chemotherapy.[251-256] The propensity of neuroblastoma to involve bone marrow has spurred development of various purging strategies, including tumor cell depletion with monoclonal antibodies or ex vivo chemotherapy, to facilitate autologous transplantation. Results with various transplantation protocols, both autologous and allogeneic, suggest a modest survival advantage for these aggressive regimens.[256]

Improvements in supportive care, including use of hematopoietic growth factors, may allow shortening of the intervals between treatment courses. They also may allow increases in the dose intensity of currently available chemotherapeutic agents in the treatment of patients with advanced-stage disease and decreases in toxicity among infants. In addition, parallel clinical studies of newer biologic therapies, such as differentiation agents and immunomodulators, in a setting of minimal residual disease or genetically engineered tumor vaccines will form the basis for future therapeutic gains.[257]

WILMS' TUMOR

Epidemiology

Wilms' tumor, or nephroblastoma, is the most common primary malignant renal neoplasm of childhood. Although relatively rare, this disease has served as a paradigm for multimodal management of childhood solid tumors. Owing to refinements in surgery, chemotherapy, and radiation therapy, the overall cure rate for Wilms' tumor exceeds 85%. Studies of Wilms' tumor genetics have laid the foundation for our understanding of tumor suppressor genes and genomic imprinting.

The annual incidence of Wilms' tumor is 8 cases per million children younger than 15 years, representing 6.3% of cases of childhood cancer.[258] In the United States, approximately 460 new cases are diagnosed each year, making Wilms' tumor the fourth most common pediatric cancer by specific histologic type.[258] The incidence of Wilms' tumor varies with race and ethnic group. The range is 2.5 cases per million Chinese children to 10.9 cases per million African American children.[259] Girls have a slightly increased risk of Wilms' tumor with a male-to-female ratio of 0.92 to 1.00. The mean age at diagnosis is 44 months for unilateral disease and 31 months for bilateral disease. According to the Knudson two-hit model of tumorigenesis, the earlier age at onset of bilateral Wilms' tumor represents a genetic predisposition to the disease. Wilms' tumor in the adult population is rare, although numerous cases have been reported.[260,261] Although results of older studies indicate that the prognosis for adult Wilms' tumor is unfavorable, newer reports demonstrate cure of both localized and advanced disease with treatment regimens similar to those used for children.[262]

Familial Wilms' tumor is uncommon, occurring in only 1.5% of affected patients.[263] Most cases of familial Wilms' tumor occur in distant relatives rather than parents or siblings. Sixteen percent of cases of familial Wilms' tumor are bilateral, compared with 7% of sporadic cases. Unlike retinoblastoma, familial Wilms' tumor is bilateral in only a small number of cases. Conversely, only a small proportion (3%) of cases of bilateral Wilms' tumor are familial. The mean ages at diagnosis of familial unilateral and bilateral disease are 35 months and 16 months, respectively.

Biology

Although Wilms' tumor was one of the original paradigms of the Knudson two-hit model of cancer formation,[264] it has become apparent that several genetic events participate in Wilms' tumorigenesis. *WT1* was the first Wilms' tumor gene identified and is the most completely characterized Wilms' tumor gene to date. The discovery of *WT1* began with the observation that patients with aniridia, genitourinary anomalies, and mental retardation are at high (>30%) risk of development of Wilms' tumor (WAGR syndrome). Cytogenetic analysis of persons with WAGR syndrome revealed large deletions at chromosome 11p13, which was later found to encompass a contiguous set of genes, including *PAX6*, the gene responsible for aniridia,[265] and *WT1*.[266-268] Patients with sporadic aniridia (*PAX6* defect with normal *WT1*) are not at increased risk of Wilms' tumor.[269] *WT1* encodes a transcription factor critical to normal kidney and gonadal development, but whose precise role in tumorigenesis is undefined. Although germinal deletions or mutations in *WT1* have been documented in almost all patients with WAGR syndrome and the related Denys-Drash syndrome, only a small number of patients with seemingly sporadic Wilms' tumor carry *WT1* mutations in the germline (5%) or in tumor tissue (6%-18%).[270-273] Although *WT1* is a bona fide tumor suppressor gene, its role in sporadic Wilms' tumor development is limited.

A second Wilms' tumor–associated condition is Beckwith-Wiedemann syndrome (BWS), which is an overgrowth disorder that manifests as high birth weight, macroglossia, organomegaly, hemihypertrophy, neonatal hypoglycemia, abdominal wall defects, and ear pits and creases. Patients with BWS have a 5% to 10% risk of development of Wilms' tumor but are also predisposed to other malignant tumors, such as hepatoblastoma, adrenocortical carcinoma, neuroblastoma, and rhabdomyosarcoma.[274] BWS maps to chromosome 11p15, sometimes called *WT2*, because loss of heterozygosity at this locus has been detected in Wilms' tumor.[275,276] Although the precise *WT2* gene is undefined, molecular characterization of the *WT2* locus has revealed several genes that may play a role in tumorigenesis. These genes are imprinted, which means they are preferentially expressed from one of the two parental alleles. Loss of imprinting, leading to aberrant messenger RNA and protein expression, has been postulated as a mechanism of tumor formation. Genes at the *WT2* locus that have been suggested to contribute to Wilms' tumorigenesis include *IGF2*, *H19*, and *p57^{Kip2}* (*CDKN1C*).[277-283]

Genes and loci other than *WT1* and *WT2* have been implicated in the molecular pathogenesis of Wilms' tumor. In two studies investigators found that approximately 15% of Wilms' tumors have activating mutations of β-catenin, a central effector of the Wnt signaling pathway.[284,285] Interestingly, the β-catenin mutations were strongly associated with *WT1* mutations, indicating that these two genes operate in distinct pathways and may collaborate in the genesis of Wilms' tumor. Genetic linkage analysis has identified two familial Wilms' tumor loci, called *FWT1* and *FWT2*, on chromosomes 17 and 19, respectively.[286,287] Identifying the pertinent genes at these loci is an area of active investigation. Loss of heterozygosity at chromosomes 1p and 16q has been found in 10% to 20% of Wilms' tumors. Loss at either of these loci has been associated with adverse prognosis and will be used for treatment stratification in a Children's Oncology Group study.[288-290] Cytogenetic and loss of heterozygosity analyses have revealed recurrent abnormalities of chromosome 7p, but the clinical and biologic significance of these findings is unknown.[291,292] Finally, mutations in the p53 gene are observed in most cases of anaplastic histologic features of Wilms' tumor, implicating a role for this gene in progression from favorable to anaplastic histologic type.[293-295]

Pathology

Classic Wilms' tumor consists of blastemal, stromal, and epithelial elements, although tumors do not necessarily contain all three (Fig. 99-11). Because Wilms' tumor can be recognized with standard hematoxylin and eosin staining, the role of ultrastructural or immunohistochemical studies is limited. Other childhood renal neoplasms that must be considered in the differential diagnosis of Wilms' tumor are clear cell sarcoma of the kidney, rhabdoid tumor of the kidney, congenital mesoblastic nephroma, renal cell carcinoma, and soft-tissue sarcoma of the kidney.

An important advance in the care of patients with Wilms' tumor has been appreciation of the prognostic importance of histologic subtype. In 1978, Beckwith and Palmer published the results of a detailed histopathologic review of the cases of patients entered in the first National Wilms' Tumor Study (NWTS).[296] Approximately 6% of the Wilms' tumor specimens contained *anaplasia*, a term used to describe nuclear enlargement and atypia with irregular mitotic figures (Fig. 99-12). The presence of anaplasia was prognostically significant; 11 (44%) of 25 patients with anaplasia died of tumor, whereas only 26 (7.1%) of 364 patients without anaplasia died of tumor. Results of subsequent studies by NWTS investigators, studies by the International Society of Pediatric Oncology (SIOP), and a United Kingdom Wilms' tumor study confirmed the adverse prognostic significance of anaplastic histologic features.[297,298]

Nephrogenic rests are foci of embryonal kidney cells that persist abnormally into postnatal life. They are present in approximately 1% of newborn kidneys and usually regress or differentiate by early childhood.[299] Because nephrogenic rests are present in the kidneys of approximately 40% of patients with Wilms' tumor, it is presumed that the rests represent Wilms' tumor precursors. Current models of Wilms' tumorigenesis propose that a mutation in a tumor suppressor gene, such as *WT1*, predisposes to nephrogenic rests, which may sustain additional mutations and transform into a Wilms' tumor.[300]

Clinical Manifestations and Patterns of Spread

Wilms' tumor typically manifests as an asymptomatic abdominal mass discovered by a parent or health care practitioner. The mass is smooth and firm, is fixed in

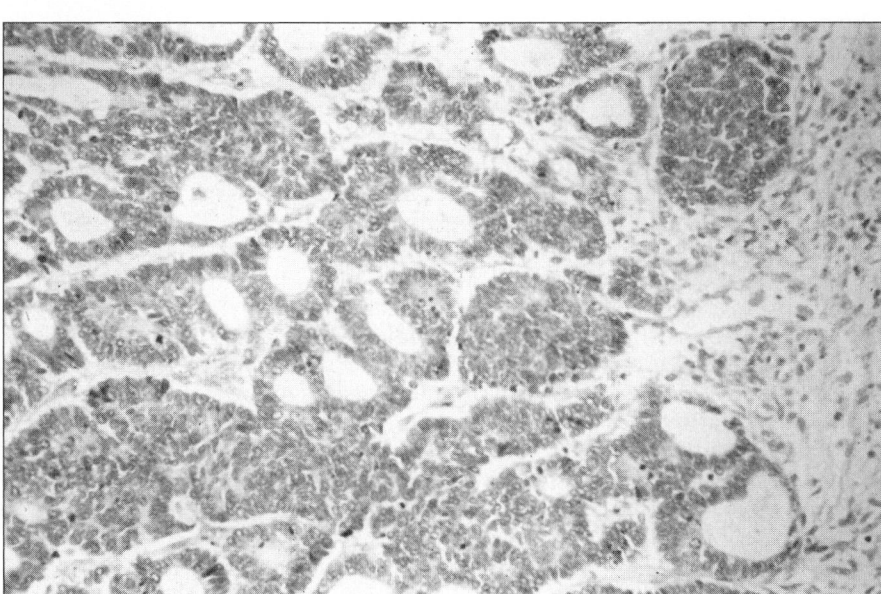

Figure 99-11. Triphasic Wilms' tumor with well-defined tubules surrounded by dense clusters of blastemal cells and zones of pale-staining stromal differentiation (×20).

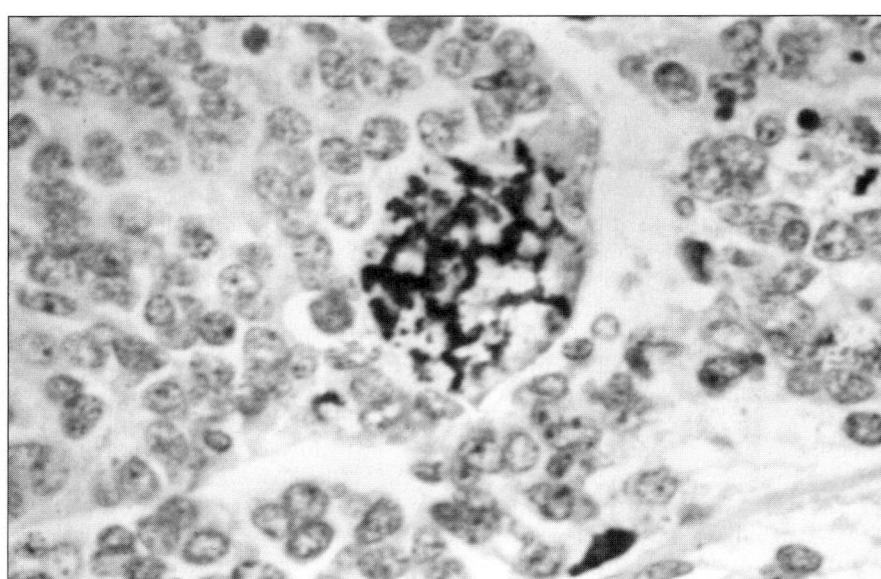

Figure 99-12. Anaplastic Wilms' tumor with several enlarged, hyperchromatic, bizarre nuclei (×60).

position, and often extends across the midline. Abdominal pain, fever, anemia, hematuria, and hypertension are other common signs and symptoms observed in 20% to 30% of children with Wilms' tumor.[301] Constitutional symptoms (e.g., weight loss, cachexia, and bone pain) are unusual manifestations of Wilms' tumor.

Wilms' tumor can spread both locally and hematogenously. Local spread typically occurs into the renal hilar structures and may penetrate the renal capsule. The tumors also have a propensity to invade the renal vein and form thrombi in the inferior vena cava, sometimes progressing as far as the right atrium. Local and distant lymph node involvement can occur. The most common sites of hematogenous metastasis are the lungs and liver.

Laboratory and Radiologic Evaluation

The goal of imaging before Wilms' tumor therapy is to define the extent of disease, assess the contralateral kidney, and determine whether tumor thrombus is present. Ultrasonography with Doppler technique is the recommended first-line study for Wilms' tumor because it allows panoramic examination of the abdomen, including the patency of the inferior vena cava, in a safe and painless manner (Fig. 99-13). CT can depict pelvic and abdominal structures as well as lymph nodes (Fig. 99-14). CT is especially useful in detection of bilateral tumors. Intravenous pyelography and MRI are not typically necessary in the evaluation of Wilms' tumor, although MRI may facilitate differentiation between nephrogenic rests and Wilms' tumor.[302] Because Wilms' tumor metastasizes to the lungs, preoperative chest radiography is imperative. Plain radiographs of the chest are the traditional evaluation. Although chest CT is more sensitive than plain radiography in the detection of pulmonary metastasis, its role in initial evaluation for Wilms' tumor is controversial because CT is associated with false-positive findings and high inter-reader variability among radiologists.[303-305]

Moreover, it is not clear whether the prognosis among patients with small pulmonary nodules detected only with chest CT is inferior to the prognosis among patients without radiologically detectable pulmonary metastasis.[306,307]

Treatment

The dramatic increase in cure rate of Wilms' tumor over the past 30 years is largely a testimony to the efforts of cooperative groups consisting of oncologists, surgeons, radiation oncologists, pathologists, and statisticians. Nearly all patients undergo surgery as the primary method

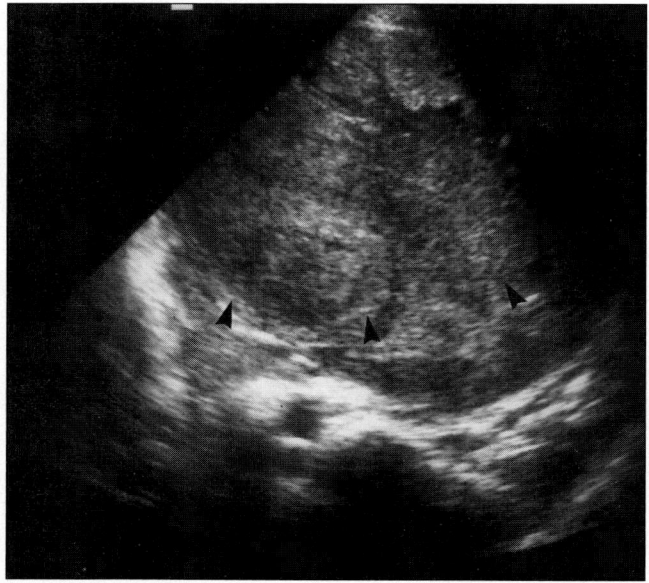

Figure 99-13. Transverse sonogram shows large Wilms' tumor with almost no remaining normal renal parenchyma.

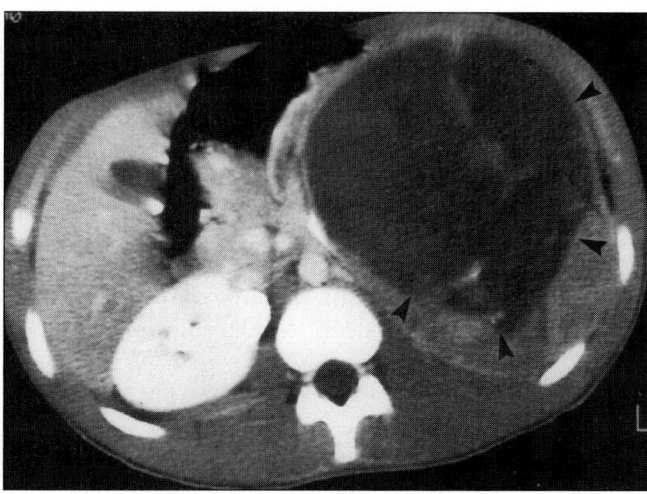

Figure 99-14. Transverse computed tomographic image of the Wilms' tumor depicted in Figure 99-13 shows a large intrarenal mass.

TABLE 99-7

National Wilms' Tumor Study Clinicopathologic Staging

STAGE	DESCRIPTION
I	Tumor limited to kidney and completely excised. No penetration of the renal capsule or involvement of renal sinus vessels.
II	Tumor extends beyond the kidney but is completely excised with negative margins and lymph nodes. At least one of the following has occurred: (a) penetration of the renal capsule, (b) invasion of the renal sinus vessels, (c) biopsy of the tumor before removal (except for fine needle aspirate, which may qualify as stage I), (d) spillage of tumor locally during removal.
III	Gross or microscopic residual tumor remains postoperatively, including inoperable tumor, positive surgical margins, diffuse tumor spillage involving peritoneal surfaces, regional lymph node metastasis, or transected tumor thrombus.
IV	Hematogenous metastasis (lung, liver, bone, brain) or lymph node metastasis outside the abdominal or pelvic cavities.
V	Bilateral renal tumors at diagnosis.

of achieving local control. The NWTS group advocates surgical resection at diagnosis, which yields the most accurate staging information. In contrast, SIOP recommends preoperative chemotherapy with the aim of decreasing tumor size, promoting fibrosis, and hence preventing intraoperative tumor spillage. Both approaches produce high rates of treatment success. The following discussion focuses on the results of the NWTS.

ST. JUDE CHILDREN'S RESEARCH HOSPITAL APPROACH TO THE MANAGEMENT OF WILMS' FAMILY TUMORS

Patients with suspected Wilms' tumor undergo nephrectomy at diagnosis unless the disease is bilateral or unresectable. We treat patients with stage I and II Wilms' tumor with favorable histologic features with 18 weeks of vincristine and actinomycin D without radiation therapy. We treat patients with stage III and IV Wilms' tumor with favorable histologic features with 24 weeks of vincristine, actinomycin D, and doxorubicin with radiation to the involved sites. Management of bilateral (stage V) Wilms' tumor is complex, and each patient needs an individualized treatment plan. In general, we perform biopsy on at least one tumor to establish the diagnosis and administer preoperative chemotherapy before definitive nephron-sparing surgery is attempted. Because patients with bilateral Wilms' tumor do not undergo lymph node sampling at diagnosis, we use three-drug chemotherapy (vincristine, actinomycin D, and doxorubicin). If the tumor margins after nephron-sparing surgery are positive for viable tumor, we administer flank radiation to the side with residual disease. Diffuse anaplastic Wilms' tumor is a therapeutic challenge. Patients with this tumor are treated with ifosfamide, carboplatin, and etoposide alternated with vincristine, doxorubicin, cyclophosphamide, and radiation to the flank and sites of metastatic disease.

Wilms' tumor surgery should be performed by an experienced pediatric surgeon through a transverse abdominal incision. The contralateral kidney, peritoneal surface, liver, and lymph nodes are inspected for tumor involvement. Biopsy is performed on suspicious lesions. A lymph node sample should be obtained whether or not the node appears involved. The tumor is then removed en bloc with the kidney, hilar structures, and a generous segment of the ureter. The adrenal gland is included in the resection if the tumor is adherent to the gland or if the tumor originates in the upper pole of the kidney. Caution should be exercised to avoid capsular rupture and tumor spillage, which could adversely influence staging and alter therapy. If a tumor is deemed inoperable owing to size or invasion of vital structures, biopsy is performed and adjuvant therapy is administered before definitive surgery. The NWTS staging system for Wilms' tumor is based on surgical and pathologic findings (Table 99-7).[308]

Consecutive trials of the NWTS beginning in the late 1960s provided critical insights into the role of adjuvant therapy for Wilms' tumor. NWTS-1 and NWTS-2 revealed that the combination of vincristine and actinomycin D is superior to treatment with either drug alone and that irradiation is not necessary in the care of patients with stage I disease. NWTS-3 showed that patients with stage II tumors with favorable histologic features can be treated without abdominal irradiation if vincristine and actinomycin D are administered. This study also revealed that the addition of doxorubicin to the two-drug regimen improves outcome in stage III and IV disease with favorable histologic features. If doxorubicin is administered, radiation doses of 1000 cGy are sufficient to eliminate residual microscopic disease in the abdomen. NWTS-3 also showed that addition of cyclophosphamide to the vincristine/actinomycin D/doxorubicin regimen improved outcome for patients with stages II through IV tumors with anaplastic histologic features but not tumors with

TABLE 99-8

Results of National Wilms' Tumor Studies 3 and 4

STAGE	4-YEAR RELAPSE-FREE SURVIVAL RATE* (%)	4-YEAR OVERALL SURVIVAL* (%)
Favorable Histologic Features		
I	89.0	95.6
II	87.4	91.1
III	82.0	90.9
IV	79.0	80.9
V	—	81.7
Anaplastic Histologic Features		
I	93.8[†]	93.3[†]
II	71.6	70.1
III	58.7	56.3
IV	16.7	16.7

*When more than one treatment was used, numbers reflect the results of the most successful regimen.
[†]Reflects 2-year rather than 4-year survival rate. Preliminary analysis of National Wilms' Tumor Study 5 data suggests that survival among patients with stage I anaplastic histologic features may not be as good as in previous studies. NWTS Data and Statistical Center, 2003, personal communication.

favorable histologic features. NWTS-4 compared the use of single-dose pulse-intensive actinomycin D and doxorubicin with the traditional divided-dose method of administration. The investigators found that pulse-intensive dosing was equally efficacious, less toxic, and more cost-effective than the conventional regimen.[309,310] NWTS-4 also revealed that 6 months of therapy for stage II through IV tumors with favorable histologic features was equivalent to 15 months of therapy. Results from the NWTS-3 and NWTS-4 are presented in Table 99-8.[310-313]

NWTS-5 study sought to capitalize on previous successes. The aim was to curtail therapy in low-risk groups, improve cure rates for high-risk groups, and identify novel prognostic markers. The treatment algorithms used in NWTS-5 are shown in Table 99-9.[308] One of the primary objectives was to evaluate whether adjuvant chemotherapy provides benefit to children

TABLE 99-9

National Wilms' Tumor Study Treatment Algorithms

STAGE TREATMENT

Favorable Histology

I and II AMD/VCR × 18 weeks, no XRT
III AMD/VCR/DOX × 24 weeks, XRT to flank or abdomen
IV AMD/VCR/DOX × 24 weeks, XRT to flank or abdomen if local stage III and to metastatic sites

Anaplastic Histology

I AMD/VCR × 18 weeks, no XRT
II–IV VCR/DOX/CPM/VP-16 for 24 weeks, XRT to flank or abdomen and to metastatic sites

AMD, dactinomycin; CPM, cyclophosphamide; DOX, doxorubicin; VCR, vincristine; VP-16, etoposide; XRT, radiation therapy.

younger than 24 months who have small stage I tumors with favorable histologic features, a group with an outstanding prognosis. Seventy-five patients who met the eligibility criteria were treated with surgical resection and close observation only. Eleven (14.7%) of these 75 patients had relapses or metachronous disease in the contralateral kidney, prompting early closure of this study arm.[314] Additional follow-up findings indicated that salvage therapy was very successful in this group. Only one patient had subsequent recurrence, and all patients were alive after a median follow-up period of 2.84 years. Future studies will reassess the need for adjuvant therapy in this group of patients.

Bilateral Wilms' Tumor

Bilateral Wilms' tumor occurs in approximately 5% to 10% of patients with Wilms' tumor. These children pose a therapeutic challenge because of difficulty in obtaining local control while sparing renal parenchyma. The approach to patients with bilateral Wilms' tumor is to administer preoperative chemotherapy to elicit tumor shrinkage and then to perform partial nephrectomy, whenever possible, or complete nephrectomy. Patients with tumors that cannot be resected with clear margins receive localized radiation therapy. The 4-year overall survival rate among patients with bilateral Wilms' tumor treated in NWTS-4 was 81.7%.[313] Compared with patients with unilateral Wilms' tumor, patients with bilateral tumors have an increased rate of renal failure, estimated to be 3.8% among patients treated in NWTS-4.[315] The most common cause of renal failure in this patient group is nephrectomy due to tumor progression or recurrence, not therapy-related effects.

Recurrent Wilms' Tumor

Despite excellent outcome among most patients with Wilms' tumor, approximately 10% to 15% of patients with disease with favorable histologic features and 50% of patients with anaplastic disease experience primary progression or tumor recurrence. The most common sites of recurrence are the lungs, liver, opposite kidney, and intra-abdominal sites, including the original tumor bed. Wilms' tumor occasionally recurs in the brain, bone, and distant lymph nodes. Most relapses are diagnosed within the first 2 years after the original diagnosis. Factors associated with favorable prognosis after recurrence include favorable histologic features, initial treatment with only vincristine and actinomycin D, relapse to the lungs only, relapse in the abdomen of a patient who did not receive abdominal irradiation, and relapse more than 12 months after the original diagnosis.[316,317] With aggressive therapy, approximately 60% to 80% of patients with favorable prognostic features can be cured. Salvage regimens are not as successful for patients with at least one unfavorable prognostic feature. Salvage regimens include ifosfamide, cyclophosphamide, carboplatin, and etoposide.[317-319] Several groups have used high-dose chemotherapy followed by autologous stem cell rescue in patients with recurrent Wilms' tumor.[320,321] Results are promising, but it is unclear whether high-dose therapy is superior to conventional-dose chemotherapy with modern agents.

Late Effects of Therapy

The late effects of Wilms' tumor treatment have received considerable attention because Wilms' tumor usually is curable, and there are a growing number of long-term survivors. Late complications can result from chemotherapy, radiation therapy, or the primary nephrectomy itself. Although most Wilms' tumor survivors have only one kidney, fewer than 1% of patients with unilateral Wilms' tumor treated in NWTS-1 through NWTS-4 were found to have renal failure.[315] The median interval from diagnosis to onset of renal failure was 21 months. Renal failure is most prevalent in patients with bilateral Wilms' tumor. Another recognized long-term effect of Wilms' tumor therapy is congestive heart failure (CHF), which was found to have a cumulative frequency of 4.4% 20 years after diagnosis of Wilms' tumor in patients initially treated with doxorubicin.[322] The frequency of CHF was higher among patients who received doxorubicin as part of a salvage chemotherapy regimen. Risk factors for CHF included increasing cumulative doxorubicin dose, female sex, and radiation to the lung and left hemiabdomen (but not right hemiabdomen). An analysis of pregnancy outcome among Wilms' tumor survivors revealed that women who received flank radiation therapy were at increased risk of fetal malposition, premature labor, low birth weight, and occurrence of congenital malformations.[323] Finally, the cumulative incidence of second malignant neoplasms in Wilms' tumor survivors was 1.6% 15 years after diagnosis of Wilms' tumor.[324]

RENAL CELL CARCINOMA

Renal cell carcinoma (RCC) is an uncommon malignant tumor of childhood. The latest Surveillance, Epidemiology and End Results statistics indicated an incidence of 0.4 cases per million persons younger than 20 years.[325] RCC represents 2% to 7% of primary renal malignant tumors of childhood.[326-328] The median age of children brought for evaluation of RCC is 9 years, considerably older than the age at manifestation of other pediatric renal malignant tumors. Unlike Wilms' tumor, clear cell sarcoma of the kidney, and rhabdoid tumor of the kidney, which have been studied by the NWTS group and SIOP, there have been no prospective clinical trials of therapy for pediatric RCC. Information about this entity is therefore limited to retrospective single-institutional case series.

Typical features of pediatric RCC include abdominal mass (24%–55%), hematuria (42%), and pain (32%). Children also may have the constitutional symptoms of hypertension, fever, weight loss, and polycythemia.[329] Approximately 25% of children with RCC have distant metastatic disease when they arrive for evaluation, most commonly to the lung, liver, and bone.

Tumors classified as childhood RCC compose a heterogeneous group of renal epithelial malignant neoplasms.

Childhood RCC may resemble the adult clear cell and papillary subtypes.[330] Although some reviews indicate that the papillary subtype is prevalent in the pediatric population,[330] other reviews indicate that the clear cell subtype is more common.[329,331] Genetic alterations at chromosome 3p, the site of the von Hippel-Lindau gene, have not been described in pediatric RCC, although few cytogenetic and molecular studies have been performed. A distinctive variant of RCC that preferentially affects children and young adults is characterized by the translocation t(X;17)(p11.2;q25), which results in a fusion product between the *TFE3* and *ASPL* genes. This same translocation is observed in alveolar soft-part sarcoma, but it is balanced in RCC and unbalanced in alveolar soft-part sarcoma.[332-334] Another variant is associated with the translocation t(6;11)(p21.1;q12).[335] The prevalence and clinical behavior of these variants have not been characterized. Another renal epithelial malignant neoplasm of childhood is renal medullary carcinoma, which is a highly aggressive tumor associated with sickle cell trait.[336]

Review of the pediatric literature from 1974 to 2000 reveals that overall survival for childhood RCC is 45%, outcome worsening with more advanced stage.[327-329,337-355] It is difficult to compare outcome of childhood RCC with that of adult RCC because different staging systems are used. Nevertheless, adult and pediatric RCC have similar stage-for-stage outcomes: very good outcome for stage I and II disease, less favorable outcome for stage III disease, and poor outcome for stage IV disease (Table 99-10). An apparent difference between adult and pediatric RCC is the prognostic significance of local lymph node involvement. Adults with RCC with lymph node involvement have a 5-year overall survival rate of approximately 20%. By contrast, a review of the published pediatric RCC experience showed that 29 (66%) of 44 patients with local lymph node involvement without distant metastatic lesions had durable survival (J. Geller and J. Dome, unpublished observations, 2003).

The optimal therapy for pediatric RCC is unknown. Nearly all patients have received chemotherapy (typically Wilms' tumor therapy) or radiation after nephrectomy. Because of the poor outcome among patients with metastatic disease and the lack of antitumor activity in

TABLE 99-10

Comparison of Outcomes for Adult* and Pediatric† Renal Cell Carcinoma

STAGE‡	NUMBER	SURVIVAL RATE (%)	NUMBER	SURVIVAL RATE (%)
I	303 (45%)	94	49 (30%)	96
II	119 (18%)	89.7	29 (17%)	72.4
III	150 (22%)	63.4	44 (27%)	54.5
IV	103 (15%)	28	43 (26%)	11.6
Total	675	74	165	45.5

*Adult data are 5-year survival estimates reported by Ficarra and colleagues.[356]
†Pediatric data are derived from a comprehensive review of the literature. J. Geller and J. Dome, 2003, unpublished observations.
‡The American Joint Committee on Cancer staging system (TNM) was used for adult staging and the modified Robson system for pediatric staging.

adult RCC, it is unlikely that chemotherapy or radiation therapy contributes significantly to improving patient outcome.[328] Several recently treated patients received interleukin-2 or interferon-α, and there have been case reports of responses.[342,343] Because of the favorable outcome among most children with localized and completely resected RCC, adjuvant therapy is not recommended for this group. On the other hand, the poor outcome associated with stage IV disease warrants the use of investigational agents. The Children's Oncology Group plans to open a childhood RCC study in which interleukin-2– and interferon-α–based therapy will be used in the treatment of children with metastatic or recurrent RCC.

RHABDOMYOSARCOMA

Epidemiology

Rhabdomyosarcoma is the most common soft-tissue sarcoma of childhood. According to population-based data from the Surveillance, Epidemiology and End Results program of the National Cancer Institute, rhabdomyosarcoma accounts for approximately 3% of pediatric malignant neoplasms.[357] The disease is slightly more common in boys than in girls, and approximately two thirds of cases occur in children younger than 10 years.[357-360] Embryonal RMS is the most common histologic subtype at all ages; however, adolescents have a higher proportion of alveolar RMS than other age groups.[357,361] In many cases, histologic features and primary site are correlated. For example, orbital and genitourinary sites are strongly associated with embryonal histologic features, whereas tumors of the extremities are most commonly of alveolar histologic type.[357,362-364]

Biology

RMS arises from primitive mesenchymal cells that retain capacity for skeletal muscle differentiation. The two main histologic subtypes of RMS, embryonal and alveolar, differ in biologic characteristics. The reciprocal translocation t(2;13)(q35;q14) is characteristic of tumors of the alveolar histologic type.[365] This translocation juxtaposes the *PAX3* gene located on chromosome 2q35 and the *FKHR* gene on chromosome 13q14 to form a novel chimeric gene that encodes an aberrant transcription factor. A less common translocation in alveolar RMS is t(1;13)(p36;q14), which fuses the *PAX7* gene located on chromosome 1p36 with the *FKHR* gene. The t(2;13) and t(1;13) translocations are found exclusively in alveolar RMS and are thus diagnostic of this histologic subtype.

Unlike alveolar RMS, embryonal RMS is not characterized by recurring chromosomal translocations. However, embryonal RMS is consistently associated with loss of heterozygosity at chromosome band 11p15.5. This association suggests the presence of a tumor suppressor gene at this location.[366] Children with Beckwith-Wiedemann syndrome, which is associated with cytogenetic alterations of chromosome band

11p15,[367] are at increased risk of RMS. This association is further evidence of a tumor suppressor gene at that locus.

A variety of other genetic alterations are associated with RMS. Li-Fraumeni syndrome, defined by germline mutation of the p53 tumor suppressor gene, is characterized by development of a variety of malignant neoplasms, including childhood RMS.[368] Sporadic mutation of the p53 gene has been identified in randomly selected tumor samples from children with RMS.[369] This finding suggests that acquired p53 alterations may play a role in development of this malignant disease. Other genetic abnormalities include amplification of the N-*myc* proto-oncogene in alveolar RMS[370] and point mutations in the N-*ras* and K-*ras* proto-oncogenes in embryonal RMS.[371]

Pathology

Although it can be difficult to establish the diagnosis and histologic subtype of RMS, diagnostic accuracy is crucial for appropriate assignment of therapy. RMS is a small round blue cell neoplasm and must be differentiated from the other small round blue cell neoplasms of childhood, including neuroblastoma, ESFT, and non-Hodgkin's lymphoma. The presence of malignant skeletal muscle differentiation, characterized by cross-striations in tumor cells at light microscopic examination confirms the diagnosis of RMS.[372] Unfortunately, cross-striations often are difficult to identify. In the absence of this highly specific finding, immunohistochemical staining often is needed to establish the diagnosis. The presence of staining for myogenin, MyoD, muscle-specific actin, myoglobin, or desmin supports the diagnosis.[373-375] The finding of sarcomeric differentiation of tumor cells at electron microscopic examination also confirms the diagnosis of RMS.

RMS comprises several histologic subtypes classified according to the modified International Classification of Rhabdomyosarcoma.[376] This system divides the disease into three prognostic categories on the basis of histologic findings: favorable (botryoid RMS, spindle cell RMS), intermediate (embryonal RMS), and unfavorable (alveolar RMS and undifferentiated sarcoma). In most cases, the histologic subtype can be determined with light microscopic examination. However, the use of RT-PCR detection of the chimeric fusion transcripts resulting from the t(2;13) and t(1;13) translocations can be useful in confirming the diagnosis of alveolar RMS in the absence of the characteristic histologic findings.[365]

Clinical Manifestations

The initial features of RMS depend on the site and size of the primary tumor and on the extent of metastatic disease. Because it is derived from primitive mesenchymal cells, RMS can arise in almost any tissue in the body. The most common sites are the head and neck (27%–37%), genitourinary tract (19%–26%), and extremities (17%–20%).[358-360] Head and neck tumors are divided by primary site into three major groups: orbital, parameningeal, and nonparameningeal. Orbital RMS, which accounts for approximately one fourth of head

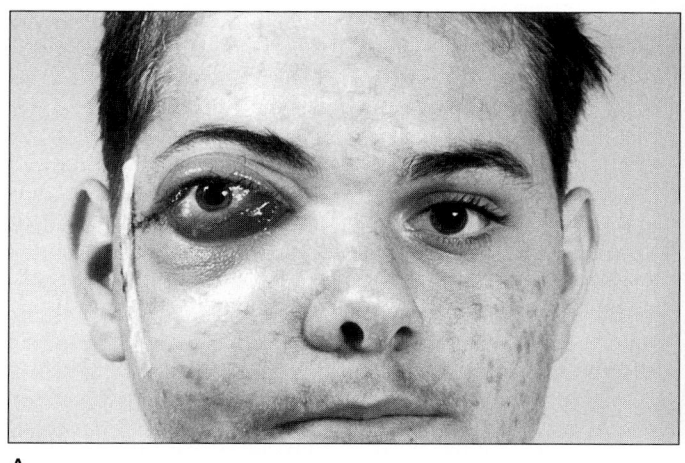
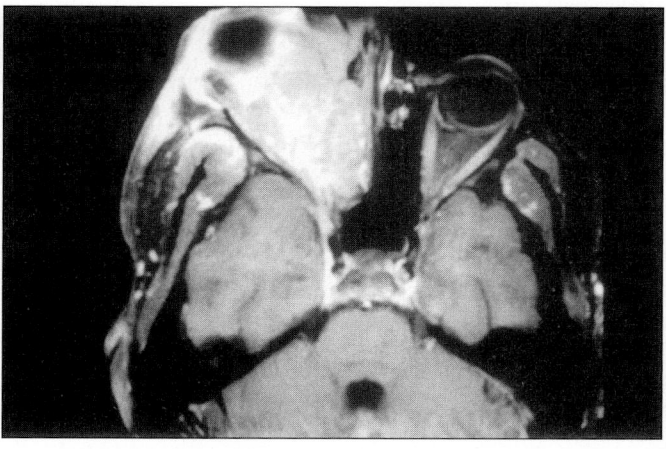

A   B

Figure 99-15. A, Rhabdomyosarcoma of the right orbit invading the paranasal sinuses and soft tissues of the face. Tumor manifested as proptosis and facial swelling with accompanying vision loss. **B,** T_1-weighted contrast-enhanced axial magnetic resonance image shows a large right intraorbital mass displacing the globe anteriorly and extending into the subcutaneous tissues overlying the right maxilla.

and neck tumors, commonly manifests as proptosis and occasionally ophthalmoplegia (Fig. 99-15). Approximately one half of cases of RMS of the head and neck arise in parameningeal sites that include the nasopharynx and paranasal sinuses, middle ear and mastoid, and pterygoid/infratemporal fossae. Tumors at these sites may produce nasal, sinus, or aural obstruction, occasionally with purulent or bloody discharge. Parameningeal tumors may be associated with cranial base erosion, cranial nerve palsy, and intracranial tumor extension. Patients with intracranial tumor extension may have signs of increased intracranial pressure and are at risk of leptomeningeal tumor spread.[377] The other one fourth of head and neck tumors arise in nonparameningeal sites, such as the scalp, face, buccal mucosa, oropharynx, and neck. A visible or palpable mass often brings these tumors to medical attention.

Genitourinary primary sites account for approximately one fourth of all cases of RMS and include the bladder, prostate, uterus, cervix, vagina, vulva, and paratesticular area. Bladder tumors often grow intraluminally and can cause hematuria or obstruct urinary outflow. Prostatic primary tumors can become large before causing appreciable clinical symptoms. Urinary retention, constipation, and a palpable pelvic mass are characteristic. Female genital tract RMS is associated with protrusion of tumor tissue from the introitus accompanied by vaginal discharge or bleeding. Patients with paratesticular tumors characteristically have a painless unilateral scrotal mass with or without back or abdominal pain related to tumor involvement of retroperitoneal lymph nodes.

RMS arises in an extremity in approximately 20% of patients. Patients typically notice an enlarging, firm mass that often is painless. Extremity tumors frequently spread into the regional lymphatic system.[364] Thus the presence of axillary or inguinal adenopathy may be the problem for which medical attention is sought.

Approximately 15% to 20% of patients with RMS have identifiable distant metastatic lesions at initial diagnosis,[358-360] and an additional 10% to 15% have regional nodal involvement.[378] Lymphatic spread is most common in genitourinary and extremity RMS. It is rare in orbital and other head and neck primary sites. The most common sites of distant metastasis are lung, bone marrow, and bone.[379]

Diagnostic Evaluation

The goals of diagnostic evaluation of children for suspected RMS are to establish a specific histologic diagnosis, assess the degree of local, regional, and distant tumor involvement, and collect baseline data against which to measure the response to treatment. A careful physical examination should be performed with particular attention to regional lymph nodes. MRI or CT is used to determine the location, size, and invasiveness of the primary tumor and the anatomic relations that influence the choice of local therapy. Imaging assessment of regional lymph nodes should be performed for patients with genitourinary or extremity tumors as well as for patients with palpable regional lymphadenopathy. Evaluation for distant metastatic disease includes CT of the chest, ^{99m}Tc bone scanning, and bilateral bone marrow aspiration and biopsy. For patients with parameningeal primary tumors, cerebrospinal fluid examination also is warranted to rule out meningeal involvement.

Open biopsy of the tumor usually is needed to obtain adequate tissue for histologic and molecular characterization. Because of the high incidence of occult nodal involvement, regional lymph node sampling is necessary for patients with extremity RMS[364] and for those older than 10 years who have paratesticular RMS.[380]

Prognostic Factors

Assessment of prognostic variables is crucial for understanding the clinical behavior of RMS and for planning therapy. The clinical group classification[358] (Table 99-11) is

TABLE 99-11

Intergroup Rhabdomyosarcoma Study Clinical Grouping

CLINICAL GROUP	CHARACTERISTICS
I	Localized disease, completely resected; regional nodes not involved a. Confined to muscle or organ of origin b. Contiguous involvement—infiltration outside the muscle or organ of origin, as through fascial planes
II	a. Grossly resected tumor with microscopic residual disease; evidence of gross residual tumor; no clinical or microscopic evidence of regional node involvement b. Regional disease, completely resected; regional nodes involved and/or extension of tumor into an adjacent organ; all tumor completely resected with no microscopic residual disease c. Regional disease with involved nodes grossly resected, but with evidence of microscopic residual disease
III	Incomplete resection or biopsy with gross residual disease
IV	Metastatic disease present at onset

based on extent of disease after initial definitive surgery, which is the most important factor predictive of outcome in RMS.[360] Patients with localized tumor that is completely excised (clinical group I) or that is excised with microscopic residual disease (clinical group II) have a favorable prognosis. Those with gross residual disease (clinical group III) have an intermediate prognosis, and patients with metastatic disease (clinical group IV) have an unfavorable outcome.

The site of the primary tumor is predictive of outcome.[360,381] Children with orbital tumors or with genitourinary tumors that do not arise in the bladder or prostate gland have the best prognosis, whereas those with parameningeal or extremity tumors have the worst outcome. Children with nonparameningeal head and neck tumors and tumors of the bladder and prostate have an intermediate prognosis. In some cases, the prognostic importance of the primary site reflects other clinical factors. For example, the favorable outcome among children with orbital RMS may be due, in part, to the small size of these tumors when they come to medical attention and to almost complete absence of regional nodal involvement. On the other hand, the less favorable outcome among patients with extremity tumors may be related to the frequency of large tumor size when the patient arrives for evaluation and to the frequency of regional tumor spread.

Treatment

Because more than two thirds of children and adolescents with RMS can be cured, this goal should be the basis of treatment, which comprises the coordinated use of chemotherapy, radiation therapy, and surgery. All patients are presumed to have micrometastatic disease; therefore systemic chemotherapy is administered universally. Agents shown to be active alone or in combination include vincristine, actinomycin D (dactinomycin), doxorubicin, cyclophosphamide, ifosfamide, melphalan, cisplatin, methotrexate, etoposide, topotecan, and irinotecan.[382-395] The standard of care in North America was established by the clinical trials of the Intergroup Rhabdomyosarcoma Study Group (IRSG), renamed the Soft Tissue Sarcoma Committee (STSC) of the Children's Oncology Group. The IRSG studies, which began in 1972, established vincristine and dactinomycin chemotherapy, with or without cyclophosphamide, as the therapeutic standard for RMS against which all other approaches are measured. Selected patients with favorable prognostic features are treated with only vincristine and dactinomycin, but patients with less favorable features need the addition of cyclophosphamide. Novel chemotherapeutic approaches under investigation by the STSC include the use of the camptothecin analogs topotecan and irinotecan. The risk stratification scheme and study design for the current series of STSC studies are shown in Table 99-12. These treatment algorithms based on risk-

---

ST. JUDE CHILDREN'S RESEARCH HOSPITAL APPROACH TO THE MANAGEMENT OF RHABDOMYOSARCOMA

We remove the tumor surgically at initial diagnosis, when the operation can be accomplished without marked functional impairment or disfigurement. Primary re-excision is considered when gross or microscopic tumor can be removed with minimal morbidity. After initial surgery, we administer systemic chemotherapy according to St. Jude or national research protocols (e.g., Children's Oncology Group). Patients with embryonal tumors in favorable sites that have been grossly resected and have no nodal involvement, those with embryonal tumors of the orbit with gross residual tumor, and those with embryonal tumors in unfavorable sites that have been resected with negative microscopic margins receive vincristine/actinomycin D chemotherapy. All other patients receive the same agents plus cyclophosphamide chemotherapy. New experimental agents such as topotecan or irinotecan may be used as part of combination therapy when a patient has unfavorable or high-risk features (e.g., stage IV alveolar histologic findings).

We prescribe radiation therapy at week 12 on the basis of histologic subtype of the tumor and extent of disease remaining after initial surgery. We do not administer radiation therapy to patients with embryonal RMS that has been resected with negative microscopic margins. All patients with microscopic residual disease, as well as those with alveolar tumors resected with negative microscopic margins, receive a radiation therapy dose of 41.4 Gy to the primary tumor. Patients with gross residual disease after initial surgery receive 50.4 Gy of radiation therapy to the tumor. The same dose is used to manage measurable metastatic disease. We decrease the dose of radiation therapy for patients who undergo second-look procedures that result in removal of all grossly evident tumor.

TABLE 99-12

Children's Oncology Group Soft tissue Sarcoma Committee Risk Stratification Scheme and Study Design

AGE	SITE*	STAGE†	CLINICAL GROUP‡	NODAL STATUS	HISTOLOGY§	CHEMOTHERAPY	RADIATION THERAPY
Low Risk Subgroup A							
Any	Favorable	I	I	N0	Embryonal		None
Any	Favorable	I	II	N0	Embryonal	VA × 45 wk	36 Gy at week 3%
Any	Orbit only	I	III	N0	Embryonal		45 Gy at week 3
Any	Unfavorable	2	I	N0, NX	Embryonal		None
Low Risk Subgroup B							
Any	Favorable	I	II	N1	Embryonal		41.4 Gy at week 3%
Any	Orbit only	I	III	N1	Embryonal		45 Gy at week 3
Any	Favorable	I	III	N0, NX, N1	Embryonal		50.4 Gy at week 12¶
Any	Unfavorable	2	II	N0, NX	Embryonal	VAC × 45 wk	36 Gy at week 3**
Any	Unfavorable	2	II	N1	Embryonal		36 Gy at week 3
Any	Unfavorable	3	I	N0, NX	Embryonal		None
Any	Unfavorable	3	II	N0, NX	Embryonal		36 Gy at week 3**
Any	Unfavorable	3	II	N1	Embryonal		41.4 Gy at week 3**
Intermediate Risk							
Any	Unfavorable	2,3	III	N0, NX, N1	Embryonal		50.4 Gy at week 12**
<10 yr	Any	4	IV	N0, NX, N1	Embryonal	Randomization to VAC or VAC/VTC × 42 wk‡‡	Primary site radiation therapy at week 12**,‡‡, 50.4 Gy to metastatic sites at week 12
Any	Any	2,3	I	N0, NX	Alveolar		36 Gy at week 12**
Any	Paratesticular region only	2,3	I	N0, NX	Alveolar		None
Any	Any	2,3	II	N0, NX	Alveolar		36 Gy at week 12**
Any	Any	2,3	II	N1	Alveolar		41.4 Gy at week 12**
Any	Any	2,3	III	N0, NX, N1	Alveolar		50.4 Gy at week 12**
High Risk							
Any	Orbit only	2,3	III	N0, NX, N1	Alveolar		45 Gy at week 12**
≥10 yr	Any	4	IV	N0, NX	Embryonal	VI window, then VAC or VAC/VI × 44 weeks‡‡	Primary site radiation therapy at week 15**,‡‡ 50.4 Gy to metastatic sites at week 15
≥10 yr	Any	4	IV	N1	Embryonal‡‡		Primary site radiation therapy at week 15**,‡‡ 41.4 Gy to nodes at week 15 50.4 Gy to metastatic sites at week 15
Any	Any	4	IV	N0, NX	Alveolar		Primary site radiation therapy at week 15**,‡‡ 50.4 Gy to metastatic sites at week 15
Any	Any	4	IV	N1	Alveolar		Primary site radiation therapy at week 15**,‡‡ 41.4 Gy to nodes at week 15** 50.4 Gy to metastatic sites at week 15

*Favorable sites include orbit, nonparameningeal head and neck sites, genitourinary sites other than bladder/prostate, and biliary tract. All other sites are classified as unfavorable.

†Stage 1, nonmetastatic tumor arising at a favorable site; stage 2, nonmetastatic tumor measuring ≤5 cm in diameter arising at an unfavorable site with regional nodes clinically negative for tumor; stage 3, nonmetastatic tumor arising at an unfavorable site that is either >5 cm in diameter or has regional nodes clinically involved by tumor; stage 4, metastatic tumor.

‡See Table 99-11 for definition of clinical group.

§Embryonal tumors include botryoid and spindle cell tumors. Alveolar tumors include undifferentiated sarcoma.

 Patients with vaginal tumors receive radiationtherapy at week 28 depending on the extent of residual disease at that time.

¶Radiation therapy dose reduced if no gross tumor evident after second-look surgery.

**Radiation therapy administered at week 0 for patients with parameningeal tumors with intracranial extension and for those who need emergency radiation therapy (e.g., for spinal cord compression).

‖Patients with parameningeal tumors with cranial base erosion receive only VAC therapy.

‡‡Dose of radiation therapy to primary site dependent on tumor histology, presence or absence of nodal involvement, and extent of disease at primary site after initial surgery: completely resected, embryonal histology, 0 Gy; completely resected, alveolar histology, 36 Gy; microscopic residual, nodes negative, 36 Gy; microscopic residual, nodes positive, 41.4 Gy; gross residual, 50.4 Gy.

N0, regional nodes negative for tumor; NX, status of regional lymph nodes unknown; N1, regional nodes positive for tumor; VA, vincristine/actinomycin D; VAC, vincristine/actinomycin D/cyclophosphamide; VI, vincristine/irinotecan; VTC, vincristine/topotecan/cyclophosphamide.

group characterization currently are the subject of clinical investigation. To date, high-dose chemotherapy with autologous stem cell or bone marrow rescue has not been shown to improve outcome in RMS.[396,397]

In addition to systemic chemotherapy, local treatment with surgery, radiation therapy, or both is necessary for all sites of gross disease. Because complete surgical excision is associated with a better outcome, the goal of surgery is complete tumor removal without significant cosmetic or functional impairment. However, fewer than 20% of tumors are completely excised with negative microscopic margins.[358-360] Re-excision of tumors arising in the extremities and trunk to achieve negative margins before initiation of systemic therapy appears to confer a local control benefit and may favorably influence survival.[398,399] Therefore the tumor bed should be re-excised before administration of chemotherapy when negative microscopic margins can be achieved. For patients with tumors not amenable to surgical excision at the time of initial diagnosis, administration of neoadjuvant chemotherapy may allow delayed surgical resection.

Radiation therapy is indicated for all patients except those who have embryonal tumors that have been completely resected (with negative microscopic margins). Radiation therapy usually is delayed until after the initial response to chemotherapy is ascertained. However, immediate initiation of radiation therapy is warranted in patients with tumors that erode the skull base, extend intracranially, or cause cranial nerve dysfunction or spinal cord compression.[377] The recommended dose of radiation therapy ranges from 36 Gy to 50.4 Gy, depending on tumor site, extent of residual tumor, and response to chemotherapy. In an effort to improve local control and decrease the late effects of conventional radiation therapy, an IRSG study evaluated a twice-daily hyperfractionation schedule. This schedule has shown no benefit.[400,401] Techniques such as brachytherapy, three-dimensional conformal radiation therapy, and intensity-modulated radiation therapy may be helpful in decreasing the late complications of radiation therapy.

Outcome and Late Sequelae

With contemporary therapy, the long-term survival rate among children with RMS exceeds 70%. For patients who have disease recurrence, however, outcome is poor. Fewer than 20% of children survive more than 5 years after recurrence, and almost all of these survivors have local recurrence of botryoid or embryonal tumors.[402]

Although long-term survival is the norm for children with RMS, the late effects of the disease and its therapy can be substantial. Long-term sequelae are site-specific in some cases. More than one half of survivors of orbital RMS have dry eye, impaired vision, or cataracts.[403,404] Dental abnormalities, including root stunting, microdontia, and hypodontia are common among survivors of head and neck RMS.[405] Other common problems in children treated for head and neck RMS include short stature (due to growth hormone deficiency), hypothyroidism, and hearing loss.[358,406,407] Children treated for RMS of the bladder or prostate are at risk of impaired bladder function, hematuria, hydronephrosis, and gonadal failure,[408] whereas those treated for paratesticular RMS may experience ejaculatory dysfunction and hypogonadism.[409] Other late effects may be caused by chemotherapy, radiation therapy, or both. The most important of these effects include infertility,[410,411] impaired bone and soft-tissue growth,[412,413] and second malignant neoplasms.[414,415]

NONRHABDOMYOSARCOMA SOFT-TISSUE SARCOMA

Epidemiology

Population-based data from the Surveillance, Epidemiology and End Results program of the National Cancer Institute indicate that approximately 4% of pediatric malignant tumors are nonrhabdomyosarcoma soft-tissue sarcoma (NRSTS). As a group these tumors occur more frequently than RMS.[357] Unlike RMS, which occurs most often in children younger than 10 years, NRSTS is found predominantly in older children and adolescents. NRSTS includes many histologically and biologically distinct entities, all of which are derived from primitive mesenchymal cells. Most tumors are named for the mature tissue that they resemble histologically. In pediatrics, the most common subtypes are synovial sarcoma, malignant fibrous histiocytoma, malignant peripheral nerve sheath tumor, and fibrosarcoma.[357,416-418] Certain subtypes that occur frequently in adults, such as leiomyosarcoma and liposarcoma, are rare in children.[419-422] Tumors unique to pediatrics include infantile hemangiopericytoma and infantile fibrosarcoma, which behave in a more benign manner than their counterparts in adults.[423-425]

Biology

Most cases of NRSTS arise sporadically. However, some of these tumors have been found in patients with constitutional p53 gene mutations (Li-Fraumeni syndrome).[426] This finding suggests that aberrant p53 gene function may contribute to pathogenesis in some cases. Patients with neurofibromatosis type I, an autosomal-dominant genetic disorder caused by abnormalities on the long arm of chromosome 17, are at increased risk of malignant peripheral nerve sheath tumor (MPNST),[427] which often arises within a preexisting neurofibroma. MPNST also occurs sporadically in patients who do not have neurofibromatosis type I.[428] An unusually high incidence of leiomyosarcoma has been found among children with human immunodeficiency virus (HIV) infection.[429] Epstein-Barr virus (EBV) infection has been found in patients with HIV-associated leiomyosarcoma. This finding suggests that EBV has an etiologic role in leiomyosarcoma in HIV-infected patients.[430] Leiomyosarcoma in HIV-negative patients is not associated with EBV infection.[431]

A variety of forms of NRSTS have been reported as secondary malignant neoplasms following radiation therapy or chemotherapy for unrelated malignant disease.[153,432] Children with bilateral retinoblastoma are at high risk of secondary NRSTS that can arise either within or outside of the radiation field used to manage retinoblastoma. This finding suggests that the *RB* gene locus may be important in the pathogenesis of some cases of NRSTS.[433]

Pathology

Because NRSTS is uncommon during childhood, these tumors can be diagnostically challenging. Procurement of an adequate tissue specimen during the initial evaluation is crucial to establishing an accurate diagnosis. Incisional biopsy is preferred, because fine-needle aspiration and biopsy may yield inadequate tissue for thorough histologic and immunohistochemical evaluation and for molecular pathologic studies. Detection of chromosomal translocations specific to certain histologic subtypes may be helpful in confirming the precise diagnosis (Table 99-13).[433-441] Identification of specific tumor-cell gene fusions also may have prognostic importance. For example, synovial sarcoma with the *SYT-SSX1* fusion gene appears to have a less favorable outcome than synovial sarcoma with the *SYT-SSX2* fusion gene.[442]

Childhood NRSTS is divided into low-, intermediate-, and high-grade categories according to a grading schema formulated by the Pediatric Oncology Group.[443] This grading system includes elements of the system devised by Costa and colleagues[444] for adult NRSTS, in which metastatic potential and necrosis are assessed, as well as elements of the system developed by Enzinger and Weiss,[445] which is based primarily on histologic criteria. The system also includes the clinical variable of patient age to account for infantile tumors, which have a highly malignant histologic appearance but behave clinically in a benign manner. Histologic grade is highly predictive of outcome. Patients with high-grade NRSTS are at substantially greater risk of distant tumor recurrence and death than are those with low- and intermediate-grade tumors.[416,417]

Clinical Manifestations

The manifestations of NRSTS depend mainly on the site of the primary tumor. Because they are derived from primitive mesenchymal cells, these tumors arise in almost any tissue. Extremity sites are most common, followed by trunk wall, head and neck, and visceral sites.[416-418,446,447] Extremity, trunk wall, and head and neck NRSTS most commonly manifests as an enlarging, painless mass. Compression of nerves by the tumor can cause pain or disturbances in sensory or motor function. Tumors in the head and neck region can cause nasal, aural, or sinus obstruction and can impinge on the airway. Retroperitoneal and visceral tumors of the abdomen and pelvis often are large at initial evaluation. These tumors characteristically cause abdominal pain with or without symptoms of gastrointestinal or urinary tract obstruction.

Regional lymph node involvement is uncommon[417,447] and is rarely clinically evident when present. Children with synovial sarcoma, epithelioid sarcoma, angiosarcoma, and clear cell sarcoma are presumed to be at the highest risk of regional nodal disease, because these histologic subtypes are most commonly associated with regional spread in adults.[448] Approximately 15% of children and adolescents with NRSTS have distant metastatic lesions at initial diagnosis. The lung is the predominant site of metastatic disease,[446] but symptoms of pulmonary metastasis are rare at initial diagnosis. Metastatic involvement of bone, skin, liver, and brain also has been reported. Pleural, peritoneal, and omental metastasis can occur in patients with tumors of the trunk wall, retroperitoneum, or viscera.

Diagnostic Evaluation

The goals of the diagnostic evaluation of children for suspected NRSTS are to establish a specific diagnosis and to assess the extent of disease to allow optimal treatment planning and measurement of response. The physical examination should be focused particularly on the local extent of the primary tumor and on the presence or absence of regional lymphadenopathy. MRI or CT aids in determining the location, size, and invasiveness of the primary tumor, as well as the anatomic relations that influence the surgical approach. Patients with synovial sarcoma, epithelioid sarcoma, angiosarcoma, and clear cell sarcoma need imaging assessment of regional lymph nodes, because regional tumor spread is most common in

TABLE 99-13

Chromosomal Translocations and Associated Fusion Proteins Described in Childhood Nonrhabdomyosarcoma Soft–Tissue Sarcoma		
TUMOR	**CHROMOSOMAL TRANSLOCATION**	**FUSION PROTEIN**
Alveolar soft-part sarcoma	der(17)t(X;17)(p11.2;q25)	ASPL-TFE3
Clear cell sarcoma	t(12;22)(q13;q12)	EWS-ATF1
Dermatofibrosarcoma protuberans	t(17;22)(q22;q13)	COL1A1-PDGFB
Desmoplastic small round cell tumor	t(11;22)(p13;q12)	EWS-WT1
Extraskeletal myxoid chondrosarcoma	t(9,22)(q22;q11–12)	EWS-CHN
	t(9;17)(q22;q11)	RBP56-CHN
Infantile fibrosarcoma	t(12;15)(p13;q25)	ETV6-NTRK3
Myxoid liposarcoma	t(12;16)(q13;p11)	FUS-CHOP
	t(12;22)(q13;q11–12)	EWS-CHOP
	t(12;22;20)(q13;q12;q11)	EWS-CHOP
Synovial sarcoma	t(X;18)(p11;q11)	SYT-SSX1 or SYT-SSX2

these subtypes of NRSTS in adults.[448] Any patient with enlarged regional lymph nodes also needs imaging of the nodal bed for definition of the extent of disease. The evaluation for distant metastatic disease should include either radiography or CT of the chest. CT is more sensitive and more expensive than radiography, but it is most cost-effective in patients with large, high-grade NRSTS.[449] Patients with tumors of the abdomen, pelvis, and retroperitoneum need CT or MRI of the liver. Routine screening for bone, bone marrow, and brain metastasis is not warranted.[450]

The best approach to ensure adequate tissue for histologic and molecular tumor characterization is open biopsy. However, core needle biopsy has been shown to provide accurate diagnostic information when the specimen is reviewed by an experienced pathologist.[451] Fine-needle aspiration is inadequate for establishing a specific diagnosis[452] but may be helpful in documentation of tumor recurrence.[453]

Prognostic Factors

Assessment of prognostic factors is important in selecting a therapeutic approach for patients with NRSTS. Few prospective studies of childhood NRSTS have been conducted, but the available results of prospective and retrospective studies suggest that the prognostic features of NRSTS are similar in children and adults. Extent of disease and histologic grade and size of the tumor appear to be the most important prognostic variables. Patients with tumors that can be excised at initial diagnosis fare significantly better than those with unresectable or metastatic tumors.[416,417,446,447,454] Among patients with tumors that are surgically resected, high histologic grade is strongly associated with development of distant metastasis and with an inferior survival rate.[416,417] Tumor diameter greater than 5 cm is a risk factor for adverse outcome among patients with nonmetastatic NRSTS.[417,447] Other variables that have been associated with reduced probability of survival include age 10 years or older and intra-abdominal primary tumor site. Local recurrence is more likely in patients who have gross residual disease or positive microscopic margins after initial surgery.

Treatment

Only three prospective multi-institutional clinical trials of therapy for pediatric NRSTS have been conducted.[416,454,455] Therefore the approach to management of childhood NRSTS depends largely on experience in managing adult NRSTS. However, the potential long-term effects of antineoplastic therapy on growth and development in the pediatric population are additional factors that must be weighed.

Children and adolescents with NRSTS can be divided into three risk categories for the purpose of treatment assignment. Low-risk disease includes resectable low-grade tumors and resectable high-grade tumors having a maximal diameter of 5 cm or less. Approximately 85% of patients with low-risk NRSTS become long-term survivors, and efforts should be made to limit the toxicity of treatment.[416,417] Wide local excision is generally adequate for cure.[416,417,456,457] When microscopic tumor remains after surgery, adjuvant radiation therapy (external beam or brachytherapy) usually is indicated.[458,459] However, selected patients with microscopic residual disease after resection of low-grade NRSTS may be observed, because only a small number of these patients experience local recurrence, and salvage therapy is almost always successful in these cases.[417,460] The intermediate-risk

---

ST. JUDE CHILDREN'S RESEARCH HOSPITAL APPROACH TO THE MANAGEMENT OF CHILDHOOD NONRHABDOMYOSARCOMA SOFT-TISSUE SARCOMA

Our primary goal in managing childhood NRSTS is to completely resect all sites of disease. Whether we also use radiation therapy or chemotherapy depends on results of assessment of the risk factors for local and distant disease recurrence and on whether the tumor is resectable at diagnosis.

For patients with localized, surgically resectable NRSTS that is either low grade or high grade and 5 cm or less in diameter, we excise the tumor when it comes to medical attention. Although the goal of surgery is wide margins, we try to avoid functional impairment or disfigurement. Primary re-excision is performed in patients who have undergone unplanned resection and in those in whom negative microscopic margins can be achieved. We administer external-beam radiation therapy or brachytherapy to patients with high-grade tumors who have microscopic residual tumor after surgery. For patients with low-grade tumors who have microscopic residual tumor after surgery, we generally avoid radiation therapy because local recurrence develops in few of these patients and is readily controllable by re-excision with or without radiation therapy. We do not give adjuvant chemotherapy to patients with localized low-grade NRSTS or to those with localized high-grade NRSTS 5 cm or less in diameter.

We administer neoadjuvant doxorubicin and ifosfamide chemotherapy to patients with high-grade NRSTS larger than 5 cm in diameter, to those with unresectable NRSTS of any grade, and to those with metastatic NRSTS. After two or three cycles of chemotherapy, we attempt to excise all tumors visible on radiographs, if possible. Postoperatively, we administer an additional two or three cycles of chemotherapy, provided the response to neoadjuvant therapy is favorable. If microscopic tumor remains after surgery, we administer external-beam radiation therapy or brachytherapy. In selected cases, we initiate radiation therapy concurrently with preoperative chemotherapy and give a postoperative radiation therapy boost only if microscopic tumor remains after surgery. For patients with NRSTS that continues to be unresectable after neoadjuvant chemotherapy, we try different chemotherapeutic approaches or radiation therapy in an effort to allow tumor resection.

category includes high-grade tumors larger than 5 cm in diameter and unresectable tumors. Patients at intermediate risk have an approximately 50% likelihood of long-term survival.[447] The optimal treatment of this subgroup is elusive. Patients with large, high-grade tumors are at substantial risk of distant disease recurrence,[417] but experience in treatment of adults suggests the available chemotherapy regimens are only modestly effective in preventing this usually fatal complication.[461-463] The most active antineoplastic agents are doxorubicin and ifosfamide; however, the rate of tumor response after neoadjuvant treatment with these agents is in the 25% to 40% range.[454,455,464,465] Dose intensification of these drugs may slightly improve the rate of response, although the effect of dose intensification on survival appears limited.[466] The late effects of high cumulative doses of doxorubicin and ifosfamide also must be considered.[467,468] Patients who have unresectable NRSTS are at risk not only of distant dissemination of disease but also of local tumor progression.[447] Local tumor growth can cause fatal complications when the tumor arises in the head and neck or intrathoracic and intra-abdominal regions. Neoadjuvant combined chemotherapy and radiation therapy may be a promising approach for improving local control in these patients.[469] Children and adolescents with metastatic NRSTS compose the high-risk subgroup. These patients have a dismal prognosis. The median duration of survival is approximately 6 months, and fewer than 10% of these patients are alive 5 years after the initial diagnosis.[446,454] Novel treatment approaches are needed for these patients. Given the poor outcome with standard chemotherapy, enrollment in phase I and II clinical trials of investigational agents should be considered.

Many aspects of the management of childhood NRSTS are controversial. Questions that have not been answered definitively include the following: (1) Which children with resected NRSTS can be treated without adjuvant therapy? (2) What minimum dose and field of radiation therapy provide adequate local control of resected NRSTS with positive microscopic margins? (3) What is the optimal systemic therapy for patients at high risk of distant metastatic disease? (4) What is the most effective local control therapy for unresectable NRSTS? Prospective clinical trials are warranted for investigation of these questions.

Outcome

The prognosis among children and adolescents with NRSTS depends on the histologic grade and size of the tumor, the resectability of the tumor, and the presence or absence of metastatic disease. Patients with low-grade and small high-grade tumors that are resectable have a favorable outcome with approximately 85% long-term survival.[419,420] Patients with large, high-grade tumors or with unresectable tumors of any grade have an intermediate prognosis. Approximately one half of these patients are alive 5 years after diagnosis.[447] Patients with metastatic disease at diagnosis have a dismal prognosis; fewer than 10% become long-term survivors.[446,454]

The likelihood of cure of patients who have tumor recurrence is difficult to ascertain given the paucity of

data on this subject. Patients who have local recurrence, particularly if the tumor is of low histologic grade and is resectable, usually have good results.[417] Development of distant metastatic disease, particularly when the tumor is of high histologic grade, is a very unfavorable prognostic sign.

Few reports have addressed the late effects of therapy for NRSTS in children and adolescents. However, like pediatric patients treated with intensive chemotherapy, surgery, and radiation therapy for other malignant diseases, those undergoing therapy for NRSTS are at risk of a number of long-term complications (Fig. 99-16). Surgical intervention can lead to permanent organ damage, disability, or disfigurement. Radiation therapy can cause disturbances of bone and soft-tissue growth,[412,413] restriction of soft-tissue mobility, neuroendocrine abnormalities,[407,470] and secondary malignant tumors.[153] Administration of anthracycline and alkylating agent chemotherapy has been associated with cardiotoxicity,[467]

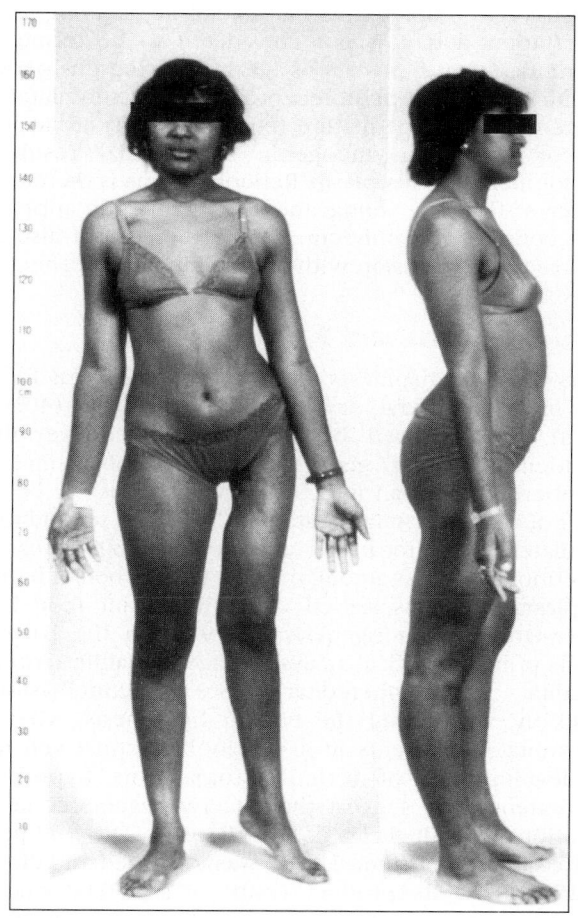

Figure 99-16. A 19-year-old patient who had been treated at age 10 years with chemotherapy, surgical resection, and 64.8-Gy external-beam radiation therapy for synovial sarcoma of the left anterior thigh. Marked soft-tissue atrophy of the left thigh and associated leg length discrepancy due to impaired skeletal growth are evident. Other late effects include avascular necrosis of the left femoral head and thoracolumbar scoliosis.

infertility,[411] nephrotoxicity,[468] and development of secondary malignant tumors.[414,471] These potential sequelae must be considered when treatment is selected for children and adolescents with NRSTS. Advances in the treatment of pediatric patients with NRSTS depend on further studies to identify more effective therapies that cause less long-term toxicity.

RETINOBLASTOMA

Epidemiology

Retinoblastoma is the most frequent neoplasm of the eye in childhood and the third most common intraocular malignant tumor in all ages, following malignant melanoma and metastatic carcinoma. Retinoblastoma represents 3% of all pediatric cancers. The average incidence of retinoblastoma in the United States is 1 in 14,000 to 18,000 live births. Thus retinoblastoma develops in an estimated 200 to 300 children each year.[4] There is no sex or racial predilection. The human retina is far from having completed its maturation at the completion of gestation, and it is not considered to be terminally differentiated until 3 years of age. It is during this period, in which primitive photoreceptor cells are stimulated to differentiate into the mature retina, that cells are at high risk of sustaining oncogenic events that result in development of a neoplasm. Retinoblastoma is therefore a cancer of the very young, and any therapeutic approach must consider not only cure of the disease but also the need to preserve vision with minimal long-term effects.

Clinical Forms and Biology

Retinoblastoma manifests in two distinct clinical forms. The first is bilateral or multifocal hereditary (40% of cases), characterized by the presence of germline mutations of the *RB1* gene. Multifocal retinoblastoma can be inherited from an affected survivor (25%) or be the result of a new germline mutation (75%). The second form is unilateral or unifocal and nonhereditary (60% of cases).

Retinoblastoma is among the best understood of human neoplasms and has served as an important model for understanding tumorigenesis. In 1971, on the basis of results of mathematical analysis of age at manifestation of hereditary and nonhereditary cases of retinoblastoma, Knudson[472] proposed the two-hit hypothesis, whereby two mutational events in a developing retinal cell lead to development of retinoblastoma. This hypothesis was extended to suggest that the two events could be mutations of both alleles of the *RB1* gene. The *RB1* gene, located in chromosome 13q14, was identified and cloned in 1986.[473,474] Its product (pRb) is a 110-kd nuclear phosphoprotein that acts by binding and inhibiting several proteins with growth-stimulatory activity. pRb is a key substrate for G_1 cyclin-cdk complexes, which phosphorylate target gene products required for transition of the cell through G_1. The active pRb is the unphosphorylated gene product, which binds to several cellular proteins, among which is transcription factor E2F,

which activates transcription of genes whose products are required for entry into the S phase of the cell cycle. During the progression through G_1, pRb undergoes additional phosphorylation. The result is a hyperphosphorylated form that persists through the S, G_2, and M phases. pRb appears to function as a tumor suppressor at least in part by inhibiting cell-cycle progression past the G_1-S restriction point. Once cells traverse the G_1-S restriction point and enter S phase, they become irreversibly committed to cell division. Thus pRb stands as the major gatekeeper to control this critical point in growth regulation. Lack of pRb or its inactivation removes the pRb constraint on cell-cycle control. The consequence is deregulated cell proliferation.[475]

The First Hit

RB1 is a large gene, containing 27 exons over approximately 200 kb of DNA, and mutations have been described in almost every exon. Nonsense and frameshift are the most common germline and somatic mutations, although deletions and duplications are also frequently encountered.[475] There are no mutational hot spots, although new germline mutations have an overwhelming preference for the paternal allele, a finding that suggests deamination of methylated CpG pairs has an important role in mutagenesis.[476]

The Second Hit

In both hereditary and nonhereditary retinoblastoma, the second tumorigenic event is chromosomal in nature, often as a result of mitotic recombination errors.[477] This second hit occurs at a much higher frequency than the first hit, and it is more sensitive to environmental factors, such as ionizing radiation, thus the increased risk of radiation-induced malignant tumors in survivors of retinoblastoma.[478] After the second hit has occurred, retinoblastoma cells rapidly accumulate additional genetic damage. It is possible that an additional mutation (*third hit*), probably involving a gene of the apoptotic pathway, is necessary for final retinal tumor formation.[475]

Genetic Counseling

Retinoblastoma is a unique neoplasm because the hereditary type has autosomal-dominant inheritance with almost complete penetrance (85%–95%).[479] However, some families have an inheritance pattern characterized by reduced penetrance and expressivity. These low-penetrance retinoblastoma mutations either cause a reduction in the amount of normal pRb produced or result in a partially functional mutant pRb.[480] The *RB1* gene mutation can occur at a late stage of embryogenesis, the result being variable expression depending on the tissue and mosaicism in 10% to 15% of family members.[481] Genetic counseling is of utmost importance for determining the heritability of a given case and to estimate the risk among relatives. However, because of the size of the *RB1* gene and the lack of mutational hot spots, exhaustive analysis of the *RB1* gene is required for clinical DNA testing.[482] These analyses are very expensive and complex and cannot be routinely performed for all patients and their families. In general, however, on the basis of inheritance pattern but in consideration of the existence of mosaicism, the following risk estimates can be made.[479]

Risk among Offspring of Survivors of Retinoblastoma

The risk of retinoblastoma arising in the offspring of survivors of bilateral (hereditary) disease is 45%. The risk is 2.5% among the offspring of survivors of unilateral retinoblastoma.

Risk among Siblings of Patients with Retinoblastoma

When there is a family history of retinoblastoma, siblings of patients with bilateral tumors have a 45% risk of development of retinoblastoma. The siblings of patients with unilateral tumors have a 30% risk. When there is a family history, the risk is 2% among siblings of patients with bilateral tumors and 1% among siblings of patients with unilateral tumors.

Pathology

Retinoblastoma arises from the photoreceptor elements of the inner layer of the retina,[483] usually extending into the vitreous cavity as a fleshy nodular mass (endophytic retinoblastoma). Less frequently, it extends externally, causing secondary retinal detachment; in this case there is no localized visible vitreous nodule (exophytic retinoblastoma). Macroscopically, retinoblastoma is soft and friable, and it tends to outgrow its blood supply; the result is necrosis and calcification. Because of the friability of the tumor, dissemination within the vitreous and retina in the form of small, white nodules (seeds) is common. In those cases, it may be difficult to differentiate multicentric primary tumor from disseminated tumor.[484]

The microscopic appearance of retinoblastoma depends on the degree of differentiation. Undifferentiated retinoblastoma is composed of small, round, densely packed cells with hypochromatic nuclei and scant cytoplasm. Several degrees of photosensory differentiation have been described and are characterized by distinctive arrangements of tumor cells. Homer-Wright rosettes are composed of irregular circlets of tumor cells arranged around a tangle of fibrils with no lumen or internal limiting membrane. These rosettes are infrequent in retinoblastoma but are most common in other neuroblastic tumors, such as neuroblastoma and medulloblastoma. Flexner-Wintersteiner rosettes, on the other hand, are specific for retinoblastoma. These structures consist of a cluster of low columnar cells arranged around a central lumen bounded by an eosinophilic membrane analogous to the external membrane of the normal retina. The lumen contains an acid mucopolysaccharide similar to that around normal rods and cones. These rosettes are present in 70% of tumors. Fleurettes are less common. If rosettes are present, the cells exhibit even more ultrastructural characteristics of photoreceptor differentiation. The tumor is composed of larger cells with abundant eosinophilic cytoplasm arranged in a distinctive *fleur-de-lis* pattern. Especially well-differentiated tumors composed almost entirely of fleurettes have been called *retinoma* or *retinocytoma*. Ultrastructurally, retino-

blastoma cells exhibit photoreceptor differentiation with the presence of the 9-0 microtubule doublet pattern, abundant cytoplasmic microtubules, synaptic ribbons, and neurosecretory granules.[484,485]

Dissemination of retinoblastoma occurs by several routes. Choroidal invasion provides access to a rich vascular network that serves as a potential route for distant metastatic lesions. In advanced cases, direct extension occurs through the sclera into the orbit. Retinoblastoma can invade the iris and the ciliary body and metastasize to regional lymph nodes. Finally, retinoblastoma can extend along the optic nerve, gaining access to the subarachnoid space and intracranial cavity.

Clinical Manifestations

Successful management of retinoblastoma depends on ability to detect the disease while it is still intraocular. Patients with bilateral retinoblastoma tend to come to medical attention at a younger age (14–16 months) than patients with unilateral disease (29–30 months).[479,486] In more than half of cases, the presenting sign is leukocoria, which occasionally is first noticed after a flash photograph (Fig. 99-17). Strabismus is the second most common sign and usually correlates with macular involvement. Very advanced intraocular tumors can become painful as a result of secondary glaucoma.[486] The differential diagnosis includes other childhood diseases that manifest as leukocoria, such as persistent hyperplastic primary vitreous, retrolental fibrodysplasia, Coats' disease, congenital cataracts, toxocariasis, and toxoplasmosis. In some series, these nonmalignant conditions account for a large proportion of enucleated eyes.[487]

Trilateral retinoblastoma is the association of bilateral retinoblastoma with an asynchronous intracranial neuroblastic tumor.[488] This association can occur in 3% to 9% of patients with hereditary disease, and the prognosis is almost uniformly fatal. Most of these tumors are

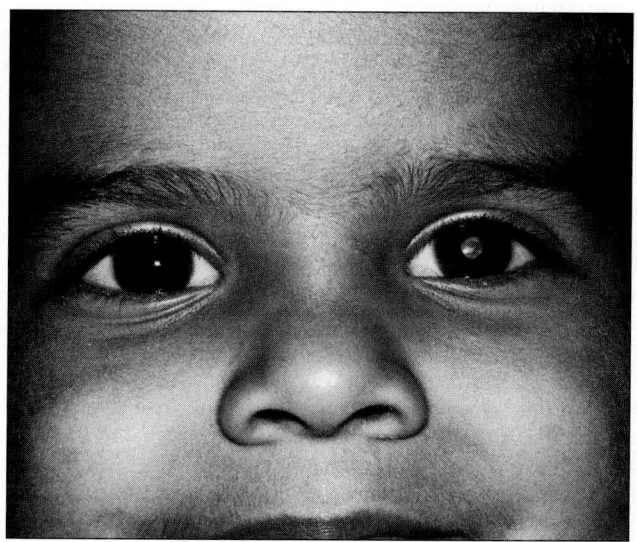

Figure 99-17. A 3-year-old boy with leukocoria of the left eye.

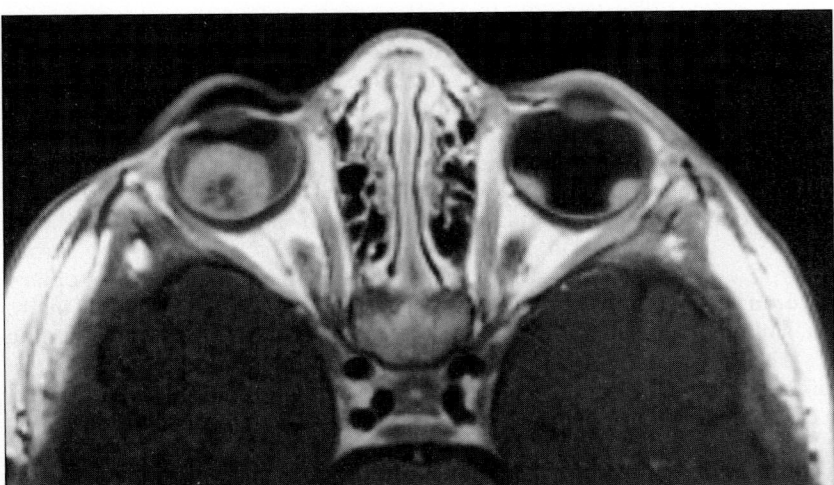

Figure 99-18. T_1-weighted image after contrast enhancement shows bilateral retinoblastoma with associated retinal detachment of the right globe.

pinealoblastoma, but suprasellar or parasellar tumors also occur. In most cases, the tumor resembles undifferentiated retinoblastoma with the more frequent formation of Homer-Wright rosettes. The median interval between diagnosis of bilateral retinoblastoma and diagnosis of the brain tumor is 35 months. In recent years, with more widespread use of chemoreduction treatment of patients with bilateral retinoblastoma, the incidence of trilateral retinoblastoma has decreased dramatically.[489]

Evaluation

The diagnosis of intraocular retinoblastoma usually is made without pathologic confirmation. Anesthesia and a maximally dilated pupil and scleral indentation are required to examine the entire retina. Retinoblastoma usually appears as a mass projecting into the vitreous, although the presence of retinal detachment or vitreous hemorrhage can make visualization difficult. Additional imaging studies that aid in the diagnosis include bidimensional ultrasonography, CT, and MRI (Fig. 99-18). These imaging studies are particularly important in evaluation of extraocular extension and differentiating retinoblastoma from other causes of leukocoria. CT is helpful in detection of calcification, and MRI is helpful in the differential diagnosis of Coats' disease and other inflammatory conditions.[490] Evaluation for the presence of metastatic disease also must be considered in a subgroup of patients. Metastatic disease occurs in approximately 10% to 15% of patients, usually in association with distinct intraocular histologic features, such as deep choroidal and scleral invasion, or with involvement of the iris–ciliary body and optic nerve beyond the lamina cribrosa.[491] In these cases, additional staging procedures, including bone scintigraphy, bone marrow aspiration and biopsy, and lumbar puncture, must be performed. These staging studies also are recommended for patients receiving chemotherapy or radiation therapy before enucleation, because proper histologic evaluation cannot be performed.

Staging

The Reese-Ellsworth grouping system has been generally accepted as the standard for intraocular disease. This grouping system was initially designed for prediction of outcome after external-beam radiation therapy. In this system, eyes are divided into five groups on the basis of size, location, and number of lesions and presence of vitreous seeding (Table 99-14).[492] For patients undergoing enucleation, we use the St. Jude staging system, a

TABLE 99-14

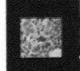 **Reese-Ellsworth Grouping of Suitability for Management of Retinoblastoma by Radiation Therapy**

STAGE	DESCRIPTION
Group I. Very Favorable	
Ia	Solitary tumor smaller than 4 dd at or behind the equator
Ib	Multiple tumors, none larger than 4 dd, all at or behind equator
Group II. Favorable	
IIa	Solitary tumor 4–10 dd, at or behind equator
IIb	Multiple tumors 4–10 dd, at or behind equator
Group III. Doubtful	
IIIa	Any lesion anterior to equator
IIIb	Solitary tumor larger than 10 dd behind equator
Group IV. Unfavorable	
IVa	Multiple tumors, some larger than 10 dd
IVb	Any lesion extending anteriorly to the ora serrata
Group V. Very Unfavorable	
Va	Massive tumors involving more than half the retina
Vb	Vitreous seeding

dd, disk diameter (1.5 mm).
Adapted from Reese AB, Ellsworth RM: The evaluation and current concept of retinoblastoma therapy. Trans Am Acad Opthalmol Otolaryngol 1963;67:164.

pathologic staging that incorporates other features known to influence modality of treatment and prognosis, such as choroidal involvement, optic nerve extension, and presence of metastatic disease (Table 99-15).[493]

Principles of Treatment

Management of retinoblastoma is aimed at saving life and preserving useful vision, and thus it must be individualized. Factors to be considered include unilaterality or bilaterality of disease, potential for vision, and intraocular and extraocular staging.

Surgery

Enucleation is indicated for large tumors filling the vitreous for which there is little or no likelihood of restoring vision and in cases of tumor present in the anterior chamber or in association with neovascular glaucoma. For optimal staging, a long section (10–15 mm) of optic nerve has to be removed with the globe. A hydroxyapatite implant usually is fitted during the same procedure, and the extraocular muscles are attached to it. The size and type of implant are important for stimulating orbital growth.[494]

Focal Therapy

Focal treatments are used for small tumors (<3–6 mm), usually in patients with bilateral disease, and in combination with chemoreduction. Photocoagulation with argon laser is used to manage tumors situated at or posterior to the equator and to manage retinal neovascularization due to radiation therapy.[495] Cryotherapy is used to manage small lesions situated in the anterior retina.[496] An important focal method is transpupillary

TABLE 99-15

St. Jude Children's Research Hospital Modified Staging

STAGE	DESCRIPTION
Group I. Tumor Confined to the Retina	
IA	Solitary, smaller than 6 dd
IB	Multiple, all smaller than 6 dd
IC	Solitary or multiple tumors, involving less than 50% of retinal surface behind equator
ID	Solitary or multiple tumors, involving more than 50% of retinal surface behind equator
IE	Solitary or multiple tumors, involving more than 50% of retinal surface anterior to equator
Group II. Tumor Confined to Globe, Extraretinal	
IIA	Extends to optic nerve head
IIB1	Extends to choroid
IIB2	Extends to choroid with replacement
IIC	Anterior chamber involvement
IID	Extends to choroid and optic nerve
Group III. Tumor with Extrachoroidal Extension (Regional)	
IIIA	Extends to emissaries
IIIB	Extends beyond cut end of optic nerve (including subarachnoid)
IIIC	Extends through sclera into orbital contents
IIID	Extends to choroid and beyond cut end of optic nerve (includes subarachnoid)
IIIE	Extends through sclera and cut end of optic nerve
Group IV. Distant Disease	
IVA	Extension through optic nerve into brain, including positive spinal fluid finding
IVB	Blood-borne metastasis to soft tissue, node, or bone
IVC	Bone marrow metastasis

dd, disk diameter (1.5 mm).
From Pratt CB, Fontanesi J, Lu X, et al: Proposal for a new staging scheme for intraocular and extraocular retinoblastoma based on an analysis of 103 globes. Oncologist 1997; 2:1–5.

ST. JUDE CHILDREN'S RESEARCH HOSPITAL APPROACH TO THE MANAGEMENT OF RETINOBLASTOMA

Most patients with unilateral, sporadic nonmetastatic retinoblastoma can be cured with enucleation alone. However, careful histologic evaluation of the enucleated eye has to be performed. We consider as risk factors for extraocular dissemination extension of the tumor to the anterior chamber, ciliary body, or iris; massive choroidal involvement or extension into the sclera; and invasion of the optic nerve beyond the lamina cribrosa. In these cases, we recommend adjuvant chemotherapy with the addition of orbital radiation for patients with scleral involvement. Patients with metastasis to bone or bone marrow and patients with tumor extension into the central nervous system (or in the optic nerve beyond the cut end) need more intensive chemotherapy and consolidation with high-dose chemotherapy and autologous hematopoietic stem cell rescue.

Patients with bilateral or multifocal disease present a challenge. Cure of the disease is the priority, but the therapeutic approach also has to consider preservation of the eye and vision. Our approach is highly conservative, and we enucleate only eyes with very advanced disease up front. Patients are treated with chemotherapy and intensive focal treatment. The aim is to delay or avoid external-beam radiation therapy and enucleation. For patients with low intraocular stage, we use a combination of vincristine and carboplatin and add etoposide for patients with more advanced disease. Because most treatment failures are caused by progression of vitreous seeds, subconjunctival carboplatin is added in cases of poor response of vitreous tumors. Patients are monitored closely with examinations under anesthesia every 4 to 6 weeks, and focal treatment is applied during the procedure. Focal treatments include cryotherapy for small anterior tumors, thermotherapy and laser photocoagulation of small posterior tumors, and brachytherapy for larger tumors. Thermotherapy often is used immediately after administration of carboplatin (thermochemotherapy). For patients who need radiation therapy, we use conformal or intensity-modulated techniques to minimize radiation to orbital bones.

thermotherapy, in which focused heat is applied at subphotocoagulation levels. Use of focal treatments is especially important in conjunction with chemotherapy, and both treatment modalities appear to have a synergistic effect. Sequential administration of thermotherapy with carboplatin enhances the antitumor effect by increasing the platinum-DNA adducts. For this reason thermochemotherapy is becoming a very important component in the management of intraocular retinoblastoma.[497,498] In addition to its effect on tumor control, cryotherapy increases intraocular penetration of carboplatin, presumably through disruption of the blood-vitreous barrier.[499,500] In general, local control rates of 70% to 80% can be achieved.[495-497]

Radiation Therapy

Retinoblastoma is a highly radiosensitive tumor. However, with increasing use of chemoreduction in conjunction with intensive focal therapy, external beam megavoltage radiation therapy usually is reserved for cases in which more conservative approaches have failed, usually because of progression of vitreous and subretinal seeding, and for tumors adjacent to the optic nerve. Because most patients undergoing radiation therapy have multifocal disease, the entire retinal surface has to be irradiated to a uniform dose. Several techniques can be used, usually through lateral fields.[501-503] The recommended total dose is 40 to 60 cGy in 180- to 200-cGy fractions, although doses of 36 cGy can be effective in conjunction with other techniques.[504] Three types of tumor regression following radiation therapy have been categorized. In type I, tumor shrinkage with calcium deposition produces a cottage-cheese pattern. In type II, the tumor is a gray, homogeneous mass characterized by partial shrinkage and loss of the pink color of capillary injection. An annulus of atrophic pigment at the base of the tumor also is present. In type III the regression pattern has features of both type I and type II. The mass has evidence of shrinkage, has lost the pink color, and has a nidus of calcium. Radiation therapy alone can cure 75% to 80% of patients. Addition of cryotherapy or photocoagulation can improve the results to 90%.[501-503]

Radioactive plaque technique is advantageous in the management of localized tumors, both because the procedure time is short and because a high dose of irradiation is delivered to the area of interest while radiation effects on the extraocular structures are minimized. Indications for plaque therapy include solitary tumors with a diameter between 6 and 15 mm, tumor thickness of 10 mm or less, and location of the lesion more than 3 mm from the optic disk or fovea. Different radioactive episcleral plaques can be used, although ^{125}I is the most widely used. A control rate of 85% to 90% can be achieved.[505]

Chemotherapy

Chemotherapy is indicated in the care of patients with extraocular disease, the subgroup of patients with intraocular disease with high-risk histologic features, and patients with bilateral disease in conjunction with aggressive focal therapy. Agents effective in the management of retinoblastoma include platinum compounds, etoposide, cyclophosphamide, doxorubicin, vincristine, and ifosfamide.[506]

Treatment in Specific Settings

Unilateral Retinoblastoma

Patients with unilateral retinoblastoma usually have advanced tumors (Reese-Ellsworth groups IV–V) when they come to medical attention, and enucleation is the treatment of choice, being curative in more than 80% of cases. Patients with high-risk histologic features, such as deep choroidal invasion, or with involvement of the anterior chamber, iris, ciliary body, or retrolaminar portion of the optic nerve need adjuvant chemotherapy.[507,508] A small number of patients have extraocular or metastatic disease and need more intensive treatment, which usually includes high-dose chemotherapy, hematopoietic stem cell rescue, and radiation therapy to the orbit and areas of bulky disease.[509,510] Except for the small group of patients with metastatic disease, particularly those with central nervous system involvement, outcome among patients with unilateral disease in developed countries is excellent, with good functional results and minimal long-term effects.[8,511] Eye salvage techniques can be used in the rare patients with Reese-Ellsworth I through III eyes. In these cases, the combination of chemoreduction with aggressive focal consolidation techniques, usually thermochemotherapy and brachytherapy, is necessary.

Bilateral Retinoblastoma

In patients with germline mutation of the *RB1* gene, multiple, bilateral retinoblastoma develops at an earlier age. These patients are at risk of development of new tumors until the completion of retinal differentiation. These patients also continue to be at risk of development of extraocular tumors throughout life.[7,8,433] In the past, treatment of patients with bilateral retinoblastoma was enucleation of eyes with advanced intraocular disease and no visual potential and use of external-beam radiation therapy for other eyes. However, several complications are associated with the use of radiation therapy. Irradiation of the orbit during a period of rapid growth results in a major decrease in orbital volume, which leads to midfacial deformities.[512,513] More important is increased risk of development of bone sarcoma in the radiation field. This risk appears to be age related and decreases as radiation is delayed.[514] These concerns have resulted in development of new and more conservative approaches. Treatment of patients with bilateral retinoblastoma has thus evolved to incorporate the use of up-front chemotherapy, which is meant to achieve maximum chemoreduction of the intraocular tumor burden early in treatment, followed by aggressive focal therapy. The goals of this approach are to avoid or delay the use of external-beam radiation therapy and to increase the ocular salvage rate. The use of systemic chemotherapy for cytoreduction, coupled with intensive use of sequential focal therapy (cryotherapy, laser photocoagulation, thermotherapy, and brachytherapy) has resulted in an increase in eye salvage rate and a decrease (and delay) in the use of radiation therapy. Different chemotherapy combinations are used, although the best results are achieved with a combination of vincristine, carboplatin, and etoposide,[497,515-518] although a less intensive regimen with vincristine and carboplatin alone appears to be effective for early intraocular stages.[519] Salvage rates for Reese-Ellsworth group I through III eyes approaches 100% when these techniques are used. For patients with advanced intraocular tumors (Reese-Ellsworth groups IV and V), ocular salvage rates are not better than 50% to 70%, and external-beam radiation therapy usually is needed.[515] However, radiation therapy usually is delayed for several months, which allows for better orbital growth and a decrease in the risk of second malignant tumors. A large proportion of failures occur because of progression of tumor in the vitreous or as subretinal implants, two areas of difficult access for antineoplastic agents.[520] Carboplatin diffuses well into the vitreous.[521] Intraocular concentrations are 7 to 10 times higher when carboplatin is administered subconjunctivally. Results of animal studies have shown dose-dependent inhibition of intraocular tumor growth by subconjuctival carboplatin.[522] These encouraging pre-clinical data, however, have led to studies of administration of subconjunctival carboplatin to patients with advanced intraocular disease.[500,523] Radiation therapy appears to be the only valid alternative for these patients. With incorporation of external-beam radiation therapy early in treatment in the case of minimal disease before disease progression occurs, ocular salvage rates for Reese-Ellsworth group V eyes may improve.[519]

Long-Term Effects

Because their orbital growth is still in progress, children treated for retinoblastoma are at risk of functionally and cosmetically significant bony orbital abnormalities. These sequelae become evident by early adolescence, when orbital growth is largely complete, and result in hourglass facial deformity.[512] Both enucleation, which causes orbital contraction, and radiation therapy, which induces arrest of bone growth, adversely affect orbital growth. In children treated for bilateral retinoblastoma, the effect of enucleation on orbital development is not different from that of irradiation. However, final orbital volume after enucleation correlates with the size of the prosthetic implant.[513]

Patients with germline mutation of the *RB1* gene are at risk of development of second tumors.[433,512,513] These patients usually have multifocal, bilateral disease and thus often are treated with radiation therapy, which further enhances susceptibility to a second tumor. The cumulative incidence of second malignant tumors is 4% at 10 years, 18% at 35 years, and 51% at 50 years.[433,513] The tumors most commonly encountered are soft-tissue sarcoma, melanoma, and osteosarcoma. There appears to be an age effect on sarcoma risk. Patients receiving radiation during the first year of life are at higher risk of development of sarcoma.[516] Patients with nonhereditary retinoblastoma are not at increased risk.[433,512]

HEPATOBLASTOMA

Epidemiology

Primary malignant tumors of the liver are rare in the pediatric population, constituting only 1.3% of malignant tumors in children younger than 15 years.[258] Of these, approximately 60% are hepatoblastoma. The median age at diagnosis of hepatoblastoma is 18 months.[524] Although more than 83% of cases occur during the first 5 years of life, the tumor occasionally is found in adolescents and adults. There is a male preponderance, with a male-to-female ratio of approximately 1.7 to 1. An intriguing association between extremely low birth weight and hepatoblastoma has been noted.[525,526] The explanation for this association is unresolved, but it has been suggested that environmental exposures in the neonatal intensive care unit, coupled with immature or genetically altered metabolic pathways, contribute to the genesis of hepatoblastoma.[526]

Biology

Insights into the genetic cause of hepatoblastoma have emerged over the past several years. In the 1980s, an association between hepatoblastoma and familial adenomatous polyposis (FAP) was found.[527] FAP is an autosomal-dominant disorder characterized by development of colorectal adenomas and nearly universal onset of colorectal carcinoma by the fifth decade of life.[528] Children of patients with FAP are at greatly increased risk of hepatoblastoma compared with the general population. In one study investigators estimated an 847-fold risk; other investigators reported an overall risk of 0.42%.[529,530] Conversely, it is estimated that 1 in 20 cases of hepatoblastoma are associated with FAP.[531] In light of these data, colorectal screening of parents of patients with hepatoblastoma and adolescent survivors of the disease should be considered. FAP is caused by a mutation in the adenomatous polyposis coli (*APC*) gene, which encodes a member of the Wnt signaling pathway. A central effector of this pathway is β-catenin, which associates with members of the Tcf family of transcription factors to promote expression of growth-related genes such as c-*myc* and the cyclin D1 gene.[532] In normal cells, APC associates with and promotes degradation of β-catenin. Mutations of *APC*, β-catenin itself, and other members of the Wnt signaling pathway lead to accumulation of β-catenin in cell nuclei, activation of Tcf target genes, and tumorigenesis. Germline *APC* mutations in hepatoblastoma patients without FAP have been reported.[533] A study of sporadic hepatoblastoma revealed loss of heterozygosity or mutations at the *APC* locus in 69% of tumor specimens.[534] Other studies have shown activating β-catenin mutations in 48% to 65% of sporadic cases of hepatoblastoma.[535,536]

Hepatoblastoma can be associated with Beckwith-Wiedemann syndrome (BWS), an overgrowth disorder that manifests as high birth weight, macroglossia, organomegaly, hemihypertrophy, neonatal hypoglycemia, abdominal wall defects, ear pits and creases, and a predisposition to development of Wilms' tumor and other malignant lesions. In a series of 183 patients with BWS followed through the first 4 years of life, hepatoblastoma developed in 5 (2.8%) of the patients.[274] BWS has been linked to chromosome 11p15.5, the site of the *IGF2* gene (see earlier, Wilms' Tumor). Loss of heterozygosity at this locus has been found in hepatoblastoma samples, implicating *IGF2* or other proximal genes in the development of this disease. As observed in Wilms' tumor, the maternal 11p15 allele is preferentially lost, indicating the presence of genomic imprinting at this site. Loss or relaxation of imprinting of *IGF2*, resulting in a double dose of the gene, has been found in some cases of hepatoblastoma.[537-539]

Cytogenetic studies of hepatoblastoma specimens have revealed that trisomy of chromosomes 20, 2, and 8 are the most frequent chromosomal aberrations in this tumor type.[540-544] A recurrent translocation, t(1;4)(q12;q34), also has been reported.[545,546] Comparative genomic hybridization of 10 hepatoblastoma samples revealed that the most common abnormalities were gains of chromosomes 1q, 2, 17, and 20 and loss of chromosomes 4 and 11.[547] The biologic and clinical significance of these cytogenetic findings is unknown.

Pathology

Hepatoblastoma represents 60% of cases of childhood liver cancer, followed by hepatocellular carcinoma (32%) and extrahepatic biliary tree sarcoma (8%).[548] Other primary malignant tumors that arise in the liver include angiosarcoma, embryonal rhabdomyosarcoma, carcinoid tumor, leiomyosarcoma, teratoma, lymphoma, and neuroblastoma. Benign liver processes in children include vascular tumors (hemangioma and hemangioendothelioma), hamartoma, adenoma, and focal nodular hyperplasia.

Hepatoblastoma is most often unifocal, arising in the right lobe of the liver. Microscopic vascular spread may be found beyond the apparently encapsulated tumor. Hepatoblastoma is classified as either purely epithelial or mixed, consisting of both epithelial and mesenchymal elements. The epithelial type contains either fetal or embryonal cells or admixtures of the two. Rare histologic variants of the epithelial type include the macrotrabecular and small cell (anaplastic) patterns.

The prognostic significance of histologic subtype in patients with hepatoblastoma is unresolved. Data from the 1970s and early 1980s first suggested that completely resected hepatoblastoma of pure fetal histologic type with low mitotic activity is associated with an excellent prognosis.[548-550] On the basis of this observation, in the first Intergroup Hepatoma Study (INT-98) doxorubicin alone was used to treat nine patients with completely resected pure fetal hepatoblastoma. All of these patients were alive without disease when the results were reported.[551] The current Children's Oncology Group protocol for hepatoblastoma provides for surgical resection alone in patients with completely resected pure fetal hepatoblastoma. By contrast, SIOP does not incorporate histologic subtype into its treatment stratification schema because it is unclear whether completely excised hepatoblastoma of pure fetal histologic type behaves differently from completely excised hepatoblastoma of other subtypes.[552] Moreover, a standardized definition of pure fetal hepatoblastoma is lacking. There is a growing consensus that the small cell variant of hepatoblastoma is associated with poor prognosis.[524,553] This variant is easily misdiagnosed because it often is associated with low α-fetoprotein (AFP) level and may be present only focally within a tumor.

Clinical Manifestations and Patterns of Spread

Hepatoblastoma most often manifests as an asymptomatic abdominal mass, but systemic symptoms, such as anorexia, weight loss, vomiting, and abdominal pain, can occur. In rare instances, the first sign is acute abdominal crisis due to tumor rupture. At physical examination, liver enlargement is found, but jaundice is rare, occurring in fewer than 5% of cases. Other infrequent features include hemihypertrophy (2% of cases) and precocious puberty (fewer than 3% of cases), which occurs in patients whose tumors secrete β human chorionic gonadotropin. Distant metastatic spread occurs most commonly to the lungs, affecting 10% of patients when the disease manifests. Spread to bone and the central nervous system occurs but is unusual.

Laboratory and Radiologic Evaluation

Ultrasonography is typically the first-line imaging procedure in evaluation of a child with an abdominal mass. For liver tumors, this modality is particularly useful in establishing the presence of a discrete mass within an enlarged liver and in delineating cystic components. CT can be used to define local extent of tumor involvement and determine important landmarks but is not always reliable in assessment of resectability.[554] MRI is more accurate in this regard and helps define vascular involvement. Although commonly used in the past, angiography plays no role in the diagnostic evaluation of childhood liver tumors. Investigation of metastatic spread includes chest CT. Bone scans are not typically recommended because skeletal metastasis is rare, and osteopenia, which is commonly associated with hepatoblastoma, can cause misleading findings.[555]

Routine blood counts frequently reveal mild normochromic normocytic anemia and marked thrombocytosis. Liver enzyme and bilirubin levels are infrequently elevated. The most valuable laboratory test for both diagnosis and monitoring of hepatoblastoma is serum AFP level. AFP levels are elevated in 80% to 90% of patients with hepatoblastoma, presumably reflecting recapitulation of fetal liver development by the tumor. After complete resection, an exponential decrease to normal range can be expected. Failure to achieve normal levels implies the presence of residual disease. Secondary elevation implies disease recurrence. Clinicians should note that AFP levels are normally elevated at birth and gradually decline to adult level over the first year of life.

TABLE 99-16

Postsurgical Staging System for Hepatoblastoma[560]

STAGE	DESCRIPTION
I, favorable histologic features	Gross total resection with clear tumor margins. Favorable histologic type is defined as pure fetal type with fewer than two mitoses per 10 high-power microscope fields.
I, unfavorable histologic features	Gross total resection with clear tumor margins and absence of favorable histology.
II	Gross total resection with microscopic residual disease at the tumor margins.
III	Gross total resection with nodal involvement or tumor spill or incomplete resection with gross residual intrahepatic disease.
IV	Distant metastatic disease.

Staging

In North America, staging for hepatoblastoma is based on postsurgical findings. Low stage is assigned to completely resected tumors and high stage to unresectable tumors and those with distant metastatic involvement (Table 99-16).[551] With the advent of preoperative chemotherapy, SIOP introduced a presurgical grouping system called *Pretext* (pretreatment extent of disease).[556] In this system, the liver is divided into four sectors on the basis of anatomic distribution of the major veins and bile ducts. Group I denotes that three adjoining sectors are tumor free; group II, that two adjoining sectors are tumor-free; group III, that one sector or two nonadjoining sectors are tumor-free; and group IV, that all sectors are involved (Fig. 99-19). Invasion of the hepatic and portal veins,

extrahepatic extension, and distant metastatic lesions are designated separately in this system.

Treatment

The survival rate for hepatoblastoma has improved markedly. Whereas the survival rate was only 30% in the 1970s, it is now 60% to 70%. This improvement may be attributed to the advent of effective adjuvant chemotherapy and to the use of liver transplantation for patients with otherwise unresectable disease. The underlying principle of hepatoblastoma treatment is that complete surgical resection is necessary to achieve long-term cure. Although complete excision is possible at diagnosis in 40% to 60% of patients,[524] preoperative chemotherapy can render most disease resectable.[557-568] Analogous to the international debate regarding the timing of Wilms' tumor resection, there are differences in opinion regarding whether preoperative chemotherapy should be delivered to all patients with hepatoblastoma. The Children's Oncology Group advocates up-front resection of the primary tumor whenever possible, because this approach allows the most accurate histologic diagnosis.[561] By contrast, SIOP favors preoperative chemotherapy for all patients to render the tumors more amenable to resection.[562] Management of hepatoblastoma unresectable after systemic neoadjuvant chemotherapy is a clinical challenge. Disease confined to the liver after primary chemotherapy has been managed with chemoembolization, which induces tumor responses and surgical resectability in some patients.[563,564] For patients with unresectable tumors, orthotopic liver transplantation seems to offer the best possibility of cure. Several groups of investigators have reported a 50% to 83% survival rate

Figure 99-19. Pretreatment staging system (Pretext) proposed by the International Society of Pediatric Oncology. The liver is broken into four sectors on the basis of the anatomy of the major vessels and bile ducts. Group I denotes one-sector involvement (three adjoining sectors are tumor free); group II, two-sector involvement (two adjoining sectors are tumor free); group III, three-sector involvement or that one sector or two nonadjoining sectors are tumor free; and group IV, that no sectors are free of tumor. Involvement can be either unifocal or multifocal, although hepatoblastoma usually is unifocal. Additional designations are given for metastasis, ingrowth into the vena cava or porta hepatis, and extrahepatic extension.

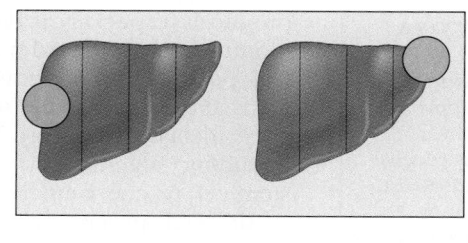

I

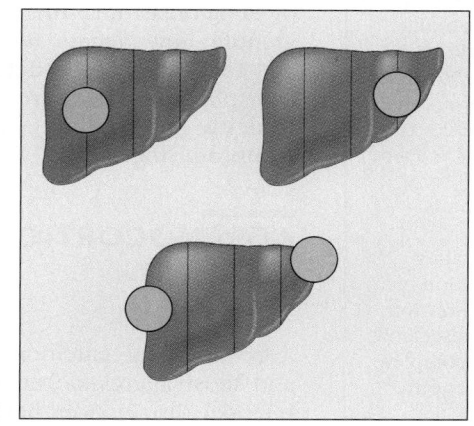

II

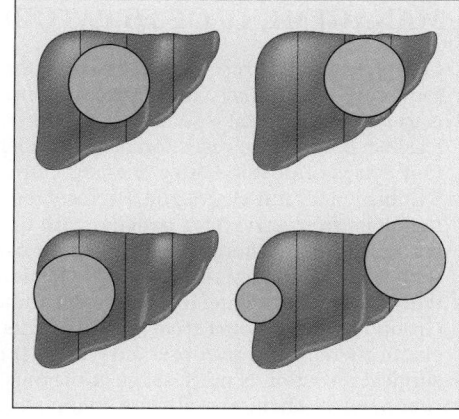

III

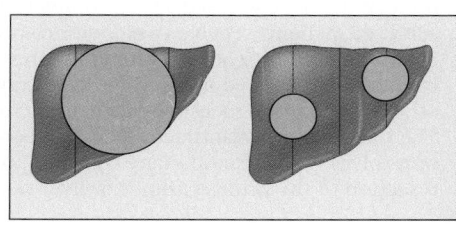

IV

Specific Malignancies

III

among children with hepatoblastoma managed with liver transplantation with or without adjuvant chemotherapy.[565-569] Cure after liver transplantation has occurred even in children with a history of pulmonary metastasis. These results are much more favorable than the experience with hepatocellular carcinoma, perhaps because of the inherent chemosensitivity of hepatoblastoma.

Even if complete resection of the primary tumor is attained, adjuvant chemotherapy is recommended to eradicate micrometastatic disease.[570] Current chemotherapy regimens for hepatoblastoma are based on several generations of clinical trials. The CCG-823F study showed that the combination of cisplatin and continuous infusion of doxorubicin led to a measurable tumor response in 75% of patients with initially unresectable disease and that 58% of these patients continued to be disease-free after treatment.[557] Contemporaneously, the POG-8697 study achieved similar results with a regimen of cisplatin, vincristine, and 5-fluorouracil.[559] The cisplatin/doxorubicin and cisplatin/vincristine/5-fluorouracil regimens were compared in a randomized trial (INT-98) that revealed 5-year EFS estimates of 69% for the doxorubicin-containing arm and 57% for the 5-fluorouracil/vincristine-containing arm ($P = .09$).[551] The EFS rate was 100% for stage I favorable histologic type, 91% for stage I unfavorable histologic type, 100% for stage II, 64% for stage III, and 25% for stage IV. Because toxicity was more frequent in the doxorubicin-containing arm, treatment with cisplatin/vincristine/5-fluorouracil emerged as the standard treatment in North America. The SIOPEL-1 study, in which a cisplatin/doxorubicin combination was used, yielded a 5-year EFS rate of 66% and a 5-year overall survival rate of 75%.[556] As in the INT-98 study, patients with metastatic disease had a 5-year EFS rate of only 28%.[571] The SIOPEL-2 study piloted a regimen of single-agent cisplatin for patients with localized hepatoblastoma confined to no more than three liver sectors (Pretext group III or lower).[562] This study showed promising results. The SIOPEL-3 study therefore was designed to compare the effectiveness of cisplatin/doxorubicin versus cisplatin alone in patients with localized hepatoblastoma.

To summarize, modern cisplatin-containing chemotherapy regimens produce very good outcome for patients with localized and completely resected hepatoblastoma. Studies have been aimed at reducing cisplatin-associated toxicity by using carboplatin up front, reserving cisplatin for patients with disease that remains unresectable after carboplatin therapy.[572] This approach yielded promising results, although in a pilot study the Italian Hepatoblastoma Study Group investigators found inferior survival rates among patients who received carboplatin/doxorubicin compared with historical controls who received cisplatin/doxorubicin.[573] The Children's Oncology Group is currently evaluating whether the drug amifostine protects against cisplatin-associated toxicity. Novel agents and approaches are needed to improve outcome among patients with metastatic disease.

The role of radiation therapy in the management of hepatoblastoma is limited and undefined. Results with small series of patients revealed that hepatoblastoma patients with microscopic or gross residual disease can achieve local control with radiation therapy and chemotherapy. These results suggested that there might be a role for irradiation in this setting.[559,574,575] Successful use of radiation therapy also has been reported for pulmonary metastatic lesions after wedge resection and chemotherapy.[574,575] However, given the effectiveness of surgery and chemotherapy, radiation therapy is not considered first-line therapy for hepatoblastoma.

Recurrence of hepatoblastoma usually confers a poor prognosis, especially if disease recurs locally or within 6 months after the initial manifestations. Long-term survival has been achieved, however, with aggressive surgical management, especially in the setting of isolated pulmonary metastatic disease.[576] The role of chemotherapy, including high-dose therapy followed by autologous stem cell rescue, is unclear.

Although progress has been made in the management of hepatoblastoma, the goal of future studies will be to identify new agents with activity against this disease and to systematically define the role of orthotopic liver transplantation. Future trials will attempt to limit toxicity and the late effects of treatment without compromising care.

ADRENOCORTICAL CARCINOMA

Epidemiology

Adrenocortical carcinoma (ACC) is one of the rarest and most aggressive endocrine neoplasms. It follows a bimodal distribution, having peaks during the first and

---

ST. JUDE CHILDREN'S RESEARCH HOSPITAL APPROACH TO THE MANAGEMENT OF HEPATOBLASTOMA

Complete surgical resection is essential for achieving long-term cure in children with hepatoblastoma. Our approach is to attempt surgical resection at diagnosis whenever feasible. If complete resection is achieved, patients receive four cycles of postoperative chemotherapy with cisplatin, 5-fluorouracil, and vincristine. Doxorubicin-containing regimens are reserved for patients with unresponsive or recurrent tumor. There is no standard of care of patients with stage I hepatoblastoma of pure fetal histologic type with a low mitotic rate. In the current Children's Oncology Group hepatoblastoma study, such patients do not receive chemotherapy and are observed closely. If complete surgical resection is not feasible at diagnosis, four cycles of preoperative chemotherapy are administered, and resectability is reassessed. Once complete resection is achieved, patients receive two additional cycles of chemotherapy. Patients with tumors unresectable after chemotherapy are considered for liver transplantation or other local control measures, such as chemoembolization. The presence of distant metastatic disease that is resectable or resolves with chemotherapy does not preclude complete resection of the primary tumor or liver transplantation.

fourth decades of life.[577] Among children, 25 new cases are expected to occur annually in the United States, for an estimated annual incidence of 0.2 to 0.3 cases per million persons. Internationally, however, the incidence of ACC appears to vary substantially. The incidence of ACC is particularly high in southern Brazil, where it is approximately 10 to 15 times that in the United States. Most cases occur in the contiguous states of Sao Paulo and Paraná. Predisposing genetic factors have been implicated in 50% of cases in the United States and in 95% of cases in Brazil. In patients in both countries, germline *P53* mutations are almost always the predisposing factors. In the United States, relatives of children with ACC often have a high incidence of cancer (Li-Fraumeni syndrome), and germline mutations occur in the p53 DNA-binding domains (exons 2 to 8). In Brazil, in contrast, patients' families do not have a high incidence of cancer, and a single mutation in axon 10 of the *P53* gene is consistently observed in these children. This mutation occurs within the tetramerization domain of p53 (p53-R337H). This mutant tetramerization domain is less stable than the wild-type domain and is highly sensitive to pH in the physiologic range. This inherited unique *P53* mutation represents a low-penetrance allele that contributes to development of ACC in a tissue-specific manner.[578,579] The incidence of R337H mutations in U.S. children with ACC is not known.

Clinical Manifestations

Patients with ACC typically have signs and symptoms of increased production of androgens (virilization) or cortisol (hypercortisolism or Cushing's syndrome). In rare instances, patients have signs of hyperestrogenism (feminization) or aldosteronism (Conn's syndrome). Mixed syndromes are frequent. In general, 40% to 80% of patients have functioning tumors,[577-586] although as many as 50% of tumors may produce mainly hormonal precursors of low bioactivity.[584] There appears to be a correlation between the degree and type of endocrine disturbance and the age of the patient.[577,582] Older patients tend to have a much higher incidence of non-functioning tumors, whereas more than 90% of children have functioning neoplasms.[582,587-589] Adults usually have mixed virilization-hypercortisolism syndromes, whereas virilization syndromes are the most common manifestations among children. Most patients (50%–60%) come to medical attention with large tumors and advanced regional or metastatic disease.[580-586,590] Distant metastatic lesions usually develop to liver, lungs, and bone, in that order.[582]

Diagnosis

The diagnosis of ACC is straightforward. Because most children have an endocrine syndrome, increased blood or urine concentration of adrenocortical hormones and a mass in the suprarenal region usually suggest a pre-operative diagnosis of adrenocortical tumor. However, the distinction between benign (adenoma) and malignant (carcinoma) tumors may not be easy. Several authors have proposed histologic criteria that may help in discriminating the two types of neoplasms.[591,592] However, the morphologic criteria used to differentiate benign from malignant pediatric adrenocortical tumors may not be reliable, especially in cases of carcinoma.

Prognostic Factors

In addition to stage at diagnosis, specific biologic and histopathologic characteristics within individual tumors appear to dictate outcome. Mitotic rate has been consistently reported as the most important determinant of aggressive behavior.[581,590,593,594] However, tumor size appears to have independent prognostic value.[590,594] Tumor size is specially important in children; tumors smaller than 200 cm^3 or 100 g have an excellent outcome with surgery alone.[587,595,596]

Treatment

Surgery is the mainstay of therapy for ACC. Curative, complete resection may be attempted in the 70% to 75% of patients with locoregional disease. Low stage and the ability to perform complete resection are the most important prognostic factors.[580,581,584,585,590,597] However, despite efforts at curative surgery, the 5-year survival rate is not better than 30% to 40%.[581,582-586] As many as 70% to 80% of patients with a localized primary tumor experience recurrence.[590] Recurrences are locoregional (15%–25%), combined local and distant (25%–30%), or distant alone (50%).[581,590,598] In children, more than 90% of patients with stage I disease are long-term survivors, compared with 10% of those with stage IV disease. Despite presumed complete tumor resection, disease recurs in 50% of patients with stage II disease.[587] Because of tumor friability, rupture of the capsule leading to tumor spillage is frequent. Large ACC tends to adhere to adjacent structures (e.g., vena cava) and have large necrotic and friable areas that make radical excision without capsule rupture very difficult.

For patients with advanced disease or with high risk of recurrence, systemic therapy with mitotane or chemotherapy is indicated, although the effect of this therapy on overall outcome is not well established. Mitotane (*o,p'*-DDD) both inhibits corticoid biosynthesis and destroys adrenocortical cells. At low doses (<3 g/day) mitotane suppresses secretion of adrenal steroids, providing symptomatic improvement and regression of some of the endocrine dysfunction. Higher doses (>3 g/day) are required for an adrenolytic effect.[580,582] In patients with advanced disease, objective responses are obtained in approximately 20% to 30% of cases.[580,582,584,599] However, these responses are transient, and the effect on prolongation of survival is uncertain.[582,584,600] In children, the use of mitotane for advanced ACC has not been evaluated systematically. There have been several reports of complete responses in children with advanced or metastatic ACC, but these appear to be rare events.[601-603] The pharmacokinetics of mitotane and the ability to maintain therapeutic levels for long periods appear to affect the antitumor effect. Serum levels plateau after 8 weeks of treatment,[582] and optimal antitumor responses occur when serum levels are maintained at more than 14 µg/mL for long periods.[597,599] A major problem, however, is the severe gastrointestinal and neurologic toxicity associated with administration of mitotane. The toxicity limits patient adherence to therapy, especially among children.[582,584,599] An alternative approach to administration of high doses of mitotane is administration of low doses (2–3 g/day) for longer periods. With the appropriate monitoring, therapeutic levels can still be achieved after 3 to 5 months.[604,605] Chemotherapeutic agents other than mitotane have been less evaluated in management of ACC. Cisplatin-based regimens induce responses in 20% to 40% of patients.[606-608] Preclinical studies have shown that mitotane reverts the multidrug resistance phenotype in vitro,[609] providing a rationale for the combination of mitotane with etoposide-containing regimens.[610,611] Responses have been observed in 53% of patients when the combination of mitotane with cisplatin, etoposide, and doxorubicin has been used.[611]

NASOPHARYNGEAL CARCINOMA

Nasopharyngeal carcinoma (NPC) is very rare in children. Only 1% of all cases of NPC occur in patients younger than 19 years.[612] In the United States, the incidence of NPC in children is approximately 1 to 1.5 cases per million persons per year. NPC represents approximately 1% of all pediatric malignant tumors, but it accounts for 35% to 50% of all nasopharyngeal malignant tumors.[613] In the United States, NPC appears to be more prevalent in the southern states and among African American children.[614] The role of EBV in the development of NPC has been well established. EBV is harbored in almost every tumor, as shown by the presence of EBV DNA, RNA, and proteins in tumor tissue samples.[615-618] The role of EBV in neoplastic transformation is further supported by the presence of clonality. In nonendemic areas of the Western hemisphere, other causative factors, such as alcohol and tobacco use, may have an important role. Information on the clinical and biologic characteristics of childhood NPC is scarce, in particular that related to the role of EBV in its pathogenesis. However, both histologic subtype and age when the tumor manifests suggest that pediatric NPC may be strongly associated with EBV infection. No studies have been aimed at characterizing or confirming the role of EBV in NPC in children.

Few studies have analyzed the clinical characteristics and outcome of NPC among children.[613,614,619-628] Almost all cases of NPC have type III histologic features and manifest at advanced stages. Most studies incorporated the use of cisplatin or doxorubicin-based neoadjuvant and adjuvant chemotherapy.[613,619-626] With this combined approach, the survival rate among patients with advanced disease is 60% to 70%. The best results have been those reported by Douglass and collaborators at St. Jude Children's Research Hospital.[629] Patients were treated with four courses of neoadjuvant chemotherapy with methotrexate, cisplatin, 5-fluorouracil, and leucovorin followed by radiation therapy (66–70 Gy). All 21 patients achieved complete remission, and 20 of them were long-term survivors. Because children are particularly sensitive to the toxicity related to therapy for NPC, alternatives aimed at decreasing toxic effects are of particular importance to this population. The alternatives include use of amifostine and investigation of carboplatin as an alternative to cisplatin.

REFERENCES

Introduction

1. Horowitz ME, Pizzo PA: Solid tumors in children. Pediatr Clin North Am 1991;38:201.
2. Crist WM, Kun LE: Common solid tumors of childhood. N Engl J Med 1991;324:461.

Osteosarcoma

3. Dorfman HD, Czerniak B: Osteosarcoma. In Dorfman HD, Czerniak B (eds): Bone Tumors. St Louis, Mosby, 1998, pp 128–252.
4. Gurney JG, Severson RK, Davis S, et al: Incidence of cancer in children in the United States. Cancer 1995;75:2186–2195.
5. Glass AG, Fraumeni JF: Epidemiology of bone cancer in children. J Natl Cancer Inst 1970;44:187–199.
6. Newton WA, Meadows AT, Shimada H, et al: Bone sarcomas as second malignant neoplasms following childhood cancer. Cancer 1991;67:193–201.
7. Mohney, BG, Robertson, DM, Schomberg, PJ, et al: Second nonocular tumors in survivors of heritable retinoblastoma and prior radiation therapy. Am J Ophthalmol 1998;126: 269–277.
8. Wong FL, Boice JD, Abramson DH, et al: Cancer incidence after retinoblastoma: Radiation dose and sarcoma risk. JAMA 1997;278:1262–1267.
9. Wadayama B, Toguchida J, Shimizu T, et al: Mutation spectrum of the retinoblastoma gene in osteosarcoma. Cancer Res 1994;54: 3042–3048.
10. Wei G, Lonardo F, Ueda T, et al: CDK4 gene amplification in osteosarcoma: Reciprocal relationship with INK4 gene alterations and mapping of 12q13 amplicons. Int J Cancer 1999;80:199–204.
11. Huang HJ, Yee JK, Shew JY, et al: Suppression of the neoplastic phenotype by replacement of the RB gene in human cancer cells. Science 1988;242:1563–1566.
12. Tebbi CK, Gaeta J: Osteosarcoma. Pediatr Ann 1988;17:285–300.
13. Gokgoz N, Wunder JS, Mousses S, et al: Comparison of p53 mutations in patients with localized osteosarcoma and metastatic osteosarcoma. Cancer 2001;92:2181–2189.
14. Ladanyi M, Cha C, Lewis R, et al: MDM2 amplification in metastatic osteosarcoma. Cancer Res 1993;53:16–18.
15. Yamaguchi T, Toguchida J, Yamamuro T, et al: Allelotype analysis in osteosarcomas: Frequent allele loss on 3q, 13q, 17p qne 18p. Cancer Res 1992;53:2419–2423.
16. Kruzelock RP, Murphy EC, Strong LC, et al: Localization of a novel tumor suppressor locus on human chromosome 3q important in osteosarcoma tumorigenesis. Cancer Res 1997;57:106–109.
17. Chavez Kappel C, Velez-Yanguas C, Hirschfeld S, et al: Human osteosarcoma cell lines are dependent on insulin-like growth factor for in vitro growth. Cancer Res 1994;54:2803–2807.
18. Rodriguez-Galindo C, Poquette CA, Daw NC, et al: Circulating concentrations of IGF-I and IGFBP-3 are not predictive of incidence or clinical behavior of pediatric steosarcoma. Med Pediatr Oncol 2001;36:605–611.
19. Bacci G, Pignatti G, Dallari D, et al: Primary chemotherapy and delayed surgery (neoadjuvant chemotherapy) for telangiectatic osteogenic sarcoma of the extremities. J Chemother 1989;1:190–196.
20. Unni KK, Dahlin DC, Beabout JW, et al: Periosteal osteogenic sarcoma. Cancer 1976;37:2476–2485.
21. Unni KK, Dahlin DC, Beabout JW, Ivins JC: Paraosteal osteogenic sarcoma. Cancer 1976;37:2466–2475.

22. Sheth DS, Yasko AW, Raymond AK, et al: Conventional and dedifferentiated paraosteal osteosarcoma: Diagnosis, treatment and outcome. Cancer 1996;78:2136-2145.

23. Parham DM, Pratt CB, Parvey LS, et al: Childhood multifocal osteosarcoma: Clinicopathologic and radiologic correlates. Cancer 1985;55:2653-2658.

24. Bielack SS, Kempf-Bielack B, Delling G, et al: Prognostic factors in high-grade osteosarcoma of the extremities or trunk: An analysis of 1,702 patients treated on neoadjuvant Cooperative Osteosarcoma Study Group Protocols. J Clin Oncol 2002;20: 776-790.

25. Marina NM, Pratt CB, Rao BN, et al: Improved prognosis of children with osteosarcoma metastatic to the lung(s) at the time of diagnosis. Cancer 1992;70:2722-2727.

26. Meyers PA, Heller G, Healey JH, et al: Osteogenic sarcoma with clinically detectable metastasis at initial presentation. J Clin Oncol 1993;11:449-453.

27. Bacci G, Picci P, Ferrari S, et al: Prognostic significance of serum alkaline phosphatase measurements in patients with osteosarcoma treated with adjuvant or neoadjuvant chemotherapy. Cancer 1993;71:1224-1230.

28. Murphy WA: Imaging of bone tumors in the 1990s. Cancer 1991;67:1169-1176.

29. Fletcher BD: Imaging pediatric bone sarcomas: Diagnosis and treatment-related issues. Radiol Clin North Am 1997;35:1477-1494.

30. Reddick WE, Taylor JA, Fletcher BD: Dynamic MR imaging (DEMRI) of microcirculation in bone sarcoma. J Magn Reson Imaging 1999;10:277-285.

31. Reddick WE, Wang S, Xiong X, et al: Dynamic magnetic resonance imaging of regional contrast access as an additional prognostic factor in pediatric osteosarcoma. Cancer 2001;91: 2230-2237.

32. Kaste SC, Billups CA, Tan M, et al: Thallium bone imaging as an indicator of response and outcome in nonmetastatic primary extremity osteosarcoma. Pediatr Radiol 2001;31:251-256.

33. Meyers PA, Heller G, Healey J, et al: Chemotherapy for nonmetastatic osteogenic sarcoma: The Memorial Sloan-Kettering Experience. J Clin Oncol 1992;10:5-15.

34. Meyers PA, Gorlick R, Heller G, et al: Intensification of preoperative chemotherapy for osteogenic sarcoma: Results of the Memorial Sloan-Kettering (T12) protocol. J Clin Oncol 1998;16:2452-2458.

35. Look AT, Douglass EC, Meyer WH: Clinical importance of near-diploid tumor stem lines in patents with osteosarcoma of an extremity. N Engl J Med 1988;318:1567-1572.

36. Baldini N, Scotlandi K, Barbanti-Brodano G, et al: Expression of P-glycoprotein in high-grade osteosarcomas in relation to clinical outcome. N Engl J Med 1995;333:1380-1385.

37. Scotlandi K, Serra M, Manara MC, et al: Clinical relevance of Ki-67 expression in bone tumors. Cancer 1995;75:806-814.

38. Ferrari S, Bertoni F, Mercuri M, et al: Predictive factors of disease-free survival for non-metastatic osteosarcoma of the extremity: An analysis of 300 patients treated at the Rizzoli Institute. Ann Oncol 2001;12:1145-1150.

39. Choong PFM, Sim FH: Limb-sparing surgery for bone tumors: New developments. Semin Surg Oncol 1997;13:64-69.

40. Meyer WH, Malawer MM: Osteosarcoma clinical features and evolving surgical and chemotherapeutic strategies. Pediatr Clin North Am 1991;38:317-348.

41. Wittig JC, Bickels J, Kellar-Graney KL, et al: Osteosarcoma of the proximal humerus: Long-term results with limb-sparing surgery. Clin Orthop 2001;397:156-176.

42. Wilkins RM, Soubeiran A: The Phenix prosthesis: Early American experience. Clin Orthop 2001;382:51-58.

43. Weeden S, Grimer RJ, Cannon SR, et al: The effect of local recurrence on survival in resected osteosarcoma. Eur J Cancer 2001;37:39-46.

44. Jaffe N, Frei E, Traggis D, et al: Adjuvant methotrexate and citrovorum-factor treatment of osteogenic sarcoma. N Engl J Med 1974;291:994-997.

45. Cortes EP, Holland JF, Wang JJ, et al: Amputation and adriamycin in primary osteosarcoma. N Engl J Med 1974;291:998-1000.

46. Rosen G, Caparros B, Huvos AG, et al: Preoperative chemotherapy for osteogenic sarcoma: Selection of postoperative adjuvant chemotherapy based on the response of the primary tumor to preoperative chemotherapy. Cancer 1982;49:1221-1230.

47. Souhami RL, Craft AW, Van der Eijken JW, et al: Randomized trial of two regimens of chemotherapy in operable osteosarcoma: A study of the European Osteosarcoma Intergroup. Lancet 1997;350: 911-917.

48. Ferrari S, Bacci G, Picci P, et al: Long-term follow-up and post-relapse survival in patients with non-metastatic osteosarcoma of the extremity treated with neoadjuvant chemotherapy. Ann Oncol 1997;8:765-771.

49. Provisor AJ, Ettinger LJ, Nachman JB, et al: Treatment of nonmetastatic osteosarcoma of the extremity with preoperative and postoperative chemotherapy: A report from the Children's Cancer Group. J Clin Oncol 1997;15:76-84.

50. Link MP, Goorin AM, Miser AW, et al: The effect of adjuvant chemotherapy on relapse-free survival in patients with osteosarcoma of the extremity. N Engl J Med 1986;314: 1600-1606.

51. Winkler K, Beron G, Delling G, et al: Neoadjuvant chemotherapy of osteosarcoma: Results of a randomized cooperative trial (COSS-82) with salvage chemotherapy based on histological tumor response. J Clin Oncol 1988;6:329-337.

52. Bramwell VHC, Burgers M, Sneath R, et al: A comparison of two short intensive adjuvant chemotherapy regimens in operable osteosarcoma of limbs in children and young adults: The first study of the European Osteosarcoma Intergroup. J Clin Oncol 1992;10:1579-1591.

53. Fuchs N, Bielack SS, Epler D, et al: Long-term results of the co-operative German-Austrian-Swiss osteosarcoma study group's protocol COSS-86 of intensive multidrug chemotherapy and surgery for osteosarcoma of the limbs. Ann Oncol 1998;9: 893-899.

54. Bowman LC, Meyer WH, Douglass EC, et al: Activity of ifosfamide in metastatic and unresectable osteosarcoma. Proc Annu Meet Am Soc Clin Oncol 1987;6:214.

55. Harris MB, Cantor AB, Goorin AM, et al: Treatment of osteosarcoma with ifosfamide: Comparison of response in pediatric patients with recurrent disease versus patients previously untreated. A Pediatric Oncology Group study. Med Pediatr Oncol 1995;24: 87-92.

56. Harris MB, Gieser P, Goorin AM, et al: Treatment of metastatic osteosarcoma at diagnosis: A Pediatric Oncology Group study. J Clin Oncol 1998;16:3641-3648.

57. Bacci G, Ferrari S, Mercuri M, et al: Neoadjuvant chemotherapy for extremity osteosarcoma. Acta Oncologica 1997;37:41-48.

58. Epelman S, Seibel N, Melaragno R, et al: Treatment of newly diagnosed high grade osteosarcoma (OS) with ifosfamide (IFOS), Adriamycin (ADR) and cisplatin (CDP) without high dose methotrexate. Proc Annu Meet Am Soc Clin Oncol 1995;14:439.

59. Meyer WH, Pratt CB, Poquette CA, et al: Carboplatin/ifosfamide window therapy for osteosarcoma: Results of the St. Jude Children's Research Hospital OS-91 trial. J Clin Oncol 2001;19:171-182.

60. Voûte PA, Souhami RL, Nooij M, et al: A phase II study of cisplatin, ifosfamide and doxorubicin in operable primary, axial skeletal and metastatic osteosarcoma. Ann Oncol 1999;10:1211-1218.

61. Yazawa Y, Takagi T, Asakura S, et al: Effects of 4-hydroperoxy ifosfamide in combination with other anticancer agents on human cancer cell lines. Orthop Sci 1999;4:231-237.

62. Miser JS, Kinsella TJ, Triche TJ, et al: Ifosfamide with mesna uroprotection and etoposide: An effective regimen in the treatment of recurrent sarcomas and other tumors of children and young adults. J Clin Oncol 1987;5:1191-1198.

63. Kung FH, Pratt CB, Vega RA, et al: Ifosfamide/etoposide combination in the treatment of recurrent malignant solid tumors of childhood. Cancer 1993;71:1898-1903.

64. Gentet JC, Brunat-Mentigny M, Demaille MC, et al: Ifosfamide and etoposide in childhood osteosarcoma: A phase II study of the French Society of Paediatric Oncology. Eur J Cancer 1997;33: 232-237.

65. Goorin AM, Cantor A, Link MP: A phase I trial of etoposide (VP) and escalating doses of ifosfamide (IFOS) plus GCSF in recurrent pediatric sarcomas. Proc Annu Meet Am Soc Clin Oncol 1994;13. Abstract 1458.

66. Ben Arush MW, Stein ME, Kuten A, et al: Postsurgical etoposide-ifosfamide regimen in poor-risk nonmetastatic osteogenic sarcoma. Am J Clin Oncol 1998;21:72–74.

67. Goorin AM, Harris MB, Bernstein M, et al: Phase II/III trial of etoposide and high-dose ifosfamide in newly diagnosed metastatic osteosarcoma: A Pediatric Oncology Group trial. J Clin Oncol 2002;20:426–433.

68. Ferguson WS, Harris MB, Goorin AM, et al: Presurgical window of carboplatin and surgery and multidrug chemotherapy for the treatment of newly diagnosed metastatic or unresectable osteosarcoma: Pediatric Oncology Group trial. J Pediatr Hematol Oncol 2001;23:340–348.

69. Bacci G, Briccoli A, Ferrari S, et al: Neoadjuvant chemotherapy for osteosarcoma of the extremity: Long-term results of the Rizzoli's 4th protocol. Eur J Cancer 2001;37:2030–2039.

70. Kleinerman ES. Biologic therapy for osteosarcoma using liposome-encapsulated muramyl tripeptide. Hematol Oncol Clin North Am 1995;9:927–938.

71. Gorlick R, Huvos AG, Heller G, et al: Expression of HER2/erbB-2 correlates with survival in osteosarcoma. J Clin Oncol 1999;17:2781–2788.

72. Kilpatrick SE, Geisinger KR, King TS, et al: Clinicopathological analysis of HER-2/neu immunoexpression among various histologic subtypes and grades of osteosarcoma. Mod Pathol 2001;14:1277–1283.

73. Maitra A, Wanzer D, Weinberg AG, et al: Amplification of the HER-2/neu oncogene is uncommon in pediatric osteosarcomas. Cancer 2001;92:677–683.

74. Anderson PM, Wiseman GA, Dispenzieri A, et al: High-dose samarium-153 ethylene diamine tetramethylene phosphonate: Low toxicity of skeletal irradiation in patients with osteosarcoma and bone metastases. J Clin Oncol 2001;20:189–196.

75. Bacci G, Ferrari S, Bertoni F, et al: Long-term outcome for patients with nonmetastatic osteosarcoma of the extremity treated at the Istituto Ortopedico Rizzoli according to the Istituto Ortopedico Rizzoli/Osteosarcoma-2 protocol: An updated report. J Clin Oncol 2000;18:4016–4027.

Ewing's Sarcoma

76. Cotterill SJ, Ahrens S, Paulussen M, et al: Prognostic factors in Ewing's tumor of bone: Analysis of 975 patients from the European Intergroup Cooperative Ewing's Sarcoma Study Group. J Clin Oncol 2000;18:3108–3114.

77. Raney RB, Asmar L, Newton WA, et al: Ewing's sarcoma of soft tissues in childhood: A report from the Intergroup Rhabdomyosarcoma Study, 1972–1991. J Clin Oncol 1997;15:574–582.

78. Bacci G, Ferrari S, Bertoni F, et al: Prognostic factors in nonmetastatic Ewing's sarcoma of bone treated with adjuvant chemotherapy: Analysis of 359 patients at the Istituto Ostopedico Rizzoli. J Clin Oncol 2000;18:4–11.

79. Dehner LP. Primitive neuroectodermal tumor and Ewing's sarcoma. Am J Surg Pathol 1993;17:1–13.

80. de Alava E, Gerald WL: Molecular biology of the Ewing's sarcoma/primitive neuroectodermal tumor family. J Clin Oncol 2000;18:204–213.

81. Delattre O, Zucman J, Melot T, GM et al: The Ewing family of tumors: A subgroup of small-round-cell tumors defined by specific chimeric transcripts. N Engl J Med 1994;331:294–299.

82. de Alava E, Panizo A, Antonescu C, et al: Association of EWS-FLI1 type 1 fusion with lower proliferative rate in Ewing's sarcoma. Am J Pathol 2000;156:849–855.

83. May WA, Gishizky ML, Lessnick SL, et al: Ewing sarcoma 11;22 translocation produces a chimeric transcription factor that requires the DNA-binding domain encoded by FLI1 for transformation. Proc Natl Acad Sci USA 1993;90:5752–5756.

84. Jeon IS, Davis JN, Braun BS, et al: D: N.A variant Ewing's sarcoma trasnlocation (7;22) fuses the EWS gene to the ETS gene ETV1. Oncogene 1995;10:1229–1234.

85. May W, Arvand A, Thompson A, et al: EWS/FLI1-induced manic fringe renders NIH 3t3 cells tumorigenic. Nat Genet 1997;17:495–497.

86. Toretsky JA, Kalebic T, Blakesley V, et al: The insulin-like growth factor-I receptor is required for EWS/FLI-1 transformation of fibroblasts. J Biol Chem 1997;272:30822–30827.

87. Benini S, Manara MC, Baldini N, et al: Inhibition of insulin-like growth factor I receptor increases the antitumor activity of doxorubicin and vincristine against Ewing's sarcoma cells. Clin Cancer Res 2001;7:1790–1797.

88. Toretsky JA, Thakar M, Eskenazi AE, et al: Phosphoinositide 3-hydroxide kinase blockade enhances apoptosis in the Ewing's sarcoma family of tumors. Cancer Res 1999;59:5745–5750.

89. Parham DM: Ewing's sarcoma, peripheral neuroepithelioma, and related tumors. In Parham DM (ed): Pediatric Neoplasia: Morphology and Biology. Philadelphia, Lippincott-Raven, 1996, pp 65–85.

90. Ambros IM, Ambros PF, Strehl S, et al: MIC2 is a specific marker for Ewing's sarcoma and peripheral primitive neuroectodermal tumors: Evidence for a common histogenesis of Ewing's sarcoma and peripheral primitive neuroectodermal tumors from MIC2 expression and specific chromosome aberration. Cancer 1991;67:1886–1893.

91. Hill, DA, O'Sullivan MJ, Zhu X, et al: Practical application of molecular genetic testing as an aid to the surgical pathologic diagnosis of sarcomas: A prospective study. Am J Surg Pathol 2002;26:965–977.

92. Widhe B, Widhe T: Initial symptoms and clinical features in osteosarcoma and Ewing sarcoma. J Bone Joint Surg Am 2000;82:667–674.

93. Maygarden SJ, Askin FB, Siegal GP, et al: Ewing sarcoma of bone in infants and toddlers: A clinicopathologic report from the Intergroup Ewing's Study. Cancer 1993;71:2109–2118.

94. Wagner LM, Neel MD, Pappo AS, et al: Fractures in pediatric Ewing sarcoma. J Pediatr Hematol Oncol 2001;23:568–571.

95. Hoffer FA: Primary skeletal neoplasms: Osteosarcoma and Ewing sarcoma. Top Magn Reson Imaging 2001;13:231–239.

96. Miller SL, Hoffer FA, Reddick WE, et al: Tumor volume or dynamic contrast-enhanced MRI for prediction of clinical outcome of Ewing sarcoma family of tumors. Pediatr Radiol 2001;31:518–523.

97. Hawkins DS, Rajendran JG, Conrad EU, et al: Evaluation of chemotherapy response in pediatric bone sarcomas by [F-18]-fluorodeoxy-D-glucose positron emission tomography. Cancer 2001;94:3277–3284.

98. Hayes FA, Thompson EI, Meyer WH, et al: Therapy for localized Ewing's sarcoma of bone. J Clin Oncol 1989;7:208–213.

99. Marina NM, Pappo AS, Parham DM, et al: Chemotherapy dose-intensification for pediatric patients with Ewing's family of tumors and desmoplastic small round cell tumor: A feasibility study at St. Jude Children's Research Hospital. J Clin Oncol 1999;17:180–190.

100. Jürgens H, Exner U, Gadner H, et al: Multidisciplinary treatment of primary Ewing's sarcoma of bone. Cancer 1988;61:23–32.

101. Ahrens S, Hoffman C, Jabar S, et al: Evaluation of prognostic factors in a tumor volume-adapted treatment strategy for localized Ewing sarcoma of bone: The CESS 86 experience. Med Pediatr Oncol 1999;32:186–195.

102. Evans R, Nesbit M, Askin F, et al: Local recurrence, rate and sites of metastases, and time to relapse as a function of treatment regimen, size of primary and surgical history in 62 patients presenting with non-metastatic Ewing's sarcoma of the pelvic bones. Int J Radiat Oncol Biol Phys 1985;11:129–136.

103. Craft AW, Cotterill SJ, Bullimore JA, et al: Long-term results from the first UKCCSG Ewing's tumour study (ET-1). Eur J Cancer 1997;33:1061–1069.

104. Burgert EO, Nesbit ME, Garnsey LA, et al: Multimodal therapy for the management of nonpelvic, localized Ewing's sarcoma of bone: Intergroup Study IESS-II. J Clin Oncol 1990;8:1514–1524.

105. Craft A, Cotterill S, Malcolm A, et al: Ifosfamide-containing chemotherapy in Ewing's sarcoma: The second United Kingdom Children's Cancer Study Group and the Medical Research Council Ewing's Tumor Study. J Clin Oncol 1998;16:3628–3633.

106. Salzer-Kuntschik M, Delling G, Beron G, et al: Morphological grades of regression in osteosarcoma after polychemotherapy: Study COSS 80. J Cancer Res Clin Oncol 1983;106(suppl):21–24.

107. Picci P, Bohling T, Bacci G, et al: Chemotherapy-induced tumor necrosis as a prognostic factor in localized Ewing's sarcoma of the extremities. J Clin Oncol 1997;15:1553–1559.

108. Paulussen M, Ahrens S, Dunst J, et al: Localized Ewing tumor of bone: Final results of the Cooperative Ewing's Sarcoma Study CESS-86. J Clin Oncol 2001;19:1818–1829.

109. Ginsberg JP, de Alava E, Ladanyi M, et al: EWS-FLI1 and EWS-ERG gene fusions are associated with similar clinical phenotypes in Ewing's sarcoma. J Clin Oncol 1999;17:1809–1814.

110. de Alava E, Kawai A, Healey JH, et al: EWS-FLI1 fusion transcript structure is an independent determinant of prognosis in Ewing's sarcoma. J Clin Oncol 1998;16:1248–1255.

111. Zoubek A, Dockhorn-Dworniczak B, Delattre O, et al: Does expression of different EWS chimeric transcripts define clinically distinct risk groups of Ewing tumor patients? J Clin Oncol 1996;14:1245–1251.

112. Terrier P, Henry-Amar M, Triche T J, et al: Is neuroectodermal differentiation of Ewing's sarcoma of bone associated with an unfavourable prognosis? Eur J Cancer 1995;31A:307–314.

113. Sandoval C, Meyer WH, Parham DM, et al: Outcome in 43 children presenting with metastatic Ewing sarcoma: The St. Jude Children's Research Hospital Experience, 1962 to 1992. Med Pediatr Oncol 1996;26:180–185.

114. Paulussen M, Ahrens S, Burdach S, et al: Primary metastatic (stage IV) Ewing tumor: Survival analysis of 171 patients from the EICESS studies. Ann Oncol 1998;9:275–281.

115. Paulussen M, Ahrens S, Craft AW, et al: Ewing's tumors with primary lung metastases: Survival analysis of 114 (European Intergroup) Cooperative Ewing's Sarcoma Studies patients. J Clin Oncol 1998;16:3044–3052.

116. West DC, Grier HE, Swallow MM, et al: Detection of circulating tumor cells in patients with Ewing's sarcoma and peripheral primitive neuroectodermal tumor. J Clin Oncol 1997;15:583–588.

117. Zoubek A, Ladenstein R, Windhager R, et al: Predictive potential of testing for bone marrow involvement in Ewing tumor patients by RT-PCR: A preliminary evaluation. Int J Cancer 1998;79:56–60.

118. Fagnou C, Michon J, Peter M, et al: Presence of tumor cells in bone marrow but not in blood is associated with adverse prognosis in patients with Ewing's tumor. J Clin Oncol 1998;16:1707–1711.

119. Zucker JM, Henry-Amar M, Sarrazin D, et al: Intensive systemic chemotherapy in localized Ewing's sarcoma in childhood: A historical trial. Cancer 1983;52:415–423.

120. Nesbit ME, Gehan EA, Burgert EO, et al: Multimodal therapy for the management of primary, nonmetastatic Ewing's sarcoma of bone: A long-term follow-up of the first intergroup study. J Clin Oncol 1990;8:1664–1674.

121. Lilley ER, Rosenberg MC, Elion GB, et al: Synergistic interactions between cyclophosphamide or melphalan and VP-16 in a human rhabdomyosarcoma xenograft. Cancer Res 1990;50:284–287.

122. Clark PI, Slevin ML, Joel SP, et al: A randomized trial of two etoposide schedules in small-cell lung cancer: The infuence of pharmacokinetics on efficacy and toxicity. J Clin Oncol 1994;12:1427–1435.

123. Kurowski V, Wagner T: Comparative pharmacokinetics of ifosfamide, 4-hydroxyifosfamide, chloroacetylaldehyde, and 2- and 3-dechloroethylifosfamide in patients on fractionated intravenous ifosfamide therapy. Cancer Chemother Pharmacol 1993;33:36–42.

124. Boddy AV, Yule SM, Wyllie R, et al: Pharmacokinetics and metabolism of ifosfamide administered as a continuous infusion in children. Cancer Res 1993;53:3758–3764.

125. Comandone A, Leone L, Oliva C, et al: Pharmacokinetics of ifosfamide administered according to three different schedules in metastatic soft tissue and bone sarcomas. J Chemother 1998;10:385–393.

126. Meyer WH, Kun L, Marina N: Ifosfamide plus etoposide in newly diagnosed Ewing's sarcoma of bone. J Clin Oncol 1992;10:1737–1742.

127. Grier H, Krailo M, Link M, et al: Improved outcome in nonmetastatic Ewing's sarcoma (EWS) and PPNET of bone with the addition of ifosfamide (I) and etoposide (E) to vincristine (V), adriamycin (Ad), cyclophosphamide (C), and actinomycin (A): A Children's Cancer Group (CCG) and Pediatric Oncology Group (POG) report. Proc Annu Meet Am Soc Clin Oncol 1994;13:421.

128. Craft AW, Paulussen M, Douglas C, et al: EICESS 92- Early results of an international Ewings tumour study. Med Pediatr Oncol 2000;35:191.

129. Shamberger RC, LaQuaglia MP, Krailo MD, et al: Ewing sarcoma of the rib: Results of an intergroup study with analysis of outcome by timing of resection. J Thorac Cardiovasc Surg 2000;119:1154–1161.

130. Kushner BH, Meyers PA, Gerald WL, et al: Very high-dose short-term chemotherapy for poor-risk peripheral primitive neuroectodermal tumors, including Ewing's sarcoma, in children and young adults. J Clin Oncol 1995;13:2796–2804.

131. Kushner BH, LaQuaglia MP, Wollner N, et al: Desmoplastic small-round cell tumor: Prolonged progression-free survival with aggressive multi-modality therapy. J Clin Oncol 1996;14:1526–1531.

132. Womer RB, Daller RT, Fenton JG, et al: Granulocyte colony stimulating factor permits dose intensification by interval compression in the treatment of Ewing's sarcomas and soft tissue sarcomas in children. Eur J Cancer 2000;36:87–94.

133. Granowetter L, Womer R, Devidas M, et al: Comparison of dose intensified and standard dose chemotherapy for the treatment of non-metastatic Ewing's sarcoma (ES) and primitive neuroectodermal tumor (PNET) of bone and soft tissue: A Pediatric Oncology Group-Children's Cancer Group phase III trial [abstract]. Med Pediatr Oncol 2001;37:172.

134. Cangir A, Vietti TJ, Gehan EA, et al: Ewing's sarcoma metastatic at diagnosis. Results and comparisons of two Intergroup Ewing's Sarcoma Studies. Cancer 1990;66:887–893.

135. Miser JS, Krailo M, Meyers P, et al: Metastatic Ewing's sarcoma (ES) and primitive neuroectodermal tumor (PNET) of bone: Failure of new regimens to improve outcome. Proc Annu Meet Am Soc Clin Oncol 1996;15:467.

136. Felgenhauer J, Hawkins D, Pendergrass T, et al: Very intensive, short-term chemotherapy for children and adolescents with metastatic sarcomas. Med Pediatr Oncol 2000;34:29–38.

137. Rodriguez-Galindo C, Poquette CA, Marina NM, et al: Hematologic abnormalities and acute myeloid leukemia in children and adolescents administered intensified chemotherapy for the Ewing sarcoma family of tumors. J Pediatr Hematol Oncol 2000;22:321–329.

138. Kushner BH, Heller G, Cheung NK, et al: High risk of leukemia after short-term dose-intensive chemotherapy in young patients with solid tumors. J Clin Oncol 1998;16:3016–3020.

139. Nitschke R, Parkhurst J, Sullivan J, et al: Topotecan in pediatric patients with recurrent and progressive solid tumors: A Pediatric Oncology Group phase II study. J Pediatr Hematol Oncol 1998;20:315–318.

140. Saylors RL, Stine KC, Sullivan J, et al: Cyclophosphamide plus topotecan in children with recurrent or refractory solid tumors: A Pediatric Oncology Group (POG) phase II study. J Clin Oncol 2001;19:3463–3469.

141. Burdach S, van Kaick B, Laws HJ, et al: Allogeneic and autologous stem-cell transplantation in advanced Ewing tumors: An update after long-term follow-up from two centers of the European Intergroup Study EICESS. Ann Oncol 2000;11:1451–1462.

142. Meyers PA, Krailo MD, Ladanyi M, et al: High-dose melphalan, etoposide, total-body irradiation, and autologous stem-cell reconstitution as consolidation therapy for high-risk Ewing's sarcoma does not improve prognosis. J Clin Oncol 2001;19:2812–2820.

143. Kushner BH, Meyers PA: How effective is dose-intensive/myeloablative therapy against Ewing's sarcoma/primitive neuroectodermal tumor metastatic to bone or bone marrow? The Memorial Sloan-Kettering Experience and a literature review. J Clin Oncol 2001;19:870–880.

144. Ladenstein R, Lasset C, Pinkerton R, et al: Impact of megatherapy in children with high-risk Ewing's tumours in complete remission: A report from the EBMT solid tumour registry. Bone Marrow Transplant 1995;15:697–705.

145. Ladenstein R, Hartmann O, Pinkerton R, et al: A multivariate and matched pair analysis on high-risk Ewing tumor (ET) patients treated by megatherapy (MGT) and stem cell reinfusion (SCR) in Europe. Proc Annu Meet Am Soc Clin Oncol 1999;18:555a.

146. Rosito P, Mancini A, Rondelli R, et al: Italian cooperative study for

the treatment of children and young adults with localized Ewing sarcoma of bone: A preliminary report of 6 years of experience. Cancer 1999;86:421–428.

147. Shankar AG, Pinkerton CR, Atra A, et al: Local therapy and other factors influencing site of relapse in patients with localised Ewing's sarcoma. Eur J Cancer 1999;35:1698–1704.

148. Evans RG, Nesbit ME, Gehan EA, et al: Multimodal therapy for the management of localized Ewing's sarcoma of pelvic and sacral bones: A report from the Second Intergroup Study. J Clin Oncol 1991;9:1173–1180.

149. Bacci G, Picci P, Ferrari S, et al: Neoadjuvant chemotherapy for Ewing's sarcoma of bone: No benefit observed after adding ifosfamide and etoposide to vincristine, actinomycin, cyclophosphamide, and doxorubicin in the maintenance phase—results of two sequential studies. Cancer 1998;82:1174–1183.

150. Hoffman C, Ahrens S, Dunst J, et al: Pelvic Ewing sarcoma: A retrospective analysis of 241 cases. Cancer 1999;85:869–877.

151. Barbieri E, Emiliani E, Zini G, et al: Combined therapy of localized Ewing's sarcoma of bone: Analysis of results in 100 patients. Int J Radiat Oncol Biol Phys 1990;19:1165–1170.

152. Ozaki T, Hillman A, Hoffman C, et al: Significance of surgical margin on the prognosis of patients with Ewing's sarcoma. Cancer 1996;78:892–900.

153. Kuttesch JF, Wexler LH, Marcus RB, et al: Second malignancies after Ewing's sarcoma: Radiation dose-dependency of secondary sarcomas. J Clin Oncol 1996;14:2818–2825.

154. Arai Y, Kun LE, Brooks T, et al: Ewing's sarcoma: Local tumor control and patterns of failure following limited-volume radiation therapy. Int J Radiat Oncol Biol Phys 1991;21:1501–1508.

Neuroblastoma

155. Wilson LMK, Draper GJ: Neuroblastoma, its natural history and prognosis: A study of 487 cases. BMJ 1974;3:301.

156. Blatt J, Lee PA, Taylor SR: Neuroblastoma associated with adrenocortical defects. Pediatrics 1988;82:790.

157. Kushner BH, Gilbert F, Helson L: Familial neuroblastoma: Case reports, literature review, and etiologic considerations. Cancer Res 1986;57:1887.

158. Kushner BH, Helson L: Monozygotic siblings discordant for neuroblastoma: Etiologic implications. J Pediatr 1985;107:405.

159. Kinney H, Faix R, Brazy J: The fetal alcohol syndrome and neuroblastoma. Pediatrics 1980;66:130.

160. Seeler RA, Israel JN, Royal JE, et al: Ganglioneuroblastoma and fetal hydantoin-alcohol syndromes. Pediatrics 1979;63:524.

161. Sawada T, Kawakatu H, Horii Y, et al: Incidental neuroblastoma. Lancet 1988;1:364.

162. Kosloske AM, Bhattacharyya N, Duncan MH: "Incidental" neuroblastoma. Lancet 1987;2:565.

163. Nishi M, Miyake H, Takeda T, et al: Effects of mass screening of neuroblastoma in Sapporo City. Cancer 1987;60:433.

164. Nishi M, Miyake H, Takeda T, et al: Cases of neuroblastoma missed by the mass screening programs. Pediatr Res 1989; 26:603.

165. McWilliams NB: Screening infants for neuroblastoma in North America. Pediatrics 1987;79:1048.

166. Woods WG, Gao RN, Shuster JJ, et al: Screening of infants and mortality due to neuroblastoma. N Engl J Med 2002;346:1041–1046.

167. Bessho F, Hashizume K, Nakajo T, et al: Mass screening in Japan increased the detection of infants with neuroblastoma without a decrease in cases in older children. J Pediatr 1991;119:237.

168. Kaneko Y, Kanda N, Maseki N, et al: Current urinary mass screening for catecholamine metabolites at 6 months of age may be detecting only a small portion of high-risk neuroblastomas: A chromosome and N-myc amplification study. J Clin Oncol 1990;8:2005.

169. Hayashi Y, Inaba T, Hanada R, et al: Chromosome findings and prognosis in 15 patients with neuroblastoma found by VMA mass screening. J Pediatr 1988;112:567.

170. Iancu TC, Shiloh H, Kedar A: Neuroblastomas contain iron-rich ferritin. Cancer 1988;61:2497.

171. Klein CE, Roberts B, Holcenberg J, et al: Cystathionine metabolism in neuroblastoma. Cancer 1988;62:291.

172. Tuchman M, Morris CL, Ramnarain ML, et al: Value of random urinary homovanillic acid and vanillylmandelic acid levels in the diagnosis and management of patients with neuroblastoma: Comparison with 24-hour urine collections. Pediatrics 1985;75:324.

173. Isiguro Y, Kato K, Ito T, et al: Nervous system-specific enolase in serum as a marker for neuroblastoma. Pediatrics 1983;72:696.

174. Tuchman M, Ramnaraine MLR, Woods WG, et al: Three years of experience with random urinary homovanillic and vanillylmandelic acid levels in the diagnosis of neuroblastoma. Pediatrics 1987;79:203.

175. Seeger RC, Seigel SE, Sidell N: Neuroblastoma: Clinical perspectives, monoclonal antibodies, and retinoic acid. Ann Intern Med 1982;97:873.

176. Cheung NKV, Lazarus H, Miraldi FD, et al: Ganglioside GD2 specific monoclonal antibody 3F8: A Phase I study in patients with neuroblastoma and malignant melanoma. J Clin Oncol 1987;5:1430.

177. Cheung NKV, von Hoff DD, Strandjord SE, et al: Detection of neuroblastoma cells in bone marrow using GD2 specific monoclonal antibodies. J Clin Oncol 1986;4:363.

178. Ladisch S, Wu ZL: Detection of a tumour-associated ganglioside in plasma of patients with neuroblastoma. Lancet 1985;1:136.

179. Zeltzer PM, Marangos PJ, Parma AM, et al: Raised neuron- specific enolase in serum of children with metastatic neuroblastoma: A report from the Children's Cancer Study Group. Lancet 1983;2:361.

180. Hann HW, Levy HM, Evans AE: Serum ferritin as a guide to therapy in neuroblastoma. Cancer 1980;40:1411.

181. Hann HW, Stahlhut MW, Evans AE: Basic and acidic isoferritins in the sera of patients with neuroblastoma. Cancer 1988;62:1179.

182. Fong CT, Dracopoli N, White PS, et al: Loss of heterozygosity for the short arm of chromosome 1 in human neuroblastoma: Correlation with N-myc amplification. Proc Natl Acad Sci USA 1989;86:3753.

183. Hayashi Y, Kanda N, Inaba T, et al: Cytogenetic findings and prognosis in neuroblastoma with emphasis on marker chromosome 1. Cancer 1989;63:126.

184. Kaneko Y, Kanda N, Maseki N, et al: Different karyotypic patterns in early and advanced stage neuroblastoma. Cancer Res 1987;47:311.

185. Brodeur GM, Green AA, Hayes FA, et al: Cytogenetic features of human neuroblastomas and cell lines. Cancer Res 1981;41:4678.

186. Ritke MK, Shah R, Valentine M, et al: Molecular analysis of chromosome 1 abnormalities in neuroblastoma. Cytogenet Cell Gent 1989;50:84.

187. Hunt JD, Tereba A: Molecular evaluation of abnormalities of the short arm of chromosome I in neuroblastoma. Genes Chromosom Cancer 1990;2:137.

188. Brodeur GM, Fong CT, Morita M, et al: Molecular analysis and clinical significance of N-myc amplification and chromosome 1 abnormalities in human neuroblastomas. Prog Clin Biol Res 1988;271:3.

189. Schneider SS, Hiemstra JL, Zehnbauer BA, et al: Isolation and structural analysis of a 1.2-megabase N-myc amplicon from a human neuroblastoma. Mol Cell Biol 1992;12:5563.

190. Seeger RC, Brodeur GM, Sather H, et al: Association of multiple copies of the N-myc oncogene with rapid progression of neuroblastomas. N Engl J Med 1985;313:111.

191. Brodeur GM, Seeger RC, Schwab M, et al: Amplification of N- myc in untreated human neuroblastomas correlates with advanced disease stage. Science 1984;224:1121.

192. Tsuda T, Obara M, Hirano H, et al: Analysis of N-myc amplification in relation to disease stage and histologic types in human neuroblastomas. Cancer 1987;60:820.

193. Taylor SR, Blatt J, Costantino JP, et al: Flow cytometric DNA analysis of neuroblastoma and ganglioneuroma: A 10-year retrospective study. Cancer 1988;62:749.

194. Taylor SR, Locker J: A comparative analysis of nuclear DNA content and N-myc gene amplification in neuroblastoma. Cancer 1990;65:1360.

195. Look AT, Hayes FA, Nitschke R, et al: Cellular DNA content as a predictor of response to chemotherapy in infants with unresectable neuroblastoma. N Engl J Med 1984;311:231.

196. Gansler T, Chatten J, Varello M, et al: Flow cytometric DNA analysis of neuroblastoma: Correlation with histology and clinical outcome. Cancer 1986;58:2453.

197. Cohn SL, Rademaker AW, Salwen HR, et al: Analysis of DNA ploidy and proliferative activity in relation to histology and N-myc amplification in neuroblastoma. Am J Pathol 1990;136:1043.

198. Look AT, Hayes FA, Shuster JJ, et al: Clinical relevance of tumor cell ploidy and N-myc gene amplification in childhood neuroblastoma: A Pediatric Oncology Group study. J Clin Oncol 1991;9:581.

199. Beckwith JB, Martin RF: Observations on the histopathology of neuroblastomas. J Pediatr Surg 1968;3:106.

200. Hughes M, Marsden HB, Palmer MK: Histologic patterns of neuroblastoma related to prognosis and clinical staging. Cancer 1974;341:1706.

201. Shimada H, Chatten J, Newton WA Jr, et al: Histopathologic prognostic factors in neuroblastic tumors: Definition of subtypes of ganglioneuroblastoma and an age-linked classification of neuroblastomas. J Natl Cancer Inst 1984;73:405.

202. Shimada H, Ambros IM, Dehner LP: The International Neuroblastoma Pathology Classification (the Shimada system). Cancer 1999;86:364–372.

203. Gitlow SE, Dziedzic SW, Strauss L, et al: Biochemical and histologic determinants in the prognosis of neuroblastoma. Cancer 1973;32:898.

204. Haas D, Ablin AR, Miller C, et al: Complete pathologic maturation and regression of stage IVS neuroblastoma without treatment. Cancer 1988;62:818.

205. Daubenton JD, Fisher RM, Karabus CD, et al: The relationship between prognosis and scintigraphic evidence of bone metastases in neuroblastoma. Cancer 1987;59:1586.

206. Heisel MA, Miller JH, Reid BS, et al: Radionuclide bone scan in neuroblastoma. Pediatrics 1983;71:206.

207. Graeve JLA, de Alarcon PA, Sato Y, et al: Miliary pulmonary neuroblastoma: A risk of autologous bone marrow transplantation. Cancer Res 1988;62:2125.

208. Cohn SL, Salwen H, Herst CV, et al: Single copies of N-myc oncogene in neuroblastomas from children presenting with the syndrome of opsoclonus-myoclonus. Cancer 1988;62:723.

209. Quinn JJ, Altman AJ, Frantz CN: Serum lactic dehydrogenase, an indicator of tumor activity in neuroblastoma. J Pediatr 1980;97:89.

210. Al Rashid RA, Cress C: Hypercalcemia associated with neuro-blastoma. Am J Dis Child 1979;133:838.

211. Scott JP, Morgan E: Coagulopathy of disseminated neuroblastoma. J Pediatr 1983;103:219.

212. Maris JM, Evans AE, McLaughlin AC, et al: 31P nuclear magnetic resonance spectroscopic investigation of human neuroblastoma in situ. N Engl J Med 1985;312:1500.

213. Punt J, Pritchard J, Pincott JR, et al: Neuroblastoma: A review of 21 cases presenting with spinal cord compression. Cancer 1980;45:3095.

214. Geatti O, Shapiro B, Sisson JC, et al: Iodine-131 metaiodobenzylguanidine scintigraphy for the location of neuroblastoma: Preliminary experience in ten cases. J Nucl Med 1985;26:736.

215. Moss TJ, Reynolds CP, Sather NH, et al: Prognostic value of immunocytologic detection of bone marrow metastases in neuroblastoma. N Engl J Med 1991;324:219.

216. Etoh T, Takahashi H, Maie M, et al: Tumor imaging by antineuroblastoma monoclonal antibody and its application to treatment. Cancer 1988;62:1282.

217. Goldman A, Vivian G, Gordon I, et al: Immunolocalization of neuroblastoma using radiolabeled monoclonal antibody UJ13A. J Pediatr 1984;105:252.

218. Moss TJ, Sanders DG: Detection of neuroblastoma cells in blood. J Clin Oncol 1990;8:736.

219. Hayes FA, Green AA, Rao BN: Clinical manifestations of ganglioneuroma. Cancer 1989;63:1211.

220. Weinblatt ME, Heisel MA, Siegel SE: Hypertension in children with neurogenic tumors. Pediatrics 1983;71:947.

221. Akhtar M, Ali MA, Sabbah RS, et al: Aspiration cytology of neuroblastoma: Light and electron microscopic correlations. Cancer 1986;57:797.

222. Evans AE, D'Angio GJ, Randolph J: A proposed staging for children with neuroblastoma: Children's Cancer Study Group A: Cancer 1971;27:374.

223. Brodeur GM, Pritchard J, Berthold F, et al: Revisions of the international criteria for neuroblastoma diagnosis, staging, and response to treatment. J Clin Oncol 1993;1:1466.

224. Evans AE, D'Angio GJ, Sather HN, et al: A comparison of four staging systems for localized and regional neuroblastoma: A report from the Childrens Cancer Study Group. J Clin Oncol 1990;8:678.

225. Smith EI, Haase GM, Seeger RC, et al: A surgical perspective on the current staging in neuroblastoma the International Neuroblastoma Staging System proposal. J Pediatr Surg 1989;24:386.

226. Brodeur GM, Seeger RC, Barrett A, et al: International criteria for diagnosis, staging, and response to treatment in patients with neuroblastoma. J Clin Oncol 1988;6:1874.

227. Evans AE: Staging and treatment of neuroblastoma. Cancer 1980;45:1799.

228. Coldman AJ, Fryer CJH, Elwood JM, et al: Neuroblastoma: Influence of age at diagnosis, stage, tumor site and sex on prognosis. Cancer 1980;46:1896.

229. Evans AE, D'Angio GJ, Propert K, et al: Prognostic factors in neuroblastoma. Cancer 1987;59:1853.

230. Pinkel D: Differences between neuroblastoma stages IV-S and IV. N Engl J Med 1981;305:1418.

231. Hann HWL, Evans AE, Cohen IJ, et al: Biologic differences between neuroblastoma stages IV-S and IV: Measurement of serum ferritin and E-Rosette inhibition in 30 children. N Engl J Med 1981;305:425.

232. Oppedal BR, Storm-Mathisen I, Lie SO, et al: Prognostic factors in neuroblastoma: Clinical, histopathologic, and immunohistochemical features and DNA ploidy in relation to prognosis. Cancer 1988;62:772.

233. Chan HSL, Haddad G, Thorner PS, et al: P-glycoprotein expression as a predictor of the outcome of therapy for neuroblastoma. N Engl J Med 1991;325:1608.

234. Brodeur GM: TRK-a expression in neuroblastomas: A new prognostic marker with biological and clinical significance. J Natl Cancer Inst 1993;85:344.

235. Nakagawara A, Arima-Nakagawara M, Scavarda NJ, et al: Association between high levels of expression of the TRK gene and favorable outcome in human neuroblastoma. N Engl J Med 1993;328:847.

236. Joshi VV, Cantor AB, Brodeur GM, et al: Correlation between morphologic and other prognostic markers of neuroblastoma: A study of histologic grade, DNA index, N-myc gene copy number, and lactic dehydrogenase in patients in the Pediatric Oncology Group. Cancer 1993;71:3173.

237. Hayes FA, Green A, Hustu HO, et al: Surgicopathologic staging of neuroblastoma: Prognostic significance of regional lymph node metastases. J Pediatr 1983;102:59.

238. Nitschke R, Smith EI, Shochat S, et al: Localized neuroblastoma treated by surgery: A Pediatric Oncology Group Study. J Clin Oncol 1988;6:1271.

239. Matthay KK, Sather HN, Seeger RC, et al: Excellent outcome of stage II neuroblastoma is independent of residual disease and radiation therapy. J Clin Oncol 1988;7:236.

240. Nitschke R, Smith EI, Altshuler G, et al: Postoperative treatment of nonmetastatic visible residual neuroblastoma: A Pediatric Oncology Group study. J Clin Oncol 1991;9:1181.

241. de Bernardi B, Rogers D, Carli M, et al: Localized neuroblastoma: Surgical and pathologic staging. Cancer 1987;60:1066.

242. Hayes FA, Green AA, O'Connor DM: Chemotherapeutic manage-ment of epidural neuroblastoma. Med Pediatr Oncol 1989;17:6.

243. Simone JV: The treatment of neuroblastoma. J Clin Oncol 1984;2:717.

244. Bowman LC, Hancock ML, Santana VM, et al: Impact of intensified therapy on clinical outcome in infants and children with neuroblastoma: The St. Jude Children's Research Hospital experience, 1962 to 1988. J Clin Oncol 1991;9:1599.

245. Rosen EM, Cassady JR, Frantz CN, et al: Neuroblastoma: The Joint Center for Radiation Therapy/Dana-Farber Cancer Institute/Children's Hospital experience. J Clin Oncol 1984;2:719.

246. Nesbit ME Jr: Advances and management of solid tumors in children. Cancer 1990;65(suppl):696.

247. Philip T, Ghalie R, Pinkerton R, et al: A Phase II study of high-dose cisplatin and VP-16 in neuroblastoma: A report from the Société Française d'Oncologie Pediatrique. J Clin Oncol 1987;5:941.

248. Shafford EA, Rogers DW, Pritchard J: Advanced neuroblastoma: Improved response rate using a multiagent regimen (OPEC) including sequential cisplatin and VM-26. J Clin Oncol 1984;2:742.

249. Green AA, Hayes FA, Hustu HO: Sequential cyclophosphamide and doxorubicin for induction of complete remission in children with disseminated neuroblastoma. Cancer 1981;48:2310.

250. Finklestein JZ, Klemperer MR, Evans A, et al: Multiagent chemotherapy for children with metastatic neuroblastoma: A report from Children's Cancer Study Group. Med Pediatr Oncol 1979;6:179-188.

251. Johnson FL, Goldman S: Role of autotransplantation in neuroblastoma. Hematol Oncol Clin North Am 1993;7:3.

252. Graham Pole J, Casper J, Elfenbein G, et al: High-dose chemoradiotherapy supported by marrow infusions for advanced neuroblastoma: A Pediatric Oncology Group study. J Clin Oncol 1991;9:152.

253. Kushner BH, O'Reilly RJ, Mandell LR, et al: Myeloablative combination chemotherapy without total body irradiation for neuroblastoma. J Clin Oncol 1991;9:274.

254. Philip T, Bernard JL, Zucker BJM, et al: High-dose chemoradio-therapy with bone marrow transplantation as consolidation treatment in neuroblastoma: An unselected group of stage IV patients over 1 year of age. J Clin Oncol 1987;5:266.

255. Matthay KK, Harris R, Reynolds CP, et al: Improved event-free survival for autologous bone marrow transplantation vs. chemotherapy in neuroblastoma: A phase III randomized Children's Cancer Group (CCG) study [abstract]. Proc Am Soc Clin Oncol 1998;17:2018. Abstract 525a.

256. Matthay KK, Villablanca JG, Seeger RC, et al: Treatment of high-risk neuroblastoma with intensive chemotherapy, radiotherapy, autologous bone marrow transplantation, and 13-cis-retinoic acid. Children's Cancer Group. N Engl J Med 1999;341:1165-1173.

257. Bowman L, Grossmann M, Rill D, Brown M, et al: IL-2 adenovector-transduced autologous tumor cells induce antitumor immune responses in patients with neuroblastoma. Blood 1998;92:1941-1949.

Wilms' Tumor

258. Miller RW, Young JLJ, Novakovic B: Childhood cancer. Cancer 1995;75:395-405.

259. Breslow N, Olshan A, Beckwith JB, et al: Epidemiology of Wilms tumor. Med Pediatr Oncol 1993;21:172-181.

260. Hentrich MU, Meister P, Brack NG, et al: Adult Wilms' tumor: Report of two cases and review of the literature. Cancer 1995;75:545-551.

261. Orditura M, De Vita F, Catalano G: Adult Wilms' tumor: A case report. Cancer 1997;80:1961-1965.

262. Abratt RP, du Preez HM, Kaschula R: Adult Wilms' tumor: Cisplatin and etoposide for relapse after adjuvant chemotherapy. Cancer 1990;65:890-892.

263. Breslow NE, Olson J, Moksness J, et al: Familial Wilms' tumor: A descriptive study. Med Pediatr Oncol 1996;27:398-403.

264. Knudson AG, Strong LC: Mutation and cancer: A model for Wilms' tumor of the kidney. J Natl Cancer Inst 1972;48:313-324.

265. Ton CCT, Hirvonen H, Miwa H, et al: Positional cloning and characterization of a paired box- and homeobox-containing gene from aniridia region. Cell 1991;67:1059-1074.

266. Call KM, Glaser T, Ito CY, et al: Isolation and characterization of a zinc finger polypeptide gene at the human chromosome 11 Wilms' tumor locus. Cell 1990;60:509-520.

267. Gessler M, Poustka A, Cavenee W, et al: GAP homozygous deletion in Wilms tumors of a zinc-finger gene identified by chromosome jumping. Nature 1990;343:774-778.

268. Bonetta L, Kuehn SE, Huang A, et al: Wilms tumor locus on 11p13 defined by multiple CpG island-associated transcripts. Science 1990;250:994-997.

269. Gronskov K, Olsen JH, Sand A, et al: Population-based risk estimates of Wilms tumor in sporadic aniridia: A comprehensive mutation screening procedure of PAX6 identifies 80% of mutations in aniridia. Hum Genet 2001;109:11-18.

270. Varanasi R, Bardeesy N, Petruzzi MJ, et al: Fine structure analysis of the WT1 gene in sporadic Wilms tumor. Proc Natl Acad Sci USA 1994;91:3554-3558.

271. Gessler M, Konig A, Arden K, et al: Infrequent mutation of the WT1 gene in 77 Wilms tumors. Hum Mutat 1994;3:212-222.

272. Huff V: Wilms' tumor genetics. Am J Med Genet 1998;79:260-267.

273. Diller L, Ghahremani M, Morgan J, et al: Constitutional WT1 mutations in Wilms' tumor patients. J Clin Oncol 1998;16:3634-3640.

274. DeBaun MR, Tucker MA: Risk of cancer during the first four years of life in children from the Beckwith-Wiedemann Syndrome Registry. J Pediatr 1998;132:398-400.

275. Koufos A, Grundy P, Morgan K, et al: Familial Wiedemann-Beckwith syndrome and a second Wilms tumor locus both map to 11p15.5. Am J Hum Genet 1989;44:711-719.

276. Ping AJ, Reeve AE, Law DJ, et al: Genetic linkage of Beckwith-Wiedemann syndrome to 11p15. Am J Hum Genet 1989;44:720-723.

277. Reeve AE, Eccles MR, Wilkins RJ, et al: Expression of insulin-like growth factor-II transcripts in Wilms' tumour. Nature 1985;317:258-260.

278. Steenman MJC, Rainier S, Dobry CJ, et al: Loss of imprinting of IGF2 is linked to reduced expression and abnormal methylation of H19 in Wilms' tumour. Nat Genet 1994;7:433-439.

279. Scott J, Cowell J, Robertson M E, et al: Insulin-like growth factor-II gene expression in Wilms' tumour and embryonic tissues. Nature 1985;317:260-262.

280. Chung WY, Yuan L, Feng L, et al: Chromosome 11p15.5 regional imprinting: Comparative analysis of KIP2 and H19 in human tissues and Wilms' tumors. Hum Mol Genet 1996;5:1101-1108.

281. Moulton T, Chung W Y, Yuan L, et al: Genomic imprinting and Wilms' tumor. Med Pediatr Oncol 1996;27:476-483.

282. Hatada I, Inazawa J, Abe T, et al: Genomic imprinting of human p57KIP2 and its reduced expression in Wilms' tumors. Hum Mol Genet 1996;5:783-788.

283. Thompson JS, Reese KJ, DeBaun MR, et al: Reduced expression of the cyclin-dependent kinase inhibitor gene p57KIP2 in Wilms' tumor. Cancer Res 1996;56:5723-5727.

284. Maiti S, Alam R, Amos CI, et al: Frequent association of beta-catenin and WT1 mutations in Wilms tumors. Cancer Res 2000;60:6288-6292.

285. Koesters R, Ridder R, Kopp-Schneider A, et al: Mutational activation of the beta-catenin proto-oncogene is a common event in the development of Wilms' tumors. Cancer Res 1999;59:3880-3882.

286. McDonald JM, Douglass EC, Fisher R, et al: Linkage of familial Wilms' tumor predisposition to chromosome 19 and a two-locus model for the etiology of familial tumors. Cancer Res 1998;58:1387-1390.

287. Rahman N, Arbour L, Tonin P, et al: Evidence for a familial Wilms' tumour gene (FWT1) on chromosome 17q12-q21. Nat Genet 1996;13:461-463.

288. Grundy PE, Telzerow PE, Breslow N, et al: Loss of heterozygosity for chromosomes 16q and 1p in Wilms' tumors predicts an adverse outcome. Cancer Res 1994;54:2331-2333.

289. Maw MA, Grundy PE, Millow LJ, et al: A third Wilms' tumor locus on chromosome 16q. Cancer Res 1992;52:3094-3098.

290. Grundy RG, Pritchard J, Scambler P, et al: Loss of heterozygosity on chromosome 16 in sporadic Wilms' tumour. Br J Cancer 1998;78:1181-1187.

291. Wilmore HP, White GFJ, Howell RT, et al: Germline and somatic abnormalities of chromosome 7 in Wilms' tumor. Cancer Genet Cytogenet 1994;77:93-98.

292. Grundy RG, Pritchard J, Scambler P, et al: Loss of heterozygosity for the short arm of chromosome 7 in sporadic Wilms tumour. Oncogene 1998;17:395-400.

293. Bardeesy N, Falkoff D, Petruzzi MJ, et al: Anaplastic Wilms' tumour, a subtype displaying poor prognosis, harbours p53 gene mutations. Nat Genet 1994;7:91-97.

294. Malkin D, Sexsmith E, Yeger H, et al: Mutations of the p53 tumor suppressor gene occur infrequently in Wilms' tumor. Cancer Res 1994;54:2077-2079.

295. Bardeesy N, Beckwith JB, Pelletier J, Clonal expansion and attenuated apoptosis in Wilms' tumors are associated with p53 gene mutations. Cancer Res 1995;55:215-219.

296. Beckwith JB, Palmer NF: Histopathology and prognosis of Wilms tumor. Cancer 1978;41:1937–1948.

297. Pritchard J, Imeson J, Barnes J, et al: Results of the United Kingdom Children's Cancer Study Group first Wilms' tumor study. J Clin Oncol 1995;13:124–133.

298. Tournade MF, Com-Nougue C, de Kraker J, et al: Optimal duration of preoperative therapy in unilateral and nonmetastatic Wilms' tumor in children older than 6 months: Results of the Ninth International Society of Pediatric Oncology Wilms' Tumor Trial and Study. J Clin Oncol 2001;19:488–500.

299. Beckwith JB, Kiviat NB, Bonadio JF: Nephrogenic rests, nephroblastomatosis, and the pathogenesis of Wilms' tumor. Pediatr Pathol 1990;10:1–36.

300. Dome JS, Coppes MJ: Recent advances in Wilms tumor genetics. Curr Opin Pediatr 2002;14:5–11.

301. Green DM: Diagnosis and management of malignant solid tumors in infants and children. Boston, Martinus Nijhoffr Publishing, 1985, pp 129–186.

302. Gylys-Morin V, Hoffer FA, Kozakewich H, et al: Wilms tumor and nephroblastomatosis: Imaging characteristics at gadolinium-enhanced MR imaging. Radiology 1993;188:517–521.

303. Cohen MD: Current controversy: Is computed tomography scan of the chest needed in patients with Wilms' tumor? Am J Pediatr Hematol Oncol 1994;16:191–193.

304. D'Angio GJ, Rosenberg H, Sharples K, et al: Position paper: Imaging methods for primary renal tumors of childhood: Costs versus benefits. Med Pediatr Oncol 1993;21:205–212.

305. Wilimas JA, Kaste SC, Kauffman WM, et al: Use of chest computed tomography in the staging of pediatric Wilms' tumor: Interobserver variability and prognostic significance. J Clin Oncol 1997;15:2631–2635.

306. Green DM, Fernbach DJ, Norkool P, et al: The treatment of Wilms' tumor patients with pulmonary metastases detected only with computed tomography: A report from the National Wilms' Tumor Study. J Clin Oncol 1991;9:1776–1781.

307. Meisel JA, Guthrie KA, Breslow NE, et al: Significance and management of computed tomography detected pulmonary nodules: A report from the National Wilms Tumor Study Group. Int J Radiat Oncol Biol Phys 1999;44:579–585.

308. Grundy PE, Green DM, Coppes MJ, et al: Renal Tumors. In Pizzo PA, Poplack DG (eds): Principles and Practice of Pediatric Oncology, 4th ed. Philadelphia, Lippincott Williams & Wilkins, 2002, pp 865–893.

309. Green DM, Breslow NE, Evans I, et al: Relationship between dose schedule and charges for treatment on National Wilms' Tumor Study-4: A report from the National Wilms' Tumor Study Group. J Natl Cancer Inst Monogr 1995;(19)21–25.

310. Green DM, Breslow NE, Beckwith JB, et al: Comparison between single-dose and divided-dose administration of dactinomycin and doxorubicin for patients with Wilms' tumor: A report from the National Wilms' Tumor Study Group. J Clin Oncol 1998;16:237–245.

311. Green DM, Beckwith JB, Breslow NE, et al: Treatment of children with stages II to IV anaplastic Wilms' tumor: A report from the National Wilms' Tumor Study Group. J Clin Oncol 1994;12:2126–2131.

312. Green DM, D'Angio G J, Beckwith JB, et al: Wilms tumor. CA Cancer J Clin 1996;46:46–63.

313. Horwitz JR, Ritchey ML, Moksness J, et al: Renal salvage procedures in patients with synchronous bilateral Wilms' tumors: A report from the National Wilms' Tumor Study Group. J Pediatr Surg 1996;31:1020–1025.

314. Green DM, Breslow NE, Beckwith JB, et al: Treatment with nephrectomy only for small, stage I/favorable histology Wilms' tumor: A report from the National Wilms' Tumor Study Group. J Clin Oncol 2001;19:3719–3724.

315. Ritchey ML, Green DM, Thomas PR, et al: Renal failure in Wilms' tumor patients: A report from the National Wilms' Tumor Study Group. Med Pediatr Oncol 1996;26:75–80.

316. Grundy P, Breslow N, Green DM, et al: Prognostic factors for children with recurrent Wilms' tumor: Results from the Second and Third National Wilms' Tumor Study. J Clin Oncol 1989;7:638–647.

317. Dome JS, Liu T, Krasin M, et al: Improved survival for patients with recurrent Wilms tumor: The experience at St. Jude Children's Research Hospital. J Pediatr Hematol Oncol 2002;24:192–198.

318. Kung FH, Desai SJ, Dockerman JD, et al: Ifosfamide/carboplatin/etoposide (ICE) for recurrent malignant solid tumors of childhood: A Pediatric Oncology Group phase I/II study. J Pediatr Hematol Oncol 1995;17:265–269.

319. Abu-Ghosh AM, Krailo MD, Goldman SC, et al: Ifosfamide, carboplatin and etoposide in children with poor-risk relapsed Wilms' tumor: A Children's Cancer Group report. Ann Oncol 2002;13:460–469.

320. Pein F, Michon J, Valteau-Couanet D, et al: High-dose melphalan, etoposide, and carboplatin followed by autologous stem-cell rescue in pediatric high-risk recurrent Wilms' tumor: A French Society of Pediatric Oncology study. J Clin Oncol 1998;16:3295–3301.

321. Garaventa A, Hartmann O, Bernard JL, et al: Autologous bone marrow transplantation for pediatric Wilms' tumor: The experience of the European Bone Marrow Transplantation Solid Tumor Registry. Med Pediatr Oncol 1994;22:11–14.

322. Green DM, Grigoriev YA, Nan B, et al: Congestive heart failure after treatment for Wilms' tumor: A report from the National Wilms' Tumor Study Group. J Clin Oncol 2001;19:1926–1934.

323. Green DM, Peabody EM, Nan B, et al: Pregnancy outcome after treatment for Wilms tumor: A report from the National Wilms Tumor Study Group. J Clin Oncol 2002;20:2506–2513.

324. Breslow NE, Takashima JR, Whitton JA, et al: Second malignant neoplasms following treatment for Wilms' tumor: A report from the National Wilms' Tumor Study Group. J Clin Oncol 1995;13:1851–1859.

Renal Cell Carcinoma

325. Ries LAG, Eisner MP, Kosary CL, et al: SEER Cancer Statistics Review, 1973–1999. Bethesda, MD, National Cancer Institute, 2002.

326. Leuschner I, Harms D, Schmidt D: Renal cell carcinoma in children: Histology, immunohistochemistry, and follow-up of 10 cases. Med Pediatr Oncol 1991;19:33–41.

327. Chan HSL, Daneman A, Gribbin M, et al: Renal cell carcinoma in the first two decades of life. Pediatr Radiol 1983;13:324–328.

328. Eckschlager T, Kodet R: Renal cell carcinoma in children: A single institution's experience. Med Pediatr Oncol 1994;23:36–39.

329. Carcao MD, Taylor GP, Greenberg ML, et al: Renal-cell carcinoma in children: A different disorder from its adult counterpart. Med Pediatr Oncol 1998;31:153–158.

330. Renshaw AA, Granter SR, Fletcher JA, et al: Renal cell carcinomas in children and young adults. Am J Surg Pathol 1999;23:795–802.

331. Dehner LP, Leestma JE, Price EB Jr: Renal cell carcinoma in children: A clinicopathologic study of 15 cases and review of the literature. J Pediatr 1970;76:358–368.

332. Tomlinson GE, Niesen PD, Timmons CF, Schneider NR: Cytogenetics of a renal cell carcinoma in a 17-month-old child. Cancer Genet Cytogenet 1991;57:11–17.

333. Ladanyi M, Lui MY, Antonescu CR, et al: The der (17) t(X; 17)(p11; q25) of human alveolar soft part sarcoma fuses the TFE3 transcription factor gene to ASPL, a novel gene at 17q25. Oncogene 2001;20:48–57.

334. Argani P, Antonescu CR, Illei PB, et al: Primary renal neoplasms with the ASPL-TFE3 gene fusion of alveolar soft part sarcoma: A distinctive tumor entity previously included among renal cell carcinomas of children and adolescents. Am J Pathol 2001;159:179–192.

335. Argani P, Hawkins A, Griffin CA, et al: A distinctive pediatric renal neoplasm characterized by epithelioid morphology, basement membrane production, focal HMB45 immunoreactivity, and t(6;11)(p21.1;q12) chromosome translocation. Am J Pathol 2001;158:2089–2096.

336. Davis CJ, Mostofi FK, Sesterhenn IA: Renal medullary carcinoma: The seventh sickle cell nephropathy. Am J Surg Pathol 1995;19:1–11.

337. Uchiyama M, Iwafuchi M, Yagi M, et al: Treatment of childhood renal cell carcinoma with lymph node metastasis: Two cases and a review of literature. J Surg Oncol 2000;75:266–269.

338. Asanuma H, Nakai H, Takeda M, et al: Renal cell carcinoma in children: Experience at a single institution in Japan. J Urol 1999;162:1402-1405.

339. Androulakakis PA, Polychronopoulou-Androulakaki S, Michael V, et al: Renal cell carcinoma in children under 14 years old: Long-term survival. BJU Int 1999;83:654-657.

340. Freedman AL, Vates TS, Stewart T, et al: Renal cell carcinoma in children: The Detroit experience. J Urol 1996;155:1708-1710.

341. Aronson DC, Medary I, Finlay J L, et al: Renal cell carcinoma in childhood and adolescence: A retrospective survey for prognostic factors in 22 cases. J Pediatr Surg 1996;31:183-186.

342. Bauer M, Reaman GH, Hank JA, et al: A phase II trial of human recombinant interleukin-2 administered as a 4-day continuous infusion for children with refractory neuroblastoma, non-Hodgkin's lymphoma, sarcoma, renal cell carcinoma, and malignant melanoma. Cancer 1995;75:2959-2964.

343. MacArthur CA, Isaacs H Jr, Miller JH, et al: Pediatric renal cell carcinoma: A complete response to recombinant interleukin-2 in a child with metastatic disease at diagnosis. Med Pediatr Oncol 1994;23:365-371.

344. Cabala JE, Shield J, Duncan A: Renal cell carcinoma in childhood. Pediatr Radiol 1992;22:203-205.

345. Brecker B: Renal cell carcinoma in children. Urology 1991;38:54-56.

346. Bruce J, Gouge DCS: Long-term follow-up of children with renal carcinoma. Br J Urol 1990;65:446-448.

347. Mancini AF, Polecki G: Renal cell carcinoma in childhood. Med Pediatr Oncol 1989;17:53-57.

348. Booth CM: Renal parenchymal carcinoma in children. Br J Surg 1986;73:313-317.

349. Gotu S, Ikea K, Nakagawa A, et al: Renal cell carcinoma in Japanese children. J Urol 1986;136:1261-1263.

350. Senga Y, Taguchi H, Asao T, et al: Undifferentiated renal cell carcinoma in infancy: Report of a case and review of literature. Pediatr Pathol 1986;5:157-165.

351. Lack EE, Cassady JR, Sallan SE: Renal cell carcinoma in childhood and adolescence: A clinical and pathological study of 17 cases. J Urol 1985;133:822-828.

352. Raney RB Jr, Palmer N, Sutow WW, et al: Renal cell carcinoma in children. Med Pediatr Oncol 1983;11:91-98.

353. Herschorn S, Hardy BE, Churchill BM: Renal cell carcinoma in children. Can J Surg 1979;22:412-418.

354. Futrell JW, Filston HC, Reid JD: Rupture of a renal cell carcinoma in a child. Cancer 1978;41:1565-1570.

355. Castellanos RD, Aron BS, Evans AT: Renal adenocarcinoma in children: Incidence, therapy and prognosis. J Urol 1974;111:534-537.

356. Ficarra V, Righetti R, Pilloni S, et al: Prognostic factors in patients with renal cell carcinoma: Retrospective analysis of 675 cases. Eur Urol 2002;41:190-198.

Rhabdomyosarcoma and Nonrhabdomyosarcoma

357. Gurney JG, Young JL Jr, Roffers SD, et al: Soft tissue sarcomas. In Ries LAG, Smith MA, Gurney JG, et al (eds): Cancer Incidence and Survival among Children and Adolescents: United States. SEER Program 1975-1995. Bethesda, MD, National Cancer Institute, SEER Program. NIH Pub. No 99-4649, 1999, pp 111-123.

358. Maurer HM, Beltangady M, Gehan EA, et al: The Intergroup Rhabdomyosarcoma Study-I: A final report. Cancer 1988;61:209-220.

359. Maurer HM, Gehan EA, Beltangady M, et al: The Intergroup Rhabdomyosarcoma Study-II. Cancer 1993;71:1904-1922.

360. Crist W, Gehan EA, Ragab AH, et al: The Third Intergroup Rhabdomyosarcoma Study. J Clin Oncol 1995;13:610-630.

361. Hays DM, Newton W Jr, Soule EH, et al: Mortality among children with rhabdomyosarcomas of the alveolar histologic subtype. J Pediatr Surg 1983;18:412-417.

362. Kodet R, Newton WA Jr, Hamoudi AB, et al: Orbital rhabdomyosarcomas and related tumors in childhood: Relationship of morphology to prognosis—an Intergroup rhabdomyosarcoma study. Med Pediatr Oncol 1997;29:51-60.

363. Raney RB Jr, Gehan EA, Hays DM, et al: Primary chemotherapy with or without radiation therapy and/or surgery for children with localized sarcoma of the bladder, prostate, vagina, uterus, and cervix. A comparison of the results in Intergroup Rhabdomyosarcoma Studies I and II. Cancer 1990;66:2072-2081.

364. Neville HL, Andrassy RJ, Lobe TE, et al: Preoperative staging, prognostic factors, and outcome for extremity rhabdomyosarcoma: A preliminary report from the Intergroup Rhabdomyosarcoma Study IV (1991-1997). J Pediatr Surg 2000;35:317-321.

365. Sorensen PH, Lynch JC, Qualman SJ, et al: PAX3-FKHR and PAX7-FKHR gene fusions are prognostic indicators in alveolar rhabdomyosarcoma: A report from the children's oncology group. J Clin Oncol 2002;20:2672-2679.

366. Scrable H, Cavenee W, Ghavimi F, et al: A model for embryonal rhabdomyosarcoma tumorigenesis that involves genome imprinting. Proc Natl Acad Sci USA 1989;86:7480-7484.

367. Turleau J, de Grouchy F, Chavin-Colin H, et al: Trisomy 11p15 and Beckwith-Wiedemann syndrome: A report of two cases. Hum Genet 1984;67:219-221.

368. Malkin D, Li FP, Strong LC, et al: Germ line p53 mutations in a familial syndrome of breast cancer, sarcomas, and other neoplasms. Science 1990;250:1233-1238.

369. Yoo HK, Lee CS, Kang WS, et al: p53 gene mutations and p53 protein expression in human soft tissue sarcomas. Arch Pathol Lab Med 1997;121:395-399.

370. Driman D, Thorner PS, Greenberg M, et al: MYCN gene amplification in rhabdomyosarcoma. Cancer 1994;73:2231-2237.

371. Stratton MR, Fisher C, Gusterson BA, et al: Detection of point mutations in N-ras and K-ras genes of human embryonal rhabdomyosarcomas using oligonucleotide probes and the polymerase chain reaction. Cancer Res 1989;49:6324-6327.

372. Horn RC, Enterline HT, et al: Rhabdomyosarcoma: A clinicopathological study and classification of 39 cases. Cancer 1958;11:181-199.

373. Parham DM, Webber B, Holt H, et al: Immunohistochemical study of childhood rhabdomyosarcomas and related neoplasms: Results of an Intergroup Rhabdomyosarcoma Study project. Cancer 1991;67:3072-3080.

374. Cessna MH, Zhou H, Perkins SL, et al: Are myogenin and myoD1 expression specific for rhabdomyosarcoma? A study of 150 cases, with emphasis on spindle cell mimics. Am J Surg Pathol 2001;25:1150-1157.

375. Dias P, Parham DM, Shapiro DN, et al: Myogenic regulatory protein (MyoD1) expression in childhood solid tumors: Diagnostic utility in rhabdomyosarcoma. Am J Pathol 1990;137:1283-1291.

376. Newton WA Jr, Gehan EA, Webber BL, et al: Classification of rhabdomyosarcomas and related sarcomas: Pathologic aspects and proposal for a new classification—an Intergroup rhabdomyosarcoma study. Cancer 1995;76:1073-1085.

377. Raney RB, Meza J, Anderson JR, et al: Treatment of children and adolescents with localized parameningeal sarcoma: Experience of the Intergroup Rhabdomyosarcoma Study Group protocols IRS-II through IV, 1978-1997. Med Pediatr Oncol 2002;38:22-32.

378. Lawrence W Jr, Hays DM, Heyn R, et al: Lymphatic metastases with childhood rhabdomyosarcoma: A report from the Intergroup Rhabdomyosarcoma Study. Cancer 1987;60:910-915.

379. Raney RB Jr, Tefft M, Maurer HM, et al: Disease patterns and survival rate in children with metastatic soft-tissue sarcoma: A report from the Intergroup Rhabdomyosarcoma Study (IRS)-I. Cancer 1988;62:1257-1266.

380. Wiener S, Anderson JR, Ojimba JI, et al: Controversies in the management of paratesticular rhabdomyosarcoma: Is staging retroperitoneal lymph node dissection necessary for adolescents with resected paratesticular rhabdomyosarcoma? Semin Pediatr Surg 2001;10:146-152.

381. Rodary EA, Gehan F, Flamant J, et al: Prognostic factors in 951 nonmetastatic rhabdomyosarcoma in children: A report from the International Rhabdomyosarcoma Workshop. Med Pediatr Oncol 1991;19:89-95.

382. Sutow WW, Berry DH, Haddy TB, et al: Vincristine sulfate therapy in children with metastatic soft tissue sarcoma. Pediatrics 1966;38:465-472.

383. James DH Jr, Hustu O, Wrenn EL Jr, et al: Childhood malignant tumors: Concurrent chemotherapy with dactinomycin and vincristine sulfate. JAMA 1966;197:1043–1045.

384. Grosfeld JL, Clatworthy HW Jr, Newton WA Jr: Combined therapy in childhood rhabdomyosarcoma: An analysis of 42 cases. J Pediatr Surg 1969;4:637–645.

385. Ragab H, Sutow WW, Komp DM, et al: Adriamycin in the treatment of childhood solid tumors. A Southwest Oncology Group study. Cancer 1975;36:1567–1576.

386. Sandler E, Lyden F, Ruymann H, et al: Efficacy of ifosfamide and doxorubicin given as a phase II "window" in children with newly diagnosed metastatic rhabdomyosarcoma: A report from the Intergroup Rhabdomyosarcoma Study Group. Med Pediatr Oncol 2001;37:442–448.

387. Pratt CB, Crom DB: Cisplatin and doxorubicin for locally recurrent and metastatic childhood rhabdomyosarcoma. Chemioterapia 1984;3:207–210.

388. Haddy TB, Nora AH, Sutow WW, et al: Cyclophosphamide treatment for metastatic soft tissue sarcoma: Intermittent large doses in the treatment of children. Am J Dis Child 1967;114:301–308.

389. Finklestein JZ, Hittle RE, Hammond GD, et al: Evaluation of a high dose cyclophosphamide regimen in childhood tumors. Cancer 1969;23:1239–1242.

390. Breitfeld PP, Lyden E, Raney RB, et al: Ifosfamide and etoposide are superior to vincristine and melphalan for pediatric metastatic rhabdomyosarcoma when administered with irradiation and combination chemotherapy: A report from the Intergroup Rhabdomyosarcoma Study Group. J Pediatr Hematol Oncol 2001;23:225–233.

391. Horowitz ME, Etcubanas E, Christensen ML, et al: Phase II testing of melphalan in children with newly diagnosed rhabdomyosarcoma: A model for anticancer drug development. J Clin Oncol 1988;6:308–314.

392. Crist WM, Raney RB, Ragab A, et al: Intensive chemotherapy including cisplatin with or without etoposide for children with soft-tissue sarcomas. Med Pediatr Oncol 1987;15:51–57.

393. Pappo AS, Bowman LC, Furman WL, et al: A phase II trial of high-dose methotrexate in previously untreated children and adolescents with high-risk unresectable or metastatic rhabdomyosarcoma. J Pediatr Hematol Oncol 1997;19:438–442.

394. Pappo AS, Lyden E, Breneman J, et al: Up-front window trial of topotecan in previously untreated children and adolescents with metastatic rhabdomyosarcoma: An intergroup rhabdomyosarcoma study. J Clin Oncol 2001;19:213–219.

395. Pappo AS, Lyden E, Breitfeld PP, et al: Irinotecan (CPT-11) is active against pediatric rhabdomyosarcoma (RMS): A phase II window trial from the Soft Tissue Sarcoma Committee (STS) of the Children's Oncology Group (COG) [abstract]. Proc Am Soc Clin Oncol 2002;21. Abstract 1570.

396. Carli M, Colombatti R, Oberlin O, et al: High-dose melphalan with autologous stem-cell rescue in metastatic rhabdomyosarcoma. J Clin Oncol 1999;17:2796–2803.

397. Weigel J, Breitfeld PP, Hawkins D, et al: Role of high-dose chemotherapy with hematopoietic stem cell rescue in the treatment of metastatic or recurrent rhabdomyosarcoma. J Pediatr Hematol Oncol 2001;23:272–276.

398. Hays DM, Lawrence W, Wharam M Jr, et al: Primary reexcision for patients with "microscopic residual" tumor following initial excision of sarcomas of trunk and extremity sites. J Pediatr Surg 1989;24:5–10.

399. Cecchetto G, Carli M, Sotti G, et al: Importance of local treatment in pediatric soft tissue sarcomas with microscopic residual after primary surgery: Results of the Italian Cooperative Study RMS-88. Med Pediatr Oncol 2000;34:97–101.

400. Donaldson SS, Asmar L, Breneman J, et al: Hyperfractionated radiation in children with rhabdomyosarcoma: Results of an Intergroup Rhabdomyosarcoma Pilot Study. Int J Radiat Oncol Biol Phys 1995;32:903–911.

401. Crist WM, Anderson JR, Meza JL, et al: Intergroup rhabdomyosarcoma study-IV: Results for patients with nonmetastatic disease. J Clin Oncol 2001;19:3091–3102.

402. Pappo AS, Anderson JR, Crist WM, et al: Survival after relapse in

403. Raney RB, Anderson JR, Kollath J, et al: Late effects of therapy in 94 patients with localized rhabdomyosarcoma of the orbit: Report from the Intergroup Rhabdomyosarcoma Study (IRS)-III, 1984–1991. Med Pediatr Oncol 2000;34:413–420.

404. Oberlin O, Rey A, Anderson J, et al: Treatment of orbital rhabdomyosarcoma: Survival and late effects of treatment—results of an international workshop. J Clin Oncol 2001;19:197–204.

405. Kaste SC, Hopkins KP, Bowman LC: Dental abnormalities in long-term survivors of head and neck rhabdomyosarcoma. Med Pediatr Oncol 1995;25:96–101.

406. Raney RB, Asmar L, Vassilopoulou-Sellin R, et al: Late complications of therapy in 213 children with localized, nonorbital soft-tissue sarcoma of the head and neck: A descriptive report from the Intergroup Rhabdomyosarcoma Studies (IRS)-II and -III. IRS Group of the Children's Cancer Group and the Pediatric Oncology Group. Med Pediatr Oncol 1999;33:362–371.

407. Paulino C, Simon JH, Zhen W, et al: Long-term effects in children treated with radiotherapy for head and neck rhabdomyosarcoma. Int J Radiat Oncol Biol Phys 2000;48:1489–1495.

408. Raney RB, Heyn R, Hays DM, et al: Sequelae of treatment in 109 patients followed for 5 to 15 years after diagnosis of sarcoma of the bladder and prostate: A report from the Intergroup Rhabdomyosarcoma Study Committee. Cancer 1993;71:2387–2394.

409. Heyn R, Raney RB, Hays DM, et al: Late effects of therapy in patients with paratesticular rhabdomyosarcoma. Intergroup Rhabdomyosarcoma Study Committee. J Clin Oncol 1992;10:614–623.

410. Goldman S, Johnson FL: Effects of chemotherapy and irradiation on the gonads. Endocrinol Metab Clin North Am 1993;22:617–629.

411. Kenney LB, Laufer MR, Grant FD, et al: High risk of infertility and long term gonadal damage in males treated with high dose cyclophosphamide for sarcoma during childhood. Cancer 2001;91:613–621.

412. Kroll SS, Woo SY, Santin A, et al: Long-term effects of radiotherapy administered in childhood for the treatment of malignant diseases. Ann Surg Oncol 1994;1:473–479.

413. Guyuron B, Dagys AP, Munro IR, et al: Effect of irradiation on facial growth: A 7- to 25-year follow-up. Ann Plast Surg 1983;11:423–427.

414. Heyn R, Haeberlen V, Newton WA, et al: Second malignant neoplasms in children treated for rhabdomyosarcoma. Intergroup Rhabdomyosarcoma Study Committee. J Clin Oncol 1993;11:262–270.

415. Spunt SL, Meza JL, Anderson JR, et al: Second malignant neoplasms (SMN) in children treated for rhabdomyosarcoma: A report from the Intergroup Rhabdomyosarcoma Studies (IRS) I-IV [abstract]. Proc Am Soc Clin Oncol 2001;20:abstract 1473.

416. Pratt B, Pappo AS, Gieser P, et al: Role of adjuvant chemotherapy in the treatment of surgically resected pediatric nonrhabdomyosarcomatous soft tissue sarcomas: A Pediatric Oncology Group study. J Clin Oncol 1999;17:1219.

417. Spunt SL, Poquette CA, Hurt YS, et al: Prognostic factors for children and adolescents with surgically resected nonrhabdomyosarcoma soft tissue sarcoma: An analysis of 121 patients treated at St Jude Children's Research Hospital. J Clin Oncol 1999;17:3697–3705.

418. Marcus KC, Grier HE, Shamberger RC, et al: Childhood soft tissue sarcoma: A 20-year experience. J Pediatr 1997;131:603–607.

419. Lack EE: Leiomyosarcomas in childhood: A clinical and pathologic study of 10 cases. Pediatr Pathol 1986;6:181–197.

420. Angel CA, Gant LL, Parham DM, et al: Leiomyosarcomas in children: Clinical and pathologic characteristics. Pediatr Surg Int 1992;7:116–120.

421. Ferrari M, Casanova F, Spreafico R, et al: Childhood liposarcoma: A single-institutional twenty-year experience. Pediatr Hematol Oncol 1999;16:415–421.

422. La Quaglia MP, Spiro SA, Ghavimi F, et al: Liposarcoma in patients younger than or equal to 22 years of age. Cancer 1993;72:3114–3119.

423. Soule H, Pritchard DJ: Fibrosarcoma in infants and children: A review of 110 cases. Cancer 1977;40:1711-1721.

424. McCarville MB, Kaste SC, Pappo AS: Soft-tissue malignancies in infancy. Am J Roentgenol 1999;173:973-977.

425. Rodriguez-Galindo C, Ramsey K, Jenkins JJ, et al: Hemangiopericytoma in children and infants. Cancer 2000;88:198-204.

426. Carnevale A, Lieberman E, Cardenas R: Li-Fraumeni syndrome in pediatric patients with soft tissue sarcoma or osteosarcoma. Arch Med Res 1997;28:383-386.

427. Korf BR: Malignancy in neurofibromatosis type 1. Oncologist 2000;5:477-485.

428. deCou JM, Rao BN, Parham DM, et al: Malignant peripheral nerve sheath tumors: The St. Jude Children's Research Hospital experience. Ann Surg Oncol 1995;2:524-529.

429. Granovsky MO, Mueller BU, Nicholson HS, et al: Cancer in human immunodeficiency virus-infected children: A case series from the Children's Cancer Group and the National Cancer Institute. J Clin Oncol 1998;16:1729-1735.

430. McClain KL, Leach CT, Jenson HB, et al: Association of Epstein-Barr virus with leiomyosarcomas in children with AIDS. N Engl J Med 1995;332:12-18.

431. Hill MA, Araya JC, Eckert MW, et al: Tumor specific Epstein-Barr virus infection is not associated with leiomyosarcoma in human immunodeficiency virus negative individuals. Cancer 1997;80:204-210.

432. Metayer CF, Lynch EA, Clarke B, et al: Second cancers among long-term survivors of Hodgkin's disease diagnosed in childhood and adolescence. J Clin Oncol 2000;18:2435-2443.

433. Eng C, Li FP, Abramson DH, et al: Mortality from second tumors among long-term survivors of retinoblastoma. J Natl Cancer Inst 1993;85:1121-1128.

434. Zucman O, Delattre C, Desmaze A, et al: EWS and ATF-1 gene fusion induced by t(12;22) translocation in malignant melanoma of soft parts. Nat Genet 1993;4:341-345.

435. Simon MP, Pedeutour F, Sirvent N, et al: Deregulation of the platelet-derived growth factor B-chain gene via fusion with collagen gene COL1A1 in dermatofibrosarcoma protuberans and giant-cell fibroblastoma. Nat Genet 1997;15:95-98.

436. Ladanyi M, Gerald W: Fusion of the EWS and WT1 genes in the desmoplastic small round cell tumor. Cancer Res 1994;54:2837-2840.

437. Panagopoulos I, Mertens F, Isaksson H, et al: Molecular genetic characterization of the EWS/CHN and RBP56/CHN fusion genes in extraskeletal myxoid chondrosarcoma. Genes Chromosomes Cancer 2002;35:340-352.

438. Knezevich SR, McFadden DE, Tao W, et al: A novel ETV6-NTRK3 gene fusion in congenital fibrosarcoma. Nat Genet 1998;18:184-187.

439. Panagopoulos C, Lassen M, Isaksson F, et al: Characteristic sequence motifs at the breakpoints of the hybrid genes FUS/CHOP, EWS/CHOP and FUS/ERG in myxoid liposarcoma and acute myeloid leukemia. Oncogene 1997;15:1357-1362.

440. Dal Cin P, Sciot R, Panagopoulos I, et al: Additional evidence of a variant translocation t(12;22) with EWS/CHOP fusion in myxoid liposarcoma: Clinicopathological features. J Pathol 1997;182:437-441.

441. Crew J, Clark J, Fisher C, et al: Fusion of SYT to two genes, SSX1 and SSX2, encoding proteins with homology to the Kruppel-associated box in human synovial sarcoma. EMBO J 1995;14:2333-2340.

442. Ladanyi M, Antonescu CR, Leung DH, et al: Impact of SYT-SSX fusion type on the clinical behavior of synovial sarcoma: A multi-institutional retrospective study of 243 patients. Cancer Res 2002;62:135-140.

443. Parham DM, Webber BL, Jenkins JJ, et al: Nonrhabdomyosarcomatous soft tissue sarcomas of childhood: Formulation of a simplified system for grading. Mod Pathol 1995;8:705-710.

444. Costa J, Wesley RA, Glatstein E, et al: The grading of soft tissue sarcomas: Results of a clinicohistopathologic correlation in a series of 163 cases. Cancer 1984;53:530-541.

445. Enzinger FM, Weiss SW: Soft Tissue Tumors. St. Louis, Mosby, 1988.

446. Pappo S, Rao BN, Jenkins JJ, et al: Metastatic nonrhabdomyosarcomatous soft-tissue sarcomas in children and adolescents: The St. Jude Children's Research Hospital

447. Spunt SL, Hill DA, Motosue AM, et al: Clinical features and outcome of initially unresected nonmetastatic pediatric nonrhabdomyosarcoma soft tissue sarcoma. J Clin Oncol 2002;20:3225-3235.

448. Fong Y, Coit DG, Woodruff JM, et al: Lymph node metastasis from soft tissue sarcoma in adults: Analysis of data from a prospective database of 1772 sarcoma patients. Ann Surg 1993;217:72-77.

449. Porter GA, Cantor SB, Ahmad SA, et al: Cost-effectiveness of staging computed tomography of the chest in patients with T2 soft tissue sarcomas. Cancer 2002;94:197-204.

450. Espat NJ, Bilsky M, Lewis JJ, et al: Soft tissue sarcoma brain metastases: Prevalence in a cohort of 3829 patients. Cancer 2002;94:2706-2711.

451. Heslin MJ, Lewis JJ, Woodruff JM, et al: Core needle biopsy for diagnosis of extremity soft tissue sarcoma. Ann Surg Oncol 1997;4:425-431.

452. Miralles TG, Gosalbez F, Menendez P, et al: Fine needle aspiration cytology of soft-tissue lesions. Acta Cytol 1986;30:671-678.

453. Trovik S, Bauer HC, Brosjo O, et al: Fine needle aspiration (FNA) cytology in the diagnosis of recurrent soft tissue sarcoma. Cytopathology 1998;9:320-328.

454. Pratt B, Maurer HM, Gieser P, et al: Treatment of unresectable or metastatic pediatric soft tissue sarcomas with surgery, irradiation, and chemotherapy: A Pediatric Oncology Group study. Med Pediatr Oncol 1998;30:201-209.

455. Pappo S, Devidas M, Jenkins J, et al: Vincristine (V), ifosfamide (I), doxorubicin (D), and G-CSF (G) for pediatric unresected and metastatic non-rhabdomyosarcomatous soft tissue sarcomas (NRSTS): A Pediatric Oncology Group (POG) study [abstract]. Proc Am Soc Clin Oncol 2001;20. Abstract 1508.

456. Baldini EH, Goldberg J, Jenner C, et al: Long-term outcomes after function-sparing surgery without radiotherapy for soft tissue sarcoma of the extremities and trunk. J Clin Oncol 1999;17:3252-3259.

457. Rydholm A, Gustafson P, Rooser B, et al: Limb-sparing surgery without radiotherapy based on anatomic location of soft tissue sarcoma. J Clin Oncol 1991;9:1757-1765.

458. Yang C, Chang AE, Baker AR, et al: Randomized prospective study of the benefit of adjuvant radiation therapy in the treatment of soft tissue sarcomas of the extremity. J Clin Oncol 1998;16:197-203.

459. Pisters PW, Harrison LB, Leung DH, et al: Long-term results of a prospective randomized trial of adjuvant brachytherapy in soft tissue sarcoma. J Clin Oncol 1996;14:859-868.

460. Brennan MF: The enigma of local recurrence. The Society of Surgical Oncology. Ann Surg Oncol 1997;4:1-12.

461. Adjuvant chemotherapy for localised resectable soft-tissue sarcoma of adults: Meta-analysis of individual data. Sarcoma Meta-analysis Collaboration. Lancet 1997;350:1647-1654.

462. Frustaci S, Gherlinzoni F, De Paoli A, et al: Adjuvant chemotherapy for adult soft tissue sarcomas of the extremities and girdles: Results of the Italian randomized cooperative trial. J Clin Oncol 2001;19:1238-1247.

463. Bramwell VH: Adjuvant chemotherapy for adult soft tissue sarcoma: Is there a standard of care? J Clin Oncol 2001;19:1235-1237.

464. Walter W, Shearer PD, Pappo AS, et al: A pilot study of vincristine, ifosfamide, and doxorubicin in the treatment of pediatric non-rhabdomyosarcoma soft tissue sarcomas. Med Pediatr Oncol 1998;30:210-216.

465. Demetri GD, Elias AD: Results of single-agent and combination chemotherapy for advanced soft tissue sarcomas. Implications for decision making in the clinic. Hematol Oncol Clin North Am 1995;9:765-785.

466. Patel SR, Vadhan-Raj S, Burgess MA, et al: Results of two consecutive trials of dose-intensive chemotherapy with doxorubicin and ifosfamide in patients with sarcomas. Am J Clin Oncol 1998;21:317-321.

467. Singal PK, Iliskovic N: Doxorubicin-induced cardiomyopathy. N Engl J Med 1998;339:900-905.

468. Pratt CB, Meyer WH, Jenkins JJ, et al: Ifosfamide, Fanconi's syndrome, and rickets. J Clin Oncol 1991;9:1495-1499.

469. Kraybill WG, Spiro I, Harris J, et al: Radiation Therapy Oncology Group (RTOG) 95-14: A phase II study of neoadjuvant chemotherapy (CT) and radiation therapy (RT) in high risk (HR), high grade, soft tissue sarcomas (STS) of the extremities and body wall—a preliminary report [abstract]. Proc Am Soc Clin Oncol 2001;20. Abstract 348a.

470. Sklar CA, Constine LS: Chronic neuroendocrinological sequelae of radiation therapy. Int J Radiat Oncol Biol Phys 1995;31: 1113-1121.

471. Meadows AT, Baum E, Fossati-Bellani F, et al: Second malignant neoplasms in children: An update from the Late Effects Study Group. J Clin Oncol 1985;3:532-538.

Retinoblastoma

472. Knudson AG: Mutation and cancer: Statistical study of retinoblastoma. Proc Natl Acad Sci USA 1971;68:820-823.

473. Lee WH, Bookstein R, Hong F, et al: Human retinoblastoma susceptibility gene: Cloning, identification, and sequence. Science 1987;235:1394-1399.

474. Friend SH, Bernards R, Rogelj S, et al: A human DNA segment with properties of the gene that predisposes to retinoblastoma and osteosarcoma. Nature 1986;323:643-646.

475. Brantley MA, Harbour JW: The molecular biology of retinoblastoma. Ocul Immunol Inflamm 2001;9:1-8.

476. Dryja TP, Mukai S, Petersen R, et al: Parental origin of mutations of the retinoblastoma gene. Nature 1989;339:556-558.

477. Zhu X, Dunn JM, Goddard AD, et al: Mechanisms of loss of heterozygosity in retinoblastoma. Cytogenet Cell Genet 1992;59:248-252.

478. Weinberg RA: The tumor suppressor genes. Science 1991;254:1138-1146.

479. Draper GJ, Sanders BM, Brownhill PA, et al: Patterns of risk of hereditary retinoblastoma and applications to genetic counselling. Br J Cancer 1992;66:211-219.

480. Harbour JW: Molecular basis of low-penetrance retinoblastoma. Arch Ophthalmol 2001;119:1699-1704.

481. Sippel KC, Fraioli RE, Smith GD, et al: Frequency of somatic and germ-line mosaicism in retinoblastoma: Implications for genetic counseling. Am J Hum Genet 1998;62:610-619.

482. Yandell DW, Campbell TA, Dayton SH, et al: Oncogenic point mutations in the human retinoblastoma gene: Their application to genetic counseling. N Engl J Med 1989;321:1689-1695.

483. Perentes E, Herbort CP, Rubinstein LJ, et al: Immunohistochemical characterization of human retinoblastomas in situ with multiple markers. Am J Ophthalmol 1987;103:647-658.

484. Sang DN, Albert DM: Retinoblastoma: Clinical and histopathologic features. Hum Pathol 1982;13:133-147.

485. Wang MX, Jenkins JJ, Cu-Unjieng AB, et al: Eye tumors. In Parham DM (ed): Pediatric Neoplasia: Morphology and Biology. Philadelphia, Lippincott-Raven, 1996, pp 405-422.

486. Abramson DH, Frank CM, Susman M, et al: Presenting signs of retinoblastoma. J Pediatr 1998;132:505-508.

487. Zelter M, Damel A, Gonzalez G, et al: A prospective study on the treatment of retinoblastoma in 72 patients. Cancer 1991;68:1685-1690.

488. Kivelä T: Trilateral retinoblastoma: A meta-analysis of hereditary retinoblastoma associated with primary ectopic intracranial retinoblastoma. J Clin Oncol 1999;17:1829-1837.

489. Shields CL, Meadows AT, Shields JA, et al: Chemoreduction for retinoblastoma may prevent intracranial neuroblastic malignancy (trilateral retinoblastoma). Arch Ophthalmol 2001;119:1269-1272.

490. Beets-Tan RG, Hendriks MJ, Ramos LM, et al: Retinoblastoma: CT and MRI. Neuroradiology 1994;36:59-62.

491. Karcioglu ZA, al-Mesfer SA, Abboud E, et al: Workup for metastatic retinoblastoma: A review of 261 patients. Ophthalmology 1997;104:307-312.

492. Reese AB, Ellsworth RM: The evaluation and current concept of retinoblastoma therapy. Trans Am Acad Ophthalmol Otolaryngol 1963;67:164-172.

493. Pratt CB, Fontanesi J, Lu X, et al: Proposal for a new staging scheme for intraocular and extraocular retinoblastoma based on an analysis of 103 globes. Oncologist 1997;2:1-5.

494. Shields JA, Shields CL, DePotter P: Enucleation technique for children with retinoblastoma. J Pediatr Ophthalmol Strabismus 1992;29:213-215.

495. Shields JA, Shields CL, DePotter P: Photocoagulation of retinoblastoma. Int Ophthalmol Clin 1993;33:95-99.

496. Shields JA, Parsons H, Shields CL, et al: The role of cryotherapy in the management of retinoblastoma. Am J Ophthalmol 1989;106:260-264.

497. Murphree AL, Villablanca JG, Deegan WF, et al: Chemotherapy plus local treatment in the management of intraocular retinoblastom. Arch Ophthalmol 1996;114:1348-1356.

498. Lumbroso L, Doz F, Urbieta M, et al: Chemothermotherapy in the management of retinoblastoma. Ophthalmology 2002;109: 1130-1136.

499. Wilson TW, Chan HSL, Moselhy GM, et al: Penetration of chemotherapy into vitreous is increased by cryotherapy and cyclosporine in rabbits. Arch Ophthalmol 1996;114:1390-1395.

500. Murray TG, Cicciarelli N, O'Brien JM, et al: Subconjunctival carboplatin therapy and cryotherapy in the treatment of transgenic murine retinoblastoma. Arch Ophthalmol 1997;115:1286-1290.

501. Scott IU, Murray TG, Feuer WJ, et al: External beam radiotherapy in retinoblastoma: Tumor control and comparison of 2 techniques. Arch Ophthalmol 1999;117:766-770.

502. Hungerford JL, Toma NMG, Plowman PN, et al: External beam radiotherapy for retinoblastoma. I. Whole eye technique. Br J Ophthalmol 1995;79:109-111.

503. Toma NMG, Hungerford JL, Plowman PN, et al: External beam radiotherapy for retinoblastoma. II. Lens sparing technique. Br J Ophthalmol 1995;79:112-117.

504. Merchant TE, Gould CJ, Hilton NE, et al: Ocular preservation after 36 Gy external beam radiation therapy for retinoblastoma. J Pediatr Hematol Oncol 2002;24:246-249.

505. Shields CL, Shields JA, Cater J, et al: Plaque radiotherapy for retinoblastoma: Long-term control and treatment complications in 208 tumors. Ophthalmology 2001;108:2116-2121.

506. Schouten-van Meeteren AYN, Moll AC, Imhof SM, et al: Chemotherapy for retinoblastoma: An expanding area of clinical research. Med Pediatr Oncol 2001;38:428-438.

507. Uusitalo MS, Van Quill KR, Scott IU, et al: Evaluation of chemoprophylaxis in patients with unilateral retinoblastoma with high-risk features on histopathologic examination. Arch Ophthalmol 2001;119:41-48.

508. Khelfaoui F, Validire P, Auperin A, et al: Histopathologic risk factors in retinoblastoma: A retrospective study of 172 patients treated in a single institution. Cancer 1996;77:1206-1213.

509. Namouni F, Doz F, Tanguy ML, et al: High-dose chemotherapy with carboplatin, etoposide and cyclophosphamide followed by a haematopoietic stem cell rescue in patients with high-risk retinoblastoma: A SFOP and SFGM study. Eur J Cancer 1997;33:2368-2375.

510. Dunkel IJ, Aledo A, Kernan NA, et al: Successful treatment of metastatic retinoblastoma. Cancer 2000;89:2117-2121.

511. Ross G, Lipper EG, Abramson D, et al: The development of young children with retinoblastoma. Arch Pediatr Adolesc Med 2001;155:80-83.

512. Yue NC, Benson ML: The hourglass deformity as a consequence of orbital irradiation for bilateral retinoblastoma. Pediatr Radiol 1996;26:421-423.

513. Kaste SC, Chen G, Fontanesi J, et al: Orbital development in long-term survivors of retinoblastoma. J Clin Oncol 1997;15:1183-1189.

514. Abramson DH, Frank CM: Second nonocular tumors in survivors of bilateral retinoblastoma: A possible age effect on radiation-related risk. Ophthalmology 1998;105:573-580.

515. Shields CL, Honavar SG, Meadows AT, et al: Chemoreduction plus focal therapy for retinoblastoma: Factors predictive of need for treatment with external beam radiotherapy or enucleation. Am J Ophthalmol 2002;133:657-664.

516. Nenadov-Beck M, Balmer A, Dessing C, et al: First-line chemotherapy with local treatment can prevent external-beam irradiation and enucleation in low-stage intraocular retinoblastoma. J Clin Oncol 2000;18:2881-2887.

517. Kingston JE, Hungerford JL, Madreperla SA, et al: Results of

combined chemotherapy and radiotherapy for advanced intraocular retinoblastoma. Arch Ophthalmol 1996;114:1339-1343.

518. Gallie BL, Budning A, DeBoer G, et al: Chemotherapy with focal therapy can cure intraocular retinoblastoma without radiotherapy. Arch Ophthalmol 1996;114:1321-1328.

519. Wilson MW, Rodriguez-Galindo C, Haik BG, et al: Multiagent chemotherapy as neoadjuvant treatment for multifocal intraocular retinoblastoma. Ophthalmology 108:2106-2115.

520. Friedman DL, Himelstein B, Shields CL, et al: Chemoreduction and local ophthalmic therapy for intraocular retinoblastoma. J Clin Oncol 2000;18:12-17.

521. Mendelsohn ME, Abramson DH, Madden T, et al: Intraocular concentrations of chemotherapeutic agents after systemic or local administration. Arch Ophthalmol 1998;116:1209-1212.

522. Hayden BH, Murray TG, Scott IU, et al: Subconjunctival carboplatin in retinoblastoma: Impact of tumor burden and dose schedule. Arch Ophthalmol 2000;118:1549-1554.

523. Abramson D, Frank CM, Dunkel IJ. A phase I/II study of subconjunctival carboplatin for intraocular retinoblastoma. Ophthalmology 1999;106:1947-1950.

Hepatoblastoma

524. Lack EE, Neave C, Vawter G F: Hepatoblastoma: A clinical and pathologic study of 54 cases. Am J Surg Pathol 1982;6:693-705.

525. Ikeda H, Matsuyama S, Tanimura M: Association between hepatoblastoma and very low birth weight: A trend or a chance? J Pediatr 1997;130:557-560.

526. Feusner J, Plaschkes J: Hepatoblastoma and low birth weight: A trend or chance observation? Med Pediatr Oncol 2002;39:508-509.

527. Kingston JE, Herbert A, Draper GJ, et al: Association between hepatoblastoma and polyposis coli. Arch Dis Child 1983;58:959-962.

528. Li FP, Thurber WA, Seddon J, et al: Hepatoblastoma in families with polyposis coli. JAMA 1987;257:2475-2477.

529. Giardiello FM, Offerhaus GJ, Krush AJ, et al: Risk of hepatoblastoma in familial adenomatous polyposis. J Pediatr 1991;119:766-768.

530. Hughes LJ, Michels VV: Risk of hepatoblastoma in familial adenomatous polyposis. Am J Med Genet 1992;43:1023-1025.

531. Phillips M, Dicks-Mireaux C, Kingston J, et al: Hepatoblastoma and polyposis coli (familial adenomatous polyposis). Med Pediatr Oncol 1989;17:441-447.

532. Goss KH, Groden J: Biology of the adenomatous polyposis coli tumor suppressor. J Clin Oncol 2000;18:1967-1979.

533. Kurahashi H, Takami K, Oue T, et al: Biallelic inactivation of the APC gene in hepatoblastoma. Cancer Res 1995;55:5007-5011.

534. Oda H, Imai Y, Nakatsuru Y, et al: Somatic mutations of the APC gene in sporadic hepatoblastomas. Cancer Res 1996;56:3320-3323.

535. Koch A, Denkhaus D, Albrecht S, et al: Childhood hepatoblastomas frequently carry a mutated degradation targeting box of the beta-catenin gene. Cancer Res 1999;59:269-273.

536. Takayasu H, Horie H, Hiyama E, et al: Frequent deletions and mutations of the beta-catenin gene are associated with overexpression of cyclin D1 and fibronectin and poorly differentiated histology in childhood hepatoblastoma. Clin Cancer Res 2001;7:901-908.

537. Albrecht S, von Schweinitz D, Waha A, et al: Loss of maternal alleles on chromosome arm 11p in hepatoblastoma. Cancer Res 1994;54:5041-5044.

538. Montagna M, Menin C, Chieco-Bianchi L, et al: Occasional loss of constitutive heterozygosity at 11p15.5 and imprinting relaxation of the IGFII maternal allele in hepatoblastoma. J Cancer Res Clin Oncol 1994;120:732-736.

539. Rainier S, Dobry CJ, Feinberg AP: Loss of imprinting in hepatoblastoma. Cancer Res 1995;55:1836-1838.

540. Fletcher JA, Kozakewich HP, Pavelka K, et al: Consistent cytogenetic aberrations in hepatoblastoma: A common pathway of genetic alterations in embryonal liver and skeletal muscle malignancies? Genes Chromosomes Cancer 1991;3:37-43.

541. Mascarello JT, Jones MC, Kadota RP, et al: Hepatoblastoma characterized by trisomy 20 and double minutes. Cancer Genet Cytogenet 1990;47:243-247.

542. Swarts S, Wisecarver J, Bridge JA: Significance of extra copies of chromosome 20 and the long arm of chromosome 2 in hepatoblastoma. Cancer Genet Cytogenet 1996;91:65-67.

543. Tonk VS, Wilson KS, Timmons CF, et al: Trisomy 2, trisomy 20, and del(17p) as sole chromosomal abnormalities in three cases of hepatoblastoma. Genes Chromosomes Cancer 1994;11:199-202.

544. Surace C, Leszl A, Perilongo G, et al: Fluorescent in situ hybridization (FISH) reveals frequent and recurrent numerical and structural abnormalities in hepatoblastoma with no informative karyotype. Med Pediatr Oncol 2002;39:536-539.

545. Schneider NR, Cooley LD, Finegold MJ, et al: The first recurring chromosome translocation in hepatoblastoma: der(4)t(1;4)(q12;q34). Genes Chromosomes Cancer 1997;19:291-294.

546. Ma SK, Cheung AN, Choy C, et al: Cytogenetic characterization of childhood hepatoblastoma. Cancer Genet Cytogenet 2000;119:32-36.

547. Hu J, Wills M, Baker BA, et al: Comparative genomic hybridization analysis of hepatoblastomas. Genes Chromosomes Cancer 2000;27:196-201.

548. Weinberg AG, Finegold MJ: Primary hepatic tumors of childhood. Hum Pathol 1983;14:512-537.

549. Watanabe I: Histopathologic features of liver cell carcinoma in infancy and childhood and their relations to surgical prognosis. J Cancer Clin 1977;23:691.

550. Haas JE, Muczynski KA, Krailo M, et al: Histopathology and prognosis in childhood hepatoblastoma and hepatocarcinoma. Cancer 1989;64:1082-1095.

551. Ortega JA, Douglass EC, Feusner JH, et al: Randomized comparison of cisplatin/vincristine/fluorouracil and cisplatin/continuous infusion doxorubicin for treatment of pediatric hepatoblastoma: A report from the Children's Cancer Group and the Pediatric Oncology Group. J Clin Oncol 2000;18:2665-2675.

552. Perilongo G, Dall'Igna P, Sainat L: Modern treatment of childhood hepatoblastoma: What do clinicians and pathologists have to say to each other? Med Pediatr Oncol 2002;39:474-477.

553. Haas JE, Feusner JH, Finegold MJ: Small cell undifferentiated histology in hepatoblastoma may be unfavorable. Cancer 2001;92:3130-3134.

554. King SJ, Babyn PS, Greenberg ML, et al: Value of CT in determining the resectability of hepatoblastoma before and after chemotherapy. AJR Am J Roentgenol 1993;160:793-798.

555. Archer D, Babyn P, Gilday D, et al: Potentially misleading bone scan findings in patients with hepatoblastoma. Clin Nucl Med 1993;18:1026-1031.

556. Pritchard J, Brown J, Shafford E, et al: Cisplatin, doxorubicin, and delayed surgery for childhood hepatoblastoma: A successful approach—results of the first prospective study of the International Society of Pediatric Oncology. J Clin Oncol 2000;18:3819-3828.

557. Ortega JA, Krailo MD, Haas JE, et al: Effective treatment of unresectable or metastatic hepatoblastoma with cisplatin and continuous infusion doxorubicin chemotherapy: A report from the Children's Cancer Study Group. J Clin Oncol 1991;9:2167-2176.

558. Filler RM, Ehrlich PF, Greenberg ML, et al: Preoperative chemotherapy in hepatoblastoma. Surgery 1991;110:591-596.

559. Douglass EC, Reynolds M, Finegold M, et al: Cisplatin, vincristine, and fluorouracil therapy for hepatoblastoma: A Pediatric Oncology Group study. J Clin Oncol 1993;11:96-99.

560. Ehrlich PF, Greenberg ML, Filler RM: Improved long-term survival with preoperative chemotherapy for hepatoblastoma. J Pediatr Surg 1997;32:999-1002.

561. Finegold MJ: Chemotherapy for suspected hepatoblastoma without efforts at surgical resection is a bad practice. Med Pediatr Oncol 2002;39:484-486.

562. Perilongo G, Shafford E, Plaschkes J: SIOPEL trials using preoperative chemotherapy in hepatoblastoma. Lancet Oncol 2000;1:94-100.

563. Malogolowkin MH, Stanley P, Steele DA, et al: Feasibility and toxicity of chemoembolization for children with liver tumors. J Clin Oncol 2000;18:1279-1284.

564. Arcement CM, Towbin RB, Meza MP, et al: Intrahepatic chemoembolization in unresectable pediatric liver malignancies. Pediatr Radiol 2000;30:779-785.

565. Koneru B, Flye MW, Busuttil RW, et al: Liver transplantation for hepatoblastoma. Ann Surg 1991;213:118-121.

566. Tagge EP, Tagge DU, Reyes J, et al: Resection, including transplantation, for hepatoblastoma and hepatocellular carcinoma: Impact on survival. J Pediatr Surg 1992;27:292-297.

567. Lockwood L, Heney D, Giles GR, et al: Cisplatin-resistant metastatic hepatoblastoma: Complete response to carboplatin, etoposide, and liver transplantation. Med Pediatr Oncol 1993;21:517-520.

568. Achilleos OA, Buist LJ, Kelly DA, et al: Unresectable hepatic tumors in childhood and the role of liver transplantation. J Pediatr Surg 1996; 31:1563-1567.

569. Pimpalwar AP, Sharif K, Ramani P, et al: Strategy for hepatoblastoma management: Transplant versus nontransplant surgery. J Pediatr Surg 2002;37:240-245.

570. Evans AE, Land VJ, Newton WA, et al: Combination chemotherapy (vincristine, adriamycin, cyclophosphamide, and 5-fluorouracil) in the treatment of children with malignant hepatoma. Cancer 1982;50:821-826.

571. Perilongo G, Brown J, Shafford E, et al: Hepatoblastoma presenting with lung metastases: Treatment results of the first cooperative, prospective study of the International Society of Paediatric Oncology on childhood liver tumors. Cancer 2000;89:1845-1853.

572. Katzenstein HM, London WB, Douglass EC, et al: Treatment of unresectable and metastatic hepatoblastoma: A pediatric oncology group phase II study. J Clin Oncol 2002;20:3438-3444.

573. Dall'Igna P, Cecchetto G, Dominici C, et al: Carboplatin and doxorubicin (CARDOX) for nonmetastatic hepatoblastoma: A discouraging pilot study. Med Pediatr Oncol 2001;36:332-334.

574. Habrand JL, Pritchard J: Role of radiotherapy in hepatoblastoma and hepatocellular carcinoma in children and adolescents: Results of a survey conducted by the SIOP Liver Tumour Study Group [letter]. Med Pediatr Oncol 1991;19:208.

575. Habrand JL, Nehme D, Kalifa C, et al: Is there a place for radiation therapy in the management of hepatoblastoma and hepatocellular carcinomas in children? Int J Radiat Oncol Biol Phys 1992;23:525-531.

576. Black CT, Luck SR, Musemeche CA, et al: Aggressive excision of pulmonary metastases is warranted in the management of childhood hepatic tumors. J Pediatr Surg 1991;26:1082-1086.

Adrenocortical Carcinoma/Nasopharygeal

577. Wooten MD, King DK: Adrenal cortical carcinoma: Epidemiology and treatment with mitotane and a review of the literature. Cancer 1993;72:3145-3155.

578. DiGiammarino EL, Lee AS, Cadwell C, et al: A novel mechanism of tumorigenesis involving pH-dependent destabilization of a mutant p53 tetramer. Nat Struct Biol 2001;9:12-16.

579. Ribeiro RC, Sandrini F, Figueiredo B, et al: An inherited p53 mutation that contributes in a tissue-specific manner to pediatric adrenal cortical carcinoma. Proc Natl Acad Sci USA 2001;98: 9330-9335.

580. Vassilopoulou-Sellin R, Schultz PN: Adrenocortical carcinoma: Clinical outcome at the end of the 20th century. Cancer 2001;92:1113-1121.

581. Kendrick ML, Lloyd R, Erickson L, et al: Adrenocortical carcinoma: Surgical progress or status quo? Arch Surg 2001;136:543-549.

582. Wajchenberg BL, Pereira MAA, Medonca BB, et al: Adrenocortical carcinoma: Clinical and laboratory observations. Cancer 2000;88:711-736.

583. Schulick RD, Brennan MF: Long-term survival after complete resection and repeat resection in patients with adrenocortical carcinoma. Ann Surg Oncol 1999;6:719-726.

584. Luton JP, Cerdas S, Billaud L, et al: Clinical features of adrenocortical carcinoma, prognostic factors, and the effect of mitotane therapy. N Engl J Med 1990;322:1195-1201.

585. Crucitti F, Bellantone R, Ferrante A, et al: The Italian Registry for Adrenal Cortical Carcinoma: Analysis of a multi-institutional series of 129 patients. The ACC Italian Registry Study Group. Surgery 1996;119:161-170.

586. Icard P, Chapuis Y, Andreassian B, et al: Adrenocortical carcinoma in surgically treated patients: A retrospective study on 156 cases by the French Association of Endocrine Surgery. Surgery 1992;112:972-979.

587. Ribeiro RC, Sandrini Neto R, Schell MJ, et al: Adrenocortical carcinoma in children: A study of 40 cases. J Clin Oncol 1990;8:67-74.

588. Ciftci AO, Senocak ME, Tanyel FC, et al: Adrenocortical tumors in children. J Pediatr Surg 2001;36:549-554.

589. Driver CP, Birch J, Gough DCS, et al: Adrenal cortical tumors in childhood. Pediatr Hematol Oncol 1998;15:527-532.

590. Stojadinovic A, Ghossein RA, Hoos A, et al: Adrenocortical carcinoma: Clinical, morphologic, and molecular characterization. J Clin Oncol 2002;20:941-950.

591. Weiss LM: Comparative histologic study of 43 metastasizing and nonmetastasizing adrenocortical tumors. Am J Surg Pathol 1984;8:163-169.

592. Slooten HV, Schaberg A, Smeenk D, et al: Morphologic characteristics of benign and malignant adrenocortical tumors. Cancer 1985;55:766-773.

593. Weiss LM, Medeiros LJ, Vickery AL: Pathologic features of prognostic significance in adrenocortical carcinoma. Am J Surg Pathol 1989;13:202-206.

594. Harrison LE, Gaudin PB, Brennan MF: Pathologic features of prognostic significance for adrenocortical carcinoma after curative resection. Arch Surg 1999;134:181-185.

595. Michalkiewicz EL, Sandrini R, Bugg MF, et al: Clinical characteristics of small functioning adrenocortical tumors in children. Med Pediatr Oncol 1997;28:175-178.

596. Bugg MF, Ribeiro RC, Roberson PK, et al: Correlation of pathologic features with clinical outcome in pediatric adrenocortical neoplasia. Am J Clin Pathol 1994;101:625-629.

597. Haak HR, Hermans J, van de Velde CJ, et al: Optimal treatment of adrenocortical carcinoma with mitotane: Results in a consecutive series of 96 patients. Br J Cancer 1994;69:947-951.

598. Bellantone R, Ferrante A, Boscherini M, et al: Role of reoperation in recurrence of adrenal cortical carcinoma: Results from 188 cases collected in the Italian national registry for adrenal cortical carcinoma. Surgery 1997;122:1212-1218.

599. Van Slooten H, Moolenaar AJ, Van Seters AP, et al: The treatment of adrenocortical carcinoma with o,p'-DDD: Prognostic implications of serum level monitoring. Eur J Cancer Clin Oncol 1984;20:47-53.

600. Vassilopoulou-Sellin R, Guinee VF, Klein MJ, et al: Impact of adjuvant mitotane on the clinical course of patients with adrenocortical cancer. Cancer 1993;71:3119-3123.

601. Coelho Netto AS, Wajchenberg BL, Ravaglia C, et al: Treatment of adrenocortical cancer with o,p'-DDD: Ann Intern Med 1963;59:74-78.

602. Fisher DA, Panos TC, Melby JC: Therapy of adrenocortical cancer with o,p'-DDD in two children. J Clin Endocrinol Metab 1963;23:218-221.

603. Ostuni JA, Roginsky MS: Metastatic adrenal cortical carcinoma: Documented cure with combined chemotherapy. Arch Intern Med 1975;135:1257-1258.

604. Dickstein G, Shechner C, Arad E, et al: Is there a role for low doses of mitotane (o,p'-DDD) as adjuvant therapy in adrenocortical carcinoma? J Clin Endocrinol Metab 1998;83:3100-3103.

605. Terzolo M, Pia A, Berruti A, et al: Low-dose monitored mitotane treatment achieves the therapeutic range with manageable side effects in patients with adrenocortical cancer. J Clin Endocrinol Metab 2000;85:2234-2238.

606. Van Slooten H, Van Oosterom AT: CAP (cyclophosphamide, doxorubicin and cisplatinum) regimen in adrenal cortical carcinoma. Cancer Treat Rep 1983;67:377-379.

607. Schlumberger M, Brugieres L, Gicquel C, et al: Fluorouracil, doxorubicin and cisplatin as treatment for adrenal cortical carcinoma. Cancer 1991;67:2997-3000.

608. Williamson SK, Lew D, Miller GJ, et al: Phase II evaluation of cisplatin and etoposide followed by mitotane at disease progression in patients with locally advanced or metastatic adrenocortical carcinoma. Cancer 2000;88:1159-1165.

609. Bates SE, Shieh CY, Mickley LA, et al: Mitotane enhances cytotoxicity of chemotherapy in cell lines expressing a multidrug

resistance gene (MDR-1/P-Glycoprotein) which is also expressed by adrenocortical carcinoma. J Clin Endocrinol Metab 1991;73:18–29.

610. Bonacci R, Gigliotti A, Baudin E, et al: Cytotoxic therapy with etoposide and cisplatin in advanced adrenocortical carcinoma. Br J Cancer 1998;78:546–549.

611. Berruti A, Terzolo M, Pia A, et al: Mitotane associated with etoposide, doxorubicin, and cisplatin in the treatment of advanced adrenocortical carcinoma. Cancer 1998;83:2194–2200.

Nasopharyngeal Carcinoma

612. Marks JE, Phillips JL, Menck HR: The National Cancer Data Base report on the relationship of race and national origin to the histology of nasopharyngeal carcinoma. Cancer 1998;83:582–588.

613. Ayan I, Altun M: Nasopharyngeal carcinoma in children: Retrospective review of 50 patients. Int J Radiat Oncol Biol Phys 1996;35:485–492.

614. Greene MH, Fraumeni JF, Hoover R: Nasopharyngeal cancer among young people in the United States: Racial variations by cell type. J Natl Cancer Inst 1977;58:1267–1270.

615. Chang YS, Tyan YS, Liu ST, et al: Detection of Epstein-Barr virus DNA sequences in nasopharyngeal carcinoma cells by enzymatic DNA amplification. J Clin Microbiol 1990;28:2398–2402.

616. Wu TC, Mann RB, Epdtein JI, et al: Abundant expression of EBER1 small nuclear RNA in nasopharyngeal carcinoma: A morphologically distinctive target for detection of Epstein-Barr virus in formalin-fixed paraffin-embedded carcinoma specimens. Am J Pathol 1991;138:1461–1469.

617. Chen CL, Wen WN, Chen JY, et al: Detection of Epstein-Barr virus genome in nasopharyngeal carcinoma by in situ DNA hybridization. Intervirology 1993;36:91–98.

618. Pathmanathan R, Prasad U, Chandrika G, et al: Undifferentiated, nonkeratinizing, and squamous cell carcinoma of the nasopharynx: Variants of Epstein-Barr virus–infected neoplasia. Am J Pathol 1995;146:1355–1367.

619. Pao WJ, Hustu HO, Douglass EC, et al: Pediatric nasopharyngeal carcinoma: Long term follow-up of 29 patients. Int J Radiat Oncol Biol Phys 1989;17:299–305.

620. Ghim TT, Briones M, Mason P, et al: Effective adjuvant chemotherapy for advanced nasopharyngeal carcinoma in children: A final update of a long-term prospective study in a single institution. J Pediatr Hematol Oncol 1998;20:131–135.

621. Lobo-Sanahuja F, Garcia I, Carranza A, et al: Treatment and outcome of undifferentiated carcinoma of the nasopharynx in childhood: A 13-year experience. Med Pediatr Oncol 1986;14:6–11.

622. Roper HP, Essex-carter A, Marsden HB, et al: Nasopharyngeal carcinoma in children. Pediatr Hematol Oncol 1986;3:143–152.

623. Gasparini M, Lombardi F, Rottoli L, et al: Combined radiotherapy and chemotherapy in stage T3 and T4 nasopharyngeal carcinoma in children. J Clin Oncol 1988;6:491–494.

624. Arush MW, Stein ME, Bosenblatt E, et al: Advanced nasopharyngeal carcinoma in the young: The Northern Israel Oncology Center experience, 1973–1991. Pediatr Hematol Oncol 1995;12:271–276.

625. Werner-Wasik M, Winkler P, Uri A, et al: Nasopharyngeal carcinoma in children. Med Pediatr Oncol 1996;26:352–358.

626. Strojan P, Benedik MD, Kragelj R, et al: Combined radiation and chemotherapy for advanced undifferentiated nasopharyngeal carcinoma in children. Med Pediatr Oncol 1997;28:366–369.

627. Ingersoll L, Woo SY, Donaldson S, et al: Nasopharyngeal carcinoma in the young: A combined M.D. Anderson and Stanford experience. Int J Radiat Oncol Biol Phys 1990;19:881–887.

628. Berberoglu S, Ilhan I, Cetindag F, et al: Nasopharyngeal carcinoma in Turkish children: Review of 33 cases. Pediatr Hematol Oncol 2001;18:309–315.

629. Douglass EC, Fontanesi J, Ribeiro RC, et al: Improved long-term disease-free survival in nasopharyngeal carcinoma (NPC) in childhood and adolescence: A multi-institution treatment protocol. Proc Annu Meet Am Soc Clin Oncol 1996;15:A1470.

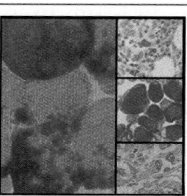

THE WORLD HEALTH ORGANIZATION CLASSIFICATION OF HEMATOLOGIC MALIGNANCIES*

Elaine S. Jaffe

SUMMARY OF KEY POINTS

- The World Health Organization (WHO) Classification of Hematologic Malignancies includes tumors of lymphoid, myeloid, histiocytic, and dendritic cell lineages.
- Each disease is defined as a distinct entity based on a constellation of morphologic, clinical, and biologic features.
- The cell of origin is the starting point of disease definition.
- Some lymphomas and leukemias can be identified by routine morphologic approaches. For many diseases, however, knowledge of the immunophenotype and molecular genetics or cytogenetics plays an important role in differential diagnosis.

- The sites of presentation and involvement are important clues to underlying biologic distinctions. Extranodal lymphomas differ in many respects from their nodal counterparts.
- Many lymphoma entities display a range in cytologic grade and clinical aggressiveness, making it difficult to stratify lymphomas according to clinical behavior. A number of prognostic factors influence clinical outcome, including stage, international prognostic index (IPI), cytologic grade, and secondary genetic events.
- The WHO classification includes four major categories of myeloid diseases, all of which are clonal stem

cell disorders leading to either effective or ineffective hematopoiesis: (1) chronic myeloproliferative diseases; (2) myelodysplastic/myeloproliferative diseases; (3) myelodysplastic syndromes; and (4) acute myeloid leukemias.
- Among myeloid leukemias, genetic features predict behavior better than morphology alone, necessitating genetic studies for accurate diagnosis.
- Acute myeloid leukemias, with or without multilineage dysplasia, appear to represent separate pathways to leukemogenesis, with clinical implications for response to therapy.

INTRODUCTION

In recent years, the discipline of hematopathology has emphasized the integration of morphology and biologic markers for diagnosis. The approaches used in hematopathologic diagnosis often have served as a model for other areas of pathology. For example, in the early 1980s, detection of rearrangements of the antigen receptor genes in lymphoid cells was used to indicate both clonality and cell lineage, long before molecular diagnostic techniques became commonplace in pathology.[1] Biologic approaches such as immunohistochemistry and molecular biology enhance diagnostic accuracy and play a critical role in the definition of disease entities.

Classification approaches for both lymphoid and myeloid neoplasms have undergone significant reappraisal over the past 40 years. These changes have resulted from insights gained through the application of immunologic and molecular techniques, as well as a better understanding of the clinical aspects of lymphoma and leukemia through advances in diagnosis, staging, and treatment.

HISTORICAL BACKGROUND

In the past, the classification of lymphomas has been controversial, and it has been difficult to establish an

internationally accepted scheme. The earliest classification systems were morphologically based on cytologic and architectural features.[2] However, insights into the complexities of the normal immune system led to attempts to relate the lymphomas to their normal cellular counterparts. In the 1970s, several European and American groups published proposals for the classification of lymphoma, and competing classification systems in use in clinical studies made it difficult to compare outcome data from different treatment centers.[3-6] The inability of the pathologists to develop consensus and agree on a common approach led to the development of the working formulation for the non-Hodgkin lymphomas, following a National Cancer Institute–directed study to evaluate the six published schemes.[7]

Constructed in large measure by clinicians, the working formulation tried to stratify lymphomas according to clinical outcome based on clinical trials conducted in the 1970s.[7] The low-grade, intermediate-grade, and high-grade groupings were intended to provide a clinical guide for patient management. The individual lymphoma categories were defined by morphologic principles, such as growth pattern and cell size, without regard to cell lineage or stage of differentiation. Therefore, most of the diagnostic categories of the working formulation were heterogeneous. For example, "diffuse mixed small and large cell lymphoma" included a variety of both B- and T-cell lymphomas. It is therefore not surprising that pathologists could not use these categories reproducibly.[8]

*This chapter is in the public domain.

The original intent of the working formulation proposal was to have it serve as a common language to translate among classifications, not to serve as a freestanding classification scheme. However, because it was a convenient guide to therapy, it quickly became popular among clinicians, and was adopted for use in many centers in the United States for clinical trials. In reality, the working formulation was in essence the Rappaport classification[2] with updated terminology from Lukes and Collins.[3] A more basic flaw in the working formulation is that it was based on treatment outcome, not on the recognition of individual disease entities or the cell of origin for a malignant neoplasm. It lumped diseases that shared a similar cell size and median survival into single categories, despite the fact that they might be of different cellular (B and T cell) origins with diverse clinical features. At the time the working formulation was proposed, immunophenotyping was felt to be beyond the reach of the routine pathology laboratory, and the classification was based on morphology alone.

A similar paradigm developed in the classification of acute myeloid and lymphoid leukemias. Earlier classification systems emphasized morphologic approaches, although the French, American, and British (FAB) classification did use enzyme cytochemistry to identify cellular lineage and degree of differentiation, at least within the myeloid and monocytic neoplasms.[9] The categories of acute lymphoblastic leukemia—L1, L2, and L3—included both mature and immature lymphoid malignancies. L3 was composed largely of mature blastic B cells similar to the cells of Burkitt's lymphoma. L1 and L2, although both of lymphoblastic origin, correlated poorly with precursor T- or B-cell lineage.

Modern immunophenotypic and molecular approaches for characterizing lymphoid cells are now readily available at even the community hospital level. The use of these new biologic approaches has transformed our understanding of lymphoid neoplasia. Immunophenotypic and genotypic studies have permitted an impartial analysis of questions that were unresolved when addressed with only routine hematoxylin and eosin–stained sections. Indeed, a broad international consensus has emerged on many topics. This consensus was embodied in the Revised European-American Classification of Lymphoid Neoplasms (the REAL classification) published by the International Lymphoma Study Group (ILSG) in 1994.[10]

THE NEXT STEPS: REAL TO WHO

The REAL classification[10] and its successor, the WHO classification,[11] represented a new paradigm in the classification of lymphoid neoplasms. The focus was on the identification of "real" diseases, rather than a global theoretical framework, such as survival (working formulation), or cellular differentiation (Kiel classification). The REAL classification was based on the building of consensus, and recognized that a comprehensive classification system was beyond the experience of any one individual. The 19 members of the ILSG contributed their diverse perspectives to achieve a unified point of view.

In addition, the ILSG made the decision to base the classification exclusively on published data. Earlier classification systems often had been based on theoretical and untested propositions. However, for an entity to be included in the REAL classification, it had to be validated in several publications (at least two, preferably three or more). In addition, a number of entities were listed as provisional, based on more limited published data.

The REAL classification departed from traditional schemes by emphasizing that each disease was a distinct entity, defined by a constellation of laboratory and clinical features, including morphology, immunophenotype, genetic features, clinical presentation, and course. The inclusion of clinical criteria was one of the most innovative aspects of the ILSG approach. The REAL classification recognized that the site of presentation often is a signpost for underlying biologic distinctions, as in extranodal lymphomas of the mucosa-associated lymphoid tissues (MALT)[12] or many forms of T-cell lymphoma.[13,14] Accurate diagnosis requires knowledge of the clinical history, because biologically distinct entities may appear cytologically similar.

The REAL classification also stressed the distinction between histologic grade and clinical aggressiveness, because these factors do not necessarily go hand in hand. For example, mantle cell lymphoma, which is composed of small to medium-sized lymphoid cells with condensed chromatin, had been considered cytologically low grade, but it is, in fact, one of the more aggressive lymphoma subtypes.[15,16] Similarly, among the T-cell lymphomas, angioimmunoblastic T-cell lymphoma has an aggressive clinical course, with a median survival of less than 3 years.[17] By contrast, anaplastic large cell lymphoma, which would appear to be of high histologic grade, has an excellent response to chemotherapy with prolonged disease-free survival.[18]

Moreover, within a given disease entity a number of prognostic factors influence the clinical outcome. Cytologic grade is one type of prognostic factor, and is used in the stratification of follicular lymphoma. Clinical features, such as the stage or International Prognostic Index (IPI), also markedly affect survival and response to treatment.[19] Finally, a variety of biologic factors, some of which may be secondary, affect the prognosis. These include secondary genetic events, such as mutations in p53 genes, which often lead to histologic and clinical progression.[20-22] Thus the WHO classification stresses the distinction between a *disease entity* and a *prognostic factor*.

For these reasons, it is not possible to stratify lymphoma subtypes according to clinical grade, as had been attempted in the working formulation. Moreover, clinical groupings for either protocol treatment or routine clinical practice usually are not feasible. In evaluating new therapies the data for each disease must be evaluated individually. Indeed, treatment approaches for one type of lymphoid malignancy are not necessarily applicable to other diseases, even of the same cell lineage. This point is exemplified by hairy cell leukemia, a rare disease for which highly effective forms of therapy have been developed.[23,24] However, the purine analogs 2′-deoxycoformycin and 2′-chlorodeoxyadenosine have not been similarly effective in treating other B-cell leukemias and lymphomas.[25]

The REAL classification was first to emphasize the importance of molecular oncology in defining disease entities. Cancer is increasingly recognized as a genetic disease.[26] For many lymphomas, there is a good correlation between the molecular pathogenesis and routine histologic and immunophenotypic features. For example, the t(14;18) involving the *BCL-2* and *JH* genes is highly associated with follicular lymphoma diagnosed by routine methods. (There appears to be no similar consistent correlation between morphology and genetics in acute leukemias.) In addition, some molecular phenotypes can be recognized by immunohistochemistry, such as cyclin D1 overexpression in the diagnosis of mantle cell lymphoma, or ALK expression in anaplastic large cell lymphoma.

However, for many lymphoma subtypes, particularly the mature T-cell malignancies, the molecular pathogenesis is not known. The REAL/WHO classifications recognized limitations in our knowledge, and created "generic groupings" for those broad categories of disease that could not be resolved with existing data; these include diffuse large B-cell lymphomas and peripheral T-cell lymphomas, unspecified. A number of morphologic variants had been described, but evidence that these delineated distinct biologic or clinical entities was lacking. Molecular profiling studies are leading to new subdivisions of diffuse large B-cell lymphomas.[27,28] Accurate disease definition is the first step in identifying the molecular pathogenesis, and it is expected that new insights will continue to be made.

Following the publication of the REAL classification, an international study directed by Dr. James Armitage sought to determine if the REAL classification could be readily applied by a group of independent expert pathologists.[18] Other goals of the International Lymphoma Classification Project were as follows: (1) to determine the role of immunophenotyping and clinical data in the diagnosis of disease entities; (2) to determine both intra- and interobserver reproducibility in the diagnosis of the various entities; (3) to investigate further the clinical features or epidemiology of the various entities; and (4) to determine if clinical groupings would be practical or useful for clinical trials or practice.

The conclusions of that study affirmed the principles of the REAL classification.[18] Virtually all cases could be classified in the published scheme. Intra- and interobserver rates of reproducibility were excellent. The use of precise disease definitions, as provided by the REAL scheme, enhanced diagnostic accuracy and reduced subjectivity on the part of pathologists. Immunophenotyping was found to be essential for some diagnostic categories, such as most of the peripheral T-cell lymphomas. Importantly, the significance of identifying individual disease entities was confirmed by overall survival and failure-free survival data.

Interestingly, this study also highlighted the importance of clinical factors such as the IPI for predicting prognosis and providing a guide to clinical management.[19] There was a wide range in survival within most disease entities

based on the risk factors identified in the IPI.[18] This result confirms that it can be misleading to stratify different diseases into risk groups based only on histologic criteria. Treatment planning must take into consideration clinical factors, as well as the histologic diagnosis. Moreover, when the diseases were grouped according to post-treatment survival, it was noted that the entities included within each group were heterogeneous, requiring markedly different treatment approaches. For example, the lymphomas in the best-risk group were anaplastic large cell lymphomas, marginal zone lymphomas of MALT type, and follicular lymphomas. Clearly, the treatment approaches for these diseases are completely different, indicating that clinical groupings by survival are not useful. One must approach each disease entity individually, considering the diagnosis, the patient's risk factors, and the known idiosyncrasies of each disease with regard to treatment.

The international classification project also confirmed previous epidemiologic observations, such as the increased frequency of extranodal NK/T-cell lymphoma, nasal type, among Hong Kong Chinese as compared with patients from North America and Western Europe.[29] The distinctive clinical features of mediastinal large B-cell lymphoma and T/null anaplastic large cell lymphoma also were confirmed.[18,30-32]

THE WHO CLASSIFICATION

In 2001 the International Agency for Research on Cancer (IARC) under the auspices of the World Health Organization (WHO) published a unified and internationally accepted classification scheme for all lymphoid, myeloid, histiocytic, and dendritic cell neoplasms (Table 100-1).[11] Part of a series by the IARC, one goal is to integrate pathology and genetics to develop biologically relevant classification systems. The WHO adopted the approach of the REAL classification for the lymphoid malignancies, because this approach had been validated, and in turn applied the same principles to tumors of other hematopoietic lineages, mainly myeloid and histiocytic tumors.

The task of developing the WHO classification was undertaken as a joint project by the Society for Hematopathology (SH) and the European Association of Hematopathology (EAHP). A Steering Committee was appointed by the two societies, which, in turn, established 10 individual committees to deal with different disease groups within hematopoietic and lymphoid malignancies.[33] More than 50 pathologists participated in this effort, leading to a broad international consensus. In addition, to ensure that the classification was clinically relevant, more than 40 expert clinicians in the field of leukemia and lymphoma were appointed to a Clinical Advisory Committee.[34] The WHO classification was developed over a period of 7 years, during which time the proposal was extensively discussed and vetted at a number of international meetings and symposia, to ensure worldwide acceptance. Approximately 100 pathologists and clinicians gathered at a clinical advisory meeting to discuss a number of questions of clinical relevance. The proposed classification was circulated in advance of the meeting, and participants

TABLE 100-1

World Health Organization Classification of the Tumors of the Hematopoietic and Lymphoid Tissues

	ICD-O*
Chronic Myeloproliferative Diseases	
Chronic myelogenous leukemia	9875/3
Chronic neutrophilic leukemia	9963/3
Chronic eosinophilic leukemia/hypereosinophilic syndrome	9964/3
Polycythemia vera	9950/3
Chronic idiopathic myelofibrosis	9961/3
Essential thrombocythemia	9962/3
Chronic myeloproliferative disease, unclassifiable	9975/3
Myelodysplastic/Myeloproliferative Diseases	
Chronic myelomonocytic leukemia	9945/3
Atypical chronic myeloid leukemia	9876/3
Juvenile myelomonocytic leukemia	9946/3
Myelodysplastic/myeloproliferative diseases, unclassifiable	9975/3
Myelodysplastic Syndromes	
Refractory anemia	9980/3
Refractory anemia with ringed sideroblasts	9982/3
Refractory cytopenia with multilineage dysplasia	9985/3
Refractory anemia with excess blasts	9983/3
Myelodysplastic syndrome associated with isolated del(5q) chromosome abnormality	9986/3
Myelodysplastic syndrome, unclassifiable	9989/3
Acute Myeloid Leukemias	
I. Acute Myeloid Leukemia with Recurrent Cytogenetic Abnormalities	
AML with t(8;21)(q22;q22) (*AML1/ETO*)	9896/3
AML with inv(16)(p13q22) or t(16;16)(p13;q22),(*CBFb//MYH11*)	9871/3
Acute promyelocytic leukemia: AML with t(15;17)(q22;q12), *PML/RARα* and variants	9866/3
AML with 11q23 (*MLL*) abnormalities	9897/3
II. Acute Myeloid Leukemia with Multilineage Dysplasia	9895/3
With prior myelodysplastic syndrome	
Without prior myelodysplastic syndrome	
III. Acute Myeloid Leukemia and Myelodysplastic Syndrome, Therapy-related	9920/3
Alkylating agent–related	
Topoisomerase II inhibitor–related	
IV. Acute Myeloid Leukemia not Otherwise Categorized	
AML, minimally differentiated	9872/3
AML without maturation	9873/3
AML with maturation	9874/3
Acute myelomonocytic leukemia	9867/3
Acute monoblastic and monocytic leukemia	9891/3
Acute erythroid leukemia	9840/3
Acute megakaryoblastic leukemia	9910/3
Acute basophilic leukemia	9870/3
Acute panmyelosis with myelofibrosis	9931/3
Myeloid sarcoma	9930/3
V. Acute Leukemia of Ambiguous Lineage	9805/3
B-Cell Neoplasms	
Precursor B-Cell Neoplasm	
Precursor B lymphoblastic leukemia[1]/lymphoma[2]	9836/3[1]
(Precursor B-cell acute lymphoblastic leukemia[1])	9728/3[2]
Mature B-Cell Neoplasms	
Chronic lymphocytic leukemia[1]/small lymphocytic lymphoma[2]	9823/3[1]
	9670/3[2]
B-cell prolymphocytic leukemia	9833/3
Lymphoplasmacytic lymphoma	9671/3
Splenic marginal zone lymphoma	9689/3
Hairy cell leukemia	9940/3
Plasma cell myeloma	9732/3
Solitary plasmacytoma of bone	9731/3
Extraosseus plasmacytoma	9734/3
Extranodal marginal zone B-cell lymphoma of mucosa-associated lymphoid tissue (MALT lymphoma)	9699/3
Nodal marginal zone B-cell lymphoma	9699/3

TABLE 100-1

World Health Organization Classification of the Tumors of the Hematopoietic and Lymphoid Tissues—cont'd

Follicular lymphoma	9690/3
Grade 1	9695/3
Grade 2	9691/3
Grade 3	9698/3
Mantle cell lymphoma	9673/3
Diffuse large B-cell lymphoma	9680/3
Mediastinal (thymic) large B-cell lymphoma	9679/3
Intravascular large B-cell lymphoma	9680/3
Primary effusion lymphoma	9678/3
Burkitt's lymphoma[1]/leukemia[2]	9687/3[1]
	9826/3[2]

T-Cell and NK-Cell Neoplams
Precursor T-cell Neoplasms

Precursor T lymphoblastic leukemia[1]/lymphoma[2]	9837/3[1]
(Precursor T-cell acute lymphoblastic leukemia[1])	9729/3[2]
Blastic NK cell lymphoma[†]	9727/3

Mature T-Cell and NK-Cell Neoplasms

T-cell prolymphocytic leukemia	9834/3
T-cell large granular lymphocytic leukemia	9831/3
Aggressive NK cell leukemia	9948/3
Adult T-cell leukemia/lymphoma	9827/3
Extranodal NK/T-cell lymphoma, nasal type	9719/3
Enteropathy-type T-cell lymphoma	9717/3
Hepatosplenic T-cell lymphoma	9716/3
Subcutaneous panniculitis-like T-cell lymphoma	9708/3
Mycosis fungoides	9700/3
Sézary syndrome	9701/3
Primary cutaneous anaplastic large cell lymphoma	9718/3
Peripheral T-cell lymphoma, unspecified	9702/3
Angioimmunoblastic T-cell lymphoma	9705/3
Anaplastic large cell lymphoma	9714/3

B-Cell Lymphoproliferations of Uncertain Malignant Potential

Lymphomatoid granulomatosis	9766/1
Polymorphic posttransplant lymphoproliferative disorder	

T-Cell Lymphoproliferation of Uncertain Malignant Potential

Lymphomatoid papulosis	9718/1

Hodgkin's Lymphoma

Nodular lymphocyte–predominant Hodgkin's lymphoma	9659/3
Classical Hodgkin's lymphoma	9650/3
Nodular sclerosis classical Hodgkin's lymphoma	9663/3
Lymphocyte-rich classical Hodgkin's lymphoma	9651/3
Mixed cellularity classical Hodgkin's lymphoma	9652/3
Lymphocyte-depleted classical Hodgkin's lymphoma	9653/3

Histiocytic and Dendritic-Cell Neoplasms
Macrophage/Histiocytic Neoplasm

Histiocytic sarcoma	9755/3

Dendritic Cell Neoplasms

Langerhans cell histiocytosis	9751/1
Langerhans cell sarcoma	9756/3
Interdigitating dendritic cell sarcoma[1]/tumor[2]	9757/3[1]/ 9757/1[2]
Follicular dendritic cell sarcoma[1]/tumor[2]	9758/3[1]/ 9758/1[2]
Dendritic cell sarcoma, not otherwise specified	9757/3

Mastocytosis

Cutaneous mastocytosis	
Indolent systemic mastocytosis	9741/1
Systemic mastocytosis with associated clonal, hematologic non–mast cell lineage disease	9741/3
Aggressive systemic mastocytosis	9741/3
Mast cell leukemia	9742/3
Mast cell sarcoma	9740/3
Extracutaneous mastocytoma	9740/1

*Morphology code of the International Classification of Diseases (ICD-O), 3rd edition. Behavior is coded /3 for malignant tumors and /1 for lesions of low or uncertain malignant potential.
[†]Neoplasm of uncertain lineage and stage of differentiation; current data indicate dendritic cell precursor.

were invited to submit topics for discussion. A consensus was achieved on most of the questions raised.[34]

The participants recognized the value of a disease-oriented approach to classification. Disease definition is the first step in elucidating the pathogenesis of diseases, and most pathogenetic insights have followed on the heels of the identification of a disease along clinical lines. Advances in therapy are best achieved when studies are conducted on a homogeneous disease entity. For example, the approaches to therapy of extranodal marginal B-cell lymphoma of MALT type differ from those for more systemic small B-cell malignancies. The ultimate goal in this model is molecularly targeted therapy, such as the use of STI571 to target the *BCR/ABL* tyrosine kinase of chronic myelogenous leukemia.[35] The committee also concluded that sorting B-cell and T-cell neoplasms into prognostic groupings would have no clear purpose, and would hamper insights into the unique characteristics of some diseases.

The Clinical Advisory Meeting, combined with data published after the REAL classification was published, led to minor revisions of the classification of lymphoid malignancies proposed by the ILSG. Entities that previously had been listed as provisional in the REAL classification were resolved; most were retained, whereas others were eliminated from the classification scheme. "Hodgkin's-like anaplastic large cell lymphoma"[36,37] was felt on further analysis to be resolvable in most cases into either an aggressive form of Hodgkin disease, or a rare variant of T/null anaplastic large cell lymphoma.[32] It was eliminated, therefore, as a category in the WHO scheme. The category "high-grade B-cell lymphoma, Burkitt-like" likewise was considered heterogeneous, resolvable in most cases into either Burkitt's lymphoma or a diffuse large B-cell lymphoma. Additionally, some minor changes in terminology were proposed for some entities.

The WHO classification applied the principles of the REAL classification to the classification of myeloid and histiocytic tumors, and expanded on the classification of

PATHOGENETIC INSIGHTS BASED ON A DISEASE-ORIENTED APPROACH TO CLASSIFICATION

DISEASE	PATHOGENETIC FACTOR
Nasal NK/T-cell lymphoma	Genetics, EBV
Adult T-cell leukemia/lymphoma	HTLV-1
Anaplastic large cell lymphoma	*ALK* kinase
Mantle cell lymphoma	*CCND1*
Follicular lymphoma	*BCL-2*
Lymphomatoid granulomatosis	EBV, immune dysfunction
Gastric MALT lymphoma	*Helicobacter pylori,* MLT
Burkitt's lymphoma	*C-MYC*
Primary effusion lymphoma	*KSHV/HHV-8*

EBV, Epstein-Barr virus; HTLV, human T-cell leukemia-lymphoma virus; MALT, mucosa-associated lymphoid tissue.

precursor lymphoid malignancies, the lymphoblastic lymphomas and leukemias, which had been touched upon only briefly in the REAL classification. For the acute leukemias, the molecular pathogenesis is a very important determinant of clinical behavior. Unfortunately, in contrast to the lymphomas, correlations among the genetic profile, morphology, and the immuno/enzymatic phenotype often are absent. Additionally, acute leukemias, because they are of stem cell origin, display significant lineage promiscuity at the genetic and phenotypic levels. Therefore, it is somewhat more difficult to achieve a classification of acute leukemias that is widely applicable in the medical community as well as biologically and clinically relevant.

The WHO classification for myeloid neoplasms departed from the FAB classification in a number of ways. For those forms of acute myeloid leukemia (AML) associated with recurrent genetic abnormalities, genetic features take precedence over morphology. However, some genetic lesions are associated with a characteristic morphologic appearance.[38] For example, the detection of the inv(16) or t(16;16) usually correlates with M4 with abnormal eosinophils in the FAB approach.[39] Recurrent genetic abnormalities can be identified with classical cytogenetics, reverse transcriptase-polymerase chain reaction (RT-PCR), or fluorescence in situ hybridization (FISH) techniques.

Based on the observation that AML arising in the setting of myelodysplastic syndrome (MDS) is associated with some distinctive clinical and biologic features, the WHO classification distinguishes two broad groups of de novo AML, with and without multilineage dysplasia.[40-42] Cases of AML with significant myelodysplastic features usually occur at an older age, respond poorly to therapy, and have high-risk cytogenetic features.[38]

The WHO classification recognizes two forms of AML that occur secondary to iatrogenic therapy. Acute myeloid leukemia following alkylating agent therapy or radiation therapy closely resembles AML with multilineage dysplasia, and many of these patients have antecedent MDS.[43] The interval to diagnosis usually is long, and the response to therapy poor. The acute leukemias arising after topoisomerase II inhibitor therapy occur after a shorter interval, do not have associated MDS, often contain a prominent monocytic component, and have characteristic translocations. These patients have a response to therapy similar to that seen in other de novo cases of AML with comparable cytogenetic features.[38]

AML, *not further categorized*, is subclassified according to the morphologic and cytochemical approaches of the FAB classification. The intent is to provide a broad framework for the classification of these disorders to facilitate future studies regarding the pathogenesis. The approach is similar to that used for diffuse large B-cell lymphomas and peripheral T-cell lymphomas, unspecified. It is recognized that these categories are heterogeneous. Morphologic variants are described, but there is no evidence yet that these variants are biologically significant or relate to underlying pathogenetic mechanisms.

The other major categories addressed in the WHO classification of myeloid neoplasms are (1) myelodysplastic syndromes; (2) myeloid disorders that have features of both MDS and myeloproliferative diseases such as chronic myelomonocytic leukemia; and (3) chronic myeloproliferative disorders. The myeloproliferative and myelodysplastic diseases are clonal stem cell disorders, with or without effective hematopoiesis, respectively. The term *chronic myelogenous leukemia* is restricted to those cases with a BCR/ABL fusion gene. The diagnosis of chronic neutrophilic leukemia requires genetic evidence of a myeloid neoplasm, other than the Ph chromosome or *BCR/ABL*.

Knowing the clonal nature of myelodysplastic syndromes and their generally poor prognosis, some have questioned the use of the term *myelodysplasia*, and suggest this nosology obscures the neoplastic nature of the process.[44] In the WHO classification, the blast threshold for the diagnosis of AML was reduced from 30% to 20% blasts in the bone marrow or peripheral blood. Moreover, in recognition of the importance of genetic abnormalities, patients with recurring cytogenetic abnormalities are considered to have acute leukemia regardless of the blast count.[38]

CONCLUSION

The WHO classification integrates morphologic classification systems with biologic data related to the pathogenesis of disease. The ultimate goal might be a genetically defined classification system in which the molecular pathogenesis of every neoplasm is known, but this aim is undoubtedly some years away. However, the recognition of carefully defined disease entities should facilitate the investigation of pathogenetic mechanism, and the development of molecularly targeted therapies. The WHO classification is a milestone, because it is the first classification system for lymphomas and leukemias universally accepted and in use on a worldwide basis. It also is a roadmap for future scientific and clinical investigations. The use of common diagnostic criteria will facilitate collaboration and synthesis of data generated from such studies.

REFERENCES

1. Arnold A, Cossman J, Bakhshi A, et al: Immunoglobulin-gene rearrangements as unique clonal markers in human lymphoid neoplasms. N Engl J Med 1983;309:1593.
2. Rappaport H: Tumors of the hematopoietic system. In: Atlas of Tumor Pathology, 1st series. Washington, DC, Armed Forces Institute of Pathology; 1966, p 10–14.
3. Lukes R, Collins R: Immunologic characterization of human malignant lymphomas. Cancer 1974;34:1488.
4. Gerard-Marchant R, Hamlin I, Lennert K, et al: Classification of non-Hodgkin's lymphomas. Lancet 1974;2:406.
5. Bennett MH, Farrer-Brown G, Henry K, Jeliffe AM: Classification of non-Hodgkin's lymphomas. Lancet 1974;2:405.
6. Dorfman RF: Classification of non-Hodgkin's lymphomas [letter]. Lancet 1974;1(7869):1295.
7. Non-Hodgkin's lymphoma pathologic classification project. National Cancer Institute sponsored study of classifications of non-Hodgkin's lymphomas: summary and description of a Working Formulation for clinical usage. Cancer 1982;49:2112.
8. NCI Non-Hodgkin's Classification Project Writing Committee.

Classification of non-Hodgkin's lymphomas. Reproducibility of major classification systems. Cancer 1985;55:91.
9. Bennett JM, Catovsky D, Daniel MT, et al: Proposals for the classification of the acute leukaemias. French-American-British (FAB) co-operative group. Br J Haematol 1976;33:451.
10. Harris NL, Jaffe ES, Stein H, et al: A revised European-American classification of lymphoid neoplasms: a proposal from the International Lymphoma Study Group. Blood 1994;84:1361.
11. Jaffe ES, Harris NL, Stein H, Vardiman J: Pathology and Genetics of Tumours of Haematopoietic and Lymphoid Tissues. Lyon, France, IARC Press, 2001.
12. Isaacson P, Spencer J: Malignant lymphoma of mucosa-associated lymphoid tissue. Histopathology 1987;11:445.
13. Jaffe ES, Krenacs L, Raffeld M: Classification of T-cell and NK-cell neoplasms based on the REAL classification. Ann Oncol 1997;8(suppl 2):S17.
14. Jaffe ES, Krenacs L, Raffeld M: Classification of cytotoxic T-cell and natural killer cell lymphomas. Semin Hematol 2003;40:175.
15. Raffeld M, Jaffe ES: bcl-1, t(11;14), and mantle cell derived neoplasms. Blood 1991;78:259.
16. Campo E, Raffeld M, Jaffe ES: Mantle-cell lymphoma. Semin Hematol 1999;36:115.
17. Siegert W, Agthe A, Griesser H, et al: Treatment of angioimmunoblastic lymphadenopathy (AILD)-type T-cell lymphoma using prednisone with or without the COPBLAM/IMVP-16 regimen. A multicenter study. Kiel Lymphoma Study Group. Ann Intern Med 1992;117:364.
18. The Non-Hodgkin's Lymphoma Classification Project: A clinical evaluation of the International Lymphoma Study Group classification of non-Hodgkin's lymphoma. Blood 1997;89:3909.
19. A predictive model for aggressive non-Hodgkin's lymphoma. The International Non-Hodgkin's Lymphoma Prognostic Factors Project. N Engl J Med 1993;329:987.
20. Sander CA, Yano T, Clark HM, et al: p53 mutation is associated with progression in follicular lymphomas. Blood 1993;82:1994.
21. Hernandez L, Fest T, Cazorla M, et al: p53 gene mutations and protein overexpression are associated with aggressive variants of mantle cell lymphomas. Blood 1996;87:3351.
22. Piris MA, Pezzella F, Martinez MJ, et al: p53 and bcl-2 expression in high-grade B-cell lymphomas: correlation with survival time. Br J Cancer 1994;69:337 [published erratum appears in Br J Cancer 1994;69:978].
23. Kraut EH, Grever MR, Bouroncle BA: Long-term follow-up of patients with hairy cell leukemia after treatment with 2'-deoxycoformycin. Blood 1994;84:4061.
24. Saven A, Piro LD: Treatment of hairy cell leukemia. Blood 1992;79:1111.
25. Saven A, Piro LD: 2-Chlorodeoxyadenosine: A newer purine analog active in the treatment of indolent lymphoid malignancies. Ann Intern Med 1994;120:784.
26. Buetow KH, Klausner RD, Fine H, et al: Cancer Molecular Analysis Project: Weaving a rich cancer research tapestry. Cancer Cell 2002;1:315.
27. Rosenwald A, Wright G, Chan WC, et al: The use of molecular profiling to predict survival after chemotherapy for diffuse large-B-cell lymphoma. N Engl J Med 2002;346:1937.
28. Shipp MA, Ross KN, Tamayo P, et al: Diffuse large B-cell lymphoma outcome prediction by gene-expression profiling and supervised machine learning. Nat Med 2002;8(1):68.
29. Jaffe ES, Chan JKC, Su IJ, et al: Report of the workshop on nasal and related extranodal angiocentric T/NK cell lymphomas: Definitions, differential diagnosis, and epidemiology. Am J Surg Pathol 1996;20:103.
30. Moller P, Moldenhauer G, Momburg F, et al: Mediastinal lymphoma of clear cell type is a tumor corresponding to terminal steps of B cell differentiation. Blood 1987;69:1087.
31. Lamarre L, Jacobson J, Aisenberg A, Harris N: Primary large cell lymphoma of the mediastinum. Am J Surg Pathol 1989;13:730.
32. Jaffe ES: Anaplastic large cell lymphoma: the shifting sands of diagnostic hematopathology. Mod Pathol 2001;14:219.
33. Jaffe ES, Harris NL, Diebold J, Muller-Hermelink HK: World Health Organization classification of neoplastic diseases of the hematopoietic and lymphoid tissues: A progress report. Am J Clin Pathol 1999;111(Suppl.1):S8.

Specific Malignancies

34. Harris NL, Jaffe ES, Diebold J, et al: World Health Organization classification of neoplastic diseases of the hematopoietic and lymphoid tissues: report of the Clinical Advisory Committee Meeting, Airlie House, Virginia, November 1997. J Clin Oncol 1999;17:3835.

35. O'Dwyer ME, Mauro MJ, Druker BJ: STI571 as a targeted therapy for CML. Cancer Invest 2003;21:429.

36. Leoncini L, Del Vecchio M, Kraft R, et al: Hodgkin's disease and CD30-positive anaplastic large cell lymphomas—a continuous spectrum of malignant disorders. Am J Pathol 1990;137:1047.

37. Pileri S, Bocchia M, Baroni C, et al: Anaplastic large cell lymphoma (CD30+/Ki-1+): results of a prospective clinicopathologic study of 69 cases. Br J Haematol 1994;86:513.

38. Vardiman JW, Harris NL, Brunning RD: The World Health Organization (WHO) classification of the myeloid neoplasms. Blood 2002;100:2292.

39. Mrozek K, Prior TW, Edwards C, et al: Comparison of cytogenetic and molecular genetic detection of t(8;21) and inv(16) in a prospective series of adults with de novo acute myeloid leukemia: A Cancer and Leukemia Group B Study. J Clin Oncol 2001;19:2482.

40. Goasguen JE, Matsuo T, Cox C, Bennett JM: Evaluation of the dysmyelopoiesis in 336 patients with de novo acute myeloid leukemia: Major importance of dysgranulopoiesis for remission and survival. Leukemia 1992;6:520.

41. Leith CP, Kopecky KJ, Godwin J, et al: Acute myeloid leukemia in the elderly: assessment of multidrug resistance (MDR1) and cytogenetics distinguishes biologic subgroups with remarkably distinct responses to standard chemotherapy. A Southwest Oncology Group study. Blood 1997;89:3323.

42. Head DR: Revised classification of acute myeloid leukemia. Leukemia 1996;10:1826.

43. Michels SD, McKenna RW, Arthur DC, Brunning RD: Therapy-related acute myeloid leukemia and myelodysplastic syndrome: A clinical and morphologic study of 65 cases. Blood 1985;65:1364.

44. Lichtman MA: Myelodysplasia or myeloneoplasia: Thoughts on the nosology of clonal myeloid diseases. Blood Cells Mol Dis 2000;26:572.

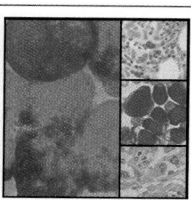

01

CHILDHOOD LEUKEMIA

Dario Campana

Ching-Hon Pui

SUMMARY OF KEY POINTS

INCIDENCE

- Leukemia is the most common childhood cancer in developed countries and is usually acute in children.
- The most common subtype, acute lymphoblastic leukemia (ALL), accounts for 75% to 80% of all cases of childhood leukemia, while acute myeloid leukemia (AML) accounts for approximately 20%.

ETIOLOGY

- Although environmental agents, such as ionizing radiation and chemical mutagens, have been implicated in the induction of leukemia, discernible etiologic factors are lacking in almost all cases of primary leukemia.
- Acquired genetic changes are believed to be central to the development of leukemia.

EPIDEMIOLOGY

- Males are generally affected by leukemia slightly more often than females in all but infants' age groups.
- In developed countries, the incidence of ALL is highest between ages 2 and 5 years.
- The incidence of AML is relatively constant during childhood, with slight peaks in the first 2 years of life and in late adolescence.

CLINICAL FINDINGS

- Physical signs and symptoms of thrombocytopenia and anemia are common.
- Neutropenia can lead to severe infection.
- Bone pain and arthralgia caused by leukemic infiltration are more common in ALL than in AML and can be especially severe in young children.
- Common sites of extramedullary involvement in ALL include liver, spleen, thymus, and lymph nodes.

- Skin, gums, and the head and neck area are typical sites of extramedullary disease in AML.
- Infiltration of the central nervous system can be found in both ALL and AML.

DIFFERENTIAL DIAGNOSIS

- The acute onset of petechiae, ecchymoses, and bleeding could suggest idiopathic thrombocytopenic purpura.
- Both acute leukemia and aplastic anemia can present with pancytopenia and complications associated with bone marrow failure.
- Infectious mononucleosis and other viral infections can be confused with ALL.
- Bone pain, arthralgia, and occasionally arthritis can mimic juvenile rheumatoid arthritis, rheumatic fever, other collagen diseases, or osteomyelitis.
- Childhood ALL should also be distinguished from pediatric small round cell tumors that involve the bone marrow.

THERAPY

- Patients with ALL undergo a relatively brief remission-induction phase followed by intensification (consolidation) therapy and then prolonged continuation treatment.
- All patients require treatment for subclinical central nervous system (CNS) involvement, which should be initiated early in the form of intrathecal chemotherapy.
- Most protocols for AML include remission induction and consolidation therapy, although other postremission therapy differs widely between studies.
- Autologous hematopoietic stem cell transplantation is not usually recommended. At present, childhood ALL with the Philadelphia

chromosome or early hematologic relapse, and T-cell ALL with poor early response or hematologic relapse are clear indications for allogeneic transplantation.
- Allogeneic transplantation appears to improve overall survival in AML, although the indications for this procedure during first remission are debated.

PROGNOSIS

- Five-year event-free survival estimates for children with newly diagnosed ALL are now as high as 83%.
- Philadelphia chromosome is an unfavorable prognostic indicator, whereas hyperdiploidy with greater than 50 chromosomes and the *TEL-AML1* gene fusion are associated with a lower risk of relapse.
- Event-free survival for infants with ALL, especially those with 11q23/*MLL* rearrangement, remains at only 20% to 35% and has not been improved by allogeneic transplantation.
- In children with AML, patients with Down syndrome or acute promyelocytic leukemia have a favorable prognosis with optimal therapy, whereas patients with acute megakaryoblastic leukemia have significantly worse outcomes than others.
- Relapse less than 18 months after the end of therapy and treatment-related AML carry a dismal prognosis.
- Patients with myelodysplastic syndrome (MDS), AML arising from MDS, or AML with monosomy 7 often have resistant disease.
- Slow response to remission induction therapy and persistent minimal residual disease are associated with a higher risk of relapse in both ALL and AML.

INTRODUCTION

Leukemia is the most common childhood cancer in developed countries. Unlike leukemia in adults, childhood leukemia is acute in the vast majority of cases. The most common subtype, acute lymphoblastic (also termed *lymphocytic* or *lymphoid*) leukemia (ALL), accounts for 75% to 80% of all cases of childhood leukemia, whereas acute myeloid (also termed *myelocytic*, *myelogenous*, or *nonlymphoblastic*) leukemia (AML) accounts for approximately 20%. The much less common chronic leukemias include chronic myelogenous leukemia (CML), juvenile chronic myelomonocytic leukemia, and extremely rare cases of chronic lymphocytic leukemia (CLL). Acute leukemia, the focus of this chapter, is a malignant proliferation and accumulation of immature lymphohematopoietic cells. The leukemic cell population is shown to be clonal by cytogenetics, glucose-6-phosphate dehydrogenase characterization, and analysis of antigen-receptor gene rearrangements and X-linked restriction fragment-length polymorphisms.[1,2]

Although leukemic cells generally do not proliferate as actively as their normal hematopoietic counterparts, they accumulate inexorably and compete successfully with normal cells.[3,4] Their inability to differentiate and their relative resistance to apoptosis could explain this phenomenon. By the time of diagnosis, leukemic cells have usually replaced normal bone marrow cells and have disseminated to various extramedullary sites. Therefore, the presenting features of leukemia typically reflect the degree of bone marrow replacement and the extent of extramedullary spread.

Both ALL and AML are heterogeneous diseases that comprise different biologic subtypes. The major morphologic and immunophenotypic divisions based on lineage association and degree of maturation are subclassified by the identification of distinct, recurrent chromosomal and molecular abnormalities and gene expression patterns.[5-10]

EPIDEMIOLOGY

Leukemia is the most common malignancy among patients less than 15 years of age. ALL is approximately five times more common than AML. Males are generally affected by leukemia slightly more often than females in all age groups, with two exceptions: Boys have a risk of T-cell leukemia that is four times that of girls, and girls have a slightly higher incidence of leukemia in the first year of life (1.5:1 ratio).[11] Rates of ALL are comparatively higher in Northern and Western Europe, North America, and Oceania than in Asia and Africa.[12] In developed countries, the incidence of ALL is highest between ages 2 and 5 years. This age peak is accounted for largely by ALL with hyperdiploidy (>50 chromosomes) or *TEL-AML1* gene fusion.[6] The incidence of ALL is higher in the white than in the black population, especially among children 2 to 5 years of age. Black children have a higher incidence of T-cell ALL and pre-B leukemia with *E2A-PBX1* fusion and are less likely than white children to have hyper-

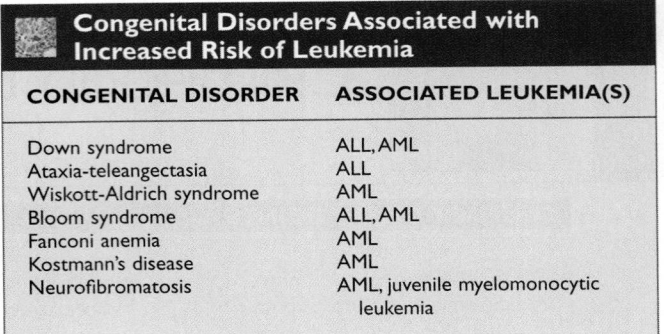

TABLE 101-1

Congenital Disorders Associated with Increased Risk of Leukemia	
CONGENITAL DISORDER	**ASSOCIATED LEUKEMIA(S)**
Down syndrome	ALL, AML
Ataxia-teleangectasia	ALL
Wiskott-Aldrich syndrome	AML
Bloom syndrome	ALL, AML
Fanconi anemia	AML
Kostmann's disease	AML
Neurofibromatosis	AML, juvenile myelomonocytic leukemia

diploid ALL with greater than 50 chromosomes. The incidence of AML in children peaks at 2 years of age, decreases to a nadir at 9 years, then peaks again at around age 16.[13] The highest incidence of pediatric AML occurs among the Maori of New Zealand, Hawaiian Americans, and Africans in Zimbabwe. In most populations of children, less than 10% of cases of AML are acute promyelocytic leukemia.[13] This figure, however, is approximately 25% in Latin American children and about 30% in Italian children.[14,15]

A small percentage (<5%) of cases of leukemia are associated with inherited genetic syndromes (Table 101-1). Children with Down syndrome have a 10- to 20-fold increased risk of leukemia (ALL and AML).[11,16] Several other genetic disorders are associated with an increased risk of ALL and AML, including ataxia-telangiectasia, Wiscott-Aldrich syndrome, Bloom syndrome, Fanconi anemia, Kostmann's disease, and neurofibromatosis.[11,13,16,17] The association between leukemia and congenital immunodeficiencies, such as X-linked agammaglobulinemia and common variable immunodeficiency, is not well supported.[17]

Fraternal twins and siblings of affected children are at a two- to fourfold greater risk of leukemia during the first decade of life than are unrelated children.[11,12] When leukemia occurs in one identical twin, the likelihood that the other twin will develop the disease is approximately 20%. On the other hand, when leukemia is diagnosed in one twin before 1 year of age, it almost invariably develops in the other twin, typically within a few months. Molecular studies have demonstrated that intrauterine metastasis of ALL from one twin to the other via the shared placental circulation is responsible for the concordant leukemia.[18-23]

ETIOLOGY AND PATHOGENESIS

Although environmental agents, such as ionizing radiation and chemical mutagens, have been implicated in the induction of leukemia, discernible etiologic factors are lacking in almost all cases of primary leukemia.[12,16] Association between leukemia and maternal exposure to various potential mutagens, neonatal administration of vitamin K, parental use of medications and drugs, and proximity to electromagnetic fields has not been authoritatively demonstrated.[12,16] Because higher socioeconomic status and social isolation are associated with an increased risk of B-lineage ALL, Greaves hypothesized that many cases of childhood B-lineage ALL are the consequence of abnormally late exposure to (and thus immune response to) common infections, a scenario that could enhance the likelihood of leukemogenic genetic mutations.[24] In line with this notion is the observation of an increased risk of childhood ALL associated with rural-urban population mixing, presumably caused by a dysregulation of host immune response to infection.[25]

Infant leukemias frequently involve the *MLL* gene, located on chromosome band 11q23.[26] *MLL* rearrangements are also common in therapy-related AML, arising shortly after treatment with topoisomerase II inhibitors.[27] The similarity of molecular genetic abnormalities in infant leukemias and topoisomerase II inhibitor-related leukemias raises the possibility that transplacental fetal exposure to substances that inhibit topoisomerase II, such as flavonoids (in food and drink), quinolone antibiotics, benzene metabolites, catechins, and estrogens, is leukemogenic.[26,28] A recent case-control study found that in utero exposure to DNA-damaging drugs, herbal medicines, or pesticides was significantly associated with infant leukemia with *MLL* rearrangements.[29] Because the functional doses received via dietary and environmental exposure are much lower than those received from anticancer chemotherapy, infant or maternal carcinogen-detoxifying enzymes might have reduced activity due to genetic polymorphism in these cases. For example, deficiency of glutathione S-transferases (GST-M1 and GST-T1), enzymes that detoxify electrophilic metabolites by catalyzing their conjugation to glutathione, is associated with infant leukemia without *MLL* rearrangement and with ALL in black children.[26,30] Polymorphisms of another enzyme, reduced nicotinamide adenine dinucleotide phosphate: quinone oxidoreductase, which converts benzoquinones to less toxic hydroxyl metabolites, have been asociated with the development of infant and childhood ALL.[31,32] Cytochrome P-450 CYP1A1*2A and NQO1*2 variant genotypes have also been linked to an increased risk of childhood ALL; children carrying both genotypes are at a particularly high risk.[33] Recent studies also have suggested that folate pathways could play a role in susceptibility to ALL and that folate supplement might reduce the risk, an intriguing finding that requires confirmation.[34-36]

Acquired genetic changes are believed to be central to the development of leukemia.[5] These changes affect the number (ploidy) and/or the structure of chromosomes; structural changes comprise translocations, inversions, deletions, point mutations, and amplifications. The dysregulation of transcription factors that regulate hematopoietic cell homeostasis is a plausible mechanism of leukemogenesis. For example, the core binding factor (CBF) family of transcription factors regulates the expression of growth factors, such as interleukin-3, granulocyte-macrophage colony stimulating factor, and macrophage colony-stimulating factor receptor, as well as the T-cell receptor β enhancer and the immunoglobulin heavy chain enhancer/promoter. CBF function is disrupted by recurrent chromosomal translocations, such

as those involving *TEL-AML1* in ALL and *AML1-ETO* and *CBFB-MYH11* in AML.[37,38] The function of homeobox (HOX) genes, an evolutionarily highly conserved family of transcription factors whose expression is tightly regulated during hematopoietic cell differentiation, can also be disrupted either by direct involvement in chromosomal translocations [e.g., the t(7;11), forming the *NUP98-HOXA9* fusion gene] or by the disruption of proteins believed to be their upstream regulators.[5,38] Among the latter, the most notable is encoded by *MLL*, a gene crucial for both embryonic development and hematopoiesis, which is involved in translocations of the 11q23 region in both ALL and AML.[5,38] Moreover, *PBX1*, a gene involved with *E2A* in the t(1;19) typical of pre-B ALL, encodes a common partner of HOX proteins.[5] Chimeric proteins encoded by fused genes can also interfere directly with normal apoptotic pathways, as has been demonstrated in the case of the E2A-HLF protein.[39] Further, cell survival requirements can be altered by the dysregulated activity of tyrosine kinases, as in the case of the *BCR-ABL* gene fusion.[40]

The expression of essential molecules also can be altered in the absence of detectable genetic abnormalities. For example, five different T-cell oncogenes (*HOX11*, *TAL1*, *LYL1*, *LMO1*, and *LMO2*) often are expressed aberrantly in T-lineage ALL in the absence of chromosomal abnormalities.[8] Abnormal expression and function of molecules that regulate apoptosis, such as BCL-2 and BAX, also have been described.[41-43] Finally, mutant tyrosine kinase receptors for growth factors could confer a growth advantage to leukemic cells. This mechanism is best exemplified by mutations of FLT3, a receptor tyrosine kinase expressed by immature hematopoietic cells, which acts synergistically with other growth factors to stimulate proliferation of hematopoietic progenitor cells.[44] Mutant FLT3 has been detected in approximately 30% of cases of AML and a small percentage of cases of ALL; these mutations typically involve small tandem duplications of amino acids that result in constitutive tyrosine kinase activity.[45] Expression of a mutant FLT3 receptor in murine bone marrow cells results in a myeloproliferative syndrome.[44]

The retrospective identification of leukemia-specific fusion genes (e.g. *MLL-AF4*, *TEL-AML1*) in the neonatal blood spots of identical twins who experienced concordant leukemia has shown that some leukemias have a prenatal origin.[22] In cases with the t(4;11) translocation and *MLL-AF4*, the high rate of concordance in identical twins (25%–100%) and the very brief latency period after birth (a few weeks to a few months) suggest that this fusion alone is either leukemogenic or able to induce changes that are directly leukemogenic.[46] In other types of leukemia—for example, those with the *TEL-AML1* fusion or T-cell phenotype—the rate of concordance is lower, the postnatal latency period is longer and is variable, and the clinical presentation and outcome of therapy can differ widely among identical twins; these facts suggest that secondary postnatal molecular events are necessary for full leukemic transformation.[46] Further insights were gained from a recent report of a set of triplets in which the two monozygotic twins developed concordant leukemia with identical *TEL-AML1* fusion at 3 years of age, while the third child, who had developed from a second zygote, was free of leukemia and of the genomic sequence.[23] In addition to the fusion transcript, the identical twins had a secondary, independent deletion of the normal unrearranged *TEL* allele, suggesting a different postnatal event. Clone-specific antigen receptor gene rearrangements were analyzed in the neonatal blood spots of five children who were aged 6 months to 4 years and 8 months, respectively, at diagnosis of B-lineage ALL and T-ALL. In all five children, the clonotypic antigen receptor gene rearrangements had been present at birth. The estimated number of clonotypic cells per blood spot was in the range of 10 to 100.[47] Recently, Mori and colleagues[48] demonstrated that the *TEL-AML1* fusion is present in the cord blood of about 1% of randomly selected newborns, a frequency about 100 times that of ALL with *TEL-AML1*. This finding further supports the notion that preleukemic clones are generated in utero at a high frequency and that secondary postnatal leukemogenic events are required for a fully malignant transformation of *TEL-AML1* cells. The prevalence of leukemias with prenatal origin is not known. Clearly, not all cases develop in utero. For example, t(1;19) *E2A-PBX1* ALL appears to have a postnatal origin in most cases.[49]

GENERAL CLINICAL AND LABORATORY FEATURES

Physical examination of children with leukemia can reveal pallor, petechiae, ecchymoses, and mucosal bleeding. If thrombocytopenia and hyperleukocytosis are severe, there can be life-threatening bleeding (e.g., intracranial hematoma). Anemia can cause fatigue and lethargy, dyspnea, angina, and dizziness. Neutropenia can lead to severe infection. Bone pain and arthralgia caused by leukemic infiltration or, less frequently, by hemorrhage is more common in ALL than in AML and can be especially severe in young children. Patients can present with fever, which could be induced by infection or by pyrogenic cytokines (e.g., interleukin-1, interleukin-6, and tumor necrosis factor) released from the leukemic cells. The liver, spleen, thymus, and lymph nodes are common sites of extramedullary involvement; in AML, however, massive hepatosplenomegaly is common only in infants. Infiltration of the central nervous system is seen in children with ALL or AML. An anterior mediastinal (thymic) mass is typical of T-cell ALL. Painless enlargement of the scrotum can be a sign of testicular leukemia or hydrocele resulting from lymphatic obstruction. Testicular involvement is rare in AML. In patients with AML, common sites of extramedullary disease include the skin, gums, and the neck and head area. Myeloblastomas (granulocytic sarcomas, chloromas) are solid tumors composed of myeloblasts that could precede overt bone marrow involvement of AML. They typically occur in the skin, soft tissue, bones, and central nervous system but can develop in virtually any tissue or organ.[50] Very rarely, acute leukemia produces no signs or symptoms and is detected during routine examination.

Anemia, neutropenia, and thrombocytopenia are common findings, and their severity reflects the degree of bone marrow replacement by leukemic cells. The presenting leukocyte count ranges from 0.1 to 1500 × 10^9/L (median, 10 to 12 × 10^9/L); hyperleukocytosis (>100 × 10^9/L) occurs in 15% to 18% of cases of ALL and AML. Most patients have circulating leukemic blast cells. A large leukemic cell burden is commonly accompanied by elevated serum lactate dehydogenase activity and elevated uric acid and phosphorous concentration. Some patients with T-cell ALL have normal red blood cell and platelet counts. In these cases, the lymphoblasts in the bone marrow usually represent the leukemic phase of an extramedullary lymphoblastic lymphoma. Not infrequently, the marrow contains a significant population of myeloblasts, which can be difficult to distinguish morphologically from the leukemic cells.

Leukemic blast cells are identified at diagnosis in the cerebrospinal fluid (CSF) of as many as one third of children with ALL (most of whom have no neurologic symptoms) and in approximately 5% of children with AML. Traditionally, central nervous system (CNS) leukemia is defined by the presence of at least five leukocytes per microliter of CSF and the detection of leukemic blast cells, or by the presence of cranial nerve palsy. Recent studies, however, have demonstrated that the presence of any amount of leukemic cells in CSF, even from iatrogenic introduction due to a traumatic lumbar puncture, is associated with an increased risk of ALL relapse and requires additional intrathecal therapy.[51]

DIFFERENTIAL DIAGNOSIS

The acute onset of petechiae, ecchymoses, and bleeding could suggest idiopathic thrombocytopenic purpura (often associated with a recent viral infection, large platelets in blood smears, and no evidence of anemia). Both acute leukemia and aplastic anemia can present with pancytopenia and complications associated with bone marrow failure, but in aplastic anemia, hepatosplenomegaly and lymphadenopathy are rare, and the skeletal changes associated with leukemia are absent.

Infectious mononucleosis and other viral infections can be confused with ALL. Detection of atypical lymphocytes or elevated viral titers aid in the diagnosis. Patients with pertussis or parapertussis can have marked lymphocytosis, but the affected cells are mature lymphocytes rather than lymphoblasts. Bone pain, arthralgia, and occasionally arthritis can mimic juvenile rheumatoid arthritis, rheumatic fever, other collagen diseases, or osteomyelitis.

Childhood ALL should also be distinguished from pediatric small round cell tumors that involve the bone marrow, which include neuroblastoma, rhabdomyosarcoma, and retinoblastoma. Generally, in such cases, a primary lesion can be found by routine diagnostic studies, and disseminated tumor cells often form clumps.

MORPHOLOGIC AND CYTOCHEMICAL ANALYSIS

Morphologic analysis of leukemic cells in smears stained with Romanowsky (Wright-Giemsa or May-Grünwald-

ALL   AML

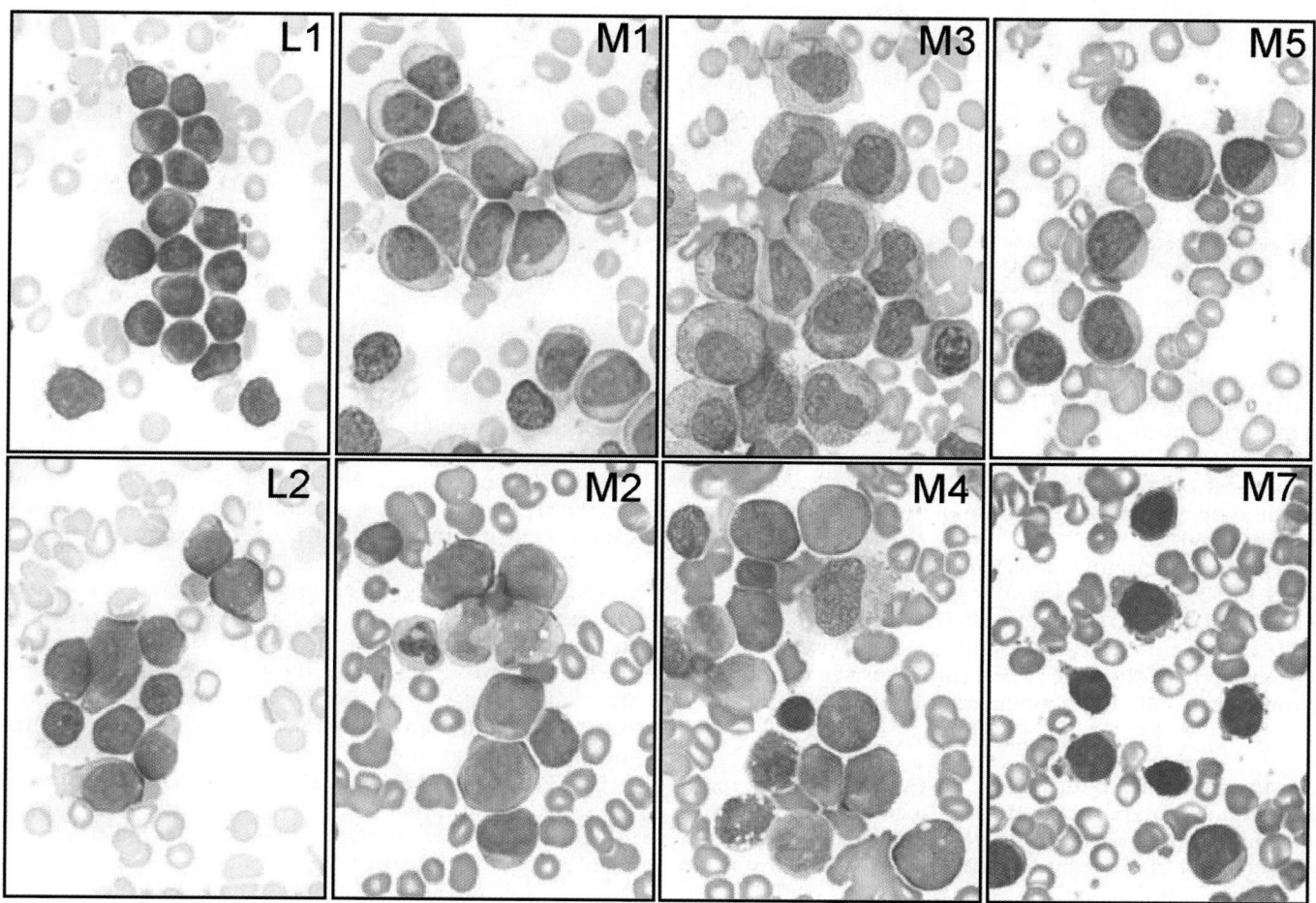

Figure 101-1. Morphology of leukemic cells. Bone marrow smears obtained at diagnosis from children with ALL or AML were stained with Wright-Giemsa. The morphologic classification according to the French-Amercan-British criteria is shown. (Courtesy of Dr. F.G. Behm, St. Jude Children's Research Hospital.)

Giemsa) stain distinguishes three subtypes of ALL (L1, L2, and L3) and eight subtypes of AML (M0–M7) as classified by the French-American-British (FAB) scheme (Fig. 101-1).[52] The term *acute myeloid leukemia* is used to designate even leukemias in which some or all cells have the morphology of monocytes (M4, M5), erythroblasts (M6), or megakaryoblasts (M7).

Analysis of a Romanowsky-stained smear cannot distinguish accurately between ALL and AML. Cytochemical stains aid in this distinction. Myeloperoxidase, Sudan black, and nonspecific esterases (including alpha naphthyl butyrate and alpha naphthyl acetate esterase) react with myeloid blast cells, while periodic acid-Schiff reagent reacts positively in more than 70% of ALL cases. Despite the traditional use of morphology and cytochemistry, however, contemporary classification of acute leukemias is based on subtypes that can be identified only by immunologic and molecular analyses.

IMMUNOLOGIC CLASSIFICATION

Acute Lymphoblastic Leukemia (ALL)

Table 101-2 summarizes antigen expression patterns in ALL.

Early Pre-B ALL

Leukemic blast cells of early pre-B ALL resemble normal marrow B-cell precursors. Although immunoglobulin heavy-chain genes usually are rearranged in these cells, immunoglobulins are not detectable. The leukemic cells of early pre-B ALL always express CD19. Almost all cases have cytoplasmic CD22 and CD79a; weak surface CD22 expression is also evident in many cases.[53-57] CD10 and terminal deoxynucleotidyl transferase (TdT) are detectable in 90% of cases, and cells in more than 75% of

Specific Malignancies

III

TABLE 101-2

Immunophenotypic Subgroups of ALL[111]

| SUBTYPE | ANTIGEN EXPRESSION (% OF CASES POSITIVE) | | | | | | | | | | FREQUENCY (%) |
	CD19	CCD22	CD79A	CD10	CD7	CD5	CCD3	CIG μ	SIG μ	SIG κ OR λ	
Early pre-B	100	>95*	>95	95	5	0	0	0	0	0	60–65
Pre-B	100	100*	100	>95	0	<2	0	100	0	0	20–25
Transitional pre-B	100	100*	100	50	0	0	0	100	100	0	1–3
B	100	100*	100	50	0	0	0	>95	>95	>95	2–3
T	<5	0	30	45	100	95	100*	0	0	0	15–18

c, cytoplasmic; clg μ, cytoplasmic immunoglobulin μ chain; slg μ, surface immunoglobulin μ chain; slg κ or λ, surface immunoglobulin κ or λ chain.
*Detectable on the cell surface membrane in some cases.

cases express CD34.[58,59] The CD20 antigen is present on a minor proportion of blast cells in one half of cases.[58] In 10% to 15% of early pre-B ALL cases, CD45 is very weakly expressed or undetectable; cells that have this immunophenotype are usually hyperdiploid (modal chromosome number >50).[60]

ALL with rearrangement of the *MLL* gene is usually early pre-B ALL.[58] Cases with t(4;11) typically are CD19+, CD22+, CD10−, CD15+, and CD65+.[61] Almost all B-lineage ALL cases and more than half of AML cases with rearrangement of the *MLL* gene express surface chondroitin protoglycan sulfate, a nonhematopoietic molecule.[62]

Pre-B ALL

About 25% of newly diagnosed cases of ALL have a pre-B immunophenotype consisting of accumulation of cytoplasmic immunoglobulin μ heavy chains with no detectable surface immunoglobulins.[58,63] Like early pre-B ALL, this subtype expresses CD19, CD22, and CD79a. Rearrangement of immunoglobulin light-chain genes is evident in some of these leukemias, but κ and λ proteins are not detectable. More than 95% of pre-B ALL express CD10 and TdT, but only two thirds express CD34.[64] In many cases of pre-B ALL, surface CD20 is absent or is weakly expressed.

Between 20% and 25% of pre-B ALL cases have either the t(1;19)(q23;p13) or the der(19)t(1;19)(q23;p13).[65] The antigen expression profile CD19+, CD22+, CD20±, CD34−, CD45+, cytoplasmic μ+ is characteristic of ALL cases with the t(1;19) but is not specific to these cases.[65,66]

Transitional (or Late) Pre-B ALL

Leukemic cells that express both cytoplasmic and surface immunoglobulin μ heavy chains without κ or λ light chains have been designated transitional pre-B ALL.[67] The surface μ chains on these leukemic cells are linked to pseudo light chains and to CD79a and CD79b. The blast cells express CD10, usually TdT, and sometimes CD34. Initial studies found this phenotype in only 1% of childhood ALL cases, but it could be more common if more sensitive reagents are used. There is no chromosomal abnormality that is characteristic of this subgroup of ALL.[67]

B-Cell ALL

In 2% to 4% of childhood ALL cases, cells express surface immunoglobulin μ heavy chains plus either κ or λ light chains. The most common type of B-cell ALL is characterized by L3 morphology according to the FAB classification; cells express CD19, CD22, CD20, and frequently CD10 and CD23; CD34 is negative. In rare cases, TdT is expressed, or sIg is absent.[68-71] Often, these cases represent the leukemic phase of Burkitt lymphoma arising in the abdomen or in the head and neck. The hallmark of this subset of B-cell ALL is the presence of a reciprocal translocation of chromosome 8 with one of the chromosomes containing an immunoglobulin gene. These translocations, which include the t(8;14)(q24;q32), t(2;8)(p12;q24), and t(8;22)(q24;q11), involve rearrangement of the c-*MYC* gene.

The less common subtype of B-cell ALL is characterized by blast cells with L1 or L2 morphology. These leukemias may express TdT and CD34, and they express CD20 only weakly.[72,73] Extramedullary masses are not seen at presentation. The t(8;14), t(2;8), and t(8;22) are absent, as are characteristic rearrangements of the c-*MYC* gene.

T-Lineage ALL

T-lineage ALL cells have surface CD7 and cytoplasmic CD3 (cCD3) antigens.[54,74-76] More than 90% of T lymphoblasts express CD2, CD5, and TdT. Surface CD1a, CD3, CD4, and CD8 are detected in fewer than 45% of cases.[77] The HLA-DR antigen is not commonly expressed, and 40% to 45% of cases are CD10+ and/or CD21+.[77,78]

T-lineage ALL can be divided into three stages of immunophenotypic differentiation: early (CD7+, cCD3+, surface CD3−, CD4−, and CD8−), mid or common (cCD3+, surface CD3−, CD4+, CD8+, and CD1+), and late (surface CD3+, CD1−, and either CD4+ or CD8+). As many as 25% of cases of T-lineage ALL have antigen patterns that do not conform to any of these maturation stages, however. Further, several studies have yielded conflicting conclusions about the prognostic significance of the expression of surface CD3 and the absence of CD2, CD5, or CD10.[77,79-81] In a study of children with T-cell ALL at our institution, expression of CD10 was associated independently with a favorable clinical outcome.[77]

T-cell receptor (TCR) proteins are heterogeneously expressed in T-lineage ALL.[82,83] In approximately two thirds of cases, membrane CD3 and TCR proteins are absent. In half of these cases, however, TCR proteins (TCRβ, TCRα, or both) are present in the cells' cytoplasm. Most cases with membrane CD3 and TCR chains express the αβ form of the TCR, whereas a minority express TCRγδ proteins.

Acute Myeloid Leukemia

Table 101-3 summarizes the patterns of antigen expression in AML. The leukemic cells in all myelocytic and monocytic subtypes of AML (M0 through M5) express various combinations of CD13, CD33, CD65, CD117, and myeloperoxidase (MPO).[84-87]

Acute Myelocytic Leukemia with Little Differentiation (M1 AML)
M1 AML cases commonly express MPO, CD13, CD33, CD34, CD65, CD117, and HLA-DR, but in variable combinations. Expression of CD4, CD11b, CD15, and CD66 is less frequent. No single antigenic profile is characteristic of M1 leukemias.

Acute Myelocytic Leukemia with Differentiation (M2 AML)
About 35% to 45% of cases of childhood M2 AML have the t(8;21)(q22;q22). Leukemic blast cells commonly express MPO, CD34, CD65, and HLA-DR, but CD13 and CD33 expression is characteristically weak and sometimes is not detectable.[88-90] Most cases weakly express CD19 and, less commonly, CD56.[88,90,91] By contrast, the leukemic myeloblasts of M2 AML without the t(8;21) can also express MPO, CD34, CD65, and HLA-DR, but the expression of CD13 and CD33 usually exceeds that of myeloblasts that have the t(8;21). In addition, the CD19 antigen is often detectable, and T-cell–associated CD2 or CD7 is commonly present in these cases.[90]

Acute Promyelocytic Leukemia (M3 AML)
This group of leukemias includes a microgranular variant referred to as M3v that morphologically can mimic acute monocytic leukemia. Cells of M3 and M3v AML strongly express MPO, CD13, CD33, and CD65 but usually do not express CD34 or HLA-DR.[84,92] Expression of CD11b and CD15 is variable, and CD4 and CD56 are seldom detected.[93,94] Atypical expression of CD2 is observed in 40% to 45% of cases but may be more prevalent in the M3v subtype.[92,95,96] Heterogeneous expression of CD13, the existence of a single primary blast cell population, and a characteristic pattern of CD34 and CD15 expression are reportedly also useful in identifying M3 AML.[97]

Acute Myelomonocytic Leukemia (M4 AML)
Blast cells of most myelomonocytic leukemias express MPO, CD4, CD11b, CD11c, CD13, CD14, CD33, CD34, CD45, CD65, and HLA-DR. In adult patients with AML, the M4 and M5 leukemias are the subtypes that most frequently express CD19.[98]

A relatively uncommon variant of M4 AML, M4Eo, is associated with increased numbers of eosinophils in the bone marrow, with or without peripheral blood eosinophilia. These cases usually express the *CBFB-MYH11* chimeric gene, which is often associated with expression of CD2.[99,100]

Acute Monocytic Leukemia (M5 AML)
Monoblasts usually express MPO, HLA-DR, CD4, CD11b, CD11c, CD33, and CD65. The cells of some monocytic leukemias express CD117, but CD34 is detected only rarely. The cells of most monocytic leukemias also express CD15, CD36, and, not infrequently, CD56. Expression of CD14 is restricted largely to cells of the monocytic lineage but is often absent in pediatric M5 cases. A variable number of monoblasts might appear to react weakly with antibodies to CD41a and CD61 because of the adhesion of platelets to their surfaces or their adsorption of glycoprotein IIb/IIIa.[101]

Acute Erythroleukemia (M6 AML) and Acute Erythroblastic Leukemia
Leukemias composed primarily of erythroid precursors are uncommon. Leukemic erythroblasts usually express CD36, CD71, and glycophorin A (GPA), and hemoglobin is detectable in late-stage erythroid precursors. Cells of the

TABLE 101-3

| Immunophenotype of AML Subtypes[111] | | | | | | | | | | | | |

FAB SUBTYPE	ANTIGEN EXPRESSION (APPROXIMATE % OF CASES POSITIVE FOR MARKER)											
	CD34	CD117	HLADR	MPO	CD13	CD33	CD15	CD65	CD14	GPA	CD36	CD41A
M0	75	75	75	>80	75	75	30	30	0	0	0	0
M1	75	75	75	>80	75	75	75	75	0	0	0	0
M2	75	75	>80	>80	>80	>80	75	75	0	0	0	0
M3	<10	30	<10	>80	>80	>80	75	75	0	0	0	0
M4	75	75	>80	>80	75	>80	75	>80	75	0	30	0
M5	<10	30	>80	>80	75	>80	75	>80	75	0	75	0
M6	30	30	75	>80	75	75	30	75	0	>80	75	0
M7	30	30	30	0	30	75	30	<10	0	<10	75	>80

FAB, French-American-British classification; GPA, glycophorin A; MPO, myeloperoxidase.

myeloid component express CD13, CD33, and MPO. M6 AML can be difficult to distinguish from M0 and M7 AML, because undifferentiated erythroblasts have few or no erythroid-associated antigens, and their antigenic and ultrastructural features could mimic those of early megakaryoblasts.

Acute Megakaryoblastic Leukemia (M7 AML)

The leukemic cells of most M7 AML cases express CD41a and CD61, and those of more than half of M7 AML cases express detectable CD42b.[102,103] Most cases are positive for CD4 and CD33; CD13, CD34, CD36, CD45, and HLA-DR are detected infrequently. The morphologic differential diagnosis of megakaryoblastic leukemia includes ALL, M0 and M5 AML, acute erythroblastic leukemia, and metastatic small-cell tumor.

Acute Myeloid Leukemia without Morphologic or Cytochemical Evidence of Differentiation (M0 AML)

The term *M0* denotes minimally differentiated myeloid leukemia.[104] In general, the expression of CD3, CD79a, or TCR proteins is strongly indicative of lymphoid lineage differentiation. In the absence of these lymphoid markers and of markers associated with the megakaryocytic lineage, the expression of CD13, CD15, CD33, CD65, or MPO is evidence of myeloid lineage commitment. Leukemias that are devoid of detectable MPO should be classified as M0 AML only in the absence of lineage-restricted lymphoid and megakaryocytic antigens. Although the cells of most M0 cases express CD13 or CD33, some MPO+ cases might lack these antigens.[105] The expression of CD117 by leukemic cells is strongly suggestive of AML. Other non-lineage–restricted antigens found on M0 AML cells include CD2, CD4, CD7, CD9, CD10, CD11b, CD19, CD34, CD71, TdT, and HLA-DR.[105]

Acute Undifferentiated or Unclassifiable Leukemia

Rare cases of leukemia remain difficult to classify even after extensive morphologic and immunophenotypic analysis; these are designated acute undifferentiated (or unclassified) leukemia (AUL). Morphologically, these leukemias might resemble ALL or AML, and immunophenotyping studies show the absence of B-lymphoid, T-lymphoid, myeloid, and megakaryocytic antigens.[106] The leukemic cells of true AUL lack surface and cytoplasmic antigens associated with B (CD19, CD22, and CD79), T (CD2, CD3, CD5, and TCR proteins), myelomonocytic (MPO, CD13, CD14, CD33, CD15, and CD65), and megakaryocytic or erythrocytic (CD36, CD41a, CD42b, CD61, and GPA) lineages. Diagnostic studies should also exclude neuroblastoma, Ewing sarcoma, and other small cell tumors.

Acute Leukemias with Aberrant Lymphoid or Myeloid Antigen Expression

Immunologic and molecular studies show that many leukemias possess features characteristic of multiple hematopoietic lineages. Acute leukemias whose blast cells simultaneously demonstrate features of more than one lineage (e.g., lymphoid plus myeloid) have been termed *acute mixed-lineage*, *hybrid*, *chimeric*, or *biphenotypic leukemias*.[107-110] The diagnosis of B-lineage ALL should be made when leukemic cells express either cytoplasmic immunoglobulin or CD79a or CD19 plus CD22, regardless of CD13, CD15, CD33, or CD65 expression.[111] The diagnosis of T-lineage ALL should be made when leukemic cells express CD7 plus either surface or cytoplasmic CD3, regardless of myeloid antigen expression. A diagnosis of AML is rendered when leukemic cells express MPO or two or more myeloid-associated antigens, including CD13, CD15, CD33, or CD65, in the absence of the lymphoid-associated markers designated previously. An immunophenotypic diagnosis of "true" mixed-lineage leukemia should be considered when leukemic blast cells co-express MPO and CD3, MPO and immunoglobulin, or MPO and CD79a. "True" mixed-lineage leukemia should not be confused with biclonal or oligoclonal leukemias, which consist of two or more morphologically or immunophenotypically distinct leukemic cell populations. The latter types of leukemia are very rare.

Expression of myeloid antigens in ALL has no independent prognostic significance in children but is associated with molecular genetic abnormalities.[112-114] Atypical expression of the myeloid-associated antigen CD15 is characteristic of B-lineage ALL with the t(4;11) translocation. Lymphoid antigen expression in AML cells also lacks prognostic significance in children.[113,115]

CYTOGENETIC AND MOLECULAR CLASSIFICATION

Acute Lymphoblastic Leukemia (Fig. 101-2)

Hyperdiploid ALL

In approximately half of ALL cases, leukemic blast cells have a modal chromosomal number greater than 46. Hyperdiploidy can be identified by conventional karyotyping or by DNA content analysis with flow cytometry.[116] In approximately 50% of hyperdiploid cases, the leukemic cells have additional structural chromosomal abnormalities, including duplication of 1q and isochromosome of 17q; however, no consistent structural abnormality has been identified. Recent data suggest that hyperdiploidy occurs early in leukemogenesis.[117]

Hyperdiploid cases with a modal chromosome number of 51 to 65 represent a distinct biologic subset with an excellent prognosis.[118,119] Leukemic lymphoblasts with this karyotype have a marked propensity to undergo apoptosis in vitro and in vivo.[120,121] In addition, they accumulate greater quantities of methotrexate and its active polyglutamate metabolites than do other leukemic lymphoblasts, and they reportedly have greater sensitivity to antimetabolites in vitro.[122,123] These features explain the relatively small presenting tumor burden and the good prognosis of this subtype of ALL. Trisomy of chromosomes 4, 10, and 17, a chromosome number of 56 or more, and the absence of chromosomal translocations have been correlated with the most favorable outcome, but no dis-

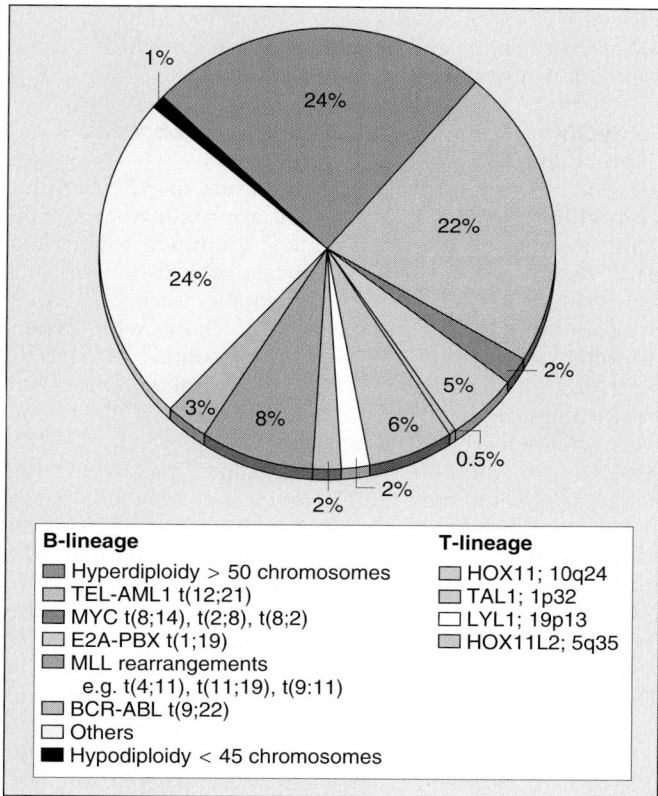

1%

24%

22%

24%

2%

5%

3%

8%

6%

0.5%

2%

2%

B-lineage
- Hyperdiploidy > 50 chromosomes
- TEL-AML1 t(12;21)
- MYC t(8;14), t(2;8), t(8;2)
- E2A-PBX t(1;19)
- MLL rearrangements
  e.g. t(4;11), t(11;19), t(9;11)
- BCR-ABL t(9;22)
- Others
- Hypodiploidy < 45 chromosomes

T-lineage
- HOX11; 10q24
- TAL1; 1p32
- LYL1; 19p13
- HOX11L2; 5q35

Figure 101-2. Cytogenetic subgroups in childhood ALL.

tinguishing biologic features were detected in this subset of hyperdiploid ALL.[120,124-127]

In contrast to the favorable prognosis of this ALL subtype, ALL cases with near-triploidy (69–81 chromosomes) have a response to therapy similar to that of nonhyperdiploid ALL; cases with near-tetraploidy (82–94 chromosomes) have a high frequency of T-cell imunophenotype.[128]

ALL with E2A-PBX1 and E2A-HLF Rearrangements
The t(1;19)(q23;p13) is found in 20% to 25% of pre-B ALL cases. The affected genes are those encoding the E2A transcription factor on chromosome 19 and the PBX1 homeodomain-containing transcription factor on chromosome 1.[129] The resulting E2A-PBX1 fusion protein contains the transcriptional activation domains of E2A linked to the DNA-binding domain of PBX1. Thus, the protein should inappropriately activate the transcription of genes normally regulated by PBX1. PBX1 is required for the maintenance of definitive hematopoiesis and contributes to the growth of subsets of hematopoietic progenitors.[130] Ectopic expression of the E2A-PBX1 chimeric protein in mice leads to the development of lymphomas and myeloid leukemias.[131,132] Some of the oncogenic potential of E2A-PBX1 could be mediated through the formation of heterocomplexes with HOX proteins. Both PBX1 and E2a-PBX1 bind to HOX proteins, and PBX1 and HOXA9 exhibit synergism in inducing leukemia in mice.[133,134]

A second E2A fusion gene is created by the t(11;17), in which E2A is fused to the gene that encodes hepatic leukemia factor (HLF).[135] HLF is a member of the bZip family of transcription factors. The E2A-HLF fusion protein contains the transcriptional activation domains of E2A linked to the DNA-binding and protein-protein interaction motifs of HLF. Thus, this chimeric protein should activate the transcription of genes normally regulated by HLF. In addition, E2A-HLF itself appears to inhibit apoptosis.[135] A zinc-finger transcriptional repressor, SLUG, which functions as an antiapoptotic factor in normal hematopoietic progenitor cells, is aberrantly upregulated by E2A-HLF.[136]

ALL with TEL-AML1 Rearrangements
The t(12;21) translocation forms a chimeric gene consisting of the 5′ portion of the TEL gene (also known as ETV6) and the nearly complete AML1 gene (also known as CBFA2).[137] This translocation can rarely be identified by conventional cytogenetic banding techniques but can frequently be detected by fluorescence in situ hybridization (FISH). The TEL-AML1 gene fusion is the most common genetic abnormality in pediatric ALL (approximately 20% of cases). In some series, the TEL-AML1 abnormality was not significantly prognostic, while in others it defined a subgroup with excellent prognosis.[138-141] ALL cells bearing this abnormality do not show a distinctive propensity to apoptosis.[120] Reportedly, however, they have an increased sensitivity to L-asparaginase in vitro.[142] It has been postulated that increased expression of CD40 and HLA-DR could render these cells more susceptible to immune surveillance.[143]

The TEL gene belongs to the Ets family of transcription factors. TEL functions as a sequence-specific DNA-binding transcription regulator. It is normally widely expressed and appears to have an essential role in yolk sac angiogenesis, neuronal development, and the establishment of bone marrow hematopoiesis.[137] AML1 encodes a transcription factor that binds DNA as a heterodimer with CBFβ and is essential for the development of definitive hematopoiesis. In addition, the TEL-AML1 protein represses AML1-mediated transcriptional activation through a dominant negative mechanism. The nontranslocated TEL allele is frequently deleted in cases with the t(12;21); this deletion could be important for leukemogenesis.[137] Retroviral transduction of murine bone marrow cells with TEL-AML1 is associated with a higher frequency of leukemia resembling ALL.[144] Notably, the TEL-AML1 fusion can be induced by apoptogenic stimuli in lymphoid cells.[145]

ALL with MLL Gene Rearrangements
Structural alterations involving band 11q23 of chromosome 11 are the most frequent cytogenetic abnormality in infant ALL.[146] In most cases, the target is a gene designated MLL, for mixed-lineage leukemia (also known as HRX, ALL-1, and HTRX1).[146] The most common 11q23 abnormality in ALL is the t(4;11), which produces a chimeric protein that contains the N-terminal portion of MLL linked in-frame to the C-terminal portion of AF-4; however, MLL has been reported in translocations with more than 40 partner genes in cases of leukemia.

MLL is crucial for embryonic development and hematopoiesis.[147] MLL normally maintains expression of specific HOX genes by binding to DNA and recruiting a histone acetylase that keeps chromatin in an open conformation, accessible to transcriptional activators.[146,148] In addition to interacting with DNA, MLL also directly interacts with the antiphosphatase SBF1, which positively regulates kinase signaling pathways.[149] The leukemia-associated alterations in MLL directly disrupt both of these crucial activities.

In a microarray analysis of gene expression in 17 cases of ALL with *MLL* rearrangement, Armstrong and coworkers[150] found expression of several genes normally expressed in hematopoietic lineages other than lymphocytes, including *FLT3* and *LMO2*. Overexpression of HOX genes, such as *HOXA9*, *HOXA5*, *HOXA4*, and *HOXC6*, was also noted. On the basis of the global pattern of gene expression, the authors concluded that despite its current designation, ALL with *MLL* rearrangement is distinct from both ALL and AML.

ALL with BCR-ABL Rearrangements

The t(9;22)(q34;q11) encodes a chimeric gene consisting of the 5′ portion of *BCR* fused to the 3′ portion of *ABL*.[151] In chronic myelogenous leukemia, breaks occur most often within the major breakpoint cluster region of *BCR* and encode a 210-kilodalton (kDa) BCR-ABL chimeric tyrosine kinase. In ALL, breaks tend to occur in the minor breakpoint cluster regions, forming a 190-kDa BCR-ABL.[152] In each fusion protein, N-terminal sequences of ABL are replaced by BCR sequences. This alteration results in a constitutively active ABL tyrosine kinase that induces aberrant signaling and activates multiple cellular pathways.[151] Expression of either chimeric protein results in malignant transformation of hematopoietic cells and causes leukemia in murine experimental systems.[153] As a group, ALL with *BCR-ABL* fusion has been consistently associated with poor response to therapy.[6]

The development of an inhibitor of the ABL kinase (known as CGP 57148B, STI571, imatinib mesylate, Gleevec, or Glivec) has provided a way to turn off molecular mechanisms that drive leukemic cell growth in this subtype of ALL.[154] Clinical results in patients with ALL and *BCR-ABL* show dramatic responses that are followed by the rapid development of resistance.[155] Shah and associates[156] identified *BCR-ABL* kinase domain mutations in 29 of 32 patients with chronic myelogenous leukemia who developed resistance to imatinib. Fifteen different amino acid substitutions affecting 13 residues in the kinase domain were found. Mutations altered either amino acids that directly contact imatinib or those postulated to prevent the inactive BCR-ABL conformational state required for imatinib binding.[156]

ALL with c-MYC Rearrangements

Most B-cell ALL cases have the t(8;14) translocation; less frequently, they have the t(2;8) or the t(8;22). These translocations juxtapose the *c-MYC* proto-oncogene on chromosome 8 with the *IgH*, *Igκ*, and *Igλ* loci on chromosomes 14, 2, and 22, respectively. These rearrangements dysregulate the expression of *c-MYC* (a transcription factor), resulting in altered cell proliferation and survival.[157] Dysregulated *c-MYC* expression in mice, in the presence of other genetic alterations, results in B-lineage leukemia/lymphoma.[158]

Subtypes of B-Lineage ALL Defined by Global Gene Expression

In gene expression microarray analysis of 327 samples from children with ALL that used approximately 12,500 gene probes, Yeoh and colleagues[9] identified expression patterns that distinguished B-lineage ALL from T-lineage ALL, confirming the results of a smaller series.[159] Moreover, among cases of B-lineage ALL, those with hyperdiploidy greater than 50 chromosomes, *BCR-ABL*, *E2A-PBX1*, *TEL-AML1*, or *MLL* gene rearrangement could be distinguished clearly.[9] Cases with *E2A-PBX1* fusion were characterized by high expression of the *C-MER* receptor tyrosine kinase (*MERTK*), a known transforming gene, suggesting that C-MER might be involved in the abnormal growth of these cells. Similarly, *HOXA9* and *MEIS1* were exclusively expressed in cases that had *MLL* rearrangements, indicating that they could be directly involved in MLL-mediated alterations in the growth of the leukemic cells. Interestingly, high expression of *MTG16*, a homolog of *ETO*, was found in cases that had the *TEL-AML1* fusion. In addition, a subgroup of 14 cases had a distinct gene expression profile but showed no consistent cytogenetic abnormality.[9] This novel subgroup of ALL had high expression of the receptor phosphatase *PTPRM* and *LHFPL2*, a gene that is a part of the *LHFP*-like gene family, the founding member of which was identified as the target of a lipoma-associated chromosomal translocation. Gene expression profiling could be used to predict relapse of ALL in this series, and, more provocatively, to predict the occurrence of treatment-related AML. These findings warrant prospective studies to validate the prognostic value of microarray analysis beyond that of conventional molecular and clinical classification.

Genetic Abnormalities in T-Cell ALL

Genes that are dysregulated in T-cell ALL include *SCL* (*TAL-1*), *LMO1* (*TTG-1*), *LMO2* (*TTG-2*), and *HOX11*.[5] As a result of the t(1;14), *SCL* (a gene involved in early hematopoiesis) is inserted into the *TCRδ* locus on chromosome 14; an internal deletion in the 5′ untranslated region of SCL is found in an additional 25% of T-lineage ALL cases.[160] This deletion juxtaposes a locus called *SIL* with the *SCL* coding region, resulting in the expression of a fused *SIL-SCL* transcript that encodes a normal SCL protein.

The t(11;14)(p15;q11) inserts *LMO1* into the *TCRA/D* locus, whereas the t(11;14)(p13;q11) places *LMO2* in this locus. The LMO1 and LMO2 proteins, which are then expressed inappropriately, contain two zinc-binding domains and participate in multiprotein DNA-binding complexes. LMO2, like SCL, plays an essential role in the development of primitive and definitive hematopoiesis.[161] Recently, activation of LMO2 by retroviral insertion in its proximity has been implicated in the development of T-cell leukemia in a patient with X-linked severe combined immunodeficiency treated with gene therapy.[162]

An additional alteration found in T-cell ALL is the deletion from chromosome 9p21 of the *INK4a* and *INK4b* genes, which encode the p16[INK4a] and p15[INK4b] inhibitors of the Cdk4 cyclin D-dependent kinase.[163] This locus, which is deleted in more than 50% of T-lineage cases, also encodes another cell cycle regulatory protein, p19[ARF], which arrests cell cycle progression through p53.[164]

In a study of 59 T-lineage ALL cases, Ferrando and coworkers[8] detected high expression of *HOX11* mRNA in 8, *TAL1* mRNA in 29, and *LYL1* mRNA in 13. Overexpression of *LMO1* or *LMO2* was observed in most samples overexpressing *TAL1*, and high levels of *LMO2* (but not of *LMO1*) were found in the *LYL1*+ samples. Ten of the 59 cases did not express abnormal levels of any of the transcription factor genes studied. By microarray analysis, *HOX11*+ cases showed increased expression of the genes associated with the early cortical thymocyte stage of differentiation, whereas the expression pattern associated with *TAL1* expression appeared to reflect the late cortical stage of thymocyte differentiation. High levels of *LYL1* expression were associated with an undifferentiated thymocyte phenotype. A number of potential associations between the expression of these genes and of molecules that regulate cell growth, leukemogenesis, and drug resistance were also disclosed.[8] A highly favorable prognosis was noted for HOX11+ cases, whose cells had a pattern of gene expression compatible with propensity to apoptosis. Expression of HOX11L2, a transcriptional regulator closely related to HOX11, is a frequent abnormality in childhood T-ALL.[8,165,166] The prognosis of this subset of T-ALL depends on the treatment, and it was associated with poor outcome in some studies.[8,166]

Acute Myeloid Leukemia (Fig. 101-3)

Acute Promyelocytic Leukemia with t(15;17)

Acute promyelocytic leukemia (APL) accounts for approximately 10% of childhood AML cases, and more than 95% of cases of APL show the presence of a t(15;17)(q22;q11) chromosomal translocation. As a result of this translocation, the retinoic acid gene (*RARA*) on chromosome 17 is fused to the *PML* gene on chromosome 15, resulting in the formation of a PML-RARA chimeric protein.[167-170] The translocation gives rise to two fusion transcripts: PML-RARA, which is expressed in all cases, and RARA-PML, which is expressed in approximately 80% of cases.[171] The t(15;17)(q22;q11) is invariably associated with APL, and the *PML-RARA* gene fusion can cause a syndrome similar to APL in transgenic mouse models.[172-174]

RARα is a ligand-regulated transcription factor that controls the transcription of many genes, some of which are involved in hematopoietic differentiation.[175] The normal function of RARα is linked to its formation of heterodimers with a member of the retinoid X receptors (RXR). Its repression is mediated through the formation of a multisubunit complex consisting of RARα, RXR, the nuclear receptor-corepressors N-CoR/SMRT and Sin3A, and a histone deacetylase.[176] Normally, retinoic acid induces a conformational change in RARα that results in the disassembly of the complex and the recruitment of transcriptional coactivators.[175] The ubiquitous protein PML resides in nuclear organelles (nuclear bodies) conjugated to the ubiquitin-like protein SUMO1.[177] PML has

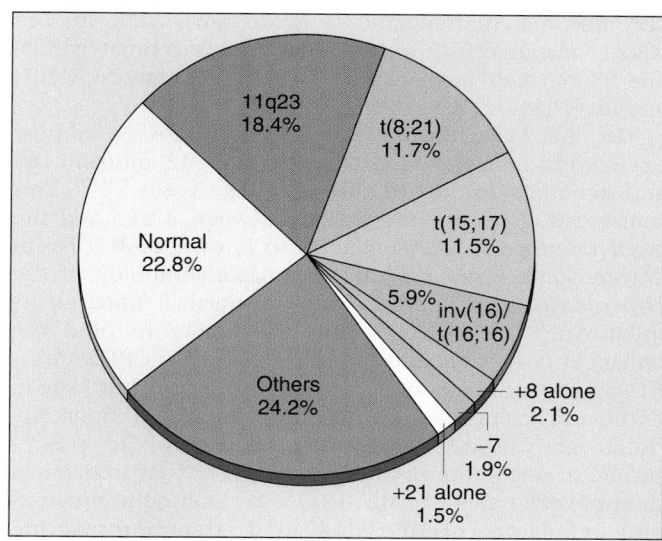

Figure 101-3. Cytogenetic subgroups in childhood AML.

been implicated in multiple cellular functions, including apoptosis, but its precise role remains undefined.[177,178] There is substantial evidence indicating that the PML-RARα fusion protein functions as a dominant negative inhibitor of both RARα and PML. PML-RARα can bind to RXR but cannot function as a ligand-induced transcriptional activator.[170,179] Physiologic doses of retinoic acid do not release the corepressor complex from the chimeric molecule. In addition, PML-RARα sequesters RXRs so that they cannot participate in other cellular functions with other nuclear hormone receptors.[180] These events could result in a block of myeloid differentiation and increased resistance to apoptosis. In addition, PML-RARα disrupts PML nuclear bodies; the redistribution of PML could interfere with the growth-regulatory activities of PML.[181,182] Unlike physiologic levels of retinoic acid, pharmacologic doses of all-*trans* retinoic acid (ATRA) lead to conformational changes in PML-RARα that are sufficient to release the nuclear corepressor complex, allowing the recruitment of transcriptional coactivators, including CBP and p300.[181,182] Mutations of the RARα binding domain can lead to resistance to ATRA, however.[183] Arsenic trioxide (As2O3), another effective treatment for APL, does not bind to RARα, but it does bind to PML and induces the degradation of PML-RARα, leading to apoptosis of leukemic cells.[184,185]

Two variants of the t(15;17) translocation have been identified—the t(5;17), which encodes an NPM-RARα fusion oncoprotein, and the t(11;17), which encodes a PLZF-RARα fusion protein.[186,187] The latter chimeric protein forms a stable complex with nuclear corepressors and histone deacetylases and is unresponsive to either retinoic acid or ATRA. Thus, cases of AML with the t(11;17) have APL morphology but are unresponsive to treatment with ATRA.

AML with Alterations of the Core Binding Factor Complex

The AML1/CBFβ transcription factor complex is essential for normal hematopoiesis.[37,188,189] The two most common chromosomal rearrangements in de novo AML are the t(8;21) and inv(16)/t(16;16), found in approximately 12% and 6% of cases, respectively.[190] The t(8;21) targets AML1, and inv(16)/t(16;16) targets CBFβ.

The t(8;21)(q22;q22) translocation is seen almost exclusively in cases of AML with FAB M2 morphology and accounts for up to 40% of these cases.[190,191] This translocation results in a fusion between *AML1* and the *eight twenty-one* (*ETO*) gene (also known as *MTG8*) on chromosome 8. *ETO* is the mammalian homolog of the *Drosophila* gene *nervy*, and its normal function is unknown.[37] AML1-ETO retains the ability to bind the enhancer core sequence and to interact with CBFβ.AML1-ETO, however, does not activate transcription, but instead dominantly represses normal AML1-mediated transcriptional activation.[37] AML1-ETO represses the p14^{ARF} promoter and reduces endogenous p14^{ARF} expression in multiple cell types.[192] AML1-ETO also can bind to the myeloid regulators c/EBPα and PU-1, thus interrupting myeloid differentiation.[193,194]

Expression of AML1-ETO during murine development through a gene targeting strategy resulted in an embryonic lethal phenotype that was almost identical to that observed with the loss of AML1 or CBFβ.[195,196] Unlike AML1- or CBFβ-deficient embryos, which lack detectable hematopoietic progenitors, AML1-ETO-expressing embryos contained dysplastic multilineage hematopoietic progenitors with an abnormally high capacity for self-renewal. In more recent experiments using a conditional "knock-in" strategy to bypass the embryonic lethality, AML-ETO did not block myeloid cell differentiation, nor was it sufficient to induce leukemia.[197] Induction of cooperating mutations, however, resulted in the development of an AML-like disease that resembled human AML1-ETO-associated leukemia.[197]

The inv(16)(p13q22) and the variant translocation t(16;16) result in the formation of a chimeric gene consisting of the 5′ portion of *CBFB* fused to a variable length of the 3′ portion of the smooth muscle myosin heavy chain gene, *MYH11*.[191,198] The encoded CBFβ-MYH11 product continues to bind to AML1.[199] The genetics of the inv(16) chromosomal rearrangement suggest that the encoded product functions in a dominant manner to induce leukemia. Further, CBFβ-MYH11 has been shown to repress AML1-mediated transcription directly by sequestering AML1 into inactive cytoplasmic complexes that are attached to actin-containing filamentous structures.[200,201]

Direct evidence that CBFβ-MYH11 functions in a dominant negative fashion comes from experiments in which *CBFB-MYH11* was expressed during murine embryogenesis.[202] Like expression of *AML1-ETO*, expression of *CBFB-MYH11* resulted in a phenotype nearly identical to that observed with the loss of *AML1* or *CBFB*. *CBFB-MYH11*, however, also resulted in an abnormal shift of primitive erythropoietic differentiation toward immature to mid-mature cells. This result suggests that the chimeric product not only inhibits normal AML1/CBFβ activity but also provides positive signals that result in abnormalities in cell growth and development. Definitive hematopoiesis can be restored in CBFβ-deficient mice by

ectopic expression of *CBFβ* transgenes but not transgenes encoding *CBFB-MYH11*.[189]

AML with Alterations of MLL

As discussed in the earlier section on ALL, translocations involving 11q23 and the *MLL* gene result in a gain of MLL function by generating novel chimeric proteins containing the amino terminus of MLL fused in-frame with one of many partner proteins of diverse function.[203] Translocations involving 11q23 are found in approximately 18% of childhood AML cases.[190] The two most common 11q23 translocations in AML, t(9;11)(p22;q23) and t(11;19)(q23;p13.3), involve AF-9 and ENL, respectively. Both molecules are homologous to proteins involved in RNA polymerization. When *MLL-AF-9* was expressed in mice through a "knock-in" strategy, mice developed AML, as did mice in which hematopoietic stem cells had been transduced with *MLL-ENL*.[204-206] Other MLL fusions involving the forkhead transcription factors FKHRL1 and AFX and the leucine zipper AF10 also can induce leukemia in mice when expressed in murine hematopoietic cells.[207,208]

CLINICAL COURSE AND PROGNOSTIC FACTORS

Relapse

Relapse is defined as the reappearance of leukemic cells at any site after remission has occurred. Most relapses occur during treatment or within the first 2 years after its completion, although ALL has been observed to relapse as late as 10 years after diagnosis.[209] The bone marrow is the most common site of relapse in both ALL and AML. In children with ALL, the frequency of relapse in extramedullary sites, such as the CNS and testes, has decreased to less than 5% and 2%, respectively. Leukemic relapse occasionally occurs at other sites, including the eye, ear, ovary, uterus, bone, muscle, tonsil, kidney, mediastinum, pleura, and paranasal sinus. Extramedullary relapse in children with ALL frequently presents as an "isolated" finding, but most occurrences are associated with minimal residual disease in the bone marrow.[210]

A small fraction of patients experience a recurrence of acute leukemia with an immunophenotype different from that determined at diagnosis. Often, these leukemias are secondary malignancies caused by the mutagenic effects of leukemia treatment.[211,212]

In some cases, recurrent leukemia has genetic features that confirm its relationship to the original leukemic clone but has the phenotype of a different lineage (lineage switch). There have been reports of leukemias morphologically and immunophenotypically characterized as ALL that relapse as AML (or vice versa) while retaining the karyotypic and molecular features of the original clone.[213-215]

Bone marrow relapse, with or without extramedullary involvement, predicts a poor outcome for most patients; patients with isolated bone marrow relapse generally fare worse than those with combined bone marrow and extramedullary relapse.[13,216] In either ALL or AML, the duration of the second remission depends on the duration of the first remission.[6,13,217] In children with relapsed ALL, factors indicating an especially poor prognosis are short initial remission and T-cell immunophenotype. Other adverse factors include t(9;22), presence of circulating blast cells, or a high leukocyte count at relapse and intensive primary therapy. Although chemotherapy might secure a prolonged second remission in children with ALL who experience late relapse (i.e., more than 6 months after cessation of therapy), allogeneic hematopoietic stem cell transplantation is the treatment of choice for patients who experience hematologic relapse during therapy or shortly thereafter and for those with T-cell ALL. In children with AML, relapse occurring at earlier than 18 months after therapy carries a dismal prognosis.[13]

Prognostic Factors in Acute Lymphoblastic Leukemia

Stringent evaluation of the risk of relapse is needed at the time of diagnosis to direct therapy so that patients are neither overtreated nor undertreated. Although age, leukocyte count, leukemic cell genotype, and response to early remission induction therapy are used commonly in risk classification, there is no consensus on the most useful criteria, and there is also no widely accepted system or terminology for defining risk groups.[125,218-224] For example, patients have been classified as lower-risk, intermediate-risk, and higher-risk by the Children's Cancer Group[125]; as standard-risk, medium-risk, or high-risk by the Berlin-Frankfurt-Münster Consortium[218]; as good-risk B-lineage, poor-risk B-lineage, or T-lineage by the Pediatric Oncology Group[221]; and as standard-risk, high-risk, or very high-risk by St. Jude Children's Research Hospital.[222] Having identified a group of patients at very low risk of relapse, the Children's Oncology Group recently proposed a four-group classification scheme: low-risk, standard-risk, high-risk, and very-high-risk.[225] In this review, we use the St. Jude risk classification system. This risk classification

based on presenting features is complemented by results of treatment response based on minimal residual disease assay for a final risk assignment. It should be noted that infants less than 12 months of age are generally treated on a separate protocol.

The type of treatment regimen remains the most important determinant of outcome. Thus, clinical and biologic variables might lose their predictive strength when treatment is changed. To date, the presenting age and leukocyte count have maintained prognostic strength in B-lineage but not in T-lineage ALL.[221,222,226] Even in B-lineage ALL, their value is limited, because as many as one third of patients who are considered at standard risk by these criteria (age 1 to 9 years with leukocyte count $<50 \times 10^9$/L) might relapse, and very-high-risk cases that require allogeneic hematopoietic stem cell transplantation cannot be distinguished reliably from high-risk cases by these criteria. For reasons still poorly understood and with rare exceptions, boys fare significantly worse than girls on most treatment protocols.[125,218-224,227] In the studies of Children's Oncology Group (COG), blacks and children of hispanic origin had a significantly worse outcome than whites, after adjustment for other prognostic features.[228,229] By contrast, blacks fared as well as whites in our single-institution protocols, a finding we attributed to equal access to effective contemporary treatment for both groups of patients.[230]

Primary genetic abnormalities of leukemic cells influence their aggressiveness and response to therapy but are not 100% predictive of outcome. For example, as many as 20% of children with favorable genetic features (*TEL-AML1* fusion and hyperdiploidy >50 chromosomes) eventually experience relapse, while approximately one third of those with high-risk abnormalities [the Philadelphia chromosome with *BCR-ABL* fusion or the t(4;11) with *MLL-AF4* fusion] can be cured with chemotherapy alone.[6] It should be noted that age between 1 and 9 years conferred a favorable prognosis in cases with the Philadelphia chromosome or the t(4;11), and a high leukocyte count was associated with a poor outcome in

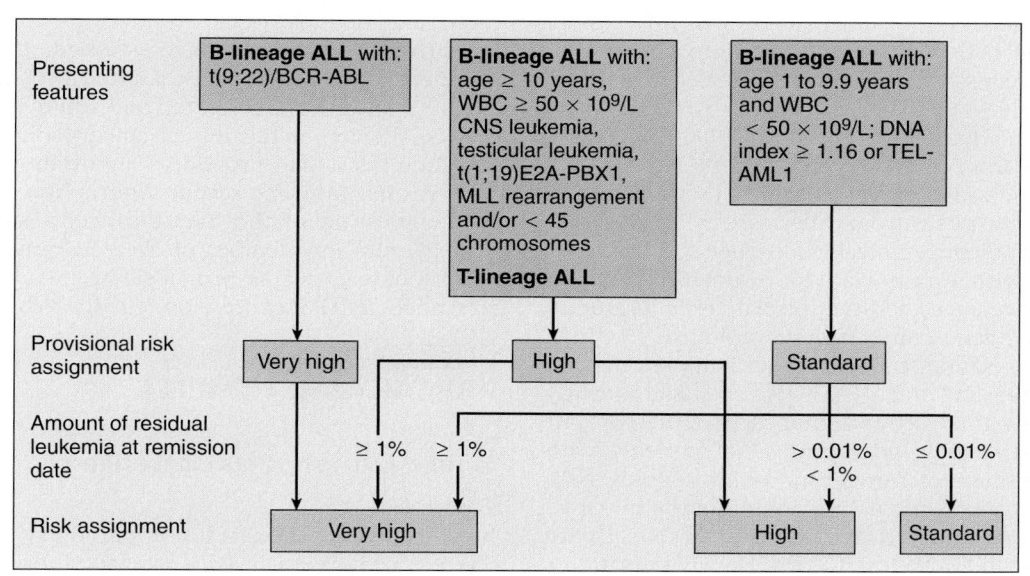

those with the former genetic feature.[225,231-233] More recently, the presence of trisomy 4, 10, or 17 has been shown to be associated with a very favorable prognosis, a finding that requires independent confirmation.[125,221]

Prognostic Factors in Acute Myeloid Leukemia

Patients with Down syndrome, AML, and APL have a favorable prognosis; however, the impact of these and other prognostic factors is highly dependent on therapy.[234] The Cancer and Leukemia Group B (CALGB) trials demonstrated that patients with AML and inv(16) or t(8;21) had a better outcome than patients with all other subtypes of AML and had a particularly good outcome when they were treated with multiple courses of high-dose cytarabine.[235,236] In the MRC AML10 trial, the 5-year overall survival estimates for patients with t(8;21) and inv(16) were 69% and 61%, respectively.[237] The POG reported 4-year overall survival estimates of 52% and 75% for children with similar karyotypes treated on the 8821 trial.[190] A similar result has been achieved at St. Jude's Hospital, with 6-year overall survival estimates of 55% for cases with t(8;21) and 70% for cases with inv(16) treated in recent trials.[238,239] Recently, the French AML Intergroup demonstrated a 5-year overall survival estimate of 59% for patients with t(8;21) and suggested that the white blood cell (WBC) index (the product of the WBC count and the ratio of bone marrow blast cells) can identify prognostic subgroups of t(8;21)-positive patients.[240]

AML patients with the t(9;11) also have had a favorable prognosis in some trials but not in others.[190,191,241-243] In the MRC AML10 trial, patients with the t(9;11) had an intermediate outcome, with a 3-year overall survival estimate of 50%, whereas patients with the t(9;11) or other 11q23 abnormalities had a rather poor outcome on POG 8821 (4-year overall survival 33%).[190,237] Among patients treated at St. Jude for AML during the past 2 decades, those with the t(9;11) had a better outcome (5-year event-free survival estimate, 65%) than patients in all other cytogenetic or molecular subgroups.[244] Favorable outcome of these patients is attributed to the use of epipodophyllotoxins, agents known to be effective against M5 leukemia, and of 2-chlorodeoxyadenosine (2-CDA), which is particularly effective against M5 AML.[245-247] In vitro, blast cells from patients with the t(9;11) are more sensitive to cytarabine, etoposide, anthracyclines, and 2-CDA than are blast cells from other cases.[248]

Certain morphologic, clinical, and genetic features are also associated with a particularly poor outcome in AML. Some studies have suggested that partial tandem duplications of the *MLL* gene confer a poor prognosis.[249,250] We and others have demonstrated that patients with acute megakaryoblastic leukemia (AMKL) have significantly worse outcomes than other subtypes of AML.[251-253] At St. Jude, the estimated 5-year survival of patients with AMKL in the absence of Down syndrome was only 10%, and no patients were cured by chemotherapy alone.[251] The outcome of treatment-related AML is also dismal, with survival rates of only 10% to 20%.[254,255] Likewise, patients

with myelodysplastic syndrome (MDS), AML arising from MDS, or AML with monosomy 7 often have resistant disease that is difficult to cure.[190,191,237,256-258]

Mutations and internal tandem duplications (ITD) of the *FLT3* gene have been associated with a poor prognosis in both adults and children with AML.[259-264] In a Japanese study of adult AML, the estimated 5-year overall survival rate was only 14% for patients with FLT3 ITD, which was the strongest prognostic factor in multivariate analysis.[259] Similarly, in an analysis of 106 adults treated on MRC AML trials, 13 of the 14 patients with FLT3 ITD died within 18 months of diagnosis.[261] A subsequent study of 854 patients treated on the MRC 10 and 12 trials revealed FLT3 ITD in 27% of cases.[262] The presence of FLT3 ITD was associated with an increased risk of relapse and with lower estimates of disease-free, event-free, and overall survival. Notably, an analysis of 91 children with ALL treated on CCG trials demonstrated an 8-year event-free survival estimate of only 7% for the 15 cases with FLT3 ITD.[263] A multivariate analysis demonstrated that FLT3 ITD was the most important prognostic factor in this study.

Recently, several studies have questioned the prognostic importance of FLT3 mutations.[265-268] In an analysis of 82 adults with AML who were treated on the CALGB 9621 protocol and who had normal cytogenetics, three leukemic-cell genotypes were detected: 59 patients had two wild-type FLT3 alleles (FLT3$^{wt/wt}$), 15 had one wt and one ITD allele (FLT3$^{ITD/wt}$), and eight had only one ITD allele (FLT3$^{ITD/-}$).[265] Interestingly, overall and event-free survival were similar in patients with the FLT3$^{wt/wt}$ and FLT3$^{ITD/wt}$ genotypes. Only patients with the FLT3$^{ITD/-}$ genotype had a significantly worse outcome. Similarly, an analysis of 979 patients revealed that those with a high FLT3 mutant:wt ratio had significantly shorter disease-free and overall survivals, whereas those with low ratios had outcomes similar to those of patients without FLT3 mutations.[267] These studies, as well as emerging data from the Children's Cancer Group (CCG), suggest that the true prognostic importance of FLT3 mutations depends on the relative amount of wt FLT3 and that only those patients with a predominance of the mutant protein are at increased risk of relapse.

Many investigators have studied the prognostic significance of ATP-binding cassette (ABC) transporters in AML.[269-271] Studies in children and adults have implicated P-glycoprotein, multidrug resistance-associated protein 1, and lung resistance protein as important mechanisms of drug resistance. Some recent reports have also suggested that expression of the breast cancer resistance protein (BCRP), another member of the ABC transporter family, might confer a worse prognosis in AML, but the clinical relevance of BCRP expression remains to be defined.[272-274]

PRIMARY TREATMENT

Acute Lymphoblastic Leukemia

Overview

In the more successful contemporary clinical trials, 5-year event-free survival estimates for children with

TABLE 101-4

Results of International Studies of Childhood ALL

				PERCENT 5-YEAR EVENT-FREE SURVIVAL (±1SE)			
				B-LINEAGE*			
STUDY	YEAR	ELIGIBLE AGE (YEARS)	NO. OF PATIENTS	OVERALL	STANDARD	HIGH	T-LINEAGE
AIEOP-91[275]	1991–1995	≤15	1194	70.8±1.3	79.9±1.5	61.5±2.9	40.4±4.1
BFM-90[218,276]	1990–1995	≤18	2178	78.0±0.9	87.4±1.0	66.3±2.1	61.1±2.9
CCG-1800[125]	1989–1995	≤21	5121	75±1	80±1	67±2	73±2
COALL-CLCG-92[219]	1992–1997	≤18	538	76.9±1.9	82.1±2.4	75.7±3.9	71.2±5.1
DCLSG-8[277]	1991–1996	≤18	467	73±2	79±2	67±5	71±6
DFCI-91-01[224,278]	1991–1995	≤18	377	83±2	85±2	82±4	79±8
EORTC-58881[220,279,280]	1989–1998	≤18	2065	70.9±1.1	78.4±1.3	57.3±2.4	64.4±2.9
NOPHO-III[281]	1992–1998	≤15	1143	77.6±1.4	85.2±1.5	67.9±3.3	61.3±4.9
POG[221]	1986–1994	≤21	3828	70.9±0.8	77.4±0.9	55.3±1.6	51.0±2.4
SJCRH-13A[222,282]	1991–1994	≤18	165	76.9±3.3	88.1±3.6	70.4±6.2	60.9±10.2
TCCSG-L92-13[223]	1992–1995	≤15	347	63.4±2.7	67.8±3.4	56.7±5.4	59.3±8.6
UKALL-XI[226,283]	1990–1997	≤15	2090	63±1.1	74±2.2	59±4.1	51±3.5

AIEOP, Associazione Italiana di Ematologia ed Oncologia Pediatrica; BFM, Berlin-Frankfurt-Münster ALL Study Group; CCG, Children's Cancer Group; COALL, Cooperative ALL Study Group; DCLSG, Dutch Childhood Leukemia Study Group; DFCI, Dana Farber Cancer Institute ALL Consortium; EORTC-CLCG, European Organization for Research and Treatment of Cancer–Children's Leukaemia Cooperative Study Group; NOPHO, Nordic Society of Pediatric Hematology and Oncology; POG, Pediatric Oncology Group; SJCRH, St. Jude Children's Research Hospital; TCCSG, Tokyo Children's Cancer Study Group; UKALL, UK Medical Research Council Working Party on Childhood Leukaemia.

*Standard-risk group: children 1 to 9 years old with leukocyte count <50 × 10⁹/L; high-risk group: all others, except infants. Differences in "overall" partly reflect the disproportion of high-risk cases referred to some institutions as compared to the others.

newly diagnosed ALL now range from 75% to 83% (Table 101-4).[125,218-224,226,275-283] The improved cure rate of ALL can be attributed mainly to the development of more effective chemotherapeutic regimens through successive clinical trials. In patients with mature B-cell ALL, short-term (2 to 8 months) regimens of intensive chemotherapy based primarily on cyclophosphamide, methotrexate, cytarabine, and intrathecal therapy currently result in cure rates of 74% to 87%.[284-286] The recent development of a highly effective uricolytic agent, recombinant urate oxidase (rasburicase, Elitek, Fasurtec), promises to improve the results of treatment still further by reducing early morbidity and mortality caused by tumor lysis syndrome and acute renal failure.[287,288]

Event-free survival estimates for infants with ALL, especially those with 11q23/*MLL* rearrangements, remain low, ranging from 20% to 35%.[26] In several recent clinical trials, high-dose cytarabine, high-dose methotrexate, and intensive consolidation/reinduction therapy appeared to improve outcome.[289,290] These results should be viewed as preliminary, however, because of the small numbers of patients studied and the absence of randomization. Intensive systemic and intrathecal treatment, without cranial irradiation, appear to provide adequate CNS protection, even in infants who have CNS leukemia at diagnosis.[291] Most investigators now treat infants as a unique subgroup with multiple drugs given at high dosages, without cranial irradiation. The use of allogeneic hematopoietic stem cell transplantation failed to improve outcome in this age group.[232,292]

For all other patients, the basic approach to therapy consists of a relatively brief remission-induction phase followed by intensification (consolidation) therapy and then prolonged continuation treatment. All patients require treatment for subclinical leukemia of the CNS, which should be initiated early in the form of intrathecal therapy.

Remission Induction

Remission induction regimens include a glucocorticoid (prednisone, prednisolone, or dexamethasone), vincristine, and at least a third agent (asparaginase or anthracycline). With improved supportive care and chemotherapy, the rate of complete remission now ranges from 96% to 99%.[125,218-224,226,275-283] Attempts have been made to intensify induction therapy, especially for patients with high-risk and very-high-risk ALL, on the premise that a more rapid and profound reduction of the leukemic cell burden could forestall the development of drug resistance in leukemic cells. Several studies, however, suggest that intensive induction therapy might not be necessary for standard-risk patients, providing that they receive post-induction intensification therapy.[125,219] Moreover, intensive induction therapy might lead to inferior overall outcome because of increased early morbidity and mortality.[293,294] Further, we found that patients who achieve minimal residual disease-negative status at week 14 after the end of remission induction therapy have a risk of relapse as low as that of patients who achieve this status earlier (at the end of remission induction).[295]

Most remission induction regimens include asparaginase; however, several clinical trials using asparaginase in the postinduction period only had an excellent remission induction rate with low morbidity (especially in terms of thrombotic complications) and excellent long-term event-free survival.[219,224] A recent randomized trial compared the relative efficacy and toxicity of asparaginase and epidoxorubicin as a third remission-induction agent in patients with standard-risk ALL. Patients treated with asparaginase had a significantly lower rate of successful remission induction due to a higher rate of fatal infection.[293] Therefore, the use of asparaginase in remission induction regimens is being challenged. It should also be noted that different forms of asparaginase have different pharmacokinetic profiles and differences in toxicity and efficacy.[293,296] Limited studies suggested that polyethylene glycol-conjugated asparaginase, a long-acting and less allergenic form, can replace native *E. coli* asparaginase in initial treatment.[296] Because of the cross-reactivity of antibodies to these two forms of asparaginase, patients with allergic reactions to either preparation should be treated subsequently with *Erwinia* asparaginase (MV Relling, C-H Pui; unpublished observation).

Perhaps because of its longer half-life and increased penetration into cerebrospinal fluid, dexamethasone has been used instead of prednisone or prednisolone in some induction and continuation regimens.[297] Although this substitution yielded an improved outcome in one randomized trial, it was implicated in excessive life-threatening infections and septic deaths in another study.[125,294] This finding underscores the importance of potential drug interactions in any complex multiagent regimen.

Intensification or Consolidation

With restoration of normal hematopoiesis, patients in remission become candidates for intensification (consolidation) therapy. There is no dispute about the importance of this phase of therapy, but there is also no consensus about the optimal regimens and their duration. Delayed intensification (or reinduction), pioneered by investigators in the Berlin-Frankfurt-Münster consortium, is perhaps the most widely used regimen.[276] It is basically a repetition of the initial induction therapy 3 months after the end of remission induction and is most beneficial for standard-risk cases. Investigators at the Children's Cancer Group showed that double delayed intensification beginning at week 32 of treatment improved the outcome of patients with high-risk (or so-called intermediate-risk) leukemia.[298] Interestingly, in this study, additional pulses of vincristine and prednisone during continuation therapy did not improve outcome, suggesting that double delayed intensification was of benefit because of the increased dose intensity of other agents (e.g., asparaginase, anthracycline, cytarabine, and cyclophosphamide) or the timing or scheduling of the intensification regimen. Extended and stronger intensification therapy also significantly benefited patients with high-risk ALL and a slow response to initial induction therapy.[299] The benefit of double delayed intensification for high-risk ALL was confirmed recently by the Italian group AIEOP.[300] Whether this approach will benefit patients at standard risk remains uncertain. Hence, it appears that reinduction or delayed intensification therapy is beneficial to all patients, and double or prolonged intensification is beneficial to those with high-risk or very-high-risk leukemia.

The use of different intensification regimens in various clinical trials also has led to the identification of effective treatment components for certain subtypes of leukemia. For example, improved outcome of T-lineage ALL in the

clinical trials of the Dana Farber Cancer Institute consortium and Children's Cancer Group has been credited to the intensive use of asparaginase, a finding that has been corroborated by a randomized study of the Pediatric Oncology Group.[224,278,301] Interestingly, in the study by the Dana Farber Cancer Institute Consortium, patients who tolerated at least 26 weekly doses of asparaginase had a significantly better outcome than those who received fewer doses.[224] Intensive asparaginase treatment is also credited for a very low rate of relapse of ALL with the *TEL-AML1* fusion on the protocols of the Dana Farber Institute Consortium.[224] In line with this clinical observation, leukemic blast cells with the *TEL-AML1* fusion are reportedly highly sensitive to asparaginase in vitro.[142]

Very high doses of methotrexate (5 g/m^2) appear to improve outcome in patients with T-lineage ALL.[218,225] This observation is consistent with the finding that T-lineage blast cells accumulate methotrexate polyglutamates (active metabolites of methotrexate) less avidly than do B-lineage blast cells, so that a higher serum concentration of methotrexate is needed for adequate response in T-lineage ALL.[302] Nonetheless, high-dose methotrexate also benefits patients with B-lineage ALL.[303] Although the optimal dosage of methotrexate for individual genetic subtypes remains to be determined, a dosage of 2.5 g/m^2 should be adequate for most of these patients.[304] High-dose intravenous 6-mercaptopurine has no clinical benefit and was associated with an inferior outcome in one study.[277,305] Consistent with this result is the finding that intravenous high-dose 6-mercaptopurine inhibited de novo purine synthesis minimally and exerted minimal antileukemic effects.[306] Similarly, high-dose cytarabine failed to improve the outcome of high-risk ALL in a randomized trial.[279]

Continuation Treatment

The most successful postremission intensification regimens generally feature continuous therapy, whereas high-dose pulse therapy with prolonged rest periods to recover from myelosuppression appears to be less effective.[224,276,299] This observation is consistent with the concept of metronomic dosing for solid tumors, which is based on the idea that continuous or frequent administration of cytotoxic drugs might improve outcome by abrogating the ability of slowly proliferating endothelial cells (which are essential for tumor cell survival) to repair and recover during the usual rest periods.[307] The role of angiogenesis in leukemia has been suggested but not conclusively demonstrated.[308] In any case, the tempo and dosage of chemotherapy could variably affect the recovery of bone marrow mesenchymal cells that provide essential survival factors for leukemic lymphoblasts.[309]

Children with ALL (except those with mature B-cell leukemia) require prolonged continuation treatment. The attempt to intensify early therapy but shorten the total duration of treatment to 1 year in a recent study resulted in inferior overall event-free survival.[223] Interestingly, the abbreviated therapy appeared to be adequate for a small subset of patients with T-cell ALL who responded well to prednisolone. Notwithstanding this result, the general rule is to continue therapy for a total duration of

2 to 2.5 years. Many investigators prefer to extend treatment for boys to 3 years because of their generally poorer outcome, although the benefit of this approach remains to be determined.[227,310]

The combination of methotrexate administered weekly and mercaptopurine administered daily constitutes the standard "backbone" of the ALL continuation regimen. Tailoring the doses to the limits of tolerance (as indicated by low neutrophil counts) has been associated with an improved clinical outcome.[311] Overzealous use of 6-mercaptopurine, however, so that neutropenia precludes further use of chemotherapy and reduces overall dose intensity, is counterproductive.[312] It is well recognized that the rare patients (1 in 300) who have an inherited deficiency of thiopurine S-methyltransferase have extreme sensitivity to mercaptopurine. Patients who are heterozygous for this deficiency (approximately 10%) and who have intermediate levels of enzyme activity might also require moderate dose reduction to avert side effects.[313] Identification of the genetic basis of this autosomal codominant trait has made the molecular diagnosis of these cases possible.[314] When patients show poor tolerance to methotrexate and mercaptopurine, studies can now be performed to identify and selectively reduce the dosage of the responsible agent, allowing full dosage of the other drug. In a recent study, 6-thioguanine did not improve outcome compared with mercaptopurine, and it has been associated with increased toxicities, such as thrombocytopenia and veno-occlusive disease.[315,316] Hence, mercaptopurine remians the preferred drug for continuation treatment.

The addition of intermittent pulses of vincristine and a glucocorticoid to the antimetabolite continuation regimen improves the results and has been adopted widely.[317] Dexamethasone has been substituted for prednisone during continuation therapy in many clinical trials because of its superior clinical efficacy.[125] Studies are needed to determine the optimal dosage and duration of dexamethasone therapy during this phase of treatment, however.

Prevention and Treatment of Central Nervous System Leukemia

Several factors are associated with the occurrence of leukemia in the CNS: presenting risk features, the quantity of leukemic blasts cells in the cerebrospinal fluid, and the types of systemic and CNS-directed therapies. Patients with high-risk genetic features, large leukemic cell burden, T-lineage ALL, and leukemic cells in the cerebrospinal fluid (even if iatrogenic from a traumatic lumbar puncture) are at increased risk of CNS relapse and require more intensive CNS-directed therapy.[51,318-320] Because of the adverse consequence of traumatic lumbar puncture at the time of diagnosis, when patients have circulating blast cells, we have routinely performed this procedure under deep sedation or general anesthesia, transfused thrombocytopenic patients with platelets, and administered intrathecal chemotherapy immediately after injection of cerebrospinal fluid. High-dose methotrexate, although useful in preventing hematologic or testicular relapse, generally has only a marginal effect on the control of CNS leukemia. In one study, however, high-dose methotrexate plus intrathecal methotrexate reduced CNS relapse, although it did not affect relapse at other sites or overall surviva1.[226] Additional analyses of the method of delivery of high-dose methotrexate and folic acid rescue are needed to explain this finding. By contrast, dexamethasone was definitely shown to improve CNS control.[125] The relative efficacy of triple intrathecal therapy with methotrexate, hydrocortisone, and cytarabine, compared with that of intrathecal methotrexate alone, is still unknown and is the subject of an ongoing randomized trial of the Children's Cancer Group.

Cranial irradiation is the most effective CNS-directed therapy; however, the concern that it can cause substantial neurotoxicity and occasional brain tumors has led to its replacement with intensive intrathecal and systemic chemotherapy for 80% to 95% of all patients. This approach, in combination with cranial irradiation for selected high-risk or very high-risk cases, has lowered the rate of CNS relapse to less than 5% in most studies.[224,276,282,299] The dose of radiation can be lowered to 12 Gy without increasing the risk of CNS relapse, provided that effective systemic chemotherapy is used.[276] It has not been established conclusively whether CNS irradiation can decrease the risk of hematologic relapse. In one study, the omission of cranial irradiation was implicated as a cause of increased CNS and hematologic relapses in T-lineage ALL with presenting leukocyte count greater than $100 \times 10^9/L$.[321] The study involved only a small number of cases, however, and inadequate systemic chemotherapy could have contributed to the increased rate of relapse. In another retrospective study of T-lineage ALL with high presenting leukocyte count ($>50 \times 10^9/L$) or CNS leukemia at diagnosis, CNS irradiation reduced the rate of CNS relapse but failed to improve event-free survival.[322]

Two studies omitted cranial irradiation altogether for all patients.[220,323] The cumulative risk of isolated CNS relapse was 4.2% and 3%, respectively, and the rate of any CNS relapse (including combined CNS and hematologic relapse) was 8.3% and 6%. Patients with a CD10⁻ B-lineage (pro-B) leukemic phenotype, CNS 2 or CNS 3 status, and leukocyte count greater than $100 \times 10^9/L$ had an increased risk of CNS relapse. Because the overall 8-year event survival estimates for the two studies were only 60.7% ± 4% (SE) and 68.4 ± 1.2%, it is still unclear whether improved systemic chemotherapy can reduce the hazard of CNS relapse. Moreover, patients with isolated CNS relapse who did not receive cranial irradiation as initial CNS-directed therapy have a very high retrieval rate; in those who had a long initial remission before the CNS event, the long-term prognosis could even be comparable to that of newly diagnosed patients.[324] At St. Jude's Hospital, cranial irradiation is reserved for salvage therapy. Although this approach is under study, most clinical trials still specify cranial irradiation for patients at particularly high risk of CNS relapse—those with CNS 3 status or T-cell ALL with high leukocyte count.

Pharmacokinetic and Pharmacogenomic Variables

There is wide variability in the rate of metabolism and systemic clearance of antileukemic agents and in the absorption of orally administered chemotherapy. Both low systemic exposure to methotrexate and low dose intensity of 6-mercaptopurine have been associated with an inferior treatment outcome.[325,326] It is important to note that concomitant administration of cytochrome P450 enzyme-inducing anticonvulsants (phenytoin, phenobarbital, carbamazepine, or a combination) significantly increases the systemic clearance rates of several antileukemic agents and is associated with lower efficacy of chemotherapy.[327] At St. Jude, other anticonvulsants that are less likely to induce the activity of drug-metabolizing enzymes (e.g., gabapentin, valproic acid) are used. Genetic polymorphisms of several drug-metabolizing enzymes are also associated with treatment outcome. Patients who have homozygous or heterozygous deficiency of thiopurine methyltransferase, the enzyme that catalyzes the S-methylation (inactivation) of mercaptopurine, tend to have better event-free survival, probably because they receive a higher effective dose intensity of 6-mercaptopurine.[326] The thiopurine methyltransferase genetic polymorphism, however, is also linked, in the context of antimetabolite-based therapy, to acute dose-limiting toxicity and the risks of irradiation-induced brain tumor and therapy-related acute myeloid leukemia.[254,328-330] Hence, therapy must be adjusted for patients who have homozygous mutant genotypes of this enzyme and in many heterozygotes. The null genotype (absence of both alleles) for *GSTM1* or *GSTT1* and the *GSTP1 Val$_{105}$/Val$_{105}$* genes are also associated with increased treatment-related toxicity and a lower risk of relapse, perhaps because of reduced detoxification of cytotoxic chemotherapy.[331-333]

Acute Myeloid Leukemia

Clinical trials of therapy for AML are characterized by dose intensification of conventional therapeutic agents. Remission induction and consolidation therapy are essential components of virtually every protocol, whereas other postremission therapy differs widely between studies.

Remission Induction

With the exception of APL, which is now treated initially with ATRA in combination with chemotherapy (generally at least an anthracycline), all cases of AML are treated with induction chemotherapy consisting of cytarabine and a topoisomerase II inhibitor (anthracycline, idarubicin, doxorubicin, or mitoxantrone) with or without a third agent (etoposide or 6-thioguanine) (see Table 101-4).[247,334-342] Rates of remission induction range from 74% to 91% among contemporary clinical trials[247,334-343] This variation is due in part to differences in the timing of remission studies (i.e., after one, two, or multiple courses of therapy). Nonetheless, many attempts have been made to modify remission induction therapy not only to increase the rate of remission but to improve its "quality" or "degree," which in turn can affect the ultimate treatment outcome favorably.

Modifications to remission induction include the use of additional agents or different topoisomerase II inhibitors, increased drug dosages, increased duration of drug exposure, and decreased intervals between treatment courses.[247,334-343] Because idarubicin has faster cellular uptake, increased cellular retention, less in vitro drug resistance, longer plasma half life of the active metabolites, and potentially less cardiotoxicity than daunorubicin, investigators of the BFM consortium compared the clinical efficacy of these two agents during remission induction in their AML93 study.[335,336,344-346] Idarubicin yielded a significantly lower bone marrow blast cell count on day 15 than did daunorubicin. Although long-term outcome did not differ significantly between the two randomized groups, the subset of patients who had more than 5% blast cells in the bone marrow on day 15 appeared to have a better outcome with idarubicin. By contrast, the Australian and New Zealand Children's Cancer Group found daunorubicin to be as effective as idarubicin and less toxic.[334] Using an "up-front window" therapy approach, investigators at our institution demonstrated that 2-CDA given as a single agent induced remission in 45% of patients after one course and in 70.6% after two courses of treatment; 2-CDA was also particularly effective against acute monoblastic leukemia.[247] In recently reported results, complete remission rates of 90% and 100% were observed in two treatment arms that used two different schedules of a 2-CDA-cytarabine combination followed by two courses of daunorubicin, cytarabine, and etoposide.[347] The long-term results of this approach remain to be determined.

The CCG pursued the approach of timed-sequential therapy (i.e., intensification of therapy) by reducing the interval between two induction courses. The intensive-timing arm had a remission induction rate comparable to that of the standard-timing arm, despite a much higher rate of early mortality (11% vs. 4%); more important, it yielded a superior overall outcome, regardless of the type of postremission therapy.[337,338] In a subsequent study, these investigators found that patients with a negative genotype (i.e., homozygous polymorphism) for glutathione S-transferase theta, a detoxifying enzyme, experienced greater toxicity and mortality than did patients with a least one wild-type allele.[348] The Pediatric Oncology Group (POG) has used high-dose cytarabine to intensify therapy. In the POG 8498 study, patients were randomized to receive two courses of DAT (daunorubicin, cytarabine and 6-thioguanine) or one course of DAT followed by a course of high-dose cytarabine.[349] The two treatment arms had comparable remission rates (both 85%), but patients who received high-dose cytarabine had a higher estimate of 3-year event-free survival (34% vs. 29%). In the POG 9421 study, patients were randomized to receive DAT induction at standard dose or DAT with cytarabine at a high dose. Remission rates were somewhat lower in the standard arm (87% vs. 91%), as were 3-year event-free survival estimates (34% vs. 40.4%, $P=0.17$).[343]

The United Kingdom Medical Research Council (MRC) used a prolonged daily exposure approach to intensify therapy. They found that prolonged treatment resulted in greater toxicity but an improved remission rate and a shorter time to remission.[350] In the MRC AML-10 trial, patients randomly assigned to receive 6-thioguanine or etoposide as the third induction agent had a comparable overall outcome.[339]

In summary, intensified remission induction in general improves long-term outcome; however, vigilance in supportive care is important to reduce early mortality. In this regard, pharmacogenetic studies could be useful in identifying patients at increased risk of early mortality. Finally, patients with Down syndrome should not receive intensified therapy, as they have more drug-sensitive disease and are more susceptible to treatment-related toxicity than the general population.[341,351-353]

Consolidation and Other Postremission Therapy

Without postremission therapy, disease relapses in nearly all cases.[217] Although more courses of consolidation therapy are thought to be better, the optimal number is uncertain. The current MRC AML-12 trial is investigating whether four or five courses of consolidation therapy is better. In most clinical trials, postremission consolidation therapy lasts for 6 to 12 months in patients who do not undergo hematopoietic stem cell transplantation.

The optimal consolidation therapy has yet to be determined but generally includes high-dose cytarabine. In the BFM AML93 study, the improved outcome of high-risk cases was attributed to intensification with high-dose cytarabine and mitoxantrone.[336] This drug combination is also an integral component of the MRC AML10 trial.[339,340] The combination of high-dose cytarabine and L-asparaginase (Capizzi II regimen) was credited for the improved outcome in the CCG-213 and CCG-213P studies.[354,355] Consolidation therapy with high-dose cytarabine alone also resulted in an improved outcome in the POG 8498 study.[349] In adult clinical trials, high-dose cytarabine appeared to be particularly beneficial to patients whose leukemia involved disruption of core-binding factor.[235,236]

The need for continuation therapy beyond consolidation therapy is less certain. Although the BFM study group achieved excellent results with continuation therapy lasting 18 to 24 months, other studies could not demonstrate the clinical benefit of this phase of therapy.[335,336,356-360] In fact, a randomized study by the CCG (213P) showed that 2 years of continuation treatment after intensification therapy resulted in a worse outcome than no continuation treatment. In a recent LAME 89/91 study, low-dose continuation treatment of 18 months also resulted in worse overall survival than no continuation treatment.[338] The investigators attributed this finding to the development of drug resistance during continuation therapy, leading to a poor salvage rate. Hence, most study groups, with the exception of the BFM group, have abandoned the use of continuation therapy in AML. It should be noted that cases of APL benefit from prolonged continuation treatment with all-trans retinoic acid and perhaps with 6-mercaptopurine and methotrexate.[361]

CNS-directed Therapy

Relatively little attention has been paid to CNS-directed therapy for AML, because control of hematologic disease remains the focus of treatment. Suboptimal systemic therapy might allow hematologic relapse to precede meningeal relapse. In most clinical trials, intrathecal cytarabine with or without methotrexate and systemic high-dose cytarabine are used as CNS prophylaxis. The

BFM AML-87 study attempted to address whether cranial irradiation is necessary in childhood AML.[358] In that randomized study, children who received cranial irradiation had longer relapse-free survival than did those receiving only intrathecal therapy, although there was only a marginal difference between the two groups in the rate of CNS relapse. The early termination of randomization in that study prevents firm conclusions; moreover, many other clinical trials have yielded similar outcomes without the use of cranial irradiation (Table 101-5). Therefore, cranial irradiation might not be necessary if systemic and intrathecal chemotherapy is adequate. Even less is known about the optimal treatment of overt CNS leukemia at presentation. In an earlier study at our institution, this factor lacked prognostic significance.[362] The results of our recent study suggested that these patients can be cured without the use of cranial irradiation (Razzouk B, Pui CH, unpublished observation).

Hematopoietic Stem Cell Transplantation

Because advances in transplantation and chemotherapy are occurring in parallel, the indications for transplantation should be re-evaluated periodically. At present, among children with ALL, those with the Philadelphia chromosome, early hematologic relapse, or T-cell ALL with poor early response or hematologic relapse are clearly candidates for transplantation.[6,231] Transplantation has not been shown to improve outcome in other types of very high-risk leukemia, including infant cases and those with *MLL* rearrangement[232,233]

Autologous stem cell transplantation has generally been associated with a high rate of relapse in childhood ALL. Excellent results have been reported in a few small series of patients with AML, but autologous transplantation has failed to show any survival benefit over chemotherapy in most studies.[363-367] The benefit of in vitro purging to rid autografts of residual leukemia cells remains unproven.[368] Hence, autologous transplantation is not recommended by most investigators.

Allogeneic transplantation in children with AML has been shown in most clinical trials to reduce the risk of relapse and to improve overall survival, compared with either autologous transplant or chemotherapy alone, despite a higher rate of morbidity and mortality.[217,337] The indications for this procedure during first remission are still debated, however. Investigators of the COG favor allogeneic transplantation for all patients who have a suitable donor because this procedure yielded a superior outcome, regardless of the risk group, in their study. Most European investigators do not recommend allogeneic transplantation for patients at lower risk, especially in view of recent improved results with chemotherapy, and instead reserve this procedure for patients with relapsed AML.[339,368] They contend that because most patients with relapsed AML can readily be salvaged with hematopoietic stem cell transplantation, others should be spared the transplant-related morbidity and mortality.

Notwithstanding the controversy of allogeneic transplantation, there is general consensus that patients with very-high-risk AML [monosomy 5 or 7, del (5q), 3q abnormalities, acute megakaryoblastic leukemia, or poor

TABLE 101-5

Results of Selected Recent Clinical Trials for Childhood AML

STUDY	YEARS	TREATMENT SCHEDULE	NO. OF PATIENTS	REMISSION RATE (%)	EARLY MORTALITY (%)	OVERALL OUTCOME	CONCLUSIONS
ANZCCSG AML2[334]	1993–1999	Remission induction 1. Ida/Ara-C/6TG 2. HD Ara-C Consolidation 1. Ida/Ara-C/VP16 2. Ara-C/Amsa Interim therapy Ara-C/6TG Postconsolidation Allo HSCT or Auto HSCT	160	91.2	5	5-yr EFS 41% 5-yr OS 55%	Idarubicin was more toxic than daunorubicin (used in preceding AML1 trial) during remission induction.
BFM AML93[335,336]	1993–1998	Remission induction Dauno/Ara-C/VP16 vs Ida/Ara-C/VP16 Consolidation 7-day 6-week consolidation plus Mito/Ara-C for high-risk patients Intensification HD Ara-C/VP16 Continuation (18 months) 6TG/Ara-C plus cranial radiation Allo HSCT for high-risk patients	471	82	7	5-yr EFS 51%±2% 5-yr OS 60%±3%	Idarubicin reduced blast cells more profoundly than daunorubicin during the first 2 weeks of remission induction in high-risk cases. Improved outcome for high-risk cases was attributed to mitoxantrone and high-dose cytarabine
CCG 2891[337,431]	1989–1995	Remission induction DCTER × 2 Consolidation DCTER × 2 Postconsolidation Allo HSCT for patients with suitable donor Others:Auto HSCT or 4 cycles chemotherapy	652	74	8	3-yr EFS Standard timing 27% Intensive timing 42% 3-yr OS Standard timing 39% Intensive timing 51%	Overall survival was improved by timing-intensive treatment. Outcome of allogeneic transplantation was superior to outcome of autologous transplant or chemotherapy. Intensive chemotherapy was as efficacious as autologous transplant.
LAME 89/91[338]	1988–1996	Remission induction Ara-C/Mito Consolidation Allo HSCT for patients with suitable donor Others: chemotherapy 1. VP16/Ara-C/Dauno 2. Amsa HD Ara-C/Asp × 2 ± Continuation (18 months) 6MP/Ara-C	268	90	5	6-yr EFS 48%±6% 6-yr OS 60%±6%	Low-dose continuation treatment had no benefit and may contribute to drug resistance and poor salvage rate after relapse.
MRC AML10[339,340]	1988–1995	Remission induction DAT vs ADE × 2 Consolidation 1. Amsa/Ara-C/VP16 2. Mito/Ara-C Postconsolidation Allo HSCT for patients with suitable donor Others:Auto HSCT or no chemotherapy.	341	92	6	7-yr EFS 48% 7-yr OS 56%	Short-term intensive chemotherapy without continuation treatment can cure 50% of patients. Transplantation reduced risk of relapse but did not improve survival.

TABLE 101-5

Results of Selected Recent Clinical Trials for Childhood AML—cont'd

STUDY	YEARS	TREATMENT SCHEDULE	NO. OF PATIENTS	REMISSION RATE (%)	EARLY MORTALITY (%)	OVERALL OUTCOME	CONCLUSIONS
NOPHO88[341]	1988–1992	Remission induction 1. 6TG/Ara-C/VP16/Doxo 2. Mito/Ara-C 3. 6TG/Ara-C/VP16/Doxo Consolidation 1. HD Ara-C/Mito 2. HD Ara-C/VP16 3. HD Ara-C 4. HD Ara-C/VP16	118	85	12	5-yr EFS 42%±5%	Addition of mitoxantrone and etoposide to consolidation therapy with high-dose cytarabine did not improve outcome due to excessive deaths in relapse.
POG 9421[343] [342]	1995–1999	Remission induction 1. DAT vs HDAT 2. HD Ara-C Consolidation Allo HSCT for patients with suitable donor Others: chemotherapy: 1. VP16/Mito±CsA 2. HD Ara-C 3. VP16/Mito±CsA	632	90	—	3-yr EFS 30.5% to 43.2% 3-yr OS 51.3% to 55.4%	High-dose cytarabine during induction did not improve complete remission rate but tended to improve EFS.
SJCRH AML91[247]	1991–1996	Remission induction 1. 2CDA 2. Dauno/Ara-C/VP16 Consolidation Dauno/Ara-C/VP16 x 2 Postconsolidation Allo HSCT for patients with suitable donor, Others: Auto HSCT	73	78	—	5-yr EFS 40%±8% 5-yr OS 53%	2-chlorodeoxyadenosine was effective treatment for monoblastic leukemia.

2CDA, 2-chlorodeoxyadenosine; 6MP, 6-mercaptopurine; 6TG, 6-thioguanine; ADE, cytarabine, daunorubicin, etoposide; doxo, doxorubicin; Allo HSCT, Allogeneic hematopoietic stem cell transplant; Amsa, amsacrine; ANZCCSG, Australian and New Zealand Children's Cancer Group; Ara-C, cytarabine; Asp, asparaginase; Auto HSCT, autologous hematopoietic stem cell transplant; BFM, Berlin-Frankfurt-Münster Study Group; CCG, Children's Cancer Group; CsA, cyclosporine; DAT, daunorubicin, cytarabine, 6-thioguanine; Dauno, daunorubicin; DCTER, decadron, cytarabine, 6-thioguanine, etoposide, rubomycin (daunorubicin); EFS, event-free survival; HD Ara-C, high-dose cytarabine; HDAT, daunorubicin, high-dose cytarabine, 6-thioguanine; Ida, idarubicin; LAME, Leucamie Aiquë Myéloide Enfant; Mito, mitoxantrone; MRC, Medical Research Council; NOPHO, Nordic Society of Paediatric Haematology and Oncology; OS, overall survival; POG, Pediatric Oncology Group; SJCRH, St Jude Children's Research Hospital; VP16, etoposide.

response to remission induction therapy] are candidates for this procedure, perhaps even if alternative or unrelated donors are the only options.[368,369] By contrast, transplantation is not recommended for patients with Down syndrome or APL in first remission, which have a favorable prognosis with current therapy.[368,369]

Treatment Sequelae

Improved supportive care reduced the rate of early death to less than 2% in the 1990s.[304] Induction therapy with prednisone, vincristine, and L-asparaginase might cause hyperglycemia and thrombosis. The intensified use of methotrexate and glucocorticoids has caused an increased frequency of neurotoxicity and, in older children and adults, aseptic necrosis of bone. High cumulative doses of anthracyclines can produce severe cardiomyopathy, especially in young children. Cranial irradiation causes neuropsychologic deficits, endocrine abnormalities that lead to obesity, short stature, precocious puberty, osteoporosis, and second neoplasms within the irradiated field.

Development of therapy-related AML has been linked to the use of topoisomerase II inhibitors (teniposide and etoposide), and the risk is apparently dependent on the treatment schedule and the concomitant use of other agents (e.g., L-asparaginase, alkylating agents, and perhaps antimetabolites).[254] Children who receive cranial irradiation at 6 years of age or younger are most susceptible to the development of brain tumors. This risk is increased by the intensive use of antimetabolite drugs before and during cranial irradiation.[370]

MINIMAL RESIDUAL DISEASE

Rationale for Studies of Minimal Residual Disease

In vivo measurement of the cytoreductive effect of therapy can provide direct information about the combined effect of clinical and cellular variables in each patient, thereby directly measuring the effectiveness of treatment rather than predicting outcome. The independent prognostic importance of a patient's gross early response to therapy (i.e., initial reduction of leukemic blasts) is well established. Sluggish or incomplete clearance of leukemic cells by remission induction therapy as determined by morphologic examination of the bone marrow or peripheral blood is associated with a poor treatment outcome.[125,218,371-374] Conventional morphologic techniques have limited sensitivity and accuracy, however; in most cases, leukemic cells can be detected in bone marrow with certainty only when they constitute 5% or more of the total cell population. Methods for detecting minimal (i.e., submicroscopic) residual disease (MRD) are at least 100 times as sensitive as conventional morphologic techniques and allow a more stringent definition of "remission" in patients with acute leukemia. This more stringent definition is rapidly becoming the standard at many cancer centers. In addition, these methods have multiple potential application in the clinical management of patients with leukemia (Table 101-6).

TABLE 101-6

Clinical Applications of MRD Studies

TIME OF STUDY	OBJECTIVE
During remission induction	Measure early response to treatment
Throughout treatment	Identify patients at a higher risk of relapse
Before autograft	Detect contaminating leukemic cells; evaluate the efficacy of "purging"
Postallogeneic transplant	Gauge effect of withdrawal of immunosuppressive therapy and of donor lymphocyte infusions
Throughout treatment	Use MRD as a surrogate endpoint to test the effect of new agents

MRD, minimal residual disease.

Methodological Options for MRD Studies

Many methods of MRD measurement have been tested.[375-381] The most reliable methods for ALL include flow cytometric profiling of aberrant immunophenotypes, polymerase chain reaction (PCR) amplification of fusion transcripts and chromosomal breakpoints, and PCR amplification of antigen-receptor genes. Only the first two can be applied AML, as most cases lack antigen-receptor gene rearrangement. The value of another PCR target, WT-1, remains controversial.[382-384] *FLT3* ITD could, in principle, be used as targets for PCR-based MRD studies in AML; however, *FLT3* ITD that are detected at diagnosis are often undetectable at the time of relapse.[385-387] Because of their limited sensitivity (approximately 1%–5%), conventional karyotyping and FISH cannot reliably detect submicroscopic leukemia but are occasionally useful in clarifying the nature of morphologically suspicious blast cells.[388] Improved image analysis technology that allows simultaneous visualization of morphologic, immunophenotypic, and FISH features might enhance the usefulness of FISH studies.[389] Only a few laboratories have reported success with methods based on the differential properties of normal and leukemic cells in culture.[390,391]

We compared flow cytometric detection of aberrant immunophenotyes and PCR amplification of *IGH* genes by studying serial dilutions of normal and leukemic cells and 62 remission samples from patients with ALL.[392] We found the two methods to be generally concordant. A study comparing the detection of MRD by flow cytometry and PCR amplification of *TCRG* and *TCRD* genes also found concordant results in most samples.[393] A study comparing flow cytometry with RT-PCR detection of BCR-ABL transcripts in 23 remission bone marrow samples from patients who had ALL with the Philadelphia-chromosome observed concordant results in 18 samples.[394]

Prognostic Value of MRD in ALL

Several prospective studies have defined the prevalence and the clinical significance of MRD at different time points during treatment of childhood ALL. In one multicenter study, MRD was measured in 178 patients by a competitive PCR assay targeting junctional sequences of

IGH and *TCR*.[395] The presence or absence and the level of residual leukemia during the first 6 months of therapy were correlated significantly with the risk of early relapse at each of the time points studied. Patients who had 1% or more leukemic cells after the completion of induction therapy or who had 0.1% or more at later time points had a particularly high risk of relapse. Another multicenter study monitored MRD in 240 children with ALL treated in the International BFM Study Group protocols.[396] This study used PCR analysis of *IGH* genes, *TCR* genes, and *TAL1* deletions. MRD-positive patients had relapse rates 5 to 10 times the relapse rate of patients who were MRD-negative at the various follow-up times. MRD levels greater than or equal to 1% at the end of induction treatment and before consolidation treatment were associated with a very high relapse rate. Combined MRD information from the first two follow-up time points was particularly informative, allowing the identification of three different risk groups: (1) A low-risk group comprising 43% of patients with a 3-year relapse rate of 2% (95% CI, 0.05%–12%); (2) a high-risk group comprising 15% of patients with a relapse rate of 75% (55%–95%); and (3) an intermediate-risk group (43%) with a 3-year relapse rate of 23% (13%–36%).

We used flow cytometry to study MRD prospectively in 195 children with newly diagnosed ALL enrolled in a single-institution chemotherapy program (Total XIII).[295,397,398] We found that detectable MRD (i.e., ≥0.01% leukemic mononuclear cells) at any of the time points studied (day 19 and end of remission induction therapy and weeks 14, 32, and 56 of continuation) had significant association with a higher relapse rate (Fig. 101-4). Patients who had high levels of MRD at the end of the induction phase (≥1%) or at week 14 of continuation therapy (≥0.1%) had a dismal outcome. The incidence of relapse among patients with MRD at the end of the induction phase was 68% ± 16% (SE) if they remained MRD-positive through week 14 of continuation therapy, but only 7% ± 7% if MRD became undetectable. The persistence of MRD until week 32 was highly predictive of relapse: All four patients who were MRD-positive at week 32 had relapses, but only two of the eight who became MRD-negative had relapses.

Of the 112 patients studied at day 19 of remission induction therapy, 53 had achieved a profound cytoreduction (MRD <0.01%) despite the brief duration of chemotherapy.[398] The outcome of treatment for this group of patients was outstanding: The 3-year cumulative incidence of relapse was 1.9% ± 1.9%, compared with 28.4% ± 6.4% for MRD-positive patients. These results are consistent with those of another study, in which bone marrow samples collected at day 15 of therapy from 68 children with ALL were assayed by PCR amplification of antigen-receptor genes.[399] The proportion of children who had the lowest levels of MRD in the two studies was different, however: 21% in this series, 46% in ours.

In the studies just outlined, the prognostic value of MRD was independent of other known clinical and biologic prognosticators of outcome. In our study, MRD remained a significant predictor in analyses that excluded patients at very high or very low risk of relapse by St. Jude criteria or that focused on patients at high risk of relapse by the National Cancer Institute criteria.[6,295] In the I-BFM study, MRD was also a strong predictor of outcome in children with features that indicated a medium risk.[400]

A recent study showed that the predictive value of MRD monitoring extends to children receiving treatment for relapsed ALL.[401] MRD detection by PCR amplification of antigen-receptor genes before or after allogeneic bone marrow transplantation was predictive of relapse in children with ALL.[402-404]

In sum, there is strong collective evidence of an association between MRD and an increased risk of relapse of ALL; however, no such association was observed in one study in which MRD was monitored by RT-PCR amplification of *E2A-PBX1* fusion transcripts at the end of consolidation treatment in children with t(1;19)-positive ALL.[405] It remains unclear whether a more precise quantitation of MRD would have identified patients at higher risk of relapse or whether MRD is uninformative in this subset of patients with ALL.

In children with ALL in first remission, a study that used PCR amplification of *IGH* genes detected MRD in 15 of 17 patients who remained in remission 2 to 35 months after completion of treatment, suggesting that eradication of all leukemic cells is not a prerequisite for cure.[406] The high frequency of detectable leukemic cells or leukemia-specific PCR products in children with ALL who enjoy prolonged complete remission has not been confirmed by other studies.[395-397,407]

In recent studies comparing MRD measurements in bone marrow and peripheral blood samples, findings in bone marrow and blood were completely concordant in the paired samples from patients with T-lineage ALL.[408]

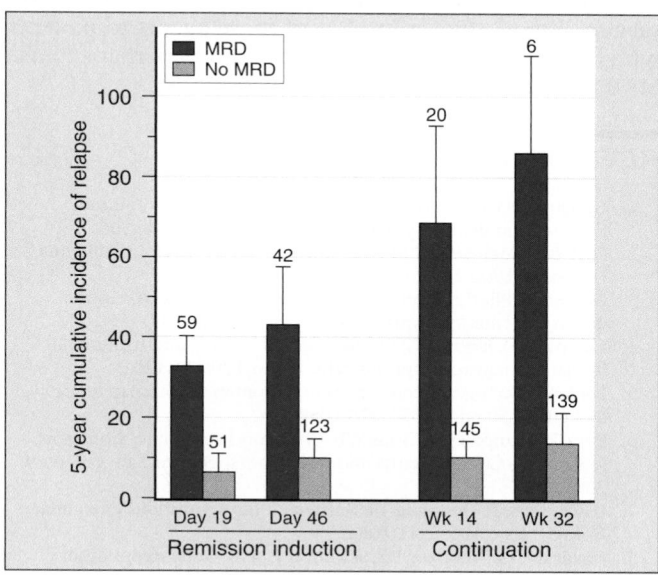

Figure 101-4. Risk of relapse according to MRD in children with ALL. The 5-year cumulative incidence of relapse according to the results of a flow cytometric MRD assay at different times during treatment is shown. (Data from Coustan-Smith E, Sancho J, Hancock ML, et al: Clinical importance of minimal residual disease in childhood acute lymphoblastic leukemia. Blood 2000;96:2691; Coustan-Smith E, Sancho J, Behm FG, et al: Prognostic importance of measuring early clearance of leukemic cells by flow cytometry in childhood acute lymphoblastic leukemia. Blood 2002;100:52.)

The results of a recently reported study using immuno-fluorescence analysis and real time RT-PCR are in agreement with these data.[409] We also observed that peripheral-blood MRD in patients with B-lineage ALL was associated with a very high risk of disease recurrence.[408] Therefore, peripheral blood can be used to monitor MRD in patients with T-lineage ALL. In B-lineage ALL, the presence of MRD in peripheral blood appears to identify patients who are at a very high risk of relapse.

MRD Studies in Patients with AML

The lack of widely expressed molecular markers in AML cells precludes the systematic study of MRD by PCR. Antigen-receptor genes are rearranged in fewer than 10% of AML cases, and fewer than half of patients have nonrandom genetic abnormalities with fusion transcripts suitable for molecular studies of MRD.[381] Thus, correlative studies between MRD and treatment outcome have been performed only in selected groups of patients, almost exclusively adults. In APL, PCR detection of *PML-RARA* and *RARA-PML* transcripts during remission generally predicts relapse.[410-412] The significance of *AML1-ETO* transcripts during remission of AML with the t(8;21) is less clear. Early studies showed that these transcripts persist for more than 5 years of remission after the completion of treatment, a finding that could be explained by the expression of *AML1-ETO* transcripts in normal monocytes, B cells, and hematopoietic colony-forming cells.[413,414] Careful quantitation of these transcripts can help to monitor MRD, however.[415,416] Productive MRD studies have also been reported in patients with AML and inv(16)/*CBFB-MYH11*.[417-420]

The presence of MRD detected by flow cytometry was associated with earlier relapse in 19 of 35 children with AML in first morphologic remission.[421] In another study including mostly adult patients, the first bone marrow sample showing morphologic remission after induction treatment was found to be very informative.[422] The 126 patients could be divided into four groups on the basis of MRD level. Eight patients had fewer than 0.01% leukemic cells, and none had relapsed at the time of the report; 37 patients had 0.01% to 0.1% leukemic cells and had a 3-year cumulative relapse rate of 14%; 64 patients had 0.1% to 1% leukemic cells and had a relapse rate of 50%; and 17 patients had more than 1% residual leukemic cells and had a relapse rate of 84%. In another study of 51 patients in whom MRD was examined after consolidation therapy, the most predictive MRD cut-off value determined retrospectively was 0.035%: 17 of 22 patients with that level of MRD or higher had a relapse, compared with 5 of 29 patients who had lower MRD levels.[423] In patients with AML who received autologous bone marrow transplants, the proportion of cells expressing an aberrant immunophenotype in the autograft was associated with disease recurrence.[424]

ISSUES FOR THE FUTURE

The current cure rates for ALL attest to the steady progress that has been made in treating this disease. A further increase in cure rates will require success in maximizing the efficacy and minimizing the toxicity of current therapy. The methods of achieving optimal treatment are the subject of intense debate, however. For example, there is considerable disagreement about the most useful risk criteria and terminology for defining prognostic subgroups. In the future, it could be possible to identify more accurate and universally acceptable indicators of risk, perhaps through the use of global gene expression analysis or proteomics studies.[8,9] MRD monitoring now allows the objective and sensitive assessment of treatment response, and it has been incorporated into treatment protocols at our institution and in BFM studies.[425]

Cure rates for children with AML and for subset of patients with ALL, such as infants and those with t(9;22), remain low. For these patients, substantial improvement in cure rates can come only from the development of new treatments. In addition to imatinib for the treatment of ALL with the t(9;22) translocation, recently developed compounds with potential clinical value include GW506U78 (a prodrug of arabinosylguanine) for the treatment of T-lineage ALL, docetaxel for the treatment of ALL, CD52 (Campath I) for the treatment of ALL, and an anti-CD33 antibody conjugated to a toxin (calicheamicin) for the treatment of AML.[426-429] Other therapeutic approaches that are being investigated include the use of T cells manipulated ex vivo to specifically recognize leukemia cells, diphteria toxin-conjugated to the granulocyte-macrophage colony-stimulating factor, and compounds that directly interfere with oncogenic molecular aberrations, such as farnesyltransferase inhibitors, proteasome, and FLT3-inhibitors.[430] Testing of these approaches could necessitate nontraditional methods. It might soon be necessary to extend efficacy studies of these agents to patients who have not yet been heavily treated, and perhaps to use MRD measurement to assess tumor response.

REFERENCES

1. Gilliland DG, Blanchard KL, Bunn HF: Clonality in acquired hematologic disorders. Annu Rev Med 1991;42:491–506.
2. Gale RE, Linch DC: Clonality studies in acute myeloid leukemia. Leukemia 1998;12:117.
3. Gavosto F, Pileri A, Bachi C, et al: Proliferation and maturation defect in acute leukemia cells. Nature 1964;203:92.
4. Campana D, Janossy G: Proliferation of normal and malignant human immature lymphoid cells. Blood 1988;71:1201.
5. Look AT: Oncogenic transcription factors in the human acute leukemias. Science 1997;278:1059.
6. Pui CH, Campana D, Evans WE: Childhood acute lymphoblastic leukemia—Current status and future perspectives. Lancet Oncol 2001;2:597.
7. Lowenberg B, Downing JR, Burnett A: Acute myeloid leukemia. N Engl J Med 1999;341:1051.
8. Ferrando AA, Neuberg DS, Staunton J, et al: Gene expression signatures define novel oncogenic pathways in T cell acute lymphoblastic leukemia. Cancer Cell 2002;1:75.
9. Yeoh EJ, Ross ME, Shurtleff SA, et al: Classification, subtype discovery, and prediction of outcome in pediatric acute lymphoblastic leukemia by gene expression profiling. Cancer Cell 2002;1:133.
10. Schoch C, Kohlmann A, Schnittger S, et al: Acute myeloid leukemias with reciprocal rearrangements can be distinguished by specific gene expression profiles. Proc Natl Acad Sci USA 2002;99:10008.
11. Sandler DP, Ross JA: Epidemiology of acute leukemia in children and adults. Semin Oncol 1997;24:3.

12. Bhatia S, Ross JA, Greaves MF, et al: Epidemiology and etiology. In Pui CH (ed): Childhood Leukemias. Cambridge, Cambridge University Press, 1999, p 38.
13. Langmuir PB, Aplenc R, Lange BJ: Acute myeloid leukaemia in children. Best Pract Res Clin Haematol 2001;14:77.
14. Douer D, Preston-Martin S, Chang E, et al: High frequency of acute promyelocytic leukemia among Latinos with acute myeloid leukemia. Blood 1996;87:308.
15. Biondi A, Rovelli A, Cantu-Rajnoldi A, et al: Acute promyelocytic leukemia in children: Experience of the Italian Pediatric Hematology and Oncology Group (AIEOP). Leukemia 1994;8:1264.
16. Bhatia S, Neglia JP: Epidemiology of childhood acute myelogenous leukemia. J Pediatr Hematol Oncol 1995;17:94.
17. Louie S, Schwartz RS: Immunodeficiency and the pathogenesis of lymphoma and leukemia. Semin Hematol 1978;15:117.
18. Ford AM, Ridge SA, Cabrera ME, et al: In utero rearrangements in the trithorax-related oncogene in infant leukaemias. Nature 1993;363:358.
19. Mahmoud HH, Ridge SA, Behm FG, et al: Intrauterine monoclonal origin of neonatal concordant acute lymphoblastic leukemia in monozygotic twins. Med Pediatr Oncol 1995;24:77.
20. Gale KB, Ford AM, Repp R, et al: Backtracking leukemia to birth: Identification of clonotypic gene fusion sequences in neonatal blood spots. Proc Natl Acad Sci USA 1997;94:13950.
21. Ford AM, Pombo-de-Oliveira MS, McCarthy KP, et al: Monoclonal origin of concordant T-cell malignancy in identical twins. Blood 1997;89:281.
22. Wiemels JL, Cazzaniga G, Daniotti M, et al: Prenatal origin of acute lymphoblastic leukaemia in children. Lancet 1999;354:1499.
23. Maia AT, Ford AM, Jalali GR, et al: Molecular tracking of leukemogenesis in a triplet pregnancy. Blood 2001;98:478.
24. Greaves MF: Aetiology of acute leukaemia. Lancet 1997;349:344.
25. Kinlen LJ: Infection and childhood leukemia. Cancer Causes Control 1998;9:237.
26. Biondi A, Cimino G, Pieters R, et al: Biological and therapeutic aspects of infant leukemia. Blood 2000;96:24.
27. Pui CH, Relling MV: Topoisomerase II inhibitor-related acute myeloid leukaemia. Br J Haematol 2000;109:13.
28. Wiemels JL, Pagnamenta A, Taylor GM, et al: A lack of a functional NAD(P)H:quinone oxidoreductase allele is selectively associated with pediatric leukemias that have MLL fusions. United Kingdom Childhood Cancer Study Investigators. Cancer Res 1999;59:4095.
29. Alexander FE, Patheal SL, Biondi A, et al: Transplacental chemical exposure and risk of infant leukemia with MLL gene fusion. Cancer Res 2001;61:2542.
30. Chen CL, Liu Q, Pui CH, et al: Higher frequency of glutathione S-transferase deletions in black children with acute lymphoblastic leukemia. Blood 1997;89:1701.
31. Krajinovic M, Sinnett H, Richer C, et al: Role of NQO1, MPO and CYP2E1 genetic polymorphisms in the susceptibility to childhood acute lymphoblastic leukemia. Int J Cancer 2002;97:230.
32. Smith MT, Wang Y, Skibola CF, et al: Low NAD(P)H:quinone oxidoreductase activity is associated with increased risk of leukemia with MLL translocations in infants and children. Blood 2002;100:4590.
33. Krajinovic M, Labuda D, Mathonnet G, et al: Polymorphisms in genes encoding drugs and xenobiotic metabolizing enzymes, DNA repair enzymes, and response to treatment of childhood acute lymphoblastic leukemia. Clin Cancer Res 2002;8:802.
34. Franco RF, Simoes BP, Tone LG, et al: The methylenetetrahydro-folate reductase C677T gene polymorphism decreases the risk of childhood acute lymphocytic leukaemia. Br J Haematol 2001;115:616.
35. Wiemels JL, Smith RN, Taylor GM, et al: Methylenetetrahydrofolate reductase (MTHFR) polymorphisms and risk of molecularly defined subtypes of childhood acute leukemia. Proc Natl Acad Sci USA 2001;98:4004.
36. Thompson JR, Gerald PF, Willoughby ML, et al: Maternal folate supplementation in pregnancy and protection against acute lymphoblastic leukaemia in childhood: A case-control study. Lancet 2001;358:1935.
37. Lorsbach RB, Downing JR: The role of the AML1 transcription factor in leukemogenesis. Int J Hematol 2001;74:258.
38. Dash A, Gilliland DG: Molecular genetics of acute myeloid leukaemia. Best Pract Res Clin Haematol 2001;14:49.
39. Inukai T, Inoue A, Kurosawa H, et al: SLUG, a ces-1-related zinc finger transcription factor gene with antiapoptotic activity, is a downstream target of the E2A-HLF oncoprotein. Mol Cell 1999;4:343.
40. Gotoh A, Broxmeyer HE: The function of BCR/ABL and related proto-oncogenes. Curr Opin Hematol 1997;4:3.
41. Campos L, Rouault JP, Sabido O, et al: High expression of bcl-2 protein in acute myeloid leukemia cells is associated with poor response to chemotherapy. Blood 1993;81:3091.
42. Coustan-Smith E, Kitanaka A, Pui CH, et al: Clinical relevance of BCL-2 overexpression in childhood acute lymphoblastic leukemia. Blood 1996;87:1140.
43. Meijerink JP, Mensink EJ, Wang K, et al: Hematopoietic malignancies demonstrate loss-of-function mutations of BAX. Blood 1998;91:2991.
44. Gilliland DG, Griffin JD: The roles of FLT3 in hematopoiesis and leukemia. Blood 2002;100:1532.
45. Griffin JD: Point mutations in the FLT3 gene in AML. Blood 2001;97:2193A.
46. Greaves M: Molecular genetics, natural history and the demise of childhood leukaemia. Eur J Cancer 1999;35:1941.
47. Fasching K, Panzer S, Haas OA, et al: Presence of clone-specific antigen receptor gene rearrangements at birth indicates an in utero origin of diverse types of early childhood acute lymphoblastic leukemia. Blood 2000;95:2722.
48. Mori H, Colman SM, Xiao Z, et al: Chromosome translocations and covert leukemic clones are generated during normal fetal development. Proc Natl Acad Sci USA 2002;99:8242.
49. Wiemels JL, Leonard BC, Wang Y, et al: Site-specific translocation and evidence of postnatal origin of the t(1;19) E2A-PBX1 fusion in childhood acute lymphoblastic leukemia. Proc Natl Acad Sci USA 2002;99:15101.
50. Bisschop MM, Revesz T, Bierings M, et al: Extramedullary infiltrates at diagnosis have no prognostic significance in children with acute myeloid leukaemia. Leukemia 2001;15:46.
51. Pui CH: Toward optimal CNS-directed treatment in childhood ALL. J Clin Oncol 2003;21:179.
52. Bennett JM, Catovsky D, Daniel MT, et al: Proposals for the classification of the acute leukaemias. French-American-British (FAB) Co-operative Group. Br J Haematol 1976;33:451.
53. Mason DY, Stein H, Gerdes J, et al: Value of monoclonal anti-CD22 (p135) antibodies for the detection of normal and neoplastic B lymphoid cells. Blood 1987;69:836.
54. Janossy G, Coustan-Smith E, Campana D: The reliability of cytoplasmic CD3 and CD22 antigen expression in the immunodiagnosis of acute leukemia: A study of 500 cases. Leukemia 1989;3:170.
55. Mason DY, Cordell JL, Tse AG, et al: The IgM-associated protein mb-1 as a marker of normal and neoplastic B cells. J Immunol 1991;147:2474.
56. Buccheri V, Mihaljevic B, Matutes E, et al: mb-1: A new marker for B-lineage lymphoblastic leukemia. Blood 1993;82:853.
57. Boue DR, LeBien TW: Expression and structure of CD22 in acute leukemia. Blood 1988;71:1480.
58. Pui CH, Behm FG, Crist WM: Clinical and biologic relevance of immunologic marker studies in childhood acute lymphoblastic leukemia. Blood 1993;82:343.
59. Borowitz MJ, Shuster JJ, Civin CI, et al: Prognostic significance of CD34 expression in childhood B-precursor acute lymphocytic leukemia: A Pediatric Oncology Group study. J Clin Oncol 1990;8:1389.
60. Behm FG, Raimondi SC, Schell MJ, et al: Lack of CD45 antigen on blast cells in childhood acute lymphoblastic leukemia is associated with chromosomal hyperdiploidy and other favorable prognostic features. Blood 1992;79:1011.
61. Pui CH, Frankel LS, Carroll AJ, et al: Clinical characteristics and treatment outcome of childhood acute lymphoblastic leukemia with the t(4;11)(q21;q23): A collaborative study of 40 cases. Blood 1991;77:440.
62. Behm FG, Smith FO, Raimondi SC, et al: Human homologue of the rat chondroitin sulfate proteoglycan, NG2, detected by monoclonal antibody 7.1, identifies childhood acute lymphoblastic leukemias with t(4;11)(q21;q23) or

t(11;19)(q23;p13) and MLL gene rearrangements. Blood 1996;87:1134.

63. Vogler LB, Crist WM, Bockman DE, et al: Pre-B-cell leukemia. A new phenotype of childhood lymphoblastic leukemia. N Engl J Med 1978;298:872.

64. Pui CH, Hancock ML, Head DR, et al: Clinical significance of CD34 expression in childhood acute lymphoblastic leukemia. Blood 1993;82:889.

65. Pui CH, Raimondi SC, Hancock ML, et al: Immunologic, cytogenetic, and clinical characterization of childhood acute lymphoblastic leukemia with the t(1;19) (q23; p13) or its derivative. J Clin Oncol 1994;12:2601.

66. Borowitz MJ, Hunger SP, Carroll AJ, et al: Predictability of the t(1;19)(q23;p13) from surface antigen phenotype: implications for screening cases of childhood acute lymphoblastic leukemia for molecular analysis: A Pediatric Oncology Group study. Blood 1993;82:1086.

67. Koehler M, Behm FG, Shuster J, et al: Transitional pre-B-cell acute lymphoblastic leukemia of childhood is associated with favorable prognostic clinical features and an excellent outcome: A Pediatric Oncology Group study. Leukemia 1993;7:2064.

68. Drexler HG, Messmore HL, Menon M, et al: A case of TdT-positive B-cell acute lymphoblastic leukemia. Am J Clin Pathol 1986; 85:735.

69. Secker-Walker L, Stewart E, Norton J, et al: Multiple chromosome abnormalities in a drug resistant TdT positive B-cell leukemia. Leuk Res 1987;11:155.

70. Mufti GJ, Hamblin TJ, Oscier DG, et al: Common ALL with pre-B-cell features showing (8;14) and (14;18) chromosome translocations. Blood 1983;62:1142.

71. Gluck WL, Bigner SH, Borowitz MJ, et al: Acute lymphoblastic leukemia of Burkitt's type (L3 ALL) with 8;22 and 14;18 translocations and absent surface immunoglobulins. Am J Clin Pathol 1986;85:636.

72. Walle AJ, Al-Katib A, Wong GY, et al: Multiparameter characterization of L3 leukemia cell populations. Leuk Res 1987;11:73.

73. Finlay JL, Borcherding W: Acute B-lymphocytic leukemia with L1 morphology: A report of two pediatric cases. Leukemia 1988;2:60.

74. Link MP, Stewart SJ, Warnke RA, et al: Discordance between surface and cytoplasmic expression of the Leu-4 (T3) antigen in thymocytes and in blast cells from childhood T lymphoblastic malignancies. J Clin Invest 1985;76:248.

75. Campana D, Thompson JS, Amlot P, et al: The cytoplasmic expression of CD3 antigens in normal and malignant cells of the T lymphoid lineage. J Immunol 1987;138:648.

76. van Dongen JJ, Krissansen GW, Wolvers-Tettero IL, et al: Cytoplasmic expression of the CD3 antigen as a diagnostic marker for immature T-cell malignancies. Blood 1988;71:603.

77. Pui CH, Behm FG, Singh B, et al: Heterogeneity of presenting features and their relation to treatment outcome in 120 children with T-cell acute lymphoblastic leukemia. Blood 1990; 75:174.

78. Pui CH, Rivera GK, Hancock ML, et al: Clinical significance of CD10 expression in childhood acute lymphoblastic leukemia. Leukemia 1993;7:35.

79. Thiel E, Kranz BR, Raghavachar A, et al: Prethymic phenotype and genotype of pre-T (CD7+/ER-)-cell leukemia and its clinical significance within adult acute lymphoblastic leukemia. Blood 1989;73:1247.

80. Shuster JJ, Falletta JM, Pullen DJ, et al: Prognostic factors in childhood T-cell acute lymphoblastic leukemia: A Pediatric Oncology Group study. Blood 1990;75:166.

81. Uckun FM, Steinherz PG, Sather H, et al: CD2 antigen expression on leukemic cells as a predictor of event-free survival after chemotherapy for T-lineage acute lymphoblastic leukemia: A Children's Cancer Group study. Blood 1996;88:4288.

82. Campana D, van Dongen JJ, Mehta A, et al: Stages of T-cell receptor protein expression in T-cell acute lymphoblastic leukemia. Blood 1991;77:1546.

83. Campana D, Coustan-Smith E, Behm FG, et al: Normal and aberrant T-cell receptor protein expression in T-cell acute lymphoblastic leukemia. In Ludwig WD, Thiel E (eds): Recent Advances in Cell Biology of Acute Leukemia. Berlin, Springer-Verlag, 1993, p 19.

84. Drexler HG: Classification of acute myeloid leukemias—a comparison of FAB and immunophenotyping. Leukemia 1987;1:697.

85. Buccheri V, Shetty V, Yoshida N, et al: The role of an anti-myeloperoxidase antibody in the diagnosis and classification of acute leukemia: A comparison with light and electron microscopy cytochemistry. Br J Haematol 1992;80:62.

86. Knapp W, Strobl H, Majdic O: Flow cytometric analysis of cell-surface and intracellular antigens in leukemia diagnosis. Cytometry 1994;18:187.

87. Rothe G, Schmitz G: Consensus protocol for the flow cytometric immunophenotyping of hematopoietic malignancies. Working Group on Flow Cytometry and Image Analysis. Leukemia 1996; 10:877.

88. Kita K, Nakase K, Miwa H, et al: Phenotypical characteristics of acute myelocytic leukemia associated with the t(8;21)(q22;q22) chromosomal abnormality: Frequent expression of immature B-cell antigen CD19 together with stem cell antigen CD34. Blood 1992;80:470.

89. Arber DA, Glackin C, Lowe G, et al: Presence of t(8;21)(q22;q22) in myeloperoxidase-positive, myeloid surface antigen-negative acute myeloid leukemia. Am J Clin Pathol 1997;107:68.

90. Hurwitz CA, Raimondi SC, Head D, et al: Distinctive immunophenotypic features of t(8;21)(q22;q22) acute myeloblastic leukemia in children. Blood 1992;80:3182.

91. Seymour JF, Pierce SA, Kantarjian HM, et al: Investigation of karyotypic, morphologic and clinical features in patients with acute myeloid leukemia blast cells expressing the neural cell adhesion molecule (CD56). Leukemia 1994;8:823.

92. Paietta E, Andersen J, Gallagher R, et al: The immunophenotype of acute promyelocytic leukemia (APL): An ECOG study. Leukemia 1994;8:1108.

93. Vidriales MB, Orfao A, Gonzalez M, et al: Expression of NK and lymphoid-associated antigens in blast cells of acute myeloblastic leukemia. Leukemia 1993;7:2026.

94. Paietta E, Andersen J, Yunis J, et al: Acute myeloid leukaemia expressing the leucocyte integrin CD11b-a new leukaemic syndrome with poor prognosis: Result of an ECOG database analysis. Eastern Cooperative Oncology Group. Br J Haematol 1998;100:265.

95. Claxton DF, Reading CL, Nagarajan L, et al: Correlation of CD2 expression with PML gene breakpoints in patients with acute promyelocytic leukemia. Blood 1992;80:582.

96. Lo Coco F, Avvisati G, Diverio D, et al: Rearrangements of the RAR-alpha gene in acute promyelocytic leukaemia: Correlations with morphology and immunophenotype. Br J Haematol 1991;78:494.

97. Orfao A, Chillon MC, Bortoluci AM, et al: The flow cytometric pattern of CD34, CD15 and CD13 expression in acute myeloblastic leukemia is highly characteristic of the presence of PML-RARa gene rearrangements. Haematologica 1999;84:405.

98. Solary E, Casasnovas RO, Campos L, et al: Surface markers in adult acute myeloblastic leukemia: correlation of CD19+, CD34+ and CD14+/DR—phenotypes with shorter survival. Groupe d'Etude Immunologique des Leucemies (GEIL). Leukemia 1992;6:393.

99. Adriaansen HJ, te Boekhorst PA, Hagemeijer AM, et al: Acute myeloid leukemia M4 with bone marrow eosinophilia (M4Eo) and inv(16)(p13q22) exhibits a specific immunophenotype with CD2 expression. Blood 1993;81:3043.

100. Paietta E, Wiernik PH, Andersen J, et al: Acute myeloid leukemia M4 with inv(16) (p13q22) exhibits a specific immunophenotype with CD2 expression. Blood 1993;82:2595.

101. Breton-Gorius J, Lewis JC, Guichard J, et al: Monoclonal antibodies specific for human platelet membrane glycoproteins bind to monocytes by focal absorption of platelet membrane fragments: an ultrastructural immunogold study. Leukemia 1987;1:131.

102. Erber WN, Breton-Gorius J, Villeval JL, et al: Detection of cells of megakaryocyte lineage in haematological malignances by immuno-alkaline phosphatase labelling cell smears with a panel of monoclonal antibodies. Br J Haematol 1987;65:87.

103. Breton-Gorius J, Villeval JL, Kieffer N, et al: Limits of phenotypic markers for the diagnosis of megakaryoblastic leukemia. Blood Cells 1989;15:259.

104. Bennett JM, Catovsky D, Daniel MT, et al: Proposal for the recognition of minimally differentiated acute myeloid leukemia (AML-MO). Br J Haematol 1991;78:325.

105. Venditti A, Del Poeta G, Buccisano F, et al: Minimally differentiated acute myeloid leukemia (AML-M0): Comparison of 25 cases with other French-American-British subtypes. Blood 1997;89:621.
106. Campana D, Hansen-Hagge TE, Matutes E, et al: Phenotypic, genotypic, cytochemical, and ultrastructural characterization of acute undifferentiated leukemia. Leukemia 1990;4:620.
107. Ben-Bassat I, Gale RP: Hybrid acute leukemia. Leuk Res 1984; 8:929.
108. Mirro J, Zipf TF, Pui CH, et al: Acute mixed lineage leukemia: Clinicopathologic correlations and prognostic significance. Blood 1985;66:1115.
109. Drexler HG, Thiel E, Ludwig WD: Review of the incidence and clinical relevance of myeloid antigen-positive acute lymphoblastic leukemia. Leukemia 1991;5:637.
110. Drexler HG, Thiel E, Ludwig WD: Acute myeloid leukemias expressing lymphoid-associated antigens: Diagnostic incidence and prognostic significance. Leukemia 1993;7:489.
111. Campana D, Behm FG: Immunophenotyping of leukemia. J Immunol Methods 2000;243:59.
112. Pui CH, Behm FG, Singh B, et al: Myeloid-associated antigen expression lacks prognostic value in childhood acute lymphoblastic leukemia treated with intensive multiagent chemotherapy. Blood 1990;75:198.
113. Pui CH, Raimondi SC, Head DR, et al: Characterization of childhood acute leukemia with multiple myeloid and lymphoid markers at diagnosis and at relapse. Blood 1991;78:1327.
114. Uckun FM, Sather HN, Gaynon PS, et al: Clinical features and treatment outcome of children with myeloid antigen positive acute lymphoblastic leukemia: A report from the Children's Cancer Group. Blood 1997;90:28.
115. Smith FO, Lampkin BC, Versteeg C, et al: Expression of lymphoid-associated cell surface antigens by childhood acute myeloid leukemia cells lacks prognostic significance. Blood 1992;79:2415.
116. Look AT, Melvin SL, Williams DL, et al: Aneuploidy and percentage of S-phase cells determined by flow cytometry correlate with cell phenotype in childhood acute leukemia. Blood 1982;60:959.
117. Panzer-Grumayer ER, Fasching K, Panzer S, et al: Nondisjunction of chromosomes leading to hyperdiploid childhood B-cell precursor acute lymphoblastic leukemia is an early event during leukemogenesis. Blood 2002;100:347.
118. Secker-Walker LM, Swansbury GJ, Hardisty RM, et al: Cytogenetics of acute lymphoblastic leukaemia in children as a factor in the prediction of long-term survival. Br J Haematol 1982;52:389.
119. Williams DL, Tsiatis A, Brodeur GM, et al: Prognostic importance of chromosome number in 136 untreated children with acute lymphoblastic leukemia. Blood 1982;60:864.
120. Ito C, Kumagai M, Manabe A, et al: Hyperdiploid acute lymphoblastic leukemia with 51 to 65 chromosomes: A distinct biological entity with a marked propensity to undergo apoptosis. Blood 1999;93:315.
121. Zhang Y, Lu J, van den Berghe J, et al: Increased incidence of spontaneous apoptosis in the bone marrow of hyperdiploid childhood acute lymphoblastic leukemia. Exp Hematol 2002;30:333.
122. Synold TW, Relling MV, Boyett JM, et al: Blast cell methotrexate-polyglutamate accumulation in vivo differs by lineage, ploidy, and methotrexate dose in acute lymphoblastic leukemia. J Clin Invest 1994;94:1996.
123. Kaspers GJ, Smets LA, Pieters R, et al: Favorable prognosis of hyperdiploid common acute lymphoblastic leukemia may be explained by sensitivity to antimetabolites and other drugs: Results of an in vitro study. Blood 1995;85:751.
124. Harris MB, Shuster JJ, Carroll A, et al: Trisomy of leukemic cell chromosomes 4 and 10 identifies children with B-progenitor cell acute lymphoblastic leukemia with a very low risk of treatment failure: A Pediatric Oncology Group study. Blood 1992;79:3316.
125. Gaynon PS, Trigg ME, Heerema NA, et al: Children's Cancer Group trials in childhood acute lymphoblastic leukemia: 1983–1995. Leukemia 2000;14:2223.
126. Raimondi SC, Pui CH, Hancock ML, et al: Heterogeneity of hyperdiploid (51–67) childhood acute lymphoblastic leukemia. Leukemia 1996;10:213.
127. Pui CH, Raimondi SC, Dodge RK, et al: Prognostic importance of structural chromosomal abnormalities in children with

128. hyperdiploid (greater than 50 chromosomes) acute lymphoblastic leukemia. Blood 1989;73:1963.
128. Pui CH, Carroll AJ, Head D, et al: Near-triploid and near-tetraploid acute lymphoblastic leukemia of childhood. Blood 1990;76:590.
129. Hunger SP: Chromosomal translocations involving the E2A gene in acute lymphoblastic leukemia: Clinical features and molecular pathogenesis. Blood 1996;87:1211.
130. DiMartino JF, Selleri L, Traver D, et al: The Hox cofactor and proto-oncogene Pbx1 is required for maintenance of definitive hematopoiesis in the fetal liver. Blood 2001;98:618.
131. Dedera DA, Waller EK, LeBrun DP, et al: Chimeric homeobox gene E2A-PBX1 induces proliferation, apoptosis, and malignant lymphomas in transgenic mice. Cell 1993;74:833.
132. Kamps MP, Baltimore D: E2A-Pbx1, the t(1;19) translocation protein of human pre-B-cell acute lymphocytic leukemia, causes acute myeloid leukemia in mice. Mol Cell Biol 1993;13:351.
133. Chang CP, Shen WF, Rozenfeld S, et al: Pbx proteins display hexapeptide-dependent cooperative DNA binding with a subset of Hox proteins. Genes Dev 1995;9:663.
134. Thorsteinsdottir U, Krosl J, Kroon E, et al: The oncoprotein E2A-Pbx1a collaborates with Hoxa9 to acutely transform primary bone marrow cells. Mol Cell Biol 1999;19:6355.
135. Inaba T, Inukai T, Yoshihara T, et al: Reversal of apoptosis by the leukaemia-associated E2A-HLF chimaeric transcription factor. Nature 1996;382:541.
136. Inoue A, Seidel MG, Wu W, et al: Slug, a highly conserved zinc finger transcriptional repressor, protects hematopoietic progenitor cells from radiation-induced apoptosis in vivo. Cancer Cell 2002;2:279.
137. Rubnitz JE, Pui CH, Downing JR: The role of TEL fusion genes in pediatric leukemias. Leukemia 1999;13:6.
138. Seeger K, Stackelberg AV, Taube T, et al: Relapse of TEL-AML1-positive acute lymphoblastic leukemia in childhood: A matched-pair analysis. J Clin Oncol 2001;19:3188.
139. Hann I, Vora A, Harrison G, et al: Determinants of outcome after intensified therapy of childhood lymphoblastic leukaemia: Results from Medical Research Council United Kingdom acute lymphoblastic leukaemia XI protocol. Br J Haematol 2001;113:103.
140. Rubnitz JE, Downing JR, Pui CH, et al: TEL gene rearrangement in acute lymphoblastic leukemia: A new genetic marker with prognostic significance. J Clin Oncol 1997;15:1150.
141. Maloney K, McGavran L, Murphy J, et al: TEL-AML1 fusion identifies a subset of children with standard risk acute lymphoblastic leukemia who have an excellent prognosis when treated with therapy that includes a single delayed intensification. Leukemia 1999;13:1708.
142. Ramakers-Van Woerden NL, Pieters R, Loonen AH, et al: TEL/AML1 gene fusion is related to in vitro drug sensitivity for L-asparaginase in childhood acute lymphoblastic leukemia. Blood 2000;96:1094.
143. Alessandri AJ, Reid GS, Bader SA, et al: ETV6 (TEL)-AML1 pre-B acute lymphoblastic leukaemia cells are associated with a distinct antigen-presenting phenotype. Br J Haematol 2002;116:266.
144. Bernardin F, Yang Y, Cleaves R, et al: TEL-AML1, expressed from t(12;21) in human acute lymphocytic leukemia, induces acute leukemia in mice. Cancer Res 2002;62:3904.
145. Eguchi-Ishimae M, Eguchi M, Ishii E, et al: Breakage and fusion of the TEL (ETV6) gene in immature B lymphocytes induced by apoptogenic signals. Blood 2001;97:737.
146. Rowley JD: The critical role of chromosome translocations in human leukemias. Annu Rev Genet 1998;32:495.
147. Hess JL, Yu BD, Li B, et al: Defects in yolk sac hematopoiesis in Mll-null embryos. Blood 1997;90:1799.
148. Yu BD, Hess JL, Horning SE, et al: Altered Hox expression and segmental identity in Mll-mutant mice. Nature 1995;378:505.
149. De Vivo I, Cui X, Domen J, et al: Growth stimulation of primary B cell precursors by the anti-phosphatase of Sbf1. Proc Natl Acad Sci USA 1998;95:9471.
150. Armstrong SA, Staunton JE, Silverman LB, et al: MLL translocations specify a distinct gene expression profile that distinguishes a unique leukemia. Nat Genet 2002;30:41.
151. Radich JP: Philadelphia chromosome-positive acute lymphocytic leukemia. Hematol Oncol Clin North Am 2001;15:21.

Specific Malignancies

III

152. Hermans A, Heisterkamp N, von Linden M, et al: Unique fusion of bcr and c-abl genes in Philadelphia chromosome positive acute lymphoblastic leukemia. Cell 1987;51:33.

153. Daley GQ, Van Etten RA, Baltimore D: Induction of chronic myelogenous leukemia in mice by the P210bcr/abl gene of the Philadelphia chromosome. Science 1990;247:824.

154. Druker BJ, Tamura S, Buchdunger E, et al: Effects of a selective inhibitor of the Abl tyrosine kinase on the growth of Bcr-Abl positive cells. Nat Med 1996;2:561.

155. Druker BJ, Sawyers CL, Kantarjian H, et al: Activity of a specific inhibitor of the BCR-ABL tyrosine kinase in the blast crisis of chronic myeloid leukemia and acute lymphoblastic leukemia with the Philadelphia chromosome. N Engl J Med 2001;344:1038.

156. Shah NP, Nicoll JM, Nagar B, et al: Multiple BCR-ABL kinase domain mutations confer polyclonal resistance to the tyrosine kinase inhibitor imatinib (STI571) in chronic phase and blast crisis chronic myeloid leukemia. Cancer Cell 2002;2:117.

157. Nowell P, Finan J, Dalla-Favera R, et al: Association of amplified oncogene c-myc with an abnormally banded chromosome 8 in a human leukaemia cell line. Nature 1983;306:494.

158. Adams JM, Harris AW, Pinkert CA, et al: The c-myc oncogene driven by immunoglobulin enhancers induces lymphoid malignancy in transgenic mice. Nature 1985;318:533.

159. Golub TR, Slonim DK, Tamayo P, et al: Molecular classification of cancer: Class discovery and class prediction by gene expression monitoring. Science 1999;286:531.

160. Brown L, Cheng JT, Chen Q, et al: Site-specific recombination of the tal-1 gene is a common occurrence in human T cell leukemia. EMBO J 1990;9:3343.

161. Rabbitts TH: LMO T-cell translocation oncogenes typify genes activated by chromosomal translocations that alter transcription and developmental processes. Genes Dev 1998;12:2651.

162. Hacein-Bey-Abina S, Le Deist F, Carlier F, et al: Sustained correction of X-linked severe combined immunodeficiency by ex vivo gene therapy. N Engl J Med 2002;346:1185.

163. Drexler HG: Review of alterations of the cyclin-dependent kinase inhibitor INK4 family genes p15, p16, p18 and p19 in human leukemia-lymphoma cells. Leukemia 1998;12:845.

164. Kamijo T, Zindy F, Roussel MF, et al: Tumor suppression at the mouse INK4a locus mediated by the alternative reading frame product p19ARF. Cell 1997;91:649.

165. Mauvieux L, Leymarie V, Helias C, et al: High incidence of Hox11L2 expression in children with T-ALL. Leukemia 2002;16:2417.

166. Ballerini P, Blaise A, Busson-Le Coniat M, et al: HOX11L2 expression defines a clinical subtype of pediatric T-ALL associated with poor prognosis. Blood 2002;100:991.

167. de The H, Chomienne C, Lanotte M, et al: The t(15;17) translocation of acute promyelocytic leukaemia fuses the retinoic acid receptor alpha gene to a novel transcribed locus. Nature 1990;347:558.

168. Borrow J, Goddard AD, Sheer D, et al: Molecular analysis of acute promyelocytic leukemia breakpoint cluster region on chromosome 17. Science 1990;249:1577.

169. Alcalay M, Zangrilli D, Pandolfi PP, et al: Translocation breakpoint of acute promyelocytic leukemia lies within the retinoic acid receptor alpha locus. Proc Natl Acad Sci USA 1991;88:1977.

170. Kakizuka A, Miller WH Jr, Umesono K, et al: Chromosomal translocation t(15;17) in human acute promyelocytic leukemia fuses RAR alpha with a novel putative transcription factor, PML. Cell 1991;66:663.

171. Biondi A, Rambaldi A, Pandolfi PP, et al: Molecular monitoring of the myl/retinoic acid receptor-alpha fusion gene in acute promyelocytic leukemia by polymerase chain reaction. Blood 192;80:492.

172. Grisolano JL, Wesselschmidt RL, Pelicci PG, et al: Altered myeloid development and acute leukemia in transgenic mice expressing PML-RAR alpha under control of cathepsin G regulatory sequences. Blood 1997;89:376.

173. He LZ, Tribioli C, Rivi R, et al: Acute leukemia with promyelocytic features in PML/RARalpha transgenic mice. Proc Natl Acad Sci USA 1997;94:5302.

174. Brown D, Kogan S, Lagasse E, et al: A PMLRARalpha transgene initiates murine acute promyelocytic leukemia. Proc Natl Acad Sci USA 1997;94:2551.

175. Piazza F, Gurrieri C, Pandolfi PP: The theory of APL. Oncogene 2001;20:7216.

176. Nagy L, Kao HY, Chakravarti D, et al: Nuclear receptor repression mediated by a complex containing SMRT, mSin3A, and histone deacetylase. Cell 1997;89:373.

177. Salomoni P, Pandolfi PP: The role of PML in tumor suppression. Cell 2002;108:165.

178. Quignon F, De Bels F, Koken M, et al: PML induces a novel caspase-independent death process. Nat Genet 1998;20:259.

179. de The H, Lavau C, Marchio A, et al: The PML-RAR alpha fusion mRNA generated by the t(15;17) translocation in acute promyelocytic leukemia encodes a functionally altered RAR. Cell 1991;66:675.

180. Guiochon-Mantel A, Savouret JF, Quignon F, et al: Effect of PML and PML-RAR on the transactivation properties and subcellular distribution of steroid hormone receptors. Mol Endocrinol 1995;9:1791.

181. Weis K, Rambaud S, Lavau C, et al: Retinoic acid regulates aberrant nuclear localization of PML-RAR alpha in acute promyelocytic leukemia cells. Cell 1994;76:345.

182. Dyck JA, Maul GG, Miller WH Jr, et al: A novel macromolecular structure is a target of the promyelocyte-retinoic acid receptor oncoprotein. Cell 1994;76:333.

183. Shao W, Benedetti L, Lamph WW, et al: A retinoid-resistant acute promyelocytic leukemia subclone expresses a dominant negative PML-RAR alpha mutation. Blood 1997;89:4282.

184. Chen GQ, Zhu J, Shi XG, et al: In vitro studies on cellular and molecular mechanisms of arsenic trioxide (As2O3) in the treatment of acute promyelocytic leukemia: As2O3 induces NB4 cell apoptosis with downregulation of Bcl-2 expression and modulation of PML-RAR alpha/PML proteins. Blood 1996; 88:1052.

185. Zhu J, Koken MH, Quignon F, et al: Arsenic-induced PML targeting onto nuclear bodies: Implications for the treatment of acute promyelocytic leukemia. Proc Natl Acad Sci USA 1997;94:3978.

186. Redner RL, Chen JD, Rush EA, et al: The t(5;17) acute promyelocytic leukemia fusion protein NPM-RAR interacts with co-repressor and co-activator proteins and exhibits both positive and negative transcriptional properties. Blood 2000;95:2683.

187. Ruthardt M, Testa U, Nervi C, et al: Opposite effects of the acute promyelocytic leukemia PML-retinoic acid receptor alpha (RAR alpha) and PLZF-RAR alpha fusion proteins on retinoic acid signalling. Mol Cell Biol 1997;17:4859.

188. Okuda T, van Deursen J, Hiebert SW, et al: AML1, the target of multiple chromosomal translocations in human leukemia, is essential for normal fetal liver hematopoiesis. Cell 1996;84:321.

189. Miller JD, Stacy T, Liu PP, et al: Core-binding factor beta (CBFbeta), but not CBFbeta-smooth muscle myosin heavy chain, rescues definitive hematopoiesis in CBFbeta-deficient embryonic stem cells. Blood 2001;97:2248.

190. Raimondi SC, Chang MN, Ravindranath Y, et al: Chromosomal abnormalities in 478 children with acute myeloid leukemia: Clinical characteristics and treatment outcome in a cooperative pediatric oncology group study-POG 8821. Blood 1999;94:3707.

191. Mrozek K, Heinonen K, de La Chapelle A, et al: Clinical significance of cytogenetics in acute myeloid leukemia. Semin Oncol 1997;24:17.

192. Linggi B, Muller-Tidow C, van de LL, et al: The t(8;21) fusion protein, AML1 ETO, specifically represses the transcription of the p14(ARF) tumor suppressor in acute myeloid leukemia. Nat Med 2002;8:743.

193. Pabst T, Mueller BU, Harakawa N, et al: AML1-ETO downregulates the granulocytic differentiation factor C/EBPalpha in t(8;21) myeloid leukemia. Nat Med 2001;7:444.

194. Vangala RK, Heiss-Neumann MS, Rangatia JS, et al: The myeloid master regulator transcription factor PU.1 is inactivated by AML1-ETO in t(8;21) myeloid leukemia. Blood 2003;101:270.

195. Yergeau DA, Hetherington CJ, Wang Q, et al: Embryonic lethality and impairment of haematopoiesis in mice heterozygous for an AML1-ETO fusion gene. Nat Genet 1997;15:303.

196. Okuda T, Cai Z, Yang S, et al: Expression of a knocked-in AML1-ETO leukemia gene inhibits the establishment of normal definitive hematopoiesis and directly generates dysplastic hematopoietic progenitors . Blood 1998;91:3134.

197. Higuchi M, O'Brien D, Kumaravelu P, et al: Expression of a conditional AML1-ETO oncogene bypasses embryonic lethality and establishes a murine model of human t(8;21) acute myeloid leukemia. Cancer Cell 2002;1:63.

198. Liu P, Tarle SA, Hajra A, et al: Fusion between transcription factor CBF beta/PEBP2 beta and a myosin heavy chain in acute myeloid leukemia. Science 1993;20;261:1041.

199. Shurtleff SA, Meyers S, Hiebert SW, et al: Heterogeneity in CBF beta/MYH11 fusion messages encoded by the inv(16)(p13q22) and the t(16;16)(p13;q22) in acute myelogenous leukemia. Blood 1995;85;3695.

200. Kanno Y, Kanno T, Sakakura C, et al: Cytoplasmic sequestration of the polyomavirus enhancer binding protein 2 (PEBP2)/core binding factor alpha (CBFalpha) subunit by the leukemia-related PEBP2/CBFbeta-SMMHC fusion protein inhibits PEBP2/CBF-mediated transactivation. Mol Cell Biol 1998;18:4252.

201. Kundu M, Liu PP: Function of the inv(16) fusion gene CBFB-MYH11. Curr Opin Hematol 2001;8:201.

202. Castilla LH, Wijmenga C, Wang Q, et al: Failure of embryonic hematopoiesis and lethal hemorrhages in mouse embryos heterozygous for a knocked-in leukemia gene CBFB-MYH11. Cell 1996;87:687.

203. Ayton PM, Cleary ML: Molecular mechanisms of leukemogenesis mediated by MLL fusion proteins. Oncogene 2001;20:5695.

204. Corral J, Lavenir I, Impey H, et al: An Mll-AF9 fusion gene made by homologous recombination causes acute leukemia in chimeric mice: A method to create fusion oncogenes. Cell 1996;85:853.

205. Dobson CL, Warren AJ, Pannell R, et al: The mll-AF9 gene fusion in mice controls myeloproliferation and specifies acute myeloid leukaemogenesis. EMBO J 1999;18:3564.

206. Lavau C, Szilvassy SJ, Slany R, et al: Immortalization and leukemic transformation of a myelomonocytic precursor by retrovirally transduced HRX-ENL. EMBO J 1997;16:4226.

207. So CW, Cleary ML: Common mechanism for oncogenic activation of MLL by forkhead family proteins. Blood 2003;101:633.

208. DiMartino JF, Ayton PM, Chen EH, et al: The AF10 leucine zipper is required for leukemic transformation of myeloid progenitors by MLL-AF10. Blood 2002;99:3780.

209. Rivera GK, Hudson MM, Liu Q, et al: Effectiveness of intensified rotational combination chemotherapy for late hematologic relapse of childhood acute lymphoblastic leukemia. Blood 1996;88:831.

210. Neale GA, Pui CH, Mahmoud HH, et al: Molecular evidence for minimal residual bone marrow disease in children with 'isolated' extra-medullary relapse of T-cell acute lymphoblastic leukemia. Leukemia 1994;8:768.

211. Neglia JP, Meadows AT, Robison LL, et al: Second neoplasms after acute lymphoblastic leukemia in childhood. N Engl J Med 1991;325:1330.

212. Pui CH, Ribeiro RC, Hancock ML, et al: Acute myeloid leukemia in children treated with epipodophyllotoxins for acute lymphoblastic leukemia. N Engl J Med 1991;325:1682.

213. Stass S, Mirro J, Melvin S, et al: Lineage switch in acute leukemia. Blood 1984;64:701.

214. Gagnon GA, Childs CC, LeMaistre A, et al: Molecular heterogeneity in acute leukemia lineage switch. Blood 1989;74:2088.

215. Beishuizen A, Verhoeven MA, Van Wering ER, et al: Analysis of Ig and T-cell receptor genes in 40 childhood acute lymphoblastic leukemias at diagnosis and subsequent relapse: Implications for the detection of minimal residual disease by polymerase chain reaction analysis. Blood 1994;83:2238.

216. Gaynon PS, Qu RP, Chappell RJ, et al: Survival after relapse in childhood acute lymphoblastic leukemia: Impact of site and time to first relapse—the Children's Cancer Group Experience. Cancer 1998;82:1387.

217. Arceci RJ: Progress and controversies in the treatment of pediatric acute myelogenous leukemia. Curr Opin Hematol 2002;9:353.

218. Schrappe M, Reiter A, Zimmermann M, et al: Long-term results of four consecutive trials in childhood ALL performed by the ALL-BFM study group from 1981 to 1995. Berlin-Frankfurt-Munster. Leukemia 2000;14:2205.

219. Harms DO, Janka-Schaub GE: Co-operative study group for childhood acute lymphoblastic leukemia (COALL): Long-term follow-up of trials 82, 85, 89 and 92. Leukemia 2000;14:2234.

220. Vilmer E, Suciu S, Ferster A, et al: Long-term results of three randomized trials (58831, 58832, 58881) in childhood acute lymphoblastic leukemia: A CLCG-EORTC report. Children Leukemia Cooperative Group. Leukemia 2000;14:2257.

221. Maloney KW, Shuster JJ, Murphy S, et al: Long-term results of treatment studies for childhood acute lymphoblastic leukemia: Pediatric Oncology Group studies from 1986–1994. Leukemia 2000;14:2276.

222. Pui CH, Boyett JM, Rivera GK, et al: Long-term results of Total Therapy studies 11, 12 and 13A for childhood acute lympho-blastic leukemia at St Jude Children's Research Hospital. Leukemia 2000;14:2286.

223. Tsuchida M, Ikuta K, Hanada R, et al: Long-term follow-up of childhood acute lymphoblastic leukemia in Tokyo Children's Cancer Study Group 1981–1995. Leukemia 2000;14:2295.

224. Silverman LB, Gelber RD, Dalton VK, et al: Improved outcome for children with acute lymphoblastic leukemia: Results of Dana-Farber Consortium Protocol 91-01. Blood 2001;97:1211.

225. Pui CH, Sallan S, Relling MV, et al: International Childhood Acute Lymphoblastic Leukemia Workshop: Sausalito, CA, 30 November–1 December 2000. Leukemia 2001;15:707.

226. Eden OB, Harrison G, Richards S, et al: Long-term follow-up of the United Kingdom Medical Research Council protocols for childhood acute lymphoblastic leukaemia, 1980–1997. Medical Research Council Childhood Leukaemia Working Party. Leukemia 2000;14:2307.

227. Pui CH, Boyett JM, Relling MV, et al: Sex differences in prognosis for children with acute lymphoblastic leukemia. J Clin Oncol 1999;17:818.

228. Pollock BH, DeBaun MR, Camitta BM, et al: Racial differences in the survival of childhood B-precursor acute lymphoblastic leukemia: A Pediatric Oncology Group study. J Clin Oncol 2000;18:813.

229. Bhatia S, Sather HN, Heerema NA, et al: Racial and ethnic differences in survival of children with acute lymphoblastic leukemia. Blood 2002;100:1957.

230. Pui CH, Boyett JM, Hancock ML, et al: Outcome of treatment for childhood cancer in black as compared with white children. The St Jude Children's Research Hospital experience, 1962 through 1992. JAMA 1995;273:633.

231. Arico M, Valsecchi MG, Camitta B, et al: Outcome of treatment in children with Philadelphia chromosome-positive acute lymphoblastic leukemia. N Engl J Med 2000;342:998.

232. Pui CH, Gaynon PS, Boyett JM, et al: Outcome of treatment in childhood acute lymphoblastic leukaemia with rearrangements of the 11q23 chromosomal region. Lancet 2002;359:1909.

233. Pui CH, Chessells JM, Camitta BA, et al: Clinical heterogeneity in childhood acute lymphoblastic leukemia with 11q23 rearrangements. Leukemia 2003;17:700.

234. Webb DK, Harrison G, Stevens RF, et al: Relationships between age at diagnosis, clinical features, and outcome of therapy in children treated in the Medical Research Council AML 10 and 12 trials for acute myeloid leukemia. Blood 2001;98:1714.

235. Bloomfield CD, Lawrence D, Byrd JC, et al: Frequency of prolonged remission duration after high-dose cytarabine intensification in acute myeloid leukemia varies by cytogenetic subtype. Cancer Res 1998;58:4173.

236. Byrd JC, Dodge RK, Carroll A, et al: Patients with t(8;21)(q22;q22) and acute myeloid leukemia have superior failure-free and overall survival when repetitive cycles of high-dose cytarabine are administered. J Clin Oncol 1999;17:3767.

237. Grimwade D, Walker H, Oliver F, et al: The importance of diagnostic cytogenetics on outcome in AML: Analysis of 1,612 patients entered into the MRC AML 10 trial. The Medical Research Council Adult and Children's Leukaemia Working Parties. Blood 1998;92:2322.

238. Rubnitz JE, Raimondi SC, Halbert AR, et al: Characteristics and outcome of t(8;21)-positive childhood acute myeloid leukemia: a single institution's experience. Leukemia 2002;16:2072.

239. Razzouk BI, Raimondi SC, Srivastava DK, et al: Impact of treatment on the outcome of acute myeloid leukemia with inversion 16: A single institution's experience. Leukemia 2001;15:1326.

240. Nguyen S, Leblanc T, Fenaux P, et al: A white blood cell index as the main prognostic factor in t(8;21) acute myeloid leukemia

(AML): A survey of 161 cases from the French AML Intergroup. Blood 2002;99:3517.

241. Kalwinsky DK, Raimondi SC, Schell MJ, et al: Prognostic importance of cytogenetic subgroups in de novo pediatric acute nonlymphocytic leukemia. J Clin Oncol 1990;8:75.

242. Sandoval C, Head DR, Mirro J Jr, et al: Translocation t(9;11)(p21;q23) in pediatric de novo and secondary acute myeloblastic leukemia. Leukemia 1992;6:513.

243. Martinez-Climent JA, Lane NJ, Rubin CM, et al: Clinical and prognostic significance of chromosomal abnormalities in childhood acute myeloid leukemia de novo. Leukemia 1995;9:95.

244. Rubnitz JE, Raimondi SC, Tong X, et al: Favorable impact of the t(9;11) in childhood acute myeloid leukemia. J Clin Oncol 2002;20:2302.

245. Odom LF, Gordon EM: Acute monoblastic leukemia in infancy and early childhood: Successful treatment with an epipodophyllotoxin. Blood 1984;64:875.

246. Nishikawa A, Nakamura Y, Nobori U, et al: Acute monocytic leukemia in children. Response to VP-16-213 as a single agent. Cancer 1987;60:2146.

247. Krance RA, Hurwitz CA, Head DR, et al: Experience with 2-chlorodeoxyadenosine in previously untreated children with newly diagnosed acute myeloid leukemia and myelodysplastic diseases. J Clin Oncol 2001;19:2804.

248. Zwaan CM, Kaspers GJ, Pieters R, et al: Cellular drug resistance in childhood acute myeloid leukemia is related to chromosomal abnormalities. Blood 2002;100:3352.

249. Dohner K, Tobis K, Ulrich R, et al: Prognostic significance of partial tandem duplications of the MLL gene in adult patients 16 to 60 years old with acute myeloid leukemia and normal cytogenetics: A study of the Acute Myeloid Leukemia Study Group Ulm. J Clin Oncol 2002;20:3254.

250. Shiah HS, Kuo YY, Tang JL, et al: Clinical and biological implications of partial tandem duplication of the MLL gene in acute myeloid leukemia without chromosomal abnormalities at 11q23. Leukemia 2002;16:196.

251. Athale UH, Razzouk BI, Raimondi SC, et al: Biology and outcome of childhood acute megakaryoblastic leukemia: A single institution's experience. Blood 2001;97:3727.

252. Pagano L, Pulsoni A, Vignetti M, et al: Acute megakaryoblastic leukemia: Experience of GIMEMA trials. Leukemia 2002;16:1622.

253. Tallman MS, Neuberg D, Bennett JM, et al: Acute megakaryocytic leukemia: The Eastern Cooperative Oncology Group experience. Blood 2000;96:2405.

254. Pui CH, Relling MV: Topoisomerase II inhibitor-related acute myeloid leukemia. Br J Haematol 2000;109:13.

255. Hale GA, Heslop HE, Bowman LC, et al: Bone marrow transplantation for therapy-induced acute myeloid leukemia in children with previous lymphoid malignancies. Bone Marrow Transplant 1999;24:735.

256. Luna-Fineman S, Shannon KM, Lange BJ: Childhood monosomy 7: Epidemiology, biology, and mechanistic implications. Blood 1995;85:1985.

257. Luna-Fineman S, Shannon KM, Atwater SK, et al: Myelodysplastic and myeloproliferative disorders of childhood: A study of 167 patients. Blood 1999;93:459.

258. Sasaki H, Manabe A, Kojima S, et al: Myelodysplastic syndrome in childhood: A retrospective study of 189 patients in Japan. Leukemia 2001;15:1713.

259. Kiyoi H, Naoe T, Nakano Y, et al: Prognostic implication of FLT3 and N-RAS gene mutations in acute myeloid leukemia. Blood 1999;93:3074.

260. Iwai T, Yokota S, Nakao M, et al: Internal tandem duplication of the FLT3 gene and clinical evaluation in childhood acute myeloid leukemia. The Children's Cancer and Leukemia Study Group, Japan. Leukemia 1999;13:38.

261. Abu-Duhier FM, Goodeve AC, Wilson GA, et al: FLT3 internal tandem duplication mutations in adult acute myeloid leukaemia define a high-risk group. Br J Haematol 2000;111:190.

262. Kottaridis PD, Gale RE, Frew ME, et al: The presence of a FLT3 internal tandem duplication in patients with acute myeloid leukemia (AML) adds important prognostic information to cytogenetic risk group and response to the first cycle of chemotherapy: Analysis of 854 patients from the United Kingdom

Medical Research Council AML 10 and 12 trials. Blood 2001;98:1752.

263. Meshinchi S, Woods WG, Stirewalt DL, et al: Prevalence and prognostic significance of Flt3 internal tandem duplication in pediatric acute myeloid leukemia. Blood 2001;97:89.

264. Frohling S, Schlenk RF, Breitruck J, et al: Prognostic significance of activating FLT3 mutations in younger adults (16 to 60 years) with acute myeloid leukemia and normal cytogenetics: A study of the AML Study Group Ulm. Blood 2002;100:4372.

265. Whitman SP, Archer KJ, Feng L, et al: Absence of the wild-type allele predicts poor prognosis in adult de novo acute myeloid leukemia with normal cytogenetics and the internal tandem duplication of FLT3: a cancer and leukemia group B study. Cancer Res 2001;61:7233.

266. Boissel N, Cayuela JM, Preudhomme C, et al: Prognostic significance of FLT3 internal tandem repeat in patients with de novo acute myeloid leukemia treated with reinforced courses of chemotherapy. Leukemia 2002;16:1699.

267. Thiede C, Steudel C, Mohr B, et al: Analysis of FLT3-activating mutations in 979 patients with acute myelogenous leukemia: Association with FAB subtypes and identification of subgroups with poor prognosis. Blood 2002;99:4326.

268. Schnittger S, Schoch C, Dugas M, et al: Analysis of FLT3 length mutations in 1003 patients with acute myeloid leukemia: correlation to cytogenetics, FAB subtype, and prognosis in the AMLCG study and usefulness as a marker for the detection of minimal residual disease. Blood 2002;100:59.

269. Leith CP, Kopecky KJ, Chen IM, et al: Frequency and clinical significance of the expression of the multidrug resistance proteins MDR1/P-glycoprotein, MRP1, and LRP in acute myeloid leukemia: A Southwest Oncology Group study. Blood 1999;94:1086.

270. Legrand O, Simonin G, Beauchamp-Nicoud A, et al: Simultaneous activity of MRP1 and Pgp is correlated with in vitro resistance to daunorubicin and with in vivo resistance in adult acute myeloid leukemia. Blood 1999;94:1046.

271. den Boer ML, Pieters R, Kazemier KM, et al: Relationship between major vault protein/lung resistance protein, multidrug resistance-associated protein, P-glycoprotein expression, and drug resistance in childhood leukemia. Blood 1998;91:2092.

272. Steinbach D, Sell W, Voigt A, et al: BCRP gene expression is associated with a poor response to remission induction therapy in childhood acute myeloid leukemia. Leukemia 2002;16:1443.

273. van den Heuvel-Eibrink MM, Wiemer EA, Prins A, et al: Increased expression of the breast cancer resistance protein (BCRP) in relapsed or refractory acute myeloid leukemia (AML). Leukemia 2002;16:833.

274. van der Kolk DM, Vellenga E, Scheffer GL, et al: Expression and activity of breast cancer resistance protein (BCRP) in de novo and relapsed acute myeloid leukemia. Blood 2002;99:3763.

275. Conter V, Arico M, Valsecchi MG, et al: Long-term results of the Italian Association of Pediatric Hematology and Oncology (AIEOP) acute lymphoblastic leukemia studies, 1982-1995. Leukemia 2000;14:2196.

276. Schrappe M, Reiter A, Ludwig WD, et al: Improved outcome in childhood acute lymphoblastic leukemia despite reduced use of anthracyclines and cranial radiotherapy: Results of trial ALL-BFM 90. German-Austrian-Swiss ALL-BFM Study Group. Blood 2000;95:3310.

277. Kamps WA, Bokkerink JP, Hakvoort-Cammel FG, et al: BFM-oriented treatment for children with acute lymphoblastic leukemia without cranial irradiation and treatment reduction for standard risk patients: results of DCLSG protocol ALL-8 (1991-1996). Leukemia 2002;16:1099.

278. Silverman LB, Declerck L, Gelber RD, et al: Results of Dana-Farber Cancer Institute Consortium protocols for children with newly diagnosed acute lymphoblastic leukemia (1981-1995). Leukemia 2000;14:2247.

279. Millot F, Suciu S, Philippe N, et al: Value of high-dose cytarabine during interval therapy of a Berlin-Frankfurt-Munster-based protocol in increased-risk children with acute lymphoblastic leukemia and lymphoblastic lymphoma: Results of the European Organization for Research and Treatment of Cancer 58881 randomized phase III trial. J Clin Oncol 2001;19:1935.

280. Duval M, Suciu S, Ferster A, et al: Comparison of Escherichia coli-asparaginase with Erwinia-asparaginase in the treatment of childhood lymphoid malignancies: Results of a randomized European Organisation for Research and Treatment of Cancer-Children's Leukemia Group phase 3 trial. Blood 2002;99:2734.

281. Gustafsson G, Schmiegelow K, Forestier E, et al: Improving outcome through two decades in childhood ALL in the Nordic countries: The impact of high-dose methotrexate in the reduction of CNS irradiation. Nordic Society of Pediatric Haematology and Oncology (NOPHO). Leukemia 2000;14:2267.

282. Pui CH, Mahmoud HH, Rivera GK, et al: Early intensification of intrathecal chemotherapy virtually eliminates central nervous system relapse in children with acute lymphoblastic leukemia. Blood 1998;92:411.

283. Chessells JM, Harrison G, Richards SM, et al: Failure of a new protocol to improve treatment results in paediatric lymphoblastic leukaemia: Lessons from the UK Medical Research Council trials UKALL X and UKALL XI. Br J Haematol 2002;118:445.

284. Reiter A, Schrappe M, Tiemann M, et al: Improved treatment results in childhood B-cell neoplasms with tailored intensification of therapy: A report of the Berlin-Frankfurt-Munster Group trial NHL-BFM 90. Blood 1999;94:3294.

285. Patte C, Auperin A, Michon J, et al: The Societe Francaise d'Oncologie Pediatrique LMB89 protocol: Highly effective multiagent chemotherapy tailored to the tumor burden and initial response in 561 unselected children with B-cell lymphomas and L3 leukemia. Blood 2001;97:3370.

286. Spreafico F, Massimino M, Luksch R, et al: Intensive, very short-term chemotherapy for advanced Burkitt's lymphoma in children. J Clin Oncol 2002;20:2783.

287. Pui CH, Mahmoud HH, Wiley JM, et al: Recombinant urate oxidase for the prophylaxis or treatment of hyperuricemia in patients With leukemia or lymphoma. J Clin Oncol 2001;19:697.

288. Pui CH: Rasburicase: A potent uricolytic agent. Expert Opin Pharmacother 2002;3:433.

289. Silverman LB, McLean TW, Gelber RD, et al: Intensified therapy for infants with acute lymphoblastic leukemia: Results from the Dana-Farber Cancer Institute Consortium. Cancer 1997;80:2285.

290. Dreyer ZE, Steuber CP, Bowman WP, et al: High risk infant ALL—improved survival with intensive chemotherapy [abstract]. Proc Am Soc Clin Oncol 1998;17:529a.

291. Reaman GH, Sposto R, Sensel MG, et al: Treatment outcome and prognostic factors for infants with acute lymphoblastic leukemia treated on two consecutive trials of the Children's Cancer Group. J Clin Oncol 1999;17:445.

292. Chessells JM, Harrison CJ, Watson SL, et al: Treatment of infants with lymphoblastic leukaemia: Results of the UK Infant Protocols 1987–1999. Br J Haematol 2002;117:306.

293. Liang DC, Hung IJ, Yang CP, et al: Unexpected mortality from the use of E. coli L-asparaginase during remission induction therapy for childhood acute lymphoblastic leukemia: A report from the Taiwan Pediatric Oncology Group. Leukemia 1999;13:155.

294. Hurwitz CA, Silverman LB, Schorin MA, et al: Substituting dexamethasone for prednisone complicates remission induction in children with acute lymphoblastic leukemia. Cancer 2000;88:1964.

295. Coustan-Smith E, Sancho J, Hancock ML, et al: Clinical importance of minimal residual disease in childhood acute lymphoblastic leukemia. Blood 2000;96:2691.

296. Avramis VI, Sencer S, Periclou AP, et al: A randomized comparison of native Escherichia coli asparaginase and polyethylene glycol conjugated asparaginase for treatment of children with newly diagnosed standard-risk acute lymphoblastic leukemia: A Children's Cancer Group study. Blood 2002;99:1986.

297. Balis FM, Lester CM, Chrousos GP, et al: Differences in cerebro-spinal fluid penetration of corticosteroids: Possible relationship to the prevention of meningeal leukemia. J Clin Oncol 1987;5:202.

298. Lange BJ, Bostrom BC, Cherlow JM, et al: Double-delayed intensification improves event-free survival for children with intermediate-risk acute lymphoblastic leukemia: A report from the Children's Cancer Group. Blood 2002;99:825.

299. Nachman JB, Sather HN, Sensel MG, et al: Augmented post-induction therapy for children with high-risk acute lymphoblastic leukemia and a slow response to initial therapy. N Engl J Med 1998;338:1663.

300. Arico M, Valsecchi MG, Conter V, et al: Improved outcome in high-risk childhood acute lymphoblastic leukemia defined by prednisone-poor response treated with double Berlin-Frankfurt-Muenster protocol II. Blood 2002;100:420.

301. Amylon MD, Shuster J, Pullen J, et al: Intensive high-dose asparaginase consolidation improves survival for pediatric patients with T cell acute lymphoblastic leukemia and advanced stage lymphoblastic lymphoma: A Pediatric Oncology Group study. Leukemia 1999;13:335.

302. Masson E, Relling MV, Synold TW, et al: Accumulation of methotrexate polyglutamates in lymphoblasts is a determinant of antileukemic effects in vivo. A rationale for high-dose methotrexate. J Clin Invest 1996;97:73.

303. Mahoney DH Jr, Shuster JJ, Nitschke R, et al: Intensification with intermediate-dose intravenous methotrexate is effective therapy for children with lower-risk B-precursor acute lymphoblastic leukemia: A Pediatric Oncology Group study. J Clin Oncol 2000;18:1285.

304. Pui CH, Evans WE: Drug therapy: Acute lymphoblastic leukemia. N Engl J Med 1998;339:605.

305. Van Der Werff ten Bosch J, Suciu S, Philippe N, et al: The value of 6-MP i.v. during maintenance treatment in childhood acute lymphoblastic leukemia and non-Hodgkin lymphoma: Results of the randomized Phase III trial 58881 of EORTC Childhood Leukemia Cooperative Group (CLCG). Blood 1999; 94(Suppl 1):628a.

306. Dervieux T, Brenner TL, Hon YY, et al: De novo purine synthesis inhibition and antileukemic effects of mercaptopurine alone or in combination with methotrexate in vivo. Blood 2002;100:1240.

307. Hanahan D, Bergers G, Bergsland E: Less is more, regularly: Metronomic dosing of cytotoxic drugs can target tumor angiogenesis in mice. J Clin Invest 2000;105:1045.

308. Perez-Atayde AR, Sallan SE, Tedrow U, et al: Spectrum of tumor angiogenesis in the bone marrow of children with acute lymphoblastic leukemia. Am J Pathol 1997;150:815.

309. Nishigaki H, Ito C, Manabe A, et al: Prevalence and growth characteristics of malignant stem cells in B-lineage acute lymphoblastic leukemia. Blood 1997;89:3735.

310. Shuster JJ, Wacker P, Pullen J, et al: Prognostic significance of sex in childhood B-precursor acute lymphoblastic leukemia: A Pediatric Oncology Group study. J Clin Oncol 1998;16:2854.

311. Chessells JM, Harrison G, Lilleyman JS, et al: Continuing (maintenance) therapy in lymphoblastic leukaemia: Lessons from MRC UKALL X. Medical Research Council Working Party in Childhood Leukaemia. Br J Haematol 1997;98:945.

312. Relling MV, Hancock ML, Boyett JM, et al: Prognostic importance of 6-mercaptopurine dose intensity in acute lymphoblastic leukemia. Blood 1999;93:2817.

313. Relling MV, Hancock ML, Rivera GK, et al: Mercaptopurine therapy intolerance and heterozygosity at the thiopurine S-methyltransferase gene locus. J Natl Cancer Inst 1999;91:2001.

314. Loennechen T, Yates CR, Fessing MY, et al: Isolation of a human thiopurine S-methyltransferase (TPMT) complementary DNA with a single nucleotide transition A719G (TPMT*3C) and its association with loss of TPMT protein and catalytic activity in humans. Clin Pharmacol Ther 1998;64:46.

315. Harms DO, Gobel U, Spaar HJ, et al: Thioguanine offers no advantage over mercaptopurine in maintenance treatment of childhood ALL: Results of the randomized trial COALL-92. Blood 2003;102:2736.

316. Richardson P, Guinan E: The pathology, diagnosis, and treatment of hepatic veno-occlusive disease: Current status and novel approaches. Br J Haematol 1999;107:485.

317. Childhood ALL Collaborative Group: Duration and intensity of maintenance chemotherapy in acute lymphoblastic leukaemia: Overview of 42 trials involving 12,000 randomised children. Childhood ALL Collaborative Group. Lancet 1996;347:1783.

318. Gajjar A, Harrison PL, Sandlund JT, et al: Traumatic lumbar puncture at diagnosis adversely affects outcome in childhood acute lymphoblastic leukemia. Blood 2000;96:3381.

319. Nachman J, Cherlow JM, Sather HN, et al: Effect of initial central nervous system status on event-free survival in children and

adolescents with acute lymphoblastic leukemia. Med Pediatr Oncol 2002;39:277.

320. Burger B, Zimmermann M, Mann G, et al: Diagnostic cerebrospinal fluid examination in children with acute lymphoblastic leukemia: Significance of low leukocyte counts with blasts or traumatic lumbar puncture. J Clin Oncol 2003;21:184.

321. Conter V, Schrappe M, Arico M, et al: Role of cranial radiotherapy for childhood T-cell acute lymphoblastic leukemia with high WBC count and good response to prednisone. Associazione Italiana Ematologia Oncologia Pediatrica and the Berlin-Frankfurt-Munster groups. J Clin Oncol 1997;15:2786.

322. Laver JH, Barredo JC, Amylon M, et al: Effects of cranial radiation in children with high risk T cell acute lymphoblastic leukemia: A Pediatric Oncology Group report. Leukemia 2000;14:369.

323. Manera R, Ramirez I, Mullins J, et al: Pilot studies of species-specific chemotherapy of childhood acute lymphoblastic leukemia using genotype and immunophenotype. Leukemia 2000;14:1354.

324. Ritchey AK, Pollock BH, Lauer SJ, et al: Improved survival of children with isolated CNS relapse of acute lymphoblastic leukemia: a Pediatric Oncology Group study. J Clin Oncol 1999;17:3745.

325. Evans WE, Relling MV, Rodman JH, et al: Conventional compared with individualized chemotherapy for childhood acute lymphoblastic leukemia. N Engl J Med 1998;338:499.

326. Relling MV, Hancock ML, Boyett JM, et al: Prognostic importance of 6-mercaptopurine dose intensity in acute lymphoblastic leukemia. Blood 1999;93:2817.

327. Relling MV, Pui CH, Sandlund JT, et al: Adverse effect of anticonvulsants on efficacy of chemotherapy for acute lymphoblastic leukaemia. Lancet 2000;356:285.

328. Relling MV, Hancock ML, Rivera GK, et al: Mercaptopurine therapy intolerance and heterozygosity at the thiopurine S-methyltransferase gene locus. J Natl Cancer Inst 1999;91:2001.

329. Relling MV, Rubnitz JE, Rivera GK, et al: High incidence of secondary brain tumours after radiotherapy and antimetabolites. Lancet 1999;354:34.

330. Bo J, Schroder H, Kristinsson J, et al: Possible carcinogenic effect of 6-mercaptopurine on bone marrow stem cells: Relation to thiopurine metabolism. Cancer 1999;86:1080.

331. Davies SM, Robison LL, Buckley JD, et al: Glutathione S-transferase polymorphisms and outcome of chemotherapy in childhood acute myeloid leukemia. J Clin Oncol 2001;19:1279.

332. Allan JM, Wild CP, Rollinson S, et al: Polymorphism in glutathione S-transferase P1 is associated with susceptibility to chemotherapy-induced leukemia. Proc Natl Acad Sci USA 2001;98:11592.

333. Stanulla M, Schrappe M, Brechlin AM, et al: Polymorphisms within glutathione S-transferase genes (GSTM1, GSTT1, GSTP1) and risk of relapse in childhood B-cell precursor acute lymphoblastic leukemia: A case-control study. Blood 2000;95:1222.

334. O'Brien TA, Russell SJ, Vowels MR, et al: Results of consecutive trials for children newly diagnosed with acute myeloid leukemia from the Australian and New Zealand Children's Cancer Study Group. Blood 2002;100:2708.

335. Creutzig U, Ritter J, Zimmermann M, et al: Idarubicin improves blast cell clearance during induction therapy in children with AML: Results of study AML-BFM 93. AML-BFM Study Group. Leukemia 2001;15:348.

336. Creutzig U, Ritter J, Zimmermann M, et al: Improved treatment results in high-risk pediatric acute myeloid leukemia patients after intensification with high-dose cytarabine and mitoxantrone: Results of Study Acute Myeloid Leukemia—Berlin-Frankfurt-Munster 93. J Clin Oncol 2001;19:2705.

337. Woods WG, Neudorf S, Gold S, et al: A comparison of allogeneic bone marrow transplantation, autologous bone marrow transplantation, and aggressive chemotherapy in children with acute myeloid leukemia in remission: A report from the Children's Cancer Group. Blood 2001;97:56.

338. Perel Y, Auvrignon A, Leblanc T, et al: Impact of addition of maintenance therapy to intensive induction and consolidation chemotherapy for childhood acute myeloblastic leukemia: Results of a prospective randomized trial, LAME 89/9. J Clin Oncol 2002;20:2774.

339. Stevens RF, Hann IM, Wheatley K, et al: Marked improvements in outcome with chemotherapy alone in paediatric acute myeloid leukaemia: Results of the United Kingdom Medical Research Council's 10th AML trial. MRC Childhood Leukaemia Working Party. Br J Haematol 1998;101:130.

340. Riley LC, Hann IM, Wheatley K, et al: Treatment-related deaths during induction and first remission of acute myeloid leukaemia in children treated on the Tenth Medical Research Council acute myeloid leukaemia trial (MRC AML10). The MCR Childhood Leukaemia Working Party. Br J Haematol 1999;106:436.

341. Lie SO, Jonmundsson G, Mellander L, et al: A population-based study of 272 children with acute myeloid leukaemia treated on two consecutive protocols with different intensity: Best outcome in girls, infants, and children with Down's syndrome. Nordic Society of Paediatric Haematology and Oncology (NOPHO). Br J Haematol 1996;94:82.

342. Lacayo NJ, Lum BL, Becton DL, et al: Pharmacokinetic interactions of cyclosporine with etoposide and mitoxantrone in children with acute myeloid leukemia. Leukemia 2002;16:920.

343. Becton D, Ravindranath Y, Dahl GV, et al: A Phase III study of intensive cytarabine induction followed by cyclosporine modulation of drug resistance in de novo pediatric AML; POG 9421 [abstract]. Blood 2001;98(Suppl 1):461a.

344. Carella AM, Berman E, Maraone MP, et al: Idarubicin in the treatment of acute leukemias. An overview of preclinical and clinical studies. Haematologica 1990;75:159.

345. Berman E, McBride M: Comparative cellular pharmacology of daunorubicin and idarubicin in human multidrug-resistant leukemia cells. Blood 1992;79:3267.

346. Hollingshead LM, Faulds D: Idarubicin. A review of its pharmacodynamic and pharmacokinetic properties, and therapeutic potential in the chemotherapy of cancer. Drugs 1991;42:690.

347. Crews KR, Gandhi V, Srivastava DK, et al: Interim comparison of a continuous infusion versus a short daily infusion of cytarabine given in combination with cladribine for pediatric acute myeloid leukemia. J Clin Oncol 2002;20:4217.

348. Davies SM, Robison LL, Buckley JD, et al: Glutathione S-transferase polymorphisms and outcome of chemotherapy in childhood acute myeloid leukemia. J Clin Oncol 2001;19:1279.

349. Ravindranath Y, Steuber CP, Krischer J, et al: High-dose cytarabine for intensification of early therapy of childhood acute myeloid leukemia: A Pediatric Oncology Group study. J Clin Oncol 1991;9:572.

350. Rees JK, Gray RG, Swirsky D, et al: Principal results of the Medical Research Council's 8th acute myeloid leukaemia trial. Lancet 1986;2:1236.

351. Creutzig U, Ritter J, Vormoor J, et al: Myelodysplasia and acute myelogenous leukemia in Down's syndrome. A report of 40 children of the AML-BFM Study Group. Leukemia 1996;10:1677.

352. Lange BJ, Kobrinsky N, Barnard DR, et al: Distinctive demography, biology, and outcome of acute myeloid leukemia and myelodysplastic syndrome in children with Down syndrome: Children's Cancer Group Studies 2861 and 2891. Blood 1998;91:608.

353. Zwaan CM, Kaspers GJ, Pieters R, et al: Different drug sensitivity profiles of acute myeloid and lymphoblastic leukemia and normal peripheral blood mononuclear cells in children with and without Down syndrome. Blood 2002;99:245.

354. Wells RJ, Woods WG, Buckley JD, et al: Treatment of newly diagnosed children and adolescents with acute myeloid leukemia: A Childrens Cancer Group study. J Clin Oncol 1994;12:2367.

355. Feig SA, Lampkin B, Nesbit ME, et al: Outcome of BMT during first complete remission of AML: A comparison of two sequential studies by the Children's Cancer Group. Bone Marrow Transplant 1993;12:65.

356. Creutzig U, Ritter J, Riehm H, et al: Improved treatment results in childhood acute myelogenous leukemia: A report of the German cooperative study AML-BFM-78. Blood 1985;65:298.

357. Creutzig U, Ritter J, Schellong G: Identification of two risk groups in childhood acute myelogenous leukemia after therapy intensification in study AML-BFM-83 as compared with study AML-BFM-78. AML-BFM Study Group. Blood 1990;75:1932.

358. Creutzig U, Ritter J, Zimmermann M, et al: Does cranial irradiation reduce the risk for bone marrow relapse in acute myelogenous

leukemia? Unexpected results of the Childhood Acute Myelogenous Leukemia Study BFM-87. J Clin Oncol 1993;11:279.

359. Dahl GV, Kalwinsky DK, Murphy S, et al: Cytokinetically based induction chemotherapy and splenectomy for childhood acute nonlymphocytic leukemia. Blood 1982;60:856.

360. Baehner RL, Kennedy A, Sather H, et al: Characteristics of children with acute nonlymphocytic leukemia in long-term continuous remission: A report for Childrens Cancer Study Group. Med Pediatr Oncol 1981;9:393.

361. Sanz M, Martinez JA, Barragan E, et al: All-trans retinoic acid and low-dose chemotherapy for acute promyelocytic leukaemia. Br J Haematol 2000;109:896.

362. Pui CH, Dahl GV, Kalwinsky DK, et al: Central nervous system leukemia in children with acute nonlymphoblastic leukemia. Blood 1985;66:1062.

363. Tiedemann K, Waters KD, Tauro GP, et al: Results of intensive therapy in childhood acute myeloid leukemia, incorporating high-dose melphalan and autologous bone marrow transplantation in first complete remission. Blood 1993;82: 3730.

364. Bonetti F, Zecca M, Pession A, et al: Total-body irradiation and melphalan is a safe and effective conditioning regimen for autologous bone marrow transplantation in children with acute myeloid leukemia in first remission. The Italian Association for Pediatric Hematology and Oncology-Bone Marrow Transplantation Group. J Clin Oncol 1999;17:3729.

365. Amadori S, Testi AM, Arico M, et al: Prospective comparative study of bone marrow transplantation and postremission chemotherapy for childhood acute myelogenous leukemia. The Associazione Italiana Ematologia ed Oncologia Pediatrica Cooperative Group. J Clin Oncol 1993;11:1046.

366. Ravindranath Y, Yeager AM, Chang MN, et al: Autologous bone marrow transplantation versus intensive consolidation chemotherapy for acute myeloid leukemia in childhood. Pediatric Oncology Group. N Engl J Med 1996;334:1428.

367. Burnett AK, Wheatley K, Goldstone AH, et al: The value of allogeneic bone marrow transplant in patients with acute myeloid leukaemia at differing risk of relapse: Results of the UK MRC AML 10 trial. Br J Haematol 2002;118:385.

368. Creutzig U, Reinhardt D: Current controversies: Which patients with acute myeloid leukaemia should receive a bone marrow transplantation?—a European view. Br J Haematol 2002;118:365.

369. Chen AR, Alonzo TA, Woods WG, et al: Current controversies: Which patients with acute myeloid leukaemia should receive a bone marrow transplantation?—an American view. Br J Haematol 2002;118:378.

370. Relling MV, Rubnitz JE, Rivera GK, et al: High incidence of secondary brain tumours after radiotherapy and antimetabolites. Lancet 1999;354:34.

371. Estey EH, Shen Y, Thall PF: Effect of time to complete remission on subsequent survival and disease-free survival time in AML, RAEB-t, and RAEB. Blood 2000;95:72.

372. Buchner T, Urbanitz D, Hiddemann W, et al: Intensified induction and consolidation with or without maintenance chemotherapy for acute myeloid leukemia (AML): Two multicenter studies of the German AML Cooperative Group. J Clin Oncol 1985; 3:1583.

373. Wheatley K, Burnett AK, Goldstone AH, et al: A simple, robust, validated and highly predictive index for the determination of risk-directed therapy in acute myeloid leukaemia derived from the MRC AML 10 trial. United Kingdom Medical Research Council's Adult and Childhood Leukaemia Working Parties. Br J Haematol 1999;107:69.

374. Kern W, Haferlach T, Schoch C, et al: Early blast clearance by remission induction therapy is a major independent prognostic factor for both achievement of complete remission and long-term outcome in acute myeloid leukemia: Data from the German AML Cooperative Group (AMLCG) 1992 Trial. Blood 2003;101:64.

375. Campana D, Pui CH: Detection of minimal residual disease in acute leukemia: Methodologic advances and clinical significance. Blood 1995;85:1416.

376. Foroni L, Harrison CJ, Hoffbrand AV, et al: Investigation of minimal residual disease in childhood and adult acute lymphoblastic leukaemia by molecular analysis. Br J Haematol 1999;105:7.

377. Lo Coco F, Diverio D, Falini B, et al: Genetic diagnosis and molecular monitoring in the management of acute promyelocytic leukemia. Blood 1999;94:12.

378. van Dongen JJ, Macintyre EA, Gabert JA, et al: Standardized RT-PCR analysis of fusion gene transcripts from chromosome aberrations in acute leukemia for detection of minimal residual disease. Report of the BIOMED-1 Concerted Action: Investigation of minimal residual disease in acute leukemia. Leukemia 1999;13:1901.

379. Campana D, Coustan-Smith E: Advances in the immunological monitoring of childhood acute lymphoblastic leukaemia. Best Pract Res Clin Haematol 2002;15:1.

380. Szczepanski T, Orfao A, van der Velden VH, et al: Minimal residual disease in leukaemia patients. Lancet Oncology 2001;2:409.

381. Liu YJ, Grimwade D: Minimal residual disease evaluation in acute myeloid leukaemia. Lancet 2002;360:160.

382. Ogawa H, Tamaki H, Ikegame K, et al: The usefulness of monitoring WT1 gene transcripts for the prediction and management of relapse following allogeneic stem cell transplantation in acute type leukemia. Blood 2003;101:1698.

383. Cilloni D, Gottardi E, De Micheli D, et al: Quantitative assessment of WT1 expression by real time quantitative PCR may be a useful tool for monitoring minimal residual disease in acute leukemia patients. Leukemia 2002;16:2115.

384. Elmaagacli AH, Beelen DW, Trenschel R, et al: The detection of wt-1 transcripts is not associated with an increased leukemic relapse rate in patients with acute leukemia after allogeneic bone marrow or peripheral blood stem cell transplantation. Bone Marrow Transplant 2000;25:91.

385. Stirewalt DL, Willman CL, Radich JP: Quantitative, real-time polymerase chain reactions for FLT3 internal tandem duplications are highly sensitive and specific. Leuk Res 2001;25:1085.

386. Shih LY, Huang CF, Wu JH, et al: Internal tandem duplication of FLT3 in relapsed acute myeloid leukemia: A comparative analysis of bone marrow samples from 108 adult patients at diagnosis and relapse. Blood 2002;100:2387.

387. Kottaridis PD, Gale RE, Langabeer SE, et al: Studies of FLT3 mutations in paired presentation and relapse samples from patients with acute myeloid leukemia: Implications for the role of FLT3 mutations in leukemogenesis, minimal residual disease detection, and possible therapy with FLT3 inhibitors. Blood 2002;100:2393.

388. Mancini M, Cedrone M, Diverio D, et al: Use of dual-color interphase FISH for the detection of inv(16) in acute myeloid leukemia at diagnosis, relapse and during follow-up: A study of 23 patients. Leukemia 2000;14:364.

389. Bielorai B, Golan H, Trakhtenbrot L, et al: Combined analysis of morphology and fluorescence in situ hybridization in follow-up of minimal residual disease in a child with Philadelphia-positive acute lymphoblastic leukemia. Cancer Genet Cytogenet 2002; 138:64.

390. Estrov Z, Grunberger T, Dube ID, et al: Detection of residual acute lymphoblastic leukemia cells in cultures of bone marrow obtained during remission. N Engl J Med 1986;315:538.

391. Uckun FM, Kersey JH, Haake R, et al: Pretransplantation burden of leukemic progenitor cells as a predictor of relapse after bone marrow transplantation for acute lymphoblastic leukemia. N Engl J Med 1993;329:1296.

392. Neale GA, Coustan-Smith E, Pan Q, et al: Tandem application of flow cytometry and polymerase chain reaction for comprehensive detection of minimal residual disease in childhood acute lymphoblastic leukemia. Leukemia 1999;13:1221.

393. Malec M, Bjorklund E, Soderhall S, et al: Flow cytometry and allele-specific oligonucleotide PCR are equally effective in detection of minimal residual disease in ALL. Leukemia 2001;15:716.

394. Munoz L, Lopez O, Martino R, et al: Combined use of reverse transcriptase polymerase chain reaction and flow cytometry to study minimal residual disease in Philadelphia positive acute lymphoblastic leukemia. Haematologica 2000;85:704.

395. Cave H, van der Werff ten Bosch, Suciu S, et al: Clinical significance of minimal residual disease in childhood acute lymphoblastic leukemia. European Organization for Research and

Specific Malignancies

III

Treatment of Cancer—Childhood Leukemia Cooperative Group. N Engl J Med 1998;339:591.

396. van Dongen JJ, Seriu T, Panzer-Grumayer ER, et al: Prognostic value of minimal residual disease in acute lymphoblastic leukaemia in childhood. Lancet 1998;352:1731.

397. Coustan-Smith E, Behm FG, Sanchez J, et al: Immunological detection of minimal residual disease in children with acute lymphoblastic leukaemia. Lancet 1998;351:550.

398. Coustan-Smith E, Sancho J, Behm FG, et al: Prognostic importance of measuring early clearance of leukemic cells by flow cytometry in childhood acute lymphoblastic leukemia. Blood 2002;100:52.

399. Panzer-Grumayer ER, Schneider M, Panzer S, et al: Rapid molecular response during early induction chemotherapy predicts a good outcome in childhood acute lymphoblastic leukemia. Blood 2000;95:790.

400. Biondi A, Valsecchi MG, Seriu T, et al: Molecular detection of minimal residual disease is a strong predictive factor of relapse in childhood B-lineage acute lymphoblastic leukemia with medium risk features. A case control study of the International BFM study group. Leukemia 2000;14:1939.

401. Eckert C, Biondi A, Seeger K, et al: Prognostic value of minimal residual disease in relapsed childhood acute lymphoblastic leukaemia. Lancet 2001;358:1239.

402. Knechtli CJC, Goulden NJ, Hancock JP, et al: Minimal residual disease status before allogeneic bone marrow transplantation is an important determinant of successful outcome for children and adolescents with acute lymphoblastic leukemia. Blood 1998; 92:4072.

403. Goulden NJ, Knechtli CJ, Garland RJ, et al: Minimal residual disease analysis for the prediction of relapse in children with standard-risk acute lymphoblastic leukaemia. Br J Haematol 1998;100:235.

404. Bader P, Hancock J, Kreyenberg H, et al: Minimal residual disease (MRD) status prior to allogeneic stem cell transplantation is a powerful predictor for post-transplant outcome in children with ALL. Leukemia 2002;16:1668.

405. Hunger SP, Fall MZ, Camitta BM, et al: E2A-PBX1 chimeric transcript status at end of consolidation is not predictive of treatment outcome in childhood acute lymphoblastic leukemias with a t(1;19)(q23;p13): A Pediatric Oncology Group study. Blood 1998;91:1021.

406. Roberts WM, Estrov Z, Ouspenskaia MV, et al: Measurement of residual leukemia during remission in childhood acute lymphoblastic leukemia. N Engl J Med 1997;336:317.

407. Gruhn B, Hongeng S, Yi H, et al: Minimal residual disease after intensive induction therapy in childhood acute lymphoblastic leukemia predicts outcome. Leukemia 1998;12:675.

408. Coustan-Smith E, Sancho J, Hancock ML, et al: Use of peripheral blood instead of bone marrow to monitor residual disease in children with acute lymphoblastic leukemia. Blood DOI 2002;10:1182.

409. van der Velden V, Jacobs DC, Wijkhuijs AJ, et al: Minimal residual disease levels in bone marrow and peripheral blood are comparable in children with T cell acute lymphoblastic leukemia (ALL), but not in precursor-B-ALL. Leukemia 2002;16:1432.

410. Grimwade D: The pathogenesis of acute promyelocytic leukaemia: Evaluation of the role of molecular diagnosis and monitoring in the management of the disease. Br J Haematol 1999;106:591.

411. Burnett AK, Grimwade D, Solomon E, et al: Presenting white blood cell count and kinetics of molecular remission predict prognosis in acute promyelocytic leukemia treated with all-trans retinoic acid: Result of the Randomized MRC Trial. Blood 1999;93:4131.

412. Diverio D, Rossi V, Avvisati G, et al: Early detection of relapse by prospective reverse transcriptase-polymerase chain reaction analysis of the PML/RARalpha fusion gene in patients with acute promyelocytic leukemia enrolled in the GIMEMA-AIEOP multicenter "AIDA" trial. GIMEMA-AIEOP Multicenter "AIDA" Trial. Blood 1998;92:784.

413. Nucifora G, Larson RA, Rowley JD: Persistence of the 8;21 translocation in patients with acute myeloid leukemia type M2 in long-term remission. Blood 1993;82:712.

414. Miyamoto T, Weissman IL, Akashi K: AML1/ETO-expressing nonleukemic stem cells in acute myelogenous leukemia with 8;21 chromosomal translocation. Proc Natl Acad Sci USA 2000;97:7521.

415. Tobal K, Newton J, Macheta M, et al: Molecular quantitation of minimal residual disease in acute myeloid leukemia with t(8;21) can identify patients in durable remission and predict clinical relapse. Blood 2000;95:815.

416. Morschhauser F, Cayuela JM, Martini S, et al: Evaluation of minimal residual disease using reverse-transcription polymerase chain reaction in t(8;21) acute myeloid leukemia: A multicenter study of 51 patients. J Clin Oncol 2000;18:788.

417. Marcucci G, Caligiuri MA, Dohner H, et al: Quantification of CBFbeta/MYH11 fusion transcript by real time RT-PCR in patients with INV(16) acute myeloid leukemia. Leukemia 2001;15:1072.

418. Laczika K, Mitterbauer G, Mitterbauer M, et al: Prospective monitoring of minimal residual disease in acute myeloid leukemia with inversion(16) by CBFbeta/MYH11 RT-PCR: Implications for a monitoring schedule and for treatment decisions. Leuk Lymphoma 2001;42:923.

419. Buonamici S, Ottaviani E, Testoni N, et al: Real-time quantitation of minimal residual disease in inv(16)-positive acute myeloid leukemia may indicate risk for clinical relapse and may identify patients in a curable state. Blood 2002;99:443.

420. Guerrasio A, Pilatrino C, De Micheli D, et al: Assessment of minimal residual disease (MRD) in CBFbeta/MYH11-positive acute myeloid leukemias by qualitative and quantitative RT-PCR amplification of fusion transcripts. Leukemia 2002;16:1176.

421. Sievers EL, Lange BJ, Buckley JD, et al: Prediction of relapse of pediatric acute myeloid leukemia by use of multidimensional flow cytometry. J Natl Cancer Inst 1996;88:1483.

422. San Miguel JF, Vidriales MB, Lopez-Berges C, et al: Early immunophenotypical evaluation of minimal residual disease in acute myeloid leukemia identifies different patient risk groups and may contribute to postinduction treatment stratification. Blood 2001;98:1746.

423. Venditti A, Buccisano F, Del Poeta G, et al: Level of minimal residual disease after consolidation therapy predicts outcome in acute myeloid leukemia. Blood 2000;96:3948.

424. Reichle A, Rothe G, Krause S, et al: Transplant characteristics: Minimal residual disease and impaired megakaryocytic colony growth as sensitive parameters for predicting relapse in acute myeloid leukemia. Leukemia 1999;13:1227.

425. Pui CH, Campana D: New definition of remission in childhood acute lymphoblastic leukemia. Leukemia 2000;14:783.

426. Gandhi V, Plunkett W, Rodriguez COJ, et al: Compound GW506U78 in refractory hematologic malignancies: Relationship between cellular pharmacokinetics and clinical response. J Clin Oncol 1998;16:3607.

427. Consolini R, Pui CH, Behm FG, et al: In vitro cytotoxicity of docetaxel in childhood acute leukemias. J Clin Oncol 1998; 16:907.

428. Mehta J, Powles R, Treleaven J, et al: Autologous transplantation with CD52 monoclonal antibody-purged marrow for acute lymphoblastic leukemia: Long-term follow-up. Leuk Lymphoma 1997;25:479.

429. Sievers EL, Appelbaum FR, Spielberger RT, et al: Selective ablation of acute myeloid leukemia using antibody-targeted chemotherapy: a phase I study of an anti-CD33 calicheamicin immunoconjugate. Blood 1999;93:3678.

430. Clark JJ, Smith FO, Arceci RJ: Update in childhood acute myeloid leukemia: Recent developments in the molecular basis of disease and novel therapies. Curr Opin Hematol 2003;10:31.

431. Woods WG, Kobrinsky N, Buckley JD, et al: Timed-sequential induction therapy improves postremission outcome in acute myeloid leukemia: A report from the Children's Cancer Group. Blood 1996;87:4979.

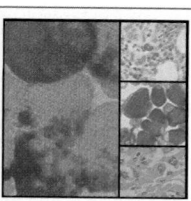

CHILDHOOD LYMPHOMA

John T. Sandlund

Frederick G. Behm

SUMMARY OF KEY POINTS

INCIDENCE

- Malignant lymphoma, which comprises both Hodgkin's disease and the non-Hodgkin's lymphoma (NHL), is the third most common malignancy in childhood.
- Among children younger than 15 years, there is a slight predominance of NHL, whereas the reverse is true among children younger than 18 years.
- Approximately 500 new cases of pediatric NHL are diagnosed in the United States each year.

ETIOLOGY/EPIDEMIOLOGY

- NHL is more common in boys than in girls and in white children than in black children.
- Geographic differences exist with respect to the frequency of histologic subtypes of NHL. Burkitt's lymphoma is the predominant subtype in equatorial Africa and northeast Brazil. Epstein-Barr virus (EBV) is associated with the majority of cases of Burkitt's lymphoma in equatorial Africa, in contrast to the infrequent association observed in the United States and Western Europe.
- Children with immunodeficiency conditions are at increased risk for NHL to develop. These include those with ataxia-telangiectasia (A-T), Wiscott-Aldrich syndrome, and X-linked lymphoproliferative syndrome (XLP). Children with acquired immunodeficiency disorders including the acquired immunodeficiency syndrome (AIDS) and those receiving immuno-suppressive therapy after bone marrow or organ transplantation also are at increased risk.

PATHOLOGY/BIOLOGY

- The three most common subtypes of NHL in children are Burkitt's, lymphoblastic, and large cell lymphoma.

- Burkitt's lymphoma has a mature B-cell immunophenotype and is characterized by one of three reciprocal chromosomal translocations involving the c-*myc* proto-oncogene and one of the immunoglobulin genes [i.e., t(8;14), t(2;8), and t(8;22)].
- Lymphoblastic lymphoma usually arises from a T-cell progenitor and may be associated with reciprocal translocations involving a T-cell receptor (TCR) gene.
- Large cell lymphomas may have either B-cell or T-cell immunophenotype. The majority of the T-cell cases are anaplastic large cell lymphomas (ALCL), which are characterized by anaplastic histology, CD30 expression, and the presence of the t(2;5)(p23;q35) translocation.

CLINICAL FINDINGS

- The clinical features at diagnosis are determined by primary sites of disease, which vary according to histologic subtype.
- Children with Burkitt's lymphoma usually are first seen with an abdominal mass and associated gastrointestinal symptoms, whereas those with advanced-stage lymphoblastic lymphoma typically have a mediastinal mass associated with a spectrum of respiratory symptoms.
- Children with large cell lymphoma or Hodgkin's disease may have disease in either the abdomen or mediastinum.

DIAGNOSIS AND DIFFERENTIAL DIAGNOSIS

- Infectious processes, such as bacterial adenitis, histoplasmosis, tuberculosis, and Epstein-Barr virus infection, may simulate lymphoma.
- A comprehensive characterization of the biologic features of tissue will help distinguish NHL from other small round blue cell tumors,

including Ewing's sarcoma, neuroblastoma, and rhabdomyosarcoma.

INITIAL WORKUP AND STAGING

- The workup should include a history and physical examination, complete blood count, chemistry panel [including electrolytes, blood urea nitrogen (BUN), creatinine, uric acid, phosphorus, calcium, and lactate dehydrogenase (LDH)]; diagnostic imaging studies [computed tomography (CT) scan of chest, abdomen, and pelvis; bone scan/gallium scan]; and human immuno-deficiency virus (HIV) screen.
- For children with NHL, stage is usually assigned according to the St. Jude system, whereas children with Hodgkin's disease are staged by using the Ann Arbor system.

PRIMARY THERAPY

- The treatment plan is determined on the basis of histology, stage, immunophenotype, and in some cases, clinical symptoms such as fever, weight loss, and night sweats.
- Children with advanced-stage Burkitt's lymphoma are generally treated with intensive cyclophosphamide-based regimens given over a relatively short period, whereas children with lymphoblastic lymphoma are generally treated with regimens derived from strategies for children with acute lymphoblastic leukemia (ALL).
- Among children with large cell lymphoma, the treatment plan varies with respect to tumor cell immunophenotype.
- Involved-field radiation therapy (IFRT) has a role in certain cases of Hodgkin's disease but is rarely indicated for children with NHL.

SALVAGE THERAPY

- Children with refractory or recurrent disease are generally

SUMMARY OF KEY POINTS—cont'd

considered to have a poor prognosis and are therefore candidates for intensive or novel salvage-treatment regimens.

- Those with chemosensitive disease are potential candidates for an intensification phase with hematopoietic stem cell rescue.

COMPLICATIONS

- The most concerning late effects of therapy include cardiac toxicity, infertility, and the development of a second malignancy.
- The risks for these complications are determined in part by the components of initial therapy.

PROGNOSIS

The most important predictors of treatment outcome for children with NHL are treatment protocol and tumor burden, as reflected by stage and serum LDH.

INTRODUCTION

Substantial clinical and laboratory advances have improved our understanding of both the pathogenesis and treatment of the malignant lymphomas of childhood and adolescence, which comprise Hodgkin's disease and the non-Hodgkin's lymphomas (NHLs).[1-3] These are the third most common type of cancer in children in the United States, comprising approximately 13% of newly diagnosed cases in this age group each year.[4-7] Among children younger than 15 years, the NHLs account for approximately 60% of cases. However, when children up to age 18 are included, a slight predominance of Hodgkin's disease is found.[8]

The NHLs of childhood are markedly different from those of adulthood.[9,10] Diffuse high-grade extranodal subtypes account for the majority of pediatric cases, whereas low- and intermediate-grade lymphomas are predominant in adults. These differences are probably due in part to age-related maturational changes in the immune system and consequently in the types of cells susceptible to malignant transformation.[2] The differences between adults and children in histologic subtype underlie the differing clinical features, staging, and treatment strategies in these age groups.[10]

The clinical presentation, staging, histologic subtypes, and treatment strategies in children and adults with Hodgkin's disease are less dissimilar; however, some differences are worth noting.[11] Epidemiologic studies have suggested three distinct forms that depend on age: the childhood form in patients aged 14 years or younger, the young adult form (ages 15 to 34 years), and an older adult form in individuals aged 55 to 74 years.[12] Among the four histologic subtypes of Hodgkin's disease described in the Rye classification system,[13] the nodular sclerosing subtype is most common in children, occurring in 40% of younger children and 70% of adolescents.[14] Mixed cellularity Hodgkin's disease occurs in approximately 30% of cases and is more common in children with human immunodeficiency virus (HIV) infection and in those younger than 10 years; it frequently is associated with an advanced stage (with extranodal extension) at presentation.[14] Lymphocyte-predominant Hodgkin's disease accounts for approximately 10% to 15% of pediatric cases, is usually associated with localized disease at presentation,

and occurs more commonly in younger patients and in boys. The fourth subtype of Hodgkin's disease, lymphocyte depletion, is very rare in children.[11]

Despite excellent event-free survival rates in Hodgkin's disease, well-recognized challenges are related to the sequelae of therapy, which include endocrine dysfunction, chemotherapy-induced sterility, radiation-induced abnormalities in bone growth, chemotherapy- and radiation-related second cancers, and late cardiac deaths.[11] Most current studies are exploring strategies that maintain an excellent treatment result while reducing late effects. For example, a combined-modality approach with low-dose radiation and combination chemotherapy may reduce the bone-growth abnormalities associated with high-dose extended-field radiation therapy.[11] However, as therapy is modified in an attempt to reduce the risk of late effects, the rates of event-free survival may be compromised.[15-18] For example, attempts at reducing alkylating agent–related late effects in patients with advanced-stage disease, by substituting other chemotherapeutic agents, have reduced event-free survival rates.[15,16] These and other issues regarding the management of Hodgkin's disease are discussed in Chapter 111. The remainder of this chapter focuses on the NHLs of childhood.

EPIDEMIOLOGY AND PATHOGENESIS

NHLs may occur at any age in childhood, but are unusual in children younger than 3 years; the median age at diagnosis is approximately 10 years.[10,19] Approximately 500 new cases of pediatric NHL are found in the United States each year.[1,5-8] In contrast to Hodgkin's disease, which has a bimodal age distribution with peaks in early and late adulthood, the incidence of NHLs increases steadily with age.[8,12] NHL occurs almost twice as commonly in whites as in blacks, and 2 to 3 times more often in boys than in girls; the explanation for these differences has yet to be elucidated.[2]

Specific populations are at increased risk for the development of NHL.[2,20-28] These include individuals with inherited immunodeficiency syndromes,[2,25,26] including ataxia-telangiectasia (AT), Wiskott-Aldrich syndrome, and X-linked lymphoproliferative syndrome (XLP). It is important that these syndromes be recognized so that appropriate therapy can be designed. For example, in the management of children with AT in whom a malignancy develops, involved-field irradiation and radiomimetics such as bleomycin should be avoided. Children with AT also are at increased risk for the development of hemorrhagic cystitis after exposure to cyclophosphamide. Boys with XLP are at increased risk to develop fatal infectious mononucleosis and/or B-cell lymphomas. XLP should be considered in any boy whose brother has had either fatal infectious mononucleosis or B-cell lymphoma, or in any boy who has had two primary B-cell lymphomas. Children who have received immunosuppressive therapy (e.g., recipients of bone marrow or organ transplants) and those with the acquired immunodeficiency syndrome (AIDS) also are at a higher risk for developing NHL.[23] The overall prevalence of lymphomas among children with HIV infection is approximately 1.6%.[23] Among pediatric HIV-positive hemophiliacs, NHL is 36 times more frequent than in HIV-negative children with factor VIII deficiency.[24] The majority of the HIV-associated NHLs have a B-cell immunophenotype with either Burkitt's or large-cell morphology. Proliferative lesions of mucosa-associated lymphoid tissue (MALT), which may be either benign or malignant, also have been described in children with HIV infection.[23] Although deficient T-cell function has been implicated in these congenital and acquired immuno-deficiency states, further study is required to clarify fully the mechanisms of pathogenesis.

Well-recognized geographic differences are found in both the incidence and the distribution of histologic subtypes of NHL.[2,4,29-32] For example, the NHLs are very rare in Japan but are very common in equatorial Africa. More specifically, Burkitt's lymphoma accounts for approximately one half of all childhood malignancies in equatorial Africa and is the predominant NHL subtype in Northeastern Brazil and areas of the Middle East.[29,30] In contrast, lymphoblastic lymphomas are the predominant histologic subtype in southern India.[31] In some parts of the world, the distribution of histologic subtypes of childhood NHL has yet to be firmly established.

Geographic differences also exist in the clinical and biologic features of some NHLs.[2,31,33] For example, Burkitt's lymphoma in equatorial Africa (endemic Burkitt's lymphoma) frequently involves the jaw, abdomen, orbit, paraspinal area, and central nervous system (CNS), whereas the common sites of involvement associated with Burkitt's lymphoma in the United States and Western Europe (sporadic Burkitt's lymphoma) include the abdomen, bone marrow, and nasopharynx.[2] The predominant chromosome 8 break points are upstream of *MYC* among endemic cases, whereas among sporadic cases, the break point is usually within the *MYC* gene.[32] The endemic cases are associated with immunoglobulin M (IgM) secretion, whereas the sporadic cases generally are not.[2] The sporadic and endemic cases also differ with respect to Epstein-Barr virus (EBV) association.[32]

The overlap of the lymphoma belt in equatorial Africa with the malaria belt prompted speculation that an infectious agent might be involved in lymphomagenesis. This led to the discovery of the association between EBV and African Burkitt's lymphoma.[2] Although a direct role in pathogenesis has not been demonstrated, the circumstantial evidence for its involvement is compelling. It has been suggested that as a B-cell mitogen, EBV increases the target pool of cells potentially susceptible to malignant transformation.[32] Supporting this hypothesis is evidence that *Rag* gene expression can be induced by EBV, theoretically increasing the likelihood of a translocation occurring in immature B cells that are about to rearrange their immunoglobulin genes.[34] The potential role of EBNA-1 in pathogenesis has been suggested by experiments demonstrating that lymphomas develop in mice transgenic for EBNA-1.[35] Moreover, an identified EBNA-1 variant has been shown to be associated with the majority of Burkitt's lymphoma cases studied, prompting investigators to speculate that this tumor-associated mutation alters EBNA-1 function in a way that directly or indirectly provides a growth advantage for the lymphoma cell.[36] A more direct role for EBV in lymphomagenesis is suggested by studies of the EBV-positive Burkitt's lymphoma cell line, Akata, which loses its malignant phenotype with spontaneous loss of EBV; however, the malignant phenotype is regained with EBV reinfection.[37] EBV association has been reported in approximately 90% of the endemic (i.e., African) Burkitt's tumors and in approximately 15% of sporadic cases (United States and Western Europe).[2] Aberrant and disrupted expression of the EBV genome has recently been reported in cases of sporadic Burkitt's lymphoma that were EBV negative by conventional EBNA screening.[38] This observation, coupled with the 50% rate of EBV association in Burkitt's tumors in other parts of the world (including Brazil, Russia, Argentina, and Chile), suggests a widespread role for this virus in lymphomagenesis.[31]

PATHOLOGY AND BIOLOGY

Various schemes have been used to classify the tumors collectively referred to as the NHLs. The National Cancer Institute (NCI) Working Formulation for clinical use, which was published in 1982,[9] divides the NHLs into three grades (low, intermediate, and high) based on their clinical aggressiveness. The NHLs of childhood are almost entirely high-grade tumors, which comprise the small noncleaved cell, lymphoblastic, and large cell subtypes (Fig. 102-1; Table 102-1). In 1994, The International Lymphoma Study Group published the Revised European-American Lymphoma (REAL) Classification, an effort to build on the currently used European and American classification systems.[39] More recently, the World Health Organization (WHO) published its Classification of Tumors of Haematopoietic and Lymphoid Tissues.[40] Both the REAL and WHO classification systems incorporate additional histopathologic features and genetic abnormalities in their descriptions of clinically relevant disease entities. The REAL and WHO systems have had more impact on the classification of the NHLs in adults than in children. Among childhood NHLs, the most significant changes have occurred in the classification of large cell lymphomas, which are designated as either T-cell or B-cell, and include entities such as anaplastic large cell

Burkitt's   Lymphoblastic   Large Cell

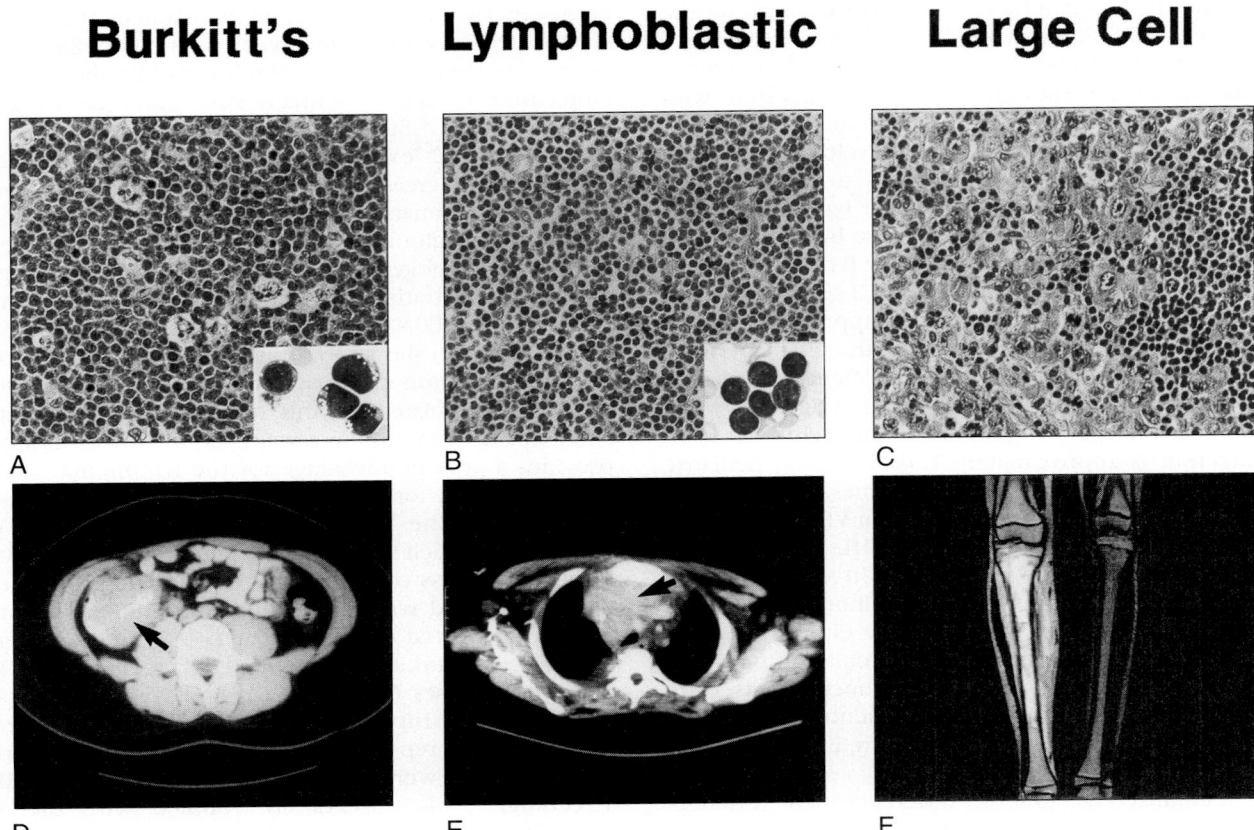

Figure 102-1. Histologic and clinical features of non-Hodgkin's lymphoma in children. The upper panels show the histologic "starry sky" appearance of small noncleaved-cell (Burkitt's) lymphoma (**A**); lymphoblastic lymphoma (**B**); anaplastic subtype of large-cell lymphoma (**C**). The inserts in (**A**) and (**B**) show the characteristic L3 blasts of Burkitt's tumors and the characteristic L1 blasts of lymphoblastic lymphoma, respectively. The lower panels show common clinical presentations of the three histologic subtypes of lymphoma: **D,** Encasement of the bowel lumen by Burkitt's lymphoma on abdominal computed tomography; **E,** Airway compression by lymphoblastic lymphoma on computed tomography of the anterior mediastinum; **F,** Bony destruction of the tibias by large-cell lymphoma.

TABLE 102-1

Clinical and Biologic Characteristics of Non-Hodgkin's Lymphoma in Children

SUBTYPE	PROPORTION OF CASES (%)*	PHENOTYPE	PRIMARY SITE	TRANSLOCATION	AFFECTED GENES
Burkitt	39	B cell	Abdomen or head and neck	t(8;14)(q24;q32) t(2;8)(p11;q24) t(8;22)(q24;q11)	IgH-cMYC Ig6-cMYC Ig8-cMYC
Lymphoblastic	28	T cell†	Mediastinum or head and neck	t(1;14)(p32;q11) t(11;14)(p13;q11) t(11;14)(p15;q11) t(10;14)(q24;q11) t(7;19)(q35;p13) t(8;14)(q24;q11) t(1;7)(p34;q34)	TCRαδ-TAL1 TCRαδ-RHOMB2 TCRαδ-RHOMB1 TCRαδ-HOX11 TCRβ-LYL1 TCRαδ-MYC TCRβ-LCK
Large cell	26	B cell, T cell‡, indeterminate‡	Mediastinum, abdomen, head and neck, or skin*	t(2;5)(p23;q35)	NPM-ALK

Ig, immunoglobulin; TCR, T-cell receptor.
*Proportion at St. Jude Children's Research Hospital; other histotypes account for ~7%.
†B-cell-progenitor variants have also been described.
‡Associated with anaplastic large cell lymphoma (ALCL) subtype: ≈10% of childhood NHL.

TABLE 102-2

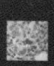

Pediatric Non-Hodgkin's Lymphoma According to the World Health Organization Classification

Common Pediatric Lymphomas

B-cell lymphomas
  Precursor B-lymphoblastic lymphoma/leukemia
  Burkitt's lymphoma
  Diffuse large B-cell lymphoma
  Mediastinal (thymic) large B-cell lymphoma
T-cell lymphomas
  Precursor T-lymphoblastic lymphoma/leukemia
  Anaplastic large cell lymphoma
  Peripheral T-cell lymphoma, unspecified

Uncommon Pediatric Lymphomas

Follicular lymphoma (grade 1, 2, or 3)
Hepatosplenic T-cell lymphoma
Extranodal marginal zone B-cell lymphoma of mucosa-associated
  lymphoid tissue (MALT lymphoma)

Rare Pediatric Lymphomas

Mycosis fungoides
Subcutaneous panniculitis-like T-cell lymphoma
Adult T-cell leukemia/lymphoma (HTLV-1–associated
  leukemia/lymphoma)
Primary cutaneous CD30-positive T-cell lymphoproliferative disorders
Extranodal natural killer (NK)/T-cell lymphoma

lymphoma (ALCL) and mediastinal large B-cell lymphoma (MLBCL), which were not featured in the NCI Working Formulation. The WHO classification of pediatric NHLs is summarized in Table 102-2.

Burkitt's Lymphoma

The REAL[39] and WHO[40] classification systems have replaced the term *small noncleaved cell lymphoma*, used in the NCI Working Formulation[9] with the term *Burkitt's lymphoma*. The L3-ALL leukemia subtype (Burkitt's leukemia) of the French-American-British classification system, also is included in the Burkitt's lymphoma designation. The primary Burkitt's lymphomas are biologically and clinically similar to Burkitt's leukemia.[41] Classic Burkitt's lymphomas are characterized histologically by a diffuse infiltrative pattern of monomorphic small to medium-sized cells with basophilic cytoplasm, round nuclei, clumped chromatin, and one to three nucleoli.[39,40] Tingible body macrophages interspersed among tumor cells in the field result in the low-power microscopic "starry sky" appearance frequently associated with this tumor.

Two morphologic variants are recognized in the WHO classification system:[40] Burkitt's lymphoma with plasmacytoid differentiation and atypical Burkitt's or Burkitt's-like lymphoma. The plasmacytoid variant, which is more frequently found among immunodeficiency-related lymphomas, contains features of plasma cells, which include eccentrically placed nuclei and a single central nucleolus.[39,40,42] No prognostic significance has been described for this variant in children. The atypical Burkitt's or Burkitt's-like lymphomas are characterized

histologically by a wider range of nuclear size and shape, and nucleoli that are larger but fewer in number.[40,43] These features may lead to difficulty in distinguishing it from large B-cell lymphomas. These lymphomas must have evidence of a *c-MYC* translocation to be considered part of the Burkitt's lymphoma family, although some large B-cell lymphomas may contain a *c-MYC* translocation. In classic Burkitt's lymphoma, the deregulation *c-MYC* results in virtually all of the tumor cells being in cycle. This high proliferative rate is detected by positive nuclear reactivity to Ki-67 antibodies in almost every tumor cell. The WHO system suggests that the "Burkitt's-like" designation should be used for lymphomas with morphologic features intermediate between diffuse large B-cell lymphoma (DLBCL) and Burkitt's lymphoma where the Ki-67 fraction of viable tumor cells is at least 99% or a *c-MYC* translocation is present.[40,44] Lymphomas with histologic features of large cell lymphoma and found to have a *c-MYC* translocation or very high Ki-67–positive fraction or Burkitt's-like lymphomas with a low Ki-67 index should be classified as DLBCL.[40,44] The clinical significance of the atypical-Burkitt's variant in children remains controversial.[45]

Burkitt's tumors are characterized by the presence of one of three reciprocal chromosomal translocations [t(8;14), t(2;8), or t(8;22)] involving the *MYC* gene located on chromosome 8 at band q24 and one of the immunoglobulin genes.[32,46-51] The classic translocation, t(8;14)(q24;q11), is identified in approximately 85% of cases and involves the heavy-chain immunoglobulin locus. The two variant translocations, t(2;8)(p11;q24) and t(8;22)(q24;q11), account for the remaining 15% of cases; each involves one of two light-chain immunoglobulin loci. Each of these three translocations juxtaposes the *MYC* proto-oncogene on chromosome 8 with one of the three immunoglobulin genes, resulting in dysregulation of the *MYC* gene.[32,46]

MYC is a transcription factor gene whose expression is increased with cellular proliferation, as in the case of mitogenic stimulation of B cells.[32,52-55] It is thought that MYC activates key target genes that induce cycle progression from G_1 into the S phase. MYC protein forms heterodimers with related proteins (e.g., MAX) through its carboxy-terminal motifs (basic helix-loop-helix and leucine zipper).[56-59] These DNA-binding heterodimers influence cell cycling. MYC:MAX heterodimers are potent transactivators,[56-61] whereas MAX:MAX dimers are transcription repressors. The deregulation of *MYC* in Burkitt's lymphoma may increase the proportion of MYC:MAX complexes, which in turn would lead to proliferation of lymphoma cells.[62]

Several explanations are given for the dysregulated expression of MYC in Burkitt's lymphoma.[32,63-65] Many stem from the observed mutations and structural abnormalities of the translocated *MYC* gene. Mutations in the MYC-inhibiting factor (MIF) binding sites located in a first intron regulatory region are associated with loss of the repressive effect of MIF binding on transcription.[66] Mutations in the coding region of *MYC* in Burkitt's lymphoma have been associated with gain-of-function activities.[64] Other data strongly implicate the role of the juxtaposed immunoglobulin gene in lymphomagenesis, leading to speculation that the immunoglobulin gene usurps control over the *MYC* gene through putative long-range enhancer elements.[63,65]

Transgenic mouse models mimicking the abnormality in Burkitt's lymphoma have provided additional important insights into the role of *MYC* in pathogenesis.[67,68] These studies have demonstrated that MYC is an essential but insufficient factor in lymphomagenesis. In this model, the programmed expression of MYC in the B-cell compartment results in the development of B-cell malignancies. However, the fact that these tumors are monoclonal and take 6 to 9 months to develop suggests that additional molecular events or factors are necessary for malignant transformation. The identity and role of other oncogenes or tumor-suppressor genes are currently under investigation.[69,70] More recent analysis of the ARF-Mdm2-p53 apoptotic pathway in Eu-myc transgenic mice has provided additional insights into pathogenesis.[71-73] In normal B cells, this pathway is activated by overexpression of c-myc. In 80% of the lymphomas that arise in the transgenic mouse, mutations of this pathway are observed, including deletions of Ink4a/ARF (25%), mutations of p53 (30%), or overexpression of Mdm2 (50%).[71] Although some data suggest that one third of primary human Burkitt's tumors have mutations in p53, limited data exist on the ARF-Mdm2-p53 pathway[74-76]; studies in human tumors are currently ongoing.

Burkitt's lymphoma has a mature B-cell immunophenotype with a characteristic but not unique profile: CD19+, CD20+, CD22+, CD79α+, and moderately strong surface expression of IgM or less commonly IgA or IgG with light-chain κ or λ restriction.[77] CD10 is expressed in more than 50% of cases. Nuclear Bcl-6 is typically present (without *BCL-6* rearrangement), and CD5, CD34, BCL2 and TdT are typically absent.[78] CD21, the receptor for EBV and the complement fragment Cd3, is more frequently detected in the endemic than in the sporadic Burkitt's subtype. In very rare cases, Burkitt's tumors have cytoplasmic mμ with no detectable surface immunoglobulin, and less commonly cases that have neither[79,80]; very rare instances are found of double κ plus λ expression.

Lymphoblastic Lymphoma

The lymphoblasts in lymphoblastic lymphoma and ALL have overlapping morphologic, immunophenotypic, and cytogenetic features, leading many to believe that the distinction between the two is largely arbitrary.[81-83] According to the WHO classification, these malignancies are considered to be either "precursor T-cell" or "precursor B-cell" neoplasms.[34,40] Clinically, some lymphoblastic lymphomas have isolated bulky mediastinal masses, whereas others have overt involvement of the bone marrow. The clinical distinction between lymphoblastic lymphoma and ALL is determined on the basis of bone marrow involvement: those with more than 25% replacement by lymphoblasts are considered to have ALL, whereas those with a lesser degree of replacement are considered to have advanced-stage lymphoblastic lymphoma with marrow involvement.[10,84]

The malignant lymphoblasts are characteristically small with round or convoluted nuclei, distinct nuclear membranes, inconspicuous nucleoli, and a scant rim of basophilic cytoplasm.[2] The nuclei of T- or B-cell types may be markedly convoluted, although this is a more common feature of T-cell lymphomas. Histologically, actively phagocytosing histiocytes in the field may result in a microscopic "starry sky" appearance similar to that seen in Burkitt's lymphoma.

The majority of lymphoblastic lymphomas are of T lineage (~90%); the remaining are primarily of B lineage,[85-94] although very rare cases of natural killer (NK) cell origin have been described.[93,95,96] Only minor antigen-expression differences are found between T- or B-lineage lymphoblastic lymphomas and their ALL counterparts. Lymphoblastic lymphomas are typically positive for TdT (terminal deoxynucleotidyl transferase)[97-101] and CD34 expression,[102] which is helpful in distinguishing them from Burkitt's lymphoma. CD10 [the common ALL antigen (CALLA)] expression also may be detected in cases of T- or B-precursor lymphoblastic lymphoma. Although a favorable clinical outcome has been associated with CALLA expression in cases of T-ALL, this association has not been described in precursor T lymphoblastic lymphoma.[93,103]

The lymphoblastic lymphomas also may be further subclassified on the basis of their intrathymic or bone marrow stage of maturation in a manner analogous to that with ALL[104-107] (Table 102-3). Attempts to separate lymphoblastic lymphoma from ALL on the basis of these immunophenotypic features, and the identification of clinically relevant immunophenotypic subtypes, have been largely unsuccessful. B-lymphoblastic lymphomas may be characterized by any of the four subtypes listed in Table 102-2.[92,108,109] The very rare case in which surface immunoglobulin is expressed without detectable TdT should not be confused with Burkitt's lymphoma.[93,110] T-ALL and T-lymphoblastic lymphoma can be subdivided according to corresponding stages on normal intrathymic T-cell maturation (see Table 102-3). The majority of T-cell lymphoblastic lymphomas correspond to a late stage of intrathymic maturation.[105-107] The expression of pan–T-cell antigens (e.g., CD7, CD2, CD5, and CD6) is retained in most T-lineage lymphoblastic lymphomas, in contrast to T large cell lymphoma in which one or more of these is undetectable. T lymphoblastic lymphomas are characterized by a more frequent expression of T-cell receptor (TCR) αβ than γδ, as compared with T-ALL.[111]

Few published studies concern on the cytogenetic abnormalities of lymphoblastic lymphoma, and those that do exist comprise small numbers of patients.[112-114] Similarities in morphology, immunophenotype, cellular origin, and clinical features have led to the tacit assumption that lymphoblastic lymphoma and T-cell ALL are different presentations of the same disease process.[115-117] In fact, most theories regarding the pathogenesis of lymphoblastic lymphoma are based on biologic studies of lymphoblasts from patients with T-cell ALL. Both entities may involve a reciprocal chromosomal translocation that affects one of the TCR genes and results in dysregulation of the reciprocal partner gene, which is often a transcrip-

TABLE 102-3

Immunophenotypic Features of Precursor B- and T-lymphoblastic Lymphomas

SUBTYPE	CD45	CD34	TDT	CD3*	CD5	CD7	CD19	CD20	CD22	CD79α*	CD10	IMMUNOGLOBULIN EXPRESSION
Early pre-B	+†	+	+	−	−	−	+	±	+	+	+‡	clgμ⁻, slgμ⁻, κ⁻, λ⁻
Pre-B	+	±	+	−	−	−	+	±	+	+	+	clgμ⁺, slgμ⁻, κ⁻, λ⁻
Late pre-B‡	+	±	±	−	−	−	+	±	+	+	+	clgμ⁺, slgμ⁻, κ⁻, λ⁻
Mature B§	+	±	±	−	−	−	+	±	+	+	+	clgμ⁺, slgμ⁺, κ⁻, λ⁻
T‖	+	±	±	+	±	+	−	−	−	±	−	clgμ⁺, slgμ⁺, κ⁺, λ±

clgμ, cytoplasmic immunoglobulin μ; κ, immunoglobulin light chain κ; λ, immunoglobulin light chain λ; slgμ, surface immunoglobulin μ; Tdt, terminal deoxynucleotidyl transferase.
*Cytoplasmic antigen expression.
†10% of cases may have very weak to no detectable CD45 antigen.
‡Also termed transitional-pre-B.
§Rare subtype not to be confused with Burkitt's lymphoma.
‖May be subclassified into early thymic stage (CD7⁺, cytoplasmic CD3⁺, CD5±, CD2±, CD1a⁻, CD4⁻, CD8⁻), mid-thymic stage (CD7⁺, CD5⁺, CD2⁺, cytoplasmic CD3⁺, surface CD3±, CD1a±, CD4±, CD8±), and late thymic stage (CD7⁺, CD5⁺, CD2⁺, surface CD3⁺, CD1a⁻, CD4⁺ or CD8⁺).

tion factor gene.[118-126] For example, *TAL1* is involved in the t(1;14)(p32;q11) chromosomal abnormality, which is present in approximately 3% of newly diagnosed cases of T-ALL. However, submicroscopic deletions of *TAL1* can be identified in up to 25% of cases of T-ALL.[119,120,125,126] suggesting that this deletion also may be the most common molecular abnormality in lymphoblastic lymphoma.[125] The *HOX11* transcription factor gene and the *RHOMB* genes, whose products are members of a family of proteins that contain a cysteine-rich (LIM) protein-protein interaction domain, also may be involved in translocations occurring in both T-ALL and lymphoblastic lymphoma.[121,123,124] The t(9;17) translocation is more commonly detected in T-lineage lymphoblastic lymphoma than in precursor T-ALL,[113] and is often associated with a mediastinal mass and aggressive disease course. The t(10;11)(p13-14;q14-21), which is relatively uncommon in pediatric lymphoblastic lymphoma cases, also has been associated with ALL and acute myelocytic leukemia (AML).[127,128] The t(8;13)(p11;q11-14) has been reported in rare cases of T-cell lymphoblastic lymphoma that are seen with eosinophilia and myeloid hyperplasia.[129-131] Cytogenetic abnormalities have not been associated with prognostic significance in children with lymphoblastic lymphoma, perhaps because of the small number of studied cases. Gene-expression profiling studies (i.e., microarray analyses), however, may identify subgroups that are at higher risk of treatment failure, as has been reported for T-ALL.[132,133]

Large Cell Lymphoma

The large cell lymphomas of childhood are heterogeneous with respect to immunophenotype, histology, and cytogenetics.[134-136] Morphologically, the large cell lymphomas are usually characterized by cells that are larger than the diameter of histiocytic nuclei or 2 to 3 times the width of small inactive-appearing lymphocytes. The immunophenotype may be T-cell, B-cell, or rarely of NK-cell origin. Those that are designated as non-T, non-B-cell (indeterminate) are usually incompletely characterized with

respect to the cell of origin and should not be considered lymphomas without lineage commitment. Large cell malignancies of dendritic or true monocytic-histiocytic immunophenotype should not be considered to be large cell lymphomas in that their biologic features, clinical course, and treatment differ. When large cell lymphomas are grouped according to the NCI Working Formulation, the majority are high-grade, large cell immunoblastic lymphomas, and a smaller percentage are intermediate-grade diffuse large cell lymphomas. Among children, no clinically significant difference is seen between these two groups with respect to presentation or treatment outcome.[134] When large cell lymphomas are grouped according to the revised REAL[39] or current WHO[40] classification systems, several different subtypes are recognized: diffuse large B-cell, anaplastic large cell, peripheral T-cell unspecified, angioimmunoblastic T-cell, adult T-cell leukemia/lymphoma, extranodal nasal NK/T-cell lymphoma, enteropathy-type T-cell lymphoma, subcutaneous panniculitis-like T-cell lymphoma, and primary cutaneous CD-30+ T-cell disorders. The two most common types of large cell lymphoma in children are ALCL (~40% to 50%)[137-147] and DLBCL (~30% to ~40%); however, rare examples of the other subtypes have been reported.[148,149] Although the morphologic and immunophenotypic features of large cell lymphomas in adults and children are quite similar, relatively few detailed biologic and laboratory studies have compared them, except for the anaplastic large cell subtype.

Anaplastic Large Cell Lymphoma

The ALCLs of childhood are recognized as a unique clinicopathologic entity among the large cell lymphomas and are usually characterized by frequent extranodal disease sites (e.g., skin, lung, soft tissue, and bone), anaplastic histology, CD30+ T-cell/null immunophenotype, and the presence of a t(2;5) translocation.[138,150,151] ALCL has a peak incidence in adolescence and is rare in very young children.[150] Approximately 20% to 25% of patients may have involvement of the bone marrow at presentation that may not be detected without special studies.[152] Histologically, lymph node architecture may be partially or totally effaced by sheets of adherent lymphoma cells, often involving the lymphoid sinuses, an appearance that mimics metastatic tumor. A variable number of small, medium-sized, and large neoplastic cells are typically identified. The hallmark cells of ALCL are large cells with eccentrically placed, horseshoe–shaped, or monocytoid nuclei with an eosinophilic Golgi region adjacent to the nucleus. Gigantic cells containing multiple nuclei forming a wreath-like appearance also are commonly observed. The large ALCL cells often resemble Reed-Sternberg cells and their variant forms.

The ALCL category includes several morphologic subtypes or variants, which include common, lymphohistiocytic, and small cell.[40,153] The common type accounts for at least 70% of cases and is characterized by the presence of the hallmark large anaplastic lymphoma cells described earlier.[154] A spectrum of small and medium-sized cells is commonly observed as well. Erythrophagocytosis is a prominent feature in some cases. The lymphohistiocytic variant, which accounts for fewer than 20% of pediatric ALCL cases, is characterized by a mixture of lymphoid cells of varying sizes and many histiocytes, which may be so numerous that they partially obscure the lymphoid cells.[155,156] Histiocytic erythrophagocytosis, simulating a hemophagocytic syndrome, may be present in some cases.[157,158] The small cell variant, which accounts for fewer than 10% of cases, may not be recognized if the hallmark ALCL cells are scarce and cytogenetic and immunophenotyping studies are not performed.[159] Rare subtypes of ALCL include the signet-ring, granulomatous, and sarcomatoid forms.[160-162] A neutrophil-rich form of ALCL has been described[163-166]; however, it is not a recognized variant in the WHO classification.

The ALCLs are primarily of T-lineage, as evidenced by surface markers and TCR gene rearrangements. Most ALCLs express one or more T-cell–associated antigens (e.g., CD2, CD3, CD4, CD7, or CD45RO; Table 102-4).[40,167] T-cell antigens CD5 and CD8 are usually not detected. Some cases do not have detectable T-cell antigens, but do have TCR gene rearrangements; they may be referred to as null/T ALCL.[40] In most cases of ALCL, expression of cytoplasmic cytotoxic cell-associated proteins TIA-1, granzyme B, or perforin are detected. CD30 expression (membranous plus Golgi pattern) is characteristic of the tumor cells of ALCL[168]; typically, the larger cells demonstrate intense reactivity to CD30 antibodies, whereas the smaller cells are weakly reactive or more often nonreactive. Most ALCLs also are positive for the epithelial membrane antigen (EMA) in a pattern similar to that of CD30.[169] The myeloid-associated antigen, CD15, may be weakly expressed in rare cases. Gene expression-profiling studies of ALK-negative ALCLs have demonstrated aberrant expression of clusterin in systemic but not primary cutaneous tumors.[170] B-cell–associated antigens (e.g., CD19, CD20, CD22, and CD79a) are not typically expressed in ALCL, except for the extremely rare case of B-lineage ALCL.

The majority (>75%) of pediatric ALCL cases contain the t(2;5)(p23;q35) chromosomal abnormality.[142,171,172] Variant translocations involving *ALK* have been described: t(1;2)(q25;p23), t(2;3)(p23;q21), inv(2)(p23;q35), t(2;22), t(2;17)(p23;q11), and t(2;19)(p23;p13).[173-176] In contrast to the translocations of Burkitt's and lymphoblastic lymphoma, which result in the dysregulated expression of a transcription factor gene by its reciprocal partner gene, the t(2;5) results in the fusion of the involved genes (the amino-terminal portion of the nucleophosmin gene, *NPM*, on chromosome 5 with the catalytic domain of the anaplastic lymphoma kinase gene, *ALK*, on chromosome 2),[144] resulting in a chimeric NPM-ALK protein product with properties unlike those of either component.[145] It is thought that the cytoplasmic localization of this product may inappropriately phosphorylate substrates involved in normal cell growth and differentiation, resulting in malignant transformation. ALK protein, a transmembrane protein, is normally expressed in some cells in the brain, but not in normal lymphoid or hematopoietic cells. The ALCL-associated ALK translocations result in aberrant expression of the chimeric ALK protein in the tumor cells. The ALCLs that have a t(2;5) translocation are character-

TABLE 102-4

Immunohistochemical Markers of Lymphomas of Children

	TDT	CD20	CD79A	IG	CD5	CD3	CD30	CD15	ALK	CTA	MUM1	BCL2	BCL6
T-LBL	+(−)	−	−(+)	−	+/−	+*	−	−	−	−	−/+	−	+/−
Burkitt's	−	+	+	+	−	−	−	−	−	−	−	−	+
ALCL†	−	−	−	−	−	−/+	+	−(+)	+	+/−	+	−	+/−
PTL	−	−	−	−	+/−	+/−	−/+	−	−	−/+	+/−	−	−/+
MLBCL	−	+	+	+/−	−	−	+/−	−	−	−	+/−	−	−
DLBCL	−	+	+	+/−	−/+	−	+/−	−	−	+/−	+/−	+/−	+/−
FL	−	+	+	+/−	−	−	−	−	−	−	−/+	+/−	−/+
HPL	−	−	−	−	−	+	−	−	−	+	−/+	−	+

+, positive; −, negative; (+), <15% of cases positive; +/−, commonly positive but may be negative; −/+, commonly negative but may be positive; (−), <15% of cases negative; ALCL, anaplastic large cell lymphoma; CTA, cytotoxic antigen (e.g., TIA-1, perforin); DLBCL, diffuse large B-cell lymphoma; FL, follicular lymphoma; HSL, hepatosplenic lymphoma; MLBCL, mediastinal large B-cell lymphoma; MUM1, interferon regulatory factor-4 (IRF4); PTL, peripheral T-cell lymphoma; T-LBL, T-lymphoblastic lymphoma.
*Cytoplasmic CD3.
†Marker features are for T-lineage ALCL with ALK gene rearrangements. Rare ALK-positive case may be B-lineage with CD20⁺/CD79a⁺/CD3-profile; ALCLs without ALK rearrangements are ALK-1 negative and may express Bcl2 protein.
Data from Falini B, Mason DY: Proteins encoded by genes involved in chromosomal alterations in lymphoma and leukemia: Clinical value of their detection by immunocytochemistry. Blood, 2002;99:409–426.

ized by both cytoplasmic and nuclear ALK expression, in contrast to those with variant translocations that display cytoplasmic expression only.[167,168] Granular cytoplasmic staining with ALK antibodies has been described in rare cases of ALCL associated with the t(2;17)(q23;q11) translocation.[177] A small percentage (~10%) of pediatric ALCL cases have no ALK translocation or ALK expression (in contrast to ALCLs in adults, among which ~50% have no ALK expression).[156] Conversely, lymphomas containing the t(2;5) but lacking anaplastic features have been described.[150] Expression of ALK proteins in tumor cells can be detected with p80 or ALK-1 antibodies in the majority (85%) of ALCL cases.[144,178,179] Therefore ALK expression is a very sensitive marker for ALCLs containing either the classic or variant ALK translocations. Lymphomas with morphologic and immunophenotypic features of ALCL but lacking ALK expression should be considered phenotypic variants of ALCL; ALK expression has prognostic significance among ALCL cases in adults.[40] Some mesenchymal tumors in children and adults such as neuroblastoma, inflammatory myofibroblastic tumor, rhabdomyosarcoma, and malignant peripheral nerve sheath tumors also may express ALK[180-182]; therefore ALK expression alone should not be used to distinguish between lymphomas and other neoplasms.

A leukemic phase of ALCL may rarely be present at diagnosis or develop at some time during the course of the disease.[176,183-188] Patients first seen with a leukemic process may have no lymphadenopathy or extranodal masses. The circulating lymphoma cells are usually small to medium size with atypical nuclear features, in contrast to the larger cell size often observed in nodal and extranodal masses. When tissue masses are present, they may have the typical features of common ALCL, although most cases resemble the small cell variant of ALCL. The peripheral white blood cell count may be very high (i.e., >10^9/L). The bone marrow may be involved with lymphoma cells like those observed in the peripheral blood or with large anaplastic cells. The circulating lymphoma cells are of T-lineage, but in contrast to precursor T-ALL, CD1a, CD34, and TdT are not expressed. EMA- and ALK-expressing cells are usually detected in the bone marrow. Detection of an *ALK* translocation is necessary to confirm the diagnosis. The t(2;5)(p23;q35) translocation is detected in most cases; however, variant *ALK* translocations may be present.[176]

Diffuse Large Cell Lymphomas of B Lineage

On the basis of both clinical and laboratory features, four types of large cell lymphomas of B-cell lineage are recognized by the WHO classification system: (1) diffuse large B-cell lymphoma, (2) MLBCL, (3) intravascular large B-cell, and (4) primary effusion lymphoma.[40] The first two account for the majority in both adults and children. The last two are very rare in adults and are very uncommon or unreported in children.

Diffuse Large B-Cell Lymphoma.

The DLBCL designation comprises four morphologic variants, which include centroblastic, immunoblastic, T-cell/histiocyte rich, and anaplastic.[40] These variants are not recognized in the WHO classification system as distinct clinicopathologic entities because of both the difficulties in morphologic reproducibility and the controversy over the clinical relevance of subdividing these lymphomas. Challenges also are found in distinguishing between Burkitt's, Burkitt's-like, and DLBCLs. In this regard, a recent study demonstrated that consensus for identifying Burkitt's and DLBCL was 88% and 80%, respectively, whereas for Burkitt's-like lymphoma, only a 42% rate was observed.[189] In many cases, this difficulty may be the result of limited quantity or quality of the tumor sample submitted.

The DLBCLs are characterized by the expression of one or more pan-B–associated markers (e.g., CD19, CD20, CD22, and CD79a). In more than half of the cases, surface or cytoplasmic immunoglobulin expression also is detected. In some cases, expression of CD5, CD10, BCL2, or BCL6 is detected. Nuclear Ki-67 expression, a measure of the proliferative index, may be elevated in some DLBCL cases, but is less than that seen in Burkitt's lymphoma. Among the DLBCL variants, the centroblastic subtype may be the most common subtype in children and is thought to arise from germinal center cells (CD20+, CD79a+ CD10+, BCL6+, MUM-1-, CD138-). The immunoblastic variant, which is characterized by a predominance of immunoblasts (>90%) with a single large centrally located nucleolus (sometimes with a plasmacytoid appearance), is rare in children. This variant is characterized by expression of CD20 and CD79a, and in some cases, CD30, MUM-1, or CD138. The B-cell anaplastic large cell lymphoma variant, which is characterized by large cohesive pleomorphic cells (CD30+, ALK-) that infiltrate the sinuses of involved lymph nodes, occurs infrequently. Among adults, full-length ALK protein has been reported in a rare DLBCL subtype characterized by plasmacytoid features but no rearrangement of the *ALK* gene.[190] Among children, rare cases of DLBCL characterized by plasmacytoid features, presence of the t(2;5), and ALK expression have been described.[191] The T-cell/histiocyte–rich large B-cell lymphomas, which may be confused with Hodgkin's lymphoma or a reactive process, occur infrequently in children.[192] This variant is characterized by expression of CD20, CD79a, BCL-6, and in some cases CD30 or EMA, but not ALK or CD15.[189,193]

Few published data exist on the genetic abnormalities associated with DLBCL in children. In one small study of DLBCL, expression of Bcl-6, c-MYC and Bcl-2 were detected in 66%, 100% and 50% of cases, respectively.[194] Among adult cases, approximately 30% have a t(14;18) translocation or express Bcl-2, suggestive of a germinal center origin. Abnormalities of chromosome 3 band q27 (locus of *BCL-6*) may be detected in another 30% of cases, and the t(8;14) translocation may be identified in a small number of cases. Gene-profiling studies of adult cases of DLBCL have identified three subgroups: germinal center B-cell–like, activated B-cell–like, and a third type not clearly corresponding to a recognized stage of B-cell differentiation.[195-197] One gene-profiling study identified patients within International Prognostic Index (IPI) risk categories who were at greater risk for treatment failure.[198] Gene-profiling studies of DLBCL cases in children have not been reported.

Mediastinal Large B-Cell Lymphoma. MLBCL is a relatively uncommon subtype of DLBCL, and accounts for fewer than 10% of all large cell lymphomas in children.[40,199-204] This type of lymphoma also has been called mediastinal clear cell lymphoma of B-cell type and mediastinal diffuse large cell lymphoma with sclerosis. Among adults, this tumor occurs more frequently in women, whereas among children and adolescents, it may occur slightly more frequently in boys.

Histologically, MLBCLs are characterized by small clusters of large lymphoid cells surrounded by thin to thick, dense fibrotic bands. These clusters of lymphoma cells can mimic metastatic undifferentiated carcinoma. In small biopsy samples, remnant thymic epithelial cells expressing cytokeratin may be confused with an epithelial tumor or thymoma. In some cases, intense fibrosis may obscure the malignant cells. The tumor may contain cells that vary in size (i.e., small, medium, or large lymphoid cells) or may consist primarily of large cells with abundant clear cytoplasm (or less commonly weakly basophilic or acidophilic cytoplasm).[205] In some cases, the presence of small benign-appearing lymphocytes or eosinophils may initially raise the question of Hodgkin's lymphoma. However, unlike classic Hodgkin's lymphoma, tumor cells in MLBCL express CD45- and B-cell–associated antigens (e.g., CD19, CD20, CD22, and CD79a). Detection of BCL-6 and CD10 in the lymphoma cells of MLBCL suggests a derivation from germinal center B cells.[206] Immunoglobulin gene expression may be weakly detectable, but is often undetectable.[207,208] Unlike in lymphoblastic lymphomas, TdT and CD34 are not expressed in MLBCL. Expression of the CD30 antigen may be weakly to strongly detected in a few or sometimes most of the lymphoma cells.[209]

Clonal immunoglobulin gene rearrangements are uniformly detected with molecular studies, even in cases in which immunoglobulins are not detected by conventional immunologic techniques. Mutated immunoglobulin V region genes are detected in lymphoma cells, consistent with a postantigen exposure or postgerminal center B cell.[210] In rare cases, evidence of clonal EBV genome may be detected in the tumor cells. In the few published studies of cytogenetic abnormalities in MLBCL, aneuploid tumor cells, often with gains of chromosome Xq or 9p, are described.[211,212] The t(14;18) translocation, which is associated with adult large cell follicular lymphomas, is infrequent.[212] Overexpression of REL or MAL may be detected in a minority of cases.[213] Rearrangements of *c-MYC*, or *BCL-6*, p53, p16/ink4 alterations may be detected.[211-215]

Uncommon Pediatric Lymphomas

Follicular Lymphoma

The follicular lymphomas are tumors arising from follicular center B cells with a follicular or nodular growth pattern. The three grades of follicular lymphomas recognized in the WHO classification system are distinguished on the basis of the ratio of centroblasts and centrocytes (noncleaved and cleaved follicular center cells, respectively).[40] Follicular lymphomas represent a much higher proportion of NHLs in adults than that seen in children

(~35% vs. <3%, respectively).[216-221] Adults with follicular lymphoma usually are first seen with advanced-stage disease, which may include node, spleen, and bone marrow.[40] In contrast, most children with follicular lymphomas have localized disease involving the tonsillar, cervical, and inguinal lymphoid tissue; cases of localized follicular large cell lymphoma of the testicle also have been reported.[221-225] In contrast to adults with follicular lymphoma, transformation to a high-grade diffuse lymphoma, or leukemic phase, is very uncommon in children. Adults with follicular lymphoma are generally not cured, in contrast to children, who have prolonged remissions with minimal chemotherapy, and in some cases, no chemotherapy. In one pediatric series, a 5-year event-free survival of 94% was reported (most receiving chemotherapy),[219] and in another study, 3 of 6 achieved complete remissions including 3 who did not receive chemotherapy.[220] In a more recent study, 15 of 19 patients with follicular lymphoma were found to have stage I disease, and 11 of 13 had sustained remissions.[221]

Although the morphologic criteria for the diagnosis of follicular lymphoma are well defined, the rarity of this lymphoma in children requires additional studies (i.e., immunophenotypic and molecular) to clearly distinguish it from benign follicular hyperplasia, which is much more frequently encountered. Although no morphologic differences exist between the follicular lymphomas in children and adults, recent studies have identified important biologic differences. Pediatric testicular follicular lymphomas have been reported to express Bcl-6 or have rearrangements of *BCL6*; however, t(14;18)(q32;q21) translocations and bcl-2 and p53 gene abnormalities are lacking.[222-225] In contrast, the majority of follicular lymphomas occurring in adults express bcl-2, and have a t(14;18) translocation involving rearrangement of *BCL-2*.[40] Bcl-2 is a mitochondrial protein that plays an important role in resistance to apoptosis. Its expression is normally detected in T cells and in mantle zone B cells, but not in germinal center cells. Aberrant expression of bcl-2 in follicular lymphomas may influence treatment outcome. In two different studies of pediatric nontesticular follicular lymphomas, *BCL-2* rearrangements were detected by polymerase chain reaction (PCR) in 2 of 16 patients studied and bcl-2 expression was detected in only 6 of 20 patients, respectively.[220,221] In the former study, all 4 patients with tumors expressing bcl-2 had advanced-stage disease or had a poor treatment outcome, in contrast to the children with bcl-2–negative lymphomas, who had limited-stage disease and an excellent treatment outcome.[221] Therefore it does not appear that bcl-2 expression contributes to the pathogenesis of most pediatric follicular lymphomas; however, it may identify a subset of pediatric follicular lymphomas associated with advanced stage and a poorer treatment outcome.

Hepatosplenic T-cell Lymphoma

The hepatosplenic T-cell lymphomas are aggressive extranodal cytotoxic T-cell neoplasms, usually of $\gamma\delta$ and less commonly $\alpha\beta$ TCR type.[40,226-231] The $\alpha\beta$ and $\gamma\delta$ subtypes are histologically, cytogenetically, and clinically similar, although children with $\alpha\beta$ hepatosplenic lymphomas tend to be younger that those with the γδ subtype.[230,232] These systemic lymphomas are relatively rare in children and in adults; a peak incidence is reported in adolescents and young adults.[40,227] These lymphomas occur more frequently in male than female patients, although the αβ subtype is more common in women.[229,230] Patients typically are first seen with significant hepatosplenomegaly, but no appreciable adenopathy. Evaluation of the peripheral smear often reveals anemia, thrombocytopenia, and circulating lymphoma cells, which may be difficult to distinguish from atypical lymphocytes. Disease progression may be associated with a more obvious leukemic phase.[229,230,233-236]

The tumor cells are typically medium-sized, with scant to moderate amounts of cytoplasm; azurophilic cytoplasmic granules have been infrequently reported. The nuclei may be either convoluted or round with dense chromatin and inconspicuous nucleoli. Mitotic figures are infrequently observed. Disease progression may be associated with a blast cell transformation, featuring cells with prominent nucleoli.[233,237,238] It may be difficult to identify lymphoma cells in bone marrow aspirate samples; however, examination of bone marrow biopsy samples frequently reveals a characteristic sinusoidal infiltrate.[230,231,238] Sinusoidal infiltrate by lymphoma cells also may be observed in the liver and spleen.[230,231] Erythrophagocytosis may be detected in splenic and bone marrow sinusoids.[230,231,239,240] The immunophenotype is usually CD2+, CD3+, CD4−, CD8+/−, CD5−, CD7+, CD16+, and CD56+/−, although variants have been reported.[40,229] The αβ subtype is similar to the γδ subtype, except for a slightly more frequent expression of CD57.[230] Flow cytometric analyses may detect TCR γδ or less commonly TCR αβ proteins.[226,231] Cytotoxic granular protein TIA-1 is detected in most cases whereas perforin or granzyme B is infrequently detected.[229,230,239,241,242]

In most cases, cytogenetic studies reveal an isochrome 7q, often with trisomy 8 and other random chromosomal abnormalities.[230,235,237,238,243-246] Studies of TCR β- and γ-chain gene rearrangements reveal reciprocal findings between αβ and γδ subtypes of hepatosplenic lymphomas and therefore cannot be used as a distinguishing feature between the two.[229,230] V delta 1 is used by the majority of γδ cytotoxic T cells in the sinuses of normal spleens. Because the majority of hepatosplenic lymphomas preferentially express V delta 1, splenic γδ cytotoxic T cells are thought to be the origin of γδ hepatosplenic lymphomas.[229,247] Although EBV has been detected in the lymphoma cells of some cases, a direct role in pathogenesis has not been demonstrated.[229,248]

Very Rare Pediatric Lymphomas

Lymphomas that occur infrequently in children and adolescents include panniculitis-like T-cell lymphoma,[249,250] mycosis fungoides,[251-258] NK lymphoma,[259-261] MALT lymphoma,[262] and human T-cell leukemia virus (HTLV-1)–associated leukemia/lymphoma.[263-265] The clinical and biologic features of these lymphomas in children are generally similar to those observed in adults; however, this conclusion is drawn from the very few reported pediatric cases.

CLINICAL PRESENTATION

The primary sites of involvement and the extent of disease spread determine the clinical features of NHL at presentation (see Fig. 102-1).[1-3] Although adults usually are first seen with nodal disease, children with NHL usually have extranodal disease, most frequently involving the abdomen (31% of cases), the mediastinum (26% of cases), or head and neck region (29% of cases).[3] These rapidly growing tumors are associated with hematogenous disease spread, and the majority of children with NHL have locally invasive or advanced-stage disease. Involvement of the CNS is characterized by the presence of cranial nerve palsies and/or cerebrospinal fluid (CSF) pleocytosis. When the bone marrow is involved, the distinction between NHL and leukemia is somewhat arbitrary: if more than 25% of the marrow is replaced by lymphoblasts, the patient is considered to have leukemia; if less than 25%, the patient is considered to have advanced-stage NHL with marrow involvement.

A striking relation exists between the histologic subtype and the presenting site of disease in the lymphoblastic and Burkitt's lymphomas.[3] Among the lymphoblastic lymphomas, the typical primary site of involvement is the mediastinum and/or head and neck region, but rarely the abdomen, whereas the Burkitt's lymphomas typically are present in the abdomen or head and neck region, but rarely the mediastinum. In contrast to patients with lymphoblastic and Burkitt's lymphomas, children with large cell lymphomas may have disease at almost any location. Involvement of the CNS at diagnosis is associated with both the Burkitt's and lymphoblastic histiotypes, but rarely with large cell histology.[134] In contrast, spread to the bone marrow may occur in any of these three histologic subtypes.[3,266,267]

Primary involvement of the abdomen, as is typical of Burkitt's lymphoma, may be associated with nausea, vomiting, or abdominal pain at presentation. These tumors usually arise from the distal ileum and result in obstruction of the bowel by either intussusception or direct compression of the lumen. Other primary sites of involvement in the abdomen include the appendix and/or large bowel. Abdominal tumors may be associated with malignant ascites; involvement of kidney, liver or lymph node; and invasion of adjacent structures, including the abdominal wall.[2,3] Involvement of the pelvis may include ureteral compression with associated hydronephrosis.

Primary involvement of the mediastinum, as is typical of advanced-stage lymphoblastic lymphoma, may be associated with respiratory symptoms ranging from mild cough to severe respiratory distress caused by direct tumor compression of the airway, requiring emergency attention (see Emergency Situations).[2,3] Associated pleural effusions may further complicate the respiratory status. Compression of the superior vena cava by the tumor may obstruct venous blood return, resulting in swelling of the neck, shoulder, and face (*superior vena cava syndrome*); this condition may predispose the patient to the development of deep venous thromboses. In rare cases, children with mediastinal masses may also have cardiac irregularities or tamponade.[2]

Involvement of the CNS may cause symptoms resulting from increased intracranial pressure, including nausea, vomiting, headache, and vision changes; neurologic abnormalities also may be found on physical examination, resulting from palsies of cranial nerves innervating the face or extraocular muscles. Involvement of the bone marrow may be associated with bone pain, pallor, neutropenia, and/or thrombocytopenia with associated bruising and bleeding. Involvement of the skin occurs in approximately 4% of children with newly diagnosed NHL. When present, it is usually associated with CD30[+] anaplastic large cell histology;[136,138,143] however, lymphoblastic lymphomas (often non–T-cell immunophenotype) also may involve the skin.[115,268]

DIAGNOSIS AND DIFFERENTIAL DIAGNOSIS

The differential diagnosis of NHL comprises both benign and malignant conditions. If no mediastinal mass is present, and if blood counts and physical examination are within normal limits except for an isolated painless enlarged peripheral lymph node, a 10- to 14-day trial of antibiotics is permissible to treat presumed bacterial adenitis.[269] Serologic and skin testing may be helpful in the diagnosis of histoplasmosis, tuberculosis, and EBV infection, which also may cause adenopathy simulating lymphoma.

The non-Hodgkin's lymphomas of childhood grow very rapidly; therefore an expeditious diagnostic workup in consultation with a pediatric oncologist is indicated if NHL is suspected. The diagnosis of NHL is most readily established by examination of tissue obtained by open biopsy of the involved site. A comprehensive characterization of the biologic features of the tissue, including histologic, immunophenotypic, cytogenetic, and molecular studies, will help to distinguish NHL from the small round blue cell tumors, including Ewing's sarcoma, neuroblastoma, and rhabdomyosarcoma. When patients (such as those with large anterior mediastinal masses and associated airway compression) are too unstable to undergo anesthesia for open biopsy, the diagnosis may be established by parasternal fine-needle aspiration or biopsy with local anesthesia.[270] Among children with an associated pleural effusion, thoracentesis with cytologic examination of pleural fluid is usually diagnostic. For children with large abdominal Burkitt's tumors, either percutaneous aspiration of the mass or paracentesis to obtain ascitic fluid often yields diagnostic cytologic and cytogenetic findings. A bone marrow and CSF examination should be performed early in the workup of a child with suspected NHL, because these studies may be diagnostic and may preclude the need for more-invasive procedures.

Initial Evaluation and Staging Workup

A prompt and meticulous staging workup is imperative, because treatment is determined in part by primary site

and degree of disease spread. A complete history and physical examination, including documentation of the presence or absence of B symptoms by history, should be completed. Computed tomographic (CT) imaging of the chest, abdomen, and pelvis, as well as bone scans should be performed on all patients. Gallium scanning also may be helpful in selected cases, particularly in following up residual masses that were gallium positive at diagnosis.[1-3] It has been suggested that thallium scanning may help to differentiate benign from malignant mediastinal disease[271]; however, further investigation of the use of this modality in children with NHL is needed. Positron emission tomography (PET) is commonly used in the evaluation of adults with Hodgkin's or NHL[272]; however, this modality is not part of the standard staging workup of children with NHL. Bilateral posterior iliac crest aspirations and biopsies increase the chance of identifying overt marrow involvement, thus reducing the possibility of underestimating the stage of disease.[273] The bone marrow samples should be submitted for cell count and differential, flow cytometric (if marrow overtly involved), cytogenetic, and molecular pathologic analyses. Magnetic resonance imaging (MRI) of the bone marrow has been shown to be effective in detecting occult disease is some studies[274]; however, it is not a standard component of the currently accepted pediatric NHL workup. A lumbar puncture should be performed for cytologic evaluation of the CSF.

The stage of disease is usually assigned according to the St. Jude Staging System described by Murphy (Table 102-5),[10] which was developed to accommodate the noncontiguous nature of disease spread, predominant extranodal involvement, and involvement of the bone marrow and CNS that characterize the pediatric NHLs.

TABLE 102-5

Stages of Non-Hodgkin's Lymphoma

Stage I

A single tumor (extranodal) or involvement of a single anatomic area (nodal), with the exclusion of the mediastinum and abdomen

Stage II

A single tumor (extranodal) with regional node involvement
Two or more nodal areas on the same side of the diaphragm
Two single (extranodal) tumors, with or without regional node involvement on the same side of the diaphragm
A primary gastrointestinal tract tumor (usually in the ileocecal area), with or without involvement of associated mesenteric nodes, that is completely resectable

Stage III

Two single tumors (extranodal) on opposite sides of the diaphragm
Two or more nodal areas above and below the diaphragm
Any primary intrathoracic tumor (mediastinal, pleural, or thymic)
Extensive primary intra-abdominal disease
Any paraspinal or epidural tumor, whether or not other sites are involved

Stage IV

Any of the above findings with initial involvement of the central nervous system, bone marrow, or both

Based on the classification proposed by Murphy.

DIAGNOSTIC WORK-UP, STAGING WORK-UP AND TREATMENT FOR PEDIATRIC NHL

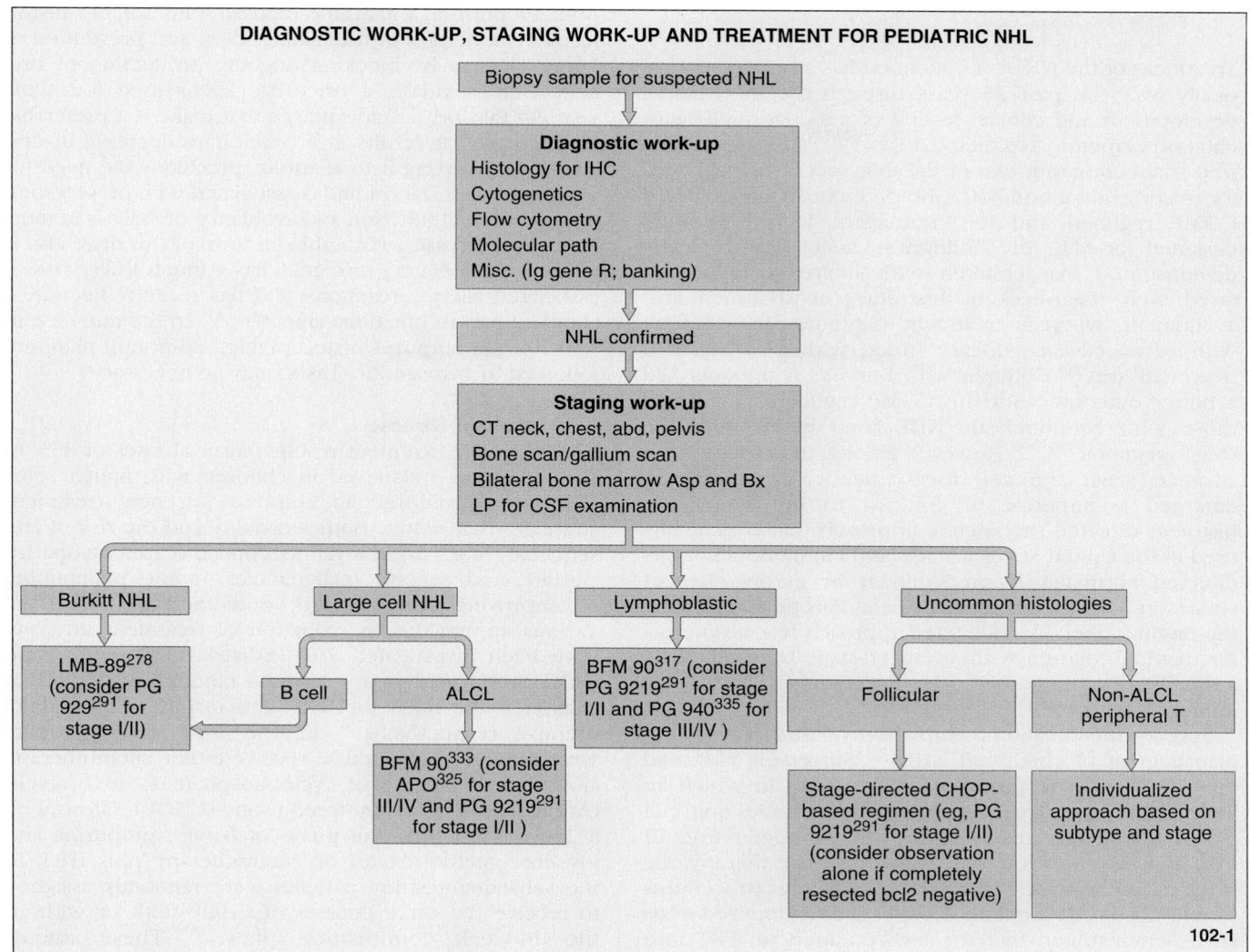

102-1

Stages I and II are considered to be limited-stage disease, whereas stages III and IV are advanced-stage disease. The initial laboratory evaluation should include a complete blood count with differential and a chemistry panel comprising electrolytes, blood urea nitrogen (BUN), creatinine, LDH, calcium, phosphorus, and uric acid. An HIV screen should be performed on all patients newly diagnosed with lymphoma. Those who test positive may be at increased risk for therapy-related toxicity, including life-threatening infections. Serologic tests for EBV infection may be helpful when lymphoproliferative disease is highly suspected in the differential diagnosis; however, positive serologic results do not rule out a malignancy.

Prognostic Factors

Tumor burden at diagnosis, reflected by both the disease stage and serum LDH, is an important predictor of outcome for children.[3] In one large single-institution study

of childhood NHL, the treatment era, disease stage, and serum LDH level all emerged as independent and significant prognostic indicators.[3] Serum interleukin-2 (IL-2) receptor levels, which reflect tumor burden, also have been shown to predict outcome.[275,276]

A poor early response to therapy is considered by some to confer a poorer prognosis, as has been demonstrated in children with ALL.[277] In the LMB-89 protocol, poor early response is a criterion for placement in the most intensive arm of therapy.[278] The current COG study for children with advanced-stage lymphoblastic lymphoma is examining the impact of early response as determined by both diagnostic imaging and flow cytometric MRD technology.

Prognostic factors also have been identified with respect to specific histologic subtypes. For example, among adults with ALCL, ALK protein expression is a favorable prognostic factor.[279-281] In a multivariate analysis of clinical features in childhood ALCL, mediastinal, visceral (lung, liver, spleen), and skin involvement were associated with adverse risk.[282,283]

Primary Treatment

Treatment of the NHLs of childhood has advanced dramatically over the past 25 years through the incremental development and clinical testing of effective multiagent chemotherapeutic regimens.[1-3,134,278,284-335] In a randomized trial comparing two of the first successful regimens for treating childhood NHL (the cyclophosphamide-based COMP regimen and the multiagent LSA_2L_2 regimen designed for ALL), the Children's Cancer Group clearly demonstrated that children with limited-stage disease fared well regardless of histology or treatment-arm assignment, whereas treatment outcomes for children with advanced-stage disease varied with histology and treatment arm.[284] Children with Burkitt's lymphoma had a better outcome with the COMP regimen,[284] whereas those with lymphoblastic NHL fared better with the LSA_2L_2 regimen.[284-286] However, among those who with advanced-stage large cell disease, neither treatment arm emerged as superior. In contrast to the stage- and histology-directed therapeutic approach that is generally used in the United States, a stage- and immunophenotype-directed approach is predominant in Europe. Recent studies in both the United States and Europe suggest that the immunophenotype-directed approach has advantages for treating children with advanced-stage large-cell NHL, a family of lymphomas whose prognoses vary with immunophenotype.[135]

Surgery and radiation therapy have minimal roles in the management of childhood NHLs.[2,3] Surgery is indicated only for diagnostic purposes and in cases in which an ileocecal mass, associated with mesenteric nodes only, can be completely resected (resulting in downstaging from III to II, which requires less intensive systemic therapy; see Staging). Otherwise, aggressive debulking procedures should not be undertaken. Prospective randomized trials have demonstrated that the incorporation of IFRT into a multiagent chemotherapy regimen does not improve outcome.[291,332] The use of radiation therapy in the management of relapse, CNS disease, and certain emergency situations is discussed in other sections.

Initial Management

The serum chemistry values should be reviewed before chemotherapy is started. Many patients with bulky Burkitt's or lymphoblastic lymphomas are first seen with hyperuricemia, hyperphosphatemia, and renal dysfunction due to the rapid turnover of lymphoblasts. These metabolic abnormalities are exacerbated by chemotherapy, which rapidly lyses tumor cells. Tumor lysis releases purines, potassium, and phosphorus into the bloodstream, resulting in the deposition of uric acid, xanthines, and phosphates in the renal tubules, which causes further renal dysfunction—a clinical condition termed *tumor lysis syndrome*.[2] This problem can be precluded or reduced if patients with advanced-stage disease are vigorously hydrated (3 to 4 L/m^2/day) before receiving chemotherapy. Alkalinization is usually necessary to maintain a urine pH of approximately 7.0. The urinary excretion of uric acid is reduced at an acidic pH, whereas the excretion of phosphorus is impaired by overalkaliniza-

tion. Allopurinol, a xanthine oxidase inhibitor, has historically been helpful in the management and prevention of hyperuricemia by blocking ongoing production of uric acid. Urate oxidase, a uricolytic agent used for many years in Europe, has advantages that make it a preferable alternative.[336] It results in a precipitate decrease in uric acid by converting it to allantoin, precludes the need for vigorous alkalinization, and is associated with preservation of normal renal function and avoidance of dialysis in most cases. Rasburicase, a recombinant form of this drug, also is effective in reducing uric acid, has a much lower risk of associated allergic reactions, and has recently become a standard part of initial management.[337] In the rare case in which urine output is unacceptable, addition of mannitol followed by furosemide (Lasix) may be necessary.

Limited-stage Disease

The excellent treatment results (survival rates of 85% to 95% at 5 years) achieved in children with limited-stage NHL have prompted an emphasis on new treatment strategies that reduce both morbidity and the risk of late sequelae (e.g., anthracycline-induced cardiomyopathy, sterility, and second malignancies) while maintaining or improving the treatment outcome.[278,290,291,309,312,313] Various approaches to reduction of treatment intensity have been investigated. The Pediatric Oncology Group (POG) performed two sequential randomized trials that examined the need for IFRT and maintenance chemotherapy, respectively.[291] In the first study, patients were randomly assigned to receive either chemotherapy alone [three courses of cyclophosphamide/doxorubicin (Adriamycin)/vincristine/prednisone (CHOP) followed by a 24-week continuation phase of 6-mercaptopurine and low-dose methotrexate] or chemotherapy plus IFRT. In the subsequent study, patients were randomly assigned to receive the three courses of CHOP with or without the 24-week continuation phase.[291] These studies demonstrated that both IFRT and the continuation phase of therapy could be safely eliminated without compromising outcome, with one exception. Children with limited-stage lymphoblastic lymphoma had lower event-free survival rates than did those with nonlymphoblastic histology. Even with the 24-week continuation phase, one third of the patients with lymphoblastic lymphoma developed recurrent disease. With salvage therapy, no difference was reported in overall survival between those with lymphoblastic and nonlymphoblastic histology. The optimal management of limited-stage lymphoblastic lymphoma remains controversial. The French Society of Pediatric Oncology (SFOP) uses a more aggressive initial approach to avoid the need for retreatment.[308] Children with limited-stage lymphoblastic lymphoma are entered on the same protocol used for advanced-stage lymphoblastic lymphoma, and children with limited-stage nonlymphoblastic lymphoma are candidates for less-intensive regimens only if complete resection of disease occurs.[278]

Advanced-stage Disease

Historically, attempts to improve the treatment result in children with advanced-stage NHL have relied on further intensification of therapy. The general approach in the

United States has been histology directed, whereas in Europe, an immunophenotype-directed approach has predominated. For example, French investigators enter patients with Burkitt's lymphoma and B-cell large cell lymphoma on the same protocol.[278,318] In this regard, some centers in the United States are now incorporating immunophenotype into their treatment planning.

Burkitt's Lymphoma. The dramatic improvements achieved in the treatment of advanced-stage Burkitt's lymphoma and B-cell ALL represent one of pediatric oncology's undisputed success stories. With current therapy, which is generally cyclophosphamide based, very intensive, and given over a relatively short period (4 to 8 months); at least 75% of patients are event-free survivors. Results achieved with the COMP regimen were first improved on by the incorporation of high-dose methotrexate and/or high-dose cytarabine.[289,292–294,296] Two studies during the same period showed that the duration of therapy could be shortened to 2 to 4 months without compromising patient outcome.[294,300] Further improvements in treatment outcome have been achieved over the past 8-year period by further intensification of therapy (escalation of cyclophosphamide, methotrexate, and cytarabine dosages) and by the addition of new active agents including etoposide and ifosfamide.[278,313,316] The LMB-89 regimen designed by the SFOP, for example, has produced one of the best results to date (Fig. 102-2).[278] In this protocol, children receive high-dose methotrexate (3 g/m²), fractionated cyclophosphamide, doxorubicin (Adriamycin), vincristine, prednisone, and low-dose cytarabine given over a period of approximately 5 months if marrow blast cells at diagnosis are less than 70%. For children with more than 70% marrow blast cells or with CNS involvement at diagnosis, therapy is intensified

(methotrexate dose is escalated to 8 g/m², high-dose cytarabine and etoposide are incorporated, and the total duration of therapy is extended to approximately 8 months).

Other equally successful treatment strategies for advanced-stage Burkitt's lymphoma and B-cell ALL have been reported (Table 102-6). Excellent results have been achieved by the BFM (Berlin-Frankfurt-Munster) cooperative group by using a regimen that incorporates high-dose methotrexate (5 g/m²), ifosfamide, etoposide, doxorubicin, and steroids.[313] Sequential NCI studies have shown that adding etoposide, high-dose cytarabine, and ifosfamide to a regimen of cyclophosphamide, doxorubicin, vincristine, and high-dose methotrexate improved the treatment result.[316] Importantly, these more aggressive approaches have shown encouraging preliminary results in adults with the same malignancies.[315,321]

Lymphoblastic Lymphoma. Most of the successful treatment plans for children with advanced-stage lymphoblastic lymphoma are derived from therapies designed to treat children with high-risk ALL (Table 102-7). These regimens, which generally use multiple chemotherapy agents (up to 10 different agents) and are given over a 15- to 32-month period, result in an approximate 65% to 90% event-free survival rate at 4 to 5 years.[284–286,302,303,308,311,317] Although the multiagent nature of these regimens makes it difficult to determine the relative merit of individual components, compelling data suggest the importance of high-dose methotrexate. The French (SFOP) achieved an excellent result by incorporating courses of high-dose methotrexate into the previously studied LSA₂L₂ regimen.[308] Moreover, the BFM group recently reported very encouraging results (3-year event-free survival of ~90%) of a regimen that features an intensive high-dose

Figure 102-2. Treatment schema for LMB-89 for Burkitt's lymphoma and B-acute lymphoblastic leukemia. (From Patte C, Auperin A, Michon J: The Société Française d'Oncologie Pédiatrique LMB89 protocol: Highly effective multiagent chemotherapy tailored to the tumor burden and initial response in 561 unselected children with B-cell lymphomas and L3 leukemia. Blood 2001;97:3370–3379.)

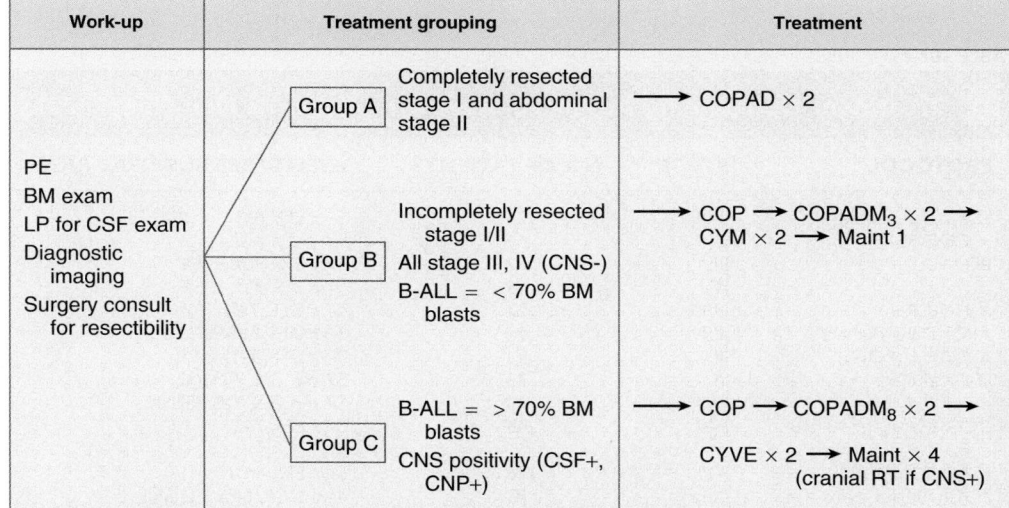

Work-up	Treatment grouping		Treatment
PE BM exam LP for CSF exam Diagnostic imaging Surgery consult for resectibility	Group A	Completely resected stage I and abdominal stage II	⟶ COPAD × 2
	Group B	Incompletely resected stage I/II All stage III, IV (CNS−) B-ALL = < 70% BM blasts	⟶ COP ⟶ COPADM₃ × 2 ⟶ CYM × 2 ⟶ Maint 1
	Group C	B-ALL = > 70% BM blasts CNS positivity (CSF+, CNP+)	⟶ COP ⟶ COPADM₈ × 2 ⟶ CYVE × 2 ⟶ Maint × 4 (cranial RT if CNS+)

Abbreviations: PE: physical examination; BM: bone marrow; LPL: lumbar puncture; RT: radiation therapy; CNS: central nervous system; CSF: cerebrospinal fluid; CNP: cranial nerve palsy; COP: cylophosphamide, vincristine, prednisone; COPADM₃: cyclophosphamide, vincristine, prednisone doxorubicin, methotrexate (3 grams vs. 8 grams); CYM: cytarabine, methotrexate; CYVE: cytarabine, etoposide; Maint: maintenance courses.

TABLE 102-6

Treatment Outcome for Advanced-Stage Burkitt's Lymphoma

PROTOCOL	STAGE	NO. OF PATIENTS	EVENT-FREE SURVIVAL RATE	REFERENCE
POG 8617	IV	34	4-yr EFS, 79 ± 9%	293
	B-ALL	47	4-yr EFS, 65 ± 8%	
LMB 89*	III	278	5-yr EFS, 91% (95%CI, 87–94%)	278
	IV	62	5-yr EFS, 87% (95%CI, 77–93%)	
	B-ALL	102	5-yr EFS, 87% (95%CI, 79–92%)	
BFM 90	III	169	6-yr EFS, 86% ± 3%	313
	IV	24	6-yr EFS, 73% ± 10%	
	B-ALL	56	6-yr EFS, 74% ± 6%	
CCG*				
Orange	III/IV/B-ALL	43	12-mo EFS, 83%	298
vs.				
LMB 86	III/IV/B-ALL	42	12-mo EFS, 84%	

*Includes patients with B-cell large-cell NHL.

methotrexate (5 g/m^2) consolidation course (Fig. 102-3).[317] Although definitive data are lacking, this result may reflect the higher levels of intracellular methotrexate polyglutamates produced in T-cell lymphoblasts by high-dose methotrexate as compared with low-dose methotrexate.[330] Preliminary data from a recent POG study suggested that high-dose methotrexate may not be needed for advanced-stage lymphoblastic lymphoma in the context of an anthracycline and L-asparaginase–rich backbone.[335] A current COG study is examining whether high-dose methotrexate can be safely eliminated if replaced by extended intrathecal therapy. L-Asparaginase also is commonly used in many successful regimens. In this regard, a POG study demonstrated a survival advantage to those randomized to receive additional L-asparaginase.[326] Efforts to improve the treatment result also included the addition of new active agents (e.g., epipodophyllotoxins)[302] and the incorporation of a reinduction[307] or late intensification phase.

Large Cell Lymphoma. The biologic heterogeneity of advanced-stage large-cell lymphoma has made it difficult to identify an optimal treatment approach (Table 102-8).[134] Histology-directed therapies in the United States, primarily CHOP based, have resulted in a 50% to 70% event-free survival rate at 3 years.[134,135,284,297,304-306] Although some studies have examined the feasibility of eliminating agents associated with significant late effects,[297,325] most current studies are examining the benefit of incorporating additional active agents (e.g., intermediate- and high-dose methotrexate, intermediate- and high-dose cytarabine, ifosfamide, and carboplatin). POG investigators reported that children with large-cell lymphoma of the B-cell immunophenotype had a better outcome than did those with a non–B-cell immunophenotype, a finding that suggested that immunophenotype-directed therapies for pediatric large-cell lymphomas should be further pursued.[135] In this regard, European trials for children with large-cell lymphoma have historically assigned

TABLE 102-7

Treatment Outcome for Advanced-Stage Lymphoblastic Non-Hodgkin's Lymphoma

PROTOCOL	STAGE	NO. OF PATIENTS	EVENT-FREE SURVIVAL RATE	REFERENCE
LSA$_2$L$_2$ (modified) CCG-551	III/IV	124	5-yr EFS, 64%	284
BFM 90	III	82	5-yr EFS, 90% ± 3%	317
	IV	19	5-yr EFS, 95% ± 5%	
X-H SJCRH	III/IV	22	4-yr DFS, 73%	302
APO (Dana Farber)	III/IV	21	3-yr DFS, 58% ± 23%	334
A-COP + (POG)	III	33	3-yr DFS, 54% ± 9%	303
SFOP LMT81	III	33	57-mo EFS, 79% (SE, 4%)	308
	IV/ALL	43	57-mo EFS, 72% (SE, 4%)	
CCG: LSA$_2$L$_2$ (modified)	I–IV	243	5-yr EFS, 74%	311
vs.				
ADCOMP	I–IV	138	5-yr EFS, 64%	
POG8704: no extra Asp	III/IV	83	4-yr CCR, 64% (SE, 6%)	326
vs.				
Extra Asp	III/IV	84	4-yr CCR, 78% (SE, 5%)	

CCR, complete continuous remission; DFS, disease-free survival.

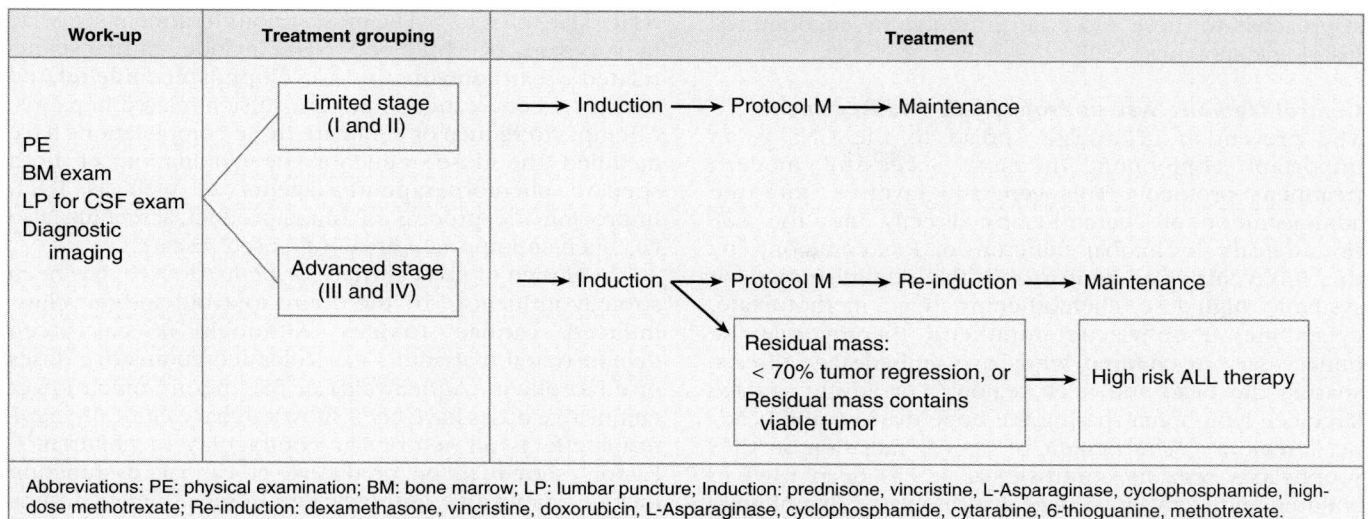

Work-up	Treatment grouping	Treatment

Figure 102-3. Treatment schema for BFM-90 for lymphoblastic lymphoma. (From Reiter A, Schrappe M, Ludwig W-D, et al: Intensive ALL-type therapy without local radiotherapy provides a 90% event-free survival for children with T-cell lymphoblastic lymphoma: A BFM group report. Blood 2000;95:416–421.)

treatment on the basis of immunophenotype (e.g., B-cell, T-cell, CD30⁺). For example, the SFOP reported equally excellent outcomes for children with either B-cell, large cell, or Burkitt's lymphoma who were treated with the same B-cell regimen (i.e., LMB-89).[278,318] Children with MLBCLs may have a slightly worse outcome compared with those with diffuse large B-cell lymphoma (DLBCL).[200,202]

The vast majority of large cell lymphomas of T lineage in children are the CD30⁺ ALCLs. The optimal approach to the treatment of children with CD30⁺ ALCL has yet to be determined.[323] In the United States, children with CD30⁺ and CD30⁻ large cell lymphoma have historically received the same therapy, whereas in the German cooperative (BFM), children with CD30⁺ ALCL are treated with a B-cell lymphoma strategy (e.g., Burkitt's lymphoma), with excellent treatment results (3-year event-free survival of ~80%).[307,333] The SFOP examined regimens designed specifically for those with CD30⁺ large cell lymphomas.[156] Further study is required to determine the optimal therapy for CD30⁺ cases. The SFOP identified vinblastine

as very active when used as a single agent in children with recurrent ALCL, even if the children were heavily pretreated.[329] Currently, a multinational European trial is examining the benefit of adding vinblastine to the very successful BFM B-cell approach, and the COG is examining the benefit of adding vinblastine to the APO regimen.[304,325]

Rare Histologies. The therapeutic approaches to the treatment of children with unusual histologic subtypes are often derived from strategies used in adults. Children with localized follicular lymphoma have been successfully treated with CHOP-based limited-stage therapeutic approaches; however, children have remained disease free after complete resection without adjuvant chemotherapy.[219-221] Children with hepatosplenic lymphomas have an aggressive disease course, and often have recurrent disease even after an initial good response to aggressive therapy.[226,229,230,246,251] Clearly a need exists for organized national trials to improve our treatment

TABLE 102-8

Treatment Outcome for Advanced-Stage Large-Cell Non-Hodgkin's Lymphoma

PROTOCOL	STAGE	NO. OF PATIENTS	EVENT-FREE SURVIVAL RATE	REFERENCE
CHOP	III & IV	21	3-yr EFS, 62% ± 11%	287
MACOP-B	III & IV	11	3-yr EFS, 55% ± 16%	306
COMP	III & IV	42	5-yr EFS, 52%	284
vs.				
LSA₂L₂	III & IV	18	5-yr EFS, 43%	
APO	III & IV	62	3-yr EFS, 72% ± 6%	325
vs.				
ACOP+	III & IV	58	4-yr EFS, 62% ± 7%	

ACOP, Adriamycin, cyclophosphamide, vincristine, prednisone; APO, Adriamycin (doxorubicin), prednisone, vincristine; CHOP, cyclophosphamide, hydroxydaunomycin, Oncorin, prednisone; COMP, cyclophosphamide, vincristine, methotrexate, prednisone.

approaches to these and other infrequently encountered histologic subtypes.

Central Nervous System Prophylaxis and Treatment

The prevention of disease spread to the CNS is an important component of most successful modern treatment protocols. This generally involves both the administration of chemotherapy directly into the CSF (intrathecally by lumbar puncture or less commonly by the intraventricular route) and the administration of systemic high-dose chemotherapy (e.g., methotrexate, cytarabine). Prophylactic intrathecal therapy may be unnecessary in children who have limited-stage disease sparing the head and neck region[291] or advanced-stage large cell lymphoma sparing the bone marrow and head/neck region.[134] The benefit of cranial radiation as CNS prophylaxis remains controversial. It has been used in children with advanced-stage lymphoblastic lymphoma, but is not widely favored.[317]

Among children first seen with overt CNS disease (cranial nerve palsies or CSF pleocytosis), intensification of both systemic and intrathecal chemotherapy is usually indicated; with the exception of Burkitt's lymphoma, cranial radiation also is usually incorporated.

Emergency Situations

Various emergencies may arise in the management of children with NHL.[2] First, children with large anterior mediastinal masses associated with severe respiratory distress require immediate attention. If significant airway compression is noted, deep sedation should be avoided. Chemotherapy should be started as soon as possible if the diagnostic samples have been obtained. If they have not, local radiation therapy may be the best approach, because it spares more-peripheral disease for subsequent biopsy and study. Steroids may be necessary in some cases, but this therapy may alter tumor histologic characteristics and preclude an accurate tissue diagnosis.

In some children with bulky Burkitt's or lymphoblastic tumors, renal failure develops secondary to tumor-lysis syndrome, despite appropriate prechemotherapy management. A nephrologist should be consulted immediately when renal dysfunction is first noted, so that dialysis can be considered. This situation may be further complicated when a large pelvic mass creates direct ureteral compression. The placement of ureteral stents or a percutaneous nephrostomy tube may help temporarily; however, the problem is most effectively dealt with by delivering appropriate chemotherapy.

A small percentage of children may have epidural tumors causing cord compression and corresponding neurologic deficits. Delivery of appropriate chemotherapy is usually all that is required; however, if no prompt recovery of neurologic function occurs, a radiation therapist should be consulted about the possible need for low-dose local irradiation.[2]

Treatment Complications

As the survival of children with malignant lymphomas has improved, increased attention has focused on treatment-related late effects.[338] The most serious treatment sequelae in survivors of childhood NHL include anthracycline-related cardiomyopathy, cyclophosphamide-related sterility, second cancers, and transfusion-related hepatitis. Attempts to reduce or eliminate these complications have included the dose reduction or elimination of both specific chemotherapeutic agents as well as IFRT. Improving the process of blood-product screening also has been an important area of focused research.

The design of clinical trials for pediatric NHL has been strongly influenced by the desire to avoid anthracycline-induced cardiac toxicity. Although it has been demonstrated that adults may tolerated cumulative doses of doxorubicin (Adriamycin) of 550 mg/m^2, much lower cumulative doses have been shown to have clinically significant effects on ventricular contractility in children.[339] Factors shown to be predictive of cardiac dysfunction include cumulative anthracycline dosage, higher anthracycline dose intensity, younger age at the time of treatment, female sex, time interval since completion of therapy, and combined-modality therapy that includes mediastinal irradiation.[340,341] Future trials that focus on the reduction of cumulative anthracycline dosage and the utility of cardioprotectant agents are indicated.[297]

The preservation of fertility is another important concern in the development of optimal therapeutic strategies for children with NHL. A dose-related depletion of germinal cells is associated with the use of alkylating agents such as cyclophosphamide and ifosfamide; these agents tend to be more gonadotoxic in boys. Studies thus far have suggested that sterility is likely at cumulative doses of cyclophosphamide greater than 7.5 g/m^2, whereas fertility is usually maintained at cumulative dosages less than 4 g/m^2.[342] In this regard, a number of pediatric NHL trials have attempted to eliminate or reduce the dosage of cyclophosphamide.[325]

Pediatric NHL trials also focused on the elimination of involved field irradiation. In the first of two POG trials for limited-stage NHL, it was demonstrated that IFRT could be safely eliminated without compromising outcome.[291] A similar observation was made for children with advanced-stage disease in a St. Jude study.[332] Although IFRT is not used in most current NHL trials, cranial irradiation is considered in the management of overt CNS involvement in children with lymphoblastic lymphoma (its use for CNS prophylaxis in children with this histologic subtype is controversial).

Follow-up

Management of Primary Treatment Failure

Children with refractory or recurrent disease, particularly after receiving modern intensive therapy, are generally considered to have a poor prognosis. Thus aggressive or novel approaches are often used to treat relapse. Current approaches generally comprise multiagent salvage chemotherapy followed by an intensification phase that may include autologous or allogeneic hematopoietic stem cell transplantation (HSCT). Multiagent salvage regimens that have been studied include DHAP[306] (dexamethasone, high-dose cytarabine, and platinum), which has been shown to be active in childhood and adult recurrent large cell lymphoma, and VIPA[343] (etoposide, ifosfamide, and high-dose cytarabine), which has been shown to be active in children with relapsed Burkitt's lymphoma. Other active salvage regimens for children with refractory or recurrent malignant lymphoma include ICE[344] (ifosfamide, carboplatin, and etoposide) and MIED (high-dose methotrexate, ifosfamide, etoposide, and dexamethasone). Children who are found to have chemosensitive recurrent disease are usually considered for an intensification phase of chemotherapy followed by an HSCT. In a recent report, however, the benefit of HSCT in this setting was questioned.[331]

Although published data on the use of HSCT in children with recurrent or refractory NHL are limited compared with those reported for adults, reported studies support its use.[313,345-354] For example, European cooperative group trials demonstrated that some children with Burkitt's lymphoma who had a poor early response to therapy could be successfully salvaged with high-dose chemotherapy followed by an autologous HSCT.[313,347,349,350,352] Moreover, the Spanish Working Party for Bone Marrow Transplantation reported a 58% event-free survival rate after HSCT in children with either recurrent/refractory NHL or high-risk NHL in first CR.[349] The SFOP reported that 8 of 24 children with NHL for whom initial therapy failed were long-term disease-free survivors after HSCT.[350] In a review of 22 children at the St. Jude Children's Research Hospital, approximately 45% were survivors after intensive chemotherapy and HSCT.[354] It is difficult to make direct comparisons between the published studies of HSCT in children because they vary with respect to type of HSCT (autologous vs. allogeneic), preparative regimen, numbers of patients, and histologic subtypes studied.

It appears, however, that histologic subtype should be considered in determining the type of HSCT (autologous vs. allogeneic) for children with refractory or recurrent NHL. Among children with Burkitt's lymphoma, an autologous approach has been shown to be beneficial for those with a poor early response.[313,345,350] For those with disseminated recurrent Burkitt's lymphoma involving the marrow, many would favor an allogeneic approach if a suitable donor can be identified. An autologous HSCT has been shown to be effective strategy for some children with recurrent large cell lymphoma[348,354]; however, for children with recurrent lymphoblastic lymphoma, the results are less encouraging.[331]

Various preparative regimens have been successfully used in the salvage of children with refractory or recurrent NHL.[313,345-354] Two of the earliest reported regimens are BACT (carmustine, cytarabine, cyclophosphamide, and thioguanine) and BEAM (carmustine, etoposide, cytarabine, and melphalan).[345,346,353] High-dose busulfan was reported as an important component of a successful SFOP preparative regimen.[350] Gordon and colleagues[348] reported the successful salvage of children with recurrent peripheral T-cell lymphoma by using a preparative regimen that featured thiotepa; however, it was associated with significant mucositis.

Currently most would consider an autologous HSCT for children with chemosensitive recurrent large cell

lymphoma and in those with Burkitt's lymphoma who have a poor early response. If a suitable donor is available, an allogenic HSCT approach would be considered for children with widely disseminated recurrent lymphoblastic lymphoma or Burkitt's lymphoma involving the bone marrow. Nevertheless, it is clear that additional prospective clinical trials must evaluate the optimal preparative regimen and HSCT approach for children with recurrent or refractory NHL. In this regard, the European Lymphoma Bone Marrow Transplantation Registry has suggested that the potential graft versus lymphoma effect of allogeneic HSCT be studied.[352]

After Completion of Therapy Clinic

It is important that all children who have completed therapy for NHL be followed up annually in an "after-completion-of-therapy" or late-effects clinic.[355,356] The purposes of these visits are both to screen for therapy-related late effects (see section on complications of therapy) and to provide education and counseling about the medical and psychosocial issues that affect cancer survivors. These clinics also provide an opportunity for children and young adults to participate in important research initiatives that focus on cancer prevention and control, psychosocial problems, and treatment-related sequelae.

FUTURE DIRECTIONS

Despite dramatic improvements in the treatment of childhood NHL, approximately 20% to 30% of patients either do not achieve a complete remission or have recurrent disease.[1-3] Treatment-related late effects that place cancer survivors at risk are of additional concern.[338] Therefore the development of more effective and less toxic therapy remains an ongoing challenge. The identification of clinical and biologic features that are predictive of treatment failure may help in the refinement of a risk-adapted treatment approach to children with NHL.

Improvement in treatment outcome may be achieved by the incorporation of new active agents or the development of novel schedules for the delivery of currently used agents. Novel therapeutic approaches include the incorporation of immunotherapeutic approaches into multiagent chemotherapeutic regimens. In this regard, trials currently being designed for children with CD20[+] B-cell lymphomas incorporate the anti-CD20 antibody, rituximab, an agent that has already been shown to be valuable in the treatment of some adults with CD20[+] B-cell lymphomas.[357,358] A radiolabeled form of this antibody also is being studied in children with recurrent disease.[359] Clinical trials for patients with CD30[+] ALCL and Hodgkin's lymphoma also have been designed to examine the safety and efficacy of a newly developed anti-CD30 antibody.[360] Novel immunotherapeutic strategies also may be used in the processing of bone marrow samples before transplantation. For example, immunotoxins directed against T-lineage antigens (CD5 and CD7) in combination with 4-hydroperoxycyclophosphamide have been used to purge autologous marrow in children with T-cell leukemia.[361] Other potential therapies include the use of protein-specific cytotoxic T lymphocytes, a strategy that has been successful in preventing and treating EBV-related post-transplantation lymphoproliferative disease.[362] Novel approaches also may include the incorporation of small-molecule inhibitors, as well as antisense and anti-idiotype strategies.[363,364]

Molecular characterization of the chromosomal abnormalities associated with the NHLs of childhood is providing us with tools that enhance diagnosis, disease classification, and monitoring of the response to therapy [detection of minimal residual disease (MRD)]. A clearer understanding of molecular pathogenesis may provide insights that permit the development of therapeutic strategies that target tumor-specific molecular lesions.

REFERENCES

1. Sandlund JT, Downing JR, Crist WM: Non-Hodgkin's lymphoma in childhood. N Engl J Med 1996;334:1238–1248.
2. Magrath IT: Malignant non-Hodgkin's lymphomas in children. In: Pizzo PA, Poplack DG, (eds): Principles and Practice of Pediatric Oncology. 2nd ed. Philadelphia, JB Lippincott, 1993, 537–575.
3. Murphy S, Fairclough DL, Hutchison RE, Berard CW: Non-Hodgkin's lymphomas of childhood: An analysis of the histology, staging, and response to treatment of 338 cases at a single institution. J Clin Oncol 1989;7:186–193.
4. Robison LL: General principles of the epidemiology of childhood cancer. In Pizzo PA, Poplack DG, (ed): Principles and Practice of Pediatric Oncology. 2nd ed. Philadelphia, JB Lippincott, 1993, pp 3–10.
5. Young JL Jr, Ries LG, Silverberg E, Horm JW, Miller RW: Cancer incidence, survival and mortality for children younger than age 15 years. Cancer 1986;58:598–602.
6. Bleyer WA: The impact of childhood cancer on the United States and the world. CA Cancer J Clin 1990;40:355–366.
7. Parker SL, Tong T, Bolden S, Wingo PA: Cancer Statistics, 1996. CA-A Cancer J Clin 1996;65:5–27.
8. Ries LAG, Miller BA, Hankey BF, Kosary CL, Harras A, Edwards BK: SEER Cancer Statistics Review, 1973–1991. Bethesda, MD, NIH, 1994.
9. National Cancer Institute: Sponsored study of classifications of non-Hodgkin's lymphoma: Summary and description of a working formulation for clinical usage. Cancer 1982;49:2112–2135.
10. Murphy SB: Classification, staging and end results of treatment of childhood non-Hodgkin's lymphomas: Dissimilarities from lymphoma in adults. Semin Oncol 1980;7:332–339.
11. Hudson MM, Donaldson S: Hodgkin's disease. Pediatr Oncol Pediatr Clin North Am 1997;44:891.
12. Grufferman SL, Delzell E: Epidemiology of Hodgkin's disease. Epidemiol Rev 1984;6:76.
13. Lukes RJ, Butler JJ: The pathology and nomenclature of Hodgkin's disease. Cancer Res 1966;26:1063.
14. Donaldson SS, Link MP: Childhood lymphomas: Hodgkin's disease and non-Hodgkin's lymphoma. In Moosa AR, Robson MC, Schimpff SC (eds): Comprehensive Textbook of Oncology. Baltimore, Williams & Wilkins, 1986, p 1161.
15. Link MP, Hudson M, Donaldson S, et al: Treatment of children with unfavorable and advanced stage Hodgkin's disease with vinblastine, etoposide, prednisone and Adriamycin (VEPA) and low-dose, involved field irradiation. Proc Am Soc Clin Oncol 1994;13:3920.
16. Schellong G, Branswig JH, Hornig-Franz I: Treatment of children with Hodgkin's disease: Results of the German Pediatric Oncology Group. Ann Oncol 1992;3:73.
17. Hudson MM, Lee J, Luo X, et al: Increased mortality after successful treatment of Hodgkin's disease. J Clin Oncol 1998;16:3592–3600.
18. Hudson MM, Donaldson SS: Hodgkin's disease. In Pizzo PA, Poplack DG (eds): Principles and Practice of Pediatric Oncology. 4th ed. Philadelphia, Lippincott Williams & Wilkins, 2002, pp 637–660.
19. Hutchison RE, et al: Non-Hodgkin's lymphoma in children younger than three years. Cancer 1988;62:1371.
20. Taylor AMR, Metcalfe JA, Thick J, Mak Y-F: Leukemia and lymphoma in ataxia telangiectasia. Blood 1996;87:423–438.
21. Ellaurie M. Lymphoma in pediatric HIV infection. Pediatr Res 1989;25:884a.
22. Murphy SB, Jenson HB, McClain KL, Leach TC, Joshi VV, Pollack BH: AIDS related tumors. Med Pediatr Oncol 1997;29:381.
23. McClain KL, Joshi VV, Murphy SB: Cancers in children with HIV infection. Hematol Oncol Clin North Am 1996;10:1189.
24. Pluda JM, Yarchoan R, Jaffe ES, et al: Development of non-Hodgkin lymphoma in a cohort of patients with severe human immunodeficiency virus (HIV) infection on long-term antiretroviral therapy. Ann Intern Med 1990;113:276.
25. Filipovich AH, Heinitz KJ, Robison LL, Frizzera G: The immunodeficiency cancer registry: A research resource. Am J Pediatr Hematol Oncol 1987;9:183–184.
26. Gatti RA, Good RA: Occurrence of malignancy in immunodeficiency disease: A literature review. Cancer 1971;28:89–98.
27. Parekh S, Ratech H, Sparano JA: Human immunodeficiency virus-associated lymphoma. Clin Adv Hematol Oncol 2003;1:295–301.
28. Levine AM, Seneviratne L, Espina BM, et al: Evolving characteristics of AIDS-related lymphoma. Blood 2000;96:4084–4090.
29. Sandlund J, Fonseca T, Leimig T, Verissimo L, Ribeiro RC, Pedrose F: Clinical and biological characteristics of childhood non-Hodgkin lymphoma (NHL) in northeast Brazil. Leukemia 1997;11:743–746.
30. Madanat FF, Amr SS, Tarawneh MS, et al: Burkitt's lymphoma in Jordanian children: epidemiological and clinical study. Trop Med Hyg 1986;89:189–191.
31. Shad A, Magrath I: Non-Hodgkin's lymphoma. Pediatr Oncol Pediatr Clin North Am 1997;44:863.
32. Magrath IT, Bhatia K: Pathogenesis of small noncleaved cell lymphomas (Burkitt's lymphoma). In Magrath IT (ed): The Non-Hodgkin Lymphomas, 2nd ed. London, Arnold, Chapter 16, pp 385–409.
33. Gutierrez MI, Bhatia K, Barriga F, Diez B, et al: Molecular epidemiology of Burkitt's lymphoma from South America: Differences in break point location and Epstein-Barr virus association from tumors in other world regions. Blood 1992;79:3261–3266.
34. Kuhn-Hallek I, Sage DR, Stein L, et al: Expression of recombination activating genes (RAG-1 and RAG-2) in Epstein-Barr virus-bearing B-cells. Blood 1995;85:1289–1299.
35. Wilson JB, Levine AJ: The oncogenic potential of Epstein-Barr virus nuclear antigen 1 in transgenic mice. Curr Top Microbiol Immunol 1992;182:375–385.
36. Bhatia K, Raj A, Gutierrez MI, et al: Variation in the sequence of Epstein Barr virus nuclear antigen 1 in normal peripheral blood lymphocytes and in Burkitt's lymphoma. Oncogene 1996;13:177–181.
37. Ruf IK, Rhyne PW, Yang H, et al: Epstein-Barr virus regulates c-MYC, apoptosis, and tumorigenicity in Burkitt lymphoma. Mol Cell Biol 1999;19:1651–1660.
38. Razzouk BI, Srinivas S, Sample CE, Singh V, Sixbey JW: Epstein-Barr virus DNA recombination and loss in sporadic Burkitt's lymphoma. J Infect Dis 1996;173:529–535.
39. Harris NL, Jaffe ES, Stein H, et al: A revised European-American classification of lymphoid neoplasms: A proposal from the International Lymphoma Study Group. Blood 1994;84:1361–1392.
40. Jaffe ES, Harris NL, Stein H, Vardiman JW (eds): World Health Organization classification of tumours: Pathology and genetics of tumours of haematopoietic and lymphoid tissues. Lyon, IARC Press, 2001.
41. Bennett JM, Catovsky D, Daniel M-T, et al: The morphologic classification of acute lymphoblastic leukemia: Concordance among observers and clinical correlations. Br J Haematol 1981;41:553–561.
42. Raphael M, Gentihomme O, Tulliez M, et al: Histolopathological features of high-grade non-Hodgkin's lymphoma in acquired immunodeficiency syndrome: The French Study Group of

Pathology for Human Immunodeficiency Virus-Associated Tumors. Arch Pathol Lab Med 1991;115:15–20.

43. Hutchison RE, Finch C, Kepner J, et al: Burkitt lymphoma is immunophenotypically different from Burkitt-like lymphoma in young persons. Ann Oncol 2000;11(suppl 1):35–38.

44. Harris NL, Jaffe ES, Diebold J, et al: The World Health Organization classification of hematological malignancies: Report of the Clinical Advisory Committee Meeting. J Clin Oncol 1999;17:3835–3849.

45. Hutchison RE, Murphy SB, Fairclough DL, et al: Diffuse small noncleaved-cell lymphoma in children, Burkitt's versus non-Burkitt's types: Results from the Pediatric Oncology Group and St. Jude Children's Research Hospital. Cancer 1989;64:23–28.

46. Taub R, Krisch I, Morton C, et al: Translocation of the c-myc gene into the immunoglobulin heavy chain locus in human Burkitt lymphoma and murine plasmacytoma cells. Proc Natl Acad Sci USA 1982;79:7837–7841.

47. Magrath IT, Bhatia K: Pathogenesis of small noncleaved cell lymphomas (Burkitt's lymphoma). In Magrath I (ed): The Non-Hodgkin Lymphomas, 2nd ed. London, Arnold, 1997, pp 385–409.

48. Dalla-Favera R, Bregni M, Erikson J, Patterson D, Gallo RC, Croce CM: Human c-myc oncogene is located on the region of chromosome 8 that is translocated in Burkitt lymphoma cells. Proc Natl Acad Sci USA 1982;79:7824–7827.

49. Kornblau SM, Goodacre A, Cabanillas F: Chromosomal abnormalities in adult non-endemic Burkitt's lymphoma and leukemia: 22 new reports and a review of 148 cases from the literature. Hematol Oncol 1991;9:63–78.

50. Krolewski JJ, Dalla-Favera R: Molecular genetic approaches in the diagnosis and classification of lymphoid malignancies. Hematol Pathol 1989;3:45–61.

51. Nishida K, Ritterbach J, Repp R, et al: Characterization of chromosome 8 abnormalities by fluorescence in situ hybridization in childhood B-acute lymphoblastic leukemia/non-Hodgkin lymphoma. Cancer Genet Cytogenet 1995;79:8–14.

52. Kelly K, Siebenlist U: Mitogenic activation of normal T-cells leads to increased initiation of transcription in the c-myc locus. J Biol Chem 1988;26:4828–4831.

53. Kelly K, Sienbenlist U: The regulation and expression of c-myc in normal and malignant cells. Annu Rev Immunol 1986;4:317–338.

54. Luscher B, Eisenman RN: New light on Myc and Myb. Part I. Myc. Genes Dev 1990;4:2025–2035.

55. Packham G, Cleveland JL: Ornithine decarboxylase is a mediator of c-Myc-induced apoptosis. Mol Cell Biol 1994;14:5741–5747.

56. Blackwood EM, Eisenman RN: Max: A helix-loop-helix zipper protein that forms a sequence-specific DNA-binding complex with Myc. Science 1991;251:1211–1217.

57. Prendergast GC, Lawe D, Ziff EB: Association of Myn, the murine homolog of Max, with c-Myc stimulates methylation-sensitive DNA binding and ras co-transformation. Cell 1991;65:395–407.

58. Ayer DE, Kretzner L, Eisenman RN: Mad: A heterodimeric partner for Max that antagonized Myc transcriptional activity. Cell 1993;72:211–222.

59. Zervox AS, Gyuris J, Brent R: Mxi1, a protein that specifically interacts with Max to bind Myc-Max recognition sites. Cell 1993;72:223–232 [Erratum, Cell 1994;79:388].

60. Amati B, Land H: Myc-Max-Mad: A transcription factor network controlling cell cycle progression, differentiation and death. Curr Opin Genet Dev 1994;4:102–118.

61. Ayer DE, Lawrence QA, Eisenman RN: Mad-Max transcriptional repression is mediated by ternary complex formation with mammalian homologs of yeast repressor Sin3. Cell 1995;80:767–776.

62. Gu S, Cechova K, Tassi V, Dalla-Favera R: Opposite regulation of gene transcription and cell proliferation by c-Myc and max. Proc Natl Acad Sci USA 1993;90:2935–2939.

63. Croce CM, Erikson J, Ar-Rushdi A, Aden D, Nishikura K: Translocated c-myc oncogene of Burkitt lymphoma is transcribed in plasma cells and repressed in lymphoblastoid cells. Proc Natl Acad Sci USA 1984;81:3170–3174.

64. Gu W, Bhatia K, Magrath IT, Dang CV, Dalla-Favera R: Binding and suppression of the Myc transcriptional activation domain by p107. Science 1994;264:251–254.

65. Sandlund JT, Neckers LM, Schneller HE, Woodruff LS, Magrath IT: Theophylline induced differentiation provides direct evidence for the deregulation of c-myc in Burkitt's lymphoma and suggests participation of immunoglobulin enhanced sequences. Cancer Res 1993;52:127–132.

66. Zajac-Kaye M, Yu B, Ben-Baruch N: Downstream regulatory elements in the c-myc gene. Curr Top Microbiol Immunol 1990;166:279–284.

67. Adams JM, Harris AW, Pinkert CA, et al: The c-myc oncogene driven by immunoglobulin enhancers induces lymphoid malignancy in transgenic mice. Nature 1985;318:533–538.

68. Cory S, Adams JM: Transgenic mice and oncogenesis. Annu Rev Immunol 1988;6:25–48.

69. Packham G, Cleveland JL: c-Myc and apoptosis. Biochim Biophys Acta 1995;1242:11–28.

70. Hendeson S, Rowe M, Gregory C, et al: Induction of bcl-2 expression by Epstein-Barr virus latent membrane protein 1 protects infected B cells from programmed cell death. Cell 1991;65:1107–1115.

71. Eischen CM, Weber JD, Roussel MF, Sherr CJ, Cleveland JL: Disruption of the ARF-Mdm2-p53 tumor suppressor pathway in Myc-induced lymphomagenesis. Genes Dev 1999;13:2658–2669.

72. Eischen CM, Roussel MF, Korsmeyer SJ, Cleveland JL: Bax loss impairs Myc-induced apoptosis and circumvents the selection of p53 mutations during Myc-mediated lymphomagenesis. Mol Cell Biol 2001;21:7653–7662.

73. Eischen CM, Woo D, Roussel MF, Cleveland JL: Apoptosis triggered by Myc-induced suppression of Bcl-X_L or Bcl-2 is bypassed during lymphomagenesis. Mol Cell Biol 2001;21:5063–5070.

74. Gaidano G, Ballerini P, Gong JZ, Inghirami G, et al: p53 mutations in human lymphoid malignancies: Association with Burkitt lymphoma and chronic lymphocytic leukemia. Proc Natl Acad Sci USA 1991;88:5413–5417.

75. Bhatia KG, Gutiérrez MI, Huppi K, Siwarski D, Magrath IT: The pattern of p53 mutations in Burkitt's lymphoma differs from that of solid tumors. Cancer Res 1992;53:4273–4276.

76. Gutierrez MI, Bhatia K, Diez B, et al: Prognostic significance of p53 mutations in small noncleaved cell lymphomas. Int J Oncol 1994;4:567–571.

77. Behm FG, Campana D: Immunophenotyping. In: Pui C-H (ed): Childhood Leukemias. New York, Cambridge University Press, 1999, pp 111–141.

78. Falini B, Fizzotti M, Pileri S, et al: Bcl-6 protein expression in normal and neoplastic lymphoid tissue. Ann Oncol 1997;8(suppl 2):101–104.

79. Navid F, Mosijczuk AD, Head DR, et al: Acute lymphoblastic leukemia with the (8;14)(q24;q32) translocation and FAB L3 morphology associated with a B-precursor immunophenotype: The Pediatric Oncology Group experience. Leukemia. 1999;13:135–141.

80. Loh ML, Samson Y, Motte E, et al: Translocation (2;8)(p12;q24) associated with a cryptic t(12;21)(p13;q22) TEL/AML1 gene rearrangement in a child with acute lymphoblastic leukemia. Cancer Genet Cytogenet 2000;122:79–82.

81. Williams AH, Taylor CR, Higgins GR, et al: Childhood lymphoma-leukemia, I: Correlation of morphology and immunological studies. Cancer 1978;42:171–181.

82. Mitchell CD, Gordon I, Chessells JM: Clinical, haematological and radiological features in T-cell lymphoblastic malignancy in childhood. Clin Radiol 1986;37:257–261.

83. Head DR, Behm FG: Acute lymphoblastic leukemia and the lymphoblastic lymphomas of childhood. Semin Diagn Pathol 1995;12:325–334.

84. Murphy SB: Childhood non-Hodgkin's lymphoma. N Engl J Med 1978;299:1446–1448.

85. Maitra A, McKenna RW, Weinberg AG, et al: Precursor B-cell lymphoblastic lymphoma: A study of nine cases lacking blood and bone marrow involvement and review of the literature. Am J Clin Pathol 2001;115:868–875.

86. Lin P, Jones D, Dorfman DM, Medeiros LJ: Precursor B-cell lymphoblastic lymphoma: A predominantly extranodal tumor with low propensity for leukemic involvement. Am J Surg Pathol 2000;24:1480–1490.

Specific Malignancies

III

87. Neth O, Seidemann K, Jansen P, et al: Precursor B-cell lymphoblastic lymphoma in childhood and adolescence: Clinical features, treatment, and results in trials NHL-BFM 86 and 90. Med Pediatr Oncol 2000;35:20–27.

88. Millot F, Robert A, Bertrand Y, et al: Cutaneous involvement in children with acute lymphoblastic leukemia or lymphoblastic lymphoma: The Children's Leukemia Cooperative Group of the European Organization of Research and Treatment of Cancer (EORTC). Pediatrics 1997;100:60–64.

89. Kahwash SB, Qualman SJ: Cutaneous lymphoblastic lymphoma in children: Report of six cases with precursor B-cell lineage. Pediatr Dev Pathol 2002;5:45–53.

90. Bernard A, Boumsell L, Reinherz EL, et al: Cell surface characterization of malignant T cells from lymphoblastic lymphoma using monoclonal antibodies: Evidence for phenotypic differences between malignant T cells from patients with acute lymphoblastic leukemia and lymphoblastic lymphoma. Blood 1981;57:1105–1110.

91. Weiss LM, Bindl JM, Picozzi VJ, et al: Lymphoblastic lymphoma: An immunophenotype study of 26 cases with comparison to T cell acute lymphoblastic leukemia. Blood 1986;67:474–478.

92. Cossmann J, Chused T, Fisher R, et al: Diversity of immunological phenotypes of lymphoblastic lymphoma. Cancer Res 1983;43: 4486–4490.

93. Sheibani K, Nathwani BN, Winberg CD, et al: Antigenically defined subgroups of lymphoblastic lymphoma: Relationship to clinical presentation and biologic behavior. Cancer 1987;60:183–190.

94. Grogan T, Spier C, Wirt DP, et al: Immunologic complexity of lymphoblastic lymphoma. Diagn Immunol 1986;4:81–88.

95. Swerdlow SH, Habeshaw JA, Richards MA, et al: T lymphoblastic lymphoma with LEU-7 positive phenotype and unusual clinical course: A multiparameter study. Leuk Res 1985;9:167–173.

96. Sheibani K, Winberg CD, Burke JS, et al: Lymphoblastic lymphoma expressing natural killer cell-associated antigens: A clinicopathologic study of six cases. Leuk Res 1987;11:371–377.

97. Braziel RM, Keneklis T, Donlan JA, et al: Terminal deoxynucleotidyl transferase in non-Hodgkin's lymphoma. Am J Clin Pathol 1983;80:655–659.

98. Kung PC, Long JC, McCaffrey RP, et al: Terminal deoxynucleotidyl transferase in the diagnosis of leukemia and malignant lymphoma. Am J Med 1978;64:788–794.

99. Murphy S, Jaffe ES: Terminal transferase activity and lymphoblastic neoplasm. N Engl J Med 1984;311:1373–1375.

100. Bearman RM, Winberg CD, Maslow WC, et al: Terminal deoxynucleotidyl transferase activity in neoplastic and nonneoplastic hematopoietic cells. Am J Clin Pathol 1981;75:794–802.

101. McCaffrey R, Smoler DF, Baltimore D: Terminal deoxynucleotidyl transferase in a case of childhood acute lymphoblastic leukemia. Proc Natl Acad Sci USA 1973;70:521–525.

102. Soslow RA, Bhargave V, Warnke RA: MIC2 Tdt, bcl-2, and CD34 expression in paraffin-embedded high-grade lymphoma/acute lymphoblastic leukemia distinguishes between distinct clinicopathologic entities. Hum Pathol 1997;28:1158–1165.

103. Pui C-H, Rivera GK, Hancock ML, et al: Clinical significance of CD10 expression in childhood acute lymphoblastic leukemia. Leukemia 1993;7:35–40.

104. Pui C-H, Behm FG, Crist WM: Clinical and biological relevance of immunologic marker studies in childhood acute lymphoblastic leukemia. Blood 1993;82:343–362.

105. Roper M, Crist WM, Metzgar R, et al: Monoclonal antibody characterization of surface antigens in childhood T-cell lymphoid malignancies. Blood 1983;61:830–837.

106. MacGrath IT: Malignant non-Hodgkin's lymphomas in children. Hematol Oncol Clin North Am 1987;1:577–602.

107. Crist WM, Shuster JJ, Falletta J, et al: Clinical features and outcome of T-cell acute lymphoblastic leukemia in childhood with respect to alterations at the TAL1 locus: A Pediatric Oncology Group study. Blood 1993;81:2110–2117.

108. Link MP, Roper M, Dorfman RF, et al: Cutaneous lymphoblastic lymphoma with pre-B markers. Blood 1983;61:838–841.

109. Borowitz MJ, Croker BP, Metzgar RS: Lymphoblastic lymphoma with the phenotype of common acute lymphoblastic leukemia. Am J Clin Pathol 1983;79:387–391.

110. Stroup R, Sheibani K, Misset JL, et al: Surface immunoglobulin-positive lymphoblastic lymphoma: A report of three cases. Cancer 1990;65:2559–2563.

111. Gouttefangeas C, Bensussan A, Boumsell L: Study of the CD3-associated T-cell receptors reveals further differences between T-cell acute lymphoblastic lymphoma and leukemia. Blood 1990;15:931–934.

112. Thomas DA, Kantarjian HM: Lymphoblastic lymphoma. Hematol Oncol Clin North Am 2001;15:51–95.

113. Shikano T, Ishikawa Y, Naito H, et al: Cytogenetic characteristics of childhood non-Hodgkin lymphoma. Cancer 1992;70:714–719.

114. Kaneko Y, Frizzera G, Shikano T, et al: Chromosomal and immunophenotypic patterns in T cell acute lymphoblastic leukemia (T ALL) and lymphoblastic lymphoma (LBL). Leukemia 1989;3:886–892.

115. Link MP, Hoper M, Dorfman RF: Cutaneous lymphoblastic lymphoma with pre-B markers. Blood 1983;61:838–841.

116. Roper M, Crist WM, Metzgar R, et al: Monoclonal antibody characterization of surface antigens in childhood T-cell lymphoid malignancies. Blood 1983;61:830–837.

117. Crist WM, Kelly DR, Ragab AH, et al: Predictive ability of Lukes-Collins classification for immunologic phenotypes of childhood non-Hodgkin's lymphoma: An institutional series and literature review. Cancer 1981;48:2070–2075.

118. Pui C, Crist WM: Cytogenetic abnormalities in childhood acute lymphoblastic leukemia correlate with clinical features and treatment outcome. Leuk Lymphoma 1992;7:259–274.

119. Xia Y, Brown L, Yang CY, et al: TAL2, a helix-loop-helix gene activated by the (7;9)(q34;q32) translocation in human T-cell leukemia. Proc Natl Acad Sci USA 1991;88:11416–11420.

120. Mellentin JD, Smith SD, Cleary ML: lyl-1, A novel gene altered by chromosomal translocation in T-cell leukemia codes for a protein with a helix-loop-helix DNA binding motif. Cell 1989;58:77–83.

121. Kennedy MA, Gonzalez-Sarmiento R, Kees UR, et al: HOX11, a homeobox-containing T-cell oncogene on human chromosome 10q24. Proc Natl Acad Sci USA 1991;88:8900–8904.

122. Lu M, Gong ZY, Shen WF, Ho AD: The tcl-3 proto-oncogene altered by chromosomal translocation in T-cell leukemia codes for a homeobox protein. EMBO J 1991;10:2905–2910.

123. Hanto M, Roberts CW, Minden M, Crist WM, Korsmeyer SJ: Deregulation of a homeobox gene, HOX11, by the t(10;14) in T-cell leukemia. Science 1991;253:79–82.

124. Boehm T, Fornoni L, Kaneko Y, Perutz MF, Rabbitts TH: The rhombotin family of cysteine-rich LIM-domain oncogenes: Distinct members are involved in T-cell translocations to human chromosome 11p15 and 11p13. Proc Natl Acad Sci USA 1991;88:4367–4371.

125. Bash RO, Crist WM, Shuster JJ, et al: Clinical features and outcome of T-cell acute lymphoblastic leukemia in childhood with respect to alterations at the TAL1 locus: A Pediatric Oncology Group Study. Blood 1993;81:2110–2117.

126. Hsu H-L, Wadman I, Baer R: Formation of in vivo complexes between the TAL1 and E2A polypeptides of leukemic T cells. Proc Natl Acad Sci USA 1994;91:3181–3185.

127. Narita M, Shimizu K, Hayashi Y, et al: Consistent detection of CALM-AF10 chimaeric transcripts in haematological malignancies with t(10;11)(p13;q14) and identification of novel transcripts. Br J Haematol 1999;105:928–937.

128. Bohlander SK, Muschinsky V, Schrader K, et al: Molecular analysis of the CALM/AF10 fusion: identical rearrangements in acute myeloid leukemia, acute lymphoblastic leukemia and malignant lymphoma patients. Leukemia 2000;14:93–99.

129. Naeem R, Singer S, Fletcher JA: Translocation t(8;13)(p11;q11-12) in stem cell leukemia/lymphoma of T-cell and myeloid lineages. Genes Chromosomes Cancer 1995;12:148–151.

130. Inhorn RC, Aster JC, Roach SA, et al: A syndrome of lymphoblastic lymphoma, eosinophilia, and myeloid hyperplasia/malignancy associated with t(8;13)(p11;q11): Description of a distinctive clinicopathologic entity. Blood 1995;85:1881–1887.

131. Xiao S, Nalabolu SR, Aster JC, et al: FGFR1 is fused with a novel zinc-finger gene, ZNF198, in the t(8;3) leukaemia/lymphoma syndrome. Nat Genet 1998;18:84–87.

132. Yeoh E-J, Ross MB, Shurtleff S, et al: Classification, subtype discovery and prediction of outcome in pediatric acute

lymphoblastic leukemia by gene expression profiling. Cancer Cell 2002;1:133–143.

133. Ferrando AA, Neuberg DS, Staunton J, et al: Gene expression signatures define novel oncogenic pathways in T cell acute lymphoblastic leukemia. Cancer Cell 2002;1:75–87.

134. Sandlund JT, Santana V, Abromowitch M, et al: Large cell non-Hodgkin lymphoma of childhood: Clinical characteristics and outcome. Leukemia 1994;8:30–34.

135. Hutchison RE, Berard CW, Shuster JJ, Link MP, Pick TE, Murphy SB: B-cell lineage confers a favorable outcome among children and adolescents with large-cell lymphoma: A Pediatric Oncology Group study. J Clin Oncol 1995;13:2023–2032.

136. Sandlund JT, Pui C, Santana VM, et al: Clinical features and treatment outcome for children with CD30 positive large cell non-Hodgkin lymphoma. J Clin Oncol 1994;12:895–898.

137. Stansifeld AG, Diebold J, Noel H, et al: Updated Kiel classification for lymphomas. Lancet 1988;1:292.

138. Kadin ME: Ki-1–positive anaplastic large-cell lymphoma: A clinicopathologic entity? J Clin Oncol 1991;9:533–536.

139. Stein H, Mason DY, Gerdes J, et al: The expression of the Hodgkin's disease associated antigen Ki-1 in reactive and neoplastic lymphoid tissue: Evidence that Reed-Sternberg cells and histiocytic malignancies are derived from activated lymphoid cells. Blood 1985;66:848–858.

140. Kaneko Y, Frizzera G. Maseki N, et al: A novel translocation, t(2;5)(p23;q35), in childhood phagocytic large T-cell lymphoma mimicking malignant histiocytosis. Leukemia 1988;2:745–748.

141. LeBeau MM, Bitter MA, Larson RA, et al: The t(2;5)(p23;q35): A recurring chromosomal abnormality in Ki-1-positive anaplastic large cell lymphoma. Leukemia 1989;3:866.

142. Sandlund JT, Pui C, Roberts M, et al: Clinicopathologic features and treatment outcome of children with large cell lymphoma and the t(2;5)(p23;q35). Blood 1994;84:2467–2471.

143. Kadin ME: Ki-1/CD30+ (anaplastic) large-cell lymphoma: maturation of a clinicopathologic entity with prospects of effective therapy. J Clin Oncol 1994;12:884–887.

144. Morris SW, Kirstein MN, Valentine MB, et al: Fusion of a kinase gene, ALK, to a nucleolar protein gene, NPM in non-Hodgkin lymphoma. Science 1994;263:1281–1284.

145. Shiota M, Makamura S, Ichinohasama R: Anaplastic large cell lymphomas expressing the novel chimeric protein p80NPM/ALK: A distinct clinicopathologic entity. Blood 1995;86:1954–1960.

146. Downing JR, Shurtleff SA, Zielenska M, et al: Molecular detection of (2;5) translocation of non-Hodgkin's lymphoma by reverse transcriptase-polymerase chain reaction. Blood 1995;85:3416–3422.

147. Uner AH, Link MP, Laver J, et al: Detection of nucleophosmin-anaplastic lymphoma kinase (NPM-ALK) in pediatric large cell lymphoma using monoclonal antibody ALK 1: SIOP XXIX. Med Pediatr Oncol 1997;29:345.

148. Mora J, Filippa DA, Thaler HT, et al: Large cell non-Hodgkin lymphoma of childhood: Analysis of 78 consecutive patients enrolled in 2 consecutive protocols at the Memorial Sloan-Kettering Cancer Center. Cancer 2000;88:186–197.

149. Wright D, McKeever P, Carter R: Childhood non-Hodgkin lymphomas in the United Kingdom: Findings from the UK Children's Cancer Study Group. J Clin Pathol 1997;50:128–134.

150. Sandlund J, Pui C-H, Santana V, et al: Clinical features and treatment outcome for children with CD30+ large-cell non-Hodgkin's lymphoma. J Clin Oncol 1994;12:895–898.

151. Rubie H, Gladieff L, Robert A, et al: Childhood anaplastic large cell lymphoma Ki-1/CD30 clinicopathologic features of 19 cases. Med Pediatr Oncol 1994;22:155–161.

152. Fraga M, Brousset P, Schlaifer D, et al: Bone marrow involvement in anaplastic large cell lymphoma: Immunohistochemical detection of minimal disease and its prognostic significance. Am J Clin Pathol 1995;103:82–89.

153. Benharroch D, Meguerian-Bedoyan Z, Lamant L, et al: ALK-positive lymphoma: A single disease with a broad spectrum of morphology. Blood 1998;91:2076–2084.

154. Stein H: Ki-1-anaplastic large cell lymphoma: Is it a discrete entity? Leuk Lymphoma 1993;10:81–84.

155. Peleri S, Falini B, Delsol G, et al: Lymphohistiocytic T-cell lymphoma (anaplastic large cell lymphoma CD30+/Ki-1+ with a high content of reactive histiocytes). Histopathology 1990;16:383–391.

156. Brugieres L, Le Deley MC, Pacquement H, et al: CD30+ anaplastic large-cell lymphoma in children: analysis of 82 patients enrolled in two consecutive studies of the French Society of Pediatric Oncology. Blood 1998;92:3591–3598.

157. Sandlund JT, Roberts WM, Pui C-H, Crist WM, Behm FG: Systemic hemophagocytosis masking the diagnosis of large cell non-Hodgkin lymphoma. Med Pediatr Oncol 1997;29:167–169.

158. Blatt J, Weston B, Belhorn T, et al: Childhood non-Hodgkin lymphoma presenting as hemophagocytic syndrome. Pediatr Hematol Oncol 2002;19:45–49.

159. Kinney MC, Collins RD, Greer JP, et al: A small-cell-predominant variant of primary Ki-1 (CD30)+ T-cell lymphoma. Am J Surg Pathol 1993;17:859–868.

160. Chan JK, Buchanan R, Fletcher CD: Saracomatoid variant of anaplastic large-cell Ki-1 lymphoma. Am J Surg Pathol 1990;14:983–988.

161. Falini B, Liso A, Pasqualucci L, et al: CD30+ anaplastic large cell lymphoma, null type, with signet-ring appearance. Histopathology 1997;30:90–92.

162. Piccaluga PP, Ascani S, Fraternali Orcioni G, et al: ALK expression as a marker of malignancy: Application to a case of anaplastic large cell lymphoma with huge granulomatous reaction. Haematologica 2000;85:978–981.

163. Mann KP, Hall B, Kamino H, et al: Neutrophil-rich, Ki-1-positive anaplastic large-cell malignant lymphoma. Am J Surg Pathol 1995;19:407–416.

164. McCluggage WG, Walsh MY, Bharucha H: Anaplastic large cell malignant lymphoma with extensive eosinophilic or neutrophilic infiltration. Histopathology 1998;32:110–115.

165. Simonart T, Kentos A, Renoirte C, et al: Cutaneous involvement by neutrophil-rich, CD30-positive anaplastic large cell lymphoma mimicking deep pustules. Am J Surg Pathol 1999;23:244–246.

166. Burg G, Kempf W, Kazakov DV, et al: Pyogenic lymphoma of the skin: A peculiar variant of primary cutaneous neutrophil-rich CD30+ anaplastic large-cell lymphoma: Clinicopathological study of four cases and review of the literature. Br J Dermatol 2003;148:580–586.

167. Falini B: Anaplastic large cell lymphoma: pathological, molecular and clinical features. Br J Haematol 2001;114:741–760.

168. Stein H, Foss HD, Durkop H, et al: CD30-positive anaplastic large cell lymphoma: A review of its histopathological, genetic, and clinical features. Blood 2000;96:3681–3695.

169. Delsol GA, Al Saati T, Gatter KC, et al: Coexpression of epithelial membrane antigen (EMA), Ki-1, and interleukin-2 receptor by anaplastic large cell lymphoma: Diagnostic value in so-called malignant histiocytosis. Am J Pathol 1998;130:59–70.

170. Wellmann A, Thieblemont C, Pittaluga S, et al: Detection of differentially expressed genes in lymphomas using cDNA arrays: Identification of clusterin as a new diagnostic marker for anaplastic large-cell lymphomas. Blood 2000;96:398–404.

171. Kaneko Y, Frizzera G, Edamura S, et al: A novel translocation, t(2;5)(p23;q35), in childhood phagocytic large T-cell lymphoma mimicking malignant histiocytosis. Blood 1989;73:806–813.

172. Mason DY, Bastard C, Rimokh R, et al: CD30-positive large cell lymphomas ('Ki-1 lymphoma') are associated with a chromosomal translocation involving 5q35. Br J Haematol 1990;74:161–168.

173. Rosenwald A, Ott G, Pullford K, et al: t(1;2)(q21;p23) And t(2;3)(p23;q21): Two novel variant translocations of the t(2;5)(p23;q35) in anaplastic large cell lymphoma. Blood 1999;94:362–364.

174. Lamant L, Dastugue N, Pullford K, et al: A new fusion gene TPM3-ALK in anaplastic large cell lymphoma created by a (1;2)(q25;p23) translocation. Blood 1999;93:3088–3095.

175. Colleoni GW, Bridge JA, Garicochea B, et al: ATIC-ALK: A novel variant ALK gene fusion in anaplastic large cell lymphoma resulting from the recurrent cryptic chromosomal inversion, inv(2)(p23q35). Am J Pathol 2000;156:781–789.

176. Meech SJ, McGavaran L, Odom LF, et al: Unusual childhood extramedullary hematologic malignancy with natural killer cell properties that contains tropomyosin 4-anaplastic lymphoma kinase gene fusion. Blood 2001;98:1209–1216.

177. Touriol C, Greenland C, Lamant L, et al: Further demonstration of the diversity of chromosomal changes involving 2p23 in ALK-positive lymphoma: 2 cases expressing ALK kinase fused to CLTCL (clathrin chain polypeptide-like). Blood 2000;95:3204–3207.

178. Lamant L, Meggetto F, Al Saati TA, et al: High incidence of the t(2;5)(p23;q35) translocation in anaplastic large cell lymphoma and its lack of detection in Hodgkin's disease: Comparison of cytogenetic analysis, reverse transcriptase-polymerase chain reaction, and P-80 immunostaining. Blood 1996;87:284–291.

179. Pulford K, Lamant L, Morris SW, et al: Detection of anaplastic lymphoma kinase (ALK) and nucleolar protein (NPM)-ALK proteins in normal and neoplastic cells with the monoclonal antibody ALK1. Blood 1997;89:1394–1404.

180. Lamant L, Pullford K, Bischof D, et al: Expression of the ALK tyrosine kinase gene in neuroblastoma. Am J Pathol 2000;156:1711–1721.

181. Lawrence B, Perez-Atayde A, Hibbard MK, et al: TPM3-ALK and TPM4-ALK oncogenes in inflammatory myofibroblastic tumors. Am J Pathol 2000;157:377–384.

182. Cessna MH, Zhoou H, Sanger WG, et al: Expression of ALK1 and p80 in inflammatory myofibroblastic tumor and its mesenchymal mimics: A study of 135 cases. Mod Pathol 2002;15:931–938.

183. van den Berg H, Noorduyn A, van Kullenburg ABP, et al: Leukaemic expression of anaplastic large cell lymphoma with 46,XX,ins(2;5)(p23;q15q35) in a child with dihydropyrimidine dehydrogenase deficiency. Leukemia 2000;4:769–770.

184. Anderson MM, Ross CW, Singleton TP, et al: Ki-1 anaplastic large cell lymphoma with a prominent leukemic phase. Hum Pathol 1996;27:1093–1095.

185. Villamor N, Rozman M, Esteve J, et al: Anaplastic large-cell lymphoma with rapid evolution to leukemic phase. Ann Hematol 1999;78:478–482.

186. Bayle C, Charpentier A, Duchayne E, et al: Leukaemic presentation of small cell variant anaplastic large cell lymphoma: Report of four cases. Br J Haematol 1999;104:680–688.

187. Chacnabhai M, Britten C, Klasa R, Gascoyne RD: t(2;5)-Positive lymphoma with peripheral blood involvement. Leuk Lymphoma 1998;28:415–422.

188. Onciu M, Behm FG, Raimondi S, Harwood EL, Pui CH, Sandlund JT: ALK-positive anaplastic large cell lymphoma (ALCL) with leukemic peripheral blood involvement: Report of three pediatric cases. Am J Clin Pathol 2003;120(4):617–625.

189. Lones MA, Auperin A, Raphael M, et al: Mature B-cell lymphoma/leukemia in children and adolescents: Intergroup pathologist consensus with the revised European-Amerian Lymphoma Classification. Ann Oncol 2000;11:47–51.

190. Delsol G, Lamant L, Mariame B, et al: A new subtype of large B-cell lymphoma expressing the ALK kinase and lacking the 2;5 translocation. Blood 1997;89:1483–1490.

191. Onciu M, Behm FG, Downing JR, et al: ALK-positive plasmablastic B-cell lymphoma with expression of the NPM-ALK fusion transcript: Report of two cases. Blood 2003;102:2642–2644.

192. Lones MA, Cairo MS, Perkins SL: T-cell-rich large B-cell lymphoma in children and adolescents: A clinicopathologic report of six cases from the Children's Cancer Group Study CCG-5961. Cancer 2000;88:2378–2386.

193. Lim MS, Beaty M, Sorbara L, et al: T-cell/histiocyte-rich large B-cell lymphoma: A heterogeneous entity with derivation from germinal center B cells. Am J Surg Pathol 2002;26:1458–1466.

194. Hutchison RE, Fairclough DL, Holt H, et al: Clinical significance of histology and immunophenotype in childhood diffuse large cell lymphoma. Am J Clin Pathol 1991;95:787–793.

195. Alizadeh AA, Eisen MB, Davis RE, et al: Distinct types of diffuse large B-cell lymphoma identified by gene expression profiling. Nature 2000;405:503–511.

196. Rosenwald A, Wright G, Chang WC, et al: The use of molecular profiling to predict survival after chemotherapy for diffuse large B-cell lymphoma. N Engl J Med 2002;346:1937–1947.

197. Davis RE, Staudt LM: Molecular diagnosis of lymphoid malignancies by gene expression profiling. Curr Opin Hematol 2002;9:333–338.

198. Shipp MA, Ross KN, Tamayo P, et al: Diffuse large B-cell lymphoma outcome prediction by gene-expression profiling and supervised machine learning. Nat Med 2002;8:68–74.

199. Lazzarino M, Orlandi E, Paulli M, et al: Treatment outcome and prognostic factors for primary mediastinal (thymic) B-cell lymphoma: A multicenter study of 106 patients. J Clin Oncol 1997;15:1646–1653.

200. Zanzani PL, Bendandi M, Frezza G, et al: Primary mediastinal B-cell lymphoma with sclerosis: Clinical and therapeutic evaluation of 22 patients. Leuk Lymphoma 1996;21:311–316.

201. Pauli M, Lazzarino M, Gianelli U, et al: Primary mediastinal B-cell lymphoma: Update of its clinicopathologic features. Leuk Lymphoma 1997;26:115–123.

202. Lones MA, Perkins SL, Sposto R, et al: Large-cell lymphoma arising in the mediastinum in children and adolescents is associated with an excellent outcome: A Children's Cancer Group report. J Clin Oncol 2000;18:3845–3853.

203. Van Besien K, Kelta M, Bahaguna P: Primary mediastinal B-cell lymphoma: A review of pathology and management. J Clin Oncol 2001;19:1855–1864.

204. Abou-Ellela AA, Weinburger DD, Vose JM, et al: Primary mediastinal large B-cell lymphoma: A clinicopathologic study of 43 patients from the Nebraska Lymphoma Study Group. J Clin Oncol 1999;17:784–790.

205. Pauli M, Strater J, Gianelli U, et al: Mediastinal B-cell lymphoma: A study of its histomorphologic spectrum based on 109 cases. Hum Pathol 1999;30:178–187.

206. de Leval L, Ferry JA, Falini B, et al: Expression of bcl-6 and CD10 in primary mediastinal large B-cell lymphoma: Evidence for derivation from germinal center B cells? Am J Surg Pathol 2001;25:1277–1282.

207. Kanavaros P, Gaulard P, Charlotte F, et al: Discordant expression of immunoglobulin and its associated molecule mb-1/CD79a is frequently found in mediastinal large B cell lymphomas. Am J Pathol 1995;146:735–741.

208. Lamarre L, Jacobson JO, Aisenberg AC, et al: Primary large cell lymphoma of the mediastinum: A histologic and immunophenotypic study of 29 cases. Am J Surg Pathol 1989;13:730–739.

209. Higgins JP, Warnke RA: CD30 expression is common in mediastinal large B-cell lymphoma. Am J Clin Pathol 1999;112:241–247.

210. Kuppers R, Rajewsky K, Hansmann ML, et al: Diffuse large cell lymphomas are derived from mature B cells carrying V region genes with a high load of somatic mutation and evidence of selection for antibody expression. Eur J Immunol 1997;27:1398–1405.

211. Bentz M, Barth TF, Bruderlein S, et al: Gain of chromosome arm 9p is characteristic of primary mediastinal B-cell lymphoma (MBL): Comprehensive molecular cytogenetic analysis and presentation of a novel MBL cell line. Genes Chromosomes Cancer 2001;30:393–401.

212. Palanisamy N, Abou-Elella AA, Chaganti SR, et al: Similar patterns of genomic alterations characterize primary mediastinal large-B-cell lymphoma and diffuse large-B-cell lymphoma. Genes Chromosomes Cancer 2002;33:114–122.

213. Joos S, Otano-Joos MI, Ziegler S, et al: Primary mediastinal (thymic) B-cell lymphoma is characterized by gains of chromosomal material including 9p and amplification of the REL gene. Blood 1996;87:1571–1578.

214. Scarpa A, Moore PS, Riguad G, et al: Molecular features of primary mediastinal B-cell lymphoma: Involvement of p16INK4A, p53, and c-myc. Br J Haematol 1999;170:106–113.

215. Tsang P, Cesarman E, Chadburn A, et al: Molecular characterization of primary mediastinal B cell lymphoma. Am J Pathol 1996;148:2017–2025.

216. Frizzera G, Murphy SB: Follicular (nodular) lymphoma in childhood: A rare clinical-pathological entity: Report of eight cases from four cancer centers. Cancer 1979;44:2218–2235.

217. Murphy SB, Fairclough DL, Hutchison RE, Berard CW: Non-Hodgkin's lymphomas of childhood: An analysis of the histology, staging, and response to treatment of 338 cases at a single institution. J Clin Oncol 1989;7:186–193.

218. Pinto A, Hutchison RE, Grant LH, et al: Follicular lymphomas I pediatric patients. Mod Pathol 1990;3:308–313.

219. Ribeiro RC, Pui C-H, Murphy SB, et al: Childhood malignant non-Hodgkin's lymphomas of uncommon histology. Leukemia 1992;6:761–765.

220. Atra A, Meller ST, Stevens RS, et al: Conservative management of follicular non-Hodgkin's lymphoma in childhood. Br J Haematol 1998;103:320–323.

221. Lorsbach RB, Shay-Seymore D, Moore J, et al: Clinicopathologic analysis of follicular lymphoma occurring in children. Blood 2002;99:1959–1964.

222. Moertel CL, Watterson J, McCormick SR, Simonton SC: Follicular large cell lymphoma of the testis in a child. Cancer 1995;75:1182–1186.

223. Finn LS, Viswanatha DS, Belasco JB, et al: Primary follicular lymphoma of the testis in childhood. Cancer 1999;85:1626–1635.

224. Lu D, Medeiros LJ, Eskenazi AE, Abruzzo LV: Primary follicular large cell lymphoma of the testis in a child. Arch Pathol Lab Med 2001;125:551–554.

225. Pakzad K, MacLennan GT, Elder JS, et al: Follicular large cell lymphoma localized to the testis in children. J Urol 2002;168:225–228.

226. Lai R, Larratt LM, Etches W, et al: Hepatosplenic T-cell lymphoma of alphabeta lineage in a 16-year-old boy presenting with hemolytic anemia and thrombocytopenia. Am J Surg Pathol 2000;24:45–63.

227. Weidmann E: Hepatosplenic T cell lymphoma: A review on 45 cases since the first report describing the disease as a distinct lymphoma entity in 1990. Leukemia 2000;14:991–997.

228. Suarez F, Wlodarska I, Rigal-Huguet F, et al: Hepatosplenic alphabeta T-cell lymphoma: An unusual case with clinical, histologic, and cytogenetic features of gammadelta hepatosplenic T-cell lymphoma. Am J Surg Pathol 2000;24:1027–1032.

229. Cooke CB, Krenacs L, Stetler-Stevenson M, et al: Hepatosplenic T-cell lymphoma: A distinct clinicopathologic entity of cytotoxic gamma delta T-cell origin. Blood 1996;88:4265–4274.

230. Macon WR, Levy NB, Kurtin PJ, et al: Hepatosplenic αβ T-cell lymphomas. Am J Surg Pathol 2001;25:285–296.

231. Farcet J, Gaulard P, Marolleau J, et al: Hepatosplenic T-cell lymphoma: Sinusal/sinusoidal localization of malignant cells expressing the T-cell receptor αβ. Blood 1990;75:2213–2219.

232. Garcia-Sanchez F, Menarguez J, Cristobal E, et al: Hepatosplenic gamma-delta T-cell malignant lymphoma: Report of the first case in childhood, including molecular minimal residual disease follow-up. Br J Haematol 1995;90:943–946.

233. Francosis A, Lesesve J-F, Stamatoullas A, et al: Hepatosplenic gamma/delta T-cell lymphoma: A report of two cases in immunocompromised patients associated with isochromosome 7q. Am J Surg Pathol 1997;21:781–790.

234. Ross CW, Schnitzer B, Scheldon S, et al: γδ T-cell posttransplantation lymphoproliferative disorder primarily in the spleen. Am J Clin Pathol 1994;102:310–315.

235. Khan WA, Yu L, Eisenbrey AB, et al: Hepatosplenic gamma/delta T-cell lymphoma in immunocompromised patients: Report of two cases and review of literature. Am J Clin Pathol 2001;116:41–50.

236. Steurer M, Stauder R, Grunewald K, et al: Hepatosplenic gammadelta-T-cell lymphoma with leukemic course after renal transplantation. Hum Pathol 2002;33:253–258.

237. Wang CC, Tien HF, Kin MT, et al: Consistent presence of isochromosome 7q in hepatosplenic T gamma/delta lymphoma: A new cytogenetic-clinicopathologic entity. Genes Chromosomes Cancer 1995;12:161–164.

238. Vega F, Medeiros LJ, Bueso-Ramos C, et al: Hepatosplenic gamma/delta T-cell lymphoma in bone marrow: A sinusoidal neoplasm with blastic cytologic features. Am J Clin Pathol 2001;116:410–419.

239. Salhany KE, Feldman M, Kahn MJ, et al: Hepatosplenic gammadelta T-cell lymphoma: Ultrastructural, immunophenotypic, and functional evidence for cytotoxic T lymphocyte differentiation. Hum Pathol 1997;28:674–685.

240. Nosari A, Oreste PL, Biondi A, et al: Hepato-splenic gammadelta T-cell lymphoma: A rare entity mimicking the hemophagocytic syndrome. Am J Hematol 1999;60:61–65.

241. Felger RE, Macon WR, Kinney MC, et al: TIA-1 expression in lymphoid neoplasma: Identification of subsets with cytotoxic T lymphocyte or natural killer cell differentiation. Am J Pathol 1997;150:1893–1900.

242. Boulland ML, Kanavaros P, Wechsler J, et al: Cytotoxic protein expression in natural killer cell lymphomas and in alpha beta and gamma delta peripheral T-cell lymphomas. J Pathol 1997;183:432–439.

243. Joneaux P, Daniel MT, Martel V, et al: Isochromosome 7q and trisomy 8 are consistent primary, non-random chromosomal abnormalities associated with hepatosplenic T gamma/delta lymphoma. Leukemia 1996;10:1453–1455.

244. Coventry S, Punnett HH, Tomeczak EZ, et al: Consistency of isochromosome 7q and trisomy 8 in hepatosplenic gammadelta T-cell lymphoma: Detection by fluorescence in situ hybridization of a splenic touch-preparation from a pediatric patient. Pediatr Dev Pathol 1999;2:478–483.

245. Wlodarska I, Martin-Garcia N, Achten R, et al: Fluorescence in situ hybridization study of chromosome 7 aberrations in hepatosplenic T-cell lymphoma: Isochromosome 7q as a common abnormality accumulating in forms with features of cytologic progression. Genes Chromosomes Cancer 2002;33:243–251.

246. Rossbach HC, Chamizo W, Dumont DP, et al: Hepatosplenic gamma/delta T-cell lymphoma with isochromosome 7q, translocation t(7;21), and tetrasomy 8 in a 9-year-old girl. J Pediatr Hematol Oncol 2002;24:154–157.

247. Przybylski GK, Wu H, Macon WR, et al: Hepatosplenic and subcutaneous panniculitis-like gamma/delta T cell lymphomas are derived from different Vdelta subsets of gamma/delta T lymphocytes. J Mol Diagn 2000;2:11–9.

248. Ohshima K, Haraoka S, Harada N, et al: Hepatosplenic gammadelta T-cell lymphoma: Relation to Epstein-Barr virus and activated cytotoxic molecules. Histopathology 2000;36:127–135.

249. Thomson AB, McKenzie KJ, Jackson R, Wallace WH: Subcutaneous panniculitic T-cell lymphoma in childhood: successful response to chemotherapy. Med Pediatr Oncol 2001;37:549–552.

250. Sen F, Rassidakis GZ, Jones D, et al: Apoptosis and proliferation in subcutaneous panniculitis-like T-cell lymphoma. Mod Pathol 2002;15:625–631.

251. Agnarrsson BA, Kadin ME: Peripheral T-cell lymphomas in children. Semin Diagn Pathol 1995;12:314–324.

252. El-Hoshy K, Hashimoto K: Adolescence mycosis fungoides: An unusual presentation with hypopigmentation. J Dermatol 1995;22:424–427.

253. Grunwald MH, Amichai B: Localized hypopigmented mycosis fungoides in a 12-year-old Caucasian boy. J Dermatol 1999;26:70–71.

254. Schmid H, Dummer R, Kempf W, et al: Mycosis fungoides with mucinous follicularis in childhood. Dermatology 1999;198:284–287.

255. Garzon MC: Cutaneous T cell lymphoma in children. Semin Cutan Med Surg 1999;18:226–232.

256. Tan E, Tay YK, Giam YC: Profile and outcome of childhood mycosis fungoides in Singapore. Pediatr Dermatol 2000;17:352–356.

257. Neuhaus IM, Ramos-Caro FA, Hassanein AM: Hypopigmented mycosis fungoides in childhood and adolescence. Pediatr Dermatol 2000;17:403–406.

258. Whittam LR, Calonje E, Orchard G, et al: CD8-positive juvenile onset mycosis fungoides: An immunohistochemical and genotypic analysis of six cases. Br J Dermatol 2000;143:1199–1204.

259. Miyazaki M, Lin Y-W, Okiada M, et al: Childhood cutaneous natural killer/T-cell lymphoma successfully treated with only one course chemotherapy and incomplete tumor resection. Haematologica 2001;86:883–884.

260. Ohnuma K, Toyada Y, Nishihira H, et al: Aggressive natural killer (NK) cell lymphoma: Report of a pediatric case and review of the literature. Leuk Lymphoma 1997;25:387–392.

261. Shaw PH, Cohn SL, Morgan ER, et al: Natural killer cell lymphoma: Report of two pediatric cases, therapeutic options, and review of the literature. Cancer 2001;91:642–646.

262. Gold BD: *Helicobacter pylori* prevalence infection in children. Curr Gastroenterol Rep 2001;3:235–247.

263. Lewis JM, Vasef MA, Seabury Stone M: HTLV-I-associated granulomatous T-cell lymphoma in a child. J Am Acad Dermatol 2001;44:525–529.

264. Broniscer A, Ribeiro RC, Srinivas RV, et al: An adolescent with HTLV-I-associated adult T cell leukemia treated with interferon-alfa and zidovudine. Leukemia 1996;10:1244–1254.

265. Pombo-de-Oliveira MS, Dobbin JA, Loureiro P, et al: Genetic mutation and early onset of T-cell leukemia in pediatric patients infected at birth with HTLV-I. Leuk Res 2002;26:155–161.

266. Sandlund JT, Ribeiro R, Lin J, et al: Factors contributing to the prognostic significance of bone marrow involvement in childhood non-Hodgkin lymphoma. Med Pediatr Oncol 1994;23:350–353.

267. Haddy TB, Adde MA, Magrath IT: CNS involvement in small noncleaved-cell lymphoma: Is CNS disease per se a poor prognostic sign? J Clin Oncol 1991;9:1973–1982.

268. Bernard A, Murphy SB, Melvin S, et al: Non-T, non-B lymphomas are rare in childhood and associated with cutaneous tumor. Blood 1982;59:549–554.

269. Murphy SB: Childhood lymphomas. In Hoffman R, Berg Jr HJ, Shattil SJ, et al (eds): Hematology, Basic Principles and Practice, 2nd ed. Philadelphia, Churchill Livingstone, 1995, pp 1299–1307.

270. Garrett KM, Hoffer FA, Behm FG, Gow KW, Hudson MM, Sandlund JT: Interventional radiology techniques for the diagnosis of lymphoma or leukemia. Pediatr Radiol 2002;32:653–662.

271. Fletcher BD, Kauffman WM, Kaste SC, et al: Use of T1-201 to detect untreated pediatric Hodgkin disease. Radiology 1995;196:851–855.

272. Naumann R, Vaic A, Beuthien-Baumann B, et al: Prognostic value of positron emission tomography in the evaluation of post-treatment residual mass in patients with Hodgkin's disease and non-Hodgkin's lymphoma. Br J Haematol 2001;115:793–800.

273. Haddy TB, Parker RI, Magrath IT: Bone marrow involvement in young patients with non-Hodgkin's lymphoma: The importance of multiple bone marrow samples for accurate staging. Med Pediatr Oncol 1989;17:418–423.

274. Carr R, Barrington SF, Madan B, et al: Detection of lymphoma in bone marrow by whole-body positron emission tomography. Blood 1998;91:3340–3346.

275. Wagner DK, Kiwanuka J, Edwards BK, Rubin LA, Nelson DL, Magrath IT: Soluble interleukin-2 receptor levels in patients with undifferentiated and lymphoblastic lymphomas: Correlation with survival. J Clin Oncol 1987;5:1262–1274.

276. Pui C-H, Ip SH, Kung P, et al: High serum interleukin-2 receptor levels are related to advanced disease and a poor outcome in childhood non-Hodgkin's lymphoma. Blood 1987;70:624–628.

277. Gaynon PS, Desai AA, Bostrom BC, et al: Early response to therapy and outcome in childhood acute lymphoblastic leukemia. Cancer 1997;80:1717–1726.

278. Patte C, Auperin A, Michon J: The Société Française d'Oncologie Pédiatrique LMB89 protocol: Highly effective multiagent chemotherapy tailored to the tumor burden and initial response in 561 unselected children with B-cell lymphomas and L3 leukemia. Blood 2001;97:3370–3379.

279. Siota M, Nakamura S, Ichinohasama R, et al: Anaplastic large cell lymphomas expressing the novel chimeric protein p80NPM/ALK: A distinct clinicopathologic entity. Blood 1995;86:1954–1960.

280. Faini B, Bigerna B, Pizzotti M, et al: ALK expression defines a distinct group of t/null lymphomas ("ALK lymphoma") with a wide morphologic spectrum. Am J Pathol 1998;153:875–886.

281. Gascoyne RD, Aoun P, Wu D, et al: Prognostic significance of anaplastic lymphoma kinase (ALK) protein expression in adults with anaplastic large cell lymphoma. Blood 1999;93:3913–3921.

282. Le Deley MC, Reiter A, Williams D, et al: Prognostic factors in childhood anaplastic large cell lymphoma: Results of the European Intergroup Study. Ann Oncol 1999;10(suppl 3):28.

283. Williams DM, Hobson R, Imeson J, et al: Anaplastic large cell lymphoma in childhood: Analysis of 72 patients treated on The United Kingdom Children's Cancer Study Group chemotherapy regimens. Br J Haematol 2002;117:812–820.

284. Anderson JR, Jenkin RDT, Wilson JF, et al: Long-term follow-up of patients treated with COMP or LSA2-L2 therapy for childhood non-Hodgkin's lymphoma: A report of CCG-551 from the Children's Cancer Group. J Clin Oncol 1993;11:1024–1032.

285. Wollner N, Burchenal JH, Liebermann PH: Non-Hodgkin's lymphoma in children: A comparative study of two modalities of therapy. Cancer 1976;37:123.

286. Sullivan MP, Boyett J, Pullen J, et al: Pediatric Oncology Group experience with modified LSA2-L2 therapy in 107 children with non-Hodgkin's lymphoma (Burkitts lymphoma excluded). Cancer 1985;55:323–336.

287. Sandlund JT, Santana V, Abromowitch M, et al: Large cell non-Hodgkin lymphoma of childhood: Clinical characteristics and outcome. Leukemia 1994;8:30–34.

288. Hutchison RE, Berard CW, Shuster JJ, Link MP, Pick TE, Murphy SB: B-cell lineage confers a favorable outcome among children and adolescents with large-cell lymphoma: A Pediatric Oncology Group study. J Clin Oncol 1995;13:2023–2032.

289. Murphy SB, Bowman WP, Abromowitch M, et al: Results of treatment of advanced-stage Burkitt's lymphoma and B cell (SIg+) acute lymphoblastic leukemia with high-dose fractionated cyclophosphamide and coordinated high-dose methotrexate and cytarabine. J Clin Oncol 1986;4:1732–1739.

290. Murphy SB, Hustu HO, Rivera G, Berard CW: End results of treating children with localized non-Hodgkin's lymphomas with a combined modality approach of lessened intensity. J Clin Oncol 1983;1:326–330.

291. Link MP, Shuster JJ, Donaldson SS, Berard CW, Murphy SB: Treatment of children and young adults with early-stage non-Hodgkin's lymphoma. N Engl J Med 1997;337:1259–1266.

292. Brecher M, Schwenn MR, Coppes MJ, et al: Fractionated cyclophosphamide and back to back high dose methotrexate and cytosine arabinoside improves outcome in patients with stage III high grade small non-cleaved cell lymphomas (SNCCL): A randomized trial of the Pediatric Oncology Group. Med Pediatr Oncol 1997;29:526–533.

293. Bowman WP, Shuster J, Cook B, et al: Improved survival for children with B-cell acute lymphoblastic leukemia and stage IV small noncleaved cell lymphoma: A Pediatric Oncology Group study. J Clin Oncol 1996;14:1252–1261.

294. Patte C, Philip T, Rodary C, et al: High survival rate in advanced-stage B-cell lymphomas and leukemias without CNS involvement with a short intensive polychemotherapy: Results from the French Pediatric Oncology Society of a randomized trial of 216 children. J Clin Oncol 1991;9:123–132.

295. Patte C, Leverger G, Perel Y, et al: Updated results of the LMB86 protocol of the French Pediatric Oncology Society (SFOP) for B-cell non-Hodgkin's lymphomas (B-NHL) with CNS involvement (CNS+) and B-ALL. Med Pediatr Oncol 1990;18:397.

296. Reiter A, Schrappe M, Ludwig W: Favorable outcome of B-cell acute lymphoblastic leukemia in childhood: A report of three consecutive studies of the BFM Group. Blood 1992;80:2471.

297. Sposto R, Meadows AT, Chilcote RR, et al: Comparison of long-term outcome of children and adolescents with disseminated non-lymphoblastic non-Hodgkin lymphoma treated with COMP or daunomycin-COMP: A report from the Children's Cancer Group. Med Pediatr Oncol 2001;37:432–441.

298. Cairo MS, Krailo M, Hutchinson R, Harris R, Meadows A, Bleyer WA: Results of a phase II trial of "French" (F) (LMB-86) or "orange" (O) (CCG-hybrid) in children with advanced non-lymphoblastic non-Hodgkin's lymphoma: An improvement in survival. Proc Am Soc Clin Oncol 1994;13:392a.

299. Magrath IT, Janus C, Edwards BK, et al: An effective therapy for both undifferentiated (including Burkitt's) lymphomas and lymphoblastic lymphomas in children and young adults. Blood 1984;63:1102–1111.

300. Schwenn MR, Blattner SR, Lynch E, Weinstein HJ: HiC-COM: A 2-month intensive chemotherapy regimen for children with stage III and IV Burkitt's lymphoma and B-cell acute lymphoblastic leukemia. J Clin Oncol 1991;9:133–138.

301. Muller-Weihrich S, Henze G, Odenwald E: BFM trials for childhood non-Hodgkin's lymphomas. In Cavalli F, Bonadonna G, Rozencweig M (eds): Malignant Lymphomas and Hodgkin's Disease: Experimental and Therapeutic Advances. Boston, Martinus Nijhoff, 1985, p 633.

302. Dahl GV: A novel treatment of childhood lymphoblastic non-Hodgkin's lymphoma: early and intermittent use of teniposide plus cytarabine. Blood 1985;66:1110–1114.

303. Hvizdala E. Lymphoblastic lymphoma in children: A randomized trial comparing LSA$_2$L$_2$ with the A-COP therapeutic regimen: A POG study. J Clin Oncol 1988;6:26–33.

304. Weinstein HJ, Lack EE, Cassady JR: APO therapy for malignant lymphoma of large cell histiocytic type of childhood: Analysis of treatment results for 29 patients. Blood 1984;64:422–426.

305. Hvizdala EV, Berard C, Callihan T: Nonlymphoblastic lymphoma in children: histology and stage-related response to therapy: A POG study. J Clin Oncol 1991;9:1189–1195.

306. Santana VM, Abromowitch M, Sandlund JT, et al: MACOP-B treatment in children and adolescents with advanced diffuse large-cell non-Hodgkin's lymphoma. Leukemia 1993;7:187–191.

307. Reiter A, Schrappe M, Tiemann M, et al: Successful treatment strategy for Ki-1 anaplastic large-cell lymphoma of childhood: A prospective analysis of 62 patients enrolled in three consecutive Berlin-Frankfurt-Munster group studies. J Clin Oncol 1994;12:899–908.

308. Patte C, Kalifa C, Flamant F, et al: Results of the LMT81 protocol, a modified LSA2L2 protocol with high dose methotrexate, in 84 children with non-B-cell (lymphoblastic) lymphoma. Med Pediatr Oncol 1992;20:105–113.

309. Meadows A, Sposto R, Jenkin R, et al: Similar efficacy of 6 and 18 months of therapy with four drugs (COMP) for localized non-Hodgkin's lymphoma of children: A report from the Children's Cancer Study Group. J Clin Oncol 1989;7:92–99.

310. Patte C, Philip T, Rodary C, et al: Improved survival rate in children with stage III and IV B cell non-Hodgkin's lymphoma and leukemia using multi-agent chemotherapy: Results of a study of 114 children from the French Pediatric Oncology Society. J Clin Oncol 1986;4:1219–1226.

311. Tubergen DG, Krailo MD, Meadows AT, et al: Comparison of treatment regimens for pediatric lymphoblastic non-Hodgkin's lymphoma: A Children's Cancer Group study. J Clin Oncol 1995;13:1368-1376.

312. Reiter A, Schrappe M, Parwaresch R, et al: Non-Hodgkin's lymphomas of childhood and adolescence: Results of a treatment stratified for biologic subtypes and stage: A report of the Berlin-Frankfurt-Munster Group. J Clin Oncol 1995;13:359–372.

313. Reiter A, Schrappe M, Tiemann M, et al: Improved treatment results in childhood B-cell neoplasm with tailored intensification of therapy: A report of the Berlin-Frankfurt-Münster Group Trial NHL-BFM 90. Blood 1999;94:3294–3306.

314. Jansen P, Schrappe M, Zimmermann M, et al: Intraventricularly applied chemotherapy and intensive systemic therapy is effective for CNS positive patients with Burkitt-type lymphomas or acute B-cell leukemia (B-ALL): SIOP XXIX. Med Pediatr Oncol 1997;29:359.

315. Magrath I, Adde M, Shad A, et al: Adult and children with small noncleaved cell lymphoma have a similar excellent outcome when treated with the same chemotherapy regimen. J Clin Oncol 1996;14:925–934.

316. Adde M, Shad A, Venzon D, et al: Additional chemotherapy agents improve treatment outcome for children and adults with advanced B-cell lymphomas. Semin Oncol 1998;25(2 suppl 4):33–39.

317. Reiter A, Schrappe M, Ludwig W-D, et al: Intensive ALL-type therapy without local radiotherapy provides a 90% event-free survival for children with T-cell lymphoblastic lymphoma: A BFM group report. Blood 2000;95:416–421.

318. Patte C, Michon J, Behrendt H, et al: B-cell large cell lymphoma in children: Description and outcome when treated with the same regimen as Burkitt: SFOP experience with the LMB 89 protocol. Ann Oncol 1996;7:abst 092.

319. Mann G, Yakisan E, Schrappe M, et al: Diffuse large B-cell lymphomas in childhood and adolescence: Favorable outcome with a Burkitt's lymphoma directed therapy in trial NHL-BFM 90: A report of the BFM group, SIOP XXIX. Med Pediatr Oncol 1997;29:358.

320. Patte C: Non-Hodgkin's lymphoma. Eur J Cancer 1998;34:359–363.

321. Soussain C, Patte C, Ostronoff M, et al: Small noncleaved cell lymphoma and leukemia in adults: A retrospective study of 65 adults treated with the LMB pediatric protocols. Blood 1995;85:664–674.

322. Asselin B, Shuster J, Amylon M, et al: Improved event-free survival (EFS) with high dose methotrexate (HDM) in T-cell lymphoblastic leukemia (T-ALL) and advanced lymphoblastic lymphoma (T-NHL): A Pediatric Oncology Group (POG) study. Pediatr Oncol 2001;1464:367a.

323. Murphy SB: Pediatric lymphomas: Recent advances and commentary on Ki-1-positive anaplastic large-cell lymphomas of childhood. Ann Oncol 1994;5(suppl 1):S31–S33.

324. Brugieres L, Le Deley MC, Pacquement H, et al: Anaplastic large cell lymphoma in children: Analysis of 63 patients enrolled in two consecutive studies of the SFOP, SIOP XXIX. Med Pediatr Oncol 1997;29:357.

325. Laver JH, Mahmoud H, Pick TE, et al: Results of a randomized phase III trial in children and adolescents with advanced stage diffuse large cell non-Hodgkin's lymphoma: A Pediatric Oncology Group study. Leuk Lymphoma 2002;43:105–109.

326. Amylon MD, Shuster J, Pullen J, et al: Intensive high-dose asparaginase consolidation improves survival for pediatric patients with T cell acute lymphoblastic leukemia and advanced stage lymphoblastic lymphoma: A Pediatric Oncology Group study. Leukemia 1999;13:335–342.

327. Williams DM, Hobson R, Imeson J, et al: Anaplastic large cell lymphoma in childhood: Analysis of 72 patients treated on The United Kingdom Children's Cancer Study Group chemotherapy regimens. Br J Haematol 2002;117:812–820.

328. Abromowitch M, Sposto R, Perkins S, et al: Outcome of Children's Cancer Group (CCG) 5941: A pilot study for the treatment of newly diagnosed pediatric patients with disseminated lymphoblastic lymphoma. Proc ASCO 2000;19:583abst 2295.

329. Brugiéres L, Quartier P, Le Deley MC, et al: Relapses of childhood anaplastic large-cell lymphoma: Treatment results in a series of 41 children: A report from the French Society of Pediatric Oncology. Ann Oncol 2000;11:53–58.

330. Synold TW, Relling MV, Boyett JM, et al: Blast cell methotrexate-poly-glutamate accumulation in vivo differs by lineage, ploidy, and methotrexate dose in acute lymphoblastic leukemia. J Clin Invest 1994;94:1996–2001.

331. Korinsky NL, Sposto R, Shah NR et al: Outcomes of treatment of children and adolescents with recurrent non-Hodgkin's lymphoma and Hodgkin's disease with dexamethasone, etoposide, cisplatin, cytarabine, and L-asparaginase, maintenance chemotherapy, and transplantation: Children's Cancer Group Study CCG-5912. J Clin Oncol 2001;19:2390–2396.

332. Murphy SB, Hustu HO: A randomized trial of combined modality therapy of childhood non-Hodgkin's lymphoma. Cancer 1980;45:630–637.

333. Seidemann K, Tiemann M, Schrappe M, et al: Short-pulse B-non-Hodgkin lymphoma-type chemotherapy is efficacious treatment for pediatric anaplastic large cell lymphoma: A report of the Berlin-Frankfurt-Münster Group Trial NHL-BFM 90. Blood 2001;97:3699–3706.

334. Weinstein HJ, Cassady JR, Levey R: Long-term results of the APO protocol [vincristine, doxorubicin (Adriamycin) and prednisone] for treatment of mediastinal lymphoblastic lymphoma. J Clin Oncol 1983;1:537–541.

335. Asselin B, Shuster J, Amylon M, et al: Improved event-free survival (EFS) with high dose methotrexate (HDM) in T-cell lymphoblastic leukemia (T-ALL) and advanced lymphoblastic lymphoma (T-NHL): A Pediatric Oncology Group (POG) study. Proc Am Soc Oncol 2001;20:367abst 1464.

336. Pui C-H, Relling MV, Lascombes F, et al: Urate oxidase in prevention and treatment of hyperuricemia associated with lymphoid malignancies. Leukemia 1997;11:1813–1816.

337. Pui C-H, Mahmoud HH, Wiley JM, et al: Recombinant urate oxidase for the prophylaxis or treatment of hyperuricemia in patients with leukemia or lymphoma. J Clin Oncol 2001;19:697–704.

338. Haddy TB, Adde MA, McCalla J, et al: Late effects in long-term survivors of high-grade non-Hodgkin's lymphomas. J Clin Oncol 1998;16:2070–2079.

339. Lipshultz SE, Colan SD, Gelber RD, Perez-Atayde AR, Sallan SE, Sanders SP: Late cardiac effects of doxorubicin therapy for acute lymphoblastic leukemia in childhood. N Engl J Med 1991;324:808–815.

340. Sorensen K, Levitt G, Bull C, Chessells J, Sullivan I: Anthracycline dose in childhood acute lymphoblastic leukemia: Issues of early survival versus late cardiotoxicity. J Clin Oncol 1997;15:61–68.

341. Nysom K, Holm K, Lipsitz SR, et al: Relationship between cumulative anthracycline dose and late cardiotoxicity in childhood acute lymphoblastic leukemia. J Clin Oncol 1998;16:545–550.

342. Meistrich ML, Wilson G, Brown BW, da Cunha MF, Lipshultz LI: Impact of cyclophosphamide on long-term reduction in sperm count in men treated with combination chemotherapy for Ewing and soft tissue sarcomas. Cancer 1992;70:2703–2712.

343. Magrath I, Adde M, Sandlund J, Jain V: Ifosfamide in the treatment of high-grade recurrent non-Hodgkin's lymphomas. Hematol Oncol 1991;9:267–274.

344. Kung FH, Harris MB, Krischer JP: Ifosfamide/carboplatin/etoposide (ICE), an effective salvaging therapy for recurrent malignant non-Hodgkin lymphoma of childhood: A Pediatric Oncology Group phase II study. Med Pediatr Oncol 1999;32:225–226.

345. Philip T, Biron P, Philip I, et al: Massive therapy and autologous bone marrow transplantation in pediatric and young adults Burkitt's lymphoma (30 courses on 28 patients: a 5-year experience). Eur J Cancer Clin Oncol 1986;22:1015–1027.

346. Philip T, Armitage JO, Spitzer G, et al: High-dose therapy and autologous bone marrow transplantation after failure of conventional cheomtherapy in adults with intermediate-grade or high-grade non-Hodgkin's lymphoma. N Engl J Med 1987;316:1493–1498.

347. Philip T, Hartmann O, Biron P, et al: High-dose therapy and autologous bone marrow transplantation in partial remission after first-line induction therapy for diffuse non-Hodgkin's lymphoma. J Clin Oncol 1988;6:1118–1124.

348. Gordon BG, Warkentin PI, Weisenburger DD, et al: Bone marrow transplantation for peripheral T-cell lymphoma in children and adolescents. Blood 1992;80:2938–2942.

349. Bureo E, Ortega JJ, Muñoz A, et al: Bone marrow transplantation in 46 pediatric patents with non-Hodgkin's lymphoma. Bone Marrow Transplant 1995;15:353–359.

350. Avet Loiseau H, Hartmann O, Valteau D, et al: High-dose chemotherapy containing busulfan followed by bone marrow transplantation in 24 children with refractory or relapsed non-Hodgkin's lymphoma. Bone Marrow Transplant 1991;8:465–472.

351. O'Leary M, Ramsay NKC, Nesbit ME, et al: Bone marrow transplantation for non-Hodgkin's lymphoma in children and young adults. Am J Med 1983;74:497.

352. Ladenstein R, Pearce R, Hartmann O, et al: High-dose chemotherapy with autologous bone marrow rescue in children with poor-risk Burkitt's lymphoma: A report from the European Lymphoma Bone Marrow Transplantation Registry. Blood 1997;90:2921–2930.

353. Appelbaum FR, Deisseroth AB, Graw RG, et al: Prolonged complete remission following high-dose chemotherapy of Burkitt's lymphoma in relapse. Cancer 1978;41:1059–1063.

354. Sandlund JT, Bowman L, Heslop HE, et al: Intensive chemotherapy with hematopoietic stem-cell support for children with recurrent or refractory NHL. Cytotherapy 2002;4:253–258.

355. Pui C, Ribeiro RC, Hancock ML, et al: Acute myeloid leukemia in children treated with epipodophyllotoxins for acute lymphoblastic leukemia. N Engl J Med 1991;325:1682–1687.

356. Leung W, Sandlund JT, Hudson MM, et al: Second malignancy after treatment of childhood non-Hodgkin lymphoma. Cancer 2001;92:1959–1966.

357. Colombat P, Salles G, Brousse N, et al: Rituximab (anti-CD20 monoclonal antibody) as single first-line therapy for patients with follicular lymphoma with a low tumor burden: Clinical and molecular evaluation. Blood 2001;97:101–106.

358. Coiffier B, Haioun C, Ketterer N, et al: Rituximab (anti-CD20 monoclonal antibody) for the treatment of patients with relapsing or refractory aggressive lymphoma: A multicenter phase II study. Blood 1998;92:1927–1932.

359. Witzig TE, White CA, Gordon LI, et al: Safety of yttrium-90 ibritumomab tiuxetan radioimmunotherapy for relapsed low-grade, follicular, or transformed non-Hodgkin's lymphoma. J Clin Oncol 2003;21:1263–1270.

360. Wahl AF, Klussman K, Thompson JD, et al: The anti-CD30 monoclonal antibody SGN-30 promotes growth arrest and DNA fragmentation in vitro and affects antitumor activity in models of Hodgkin's disease. Cancer Res 2002;62:3736–3742.

361. Uckun FM, Reaman GH: Immunotoxins for treatment of leukemia and lymphoma. Leuk Lymphoma 1995;18:195–201.

362. Rooney CM, Smith CA, Ng CYC, et al: Use of virus-specific gene modified T lymphocytes to control Epstein-Barr virus-related lymphoproliferation. Lancet 1995;345:9–13.

363. McManaway ME, Neckers LM, Loke SL, et al: Tumour-specific inhibition of lymphoma growth by an antisense oligodeoxynucleotide. Lancet 1990;335:808–811.

364. Magrath IT: Prospects for the therapeutic use of antisense oligonucleotides in malignant lymphomas. Ann Oncol 1994;5(suppl 1):S67–S70.

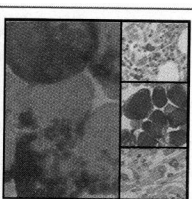

03

ACUTE LYMPHOID LEUKEMIA IN ADULTS

Hagop M. Kantarjian

Stefan Faderl

SUMMARY OF KEY POINTS

INCIDENCE

- Between 3000 and 4000 new cases of acute lymphoid leukemia (ALL) are diagnosed in the United States yearly; about two thirds of them are children.
- The overall incidence of ALL is 1 to 1.5 per 100,000 population but can range as high as four to five per 100,000 population from ages 2 to 4 and 2 per 100,000 population during its second peak among patients age 50 and older.
- ALL comprises 25% of all childhood cancers but represents only 20% of adult leukemias.

ETIOLOGY

- Associations of ALL with environmental, socioeconomic, infectious, and genetic events are being studied extensively, but few causal links have been established thus far.
- A higher incidence of ALL is observed among mono- and dizygotic twins and among patients with other inherited and congenital conditions such as trisomy 21 (Down syndrome).
- Among the more established viral etiologies of acute leukemias, HTLV-1 has been identified as the etiologic agent of adult T-cell leukemia/lymphoma (ATLL), while Epstein-Barr virus (EBV) is associated with mature B-cell ALL.

PATHOLOGY AND BIOLOGY

- The diagnostic work-up of ALL requires integration of French-American-British (FAB) criteria (morphology and cytochemistry) with immunophenotyping and identification of cytogenetic-molecular abnormalities.
- Immunophenotyping by flow cytometry has improved diagnostic accuracy vastly and makes it possible to distinguish B-lineage ALL from T-lineage ALL.

- In a minority of cases, mixed-lineage leukemias can originate from two distinct blast populations or from one blast population that coexpresses markers of more than one lineage.
- Recurrent cytogenetic-molecular abnormalities occur in most patients with ALL.
- Detection and further characterization of these abnormalities has become increasingly important for two reasons:
  1. Further dissection of molecular derangements will lead to a better understanding of pathogenetic pathways that are operative in ALL blasts.
  2. It has been clearly established that detection of these abnormalities has a direct impact on the prognosis of patients with ALL. Notably, poor-prognosis cytogenetic-molecular abnormalities that influence the clinical decision-making process include the presence of the Philadelphia translocation and cases with 11q23 rearrangements.

CLINICAL FINDINGS

- Most signs and symptoms of ALL are nonspecific and derive predominantly from those of anemia, thrombocytopenia, and neutropenia. Fatigue, lack of energy, dyspnea, dizziness, bleeding and easy bruisiability, and a history of recurrent infections are observed most frequently.
- Physical examination can reveal pallor and the presence of ecchymoses or petechiae.
- Lymphadenopathy and hepatosplenomegaly are rare and, if present, rarely symptomatic.
- Involvement of other extramedullary sites, such as the

central nervous system (CNS), is infrequent at presentation.

DIFFERENTIAL DIAGNOSIS

- Once the diagnosis of acute leukemia is established, the major challenge is to distinguish ALL from acute myeloid leukemias and other non-neoplastic conditions that are accompanied by lymphoid hyperplasia.
- Disorders with reactive lympho-cytosis, such as infectious mono-nucleosis, EBV, or cytomegalovirus (CMV) infections, can be confused with ALL, especially in children.
- Hematogones in regenerating bone marrows can sometimes be misdiagnosed as leukemic blasts.
- Metastatic small cell tumors in the bone marrow of adults also can resemble ALL and must be excluded by specific stains.

PRIMARY THERAPY OF ALL

- Current adult treatment regimens have been patterned after successful pediatric treatment programs and incorporate a multitude of drugs into regimen-specific sequences of increased dose and time intensity.
- The goal of therapy is rapid restoration of normal hematopoiesis using multiagent, dose-intense treatments, prevention of the emergence of resistant sublcones, adequate prophylaxis of sanctuary sites such as the CNS, and elimination of minimal residual disease.
- ALL therapy is typically divided into three phases: induction, consolidation, and maintenance therapy. Additional therapy for the CNS is required. Following current induction regimens, more than 80% of patients achieve a complete remission. Unlike children, however, only 30% to 40% of adults can be considered cured.

SUMMARY OF KEY POINTS—cont'd

- More intensive therapy in the form of stem cell transplantation is usually recommended for patients who have features of poor prognosis at presentation, notably the presence of cytogenetic abnormalities such as translocations t(9;22) or t(4;11).

SALVAGE THERAPY
- Outcomes of patients who relapse are unsatisfactory.
- Although complete resmissions can be obtained again in about 30% to 50% of the patients, long-term disease-free survival remains extremely poor. Stem cell transplantation should be pursued aggressively in this setting.
- New agents are continuously being assessed and are incorporated into new or existing salvage strategies.

PROGNOSIS
- The prognosis of adult patients with ALL has improved, especially among well-defined subtypes. Whereas patients with mature B-cell ALL and T-lineage leukemias did poorly in the past, current long-term disease-free survival rates are now superior even to patients with other forms of standard-risk ALL.
- Further dissection of ALL into subgroups based on distinct cytogenetic-molecular abnormalities will continue to refine risk-adapted treatment strategies and, it is hoped, improve outcomes for the majority of patients with ALL in the future.

INTRODUCTION

Acute lymphoid leukemia (ALL) results from a monoclonal proliferation and expansion of immature lymphoid cells in the bone marrow, peripheral blood, and other organs such as the lymph nodes, liver, spleen, or the central nervous system (CNS). Since the clinical picture of acute leukemias was first recognized about 150 years ago, much progress has been made in our understanding of the biology of ALL. The specificity of diagnosis, historically based on morphology and staining of bone marrow slides, now incorporates cytogenetic-molecular markers and, most recently, recognized distinct gene expression patterns in patient subgroups with ALL. We have therefore come to recognize ALL as a heterogeneous group of disorders that appear to be ever expanding as our knowledge of pathogenetic pathways on a molecular level increases.

Progress in the pathologic classification of ALL has therapeutic implications. Accurate definition of prognostic subgroups has permitted the institution of risk-oriented therapies. Adaptation of successful pediatric ALL treatment strategies to the therapeutic algorithms of adult ALL has resulted in response rates similar to those achieved in children. This improvement has been particularly evident in subgroups with mature B-cell ALL or ALL with T-cell immunophenotypes. Whereas almost 80% of children are now cured from ALL, however, only about 30% to 40% of adults achieve long-term disease-free survival. As will be discussed later in this chapter, intense clinical and laboratory research have attempted to close this gap and have focused on the following:

- Refinement of the basic treatment stratagem of induction, consolidation, and maintenance.
- Expansion of risk- and subgroup-oriented therapies.
- Definition of the role of stem cell transplantation in ALL.
- Quantification of residual disease, assessment of its impact on disease recurrence, and definition of its effect in clinical practice.
- Salvage strategies.
- Development of new drugs based on a clear understanding of disease pathogenesis, an example of which is the recent introduction of imatinib (STI571; Gleevec) for Philadelphia chromosome-positive leukemias.

EPIDEMIOLOGY

Acute leukemias are rare diseases. Among approximately 1,300,000 new cancer cases in the United States in 2001, only 13,500 were acute leukemias.[1] However small the proportion appears to be, acute leukemias disproportionately affect cancer survival statistics of adults and children and are among the leading causes of death in patients over age 35.[1] About 5000 new cases of ALL are diagnosed in the United States yearly; about two thirds of them are children.[2] ALL is the most frequently diagnosed childhood acute leukemia and constitutes 25% of childhood cancers. In contrast, adult ALL represents only 20% of adult leukemias and only 1% to 2% of all cancers combined. ALL has a bimodal distribution. Overall, 1 to 1.5 per 100,000 population will be diagnosed with ALL, and the incidence is as high as 4 to 5 persons per 100,000 population during the first peak between 2 to 4 years of age. Incidence rates then decrease during later childhood, adolescence, and young adulthood but manifest a second (albeit smaller) peak among patients older than 50 years; within this group, the incidence is approximately 2 per 100,000 population.

Among children, whites are affected more frequently than African Americans. Although there is little difference in incidence rates among children of either gender, ALL in patients older than 20 years is consistently more predominant among males. Although incidence rates for ALL remained stable worldwide for decades, a small and unexplained increase of cases diagnosed as ALL has been observed recently.[3]

ETIOLOGY

The phenotype of ALL is the result of cytogenetic-molecular alterations of the leukemic cell. The cause of these changes is unknown in most cases. Although associations with environmental, socioeconomic, infectious, and genetic events are being studied extensively, few causal links have been established thus far.[4]

A role for genetic factors in the etiology of ALL is suggested by several observations. The diagnosis of ALL in a monozygotic twin is associated with a 20% to 25% likelihood that the second twin will also develop ALL within 1 year.[5] Even among dizygotic siblings with acute leukemia, there is up to a fourfold higher risk of leukemia compared with the general population.[6,7] Based on the identification of concordant gene rearrangements in leukemic cells (but not in other somatic cell types) of infant twins with ALL, the possibility of intraplacental metastasis has been raised to explain the occurrence of leukemia in twins in some of these situations.[8] As ALL cases might cluster within families, however, it is not always possible to distinguish the etiologic impact of genetic factors from environmental ones.[9] The association of certain congenital and inherited conditions with ALL lends further weight to the influence of genetic abnormalities in the pathogenesis of ALL, as exemplified by patients with trisomy 21 (Down syndrome), the only autosomal trisomy compatible with survival beyond infancy.[10] Patients with trisomy 21 have a 20-fold higher risk than the general population of developing acute leukemias at any age.[11-14] Younger individuals with trisomy 21 are more likely to develop ALL than myeloid leukemias, and thus, these account for nearly 2% of childhood ALL cases. Other associations of ALL with genetic disorders include Klinefelter syndrome and inherited diseases with excessive chromosomal fragility, such as Fanconi's anemia, Bloom's syndrome, and ataxia-telangiectasia.[10,15-17]

Environmental factors also have been linked with a heightened risk of developing ALL. Exposure to radiation is among the most well-established etiologic factors in the development of acute leukemias. Although most frequently associated with acute myeloid leukemia (AML), cases of ALL associated with radiation have been reported and include survivors of the atomic bomb explosions, survivors of other nuclear exposures such as the Chernobyl accident, persons who were possibly exposed to therapeutic radiotherapy, and cases of in utero exposure.[18-21] Exposure to chemicals has also been related to an increased risk of ALL and might be more important than previously appreciated. Residence within 5 miles of an industrial site seems to predict for a higher risk of developing ALL.[22] Exposure to petroleum products—gasoline, diesel, and motor exhausts—was linked to an excess risk of acute leukemia in professional drivers, with an odds ratio of 5.0 for those exposed for longer than 5 years in their life time or longer than 1 year during the 5 to 20 years prior to the diagnosis.[23] Smoking has been found to increase the risk of ALL, particularly among patients older than 60 years who have a threefold higher risk of developing ALL compared with nonsmoking matched controls.[24] Use of hair dyes has been linked to the development of ALL, especially among persons exposed to hair dyes for more than 15 years.[25] A large case-control study conducted by the Children's Cancer Group found an association between maternal and paternal use of medication and the risk of ALL in offspring.[26] Whereas maternal use of vitamins and iron supplements was

associated with a decreased risk of ALL, paternal use of amphetamines, diet pills, and mind-altering drugs before and during the pregnancy was related to an increased risk of childhood ALL; the risk was higher if both parents were using these drugs. Employment in electrical occupations with exposure to electromagnetic fields has been associated with an increased risk of acute leukemias. In a case-control study including 110 leukemia cases and 199 controls in New Zealand, an odds ratio of 1.9 was found for subjects who had ever worked in an electrical occupation. Significantly increased risks for leukemia were seen in welders, flame cutters, and telephone line workers.[27]

Some epidemiologic data has suggested an increased incidence of ALL with higher socioeconomic status. This observation might relate to confounding variables such as better hygiene and less social contact in early infancy, and thus a differing exposure to infectious agents.[28] Other studies have established a link between the onset of ALL and seasonality, which could provide an indirect association with infectious etiologies.[29,30] In one study, a significant excess of winter births was found among infants diagnosed with acute leukemia.[29] In another study, significantly more ALL and de novo leukemias were diagnosed in the dark and cold compared with the light and warm period of the year, and also during influenza epidemics compared with nonepidemic periods.[30]

Among the more established viral etiologies in acute leukemias, retroviruses are associated with most of the known leukemia viruses in animals and might cause many neoplasms, including leukemia of mice and cats. A human retrovirus, HTLV-1, has been identified as the etiologic agent of adult T-cell leukemia/lymphoma (ATLL).[31] Epstein-Barr virus, a DNA virus causing infectious mononucleosis, is associated with Burkitt's lymphoma as well as with its leukemic counterpart, mature B-cell ALL, and is also found in many human immunodeficiency virus (HIV)-related lymphoproliferative disorders.[32] In addition to the link between seasonality and the diagnosis of ALL, further evidence for an infectious etiology could stem from the observation of increased rates of ALL among farming and slaughterhouse workers.[33,34] Although exposure to viruses such as bovine leukemia viruses is possible under these circumstances, other environmental hazards, such as exposure to pesticides, might be involved.

Secondary acute leukemias are predominantly myeloid in origin and evolve in patients with antecedent hematologic disorders or those with past exposure to chemotherapy agents (notably, alkylating agents and epidophyllotoxins) for treatment of other malignancies. Few cases of ALL have been described under similar circumstances, however. Translocation t(4;11)(q21;q23) has been demonstrated in ALL following treatment with topoisomerase II inhibitors up to 2 years after administration of the agents.[35] Cases of ALL in the context of other hematologic and solid tumors have been reported.[36-39]

PATHOLOGY

Since the early studies by Paul Ehrlich, assessment of morphology and cytochemical stains of bone marrow and peripheral blood smears have laid the foundations for the diagnosis and classification of ALL.[40] Although they remain essential components in the initial work-up of ALL to the present day, morphology and cytochemistry alone only crudely reflect the biologic heterogeneity of the disease and provide only limited prognostic information for stratifying patients to various treatments. Identification of distinct immunophenotypes and detection of cytogenetic-molecular abnormalities have contributed to a more complex view of the leukemic blasts in ALL and have made possible a more accurate assessment of several features of the disease:

- Lineage, differentiation, and stage of maturation of the leukemic cell within the sequence of its biological development.
- Identification of the genotype and cytogenetic-molecular abnormalities.
- Association of expression of cytogenetic-molecular markers with response to therapy and prognosis.

Current research is focused not only on extensive immunophenotyping and identification of cytogenetic-molecular abnormalities but also on genomic profiling that might lead to a better understanding of the complexity of ALL and to the identification of subgroups of patients with different treatment outcomes and prognosis. Such subgroups are not well discriminated by the diagnostic tools that are currently available.

Morphology and Cytochemistry—the FAB Classification

For all newly diagnosed cases of ALL, a bone marrow core biopsy with touch imprints and marrow aspirate clots should be obtained. The bone marrow is generally hypercellular and characterized by massive replacement of the marrow space by a homogenous-appearing population of leukemic blasts. Focal involvement of the bone marrow is rare in ALL but more common in AML. Hypoplastic ALL with significant marrow hypocellularity and increased numbers of lymphoblasts is infrequent.[41] Marrow necrosis with ALL is uncommon, can occur without a history of prior chemotherapy, can involve large areas of the marrow section, and might be associated with

pancytopenia, leukoerythroblastic anemia, and elevated serum lactate dehydrogenase and alkaline phosphatase values.[42-44]

Based on the lymphoblast morphology on Romanovsky stained smears, the French-American-British (FAB) Cooperative Group has recognized three distinct ALL subsets—L1, L2, and L3.[45] Distinguishing criteria include cell size, amount of cytoplasm, prominence of nucleoli, degree of cytoplasmic basophilia, and vacuolation (Fig. 103-1; Table 103-1). L1 Lymphoblasts are typically small (approximately twice the size of normal lymphocytes) and have a high nuclear-to-cytoplasmic ratio and inconspicuous nucleoli. The cytoplasm is sparse and variably basophilic. L2 lymphoblasts are larger and more pleomorphic and have moderately abundant cytoplasm, a lower nuclear-to-cytoplasmic ratio, and more prominent nucleoli.[46,47] L3 morphology is linked to a specific subgroup of patients with ALL. It has the same features as small noncleaved cell lymphoma and is typically associated with Burkitt's leukemia/lymphoma. L3 blasts are homogenous and medium sized, with dispersed chromatin and two to four prominent nucleoli. The cytoplasm is moderately abundant, with a deep blue cytoplasm and sharply defined vacuoles.

For ALL, unlike AML, no single cytochemical reactivity is uniquely specific. By definition, ALL blasts are negative for myeloperoxidase by cytochemistry and lack staining for the myeloperoxidase protein. AML is diagnosed if 3% or more of the blasts stain positive for myeloperoxidase. Low-level (3%–5%) expression of myeloperoxidase, however, has been described in rare cases that are otherwise unequivocally diagnosed as ALL and lack expression of other myeloid markers by flow cytometry.[48,49] Sudan black B stains the lipid membrane of the myeloperoxidase granule. Its reactivity patterns closely resembles that of myeloperoxidase itself, but lack of specificity and the ease with which myeloperoxidase stains can be applied has limited its use.[50] Terminal deoxynucleotidyl transferase (TdT) is a DNA polymerase that contributes to the heterogeneity of the recombinant event of immunoglobulins by inserting nucleotide sequences at splice sites required for the recombination of immunoglobulin and T-cell receptor genes.[51] Although TdT can be found in up to 20% of patients with AML and is thus not uniquely specific for

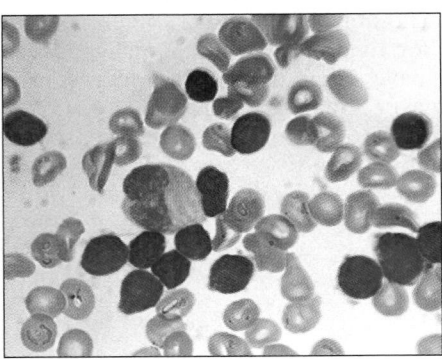
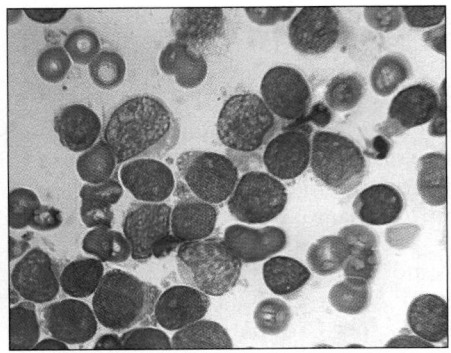
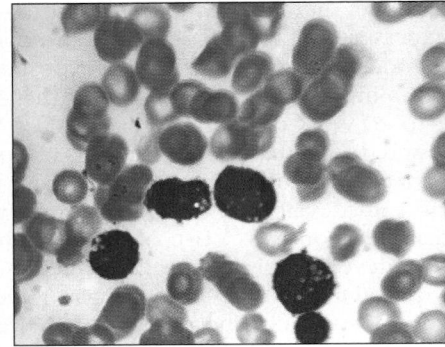

Figure 103-1. ALL cells by FAB classification.

TABLE 103-1

FAB Classification of ALL

FAB	MORPHOLOGY	SCORING CRITERIA	INCIDENCE (%)		CYTOCHEMISTRY			
			ADULTS	CHILDREN	MPO	NSE	PAS	AP
L1	Cells small in size and homogenous. Moderate basophilia. ↑ N/C ratio. Inconspicuous nucleoli.	↑ N/C ratio in > 75% of cells (+1) Nucleoli: 0–1 (small) (+1) Regular nuclear membrane Large cells < 50%	30	85	–	+/–	+	+
L2	Cells pleomorphic and often larger in size. ↓ N/C ratio. Abundant cytoplasm. Prominent nucleoli.	↓ N/C ratio in > 25% of cells (–1) Nucleoli: ≥ 1 (–1) Irregular nuclear membrane (–1) Large cells ≥ 50% (–2)	60	14	–	+/–	+	+
		Subtype **Score** L1 0 to 2 L2 –1 to –4						
L3	Cells homogenous of medium size with dispersed chromatin. Multiple nucleoli. Deep blue cytoplasm with sharply defined vacuoles.	N/A	10	1	–	–	–	–

AP, acid phosphatase; MPO, myeloperoxidase; N/A, not applicable; N/C, nuclear-to-cytoplasmic; NSE, nonspecific esterase; PAS, periodic acid-Schiff.

ALL, it is a useful marker to distinguish between reactive vs. malignant lymphocytosis, especially in cases with predominantly L1 morphology. L3 ALL is typically TdT-negative.[52-54] Periodic acid-Schiff (PAS) primarily identifies glycogen in blood cells. PAS staining patterns in ALL, referred to as "block" staining, result from disturbances in glycogen metabolism. Only around 10% of ALL blasts are strongly positive for PAS, however, and block PAS reactivity can also be seen in some cases of AML, especially erythroblastic leukemia. Reactivity for nonspecific esterase can be detected in some patients with ALL but is usually weaker than in cases of AML. Among cases of ALL, the acid phosphatase and α-naphthyl-acetate-esterase reactions are demonstrated in almost 80% of T-lineage ALL blasts, where (in contrast to non–T-cell ALL blasts) they exhibit a strong reaction in the Golgi region of the cytoplasm.

Although the FAB classification represents a milestone in the development of the classification of ALL, it is purely morphology-based and fails to integrate immunophenotypic differences and other novel biologic variables.[55] Neither the immunophenotype nor the presence or absence of cytogenetic-molecular abnormalities correlates well with L1 or L2 morphology. Even the morphologic distinction between L1/L2 and L3 might be obscured, as L1/L2 blasts might contain vacuoles and, conversely, L3 blasts might have very few vacuoles. Given current treatment modalities, no significant difference in prognosis exists between L1 and L2 varieties of ALL. Furthermore, the designation of L1 vs. L2 remains subjective; concordance rates among observers depend on the experience of the pathologist and factors such as the quality of the diagnostic slides. Unusual morphologic types of ALL that do not fit the FAB system are occasionally diagnosed—for example, ALL blasts with azurophilic granules (granular

ALL), or ALL with accompanying eosinophilia that closely resembles myeloproliferative syndromes in blast transformation.

Immunophenotype

Immunophenotype has improved the diagnostic accuracy of ALL. Immunophenotypic analysis by flow cytometry involves the use of monoclonal antibodies with high specificity for distinct epitopes of surface and intracellular antigens.[56] About 160 antigens have been identified and are grouped into so-called *clusters of differentiation* based on their reactivity with the same class of antibodies. Flow cytometry is a rapid and reliable method for diagnosis and for assessment of residual disease. Detection rates as high as 10^{-4} to 10^{-5} leukemic cells can be achieved with the help of multicolor immunofluorescence or fluorescence microscopy.[57,58]

Conventionally, any marker expressed in more than 20% of blasts is considered positive, whether the detection method involves indirect immunofluorescence, flow cytometry, or immunocyotchemical techniques. For markers with high specificity (such as anti-MPO, CD3, CD79, and TdT), the cutoff point is set to at least 10% blast positivity.[59-64]

Due to its ease of application, accuracy in diagnosis, and quantifiability of results, flow cytometry has become the preferred method for lineage assignment and analysis of maturation in ALL.[62] Multiparameter immunophenotype analysis has contributed substantial information to the diagnosis of ALL, to detection of aberrant antigen expression, and to analysis of the heterogeneity and clonality of the leukemic blasts. According to the patterns of normal expression of B, T, and myeloid markers, the most relevant antigen clusters for ALL diagnosis have been identified

Specific Malignancies

III

TABLE 103-2

Immunologic Markers Used in the Classification of ALL

B-LINEAGE	TDT	HLA-DR	CD34	CD19	CD22	CD79A	CD10	CYμ	CYκ/λ	SIGH	SIGL
Pro-B-ALL	✓	✓	✓	✓	✓	✓					
cALL (CALLA)	✓	✓		✓	✓		(✓)				
Pre-B-ALL	✓	✓		✓	✓		(✓)	✓			
Transitional pre-B-ALL	(✓)	✓		✓	✓					✓	
Mature B-ALL		✓			✓				(✓)	✓	✓

T-LINEAGE	TDT	HLA-DR	CD34	CYCD3	CD7	CD1A	CD2	CD5	SCD3
Pro-T-ALL	✓	(✓)	(✓)	✓	✓				
Pre-T-ALL	✓	(✓)	(✓)	✓	✓		✓	✓	
Cortical T-ALL	✓			✓	✓	✓	✓	✓	✓
Mature T-ALL	✓			✓	✓		✓	✓	✓

(Table 103-2).[65,66] A distinct lineage determination is possible in greater than 98% of the leukemic blasts. Although ALL can be divided into several immunophenotypically recognizable categories, the only distinction of clinical importance is among precursor B-cell, mature B-cell, and T-cell ALL. Identification of ALL subtypes rests on two broad types of antigen clusters:

1. Those that are maturation-specific in that their pattern of expression is restricted to earlier or more mature hematopoietic progenitors.
2. Those that indicate lineage commitment in that they allow distinction among B-, T-, and myeloid-lineage–associated blasts. Figure 103-2 provides an example for the diagnostic workup of ALL, integrating FAB criteria with immunophenotyping and cytogenetic-molecular abnormalities.

B-Lineage ALL

Four categories of B-lineage ALL have been established according to the degree of differentiation of the B lymphoblasts.[59]

Expression of CD19, CD79a, or CD22 with absence of any other B-cell differentiation antigen characterizes the most immature lineage association of ALL blasts and is referred to as *pre-pre-B-ALL* (or *pro-B-ALL*). It occurs with a frequency of 5% to 10% and is more common in adult ALL.[67] Expression of TdT, HLA-DR, and CD34 is found frequently on these early lymphoid progenitors. Although neither CD34 nor HLA-DR is lineage-specific, positive staining for either antigen favors the diagnosis of B-lineage ALL.[68,69] A sizable proportion of cases referred to in the past as *null ALL* or *non-B, non-T-ALL* express TdT and HLA-DR, but none of the more mature differentiation antigens such as CD10 or cytoplasmic immunoglobulins (cyIg).[70] Coexpression of early B-cell antigens such as CD19 or rearrangement of immunoglobulin heavy-chain genes confirms the lymphoid origin of these blasts. CD19-positive, CD10-negative, cyIg-negative B-lineage ALL is a common variant among infants with ALL, in which myeloid marker coexpression is frequent and in which a significant association exists with translocation t(4;11)

and MLL gene rearrangements, presentation with leukocytosis, massive hepatosplenomegaly, CNS disease, and poor response to therapy.[71]

Common ALL (cALL, early pre-B-ALL) is the most common ALL subtype, representing up to 70% of ALL cases in children and 40% to 50% in adults.[67] The immunophenotypic hallmark of cALL is expression of CD10 (common ALL antigen, CALLA), with or without expression of CD19 and usually without expression of markers that indicate more advanced maturation, such as cytoplasmic and surface immunoglobulins. Expression of CD10 is found in 80% to 90% of children between the ages of 1 and 9 years, but in only 40% to 50% of infants below 1 year of age and in adults.[72] It is also frequent in Philadelphia chromosome-positive ALL (50%), accounting for the worse prognosis of CD10-positive ALL in adults compared with children.

Expression of cytoplasmic immunoglobulins (pre-B-ALL) occurs in up to 10% of adults and 20% of children.[67] The blasts are somewhat more differentiated than in pre-pre-B-ALL.[73] Associations with higher hemoglobin levels and leukocyte counts have been described. Relatively more cases exhibit translocation t(1;19).[74] In children and adolescents (but not in adults), identification of this cytogenetic abnormality has been linked to a worse prognosis in pre-B-ALL than in pre-pre-B-ALL.[75]

Transitional pre-B-ALL is a rare subtype of ALL (about 1%) that expresses cytoplasmic and surface μ heavy chains but lacks surface light-chain expression.[76,77]

Mature B-cell ALL occurs in 5% of patients. It is distinguished by expression of surface immunoglobulins (sIg), by IgM in many cases, and by absence of staining for TdT. Mature B-cell ALL is associated with the FAB L3 subtype, although in some cases L1 or L2 morphology has been described.[78] Patients with mature B-cell ALL frequently present with lymphoma-like features; this presentation constitutes the leukemic phase of Burkitt's lymphoma. Patients tend to be older and are predominantly male, with a higher incidence of CNS disease and more frequent development of bulky abdominal and (particularly in children) testicular masses.[79] Characteristically, leukemic blasts demonstrate translocations

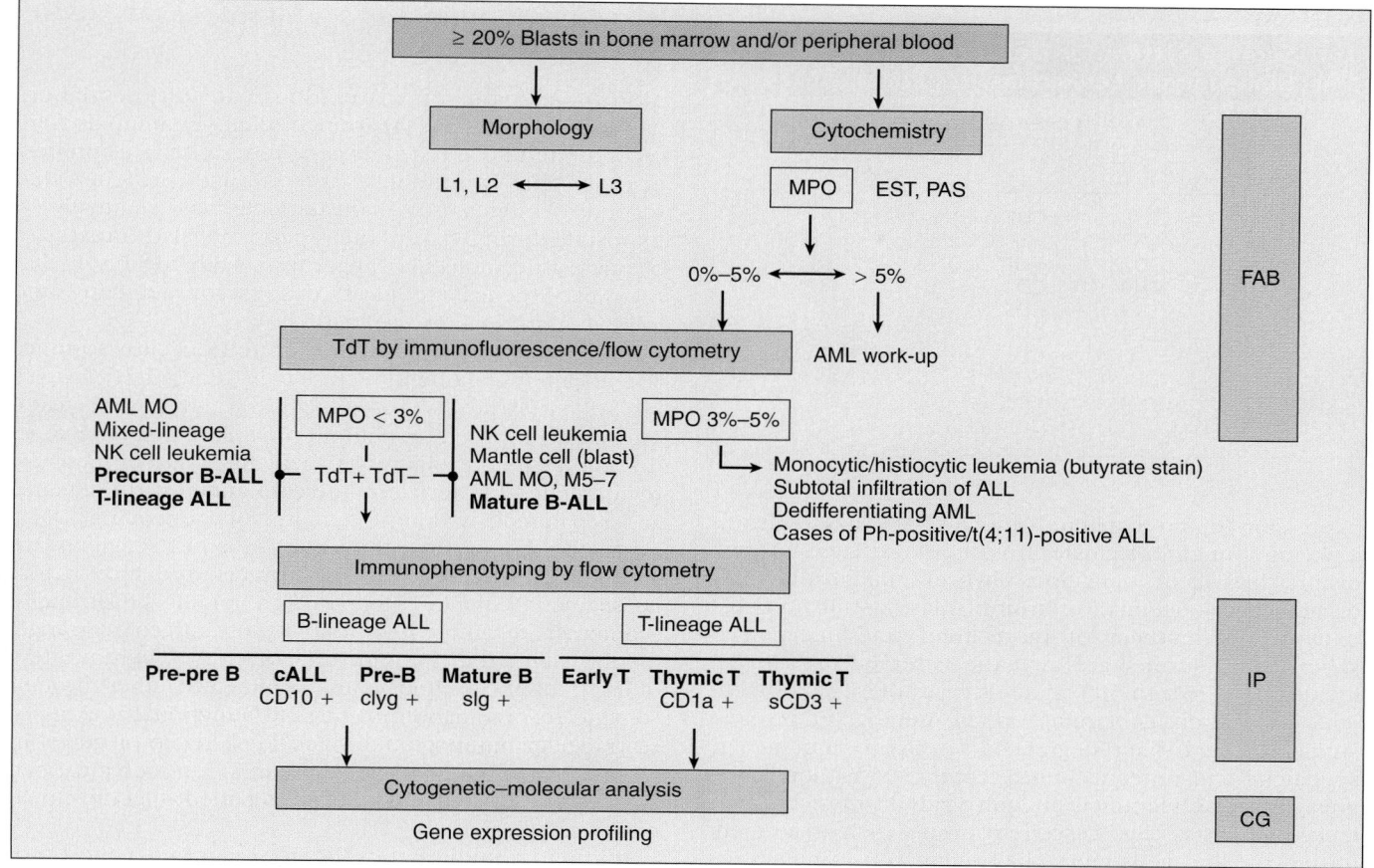

Figure 103-2. Diagnostic approach to patients with acute lymphoblastic leukemia (ALL). CG, cytogenetics; IP, immunophenotype; MPO, myeloperoxidase.

between the c-myc locus on chromosome 8q24 and one of the loci for the immunoglobulin heavy- or light-chain genes, including 14q32, 2p12, and 22q11.[80]

T-Lineage ALL

About 15% of ALL patients have a T-cell phenotype. The incidence is higher among adults than children and increases with age among children as well. Similar to B-lineage ALL, different T-lineage ALL (T-ALL) subtypes can be distinguished according to the stage of normal thymocyte development. Four subtypes are recognized in children, but only two subtypes are relevant for ALL in adults.[81] The early subtype is negative for expression of surface CD3 (sCD3) but stains positive for cytoplasmic CD3 (cCD3); CD4 and CD8 are either double-positive or double-negative; CD2 is negative. More mature subtypes of T-lineage ALL are positive for both sCD3 and cCD3, CD2, and either CD4 or CD8 but not both.[82] CD7 is the most sensitive T-cell marker but lacks specificity, as cases of AML or natural killer (NK)-cell leukemia are sometimes CD7-positive also. cCD3 is considered the most lineage-specific marker for T-cell differentiation. Expression of B-cell markers, such as CD10 and CD21, occurs in some cases.[83] At least in childhood T-lineage ALL, lack of CD10 expression has been linked with a worse prognosis. T-cell

ALL has been associated with male gender, older age, high leukocyte counts, extramedullary disease (e.g., CNS involvement), a higher tendency for testicular relapse, and development of mediastinal masses. Patients with mature T-cell immunophenotypes are more likely to present with lymphadenopathy, mediastinal mass, and thrombocytopenia.[84] In older studies, T-cell ALL in adults had a distinctly poor prognosis. With recent advances in treatment programs—possibly through the use of L-asparaginase, higher doses of ara-C, and cyclophosphamide—the remission rates are very high, and overall, survival surpasses that for other subtypes. Improvement in prognosis is particularly evident for mature T-cell ALL but not for pre-T-cell ALL.

Mixed-Lineage ALL

Although ALL lymphoblasts are considered malignant counterparts of normal lymphocytes in various stages of their maturation, pathways of antigen expression are frequently aberrant in the leukemic cells, leading to lineage infidelity. Infidelity of antigen expression includes expression of an antigen of the wrong lineage (such as expression of myeloid markers on blast cells that are morphologically lymphoblasts and that are negative for myeloperoxidase), the simultaneous expression of antigens of different stages of maturation, or the lack of

TABLE 103-3

	LINEAGE MARKER		
POINTS	**B**	**T**	**MYELOID**
2	CD79a	CD3 (s/cy)	MPO
	clgM	anti-TCR α/β	
	cCD22	anti-TCR γ/δ	
1	CD10	CD2	CD13
	CD19	CD5	CD33
	CD20	CD8	CD65s
		CD10	CD117 (c-kit)
0.5	TdT	TdT	CD14
	CD24	CD1a	CD15
		CD7	CD65

Scoring System for Definition of Biphenotypic Leukemias

expression of an expected antigen.[85,86] Mixed lineage leukemias might originate from the presence of two distinct blast cell populations (hybrid leukemia, biclonal or bilineage leukemia), or from a blast population that coexpresses markers of more than one lineage.[59,87] Whereas the former are rare, the latter occur with an incidence of 15% to 50% in adult cases of ALL and 5% to 35% in children, depending on the number of myeloid antigens tested, their degree of sensitivity and lineage specificity, and other technical factors.[88–90] Although the lineage can be identified unequivocally in most cases of leukemic blasts, a few cases remain in which assignment of the true lineage is more challenging. A scoring system has been developed for these circumstances, in which lineage-specific markers are weighed according to their discriminatory value of myeloid vs. lymphoid (Table 103-3).[59,91,92] Myeloid marker coexpression is more frequent in precursor B-cell ALL (40%–50%) than in T-lineage ALL (30%). Frequently coexpressed myeloid markers include CD13 and CD33, followed by CD14, CD15, and CDw65.[93–95] There is no association between myeloid marker expression and FAB group or karyotype except for a higher frequency with translocation t(9;22) and t(4;11).[88] Although earlier studies had shown a worse outcome for patients whose ALL blasts coexpressed myeloid markers, recent studies have not shown any prognostic significance with modern programs.[89,90,96–100]

WHO Classification of ALL

The World Health Organization (WHO) recently proposed new guidelines for the diagnosis of Neoplastic Diseases of Hematopoietic and Lymphoid Tissues or Lymphomas.[101] In addition to establishing a blast count of 20% or greater as sufficient for the diagnosis of ALL, the FAB classification into L1, L2, and L3 morphologies is abandoned as no longer relevant, as L1 and L2 morphology do not predict immunophenotype, genetic aberrations, or clinical behavior, and because L3 is typically associated with Burkitt's lymphoma in leukemic phase. Furthermore, the WHO classification strongly advocates including cytogenetics in the classification as prognostic factors within each subtype.

Immunoglobulin and T-Cell Receptor Gene Rearrangements

Along the path of maturation and differentiation, lymphoid precursors rearrange their immunoglobulin receptor and T-cell receptor gene repertoire. This process enables the lymphoblast to produce proteins that recognize antigens to which the cells will eventually be exposed during their life spans. It also creates a characteristic molecular fingerprint, with the result that rearranged genes are ideal markers for detecting and following residual disease in ALL.

Antigen receptor genes are located on chromosomes 14q32 (immunoglobulin heavy chain genes [IgH]), 14q11 (TCRα and TCRδ), 7q32–36 (TCRβ), and 7p15 (TCRγ). They are composed of multiple variable region (V) exons, diversity (D) and joining (J) segments, and constant (C) region genes. In their germline configuration, these genes are separated by long segments of noncoding DNA. Through recombinatorial events, V, D, and J segments are juxtaposed to one another in a precise order, by which DJ segments join first, followed by joining of DJ and V segments. The immense variability of antigen rearrangements results from combinatorial diversity, whereby a few of the pool of germline genes are joined together through somatic recombination events. The junctional regions of rearranged immunoglobulin and T-cell receptor genes in ALL are thus uniquely characteristic for an individual cell and its progeny and can be used as patient-specific clonal markers.[102,103]

Immunoglobulin and T-cell receptor genes are rearranged in ALL with high frequency in at least one locus. IgH genes are rearranged in almost all cases of pre-B-ALL, while immunoglobulin light genes are rearranged in about 50% (kappa) and 25% (lambda) of cases, respectively. Likewise, T-cell receptor genes are found to be rearranged in about 60% to 90% of cases of T-cell ALL.[104–106] The distinction between B-lineage and T-lineage ALL is sometimes difficult because of cross-lineage immunoglobulin and T-cell receptor gene rearrangements. TCRγ and –δ gene rearrangements have been described in up to 55% of patients with pre-B-ALL, and IgH gene rearrangements are observed in up to 15% of patients with T-lineage ALL.[104]

BIOLOGY

In childhood ALL, complete remission rates exceed 90%, and cure rates are attained in 70% to 80% of cases.[107] In adult ALL, even though complete remission rates are comparable, long-term survival is achieved in only 30% to 40% of cases. Many explanations for this phenomenon have been offered: older age and other medical problems, unfavorable distribution of prognostic factors in older patients (immunophenotype, elevation of the leukocyte count, response to induction chemotherapy, cytogenetic markers), different mechanisms of drug resistance and sensitivity to steroids, and lower tolerance to dose-intense chemotherapy programs. Most of the prognostic difference, however, is explained by different cytogenetic-

TABLE 103-4

Cytogenetic Abnormalities in Adult ALL

LINEAGE	KARYOTYPE	INVOLVED GENES	FREQUENCY (%)
B-lineage	t(9;22)(q34;q11)	BCR-ABL	15–30
	t(8;14)(q24;q32)	C-MYC/IgH	< 5
	t(8;22)(q24;q11)	C-MYC/Igλ	< 5
	t(2;8)(p12;q24)	Igk/C-MYC	< 5
	t(9;12)(p11-12;q11-13)	?	< 5
	t(4;11)(q21;q23)	MLL-AF1	< 5
	t(9;12)(Q34;P13)	ABL-TEL	< 5
	t(12;21)(p11-12;q22)	TEL-AML1	< 5
	i(17q)	?	7–9
	t(1;19)(q23;p13)	PBX1-E2A	< 5
	t(17;19)(q22;p13)	HLF-E2A	< 5
	i(21q)	?	< 5
T-lineage	del(9q(p21-22)	p16^{INK4a}/p14^{ARF}	7–15
	t(1;7)(p32;q35)	TAL1-TCR-β	< 5
	t(1;7)(p34;q34)	LCK-TCR-β	< 5
	t(7;9)(q34;q32)	TAL2-TCR-β	< 5
	t(7;10)(q35;q24)	Rhom2-TCR-β	< 5
	t(7;11)(q35;p13)	Rhom2-TCR-β	< 5
	t(1;14)(p32-34;q11)	TAL1-TCR-δ	20
	t(10;14)((q24;q11)	HOX11-TCR-δ	3–7
	t(11;14)(p13;q11)	RHOM2-TCR-δ	5–7
	Inv(14)(q11;q32.1)	RHOM1-TCR-δ	1

molecular abnormalities in adult-onset ALL compared with childhood ALL and by their effects on the pathogenesis of the leukemic cells—for example, cell cycle regulation, induction of programmed cell death (apoptosis), intracellular signaling pathways, or angiogenesis. Philadelphia chromosome-positive ALL, a disease that carries a very poor prognosis, occurs in 25% of adult ALL cases but in less than 5% of childhood ALL cases. The cryptic cytogenetic abnormality, translocation t(12;21), is detected molecularly in 25% of children but in fewer than 5% of adults. Children with *TEL* rearrangements have a cure rate of 90% vs. 60% among cases with other types of rearrangements. Hyperdiploid karyotype ALL (more than 50 chromosomes), a favorable ALL subtype, is found in 25% of children but in 5% of adults.

Recurrent cytogenetic abnormalities occur in up to 80% of children and 60% to 70% of adults (Table 103-4).[108] These discoveries have provided insights into the pathophysiology of ALL and its underlying molecular events, including the roles of fusion transcripts from translocations, tumor suppressor genes from deletions, or the control of cell cycle regulatory genes. Many of these defects have profound effects on proliferation, differentiation, maturation, and apoptosis of the hematopoietic progenitor cells. In addition, clinically distinct subsets of ALL can now be identified based on molecular abnormalities and have effects on prognosis and on the choice of therapy for an increasing number of patients.

Numerical Chromosome Abnormalities

Numerical abnormalities denote gains or losses of individual chromosomes. Among hyperdiploid ALL types, two groups are usually distinguished: those with 47 to 51

chromosomes and those with more than 51 (high hyperdiploid) chromosomes. Hyperdiploidy of more than 50 chromosomes is associated with a good prognosis and an event-free survival of 80% at 5 years and is particularly favorable among children with an additional chromosome 4, 6, 10, or 17.[108-111] Gain of chromosome 5 and isochromosome i(17)(q10), on the other hand, have been linked to a less favorable prognosis.[112] Hyperdiploidy is commonly associated with favorable prognostic features and pre-B-cell surface markers. Hyperdiploid leukemic cell clones accumulate methotrexate polyglutamates more easily and are more sensitive to the effects of mercaptopurine, L-asparaginase, thioguanine, and cytarabine.[113] Some studies indicate more stringent growth requirements and more rapid induction of apoptosis in hyperdiploid vs. nonhyperdiploid ALL blasts, which could explain their higher sensitivity to antileukemic agents.[114] The association with favorable outcome is weaker in adult ALL, in which hyperdiploidy is frequently linked to poor-prognosis karyotypes, different paths of drug accumulation or resistance, and possibly different sensitivities to activation of apoptosis. Leukemic blasts with less than 46 chromosomes are referred to as hypodiploid. Hypodiploid blasts are found in 4% to 9% of adults with ALL. Hypodiploidy is frequently associated with other structural abnormalities, but the influence of these defects on prognosis is unknown. Cases with 23 to 29 chromosomes (near-haploid) have a poor prognosis independent of other variables such as age, gender, and leukocytosis.[115]

Structural Chromosomal Abnormalities

Structural chromosomal abnormalities are described in up to 70% of patients with ALL. Their incidence varies by immunophenotype and age.[108] Most of the more than 30 identified recurring karyotype abnormalities are usually found in less than 2% to 5% of patients, but some stand out in terms of either higher incidence or prognostic significance. The most important structural cytogenetic abnormalities are discussed in the sections that follow.

t(9;22)(q34;q11)—the Philadelphia Chromosome

The Philadelphia (Ph) chromosome results from a reciprocal translocation between the long arms of chromosomes 9 and 22. It is the most common cytogenetic-molecular abnormality in adult ALL, with a frequency of 15% to 30%.[108] At the molecular level, the translocation moves a large segment of the *ABL* gene from 9q34 into one of several breakpoint cluster regions of the *BCR* gene on chromosome 22q11. The chimeric *BCR-ABL* gene is then translated into hybrid BCR-ABL oncoproteins of different molecular weights, depending on the exact location of the breakpoint area in the *BCR* gene.[116] The breakpoint location along the *ABL* gene is fairly constant (usually just upstream of exon a2). Several breakpoint locations have been identified on BCR. The first breakpoint identified is located between exons 12 and 16 (also referred to as b1 to b5) and is called the *major breakpoint cluster region* (M-BCR). Involvement of M-BCR results in a *BCR-ABL* fusion gene with a b2a2 or b2a3 junction. The fusion mRNA is translated into a chimeric protein of 210 kDa (p210$^{BCR-ABL}$). Whereas p210$^{BCR-ABL}$ is typically found in chronic myeloid leukemia (CML), a shorter version predominates in Ph-positive ALL. In about 60% of adults and 80% of children with the Ph translocation, the breakpoint on *BCR* is upstream of M-BCR, adjacent to exon e1, and is called the *minor breakpoint cluster region* (m-BCR).[117,118] Transposition of *ABL* sequences into m-BCR generates a more truncated version of *BCR-ABL*, which translates into a smaller protein of 190 kDa, p190$^{BCR-ABL}$. Both fusion proteins are characterized by deregulated and abnormally increased tyrosine kinase activity located in the SH1 domain of the ABL part of the fusion gene, leading to the involvement of downstream signaling pathways which, in turn, eventually result in abnormal gene expression and expression of the leukemic phenotype. Patients with t(9;22) are usually older and frequently have higher white blood cell and blast counts at diagnosis than patients with normal karyotypes.[119] A pre-B-cell immunophenotype and expression of CD10 and myeloid markers such as CD13 and CD33 are typically associated with the t(9;22) translocation. Additional chromosomal abnormalities are described in 40% to 80% of patients and include, in decreasing frequency:

- Monosomy 7
- An additional Philadelphia chromosome
- 9p abnormalities
- Trisomy 8
- Hyperdiploidy[120,121]

Variant and complex Philadelphia translocations and novel BCR-ABL transcripts with unusual breakpoints have been described. The prognostic significance of additional abnormalities is unclear. Overall, the presence of Ph is associated with a poor prognosis. Clarification of the molecular events triggered by the Ph translocation and of the way in which these events influence intracellular signaling pathways has resulted in new and targeted therapies, such as imatinib mesylate (to be discussed shortly).

Abnormalities of 9p

Abnormalities of the short arm of chromosome 9 (in particular 9p21) occur in up to 15% of ALL cases.[122] Most abnormalities of 9p21 result in deletions. The cyclin-dependent kinase inhibitor (CDKI) molecules p16^{INK4a}/p14^{ARF} and p15^{INK4b} have been localized to chromosome 9p21, and deletions of these genes, rather than silencing of gene expression by hypermethylation, appear to be their major mode of inactivation.[123] The main target is the p16^{INK4a} gene. When analyzed by fluorescence in situ hybridization (FISH) or molecular tools, deletions of p16^{INK4a} have been described in up to 80% of children with T-ALL and in 20% of children with pre-B-ALL, more frequently than by conventional karyotype analysis. Anomalies of 9p21 are associated with other clonal abnormalities in almost 90% of patients, suggesting that abnormalities of 9p21 are secondary cytogenetic events.[121] In some cases, chromosome 9 has been involved in the formation of dicentric chromosomes—namely, with chromosome 12 and 20, which leads to deletions of 9p. Usually, FISH with centromeric and/or whole chromosome painting probes is required to detect these aberrations, as they frequently remain undetected by conventional cytogenetic studies.[124] Patients with 9p21 abnormalities are a prognostically heterogeneous group. Deletions of 9p are an adverse risk factor in B-lineage (but not T-cell) ALL; exceptions include homozygous deletions, which are associated with a significantly poorer survival in T-cell ALL as well.[125] Prognostic associations are usually stronger in children and are less clear in adult ALL.[126-128]

11q23 Rearrangements

The common denominator of abnormalities of 11q23 is involvement of the mixed-lineage leukemia gene *MLL* (previously known as *ALL-1*, *HRX*, or *HTRX1*). More than 20 chromosomal loci are known to participate in reciprocal rearrangements with 11q23, including 4q21, 9p22, 19p13, and 1p32.[129,130] The most common translocation involving 11q23 is t(4;11)(q21;23). It is specifically associated with ALL in infants, accounting for up to 85% of such cases, and it is found in 3% to 8% of adults.[120,129] Similar to patients with t(9;22), adults with this translocation tend to be older and have higher white blood cell counts and organomegaly; sanctuary sites such as the CNS are involved. The immunophenotype is pre-pre-B-ALL and is positive for TdT, HLA-DR, CD19, and variably negative for CD10. Myeloid antigen coexpression is common. The prognosis of adults with 11q23 rearrangements remains poor, and allogeneic stem cell transplantation (SCT) in first remission is currently the treatment of choice.[131]

Abnormalities Involving 19p13

The two known translocations involving 19p13 are t(1;19)(q23;p13) and its rare variant, t(17;19)(q21;p13). Translocation t(1;19) has a strong association with pre-B-ALL phenotype expressing cytoplasmic immunoglobulin.[132] Its overall frequency is approximately 5% in childhood ALL and 25% in pre-B-cell ALL. A rare variant of t(1;19)-positive ALL is seen in early childhood cases of pre-pre-B-cell ALL with lack of expression of cytoplasmic immunoglobulins. This abnormality is less common in adult ALL (3%).[133] The translocation juxtaposes the *E2A* gene on chromosome 19 with homeobox-containing gene *PBX1* to generate the *E2A-PBX1* fusion gene. It functions as a potent transcriptional activator and transforms a variety of cell types in vitro, including fibroblasts, myeloid progenitors, and lymphoblasts.[133] Patients with ALL who express *E2A-PBX1* do poorly with standard or less aggressive therapy but have a better prognosis with more aggressive approaches. In contrast to the unfavorable prognosis of patients with pre-B-ALL and t(1;19), patients with pre-pre-B-ALL and t(1;19) have a better prognosis.[134]

Translocation t(12;21)

Translocation t(12;21) is largely undetectable by routine cytogenetics and for this reason was considered rare (2%–3%) until recently. Application of more sensitive molecular tools (polymerase chain reaction [PCR]) has identified this translocation in up to 30% of children with ALL, making it the most frequently recurring cytogenetic-molecular abnormality in pediatric ALL. It remains rare in adults (1%–3%).[135,136] The translocation involves *TEL* (or *ETV6*), a transcription-regulating gene of the Ets family of transcription factors on 12p11, and *AML1* on 21q22, forming a *TEL-AML1* fusion gene.[137] The outcome of patients with a *TEL-AML1* fusion is favorable in children with pre-B-ALL, independent of age or white blood cell count at presentation. One study, however, suggested that the favorable outcome was due to exclusion of patients with other poor-risk cytogenetic abnormalities and to the younger ages of these patients compared with patients having normal karyotypes.[121] Translocation t(12;21) could be associated with late relapses.[138,139] Due to its rarity, its prognostic significance is undetermined in adults.

Translocation t(8;14) and Its Variants

Translocation t(8;14)(q24;q32) and its less common variants t(8;22)(q24;q11) and t(2;8)(p12;q24) are characteristic of mature B-cell ALL. Mature B-cell ALL represents the leukemic phase of Burkitt's lymphoma and accounts for 5% of all cases of ALL in children or adults.[108] Patients with mature B-cell ALL present with bulky extramedullary disease, frequent and early CNS involvement, and, unless treatment is instituted rapidly, a relentlessly progressive clinical course due to an unusually high blast cell proliferative rate. The translocations involving 8q24 lead to rearrangement and inappropriate overexpression of the proto-oncogene *C-MYC* at that location. In 80% of the cases, band 8q24 is juxtaposed to the immunoglobulin heavy-chain (IgH) gene locus on 14q32, whereas the Ig lamba gene locus on 22q11 is involved in 15% of cases, and the Ig kappa gene locus on 2p12 is involved in 5% of cases.[140] All three translocations result in deregulation, increased transcription, and overexpression of *C-MYC* leading to uncontrolled cell proliferation. In about 30% of cases, 8q24 rearrangements are the single defining karyotype abnormality. Additional recurrent genetic aberrations include t(14;18), t(11;14); translocations of *BCL-6* on chromosome 3q27; deletions and rearrangements of 1q11-26 and 6q; and trisomy 7, 8, 12, and 18. The increased frequency of chromosome 6q abnormalities suggests that this locus might harbor an important tumor suppressor gene.[141-144] The diagnosis of mature B-cell ALL was long associated with a poor prognosis; however, the introduction of short-term dose-intensive regimens has improved clinical outcomes significantly, with long-term disease-free survival occurring in up to 50% to 80% of patients.[145]

T-Cell Receptor Gene Rearrangements

Unlike the high frequency of recurrent translocations in B-lineage ALL, only about 30% of T-cell ALL cases feature chromosomal translocations.[108] Among them, T-cell receptor (TCR) gene rearrangements are the most common. They involve chromosome 14q11 (TCR-α and -δ genes), 7q32-36 (TCR-β), and 7p15 (TCR-γ).[146] The β-chain locus on 7q32-36 is less frequently rearranged than the α–δ chain locus on 14q. Rearrangements of TCR-γ on 7q15 are very infrequent. T-cell ALL is characterized by male gender, increased age in children, and leukocytosis at presentation. The clinical course is usually aggressive, and the prognosis used to be poor. With current dose-intensive induction/consolidation regimens and incorporation of higher doses of ara-C and cyclophosphamide, however, the outcome for patients has improved

dramatically. Although no specific cytogenetic abnormality can be linked to a specific clinical subtype of T-cell ALL, a number of distinct chromosomal translocations have been identified (see Table 103-4).

Gene Expression Profiling in ALL

The current approach to the diagnosis of ALL includes an extensive range of procedures—morphology, immunophenotyping, karyotype analysis, and assays for the detection of molecular abnormalities. The information thus obtained has made it possible to dissect ALL into a cluster of subtypes, each with a unique biological behavior and a different therapeutic outcome. A large part of the success in treatment, especially in cases of pediatric ALL, has been achieved by recognizing ALL as a heterogeneous disease and using risk-adapted therapies, which means tailoring the intensity of treatment to each patient's risk of relapse.[146] Assignment of risk accounts for a number of clinical and laboratory parameters, but cytogenetic-molecular alterations are emerging as the defining prognostic features in ALL.[147] The development of oligonucleotide microarray technology has made it possible to quantify the expression of thousands of individual genes simultaneously and thus establish a gene expression profile in well-defined subgroups of patients. This development will have a profound impact on both future definitions of disease subtypes and approaches to therapy. The major goals of gene expression profiling in ALL are as follows:

1. Definition of lineage affiliation and, by extension, of distinct molecular subtypes that might defy current classification schemes.
2. Association of gene expression with chromosomal abnormalities, including the possibility of identifying cases with cryptic translocations.
3. Identification of genetic alterations that underlie the pathogenesis of individual leukemia subypes.
4. Detection of gene expression clusters that characterize patients with distinct responses to therapy, thus providing prognostic information.
5. Establishment of gene expression clusters in relapse and those associated with development of secondary myeloid leukemias.

Most progress to date with the integration of DNA microarray technology into diagnostic procedures of ALL has been achieved in childhood ALL. Using oligonucleotide microarrays targeting 12,600 genes, Yeoh and collaborators[146] analyzed the pattern of gene expression in leukemic blasts from 360 children with ALL. They identified a characteristic gene expression signature composed of a large number of individual genes for ALL blasts with T-cell lineage, hyperdiploid chromosome sets (> 50), *BCR-ABL*, *E2A-PBX1*, *TEL-AML1*, and *MLL* gene rearrangements. The differentially expressed genes predicted for each leukemia subtype with high accuracy. The assignment of leukemic samples to a specific biologic subgroup was more distinctly reflected by its gene expression profile than by identification of the molecular abnormality per se, and the differences in expression among individual

ALL subtypes were even more robust than among various types of epithelial cancers. Identification of novel subtypes of ALL outside cytogenetically recognizable subgroups, development of genetic expression profiling to monitor minimal residual disease, and detection of expression profiles that might indicate underlying mechanisms of relapse or transformation are further steps in the development of this technique for clinical use. The dissection of human T-cell leukemias by gene expression profiling has generated further insights into the deregulation of oncogenes as a central motif of leukemogenesis.[148] Recurrent chromosomal abnormalities and intrachromosomal rearrangements in T-cell ALL typically result in the juxtaposition of strong promoter and enhancer elements of TCR genes next to a small number of developmentally important transcription factor genes, including *HOX11*, *TAL1*, and *LYL1*. Several gene expression signatures have recently been identified that were related to specific stages of thymocyte development. *HOX11* clusters correlating with early cortical thymocytes were found to be associated with a favorable prognosis, whereas expression of *TAL1* (late cortical thymocyte) and *LYL1* (pro-T-cell ALL) groups conferred a worse prognosis.

In this way, gene expression analysis using oligonucleotide or cDNA microarrays is being established as a viable alternative to conventional karyotyping and FISH in the diagnosis of leukemia subtypes, and to recognize previously unrecognized molecular subtypes of ALL.[149] Further applications will include comparisons of gene expression profiles of adults with ALL with those of children with ALL, as within the same recurrent translocation (e.g., Ph abnormality), adults fare much worse than children. New therapies targeting specific molecular abnormalities that have been identified recently could increase the effectiveness of current therapies.

CLINICAL PRESENTATION AND EVALUATION OF THE PATIENT WITH ALL

Clinical Manifestations

The onset of clinical manifestations can be acute or insidious. Most symptoms derive from expansion of the leukemic clone in the medullary space, involvement of the peripheral blood and extramedullary sites such as lymph nodes, liver, spleen, and the CNS, and suppression of normal hematopoiesis. Presenting signs and symptoms are dominated by anemia, thrombocytopenia, fever, and neutropenia. Fatigue, lack of energy, dyspnea, dizziness, bleeding and easy bruisiability, and infections are common. Among children, extremity and joint pain are frequent complaints at diagnosis. The most frequent findings on physical examination are pallor and ecchymoses or petechiae. Lymphadenopathy and hepatosplenomegaly are rarely symptomatic.[150] Involvement of other extramedullary sites, such as skin, testicles, kidneys, joints, and bones, is infrequent.[151,152] CNS involvement at diagnosis occurs in less than 10% of patients and can

present with cranial nerve deficiencies (especially cranial nerves VI, III, IV, and VII) leading to double vision, abnormal ocular movements, facial dysesthesias, and facial droop.[153] CNS involvement is especially frequent in mature B-cell ALL (50%–60%); chin numbness due to mental nerve involvement is also common when the patient is solicited about this symptom. About 10% of patients, especially those with T-lineage ALL, present with a mediastinal mass on chest x-ray, which, if sufficiently enlarged, can give rise to stridor and wheezing, pericardial effusions, and superior vena cava syndrome.[154-156] Patients with a diagnosis of mature B-cell ALL typically present with signs and symptoms of a rapidly proliferating tumor and metabolic hyperactivation, including profound constitutional symptoms, weight loss, and often large abdominal and (mainly in children) testicular masses leading to obstructive hydronephrosis with renal insufficiency in some cases.[157,158] Involvement of the gastrointestinal tract under these circumstances is frequent and can cause additional problems, such as bleeding or rupture.

Evaluation of the Patient

The main goal of the initial workup is threefold:

1. To establish the correct diagnosis.
2. To assess carefully the function of vital organs and apprehend potential complications.
3. To assign patients to appropriate treatment.

In addition to the complex, disease-specific workup, which includes a thorough bone marrow evaluation, immunophenotyping, karyotype analysis, and molecular diagnosis, the evaluation of the patient will focus on the integrity of the cardiovascular, pulmonary, renal, and hepatic systems.[150] Table 103-5 summarizes the essential components of the workup of a patient with ALL.

Differential Diagnosis

The major challenge in making the diagnosis of ALL is to distinguish it from myeloid leukemias and to separate if from non-neoplastic conditions that are accompanied by lymphoid hyperplasia (Table 103-6). In the presence of prominent lymphadenopathy, other forms of non-Hodgkin's lymphoma should be considered. The distinctions between T-cell ALL and lymphoblastic lymphoma and between mature B-cell ALL and Burkitt's lymphoma or small noncleaved cell lymphoma are mostly semantic, and the treatments for these conditions are nearly identical. If the lymphoid blast count is less than 25% in the marrow at the time of diagnosis, the lymphoma diagnosis is usually preferred.[45,159]

Disorders with reactive lymphocytosis, such as infectious mononucleosis, Epstein-Barr virus (EBV), or cytomegalovirus (CMV) infections can be confused with ALL, especially in children.[160] Marrow samples with increased numbers of lymphocyte progenitor cells (hematogones) are found in a number of disease processes, including iron deficiency, congenital neutropenia, red blood cell aplasia, or immune thrombocytopenia (ITP) and can sometimes give the appearance of involvement of the marrow with

TABLE 103-5

Components of the Work-up of a Patient with ALL

History	Symptoms of cytopenias (anemia, thrombocytopenia, neutropenia)
	Recurrent infectious episodes
	Prior malignancy or treatment with chemotherapy
	Prior radiation therapy
	Exposure to environemental toxins and pollutants
	Tobacco use
	Family history of ALL
Physical examination	Vital sign assessment
	Lymphadenopathy, hepatosplenomegaly
	Skin infiltrations
	Ecchymoses and petechiae
	Abdominal or testicular masses
	Neurological assessment
Laboratory testing	CBC with differential and platelet count
	Chemistry profile (liver, renal, uric acid, lactic dehydrogenase, electrolytes)
	Coagulation profile (PT, PTT, fibrinogen, D-dimers)
	HLA-typing
	Bone marrow aspirate and biopsy for morphology, cytochemical stains, immunophenotyping, chromosome analysis, FISH, PCR for t(9;22), other molecular studies
Imaging studies	Chest x-ray
	Echocardiogram/Gated cardiac scan and/or EKG (if clinically indicated)

leukemic lymphoblasts. Increased lymphoid progenitor cells are also found frequently in regenerating marrows following chemotherapy for ALL.[161,162] Other hematologic and nonhematologic conditions must sometimes be excluded. Among the latter, metastatic small cell tumors in the bone marrow, such as those from neuroblastomas, embryonal rhabdomyosarcoma, retinoblastoma, Ewing sarcoma, medulloblastoma, or small cell carcinoma in adults, can resemble ALL.[163]

TABLE 103-6

Differential Diagnosis of ALL

Reactive lymphocytosis
 Infectious mononucleosis
 CMV
 EBV
Autoimmune diseases
Hypoplastic anemias
Hematogones
 Iron deficiency anemia
 ITP
 Regenerating bone marrow
Hematologic malignancies
 Acute myeloid leukemia
 Non–Hodgkin's lymphomas
Metastatic small cell tumors
 Neuroblastoma
 Retinoblastoma
 Medulloblastoma
 Embryonal rhabdomyosarcoma

CMV, cytomegalovirus; EBV, Epstein-Barr virus; ITP, idiopathic thrombocytopenic purpura.

PROGNOSIS

Prognostic factors assign patients to well-defined risk groups and to risk-adapted therapies that avoid both under- and overtreatment. Advances in ALL therapy have changed the risk assignment of some subgroups. Whereas the complete remission (CR) rate in T-lineage ALL was 40% to 60% and the expected disease-free survival (DFS) was less than 10%, recent treatment regimens incorporating cyclophosphamide and cytarabine have increased CR rates to 80% and DFS rates to 50%. Likewise, patients with mature B-cell ALL had a similarly dismal outcome in the past. The introduction of short-term, dose-intense treatment regimens in mature B-cell ALL have improved the CR rates from 50% to more than 80% and have improved the long-term DFS from 10% to greater than 50%. Thus, some clinical, laboratory, or biological variables thought to be useful prognostic predictors now have little value, as the treatment for patients with ALL has improved dramatically over the last two decades.[145,164,165] Other prognostic variables can be explained by superceding genetic-molecular abnormalities that are recognized increasingly as powerful predictors of outcome.[108]

Persistent adverse prognostic features include older age, elevated white blood cell (WBC) count at presentation, delayed response to therapy, specific cytogenetic abnormalities, and—with some limitations—immunophenotype.

There is a continuous decrease of CR rates with increasing age, starting from 95% in children to 40% to 60% in patients older than 60 years of age.[166] The prognostic significance is due partly to decreased tolerance to intensive induction/consolidation regimens in older patients, but it is mostly due to biologic differences [higher incidence of poor-prognosis cytogenetic abnormalities, e.g., Ph-positive ALL; lower incidence of favorable karyotypes, e.g., hypderdiploidy, t(12;21)] and to differences in drug metabolism and cellular pharmacokinetics).[167,168]

Like age, leukocyte count at presentation is a reliable predictor of CR rate and duration. The cutoff point varies between 5×10^9/L to 100×10^9/L, depending on the study and whether age is incorporated as a poor-prognosis factor into the particular model.[2] An inverse relationship between age and leukocytosis has been suggested, and a higher leukocyte cutoff point is used if age is factored into the prognostic model. In general, the critical level of leukocyte elevation is between 25 and 35×10^9/L, similar to what has been defined for childhood ALL.[169] An exception is T-lineage ALL, in which a higher WBC at diagnosis is typically observed, and in which a cutoff point of 100×10^9/L is more predictive of relapse than are lower levels.

The rapidity of clearance of blasts and reconstitution of normal hematopoiesis correlates inversely with duration of remission.[170] Patients who respond within 4 to 5 weeks after one course of induction have a superior DFS.[169] Time to platelet recovery is a sensitive marker of marrow recovery and a reliable predictor of outcome, even within the group of patients carrying translocation t(9;22).[171] Clearance of peripheral blasts by day 7 and of marrow blasts by day 14 both correlate with improved prognosis in childhood and adult ALL.

Distinct cytogenetic-molecular subgroups show clinical differences in response to therapy and prognosis. The most important ones are t(9;22), 11q23 rearrangements, t(1;19), t(8;14) and variants, t(12;21), and, possibly, abnormalities of the short arm of chromosome 9. Rearrangements involving chromosome band 14q11-13 are associated with T-lineage ALL and with an excellent prognosis using conventional multiagent regimens.[108]

Immunophenotype has become less relevant since the introduction of contemporary dose-intensive multiagent treatment regimens, but differences in response to therapy and outcome still exist in some immunophenotypic subtypes.[97] In a GMALL (German ALL study group) study, patients with early and mature T-cell ALL had an inferior DFS of less than 30% compared with patients with cortical T-cell ALL, who achieved a DFS of greater than 50%.[172] Similarly, among B-lineage ALL, pre-pre-B-ALL (pro-ALL) has been associated with a poor outcome in children and in adults.[173]

In current prognostic models of adult ALL, up to 75% of patients are considered poor risk with an expected DFS of 25%, and only one quarter constitute good-risk patients with a projected DFS of greater than 50%. Thus, most adults are still considered high-risk patients when compared with children. Several variables have been identified recently to predict prognosis. The dynamics of blast clearance in response to steroids, assessed within 1 to 2 weeks, have prognostic value in adults also.[174] Markers of drug resistance, such as expression of MDR-1, were reported to be prognostic by the Italian GIMEMA group.[175] Finally, assessment of minimal residual disease is emerging as a highly important new prognostic factor for relapse risk in individual patients and will be discussed shortly.

PRIMARY THERAPY FOR ALL

The treatment of ALL has witnessed an astonishing metamorphosis—from the use of a relatively small number of agents to the design of ever more complex treatment schemes that incorporate multiple drugs into regimen-specific sequences of increased dose- and time-intensity (Table 103-7).[165,174,176-185] This has led to one of the most remarkable success stories in cancer medicine—namely, a cure rate of greater than 80% for children with ALL—and the creation of a template after which current adult programs are patterned. ALL is rare, and the increasing complexities associated with its therapy emphasize the role of specialized tertiary care centers that can deliver high-dose intensity treatment with minimal mortality and maximum supportive care. Refining treatment further mandates an integrated treatment approach that includes stem cell transplantation and risk-adapted therapies based on emergence of novel prognostic markers such as cytogenetic-molecular abnormalities.

Chemotherapy

The goal of chemotherapy treatment is rapid restoration of normal hematopoiesis using multiagent, dose-intense treatments; prevention of the emergence of resistant subclones; adequate prophylaxis of sanctuary sites, such as the CNS; and elimination of minimal residual disease through postremission consolidation strategies. Therapy is thus divided into several phases. Induction aims at achieving CR, defined as recovery of normal hematopoiesis and reduction of bone marrow blasts to less than 5% in a normocellular marrow. Postremission therapy is divided into consolidation, intensification, and maintenance phases. CNS prophylaxis is part of both induction and postremission therapy.

Induction

Vincristine and corticosteroids (previously prednisone, more recently dexamethasone) form the backbone of ALL induction therapy. These two drugs achieve CR rates of 40% to 65%, but the median remission duration is only 3 to 7 months. Incorporation of anthracyclines has increased the CR rate to 72% to 92% and improved the median remission duration to around 18 months.[186] The combination of vincristine-anthracycline-steroids now constitutes the standard regimen for remission induction.[187,188] Although daunorubicin has been used most frequently in this combination, both doxorubicin and daunorubicin have produced similar results. Dexamethasone has been substituted for prednisone based on better in vitro antileukemic activity and achievement of higher drug levels in the cerebrospinal fluid (CSF). Although in a randomized childhood ALL study conducted by the EORTC, the rate of CNS relapse was significantly reduced with dexamethasone compared with prednisone, dexamethasone was associated with an increased risk of septicemia and fungal infections.[189,190] Intensification with preparations of asparaginase, cyclophosphamide, cytarabine, and other agents have been the next steps in the evolution of induction regimens. Given the already high CR rates of up to 90%, it has been difficult to demonstrate further improvements of remission induction. Intensification of induction, however, could have a positive effect on the duratin of remission and survival time. Specific immunophenotypic subtypes have benefited from additional drugs during induction; for example, T-lineage ALL with ara-C and cyclophosphamide and mature B-cell ALL with fractionated doses of cyclophosphamide. Methotrexate for treatment of childhood ALL has resulted in improved 9-year survival, improved disease-free survival, and lower rates of CNS relapse.

The role of cyclophosphamide during remission induction has been studied in several trials. The GIMEMA ALL 0288 study randomized 778 patients to induction with a four-drug combination of vincristine, daunorubicin, L-asparaginase, and prednisone alone or with cyclophosphamide.[174] No difference between the two randomized induction arms was found with respect to CR rates, overall survival, and rates of continuous complete remissions. The CALGB (8811) used a five-drug induction regimen with cyclophosphamide as a single dose on day 1 and L-asparaginase in addition to the combination of vincristine, daunorubicin, and prednisone.[165] The overall CR rate in 197 patients was 85%. The CR rate was 94% in patients younger than 30 years and 100% in those

TABLE 103-7

Results of Chemotherapy Studies in Adult ALL

STUDY	YEAR	N	AGE, YRS. (MEDIAN, RANGE)	CR (%)	IM (%)	PROGNOSIS	COMMENTS
Annino et al.[174]	2002	794	27.5 (12–59.9)	82	7	2 yrs. (median DFS)	The study had three objectives: (1) influence of prednisone pretreatment on CR; (2) impact of addition of cyclophosphamide to induction; and (3) impact of post-CR intensification on CR duration.
Linker et al.[183]	2002	84	27 (18–59)	93	NA	48% at 5 yrs. (EFS)	Intensified and shortened cyclical chemotherapy followed by maitense. 5-yr. EFS 63% in patients ≤30 yrs. of age.
Goekbuget et al.[198]	2001	1200	35 (15–65)	86	5	47% at 5 yrs. (OS)	The goal of this study was to improve outcome by intensification of induction and consolidation and application of a risk-adapted strategy.
Bassan et al.*	2001	121	35 (unknown)	84		49% at 3 yrs. (LFS)	Application of risk-oriented postremission strategies, role of anthracyclines in standard risk ALL, and role of SCT in high-risk ALL.
Dekker et al.†	2001	193	33 (15–60)	82	NA	35% at 5 yrs. (DFS)	Study evaluates role of auto-SCT vs allo-SCT as postinduction treatment for ALL.
Kantarjian et al.[179]	2000	203	39.5 (16–79)	91	6	39% at 5 yrs. (survival)	Study establishes superior activity of dose-intensive regimen to previous regimens, such as VAD.
Thiebault et al.[233]	2000	572	33 (15–60)	76	9	27% at 10 yrs. (survival)	LALA87 trial assessing role of allogeneic and autologous SCT in postremission therapy of ALL.
Rowe et al.[227]	1999	920	29 (14–60)	89	4.5	39% at 3 yrs. (EFS)	Study examines role of allogeneic SCT as postremission consolidation vs chemotherapy/autologous SCT. 3-yr. EFS in allogeneic SCT group was 58%.
Hallbook et al.‡	1999	120	44 (16–82)	85	5	36% at 3 yrs. (CCR)	Induction course included high-dose ara-C. Patients with standard risk continued with 2.5 yrs. of maintenance. High-risk patients are referred for SCT.
Todeschini et al.[185]	1998	60	34 (14–71)	93	5	55% at 6yrs. (EFS)	Regimen characterized by inclusion of high-dose daunorubicin in induction and high-dose ara-C in postremission.
Ribera et al.[199]	1998	108	28 (15–74)	86	5	41% at 5 yrs. (LFS)	Late intensification chemotherapy has not improved results.
Larson et al.[197]	1998	198	35 (16–83)	82	8	23 mos median survival	G-CSF during induction increases CR rate but not overall survival.
Durrant et al.[184]	1997	618	>15	88	9	28% at 5 yrs.	Intensification of ALL therapy may increase DFS; however, compliance with intensification is poor.
Larson et al.[165]	1995	197	32 (16–80)	85	9	36 mos median survival	Intensive chemotherapy regimen produces high rate of remissions and durable responses in adults with ALL.
Gökbuget et al.[176]	1993§	569	27 (15–65)	75	< 10	39% at 7 yrs. (CCR)	Consolidation therapy with teniposide and cytarabine is feasible and improves outcome for patients with high-risk ALL.
Hussein et al.[181]	1989	168	28 (15–85)	68	17	17.7 mos median survival	
GIMEMA[182]	1989	358	31 (15–64)	79	7	21.7 mos median survival	

CCR, continued complete remission; CR, complete remission; DFS, disease-free survival; EFS, event-free survival; G-CSF, granulocyte colony-stimulating factor; IM, induction mortality; LFS, leukemia-free survival; OS, overall survival; SCT, stem cell transplantation; VAD, vincristine, adriamycin, dexamethasone.
*Bassan R, Pogliani E, Casula P, et al: Risk-oriented postremission strategies in adult acute lymphoblastic leukemia: Prospective confirmation of anthracycline activity in standard-risk class and role of hematoiopoietic stem cell transplants in high-risk groups. Hematology J 2001;2:117.
†Dekker AW, van't Veer MB, van der Holt B, et al: Postremission treatment with autologous stem cell transplantation (Auto-SCT) or allogeneic stem cell transplantation (Allo-SCT) in adults with acute lymphoblastic leukemia (ALL). A phase II clinical trial (HOVON 18 ALL). Blood 2001;98:859a.
‡Hallbook H, Simonsson B, Bjorkholm M, et al: High dose ara-C as upfront therapy for adult patients with acute lymphoblastic leukemia (ALL). Blood 1999;94:297a.
§Reference from 2000.

who presented with a mediastinal mass or blasts with a T-cell immunophenotype. The hyper-CVAD regimen has reported a CR rate of 91% using hyperfractionated cyclophosphamide.[179] This regimen proved superior in CR rate and survival when compared with induction with vincristine, dexamethasone, and doxorubicin only.

Inclusion of L-asparaginase has been shown to improve the CR rate in children with ALL when it is added to vincristine and prednisone, and to prolong DFS when given during consolidation. Its usefulness in adult ALL is less clear, as many regimens consist of a combination of L-asparaginase with anthracyclines and cyclophosphamide. Linker and colleagues[191] induced 109 patients with adult ALL with a four-drug combination of vincristine, prednisone, daunorubicin, and L-asparaginase, which was also part of further consolidation cycles. The CR rate of 88% and 5-year DFS survival rate of 42% are in accordance with results from comparable studies. In one randomized trial of L-asparaginase in induction therapy, intensification of induction might have contributed to a longer duration of remission, although CR rate was not improved.[192]

As it appears unlikely that further variations of vincristine, prednisone, and anthracyclin-based induction regimens will lead to improved results, some investigators have suggested an intensive induction regimen consisting of high-dose cytarabine with a single high dose of mitoxantrone. In a phase II study of 37 patients, induction treatment with cytarabine at a dose of 3 g/m^2/day for 5 days and mitoxantrone at a dose of 80 mg/m^2 given once on day 3 with G-CSF support has achieved a CR rate of 84%, maintaining an induction mortality of less than 10%.[193] The impact of omission of the traditional "backbone" drugs in favor of a high-dose cyarabine induction on remission duration, overall survival, and response of ALL subtypes remains to be determined.

Based on retrospective studies showing that daunorubicin dose-intensity during induction was an independent prognostic factor in adult ALL, Todeschini and associates designed a regimen with high doses of daunorubicin (total of 270 mg/m^2) during induction and with high-dose cytarabine during consolidation.[185] The CR rate was 93%, the induction mortality was 8%, and the 6-year event-free survival was 55% in 60 patients with adult ALL. A larger Italian cooperative study is ongoing to confirm these results. High doses of liposomal daunorubicin (daunoxome) during induction might achieve the same goals with lower rates of cardiotoxicity and mucositis.

Other agents, such as mitoxantrone, etoposide, teniposide, and m-amsacrine, have also been studied.[194] No further benefit, at least in terms of CR rate, has been established, and their value for improvement of remission quality is largely untested. Intensifying induction has led to more rapid cytoreduction and more profound myelosuppression. In this context, the use of hematopoietic growth factors has become increasingly important.[195,196] Rapid recovery of bone marrow function following chemotherapy is a prerequisite to propitious administration of dose-intense treatment regimens. In a double-blinded, randomized trial (CALGB 9111), the use of G-CSF during induction was associated with faster neutrophil recovery to greater than 1×10^9/L ($p < .0001$), faster platelet recovery, and reduction in the duration of hospital stay ($p = .02$).[197] In addition, the CR rate was higher for patients who received G-CSF (90% vs. 81%; $p=.10$), an effect that was even more pronounced among elderly patients. Induction mortality was also improved, both overall and among elderly patients. Induction mortality was also reduced overall, with a higher-than-expected proportion of deaths in the placebo group compared with the G-CSF treated group (11% vs. 4%, $p=.04$) and among patients 60 years of age or older (25% vs. 10%, $p=.24$). Use of G-CSF during induction and consolidation has not, however, been shown to prolong either remission duration or overall survival.

Consolidation

The purpose of consolidation therapy is to eradicate subclinical disease in CR. It includes rotational consolidation programs, repetition of a modified induction treatment, and, in some cases, stem cell transplantation. It is difficult to assess the value of individual components of consolidation approaches, as the number, schedule, and combination of cytostatic drugs vary considerably between studies. The overall strategy of intensive therapy, however—including high-dose methotrexate and high-dose cytarabine—is beneficial, as established in various randomized studies and compared with historical data. Future strategies will address subtype- and risk-oriented approaches to consolidation programs.

The hyper-CVAD program by the M.D. Anderson group is a dose-intensive regimen with alternating hyperfractionated cyclophosphamide therapy and high doses of cytarabine and methotrexate.[179] Compared with the earlier and less intense VAD program, CR rate (91% versus 75%, $p<.01$) and survival ($p<.01$) have been superior with hyper-CVAD.

In CALGB study 8811, patients underwent early and late intensification courses with eight drugs following a five-drug induction regimen.[165] A prolonged maintenance therapy then continued until 2 years after diagnosis. The median remission duration was 29 months and the median survival 36 months, both of which are considerably better than the outcome observed with earlier, less intense trials.

In the MRC UKALL XA, patients were randomized to receive early intensification at 5 weeks, late intensification at 20 weeks, both, or neither.[184] The trial showed that the early block of intensive treatment prevented relapses, although DFS at 5 years was increased only slightly. The study highlights the question of the degree of intensification necessary to improve survival, as the toxicity in the MRC study was low, with only six deaths in remission related to the intensive block.

The German multicenter trial of May 1993 increased the intensity and combinations of consolidation therapy in a subtype-specific manner as follows:[198]

- High-dose methotrexate in standard risk B-lineage ALL
- Cyclophosphamide and cytarabine in T-lineage ALL
- High-dose methotrexate and high-dose cytarabine in high-risk B-lineage ALL

Risk factors included translocation t(9;22)/BCR-ABL and t(4;11)/ALL1-AF4, pre-pre-B-ALL, white blood cell count $\geq 30 \times 10^9$/L, and time to CR of 4 weeks or greater. For high-risk patients, intensified induction with high-dose cytarabine ($3 \text{ g/m}^2 \times 4$ doses) and mitoxantrone was administered instead of the phase II induction. Standard-risk patients achieved a CR rate of 87% with a long median remission duration of 57 months and a 5-year survival probability of 55%. Intensified induction/consolidation, however, did not improve CR rate and DFS in high-risk patients, with the exception of pre-pre-B-ALL cases, in which a continuous CR rate of 41% (compared with 19% in other high-risk patients) was achieved.

Two randomized studies have evaluated the value of intensified consolidation therapy. The GIMEMA study randomized patients to an early post-CR intensification or to maintenance therapy.[174] Of 388 patients, 201 had maintenance alone, whereas 187 received consolidation followed by maintenance. Intensification of post-CR treatment did not show any influence on continuous CR rate. At 8 years, 36% of patients on consolidation-maintenance and 37% of patients on maintenance remained in CR. Furthermore, only 35% of the patients who were randomized to the intensified consolidation completed their treatment within the expected time frame, raising doubts about the feasibility of prolonged intensified consolidation in adults because of toxicities and compliance problems. In the PETHEMA ALL-89 trial, patients in remission at the end of the first year were randomized to receive one 6-week cycle of late intensification therapy.[199] There was no difference in survival and DFS between patients who did and who did not receive late intensification.

Maintenance

Maintenance therapy consists of 6-mercaptopurine and methotrexate, usually augmented by monthly pulses of vincristine and prednisone. Although clearly effective, its biological rationale remains obscure. Continuous presence of the antimetabolites might be necessary to kill slowly dividing leukemia cells that reenter the cell cycle, or modulation of the host immune system might be necessary to suppress leukemic cell growth and allow apoptosis to occur.[200] Maintenance therapy typically extends over 2 to 3 years. Prolongation of maintenance therapy beyond 3 years has not shown any additional benefits. Omission of maintenance therapy altogether has been associated with significantly shorter DFS rates.[194,201,202] No clear advantage has been demonstrated for patients treated with intensified maintenance programs compared with conventional maintenance doses, an observation that has led some investigators to revisit shorter maintenance strategies.[203] In T-cell ALL, the benefit of maintenance chemotherapy has also been questioned. As accumulation of higher intracellular concentrations of the active metabolites of 6-mecaptopurine and methotrexate have been associated with improved clinical outcome, administration of this combination to the limits of tolerance (as reflected in low leukocyte counts) should be pursued.[204] No maintenance therapy is usually given in mature B-cell ALL, as these patients respond well to short-term, dose-intense regimens and because relapses after 1 year in remission are rare. Standard maintenance is probably not beneficial for patients with Philadelphia chromosome-positive ALL, for whom stem cell transplantation or novel strategies with targeted therapies such as imatinib mesylate probably offer better chances for improving DFS rates.

Central Nervous System Prophylaxis

Central nervous system (CNS) prophylaxis is essential in any therapeutic regimen for ALL. The CNS is a common sanctuary for ALL cells. At time of diagnosis, the incidence of CNS disease is less than 10% but increases to 50% to 75% after 1 year in the absence of CNS-directed therapy.[169,179,205-207] CNS involvement by ALL may result in cranial neuropathies and symptoms associated with increased intracranial pressure, including headaches, nausea and vomiting, lethargy, visual blurring, irritability, and nuchal rigidity. The diagnosis of CNS leukemia requires the presence of more than five WBCs per microliter in the cerebrospinal fluid (CSF) and unequivocal identification of lymphoblasts in the CSF differential.[208] The presence of blasts in a CSF sample with less than five WBCs per microliter might still signify CNS disease.[209] During maintenance therapy, the appearance of blasts and fewer than five WBCs per microliter in the CSF of children with intermediate-risk ALL in complete bone marrow remission has been associated with earlier CNS relapse. False-negative CSF results can occur in cases with predominantly cranial nerve involvement.

The value of CNS prophylaxis has been established in a randomized trial of 62 evaluable patients, in which CNS prophylaxis with cranial irradiation and intrathecal (IT) methotrexate was compared with no CNS prophylaxis.[210] With CNS prophylaxis, the rate of CNS relapse was 11%; without CNS prophylaxis, it was 32%. With current CNS prophylaxis, the incidence of CNS disease is usually less than 10%. Effective means of CNS prophylaxis include IT chemotherapy (methotrexate, cytarabine, steroids), high-dose systemic chemotherapy (methotrexate, cytarabine, L-asparaginase), and craniospinal irradiation (18–24 Gy).[153] The best results are probably achieved with IT prophylaxis and high-dose systemic chemotherapy. The role of cranial XRT (radiation therapy) has become controversial. Prophylaxis can result in neurological adverse events, including seizures, dementia, intellectual dysfunction, and other complications, particularly growth retardation in children. Complications of XRT could be more common in children. Several reports have identified risk factors for the development of CNS leukemia.[211,212] Among children, a higher incidence of CNS disease has been described in infants, and with high leukocyte counts, T-lineage and mature B-cell ALL, lymphadenopathy, thrombocytopenia, hepatomegaly, and splenomegaly. In a multivariate analysis in adults, mature B-cell ALL, serum lactate dehydrogenase (LDH) levels, and a high proportion of bone marrow cells in a proliferative state (more than 14% of cells in S+G2M phase of the cell cycle) had independent prognostic value and were used to determine the intensity of CNS prophylaxis.[213] In children with low-risk ALL, IT chemotherapy alone can prevent CNS disease effectively, with relapse rates of less than 5% in most studies.[107] In intermediate-risk patients, the combination of IT chemotherapy with either high-dose systemic chemotherapy or low doses of CNS irradiation (12 Gy) have achieved similar results, with CNS disease-free survival rates of greater than 90%.[214,215] Cranial irradiation at higher doses is used most frequently for high-risk patients.[214] CNS prophylaxis in adult trials includes cranial irradiation in some studies but not in others. A recently published analysis of several nonradiation approaches for CNS prophylaxis has suggested that effective CNS prophylaxis can be achieved with a combination of IT chemotherapy and high-dose systemic chemotherapy without cranial irradiation, even in patients with high risk for CNS disease.[207] For patients with low risk for CNS leukemia, high-dose systemic chemotherapy improved the 5-year CNS event-free rate from 65% (with no prophylaxis) to 85% (p=.05). Patients with high risk for CNS leukemia had a 5-year CNS event-free rate of 28% with no prophylaxis, 67% with high-dose systemic chemotherapy, 70% with high-dose systemic chemotherapy and late IT chemotherapy (at CR), but 98% for patients receiving high-dose systemic chemotherapy and IT chemotherapy starting early during the induction phase. In general, a risk-adapted approach should be developed to minimize risks and optimize efficacy.[213] Based on the experience with the hyper-CVAD regimen of the MD Anderson group, CNS prophylaxis (in addition to systemic high-dose chemotherapy) consists of four intrathecal treatments for patients in the low-risk category (based on a normal LDH and low proliferative index), eight intrathecal treatments for patients with high-risk disease, and 16 intrathecal treatments for patients with mature B-cell ALL or Burkitt's disease. Patients with cranial nerve root involvement might benefit from selective irradiation to the base of the skull.

Stem Cell Transplantation

Stem cell transplantation (SCT) from marrow and peripheral stem cells is essential for consolidation treatment, especially for patients with high-risk ALL. SCT enables delivery of high doses of chemotherapy with or without radiotherapy and provides immunology-based antileukemia activity through graft-vs.-leukemia (GVL) effect.[216,217] In a retrospective analysis of 267 patients with ALL who were in first remission, significantly fewer relapses were seen among patients who developed acute and chronic graft-vs.-host disease (GVHD), a phenomenon that highlights the role of the GVL effect.[218] Autologous transplants, transplants from alternative donor sources (matched unrelated donor SCT, haplotype transplantations, umbilical cord SCT), and reduced-intensity regimens (nonmyeloablative SCT or mini-SCT) are increasingly being investigated.[219]

Allogeneic Sibling Stem Cell Transplantation

Success of SCT in relapsed and refractory ALL led researchers to explore it in first remission. Survival in adult ALL with allogeneic SCT from related donors in first CR is around 50% (range, 20%–81%).[220-222] The wide range observed is due to patient selection. Typically, patients referred for SCT are younger and lack significant comorbidities. Other factors, such as ALL phenotype, sex mismatch, CMV status at time of transplant, and the type of GVHD prophylaxis influence transplant outcome. Several studies have tried to compare outcomes of SCT vs. chemotherapy among patients with ALL in first CR.

In a large French multicenter trial (LALA 87), allogeneic SCT was compared with chemotherapy or autologous SCT in first CR.[223] Of 257 randomized patients, 116 were allocated to allogeneic SCT and 114 to the control group (chemotherapy and autologous SCT). The 5-year survival rates between both arms were not significantly different

(48% vs. 35%, p=.08). When patients with high-risk ALL were considered, however, the 5-year overall survival (44% vs. 20%, p=.03) and 5-year disease-free survival (39% vs. 14%, p=.01) were more favorable in the allogeneic SCT group compared with the control group. The study concluded that allogeneic SCT in first CR does not improve survival in patients with standard-risk ALL but should be recommended for patients with adverse prognostic features.

In a similarly designed Spanish multicenter trial (PETHEMA ALL-93), patients were genetically randomized to receive allogeneic SCT in first CR if a sibling donor was identified, or to autologous SCT or further consolidation therapy followed by maintenance treatment.[224] No differences were found in CR rate, 5-year event-free survival, and overall survival except for patients with Ph-positive ALL, in whom CR rate, event-free survival, and overall survival were significantly lower than for the remaining patients. It is not clear from these preliminary data whether allogeneic SCT specifically benefited patients with Ph-positive ALL.

The International Bone Marrow Transplant Registry (IBMTR) compared the efficacy of intensive postremission chemotherapy in 484 patients with allogeneic SCT in 251 patients for whom a matched related sibling donor could be identified. After adjustments for differences in disease characteristics and time to treatment, the 9-year DFS rates were 32% for chemotherapy and 34% for allogeneic SCT.[225] The causes of treatment failure were different for the two groups: Actuarial relapse probabilities at 9 years were 66% for chemotherapy but only 30% for transplantation, and treatment-related mortality was the main cause of failure in transplanted patients.[226]

In the international ALL trial (MRC UKALL XII/ECOG E2993), all patients received two phases of induction therapy and were then assigned in CR to allogeneic SCT if they had histocompatible donors.[227] The remaining patients received either standard consolidation/maintenance for another 2.5 years or a single autologous SCT. Early results have been presented for 173 patients receiving allogeneic SCT and 426 patients who were eligible for randomization. The 3-year overall survival was 60% for the allogeneic group and 48% for the randomized group. In the standard-risk group, the 3-year survival was 75% with allogeneic SCT treatment and 67% for the randomized group. The rates were 58% and 38%, respectively, for high-risk patients (mainly defined by the presence of the Philadelphia chromosome). Contrary to most other studies, the data suggested that allogeneic SCT was beneficial for patients in first CR irrespective of risk group. Overall results and comparison of autologous SCT and chemotherapy from this trial are not yet available, however.

Currently, it is accepted that allogeneic SCT offers a definite advantage over chemotherapy in high-risk ALL, which is defined by the presence of unfavorable cytogenetic abnormalities [e.g., Ph-positive and t(4;11)]. Most adults (70%) cannot be allocated to SCT because of lack of a matched related sibling, comorbidities, or severe infections. Thus, an objective and unbiased comparison among treatments is difficult.[219]

Allogeneic SCT is the treatment of choice for patients with refractory and relapsed ALL or with ALL in a second CR. Long-term DFS rates in primary refractory ALL of 20% to 35% have been reported with SCT, higher than expected with any salvage chemotherapy.[228] Patients whose disease relapses after allogeneic SCT are candidates for salvage chemotherapy, donor lymphocyte infusions, or a second allogeneic SCT if they have had a remission for at least 1 year.[229] Overall, only few patients who relapse from allogeneic SCT are long-term survivors.

Autologous Stem Cell Transplantation

Although autologous SCT results in a lower rate of treatment-related complications and mortality, the absence of the GVL effect, potential leukemia cell contamination of the autologous marrow, and limited ability to eliminate minimal residual disease following the procedure raise barriers to the effectiveness of autologous SCT. In most studies, autologous SCT results are inferior to those for allogeneic SCT.[219]

Attal and colleagues[230] conducted a randomized trial of allogeneic SCT vs. autologous SCT in adult patients with ALL in first CR. Patients with an HLA-identical sibling received an allogeneic transplant; the others received autologous SCT. The 3-year DFS rate was significantly higher for the allogeneic SCT group (68% vs. 26%, $p<.001$). The authors concluded that early allogeneic SCT is superior to autologous SCT. Reasons for the poor results seen with autologous SCT in contrast to other studies oculd include differences in patient selection, analysis on an intent-to-treat basis in the Attal study, and the use of unpurged marrow grafts for the autologous SCT procedure.

Vey and associates[231] compared the results of 63 patients undergoing allogeneic or autologous SCT. At 6 years, the DFS rates (62% vs. 27%, $p<.06$) and relapse rates (10% vs. 65%, $p<.05$) favored allogeneic SCT significantly.

No advantage in terms of DFS has been demonstrated for patients receiving autologous SCT compared with chemotherapy alone. In a trial of the French Group on Therapy for ALL, chemotherapy and autologous SCT produced similar DFS rates at 3 years (39% vs. 32%, $p=.08$).[232] In an updated trial (LALA87), there was a trend for better results in the autologous SCT arm. The results were still not significant, even when comparing high-risk and standard-risk patients.[233] Investigators at MD Anderson found no significant difference in 3-year DFS and overall survival between patients who underwent autologous SCT in first CR and those who continued with postremission chemotherapy (60% vs. 49% and 58% vs. 62%, respectively).[234]

For patients with refractory or relapsed ALL, autologous SCT can result in long-term DFS of 5% to 30%.[235] Strategies to enhance the efficacy of autologous SCT include improved purging techniques and preparative regimens and developing post-transplant therapy to eliminate residual disease.

Alternative Donor Stem Cell Transplantation

Fewer than 30% of adults with ALL have a matched-related sibling. Other donor sources include matched unrelated donors, haplotype transplantations, and umbilical cord transplants. SCT from matched unrelated donors results in a DFS rate of 40%, a relapse probability of 22%, and higher risks of graft rejection, GVHD, and transplant-related mortality (about 50%).[236,237] In a study by Cornelissen and associates,[238] 127 patients with poor-risk ALL in either first CR, second or higher CR, or primary refractory and relapsed disease received a matched unrelated donor SCT. Overall survival from SCT at 2 years was 40% for patients in first CR, 17% for patients in subsequent remissions, and 5% in primary induction failures. Treatment-related mortality ranged from 54% to 75%. Multivariate analysis showed that transplantation in first CR, shorter interval from diagnosis to transplantation, DRB1 match, negative cytomegalovirus serology, and presence of the Philadelphia chromosome were independently associated with better DFS. Treatment-related mortality with matched unrelated donors is excessive, and a careful selection of patients should be undertaken for this procedure.

Minimal Residual Disease in Adult ALL

Patients in remission still can harbor up to 10^{10} malignant cells even though they are apparently disease-free by morphologic criteria.[239] Relapse thus occurs most frequently from residual leukemic cells that are below the limits of detection using conventional morphologic marrow assessment. Several techniques are available to determine the state and course of residual disease. Multicolor flow cytometry, FISH, and PCR assays detect up to 1 leukemic cell in 10^4 to 10^5 normal hematopoietic cells.[240] Measurement of minimal residual disease (MRD) in ALL has become a new and increasingly important prognostic factor for assessing the risk of relapse, thus facilitating the evaluation of future treatment strategies targeted at MRD. The extent to which minimal residual disease needs to be controlled or eliminated to prevent leukemic relapse remains uncertain.

Cavé and colleagues[241] used quantitative PCR for junctional sequences of T-cell receptor or immunoglobulin gene rearrangements in 246 children with ALL to determine the predictive value of the presence or absence of residual disease at various time points during the first 6 months following remission induction. There was a significant correlation between the presence of MRD and risk of early relapse at each of the time points studied, particularly in patients with 10^{-2} or more residual blasts/ 2×10^5 mononuclear marrow cells immediately following remission induction, or with 10^{-3} or more at later time points. The study concluded that residual leukemia after induction is a powerful prognostic factor in childhood ALL.

Fewer data exist on MRD in adult ALL. Furthermore, differences in pattern and dynamics of clearance of residual disease exist between adult and childhood ALL. Foroni and colleagues[242] analyzed marrow samples from 33 adults and 21 children by PCR for immunoglobulin heavy chain gene rearrangements at specific time points after diagnosis. Among patients who remained in CR, a decrease in the MRD positivity occurred during the first

12 months. The proportion of positive tests decreased faster in children than in adults, however, suggesting more rapid resolution of MRD among children, particularly during the first 6 months of CR. Other investigators established a threshold level of residual disease for relapse in adults similar to that described in children. Using quantitative PCR for 27 adults with ALL, Brisco and coworkers[243] found a significantly higher probability of relapse (89%) if residual disease persisted above a level of 10^{-3} leukemic cells per marrow cell. Even among patients with lower levels of residual disease, however, the risk of relapse was still high (46%). Beyond the issue of reservations about the predictive threshold of residual disease, the optimal time point to measure residual disease is not clear. In a study of 85 adult patients with B-lineage ALL, residual disease was assessed by semiquantitative immunoglobulin H gene analysis during four time bands in the first 24 months of treatment.[244] Even though MRD positivity was associated with increased relapse rates at all times, the association was most significant at 3 to 5 months after induction and beyond. The association between residual disease and DFS was independent of and greater than other standard predictors of outcome. Analysis of MRD thus allows further identification of high-risk patients for relapse. Although data from analysis of minimal residual disease are increasingly applied in study protocols and integrated into clinical decision making, important issues remain to be solved by larger randomized studies in the future. Even if early detection of residual disease by sensitive techniques predicts relapse, how can early detection of molecular relapse guide therapy, and does treatment of molecular relapse indeed improve survival? Finally, it might not be necessary to eliminate residual disease completely to achieve cure, and other homeostatic mechanisms might modulate growth of the leukemic clones that are currently not identifiable with the assays applied to residual disease studies.[239]

SALVAGE THERAPY OF ALL

Outcome with salvage therapy remains unsatisfactory, with CR rates of 10% to 50% and poor long-term DFS even when patients are consolidated with allogeneic or autologous SCT. Salvage regimens are patterned according to promising leads from frontline therapy. Regimens are divided into those that use the combination of vincristine, steroids, and anthracyclines; combinations of asparaginase and methotrexate; programs that integrate high-dose ara-C; and allogeneic and autolgogous SCT procedures.[245] New agents are continuously being assessed and incorporated into salvage strategies.

Prognostic Factors in ALL Salvage

The risk factors that influence outcome are similar to de novo ALL. The MD Anderson group reviewed their experiences with 314 adults with ALL in first relapse.[246] The overall CR rate was 31%. A significant difference in CR rates was demonstrated among patients "refractory" to induction therapy at M.D. Anderson, compared with those who were referred from outside programs with "refractory" disease (CR rate 34% vs. 68%, respectively). The median time in second remission was 6 months, the median survival 5 months, and the projected survival was 24% at 1 year and only 3% at 5 years. Favorable predictors of outcome by multivariate analysis included age less than 40 years, no circulating blasts, and a first CR duration of greater than 1 year. Based on these characteristics, patients could be divided into four different prognostic groups, with median survival times ranging from 11 months in the absence of unfavorable features to 2 months in the presence of all three poor-prognosis variables.

The significance of the duration of first CR has been emphasized in several studies. In an update of the M.D. Anderson group of 404 adults with relapsed or primary refractory ALL, 43 patients had a first CR duration of greater than 2 years (median 3 years; range 2 to 12 years).[247] The CR rate following first salvage therapy was 60%, the median second CR duration was 2 years, and the median survival was 4.6 years (range, 2.6 to 23 years). Seven of these patients remain alive in CR with a median follow-up time of 9.7 years. Relapses more than 10 years after successful completion of therapy are rare but can occur. Vora and colleagues[248] evaluated children with ALL who relapsed 10 years or later after first CR by PCR analysis of immunoglobulin heavy-chain genes or T-cell receptor genes at diagnosis and relapse. In all cases, the molecular markers were identical, suggesting long-term dormant leukemia and resurgence of the original clone. All of the 12 children achieved a second CR following retreatment, and 8 remained in a continuous CR at a median of 52+ months (range, 12+ to 108+ months).

Differences in salvage outcomes have been observed by site of relapse. This information is derived largely from large series of childhood ALL, and little information is available from adult ALL cases. Gaynon and associates[249] identified 1144 relapses among 3712 children with ALL enrolled in various trials. Long-term DFS was more favorable with longer durations of first remission. Site of relapse had an additional impact on survival, however. The 6-year survival rate of patients with bone marrow relapse, either isolated or in combination with any other site, ranged from 6% to 9% if the first CR duration was less than 18 months, up to 42% to 49% if duration of the first CR was 36 months of longer. In contrast, the 6-year survival rates were 33% to 72% with isolated CNS relapses and 52% to 81% with isolated testicular relapses. These data indicate that substantial long-term DFS rates could still be obtained in children who relapse after 36 months in the bone marrow, or those with isolated extramedullary relapses at any time. In adult ALL, however, 80% of relapses occur in the bone marrow, extramedullary relapse is followed by marrow relapse, and prognosis is poor. Patients should receive systemic chemotherapy in addition to site-directed therapy.

Karyotypic changes and clonal evolution are observed at relapse with a frequency ranging from 30% to 96%.[250,251] Chucrallah and coworkers[252] examined the type and frequency of cytogenetic, immunophenotypic, and molecular changes at relapse compared with presentation in 53 adults with ALL. Clonal evolution occurred in 28% and was an adverse variable for survival. Clonal evolution at relapse in the setting of unfavorable cytogenetic abnormalities at diagnosis [e.g., t(9;22)] did not impact survival significantly, however. Changes in expression of immunophenotype at relapse were observed in 24% of the patients but did not influence outcome.

Drug resistance could be an important factor in determining treatment failure and outcome. In childhood ALL, the prognostic value of drug resistance profiles has been demonstrated in several studies, but few results are available in adult ALL. Drug resistance can be assessed using the methyl-thiazol-tetrazolium (MTT) assay. In adults with Ph-positive ALL, a lower CR rate has been associated with resistance to daunorubicin and prednisone but not to asparaginase and vincristine.[253,254] Drug resistance is frequently related to abnormalities in the expression of the multidrug resistance gene (MDR-1) or its protein product, gp170. This generates resistance to chemotherapeutic agents such as vinca alkaloids, anthracyclines, epipodophylotoxins, and alkylating agents. In adult ALL, the incidence of MDR-1 positivity increases from 10% at diagnosis to about 50% at relapse. Expression of MDR-1 has been associated with lower CR and higher relapse rates.[255]

Salvage Regimens

Chemotherapy

The choice of salvage therapy is influenced by the initial induction regimen, the duration of first remission, disease features at relapse, and feasibility of SCT. It is difficult to compare the various regimens, as differences exist in the preceding factors.

With VAD (vincristine, doxorubicin, and dexamethasone) therapy in 64 patients with relapsed or refractory ALL, the overall CR rate was 39%, and the median CR duration and survival 7 and 6 months, respectively.[188] DFS at 2 years and overall survival rates were 20% and 8%, respectively. Koller and colleagues[256] compared the more intensive hyper-CVAD (fractionated cyclophosphamide, vincristine, doxorubicin, and dexamethasone alternating with high-dose methotrexate and ara-C) program with a high-dose cytarabine-based treatment (mitoxantrone, high-dose cytarabine plus GM-CSF). Patient characteristics were similar. The CR rates were similar for both regimens (44% vs. 38%), but a survival advantage was observed with hyper-CVAD.

Synergistic and schedule-dependent antileukemic activity is observed when L-asparaginase is administered in combination with methotrexate, with response rates ranging from 33% to 79%.[257] Anthracyclines, vinca alkaloids, and prednisone have been combined L-asparaginase in several regimens. Reported CR rates range from 64% to 69%, with median DFS rates of 3 to 6 months. The MOAD regimen (methotrexate 100 mg/m^2 on day 1, vincristine 2 mg on day 1, L-asparaginase 500 IU/kg on day 2, dexamethasone 6 mg/m^2 on days 2 through 10) was investigated in untreated and previously treated adult ALL.[258] Courses were repeated every 10 days. The CR rate in 14 previously treated patients was 79%, with a

median CR duration and survival of 7.5 and 11.2 months, respectively. In a similar combination to MOAD with polyethylene-glycol conjugated (PEG) asparaginase, only 7 of 32 patients (22%) achieved a CR.[259] Abshire and associates[260] observed a higher remission induction rate in children with relapsed ALL given weekly PEG-asparaginase compared with biweekly administration (97% vs. 82%, p=.003); response rates correlated with higher serum asparaginase levels, suggesting that further pharmacologic evaluation in adult ALL is necessary to improve outcomes.

Remission rates of 17% to 70% have been reported with high-dose cytarabine-based regimens.[261] Suki and colleagues[262] used a combination of cytarabine (1 g/m^2 over 2 hours daily on days 1 through 6) and fludarabine (30 mg/m^2 daily over 30 minutes 4 hours prior to cytarabine on days 2 to 6) in 30 adult patients with relapsed or refractory ALL. About one third of patients had Ph-postive disease. The CR rate was 30%, and the median CR duration was 42 months. Other investigators have reported CR rates of 67% to 87% with higher doses of cytarabine (2 versus 1 g/m^2) given with fludarabine and G-CSF.[263]

Stem Cell Transplantation

The results of SCT are superior to those for chemotherapy, with long-term DFS rates of 20% to 40%.[264,265] Outcome of allogeneic SCT is influenced by the duration of first CR, disease status at transplant, and patient age. High-risk ALL patients in the International Bone Marrow Transplant Registry (IBMTR) who received a matched related allogeneic BMT in their second remission had a 4-year survival probability of 22% compared with 36% in standard-risk patients.[266] These figures do not account for biases related to patient selection and time to transplant. Of 30% to 40% of patients who achieve a second CR and become eligible for SCT, fewer than half would have enough time prior to relapse to undergo SCT. Considering a DFS rate of around 25%, only a fraction of the total population at risk would thus benefit from transplant. When no sibling donor is available, identifying an unrelated donor in a timely fashion can be difficult. Davies and coworkers[267] studied the outcome of 115 consecutive relapsed ALL referrals over a 2-year period to determine the success rate of identifying a matched related or unrelated donor and the feasibility of performing SCT under these circumstances. A matched related donor could be identified in 35% of cases, and 75% of these patients received SCT. Of 58 patients for whom an unrelated donor search was initiated, a donor was identified for 22 patients, and 15 proceeded to a matched unrelated donor SCT.

With autologous transplantation, the relapse rate is comparable to that for chemotherapy. Uckun and colleagues[268] demonstrated that DFS following autologous SCT in second or later remission is related to the number of leukemia cells reinfused. Eradication of leukemic cells has been attempted with purging methods using monoclonal antibodies such as rituximab and alemtuzumab, magnetobeads, or ex vivo incubation of the graft with chemotherapeutic agents. Weisdorf and associates[269] compared the results of autologous SCT with matched unrelated donor SCT for patients with ALL in second or later remissions. The DFS rates were superior for patients receiving a matched, unrelated SCT (42% vs. 20%, p=0.02).

SPECIAL TREATMENT CONSIDERATIONS

Mature B-Cell ALL (Burkitt's ALL, ALL FAB L3)

Mature B-cell ALL is defined as greater than 25% marrow involvement with lymphoblasts of the L3 morphologic subtype of the FAB classification; it accounts for 3% to 5% of adult ALL cases.[45,212] The distinction between Burkitt's lymphoma with marrow involvement and mature B-cell ALL is arbitrary, although absence of extramedullary disease favors the latter. Mature B-cell ALL is typically characterized by FAB L3 morphology, expression of surface immunoglobulins, and the characteristic chromosomal abnormalities of translocation t(8;14)(q24;q32), or one of its variants (see the discussion earlier in this chapter). Cases with typical immunophenotype and karyotype abnormalities but FAB L1 or L2 morphology, or typical FAB L3 morphology without the associated cytogenetic findings or surface immunoglobulin expression, have been described.[270,271] These are treated as cases of mature B-cell ALL.

Mature B-cell ALL is more frequent in men (3:1 male-to-female ratio); the median age of patients is 25 to 30 years in most published series. In the study from M.D. Anderson, the median age was 56 years; this is important in evaluating the comparative regimen efficiencies, as prognosis is significantly worse in elderly patients (age 60 years or greater). Leukocytosis greater than 50×10^9/L is seen in 20% to 30% of patients. Nearly all patients present with elevated serum LDH levels and other signs and symptoms of a rapid tumor cell turnover. Adenopathy and/or hepatosplenomegaly occur in two thirds of patients. CNS involvement at presentation is frequent (12% to 70%). Frequently, CNS disease manifests as cranial nerve palsies without detectable blasts in the cerebrospinal fluid; mental nerve involvement with chin numbness is elicited frequently.[212]

Therapy
Historically, outcome for mature B-cell ALL with conventional ALL therapy was historically poor, with long-term disease-free survival rates of only 0% to 10%.[158] Recent short-term, dose-intensive, alternating multiagent chemotherapy programs have incorporated high doses of cyclophosphamide, cytarabine, and methotrexate. Maximizing exposure of rapidly proliferating B-ALL blasts to drug by hyperfractionation of the alkylating agent, and use of different non–cross-resistant agents in tandem, has formed the basis of many dose-intensive programs.[272-275] In recent studies, complete remission was attained in 89% to 92% of patients, and 2-year DFS rates increased to 60% to 80%; relapses were rare after the first year in remission. Intensive early prophylactic intrathecal therapy (with or without cranial irradiation), in addition to intensive

systemic administration of methotrexate and ara-C, significantly reduced the CNS relapse rate.

Similar programs for treating adult mature B-cell ALL have resulted in improved outcome, with long-term disease-free survival rates of 50% to 65%.[145,276-278] These favorable results have been attributed to the fractionation and use of higher doses of alkylating agents and higher doses of methotrexate and cytarabine. Review of the childhood data suggests that higher doses of methotrexate correlates with higher DFS rates, particularly for patients presenting with CNS involvement. The French protocol LMB84 used methotrexate doses of 3 g/m^2 compared with 8 g/m^2 in the LMB86 protocol; disease-free survival rates were 46% and 77%, respectively.[272] Similar results were observed in the BFM trials, with an increase in DFS rates from 50% to 78% when the dose of methotrexate was increased.[279]

The recent M.D. Anderson experience with hyper-CVAD—a dose-intensive multiagent chemotherapy program modeled after the Total Therapy B designed by Murphy and colleagues[274] for childhood mature B-cell ALL—has been favorable. The program consists of fractionated cyclophosphamide, vincristine, doxorubicin, and dexamethasone alternating with high doses of methotrexate and ara-C every 3 weeks. CNS prophylaxis involved 16 intrathecal treatments with methotrexate and cytarabine. Of the 26 patients, almost half were age 60 or older, with a median age of 58 years; in the majority of reported clinical trials, by comparison, median ages have ranged from 25 to 36 years. The overall CR rate was 81%, comparable to those reported by other groups that included predominantly younger patients.[145,276] Long-term DFS was 83% for patients under the age of 60 years and 16% for those 60 years or older. The sharp decrease in DFS among older patients was due to both induction mortality and relapses in this age group. The induction mortality of 19% was related to deaths from infectious complications in the older age group. By multivariate analysis, older age, hemoglobin levels below 10 g/dL, and circulating blasts at presentation were independent predictors of poor outcome. The 3-year survival rate was 89% for patients with none or only one of these adverse features, 47% for those with two, and 0% for those with all three. Recent programs have included rituximab with hyper-CVAD in an attempt to improve survival.

Cortes and associates[280] extended the experience of the hyper-CVAD program for newly diagnosed patients with HIV-related mature B-cell ALL, including the anti-CD20 monoclonal antibody Rituximab combined with highly active antiretroviral treatment (HAART). The CR rate in 13 patients was 92%, with a median survival of 12 months and nearly 50% of the patients alive longer than 2 years after diagnosis. Outcome was better in the group receiving HAART early in the course of therapy (Dr. Jorge Cortes, personal communication).

The role of autologous or allogeneic SCT in patients with mature B-cell ALL is difficult to assess. Sweetenham and associates[281] reported a favorable outcome after autologous SCT in CR for 70 adults with Burkitt's or Burkitt's-like lymphoma following various induction regimens. The 3-year actuarial survival rate was 72%. All

THE MDACC APPROACH TO NEWLY DIAGNOSED PATIENTS WITH ALL

For patients with newly diagnosed ALL, we use the hyper-CVAD regimen. The hyper-CVAD program has been patterned after a similar chemotherapy program that has been developed for the treatment of children with mature B-cell ALL. After exclusion of Philadelphia chromosome-positive disease (Philadelphia chromosome quick screen by the cytogenetics laboratory facility), patients receive eight courses of chemotherapy, alternating between hyper-CVAD (intravenous cyclphosphamide, 300 mg/m^2 over a 3-hour period every 12 hours for six doses on days 1 through 3 with concomitant administration of Mesna; intravenous doxorubicin, 50 mg/m^2 on day 4; intravenous vincristine, 2 mg on days 4 and 11; and dexamethasone, 40 mg/day on days 1 through 4 and again on days 11 through 14) during courses 1, 3, 5, and 7, and methotrexate (200 mg/m^2 intravenously over 2 hours, followed by 800 mg/m^2 intravenously over 22 hours on day 1) and high-dose cytarabine (3 g/m^2 intravenously over 2 hours every 12 hours for four doses on days 2 and 3) during courses 2, 4, 6, and 8. Although there is no fixed-time interval between the courses, and although subsequent cycles should start as soon as the peripheral blood recovery is indicated by an increase of the absolute neutrophil count to 1×10^9/L or greater and the platelet count to 60×10^9/L or greater, courses are typically spaced approximately 21 days apart.

We stratify patients without CNS involvement according to the predicted risk of CNS relapse, which is based on lactate dehyrogenase (LDH) levels of greater than × 3 ULN, a proliferative index (% S+G$_2$M) of 14% or greater, and a diagnosis of mature B-cell ALL. Patients with low risk of CNS disease (absence of any risk factor) receive a total of four intrathecal treatments (two with the first two courses each) of methotrexate, 12 mg alternating with cytarabine, 100 mg. Although we rarely use and do not recommend Omaya reservoirs for most of our patients, the dose of intrathecal methotrexate should be adjusted to 6 mg if this route of administration is chosen. Patients with high risk for CNS disease receive a total of eight intrathecal administrations accompanying the first four courses, and all other patients receive six treatments. We avoid cranial radiation, as in our opinion and based on available data, effective CNS prophylaxis is possible with intrathecal chemotherapy agents in association with high doses of systemic methotrexate and cytarabine.

Following induction and the intensified consolidation, we continue maintenance therapy for a total of 2 years. The backbone of the maintenance program consists of methotrexate at a dose of 20 mg/m^2 orally every week, 6-mercaptopurine at a dose of 50 mg orally three times daily, vincristine intravenously at a dose of 2 mg once a month, and prednisone at a dose of 200 mg orally daily for 5 days every month (POMP). The doses are adjusted frequently depending on the degree of myelosuppression and occurrence of other toxicities (primarily mucositis and hepatic dysfunction). The POMP courses are usually interrupted twice for intensification with intravenously administered methotrexate and L-asparaginase. We continue antibiotic prophylaxis with trimethoprim/sulfamethoxazole twice daily on Saturdays and Sundays and valacyclovir at a dose of 500 mg orally daily (or equivalent antiviral).

Patients who test Philadelphia chromosome- or BCR-ABL-positive after at least the first two cycles of therapy are treated via a separate protocol. In such cases, we give imatinib at a dose of 600 mg orally daily for the first 14 days together with each course of the induction and induction/consolidation phase according to the hyper-CVAD regimen. The maintenance therapy for these patients consists of imatinib with vincristine and prednisone only for another 12 months. The hyper-CVAD regimen has proved to be an active program for adult patients with ALL. Current modifications of this program include the following:

- Inclusion of high-dose anthracyclines early during the induction/consolidation phase.
- Addition of rituximab to the treatment regimen of patients whose blasts test positive for CD20.
- Development of early and late intensifications with two courses of hyper-CVAD and methotrexate/L-asparaginase, respectively, at months 6 and 18 during the POMP maintenance.
- Prolongation of the maintenance phase to 3 years instead of 2 years.

In addition, patients older than 60 years of age are offered laminar air flow rooms during the induction period.

---

relapses occurred within 6 months of transplant. Disease bulk at presentation influenced outcome, with progression-free survival rates declining with increasing tumor dimensions of less than 5 cm (100%), 5 to 10 cm (80%), and greater than 10 cm (61%). The overall survival rate was 37% for patients undergoing autologous SCT in chemosensitive relapse.

When concurrently applying short-term, dose-intensive chemotherapy programs, most patients are either cured or relapse with rapidly progressive disease that is usually not amenable to successful tumor reduction to allow consolidation with SCT. The selection and time bias of SCT could influence outcome, as most relapses occur within the first year. Patients who remain in CR long enough to proceed to transplant undergo a natural selection, which might result in a falsely superior outcome, with high dose chemotherapy followed by autologous intensification.

Lymphoblastic Lymphoma

With an incidence of 3% to 5%, lymphoblastic lymphoma is rare in adults but accounts for up to 40% of childhood non-Hodgkin's lymphoma (NHL) cases. Most patients present with advanced disease and can be classified as T-cell T-ALL when there are more than 25% marrow blasts. The outcome of lymphoblastic lymphoma was historically dismal, with low CR rates and few long-term survivors. As with other variants of ALL, the use of intensive chemotherapy programs incorporating anthracyclines, cyclophosphamide, cytosine arabinoside, epipodophyllotoxins, and/or high-dose methotrexate has improved prognosis dramatically. Early CNS prophylaxis, application of risk-adapted treatment strategies, and advances in supportive care measures also have contributed.[159]

Patients with lymphoblastic lymphoma typically present with symptomatic supradiaphragmatic adenopathy, with lymphoblasts commonly found in the mediastinum, bone marrow, CNS, skin, and other extramedullary sites. Frequent symptoms include cough, wheezing, and shortness of breath. Superior vena cava (SVC) syndrome, tracheal obstruction, and cardiac tamponade can occur. Occasionally, bone pain and hypercalcemia could be manifestations of lytic bone disease. Primary intraabdominal adenopathy is unusual. Marrow involvement is seen in about 50% of patients, and even if absent on initial evaluation, a leukemic phase can be observed as disease progresses. For patients with SVC syndrome, treatment with steroids can alleviate signs and symptoms rapidly; early mediastinal irradiation is only rarely needed.[282,283]

Therapy

The early programs were modeled after non-Hodgkin's lymphoma regimens incorporating cyclical and multiagent therapy. Coleman and coworkers[283] treated lymphoblastic lymphomas (n=44) with a 1-year program of CHOP and L-asparaginase, CNS prophylaxis, and maintenance with 6-mercaptopurine and methotrexate. The CR rate was 95%, with a 3-year actuarial DFS rate of 56% (median follow-up 26 months). Most relapses occurred at distant sites, including bone marrow and CNS. In a pilot study by the same investigators, the incidence of CNS relapse was 29%. CNS prophylaxis with methotrexate was not administered until week 8 or 9 following induction therapy and was given concurrently with systemic methotrexate at a dose of 1 g/m^2. In the later series, earlier administration of intrathecal methotrexate and the addition of prophylactic cranial irradiation reduced the incidence of CNS relapse to 3%. No improvement of survival was observed.

Morel and colleagues[284] compared outcomes for 80 adults treated with either non-Hodgkin's lymphoma programs (CHOP followed by 12 months of COP, or LNH-84 [ACVBP]), or conventional ALL regimens (FRALLE or LALA). The overall CR rate was 82% without significant differences among the various regimens, although a trend for a higher CR was seen with ALL therapy. Disease-free and overall survival rates were 46% and 51%, respectively, and no differences were observed among the regimens. Thirty-seven of 56 responders (56%) relapsed, most within 2 years. Mediastinal relapse was observed in 5 patients (14%) and CNS relapse in 12 (32%) despite CNS prophylaxis.

Other investigators using ALL induction/consolidation and maintenance regimens have reported similar results.[285-287] Investigators from MD Anderson reported their results with the hyper-CVAD regimen, incorporating CNS risk-oriented prophylaxis, mediastinal irradiation, and maintenance therapy.[288] The CR rate for 24 consecutive adults treated was 96%. Most patients had advanced-stage disease. None received autologous or allogeneic SCT in first remission. Six patients (26%) relapsed, with a median CR duration of 14 months (range, 12 to 38 months). Three patients were salvaged successfully with allogeneic SCT and remained alive without disease at 3+, 4, and 4+ years. The 3-year overall and disease-free survival rates were

80% and 72%, respectively, with median follow-up of 3 years.

Overall, intensive chemotherapy regimens with or without irradiation have improved the CR rate to 75% to 90%; the long-term DFS rate is 40% to 60% in responders. Direct comparisons between the multitude of treatment programs applied are difficult, but current experience suggests the following:

- Intensive ALL-type chemotherapy programs are superior to lymphoma-type regimens or conventional ALL regimens.
- Shorter-term chemotherapy without a maintenance phase appears to increase the risk of relapse.
- An intensive intrathecal chemotherapy prophylaxis is required to reduce the incidence of CNS relapse.[289]

The role of mediastinal irradiation and duration of maintenance therapy remain controversial.

Unfavorable outcome appears to be determined by the following clinical features at presentation:

- Older age
- High tumor burden with hyperleukocytosis
- Ann Arbor stage IV disease with bone marrow or CNS involvement
- Elevated LDH levels, and B symptoms
- Failure to achieve CR with chemotherapy, anemia, circulating blasts, and bulky mediastinal lymphadenopathy

Coleman and coworkers[283] conducted a multivariate analysis of pretreatment features in 44 patients, devising a risk stratification system based on bone marrow involvement, CNS disease, and serum LDH level. Good-risk lymphoblastic lymphomas (Ann Arbor stage less than IV, or stage IV with no marrow or CNS involvement, and LDH below 300 IU/L) had a 5-year relapse-free survival rate of 94% compared with 19% for the poor-risk group (p=.0006).

The European Bone Marrow Transplantation Group (EBMTG)[290] reported a retrospective series of 214 patients with lymphoblastic lymphoma who received autologous SCT in first CR (49%) or in second or later CR (15%). The actuarial 6-year survival rate was 42% overall, 63% for those transplanted in first CR, and 15% for refractory or relapsed disease. The survival rate in second CR was 31%. Sweetenham and colleagues[291] of the EBMTG then conducted a randomized study of autologous SCT compared with conventional-dose consolidation therapy in first remission. Of 119 adults who received standard remission induction chemotherapy, 65 patients were randomized. Disease-free survival favored autologous SCT, but overall survival was similar for both groups, suggesting either that SCT might improve outcome in second remission or that other salvage strategies were effective.

Only few studies have reported the use of allogeneic SCT as postremission therapy in lymphoblastic lymphoma. Selection bias, differences in the choice of induction chemotherapy, and disease heterogeneity limit firm conclusions regarding the benefit of postremission therapy with allogeneic SCT.

Philadelphia Chromosome-Positive ALL

Using current dose-intensive induction regimens, remission rates for patients with Philadelphia chromosome (Ph)-positive ALL are similar to those for Ph-negative ALL, but long-term DFS remains less than 10%.[292] The CALGB[121] reported on the outcome of 67 patients out of 256 (28.6%) who had the Ph translocation. The Ph chromosome was the sole abnormality in one third of the patients; additional chromosomal abnormalities were detected in the remaining two thirds. The CR rate was 79% for the Ph-positive group compared with 80% overall. The median DFS was only 11 months, and the 5-year continuous CR rate was 8% in Ph-positive ALL, compared with a median DFS of 2.3 years and a 5-year continuous CR rate of 38% for diploid karyotype ALL. Survival of Ph-positive ALL was 11%, compared with 37% for other types of ALL. A multivariate analysis confirmed the presence of Ph karyotype as the most significant factor associated with worse remission duration and survival.

Given the disappointing results of chemotherapy programs for Ph-positive ALL, high-dose chemotherapy followed by SCT is recommended after achieving a first CR. The International ALL Trial group compared the outcomes of 167 patients with Ph-positive ALL who received one of the following forms of treatment:

- A matched related SCT (*n*=49)
- A matched unrelated donor transplant (*n*=23)
- An autologous SCT (*n*=7)
- Continuation with chemotherapy alone (*n*=77)[293]

The treatment-related mortality was higher for patients receiving SCT (37% for matched sibling transplants, 43% for matched unrelated donor transplants, 14% with autologous SCT, 8% with chemotherapy). The risk of relapse at 5 years was lower for patients receiving allogeneic SCT (29%) compared with autologous SCT/chemotherapy (81%). Likewise, the 5-year survival probability was 43% for patients receiving allogeneic SCT and 19% for patients receiving autologous SCT or chemotherapy only. Some studies suggest a benefit only for patients receiving matched related sibling SCT rather than matched unrelated transplant procedures or autologous SCT.

Imatinib mesylate (STI571, Gleevec), a small molecule of the group of 2-phenylaminopyrimidines, is a potent and selective inhibitor of the BCR-ABL tyrosine kinase.[294] The M.D. Anderson studies combined imatinib mesylate with hyper-CVAD for newly diagnosed patients with Ph-positive ALL.[295] A total of eight induction/consolidation courses (hyper-CVAD alternating with high-dose methotrexate and cytarabine), during which imatinib is given for 14 days of each treament cycle, was followed by a 1-year maintenance program using imatinib at a daily dose of 600 mg orally. Preliminary results show this combination to be safe, and remission rates are high. The effect on long-term DFS is still unclear. Limited experience exists with imatinib in Ph-positive ALL transplant failures.[296] In a study of 20 consecutive Ph-positive ALL patients who relapsed after allogeneic SCT, imatinib mesylate induced CR in 11 patients (55%).

CONCLUSIONS AND FUTURE DIRECTIONS FOR TREATMENT OF ADULT ALL

Improvements in chemotherapy programs for adult ALL have achieved CR rates of approximately 90% and long-term DFS of 30% to 40%. Prognosis has improved remarkably in subsets of T-lineage ALL and mature B-cell ALL; about 50% of these patients can be cured with chemotherapy alone. On the other hand, Ph-positive ALL or other high-risk cytogenetic abnormalities continue to do poorly. Improving the outcomes of patients within these subsets is the major challenge in the treatment of adult ALL.

How can the prognosis of these patients be improved? Better knowledge of biological subtleties of leukemic blasts is and pathophysiology of ALL will allow therapy-oriented discoveries (e.g., imatinib mesylate for Ph-positive ALL). The ultimate goal in ALL therapy will be to devise risk group- and disease-specific directed therapies.

Many investigational approaches appear promising. Novel chemotherapy agents (e.g., compound 506U, liposomal vincristine), use of monoclonal antibodies (rituximab for CD20-positive ALL, alemtuzumab, or anti-CD22 monoclonal antibodies), or immunomodulatory strategies are being explored. Even though progress in the treatment of ALL in adults lags behind that achieved in childhood programs, the gap is starting to narrow.

REFERENCES

1. Greenlee RT, Hill-Harmon MB, Taylor M, Thun M: Cancer Statistics, 2001. CA Cancer J Clin 2001;51:15.
2. Cortes J, Kantarjian HM: Acute lymphoblastic leukemia: A comprehensive review with emphasis on biology and therapy. Cancer 1995;76:2393.
3. Groves FD, Linet MS, Devesa SS: Epidemiology of leukemia: Overview of patterns of occurrence. In Henderson ES, Lister TA, Greaves MF (eds): Leukemia, 6th ed. Philadelphia, WB Saunders, 1996, p 145.
4. Sandler DP: Epidemiology and etiology of leukemia. Curr Opin Oncol 1990;2:3.
5. De Oliveira MSP, El Seed FERA, Foroni L, et al: Lymphoblastic leukaemia in Siamese twins: evidence for identity. Lancet 1986;2:969.
6. Schmitt TA, Degos L: Leucemies familiales. Bull Cancer 1978;65:83.
7. Li FP: Epidemiology of cancer in childhood. In Nathan DG, Oski FA (eds): Hematology of Infancy and Childhood, 4th ed. WB Saunders, Philadelphia, 1993, p 1102.
8. Ford AM, Ridge SA, Cabrera ME, et al: In utero rearrangements in the trithorax-related oncogene in infant leukemias. Nature 1993;363:358.
9. Mulvihill JJ: Childhood cancer, the environment and heredity. In Pizzo PA, Poplacle (eds): Principles and Practice of Pediatric Oncology. JP Lippincott, Philadelphia, 1993, p 11.
10. Mertens AC, Wen W, Davies SM, et al: Congenital abnormalities in children with acute leukemia: A report from the Children's Cancer Group. J Pediatr 1998;133:617.
11. Robison LL, Nesbit ME, Sather HN, et al: Down syndrome and acute leukemia in children: A 10 year retrospective survey from Childrens Cancer Study Group. J Pediatr 1984;105:235.
12. Fong C, Brodeur GM: Down's syndrome and leukemia: Epidemiology, genetics, cytogenetics, and mechanisms of leukemogenesis. Cancer Genet Cytogenet 1987;28:55.

13. Chessells JM, Harrison G, Richards SM, et al: Down's syndrome and acute lymphoblastic leukaemia: Clinical features and response to treatment. Arch Dis Child 2001;85:321.

14. Taub JW: Relationship of chromosome 21 and acute leukemia in children with Down syndrome. J Pediatr Hematol Oncol 2001;23:175.

15. Shaw MP, Eden OB, Grace E, Ellis PM: Acute lymphoblastic leukemia and Klinefelter's syndrome. Pediatr Hematol Oncol 1992;9:81.

16. Janik-Moszat A, Bubala H, Stojewska M, Sonta-Jakimczyk D: Acute lymphoblastic leukemia in children with Fanconi anemia. Wiad Lek 1998;51(Suppl 4):285.

17. Toledano SR, Lange BJ: Ataxia-telangiectasia and acute lymphoblastic leukemia. Cancer 1980;45:1675.

18. Ichimura M, Ishimura T, Belsky JL: Incidence of leukemia in atomic bomb survivors belonging to a fixed cohort in Hiroshima and Nagasaki, 1950–1971: Radiation dose, years after exposure, age at exposure, and type of leukemia. J Radiat Res (Tokyo) 1978;19:262.

19. Mukhin VN: Acute leukemia in adults: Morbidity in Donetsk region of Ukraine before and after Chernobyl's accident. Ter Arkh 2000;72:60.

20. Court Brown WM, Doll R: Mortality from cancer and other causes after radiotherapy for ankylosing spondylitis. BMJ 1986;ii:1327.

21. Stewart A, Kneale GW: Radiation dose effects in relation to obstetric x-rays and childhood cancer. Lancet 1970;1:1185.

22. Shore DL, Sandler DP, Davey FR, et al: Acute leukemia and residential proximity to potential sources of environmental pollutants. Arch Environ Health 1993;48:414.

23. Lindquist R, Nilsson B, Eklund G, Gahrton G: Acute leukemia in professional drivers exposed to gasoline and diesel. Eur J Heamatol 1991;47:98.

24. Brownson RC, Novotny TE, Perry MC: Cigarette smoking and adult leukemia: A meta-analysis. Arch Intern Med 1993;153:469.

25. Sandler DP, Shore DL, Bloomfield CD: Hair dye use and leukemia. Am J Epidemiol 1993;138:636.

26. Wen W, Shu XO, Potter JD, et al: Parental medication use and risk of childhood acute lymphoblastic leukemia. Cancer 2002;95:1786.

27. Bethwaite P, Cook A, Kennedy J, Pearce N: Acute leukemia in electrical workers: A New Zealand case-control study. Cancer Causes Control 2001;12:683.

28. Greaves MF, Alexander FE: An infectious etiology for common acute lymphoblastic leukemia in childhood? Leukemia 1993;7:349.

29. Meltzer AA, Spitz MR, Johnson CC, Culbert SJ: Seaon-of-birth and acute leukemia of infancy. Chronobiol Int 1989;6:285.

30. Timonen TT: A hypothesis concerning deficiency of sunlight, cold temperature, and influenza epidemics associated with the onset of acute lymphoblastic leukemia in northern Finland. Ann Hematol 1999;78:408.

31. Sarma PS, Graber J: Human lymphotropic viruses in human diseases. J Natl Cancer Inst 1990;82:1100.

32. Lombardi L, Newcomb EW, Dalla-Favera R: Pathogenesis of Burkitt's lymphoma: Expression of an activated *c-myc* oncogene causes the tumorigenic conversion of EBV-infected B lymphoblasts. Cell 1987;49:161.

33. Whitaker JA: Acute lymphoblastic leukemia in butchers and abattoir workers. Br J Haematol 1991;79:649.

34. Blair A, Mulker G, Cantor K, et al: Cancer among farmers: A review. Scand J Work Environ Health 1985;11:397.

35. Pederson-Bjergaard J: Acute lymphoid leukemia with t(4;11)(q21;q23) following chemotherapy with cytostatic agents targeting at DNA-topoisomerase II (editorial). Leuk Res 1992;16:733.

36. Rafsanjani KA, Vossough P: Acute lymphoblastic leukemia and hepatoblastoma in a family. Pediatr Hematol Oncol 2002;19:521.

37. Karauzum SB, Hazar V, Acikbas I, et al: Existence of acute lymphoblastic leukemia and osteosarcoma in a child. J Pediatr Hematol Oncol 2002;24:572.

38. Liou MC, Lin KH, Lu MY, Lin DT: Acute lymphoblastic leukemia occurring as a second malignant neoplasm in a child. J Formos Med Assoc 2002;101:502.

39. Sun X, Gordon LI, Peterson LC: Transformation of follicular lymphoma to acute lymphoblastic leukemia. Arch Pathol Lab Med 2002;126:997.

40. Ehrlich P, Lazarus P, Pinkus F: Leukämie, Pseudoleukämie, Hämoglobinämie. Vienna, A Hölder, 1901.

41. Wegelius R: Preleukemic states in children. Scand J Haematol 1986;45:133.

42. Kiraly JF, Brooks JSJ: Bone marrow necrosis. Am J Med 1976;60:361.

43. Shibata K, Watanabe M, Yamaguchi M: Two cases of acute lymphocytic leukemia associated with bone marrow necrosis: A brief review of the literature. Eur J Haematol 1994;52:115.

44. Paydas S, Ergin M, Baslamisli F, et al: Bone marrow necrosis: Clinicopathologic analysis of 20 cases and review of the literature. Am J Hematol 2002;70:300.

45. Bennett JM, Catovsky D, Daniel MT, et al: Proposals for the classification of acute leukemia. French-American-British Cooperative Group. Br J Haematol 1976;33:451.

46. Bennett JM, Catovsky D, Daniel MT, et al: The morphologic classification of acute lymphoblastic leukemia: Concordance among observers and clinical correlations. Br J Haematol 1981;47:553.

47. Davey FR, Castella A, Lauenstein, et al: Prognostic significance of the revised French-American-British classification for acute lymphoblastic leukemia. Clin Lab Haematol 1983;5:343.

48. Ferrari S, Mariano MT, Tagliafico E, et al: Myeloperoxidase gene expression in blast cells with a lymphoid phenotype in cases of acute lymphoblastic leukemia. Blood 1988;72:873.

49. Serrano J, Roman J, Sanchez J, et al: Myeloperoxidase gene expression in acute lymphoblastic leukemia. Br J Haematol 1997;97:841.

50. Ho FCS, Chan GTC, Todd D: Non-specificity of Sudan black B in the diagnosis of acute myeloid leukemia. Br J Haematol 1993;53:171.

51. McCaffrey R, Harrison TA, Parkman P, et al: Terminal deoxynucleotidyl transferase activity in human leukemic cells and in normal thymocytes. N Engl J Med 1975;292:775.

52. Janossy G, Hoffbrand AV, Greaves MF, et al: Terminal transferase enzyme assay and immunological membrane markers in the diagnosis of leukemia: A multiparameter analysis of 300 cases. Br J Haematol 1980;44:221.

53. Meenan B, Heavey C, Lichtenstein A, et al: Terminal transferase expression in the differential diagnosis of acute leukemias. Eastern Cooperative Oncology Group. Leuk Lymphoma 1996;22:265.

54. Huh YO, Smith TL, Collins P, et al: Terminal deoxynucleotidyl transferase expression in acute myelogenous leukemia and myelodysplasia as determined by flow cytometry. Leuk Lymphoma 2000;37:319.

55. Foa R, Vitale A: Towards an integrated classification of adult acute lymphoblastic leukemia. Rev Clin Exp Hematol 2002;6:181.

56. Paredes-Aguilera R, Romero-Guzman L, Lopez-Santiago N, et al: Flow cytometric analysis of cell-surface and intracellular antigens in the diagnosis of acute leukemia. Am J Hematol 2001;68:69.

57. Campana D, Pui CH: Detection of minimal residual disease in acute leukemia: Methodologic advances and clinical significance. Blood 1995;86:1416.

58. Huh YO, Ibrahim S: Immunophenotypes in adult acute lymphoblastic leukemia. Role of flow cytometry in diagnosis and monitoring of disease. Hematol Oncol Clin North Am 2000;14:1251.

59. Bene MC, Castoldi G, Knapp W, et al: Proposals for the immunological classification of acute leukemias. Leukemia 1995;9:1783.

60. Janossy G, Bollum FJ, Bradstock KF, et al: Cellular phenotypes of normal and leukemic hemopoietic cells determined by analysis with selected antibody combinations. Blood 1980;56:430.

61. Greaves MF: Differentiation-linked leukemogenesis in lymphocytes. Science 1986;234:697.

62. Rothe G, Schmitz G: Consensus protocol for the flow cytometric immunophenotyping of hematopoietic malignances. Working Group on Flow Cytometry and Image Analysis. Leukemia 1996;14:877.

63. Farahat N, Morilla A, Owusu-Ankomah K, et al: Detection of minimal residual disease in B-lineage acute lymphoblastic leumkaemia by quantitative flow cytometry. Br J Haematol 1998;101:158.

64. Farahat N, Lens D, Zomas A, et al: Quantitative flow cytometry can distinguish between normal and leukaemic B-cell precursors. Br J Haematol 1995;91:640.

65. Terstappen LWMM, Huang S, Picker LJ: Flow cytometric assessment of human T-cell differentiation in thymus and bone marrow. Blood 1992;79:666.

66. Wormann B, Safford M, Konemann S, et al: Detection of aberrant antigen expression in acute myeloid leukemia by multiparameter flow cytometry. Recent Results Cancer Res 1993;131:185.

67. Ludwig W-D, Raghavachar A, Thiel E: Immunophenotypic classification of acute lymphoblastic leukaemia. Baillieres Clin Haematol 1994;7:235.

68. Gores SD, Kastan MG, Civin CI: Normal human bone marrow precursors that express terminal deoxynucleotidyl transferase include T-cell precursors and possible lymphoid stem cells. Blood 1991;77:1681.

69. Borowitz MJ: Immunologic markers in childhood acute lymphoblastic leukemia. Hematol Oncol Clin North Am 1990;4:743.

70. Batinic D, Tindle R, Boban D, et al: Expression of haematopoietic progenitor cell-associated antigen BI-3C5/CD34 in leukaemia. Leukemia Res 1989;13:83.

71. Pui C-H, Evans WE: Acute lymphoblastic leukemia. N Engl J Med 1998;339:605.

72. Crist W, Pullen J, Boyett J, et al: Clinical and biologic features predict a poor prognosis in acute lymphoid leukemias in infants: A Pediatric Oncology Group study. Blood 1986;67:135.

73. Vogler LB, Crist WM, Bockman DE, et al: Pre-B-leukemia: A new phenotype of childhood lymphoblastic leukemia. N Engl J Med 1978;298:872.

74. Crist WM, Carroll AJ, Shuster JJ, et al: Poor prognosis of children with pre-B acute lymphoblastic leukemia is associated with the t(1;19)(q23;p13). A Pediatric Oncology Group study. Blood 1990;76:117.

75. Crist W, Pullen J, Boyett J, et al: Acute lymphoid leukemia in adolescents: Clinical and biological features predict a poor prognosis—A Pediatric Oncology Group study. J Clin Oncol 1988;6:34.

76. Koehler M, Behm FG, Shuster J, et al: Transitional pre-B-cell acute lymphoblastic leukemia of childhood is associated with favorable prognostic clinical features and an excellent outcome: A Pediatric Oncology Group study. Leukemia 1993;7:2064.

77. Rivera-Luna R, Cardenas-Cardos R, Leal-Leal C, et al: B-lineage acute lymphoblastic leukemia of childhood. An institutional experience. Arch Med Res 1997;28:233.

78. Vasef MA, Brynes RK, Murata-Collins JL, et al: Surface immuno-globulin light chain-positive acute lymphoblastic leukemia of FAB L1 or L2 type: A report of 6 cases in adults. Am J Clin Pathol 1998;110:143.

79. Evens AM, Gordon LI: Burkitt's and Burkitt-like lymphoma. Curr Treat Options Oncol 2002;3:291.

80. Lai JL, Fenaux P, Zandecki M, et al: Cytogenetic studies in 30 patients with Burkitt's lymphoma or L3 acute lymphoblastic leukemia with special reference to additional chromosome abnormalities. Ann Genet 1989;32:26.

81. Pui C-H, Behm FG, Crist WM: Clinical and biological relevance of immunologic marker studies in childhood acute lymphoblastic leukemia. Blood 1993;82:343.

82. Lai R, Hirsch-Ginsberg CF, Bueso-Ramos C: Pathologic diagnosis of acute lymphocytic leukemia. Hematol Oncol Clin North Am 2000;14:1209.

83. Thalhammer-Scherrer R, Mitterbauer G, Simonitsch I, et al: The immunophenotype or 325 adult acute leukemias: Relationship to morphologic and molecular classification and proposal for a minimal screening program highly predictive for lineage discrimination. Am J Clin Pathol 2002;117:380.

84. Onciu M, Lai R, Vega F, et al: Precursor T-cell acute lymphoblastic leukemia in adults: Age-related immunophenotypic, cytogenetic, and molecular subsets. Am J Clin Pathol 2002;117:252.

85. Greaves MF, Chan LC, Furley AJW, et al: Lineage promiscuity in hematopoietic differentiation and leukemia. Blood 1986;67:1.

86. Ferrara F, Del Vecchio L: Clinical relevance of acute mixed-lineage leukemias. Leukemia Lymph 193;12:11.

87. Matutes E, Morilla R, Farahat N, et al: Definition of acute biphenotypic leukemia. Haematologica 1997;82:64.

88. Khalidi HS, Chang KL, Medeiros LJ, et al: Acute lymphoblastic leukemia. Survey of immunophenotype, French-American-British classification, frequency of myeloid antigen expression, and karyotype abnormalities in 210 pediatric and adult cases. Hematopathology 1999;111:467.

89. Pui CH, Rubnitz JE, Hancock ML, et al: Reappraisal of the clinical and biologic significance of myeloid-associated antigen expression in childhood acute lymphoblastic leukemia. J Clin Oncol 1998;16:3768.

90. Den Boer ML, Kapaun P, Pieters R, et al: Myeloid antigen co-expression in childhood acute lymphoblastic leukaemia: Relationship with in vitro drug resistance. Br J Haematol 1999;105:876.

91. Bene MD, Bernier M, Casasnovas RO, et al: The reliability and specificity of c-kit for the diagnosis of acute myeloid leukemias and undifferentiated leukemias. Blood 1998;92:596.

92. EGIL (European Group for the Immunological Classification of Leukemias): The value of c-kit in the diagnosis of biphenotypic acute leukemia. Leukemia 1998;12:2038.

93. Nakase K, Kenkichi K, Shiku H, et al: Myeloid antigen, CD13, CD14, and/or CD33 expression in adult acute lymphoblastic leukemia patients: Diagnostic and prognostic implication. Am J Clin Pathol 1996;105:761.

94. Guyotat D, Campos L, Shi ZH, et al: Myeloid surface antigen expression in adult acute lymphoblastic leukemia. Leukemia 1990;4:664.

95. Wells SJ, Bray RA, Stempora LI, et al: CD117/CD34 expression in leukemic blasts. Am J Clin Pathol 196;106:192.

96. Cascavilla N, Musto P, Melillo L, et al: Is the scoring system an effective clinico-biological tool in myeloid antigen positive adult acute lymphoblastic leukemia? Results of a longterm study. Hematol J 2002;3:251.

97. Czuzcman MS, Dodge RK, Stewart CC, et al: Value of immunopheno-type in intensively treated adult acute lymphoblastic leukemia: Cancer and leukemia Group B study 8364. Blood 1999;93:3931.

98. Putti MC, Rondelli R, Cocito MG, et al: Expression of myeloid markers lacks prognostic impact in children treated for acute lymphoblastic leukemia: Italian experience in AIEOP-ALL 88-91 studies. Blood 1998;92:795.

99. Uckun FM, Sather HN, Gaynon PS, et al: Clinical features and treatment outcome of children with myeloid antigen positive acute lymphoblastic leukemia: A report from the Children's Cancer Group. Blood 1997;90:28.

100. Preti HA, Huh YO, O'Brien SM, et al: Myeloid markers in adult acute lymphoblastic leukemia. Correlations with patient and disease characteristics and with prognosis. Cancer 1995;76:1564.

101. Harris NL, Jaffe ES, Diebold J, et al: World Health Organization Classification of Neoplastic Diseases of the Hematopoietic and Lymphoid Tissues: Report of the Clinical Advisory Committee Meeting—Airlie House, Virginia, November 1997. J Clin Oncol 1999;17:3835.

102. Tonegawa S: Somatic generation of antibody diversity. Nature 1983;302:575.

103. Ichihara Y, Matsuoka H, Kurosawa Y: Organization of human immunoglobulin heavy chain diversity gene loci. EMBO J 1988;7:4141.

104. Van Dongen JJM, Wovlers-Tettero ILM: Analysis of immunoglobulin and T cell receptor genes. Part II: possibilities and limitations in the diagnosis and management of lymphoproliferative diseases and related disorders. Clin Chim Acta 1991;198:93.

105. Felix CA, Poplack DG, Reaman GH, et al: Characterization of immunoglobulin and T-cell receptor gene patterns in B-cell precursor acute lymphoblastic leukemia of childhood. J Clin Oncol 1990;8:431.

106. Breit TM, Wovlers-Tettero ILM, Beishuizen A, et al: Southern blot patterns, frequencies and junctional diversity of T-cell receptor δ gene rearrangements in acute lymphoblastic leukemia. Blood 1993;82:3063.

107. Pui CH: Acute lymphoblastic leukemia in children. Curr Opin Oncol 2000;12:3.

Specific Malignancies

III

108. Faderl S, Kantarjian HM, Talpaz M, Estrov Z: Clinical significance of cytogenetic abnormalities in adult acute lymphoblastic leukemia. Blood 1998;91:3995.

109. Harris MB, Shuster JJ, Carroll A, et al: Trisomy of leukemic cell chromosomes 4 and 10 identifies children with B-progenitor cell acute lymphoblastic leukemia with a very low risk of treatment failure: A Pediatric Oncology Group study. Blood 1992;79:3316.

110. Jackson JF, Boyett J, Pullen J, et al: Favorable prognosis associated with hyperdiploidy in children with acute lymphocytic leukemia correlates with extrachromosome 6. Cancer 1990;66:1184.

111. Heerema NH, Sather HN, Sensel MG, et al: Prognostic impact of trisomies of chromosomes 10, 17, and 5 among children with acute lymphoblastic leukemia and high hyperdiploidy (> 50 chromosomes). J Clin Oncol 2000;18:1876.

112. Pui CH, Raimondi SC, Williams DL: Isochromosome 17q in childhood acute lymphoblastic leukemia: An adverse cytogenetic feature in association with hyperdiploidy? Leukemia 1988;2:222.

113. Kaspers GJ, Smets LA, Pieters R, et al: Favorable prognosis of hyperdiploid common acute lymphoblastic leukemia may be explained by sensitivity to antimetabolites and other drugs: Results of an in vitro study. Blood 1995;87:751.

114. Ito C, Kumagai M, Manabe A, et al: Hyperdiploid acute lymphoblastic leukemia with 51 to 65 chromosomes: A distinct biological entity with a marked propensity to undergo apoptosis. Blood 1999;93:315.

115. Gibbons B, MacCallum P, Watts E, et al: Near haploid acute lymphoblastic leukemia: Seven new cases and a review of the literature. Leukemia 1991;5:783.

116. Faderl S, Talpaz M, Estrov Z, et al: The biology of chronic myeloid leukemia. N Engl J Med 1999;341:164.

117. Kurzrock R, Shtalrid M, Romero P, et al: A novel c-abl protein product in Philadephia-positive acute lymphoblastic leukemia. Nature 1987;325:631.

118. Specchia G, Mininni D, Guerrasio A, et al: Ph positive acute lymphoblastic leukemia in adults: Molecular and clinical studies. Leuk Lymphoma 1995;18(Suppl 1):37.

119. Preti HA, O'Brien S, Giralt S, et al: Philadelphia chromosome-positive adult acute lymphocytic leukemia: Characteristics, treatment results, and prognosis in 41 patients. Am J Med 1994;97:60.

120. The Groupe Francais de Cytogenetique Hematologique: Cytogenetic abnormalities in adult acute lymphoblastic leukemia: Correlations with the hematologic findings and outcome. A collaborative study of the Groupe Francais de Cytogenetique Hematologique. Blood 1996;87:3135.

121. Wetzler M, Dodge RK, Mrozek K, et al: Prospective karyotype analysis in adult acute lymphoblastic leukemia: The Cancer and Leukemia Group B experience. Blood 1999;93:383.

122. Zhou M, Gu L, Yeager AM, et al: Incidence and clinical significance of CDKN2/MTS1/P16ink4A and MTS2/P15ink4b gene deletions in childhood acute lymphoblastic leukemia. Pediatr Hematol Oncol 1997;14:141.

123. Rubnitz JE, Behm FG, Pui CH, et al: Genetic studies of childhood acute lymphoblastic leukemia with emphasis on p16, MLL, and ETV6 gene abnormalities: Results of St Jude Total Therapy Study XII. Leukemia 1997;11:1201.

124. Behrendt B, Charrin C, Gibbons B, et al: Dicentric (9;12) in acute lymphocytic leukaemia and other haemtological malignancies: Report from a dic(9;12) study group. Leukemia 1995;9:102.

125. Heerema NA, Sather HN, Sensel MG, et al: Association of chromosome arm 9p abnormalities with adverse risk in childhood acute lymphoblastic leukemia: A report from the Children's Cancer Group. Blood 1999;94:1537.

126. Secker-Walker LM, Prentice HG, Durrant J, et al; On behalf of the MRC Adult Leukaemia Working Party: Cytogenetics adds independent prognostic information in adults with acute lymphoblastic leukaemia on MRC trial UKALL XA. Br J Haematol 1997;96:601.

127. Faderl S, Kantarjian HM, Manshouri T, et al: The prognostic significance of p16INK4a/p14ARF and p15INK4b deletions in adult acute lymphoblastic leukemia. Clin Cancer Res 1999;5:1855.

128. Hoshino K, Asou N, Okubo T, et al: The absence of the p15INK4B gene alterations in adult patients with precursor B-cell acute lymphoblastic leukaemia is a favourable prognostic factor. Br J Haematol 2002;117:531.

129. Secker-Walker LM, on behalf of the European 11q23 Workshop Participants: General Report on the European Union Concerted Action Workshop on 11q23. Leukemia 198;12:776.

130. Harrison CJ, Cuneo A, Clark R, et al: Ten novel 11q23 chromosomal partner sites. Leukemia 1998;12:811.

131. Heerema NA, Arthur DC, Sather H, et al: Cytogenetic features of infants less than 12 months of age at diagnosis of acute lymphoblastic leukemia: impact of the 11q23 breakpoint on outcome: A report of the Childrens Cancer Group. Blood 1994;83:2274.

132. Carroll AJ, Crist WM, Parmley RT, et al: Pre-B cell leukemia associated with chromosome translocation 1;19. Blood 1984;63:721.

133. Hunger SP: Chromosomal translocations involving the E2A gene in acute lymphoblastic leukemia: Clinical features and molecular pathogenesis. Blood 1996;87:1211.

134. Crist WM, Carroll AJ, Shuster JJ, et al: Poor prognosis of children with pre-B acute lymphoblastic leukemia is associated with the t(1;19)(q23;p13). A Pediatric Oncology Group study. Blood 1990;76:117.

135. Aguiar RC, Sohal J, van Rhee F, et al: TEL-AML1 fusion in acute lymphoblastic leukaemia of adults. M.R.C. Adult Leukaemia Working Party. Br J Haematol 1996;95:673.

136. Raynaud S, Mauvieux L, Cayuela JM, et al: TEL/AML1 fusion gene is a rare event in adult acute lymphoblastic leukemia. Leukemia 1996;10:529.

137. Romana SP, Mauchauffee M, Le Coniat M, et al: The t(12;21) of acute lymphoblastic leukemia results in TEL-AML1 gene fusion. Blood 1995;85:3662.

138. Harbott J, Viehmann S, Borkhardt A, et al: Incidence of TEL/AML1 fusion gene analyzed consecutively in children with acute lymphoblastic leukemia in relapse. Blood 1997;90:4933.

139. Seeger K, Adams HP, Buchwald D, et al: TEL-AML1 fusion transcript in relapsed childhood acute lymphoblastic leukemia. The Berlin-Frankfurt-Munster Study Group. Blood 1998;91:1716.

140. Rabbitts TH: Chromosomal translocations in human cancer. Nature 1994;372:143.

141. Capello D, Carbone A, Pastore C, et al: Point mutations of the BCL-6 gene in Burkitt's lymphoma. Br J Haematol 1997;99:168.

142. Lai JL, Fenaux P, Zandecki M, et al: Cytogenetic studies in 30 patients with Burkitt's lymphoma or L3 acute lymphoblastic leukemia with special reference to additional chromosome abnormalitites. Ann Genet 1989;32:26.

143. Parsa NZ, Gaidano G, Mukherjee AB, et al: Cytogenetic and molecular analysis of 6q deletions in Burkitt's lymphoma cell lines. Genes Chromosomes Cancer 1994;9:13.

144. Kornblau SM, Goodacre A, Cabanillas F: Chromosomal abnormalities in adult non-endemic Burkitt's lymphoma and leukemia: 22 new reports and a review of 148 cases from the literature. Hematol Oncol 1991;9:63.

145. Hoelzer D, Ludwig W-D, Eckhard E, et al: Improved outcome in adult B-cell acute lymphoblastic leukemia. Blood 1996;87:495.

146. Yeoh E-J, Ross ME, Shurtleff SA, et al: Classification, subtype discovery, and prediction of outcome in pediatric acute lymphoblastic leukemia by gene expression profiling. Cancer Cell 2002;1:133.

147. Staudt LM: It's ALL in the diagnosis. Cancer Cell 2002;1:109.

148. Ferrando AA, Neuberg DS, Staunton J, et al: Gene expression signatures define novel oncogenic pathways in T cell acute lymphoblastic leukemia. Cancer Cell 2002;1:75.

149. Golub TR, Slonim DK, Tamayo P, et al: Molecular classification of cancer: Class discovery and class prediction by gene expression monitoring. Science 1999;286:531.

150. Frankel SR, Herzig GP, Bloomfield CD: Acute lymphoid leukemia in adults. In Abeloff MD, Armitage JO, Lichter AS, Niederhuber JE (eds): Clinical Oncology, 1st ed. New York, Churchill Livingstone, 1995, p 1925.

151. Jaing TH, Hsueh C, Chiu CH, et al: Cutaneous lymphocytic vasculitis as the presenting feature of acute lymphoblastic leukemia. J Pediatr Hematol Oncol 2002;24:555.

152. Mayo GL, Carter JE, McKinnon SJ: Bilateral optic disk edema and blindness as initial presentation of acute lymphocytic leukemia. Am J Ophthalmol 2002;134:141.

153. Cortes J: Central nervous system involvement in adult acute lymphocytic leukemia. Hematol Oncol Clin North Am 2001; 15:145.

154. Ye CC, Echeverri C, Anderson JE, et al: T-cell blast crisis of chronic myelogenous leukemia manifesting as a large mediastinal tumor. Hum Pathol 2002;33:770.

155. Attarbaschi A, Mann G, Dworzak M, et al: Mediastinal mass in childhood T-cell acute lymphoblastic leukemia: Significance and therapy response. Med Pediatr Oncol 2002;39:558.

156. Picozzi VJ Jr, Coleman CN: Lymphoblastic lymphoma. Semin Oncol 1990;17:96.

157. Gill PS, Meyer PR, Pavlova Z, et al: B cell acute lymphoblastic leukemia in adults. Clinical, morphological, and immunologic findings. J Clin Oncol 1986;4:737.

158. Fenaux P, Bourhuis JH, Ribrag V: Burkitt's acute lymphocytic leukemia (L3 ALL) in adults. Hematol Oncol Clin North Am 2001; 15:37.

159. Thomas DA, Cortes J, Kantarjian HM, et al: High grade non-Hodgkin's lymphomas. In Grossbard ML (ed): American Cancer Society Atlas of Clinical Oncology, Malignant Lymphomas. Hamilton, Ont., B.C. Decker, 2002, p 152.

160. Kubic VL, Kubic PT, Brunning RD: The morphologic and immunphenotypic assessment of the lymphocytosis accompanying Bordetella pertussis infection. Am J Clin Pathol 1991;95:809.

161. Longacre TA, Foucar K, Crago S, et al: Hematogones: A multi-parameter analysis of bone marrow precursor cells. Blood 1989;73:543.

162. van den Doel LJ, Pieters R, Huisman Dr, et al: Immunological phenotype of lymphoid cells in regenerating bone marrow of children after treatment for acute lymphoblastic leukemia. Eur J Haematol 1988;41:170.

163. Acute Leukemias. In Brunning RD, McKennan RW (eds): Atlas of Tumor Pathology—Tumors of the Bone Marrow, 3rd series, fascicle 9. Washington, DC, Armed Forces Institute of Pathology, 1994, p 19.

164. Laport GF, Larson RA: Treatment of adult acute lymphoblastic leukemia. Semin Oncol 1997;24:70.

165. Larson RA, Dodge RK, Burns CP, et al: A five-drug remission induction regimen with intensive consolidation for adults with acute lymphoblastic leukemia: Cancer and Leukemia Group B Study 8811. Blood 1995;85:2025.

166. Hoelzer D: Which factors influence the different outcome of therapy in adults and children with ALL. Bone Marrow Transplant (Suppl 1) 1989;4:98.

167. Goekbuget N, Hoelzer D, Arnold R, et al: Subtypes and treatment outcome in adult acute lymphoblastic leukemia (ALL) < 55 yrs. The Hematol J 2001;1:694a.

168. Faderl S, Albitar M: Insights into the biologic and molecular abnormalities in adult acute lymphocytic leukemia. Hematol Oncol Clin North Am 2000;14:1267.

169. Hoelzer D, Thiel E, Löffler H, et al: Prognostic factors in a multicenter study for treatment of acute lymphoblastic leukemia in adults. Blood 1994;71:123.

170. Miller DR, Coccia PF, Bleyer WA et al: Early response to induction therapy as a predictor of disease-free survival and late recurrence of childhood acute lymphoblastic leukemia: A report from the Children's Cancer Study Group. J Clin Oncol 1989;7:1807.

171. Faderl S, Thall PF, Kantarjian HM, Estrov Z: Time to platelet recovery predicts outcome of patients with de novo acute lymphoblastic leukaemia who have achieved a complete remission. Br J Haematol 2002;117:869.

172. Hoelzer D, Arnold R, Freund M, et al: Characteristics, outcome and risk factors in adult T-lineage acute lymphoblastic leukemia (ALL). Blood 1999;94:2926a.

173. Ludwig W-D, Rieder H, Bartram CR, et al: Immunophenotypic and genotypic features, clinical characteristics, and treatment outcome of adult pro-B acute lymphoblastic leukemia: Results of German multicenter trials GMALL 03/87 and 04/89. Blood 1998;92:1898.

174. Annino L, Vegna ML, Camera A, et al: Treatment of adult acute lymphoblastic leukemia (ALL): Long-term follow-up of the GIMEMA ALL 0288 randomized study. Blood 2002;99:863.

175. Tafuri A, on behalf of the GIMEMA Cooperative Study Group: Multidrug resistance proteins MDR1/P-gp, MRP1, and LRP in adult ALL patients uniformly treated according to the GIMEMA 0496 protocol: Poor prognostic impact of MDR1/P-gp. Blood 1999;94:1265a.

176. Gökbuget N, Hoelzer D, Arnold R, et al: Treatment of adult ALL according to protocols of the German Multicenter Study Group for Adult ALL (GMALL). Hematol Oncol Clin North Am 2000; 14:1307.

177. Durrant IJ, Richards SM, Prentice HG, et al: The Medical Research Council trials in adult acute lymphocytic leukemia. Hematol Oncol Clin North Am 2000;14:1327.

178. Larson RA: Recent clinical trials in acute lymphocytic leukemia by the Cancer and Leukemia Group B. Hematol Oncol Clin North Am 2000;14:1367.

179. Kantarjian HM, O'Brien S, Smith TL, et al: Results of treatment with hyper-CVAD, a dose-intensive regimen, in adult acute lymphocytic leukemia. J Clin Oncol 2000;18:547.

180. Schaison G, Sommelet D, Bancillon A, et al: Treatment of acute lymphoblastic leukemia French protocol Fralle 83-87. Leukemia 1992;6(Suppl 2):148.

181. Hussein KK, Dahlberg S, Head D, et al: Treatment of acute lymphoblastic leukemia in adults with intensive induction, consolidation, and maintenance chemotherapy. Blood 1989;73:57.

182. GIMEMA Cooperative Group: GIMEMA ALL 0183: A multicentric study on adult acute lymphoblastic leukaemia in Italy. Br J Haematol 1989;71:377.

183. Linker C, Damon L, Ries C, Navarro W: Intensified and shortened cyclical chemotherapy for adult acute lymphoblastic leukemia. J Clin Oncol 2002;20:2464.

184. Durrant IJ, Prentice HG, Richards SM: Intensification of treatment for adults with acute lymphoblastic leukaemia: Results of U.K. Medical Research Council randomized trial UKALL XA. Br J Haematol 1997;99:84.

185. Todeschini G, Tecchio C, Meneghini V, et al: Estimated 6-year event-free survival of 55% in 60 consecutive adult acute lymphoblatsic leukemia patients treated with an intensive phase II protocol based on high induction dose of daunorubicin. Leukemia 1998;12:144.

186. Stryckmans P, Debusscher L: Chemotherapy of adult acute lymphoblastic leukaemia. Baillieres Clin Haematol 1991;4:115.

187. Kantarjian HM, O'Brien S, Smith T, et al: Acute lymphocytic leukaemia in the elderly: Characteristics and outcome with the vincristine-adriamycin-dexamethasone (VAD) regimen. Br J Haematol 194;88:94.

188. Kantarjian HM, Walters RS, Keating MJ, et al: Experience with vincristine, doxorubicin, and dexamethasone (VAD) chemotherapy in adults with refractory acute lymphocytic leukemia. Cancer 1989;64:16.

189. Jones B, Freeman Aik, Shuster JJ, et al: Lower incidence of meningeal leukemia when prednisone is replaced by dexamethasone in the treatment of acute lymphocytic leukemia. Med Pediatr Oncol 1991;19:269.

190. Hurwitz CA, Silverman LB, Schorin MA, et al: Substituting dexamethasone for prednisone complicates remission induction in children with acute lymphoblastic leukemia. Cancer 2000; 88:1964.

191. Linker CA, Levitt LJ, O'Donnell M, et al: Treatment of adult acute lymphoblastic leukemia with intensive cyclical chemotherapy: A follow-up report. Blood 1991;78:2814.

192. Nagura E: Nation-wide randomized comparative study of doxorubicin, vincristine and prednisolone combination therapy with and without L-asparaginase for adult acute lymphoblastic leukemia. Cancer Chemother Pharmacol 1994;33:359.

193. Weiss M, Maslak P, Feldman E, et al: Cytarabine with high dose mitoxantrone induces rapid complete remissions in adult acute lymphoblastic leukemia (ALL) without the use of vincristine or prednisone. J Clin Oncol 1996;14:2480.

194. Cuttner J, Mick R, Budman DR, et al: Phase III trial of brief intensive treatment of adult acute lymphocytic leukemia comparing daunorubicin and mitoxantrone: A CALGB study. Leukemia 1991;5:425.

195. Ottman OG, Hoelzer D, Gracien E, et al: Concomitant granulocyte colony-stimulating factor and induction chemoradiotherapy in adult acute lymphoblastic leukemia: A randomized phase III trial. Blood 1995;86:444.

196. Scherrer R, Bettelheim P, Gaissler K, et al: High efficiency of the German multicenter ALL (GMALL) protocol for treatment of adult acute lymphoblastic leukemia (ALL)—a single institution study. Ann Hematol 1994;69:181.

197. Larson RA, Dodge RK, Linker CA, et al: A randomized controlled trial of filgrastim during remission induction and consolidation chemotherapy for adults with acute lymphoblastic leukemia: CALGB Study 9111. Blood 198;92:1556.

198. Goekbuget N, Arnold R, Buechner T, et al: Intensification of induction and consolidation improves only subgroups of adult ALL: Analysis of 1200 patients in GMALL Study 05/93. Blood 2001;98:802a.

199. Ribera J-M, Ortega JJ, Oriol A, et al: Late intensification chemotherapy has not improved the results of intensive chemotherapy in adult acute lymphoblastic leukemia. Results of a prospective multicenter randomized trial (PETHEMA ALL-89). Haematologica 1998;83:222.

200. Laport GJ, Larson RA: Treatment of adult acute lymphoblastic leukemia. Semin Oncol 1997;24:70.

201. Cassileth PA, Andersen JW, Bennett JM, et al: Adult acute lymphocytic leukemia. The Eastern Cooperative Oncology Group experience. Leukemia 1992;62:178.

202. Childhood ALL Collaborative Group: Duration and intensity of maintenance chemotherapy in acute lymphoblastic leukaemia: Overview of 42 trials involving 12 000 randomized children. Lancet 1996;347:1783.

203. Mandelli F, Annino L, Rotoli B: The GIMEMA ALL 0183 trial: Analysis of 10-year follow-up. Br J Haematol 1996;92:665.

204. Chessells JM, Harrison G, Lilleyman JS, et al: Continuing (maintenance) therapy in lymphoblastic leukaemia: Lessons from MRC UKALL X. Br J Haematol 1997;98:945.

205. Cortes J, O'Brien SM, Pierce S, et al: The value of high-dose systemic chemotherapy and intrathecal therapy for central nervous system prophylaxis in different risk groups of adult acute lymphoblastic leukemia. Blood 1995;86:2091.

206. Bleyer WA, Poplack DA: Prophylaxis and treatment of leukemia in the central nervous system and other sanctuaries. Semin Oncol 1985;12:131.

207. Evans AE, Gilbert ES, Zandstra R: The increasing incidence of central nervous system leukemia in children. Children's Cancer Study Group A. Cancer 1970;26:404.

208. Matrangelo R, Poplack D, Bleyer A, et al: Report and recommendation from the Rome workshop concerning poor-prognosis acute lymphoblastic leukemia in children: Biologic bases for staging, stratification, and treatment. Med Pediatr Oncol 1986;14:191.

209. Mahmoud DH Jr, Rivera GK, Hancock ML, et al: Low leukocyte counts with blast cells in cerebrospinal fluid of children with newly diagnosed acute lymphoblastic leukemia. N Engl J Med 1993;329:314.

210. Omura GA, Moffitt S, Vogler WR, et al: Combination chemotherapy of adult acute lymphoblastic leukemia with randomized central nervous system prophylaxis. Blood 1980;55:199.

211. Pavlovsky S, Eppinger-Helft M, Sackmann MF: Factors that influence the appearance of central nervous system leukemia. Blood 1973;42:935.

212. Thomas DA, Cortes J, O'Brien S, et al: Hyper-CVAD program in Burkitt's-type adult acute lymphoblastic leukemia. J Clin Oncol 1999;17:2461.

213. Kantarjian HM, Walters RS, Smith TL, et al: Identification of risk groups for development of central nervous system leukemia in adults with acute lymphocytic leukemia. Blood 1988;72:1784.

214. Schrappe M, Reiter A, Ludwig WD, et al: Improved outcome in childhood acute lymphoblastic leukemia despite reduced dose of anthracyclines an cranial radiotherapy: Results of trial ALL-BFM 90. Blood 2000;95:3310.

215. Tubergen DG, Gilchrist GS, O'Brien RT, et al: Prevention of CNS disease in intermediate-risk acute lymphoblastic leukemia: Comparison of cranial radiation and intrathecal methotrexate and the importance of systemic therapy: A Children's Cancer Group report. J Clin Oncol 1993;11:520.

216. Chester S, Esparza A, Flinton L, et al: Further development of a successful protocol of graft versus leukemia without fatal graft-versus-host disease in AKR mice. Cancer Res 1977;37:3494.

217. Fefer A, Einstein A, Cheever M: Adoptive chemoimmunotherapy of cancer in animals: A review of results, principles and problems. Ann N Y Acad Sci 1976;277:492.

218. Ringden O, Horowitz M: Graft-versus-leukemia reactions in humans. Transplant Proc 1989;21:2989.

219. Martin TG, Gajewski JL: Allogeneic stem cell transplantation for acute lymphocytic leukemia in adults. Hematol Oncol Clin North Am 2001;15:97.

220. Blume K, Forman S, Snyder D, et al: Allogeneic bone marrow transplantation for acute lymphoblastic leukemia during first complete remission. Transplantation 1987;43:389.

221. Chao N, Formen S, Schmidt G, et al: Allogeneic bone marrow transplantation for high-risk acute lymphoblastic leukemia during first complete remission. Blood 1995;85:3353.

222. DeWitte T, Awwad B, Boezeman J, et al: Role of allogeneic bone marrow transplantation in adolescent or adult patients with acute lymphoblastic leukemia or lymphoblastic lymphoma in first remission. Bone Marrow Transplant 1994;14:767.

223. Sebban C, Lepage E, Vernant J, et al: Allogeneic bone marrow transplantation in adult acute lymphoblastic leukemia in first complete remission: A comparative study. J Clin Oncol 1994;12:2580.

224. Ribera JM, Ortega JJ, Oriol A, et al: Intensive chemotherapy (CHT), allogeneic (allo) or autologous (auto) stem cell transplantation (SCT) for high-risk ALL (HRALL). Results of the ongoing protocol PETHEMA ALL-93. Blood 1999;94:168a.

225. Horowitz M, Messere D, Hoelzer D, et al: Chemotherapy compared with bone marrow transplantation for adults with acute lymphoblastic leukemia in first remission. Ann Intern Med 1991;115:13.

226. Zhang M, Hoelzer D, Horowitz M, et al: Long-term follow-up of adults with acute lymphoblastic leukemia in first remission treated with chemotherapy or bone marrow transplantation. Ann Intern Med 1995;123:428.

227. Rowe JM, Richards S, Wiernik PH, et al: Allogeneic bone marrow transplantation (BMT) for adults with acute lymphoblastic leukemia (ALL) if first complete remission (CR): Early results from the International ALL trial (MRC UKALL XII/ECOG E2993). Blood 1999;94:168a.

228. Biggs JC, Horowitz MM, Gale RP, et al: Bone marrow transplants may cure patients with acute leukemia never achieving remission with chemotherapy. Blood 1992;80:1090.

229. Mortimer J, Blinder M, Schulman S, et al: Relapse of acute leukemia after marrow transplantation: Natural history and results of subsequent therapy. J Clin Oncol 1989;7:50.

230. Attal M, Blaise D, Marit G, et al: Consolidative treatment of adult acute lymphoblastic leukemia: A prospective, randomized trial comparing allogeneic versus autologous bone marrow transplantation and testing the impact of recombinant interleukin-2 after autologous bone marrow transplantation. Blood 1995;86:1619.

231. Vey N, Blaise D, Stoppa A, et al: Bone marrow transplantation in 63 adult patients with acute lymphoblastic leukemia in first complete remission. Bone Marrow Transplant 1994;14:383.

232. Fiere D, Lepage E, Sebban C, et al: Adult acute lymphoblastic leukemia: a multicentric randomized trial testing bone marrow transplantation as postremission therapy. J Clin Oncol 1993;11:1990.

233. Thiebault A, Vernant JP, Degos L, et al: Adult acute lymphocytic leukemia study testing chemotherapy and autologous and allogeneic transplantation. A follow-up report of the French protocol LALA 87. Hematol Oncol Clin North Am 2000;14:1353.

234. Kantarjian HM, Walters RS, Keating MJ, et al: Results of the vincristine, doxorubicin, and dexamethasone regimen in adults with standard- and high-risk acute lymphocytic leukemia. J Clin Oncol 1990;8:994.

235. Hoelzer D, Gale R: Acute lymphoblastic leukemia in adults: Recent progress, future directions. Semin Hematol 1987;24:27.

236. Hoelzer D, Gökbuget N: Recent approaches in acute lymphoblastic leukemia in adults. Crit Rev Oncol Hematol 2000;36:49.

237. Szydlo R, Goldman J, Klein J, et al: Results of allogeneic bone marrow transplants for leukemia using donors other than HLA-identical siblings. J Clin Oncol 1997;15:1767.

238. Cornelissen JJ, Carston M, Kollman C, et al: Unrelated marrow transplantation for adult patients with poor-risk acute lymphoblastic leukemia: Strong graft-versus-leukemia effect and risk factors determining outcome. Blood 2001;97:1572.

239. Faderl S, Estrov Z: The clinical significance of detection of residual disease in childhood ALL. Crit Rev Oncol Hematol 1998;28:31.

240. Stock W, Estrov Z: Studies of minimal residual disease in acute lymphocytic leukemia. Hematol Oncol Clin North Am 2000;14:1289.

241. Cavé H, van der Werff ten Bosch J, Suciu S, et al: Clinical significance of minimal residual disease in childhood acute lymphoblastic leukemia. N Engl J Med 19998;339:591.

242. Foroni L, Coyle LA, Papaioannou M, et al: Molecular detection of minimal residual disease in adult and childhood acute lymphoblastic leukaemia reveals differences in treatment response. Leukemia 1997;11:1732.

243. Brisco MJ, Hughes E, Neoh SH, et al: Relationship between minimal residual disease and outcome in adult acute lymphoblastic leukemia. Blood 1996;87:5251.

244. Mortuza FY, Papaioannou M, Moreira IM, et al: Minimal residual disease tests provide an independent predictor of clinical outcome in adult acute lymphoblastic leukemia. J Clin Oncol 2002;20:1094.

245. Garcia-Manero G, Thomas DA: Salvage therapy for refractory or relapsed acute lymphocytic leukemia. Hematol Oncol Clin North Am 2001;15:163.

246. Larson RA, Stock W, Hoelzer DF, Kantarjian HM: Acute lympho-blastic leukemia in adults. Hematology 1998. Washington DC, American Society of Hematology Education Program Book, 1998, p 44.

247. Thomas DA, Kantarjian H, Smith TL, et al: Primary refractory and relapsed acute lymphoblastic leukemia: Characteristics, treatment results, and prognosis with salvage therapy. Cancer 1999;86:1216.

248. Vora A, Frost L, Goodeve A, et al: Late relapsing childhood lymphoblastic leukemia. Blood 1998;92:2334.

249. Gaynon PS, Qu RP, Chappell RJ, et al: Survival after relapse in childhood acute lymphoblastic leukemia: Impact of site and time to first relapse—the Children's Cancer Group experience. Cancer 1998;82:1387.

250. Abshire TC, Buchanan GR, Jackson JF, et al: Morphologic, immunologic and cytogenetic studies in children with acute lymphoblastic leukemia at diagnosis and relapse: A Pediatric Oncology Group study. Leukemia 1992;6:357.

251. Raimondi SC, Pui CH, Head DR, et al: Cytogenetically different leukemic clones at relapse of childhood acute lymphoblastic leukemia. Blood 1993;82:576.

252. Chucrallah AE, Stass SA, Huh YO, et al: Adult acute lymphoblastic leukemia at relapse: Cytongenetic, immunophenotypic, and molecular changes. Cancer 1995;76:985.

253. Tosi P, Visani G, Ottaviani E, et al: Biological and clinical significance of in vitro prednisolone resistance in adult acute lymphoblastic leukaemia. Eur J Haematol 1996;57:134.

254. Ramakers-van-Woerden NL, Pieters R, Kaspers GJL, et al: The Philadelphia chromosome t(9;22) is associated with in vitro prednisolone and daunorubicin resistance in adult acute lymphoblastic leukemia. Ann Hematol 1997;74:A38.

255. Goasguen JE, Dossot JM, Fardel O, et al: Expression of the multidrug resistance-associated P-glycoprotein (P-170) in 59 cases of de novo acute lymphoblastic leukemia: Prognostic implications. Blood 1993;81:2394.

256. Koller CA, Kantarjian HM, Thomas D, et al: The hyper-CVAD regimen improves outcome in relapsed acute lymphoblastic leukemia. Leukemia 1997;11:2039.

257. Sur P, Fernandes DJ, Kute TE, et al: L-Asparaginase-induced modulation of methotrexate polyglutamylation in murine leukemia L5178Y. Cancer Res 1987;47:1313.

258. Esterhay RJ Jr, Wiernik PH, Grove WR, et al: Moderate dose metho-trexate, vincristine, asparaginase, and dexamethasone for treatment of adult acute lymphocytic leukemia. Blood 1982;59:334.

259. Aguayo A, Cortes J, Thomas D, et al: Combination therapy with methotrexate, vincristine, polyethylene-glycol conjugated-asparaginase, and prednisone in the treatment of patients with refractory or recurrent acute lymphoblastic leukemia. Cancer 1999;86:1203.

260. Abshire TC, Pollock BH, Billett AL, Bradley P, Buchanan GR: Weekly polyethylene glycol conjugated L-asparaginase compared with biweekly dosing produces superior induction remission rates in a childhood relapsed acute lymphoblastic leukemia: A Pediatric Oncology Group Study. Blood 2000;96:1709–1715.

261. Willemze R, Peters WG, Colly LP: Short-term intensive treatment (VAAP) of adult acute lymphoblastic leukemia and lymphoblastic lymphoma. Eur J Haematol 1988;41:489.

262. Suki S, Kantarjian H, Gandhi V, et al: Fludarabine and cytosine arabinoside in the treatment of refractory or relapsed acute lymphocytic leukemia. Cancer 1993;72:2155.

263. Deane M, Koh M, Foroni L, et al: FLAG-idarubicin and allogeneic stem cell transplantation for Ph-positive ALL beyond frist remission. Bone Marrow Transplant 1998;22:1137.

264. Fleming DR, Henslee-Downey PJ, Romond EH, et al: Allogeneic bone marrow transplantation with T cell-depleted partially matched related donors for advanced acute lymphoblastic leukemia in children and adults: A comparative matched cohort study. Bone Marrow Transplant 1996;17:917.

265. Herzig RH, Bortin MM, Barrett AJ, et al: Bone-marrow transplantation in high-risk acute lymphoblastic leukaemia in first and second remission. Lancet 1987;1:786.

266. Advisory Committee of IBMTR: Report from the International Bone Marrow Transplant Registry. Bone Marrow Transplant 1989;4:221.

267. Davies SM, Ramsay NK, Weisdorf DJ: Feasibility and timing of unrelated donor identification for patienst with ALL. Bone Marrow Transplant 1996;17:737.

268. Uckun FM, Kersey HJ, Haake R, et al: Pretransplantation burden of leukemic progenitor cells as a predictor of relapse after bone marrow transplantation for acute lymphoblastic leukemia. N Engl J Med 1993;329:1296.

269. Weisdorf DJ, Billett AL, Hannan P, et al: Autologous versus unrelated donor allogeneic marrow transplantation for acute lymphoblastic leukemia. Blood 1997;90:2962.

270. Gluck WL, Bigner SH, Borowitz MJ, Brenckman WD Jr: Acute lymphoblastic leukemia of Burkitt's type (L3 ALL) with 8;22 and 14;18 translocations and absent surface immunoglobulins. Am J Clin Pathol 1986;85:636.

271. Imamura N, Mtasiwa DM, Ota H, et al: FAB L3 type of B-cell acute lymphoblastic leukemia (B-ALL) without chromosome abnormal-ities. Am J Hematol 1990;35:216.

272. Patte C, Philip T, Rodary C, et al: Improved survival rate in children with stage III and stage IV B cell non-Hodgkin's lymphoma and leukemia using multi-agent chemotherapy: Results of a study of 114 children from the French Pediatric Oncology Society. J Clin Oncol 1986;4:1219.

273. Reiter A, Schrappe M, Ludwig W-D, et al: Favourable outcome of B-cell acute lymphoblastic leukemia in childhood: A report of three consecutive studies of the BFM group. Blood 1992;80:2471.

274. Murphy SB, Bowman WP, Abromowitch M, et al: Results of treatment of advanced-stage Burkitt's lymphoma and B cell (sIg+) acute lymphoblastic leukemia with high-dose fractionated cyclosphosphamide and coordinated high-dose methotrexate and cytarabine. J Clin Oncol 1986;4:1732.

275. Bowman PW, Shuster JJ, Cook B, et al: Improved survival for children with B cell acute lymphoblastic leukemia and stage IV small noncleaved cell lymphoma: A Pediatric Oncology Group Study. J Clin Oncol 1996;14:1252.

276. Soussain C, Patte C, Ostronoff M, et al: Small noncleaved cell lymphoma and leukemia in adults. A retrospective study of 65 adults treated with the LMB pediatric protocols. Blood 1995;85:664.

277. Pees HW, Radtke H, Schwamborn J, Graf N: The BFM-protocol for HIV-negative Burkitt's lymphomas and L3 ALL in adult patients: A high chance for cure. Ann Hematol 1992;65:201.

278. Todeschini G, Tecchio C, Degani D, et al: Eight-one percent event-free survival in advanced Burkitt's lymphoma/leukemia: No differences in outcome between pediatric and adult patients treated with the same intensive pediatric protocol. Ann Oncol 1997;8(Suppl 1):77.

279. Reiter A, Schrappe M, Parwaresch R, et al: Non-Hodgkin's lymphomas of childhood and adolescence: Results of a treatment stratified for biologic subtypes and stage. A report of the Berlin-Frankfurt-Munster Group. J Clin Oncol 1995;13:359.

280. Cortes J, Koller C, Thomas D, et al: Treatment of AIDS-related Burkitt's leukemia or lymphoma with the hyper-CVAD regimen. Blood 1998;92:401a.

281. Sweetenham JW, Pearce R, Taghipour G, et al: Adult Burkitt's and Burkitt-like non-Hodgkin's lymphoma—Outcome for patients treated with high-dose therapy and autologous stem-cell transplantation in first remission or at relapse: Results from the European Group for Blood and Bone Marrow Transplantation. J Clin Oncol 1996;14:2465.

282. Nathwani BN, Diamond LW, Winberg CD, et al: Lymphoblastic lymphoma: A clinicopathologic study of 95 patients. Cancer 1981;48:2347.

283. Coleman CN, Picozzi VJ, Cox RS, et al: Treatment of lymphoblastic lymphoma in adults. J Clin Oncol 1986;4:1628.

284. Morel P, Lepage E, Brice P, et al: Prognosis and treatment of lymphoblastic lymphoma in adults: A report on 80 patients. J Clin Oncol 1992;10:1078.

285. Bernasconi C, Brusamolino E, Lazzarino M, et al: Lymphoblastic lymphoma in adult patients: Clinicopathological features and response to intensive multiagent chemotherapy analogous to that used in acute lymphoblastic leukemia. Ann Oncol 1990;1:141.

286. Slater DE, Mertelsmann R, Koziner B, et al: Lymphoblastic lymphoma in adults. J Clin Oncol 1986;4:57.

287. Salloum E, Henry-Amar M, Caillou B, et al: Lymphoblastic lymphoma in adults: A clinico-pathologic study of 34 cases treated at the Institute Gustave Roussy. Cancer Clin Oncol 1988;24:1609.

288. Thomas DA, Kantarjian H, O'Brien S, et al: Outcome with the hyper-CVAD regimen in lymphoblastic lymphoma (LL). Proc Am Soc Clin Oncol 1999;18:11a.

289. Thomas DA, Kantarjian HM: Lymphoblastic lymphoma. Hematol Oncol Clin North Am 2001;15:51.

290. Sweetenham JW, Liberti G, Pearce R, et al: High-dose therapy and autologous bone marrow transplantation for adult patients with lymphoblastic lymphoma: Results of the European Group for Bone Marrow Transplantation. J Clin Oncol 1994;12:1358.

291. Sweetenham JW, Santini G, Simnett S, et al: Autologous stem cell transplantation (ASCT) in 1st remission improves relapse free survival (RFS) in adult patients (pts) with lymphoblastic lymphoma (LBL): Results from a randomized trial of the European Group for Blood and Marrow Transplantation (EBMT) and the UK Lymphoma Group (UKLG). Proc Am Soc Clin Oncol 1998;17:17a.

292. Faderl S, Garcia-Manero G, Thomas DA, Kantarjian HM: Philadelphia chromosome-positive acute lymphoblastic leukemia—Current concepts and future perspectives. Rev Clin Exp Hematol 2002;6:142.

293. Goldstone AH, Prentice HG, Durant J, et al: Allogeneic transplant (related or unrelated donor) is the preferred treatment for adult Philadelphia chromosome positive (Ph+) acute lymphoblastic leukemia (ALL). Results from the International ALL Trial (MRC UKALLXII/ECOG E2993). Blood 2001;98:856a.

294. Druker BJ, Tamura S, Buchdunger E, et al: Effects of a selective inhibitor of the ABL tyrosine kinase on the growth of BCR-ABL positive cells. Nat Med 1996;2:561.

295. Thomas DA, Cortes J, Giles FJ, et al: Combination of Hyper-CVAD with imatinib mesylate (STI571) for Philadelphia (Ph)-positive adult acute lymphoblastic leukemia (ALL) or chronic myelogenous leukemia in lymphoid blast phase (CML-LBP). Blood 2001;98:803a.

296. Ottmann OG, Wassmann B, Pfeifer H, et al: Activity of the ABL-tyrosine kinase inhibitor Glivec (STI571) in Philadelphia chromosome positive acute lymphoblastic leukemia (PH+ ALL) relapsing after allogeneic stem cell transplantation (allo-SCT). Blood 2001;98:589a.

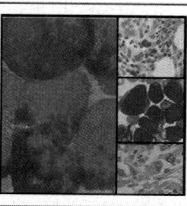

04

ACUTE MYELOID LEUKEMIA IN ADULTS

Frederick R. Appelbaum

SUMMARY OF KEY POINTS

EPIDEMIOLOGY AND ETIOLOGY

- Incidence: 3/100,000/year in the United States.
- Increased incidence with age; median age, 60.
- Known causes include exposure to benzene or ionizing radiation, prior exposure to chemotherapy, and a few uncommon inherited syndromes.

BIOLOGY

- AML is a clonal disease arising in a primitive hematopoietic progenitor cell.
- Leukemogenesis is a multistep process requiring some mutations that block differentiation and others that promote proliferation.

DIAGNOSIS AND CLASSIFICATION

- Diagnosis requires greater than 20% blasts of myeloid origin in marrow or peripheral blood.

- New WHO classification recognizes four categories of AML: (1) AML with recurrent genetic abnormalities; (2) AML with multilineage dysplasia; (3) AML and MDS, therapy related; (4) AML not otherwise categorized.
- Cytogenetics are the most powerful single indicator of outcome, and cases can be defined as favorable, intermediate, or unfavorable according to cytogenetic subtype. Translocation t(15;17) is diagnostic of acute promyelocytic leukemia, the M3 subtype of AML that requires a very specific form of therapy.

TREATMENT

- Younger patients with non-M3 AML: Induction—Anthracycline plus cytarabine induces complete remission in approximately 70% of patients.

Postinduction therapy—Patients with good-risk disease can be treated with repetitive doses of cytarabine with a greater than 50% expectation of cure. Patients with intermediate-risk disease can be treated with either continued chemotherapy or hematopoietic cell transplantation. Patients with poor-risk disease should receive transplantation in first remission if possible.
- Older patients with non-M3 AML: Induction—Anthracyclines plus cytarabine induce complete remission in 50% of patients. Postinduction therapy—Continued chemotherapy might cure 15% of patients.
- Acute promyelocytic leukemia.
- ATRA should be added to induction and used as maintenance, with an expectation of cure in two-thirds of patients.

INTRODUCTION

Acute myeloid leukemia (AML) is the result of a genetic event or series of events occurring in an early hematopoietic precursor that both blocks differentiation and allows uncontrolled proliferation. The abnormally proliferating leukemic cells accumulate in the marrow space, eventually replacing normal marrow progenitors and resulting in diminished production of red cells, white cells, and platelets. This, in turn, causes the common clinical manifestations of AML—namely, anemia, infection, and bleeding. As the disease progresses, leukemic blasts pour out into the bloodstream, leading to the "weisses Blut" described by Virchow in 1845.[1] Eventually, the leukemic cells accumulate in the spleen, lung, brain, and other vital organs. If left untreated, AML rapidly becomes fatal, with most patients dying within a few months of diagnosis. If treated appropriately, however, a substantial proportion of patients can be cured. There has been remarkable growth in our understanding of AML over the past decade. One of the major lessons arising from this new knowledge is the complexity of the leukemic process—a lesson that can be daunting but one that also provides multiple new targets for prevention, detection, and treatment.

EPIDEMIOLOGY AND ETIOLOGY

Incidence

Approximately 32,000 Americans developed leukemia in 2001.[2] Of these, 32% developed AML, 26% chronic lymphocytic leukemia (CLL), 15% chronic myeloid leukemia (CML), 11% acute lymphocytic leukemia (ALL), and the remaining 16% had unclassified types. The male-to-female ratio is approximately 1.3:1. The incidence of AML is constant during the first 30 years of life but then begins to increase almost exponentially (Fig. 104-1). The overall incidence of leukemia in the United States has remained stable over the last 30 years.[3]

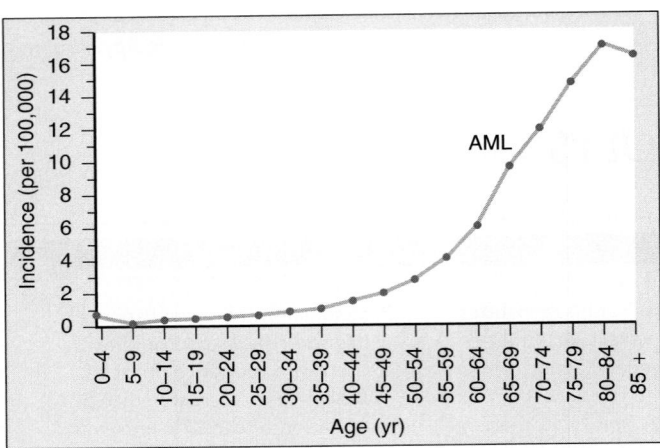

Figure 104-1. Age-related incidence of AML. The incidence is relatively stable until age 30 and then increases dramatically.

Geographic Clustering

Although there have been occasional reports of leukemic clusters within a given geographic area, no compelling studies suggest that these are more than chance events.

Viruses

There is a clear association between infection with human T-cell leukemia virus and an adult form of T-cell leukemia. There is, however, no known association between any viral infection and the development of AML.

Carcinogens

Heavy benzene exposure is associated with the development of aplastic anemia, myelodysplasia, and AML.[4] Most studies examining the issue find a small but consistent increase in AML among cigarette smokers.[5] Survivors of the atomic bomb explosions of Hiroshima and Nagasaki in 1945 demonstrated an increased risk of all leukemias except CLL, which began as early as 1.5 years after the explosions, peaked at around 7 years, and returned to baseline by 1970.[6] Other evidence that ionizing radiation is leukemogenic comes from the tenfold increased risk of AML among individuals receiving radiation treatment for ankylosing spondylitis in the 1930s and the 1940s.[7]

Treatment-related AML

With the increasing use of radiation and chemotherapy to treat malignancies, the incidence of treatment-related AML has grown. It is estimated that perhaps 6% to 10% of AML cases are treatment-related.[8] These can be grouped in several relatively distinct syndromes. AML developing after exposure to alkylating agents has a latency of 5 to 6 years, often first appears as a myelodysplastic syndrome (MDS), and is frequently associated with chromosomal abnormalities involving the long arms of chromosomes 5 or 7. This association was first appre-

ciated in the 1970s in patients previously treated for lymphoma with alkylating agents with or without radiation.[9] Patients treated for Hodgkin's disease with combination chemotherapy (including nitrogen mustard) could have a cumulative incidence of secondary AML as high as 10% at 10 years, particularly if they are older.[10-12] It is uncertain whether the addition of radiation therapy further increases the risk of AML.[13] Both melphalan and cyclophosphamide have been associated with the development of AML in women treated for ovarian cancer.[14,15] Patients receiving chloroethylnitrosoureas for colorectal cancer have likewise been shown to be at increased risk.[16] Likely, all alkylating agents are leukemogenic, with risk increasing with cumulative dose.[17]

Patients treated with topoisomerase II inhibitors are also at risk for developing therapy-related AML. In contrast to the leukemias seen after exposure to alkylating agents, these leukemias develop relatively rapidly (often within 2 years), are not generally preceded by a myelodysplastic phase, and frequently have rearrangements involving 11q23, the locus for MLL (the mixed-lineage leukemia gene) or 21q22.[18] The epipodophyllotoxins etoposide and teniposide fall in this category; with these drugs, the risk of developing secondary AML appears to be dose-related and might increase when methotrexate or cisplatin is also administered.[19,20] The anthracyclines also are topoisomerase II inhibitors, and their use—particularly when given with cyclophosphamide in dose-intense regimens—has been associated with secondary AML.[21]

Patients treated for non-Hodgkin's lymphoma using autologous hematopoietic cell transplantation (HCT) appear to be at increased risk for the development of secondary AML, with cumulative incidences as high as 15% reported in some series.[22,23] Leukemias typical of exposure to both a prior alkylating agent and a prior topoisomerase II inhibitor have been reported. Recent registry data demonstrate that the risk of MDS/AML after autologous HCT is predicted largely by the type and intensity of chemotherapy received by the patient before referral for transplantation. This observation raises some questions about the exact contribution of the transplant procedure itself to the development of secondary AML.[24]

Bimolane, a dioxopiperazine derivative used for the treatment of psoriasis, has been associated with the development of acute promyelocytic leukemia.

Not all secondary leukemias fall into the discrete categories described here. Secondary leukemias with inv 16, t(9;22) and abnormalities involving 3q21 have been reported.[25] Not every leukemia developing in patients who have received radiation or chemotherapy is necessarily due to that therapy. In fact, there is a significant elevation in risk for AML among individuals with a prior malignancy treated only with surgery, suggesting a genetic or other predisposition.[26]

Ethnic Differences

Acute promyelocytic leukemia has been reported to be more common among Hispanic populations in the Los Angeles area than in the general population.[27] A similar increased incidence has been reported in Spain.[28]

Familial Clustering

The concordance rate of leukemia in identical twins is virtually 100% if one twin develops leukemia before the first year of life, but the rate then declines with age.[29] A large comprehensive study of proband effects in Utah using data from 125,000 cancer patients found that the relative risk of leukemia among first-degree relatives of probands with leukemia was 5.69, strongly suggesting that complex genetic factors could influence the development of leukemia in later life.[30] Several single-gene leukemia syndromes have also been described, including an autosomal recessive syndrome of childhood-onset myelodysplasia with monosomy 7 and a familial syndrome of erythroleukemia.[31,32] A familial syndrome of an aspirin-like platelet disorder with thrombocytopenia and propensity for the development of AML has recently been shown to be due to germline mutations in the AML-1 gene.[33] Nearly all of these autosomal dominant leukemia syndromes (with the exception of the AML-1 syndrome) demonstrate anticipation with declining age of onset with each generation.

Constitutional Chromosomal Abnormalities

Children with trisomy 21 (Down syndrome) have an increased risk of leukemia, with M7 AML seen in early childhood and ALL predominating in later years. Trisomy 8 mosaicism is a rare constitutional abnormality with mental retardation, multiple developmental defects, and an increased incidence of myeloid leukemias.

Genetic Syndromes Associated with AML

Several DNA-repair syndromes are associated with an increased incidence of AML. Bloom's syndrome is an autosomal recessive disorder resulting from mutations in a DNA helicase at 15q21.1 and is characterized by growth retardation, characteristic facial appearance, immuno-deficiency, and in 25% of patients, hematologic malignancies including AML.[34] Ataxia telangiectasia is an autosomal recessive disease due to mutations in the ATM gene at 11q22-23, which results in deficiencies in the G1-S checkpoint. Patients with this disorder can develop progressive cerebellar ataxia, telangiectatic skin lesions, and malignancies that are more often of lymphoid than myeloid origin.[35] Fanconi anemia is an autosomal recessive syndrome characterized by pancytopenia and a variety of developmental disorders that include skeletal abnormalities (most notably, hypoplastic thumbs) and short stature. Exposure of cells from Fanconi patients to mitomycin C or diepoxybutane results in excess chromosome breaks. Almost 50% of patients with Fanconi anemia develop myelodysplasia or AML by age 40 if they do not die of other causes first.[36] Based on chromosome complementation studies, at least eight different genes can result in this syndrome.

The tumor suppressor gene syndromes Li-Fraumeni and Neurofibromatosis 1 could be associated with an increased risk of AML, but the exact extent of increased risk is unclear.

Several congenital cytopenia syndromes are associated with a definite increased risk of AML. Blackfan-Diamond syndrome is characterized by congenital hypoplastic anemia, growth retardation, and a definite increase in AML. Severe congenital neutropenia, also sometimes called Kostmann's syndrome, results in myelodysplasia or AML in 10% to 20% of individuals who do not first succumb to infection.[37] Schwachman syndrome is an autosomal recessive disease with pancreatic insufficiency, moderate dwarfism, and a hematologic picture resembling Fanconi anemia.[38]

BIOLOGY

Pathophysiology

Clonality

AML is a clonal disorder, with all leukemic cells in a given patient descending from a common progenitor. The initial proof of the clonality of AML came from studies of the disease in females who were heterozygotic for the x-linked glucose-6-phosphate dehydrogenase isoenzymes. In normal heterozygotic women, because of random x-chromosome inactivation, any single blood cell will express one or the other isoenzyme, and hematopoietic cells overall will be a 50-50 mix. Leukemia cells in G6PD heterozygotic females, however, were found in every case to be all of one isoenzyme or the other, indicating their origin from a single precursor.[39] With the development of methods to detect x-chromosome-linked DNA polymorphisms more broadly, it has since become possible to assess the clonality of leukemia in virtually any female patient. These studies have demonstrated differing patterns of clonal involvement among patients so that in some (generally younger) patients, only the frankly myeloid leukemic blasts are clonal, whereas in other (often older) patients, normal appearing monocytes, platelets, and red cell precursors might also be of clonal origin.[40] Studies of clonality have also given the surprising result that some patients treated to complete remission with recovery of entirely normal-looking hematopoiesis—including loss of a leukemic chromosome marker—might still have clonal hematopoiesis, a result consistent with the hypothesis of a multistep pathogenesis for AML.[41,42]

Cell of Origin

The clonal nature of AML also suggests that there is a leukemic stem cell capable of both self-renewal and proliferation. Identification of the AML stem cell is of considerable interest both for aiding in our understanding of the disease and because this cell would represent the ideal target of therapy. The existence of AML cases with blasts of varying degrees of differentiation has given rise to two general hypotheses. In one model, progenitor cells at various levels of commitment and differentiation are all susceptible to transformation, leading to considerable heterogeneity in AML stem cells. In an alternative model, only very undifferentiated hematopoietic stem cells are capable of being transformed, but based on the particular mutations involved, some degree of further commitment and differentiation of the leukemic cell is possible. Recent studies attempting to identify the AML stem cell based on the cell's ability to transfer human leukemia to an immunodeficient (NOD-SCID) mouse are more consistent with the latter hypothesis. When human AML cases are tested to determine which fraction of cells are able to initiate leukemia in the NOD-SCID mouse, it is only the primitive CD34++ CD38- fraction that is able to do so, regardless of the differentiative stage of leukemic blasts.[43,44] The leukemias that subsequently develop in the animals have the same level of differentiation as the leukemias from which the CD34++ CD38- blasts are derived, a finding that suggests that these leukemic clones are capable of some genetically determined degree of differentiation. The CD34++ CD38- AML stem cells are at the same level of differentiation as the normal hematopoietic stem cell capable of engrafting NOD-SCID mice and are rare cells among the leukemic mass, with a frequency of $0.2-100/10^6$. APL could be an exception to this general model, and APL blasts do not easily engraft in NOD-SCID mice.[44]

Cell Kinetics

Available data suggest that it is the persistence rather than the speed of proliferation that leads to the outgrowth of AML. Only a small fraction of leukemic cells are in cycle at any given time, and the cell cycle duration is, in fact, longer than that of normal hematopoietic cells.[45] An unfortunate but instructive case involved a woman with CML who, after an ablative preparative regimen, was transplanted from her HLA-matched brother. Although the brother's routine pretransplant workup was negative, the transplanted marrow contained 38% AML blasts with t(1;5). Somewhat surprisingly, the patient engrafted with normal male hematopoiesis and did not show evidence of the transplanted AML until 6 months after the transplant.[46]

Marrow Failure

Although the persistent growth of the AML clone leads to marrow failure at least in part by physically crowding out normal progenitors, other mechanisms of suppression of normal marrow probably exist. Frequently, peripheral blood counts start to fall weeks or months before the appearance of leukemic blasts in the marrow, and cases of hypoplastic AML are not uncommon. The mechanisms by which suppression of normal hematopoiesis occurs are not well understood.

MOLECULAR PATHOLOGY

The identification of recurrent chromosomal abnormalities—which can include translocations, point mutations, and gene duplications in AML cases—followed by the cloning of many of the involved genes has provided important insights into the pathogenesis of AML. The number of recurrent abnormalities so far identified is in the hundreds, a fact that would make it seem almost futile to attempt to make sense of such a wide range of abnormalities. With further investigation, however, it is becoming clear that many of these abnormalities tend to

affect a limited number of transcriptional or signal transduction pathways. Of those abnormalities that have been studied extensively, most are pro-oncogenic and are not simply innocent bystanders in the leukemic process. Only a few of these abnormalities are both necessary and sufficient to cause leukemia in murine models, however, a finding that suggests that multiple mutations are required to develop overt leukemia. The following section describes some of the more common and better understood molecular categories of AML.

Core Binding Factor Translocations

Core binding factor (CBF) is a heterodimeric transcription factor made up of two subunits, CBFα (also known as AML-1) and CBFβ. CBF plays an important role in the transcriptional activation of a number of genes required for normal hematopoietic differentiation (Fig. 104-2). A number of leukemias are associated with translocations or mutations that involve the components of CBF.

AML 1/ETO

The t(8;21) abnormality seen in approximately 8% of adult AML cases results in the fusion of the AML-1 (CBFα) gene

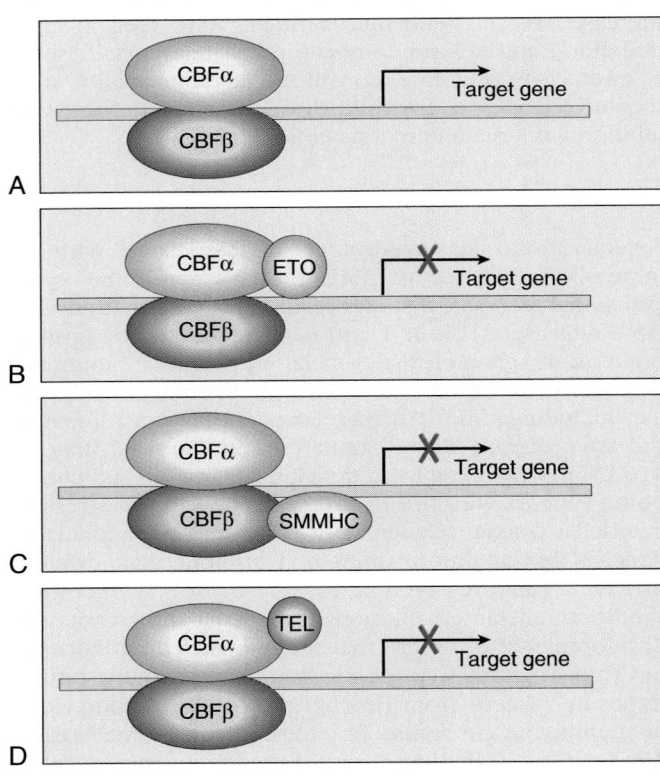

Figure 104-2. A, CBFα and CBFβ form a heterodimeric transcription factor that regulates a spectrum of genes important in hematopoiesis including IL-3, GM-CSF, and others. **B,** If instead of normal CBFα, a fusion product of CBFα-ETO dimerizes with CBFβ, the transcription factor does not function, and target genes are not transcribed. **C,** The fusion product CBFβ-SMMHC is a dominant negative regulator of gene transcription. **D,** Analogous to the situation with CBFα-ETO, the fusion product CBFα-TEL is a dominant negative regulator of normal CBF function.

on chromosome 21 to the ETO (8;21) gene on chromosome 8.[47] The AML-1/ETO fusion protein acts as a dominant negative inhibitor of the wild-type AML-1 gene, meaning that presence of the AML-1/ETO fusion protein blocks the ability of the wild-type AML-1 from the remaining nontranslocated chromosome to activate appropriately the transcription required for normal hematopoietic differentiation (see Fig. 104-2).[48] The AML-1 "knockout" mouse and the AML-1/ETO "knock-in" mouse have identical phenotypes, with embryonic death at day 11.5 and a characteristic pattern of central nervous system hemorrhage and lack of hematopoiesis. AML1 characterized by t(8;21) has a favorable prognosis.

INV 16

Inv (16) (p13;q22) and t(16;16) (p13;q22) both result in the fusion of CBFβ at 16q22 to the smooth-muscle myosin heavy chain (SMMHC) gene at 16p13 (see Fig. 104-2).[49] As in the case of t(8;21), the resultant fusion protein acts as a dominant negative regulator of transcription. CBFβ/SMMHC "knock-in" mice have a phenotype identical to those noted for AML-1 "knockouts" and AML-1/ETO "knock-ins". AML cases with involvement of 16q22 account for approximately 9% of adult AML cases, have a unique myelomonocytic morphology, and, like t(8;21) leukemias, have a favorable prognosis.

TEL-AML-1

In up to 25% of cases of pediatric pre-B-cell ALL, a t(12;21) abnormality fusing the TEL gene with AML1 can be found (see Fig. 104-2).[50] The resultant fusion protein appears to function as a dominant negative regulator of transcription. In general, this translocation is associated with a favorable prognosis in childhood ALL.

Point Mutations

Point mutations in AML1 occur in 3% to 5% of sporadic cases of adult AML.[51,52] In addition, as noted earlier, inherited point mutations resulting in AML1 haplo-insufficiency are found in families with familial platelet disorder and a high prevalence of subsequent AML.[33] The fact that these patients do not always develop AML or do so only after years suggests that subsequent mutational events are required.

The mechanisms by which t(8;21), inv (16), and t(12;21) fusion proteins exert their dominant negative effects are only now becoming understood. Recent data suggest that segments of the fusion protein recruit nuclear co-repressor (NCoR)-histone deacetylase (HD) complexes in a matter analogous to that seen in APL, as will be discussed shortly. The specific pattern of transcriptional suppression likely differs for each fusion product, given the somewhat different phenotypes associated with each.

Retinoic Acid Receptor α Translocations

APL, which accounts for approximately 8% of adult AML cases, is almost always associated with t(15;17) (q22;q11.2), a translocation that fuses the promyelocytic leukemia (PML) gene on chromosome 15 to the retinoic acid receptor gene on chromosome 17. The resultant

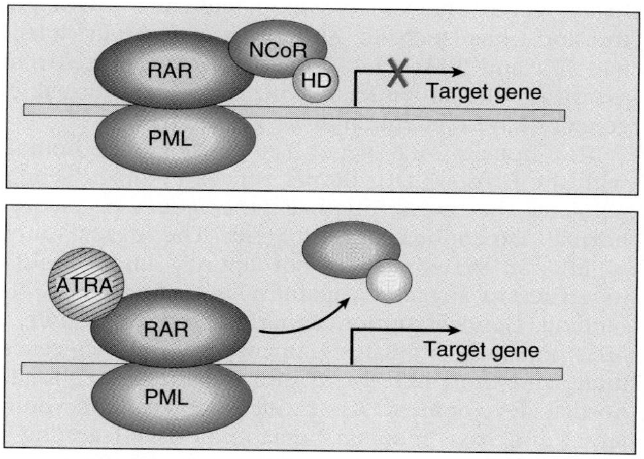

Figure 104-3. A, The abnormal fusion product RAR-PML binds a nuclear co-repressor (NCoR) Histone Deacetylase (HD) complex. This deacetylates histones in the region, leading to inhibition of transcription. **B,** When ATRA binds to RAR, a change in confirmation leads to release of the NCoR-HD complex, acetylation of histones, and resumption of transcription.

PML/RARα fusion product acts as a dominant negative inhibitor of normal PML function and of the function of RXRα, an important heterodimeric partner of RARα (Fig. 104-3).[53] PML/RARα recruits a nuclear co-repressor (NCoR) and the molecules sin3 and histone deacetylase (HD). HD deacetylases histones, a process which, in turn, inhibits binding of transcription factors, thus inhibiting the expression of genes required for hematopoietic differentiation. The unique activity of all-transretinoic acid (ATRA) in APL appears to be explained by its ability to bind to the PML/RARα fusion, changing its configuration and releasing the attached nuclear co-repressor (see Fig. 104-3). This then allows subsequent transcription and gene expression. Transgenic expression of PML/RARα in mice results in APL in a fraction of animals after a latency period of some months. The relatively long latency and incomplete penetration suggest that, like many other leukemias, multiple mutations are required for the full development of overt APL.

A number of other translocations, including t(5;17) and t(11;17), involve RARα and result in the APL phenotype. These leukemias are generally unresponsive to ATRA because clinically achievable concentrations of the drug do not result in release of the NCoR-HD complex.

Mixed-Lineage Leukemia Mutations

Most nonrandom chromosomal abnormalities are associated with specific lineages or subtypes of leukemia, but abnormalities involving the mixed-lineage leukemia gene (MLL) located on 11q23 are exceptions, with many partner genes and many forms of hematologic malignancy including ALL, AML, and lymphoma. All together, translocations involving 11q23 comprise about 7% of adult AML cases, and among these, t(9;11) (p22;q23), associated with acute monoblastic leukemia, is the most common.[54,55] The translocation fuses MLL with AF9, and mice with this fusion gene "knock-in" develop leukemia.[56] Other MLL translocations seen in AML include t(6;11), t(10;11), t(11;17), and t(11;19). It has also been reported that as many as 10% of patients with AML and normal cytogenetics have tandem duplications of MLL.[57]

The human MLL gene has considerable homology with the Drosophila trithorax gene, a complex gene that regulates the transcription of other genes necessary for normal Drosophila development. The exact function of MLL in vertebrates is not entirely understood, but its structure suggests capability of minor groove DNA binding. Gene-disruption experiments have shown that MLL positively regulates homeodomain (Hox) genes in mice, and thus, like the trithorax gene, is required for normal development. Knockout mice are embryonically lethal and have reduced hematopoiesis, suggesting that the gene has, as one of its functions, a broad effect on early hematopoiesis.[58-60] The precise mechanisms by which translocations affecting MLL give rise to hematologic malignancies are not entirely understood.

Tyrosine Kinase Receptor Mutations

FLT1, FLT3, FMS, KIT, and PDGF are members of a family of genes encoding receptor tyrosine kinases, each with an extracellular ligand binding domain, transmembrane and juxtamembrane domains, and an intracellular domain with tyrosine kinase activity. In general, ligand binding with the receptor causes receptor dimerization, autophosphorylation, and then subsequent phosphorylation activation of adaptive proteins (including GRB-2), which in turn activate RAS and other proteins.

FLT3 is mutated in 30% to 35% of patients with AML.[61,62] The majority of these are internal tandem duplications, but approximately one-fourth of the mutations are in the form of point mutations. Both forms of mutations are activating. When inserted into murine cell lines, these mutations result in factor-independent growth.[63] Retroviral transmission of these mutations into mouse marrow is not, by itself, sufficient to cause overt AML but does lead to a myeloproliferative phenotype.[64] In clinical studies, the incidence of FLT3 mutations in AML appears to increase with age and to be associated with high white counts at diagnosis and, perhaps, poorer clinical outcome.[62,65,66] Clinical trials of small-molecule inhibitors of FLT3 are being performed.

Mutations in other receptor tyrosine kinase genes are also sometimes seen in AML. Point mutations in FMS have been reported in 10% to 20% of cases.[67] Point mutations, deletions, or insertions of KIT have also been reported in a small percentage of patients.[68] Mutations in one or another receptor tyrosine kinase exist in almost half of all AML cases.

RAS Mutations

RAS is a monomeric guanosine diphosphate binding protein activated by various tyrosine kinases. Activation of RAS has multiple and varied effects which, depending on the target cell and its particular state, can result in proliferation, transformation, or differentiation. RAS

mutations have been identified in 15% to 30% of cases of AML.[69,70] In most cases, these mutations result in prevention of hydrolysis of RAS-GTP, effectively keeping RAS in the "on" position. Thus, therapies to inhibit RAS function have been developed. To function normally, newly transcribed RAS must have a farnesyl or geranyl-geranyl lipid attached, and for this reason farnesyl transferase inhibitors have been explored as therapeutic agents in AML.[71]

Mutations Involving 5q, 7q, and 20q

AML evolving from myelodysplasia or developing from exposure to alkylating agent therapy frequently is associated with partial or complete loss of chromosomes 5, 7, and 20. The frequent loss of 5q, 7q, or 20q has led a number of investigators to hypothesize that a classic tumor suppressor gene might exist in these areas. With classic tumor suppressor genes like Rb, when one allele is deleted, a mutation in the second results in disease. Despite considerable efforts to identify such genes, however, no classic tumor suppressor of AML in these regions has been reported. It is possible that such genes do not exist and that instead, haploinsufficiency of one or more genes is sufficient for one of the multiple steps in the progression of myelodysplasia to overt leukemia.

PATHOLOGY

Morphology

The diagnosis of AML generally is made by the examination of well prepared peripheral blood and bone marrow specimens. For more than 3 decades, the French-American-British (FAB) system was used to describe and classify AML, and according to this system, a finding of 30% blasts in marrow or peripheral blood was required to make the diagnosis.[72] More recently, a World Health Organization (WHO) classification suggests that a finding of 20% blasts is sufficient to make the diagnosis.[73] AML blasts can be placed into the following categories based on their appearance (Fig. 104-4):

- Minimally differentiated AML (FAB M0) blasts are nondescript. Without immunophenotyping, it is very difficult to identify these cells as being of myeloid origin.
- AML with differentiation (FAB M1) defines cases with sparse cytoplasmic granules, only occasional Auer rods, and positive myeloperoxidase staining.
- Cases of AML with maturation (FAB M2) are more clearly myeloid in origin, with increased cytoplasmic granules, clear myeloperoxidase positivity, and the frequent presence of Auer rods.
- Acute promyelocytic leukemia (FAB M3) is characterized by intense cytoplasmic granulation that often obscures the nucleus. A microgranular variant exists with marked nuclear folding and only subtle cytoplasmic granulations. Both subtypes stain intensely with Sudan black or myeloperoxidase. M3 AML is invariably associated with t(15;17) or one of its variants.

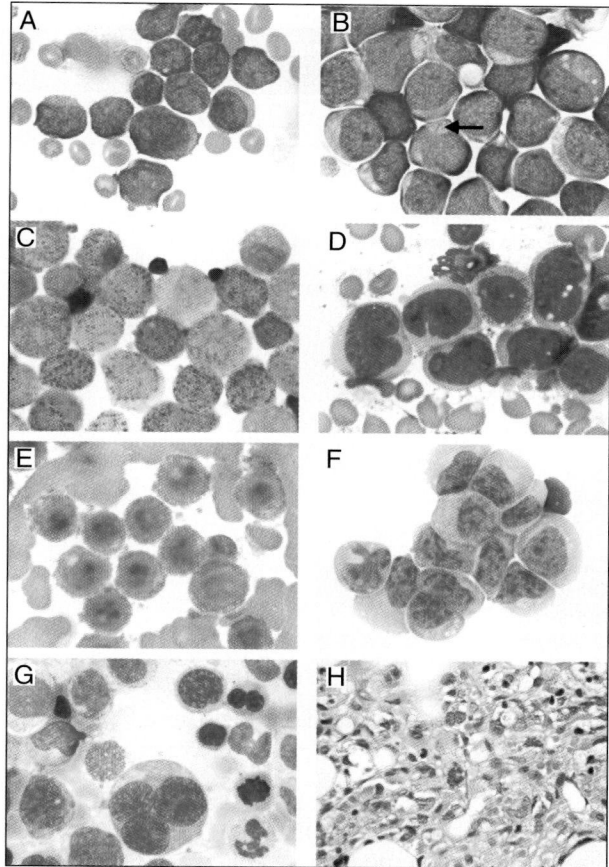

Figure 104-4. The morphological spectrum of the acute myeloid leukemias in bone marrow aspirates (**A–G**) and a marrow biopsy (**H**). **A,** Acute myeloblastic leukemia with minimal (FAB AML-M0) or no (FAB AML-M1) maturation. The cells are myeloblasts with dispersed chromatin and variable amounts of agranular cytoplasm. Some display medium-sized, poorly defined nucleoli. **B,** Acute myeloblastic leukemia with maturation (FAB AML-M2). Some of the blasts contain azurophilic granules, and there are promyelocytes. More mature neutrophils were present in other fields. Note the Auer rod (*arrow*). **C,** Acute promyelocytic leukemia (FAB AML-M3). All of these cells are promyelocytes containing coarse cytoplasmic granules, which sometimes obscure the nuclei. **D,** Acute myelomonocytic leukemia (FAB AML-M4). Promonocytes with indented nuclei are present with myeloblasts. The dense nuclear staining is unusual. **E,** Acute monoblastic leukemia (FAB AML-M5a). These characteristic monoblasts have round nuclei with delicate chromatin and prominent nucleoli. Cytoplasm is abundant. Nonspecific esterase staining was intense (not shown). **F,** Acute monocytic leukemia (FAB AML-M5b). Most of the cells in this field are promonocytes. Monoblasts and an abnormal monocyte are also present. **G,** Acute erythroid leukemia (FAB AML-M6). Dysplastic multinucleated erythroid precursors with megaloblastoid nuclei are present. **H,** Acute megakaryoblastic leukemia (FAB AML-M7). In this marrow biopsy, there are large and small blasts and atypical megakaryocytes.

- AML with myelomonocytic differentiation (FAB M4) is often characterized by dysplastic features, such as hypogranular cytoplasm and nuclear hyposegmentation. One subset associated with inv (16) (p13q22) is characterized by increased eosinophilia. M4 AML stains positively with both myeloperoxidase and nonspecific esterase. Diagnosis of M4 AML is further strengthened

by immunophenotyping demonstrating both myeloid and monocytic antigens.

- Acute monocytic leukemia (FAB M5) is characterized by blasts with folded nuclei and abundant cytoplasm that stains positively with nonspecific esterase but is myeloperoxidase negative.
- AML FAB M6, acute erythroid leukemia, can have a variable appearance but usually is accompanied by dysplastic erythroid elements which, on occasion, can become the predominant cell type.
- The diagnosis of acute megakaryocytic leukemia (FAB M7) requires that more than 30% of blasts are of the megakaryocytic lineage. These blasts often display clumping, multinucleation, and cytoplasmic blebbing, but immunophenotyping is usually required to make the diagnosis.

Although in the past, considerable time and effort went into categorizing AML cases among these morphologic categories, morphology in fact has almost no significance once cytogenetic and (to a lesser extent) immunophenotypic information is taken into consideration.

Immunophenotype

AML cases can be categorized according to the combinations of myeloid-associated antigens displayed on the surface of the malignant blast. Undifferentiated AML cases, including FAB M0 cases, express CD34, CD117, and CD33 but tend not to express CD65s. More mature AML types—including most FAB M1 and M2 cases—express CD34, CD33, CD13, and CD65s. Leukemias associated with t(8;21), often of M2 morphology, have an immunophenotype similar to other M2 AML types but also express the NK marker CD56 and the B lymphoid marker CD19. Acute promyelocytic leukemias uniquely stain strongly with CD15s and weakly with CD15. In addition, they usually do not express CD34 or HLA-DR. Acute myelomonocytic and monocytic leukemias express CD14, the prototypic monocytic antigen. Early myeloid markers, including CD34 and CD117, are generally absent. Myelomonocytic leukemias associated with inv (16) frequently express the T-cell antigen, CD2. Most acute erythroid leukemias fail to express early myeloid markers (e.g., CD34) but do express CD36 and CD71 and often express blood group H antigen, the precursor to ABO. Acute megakaryocytic leukemias react with antibodies to CD41a/CD61 (GPIIb/IIIa). Mature platelets can sometimes adhere to the surface of M5 AML types, making them appear as M7 leukemias. True M7 AML types do not express CD14, however.

Cytogenetics

Cytogenetic analysis of human leukemias has been absolutely central to the identification of the genetic events involved in leukemogenesis. In addition, cytogenetics has emerged as by far the single most important diagnostic factor in AML.

Conventional cytogenetics involves the staining of metaphase cells and thus requires dividing cells. Because malignant cells in the marrow are more frequent and have a higher mitotic rate, marrow, rather than peripheral blood, is the preferred source for cytogenetic analysis. Cells are usually cultured for 24 hours, arrested by short-term incubation with colchicine, and then, typically, 20 metaphases are analyzed. The abnormalities detected include changes in chromosome number, gains or losses of portions of chromosomes, and reciprocal exchange of genetic material either between two or more chromosomes (translocations) or within a single chromosome (inversions).

Two other molecular techniques are sometimes used. Fluorescent in situ hybridization (FISH) techniques involve hybridization of single-stranded DNA probes to homologous single-stranded sequences in chromosomes of metaphase or interphase cells. FISH has the advantage of being able to analyze large numbers of dividing (metaphase FISH) or nondividing (interphase FISH) cells with relatively little effort. Only those abnormalities targeted by the specific probe being applied will be detected, however. Thus, FISH is very useful for monitoring the disappearance or reappearance of a specific translocation [for example, t(9;22) in CML] but is not a substitute for conventional cytogenetics for initial evaluation of AML. Polymerase chain reaction (PCR) is a method capable of amplifying selected regions of DNA through repeated cycles of DNA synthesis, denaturation, and hybridization. To use PCR analysis, the specific gene sequences to be amplified must be known. Standardized PCR analyses of several of the more common fusion gene transcripts have been developed and are proving useful for monitoring minimal residual disease.

A listing of the most common cytogenetic abnormalities seen in adult AML is provided in Table 104-1. These abnormalities can be categorized according to their underlying biology and according to their prognostic significance (Fig. 104-5). Table 104-1 organizes these abnormalities according to biologic subgroups. Thus, t(8;21), t(16;21), inv (16), and t(16;16) all belong to the core binding factor leukemias. The abnormalities t(4;11), t(9;11), and del (11)(q23) comprise most of the MLL family of AML types. Leukemias involving RARα include t(15;17), t(11;17), and t(5;17), while t(6;9) involves the fusion of the DEK and CAN genes. The EVI 1 gene is involved in inv (3) and t(3;3). Monosomy or interstitial deletions of chromosomes 5, 7, 17, and 20 are typical of AML evolving from MDS or from prior alkylating agent exposure. Trisomy 8 is quite common in AML and can appear as a sole abnormality or in combination with other abnormalities. By itself, trisomy 8 does not appear to influence prognosis, but when present it is often accompanied by other unfavorable cytogenetic abnormalities.[74] Trisomy 11, 13, and 21 are also often seen in AML.

A number of studies have analyzed the outcomes of patients with AML according to cytogenetics and have demonstrated that both complete remission rates and duration are highly associated with pretreatment cytogenetics. In general, patients can be categorized as having a favorable, intermediate, or unfavorable cytogenetic risk status. Two of the largest prospective studies in adult AML were published by the Medical Research Council

TABLE 104-1

Cytogenetic Abnormalities in Acute Myeloid Leukemia

ABNORMALITY	INCIDENCE (%)*
Core binding factor translocations	
t(8;21)	8
Inv (16) or t(16;16)	9
Retinoic acid receptor translocations	
t(15;17)	10
Mixed lineage leukemia translocations	
t(9;11)	2
t(10;11)	1
Other MLL	3
Trisomies	
+8	9
+21	3
Other trisomy	6
Deletions	
-5 or 5q-	6
-7 or 7q-	8
-9 or 9q-	3
Complex†	10
Other	17
Normal	40

*All patients with a specific abnormality are considered whether or not an additional cytogenetic change is present. Thus, because some patients are counted twice, the total incidence is greater than 100%.
†Complex is defined as a clone with at least five abnormalities.

(MRC) and the Southwest Oncology Group (SWOG).[54,55] These studies concerned adults below age 60 with newly diagnosed AML who were treated using contemporary chemotherapy and transplant approaches. As noted in Table 104-2, the two groups reached very similar categorizations, with CBF and RARα leukemias comprising the favorable group, normal leukemias and trisomy 8 the intermediate group, and abnormalities of 5, 7, and complex abnormalities defining the poor risk group. Some controversy remains about whether 11q23 leukemias are considered intermediate or unfavorable. Overall, as noted in Table 104-2, 85% to 90% of favorable-risk, 75% to 80% of intermediate-risk, and 55% to 60% of poor-risk patients are predicted to achieve complete remission. Survival at 5 years is also highly associated with risk group, with 55% to 65% of good-risk, 38% to 41% of intermediate-risk, and only 11% to 15% of poor-risk patients predicted to be alive. As will be discussed later under "Primary Treatment," some of these outcomes are dependent on the particular treatment used. For example, the favorable outcomes seen in CBF leukemias might particularly depend on the use of high-dose cytarabine in the treatment regimen, while the use of allogeneic transplantation might overcome to some extent the impact of having unfavorable cytogenetics.[54,75]

CLASSIFICATION

The FAB classification schema for AML is presented in Table 104-3.[72] This system, which has been in use for several decades, relies totally on morphology and is of only

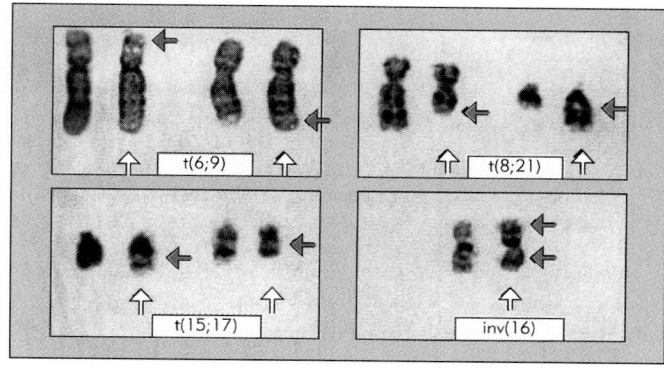

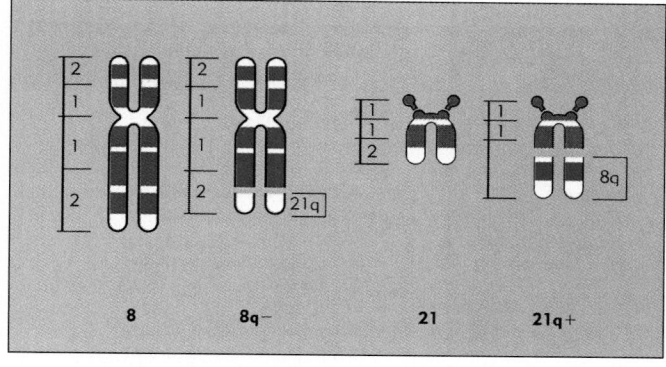

Figure 104-5. Common cytogenetic abnormalities in adult AML. **A**, Red arrows mark the regions of chromosome breakage and rejoining. **B**, M2 subtype: diagrammatic systematized description of the structural aberration t(8;21). **C**, M3 subtype (acute promyelocytic leukemia, APL): systematized description of the structural aberration t(15; 17). (Courtesy of Prof. LM Secker-Walker.)

limited therapeutic or prognostic utility. More recently, the WHO has offered an alternative schema (Table 104-4).[73] This schema includes, as subgroups, AML with the most common recurrent genetic abnormalities, AML types that evolve from MDS, AML types that are clearly therapy related, and for those that fail to fall into the other three categories, the system resorts to a morphologic categorization similar to the previous FAB system.

CLINICAL MANIFESTATIONS

The initial clinical manifestations of AML are usually nonspecific and relate to the diminished production of normal blood cells. The onset is most often insidious over the course of several weeks to months, and it is not uncommon for a patient to be seen several times before a

TABLE 104-2

Impact of Cytogenetics on Complete Response and Survival*

RISK STATUS	INCIDENCE (%)		CR RATES (%)		5-YEAR SURVIVAL (%)	
	SWOG	MRC	SWOG	MRC	SWOG	MRC
Favorable	20	23	84	91	55	65
Inv (16), t(16;16),						
t(8;21), t(15;17)						
Intermediate	46	66	76	86	38	41
Normal, +8, +6, -y						
Unfavorable						
Del 5q, -5, del 7q, -7, complex	30	10	55	63	11	14
Unknown Risk	4	—	54	—	24	—

*The SWOG study includes only adults and does not exclude secondary AML, whereas the MRC data refer to both children and adults and exclude cases of secondary AML. In the SWOG data, 11q23 is defined as unfavorable, whereas in the MRC data, 11q23 is considered intermediate risk.

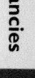

TABLE 104-3

FAB Classifications of Acute Myeloid Leukemia

SUBTYPES	DEFINITION
M0, acute undifferentiated leukemia	≥ 30% blasts < 3% myeloperoxidase positive Myeloid antigen expression
M1, AML with minimal differentiation	> 30% blasts ≥ 3% myeloperoxidase positive < 10% cells mature beyond blast stage
M2, AML with differentiation	> 30% blasts ≥ 3% myeloperoxidase positive > 10% myeloid cells mature beyond blast stage
M3, acute promyelocytic leukemia	> 30% blasts plus hypergranular promyelocytes Intense myeloperoxidase positivity
M4, acute myelomonocyte leukemia	Monocytosis > 30% myeloblasts + monoblasts + promonocytes > 20% myeloperoxidase positive > 20% nonspecific esterase positive
M5, acute monoblastic leukemia	> 30% myeloblasts + monoblasts + promonocytes < 20% myeloperoxidase positive > 80% nonspecific esterase positive
M6, acute erythroid leukemia	≥ 30% of nonerythroid cells are myeloblasts > 50% erythroid elements
M7, acute megakaryocytic leukemia	> 30% blasts (myeloblasts + megakaryoblasts) > 30% megakaryocytic elements defined by immunophenotyping or electron microscopy

TABLE 104-4

WHO Classification of Acute Myeloid Leukemia

Acute myeloid leukemia with recurrent genetic abnormalities
  Acute myeloid leukemia with t(8;21)(q22;q22), (AML1/ETO)
  Acute myeloid leukemia with abnormal bone marrow eosinophils and inv (16)(p13q22) or t(16;16)(q13;q22), (CBFβ/MYH11)
  Acute promyelocytic leukemia with t(15;17)(q22q12), (PML/RARα) and variants
  Acute myeloid leukemia with 11q23 (MLL) abnormalities
Acute myeloid leukemia with multilineage dysplasia
  Following MDS or MDS/MPD
  Without antecedent MDS or MDS/MPD, but with dysplasia in at least 50% of cells in two or more myeloid lineages
Acute myeloid leukemia and myelodysplastic syndromes, therapy related
  Alkylating agent/irradiation-related type
  Topoisomerase II inhibitor-related type (some may be lymphoid)
  Others
Acute myeloid leukemia, not otherwise categorized
  Classify as:
    Acute myeloid leukemia, minimally differentiated
    Acute myeloid leukemia without maturation
    Acute myeloid leukemia with maturation
    Acute myelomonocytic leukemia
    Acute monoblastic leukemia
    Acute monoblastic/acute monocytic leukemia
    Acute erythroid leukemia (erythroid/myeloid and pure erythroleukemia)
    Acute megakaryocytic leukemia
    Acute basophilic leukemia
    Acute panmyelosis with myelofibrosis
    Myeloid sarcoma

LABORATORY MANIFESTATIONS

blood count is finally taken and the diagnosis of leukemia is suspected. Most patients complain of a brief, virus-like illness with fatigue and malaise. Some patients present with a chief complaint of easy bruising, and occasionally, a nonhealing skin wound brings the patient to a doctor's attention. Anemia is present at diagnosis in most patients, causing fatigue, pallor, headache, and, in the predisposed patient, angina. Thrombocytopenia is usually present and, when asked, approximately one-third of patients note easy bruising, bleeding gums, epistaxis, or other evidence of bleeding at diagnosis. Approximately one-third of patients with AML have significant infections (most often of bacterial origin) when the diagnosis is finally made.

In addition to suppressing normal blood production, leukemia can infiltrate normal organs. Diffuse bone tenderness is seen in approximately 25% of patients. Chloromas, which are local collections of blasts, can present as rubbery, fast-growing, soft tissue masses. Gingival hyperplasia due to leukemic infiltration of the gums is sometimes seen, particularly with M5 AML (Fig. 104-6). Leukemia sometimes infiltrates the skin and results in a raised, nonpruritic rash termed leukemia cutis (Fig. 104-7). Although uncommon, an occasional patient might present with meningeal signs or cranial neuropathies (most often affecting cranial nerves IV or VII) due to infiltration of the central nervous system with leukemia.

Peripheral blood counts are abnormal at diagnosis in virtually every case of AML. Most patients have a normochromic, normocytic anemia. Most are thrombocytopenic, with 50% of patients having less than 50,000 platelets/mm^3 and 25% having below 20,000. Most patients are granulocytopenic, but the total white blood cell (WBC) count is more variable. Approximately 25% have very high WBC counts (greater than 50,000/mm^3), approximately 25% have low WBC counts (less than 5000/mm^3), and the remainder are in between. Blasts can usually be seen in the peripheral blood.

Bone marrow examination generally reveals a hypercellular marrow containing 20% to 100% blast cells largely

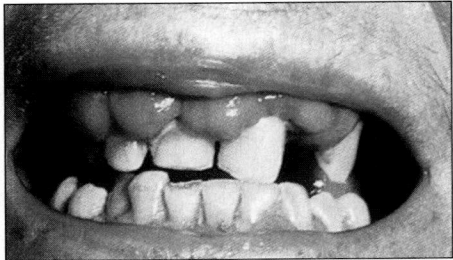

Figure 104-6. Leukemic infiltration of the gums results in their expansion and thickening and in partial covering of the teeth.

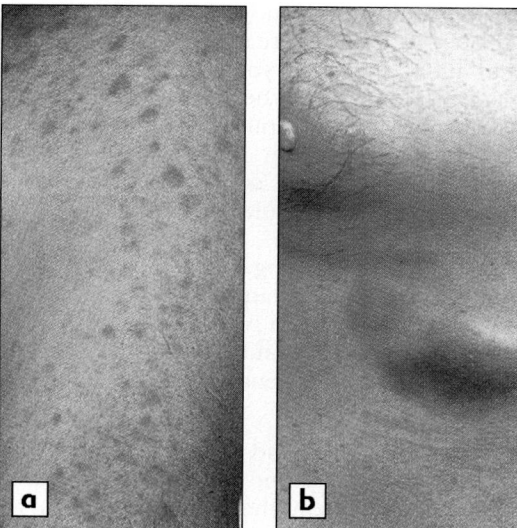

Figure 104-7. Acute myeloid leukemia, M5 subtype. **A,** Multiple, raised, erythematous skin lesions caused by leukemic infiltration. **B,** Close-up view of nodular skin lesion. (From Hoffbrand AV, Pettit JE: Color Atlas of Clinical Hematology, 3rd ed. St. Louis, Mosby, 2000.)

replacing the normal marrow. The morphologic, immunologic, and cytogenetic characteristics of AML have been described in earlier sections of this chapter.

The partial thromboplastin and prothrombin times can be prolonged, and in APL, reduced fibrinogen and other evidence of disseminated intervascular coagulation (DIC) are not infrequent. Blood chemistries are usually normal, although in patients presenting with very aggressive and advanced disease, there could be some evidence of tumor lysis syndrome at presentation with hyperkalemia, hyperphosphatemia, hyperuricemia, hypocalcemia, increased lactate dehydrogenase, and renal insufficiency. This syndrome more often presents shortly after therapy is initiated and can become fatal rapidly if untreated. Occasional patients with monocytic leukemia might have tumor infiltration of the kidneys sufficient to cause renal impairment. Lumbar puncture will reveal unsuspected involvement with leukemia in approximately 5% of patients.[76]

DIFFERENTIAL DIAGNOSIS

The diagnosis of AML is usually straightforward. The major difficulties involve distinguishing AML from other malignant hematologic disorders. The distinction between AML and advanced MDS is made by percentage of blasts and is often an arbitrary distinction with little clinical relevance. Distinguishing AML from ALL can virtually always be accomplished using immunophenotyping. CML in myeloid blast crisis can mimic AML, but the presence of the Ph chromosome, splenomegaly, and myeloid cells at all levels of differentiation distinguish CML from AML. Other small round cell neoplasms can infiltrate the marrow, sometimes mimicking leukemia, but immunologic markers easily differentiate between the two conditions. Leukemoid reactions are sometimes seen in infections

such as tuberculosis, but the proportion of blasts in the marrow in nonmalignant diseases virtually never reaches the 20% to 30% required for a diagnosis of AML. Infectious mononucleosis and other viral infections can sometime resemble ALL but are almost never confused with AML.

PRIMARY TREATMENT

Advances in chemotherapy, hematopoietic cell transplantation, and supportive care now enable many patients with AML to be cured. These therapeutic measures are complex, however, and so they are best conducted at centers with appropriate experience and support services. Leukemia is often a rapidly progressive disease, and therefore, specific therapy should be initiated soon after diagnosis—usually within 48 hours if possible. Before therapy is initiated, acute hemorrhage and infection should be brought under control if at all possible. Patients should be hydrated and given allopurinol, 100–200 mg orally three times a day to prevent uric acid nephropathy. Ideally, stable venous access should be established by placing a Hickman or similar catheter. The diagnosis of leukemia causes a profound shock to the patient and family and has far-reaching implications. Thus, in addition to stabilizing the patient medically, many practitioners find it valuable to have at least one formalized conference at which the patient and family can be instructed about the nature of leukemia, the immediate plans for therapy, and the likely consequences of treatment.

Management of Emergencies

A number of treatable emergencies might need to be managed before specific antileukemic therapy can begin. Severe bleeding from thrombocytopenia can usually be controlled with platelet transfusions. DIC is typically associated with a diagnosis of APL. This coagulopathy rapidly abates with the institution of ATRA therapy and, thus, many of the measures used in the past to attempt control of DIC (i.e., low-dose heparin, fresh-frozen plasma, and fibrinogen) are now no longer needed. Patients with fever and granulocytopenia should have blood cultures taken but should be placed on broad-spectrum antibiotics empirically. Patients with very high WBC counts might have early evidence of tumor lysis syndrome and should be hydrated, placed on allopurinol to prevent further uric acid production, and be given acetazolamide (500 mg daily) to alkalinize the urine. Patients presenting with very high WBC counts (greater than $100,000/mm^3$) are also at risk for hemorrhage or microinfarctions of small vessels, presumably due to leukostasis. Lung involvement can result in pulmonary infiltrates and hypoxia, while central nervous system (CNS) leukostasis can lead to mental status changes, seizures, and sudden death. Pulmonary or CNS leukostasis is a medical emergency requiring intravenous hydration and measures to lower the blast count immediately. Although oral hydroxyurea is often used, whether it lowers counts any faster than intravenous cyclophosphamide, daunorubicin, or cytarabine is unknown. Leukapheresis is of short-term benefit.[77] Patients with CNS symptoms should be given whole-brain irradiation emergently. Leukostasis has been associated with the expression of the adhesion molecule CD14 on malignant blasts; this might explain why the syndrome is almost never seen in lymphoid leukemias, which lack this antigen.[78]

Remission Induction

General Principles

Without therapy, AML is a rapidly fatal disease; therefore, prompt initiation of antileukemic therapy is appropriate for the vast majority of patients. Some patients, however, might have a more smoldering variant of AML, often arising from a prior myelodysplastic syndrome. If such patients are elderly or have other serious medical problems, supportive care measures without attempts at remission induction might be more appropriate. The large majority of patients, however, should be treated with combination chemotherapy in an effort to eradicate the bulk of leukemic cells and allow the regrowth of normal marrow, resulting in a complete remission. In the United States, there is general agreement that the definition of complete remission requires recovery of peripheral neutrophils to counts greater than 1500/mm³, platelets to counts greater than 100,000/mm³, no evidence of extramedullary leukemia, and bone marrow with fewer than 5% blasts. This status must be maintained for a minimum of one month to be called a complete remission. Not all studies have identical requirements. For example, the British Medical Research Council (MRC) has no requirement for platelet recovery and so, conceivably, some differences in study outcomes might be explainable by differences in definition. Complete remission does not imply complete eradication of disease and, as will be discussed, if patients are given only induction therapy, disease will recur in essentially every patient. Induction chemotherapy is generally given at relatively high doses and is followed by a period of significant pancytopenia before recovery of normal hematopoiesis. There are essentially no reports of successful approaches using lower-dose therapy given at longer intervals designed to "chip away" at the disease. As will be discussed, most regimens include 3 days of an anthracycline and 7 days of cytarabine. The usual practice is to check the marrow status at day 14 after beginning induction and, if residual leukemic cells remain, to give a second course of therapy. Sometimes it is difficult to distinguish between residual leukemic cells and early recovery of normal hematopoiesis. In these cases, it is advisable to repeat the check of marrow status in a few days.

In order to better understand the reasons for the success or failure of treatment, a number of systems have been proposed to define the outcome of induction therapy. One simple but helpful system offers three categories for treatment failure.[79] One group of patients fail because they clearly have resistant leukemia. A second group includes those who die early of toxicities with an aplastic marrow. A final category of patients are those for whom adequate information is unavailable to distinguish between resistant leukemia and early death.

Some studies of remission induction conducted in the 1970s suggested that the reasons for treatment failure tended to differ between younger and older patients, with relatively few patients below age 50 or 55 dying of early treatment-related complications but a much higher incidence of this problem among older individuals. Accordingly, more recently, separate studies have been conducted for younger and older patients.

Remission Induction in Younger Patients

For more than 2 decades, standard induction therapy for patients below age 60 with AML has generally included 3 days of an anthracycline and 7 days of cytarabine. Four general questions have dominated recent clinical trials of induction therapy:

1. What are the best type and dose of anthracycline?
2. What are the best dose and schedule of cytarabine?
3. Should additional chemotherapeutic agents be added?
4. Is there a role for hematopoietic growth factors?

Daunorubicin, 45 mg/m² for 3 days, generally has been viewed as the standard anthracycline component of therapy. Four randomized trials have compared idarubicin, 12 mg/m² for 3 days to daunorubicin, 45 mg/m² for 3 days, both with standard-dose cytarabine.[80-83] The complete response rates were higher with idarubicin in three of the four trials, particularly in patients below age 50. A problem with these studies is that idarubicin and daunorubicin were not compared at equitoxic doses. For example, the degree of myelosuppression during consolidation was considerably greater with idarubicin. No prospective randomized trial has yet been completed comparing daunorubicin, 45 mg/m² to daunorubicin at 60 or 70 mg/m²—doses which have been shown to be well tolerated by patients below age 60. Nor have randomized trials been reported comparing idarubicin to the higher-dose daunorubicin regimens. On the other hand, sequential trials from both the Southwest Oncology Group (SWOG) and the Eastern Cooperative Oncology Group (ECOG) suggest that in patients below age 60, complete response rates are higher with higher doses of daunorubicin (i.e., 60 or 70 mg/m² for 3 days) than with lower doses (i.e., 45 mg/kg/m² for 3 days).[84-87]

Cytarabine is generally given intravenously at a dose of 100–200 mg/m² per day by bolus or by continuous infusion. Much higher doses of cytarabine are tolerable, and two prospective randomized trials compared a combination of daunorubicin and standard cytarabine with daunorubicin and cytarabine at 2 g/m²/day for 6 days.[85,88] In neither study was the complete response rate increased, although in the SWOG study, the group randomized to high-dose induction tended to have an improved disease-free survival. The use of high-dose cytarabine is associated with increased toxicities, including more nausea, vomiting, and conjunctivitis. An occasional patient can develop a disabling cerebellar toxicity.

Whether the addition of a third drug to the standard daunorubicin-plus-cytarabine regimen is beneficial is uncertain. Many regimens add 6-thioguanine, but no randomized trial exists showing a benefit. The addition of etoposide was studied by the Australian Leukemia Study Group and did not increase complete response rates but might have lengthened disease-free survival without benefitting overall survival.[89]

Because profound myelosuppression always follows administration of induction chemotherapy, a large number of trials have asked whether administration of a myeloid growth factor immediately after completion of induction chemotherapy might hasten marrow recovery, thereby preventing serious and potentially lethal infections and improving complete response rates.[90-94] In general, these studies found that administration of a myeloid growth factor after completion of induction chemotherapy accelerates subsequent myeloid recovery. In only a minority of studies, however, did this accelerated recovery result in fewer documented infections, and in only the rare study was the complete response rate or survival affected. In those studies where it was assessed, the dollars saved by shorter hospitalizations with the use of growth factors were approximately balanced by the cost of the agent.[95,96]

In summary, standard induction therapy for younger patients with AML continues to be 3 days of an anthracycline at an intensity approximately equal to daunorubicin 60 mg/m^2/day and 7 days of cytarabine. There is a lack of convincing evidence that alternatives in the dosing of cytarabine, inclusion of other chemotherapeutic agents, or the addition of hematopoietic growth factors consistently improves complete response rates or prolongs survival.

Despite optimal therapy, as many as 30% of younger adults fail to achieve a complete remission with initial induction therapy—some because they die of treatment complications, others because they have resistant leukemia. Allogeneic hematopoietic cell transplantation can cure 15% to 20% of patients who fail initial induction attempts, but the logistics of identifying a donor and initiating a transplant in a timely matter for such patients are often challenging. To facilitate this process, it is reasonable to obtain HLA typing on all younger patients with AML and siblings shortly after diagnosis rather than waiting until induction has failed and patients have only a very narrow window of opportunity in which to receive potentially curative therapy.

Remission Induction in Older Patients

The advantages seen with more intensive anthracycline dosing—daunorubicin doses above 45 mg/m^2 for 3 days or the equivalent—have generally been restricted to younger patients. For patients over age 55, most experts suggest limiting the anthracycline to a dose equivalent to daunorubicin 45 mg/m^2 for 3 days. As for younger patients, there is no clear advantage to one anthracycline over another when given at relatively equitoxic doses. A recent ECOG study compared daunorubicin with mitoxantrone or idarubicin (all given with standard-dose cytarabine) and found no advantage for any single arm.[87] As with younger patients, there is no evidence for an advantage of high-dose cytarabine or for the addition of further chemotherapeutic agents to the induction regimen for older patients. Many of the studies of the addi-

tion of hematopoietic growth factors to AML induction have been restricted to older patients, but, as with younger patients, the advantages of the addition of growth factor appear limited to faster hematopoietic recovery and fewer days with neutropenic fever, but no consistent improvement in complete response rates or overall survival.

In virtually every study conducted to date, the complete response rate drops as the age of patients increases. Although some of this effect could be due to a diminished ability of patients to tolerate therapy and to a tendency of physicians to reduce doses in older patients, even when identical doses of drugs are used and toxic deaths are censored, the incidence of remission failures increases with age. AML among older patients is much more likely to evolve from a myelodysplastic syndrome, to be accompanied by unfavorable-risk cytogenetics, and to express the multidrug resistance gene.[97,98] All three of these have been found to be independent risk factors mitigating against the likelihood of achieving a complete remission. Thus, in a recent SWOG study of remission induction in patients over age 55 with AML, the overall complete response rate using a standard preparative regimen was 45%. If patients had none of these three factors, their complete response rate was 81%, whereas if all three factors were present, the complete response rate was less than 15%.[97] Similar results have been reported by the M.D. Anderson group.[99]

Postremission Therapy

General Principles

If no further therapy is given after patients enter remission, all will inevitably relapse and do so rapidly (on average in about 4 months), demonstrating the need for further therapy.[100] Three types of postremission therapy are in general use: chemotherapy, autologous hematopoietic cell transplantation (HCT), and allogeneic HCT.

Postremission Chemotherapy

Postremission chemotherapy usually consists of several cycles of combination chemotherapy given at doses similar to those used for induction. This form of therapy is often termed "consolidation" when given within a few months of induction or "late intensification" if given after a greater delay. Some trials also have explored the use of low-dose "maintenance" chemotherapy.

Most contemporary protocols include several consolidation cycles of high-dose cytarabine. The original idea behind the use of high-dose cytarabine came from studies suggesting that at higher doses, the drug is able to saturate deaminating enzymes resulting in production of higher levels of the active intracellular metabolite ARA-CTP, which in turn leads to enhanced inhibition of DNA synthesis.[101] Early phase I and II trials suggested that high-dose cytarabine regimens were tolerated and could result in complete remissions in patients with relapsed AML.[102,103] These observations led to the use of high-dose cytarabine as consolidation therapy after initial remission induction, with several phase II studies reporting sustained remissions in 30% to 40% of adults.[104,105] Ultimately, several large randomized trials have explored the value of high-dose cytarabine as postremission therapy in adult cases of AML.[85,106] The Cancer and Leukemia Group B (CALGB) randomly assigned 596 patients in complete remission to receive four courses of cytarabine at one of three doses:

1. 100 mg/m^2/day by continuous infusion for 5 days.
2. 400 mg/m^2/day by continuous infusion for 5 days.
3. 3 g/m^2 as a 3-hour intravenous infusion twice daily on days 1, 3, and 5.

High rates of CNS toxicity were observed among patients over age 60, and subsequent randomizations were limited to younger patients. At 3 years, disease-free-survival (DFS) was 21% in the 100 mg group, 25% in the 400 mg group, and 39% in the 3 g group. This trial established 3 or 4 doses of cytarabine at 3 g every 12 hours on days 1, 3, and 5 as among the most widely used consolidation regimens for younger patients with AML in first remission. Subsequent analyses have demonstrated that the advantage of the highest-dose arm was restricted to patients with favorable cytogenetics and thus, the intermediate-dose regimen might be as appropriate for patients with intermediate or unfavorable cytogenetics.[75] A SWOG trial randomized patients to conventional or high-dose cytarabine both during induction and consolidation.[85] The best result (52% 4-year survival) was seen among patients who received high-dose cytarabine at both induction and consolidation, a result consistent with those of the CALGB study. A number of other multiagent postremission chemotherapy regimens have been developed. For example, the MRC has reported on a regimen that uses as consolidation a cycle of standard anthracycline plus cytarabine, a cycle of "MACE" combining amsacrine, conventional dose cytarabine and etoposide, and a cycle of high-dose cytarabine plus mitoxantrone. The reported results looked generally similar to those reported by CALGB and SWOG.[107] No large randomized trials have been conducted comparing the various more commonly used consolidation regimens. These regimens, which include repetitive cycles of high-dose therapy, are generally inappropriate for patients over age 60. Most older patients are treated with several cycles of combination chemotherapy at moderate dosing, such as 2 days of daunorubicin plus 5 days of conventional-dose cytarabine. There are almost no data suggesting superiority of any particular consolidation regimen for older patients with AML.

With the increasing acceptance of short-term intensive consolidation chemotherapy as the standard for younger patients with AML, the concept of low-dose maintenance has fallen into disuse. There are data for both younger and older patients from randomized trials, however, demonstrating that maintenance therapy can prolong the duration of first remission, although an impact on overall survival has not been seen.[84,108,109]

Autologous Hematopoietic Cell Transplantation

The principles underlying the concept of autologous HCT and the general technique are outlined in other chapters in this book and will not be repeated here. Based on encouraging results in patients in second or subsequent remission, a number of single-center phase II trials of autologous HCT for AML in first remission were conducted and reported in the mid-1980s.[110-112] These small trials provided encouraging results, leading to wider use of the technique. Registry data describing results in hundreds of patients soon became available and suggested leukemia-free survival rates of approximately 45% at 5 years.[113] In an effort to minimize the possible impact of treatment selection bias, several large prospective randomized trials have been conducted in which adults in first remission with matched siblings have been assigned to allogeneic transplantation, while those without have been randomized to either autologous HCT or postremission chemotherapy. As noted in Table 104-5, relapse rates were reduced in all four trials with the use of autologous transplantation compared with chemotherapy.[107,114-116] In two of these four studies, autologous transplantation resulted in an improvement in disease-free survival, while in the other two it did not. A discussion about who might best benefit from autologous HCT in first remission is provided in the ensuing discussion, after the presentation of data related to studies of allogeneic transplantation.

A large number of questions exist about how best to conduct autologous HCT for AML. The most commonly used preparative regimens are combinations of busulfan plus cyclophosphamide, busulfan plus etoposide, or cyclophosphamide plus total body irradiation (TBI), but few randomized trials have been conducted.[117,118] Registry data suggest relative equivalence among regimens. Although gene-marking studies have provided unequivocal evidence that occult tumor cells in remission marrow can contribute to the risk of relapse, there are no published comparative clinical trials to confirm that

TABLE 104-5

	ALLOGENEIC HCT		**AUTOLOGOUS HCT**		**CHEMOTHERAPY**	
Results of Allogeneic HCT, Autologous HCT, or Chemotherapy for AML	**RELAPSE (%)**	**DFS (%)**	**RELAPSE (%)**	**DFS (%)**	**RELAPSE (%)**	**DFS (%)**
EORTC[116]	24	55	40	48	57	30
GOELAM[114]	28	49	45	48	55	43
MRC[107]	—	—	35	54	53	40
ECOG/SWOG[115]	29	43	48	34	61	34

the methods of ex vivo purging are of any clinical benefit.[119,120] The four randomized clinical studies described in the foregoing paragraphs used a variety of preparative regimens, approaches to in vitro stem cell treatment, and applied transplantation at different times in the therapy. The study that showed the greatest benefit of the procedure used it after three or four cycles of intensive therapy, while the studies that showed the least benefit applied the treatment almost immediately after induction. As these were randomized trials, effects of patient selection on lead time bias should have been minimized, suggesting that autologous transplantation is of greatest differential benefit if applied after consolidation therapy rather than as a substitute for it.

Allogeneic Hematopoietic Cell Transplantation

The initial application of allogeneic HCT to treat AML was published by Thomas and colleagues[121] in 1977, when they reported on 54 patients with recurrent or refractory AML treated with TBI-containing regimens and allogeneic HCT. At the time of the report, seven of these patients were alive in remission, and a subsequent follow-up more than 13 years later showed that 6 of the 54 remained alive and disease free.[122] In 1979, Thomas and associates[123] published the initial results of allogeneic HCT for patients in first remission, reporting for a small group of patients a 5-year disease free survival in excess of 50%. Similar results were soon reported by others as well.[124,125] The results reported in these small, uncontrolled, single-institution series were far superior to anything achieved at the time with conventional chemotherapy, but the potential impact of patient selection bias was unknown. Accordingly, these small, single-institution series were soon followed by a substantial number of single-institution or group trials comparing allogeneic transplantation for patients with donors to conventional chemotherapy for patients without donors. Studies published in the mid-1980s from the Royal Marsden, Seattle, UCLA, and Genova all showed a markedly diminished risk of relapse with transplantation, a higher risk of treatment-related death with transplantation, and, in all four studies, improved disease-free survival with transplantation.[126–129]

Since the mid-1980s, there have, of course, been significant changes in both chemotherapy and the practice of allogeneic HCT, and so comparisons of these techniques continue to be made. Four of the more recent large comparative trials are listed in Table 104-5. In all four trials, use of allogeneic transplantation was associated with the lowest risk of leukemic relapse.[107,114–116] On the other hand, allogeneic transplantation was also associated with a higher treatment-related mortality. In all four trials, the DFS was highest in the allogeneic arm, but only in the EORTC trial did this reach statistical significance. These studies, although useful, also have a significant number of shortcomings. One of the more obvious is that patients with allogeneic donors are assigned to HCT in first remission, and thus a strategy of chemotherapy first, followed by allogeneic HCT as salvage therapy, is not tested, although this is a logical alternative for the patient with AML and a matched sibling. Second, the studies were not sized to study the impact of these alternative

approaches among the different risk groups of AML. For example, the ECOG/SWOG trial suggests a particular advantage of allogeneic transplantation among patients with unfavorable-risk cytogenetics, but because of the size of these studies, questions about specific interactions of disease and treatment remain.

The general technique of allogeneic HCT is described in Chapter 28 and will not be repeated here, except for the following few points specifically relevant to AML. The optimal preparative regimen for transplantation of AML in first CR is arguable. One prospective randomized trial demonstrates superiority of cyclophosphamide plus TBI over busulfan plus cyclophosphamide.[130] A subsequent large registry study, however, found equivalence between the two approaches.[117] Although bone marrow has been the usual source of stem cells, three recent randomized trials have shown faster engraftment with the use of G-CSF mobilized peripheral blood without increasing acute graft-vs.-host disease (GVHD).[131–133] In all three studies, there was a trend toward more chronic GVHD with the use of peripheral blood, but in two of three trials, overall survival was improved with the use of peripheral blood as a source of stem cells. The combination of cyclosporine plus methotrexate is the most commonly used form of GVHD prophylaxis. Although some encouraging phase I/II studies of T-cell depletion have been published, there are no randomized trials showing an advantage of T-cell depletion for patients with AML in first remission.[134] Recent trials using unrelated donors have shown results approaching those achieved with fully matched siblings.

Selection of Appropriate Postremission Therapy

Postremission chemotherapy, autologous transplantation, and allogeneic transplantation all represent viable treatment options for the younger patient with AML in first remission. Opinions vary among experts but in general, most would recommend allogeneic transplantation using a matched sibling or an unrelated donor for patients with AML and unfavorable-risk cytogenetics. For patients with favorable-risk cytogenetics, most experts would recommend consolidation chemotherapy with repetitive cycles of high-dose cytarabine. Opinions for patients with intermediate-risk cytogenetics are more varied and might be influenced by subtle risk factors such as the age of the patient and the WBC count at diagnosis, with transplantation being favored for younger patients with higher WBC counts. Of course, many other patient-specific factors enter into this difficult decision-making process. The foregoing recommendations are consistent with those of the National Comprehensive Cancer Network.[135]

For patients over age 55, conventional myeloablative transplantation is not normally used, although recent studies of nonmyeloablative transplantation for patients over age 55 are showing promise.[136] The advantages of autologous transplantation seen in randomized trials were restricted to patients less than age 60. Thus, for most older patients with AML, standard consolidation chemotherapy is recommended. For these patients as for all patients with AML, however, participation in well designed clinical trials is appropriate and should be pursued actively.

TREATMENT OF RECURRENT ACUTE MYELOID LEUKEMIA

General Principles

Allogeneic or autologous HCT is the only therapy able to cure substantial proportions of patients with recurrent AML. For those patients who are transplant candidates, who are found to be in early first relapse and who have a previously identified source of stem cells, it could be appropriate to proceed directly to transplantation.[137,138] For all other patients, an initial trial of chemotherapy in an attempt to obtain a second remission is appropriate.

Reinduction Chemotherapy

A number of large observational studies of reinduction chemotherapy have been published over the last 15 years.[139-143] In general, CR rates have ranged from 30% to 50%, and the mortality rates associated with reinduction have been 15% to 25%. Three prognostic factors have consistently been identified with an improved outcome: younger age, favorable cytogenetic risk group, and longer duration of first remission.

A limited number of randomized trials has been conducted in this group of patients. Vogler[144] found that adding etoposide to high-dose cytarabine was of no advantage, whereas Karanes[145] did show a benefit of adding mitoxantrone to high-dose cytarabine. More recently, List and associates[146] performed a large randomized trial testing whether the addition of cyclosporine to a regimen of high-dose cytarabine plus infusional daunorubicin would be of benefit. This study was based on the high incidence of multidrug resistance in recurrent AML and the ability of cyclosporine at clinically achievable levels to reverse this phenotype. In this randomized trial, the investigators found a significantly reduced incidence of resistant leukemia with the addition of cyclosporine and a resulting improvement in both disease-free and overall survival.

Gemtuzumab ozogamicin combines a humanized anti-CD33 antibody with the potent antitumor agent, calicheamicin. Gemtuzumab ozogamicin was developed based on the observation that CD33 is expressed by virtually all cases of AML but not in normal hematopoietic stem cells or in nonhematopoietic tissues and on the conclusion that by targeting CD33, a less toxic, effective therapeutic might result. Phase I studies showed saturation of CD33 antigenic sites at 9 mg/m^2 and clearing of leukemic blasts in many patients at this dose.[147] Subsequent phase II trials showed a CR rate of 30% with less toxicity than might be expected with aggressive combination chemotherapy.[148] Based on this result, gemtuzumab ozogamicin was approved by the FDA for the treatment of older patients with recurrent AML.

Hematopoietic Cell Transplantation for Recurrent AML

Approximately 30% of patients with AML who are transplanted in untreated first relapse from matched siblings can expect to become long-term disease-free survivors.[149-152] Autologous transplantation using marrow previously stored in first remission has resulted in a 26% 5-year disease-free survival.[151] These outcomes are not markedly less than what might be expected for transplantation in second remission, and so, for those patients in early relapse with an identified source of stem cells, immediate stem cell transplantation is a reasonable option.

The majority of patients will require reinduction, however. For those patients who achieve a second remission, have a matched sibling, and are below age 55, allogeneic transplantation is the preferred form of therapy, and cure can be expected in 35% of cases.[152] For patients without matched siblings, either autologous or matched unrelated transplantation should be considered. There have been no randomized trials comparing either approach to further chemotherapy or the two approaches to one another. A retrospective case-controlled study was conducted by the European Bone Marrow Transplant Group, and no statistically significant difference in disease-free survival or overall survival was found between autologous and matched unrelated donor transplantation.[153] Without further outcome data, the choice of autologous vs. unrelated transplantation for AML in second remission is difficult, but an allogeneic approach might be favored for younger patients with poor-risk disease characteristics (e.g., a short remission duration and unfavorable cytogenetics), while autologous transplantation might be favored for older patients with more favorable disease characteristics, including a long first remission.

The results of transplantation for patients who fail reinduction are less favorable, and long-term survival can

---

MANAGEMENT OF NEWLY DIAGNOSED ACUTE MYELOID LEUKEMIA IN PATIENTS BELOW AGE 55 YEARS

INDUCTION	Daunorubicin, 60 mg/m^2/day for 3 days (or idarubicin, 12 mg/m^2/day for 3 days) and cytarabine, 200 mg/m^2/day for 7 days
POSTREMISSION	
Favorable risk	Cytarabine, 3 g/m^2 over 3 hours every 12 hours on days 1, 3, and 5 for four courses; store autologous stem cells if no HLA-matched sibling donor
Intermediate risk	If HLA-matched sibling, allogeneic transplantation. If no HLA-matched sibling, cytarabine, 3 g/m^2 over 3 hours every 12 hours on days 1, 3, and 5 for two courses, followed by autologous transplantation
Unfavorable risk	If HLA-matched sibling or HLA-matched unrelated donor available, go to allogeneic transplant. If not, as for intermediate-risk disease.

be expected in only 10% to 20% of patients undergoing allogeneic transplant for refractory AML.[154]

TREATMENT OF ACUTE PROMYELOCYTIC LEUKEMIA

Acute promyelocytic leukemia (APL) is distinguished by both the t(15;17) translocation and a unique pattern of drug sensitivity demanding a different treatment strategy from other categories of AML. Specifically, APL is particularly sensitive to anthracyclines and to all-trans retinoic acid (ATRA), and by using both drugs appropriately, a high percentage of APL patients can expect to be cured.

The evidence for the unique sensitivity of APL to anthracyclines comes both from studies showing complete response rates as high as 75% using idarubicin as a single agent and from studies showing that the percentage of patients cured with chemotherapy is directly proportional to the dose of anthracycline used.[155,156]

In the late 1980s, ATRA, when used as a single agent, was found to be able to induce complete remissions in most patients, with rapid resolution of the often-seen coagulopathy.[157] The duration of complete remission was brief when ATRA was used as a single agent, however.

Initial Therapy

A number of studies have been conducted in the attempt to define the best ways to incorporate high-dose anthracyclines plus ATRA into the management of the patient newly diagnosed with APL. The use of ATRA as a single agent for induction results in CR rates as high as those achieved with conventional anthracycline-containing chemotherapy and an improved overall survival.[158] A European APL study has since shown that concurrent administration of ATRA plus chemotherapy might result in a slight improvement in overall event-free survival (84% vs. 77% at 2 years).[159] Combining chemotherapy and ATRA during induction has the added benefit of reducing the incidence of the retinoic acid syndrome (to be discussed shortly) from 25% down to less than 10%, and this is now considered standard therapy.

Consolidation chemotherapy for APL generally involves giving repeated cycles of a regimen consisting of an anthracycline and ATRA. There does not appear to be any benefit for the use of high-dose cytarabine in this disease, and some question whether there is any role for cytarabine at any dose.[160] The appropriate number of cycles of consolidation is unknown.

There is a clear role for maintenance therapy in APL. In a large North American Cooperative Group study, patients were randomized to maintenance with daily ATRA or to observation. Those randomized to ATRA had an improved DFS.[158,161] Because ATRA induces enzymes that enhance its metabolism, many have suggested that intermittent ATRA therapy might be advantageous. The European APL 93 trial randomized patients to intermittent ATRA, 6-mercaptopurine plus methotrexate or a combination of intermittent ATRA plus the combination chemo-

MANAGEMENT OF ACUTE PROMYELOCYTIC LEUKEMIA	
NEWLY DIAGNOSED DISEASE	
Induction	ATRA, 45 mg/m^2/day until CR plus daunorubicin, 60 mg/m^2/day for 3 days and cytarabine, 200 mg/m^2/day for 7 days
Consolidation	Two cycles each consisting of ATRA, 45 mg/m^2/day for 7 days and daunorubicin, 50 mg/m^2/day for 3 days
Maintenance	ATRA, 45 mg/m^2/ daily for 15 days every 3 months plus 6MP, 100 mg/m^2/day and MTX, 10 mg/m^2 per week for 2 years
RECURRENT DISEASE	
Induction	Arsenic trioxide, 0.15 mg/kg daily until second CR
Consolidation	Autologous transplant if PCR-negative stem cells available, otherwise allogeneic transplant if suitable donor available

therapy. The maintenance arm combining ATRA plus chemotherapy had the best overall survival.[159]

With current management, the prognosis for patients with APL has improved remarkably from what it was in the 1980s. For example, in the North American Intergroup Trial, the 5-year survival rate for patients randomized to ATRA induction and maintenance was 69%.[158,161] A few factors might alter the prognosis of APL slightly. An improved survival has been seen among patients presenting with lower WBC counts and among females.[162] Because of the excellent outcome with current regimens, there is no generally accepted role for transplantation during first remission of APL.

Treatment of Recurrent APL

In addition to its unique sensitivity to ATRA, APL is also remarkably sensitive to treatment with arsenic trioxide, as first reported by investigators from China.[163,164] A more recent multicenter study has reported an 85% CR rate among patients with recurrent APL using arsenic trioxide.[165] The most important toxicities include prolongation of the QT interval and a syndrome essentially identical to the retinoic acid syndrome to be discussed shortly. The QT prolongation requires careful monitoring, as two recent reports have documented sudden deaths associated with the use of arsenic trioxide.[166,167] Thus, metabolic abnormalities that also prolong the QT interval, such as hypokalemia, hypophosphatemia, and hypomagnesemia, should be connected before therapy is initiated. Currently, reinduction with arsenic trioxide is generally considered as the initial treatment of choice for patients with APL who have failed first-line therapy, particularly if that failure is within 12 months of receiving ATRA.

There is only sparse data about the expected duration of second remission induced with arsenic trioxide.

Although some patients might remain in remission for some time if given arsenic plus chemotherapy, most experts would recommend either autologous or allogeneic HCT for patients with APL in second remission. Sanz and associates[168] presented results from the European Blood and Marrow Transplant Group for patients with APL in second remission and reported overall survival rates of 58% for allogeneic transplantation vs. 40% for autologous transplantation. The choice of autologous or allogeneic HCT might be influenced by the status of the autologous stem cell source. In a small but provocative study, Meloni reported on 15 patients with APL in second remission undergoing autologous transplantation. Only one of eight patients transplanted with marrow that was PCR-negative subsequently relapsed, whereas all seven who were transplanted using PCR-positive marrow did so.[169]

Retinoic Acid Syndrome

After therapy with ATRA, a proportion of APL patients develop a syndrome manifested by fever, weight gain, respiratory distress, pulmonary infiltrates and effusions, episodic hypotension, and renal failure.[170] When ATRA is used as a single agent, this syndrome can be seen in as many as 25% of cases. Risk factors for the development of the syndrome are not obvious, but the simultaneous administration of chemotherapy during induction has seemed to diminish the risk of its development. The mortality rate of this syndrome, when first described, was about 30%, but with the recognition that the syndrome responds dramatically to the institution of dexamethasone, mortality rates have fallen to less than 5%. The observation that an identical syndrome can be seen with arsenic trioxide suggests that the syndrome is likely associated with the differentiation of APL cells and is poorly named.

SUPPORTIVE CARE

The treatment of AML is accompanied by a substantial number of complications and thus is best conducted at a center experienced in the management of these sometimes complex patients. During the granulocytopenic period after intensive induction and consolidation chemotherapy, most patients become febrile, and bacterial infections can be documented in roughly 50%. Gram-positive organisms (e.g., *Staphylococcus epidermidis*) and gram-negative enteric organisms (e.g., *Escherichia coli* and *Klebsiella/Aerobacter*) are common, but the experience can vary by medical center. Reactivation of herpes simplex infections can add to mucositis, and fungal infections can develop in patients on antibiotics. Thus, we generally recommend starting the following antimicrobial prophylaxis before initiating therapy: ciprofloxacin, 500 mg every 12 hours; fluconazole, 200 mg daily; and acyclovir, 800 mg every 12 hours orally. Patients who become febrile while neutropenic should start on broad-spectrum antibiotics, such as monotherapy with imipenem, or a combination of an antipseudomonal penicillin and a third-generation cephalosporin. If patients are persistently febrile after 72 hours of broad-spectrum

antibiotics, additional antibiotics or antifungal coverage should be considered. The choice should be dictated by the unique clinical circumstances of the patient. Patients should continue on broad-spectrum antibiotics until recovery of granulocyte counts and defervescence.

The hemoglobin of patients should be maintained above 8 to 10 g/dL, and platelet counts should be kept above 10,000/mm^3 in asymptomatic patients and above 20,000/mm^3 in the presence of fever or hypertension. Many patients might become candidates for hematopoietic cell transplantation, and so if patients are CMV seronegative at the start of induction, every effort should be made to assure that they continue to receive either CMV seronegative or filtered blood products.

Malnutrition can be a significant problem, particularly in the older, frailer patient. Early institution of hyperalimentation should be considered if oral intake becomes inadequate.

MONITORING RESPONSE TO THERAPY

Substantial effort has been made to develop assays of leukemic burden that are more sensitive than the admittedly gross estimates afforded by morphologic examination.[171] Such assays, if sensitive, specific, and predictive of outcome, could be used to guide therapy so that, as one example, a patient in first remission could be taken immediately to transplantation if the response to initial chemotherapy predicted a high probability of relapse, or the patient might be spared the toxicities of transplantation if the extent of response to initial therapy was so favorable as to predict a high probability of cure. Efforts to develop such assays have, to date, focused on PCR detection of leukemia-specific translocations and multidimensional flow cytometry.

The major attraction of PCR-based assays is their high level of sensitivity and specificity. In AML there are no universal translocations, however, and so separate studies, each involving only a small subset of AML cases, have been required. The most encouraging results have come from the study of APL, in which PCR-based assays for t(15;17) conducted after induction and consolidation were predictive of outcome.[172] More recent studies suggest that more precise information might be available by use of a semiquantitative PCR assay in this disease.[173] The results with other translocations have been more perplexing. PCR-based assays of t(8;21) do not appear to predict relapse, and many patients show persisting positive PCR assays while remaining in complete remission for years after completing all therapy. Miyamoto and colleagues[174] studied 18 patients off therapy for 1 to 12 years, all of whom remained PCR-positive for the AML/ETO chimeric transcript. The positive signal could be found in CD34+ marrow cells, and analyses of the PCR-positive colonies demonstrated them to be clonal. These results help explain why, at present, there are no easy PCR-based methods to monitor response to therapy of most patients with AML.

An alternative approach to monitoring response to therapy is the use of multidimensional flow cytometry.

This approach is not nearly as sensitive as PCR and has a sensitivity of, at best, one in 500 cells. Flow cytometry does has the advantage that it might be broadly applicable to virtually all cases of AML. There are several studies, one in pediatric AML and a second in adult AML, that suggest that a flow-based assessment of the initial remission marrow sample could be useful in adding information beyond that of routine prognostic factors about which patients are likely to relapse within the first several years after diagnosis.[175,176]

FUTURE DIRECTIONS IN TREATMENT

With increased understanding of the molecular events involved in the development of AML, the number of potential therapeutic targets has grown. These targets can be categorized into three general categories:

- Those that are the immediate consequences of the mutational events leading to AML.
- Those that are the adaptive changes a leukemic cell must make to stay alive given the initial mutational event.
- Those that immunologically distinguish AML cells from normal hematopoietic stem cells.

The most common mutations in AML involve FLT-3, and because these mutations are activating, clinical trials are beginning to explore the use of a number of inhibitors of FLT-3 tyrosine kinase, including CEP-701, PKC-412, SU11248, and CT53518. RAS molecules are downstream from tyrosine kinase receptors and themselves can be mutated in AML. Because farnesylation is required for RAS function, trials of several farnesyl transferase inhibitors (including R11597 and BMS214662) are underway. The CBF and retinoic acid receptor translocations result in recruitment of histone deacetylases, which are thought to inhibit transcription, thereby contributing to the malignant phenotype. Thus, a number of histone deacetylase inhibitors (including phenylbutyrate, trichostatin, depsipeptide, and MS-275) are being studied in AML.

The mutational event or events giving rise to AML could require the cell to make other adaptive changes not required of normal cells in order to survive. Such responses might be particularly required during moments of cell stress. One example is BCL-2, which is overexpressed in almost all AML samples compared to normal marrow and might be further overexpressed when cells are exposed to chemotherapy. Thus, agents that inhibit BCL-2, such as BCL-2 antisense, are being studied alone and with chemotherapy for AML.

Cell surface antigens are being increasingly explored as targets for antibody and cellular-based therapies. As noted earlier, the anti-CD33 calicheamicin conjugate gemtuzumab ozogamicin is an active agent for patients with recurrent AML. Recent studies combining it with standard-dose daunorubicin and cytarabine as initial induction therapy have reported encouraging results, with 85% and 86% CR rates, respectively, in two phase II trials.[177,178] Studies using antibodies to target radionuclides to marrow in efforts to develop improved preparative regimens for transplantation are also yielding encouraging outcomes.[179]

The markedly lower rates of disease recurrence after allogeneic transplants compared with identical twin transplants have encouraged further research into the development of cell-based immunotherapies. Some of these approaches, such as the further development of nonablative allogeneic transplants, attempt to make use of polymorphic minor histocompatability differences between donor and host. Other investigators are exploring the possibility of targeting T cells to either mutational fusion proteins, such as the AML/ETO protein, or to overexpressed self-antigens, such as PR3 and WT1. This long list of therapies currently in development offers great hope that the outcomes of treatment for patients with AML will continue to improve.

REFERENCES

1. Virchow R: Weisses blut. Frorieps Notizen 36:151.
2. Greenlee RT, Hill-Harmon MB, Murray T, et al: Cancer statistics, 2001 [erratum appears in CA Cancer J Clin 2001 Mar-Apr;51(2):144]. CA Cancer J Clin 2001;51:15–36.
3. Wingo PA, Ries LA, Giovino GA, et al: Annual report to the nation on the status of cancer, 1973–1996, with a special section on lung cancer and tobacco smoking. J Natl Cancer Inst 1999;91:675–690.
4. Cronkite EP: Chemical leukemogenesis: benzene as a model [review]. Semin Hematol 1987;24:2–11.
5. Brownson RC, Novotny TE, Perry MC: Cigarette smoking and adult leukemia. A meta-analysis. Arch Intern Med 1993;153:469–475.
6. Cronkite EP, Moloney W, Bond VP: Radiation leukemogenesis. An analysis of the problem. Am J Med 1960;28:673.
7. Darby SC, Doll R, Gill SK, et al: Long term mortality after a single treatment course with X-rays in patients treated for ankylosing spondylitis. Br J Cancer 1987;55:179–190.
8. Leone G, Mele L, Pulsoni A, et al: The incidence of secondary leukemias [review]. Haematologica 1999;84:937–945.
9. Rowley JD, Golomb HM, Vardiman J: Acute leukemia after treatment of lymphoma. N Engl J Med 1977;297:1013.
10. Coltman CA Jr, Dixon DO: Second malignancies complicating Hodgkin's disease: A Southwest Oncology Group 10-year follow-up. Cancer Treat Rep 1982;66:1023–1033.
11. Pedersen-Bjergaard J, Larsen SO: Incidence of acute nonlymphocytic leukemia, preleukemia, and acute myeloproliferative syndrome up to 10 years after treatment of Hodgkin's disease. N Engl J Med 1982;307:965–971.
12. Tucker MA, Coleman CN, Cox RS, et al: Risk of second cancers after treatment for Hodgkin's disease. N Engl J Med 1988;318:76–81.
13. Andrieu JM, Ifrah N, Payen C, et al: Increased risk of secondary acute nonlymphocytic leukemia after extended-field radiation therapy combined with MOPP chemotherapy for Hodgkin's disease [review]. J Clin Oncol 1990;8:1148–1154.
14. Greene MH, Harris EL, Gershenson DM, et al: Melphalan may be a more potent leukemogen than cyclophosphamide. Ann Intern Med 1986;105:360–367.
15. Kaldor JM, Day NE, Pettersson F, et al: Leukemia following chemotherapy for ovarian cancer. N Engl J Med 1990;322:1–6.
16. Boice JD Jr, Greene MH, Killen JY, et al: Leukemia and preleukemia after adjuvant treatment of gastrointestinal cancer with semustine (methyl-ccnu). N Engl J Med 1983;309:1079–1084.
17. Pedersen-Bjergaard J, Specht L, Larsen SO, et al: Risk of therapy-related leukaemia and preleukaemia after Hodgkin's disease. Relation to age, cumulative dose of alkylating agents, and time from chemotherapy. Lancet 1987;2:83–88.
18. Larson RA, Le Beau MM, Ratain MJ, et al: Balanced translocations involving chromosome bands 11q23 and 21q22 in therapy-related leukemia. Blood 1992;79:1892–1893.
19. Hawkins MM, Wilson LM, Stovall MA, et al: Epipodophyllotoxins, alkylating agents, and radiation and risk of secondary leukaemia after childhood cancer. BMJ 1992;304:951–958.

20. Pedersen-Bjergaard J, Philip P, Larsen SO, et al: Therapy-related myelodysplasia and acute myeloid leukemia. Cytogenetic characteristics of 115 consecutive cases and risk in seven cohorts of patients treated intensively for malignant diseases in the Copenhagen series. Leukemia 1993;7:1975–1986.

21. Shepherd L, Ottaway J, Myles J, et al: Therapy-related leukemia associated with high-dose 4-epi-doxorubicin and cyclophosphamide used as adjuvant chemotherapy for breast cancer. J Clin Oncol 1994;12:2514–2515.

22. Miller JS, Arthur DC, Litz CE, et al: Myelodysplastic syndrome after autologous bone marrow transplantation: An additional late complication of curative cancer therapy. Blood 1994;83:3780–3786.

23. Darrington DL, Vose JM, Anderson JR, et al: Incidence and characterization of secondary myelodysplastic syndrome and acute myelogenous leukemia following high-dose chemoradiotherapy and autologous stem-cell transplantation for lymphoid malignancies. J Clin Oncol 1994;12:2527–2534.

24. Metayer C, Curtis RE, Vose J, et al: Myelodysplastic syndrome and acute myeloid leukemia after autotransplantation for lymphoma: A multicenter case-control study. Blood 2003;100:2015–2023.

25. Rowley JD, Olney HJ: International workshop on the relationship of prior therapy to balanced chromosome aberrations in therapy-related myelodysplastic syndromes and acute leukemia: Overview report. Genes Chromosomes Cancer 2002;33:331–345.

26. Pagano L, Pulsoni A, Tosti ME, et al: Acute lymphoblastic leukaemia occurring as second malignancy: Report of the GIMEMA archive of adult acute leukaemia. Gruppo Italiano Malattie Ematologiche Maligne dell'Adulto. Br J Haematol 1999;106:1037–1040.

27. Douer D, Preston-Martin S, Chang E, et al: High frequency of acute promyelocytic leukemia among Latinos with acute myeloid leukemia. Blood 1996;87:308–313.

28. Tomas JF, Fernandez-Ranada JM: About the increased frequency of acute promyelocytic leukemia among Latinos: The experience from a center in Spain. Blood 1996;88:2357–2358.

29. Buckley JD, Buckley CM, Breslow NE, et al: Concordance for childhood cancer in twins. Med Pediatr Oncol 1996;26:223–229.

30. Goldgar DE, Easton DF, Cannon-Albright LA, et al: Systematic population-based assessment of cancer risk in first-degree relatives of cancer probands. J Natl Cancer Inst 1994;86:1600–1608.

31. Paul B, Reid MM, Davison EV, et al: Familial myelodysplasia: Progressive disease associated with emergence of monosomy 7. Br J Haematol 1987;65:321–323.

32. Lee EJ, Schiffer CA, Misawa S, et al: Clinical and cytogenetic features of familial erythroleukaemia. Br J Haematol 1987;65:313–320.

33. Song WJ, Sullivan MG, Legare RD, et al: Haploinsufficiency of CBFA2 causes familial thrombocytopenia with propensity to develop acute myelogenous leukaemia. Nat Genet 1999;23:166–175.

34. Ellis NA, Groden J, Ye TZ, et al: The Bloom's syndrome gene product is homologous to RecQ helicases. Cell 1995;83:655–666.

35. Taylor AM, Metcalfe JA, Thick J, et al: Leukemia and lymphoma in ataxia telangiectasia [review]. Blood 1996;87:423–438.

36. Butturini A, Gale RP, Verlander PC, et al: Hematologic abnormalities in Fanconi anemia: An International Fanconi Anemia Registry Study. Blood 1994;84:1650–1655.

37. Welte K, Dale D: Pathophysiology and treatment of severe chronic neutropenia [review]. Ann Hematol 1996;72:158–165.

38. Woods WG, Roloff JS, Lukens JN, et al: The occurrence of leukemia in patients with the Shwachman syndrome. J Pediatr 1981;99:425–428.

39. Fialkow PJ: Clonal origin of human tumors. Biochim Biophys Acta 1976;458:283–321.

40. Fialkow PJ, Singer JW, Adamson JW, et al: Acute nonlymphocytic leukemia: Heterogeneity of stem cell origin. Blood 1981;57:1068–1073.

41. Jacobson RJ, Temple MJ, Singer JW, et al: A clonal complete clinical remission in acute nonlymphocytic leukemia originating in a multipotent stem cell. N Engl J Med 1984;310:1513–1517.

42. Fialkow PJ, Janssen JWG, Bartram CR: Clonal remissions in acute nonlymphocytic leukemia: Evidence for a multistep pathogenesis of the malignancy. Blood 1991;77:1415–1517.

43. Bonnet D, Dick JE: Human acute myeloid leukemia is organized as a hierarchy that originates from a primitive hematopoietic cell. Nat Med 1997;3:730–737.

44. Lapidot T, Sirard C, Vormoor J, et al: A cell initiating human acute myeloid leukaemia after transplantation into SCID mice. Nature 1994;367:645–648.

45. Sjogren U: Mitotic activity in myeloid leukaemias. A study of 277 cases. Scand J Haematol 1978;20:159–167.

46. Niederwieser DW, Appelbaum FR, Gastl G, et al: Inadvertent transmission of a donor's acute myeloid leukemia in bone marrow transplantation for chronic myelocytic leukemia. N Engl J Med 1990;322:1794–1796.

47. Nucifora G, Birn DJ, Erickson P, et al: Detection of DNA rearrangements in the AML1 and ETO loci and of an AML1/ETO fusion mRNA in patients with t(8;21) acute myeloid leukemia. Blood 1993;81:883–888.

48. Meyers S, Lenny N, Hiebert SW: The t(8;21) fusion protein interferes with AML-1B-dependent transcriptional activation. Mol Cell Biol 1995;15:1974–1982.

49. Liu P, Tarle SA, Hajra A, et al: Fusion between transcription factor CBF beta/PEBP2 beta and a myosin heavy chain in acute myeloid leukemia. Science 1993;261:1041–1044.

50. Golub TR, Barker GF, Bohlander SK, et al: Fusion of the TEL gene on 12p13 to the AML1 gene on 21q22 in acute lymphoblastic leukemia. Proc Natl Acad Sci USA 1995;92:4917–4921.

51. Osato M, Asou N, Abdalla E, et al: Biallelic and heterozygous point mutations in the runt domain of the AML1/PEBP2alphaB gene associated with myeloblastic leukemias. Blood 1999;93:1817–1824.

52. Preudhomme C, Warot-Loze D, Roumier C, et al: High incidence of biallelic point mutations in the Runt domain of the AML1/PEBP2 alpha B gene in Mo acute myeloid leukemia and in myeloid malignancies with acquired trisomy 21. Blood 2000;96:2862–2869.

53. De The H, Lavau C, Marchio A, et al: The PML-RAR alpha fusion mRNA generated by the t(15;17) translocation in acute promyelocytic leukemia encodes a functionally altered RAR. Cell 1991;66:675–684.

54. Slovak ML, Kopecky KJ, Cassileth PA, et al: Karyotypic analysis predicts outcome of preremission and postremission therapy in adult acute myeloid leukemia: A Southwest Oncology Group/Eastern Cooperative Oncology Group study. Blood 2000;96:4075–4083.

55. Grimwade D, Walker H, Oliver F, et al: The importance of diagnostic cytogenetics on outcome in AML: Analysis of 1,612 patients entered into the MRC AML 10 trial. The Medical Research Council Adult and Children's Leukaemia Working Parties. Blood 1998;92:2322–2333.

56. Corral J, Lavenir I, Impey H, et al: An MLL-AF9 fusion gene made by homologous recombination causes acute leukemia in chimeric mice: A method to create fusion oncogenes. Cell 1996;85:853–861.

57. Caligiuri MA, Strout MP, Schichman SA, et al: Partial tandem duplication of MLL1 as a recurrent molecular defect in acute myeloid leukemia with trisomy 11. Cancer Res 1996;56:1418–1425.

58. Ernst P, Wang J, Korsmeyer SJ: The role of MLL in hematopoiesis and leukemia [review]. Curr Opin Hematol 2002;9:282–287.

59. Yagi H, Deguchi K, Aono A, et al: Growth disturbance in fetal liver hematopoiesis of MLL-mutant mice. Blood 1998;92:108–117.

60. Ayton P, Sneddon SF, Palmer DB, et al: Truncation of the MLL gene in exon 5 by gene targeting leads to early preimplantation lethality of homozygous embryos. Genesis 2001;30:201–212.

61. Nakao M, Yokota S, Iwai T, et al: Internal tandem duplication of the flt3 gene found in acute myeloid leukemia. Leukemia 1996;10:1911–1918.

62. Stirewalt DL, Kopecky KJ, Meshinchi S, et al: FLT3, RAS, and TP53 mutations in elderly patients with acute myeloid leukemia. Blood 2001;97:3589–3595.

63. Hayakawa F, Towatari M, Kiyoi H, et al: Tandem-duplicated Flt3 constitutively activates STAT5 and MAP kinase and introduces autonomous cell growth in IL-3-dependent cell lines. Oncogene 2000;19:624–631.

64. Kelly LM, Liu Q, Kutok JL, et al: FLT3 internal tandem duplication mutations associated with human acute myeloid leukemias induce myeloproliferative disease in a murine bone marrow transplant model. Blood 2002;99:310–318.

65. Kottaridis PD, Gale RE, Frew ME, et al: The presence of a FLT3 internal tandem duplication in patients with acute myeloid leukemia (AML) adds important prognostic information to cytogenetic risk group and response to the first cycle of chemotherapy: Analysis of 854 patients from the United Kingdom Medical Research Council AML 10 and 12 trials. Blood 2001;98: 1752–1759.

66. Whitman SP, Archer KJ, Feng L, et al: Absence of the wild-type allele predicts poor prognosis in adult de novo acute myeloid leukemia with normal cytogenetics and the internal tandem duplication of FLT3: A cancer and leukemia group B study. Cancer Res 2001;61:7233–7239.

67. Farr CJ, Saiki RK, Erlich HA, et al: Analysis of RAS gene mutations in acute myeloid leukemia by polymerase chain reaction and oligonucleotide probes. Proc Natl Acad Sci USA 1988;85: 1629–1633.

68. Gari M, Goodeve A, Wilson G, et al: c-kit proto-oncogene exon 8 in-frame deletion plus insertion mutations in acute myeloid leukaemia. Br J Haematol 1999;105:894–900.

69. Radich JP, Kopecky KJ, Willman CL, et al: N-ras mutations in adult de novo acute myelogenous leukemia: Prevalence and clinical significance. Blood 1990;76:801–807.

70. Bos JL, Verlaan-de VM, van der Eb AJ, et al: Mutations in N-ras predominate in acute myeloid leukemia. Blood 1987;69: 1237–1241.

71. Karp JE, Lancet JE, Kaufmann SH, et al: Clinical and biologic activity of the farnesyltransferase inhibitor R115777 in adults with refractory and relapsed acute leukemias: A phase I clinical-laboratory correlative trial. Blood 2001;97: 3361–3369.

72. Bennett JM, Catovsky D, Daniel MT, et al: Proposals for the classification of the acute leukaemias. French-American-British (FAB) co-operative group. Br J Haematol 1976;33:451–458.

73. Vardiman JW, Harris NL, Brunning RD: The World Health Organization (WHO) classification of the myeloid neoplasms [review]. Blood 2002;100:2292–2302.

74. Wolman SR, Gundacker H, Appelbaum FR, et al: Impact of trisomy 8 (+8) on clinical presentation, treatment response, and survival in acute myeloid leukemia: A Southwest Oncology Group study. Blood 2002;100:29–35.

75. Bloomfield CD, Lawrence D, Byrd JC, et al: Frequency of prolonged remission duration after high-dose cytarabine intensification in acute myeloid leukemia varies by cytogenetic subtype. Cancer Res 1998;58:4173–4179.

76. Morrison FS, Kopecky KJ, Head DR, et al: Late intensification with POMP chemotherapy prolongs survival in acute myelogenous leukemia—Results of a Southwest oncology group study of rubidazone vs. adriamycin for remission induction, prophylactic intrathecal therapy, late intensification, and levamisole maintenance. Leukemia 1992;6:708–714.

77. Cuttner J, Holland JF, Norton L, et al: Therapeutic leukapheresis for hyperleukocytosis in acute myelocytic leukemia. Med Pediatr Oncol 1983;11:76–78.

78. Campos L, Guyotat D, Archimbaud E, et al: Surface marker expression in adult acute myeloid leukaemia: Correlations with initial characteristics, morphology and response to therapy. Br J Haematol 1989;72:161–166.

79. Preisler H, Bjornsson S, Henderson ES, et al: Remission induction in acute nonlymphocytic leukemia: Comparison of a seven-day and ten-day infusion of cytosine arabinoside in combination with adriamycin. Med Pediatr Oncol 1979;7:269–275.

80. Berman E, Heller G, Santorsa J, et al: Results of a randomized trial comparing idarubicin and cytosine arabinoside with daunorubicin and cytosine arabinoside in adult patients with newly diagnosed acute myelogenous leukemia. Blood 1991;77(8):1666–1674.

81. Vogler WR, Velez-Garcia E, Weiner RS, et al: A phase III trial comparing idarubicin and daunorubicin in combination with cytarabine in acute myelogenous leukemia: A Southeastern Cancer Study Group Study. J Clin Oncol 1992;10(7):1103–1111.

82. Wiernik PH, Banks PL, Case DC Jr, et al: Cytarabine plus idarubicin or daunorubicin as induction and consolidation therapy for previously untreated adult patients with acute myeloid leukemia. Blood 1992;79(2):313–319.

83. Mandelli F, Petti MC, Ardia A, et al: A randomized clinical trial comparing idarubicin and cytarabine to daunorubicin and cytarabine in the treatment of acute non-lymphoid leukemia. A multicentric study from the Italian Co-operative Group GIMEMA. Eur J Cancer 1991;27:750–755.

84. Hewlett J, Kopecky KJ, Head D, et al: A prospective evaluation of the roles of allogeneic marrow transplantation and low-dose monthly maintenance chemotherapy in the treatment of adult acute myelogenous leukemia (AML): A Southwest Oncology Group study. Leukemia 1995;9:562–569.

85. Weick JK, Kopecky KJ, Appelbaum FR, et al: A randomized investigation of high-dose versus standard-dose cytosine arabinoside with daunorubicin in patients with previously untreated acute myeloid leukemia: A Southwest Oncology Group Study. Blood 1996;88:2841–2851.

86. Rowe JM, Andersen JW, Mazza JJ, et al: A randomized placebo-controlled phase III study of granulocyte-macrophage colony-stimulating factor in adult patients (> 55 to 70 years of age) with acute myelogenous leukemia: A study of the Eastern Cooperative Oncology Group (E1490). Blood 1995;86:457–462.

87. Rowe JM, Neuberg D, Friedenberg W, et al: A phase III study of daunorubicin vs idarubicin vs mitoxantrone for older adult patients (>55 yrs) with acute myelogenous leukemia (AML): A study of the Eastern Cooperative Oncology Group (E3993) [abstract]. Blood 1998;92 (Part 1):313a.

88. Bishop JF, Matthews JP, Young GA, et al: A randomized study of high-dose cytarabine in induction in acute myeloid leukemia. Blood 1996;87:1710–1717.

89. Bishop JF, Lowenthal RM, Joshua D, et al: Etoposide in acute nonlymphocytic leukemia. Blood 1990;75:27–32.

90. Godwin JE, Kopecky KJ, Head DR, et al: A double-blind placebo-controlled trial of granulocyte colony-stimulating factor in elderly patients with previously untreated acute myeloid leukemia: A Southwest Oncology Group Study (9031). Blood 1998;91:3607–3615.

91. Stone RM, Berg DT, George SL, et al: Granulocyte-macrophage colony-stimulating factor after initial chemotherapy for elderly patients with primary acute myelogenous leukemia. N Engl J Med 1995;332:1671–1677.

92. Lowenberg B, Suciu S, Archimbaud E, et al: Use of recombinant GM-CSF during and after remission induction chemotherapy in patients aged 61 years and older with acute myeloid leukemia: Final report of AML-11, a phase III randomized study of the Leukemia Cooperative Group of European Organisation for the Research and Treatment of Cancer and the Dutch Belgian Hemato-Oncology Cooperative Group. Blood 1997;90:2952–2961.

93. Estey E, Thall P, Andreeff M, et al: Use of granulocyte colony-stimulating factor before, during, and after fludarabine plus cytarabine induction therapy of newly diagnosed acute myelogenous leukemia or myelodysplastic syndromes: Comparison with fludarabine plus cytarabine without granulocyte colony-stimulating factor. J Clin Oncol 1994;12:671–678.

94. Heil G, Hoelzer D, Sanz MA, et al: A randomized, double-blind, placebo-controlled, phase III study of filgrastim in remission induction and consolidation therapy for adults with de novo acute myeloid leukemia. Blood 197;90:4710–4718.

95. Bennett CL, Stinson TJ, Tallman MS, et al: Economic analysis of a randomized placebo-controlled phase III study of granulocyte macrophage colony stimulating factor in adult patients (> 55 to 70 years of age) with acute myelogenous leukemia. Eastern Cooperative Oncology Group (E1490). Ann Oncol 1999;10:177–182.

96. Bennett CL, Hynes D, Godwin J, et al: Economic analysis of granulocyte colony stimulating factor as adjunct therapy for older patients with acute myelogenous leukemia (AML): Estimates from a Southwest Oncology Group clinical trial. Cancer Invest 2001;19:603–610.

97. Leith CP, Chir B, Kopecky KJ, et al: Acute myeloid leukemia in the elderly: Assessment of multidrug resistance (MDR1) and

cytogenetics distinguishes biologic subgroups with remarkably distinct responses to standard chemotherapy. A Southwest Oncology Group Study. Blood 1997;89:3323–3329.

98. Leith CP, Kopecky KJ, Chen I-M, et al: Frequency and clinical significance of the expression of the multidrug resistance proteins MDR1/P-glycoprotein, MRP1, and LRP in acute myeloid leukemia. A Southwest Oncology Group study. Blood 1999;94: 1086–1099.

99. Estey EH: How I treat older patients with AML. Blood 2000;96: 1670–1673.

100. Cassileth PA, Hines JD, Oken MM, et al: Maintenance chemotherapy prolongs remission duration in adult acute nonlymphocytic leukemia. J Clin Oncol 1988;6(4):583–587.

101. Kufe DW, Major PP, Egan EM, et al: Correlation of cytotoxicity with incorporation of ara-C into DNA. J Biol Chem 1980;255: 8997–9000.

102. Rudnick SA, Cadman EC, Capizzi RL, et al: High dose cytosine arabinoside (HDARAC) in refractory acute leukemia. Cancer 1979;44:1189–1193.

103. Herzig RH, Lazarus HM, Wolff SN, et al: High-dose cytosine arabinoside therapy with and without anthracycline antibiotics for remission reinduction of acute nonlymphoblastic leukemia. J Clin Oncol 1985;3:992–997.

104. Wolff SN, Herzig RH, Fay JW, et al: High-dose cytarabine and daunorubicin as consolidation therapy for acute myeloid leukemia in first remission: Long-term follow-up and results. J Clin Oncol 1989;7:1260–1267.

105. Phillips GL, Reece DE, Shepherd JD, et al: High-dose cytarabine and daunorubicin induction and postremission chemotherapy for the treatment of acute myelogenous leukemia in adults. Blood 1991;77:1429–1435.

106. Mayer RJ, Davis RB, Schiffer CA, et al: Intensive post-remission chemotherapy in adults with acute myeloid leukemia. N Engl J Med 1994;331:896–903.

107. Burnett AK, Goldstone AH, Stevens RM, et al: Randomised comparison of addition of autologous bone-marrow transplantation to intensive chemotherapy for acute myeloid leukaemia in first remission: Results of MRC AML 10 trial. UK Medical Research Council Adult and Children's Leukaemia Working Parties. Lancet 1998;351:700–708.

108. Rees JK, Gray RG, Wheatley K: Dose intensification in acute myeloid leukaemia: Greater effectiveness at lower cost. Principal report of the Medical Research Council's AML9 study. MRC Leukaemia in Adults Working Party. Br J Haematol 1996;94: 89–98.

109. Lowenberg B, Suciu S, Archimbaud E, et al: Mitoxantrone versus daunorubicin in induction-consolidation chemotherapy—The value of low-dose cytarabine for maintenance of remission, and an assessment of prognostic factors in acute myeloid leukemia in the elderly: final report. European Organization for the Research and Treatment of Cancer and the Dutch-Belgian Hemato-Oncology Cooperative Hovon Group. J Clin Oncol 1998;16:872–881.

110. Stewart P, Buckner CD, Bensinger W, et al: Autologous marrow transplantation in patients with acute nonlymphocytic leukemia in first remission. Exp Hematol 1985;13:267–272.

111. Löwenberg B, Abels J, Dirk W, et al: Transplantation of non-purified autologous bone marrow in patients with AML in first remission. Cancer 1984;54:2840–2843.

112. Burnett AK, Tansey P, Watkins R, et al: Transplantation of unpurged autologous bone-marrow in acute myeloid leukaemia in first remission. Lancet 1984;2:1068–1070.

113. Gorin NC, Labopin M, Fouillard L, et al: Retrospective evaluation of autologous bone marrow transplantation vs allogeneic bone marrow transplantation from an HLA identical related donor in acute myelocytic leukemia. Bone Marrow Transplant 1996;18: 111–117.

114. Harousseau J-L, Cahn J-Y, Pignon B, et al: Comparison of autologous bone marrow transplantation and intensive chemotherapy as postremission therapy in adult acute myeloid leukemia. Blood 1997;90:2978–2986.

115. Cassileth PA, Harrington DP, Appelbaum FR, et al: Chemotherapy compared with autologous or allogeneic bone marrow transplantation in the management of acute myeloid leukemia in first remission. N Engl J Med 1998;339:1649–1656.

116. Zittoun RA, Mandelli F, Willemze R, et al: Autologous or allogeneic bone marrow transplantation compared with intensive chemotherapy in acute myelogenous leukemia. N Engl J Med 1995;332:217–223.

117. Ringden O, Labopin M, Tura S, et al: A comparison of busulphan versus total body irradiation combined with cyclophosphamide as conditioning for autograft or allograft bone marrow transplantation in patients with acute leukaemia. Acute Leukaemia Working Party of the European Group for Blood and Marrow Transplantation (EBMT). Br J Haematol 1996;93:637–645.

118. Dusenbery KE, Daniels KA, McClure JS, et al: Randomized comparison of cyclophosphamide-total body irradiation versus busulfan-cyclophosphamide conditioning in autologous bone marrow transplantation for acute myeloid leukemia. Int J Radiat Oncol Biol Phys 1995;31:119–128.

119. Brenner MK, Rill DR, Moen RC, et al: Gene-marking to trace origin of relapse after autologous bone-marrow transplantation. Lancet 1993;341:85–86.

120. Gorin NC: Autologous stem cell transplantation in acute myelocytic leukemia [review]. Blood 1998;92:1073–1090.

121. Thomas ED, Buckner CD, Banaji M, et al: One hundred patients with acute leukemia treated by chemotherapy, total body irradiation, and allogeneic marrow transplantation. Blood 1977;49:511–533.

122. Fefer A, Thomas ED: Marrow transplantation in the treatment of leukemia. In Henderson ES, Lister TA. (eds): Leukemia, 5th ed. Philadelphia, WB Saunders, 1990, pp 431–441.

123. Thomas ED, Buckner CD, Clift RA, et al: Marrow transplantation for acute nonlymphoblastic leukemia in first remission. N Engl J Med 1979;301:597–599.

124. Blume KG, Beutler E, Bross KJ, et al: Bone-marrow ablation and allogeneic marrow transplantation in acute leukemia. N Engl J Med 1980;302:1041–1046.

125. Forman SJ, Spruce WE, Farbstein MJ, et al: Bone marrow ablation followed by allogeneic marrow grafting during first complete remission of acute nonlymphocytic leukemia. Blood 1983;61: 439–442.

126. Powles RL, Watson JG, Morgenstern GR, et al: Bone-marrow transplantation in leukaemia remission. Lancet 1982;1:336–337.

127. Appelbaum FR, Dahlberg S, Thomas ED, et al: Bone marrow transplantation or chemotherapy after remission induction for adults with acute nonlymphoblastic leukemia—A prospective comparison. Ann Intern Med 1984;101:581–588.

128. Champlin RE, Ho WG, Gale RP, et al: Treatment of acute myelogenous leukemia. A prospective controlled trial of bone marrow transplantation versus consolidation chemotherapy. Ann Intern Med 1985;102:285–291.

129. Marmont A, Bacigalupo A, Van Lint MT, et al: Bone marrow transplantation versus chemotherapy alone for acute nonlymphoblastic leukemia. Exp Hematol 1985;13:40.

130. Blaise D, Maraninchi D, Archimbaud E, et al: Allogeneic bone marrow transplantation for acute myeloid leukemia in first remission: A randomized trial of a busulfan-cytoxan versus cytoxan-total body irradiation as preparative regimen: A report from the Groupe d'Etudes de la Greffe de Moelle Osseuse. Blood 1992;79:2578–2582.

131. Bensinger WI, Martin PJ, Storer B, et al: Transplantation of bone marrow as compared with peripheral-blood cells from HLA-identical relatives in patients with hematologic cancers. N Engl J Med 2001;344:175–181.

132. Schmitz N, Beksac M, Hasenclever D, et al: Transplantation of mobilized peripheral blood cells to HLA-identical siblings with standard-risk leukemia. Blood 2002;100:761–767.

133. Couban S, Simpson DR, Barnett MJ, et al: A randomized multicenter comparison of bone marrow and peripheral blood in recipients of matched sibling allogeneic transplants for myeloid malignancies. Blood 2002;100:1525–1531.

134. Papadopoulos EB, Carabasi MH, Castro-Malaspina H, et al: T-cell-depleted allogeneic bone marrow transplantation as postremission therapy for acute myelogenous leukemia: Freedom from relapse in the absence of graft-versus-host disease. Blood 1998;91:1083–1090.

135. O'Donnell MR, Appelbaum FR, Baer MR, et al: NCCN practice guidelines for acute myelogenous leukemia. Oncology NCCN Proc 2000;14:53–61.

136. McSweeney PA, Niederwieser D, Shizuru JA, et al: Hematopoietic cell transplantation in older patients with hematologic malignancies: Replacing high-dose cytotoxic therapy with graft-versus-tumor effects. Blood 2001;97:3390–3400.

137. Appelbaum FR: Who should be transplanted for AML? [editorial]. Leukemia 2001;15:680–682.

138. Appelbaum FR: Hematopoietic cell transplantation beyond first remission [keynote Address]. Leukemia 2002;16:157–159.

139. Rees JK, Gray RG, Swirsky D, et al: Principal results of the Medical Research Council's 8th acute myeloid leukaemia trial. Lancet 1986;2:1236–1241.

140. Keating MJ, Kantarjian H, Smith TL, et al: Response to salvage therapy and survival after relapse in acute myelogenous leukemia. J Clin Oncol 1989;7:1071–1080.

141. Thalhammer F, Geissler K, Jager U, et al: Duration of second complete remission in patients with acute myeloid leukemia treated with chemotherapy: A retrospective single-center study. Ann Hematol 1996;72:216–222.

142. Hiddemann W, Martin WR, Sauerland CM, et al: Definition of refractoriness against conventional chemotherapy in acute myeloid leukemia: A proposal based on the results of retreatment by thioguanine, cytosine arabinoside, and daunorubicin (TAD 9) in 150 patients with relapse after standardized first line therapy. Leukemia 1990;4:184–188.

143. Davis CL, Rohatiner AZ, Lim J, et al: The management of recurrent acute myelogenous leukaemia at a single centre over a fifteen-year period. Br J Haematol 1993;83:404–411.

144. Vogler WR: High-dose carboplatin in the treatment of hematologic malignancies. Oncology 1993;50:42–46.

145. Karanes C, Kopecky KJ, Grever MR, et al: A phase III comparison of high dose ARA-C (HIDAC) versus HIDAC plus mitoxantrone in the treatment of first relapsed or refractory acute myeloid leukemia. Southwest Oncology Group Study. Leuk Res 1999;23:787–794.

146. List AF, Kopecky KJ, Willman CL, et al: Benefit of cyclosporine modulation of drug resistance in patients with poor-risk acute myeloid leukemia: A Southwest Oncology Group study. Blood 2001;98:3212–3220.

147. Sievers EL, Appelbaum FR, Spielberger RT, et al: Selective ablation of acute myeloid leukemia using antibody-targeted chemotherapy: A phase I study of an anti-CD33 calicheamicin immunoconjugate. Blood 1999;93:3678–3684.

148. Sievers EL, Larson RA, Stadmauer EA, et al: Efficacy and safety of gemtuzumab ozogamicin in patients with CD33-positive acute myeloid leukemia in first relapse. J Clin Oncol 2001;19:3244–3254.

149. Appelbaum FR, Clift RA, Buckner CD, et al: Allogeneic marrow transplantation for acute nonlymphoblastic leukemia after first relapse. Blood 1983;61:949–953.

150. Clift RA, Buckner CD, Appelbaum FR, et al: Allogeneic marrow transplantation during untreated first relapse of acute myeloid leukemia. J Clin Oncol 1992;10:1723–1729.

151. Schiffman K, Clift R, Appelbaum FR, et al: Consequences of cryopreserving first remission autologous marrow for use after relapse in patients with acute myeloid leukemia. Bone Marrow Transplant 1993;11:227–232.

152. Reiffers J: HLA-identical sibling hematopoietic stem cell transplantation for acute myeloid leukemia. In Atkinson K. (ed): Clinical Bone Marrow and Blood Stem Cell Transplantation, 2nd ed. Cambridge, Cambridge University Press, 2000, pp 433–445.

153. Ringden O, Labopin M, Gluckman E, et al: Donor search or autografting in patients with acute leukaemia who lack an HLA-identical sibling? A matched-pair analysis. Bone Marrow Transplant 1997;19:963–968.

154. Clift RA, Buckner CD, Thomas ED, et al: The treatment of acute non-lymphoblastic leukemia by allogeneic marrow transplantation. Bone Marrow Transplant 1987;2:243–258.

155. Avvisati G: Event free survival (EFS) duration in newly diagnosed acute promyelocytic leukemia (APL) is favorably influenced by induction treatment with idarubicin alone: Final results of the Gimema randomized study "LAP0389" comparing IDA vs IDA + ARA-C in newly diagnosed APL [abstract]. Blood 1999;94(Part 1):505a.

156. Head D, Kopecky KJ, Weick J, et al: Effect of aggressive daunomycin therapy on survival in acute promyelocytic leukemia. Blood 1995;86:1717–1728.

157. Huang ME, Ye YC, Chen SR, et al: Use of all-trans retinoic acid in the treatment of acute promyelocytic leukemia. Blood 1988;72:567–572.

158. Tallman MS, Anderson JW, Schiffer CA, et al: All-trans-retinoic acid in acute promyelocytic leukemia. N Engl J Med 1997;337:1021–1028.

159. Fenaux P, Chastang C, Chevret S, et al: A randomized comparison of all transretinoic acid (ATRA) followed by chemotherapy and ATRA plus chemotherapy and the role of maintenance therapy in newly diagnosed acute promyelocytic leukemia. The European APL Group. Blood 1999;94:1192–1200.

160. Sanz MA, Martin G, Rayon C, et al: A modified AIDA protocol with anthracycline-based consolidation results in high antileukemic efficacy and reduced toxicity in newly diagnosed PML/RARalpha-positive acute promyelocytic leukemia. PETHEMA group. Blood 1999;94:3015–3021.

161. Tallman MS, Andersen JW, Schiffer CA, et al: All-*trans* retinoic acid in acute promyelocytic leukemia: Long-term outcome and prognostic factor analysis from the North American Intergroup protocol. Blood 2002;100:4298–4302.

162. Tallman MS, Nabhan C, Feusner JH, et al: Acute promyelocytic leukemia: Evolving therapeutic strategies. Blood 2002;99:759–767.

163. Shen ZX, Chen GQ, Ni JH, et al: Use of arsenic trioxide (As2O3) in the treatment of acute promyelocytic leukemia (APL): II. Clinical efficacy and pharmacokinetics in relapsed patients. Blood 1997;89:3354–3360.

164. Niu C, Yan H, Yu T, et al: Studies on treatment of acute promyelocytic leukemia with arsenic trioxide: Remission induction, follow-up, and molecular monitoring in 11 newly diagnosed and 47 relapsed acute promyelocytic leukemia patients. Blood 1999;94:3315–3324.

165. Soignet SL, Frankel SR, Douer D, et al: United States multicenter study of arsenic trioxide in relapsed acute promyelocytic leukemia. J Clin Oncol 2001;19:3852–3860.

166. Unnikrishnan D, Dutcher JP, Varshneya N, et al: Torsades de pointes in 3 patients with leukemia treated with arsenic trioxide. Blood 2001;97:1514–1516.

167. Westervelt P, Brown RA, Adkins DR, et al: Sudden death among patients with acute promyelocytic leukemia treated with arsenic trioxide. Blood 2001;98:266–271.

168. Sanz MA, Arcese W, de la Rubia J, et al: Stem cell transplantation (SCT) for acute promyelocytic leukemia (APL) in the atra era: A survey of the European Blood and Marrow Transplantation Group (EBMT) [abstract]. Blood 2000;96(Part 1):522a.

169. Meloni G, Diverio D, Vignetti M, et al: Autologous bone marrow transplantation for acute promyelocytic leukemia in second remission: Prognostic relevance of pretransplant minimal residual disease assessment by reverse-transcription polymerase chain reaction of the PML/RAR alpha fusion gene. Blood 1997;90:1321–1325.

170. Frankel SR, Eardley A, Heller G, et al: All-trans retinoic acid for acute promyelocytic leukemia. Results of the New York Study. Ann Intern Med 1994;120:278–286.

171. Appelbaum FR: Molecular diagnosis and clinical decisions in adult acute leukemia. Semin Hematol 1999;36:401–410.

172. Diverio D, Rossi V, Avvisati G, et al: Early detection of relapse by prospective reverse transcriptase-polymerase chain reaction analysis of the PML/RARalpha fusion gene in patients with acute promyelocytic leukemia enrolled in the GIMEMA-AIEOP multicenter "AIDA" trial. GIMEMA-AIEOP Multicenter "AIDA" Trial. Blood 1998;92:784–789.

173. Gallagher RE, Yeap BY, Bi W, et al: Quantitative real-time RT-PCR analysis of PML-RARa mRNA levels in acute promyelocytic leukemia: Assessment of prognostic significance in adult patients from intergroup protocol 0129. Blood 2003;101:2521–2528.

174. Miyamoto T, Nagafuji K, Akashi K, et al: Persistence of multipotent progenitors expressing AML1/ETO transcripts in long-term remission patients with t(8;21) acute myelogenous leukemia. Blood 1996;87:4789–4796.

175. Sievers EL, Radich JP: Detection of minimal residual disease in acute leukemia. Curr Opin Hematol 2000;7:212–216.

Specific Malignancies

III

176. San Miguel JF, Vidriales MB, Lopez-Berges C, et al: Early immunophenotypical evaluation of minimal residual disease in acute myeloid leukemia identifies different patient risk groups and may contribute to postinduction treatment stratification. Blood 2001;98:1746–1751.

177. De Angelo DJ, Schiffer C, Stone R, et al: Interim analysis of a phase II study of the safety and efficacy of gemtuzumab ozogamicin (Mylotarg®) given in combination with cytarabine and daunorubicin in patients <60 years old with untreated acute myeloid leukemia [abstract]. Blood 2002;100(Part 1): 198a–199a.

178. Kell JW, Burnett AK, Chopra R, et al: Mylotarg (gemtuzumab ozogomycin: GO) given simultaneously with intensive induction and/or consolidation therapy for AML is feasible and may improve the response rate [abstract]. Blood 2002;100(Part 1):199a.

179. Pagel JM, Matthews DC, Appelbaum FR, et al: The use of radioimmunoconjugates in stem cell transplantation [mini-review]. Bone Marrow Transplant 2002;29:807–816.

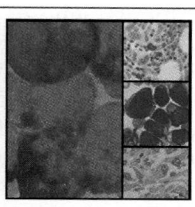

05

THE MYELODYSPLASTIC SYNDROMES

John M. Bennett

Rami Komrokji

Peter A. Kouides

SUMMARY OF KEY POINTS

ETIOLOGY

- Myelodsyplastic syndromes are not true dysplastic disorders but rather are clonal disorders of hematopoiesis with site of transformation at a pluripotent stem cell or early myeloid progenitor cell.
- 50%–90% of cases associated with chromosomal abnormalities are often in proximity to oncogenes—partial deletion of the long arm of chromosome 5 (5q-) and the *fms* gene, monosmy 7 (7-) and the *met* oncogene—and hematopoietic growth factor genes [5q- and genes for granulocyte-macrophage colony-stimulating factor (GM-CSF), interleukin-3 (IL-3), IL-5, macrophage colony-stimulating factor (M-CSF); 7- and erythropoietin gene].
- These resultant genetic alterations can manifest by increased apoptosis, which explains the seemingly opposing findings of marrow hypercellularity but peripheral blood cytopenia in patients with myelodysplastic syndrome (MDS).

EPIDEMIOLOGY

- The therapy-related subset of MDS is secondary to prior use of alkylating agents (typically associated with monosomy 7 and 5q-), with an increasing number of cases secondary to prior use of DNA-topoisomerase II targeting agents (epipodophyllotoxins), which are typically associated with translocation involving band 11q23 or band 21q22.
- Chronic exposure to benzene (above the level set by national guidelines) is the most important environmental exposure risk.

PATHOLOGY

- The new WHO classification is a revision of the FAB system and recognizes the following subtypes: refractory anemia (RA), refractory anemia with ring sideroblasts (RARS), refractory cytopenia with multilineage dysplasia (RCMD), refractory cytopenia with multilineage dysplasia and ring sideroblasts (RCMD-RS), refractory anemia with excess blasts type I and II (RAEB I and II), 5 q syndrome, and unclassified MDS. Refractory anemia with excess blasts in transformation was eliminated from the WHO classification. Chronic myelomonocytic leukemia (CMML) has been reclassified into a new separate category as myelodysplastic/myeloproliferative disorders, along with juvenile myelomonocytic leukemia (JMML) and atypical chronic myelogenous leukemia (aCML).

INCIDENCE

- About four per 100,000 population; primarily a disease of the elderly.
- Twenty per 100,000 over the age of 70, with only 10%–20% of patients under age 60, though patients in the therapy-related subset are 10 to 20 years younger.

DIFFERENTIAL DIAGNOSIS

- MDS is often a diagnosis of exclusion after ruling out other disorders associated with cytopenia and hematopoietic dysplasia: vitamin B_{12} and/or folate deficiency, recent cytotoxic therapy, heavy-metal intoxication, chronic liver disease, and chronic inflammation, which includes human immunodeficiency virus (HIV) infection.

PROGNOSIS

- Using the International Prognostic Scoring System, patients can be categorized into distinctive sub-groups with respect to both median survival and the risk for the respective subgroup to undergo acute leukemic transformation based on four variables—age, percentage of bone marrow blasts, number and/or type of chromosomal abnormalities, and degree of cytopenia.

PRIMARY THERAPY

- Usually a "wait and watch" approach is followed, given the poor risk/benefit ratio of intensive (acute myelogenous leukemia [AML] type) chemotherapy for the majority of patients over 60 years of age, though intensive chemotherapy at the time of blast progression is appropriate and might benefit up to half of patients, albeit transiently. A minority of patients (those under age 55 years) might be long-term survivors if they undergo allogeneic bone marrow transplantation. The nonmyeloablative "minitransplant" procedure could increase the upper age limit of transplant in the future.
- Erythropoeitin could reduce requirements for blood transfusion, its efficacy might be augmented by cotreatment with G-CSF.

EFFECTIVE SECOND- OR THIRD-LINE THERAPIES

- No consistently effective therapies are available, but one-quarter to one-third of patients respond to agents such as 5-azacytidine, decitabine, thalidomide, amifostine, low dose ara-c, and topotecan. The use of novel targeted therapies for MDS is in various phases of clinical trials.

INTRODUCTION

For decades, the myelodysplastic syndromes (MDS) have been a most challenging set of diseases for hematologists and oncologists in terms of diagnosis and management.[1-7] The definition of MDS also has two parts, as it is essentially a clinical-pathologic description. MDS can be defined as a clonal disease of the bone marrow with the following:

- The clinical manifestation of bone marrow failure together with a tendency to transform into an acute leukemic phase
- The pathologic manifestation of morphologic abnormalities (termed *dysplasia* although MDS is a clonal disorder and thus neoplastic) of the peripheral blood and bone marrow cells, such as ringed sideroblasts, megaloblastic erythroid precursors, hypogranulation/hyposegmentation of the granulocytes, and micromegakaryocytes.[1,2,8]

The foregoing description serves as a clinical-pathologic definition of MDS; the pathologic manifestation reminds the reader that for lack of a dependable "gold standard" (i.e., a reproducible marker of clonality), the diagnosis of MDS is based on the detection of abnormal hematopoietic cell morphology after excluding other conditions that cause cytopenias with blood-cell dysplasia. The clinical description reminds the reader that the typical presentation is one of anemia with or without thrombocytopenia and/or neutropenia. The correlation of the biology of this clonal disorder with its clinical presentation of cytopenias is extremely varied, ranging from an incidental mild anemia that has been stable for over a decade to a rapidly evolving leukemia that becomes fatal within weeks. It is not surprising, then, that this disease has defied proper classification over the years. The medical literature is replete with many descriptive terms prior to the widespread use of the term *MDS*: herald state of leukemia, refractory anemia, preleukemic anemia, preleukemic syndrome, preleukemia, refractory anemia with ringed sideroblasts, refractory normoblastic anemia, refractory anemia with excess myeloblasts, smoldering acute leukemia, chronic erythemic myelosis, subacute myelomonocytic leukemia, hypoplastic acute myelogenous leukemia, hematopoietic dysplasia, subacute myeloid leukemia, for example.[8]

Recognition of this disease began early in the 20th century, when reports described anemia that was refractory to treatment.[9] In 1938, an analysis of 100 cases of refractory anemia was published.[10] In 1949, Hamilton-Paterson[11] applied the term *preleukemia anemia*. In 1956, Block and coworkers[12] expanded the definition of the disease to include multilineage cytopenias, reporting 12 cases with refractory cytopenias that evolved into acute leukemia. In 1973, based on their review, Saarni and Linman[13] suggested that preleukemic anemia is a primary bone marrow disease characterized by peripheral cytopenias, marrow hypercellularity, disordered precursor maturation, and ultimate transformation to acute myeloid leukemia (AML). The first series of patients described in the literature included mostly patients whose disease courses culminated in AML. In general, however, only 20%–30% of all patients with MDS progress to overt, acute leukemia.[14-20] In 1975, the French-American-British (FAB) group, in their initial proposals for the morphologic classification of the acute leukemias, acknowledged that not all patients with MDS progress to acute leukemia.[21] A distinction was made between acute leukemia, with its rapid onset of signs and symptoms requiring immediate treatment, and a group of disorders that showed some of the characteristics of AML but were subacute or chronic in nature. The FAB group chose the term *dysmyelopoietic* or *myelodysplastic syndromes* for this group of disorders; unlike AML, this group of disorders rarely required immediate treatment, and affected patients were typically 65 years of age or older.[21] Initially, the FAB group recognized two categories of MDS: refractory anemia with excess blasts (RAEB) and chronic myelomonocytic leukemia (CMML). It was noted that a variable progression of these cases evolved to overt acute leukemia associated with an increase in blasts to approximately greater than 30%. In 1980, a larger number of cases were reviewed with the intent to determine whether specific morphologic abnormalities, singly or in groups, would predict for a different biologic outcome. This larger review of cases led to an expanded definition of the myelodysplastic syndromes into five subgroups with dysplastic features in common.[22] The subgroups were refractory anemia (RA), refractory anemia with ring sideroblasts (RARS), refractory anemia with excess blasts (RAEB), refractory anemia with excess blasts in transformation (RAEB-T), and chronic myelomonocytic leukemia CMML). The need to predict the risk of transformation to AML and the overall survival of patients with MDS led to the development of the International Prognostic Scoring System (IPSS) for MDS, which uses percentage of marrow blasts, number of cytopenias, and cytogenetics as the main prognostic features.[23] The worldwide experience applying the FAB classification and the IPSS showed that FAB subgroups are heterogeneous and overlap in predicting the survival of patients with MDS and estimating the rate of progression to AML. To better understand the disease and be able to assign patients to homogeneous subgroups with similar behavior and outcome, a distinguished panel of hematologists and hematopathologists under the auspices of WHO recently issued the new WHO MDS classification system.[24] It is hoped that the WHO classification system will be used in conjunction with the IPSS, thus improving the identification, clinicopathological correlation, and ultimately, the treatment of patients with MDS.

INCIDENCE

The best studies on incidence to date are from Europe.[25-27] The overall incidence of MDS is approximately three to four persons out of 100,000 annually; the incidence rises to approximately 20 of 100,000 annually over the age of 70 years. Only 10%–20% of patients with MDS are under the age of 60 years.[26] There also appears to be a slight male preponderance. Unfortunately, incidence has not been established in the United States. In general, the overall incidence of MDS appears to be increasing over the past decade.[28] It is estimated that for every known case of MDS, there are perhaps two other asymptomatic cases that remain undiagnosed.[29]

ETIOLOGY AND EPIDEMIOLOGY

Though we use the term *dysplasia* in describing the morphologic abnormalities of MDS, it must be emphasized that the underlying process is neoplastic, not dysplastic in the strict sense of the term. This was first suggested by Dacie,[30] who noted a dimorphic population of red cells consistent with a clonal disorder. Evidence of clonality is supported by studies of glucose-6-phosphate dehydrogenase mosaicism and by cytogenetic studies that have demonstrated an abnormal karyotype in the dysplastic cells coexisting with residual marrow cells that have a normal karyotype.[31,32] The abnormal clone of MDS might arise from a pluripotent stem cell that is capable of both myeloid and lymphoid differentiation.[33-35] Several studies have demonstrated clonality in the lymphoid lineage by cytogenetics, oncogene analysis, or analysis of X-linked restriction fragment length polymorphisms (RFLPs).[36-38] Yet, other studies suggest that the origin of the transformed clone could be derived at a committed myeloid progenitor cell rather than at a less committed stem cell. All of these studies might be consistent with the hypothesis that MDS involves a pluripotent stem cell with preferential myeloid commitment.

The development of a clonal population of hematopoietic cells that characterizes MDS can be viewed within the framework of the multi-hit theory of carcinogenesis, "one cell, multiple hits."[39,40] The fact that MDS is rare among patients under 50 years of age is consistent with this theory, given the increased probability over time of spontaneous genetic mutations and genetic "insults" from the environment. Epidemiologic studies of MDS and acute leukemia suggest many factors that could be the "first hit" or subsequent "hit."[41] These factors include genetic predisposition, immunologic, occupational or environmental exposure, and iatrogenic causes, each of which is briefly discussed here.

Genetic Predisposition

In adult-onset MDS, several familial cases of MDS have been reported.[42,43] In childhood-onset MDS, about one-third of pediatric patients with MDS had a constitutional genetic disorder such as Down syndrome, neurofibromatosis, Fanconi anemia, or Kostman's syndrome.[44]

Immunologic

The immune system is clearly impaired in MDS, with abnormalities of B cells, T cells, natural killer (NK) cells, and monocytes described.[45,46] It is unclear to what degree these abnormalities are a cause or effect of MDS.

Occupational/Environmental Exposure

It is well known that exposure to benzene is a risk factor for AML, which often is preceded by a pancytopenic phase with morphologic abnormalities consistent with MDS.[47] The risk is proportional to the cumulative exposure of benzene. Patients with primary MDS or de novo AML with an occupational exposure to chemical solvents, insecticides, or petroleum products can have the same nonrandomly occurring abnormalities of chromosomes 5 and 7 that are seen in chemotherapy-related MDS and AML.[48] Yet, the association of specific chemical mutagens other than benzene with the development of MDS or AML is not as well established, given conflicting case-controlled studies.[49] In the case of radiation exposure, low doses of ionizing radiation appear to be more leukemogenic than high doses.[50] Smoking was reported as a risk factor for MDS, with the degree of risk related to the duration and intensity of smoking.[51] A recent French case-control study suggested that agricultural workers, textile operators, health professionals, machine operators, and commercial and technical representatives were among the occupations with higher risk for MDS; other higher-risk factors included living next to an industrial plant, smoking, and lifetime exposure to oil.[52]

Iatrogenic (Therapy-related MDS)

Chemotherapy and (less so) radiotherapy have been associated with the risk of developing AML; the relative risk is 100- to 300-fold for chemotherapy and two- to tenfold for radiotherapy.[53-55] Among 560 patients examined with therapy-related MDS or leukemia, the primary disease was a solid tumor in 52%, hematologic malignancy in 47%, and nonmalignant disorders in 1.3%.[56]

Historically, the type of chemotherapy associated with iatrogenic MDS has been primarily alkylating agents (Table 105-1), ranging from mechlorethamine in the treatment of Hodgkin's disease (HD) to semustine in colon cancer.[55] The risk of developing therapy-related MDS/AML (t- MDS/AML) begins from the start of therapy, with a peak incidence at four years, and with the risk beginning to disappear after 10 years. The MDS phase usually precedes AML by six to 12 months.[55] The best-studied time frame of t-MDS/AML is among patients receiving the alkylating agents mechlorethamine and procarbazine as part of MOPP (mechlorethamine, oncovin {vincristine}, prednisone, and procarbazine) in Hodgkin's disease. The risk is 0.5%–2.2% per year, with a cumulative incidence of 3.3%–10% at 10 years.[57] It is not surprising, given the previously mentioned multi-hit theory of carcinogenesis, that the risk in general is proportional to the patient's age and cumulative dose.[55]

The underlying disease necessitating the use of the alkylating agent does not appear to be a risk factor for developing t-MDS/AML.[50] Within Hodgkin's disease, however, there could be a higher risk among splenectomized patients, particularly those over the age of 40 years.[58] The specific alkylating agent does not appear to be important except for cyclophosphamide, which

TABLE 105-1

Alkylating Agents as Leukemogens in Various Diseases

ALKYLATING AGENT	HD	NHL	MM	PV	BC	GI	OC	LC
Busulfan								x
Carmustine	x		x					
Chlorambucil	x			x	x		x	
Cyclophosphamide	x	x	x				x	x
Dihydroxybusulfan							x	
Lomustine	x		x					x
Mechlorethamine	x							
Melphalan			x		x		x	
Semustine						x		

BC, breast cancer; GI, gastrointestinal cancer; HD, Hodgkin's disease; LC, lung cancer; MM, multiple myeloma; NHL, non-Hodgkin's lymphoma; OC, ovarian cancer; PV, polycythemia.
Adapted from Pedersen-Bjergaard J: Radiotherapy- and chemotherapy-induced myelodysplasia and acute myeloid leukemia. A review. Leuk Res 1992;16:61.

appears to be less leukemogenic than melphalan.[59] Other factors potentially increasing the risk of t-MDS include the schedule of administration of the alkylating agent, the addition of radiotherapy to alkylating agent therapy, and the use of more than one alkylating agent.[55] None of these factors has been shown to increase the incidence of t-MDS/AML unequivocally except for the use of multiple alkylating agents, which probably is due to an additive effect (increased cumulative dose) rather than a synergistic effect.[55] Therapy-related MDS is being increasingly reported after autologous bone marrow transplantation, but this could reflect primarily prior exposure to alkylating agents and not primarily the conditioning regimen itself.[60-62]

In the past decade, another class of chemotherapeutic agents has emerged as clearly leukemogenic, the epipodophyllotoxins—etoposide and teniposide.[63-65] The risk of t-MDS/AML after a high cumulative dose appears to be in the 5% range, within five years of treatment. Treatment with the epipodophyllotoxins has included either cisplatinum or alkylating agents. The direct damage of DNA by cisplatinum and/or the alkylators is probably coupled with the indirect effect on DNA by epipodophyllotoxin stimulation of DNA-topoisomerase II.[63,64]

Several pertinent differences exist between the class of agents targeting topoisomerase II and the class of alkylating agents (Table 105-2).[65,66] These patients usually present with overt leukemia without a preceding MDS phase. The latency period is shorter (less than 5 years). The morphology can usually be classified by a FAB subtype (M3 with the dioxopiperazines, M4 or M5 with the epipodophyllotoxins). The latency period of development to AML is shorter. The cytogenetic aberration is typically balanced as opposed to an unbalanced aberration involving chromosome 5 or 7 in alkylating agent–induced MDS/AML. The balanced aberration in the case of the epipodophyllotoxins is typically a translocation involving either band 11q23 or band 21q22.[66,67] The schedule of administration could be critical. Weekly or biweekly epipodophyllotoxin therapy markedly increases the risk of MDS/AML.[65] Finally, the complete remission

rate is higher after intensive chemotherapy for epipodophyllotoxin-induced MDS/AML[66] but, not surprisingly, long-term disease control is poor.[63]

Radiolabeled monoclonal antibodies are probably not leukemogenic. In a review of 773 patients from seven tositumomab (Bexxar, anti CD 20 conjugated with iodine 131) studies of low-grade non–Hodgkin's lymphoma (NHL), the overall incidence of MDS was similar to those reported from pre-Bexxar chemotherapy and radiotherapy t-MDS/leukemia rates in low-grade NHL. No t-MDS/leukemia was reported among previously untreated patients who received Bexxar as first-line treatment.[68] Long-term follow-up is warranted to verify the effect of these antibodies on bone marrow.

It is not yet clear whether it is possible to identify patients at higher risk for t-MDS/leukemia. Some data suggest that certain coexisting gene mutations increase the susceptibility to develop MDS. NQO1 gene mutation (NQO1 is a quinone oxireductase required for detoxifying benzene derivatives) increases the risk for t-MDS in both the homozygotic and heterozygotic states. Other described gene mutations include mutations in CYP3a, P53, and MDR genes.[69,70]

TABLE 105-2

Two Classes of Therapy-related MDS/AML

	CLASS I	CLASS II
Type of leukemogen	Alkylating agent	Topoisomerase II targeting agent
Age	Older	Younger
Classifiable by FAB	No	Yes
Cytogenetics	Unbalanced aberration	Balanced aberration
MDS phase	Yes	No
Response to therapy	CR ±	CR likely

AML, acute myeloid leukemia; CR, complete response; FAB, French-American-British; MDS, myelodysplastic syndrome.

Pathogenesis Model

The numerous epidemiologic factors just discussed can be viewed as genetic "hits" that invariably trigger cellular oncogenes, suppressor genes, and/or genes that normally encode hematopoietic growth factors and receptors. These alterations appear to be manifest in part by extensive apoptosis in the marrow of patients with MDS.[71] Raza/Preisler and colleagues[72-74] have carried out cell kinetic studies from MDS bone marrow biopsies using intravenous infusions of either iododeoxyuridine or bromodeoxyuridine or both and estimating the degree of apoptosis by in situ end-labeling of DNA.[73,74] Virtually all marrows studied demonstrated both apoptosis and rapid cell proliferation. Whether apoptosis is this extensive in all cases of MDS and whether it is specific for MDS and no other marrow disease is unclear at this time.[75,76] Nonetheless, the observation of increased apoptosis nicely explains the seemingly opposing findings of marrow hypercellularity but peripheral blood pancytopenia in patients with MDS.[77] Intuitively, this would appear to be related to levels of apoptosis-related oncogene products such as c-*myc*, which enhances apoptosis, and *bcl*-2, which diminishes apoptosis, as suggested by a study by Rajapaksa and associates.[78] The proportion of CD34 cells with apoptosis was higher in the early stages of MDS than in advanced MDS, AML, or normal individuals.[78] The oncoprotein ratio c-*myc*/ *BCL2* was higher in RA than RAEB or AML, indicating that apoptosis decreases as MDS progress to AML. Interestingly, in the Rajapaksa study,[78] patients treated with erythropoietin and granulocyte colony-stimulating factor (G-CSF) had reduced apoptosis

within CD34+ marrow cells. The neoplastic MDS clone is recognized by T-cells, probably due to changed antigenic representation leading to clonal T-cell expansion. Cytotoxic T-cells, as in aplastic anemia, suppress bone marrow production—an effect seen more on the normal stem cells than on the clonal MDS cells, leading to preferential proliferation of the abnormal clone.[79-83] The proliferating MDS clone is susceptible to increased apoptosis, due not only to the aforementioned intrinsic changes of DNA damage but also to the production of aberrant cytokines, the altered microenvironment, and interaction with the stromal cells. Chronic immunosuppression and other factors cause release of cytokines such as tumor necrosis factor-α (TNF-α), transforming growth factor-β (TGF-β), and interleukin-1 β–converting enzyme, all of which are elevated in patients with MDS.[84-87] These cytokines might exert a dual effect of stimulating proliferation of the early CD34+ MDS progenitors while inducing apoptosis in their progeny.[74,87] Neovascularization of the bone marrow is increased and could contribute to the progression to AML.[88,89] The exact mechanism by which transformation to AML occurs is not known. Figure 105-1 summarizes the pathogenesis module in MDS.

PATHOLOGY/CLASSIFICATION

The FAB classification system for AML and MDS served as the standard classification system for more than 20 years. The FAB classification system has recently been revised under the WHO Classification for Leukemias and Lymphomas, which represents the culmination of a three-

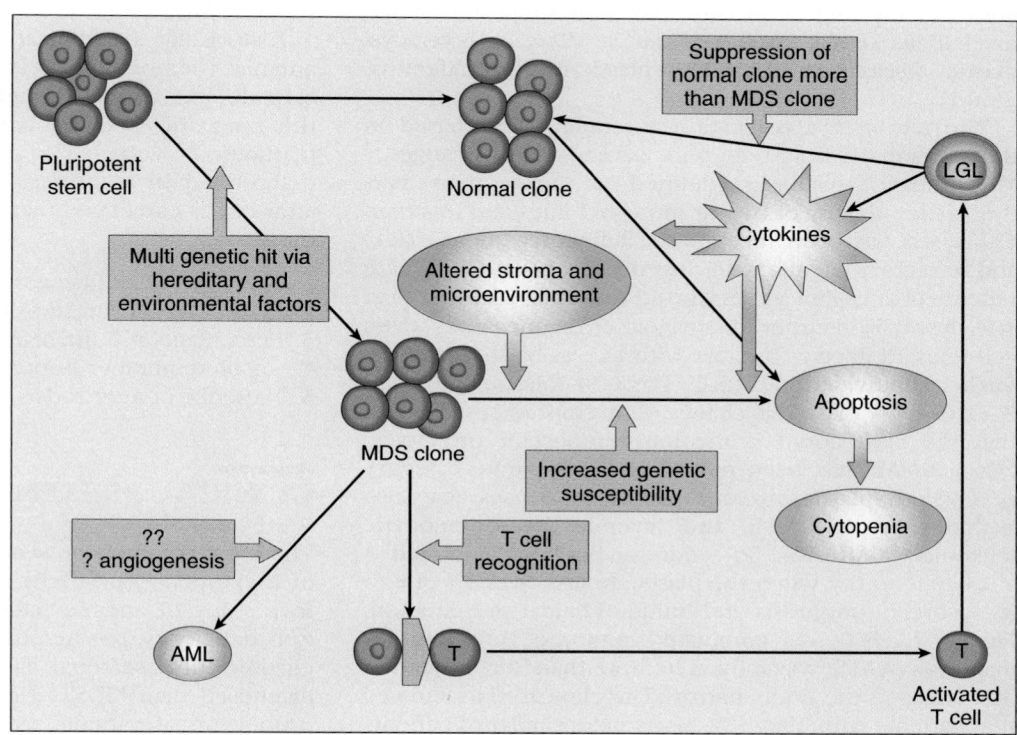

Figure 105-1. Pathogenesis model of MDS.

TABLE 105-3

The WHO Classification of MDS

CATEGORY	MDS CASES (%)	PERIPHERAL BLOOD	BONE MARROW	CYTOGENETICS ABNORMALITIES DETECTED (%)	RATE OF PROGRESSION TO AML (%)
Refractory anemia (RA)	5–10	Anemia <1% blasts <1×10^9 monocytes	Erythroid dysplasia <10% myeloid or megakaryocytic dysplasia <5% blasts <15% sideroblasts	25	6
Refractory anemia with ring sideroblasts (RARS)	10–15	Anemia <1% blasts <1×10^9 monocytes	Erythroid dysplasia <10% myeloid or megakaryocytic dysplasia <5% blasts >15% sideroblasts	10	1–2
Refractory cytopenia with multilineage dysplasia (RCMD)	24	Bi- or pancytopenia <1% blasts <1×10^9 monocytes	Dysplasia in >10% of the cells in 2 or more cell lines <5% blasts in BM <15% sideroblasts	50	11
Refractory anemia with multilineage dysplasia and ring sideroblasts (RCMD-RS)	15	Bi- or pancytopenia <1% blasts <1×10^9 monocytes	Dysplasia in >10% of the cells in 2 or more cell lines <5% blasts in BM >15% sideroblasts	50	11
Refractory anemia with excess blasts type I and II (RAEB-1 & RAEB-II)	40	Cytopenia Type I: 1–5% blasts Type II: 5–19% blasts	Uni or multilineage dysplasia Type I 5–9% blasts Type II 10–19% blasts	30–50	RAEB I 25 RAEB II 33
5q- syndrome	?	Anemia Normal or elevated platelets <5% blasts	Normal or increased megakaryocytes <5% blasts	Deletion between bands q31 and 33 on chromosome 5	Uncommon
MDS unclassified (MDS-U)	?	Cytopenia <1% blasts	Unilineage dyplasia of myeloid or megakaryocytic line <5% blasts	No known cytogenetic abnormalities	Unknown

year effort by working committees worldwide.[90] The WHO classification system recognizes four broad categories of myeloid neoplasms and their subgroups: acute myeloid leukemia, myeloproliferative diseases, myelodysplastic diseases, and myelodysplastic/myeloproliferative group.

The new WHO classification system for MDS is based on the previous FAB system, with several major changes.[24] Multilineage dysplasia (defined as more than 10% dysplastic progeny of two or more cell lines and less than 5% blasts) has been recognized. Refractory anemia (RA) and refractory anemia with ringed sideroblasts (RARS) are redefined as unilineage erythroid dysplasia and less than 10% dysplasia in either the myeloid or the megakaryocytic cell lines. Refractory anemia with excess blasts (RAEB) is further subdivided into RAEB I (5%–9% blasts) and RAEB II (10%–19% blasts), a change that emphasizes the fact that the blast count is the most important prognostic factor. CMML has been moved into a separate category of myelodysplastic/myeloproliferative diseases that also includes atypical CML and juvenile myelomonocytic leukemia (JMML). The 5q- syndrome has been identified as a separate entity when the blasts are less than 5% due to its favorable prognosis and unique clinical presentation. Finally, RAEB-T was eliminated, and the threshold for diagnosis of AML was moved to more than 20% instead of 30% blasts in the bone marrow. The clinical trials showed that patients with 20%–30% blasts were similar to patients

with AML with regard to outcome and response to treatment.[91,92] Table 105-3 summarizes characteristics of the new MDS subgroups.

Historically, the clinical starting point for diagnosis is anemia (hemoglobin less than 11 g/dL) with a low reticulocyte count, though marked reticulocytosis in the range of 30% has been reported on the basis of maturational delay.[93] The actual subgroup of MDS can be determined by considering the following five features after one is convinced that there is an adequate degree of dysplasia:

1. Number of cell lineages involved with dysplasia
2. Percentage of ringed sideroblasts
3. Percentage of bone marrow blasts
4. Absolute number of peripheral blood monocytes
5. Presence of Auer rods

CLINICAL PRESENTATION

The most common presentation of MDS is the discovery of a cytopenia (primarily anemia) in an elderly patient. In a study of anemic patients in a geriatric ward, only iron deficiency, posthemorrhagic anemia, and anemia of chronic disease/renal failure were more commonly diagnosed than MDS.[94] Unlike the case with AML, a fair proportion of patients with MDS, though often anemic,

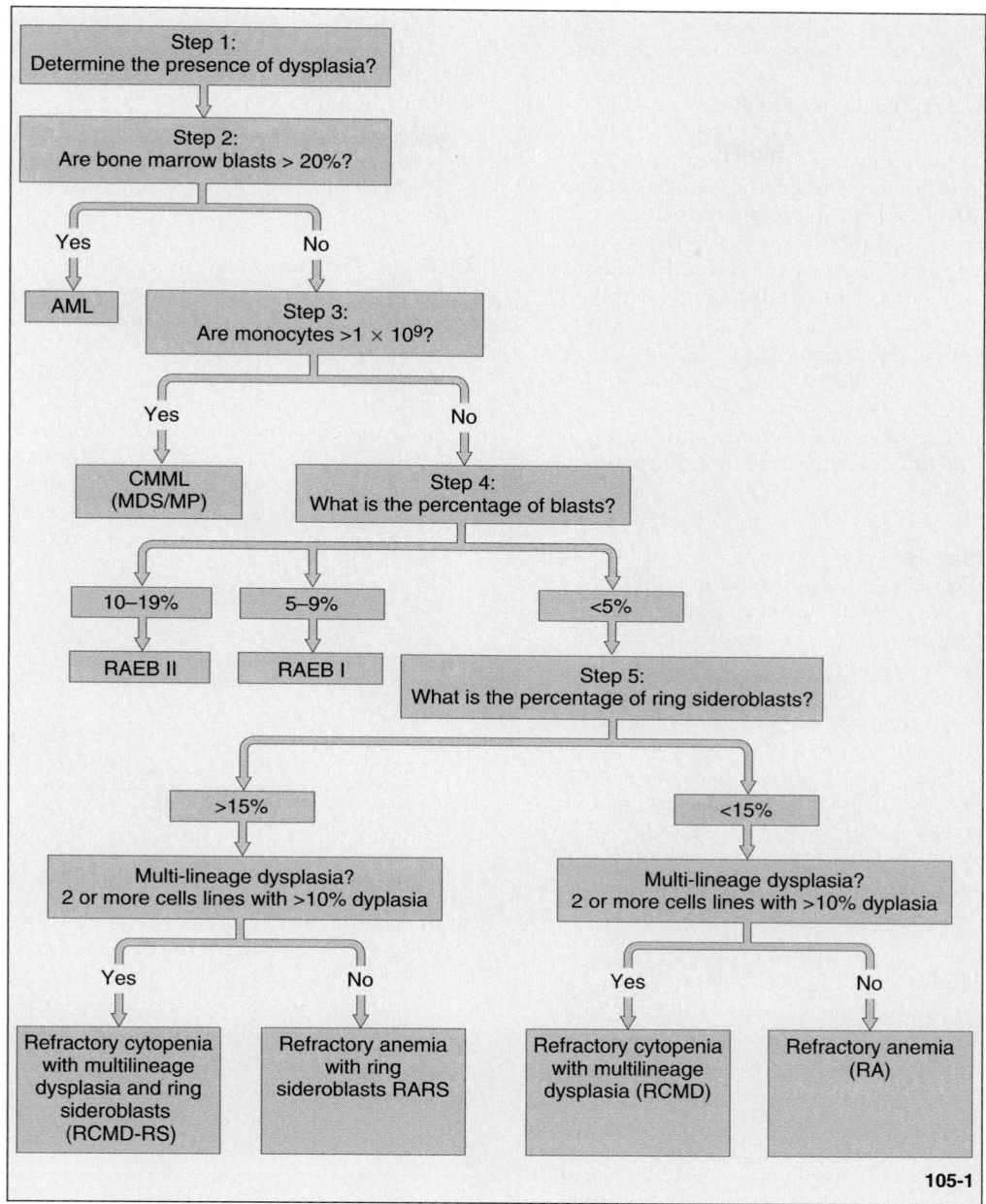

Step 1:
Determine the presence of dysplasia?

Step 2:
Are bone marrow blasts > 20%?

Yes → AML

No → **Step 3:**
Are monocytes >1 × 10⁹?

Yes → CMML (MDS/MP)

No → **Step 4:**
What is the percentage of blasts?

10–19% → RAEB II

5–9% → RAEB I

<5% → **Step 5:**
What is the percentage of ring sideroblasts?

>15% → Multi-lineage dysplasia? 2 or more cells lines with >10% dyplasia

Yes → Refractory cytopenia with multilineage dysplasia and ring sideroblasts (RCMD-RS)

No → Refractory anemia with ring sideroblasts RARS

<15% → Multi-lineage dysplasia? 2 or more cells lines with >10% dyplasia

Yes → Refractory cytopenia with multilineage dysplasia (RCMD)

No → Refractory anemia (RA)

105-1

are asymptomatic. A small proportion (10%) present with infection and probably even a lesser proportion with bleeding.[95] Abnormalities detected on physical examination are not common with MDS. It is not unusual, then, that the patient often is diagnosed because of an incidental hemogram.[95] Anemia (hemoglobin less than 11 g/dL) is the most common finding (typically isolated), but occasionally, isolated thrombocytopenia and even less commonly, isolated neutropenia have been noted. Isolated thrombocytopenia can precede by two to ten years the development of the features (to be discussed shortly) that permit classification as MDS.[96,97] Thrombocytosis, particularly in association with refractory anemia or refractory anemia with ringed sideroblasts (in turn in

association often with partial deletion of the long arm of chromosome 5 [termed 5q-]) could be the presenting abnormality.[98-100]

Patient Subsets

Elderly
As noted previously, MDS is a relatively common cause of anemia in the elderly.[94,101]

Therapy-related MDS
These patients are typically younger and more symptomatic (particularly in terms of fatigue and fevers) than patients with primary MDS.[102] In the initial FAB classifi-

cation, it was felt that this entity could be indistinguishable from primary MDS.[22] Macrocytic anemia is an early sign of t-MDS. Trilineage dysplasia is a hallmark of t-MDS. Also, the marrow is typically hypocellular with increased fibrosis.[103] The bone marrow biopsy can be invaluable in such cases, given the relatively high frequency of "dry" aspirates.[103] As mentioned earlier, the clinical course of therapy-related MDS is less stable than that of primary MDS, with inevitable progression to AML. The new WHO classification recognizes therapy-related AML and myelodysplastic syndrome as separate entities under AML.[24]

AML with Trilineage Dysplasia. Cases of de novo AML with trilineage myelodysplastic features could represent either progression of clinically occult MDS or simultaneous occurrence.[95] Several studies have shown an approximately 20% lower induction-remission rate among such patients.[104-106]

MDS of Childhood. MDS is rare among children; the annual incidence is 1.8 per million children. MDS accounts for 4% of all hematologic malignancies in childhood.[107,108] Constitutional abnormalities are present in up to one-third of children with MDS.[107,108] Monosomy 7 is the most common cytogenetic abnormality seen in pediatric MDS.[109] Compared with adult MDS, two striking differences are the paucity of ringed sideroblasts and the much higher rate of progression to acute leukemia.[110] Both MDS and AML associated with Down's syndrome are highly chemosensitive and have good prognosis with treatment.[111] Juvenile myelomonocyitc leukemia (JMML) is now classified under myelodysplastic/myeloproliferative disorders and will be discussed later in this chapter.

HIV-related MDS. Myelodysplasia has frequently been described in the literature on HIV in adults.[112-119] Typically, this occurs in the setting of cytopenias with the discordant marrow finding of hypercellularity as seen in primary MDS. There is clearly more than one mechanism responsible for dysplasia in HIV disease—antiretroviral therapy, direct infection by HIV, or opportunistic infections, for example. Harris and coworkers[114] found dyserythropoiesis in all patients on azidothymidine (AZT).

In the series by Karcher and Frost,[113] dysplastic features of at least one lineage in 105 of 152 patients were noted—the same features that were mentioned for the former FAB criteria of MDS. Dyserythropoiesis was most common (in 56% of these patients), followed by dysmegakaryopoiesis (31%), then dysgranulopoiesis (18%). Although the morphologic features might resemble those of primary MDS, a major difference is that progression to overt acute leukemia is highly unlikely.[114] In a recent study of 158 hemophilic patients with HIV, 44 patients (27.8%) met the criteria for myelodysplastic features. The mean time under AZT treatment was 44 months. The results of the 44 hemophilic HIV patients with MDS were compared with those for 61 patients with primary MDS. Hypocellularity, plasmacytosis, and eosinophilia were more pronounced in HIV patients. Neither blasts greater than 5% nor progression to AML was seen among HIV patients

with MDS. Cytogenetics were normal in HIV patients, compared with 43% abnormal cytogenetics seen in patients with primary MDS. Finally, responses to erythropoietin injections were better among HIV patients (84% vs. 20% response rate).[120] This observation might suggest, as mentioned previously, that HIV-related myelodysplastic features could be a different entity, referred to as HIV myelopathy.[117]

MDS in Pregnancy. A macrocytic anemia developing during pregnancy is invariably due to folate deficiency. MDS is very rare during pregnancy. Fewer than 25 cases have been reported. Five cases of MDS during pregnancy were noted in a five-year period at a university hospital.[121] Four of the five cases had macrocytic erythrocyte indices and/or megaloblastoid changes in the bone marrow. Outcomes of seven pregnancies in four women with MDS were reported from the Mayo clinic over a 15-year period. Three were diagnosed by abnormal blood counts during pregnancy, while the fourth had preexisting MDS and suffered from recurrent abortions.[122]

Clinical Manifestations/Natural History

There is a wide range of clinical manifestations in primary MDS (Fig. 105-2). Because this is a disease of the elderly, there are often comorbid conditions that ultimately might shorten the patient's life expectancy, with the result that about 20% of patients with MDS will not succumb to MDS.[123] Approximately one-third of patients will undergo transformation into AML, which is ultimately fatal. In the remaining patients, the majority will succumb to infection, in part from neutropenia (in one series, 60% of patients with MDS had a neutrophil count below $2500/\mu L^{11}$) and in part from granulocyte dysfunction, as the MDS clone can have impairment in phagocytic adhesion, chemotaxis, and microcidal killing.[124,125] The decreased neutrophil count and neutrophil dysfunction also might account for slowly resolving abscesses and for the lack of fever, with such patients often manifesting

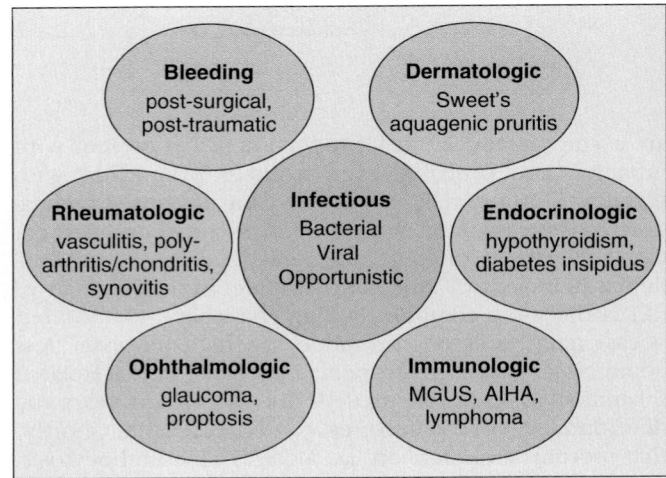

Figure 105-2. The spectrum of clinical manifestations in MDS.

malaise only.[126] In a study by Pomeroy and colleagues[123] of 86 patients with MDS, infection accounted for 64% of deaths. The risk for infection was about one infection per patient per year.[123] Bacterial pneumonias and skin abscesses were the most common infections, but unusual or opportunistic-type infections have also been reported, such as disseminated *Mycobacterium avium-intracellulare*, *Aeromonas hydrophila* endocarditis, bacterial thyroiditis, and Epstein-Barr virus hepatitis.[123,127,128] The course of these infections can be quite prolonged, in part because of the underlying defects in neutrophil function. Prophylactic antibiotic therapy, such as daily trimethoprim-sulfamethoxazole as piloted in other hematologic malignancies, has not been systematically studied in MDS.[129] Neither has the use of intravenous gammaglobulin. As for the use of hematopoietic growth factors, they predictably lead to resolution of the neutropenia (80%–90% efficacy with G-CSF or GM-CSF).[130] On the other hand, they have not yet been proven in randomized, placebo-controlled, double-blind studies to prolong survival when given prophylactically.[131,132]

Less common than infection but potentially life threatening is the risk of bleeding among patients with MDS. Bleeding can occur even in the absence of thrombocytopenia attributable to platelet dysfunction, as evidenced by a prolonged bleeding time that corresponds to an increase in atypical megakaryocytes.[133,134]

Patients with MDS also can manifest a wide range of autoimmune phenomena such as cutaneous vasculitis, polymyalgia rheumatica, necrotizing panniculitis, Coombs'-positive autoimmune hemolytic anemia, remitting seronegative symmetric synovitis with pitting edema, and inflammatory seronegative arthritis.[135-142] Acute manifestations of a systemic autoimmune disease, as described in a study by Enright and associates,[143] include pericarditis, pleural effusions, skin ulceration, seizures, myositis, and peripheral neuropathy. They also reported the following chronic or isolated autoimmune manifestations: glomerulonephritis, polyneuropathy, pyoderma gangrenosum, polyarthritis, and ulcerative colitis.[143] An association of inflammatory bowel disease with MDS had also been reported by other groups.[144-146] It does appear that management of the autoimmune manifestations with immunosuppressive therapy is effective; it might also improve the associated cytopenias.[143]

Another clinical feature peculiar to MDS is that these patients have a higher incidence of malignant tumors and lymphoma than the general population.[147,148] It has been hypothesized that the increased risk of developing malignant tumors reflects an underlying defect in immune surveillance that initially leads to the emergence of the MDS clone in the first place.[46]

LABORATORY EVALUATION

Peripheral Blood and Bone Marrow

The diagnosis of MDS can be made only after careful examination of the peripheral blood smear, bone marrow aspirate, and biopsy. No single morphologic finding is diagnostic; rather, a combination of dysplastic features in the peripheral blood and bone marrow is necessary. It must be emphasized that the diagnosis of MDS is a diagnosis of exclusion, as will be reviewed in the section on differential diagnosis. Even after ruling out various conditions of cytopenia with peripheral/bone marrow dysplasia, the diagnosis of MDS can be elusive, given the variability in the following factors:

- Sampling of the sternal site vs. the iliac site
- Cellularity that can even be noted in adjacent marrow spaces of the same core biopsy
- Differences over time in the same patient
- Involvement of the erythroid, myeloid, and megakaryo-cytic lineages[149]

The general recommendations for diagnosis of MDS are the same in the WHO system as in the FAB system.[90] The variant morphologic dysplastic features in the peripheral blood and bone marrow are summarized in Figures 105-3 and 105-4. To determine the blast percentage, a 500-cell differential should be performed in the marrow and a 200-cell differential in the peripheral blood. Abnormal sideroblasts are defined by five or more iron granules (from the Greek *sidero*). When the granules encircle one-third or more of the nucleus in iron-stained smears, the term *ringed sideroblast* is applied.

The standard stains (Romanowsky, hematoxylin, and eosin) should be done, as should the Prussian blue stain for iron and the reticulin stain for fibrosis. If the patient is iron deficient based on the Prussian blue stain, a silver stain might reveal ringed sideroblasts that would otherwise be masked by iron deficiency, as the silver stain demonstrates only the phosphate moiety.[150]

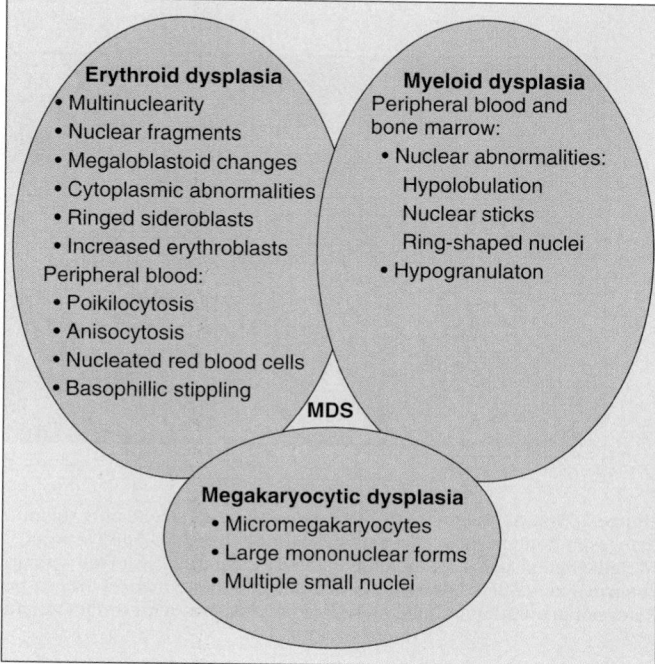

Figure 105-3. Dysplastic bone marrow features of MDS.

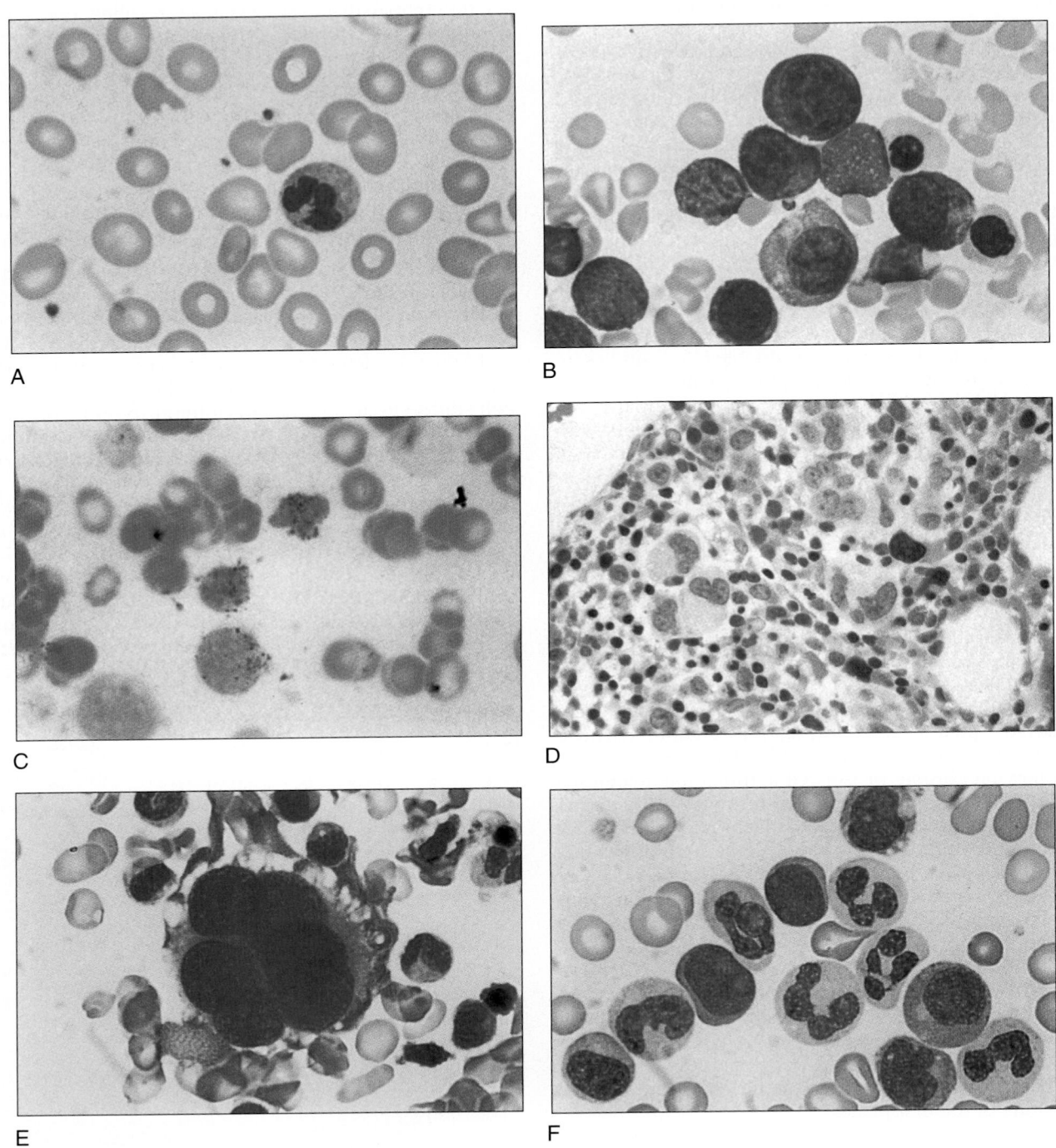

Figure 105-4. A, Macrocytosis of pseudo-Pelger stab from; note the nuclear projections. Peripheral blood (Wright-Giemsa stain). **B,** Megaloblastoid changes in bone marrow of a patient with RA (Wright-Giemsa stain). **C,** Abnormal sideroblasts with ringed forms in bone marrow of a patient RARS (Wright-Giemsa stain). **D,** Increase in dysplastic megakaryocytes with apoptosis in bone marrow from a patient with RAEB (H & E stain). **E,** Abnormal megakaryocyte with several nuclei in bone marrow from a patient with RAEB (Wright-Giemsa stain). **F,** Increase in type I blasts and abnormal maturation in bone marrow from a patient with RAEB (Wright-Giemsa stain).

Continued

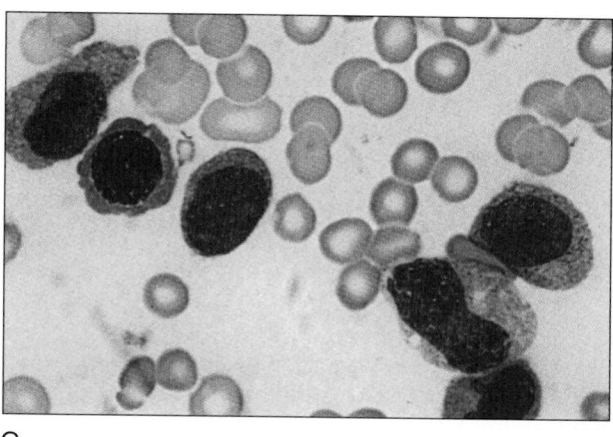
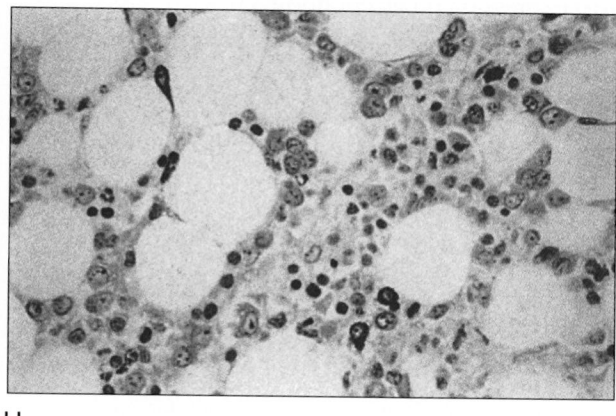

Figure 105-4, *cont'd.* **G,** Increase in immature monocytes in bone marrow from a patient with CMML (Wright-Giemsa stain). **H,** Cluster of blasts in a bone marrow biopsy from a patient with RAEB (Giemsa stain; ALIP).

Several cytochemical and immunologic techniques exist that can supplement the preceding standard stains.[3] The myeloid origin of the blast cells can usually be confirmed by the peroxidase and Sudan black B stains, while the nonspecific esterase or double-esterase stain often can distinguish early monocytic precursors from poorly granulated myelocytes. The double-esterase stain might also identify a population of early myeloid/monocytic cells (presence of both granulocytic and monocyte esterase) in the marrow.[151] In one study, the iron stain was the most useful cytochemical stain in distinguishing certain types of MDS cases from cases in the non-MDS and nondiagnostic groups.[152] It should be noted that the peroxidase decreases in each cell and in amount over the course of MDS.[14,152]

The application of immune-marker analysis of lymphoid and myeloid cells in the diagnosis of the acute leukemias has naturally found use in the diagnosis of the myelodysplastic syndromes. Several immunologic phenotypes have been described using a battery of monoclonal antibodies: The most common is "myeloid" (CD13+, CD14+, CD33+, peroxidase+) but both pure lymphoid blast types (TdT+, CD19+, CD10+) and biphenotypic patterns have been noted.[34] Immunologic techniques have also been applied toward characterization of megakaryocytes in MDS. Occasionally in MDS, the megakaryocytes cannot easily be identified by light microscopy. In particular, the abnormally small megakaryoblasts (*dwarf cells*) might resemble lymphoid precursors similar to FAB L2 lymphoblasts. In such cases, staining the megakaryocytes for GP IIb/IIIa, "CDw41" by the alkaline-phosphatase anti-alkaline phosphatase technique can be helpful.[154] Other immunostains that can identify megakaryocytes on air dried smears easily include an antibody prepared against platelet-specific gp IIIa alone (CD61) or by histologic bone marrow reactions with an antibody against factor VIII or fibronectin.[3,155,156] Erythroid progenitors also can be identified by a variety of immunostains with antibodies against glycophorin A, hemoglobin, CD45, and transferrin receptor CD71.[3] The identification of erythroblasts by

immunostaining could be of prognostic significance, as they could portend a higher incidence of transformation to erythroleukemia.[157]

Several flow cytometric studies of bone marrow aspirates in MDS have assayed for the early marker of stem cell/myeloid differentiation, CD34.[158,159] Immunohistochemical staining of the bone marrow biopsy can also be done for CD34 expression.[160-162] In these studies, there has been a correlation of CD34 positivity with RAEB and RAEB-T subtypes (former FAB system), with CD34 positivity significantly associated with progression to leukemia and shorter survival. In a study by Oertel and associates,[161] the blasts in the RAEB subtype were predominantly CD34−, with an emergence of CD34+ blasts in the RAEB-T (refractory anemia with excess blasts in transformation) subtype (former FAB system). Along those lines, the finding of CD34 positivity or a phenotype such as the coexpression of CD33/CD13 might prompt the clinician to consider induction-remission therapy similar to that used for de novo AML. Another aggressive clinical subset of MDS with an immunophenotypic correlate are those cases of MDS clearly related to organo-chemical exposure. Such cases have a high expression of glycoprotein (GP) p-170, the product of the multidrug resistance gene-1 (as well as CD34 positivity).[163] In these cases of p-170 expression or, for that matter, CD34 positivity, intensive chemotherapy, though possibly achieving a complete remission, is usually not curative; the "remission" hematopoiesis will most likely still be clonal, as the MDS phenotype typically involves an early stem cell (i.e., CD34+).[164]

Flow cytometric immunophenotyping has not been established as a tool in the diagnosis of MDS. Flow cytometry could have a role in cases in which morphology and cytogenetics are nonconclusive and repeat analysis remains noninformative. Immunophenotypic myeloid dysplasia features could include hypogranular neutrophils based on orthogonal scatter, CD64−, and low CD11b, CD16, and CD13 expression. Erythroid immunophenotypic dysplasia could include decreased Cd71 (transferrin receptor) expression on glycophorin A-positive precursors. Currently, megakaryocytic lineage dysplasia is difficult to recognize immunophenotypically.[165]

Despite the many cytoimmunologic tests available on the marrow aspirate, the need for careful examination of the bone marrow biopsy by routine light microscopy should not be trivialized. The definition of dysplasia as defined by Bartl and colleagues[149] as "a loss in uniformity of the individual cells, as well as a loss in the their architectural orientation" reminds one that biopsy is necessary for the full delineation of MDS. The core biopsy can complement examination of the aspirate in both the diagnosis and the prognosis of MDS in several ways:[166]

1. In cases of inadequate marrow aspiration, the core biopsy still usually allows for determination of the subgroups of MDS.[167,168]
2. Identification of clusters of immature cells (myeloid in origin by cyto- or immunohistochemistry)—myeloblasts or promyelocytes—displaced from the paratrabecular area to the intertrabecular areas and referred to as abnormal localization of immature precursors (ALIP).[169] The presence of three or more foci in the section is considered positive. The finding of ALIP might possibly confer a poor prognosis.[169] ALIP is frequently present in RAEB; its presence in other subtypes could denote rapid progression to AML, or it should at least prompt review of the slides to exclude higher-grade disease.[170,171]
3. Easier identification of dysmegakaryopoiesis than by the marrow aspirate.
4. Ability by core biopsy to determine the degree of marrow fibrosis. Approximately 50% of cases have a mild-to-moderate increase in marrow reticulin.[168,172] Cases with marked fibrosis might connote a poor prognosis; on the other hand, such cases might respond to steroids.[173-178]
5. Accurate assessment of the marrow cellularity. The bone marrow cellularity should be at least normocellular for the age of the patient. Typically, it is hypercellular, particularly in RAEB.[179] There are cases of hypoplastic MDS, however.[180-186] The core biopsy also can help in distinguishing this from cases of a hypocellular marrow with foci of blasts ("hypocellular AML").[187,188]

Cytogenetics

Given that MDS is by definition a clonal disorder, it might be surprising that the karyotype is normal in 30%-50% of cases, particularly in primary MDS.[189] One reason is the technical causes of failure to obtain an adequate number of metaphases for analysis.[190] The expanding use of fluorescent in situ hybridization (FISH) will be one way to overcome this technical issue.[191] The karyotypic abnormality can also appear and disappear over time.[192,193] Another reason is that the chromosomal abnormality can be submicroscopic, and only over time, with progressive genomic instability, will there be a gross karyotypic abnormality.[190,194] Logically, then, those subgroups of "early" MDS (RA, RARS) have a much lower probability of

a detectable karyotypic abnormality (7%-30%) compared with subgroups of "advanced" MDS (RCMD, RAEB), in which there is a greater than 50% probability of a detectable karyotypic abnormality. Understandably, the highest probability (80%-90%)[189] is in t-MDS.[191,195]

In general, three karyotypic abnormalities are noted: deletions (the most common), chromosomal loss or gain, and translocations.[190] Among these categories, there is variation between primary vs. t-MDS and geographic variation also.[196]

Cytogenetic Abnormalities in Primary MDS

The most common abnormalities are 5q- (30% of those with a detectable karyotype), trisomy 8 (19%), and monosomy 7 (15%).[190] Less commonly, there is loss of chromosome Y, 17 p-, interstitial deletions of chromosomes 3, 11, 12, 13, or 20, and isochromosome 17q.[189,197,198] Least common, comprising only 3%-5% of cases, are translocations involving t(3; 3), t(1;7), t(3;21), t(5;7), t(6;9), or t(5;17).[189,190] Complex karyotypes are seen in 10%-20% of patients with primary MDS.

Cytogenetic Abnormalities in Therapy-related MDS

All of the previously mentioned abnormalities in primary MDS can be noted, but monosomy 7/7q- and monosomy 5/5q- are the most prevalent. As previously mentioned, translocations/rearrangements involving band 11q23 or 21q22 are unique to t-MDS and are related to epipodophyllotoxin therapy.

The 5q- Syndrome

A subset of patients with isolated partial deletion of 5q has peculiar clinicopathologic features that have prompted its recognition in the new WHO classification as a separate subgroup. Patients with the 5q- syndrome are usually upper-middle-aged females with isolated macrocytic anemia. Surprisingly, they often have thrombocytosis in the 500,000/μL to 1 million/μL range. They often become red cell transfusion-dependent, but otherwise the clinical course is stable. The cytogenetic abnormality involves deletion between bands q31 and 33, where the size of the deletion and the breakpoint are variable.[98,99,199]

Gene Mutations

The aforementioned cytogenetic chromosomal abnormalities ultimately lead to loss or alteration of certain genes they carry. These genes can be tumor suppressor genes, pro-oncogenes, or genes that carry other functions. It is known now that multiple gene mutations contribute to the pathogenesis and development of MDS. The RAS gene family is the one most studied in MDS. Ten percent to 40% of patients with MDS (including CMML by the former FAB classification) have RAS mutation.[200,201] The most common mutation is single base change at codon 12 of the N-RAS family. The resultant mutated N-RAS protein retains active GTP form, promoting continuous signaling to the nucleus. Patients with MDS who have the RAS mutation carry a worse prognosis and have a higher rate of progression to AML. The RAS protein is now a target for a group of medications known as Farnesyl transferase inhibitors (see later sections relating to treatment).[202]

Other gene mutations involved in MDS include P53 tumor suppression gene (5%–10% of cases), FLT3 oncogene receptor kinase (5% of cases), P15 ink4b-a cyclin dependent kinase inhibitor, and hypermethylation genes that can be present in up to 50% of high-risk cases. We hope that as we learn more about these mutations and their altered signaling pathways that we will be able to develop a new generation of targeted therapy.

In vitro Bone Marrow Cultures

The literature is replete with studies of in vitro bone marrow growth from patients with MDS, yet no one consistent diagnostic abnormality has been detected. This is probably in part due to a lack of standardized methods.[203] Common abnormalities are absent or decreased colony growth, progressive decrease in cloning efficiency on sequential plating, abortive cluster formation, and defective maturation within colonies.[203]

DIFFERENTIAL DIAGNOSIS

Before proceeding with a bone marrow aspirate and biopsy in a patient suspected to have MDS (e.g., an elderly patient with a non–iron deficiency anemia and borderline low WBC and/or platelet count with hypogranular/hypolobulated white blood cells and red cells with basophilic stippling on the peripheral blood smear), it is incumbent on the clinician to consider the possibility of the following five conditions that might also be associated with cytopenia and peripheral blood cell dysplasia:

1. Vitamin B_{12} and/or folate deficiency, as low B_{12} levels are not that uncommon in the elderly and because hyperlobulation of the neutrophils can be seen as a dysplastic feature in MDS.[204]
2. Proven exposure to heavy metals.[205]
3. Recent cytotoxic therapy, especially among patients who are receiving agents such as methotrexate and azathioprine for rheumatologic diseases.
4. Ongoing inflammatory conditions, including HIV and cancer.[112-117,148,206]
5. Chronic liver disease, as macrocytosis is common in both entities.[207,208]

Above all, the first three conditions must be excluded. The latter two could be considered to be relative exclusions, as some patients will have both MDS and a coincidental inflammatory state (such as cancer or rheumatoid arthritis) or MDS with coincidental chronic liver disease and/or alcohol use. That MDS is a diagnosis of exclusion is illustrated by the not-uncommon scenario of a patient referred to the hematologist for further evaluation of a persistent macrocytic anemia despite a trial of vitamin B_{12} injections. Such occurrences are a reminder of why historically the term "refractory anemia" was coined.

Finally, what about cases lacking overt dysplasia in which all of the preceding disorders and the various medical conditions associated with dysplasia have been excluded, but there persists an unexplainable abnormality in the peripheral blood, such as a macrocytosis without anemia or monocytosis? These are cases to which Hamblin[209] has referred, perhaps tongue in cheek, as NYMDS (not yet MDS) or NQMDS (not quite MDS). Anttila and associates[211] studied a group of elderly patients with macrocytic anemia that did not fulfill the FAB criteria for MDS. Four molecular markers for indirect/direct evidence of clonality were applied—DNA hypermethylation at the calcitonin A gene 5′ area, N-RAS point mutations at codon 12 and 13, in vitro colony formation of peripheral blood progenitor cells, and cytogenetics of the bone marrow cells. In eight of nine of these cases that did not fulfill the FAB criteria for MDS, at least one molecular study was abnormal, consistent with an early stage of MDS. It thus seems that in cases without overt dysplastic morphology, the demonstration of a clonal cytogenetic abnormality or monoclonality by other methods could conceivably lead to a provisional diagnosis of MDS.[211]

PROGNOSIS

Since the advent of the FAB classification of MDS, numerous clinical, pathologic, and biologic factors have been studied in the hope of best predicting the overall survival and acute leukemic transformation risk in patients with MDS.[210-212] These factors include the degree of cytopenia, percentage of bone marrow (BM) blasts, BM cytogenetics, serum lactate dehydrogenase level, BM histology for abnormal localization of immature precursors, the marrow immunophenotype, and in vitro bone marrow culture characteristics.[210,212] None of these factors, either singly or in combination, have led clearly to a prognostic index with adequate precision. The search for such an index led to the development of the International Prognostic Scoring System (IPSS) for MDS, wherein combined data from seven previously reported studies was analyzed.[213] It was determined that patients could be separated into four distinctive risk subgroups (low, intermediate-1, intermediate-2, and high) for both median survival and time to 25% of the patients to evolve to acute myeloid leukemia (Table 105-4). These designations based on three prognostic variables: the percentage of marrow blasts, the degree of karyotypic abnormalities, and the degree of cytopenias. Stratification by age (less than or greater than 60 years) separates patients further within the low-risk and intermediate-1 subgroups. The IPSS was able to discriminate between the subgroups of other categorization systems.

In a recent retrospective analysis, Germing and colleagues[92] validated the WHO classification system regarding to its prognostic relevance. They applied the WHO classification categories to 1600 patients from the Dusseldorf MDS registry. The reclassified registry was then subjected to evaluation by four different scoring systems, including the IPSS. The results confirmed a significant prognostic difference between RAEB I and RAEB II (median survival 18 months and 10 months, respectively). Also, there was a significant prognostic difference between RA/RARS without dysplasia and the new refractory cytopenia with multilineage dysplasia subtype (RCMD); the

TABLE 105-4

The International Prognostic Scoring System

RISK SUBGROUP	SCORE	MEDIAN SURVIVAL (YRS)	AMLS RISK*
Low	0	5.7	9.4
Intermediate-1	0.5–1.0	3.5	3.3
Intermediate-2	1.5–2.0	1.2	1.1
High	≥2.5	0.4	0.2

The score is based on the following parameters:

Prognostic Variable	0	0.5	1.0	1.5	2.0
BM blasts (%)	<5	5–10	—	11–20	21–30
Karyotype	Good (normal or 5q- or 20q- or -Y)	Intermediate	Poor (≥3 abnormalities or monosomy 7)		
Cytopenias (hemoglobin <10 g/dL, ANC <1,500/μL, platelet count <100,000/μL)	0/1	2/3			

AML, acute myelogenous leukemia; ANC, absolute neutrophil count.
*Number of years for a quarter of the group to evolve into acute myelogenous leukemia.
From Greenberg P, Cox C, LeBeau MM, et al: International scoring system for evaluating prognosis in myelodysplastic syndromes. Blood 1997;89:2079.

median survival time was 69 month for RA/RARS but 33 month for RCMD, and 32 months for RCMD-RS. The rate of progression to AML was higher for RAEB II compared with RAEB I and for RCMD compared with RA/RARS. It is hoped that the WHO system will be an adjunct tool with the IPSS for predicting prognosis. Prospective studies are needed to validate the new classification system.

THERAPY

Treatment of MDS can be categorized conceptually into three main approaches, as diagrammed in Figure 105-5. These approaches include:

1. Differentiation of the abnormal clone by differentiation-induction agents or perhaps by cytokine therapy.

2. Suppression of the abnormal clone by low-dose or standard-dose chemotherapy, or perhaps by cytokine therapy via stimulation of residual normal hematopoiesis with subsequent suppression of the malignant hematopoiesis, or by activation of the residual normal host immune system by cytokines or cytokine-activated lymphocytes ("immunotherapy").

3. Ablation of the abnormal clone by more intensive therapy via an allogeneic bone marrow transplant (BMT).

The appropriate approach, if any, should depend primarily on three clinical and biologic factors:

1. Severity of the patient's cytopenia
2. The patient's age
3. The degree of leukemic progression (percent marrow blasts)

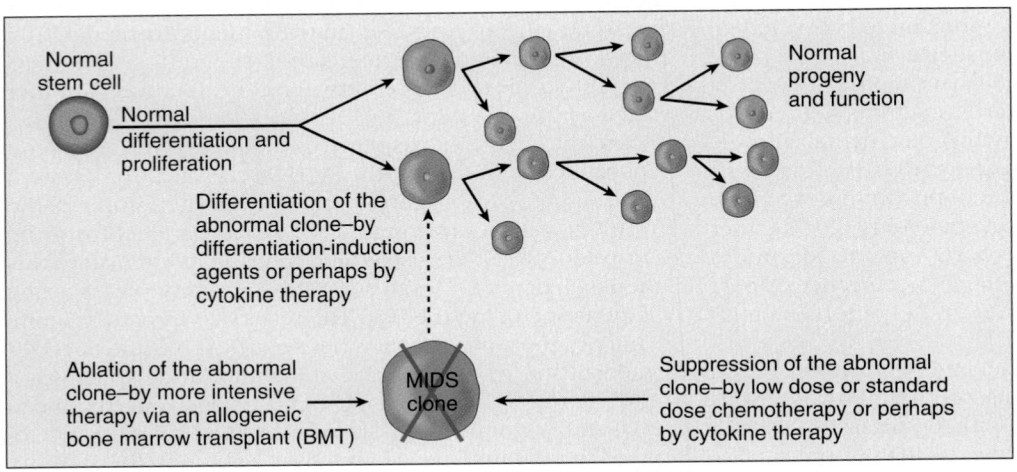

Figure 105-5. Schema of the various therapeutic approaches in MDS.

These factors, in turn, are reflected in the IPSS described previously.[197] The main aim for elderly patients should be to ameliorate the cytopenias when they become transfusion dependent. For younger patients, on the other hand, the aim could be curative therapy via an allogeneic BMT.

Therapeutic options for patients with MDS that target the aforementioned mechanisms and serve the approaches just outlined include:

- Noncytotoxic therapy: hematopoietic growth factors, immune therapy, cytokine inhibitors, antiangiogenesis, differentiating agents
- Cytotoxic therapy: low-dose chemotherapy, high-dose chemotherapy
- Bone marrow transplantation: allogenic stem cell transplant, autologous stem cell transplant
- Novel targeted strategies
- Palliative treatment

An international working group has standardized the response criteria to treatment.[214] Complete remission has been defined by bone marrow criteria (less than 5% myeloblasts with normal maturation of all cell lines and no evidence for dysplasia) and peipheral blood criteria (hemoglobin 11 g/dL or more, neutrophils 1500/mm^3 or more, and platelets 100,000/mm^3 or more, with no evidence of dysplasia or blasts). A major erythroid response has been defined as 2 g/dL increase in hemoglobin or transfusion independence for patients with hemoglobin less than 11 g/dL. A minor erythroid response has been defined as 1–2 g/dL increase in hemoglobin or 50% reduction in transfusion requirements among patients with less than 11 g/dL hemoglobin level. Platelets major response is defined by increased platelets by 30,000/mm^3 or transfusion independence, whereas a platelets minor response is defined by a 10,000/mm^3 to 30,000/mm^3 increase or by a 50% or greater increase in platelets. Finally, major neutrophils response is shown by an absolute increase of more than 500/mm^3 or a 100% increase in neutrophils in patients with less than 1500/mm^3. Following these standardized criteria makes the comparison of various clinical therapeutic trials both easier and more uniform.

Hematopoietic Growth Factors

G-CSF/GM-CSF

Currently, there is no evidence to support use of either GCSF or GMCSF as a single therapy for patients with MDS. Ganser and Hoelzer[130] showed that G-CSF and GM-CSF can raise the neutrophil counts in patients with MDS. Of a total of 78 patients receiving G-CSF and 263 receiving GM-CSF, a sufficient rise in the neutrophil count was noted in 76% of the patients treated with GM-CSF (two-thirds of patients responded to very low doses of GM-CSF) and in 90% of the patients treated with G-CSF.[215] On the other hand, GM-CSF therapy affected neither hemoglobin levels nor the transformation to AML in two randomized clinical trials published in abstract form.[216,217] In a randomized trial, GCSF had no effect on survival, transformation to AML, or hemoglobin levels.[218]

Erythropoeitin

The role of erythropoeitin (EPO) in MDS has been explored in multiple studies.[219-221] Two meta-analyses have been published covering trials of EPO alone in MDS. The first meta-analysis by Hellström-Lindberg in 1995[219] included 205 patients from 17 trials. The overall response rate (defined as no requirement for transfusion) was 16%. Predictors for good response were serum EPO level below 200 U/L, nonrefractory anemia with ring sideroblasts (RARS) subtype, and lack of previous need for transfusion. The second meta-analysis, by Rodriguez and coworkers,[222] included 114 patients from 10 trials. The overall response rate was 23.5%, with RAEB as as negative predictor for response. The Italian cooperative group study[221] is the only randomized, double-blind, placebo-controlled study of EPO treatment in MDS. The response rate (defined as more than 50% reduction in transfusion requirement) was 37% vs. 11% for the group receiving placebo. Again, refractory anemia and no need for transfusion were favorable predictors of response.

On occasion, trilineage responses have been noted with G-CSF and GM-CSF, and in vitro there can be synergism of HGFs on normal and MDS progenitors.[130, 223-225] These two observations have prompted studies of either of these cytokines with erythropoietin. By and large, the response rate for combined EPO and G-CSF treatment is approximately 40%, double the response rate for therapy with EPO alone.[226,227] The synergistic effect is most pronounced in patients with refractory anemia with ring sideroblasts (RARS) (50% response rate). A predictive model of the response rate to combined EPO+ G-CSF treatment was developed using serum EPO level and need for transfusion as the criteria; patients with a high score (low level of EPO below 100, fewer than two units per month blood transfusion) had a 74% response rate, while patients with a low score (serum EPO above 500 or more than two units per month transfusion) had only a 7% response rate.[228] There is little evidence to support use of EPO with GM-CSF or EPO with IL3.[229,230]

Regarding thrombocytopenia in MDS, IL-11 could become an effective therapy. Low-dose IL-11 was tested in 16 patients with bone marrow failure, 11 of whom had MDS. Five out of the 11 patients with MDS showed response to IL-11, with 95×10(9)/L median increase in peak platelet counts.[231]

Immune Therapy

Immune system abnormality might, as mentioned, be involved in both the etiology and the pathogenesis of MDS; in these processes, cytotoxic T-cells play a role in bone marrow suppression and also enhance cytokine production.

Steroids

Bagby[232] studied steroids as MDS therapy in 1980; a minority of patients experienced improvements in their low blood counts. An effect correlated in vitro with increased CFU-GM growth. Subsequent clinical use of steroids, however, showed low response rate and high potential risk of infection.

Specific Malignancies

Anti-thymocyte Globulin

Another immune therapy, anti-thymocyte globulin (ATG), was studied in 61 patients with MDS.[233] Patients were transfusion dependent, not receiving concurrent therapy, but most had failed previous treatments. Thirty-three percent of patients became red cell transfusion independent, an effect maintained in two-thirds of the patients for a median of 32 months. Fifty-six percent of patients experienced a sustained increase in platelets count and 44% a sustained increase in neutrophils count. A multivariate analysis showed that young age, shorter duration of transfusion dependence, and HLA DR 15 are predictors of better outcome.

Cyclosporine

Cyclosporine therapy was studied in 16 patients with refractory anemia and one patient with refractory anemia with excess blasts. Twelve patients were transfusion dependent. All 12 patients became transfusion independent, and increases in platelets and neutrophil counts were observed also.[234] Finally, trials with immune therapy are ongoing in the United States and Europe.

Cytokine Inhibitors

Pentoxifylline

Pentoxifylline is a xanthine derivative that blocks the lipid-signaling pathway used by TNFα, TGFβ, and IL-1β. It was studied in patients with MDS combined with ciprofloxacin (which decreases hepatic degradation of pentoxifylline) and with dexamethasone (which down regulates TNFα production). Unfortunately, responses were neither sustained nor complete.[235,236]

Amifostine

Amifostine is a phosphorylated aminothiol used as cytoprotective agent; it has an antioxidant activity and suppresses cytokine release. The drug initially was developed by Walter Reed Army Medical Center during the cold war as a protective agent against radiation for military personnel. In vitro, amifostine improved colony growth of MDS marrow cells.[237] List and coworkers[238] reported results for 117 patients with MDS treated with amifostine. One hundred four patients were evaluable at time of presentation of this study. Of this group, 66 patients were evaluable for red cell response, seven patients had a major response, and three had a minor response. Twenty-seven patients had major improvement in platelet counts, and 10 out of 30 patients experienced a neutrophil response. Other reports showed disappointing results. Trials combining amifostine with chemotherapy and growth factors are ongoing.

Enbrel

Enbrel is a TNF-α fusion protein (soluble receptor). Theoretically, it neutralizes TNF-α production by binding it. Deeg and coworkers[239] reported use of Etarncept, 25 mg subcutaneously twice weekly for 14 patients with MDS. Among 12 evaluable patients, four had rises in hemoglobin by 1–1.5 g/dL (three patients) or decreased transfusion requirements (one patient). Two patients had increased platelet counts, and two had increased neutrophils. Baseline TNF-α levels, determined in all patients, did not correlate with responses. Among eight marrows available for sequential in vitro assays, four showed increases in CFU-GM of 1.5- to fivefold at eight weeks, whereas three showed three- to tenfold decrements relative to baseline. In a recent study, sixteen patients participated in a pilot study of Enbrel; one became (temporarily) transfusion independent and in one patient, absolute neutrophilic count (ANC) increased.[240] No significant increase on haematopoietic colony formation was seen, and there was no correlation with TNF-α levels.

Thalidomide

Thalidomide is a potent antiangiogenic drug.[241] Angiogenesis is increased in MDS bone marrow biopsies.[242] Thalidomide inhibits TNF-α production by inducing Th2 cells and inhibiting Th1 cytokine production. It also inhibits direct TNF-α production via monocytes.[243,244] Theoretically, thalidomide is an ideal drug for treating MDS, as it appears to target the major pathways incriminated in the pathogenesis of MDS, including immune, cytokine, and angiogenesis pathways.

Raza and associates[245] treated 83 patients with MDS with thalidomide. Fifty-one patients completed 12 weeks of treatment. Sixteen patients had a partial response, whereby 10 erythroid responders became transfusion independent. By intention to treat, 19% of all patients (16 of 83) and 31% of patients who were able to complete 12 weeks of treatment achieved response. The majority of patients were maintained on doses between 150 mg to 200 mg; only eight patients could continue the full 400 mg dose for 8 weeks. The major side effects were fatigue, constipation, shortness of breath, fluid retention, dizziness, rash, numbness and tingling, fever, headache, and nausea. The conclusion was that thalidomide is effective in improving cytopenia among certain patients with MDS, especially those with high blasts. Dourado and colleagues[246] reported that six out of nine patients treated with thalidomide for MDS responded (two achieving complete response and four partial response). Thomas and coworkers[247] reported one out of seven patients achieving complete response to thalidomide. Finally, in a recent study, Strupp and associates[248] reported hematological response in 19 out of 29 evaluable patients. Nine patients had partial response, with granulocytes more than 1500/mm^3, hemoglobin more than 11 g/dL, and platelets more than 100,000/mm^3. The responders became transfusion independent over a two-month period of treatment. Interestingly, a reduction in the proportion of blast cells was seen in the bone marrow of five patients with RAEB and RAEB-T. Three patients achieved normal blast counts, suggesting that thalidomide might alter the course of the disease and its progression.

Early reports of combining thalidomide with agents such as amifostine, pentoxifylline, or Enbrel are showing results superior to the use of either single agent.[249-251]

Finally, thalidomide analogues selective cytokine inhibitory drugs (SelCID) and immunomodulatory drugs (IMiD) are currently being studied in patients with

MDS. Those drugs are probably more potent and less toxic then thalidomide. Revimid (CC-5013), the lead IMiD compound, was tested in a phase I/II study of 25 patients with MDS. Most patients had RA or RARS with low or intermediate-1 IPSS. Erythroid responses were seen in 64% of patients with a median duration of response of 36 weeks; major platelet response was seen in 25%. Interestingly, a 50% or greater decrease in the excess bone marrow blasts was seen in 33% of patients. A complete cytogenetic response was seen in 62% of patients that had abnormal karyotype originally mostly with 5q syndrome (A. List, personal communication). Ongoing studies will further define the role of those compounds in treatment of patients with MDS.

Other Differentiating Agents

Cis-retinoic acid follow-up studies have not shown this agent to be effective as therapy for MDS.[252,253] The same disappointing results were found with all-trans retinoic acid (ATRA).[254,255] Hexamethylene bisacetamide (HMBA) demonstrated a limited degree of efficacy but has not been studied further.[256,257] The use of phenylbutrate for MDS has not been encouraging, although it has shown itself to be a potent differentiating agent in vitro; better results via prolonged continuous IV infusion (as shown in phase I studies) might need to be confirmed.[258,259] Heme arginate (heme infusion) has not been pursued therapeutically for MDS.[260] Interferon, in spite of the "twist" using α as well as γ, has not been shown helpful.[261] Pyridoxine (50 mg three times a day) might be useful in cases of RARS with low MCV.[262]

Low-Dose Chemotherapy

Historically the efficacy of low-dose chemotherapy, particularly that of ara-C, was considered to be due to a differentiative effect.[263] Further studies have demonstrated a predominantly cytotoxic effect, with marrow aplasia noted.[264] Given the baseline of a total response rate with low-dose ara-C (LDAC) in up to one-third of patients (16% CR, 21% PR as reviewed by Cheson[265]), further studies have attempted to improve on this by adding additional cytotoxic agents (e.g., etoposide, 6-TG, G-CSF, or IL-3) at low doses. In all cases, the response rate has been higher than that seen with LDAC alone but typically not significantly greater and such response is usually of short duration.[266–269] One study of ara-C alone deserves particular attention, as all five patients achieved a complete hematologic response with low-dose ara-C. These patients all had deletion of 5q- and were red cell transfusion dependent.[199] Notably, the dysplasia continued to persist in the follow-up marrows, as did usually the 5q- abnormality. The authors of this study as well as ourselves have no logical explanation to offer as to why there is specificity for response to ara-C in patients with 5q-. Low-dose ara-c, however, did not show improvement in terms of overall survival time when compared with the best supportive care in the only phase III prospective randomized study for this agent.[264] Low-dose melphalan had a response rate of approximately 40%, with a better response in a group of patients with hypocellular marrow (hypocellular MDS compromises only 10%–20% of MDS cases).[8,270,271] The use of homoharringtonine (HHT), a plant alkaloid, has been studied in patients with MDS and has achieved a relatively good response, but with severe cytopenia resulting in death. The use of lower doses or of HHT derivatives could have some promise in the future.[272]

Intensive Chemotherapy

Studies employing intensive AML-type induction regimens for MDS continue to be associated with a lower complete remission rate and shorter remission duration than in de novo AML, though there have been some studies with comparable CR rates and duration of remission.[273–278] Because one major negative factor for intensive chemotherapy in MDS—age—cannot be manipulated, investigators have attempted to manipulate two other factors:

1. The longer duration of aplasia/hypoplasia, by administering G-CSF or GM-CSF.[273,274]
2. Multidrug resistance, by adding additional agents such as etoposide and administering IL-2 post-CR to lengthen the duration of CR by stimulating immune surveillance.[273]

Beyond intensive AML-type regimens, investigators have tried novel agents not previously administered in MDS therapy. Topotecan, a topoisomerase-I inhibitor, is the most promising agent, having one of the highest CR rates for single-agent therapy in MDS (31% CR in 19 of 60 patients). Clinicians' enthusiasm is tempered, however, by the fact that 20% of the patients died during the induction period.[279] Topotecan was combined with cytarabine (ara-c) in 59 patients with MDS and in 27 patients with CMML. Fifty-six percent had a complete remission, 7% died during induction; and the average duration of complete remission was 8 months.[280] A retrospective analysis of 394 patients with MDS who were treated with multiple high-dose chemotherapy regimens from the MD Anderson cancer center was published recently. Regimens were idarubicin/ara-c (AI), topotecan/ara-c (TA), topotecan/ara-c/cyclophosphamide (CAT), and fludarabine/araC/idarubicin (FAI). The overall response rate was 58%, with no statistical difference between various regimens. Induction death rates were lowest among patients receiving TA (5.4%) and highest among those receiving FAI (20.7%). After adjusting for covariates, AI was found to be superior to CAT and FAI but no different from TA.[281] Topotecan with araC and idarubicin was then tested in 10 patients with MDS. Four patients experienced complete remission with a median survival time of 15 months.[282] A phase I study of oral topotecan showed that 1.4 mg/m^2 daily was the maximum tolerated dose. Nausea, vomiting, and diarrhea were dose-limiting toxicities. Complete remission was seen in two out of 12 patients with MDS and in two out of seven patients with CMML.[283]

Ongoing studies are evaluating the effects of other agents such as irinotecan, gemcitabine, and temozolomide. High-dose chemotherapy is reserved for high-risk patients with MDS. Complete remission rates are improving but have yet to translate into improved survival times.

Allogeneic Stem Cell Transplantation

Allogenic stem cell transplantation (allo-SCT) is recognized as a curative option for patients with MDS. Overall, studies show that approximately 40% of patients with MDS will be cured with allo-SCT. The best results are obtained for patients with RA who receive matched-related donor (MRD) transplantation; 75% of these patients have long-term disease-free survival (DFS). Treatment-related mortality (TRM) associated with allogeneic bone marrow transplantation for MDS ranges from 30% to 50%. Predictors of disease relapse are percentage of blasts and cytogenetics.[284] Longer disease duration, male sex, non–matched-related donor, and therapy-related MDS (tMDS) are factors associated with increased non–relapse mortality.[285] Table 105-5 summarizes the major studies of allo-SCT in MDS.[239] There remain many questions concerning allo-SCT for MDS, the most important of which we discuss next.

What Should Be the Upper Age Limit for Allo-transplant?

The median age at diagnosis of MDS is 65 years. Results for allo-SCT are more favorable with younger patients (under 40 years of age). Higher non–relapse mortality and relapse rates are seen among patients who are older than this. Overall DFS is 48% for patients younger than age 40 years, whereas it is 17% for those older than 40 years, according to a Seattle study.[286] Most transplant centers exclude patients older than age 55 years from their protocols. Deeg and colleagues[287] have published data of patients with MDS between the ages of 55 and 65 years. Of 55 patients, 36 underwent match-related donor transplantation, four underwent syngeneic transplantation, four underwent mismatched-related donor transplantation, and four underwent matched-unrelated donor transplantation. Total-body irradiation was used for 23 patients, while chemotherapy alone was used for 27 patients. The actuarial DFS was 42%, the relapse rate was 22%, and TRM was 40%. Allo-SCT can be offered selectively to patients between 55 and 65 years of age. The "age" obstacle, as we will discuss shortly, is becoming less critical with the introduction of "mini" bone marrow transplantation.

At What Stage Should Allo-SCT Be Offered to Patients with MDS?

In appropriately selected patients, allo-SCT should be offered early. Data about the disease duration and outcome are controversial. The Seattle group[288] reported a higher incidence of non–relapse mortality among patients having a longer duration of disease. Two other studies found no correlation between duration of disease and non–relapse mortality.[289,290] The European Bone Marrow Transplant Group (EBMT) confirmed that shorter disease duration is associated with lower non–relapse mortality.

There are no randomized clinical trials examining transplantation in comparison with other options according to the IPSS; however, long-term DFS for intermediate-1, intermediate-2, and high-risk groups appeared to be better with allo-SCT when compared with historical cohorts from IPSS data. There was no difference in TRM in patients with advanced IPSS, but there was a statistically significant higher relapse rate among those patients (2% for intermediate-1, 17% for intermediate-2, and 38% for high-risk MDS).[284]

Should the Patient Receive Induction Chemotherapy Before Allo-SCT?

The rationale for induction chemotherapy includes hope for better transplantation outcome while the patients are in complete remission, improving symptomatic cytopenia, and buying time until SCT can be arranged. On the other hand, the rationale for not using induction chemotherapy includes considerations of higher toxicity, potential delay of transplantation secondary to chemotherapy-related toxicity, and a nonguaranteed response rate with induction (around 50%).

There are no prospective randomized trials comparing induction chemotherapy followed by allo-SCT with allo-SCT alone. Some studies have shown no statistically significant difference in DFS at five years; others have demonstrated better outcome in complete responders, only related to non–relapse mortality.[286,291,292]

If a complete remission can be obtained in 50% of patients with induction chemotherapy, and if 40%–50% DFS can be obtained with allo-SCT, then the overall DFS is about 25%, which is similar to the outcome of allo-SCT for untreated patients or for de novo AML. A prospective study is needed to address this issue further.

Is Unrelated Bone Marrow Transplantation a Viable Option for Young Patients?

It seems that unrelated bone marrow transplantation (MUD) is a feasible option. Overall, 30% of patients undergoing such transplantations are cured. The lower relapse rates obtained are at the expense of higher non–relapse-related mortality. The largest published series is from the EBMT group;[290] in this series, 118 patients received one to two minor HLA-mismatched donor transplantations. DFS was 28% at two years, the relapse rate was 35%, and TRM was 58%. The National Marrow Donor Program (NMDP) published a report of 510 patients. DFS was 29% at two years, the relapse rate was 14%, and TRM was 54%.[293]

What Is the Best Conditioning Regimen?

Historically, cyclophosphamide with total body irradiation (TBI) has been the standard. A recent study of 26 patients evaluating TBI (12 Gy) and busulfan (7 mg/kg) showed better DFS and a lower relapse rate than the cyclophosphamide and TBI protocol.[294] Those results are now being confirmed by a phase III study by the Southwest Oncology Group (SWOG). There is no difference in outcome between TBI-based regimens and chemotherapy-based regimens.

What Is the Role of T-Cell–depleted Technique?

Theoretically, this technique offers a lower rate of graft-vs.-host disease (GVHD) and TRM. Data are controversial; however, one study showed good results, while the other failed.[295,296]

TABLE 105-5

Compilation of SCT Studies: Allogenic Stem Cell Transplantation

STUDY/ (FOLLOW-UP)	NO.	MEDIAN AGE	TYPE	CONDITIONING REGIMEN	DFS	RELAPSE	TRM
Copelan, 2000 (1984–1999)[a]	42	46 (11–62)	35 = MRD 3 = mMRD 4 = MUD	Bu-Cy Bu-Cy-Ep	35% at 4 years	21%	36%
De witte, 2000 (1983–1998)[b]	1378	Majority between 20–40	885 = MRD 198 = MUD 91 = mMRD 173 = autologous	NA	At 3 years MRD=36% with OS 41% MUD=25% with OS 26% mMRD=28% with 31% OS auto-SCT=30% with 32% OS	MRD =36% 43–43% for RAEB 49% for MDS/AML MUD = 41% mMRD =18% auto-SCT= 58%	MRD= 43% MUD =58% mMRD =66% auto-SCT=29%
Deeg, 2000 (26 mo)[c]	50	59 (55–66)	34 = MRD 4 = mMRD 6 = MUD 6 = mMUD (4 = twins)	CY-TBI CY-TBI (with lung and liver shielding) Bu-TBI Bu-CY	42% at 3 year DFS in RA 53%	22%	39%
Appelbaum, 1998 (1981–1996)[d]	251	38	59 MRD 13 mMRD 28 MUD	Bu-Cy Cy-TBI	40%	18%	20% age <20 50% age >50
Nevill, 1998 (1986–1996)[e]	60	40 (15–55)	37 = MRD 1 = mMRD 22 = MUD	Bu-Cy Bu-Cy + other Cy-TBI Cy-TBI + other	29% at 7 year 32% for MUD at median of 70 mo	42% 23% for MUD at median of 70 mo	50%
Runde, 1998 (27 mo)[f]	131	33 (2–55)	MRD	Chemo +/– TBI	41% OS at 5 years 34% DFS	21% 39% actuarial relapse at 5 years	38%
Arnold, 1998 (24 mo)[g]	118	24 (.3–53)	MUD	Chemo +/– TBI Chemo +/– serotherapy	28% 2-year actuarial	35%	58%
Mattijsen, 1997 (20 mo)[h]	35	41 (23–60)	32 = MRD 1 = mMRD 2 = MUD	Cy-TBI = /–Ida	39% at 2 years	20%	40%
Anderson, 1996 (24 mo)[i]	52	33 (1–53)	MUD	Bu-Cy Bu-Cy-TBI Cy-TBI	38% 2-year actuarial survival 40%	28%	48%
Sutton, 1996 (72 mo)[j]	71	37 (5–55)	MRD	Majority TBI	32% at 7 years	48%	39%
O'Donnell, 1995 (60 mo)[k]	38	35 (5–55)	MRD	Bu-Cy	37% at 2 years OS at 2 years 45%	24%	50%
Ratanatharathorn, 1993 (20 mo)[l]	27	33 (4–54)	24 = MRD 3 = MUD	Bu + /-ara-c/Cy	63%	4%	33%

auto-SCT, autologous stem cell transplant; Bu, busulfan; Cy, cyclophosphamide; DFS, disease-free survival; EP, etoposide; mMRD, mismatched related donor; MRD, matched related donor; MUD, matched unrelated donor; OS, overall survival; SCT, stem cell transplant; TBI, total body irradiation; TRM, transplant-related mortality.

[a]Copelan EA, Penza SL, Elder PJ, et al: Analysis of prognostic factors for allogeneic marrow transplantation following busulfan and cyclophosphamide in myelodysplastic syndrome and after leukemic transformation. Bone Marrow Transplant 2000;25(12):1219–1222.

[b]DeWitte T, Hermans J, Vossen J, et al: Haematopoietic stem cell transplantation for patients with myelo-dysplastic syndromes and secondary acute myeloid leukaemias: A report on behalf of the Chronic Leukemia Working Party of the European Group for Blood and Marrow Transplantation. Br J Haematol 2000;110:620–630.

[c]Deeg HJ, Shulman HM, Andersen JE, et al: Allogeneic and syngeneic marrow transplantation for myelodysplastic syndromes in patients 55 to 66 years of age. Blood 2000;95:1188–1194.

[d]Appelbaum FR, Anderson J: Allogenic bone marrow transplantation for myelodysplastic syndromes: Outcomes analysis according to IPSS score. Leukemia 1998;12(Suppl 1):25–29.

[e]Nevill TJ, Fung HC, Sheperd JD, et al: Cytogenetic abnormalities in primary myelodysplastic syndromes are highly predictive of outcome after allogeneic bone marrow transplantation. Blood 1998;92:1910–1917.

[f]Runde V, de Witte T, Arnold R, et al: Bone marrow transplantation from HLA-identical siblings as first-line treatment in patients with myelodysplastic syndromes: Early transplantation is associated with improved outcome. Chronic Leukemia Working Party of the European Group for Blood and Marrow Transplantation. Bone Marrow Transplant 1998;21(3):255–261.

[g]Arnold R, de Witte T, van Biezen A, et al: Unrelated bone marrow transplantation in patients with myelodysplastic syndromes and secondary acute myeloid leukemia: An EBMT survey. European Blood and Marrow Transplantation Group. Bone Marrow Transplant 1998;21(12):1213–1216.

[h]Mattijssen V, Schattenberg A, Schaap N, et al: Outcome of allogeneic bone marrow transplantation with lymphocyte-depleted marrow grafts in adult patients with myelodysplastic syndromes. Bone Marrow Transplant 1997;19(8):791–794.

[i]Anderson JE, Appelbaum FR, Schoch G, et al: Allogeneic marrow transplantation for refractory anemia: A comparison of two preparative regimens and analysis of prognostic factors. Blood 1996;87:51.

[j]Sutton L, Chastang C, Ribaud P, et al: Factors influencing outcome in de novo myelodysplastic syndromes treated by allogeneic bone marrow transplantation: A long-term study of 71 patients. Societe Francaise de Greffe de Moelle. Blood 1996;88:358.

[k]O'Donnell MR, Long GD, Parker PM, et al: Busulfan/cyclophosphamide as conditioning regimen for allogeneic bone marrow transplantation for myelodysplasia. J Clin Oncol 1995;13:2973.

[l]Ratanatharathorn V, Karanes C, Uberti J, et al: Busulfan-based regimens and allogeneic bone marrow transplantation in patients with myelodysplastic syndromes. Blood 1993;81:2194.

Autologous Stem Cell Transplantation

Autologous stem cell transplantation (auto-SCT) could be an alternative to allo-SCT for patients with MDS for whom no suitable donor is available or for whom allo-SCT is not feasible. The presence of polyclonal hematopoeisis in the peripheral blood stem cell harvests is the theoretical basis for the use of auto-SCT.[297] Most auto-SCT studies are of patients with MDS/sAML who achieved a complete remission. Approximately 30% have DFS at two to three years, but there are also high relapse rates in the first two years (greater than 50%). Transplant-related mortality is lower than expected. Table 105-6 summarizes major auto-SCT studies of patients with MDS.

Nonmyeloablative Stem Cell Transplantation ("Minitransplant")

This form of stem cell transplantation is emerging for various types of malignancies; its goal is to reduce the nonselective toxicity to various body organs of the ablative conditioning regimens. Minitransplant uses conditioning regimens as immune system modifiers to accept the stem cell transplant and then depends on the graft-vs.-leukemia/tumor effect for curing the disease. This concept draws a fine balance between GVHD and graft-vs.-leukemia disease.

Early reports on treating patients with MDS with this modality are emerging. Nonmyeloablative transplant could offer hope to more patients with MDS, especially elderly patients or those with medical comorbidities who are not candidates for regular stem cell transplantation. In one study of 46 patients with MDS, 20 received a nonmyeloablative regimen due to age or other medical conditions. Transplant-related mortality at 100 days was 5% compared with 23% of 26 patients with MDS in the myeloablative arm; the three-year survival rate was 49% for the nonmyeloablative group compared to 54% for the control group.[298] In another study, 18 patients with MDS or MDS/sAML received nonmyeloablative SCT with fludarabine and TBI as a conditioning regimen. Three patients died due to transplant-related mortality, eight remained in complete remission at a median of 246 days, and two patients were in partial remission.[299] Larger studies with longer follow-up are warranted to address the promising role of "minitransplant" for patients with MDS.

In summary, all patients with MDS below the age of 55 years should be evaluated for SCT. According to the IPSS, patients classified as having intermediate-1, intermediate-2, and high-risk disease who have a matched related donor can be offered an allo-SCT option in experienced institutions. Younger patients with intermediate-2 and high-risk IPSS disease who have no matched donor can be offered matched nonrelated allo-SCT, and the same applies for patients with intermediate-1 disease with progressive cytopenia and unstable disease. Low-risk patients could be observed or offered SCT in the presence of MRD and progressive or life-threatening cytopenia or very young age. Patients between ages of 55 to 65 years should be selected carefully, preferably in clinical trials. Nonmyeloablative SCT might become a viable option for patients older than 55 years with poor prognostic disease (intermediate-2, high-risk, and certain intermediate-1 patients). Auto-SCT may be considered in the absence of a matched donor after achievement of CR in intermediate-2 or high-risk IPSS patients.

Novel Targeted Strategies

Gene Transcription Agents

Gene transcription is regulated by various activation and repression mechanisms. Two mechanisms for gene silencing (repression of transcription) are DNA hypermethylation and histone deacytalation.[300]

The interest in using hypomethylating agents was generated by the fact that several abnormal gene methylations had been described in leukemia and MDS.[300] The pyrimidine nucleoside cytosine analogue 5-azacytidine (5-AZA) acts as a hypomethylating agent.[301] It inhibits DNA methyltransferase, which is needed for methylation of cytosine-guanosine dinucleotides (CpG); inhibiting this methylation leads to activation of the gene transcription of previously silenced genes.[302,303] Silverman[304] reported a 49% response rate among RAEB and RAEB-T patients with MDS treated with 5-AZA. It was given as 75 mg/m^2 daily as a continuous infusion for seven days every four weeks. The most frequent side effects were nausea and vomiting. The CALGB group[305] carried these good results into a large phase III randomized trial of 191 patients using 75 mg/m^2 5-AZA subcutaneously for seven days every four weeks for four complete cycles. The overall response rate was 60% in the treatment group compared with 5% in the group receiving best supportive care. The median time to leukemic transformation for patients receiving 5-AZA was 21 months, compared with 12 months for the control arm. Quality of life was also enhanced for the 5-AZA treatment group. There was a trend toward improved survival in the azacitidine arm. This is the first randomized trial to show that treatment of MDS is better than supportive care. The study, however, has been criticized for allowing crossover from the supportive arm to the AZA arm and for less-defined criteria of hematological improvement.

Decitabine (5-aza-2′-deoxycytidine), a more potent hypomethylating agent, has also been used in phase II trials. The overall response rate was 49%, and the actuarial median survival time was 15 months.[306] Myelosuppression was the most common side effect. Decitabine might be more effective than azacitidine but is definitely more toxic.

Histone deacetylase removes an acetyl group from histone protein, causing a conformational change that creates an unfavorable environment for transcription, thus silencing the gene. Histone deacetylase forms a complex with a nuclear corepressor complex that is present on promotor regions (NCHDC). NCHDC plays a role in acute promyelocytic leukemia and AML. Inhibition of histone deacetylase overcomes the gene silencing. Agents that act as histone deacetylase inhibitors include phenylbutrate and hybrid polar compounds such as hexamethylene bisacetamide (HMBA), depsipeptide, and MS27-275. Unfortunately, phenylbutrate and HMBA, as mentioned

TABLE 105-6

Compilation of SCT Studies: Autologous Stem Cell Transplantation

STUDY	NO. OF PATIENTS	MEDIAN AGE	CONDITIONING REGIMEN	DFS	RELAPSE/TRM	COMMENTS
de Witte, 2001*	35	47	TBI-Cy Bu-Cy Other non-TBI	12 remained in CR 4-year DFS in patients with CR 7.3% 4-year OS in patients with CR 32.7%	19 out 35, 4 out 35	197 patients from 35 institutions with MDS or sAML were registered, 184 were evaluable. 100 patients (54%) entered CR after 1 or 2 induction treatments. Ninety patients received one consolidation treatment. Out of 56 patients with a HLA-identical sibling, 33 achieved CR; 26 of these received allo-SCT. Out of 128 patients with no donor, 61 patients achieved CR; 35 of these received auto-SCT. Analysis was based on intention to treat so all patients who achieved complete remission were considered candidates for SCT. 4-year DFS in the group of patients with (allo-SCT) or without donor (auto-SCT) was 30.8%, and 27.3%. 4-yr OS was 36.4% vs. 32.7%.
Wattel, 1999†	24	<55	Bu-Cy	12 (50%) still in CR after 8–55 mo	9 out of 24, 3 out of 24	Out of 83 patients, 42 achieved CR after chemotherapy induction. Three patients received allo-SCT, and 24 received auto-SCT, where 16 received ABMT and 8 APSCT. In autografted patients, median Kaplan-Meier DFS and survival were 29 and 33 months from the autograft, respectively.
de Witte, 1997 (EBMT)‡	79	39	NA	34% at 2 years 39% 2-year OS	64%, <10%	Patients were sAML/MDS in CR, 39% DFS for age <40 yr. A cohort of 55 patients within the study were compared to 110 patients with de novo AML. DFS at 2 years was 28% for MDS/AML patients compared with 51% for de novo AML (p = 0.025). the relapse rate was 69% for MDS/AML vs. 40% for de novo AML (p = 0.007)
Demuynck, 1996§	5		Bu-Cy			No long-term survivial results. ANC recovery to 500 in 14 days, platelet recovery in 41 days, one case of marrow failure
Laporte, 1993¶	7	44	Cy + TBI	2/7 alive and well at 10+ and 28 mo	1 died periSCT	Despite prolonged thrombocytopenias regeneration occurred in all patients

ABMT, autologous bone marrow transplant; allo-SCT, allogenic stem cell transplant; APSCT, autologous peripheral stem cell transplant; auto-SCT, autologous stem cell transplant; Bu, busulfan; CR, complete remission; Cy, cyclophosphamide; DFS, disease-free survival; OS, overall survival; SCT, stem cell transplant; TBI, total body irradiation; TRM, transplant-related mortality.

*de Witte T, Suciu S, Verhoef G, et al: Intensive chemotherapy followed by allogeneic or autologous stem cell transplantation for patients with myelodysplastic syndromes (MDSs) and acute myeloid leukemia following MDS. Blood 2001;98(8):2326–2331.

†Wattel E, Solary E, Leleu X, et al: A prospective study of autologous bone marrow or peripheral blood stem cell transplantation after intensive chemotherapy in myelodysplastic syndromes. Groupe Francais des Myelodysplasies. Group Ouest-Est d'etude des Leucemies aigues myeloides. Leukemia 1999;13(4):524–529.

‡de Witte T, Van Biezen A, Hermans J, et al: Autologous bone marrow transplantation for patients with myelodysplastic syndrome (MDS) or acute myeloid leukemia following MDS. Chronic and Acute Leukemia Working Parties of the European Group for Blood and Marrow Transplantation. Blood 1997;90(10):3853–3857.

§Demuynck H, Verhoef GE, Zachee P, et al: Treatment of patients with myelodysplastic syndromes with allogeneic bone marrow transplantation from genotypically HLA-identical sibling and alternative donors. Bone Marrow Transplant 1996;17:745.

¶Laporte JP, Isnard F, Lesage S, et al: Autologous bone marrow transplantation with marrow purged by mafosfamide in seven patients with myelodysplastic syndromes in transformation (AML-MDS): A pilot study. Leukemia 1993;7:2030.

previously, did not have impressive results for treatment of MDS. Depsipeptides and MS27-275 are currently being evaluated in phase I trials.[300]

Monoclonal Antibodies

Gemtuzumab ozogamicin (Mylotarg) is a humanized anti-CD33 monoclonal antibody linked to calicheamicin—a novel, highly potent cytotoxic agent. CD33 is expressed in more than 90% of AML cases and is absent from normal stem cells. The FDA has approved Mylotarg for the treatment of relapsed AML in patients over the age of 60 years. The overall response rate is approximately 30%.[307]

MDS is second to AML in expression of CD33 among hematological malignancies. Interestingly, patients younger than than age 60 years with secondary AML have a higher intensity of CD33 expression than do elderly patients. There was no correlation, however, between the clinical response and the intensity of CD33 expression among 45 patients treated with various Mylotarg protocols.[308]

In a study of Mylotarg as front-line treatment for AML and high-risk MDS, 14 patients with MDS were included. CR was achieved in 25% of patients with diploid karyotype. No complete remission was achieved in patients with abnormal karyotype. The mortality rate for all patients, however, was very high.[309] Ongoing trials are evaluating the use of Mylotarg with various chemotherapy combinations, including a 3 plus 7 AML regimen, high-dose ara-c, topotecan, troxacitabine, anti-BCL2, and MDR blockers. Also, a regimen of Fludarabine, ara-c, Mylotarg, and cyclosporine is being tested.

Farnesyl Transferase Inhibitors

RAS is a protein group involved in signal transduction. Activation of the RAS protein occurs in response to the binding of variety of growth factors and hormones to tyrosine kinase receptors. GDP RAS is converted to GTP RAS, leading to a downstream of signaling. Mutated RAS results from single amino acid substitution, whereby the GTP form is nonhydrolyzed, leading to continuous activation of RAS.[202,310] R1157 is a methylquinolone analog that is a competitive inhibitor of the farnesyl transferase enzyme needed for prenylation of RAS protein, thus anchoring the RAS protein to the membrane.[202] Farnesyl transferase inhibitors (FTI) activity could also be independent of the presence of RAS mutation.[202,310] RAS mutation is described in 20%–40% of patients with MDS, particularly in cases of patients with CMML.[200,201]

Forty-two patients with MDS were treated in phase I and II studies of FTI. The maximum tolerated dose was 300 mg given twice daily for three to four weeks, and the dose-limiting toxicity was neurological. Overall, 24% of patients with MDS experienced CR with FTI treatment.[311,312] Additional studies are further evaluating the role of this agent in treating AML and MDS.

Miscellaneous Therapies

Androgens have been tried for years in anemic patients with MDS without much success; nonetheless, there continue to be studies of its use for MDS.[313,314] There also continue to be studies of danazol, including two studies of a combined 110 patients; a partial response was noted in only four of these patients.[252,315] Generally, these patients did not have platelet counts less than 50,000/μL. Based on previous studies that appeared to show some degree of response in the platelet count of thrombocytopenic patients, a study by Wattel and associates[313] included only patients with platelet counts below 50,000/μL and less than 10% marrow blasts. Either danazol or fluoxymestrone was administered, with 11 of 20 patients having at least a 30,000/μL incremental rise in their platelet counts; of the six patients who had bleeding before therapy, all had resolution of bleeding. In another study by this same group, in which 9 of 26 evaluable patients responded to danazol, there was no correlation of the responders with antiplatelet antibodies or platelet lifespan.[316] Previously, there had been a study of thrombocytopenic patients with MDS responding to danazol, providing evidence for an autoimmune component of MDS.[317]

Interestingly, transfusion dependence might be lessened by subcutaneous desferrioxamine.[318] This is a reminder, particularly for low-risk patients with MDS, that their iron stores should be assessed and consideration given for iron chelation therapy, not only to reduce the morbidity of iron overload (which in time might come into play given the relatively long overall survival in that IPSS subgroup) but also (as demonstrated by Jensen and colleagues[318]) to reduce the transfusion requirement in the majority of these "de-ironed" patients.

PALLIATION OF THE INCURABLE PATIENT

Despite the many therapeutic options mentioned in the foregoing discussion, MDS is essentially a terminal disease. Red cell and platelet transfusions and appropriate use of antibiotics remain a mainstay of therapy.

PREVENTION AND EARLY DETECTION

As the majority of cases of MDS are not secondary to chemotherapy, there are no firm preventive measures to be promulgated save for direct monitoring of exposure to benzene in the workplace where applicable. It should be emphasized that presumably less hazardous solvents, such as toluene and xylene, might contain impurities of benzene at concentrations that could still be leukemogenic.[319] Indirect monitoring by a routine hemogram in the workplace does not appear to be helpful.[320]

MYELODYSPLASTIC/MYELOPROLIFERATIVE DISEASES

The category of myelodysplastic/myeloproliferative diseases is new to the recent WHO classification. It includes myeloid disorders which, at initial time of presentation, combine features of both dysplastic and proliferative myeloid disorders. This categorization recognizes a group of diseases that do not fit a distinct stem cell disorder and indicates our need to better understand the molecular pathogenesis of these disorders that lead to dysplastic and proliferative abnormalities. The new category includes the following disorders:

- Chronic myelomonocytic leukemia (CMML)
- Juvenile myelomonocytic leukemia (JMML)
- Atypical chronic myeloid leukemia (aCML)
- Myelodysplastic/myeloproliferative disease, unclassifiable

A detailed description of JMML and aCML is beyond the scope of this chapter.

Chronic Myelomonocytic Leukemia

Definition

Chronic myelomonocytic leukemia (CMML) is a neoplastic clonal stem cell disorder characterized by persistent monocytosis (more than 1×10^9/L monocytes in the peripheral blood and in the marrow) as a defining feature. Bone marrow blasts should be less than 20%, and BCR/ABL (Philadelphia chromosome) should be absent.[91] In most cases, some degree of dysplasia is present.[22,321] Diagnosis in the absence of dysplasia can still be made if the other requirements are met and if an acquired clonal cytogenetic abnormality is present in the marrow cells, or if monocytosis is present for more than three months and other causes of monocytosis have been excluded.

Epidemiology

The incidence of CMML is around 1 to 2 per 100,000 population. CMML is a disease of older adults, with a median age at onset of 70 years. It also shows a male predominance (1.6–2.1:1).[322-324]

Etiology and Pathogenesis

The exact etiology of CMML is not known. CMML is a neoplastic clonal stem cell disorder with a multipotent stem cell as the cell of origin. Environmental carcinogens, occupational carcinogens, cytotoxic agents, and radiation could all be possible causative agents.[324]

Cytogenetic abnormalities are seen in 20%–40% of patients with CMML. The most common are +8,-7, and 12p structural abnormalities.[201,322,325] Chromosomal translocations, including the platelet-derived growth factor β receptor gene (PDGFβR), are described in a minority of CMML patients (the PDGFβR gene is located on 5q33). The protein is a well characterized plasma membrane receptor with tyrosine kinase activity. Autophosphorylation of the receptor leads to a variety of downstream signaling events involved in variable biological responses. Chromosomal translocations lead to fusion oncogenes between the PDGFβR gene and other genes, resulting in an auto-activated PDGFβR retaining its tyrosine kinase activity without the ligand binding the receptor. The following translocations have been described in CMML:

- t(5;12)(q33;p13) TEL/PDGFβR. TEL is a transcription factor gene involved in angiogenesis and hematopoiesis. TEL fuses to the transmembrane and cytoplasmic domains of PDGFβR, replacing the ligand binding site and leading to autoactivation. This abnormality occurs in 2%–3% of CMML cases, but it could be a potential target for tyrosine kinase inhibitors.[326,327]
- t(5;7)(q33;p13) Rabaptin/PDGFβR.[330] The fusion oncogene causes IL-3–independent cell growth.
- t(5;7)(q33;p11.2) HIP1/PDGFβR.[329]
- t(5;10)(q33;q21) H4-D10S170/PDGFβR.[330]

In addition to the chromosomal translocations just described, RAS mutation, as mentioned previously, occurs in up to 57% of CMML patients, with point mutations in which aspartic acid is substituted for glycine.[331]

Clinical Presentation

CMML presentation can be divided into two subgroups:[332]

1. Nonproliferative CMML (WBC less than 13,000/μL), which presents in a fashion similar to MDS.
2. Proliferative CMML (WBC greater than 13,000/μL), which presents more like a myeloproliferative pattern with hepatosplenomegaly.

Extramedullary involvement includes skin and gums. Pleural effusions and pericardial effusions are always serous.[333] Hypergammaglobulinemia occurs in one-third of the patients. Monoclonal gammopathy occurs in 5%–10% of patients. Immunophenotyping usually reveals a myelomonocytic pattern. Plasmacytoid monocytes associated with CMML have a characteristic pattern, with CD14, CD43, CD56, CD68, CD4, T-cell Ag CD2, and CD5 often present.[332]

Treatment

Nonproliferative CMML can be treated in a way similar to MDS. Proliferative CMML treatment options include conventional therapies, stem cell transplantation, and certain novel therapies, each of which we discuss next.

Conventional Therapies

Hydroxyurea. Hydroxyurea was compared with VP16 in 105 patients who had visceral disease or a neutrophils count greater than 16,000, a platelet count less than 100,000, spleen enlarged more than 5 cm, and bone marrow blasts less than 5%. The dose ranged from 1 g to 4 g daily for hydroxyurea and from 150 mg to 1600 mg weekly for VP16. Sixty percent of the hydroxyurea patients showed a response compared with 36% in the VP16 arm (P = 0.02). The time to response was 2.1 months for hydroxyurea vs. 9 months for VP16. The median survival time was 20 months for the patients receiving hydroxyurea vs. 9 months in the VP16 arm (P = 0.004). The rate to progression to AML and the effects on platelets, hemoglobin, and splenomegaly were similar for both treatment groups.[334]

Topotecan. Administration of topotecan was studied in a group of 25 CMML patients. The dose was 2 mg/m^2 as a continuous intravenous infusion for five days. Of these patients, 28% had a CR with a median duration of 7.5 months; median survival time was 10.5 months.[335]

High-Dose Chemotherapy. High-dose ara-c, Idarubicin plus ara-c, topotecan plus ara-c, and VP16 plus carboplatin were tested in CMML. Complete remission rates ranged from 27% to 41%. Topotecan plus ara-c had a higher CR but not a statistically significant one. It is not known whether CR translates to improved survival.[336]

Stem Cell Transplantation. Results of 50 allo-SCT cases from 43 European centers for CMML patients were reported. The median age in this patient group was 44 years, and the median time since diagnosis was nine months. Eighteen patients had excess blasts. Thirty-eight cases received matched related donor SCT, while six cases received matched unrelated donor SCT. In this study, 26% developed grade II to IV GVHD, and 47% died of transplant-related mortality. The median follow-up time was 24 months. The five-year overall survival rate was 21%, and the DFS rate was 16%. Earlier timing of transplant, male donor gender, non–T-cell depletion, and occurrence of acute GVHD were favorable for better DFS but not statistically significant.[337]

Specific Malignancies

Novel Therapy. STI-571 (imatinib mesylate) (Gleevec) use was reported for a 29-year-old CMML male patient with a t (5; 17) translocation with persistent positive RT-PCR after stem cell transplantation, and donor lymphocyte infusion. The patient attained a molecular remission after six weeks of treatment with imatinib, 400 mg.[338] In another report, however, 15 patients with CMML were treated with imatinib. No effect was observed, but none of the patients had the PDGFβR translocation.[339] Imatinib should be studied in the setting of the rare chromosomal translocations mentioned previously.

Farnesyl transferase inhibitors are in Phase II studies that include CMML patients.[311,312]

Prognosis

The median survival time for CMML patients is 20–40 months overall. Progression to AML occurs in 15%–30% of cases.

The percentage of blasts is the most important prognostic factor. Degree of anemia, leukocytosis, and splenomegaly are other possibly prognostic factors.[332]

Juvenile Myelomonocytic Leukemia

Juvenile myelomonocytic leukemia (JMML) is a clonal stem cell disorder characterized mainly by granulocytic and monocytic proliferation. It makes up less than 2%–3% of childhood leukemia cases but accounts for 20%–30% of myelodysplastic and myeloproliferative disorders under the age of 14 years. The exact etiology is unknown, but a strong association with neurofibromatosis type 1 (NF1) exists (10% of JMML cases occur in children with NF1). Cytogenetic abnormalities occur in 30%–40% of cases, but none is specific for JMML. RAS mutation occurs in 20% of patients. Interestingly, neurofibromatosis protein is important for the regulation of the RAS family. Diagnostic criteria include peripheral blood monocytosis greater than 1×10^9/L, less than 20% blasts, absent BCR/ABL oncogene, or Ph chromosome plus two or more of the following: Hgb F being increased for age, presence of immature granulocytes in the peripheral blood, WBC greater than 10×10^9/L, presence of chromosomal clonal abnormality, and GM-CSF hypersensitivity of myeloid progenitors in vitro. Clinical presentation includes malaise, fever, infection, maculopapular rash, and bleeding. Stem cell transplant is the only treatment that improves survival. Untreated, 30% of patients die within one year, while 10%–20% of cases evolve into acute leukemia. Poor prognostic factors include age greater than two years, platelet count less than 33,000/mm^3, and Hgb F greater than 15%.[340]

Atypical Chronic Myeloid Leukemia

Atypical chronic myeloid leukemia (aCML) is also a clonal stem cell disorder characterized by leukocytosis (mainly mature neutrophils and multilineage dysplasia). BCR/ABL or Ph chromosome is absent. Neutrophil precursors are higher than 10% with no or minimal basophilia or monocytosis, and blasts are less than 20%. aCML tends to occur in elderly patients. Cytogenetic abnormailties can occur in up to 80% of cases. Prognosis is poor, with 24%–40% of cases evolving into AML and a median survival time of 20 months.[341]

MYELODYSPLASTIC/MYELOPROLIFERA-TIVE DISEASE, UNCLASSIFIABLE

This category is a designation for disorders that combine clinical, laboratory, and morphological features of both myelodysplastic and myeloproliferative diseases but do not fit the strict criteria of the other MDS/MP diseases. An example of this type of disorder is refractory anemia with ring sideroblasts, with thrombocytosis more than 600,000 μL.[342]

THE FUTURE

This chapter is a testament to the advances already made in the field of molecular biology. The relatively prompt translation of results from the bench to the bedside is astounding. Future advances will encompass all aspects of MDS and related disorders.

Epidemiology

Further identification and understanding of the predisposing genetic, immunological, occupational, and environmental factors involved in MDS should take place. The interaction between these factors and pathogenesis of the disease will be dissected further at the molecular level. Therapy-related MDS will be explored further in the hope of designing less leukemogenic congeners.

Pathology

We expect that the new WHO classification will be applied worldwide with further refinements as we learn more about the disease. It is hoped that the new classification will define more homogenous subsets of patients with MDS, allowing better understanding, study, and treatment of the disease and serving as a prognostic adjunct to IPSS.

Therapy

The multistep process of leukemogenesis will be further elucidated, particularly in terms of activation of oncogenes and inactivation of suppressor genes involved in apoptosis. Such advancement could lead to the design and application of antisense oligonucleotides, antiapoptotic agents, and gene transcription agents as part of a rational approach to therapy.

The study of the cytokines at the cellular and molecular levels could lead to more effective trials of combination therapy with differentiation-induction agents, chemotherapy, and/or early-acting cytokines. Further study of the immune pathogenesis module will allow clinicians to apply various immune modulators and test them in clinical trials. It is hoped that the role of "mini" trans-

CLINICAL CARE OF THE MDS PATIENT: NO DOSE, LOW DOSE OR HIGH DOSE?

The judgment weighs heavy on the physician, as no proven approach definitely prolongs survival in the majority of patients. At our institution, since the development of the International Prognostic Scoring System (IPSS) for MDS, we aim to guide therapy based on the patient's respective prognostic group. Also, whenever there is a clinical trial available, we encourage patients to enroll.

Is the patient in the IPSS high-risk, intermediate-2, or intermediate-1 risk group?
If yes:
Is the patient younger than age 50 years with a haploidentical sibling?
If yes:
Consider allogeneic stem cell transplant (SCT), perhaps with an attempt of AML-type induction therapy before SCT if the patient is in the high-risk or intermediate-2 risk group.
If no:

- Patients less than 40 years old with high-risk or intermediate-2 risk IPSS disease or with intermediate-1 risk accompanied by progressive cytopenia can be offered matched nonrelated allogenic stem cell transplant in the absence of a matched donor.
- Consider a trial of topotecan or AML-type induction therapy.
- Patients between the ages of 50 and 65 could be offered clinical trials with nonmyeloablative "mini" transplantation.

If no:

- Is the patient moderately to severely cytopenic?

If yes:

- Suggest a trial of erythropoietin, 50,000–70,000 U weekly if serum erythropoietin level is below 500 U/L and red cell transfusion requirements are less than 2 U per month; if there is no response after eight weeks, then a trial of erythropoietin with G-CSF is in order.
- Consider a trial of thalidomide.
- Consider a trial of azacitidine.
- Consider a trial of ATG and/or cyclosporine.
- Therapy can include subcutaneous desferal if serum ferritin is greater than 500 ng/mL and iron saturation is greater than 60%.
- If the patient is thrombocytopenic (platelets less than 50,000/μL), consider a trial of danazol, 200 mg orally three times daily.
- If the patient is neutropenic (less than 1000 ANC) with recurrent infections, use G- or GM-CSF subcutaneously, titrating from weeks 1 through 7.
- If the bone marrow is hypoplastic, consider a trial of low-dose daily melphalan, 2 mg qd (once a day) orally, or oral cyclosporine ± antithymocyte globulin.

If no:

- Watch and wait.

plantation will be explored further, thereby increasing the upper age limit for stem cell transplantation. It is hoped also that further refinement of stem cell transplantation methods will permit a more selective graft-vs.-leukemia/ MDS effect while decreasing graft-vs.-host disease.

Most important, the coming years will be the era of biological targeted therapy. As we come to better understand the molecular biology of this disease, we should be able to target more specific pathways involved in its pathogenesis, probably using combinations of biological agents with one other as well as with chemotherapy. Finally, the key to the future of medicine remains with continuing dedicated research and carrying it from the bench to clinical trials.

Presently, we can tailor the approach to patients with MDS based on their IPSS risk stratifications, the degree of cytopenia, and patient age, as outlined in "Clinical Care of the MDS Patient: No Dose, Low Dose, or High Dose?"

PREVENTION OF THERAPY-RELATED MDS/AML

Some general principles can be enumerated for minimizing the risk of t-MDS when using alkylating agents:

1. Shorter duration of induction and maintenance (if any) should reduce the risk by reducing the cumulative dose of the chemotherapeutic agent. A good example would be to cease alkylating agent therapy within a year after achieving a stable paraprotein level in myeloma.
2. Older patients should receive the less leukemogenic of equally effective regimens, given the age-related incidence of t-MDS. For example, myeloma patients of advanced age needing treatment should receive cyclophosphamide instead of melphalan.[43]
3. Pulse therapy appears to be preferable to daily therapy, provided that dose intensity is not an important issue. In chronic lymphocytic leukemia (CLL), for example, it is not an issue, so bimonthly chlorambucil would be preferable to daily chlorambucil. In an adjuvant therapy setting for certain solid tumors, however, the risk of t-MDS is probably much less than the potential benefit of dose intensity.

REFERENCES

1. Farhi DC: Myelodysplastic syndromes and acute myeloid leukemia. Diagnostic criteria and pitfalls [review]. Pathol Ann 1995;30:29.
2. Galton DA: The myelodysplastic syndromes. Part I. What are they? Part II. Classification [review]. Scand J Haematol Suppl 1986;45:11.
3. Schumacher HR, Nand S: Myelodysplastic Syndromes: Approach to Diagnosis and Treatment. New York, Igaku-Shoin, 1995.
4. Hofmann WK, Ottmann OG, Ganser A, Hoelzer D: Myelodysplastic syndromes: Clinical features [review]. Semin Hematol 1996; 33:177.
5. Fenaux P: Myelodysplastic syndromes [review]. Hematol Cell Ther 196;38:363.
6. Oscier DG: ABC of clinical haematology. The myelodysplastic syndromes [review]. BMJ 1997;314:883.
7. Lowenthal RM, Marsden KA: Myelodysplastic syndromes [review] Int J Hematol 1997;65:319.
8. Kouides PA, Bennett JM: Morphology and classification of the myelodysplastic syndromes and their pathologic variants [review]. Semin Hematol 1996;33:95.
9. Layton DM, Mufti GJ: Myelodysplastic syndromes: Their history, evolution and relation to acute myeloid leukaemia [review]. Blut 1986;53(6):423-436.
10. Rhoades CP, Barker WH: Refractory anemia: An analysis of one hundred cases. JAMA 1938;110:794.
11. Hamilton-Paterson JL: Pre-leukemia anemia. Acta Haematol 1949;2:309.
12. Block M, Jacobson LO, Bethard WF: Preleukemic acute human leukemia. JAMA 1953;152:1018.
13. Saarni MI, Linman JW: Preleukemia: The hematological syndrome preceding acute leukemia. Am J Med 1973;55:38-48.
14. Sanz GF, Sanz MA, Vallespi T, et al: Two regression models and a scoring system for predicting survival and planning treatment in myelodysplastic syndromes: A multivariate analysis of prognostic factors in 370 patients. Blood 1989;74:395.
15. Coiffier B, Adeleine P, Gentilhomme O, et al: Myelodysplastic syndromes. A multiparametric study of prognostic factors in 336 patients. Cancer 1987;60:3029.
16. Mufti GJ, Stevens JR, Oscier DG, et al: Myelodysplastic syndromes: A scoring system with prognostic significance. Br J Haematol 1985;59:425.
17. Goasguen JE, Garand R, Bizet M, et al: Prognostic factors of myelodysplastic syndromes—A simplified 3-D scoring system. Leuk Res 1990;14:255.
18. Varela BL, Chuang C, Woll JE, Bennett JM: Modifications in the classification of primary myelodysplastic syndromes: The addition of a scoring system. Hematol Oncol 1985;3:55.
19. Anonymous: Recommendations for a morphologic, immunologic, and cytogenetic (MIC) working classification of the primary and therapy-related myelodysplastic disorders. Report of the workshop held in Scottsdale, Arizona, USA, on February 23-25, 1987. Third MIC Cooperative Study Group. Cancer Genet Cytogenet 1988;32:1.
20. Kerkhofs H, Hermans J, Haak HL, Leeksma CH: Utility of the FAB classification for myelodysplastic syndromes: Investigation of prognostic factors in 237 cases. Br J Haematol 1987;65:73.
21. Bennett JM, Catovsky D, Daniel MT, et al: Proposals for the classification of the acute leukaemias. French-American-British (FAB) cooperative group. Br J Haematol 1976;33:451.
22. Bennett JM, Catovsky D, Daniel MT, et al: Proposals for the classification of the myelodysplastic syndromes. Br J Haematol 1982;51:189.
23. Greenberg P, Cox C, LeBeau MM, et al: International scoring system for evaluating prognosis in myelodysplastic syndromes. Blood 1997;89(6):2079-2088.
24. Harris NL, Jaffe ES, Diebold J, et al: World Health Organization classification of neoplastic diseases of the hematopoietic and lymphoid tissues: Report of the Clinical Advisory Committee meeting-Airlie House, Virginia, November 1997. J Clin Oncol 1999;17(12):3835-8349.
25. Maynadie M, Verret C, Moskovtchenko P, et al: Epidemiological characteristics of myelodysplastic syndrome in a well-defined French population. Br J Cancer 1996;74:288.
26. Aul C, Gattermann N, Schneider W: Age-related incidence and other epidemiological aspects of myelodysplastic syndromes. Br J Haematol 1992;82:358.
27. Cartwright RA: Incidence and epidemiology of the myelodysplastic syndromes. In Mufti GJ, Galton DAG (eds): The Myelodysplastic Syndromes. Edinburgh, Churchill Livingstone, 1992, p 23.
28. Reizenstein P, Dabrowski L: Increasing prevalence of the myelodysplastic syndrome. An international Delphi study. Anticancer Res 1991;11:1069.
29. Williamson PJ, Kruger AR, Reynolds PJ, et al: Establishing the incidence of myelodysplastic syndrome. Br J Haematol 1994;87(4):743-745.
30. Dacie JV, Smith MD, White JC, Mollin DL: Refractory normoblastic anaemia: A clinical and haematological study of seven cases. Br J Haematol 1959;5:56.
31. Prchal JT, Throckmorton DW, Carroll AJ III, et al: A common progenitor for human myeloid and lymphoid cells. Nature 1978;274:590.
32. Amenomori T, Tomonaga M, Jinnai I, et al: Cytogenetic and cytochemical studies on progenitor cells of primary acquired sideroblastic anemia (PASA): Involvement of multipotent myeloid stem cells in PASA clone and mosaicism with normal clone. Blood 1987;70:1367.
33. Abruzzese E, Buss D, Rainer R, et al: Study of clonality in myelodysplastic syndromes: Detection of trisomy 8 in bone marrow cell smears by fluorescence in situ hybridization [see comments]. Leuk Res 1996;20:551.
34. Kouides PA, Bennett JM: Transformation of chronic myelomonocytic leukemia to acute lymphoblastic leukemia: Case report and review of the literature of lymphoblastic transformation of myelodysplastic syndrome [review]. Am J Hematol 1995;49:157.
35. Inoue T, Hirabayashi Y, Sasaki H, et al: Model of myelodysplastic syndrome-like myelodysplasia that transforms into single lineage hemopoietic malignancies upon transplantation—Implications for pediatric myelodysplastic syndrome. Int J Pediatr Hematol Oncol 1997;4:221.
36. Lawrence HJ, Broudy VC, Magenis RE, et al: Cytogenetic evidence for involvement of B lymphocytes in acquired idiopathic sideroblastic anemias. Blood 1987;70:1003.
37. Janssen JW, Buschle M, Layton M, et al: Clonal analysis of myelodysplastic syndromes: Evidence of multipotent stem cell origin. Blood 1989;73:248.
38. Tefferi A, Thibodeau SN, Solberg LA Jr: Clonal studies in the myelodysplastic syndrome using X-linked restriction fragment length polymorphisms. Blood 1990;75:1770.
39. Gallagher A, Darley RL, Padua RA: The molecular basis of myelodysplastic syndromes [review]. Haematologica 1997;82:191.
40. Scott RE, Wille JJ Jr, Wier ML: Mechanisms for the initiation and promotion of carcinogenesis: A review and a new concept [review]. Mayo Clin Proc 1984;59:107.
41. Cole P, Sateren W, Delzell E: Epidemiologic perspectives on myelodysplastic syndromes and leukemia [review]. Leuk Res 1995;19:361.
42. Rosoff PM: Congenital bone marrow failure with myelodysplasia in siblings. J Pediatr Hematol/Oncol 1995;17:56.
43. Paul B, Reid MM, Davison EV, et al: Familial myelodysplasia: Progressive disease associated with emergency of monosomy 7. Br J Haematol 1987;65:321.
44. Luna-Fineman S, Shannon KM, Atwater SK, et al: Myelodysplastic and myeloproliferative disorders of childhood: A study of 167 patients. Blood 1999;93(2):459-466.
45. Okamoto T, Okada M, Mori A, et al: Correlation between immunological abnormalities and prognosis in myelodysplastic syndrome patients. Int J Hematol 1997;66:345.
46. Hamblin TJ: Immunological abnormalities in myelodysplastic syndromes [review]. Semin Hematol 1996;33:150.
47. Smith MT, Fanning EW: Report on the workshop entitled: Modeling chemically induced leukemia—Implications for benzene risk assessment. Leuk Res 1997;21:361.

48. Mitelman F, Nilsson PG, Brandt L: Fourth International Workshop on Chromosomes in Leukemia 1982: Correlation of karyotype and occupational exposure to potential mutagenic/carcinogenic agents in acute nonlymphocytic leukemia. Cancer Genet Cytogenet 1984;11:326.

49. Pasqualetti P, Casale R, Colantonio D, Collacciani A: Occupational risk for hematological malignancies. Am J Hematol 1991;38:147.

50. Pedersen-Bjergaard J: Radiotherapy- and chemotherapy-induced myelodysplasia and acute myeloid leukemia [review]. Leuk Res 1992;16:61.

51. Bjork J, Albin M, Mauritzson N, et al: Smoking and myelodysplastic syndromes. Epidemiology 2000;11(3):285–291.

52. Nisse C, Haguenoer JM, Grandbastien B, et al: Occupational and environmental risk factors of the myelodysplastic syndromes in the North of France. Br J Haematol 2001;112(4):927–935.

53. Karp JE, Smith MA: The molecular pathogenesis of treatment-induced (secondary) leukemias: Foundations for treatment and prevention [review]. Semin Oncol 1997;24:103.

54. van Leeuwen FE: Risk of acute myelogenous leukaemia and myelodysplasia following cancer treatment [review]. Baillieres Clin Haematol 1996;9:57.

55. Park DJ, Koeffler HP: Therapy-related myelodysplastic syndromes [review]. Semin Hematol 1996;33:256.

56. Rowley JD, Espinosa R, Wen M, et al: The relationship of prior therapy to balanced translocations in treatment related leukemia and myelodysplastic syndrome, Report of an international workshop. Blood(Suppl 1) 2000;96:826a,[abstract # 3571].

57. Urba WJ, Longo DL: Hodgkin's disease [review]. N Engl J Med 1992;326:678.

58. van Leeuwen FE, Somers R, Hart AA: Splenectomy in Hodgkin's disease and second leukaemias [letter]. Lancet 1987;2:210.

59. Cuzick J, Erskine S, Edelman D, Galton DA: A comparison of the incidence of the myelodysplastic syndrome and acute myeloid leukaemia following melphalan and cyclophosphamide treatment for myelomatosis. A report to the Medical Research Council's working party on leukaemia in adults. Br J Cancer 1987;55:523.

60. Taylor PR, Jackson GH, Lennard AL, et al: Low incidence of myelodysplastic syndrome following transplantation using autologous non-cryopreserved bone marrow. Leukemia 1997;11:1650.

61. Traweek ST, Slovak ML, Nademanee AP, et al: Myelodysplasia and acute myeloid leukemia occurring after autologous bone marrow transplantation for lymphoma [review]. Leuk Lymphoma 1996;20:365.

62. Shounan Y, MacKenzie K, Dolnikov A, et al: Myeloproliferative disease and myelodysplastic syndrome induced by transplantation of bone marrow cells expressing mutant p53. Leukemia 1997;11:1641.

63. Sandler ES, Friedman DJ, Mustafa MM, et al: Treatment of children with epipodophyllotoxin-induced secondary acute myeloid leukemia. Cancer 1997;79:1049.

64. Stine KC, Saylors RL, Sawyer JR, Becton DL: Secondary acute myelogenous leukemia following safe exposure to etoposide. J Clin Oncol 197;15:1583.

65. Pui CH, Ribeiro RC, Hancock ML, et al: Acute myeloid leukemia in children treated with epipodophyllotoxins for acute lymphoblastic leukemia. N Engl J Med 191;325:1682.

66. Pedersen-Bjergaard J, Philip P: Two different classes of therapy-related and de-novo acute myeloid leukemia? [review]. Cancer Genet Cytogenet 1991;55:119.

67. Pedersen-Bjergaard J, Pedersen M, Roulston D, Philip P: Different genetic pathways in leukemogenesis for patients presenting with therapy-related myelodysplasia and therapy-related acute myeloid leukemia. Blood 1995;86:3542.

68. Bennett JM, Zelenetz AD, Press OW, et al: Incidence of myelodysplastic syndromes (tMDS) and acute myeloid leukemia (tAML) in patients with low-grade non–Hodgkin's lymphoma (LG-NHL) treated with Bexxar™. Abstract # [1416]. Blood 2001;98(11):335a.

69. Larson RA, Wang Y, Banerjee M, et al: Prevalence of the inactivating 609C—>T polymorphism in the NAD(P)H:quinone oxidoreductase (NQO1) gene in patients with primary and therapy-related myeloid leukemia. Blood 1999;.94(2):803–807.

70. Naoe T, Takeyama K, Yokozawa T, et al: Analysis of genetic polymorphism in NQO1, GST-M1, GST-T1, and CYP3A4 in 469 Japanese patients with therapy-related leukemia/ myelodysplastic syndrome and de novo acute myeloid leukemia. Clin Cancer Res 2000;6(10):4091–4095.

71. Bogdanovic AD, Trpinac DP, Jankovic GM, et al: Incidence and role of apoptosis in myelodysplastic syndrome—Morphological and ultrastructural assessment. Leukemia 1997;11:656.

72. Raza A, Gezer S, Mundle S, et al: Apoptosis in bone marrow biopsy samples involving stromal and hematopoietic cells in 50 patients with myelodysplastic syndromes. Blood 1995;86:268.

73. Raza A, Mundle S, Iftikhar A, et al: Simultaneous assessment of cell kinetics and programmed cell death in bone marrow biopsies of myelodysplastics reveals extensive apoptosis as the probable basis for ineffective hematopoiesis. Am J Hematol 1995;48:143.

74. Raza A, Mundle S, Shetty V, et al: A paradigm shift in myelodysplastic syndromes [review]. Leukemia 1996; 10:1648.

75. Lepelley P, Campergue L, Grardel N, et al: Is apoptosis a massive process in myelodysplastic syndromes? Br J Haematol 1996;95: 368.

76. Magill MK, Macfarlane E, McMullin MF: Intramedullary apoptosis may simply be a correlate of ineffective hematopoiesis. Br J Haematol 1997;97(Suppl 1):17.

77. Yoshida Y, Anzai N, Kawabata H: Apoptosis in myelodysplasia: A paradox or paradigm [review]. Leuk Res 1995;19:887.

78. Rajapaksa R, Ginzton N, Rott LS, Greenberg PL: Altered oncoprotein expression and apoptosis in myelodysplastic syndrome marrow cells. Blood 1996;88:4275.

79. Culligan DJ, Cachia P, Whittaker J, Jacobs A, Padua RA: Clonal lymphocytes are detectable in only some cases of MDS. Br J Haematol 1992;81:346–352.

80. Barrett AJ, Saunthararajah Y, Molldrem J: Myelodysplastic syndrome and aplastic anemia—Distinct entities or diseases linked by a common pathophysiology? Semin Hematol 2000;37:15–29.

81. Smith MA, Smith JG. The occurrence subtype and significance of hematopoietic inhibitory T cells (HIT cells) in myelodysplasia: An in vitro study. Leuk Res 1991;5:597–601.

82. Molldrem JJ, Jiang YZ, Stetler-Stevenson MA, et al: Haematological response of patients with myelodysplastic syndrome to antithymocyte globulin is associated with a loss of lymphocyte-mediated inhibition of CFU-GM and alterations in T-cell receptor V beta profiles. Br J Haematol 1998;102:1314–1322.

83. Sugarawa T, Endo K, Shishido T, et al: T-cell mediated inhibition of erythropoiesis in myelodysplastic syndromes. Am J Hematol 1992;41:304–305.

84. Kitagawa M, Saito I, Kuwata T, et al: Overexpression of tumor necrosis factor (TNF)-alpha and interferon (IFN)-gamma by bone marrow cells from patients with myelodysplastic syndromes. Leukemia 1997;11:2049–2054.

85. Deeg HJ, Beckham C, Loken MR, et al: Negative regulators of hemopoiesis and stroma function in patients with myelodysplastic syndrome. Leuk Lymphoma 2000;37:405–414.

86. Verhoef GEG, De Schouwer P. Ceuppens JL, Van Damme J, Goossens W, Boogaerts MA. Measurement of serum cytokines levels in patients with myelodysplastic syndromes. Leukemia 1992;2:1268–1272.

87. Mundle SD, Venugopal P, Cartlidge JD, et al: Indication of an involvement of interleukin-1 beta converting enzyme-like protease in intramedullary apoptotic cell death in the bone marrow of patients with myelodysplastic syndromes. Blood 1996;88:2640.

88. Pruneri G, Bertolini F, Soligo D, et al: Angiogenesis in myelodysplastic syndromes. Br J Cancer 1999;81:1398–1401.

89. Bellamy WT, Richter L, Frutiger Y, Grogan TM: Expression of vascular endothelial growth factor and its receptors in hematopoietic malignancies. Cancer Res 1999;59:728–733.

90. Brunning RD, Bennett JM, Flandrin G, et al: Myelodysplastic syndromes. In Jaffe E, Harris N, Stein H (eds): Pathology and Genetics of Tumors of Haematopoietic and Lymphoid Tissue. Lyon, France, IARC Press, 2001, p 61.

91. Bennett JM: World Health Organization classification of the acute leukemias and myelodysplastic syndrome [review]. Int J Hematol 2000;72(2):131–133.

Specific Malignancies

III

92. Germing U, Gattermann N, Strupp C, et al: Validation of the WHO proposals for a new classification of primary myelodysplastic syndromes: A retrospective analysis of 1600 patients. Leuk Res 2000;24(12):983–992.

93. de Pree C, Cabrol C, Frossard JL, Beris P: Pseudoreticulocytosis in a case of myelodysplastic syndrome with translocation t(1; 14) (q42;<+>q32). Semin Hematol 1995;32:232.

94. Joosten E, Pelemans W, Hiele M, et al: Prevalence and causes of anaemia in a geriatric hospitalized population. Gerontology 1992;38:111.

95. Hamblin T: Clinical features of MDS [review]. Leuk Res 1992;16:89.

96. Najean Y, Lecompte T: Chronic pure thrombocytopenia in elderly patients. An aspect of the myelodysplastic syndrome. Cancer 1989;64:2506.

97. Menke DM, Colon-Otero G, Cockerill KJ, et al: Refractory thrombocytopenia. A myelodysplastic syndrome that may mimic immune thrombocytopenic purpura {see comments}. Am J Clin Pathol 1992;98:502.

98. Mathew P, Tefferi A, Dewald GW, et al: The 5q- syndrome: A single-institution study of 43 consecutive patients. Blood 1992;81:1040.

99. Van den Berghe H: The 5q- syndrome. Scand J Haematol 1986;45(Suppl):78.

100. Patel K, Kelsey P: Primary acquired sideroblastic anemia, thrombocytosis, and trisomy 8. Ann Hematol 1997;74:199.

101. Mansouri A, Lipschitz DA: Myelodysplastic syndromes in the elderly [review]. J Am Geriatr Soc 1992;40:386.

102. Michels SD, McKenna RW, Arthur DC, Brunning RD: Therapy-related acute myeloid leukemia and myelodysplastic syndrome: A clinical and morphologic study of 65 cases. Blood 1985;65:1364.

103. Bennett JM, Moloney WC, Greene MH, Boice JD Jr: Acute myeloid leukemia and other myelopathic disorders following treatment with alkylating agents. Hematol Pathol 1987;1:99.

104. Brito-Babapulle F, Catovsky D, Galton DA: Myelodysplastic relapse of de novo acute myeloid leukaemia with trilineage myelodysplasia: A previously unrecognized correlation. Br J Haematol 1988;68:411.

105. Goasguen JE, Matsuo T, Cox C, Bennett JM: Evaluation of the dysmyelopoiesis in 336 patients with de novo acute myeloid leukemia: Major importance of dysgranulopoiesis for remission and survival. Leukemia 1992;6:520.

106. Lima CSP, Vassalo J, Lorandmetze I, et al: The significance of trilineage myelodysplasia in de novo acute myeloblastic—Clinical and laboratory features. Haematologica 1997;28:85.

107. Hasle H, Kerndrup G, Jacobsen BB: Childhood myelodysplastic syndrome in Denmark: Incidence and predisposing conditions. Leukemia. 1995;9(9):1569–1572.

108. Hasle H, Wadsworth LD, Massing BG, et al: A population-based study of childhood myelodysplastic syndrome in British Columbia, Canada. Br J Haematol 1999;106(4):1027–1032.

109. Hasle H, Arico M, Basso G, et al: Myelodysplastic syndrome, juvenile myelomonocytic leukemia, and acute myeloid leukemia associated with complete or partial monosomy 7. European Working Group on MDS in Childhood (EWOG-MDS). Leukemia 1999;13(3):376–385.

110. Haas OA, Gadner H: Pathogenesis, biology, and management of myelodysplastic syndromes in children [review]. Semin Hematol 1996;33:225.

111. Lange BJ, Kobrinsky N, Barnard DR, et al: Distinctive demography, biology, and outcome of acute myeloid leukemia and myelodysplastic syndrome in children with Down syndrome: Children's Cancer Group Studies 2861 and 2891. Blood 1998;91(2):608–615.

112. Kaloutsi V, Kohlmeyer U, Maschek H, et al: Comparison of bone marrow and hematologic findings in patients with human immunodeficiency virus infection and those with myelodysplastic syndromes and infectious diseases. Am J Clin Pathol 1994;101:123.

113. Karcher DS, Frost AR: The bone marrow in human immunodeficiency virus (HIV)-related disease. Morphology and clinical correlation. Am J Clin Pathol 1991;95:63.

114. Harris CE, Biggs JC, Concannon AJ, Dodds AJ: Peripheral blood and bone marrow findings in patients with acquired immune deficiency syndrome. Pathology 1990;22:206.

115. Treacy M, Lai L, Costello C, Clark A: Peripheral blood and bone marrow abnormalities in patients with HIV related disease. Br J Haematol 1987;65:289.

116. Moreno Garcia M: Bone marrow in human immunodeficiency virus (HIV) infection: Morphological changes in the bone marrow in HIV infection [review] [in Spanish]. Sangre 1996;41:231.

117. Thiele J, Zirbes TK, Bertsch HP, et al: AIDS-related bone marrow lesions—Myelodysplastic features or predominant inflammatory-reactive changes (HIV-myelopathy)? A comparative morphometric study by immunohistochemistry with special emphasis on apoptosis and PCNA-labeling. Anal Cell Pathol 1996;11:141.

118. Rodriguez JN, Dieguez JC, Moreno MV, et al: Usefulness of bone marrow examination in patients with advanced HIV infection {in Spanish}. Rev Clin Esp 1996;196:213.

119. Moller T, Hasselbalch HC: Hematological changes associated with human immunodeficiency virus (HIV-1) infection [review] [in Danish]. Ugeskr Laeger 1993;155:1442.

120. Katsarou O, Terpos E, Patsouris E, et al: Myelodysplastic features in patients with long-term HIV infection and haemophilia. Haemophilia 2001;7(1):47–52.

121. Siddiqui T, Elfenbein GJ, Noyes WD, et al: Myelodysplastic syndromes presenting in pregnancy. A report of five cases and the clinical outcome. Cancer 1990;66:377.

122. Steensma DP, Tefferi A: Myelodysplastic syndrome and pregnancy: The Mayo Clinic experience. Leuk Lymphoma 2001;42(6):1229–1234.

123. Pomeroy C, Oken MM, Rydell RE, Filice GA: Infection in the myelodysplastic syndromes. Am J Med 1991;90:338.

124. Ruutu P: Granulocyte function in myelodysplastic syndromes [review]. Scand J Haematol Suppl 1986;45:66.

125. Boogaerts MA, Nelissen V, Roelant C, Goossens W: Blood neutrophil function in primary myelodysplastic syndromes. Br J Haematol 1983;55:217.

126. Williamson PJ, Oscier DG, Mufti GJ, Hamblin TJ: Pyogenic abscesses in the myelodysplastic syndrome. BMJ 1989;299:375.

127. Tsukada H, Chou T, Ishizuka Y, et al: Disseminated *Mycobacterium avium-intracellulare* infection in a patient with myelodysplastic syndrome (refractory anemia). Am J Hematol 1994;45:325.

128. Ong KR, Sordillo E, Frankel E: Unusual case of *Aeromonas hydrophila* endocarditis. J Clin Microbiol 1991;29:1056.

129. Oken MM, Pomeroy C, Weisdorf D, Bennett JM: Prophylactic antibiotics for the prevention of early infection in multiple myeloma. Am J Med 1996;100:624.

130. Ganser A, Hoelzer D: Clinical use of hematopoietic growth factors in the myelodysplastic syndromes [review]. Semin Hematol 1996;33:186.

131. Schuster MW, Thompson JA, Larson R, et al: Randomized trial of subcutaneous granulocyte-macrophage colony stimulating factor versus observation in patients with myelodysplastic syndrome or aplastic anemia. Proc Am Soc Clin Oncol 1990;9:205a.

132. Greenberg P, Taylor K, Koeffler P, et al: Phase III randomized multicenter trial of G-CSF vs. observation for myelodysplastic syndromes. Blood 1993;82(Suppl 1):196a.

133. Raman BK, Van Slyck EJ, Riddle J, et al: Platelet function and structure in myeloproliferative disease, myelodysplastic syndrome, and secondary thrombocytosis. Am J Clin Pathol 1989;91:64.

134. Mori H, Niikura H, Terada H, Fujita K: Morphological analysis of the megakaryocytes in myelodysplastic syndrome [in Japanese]. Rinsho Byori 1990;38:1347.

135. Green AR, Shuttleworth D, Bowen DT, Bentley DP: Cutaneous vasculitis in patients with myelodysplasia [see comments]. Br J Haematol 1990;74:364.

136. Kohli M, Bennett RM: An association of polymyalgia rheumatica with myelodysplastic syndromes. J Rheumatol 1994;21:1357.

137. Billstrom R, Johansson H, Johansson B, Mitelman F: Immune-mediated complications in patients with myelodysplastic syndromes—Clinical and cytogenetic features. Eur J Haematol 1995;55:42.

138. Pendry K, Harrison C, Geary CG: Myelodysplasia presenting as autoimmune haemolytic anaemia [letter]. Br J Haematol 1991;79:133.

139. Mufti GJ, Figes A, Hamblin TJ, et al: Immunological abnormalities in myelodysplastic syndromes. I. Serum immunoglobulins and autoantibodies. Br J Haematol 1986;63:143.

140. Olive A, del Blanco J, Pons M, et al: The clinical spectrum of remitting seronegative symmetrical synovitis with pitting edema. The Catalan Group for the Study of RS3PE [see comments]. J Rheumatol 1997;24:333.

141. Chandran G, Ahern MJ, Seshadri P, Coghlan D: Rheumatic manifestations of the myelodysplastic syndromes: A comparative study. Aust N Z J Med 1996;26:683.

142. George SW, Newman ED: Seronegative inflammatory arthritis in the myelodysplastic syndromes [review]. Semin Arthritis Rheum 1992;21:345.

143. Enright H, Jacob HS, Vercellotti G, et al: Paraneoplastic autoimmune phenomena in patients with myelodysplastic syndromes: Response to immunosuppressive therapy. Br J Haematol 1995;91:403.

144. Castellote J, Porta F, Tuset E, Salinas R: Crohns-disease and the myelodysplastic syndrome. J Clin Gastroenterol 1997;24:286.

145. Eng C, Farraye FA, Shulman LN, et al: The association between the myelodysplastic syndromes and Crohn disease. Ann Intern Med 1992;117:661.

146. Sahay R, Prangnell DR, Scott BB: Inflammatory bowel disease and refractory anaemia (myelodysplasia). Gut 1993;34:1630.

147. Copplestone JA, Mufti GJ, Hamblin TJ, Oscier DG: Immunological abnormalities in myelodysplastic syndromes. II. Coexistent lymphoid or plasma cell neoplasms: A report of 20 cases unrelated to chemotherapy. Br J Haematol 1986;63:149.

148. Sans-Sabrafen J, Buxo-Costa J, Woessner S, et al: Myelodysplastic syndromes and malignant solid tumors: Analysis of 21 cases. Am J Hematol 1992;41:1.

149. Bartl R, Frisch B, Baumgart R: Morphologic classification of the myelodysplastic syndromes (MDS): Combined utilization of bone marrow aspirates and trephine biopsies. Leuk Res 1992;16:15.

150. Tham KT, Cousar JB, Macon WR: Silver stain for ringed sideroblasts. A sensitive method that differs from Perls' reaction in mechanism and clinical application. Am J Clin Pathol 1990;94:73.

151. Scott CS, Cahill A, Bynoe AG, et al: Esterase cytochemistry in primary myelodysplastic syndromes and megaloblastic anaemias: Demonstration of abnormal staining patterns associated with dysmyelopoiesis. Br J Haematol 1983;55:411.

152. Seo IS, Li CY, Yam LT: Myelodysplastic syndrome: Diagnostic implications of cytochemical and immunocytochemical studies. Mayo Clin Proc 1993;8:47.

153. Davey FR, Erber WN, Gatter KC, Mason DY: Abnormal neutrophils in acute myeloid leukemia and myelodysplastic syndrome. Hum Pathol 1988;19:454.

154. Kawaguchi M, Nehashi Y, Aizawa S, Toyama K: Comparative study of immunocytochemical staining versus Giemsa stain for detecting dysmegakaryopoiesis in myelodysplastic syndromes (MDS) [published erratum appears in Eur J Haematol 45(2):125]. Eur J Haematol 1990;44:89.

155. Thiele J, Hoffmann I, Bertsch HP, Fischer R: Myelodysplastic syndromes: Immunohistochemical and morphometric evaluation of proliferative activity in erythropoiesis and endoreduplicative capacity of megakaryocytes. Virchows Arch A Pathol Anat Histopathol 1993;423:33.

156. Bennett JM, Catovsky D, Daniel MT, et al: Criteria for the diagnosis of acute leukemia of megakaryocyte lineage (M7). A report of the French-American-British Cooperative Group. Ann Intern Med 1985;103:460.

157. Cuneo A, Fagioli F, Pazzi I, et al: Morphologic, immunologic and cytogenetic studies in acute myeloid leukemia following occupational exposure to pesticides and organic solvents. Leuk Res 1992;16:789.

158. Jensen IM, Hokland P: The proliferative activity of myelopoiesis in myelodysplasia evaluated by multiparameter flow cytometry. Br J Haematol 1994;87:477.

159. Guyotat D, Campos L, Thomas X, et al: Myelodysplastic syndromes: A study of surface markers and in vitro growth patterns. Am J Hematol 1990;34:26.

160. Soligo DA, Oriani A, Annaloro C, et al: CD34 immunohisto-chemistry of bone marrow biopsies: Prognostic significance in primary myelodysplastic syndromes. Am J Hematol 1994; 46:9.

161. Oertel J, Oertel B, Beyer J, Huhn D: CD 34 immunotyping of blasts in myelodysplasia. Ann Hematol 1994;68:77.

162. Min YH, Lee ST, Min DW, et al: CD34 immunohistochemical staining of bone marrow biopsies in myelodysplastic syndromes. Yonsei Med 195;J36:1.

163. Sonneveld P, van Dongen JJ, Hagemeijer A, et al: High expression of the multidrug resistance P-glycoprotein in high-risk myelodysplasia is associated with immature phenotype. Leukemia 1993;7:963.

164. List AF, Spier CM, Cline A, et al: Expression of the multidrug resistance gene product (P-glycoprotein) in myelodysplasia is associated with a stem cell phenotype. Br J Haematol 1991;78:28.

165. Stetler-Stevenson M, Arthur DC, Jabbour N, et al: Diagnostic utility of flow cytometric immunophenotyping in myelodysplastic syndrome. Blood 2001;98(4):979–987.

166. Maschek H, Gutzmer R, Choritz H, Georgii A: Life expectancy in primary myelodysplastic syndromes: A prognostic score based upon histopathology from bone marrow biopsies of 569 patients. Eur J Haematol 1994;53:280.

167. Winfield DA, Polacarz SV: Bone marrow histology 3: Value of bone marrow core biopsy in acute leukaemia, myelodysplastic syndromes, and chronic myeloid leukaemia [see comments]. J Clin Pathol 1992;45:855.

168. Tricot G, De Wolf-Peeters C, Hendrickx B, Verwilghen RL: Bone marrow histology in myelodysplastic syndromes. I. Histological findings in myelodysplastic syndromes and comparison with bone marrow smears. Br J Haematol 1984;57:423.

169. Tricot G, De Wolf-Peeters C, Vlietinck R, Verwilghen RL: Bone marrow histology in myelodysplastic syndromes. II. Prognostic value of abnormal localization of immature precursors in MDS. Br J Haematol 1984;58:217.

170. Brunning RD, McKenna RW, Rosai J, et al: Tumors of the bone marrow. Washington, DC, Armed Forces Institute of Pathology, 1994.

171. Bellamy WT, Richter L, Sirjani D, et al: Vascular endothelial cell growth factor is an autocrine promoter of abnormal localized immature myeloid precursors and leukemia progenitor formation in myelodysplastic syndromes. Blood 2001;97(5):1427–1434.

172. Rios A, Canizo MC, Sanz MA, et al: Bone marrow biopsy in myelodysplastic syndromes: Morphological characteristics and contribution to the study of prognostic factors. Br J Haematol 1990;75:26.

173. Lambertenghi-Deliliers G, Orazi A, Luksch R, et al: Myelodysplastic syndrome with increased marrow fibrosis: A distinct clinico-pathological entity [see comments]. Br J Haematol 1991;78:161.

174. Ohyashiki K, Sasao I, Ohyashiki JH, et al: Clinical and cytogenetic characteristics of myelodysplastic syndromes developing myelofibrosis. Cancer 1991;68:178.

175. Takahashi M, Koike T, Nagayama R, et al: Myelodysplastic syndrome with myelofibrosis: Myelodysplastic syndrome as a major primary disorder for acute myelofibrosis. Clin Lab Haematol 1991;13:17.

176. Maschek H, Georgii A, Kaloutsi V, et al: Myelofibrosis in primary myelodysplastic syndromes: A retrospective study of 352 patients. Eur J Haematol 1992;48:208.

177. Pagliuca A, Layton DM, Manoharan A, et al: Myelofibrosis in primary myelodysplastic syndromes: A clinico-morphological study of 10 cases [see comments]. Br J Haematol 1989;71:499.

178. Watts EJ, Majer RV, Green PJ, Mavor WO: Hyperfibrotic myelodysplasia: A report of three cases showing haematological remission following treatment with prednisolone [see comments]. Br J Haematol 1991;78:120.

179. Ho PJ, Gibson J, Vincent P, Joshua D: The myelodysplastic syndromes: Diagnostic criteria and laboratory evaluation [review]. Pathology 1993;25:297.

180. Maschek H, Kaloutsi V, Rodriguez-Kaiser M, et al: Hypoplastic myelodysplastic syndrome: Incidence, morphology, cytogenetics, and prognosis. Ann Hematol 1993;66:117.

181. Toyama K, Ohyashiki K, Yoshida Y, et al: Clinical and cytogenetic findings of myelodysplastic syndromes showing hypocellular bone marrow or minimal dysplasia, in comparison with typical myelodysplastic syndromes. Int J Hematol 1993;58:53.

182. Nand S, Godwin JE: Hypoplastic myelodysplastic syndrome. Cancer 1988;62:958.

183. Fohlmeister I, Fischer R, Modder B, et al: Aplastic anaemia and the hypocellular myelodysplastic syndrome: Histomorphological, diagnostic, and prognostic features. J Clin Pathol 1985;38:1218.

184. Tuzuner N, Cox C, Rowe JM, et al: Hypocellular myelodysplastic syndromes (MDS): New proposals. Br J Haematol 1995;91:612.

185. Yoshida Y, Oguma H, Maekawa T: Refractory myelodysplastic anemias with hypocellular bone marrow. J Clin Pathol 1995;41:763.

186. Orazi A, Albitar M, Heerema NA, et al: Hypoplastic myelodysplastic syndromes can be distinguished from acquired aplastic anemia by CD34 and PCNA immunostaining of bone marrow biopsy specimens [see comments]. Am J Clin Pathol 1997;107:268.

187. Howe RB, Bloomfield CD, McKenna RW: Hypocellular acute leukemia. Am J Med 1982;72:391.

188. Nagai K, Kohno T, Chen YX, et al: Diagnostic criteria for hypocellular acute leukemia: A clinical entity distinct from overt acute leukemia and myelodysplastic syndrome. Leuk Res 1996;20:563.

189. Fenaux P, Morel P, Lai JL: Cytogenetics of myelodysplastic syndromes [review]. Semin in Hematol 1996;33:127.

190. Mufti GJ: Chromosomal deletions in the myelodysplastic syndrome [review]. Leuk Res 1992;16:35.

191. Anastasi J: Molecular cytogenetics and the myelodysplastic syndromes [comment] [review]. Leuk Res 1996;20:559.

192. Iwabuchi A, Ohyashiki K, Ohyashiki JH, et al: Trisomy of chromosome 8 in myelodysplastic syndrome. Significance of the fluctuating trisomy 8 population. Cancer Genet Cytogenet 1992;62:70.

193. Broun ER, Heerema NA, Tricot G: Spontaneous remission in myelodysplastic syndrome. A case report. Cancer Genet Cytogenet 1990;46:125.

194. Shepherd L, Cameron C, Galbraith P, et al: Absence of allelic loss on chromosome 5q by RFLP analysis in preleukemia. Leuk Res 1991;15:297.

195. Ohyashiki K, Ohyashiki JH, Iwabuchi A, Toyama K: Clinical aspects, cytogenetics and disease evolution in myelodysplastic syndromes [review]. Leuk Lymphoma 1996;23:409.

196. Johansson B, Mertens F, Mitelman F: Geographic heterogeneity of neoplasia-associated chromosome aberrations [see comments]. Genes Chromosomes Cancer 1991;3:1.

197. Johansson B, Billstrom R, Kristoffersson U, et al: Deletion of chromosome arm 3p in hematologic malignancies. Leukemia 1997;11:1207.

198. Kurtin PJ, Dewald GW, Shields DJ, Hanson CA: Hematologic disorders associated with deletions of chromosome 20q: A clinicopathologic study of 107 patients. Am J Clin Pathol 1996;106:680.

199. Juneja HS, Jodhani M, Gardner FH, et al: Low-dose ARA-C consistently induces hematologic responses in the clinical 5q- syndrome. Am J Hematol 1994;46:338.

200. Gallagher A, Darley R, Padua RA: RAS and the myelodysplastic syndromes {review}. Pathol Biol 1997;45(7):561–568.

201. Fenaux P, Preudhomme C: Molecular abnormalities and clonality in myelodysplastic syndromes [review]. Pathol Biol 1997;45(7):556–560.

202. Rowinsky EK, Windle JJ, Von Hoff DD: Ras protein farnesyltransferase: A strategic target for anticancer therapeutic development. J Clin Oncol 1999;17:3631–3652.

203. Greenberg PL: Biologic and clinical implications of marrow culture studies in the myelodysplastic syndromes [review]. Semin Hematol 1996;33:163.

204. Allen RH, Lindenbaum J, Stabler SP: High prevalence of cobalamin deficiency in the elderly [review]. Trans Am Clin Climatol Assoc 1995;107:37.

205. Rezuke WN, Anderson C, Pastuszak WT, et al: Arsenic intoxication presenting as a myelodysplastic syndrome: A case report. Am J Hematol 1991;36:291.

206. Castello A, Coci A, Magrini U: Paraneoplastic marrow alterations in patients with cancer. Haematologica 1992;77:392.

207. Clatch RJ, Krigman HR, Peters MG, Zutter MM: Dysplastic haemopoiesis following orthotopic liver transplantation: Comparison with similar changes in HIV infection and primary myelodysplasia. Br J Haematol 1994;88:685.

208. Hadnagy C, Laszlo GA: Acquired dyserythropoiesis in liver disease. Br J Haematol 1991;78:283.

209. Hamblin T: Minimal diagnostic criteria for the myelodysplastic syndrome in clinical practice. Leuk Res 1992;16:3.

210. Boogaerts MA, Verhoef GE, Demuynck H: Treatment and prognostic factors in myelodysplastic syndromes [review]. Baillieres Clin Haematol 1996;9:161.

211. Anttila P, Ihalainen J, Salo A, et al: Idiopathic macrocytic anaemia in the aged: Molecular and cytogenetic findings. Br J Haematol 1995;90:797.

212. Mufti GJ: A guide to risk assessment in the primary myelodysplastic syndrome [review]. Hematol Oncol Clin North Am 1992;6:587.

213. Greenberg P, Cox C, LeBeau MM, et al: International scoring system for evaluating prognosis in myelodysplastic syndromes. Blood 1997;89:2079.

214. Cheson BD, Bennett JM, Kantarjian H, et al: Report of an international working group to standardize response criteria for myelodysplastic syndromes. Blood 2000;96(12):3671–3674.

215. Rose C, Wattel E, Bastion Y, et al: Treatment with very low-dose GM-CSF in myelodysplastic syndromes with neutropenia. A report on 28 cases. Leukemia 1994;8:1458.

216. Shuster MW, Larson RA, Thompson JA, et al: GM-CSF for myelodyplastic syndrome: Results of multicenter randomized controlled trial [abstract]. Blood 1990;76:318.

217. Shuster MW, Thompson JA, Larson B, et al: Randomized phase II study of recombinant human GMCSF in patients with neutropenia secondary to MDS [abstract]. Blood 1995;86(Suppl 1):338.

218. Greenberg P, Taylor K, Larson et al: Phase III randomized multicenter trial of G-CSF Vs observation for MDS [abstract]. Blood 1994;82 (Suppl):196.

219. Hellström-Lindberg E: Efficacy of erythropoietin in the myelodysplastic syndromes. An analysis of 205 patients in 17 studies. Br J Haematol 1995;89:67–71.

220. Rose EH, Abels RI, Nelson RA, McCullough DM, Lessin L: The use of r-HuEpo in the treatment of anemia related to myelodysplasia (MDS). Br J Haematol 1995;89:831–837.

221. Italian Cooperative Study Group for rHuEpo in Myelodysplastic Syndromes: A randomized double-blind placebo-controlled study with subcutaneous recombinant human erythropoietin in patients with low-risk myelodyplastic syndromes. Br J Haematol 1998;103:1070–1074.

222. Rodriguez JN, Dieguez JC, Muniz R, et al: Human recombinant erythropoietin in the treatment of myelodysplastic syndromes anemia [in Spanish]. Sangre 1994;39:435–439.

223. Chiba S, Inamori K, Mitani K, et al: Marked and reproducible increase in trilineage blood cell counts by administration of granulocyte colony-stimulating factor in a patient with refractory anaemia with excess blasts in transformation. Br J Haematol 1994;86:665.

224. Perugini O, Montanari G, Nalli G: Trilineage response to granulocyte colony-stimulating factor administration in a patient with myelodysplastic syndrome. Haematologica 1995;80:234.

225. Takahashi M, Yoshida Y, Kaku K, et al: Phase II study of recombinant human granulocyte-macrophage colony-stimulating factor in myelodysplastic syndrome and aplastic anemia. Acta Haematol 1993;89:189.

226. Negrin RS, Stein R, Doherty K, et al: Maintenance treatment of the anemia of myelodysplastic syndromes with recombinant human granulocyte colony-stimulating factor and erythropoietin: Evidence for in vivo synergy. Blood 1996;87:4076–4081.

227. Hellström-Lindberg E, Tangen JM, Grimfors G, et al: Treatment of the anemia in myelodysplastic syndromes with granulocyte-CSF plus erythropoietin: Results from a randomized phase II study and long-term follow-up on 71 patients. Blood 1998;2:68–75.

228. Remacha AF, Arrizabalaga B, Villegas A, et al: Erythropoietin plus granulocyte colony-stimulating factor in the treatment of myelodysplastic syndromes. Identification of a subgroup of responders. The Spanish Erythropathology Group. Haematologica 1999;84:1058–1064.

229. Thompson JA, Gilliland DG, Prchal JT, et al: Effect of recombinant human erythropoietin combined with granulocyte/macrophage colony-stimulating factor in the treatment of patients with myelodysplastic syndromes. Blood 2000;95:1175–1179.

230. Miller AM, Noyes WE, Taetle R, List AF. Limited erythropoietic response to combined treatment with recombinant human interleukin 3 and erythropoietin in myelodysplastic syndromes. Leukemia Res 1999;23:77–83.

231. Kuzrock R, Cortes J, Thomas DA, et al: Pilot study of low dose interleukin 11 in patients with bone marrow failure. JCO 2001;19(21):4165–4172.

232. Bagby GC Jr, Gabourel JD, Linman JW: Glucocorticoid therapy in the preleukemic syndrome (hemopoietic dysplasia): Identification of responsive patients using in-vitro techniques. Ann Intern Med 1980;92:55–58.

233. Molldrem JJ, Caples M, Mavroudis D, et al: Antithymocyte globulin for patients with myelodysplastic syndrome. Br J Haematol 1997;99:690–705.

234. Jonasova A, Neuwirtova R, Cermak J, et al: Cyclosporin A therapy in hypoplastic patients with MDS and certain refractory anaemias without hypoplastic bone marrow. Br J Haematol 1998;100:304–309.

235. Raza A, Qawi H, Lisak L, et al: Patients with myelodysplastic syndromes benefit from palliative therapy with amifostine, pentoxifylline, and ciprofloxacin with or without dexamethasone. Blood 2000;95:1580–1587.

236. Nemunaitis J, Rosenfeld C, Getty L, et al: Rentoxifylline and ciproloxacin in patients with myelodysplastic syndrome. A phase II trial. Am J Clin Oncol 1995;18:189–193.

237. List AF, Brasfield F, Heaton R, et al: Stimulation of hematopoiesis by amifostine in patients with myelodysplastic syndrome. Blood 1997;90:3364–3369.

238. List AF, Holmes H, Greenberg PL, Bennett JM, Oster W: Phase II study of amifostine in patients with myelodysplastic syndromes (MDS) {abstract}. Blood 1999;94:305a.

239. Deeg HJ, Gotlib J, Beckham C, et al: Soluble TNF receptor fusion protein (etanercept) for the treatment of myelodysplastic syndrome: A pilot study. Leukemia 2000;16(2):162–164.

240. Maciejewski JP, Ristiano AM, Sloand EM, et al: A pilot study of the recombinant soluble human tumour necrosis factor receptor (p75)-Fc fusion protein in patients with myelodysplastic syndrome. Br J Haematol 2002;117(1):119–126.

241. Amato RJ, Loughnan MS, Flynn E, Folkman J: Thalidomide is an inhibitor of angiogenesis. Proc Nat Acad Sci USA 1994;91:4082–4085.

242. Aguayo A, Kantarjian H, Manshouri T, et al: Angiogenesis in acute and chronic leukemias and myelodysplastic syndromes. Blood 2000;96(6):2240–2245.

243. Hugh SM, Rifkin IR, Deighton J, et al: The immunosuppressive drug thalidomide induces T-helper cell type 2 (Th2) and concomitantly inhibits Th1 cytokine production in mito-gen and antigen stimulated human peripheral blood mononuclear cell cultures. Clin Exp Immunol 1995;99:160–167.

244. Sampaio EP, Sarno EN, Galilly R, Cohn ZA, Kaplan G: Thalidomide selectively inhibits tumor necrosis factor alpha production by stimulated human monocytes [abstract]. J Exp Med 1991;173:699–703.

245. Raza A, Meyer P, Lisak L, et al: Thalidomide produces transfusion independence in long-standing refractory anemias of patients with myelodysplastic syndromes. Blood 2001;98(4):958–965.

246. Dourado CMC, Seixas-Silva J, Besa EC: Response to thalidomide in 9 patients with myelodysplastic syndrome: A promising treatment for early and post chemotherapy in late froms of MDS. Blood 2000;96:260b.

247. Thomas DA, Aguayo A, Estey E, et al: thalidomide as anti-angiogenesis therapy (RX) in refractory and relapsed leukemias. Blood 1999;94:2269a.

248. Strupp C, Germing U, Aivado M, Misgeld E, et al: Thalidomide for the treatment of patients with myelodysplastic syndromes. Leukemia 2002;16(1):1–6.

249. Raza A, Dutt D, Lisak L, et al: Combination of thalidomide and enbrel for the treatment of patients with myelodysplastic syndromes (MDS) [abstract]. Blood 2001;98(11):273–274b.

250. Fabbri A, Biscardi M, Innocenti F, et al: Thalidomide in combination with amifostine in the treatment of MDS: evaluation of clinical and laboratory findings [abstract]. Blood 2001;98(11):271b.

251. Raza A, Lisak L, Dutt D, et al: Combination of thalidomide with pentoxifylline, ciprofloxacin, and dexamethasone (pcd) in patients with myelodysplastic syndromes (MDS) [abstract]. Blood 2001;98(11):273b.

252. Letendre L, Levitt R, Pierre RV, et al: Myelodysplastic syndrome treatment with danazol and cis-retinoic acid. Am J Hematol 1995;48:233.

253. Bourantas KL, Tsiara S, Christou L: Treatment of 34 patients with myelodysplastic syndromes with 13-CIS retinoic acid. Eur J Haematol 1995;55:235.

254. Kurzrock R, Estey E, Talpaz M: All-trans retinoic acid: Tolerance and biologic effects in myelodysplastic syndrome. J Clin Oncol 1993;11:1489.

255. Cambier N, Wattel E, Menot ML, et al: All-trans retinoic acid in adult chronic myelomonocytic leukemia: Results of a pilot study. Leukemia 1996;10:1164.

256. Andreeff M, Stone R, Michaeli J, et al: Hexamethylene bisacetamide in myelodysplastic syndrome and acute myelogenous leukemia: A phase II clinical trial with a differentiation-inducing agent. Blood 1992;80:2604.

257. Rowinsky EK, Donehower RC, Spivak JL, et al: Effects of the differentiating agent hexamethylene bisacetamide on normal and myelodysplastic hematopoietic progenitors. J Natl Cancer Inst 1990;82:1926.

258. Gore SD, Samid D, Weng LJ: Impact of the putative differentiating agents sodium phenylbutyrate and sodium phenylacetate on proliferation, differentiation, and apoptosis of primary neoplastic myeloid cells. Clin Cancer Res 1997;3(10):1755–1762.

259. Gore SD, Weng LJ, Figg WD, et al: Impact of prolonged infusions of the putative differentiating agent sodium phenylbutyrate on myelodysplastic syndromes and acute myeloid leukemia. Clin Cancer Res 2002;8(4):963–970.

260. Timonen TT, Kauma H. Therapeutic effect of heme arginate in myelodysplastic syndromes. Eur J Haematol 1992;49(5):234–238.

261. Petti MC, Latagliata R, Avvisati G, et al: Treatment of high-risk myelodysplastic syndromes with lymphoblastoid alpha interferon. Br J Haematol 1996;95:364.

262. Takeda Y, Sawada H, Sawai H, et al: Acquired hypochromic and microcytic sideroblastic anaemia responsive to pyridoxine with low value of free erythrocyte protoporphyrin: A possible subgroup of idiopathic acquired sideroblastic anaemia (IASA). Br J Haematol 1995;90(1):207–209.

263. Januszewicz EH, Firkin FC: Differentiation in acute myeloid leukemia and myelodysplastic disorders. Is differentiation-induction therapy possible? [review]. Aust N Z J Med 1988;18:705.

264. Miller KB, Kim K, Morrison FS, et al: The evaluation of low-dose cytarabine in the treatment of myelodysplastic syndromes: A phase-III intergroup study [published erratum appears in Ann Hematol 1993;66(3):164]. Ann Hematol 1992;65:162.

265. Cheson BD, Jasperse DM, Simon R, Friedman MA: A critical appraisal of low-dose cytosine arabinoside in patients with acute non-lymphocytic leukemia and myelodysplastic syndromes [review]. J Clin Oncol 1986;4:1857.

266. Kuriya S, Murai K, Miyairi Y, et al: A combination chemotherapy with low doses of cytarabine and etoposide for high risk myelodysplastic syndromes and their leukemic stage. A pilot study. Cancer 1996;78:422.

267. Munshi NC, Tricot GJ: Single weekly cytosine arabinoside and oral 6-thioguanine in patients with myelodysplastic syndrome and acute myeloid leukemia. Ann Hematol 1997;74:111.

268. Im T, Yamane T, Mugitani A, et al: Treatment with cytosine arabinoside and granulocyte colony-stimulating factor in patients with myelodysplastic syndrome and its leukemic phase. Int J Hematol 1994;60:215.

269. Gerhartz HH, Zwierzina HH, Walther J, et al: Interleukin-3 plus low-dose cytosine arabinoside for advanced myelodysplasia: A pilot study. EORTC Leukemia Group. Cancer Invest 1996;14:299.

270. Omoto E, Deguchi S, Takaba S, et al: Low-dose melphalan for treatment of high-risk myelodysplastic syndromes. Leukemia 1996;10:609–614.

271. Denzlinger C, Benz D, Bowen D, Gelly K, Brugger W, Kanz L: Low-dose melphalan induces favourable responses in elderly patients with high risk myelodysplastic syndromes or secondary leukemia. Br J Haem 2000;108:93–95.

272. Feldman FJ, Seiter KP, Ahmed T, et al: Homoharringtonine in patients with myelodysplastic syndrome (MDS) and MDS evolving to acute myeloid leukemia. Leukemia 1996;10:40–42.

Specific Malignancies

III

273. Ganser A, Heil G, Kolbe K, et al: Aggressive chemotherapy combined with G-CSF and maintenance therapy with interleukin-2 for patients with advanced myelodysplastic syndrome, subacute or secondary acute myeloid leukemia—Initial results. Ann Hematol 1993;66:123.

274. Economopoulos T, Papageorgiou E, Stathakis N, et al: Treatment of high risk myelodysplastic syndrome with idarubicin and cytosine arabinoside supported by granulocyte-macrophage colony-stimulating factor (GM-CSF). Leuk Res 1996;20:385.

275. Gassmann W, Schmitz N, Loffler H, De Witte T: Intensive chemotherapy and bone marrow transplantation for myelodysplastic syndromes [review]. Semin Hematol 1996;33:196.

276. Estey E, Thall P, Beran M, et al: Effect of diagnosis refractory anemia with excess blasts, refractory anemia with excess blasts in transformation, or acute myeloid leukemia [AML] on outcome of AML-type chemotherapy. Blood 1997;90:2969.

277. Bernstein SH, Brunetto VL, Davey FR, et al: Acute myeloid leukemia-type chemotherapy for newly diagnosed patients without antecedent cytopenias having myelodysplastic syndrome as defined by French-American-British criteria: A Cancer and Leukemia Group B Study. J Clin Oncol 1996;14:2486.

278. Ruutu T, Hanninen A, Jarventie G, et al: Intensive chemotherapy of poor prognosis myelodysplastic syndrome (MDS) and acute myeloid leukemia following MDS with idarubicin and cytarabine. Leuk Res 1997;21:133.

279. Beran M, Estey E, O'Brien SM, et al: Results of topotecan single-agent therapy in patients with myelodysplastic syndromes and chronic myelomonocytic leukemia. Leuk Lymphoma 1998; 31(5–6):521–531.

280. Beran M, Estey E, O'Brien S, et al: Topotecan and cytarabine is an active combination regimen in myelodysplastic syndromes and chronic myelomonocytic leukemia. J Clin Oncol 1999;17(9): 2819–2830.

281. Beran M, Shen Y, Kantarjian H, et al: High-dose chemotherapy in high-risk myelodysplastic syndrome: Covariate-adjusted comparison of five regimens. Cancer 2001;92(8):1999–2015.

282. Lee ST, Hahn JS, Ko YW, et al: Idarubicin, cytarabine, and topotecan in patients with refractory or relapsed acute myelogenous leukemia and high-risk myelodysplastic syndrome [abstract]. Blood 2001;98(11):215b.

283. Beran M, Cortes JE, O'Brien S, et al: Phase I study of prolonged administration of oral topotecan in hematological malignancies [abstract]. Blood 2001;98(11):624a.

284. Appelbaum FR, Anderson J: Allogeneic bone marrow transplantation for myelodysplastic syndromes: Outcomes analysis according to IPSS score. Leukemia 1998;12(Suppl 1):25–29.

285. Anderson JE, Appelbaum FR, Schoch G, et al: Allogeneic marrow transplantation for refractory anemia: A comparison of two preparative regimens and analysis of prognostic factors. Blood 1996;87:51.

286. Anderson JE, Appelbaum FR, Fisher LD, et al: Allogeneic bone marrow transplantation for 93 patients with myelodysplastic syndrome. Blood 1993;82:677.

287. Deeg HJ, Shulman HM, Anderson JE, et al: Allogeneic and syngeneic marrow transplantation for myelodysplastic syndrome in patients 55 to 66 years of age. Blood 2000;15;95(4):1188–1194.

288. Anderson JE, Anasetti C, Appelbaum FR, et al: Unrelated donor marrow transplantation for myelodysplasia (MDS) and MDS-related acute myeloid leukaemia. Br J Haematol 1996;93(1):59–67.

289. Runde V, de Witte T, Arnold R, et al: Bone marrow transplantation from HLA-identical siblings as first-line treatment in patients with myelodysplastic syndromes: Early transplantation is associated with improved outcome. Chronic Leukemia Working Party of the European Group for Blood and Marrow Transplantation. Bone Marrow Transplant 1998;21(3):255–261.

290. Arnold R, de Witte T, van Biezen A, et al: Unrelated bone marrow transplantation in patients with myelodysplastic syndromes and secondary acute myeloid leukemia: An EBMT survey. European Blood and Marrow Transplantation Group. Bone Marrow Transplant 1998;21(12):1213–1216.

291. Anderson JE, Gooley TA, Schoch G, et al: Stem cell transplantation for secondary acute myeloid leukemia: Evaluation of transplantation as initial therapy or following induction chemotherapy [review]. Blood 1997;89:2578–2585.

292. Sutton L, Chastang C, Ribaud P, et al: Factors influencing outcome in de novo myelodysplastic syndromes treated by allogeneic bone marrow transplantation: A long-term study of 71 patients. Societe Francaise de Greffe de Moelle. Blood 1996;88:358.

293. Castro-Malaspina H, Harris RE, Gajewski J, et al: Unrelated donor marrow transplantation for myelodysplastic syndromes: Outcome analysis in 510 transplants facilitated by the National Marrow Donor Program. Blood 2002;99(6):1943–1951.

294. Anderson JE, Applebaum FR, Deeg HJ, et al: Phase II study of busulphan and total body irradiation as novel preparation regimen in allogenic BMT for advanced MDS [abstract]. Leukemia Res 1999;23(Suppl 1):583.

295. O'Donnell PV, Noga SJ, Grever M, et al: Using engineered allografts to improve transplant outcome in myelodysplastic syndrome (MDS) [abstract]. Blood 1997;90(Suppl):229a.

296. Castro-Malaspina H, Childs B, Papadopoulos E, et al: T-cell depleted (SBA-E-) bone marrow transplantation for myelodysplastic syndrome [abstract]. Leukemia Res 1997;21(Suppl):S51.

297. Delforge M, Demuynck H, Vandenberghe P, et al: Polyclonal primitive hematopoietic progenitors can be detected in mobilized peripheral blood from patients with high-risk myelodysplastic syndromes. Blood 1995;86:3660.

298. Parker JE, Shafi T, Mijovic A, et al: Allogenic stem cell transplantation (SCT) in MDS: Interim results of outcome following non-myeloablative conditioning compared to standards preparative regimens [abstract]. Blood 2000;96(Suppl):554a.

299. Cao TM, McSweeney PA, Niederwieser D, et al: Non-myeloablative allogenic hematopoietic cell transplantation (AHCT) for patients with myelodysplastic syndrome (MDS) and myeloproliferative disorders (MPD) [abstract]. Blood 2000;96(Suppl):170a.

300. Cheson BD, Zwiebel JA, Dancey J, et al: Novel therapeutic agents for the treatment of myelodysplastic syndromes [review]. Semin Oncol 2000;27(5):560–577.

301. Li L, Olin E, Buskirk H, et al: Cytotoxicity and mode of action of 5-azacytidine on l1210 leukemia. Cancer Res 1970;30: 2760–2769.

302. Creusot F, Acs G, Christman J: Inhibition of DNA methyltransferase and induction of Friend erythroleukemia cell differentiation by 5-azacytidine and 5-aza-2′deoxycytidine. J Biol Chem 1982;257:2041–2048.

303. Christman J, Mendelsohn N, Herzog D, et al: Effect of 5-azacytidine on differentiation and DNA methylation in human promyelocytic leukemia cells (HL-60). Cancer Res 1983;43:763–769.

304. Silverman LR, Holland JF, Weinberg RS, et al: Effects of treatment with 5-azacytidine on the in vivo and in vitro hematopoiesis in patients with myelodysplastic syndromes. Leukemia 1993; 7(Suppl):21–29.

305. Silverman L, Demakos EP, Peterson BL, et al: Randomized controlled trial of azacitidine in patients with the myelodysplastic syndrome: A study of the Cancer and Leukemia Group B. J Clin Oncol 2002;20:2429–2440.

306. Wijermans P, Lubbert M, Verhoef G, et al: Low-dose 5-aza-2′-deoxycytidine, a DNA hypomethylating agent, for the treatment of high-risk myelodysplastic syndrome: A multicenter phase II study in elderly patients. J Clin Oncol 2000;18(5):956–962.

307. Sievers EL, Larson RA, Stadtmauer EA, et al: Efficacy and safety of gemtuzumab ozogamicin in patients with CD33-positive acute myeloid leukemia in first relapse. J Clin Oncol 2001;19(13):3244–3254.

308. Jilani I, Estey E, Huh YO, et al: Quantitative differences in CD33 intensity between various myeloid neoplasms [abstract]. Blood 2001;98(11):586a.

309. Estey E, Cortes J, Thall P, et al: Mylotarg +/- IL-11 in patients age ≥65 with newly-diagnosed AML/MDS: Comparison with idarubicin + ara-c [abstract]. Blood 2001;98 (11):720–721a.

310. Gibbs JB, Graham SL, Hartman GD, et al: Farnesyltransferase inhibitors versus RAS inhibitors. Curr Opin Chem Biol 1997;1:197–203.

311. Kurzrock R, Sebti SM, Kantarjian H, et al: Phase I study of a farnesyl transferase inhibitor, R115777, in patients with myelodysplastic syndrome [abstract]. Blood 2001;98(11):623a.

312. Kurzrock R, Cortes J, Ryback ME: Phase II study of R115777, a farnesyltransferase inhibitor, in myelodysplastic syndrome [abstract]. Blood 2001;98(11):848a.

313. Wattel E, Cambier N, Caulier MT, et al: Androgen therapy in myelodysplastic syndromes with thrombocytopenia: A report on 20 cases [see comments]. Br J Haematol 1994;87:205.

314. Katayama Y, Kojima K, Omoto E, Harada M: Androgen therapy in combination with granulocyte colony-stimulating factor and erythropoietin in a patient with refractory anemia. Int J Hematol 1996;65:89.

315. Chabannon C, Molina L, Pegourie-Bandelier B, et al: A review of 76 patients with myelodysplastic syndromes treated with danazol [see comments]. Cancer 1994;73:3073.

316. Hebbar M, Kaplan C, Caulier MT, et al: Low incidence of specific anti-platelet antibodies detected by the MAIPA assay in the serum of thrombocytopenic patients with MDS and lack of correlation between platelet autoantibodies, platelet lifespan and response to danazol therapy. Br J Haematol 1996;94:112.

317. Stadtmauer EA, Cassileth PA, Edelstein M, et al: Danazol treatment of myelodysplastic syndromes [see comments]. Br J Haematol 1991;77:502.

318. Jensen PD, Heickendorff L, Pedersen B, et al: The effect of iron chelation on haemopoiesis in patients with MDS with transfusional iron overload. Br J Haematol 1996;94:288.

319. Brandt L: Exposure to organic solvents and risk of haematological malignancies [review]. Leuk Res 1992;16:67.

320. Cowles SR, Bennett JM, Ross CE: Medical surveillance for leukemia at a petrochemical manufacturing complex: Four-year summary. J Occup Med 1991;3:808.

321. Cowles SR, Bennett JM, Ross CE: The chronic myeloid leukemias: Guidelines for distinguishing chronic granulocytic leukemia, atypical myeloid leukemia, and chronic myelomonocytic leukemia: Proposal by the French-American-British Cooperative Leukemia Group. Br J Hematol 1994;87:746–754.

322. Germing U, Gattermann N, Minning H, et al: Problems in the classification of CMML—Dysplastic versus proliferative type. Leuk Res 1998;22(10):871–878.

323. Solal-Celigny P, Desaint B, Herrera A, et al: Chronic myelomonocytic leukemia according to FAB classification: Analysis of 35 cases. Blood 1984;63(3):634–638.

324. Storniolo AM, Moloney WC, Rosenthal DS, et al: Chronic myelomonocytic leukemia. Leukemia 1990;4(11):766–770.

325. Aul C, Bowen DT, Yoshida Y. Pathogenesis, etiology and epidemiology of myelodysplastic syndromes [review]. Haematologica 1998;83(1):71–86.

326. Pear WS: Signaling in leukemia: Which messenger to kill? J Clin Invest 2000;105(4):419–422.

327. Tomasson MH, Sternberg DW, Williams IR, et al: Fatal myeloproliferation, induced in mice by TEL/PDGFbetaR expression, depends on PDGFbetaR tyrosines 579/581. J Clin Invest 2000;105(4):423–432.

328. Magnusson MK, Meade KE, Brown KE, et al: Rabaptin-5 is a novel fusion partner to platelet-derived growth factor beta receptor in chronic myelomonocytic leukemia. Blood 2001;15;98(8):2518–2125.

329. Saint-Dic D, Chang SC, Taylor GS, Provot MM, Ross TS: Regulation of the Src homology 2-containing inositol 5-phosphatase SHIP1 in

330. HIP1/PDGFbeta R-transformed cells. J Biol Chem 2001;276:21192–21198.

330. Schwaller J, Anastasiadou E, Cain D, et al: H4 (D10S170), a gene frequently rearranged in papillary thyroid carcinoma, is fused to the platelet-derived growth factor receptor [beta] gene in atypical chronic myeloid leukemia with t(5;10)(q33;q22). Blood 2001;97:3910–3918.

331. Hirsch-Ginsberg C, LeMaistre AC, Kantarjian H, et al: RAS mutations are rare events in Philadelphia chromosome-negative/bcr gene rearrangement-negative chronic myelogenous leukemia, but are prevalent in chronic myelomonocytic leukemia. Blood 1990;76:1214–1219.

332. Vardiman JW, Pierre R, Bain B, Bennett JM: Chronic myelomoncytic leukaemia. In Jaffe E, Harris N, Stein H (eds): Pathology and Genetics of Tumors of Haematopoietic and Lymphoid Tissue. Lyon, France, IARC Press, 2001, p 49.

333. Bourantas KL, Tsiara S, Panteli A, et al: Pleural effusion in chronic myelomonocytic leukemia. Acta Haematol 1998;99(1):34–37.

334. Wattel E, Guerci A, Hecquet B, et al: A randomized trial of hydroxyurea versus VP16 in adult chronic myelomonocytic leukemia. Groupe Francais des Myelodysplasies and European CMML Group. Blood 1996;88(7):2480–2487.

335. Beran M, Kantarjian H, O'Brien S, et al: Topotecan, a topoisomerase I inhibitor, is active in the treatment of myelodysplastic syndrome and chronic myelomonocytic leukemia. Blood 1996;1;88(7):2473–2479.

336. Beran M, Onida F, Cortes JE, et al: Chemotherapy of increasing intensity in the treatment of chronic myelomonocytic leukemia (CMML) [abstract]. Blood 2001;98(11):624a.

337. Kroger N, Zabelina T, Guardiola P, et al: Allogeneic stem cell transplantation for adult chronic myelomonocytic leukaemia. A report on behalf of the chronic leukaemia Working Party of the European Group for Blood and Marrow Transplantation (EBMT) [abstract]. Blood 2001;98(11):620a.

338. Magnusson MK, Meade KE, Nakamura R, et al: Molecular evidence for efficacy of STI-571 in chronic myelomonocytic leukemia (CMML) with a platelet-derived growth factor β-receptor (PDGFβR) fusion oncogene [abstract]. Blood 2001;98(11):631a.

339. Raza A, Lisak L, Dutt D, et al: Gleevec (imatinib mesylate) in 16 patients with chronic myelomonocytic leukemia (CMMoL) [abstract]. Blood 2001;98(11):273b.

340. Vardiman JW, Pierre R, Imbert R: Juvenile myelomonocytic leukaemia. In Jaffe E, Harris N, Stein H (eds): Pathology and Genetics of Tumors of Haematopoietic and Lymphoid Tissue. Lyon, France, IARC Press, 2001, p 55.

341. Vardiman JW, Imbert R, Pierre R: Atypical chronic myeloid leukaemia. In Jaffe E, Harris N, Stein H (eds): Pathology and Genetics of Tumors of Haematopoietic and Lymphoid Tissue. Lyon, France, IARC Press, 2001, p 53.

342. Bain B, Vardiman JW, Imbert R: Myelodysplastic/myeloproliferative disease, unclassifiable. In Jaffe E, Harris N, Stein H (eds): Pathology and Genetics of Tumors of Haematopoietic and Lymphoid Tissue. Lyon, France, IARC Press, 2001, p 58.

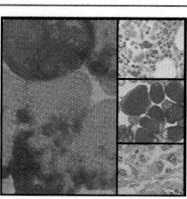

CHRONIC MYELOPROLIFERATIVE DISEASES

06

Ayalew Tefferi

SUMMARY OF KEY POINTS

INCIDENCE

- Three chronic myeloproliferative disorders (CMPDs) have been identified: polycythemia vera (PV), essential thrombocythemia (ET), and myelofibrosis with myeloid metaplasia (MMM).
- Each type is estimated to occur at the rate of 1 to 2.5/100,000/year.

DIFFERENTIAL DIAGNOSIS

- All three CMPDs may be considered diagnoses of exclusion because a specific diagnostic marker is currently lacking.
- A working diagnosis of PV requires the exclusion of apparent and secondary polycythemia.
- Before the diagnosis of ET is made, both reactive thrombocytosis and primary thrombocythemia associated with other chronic myeloid disorders must be considered.
- Myelofibrosis is nonspecific and can accompany chronic myeloid leukemia, myelodysplastic syndrome, or other chronic myeloid disorders, in addition to MMM.

DIAGNOSTIC EVALUATION

- Bone marrow examination is essential in the diagnosis of all three

chronic myeloproliferative disorders; the diagnosis is primarily based on morphologic assessment of the bone marrow.
- There are no specific cytogenetic markers for chronic myeloproliferative disorder.
- Bone marrow examination may be avoided if there is adequate clinical evidence of reactive erythrocytosis or thrombocytosis.
- Specialized tests, including endogenous erythroid colony assays, are rarely needed to make a working diagnosis of chronic myeloproliferative disorder.

RISK STRATIFICATION

- For both PV and ET, life expectancy is nearly normal in the first decade of disease.
- The major problem during this period is thrombosis, which may occur in up to 30% of patients.
- A history of thrombosis or age older than 60 years is associated with a high risk of thrombosis.
- Platelet count by itself has not been significantly associated with thrombosis in either PV or ET.
- In MMM, adverse risk factors include anemia, either leukopenia or

leukocytosis; severe constitutional symptoms; and circulating blasts.

TREATMENT

- Phlebotomy is the mainstay of treatment in PV.
- Low-risk patients (younger than 60 years, with no history of thrombosis) with either PV or ET have not been shown to benefit from cytoreductive therapy.
- Treatment with hydroxyurea reduces the risk of thrombosis in high-risk patients with both ET and PV.
- Microvascular symptoms, including headache and erythromelalgia, are easily treated with low-dose aspirin therapy, which is indicated in the absence of extreme thrombocytosis.
- Drug therapy in MMM is currently palliative, and effective agents include corticosteroids, erythropoietin, androgen preparations, thalidomide, and hydroxyurea.
- Splenectomy continues to have a palliative role in MMM.
- The therapeutic value of hematopoietic stem cell transplantation in MMM is being investigated.

INTRODUCTION

Hematologic malignancies are generally organized into myeloid and lymphoid disorders, depending on the phenotype of the predominantly proliferative cell lineage. Myeloid disorders, in turn, are classified into acute myeloid leukemia and chronic myeloid disorders (CMDs), based on whether bone marrow biopsy specimens show greater than 20% to 30% immature myeloid progenitors (blasts or promyelocytes). CMDs are further subclassified into four operational categories, including chronic myeloproliferative disorders, chronic myeloid leukemia (CML), myelodysplastic syndrome (MDS), and atypical CMD (Fig. 106-1). Although CML was traditionally considered a chronic

myeloproliferative disorder,[1] it is now classified as a separate entity because of its specific association with the Philadelphia (Ph[1]) translocation (bcr-abl) as well as its unique treatment response to both interferon-alfa and imatinib mesylate. Therefore, currently, chronic myeloproliferative disorder refers only to polycythemia vera (PV), essential thrombocythemia (ET), and myelofibrosis with myeloid metaplasia (MMM).

Chronic myeloproliferative disorders (PV, ET, and MMM) are pathogenetically similar to the other CMD subgroups (CML, MDS, and atypical CMD) in that they represent clonal myeloproliferation that originates at the stem cell level.[2] Atypical CMD is an arbitrary designation for a myriad of bcr-abl–negative hematologic disorders that are not easily classified as either MDS or chronic myelopro-

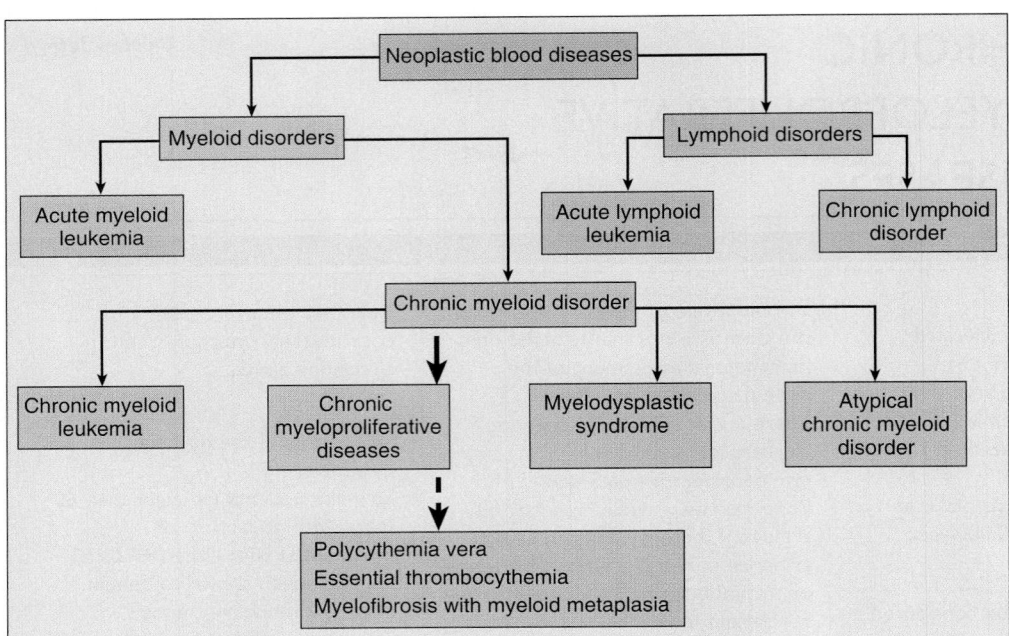

Figure 106-1. A working classification of hematologic malignancies.

liferative disorders but have been shown to be clonal myeloid disorders. These include hybrid myeloproliferative and myelodysplastic disorders, chronic myelomonocytic leukemia, juvenile myelomonocytic leukemia, chronic neutrophilic leukemia, hypereosinophilic syndrome and eosinophilic leukemia, and systemic mast cell disease.[3-7]

POLYCYTHEMIA VERA

Vaquez and Osler[8,9] are credited for the initial descriptions of PV as a primary erythrocythemic process in 1892 and 1903, respectively. The reported incidence of PV is approximately 0.5 to 2.6/100,000.[10,11] A higher incidence of disease has been suggested in persons of Jewish ancestry[12] as well as among parent–offspring pairs.[13] The median age at diagnosis of PV is approximately 60 years, with a slight (1.2:1) male preponderance.[14] Approximately 7% of patients are diagnosed before 40 years of age,[14] and there are rare cases of children with PV.[15]

Pathogenesis

Polycythemia vera is a clonal stem cell disease with trilineage myeloid involvement.[16] In addition, some studies have suggested clonal heterogeneity, including clonal involvement of B lymphocytes,[17] as well as polyclonal granulopoiesis in certain cases.[18] Unlike with CML, the disease-causing molecular lesion in PV has not been identified.

In vitro, erythroid colony formation in patients with PV does not require the addition of exogenous erythropoietin (EPO).[19] This phenomenon, known as endogenous erythroid colony growth, does not occur in normal control subjects or in patients with nonclonal polycythemia. In addition, erythroid progenitor cells in PV display growth factor hypersensitivity to insulin-like growth factor (IGF)-1[20] and other cytokines.[21] The consistently observed IGF-1 hypersensitivity of erythroid cells in PV has been attributed to alterations in IGF-1 binding proteins.[22] However, several studies show that growth factor–independent or growth factor–hypersensitive colony formation is specific to neither PV nor erythroid progenitor cells.[21]

The EPO receptor gene and its protein are intact in PV.[23] On the other hand, several postreceptor molecular abnormalities have been reported, including increased baseline phosphorylation of the IGF-1 receptor,[24] decreased activity of SH-PTP1 (a tyrosine phosphatase),[25] increased activity of membrane-associated SH-PTP,[26] constitutive activation of STAT3,[27] upregulation of negative control elements of the cell cycle (p16/p14),[28] and abundance of antiapoptotic proteins (Bcl-x_L) in erythroid precursors.[29] However, these observations have not been always reproducible, and none of them have been shown to be specific to PV.

Diagnosis

In clinical practice, the term *polycythemia* is used to indicate possible increased erythrocyte volume (i.e., red blood cell mass). This perception may be real (true polycythemia) or spurious (apparent polycythemia; Fig. 106-2).[21] True polycythemia may represent either PV or a nonclonal increase in red cell mass (RCM) that is often, but not always, mediated by EPO (secondary polycythemia; Table 106-1). Apparent polycythemia may result from either a reduction in plasma volume (relative polycythemia) or an inaccurate perception of an elevated

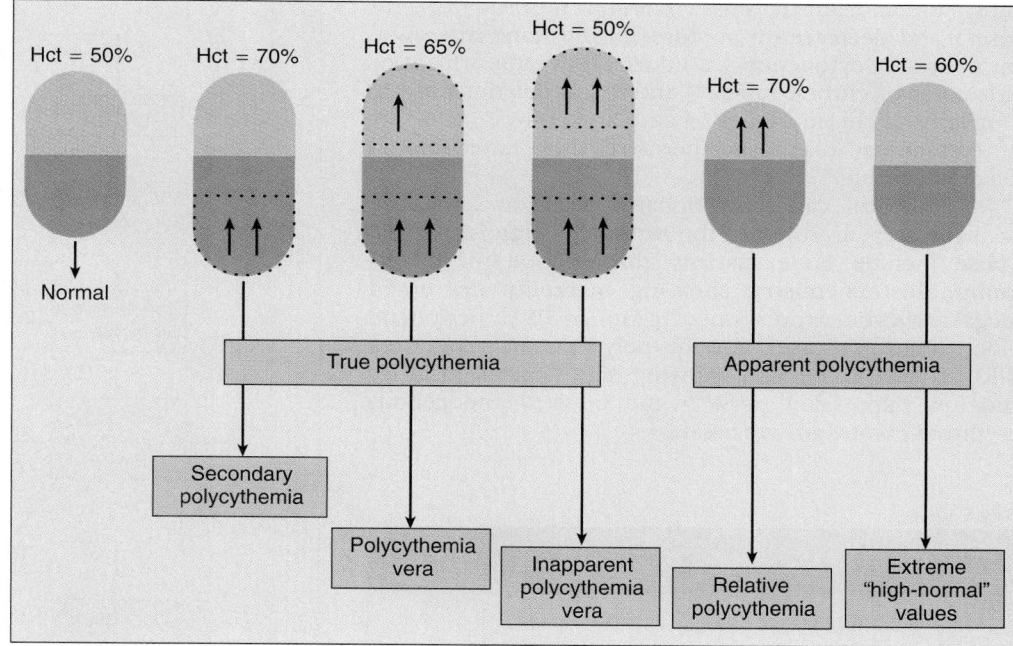

Figure 106-2. An operational classification of polycythemias. (From Tefferi A: Polycythemia vera: A comprehensive review and clinical recommendations. Mayo Clin Proc 2003;78:174–194.)

RCM that occurs when high-normal values of hemoglobin or hematocrit are not recognized.[30]

Inapparent polycythemia is the converse of apparent polycythemia and indicates a true increase in RCM that is masked by a normal hemoglobin or hematocrit value as a result of a concomitant increase in plasma volume (see Fig. 106-2).[31]

In 1975, the Polycythemia Vera Study Group published a set of diagnostic criteria that were primarily used to ensure that patients with secondary or apparent polycythemia were excluded from treatment protocols.[32] These criteria required the finding of increased red cell mass by measurement of blood volume with labeled erythrocytes as well as the finding of normal hemoglobin oxygen saturation. Unfortunately, these "study inclusion criteria" have been adopted by many as "diagnostic criteria," despite well-documented instances of inadequacy in diagnostic sensitivity and specificity. Similarly, some investigators strongly advocate the routine use of measuring red cell mass, although it represents another laboratory test, with unavoidable false-positive and false-negative findings. The recent identification of PV-specific biologic parameters has allowed further refinement of the original Polycythemia Vera Study Group diagnostic criteria. These revised Polycythemia Vera Study Group criteria have increased diagnostic accuracy, but have added complexity to the diagnostic process.[33-35]

For these reasons, I do not use either the Polycythemia Vera Study Group diagnostic criteria or red cell mass measurement during the workup of a patient with suspected PV. Instead, I rely on the characteristic biologic and histologic features to formulate a diagnostic algorithm (discussed later) that does not require the information from red cell mass measurement (Fig. 106-3).[21]

Stepwise Diagnostic Workup

The diagnostic possibility of PV should be entertained only if the hemoglobin or hematocrit level is greater than the 95th percentile of the normal distribution adjusted for sex and race; there is a documented increase in the hemoglobin or hematocrit level above the baseline for an individual patient, regardless of where the specific hematocrit level lies within the reference range; or a PV-related feature (i.e., splenomegaly, leukocytosis, thrombocytosis, thrombosis, pruritus) accompanies a borderline high hematocrit value.

In one of these three scenarios, it is reasonable to start the diagnostic workup by determining the serum EPO level (see Fig. 106-3). In general, serum EPO levels are low in patients with PV, even when they are treated with phlebotomy.[36] However, the level also may be low in other chronic myeloproliferative disorders, including ET,[37] as well as rare cases of congenital polycythemia with activating mutation of the EPO receptor (EPOR).[38] Therefore a low serum EPO level is highly suggestive, but not diagnostic, of PV (estimated specificity >90%).[39] On the other hand, the serum EPO level may lie within the normal reference range in patients with a definite diagnosis of PV. The sensitivity of a low serum EPO level for PV is estimated at less than 70%.[39,40] However, PV is unlikely to be associated with an increased serum EPO level.[39] Therefore PV remains a diagnostic consideration in the presence of either a low or "normal" serum EPO level.

The next step is cytogenic examination of the bone marrow (see Fig. 106-3). To the experienced hematopathologist, the histologic features of the bone marrow often show characteristic changes. These may include hypercellularity; an increased number of megakaryocytes, including cluster formation; giant megakaryocytes that show pleomorphism; mild reticulin fibrosis (12% of cases); and decreased iron stores in the bone marrow.[41] In contrast, cytogenetic studies show abnormalities (trisomies of chromosomes 9 and 8 and deletions of the long arms of chromosomes 13 and 20) in only 13% to 18% of patients at diagnosis; therefore they have limited diagnostic value.[42]

In equivocal cases, additional specialized tests may be necessary to support the working diagnosis of PV. These include bone marrow thrombopoietin (c-Mpl) immunohistochemistry, showing markedly decreased megakaryocytic expression of c-Mpl in PV[43]; peripheral blood neutrophil assay for the polycythemia rubra vera (PRV)-1 gene expression; showing high expression in PV and low expression in SP[44]; and in vitro endogenous erythroid colony growth assay.

TABLE 106-1

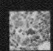 **Causes of Secondary Polycythemia**

Erythropoietin (EPO)-Mediated

Hypoxia-driven

Central hypoxic process
 Chronic lung disease
 Right-to-left cardiopulmonary vascular shunts
 High-altitude habitat
 Carbon monoxide poisoning
 Smoker's polycythemia (chronic carbon monoxide exposure)
 Hypoventilation syndromes, including sleep apnea
Peripheral hypoxic process
 Localized
  Renal artery stenosis
 Diffuse
  High-oxygen-affinity hemoglobinopathy (congenital; autosomal-dominant)
  2,3-Diphosphoglycerate mutase deficiency (congenital; autosomal-recessive)

Hypoxia-independent (pathologic EPO production)

Malignant tumors
 Hepatocellular carcinoma
 Renal cell cancer
 Cerebellar hemangioblastoma
 Parathyroid carcinoma
Nonmalignant conditions
 Uterine leiomyomas
 Renal cysts (polycystic kidney disease)
 Pheochromocytoma
 Meningioma
 Abnormally elevated set point for EPO production (congenital)
 Chuvash polycythemia (congenital; abnormal oxygen homeostasis?)

EPO Receptor-Mediated

Activating mutation of the erythropoietin receptor

Some cases of autosomal-dominant congenital polycythemia

Drug-Associated

EPO doping

Treatment with androgen preparations

Unknown Mechanisms

Most cases of autosomal-dominant congenital polycythemia

Some forms of autosomal-recessive congenital polycythemia

Post-renal-transplant erythrocytosis

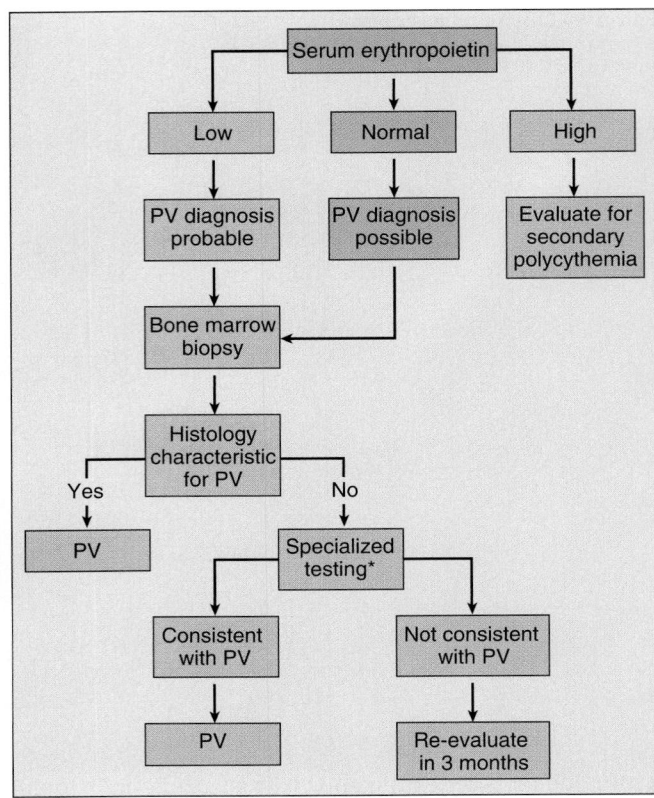

Figure 106-3. A practical algorithm for the diagnosis of polycythemia vera (PV). *Specialized testing includes bone marrow immunohistochemistry for the thrombopoietin receptor, reverse transcriptase-polymerase chain reaction for neutrophil expression of polycythemia rubra vera-1 gene, and spontaneous erythroid colony assay. (From Tefferi A: Polycythemia vera: A comprehensive review and clinical recommendations. Mayo Clin Proc 2003;78:174–194.)

Treatment

The natural history of PV is characterized by a lifelong propensity for thrombohemorrhagic complications, late-onset disease transformation into both MMM and acute myeloid leukemia (AML), and a shortened life expectancy. Specific treatment positively affects the risk of both macrovascular and microvascular complications, but not that of clonal evolution to MMM or AML.

Phlebotomy is the cornerstone of therapy for PV, and is the only treatment modality that has improved survival in affected patients. Median survival may be as low as 2 years in the absence of this treatment.[45] Based on limited retrospective studies of PV that showed a progressive increase in the incidence of vascular occlusive episodes above a hematocrit level of 44%[46] as well as other studies that showed suboptimal cerebral blood flow when hematocrit values were between 46% and 52%,[47] the therapeutic target hematocrit level is currently 45% or lower. Furthermore, because of the physiologic difference in hematocrit values in men and women as well as among persons of different races, it is reasonable, although not evidence-based, to target an even lower hematocrit level (i.e., 42%) in women and African Americans.

Role of Drug Therapy in Polycythemia Vera: Observations from Randomized Studies

In the first controlled study of PV, the Polycythemia Vera Study Group randomized 431 patients to receive treatment with either phlebotomy alone or phlebotomy accompanied by treatment with either oral chlorambucil or intravenous radioactive phosphorus (^{32}P). The results favored treatment with phlebotomy alone, with a median survival of 12.6 years compared with 10.9 and 9.1 years for treatment with ^{32}P and chlorambucil, respectively ($P = 0.008$). The difference in survival was attributed to an increased incidence of acute leukemia in patients treated with chlorambucil or ^{32}P compared with those treated with phlebotomy alone (13.2% vs. 9.6% vs. 1.5% over 13 to 19 years).[48] Furthermore, large cell lymphoma developed in 3.5% of patients treated with chlorambucil, and the incidence of gastrointestinal and skin cancer was increased in patients treated with either chlorambucil or ^{32}P.

In another controlled study, the European Organization for Research on Treatment of Cancer (EORTC) randomized 293 patients to receive treatment with either ^{32}P or oral busulfan. The results favored busulfan in terms of both duration of first remission (median, 4 years vs. 2 years) and overall survival (10-year survival rates of 70% vs. 55%; $P = 0.02$). At a median follow-up of 8 years, there was no significant difference in the risk of leukemic transformation (2% vs. 1.4%), nonhematologic malignancy (2.8% vs. 5%), vascular complications (27% vs. 37%), or transformation into MMM (4.8% vs. 4.1%) between the busulfan and ^{32}P arms, respectively.[49]

Other randomized studies of PV compared hydroxyurea with pipobroman and showed a significant difference favoring pipobroman in the incidence of transformation into MMM, but found no difference in survival, the incidence of thrombosis, or the rate of leukemic conversion.[50] Studies comparing ^{32}P alone with ^{32}P plus HU (hydroxyurea) found no difference in survival, the incidence of thrombosis, or the risk of transformation into MMM. However, ^{32}P alone was associated with a significantly lower incidence of acute leukemia and other cancers.[51] In a study of ^{32}P plus phlebotomy vs. phlebotomy plus high-dose aspirin (900 mg daily) in combination with dipyridamole 225 mg daily, the addition of antiplatelet agents provided no benefit in terms of thrombosis prevention, but increased the risk of gastrointestinal bleeding.[52]

However, a more recent randomized study of PV (112 patients) using lower doses of aspirin (40 mg daily) did not show an increased incidence of bleeding diathesis.[53] Furthermore, the results of the Polycythemia Vera Study Group aspirin study may have been influenced by the fact that 27% of the patients who were randomized to receive treatment with phlebotomy, aspirin, and dipyridamole had a history of thrombosis compared with 13% of patients in the other arm. An ongoing European Collaboration on Low Dose Aspirin study is expected to further clarify the role of low-dose aspirin in the treatment of PV.

Role of Drug Therapy in Polycythemia Vera: Observations from Nonrandomized Studies

In a nonrandomized Polycythemia Vera Study Group study, treatment with hydroxyurea was associated with a lower incidence of early thrombosis compared with a historical cohort treated with phlebotomy alone (6.6% vs. 14% at 2 years). Similarly, the incidence of acute leukemia in patients treated with hydroxyurea compared with historical control subjects treated with either chlorambucil or ^{32}P was significantly lower (5.9 % vs. 10.6% vs. 8.3%, respectively, in the first 11 years of treatment).[54] Other studies confirmed the low incidence of AML in patients with PV who were treated with hydroxyurea (1% to 5.6%).[55,56]

Many studies have reported the use of pipobroman as a single agent in PV.[57,58] In one of these studies involving 163 patients, the drug was effective in more than 90% of patients and median survival exceeded 17 years.[57] In the first 10 years, the incidences of thrombotic events, acute leukemia, MMM, and other malignancies were 16%, 5%, 4%, and 8%, respectively. Favorable outcome was also reported in single-arm studies with oral busulfan.[59,60] In 65 busulfan-treated patients with PV who were followed between 1962 and 1983, overall median survival was 11.1 years; it was 19 years in patients whose disease was diagnosed before 60 years of age.[59] Acute leukemia developed in only two patients (3.5%) who were treated with busulfan alone.

Most recently, interferon-alfa was shown to control erythrocytosis in approximately 76% of patients with PV receiving subcutaneous drug in doses of 4.5 to 27 million units per week. The usual dose is 3 million units subcutaneously three times a week.[61,62] A similar benefit is seen in reduction in spleen size or relief from intractable pruritus. Anagrelide is an oral imidazole quinazoline derivative that inhibits platelet aggregation at higher than therapeutic drug concentrations, but shows a species-specific platelet-lowering effect in humans at therapeutic concentrations.[63] Anagrelide is capable of substantially reducing the platelet count in more than 80% of patients with PV.[64]

In summary, the results of single-arm studies support those of the randomized studies, and show that pipobroman and busulfan are valuable therapeutic agents in PV and may be considered as alternatives to hydroxyurea. Pipobroman is not available in the United States. It is not clear what additional value is gained by substituting newer drugs (i.e., interferon-alfa and anagrelide) for the traditional cytoreductive agents, especially in view of their unfavorable toxicity and cost profile (Table 106-2).[65]

Thrombohemorrhagic Risk Factors in Polycythemia Vera

The series of Polycythemia Vera Study Group studies showed the following: (1) a significantly greater incidence of thrombotic events in the first 3 years in patients treated with phlebotomy alone; (2) a lack of correlation between thrombosis and either platelet count or hematocrit value; and (3) a significant association between the risk of thrombosis and either age older than 70 years or a history of thrombosis. In addition, in patients treated with phlebotomy alone, the risk of thrombosis was associated with increased frequency of phlebotomy (maintenance phlebotomy more than once every 3 months). Other studies confirmed the detrimental effect of advanced age (>60 years) and history of thrombosis on patients with

TABLE 106-2

Clinical Properties of Popular Cytoreductive Agents used in Polycythemia Vera or Essential Thrombocythemia

DRUG (CLASS)	HYDROXYUREA	ANAGRELIDE	INTERFERON-ALFA	PHOSPHOROUS-32	PIPOBROMAN
Mechanism of Action	Myelosuppressive Antimetabolite	Platelet-specific Unknown	Myelosuppressive Biologic agent	Myelosuppressive Radionuclide	Myelosuppressive Alkylating agent
Pharmacology	Half-life ≈ 5 hr, renal excretion	Half-life ≈ 1.5 hr, renal excretion	Kidney is main site of metabolism	Half-life ≈ 14 days	Insufficient information
Starting Dose	500 mg PO BID	0.5 mg PO TID	5 million units SC TIW	2.3 mCi/m^2 IV	1 mg/kg/day PO
Onset of Action	≈ 3–5 days	≈ 6–10 days	1–3 wk	4–8 wk	≈ 16 days
Frequent Side Effects	Leukopenia, oral ulcers, anemia, hyperpigmentation, nail discoloration, xerodermia	Headache, palpitations, diarrhea, fluid retention, anemia	Flulike syndrome, fatigue, anorexia, weight loss, lack of ambition, alopecia	Transient mild cytopenia	Nausea, abdominal pain, diarrhea
Infrequent Side Effects	Leg ulcers, nausea, diarrhea, alopecia, skin atrophy	Arrhythmias, lightheadedness, nausea	Confusion, depression, autoimmune thyroiditis, myalgia, arthritis	Prolonged pancytopenia in elderly patients	Leukopenia, thrombocytopenia, hemolysis
Rare Side Effects	Fever, cystitis, platelet oscillations	Cardiomyopathy	Pruritus, hyperlipidemia, transaminasemia	Leukemogenic	
Cost	Annual $1714, for 500-mg TID dose	Annual $8500, for 0.5-mg QID dose	Annual $10,500, for 3 million units 5 days/wk	Approximately $1025 for 4 mCi	Not available in US

PV.[21] Patients 60 years of age or older and those with a history of thrombosis are considered at high risk (Table 106-3). In contrast, the degree of thrombocytosis has never been correlated with the risk of thrombosis. However, some patients with extreme thrombocytosis (platelet count >1 to 1.5 million/mL) have an acquired bleeding diathesis that results from abnormal adsorption and catabolism of large-molecular-weight von Willebrand factor (vWf).[66] The prognostic effect of extreme thrombocytosis, in the absence of acquired von Willebrand disease, is unknown. Equally uncertain is the prognostic relevance

TABLE 106-3

Risk Stratification in Polycythemia Vera and Essential Thrombocythemia

RISK CATEGORY	PATIENT CHARACTERISTICS
Low-risk	Age <60 yr, and no history of thrombocytosis, and platelet count <1.5 million/μL, and absence of cardiovascular risk factors*
Indeterminate	Age <60 yr, and no history of thrombocytosis, and either platelet count >1.5 million/μL, or presence of cardiovascular risk factors
High	Age ≥60 yr or older, or history of thrombosis

*Risk factors include tobacco use, diabetes, hypertension, coronary artery disease, and obesity.

of cardiovascular risk factors. Patients who are at not high risk, but have either extreme thrombocytosis or cardiovascular risk factors, are grouped in an indeterminate-risk category. All other patients are considered to be at low risk (see Table 106-3).

Current Treatment Recommendations

The mainstay of therapy in patients with PV remains phlebotomy for all patients to keep hematocrit at 45% or less in white men and at the appropriate corresponding value for women and persons of other races. Additional drug therapy depends on an individual patient's risk for thrombohemorrhagic complications (see Table 106-3). In general, there is good evidence to advocate the use of cytoreductive agents in high-risk patients (Table 106-4).[48] In this regard, and based on the results of these studies, my current choice of chemotherapy is hydroxyurea, at a starting dose of 500 mg twice daily, or busulfan, at a starting dose of 4 mg daily, in patients who cannot tolerate hydroxyurea. Side effects of hydroxyurea that may necessitate the use of an alternative agent include neutropenia and mucocutaneous changes. When busulfan is used, it is important to recognize the potential, but infrequent, toxicity to the lungs (pulmonary fibrosis)[67] and bone marrow (aplasia).[68] Intermittent treatment, with drug holidays, and withholding treatment for impending cytopenia are recommended.

In younger high-risk patients, some investigators are concerned about drug leukemogenicity associated with long-term treatment with either hydroxyurea or busulfan. However, there is currently no hard evidence to support

TABLE 106-4

| **Treatment Algorithm for Polycythemia Vera** | | | |
RISK CATEGORY	AGE <60 YR	AGE ≥60 YR	WOMEN OF CHILDBEARING AGE
Low	Phlebotomy alone ± low-dose aspirin*	Not applicable	Phlebotomy alone ± low-dose aspirin*
Indeterminate	Phlebotomy alone[†]	Not applicable	Phlebotomy alone[†]
High	Phlebotomy + hydroxyurea *or* interferon-alfa + low-dose aspirin*	Phlebotomy + hydroxyurea + low-dose aspirin*	Phlebotomy + interferon-alfa* + low-dose aspirin*

*Not evidence-based.
[†]Use of aspirin is discouraged if the platelet count is >1 million/μL, but encouraged otherwise.

this concern. Regardless, interferon-alfa, at a starting dose of 3 million units subcutaneously three times weekly, is a reasonable alternative in this case (see Table 106-4).[61] Interferon-alfa is also the treatment of choice in women of childbearing age, because of the theoretical risk of teratogenicity associated with the other cytoreductive agents.[62]

Because ^{32}P-associated leukemia in PV peaks after the first 7 years of treatment, it is reasonable to advocate the use of ^{32}P in elderly patients who have issues of treatment compliance and convenience, especially if life expectancy is less than 10 years (intravenous ^{32}P at 2.3 mCi/m^2, repeated every 3 months if necessary).[48] The lack of evidence that correlates thrombocytosis with thrombosis in patients with PV argues against the potential therapeutic value of anagrelide in PV.

It is unclear whether any specific drug therapy affects clonal evolution in PV. Under current treatment strategies, the incidence of transformation into MMM or acute leukemia, in the first decade of disease, is estimated at 10% and 5%, respectively.[48] The risk beyond the first decade increases progressively.[69]

Treatment of Non–Life-Threatening Complications in Polycythemia Vera

Additional clinical features of PV include microvascular disturbances, aquagenic pruritus, and constitutional symptoms. Microvascular disturbances in PV and related disorders are believed to represent a transient inflammation-based occlusive phenomenon that is a result of interaction between clonal platelets and the endothelium of arterioles. Corresponding clinical manifestations include headache, lightheadedness, transient neurologic or ocular disturbances, tinnitus, atypical chest discomfort, paresthesias, and erythromelalgia (painful and burning sensation of the feet or hands associated with erythema and warmth). Aspirin promptly (within hours) alleviates symptoms in most patients with PV-associated microvascular disturbances.

Generalized pruritus that is often exacerbated by a hot bath is a characteristic feature of PV and occurs in 48% of patients, either at diagnosis or at a later stage of disease.[70] The etiology of PV-associated pruritus remains to be determined, and treatment responses to antihistamines have been both unpredictable and variable.[70] Interestingly, a recent study showed a greater than 80% response rate in

PV-associated pruritus treated with paroxetine, which is a selective serotonin reuptake inhibitor.[71] Other treatment modalities that have been used in PV-associated pruritus include interferon-alfa, psoralen photochemotherapy, and cholestyramine.[21]

ESSENTIAL THROMBOCYTHEMIA

Among the chronic myeloproliferative disorders, ET is the most recently described.[72] Reported incidence figures range from 0.2 to 2.5.[12,73-75] With a median age at diagnosis of 60 years, approximately 20% of patients with ET are diagnosed before 40 years of age; in younger patients, the incidence is higher in women than in men.[76,77] There are well-documented cases of ET in children, although some reported cases may represent familial thrombocytosis.[78,79]

POLYCYTHEMIA VERA

The Polycythemia Vera Study Group diagnostic criteria, including laboratory measurement of red cell mass, are neither essential nor practical for the diagnosis of polycythemia vera in routine clinical practice.

A contemporary algorithm based on disease-characteristic biologic parameters as well as the histologic features of bone marrow can be formulated to make a working diagnosis of polycythemia vera.

All patients with polycythemia vera should be treated with phlebotomy to maintain the hematocrit at 45% or less.

In addition to phlebotomy, patients with polycythemia vera who are older than 60 years of age or have a history of thrombosis should receive myelosuppressive treatment.

Hydroxyurea remains the myelosuppressive treatment of choice in polycythemia vera; interferon-alfa is a reasonable alternative treatment agent.

There is no good evidence to implicate thrombocytosis as a prothrombotic risk factor in polycythemia vera.

Although it is probably safe to use, the antithrombotic value of low-dose aspirin (81 to 325 mg daily) in polycythemia vera is unknown.

It is unclear whether drugs that are currently used to treat polycythemia vera affect the transformation of disease into either myelofibrosis with myeloid metaplasia or acute leukemia.

Pathogenesis

Trilineage clonal myeloproliferation has been shown in most patients with ET using X-chromosome–linked DNA or gene product analysis.[80,81] However, X-linked clonal assays have shown both polyclonal hematopoiesis in a substantial minority of patients with ET and "monoclonal" hematopoiesis in normal elderly control subjects.[82] Furthermore, in some cases, the clonal process in ET included lymphocytes[17] or was restricted to megakaryocytes.[81] Although these observations strongly suggest biologic heterogeneity, they have not clarified the issue of clonality in ET. Furthermore, as with both PV and MMM, the primary oncogenic event in ET remains elusive.

Several studies have evaluated the potential pathogenetic role of both thrombopoietin (TPO) and its receptor (c-Mpl) in ET. Serum TPO levels in ET are usually normal or only slightly elevated,[83] and are not significantly different from those of secondary thrombocytosis.[84] Similarly, mutation studies showed intact TPO and c-Mpl genes in ET and other chronic myeloproliferative disorders.[85,86] On the other hand, megakaryocyte progenitors in ET may be hypersensitive to TPO[87] as well as to other cytokines,[88] suggesting altered signal transduction as part of the pathogenetic process.

Diagnosis

Although thrombocytosis is the hallmark of ET, more than 85% of patients with thrombocytosis who are seen in routine clinical practice show reactivity (secondary thrombocytosis) and have another comorbid condition (Table 106-5).[89] The degree of thrombocytosis does not differentiate between ET and secondary thrombocytosis (ST). However, the clinical scenario is often helpful in

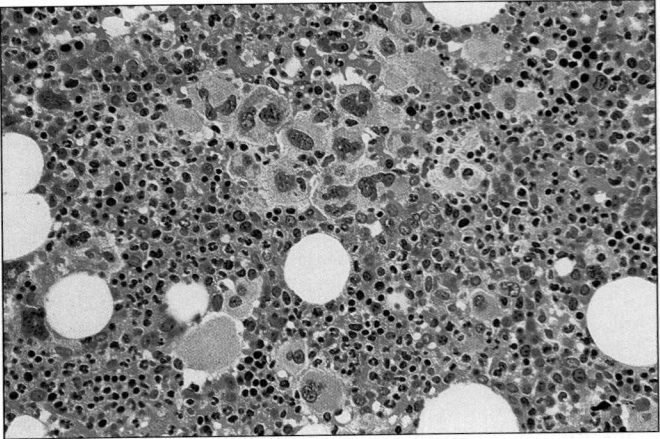

Figure 106-4. Bone marrow megakaryocyte clusters in essential thrombocythemia.

distinguishing ET from ST. In routine clinical practice, it is important to exclude the contribution of either iron deficiency anemia or hyposplenia as a possible cause of unexplained thrombocytosis. This is accomplished by the measurement of serum ferritin concentration and examination of a peripheral blood smear looking for Howell-Jolly bodies, respectively. The possibility of ST associated with an occult inflammatory or malignant process is addressed by the measurement of C-reactive protein or other acute-phase reactants.[90] In other words, uncomplicated ET should be accompanied by a normal serum ferritin concentration, a mostly unremarkable peripheral smear, and a normal serum C-reactive protein level. In general, plasma TPO levels are not helpful in distinguishing ST from ET.[83]

The typical bone marrow finding in ET is a mild to moderate increase in cellularity and the presence of megakaryocyte clusters that are often absent in ST (Fig. 106-4). On the other hand, many studies show markedly decreased c-Mpl surface expression in both megakaryocytes[91] and platelets.[92] Therefore bone marrow c-Mpl immunohistochemistry may complement the histologic distinction between ET and ST.[93] Other specialized tests that may be used in this regard include in vitro myeloid colony assays (both spontaneous and TPO-hypersensitive megakaryocyte growth is not seen in ET, but not in ST)[87] and PRV-1 expression assay in peripheral blood granulocytes (the level is high in ET, but is not detectable in ST).[94] However, these assays are available only in research laboratories and may not be suitable for widespread use. Furthermore, none of the currently available specialized tests, including endogenous erythroid colony growth and PRV-1 assay, can distinguish ET from PV.

CML and the cellular phase of MMM can both mimic ET in presentation.[95] With CML, a peripheral blood or bone marrow fluorescence in situ hybridization (FISH) study may be needed, in addition to cytogenetic analysis, to exclude karyotypically occult CML.[96] Similarly, the histologic features of the bone marrow should be scrutinized to detect intense marrow cellularity with

TABLE 106-5

Causes of Thrombocytosis

Secondary

Acute

Postsurgery
Bleeding
Hemolysis
Infection
Tissue damage
Chemotherapy rebound effect
Coronary artery bypass surgery

Chronic

Iron deficiency anemia
Surgical or functional asplenia
Metastatic cancer or lymphoma
Chronic inflammatory process
Renal failure, nephrotic syndrome

Primary

Essential thrombocythemia
Polycythemia vera
Agnogenic myeloid metaplasia
Chronic myeloid leukemia
Myelodysplastic syndrome

TABLE 106-6

Treatment Algorithm for Essential Thrombocythemia

RISK CATEGORY	AGE <60 YR	AGE ≥60 YR	WOMEN OF CHILDBEARING AGE
Low	± Low-dose aspirin*	Not applicable	± Low-dose aspirin*
Indeterminate	Individualized[†]	Not applicable	Individualized[†]
High	Hydroxyurea or anagrelide[‡] + low-dose aspirin*	Hydroxyurea[‡] + low-dose aspirin*	Interferon-alfa[§] + low-dose aspirin*

*Not evidence-based.
[†]Use of aspirin is discouraged if the platelet count is >1 million/μL, unless acquired von Willebrand disease is excluded. In the presence of symptomatic acquired von Willebrand disease, it is reasonable to use a cytoreductive agent to correct the abnormality.
[‡]In high-risk patients, these cytoreductive agents reflect the authors' preferred first-line treatment. Alternative cytoreductive agents may be used (see text).
[§]Based on anecdotal evidence of safety.

florid atypical megakaryocytic hyperplasia, which suggests cellular-phase MMM. Cytogenetic abnormalities are rare in ET (<5%).[97]

Treatment

Most patients with ET either are asymptomatic or have non–life-threatening microvascular symptoms (headache, visual symptoms, lightheadedness, atypical chest pain, acral dysesthesia, erythromelalgia) that are effectively treated with low-dose aspirin.[98] Erythromelalgia is painful acral erythema associated with warmth and mild edema.

Approximately 20% of patients have nonfatal thrombohemorrhagic complications, and only 5% progress to AML or MMM during the first decade of disease.[99-101] Therefore it is reasonable to expect long survival in most patients with ET. The relatively low incidence of thrombosis and hemorrhage as well as the occurrence of both short-term and long-term drug side effects are the basis for carefully selecting patients with ET who require specific treatment. Risk stratification in ET is similar to that in PV (see Table 106-3). Table 106-6 outlines the risk-adjusted treatment guidelines in patients with ET (described later).

Antiplatelet Therapy

Unlike with higher doses (≥500 mg daily), low-dose aspirin (81 to 325 mg daily) may not increase bleeding diathesis in patients with ET, and it is currently recommended as a supplement to cytoreductive therapy in high-risk patients as well as an optional consideration in most patients with ET (see Table 106-6).[102] However, acquired von Willebrand disease must be excluded before aspirin is used in patients with a platelet count of more than 1 million/mL.

Cytoreductive Therapy

The use of cytoreductive therapy to reduce the risk of thrombosis in ET is appropriate and evidence-based as long as it is applied to patients with an increased risk of thrombosis (see Tables 106-3 and 106-6).[103] In this instance, the platelet count may need to be reduced to 400,000/mL or lower.[104] Less aggressive platelet control with a cytoreductive drug may also be indicated in patients who have either aspirin-resistant microvascular disturbances or symptomatic acquired von Willebrand

disease.[66,105] In all other cases, the decision to use a platelet-lowering agent in ET is not supported by hard data. Specifically, neither the degree of thrombocytosis nor the presence of cardiovascular risk factors has consistently been correlated with increased thrombotic risk in ET.[98] The frequently cited association of extreme thrombocytosis and increased gastrointestinal bleeding is based on anecdotal observation and, in some instances, may be attributed to occult acquired von Willebrand disease.

Table 106-2 summarizes the practical pharmacologic and clinical information about current platelet-lowering agents in ET. Only hydroxyurea, as a treatment agent, has been shown in a prospective study to be associated with a reduced risk of thrombosis in ET.[103] Additional

ESSENTIAL THROMBOCYTHEMIA

Essential thrombocythemia remains a diagnosis of exclusion; both secondary thrombocytosis and clonal thrombocytosis associated with other chronic myeloid disorders must be excluded before a working diagnosis of essential thrombocythemia is made.

Not all patients with essential thrombocythemia need specific therapy.

Observation alone is a reasonable option in asymptomatic patients with essential thrombocythemia who are younger than 60 years of age and do not have a history of thrombosis; cytoreductive therapy in essential thrombocythemia benefits patients who are at high risk for thrombosis.

There is no good evidence to implicate thrombocytosis as a prothrombotic risk factor in "low-risk" and "indeterminate-risk" patients with essential thrombocythemia.

Although it is probably safe to use, the antithrombotic value of low-dose aspirin (81 to 325 mg daily) in essential thrombocythemia is unknown.

There is no good evidence to implicate hydroxyurea as a leukemogenic drug in essential thrombocythemia.

Pregnancy is not contraindicated in patients with essential thrombocythemia; the maternal morbidity rate is very low, whereas the first-trimester miscarriage rate is significantly higher than that of the general population.

No specific treatment is recommended for the pregnant low-risk or indeterminate-risk patient with essential thrombocythemia.

prospective studies, in a randomized setting, are currently ongoing and may clarify the comparative advantages and disadvantages of other platelet-lowering agents. In this regard, the concern about drug leukemogenicity in ET is unsubstantiated and the indiscriminate use of new drugs that are not tested in a controlled setting is unwarranted.

Pregnancy and Essential Thrombocythemia

The rate of first-trimester spontaneous abortion in ET (37%) is significantly higher than the 15% rate expected in the control population, and does not appear to be affected by specific treatment.[106] Late obstetric complications and maternal thrombohemorrhagic events are relatively infrequent. Neither the platelet count nor treatment with aspirin appears to affect either maternal morbidity or pregnancy outcome. Several studies show a spontaneous lowering of platelet counts during pregnancy in patients with ET. Therefore cytoreductive treatment is currently not recommended for low-risk women with ET who are pregnant or wish to become pregnant. In contrast, high-risk women require cytoreductive therapy to minimize the risk of recurrent thrombosis. Anecdotal evidence of safety has encouraged a preference for the use of interferon-alfa in case of pregnancy in these patients.

MYELOFIBROSIS WITH MYELOID METAPLASIA

MMM, also known as agnogenic myeloid metaplasia, or idiopathic myelofibrosis, was first described in 1879.[107] The clinical course of MMM is characterized by progressive anemia, marked hepatosplenomegaly, cachexia, nonhepatosplenic extramedullary hematopoiesis, and evolution into acute leukemia.[108] Similar to the situation in both PV and ET, the disease-initiating genetic lesion in MMM has not been identified. Currently, the diagnosis is based on characteristic, but not specific, clinical and laboratory features that include bone marrow fibrosis and osteosclerosis.[108] Among the chronic myeloproliferative disorders, MMM is the least frequent, with an incidence of 0.3 to 1.5/100,000.[74,75] The median age at diagnosis is 60 years, and approximately 10% of patients are diagnosed by 45 years of age.[109] Children are affected by MMM, but their clinical course may be less aggressive.[110]

Pathogenesis

It is now well established that MMM is a clonal stem cell disease involving both myeloid and lymphoid lineage.[111,112] In addition to clonal myeloproliferation, the bone marrow in MMM displays excess collagen fibrosis, new bone formation (osteosclerosis), and angiogenesis. These changes have been associated with alterations in both cellular and extracellular levels of various fibrogenic and angiogenic cytokines, including transforming growth factor-β, basic fibroblast growth factor, and platelet-derived growth factor.[113] The finding of polyclonal fibroblast proliferation in MMM is the basis for the current assumption that the bone marrow stromal aberration in MMM is reactive[114] and is mediated by the cytokines

derived from the resident clonal megakaryocytes and monocytes.[115]

An animal model of MMM has been established in mice that are chronically overexposed to TPO[116] or are carriers of a mutant GATA-1 gene that results in reduced expression of a transcription factor that plays a role in erythroid and megakaryocyte differentiation.[117] These mice show the characteristic features of MMM, including megakaryocytic hyperplasia, bone marrow fibrosis, osteosclerosis, and extramedullary hematopoiesis. The increased accumulation of megakaryocytes in these experimental animals has been attributed to either a direct effect of TPO or the lack of negative feedback from mature elements as a result of impaired megakaryocyte differentiation, respectively. In both instances, the abnormal accumulation of megakaryocytes and their sequestered cytokines mat be central to the pathogenesis of the associated stromal reaction. In this regard, the development of TPO-induced bone marrow fibrosis in mice has been temporally associated with elevated levels of transforming growth factor-β,[118] whereas it was abrogated in transforming growth factor-β knockout experiments.[119] Similar experiments may show the individual roles of other cytokines, including basic fibroblast growth factor and platelet-derived growth factor, that have been implicated in MMM.[120]

It is not clear whether animal models of MMM involve pathogenetic mechanisms that operate in the human form of the disease. For example, in human MMM, there is no evidence of either excess TPO production[121] or a genetic mutation involving the genes for TPO and c-Mpl.[85,121] Alternatively, the stromal reaction in human MMM may involve either a different process that drives megakaryocyte proliferation or a different source (e.g., monocytes) of fibrogenic cytokines.[122]

Diagnosis

The typical presentation of MMM includes anemia (from ineffective erythropoiesis), marked splenomegaly (from extramedullary hematopoiesis), and a myelophthisic peripheral blood smear. Myelophthisis (nucleated red blood cells, granulocyte precursors, and teardrop-shaped erythrocytes) suggests a bone marrow infiltrative process. The differential diagnosis includes bone marrow fibrosis, metastatic cancer, granulomatous infection, and lymphoma. In MMM, peripheral blood myelophthisis is associated with bone marrow megakaryocytic hyperplasia, collagen fibrosis, osteosclerosis, and intramedullary sinusoidal hematopoiesis (Fig. 106-5). However, bone marrow fibrosis may accompany MMM as well as other hematologic and nonhematologic disorders, including CML, MDS, systemic mast cell disease, eosinophilic disorders, and hairy cell leukemia (Table 106-7). Therefore, before making treatment recommendations, the clinician must consult with an experienced hematopathologist to confirm a specific diagnosis. Caution should be taken not to misdiagnose CML or hairy cell leukemia as MMM.

In cellular-phase MMM, the degree of bone marrow fibrosis may be minimal, but splenomegaly and myelophthisis are often present. MMM may develop de novo

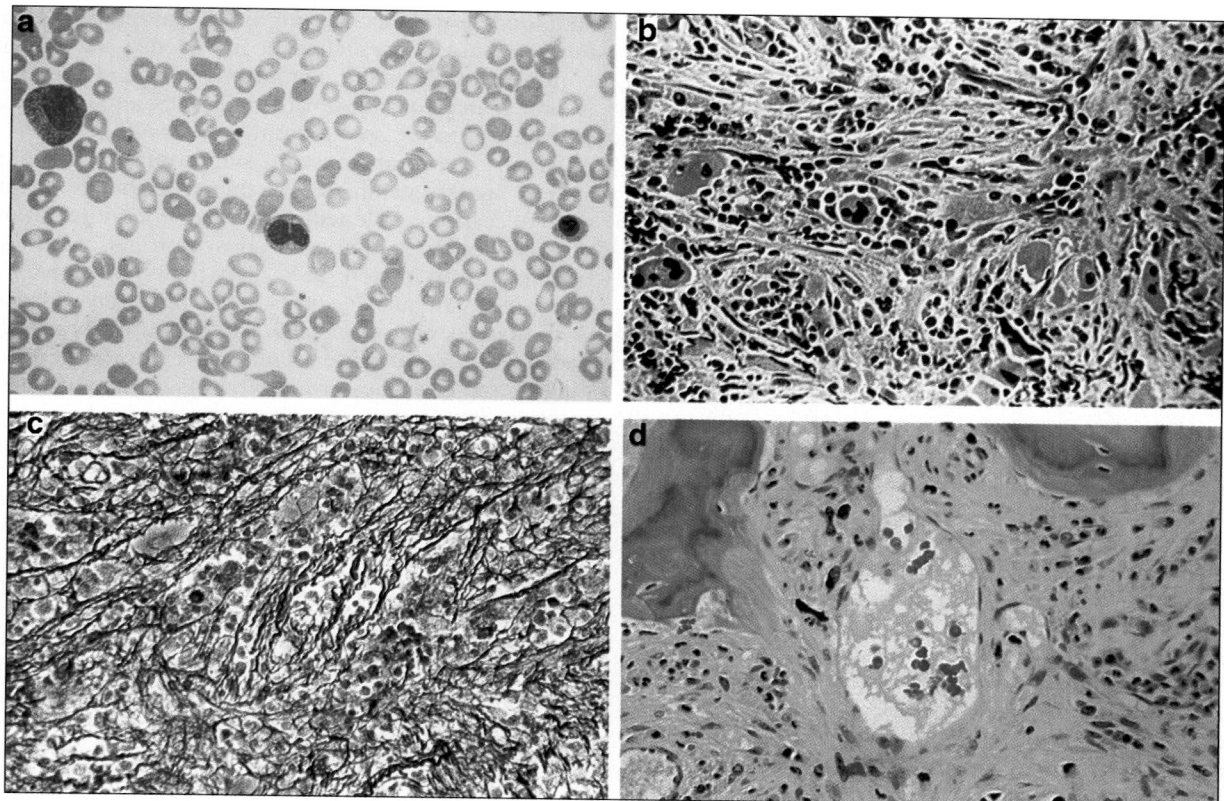

Figure 106-5. Peripheral blood myelophthisis (**A**), bone marrow fibrosis (**B** and **C**), and osteosclerosis and sinusoidal hematopoiesis (**D**) in myelofibrosis with myeloid metaplasia. (From Tefferi A: Myelofibrosis with myeloid metaplasia. N Engl J Med 2000;342:1255.)

TABLE 106-7

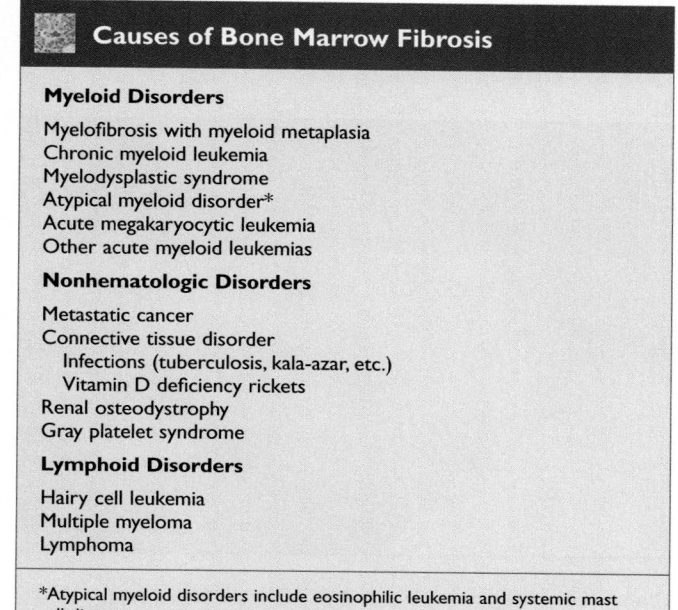

Causes of Bone Marrow Fibrosis

Myeloid Disorders

Myelofibrosis with myeloid metaplasia
Chronic myeloid leukemia
Myelodysplastic syndrome
Atypical myeloid disorder*
Acute megakaryocytic leukemia
Other acute myeloid leukemias

Nonhematologic Disorders

Metastatic cancer
Connective tissue disorder
  Infections (tuberculosis, kala-azar, etc.)
  Vitamin D deficiency rickets
Renal osteodystrophy
Gray platelet syndrome

Lymphoid Disorders

Hairy cell leukemia
Multiple myeloma
Lymphoma

*Atypical myeloid disorders include eosinophilic leukemia and systemic mast cell disease.

(agnogenic myeloid metaplasia) or during the latter stages of PV (postpolycythemic myeloid metaplasia) or ET (post-thrombocythemic myeloid metaplasia). Clonal cytogenetic abnormalities occur in approximately 50% of patients with MMM, and include 13q-, 20q-, +8, +9, and abnormalities of chromosomes 1, 7, and 12.[123] None of these cytogenetic markers are specific for MMM, and they are also seen in other myeloid and lymphoid disorders.

Treatment

Prognostic Factors

Among the chronic myeloproliferative disorders, MMM has the worst prognosis, with an approximate median survival of 5 years.[124] However, several studies identified both clinical and laboratory parameters that are used to identify low-risk as well as high-risk patient categories.[108] The most important indicators of adverse prognosis are anemia (hemoglobin <10 g/dL), advanced age (>64 years), hypercatabolic symptoms (weight loss, profound fatigue, night sweats, low-grade fever), leukocytosis (>30,000/μL) or leukopenia (<4000/μL), circulating blasts (≥1%), and high-risk cytogenetic abnormalities (+8, 12p-).[123-125] In the absence of these poor prognostic factors, median survival exceeds 10 years, whereas it may be less than 3 years in patients with two or more of these factors. Preliminary observations suggest that a high degree of bone marrow angiogenesis[126] and an increased circulating CD34 count may contribute to poor prognosis.[127]

Hematopoietic Stem Cell Transplantation

The only potentially curative therapy for MMM is allogeneic hematopoietic stem cell transplantation (HSCT).[128] In a retrospective, multicenter study of 66 consecutive patients, engraftment was not a major obstacle (84% rate of 30-day recovery of neutrophils), although it was delayed in patients with pretransplant anemia (hemoglobin <10 g/dL) and osteosclerosis.[129] In contrast, pretransplant splenectomy and higher doses of nucleated cells in the stem cell infusate were associated with more rapid engraftment. The 5-year survival rate was 62% in patients younger than 45 years of age and 14% in those who were older. Other investigators reported better survival figures in patients older than 44 years of age,[130] and preliminary data suggest that transplant-related morbidity in older patients may be positively influenced by the use of reduced-intensity conditioning regimens.[131]

Nevertheless, current information does not allow definitive comments about the role of allogeneic HSCT in MMM. I am not convinced that the risk of death or chronic graft-versus-host disease associated with allogeneic HSCT is justified in the setting of low-risk disease (<2 adverse features), even though the outcome may be better when allogeneic HSCT is performed in patients with early-stage disease.[128] In the presence of two or more adverse risk factors, it is reasonable to consider the procedure in high-risk patients younger than 45 years of age who have an HLA-identical sibling donor. The decision in all other cases should be individualized, unless there is new information that dictates otherwise.

Finally, limited information about autologous HSCT suggests improvement in both anemia and splenomegaly in most patients in the absence of leukemic transformation.[132]

Conventional Drug Treatment of Anemia

Conventional drug therapy for anemia includes a combination of an androgen preparation (fluoxymesterone [Halotestin] 10 mg twice daily) and prednisone (0.5 mg/kg daily),[133] exogenous EPO administration (40,000 units weekly subcutaneously) in the presence of an endogenous EPO level of less than 100 mU/mL,[134] and danazol (200 to 800 mg daily).[135] This therapy is not expected to alleviate splenomegaly and, in some cases, may further increase spleen size. Furthermore, cytoreductive treatment to control splenomegaly may be combined with EPO administration in an effort to offset drug-induced anemia.

Management of Splenomegaly and Other Extramedullary Hematopoieses

Hydroxyurea is the drug of choice for controlling splenomegaly, leukocytosis, or thrombocytosis.[136] Other drugs that have been used in a similar setting include busulfan,[137] melphalan,[138] and 2-chlorodeoxyadenosine.[139] In contrast, interferon-alfa has limited therapeutic value in MMM.[140] Many patients with MMM have recurrent splenic infarcts that may be associated with debilitating left upper quadrant pain that may be preceded by referred left

shoulder discomfort. A computed tomography scan may, but does not always, show a hypodense region without contrast enhancement. Symptoms of splenic infarcts are usually managed with opiate analgesics, and drug-resistant cases may require splenectomy.

Drug-resistant anemia and symptomatic splenomegaly (portal hypertension, severe hypercatabolic symptoms) may necessitate splenectomy. This procedure often alleviates splenomegaly-associated symptoms and may also benefit approximately 25% of patients with transfusion-dependent anemia (Fig. 106-6).[141] The surgical procedure is associated with a mortality rate of approximately 9%, and up to 25% of patients may have accelerated hepatomegaly and extreme thrombocytosis or leucocytosis after splenectomy. In patients with severe portal hypertension, which is primarily caused by intrahepatic obstruction rather than by increased portal flow as a result of marked splenomegaly, portal-systemic shunt surgery may be performed concomitantly with splenectomy. This has been shown to be a useful therapeutic option.[142]

In patients with mechanical splenic discomfort, splenic irradiation (100 to 500 cGy in 5 to 10 fractions) may be considered as an alternative to splenectomy.[143] However, the benefit of splenic irradiation is transient (median duration of response, 6 months), and the procedure has a mortality rate of more than 10% as a result of severe, prolonged cytopenias that occur in up to 25% of treated patients. The outcome from hepatic irradiation is even worse, and the procedure is generally not recommended.[144]

Radiation therapy is most useful in the treatment of non-hepatosplenic extramedullary hematopoiesis (EMH).[145] Symptomatic pulmonary hypertension that is not the result of a thromboembolic process has been associated with MMM, and is believed to arise from diffuse pulmonary EMH. The diagnosis is confirmed by ^{99m}Tc sulfur colloid scintigraphy, which shows diffuse pulmonary uptake, and treatment with single-fraction (100 cGy) whole-lung irradiation has been shown to be effective.[146,147] Low-dose irradiation is also effective for the treatment of

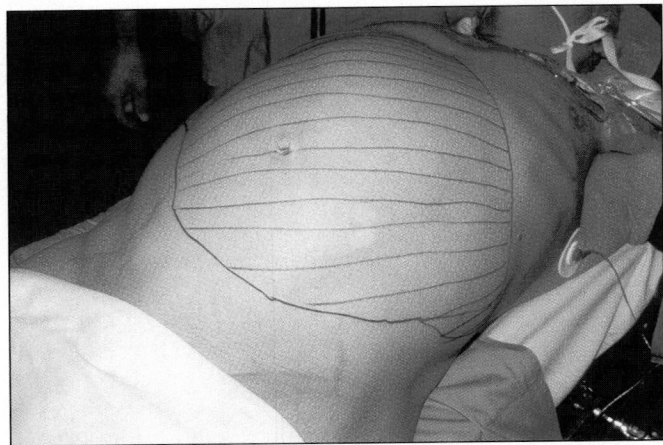

Figure 106-6. In a retrospective study of 223 splenectomies performed in patients with myelofibrosis with myeloid metaplasia, the average spleen weight was 2.7 kg (range, 380 g to 7.7 kg).

MYELOFIBROSIS WITH MYELOID METAPLASIA

The diagnosis of myelofibrosis with myeloid metaplasia requires consultation with an experienced hematopathologist; caution must be taken to exclude chronic myeloid leukemia, hairy cell leukemia, myelodysplastic syndrome with myelofibrosis, and acute myelofibrosis.

Drug therapy in myelofibrosis with myeloid metaplasia is palliative and may not prolong life.

The place of hematopoietic stem cell transplantation in the treatment of myelofibrosis with myeloid metaplasia is being defined, and specific decisions require consultation with disease experts and experienced transplant physicians.

The indications for splenectomy in myelofibrosis with myeloid metaplasia include symptomatic portal hypertension, severe mechanical discomfort that is often associated with cachexia, and treatment-resistant anemia with heavy transfusion requirements.

Low-dose radiation therapy is effective in the treatment of nonhepatosplenic extramedullary hematopoiesis in patients with myelofibrosis with myeloid metaplasia.

paraspinal or epidural EMH (1000 cGy in 5 to 10 fractions) and EMH causing pleural and peritoneal effusions (100 to 500 cGy in 5 to 10 fractions).[145,148]

Investigational Treatment

The finding of intense bone marrow angiogenesis in MMM prompted a series of studies of thalidomide as a therapeutic agent. When used as a single agent and at doses that average approximately 200 mg daily, thalidomide results in clinically relevant improvement of anemia (20%), splenomegaly (23%), and thrombocytopenia (71%).[149] However, approximately 20% of patients have substantial thrombocytosis or leukocytosis in addition to the usual side effects of thalidomide. The use of low-dose thalidomide (50 mg daily) in combination with a tapering dose of prednisone (0.5 mg/kg daily) has been associated with a higher rate of response in both anemia (62%) and clinically relevant thrombocytopenia (75%) as well as a better toxicity profile.[150] These favorable responses to thalidomide were not associated with reduced bone marrow angiogenesis, and the mechanism of action may involve other effects of thalidomide, including immune modulation and tumor necrosis factor antagonism. The latter possibility is supported by another study that showed a favorable effect on constitutional symptoms with the use of a soluble tumor necrosis factor receptor, etanercept.[151] Immunomodulatory thalidomide analogs and the combination of thalidomide and etanercept are currently being tested.

REFERENCES

1. Dameshek W: Some speculations on the myeloproliferative syndromes. Blood 1951;6:372–375.
2. Raskind WH, Steinmann L, Najfeld V: Clonal development of myeloproliferative disorders: Clues to hematopoietic differentiation and multistep pathogenesis of cancer. Leukemia 1998;12:108–116.
3. Janssen JW, Buschle M, Layton M, et al: Clonal analysis of myelodysplastic syndromes: Evidence of multipotent stem cell origin. Blood 1989;73:248–254.
4. Flotho C, Valcamonica S, Mach-Pascual S, et al: RAS mutations and clonality analysis in children with juvenile myelomonocytic leukemia (JMML). Leukemia 1999;13:32–37.
5. Froberg MK, Brunning RD, Dorion P, Litz CE, Torlakovic E: Demonstration of clonality in neutrophils using FISH in a case of chronic neutrophilic leukemia. Leukemia 1998;12:623–626.
6. Chang HW, Leong KH, Koh DR, Lee SH: Clonality of isolated eosinophils in the hypereosinophilic syndrome. Blood 1999;93:1651–1657.
7. Yavuz AS, Lipsky PE, Yavuz S, Metcalfe DD, Akin C: Evidence for the involvement of a hematopoietic progenitor cell in systemic mastocytosis from single-cell analysis of mutations in the c-kit gene. Blood 2002;100:661–665.
8. Vaquez MH: Sur une forme speciale de cyanose s'accompagnant d'hyperglobulie excessive et persistante. C R Soc Biol (Paris) 1892;44:384–388.
9. Osler W: Chronic cyanosis, with polycythemia and enlarged spleen: A new clinical entity. Am J Med Sci 1903;126:187–201.
10. Ania BJ, Suman VJ, Sobell JL, Codd MB, Silverstein MN, Melton LJ III: Trends in the incidence of polycythemia vera among Olmsted County, Minnesota residents, 1935–1989. Am J Hematol 1994;47:89–93.
11. Berglund S, Zettervall O: Incidence of polycythemia vera in a defined population. Eur J Haematol 1992;48:20–26.
12. Chaiter Y, Brenner B, Aghai E, Tatarsky I: High incidence of myeloproliferative disorders in Ashkenazi Jews in northern Israel. Leuk Lymphoma 1992;7:251–255.
13. Hemminki K, Jiang Y: Familial polycythemia vera: Results from the Swedish Family-Cancer Database. Leukemia 2001;15:1313–1315.
14. Anonymous: Polycythemia vera: The natural history of 1213 patients followed for 20 year: Gruppo Italiano Studio Policitemia. Ann Intern Med 1995;123:656–664.
15. Heilmann E, Klein CE, Beck JD: Primary polycythaemia in childhood and adolescence. Folia Haematol Int Mag Klin Morphol Blutforsch 1983;110:935–941.
16. Adamson JW, Fialkow PJ, Murphy S, Prchal JF, Steinmann: Polycythemia vera: Stem-cell and probable clonal origin of the disease. N Engl J Med 1976;295:913–916.
17. Raskind WH, Jacobson R, Murphy S, Adamson JW, Fialkow PJ: Evidence for the involvement of B lymphoid cells in polycythemia vera and essential thrombocythemia. J Clin Invest 1985;75:1388–1390.
18. Gilliland DG, Blanchard KL, Levy J, Perrin S, Bunn HF: Clonality in myeloproliferative disorders: Analysis by means of the polymerase chain reaction. Proc Natl Acad Sci USA 1991;88:6848–6852.
19. Prchal JF, Axelrad AA: Bone-marrow responses in polycythemia vera (letter). N Engl J Med 1974;290:1382.
20. Correa PN, Eskinazi D, Axelrad AA: Circulating erythroid progenitors in polycythemia vera are hypersensitive to insulin-like growth factor-1 in vitro: Studies in an improved serum-free medium (see comments). Blood 1994;83:99–112.
21. Tefferi A: Polycythemia vera: A comprehensive review and clinical recommendations. Mayo Clin Proc 2003;78:174–194.
22. Michl P, Spoettl G, Engelhardt D, Weber MM: Alterations of the insulin-like growth factor system in patients with polycythemia vera. Mol Cell Endocrinol 2001;181:189–197.
23. Hess G, Rose P, Gamm H, Papadileris S, Huber C, Seliger B: Molecular analysis of the erythropoietin receptor system in patients with polycythaemia vera. Br J Haematol 1994;88:794–802.
24. Mirza AM, Correa PN, Axelrad AA: Increased basal and induced tyrosine phosphorylation of the insulin-like growth factor I receptor beta subunit in circulating mononuclear cells of patients with polycythemia vera. Blood 1995;86:877–882.
25. Wickrema A, Chen F, Namin F, et al: Defective expression of the SHP-1 phosphatase in polycythemia vera. Exp Hematol 1999;27:1124–1132.
26. Sui XW, Krantz SB, Zhao ZH: Identification of increased protein tyrosine phosphatase activity in polycythemia vera erythroid progenitor cells. Blood 1997;90:651–657.

27. Roder S, Steimle C, Meinhardt G, Pahl HL: STAT3 is constitutively active in some patients with polycythemia rubra vera. Exp Hematol 2001;29:694–702.

28. Dai C, Krantz SB: Increased expression of the INK4a/ARF locus in polycythemia vera. Blood 2001;97:3424–3432.

29. Silva M, Richard C, Benito A, Sanz C, Olalla I, Fernandez-Luna JL: Expression of Bcl-x in erythroid precursors from patients with polycythemia vera (see comments). N Engl J Med 1998;338:564–571.

30. Fairbanks VF, Tefferi A: Normal ranges for packed cell volume and hemoglobin concentration in adults: Relevance to 'apparent polycythemia.' Eur J Haematol 2000;65:285–296.

31. Lamy T, Devillers A, Bernard M, et al: Inapparent polycythemia vera: An unrecognized diagnosis. Am J Med 1997;102:14–20.

32. Berlin NI: Diagnosis and classification of the polycythemias. Semin Hematol 1975;12:339–351.

33. Murphy S: Diagnostic criteria and prognosis in polycythemia vera and essential thrombocythemia. Semin Hematol 1999;36(1 Suppl 2):9–13.

34. Pearson TC: Diagnosis and classification of erythrocytoses and thrombocytoses. Baillieres Clin Haematol 1998;11:695–720.

35. Michiels JJ, Juvonen E: Proposal for revised diagnostic criteria of essential thrombocythemia and polycythemia vera by the Thrombocythemia Vera Study Group. Semin Thromb Hemost 1997;23:339–347.

36. Birgegard G, Wide L: Serum erythropoietin in the diagnosis of polycythaemia and after phlebotomy treatment. Br J Haematol 1992;81:603–606.

37. Andreasson B, Lindstedt G, Stockelberg D, Wadenvik H, Kutti J: The relation between plasma thrombopoietin and erythropoietin concentrations in polycythaemia vera and essential thrombocythaemia. Leuk Lymphoma 2001;41:579–84.

38. Kralovics R, Indrak K, Stopka T, Berman BW, Prchal JF, Prchal JT: Two new Epo receptor mutations: Truncated Epo receptors are most frequently associated with primary familial and congenital polycythemias. Blood 1997;90:2057–2061.

39. Messinezy M, Westwood NB, El-Hemaidi I, Marsden JT, Sherwood RS, Pearson TC: Serum erythropoietin values in erythrocytoses and in primary thrombocythaemia. Br J Haematol 2002;117:47–53.

40. Cotes PM, Dore CJ, Yin JA, et al: Determination of serum immunoreactive erythropoietin in the investigation of erythrocytosis. N Engl J Med 1986;315:283–287.

41. Thiele J, Kvasnicka HM, Zankovich R, Diehl V: The value of bone marrow histology in differentiating between early stage polycythemia vera and secondary (reactive) polycythemias. Haematologica 2001;86:368–374.

42. Diez-Martin JL, Graham DL, Petitt RM, Dewald GW: Chromosome studies in 104 patients with polycythemia vera. Mayo Clin Proc 1991;66:287–299.

43. Tefferi A, Yoon SY, Li CY: Immunohistochemical staining for megakaryocyte c-Mpl may complement morphologic distinction between polycythemia vera and secondary erythrocytosis. Blood 2000;96:771–772.

44. Temerinac S, Klippel S, Strunck E, et al: Cloning of PRV-1, a novel member of the uPAR receptor superfamily, which is overexpressed in polycythemia rubra vera. Blood 2000;95:2569–2576.

45. Chievitz E, Thiede T: Complications and causes of death in polycythemia vera. Acta Med Scand 1962;172:513–523.

46. Pearson TC, Wetherley-Mein G: Vascular occlusive episodes and venous haematocrit in primary proliferative polycythaemia. Lancet 1978;2(8102):1219–1222.

47. Thomas DJ, et al: Cerebral blood flow in polycythemia. Lancet 1977;2(8030):161–163.

48. Berk PD, Wasserman LR, Fruchtman SM, Goldberg JD: Treatment of polycythemia vera: A summary of clinical trials conducted by the Polycythemia Vera Study Group. In Wasserman LR, et al (eds): Polycythemia vera and the myeloproliferative disorders. Philadelphia, WB Saunders, 1995, pp 166–194.

49. Anonymous: Treatment of polycythaemia vera by radiophosphorus or busulphan: A randomized trial. "Leukemia and Hematosarcoma" Cooperative Group, European Organization for Research on Treatment of Cancer (E.O.R.T.C.). Br J Cancer 1981;44:75–80.

50. Najean Y, Rain JD: Treatment of polycythemia vera: The use of hydroxyurea and pipobroman in 292 patients under the age of 65 years. Blood 1997;90:3370–3377.

51. Najean Y, Rain JD: Treatment of polycythemia vera: Use of 32P alone or in combination with maintenance therapy using hydroxyurea in 461 patients greater than 65 years of age. The French Polycythemia Study Group. Blood 1997;89:2319–2327.

52. Tartaglia AP, Goldberg JD, Berk PD, Wasserman LR: Adverse effects of antiaggregating platelet therapy in the treatment of polycythemia vera. Semin Hematol 1986;23:172–176.

53. Landolfi R, Marchioli R: European Collaboration on Low-dose Aspirin in Polycythemia Vera (ECLAP): A randomized trial. Semin Thromb Hemost 1997;23:473–478.

54. Fruchtman SM, Mack K, Kaplan ME, Peterson P, Berk PD, Wasserman LR: From efficacy to safety: A Polycythemia Vera Study Group report on hydroxyurea in patients with polycythemia vera. Semin Hematol 1997;34:17–23.

55. West WO: Hydroxyurea in the treatment of polycythemia vera: A prospective study of 100 patients over a 20-year period. South Med J 1987;80:323–327.

56. Tatarsky I, Sharon R: Management of polycythemia vera with hydroxyurea. Semin Hematol 1997;34:24–28.

57. Passamonti F, Brusamolino E, Lazzarino M, et al: Efficacy of pipobroman in the treatment of polycythemia vera: Long-term results in 163 patients. Haematologica 2000;85:1011–1018.

58. Petti MC, Spadea A, Avvisati G, et al: Polycythemia vera treated with pipobroman as single agent: Low incidence of secondary leukemia in a cohort of patients observed during 20 years (1971–1991). Leukemia 1998;12:869–874.

59. Messinezy M, Pearson TC, Prochazka A, Wetherley-Mein G: Treatment of primary proliferative polycythaemia by venesection and low dose busulphan: Retrospective study from one centre. Br J Haematol 1985;61:657–666.

60. D'Emilio A, Battista R, Dini E: Treatment of primary proliferative polycythaemia by venesection and busulphan. Br J Haematol 1987;65:121–122.

61. Silver RT: Interferon alfa: Effects of long-term treatment for polycythemia vera. Semin Hematol 1997;34:40–50.

62. Elliott MA, Tefferi A: Interferon-alpha therapy in polycythemia vera and essential thrombocythemia. Semin Thromb Hemost 1997;23:463.

63. Tefferi A, Silverstein MN, Petitt RM, Mesa RA, Solberg LA: Anagrelide as a new platelet-lowering agent in essential thrombocythemia: Mechanism of action, efficacy, toxicity, current indications. Semin Thromb Hemost 1997;23:379.

64. Anonymous: Anagrelide: A therapy for thrombocythemic states. Experience in 577 patients: Anagrelide Study Group. Am J Med 1992;92:69–76.

65. Tefferi A, Elliott MA, Solberg LA Jr, Silverstein MN: New drugs in essential thrombocythemia and polycythemia vera. Blood Rev 1997;11:1–7.

66. Budde U, Schaefer G, Mueller N, et al: Acquired von Willebrand's disease in the myeloproliferative syndrome. Blood 1984;64:981–985.

67. Rosenow EC III, Limper AH: Drug-induced pulmonary disease. Semin Respir Infect 1995;10:86–95.

68. Stuart JJ, Crocker DL, Roberts HR: Treatment of busulfan-induced pancytopenia. Arch Intern Med 1976;136:1181–1183.

69. Najean Y, Dresch C, Rain JD: The very-long-term course of polycythaemia: A complement to the previously published data of the Polycythaemia Vera Study Group (see comments). Br J Haematol 1994;86:233–235.

70. Diehn F, Tefferi A: Pruritus in polycythaemia vera: Prevalence, laboratory correlates and management. Br J Haematol 2001;115:619–621.

71. Tefferi A, Fonseca: Selective serotonin reuptake inhibitors are effective in the treatment of polycythemia vera-associated pruritus. Blood 2002;99:2627.

72. Epstein E, Goedel A: Hamorrhagische thrombozythamie bei vascularer schrumpfmilz. Virchows Archiv A Pathol Anat Histopathol 1934;293:233.

73. Jensen MK, de Nully Brown P, Nielsen OJ, Hasselbalch HC: Incidence, clinical features and outcome of essential

thrombocythaemia in a well defined geographical area. Eur J
Haematol 2000;65:132–139.

74. Ridell B, Carneskog J, Wedel H, et al: Incidence of chronic
myeloproliferative disorders in the city of Goteborg, Sweden
1983–1992. Eur J Haematol 2000;65:267–271.

75. Mesa RA, Silverstein MN, Jacobsen SJ, Wollan PC, Tefferi A:
Population-based incidence and survival figures in essential
thrombocythemia and agnogenic myeloid metaplasia: An Olmsted
County study, 1976–1995. Am J Hematol 1999;61:10–15.

76. Gugliotta L: Epidemiological, diagnostic, therapeutic, and
prognostic aspects of essential thrombocythemia in a
retrospective study of the GIMMC group in two thousand
patients (abstract 1551). Blood 1997;90:348a.

77. McNally RJ, Rowland D, Roman E, Cartwright RA: Age and sex
distributions of hematological malignancies in the UK. Hematol
Oncol 1997;15:173–189.

78. Randi ML, Putti MC, Fabris F, Sainati L, Zanesco L, Girolami A:
Features of essential thrombocythaemia in childhood: A study of
five children. Br J Haematol 2000;108:86–89.

79. Dror Y, Zipursky A, Blanchette VS: Essential thrombocythemia in
children. J Pediatr Hematol Oncol 1999;21:356–363.

80. Fialkow PJ, Faguet GB, Jacobson RJ, Vaidya K, Murphy S: Evidence
that essential thrombocythemia is a clonal disorder with origin in
a multipotent stem cell. Blood 1981;58:916–919.

81. Elkassar N, Hetet G, Briere J, Grandchamp B: Clonality analysis of
hematopoiesis in essential thrombocythemia: Advantages of
studying T lymphocytes and platelets. Blood 1997;89:128–134.

82. Champion KM, Gilbert JG, Asimakopoulos FA, Hinshelwood S,
Green AR: Clonal haemopoiesis in normal elderly women:
Implications for the myeloproliferative disorders and
myelodysplastic syndromes. Br J Haematol 1997;97:920–926.

83. Wang JC, Chen C, Novetsky AD, Lichter SM, Ahmed F, Friedberg
NM: Blood thrombopoietin levels in clonal thrombocytosis and
reactive thrombocytosis. Am J Med 1998;104:451–455.

84. Espanol I, Hernandez A, Cortes M, Mateo J, Pujol-Moix N: Patients
with thrombocytosis have normal or slightly elevated
thrombopoietin levels. Haematologica 1999;84:312–316.

85. Harrison CN, Gale RE, Wiestner AC, Skoda RC, Linch DC: The
activating splice mutation in intron 3 of the thrombopoietin gene
is not found in patients with non-familial essential
thrombocythaemia. Br J Haematol 1998;102:1341–1343.

86. Kiladjian JJ, Elkassar N, Hetet G, Briere J, Grandchamp B, Gardin C:
Study of the thrombopoietin receptor in essential
thrombocythemia. Leukemia 1997;11:1821–1826.

87. Axelrad AA, Eskinazi D, Correa PN, Amato D: Hypersensitivity of
circulating progenitor cells to megakaryocyte growth and
development factor (PEG-rHu MGDF) in essential
thrombocythemia. Blood 2000;96:3310–3321.

88. Kobayashi S, Teramura M, Hoshino S, Motoji T, Oshimi K,
Mizoguchi H: Circulating megakaryocyte progenitors in
myeloproliferative disorders are hypersensitive to interleukin-3.
Br J Haematol 1993;83:539–544.

89. Griesshammer M, Bangerter M, Sauer T, Wennauer R, Bergmann L,
Heimpel H: Aetiology and clinical significance of thrombocytosis:
Analysis of 732 patients with an elevated platelet count. J Intern
Med 1999;245:295–300.

90. Tefferi A, Ho TC, Ahmann GJ, Katzmann JA, Greipp PR: Plasma
interleukin-6 and C-reactive protein levels in reactive versus
clonal thrombocytosis (see comments). Am J Med 1994;97:
374–378.

91. Yoon SY, Li CY, Tefferi A: Megakaryocyte c-Mpl expression in
chronic myeloproliferative disorders and the myelodysplastic
syndrome: Immunoperoxidase staining patterns and clinical
correlates. Eur J Haematol 2000;65:170–174.

92. Horikawa Y, Matsumura I, Hashimoto K, et al: Markedly reduced
expression of platelet C-Mpl receptor in essential thrombocythemia. Blood 1997;90:4031–4038.

93. Mesa RA, Hanson CA, Li CY, et al: Diagnostic and prognostic value
of bone marrow pathogenesis and megakaryocyte C-Mpl
expression in essential thrombocythemia. Blood 2002;99:
4131–4137.

94. Teofili L, Martini M, Luongo M, et al: Overexpression of the
polycythemia rubra vera-1 gene in essential thrombocythemia.
J Clin Oncol 2002;20:4249–4254.

95. Thiele J, Kvasnicka HM, Diehl V, Fischer R, Michiels JJ:
Clinicopathological diagnosis and differential criteria of
thrombocythemias in various myeloproliferative disorders by
histopathology, histochemistry and immunostaining from bone
marrow biopsies. Leuk Lymphoma 1999;33:207–218.

96. Dewald GW, Wyatt WA, Juneau AL, et al: Highly sensitive
fluorescence in situ hybridization method to detect double
BCR/ABL fusion and monitor response to therapy in chronic
myeloid leukemia. Blood 1998;91:3357–3365.

97. Sessarego M, Defferrari R, Dejana AM, et al: Cytogenetic analysis in
essential thrombocythemia at diagnosis and at transformation:
A 12-year study. Cancer Genet Cytogenet 1989;43:57–65.

98. Tefferi A, Murphy S: Current opinion in essential thrombocythemia: Pathogenesis, diagnosis, and management. Blood Rev
2001;15:121–131.

99. Fenaux P, Simon M, Caulier MT, Lai JL, Goudemand J, Bauters F:
Clinical course of essential thrombocythemia in 147 cases. Cancer
1990;66:549–556.

100. Besses C, Cervantes F, Pereira A, et al: Major vascular complications
in essential thrombocythemia: A study of the predictive factors in
a series of 148 patients. Leukemia 1999;13:150–154.

101. Tefferi A, Fonseca R, Pereira DL, Hoagland HC: A long-term
retrospective study of young women with essential
thrombocythemia. Mayo Clin Proc 2001;76:22–28.

102. van Genderen PJ, Mulder PG, Waleboer M, van de Moesdijk D,
Michiels JJ: Prevention and treatment of thrombotic
complications in essential thrombocythaemia: Efficacy and safety
of aspirin. Br J Haematol 1997;97:179–184.

103. Cortelazzo S, Finazzi G, Ruggeri M, et al: Hydroxyurea for patients
with essential thrombocythemia and a high risk of thrombosis
(see comments). N Engl J Med 1995;332:1132–1136.

104. Storen EC, Tefferi A: Long-term use of anagrelide in young patients
with essential thrombocythemia. Blood 2001;97:863–866.

105. Mazzucconi MG, Ferrari A, Solinas S, et al: Studies of von
Willebrand factor in essential thrombocythemia patients treated
with alpha-2b recombinant interferon. Haemostasis 1991;21:
135–140.

106. Wright CA, Tefferi A: A single institutional experience with 43
pregnancies in essential thrombocythemia. Eur J Haematol
2001;66:152–159.

107. Heuck G: Zwei Falle von Leukamie mit eigenthumlichem Blut:
Resp Knochenmarksbefund. Virchows Arch Pathol Anat Physiol
1879;78:475–496.

108. Tefferi A: Myelofibrosis with myeloid metaplasia. N Engl J Med
2000;342:1255–1265.

109. Cervantes F, Barosi G, Demory JL, et al: Myelofibrosis with myeloid
metaplasia in young individuals: Disease characteristics,
prognostic factors and identification of risk groups. Br J Haematol
1998;102:684–690.

110. Altura RA, Head DR, Wang WC: Long-term survival of infants with
idiopathic myelofibrosis. Br J Haematol 2000;109:459–462.

111. Jacobson RJ, Salo A, Fialkow PJ: Agnogenic myeloid metaplasia: A
clonal proliferation of hematopoietic stem cells with secondary
myelofibrosis. Blood 1978;51:189–194.

112. Reeder TL, Bailey RJ, Dewald GW, Tefferi A: Both B and T
lymphocytes may be clonally involved in myelofibrosis with
myeloid metaplasia. Blood 2002;24:24.

113. Reilly JT: Pathogenesis and management of idiopathic
myelofibrosis. Baillieres Clin Haematol 1998;11:751–767.

114. Castro-Malaspina H, Gay RE, Jhanwar SC, et al: Characteristics of
bone marrow fibroblast colony-forming cells (CFU-F) and their
progeny in patients with myeloproliferative disorders. Blood
1982;59:1046–1054.

115. Rameshwar P, Denny TN, Stein D, Gascon P: Monocyte adhesion in
patients with bone marrow fibrosis is required for the production
of fibrogenic cytokines: Potential role for interleukin-1 and
TGF-beta. J Immunol 1994;153:2819–2830.

116. Yan XQ, Lacey D, Hill D, et al: A model of myelofibrosis and
osteosclerosis in mice induced by overexpressing thrombopoietin
(Mpl ligand): Reversal of disease by bone marrow transplantation.
Blood 1996;88:402–409.

117. Vannucchi AM, Bianchi L, Cellai C, et al: Development of
myelofibrosis in mice genetically impaired for GATA-1 expression
(GATA-1 [low] mice). Blood 2002;100:1123–1132.

Specific Malignancies

III

118. Yanagida M, Ide Y, Imai A, et al: The role of transforming growth factor-beta in PEG-rHuMGDF-induced reversible myelofibrosis in rats. Br J Haematol 1997;99:739–745.

119. Chagraoui H, Komura E, Tulliez M, Giraudier S, Vainchenker W, Wendling F: Prominent role of TGF-beta 1 in thrombopoietin-induced myelofibrosis in mice. Blood 2002;100:3495–3503.

120. Martyre MC, Le Bousse-Kerdiles MC, Romquin N, et al: Elevated levels of basic fibroblast growth factor in megakaryocytes and platelets from patients with idiopathic myelofibrosis (see comments). Br J Haematol 1997;97:441–448.

121. Taksin AL, Couedic JPL, Dusanter-Fourt I, et al: Autonomous megakaryocyte growth in essential thrombocythemia and idiopathic myelofibrosis is not related to a c-Mpl mutation or to an autocrine stimulation by Mpl-L. Blood 1999;93:125–139.

122. Rameshwar P, Narayanan R, Qian J, Denny TN, Colon C, Gascon P: NF-kappa B as a central mediator in the induction of TGF-beta in monocytes from patients with idiopathic myelofibrosis: An inflammatory response beyond the realm of homeostasis. J Immunol 2000;165:2271–2277.

123. Tefferi A, Mesa RA, Schroeder G, Hanson CA, Li CY, Dewald GW: Cytogenetic findings and their clinical relevance in myelofibrosis with myeloid metaplasia. Br J Haematol 2001;113:763–771.

124. Cervantes F, Pereira A, Esteve J, et al: Identification of 'short-lived' and 'long-lived' patients at presentation of idiopathic myelofibrosis. Br J Haematol 1997;97:635–640.

125. Dupriez B, Morel P, Demory JL, et al: Prognostic factors in agnogenic myeloid metaplasia: A report on 195 cases with a new scoring system (see comments). Blood 1996;88:1013–1018.

126. Mesa RA, Hanson CA, Rajkumar SV, Schroeder G, Tefferi A: Evaluation and clinical correlations of bone marrow angiogenesis in myelofibrosis with myeloid metaplasia. Blood 2000;96: 3374–3380.

127. Barosi G, Viarengo G, Pecci A, et al: Diagnostic and clinical relevance of the number of circulating CD34(+) cells in myelofibrosis with myeloid metaplasia. Blood 2001;98:3249–3255.

128. Guardiola P, Anderson JE, Bandini G, et al: Allogeneic stem cell transplantation for agnogenic myeloid metaplasia: A European group for blood and marrow transplantation. Societe Francaise de Greffe de Moelle, Gruppo Italiano per il Trapianto del Midollo Osseo, and Fred Hutchinson Cancer Research Center collaborative study. Blood 1999;93:2831–2838.

129. Guardiola P, Anderson JE, Gluckman E: Myelofibrosis with myeloid metaplasia. N Engl J Med 2000;343:659; discussion 659–660.

130. Deeg HJ, Appelbaum FR: Stem-cell transplantation for myelofibrosis. N Engl J Med 2001;344:775–776.

131. Devine SM, Hoffman R, Verma A, et al: Allogeneic blood cell transplantation following reduced-intensity conditioning is effective therapy for older patients with myelofibrosis with myeloid metaplasia. Blood 2002;99:2255–2258.

132. Anderson JE, Tefferi A, Craig F, et al: Myeloablation and autologous peripheral blood stem cell rescue results in hematologic and clinical responses in patients with myeloid metaplasia with myelofibrosis. Blood 2001;98:586–593.

133. Silverstein MN: Agnogenic myeloid metaplasia. Acton, Mass, Publishing Science Group, 1975, p 126.

134. Rodriguez JN, Martino ML, Dieguez JC, Prados D: rHuEpo for the treatment of anemia in myelofibrosis with myeloid metaplasia:

135. Cervantes F, Hernandez-Boluda JC, Alvarez A, Nadal E, Montserrat E: Danazol treatment of idiopathic myelofibrosis with severe anemia. Haematologica 2000;85:595–599.

136. Lofvenberg E, Wahlin A: Management of polycythaemia vera, essential thrombocythaemia and myelofibrosis with hydroxyurea. Eur J Haematol 1988;41:375–381.

137. Naqvi T, Baumann MA: Myelofibrosis: Response to busulfan after hydroxyurea failure. Int J Clin Pract 2002;56:312–313.

138. Petti MC, Latagliata R, Spadea T, et al: Melphalan treatment in patients with myelofibrosis with myeloid metaplasia. Br J Haematol 2002;116:576–581.

139. Tefferi A, Silverstein MN, Li CY: 2-Chlorodeoxyadenosine treatment after splenectomy in patients who have myelofibrosis with myeloid metaplasia. Br J Haematol 1997;99:352–357.

140. Tefferi A, et al: Clinical and bone marrow effects of interferon alfa therapy in myelofibrosis with myeloid metaplasia. Blood 2001;97:1896.

141. Tefferi A, Mesa RA, Nagorney DM, Schroeder G, Silverstein MN: Splenectomy in myelofibrosis with myeloid metaplasia: A single-institution experience with 223 patients. Blood 2000;95: 2226–2233.

142. Tefferi A, Barrett SM, Silverstein MN, Nagorney DM: Outcome of portal-systemic shunt surgery for portal hypertension associated with intrahepatic obstruction in patients with agnogenic myeloid metaplasia. Am J Hematol 1994;46:325–328.

143. Elliott M, et al: Splenic irradiation for symptomatic splenomegaly associated with myelofibrosis with myeloid metaplasia. Br J Haematol 1997;103:505.

144. Tefferi A, Jimenez T, Gray LA, Mesa RA, Chen MG: Radiation therapy for symptomatic hepatomegaly in myelofibrosis with myeloid metaplasia. Eur J Haematol 2001;66:37–42.

145. Houck WA, Mesa RA, Tefferi A: Antemortem presentation and management of non-hepatosplenic extramedullary hematopoiesis in myelofibrosis with myeloid metaplasia. Blood 2000;96:747a.

146. Dingli D, Utz JP, Krowka MJ, Oberg AL, Tefferi A: Unexplained pulmonary hypertension in chronic myeloproliferative disorders. Chest 2001;120:801–808.

147. Steensma DP, Hook CC, Stafford SL, Tefferi A: Low-dose, single-fraction, whole-lung radiotherapy for pulmonary hypertension associated with myelofibrosis with myeloid metaplasia. Br J Haematol 2002;118:813–816.

148. Bartlett RP, Greipp PR, Tefferi A, Cupps RE, Mullan BP, Trastek VF: Extramedullary hematopoiesis manifesting as a symptomatic pleural effusion. Mayo Clin Proc 1995;70:1161–1164.

149. Elliott MA, Mesa RA, Li CY, et al: Thalidomide treatment in myelofibrosis with myeloid metaplasia. Br J Haematol 2002;117:288–296.

150. Mesa RA, Steesma DP, Pardanan A, et al: A phase 2 trial of combination low-dose thalidomide and prednisone for the treatment of myelofibrosis with myeloid metaplasia. Blood 2003;101:2534–2541.

151. Steensma DP, Mesa RA, Li CY, Gray L, Tefferi A: Etanercept, a soluble tumor necrosis factor receptor, palliates constitutional symptoms in patients with myelofibrosis with myeloid metaplasia: Results of a pilot study. Blood 2002;99:2252–2254.

Experience in 6 patients and meta-analytical approach. Haematologica 1998;83:616–621.

CHRONIC MYELOID LEUKEMIA

Brian J. Druker

John M. Goldman

SUMMARY OF KEY POINTS

INCIDENCE

- More than 4000 cases per year in the United States, accounting for approximately 15% of all leukemias
- Most patients are older than 60 years at diagnosis
- A slight male predominance exists

CLINICAL FINDINGS

- Common symptoms include fatigue, night sweats, and abdominal discomfort as a result of splenomegaly
- Many patients are asymptomatic at diagnosis
- White blood cell count is usually greater than 50×10^9/L, with a left-shifted differential

- Basophilia is present, and blast percentage is usually less than 5%
- Platelet count is increased in 50% of patients

DIFFERENTIAL DIAGNOSIS

- Chronic myelomonocytic leukemia
- Other myeloproliferative disorders
- Leukemoid reaction

EVALUATION

- Complete history and physical examination, complete blood count with differential and platelet count, and chemistries
- Bone marrow aspiration and biopsy
- Testing for the presence of the Philadelphia (Ph) chromosome by

cytogenetic analysis or for the presence of the *BCR-ABL* fusion gene by fluorescence in situ hybridization (FISH) or by reverse-transcription polymerase chain reaction (RT-PCR)

THERAPY

- Hydroxyurea or imatinib mesylate to control leukocyte and platelet counts initially
- Imatinib induces a complete hematologic and cytogenetic response in most patients, but long-term-survival data are not available
- Allogeneic stem cell transplantation is often curative, but is associated with considerable morbidity and mortality

INTRODUCTION

Chronic myeloid leukemia (CML), also chronic myelogenous leukemia or chronic granulocytic leukemia, is a clonal hematopoietic disorder caused by an acquired genetic defect in a pluripotent stem cell. Leukemia was first recognized in the 1840s, but CML was clearly distinguished from other types of leukemia only with the advent of staining methods for blood cells in the late 1800s.[1] In 1960, the Philadelphia (Ph) chromosome was discovered in CML cells,[2] making CML the first human neoplasm to be characterized by a consistent cytogenetic marker. In 1973, the Ph chromosome was shown to be the result of a balanced, reciprocal translocation involving chromosomes 9 and 22.[3] In the 1980s, the *BCR-ABL* chimeric gene and protein formed as a result of the (9;22) translocation was characterized.[4,5] It is now known that the BCR-ABL protein, which functions as a constitutively activated tyrosine kinase, has a central role in the pathogenesis of CML.

CML behaves as a biphasic or triphasic illness. Most patients are diagnosed in a relatively indolent chronic or stable phase that lasts an average of 4 to 6 years, until a more aggressive, advanced phase intervenes. The advanced phase may be further subdivided into accelerated phase and blastic phase, with survival in the blastic phase measured in months.

Allogeneic stem cell transplantation (SCT) is the only curative therapy for patients with CML but is associated with substantial morbidity and mortality. For patients not undergoing transplantation, treatment with interferon-alfa (IFN-alfa) results in longer survival compared with that of patients treated with hydroxyurea or busulfan. However, IFN-alfa has largely been replaced by imatinib mesylate (Gleevec, Glivec, formerly STI571), an agent that specifically inhibits the tyrosine kinase activity of the BCR-ABL protein. Integration of these various treatment modalities is evolving.

INCIDENCE, EPIDEMIOLOGY, AND ETIOLOGY

CML accounts for approximately 15% of all leukemias and has an incidence of 1.6 to 2.0 cases per 100,000 persons per year.[6] Although CML occurs in all age groups, its incidence increases with each decade of life, making CML primarily a disease of adults, with a median age at diagnosis of 66 years.[6] CML accounts for 3% of all childhood leukemias.[7] The disease has a slight male predominance (2.2:1.3).[6]

The etiology of CML is unknown in most patients. However, the risk of CML is higher after exposure to radiation. This is evident from studies of survivors of

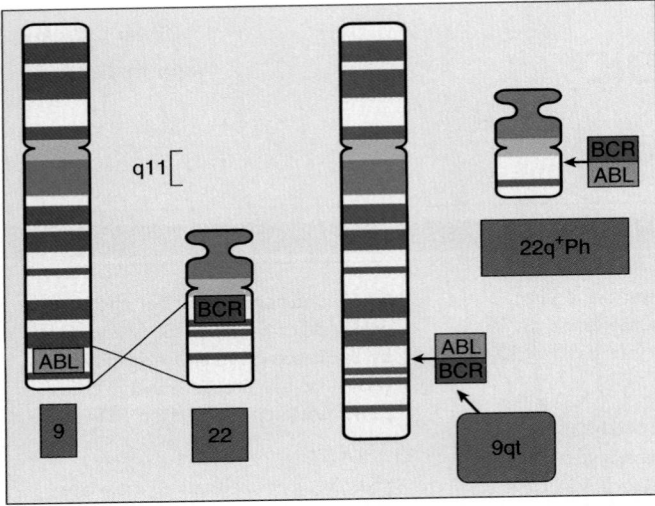

Figure 107-1. Diagrammatic representation of the formation of the Ph chromosome. The normal chromosomes 9 and 22 are shown along with the derivative chromosomes 9q+ and 22q- (Ph). The approximate positions of the normal *ABL* gene at 9q34 and *BCR* at 22q11, and the two fusion genes, formed as a result of the translocation, *BCR-ABL* on chromosome 22q- and *ABL-BCR* and chromosome 9q+, also are shown.

the atom bomb explosions in Japan in 1945 and from follow-up of patients treated with radiation for ankylosing spondylitis and cervical cancer.[8–10] CML has no known association with any infectious agent or chemical exposures. No familial predisposition has been implicated; however, isolated reports are found of CML in first-degree relatives of patients,[11] and relapse of CML originating in donor cells after related allogeneic SCT has been recorded.[12] Individuals expressing human leukocyte antigen (HLA)-B8, HLA-A3, and HLA-DR4 have a decreased risk of CML.[13,14]

PATHOGENESIS

Molecular Biology

The Ph chromosome is an acquired cytogenetic abnormality that is present in all CML cells.[2,3] It is found in cells of the myeloid, erythroid, and megakaryocytic lineages, in some B cells, and in a small proportion of T cells, but is absent from other cells of the body. These data establish CML as a clonal disorder that originates in a pluripotent hematopoietic stem cell. The Ph chromosome is a shortened chromosome 22 (22q-) that usually results from a balanced, reciprocal translocation between the long arms of chromosomes 9 and 22 t(9;22)(q34;q11) (Fig. 107-1). As a result of this translocation, the *ABL* (Abelson) proto-oncogene normally found on chromosome 9 is translocated into a relatively small, 5.8-Kb genomic region on chromosome 22 that was appropriately named the breakpoint cluster region (bcr).[15] This region is now known to form the central part of a relatively large gene of unknown function, the *BCR* gene. In the *ABL* gene, the position of the genomic breakpoint is highly variable but always occurs upstream of the second exon (a2). Thus the (9;22) translocation results in juxtaposition of 5′ sequences of the *BCR* gene with 3′ *ABL* sequences (Fig. 107-2). This event leads to the generation of a chimeric *BCR-ABL* fusion gene that is transcribed into an 8.5-Kb messenger RNA (mRNA) and encodes a protein of 210 kd (p210). The BCR-ABL fusion protein has constitutive tyrosine kinase activity compared with the tightly regulated tyrosine kinase activity of the normal *ABL* product (p145).[16,17]

Two slightly different chimeric *BCR-ABL* genes are present in patients with CML, depending on the precise location of the breakpoint in the *BCR* gene. A break occurring between exons b2 and b3 yields a b2a2 fusion mRNA, whereas a break occurring between exons b3 and b4 produces a b3a2 fusion mRNA (see Fig. 107-2).[5]

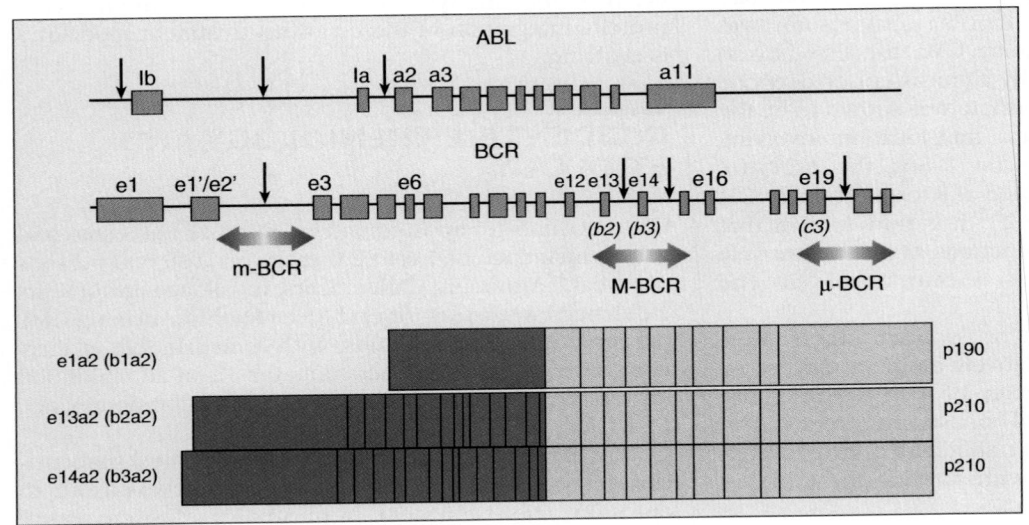

Figure 107-2. Schematic representation of the genomic structure of the normal *ABL* and *BCR* genes (*top*) and various fusion transcripts generated by the different *BCR-ABL* fusion genes. The b2a2 or the b3a2 transcript is found in the majority of patients with chronic myeloid leukemia. See text for details.

Historically this was referred to as the major breakpoint cluster region (M-BCR). More recently, with a complete map of the exon and intron structure of *BCR*, all exons of the *BCR* gene have been designated e1 through e21, with b2 and b3 corresponding to e13 and 14. Most patients have either b2a2 or b3a2 transcripts, but some patients have both transcripts in their leukemia cells. Although the b3a2 mRNA encodes a BCR-ABL protein that is 25 amino acids larger than that encoded by the b2a2 transcript, both are referred to as p210BCR-ABL. The type of *BCR-ABL* transcript has no known prognostic significance, although some, but not all, studies have shown that patients with a b3a2 fusion may have a higher platelet count than patients with a b2a2 fusion.[18]

The *BCR-ABL* fusion gene is not specific to CML and may be found in other forms of leukemia.[19] In adults with Ph chromosome–positive acute lymphoblastic leukemia (ALL), one third of patients have *BCR-ABL* transcripts indistinguishable from those found in CML. In two thirds, the genomic breakpoint on chromosome 22 occurs in the first intron of the *BCR* gene (between e1 and e2) in an area known as the minor breakpoint cluster region (m-BCR) (see Fig. 107-2). The mRNA product, designated e1a2, encodes a protein of 190 kDa (p190), also referred to as p185. In children with Ph chromosome–positive ALL, 95% have the p190 form of BCR-ABL. This transcript is rarely found in patients with CML. Very rarely, patients with Ph chromosome–positive chronic neutrophilic leukemia have a chimeric *BCR-ABL* gene with an e19a2 mRNA product that encodes a 230-kDa protein (p230). The genomic breakpoint of the *BCR* gene at e19 also is referred to as the micro-breakpoint cluster region (m-BCR). Other types of fusions have been observed in isolated cases.

Animal Models of Chronic Myeloid Leukemia

Several experimental approaches have shown the ability of *BCR-ABL* to cause leukemia. In one set of experiments, transgenic mice that express *BCR-ABL* had rapidly fatal acute leukemia.[20] With a different approach, a *BCR-ABL*–expressing retrovirus was used to infect murine bone marrow. These *BCR-ABL*–expressing marrow cells were used to repopulate irradiated mice. The transplanted mice had a variety of myeloproliferative disorders, including a CML-like syndrome.[21,22] Although these approaches show the leukemogenic potential of *BCR-ABL*, it is possible that secondary changes are required for leukemia to develop. Recently, Huettner and colleagues[23] placed *BCR-ABL* under the control of a tetracycline repressible promoter. In mice expressing this transgene, a lymphoid leukemia develops that is reversed in the presence of tetracycline, showing the leukemic potential of *BCR-ABL* as a sole oncogenic abnormality.

BCR-ABL Signaling and Chronic Myeloid Leukemia Pathogenesis

Significant advances have been made in determining the signaling pathways that are activated by BCR-ABL kinase activity. Numerous substrates and binding partners have been identified, and current efforts are directed at linking these pathways to the specific pathologic defects that characterize CML.[5] The pathologic defects identified in CML cells include increased proliferation or decreased apoptosis of a hematopoietic stem or progenitor cell, leading to a massive increase in myeloid cell numbers. An example of a cellular pathway that links to an increased proliferative rate is activation of the RAS pathway. STAT-5–mediated upregulation of the antiapoptotic molecule BCL_{XL} and phosphorylation of and inactivation of the proapoptotic molecule BAD by AKT are postulated to lead to a protection from programmed cell death.[5] Because patients with CML have circulating immature myeloid progenitors, it has been postulated that a defect exists in adherence of myeloid progenitors to marrow stroma. CML cells exhibit reduced adhesion to fibronectin, possibly as a downstream effect of CRKL phosphorylation.[5] Despite the seemingly endless expansion of the list of pathways activated by *BCR-ABL* and the increasing complexity that is being revealed in these pathways, all of the transforming functions of *BCR-ABL* are dependent on its tyrosine kinase activity.[17]

Molecular Diagnosis of Chronic Myeloid Leukemia

Classic or typical CML is defined by the presence of the *BCR-ABL* fusion gene and accounts for 95% of patients who have a hematologic profile resembling that of CML. In 90% of patients, the presence of the *BCR-ABL* gene can be inferred from the presence of the Ph chromosome by using standard cytogenetic analysis of bone marrow metaphases. In patients with CML, 85% have a typical t(9;22), and 5% have variant translocations. These variant translocations may be simple, involving chromosome 22 and a chromosome other than chromosome 9, or they may be complex, involving one or more chromosomes in addition to chromosomes 9 and 22.[24] In the 10% of patients with hematologic features resembling CML who lack a detectable Ph chromosome, at least half of these patients have a *BCR-ABL* fusion detectable by fluorescence in situ hybridization (FISH) or reverse transcription polymerase chain reaction (RT-PCR). These Ph-chromosome-negative, *BCR-ABL*–positive patients and patients with variant translocations have a clinical course that is indistinguishable from that of Ph-chromosome–positive, *BCR-ABL*–positive patients.[25]

A FISH analysis relies on the colocalization of large genomic probes specific to the *BCR* and *ABL* genes. FISH has several advantages over conventional cytogenetics. It can be performed on metaphase or interphase cells as well as on peripheral blood. Comparison of marrow and blood samples by FISH analysis shows high concordance, at least in IFN-alfa–treated patients.[26] One potential problem with FISH is the random colocalization of the signals from the *BCR* and *ABL* probes such that 8% to 10% of normal cells appear positive. This has been circumvented, in part, with D-FISH, which uses probes that span the breakpoint region.[27] However, at diagnosis, where typically more than 90% of cells are *BCR-ABL* positive,

Specific Malignancies

III

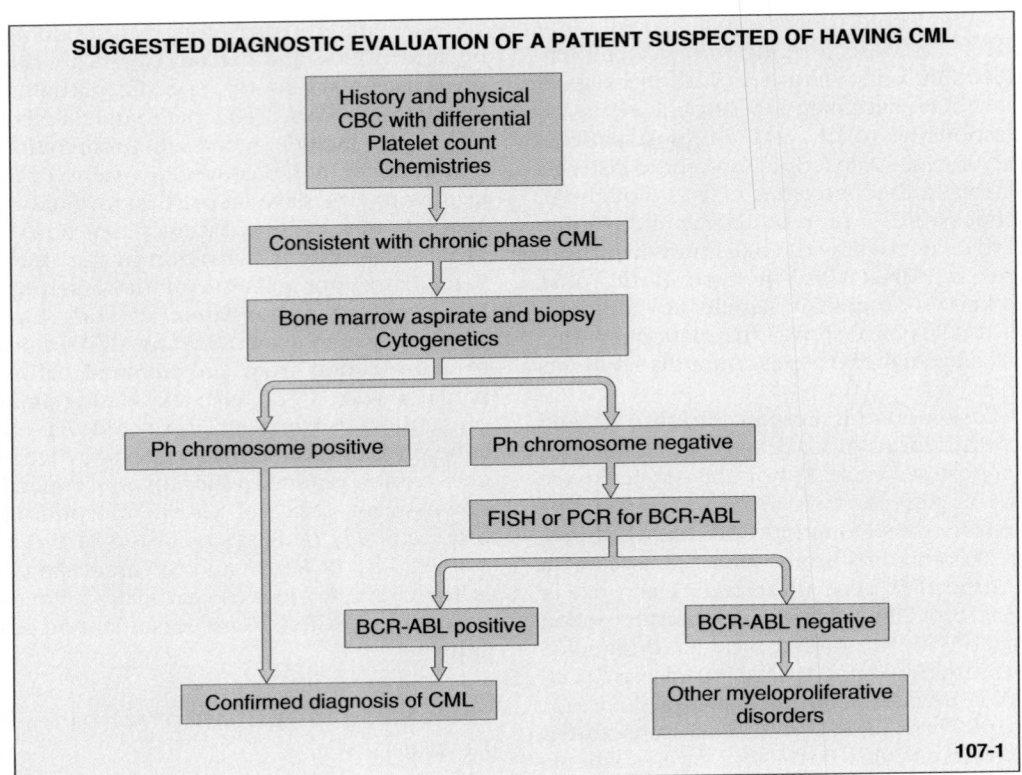

SUGGESTED DIAGNOSTIC EVALUATION OF A PATIENT SUSPECTED OF HAVING CML

History and physical
CBC with differential
Platelet count
Chemistries

↓

Consistent with chronic phase CML

↓

Bone marrow aspirate and biopsy
Cytogenetics

Ph chromosome positive   Ph chromosome negative

↓

FISH or PCR for BCR-ABL

BCR-ABL positive   BCR-ABL negative

Confirmed diagnosis of CML   Other myeloproliferative disorders

107-1

FISH is a highly accurate diagnostic test because false-negative results are rare. FISH on peripheral blood or marrow may be the most accurate diagnostic test for *BCR-ABL* fusion genes.[28]

RT-PCR can be used to amplify the region around the splice junction between *BCR* and *ABL*. The high sensitivity of this technique makes it ideal for the detection of minimal residual disease.[28] PCR testing can either be qualitative, providing information about the presence of the *BCR-ABL* transcript, or quantitative, assessing the amount of *BCR-ABL* message. Qualitative PCR is particularly useful in the diagnosis of CML, whereas quantitative PCR is preferred for monitoring residual disease, because serial quantitative analyses may allow detection of upward trends, predictive of relapse.[28]

Similar to FISH, peripheral blood and marrow RT-PCR values show a high level of concordance. Both false-positive and false-negative results are possible with RT-PCR, and rigorous controls are required to detect these events. False-negative results can be the result of poor-quality RNA or failure of the reaction, whereas false-positive results are usually caused by contamination.

In the 10% of patients with hematologic features resembling those of CML without the Ph chromosome, half also lack the *BCR-ABL* fusion gene These Ph chromosome–negative, *BCR-ABL*–negative patients encompass a heterogeneous spectrum of conditions, some of which may have a more aggressive clinical course than that in those with *BCR-ABL*–positive disease.[29] Although the molecular pathogenesis of these *BCR-ABL*–negative myeloproliferative disorders is not well understood,

subsets of these patients have chromosomal rearrangements that activate tyrosine kinases, such as the platelet-derived growth factor receptor (PDGF-R), the fibroblast growth factor receptor (FGF-R), or JAK-2.[30]

CLINICAL PRESENTATION

Chronic Phase

Ninety percent of patients with CML are diagnosed in the chronic or stable phase. Thirty to fifty percent of patients are asymptomatic and are diagnosed when an elevated white blood cell (WBC) count is found on routine blood sampling. The most common symptoms of CML are related to anemia, splenomegaly, and increased cell turnover. These symptoms include fatigue, left upper quadrant pain, abdominal fullness or discomfort, early satiety, weight loss, and night sweats.[31] Occasionally, patients have hyperviscosity syndrome, with manifestations such as stroke, priapism, stupor, or visual changes caused by retinal hemorrhage (Table 107-1). These patients may require leukapheresis to reduce the WBC count.

The most common physical finding in patients with CML is splenomegaly, which is present in up to 75% of patients (Table 107-2). The tip of the spleen extends more than 10 cm below the left costal margin in half of these patients. The magnitude of splenomegaly correlates well with the degree of leukocytosis. The larger the spleen, the more susceptible it is to infarction. Ecchymoses are relatively common, but spontaneous bleeding is un-

TABLE 107-1

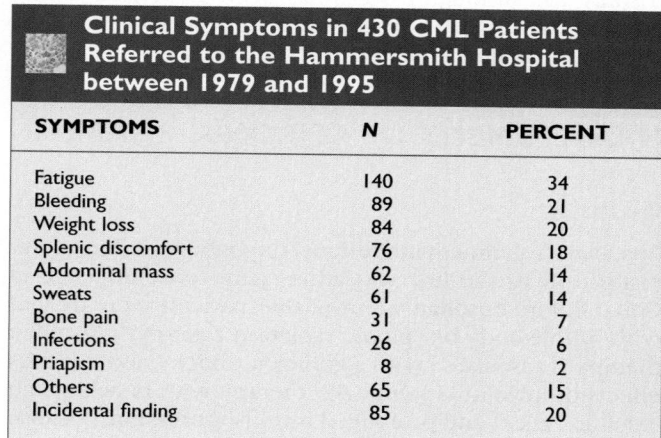

SYMPTOMS	N	PERCENT
Fatigue	140	34
Bleeding	89	21
Weight loss	84	20
Splenic discomfort	76	18
Abdominal mass	62	14
Sweats	61	14
Bone pain	31	7
Infections	26	6
Priapism	8	2
Others	65	15
Incidental finding	85	20

Clinical Symptoms in 430 CML Patients Referred to the Hammersmith Hospital between 1979 and 1995

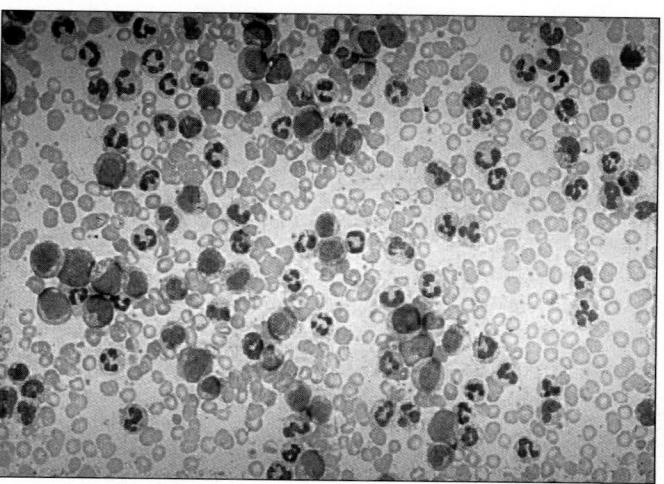

Figure 107-3. Peripheral blood smear of chronic-phase chronic myeloid leukemia. Note the prominent neutrophilia, myelocytes, and basophilia.

common and may be related to concomitant thrombocytosis. Lymphadenopathy is uncommon. Twenty percent of patients have no physical signs at diagnosis.

Hematologic Findings

The diagnosis of CML is commonly made by the typical appearance of the peripheral blood and bone marrow. The WBC count in stable-phase CML is usually greater than 50×10^9/L at the time of diagnosis, with a range from 20×10^9/L to 800×10^9/L. During the chronic phase, leukemic cells retain the capacity to differentiate normally, and the peripheral blood smear shows a full spectrum of myeloid cells, from blasts to neutrophils. Neutrophils and myelocytes are the most predominant cells in the peripheral blood smear; blasts compose less than 15% and usually less than 5% of the WBC differential (Fig. 107-3). Basophilia is an important diagnostic feature, and its absence suggests other myeloproliferative disorders, particularly if *BCR-ABL* also is absent. Eosinophilia is commonly present. Most patients have thrombocytosis with platelet anisocytosis. Occasionally, the platelet count may be more than 1000×10^9/L. Most patients with CML have normochromic, normocytic anemia that is inversely proportional to the degree of leukocytosis. Nucleated red cells may be present.

The bone marrow in patients with CML is markedly hypercellular, with a predominance of myeloid cells with full maturation. Myeloblasts compose less than 15% and

most commonly, less than 5% of marrow elements. The basophilia seen in the peripheral blood also is present in the marrow. Megakaryocytes are usually increased and may form clusters that are more apparent in the biopsy specimen. These clusters are less striking than are those seen in essential thrombocythemia. Occasionally, micro-megakaryocytes may be present. Because of the increased myeloid/erythroid ratio, apparent erythroid hypoplasia is noted. Erythroid precursors are otherwise unremarkable morphologically. Reticulin fibrosis is usually absent or mild. Excessive reticulin fibrosis is associated with more advanced disease, with massive splenomegaly and increased blast cell counts.

Other Laboratory Abnormalities

Leukocyte alkaline phosphatase (LAP) levels are low or undetectable in the blood of most patients with CML. Transcobalamin I is produced by granulocytes; thus serum B_{12} levels are increased in proportion to the total WBC count. Uric acid and lactate dehydrogenase (LDH) levels also are frequently elevated, reflecting the increased WBC mass and increased cell turnover.

DIFFERENTIAL DIAGNOSIS

Anyone with a WBC count greater than 50×10^9/L and a peripheral blood smear showing a full spectrum of myeloid lineage cells plus basophilia should be suspected of having CML. This diagnosis can be confirmed by the presence of the *BCR-ABL* gene, as described earlier. The differential diagnosis includes a leukemoid reaction, which is typically seen in patients with underlying infections. In patients with a leukemoid reaction, the WBC count is usually less than 50×10^9/L, and the peripheral blood smear consists predominantly of segmented neutrophils and bands, often with toxic granulations. Less mature myeloid cells are rarely seen, there is no basophilia, the leukocyte alkaline phosphatase is elevated, and the Ph chromosome is absent.

TABLE 107-2

Clinical Signs in 430 CML Patients Referred to the Hammersmith Hospital between 1979 and 1995

SIGNS	N	PERCENT
Spleen palpable	314	76
1–10 cm	153	37
>10 cm	161	39
Spleen not palpable	100	24
Purpura	66	16
Palpable liver	9	2
No signs	85	20

Approximately 5% of patients with CML have extreme thrombocytosis and a minimally elevated WBC count, resembling essential thrombocytosis (ET), but this can be distinguished from ET by the presence of the *BCR-ABL* gene. Although patients with CML may have an increase in monocyte numbers, corresponding to the leukocytosis, relative monocytopenia is found, which differentiates CML from chronic myelomonocytic leukemia (CMML). In addition, patients with CMML and other myeloproliferative disorders often lack the basophilia seen with CML and lack the *BCR-ABL* gene.

PROGNOSIS

Various staging systems have been developed to predict the probability of chronic-phase disease progressing to the advanced phase and to assist in the decision-making process about appropriate treatment options. The prognostic scoring system proposed by Sokal[32] reproducibly segregates chemotherapy-treated patients into high- and low-risk groups for disease progression. Sokal's model identified four independent prognostic factors: older age, splenomegaly, higher platelet count, and higher peripheral blast percentage (Table 107-3). Sokal's index is less efficient in discriminating outcome in IFN-alfa–treated patients. However, a revised score, the Euro score, which also incorporates peripheral blood eosinophils and basophils, can identify risk groups in patients treated with IFN-alfa (see Table 107-3).[33] Whether either of these scores will discriminate outcome for patients treated with imatinib is unknown.

Recent data suggest that genomic deletions in the *ABL* gene on chromosome 9q+ may have prognostic significance.[34] Moreover, telomere length may correlate with survival.[35] These later two findings must be validated in larger clinical trials. Clonal cytogenetic abnormalities in addition to the Ph chromosome are present at diagnosis in some patients, with the most common being duplication of the Ph chromosome, trisomy 8, iso-17q, and trisomy 19. Although iso-17q has been associated with a poorer prognosis, the prognostic significance of the other chromosomal abnormalities is less clear.[36,37]

MANAGEMENT OF CHRONIC PHASE

Busulfan

Busulfan (1,4-dimethane-sulfonyl-oxybutane) is important historically as the first alkylating agent to be effective in CML.[1] Before busulfan was available, patients were treated with whole-body or splenic radiation therapy.[38] Busulfan therapy is associated with significant toxicity, and given its effects on primitive stem cells, therapy with busulfan can result in severe and prolonged myelosuppression. Because of these concerns, plus the availability of more effective therapies, the use of busulfan should be limited to those patients who are intolerant of or resistant to other available therapies. Busulfan is used as part of some conditioning regimens in allogeneic SCT, but it should not be used in patients awaiting allogeneic SCT, because its use is associated with an adverse outcome.[39]

Hydroxyurea

Hydroxyurea is a well-tolerated, oral cytotoxic agent that can effectively and rapidly control blood counts in most patients with CML. Hydroxyurea is a ribonucleotide reductase inhibitor that acts on relatively late myeloid progenitors compared with busulfan. This accounts for the prompt increase of the leukocyte count on discontinuation of the drug. Treatment with hydroxyurea requires close monitoring, because excessive reduction of the WBC count often occurs, particularly in the initial stages of therapy, until the WBC count is stabilized. Rare side effects include nausea, rashes, and mouth ulcers. Leg ulcers limit clinical utility in a small number of patients.[40] Initial treatment with hydroxyurea is usually with a daily dose of 1 to 4 g, depending on the WBC count, presence of

TABLE 107-3

Prognostic Models in Chronic Myeloid Leukemia		
	SOKAL MODEL*	**EURO MODEL**
Characteristics	Age	Age
	Platelet count	Platelet count
	Spleen size	Spleen size
	Percentage blood blasts	Percentage blood blasts
		Percentage blood basophils
		Percentage blood eosinophils
Online Calculator	http://www.nrhg.ncl.ac.uk/cgi-bin/cml/sokal.pl	http://www.pharmacoepi.de/cmlscore.html
Risk Groups and (Median Survival)		
Low	<0.8 (60 mo)	≤780 (98 mo)
Intermediate	0.8–1.2 (45 mo)	781–1480 (65 mo)
High	>1.2 (30 mo)	>1481 (42 mo)

*The Sokal index was derived from data for patients treated with busulfan and hydroxyurea, and the Euro score, from patients treated with IFN-alfa. A statistically significant correlation was found in the various indices to risk groups. However, these scores are limited in their ability to predict survival in any particular patient.

symptoms, and urgency to reduce the WBC count. The maintenance dose usually is 0.5 and 2.0 g daily and is titrated to keep the WBC count between 5 and 20×10^9/L.

Although hydroxyurea is effective in controlling the WBC count and reducing splenomegaly, it rarely results in a decrease in the percentage of Ph-chromosome–positive metaphases in the marrow (cytogenetic response) and does not prevent disease progression. It is better tolerated than busulfan, and its superiority to busulfan was shown in a multicenter randomized trial in Germany.[41] The median survival of patients treated with busulfan was 3.8 years compared with that of hydroxyurea at 4.7 years ($P = .008$). This survival advantage was seen in all Sokal prognostic groups.

Interferon-alfa

IFN-alfa belongs to a family of glycoproteins that have antiviral and antiproliferative properties. It was first shown to be an active agent in CML in the early 1980s.[42] Multiple studies show that IFN-alfa induces complete or partial hematologic remissions in 50% to 80% of untreated patients with CML.[43] In contrast to hydroxyurea or busulfan, cytogenetic responses are observed in 40% to 60% of IFN-alfa–treated patients. This includes 10% to 38% major cytogenetic responses (<35% Ph chromosome positivity) and 7% to 26% complete cytogenetic responses.[43]

In a meta-analysis of 1554 patients with CML enrolled in seven prospective, randomized trials, those treated with IFN-alfa had a statistically significant better survival than that of patients treated with hydroxyurea ($P = .001$) or busulfan ($P = .00007$) alone.[44] Patient survival at 5 years was 57% for patients treated with IFN-alfa versus 42% in the chemotherapy-treated groups ($P < .00001$).[44] With the Euro score to segregate patients into different risk categories for response to IFN-alfa, "low-risk" patients have an expected median survival of 96 to 104 months,[33] and an expected major cytogenetic response rate of about 50%.[45] In contrast, patients with "high-risk" disease can be expected to have a median survival of 42 months[33] and a major cytogenetic response rate of no more than 20%.[45] Consistent with this trend, IFN-alfa has minimal activity in accelerated-phase or blastic-phase CML.[46]

Unfortunately, the clinical utility of IFN-alfa is limited by its toxicity profile. Between 15% and 25% of patients discontinue treatment with IFN-alfa because of intolerable side effects, and another 30% to 50% of patients in various trials have required dose reductions because of poor treatment tolerance. Toxicity of IFN-alfa increases with increasing dose and patient age.[47] Side effects commonly encountered early in treatment include flulike symptoms, with fevers, chills, myalgias, and fatigue. With ongoing therapy, patients may have chronic fatigue, depression, insomnia, weight loss, peripheral neuropathy, alopecia, stomatitis, diarrhea, and loss of recent memory.[48] Immune-mediated complications, including autoimmune hemolytic anemia, hypothyroidism, immune-mediated thrombo-cytopenia, and collagen vascular disorders, occur in approximately 5% of patients. Transient increases in transaminases or alkaline phosphatase may be seen in up to 50% of patients treated with IFN-alfa, but severe liver enzyme abnormalities requiring discontinuation of therapy are uncommon.

Thrombocytopenia, leukopenia, and mild anemia (hemoglobin, 10 to 12 g/dL) are common with IFN-alfa therapy. Leukopenia may be necessary to achieve optimal clinical benefit from INF-alfa. In a single-institution trial in which the IFN-alfa dose was titrated to maintain a WBC count between 1.5 and 5×10^9/L, a major cytogenetic response rate of 44% was reported.[49]

The appropriate dose of IFN-alfa is the subject of debate. In some studies, a higher dose of IFN-alfa (5 million units/m^2) was associated with a higher rate of major cytogenetic response. However, in a randomized study, 3 million units given 3 times per week was as effective as full-dose IFN-alfa.[50] An individual's response to IFN-alfa is an important prognostic factor. Median time to achieve a hematologic remission is 6 to 8 months.[51] Patients who achieve a complete hematologic response after 3 to 6 months of IFN-alfa therapy have a statistically better outcome.[51,52] The median time to complete cytogenetic response is 22 to 24 months, and the median time to partial response is 12 to 18 months.[51] Achievement of a cytogenetic response has been associated with a survival advantage in most studies; however, a cytogenetic response in high-risk patients does not seem to confer the same good prognosis as that in low-risk patients.[53]

Investigators have sought to improve on the success of treatment with IFN-alfa by adding cytosine arabinoside (Ara-C), another agent with antileukemic activity. One randomized trial of the combination showed significantly improved hematologic and cytogenetic response rates over those of IFN-alfa alone, which translated into an overall survival advantage.[54] A subsequent study confirmed the improved response rates but found no survival advantage for the combination.[55] In addition, the combination of IFN-alfa and cytarabine is associated with increased gastrointestinal and marrow toxicity, and not surprisingly, many patients tolerate it poorly. Another potential problem with the use of IFN-alfa is that it may compromise the outcome of subsequent transplantation because of an increase in graft rejection or graft-versus-host disease. However, conflicting data are found on this issue, and many recommend discontinuing IFN-alfa at least 3 months before transplantation.[56]

New formulations of IFN-alfa may improve tolerance and efficacy. Attachment of IFN-alfa to polyethylene glycol (PEG) prolongs the half-life of IFN-alfa, allowing weekly administration. In one randomized study comparing regular IFN-alfa with pegylated IFN-alfa, a suggestion of improved cytogenetic responses was noted with the pegylated IFN-alfa (Roche, Pegasys).[57] These results may be preparation dependent, as an IFN-alfa product pegylated in a different fashion (Peg-Intron) did not show improved responses compared with those of regular IFN-alfa.[58]

Imatinib

Imatinib mesylate (Gleevec, Glivec, formerly STI571) has rapidly become the treatment of choice for patients with chronic-phase CML who are not candidates for immediate

SCT.[59] Imatinib is an orally administered inhibitor of the BCR-ABL tyrosine kinase. Other tyrosine kinases inhibited by imatinib include the PDGF-R, KIT and ARG (ABL-related gene). Preclinical data showed significant specific activity against BCR-ABL–expressing cells lines in vitro and in vivo. In addition, imatinib could select for the growth of BCR-ABL–negative hematopoietic cells from CML patient samples in colony-forming assays and long-term marrow cultures.[60]

Based on the favorable preclinical data, imatinib was tested in phase I clinical trials in chronic-phase patients with CML who were refractory to or intolerant of IFN-alfa. In the phase I study, significant therapeutic benefits and minimal side effects were seen at doses of 300 mg daily and greater.[61] Based on these data, a phase II trial enrolled 454 patients with confirmed chronic-phase disease who were refractory to or intolerant of IFN-alfa. Patients were treated with an imatinib dose of 400 mg by mouth daily.

Eligibility criteria in this study allowed inclusion of patients with up to 15% blasts and 15% basophils in the marrow or peripheral blood. Median duration of disease was 34 months, and median duration of previous IFN-alfa therapy was 14 months.[62] With a median follow-up of 29 months, 96% of patients achieved a complete hematologic response (CHR), with a median time to CHR of less than 1 month. Imatinib induced major cytogenetic responses in 64% of patients, with a complete cytogenetic response rate of 48%. The estimated progression-free survival at 24 months was 87% (Table 107-4).

In this phase II study, cytogenetic responses have been durable thus far and correlate with improved progression-free and overall survival. Thus once a patient achieves a major cytogenetic response, it is estimated that 24 months later, 91% of these patients will not show disease progression. Achievement of a major cytogenetic response at 3, 6, or within 12 months was associated with a statistically significant improvement in overall survival. For example, if patients achieve a major cytogenetic response within 12 months, the estimated survival at 24 months is 99% compared with 86% for patients with less than a major cytogenetic response ($P < .001$). Baseline features that independently predicted a high rate of major cytogenetic responses were the absence of blasts in the peripheral blood, a hemoglobin greater than 12 g/dL, less

TABLE 107-4

Phase II Results with Imatinib

	CHRONIC PHASE (IFN FAILURE)[62]	ACCELERATED PHASE[131]	BLAST CRISIS[132]
CHR	96%	40%	9%
MCR	64%	28%	16%
CCR	48%	20%	7%
Disease progression	13%	50%	90%

CCR, complete cytogenetic response; CHR, complete hematologic response; IFN, interferon; MCR, major cytogenetic response (Philadelphia chromosome–positive metaphases ≤35%).

TABLE 107-5

Phase III Results of Imatinib versus IFN-Alfa Plus Cytarabine for Newly Diagnosed Chronic-Phase CML Patients[63]

	IMATINIB 400 MG	IFN-ALFA + ARA-C
CHR	97%	69%
MCR	87%	35%
CCR	76%	14%
Intolerance	3%	31%
Progressive disease	3%	8.5%

CCR, complete cytogenetic response; CHR, complete hematologic response; IFN, interferon; MCR, major cytogenetic response (Philadelphia chromosome positive metaphases <35%). Intolerance leading to discontinuation of first-line therapy. Progressive disease to accelerated phase or blast crisis. (All of these differences are highly statistically significant with $P < .001$).

than 5% blasts in the marrow, CML disease duration of less than 1 year, and a previous cytogenetic response to IFN-alfa.[62]

A phase III randomized study, comparing imatinib at 400 mg daily with IFN-alfa plus Ara-C in newly diagnosed patients with chronic-phase CML, enrolled 1106 patients from June 2000 to January 2001. Five hundred fifty-three patients were randomized to each treatment. Baseline characteristics were well balanced for all features evaluated, including age, WBC count, Sokal and Euro scores, and time from diagnosis. With a median follow-up of 19 months, patients randomized to imatinib had statistically significantly better results than did patients treated with IFN-alfa plus Ara-C in all parameters measured (Table 107-5) including rates of CHR (97% vs. 56%; $P < .001$), major and complete cytogenetic responses (85% and 74% vs. 22% and 8%; $P < .001$), discontinuation of assigned therapy because of intolerance (3% vs. 31%), and progression to accelerated-phase disease or blast crisis (3% vs. 8%; $P < .001$).[63] Although 74% of patients randomized to receive imatinib achieved a complete cytogenetic response, most of these patients had detectable leukemia, as analyzed by RT-PCR for BCR-ABL transcripts.[64]

Imatinib therapy may be instituted as soon as the diagnosis of Ph-positive CML has been established, even if the WBC count is dramatically elevated.[65] For patients with a WBC count of greater than 20,000/mm^3, concomitant therapy with allopurinol is recommended until the WBC count is consistently less than 20,000/mm^3. Tumor lysis syndrome has been rare, even in patients with advanced-phase disease; however, maintaining adequate hydration is essential, and patients with advanced-phase disease should be monitored for this complication. After treatment with imatinib is initiated, the WBC count should begin to decrease within the first 2 weeks and usually normalizes within 4 to 6 weeks. The decline in the platelet count is typically delayed by 1 to 2 weeks.

Complete blood counts (CBCs) should be monitored weekly in patients with chronic-phase disease during the first month of imatinib therapy. In patients without significant myelosuppression [absolute neutrophil count (ANC), $<1.5 \times 10^9$/L or platelet count $<100 \times 10^9$/L], hematologic monitoring can be reduced to every 2 weeks until 12 weeks of therapy is reached. Thereafter, the frequency of monitoring can be lengthened to monthly or even longer, depending on the stability of the counts and the cytogenetic status. For patients with accelerated-phase disease or blast crisis, CBCs should initially be performed at least weekly, depending on the clinical situation.

Bone marrow cytogenetics should be monitored every 6 months in patients who have not achieved a complete cytogenetic response. Even in patients without a cytogenetic response, most patients treated with imatinib will have marrow morphologies revert to normal.[66] In patients with a complete cytogenetic response, bone marrow should still be monitored yearly, as some patients have new cytogenetic abnormalities in Ph-chromosome–negative clones.[67] Although the significance of these abnormalities is unclear, reports exist of some of these patients having myelodysplasia. In patients with a complete cytogenetic response, quantitative RT-PCR for *BCR-ABL* should be performed on peripheral blood every 3 months, if available, because this may allow detection of early relapse.

Myelosuppression is particularly common in patients with CML treated with imatinib and is more common in patients with advanced disease (Table 107-6).[65] In the phase III randomized trial of newly diagnosed patients in the chronic phase, grade 3 neutropenia (ANC, $<1.0 \times 10^9$/L) was experienced by 11% of patients; grade 4 neutropenia (ANC, $<0.5 \times 10^9$/L) occurred in 2% of patients; grade 3 thrombocytopenia (platelets, $<50 \times 10^9$/L) occurred in 6.9% of patients, and grade 4 (platelets, $<10 \times 10^9$/L) in fewer than 1% of patients.[63] Myelosuppression can occur at any time during imatinib therapy, but usually begins within the first 2 to 4 weeks of the initiation of therapy for blast crisis, with a slightly later onset in patients in accelerated or chronic phase. Clinical features associated with a greater risk of myelosuppression include an increased percentage of bone marrow blasts, a lower hemoglobin level, a longer time from diagnosis, a history of cytopenias induced by IFN-alfa, and previous busulfan therapy.[63] It is wise to monitor patients with these risk factors more closely, particularly during the early phases of treatment. A few patients (<5%) have repeated episodes of severe myelosuppression, and prolonged interruptions of therapy may be required.

Myelosuppression induced by imatinib is probably a therapeutic effect on the Ph-positive leukemic clone, as most hematopoiesis is derived from Ph-positive stem cells. With disease progression from early chronic phase to advanced disease, the progenitor cell compartment gradually becomes dominated by Ph-positive cells.[68] A guiding principle in the management of imatinib-induced myelosuppression is to match the aggressiveness of therapy with the phase of disease. Based on dose–response considerations, daily doses less than 300 mg should rarely, if ever, be used. Because minimal suppression of normal hematopoiesis occurs with imatinib, dose reductions less than 300 mg daily are unlikely to assist in the recovery of normal hematopoiesis, but may allow emergence of imatinib-resistant leukemic clones. The primary goal in treating otherwise healthy patients with chronic-phase disease is to avoid the risk of potentially dangerous neutropenia and platelet-transfusion dependence. Among possible approaches to managing myelosuppression, interruption of treatment, not dose reduction, is the preferred course of action. For myelosuppression of grade 3 or higher severity (ANC, $<1.0 \times 10^9$/L, or platelets, $<50 \times 10^9$/L), imatinib should be withheld until blood counts recover (ANC, $>1.5 \times 10^9$/L, or platelets, $>100 \times 10$/L). This generally occurs within 2 to 4 weeks, and when it does, imatinib may be resumed at full dose. In patients with recurrent episodes of myelosuppression, it might be reasonable to decrease the dose to 300 mg daily. These recommendations may be modified slightly for patients with features associated with advanced disease (e.g., higher percentage of blasts or basophils, or clonal evolution). Several small studies showed that myeloid growth factors may accelerate recovery from myelosuppression, allowing imatinib to be continued.[69,70] However, the long-term safety of this approach is not known.

The most common nonhematologic adverse events of imatinib are nausea; muscle cramps; fluid retention, particularly periorbital edema; diarrhea; musculoskeletal pain; fatigue; and rashes. Few patients had grade 3/4 toxicity, and most side effects can be managed successfully with supportive measures.[65] The most common side effect resulting in discontinuation of imatinib therapy was rash; however, in most cases, rashes are mild, self-limiting, and easily manageable with antihistamines or topical

TABLE 107-6

Myelosuppression in the Phase II and III Studies with Imatinib

	NEUTROPENIA		THROMBOCYTOPENIA	
	GRADE 3	GRADE 4	GRADE 3	GRADE 4
	ANC, $<1.0 \times 10^9$/L	ANC, $<0.5 \times 10^9$/L	$<50 \times 10^9$/L	$<10 \times 10^9$/L
Chronic phase (newly dx'd)	11%	2%	7%	0.5%
Chronic phase (IFN failure)	27%	8%	19%	1%
Accelerated phase	23%	35%	31%	12%
Blast crisis	16%	48%	29%	33%

ANC, absolute neutrophil count; dx'd, diagnosed; IFN, interferon.

Specific Malignancies

III

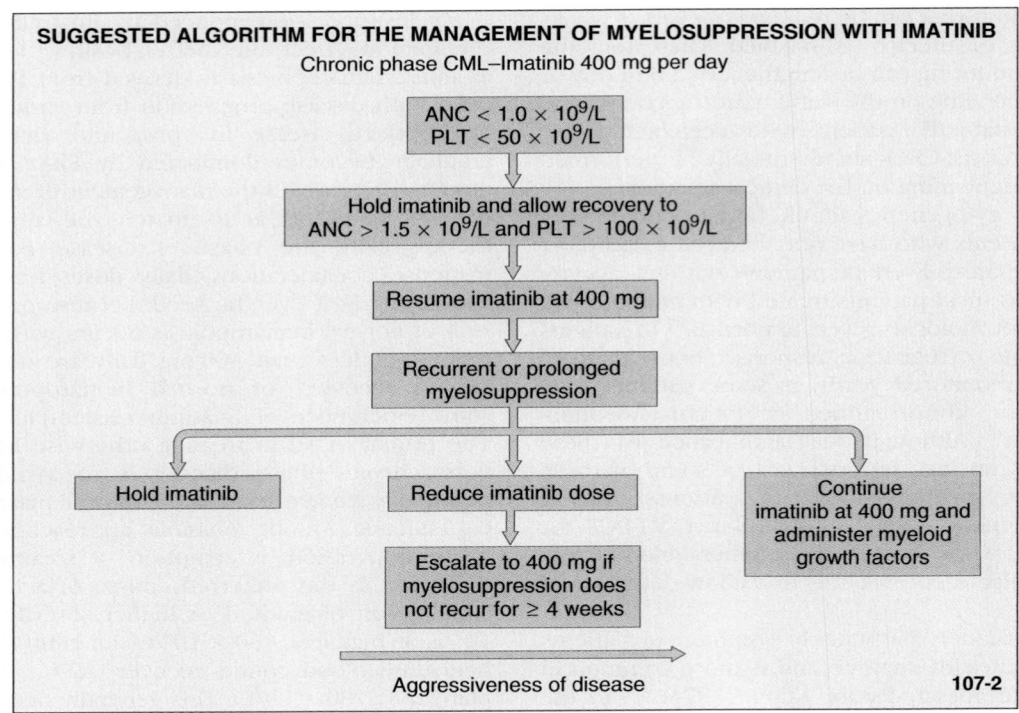

SUGGESTED ALGORITHM FOR THE MANAGEMENT OF MYELOSUPPRESSION WITH IMATINIB
Chronic phase CML–Imatinib 400 mg per day

ANC < 1.0×10^9/L
PLT < 50×10^9/L

Hold imatinib and allow recovery to
ANC > 1.5×10^9/L and PLT > 100×10^9/L

Resume imatinib at 400 mg

Recurrent or prolonged myelosuppression

Hold imatinib

Reduce imatinib dose

Continue imatinib at 400 mg and administer myeloid growth factors

Escalate to 400 mg if myelosuppression does not recur for ≥ 4 weeks

Aggressiveness of disease

107-2

steroids, whereas a short course of oral steroids can be used to treat more severe cases. Although hepatoxicity is uncommon, it is the second most common reason for permanent discontinuation of imatinib therapy, applying to fewer than 1% of patients. Because of concerns about hepatotoxicity, liver function tests should be obtained before treatment is started, every other week during the first month of therapy, and at least monthly thereafter.

Resistance to Imatinib Therapy

In evaluating relapse mechanisms, patients can be separated into two categories, those with persistent inhibition of the *BCR-ABL* kinase (*BCR-ABL* independent) and those with reactivation of the *BCR-ABL* kinase (*BCR-ABL* dependent) at relapse. In the largest studies of resistance or relapse, several consistent themes emerge. In patients with primary resistance, that is, patients who do not respond to imatinib therapy, *BCR-ABL*–independent mechanisms are most common.[71] In contrast, most patients who have a relapse while receiving therapy with imatinib reactivate the *BCR-ABL* kinase. In these studies, more than 50% and perhaps as many as 90% of patients with hematologic relapse have *BCR-ABL* point mutations in at least 13 different amino acids scattered throughout the *ABL* kinase domain.[71-73] Other patients have amplification of *BCR-ABL* at the genomic or transcript level.[71] In patients with chronic-phase disease who have a relapse while receiving imatinib or who do not achieve a complete hematologic response or who do not have a cytogenetic response, dose escalation to 800 mg daily has resulted in an improved response in approximately one third of patients.[74] Alternatively, patients who have a relapse while receiving imatinib should be considered as candidates

for allogeneic SCT or could be treated in clinical trials of combinations of imatinib with other agents such as IFN-alfa, Ara-C, a variety of investigational agents, or autologous SCT.

Allogeneic Stem Cell Transplantation

Currently the only approach that can unequivocally cure patients with CML is SCT from a suitably matched donor. This conclusion is based primarily on the observation that patients who survive 5 years after SCT without evidence of disease at the molecular level have an extremely low risk of relapse.[75] It was previously believed that the principal component of the transplant that contributed to cure was the intensive chemotherapy with or without radiation that preceded the infusion of hematopoietic stem cells; however, it has become clear that the so-called graft-versus-leukemia (GVL) effect, whereby the leukemia cells in the patient are destroyed by donor-derived T cells, is the most important component of the transplant.[76] The evidence for this statement comes from the observation that all methods that reduce the risk of graft-versus-host disease (GVHD) increase the risk of relapse after SCT for CML. This is well exemplified by T-cell depletion of the donor inoculum, which greatly increases the risk of relapse.[77] In contrast, administration of donor-derived lymphocytes to patients who relapse frequently restores remission.[78,79] The biologic basis for the GVL effect is not well defined.[76] Donor-derived CD4 T cells are central to the GVL effect, but natural killer (NK) cells also may contribute. The target antigens also are not well defined, but may be leukemia specific, such as peptides derived from the BCR-ABL fusion protein,[80] tissue-specific peptides, such as those derived from proteinase 3 or the Wilms' tumor protein, or minor histocompatibility peptides such as HA-1, HA-2 or HY-1.

Results of Allogeneic Transplant in Chronic Myeloid Leukemia

Sibling Donors. The results of allogeneic SCT from sibling donors in patients with chronic-phase CML are fairly consistent. In various transplant centers worldwide, the probability of 5-year overall survival and leukemia-free survival are 60% to 80% and 55% to 70%, respectively, with a 10% to 20% relapse rate. A recent report from the International Bone Marrow Transplant Registry (IBMTR), compiling data from 1699 patients transplanted between 1987 and 1994, showed a 3-year leukemia-free survival rate of 57% (Fig. 107-4).[81] After allogeneic SCT, most patients are Ph chromosome negative and have no detectable *BCR-ABL* transcripts by RT-PCR testing (molecular remission). Most patients who are destined to relapse, especially those transplanted in the chronic phase, do so within the first 3 years after SCT, although occasional late relapses occur.

Unrelated Donors. The results of SCT from volunteer, matched unrelated donors are inferior to those of sibling SCT because of the increased risk of mortality from graft failure and GVHD (see Fig. 107-4). This is probably caused by undetected disparities of minor histocompatibility antigens despite accurate matching of the major histocompatibility antigens. The rate of GVHD can be reduced significantly by T-cell depletion of the graft, but graft failure is more prevalent, and there is also increased morbidity and mortality from infections, particularly viral and fungal, after transplant. In the 1992 IBMTR analysis of unrelated donors SCT, the 2-year overall and leukemia-free survival rates were 38% and 35%, respectively.[82] Better

results have been reported from individual centers. For example, the Fred Hutchinson Cancer Research Center reported that for 196 patients undergoing unrelated donor SCT over a 10-year period, the overall survival at 5 years was 57%.[83] Subset analysis showed that patients younger than 50 years who underwent transplantation within 1 year of diagnosis had an overall survival rate of 74%, which is equivalent to results achieved in sibling SCT. Thus results of unrelated donor SCT can be improved with better selection of patient and donor.

Prognostic Factors for Allogeneic Stem Cell Transplantation

The results of allogeneic SCT are best if the patient is relatively young and the donor is an HLA-identical sibling donor.[84,85] However, improvements in molecular characterization of the HLA phenotype and genotype led to improved matching of patients with unrelated donors. This has been partly responsible for the improvement of the results from unrelated donor SCT in the last 10 years.[82,83,86] A better understanding has been reached of the causes of transplant-related mortality (TRM), which has aided the selection of patients deemed suitable for this treatment, as exemplified by the risk-scoring system discussed later. In addition, advances in management of complications, including diagnosis, prevention, and treatment for viral infections, in particular cytomegalovirus (CMV), have contributed to improved results of unrelated-donor SCT procedures. In general, factors that affect the outcome of transplant for CML can be considered under three headings: (1) those that can be defined before transplant, (2) those directly related to the transplant procedure, and (3) those that operate in the months or years after the transplant.

Prognostic Factors Defined before Transplant. Patient age is an important risk factor, regardless of the donor type and stem cell source.[87] The risk of treatment-related mortality is a continuous variable that appears to increase by approximately 5% for each decade. For this reason, one cannot reliably set an upper age limit for allografting, and each case must be considered on its merits. Patients undergoing transplantation early after diagnosis have a higher survival rate than do comparable patients who have been in chronic phase for many years (see Fig. 107-4).[39,87,88] Interestingly, patients who undergo transplant after longer intervals have a higher TRM rate as opposed to a higher relapse rate. Stage of disease is perhaps the most important factor affecting survival after transplant. As noted, the overall survival for patients undergoing transplantation in chronic phase is 60% to 80%, compared with 25% to 40% for patients treated in the accelerated phase, and less than 10% for patients undergoing transplantation in blast phase.[89] Patients who are seropositive for CMV before transplant have a greater risk of reactivating CMV than do seronegative patients who receive stem cells from seronegative donors. This can lead to increased morbidity and mortality, especially in recipients of stem cells from unrelated donors. CMV seropositivity may be the most important adverse prognostic factor in older patients undergoing unrelated-donor SCT.[90]

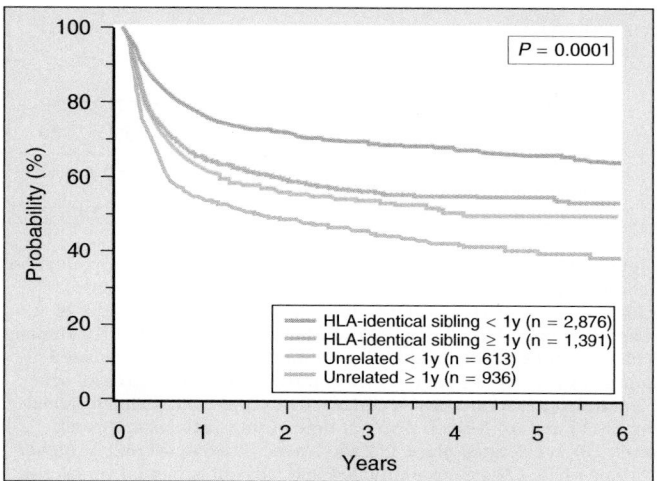

Figure 107-4. The International Bone Marrow Transplant Registry experience in patients with chronic-phase chronic myeloid leukemia. The curves show both the effect of a related versus unrelated donor and the benefit of early transplantation on survival.

Specific Malignancies

Transplant Procedure–Related Factors. One of the most important factors affecting the result of a transplant is the degree of histocompatibility between donor and recipient.[86] In terms of TRM, the best donor would be a genetically identical twin, because the TRM rate after syngeneic transplants for CML in chronic phase is extremely low (<5%). However, syngeneic transplants are associated with a relatively high risk of relapse, which offsets the survival advantage from a lower TRM. Because most patients lack identical twins, the optimal donor is an HLA-identical sibling. With typical family size in the western world, 20% to 30% of patients will have matched siblings. In the absence of a matched sibling, it is reasonable to consider a phenotypically HLA-matched family member or matched unrelated donor identified through one of the volunteer donor registries. A small number of transplants for CML have been performed by using stem cells from the umbilical cords of unrelated neonates. Cord blood SCTs are often associated with relatively slow engraftment, and identifying suitable cords with sufficient numbers of stem cells for larger adults is somewhat more difficult, thus limiting the applicability of this procedure.

The objectives of conditioning before transfusion of allogeneic stem cells are to reduce the bulk of disease in the patient and to suppress the patient's capacity to reject the incoming graft. The classic approach to conditioning has been high-dose cyclophosphamide followed by total body irradiation at "supralethal" or "myeloablative" dosage (typically 900 to 1600 cGy). Recent experience suggests that the same or perhaps better results can be obtained by replacing the radiation therapy with busulfan.[91] A single-institution report suggested that relapses may be further reduced by targeting a plasma busulfan level greater than 900 ng/mL.[92] Many other conditioning regimens have been studied in relatively small patient series.

Stem cells may be obtained from the bone marrow or the peripheral blood of the donor. For transplant using marrow-derived stem cells, survival seems to be improved when the absolute number of nucleated cells or CD34+ cells is relatively high, especially with unrelated donors.[93] Engraftment is more rapid when peripheral blood stem cells are used, but the risk of GVHD, especially chronic GVHD, may be greater than with stem cells collected from the marrow.[94-96] This may reflect the fact that peripheral blood stem cell (PBSC) allografts contain, on average, 10 times more T lymphocytes than do marrow-derived collections. Conversely the GVL effect of a PBSC transplant may be greater than that of a marrow transplant. At present, many transplant centers perform conventional marrow-derived SCTs for patients with CML in chronic phase, but prefer to use PBSCs for patients with CML in more advanced phases.

Factors Operating after Transplant. The occurrence of GVHD after transplant is more likely in older patients and in the presence of increasing degrees of HLA disparity. GVHD can be abrogated entirely by effective depletion of T lymphocytes from the donor inoculum, but unfortunately such T-cell depletion brings with it three important complications: increased risk of graft failure, impaired immune reconstitution, and increased risk of relapse, approaching 60% to 80% for a full T-cell depletion. This means that full T-cell depletion is not commonly used in CML transplants. Severe GVHD resistant to standard therapy is therefore still seen on occasion and is associated with a high risk of mortality.

European Group for Blood and Marrow Transplantation/Gratwohl Risk Score. To predict the probability of survival after allografting for a given CML patient, Gratwohl and colleagues[87] devised a scoring system based on an analysis of the outcome with CML patients whose clinical data were reported to the European Group for Blood and Marrow Transplantation (EGBMT). The analysis identified five major prognostic factors: patient age, disease duration, disease phase, degree of patient–donor histocompatibility, and patient–donor sex combination. It attributes a score of 0 (most favorable), 1, or 2 (least favorable) to each factor according to the patient's status. Patients with low total scores may expect to do relatively well, and patients with high total scores have relatively high probabilities of TRM (Fig. 107-5). This scoring system has been validated with an independent patient population.[97]

Reduced-Intensity Conditioning Allografts

Much interest is now expressed in reducing TRM by reducing the intensity of the conditioning regimen and emphasizing the role of GVL.[76] These transplants are

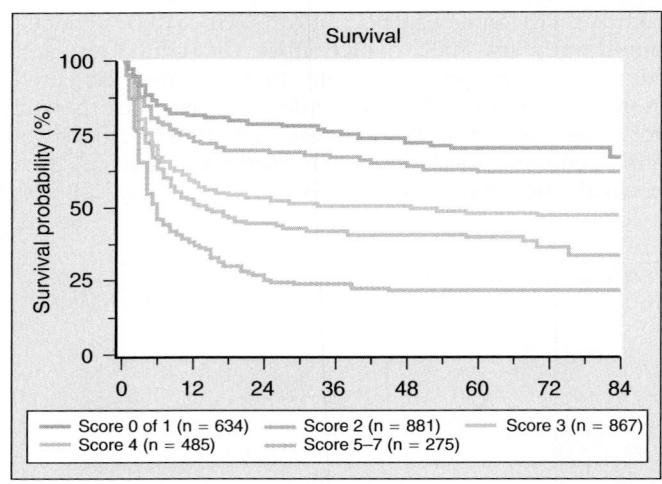

Figure 107-5. Survival of patients undergoing stem cell transplantation according to risk score calculated as follows: Zero, 1, or 2 points are allocated respectively to each feature: (a) patients younger than 20 years (0), from 20 to 40 years (1), or older than 40 years (2); (b) Human leukocyte antigen–identical sibling donor (0) or matched unrelated donor (1); (c) Disease duration <1 year (0) or >1 year (1); (d) All sex combinations of donor and recipient (0), except male recipient/female donor (1); and (e) Disease phase at time of transplant, first chronic phase (0), accelerated phase (1), and blastic phase or second or higher chronic phase (2). Points are totaled, and survival is plotted versus risk score. (From Gratwohl A, Hermans J, Goldman JM, et al: Risk assessment for patients with chronic myeloid leukaemia before allogeneic blood or marrow transplantation: Chronic Leukemia Working Party of the European Group for Blood and Marrow Transplantation. Lancet 1998;352:1087.)

known as nonmyeloablative, or reduced-intensity, conditioning transplants. The results of reduced-intensity conditioning transplants vary widely and may reflect the variability in the transplant regimens. With low-dose total body irradiation, a high incidence of graft failure was reported, but this was overcome by adding fludarabine to the regimen.[98] With a regimen of fludarabine, busulfan, and antithymocyte globulin (ATG), projected leukemia-free survival at 5 years of 85% was reported in 24 patients with CML in chronic phase[99] and confirmed in 15 patients using a similar conditioning regimen.[100] A novel transplant regimen may be identified that reduces the risk of TRM and yet retains the potent GVL effect associated with conventional allogeneic SCT.

Monitoring for Relapse after Transplant

In most patients who have a relapse of CML after SCT, the relapse occurs in the first 3 years. Thereafter, the actuarial probability of relapse is 1% to 3% per annum until 6.5 years, with rare relapses at later times. Although relapses directly into advanced phase occur, most patients relapse in a more orderly manner. Thus patients initially test positive for *BCR-ABL* transcripts by RT-PCR (molecular relapse), then progress to a cytogenetic relapse, when the Ph chromosome is found in bone marrow metaphases, and ultimately progress to a hematologic relapse, in which leukocytosis and splenomegaly are found, reminiscent of the features found at diagnosis.[101-103] Therefore monitoring by RT-PCR for *BCR-ABL* transcripts in the peripheral blood is a valuable technique to detect early molecular relapse. This is accurate, reproducible, and quantifiable by real-time RT-PCR techniques. RT-PCR for *BCR-ABL* should be performed 3 months after SCT, and then at 3- to 6-month intervals, depending on the results. Patients who have had persistently negative PCR results can have monitoring yearly. Increasing *BCR-ABL* transcript levels usually predict cytogenetic and subsequently hematologic relapse.[104,105]

Treatment of Relapse of Chronic Myeloid Leukemia after Transplant

In patients who relapse after allogeneic SCT, withdrawal of immunosuppression can lead to remission, especially patients in molecular relapse. This is likely due to increased GVL and has led to the development of various techniques to manipulate or "harness" this GVL effect. The most promising of these is donor lymphocyte infusions (DLIs).[78,79,106] The initial management of CML in relapse involves reducing and if possible stopping immunosuppressive agents such as prednisone or cyclosporine. This must be done cautiously because it could exacerbate GVHD. If this does not reverse the features of relapse, the choice of further management lies between DLI and imatinib. It is not clear which approach is preferable. If imatinib is chosen, it would be reasonable to start treatment at a dose of 400 mg daily. Treatment might be interrupted if *BCR-ABL* transcripts are persistently undetectable in the blood. If DLI is selected, the original transplant donor should be contacted and asked to provide lymphocytes that are collected by leukapheresis. Other possible treatments for relapse are IFN-alfa or a

second SCT. The latter carries a relatively high risk of transplant mortality.

Donor Lymphocyte Infusions. DLIs can induce remission in 60% to 80% of patients with molecular or cytogenetic relapse.[78,79] DLI can be given as an outpatient procedure with few immediate side effects. Responses are usually seen within 1 to 9 months. Remissions induced by DLI are usually durable, but novel statistical methods may be required to reflect this fact.[107] The major adverse effect of DLI is exacerbation of GVHD, which can be fatal. The severity and frequency of GVHD depends on the dose of DLI. However, smaller doses of DLI, which are less likely to induce GVHD, also are less efficacious in inducing remission. An intense effort is being made to separate the harmful effects of GVHD from the desired GVL. Both reside in T cells and may be functions of different T-cell subsets. Depletion of CD8$^+$ T cells confers satisfactory GVL without excessive GVHD. Pancytopenia caused by marrow aplasia occurs in 10% to 20% of DLI-treated patients. It is more common in patients in hematologic relapse because limited donor stem cells remain. This aplasia can recover spontaneously, but occasionally requires donor stem cell infusion to re-establish adequate hematopoiesis.

The risk of GVHD and marrow aplasia can be reduced or eliminated by administering DLI in escalating doses, starting with a relatively low dose and repeating the infusion with a somewhat larger dose at 4- to 12-week intervals in accordance with the patient's response.[108-110] Using DLI in this manner, most patients regain cytogenetic or molecular remissions before they experience any significant degree of GVHD. For patients who do not respond to three or more doses of DLI, the administration of imatinib may induce cytogenetic or even molecular remission.[111]

Autologous Stem Cell Transplantation (Autografting)

It is not clear what role autologous transplants have in the treatment of patients with CML. Autografting after high-dose chemotherapy has a lower TRM rate than does allografting and can induce Ph chromosome negativity in some patients.[112,113] Thus autografting may be a consideration for patients not responding to or relapsing on therapy with imatinib. It also has been proposed as a means of decreasing disease burden in patients with molecular positivity on imatinib therapy. The autologous stem cells can be a leukapheresed product collected at the time of diagnosis, or cells collected at a later stage after mobilization with granulocyte–colony-stimulating factor (G-CSF) alone or G-CSF in combination with chemotherapy.

Cytoreduction before Autografting

No consensus is found about the best conditioning regimen for autografting in CML. Some centers use the standard regimens for allogeneic SCT, such as cyclophosphamide and total body irradiation or busulfan and cyclophosphamide. However, because autografting is noncurative, less toxic and immunosuppressive regimens may be preferable. Single-agent conditioning with busulfan is advantageous because its myelosuppressive effect is delayed for up to 2 weeks, and the patient can be effectively treated as an outpatient until pancytopenia occurs.

Purging

In an effort to increase the number of Ph chromosome–negative stem cells, various purging methods have been used.[114] The process of stem cell cryopreservation confers a proliferative or survival advantage to Ph chromosome–negative cells. High-dose combination chemotherapy also eliminates Ph chromosome–positive cells, and leukapheresis on recovery has yielded Ph chromosome–negative enriched stem cells.[115]

An autograft can then be performed after myeloablative chemotherapy with these cells. Alternative efforts have been made to reduce or eliminate Ph chromosome–positive cells in vitro before transfusion to the patient. For example, long-term culture of blood or marrow cells over a 10-day period favors Ph chromosome–negative cell growth.[116] These cultured cells are autografted and produced cytogenetic remission of more than 1 year in highly selected patients. Other centers have cultured marrow in cytotoxic drugs, such as mafosfamide (hydroperoxycyclophosphamide) or IFN-alfa, and yet others have used antisense oligomers targeting the *BCR-ABL* junction or *MYB* proto-oncogene. The use of these manipulations is not clearly superior to standard treatment.

Results of Autografting

Autograft is best performed in chronic phase. It is known that autografts of unmanipulated bone marrow or PBSC can induce hematologic and complete cytogenetic remissions in CML. Partial or transient Ph chromosome negativity is achieved in about 50% of patients, with most reverting to Ph chromosome positivity by 6 to 9 months. Retrospective analysis of data from eight centers shows a progression-free survival of 60% at 5 years after autograft.[113] However, these results are in a highly selected patient group. Results of prospective trials would be required to establish a definite survival advantage for autografts in CML.

INTEGRATION OF TREATMENT OPTIONS FOR NEWLY DIAGNOSED PATIENTS IN THE CHRONIC PHASE OF DISEASE

In patients with newly diagnosed chronic-phase CML, imatinib offers the best balance between safety and efficacy, and imatinib should be initiated or patients should be enrolled in a clinical trial with an imatinib-containing regimen as soon as the diagnosis is confirmed. The only exception might be patients for whom SCT is considered as initial therapy. Even in these patients, as imatinib can achieve a rapid and reliable cytoreduction, it is possible that treatment with imatinib before transplant could improve the outcome from SCT by decreasing the rate of post-transplant relapse. Although preliminary studies have suggested no increase in TRM in patients

receiving less than 1 year of therapy with imatinib, the possibility that imatinib could increase TRM must be considered until additional, larger studies are performed. Thus the major questions are whether any patients should be considered for immediate SCT, or for patients treated with imatinib, what parameters should be used in deciding when to consider transplant. Regardless of the approach, any patient for whom an SCT would be considered should undergo HLA typing, and for patients without a sibling match, a preliminary bone marrow donor registry search should be performed.

In weighing SCT versus imatinib, the obvious issue is the probability of long-term survival balanced against the risks associated with each therapy. With SCT, patients must weigh the statistical risk of mortality against the known cure rate from this procedure. With imatinib, patients must weigh the excellent short-term results against the unknown probability of long-term survival and the unknown risk of disease progression over time. Although the survival for patients treated with imatinib in the first year of therapy is greater than 99%, the durability of these responses in unknown. Whether imatinib therapy itself or a delay in transplant while undergoing a trial of imatinib affects the survival from transplant is unknown. Although previous algorithms suggested that delaying SCT beyond 1 year from increased TRM, whether the same will be true with imatinib also is unknown. The likelihood of obtaining a molecular remission with imatinib is less than 5%, and it is currently recommended that imatinib therapy be continued indefinitely. For some patients, the option of remaining on a therapy indefinitely with a small chance of cure is not preferred. Thus for younger patients with an HLA-matched sibling, immediate transplant or transplant after a short course of imatinib might be the most reasonable option. However, in most other patients, treatment with imatinib, reserving SCT for failure of imatinib, would seem a more attractive option.[59,117,118]

For patients who opt not to undergo transplant as initial therapy, the major issue is how best to define a less than optimal response to imatinib. Several categories clearly impart a poorer prognosis, such as the lack of a CHR after 3 months of imatinib, as would loss of a response, whether that be loss of a CHR, loss of a cytogenetic response, or an increase in *BCR-ABL* levels by quantitative RT-PCR. Similarly, if a major cytogenetic response is not achieved after 12 months of therapy with imatinib, a low likelihood exists that a complete cytogenic response will be achieved. In newly diagnosed chronic-phase patients, 80% of patients achieved a major cytogenetic response in the first 12 months of therapy with imatinib. At later times, only an additional 10% of patients obtained a major or complete cytogenetic response.[63] This low probability of an improved response might be unacceptable for a young patient with a sibling transplant donor; however, it might be acceptable for an older patient with only an unrelated transplant option who could be offered dose escalation of imatinib or experimental options, including combinations of imatinib with other agents. For the future, we need a more detailed analysis of the prognosis imparted by specific levels of cytogenetic or molecular response to aid in these decisions. In patients who do not achieve a

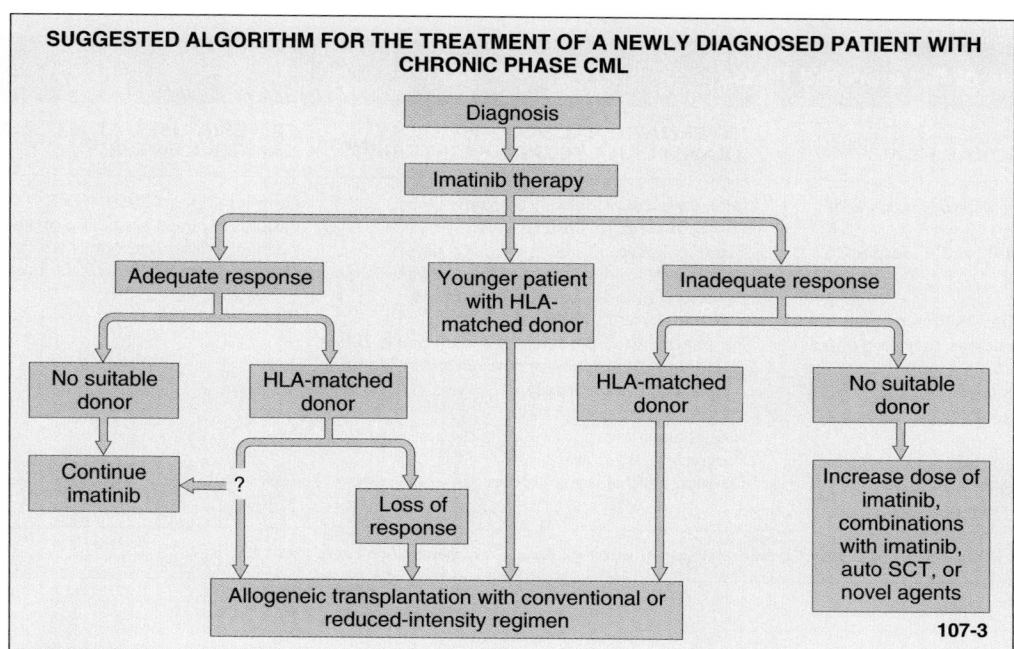

SUGGESTED ALGORITHM FOR THE TREATMENT OF A NEWLY DIAGNOSED PATIENT WITH CHRONIC PHASE CML

107-3

complete hematologic response at 3 months, have no cytogenic response at 6 months, or have a major cytogenetic response after 12 months of therapy with imatinib, it would be reasonable to readdress transplant options. Because most patients achieve complete cytogenetic remission, it would be advisable to monitor quantitative RT-PCR for *BCR-ABL* and to reconsider transplant in patients who show a confirmed one-log or greater increase in these levels. It is hoped that, as additional follow-up data for imatinib become available, these issues will be clarified.

ADVANCED DISEASE

Natural History

Historically, the median duration of the chronic phase of CML was 4 to 6 years, with progression to advanced phases occurring at a rate of approximately 5% for the first year and 20% to 25% for each subsequent year after diagnosis.[119] With imatinib, the rate of progression to accelerated or blast phase was 1.5% at 1 year and 3% at 18 months.[63] Whether these trends will hold remains unknown.

Clinical Features

In 20% to 40% of patients in chronic phase, the disease transforms abruptly into an acute leukemia. This is called *blast crisis* or *blastic transformation*. Symptoms resemble those in patients with acute leukemia and include fever, bone pain, or bleeding.

Morphologically, the bone marrow of blastic-phase CML fulfills the criteria for acute leukemia, with greater than 30% blasts. Approximately 65% of patients evolve to

blastic crisis with myeloid lineage blasts, 30% have blasts of pre-B lymphoid origin, and 5% of patients have undifferentiated or T-cell blasts.[120,121] The median survival of patients in blastic phase is 3 to 6 months, although patients with lymphoid blast crisis have a somewhat better outcome.[122] Occasionally, an isolated blast phase of extramedullary origin may occur, with the patient's blood or marrow meeting criteria for chronic-phase disease.

In most patients, the transformation to advanced phase is more insidious, and the disease gradually becomes more difficult to control with medical therapy. The intermediate period in which the patient is no longer in chronic phase but not yet clearly in blastic transformation has been termed the *accelerated phase*. The criteria for defining accelerated phase, summarized in Table 107-7, are highly variable and do not necessarily correlate with survival. WBC count, platelet count, and spleen size may escape the control of previously adequate treatment with hydroxyurea, imatinib, or IFN-alfa. A slow but perceptible increase in the blast cell population or increasing basophilia may be noted against a background of a chronic-phase blood picture. Other clues are increasing anemia and thrombocytopenia. In one series, features that correlated with a median survival of 18 months or less included blast percentage greater than 15%, blasts plus promyelocytes greater than 30%, basophils greater than 20%, and a platelet count less than 100×10^9/L unrelated to therapy.[123] In some patients, a myelofibrotic picture characterizes the accelerated phase, in which massive splenomegaly with extensive marrow fibrosis and extramedullary hematopoiesis is found.

Molecular Biology of Disease Progression

Clonal cytogenetic abnormalities besides a single Ph chromosome may be acquired in patients with CML as

Specific Malignancies

III

TABLE 107-7

Definitions of Accelerated Phase

CRITERIA OF SOKAL ET AL.[147]	INTERNATIONAL BONE MARROW TRANSPLANT REGISTRY CRITERIA[148]	CRITERIA USED AT M.D. ANDERSON CANCER CENTER[123]
Peripheral blood or marrow blasts ≥5% Basophils >20% Platelet count >1000 × 10⁹/L despite adequate therapy Clonal evolution Frequent Pelger-Huet–like neutrophils, nucleated erythrocytes, megakaryocyte nuclear fragments Marrow collagen fibrosis Anemia or thrombocytopenia unrelated to therapy Progressive splenomegaly Leukocyte doubling time <5 days Fever of unknown origin	Leukocyte count difficult to control with hydroxyurea or busulfan Rapid leukocyte doubling time (<5 days) Peripheral blood or marrow blasts ≥10% Peripheral blood or marrow blasts and promyelocytes ≥20% Peripheral blood basophils and eosinophils 20% Anemia or thrombocytopenia unresponsive to hydroxyurea or busulfan Persistent thrombocytosis Clonal evolution Progressive splenomegaly Development of myelofibrosis	Peripheral blood blasts ≥15% Peripheral blood blasts and promyelocytes ≥30% Peripheral blood basophils ≥20% Platelet count ≤100 × 10⁹/L unrelated to therapy Clonal evolution

Adapted from Faderl S, Talpaz M, Estrov Z, et al: Chronic myelogenous leukemia? Biology and therapy. Ann Intern Med 1999;131:207.

their disease progresses, and up to 80% of patients with overt blastic transformation have additional cytogenetic abnormalities.[124] The molecular basis of disease progression is poorly defined in most patients. Up to 25% of patients with myeloid blastic transformation of CML have point mutations or deletions in the *p53* tumor-suppressor gene.[125,126] As many as 50% of patients with lymphoid transformation show homozygous deletion in the *p16* tumor-suppressor gene.[127]

Alteration of the retinoblastoma (*Rb*) tumor-suppressor gene is associated with the rare megakaryoblastic transformation.[128,129] Amplification of the *MYC* proto-oncogene appears to be rare.[130] However, none of these lesions explains the loss of differentiation that is the most striking feature of transformation to blast crisis.

Treatment

Imatinib has single-agent activity in both accelerated and blast crisis (see Table 107-4). In a phase II trial in accelerated-phase disease, patients were required to have 15% to 30% blasts or greater than 30% blasts plus promyelocytes in the peripheral blood or marrow, greater than 20% peripheral basophils, or a platelet count less than 100 × 10⁹/L, unrelated to therapy. With follow-up of 3 years or less, 83% of patients showed some form of hematologic response, with 40% of patients achieving a CHR.[131] Twenty-eight percent of patients achieved a major cytogenetic response, with 20% achieving complete responses. In this study, significantly improved outcomes for response and survival were observed for patients treated with imatinib, 600 mg daily, compared with patients treated with 400 mg daily[131]; however, this was a retrospective subgroup analysis. Based on these data, 600 mg/day is the recommended dose of imatinib for advanced-phase patients.

In patients with myeloid blast crisis, most have been treated with an imatinib dose of 600 mg daily, with an overall response rate of 52%.[132] Sustained hematologic responses lasting at least 4 weeks were observed in 31% of patients. Nine percent of patients achieved a complete remission (CR, <5% blasts) with peripheral blood recovery, and another 4% of patients cleared their marrows to less than 5% blasts but did not meet the criteria for CR because of persistent cytopenias. Finally, 18% of patients either returned to chronic phase or had partial responses. Major cytogenetic responses were seen in 16% of patients, with 7% having complete responses. Median survival was 6.9 months, with an estimated survival of 17% at 24 months.[132] The baseline features predictive of prolonged survival were a platelet count of 100 × 10⁹/L or more, peripheral blood blasts less than 50%, and a hemoglobin of 10 g/dL or greater. For patients with all three of these features, the median survival was 21 months. However, for patients with none of these features, the median survival was only 4 months. Patients with a CHR or marrow blasts less than 5% at 2 months had a median survival of more than 24 months, and their survival was significantly longer than that of patients who returned to chronic phase or had no response. These results with single-agent imatinib compare favorably with historical control subjects treated with chemotherapy for myeloid blast crisis, in whom the median survival is approximately 3 months. However, the high relapse rates suggest that imatinib should be viewed as either a bridge to allogeneic SCT or that patients should be enrolled in clinical trials combining imatinib with other agents.

Patients in blastic transformation also may be given combination chemotherapy similar to that for acute leukemia. Approximately 20% of patients in myeloid transformation will achieve a second chronic phase with AML regimens containing an anthracycline and cytarabine with or without 6-thioguanine or etoposide.[133] Patients in lymphoid blastic transformation have a 50% chance of attaining second chronic phase with standard ALL treatment.[134] Central nervous system (CNS) prophylaxis should be given to patients with lymphoid transformation because leukemic meningitis may develop. Intrathecal methotrexate or cytarabine is preferable to cranial irradiation. Imatinib does not penetrate the CNS, and because of local irritant properties, intrathecal administration of imatinib is contraindicated.

The results of allogeneic SCT in accelerated phase show a 15% to 20% leukemia-free survival at 5 years.[135] Patients who receive SCT after obtaining a second chronic phase after blast transformation have a survival superior to that of those patients transplanted in blastic phase, in whom the survival is less than 10% because of a high mortality rate and a relapse rate of greater than 60%.[136]

FUTURE DIRECTIONS

One issue for the future is whether it will be possible to improve on the results with imatinib, 400 mg daily, for newly diagnosed patients with chronic-phase CML. To accomplish this, various groups have tried higher doses of imatinib, and combinations of imatinib with low doses of IFN-alfa or Ara-C. Each of these studies used cytogenetic responses as the major end point. Due in part to the extremely high rate of cytogenetic responses with 400 mg imatinib, it has been difficult to show a compelling improvement for any of these therapies. Although each of these therapies can be given safely, increased toxicity occurs, as compared with 400 mg imatinib alone.[137] Therefore various groups are initiating randomized studies comparing 400 mg daily of imatinib for newly diagnosed chronic-phase patients with CML to higher doses of imatinib to combinations of imatinib with IFN-alfa or Ara-C. The end points of these studies will be molecular response rates at 1 year and survival.

Other agents in development include second-generation *ABL* kinase inhibitors that have increased potency or specificity compared with imatinib, or are capable of inhibiting some of the mutant forms of *BCR-ABL* that are observed in patients who have developed resistance to imatinib.[138,139] A variety of signal-transduction inhibitors that affect pathways downstream of imatinib also are under development. These include farnesyl transferase inhibitors, RAF, and MEK inhibitors. Arsenic trioxide, historically the first clinically useful therapy for CML, has seen a resurgence in interest, with in vitro data showing that arsenic trioxide can downregulate BCR-ABL protein expression.[140,141] Similarly, geldanamycin analogs downregulate *BCR-ABL* expression.[142,143] Many of these agents have additive to synergistic effects when combined with imatinib, and combination clinical trials are envisioned. A number of novel chemotherapeutic agents are being developed, including homoharringtonine, decitabine, and troxacitabine, which have shown some activity in patients with CML.[137] Finally, vaccine strategies are undergoing investigation. These include vaccinations with BCR-ABL junction peptides,[144] generation of specific, cytotoxic T cells,[145] or vaccination with autologous proteins, such as heat shock protein 70.[146] If these immune strategies show promise, they may be most useful in eliminating residual disease after therapy with imatinib.

An additional direction for the future is to predict more accurately the outcome with molecularly defined risk groups, as opposed to the clinically defined criteria in the Sokal or Euro scores. Radich and colleagues[137] compared a pool of blast-crisis samples with a pool of chronic-phase samples and found approximately 500 genes that are significantly different between the two disease states. Blast-crisis and chronic-phase patients show clear differences in gene expression, and occasional cases occur in which the clinical and pathologic diagnosis is quite discordant from the gene expression pattern. Ultimately, the goal of these studies is to predict response to various therapies to aid in the decision-making process at diagnosis.

REFERENCES

1. Geary CG: The story of chronic myeloid leukaemia. Br J Haematol 2000;10:2.
2. Nowell PC, Hungerford DA: A minute chromosome in human chronic granulocytic leukemia. Science 1960;132:1497.
3. Rowley JD: A new consistent abnormality in chronic myelogenous leukaemia identified by quinacrine fluorescence and Giemsa staining. Nature 1973;243:290.
4. de Klein A, van Kessel AG, Grosveld G, et al: A cellular oncogene is translocated to the Philadelphia chromosome in chronic myelocytic leukemia. Nature 1982;300:765.
5. Deininger MW, Goldman JM, Melo JV: The molecular biology of chronic myeloid leukemia. Blood 2000;96:3343.
6. Ries LAG, Eisner MP, Kosary CL, et al: SEER Cancer Statistics Review, 1975–2000. Bethesda, MD, National Cancer Institute, 2003.
7. Rowe JM, Lichtman MA: Hyperleukocytosis and leukostasis: Common features of childhood chronic myelogenous leukemia. Blood 1984;63:1230.
8. Brown WM, Doll R: Mortality from cancer and other causes after radiotherapy for ankylosing spondylitis. BMJ 1965;5474:1327.
9. Boice JD Jr, Day NE, Andersen A, et al: Second cancers following radiation treatment for cervical cancer: An international collaboration among cancer registries. J Natl Cancer Inst 1985;74:955.
10. Kato H, Schull WJ: Studies of the mortality of A-bomb survivors: 7. Mortality, 1950–1978: Part I. Cancer mortality. Radiat Res 1982;90:395.
11. Hirschhorn K: Cytogenetic alterations in leukemia. In Dameshek W, Dutcher RM, (eds): Perspectives in Leukemia. Orlando, FL, Grune & Stratton, 1968, p 113.
12. Marmont A, Frassoni F, Bacigalupo A, et al: Recurrence of Ph'-positive leukemia in donor cells after marrow transplantation for chronic granulocytic leukemia. N Engl J Med 1984;310:903.
13. Posthuma EF, Falkenburg JH, Apperley JF, et al: HLA-DR4 is associated with a diminished risk of the development of chronic myeloid leukemia (CML): Chronic Leukemia Working Party of the European Blood and Marrow Transplant Registry. Leukemia 2000;14:859.
14. Posthuma EF, Falkenburg JH, Apperley JF, et al: HLA-B8 and HLA-A3 coexpressed with HLA-B8 are associated with a reduced risk of the development of chronic myeloid leukemia: The Chronic Leukemia Working Party of the EBMT. Blood 1999;93:3863.
15. Groffen J, Stephenson JR, Heisterkamp N, et al: Philadelphia chromosome breakpoints are clustered within a limited region, bcr, on chromosome 22. Cell 1984;36:93.
16. Konopka JB, Watanabe SM, Witte ON: An alteration of the human c-abl protein in K562 unmasks associated tyrosine kinase activity. Cell 1984;37:1035.
17. Lugo TG, Pendergast AM, Muller AJ, et al: Tyrosine kinase activity and transformation potency of bcr-abl oncogene products. Science 1990;247:1079.

18. Mills KL: The relationship between the location of the breakpoint within the M-bcr and clinical parameters. Leuk Lymphoma 1993;11(Suppl 1):73.

19. Melo JV: The diversity of BCR-ABL fusion proteins and their relationship to leukemia phenotype. Blood 1996;88:2375.

20. Heisterkamp N, Jenster G, ten Hoeve J, et al: Acute leukaemia in bcr/abl transgenic mice. Nature 1990;344:251.

21. Daley GQ, Van Etten RA, Baltimore D: Induction of chronic myelogenous leukemia in mice by the P210bcr/abl gene of the Philadelphia chromosome. Science 1990;247:824.

22. Kelliher MA, McLaughlin J, Witte ON, et al: Induction of a chronic myelogenous leukemia-like syndrome in mice with v-abl and BCR/ABL. Proc Natl Acad Sci USA 1990;87:6649.

23. Huettner CS, Zhang P, Van Etten RA, et al: Reversibility of acute B-cell leukaemia induced by BCR-ABL1. Nat Genet 2000; 24:57.

24. Mitelman F: The cytogenetic scenario of chronic myeloid leukemia. Leuk Lymphoma 1993;11(Suppl 1):11.

25. Cortes JE, Talpaz M, Beran M, et al: Philadelphia chromosome-negative chronic myelogenous leukemia with rearrangement of the breakpoint cluster region: Long-term follow-up results. Cancer 1995;75:464.

26. Schoch C, Schnittger S, Bursch S, et al: Comparison of chromosome banding analysis, interphase- and hypermetaphase-FISH, qualitative and quantitative PCR for diagnosis and for follow-up in chronic myeloid leukemia: a study on 350 cases. Leukemia 2002;16:53.

27. Dewald GW, Wyatt WA, Juneau AL, et al: Highly sensitive fluorescence in situ hybridization method to detect double BCR/ABL fusion and monitor response to therapy in chronic myeloid leukemia. Blood 1998;91:3357.

28. Wang YL, Bagg A, Pear W, et al: Chronic myelogenous leukemia: Laboratory diagnosis and monitoring. Genes Chromosomes Cancer 2001;32:97.

29. Kurzrock R, Bueso-Ramos CE, Kantarjian H, et al: BCR rearrangement-negative chronic myelogenous leukemia revisited. J Clin Oncol 2001;19:2915.

30. Cross NC, Reiter A: Tyrosine kinase fusion genes in chronic myeloproliferative diseases. Leukemia 2002;16:1207.

31. Savage DG, Szydlo RM, Goldman JM: Clinical features at diagnosis in 430 patients with chronic myeloid leukaemia seen at a referral centre over a 16-year period. Br J Haematol 1997;96:111.

32. Sokal JE, Cox EB, Baccarani M, et al: Prognostic discrimination in "good-risk" chronic granulocytic leukemia. Blood 1984;63:789.

33. Hasford J, Pfirrmann M, Hehlmann R, et al: A new prognostic score for survival of patients with chronic myeloid leukemia treated with interferon alfa: Writing Committee for the Collaborative CML Prognostic Factors Project Group. J Natl Cancer Inst 1998;90:850.

34. Huntly BJ, Bench A, Green AR: Double jeopardy from a single translocation: Deletions of the derivative chromosome 9 in chronic myeloid leukemia. Blood 2003;102:1160.

35. Brummendorf TH, Holyoake TL, Rufer N, et al: Prognostic implications of differences in telomere length between normal and malignant cells from patients with chronic myeloid leukemia measured by flow cytometry. Blood 2000;95:1883.

36. Kantarjian HM, Smith TL, McCredie KB, et al: Chronic myelogenous leukemia: A multivariate analysis of the associations of patient characteristics and therapy with survival. Blood 1985;66:1326.

37. Sokal JE, Gomez GA, Baccarani M, et al: Prognostic significance of additional cytogenetic abnormalities at diagnosis of Philadelphia chromosome-positive chronic granulocytic leukemia. Blood 1988;72:294.

38. Minot G, Buckman T, Isaccs R: Chronic myelogenous leukemia. JAMA 1924;82:1489.

39. Goldman JM, Szydlo R, Horowitz MM, et al: Choice of pretransplant treatment and timing of transplants for chronic myelogenous leukemia in chronic phase. Blood 1993;82:2235.

40. Best PJ, Daoud MS, Pittelkow MR, et al: Hydroxyurea-induced leg ulceration in 14 patients. Ann Intern Med 1998;128:29.

41. Hehlmann R, Heimpel H, Hasford J, et al: Randomized comparison of interferon-alpha with busulfan and hydroxyurea in chronic myelogenous leukemia: The German CML Study Group. Blood 1994;84:4064.

42. Talpaz M, McCredie KB, Mavligit GM, et al: Leukocyte interferon-induced myeloid cytoreduction in chronic myelogenous leukemia. Blood 1983;62:689.

43. Silver RT, Woolf SH, Hehlmann R, et al: An evidence-based analysis of the effect of busulfan, hydroxyurea, interferon, and allogeneic bone marrow transplantation in treating the chronic phase of chronic myeloid leukemia: Developed for the American Society of Hematology. Blood 1999;94:1517.

44. Chronic Myeloid Leukemia Trialists' Collaborative Group: Interferon alfa versus chemotherapy for chronic myeloid leukemia: A meta-analysis of seven randomized trials. J Natl Cancer Inst 1997;89:1616.

45. Kantarjian HM, Smith TL, O'Brien S, et al: Prolonged survival in chronic myelogenous leukemia after cytogenetic response to interferon-alpha therapy: The Leukemia Service. Ann Intern Med 1995;122:254.

46. Kantarjian HM, O'Brien S, Anderlini P, et al: Treatment of myelogenous leukemia: Current status and investigational options. Blood 1996;87:3069.

47. Cortes J, Kantarjian H, O'Brien S, et al: Result of interferon-alpha therapy in patients with chronic myelogenous leukemia 60 years of age and older. Am J Med 1996;100:452.

48. O'Brien S, Kantarjian H, Talpaz M: Practical guidelines for the management of chronic myelogenous leukemia with interferon alpha. Leuk Lymphoma 1996;23:247.

49. Mahon FX, Faberes C, Montastruc M, et al: High response rate using recombinant interferon-alpha in patients with newly diagnosed chronic myeloid leukemia. Bone Marrow Transplant 1996;17(Suppl 3):S33.

50. Shepherd P, Kluin-Nelemans H, Richards S, et al: A randomised comparison of low or high dose IFN-α in newly diagnosed CML patients shows no difference in major cytogenetic response rate or survival between the two groups: Results of MRC CML V and HOVON 20 trials. Blood 2001;98:727a.

51. Sacchi S, Kantarjian HM, Smith TL, et al: Early treatment decisions with interferon-alfa therapy in early chronic-phase chronic myelogenous leukemia. J Clin Oncol 1998;16:882.

52. Mahon FX, Faberes C, Pueyo S, et al: Response at three months is a good predictive factor for newly diagnosed chronic myeloid leukemia patients treated by recombinant interferon-alpha. Blood 1998;92:4059.

53. Bonifazi F, de Vivo A, Rosti G, et al: Chronic myeloid leukemia and interferon-alpha: A study of complete cytogenetic responders. Blood 2001;98:3974.

54. Guilhot F, Chastang C, Michallet M, et al: Interferon alfa-2B combined with cytarabine versus interferon alone in chronic myelogenous leukemia: French Chronic Myeloid Leukemia Study Group. N Engl J Med 1997;337:223.

55. Baccarani M, Rosti G, de Vivo A, et al: A randomized study of interferon-alpha versus interferon-alpha and low-dose arabinosyl cytosine in chronic myeloid leukemia. Blood 2002;99:1527.

56. Hehlmann R, Hochhaus A, Kolb HJ, et al: Interferon-alpha before allogeneic bone marrow transplantation in chronic myelogenous leukemia does not affect outcome adversely, provided it is discontinued at least 90 days before the procedure. Blood 1999;94:3668.

57. Lipton JH, Khoroshko ND, Golenkov AK, et al: A randomized multicenter comparative study of peginterferon alfa-2a (40kD) vs interferon-alfa-2a in patients with treatment naive chronic-phase chronic myelogenous leukemia. Blood 2002;100:782a.

58. Michallet M, Delain M, Maloisel F, et al: Phase III trial of PEG intron vs interferon alfa-2b for the initial treatment of chronic myelogenous leukemia. Blood 2001;98:348a.

59. Peggs K, Mackinnon S: Imatinib mesylate: The new gold standard for treatment of chronic myeloid leukemia. N Engl J Med 2003;348:1048.

60. Druker BJ, Lydon NB: Lessons learned from the development of an abl tyrosine kinase inhibitor for chronic myelogenous leukemia. J Clin Invest 2000;105:3.

61. Druker BJ, Talpaz M, Resta D, et al: Efficacy and safety of a specific inhibitor of the Bcr-Abl tyrosine kinase in chronic myeloid leukemia. N Engl J Med 2001;344:1031.

62. Kantarjian H, Sawyers C, Hochhaus A, et al: Hematologic and cytogenetic responses to imatinib mesylate in chronic myelogenous leukemia. N Engl J Med 2002;346:645.

63. O'Brien SG, Guilhot F, Larson RA, et al: Imatinib compared with interferon and low-dose cytarabine for newly diagnosed chronic-phase chronic myeloid leukemia. N Engl J Med 2003;348:994.

64. Hughes T, Kaeda J, Branford S, et al: Molecular responses to imatinib (STI571) or interferon + Ara-C as initial therapy for CML: Results in the IRIS study. Blood 2002;100:93a.

65. Deininger MW, O'Brien SG, Ford JM, et al: Practical management of patients with chronic myeloid leukemia receiving imatinib. J Clin Oncol 2003;21:1637.

66. Braziel RM, Launder TM, Druker BJ, et al: Hematopathologic and cytogenetic findings in imatinib mesylate-treated chronic myelogenous leukemia patients: 14 months' experience. Blood 2002;100:435.

67. Bumm T, Muller C, Al-Ali HK, et al: Emergence of clonal cytogenetic abnormalities in Ph-cells in some CML patients in cytogenetic remission to imatinib but restoration of polyclonal hematopoiesis in the majority. Blood 2003;101:1941.

68. Petzer AL, Eaves CJ, Lansdorp PM, et al: Characterization of primitive subpopulations of normal and leukemic cells present in the blood of patients with newly diagnosed as well as established chronic myeloid leukemia. Blood 1996;88:2162.

69. Marin D, Marktel S, Foot N, et al: Granulocyte colony-stimulating factor reverses cytopenia and may permit cytogenetic responses in patients with chronic myeloid leukemia treated with imatinib mesylate. Haematologica 2003;88:227.

70. Mauro MJ, Kurilik G, Balleisen S, et al: Myeloid growth factors for neutropenia during imatinib mesylate (STI571) therapy for CML: Preliminary evidence of safety and efficacy. Blood 2001;98:139a.

71. Hochhaus A, Kreil S, Corbin AS, et al: Molecular and chromosomal mechanisms of resistance to imatinib (STI571) therapy. Leukemia 2002;16:2190.

72. Gambacorti-Passerini CB, Gunby RH, Piazza R, et al: Molecular mechanisms of resistance to imatinib in Philadelphia-chromosome-positive leukemias. Lancet Oncol 2003;4:75.

73. Shah NP, Nicoll JM, Nagar B, et al: Multiple BCR-ABL kinase domain mutations confer polyclonal resistance to the tyrosine kinase inhibitor imatinib (STI571) in chronic phase and blast crisis chronic myeloid leukemia. Cancer Cell 2002;2:117.

74. Kantarjian HM, Talpaz M, O'Brien S, et al: Dose escalation of imatinib mesylate can overcome resistance to standard-dose therapy in patients with chronic myelogenous leukemia. Blood 2003;101:473.

75. Mughal TI, Yong A, Szydlo RM, et al: Molecular studies in patients with chronic myeloid leukaemia in remission 5 years after allogeneic stem cell transplant define the risk of subsequent relapse. Br J Haematol 2001;115:569.

76. Barrett J: Allogeneic stem cell transplantation for chronic myeloid leukemia. Semin Hematol 2003;40:59.

77. Goldman JM, Gale RP, Horowitz MM, et al: Bone marrow transplantation for chronic myelogenous leukemia in chronic phase: Increased risk for relapse associated with T-cell depletion. Ann Intern Med 1988;108:806.

78. Kolb HJ, Mittermuller J, Clemm C, et al: Donor leukocyte transfusions for treatment of recurrent chronic myelogenous leukemia in marrow transplant patients. Blood 1990;76:2462.

79. Kolb HJ, Schattenberg A, Goldman JM, et al: Graft-versus-leukemia effect of donor lymphocyte transfusions in marrow grafted patients: European Group for Blood and Marrow Transplantation Working Party Chronic Leukemia. Blood 1995;86:2041.

80. Clark RE, Dodi IA, Hill SC, et al: Direct evidence that leukemic cells present HLA-associated immunogenic peptides derived from the BCR-ABL b3a2 fusion protein. Blood 2001;98:2887.

81. Horowitz MM, Rowlings PA, Passweg JR: Allogeneic bone marrow transplantation for CML: A report from the International Bone Marrow Transplant Registry. Bone Marrow Transplant 1996;17(Suppl 3):S5.

82. Szydlo R, Goldman JM, Klein JP, et al: Results of allogeneic bone marrow transplants for leukemia using donors other than HLA-identical siblings. J Clin Oncol 1997;15:1767.

83. Hansen JA, Gooley TA, Martin PJ, et al: Bone marrow transplants from unrelated donors for patients with chronic myeloid leukemia. N Engl J Med 1998;338:962.

84. Thomas ED, Clift RA, Fefer A, et al: Marrow transplantation for the treatment of chronic myelogenous leukemia. Ann Intern Med 1986;104:155.

85. Goldman JM, Apperley JF, Jones L, et al: Bone marrow transplantation for patients with chronic myeloid leukemia. N Engl J Med 1986;314:202.

86. Weisdorf DJ, Anasetti C, Antin JH, et al: Allogeneic bone marrow transplantation for chronic myelogenous leukemia: Comparative analysis of unrelated versus matched sibling donor transplantation. Blood 2002;99:1971.

87. Gratwohl A, Hermans J, Goldman JM, et al: Risk assessment for patients with chronic myeloid leukaemia before allogeneic blood or marrow transplantation: Chronic Leukemia Working Party of the European Group for Blood and Marrow Transplantation. Lancet 1998;352:1087.

88. Gale RP, Hehlmann R, Zhang MJ, et al: Survival with bone marrow transplantation versus hydroxyurea or interferon for chronic myelogenous leukemia: The German CML Study Group. Blood 1998;91:1810.

89. Gratwohl A, Hermans J: Allogeneic bone marrow transplantation for chronic myeloid leukemia: Working Party Chronic Leukemia of the European Group for Blood and Marrow Transplantation (EBMT). Bone Marrow Transplant 1996;17:S7.

90. Craddock C, Szydlo RM, Dazzi F, et al: Cytomegalovirus seropositivity adversely influences outcome after T-depleted unrelated donor transplant in patients with chronic myeloid leukaemia: The case for tailored graft-versus-host disease prophylaxis. Br J Haematol 2001;112:228.

91. Clift RA, Buckner CD, Thomas ED, et al: Marrow transplantation for chronic myeloid leukemia: A randomized study comparing cyclophosphamide and total body irradiation with busulfan and cyclophosphamide. Blood 1994;84:2036.

92. Slattery JT, Clift RA, Buckner CD, et al: Marrow transplantation for chronic myeloid leukemia: The influence of plasma busulfan levels on the outcome of transplantation. Blood 1997;89:3055.

93. Sierra J, Storer B, Hansen JA, et al: Transplantation of marrow cells from unrelated donors for treatment of high-risk acute leukemia: The effect of leukemic burden, donor HLA-matching, and marrow cell dose. Blood 1997;89:4226.

94. Champlin RE, Schmitz N, Horowitz MM, et al: Blood stem cells compared with bone marrow as a source of hematopoietic cells for allogeneic transplantation: IBMTR Histocompatibility and Stem Cell Sources Working Committee and the European Group for Blood and Marrow Transplantation (EBMT). Blood 2000;95:3702.

95. Flowers ME, Parker PM, Johnston LJ, et al: Comparison of chronic graft-versus-host disease after transplantation of peripheral blood stem cells versus bone marrow in allogeneic recipients: Long-term follow-up of a randomized trial. Blood 2002;100:415.

96. Schmitz N, Beksac M, Hasenclever D, et al: Transplantation of mobilized peripheral blood cells to HLA-identical siblings with standard-risk leukemia. Blood 2002;100:761.

97. Passweg J, Walker I, Sobocinski K: Validation of the EBMT risk score for recipients of allogeneic hematopoietic stem cell transplants for chronic myeloid leukemia (CML). Bone Marrow Transplant 2002;29:S33.

98. McSweeney PA, Niederwieser D, Shizuru JA, et al: Hematopoietic cell transplantation in older patients with hematologic malignancies: Replacing high-dose cytotoxic therapy with graft-versus-tumor effects. Blood 2001;97:3390.

99. Or R, Shapira MY, Resnick I, et al: Nonmyeloablative allogeneic stem cell transplantation for the treatment of chronic myeloid leukemia in first chronic phase. Blood 2003;101:441.

100. Uzunel M, Mattsson J, Brune M, et al: Kinetics of minimal residual disease and chimerism in patients with chronic myeloid leukemia

after nonmyeloablative conditioning and allogeneic stem cell transplantation. Blood 2003;101:469.

101. Cross NC, Feng L, Chase A, et al: Competitive polymerase chain reaction to estimate the number of BCR-ABL transcripts in chronic myeloid leukemia patients after bone marrow transplantation. Blood 1993;82:1929.

102. Lin F, van Rhee F, Goldman JM, et al: Kinetics of increasing BCR-ABL transcript numbers in chronic myeloid leukemia patients who relapse after bone marrow transplantation. Blood 1996;87:4473.

103. Radich JP, Gehly G, Gooley T, et al: Polymerase chain reaction detection of the BCR-ABL fusion transcript after allogeneic marrow transplantation for chronic myeloid leukemia: Results and implications in 346 patients. Blood 1995;85:2632.

104. Radich JP, Gooley T, Bryant E, et al: The significance of bcr-abl molecular detection in chronic myeloid leukemia patients "late," 18 months or more after transplantation. Blood 2001;98:1701.

105. Olavarria E, Kanfer E, Szydlo R, et al: Early detection of BCR-ABL transcripts by quantitative reverse transcriptase-polymerase chain reaction predicts outcome after allogeneic stem cell transplantation for chronic myeloid leukemia. Blood 2001; 97:1560.

106. van Rhee F, Lin F, Cullis JO, et al: Relapse of chronic myeloid leukemia after allogeneic bone marrow transplant: The case for giving donor leukocyte transfusions before the onset of hematologic relapse. Blood 1994;83:3377.

107. Craddock C, Szydlo RM, Klein JP, et al: Estimating leukemia-free survival after allografting for chronic myeloid leukemia: A new method that takes into account patients who relapse and are restored to complete remission. Blood 2000;96:86.

108. Mackinnon S, Papadopoulos EB, Carabasi MH, et al: Adoptive immunotherapy evaluating escalating doses of donor leukocytes for relapse of chronic myeloid leukemia after bone marrow transplantation: Separation of graft-versus-leukemia responses from graft-versus-host disease. Blood 1995;86:1261.

109. Dazzi F, Szydlo RM, Craddock C, et al: Comparison of single-dose and escalating-dose regimens of donor lymphocyte infusion for relapse after allografting for chronic myeloid leukemia. Blood 2000;95:67.

110. Guglielmi C, Arcese W, Dazzi F, et al: Donor lymphocyte infusion for relapsed chronic myelogenous leukemia: Prognostic relevance of the initial cell dose. Blood 2002;100:397.

111. Olavarria E, Craddock C, Dazzi F, et al: Imatinib mesylate (STI571) in the treatment of relapse of chronic myeloid leukemia after allogeneic stem cell transplantation. Blood 2002;99:3861.

112. Haines ME, Goldman JM, Worsley AM, et al: Chemotherapy and autografting for chronic granulocytic leukaemia in transformation: Probable prolongation of survival for some patients. Br J Haematol 1984;58:711.

113. McGlave PB, De Fabritiis P, Deisseroth A, et al: Autologous transplants for chronic myelogenous leukaemia: Results from eight transplant groups. Lancet 1994;343:1486.

114. O'Brien SG, Goldman JM: Current approaches to hematopoietic stem-cell purging in chronic myeloid leukemia. J Clin Oncol 1995;13:541.

115. Carella AM, Cunningham I, Lerma E, et al: Mobilization and transplantation of Philadelphia-negative peripheral-blood progenitor cells early in chronic myelogenous leukemia. J Clin Oncol 1997;15:1575.

116. Barnett MJ, Eaves CJ, Phillips GL, et al: Autografting with cultured marrow in chronic myeloid leukemia: Results of a pilot study. Blood 1994;84:724.

117. Goldman JM, Druker BJ: Chronic myeloid leukemia: Current treatment options. Blood 2001;98:2039.

118. Goldman JM, Marin D: Management decisions in chronic myeloid leukemia. Semin Hematol 2003;40:97.

119. Kardinal CG, Bateman JR, Weiner J: Chronic granulocytic leukemia: Review of 536 cases. Arch Intern Med 1976; 136:305.

120. Bettelheim P, Lutz D, Majdic O, et al: Cell lineage heterogeneity in blast crisis of chronic myeloid leukaemia. Br J Haematol 1985;59:395.

121. Griffin JD, Todd RF III, Ritz J, et al: Differentiation patterns in the blastic phase of chronic myeloid leukemia. Blood 1983;61:85.

122. Kantarjian HM, Keating MJ, Talpaz M, et al: Chronic myelogenous leukemia in blast crisis: Analysis of 242 patients. Am J Med 1987;83:445.

123. Kantarjian HM, Dixon D, Keating MJ, et al: Characteristics of accelerated disease in chronic myelogenous leukemia. Cancer 1988;61:1441.

124. O'Brien S, Thall PF, Siciliano MJ: Cytogenetics of chronic myelogenous leukaemia. Baillieres Clin Haematol 1997;10:259.

125. Mashal R, Shtalrid M, Talpaz M, et al: Rearrangement and expression of p53 in the chronic phase and blast crisis of chronic myelogenous leukemia. Blood 1990;75:180.

126. Ahuja H, Bar-Eli M, Advani SH, et al: Alterations in the p53 gene and the clonal evolution of the blast crisis of chronic myelocytic leukemia. Proc Natl Acad Sci USA 1989;86:6783.

127. Sill H, Aguiar RC, Schmidt H, et al: Mutational analysis of the p15 and p16 genes in acute leukaemias. Br J Haematol 1996;92:681.

128. Towatari M, Adachi K, Kato H, et al: Absence of the human retinoblastoma gene product in the megakaryoblastic crisis of chronic myelogenous leukemia. Blood 1991;78:2178.

129. Ahuja HG, Jat PS, Foti A, et al: Abnormalities of the retinoblastoma gene in the pathogenesis of acute leukemia. Blood 1991;78: 3259–3268.

130. McCarthy DM, Rassool FV, Goldman JM, et al: Genomic alterations involving the c-myc proto-oncogene locus during the evolution of a case of chronic granulocytic leukaemia. Lancet 1984;2:1362.

131. Talpaz M, Silver RT, Druker BJ, et al: Imatinib induces durable hematologic and cytogenetic responses in patients with accelerated phase chronic myeloid leukemia: results of a phase II study. Blood 2002;99:1928.

132. Sawyers CL, Hochhaus A, Feldman E, et al: Imatinib induces hematologic and cytogenetic responses in patients with chronic myeloid leukemia in myeloid blast crisis: Results of a phase II study. Blood 2002;99:3530.

133. Sacchi S, Kantarjian HM, O'Brien S, et al: Chronic myelogenous leukemia in nonlymphoid blastic phase: Analysis of the results of first salvage therapy with three different treatment approaches for 162 patients. Cancer 1999;86:2632.

134. Derderian PM, Kantarjian HM, Talpaz M, et al: Chronic myelogenous leukemia in the lymphoid blastic phase: Characteristics, treatment response, and prognosis. Am J Med 1993;94:69.

135. Clift RA, Buckner CD, Thomas ED, et al: Marrow transplantation for patients in accelerated phase of chronic myeloid leukemia. Blood 1994;84:4368.

136. Gratwohl A, Hermans J, Niederwieser D, et al: Bone marrow transplantation for chronic myeloid leukemia: Long-term results: Chronic Leukemia Working Party of the European Group for Bone Marrow Transplantation. Bone Marrow Transplant 1993;12: 509.

137. Druker BJ, O'Brien SG, Cortes J, Radich J: Chronic myelogenous leukemia. Hematology (Am Soc Hematol Educ Program) 2002;111–135.

138. Huron DR, Gorre ME, Kraker AJ, et al: A novel pyridopyrimidine inhibitor of Abl kinase is a picomolar inhibitor of Bcr-abl-driven K562 cells and is effective against STI571-resistant Bcr-abl mutants. Clin Cancer Res 2003;9:1267.

139. La Rosee P, Corbin AS, Stoffregen EP, et al: Activity of the Bcr-Abl kinase inhibitor PD180970 against clinically relevant Bcr-Abl isoforms that cause resistance to imatinib mesylate (Gleevec, STI571). Cancer Res 2002;62:7149.

140. La Rosee P, Johnson K, O'Dwyer ME, et al: In vitro studies of the combination of imatinib mesylate (Gleevec) and arsenic trioxide (Trisenox) in chronic myelogenous leukemia. Exp Hematol 2002;30:729.

141. Perkins C, Kim CN, Fang G, et al: Arsenic induces apoptosis of multidrug-resistant human myeloid leukemia cells that express Bcr-Abl or overexpress MDR, MRP, Bcl-2, or Bcl-x(L). Blood 2000;95:1014.

142. Nimmanapalli R, O'Bryan E, Huang M, et al: Molecular characterization and sensitivity of STI-571 (imatinib mesylate, Gleevec)-resistant, Bcr-Abl-positive, human acute leukemia cells to

SRC kinase inhibitor PD180970 and 17-allylamino-17-demethoxygeldanamycin. Cancer Res 2002;62:5761.

143. Gorre ME, Ellwood-Yen K, Chiosis G, et al: BCR-ABL point mutants isolated from patients with imatinib mesylate-resistant chronic myeloid leukemia remain sensitive to inhibitors of the BCR-ABL chaperone heat shock protein 90. Blood 2002;100:3041.

144. Pinilla-Ibarz J, Cathcart K, Korontsvit T, et al: Vaccination of patients with chronic myelogenous leukemia with bcr-abl oncogene breakpoint fusion peptides generates specific immune responses. Blood 2000;95:1781.

145. Molldrem JJ, Kant S, Jiang W, et al: The basis of T-cell-mediated immunity to chronic myelogenous leukemia. Oncogene 2002;21:8668.

146. Liu B, DeFilippo AM, Li Z: Overcoming immune tolerance to cancer by heat shock protein vaccines. Mol Cancer Ther 2002;1:1147.

147. Sokal JE, Baccarani M, Russo D, et al: Staging and prognosis in chronic myelogenous leukemia. Semin Hematol 1988;25:49.

148. Savage DG, Szydlo RM, Chase A, et al: Bone marrow transplantation for chronic myeloid leukaemia: The effects of differing criteria for defining chronic phase on probabilities of survival and relapse. Br J Haematol 1997;99:30.

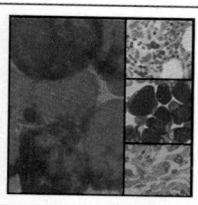

08 CHRONIC LYMPHOID LEUKEMIAS

Bruce D. Cheson

SUMMARY OF KEY POINTS

INCIDENCE

- Chronic lymphoid leukemias are the most common leukemias in Western countries, with approximately 7300 new cases per year in the United States in 2003. More common in men, with median age at onset older than 60 years.

DIFFERENTIAL DIAGNOSIS

- Chronic lymphocytic leukemia (CLL) requires the presence of more than 5000 mature-appearing lymphocytes/mm^3 in the peripheral blood. Included in the differential diagnosis are other chronic B-cell malignancies, including prolymphocytic leukemia, hairy cell leukemia, and a leukemic form of non-Hodgkin's lymphoma.
- Careful examination of the peripheral blood smear, in conjunction with immunophenotyping of peripheral blood lymphocytes, facilitates distinction among these disorders. CLL cells are positive for CD19, CD20, CD5, and CD23.

STAGING AND PROGNOSIS

- A complete history and physical examination, with particular attention to the size and distribution of lymph nodes, and presence of hepatosplenomegaly, complete blood count (CBC), and careful evaluation of the peripheral blood should be included in the staging and evaluation. If anemia or thrombocytopenia is present, a bone marrow is indicated. A Coombs' test should be performed to evaluate possible hemolysis.
- A bone marrow aspirate and biopsy

are generally not required to make the diagnosis but are needed before therapy to assess prognosis and response to treatment.
- Radiographic procedures, such as computed tomography (CT) scans, are not routinely warranted but should be considered for further evaluation of symptoms or abnormal laboratory findings.
- Cytogenetics studies are strongly predictive of outcome; however, because they do not as yet direct treatment, these expensive studies are not part of routine care. Additional studies that should be considered include quantitative immunoglobulins and β_2-microglobulin. Newer studies that are still investigational include CD38, immunoglobulin gene mutational status, and ZAP-70.

PRIMARY THERAPY

- CLL is currently not a curable disease. Therefore therapy is usually reserved for patients with disease-related symptoms, anemia or thrombocytopenia, massive or progressive lymphadenopathy or hepatosplenomegaly, or recurrent infections and may be supported by a rapid lymphocyte-doubling time.
- Fludarabine has become the standard of care because it has a higher complete and overall response rate when compared with alkylating agents, with complete response rates of 20% to 30% and overall responses in 70% to 80% of patients. Fludarabine also is associated with longer responses than those with alkylating agent regimens. Nevertheless, prolongation

of survival has been difficult to detect. Newer regimens adding cyclophosphamide, rituximab, or both are being studied in clinical trials, with impressive preliminary results.
- No effective therapy exists for prolymphocytic leukemia. Patients are generally treated with fludarabine or pentostatin. Encouraging results with alemtuzumab have been reported.

TREATMENT OF RELAPSED OR REFRACTORY DISEASE

- For patients relapsing after fludarabine therapy, retreatment is successful in approximately half of cases. Responses are infrequent with alkylating agents. Combinations of fludarabine with cyclophosphamide may achieve responses. Alemtuzumab is effective, but less so in patients with bulky lymphadenopathy. Rituximab as a single agent has limited activity in this setting but may be more effective in combination with other agents.
- The use of autologous stem cell transplantation has been disappointing. Allogeneic stem cell transplantation may be effective in selected patients, but it is associated with high rates of morbidity and mortality. Whether submyeloablative stem cell transplantation provides an effective alternative is under investigation.
- Additional approaches to fludarabine failures include the use of BCL-2 antisense oligonucleotides and other monoclonal antibodies.

EPIDEMIOLOGY

The chronic lymphoid leukemias are a group of relatively indolent clonal lymphoid disorders, primarily of B-cell lineage, including chronic lymphocytic leukemia (CLL), prolymphocytic leukemia (PLL), hairy cell leukemia (HCL), and the leukemic phase of the various non-Hodgkin's lymphomas (NHLs).

CLL is the most common adult leukemia in Western countries, with approximately 7300 new cases diagnosed in the United States each year.[1] CLL is more common in men than in women (1.7:1), with a steep age-specific incidence rate. A higher incidence seems to occur in Jewish people of Russian or Eastern European ancestry, but it is rare in Asian countries.

No known risk factors have been found for CLL. Indeed, CLL is one of the few leukemias that do not appear to be associated with exposure to ionizing radiation, chemicals, or drugs with the possible exception of Agent Orange.[2-5] Although no clear genetic factors have been identified, there is clearly an increased familial incidence of CLL, with rare sets of affected twins.[6-9] A number of chromosomal imbalances have been noted, more commonly in familial CLL than in sporadic cases.[10] A lack of concordance of oncogene expression was reported in monozygous twin sisters who both had CLL.[11] Immigrants from Japan to the United States maintain their low incidence of CLL. The occurrence in spouses has been observed.[12]

CHRONIC LYMPHOCYTIC LEUKEMIA

Cell of Origin

The precise origin of the CLL lymphocyte is controversial. CLL cells express pan-B antigens (e.g., human leukocyte antigen (HLA)-class II, CD19, CD20), as well as activation antigens (e.g., CD5, CD23, CD25, CD71) but not the terminal differentiation antigens exhibited by plasma cells. This profile supports the hypothesis that the B-CLL cell is an "activated" B lymphocyte, meaning that the cells can be activated without dividing, but does not suggest that they are in a state of active proliferation.[13]

Two of the features that distinguish CLL cells from normal B cells are that they express CD5, but surface immunoglobulins are barely detectable. CD5+ B cells are normally present in the mantle zone of normal lymph nodes and in small numbers in the peripheral blood of normal individuals. CD5+ B cells also are found in increased numbers in patients with autoimmune disorders, such as rheumatoid arthritis, Sjögren's syndrome, systemic lupus erythematosus, immune thrombocytopenic purpura, and after allogeneic bone marrow transplantation (BMT).[14,15] These observations have led to the current theory that B-CLL is a monoclonal proliferation of mantle-zone–based anergic CD5+ self-reactive B cells devoted to the production of polyreactive autoantibodies.[13]

Cytogenetic and Molecular Abnormalities

Conventional banding techniques detect cytogenetic abnormalities in more than 50% of cases of CLL.[16-18] More recently, fluorescence in situ hybridization (FISH) has increased the sensitivity of detection so that cytogenetic abnormalities can be identified in more than 80% of cases.[19,20] The most common cytogenetic abnormality in CLL is del 13q, which is present in 55% of cases, either alone or in combination with other abnormalities. Patients with 13q14 abnormalities tend to have a more benign course, often with a normal life span. Next in frequency are deletions of 11q, which are identified in 15% to 20% of cases. Deletions of 11q23 are associated with massive lymphadenopathy that is often out of proportion to the increase in peripheral blood lymphocyte count. Trisomy 12 can be detected in 15% to 20% of cases. Structural abnormalities of chromosome 17 detected by FISH occur in at least 15% of patients. The 17p13 deletions lead to disruption of the p53 gene. Chromosome 17 abnormalities are found more frequently in cases of atypical CLL, are associated with a higher likelihood of Richter's transformation, more prolymphocytes, advanced stage, chemoresistance, and a poor prognosis.[21-24]

More than one third of patients have complex abnormalities. Of note is the lack of translocations in patients with CLL. Genetic aberrations are detected in more than 80% of cases.[25] Nevertheless, no single oncogene has been implicated in the pathogenesis of CLL. Early reports of cases with the *BCL-1* translocation were more likely mantle cell lymphoma.[26,27] The translocations associated with *BCL-2* [t(14;18)(q32;q21)] and *BCL-3* [t(14;19)(q32;q13.1)] have been detected in only 5% to 10% of cases.[28,29] However, overexpression of the *BCL-2* gene is present in more than 70% of cases, even in the absence of the chromosome rearrangement.[30] The ratio of the antiapoptotic gene *BCL-2* to the proapoptotic gene, *BAX*, is increased in CLL cells, which favors cell survival. These findings support the concept that CLL is not a disorder resulting from abnormal proliferation of lymphocytes, but rather one of an accumulation of malignant B cells.

Deletions of 13q have been identified by using molecular techniques, even in cases without cytogenetic changes. This abnormality was believed to be at the site of the retinoblastoma suppressor gene, but has since been shown to be telomeric to that region with a novel suppressor gene referred to as *DBM* (disrupted in B-cell malignancy).[31] An apparent correlation is noted between the antiapoptotic protein Mcl-1 and resistance to chemotherapy.[32]

Studies of gene use in CLL have indicated that there may be nonrandom differential use of *Vb* and *Vl* genes used in the cell of origin, with an apparent increase in the use of the VH_1-69 (51p1) gene from the VH_1 family.[33,34]

BCL-3 translocations, t(14;19)(q32.3;q13.2), are uncommon, and in approximately half of cases, occur in association with trisomy 12. These patients tend to be young and to have rapidly progressive disease.

The *ATM* gene is located at chromosome 11q22-23 and encodes for a high-molecular-weight protein that is involved in cell-cycle control, DNA repair, and DNA recombination. It is mutated in patients with ataxia telangiectasia (AT), who are at an increased risk for lymphoid neoplasms. However, only a subset of patients with del 11q22-23 show mutations in the coding region of the remaining *ATM* allele,[35] suggesting a pathogenetic role for other genes.

Several recent studies suggested that two basic types of CLL exist. Lymphocytes from approximately half of patients with CLL contain V_H genes, which are mutated post–germinal center B cells (IgD⁻), whereas the other half are naive, unmutated (IgD⁺/IgM⁺).[36-38] These two populations are characterized by markedly different clinical outcomes; the unmutated group have a significantly shorter survival. DNA microarray analyses have suggested that CLL is a single disease with two different expressions, rather than two different diseases. DNA microarray studies have shown that *ZAP-70* distinguishes mutated from the unmutated populations of CLL patients.[39] *ZAP-70* is associated with enhanced signal transduction via *BCR* complex, which may contribute to an aggressive course.[40] The overall incidence of genomic aberrations is similar in the mutated and unmutated groups; however, unfavorable cytogenetic abnormalities (e.g., 17p- and 11q-) occur in the unmutated group, whereas more favorable mutations (e.g., 13q-) occur in the mutated group.[41] Lymphocytes with trisomy 12 tend to have unmutated immunoglobulin variable (V_H) genes, whereas those with 13q14 have evidence of somatic mutations.[34]

Diagnosis

CLL should be suspected in patients who have a sustained increase to more than 5000/mm³ in the number of small, mature-appearing lymphocytes circulating in the peripheral blood, unexplained by other clinical disorders.[42,43]

The morphologic appearance of the lymphocytes may help to distinguish CLL from other diseases, notably HCL or the leukemic phase of marginal zone lymphoma or mantle cell lymphoma. Up to 55% circulating prolymphocytes is considered consistent with the diagnosis of CLL.[44] The routine use of immunophenotyping has made the diagnosis of CLL considerably easier (Table 108-1).

The bone marrow in CLL is infiltrated by at least 30% lymphocytes. Nevertheless, a bone marrow aspirate and biopsy are generally not required to make the diagnosis of CLL; however, they are strongly recommended to assess prognosis (e.g., diffuse involvement associated with a poorer outcome than a nondiffuse pattern of infiltration[45]) and to evaluate erythroid precursors and megakaryocytes. Conversely, examination of the bone marrow is essential before therapy to provide a baseline for subsequent response assessment. Lymph node biopsy is needed only to confirm the clinical impression of a Richter's transformation. Computed tomography (CT) scans are usually not necessary in the initial evaluation and should be performed only when clinically indicated.

Staging and Prognosis

Patients with CLL may not require therapy for many years and eventually die of apparently unrelated causes, whereas others may die of disease-related complications within a few months of diagnosis, despite appropriate therapy. A number of characteristics have been used to separate patients with CLL into groups with differing clinical outcomes that may require different therapeutic approaches.

The first widely accepted prognostic grouping of patients was the five-stage Rai classification (Table 108-2)[46]: stage 0 includes patients with only lymphocytosis (median survival, >12.5 years); stage I, with lymphadenopathy (8.5 years); stage II, splenomegaly with or without hepatomegaly (6 years); stage III, anemia (1.5 years); and stage IV, thrombocytopenia (1.5 years). For the patient to be stage III or IV, the anemia or thrombocytopenia cannot be immune mediated. This system has subsequently been simplified to three stages[47]: low risk (stage 0), intermediate risk (stages I–II), and high risk (stages III–IV) (see Table 108-2). The Binet system designates stage A as fewer than three node-bearing areas (median survival, >10 years); stage B, three or more node-bearing areas (5 years); and stage C, anemia or thrombocytopenia (2 years) (Table

TABLE 108-1

Immunophenotypic Differentiation of CLL from Other Chronic B-Lymphoid Disorders

ANTIGEN/MARKER	CLL	MCL	MZL	B-PLL
sIg intensity	Weak	Strong	Strong	Strong
CD19/CD20	+	+	+	+
CD5	+	+	V	–
CD23	+	–	V	V
CD11c	V	–	V	–
CD79b	–	+	V	+
CD22	–	V	+	–

CLL, chronic lymphocytic leukemia; MCL, mantle cell lymphoma; MZL, marginal zone lymphoma; sIg, surface immunoglobulin; V, variably expressed.

TABLE 108-2

Rai System for CLL

STAGE	SIMPLIFIED 3-STAGE SYSTEM	CLINICAL FEATURES	MEDIAN SURVIVAL (YR)
0	Low risk	Lymphocytosis in blood and marrow only	>10
I	Intermediate risk	Lymphocytosis + lymphadenopathy	7
II		Splenomegaly ± hepatomegaly	
III	High risk	Lymphocytosis + anemia	1.5–4
		Thrombocytopenia	

CLL, chronic lymphocytic leukemia.
From Rai et al: Clinical staging of chronic lymphocytic leukemia. Blood 1975;46:219–234.

TABLE 108-3

	Binet System for Staging CLL	
GROUP	**CLINICAL FEATURES**	**MEDIAN SURVIVAL (YR)**
A	<3 areas of lymphadenopathy; no anemia or thrombocytopenia	12
B	≥3 involved node areas; no anemia or thrombocytopenia	7
C	Hemoglobin <10 g/dL and/or platelets <100,000/μL	2–4

CLL, chronic lymphocytic leukemia.

108-3).[48] The Rai classification is most commonly used in the United States, and the Binet system is most often applied in Europe. A major difference between the two is that the Binet system does not identify Rai stage 0 patients. Binet stage A patients include all Rai 0, two thirds of Rai I, and one third of Rai II. Nevertheless, the two systems have similar prognostic value and have been validated by other groups of investigators.

Approximately 10% to 15% of patients with CLL are younger than 50 years, and 20% are younger than 55 years.[49-51] Although younger patients with stage 0 disease may survive as long as an age-matched population, those with more advanced stages have a median survival of only 6 to 7 years. Younger patients are more likely to die of CLL-related events, whereas older patients more often die of secondary malignancies and non-CLL causes.[51]

Variability within stage has led to a continued search for new disease- and patient-related prognostic factors to separate patients into clinically meaningful risk groups. Recent studies suggest that two distinct types of CLL may exist: those with unmutated heavy-chain genes and expression of CD38 who have a poor outcome, irrespective of clinical stage, and those with mutated genes and CD38⁻ who have a more indolent clinical course.[38,52]

Whether CD38 and gene mutational status are independent factors is controversial.[53] Favorable cytogenetic abnormalities tend to occur in patients with mutated immunoglobulin genes and those who are CD38⁻, whereas unfavorable abnormalities occur with unmutated genes and CD38 positivity (Fig. 108-1).[41,53]

Other potential prognostic factors include sex, race, performance status, cellular morphology, pattern of bone marrow infiltration, lymphocyte doubling time,[37,38,54] serum β_2-microglobulin,[55] soluble CD23,[56,57] and plasma tumor necrosis factor-α (TNF-α).[58]

Clinical Features

Clinical Presentation

Patients with CLL are usually asymptomatic at presentation, and the diagnosis is often made incidentally when lymphocytosis is noted on routine evaluation. Findings on physical examination are normal in 20% to 30% of patients, with lymphadenopathy or hepatosplenomegaly found in an additional 40% to 50% of patients. However, as the disease progresses, generalized lymphadenopathy and splenomegaly are common features of this disease. Involvement of other organs is unusual and should suggest the possibility of Richter's transformation (see later).

Infections

Hypogammaglobulinemia is a common occurrence in CLL, especially in patients with advanced disease. The increased susceptibility to infections reflects an inability to produce specific antibodies and abnormal activation of the complement system.[59] Historically, the most common pathogens were those that require opsonization for bacterial killing, such as *Streptococcus pneumoniae, Staphylococcus aureus,* and *Haemophilus influenzae.* The increased use of immunosuppressive agents such as fludarabine, 2-chlorodeoxyadenosine (2-CdA), 2′-deoxycoformycin (DCF; pentostatin), and alemtuzumab has markedly increased the number of infections with opportunistic organisms, such as *Candida, Listeria, Pneumo-*

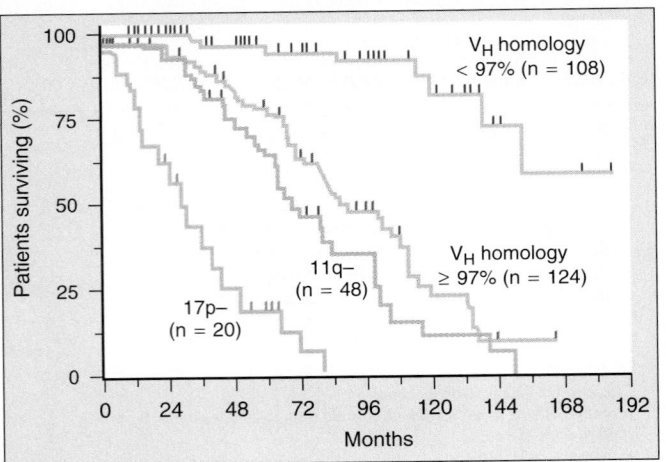

Figure 108-1. Cytogenetics and immunoglobulin V gene mutations are strong, independent predictors of outcome in patients with chronic lymphocytic leukemia. (From Kröber A, Seiler T, Brenner A, et al: V_H mutation status, CD38 expression level, genomic aberrations, and survival in chronic lymphocytic leukemia. Blood 2002;100:1410–1416.)

cystis carinii, cytomegalovirus, *Aspergillus*, herpes infections, and others that were rarely encountered before the widespread use of these agents.[60-62] A febrile patient receiving a nucleoside analog or alemtuzumab can no longer be assumed to have a common bacterial pathogen, and aggressive diagnostic measures may be required.

High-dose intravenous immunoglobulins reduce the total number of trivial to moderately severe bacterial infections, with no decrease in major infections, viral or fungal infections, the number of patients having an infection, or overall survival.[63] The prophylactic use of intravenous immunoglobulins is not cost-effective[64] and should be reserved for select patients with documented, repeated bacterial infections.[65] Myeloid growth factors do not clearly protect against chemotherapy-induced myelosuppression.[66,67]

Aggressive Transformation

In between 3% and 15% of patients, CLL evolves into a more aggressive lymphoid malignancy. The most common of these is Richter's syndrome, which was initially described in 1928 by Maurice Richter, who reported a 46-year-old man with CLL who had rapid clinical deterioration characterized by lymphocytosis, massive and diffuse adenopathy, hepatosplenomegaly, and abdominal discomfort.[68] At autopsy, large abdominal and retroperitoneal lymph nodes were infiltrated not only by small lymphocytes, but also with larger lymphoma cells. Patients with Richter's transformation characteristically have increasing lymphadenopathy, hepatosplenomegaly, fever, abdominal pain, weight loss, progressive anemia, and thrombocytopenia, with a rapid increase in the peripheral blood lymphocyte count, and an increased serum lactate dehydrogenase (LDH). Lymph node biopsy shows large cell lymphoma. This transformation is not clearly related to either the nature or extent of previous therapy. The large cell lymphoma shares immunologic, cytogenetic, and molecular features with the original CLL clone in half of patients.[69,70] Recent studies implicated a moderate to strong expression of p21[WAF1] and loss of p27 expression, with cyclin D1 overexpression.[71] Response of patients with Richter's syndrome to systemic therapy is poor, with a median survival of 4 to 5 months by using alkylating agents, but may be longer with nucleoside analog–based regimens.[72,73]

CLL also may evolve into PLL, associated with progressive anemia, thrombocytopenia, with at least 55% prolymphocytes in the peripheral blood.[44] Clinical features include lymphadenopathy, hepatosplenomegaly, wasting syndrome, and increasing resistance to therapy.

Anecdotal reports have been published of a transformation to acute lymphoblastic leukemia, plasma cell leukemia, multiple myeloma, or Hodgkin's disease.[44,74,75]

Autoimmunity

A positive Coombs' antiglobulin test may be present in 20% to 30% of cases of CLL, with clinical hemolysis in 10% to 25% of patients.[76,77] The frequency of immune thrombocytopenia appears to be approximately 2%.[76,77] The immune hemolysis is more often related to a warm-reactive than to a cold-reactive antibody. In most cases, these antibodies are polyclonal and therefore not produced by the malignant B cells.[13,78] This phenomenon probably reflects impaired interactions among malignant B cells, normal B cells, and T cells.[13] However, two VH genes are preferentially expressed in cells from CLL patients with warm-reacting antibodies; 51pl/DP-10 gene and a DP-50 gene.[79,80] Thus whereas the antibodies that are produced by the CLL are not involved in the red cell destruction, they may still be involved in the pathogenesis of the autoimmune hemolytic anemia (AIHA).

Autoimmune anemia or thrombocytopenia usually responds to corticosteroids such as prednisone, 60 to 100 mg daily, which may be tapered after a week or two after evidence of response. Patients who are unresponsive to corticosteroids may respond to high-dose intravenous immunoglobulins (IVIGs), with an initial loading dose daily for 5 days followed by 0.4 g/kg every 3 weeks. Impressive results have been seen after therapy with rituximab.[81,82] Splenectomy may be considered when systemic approaches fail.[83] Splenic irradiation induces only transient responses.

Pure Red Cell Aplasia

Pure red cell aplasia is relatively uncommon in CLL. This complication is characterized by severe anemia without a reticulocyte response or bone marrow normoblasts and in the absence of neutropenia or thrombocytopenia. Corticosteroids may induce transient responses. Chemotherapy increases the hematocrit in most patients with a response of the CLL. Cyclosporine (Cyclosporin A), with or without concurrent corticosteroids, also may achieve responses, often within 2 to 3 weeks, and may itself induce a reduction in tumor mass.[84] Anecdotal reports suggest activity for rituximab.[85]

Second Malignancies

Secondary malignancies occur with increased frequency in patients with CLL, related both to the immune defects of this disease and to the consequences of therapy.[86,87] The most frequent tumors are skin cancer, lung cancers, and melanomas; others include Hodgkin's disease, essential thrombocythemia, multiple myeloma, and acute myeloid leukemia.

Therapy

The approach to patients with CLL is determined by the stage of disease. A small proportion of patients with low-risk disease are classified as having "smoldering CLL" on the basis of a hemoglobin of 13 g/dL or greater, lymphocyte count less than 30,000/mm³, platelet count greater than 150,000/mm³, and a nondiffuse pattern of bone marrow involvement with fewer than 80% bone marrow lymphocytes.[88,89] These patients are unlikely to have disease progression and may live a normal life span without requiring therapy.

However, the outlook for patients with advanced-stage CLL has improved only modestly over the last few years as a result of earlier diagnosis and improved supportive care

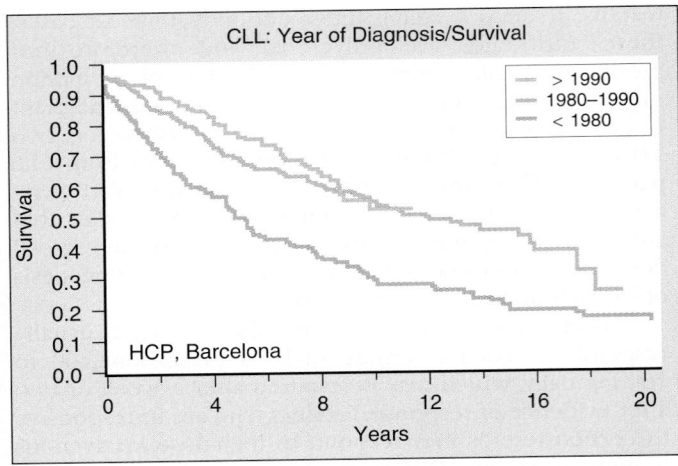

Figure 108-2. Apparent improvement in the outcome of patients with chronic lymphocytic leukemia over a series of decades reflects earlier diagnosis and better supportive care. The role of newer treatments is less clear.

(Fig. 108-2). Nevertheless, no plateau is seen in the survival curve, showing that currently available therapies are not curative. Therefore the decision as to the optimal time to initiate therapy is important. The French Cooperative Group on CLL conducted two studies in patients with Binet stage A disease; in the first, patients were randomized to receive either daily oral chlorambucil or observation.[90] In the second trial, patients received either intermittent chlorambucil plus prednisone or no initial treatment. Neither study detected an advantage in the time to progression (TTP) or survival from early initiation of treatment. Indeed, in the first trial, a survival advantage was found for delayed intervention. One con-

tributing factor was a greater number of fatal, secondary solid tumors, which was not noted in the second study.[90] Other series and a meta-analysis of international studies also did not support early intervention.[91,92]

Therefore therapy for patients with early-stage CLL should not be initiated without specific indications, including disease-related symptoms (e.g., fevers, chills, weight loss, pronounced fatigue), increasing bone marrow failure with anemia or thrombocytopenia, autoimmune anemia or thrombocytopenia, massive or progressive hepatosplenomegaly or lymphadenopathy, or recurrent infections. A rapid lymphocyte-doubling time (<6 months) may support the decision to treat.[43]

Chemotherapy agents active against CLL include the alkylating agents chlorambucil and cyclophosphamide, the nucleoside analogs fludarabine, 2CdA, and the adenosine deaminase inhibitor 2′-deoxycoformycin (pentostatin; DCF).[93-98] Corticosteroids are most useful in the treatment of autoimmune complications.

Initial Therapy

Fludarabine. Fludarabine (2-fluoro-ara-AMP) is the most active chemotherapy agent for the treatment of CLL and has replaced chlorambucil as the initial drug of choice for most patients. The response rate to fludarabine as initial treatment is 70%, including 30% complete remissions (CRs).[99-102] Fludarabine has been successfully compared with an alkylating agent–based regimen in several phase III trials.[99,101,102]

The Cancer and Leukemia Group B (CALGB), Southwest Oncology Group (SWOG), Eastern Cooperative Oncology Group (ECOG), and National Cancer Institute of Canada Clinical Trials Group (NCIC-CTG) collaborated to randomize 544 untreated patients with advanced-stage,

MANAGEMENT APPROACH

Patients with CLL usually require therapy in the presence of disease-related symptoms (e.g., fevers, chills, night sweats, weight loss), massive or progressive hepatosplenomegaly or lymphadenopathy, recurrent infections, impaired bone marrow function, and rapid doubling of the peripheral blood lymphocyte count. Fludarabine has become the standard initial therapy for most patients with CLL at a dose of 25 mg/m² daily for 5 days, generally for six monthly cycles. Alternatives being explored include the combination of fludarabine plus either cyclophosphamide or rituximab, and the three agents together. Because fludarabine is associated with modest myelosuppression and profound immunosuppression, the diagnosis of a fever should be pursued aggressively. Hematopoietic growth factors are not routinely administered because of a lack of demonstrated efficacy in patients with CLL. A bone marrow examination is performed before therapy and 1 to 2 months after the completion of therapy in patients whose peripheral blood counts and findings on physical examination have

normalized. Additional fludarabine is not usually administered if residual disease is present because CLL is an incurable disorder and the potential risks outweigh the benefits.

In patients whose disease is resistant to therapy or who have a relapse after initial therapy, subsequent treatment is guided by the nature of and response to initial treatment. For those who received an alkylating agent, fludarabine is the treatment of choice. Those who received initial treatment with fludarabine may be re-treated with the same drug if the duration of response was 1 year or longer. Other options include fludarabine, 30 mg/m² daily for 3 days, plus cyclophosphamide, 300 mg/m² daily for 3 days, or alemtuzumab for those without bulky disease. Autologous stem cell transplantation is not clearly effective in this setting. Allogeneic stem cell transplantation is associated with significant mortality and should be reserved for younger patients with refractory disease. Submyeloablative transplants are still investigational. Whenever possible, patients should be entered into clinical research studies.

active disease to either fludarabine (25 mg/m^2 daily for 5 days), chlorambucil (40 mg/m^2 as a single dose), or a combination of the two agents (fludarabine, 20 mg/m^2 daily for 5 days; chlorambucil, 20 mg/m^2 on day 1) every 4 weeks for up to 12 months.[102] Patients who were treated unsuccessfully with one agent were crossed over to receive the alternate drug. The overall response rate with fludarabine was 64% including 20% CRs, which was significantly higher than the results with chlorambucil (39% responses, 5% CRs; $P < .0001$). The duration of response was 28 months with fludarabine versus 19 months with chlorambucil, with a median progression-free survival of 20 months and 14 months for chlorambucil ($P < .0001$), respectively. No apparent prolongation of survival was seen, related in part to the crossover design of the study. The combination arm was terminated during the conduct of the trial because it was more toxic with no statistical probability of providing better results than fludarabine alone.

The French Cooperative Group on CLL and international collaborators randomized 196 with stage A (2), stage B (104) or C (89) to either fludarabine or one of two anthracycline-based regimens [CAP or cyclophosphamide, hydroxydaunomycin, vincristine (Oncovin), and prednisone (CHOP)].[99] A higher response rate was attained with fludarabine in both treated and untreated patients, although the difference was significant only in the pre-treated patients. Although the remission duration and survival in pretreated patients were longer with fludarabine, the differences were not significant. In the untreated patients, the advantage for fludarabine was significant for remission duration, with a trend toward a survival advantage ($P = .087$). In a subsequent trial by the IWCLL that included 651 patients with stage B disease and 287 patients with stage C disease,[101] a complete hematologic remission was observed in 40% of the fludarabine group, 30% of the CHOP group, and 15% of the cyclophosphamide, doxorubicin (Adriamycin), and prednisone (CAP)-treated patients. The differences were significant between fludarabine and CAP and between CHOP and CAP ($P < .0001$) in response and survival, but not between fludarabine and CHOP. Fludarabine was favored because it was the best tolerated.

For elderly patients who have a reduced performance status or who have an active infection, alternative approaches include chlorambucil or a 3-day schedule of fludarabine that appears to be almost as active, but with fewer toxicities.[103]

The major toxicities associated with fludarabine are moderate myelosuppression and severe immunosuppression, with occasional neurotoxicity, particularly at higher-than-recommended doses, and rare cases of cortical blindness.[60,104,105] Lymphocyte counts decrease within weeks, particularly CD4 cells, which do not return to normal for 1 year or longer after treatment is discontinued.[60,106] Fludarabine has not been found to be more myelotoxic but has been associated with more opportunistic infections than have alkylating agent regimens.[99,102,107]

The use of prophylactic antimicrobial therapy is not justified in most patients treated with fludarabine unless they are considered to be at a higher risk for infection, have advanced-stage disease, extensive previous therapy, concurrent steroids, or a history of infections.[60,61]

Tumor lysis syndrome is uncommon in CLL patients treated with alkylating agents and occurs in fewer than 0.4% of CLL patients treated with fludarabine.[108] Nevertheless, this complication is often fatal and is not consistently preventable with the use of prophylactic allopurinol or hydration.[108] Fludarabine may be associated with autoimmune hemolytic anemia and thrombocytopenia.[82,109,110] Whether the drug can be continued in these patients is controversial.

Despite the profound immunosuppression, secondary malignancies do not appear to be increased with single-agent fludarabine compared with what is expected in patients with CLL not treated with fludarabine.[87,111]

The currently recommended schedule of administration of fludarabine is as an intravenous bolus of 25 mg/m^2 daily for 5 consecutive days once a month. Patients who do not respond to two to three courses should be offered an alternate treatment. For patients with a partial remission (PR), therapy is generally continued to best response plus two additional courses, not exceeding 1 year of therapy, because of concerns about cumulative myelotoxicity. The oral bioavailability of fludarabine is approximately 50%, and an oral formulation is available outside of the United States.[112,113]

2-Chlorodeoxyadenosine (Cladribine). 2-Chlorodeoxyadenosine (CdA) has been most often administered as a continuous infusion over a 5- to 7–day period (0.1 mg/kg daily), although similar results can be achieved with a 2-hour bolus daily for 5 to 7 days[95,114,115] or with subcutaneous administration. The oral bioavailability of CdA is 40% to 50%, and reports suggest that this route of administration has activity comparable to that of intravenous or subcutaneous delivery.[116,117]

Variation in schedules and routes of administration, small numbers of patients, and different response criteria make the response data difficult to evaluate.[95,114,115,118–121] Approximately 55% to 85% of patients achieve a CR with CdA as up-front therapy, but with only 10% to 15% CRs and with a duration of response that appears to be shorter than that achievable with fludarabine.

Unlike the treatment of hairy cell leukemia, in which a single course of CdA may be sufficient,[122] repeated courses of this agent are required in CLL. Major toxicities include myelosuppression with neutropenic fevers, and immunosuppression, with neurotoxicity at higher doses.[123,124] As with fludarabine, no apparent increase is noted in secondary solid tumors or hematologic malignancies.[87]

2′-Deoxycoformycin (Pentostatin). DCF achieves responses in 25% to 30% of previously treated or untreated patients with CLL, although few of these responses are complete or durable.[96,125–130]

The currently recommended schedule of administration of DCF is 4 mg/m^2 IV every other week for 4 to 5 months. Toxicities include myelosuppression, immunosuppression, nausea, vomiting, fever, rash, renal toxicity, and neurotoxicity, but without an apparent increase in secondary tumors.[87,129-134]

Alkylating Agents. Administration of oral chlorambucil, either at a dose of 4 to 8 mg/m^2 daily for 4 to 8 weeks or as pulses of 15 to 30 mg/m^2 every 2 to 4 weeks, achieves responses in approximately 30% to 70% of previously untreated patients, although few of these responses are complete.[135,136]

Combination Chemotherapy. Combinations of alkylating-based regimens are not clearly superior to single-agent therapy for CLL.[99,135,137-144] The most commonly used multiple-agent regimens include chlorambucil plus prednisone (CP) or CVP (cyclophosphamide, vincristine, prednisone). CP and CVP induce responses in fewer than 10% to more than 60% of previously untreated patients, although few of these are complete, and the median survival is shorter than 2 years.[135,137-139] The French Cooperative Group randomized 151 patients with Binet stage B CLL to indefinite daily oral chlorambucil and 140 to COP. No difference was found in response rate, reduction in clinical stage, or overall survival.[145]

Regimens that include anthracyclines also did not show an advantage.[144] One small randomized trial suggested a survival advantage for an attenuated CHOP regimen (including doxorubicin at 25 mg/m^2 every 4 weeks) over COP in a small number of patients with stage C disease.[140] Moreover, data from the same investigators suggest an advantage for CHOP over CAP (cyclophosphamide, doxorubicin, prednisone).[101] However, several other randomized trials and a meta-analysis did not confirm the superiority of anthracycline-containing regimens.[135,139,141,144]

Combinations of fludarabine with a variety of other agents did not show superiority over fludarabine alone.[136,146-148] The addition of prednisone to fludarabine does not increase the response rate but is associated with more frequent opportunistic infections.[61,106] Preliminary data with various combinations of fludarabine and cyclophosphamide[149,150] suggest that overall response and complete response rates do not appear to be better than those with fludarabine alone. However, comparisons with historical controls suggest a possible advantage in survival. Two phase III trials conducted by ECOG and CALGB and by the German CLL Study Group are comparing fludarabine with the combination of fludarabine and cyclophosphamide. DCF has been combined with alkylating agents and steroids with high response rates but considerable toxicity.[151]

Treatment of Relapsed or Refractory Disease

As with initial treatment, patients with CLL should not be treated unless therapy is indicated.[43] The most appropriate treatment for patients with CLL who have a relapse after initial treatment or are refractory to initial treatment is referral to a clinical research study. For patients who are not eligible for or are unwilling to participate in clinical research, salvage therapy is determined by the choice of and response to initial treatment.

Re-treatment with an alkylating agent is associated with a lower response rate with shorter responses. The median survival after salvage chemotherapy is only 14 to 15 months.

Purine Analogs. Fludarabine is the standard agent for patients who have a relapse after treatment with an alkylating agent–based regimen.[97,106,152,153] With the NCI-Working Group response guidelines,[43] complete clinical and hematologic remissions are achieved in 3% to 13% of patients, with an overall response rate of 40% to 50%. Results vary with patient age, stage, performance status, and other factors. The median TTP is about 18 months for patients whose disease was refractory to alkylating agents, and 17 months for patients who had a relapse after a previous response; the median survival is 29 months for the relapsed patients and 9 months for the refractory patients. The lower response rates and durability of response in some series reflect the advanced stage, extensive prior therapy, and poor performance status of the treated patients.[97,154]

Retreatment with fludarabine is successful in half of patients whose initial response to fludarabine lasted 1 year or longer.[100,155] Other than alemtuzumab (see following discussion), few effective therapeutic options are available to patients whose disease is refractory to fludarabine.[136,155] The fludarabine and cyclophosphamide combination has shown promise in patients whose disease was not refractory to fludarabine.[156] CdA is also active in alkylating-agent failures, but cross-resistance occurs with fludarabine.[95,157]

Biologic Therapy

A number of monoclonal antibodies have become widely used in the treatment of CLL.

Alemtuzumab. Alemtuzumab (Campath-1H) is a humanized anti-CD52 monoclonal antibody that has been approved by the Food and Drug Administration (FDA) for the treatment of fludarabine-refractory CLL (Tables 108-4 and 108-5). CD52 is expressed on virtually all lymphocytes at various stages of differentiation, as well as on monocytes, macrophages, and eosinophils,[158] although the function of this antigen is unknown. The only other site of expression is the male reproductive tract. Hematopoietic stem cells, erythrocytes, and platelets do not express this antigen.

Alemtuzumab is generally administered at a dose of 3 mg on day 1, 10 mg on day 2, and 30 mg 3 times per week as soon as the infusion-related reactions are tolerable. Treatment is generally administered for at least 4 weeks and for as long as 12 weeks, although some studies suggested additional benefit by extending therapy to 18 weeks.[159] Antimicrobial prophylaxis should include trimethoprim-sulfamethoxazole and acyclovir. The activity of alemtuzumab is shown in Table 108-5.

The pivotal trial included 93 patients treated at 21 centers in the United States and Europe for whom previous therapy with fludarabine had failed and who had also received alkylating agents[62,160-167] (see Table 108-5).

TABLE 108-4

Monoclonal Antibodies for CLL

ANTIBODY	ANTIGEN	CONJUGATE
Alemtuzumab (Campath-1H)	CD52	None
Rituximab (C2B8, Rituxan, MabThera)	CD20	None
Epratuzumab (Lymphocide)	CD22	None
Hu-1D10 (Aplizumab)	HLA-DR	None
IDEC-152	CD23	None
IDEC-114	CD80	None
Bevacizumab (Avastin)	VEG-F	None

The median age was 66 years, and 76% had Rai stage II or IV disease. Nearly half of the patients had never responded to any nucleoside analog. Seventy percent completed the planned 12 weeks of treatment. The response rate was 33%, including 2% CR. An additional 6 patients had clearing of CLL from all sites but had persistent anemia or thrombocytopenia that improved on long-term follow-up. The median duration of response was 8.7 months. The median survival was 16 months, with 32 months in responders. Causes of death included progressive disease in 37, with 2 due to AIHA or ITP (immune mediated thrombocytopenia).

Death was due to or complicated by infection in 17 patients. Cytomegalovirus (CMV) reactivation was documented in 7 patients.

Because of the severity of infusion-related reactions, alternate modes of delivery have been explored. Lundin and colleagues[159] reported 41 patients with previously untreated CLL who received alemtuzumab by the subcutaneous route. The overall response rate was 87%, including 19% CRs. Local reactions were impressive, but generally disappeared within 2 weeks, despite continued therapy. Of note was that infusion-related reactions generally were relatively mild.

The combination or sequence of fludarabine and alemtuzumab also is being studied.[167,168]

Toxicity. Toxicities associated with alemtuzumab can be either immediate and related to the infusions or delayed

TABLE 108-5

Alemtuzumab in CLL

INVESTIGATOR	NO. OF PATIENTS	PRIOR THERAPY	CR (%)	RR (%)
Österborg et al.[160]	29	+	4	42
Bowen et al.[161]	6	+	50	50
Rawstron et al.[162]	17	+	50	70
Stilgenbauer et al.[163]	11	+	18	55
McCune et al.[164]	13	+	31	46
Keating et al.[62]	92	+	2	33
Rai et al.[165]	152	+	5	43
Österborg et al.[166]	11	−	33	89
Lundin et al.[159]	41	−	19	87

CLL, chronic lymphocytic leukemia; CR, complete response; RR, relative risk.

TABLE 108-6

Rituximab in CLL/SLL

INVESTIGATOR	NO. OF PATIENTS	PRIOR TX	CR (%)	RR (%)
Maloney[170]	3	Yes	0	0
McLaughlin[169]	33	Yes	0	13
Nguyen[171]	15	Yes	0	7
Piro[172]*	7	Yes	0	14
Winkler[173]	9	Yes	0	11
Foran[174]	29	Yes	0	14
Huhn[175]	28	Yes	0	25
Byrd[176]†	33	Yes/No	3	45
O'Brien[177]‡	40	Yes	0	36
Hainsworth[178]	15	No	NA	57
Thomas[179]	21	No	90	19

CLL, chronic lymphocytic leukemia; CR, complete response; NA, not available; RR, relative risk; SLL, small lymphocytic lymphoma; Tx, treatment.
*Eight infusions.
†3 times weekly.
‡Phase I dose escalation.

because of the myelosuppression and immunosuppression. In the pivotal trial,[62] the most frequent adverse events were infusion related, including rigors in 90% of patients, grade III in only 14%, fever in 85% (17%, grade III; 3%, grade IV). Nausea occurred in 53%, all grade I or II, vomiting in 38% (1% grade III), and rash in a third, all mild to moderate. These events decreased over the duration of treatment.

Rituximab. Rituximab is a chimeric monoclonal antibody directed against the CD20 antigen on B cells (Tables 108-4 and 108-6). Possible mechanisms of action include antibody-dependent cellular cytotoxicity, complement-mediated toxicity, and induction of apoptosis. Rituximab has been rapidly adopted for a wide range of B-cell malignancies because of its activity, its non–cross-resistance with chemotherapy, and its minimal side effects. It was approved by regulatory agencies because of its activity in relapsed and refractory follicular, low-grade NHL.[169] Response rates in this study were higher in follicular histologies than in small lymphocytic lymphoma (SLL). Single-agent activity for rituximab has been disappointing in relapsed and refractory SLL/CLL (see Table 108-6).[169-179] Potential explanations include the low density of CD20 expression on malignant cells in these patients and a shorter half-life in patients with high white blood cell counts.

A higher response rate is reported when rituximab is used as the initial treatment of patients with SLL or CLL.[179-181] Hainsworth and colleagues[181] included 15 patients with SLL among their 41 patients and reported that the response rate of 57% was comparable to those patients with a follicular histology (52%). In a subsequent study by the same investigators, 70 previously untreated patients with advanced CLL were treated with single-agent rituximab.[180] Patients who achieved a response by the sixth week received an additional 4 weeks of antibody therapy every 6 months. The 44% who responded by 6 weeks included 9% CR, but no additional benefit was derived from the maintenance therapy. Thomas and associates[179] reported an overall response rate of 90% with 19% CRs in 21 patients.

More intensive doses and schedules of administration have been explored in an attempt at improving the response rate with rituximab in CLL. Byrd and coworkers[176] used a thrice-weekly schedule in 33 treated and previously untreated patients. Thirteen patients had transient hypoxemia, hypotension, or dyspnea associated with changes in interleukin-6 (IL-6), IL-8, TNF, and IFN-γ. The overall response rate was 45%, including 3% CRs. One patient died on day 3 of a pulmonary hemorrhage, one of a septic arthritis during week 2, and one a month later of sepsis and a gastrointestinal bleed; another had ITP and required alternative therapy. The overall median duration of response was 10 months, but only 6 months in fludarabine failures. The median TTP was only 6 months. Higher response rates were obtained in the six previously untreated patients and in those who had relapsed after fludarabine compared with those with refractory disease.

O'Brien and colleagues[177] conducted a phase I trial in which the dose of rituximab was escalated to 2250 mg/m^2. The dose-limiting toxicity had not been reached; however, the expense of such an approach could not be justified by the expense, given that the only responses noted were a few partial remissions with a TTP of 8 months.

The CALGB[182] conducted a randomized phase II trial of concurrent versus sequential fludarabine and rituximab with 51 and 53 patients per arm, respectively. This approach was based on observations suggesting that antibodies might sensitize the tumor cells to the effects of subsequent administration of chemotherapy.[183-187] The overall response rate in the concurrent arm was 90% including 43% CRs, and, in the sequential arm, 77% with 28% CRs. The median disease-free and overall survival have yet to be reached, although with relatively short follow-up. Of note was that grade III and IV neutropenia were more common in the concurrent arm (37% vs. 18%). Opportunistic infections were diagnosed in 8 patients in the concurrent arm and 14 on the sequential arm. A similar regimen was reported by Schulz and associates,[188] with comparable findings.

Rituximab also has been combined with fludarabine and cyclophosphamide[189,190] to treat 79 patients, only 39% of whom had advanced-stage disease (Rai III, IV). There were 66% CRs, 14% nodular PRs, and 15% PRs. Grade IV neutropenia was seen in 20% of cycles, with grade III or IV thrombocytopenia in 4%. Only 3% of cycles were associated with a major infection. This regimen also has been used in previously treated patients with greater toxicity and limited activity in fludarabine-refractory disease.[191]

Rituximab also has been used successfully to treat the complications of CLL or its therapy, including pure red cell aplasia[85] and fludarabine-induced immune thrombocytopenia.[82]

The combination of rituximab plus alemtuzumab has been studied by several groups, although in vitro synergy data are lacking.[192,193] Faderl and coworkers[193] presented their results with this combination in a variety of relapsed and refractory chronic lymphoid malignancies, primarily CLL. Of the 47 patients eligible for response, the median number of previous regimens was four, and 79% had advanced-stage disease. Actual response rates are difficult to extract from the abstract; however, 90% of patients experienced a peripheral blood CR. Unfortunately, rates were lower in other sites. More than half (14 of 26) patients had an infection.

Toxicity. Rituximab has a favorable safety profile. Nevertheless, more than 90% of patients experience a generally mild to moderate infusion-related reaction. However, patients with CLL and high lymphocyte counts may be at an increased risk of more serious complications, including a rapid-tumor-clearance syndrome,[173,194] beginning within 30 to 60 minutes of the initial infusion, characterized clinically by fevers, rigors, dyspnea, hypoxia, and hypotension, and may progress despite interruption of the infusion. Thrombocytopenia has been common with abnormal coagulation studies in several cases. The rapid-tumor-clearance syndrome differs from typical "tumor lysis syndrome" in that, in the former, the abnormalities of potassium, calcium, and phosphorus tend to be milder, and renal insufficiency is usually not so severe.[108,173,194] Management of this complication includes interruption of the antibody infusion, hydration, allopurinol, oxygen, and bronchodilators. None of the patients who received subsequent infusions of the antibody had a recurrence of this adverse event. Patients with high white blood cell counts should be considered for prophylactic hydration, allopurinol, and in some cases, alkalinization of the urine.

Other Antibodies

Anti-CD23. IDEC-152 is a primatized anti-CD23 monoclonal antibody that inhibits IgE secretion in vitro and induces apoptosis of lymphoma cell lines.[195] It binds complement and mediates antibody-dependent, cell-mediated cytotoxicity (ADCC) by binding FcγRI and RII. In vitro data suggest a favorable interaction with rituximab.[195] Phase I and II clinical trials are under way.

Apolizumab. Apolizumab (Hu1D10) is a monoclonal antibody directed against a polymorphic determinant of HLA-DR present on both normal B cells and on malignant B cells from approximately half of patients with lymphoid malignancies. This antibody has been evaluated in patients with relapsed or refractory indolent NHL,[196,197] with activity noted in the phase I trial, but with disappointing results in the phase II study. Toxicities have included infusional and allergic reactions as well as hemolytic uremic syndrome.[198] Six of 14 evaluable patients responded, including 4 who were rituximab naïve; one of two CLL patients treated achieved a CR. However, accrual was suspended because of treatment-related complications.

Immunotoxins. Denileukin diftitox (Ontak) is an anti-CD25 diphtheria–IL-2 fusion protein approved for the treatment of cutaneous T-cell lymphoma. This immunotoxin induces partial remissions in fludarabine-refractory CLL disease.[199-201]

Radioimmunotherapy

The use of radioimmunotherapy (RIT) for the treatment of CLL has been limited by the frequent extensive bone marrow involvement. Lym-1 is a radioimmunoconjugate consisting of an ^{131}I-labeled mouse IgGκ. The antibody recognizes a 31- to 35-kd antigen, presumed to be a polymorphic variant of the HLA-DR antigen, and thought to be specific for B cells, with a particular avidity for malignant B cells.[202-206] Although responses were reported in patients with NHL and CLL, the failure to use standardized criteria for response made the data difficult to interpret. The future of this antibody is unclear.

Kaminski and colleagues[207] reported 14 patients with SLL and a median of four prior regimens. Responses occurred in 64% of patients, including 21% complete remissions. The median duration of response was 24.7+ months. Because RIT with either yttrium-90 ibritumomab tiuxetan (Zevalin) or ^{131}I-labeled tositumomab is restricted to patients with less than 25% bone marrow involvement by lymphoma, strategies are needed to reduce bone marrow involvement before RIT for patients with CLL.

Interferon-alfa

Interferon-alfa (IFN) achieves a few brief partial responses[208-212] and is of no benefit as maintenance therapy after chemotherapy.[213,214]

Stem Cell Transplantation

The data on allogeneic BMT are limited in CLL, primarily because the median age at diagnosis is older than 60 years, and it has been difficult to eradicate CLL in the patient. The European Bone Marrow Transplant Group and the International Bone Marrow Transplant Registry published their experience with 54 patients with CLL who received an allogeneic BMT.[215] The median age was 41 years, most patients were of advanced clinical stage, and all but six had received previous therapy. With a variety of preparative regimens, 70% achieved a CR. The projected leukemia-free survival at 3 years was 46%. Unfortunately, the treatment-related death rate is 25% to 50%.[215-218] In general, approximately half of transplanted patients may remain disease free for prolonged periods; however, because of late relapses, it is not clear whether they are cured.

Submyeloablative preparative regimens may achieve successful engraftment without substantial acute graft-versus-host disease (GVHD); however, chronic GVHD has been a serious problem.[219,220] Autologous stem cell transplantation for patients with CLL is still investigational.[216,217,221-224]

Gene Therapy

Genetic approaches to CLL include modification of the B-CLL phenotype to render it capable of stimulating T cells to respond to presented CLL antigens. The interaction of CD40 and its ligand CD40L (or CD154) on activated T cells plays a key role in B-cell activation, survival, and differentiation. CD40 activation of B-CLL cells may reverse the T-cell anergy against the leukemic clone.[225] A preliminary report of a phase I study with three B-CLL

patients showed anorexia, fatigue, malaise, and fever to be the major side effects. Two chemotherapy-naive patients had a greater than 50% decrease in peripheral blood lymphocytosis.[226]

Antisense

G3139 (oblimersen sodium; Genta, Berkeley Heights, NJ) is the first antisense molecule to be widely tested in the clinic. G3139 is a phosphorothioate oligonucleotide consisting of 18 modified DNA bases (i.e., 18-mer) that targets the first six codons of Bcl-2 messenger RNA (mRNA) to form a DNA/RNA duplex.[227] RNAse-H recognizes the DNA/RNA duplex, cleaves the Bcl-2 mRNA strand, and renders the message nontranslatable. Bcl-2 mRNA fragments are subsequently destroyed by ribonucleases. In a summary of the phase I and II data study of 20 patients with CLL,[228] doses of G3139 at 4, 5, or 7 mg/kg daily for 5 to 7 days were poorly tolerated, with fever, hypotension, back pain, and thrombocytopenia. Of the 19 patients evaluable for response, 2 PRs were found. However, reductions in lymphocyte counts occurred in 63%, with a reduction in lymphadenopathy in 35% and hepatosplenomegaly in 33%. Adverse events included fever, hypotension, and transient thrombocytopenia. The maximum tolerated dose (MTD) for cycle 1 in CLL as monotherapy is 3 mg/kg daily, although patients could be safely escalated to 4 mg/kg daily in subsequent cycles. A phase III trial comparing fludarabine plus cyclophosphamide with or without G3139 in patients who underwent previous unsuccessful fludarabine therapy was completed recently and is undergoing analysis. In vitro study of NHL cell lines showing marked synergy between G3139 and rituximab[229] led to clinical trials in CLL and NHL evaluating the combination of these two agents.

Other Therapeutic Measures

Splenectomy. Splenectomy may provide important palliation for patients with CLL who underwent unsuccessful systemic treatment with persistent splenomegaly or who have cytopenia precluding chemotherapy.[83] Thrombocytopenia is the most likely to respond. When performed by an experienced surgeon, the procedure has a mortality of less than 10%.

Leukopheresis. Leukopheresis is associated only with transient reductions in circulating lymphocytes and is not recommended for general practice.

Erythropoietin. Erythropoietin (EPO) may reduce transfusion requirements in approximately two thirds of patients with CLL, and a trial of this agent can be considered in anemic CLL patients with no other obvious correctable cause.[230,231]

Assessment of Response to Therapy

The NCI-WG standardized eligibility, response, and toxicity criteria and provided dose modifications for drug-related myelosuppression and provided a grading system for infectious complications[43] (Table 108-7). These

TABLE 108-7

NCI-WG Response Criteria for CLL

PARAMETER	CR*	PR*
Lymphocytes	≤4000/μL	≥50%↓
Lymph nodes (liver/spleen)	No palpable disease	≥50%↓
Neutrophils improvement	≥1500/μL	≥1500/μL or ≥50%
Platelets improvement	>100,000/μL	>100,000/μL or ≥50%
Hemoglobin improvement	>11.0 g/dL	>11.0 g/dL or ≥50%
Bone marrow	<30% lymphocytes	±Nodules
Symptoms	None	Variable

CLL, chronic lymphocytic leukemia; CR, complete response; NCI-WG, National Cancer Institute Working Group; PR, partial response.
*2 months' duration.

guidelines are currently used worldwide for clinical trials in CLL.

RELATED B-CELL LEUKEMIAS

Prolymphocytic Leukemia

Patients with PLL tend to be older than those with CLL, with a median age of 70 years. At presentation, the main symptoms include abdominal discomfort, fevers, and weight loss. Virtually all have advanced-stage disease at presentation, with a larger spleen and a higher white blood cell count, but less lymphadenopathy than those with CLL. PLL cells are large, with a round nucleus and a prominent nucleolus.[75,232,233] In de novo PLL, most of the peripheral blood mononuclear cells tend to be prolymphocytes; in the setting of an aggressive transformation from CLL, a dimorphic population is found in the peripheral blood. The immunophenotype is different from that of CLL; the cells are positive for CD19, CD20, and CD24, and strongly express CD22, surface immunoglobulins, and FMC7. Fewer than one third express CD5 or CD23. The presence of the t(11;14) in 25% of cases suggests that these may have actually been mantle cell lymphoma.

Patients with PLL tend to respond poorly to either single-agent or combination chemotherapy, with overall response rates of less than 25% and rare CRs. The median survival for de novo PLL is 3 years. Small series and anecdotal cases suggest impressive activity for nucleoside analogs in PLL.[126,234–237]

Hairy Cell Leukemia

HCL occurs in about 500 new patients each year in the United States, usually in older persons, with a strong male predominance. Patients usually have symptoms referable to cytopenias including infections in 29% and weakness or fatigue in 27%; less common presentations include left upper quadrant pain related to splenomegaly (5%) and bleeding related to thrombocytopenia (4%). An increased incidence of second malignancies is noted. The most common signs include palpable splenomegaly (72% to 86%), hepatomegaly (13% to 20%), hairy cells in the peripheral blood (85% to 89%), thrombocytopenia (<100,000/mm³; 53%), anemia (Hgb, <12 g/dL; 71% to 77%), and neutropenia (absolute neutrophil count, <500/mm³; 32% to 39%).

The cells in the peripheral blood generally have an eccentric, spongiform, kidney-shaped nucleus, with characteristic filamentous cytoplasmic projections. Bone marrow biopsy is usually required to make the diagnosis, because the aspirate is often not obtainable. The malignant cells are of B-cell origin, expressing CD19, CD20, as well as the monocyte antigen CD11c. The most specific marker is CD103. It is most difficult to distinguish HCL from hairy cell variant (HCL$_v$); the latter is often associated with a high circulating white blood cell count, cells containing bilobed nuclei with prominent nucleoli, a bone marrow with interstitial infiltration of clumped cells,[238] and resistance to treatment with IFN-alfa, CdA, and pentostatin.[238]

Treatment is indicated in the setting of massive or progressive splenomegaly, worsening blood counts, recurrent infections, more than 20,000 hairy cells/mm³ of peripheral blood, or bulky lymphadenopathy. Until the early 1980s, splenectomy was the standard treatment for HCL. This procedure improves symptoms related to splenomegaly and peripheral blood counts, often for prolonged periods, but it does not affect the disease itself. Splenectomy is now reserved for the rare patient whose disease is refractory to treatment and who has splenomegaly that is either symptomatic or is resulting in cytopenias.

IFN was the first systemic therapy to show activity in HCL. At doses of 2×10^6 U/m² daily or 3×10^6 U, 3 times per week, IFN induces responses in 80% of patients; however, only 10% of these are CRs. Although responses generally occur within 3 to 4 months, it may take more than 1 year of therapy to achieve the maximal effect. The leukemia invariably recurs after IFN therapy is discontinued, and maintenance therapy is associated with excessive toxicity and expense without any apparent survival benefit.

The purine analogs revolutionized the treatment of patients with HCL.[122,239] DCF, at doses of 4 mg/m² IV every other week for 4 to 6 months, achieves CRs in 60% to 89% of previously treated or untreated patients, including those for whom IFN failed, with overall response rates of 80% to 90%. Approximately 25% of patients have relapsed with more than 5 years of follow-up. In an intergroup trial, 350 previously untreated patients with HCL were randomized to IFN or DCF; the CR rate was approximately 11% for IFN compared with 76% for DCF, with a significant advantage to DCF in the durability of response.[134,239] The lack of a survival advantage reflects the high rate of IFN patients salvaged with pentostatin.

CdA also is highly effective for HCL. Using a 7-day infusion or a 2-hour infusion for 5 to 7 days achieves responses in 80% to more than 90% of patients, including 65% to 80% CRs. These responses tend to be durable, with 20% to 30% of patients relapsing with prolonged follow-up. In many cases, relapse is characterized only by an increase in bone marrow hairy cells, with no indication for treatment. Most patients who require re-treatment achieve a second durable response.

The results with DCF are equivalent to those with CdA. The shorter duration of treatment makes CdA somewhat more attractive, although it may be associated with greater toxicity.

An anti-CD22 *Pseudomonas* exotoxin immunoconjugate induces responses in most patients for whom purine analog therapy fails.[240] Rituximab also has shown promise for patients with HCL for whom purine analog therapy fails or for those with HCL$_v$.[241,242]

CHRONIC T-CELL LEUKEMIAS

The chronic T-cell leukemias consist of mycosis fungoides, T-PLL, adult T-cell leukemia/lymphoma (ATLL), and the various subtypes of large granular lymphocytosis (LGL), and natural killer (NK) cell leukemia. T-PLL tends to occur in older persons, with a median age of 63 years. The presenting features include widespread lymphadenopathy in half of patients, splenomegaly in almost 80% of patients, and a lymphocyte count often in excess of 100,000/mm^3. Anemia and thrombocytopenia also are common.[243] T-PLL is associated with recurrent chromosomal abnormalities, notably inversion of chromosome 14, with breakpoints at the long arm at q11 and q32, in 80% of patients. In more than half of cases, abnormalities of chromosome 8 can be identified [i(8q), trisomy 8, t(8;8)(p11;q32), or add(8)(p11)].[244] Treatment is, in general, unsatisfactory. Alemtuzumab has shown impressive activity in T-PLL, with response rates of 50% to 70%.[161,245,246] Keating and associates[247] published a retrospective analysis of 76 patients, including 4 who were chemotherapy naïve.

LGL can be divided into two major subsets, those that are CD3$^+$, representing in vivo activated cytotoxic T cells, and NK-LGL that are CD3$^-$.[248,249] T-LGL tends to occur in older persons, and most patients (60%) are symptomatic at diagnosis. An association with recurrent infections is related in part to chronic neutropenia, as well as anemia, and rheumatoid arthritis with Felty's syndrome. The phenotype includes CD3$^+$, CD8$^+$, and CD57$^+$ with clonal rearrangement of T-cell receptor (TCR) genes. NK-LGL accounts for about 15% of LGL and includes aggressive NK cell leukemia and a more indolent NK lymphocytosis. The cells are CD3$^-$, CD8$^+$, CD16$^+$, CD56$^+$, and CD57$^{+/-}$. Rearrangements of *TCR* genes are absent. In the aggressive form of the disease, patients tend to be younger without rheumatoid arthritis. Infiltration of the gastrointestinal tract and bone marrow are common.[250] Neutropenia is modest in comparison to the severity of anemia and thrombocytopenia. Patients often die of multiple-organ failure with coagulopathy, generally within a few months of diagnosis, despite aggressive chemotherapy. Approximately 5% of LGL is a nonclonal expansion of CD3$^+$ LGL that is usually unaccompanied by lymphadenopathy or hepatosplenomegaly. The features of the cells are CD3$^-$, CD4$^-$, CD8$^-$, CD16^{++} and CD56$^+$. The disease is indolent, rarely requiring intervention unless accompanied by neutropenia. Prednisone and immunosuppressive agents have been used. It is not clear whether this disorder is actually neoplastic.

ATLL is endemic in Japan, the Caribbean, and parts of Central Africa and the southeastern United States. It is linked to the prevalence of human T-cell leukemia virus (HTLV-1). A number of clinical variants range from a chronic, smoldering disorder to an aggressive, leukemic disease.[251,252] Serum calcium and LDH are prognostic for outcome. The major causes of death are infectious. Combination chemotherapy and pentostatin have been attempted, with limited success.[253]

REFERENCES

1. Jemal A, Murray T, Samuels A, et al: Cancer statistics, 2003. CA Cancer J Clin 2003;53:5–26.
2. Bizzozero JOJ, Johnson KG, Ciocco A, et al: Radiation-related leukemia in Hiroshima and Nagasaki 1946–1964. Ann Intern Med 1967;55:522–530.
3. Arp JEW, Wolf PH, Checkoway H: Lymphocytic leukemia and exposure to benzene and other solvents in the rubber industry. J Occup Med 1983;25:598–602.
4. Zahm SH, Weisenburger DD, Babbitt PA, et al: Use of hair coloring products and the risk of lymphoma, multiple myeloma, and chronic lymphocytic leukemia. Am J Public Health 1992;82:990–997.
5. Inskip PD, Kleinerman RA, Stovall M, et al: Leukemia, lymphoma, and multiple myeloma after pelvic radiotherapy for benign disease. Radiat Res 1993;135:108–124.
6. Linet MS, Van Natta MI, Brookmeyer R, et al: Familial cancer history and chronic lymphocytic leukemia. Am J Epidemiol 1989;130:655–664.
7. Blattner WA, Strober W, Muchmore AV, et al: Familial chronic lymphocytic leukemia: Immunologic and cellular characterization. Ann Intern Med 1976;84:554–557.
8. Yuille MR, Marossy A, Hilditch B, et al: Prevalence of familial B-CLL [abstract P034]. Proceedings of the VIII International Workshop on CLL, San Diego, CA. 1999;36.
9. Yuille MR, Matutes E, Marossy A, et al: Familial chronic lymphocytic leukaemia: A survey and review of published studies. Br J Haematol 2000;109:794–799.
10. Summersgill B, Thornton P, Atkinson S, et al: Chromosomal imbalances in familial chronic lymphocytic leukemia: A comparative genomic hybridization analysis. Leukemia 2002;16:1229–1232.
11. Brok-Simoni F, Rechavi G, Katzir N, et al: Chronic lymphocytic leukaemia in twin sisters: Monozygous but not identical. Lancet 1987;1:329–330.
12. Cuttner J: Increased incidence of hematologic malignancies in first-degree relatives of patients with chronic lymphocytic leukemia. Cancer Invest 1992;10:103–109.
13. Caligaris-Cappio F, Hamblin TJ: B-cell chronic lymphocytic leukemia: A bird of a different feather. J Clin Oncol 1999;17:399–408.
14. Plater-Zyberk C, Maini RN, Lam K, et al: A rheumatoid arthritis B cell subset expresses a phenotype similar to that in chronic lymphocytic leukemia. Arthritis Rheum 1985;28:971–976.
15. Mizutani H, Furubayashi T, Kashiwagi H, et al: B cells expressing CD5 antigen are markedly increased in peripheral blood and spleen lymphocytes from patients with immune thrombocytopenic purpura. Br J Haematol 1991;78:474–479.
16. Bird ML, Ueshima Y, Rowley JD, et al: Chromosome abnormalities in B cell chronic lymphocytic leukemia and their clinical correlations. Leukemia 1989;3:182.
17. Oscier D, Fitchett M, Herbert T, et al: Karyotypic evolution in B-cell chronic lymphocytic leukaemia. Genes Chromosomes Cancer 1991;3:16.
18. Juliusson G, Gahrton G: Chromosome abnormalities in B-cell chronic lymphocytic leukemia. In Cheson BD (ed): Chronic Lymphocytic Leukemia: Scientific Advances and Clinical

Developments: Basic and Clinical Oncology. New York, Marcel Dekker, 1993, pp 83–103.

19. Escudier SM, Pereira-Leahy JM, Drach JW, et al: Fluorescent in situ hybridization and cytogenetic studies of trisomy 12 in chronic lymphocytic leukemia. Blood 1993;81:2702–2707.

20. Döhner H, Stilgenbauer S, Benner A, et al: Genomic aberrations and survival in chronic lymphocytic leukemia. N Engl J Med 2000;343:1910–1916.

21. Geisler CH, Philip P, Christensen BE, et al: In B-cell chronic lymphocytic leukaemia chromosome 17 abnormalities and not trisomy 12 are the single most important cytogenetic abnormalities for the prognosis: A cytogenetic and immunophenotypic study of 480 unselected newly diagnosed patients. Leuk Res 1997;21:1011–1023.

22. Cordone I, Masi S, Mauro FR, et al: p53 expression in B-cell chronic lymphocytic leukemia: A marker of disease progression and poor prognosis. Blood 1998;91:4342–4349.

23. Döhner H, Fischer K, Bentz M, et al: p53 gene deletion predicts for poor survival and non-response to therapy with purine analogs in chronic B-cell leukemias. Blood 1995;85:1580–1589.

24. Bea S, Lopez Guillermo A, Ribas M, et al: Genetic imbalances in progressed B-cell chronic lymphocytic leukemia and transformed large-cell lymphoma (Richter's syndrome). Am J Pathol 2002;161:957–968.

25. Stilgenbauer S, Bullinger L, Lichter P, et al: Genetics of chronic lymphocytic leukemia: Genomic aberrations and V_h gene mutation status in pathogenesis and clinical course. Leukemia 2002;16:993–1007.

26. Tsujimoto Y, Yunis JJ, Onorato-Showe L, et al: Molecular cloning of the chromosomal breakpoint of B-cell lymphomas and leukemias with the t(11;14) chromosome translocation. Science 1984;224:1403.

27. Williams ME, Whitefield M, Swerdlow SH: Analysis of the cyclin-dependent kinase inhibitors p18 and p19 in mantle-cell lymphoma and chronic lymphocytic leukemia. Ann Oncol 1997;8:S71–S73.

28. McKeithan TW, Ohno H, Diaz MO: Identification of a transcriptional unit adjacent to the breakpoint in the 14;19 translocation of chronic lymphocytic leukemia. Genes Chromosomes Cancer 1990;1:247.

29. Dyer MJS, Zani VJ, Lu WZ, et al: BCL2 translocations in leukemias of mature B cells. Blood 1994;83:3682–3688.

30. Hanada M, Delia D, Aiello A, et al: bcl-2 gene hypomethylation and high-level expression in B-cell chronic lymphocytic leukemia. Blood 1993;82:1820–1828.

31. Bullrich F, Veronese ML, Kitada S, et al: Minimal region of loss at 13q14 in B-cell chronic lymphocytic leukemia. Blood 1996;88:3109–3115.

32. Kitada S, Andersen J, Akar S, et al: Expression of apoptosis-regulating proteins in chronic lymphocytic leukemia: Correlations with in vitro and in vivo chemoresponses. Blood 1998;91:3379–3389.

33. Kipps TJ: Immunoglobulin genes in chronic lymphocytic leukemia. Blood Cells 1993;19:615–625.

34. Oscier D, Thompsett A, Zhu D, et al: Differential rates of somatic hypermutation in V_h genes among subsets of chronic lymphocytic leukemia defined by chromosome abnormalities. Blood 1997;89:4153–4160.

35. Schaffner C, Stilgenbauer S, Rappold GA, et al: Somatic ATM mutations indicate a pathogenic role of ATM in B-cell chronic lymphocytic leukemia. Blood 1999;94:748–753.

36. Fais F, Ghiotto F, Hashimoto S, et al: Chronic lymphocytic leukemia B cells express restricted sets of mutated and unmutated antigen receptors. J Clin Invest 1998;102:1515–1525.

37. Hamblin T, Davis Z, Gardiner A, et al: Unmutated Ig V_h genes are associated with a more aggressive form of chronic lymphocytic leukemia. Blood 1999;94:1848–1854.

38. Damle RN, Wasil T, Fais F, et al: Ig V gene mutation status and CD38 expression as novel prognostic indicators in chronic lymphocytic leukemia. Blood 1999;94:1840–1847.

39. Rosenwald A, Alizadeh AA, Widhopf G, et al: Relation of gene expression phenotype to immunoglobulin mutation genotype in B cell chronic lymphocytic leukemia. J Exp Med 2001;194:1639–1647.

40. Chen L, Widhopf G, Huynh L, et al: Expression of ZAP-70 is associated with increased B-cell receptor signaling in chronic lymphocytic leukemia. Blood 2002;100:4609–4614.

41. Kröber A, Seiler T, Benner A, et al: V_h mutation status, CD38 expression level, genomic aberrations, and survival in chronic lymphocytic leukemia. Blood 2002;100:1410–1416.

42. Cheson BD, Bennett JM, Rai KR, et al: Guidelines for clinical protocols for chronic lymphocytic leukemia: Report of the NCI-sponsored Working Group. Am J Hematol 1988;29:152–163.

43. Cheson BD, Bennett JM, Grever M, et al: National Cancer Institute-sponsored Working Group guidelines for chronic lymphocytic leukemia: Revised guidelines for diagnosis and treatment. Blood 1996;87:4990–4997.

44. Melo JV, Catovsky D, Galton DAG: The relationship between chronic lymphocytic leukaemia and prolymphocytic leukaemia: I. Clinical and laboratory features of 300 patients and characterization of an intermediate group. Br J Haematol 1986;63:377–387.

45. Rozman C, Montserrat E, Rodríguez-Fernández JM, et al: Bone marrow histologic pattern: The best single prognostic parameter in chronic lymphocytic leukemia: A multivariate survival analysis of 329 cases. Blood 1984;64:642–648.

46. Rai KR, Sawitsky A, Cronkite EP, et al: Clinical staging of chronic lymphocytic leukemia. Blood 1975;46:219–234.

47. Rai KR: A critical analysis of staging in CLL. In Gale RP, Rai KR (eds): Chronic Lymphocytic Leukemia: Recent Progress and Future Direction. New York, Alan R. Liss, 1987, p 253.

48. Binet JL, Auquier A, Dighiero G, et al: A new prognostic classification of chronic lymphocytic leukemia derived from a multivariate survival analysis. Cancer 1981;48:198–206.

49. DeRossi G, Mandelli F, Covelli A, et al: Chronic lymphocytic leukemia (CLL) in younger adults: A retrospective study of 133 cases. Hematol Oncol 1989;7:127–137.

50. Montserrat E, Gomis F, Vallespí T, et al: Presenting features and prognosis of chronic lymphocytic leukemia in younger adults. Blood 1991;78:1545–1551.

51. Mauro FR, Foa R, Gianarelli D, et al: Clinical characteristics and outcome of young chronic lymphocytic leukemia patients: A single institution study of 204 cases. Blood 1999;94:448–454.

52. Ibrahim S, Keating M, Do KA, et al: CD38 expression as an important prognostic factor in B-cell chronic lymphocytic leukemia. Blood 2001;98:181–186.

53. Oscier D, Gardiner AC, Mould SJ, et al: Multivariate analysis of prognostic factors in CLL: Clinical stage, IVGH gene mutational status, and loss or mutation of the p53 gene are independent prognostic factors. Blood 2002;100:1177–1184.

54. Zwiebel J, Cheson BD: Prognostic factors in chronic lymphocytic leukemia. Semin Oncol 1998;25:42–59.

55. Keating MJ, Lerner S, Kantarjian H, et al: The serum β_2-microglobulin ($\beta_2 M$) level is more powerful than stage in predicting response and survival in chronic lymphocytic leukemia (CLL) [abstract 2412]. Blood 1995;86:606.

56. Reinish W, Willheim M, Hilgarth M, et al: Soluble CD23 reliably reflects disease activity in B-cell chronic lymphocytic leukemia. J Clin Oncol 1994;12:2146–2152.

57. Sarfati M, Chevret S, Chastang C, et al: Prognostic importance of serum soluble CD23 level in chronic lymphocytic leukemia. Blood 1996;88:4259–4264.

58. Ferragoli A, Keating MJ, Manshouri T, et al: The clinical significance of tumor necrosis factor-α plasma level in patients having chronic lymphocytic leukemia. Blood 2002;100:1215–1219.

59. Heath ME, Cheson BD: Defective complement activity in chronic lymphocytic leukemia. Am J Hematol 1985;19:63–73.

60. Cheson BD: Immunologic and immunosuppressive complications of purine analogue therapy. J Clin Oncol 1995;13:2431–2448.

61. Anaissie EJ, Kontoyiannis DP, O'Brien S, et al: Infections in patients with chronic lymphocytic leukemia treated with fludarabine. Ann Intern Med 1998;129:559–566.

62. Keating MJ, Flinn I, Jain V, et al: Therapeutic role of alemtuzumab (CAMPATH-1H) in patients who have failed fludarabine: Results of a large international study. Blood 2002;99:3554–3561.

63. Cooperative Group for the Study of Immunoglobulin in Chronic Lymphocytic Leukemia: Intravenous immunoglobulin for the prevention of infection in chronic lymphocytic leukemia: A

randomized, controlled clinical trial. N Engl J Med 1988;319: 902-907.

64. Weeks JC, Tierney MR, Weinstein MC: Cost effectiveness of prophylactic intravenous immune globulin in chronic lymphocytic leukemia. N Engl J Med 1991;325:81-86.

65. Molica S, Musto P, Chiurazzi F, et al: Prophylaxis against infections with low-dose intravenous immunoglobulins (IVIG) in chronic lymphocytic leukemia: Results of a crossover study. Haematologica 1996;81:121-126.

66. Vadhan-Raj S, Velasquez WS, Butler JJ, et al: Stimulation of myelopoiesis in chronic lymphocytic leukemia and in other lymphoproliferative disorders by recombinant human granulocyte-macrophage colony-stimulating factor. Am J Hematol 1990;33:189-197.

67. O'Brien S, Kantarjian H, Beran M, et al: Fludarabine and granulocyte colony-stimulating factor (G-CSF) in patients with chronic lymphocytic leukemia. Leukemia 1997;11:1631-1635.

68. Richter MN: Generalized reticular cell sarcoma of lymph nodes associated with lymphocytic leukemia. Am J Pathol 1928;4: 285-292.

69. Cherepakhin V, Baird SM, Meisenholder GW, et al: Common clonal origin of chronic lymphocytic leukemia and high-grade lymphoma of Richter's syndrome. Blood 1993;82:3141-3147.

70. Bessudo A, Kipps TJ: Origin of high-grade lymphomas in Richter syndrome. Leuk Lymphoma 1995;18:367-372.

71. Cobo F, Martínez A, Pinyol M, et al: Multiple cell cycle regulator alterations in Richter's transformation of chronic lymphocytic leukemia. Leukemia 2002;16:1028-1034.

72. Robertson LE, Pugh W, O'Brien S, et al: Richter's syndrome: A report on 39 patients. J Clin Oncol 1993;11:1985-1989.

73. Giles FJ, O'Brien S, Kantarjian HM, et al: Sequential cis-platinum, fludarabine, and arabinosyl cytosine (PFA) or cyclophosphamide, fludarabine and arabinosyl cytosine (CFA) in patients with Richter's syndrome. Blood 1996;88:93a.

74. Melo JV, Catovsky D, Galton DAG: The relationship between chronic lymphocytic leukaemia and prolymphocytic leukaemia: IV. Patterns of evolution of "prolymphocytoid" transformation. Br J Haematol 1986;64:77-86.

75. Melo JV, Catovsky D, Gregory WM, et al: The relationship between chronic lymphocytic leukaemia and prolymphocytic leukaemia: IV. Analysis of survival and prognostic features. Br J Haematol 1987;65:2329.

76. Hamblin TJ, Oscier DJ, Young BJ: Autoimmunity in chronic lymphocytic leukemia. J Clin Pathol 1986;39:713.

77. Duhrsen U, Augener W, Zwingers T, et al: Spectrum and frequency of autoimmune derangements in lymphoproliferative disorders: Analysis of 637 cases and comparison with myeloproliferative diseases. Br J Haematol 1987;67:235-239.

78. Kipps TJ, Carson DA: Autoantibodies in chronic lymphocytic leukemia and related systemic autoimmune diseases. Blood 1993;81:2475-2487.

79. Efremov DG, Ivanovski M, Siljanovski N, et al: Restricted immunoglobulin VH region repertoire in chronic lymphocytic leukemia patients with autoimmune hemolytic anemia. Blood 1996;87:3869-3876.

80. Efremov DG, Ivanovski M, Burrone OR: The pathologic significance of the immunoglobulins expressed by chronic lymphocytic leukemia B-cells in the development of autoimmune hemolytic anemia. Leuk Lymphoma 1998;28:285-293.

81. Seipelt G, Bohme A, Koschmieder S, et al: Effective treatment with rituximab in a patient with refractory prolymphocytoid transformed B-chronic lymphocytic leukemia and Evan's syndrome. Ann Hematol 2001;80:170-173.

82. Hegde UP, Wilson WH, White T, et al: Rituximab treatment of refractory fludarabine-associated immune thrombocytopenia in chronic lymphocytic leukemia. Blood 2002;100:2260-2262.

83. Seymour JF, Cusack JD, Lerner SA, et al: Case/control study of the role of splenectomy in chronic lymphocytic leukemia. J Clin Oncol 1997;15:52-60.

84. Chikkappa G, Pasquale D, Zarrabi MH, et al: Cyclosporine and prednisone therapy for pure red cell aplasia in patients with chronic lymphocytic leukemia. Am J Hematol 1992;41:5-12.

85. Ghazal HH: Successful treatment of pure red cell aplasia (PRA) with rituxan in patients with CLL [abstract 914]. Blood 2001;98:219a.

86. French Cooperative Group on Chronic Lymphocytic Leukemia: Effects of chlorambucil and therapeutic decision in initial forms of chronic lymphocytic leukemia (stage A): Results of a randomized trial on 612 patients. Blood 1990;75:1414-1421.

87. Cheson BD, Vena D, Barrett J, et al: Second malignancies as a consequence of nucleoside analog therapy of chronic lymphoid leukemias. J Clin Oncol 1999;17:2454-2460.

88. Montserrat E, Viñolas N, Reverer JC, et al: Natural history of chronic lymphocytic leukemia: On the progression and prognosis of early stages. Nouv Rev Fr Hematol 1988;30:359-361.

89. French Cooperative Group on Chronic Lymphocytic Leukaemia: Natural history of stage A chronic lymphocytic leukaemia untreated patients. Br J Haematol 1990;76:45-57.

90. Dighiero G, Maloum K, Desablens B, et al: Chlorambucil in indolent chronic lymphocytic leukemia: French Cooperative Group on Chronic Lymphocytic Leukemia. N Engl J Med 1998;338:1506-1514.

91. Shustik C, Mick R, Silver R, et al: Treatment of early chronic lymphocytic leukemia: Intermittent chlorambucil versus observation. Hematol Oncol 1988;6:7-12.

92. Richards S, Clarke M: CLL Trialists' Cooperative Group: Meta-analysis of results. Hematol Cell Ther 1997;39:S53-S102.

93. Cheson BD: New antimetabolites in the treatment of human malignancies. Semin Oncol 1992;19:695-706.

94. Keating MJ: Chemotherapy of chronic lymphocytic leukemia. In Cheson BD (ed): Chronic Lymphocytic Leukemia: Scientific Advances and Clinical Developments: Basic and Clinical Oncology. New York, Marcel Dekker, 1993, pp 297-336.

95. Saven A, Carrera CJ, Carson DA, et al: 2-Chlorodeoxyadenosine treatment of refractory chronic lymphocytic leukemia. Leuk Lymphoma 1991;5:133-138.

96. Dillman RO, Mick R, McIntyre OR: Pentostatin in chronic lymphocytic leukemia: A phase II trial of Cancer and Leukemia Group B. J Clin Oncol 1989;7:433-438.

97. Sorensen JM, Vena D, Fallavollita A, et al: Treatment of refractory chronic lymphocytic leukemia with fludarabine phosphate via the Group C mechanism of the National Cancer Institute: 5-year follow-up report. J Clin Oncol 1997;15:458-465.

98. Cheson BD: Therapy for previously untreated chronic lymphocytic leukemia: A reevaluation. Semin Hematol 1998;35:14-21.

99. French Cooperative Group on CLL, Johnson S, Smith AG, et al: Multicentre prospective randomised trial of fludarabine versus cyclophosphamide, doxorubicin, and prednisone (CAP) for treatment of advanced-stage chronic lymphocytic leukemia. Lancet 1996;347:1432-1438.

100. Keating MJ, O'Brien S, Lerner S, et al: Long-term follow-up of patients with chronic lymphocytic leukemia (CLL) receiving fludarabine regimens as initial therapy. Blood 1998;92:1165-1171.

101. Leporrier M, Chevret S, Cazin B, et al: Randomized comparison of fludarabine, CAP, and ChOP in 938 previously treated stage B and C-chronic lymphocytic leukemia. Blood 2001;98:2319-2325.

102. Rai KR, Peterson BL, Kolitz J, et al: Fludarabine compared with chlorambucil as primary therapy for chronic lymphocytic leukemia. N Engl J Med 2000;343:1750-1757.

103. Robertson LE, O'Brien S, Kantarjian H, et al: A 3-day schedule of fludarabine in previously treated chronic lymphocytic leukemia. Leukemia 1995;9:1444-1449.

104. Cheson BD, Vena D, Foss F, et al: Neurotoxicity of purine analogs: A review. J Clin Oncol 1994;12:2216-2228.

105. Cheson BD: Toxicities associated with nucleoside analog therapy. In Cheson BD, Keating MJ, Plunkett W (eds): Nucleoside Analogs in Cancer Therapy: Basic and Clinical Oncology. New York, Marcel Dekker, 1997, pp 415-459.

106. O'Brien S, Kantarjian H, Beran M, et al: Results of fludarabine and prednisone therapy in 264 patients with chronic lymphocytic leukemia with multivariate analysis-derived prognostic model for response to treatment. Blood 1993;82:1695-1700.

107. Morrison VA, Rai KR, Peterson BL, et al: Impact of therapy with chlorambucil, fludarabine, or fludarabine plus chlorambucil on infections in patients with chronic lymphocytic leukemia: Intergroup study: Cancer and Leukemia Group B 9011. J Clin Oncol 2001;19:3611-3621.

108. Cheson BD, Frame JN, Vena D, et al: Tumor lysis syndrome: An

uncommon complication of fludarabine therapy of chronic lymphocytic leukemia. J Clin Oncol 1998;16:2313–2320.

109. Tertian G, Cartron J, Bayle C, et al: Fatal intravascular autoimmune hemolytic anemia after fludarabine treatment for chronic lymphocytic leukemia. Hematol Cell Ther 1996;38:359–360.

110. Weiss RB, Freiman J, Kweder SL, et al: Hemolytic anemia after fludarabine therapy for chronic lymphocytic leukemia. J Clin Oncol 1998;16:1885–1889.

111. Morrison VA, Rai KR, Peterson BL, et al: Therapy-related myeloid leukemias are observed in patients with chronic lymphocytic leukemia after treatment with fludarabine and chlorambucil: Results of an intergroup study: Cancer and Leukemia Group B 9011. J Clin Oncol 2002;20:3878–3884.

112. Foran JM, Oscier D, Orchard J, et al: Pharmacokinetic study of single doses of oral fludarabine phosphate. J Clin Oncol 1999;17:1574–1579.

113. Boogaerts MA, Van Hoof A, Catovsky D, et al: Activity of oral fludarabine phosphate in previously treated chronic lymphocytic leukemia. J Clin Oncol 2001;19:4252–4258.

114. Juliusson G, Lilliemark J: High complete remission rate from 2-chloro-2′-deoxyadenosine in previously treated patients with B-cell chronic lymphocytic leukemia: Response predicted by rapid decrease in blood lymphocyte count. J Clin Oncol 1993;11:679–689.

115. Robak T, Blasinka-Morawiec M, Krykowski E, et al: Intermittent 2-hour intravenous infusions of 2-chlorodeoxyadenosine in the treatment of 110 patients with refractory or previously untreated B-cell chronic lymphocytic leukemia. Leuk Lymphoma 1996;22:509–514.

116. Lilliemark JO, Albertioni F, Pettersson B, et al: Bioavailability of oral and subcutaneous 2-chloro-2′-deoxyadenosine (CdA) [abstract 270]. Proc Am Soc Clin Oncol 1992;11:112.

117. Juliusson G, Christiansen I, Hansen MM, et al: Oral cladribine as primary therapy for patients with B-cell chronic lymphocytic leukemia. J Clin Oncol 1996;14:2160–2166.

118. Tallman MS, Hakimian D, Zonzig C, et al: Cladribine in the treatment of relapsed or refractory chronic lymphocytic leukemia. J Clin Oncol 1995;13:983–988.

119. Saven A, Lemon RH, Kosty M, et al: 2-Chlorodeoxyadenosine activity in patients with untreated chronic lymphocytic leukemia. J Clin Oncol 1995;13:570–574.

120. Delannoy A, Martiat P, Gala JL, et al: 2-Chlorodeoxyadenosine (CdA) for patients with previously untreated chronic lymphocytic leukemia (CLL). Leukemia 1995;9:1130–1135.

121. Rondelli D, Lauria F, Zinzani PL, et al: 2-Chlorodeoxyadenosine in the treatment of relapsed/refractory chronic lymphoproliferative disorders. Eur J Haematol 1997;58:46–50.

122. Piro LD, Carrera CJ, Carson DA, et al: Lasting remissions in hairy cell leukemia induced by a single infusion of 2-chlorodeoxyadenosine. N Engl J Med 1990;322:1117–1121.

123. Saven A, Kawasaki H, Carrera CJ, et al: 2-Chlorodeoxyadenosine dose escalation in nonhematologic malignancies. J Clin Oncol 1993;11:671–678.

124. Spielberger RT, Stock W, Larson RA: Listeriosis after 2-chlorodeoxyadenosine treatment [letter]. N Engl J Med 1993;328:813–814.

125. Kefford RF, Fox RM: Deoxycoformycin-induced response in chronic lymphocytic leukaemia: Deoxyadenosine toxicity in non-replicating lymphocytes. Br J Haematol 1982;50:627–636.

126. Dearden C, Catovsky D: Deoxycoformycin in the treatment of mature B-cell malignancies. Br J Cancer 1990;62:4–5.

127. Grever MR, Siaw MFE, Jacob WF, et al: The biochemical and clinical consequences of 2′-deoxycoformycin in refractory lymphoproliferative malignancy. Blood 1981;57:406–417.

128. Ho AD, Ganeshaguru K, Knauf WU, et al: Clinical response to deoxycoformycin in chronic lymphoid neoplasms and biochemical changes in circulating malignant cells in vivo. Blood 1988;72:1884–1890.

129. Grever MR, Leiby JM, Kraut EH, et al: Low-dose deoxycoformycin in lymphoid malignancy. J Clin Oncol 1985;3:1196–1201.

130. Ho AD, Thaler J, Strykmans P, et al: Pentostatin in refractory chronic lymphocytic leukemia: A phase II trial of the European Organization for Research and Treatment of Cancer. J Natl Cancer Inst 1990;82:1416–1420.

131. Grever MR, Coleman MS, Gray DP, et al: Definition of safe, effective, dosing regimen of 2′-deoxycoformycin with biochemical investigation. Cancer Treat Symp 1984;2:43–49.

132. O'Dwyer PJ, Spiers ASD, Marsoni S: Association of severe and fatal infections and treatment with pentostatin. Cancer Treat Rep 1986;70:1117–1120.

133. O'Dwyer PJ, Wagner B, Leyland-Jones B, et al: 2′-Deoxycoformycin (pentostatin) for lymphoid malignancies. Ann Intern Med 1988;108:733–743.

134. Flinn IW, Kopecky KJ, Foucar MK, et al: Long-term follow-up of remission duration, mortality, and second malignancies in hairy cell leukemia patients treated with pentostatin. Blood 2000;96:2981–2986.

135. Spanish Cooperative Group P: Treatment of chronic lymphocytic leukemia: A preliminary report of Spanish (PETHEMA) trials. Leuk Lymphoma 1991;5:89–91.

136. Rai KR, Peterson B, Elias L, et al: A randomized comparison of fludarabine and chlorambucil for patients with previously untreated chronic lymphocytic leukemia: A CALGB, SWOG, CTC/NCI-C and ECOG inter-group study [abstract 552]. Blood 1996;88:141a.

137. Montserrat E, Alcala A, Parody R, et al: Treatment of chronic lymphocytic leukemia in advanced stages: A randomized trial comparing chlorambucil plus prednisone versus cyclophosphamide, vincristine, and prednisone. Cancer 1985;56:2369–2375.

138. Raphael B, Andersen JW, Silber R, et al: Comparison of chlorambucil and prednisone versus cyclophosphamide, vincristine, and prednisone as initial treatment for chronic lymphocytic leukemia: Long-term follow-up of an Eastern Cooperative Oncology Group randomized clinical trial. J Clin Oncol 1991;9:770–776.

139. Hansen MM, Andersen E, Birgens H, et al: CHOP versus chlorambucil + prednisolone in chronic lymphocytic leukemia. Leuk Lymphoma 1991;5:97.

140. French Cooperative Group on Chronic Lymphocytic Leukemia: Long-term results of the CHOP regimen in stage C chronic lymphocytic leukaemia. Br J Haematol 1989;73:334–340.

141. Kimby E, Millstedt H: Chlorambucil/prednisone versus CHOP in symptomatic chronic lymphocytic leukemias of B-cell type: A randomized trial. Leuk Lymphoma 1991;5:93–96.

142. Keating MJ, Scouros M, Murphy S, et al: Multiple agent chemotherapy (POACH) in previously treated and untreated patients with chronic lymphocytic leukemia. Leukemia 1988;2:157–164.

143. Keating MJ, Hester JP, McCredie KB, et al: Long-term results of CAP therapy in chronic lymphocytic leukemia. Leuk Lymphoma 1990;2:391–397.

144. CLL Trialists' Collaborative Group: Chemotherapeutic options in chronic lymphocytic leukemia: A meta-analysis of the randomized trials. CLL Trialists' Collaborative group. J Natl Cancer Inst 1999;91:861–868.

145. French Cooperative Group on Chronic Lymphocytic Leukemia: A randomized clinical trial of chlorambucil versus COP in stage B chronic lymphocytic leukemia. Blood 1990;75:1422–1425.

146. O'Brien S, Kantarjian H, Koller C, et al: Fludarabine-prednisone: A highly effective regimen in chronic lymphocytic leukemia (CLL) [abstract 850]. Proc Am Soc Clin Oncol 1992;11:260.

147. Rummel M, Schenk M, Renner C, et al: Fludarabine and epirubicin in the treatment of CLL as first line therapy or in first relapse: Results of a phase-II-study [abstract 2359]. Blood 1997;90:530a.

148. Bosch F, Perales M, Cobo F, et al: Fludarabine, cyclophosphamide and mitoxantrone (FCM) therapy in resistant or relapsed chronic lymphocytic leukemia (CLL) or follicular lymphoma (FL) [abstract 2360]. Blood 1997;90:530a.

149. O'Brien S, Kantarjian H, Beran M, et al: Fludarabine (FAMP) and cyclophosphamide (CTX) therapy in chronic lymphocytic leukemia (CLL) [abstract 214]. Int J Hematol 1996;64:S56.

150. Flinn IW, Byrd JC, Morrison C, et al: Fludarabine and cyclophosphamide: A highly active and well tolerated regimen in patients with previously untreated chronic lymphocytic leukemia [abstract 424]. Blood 1998;92:104a.

151. Oken MM, Lee S, Cassileth PA, et al: Pentostatin, chlorambucil and prednisone for the treatment of chronic lymphocytic leukemia

(CLL): Eastern Cooperative Oncology Group (ECOG) protocol E1488 [abstract 22]. Proc ASCO 1998;17:6a.

152. Grever MR, Kopecky KJ, Coltman CA, et al: Fludarabine monophosphate: A potentially useful agent in chronic lymphocytic leukemia. Nouv Rev Fr Hematol 1988;30:457–459.

153. Keating MJ, Kantarjian H, Talpaz M, et al: Fludarabine: A new agent with major activity against chronic lymphocytic leukemia. Blood 1989;74:19–25.

154. Montserrat E, López-Lorenzo JL, Manso F, et al: Fludarabine in resistant or relapsing B-cell chronic lymphocytic leukemia: The Spanish Group experience. Leuk Lymph 1996;21:467–472.

155. Keating MJ, O'Brien S, Kantarjian H, et al: Long-term follow-up of patients with chronic lymphocytic leukemia treated with fludarabine as a single agent. Blood 1993;81:2878–2884.

156. O'Brien SM, Kantarjian HM, Cortes J, et al: Results of the fludarabine and cyclophosphamide combination regimen in chronic lymphocytic leukemia. J Clin Oncol 2001;19:1414–1420.

157. O'Brien S, Kantarjian H, Estey E, et al: Lack of effect of 2-chlorodeoxyadenosine therapy in patients with chronic lymphocytic leukemia refractory to fludarabine therapy. N Engl J Med 1994;330:319–322.

158. Hale G, Xia M-Q, Tighe HP, et al: The CAMPATH-1 antigen (CDw52). Tissue Antigens 1990;35:118–127.

159. Lundin J, Kimby E, Björkholm M, et al: Phase II trial of subcutaneous anti-CD52 monoclonal antibody alemtuzumab (CAMPATH-1H) as first-line treatment for patients with B-cell chronic lymphocytic leukemia (BCLL). Blood 2002;100:768–773.

160. Österborg A, Dyer MJS, Bunjes D, et al: Phase II multicenter study of human CD52 antibody in previously treated chronic lymphocytic leukemia. J Clin Oncol 1997;15:1567–1574.

161. Bowen AL, Zomas A, Emmett E, et al: Subcutaneous CAMPATH-1H in fludarabine-resistant/relapsed chronic lymphocytic and B-prolymphocytic leukaemia. Br J Haematol 1997;96:617–619.

162. Rawstron AC, Davies FE, Evans P, et al: CAMPATH-1H therapy for patients with refractory chronic lymphocytic leukemia (CLL) [abstract 2356]. Blood 1997;90:529a.

163. Stilgenbauer S, Döhner H: Campath-1H-induced complete remission of chronic lymphocytic leukemia despite p53 gene mutation and resistance to chemotherapy [letter]. N Engl J Med 2002;347:452–453.

164. McCune SL, Gockerman JP, Moore JO, et al: Alemtuzumab in relapsed or refractory chronic lymphocytic leukemia and prolymphocytic leukemia. Leuk Lymphoma 2002;43:1007–1011.

165. Rai KR, Coutré S, Rizzieri D, et al: Efficacy and safety of alemtuzumab (CAMPATH-1H) in refractory B-CLL patients treated on a compassionate basis [abstract 1538]. Blood 2001;98:365a.

166. Österborg A, Fassas AS, Anagnostopoulos A, et al: Humanized CD52 monoclonal antibody Campath-1H as first-line treatment in chronic lymphocytic leukaemia. Br J Haematol 1996;93:151–153.

167. Rai KR, Byrd JC, Peterson B, et al: A phase II trial of fludarabine followed by alemtuzumab (CAMPATH-1H) in previously untreated chronic lymphocytic leukemia (CLL) patients with active disease: Cancer and Leukemia Group B (CALGB) Study 19901 [abstract 772]. Blood 2002;100:205a.

168. Kennedy B, Rawstron A, Carter C, et al: CAMPATH-1H and fludarabine in combination are highly active in refractory chronic lymphocytic leukemia. Blood 2002;99:2245–2247.

169. McLaughlin P, Grillo-López AJ, Link BK, et al: Rituximab chimeric anti-CD20 monoclonal antibody therapy of relapsed indolent lymphoma: Half of patients respond to a four-dose treatment program. J Clin Oncol 1998;16:2825–2833.

170. Maloney DG, Grillo-López AJ, White CA, et al: IDEC-C2B8 (Rituximab) anti-CD20- monoclonal antibody therapy in patients with relapsed low-grade non-Hodgkin's lymphoma. Blood 1997;90:2188–2195.

171. Nguyen DT, Amess JA, Doughty H, et al: IDEC-C2B8 anti-CD20 (rituximab) immunotherapy in patients with low-grade non-Hodgkin's lymphoma and lymphoproliferative disorders: Evaluation of response on 48 patients. Eur J Haematol 1999;62:76–82.

172. Piro LD, White CA, Grillo-López AJ, et al: Extended rituximab (anti-CD20 monoclonal antibody) therapy for relapsed or refractory low-grade or follicular non-Hodgkin's lymphoma. Ann Oncol 1999;10:655–661.

173. Winkler U, Jensen M, Manzke O, et al: Cytokine-release syndrome in patients with B-cell chronic lymphocytic leukemia and high lymphocyte counts after treatment with an anti-CD20 monoclonal antibody (rituximab, IDEC-C2B8). Blood 1999;94:2217–2224.

174. Foran JM, Rohatiner AZ, Cunningham D, et al: European phase II study of rituximab (chimeric anti-CD20 monoclonal antibody) for patients with newly diagnosed mantle-cell lymphoma and previously treated mantle-cell lymphoma, immunocytoma, and small B-cell lymphocytic lymphoma. J Clin Oncol 2000;18:317.

175. Huhn D, von Schilling C, Wilhelm M, et al: Rituximab therapy of patients with B-cell chronic lymphocytic leukemia. Blood 2001;98:1326–1331.

176. Byrd JC, Murphy T, Howard RS, et al: Rituximab using a thrice weekly dosing schedule in B-cell chronic lymphocytic leukemia and small lymphocytic lymphoma demonstrates clinical activity and acceptable toxicity. J Clin Oncol 2001;19:2153–2164.

177. O'Brien SM, Kantarjian H, Thomas DA, et al: Rituximab dose-escalation trial in chronic lymphocytic leukemia. J Clin Oncol 2001;19:2165–2170.

178. Hainsworth JD, Litchy S, Burris HA, et al: Rituximab as first-line and maintenance therapy for patients with small lymphocytic lymphoma (SLL) and chronic lymphocytic leukemia (CLL) [abstract 1530]. Blood 2001;98:363a.

179. Thomas DA, O'Brien S, Giles FJ, et al: Single agent rituxan in early stage chronic lymphocytic leukemia (CLL) [abstract 1533]. Blood 2001;98:364a.

180. Hainsworth JD, Litchy S, Barton JH, et al: Single-agent rituximab as first-line and maintenance treatment for patients with chronic lymphocytic leukemia or small lymphocytic lymphoma: A phase II trial of the Minnie Pearl Cancer Research Network. J Clin Oncol 2003;21:1746–1751.

181. Hainsworth JD, Burris HA III, Morrissey LH, et al: Rituximab monoclonal antibody as initial systemic therapy for patients with low-grade non-Hodgkin's lymphoma. Blood 2000;95:3052–3056.

182. Byrd JC, Peterson B, Morrison VA, et al: Randomized phase 2 study of fludarabine with concurrent versus sequential treatment with rituximab in symptomatic, untreated patients with B-cell chronic lymphocytic leukemia: Results from Cancer and Leukemia Group B 9712 (CALGB 9712). Blood 2003;101:6–14.

183. Demidem A, Lam T, Alas S, et al: Chimeric anti-CD20 (IDEC-C2B8) monoclonal antibody sensitizes a B cell lymphoma cell line to cell killing by cytotoxic drugs. Cancer Biother Radiopharm 1997;12: 177–186.

184. Alas S, Emmanouilides C, Bonavida B: Inhibition of interleukin 10 by rituximab results in down-regulation of bcl-2 and sensitization of B-cell non-Hodgkin's lymphoma to apoptosis. Clin Cancer Res 2001;7:709–723.

185. Alas S, Bonavida B: Rituximab inactivates signal transducer and activator of transcription 3 (STAT3) activity in B-non-Hodgkin's lymphoma through inhibition of the interleukin 10 autocrine/ paracrine loop and results in down-regulation of bcl-2 and sensitization to cytotoxic drugs. Cancer Res 2001;61:5137–5144.

186. Johnson TA, Press OW: Synergistic cytotoxicity of iodine-131-anti-CD20 antibodies and chemotherapy for treatment of B-cell lymphomas. Int J Cancer 2000;85:104–112.

187. Shan D, Ledbetter JA, Press OW: Signaling events involved in anti-CD20-induced apoptosis of malignant human B cells. Cancer Immunol Immunother 2000;48:673–683.

188. Schulz H, Klein SK, Rehwald U, et al: Phase II-study of rituximab in combination with fludarabine in patients (pts) with chronic lymphocytic leukemia (CLL) [abstract 1534]. Blood 2001;98:364a.

189. Wierda W, O'Brien S, Albitar M, et al: Combined fludarabine, cyclophosphamide, and rituximab achieves a high complete remission rate as initial treatment for chronic lymphocytic leukemia [abstract 3210]. Blood 2001;98:771a.

190. Keating M, Manshouri T, O'Brien S, et al: A high proportion of molecular remission can be obtained with a fludarabine, cyclophosphamide, rituximab (FCR) combination in chronic lymphocytic leukemia (CLL) [abstract 771]. Blood 2002;100:205a.

191. Garcia-Manero G, O'Brien S, Cortes J, et al: Update of results of the combination of fludarabine, cyclophosphamide and rituximab for previously treated patients with chronic lymphocytic leukemia (CLL) [abstract 2650]. Blood 2001;98:633a.

192. Nabhan C, Tallman MS, Riley MB, et al: Phase I study of rituximab and CAMPATH-1H in patients with relapsed or refractory chronic lymphocytic leukemia [abstract 1536]. Blood 2001;98:365a.

193. Faderl S, Thomas DA, O'Brien S, et al: Experience with alemtuzumab plus rituximab in patients with relapsed and refractory lymphoid malignancies. Blood 2003;101:3413–3415.

194. Byrd JC, Waselenko JK, Maneatis T, et al: Rituximab therapy in hematologic malignancy patients with circulating tumor cells: Association with increased infusion-related side effects and rapid blood tumor clearance. J Clin Oncol 1999;17:791–795.

195. Pathan N, Hariharan K, Hopkins M, et al: Induction of apoptosis by IDEC-152 (anti-CD23) in lymphoma cells [abstract 1545]. Blood 2001;98:367a.

196. Link BK, Wang H, Byrd JC, et al: Phase I trial of humanized 1D10 (Hu1D10) monoclonal antibody targeting class II molecules in patients with relapsed lymphoma [abstract 86]. Proc ASCO 2000;19:24a.

197. Link BK, Kahl B, Czuczman M, et al: A phase II study of Remitogen™ (Hu1D10), a humanized monoclonal antibody in patients with relapsed or refractory follicular, small lymphocytic, or marginal zone/MALT B-cell lymphomas [abstract 2540]. Blood 2001;98:606a.

198. Hegde U, White T, Stetler-Stevenson M, et al: Phase I study of combination rituximab (CD20) and apolizumab (Hu1D10) monoclonal antibody therapy in previously treated B-cell lymphoma and chronic lymphocytic leukemia [abstract 1389]. Blood 2002;100:358a.

199. LeMaistre CF, Meneghetti C, Rosenblum M, et al: Phase I trial of an interleukin-2 (IL-2) fusion toxin (DAB486IL-2) in hematologic malignancies expressing the IL-2 receptor. Blood 1992;79:2547–2554.

200. Fleming DR, Powell BL, Patrick CL, et al: Diphtheria fusion protein ONTAK therapy of patients with fludarabine refractory chronic lymphocytic leukemia [abstract 1071]. Proc Am Soc Clin Oncol 2002;19:268a.

201. Frankel AE, Patrick CL, Powell BL: Phase II trial of the diphtheria fusion protein ONTAK in patients with fludarabine refractory chronic lymphocytic leukemia (CLL) [abstract 4901]. Blood 2001;98:289b.

202. Epstein AL, Marder RJ, Winter JN, et al: Two new monoclonal antibodies, Lym-1 and Lym-2, reactive with human B-lymphocytes and derived tumors, with immunodiagnostic and immunotherapeutic potential. Cancer Res 1987;47:830–840.

203. DeNardo SJ, DeNardo GL, O'Grady LF, et al: Pilot studies of radioimmunotherapy of B cell lymphoma and leukemia using I-131 Lym-1 monoclonal antibody. Antibody Immunoconjugates Radiopharm 1988;1:17–33.

204. DeNardo GL, DeNardo SJ, O'Grady LF, et al: Fractionated radioimmunotherapy of B-cell malignancies with ^{131}I-Lym-1. Cancer Res 1990;50:1014s–1016s.

205. Lewis JP, DeNardo GL, DeNardo SJ, et al: Impact of Lym-1 radioimmunoconjugate on refractory chronic lymphocytic leukemia (CLL) [abstract 1171]. Blood 1990;76:295a.

206. DeNardo GL, Lewis JP, DeNardo SJ, et al: Effect of Lym-1 radioimmunoconjugate on refractory chronic lymphocytic leukemia. Cancer 1993;73:1425–1432.

207. Kaminski MS, Press OW, Lister TA, et al: Iodine I131 tositumomab for patients with small lymphocytic lymphoma (SLL) [abstract 386]: Overall clinical trial experience. Blood 1999;94:88a.

208. Foon KA, Bottino GC, Abrams PG, et al: Phase II trial of recombinant leukocyte A interferon in patients with advanced chronic lymphocytic leukemia. Am J Med 1985;78:216–220.

209. O'Connell MJ, Colgan JP, Oken MM, et al: Clinical trial of recombinant leukocyte A interferon as initial therapy for favorable histology non-Hodgkin's lymphomas and chronic lymphocytic leukemia: An Eastern Cooperative Oncology Group pilot study. J Clin Oncol 1986;4:128–136.

210. Rozman C, Montserrat E, Viñolas N, et al: Recombinant α2-interferon in the treatment of B chronic lymphocytic leukemia in early stages. Blood 1988;71:1295–1298.

211. Molica S, Alberti A: Recombinant alpha-2a interferon in treatment of B-chronic lymphocytic leukemia: A preliminary report with emphasis on previously untreated patients in early stage of disease. Haematologica 1990;75:75–78.

212. Ferrara F, Rametta V, Mele G, et al: Recombinant interferon-alpha2A as maintenance treatment for patients with advanced stage chronic lymphocytic leukemia responding to chemotherapy. Am J Hematol 1992;41:45–49.

213. O'Brien S, Kantarjian H, Beran M, et al: Interferon maintenance therapy for patients with chronic lymphocytic leukemia in remission after fludarabine. Blood 1995;86:1296–1300.

214. Zinzani PL, Bendandi M, Magagnoli M, et al: Results with fludarabine induction and alpha-interferon maintenance protocol in pretreated patients with chronic lymphocytic leukemia and low-grade non-Hodgkin's lymphoma. Eur J Haematol 1997;59:82–88.

215. Michallet M, Archimbaud E, Bandini G, et al: HLA-identical sibling bone marrow transplantation in younger patients with chronic lymphocytic leukemia. Ann Intern Med 1996;124:311–315.

216. Rabinowe SN, Soiffer RJ, Gribben JG, et al: Autologous and allogeneic bone marrow transplantation for poor prognosis patients with B-cell chronic lymphocytic leukemia. Blood 1993;82:1366–1376.

217. Khouri IF, Keating MJ, Vriesendorp HM, et al: Autologous and allogeneic bone marrow transplantation for chronic lymphocytic leukemia: Preliminary results. J Clin Oncol 1994;12:748–758.

218. Khouri IF, Przepiorka D, van Besien K, et al: Allogeneic blood or marrow transplantation for chronic lymphocytic leukaemia: Timing of transplantation and potential effect of fludarabine on acute graft-versus-host disease. Br J Haematol 1997;97:466–473.

219. Slavin S, Nagler A, Naparstek E, et al: Nonmyeloablative stem cell transplantation and cell therapy as an alternative to conventional bone marrow transplantation with lethal cytoreduction for the treatment of malignant and nonmalignant hematologic diseases. Blood 1998;91:756–763.

220. Khouri IF, Keating M, Körbling M, et al: Transplant-lite: Induction of graft-versus malignancy using fludarabine-based nonablative chemotherapy and allogeneic blood progenitor-cell transplantation as treatment for lymphoid malignancies. J Clin Oncol 1998;16:2817–2824.

221. Itälä M, Pelliniemi T-T, Rajamäki A, et al: Autologous blood cell transplantation in B-CLL: Response to chemotherapy prior to mobilization predicts the stem cell yield. Bone Marrow Transplant 1998;19:647–651.

222. Khouri I, Keating MJ, Przepiorka D, et al: Stem cell transplantation (SCT) for chronic lymphocytic leukemia (CLL): Graft-versus-leukemia (GVL) without acute graft-versus-host disease (GVHD) [abstract 1814]. Blood 1995;86:457a.

223. Pavletic ZS, Bierman PJ, Vose JM, et al: High incidence of relapse after autologous stem-cell transplantation for B-cell chronic lymphocytic leukemia or small lymphocytic lymphoma. Ann Oncol 1998;9:1023–1026.

224. Sutton L, Maloum K, Gonzalez H, et al: Autologous hematopoietic stem cell transplantation as salvage treatment for advanced B cell chronic lymphocytic leukemia. Leukemia 1998;12:1699–1707.

225. Buhmann R, Nolte A, Westhaus D, et al: CD40-activated B-cell chronic lymphocytic leukemia cells for tumor immunotherapy: Stimulation of allogeneic versus autologous T cells generates different types of effector cells. Blood 1999;93:1992–2002.

226. Wierda WG, Cantwell MJ, Rassenti LZ, et al: CD154 (CD40-ligand) gene immunization of chronic lymphocytic leukemia: A phase I study [abstract 2018]. Blood 1998;92:489a.

227. Waters JS, Webb A, Cunningham D, et al: Phase I clinical and pharmacokinetic study of bcl-2 antisense oligonucleotide therapy in patients with non-Hodgkin's lymphoma. J Clin Oncol 2000;18:1809–1811.

228. Rai KR, O'Brien S, Cunningham C, et al: Genasense (Bcl-2 antisense) monotherapy in patients with relapsed or refractory chronic lymphocytic leukemia: Phase I and II results [abstract 1490]. Blood 2002;100:384a.

229. Smith M, Joshi I, Jin F: Combined therapy with antisense BCL-2 oligonucleotides (AS-BCL2-ODN) + αCD20 monoclonal antibody in scid/human lymphoma xenografts [abstract 1458]. Blood 2000;96:338a.

230. Pangalis GA, Poziopoulos C, Angelopoulou MK, et al: Effective treatment of disease-related anemia in B-chronic lymphocytic leukaemia patients with recombinant human erythropoietin. Br J Haematol 1995;89:627–629.

231. Österborg A, Brandberg Y, Molostova V, et al: Randomized, double-blind, placebo-controlled trial of recombinant human erythropoietin, epoetin beta, in hematologic malignancies. J Clin Oncol 2002;20:2486–2494.

232. Melo JV, Wardle J, Chetty M, et al: The relationship between chronic lymphocytic leukaemia and prolymphocytic leukaemia: III. Evaluation of cell size by morphology and volume measurements. Br J Haematol 1986;64:469–478.

233. Bennett JM, Catovsky D, Daniel M-T, et al: Proposals for the classification of chronic (mature) B and T lymphoid leukaemias. J Clin Pathol 1989;42:567–584.

234. Kantarjian HM, Childs C, O'Brien S, et al: Efficacy of fludarabine, a new adenine nucleoside analogue, in patients with prolymphocytic leukemia and the prolymphocytoid variant of chronic lymphocytic leukemia. Am J Med 1991;90: 223–228.

235. Sporn JR: Sustained response of refractory prolymphocytic leukemia to fludarabine. Acta Haematol 1991;85:209–211.

236. Saven A, Lee T, Schlutz M, et al: Major activity of cladribine in patients with de novo B-cell prolymphocytic leukemia. Blood 1997;15:37–43.

237. Döhner H, Ho AD, Thaler J, et al: Pentostatin in prolymphocytic leukemia: Phase II trial of the European Organization for Research and Treatment of Cancer Leukemia Cooperative Study Group. J Natl Cancer Inst 1993;85:658–662.

238. Sainati L, Matutes E, Mulligan S, et al: A variant of hairy cell leukemia resistant to alpha-interferon: Clinical and phenotypic characteristics of 17 patients. Blood 1990;76:157–162.

239. Grever M, Kopecky K, Foucar MK, et al: A randomized comparison of pentostatin vs alpha-interferon in previously untreated patients with hairy cell leukemia: An intergroup study. J Clin Oncol 1995;13:974–982.

240. Kreitman RJ, Wilson WH, Bergeron K, et al: Efficacy of the anti-CD22 recombinant immunotoxin BL22 in chemotherapy-resistant hairy-cell leukemia. N Engl J Med 2001;345: 241–247.

241. Thomas DA, O'Brien S, Cortes J, et al: Pilot study of rituximab in refractory or relapsed hairy cell leukemia [abstract 3116]. Blood 1999;94:705a.

242. Nieva J, Bethel K, Baker T, et al: Phase II study of rituximab in the treatment of cladribine-failed patients (pts) with hairy cell leukemia (HCL) [abstract 1535]. Blood 2001;98:364a.

243. Matutes E, Brito-Bapapulle V, Swansbury J, et al: Clinical and laboratory features of 78 cases of T-prolymphocytic leukemia. Blood 1991;78:3269–3274.

244. Maljaei SH, Brito-Babapulle V, Hiorns LR, et al: Abnormalities of chromosomes 8, 11, 14 and X in T-prolymphocytic leukemia studies by fluorescence in situ hybridization. Cancer Genet Cytogenet 1998;103:110–116.

245. Pawson R, Dyer MJS, Barge R, et al: Treatment of T-cell prolymphocytic leukemia with human CD52 antibody. J Clin Oncol 1997;15:2667–2672.

246. Dearden C, Matutes E, Cazin B, et al: High remission rate in T-cell prolymphocytic leukemia with CAMPATH-1H. Blood 2001;98:1721–1726.

247. Keating MJ, Cazin B, Coutré S, et al: Campath-1H treatment of T-cell prolymphocytic leukemia in patients for whom at least one prior chemotherapy regimen has failed. J Clin Oncol 2002;20:205–213.

248. Nash R, McSweeney P, Zambello R, et al: Clonal studies of CD3-lymphoproliferative disease of granular lymphocytes. Blood 1993;81:2362–2368.

249. Tefferi A, Li C-Y, Witzig TE, et al: Chronic natural killer cell lymphocytosis: A descriptive clinical study. Blood 1994;84:2721–2725.

250. Chan JK, Sin VC, Wong KF, et al: Nonnasal lymphoma expressing the natural killer cell marker CD56: A clinicopathologic study of 49 cases of an uncommon aggressive neoplasm. Blood 1997;89:4501–4513.

251. Yamaguchi K, Nishimura H, Kohrogi H, et al: A proposal for smoldering adult T-cell leukemia: A clinicopathologic study of five cases. Blood 1983;62:758–766.

252. Shimoyama M: Diagnostic criteria and classification of clinical subtypes of adult T-cell leukaemia-lymphoma: A report from the Lymphoma Study Group (1984–87). Br J Haematol 1991;79:428–437.

253. Lofters W, Campbell M, Gibbs WN, et al: 2'-Deoxycoformycin therapy in adult T-cell leukemia/lymphoma. Cancer 1987;60:2605–2608.

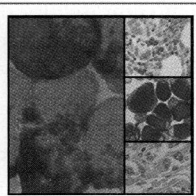

09

HAIRY CELL LEUKEMIA

Martin S. Tallman

Anaadriana Zakarija

LoAnn C. Peterson

SUMMARY OF KEY POINTS

- HCL is an uncommon clonal B-cell lymphoproliferative disorder.
- Physical findings are generally confined to splenomegaly.

- The purine analogs are the treatment of choice.

- Most patients treated with cladribine or pentostatin enjoy prolonged survival.

INTRODUCTION

Hairy cell leukemia (HCL) is a rare chronic lymphoproliferative disorder initially described as a distinct clinical entity by Bouroncle and colleagues in 1958.[1] HCL is characterized by splenomegaly, pancytopenia, and infiltration of the bone marrow with lymphocytes that have irregular cytoplasmic projections when identified in the peripheral blood.[2,3] Immunoglobulin gene rearrangements have established that the disease is a clonal B-cell malignancy.[4-6] The pattern of expression of B-cell–associated surface antigens reflects a degree of differentiation between the immature B cell of chronic lymphocytic leukemia and the plasma cell of multiple myeloma.[7,8] The majority of patients have few symptoms. However, others may develop life-threatening pancytopenia, symptomatic splenomegaly, serious infections, or constitutional symptoms precipitating treatment.[9,10]

Treatment strategies have evolved relatively rapidly as therapy has become more targeted. Splenectomy was the treatment of choice for many years and leads to normalization of the peripheral blood counts in approximately one half of all patients.[11-14] Interferon-α induces a high overall response rate; however, most responses are partial.[14-21] Remarkable progress has occurred with the introduction of the two purine analogs, 2′-deoxycoformycin (2′-DCF)[22-33] and 2-chlorodeoxyadenosine (2-CdA).[24,34-44] Most patients with both previously treated and untreated HCL achieve durable complete remission (CR) with either of these agents, although by molecular techniques, cryptic residual disease can be identified in most, if not all, patients.

EPIDEMIOLOGY

Relatively little is known about the epidemiology of HCL. In the United States, HCL represents only 2% of adult leukemias with approximately 600 to 800 new patients diagnosed each year.[45,46] Although there have been anecdotal reports of familial HCL, there is no clear genetic predisposition.[47-53] The median age of diagnosis is 52 years and the disease occurs in men more often than in women by a ratio of approximately four to one.[54] Although the incidence is similar in the United States and Great Britain,[45,46] classic HCL is reported to be rare in Japan, where a distinct variant form may occur.[55-57]

ETIOLOGY AND PATHOGENESIS

The etiology of HCL has not been determined. There may be an association with exposure to benzene,[58,59] organophosphorus insecticides,[60] or other solvents,[61] but this has not been confirmed.[62] Exposure to radiation,[63] agricultural chemicals,[59] wood dust,[46] and a previous history of infectious mononucleosis[61] have also been suggested as potential associations. The majority of patients have no such exposure identified.

Cyclin D1, an important cell cycle regulator, may play a role in the molecular pathogenesis of HCL. Overexpression of the cyclin D1 protein has been described in HCL patients.[64,65] Unlike mantle cell lymphoma, 11q13 rearrangements are not detected in most cases, suggesting other mechanisms of gene deregulation.[65]

CLINICAL PRESENTATION

The typical presentation is that of a middle-aged man with splenomegaly and pancytopenia. Circulating hairy cells are usually present in the peripheral blood. The initial evaluation of a patient with HCL includes a history and physical examination, a complete blood count with differential count, review of the peripheral blood smear, routine serum electrolytes, blood urea nitrogen and creatinine, hepatic transaminases, a bone marrow aspirate and core biopsy, and immunophenotyping of peripheral blood or bone marrow aspirate by flow cytometry.

At the time of diagnosis, most patients present with symptoms related to anemia, neutropenia, thrombocytopenia, or splenomegaly. Approximately 25% of patients present with fatigue or weakness, 25% with infection, and 25% because of incidental discovery of splenomegaly or an abnormal peripheral blood count.[54]

The majority of patients are relatively well at the time of diagnosis. The most common and often only physical finding is splenomegaly, occurring in approximately 80% of patients.[3,54] The spleen is palpable 5 cm below the left costal margin in approximately 60% of patients. Hepatomegaly occurs in approximately 20% of patients. Unlike many other lymphoproliferative disorders, peripheral adenopathy is uncommon at diagnosis, with less than 10% of patients presenting with peripheral nodes larger than 2 cm. Although adenopathy is not common at diagnosis, internal adenopathy may develop after a prolonged disease course,[66,67] and is present in 75% of patients at autopsy.[68] The characteristic distribution in HCL is likely due to the expression of the integrin receptor, $\alpha 4\beta 1$, by the hairy cells and its interaction with the vascular cell adhesion molecule-I (VCAM-1) found on splenic and hepatic endothelia, bone marrow, and splenic stroma.[69]

Patients with HCL are susceptible to both gram-positive and gram-negative bacterial infections.[70] In addition, patients are also susceptible to atypical mycobacterial infections,[71] particularly *Mycobacterium kansasii*, as well as invasive fungal infections.[70] Other opportunistic infections that have been reported include Legionnaires' disease,[72] toxoplasmosis,[73] and *Listeria monocytogenes* infection.[74] The milieu making patients susceptible to infections is attributable to granulocytopenia, monocytopenia, poor granulocyte reserve and abnormal mobilization,[75] T-cell dysfunction[76] and decreased numbers of dendritic cells and antigen presenting cells.[77]

Patients with HCL may have associated systemic immunologic disorders[78] including scleroderma and polymyositis,[79] and polyarteritis nodosa.[80] HCL has been associated with other cutaneous lesions such as erythematous maculopapules[81] and pyoderma gangrenosum.[82,83] An associated coagulopathy manifested by factor VIII antibodies has been reported.[84] Osseous involvement has also been described, primarily lytic lesions in the axial skeleton, usually the proximal femur.[85,86] Rarely, osteolytic lesions may be associated with paraproteinemia.[87] A rare case of HCL occurring with systemic mast cell disease has been reported.[88]

LABORATORY EVALUATION

Pancytopenia is present in approximately 50% of patients with HCL at diagnosis; most other patients present with suppression of one or two cell lines.[3,54] Most patients with HCL present with leukopenia, although 10% to 20% of patients exhibit a "leukemic phase" with a white blood cell count above $10–20 \times 10^9$ per liter. Monocytopenia is a frequent, but often overlooked finding.[1,3,54] Other laboratory findings include abnormal hepatic transaminases (19%), azotemia (27%), and hypergammaglobulinemia (18%), which is rarely monoclonal.[3,87,89] Unlike chronic lymphocytic leukemia, hypogammaglobulinemia is uncommon.

Hairy cells can be identified in Wright's-stained blood smears from almost all patients with HCL although the number of circulating hairy cells is usually low. Bone marrows are often inaspirable, resulting in a "dry tap." When aspiration is successful, however, hairy cells morphologically similar to those in the blood can be found.

The morphologic features of hairy cells are distinctive (Fig. 109-1). The neoplastic cells are approximately one to two times the size of a small lymphocyte. The nuclei are round, oval, indented, or monocytoid; rarely, they appear convoluted.[90] The nuclei are located in a central or eccentric position. The chromatin pattern is netlike in appearance and nucleoli are indistinct or absent. The amount of cytoplasm varies from scant to abundant and is pale blue-gray in color. The cytoplasmic borders are irregular and exhibit fine, hairlike projections or ruffled borders. Occasionally, cytoplasmic granules are present. Rarely, the cytoplasm exhibits basophilia rod-shaped inclusions that correspond to ribosomal lamellar complexes, observed ultrastructurally in about 40% of cases.[91]

Examination of the bone marrow core biopsy is important in the diagnosis of HCL because of its characteristic histopathology[92-95] (Figs. 109-2 and 109-3). Bone marrow cellularity is variable but is hypercellular in most patients. Hairy cell infiltration may be diffuse, patchy or interstitial, or a combination of these patterns. In patients with diffuse involvement, large areas of the bone marrow are replaced by hairy cells, with complete effacement of marrow in some patients. With patchy infiltration, small subtle clusters of hairy cells are present focally or scattered throughout the bone marrow. Unlike lymphomas, the hairy cells do not form well-defined, discrete aggregates; instead, they merge subtly with the surrounding residual hematopoietic tissue. In the interstitial pattern of involvement, variable numbers of hairy

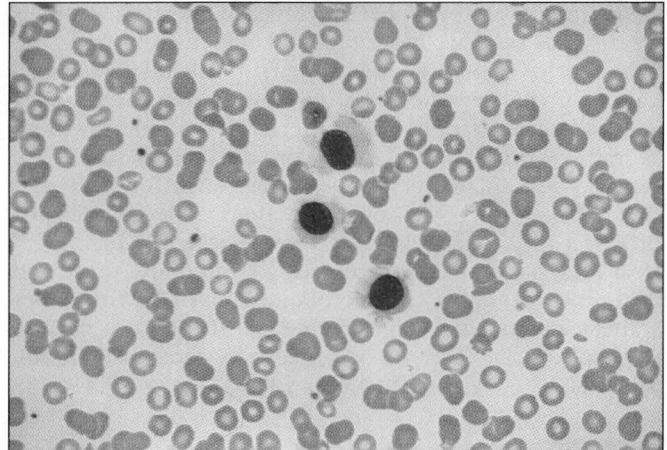

Figure 109-1. Peripheral blood smear from a patient with hairy cell leukemia. The patient was unusual in that he presented with leukocytosis. The hemoglobin and platelet count were reduced. The nuclei of the hairy cells are eccentrically located and exhibit a reticular chromatin. The cytoplasm is abundant and the cytoplasmic borders are irregular, with fine, hairlike projections. (Wright-Giemsa stain)

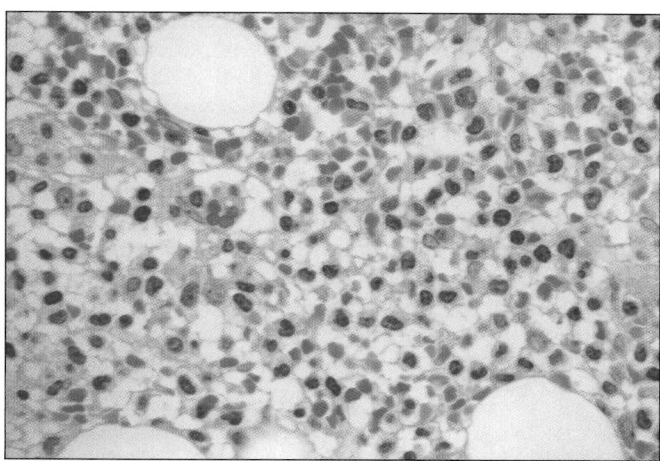

Figure 109-2. Bone marrow trephine biopsy section from a patient with hairy cell leukemia. The bone marrow is hypercellular with a diffuse infiltration by hairy cells. The hairy cell nuclei are widely spaced, separated from each other by a pale, lightly eosinophilic cytoplasm. Many extravasated red blood cells are present between the hairy cells. (Hematoxylin and eosin stain)

cells infiltrate between normal hematopoietic cells and fat with the overall bone marrow architecture preserved. Hairy cell nuclei in sections are round, oval, or indented and widely separated from each other by abundant clear or lightly eosinophilic cytoplasm; rarely the cells are convoluted or spindle shaped. The nuclear chromatin is lightly condensed, nucleoli are inconspicuous, and mitotic figures are rare or absent. Extravasated red blood cells are often seen and blood lakes, similar to those observed in the spleen, may also be observed. Reticulin stains of the bone marrow trephine biopsy in HCL show a moderate to marked increase in reticulin fibers.

Normal hematopoietic cells are usually decreased in HCL; granulocytes are typically more severely reduced

than are erythroid precursors and megakaryocytes. In about 10% to 20% of patients with HCL, the bone marrow is hypocellular. The hypocellularity may be severe[96] and strongly resemble aplastic anemia.

Cytochemical demonstration of TRAP activity has been traditionally used to confirm the diagnosis of HCL.[97] TRAP-positive cells are found in most cases of HCL at diagnosis, although the percentage of positive cells varies greatly among patients. A positive TRAP stain in conjunction with characteristic histopathology is essentially diagnostic of HCL. The routine use of immunophenotyping for the diagnosis of chronic lymphoproliferative disorders has made reliance on the TRAP stain less important.

Flow cytometric immunophenotyping is a critical part of the diagnostic evaluation, both to identify the characteristic immunophenotypic profile of HCL and to distinguish it from other lymphoproliferative disorders. Since hairy cells exhibit distinctive light scatter characteristics and immunophenotype, they can be identified even in very low levels (<1% of lymphocytes) in either the peripheral blood or bone marrow aspirate.[98] This property is useful not only at the time of diagnosis, but also after therapy to assess for residual disease.[99]

Hairy cells show bright CD45 expression with increased forward and side scatter resembling that of large lymphocytes or monocytes. They exhibit a mature B-cell phenotype and express one or more heavy chains and monotypic light chains. The number of cases expressing either kappa or lambda light chains is approximately equal. Surface immunoglobulin is of moderate to bright intensity. Hairy cells strongly express pan–B-cell antigens, including CD19, CD20, CD22, and CD79b. They are usually negative for CD5, CD10, and CD23. They strongly express CD11c, CD25, and FMC7. CD103, an antigen expressed on mucosal T cells and some activated T cells, is expressed in the majority of cases of HCL.[98,100]

Several B-cell–associated antibodies, including CD20, CD79a, and DBA.44, react with hairy cells in fixed, routinely processed tissue sections. Although these antibodies are not specific for HCL, they are useful in documenting the B-cell nature of the infiltrate and highlighting the extent of bone marrow infiltration at the time of diagnosis and after therapy.[101-104]

Splenic involvement in HCL is characterized by diffuse infiltration of the red pulp cords and sinuses, with atrophy or replacement of the white pulp. Blood-filled sinuses, lined by hairy cells, are often present but they are not pathognomonic of HCL; they have been referred to as "pseudosinuses."[105] The liver shows both sinusoidal and portal infiltration by hairy cells. Involved lymph nodes commonly exhibit partial effacement, with hairy cells infiltrating the paracortex and medulla in a leukemic pattern. The leukemic cells often surround residual lymphoid follicles and extend through the capsule.

Clonal cytogenetic abnormalities are present in approximately two thirds of patients with HCL. The most frequently involved chromosomes include chromosomes 1, 2, 5, 6, 11, 14, 19, and 20. In particular, chromosome 5 is altered in 40% of patients, most commonly as trisomy 5, pericentric inversions, and interstitial deletions involving band 5q13.[106-108]

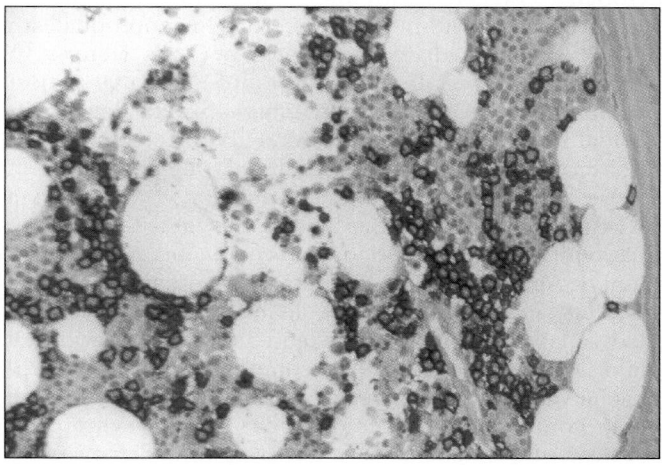

Figure 109-3. The patchy infiltration of hairy cells in this biopsy are accentuated by immunostaining for the B-cell antigen CD20. Residual hematopoietic precursors are negative for CD20. (Immunohistochemical stain for CD20)

Specific Malignancies

III

Differential Diagnosis of Hairy Cell Leukemia

Prolymphocytic leukemia
Splenic marginal zone lymphoma
Hairy cell leukemia variant
Chronic lymphocytic leukemia
Low-grade lymphoma
Agnogenic myeloid metaplasia
Systemic mastocytosis

DIFFERENTIAL DIAGNOSIS

The differential diagnosis of HCL includes other B-cell lymphoproliferative disorders associated with splenomegaly, including prolymphocytic leukemia, splenic marginal zone lymphoma, and hairy cell variant (Table 109-1). Patients with prolymphocytic leukemia typically present with splenomegaly, but this disorder can usually be distinguished from HCL by the marked leukocytosis, the characteristic morphology of the prolymphocytes, and an immunophenotypic profile that differs from HCL.[109-112] Splenic marginal zone lymphoma exhibits some clinical and morphologic features similar to HCL but, in contrast, the bone marrow infiltrates are sharply demarcated from the surrounding normal tissue and intrasinusoidal infiltration is often prominent. In addition, the immunophenotypic profile differs from HCL, including negativity for CD103.[113-116] Hairy cell variant exhibits morphologic features that are intermediate between hairy cell leukemia and prolymphocytic leukemia. Unlike HCL, hairy cell variant is associated with prominent leukocytosis, lack of monocytopenia, and absence of CD25 expression.[117-121] Finally, infiltrates of systemic mastocytosis in the bone marrow may closely resemble HCL. However, immunohistochemical studies show the mast cells, unlike hairy cells, to be negative for B-cell antigens and positive for tryptase.[122]

TREATMENT

Indications

Hairy cell leukemia almost always has an indolent course with some patients surviving 10 years without need for therapy.[123] However, progressive disease eventually leads to complications resulting from anemia, bleeding, splenomegaly, or recurrent infections. Therapy is indicated when the patient has significant cytopenias; symptomatic organomegaly or adenopathy; infections or constitutional symptoms such as fever, night sweats, or fatigue. Persistent blood counts of an absolute neutrophil count less than 1000/μL, a hemoglobin less than 11.0 g/dL, or a platelet count below 100,000/μL, are indications for therapy.

Role of Splenectomy

Splenectomy was the first effective therapy for HCL and remained the initial treatment of choice until 15 years ago.[11-14] After splenectomy, all three cell lines return to normal in approximately 40% to 70% of patients.[13,124] This response is maintained for a median of 20 months in approximately two thirds of patients, and the overall 5-year survival rate is approximately 70%.[124] There appears to be no correlation between spleen size and response to splenectomy. There may be a role for splenectomy in rare selected patients to establish the diagnosis, in rare cases of splenic rupture, or when thrombocytopenia and significant bleeding diathesis exist, as splenectomy can lead to a rapid rise in the platelet count. With these rare exceptions, however, there is little, if any, role for splenectomy since the introduction of the purine analogs.

Chemotherapeutic Approaches

Cytotoxic chemotherapy was given before the advent of more effective therapies in the early 1980s. A variety of agents including anthracyclines,[125] alkylating agents (chlorambucil),[126] and high-dose methotrexate[127] demonstrated activity. Combination chemotherapy, such as CHOP, produces long-lasting normalization of peripheral blood counts.[128] There is one report in the literature of a successful syngeneic (identical twin) bone marrow transplant, in which the patient remained free of disease at least 15 years later.[123] While HCL is sensitive to chemotherapy, there is associated significant myelosuppression and toxicity. Therefore, conventional chemotherapy is now a therapy of primarily historical interest.

Interferon

Interferon was first reported in 1984 to be an effective therapy for patients with HCL,[15] and since then numerous large studies have confirmed its activity.[15-21] The precise mechanism of action of interferon is not known, but may be due to a reduction in the production of cytokines such as granulocyte colony-stimulating factor, granulocyte–macrophage colony-stimulating factor, interleukin-3, and interleukin-6, perhaps related to the characteristic monocytopenia associated with interferon treatment.[129] Recent studies suggest that interferon-α results in apoptotic death of hairy cells, mediated by tumor necrosis factor-α.[130] Despite a high overall response rate of 75% to 90%, most patients achieve only partial remission (PR; defined as normalization of all peripheral blood counts).[18,19] Interferon is commonly administered subcutaneously at a dose of 2 million international units/m^2 three times a week for 12 to 18 months. During the first 2 months of treatment, the white blood cell count and hemoglobin often decrease, occasionally precipitating transfusion. The platelets normalize earliest in responding patients, followed by the hemoglobin and the white blood cell count. An absolute neutrophil count greater than 1500/μl is achieved after a median of 5 months of therapy. The most common toxicities include flu-like symptoms, anorexia and fatigue, nausea and vomiting, diarrhea, dry skin, peripheral neuropathies, and central nervous system dysfunction, usually manifested as depression or memory loss. Elevated hepatic transaminases are the most common laboratory abnormality, other than myelosuppression. The median failure-free survival after discontinuing interferon ranges from 6 to 25 months in different series.[18-20,131] Patients with more than 30% hairy cells in the marrow or a platelet count of less than 160,000μl at the end of treatment have a higher risk of early relapse.[18-20] In addition, patients who express the CD5 antigen appear to respond poorly to interferon.[132] Patients can be maintained on long-term interferon at a dose of 3 million units subcutaneously given three times a week with minimal toxicity. Sixty percent of patients have sustained their initial response for a median of 5 years, 9% discontinued therapy early because of unexpected neurologic toxicity, and only 13% stopped therapy because of progressive disease.[21] Although treatment of HCL with interferon is effective, complete remissions are uncommon, and failure-free survival is usually short after discontinuation of treatment.

Purine Analog Therapy

Twenty-five years ago, Giblett and colleagues observed that 30% of children with severe combined immunodeficiency syndrome lacked the enzyme adenosine deaminase (ADA).[133] It appeared that the accumulation of the triphosphorylated form of deoxyadenosine was responsible for lymphocyte destruction.[134] Therefore, the deliberate inhibition of ADA emerged as a potentially useful antileukemic strategy. The methods to accomplish this included the development of agents to bind irreversibly to ADA or to resist the action of the enzyme. These agents affect both dividing and nondividing cells.[135] After purine analog therapy, accumulation of deoxyadenosine triphosphates leads to DNA strand breaks and inhibition of DNA repair, which ultimately results in cell apoptosis.

Pentostatin (2′Deoxycoformycin)

Pentostatin or 2′-Deoxycoformycin (2′-DCF) was the first agent found to induce a significant number of complete responses in HCL.[22,136] This drug binds to ADA resulting in irreversible inhibition of the enzyme,[137] which is found in all lymphoid cells and is important in purine metabolism. In most studies complete remission (CR) is defined by disappearance of hairy cells in the blood and bone marrow, complete normalization of peripheral counts (hemoglobin > 120 g/L, platelets > 100 × 10⁹/L and absolute neutrophil count > 1.5 × 10⁹/L), and resolution of splenomegaly and lymphadenopathy. A partial remission (PR) requires normalization of blood counts, greater than 50% reduction in hairy cells in the bone marrow, and greater than 50% reduction in splenomegaly.

A number of studies have been published that demonstrate the efficacy of 2′-DCF in patients with HCL (Table 109-2).[23-33] A large prospective, randomized study showed that the complete remission rate and relapse-free survival rate are significantly better with 2′-DCF than with interferon.[31] Various dosing schedules were utilized in early studies, but the current convention is 4 mg/m² IV infusion every 2 weeks until maximum response. The median number of cycles required by patients until best response has been from 6 to 12 cycles.[24,27,29,33] In one of the earlier studies conducted by the Eastern Cooperative Oncology Group, most patients achieved maximal response within the first 6 months.[27] Therapy is relatively well-tolerated, with neutropenia, fever, or infections being the most frequent toxicities.[25,27,32] One of the largest published series providing long-term evaluation was reported by the Southwest Oncology Group.[25] A total of 241 patients received 2′-DCF on a phase III trial comparing interferon to 2′-DCF; 154 were randomized to 2′-DCF initially, while 87 crossed over after failing interferon. Seventy-two percent of patients achieved a complete remission with 2′-DCF. Long-term survival was not statistically different based on initial treatment; in both groups overall survival was 90% at 5 years, and 81% at 10 years (Fig. 109-4). With longer follow-up, 2′-DCF does not appear curative in all patients. Studies with follow-up longer than 5 years after treatment report relapses in 15% to 48% of patients.[23-25,30]

TABLE 109-2

Activity of 2′-DCF in Hairy Cell Leukemia

REF	NO. OF PATIENTS	PREVIOUSLY UNTREATED	MEDIAN NO. OF CYCLES	CR (%)	PR (%)	NR (%)	MEDIAN FOLLOW-UP (MOS)	RELAPSE (%)	MEDIAN TIME TO RELAPSE (MOS)
Johnston[26]	28	18	NA	89	11	0	14	4	13.8
Ho[28]	33	0	NA	33.3	45.5	—	14.5	8	10
Rafel[32]	78	35	7	72	16	1	31	33	29
Cassileth[27]	50	19	6	64	20	16	39	14	CR:13 PR:31
Catovsky[29]	148	23	9	74.3	22.3	3.4	42	8	22
Ribeiro[33]	50	18	12	44	52	0	47	10	22
Grever[31]	154	154	NA	76	3	—	57	9	NA
Maloisel[23]	238	NA	9	79	16.6	—	63.5	15	NA
Dearden[24]	165	38	9	82	15	—	71	24	51.5
Kraut[30]	24	NA	NA	100	0	0	82	48	30
Flinn[25]	241	241	NA	72	—	—	112	18	NA

CR, complete response; NA, not available; NR, no response; PR, partial response.

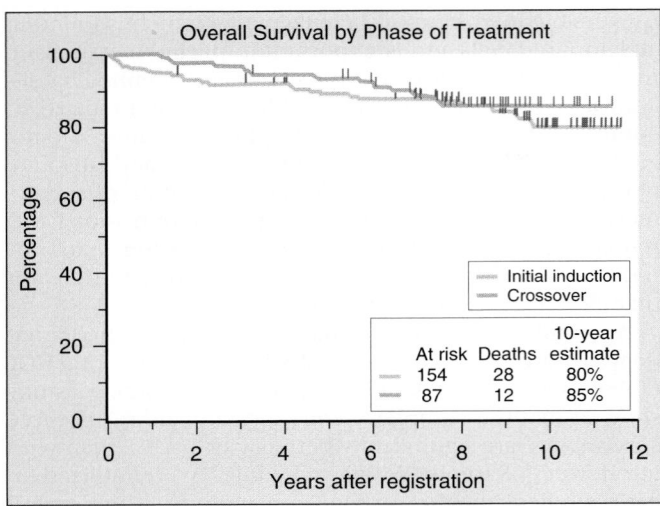

Figure 109-4. Overall survival of 241 HCL patients treated with 2'-DCF, stratified by treatment up front or after failure on interferon. (Reprinted with permission from Flinn IW, Kopecky KJ, Foucar MK, et al: Long-term follow-up of remission duration, mortality, and second malignancies in hairy cell leukemia patients treated with pentostatin. Blood 2000;96:2981.)

Cladribine (2-Chlorodeoxyadenosine)

Cladribine or 2-Chlorodeoxyadenosine (2-CdA) is a purine analog that is resistant to the action of ADA. This agent accumulates in the lymphoid cells possibly because they are rich in the enzyme deoxycytidine kinase.[134] This enzyme phosphorylates 2-CdA to the active 5'-triphosphate form, creating a deoxynucleotide that cannot readily exit the cell. This compound inhibits ribonucleotide reductase, which results in decreased synthesis of deoxynucleotides. Both DNA synthesis and repair is impaired.

The first report showing 2-CdA to be effective for patients with HCL was by Piro and colleagues in 1990.[34] Twelve patients were treated with a single cycle of 2-CdA at a dose of 0.1 mg/kg/day by continuous infusion for 7 days; a complete pathologic remission was obtained in 11 of the 12 patients within 8 weeks of treatment. A number of subsequent studies have shown similar efficacy (Table 109-3).[24,34-44] Clear orders for the 7-day infusion pump are critical since poor response to therapy has been attributed to underdosing of drug when 1 day's dose was administered over 7 days.[138] Alternative dosing schedules and routes have been reported with excellent results (Table 109-4).[139-142] The study conducted by Von Rohr and colleagues administered 2-CdA via subcutaneous bolus injection of 0.14 mg/kg/day for 5 days to 62 patients.[142] The results were similar to previous studies, with 76% of patients achieving a complete remission and an overall response rate of 97%.

The most common toxicities in patients treated with 2-CdA are neutropenia and fever. Investigators at the Scripps Clinic reported the largest collection of patients treated with 2-CdA. In 349 patients who received a single cycle of 2-CdA, 87% had grade 3-4 neutropenia, 42% had a neutropenic fever, but only 13% had a documented infection, none of which were opportunistic infections.[38] Most of the fevers seen with administration of 2CdA do not reflect infection but are likely due to release of cytokines. Due to the high incidence of neutropenic fever, these investigators conducted a prospective trial on the effect of filgrastim in 35 patients treated with 2-CdA.[143] Filgrastim was administered on days -3 through -1, and again after completion of 2-CdA until the absolute neutrophil count was over 2×10^9/L on two consecutive days. When compared to historical controls, the filgrastim-treated group more rapidly achieved an absolute neutrophil count (ANC) of greater than 1.0×10^9/L, in 9 days versus 22 days. The incidence of fever and admission

TABLE 109-3

Activity of 2-CdA in Hairy Cell Leukemia

REF	NO. OF PATIENTS	PREVIOUSLY UNTREATED	CR (%)	PR (%)	NR (%)	MEDIAN FOLLOW-UP (MOS)	RELAPSE (%)	MEDIAN TIME TO RELAPSE (MOS)
Estey[40]	46	27	78	11	11	9	2	17.8
Juliusson[41]	16	3	75	—	13	12	0	
Tallman[42]	20	12	80	20	0	12	5	NA
Piro[44]	144	69	85	12	2	14	3	36
Piro[34]	12	3	92	8	0	15.5	0	
Seymour[35]	46	27	78	11	11	30	20	16
Tallman[36]	50	27	80	18	2	33	14	24
Jehn[37]	42	32	98	2	0	33	14	29
Dearden[24]	45	12	84	16	0	45	29	23.5
Von Rohr[142]	62	33	76	21	3	46	24	38
Hoffman[43]	49	21	76	24	0	55	24	NA
Saven[38]	349	179	91	7	2	58	26	CR:30 PR:24
Goodman[39]	207	119	95	5	0	108	37	42

CR, complete response; NA, not available; NR, no response; PR, partial response.
2-CdA dose: 0.1 mg/kg/d × 7 days by continuous infusion.

TABLE 109-4

Alternate Schedules of 2-CdA Therapy

REFERENCE	DOSING	ROUTE OF ADMINISTRATION	RESPONSES
Juliusson[139]	3.4 mg/m²/d × 7 days	Subcutaneous injection	CR: 75% after 1 cycle 85% after 2 cycles
Robak[140]	0.14 mg/kg/d × 5 days	2 hour IV bolus	CR: 82%; PR: 17.4%
Chacko[141]	0.15 mg/kg/week × 6 weeks	3 hour infusion	CR: 100%
Von Rohr[142]	0.14 mg/kg/d × 5 days	Subcutaneous injection	CR: 76%; PR: 21%

CR, complete response; PR, partial response.

to the hospital, however, was not different in the two groups. Therefore routine use of prophylactic filgrastim is not indicated in this group.

Although response rates are very high with 2-CdA, they are not sustained in all patients. Follow-up after 2-CdA has been shorter than with 2'-DCF, but the experience is similar; that is, relapses have appeared with longer follow-up (see Table 109-3). Investigators at the Scripps Clinic have reported the longest follow-up to date. After a median follow-up of 108 months, 37% of patients have relapsed, with a median time to relapse of 42 months.[39] Initial partial remission is associated with a shorter duration of remission (Fig. 109-5A and B). The response to retreatment remains very good; 79% of relapsed patients were retreated with 2-CdA. The overall response was 92%, including 75% with a complete remission.[39] One retrospective study has suggested that durability of response is greater with 2'-DCF than with 2-CdA; at 45 months of follow-up for each, relapse was 9.7% versus 29%, respectively.[24] There are no randomized trials between the two agents that could resolve this issue. Thus far no plateau has been reached with either agent and relapses continue to occur after initial treatment.

Immunosuppression with Purine Analogs

Both 2'-DCF and 2-CdA produce prolonged immuno-suppression.[41,144-146] A decrease in the total lymphocyte count occurs with 2'-DCF, with a greater reduction in T cells than B cells or natural killer cells.[145] The levels of CD4+ and CD8+ cells decrease to fewer than 200 cells/μl for at least 6 months after 2'-DCF treatment is discontinued. In a series of 15 patients treated with 2'-DCF with long follow-up, the median time to recovery of CD4+ lymphocyte counts to normal was 54 months.[146] Treatment with 2-CdA induces similar suppression of CD4+ lymphocyte counts.[35] The median time to recovery of CD4+ lymphocyte counts to normal after 2-CdA was 40 months. Treatment with 2-CdA affects two distinct subsets of CD4+ T cells. The CD4+/CD45RA+ subset is significantly reduced for up to 5 years, while the CD4+/CD45RO+ T cells, which secrete cytokines and enhance B cell function, are not suppressed.[147] In addition, recovery of CD8 and NK cells is more rapid; they normalize within 3 months of treatment with 2-CdA.[148] This may explain why opportunistic infections, other than an occasional case of herpes zoster, are surprisingly uncommon.[33,38,41,147]

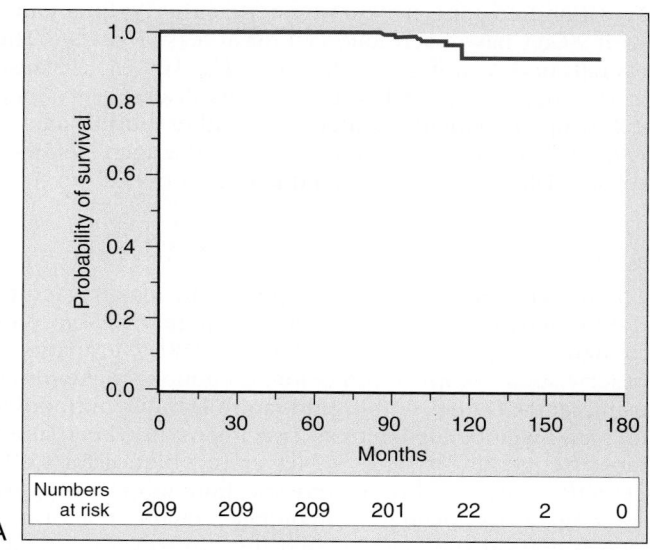

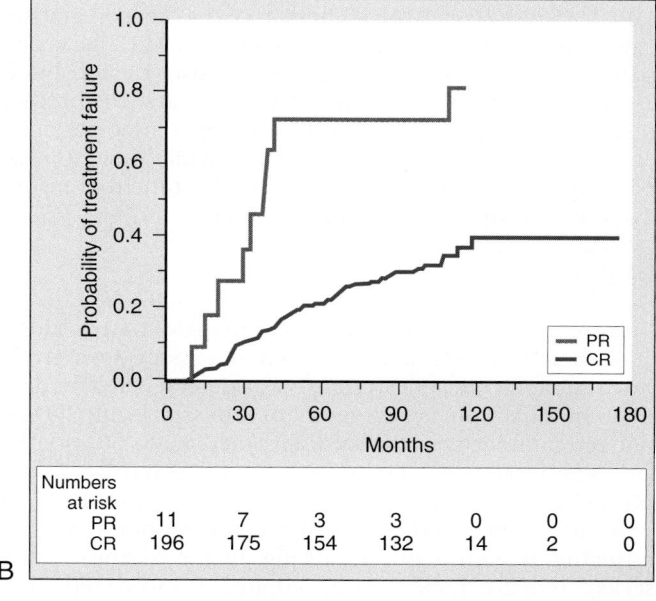

Figure 109-5. A, Kaplan-Meier survival curves for 209 HCL patients treated with 2-CdA and followed for at least 7 years. **B,** Time to treatment failure of 207 HCL after the first course of 2-CdA, stratified by response to first course of therapy. CR, complete response; PR, partial response. (**B,** Reprinted with permission from Goodman GR, Burian C, Koziol JA, Saven A: Extended follow-up of patients with hairy cell leukemia after treatment with cladribine. J Clin Oncol 2003;21:891.)

PROGNOSIS

Before the advent of interferon therapy survival at 4 years was reported to be 68%.[149] With the use of purine analogues durable remissions are attained, and even after relapse retreatment results in good responses. Therefore the 5-year survival rates are over 85%.[24,25,29,33,38,39] Flinn and colleagues report long-term results for 241 patients treated with 2'-DCF; overall survival was 90% at 5 years and 81% at 10 years (see Fig. 109-4).[25] The leading causes of death were second malignancies and infection. Only 2 of 40 deaths were attributable to hairy cell leukemia. Two hundred nine patients treated at the Scripps clinic with 2-CdA have been followed for at least 7 years.[39] The overall survival at 9 years is 97% (see Fig. 109-5A). Because of the indolent natural history of this disease, very long follow-up of patients treated with either purine analog will be required to determine if one of the agents offers a substantially longer remission duration or overall survival.

Evaluation of Minimal Residual Disease

The remarkable activity of the purine analogs has led to the examination of post-treatment bone marrow biopsies to detect minimal residual disease (MRD) in patients otherwise in complete remission. Immunohistochemistry using anti-CD20, DBA.44, and anti-CD45RO antibodies in paraffin-embedded biopsy specimens has been used most frequently.[101-104,150-152] Newer techniques for MRD detection include flow cytometric immunophenotyping or consensus primer polymerase chain reaction.[99] Depending on the criteria used, 13% to 51% of patients in apparent complete remission have evidence of MRD[101-104,153] (Fig. 109-6). There has not been a statistically significant difference in incidence of MRD between patients treated with 2'-DCF and those treated with 2-CdA.[153] The presence of MRD appears to predict relapse.[103,153] In one study evaluating MRD in 66 patients, 50% of those with MRD relapsed, while only 6% of patients without MRD relapsed.[153] At this time there is no evidence to support treatment of MRD.

Treatment of Relapse

Relapse is often detected on bone marrow biopsy alone and immediate retreatment is not necessary. In a study by Kraut and colleagues, relapse was detected at a median of 30 months from achievement of remission with 2'-DCF, but retreatment was initiated at a median of 60 months after first remission.[30] Five of seven patients retreated with purine analogs attained a complete remission. Patients with an initial response to 2-CdA also respond well to retreatment with a purine analog. In the Scripps Clinic series, 76 of 207 patients relapsed, and 79% were retreated with 2-CdA. The overall response was 92%, including 75% with a complete remission.[39] The median duration of the second response was 35 months, which is comparable to the 42-month duration of first response. Responses continue to be seen even with a third cycle of 2-CdA in 80% of retreated patients. Patients who relapse after

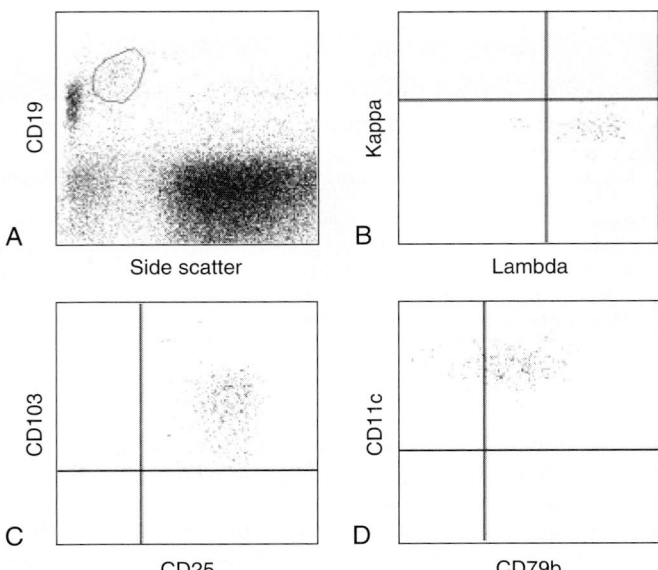

Figure 109-6. Representative example of flow cytometric detection of hairy cell leukemia, comprising 0.2% of peripheral blood sample. **A,** Distribution of CD19 staining versus side scattered light intensity. The circled population represents the hairy cell population. Note the increased side scattered light intensity that is characteristic of hairy cell leukemia. **B,** Distribution of kappa versus lambda staining for this hairy cell population, showing that it is lambda positive and kappa negative, which is indicative of its clonal nature. **C,** Distribution of CD25 versus CD103. **D,** Distribution of CD79b versus CD11c. These histograms demonstrate the characteristic CD19-, CD103-, CD11c-, and CD25-positive staining of hairy cell leukemia.

purine analog therapy may be retreated with either 2-CdA or 2'-DCF. Alternative treatments in relapsed or refractory patients include either BL22 or rituximab (see "Promising New Therapies").

Risk of Second Malignancies

An association has been noted between HCL and second malignancies, although such a relationship is difficult to determine with certainty. Malignancies which have been observed in HCL patients include melanoma, prostate cancer, gastrointestinal cancers, non-Hodgkin's lymphoma, nonmelanomatous skin cancers. It is not clear whether HCL itself increases risk or whether the type of therapy may play a role. Kampmeier and colleagues reported a significantly increased incidence of second malignancies in HCL patients treated with interferon.[154] The British Columbia Cancer Agency reported a 20-year follow-up of 117 patients; 31% developed a second malignancy, of which 30% were diagnosed before the diagnosis of HCL.[155] The risk was elevated regardless of the type of therapy. This association has not been uniformly observed, however.[156,157] Investigators at the M.D. Anderson Cancer Center reported no excess of second malignancies among 350 patients treated with either interferon, 2-CdA, or 2'-DCF.[158] The immunosuppression due to the purine analogs may play a role in the increased malignancy incidence, but the evidence is not clear. Long-term follow-up studies of patients treated with 2'-DCF have not demonstrated a statistically significant increased risk of second malignancies.[23,25] Other studies have suggested that treatment with 2-CdA is associated with an increased cancer risk.[38,39,159] In a review of the Scripps Clinic experience with 349 patients, 8% of patients had a second malignancy that developed at a median time of 62 months after the diagnosis of HCL, and 21 months after treatment with 2-CdA.[38] Of note 11% of the patients in this study had a diagnosis of malignancy before the diagnosis of HCL. Therefore it is not clear that therapy increases risk; HCL itself may have an inherent predisposition to malignancy.

Promising New Therapies

The anti-CD-20 monoclonal antibody, rituximab, has been tested in patients with hairy cell leukemia refractory to other treatments.[160,161] Hagberg and colleagues treated 11 patients with rituximab and report an overall response rate of 64% (Table 109-5).[162] The median duration of response in this group was 14 months. The largest published report describes 24 patients treated with four weekly doses of Rituximab.[163] All the patients had relapsed after prior treatment with 2-CdA, and the median time since treatment was 73 months. Thirteen percent of patients had a complete response, while 13% had a partial response, for an overall response of 26%. One third of responders relapsed after a median follow-up of 14.6 months. It appears that rituximab has activity in some patients with HCL. Thomas and colleagues[164] treated 15 patients with relapsed or refractory disease and observed an overall response rate of 60%.

CD-25, also known as Tac, is the α subunit of the IL2R, and is expressed in 80% of patients with HCL.[165] LMB-2, anti-Tac(Fv)-PE38, is an immunotoxin that contains the variable heavy domain of anti-Tac fused to the amino terminus of a 38 kD truncated form of the *Pseudomonas* exotoxin.[166] It has demonstrated some efficacy in patients with CD25+ hematologic malignancies. After binding to CD25, the compound is internalized and leads to apoptosis and cell death. In four patients who were refractory to standard therapies, including 2-CDA and interferon, all had a response to LMB-2, with one complete response.[166] This treatment is well tolerated and appears to have no hematologic toxicity. Larger studies need to be conducted to better determine the safety and efficacy of this treatment.

Another promising immunotoxin under investigation is BL22, a recombinant immunotoxin containing anti-CD22 monoclonal antibody and PE38, the *Pseudomonas* exotoxin. CD22 is expressed by normal B cells and B-cell leukemias and lymphomas, including HCL, but is not found on stem cells.[167] Kreitman and colleagues recently updated their original study,[168] and presented the results of 23 HCL patients treated with BL22.[169] The overall response was 83%, with 65% of patients attaining a complete response. Of the complete responders, only one had minimal residual disease (MRD) determined by immunohistochemistry of the bone marrow, and none had MRD when peripheral blood was tested by polymerase chain reaction (PCR). The median follow-up was 12 months, and in four patients that relapsed, retreatment resulted in a complete response in three patients. This therapy appears to be well tolerated, although two patients did have a reversible hemolytic-uremic syndrome. No other hematologic toxicity or decrease in T-cell count was observed.[168] This is the first therapy since the purine analogs to show a high complete response. These new therapies have efficacy in patients who are resistant or refractory to the purine analogues, and therefore offer another option for therapy. The durability of effect remains to be determined in larger studies with longer follow-up.

Increased angiogenesis has been reported in patients with HCL.[170-172] Microvessel density is higher in the marrow of patients with active HCL than in normal controls. Treatment with both interferon-α or 2-CdA is associated with a decrease in microvessel density.[170-172] These observations suggest the potential for antiangiogenesis agents.

MANAGEMENT

For patients with newly diagnosed HCL who require treatment (absolute neutrophil count < 1000/μl, hemoglobin < 11.0 g/dl, and platelet count < 100,000/μl or symptomatic organomegaly), we administer 2-chlorodeoxyadenosine (2-CdA) 0.1 mg/kg/day by continuous IV infusion for 7 days as an outpatient procedure by portable pump using a midline percutaneous intravenous central catheter (PICC). If fever of 100.5°F or higher develops while the patient is neutropenic, blood cultures are drawn, urine culture and chest radiography are done, and oral cipro-

TABLE 109-5

Antibody and Immunoconjugate Therapy						
REF	TREATMENT	NO. OF PATIENTS	PREVIOUSLY TREATED	CR (%)	PR (%)	OR (%)
Lauria[161]	Rituximab	10	10	10	40	50
Hagberg[162]	Rituximab	11	11	55	9	64
Nieva[163]	Rituximab	24	24	13	13	26
Thomas[164]	Rituximab	15	15	53	13	66
Kreitman[166]	LMB-2	4	4	25	75	100
Kreitman[169]	BL22	23	23	65	18	83

CR, complete response; OR, overall response; PR, partial response.

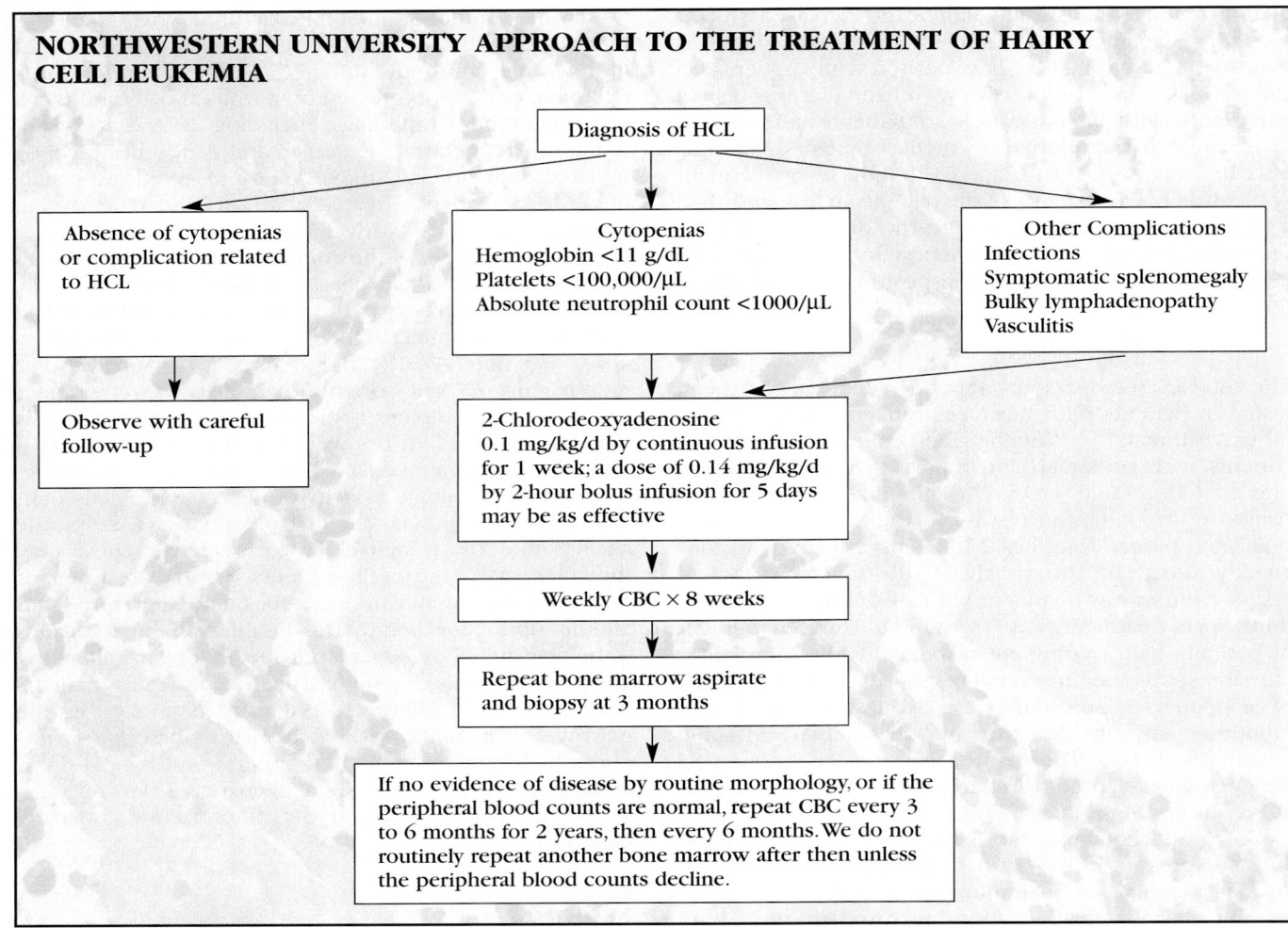

NORTHWESTERN UNIVERSITY APPROACH TO THE TREATMENT OF HAIRY CELL LEUKEMIA

Diagnosis of HCL

Absence of cytopenias or complication related to HCL

Observe with careful follow-up

Cytopenias
Hemoglobin <11 g/dL
Platelets <100,000/μL
Absolute neutrophil count <1000/μL

Other Complications
Infections
Symptomatic splenomegaly
Bulky lymphadenopathy
Vasculitis

2-Chlorodeoxyadenosine 0.1 mg/kg/d by continuous infusion for 1 week; a dose of 0.14 mg/kg/d by 2-hour bolus infusion for 5 days may be as effective

Weekly CBC × 8 weeks

Repeat bone marrow aspirate and biopsy at 3 months

If no evidence of disease by routine morphology, or if the peripheral blood counts are normal, repeat CBC every 3 to 6 months for 2 years, then every 6 months. We do not routinely repeat another bone marrow after then unless the peripheral blood counts decline.

floxacin 750 mg po bid is administered. If cultures are sterile at 24 to 48 hours, naproxen 250 mg PO twice daily is added for 2 to 4 days; 2-CdA is not discontinued. Hematopoietic growth factors are not routinely given. The platelet count is usually the first cell line to recover (within 2 to 4 weeks), followed by the white blood cell count, and finally the hemoglobin. We repeat the bone marrow at 3 months to assess remission status. We currently do not administer a second cycle of 2-CdA for patients with MRD. If the repeat bone marrow at 3 months shows evidence of MRD by either routine morphology or histochemistry, as long as the peripheral blood counts are normal, the patient is followed without further therapy.

For patients with relapsed HCL who have been previously treated with either splenectomy, interferon, or pentostatin (2′-DCF), we administer a repeat cycle of 2-CdA as described previously. For patients who relapse after a single cycle of 2-CdA, we give a second cycle of 2-CdA. For patients with a relapsed HCL previously treated with at least two prior cycles of 2-CdA, we prefer BL22 if available. If BL22 is not available, we consider rituximab. Alternatives include 2′-DCF 4 mg/m^2 IV every 2 weeks for 3 to 6 months or interferon 2×10^6 units/m^2 three times each week for 12 to 18 months.

REFERENCES

1. Bouroncle BA: Leukemic reticuloendotheliosis. Blood 1958;13:609.
2. Catovsky D: Hairy-cell leukaemia and prolymphocytic leukaemia. Clin Haematol 1977;6:245.
3. Golomb HM, Catovsky D, Golde DW: Hairy cell leukemia: A clinical review based on 71 cases. Ann Intern Med 1978;89:677.
4. Korsmeyer SJ, Greene WC, Cossman J, et al: Rearrangement and expression of immunoglobulin genes and expression of Tac antigen in hairy cell leukemia. Proc Natl Acad Sci USA 1983;80:4522.
5. Cleary ML, Wood GS, Warnke R, et al: Immunoglobulin gene rearrangements in hairy cell leukemia. Blood 1984;64:99.
6. Foroni L, Catovsky D, Luzzatto L: Immunoglobulin gene rearrangements in hairy cell leukemia and other chronic B cell lymphoproliferative disorders. Leukemia 1987;1:389.
7. Anderson KC, Boyd AW, Fisher DC, et al: Hairy cell leukemia: A tumor of pre-plasma cells. Blood 1985;65:620.
8. Jansen J, den Ottolander GJ, Schuit HR, et al: Hairy cell leukemia: Its place among the chronic B cell leukemias. Semin Oncol 1984;11:386.
9. Golde DW: Therapy of hairy-cell leukemia. N Engl J Med 1982;307:495.
10. Golomb HM, Catovsky D, Golde DW: Hairy cell leukemia: A five-year update on 71 patients. Ann Intern Med 1983;99:485.
11. Mintz U, Golomb HM: Splenectomy as initial therapy in 26 patients with leukemic reticuloendotheliosis (hairy cell leukemia). Cancer Res 1979;39:2366.

12. Jansen J, Hermans J: Splenectomy in hairy cell leukemia: A retrospective multicenter analysis. Cancer 1981;47:2066.

13. Golomb HM, Vardiman JW: Response to splenectomy in 65 patients with hairy cell leukemia: An evaluation of spleen weight and bone marrow involvement. Blood 1983;61:349.

14. Van Norman AS, Nagorney DM, Martin JK, et al: Splenectomy for hairy cell leukemia: A clinical review of 63 patients. Cancer 1986;57:644.

15. Quesada JR, Reuben J, Manning JT, et al: Alpha interferon for induction of remission in hairy-cell leukemia. N Engl J Med 1984;310:15.

16. Golomb HM, Jacobs A, Fefer A, et al: Alpha-2 interferon therapy of hairy-cell leukemia: A multicenter study of 64 patients. J Clin Oncol 1986;4:900.

17. Quesada JR, Hersh EM, Manning J, et al: Treatment of hairy cell leukemia with recombinant alpha-interferon. Blood 1986;68:493.

18. Ratain MJ, Golomb HM, Vardiman JW, et al: Relapse after interferon alfa-2b therapy for hairy-cell leukemia: Analysis of prognostic variables. J Clin Oncol 1988;6:1714.

19. Golomb HM, Ratain MJ, Fefer A, et al: Randomized study of the duration of treatment with interferon alfa-2B in patients with hairy cell leukemia. J Natl Cancer Inst 1988;80:369.

20. Berman E, Heller G, Kempin S, et al: Incidence of response and long-term follow-up in patients with hairy cell leukemia treated with recombinant interferon alfa-2a. Blood 1990;75:839.

21. Smith JW II, Longo DL, Urba WJ, et al: Prolonged, continuous treatment of hairy cell leukemia patients with recombinant interferon-alpha 2a. Blood 1991;78:1664.

22. Spiers A, Moore D, Cassileth P, et al: Remissions in hairy cell leukemia with pentostatin (2'-deoxycoformycin). N Engl J Med 1987;316:825.

23. Maloisel F, Benboubker L, Gardembas M, et al: Long-term outcome with pentostatin treatment in hairy cell leukemia patients. A French retrospective study of 238 patients. Leukemia 2003;17:45.

24. Dearden CE, Matutes E, Hilditch BL, et al: Long-term follow-up of patients with hairy cell leukaemia after treatment with pentostatin or cladribine. Br J Haematol 1999;106:515.

25. Flinn IW, Kopecky KJ, Foucar MK, et al: Long-term follow-up of remission duration, mortality, and second malignancies in hairy cell leukemia patients treated with pentostatin. Blood 2000;96:2981.

26. Johnston JB, Eisenhauer E, Corbett WE, et al: Efficacy of 2'-deoxycoformycin in hairy-cell leukemia: A study of the National Cancer Institute of Canada Clinical Trials Group. J Natl Cancer Inst 1988;80:765.

27. Cassileth PA, Cheuvart B, Spiers AS, et al: Pentostatin induces durable remissions in hairy cell leukemia. J Clin Oncol 1991;9:243.

28. Ho AD, Thaler J, Mandelli F, et al: Response to pentostatin in hairy-cell leukemia refractory to interferon-alpha. The European Organization for Research and Treatment of Cancer Leukemia Cooperative Group. J Clin Oncol 1989;7:1533.

29. Catovsky D, Matutes E, Talavera JG, et al: Long term results with 2'deoxycoformycin in hairy cell leukemia. Leuk Lymphoma 1994;1(14 Suppl):109.

30. Kraut EH, Grever MR, Bouroncle BA: Long-term follow-up of patients with hairy cell leukemia after treatment with 2'-deoxycoformycin. Blood 1994;84:4061.

31. Grever M, Kopecky K, Foucar MK, et al: Randomized comparison of pentostatin versus interferon alfa-2a in previously untreated patients with hairy cell leukemia: An intergroup study. J Clin Oncol 1995;13:974.

32. Rafel M, Cervantes F, Beltran JM, et al: Deoxycoformycin in the treatment of patients with hairy cell leukemia: Results of a Spanish collaborative study of 80 patients. Cancer 2000;88:352.

33. Ribeiro P, Bouaffia F, Peaud PY, et al: Long term outcome of patients with hairy cell leukemia treated with pentostatin. Cancer 1999;85:65.

34. Piro LD, Carrera CJ, Carson DA, Beutler E: Lasting remissions in hairy-cell leukemia induced by a single infusion of 2-chlorodeoxyadenosine. N Engl J Med 1990;322:1117.

35. Seymour JF, Kurzrock R, Freireich EJ, Estey EH: 2-chlorodeoxyadenosine induces durable remissions and prolonged suppression of CD4+ lymphocyte counts in patients with hairy cell leukemia. Blood 1994;83:2906.

36. Tallman MS, Hakimian D, Rademaker AW, et al: Relapse of hairy cell leukemia after 2-chlorodeoxyadenosine: Long-term follow-up of the Northwestern University experience. Blood 1996;88:1954.

37. Jehn U, Bartl R, Dietzfelbinger H, et al: Long-term outcome of hairy cell leukemia treated with 2-chlorodeoxyadenosine. Ann Hematol 1999;78:139.

38. Saven A, Burian C, Koziol JA, Piro LD: Long-term follow-up of patients with hairy cell leukemia after cladribine treatment. Blood 1998;92:1918.

39. Goodman GR, Burian C, Koziol JA, Saven A: Extended follow-up of patients with hairy cell leukemia after treatment with cladribine. J Clin Oncol 2003;21:891.

40. Estey EH, Kurzrock R, Kantarjian HM, et al: Treatment of hairy cell leukemia with 2-chlorodeoxyadenosine (2-CdA). Blood 1992;79:882.

41. Juliusson G, Liliemark J: Rapid recovery from cytopenia in hairy cell leukemia after treatment with 2-chloro-2'-deoxyadenosine (CdA): Relation to opportunistic infections. Blood 1992;79:888.

42. Tallman MS, Hakimian D, Variakojis D, et al: A single cycle of 2-chlorodeoxyadenosine results in complete remission in the majority of patients with hairy cell leukemia. Blood 1992;80:2203.

43. Hoffman MA, Janson D, Rose E, Rai KR: Treatment of hairy-cell leukemia with cladribine: Response, toxicity, and long-term follow-up. J Clin Oncol 1997;15:1138.

44. Piro LD, Ellison DJ, Saven A: The Scripps Clinic experience with 2-chlorodeoxyadenosine in the treatment of hairy cell leukemia. Leuk Lymphoma 14 Suppl 1994;1:121.

45. Bernstein L, Newton P, Ross RK: Epidemiology of hairy cell leukemia in Los Angeles County. Cancer Res 1990;50:3605.

46. Staines A, Cartwright RA: Hairy cell leukaemia: Descriptive epidemiology and a case-control study. Br J Haematol 1993;85:714.

47. Ward FT, Baker J, Krishnan J, et al: Hairy cell leukemia in two siblings: A human leukocyte antigen-linked disease? Cancer 1990;65:319.

48. Gramatovici M, Bennett JM, Hiscock JG, Grewal KS: Three cases of familial hairy cell leukemia. Am J Hematol 1993;42:337.

49. Begley CG, Tait B, Crapper RM, et al: Familial hairy cell leukemia. Leuk Res 1987;11:1027.

50. Mantovani G, Piso A, Santa Cruz G, et al: Familial chronic B-cell malignancy: Hairy cell leukaemia in mother and daughter. Haematologia (Budap) 1988;21:205.

51. Wylin RF, Greene MH, Palutke M, et al: Hairy cell leukemia in three siblings: An apparent HLA-linked disease. Cancer 1982;49:538.

52. Ramseur WL, Golomb HM, Vardiman JW, et al: Hairy cell leukemia in father and son. Cancer 1981;48:1825.

53. Milligan DW, Stark AN, Bynoe AG: Hairy cell leukaemia in two brothers. Clin Lab Haematol 1987;9:321.

54. Flandrin G, Sigaux F, Sebahoun G, Bouffette P: Hairy cell leukemia: Clinical presentation and follow-up of 211 patients. Semin Oncol 1984;11:458.

55. Katayama I, Mochino T, Honma T, Fukuda M: Hairy cell leukemia: a comparative study of Japanese and non-Japanese patients. Semin Oncol 1984;11:486.

56. Machii T, Tokumine Y, Inoue R, Kitani T: Predominance of a distinct subtype of hairy cell leukemia in Japan. Leukemia 1993;7:181.

57. Yamaguchi M, Machii T, Shibayama H, et al: Immunophenotypic features and configuration of immunoglobulin genes in hairy cell leukemia-Japanese variant. Leukemia 1996;10:1390.

58. Aksoy M: Chronic lymphoid leukaemia and hairy cell leukaemia due to chronic exposure to benzene: Report of three cases. Br J Haematol 1987;66:209.

59. Flandrin G, Collado S: Is male predominance (4:1) in hairy cell leukaemia related to occupational exposure to ionizing radiation, benzene and other solvents? Br J Haematol 1987;67:119.

60. Clavel J, Conso F, Limasset JC, et al: Hairy cell leukaemia and occupational exposure to benzene. Occup Environ Med 1996;53:533.

61. Oleske D, Golomb HM, Farber MD, Levy PS: A case-control inquiry into the etiology of hairy cell leukemia. Am J Epidemiol 1985;121:675.

62. McKinney PA, Cartwright RA, Pearlman B: Hairy cell leukemia and occupational exposures. Br J Haematol 1988;68:142.

63. Stewart DJ, Keating MJ: Radiation exposure as a possible etiologic factor in hairy cell leukemia (leukemic reticuloendotheliosis). Cancer 1980;46:1577.

64. Ishida F, Kitano K, Ichikawa N, et al: Hairy cell leukemia with translocation (11;20)(q13;q11) and overexpression of cyclin D1. Leuk Res 1999;23:763.

65. de Boer CJ, Kluin-Nelemans JC, Dreef E, et al: Involvement of the CCND1 gene in hairy cell leukemia. Ann Oncol 1996;7:251.

66. Mercieca J, Matutes E, Moskovic E, et al: Massive abdominal lymphadenopathy in hairy cell leukaemia: A report of 12 cases. Br J Haematol 1992;82:547.

67. Hakimian D, Tallman MS, Hogan DK, et al: Prospective evaluation of internal adenopathy in a cohort of 43 patients with hairy cell leukemia. J Clin Oncol 1994;12:268.

68. Vardiman JW, Golomb HM: Autopsy findings in hairy cell leukemia. Semin Oncol 1984;11:370.

69. Vincent AM, Burthem J, Brew R, Cawley JC: Endothelial interactions of hairy cells: The importance of alpha 4 beta 1 in the unusual tissue distribution of the disorder. Blood 1996;88:3945.

70. Bouza E, Burgaleta C, Golde DW: Infections in hairy-cell leukemia. Blood 1978;51:851.

71. Marie J, Degos L, Flandrin G: Hairy-cell leukemia and tuberculosis. N Engl J Med 1977;297:1354.

72. Cordonnier C, Farcet JP, Desforges L, et al: Legionnaires' disease and hairy-cell leukemia. An unfortuitous association? Arch Intern Med 1984;144:2373.

73. Knecht H, Rhyner K, Streuli RA: Toxoplasmosis in hairy-cell leukaemia. Br J Haematol 1986;62:65.

74. Guerin JM, Meyer P, Habib Y: Listeria monocytogenes infection and hairy cell leukemia. Am J Med 1987;83:188.

75. Yam LT, Chaudhry AA, Janckila AJ: Impaired marrow granulocyte reserve and leukocyte mobilization in leukemic reticuloendotheliosis. Ann Intern Med 1977;87:444.

76. Van De Corput L, Falkenburg JH, Kluin-Nelemans JC: T-cell dysfunction in hairy cell leukemia: An updated review. Leuk Lymphoma 1998;30:31.

77. Bourguin-Plonquet A, Rouard H, Roudot-Thoraval F, et al: Severe decrease in peripheral blood dendritic cells in hairy cell leukaemia. Br J Haematol 2002;116:595.

78. Dorsey JK, Penick GD: The association of hairy cell leukemia with unusual immunologic disorders. Arch Intern Med 1982;142:902.

79. Blanche P, Bachmeyer C, Mikdame M, et al: Scleroderma, polymyositis, and hairy cell leukemia. J Rheumatol 1995;22:1384.

80. Elkon KB, Hughes GR, Catovsky D, et al: Hairy-cell leukaemia with polyarteritis nodosa. Lancet 1979;2:280.

81. Lawrence DM, Sun NC, Mena R, Moss R: Cutaneous lesions in hairy-cell leukemia: Case report and review of the literature. Arch Dermatol 1983;119:322.

82. Kaplan RP, Newman G, Saperia D: Pyoderma gangrenosum and hairy cell leukemia. J Dermatol Surg Oncol 1987;13:1029.

83. Cartwright PH, Rowell NR: Hairy-cell leukaemia presenting with pyoderma gangrenosum. Clin Exp Dermatol 1987;12:451.

84. Moses J, Lichtman SM, Brody J, et al: Hairy cell leukemia in association with thrombotic thrombocytopenic purpura and factor VIII antibodies. Leuk Lymphoma 1996;22:351.

85. Quesada JR, Keating MJ, Libshitz HI, Llamas L: Bone involvement in hairy cell leukemia. Am J Med 1983;74:228.

86. Lembersky BC, Ratain MJ, Golomb HM: Skeletal complications in hairy cell leukemia: diagnosis and therapy. J Clin Oncol 1988;6:1280.

87. Jansen J, Bolhuis RL, van Nieuwkoop JA, et al: Paraproteinaemia plus osteolytic lesions in typical hairy-cell leukaemia. Br J Haematol 1983;54:531.

88. Petrella T, Depret O, Arnould L, et al: Systemic mast cell disease associated with hairy cell leukemia. Leuk Lymphoma 1997;25:593.

89. Turner A, Kjeldsberg CR: Hairy cell leukemia: A review. Medicine (Baltimore) 1978;57:477.

90. Hanson CA, Ward PC, Schnitzer B: A multilobular variant of hairy cell leukemia with morphologic similarities to T-cell lymphoma. Am J Surg Pathol 1989;13:671.

91. Brunning RD, McKenna RW: Tumors of the Bone Marrow. Atlas of Tumor Pathology, Third Series, Fascicle 9. Washington, DC: Amed Forces Institute of Pathology, 1994, pp 277-278.

92. Burke JS: The value of the bone-marrow biopsy in the diagnosis of hairy cell leukemia. Am J Clin Pathol 1978;70:876.

93. Bartl R, Frisch B, Hill W, et al: Bone marrow histology in hairy cell leukemia. Identification of subtypes and their prognostic significance. Am J Clin Pathol 1983;79:531.

94. Burke JS, Rappaport H: The diagnosis and differential diagnosis of hairy cell leukemia in bone marrow and spleen. Semin Oncol 1984;11:334.

95. Katayama I: Bone marrow in hairy cell leukemia. Hematol Oncol Clin North Am 1988;2:585.

96. Lee WM, Beckstead JH: Hairy cell leukemia with bone marrow hypoplasia. Cancer 1982;50:2207.

97. Yam LT, Li CY, Lam KW: Tartrate-resistant acid phosphatase isoenzyme in the reticulum cells of leukemic reticuloendotheliosis. N Engl J Med 1971;284:357.

98. Cornfield DB, Mitchell Nelson DM, Rimsza LM, et al: The diagnosis of hairy cell leukemia can be established by flow cytometric analysis of peripheral blood, even in patients with low levels of circulating malignant cells. Am J Hematol 2001;67:223.

99. Sausville JE, Salloum RG, Sorbara L, et al: Minimal residual disease detection in hairy cell leukemia: Comparison of flow cytometric immunophenotyping with clonal analysis using consensus primer polymerase chain reaction for the heavy chain gene. Am J Clin Pathol 2003;119:213.

100. Robbins BA, Ellison DJ, Spinosa JC, et al: Diagnostic application of two-color flow cytometry in 161 cases of hairy cell leukemia. Blood 1993;82:1277.

101. Hounieu H, Chittal SM, al Saati T, et al: Hairy cell leukemia: Diagnosis of bone marrow involvement in paraffin-embedded sections with monoclonal antibody DBA.44. Am J Clin Pathol 1992;98:26.

102. Hakimian D, Tallman MS, Kiley C, Peterson L: Detection of minimal residual disease by immunostaining of bone marrow biopsies after 2-chlorodeoxyadenosine for hairy cell leukemia. Blood 1993;82:1798.

103. Wheaton S, Tallman MS, Hakimian D, Peterson L: Minimal residual disease may predict bone marrow relapse in patients with hairy cell leukemia treated with 2-chlorodeoxyadenosine. Blood 1996;87:1556.

104. Ellison DJ, Sharpe RW, Robbins BA, et al: Immunomorphologic analysis of bone marrow biopsies after treatment with 2-chloro-deoxyadenosine for hairy cell leukemia. Blood 1994;84:4310.

105. Nanba K, Soban EJ, Bowling MC, Berard CW: Splenic pseudosinuses and hepatic angiomatous lesions. Distinctive features of hairy cell leukemia. Am J Clin Pathol 1977;67:415.

106. Haglund U, Juliusson G, Stellan B, Gahrton G: Hairy cell leukemia is characterized by clonal chromosome abnormalities clustered to specific regions. Blood 1994;83:2637.

107. Kluin-Nelemans HC, Beverstock GC, Mollevanger P, et al: Proliferation and cytogenetic analysis of hairy cell leukemia upon stimulation via the CD40 antigen. Blood 1994;84:3134.

108. Sambani C, Trafalis DT, Mitsoulis-Mentzikoff C, et al: Clonal chromosome rearrangements in hairy cell leukemia: Personal experience and review of literature. Cancer Genet Cytogenet 2001;129:138.

109. Kroft SH, Finn WG, Peterson LC: The pathology of the chronic lymphoid leukaemias. Blood Rev 1995;9:234.

110. Galton DA, Goldman JM, Wiltshaw E, et al: Prolymphocytic leukaemia. Br J Haematol 1974;27:7.

111. Melo JV, Catovsky D, Galton DA: The relationship between chronic lymphocytic leukaemia and prolymphocytic leukaemia. I. Clinical and laboratory features of 300 patients and characterization of an intermediate group. Br J Haematol 1986;63:377.

112. Melo JV, Catovsky D, Gregory WM, Galton DA: The relationship between chronic lymphocytic leukaemia and prolymphocytic leukaemia. IV. Analysis of survival and prognostic features. Br J Haematol 1987;65:23.

113. Matutes E, Morilla R, Owusu-Ankomah K, et al: The immunophenotype of splenic lymphoma with villous lymphocytes and its relevance to the differential diagnosis with other B-cell disorders. Blood 1994;83:1558.

114. Mulligan SP, Matutes E, Dearden C, Catovsky D: Splenic lymphoma with villous lymphocytes: Natural history and response to therapy in 50 cases. Br J Haematol 1991;78:206.

115. Troussard X, Valensi F, Duchayne E, et al: Splenic lymphoma with villous lymphocytes: Clinical presentation, biology and prognostic factors in a series of 100 patients. Groupe Francais d'Hematologie Cellulaire (GFHC). Br J Haematol 1996;93:731.

116. Isaacson PG, Matutes E, Burke M, Catovsky D: The histopathology of splenic lymphoma with villous lymphocytes. Blood 1994;84:3828.

117. de Totero D, Tazzari PL, Lauria F, et al: Phenotypic analysis of hairy cell leukemia: "Variant" cases express the interleukin-2 receptor beta chain, but not the alpha chain (CD25). Blood 1993;82:528.

118. Cawley JC, Burns GF, Hayhoe FG: A chronic lymphoproliferative disorder with distinctive features: A distinct variant of hairy-cell leukaemia. Leuk Res 1980;4:547.

119. Catovsky D, O'Brien M, Melo JV, et al: Hairy cell leukemia (HCL) variant: An intermediate disease between HCL and B prolymphocytic leukemia. Semin Oncol 1984;11:362.

120. Sainati L, Matutes E, Mulligan S, et al: A variant form of hairy cell leukemia resistant to alpha-interferon: clinical and phenotypic characteristics of 17 patients. Blood 1990;76:157.

121. Matutes E, Wotherspoon A, Brito-Babapulle V, Catovsky D: The natural history and clinico-pathological features of the variant form of hairy cell leukemia. Leukemia 2001;15:184.

122. Horny HP, Reimann O, Kaiserling E: Immunoreactivity of normal and neoplastic human tissue mast cells. Am J Clin Pathol 1988;89:335.

123. Bouroncle BA: Thirty-five years in the progress of hairy cell leukemia. Leuk Lymphoma 1994;14(Suppl 1):1.

124. Magee MJ, McKenzie S, Filippa DA, et al: Hairy cell leukemia: Durability of response to splenectomy in 26 patients and treatment of relapse with androgens in six patients. Cancer 1985;56:2557.

125. Stewart DJ, Benjamin RS, McCredie KB, et al: The effectiveness of rubidazone in hairy cell leukemia (leukemic reticuloendotheliosis). Blood 1979;54:298.

126. Golomb HM: Progress report on chlorambucil therapy in postsplenectomy patients with progressive hairy cell leukemia. Blood 1981;57:464.

127. Joosten P, Hagenbeek A, Lowenberg B, Sizoo W: High-dose methotrexate with leucovorin rescue: Effectiveness in relapsed hairy cell leukemia. Blood 1985;66:241.

128. Cold S, Brincker H: Chemotherapy of progressive hairy-cell leukaemia. Eur J Haematol 1987;38:251.

129. Schwarzmeier JD, Hilgarth M, Nguyen ST, et al: Inadequate production of hematopoietic growth factors in hairy cell leukemia: Up-regulation of interleukin 6 by recombinant IFN-alpha in vitro. Cancer Res 1996;56:4679.

130. Baker PK, Pettitt AR, Slupsky JR, et al: Response of hairy cells to IFN-alpha involves induction of apoptosis through autocrine TNF-alpha and protection by adhesion. Blood 2002;100:647.

131. Ratain MJ, Golomb HM, Bardawil RG, et al: Durability of responses to interferon alfa-2b in advanced hairy cell leukemia. Blood 1987;69:872.

132. Lauria F, Raspadori D, Foa R, et al: Reduced hematologic response to alpha-interferon therapy in patients with hairy cell leukemia showing a peculiar immunologic phenotype. Cancer 1990;65:2233.

133. Giblett ER, Anderson JE, Cohen F, et al: Adenosine-deaminase deficiency in two patients with severely impaired cellular immunity. Lancet 1972;2:1067.

134. Cohen A, Hirschhorn R, Horowitz SD, et al: Deoxyadenosine triphosphate as a potentially toxic metabolite in adenosine deaminase deficiency. Proc Natl Acad Sci USA 1978;75:472.

135. Tallman MS, Hakimian D: Purine nucleoside analogs: Emerging roles in indolent lymphoproliferative disorders. Blood 1995;86:2463.

136. Johnston J, Glazer R, Pugh L, et al: The treatment of hairy cell leukemia with 2-deoxycoformycin. Br J Haematol 1986;63:525.

137. Fox R, Mann C, Kefford R: Deoxyadenosine toxicity to human peripheral blood lymphocytes: Implications for 2-deoxyadenosine as a potential immunosuppressive drug. Cancer Treat Symp 1984;2:33.

138. Golde DW, Jakubowiak A, Caggiano J, Heaney ML: Cladribine underdosing in hairy-cell leukemia: A cause for apparent response failure. Leuk Lymphoma 2002;43:365.

139. Juliusson G, Heldal D, Hippe E, et al: Subcutaneous injections of 2-chlorodeoxyadenosine for symptomatic hairy cell leukemia. J Clin Oncol 1995;13:989.

140. Robak T, Blasinska-Morawiec M, Krykowski E, et al: 2-chlorodeoxyadenosine (2-CdA) in 2-hour versus 24-hour intravenous infusion in the treatment of patients with hairy cell leukemia. Leuk Lymphoma 1996;22:107.

141. Chacko J, Murphy C, Duggan C, et al: Weekly intermittent 2-CdA is less toxic and equally efficacious when compared to continuous infusion in hairy cell leukaemia. Br J Haematol 1999;105:1145.

142. Von Rohr A, Schmitz SF, Tichelli A, et al: Treatment of hairy cell leukemia with cladribine (2-chlorodeoxyadenosine) by subcutaneous bolus injection: A phase II study. Ann Oncol 2002;13:1641.

143. Saven A, Burian C, Adusumalli J, Koziol JA: Filgrastim for cladribine-induced neutropenic fever in patients with hairy cell leukemia. Blood 1999;93:2471.

144. Urba W, Beseler M, Kopp W, et al: Deoxycoformycin-induced immunosuppression in patients with hairy cell leukemia. Blood 1989;73:38.

145. Steis R, Urba W, Kopp W, et al: Kinetics of recovery of CD4+ T-cells in peripheral blood of deoxycoformycin treated patients. J Natl Cancer Inst 1991;83:1678.

146. Seymour J, Talpaz M, Kurzrock R: Response duration and recovery of CD4+ lymphocytes following deoxycoformycin in interferon-α-resistant hairy cell leukemia: 7-year follow-up. Leukemia 1997;11:42.

147. Raspadori D, Rondelli D, Birtolo S, et al: Long-lasting decrease of CD4+/CD45RA+ T cells in HCL patients after 2-chlorodeoxy-adenosine (2-CdA) treatment. Leukemia 1999;13:1254.

148. Juliusson G, Lenkei R, Liliemark J: Flow cytometry of blood and bone marrow cells from patients with hairy cell leukemia: Phenotype of hairy cells and lymphocyte subsets after treatment with 2-chlorodeoxyadenosine. Blood 1994;83:3672.

149. Ratain MJ, Vardiman JW, Barker CM, Golomb HM: Prognostic variables in hairy cell leukemia after splenectomy as initial therapy. Cancer 1988;62:2420.

150. Thaler J, Dietze O, Faber V, et al: Monoclonal antibody B-ly7: A sensitive marker for detection of minimal residual disease in hairy cell leukemia. Leukemia 1990;4:170.

151. Konwalinka G, Schirmer M, Hilbe W, et al: Minimal residual disease in hairy-cell leukemia after treatment with 2-chlorodeoxy-adenosine. Blood Cells Mol Dis 1995;21:142.

152. Matutes E, Meeus P, McLennan K, Catovsky D: The significance of minimal residual disease in hairy cell leukaemia treated with deoxycoformycin: A long-term follow-up study. Br J Haematol 1997;98:375.

153. Tallman MS, Hakimian D, Kopecky KJ, et al: Minimal residual disease in patients with hairy cell leukemia in complete remission treated with 2-chlorodeoxyadenosine or 2-deoxycoformycin and prediction of early relapse. Clin Cancer Res 1999;5:1665.

154. Kampmeier P, Spielberger R, Dickstein J, et al: Increased incidence of second neoplasms in patients treated with interferon alpha 2b for hairy cell leukemia: A clinicopathologic assessment. Blood 1994;83:2931.

155. Au WY, Klasa RJ, Gallagher R, et al: Second malignancies in patients with hairy cell leukemia in British Columbia: A 20-year experience. Blood 1998;92:1160.

156. Federico M, Zinzani PL, Frassoldati A, et al: Risk of second cancer in patients with hairy cell leukemia: Long-term follow-up. J Clin Oncol 2002;20:638.

157. Troussard X, Henry-Amar M, Flandrin G: Second cancer risk after interferon therapy? Blood 1994;84:3242.

158. Kurzrock R, Strom SS, Estey E, et al: Second cancer risk in hairy cell leukemia: Analysis of 350 patients. J Clin Oncol 1997;15:1803.

159. Cheson BD, Vena DA, Barrett J, Freidlin B: Second malignancies as a consequence of nucleoside analog therapy for chronic lymphoid leukemias. J Clin Oncol 1999;17:2454.

160. Pollio F, Pocali B, Palmieri S, et al: Rituximab: A useful drug for a repeatedly relapsed hairy cell leukemia patient. Ann Hematol 2002;81:736.

161. Lauria F, Lenoci M, Annino L, et al: Efficacy of anti-CD20 monoclonal antibodies (Mabthera) in patients with progressed hairy cell leukemia. Haematologica 2001;86:1046.

162. Hagberg H, Lundholm L: Rituximab, a chimaeric anti-CD20 monoclonal antibody, in the treatment of hairy cell leukaemia. Br J Haematol 2001;115:609.

163. Nieva J, Bethel K, Saven A: Phase II study of rituximab in the treatment of cladribine-failed patients with hairy cell leukemia. Blood 2003; 102:810.

164. Thomas DA, O'Brien S, Bueso-Ramos C, et al: Rituximab in relapsed or refractory hairy cell leukemia. Blood 2003;102:3906.

165. Robbins DH, Margulies I, Stetler-Stevenson M, Kreitman RJ: Hairy cell leukemia, a B-cell neoplasm that is particularly sensitive to the cytotoxic effect of anti-Tac(Fv)-PE38 (LMB-2). Clin Cancer Res 2000;6:693.

166. Kreitman RJ, Wilson WH, Robbins D, et al: Responses in refractory hairy cell leukemia to a recombinant immunotoxin. Blood 1999;94:3340.

167. Kreitman RJ, Pastan I: Immunobiological treatments of hairy-cell leukaemia. Best Pract Res Clin Haematol 2003;16:117.

168. Kreitman RJ, Wilson W, Bergeron K, et al: Efficacy of the anti-CD22 recombinant immunotoxin BL22 in chemotherapy-resistant hairy-cell leukemia. N Engl J Med 2001;345:241.

169. Kreitman RJ, Wilson WH, Noel P, et al: Complete remission of chemoresistant hairy cell leukemia with recombinant anti-CD22 immunotoxin BL22, relapse, and status of minimal residual disease in the blood and bone marrow. Blood 2001;98:2662a.

170. Korkolopoulou P, Gribabis DA, Kavantzas N, et al: A morphometric study of bone marrow angiogenesis in hairy cell leukemia with clinicopathological corrections. Br J Haematol 2003;122: 900.

171. Kini AR, Tallman MS, Peterson LC: Abnormal angiogenesis in the bone marrow of patients with hairy cell leukemia (HCL). Lab Invest 1999;79:819.

172. Pruneri G, Bertolini F, Baldini L, et al: Angiogenesis occurs in hairy cell leukaemia (HCL) and in NOD/SCID mice transplanted with the HCL line Bonna-12. Br J Haematol 2003;120:695.

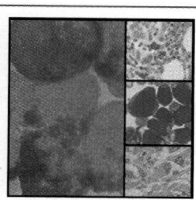

10

MULTIPLE MYELOMA AND RELATED DISORDERS

Paul Richardson

Teru Hideshima

Kenneth C. Anderson

SUMMARY OF KEY POINTS

EPIDEMIOLOGY

- The incidence rate is 4 per 100,000 per year.
- Approximately 15,000 new cases are diagnosed each year in the United States.
- The current prevalence of myeloma in the United States is about 50,000 and there were 10,800 deaths from the disease reported in 2001. Worldwide, it is estimated that there are at least 32,000 new cases reported and 24,000 deaths each year.
- Myeloma is twice as common among African Americans as compared to whites, and affects men more than women.

DIAGNOSIS AND DIFFERENTIAL DIAGNOSIS

- The criteria for diagnosis include presence of monoclonal protein in serum or urine, increased monoclonal plasma cells in bone marrow, plasmacytoma, and/or lytic bone lesions, often with associated osteopenia.
- The disease must be differentiated from monoclonal gammopathy of undetermined significance (MGUS). Smoldering myeloma or indolent multiple myeloma also needs to be defined as therapy for this can be minimal (e.g., bisphosphonates alone), with observation as the standard of care.
- Adverse prognostic factors in patients with multiple myeloma include elevation of uncorrected β_2-microglobulin level, renal failure, hypercalcemia, advanced bone disease, elevated plasma cell labeling index, and abnormal cytogenetics.
- Other unfavorable prognostic factors include elevated lactate dehydrogenase (LDH), thymidine kinase and C-reactive protein values, the presence of circulating plasma cells, plasmablastic morphology in the bone marrow, hypoalbuminemia,

Bence Jones proteinuria, and advanced age.

PRIMARY TREATMENT

- Combinations of alkylating agents produce a higher response rate in myeloma patients than melphalan-prednisone, but the duration of survival is not significantly different.
- Single-agent dexamethasone is active and convenient; combinations of thalidomide and dexamethasone show particular promise, replacing the need for more cumbersome combination chemotherapy.
- Autologous bone marrow or peripheral blood stem cell transplantation (SCT) after high-dose melphalan conditioning is now a standard of care in younger patients in response to initial therapy. The timing of SCT (either early or late) does not affect overall survival, but earlier SCT may have significant advantages in quality of life and event-free survival.
- The role of allogeneic bone marrow or peripheral blood stem cell transplantation in patients under the age of 55 with matched sibling donors is being evaluated in clinical trials. Unrelated donor transplant and allogeneic approaches in older patients remain highly investigational.

SECOND- OR THIRD-LINE THERAPY

- VAD (continuous infusion of vincristine and doxorubicin [Adriamycin] for 96 hours plus dexamethasone, 40 mg orally on days 1 to 4, 9 to 12, and 17 to 20), which can also be used as initial therapy.
- VBAP (vincristine, carmustine [BCNU], doxorubicin [Adriamycin], and prednisone) has been used as combination chemotherapy but is not superior to melphalan and prednisone in combination in terms of overall survival.

- Pulse-dose cyclophosphamide every 2 to 3 weeks with or without steroids such as alternate-day prednisone is useful in patients unresponsive to other therapies.
- High-dose dexamethasone or methylprednisolone (2 g IV three times weekly) is effective as salvage in patients with steroid-sensitive disease.
- Newer chemotherapeutic agents, including liposomally encapsulated doxorubicin, appear active and can be used in the relapsed setting, with its use in earlier disease under study.
- Novel biologically derived therapies including thalidomide, thalidomide and dexamethasone in combination, the thalidomide analog, Revimid, and the recently approved first-in-class proteasome inhibitor bortezomib (also known as PS-341). These agents have transformed the management of relapsed and refractory myeloma, and offer patients more targeted, less toxic, and more effective treatment options. Numerous other agents in the small molecule class are now under study.

SUPPORTIVE CARE

- The management of bone disease has been transformed with the advent of the potent intravenous amino-bisphosphonates, including pamidronate and zolendronic acid. The role of an important new inhibitor of osteoclast activation, osteoprotegrin (OPG) is under study. Other strategies in the management of bone disease include kyphoplasty.
- The use of growth factors, including erythropoietin for the treatment of anemia and granulocyte colony-stimulating factor for therapy-related neutropenia has improved patient management.

INTRODUCTION

The monocolonal gammopathies (paraproteinemias, dysproteinemias) are a group of diseases characterized by the proliferation of a single clone of plasma cells, which produces an electrophoretically and immunologically homogeneous (monoclonal) protein (M component, M protein, or paraprotein). Each M protein consists of two heavy (H) polypeptide chains of the same class and subclass and two light (L) polypeptide chains of the same type. The heavy chains are designated by Greek letters: γ in immunoglobulin G (IgG), α in immunoglobulin A (IgA), μ in immunoglobulin M (IgM), δ in immunoglobulin D (IgD), and ε in immunoglobulin E (IgE). The subclasses of IgG are IgG1, IgG2, IgG3, and IgG4. There are two subclasses of IgA: IgA1 and IgA2. The light chains are kappa (κ) and lambda (λ).

A complete classification of monoclonal gammopathies is given in Table 110-1. The distribution of serum monoclonal proteins in 993 new cases at the Mayo Clinic during 1996 reported by Kyle and colleagues and the diagnoses associated with the detection of a monoclonal gammopathy in the same period are shown in Figures 110-1 and 110-2, respectively.

MULTIPLE MYELOMA

Multiple myeloma (also described as plasma cell myeloma, myelomatosis, or Kahler's disease) is characterized by the neoplastic proliferation of a single clone of plasma cells

TABLE 110-1

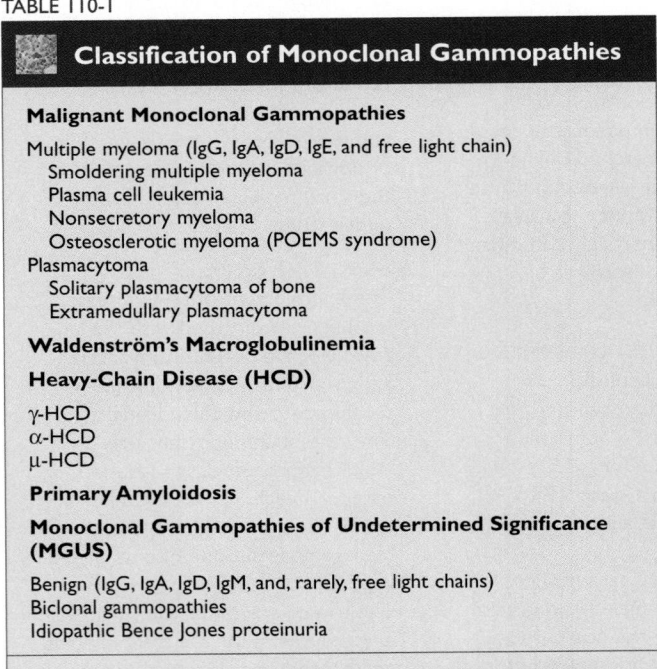

Classification of Monoclonal Gammopathies

Malignant Monoclonal Gammopathies

Multiple myeloma (IgG, IgA, IgD, IgE, and free light chain)
  Smoldering multiple myeloma
  Plasma cell leukemia
  Nonsecretory myeloma
  Osteosclerotic myeloma (POEMS syndrome)
Plasmacytoma
  Solitary plasmacytoma of bone
  Extramedullary plasmacytoma

Waldenström's Macroglobulinemia

Heavy-Chain Disease (HCD)

γ-HCD
α-HCD
μ-HCD

Primary Amyloidosis

Monoclonal Gammopathies of Undetermined Significance (MGUS)

Benign (IgG, IgA, IgD, IgM, and, rarely, free light chains)
Biclonal gammopathies
Idiopathic Bence Jones proteinuria

From Kyle RA: Classification and diagnosis of monoclonal gammopathies. In Rose NR, Friedman H, Fahey JL (eds): Manual of Clinical Laboratory Immunology, 3rd ed. Washington, DC, American Society for Microbiology, 1986, p 152.

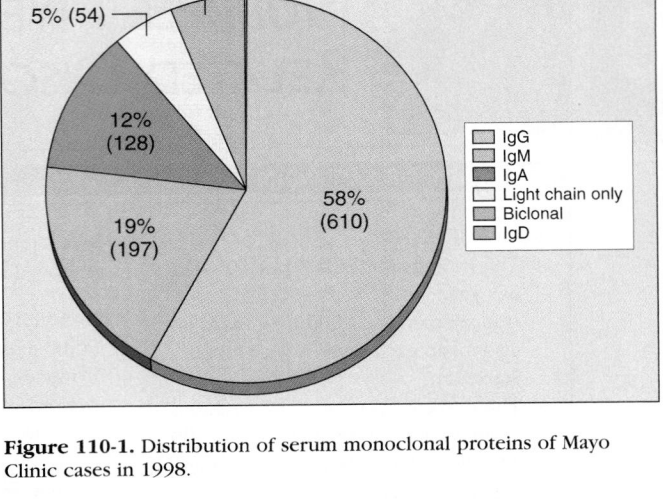

Figure 110-1. Distribution of serum monoclonal proteins of Mayo Clinic cases in 1998.

and plasmacytoid cells, almost always producing a monoclonal immunoglobulin (Ig) or Ig fragment. The plasma cell proliferation usually results in extensive skeletal destruction with osteopenia, osteolytic lesions, hypercalcemia, anemia, and, occasionally, plasma cell infiltration in different organs and soft tissues. The excessive production of M protein can lead to recurrent bacterial infections, renal failure, or less commonly hyperviscosity syndrome. Although multiple myeloma was first described in 1844 by Solly and subsequently in 1850 by MacIntyre, it was only occasionally recognized until 1889, when Kahler reported the case history of a patient named Dr. Loos. Kahler recognized the unique protein in the patient's urine, which had in fact been described by Henry Bence Jones almost 50 years earlier, and correlated this finding with the clinical syndrome. In 1890 the plasma

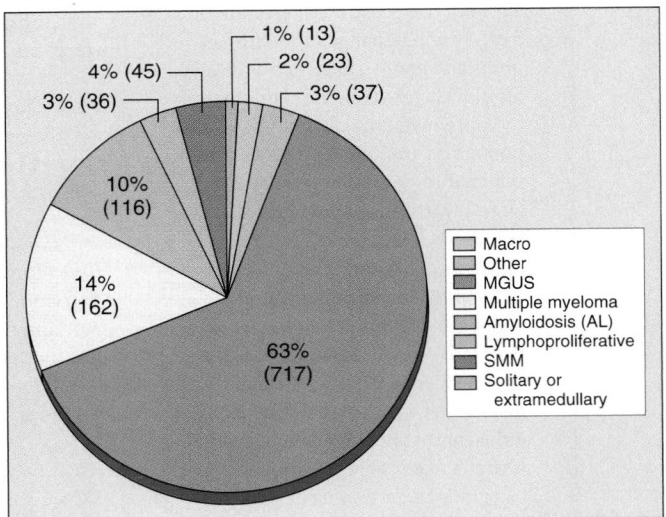

Figure 110-2. Types of monoclonal gammopathies in Mayo Clinic cases in 1998. The total number of patients differs in Figures 110-1 and 110-2 because not all patients have a serum monoclonal protein. Macro, macroglobulinemia; MGUS, monoclonal gammopathy of undetermined significance; SMM, smoldering multiple myeloma.

cell was discovered and by 1900 multiple myeloma was associated with plasmacytosis in the bone marrow. Electrophoresis of serum and urine Ig was accomplished in 1939 and immunoelectrophoresis followed in 1953.[1,2]

Etiology and Epidemiology

The cause of multiple myeloma (MM) is not established. Radiation exposure may play a role in some patients. Thus an increased risk of MM has been reported in atomic bomb survivors exposed to more than 50 Gy,[3] as well as in radiologists exposed to relatively large doses of long-term radiation. While one study suggested that workers in nuclear plants were at a higher risk of the development of MM, people living nearby had no increased risk.[4] Increased risk has been reported in farmers, especially in those who extensively use herbicides and insecticides, woodworkers and furniture manufacturers, presumably from exposure to chemical resins, paper producers, and in people exposed to organic solvents, although unlike leukemia, there is no increased risk of MM with benzene exposure.[4,5]

MM has been reported in familial clusters of two or more first-degree relatives and in identical twins. A relationship between MM and preexisting chronic inflammatory diseases has been suggested, and in experimental studies plasma cell dyscrasias associated with protracted stimulation of the reticuloendothelial system have been well demonstrated.[6] These reports raised the hypothesis that repeated chronic antigenic stimulation could contribute to the development of MM, although a case control study provided no support for the role of chronic antigenic stimulation.[7] Kaposi's sarcoma–associated herpes virus (KSHV; also known as human herpes virus-8 [HHV-8]) was found in patients with MM in bone marrow dendritic cells, and in some patients with monoclonal gammopathy of undetermined significance (MGUS), which suggested that KSHV may be required for transformation from MGUS to MM and perpetuate the growth of malignant plasma cells, but subsequent studies have failed to reproduce this observation.[8]

The annual incidence of MM is approximately 4 per 100,000.[5,9] The apparent increase during the past decades is probably in part related to increased screening with measurement of serum protein and the use of better diagnostic techniques, although an actual increase is also likely to be contributing, paralleling that seen with non-Hodgkin's lymphoma, and may be related to environmental toxins.[9,10] MM represents 1% of all malignant diseases and about 10% of hematologic malignancies, but as such constitutes the second most common hematologic malignancy after the non-Hodgkin's lymphomas. MM occurs in all races and all geographic areas, although rates are lower in Asian populations. The incidence among African Americans is twice that of white Americans, is higher in Pacific islanders, and is slightly more frequent in men than in women. The median age at diagnosis is 60 years, and while in the past only 18% and 3% of patients were younger than 50 and 40 years, respectively, the percentages among younger patients appear to be increasing.[11]

Biologic Characteristics

MM is a B-cell malignancy with mature plasma cell morphology. In most cases, malignant plasma cells are phenotypically cIg+, CD38+, PCA-1+, CD56+, and BB-4+ (CD138+), and only a minority express CD10, HLA-DR, and CD20.[12] The clonogenic cell in MM appears to be a relatively mature cell, already committed to idiotypic production of immunoglobulins but sometimes expressing aberrant markers, and studies identifying translocations involving switch regions have confirmed that the final oncogenic event occurs relatively late in B cell development in the lymph node.[13,14] There is also evidence that plasma cell precursors of myeloma circulate in peripheral blood.[15] MM Ig gene sequence analysis has revealed frequent somatic mutations, antigenic selection, and lack of intraclonal diversity or clonal progression, with the Ig VDJ gene rearrangement sequence appearing to be an important tumor marker.[12,15,16] In these studies, Ig variable (VH) gene sequence analysis has shown MM tumor cells to be postfollicular, with the mutated homogenous clonal sequences indicating no continuing exposure to somatic hypermutation.[15] Thus abnormalities of 14 q (the location of IgH) are most common in MM. Since proto-oncogenes are translocated to this region and overexpressed in B cell malignancies, they may also play a role in the oncogenesis of MM.

Cytogenetic studies in MM are difficult because of the low proliferative activity of plasma cells. Thus conventional cytogenetic studies show abnormal karyotypes in 30% to 40% of patients, when the percentage is now recognized to be actually much higher.[17] Cytogenetic analysis of bone marrow cultures stimulated with cytokines improves the results, identifying chromosome abnormalities in about 50% of patients with newly diagnosed MM.[18] Commensurate with this, between 50% and 70% of patients with myeloma have DNA aneuploidy when studied by flow cytometry. In a recent large study, 56% (142 of 257) of patients had DNA aneuploidy (53% hyperdiploid, 3% hypodiploid).[19] Moreover, fluorescence in situ hybridization analysis (FISH) using chromosome-specific probes identifies chromosome abnormalities in up to 80% of patients with MM.[20] With more sophisticated techniques such as spectral karyotyping (SKY) the incidence of significant cytogenetic abnormalities increases to almost 100%. In addition, approximately 50% of persons with MGUS already have the chromosome characteristics of a plasma cell malignancy at FISH analysis.[21] The clinical significance of this cytogenetic finding in MGUS is still unknown but does not appear to predict for progression.[3]

The incidence of chromosomal alterations varies depending upon the methodology used. Specific chromosome changes involve 14q32 in the majority of cases, with partner chromosomes at gene loci encoding transcription and growth factors[12,14,22] (Fig. 110-3). C-myc mRNA and c-myc gene rearrangement have been reported in isolated cases.[22] Increased levels of p21 (H-ras product) were found in 74% of patients with DNA aneuploidy; the presence of increased p21 was associated with a shorter survival.[23] In one study, ras mutations were found in

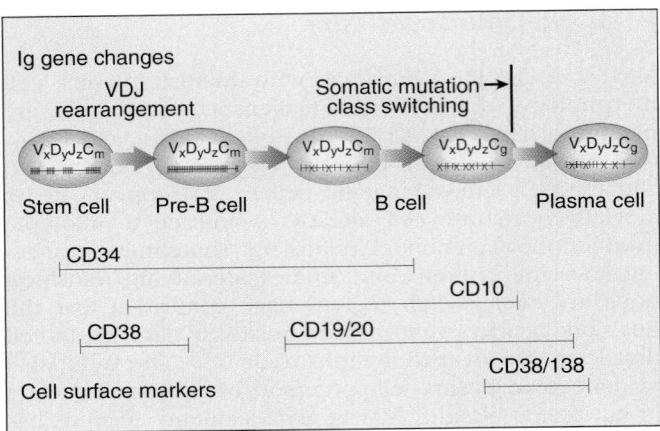

Figure 110-3. Identification of the tumor cell in MM. (From Kuehl WM: Multiple myeloma: Evolving genetic events and host interactions. Nat Rev Cancer 2002;3:175.)

47% (14 of 30) of patients with MM.[24] Patients with ras mutations usually have advanced or terminal disease and resistance to chemotherapy. Point mutations of the tumor suppressor gene p53 in myeloma cell lines have been reported.[25] Specifically, in three studies, 3% (1 of 37),[26] 20% (6 of 30),[23] and 13% (7 of 52)[27] of patients with MM had point mutations of the p53 gene. Deletion of the retinoblastoma gene (Rb-1) has been reported to occur in about 50% (12 of 23) of patients with MM studied by FISH.[28] Finally, deletions of p15, p16, and p18 recently were identified in 2 of 17 patients with MM.[29]

T cells play an important role in normal B-cell differentiation. In patients with MM, CD4 T cells often are reduced in both percentage and absolute numbers.[30] Overproduction of interleukin-1 (IL-1) and tumor necrosis factor (TNF), which have bone-resorbing activity, has been found in patients with MM.[31] It is now well established that interleukin-6 (IL-6) is a potent myeloma cell growth factor.[32] Serum IL-6 levels have been shown to correlate with disease activity and tumor cell mass in patients with MM. The increased IL-6 serum levels described in patients with an aggressive terminal phase of MM resistant to chemotherapy, as well as in those with plasma cell leukemia, support the concept that this cytokine is an important factor in the growth and progression of MM.[33] Its key role in the tumor microenvironment is elaborated in the following section.

Role of Bone Marrow in MM Pathogenesis

The hypothesis that circulating clonogenic premyeloma cells, by means of adhesion molecules, home to the bone marrow (BM), where they find an appropriate microenvironment (cytokine network) to differentiate and further expand the disease, has been supported by the results of a number of recent studies.[14] We have characterized the mechanisms whereby MM cells home to the host bone marrow and adhere to bone marrow stromal cells (BMSCs) and extracellular matrix (ECM) proteins, as well as the functional sequelae of this binding, in order to identify targets for novel therapies (Fig. 110-4). Of

importance, our past studies have identified those adhesion molecules mediating MM cell binding to fibronectin and BMSCs, as well as the MM cell growth and survival advantage conferred by this binding.[24-27]

Our studies show that BMSCs secrete cytokines, such as interleukin-6 (IL-6)[28] and insulin-like growth factor 1 (IGF-1),[29] which augment MM cell growth, survival, and drug resistance of MM cells in the bone marrow milieu. Besides localizing tumor cells in the bone marrow microenvironment, our studies demonstrate that adhesion of MM cells to BMSCs also triggers the paracrine NF-kB–dependent transcription and secretion in BMSCs of IL-6, the major cytokine mediating MM cell growth, survival, and resistance to drug (dexamethasone [Dex])-induced apoptosis via MAPK and PI3-K/Akt, Jak/STAT, and PI3-K/Akt signaling cascades, respectively.[25,29,34-46] More recently, we have shown that vascular endothelial growth factor (VEGF) is secreted by both MM cells and BMSCs, that its secretion is similarly upregulated by binding of MM cells to BMSCs, and that it augments MM cell growth (MAPK signaling) and migration (PKC-dependent cascade).[47-49] It stimulates angiogenesis, although the pathophysiologic significance of angiogenesis in MM bone marrow is undefined.[50,51]

Although tumor necrosis factor-alpha (TNF-α) does not directly alter MM cell growth and survival, our recent studies show that it induces NF-kB–dependent upregulation in cell surface expression of adhesion molecules (ICAM-1, VCAM-1) on both MM cells and BMSCs, resulting in increased binding and related induction of IL-6 transcription and secretion in BMSCs[52] (Fig. 110-5). Others have shown that MM cell adhesion to fibronectin confers conventional drug resistance with induction of p27 and G1 growth arrest.[53] Excitingly, novel agents including thalidomide (Thal) and its immunomodulatory derivatives (IMiDs),[49,54] as well as proteasome inhibitor PS-341,[52,55] can target both the tumor cell and its bone marrow microenvironment and thereby overcome cell adhesion–mediated (CAM) drug resistance (Figs. 110-6 and 110-7).

Recombinant IL-1β stimulates MM cells to produce IL-6, which consequently augments proliferation of MM cells.[56] Transforming growth factor-β (TGF-β) is secreted by MM cells and triggers IL-6 secretion in BMSCs,[57] augmenting that paracrine IL-6–mediated tumor cell growth. TGF-β secreted by MM cells likely also contributes to the immunodeficiency characteristic of MM by downregulating B cells, T cells, and natural killer cells, without similarly inhibiting the growth of MM cells. IL-10 is a proliferation factor, but not a differentiation factor, for human MM cells.[58] Insulin-like growth factor (IGF-1) has been shown to augment MM cell growth, survival, and drug resistance.[29] Macrophage inflammatory protein-1α (MIP-1α) is a potential osteoclast stimulatory factor in MM.[59] Autocrine growth mediated by IL-15,[60] and most recently IL-21,[61] has been demonstrated in both MM cell lines and patient cells.

Clinical Manifestations

The clinical manifestations and laboratory findings of patients with multiple myeloma are broad and reflect the

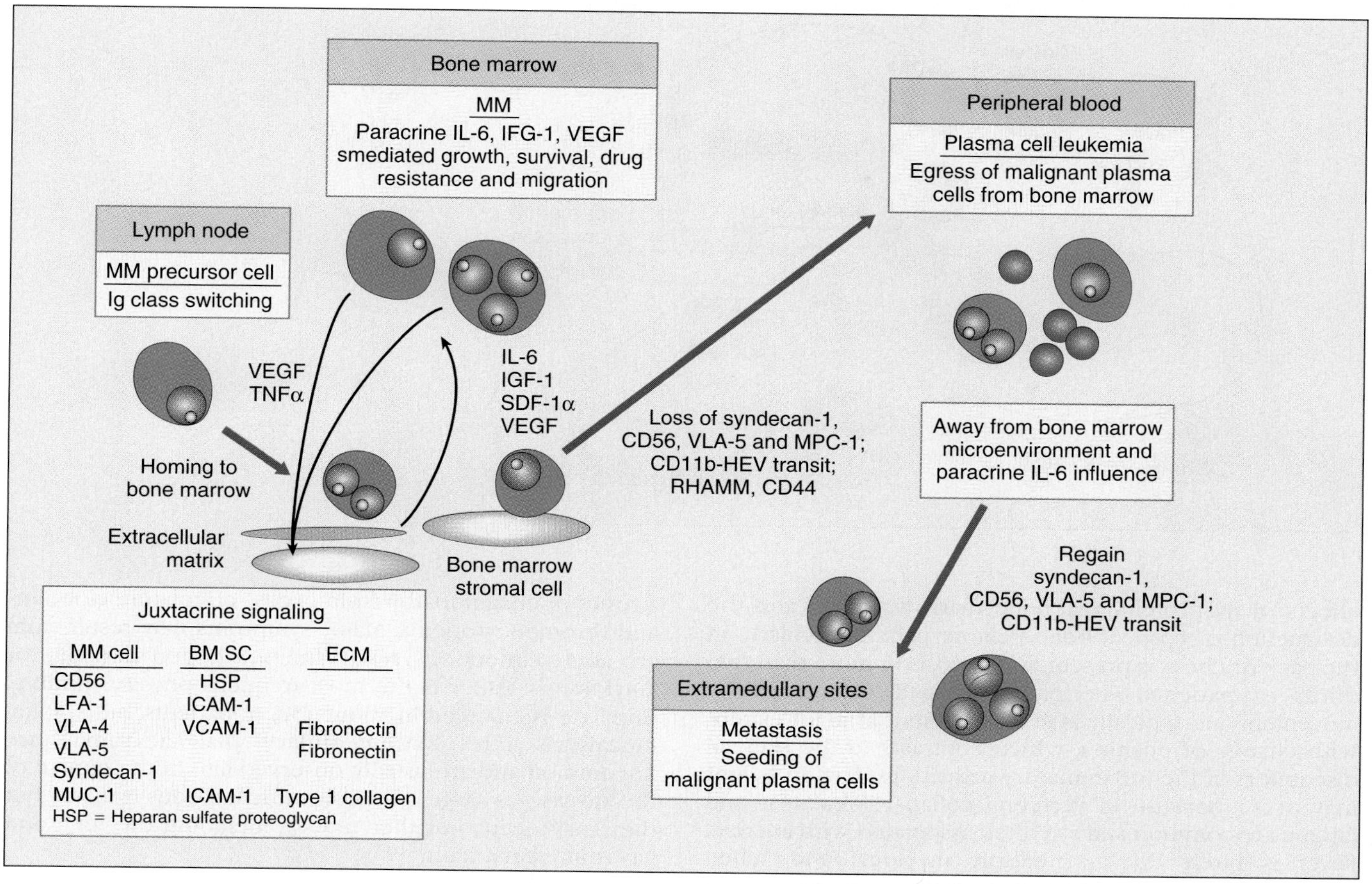

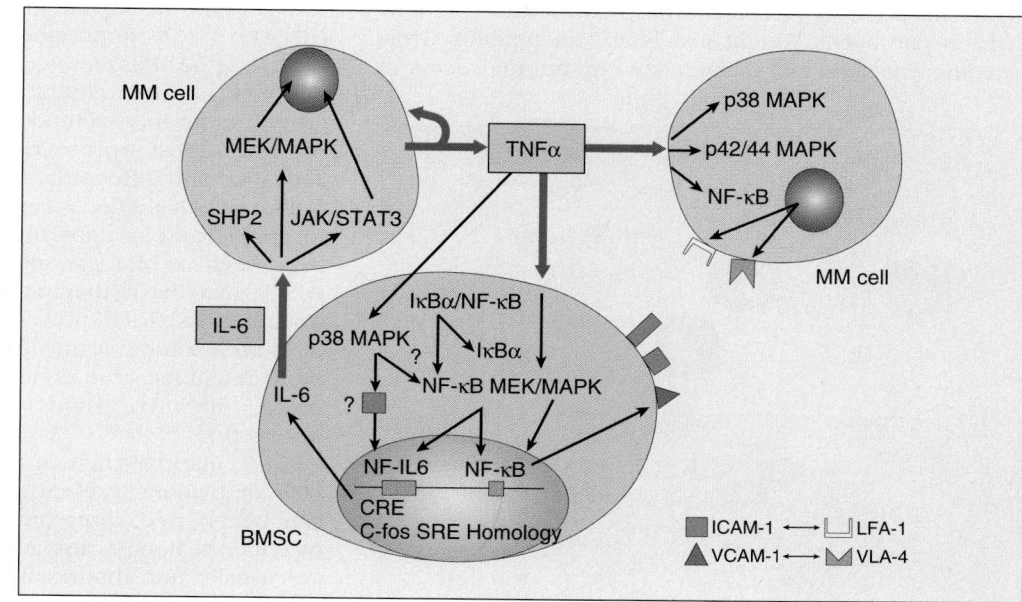

Figure 110-4. MM progression: Role of adhesion molecules. (From Teoh G: Interaction of tumor and host cells with adhesion and extracellular matrix molecules in the development of multiple myeloma. Hematol Oncol Clin North Am 1997;11:27.)

Figure 110-5. Role of TNF-α in the pathophysiology of MM.

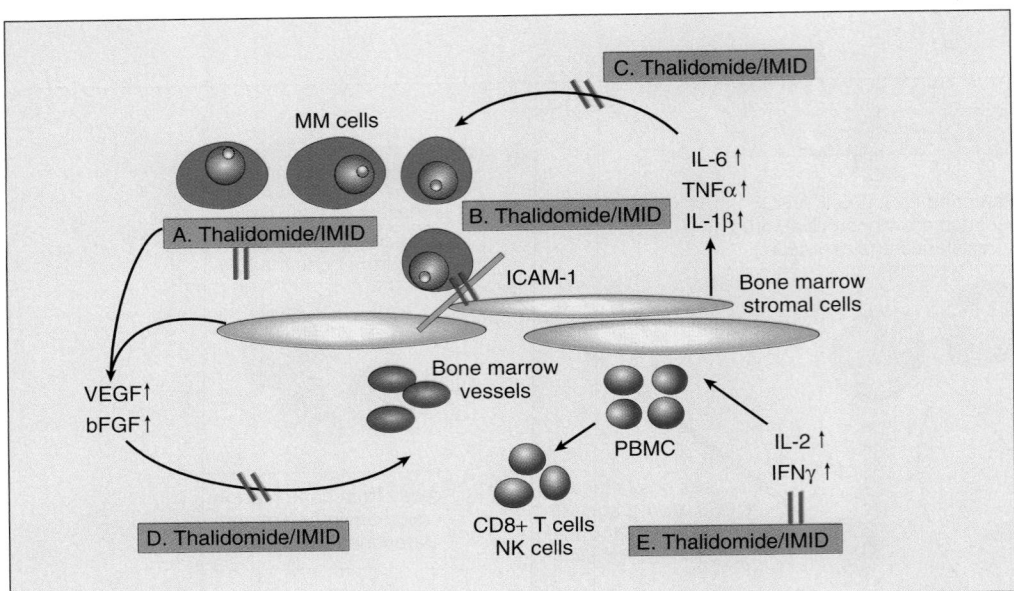

Figure 110-6. Thal/IMiDs target MM cells in the BM microenvironment.

effects of dysproteinemia, bone marrow failure, and the destruction of cortical bone.[34] Bone pain, particularly in the back or chest, is present at diagnosis in more than two thirds of patients. The pain is usually worsened by movement and typically is less prominent at night except with change of position, which contrasts to the skeletal discomfort of the inflammatory arthritides. Loss in height may occur because of vertebral collapse. Weakness and fatigue are common and are often associated with anemia. Fever is rarely due to multiple myeloma and, when present, is most often from an infectious process, which occur frequently as the immune dysfunction caused by the suppression of normal immunoglobulin production and function is profound. Upper respiratory tract and sinus infections are the most common, and encapsulated organisms such as *Streptococcus pneumoniae* predominate as pathogens. Weight loss is not uncommon. Gross bleeding, epistaxis, and purpura are rare but may occur as

a result of coagulopathy from excess circulating globulins and thrombocytopenia. Major symptoms may result from an acute infection, renal failure, hypercalcemia, or amyloidosis. Pallor is the most frequent physical finding. The liver is enlarged in about 15% of patients, but splenomegaly is rare. Extramedullary plasmacytomas are uncommon and are usually observed late in the course of the disease as large, purplish, subcutaneous masses, but they may occur in other tissues, including the lung and gastrointestinal tract.

Bone Disease and Hypercalcemia

Proposed osteoclast-activating factors in MM include lymphotoxin (LT), TNF-α, hepatocyte growth factor (HGF), IL-6, IL-1, metalloproteinases (MMP1, MMP2, MMP9), RANKL, and insulin-like growth factor binding protein 4 (IGF4).[62-66] Of importance, macrophage inflammatory protein-1α (MIP-Ia) induces OCL formation in human BM cultures[67]; conversely, blocking MIP-1α inhibits tumor growth in an in vivo model of bone disease.[59] The levels of RANKL/osteoprotegrin ligand (OPGL), an OCL activation and differentiation factor, and of osteoprotegrin (OPG), which is a decoy receptor for OPGL, modulate OCL formation; and an imbalance favoring OCL activation has been seen in MM patients.[68-70] OPG, which neutralizes OPGL, may have therapeutic application in MM bone disease.[66] RANK-Fc molecule, a fusion of the Fc portion of Ig to a soluble form of the RANK receptor, has been evaluated alone or in combination with bisphosphonates using in vivo models, and also blocks bone destruction.[71,72]

Emblematic of the central role of bone disease in MM, 80% of patients present with bone pain. Bone lesions can be isolated, discrete lytic abnormalities, or diffuse osteopenia. Bone scans and serum alkaline phosphatase are usually not abnormal, but conventional radiographs show abnormalities consisting of punched-out lytic lesions (Fig. 110-8), osteoporosis, or fractures in up to 75%

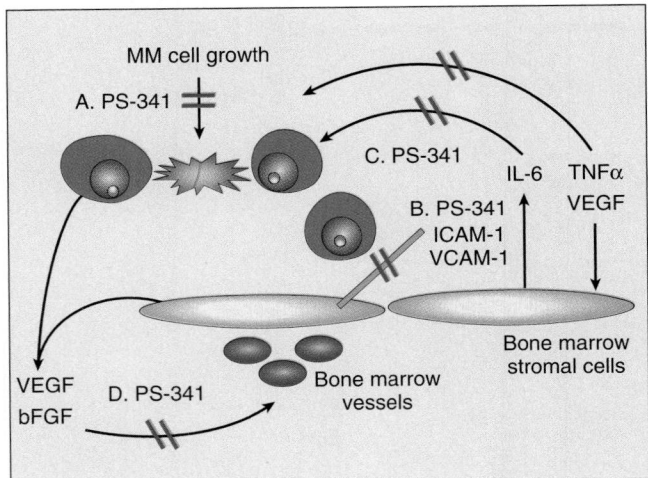

Figure 110-7. PS-341 targets MM cells in the BM microenvironment.

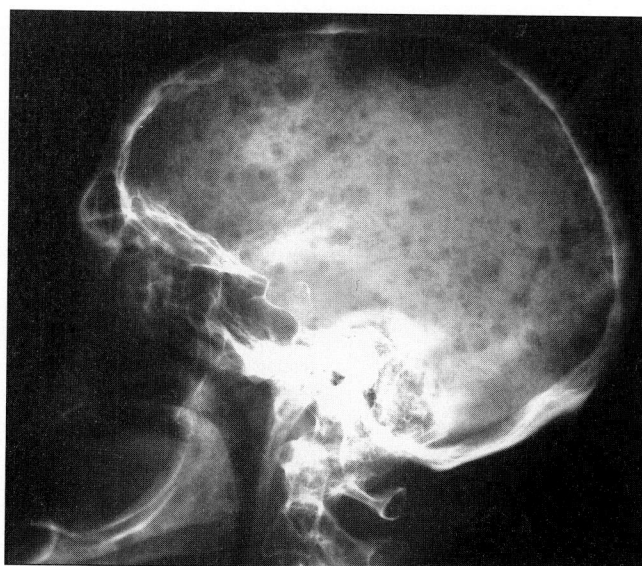

Figure 110-8. Radiograph of a skull from a patient with multiple myeloma, showing punched-out lytic lesions.

of patients at diagnosis. The axial skeleton including the vertebrae, skull, thoracic cage, pelvis, and proximal humeri and femora are most frequently involved. Osteosclerotic lesions are rare and can be seen in the MM variant, POEMS. Technetium-99m (^{99m}Tc) bone scanning is inferior to conventional radiography and should not be routinely used, as abnormalities on bone scan only correlate with sites of blastic change and thus lytic disease can be missed. Computed tomography (CT),[73] without IV contrast, or magnetic resonance imaging (MRI) may be helpful in patients who have bone pain but no abnormalities on radiograms. MRI has emerged as an important tool in the assessment of patients, in particular those with back pain and no gross abnormality on plain films as a means of not only detecting bone destruction and early cord compression but also demonstrating marrow involvement. MRI is more sensitive and demonstrates bone healing with bisphosphonate therapy. Hypercalcemia is more likely to occur in the setting of Bence Jones proteinuria, myeloma kidney, chronic infection, or uric acid nephropathy, and overall occurs in 20% to 40% of patients with MM.[74]

Renal Involvement

The serum creatinine value is initially increased ($\geq$2 mg/dL) in up to 25% of patients. The major causes of renal failure are "myeloma kidney" (also known as light-chain nephropathy), dehydration, and hypercalcemia. Myeloma kidney is characterized by the presence of large, waxy, laminated casts in the distal and collecting tubules. The casts are mainly composed of precipitated monoclonal light chains. The extent of cast formation correlates with the amount of free urinary light chains and with the severity of renal insufficiency. Dehydration contributes to acute renal failure both in this setting and in hypercalcemia, which is present in about 20% of patients

initially and is a major and treatable cause of renal insufficiency. Hyperuricemia may also contribute to renal dysfunction. Patients with MM may present with acute renal failure of other cause, however. Amyloidosis occurs in 10% to 15% of patients and may cause nephrotic syndrome or renal insufficiency, or both. Acquired Fanconi's syndrome, characterized by proximal tubular dysfunction, results in glycosuria, phosphaturia, and aminoaciduria. Deposition of monoclonal light chains, especially κ, in the renal glomeruli (light-chain deposition disease) may produce renal insufficiency or nephrotic syndrome.[75]

Neurologic Involvement

Radiculopathy is the single most frequent neurologic complication. It results from compression of the nerve by the expansion of the vertebral lesion or by the collapse of bone, and is usually in the thoracic or lumbosacral area. Compression of the spinal cord occurs in approximately 5% to 10% of patients. Peripheral neuropathy due to disease itself is relatively uncommon in MM; when present, it is usually due to amyloidosis, although treatment-related neuropathy is frequent as a result of side effects from the use of therapeutic agents, such as vinca alkaloids and thalidomide. Intracranial plasmacytomas are rare but lesions arising from the base of the skull and other parts of the calvaria are more common. Leptomeningeal myelomatosis is uncommon but is being recognized more frequently, possibly as a result of patients living longer with more successful therapies and an increase in extramedullary manifestations of multiple myeloma, as the disease evolves into a more chronic illness.[76]

Other Systemic Complications

The incidence of infections is increased in multiple myeloma; *Streptococcus pneumoniae* and gram-negative organisms are the most frequent pathogens.[77] Propensity to infection results from impairment of antibody response, reduction of normal immunoglobulins, neutropenia, and treatment with glucocorticoids, particularly when high doses of dexamethasone are used. Occasionally, the tendency to thrombosis may lead to deep vein thrombosis and pulmonary embolism in about 5% of patients, and treatment, including steroids and thalidomide, can increase this risk to between 10% to 15%.[78,79] Plasmacytomas of the ribs have been reported in 12% of cases and may present either as expanding costal lesions or as soft tissue masses.[80] Hepatomegaly, pleural effusion, and pulmonary involvement from plasma cell infiltration is relatively uncommon, but does occur.[80]

Laboratory Findings

A normocytic normochromic anemia is initially present in almost 70% of cases. The leukocyte count is usually normal. Thrombocytopenia is observed in approximately 15% of patients at diagnosis. The presence of plasma cells in the peripheral smear is infrequent; when observed, the proportion of plasma cells rarely exceeds 5%, except in patients with plasma cell leukemia. Rouleaux formation is

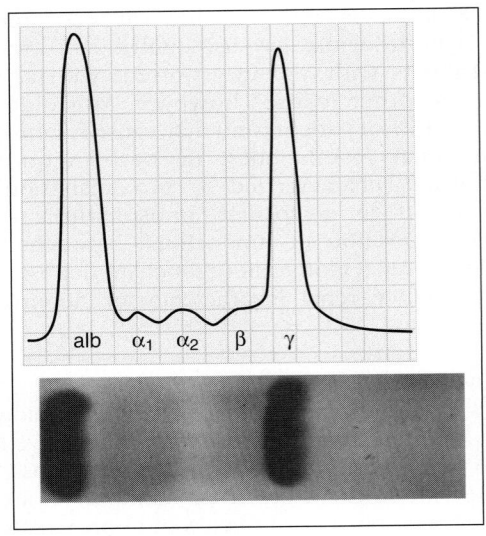

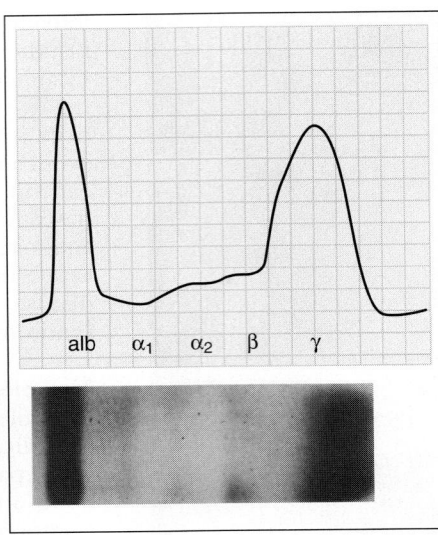

Figure 110-9. A, Monoclonal pattern of serum protein from densitometer tracing after electrophoresis of serum on cellulose acetate (anode on *left*): tall, narrow-based peak of γ mobility; dense, localized band representing monoclonal protein in γ area. **B,** Polyclonal pattern of serum protein from densitometer tracing after electrophoresis on cellulose acetate (anode on *left*): broad-based peak of γ mobility; γ band is broad. (From Kyle RA, Greipp PR: Series on clinical testing 3. The laboratory investigation of monoclonal gammopathies. Mayo Clin Proc 1978;53:719.)

present in about 60% of patients. Hypercalcemia is present at diagnosis in 30% of cases. Between one fourth and one half of patients will have impairment of renal function at diagnosis, and while up to 80% of patients may have proteinuria, about 50% have Bence Jones proteinuria confirmed by immunoelectrophoresis or immunofixation, with the κ/λ ratio seen being approximately 2:1.[6]

The serum protein electrophoretic pattern shows a peak or localized band in 80% of patients (Fig. 110-9). In the remaining 20%, hypogammaglobulinemia or a normal pattern is seen. The distribution according to the immunoglobulin type is shown in Figure 110-10. An M protein is found in the serum or urine in 99% of patients during the course of their MM. Patients with IgG and IgA myeloma have similar clinical and laboratory features at diagnosis. Patients with light-chain (Bence Jones) and IgD myeloma have a higher incidence of renal failure, higher frequency of associated amyloidosis, smaller serum M component, and greater light-chain protein excretion than those with IgG and IgA myeloma.[81]

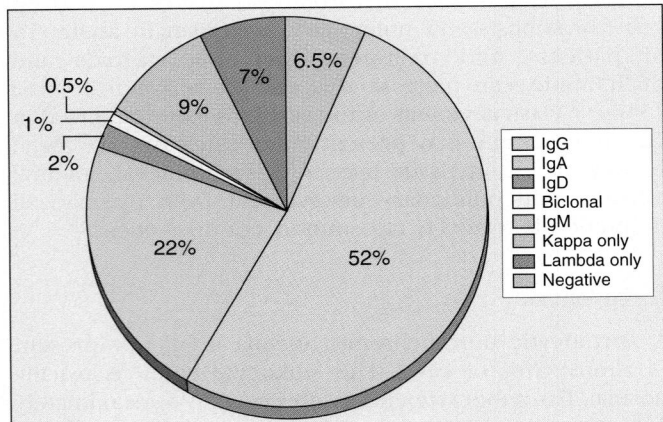

Figure 110-10. Distribution of serum monoclonal protein, according to immunoglobulin type, in 984 patients with multiple myeloma at the Mayo Clinic, 1982–1994.

In the bone marrow of patients with MM, plasma cells usually compose more than 10% of all nucleated cells, but they may range from less than 5% to almost 100% (Fig. 110-11). Bone marrow involvement may be more focal than diffuse, and some patients may require repeat bone marrow examinations for diagnosis. Identification of a monoclonal immunoglobulin in the cytoplasm of plasma cells with immunoperoxidase staining is helpful in differentiating monoclonal plasma cell proliferation in monoclonal gammopathies from reactive plasmacytosis due to autoimmune diseases, metastatic carcinoma, liver disease, acquired immunodeficiency syndrome (AIDS), or infections.

Diagnosis and Differential Diagnosis

Suggested tests for patients in whom multiple myeloma is suspected are listed in Table 110-2. The diagnosis of MM is often clear because most patients present with typical symptoms or laboratory abnormalities, including the following important triad: (1) serum or urinary M protein (in 99% of cases); (2) increased number of bone marrow plasma cells; and (3) osteolytic lesions and other roentographic abnormalities in bone. Minimal criteria for the diagnosis of MM are presented in Table 110-3.

The main conditions to consider in the differential diagnosis are MGUS, smoldering myeloma, primary amyloidosis, and metastatic carcinoma. The differentiation of a patient with MGUS (benign monoclonal gammopathy) from one in whom MM will develop is difficult when the M protein is initially recognized. In asymptomatic patients, an M component of less than 3 g/dL, less than 10% bone marrow plasma cells, and absence of osteolytic lesions, anemia, hypercalcemia, or renal insufficiency are characteristic of MGUS. Also in asymptomatic patients, an M-protein value of greater than 3 g/dL and more than 10% bone marrow plasma cells fulfills the diagnostic criteria for smoldering myeloma.[82] In asymptomatic patients with an M-protein value of greater than 3 g/dL and a monoclonal light chain in the urine,

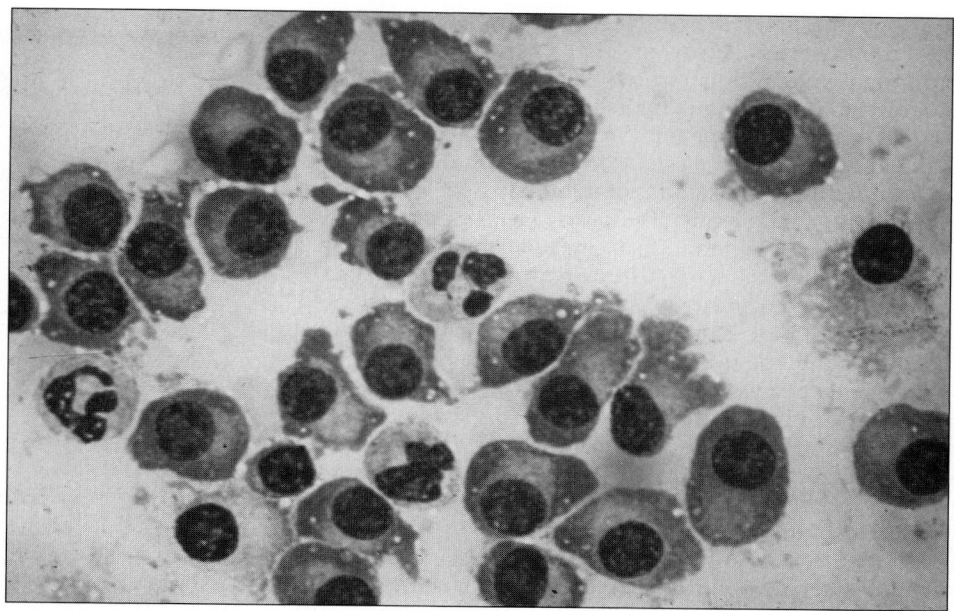

Figure 110-11. Plasma cells in bone marrow of patient with multiple myeloma. (From Kyle RA: Multiple myeloma, macroglobulinemia, and the monoclonal gammopathies. In Bone R [ed]: Current Practice of Medicine, Vol 3. Philadelphia, Current Medicine, 1996, p 19.1.)

symptomatic MM is more likely to develop.[83] Levels of uninvolved immunoglobulins are usually decreased in MM and macroglobulinemia, but this factor is not useful in the differential diagnosis because a reduction of uninvolved immunoglobulins is also observed in almost 30% of patients with MGUS.[84,85]

Elevated erythrocyte sedimentation rate and Bence Jones proteinuria have been reported as independent prognostic factors associated with MGUS transformation.[4] Other laboratory determinations, such as β_2-microglobulin level, presence of J chains in plasma cells, elevated plasma cell acid phosphatase value, a reduced number of CD4 T lymphocytes, an increased number of monoclonal idiotype-bearing peripheral blood lymphocytes, or chromosome abnormalities at FISH analysis, are unreliable for differentiation.[86]

The plasma cell labeling index (PCLI) may help differentiate patients with MGUS or smoldering myeloma

from those with MM.[87] A monoclonal antibody (BU-1) reactive with 5-bromo-2-deoxyuridine identifies the cells that synthesize DNA. The BU-1 antibody does not require denaturation, and consequently fluorescein-conjugated immunoglobulin antisera (κ and λ) identify monoclonal plasma cells and plasmacytoid lymphocytes. The PCLI of peripheral blood appears to correlate well with the bone marrow labeling index.[88] An elevated value suggests that the patient has, or will soon have, symptomatic disease, but such a finding is noted in only a minority of patients with MGUS. It must be emphasized that patients with overt MM can have a normal plasma cell labeling index and so PCLI has limitations in this respect.

Monoclonal plasma cells can be detected in the peripheral blood of 80% of patients who have active MM and in more than 90% of those with relapsed or refractory MM. Patients with MGUS or smoldering myeloma have very few or no circulating plasma cells.[89]

Recently, Kyle and colleagues identified that the height of the M component at diagnosis was the single factor that can best differentiate a patient with a benign monoclonal gammopathy from one in whom MM or other malignant disease will subsequently develop, with values less than 1 g/dL associated with least risk and those above 2 to

TABLE 110-2

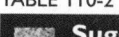 **Suggested Tests for Patients in Whom Multiple Myeloma Is Suspected**

Complete history and physical examination
Complete blood cell count and differential; peripheral blood smear
Chemistry screen (including albumin, calcium, and creatinine determinations)
Serum protein electrophoresis, immunofixation, quantitation of immunoglobulins
Serum viscosity if IgG value >6 g/dL, IgA value >5 g/dL, or symptoms of hyperviscosity are present
Routine urinalysis, 24-hour urine collection for electrophoresis and immunofixation
Bone marrow aspiration, biopsy, and plasma cell labeling index
Metastatic bone survey, including single views of humeri and femurs
β_2-Microglobulin, C-reactive protein, and lactate dehydrogenase determinations
Cytogenetics

TABLE 110-3

 Minimal Criteria for the Diagnosis of Multiple Myeloma*

Bone marrow with >10% plasma cells *or* plasmacytoma plus one of the following:
　Monoclonal protein in serum (usually >3 g/dL)
　Monoclonal protein in urine
　Lytic bone lesions

*The patient must have the usual clinical features of multiple myeloma. Connective tissue disorders, metastatic carcinoma, lymphoma, leukemia, and chronic infections must be excluded.

3 g/dL with greatest risk.[3] Overall, they reported that 1% progressed each year, the majority to multiple myeloma and Waldenström's disease, with a smaller number developing amyloidosis and plasmacytoma, and very few developing lymphoma or chronic lymphocytic leukemia.[3]

From a practical standpoint, for patients in whom MGUS has been recently diagnosed, serum electrophoresis can be repeated in 3 months to exclude an early myeloma; if the condition is stable, the test can be repeated in 6 months. If there is no progression, electrophoresis and clinical evaluation can be performed annually thereafter. Patients should be told that the risk of the development of a serious disease is only 25% and usually constitutes a late event, but they should also know that the evolution from MGUS to MM is sometimes abrupt; they should therefore be advised to follow up with periodic laboratory testing and to be reexamined promptly if clinical symptoms occur.

The differentiation between amyloidosis and MM is arbitrary because both diseases are plasma cell proliferative disorders with different manifestations but overlapping features. In amyloidosis, the proportion of bone marrow plasma cells is usually less than 20%, there are no osteolytic lesions, and the amount of Bence Jones proteinuria is modest. For patients in whom no M component is found in the serum or urine, but a lytic lesion is identified, a metastatic carcinoma, such as hypernephroma, should be ruled out before the diagnosis of nonsecretory myeloma is considered. Alternatively, for a patient with other constitutional symptoms, widespread osteolytic lesions, a modest M component, and less than 10% bone marrow plasma cells, metastatic carcinoma with an unrelated MGUS needs to be ruled out.

Prognosis and Staging

Multiple attempts have been made to define clinical and laboratory parameters that have prognostic significance.[90-93] Of the many staging systems, the Durie-Salmon system is most commonly utilized (Table 110-4).[91] Tumor

TABLE 110-4

Clinical Staging System for Multiple Myeloma

STAGE	FACTORS
I	Low cell mass ($<0.6 \times 10^{12}/m^2$)
	All of the following:
	Hemoglobin value >10 g/dL, IgG level <5 g/dL, IgA level <3 g/dL, calcium value normal
	Urinary monoclonal protein value <4 g/24 h
	No generalized lytic lesions
II	Intermediate (neither stage I nor stage III)
III	High cell mass ($>1.2 \times 10^{12}/m^2$)
	Any one of the following:
	Hemoglobin value <8.5 g/dL, IgG level >7 g/dL, IgA level >5 g/dL, calcium value >12 mg/dL
	Urinary monoclonal protein value >12 g/24 h
	Advanced lytic bone lesions
Subclasses	A, if creatinine level is <2 mg/dL; B, if level is ≥2 mg/dL

TABLE 110-5

Adverse Prognostic Factors in Multiple Myeloma

Elevated β₂-microglobulin
Hypoalbuminemia
Elevated lactate dehydrogenase
High C-reactive protein
Plasmablastic morphology
High plasma cell labeling index
Advanced age
Elevated creatinine
Hypodiploidy, low RNA content of plasma cells
Anemia, hypercalcemia, thrombocytopenia
Primary resistance to therapy with progressive disease
Unfavorable cytogenetics

cell mass for patients in stage I is low at $<0.6 \times 10^{12}$ cells/m² intermediate for patients with stage II disease at 0.6 to 1.2×10^{12} cells/m², and high for patients with stage III disease with $>1.2 \times 10^{12}$ cells/m². In this system, survival duration is 61.2, 54.5, 30.1, and 14.7 months for patients with stage IA, stage IB + IIA + IIB, stage IIIA, and stage IIIB disease, respectively. The median duration of survival for patients with MM was until recently approximately 3 years; with the advent of transplant and newer, more effective treatments this has improved to 5 years, but there is also considerable variability from one patient to another. The most important prognostic factors are listed in Table 110-5.[94-98]

The uncorrected β₂-microglobulin level is one of the most powerful prognostic factors, with serum β₂M representing the light chain of the major histocompatibility complex of the cell membrane, and increased levels resulting from release by MM with high growth fraction and cell turnover rates, such that in patients with MM and normal renal function, rising serum β₂M predicts for progression.[99] The level of C-reactive protein (CRP) correlates with the serum interleukin-6 (IL-6) level, a major growth factor for plasma cells.[100] An elevated lactate dehydrogenase level is also a predictor of poor prognosis.[98] Higher labeling indices, serum IL-6 receptor levels, more ras mutations, more aggressive disease, and shortened survival are seen in patients with plasmablast morphology.[101] The labeling index (LI), a measure of DNA synthesis by MM cells, predicts for survival. It is usually low (<1%) at diagnosis, higher at relapse, and lower in MGUS and indolent MM.[93] Chromosome 13 deletions are present in over 40% of MM and are associated with poor prognosis[21,23,102,103]; however, these deletions are also associated with MGUS,[103-105] and their role in transformation to MM is therefore at present undefined. Gene expression will define disease pathogenesis, and identify novel prognostic factors and potential therapeutic targets.[106,107] These studies will also identify mechanisms of sensitivity versus resistance to conventional and novel MM therapies.[108,109] Serum IL-6 levels in some studies appear to correlate with both stage of disease and survival.[110,111] IL-6 stimulates hepatocytes to produce acute-phase proteins, such as CRP; CRP therefore may reflect the IL-6 level and proliferative status of BM plasma cells. Indeed, CRP levels are significantly lower in patients with MGUS than in those with MM, and survival can be correlated with serum CRP level.[100] High serum soluble IL-6 receptor (sIL-6R),[112] hepatocyte growth factor,[113] and syndecan-1[114] levels, as well as low serum hyaluronate levels,[115] are independent prognostic factors predicting poor outcome. The percentage of circulating plasma cells in peripheral blood and their labeling indices are independent prognostic factors for survival in MM after both conventional and high-dose therapy.[89,116]

Except for a few cases in which long-term remission has been achieved with conventional chemotherapy,[58,59] most patients will eventually relapse with progressive MM and become refractory to systemic therapy. The most important feature of relapse is an increase in the M-protein value, along with clinical and laboratory characteristics of progressive disease. Occasionally, relapse consists of an increase in either Bence Jones proteinuria or osteolytic lesions without an increase in the serum M-protein level. In patients with advanced MM, the so-called acute or aggressive terminal phase develops, characterized by rapid tumor growth, pancytopenia, and, often, rapidly enlarging soft tissue masses, decreasing levels of M protein, and/or fever.[117] These patients do not respond satisfactorily to standard chemotherapy, and their median duration of survival is typically at most 4 to 6 months.

Treatment

General Considerations and Criteria of Response

Most patients with MM have symptomatic disease at diagnosis and require therapy. Not all patients fulfilling the diagnostic criteria for MM should be treated, however. Thus even if the M-component level and the proportion of bone marrow plasma cells are high, patients with smoldering myeloma or indolent MM should not be treated, unless myeloma-related bone pain, anemia, hypercalcemia, renal impairment, hyperviscosity, or recurrent bacterial infection develops. Bisphosphonates can be used in early disease but other agents such as thalidomide remain investigational at this time. If there is doubt about whether to begin more intensive therapy, the most reasonable approach is to reevaluate the patient in 1 to 2 months and to start therapy when progressive disease is evident.

Patients undergoing therapy for MM should have clinical and laboratory assessment to ensure both safety and efficacy of treatment. Before each course of treatment, a complete blood count including differential and platelets should be done. Serum chemistries should be measured at least every three months or more often if clinically indicated. Concomitantly, monoclonal protein in the serum and/or urine should be measured by immuno-electrophoresis, or preferably using more sensitive immunofixation techniques. A skeletal survey should be done annually, with bone marrow examination reserved for diagnosis and time of subsequent change in clinical status, in monoclonal Ig, or in hemogram. It is important to remember that reduction of serum or urine M component as objective evidence of tumor response could reflect either increased protein catabolism, decreased protein production, or both. Moreover non-M-protein-secreting MM clones may emerge during treatment, so that even a marked reduction in monoclonal Ig may not correlate with decrease in tumor burden.

In contrast with treatment of most hematologic malignancies, conventional chemotherapy for MM rarely results in complete remission but in different degrees of partial response. Objective response has generally been defined either by a 50% decrease in the serum M component or urinary M-protein excretion or by a 75% reduction in the M-component synthetic rate, along with clinical improvement. As the duration of survival in patients with myeloma who achieve disease stabilization is similar, irrespective of whether they fulfill the objective response criteria, patients who achieve a partial response should also be considered responders.[118,119] In fact, the concept of a plateau phase (consisting of a period of disease stability after chemotherapy lasting at least 4 to 6 months in which tumor progression does not occur) has been introduced.[120]

There are multiple criteria for response assessment. Perhaps the most commonly utilized is the Southwest Oncology Group (SWOG) criteria.[121] Most recently, criteria to develop more sensitive techniques for detection of residual myeloma to parallel the advent of more aggressive therapy utilizing allogeneic and autologous bone marrow/peripheral blood stem cell transplantation (SCT) were developed for the European Group for Blood and Marrow Transplant (EBMT), the International Bone Marrow Transplant Registry (IBMTR), and the Autologous Blood and Marrow Transplant Registry (ABMTR), which provide a more sensitive and rigorous definition of complete response, including absence of paraprotein assayed by immunofixation, and exclude transient responses.[122] These criteria were based upon the SWOG criteria but were amended to include immunofixation and a requirement that if no M protein is found in the serum or urine with immunofixation, the bone marrow should be examined carefully for evidence of a monoclonal proliferation of plasma cells, and if absent and repeated at 6 weeks then complete response can be confirmed (Table 110-6). If no identifiable myeloma cells are found, the polymerase chain reaction (PCR), in which oligonucleotide primers are used to amplify regions of rearranged heavy chain alleles, has been studied.[123]

Initial Therapy

If the patient is younger than 70 years, autologous SCT should be considered and, ideally, peripheral stem cells should be collected before the patient is exposed to alkylating agents. Chemotherapy is the preferred initial treatment for overt, symptomatic MM in patients older than 70 years or in younger patients in whom SCT is not feasible. Palliative radiation, at doses of 20 to 30 Gy, should be limited to patients with severe and persistent pain from a localized lesion that does not respond to chemotherapy, as analgesics and chemotherapy usually control the pain of MM.

Radiation therapy for MM is used for treatment of localized disease, including plasmacytoma or spinal cord

TABLE 110-6

Response Comparison of EBMT+ and SWOG Criteria

RESPONSE CRITERIA	SPEP REDUCTION	IF (SERUM AND URINE)	UPEP REDUCTION	BONE MARROW	BONE DISEASE	CALCIUM	CONFIRMATION
CR							
SWOG	75%	Not required	90%	Not required	Not required	Not required	Yes (3 weeks)
SWOG	100%	Negative	100%	<5% PC	Stable	Normal	Yes (6 weeks)
PR							
SWOG	50%	Not required	Not required	Not required	Not required	Not required	Yes (3 weeks)
SWOG	50%	Not required	90% or <200 mg	Not required	Normal	Normal	Yes (6 weeks)

IF, immunofixation; PC, plasma cells; SPEP, serum protein electrophoresis; UPEP, urine protein electrophoresis.
From Alexanian R, Bonnet J, Gehan E, et al: Combination chemotherapy for multiple myeloma. Cancer 1972;30:382; and Blade J, Samson D, Reece D, et al: Criteria for evaluating disease response and progression in patients with multiple myeloma treated by high-dose therapy and haemopoietic stem cell transplantation. Myeloma Subcommittee of the EMBT. Br J Hematol 1998;102:115.

compression syndrome, and is frequently used for palliation. Hemibody radiation therapy has been utilized, either as a consolidation after induction combination chemotherapy or as salvage therapy for chemotherapy-resistant MM.[124,125] Total body irradiation (TBI) can be used as a component of ablative therapy before hematopoietic stem cell grafting, but its use has diminished since a randomized trial in SCT comparing melphalan alone versus melphalan and TBI showed no benefit and more toxicity in the TBI-containing arm.[126]

Conventional Therapy

Oral administration of melphalan and prednisone (MP) is a standard form of therapy that produces objective response in 50% to 60% of patients and has constituted standard therapy for patients with MM for 25 years.[127,128] With this regimen, the median duration of survival ranges from 2 to 3 years. The dosage of melphalan, due to the variability of absorption, should be modified if necessary so that some reduction in leukocytes and platelets occurs 3 to 4 weeks after the beginning of each cycle. Unless there is disease progression, MP should be given for at least 1 year until the monoclonal Ig levels in the serum and/or urine have been stable for at least 6 months (plateau state), and then discontinued if the patient has no other evidence of active disease. Typical doses are melphalan daily in a dosage of a 0.15 mg/kg daily for 7 days (8 to 10 mg per day) and 20 mg of prednisone three times daily for the same period. Melphalan must be given before meals because food reduces absorption. It is important to remember that the natural course of MM is one of progression, so that alleviation of pain and lack of progressive disease may be beneficial even in the absence of an objective response. Leukocyte and platelet counts must be determined at 3-week intervals, and the melphalan and prednisone regimen is repeated every 6 weeks. Melphalan can also be administered at a dosage of 0.25 mg/kg daily for 4 days, in addition to prednisone, every 4 to 6 weeks, depending on hematologic tolerance. In patients with renal failure, the initial dosage of oral melphalan should be reduced by 25% initially to prevent severe myelotoxicity. If no excessive toxicity is observed, increased dosages must be administered in the subsequent courses.

Although the introduction of melphalan constituted an important advance in the management of MM, the survival of patients with this disease remains unsatisfactory, and a major controversy in treatment of MM is whether MP is as effective as combination chemotherapy (CCT). One of the best-known combinations, the M2 protocol,[129] consists of vincristine, carmustine (BCNU), melphalan, cyclophosphamide, and prednisone (VBMCP). This produces an objective response in approximately 70% of patients, but the median duration of survival is not significantly different from that obtained with melphalan and prednisone. The Southwest Oncology Group (SWOG) reported that patients treated with a combination of alkylating agents (VCMP/VBAP or VCMP/VCAP) had a better response rate and longer survival than those who received melphalan and prednisone[121] (A, Adriamycin [doxorubicin]; B, BCNU [carmustine]; C, cyclophosphamide; M, melphalan; P, prednisone; V, vincristine). In a recent large series reported by the Medical Research Council (MRC), the ABCM regimen (Adriamycin, BCNU, cyclophosphamide, and melphalan) also increased both the proportion of patients reaching the plateau phase and the survival in comparison with melphalan alone.[130] However, other studies failed to show any significant survival advantage for VCMP/VBAP alternating chemotherapy over melphalan and prednisone.[131,132] In an attempt to determine which patients, if any, do better with more aggressive therapy, Gregory and colleagues examined published reports of 18 randomized controlled trials comparing MP with CCT in the primary treatment of 3814 patients.[133] The overall results suggested that there was no difference in efficacy between these treatment modalities.

Those studies with a high MP two-year survival rate showed a survival difference in favor of MP, whereas those with a low rate suggested a difference in favor of CCT. These results imply that, rather than there being no difference between MP and CCT, MP is superior for patients with an intrinsically good prognosis and inferior for those patients with a poor prognosis. A second overview of 6633 patients from 27 randomized trials of CCT versus MP confirmed higher response rates to CCT, but equivalent mortality and survival.[134]

A meta-analysis of 18 published trials found no difference in overall duration of survival in a comparison of multiple and single alkylating agents.[133] It was concluded that patients with good-risk prognostic variables seemed to fare better when treated with melphalan and prednisone, whereas those with poor prognostic factors did better with combination chemotherapy. In addition, a large meta-analysis based on the individual patient data of more than 6000 patients with MM by the Myeloma Trialists' Collaborative Group in Oxford show no difference in survival. Chemotherapy should be continued until the patient reaches a plateau state, defined as a stable M-protein value in the serum and urine and no evidence of progression of MM.

Almost all patients with MM who initially respond to chemotherapy eventually relapse. Patients who progress with initial therapy have a 40% response to high-dose or pulsed corticosteroid therapy.[135] Patients who relapse during therapy or within 6 months of stopping initial treatment have a 75% response rate to VAD chemotherapy.[135-137] Patients who relapse more than 6 months after stopping therapy have a 60% to 70% response rate when initial therapy is reinstituted[128]; if no response is achieved, then VAD or alternate regimens can be used. Unfortunately, even in those patients who respond to salvage therapy, the duration of response is limited.

Plateau Phase and Maintenance Treatment

Both clinically and biologically, the plateau phase is near the quiescent state observed in smoldering myeloma or MGUS. The crucial difference is that in multiple myeloma, the residual malignant cells lead to relapse in virtually all cases, whereas MM or related disorders develop in only one fourth of patients with MGUS. There is no evidence that continued chemotherapy is of benefit after the attainment of a plateau phase. In fact, continued chemotherapy may lead to a greater number of myeloma cells resistant to chemotherapy or to the development of myelodysplasia or acute leukemia.

The role of interferon-alpha-2 maintenance on response duration and survival in patients responding to chemotherapy is still controversial. The potential mechanisms of action of interferon-alpha-2b (IFN-α) include direct cytotoxicity on MM cells; synergism with chemotherapy; a change in the pharmacokinetics of melphalan; inhibition of IL-6; downregulation of IL-6 receptor on MM cells; downregulation of activated oncogenes; an increase in natural killer cells; and an increase in tumor cell surface antigens and/or expansion of specific cytotoxic T cells.[138] A meta-analysis of 16 randomized trials involving 2286 patients receiving combined IFN-α chemotherapy for induction treatment yielded higher response rates in the IFN-α arms, but the average gain was only approximately 10%.[139] Similarly, significant but only marginal gains were detected in the arms in remission duration (median, 7 months) and survival (median, 5 months). Moreover, a survey of U.S. patients found a 6-month risk/benefit trade-off preferred by the majority of interviewed MM patients

with regard to IFN-α treatment.[140] Quality Adjusted Time Without Symptoms or Toxicity (Q-TWIST) analysis showed that patients treated with maintenance IFN-α gained an average of 9.8 months without disease relapse and 5.8 months of overall survival (OS) versus the control groups; however, the IFN-α group suffered an average of 4.1 months of moderate or worse toxicity.[141] IFN-α maintenance treatment therefore appears to benefit a subset of patients who have achieved low tumor burden, and its marginal benefit needs to be balanced against side effects even in this patient group. In a recent SWOG study alternate-day prednisone at a dose of 50 mg was noted to improve OS and event-free survival (EFS) after induction treatment with a VAD-like induction regimen.[142]

Refractory MM

As described, patients with MM who either fail to respond or who become refractory to the initial alkylating therapy have a low response rate to subsequent chemotherapy and a progressively shorter survival. The highest response rates reported for patients with MM resistant to alkylating agents have been with VAD: vincristine plus doxorubicin (Adriamycin), given by continuous infusion for 4 days, and dexamethasone, 40 mg daily, on days 1 to 4, days 9 to 12, and days 17 to 20 of each 28-day cycle.[135] Dexamethasone is usually given only on days 1 to 4 in even-numbered cycles because of toxicity. Most VAD activity is from dexamethasone. The major shortcomings of VAD are that vincristine and Adriamycin have to be given by a central venous catheter; significant steroid toxicity is manifested by infection, myopathy, and gastrointestinal bleeding. In addition, the median duration of response is less than 1 year.

High-dose dexamethasone also can be tried for resistant or relapsing disease. Methylprednisolone is an alternative and at a dosage of 2 g IV three times weekly for a minimum of 4 weeks produced an objective response in 25% of patients refractory to alkylating agents, with a median duration of survival of 70 weeks in patients who responded.[143] Cyclophosphamide, 600 mg/m^2 daily IV for 4 days (days 1 to 4), plus prednisone, 50 mg PO twice daily for the same 4-day period, followed by granulocyte colony-stimulating factor (G-CSF), has been a beneficial treatment in refractory patients with advanced disease. The use of interferon as a single agent for refractory patients has been disappointing; response rates have ranged from 10% to 20%.[144] Other approaches include alternate-day prednisone (50 to 100 mg) and cyclophosphamide (150 to 300 mg/m^2) orally weekly or along with pulse-dose cyclophosphamide (800 to 1200 mg IV) every 2 to 3 weeks, as a palliative treatment that can temporarily control the disease with a very low toxicity.[145]

A combination of alternating cycles of VBMCP (vincristine, BCNU [carmustine], melphalan, cyclophosphamide, prednisone) and IFN-α produced encouraging results in a pilot study.[146] In three large cooperative studies, however, the combination of IFN-α with MP[147,148] or with VBMCP[149] did not show any survival advantage when compared with MP or VBMCP alone. The multidrug-resistant phenotype is characterized by the expression of glycoprotein p-170. Cells with p-170 glycoprotein expression tend to achieve lower intracellular drug concentration. Attempts to prevent or overcome the multidrug resistance in resistant MM with a calcium channel blocker such as verapamil have been disappointing.[150] A combination of cyclosporine and VAD produced a response in 10 of 21 patients with MM who were refractory to chemotherapy.[151] The efficacy of the association of VAD with the cyclosporine analog PSC 833 in refractory MM is being investigated. The administration of anti–IL-6 antibodies to 10 patients with advanced MM resulted in inhibition of the production of C-reactive protein and a decrease in the plasma cell labeling index. However, this treatment had no long-lasting effect on the patient's clinical status or on the M-component size.[152]

A major advance in the treatment of resistant MM has been the emergence of thalidomide (Thal) as an effective therapy[50,153]; it achieves an overall 32% response rate in patients with advanced and refractory MM. The 2-year event-free survival (EFS) and overall survival (OS) were 20% and 48%, respectively; low PCLI, normal cytogenetics, and a β2-microglobulin of less than 3 mg/dL were good prognostic factors for survival. Based on the impressive results of single-agent Thal in refractory relapsed MM and in vitro data suggesting its synergy with Dex, Thal has been coupled with Dex to treat patients with disease refractory to either agent alone; even in this setting, half of patients treated respond.[79] Thal has also been combined with chemotherapy and bisphosphonates in the treatment of refractory MM,[154,155] and is now under evaluation to treat patients earlier in their disease course.

High-Dose Therapy Followed by Stem Cell Transplantation

High-dose therapy followed by autologous marrow or peripheral blood stem cell transplantation (SCT) is now a standard approach for younger patients with MM, while allogeneic SCT remains experimental.

The rationale for the administration of alkylating agents (melphalan, cyclophosphamide, busulfan) in a higher-than-conventional dose with or without total body irradiation (TBI), followed by transplantation of syngeneic, allogeneic, and autologous bone marrow or peripheral blood progenitor cells (PBPCs) is as follows: plasma cell dyscrasias remain uniformly fatal; multiple studies document sensitivity of MM cells to chemotherapy and radiotherapy; and complete remission (CR) can be obtained with high-dose therapy.

Autologous SCT. High-dose chemoradiotherapy followed by transplantation of either autologous BM or PBPCs has also achieved high (40%) CR rates, but the median duration of these responses has unfortunately only been 24 to 36 months.[156,157] Patients with sensitive disease and who are less heavily pretreated have the most favorable outcomes. Most important, a national French trial of 200 patients with MM who received two courses of VMCP alternating with VBAP were then randomized to receive either conventional chemotherapy (eight additional courses of VMCP/VBAP) or high-dose therapy (melphalan and TBI) followed by autologous BMT has demonstrated significantly higher response rates in EFS and OS for those patients treated with high dose compared to those receiving conventional therapy.[158] A second randomized trial in MM examined the relative merits of high-dose therapy either early versus late as salvage therapy for relapse after conventional therapy.[159] The OS was 64 months in both groups, but the Q-TWIST strongly favored the early transplant cohort. The Intergroupe Francophone Myeloma (IFM) has subsequently conducted a randomized trial comparing high-dose melphalan at 200 mg/m² versus melphalan at 140 mg/m² plus TBI as ablative therapies.[126] Although response rates and EFS were comparable, toxicity and OS was superior in the arm of high-dose melphalan alone, suggesting that TBI should not be considered part of the ablation regimen. A Scandinavian population-based study demonstrated prolonged survival for patients with MM who were younger than 60 years of age treated with intensive therapy compared with historical controls who received conventional therapy.[160] Although these studies are encouraging and additional randomized trials in the United States, Scandinavia, and Spain are comparing the outcome of conventional therapy versus high-dose therapy and autografting, it is unlikely that patients are cured after a single high-dose and stem cell autografting regimen. This was confirmed in a large (407 patients) recently published Medical Research Council randomized trial from the United Kingdom, where, while the rates of CR were higher and there was a higher rate of overall survival and progression-free survival in the intensive therapy group, the median survival was prolonged to 54.1 months in the SCT patients, as compared to 42.3 months in the standard therapy group, but long-term survivorship (>80 months) was seen only in a minority.[161]

Improving Outcome of Autografting. Attempts to improve the outcome of high-dose therapy followed by autografting include the use of autologous BM or PBPCs either depleted of tumor cells[162-164] or processed to select normal hematopoietic progenitor cells by virtue of CD34 expression.[165,166] These have not translated to improved outcome. Barlogie and colleagues are performing multiple high-dose therapies and stem cell transplantation.[167-169] Response rates are higher relative to historically matched controls, but the impact on long-term disease-free survival requires further follow-up. In a French randomized trial comparing a single versus double high-dose therapy and stem cell transplantation, there was no significant difference in the CR rate between single and double transplantation arms, and EFS and OS curves separated only after 3 years.[170] A second French trial found no difference in EFS or OS in patients receiving single versus double autotransplants.[171] Champlin and colleagues have reported on the use of cyclosporine to induce graft-versus-host disease after autografting in an attempt to generate associated autologous graft versus MM effect.[172] Finally, it may be possible to stimulate autologous immunity to MM to treat minimal residual disease (MRD) after autografting and thereby improve outcome. Multiple reports suggest that patients may mount an anti-MM immune response.[173-175] Further studies are needed to optimize the immunization schedule to achieve long-lasting T-cell immunity against idiotypic and other determinants on the MM cell and determine its effect on clinical outcome.

Allogeneic Stem Cell Transplantation. Syngeneic transplantation has been done infrequently in MM, but some patients reported from Seattle[176] and in the European Bone Marrow Transplant Group (EBMT)[177] remain progression free at long intervals after allogeneic bone marrow transplant (BMT). The EBMT has reported on allografting in MM.[178-180] Actuarial OS was 32% at 4 years, and 28% at 7 years for the 72 (44%) patients who achieved complete remission after BMT. Overall progression-free survival (PFS) was 34% at 6 years, however, and few patients remain in continuing CR at more than 4 years after allograft. Favorable pre-BMT prognostic factors for both response to and survival after BMT were female sex, IgA MM, low serum β_2M, stage I disease at diagnosis, one line of previous treatment, and being in CR before BMT. Of major concern is the early 40% transplant-related mortality (50% in males) in the EBMT report,[181] which has subsequently been reduced to 20% to 30% due to better patient selection, early transplantation, and less pretransplant treatment.[180]

In the allografting experience in Seattle, actuarial probabilities of OS and EFS for the 36% of patients achieving CR were 0.50 ± 0.21 and 43 ± 0.17, respectively, at 4.5 years. Adverse prognostic factors included: BMT more than 1 year from diagnosis; serum β_2M greater than 2.5 mg/dL at BMT; female patients transplanted from male donors; having received more than eight cycles of chemotherapy, and Durie-Salmon stage III disease at presentation. Again toxicity was common, with 35 (44%) patients dying of transplant-related causes within 100 days of bone marrow transplant.[176,182] In an attempt to improve the outcome of allografting in MM by avoiding treatment-related mortality (TRM), we carried out T (CD6) depleted allografting using histocompatible sibling donors in 61 patients with MM whose disease remained sensitive to conventional chemotherapy.[164,183-186] There were 17 (28%) complete relapse, 34 (57%) partial relapse, 2 (3%) no relapse, and only 3 (5%) treatment-related mortality. However, disease-free survival (DFS) after allo-BMT was 1 year, with only 20% patients disease free at 4 or more years after transplant.

Molecular remissions are more common after allografting than after autografting,[187-190] and donor lymphocyte infusions (DLI) can treat relapsed MM after allografting,[191-193] indicating clinically significant graft-versus-MM (GVM) effects. At our center, relapses after autografting versus the higher toxicity and lower relapse rates in allograft recipients result in equivalent long-term outcomes.[194] In an effort to reduce toxicity and exploit GVM, we have utilized CD4$^+$ DLI at 6 months after CD6-depleted BM allografting in order to enhance GVM and thereby improve outcome.[186] Although prophylactic DLI induces significant GVM responses after allogeneic BMT, only 58% of patients were able to receive DLI despite T-cell-depleted BMT.

The use of nonmyeloablative transplantation is an alternative strategy to preserve GVM while avoiding the toxicity of allografting. Melphalan at a dose of 100 mg/m^2 has been used in combination with DLI in high-risk MM patients.[195] Although disease control was achieved in some patients, significant GVHD was noted in this group of patients. Autografting has been performed before nonmyeloablative transplant by several investigators, demonstrating the feasibility of this approach to cytoreduce tumor and then enhance anti-MM immunity.[196,197] Although preliminary results are encouraging, follow-up is short and chronic GVHD may remain a problem.

Management of Complications

Hypercalcemia

Hypercalcemia should be suspected in the presence of anorexia, nausea, vomiting, polyuria, polydipsia, constipation, confusion, or stupor. Left untreated, renal insufficiency usually develops. Therapeutic recommendations for hypercalcemia at present include cytotoxic therapy for MM, cautious forced saline diuresis, and bisphosphonate therapy using pamidronate, with the use of calcitonin, prednisone, or mithramycin only for nonresponders to these first-line treatments. In a randomized trial of patients with hypercalcemia of malignancy, the more potent bisphosphonate zoledronate was found to be superior to pamidronate.[198] A prominent problem exacerbating hypercalcemia relates to patients becoming immobile because of bone pain or other reasons. Therefore an important approach is to keep the patient, whenever possible, physically active.

Renal Insufficiency

Reduction in renal function occurs in one fourth of patients initially and may develop insidiously or acutely. Maintenance of a high urine output (3 L/day) is important for preventing renal failure in patients with Bence Jones proteinuria. Allopurinol is effective for the prevention and treatment of hyperuricemia. Hemodialysis is necessary in patients with symptomatic azotemia. In one series, 6 of 20 patients with nonreversible renal failure who were undergoing chronic hemodialysis survived more than 3 years.[199] Plasmapheresis may be helpful in acute renal failure, but patients with severe myeloma cast formation or other irreversible changes are unlikely to benefit.[200] Unfortunately, severe renal failure is usually irreversible. Renal transplantation for myeloma kidney has been followed by prolonged survival.

Infections

Prompt and appropriate therapy for bacterial infections is essential. Prophylactic daily penicillin (orally) often benefits patients with recurrent streptococcal pneumonia infections. Pneumococcal and influenza vaccine should be given to all patients despite their suboptimal antibody response. Intravenously administered gamma globulin may be helpful for patients with recurrent infections, but it is very expensive.

Skeletal Lesions

Patients should be encouraged to be as active as possible, but they must avoid undue trauma. Fixation of fractures or impending fractures of long bones with an intramedullary rod and methyl methacrylate has produced good results. Patients in a prospective study receiving the bisphosphonate clodronate had fewer new lytic lesions, fewer vertebral fractures, and less hypercalcemia than those in the placebo group.[201] Monthly infusion of pamidronate had a significant effect on skeletal complications and improved the quality of life in a prospective randomized trial with a reduction in skeletal-related events, including pathologic fractures, radiation therapy to bone, and spinal cord compression in patients with Durie-Salmon stage III MM and more than one lytic bone lesion.[202] The potent bisphosphonate zoledronate has undergone clinical evaluation and offers the benefit of shorter infusion times than those of pamidronate with equivalent benefit.[203-205] Recent evidence supports the view that bisphosphonates may down regulate IL-6 production from BMSCs, as well as induce apoptosis of both osteoclasts and tumor cells.[206]

Others

Hyperviscosity is characterized by oronasal bleeding, blurred vision, neurologic symptoms, and congestive heart failure. Serum viscosity levels do not correlate well with the symptoms or the clinical findings. Plasmapheresis promptly relieves the symptoms and should be done regardless of the viscosity level when the patient is symptomatic. Spinal cord compression should be suspected in patients with severe back pain, the development of weakness or paresthesias of the lower extremities, or bladder or bowel dysfunction. MRI, CT, or myelography must be done immediately. Radiation therapy and dexamethasone are usually helpful. If the neurologic deficit worsens, surgical decompression is necessary. Symptomatic anemia during the plateau phase is often benefited by the administration of erythropoietin.[207,208]

VARIANTS OF MULTIPLE MYELOMA

Smoldering Myeloma

The diagnosis of smoldering myeloma depends on the presence of both an M-protein value of more than 3 g/dL and more than 10% plasma cells in the bone marrow, but no evidence of anemia, renal insufficiency, hypercalcemia, skeletal lesions, or clinical manifestations of myeloma.[82] Often, a small amount of M protein is found in the urine, and the concentration of uninvolved immunoglobulins is usually reduced. Clusters or aggregates of plasma cells are often seen in the bone marrow. The plasma cell labeling index is low. Biologically, these patients have a benign monoclonal gammopathy, but they must be followed because symptomatic MM will develop in many. The recognition of this subset of patients is crucial because they should not be treated unless progression occurs.

Plasma Cell Leukemia

Plasma cell leukemia is defined as the presence of more than 20% plasma cells in the peripheral blood and an absolute plasma cell count of greater than 2×10^9/L. It is classified as primary when it presents de novo (60% of cases) and as secondary when it is a leukemic transformation of a previously recognized MM (40%).[209] Patients with primary plasma cell leukemia are younger and have a greater incidence of hepatosplenomegaly and lymphadenopathy, a higher platelet count, fewer bone lesions, a smaller serum M component, and a longer duration of survival than patients with secondary plasma cell leukemia. Patients with plasma cell leukemia have more cytogenetic abnormalities and higher levels of serum IL-6 than do patients with classic MM. Treatment of primary plasma cell leukemia is unsatisfactory. Although the response rate is higher with combination chemotherapy than with single alkylating agents, the duration of response is short. Secondary plasma cell leukemia, which constitutes the terminal event in 1% to 2% of patients with MM, rarely responds to treatment.

Nonsecretory Myeloma

Patients with nonsecretory myeloma have no M component in either the serum or the urine and constitute 2% of patients with myeloma. The diagnosis is established by identification of an M protein in the plasma cells by immunoperoxidase or immunofluorescence methods. Cases in which no M protein could be found within the myeloma cells have been reported, however. The clinical picture, response to therapy, and survival rate of patients with nonsecretory myeloma are similar to those in patients with a serum or urinary M component, except that they have less renal involvement.[210]

Osteosclerotic Myeloma

Osteosclerotic myeloma, or POEMS syndrome, is characterized by polyneuropathy, organomegaly, endocrinopathy, M protein, and skin changes (POEMS).[211,212]

The major clinical findings are a chronic inflammatory-demyelinating polyneuropathy with predominantly motor disability and sclerotic skeletal lesions. Except for the frequent presence of papilledema, the cranial nerves are not involved. The autonomic nervous system is intact. Hepatomegaly occurs in almost one half of cases, but splenomegaly and lymphadenopathy occur in a minority. Skin hyperpigmentation and hypertrichosis may be prominent. Gynecomastia, testicular atrophy, and clubbing of the fingers and toes may occur. Angiomatous lesions on the trunk may be prominent. Moderate pedal edema is common and may be associated with ascites and pleural effusion. In contrast to MM, the hemoglobin level is usually normal or elevated, and thrombocytosis is common. The bone marrow usually contains less than 5% plasma cells, and hypercalcemia and renal insufficiency rarely occur. Most patients have a λ M protein; IgA is common. The diagnosis is confirmed by the identification of monoclonal plasma cells obtained at biopsy of an osteosclerotic lesion. If the lesions are in a limited area, radiation usually produces substantial improvement of neuropathy. If the patient has widespread osteosclerotic lesions, chemotherapy may be helpful.

Plasmacytoma

Plasmacytomas are collections of monoclonal plasma cells originating either in bone (solitary osseous plasmacytoma, SOP) or in soft tissue (extramedullary plasmacytoma, EMP). They comprise less than 10% of plasma cell dyscrasias. The persistence of stable monoclonal Ig in serum and/or urine after primary treatment for plasmacytoma does not necessitate additional therapy, since it does not influence overall survival or disease-free survival.[213] In contrast, rising monoclonal Ig levels in a patient with a history of either SOP or EMP should trigger a workup for either recurrent plasmacytoma or MM. Disappearance of protein after involved-field radiotherapy predicts for long-term disease-free survival and possible cure.[214]

Solitary Plasmacytoma of Bone

The diagnosis of solitary plasmacytoma, or solitary myeloma, is based on histologic evidence of a plasma cell tumor. In addition, complete skeletal radiographs must show no other lesions, the bone marrow aspirate must contain no evidence of MM, and immunoelectrophoresis or immunofixation of the serum and concentrated urine should show no M protein. Exceptions to the last criterion occur, but therapy of the solitary lesion usually results in disappearance of the M protein. Solitary plasmacytomas are usually located in the spine or long bones of the extremities. Treatment consists of radiation in the range of 40 to 50 Gy. There is no evidence that chemotherapy affects the incidence of conversion to MM.[215] Overt MM develops in approximately 55% of patients, and new bone lesions or local recurrence develops in about 10%.[213] Progression usually occurs within 3 to 4 years.

Extramedullary Plasmacytoma

Extramedullary plasmacytoma is a plasma cell tumor that arises outside the bone marrow. The tumor is located in the upper respiratory tract in approximately 80% of cases, especially in the nasal cavity and sinuses, nasopharynx, and larynx. Extramedullary plasmacytomas may also occur in the gastrointestinal tract, central nervous system, urinary bladder, thyroid, breast, testes, parotid gland, and lymph nodes. There is a predominance of IgA M protein in extramedullary plasmacytomas. The diagnosis is based on the finding of a plasma cell tumor in an extramedullary location and the absence of MM on bone marrow examination, radiography, and appropriate studies of serum and urine. Treatment consists of tumoricidal radiation. The prognosis is favorable. Regional recurrences develop in approximately 25% of patients, but the development of typical MM is uncommon.[216]

IgM MONOCLONAL GAMMOPATHY

Excess monoclonal IgM in the serum can occur in a variety of diseases including MGUS (56%), Waldenström's macroglobulinemia (17%), lymphoma (7%), chronic lymphocytic leukemia (5%), amyloidosis (1%), and other disease states (14%).[217]

WALDENSTRÖM'S MACROGLOBULINEMIA

Macroglobulinemia was first described by Waldenström in 1944.[218] This condition consists of a monoclonal proliferation of plasma cells and B lymphocytes producing IgM. It is an uncommon disease, and in our practice it is one fifth as common as MM. The median age at diagnosis is 63 years, and there is a slight male predominance.[217] The diagnosis of Waldenström's macroglobulinemia (WM) requires an IgM serum level of at least 3.0 gm/dL in association with an increase in lymphocytes or plasmacytoid lymphocytes in BM.[217,219-221] WM corresponds most closely to the lymphoplasmacytic lymphoma (LPA) under the WHO classification of lymphoid tumors (LPL/immunocytoma of the REAL classification of lymphoma). Cytogenetic abnormalities occur in 15% to 90% of cases, but none are specific for WM.[222,223] WM likely originates from a postgerminal center B cell, which has undergone somatic mutations and antigenic selection in the lymphoid follicle[224,225] and has the characteristics of an IgM-bearing memory B cell.[226]

Clinical Manifestations

Weakness, fatigue, oronasal bleeding, weight loss, and visual or neurologic disturbances are the most common presenting symptoms.[227] Many clinical manifestations result from hyperviscosity syndrome, consisting of: (1) diffuse bleeding (epistaxis, purpura, and oozing from the oral mucosa); (2) visual disturbances such as blurring or loss of vision, retinal hemorrhages, exudates, and venous congestion with vascular segmentation (sausage formation); (3) neurologic conditions (dizziness, headache, vertigo, nystagmus, hearing loss, ataxia, paresthesias, somnolence, and even coma); and (4) cardiovascular disorders (hypervolemia and congestive heart failure). Approximately one third of patients have a serum viscosity value of higher than 4 centipoises (cp). Although the relationship between serum viscosity and clinical manifestations varies from patient to patient, most have symptoms when the relative viscosity value is greater than 4 cp.

Physical examination may reveal pallor, hepatosplenomegaly, and lymphadenopathy. Pleuropulmonary involvement is infrequent and consists of diffuse pulmonary infiltrates, isolated masses, or pleural effusions. Lesions are composed of plasmacytoid lymphocytes. Small bowel and skin infiltration are uncommon. Peripheral neuropathy usually involves both sensory and motor modalities. Sudden deafness, progressive spinal muscle atrophy, and multifocal leukoencephalopathy have been noted. Renal failure rarely occurs. In contrast with MM, osteolytic lesions and amyloidosis are rare.

Laboratory Features

Almost all patients have a moderate normochromic normocytic anemia. The frequently increased plasma volume spuriously reduces the hemoglobin and hematocrit levels.

Lymphocytosis is present in 30% of cases and moderate thrombocytopenia in 20%. The serum cholesterol value is often low. The serum electrophoretic pattern is characterized by a tall narrow peak or dense band, almost always of γ mobility. Of the IgM proteins, 75% have a κ light chain. Both 7S and 19S IgM are present. About 10% of macroglobulins are cryoprecipitable. A monoclonal light chain is found in the urine in almost 80% of patients. Rouleaux formation is frequent, and the erythrocyte sedimentation rate is generally increased. The bone marrow aspirate is often hypocellular, but a biopsy specimen shows hypercellularity and extensive infiltration by lymphocytes, plasma cells, and lymphoplasmacytoid cells, along with an increase in mast cells, which helps differentiate it from lymphoma and myeloma.

Differential Diagnosis

The diagnosis is made on the basis of the typical symptoms and physical findings, the presence of an IgM M protein in the serum, and lymphoplasma cell proliferation in the bone marrow. Macroglobulinemia shares features with MM, chronic lymphoid leukemia, lymphoma, undifferentiated lymphoproliferative processes, and MGUS of the IgM type. The patient must be carefully observed for an indefinite period to differentiate MGUS of the IgM class from early Waldenström's macroglobulinemia.

Treatment

The median survival is approximately 50 months, not that dissimilar from the best reported series of patients with MM. In contrast to persons with MM, however, many individuals with WM have indolent disease requiring no therapy for long periods of time, with survivals in excess of 20 years. Therapy should thus be withheld until the patient is symptomatic; features requiring therapy consist of constitutional symptoms such as weakness, fatigue, night sweats, or weight loss and anemia, hyperviscosity symptoms, hepatosplenomegaly, or lymphadenopathy.

Pretreatment parameters including older age, male sex, general symptoms, and cytopenias define a high-risk population.[228,229] Nucleoside analogues fludarabine and 2-chlorodeoxyadenosine, combination chemotherapy, stem cell transplantation, and most recently Rituxan (rituximab) have achieved responses, but no cures.[221,230-237] The nucleoside analogs have been effective in 40% of patients with primary resistance from chlorambucil-prednisone and in about 80% of patients with newly diagnosed disease.[219] Ongoing studies are combining Rituxan with fludarabine in the treatment of WM. Other treatments include orally administered chlorambucil at a dosage of 6 to 8 mg daily, which is reduced when the leukocyte or platelet counts decrease. Intermittent administration of chlorambucil and prednisone every 4 to 6 weeks is also effective. Cyclophosphamide or combinations of alkylating agents such as the M2 protocol (vincristine, BCNU, melphalan, cyclophosphamide, and prednisone) have also been beneficial. Patients should be treated until the plateau phase is achieved and then followed without maintenance chemotherapy. Transfusion of packed red blood cells should be used only for patients with symptomatic anemia. Erythropoietin may be of benefit for patients in the plateau state with symptomatic anemia. Patients with symptomatic hyperviscosity syndrome should be managed with plasmapheresis.

HEAVY CHAIN DISEASES

The heavy chain diseases (HCD) are lymphoplasma cell proliferative disorders characterized by the presence of an M protein consisting of an incomplete heavy chain. There are three major types: γ, α, and μ.

γ-Heavy Chain Disease

The γ-chain is incomplete with significant deletions of amino acids, including the entire C_{H1} domain and a portion of the variable region. Although several patients younger than 20 years have been described, the median age at diagnosis of patients with γ-HCD is approximately 60 years, and its clinical picture is consistent with a chronic lymphoproliferative disorder.[238-240]

The most frequent presenting symptoms are weakness and fatigue, fever, and lymphadenopathy, but other symptoms, such as parotid gland swelling, severe soreness of the tongue, edema of the uvula and palate due to Waldeyer's ring involvement, skin infiltration, and rapid enlargement of the thyroid gland, have been reported. Hepatosplenomegaly and lymphadenopathy occur in about 60% of patients. Cervical lymph nodes are the most commonly involved, and waxing and waning of the lymphadenopathy may occur without an apparent reason.

Normochromic normocytic anemia is found in 80% of cases. Coombs'-positive autoimmune hemolytic anemia has also been observed in several instances. The serum protein electrophoretic pattern is variable and often does not suggest a monoclonal gammopathy. Some patients have hypogammaglobulinemia or a normal electrophoretic pattern, whereas others have a broad-based increase of gamma globulins or a discrete localized band. The urinary heavy chain protein concentration ranges from traces to 20 g in 24 hours, but more than one half of patients excrete less than 1 g of protein in 24 hours. Bence Jones proteinuria is not found. Histopathologic examination of the bone marrow and lymph nodes usually reveals an increased number of plasma cells, lymphocytes, and lymphoplasmacytoid cells.

The prognosis of γ-HCD is variable because the clinical course may range from an asymptomatic state to a rapidly progressive disease. The median duration of survival in 49 patients for whom such data were available was 12 months (range, 1 to 264 months).[241] Treatment with cytostatic agents should be limited to symptomatic patients. Many different drugs have been used, generally with disappointing results. Therapy with cyclophosphamide, vincristine, and prednisone seems a reasonable approach. If there is no response, a doxorubicin-containing regimen should be tried.

α-Heavy-Chain Disease

α-HCD is the most common type of heavy-chain disease; there are more than 200 reported cases.[239,242] In contrast to other monoclonal gammopathies, this disorder usually develops in the second or third decade of life. About 60% of patients are male. This disease has two major clinical variants: (1) gastrointestinal tract involvement manifested by severe malabsorption with loss of weight, diarrhea, and steatorrhea; and (2) infrequently, respiratory tract involvement. The term *immunoproliferative small intestinal disease* (IPSID) is restricted to patients with small intestinal lesions that have the same pathologic pattern as that of α-HCD, but these patients do not synthesize α heavy chains.[243]

The serum electrophoretic pattern is normal in one half of patients, whereas in the remainder a broad band in the α_2 or β regions may be observed. The diagnosis depends on the recognition of a monoclonal α-heavy chain in the serum or jejunal fluid. Occasionally, α-heavy chains may be recognized only in the small bowel or nodes (nonsecretory). The amount of α-chain in the urine is small, and Bence Jones proteinuria is always absent. The bone marrow is also normal. Untreated α-HCD is usually progressive and fatal. There have been several cases in which remissions have been obtained only with antibiotics.[244] In patients who do not respond to antibiotics and in those with initially extensive intestinal or mesentric involvement, combination chemotherapy with cyclophosphamide, Adriamycin, vincristine, and prednisone should be given.[245]

μ-Heavy-Chain Disease

μ-HCD, first reported in 1970, is characterized by a monoclonal μ-chain fragment in the serum. The clinical spectrum of the 28 cases of μ-HCD reported so far has been reviewed.[246] Most patients have an associated chronic lymphoproliferative process, mainly chronic lymphoid leukemia or lymphoma. The serum protein electrophoretic pattern shows a monoclonal spike in about 40% of patients. Two thirds have Bence Jones proteinuria, usually of the κ type. The bone marrow generally reveals an increase in lymphocytes, plasma cells, and lymphoplasmacytoid cells. In two thirds of patients, vacuolization of the plasma cells is observed. Thus μ-HCD should be suspected in patients with a chronic lymphoproliferative disorder, Bence Jones proteinuria, and vacuolated plasma cells in the bone marrow. The course of μ-HCD is variable; the duration of survival ranges from less than 1 month to 11 years (median, 24 months). There is no specific treatment for this disease. Therapy for symptomatic patients should be similar to that used in chronic lymphocytic leukemia (CLL) or lymphoma and will depend on the aggressiveness of the disease.

PRIMARY AMYLOIDOSIS

Amyloid is a substance that appears homogeneous and amorphous with light microscopy. Under polarized light,

amyloid stained with Congo red produces an apple-green birefringence. Amyloid fibrils in primary amyloidosis (AL) consist of the variable portion of a monoclonal light chain or, in some instances, the intact light chain. The light chain class is more frequently λ than κ (2:1 ratio). Patients with amyloidosis may have aberrant de novo synthesis or abnormal proteolysis of light chains. Three overviews on systemic amyloidosis have recently been published.[247-249]

Amyloidosis is relatively rare as a clinically significant disease. It has been classified into five categories. These include: (1) primary, with or without plasma cell and lymphoid neoplasms; (2) secondary, associated with chronic infections or autoimmune disease; (3) hereditary, associated with familial Mediterranean fever, Portuguese lower limb neuropathy, and others; (4) amyloidosis associated with aging; and (5) amyloidosis of endocrine glands, with medullary thyroid carcinoma and multiple endocrine neoplasia, type 2.[250,251] The amyloid found in most cases of amyloidosis can be assigned to one of two types, according to whether the fibrils consist mainly of the variable region of Ig light chains (AL, or primary amyloidosis) or protein A (AA, or secondary amyloidosis). Protein A has a molecular weight of 8500 daltons and consists of 76 amino acids; it is not related to any known immunoglobulin. In AL, amyloid primarily involves the heart, tongue, gastrointestinal tract, and skin, whereas AA primarily results in fibril deposition in liver, kidney, and spleen. A review of 229 patients with AL documented MM in 47 patients (21%).[251] Initial presenting symptoms were fatigue and weight loss, with pain more common in those who also had MM. Hepatomegaly and macroglossia were present in up to one third of patients with AL; renal insufficiency was present in one half of patients, and proteinuria (defined as albuminuria with immune globulin seen only in MM) was documented in 82% of patients. Nephrotic syndrome, congestive heart failure (CHF), orthostatic hypotension, carpal tunnel syndrome, and peripheral neuropathy were all more common in those without MM (30% to 70% of patients studied) than persons with (<20%) MM. Overall survival was 12 months, 5 months for those with MM in contrast to 13 months for individuals without MM. Treatment with alkylating agents, colchicines, and stem cell transplant achieves responses, but no cures; only 5% patients with primary AL survive[252] 10 years.[250,253-260] Attempts to improve outcomes for patients with symptomatic and advanced multisystem disease may require both solid and stem cell transplantation, as well as the use of less intensive conditioning regimens.[258] Novel drugs with promise in the treatment of MM, including Thal, its more potent immunomodulatory analogs (IMiDs), and PS-341, are also being tested in patients with amyloidosis.

Clinical Manifestations

The median age at diagnosis is 61 years, and two thirds of patients are male.[261] The annual incidence is 0.89 per 100,000.[262] Weakness, fatigue, and weight loss are the most frequent symptoms. Dyspnea and pedal edema are frequent in patients with congestive heart failure.

Specific Malignancies

Paresthesias, lightheadedness, and syncope occur in patients with peripheral or autonomic neuropathy. Hoarseness or change of voice should alert the physician to the possibility of amyloidosis.

The liver is palpable in 20% of patients, and spleno-megaly occurs in 5%. Macroglossia is observed in one tenth of patients. The consistency of the tongue (firmer than usual) and the presence of dental indentations are helpful in the recognition of macroglossia. Enlargement of submandibular structures, often confused with adenopathy, may occur. Purpura is common and usually involves the neck and face, particularly the upper eyelids. Ankle edema is frequent, often resulting from congestive heart failure or nephrotic syndrome.

Almost one third of patients have the nephrotic syndrome at diagnosis. Other syndromes associated with primary amyloidosis (AL) are carpal tunnel syndrome, congestive heart failure, peripheral neuropathy, and orthostatic hypotension. The presence of one of these syndromes and an M protein in the serum or urine is a strong indication of primary amyloidosis.

Cardiac and Circulatory Involvement

Congestive heart failure is present in about 20% of patients at diagnosis and develops in an additional 10% during the course of the disease. The electrocardiogram frequently shows low voltage in the limb leads or characteristics consistent with anterior septal infarction (loss of anterior forces), but there is no evidence of myocardial infarction at autopsy. Arrhythmias, including atrial fibrillation, ventricular premature complexes, atrial or junctional tachycardia, or heart block, are common features. Echocardiography is a reliable technique in the assessment of amyloid heart disease. There is a relationship between the thickness of the ventricular wall and septum and the incidence and severity of congestive heart failure.[263]

Early cardiac amyloidosis is characterized by abnormal relaxation, whereas advanced involvement is consistent with restrictive cardiomyopathy. Constrictive pericarditis and hypertrophic obstructive cardiomyopathy may be difficult to differentiate from amyloid heart disease. If there is doubt, endomyocardial biopsy is useful. Intermittent claudication of the jaw as well as of the upper and lower extremities may be features of amyloidosis.[264] Orthostatic hypotension is found in approximately one sixth of patients with amyloidosis.[265]

Other Organ Involvement

Nephrotic syndrome is present in one third of patients at diagnosis, but it rarely develops during the course of the disease. The nephrotic syndrome usually persists even if renal failure develops. Other organ involvement includes the gastrointestinal tract, but it is usually asymptomatic. Malabsorption occurs in less than 5% of cases. Ascites and gastrointestinal bleeding may also occur. Hepatic involvement is common, and amyloid deposition is usually in the periportal areas,[266] although centrilobular deposition may occur. Intrahepatic cholestasis with jaundice is an ominous finding, and death occurs within a few weeks.

Spontaneous splenic rupture resulting in hypovolemic shock has been the presenting feature of amyloidosis in several instances. Although the development of overwhelming pneumococcal sepsis is rare, functional hyposplenism is common. One sixth of patients have peripheral neuropathy at diagnosis. The neuropathy is more sensory than motor, and it is usually distal, symmetric, and progressive. Autonomic dysfunction may be a prominent feature, and it is often manifested by orthostatic hypotension, diarrhea, and impotence. Amyloidosis can involve the periarticular structures and produce the shoulder pad syndrome. Rarely, large amyloid deposits (amyloidomas) may cause osteolytic lesions and pathologic fractures. Involvement of the skin results in petechiae, ecchymoses, papules, plaques, nodules, bullous lesions, alopecia, or skin thickening.

Laboratory Findings

Anemia is not a prominent feature of primary amyloidosis (AL); when present, it is usually due to MM, renal insufficiency, or gastrointestinal bleeding. Thrombocytosis occurs in 10% of patients. Howell-Jolly bodies may be observed in the peripheral blood smear. Proteinuria is present in about 70% of cases. One fourth of patients have a serum creatinine value of 2 mg/dL or greater at diagnosis. Hypoalbuminemia and elevation of cholesterol and triglyceride levels are often associated with the nephrotic syndrome. The prothrombin time is increased in about 15% of patients, and the thrombin time is prolonged in 60%. The factor X level is decreased in about 15% of patients, but it is rarely the cause of bleeding. Carotene and serum B_{12} vitamin levels are each decreased in approximately 5% of patients.

The serum protein electrophoretic pattern shows a localized band or spike in almost half of the patients. Hypogammaglobulinemia occurs in one fourth of patients, and the remainder have a normal-appearing pattern. Immunoelectrophoresis or immunofixation of the serum reveals an M protein in two thirds of patients, and almost 20% have a free monoclonal light chain (Bence Jones proteinemia). An M protein is found in the serum or urine in 90% of patients.

Bone marrow plasma cells are only slightly increased. The median percentage in the Mayo Clinic series was 6%, and only 15% of the patients had more than 20% plasma cells in their bone marrow. Radiographs of the bones are normal, unless the patient has MM or an amyloidoma.

Diagnosis

The diagnosis of amyloidosis depends on the demonstration of amyloid deposits in tissues. The possibility of amyloidosis must be considered in every patient who has an M protein in the serum or urine and who also has nephrotic syndrome, congestive heart failure, sensorimotor peripheral neuropathy, carpal tunnel syndrome, giant hepatomegaly, or idiopathic malabsorption. In 98% of patients, there is an M protein in the serum or urine or a monoclonal proliferation of plasma cells in the bone marrow.[267]

The initial diagnostic procedure should be abdominal fat aspiration, which is positive in about 80% of patients. A bone marrow aspiration and biopsy should be done to determine the degree of plasmacytosis; it is also positive for amyloid in more than one half of patients. If the abdominal fat and bone marrow biopsy are negative, a rectal biopsy (including submucosa), which is positive in more than 75% of cases, should be performed. If these sites are nondiagnostic, tissue should be obtained from a suspected involved organ. Specific antisera to κ, λ, protein A, transthyretin (prealbumin), and β₂M are helpful in identifying the type of systemic amyloidosis. Iodine-123 (¹²³I)-labeled purified human serum amyloid P component is useful for detecting amyloid deposition.[249]

Prognosis

The current median duration of survival for patients with amyloidosis is approximately 13 months. Survival depends mainly on the associated syndrome. Thus the duration is about 4 months from the onset of CHF, whereas it is longer than 2 years in patients with only peripheral neuropathy. In a multivariate analysis, the initial prognostic factors influencing survival during the first year were CHF, presence of urinary light chain, hepatomegaly, and the degree of weight loss.[268] As in patients with multiple myeloma, β₂M serum levels and plasma cell labeling index are also prognostic factors.[261] Cardiac involvement is the cause of death in at least one half of patients.

Treatment

Treatment for amyloidosis is unsatisfactory. As the amyloid fibrils consist of the variable portion of a monoclonal immunoglobulin light chain that is synthesized by plasma cells, it is reasonable to attempt treatment with alkylating agents. In a placebo-controlled double-blind study of 55 patients with amyloidosis, patients randomized to melphalan-prednisone therapy continued treatment longer and received larger doses than did patients in the placebo group before the code was broken because of progressive disease. The duration of survival was not significantly different between the two groups, however.[269]

In another prospective randomized study comparing melphalan-prednisone with colchicine, no significant differences in the duration of survival were found (25 months versus 18 months), but when the duration of survival in patients who received only one regimen was analyzed or the duration was determined from the time of entry into the study until the time of death or disease progression, significant differences in favor of melphalan-prednisone were observed.[270] Furthermore, the results of a prospective trial done at the Mayo Clinic, comparing the effectiveness of three regimens for primary amyloidosis (melphalan-prednisone versus colchicine versus melphalan-prednisone plus colchicine, without crossover provision), was recently published.[255] The median duration of survival after randomization was 8.5 months in the colchicine group; 18 months in the group assigned to melphalan and prednisone; and 17 months

in the group assigned to melphalan, prednisone, and colchicine. Obviously, the differences observed in that study were statistically significant and demonstrated that treatment with melphalan and prednisone results in survival prolongation as compared with colchicine in patients with primary amyloidosis.

In a series of 153 patients with amyloidosis treated with melphalan-prednisone, the overall response rate was nearly 20%. In patients with nephrotic syndrome, a normal serum creatinine level, and no cardiac involvement, the response rate was almost 40%. It is of particular interest that the median duration of survival for responding patients was longer than 7 years.[271] A myelodysplastic syndrome or overt acute leukemia developed in 6.5% of patients treated with melphalan, with the actuarial risk at 3.5 years as high as 21%.[272]

Despite the results obtained with melphalan and prednisone, treatment of primary amyloidosis is still unsatisfactory. Substantial clinical improvement with the administration of 4'-iodo-4'-deoxyrubicin (I-DOX) has been observed in patients with primary amyloidosis.[273] This new agent may act by binding to amyloid fibrils and contribute to the resolution of amyloid deposits.

Encouraging results have recently been reported with high-dose intravenous melphalan (200 mg/m²) followed by autologous peripheral blood stem cell transplantation (SCT). In this regard, improvement in hepatic, gastrointestinal, neurologic, renal, or cardiac amyloid involvement has been reported, with decreased proteinuria and stable or improved performance status.[248] Moreover, remission of plasma cell dyscrasia (disappearance of serum or urine M protein plus absence of monoclonal bone marrow plasma cells) after high-dose melphalan has been documented.[257,274] Due to the short follow-up, however, the impact of this new treatment approach on response duration and survival is still unknown. Although high-dose melphalan in patients with primary amyloidosis can be safely administered in selected cases, there are limitations to this procedure, particularly age, performance status, and extensive cardiac or renal involvement.[248] In summary, intensive treatment followed by stem cell rescue constitutes a hope for selected patients with primary systemic amyloidosis.

The nephrotic syndrome should be managed with salt restriction and diuretics. If symptomatic azotemia develops, chronic renal dialysis is necessary.[275] Patients with congestive heart failure must also be treated with salt restriction and diuretics. In selected patients, cardiac transplantation may be performed, particularly in those in whom the disease is clinically limited to the heart. Digitalis must be used with care because patients with amyloidosis are unusually sensitive to this drug, and heart block and arrhythmias are common. Elastic stockings or leotards may be useful in the management of orthostatic hypotension.

MONOCLONAL GAMMOPATHY OF UNDETERMINED SIGNIFICANCE

Monoclonal gammopathy of undetermined significance (MGUS) denotes the presence of an M protein in persons without evidence of MM, Waldenström's macroglobulinemia, amyloidosis, or other related disorders.[276] For many years this disorder was considered of benign nature and often called benign monoclonal gammopathy. It is now known, however, that a proportion of cases will evolve to a symptomatic monoclonal gammopathy, and for this reason the term *MGUS* seems more appropriate.[277]

The frequency of MGUS is age-related; it occurs in 1% of people older than 50 years and in 3% of those older than 70 years[278,279]; the rates are even higher if more sensitive techniques are used.[280,281] Because of its high prevalence and the different fields of clinical practice in which these patients are seen, it is of great importance to know whether the M protein will remain stable and benign or, on the contrary, will progress to a symptomatic disease.

Follow-up Studies

At the Mayo Clinic, a long-term study of 241 patients with MGUS was recently updated.[41] There were 140 male and 101 female patients with a median age of 64 years. Abnormal findings at physical examination (hepatomegaly, splenomegaly) or laboratory abnormalities such as anemia, thrombocytopenia, or impairment of renal function observed in some patients were due to nonrelated disorders. The initial M-protein level ranged from 0.3 to 3.2 g/dL (median, 1.7) and consisted of IgG (74%), IgA (10%), and IgM (16%). The median percentage of bone marrow plasma cells at diagnosis was 3% (range, 1% to 10%) among the patients in whom a bone marrow aspirate was obtained. All patients were followed for more than 20 years or until death.

After 25 to 39 years of follow-up, the 241 patients were divided into four groups. In group 1 (24 patients, 10%), the M protein remained stable, and these patients were classified as having a benign monoclonal gammopathy but still being at risk for the development of malignant transformation. In group 2, despite the increase in the M component to 3 g/dL or greater, symptomatic monoclonal gammopathy did not develop, and the patients did not require therapy. More than half of patients died of unrelated diseases. In one fourth of the patients, malignant transformation developed: MM (42 cases), primary amyloidosis (8 cases), macroglobulinemia (7 cases), and malignant lymphoproliferative disorders (5 cases).

The actuarial risk of malignant transformation in the overall series was 17% at 10 years and 33% at 20 years. The interval between the recognition of the M protein and the diagnosis of a serious disease ranged from 2 to 29 years (median, 10 years). In an update of this analysis, the only feature at diagnosis that proved useful for distinguishing patients who did not progress from those in whom a malignant change developed was the height of the M spike at presentation.[3]

Similar findings were recently reported in another series[85] composed of 128 patients with MGUS who were followed for a median of 56 months (range, 12 to 216 months). In 13 cases (10.2%), malignant transformation developed: MM (10 cases), primary amyloidosis (2 cases), and macroglobulinemia (1 case). The actuarial probability

for development of a serious disease was 8.5% at 5 years and 19.2% at 10 years. The median interval from the recognition of the M protein to the diagnosis of malignant transformation was 41.6 months (range, 12 to 155 months). Patients with IgA-type MGUS had a higher probability for development of a malignant disease than the remainder.

The 20-year follow-up in the series of Axelsson[282] disclosed that 11% of the patients had progression of their benign monoclonal gammopathy. Finally, Baldini and colleagues[283] reported that in a series of 335 patients the frequency of progression, after a median follow-up of 70 months, was 6.8%. Of interest, that study identified a subset of patients with MGUS of IgG type with a low probability of progression to MM: no reduction in polyclonal immunoglobulins, no light-chain proteinuria, bone marrow plasma cells less than 5%, and IgG 1.5 g/dL or less.

In the subset of patients whose condition evolves to MM, MGUS clearly constitutes a frequent initial phase. After a long period of stability, the plasma cell clone escapes control and MM develops. In fact, in all cases of malignant transformation the M-component type in MGUS and MM has been the same. Interestingly, 58% (32 of 55) of the patients with MM in Olmsted County, Minnesota, in the past 13 years had a monoclonal plasma cell disorder (MGUS, smoldering myeloma, or plasmacytoma) before the diagnosis of MM.[10] These data suggest that a considerable proportion of patients with MM have a preceding monoclonal gammopathy.

Although MGUS frequently exists without any other abnormalities, certain diseases are associated with it, as would be expected in an older population. Therefore studies of such an association must include a control group to determine whether the association is merely a coincidence. M proteins have been noted in lymphoproliferative disorders, leukemia, other hematologic diseases, connective tissue disorders, and neurologic conditions such as peripheral neuropathy. Dermatologic diseases such as lichen myxedematosus, pyoderma gangrenosum, necrobiotic xanthogranuloma, and plane xanthomatosis have been associated with an M protein.[86]

An M protein may exhibit high specificity to riboflavin, von Willebrand's factor, dextran, antistreptolysin O, antinuclear activity, calcium, copper, and phosphates. M proteins have also been found in acquired immunodeficiency syndrome (AIDS) and in immunosuppression after renal, bone marrow, and liver transplantation.

Biclonal Gammopathies

Biclonal gammopathies occur in 3% to 4% of patients with monoclonal gammopathies. The clinical findings are similar to those of monoclonal gammopathies. Two thirds of patients with a biclonal gammopathy have biclonal gammopathies of undetermined significance.[284] The remainder have multiple myeloma, amyloidosis, macroglobulinemia, or other lymphoproliferative disorders. In many cases, the serum protein electrophoretic pattern shows only a single band, and the biclonal gammopathy is unrecognized until immunoelectrophoresis or immunofixation is performed. A few patients with triclonal gammopathy have been reported.

Idiopathic Bence Jones Proteinuria

Although Bence Jones proteinuria is most frequently associated with multiple myeloma, primary amyloidosis, Waldenström's macroglobulinemia, or other lympho-proliferative disorders, it may be "benign." Small amounts of monoclonal light chains (Bence Jones proteinuria) are not uncommon. In most patients who excrete more than 1 g of Bence Jones protein in 24 hours without evidence of malignant plasma cell proliferation, MM or amyloidosis will eventually develop. This change may not occur, however, for up to 20 years. Therefore these patients with "idiopathic" Bence Jones proteinuria should be observed indefinitely.[285]

FUTURE DIRECTIONS

Identification and Validation of Novel Targeted Multiple Myeloma Therapies

In order to overcome resistance to current therapies and improve patient outcome, novel biologically based treatment approaches that target mechanisms whereby MM cells grow and survive in bone marrow are needed.[286] To achieve this goal, we have developed systems for studying growth, survival, and drug resistance mechanisms intrinsic to MM cells. Of importance, we have also developed both in vitro systems and in vivo animal models to characterize mechanisms of MM cell homing to bone marrow, as well as factors (MM cell–BMSC interactions, cytokines, angiogenesis) promoting MM cell growth, survival, drug resistance, and migration in the bone marrow microenvironment.[36,42,44,47,287-289] These model systems have allowed for the development of several promising biologically based therapies that can target the MM cell in its bone marrow microenvironment and thereby overcome classical drug resistance in vitro, including Thal/IMiDs,[54] the proteasome inhibitor PS-341,[55] and As2O3.[290] Once in vitro promise of these novel agents is demonstrated, we have rapidly tested their efficacy is tested in murine models. Thalidomide and the ImiDs,[291] 3-amino-phthalimido-glutaramide,[292] and PS-341[293] all inhibit human MM cell growth, decrease associated angiogenesis, and prolong host survival in our model in which human MM cells and matrigel are injected subcutaneously into SCID mice. We have translated our laboratory studies to phase I and II clinical trials to evaluate their clinical utility and toxicity. Most exciting, IMiDs[294] and PS-341 (also known as bortezumib)[295] have already demonstrated marked clinical anti-MM activity even in patients with refractory relapsed MM, confirming the utility of the preclinical models to identify and validate novel therapeutics. Final results from the pivotal multi-center phase II study of PS-341 in relapsed and refractory MM led to its expedited approval in 2003.[296]

Of importance, as carried out in in vitro gene array studies with conventional Dex[108] and novel (PS-341)[109]

therapies, samples obtained from patients treated on these protocols will help identify in vivo targets and mechanisms of novel drug action on the one hand, versus mechanisms of drug resistance on the other, and also aid in determining whether in vivo targets of these novel therapies correlate with their in vitro anti-MM activities. Excitingly, preclinical studies suggest enhanced acivity when these novel agents are combined with conventional agents or with each other. These studies have established a new treatment paradigm targeting the MM cell in its bone marrow microenvironment to further elucidate MM pathogenesis as well as overcome drug resistance and improve patient outcome.

REFERENCES

1. Durie BGM: Staging and kinetics of multiple myeloma. Semin Oncol 1986;13:300–309.
2. Kyle RA: Multiple myeloma: How did it begin? Mayo Clin Proc 1994;69:680–683.
3. Kyle RA, Therneau TM, Rajkumar SV, et al: A long-term study of prognosis in monoclonal gammopathy of undetermined significance. N Engl J Med 2002;346:564–569.
4. Cesana C, Klersy C, Barbarano L, et al: Prognostic factors for malignant transformation in monoclonal gammopathy of undetermined significance and smoldering multiple myeloma. J Clin Oncol 2002;20:1625–1634.
5. Bergsagel DE, Wong O, Bergsagel PL, et al: Benzene and multiple myeloma: Appraisal of the scientific evidence. Blood 1999;94:1174–1182.
6. Kyle RA: Multiple myeloma: Review of 869 cases. Mayo Clin Proc 1975;50:29–40.
7. Herrinton LJ, Weiss NS, Olshan AF: Epidemiology of myeloma. In Malpas JS, Bergsagel DE, Kyle R, Anderson K, eds: Myeloma: Biology and Management. Oxford, Oxford Medical Publications, 1997, p 150.
8. Greenlee R, Hill-Harmon M, Murray T, Thun M: Cancer Statistics, 2001. CA Cancer J Clin 2000;51:15–36.
9. Bourguet CC, Grufferman S, Delzell E, et al: Multiple myeloma and family history of cancer. Cancer 1985;56:2133–2139.
10. Kyle RA, Beard MC, O'Fallon WM, Kurland LT: Incidence of multiple myeloma in Olmsted County, Minnesota: 1978 through 1990, with a review of the trend since 1945. J Clin Oncol 1994;12:1577–1183.
11. Pruzanski W, Ogrylo MA: Abnormal proteinuria in malignant diseases. Adv Clin Chem 1970;13:335–382.
12. Kuehl WM, Bergsagel PL: Multiple myeloma: Evolving genetic events and host interactions. Nat Rev Cancer 2002;2:175–187.
13. Bakkus MHC, Heirman C, Van Riet I, Van Camp B, Thielemans K: Evidence that multiple myeloma Ig heavy chain VDJ genes contain somatic mutations but show no intraclonal variation. Blood 1992;80:2326–2335.
14. Bergsagel PL, Chesi M, Nardini E, Brents LA, Kirby SL, Kuehl WM: Promiscuous translocations into immunoglobulin heavy chain switch regions in multiple myeloma. Proc Natl Acad Sci USA 1996;93:13931–13936.
15. Vescio RA, Cao J, Hong CH, et al: Myeloma Ig heavy chain V region sequences reveal prior antigenic selection and marked somatic mutation but no intraclonal diversity. J Immunol 1995;155:2487–2497.
16. Kubagawa H, Vogler LB, Capra JD, et al: Studies on the clonal origin of multiple myeloma: Use of individually specific (idiotypic) antibodies to trace the oncogenic event to its earliest point of expression in B cell differentiation. J Exp Med 1979;150:792–807.
17. San Miguel JF, Caballero MD, Gonzales M, Zola H, Lopez Borrasca A: Immunological phenotype of neoplasms involving the B cell in the last step of differentiation. Br J Haematol 1986;62:75–83.
18. Van Camp B, Durie BG, Spier C, et al: Plasma cells in multiple

myeloma express natural killer cell–associated antigen: CD56 (NKH-1; Leu-19). Blood 1990;76:377–382.

19. Treon SP, Mollick JA, Urashima M, et al: Muc-1 core protein is expressed on multiple myeloma cells and is induced by dexamethasone. Blood 1999;93:1287–1298.

20. Harada H, Kawano MM, Huang N, et al: Phenotypic difference of normal plasma cells from mature myeloma cells. Blood 1993;81:2658–2663.

21. Facon T, Avet-Loiseau H, Guillerm G, et al: Chromosome 13 abnormalities identified by FISH analysis and serum beta2-microglobulin produce a powerful myeloma staging system for patients receiving high-dose therapy. Blood 2001;97:1566–1571.

22. Fonseca R, Harrington D, Oken MM, et al: Biological and prognostic significance of interphase fluorescence in situ hybridization detection of chromosome 13 abnormalities (delta13) in multiple myeloma: An Eastern Cooperative Oncology Group study. Cancer Res 2002;62:715–720.

23. Tricot G, Spencer T, Sawyer J, et al: Predicting long-term (≥5 years) event-free survival in multiple myeloma patients following planned tandem autotransplants. Br J Haematol 2002;116:211–217.

24. Uchiyama H, Barut BA, Chauhan D, Cannistra SA, Anderson KC: Characterization of adhesion molecules on human myeloma cell lines. Blood 1992;80:2306–2314.

25. Uchiyama H, Barut BA, Mohrbacher AF, Chauhan D, Anderson KC: Adhesion of human myeloma–derived cell lines to bone marrow stromal cells stimulates IL-6 secretion. Blood 1993;82:3712–3720.

26. Uchiyama H, Anderson KC: Cellular adhesion molecules. Transfus Med Rev 1994;8:84–95.

27. Teoh G, Anderson KC: Interaction of tumor and host cells with adhesion and extracellular matrix molecules in the development of multiple myeloma. Hematol Oncol Clin North Am 1997;11:27–42.

28. Hallek M, Bergsagel PL, Anderson KC: Multiple myeloma: Increasing evidence for a multistep transformation process. Blood 1998;91:3–21.

29. Mitsiades CS, Mitsiades N, Poulaki V, et al: Activation of NF-kappaB and upregulation of intracellular anti-apoptotic proteins via the IGF-1/Akt signaling in human multiple myeloma cells: Therapeutic implications. Oncogene 2002;21:5673–5683.

30. Anderson KC, Park EK, Bates MP, et al: Antigens on human plasma cells identified by monoclonal antibodies. J Immunol 1983;130:1132–1138.

31. Epstein J, Barlogie B, Katzmann J, Alexanian R: Phenotypic heterogeneity in aneuploid multiple myeloma indicates pre-B cell involvement. Blood 1988;71:861–865.

32. Grogan TM, Durie BGM, Lomen C, et al: Delineation of a novel pre-B cell component in plasma cell myeloma: Immunochemical, immunophenotypic, genotypic, cytologic, cell culture, and kinetic features. Blood 1987;70:932–942.

33. Jensen GS, Mant MJ, Belch AJ, Berenson JR, Ruether BA, Pilarski LM: Selective expression of CD45 isoforms defines CALLA+ monoclonal B lineage cells in peripheral blood from myeloma patients as late stage B cells. Blood 1991;78:711–719.

34. Urashima M, Ogata A, Chauhan D, et al: Interleukin-6 promotes multiple myeloma cell growth via phosphorylation of retinoblastoma protein. Blood 1996;88:2219–2227.

35. Chauhan D, Kharbanda S, Ogata A, et al: Interleukin-6 inhibits Fas-induced apoptosis and stress-activated protein kinase activation in multiple myeloma cells. Blood 1997;89:227–234.

36. Ogata A, Chauhan D, Teoh G, et al: Interleukin-6 triggers cell growth via the *ras*-dependent mitogen-activated protein kinase cascade. J Immunol 1997;159:2212–2221.

37. Ogata A, Chauhan D, Urashima M, Teoh G, Treon SP, Anderson KC: Blockade of mitogen-activated protein kinase cascade signaling in interleukin-6 independent multiple myeloma cells. Clin Cancer Res 1997;3:1017–1022.

38. Chauhan D, Uchiyama H, Akbarali Y, et al: Multiple myeloma cell adhesion-induced interleukin-6 expression in bone marrow stromal cells involves activation of NF-kB. Blood 1996;87:1104–1112.

39. Urashima M, Teoh G, Chauhan D, et al: Interleukin-6 overcomes p21^WAF1 upregulation and G1 growth arrest induced by dexamethasone and interferon-γ in multiple myeloma cells. Blood 1997;90:279–289.

40. Urashima M, Teoh G, Ogata A, et al: Role of CDK4 and p16^INK4A in interleukin-6-mediated growth of multiple myeloma. Leukemia 1997;11:1957–1963.

41. Chauhan D, Hideshima T, Treon SP, et al: Functional interaction between retinoblastoma protein and stress activated protein kinase in multiple myeloma cells. Cancer Res 1999;59:1192–1195.

42. Chauhan D, Hideshima T, Pandey P, et al: RAFTK/PYK2-dependent and independent apoptosis in multiple myeloma cells. Oncogene 1999;18:6733–6740.

43. Chauhan D, Pandey P, Hideshima T, et al: SHP2 mediates the protective effect of interleukin-6 against dexamethasone-induced apoptosis in multiple myeloma cells. J Biol Chem 2000;275:27845–27850.

44. Chauhan D, Hideshima T, Rosen S, et al: Apaf-1/cytochrome-c independent and Smac dependent induction of apoptosis in multiple myeloma cells. J Biol Chem 2001;276:24453–24456.

45. Hideshima T, Nakamura N, Chauhan D, Anderson KC: Biologic sequelae of interleukin-6 induced PI3-K/Akt signaling in multiple myeloma. Oncogene 2001;20:5991–6000.

46. Akiyama M, Hideshima T, Hayashi T, et al: Cytokines modulate telomerase activity in a human multiple myeloma cell line. Cancer Res 2002;62:3876–3882.

47. Podar K, Tai YT, Davies FE, et al: Vascular endothelial growth factor triggers signaling cascades mediating multiple myeloma cell growth and migration. Blood 2001;98:428–435.

48. Podar K, Tai YT, Lin BK, et al: Vascular endothelial growth factor-induced migration of multiple myeloma cells is associated with beta 1 integrin- and phosphatidylinositol 3-kinase-dependent PKC alpha activation. J Biol Chem 2002;277:7875–7881.

49. Gupta D, Treon SP, Shima Y, et al: Adherence of multiple myeloma cells to bone marrow stromal cells upregulates vascular endothelial growth factor secretion: Therapeutic applications. Leukemia 2001;15:1950–1561.

50. Singhal S, Mehta J, Desikan R, et al: Antitumor activity of thalidomide in refractory multiple myeloma. N Engl J Med 1999;341:1565–1571 [published erratum appears in N Engl J Med 2000;342(5):364].

51. Rajkumar SV, Fonseca R, Witzig TE, Gertz MA, Greipp PR: Bone marrow angiogenesis in patients achieving complete response after stem cell transplantation for multiple myeloma. Leukemia 1999;13:469–472.

52. Hideshima T, Chauhan D, Schlossman RL, Richardson PR, Anderson KC: Role of TNF-α in the pathophysiology of human multiple myeloma: Therapeutic applications. Oncogene 2001;20:4519–4527.

53. Damiano JS, Cress AE, Hazlehurst LA, Shtil AA, Dalton WS: Cell adhesion mediated drug resistance (CAM-DR): Role of integrins and resistance to apoptosis in human myeloma cell lines. Blood 1999;93:1658–1667.

54. Hideshima T, Chauhan D, Shima Y, et al: Thalidomide and its analogues overcome drug resistance of human multiple myeloma cells to conventional therapy. Blood 2000;96:2943–2950.

55. Hideshima T, Richardson P, Chauhan D, et al: The proteosome inhibitor PS341 inhibits growth, induces apoptosis, and overcomes drug resistance in human multiple myeloma cells. Cancer Res 2001;61:3071–3076.

56. Kawano M, Tanaka H, Ishikawa H, et al: Interleukin-1 accelerates autocrine growth of myeloma cells through interleukin-6 in human myeloma. Blood 1989;73:2145–2148.

57. Urashima M, Ogata A, Chauhan D, et al: Transforming growth factor b1: Differential effects on multiple myeloma versus normal B cells. Blood 1996;87:1928–1938.

58. Lu ZY, Zhang XG, Rodriguez C, et al: Interleukin-10 is a proliferation factor but not a differentiation factor for human myeloma cells. Blood 1995;85:2521–2527.

59. Choi SJ, Cruz JC, Craig F, et al: Macrophage inflammatory protein 1-alpha is a potential osteoclast stimulatory factor in multiple myeloma. Blood 2000;96:671–675.

60. Tinhofer I, Marschitz I, Henn T, Egle A, Greil R: Expression of functional interleukin-15 receptor and autocrine production of interleukin-15 as mechanisms of tumor propagation in multiple myeloma. Blood 2000;95:610–618.

61. Brenne AT, Baade Ro T, Waage A, Sundan A, Borset M, Hjorth-Hansen H: Interleukin-21 is a growth and survival factor for human myeloma cells. Blood 2002;99:3756–3762.

62. Cozzolino F, Torcia M, Aldinucci D, et al: Production of interleukin-1 by bone marrow myeloma cells. Blood 1989;74:380-387.
63. Garrett IR, Durie BG, Nedwin GE, et al: Production of lymphotoxin, a bone-resorbing cytokine, by cultured human myeloma cells. N Engl J Med 1987;317:526-532.
64. Barille S, Bataille R, Rapp MJ, Harousseau JL, Amiot M: Production of metalloproteinase-7 (matrilysin) by human myeloma cells and its potential involvement in metalloproteinase-2 activation. J Immunol 1999;163:5723-5728.
65. Hjertner O, Torgersen ML, Seidel C, et al: Hepatocyte growth factor (HGF) induces interleukin-11 secretion from osteoblasts: A possible role for HGF in myeloma-associated osteolytic bone disease. Blood 1999;94:3883-3888.
66. Lacey DL, Timms E, Tan H-L, et al: Osteoprotegerin ligand is a cytokine that regulates osteoclast differentiation and activation. Cell 1998;93:165-176.
67. Han JH, Choi SJ, Kurihara N, Koide M, Oba Y, Roodman GD: Macrophage inflammatory protein-1a is an osteoclastogenic factor in myeloma that is independent of receptor activator of nuclear factor kappaB ligand. Blood 2001;97:3349-3353.
68. Giuliani N, Bataille R, Mancini C, Lazzaretti M, Barille S: Myeloma cells induce imbalance in the osteoprotegrin/osteoprotegrin ligand system in the human bone marrow environment. Blood 2001;98:3527-3533.
69. Pearse RN, Sordillo EM, Yaccoby S, et al: Multiple myeloma disrupts the TRANCE/osteoprotegrin cytokine axis to trigger bone destruction and promote tumor progression. Proc Natl Acad Sci USA 2001;98:11581-11586.
70. Seidel C, Hjertner O, Abildgaard N, Heickendorff L, et al: Serum osteoprotegrin levels are reduced in patients with multiple myeloma with lytic bone disease. Blood 2001;98:2269-2271.
71. Oyajobi BO, Anderson DM, Traianedes K, Williams PJ, Yoneda T, Mundy GR: Therapeutic efficacy of a soluble receptor activator of nuclear factor kappaB-IgG Fc fusion protein in suppressing bone resorption and hypercalcemia in a model of humoral hypercalcemia of malignancy. Cancer Res 2001;61:2572-2578.
72. Yaccoby S, Barlogie B, Epstein J: Primary myeloma cells growing in SCID-hu mice: A model for studying the biology and treatment of myeloma and its manifestations. Blood 1998;92:2908-2913.
73. Kyle RA, Schreiman JS, McLeod RA, Beabout JW: Computed tomography in diagnosis and management of multiple myeloma and its variants. Arch Intern Med 1985;145:1451-1452.
74. Mundy GR, Bertolini DR: Bone destruction and hypercalcemia in plasma cell myeloma. Semin Oncol 1986;13:291-299.
75. Heilman RL, Velosa JA, Holley KE, Offord KP, Kyle RA: Long-term follow-up and response to chemotherapy in patients with light-chain deposition disease. Am J Kidney Dis 1992;20:34-41.
76. Leifer D, Grabowski T, Simonian N, Demirjian ZN: Leptomeningeal myelomatosis presenting with mental status changes and other neurologic findings. Cancer 1992;70:1899-1904.
77. Savage DG, Lindenbaum J, Garrett TJ: Biphasic pattern of bacterial infection in multiple myeloma. Ann Intern Med 1982;96:47-50.
78. Rajkumar SV, Hayman S, Gertz MA, et al: Combination therapy with thalidomide plus dexamethasone for newly diagnosed myeloma. J Clin Oncol 2002;20:4319-4323.
79. Weber D, Rankin K, Gavino M, Delasalle K, Alexanian R: Thalidomide alone or with dexamethasone for previously untreated multiple myeloma. J Clin Oncol 2003;21:16-19.
80. Kintzer JSJ, Rosenow ECI, Kyle RA: Thoracic and pulmonary abnormalities in multiple myeloma: A review of 958 cases. Arch Intern Med 1978;138:727-730.
81. Blade J, Lust JA, Kyle RA: Immunoglobulin D multiple myeloma: Presenting features, response to therapy, and survival in a series of 53 cases. J Clin Oncol 1994;12:2398-2404.
82. Kyle RA, Greipp PR: Smoldering multiple myeloma. N Engl J Med 1980;302:1347-1349.
83. Dimopoulos MA, Moulopoulos A, Smith T, Delasalle KB, Alexanian R. Risk of disease progression in asymptomatic multiple myeloma. Am J Med 1993;94:57-61.
84. Kyle RA: "Benign" monoclonal gammopathy—after 20 to 35 years of follow-up. Mayo Clin Proc 1993;68:26-36.
85. Blade J, Lopez-Guillermo A, Rozman C, et al: Malignant transformation and life expectancy in monoclonal gammopathy of undetermined significance. Br J Haematol 1992;81:391-394.
86. Blade J, Kyle RA: Monoclonal gammopathy of undetermined significance. In Malpas JS, Bergsgagel DE, Kyle R, Anderson K (eds): Myeloma: Biology and Management, 2nd ed, Oxford, Oxford Medical Publications 1998, pp 513-544.
87. Greipp PR, Witzig TE, Gonchoroff NJ, et al: Immunofluorescence labeling indices in myeloma and related monoclonal gammopathies. Mayo Clin Proc 1987;62:969-977.
88. Witzig TE, Gonchoroff NJ, Katzmann JA, Therneau T, Kyle RA, Greipp PR: Peripheral blood B cell labeling indices are a measure of disease activity in patients with monoclonal gammopathies. J Clin Oncol 1988;6:1041-1046.
89. Witzig TE, Gertz MA, Lust JA, Kyle RA, O'Fallon WM, Greipp PR: Peripheral blood monoclonal plasma cells as a predictor of survival in patients with multiple myeloma. Blood 1996;88:1780-1787.
90. Bataille R, Durie BGM, Grenier J, Sany J: Prognostic factors and staging in multiple myeloma: A reappraisal. J Clin Oncol 1986;4:80-87.
91. Durie BGM, Salmon SE: A clinical staging system for multiple myeloma: Correlation of measured cell mass with presenting clinical features, response to treatment and survival. Cancer 1975;36:842-854.
92. Gassmann W, Pralle H, Haferlach T, et al: Staging systems for multiple myeloma: A comparison. Br J Haematol 1985;59:703-711.
93. Greipp PR: Prognosis in myeloma. Mayo Clin Proc 1994;69:895-902.
94. Greipp PR, Raymond NM, Kyle RA, O'Fallon WM: Multiple myeloma: Significance of plasmablastic subtype in morphological classification. Blood 1985;65:305-310.
95. Cuzick J, Cooper EH, MacLennan IC: The prognostic value of serum beta 2 microglobulin compared with other presentation features in myelomatosis. Br J Cancer 1985;52:1-6.
96. Blade J, Rozman C, Cervantes F, Reverter JC, Montserrat E: A new prognostic system for multiple myeloma based on easily available parameters. Br J Haematol 1989;72:507-511.
97. Dimopoulos MA, Barlogie B, Smith TL, Alexanian R: High serum lactate dehydrogenase level as a marker for drug resistance and short survival in multiple myeloma. Ann Intern Med 1991;115:931-935.
98. Greipp P, Lust J, O'Fallon M, Katzmann J, Witzig T, Kyle R: Plasma cell labeling index and b2-microglobulin predict survival independent of thymidine kinase and C-reactive protein in multiple myeloma. Blood 1993;81:3382-3387.
99. Durie BG, Stock-Novack D, Salmon SE, et al: Prognostic value of pretreatment serum beta 2 microglobulin in myeloma: A Southwest Oncology Group Study. Blood 1990;75:823-830.
100. Bataille R, Boccadoro M, Klein B, Durie B, Pileri A: C-reactive protein and β-2 microglobulin produce a simple and powerful myeloma staging system. Blood 1992;80:733-737.
101. Greipp PR, Leong T, Bennett JM, et al: Plasmablastic morphology—an independent prognostic factor with clinical and laboratory correlates: Eastern Cooperative Oncology Group (ECOG) myeloma trial E9486 report by the ECOG Myeloma Laboratory Group. Blood 1998;91:2501-2507.
102. Tricot G, Barlogie B, Jagannath S, et al: Poor prognosis in multiple myeloma is associated only with partial or complete deletions of chromosome 13 or abnormalities involving 11q and not with other karyotype abnormalities. Blood 1995;86:4250-4256.
103. Fonseca R, Bailey RJ, Ahmann GJ, et al: Genomic abnormalities in monoclonal gammopathy of undetermined significance. Blood 2002;100:1417-1424.
104. Konigsberg R, Zojer N, Ackermann J, et al: Predictive role of interphase cytogenetics for survival of patients with multiple myeloma. J Clin Oncol 2000;18:804-812.
105. Avet-Loiseau H, Li JY, Morineau N, et al: Monosomy 13 is associated with the transition of monoclonal gammopathy of undetermined significance to multiple myeloma. Intergroupe Francophone du Myelome. Blood 1999;94:2583-2589.
106. Zhan F, Hardin J, Kordsmeier B, et al: Global gene expression profiling of multiple myeloma, monoclonal gammopathy of undetermined significance, and normal bone marrow plasma cells. Blood 2002;99:1745-1757.
107. Plowright EE, Li Z, Bergsagel PL, et al: Ectopic expression of fibroblast growth factor receptor 3 promotes myeloma cell proliferation and prevents apoptosis. Blood 2000;95:992-998.

108. Chauhan D, Auclair D, Robinson EK, et al: Identification of genes regulated by dexamethasone in multiple myeloma cells using oligonucleotide arrays. Oncogene 2002;21:1346-1358.

109. Mitsiades N, Mitsiades CS, Poulaki V, et al: Molecular sequelae of proteasome inhibition in human multiple myeloma cells. Proc Natl Acad Sci USA 2002;99:14374-14379.

110. Bataille R, Jourdan M, Zhang XG, Klein B: Serum levels of interleukin 6, a potent myeloma cell growth factor, as a reflect of disease severity in plasma cell dyscrasias. J Clin Invest 1989;84:2008-2011.

111. Ludwig H, Nachbaur DM, Fritz E, Krainer M, Huber H: Interleukin-6 is a prognostic factor in multiple myeloma. Blood 1991;77:2794-2795.

112. Greipp PR, Gaillard JP, Kalish LA, et al: Independent prognostic value for serum soluble interleukin-6 receptor (sIL-6R) in Eastern Cooperative Oncology Group (ECOG) myeloma trial E9487. Proc Am Soc Clin Oncol 1993;12:404.

113. Seidel C, Borset M, Turesson I, Abildgaard N, Sundan A, Waage A: Elevated serum concentrations of hepatocyte growth factor in patients with multiple myeloma. The Nordic Myeloma Study Group. Blood 1998;91:806-812.

114. Seidel C, Sundan A, Hjorth M, et al: Serum syndecan-1: A new independent prognostic marker in multiple myeloma. Blood 2000;95:388-392.

115. Dahl IM, Turesson I, Holmberg E, Lilja K: Serum hyaluronan in patients with multiple myeloma: Correlation with survival and Ig concentration. Blood 1999;93:4144-4148.

116. Rajkumar SV, Fonseca R, Lacy MQ, et al: Plasmablastic morphology is an independent predictor of poor survival after autologous stem-cell transplantation for multiple myeloma. J Clin Oncol 1999;17:1551-1557.

117. Suchman AL, Coleman M, Mouradian JA, Wolf DJ, Saletan S: Aggressive plasma cell myeloma: A terminal phase. Arch Intern Med 1981;141:1315-1320.

118. Palmer M, Belch A, Hanson J, Brox L: Reassessment of the relationship between M-protein decrement and survival in multiple myeloma. Br J Cancer 1989;59:110-112.

119. Blade J, Lopez-Guillermo A, Bosch F, et al: Impact of response to treatment on survival in multiple myeloma: Results in a series of 243 patients. Br J Haematol 1994;88:117-121.

120. Durie BG, Russell DH, Salmon SE: Reappraisal of plateau phase in myeloma. Lancet 1980;2:65-68.

121. Salmon SE, Haut A, Bonnet JD, et al: Alternating combination chemotherapy and levamisole improves survival in multiple myeloma: A Southwest Oncology Group Study. J Clin Oncol 1983;1:453-461.

122. Blade J, Samson D, Reece D, et al: Criteria for evaluating disease response and progression in patients with multiple myeloma treated by high-dose therapy and haemopoietic stem cell transplantation. Myeloma Subcommittee of the EBMT, European Group for Blood and Marrow Transplant. Br J Haematol 1998;102:1115-1123.

123. Billadeau D, Blackstadt M, Greipp P, et al: Analysis of B-lymphoid malignancies using allele-specific polymerase chain reaction: A technique for sequential quantitation of residual disease. Blood 1991;78:3021-3029.

124. MacKenzie MR, Wold H, George C, et al: Consolidation hemibody radiotherapy following induction combination chemotherapy in high-tumor-burden multiple myeloma. J Clin Oncol 1992;10:1769-1774.

125. Thomas PJ, Daban A, Bontoux D: Double hemibody irradiation in chemotherapy-resistant multiple myeloma. Cancer Treat Rep 1984;68:1173-1175.

126. Moreau P, Facon T, Attal M, et al: Comparison of 200 mg/m(2) melphalan and 8 Gy total body irradiation plus 140 mg/m(2) melphalan as conditioning regimens for peripheral blood stem cell transplantation in patients with newly diagnosed multiple myeloma: Final analysis of the Intergroupe Francophone du Myelome 9502 randomized trial. Blood 2002;99:731-735.

127. Alexanian R, Dimopoulos M: The treatment of multiple myeloma. New Engl J Med 1994;330:484-489.

128. Kyle RA: Newer approaches to the therapy of multiple myeloma. Blood 1990;76:1678-1679.

129. Case DCJ, Lee DJI, Clarkson BD: Improved survival times in multiple myeloma treated with melphalan, prednisone, cyclophosphamide, vincristine and BCNU: M-2 protocol. Am J Med 1977;63:897-903.

130. MacLennan I, C., Chapman C, Dunn J, Kelly K: Combined chemotherapy with ABCM versus melphalan for treatment of myelomatosis. The Medical Research Council Working Party for Leukaemia in Adults. Lancet 1992;339:200-205.

131. Boccadoro M, Marmont F, Tribalto M, et al: Multiple myeloma: VMCP/VBAP alternating combination chemotherapy is not superior to melphalan and prednisone even in high-risk patients. J Clin Oncol 1991;9:444-448.

132. Blade J, San Miguel JF, Alcala A, et al: Alternating combination VCMP/VBAP chemotherapy versus melphalan/prednisone in the treatment of multiple myeloma: A randomized multicentric study of 487 patients. J Clin Oncol 1993;11:1165-1171.

133. Gregory WM, Richards MA, Malpas JS: Combination chemotherapy versus melphalan and prednisolone in the treatment of multiple myeloma: An overview of published trials. J Clin Oncol 1992;10:334-342.

134. Myeloma Trialists' Collaborative Group: Combination chemotherapy versus melphalan plus prednisone as treatment for multiple myeloma: An overview of 6633 patients from 27 randomized trials. J Clin Oncol 1998;16:3832-3842.

135. Barlogie B, Smith L, Alexanian R: Effective treatment of advanced multiple myeloma refractory to alkylating agents. N Engl J Med 1984;310:1353-1356.

136. Monconduit M, Le Loet X, Bernard JF, Michaux JL: Combination chemotherapy with vincristine, doxurubicin, dexamethasone for refractory or relapsing multiple myeloma. Br J Haematol 1986;63:599-601.

137. Sheehan T, Judge M, Parker AC: The efficacy and toxicity of VAD in the treatment of myeloma and related disorders. Scand J Haematol 1986;37:425-428.

138. Portier M, Zhang XG, Caron E, Lu ZY, Bataille R, Klein B: Gamma-interferon in multiple myeloma: Inhibition of interleukin-6 dependent myeloma cell growth and downregulation of IL-6 receptor expression in vitro. Blood 1993;81:3076-3082.

139. Ludwig H, Cohen AM, Polliack A, et al: Interferon-a for induction and maintenance in multiple myeloma: Results of two multicenter randomized trials and summary of other studies. Ann Oncol 1995;6:467-476.

140. Ludwig H, Fritz E, Neuda J, Durie BGM: Patient preferences for interferon-a in multiple myeloma. J Clin Oncol 1997;15:1672-1679.

141. Zee B, Cole B, Li T, et al: Quality-adjusted time without symptoms or toxicity analysis of interferon maintenance in multiple myeloma. J Clin Oncol 1998;16:2834-2839.

142. Berenson JR, Crowley JJ, Grogan TM, et al: Maintenance therapy with alternate-day prednisone improves survival in multiple myeloma patients. Blood 2002;99:3163-3168.

143. Gertz MA, Garton JP, Greipp PR, Witzig TE, Kyle RA: A phase II study of high-dose methylprednisolone in refractory or relapsed multiple myeloma. Leukemia 1995;9:2115-2118.

144. Avvisati G, Mandelli F: The role of interferon-alpha in the management of myelomatosis. Hematol Oncol Clin North Am 1992;6:395-405.

145. Brandes LJ, Israels LG: Weekly low-dose cyclophosphamide and alternate-day prednisone: An effective low toxicity regimen for advanced myeloma. Eur J Haematol 1987;39:362-368.

146. Oken MM, Kyle RA, Greipp PR, et al: Complete remission induction with combined VBMCP chemotherapy plus interferon (rIFN alpha 2b) in patients with multiple myeloma. Leuk Lymphoma 1996;20:447-452.

147. Cooper JA, Howell B: The when and how of Src regulation. Cell 1993;73:1051-1054.

148. Osterborg A, Bjorkholm M, Bjoreman M, et al: Natural interferon-α in combination with melphalan/prednisone versus melphalan/prednisone in the treatment of multiple myeloma stages II and III: A randomized study from the Myeloma Group of Central Sweden. Blood 1993;81:1428-1434.

149. Oken MM, Leong T, Kay NE, et al: The effect of adding interferon (rIFNa2) or high-dose cyclophosphamide to VBMCP to treat multiple myeloma: Result from an ECOG phase II trial (abstract). Blood 1995;86:441a.

150. Grogan TM, Spier CM, Salmon SE, et al: P-glycoprotein expression in human plasma cell myeloma: Correlation with prior chemotherapy. Blood 1993;81:490–495.
151. Salmon SE, Dalton WS, Grogan TM, et al: Multidrug-resistant myeloma: Laboratory and clinical effects of verapamil as a chemosensitizer. Blood 1991;78:44–50.
152. Bataille R, Barlogie B, Yang Z, et al: Biologic effects of anti-interleukin-6 murine monoclonal antibody in advanced multiple myeloma. Blood 1995;86:685–691.
153. Barlogie B, Desikan R, Eddlemon P, et al: Extended survival in advanced and refractory multiple myeloma after single-agent thalidomide: Identification of prognostic factors in a phase 2 study of 169 patients. Blood 2001;98:492–494.
154. Moehler TM, Neben K, Benner A, et al: Salvage therapy for multiple myeloma with thalidomide and CED chemotherapy. Blood 2001;98:3846–3848.
155. Garcia-Sanz R, Gonzalez-Fraile MI, Sierra M, Lopez C, Gonzalez M, San Miguel JF: The combination of thalidomide, cyclophospha-mide and dexamethasone (ThaCyDex) is feasible and can be an option for relapsed/refractory multiple myeloma. Hematol J 2002; 3:43–48.
156. Anderson KC: Who benefits from high dose therapy for multiple myeloma? J Clin Oncol 1995;13:1291–1296.
157. Harousseau JL, Attal M: The role of autologous hematopoietic stem cell transplantation in multiple myeloma. Semin Hemat 1997;34:61–66.
158. Attal M, Harousseau JL, Stoppa AM, et al: Autologous bone marrow transplantation versus conventional chemotherapy in multiple myeloma: A prospective, randomized trial. New Engl J Med 1996;335:91–97.
159. Fermand JP, Ravaud P, Chevret S, et al: High-dose therapy and autologous peripheral blood stem cell transplantation in multiple myeloma: Up-front or rescue treatment? Results of a multicenter sequential randomized clinical trial. Blood 1998;92:3131–3136.
160. Lenhoff S, Hjorth M, Holmberg E, et al: Impact on survival of high-dose therapy with autologous stem cell support in patients younger than 60 years with newly diagnosed multiple myeloma: A population-based study. Blood 2000;95:7–11.
161. Child JA, Morgan GJ, Davies FE, et al: High-dose chemotherapy with hematopoietic stem-cell rescue for multiple myeloma. N Engl J Med 2003;348:1875–1883.
162. Anderson KC, Barut BA, Ritz J, et al: Monoclonal antibody-purged autologous bone marrow transplantation therapy for multiple myeloma. Blood 1991;77:712–720.
163. Anderson KC, Anderson J, Soiffer R, et al: Monoclonal antibody-purged bone marrow transplantation therapy for multiple myeloma. Blood 1993;82:2568–2576.
164. Seiden M, Schlossman R, Andersen J, et al: Monoclonal antibody-purged bone marrow transplantation therapy for multiple myeloma. Leuk Lymphoma 1995;17:87–93.
165. Schiller G, Vescio R, Freytes C, et al: Transplantation of CD34 positive peripheral blood progenitor cells following high dose chemotherapy for patients with advanced multiple myeloma. Blood 1995;86:390–397.
166. Stewart AK, Vescio R, Schiller G, et al: Purging of autologous peripheral-blood stem cells using CD34 selection does not improve overall or progression-free survival after high-dose chemotherapy for multiple myeloma: Results of a multicenter randomized controlled trial. J Clin Oncol 2001;19:3771–3779.
167. Barlogie B, Jagannath S, Desikan KR, et al: Total therapy with tandem transplants for newly diagnosed multiple myeloma. Blood 1999;93:55–65.
168. Vesole DH, Tricot G, Jagannath S, et al: Autotransplants in multiple myeloma: What have we learned? Blood 1996;88:838–847.
169. Desikan R, Barlogie B, Sawyer J, et al: Results of high-dose therapy for 1000 patients with multiple myeloma: Durable complete remissions and superior survival in the absence of chromosome 13 abnormalities. Blood 2000;95:4008–4010.
170. Attal M, Payen C, Facon T, et al: Single versus double transplant in myeloma: A randomized trial of the Inter Groupe Francais du Myeloma (IMF). Blood 2002;100:418a.
171. Fermand JP, Marolleau JP, Alberti C, et al: Single versus tandem high dose therapy (HDT) supported with autologous blood stem cell (ABSC) transplantation using unselected or CD34 enriched
172. Giralt S, Weber D, Colome M, et al: Phase I trial of cyclosporine-induced autologous graft-versus-host disease in patients with multiple myeloma undergoing high-dose chemotherapy with autologous stem-cell rescue. J Clin Oncol 1997;15:667–673.
173. Qing Y, Osterborg A: Idiotype-specific T cells in multiple myeloma: Targets for an immunotherapeutic intervention? Med Oncol 1996;13:1–7.
174. Bergenbrant B, Yiu Q, Osterborg A, et al: Modulation of anti-idiotypic immune response by immunization with the autologous M component protein multiple myeloma patients. Br J Haematol 1996;92:840–846.
175. Hsu FJ, Benike C, Fagnoni F, et al: Vaccination of patients with B-cell lymphoma using autologous antigen-pulsed dendritic cells. Nat Med 1996;2:52–58.
176. Bensinger WI, Buchner CD, Anasetti C, et al: Allogeneic marrow transplantation for multiple myeloma: An analysis of risk factors on outcome. Blood 1996;88:2787–2793.
177. Gahrton G, Svensson H, Bjorkstrand B, et al: Syngeneic transplantation in multiple myeloma: A case-matched comparison with autologous and allogeneic transplantation. European Group for Blood and Marrow Transplantation. Bone Marrow Transplant 1999;24:741–745.
178. Gahrton G, Tura S, Ljungman P, et al: Allogeneic bone marrow transplantation in multiple myeloma. New Engl J Med 1991;325:1267–1273.
179. Gahrton G, Tura S, Ljungman P, et al: Prognostic factors in allogeneic bone marrow transplantation for multiple myeloma. J Clin Oncol 1995;13:1312–1322.
180. Gahrton G, Svensson H, Cavo M, et al: Progress in allogeneic bone marrow and peripheral blood stem cell transplantation for multiple myeloma: A comparison between transplants performed 1983–1993 and 1994–1998 at European Group for Blood and Marrow centers. Brit J Haematol 2001;113:209–216.
181. Bjorkstrand BB, Ljungman P, Svensson H, et al: Allogeneic bone marrow transplantation versus autologous stem cell transplantation in multiple myeloma: A retrospective case-matched study from the European Group for Blood and Marrow Transplantation. Blood 1996;88:4711–4718.
182. Bensinger WI, Maloney D, Storb R: Allogeneic hematopoietic cell transplantation for multiple myeloma. Semin Hematol 2001;38:243–249.
183. Schlossman SF, Alyea E, Orsini E, et al: Immune based strategies to improve hematopoietic stem cell transplantation in multiple myeloma. In Dicke KA, Keating A, eds. Autologous Marrow and Blood Transplantation. Charlottesville, Virginia, Carden, Jennings Publishing, 1999, pp 207–221.
184. Schlossman SF, Anderson KC: Bone marrow transplantation in multiple myeloma. In Jones R (ed) Current Opinions in Oncology, Vol 11. Philadelphia, Lippincott Williams & Wilkins, 1999, pp 102–108.
185. Soiffer RJ, Murray C, Mauch P, et al: Prevention of graft-versus-host disease by selective depletion of CD6-positive T lymphocytes from donor bone marrow. J Clin Oncol 1992;10:1191–1200.
186. Alyea E, Weller E, Schlossman R, et al: T-cell-depleted allogeneic bone marrow transplantation followed by donor lymphocyte infusion in patients with multiple myeloma: induction of graft-versus-myeloma effect. Blood 2001;98:934–939.
187. Corradini P, Voena C, Tarella C, et al: Molecular and clinical remissions in multiple myeloma: Role of autologous and allogeneic transplantation of hematopoietic cells. J Clin Oncol 1999;17:208–215.
188. Martinelli G, Terragna C, Zamagni E, et al: Molecular remission after allogeneic or autologous transplantation of hematopoietic stem cells for multiple myeloma. J Clin Oncol 2000;18:2273–2281.
189. Cavo M, Terragna C, Martinelli G, et al: Molecular monitoring of minimal residual disease in patients in long-term complete remission after allogeneic stem cell transplantation for multiple myeloma. Blood 2000;96:355–357.
190. Willems P, Verhagen O, Segeren C, et al: Consensus strategy to quantitate malignant cells in myeloma patients is validated in a multicenter study. Blood 2000;96:63–70.
ABSC: Preliminary results of a two by two designed randomized trial in 230 young patients with multiple myeloma. Blood 2002;100:815a.

191. Tricot G, Vesole DH, Jagannath S, et al: Graft-versus-myeloma effect: Proof of principle. Blood 1996;87:1196–1198.

192. Verdonck LF, Lokhorst HM, Dekker AW, Nieuwenhuis HK, Petersen EJ: Graft-versus-myeloma effect in two cases. Lancet 1996;347:800–801.

193. Alyea EP, Soiffer RJ, Canning C, et al: Toxicity and efficacy of defined doses of CD4+ donor lymphocytes for treatment of relapse after allogeneic bone marrow transplant. Blood 1998;91:3671–3680.

194. Alyea E, Weller E, Schlossman R, et al: Outcome after autologous and allogeneic stem cell transplantation for patients with multiple myeloma: Impact of graft versus myeloma effect. Bone Marrow Transplant 2003;32:1145–1151.

195. Badros A, Barlogie B, Morris C, et al: High response rate in refractory and poor-risk multiple myeloma after allotransplantation using a nonmyeloablative conditioning regimen and donor lymphocyte infusions. Blood 2001;97:2574–2579.

196. Kroger N, Schwerdtfeger R, Kiehl M, et al: Autologous stem cell transplantation followed by a dose-reduced allograft induces high complete remission rate in multiple myeloma. Blood 2002;100:755–760.

197. Maloney D, Sahebi F, Srockerl-Goldstein KE, et al: Combining an allogeneic graft versus myeloma effect with high dose autologous stem cell rescue in the treatment of multiple myeloma. Blood 2001;98:434a.

198. Major P, Lortholary A, Hon J, et al: Zoledronic acid is superior to pamidronate in the treatment of hypercalcemia of malignancy: A pooled analysis of two randomized, controlled clinical trials. J Clin Oncol 2001;19:558–567.

199. Torra R, Blade J, Cases A, et al: Patient with multiple myeloma requiring long-term dialysis: Presenting features, response to therapy, and outcome in a series of 20 patients. Br J Haematol 1995;91:854–859.

200. Johnson WJ, Kyle RA, Pineda AA, O'Brien PC, Holley KE: Treatment of renal failure associated with multiple myeloma: Plasmapheresis, hemodialysis, and chemotherapy. Arch Intern Med 1990;150:863–869.

201. Lahtinen R, Laasko M, Palva I, Virkkunen P, Elomaa I: Randomised, placebo-controlled multicentre trial of clodronate in multiple myeloma. Lancet 1992;340:1049–1052.

202. Berenson J, Lichtenstein A, Porter L, et al: Pamidronate disodium reduces the occurrence of skeletal events in patients with advanced multiple myeloma. N Engl J Med 1996;334:488–493.

203. Berenson JR, et al: Phase-1 clinical study of a new bisphosphonate, zoledronate (CGP-42446), in patients with osteolytic bone metastases. Blood 1996;88(Suppl 1):586a.

204. Lipton A, et al: The effects of the bisphosphonate, zoledronic acid, when administered as a short intravenous infusion in patients with bone metastases: A phase-1 study. Paper (abstract 848) presented at the American Society of Clinical Oncology Annual Meeting, May 17–20, 1997, Denver, Colorado.

205. Lipton A, et al: Phase II study of the bisphosphonate, zoledronate in patients with osteolytic lesions. Paper (abstract 48) presented at the Secondary International Conference: Cancer-Induced Bone Diseases, March 27–29, 1999, Davos, Switzerland.

206. Savage AD, Belson DJ, Vescio RA, et al: Pamidronate reduces IL-6 production by bone marrow stroma from multiple myeloma patients. Blood 1996;88:105a.

207. Garton JP, Gertz MA, Witzig TE, et al: Epoetin-α for the treatment of the anemia of multiple myeloma: A prospective, randomized, placebo-controlled, double-blind trial. Arch Intern Med 1995;155:2069–2074.

208. Osterborg A, Boogaerts MA, Cimino R, et al: Recombinant human erythropoietin in transfusion-dependent anemic patients with multiple myeloma and non-Hodgkin's lymphoma: A randomized multicenter study. Blood 1996;87:2675–2682.

209. Noel P, Kyle RA: Plasma cell leukemia: An evaluation of response to therapy. Am J Med 1987;83:1062–1068.

210. Cavo M, Galieni P, Gobbi M, et al: Nonsecretory multiple myeloma : Presenting findings, clinical course and prognosis. Acta Haematol 1985;74:27–30.

211. Bardwick PA, Zvaifler NJ, Gill GN, Newman D, Greenway GD, Resnick DL: Plasma cell dyscrasia with polyneuropathy, organomegaly, endocrinopathy, M protein, and skin changes: The POEMS syndrome. Report on two cases and a review of the literature. Medicine (Baltimore) 1980;59:311–322.

212. Waldenstrom JG: POEMS: a multifactorial syndrome. Haematologica 1992;77:197–203.

213. Frassica DA, Frassica FJ, Schray MF, Sim FH, Kyle RA: Solitary plasmactyoma of bone: Mayo Clinic Experience. Int J Radiat Oncol Biol Phys 1989;16:43–48.

214. Dimopoulos MA, Goldstein J, Fuller L, Delasalle K, Alexanian R: Curability of solitary bone plasmacytoma. J Clin Oncol 1992;10:587–590.

215. Holland J, Trenkner DA, Wasserman TH, Fineberg B: Plasmacytoma. Treatment results and conversion to myeloma. Cancer 1992;69:1513–1517.

216. Ganjoo RK, Malpas JS: Plasmacytoma. In Malpas JS, Bergsgagel DE, Kyle R, Anderson K (eds): Myeloma: Biology and Management, 2nd ed, Oxford, Oxford Medical Publications 1998, p 545.

217. Kyle RA, Garton JP: The spectrum of IgM monoclonal gammopathy in 430 cases. Mayo Clin Proc 1987;62:719–731.

218. Waldenstrom J: Incipient myelomatosis or "essential" hyperglobulinemia with fibrinogenopenia: A new syndrome? Acta Med Scand 1944;117:216.

219. Dimopoulos MA, Alexanian R: Waldenström's macroglobulinemia. Blood 1994;83:1452–1159.

220. Kyle RA, Anderson KC: A tribute to Jan Waldenström. Blood 1997;89:4245–4247.

221. Dimopoulos MA, Zervas C, Zomas A, et al: Treatment of Waldenström's macroglobulinemia with rituximab. J Clin Oncol 2002;20:2327–2333.

222. Calasanz MJ, Cigudosa JC, Odero MD, et al: Cytogenetic analysis of 280 patients with multiple myeloma and related disorders: Primary breakpoints and clinical correlations. Genes Chromosomes Cancer 1997;18:84–93.

223. Palka G, Spadano A, Geraci L, et al: Chromosome changes in 19 patients with Waldenström's macroglobulinemia. Cancer Genet Cytogenet 1987;29:261–269.

224. Wagner SD, Martinelli V, Luzzatto L: Similar patterns of V kappa gene usage but different degrees of somatic mutation in hairy cell leukemia, prolymphocytic leukemia, Waldenström's macroglobulinemia, and myeloma. Blood 1994;83:3647–3653.

225. Aoki H, Takishita M, Kosaka M, Saito S: Frequent somatic mutations in D and/or JH segments of Ig gene in Waldenström's macroglobulinemia and chronic lymphocytic leukemia (CLL) with Richter's syndrome but not in common CLL. Blood 1995;85:1913–1919.

226. Klein U, Goossens T, Fischer M, et al: Somatic hypermutation in normal and transformed human B cells. Immunol Rev 1998;162:261–280.

227. Kyle RA: Waldenström's macroglobulinemia. In Malpas JS, Bergsgagel DE, Kyle R, Anderson K (eds): Myeloma: Biology and Management, 2nd ed, Oxford, Oxford Medical Publications 1998, p 639.

228. Facon T, Brouillard M, Duhamel A, et al: Prognostic factors in Waldenström's macroglobulinemia: A report of 167 cases. J Clin Oncol 1993;11:1553–1558.

229. Gobbi PG, Bettini R, Montecucco C, et al: Study of prognosis in Waldenström's macroglobulinemia: A proposal for a simple binary classification with clinical and investigational utility. Blood 1994;83:2939–2945.

230. Dimopoulos MA, Kantarjian H, Weber D, et al: Primary therapy of Waldenström's macroglobulinemia with 2-chlorodeoxyadenosine. J Clin Oncol 1994;12:2694–2698.

231. Dimopoulos MA, Kantarjian H, Estey E, et al: Treatment of Waldenström's macroglobulinemia with 2-chlorodeoxyadenosine. Ann Int Med 1993;118:195–198.

232. Foran J, Rohatiner AZS, Coiffier B, et al: Multicenter phase II study of fludarabine phosphate for patients with newly diagnosed lymphoplasmacytoid lymphoma, Waldenström's macroglobulinemia and mantle cell lymphoma. J Clin Oncol 1999;17:546–553.

233. Leblond V, Ben-Othman T, Deconinck E, et al: Activity of fludarabine in previously treated Waldenström's macroglobulinemia: A report of 71 cases. J Clin Oncol 1998;16:2060–2064.

234. Leblond V, Levy V, Maloisel F, et al: Multicenter, randomized comparative trial of fludarabine and the combination of cyclophosphamide-doxorubicin-prednisone in 92 patients with Waldenström's macroglobulinemia in first relapse or with primary refractory disease. Blood 2001;98:2640–2644.

235. Legouffe E, Rossi JF, Laporte JP, et al: Treatment of Waldenström's macroglobulinemia with very low doses of alpha interferon. Leuk Lymphoma 1995;19:337–342.

236. Desikan R, Dhodapkar M, Siegel D, et al: High-dose therapy with autologous haemopoietic stem cell support for Waldenström's macroglobulinaemia. Br J Haematol 1999;105:993–996.

237. Byrd JC, White CA, Link B, et al: Rituximab therapy in previously treated Waldenström's macroglobulinemia: Preliminary evidence of activity [abstract]. Blood 1998;(Suppl 1):106a.

238. Franklin EC, Lowenstein J, Bigelow B, Meltzer M: Heavy chain disease, a new disorder of serum g-globulins: Report of the first case. Am J Med 1964;37:332.

239. Kyle RA, Wahner-Roedler DL: Heavy chain diseases: Neoplastic diseases of the blood, 3rd ed. New York, Churchill Livingstone, 1996.

240. Fermand JP, Brouet JC, Danon F, Seligmann M: Gamma heavy chain "disease": Heterogeneity of the clinicopathologic features. Report of 16 cases and review of the literature. Medicine (Baltimore) 1989;68:321–335.

241. Kyle RA, Greipp PR, Banks PM: The diverse picture of γ heavy-chain disease: Report of seven cases and review of literature. Mayo Clin Proc 1981;56:439–451.

242. Seligmann M, Danon F, Hurez D, Mihaesco E, Preud'homme JL: Alpha-chain disease: A new immunoglobulin abnormality. Science 1968;162:1396–1397.

243. Rambaud JC, Halphen M, Galian A, Tsapis A: Immunoproliferative small intestinal disease (IPSID): Relationships with a-chain disease and "Mediterranean" lymphomas. Springer Semin Immunopathol 1990;12:239–250.

244. O'Keefe SJ, Winter TA, Newton KA, Ogden JM, Young GO, Price SK: Severe malnutrition associated with alpha-heavy chain disease: response to tetracycline and intensive nutritional support. Am J Gastroenterol 1988;83:995–1001.

245. Ben-Ayed F, Halphen M, Najjar T, et al: Treatment of alpha chain disease: Results of a prospective study in 21 Tunisian patients by the Tunisian-French Intestinal Lymphoma Study Group. Cancer 1989;63:1251–1256.

246. Wahner-Roedler DL, Kyle RA: M-heavy chain disease: Presentation as a benign monoclonal gammopathy. Am J Hematol 1992;40:56–60.

247. Kyle RA: Amyloidosis: Introduction and overview. J Intern Med 1992;232:507–508.

248. Falk RH, Comenzo RL, Skinner M: The systemic amyloidoses. N Engl J Med 1997;337:898–909.

249. Gillmore JD, Hawkins PN, Pepys MB: Amyloidosis: A review of recent diagnostic and therapeutic developments. Br J Haematol 1997;99:245–256.

250. Gertz MA, Kyle RA, Noel P: Primary systemic amyloidosis: A rare complication of immunoglobulin M monoclonal gammopathies and Waldenström's macroblobulinemia. J Clin Oncol 1993;11:914–920.

251. Kyle RA, Greipp PR: Amyloidosis (AL): Clinical and laboratory features in 229 cases. Mayo Clin Proc 1983;58:665–683.

252. Riedel DA, Pottern LM: The epidemiology of multiple myeloma. Hematol Oncol Clin North Am 1992;6:225–247.

253. Kyle RA, Gertz MA, Greipp PR, et al: Long-term survival (10 years or more) in 30 patients with primary amyloidosis. Blood 1999;93:1062–1066.

254. Cohen AS, Rubinow A, Anderson JJ, et al: Survival of patients with primary (AL) amyloidosis: Colchicine-treated cases from 1976 to 1983 compared with cases seen in previous years (1961 to 1973). Am J Med 1987;82:1182–1190.

255. Kyle RA, Gertz MA, Greipp PR, et al: A trial of three regimens for primary amyloidosis: Colchicine alone, melphalan and prednisone, and melphalan, prednisone, and colchicine. N Engl J Med 1997;336:1200–1207.

256. Gertz MA, Lacy MQ, Lust JA, Greipp PR, Witzig TE, Kyle RA: Prospective randomized trial of melphalan and prednisone versus vincristine, carmustine, melphalan, cyclophosphamide, and prednisone in the treatment of primary systemic amyloidosis. J Clin Oncol 1999;17:262–267.

257. Comenzo RL, Vosburgh E, Simms RW, et al: Dose-intensive melphalan with blood stem cell support for the treatment of AL amyloidosis: One-year follow-up in five patients. Blood 1996;88:2801–2806.

258. Comenzo RL, Vosburgh E, Falk RH, et al: Dose-intensive melphalan with blood stem-cell support for the treatment of AL (amyloid light-chain) amyloidosis: Survival and responses in 25 patients. Blood 1998;91:3662–3670.

259. Comenzo RL, Gertz MA: Autologous stem cell transplantation for primary systemic amyloidosis. Blood 2002;99:4276–4282.

260. Dispenzieri A, Lacy MQ, Kyle RA, et al: Eligibility for hematopoietic stem-cell transplantation for primary systemic amyloidosis is a favorable prognostic factor for survival. J Clin Oncol 2001;19:3350–3356.

261. Kyle RA, Gertz MA: Primary systemic amyloidosis: Clinical and laboratory features in 474 cases. Semin Hematol 1995;32:45–59.

262. Kyle RA, Linos A, Beard CM, et al: Incidence and natural history of primary systemic amyloidosis in Olmsted County, Minnesota, 1950 through 1989. Blood 1992;79:1817–1822.

263. Cueto-Garcia L, Reeder GS, Kyle RA, et al: Echocardiographic findings in systemic amyloidosis: Spectrum of cardiac involvement and relation to survival. J Am Coll Cardiol 1985;6:737–743.

264. Gertz MA, Kyle RA, Griffing WL, Hunder GG: Jaw claudication in primary systemic amyloidosis. Medicine (Baltimore) 1986;65:173–179.

265. Kyle RA, Kottke BA, Schirger A: Orthostatic hypotension as a clue to primary systemic amyloidosis. Circulation 1966;34:83–88.

266. Gertz MA, Kyle RA: Hepatic amyloidosis (primary [AL], immunoglobulin light chain): The natural history in 80 patients. Am J Med 1988;85:73–80.

267. Gertz MA, Greipp PR, Kyle RA: Classification of amyloidosis by the detection of clonal excess of plasma cells in the bone marrow. J Lab Clin Med 1991;118:33–39.

268. Kyle RA, Greipp PR, O'Fallon WM: Primary systemic amyloidosis: Multivariate analysis for prognostic factors in 168 cases. Blood 1986;68:220–224.

269. Kyle RA, Greipp PR: Primary systemic amyloidosis: Comparison of melphalan and prednisone versus placebo. Blood 1978;52:818–827.

270. Kyle RA, Greipp PR, Garton JP, Gertz MA: Primary systemic amyloidosis: Comparison of melphalan/prednisone versus colchicine. Am J Med 1985;79:708–716.

271. Gertz MA, Kyle RA, Greipp PR: Response rates and survival in primary systemic amyloidosis. Blood 1991;77:257–262.

272. Gertz MA, Kyle RA: Acute leukemia and cytogenetic abnormalities complicating melphalan treatment of primary systemic amyloidosis. Arch Intern Med 1990;150:629–633.

273. Gianni L, Bellotti V, Gianni AM, Merlini G: New drug therapy of amyloidoses: Resorption of AL-type deposits with 4′-iodo-4′-deoxydoxorubicin. Blood 1995;86:855–861.

274. Van Buren M, Hene RJ, Verdonck LF, Verzijlbergen FJ, Lokhorst HM: Clinical remission after syngeneic bone marrow transplantation in a patient with AL amyloidosis. Ann Intern Med 1995;122:508–510.

275. Gertz MA, Kyle RA, O'Fallon WM: Dialysis support of patients with primary systemic amyloidosis: A study of 211 patients. Arch Intern Med 1992;152:2245–2250.

276. Kyle RA: Monoclonal gammopathy of undetermined significance: Natural history in 241 cases. Am J Med 1978;64:814–826.

277. Kyle RA: 'Benign' monoclonal gammopathy: A misnomer? JAMA 1984;251:1849–1854.

278. Axelsson U, Bachmann R, Hallen J: Frequency of pathological proteins (M-components) in 6995 sera from an adult population. Acta Med Scand 1966;179:235–247.

279. Kyle RA, Finkelstein S, Elveback LR, Kurland LT: Incidence of monoclonal proteins in a Minnesota community with a cluster of multiple myeloma. Blood 1972;40:719–724.

280. Crawford J, Eye MK, Cohen HJ: Evaluation of monoclonal gammopathies in the "well" elderly. Am J Med 1987;82:39–45.

281. Papadopoulos NM, Elin RJ, Wilson DM: Incidence of gamma-globulin banding in a healthy population by high-resolution electrophoresis. Clin Chem 1982;28:707–708.

282. Axelsson U: A 20-year follow-up study of 64 subjects with M-components. Acta Med Scand 1986;219:519–522.

283. Baldini L, Guffanti A, Cesana BM, et al: Role of different hematologic variables in defining the risk of malignant transformation in monoclonal gammopathy. Blood 1996;87(3):912–918.

284. Kyle RA, Robinson RA, Katzmann JA: The clinical aspects of biclonal gammopathies: Review of 57 cases. Am J Med 1981;71:999–1008.

285. Kyle RA, Greipp PR: "Idiopathic" Bence Jones proteinuria: Long-term follow-up in seven patients. N Engl J Med 1982;306:564–567.

286. Anderson KC: Targeted therapy for multiple myeloma. Semin Hematol 2001;38:286–294.

287. Chauhan D, Anderson KC: Apoptosis in multiple myeloma: Therapeutic implications. Apoptosis 2001;6:47–55.

288. Chauhan D, Pandey P, Ogata A, et al: Dexamethasone induces apoptosis of multiple myeloma cells in a JNK/SAP kinase independent mechanism. Oncogene 1997;15:837–843.

289. Chauhan D, Pandey P, Ogata A, et al: Cytochrome-c dependent and independent induction of apoptosis in multiple myeloma cells. J Biol Chem 1997;272:29995–29997.

290. Hayashi T, Hideshima T, Akiyama M, et al: Arsenic trioxide inhibits growth of human multiple myeloma cells in the bone marrow microenvironment. Mol Cancer Ther 2002;1:851–860.

291. Lentsch S, LeBlanc R, Podar K, et al: Immunodulatory analogs of thalidomide inhibit growth of HS Sultan cells and angiogenesis in vivo. Leukemia 2003;17:41–44.

292. Lentzsch S, Rogers MS, LeBlanc R, et al: S-3-Amino-phthalimido-glutarimide inhibits angiogenesis and growth of B-cell neoplasias in mice. Cancer Res 2002;62:2300–2305.

293. LeBlanc R, Catley L, Hideshima T, et al: Proteasome inhibitor PS-341 inhibits human myeloma cell growth in vivo and prolongs survival in a murine model. Cancer Res 2002;62:4996–5000.

294. Richardson PG, Schlossman RL, Weller E, et al: Immunomodulatory drug CC-5013 overcomes drug resistance and is well tolerated in patients with relapsed multiple myeloma. Blood 2002;100:3063–3067.

295. Richardson P, Berenson J, Irwin D, et al: Phase II trial of pS-341, a novel proteasome inhibitor, alone or in combination with dexamethasone, in patients with multiple myeloma who have relapsed following frontline therapy and are refractory to their most recent therapy. Blood 2001;98:774a.

296. Richardson P, Barlogie B, Berenson J, et al: A phase II study of bortezomib in relapsed refractory myeloma. N Engl J Med 2003;348:2609–2617.

Joseph M. Connors

HODGKIN'S LYMPHOMA

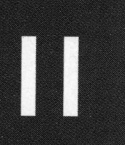
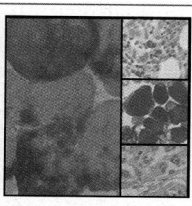

SUMMARY OF KEY POINTS

INCIDENCE
- 2.7 per 100,000 per year, falling slowly in recent decades
- Lower in Asian and native North American populations, intermediate in eastern Europe

ETIOLOGY/EPIDEMIOLOGY
- Cause unknown
- Epstein-Barr virus likely plays a role in etiology but mechanism is unclear
- Neoplastic cell is a B-cell that has lost ability to produce antibody but does not undergo expected cell death due to defective or blocked apoptosis

PATHOLOGY/BIOLOGY
- Diagnosis requires Hodgkin's/Reed-Sternberg cells in appropriate inflammatory cell background
- Classical Hodgkin's lymphoma is positive for CD30 and CD15, negative for CD45 and CD79a
- Nodular lymphocyte predominant Hodgkin's lymphoma is negative for CD30 and CD15, positive for CD45 and CD79a and also CD20

CLINICAL PRESENTATION
- Usual first sign is supradiaphragmatic lymphadenopathy
- B-symptoms (weight loss, fever, night sweats) present in approximately 25% of patients

STAGING
- Physical exam, chest radiograph, blood counts, computed tomography (CT) scan of chest, abdomen, and pelvis
- Bone marrow biopsy for patients with B symptoms or lower-than-normal blood counts

PRIMARY TREATMENT
- Limited-stage disease: brief chemotherapy and involved field radiation
- Advanced stage disease: multiagent chemotherapy for six to eight cycles, current best choice ABVD (doxorubicin, bleomycin, vinblastine, and dacarbazine)

SECONDARY TREATMENT
- Relapse after brief chemotherapy and involved field radiation for limited-stage disease is very rare and treatment must be individualized
- Relapse after extended chemotherapy for advanced disease should be treated with high-dose chemoradiotherapy followed by autologous hematopoietic stem cell transplantation

LATE COMPLICATIONS
- Treatable: psychological impact, dental caries, hypothyroidism, impaired immunity
- Irreversible: infertility (rare after ABVD)
- Major: second neoplasms of skin, thyroid, lung, breast, upper aerodigestive tract, leukemia (the latter rare after ABVD)

PROGNOSIS
- Limited disease: cure in more than 95% of patients
- Advanced disease: cure in more than 65% with primary treatment
- Relapsed disease: cure in more than 40% to 50% with high-dose chemoradiotherapy

INTRODUCTION

Incidence and Epidemiology

Hodgkin's lymphoma is an uncommon but not rare disease seen primarily in younger patients. Approximately 8400 new cases will be seen in the United States and Canada in 2004. The age-adjusted incidence of Hodgkin's lymphoma has declined modestly but significantly over the past 20 years at a rate of approximately 0.9% annually. Within these same jurisdictions, the age-adjusted annual incidence is approximately 2.7 per 100,000, which stands in clear contrast with an age-adjusted annual mortality of only 0.5 per 100,000. This lymphoma occurs slightly more often in men and is seen more frequently in whites and much less frequently in populations derived from southeastern Asia (e.g., China, Japan). Much of the difference in incidence between whites and blacks in North America can be attributed to the higher incidence seen among those of higher socioeconomic status. The cumulative lifetime risk of developing Hodgkin's lymphoma in North America is approximately 1 in 250 to 1 in 300.

The incidence of Hodgkin's lymphoma varies substantially around the world. The highest rates are seen in the United States, Canada, Switzerland, and northern Europe. Intermediate rates are seen in southern and eastern Europe, while low rates are seen in Japan, China, and elsewhere in Asia. Figure 111-1 shows age-related incidences in four representative countries. No clear explanation for this variation in incidence has been found. Postulated reasons include differences in incidence, age of onset, or genotype of Epstein-Barr virus infection; crowding during childhood as a result of lower socioeconomic status, predisposing to passage of an as yet undiscovered infectious vector causing the disease; or intrinsic genetic differences in susceptibility.

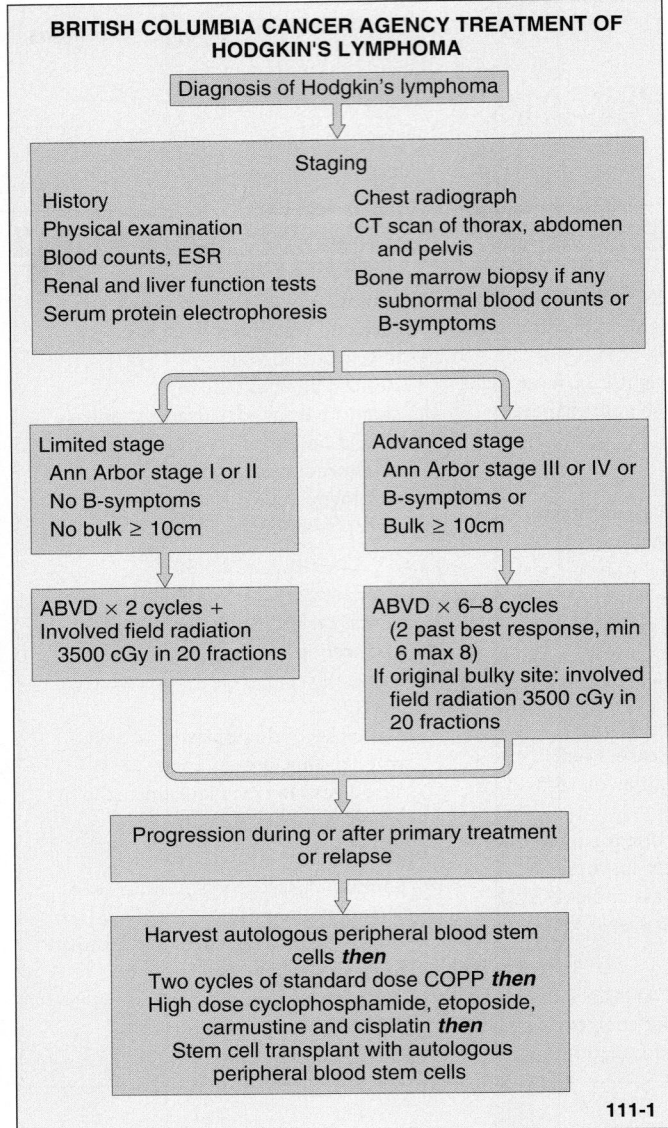

BRITISH COLUMBIA CANCER AGENCY TREATMENT OF HODGKIN'S LYMPHOMA

Diagnosis of Hodgkin's lymphoma

Staging

History
Physical examination
Blood counts, ESR
Renal and liver function tests
Serum protein electrophoresis

Chest radiograph
CT scan of thorax, abdomen and pelvis
Bone marrow biopsy if any subnormal blood counts or B-symptoms

Limited stage
Ann Arbor stage I or II
No B-symptoms
No bulk ≥ 10cm

Advanced stage
Ann Arbor stage III or IV or
B-symptoms or
Bulk ≥ 10cm

ABVD × 2 cycles +
Involved field radiation
3500 cGy in 20 fractions

ABVD × 6–8 cycles
(2 past best response, min 6 max 8)
If original bulky site: involved field radiation 3500 cGy in 20 fractions

Progression during or after primary treatment or relapse

Harvest autologous peripheral blood stem cells **then**
Two cycles of standard dose COPP **then**
High dose cyclophosphamide, etoposide, carmustine and cisplatin **then**
Stem cell transplant with autologous peripheral blood stem cells

111-1

similar illnesses causing lymphadenopathy both before and after him, Thomas Hodgkin's 1832 publication, "On some morbid appearances of the absorbent glands and spleen,"[3] in which he described a small series of cases of lymph node or splenic enlargement, is an obvious early landmark. Throughout the rest of the 1800s, other keen observers eventually took advantage of the progress in microscopic anatomic techniques to describe the histologic details of the neoplastic process within the lymph nodes and spleen. This culminated in the work of Carl Sternberg[4] and Dorothy Reed,[5] with their elegant drawings of the distinctive giant cell that came to bear their names. By the 1930s, specific descriptions by Jackson and Parker led to wide acceptance of their system of

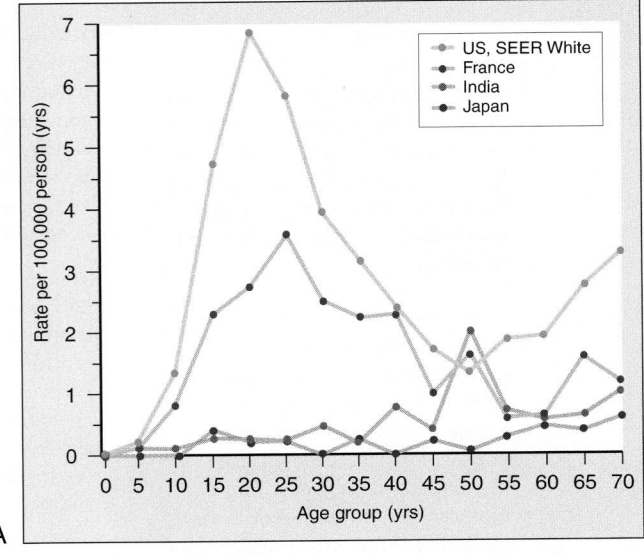

A

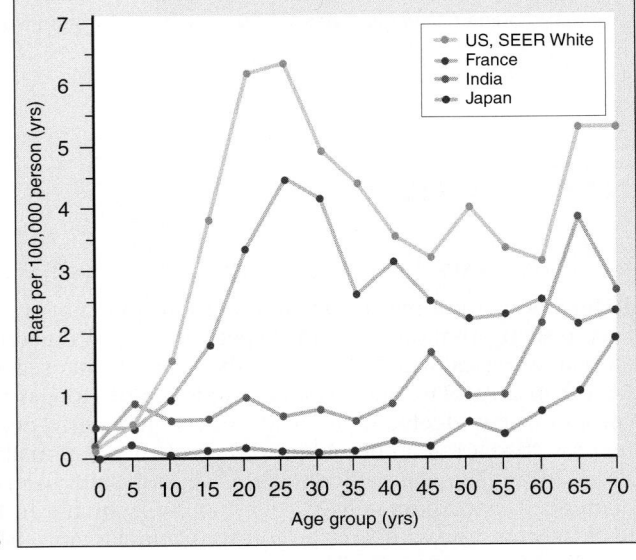

B

Figure 111-1. Female and male age-related incidence rates of Hodgkin's lymphoma per 100,000 in four countries. (From Mueller NE, Grufferman S: The epidemiology of Hodgkin's Disease. In Mauch PM, Armitage JO, Diehl V, Hoppe RT, Weiss LM [ed]: Hodgkin's Disease. Philadelphia, Lippincott Williams & Wilkins, 1999, p 64.)

Most, but not all, authors have found a peculiar bimodal age-related distribution of incidence of Hodgkin's lymphoma, with a first peak occurring in the 20s and a second after the age of 55. As recently as the 1990s, this bimodal distribution has been verified in the United States SEER (Surveillance, Epidemiology, and End Results) data.[1] Some authors, however, have found that much of the late rise in incidence after the age of 55 could be due to misdiagnosis of non-Hodgkin's lymphomas.[2] What is clear about the age distribution of Hodgkin's lymphoma is that in the western world, it is quite unusual to encounter the disease among young children or the elderly, with only about 5% of cases occurring below the age of 15 and 5% over the age of 70 years.

History

The history of Hodgkin's lymphoma is rich and extends back almost 2 centuries. Although others described classification into three subtypes: paragranuloma, granuloma, and sarcoma.[6,7] Dissatisfaction with the lumping together of most cases into the heterogenous category of granuloma encouraged pathologists to continue to seek a more reproducible and clinically relevant classification scheme. The work of Lukes and Butler[8-10] eventually led to the system still in wide use today, in which Hodgkin's lymphoma is divided into four types including, in order of frequency of diagnosis, nodular sclerosing, mixed cellularity, lymphocyte predominant, and lymphocyte depleted. The most recent refinements to this system have focused on the lymphocyte-predominant subtype and are discussed in detail in the special section on that subtype later in this chapter.

Between the first years of the 20th century and the 1960s, in parallel with the progress in classification of Hodgkin's lymphoma, remarkable strides were made in the development of therapeutic irradiation; however, initial progress was slow. Soon after the description of x-rays by the Curies and Roentgen, Pusey[11] and Senn[12] both described dramatic regression of far-advanced lymph nodal disease in response to exposure to fractionated irradiation. Eventual regrowth and appearance of disease at other sites soon led to the disappointing realization that such treatment was not curative, and throughout the 1950s, Hodgkin's lymphoma was thought to be incurable. The pioneering work of Vera Peters,[13] Henry Kaplan,[14,15] and others during the 1940s and 1950s changed that perspective forever, as these researchers demonstrated that even relatively widespread nodal disease could be cured with wide-field irradiation. Today, meticulous dosimetry, computer-assisted simulation, reliable megavoltage irradiation generated from linear accelerators, and integration of radiation treatment into a carefully planned program of combined modality treatment with chemotherapy all contribute to the central role of radiation in the cure of many patients.

Chemotherapy has come late to the field of Hodgkin's lymphoma but has had a profound therapeutic effect. By the 1950s, the palliative benefit of alkylating agents such as mechlorethamine, corticosteroids, vinca alkyloids, and antimetabolites for Hodgkin's lymphoma and related hematologic neoplasms was clear.[16-21] The real potential of chemotherapy, however, was not realized until combinations were explored. These were first demonstrated by Vincent DeVita, Jr. and his colleagues,[22,23] who described the curative potential of MOPP (mechlorethamine, vincristine, procarbazine, and prednisone) for patients with advanced disease and disease that had recurred after irradiation. Many variations of the MOPP regimen, with addition or substitution of one or two drugs or maintenance treatments, were tried without obviously better results. Further progress awaited newer chemotherapeutic agents, including the antineoplastic antibiotics doxorubicin and bleomycin and imidazole derivatives such as dacarbazine.[24-28] By the 1970s, another landmark had been reached: the cure of Hodgkin's lymphoma that was resistant to MOPP by the use of a new combination employing these new agents, ABVD (doxorubicin, bleomycin, vinblastine, and dacarbazine).[29] The most recent major contribution based on chemotherapy has been the demonstration that the use of very high doses of agents no longer effective at standard doses can overcome chemotherapy resistance and can be delivered safely with the support of hematopoietic stem cells.[30,31] This technique of high-dose chemotherapy with stem cell rescue has been shown to be more effective than standard-dose chemotherapy for the treatment of disease that has recurred despite primary chemotherapy.[32,33] This topic will be explored in greater detail in the section on treatment of recurrent disease.

The progress made in the treatment of Hodgkin's lymphoma exemplifies the fundamental dependence of clinical practice on the basic research able to produce refined techniques of radiation therapy delivery, new chemotherapeutic drugs, and definitive diagnostic methods. This progress, however, has depended equally on the development of a team approach to multimodality combination treatment, with contributions from hematopathologists, diagnostic radiologists, and radiation and medical oncologists. Finally, proof of improvement has resulted only from careful conduct of serial clinical trials involving thousands of patients in dozens of countries. The history of Hodgkin's lymphoma, encompassing as it does these contributions of research in radiation treatments, chemotherapy, hematopathology, and clinical trials, all conducted by increasingly sophisticated multimodality teams, is a very instructive example of the potential of oncologic research.

ETIOLOGY AND PATHOGENESIS

The cause of Hodgkin's lymphoma remains unclear, as it does for almost all of the lymphoid neoplasms. The peculiar rapid rise in incidence between childhood and early adulthood, the increased childhood incidence in those parts of the world where crowding should contribute to enhanced exposure to etiologic infectious agents, and the modest increase in incidence of the disease in siblings of index cases suggest that an infectious organism could contribute to causation of Hodgkin's lymphoma. No candidate virus or any other known human pathogen has been implicated clearly, however. After much suggestive evidence, the leading candidate remains Epstein-Barr virus (EBV), but no definitive proof has been uncovered. This virus is associated with the development of lymphomas of several types, with a tantalizingly suggestive collection of circumstantial observations linking it to Hodgkin's lymphoma.

EBV is a large B-cell tropic herpesvirus. Approximately 90% of the general population acquire infection with EBV by the age of early adulthood. In the developing world, this infection tends to occur in childhood, but in the developed countries, infection is often delayed into the teens, when it is associated with the syndrome of infectious mononucleosis in up to 30% of new cases. A history of infectious mononucleosis increases the likelihood of developing Hodgkin's lymphoma threefold.[34,35] Antibodies to the viral capsid antigen reach higher levels in patients with Hodgkin's lymphoma than in controls, and these higher levels appear several years before the neoplasm.[36] EBV readily infects Reed-Sternberg cells, and clonality studies confirm that this infection precedes initiation of the malignant clone.[37-39] The EBV genome is amplified 50-fold or more in Reed-Sternberg cells and is monoclonal in that patient's Reed-Sternberg cells.[40] In situ hybridization studies have demonstrated that the Reed-Sternberg cells of approximately 50% of cases of Hodgkin's lymphoma contain EBV-encoded small RNA (EBER), and in these cases virtually all of the Reed-Sternberg cells are positive for the virus.[41-43] Prior EBV infection proven by serologic tests has been variably associated with the development of Hodgkin's lymphoma (this information is summarized in Ambinder and Weiss[44]). In some populations, virtually all cases of the lymphoma occur in EBV-positive individuals; however, the high background rate of infection in these same populations and the recognition that up to 50% of cases in developed countries are not associated with demonstration of EBV in the Reed-Sternberg cells make it clear that EBV cannot be the exclusive cause of this disease. It appears likely that EBV plays an important role in the development of Hodgkin's lymphoma, but that its role is neither straightforward nor ubiquitous. Elucidation of this role remains one of the major challenges in Hodgkin's lymphoma research.

No clear-cut association with occupational or environmental factors has been found for Hodgkin's lymphoma. Indeed, a surprising lack of association has been shown for exposure to radiation.[45] Likewise, no consistent risk from chemicals, biocidal agents, working in health care related professions, or prior tonsillectomy has been discerned.[46] Although lack of evidence can never settle a question such as this, no promising lead has emerged from the epidemiologic studies so far completed, suggesting that no single environmental factor is likely to play a major role in the etiology of Hodgkin's lymphoma. Given the observation of increased risk in siblings of cases, this lack of an environmental clue suggests that a genetic factor could be at play.

Circumstantial evidence for a genetic contribution to the etiology of Hodgkin's lymphoma is readily available. First-degree relatives of individuals with the disease have up to a fivefold increased risk of developing the lymphoma.[47,48] Monozygotic twins are almost 100-fold more likely to develop Hodgkin's lymphoma compared with dizygotic twins of an affected individual.[49] This level of genetic influence cannot be ignored and clearly indicates that genetic mechanisms must be in play. Perhaps the themes of EBV infection and this genetic susceptibility can be knit together. Because exposure to the virus is nearly ubiquitous, genetically predisposed individuals could react differently to the virus, increasing their chances that a lymphoid neoplasm might be induced. With increased understanding of the molecular consequences of EBV infection and the ability to profile expression of many genes at once using techniques such as micro-array based gene expression analyses or high throughput gene sequencing, there could soon be a confluence of research in these two areas and improved insight into the molecular genesis of this unusual lymphoma.

PATHOLOGY (INCLUDING MOLECULAR DIAGNOSIS)

The diagnosis of Hodgkin's lymphoma is based on the recognition of Reed-Sternberg cells and/or Hodgkin's cells in an appropriate cellular background in tissue sections from a lymph node or extralymphatic organ such as the bone marrow, lung, or bone. Fine-needle aspiration biopsy can be suggestive but is not adequate for the diagnosis of Hodgkin's lymphoma. Open biopsy is required because of the need to establish the diagnosis unequivocally and to determine the histologic subtype. Histochemical staining of properly prepared specimens from an adequate biopsy should be sufficient for recognition of the large majority of cases with minimal error. Immunohistochemical studies can prove complementary and helpful in difficult cases or for convincing distinction of special subtypes, such as lymphocyte-rich classical Hodgkin's lymphoma and nodular lymphocyte predominant type. In classic Hodgkin's lymphoma, these histologic techniques should reveal the presence of scattered, large Reed-Sternberg cells that are either multinucleated or have large polyploid nuclei. Variations can include mononuclear cells which, though similar to the usual polylobated or multinuclear cells, have only one large nucleus with a prominent nucleolus, or lacunar cells that are Reed-Sternberg variants in which the abundant cytoplasm has retracted as an artifact of formalin fixation. The infrequent Reed-Sternberg cells are usually present in a background mixture of polyclonal lymphocytes, eosinophils, neutrophils, plasma cells, fibroblasts, and histiocytes. Occasionally, granulomas form with a prominent histiocytic component.

Hodgkin's lymphoma typically presents as one of a small number of well-described subtypes (Table 111-1). The reproducibility of the distinctions among these subtypes has been reaffirmed in the current widely accepted World Health Organization classification of the lymphoid neoplasms.[50,51] With the addition of one new category—

TABLE 111-1

World Health Organization of Hodgkin's Lymphoma Subtypes		
SUBTYPE NAME	**FREQUENCY (%)***	**ICD-O†**
Classic Hodgkin's lymphoma		
Nodular sclerosing	65	9663/3
Lymphocyte rich	3	9651/3
Mixed cellularity	12	9652/3
Lymphocyte depleted	2	9653/3
Nodular lymphocyte-predominant Hodgkin's lymphoma	6	9659/3
Hodgkin's lymphoma, not otherwise classifiable	12	9650/3

*Frequency based on all new cases (n = 272) seen in British Columbia since January 1998, when the category of lymphocyte-rich classical Hodgkin's lymphoma started to be used.
†ICD-O, International Classification of Diseases, Oncology, 3rd ed., morphology code numbers.

TABLE 111-2

MARKER	CLASSICAL	NODULAR LYMPHOCYTE PREDOMINANT
Typical Immunophenotypic Characteristics of Classical and Nodular Lymphocyte-Predominant Hodgkin's Lymphoma		
CD30	+	–
CD15	+	–
CD20	–/+*	+
CD45	–	+
CD79a	–	+
EMA	–	+
ALK	–	–

+, >90% of cases positive; +/–, majority of cases positive; –/+, minority of cases positive; –, <10% of cases positive.
*CD20 positivity in classical Hodgkin's lymphoma is quite heterogeneous, with a wide range in brightness of staining.

lymphocyte-rich classical Hodgkin's lymphoma—this newest classification scheme permits confident identification of nodular lymphocyte-predominant Hodgkin lymphoma as a separate entity, which is discussed later in the special section on this subtype. The most common subtype is the nodular sclerosing subtype, with its characteristic course bands of sclerosis surrounding nodules composed of typical Reed-Sternberg cells in the usual background mixture of reactive and inflammatory cells.

BIOLOGY

Until the mid-1990s, the cell of origin of Hodgkin's lymphoma remained obscure; however, techniques based on single-cell isolation and polymerase chain reaction (PCR) based genotypic analyses have finally clarified the issue. Working from fresh specimens from patients with new and relapsed disease (including serial specimens), investigators have definitively demonstrated the clonal

derivation of the Reed-Sternberg cell in a series of elegant steps. First came the identification of identical p53 mutations from multiple Reed-Sternberg cells extracted from single biopsy specimens unequivocally establishing clonality.[52] Next, clonal immunoglobulin gene rearrangements from multiple cells in the same biopsy confirmed both the clonal origin of the cells and further demonstrated their B-cell nature.[53] The presence of clonal somatic mutations provided proof of the germinal center origin of the neoplastic cells.[54] Finally, identification of cells with identical immunoglobulin gene rearrangements both at diagnosis and at relapse verified that the B-cell clonality of the disease is preserved over time.[55]

Immunology

The immunophenotype of the neoplastic cells in Hodgkin's lymphoma can be helpful in distinguishing it from other neoplastic processes and in identifying the specific subtype.[51] Typically, the Hodgkin's/Reed-Sternberg cells stain positively for CD30 (80%–100% of cases), CD15 (75%–85% of cases), and B-cell-specific activating protein (BSAP), the product of the PAX5 gene (>90% of cases). Even in clearly positive cases, however, often only a minority of the malignant cells stains positively for the CD15 and BSAP markers. CD20, a generally reliable marker of B-cell lineage, is positive in about 40% of cases of classic Hodgkin's lymphoma but usually only in a minority of the cells, and the staining can be weak. In contrast, nodular lymphocyte-predominant Hodgkin's lymphoma almost always stains positively for CD20 and the specialized B-cell markers CD79a and CD45 but is negative for CD30 and CD15. Table 111-2 shows a comparison of the typical immunophenotypic markers seen in classical and nodular lymphocyte-predominant Hodgkin's lymphoma.

In difficult cases, the immunophenotype can be very helpful in distinguishing Hodgkin's lymphoma from other diseases.[51] Selected immunophenotypic markers and histologic characteristics useful for this purpose are listed in Table 111-3. In particular, classical Hodgkin's lymphoma is positive for CD30 and CD15 but negative for

TABLE 111-3

Selected Immunophenotypic Markers and Histologic Characteristics of Use in the Differential Diagnosis of Hodgkin's Lymphoma and Other Lymphoid Neoplasms

MARKER	CLASSICAL HL	NODULAR LYMPHOCYTE PREDOMINANT HL	TCRBCL	ALCL
CD30	+	–	–	+
CD15	+	–	–	–
CD20	–/+*	+	+	–
CD45	–	+	+	+/–
CD79a	–	+	+	–
ALK	–	–	–	+/–
EMA	–	+	+	+
Nodular growth protein	+/–†	+	–	–

+, >90% of cases positive; +/–, majority of cases positive; –/+, minority of cases positive; –, <10% of cases positive; ALCL, anaplastic large cell lymphoma; HL, Hodgkin's lymphoma; TCRBCL, T-cell rich B-cell lymphoma.
*CD20 positivity in classical Hodgkin's lymphoma is quite heterogeneous, with a wide range in brightness of staining.
†In classical Hodgkin's lymphoma, a nodular growth pattern is confined to the nodular sclerosing subtype.

CD45, while nodular lymphocyte-predominant Hodgkin's lymphoma shows the opposite pattern, being negative for CD30 and CD15 but positive for CD45. T-cell-rich B-cell lymphoma is straightforward to distinguish from classical Hodgkin's lymphoma, being CD30 and CD15 negative but positive for CD20 and CD45. On the other hand, T-cell-rich B-cell lymphoma can be very difficult to separate from nodular lymphocyte-predominant Hodgkin's lymphoma because the immunophenotypic patterns are virtually identical. This distinction is best made by focusing on the histologic pattern of distribution of the neoplastic cells with the presence of nodularity, signaling the diagnosis of nodular lymphocyte-predominant Hodgkin's lymphoma. Finally, anaplastic large-cell lymphoma is reliably negative for CD15, CD20, and CD79a but frequently positive for anaplastic lymphoma kinase (ALK), allowing distinction from both classical and nodular lymphocyte predominant forms of Hodgkin's lymphoma.

Genetics

The neoplastic cells found in Hodgkin's lymphoma demonstrate monoclonal immunoglobulin gene rearrangements in virtually all cases, proving both their monoclonality and their B-cell lineage.[51] A few rare cases with a T-cell genotype have been reported but are obviously exceptional.[56] Despite their B-cell origin, the neoplastic cells of Hodgkin's lymphoma are incapable of making intact antibodies, apparently due to lack of ability to make necessary transcription factors to activate the immunoglobulin promoter.[57] Because B cells that are incapable of manufacturing antibody should be prone to apoptosis yet the Hodgkin's/Reed-Sternberg cells obviously avoid this self-destruction, it has been postulated that apoptosis is blocked abnormally in these cells. The observation that the antiapoptotic nuclear transcription factor NFκB is constitutively activated in these cells is consistent with this hypothesis.[58]

Classic cytogenetics have been unrevealing in Hodgkin's lymphoma. Aneuploidy and hyperploidy consistent with the multinucleated nature of the Hodgkin's/Reed-Sternberg cells are frequent, but no consistent translocation has been detected. Routine cytogenetic analysis of biopsies from patients with Hodgkin's lymphoma is not clinically useful.

CLINICAL PRESENTATION/PATIENT EVALUATION

The large majority of patients who develop Hodgkin's lymphoma present with lymphadenopathy, typically in the cervical, axillary, or mediastinal areas. In only approximately 10% of patients does the nodal disease present initially below the diaphragm.[59,60] Although peripherally located nodes seldom reach a large size except in neglected cases, very large mediastinal masses can develop with only modest symptoms. Bulky retroperitoneal nodal disease is more common among older patients. Lymph nodes involved with Hodgkin's lymphoma are usually painless, but an occasional patient notes discomfort in involved nodal sites immediately after drinking alcohol.

Approximately 25% of patients with Hodgkin's lymphoma notice constitutional symptoms of significant weight loss (greater than 10% of baseline), night sweats, or persistent fever. These classic B symptoms usually signal widespread or locally extensive disease and the need for at least some systemic treatment as part of the therapeutic plan. Pruritus, occasionally severe, can antedate the diagnosis of the Hodgkin's lymphoma by up to several years. Some patients present troubled by the consequences of growing mass lesions, such as cough or stridor due to tracheobronchial compression from mediastinal disease or bone pain secondary to metastatic involvement. Because Hodgkin's lymphoma can involve the bone marrow extensively, an occasional patient presents with symptomatic anemia or incidentally noted pancytopenia. Paraneoplastic neurologic or endocrine syndromes have been reported with Hodgkin's lymphoma but are very rare.

Previously, Hodgkin's lymphoma was a not infrequent cause of fever of unknown origin. With the widespread availability of computerized tomographic (CT) scanning and appropriate biopsy procedures to investigate enlarged intra-abdominal lymph nodes, however, the diagnosis of Hodgkin's lymphoma seldom presents difficulty once the possibility has been entertained. Likewise, as described in the later sections on pathology and immunophenotyping, appropriate immunohistopathologic evaluation and assessment by a trained hematopathologist have virtually eliminated difficulties with differential diagnosis. Problems arise mostly when inadequate material is biopsied or when it is improperly processed. Such problems are usually readily addressed by obtaining another biopsy.

LABORATORY AND IMAGING STUDIES

Once a diagnosis of Hodgkin's lymphoma has been made, investigation is needed to establish the stage or extent of disease. Three aspects of this evaluation deserve emphasis in the assessment of patients with Hodgkin's lymphoma:

1. First, the extent of disease within lymph nodes must be determined.
2. Second, because Hodgkin's lymphoma only spreads outside of the lymphatic system into four extranodal sites (bone marrow, liver, lungs, and bones), these organs must be evaluated for involvement.
3. Finally, because treatment is likely to involve radiation, chemotherapy, or both, organs such as the lungs, heart, and bone marrow might require assessment to determine their tolerance for injury from the treatment, and the excretory capability of organs such as the liver and kidneys must be determined so that the doses of therapeutic agents can be adjusted appropriately.

These three goals can be accomplished efficiently by combining standard, readily available clinical, laboratory, and imaging tests (Table 111-4).

The evaluation should start with a careful history that probes for the presence of localizing signs such as bone

TABLE 111-4

Tests for Evaluation of a Patient with Hodgkin's Lymphoma

- Pathology review
- Complete history searching for B symptoms or other symptomatic problems suggesting more advanced disease
- Physical examination for lymphadenopathy or organomegaly
- Laboratory tests
  - Complete blood cell counts plus erythrocyte sedimentation rate (ESR)
  - Serum creatinine, alkaline phosphatase, lactate dehydrogenase, bilirubin, calcium, AST, serum protein electrophoresis (including albumin level)
  - Hepatitis B surface antigen
- Chest radiograph, PA, and lateral views
- CT scan of the thorax, abdomen, and pelvis
- Certain tests are only required for specific Hodgkin's lymphoma presentations or clinical circumstances

Test	Presentation/Condition
Bone marrow biopsy and aspiration	B symptoms or WBC <4.0 x 10⁹/L or Hgb <120 g/L (women), 130 g/L (men) or Platelets <125 × 10⁹/L
ENT examination	Stage IA or IIA disease with upper cervical lymph node involvement (supra-hyoid)
Plain radiographs of bones	Localized bone pain, especially in the spine or pelvis
HIV antibody	History of lifestyle or behavioral risk Presentation in unusual extranodal sites

pain or constitutional symptoms of fever, weight loss, or night sweats, and cataloging any comorbid conditions that could affect safe delivery of planned treatment. The physical examination should search in particular for lymphadenopathy or organomegaly. Laboratory testing should include blood cell counts and erythrocyte sedimentation rate; assessment of liver and renal function; serologic testing for hepatitis B in all patients (and hepatitis C if liver enzyme abnormalities are detected); human immunodeficiency virus (HIV) antibody if the history indicates increased risk or if the sites of disease are unusual; and serum protein electrophoresis, including albumin level. Bone marrow assessment with aspirate and biopsy is necessary only for the minority of patients with B symptoms or with a lower than normal peripheral blood count at presentation. As will be discussed in the section on treatment of limited-stage disease, a major change in the staging of patients with Hodgkin's lymphoma during the last two decades has been the abandonment of the staging laparotomy.

The major innovation in assessment of patients with Hodgkin's lymphoma in the past two decades has been the refinement of imaging techniques. Current-generation CT scanning has replaced inferior venacavography, lymphangiography, nuclear medicine scans of the liver and spleen, and standard radiographs of the abdomen. All patients should undergo CT scanning of the thorax, abdomen, and pelvis at intervals of 1 cm or less. Although still often performed, gallium scanning adds little to what can be learned with such detailed CT scanning and is too prone to false-negative and -positive results to be useful for most patients. Magnetic resonance imaging adds little to the evaluation of patients with Hodgkin's lymphoma

except in the unusual circumstance of bone involvement, in which case it can be the best technique to describe the full extent of disease.

The impact on the staging and treatment of patients with Hodgkin's lymphoma of positron emission tomography (PET) is currently being assessed actively. It is already clear that PET is more sensitive and specific than CT or gallium scanning, both for staging and for assessment of residual masses after treatment.[61-64] Given the incorporation of systemic treatment into the management of patients with even limited-stage disease and the greater than 95% cure rate with such approaches, however, it is not clear whether the addition of PET to standard staging for Hodgkin's lymphoma will actually add materially to improvement of outcome. It appears much more likely that the greatest usefulness of PET will be in the assessment of residual masses during or after planned treatment to identify the minority who should receive altered or additional therapy.[61,62,64-69]

STAGING

The staging scheme used for Hodgkin's lymphoma is entitled the Ann Arbor system, recognizing the city where the experts of the day met to establish consistent criteria and definitions.[70] This system has weathered well and is still used today (Table 111-5). It very usefully categorizes

TABLE 111-5

Modified Ann Arbor Staging System for Hodgkin's Lymphoma

STAGE	INVOLVEMENT
I	Single lymph node region (I) or one extralymphatic site (I$_E$).
II	Two or more lymph node regions, same side of the diaphragm (II) or local extralymphatic extension plus one or more lymph node regions or same side of the diaphragm (II$_E$).
III	Lymph node regions on both sides of the diaphragm (III), which may be accompanied by local extralymphatic extension (III$_E$).
IV	Diffuse involvement of one or more extralymphatic organs or sites.

Symptoms

AA=	No B symptoms
B =	Presence of at least one of the following symptoms:
	1. Unexplained weight loss >10 percent baseline during 6 months prior to staging
	2. Recurrent unexplained fever >38°C
	3. Recurrent night sweats

Bulky tumor is defined as either a single mass of tumor tissue exceeding 10 cm in largest diameter or a mediastinal mass exceeding one third of the maximum transverse transthoracic diameter measured to the inside of the ribs on a standard PA chest radiograph.
E lesion. Localized extranodal extension of Hodgkin's lymphoma from a contiguous or nearby nodal site is noted with the designation E, for example, stage II$_E$A for asymptomatic disease in the mediastinum with contiguous extension into nearby lung.
From Carbone PP, Kaplan HS, Musshoff K, Smithers DW, Tubiana M: Report of the Committee on Hodgkin's Disease Staging Classification. Cancer Res 1971;31(11):1860–1861.

TABLE 111-6

Systems for Subgrouping of Patients with Hodgkin's Lymphoma

EXTENT OF DISEASE	NORTH AMERICA	EUROPE
Limited (Localized-favorable)	Ann Arbor I, II and bulk <10 cm and no B symptoms	Ann Arbor I, II and ≤3 nodal areas of disease and age <50 years and ESR <50 mm/hr if no B symptoms and ESR <30 mm/hr if B symptoms and no bulky mediastinal disease
Intermediate (Localized-unfavorable)	Not used	Ann Arbor I, II and >3 nodal areas of disease or age >50 years or ESR >50 mm/hr if no B symptoms or ESR >30 mm/hr if B symptoms or bulky mediastinal disease
Advanced	Ann Arbor III, IV or bulk >10 cm or B symptoms	Ann Arbor stage III or IV

ESR, erythrocyte sedimentation rate.

patients into four stages. The first three essentially represent expanding extents of lymph node disease:

1. Stage I involves a single nodal area.
2. Stage II involves two or more nodal areas but still on one side of the diaphragm.
3. Stage III represents nodal disease on both sides of the diaphragm. Waldeyer's ring of lymphoid tissue in the oropharynx and the spleen both count as nodal sites in this system.

Stage IV is reserved for extranodal disease, which for all practical purposes is disease in the bone marrow, lung, bone, or liver. Extranodal Hodgkin's lymphoma at any site other than those four should prompt questioning of the diagnosis or a search for HIV infection.

After determination of extent of disease into stages I though IV, patients are further subdivided into those with or without fever, night sweats, or weight loss (B symptoms). When the use of wide-field irradiation was more common, it was useful to distinguish between stage III A_1 (disease confined to portal, splenic hilar, or celiac nodes) and stage III A_2 (nodal disease in para-aortic, iliac, inguinal, or femoral nodes); however, this distinction is of little clinical relevance today. Likewise, the distinction between clinical and pathologic staging is no longer relevant with the universal abandonment of staging laparotomy. Today, all patients are staged on the basis of physical examination, imaging assessment, and bone marrow biopsy and thus technically have a clinical stage.

The major shortcoming of the Ann Arbor system has been its lack of acknowledgment of the impact of bulky sites of disease. This was corrected by the Cotswold modifications published in 1989.[71] Bulky disease is defined as the presence of any tumor mass with a largest diameter greater than 10 cm or as a mediastinal mass with a transverse diameter exceeding one third of the largest transverse transthoracic diameter. In practical terms, now that CT scanning is widely available, the latter portion of that definition is obsolete, and the term bulky is best assigned to any tumor exceeding 10 cm in largest single diameter.

Some confusion can arise in staging Hodgkin's lymphoma when applying the E-lesion designation.[72] It is useful to remember the intent of the original designers of the Ann Arbor system.[70] The E-lesion designation was intended to identify patients with such limited extranodal extension of Hodgkin's lymphoma that the disease could still be included in a reasonably modified involved field of irradiation. If this is kept in mind, it is straightforward to separate those patients with an E lesion from those with stage IV disease.

It is useful to have a practical system for subdividing patients by extent of disease for purposes of planning treatment and interpretating clinical trials. The two most common approaches to such subdivision are shown in Table 111-6. Generally, two groups have been distinguished in North America: limited and advanced. The presence of Ann Arbor stage III or IV, bulky disease or B symptoms is enough to characterize the patient as having advanced disease. Patients with none of those characteristics have limited-stage disease. Using these definitions, approximately 40% of patients have limited and 60% have advanced disease. The Europeans have divided patients into three groups: two with increasing extent of localized disease and one with advanced disease.

PROGNOSIS

The prognosis of patients with Hodgkin's lymphoma has improved steadily over the past half-century. As an example, Figures 111-2 and 111-3 show the disease-specific and overall survival of all 2170 patients found to have Hodgkin's lymphoma in the Canadian province of British Columbia since 1961, grouped by decade of diagnosis. All patients are included regardless of age, stage, comorbid conditions, or treatment. The dramatic improvement in prognosis is obvious and reflects the combined impact of better diagnosis, staging, and especially treatment.

Two factors dominate the prognosis for patients with Hodgkin's lymphoma: age and stage. Elderly patients—those over the age of 65 to 70 years—constitute only about 5% of all patients with Hodgkin's lymphoma, but they have a likelihood of being cured that is only approximately one half that of younger patients.[73-80] This

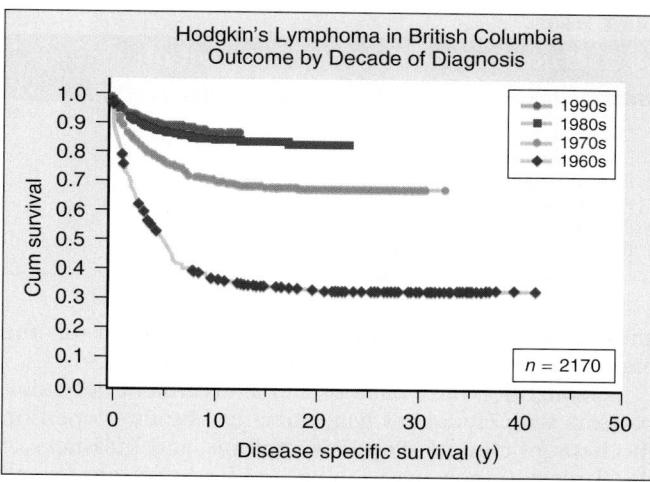

Figure 111-2. Disease-specific survival of all 2170 patients diagnosed with Hodgkin's lymphoma in the Canadian province of British Columbia during the four decades from the 1960s through the 1990s.

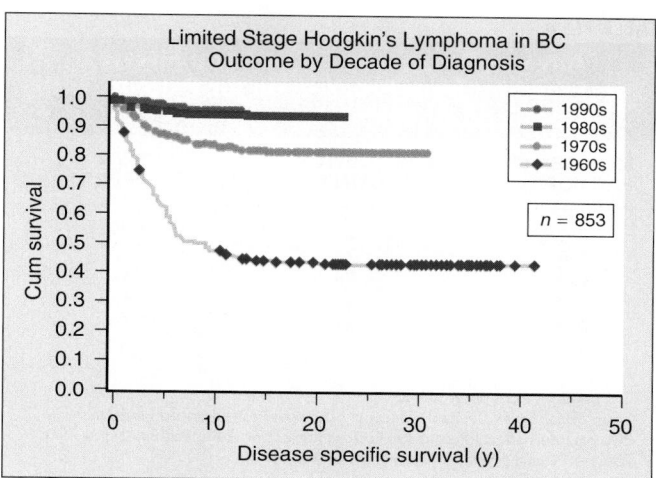

Figure 111-4. Disease-specific survival of all 853 patients with limited-stage Hodgkin's lymphoma in the Canadian province of British Columbia during the four decades from the 1960s through the 1990s.

fact appears to reflect the difficulty in delivery of full-dose treatment due to comorbid conditions, the loss of organ reserve with aging, and intrinsic resistance in the disease as it presents in older patients. The other dominant prognostic factor is stage. Whereas the typical patient with limited-stage disease has at least a 90% to 95% likelihood of cure with current approaches, the average patient with advanced disease has only an approximately 65% to 70% chance of cure with the initial course of treatment. Thus, stage and age remain the two most dominant prognostic factors for patients with Hodgkin's lymphoma.

Attempts to identify additional prognostic factors have been variously successful. Many factors, including histologic subtype, performance status, gender, number of nodal sites, symptoms such as pruritus, and numerous laboratory tests have been found significant in univariate analyses. The importance of these factors, however, must be considered in the context of expected outcome. In

patients with limited Hodgkin's lymphoma, the likelihood of cure is greater than 95%, as can be seen with our experience with all patients seen in British Columbia in the past two decades (Figure 111-4). Unless a candidate's prognostic factor can specifically identify the rare patient who is destined to relapse, focusing on other, less discriminatory factors is of little use. On the other hand, a robust prognostic model has been developed for patients with advanced disease; it has clear utility for interpretation of the results of clinical trials and possible usefulness for treatment planning. The International Prognostic Factors Project on Advanced Hodgkin's Disease has identified seven factors with approximately equal impact on probability of cure and survival for patients with advanced Hodgkin's lymphoma (Table 111-7).[81] This project is of particular relevance because more than 90% of patients were treated with regimens equivalent in efficacy to ABVD (doxorubicin, bleomycin, vinblastine, and dacarbazine).[82-84] Five-year freedom from progression varied from almost 80% for patients with only zero or one adverse factor to less than 50% for those with four or more adverse factors (Table 111-8). This prognostic factor score is very helpful in interpreting the results of clinical trials,

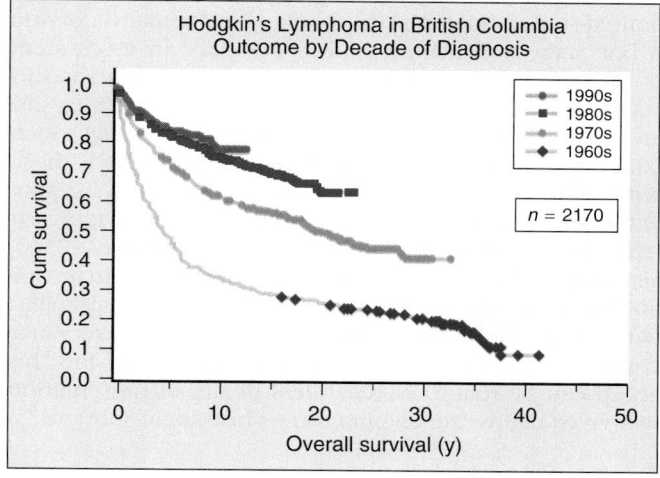

Figure 111-3. Overall survival of all 2170 patients diagnosed with Hodgkin's lymphoma in the Canadian province of British Columbia during the four decades from the 1960s through the 1990s.

TABLE 111-7

Prognostic Factors of Importance in Advanced Hodgkin's Lymphoma*	
GENDER	**MALE**
Age	>45 years
Stage	IV
Hemoglobin	<105 g/L
White blood cell count	>15 × 10⁹/L
Lymphocyte count	<0.6 × 10⁹/L or <8% of the white cell differential
Serum albumin	<40 g/L

*Identified by the International Prognostic Factors Project on Advanced Hodgkin's Disease.

TABLE 111-8

	Adverse Prognostic Factors and Five-year Freedom from Progression for Patients with Advanced Hodgkin's Lymphoma	
NUMBER OF FACTORS	**FREQUENCY ENCOUNTERED (%)**	**5-YR FFP (%)**
0–1	29	79
2–7	71	60
0–2	58	74
3–7	42	55
0–3	81	70
4–7	19	47

FFP, freedom from progression.
From Hasenclever D, Diehl V: A prognostic score for advanced Hodgkin's disease. International Prognostic Factors Project on Advanced Hodgkin's Disease. N Engl J Med 1998;339(21):1506–1514.

as is evident in the section on new chemotherapy regimens later in this chapter.

PRIMARY TREATMENT

At present, most patients with Hodgkin's lymphoma are cured. With this success has come the necessity of minimizing long-term consequences of treatment. As can be seen clearly by comparison of Figures 111-2 and 111-3, although the likelihood of being cured of the Hodgkin's lymphoma is high, overall expectation of survival is not normal. Patients cured of Hodgkin's lymphoma continue to die at excess rates several decades after being cured, and at least a part of this excess risk is due to treatment. Thus, the challenge in treating patients with Hodgkin's lymphoma is not curing the disease but rather doing so while holding the potential for long-term toxicity to a minimum. This might well mean choosing an initial approach that will cure the majority of patients and relying on secondary treatment for the minority who relapse. Further focus on how to maintain this balance between reliance on primary and secondary treatments is

TABLE 111-9

	Overview of Treatment of Hodgkin's Lymphoma	
STAGE	**BULK***	**TREATMENT**
IA, IIA	Low	ABVD × 2 + IRRT
Any stage with B symptoms or III or IV	Low	ABVD until 2 cycles past CR minimum 6 cycles, maximum 8 cycles
Any stage	Bulky	ABVD × 6 + IRRT

Special Exceptions and Their Treatment

IA low bulk mediastinal nodular sclerosing disease: mantle irradiation only

IA high neck (suprahyoid), epitrochlear, or inguinal nodular lymphocyte predominant disease: IRRT only

IRRT, involved region radiotherapy.
*Bulky ≥10 cm largest diameter of any single mass or mediastinal mass ratio >1/3 largest transthoracic diameter.

TABLE 111-10

	Major Issues Affecting Treatment of Limited-Stage Hodgkin's Lymphoma

Definition of limited stage
Staging tests and prognostic factors
Role of staging laparotomy
Role, choice of regimen, and duration of chemotherapy
Prognostic models and special cases
Role and extent of radiation therapy

an important part of our ensuing discussion of the management of patients with advanced disease.

A straightforward plan of initial treatment for adult patients with Hodgkin's lymphoma can be developed on the basis of clinical stage, B symptoms, and bulkiness of the largest tumor mass. Table 111-9 shows an overall approach based on this simple categorization of patients. The following sections discuss the rationale for these approaches by stage in greater detail.

Treatment of Limited-Stage Hodgkin's Lymphoma

Approximately 20,000 new cases of Hodgkin's lymphoma are diagnosed each year in the United States, Canada, and Europe, and of these patients, about 6000 to 7000 have limited-stage disease. Most patients with limited-stage disease can be cured, and the contemporary challenge is to optimize treatment so that this is accomplished with the least toxicity, lowest cost, and greatest efficiency possible. Currently available approaches can be reasonably expected to almost completely eliminate the risk of relapse and still minimize long-term toxicity and complications. Several crucial issues must be addressed to accomplish these desirable goals (Table 111-10).

Definition of Limited-Stage Hodgkin's Lymphoma

Table 111-6 lists the characteristics of patients with limited-stage Hodgkin's lymphoma. A combination of Ann Arbor stage and symptomatic state plus an assessment of tumor mass is generally all that is needed to define this stage. Patients with B symptoms are excluded from this group because even when one tries to manage such patients with staging laparotomy and irradiation, those with clinical stage IB or IIB disease still usually require extended chemotherapy either due to upstaging at laparotomy (40%–50%) or to eventual relapse (25%). Similarly, bulky disease indicates that more than unimodality therapy is required to control disease optimally. Once stage, bulk, and symptoms have been taken into consideration, treatment strategies appropriate for this group can be relied on, regardless of site of presentation (above or below the diaphragm) or histologic subtype.[60]

Staging Tests and Prognostic Factors

The goal of staging is to separate patients with limited disease from those with advanced disease. Thus, the tests employed need only focus on findings necessary to make this distinction. Table 111-4 lists those tests required to adequately determine the stage of Hodgkin's lymphoma for treatment planning purposes. Several tests that might in the past have been considered mandatory are no longer necessary if, as will be outlined shortly, an optimal strategy integrating chemotherapy into the management of these patients is employed. Thus, if multiagent chemotherapy is part of the standard approach, lymphangiography is unnecessary. Any disease so subtle that it would be found only by lymphangiography but be overlooked by CT scanning is minimal enough to be dealt with by the chemotherapy. Likewise, several tests known to have prognostic importance when radiation is used alone (e.g., erythrocyte sedimentation rate, lactate dehydrogenase, or serum copper) are not needed when chemotherapy will be included for all patients.[85-91] On the other hand, optimal shaping of irradiation ports requires the detail revealed with CT scanning, hence the inclusion of thoracic CT scanning to add to what is learned from the chest radiograph.[92]

Role of Staging Laparotomy

One of the most controversial areas of Hodgkin's lymphoma management until recently was the role of staging laparotomy. Attempts to test its utility definitively in randomized trials were few and difficult to interpret.[90-93] Decision-tree analysis likewise failed to resolve whether it was necessary.[94] Recent trials using optimal patient selection and superior chemotherapy, however, have provided enough information to settle the issue.[95-97] Using the results from these trials and the extensive data from laparotomy-based series, two strategies for the management of clinical stage IA and IIA nonbulky disease can be compared:

- Staging laparotomy followed by irradiation, reserving chemotherapy for those initially upstaged or who relapse; or
- Brief chemotherapy followed by irradiation.

When laparotomy and irradiation are compared to brief chemotherapy and irradiation, it is important to remember that at least 40% of the patients who start with clinical stage IA or IIA (nonbulky disease) and then undergo laparotomy will still eventually require an extended course of chemotherapy: 20% who are upstaged and 20% who relapse. The overwhelming advantages of using brief chemotherapy make the argument compelling that laparotomy should be omitted but only if we have sufficient data to be confident that this approach is highly effective at controlling the lymphoma. Fortunately, just such data are available.

Chemotherapy for Limited-Stage Hodgkin's Lymphoma

Although more than 20 randomized trials have addressed the role of chemotherapy in limited-stage Hodgkin's lymphoma, most are of only historic interest. Why are they not relevant today? Many included patients with bulky

TABLE 111-11

Brief ABVD Chemotherapy Followed by Irradiation for Limited Stage Hodgkin's Lymphoma

ELIGIBLE STAGES	MILAN IA, IB, IIA	VANCOUVER IA, IIA	GHSG IA, IIA*
Number of patients	114	170	204
Median follow-up (mo)	38	42	22
Months of ABVD	4	2	2
RT field	Involved or extended	Extended	Extended
Disease-free survival (%)	94	96	96
Overall survival (%)	100	97	98
Tumor-specific survival (%)	100	99	98
Reference	95	96	97

*Only patients with absence of unfavorable prognostic factors were included in the GHSG study.

disease. Staging often consisted of a mixture of clinical and pathologic testing, employing laparotomy selectively but often without the benefit of modern-generation CT scanning. The chemotherapy was often less effective than ABVD, which has been shown to be the regimen that is most effective and least toxic for advanced-stage disease.[83,84] Despite the fact that the chemotherapy's major role is to eradicate the subclinical disease outside the planned radiation field, its duration was often prolonged, inviting substantial acute and long-term toxicity. Today, we are most interested in data from trials based on a strategy of brief-duration ABVD followed by irradiation. Such an approach eliminates any substantial risk of infertility, premature menopause, or leukemia and holds to a minimum concerns about cardiopulmonary toxicity. Three groups have reported the results of using brief ABVD and irradiation for clinical stage IA or IIA nonbulky Hodgkin's lymphoma in adult patients: one in Milan and another in Vancouver and, more recently, the German Hodgkin's Study Group (GHSG) (Table 111-11).[95-97] The Milan trial included a randomization to involved vs. extended-field radiation therapy after 4 months of ABVD but has shown no difference in the groups using involved or extended-field irradiation. Therefore, the results from that center have been pooled in Table 111-11. These data make it clear that brief chemotherapy with ABVD followed by irradiation is highly effective at eradicating limited-stage Hodgkin's lymphoma. Combined with its other advantages over laparotomy-based treatment, the efficacy of such an approach makes it the best currently available and raises the standard of treatment for such patients to the level at which relapse is quite rare and death from Hodgkin's lymphoma is very unlikely.

Prognostic Models and Special Cases

There is another advantage to the inclusion of brief chemotherapy for all limited-stage Hodgkin's lymphoma patients. One can eliminate reliance on complex prognostic factor models, which itself can increase the risk of recurrence.[98] A substantial literature documents the importance of factors such as erythrocyte sedimentation rate, number of sites of disease, and other factors such as gender or age when staging laparotomy and irradiation are used.[85-91] Routine substitution of brief chemotherapy for the laparotomy, however, eliminates the importance of such factors, thus simplifying treatment. This approach reduces the need for elaborate, error-prone testing and removes the potential for mistakes in assigning prognosis. Not unexpectedly, improvements in the effectiveness of treatment have led to elimination of the impact of previously important prognostic factors. Such complex models are no longer necessary.

Two quite unusual and special presentations of Hodgkin's lymphoma deserve individualized approaches. When lymphocyte-predominant disease presents confined to unilateral high neck, epitrochlear, or inguinal lymph nodes, the risk of disease elsewhere is very small, and the prognosis after only localized irradiation is excellent.[98] Such patients should be staged meticulously but require only involved-field irradiation. Another similarly special case is that of nonbulky stage IA nodular sclerosing Hodgkin's lymphoma of the anterior mediastinum.[88] Such disease is also virtually always confined to the site of presentation and, if its limited extent is confirmed with full staging, it requires only regional irradiation. At the Vancouver center, we use mantle irradiation with a lower border of T_{10} for this presentation, and in the six cases we have seen in the past 21 years, no relapses have occurred. Thus, although complex prognostic models are unnecessary, recognition of certain quite rare and special presentations of Hodgkin's lymphoma occasionally can allow further reduction of planned treatment.

Radiation for Limited-Stage Hodgkin's Lymphoma

With the identification of an approach that virtually eliminates relapses for patients with limited-stage Hodgkin's lymphoma, the focus of further modifications to treatment must be on the reduction of toxicity while maintaining effectiveness. The chemotherapy in the combined-modality approach should eradicate subclinical

TABLE 111-12

Schedule and Doses of the MOPP and ABVD Regimens for Hodgkin's Lymphoma

	DOSE (MG/M²)	ROUTE	DAY(S)
MOPP (cycle length 28 days)			
Mechlorethamine	6	IV	1,8
Vincristine	1.4 (dose cap 2.0 mg)	IV	1,8
Procarbazine	100	PO	1–14
Prednisone	45	PO	1–14
ABVD (cycle length 28 days)			
Doxorubicin	25	IV	1,15
Bleomycin	10	IV	1,15
Vinblastine	6	IV	1,15
Dacarbazine	375	IV	1,15

IV, intravenous; PO, oral.

TABLE 111-13

Characteristics of the MOPP Regimen

- Agents: mechlorethamine, vincristine, procarbazine, prednisone
- 80% complete response rate
- 20% primary refractory disease
- 50% overall disease-free survival
- Most relapses occur within the first 4 years; however, about 10% of all relapses occur beyond 5 years
- Prognostic variables include B symptoms, age, time to CR, and number of extranodal sites of disease
- Major side effects are nausea, phlebitis, myelosuppression, neurotoxicity, infertility, leukemogenesis, and other secondary neoplasms

disease and allow smaller fields of irradiation to be used. Indeed, randomized trials with MOPP (mechlorethamine, vincristine, procarbazine, prednisone), VBM (vinblastine, bleomycin, methotrexate), and ABVD all have demonstrated that the extent of radiation can be reduced safely when chemotherapy is added.[95,99-101] The value of the Milan trial comparing 4 months of ABVD followed by either involved or extended-field irradiation is that it shows that 4 months of ABVD chemotherapy is sufficient to eradicate all unirradiated disease, even when only involved-field irradiation is used.[95] Thus, brief chemotherapy followed by involved-field irradiation emerges as the best current choice for the management of nonbulky, clinical stage IA and IIA Hodgkin's lymphoma.

Advanced Hodgkin's Lymphoma

Advanced Hodgkin's lymphoma was nearly always fatal until the development of combination chemotherapy, even though certain stage IIIA patients could be cured with wide-field irradiation. The first widely used multi-agent program, MOPP (mechlorethamine, vincristine, procarbazine, and prednisone) (Table 111-12), produced a response rate of 80% and long-term disease-free survival of about 50%.[23,102] The major characteristics of the MOPP regimen are listed in Table 111-13. Other four- or five-drug combinations, including MVPP (V = vinblastine), ChlVPP (Chl = chlorambucil), BCVPP (B = carmustine, C = cyclophosphamide), COPP (C = cyclophosphamide), and

TABLE 111-14

Characteristics of the ABVD Regimen

- Agents: doxorubicin, bleomycin, vinblastine, dacarbazine
- All intravenous, total compliance
- 80% complete response rate
- 10% primary refractory disease
- 60%–65% overall disease-free survival
- Most relapses occur within the first 4 years; however, about 10% of all relapses occur beyond 5 years
- Major side effects are nausea, phlebitis, myelosuppression, less cumulative myelotoxicity than MOPP
- No infertility
- No leukemia

TABLE 111-15

Results of a Trial Comparing ABVD and MOPP*

	ABVD	MOPP	P
CR (%)	92	82	<0.02
7-yr freedom from progression (%)	91	63	<0.002
7-yr overall survival (%)	77	68	0.003

Patients with stage IIA, IIB, and IIIA Hodgkin's lymphoma used a schedule of three cycles of chemotherapy before and after extended field radiation to all sites of nodal disease.
From Santoro A, Bonadonna G, Valagussa P, et al: Long-term results of combined chemotherapy-radiotherapy approach in Hodgkin's disease: Superiority of ABVD plus radiotherapy versus MOPP plus radiotherapy. J Clin Oncol 1987;5(1):27–37.

others with one or two drug substitutions in the original MOPP regimen were tested but ultimately proved to have only modestly different toxicity profiles and did not cure more patients.

ABVD was developed by the Milan group in the early 1970s.[82] It has partial non–cross resistance with MOPP and can cure about 20% of patients not cured with that regimen.[29] ABVD also has less pronounced long-term toxicity, very infrequently causing either sterility or premature menopause and being less leukemogenic (Tables 111-12 and 111-14).[103,104] It is important to remember that temporary infertility and irregular or absent menses occur commonly with ABVD but usually resolve within 1 to 2 years. ABVD has been compared with MOPP as initial therapy for advanced-stage disease, followed by irradiation to sites of nodal disease. ABVD produced a complete response (CR) rate of 71% compared with 63% for MOPP. Even more encouragingly, these investigators found a 10-year progression-free survival of 63% for ABVD followed by radiation vs. 50% for MOPP followed by radiation.[82,105] In a subsequent large trial of 232 patients with stage IIA, IIB, or IIIB disease, three cycles of MOPP before and after radiotherapy were compared with three cycles of ABVD before and after radiotherapy; the results are shown in Table 111-15.[106] This latter trial clearly suggests that ABVD is the more potent of the two major four-drug regimens for Hodgkin's lymphoma.

Hybrid or alternating combinations of MOPP and ABVD were widely tested in the 1980s and appeared to be superior to MOPP by virtue of curing approximately 10% to 15% more patients.[107–109] A number of randomized trials comparing MOPP or MOPP-like regimens with hybrid or alternating MOPP/ABVD regimens were then conducted.[84,110-116] These trials consistently demonstrated superiority of MOPP/ABVD over MOPP (5-year progression-free survival approximately 65% for MOPP/ABVD vs. 50% for MOPP alone) as long as the dose intensity of the drugs was maintained. On the other hand, no significant differences in toxicity or effectiveness emerged among the various seven to eight drug regimens.

The observation that ABVD could sometimes cure patients when MOPP had failed to do so and the trend to better outcome when ABVD was compared with MOPP in combined-modality programs provided provocative evidence that at least some of the apparent superiority of hybrid or alternating MOPP/ABVD regimens over MOPP alone might be due to the inherent superiority of ABVD and not to the seven- or eight-drug combination.[29,105,106,117,118] This superiority was confirmed in a landmark randomized trial performed by the Cancer and Leukemia Group B (CALGB) that compared MOPP with ABVD and MOPP/ABVD in advanced-stage Hodgkin's lymphoma (stages IIIA, IIIB, IVA, IVB) (Table 111-16).[84] Both ABVD-containing arms produced a significantly better progression-free survival. Although there was no statistically significant difference in overall survival across the three arms, that endpoint is obscured by secondary treatment. These results were even more solidly confirmed in a large North American intergroup study in which the MOPP/ABV hybrid regimen was tested against ABVD (Table 111-17).[83] This trial enrolled 852 evaluable patients and found no differences in CR, freedom from treatment failure, or overall survival between the two arms. Although this study was closed slightly earlier than planned on the basis of possible excess toxicity in the hybrid arm, no statistically significant difference in severe toxicity was detected in the final analysis. The most reasonable conclusion to draw from this series of trials extending over more than 2 decades is that ABVD presently demonstrates the best combination of efficacy and toxicity and should be considered the current standard of care for advanced-stage Hodgkin's lymphoma. This conclusion is especially attractive because the ABVD regimen causes no more than minimal rates of leukemia, infertility, or premature menopause and induces less cumulative myelotoxicity.

TABLE 111-16

Results of a CALGB Trial Comparing MOPP or ABVD*

	MOPP × 6–8	ABVD × 6–8	MOPP/ABVD × 12	P
n	123	115	123	
CR (%)	67	82	83	0.006
5-yr failure free survival (%)	50	61	65	0.04
5-yr overall survival (%)	66	73	75	NS

NS, not significant.
Study compared six to eight cycles to alternating MOPP/ABVD for 12 cycles for patients with advanced-stage Hodgkin's lymphoma.
From Santoro A, Bonadonna G, Bonfante V, Valagussa P: Alternating drug combinations in the treatment of advanced Hodgkin's disease. N Engl J Med 1982;306:770–775.

TABLE 111-17

Results of the North American Intergroup Trial Comparing MOPP/ABV Hybrid to ABVD for Patients with Advanced-Stage Hodgkin's Lymphoma

	ABVD	MOPP/ABV	P
N	433	419	
CR (%)	76	80	0.16
Progression during treatment (%)	10	11	
5-yr failure free survival (%)	63	66	0.42
5-yr overall survival (%)	82	81	0.82

From Duggan DB, Petroni GR, Johnson JL, et al: Randomized comparison of ABVD and MOPP/ABV hybrid for the treatment of advanced Hodgkin's disease: Report of an intergroup trial. J Clin Oncol 2003;21(4):607–614.

Role of Irradiation in Advanced-Stage Hodgkin's Lymphoma

The usefulness of irradiation in the treatment of limited-stage Hodgkin's lymphoma has led to its testing in a variety of treatment programs for patients with advanced disease; however, a clear role has yet to be defined for it in this setting. A highly valuable examination of the available data on this topic was undertaken in a meta-analysis performed by Loeffler and colleagues[119] for the International Database on Hodgkin's Disease Overview Study Group. It examined the results from 14 clinical trials including 1740 patients. Although radiotherapy resulted in a significantly improved tumor control rate after 10 years, it did not improve overall survival. On a cautionary note, more deaths unrelated to Hodgkin's lymphoma were observed in patients after radiotherapy, resulting in a significantly worse survival in the set of trials comparing the strategy of chemotherapy 1 followed by chemotherapy 2 to that of chemotherapy 1 followed by irradiation. Since that publication, three additional studies have been reported examining the impact of adding radiation after achievement of a complete remission from primary chemotherapy.[120-122] All are negative and provide no evidence that such additional radiation improves outcome for such patients. The adverse long-term effects of radiation probably outweigh any benefits for the usual patient with advanced-stage disease. Whether there is a role for localized irradiation for patients who start with a bulky site of disease remains to be determined; based on intuitive appeal, however, it is commonly added to the chemotherapy. It is likely that the powerful ability of PET to identify patients likely to relapse after primary chemotherapy will finally lay this question to rest by identifying the small subgroup of patients who might profit from postchemotherapy irradiation and allowing the rest to avoid treatment with this modality.[61,62,64,65,67,69,123]

Prognostic Factors in Advanced-Stage Hodgkin's Lymphoma

Recently, the whole approach to advanced Hodgkin's lymphoma has been placed on a more rational footing by the development of a robust prognostic model that identifies patients with differing risks of primary treatment failure. In a study identifying prognostic factors in a group of more than 5000 patients with advanced-stage Hodgkin's lymphoma, most of whom were treated with ABVD or an equivalently effective regimen, the investigators identified seven independent predictors of decreased likelihood of freedom from progression (see Tables 111-7 and 111-8).[81] Subgroups of patients with varying likelihood of freedom from progression were identified on the basis of the number of these factors present at diagnosis. For the 80% of patients with up to three of these factors, the likelihood of progression-free survival was 70%. For the 20% who have four or more of these factors, the progression-free survival rate fell to less than 50%. It is necessary to keep these likely outcomes in mind when examining the results of new regimens.

New Regimens

Two new regimens have recently been described for the treatment of patients with advanced Hodgkin's lymphoma that could hold the potential to improve on what can be achieved with standard ABVD chemotherapy. In the Stanford V regimen, the chemotherapy drugs (Table 111-18) are administered weekly for 12 weeks followed by planned irradiation with 36 Gy to sites of initial tumor bulk (≥5 cm).[124-127] The updated results of the pilot study

TABLE 111-18

Schedule and Doses of Chemotherapy in the Stanford V Regimen for Patients with Advanced-Stage Hodgkin's Lymphoma

	DOSE (mg/m²)	WEEK											
		1	2	3	4	5	6	7	8	9	10	11	12
Doxorubicin	25	x		x		x		x		x		x	
Vinblastine	6	x		x		x		x		x		x	
Mustard	6	x				x				x			
Etoposide	60 × 2			x				x				x	
Vincristine	1.4		x		x		x		x		x		x
Bleomycin	5		x		x		x		x		x		x
Prednisone	40 q2d												Taper

Filgrastim (G-CSF) added after first-dose reduction or delay for myelosuppression.

TABLE 111-19

Schedule and Doses of Chemotherapy in the Escalated BEACOPP Regimen for Patients with Advanced-Stage Hodgkin's Lymphoma

Escalated BEACOPP (cycle length 21 days)

	DOSE (mg/m^2)	ROUTE	DAY(S)
Bleomycin	10	IV	8
Etoposide	200 qd × 3d	IV	1, 2, 3
Doxorubicin	35	IV	1
Cyclophosphamide	1250	IV	1, 8
Vincristine	1.4	IV	8
Procarbazine	100	PO	1–7
Prednisone	45	PO	1–14

IV, intravenous; PO, oral.
Filgrastim (G-CSF) planned with each cycle for 8 to 14 days starting day 8.

of Stanford V and radiation included 142 patients, of whom approximately 70% received consolidative irradiation. With a median follow-up of 5.4 years, the actuarial 5-year overall survival was 96%, and freedom from progression was 89%. Fertility was apparently maintained, and there were no treatment-related deaths. Stanford V is now being compared with standard ABVD in a large North American intergroup trial for patients with advanced Hodgkin's lymphoma of all prognostic subgroups. Preliminary results from an Italian study of Stanford V compared with ABVD and a complex 10-drug regimen, MEC (mechlorethamine, lomustine, vindesine, melphalan, prednisone, epirubicin, vincristine, procarbazine, vinblastine, bleomycin), have failed to show any overall survival advantage to any of the tested regimens.[128] Possible inferiority of Stanford V compared with the other two regimens in terms of failure-free survival is difficult to interpret given the equivalence in overall survival; however, mature results will be needed to interpret this important trial fully.

The German Hodgkin Lymphoma Study Group has developed a dose-escalated and accelerated combined-modality program, BEACOPP + RT (bleomycin, etoposide, doxorubicin, cyclophosphamide, vincristine, procarbazine, and prednisone plus involved-field radiation to sites of initially bulky or residual lymphadenopathy; Table 111-19). A randomized trial has been performed comparing COPP/ABVD + RT with standard dose BEACOPP + RT and escalated dose BEACOPP + RT. Irradiation was given to approximately 70% of patients on all three arms. A fifth interim analysis with 1180 evaluable patients and a median follow-up of 36 months showed the results described in Table 111-20. BEACOPP in escalated dose showed a higher but manageable rate of hematologic toxicity, with a treatment-related lethal toxicity of 3%. Longer follow-up will be required to determine the true usefulness of escalated BEACOPP + RT. Whether the increased toxicity of this regimen (3% treatment-induced mortality; 100% infertility in men; 100% infertility plus premature menopause in most women over the age of 25; increased risk of second neoplasms) can be justified remains to be determined.

As will be described in the section on the use of high-dose chemoradiotherapy and hematopoietic stem cell transplantation (HDC/HSCT) for refractory or relapsed disease, this intensive treatment technique is capable of overcoming treatment resistance in selected patients. This efficacy as secondary treatment has prompted interest in using this technique for patients with poor-prognosis disease at diagnosis. In theory, using such a highly intensive treatment early in overall treatment should enhance its effectiveness. In practice, this promise has not been realized. Two randomized prospective trials, although only modest in size, have failed to show that early use of HDC/HSCT improves outcome compared with standard chemotherapy.[129,130]

Overall Treatment Strategy and Future Directions

The information from the prognostic factors analysis in Table 111-20 can be put together with the documentation that approximately one half of patients who are not cured

TABLE 111-20

Results of the Fifth Interim Analysis of the German Hodgkin's Study Group HD10 Trial*

	COPP/ABVD (ARM A)	STD BEACOPP (ARM B)	ESC BEACOPP (ARM C)	P (A VS. C)
CR (%)	84	88	96	
prog during Tx (%)	12	8	2	
5-yr FFTF (%)	67	75	89	< 0.0001
5-yr OS (%)	79	90	90	0.0014
5-yr OS (%)				
IPFP 0,1	91	91	95	NS
IPFP 2,3	81	90	90	NS
IPFP 4–7	87	85	77	< 0.0099

CR, complete response; FFTF, freedom from treatment failure; IDHD, International Database on Hodgkin's Disease Prognostic Factors Project score; NS, not significant; prog, progression; Tx, treatment.
*Trial compares COPP/ABVD, standard dose BEACOPP, and escalated dose BEACOPP for the treatment of 1180 patients with advanced-stage Hodgkin's lymphoma. Approximately 70% of patients on each arm received consolidative irradiation as called for in the protocol.

by primary chemotherapy such as ABVD can be treated effectively with high-dose chemotherapy and autologous hematopoietic stem cell transplantation (see later discussion). We can then evaluate whole strategies to determine which strikes the best balance of efficacy and toxicity for an individual patient. The 80% of patients who have zero to three of the IPFP prognostic factors (see Table 111-8) have a 70% chance of cure with primary chemotherapy using ABVD.[81] Thus, the best currently definable strategy is to start with ABVD. That will fail to cure 30%, and that subgroup should be given high-dose chemotherapy and hematopoietic stem cell transplantation. Such a strategy will confine the high cost and toxicity of intensified treatment (including infertility and risk of leukemia) to the minority whose disease demands it. On the other hand, the 20% of patients with a less than 50% likelihood of cure with primary chemotherapy have disease that is so difficult to eradicate that programs employing intensified treatment from the beginning should be considered. The newer, more intensified combined-modality regimens such as escalated BEACOPP and Stanford V might well fit this role. Mature data from ongoing trials will address and settle at least some of the issues relevant to this choice.

TREATMENT COMPLICATIONS

All antineoplastic interventions have at least some undesirable side effects; however, many of these toxicities (e.g., alopecia) are temporary, not life threatening, and entirely reversible. Even when the side effect is uncomfortable, inconvenient, or modestly dangerous as in the cases of vomiting, mucositis, or neutropenia, complete reversibility and supportive medications keep these toxicities within reasonably acceptable bounds for curative treatment of a potentially lethal disease. On the other hand, some toxicities can be permanent after chemotherapy or radiation and prove troublesome or life threatening long after the primary neoplasm has cured. Table 111-21 lists the major late toxicities seen after effective treatment of Hodgkin's lymphoma. Other than infertility, none of these late toxicities occurs in more than 5% of patients and, thus, they do not constitute absolute contraindications to the use of these agents, associated as they are with a high likelihood of cure. When equally effective choices are available, however—for example, ABVD, reducing the risk of major late toxicity (e.g., infertility, premature menopause, or leukemia/myelodysplasia) —ABVD obviously becomes more desirable.[82-84,103,131,132]

The effects of therapeutic irradiation on normal tissues are only partially reversible. In particular, certain organs such as the lungs, liver, testes, or ovaries have limited ability to recover from radiation exposure and cannot be included in treatment fields for Hodgkin's lymphoma without anticipating loss of function. In addition, irradiation induces genetic damage that enhances the likelihood of later development of secondary neoplasms, the major cause of excess mortality in patients with Hodgkin's lymphoma more than 10 to 15 years after treatment.[133-146] These two long-term toxicities of radiation—direct organ

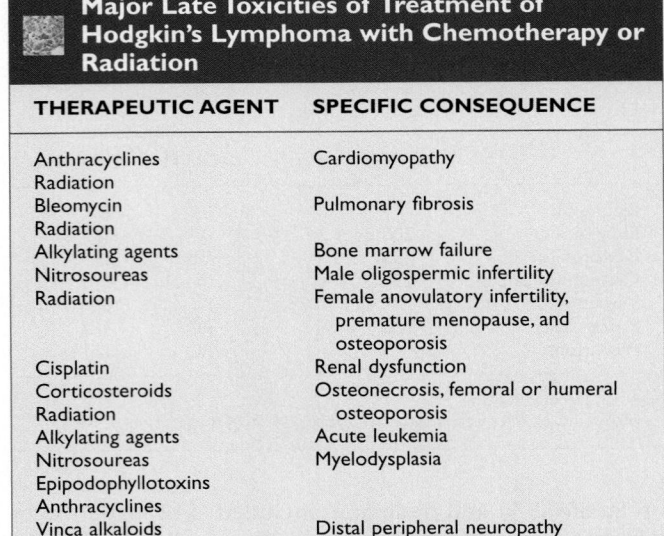

TABLE 111-21

Major Late Toxicities of Treatment of Hodgkin's Lymphoma with Chemotherapy or Radiation

THERAPEUTIC AGENT	SPECIFIC CONSEQUENCE
Anthracyclines Radiation	Cardiomyopathy
Bleomycin Radiation	Pulmonary fibrosis
Alkylating agents	Bone marrow failure
Nitrosoureas	Male oligospermic infertility
Radiation	Female anovulatory infertility, premature menopause, and osteoporosis
Cisplatin	Renal dysfunction
Corticosteroids Radiation	Osteonecrosis, femoral or humeral osteoporosis
Alkylating agents	Acute leukemia
Nitrosoureas Epipodophyllotoxins Anthracyclines	Myelodysplasia
Vinca alkaloids	Distal peripheral neuropathy
Radiation	Hypothyroidism

damage and induction of second neoplasms—provide clear justification for minimizing exposure of patients to this modality. On the other hand, therapy must not be reduced to the point that the reduction compromises overall effectiveness. In practical terms, this means reduction of the size of the field of radiation for patients with limited-stage disease who are being treated with combined modality treatment and omission of radiation for patients with advanced disease unless localized persistence of viable disease requires the use of consolidative involved-field irradiation.

FOLLOW-UP

Management of Primary Treatment Failure

Over the past two decades, high-dose chemotherapy and irradiation plus autologous hematopoietic stem cell transplantation (HDC/HSCT) has become established as the most effective treatment for patients whose Hodgkin's lymphoma has proven incurable with standard chemotherapy and radiation. Phase II trials, collected series from bone marrow transplantation registries, and two phase III randomized trials have demonstrated that the effectiveness of HDC/HSCT is sufficiently clear that it has become widely accepted as the best treatment approach for most patients who are not cured by primary treatment programs based on multiagent chemotherapy.[30,31-33,147-167]

Identification of Candidates for HDC/HSCT

The high levels of toxicity and cost associated with HDC/HSCT demand that it be reserved for patients for whom it clearly increases the chance of cure compared with alternative treatments. This describes two groups of patients: first, those whose disease progresses or

TABLE 111-22

> ### Characteristics of Patients Best Treated with HDC/HSCT for Relapse or Progression of Hodgkin's Lymphoma after Chemotherapy for Advanced Disease
>
> **Definite**
>
> Relapse <1 yr after completion of primary chemotherapy
> Relapse with B symptoms
> Relapse in one or more extranodal sites
> Relapse in previously irradiated sites
>
> **Controversial but Probably Indicated**
>
> Relapse only in previously unirradiated lymph nodes, in the absence of B symptoms, occurring >1 yr after completion of primary chemotherapy

persists despite primary chemotherapy; second, patients who relapse after a full course of multiagent chemotherapy with or without radiation. The first group, usually referred to as having refractory or chemotherapy-resistant disease, have very little chance of cure with any program of standard-dose chemotherapy with or without irradiation.[104,168,169] This group, lacking reliably curative alternatives, is best treated with HDC/HSCT because it offers a definite chance of cure.

The use of HDC/HSCT for patients in first relapse after primary chemotherapy is somewhat more controversial, especially if the relapse occurs more than 1 year after completion of the primary treatment or in an area easily amenable to irradiation. On the other hand, when relapse occurs after primary chemotherapy consisting of a regimen as effective as ABVD, the chance of inducing long-term disease-free survival with standard-dose chemotherapy is small, probably less than 20%.[104,168,170] It has been argued that two special subgroups do not share this poor prognosis: those who relapse solely in originally involved but unirradiated lymph node groups, and those who relapse more than 1 year after completion of the primary chemotherapy.[104,152,168,171-181] In the first of these two subgroups, wide-field irradiation with or without additional chemotherapy might cure 40% to 50% of very carefully selected patients.[171-180] Very few patients, however, fit the ideal pattern of nonbulky disease confined to lymph nodes at diagnosis and relapse, absence of B symptoms at diagnosis and relapse and, preferably, a long interval from primary treatment to relapse. In the second subgroup, those relapsing more than a year after completion of primary chemotherapy, switching to potentially non–cross-resistant chemotherapy with or without irradiation might cure 20% to 40% of these special selected patients.[104,152,168,181] Both of these special subgroups also are among those who have the very best outcome with HDC/HSCT. Of particular relevance is the experience of the German Hodgkin's Study Group.[33] This group found not only that HDC/HSCT produced a superior progression-free survival for all patients in their study but also that this was true both for those who relapsed early and for those who relapsed late. Table 111-22 shows the characteristics of patients who should receive HDC/HSCT for relapse of Hodgkin's lymphoma after primary chemotherapy for advanced disease.

Relatively few patients fall in the controversial group, and even among those, the case for use of HDC/HSCT is strong. Thus, the current standard treatment for relapse of Hodgkin's lymphoma after primary chemotherapy for advanced disease should be HDC/HSCT.

Technique of HDC/HSCT

Although most of the initial experience employing HDC/HSCT for Hodgkin's lymphoma was acquired using autologous bone marrow cells, most groups now use autologous peripheral blood stem cells for the reasons shown in Table 111-23.[167,182-184] Although no clear role has been defined for chemotherapy before the HDC/HSCT procedure, most groups currently employ at least some standard-dose chemotherapy in this role for two reasons:

1. It brings the Hodgkin's lymphoma under control while the logistics of stem cell collection and the hospitalization for HDC/HSCT are being arranged.
2. It provides priming for the peripheral blood stem cell collection, enhancing the effectiveness of hematopoietic growth factors.

It is important to remember, however, that the purpose of this pre-HDC/HSCT chemotherapy is not to test for chemosensitivity. Hodgkin's lymphoma, almost uniquely among human neoplasms, can be cured with the use of HDC/HSCT even when disease does not respond to standard-dose chemotherapy.

Although a variety of HDC regimens have been described, no one regimen has been shown to be clearly superior. Currently popular regimens include CBV (cyclophosphamide, carmustine, and etoposide), BEAM (carmustine, etoposide, cytarabine, and melphalan), or high-dose melphalan with or without total body irradiation.[30,33,160,162-164,167,185-189] Because none of these regimens has been shown to be superior, it is more important for investigators at an individual center to master the management of the acute and chronic toxicities of their chosen regimen than to switch from one to another seeking some modest but unproved advantage. As most patients with Hodgkin's lymphoma have previously been exposed to thoracic irradiation, bleomycin, nitrosoureas, or other agents with potential pulmonary toxicity, it is best to avoid HDC regimens that incorporate total body irradiation.[161,164] Some groups have found them

TABLE 111-23

> ### Reasons for Preference of Growth Factor–Mobilized Peripheral Blood Stem Cells for HDC/HSCT in Hodgkin's Lymphoma
>
> Ease of procurement
> Avoidance of general anesthesia
> Avoidance of hospitalization for stem cell collection
> More rapid neutrophil and platelet recovery
> Lower net cost of procurement
> Lower net cost of transplant hospitalization due to more rapid engraftment
> Applicability for patients with prior pelvic irradiation or prior or current bone marrow involvement

Specific Malignancies

III

TABLE 111-24

Results of HDC/HSCT in Patients with Disease Refractory to Primary Chemotherapy

HIGH-DOSE CHEMORADIOTHERAPY	N	~ 5 YR* PFS (%)	REFERENCE
Sequential program with melphalan + TBI or IFRT	16	31	182
BEAM	46	33	167
CBV±P	30	42	183
Etoposide + melphalan	30	34	184
BEAM (47%)			
CBV (23%)			
Other (20%)			
TBI-based (5%)	290	30	249
fTBI/ETOP/Cy			
BCNU/ETOP/Cy			
CCNU/ETOP/Cy	29	50	Reece and Phillips*
Variable	75	32	148
Variable	25	40	Josting et al[†]
BEAM	43	20	147
Variable	62	15	Constans et al[‡]
CBV (n = 47)			
Variable	122	38	149

BCNU, carmustine; ; BEAM, carmustine, etoposide, cytosine arabinoside, melphalan; CBV ± P, cyclophosphamide, carmustine, etoposide ± cisplatin; CCNU, lomustine; fTBI/ETOP/Cy, fractionated TBI, etoposide, cyclophosphamide; HDC, high-dose radiochemotherapy; IFRT, involved field radiation therapy; PFS, progression-free survival (*range 4 to 6 years to estimate); TBI, total body irradiation.
*Reece DE, Phillips GL: Intensive therapy and autotransplantation in Hodgkin's disease. Stem Cells 1994;12(5):477–493.
[†]Josting A, Reiser M, Rueffer U, Salzberger B, Diehl V, Engert A: Treatment of primary progressive Hodgkin's and aggressive non-Hodgkin's lymphoma: Is there a chance for cure? J Clin Oncol 2000;18(2):332–339.
[‡]Constans M, Sureda A, Terol MJ, et al: Autologous stem cell transplantation for primary refractory Hodgkin's disease: Results and clinical variables affecting outcome. Ann Oncol 2003;14(5):745–751.

unacceptably more toxic than the purely chemotherapeutic CBV and BEAM regimens. Whatever the reason, the use of total body irradiation for these patients could be associated with a high risk of life-threatening or fatal interstitial pneumonitis and should be avoided. Selected results achieved using HDC/HSCT for refractory or relapsed Hodgkin's lymphoma are summarized in Tables 111-24 and 111-25, respectively.

In theory, the use of allogeneic stem cells, with their potential to add an immunologic attack on the malignant cells, should be even more effective than autologous stem cell transplantation after HDC for Hodgkin's lymphoma. This improved potency, however, might be offset by increased toxicity, leaving no net gain for the patient. A modest experience has accumulated in the medical literature that seems to document just such a counterbalancing effect.[190-194] Any gain in disease control seems to have been overshadowed by increased toxicity (including lethal toxicity) from graft-vs.-host disease and interstitial pneumonitis. Presently, issues of ready availability, proven efficacy, and lower toxicity make autologous stem cells the source of choice for hematologic engraftment when HDC/HSCT is used for Hodgkin's lymphoma.

Follow-up and Late Complications of Treatment

Most patients with Hodgkin's lymphoma, especially those below the age of 65 years at diagnosis, can be cured. Most of these cured patients experience minimal long-term toxicity from the treatments; however, common predictable and occasional less common and unpredictable late effects can occur and require preventive measures or recognition and treatment. Certain late effects of treatment for Hodgkin's lymphoma should be considered when patients are reviewed in follow-up. Table 111-26 lists the common late effects and reasonable clinical responses to minimize their impact. Immunizations for pneumococcus, influenza, diphtheria, and tetanus should be updated regularly.

Table 111-27 lists the types of second neoplasms that have been reported to occur with greater frequency in patients cured of Hodgkin's lymphoma.[131-134,136,138-140,142-146,195-201] Knowledge of these possible second cancers should guide screening and follow-up procedures. At the times of planned follow-up, all patients should be examined for masses in the thyroid, breasts, abdomen, or lymph nodes; the oropharynx should be examined for mucosal abnormalities; and the skin should be inspected for pigmented lesions. Patients should be strongly discouraged from smoking and encouraged to perform careful breast and skin examination on a regular basis. Annual pap smears should be performed, and at age 40 years or 10 years after completion of treatment for the Hodgkin's lymphoma, whichever comes earlier, women should begin annual mammography.

Special Problems in Hodgkin's Lymphoma Management

Lymphocyte-Predominant Hodgkin's Lymphoma and Progressive Transformation of Germinal Centers

The wide availability of reliable, reproducible immunohistochemical tests that detect the presence of individual

TABLE 111-25

Results of HDC/HSCT for Patients in First Relapse of Hodgkin's Lymphoma after Chemotherapy for Advanced Disease

HIGH-DOSE CHEMORADIOTHERAPY	N	~ 5 YR* PFS (%)	REFERENCE
BEAM	52	47	167
BCNU/ETOP/Cy			
fTBI/ETOP/Cy	43	~40	Pecego et al*
CBV	85	40	Ager et al†
CBV±P	58	61	Rubio et al‡
BCNU/ETOP/Cy			
fTBI/ETOP/Cy			
	47	~50	Goldstone et al§
CBV	42	44	Stewart et al‖
BEAM (n = 81)			
CBV (n = 28)			
Other (n = 19)			
fTBI-containing (n = 11)	139	45	249
CBV (n = 40)			
fTBI/ETOP/Cy (n = 20)	60	50	152
CBV (50%)			
BEAM (20%)			
BEAC (14%)			
fTBI + variable chemotherapies (10%)	216	37	Sureda et al#

BCNU/ETOP/Cy, carmustine, etoposide, cyclophosphamide; BEAC, carmustine, etoposide, cytosine arabinoside, cyclophosphamide; BEAM, carmustine, etoposide, cytosine arabinoside, melphalan; CBV±P, cyclophosphamide, carmustine, etoposide ± cisplatin; CR, complete remission; Cy, cyclophosphamide; ETOP, etoposide; fTBI, fractionated TBI; HDC, high-dose chemoradiotherapy; PFS, progression-free survival.

*Pecego R, Hill R, Appelbaum FR, et al: Interstitial pneumonitis following autologous bone marrow transplantation. Transplantation 1986;42(5):515–517.
†Ager S. Mahendra P, Richards EM, Bass G, Baglin TP, Marcus RE: High-dose carmustine, eteoposide and melphalan ('BEM') with autologous stem cell transplantation: A dose-toxicity study. Bone Marrow Transplant 1996;17(3):335–340.
‡Rubio C, Hill ME, Milan S, O'Brien ME, Cunningham D: Idiopathic pneumonia syndrome after high-dose chemotherapy for relapsed Hodgkin's disease. Br J Cancer 1997;75(7):1044–1048.
§Goldstone AH, McMillan AK: The place of high-dose therapy with haemopoietic stem cell transplantation in relapsed and refractory Hodgkin's disease. Ann Oncol 1993;4(Suppl 1):21–27.
‖Stewart DA, Guo D, Sutherland JA, et al: Single-agent high-dose melphalan salvage therapy for Hodgkin's disease: Cost, safety, and long-term efficacy. Ann Oncol 1997;8(12):1277–1279.
#Sureda A, Arranz R, Iriondo A, et al: Autologous stem-cell transplantation for Hodgkin's disease: Results and prognostic factors in 494 patients from the Grupo Espanol de Linfomas/Transplante Autologo de Medula Osea Spanish Cooperative Group. J Clin Oncol 2001;19(5):1395–1404.

TABLE 111-26

Potential Late Complications Hodgkin's Lymphoma Treatment and Appropriate Clinical Responses and Preventive Strategies

RISK/PROBLEM	INCIDENCE/RESPONSE
Dental caries	Neck or oropharyngeal irradiation can cause decreased salivation. Patients should have careful dental care follow-up and should make their dentist aware of the previous irradiation.
Hypothyroidism	After external beam irradiation that encompasses the thyroid with doses sufficient to cure Hodgkin's lymphoma, at least 50% of patients will eventually become hypothyroid. All patients whose TSH level becomes elevated should be treated with lifelong thyroxine replacement in doses sufficient to suppress thyroid stimulating hormone (TSH) levels to low normal. This is also necessary to assure that the radiation-damaged thyroid is not subjected to long-term stimulation by thyroid stimulating hormone, which can increase the risk of thyroid neoplasm.
Infertility	ABVD is not known to cause any permanent gonadal toxicity, although oligospermia for 1 to 2 years after treatment is common. Direct or scatter radiation to gonadal tissue can cause infertility, amenorrhea, or premature menopause, but this seldom occurs with the current fields used for the treatment of Hodgkin's lymphoma. Thus, with the current chemotherapy regimens and radiation fields used, most patients will not develop these problems. In general, after treatment, women who continue menstruating are fertile, but men require semen analysis to provide a specific answer. High-dose chemoradiotherapy and hematopoietic stem cell transplantation almost always cause permanent infertility in both genders, although some young women occasionally recover fertility.
Impaired immunity to infections	Hodgkin's lymphoma and its treatment can lead to lifelong impairment of full immunity to infection. All patients should be given annual influenza immunization and pneumococcal immunization every five years. Patients whose spleen has been irradiated or removed should also be immunized against meningococcal types A and C and *Hemophilus influenza* type B. As for all adults, diphtheria and tetanus immunizations should be kept up-to-date.
Secondary neoplasms	Although uncommon, certain secondary neoplasms occur with increased frequency in patients who have been treated for Hodgkin's lymphoma. These include acute myelogenous leukemia, thyroid, breast, lung, and upper gastrointestinal carcinoma and melanoma and cervical carcinoma in situ. It is appropriate to screen for these neoplasms for the rest of the patient's life because they might have lengthy induction periods.

Specific Malignancies

III

TABLE 111-27

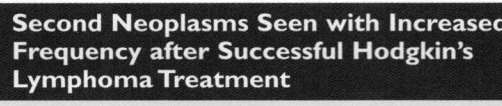

Second Neoplasms Seen with Increased Frequency after Successful Hodgkin's Lymphoma Treatment

Acute myelogenous leukemia/myelodysplasia
Non-Hodgkin's lymphoma
Melanoma
Soft tissue sarcoma
Adenocarcinoma
    Breast
    Thyroid
    Lung
    Stomach and esophagus
Squamous cell carcinoma
    Skin
    Uterine cervix
    Head and neck

cell surface antigens has transformed the field of hematopathology over the past 2 decades, ever since the development of monoclonal antibody-based technology has allowed the production and wide availability of standardized antigen-specific reagents. The classification of the lymphoproliferative diseases is a prime example of this transformation. The accurate identification of many of the entities listed in the Revised European-American Lymphoma (REAL) and World Health Organization (WHO) classification schemes can be accomplished only with the aid of these sophisticated new tools.[50,51,202] In the special area of Hodgkin's lymphoma, understanding the entity of lymphocyte-predominant Hodgkin's lymphoma has been particularly helped by application of these new immunohistochemical techniques.

Lymphocyte-predominant Hodgkin's lymphoma (LPHL) was initially recognized under other names more than 50 years ago. This designation was used to identify a subtype of Hodgkin's lymphoma with an extensive lymphocytic background infiltration and peculiar scattered larger cells, often later referred to as "L & H" or "popcorn" cells without classic Reed-Sternberg cells.[203] In the Rye classification, the nodular and diffuse types were collapsed into one entity, LPHL.[10] Results from individual centers and multi-institutional clinical trials established that LPHL often differed in presenting findings and followed a more indolent course compared with the other types of Hodgkin's lymphoma.[204] Attempts to understand whether differences distinguishing nodular and diffuse subtypes are clinically important have yielded inconsistent results.[205-209] Some authors have found a different long-term outcome, while others have not.[205-209] Fortunately, recent improvements in reproducibility of classification brought about by improved immunohistochemic testing have allowed resolution of these issues.

The pioneering work of the International Lymphoma Study Group, which proposed the REAL classification,[202] included an attempt to address the problem of LPHL. This group proposed that Hodgkin's lymphoma be subdivided into a classical variety including the familiar nodular sclerosing, mixed cellularity, and lymphocyte-depleted subtypes and, in addition, a new entity, lymphocyte-rich classical Hodgkin's lymphoma. In addition, a form of Hodgkin's lymphoma separate from the classical types should be recognized: the nodular lymphocyte-predominant subtype. Most important, specific phenotypic and immunohistochemical criteria for the diagnosis of this new entity called nodular lymphocytic predominant Hodgkin's lymphoma were developed (see Table 111-2). The neoplastic cells exhibit characteristic folded, lobulated nuclei ("popcorn" cells) and inconspicuous nucleoli and are usually positive for CD20, negative for CD30 (which is commonly positive in classical Hodgkin's lymphoma), and negative for CD15.[210] Thus, this type of Hodgkin's lymphoma can be identified reliably by its typical immunophenotypic pattern (CD20 positive, CD15 negative, CD30 negative), which clearly distinguishes it from classical forms of Hodgkin's lymphoma (CD20 negative or, if positive, quite variably so in different cells in the same biopsy—CD15 positive, CD30 positive).

The pivotal study that has transformed our understanding of LPHL was undertaken by the European Task Force on Lymphoma (ETFL).[204,210] This group assembled paraffin blocks and clinical information on 388 adult cases (age greater than 15 years). A panel of expert hematopathologists who were blinded to the clinical outcome data reclassified each case. Table 111-28 shows the outcome of the reclassification based on the full immunophenotypic profiling. Several themes emerge. First, without reliable, objective measures such as immunophenotypic profiling, accurate diagnosis of LPHL is impossible. Only 56% (219/388) of cases submitted as LPHL from centers or groups with special expertise in lymphoma management ultimately proved to have this disease. Second, most of the cases reassigned to diagnoses other than LPHL were found to have the new variety of classical disease called lymphocyte-rich classic Hodgkin's lymphoma, making up 115 of the 169 reassigned cases (68%). Third, almost all cases definitely identified as LPHL had the nodular form of the disease (206/219, 94%), and most of the diffuse cases from the original 388 actually had diagnoses other than LPHL, including 35 with lymphocyte-rich classical Hodgkin's lymphoma.

TABLE 111-28

Final Diagnosis Based on Reclassification of 388 Cases Initially Diagnosed as Lymphocyte-Predominant Hodgkin's Lymphoma

Total	**388**
Final Diagnoses	
Non-Hodgkin's lymphoma	12
Reactive hyperplasia	14
Unclassifiable	9
Classic Hodgkin's lymphoma	134
Nodular sclerosing/mixed cellularity	19
Lymphocyte rich	115
Lymphocyte-predominant Hodgkin's lymphoma	219

From Diehl V, Sextro M, Franklin J, et al: Clinical presentation, course, and prognostic factors in lymphocyte predominant Hodgkin's disease and lymphocyte-rich classical Hodgkin's disease: Report from the European Task Force on Lymphoma Project on Lymphocyte-Predominant Hodgkin's Disease. J Clin Oncol 1999;17(3):776–783.

TABLE 111-29

Clinical Characteristics of Patients with Lymphocyte-Predominant Hodgkin's Lymphoma from Representative Larger Series						
Number of cases	110	50	73	64	68	219
Age, median (yr)	39	36	29	29	35	35
Males (%)	75	86	84	81	68	74
Stage I (%)	59	52	40	55	51	53
II	11	26	36	27	24	28
III	21	16	23	17	13	14
IV	9	6	1	1	12	6
B symptoms (%)	12	6	NR	9	15	10
Reference	206	208	205	207	Orlandi et al*	204

NR, not reported.
*Orlandi E, Lazzarino M, Brusamolino E, et al: Nodular lymphocyte predominance Hodgkin's disease: Long-term observation reveals a continuous pattern of recurrence. Leuk Lymphoma 1997;26(3–4):359–368.

Understanding these findings is essential for the useful interpretation of past and future studies of LPHL.

Lymphocyte-predominant Hodgkin's lymphoma has long been recognized as an uncommon indolent disease seen more frequently in males, with a tendency to present with limited nodal disease and infrequent constitutional symptoms. Table 111-29 shows the typical presenting findings. From these studies, it is clear that LPHL usually presents without constitutional symptoms or extranodal disease. There is a 2:1–3:1 predominance of males, and the median age of adult patients is similar to that seen in Hodgkin's lymphoma in general—35 years. Mediastinal involvement is unusual (~7%). In the rare patients with stage IV disease (~6%), extranodal involvement is usually seen in sites typical of Hodgkin's lymphoma: liver (~3%), bone marrow (~1%), or lung (~1%). Bulky disease is seen in only ~13% of patients. Thus, LPHL is usually confined to nonbulky peripheral lymph nodes, seldom causes constitutional symptoms, and is more often seen in men.

LPHL has most often been treated with irradiation, with chemotherapy reserved for the uncommon cases with advanced-stage disease or as an adjuvant to the primary irradiation. No prospective randomized trials have addressed LPHL exclusively, but some conclusions can be drawn from available descriptive studies. Table 111-30 shows the range of long-term survivals reported in representative larger institutional or group experiences. Reported long-term overall survivals have been generally consistent at about 80% to 90%. Several studies have noted a pattern of late relapse that seems modestly different from classic Hodgkin's lymphoma. For example, among the 115 patients in the ETFL study reclassified to lymphocyte-rich classical Hodgkin's lymphoma, only 2 of the 20 relapses (10%) occurred after 10 years and none after 13 years. On the other hand, in the 219 patients with LPHL, 7 of 45 relapses (16%) occurred after 10 years, and 5 of these were after 13 years. Although no plateau in was seen in failure-free survival in the LPHL cases, the number of late events was small, and the patients were highly selected. Overall, the data that indicate a major difference in treatment outcome between patients with LPHL and classical forms of Hodgkin's lymphoma are interesting but not sufficiently compelling to affect treatment choices.

Several authors have noted a connection between progressively transformed germinal centers (PTGC) and LPHL, finding that PTGC can be seen before, coincident with, or after LPHL.[203,211,212] Although anecdotal case reports have linked PTGC with later development of LPHL, no convincing data have confirmed a definite increase in such risk. Presently, the major importance of PTGC is that it be recognized as a reactive, usually benign, lesion and not mistaken for a lymphoproliferative neoplasm.

Most of the larger series of cases of LPHL have noted a risk of later non-Hodgkin's lymphoma, usually diffuse large B-cell type. In the 219 confirmed LPHL cases in the ETFL study, at least six patients eventually developed

TABLE 111-30

Results of Treatment of Lymphocyte Predominant Hodgkin's Lymphoma						
	SURVIVAL (%)					
N	RELAPSE FREE		PROGRESSION FREE		OVERALL		REFERENCE
	5 yr	10 yr	5 yr	10 yr	5 yr	10 yr	
110	88			80			206
145				90			Hansmann et al*
75		80				93	209
73		60				82	205
68				45		71	Orlandi et al†
64				74		85	207
219				70		92	204

*Hansmann ML, Zwingers T, Boske A, Loffler H, Lennert K: Clinical features of nodular paragranuloma (Hodgkin's disease, lymphocyte predominance type, nodular). J Cancer Res Clin Oncol 1984;108(3):321–330.
†Orlandi E, Lazzarino M, Brusamolino E, Paulli M, Astori C, Magrini U, et al: Nodular lymphocyte predominance Hodgkin's disease: Long-term observation reveals a continuous pattern of recurrence. Leuk Lymphoma 1997;26(3–4):359–368.

non-Hodgkin's lymphoma (2.9%). In a review of 567 cases of LPHL from the medical literature, Diehl and his co-authors[213] found 15 cases of non-Hodgkin's lymphoma reported, for an incidence of 2.6%. In comparison, among the 12,411 cases recorded in the International Database on Hodgkin's Disease, only 0.9% of patients were noted to develop subsequent non-Hodgkin's lymphoma. It is reasonable to conclude that there is a two- to threefold increased risk of developing a secondary non-Hodgkin's lymphoma, usually diffuse large B-cell type, after LPHL in comparison to the rate seen after classic Hodgkin's lymphoma. The absolute risk of such secondary non-Hodgkin's lymphoma is low, however, and in a patient population already being followed carefully for possible Hodgkin's lymphoma recurrence, it does not have any clinical implication other than to make clear the necessity to obtain biopsy proof of the nature of any suspected recurrence.

Several specific questions must be answered for patients with LPHL. Should patients with LPHL be treated differently? The answer depends on one's choice of standard treatment for Hodgkin's lymphoma. Most patients with LPHL present with limited-stage disease. Cumulative evidence from extensive clinical trials and single-center experiences indicates that Hodgkin's lymphoma patients with limited-stage disease should, in general, be treated with an optimized mix of brief chemotherapy and irradiation of modest extent. Such treatment is entirely appropriate for patients with limited-stage LPHL and can reasonably be expected to produce 10- and 20-year overall survivals exceeding 90% while minimizing the risks of secondary neoplasms. Some authorities, however, would omit the chemotherapy, and to date there are no compelling data that it must be included. Patients with advanced-stage LPHL seldom have clinical or laboratory features predicting a poor outcome and, therefore, should be treated with regimens such as ABVD that minimize exposure to the more potently carcinogenic antineoplastic agents. Overtreatment should be avoided, and attention to this principle should reduce as much as possible the risk of potentially fatal late complications.

Hodgkin's Lymphoma during Pregnancy

Occurring as it does in younger patients, it is not surprising that Hodgkin's lymphoma sometimes is found while a patient is pregnant. In such a case, attention must be focused on the welfare of both the patient and the developing fetus. Fortunately, even when the Hodgkin's lymphoma is not discovered relatively early in the pregnancy, it is almost always possible to deal effectively with the disease and allow the pregnancy to go successfully to full term. Some guidance is available from small series and anecdotal experience, which can be complemented by careful clinical judgment and knowledge of the usual natural history of Hodgkin's lymphoma.[214-222]

Standard staging tests should be completed (see Table 111-4) when Hodgkin's lymphoma is discovered during pregnancy, except that imaging requiring radiation must be avoided as much as possible. Abdominal ultrasonography is very useful to identify bulky retroperitoneal disease or nodular disease in the spleen and to rule out hydronephrosis. With proper shielding, a single PA radiograph of the chest should be obtained to detect mediastinal disease. The point of this assessment is not to catalog all sites of disease exhaustively but rather to search for any sites that seriously threaten the immediate well-being of either mother or child.

The majority of patients found to have Hodgkin's lymphoma during pregnancy do not require immediate intervention. Asymptomatic or minimally symptomatic patients can be followed carefully, with treatment reserved for threatening or more symptomatic disease. As many as 50% of patients thus observed can carry the pregnancy to term without any treatment becoming necessary for the lymphoma. Patients should be seen at least monthly and questioned for B symptoms, cough, or other discomfort that can be traced to the Hodgkin's lymphoma. Blood counts should be monitored along with routine tests of renal and hepatic function. If symptomatic or threatening disease develops, some authorities have recommended irradiation with special shielding.[214,215,218,219,221,222] This procedure might endanger the fetus unnecessarily, however, and a better choice is systemic chemotherapy with vinblastine. Vinblastine is neither teratogenic nor carcinogenic and is very effective in treatment-naive patients, almost always inducing at least some disease regression. Infrequent doses can be given to keep the Hodgkin's lymphoma under control until delivery at term, minimizing risks to mother or child. Patients who have been able to complete the pregnancy without treatment for the lymphoma can be fully staged and treated appropriately after delivery. Patients who required vinblastine cannot be accurately staged after it has been given and so should be treated with multiagent chemotherapy regardless of apparent stage at the end of the pregnancy. We have managed the 12 women coincidentally found to have Hodgkin's lymphoma and to be pregnant at our center over the past 20 years with this approach. Six required vinblastine, and six were observed. All delivered healthy infants at term. One patient has died after multiple relapses of Hodgkin's lymphoma and one has died of acute leukemia 8 years after diagnosis, 6 years after successful HDC/HSCT for relapsed disease. The other 10 are alive and well, with a median follow-up of more than 6 years. These and similar data from the literature document that it is feasible to manage Hodgkin's lymphoma successfully even when it is discovered during pregnancy.

Hodgkin's Lymphoma and AIDS

Given the frequency with which young men are affected with acquired immunodeficiency syndrome (AIDS) and the young age of patients with Hodgkin's lymphoma in general, a certain number of cases of coincident disease should arise. Current best estimates, however, indicate that the incidence of Hodgkin's lymphoma in patients with HIV infection is increased as much as 5- to 10-fold above expected rates.[223,224] In addition, when present in an HIV-infected individual, Hodgkin's lymphoma presents differently and pursues a different natural history. It is now well documented that Hodgkin's lymphoma in HIV-positive individuals is almost always associated with

Epstein-Barr virus within the Hodgkin's/Reed-Sternberg cells.[224-227] In addition, it is much more likely to be of mixed cellularity or lymphocyte-depleted histology and to present in extranodal sites, especially the bone marrow, where involvement rates have been found to be as high as 50% or more.[223-229] Advanced stage is present in more than 80% of patients, and most patients have B symptoms.[224,227,229]

The treatment of coincident HIV infection and Hodgkin's lymphoma is challenging. Almost all patients have advanced-stage lymphoma and require multiagent chemotherapy. They are prone to opportunistic infections and other manifestations of AIDS, and their ability to tolerate myelosuppressive treatment is compromised. The best approach appears to be a combination of vigorous supportive care with antiviral and antifungal agents, neutrophil-stimulating growth factors, and highly active antiretroviral agents along with multiagent chemotherapy. With appropriate supportive care, multiagent regimens such as ABVD and EBVP (epirubicin, bleomycin, vinblastine, and prednisone) can be delivered; however, much greater than normal toxicity must be anticipated.[227,229] Disappointingly, even with intensive supportive care and proper multiagent chemotherapy, response rates are lower and cure rates are much lower than in the non–HIV-infected population. Most investigators have found median survivals of 1 to 2 years to be the rule. Even in the most recent era, when highly active antiretroviral treatment might be lowering the incidence of coincident HIV infection and Hodgkin's lymphoma, cure rates for the lymphoma remain low.[230]

ISSUES FOR THE FUTURE

The reliance on irradiation to treat limited-stage Hodgkin's lymphoma is an historic accident, not the result of rigorous clinical research. Radiation therapy came first and works well, as has been demonstrated over the past half century. Chemotherapy alone might work just as well, however, and the eventual choice between the two will more likely revolve around differences in toxicity rather than efficacy. The realization that a substantial proportion of the excess mortality eventually experienced by patients with limited-stage Hodgkin's lymphoma is due to cardiovascular disease and second neoplasms arising in the skin, thyroid, breast, lung, gastrointestinal tract, and connective tissue and that the incidence of these late complications is closely related to the use of irradiation, has made this an important area of clinical research.[133-146] A few trials have attempted to address this issue by eliminating irradiation but are not relevant today because of reliance on staging laparotomy, inclusion of some patients with more than limited-stage disease, and suboptimal chemotherapy.[231,232] With the identification of ABVD as the regimen best combining high efficacy with low toxicity, a test of chemotherapy vs. combined-modality therapy for limited-stage Hodgkin's lymphoma is appropriate. A cooperative trial comparing these two approaches has been conducted by the National Cancer Institute of Canada Clinical Trials Group and the Eastern Cooperative Oncology Group and should prove helpful in guiding treatment in the future.

No new chemotherapeutic agents have been introduced into the management of Hodgkin's lymphoma for several years. With more than 15% of patients still dying of lymphoma, there is a clear need to find effective new agents. Perhaps the most promising of traditional chemotherapeutic agents currently under investigation for Hodgkin's lymphoma is gemcitabine.[233-238] In small series of patients who previously were heavily treated, an overall response rate of approximately 50% has been found, with 10% to 20% complete responses. Even more encouraging, two groups have found an overall response rate of greater than 75% when gemcitabine is combined with cisplatin and a corticosteroid.[233,238] This promising new agent will need further testing and integration into combinations with standard or other novel agents to exert its ultimate impact in the management of Hodgkin's lymphoma.

One of the most promising types of new treatments for lymphoma is that of targeted immunotherapy. The anti-CD20 monoclonal antibody rituximab has proven useful for several different types of B-cell lymphomas. The nearly universal expression of CD20 on the neoplastic cells of lymphocyte predominant Hodgkin's lymphoma suggests that this lymphoma might be treated usefully with rituximab. Preliminary data from several small series show response rates exceeding 50%; however, the durability of these responses seems limited.[239-243] Treatment with rituximab is attractive for this disease because of the lack of cumulative or late toxicity with this agent, but it will need to be integrated with conventional treatments to have a substantial impact.

Efficacy of one type of targeted immunotherapy hints that others could also be useful. Monoclonal antibodies aimed at other B-cell or lymphocytic antigens, radioimmunoconjugates, and immunotoxin molecules (including bi-specific antibodies and tumor-specific immunization strategies) all hold promise.[244-248] The specificity of each of these techniques is especially attractive as we try to improve treatment effectiveness while holding acute and especially late toxicity to a minimum. Hodgkin's lymphoma is already a highly treatable, often curable disease. It should be possible to build on the sound foundation of more than three decades of careful clinical and basic research to assemble even more effective, less toxic treatments in the future.

REFERENCES

1. Gloeckler Ries LA, Kosary CL, Hankey BF, Miller BA, Harras A, Edwards BK (eds): SEER cancer statistics review, 1973-1994. Bethesda, MD: US Department of Health and Human Services, Public Health Service, National Institutes of Health, 1997. NIH Publication No. 97-2789, p 198.
2. Miller TP, LeBlanc M, Braziel R, Grogan TM, Press OW, Fisher RI: Was the bimodal age incidence of Hodgkin's lymphoma a result of mistaken diagnosis of non-Hodgkin's lymphoma? [abstract]. Blood 2002;100:771a.
3. Hodgkin T: On some morbid appearances of the absorbent glands and spleen. Medico-Chirurgical Transact 1832;17:68–114.
4. Sternberg C: Über eine eigenartige unter dem Bilde der

Pseudoleukämie verlaufende Tuberculose des lymphatischen Apperates. Ztschr Heilk 1898;31:21–90.

5. Reed DM: On the pathologic changes in Hodgkin's disease, with especial reference to its relation to tuberculosis. Johns Hopkins Hosp Rep 1902;10:133–196.

6. Jackson H Jr, Parker F Jr: Hodgkin's disease I. General considerations. N Engl J Med 1944;230:1–8.

7. Jackson H Jr, Parker F Jr: Hodgkin's disease I. Pathology. N Engl J Med 1944;230:35–42.

8. Lukes RJ, Butler JJ: The pathology and nomenclature of Hodgkin's disease. Cancer Res 1966;26(6):1063–1083.

9. Lukes RJ, Butler JJ, Hicks EB: Natural history of Hodgkin's disease as related to its pathologic picture. Cancer 1966;19:317–324.

10. Lukes RJ, Craver LF, Hall TC, Rappaport H, Ruben P: Report of the nomenclature committee. Cancer Res 1966;26:1311–1316.

11. Pusey WA: Cases of sarcoma and of Hodgkin's disease treated by exposure to X-rays: A preliminary report. JAMA 1902;38:166–169.

12. Senn N: Therapeutical value of roentgen ray in the treatment of pseudoleukemia. New York Med J 1903;77:665–668.

13. Peters MV: A study in survival of Hodgkin's disease treated radiologically. Am J Roentgenol 1950;63:299–311.

14. Kaplan HS: The radical radiotherapy of regionally localized Hodgkin's disease. Radiology 1962;78:553–561.

15. Kaplan HS: Evidence for a tumoricidal dose level in the radiotherapy of Hodgkin's disease. Cancer Res 1966;26:1221–1224.

16. Goodman LS, Wintrobe MM, Dameshek W, Goodman MJ, Gilman AZ, McLennan MT: Nitrogen mustard therapy. Use of methyl-bis-(beta-chloroethyl)amine hydrochloride and tris-(beta-chloroethyl)amine hydrochloride for Hodgkin's disease, lymphsarcoma, leukemia and certain allied and miscellaneous disorders. JAMA 1946;132:126–132.

17. Dougherty T, White A: Influence of hormones on lymphoid tissue structure and function. Role of pituitary adrenotrophic hormone in regulation of lymphocytes and other cellular elements of the blood. Endocrinology 1944;35:1–35.

18. Claman HN: Corticosteroids and lymphoid cells. N Engl J Med 1972;287(8):388–397.

19. Johnson IS, Armstrong JG, Gorman M: The vinca alkyloids: A new class of oncolytic agents. Cancer Res 1963;23:1390–1427.

20. Farber S, Diamond LK, Mercer RD, et al: Temporary remissions in acute leukemia in children produced by folic antagonist 4-amethopteroylglutamic acid (aminopterin). N Engl J Med 1948;238:787–798.

21. Krivit W, Brubaker C, Hartmann J, Murphy ML, Pierce M, Thatcher G: Induction of remission in acute leukemia of childhood by combination of prednisone and either 6-mercaptopurine or methotrexate. J Pediatr 1966;68(6):965–968.

22. DeVita VT, Serpick A, Carbone PP: Combination chemotherapy in the treatment of Hodgkin's disease. Ann Intern Med 1970;73:881–895.

23. Longo DL, Young RC, Wesley M, et al: Twenty years of MOPP therapy for Hodgkin's disease. J Clin Oncol 1986;4(9):1295–1306.

24. Zunino F, Gambetta R, Di Marco A, Zaccara A, Luoni G: A comparison of the effects of daunomycin and adriamycin on various DNA polymerases. Cancer Res 1975;35(3):754–760.

25. McKelvey EM, Gottlieb JA, Wilson HE, et al: Hydroxyldaunomycin (Adriamycin) combination chemotherapy in malignant lymphoma. Cancer 1976;38(4):1484–1493.

26. Umezawa H, Maeda K, Takeuchi T, Okami Y: New antibiotics, bleomycin A and B. J Antibiot (Tokyo) 1966;19(5):200–209.

27. Blum RH, Carter SK, Agre K: A clinical review of bleomycin—A new antineoplastic agent. Cancer 1973;31(4):903–914.

28. Frei E III, Luce JK, Talley RW, Vaitkevicius VK, Wilson HE: 5-(3,3-dimethyl-1-triazeno)imidazole-4-carboxamide (NSC-45388) in the treatment of lymphoma. Cancer Chemother Rep 1972;56(5):667–670.

29. Santoro A, Bonadonna G: Prolonged disease-free survival in MOPP-resistant Hodgkin's disease after treatment with adriamycin, bleomycin, vinblastine and dacarbazine (ABVD). Cancer Chemother Pharmacol 1979;2(2):101–105.

30. Jagannath S, Dicke KA, Armitage JO, Cabanillas FF, Horwitz LJ, Vellekoop L, Zander AR, Spitzer G: High-dose cyclophosphamide, carmustine, and etoposide and autologous bone marrow

transplantation for relapsed Hodgkin's disease. Ann Intern Med 1986;104(2):163–168.

31. Phillips GL, Wolff SN, Herzig RH, et al: Treatment of progressive Hodgkin's disease with intensive chemoradiotherapy and autologous bone marrow transplantation. Blood 1989;73(8):2086–2092.

32. Linch DC, Winfield D, Goldstone AH, et al: Dose intensification with autologous bone-marrow transplantation in relapsed and resistant Hodgkin's disease: Results of a BNLI randomised trial. Lancet 1993;341(8852):1051–1054.

33. Schmitz N, Pfistner B, Sextro M, et al: Aggressive conventional chemotherapy compared with high-dose chemotherapy with autologous haemopoietic stem-cell transplantation for relapsed chemosensitive Hodgkin's disease: A randomised trial. Lancet 2002;359(9323):2065–2071.

34. Kvale G, Hoiby EA, Pedersen E: Hodgkin's disease in patients with previous infectious mononucleosis. Int J Cancer 1979;23(5):593–597.

35. Miller RW, Beebe GW: Infectious mononucleosis and the empirical risk of cancer. J Natl Cancer Inst 1973;50(2):315–321.

36. Mueller N, Evans A, Harris NL, et al: Hodgkin's disease and Epstein-Barr virus. Altered antibody pattern before diagnosis. N Engl J Med 1989;320(11):689–695.

37. Staal SP, Ambinder R, Beschorner WE, Hayward GS, Mann R: A survey of Epstein-Barr virus DNA in lymphoid tissue. Frequent detection in Hodgkin's disease. Am J Clin Pathol 1989;91(1):1–5.

38. Anagnostopoulos I, Herbst H, Niedobitek G, Stein H: Demonstration of monoclonal EBV genomes in Hodgkin's disease and Ki-1-positive anaplastic large cell lymphoma by combined Southern blot and in situ hybridization. Blood 1989;74(2):810–816.

39. Herbst H, Niedobitek G, Kneba M, et al: High incidence of Epstein-Barr virus genomes in Hodgkin's disease. Am J Pathol 1990;137(1):13–18.

40. Gulley ML, Eagan PA, Quintanilla-Martinez L, et al: Epstein-Barr virus DNA is abundant and monoclonal in the Reed-Sternberg cells of Hodgkin's disease: Association with mixed cellularity subtype and Hispanic American ethnicity. Blood 1994;83(6):1595–1602.

41. Brousset P, Chittal S, Schlaifer D, et al: Detection of Epstein-Barr virus messenger RNA in Reed-Sternberg cells of Hodgkin's disease by in situ hybridization with biotinylated probes on specially processed modified acetone methyl benzoate xylene (ModAMeX) sections. Blood 1991;77(8):1781–1786.

42. Weiss LM, Chen YY, Liu XF, Shibata D: Epstein-Barr virus and Hodgkin's disease. A correlative in situ hybridization and polymerase chain reaction study. Am J Pathol 1991;139(6):1259–1265.

43. Lauritzen AF, Hording U, Nielsen HW: Epstein-Barr virus and Hodgkin's disease: A comparative immunological, in situ hybridization, and polymerase chain reaction study. APMIS 1994;102(7):495–500.

44. Ambinder RF, Weiss LM. Association of Epstein Barr virus with Hodgkin's disease. In Mauch PM, Armitage JO, Diehl V, Hoppe RT, Weiss LM (ed): Hodgkin's Disease. Philadelphia, Lippincott Williams & Wilkins, 1999, pp 79–98.

45. Boice Jr JD, Land CE, Preston DE: Ionizing radiation. In Schottenfeld D, Fraumeni Jr JF (ed): Cancer Epidemiology and Prevention, 2nd ed. Oxford, Oxford University Press, 1996, pp 319–345.

46. Grufferman S, Duong T, Cole P: Occupation and Hodgkin's disease. J Natl Cancer Inst 1976;57(5):1193–1195.

47. Razis DV, Diamond HD, Craver LF: Familial Hodgkin's disease: Its significance and implications. Ann Intern Med 1959;1959:933–939.

48. Grufferman S, Cole P, Smith PG, Lukes RJ: Hodgkin's disease in siblings. N Engl J Med 1977;296(5):248–250.

49. Mack TM, Cozen W, Shibata DK, et al: Concordance for Hodgkin's disease in identical twins suggesting genetic susceptibility to the young-adult form of the disease. N Engl J Med 1995;332(7):413–418.

50. Anonymous. A clinical evaluation of the International Lymphoma Study Group classification of non-Hodgkin's lymphoma. The Non-Hodgkin's Lymphoma Classification Project. Blood 1997;89(11):3909–3918.

51. Jaffe ES, Harris NL, Stein H, Vardiman JW (eds): Pathology and Genetics of Tumours of Haematopoietic and Lymphoid Tissues. Lyon, France, IARC Press, 2001.

52. Trumper LH, Brady G, Bagg A, et al: Single-cell analysis of Hodgkin and Reed-Sternberg cells: Molecular heterogeneity of gene expression and p53 mutations. Blood 1993;81(11):3097–3115.

53. Kuppers R, Rajewsky K, Zhao M, et al: Hodgkin disease: Hodgkin and Reed-Sternberg cells picked from histological sections show clonal immunoglobulin gene rearrangements and appear to be derived from B cells at various stages of development. Proc Natl Acad Sci USA 1994;91(23):10962–10966.

54. Kanzler H, Kuppers R, Hansmann ML, Rajewsky K: Hodgkin and Reed-Sternberg cells in Hodgkin's disease represent the outgrowth of a dominant tumor clone derived from (crippled) germinal center B cells. J Exp Med 1996;184(4):1495–1505.

55. Jox A, Zander T, Kornacker M, et al: Detection of identical Hodgkin-Reed Sternberg cell specific immunoglobulin gene rearrangements in a patient with Hodgkin's disease of mixed cellularity subtype at primary diagnosis and in relapse two and a half years later. Ann Oncol 1998;9(3):283–287.

56. Muschen M, Rajewsky K, Brauninger A, et al: Rare occurrence of classical Hodgkin's disease as a T cell lymphoma. J Exp Med 2000;191(2):387–394.

57. Marafioti T, Hummel M, Foss HD, et al: Hodgkin and Reed-Sternberg cells represent an expansion of a single clone originating from a germinal center B-cell with functional immunoglobulin gene rearrangements but defective immunoglobulin transcription. Blood 2000;95(4):1443–1450.

58. Bargou RC, Leng C, Krappmann D, et al: High-level nuclear NF-kappa B and Oct-2 is a common feature of cultured Hodgkin/Reed-Sternberg cells. Blood 1996;87(10):4340–4347.

59. Gospodarowicz MK, Sutcliffe SB, Clark RM, et al: Analysis of supradiaphragmatic clinical stage I and II Hodgkin's disease treated with radiation alone. Int J Radiat Oncol Biol Phys 1992;22(5):859–865.

60. Krikorian JG, Portlock CS, Rosenberg SA, Kaplan HS: Hodgkin's disease, stages I and II occurring below the diaphragm. Cancer 1979;43(5):1866–1871.

61. Hueltenschmidt B, Sautter-Bihl ML, Lang O, et al: Whole body positron emission tomography in the treatment of Hodgkin disease. Cancer 2001;91(2):302–310.

62. Jerusalem G, Beguin Y, Fassotte MF, et al: Whole-body positron emission tomography using 18F-fluorodeoxyglucose for posttreatment evaluation in Hodgkin's disease and non-Hodgkin's lymphoma has higher diagnostic and prognostic value than classical computed tomography scan imaging. Blood 1999;94(2):429–433.

63. Jerusalem G, Beguin Y, Fassotte MF, et al: Whole-body positron emission tomography using 18F-fluorodeoxyglucose compared to standard procedures for staging patients with Hodgkin's disease. Haematologica 2001;86(3):266–273.

64. Zinzani PL, Magagnoli M, Chierichetti F, et al: The role of positron emission tomography (PET) in the management of lymphoma patients. Ann Oncol 1999;10(10):1181–1184.

65. de Wit M, Bohuslavizki KH, Buchert R, Bumann D, Clausen M, Hossfeld DK: 18FDG-PET following treatment as valid predictor for disease-free survival in Hodgkin's lymphoma. Ann Oncol 2001;12(1):29–37.

66. Jerusalem G, Beguin Y, Fassotte MF, et al: Persistent tumor 18F-FDG uptake after a few cycles of polychemotherapy is predictive of treatment failure in non-Hodgkin's lymphoma. Haematologica 2000;85(6):613–618.

67. Mikhaeel NG, Timothy AR, Hain SF, O'Doherty MJ: 18-FDG-PET for the assessment of residual masses on CT following treatment of lymphomas. Ann Oncol 2000;11(Suppl 1):147–150.

68. Spaepen K, Stroobants S, Dupont P, et al: Prognostic value of positron emission tomography (PET) with fluorine-18 fluorodeoxy-glucose ([18F]FDG) after first-line chemotherapy in non-Hodgkin's lymphoma: is [18F]FDG-PET a valid alternative to conventional diagnostic methods? J Clin Oncol 2001;19(2):414–419.

69. Spaepen K, Stroobants S, Dupont P, et al: Early restaging positron emmision tomography (PET) with 18F-fluorodeoxyglucose (18FDG) predicts outcome in patients with aggressive non-Hodgkin's lymphoma [abstract]. Blood 2001;98:726a.

70. Carbone PP, Kaplan HS, Musshoff K, Smithers DW, Tubiana M: Report of the Committee on Hodgkin's Disease Staging Classification. Cancer Res 1971;31(11):1860–1861.

71. Lister TA, Crowther D, Sutcliffe SB, et al: Report of a committee convened to discuss the evaluation and staging of patients with Hodgkin's disease: Cotswolds meeting. J Clin Oncol 1989;7(11):1630–1636.

72. Connors JM, Klimo P: Is it an E lesion or stage IV? An unsettled issue in Hodgkin's disease staging. J Clin Oncol 1984;2(12):1421–1423.

73. Levis A, Depaoli L, Bertini M, et al: Results of a low aggressivity chemotherapy regimen (CVP/CEB) in elderly Hodgkin's disease patients. Haematologica 1996;81(5):450–456.

74. Macpherson N, Klasa RJ, Gascoyne R, O'Reilly SE, Voss N, Connors JM: Treatment of elderly Hodgkin's lymphoma patients with a novel 5-drug regimen (ODBEP): A phase II study. Leuk Lymphoma 2002;43(7):1395–1402.

75. Weekes CD, Vose JM, Lynch JC, et al: Hodgkin's disease in the elderly: Improved treatment outcome with a doxorubicin-containing regimen. J Clin Oncol 2002;20:1087–1093.

76. Landgren O, Algernon C, Axdorph U, et al: Hodgkin's lymphoma in the elderly with special reference to type and intensity of chemotherapy in relation to prognosis. Haematologica 2003;88(4):438–444.

77. Stark GL, Wood KM, Jack F, Angus B, Proctor SJ, Taylor PR: Hodgkin's disease in the elderly: A population-based study. Br J Haematol 2002;119(2):432–440.

78. Proctor SJ, Rueffer JU, Angus B, et al: Hodgkin's disease in the elderly: Current status and future directions. Ann Oncol 2002;13(Suppl 1):133–137.

79. Levis A, Pietrasanta D, Anselmo AP, Ambrosetti A, Bertini M: Treatment of elderly Hodgkin's lymphoma patients. The experience of the Italian Lymphoma Intergroup. Tumori 2002;88(1 Suppl 1):S29–S31.

80. Illes A, Vadasz G, Gergely L, Szegedi G: Hodgkin's disease in the elderly: A single institution retrospective study of 40 patients aged 65 or over. Haematologia 2000;30(4):263–269.

81. Hasenclever D, Diehl V: A prognostic score for advanced Hodgkin's disease. International Prognostic Factors Project on Advanced Hodgkin's Disease. N Engl J Med 1998;339(21):1506–1514.

82. Bonadonna G, Zucali R, Monfardini S, De Lena M, Uslenghi C: Combination chemotherapy of Hodgkin's disease with Adriamycin, bleomycin, vinblastine, and imidazole carboxamide versus MOPP. Cancer 1975;36(1):252–259.

83. Duggan DB, Petroni GR, Johnson JL, et al: Randomized comparison of ABVD and MOPP/ABV hybrid for the treatment of advanced Hodgkin's disease: Report of an intergroup trial. J Clin Oncol 2003;21(4):607–614.

84. Canellos GP, Anderson JR, Propert KJ, et al: Chemotherapy of advanced Hodgkin's disease with MOPP, ABVD, or MOPP alternating with ABVD. N Engl J Med 1992;327(21):1478–1484.

85. Gobbi PG, Comelli M, Grignani GE, Pieresca C, Bertoloni D, Ascari E: Estimate of expected survival at diagnosis in Hodgkin's disease: A means of weighting prognostic factors and a tool for treatment choice and clinical research. A report from the International Database on Hodgkin's Disease (IDHD). Haematologica 1994;79(3):241–255.

86. Mauch P, Larson D, Osteen R, et al: Prognostic factors for positive surgical staging in patients with Hodgkin's disease. J Clin Oncol 1990;8(2):257–265.

87. Tubiana M, Henry-Amar M, Carde P, et al: Toward comprehensive management tailored to prognostic factors of patients with clinical stages I and II in Hodgkin's disease. The EORTC Lymphoma Group controlled clinical trials: 1964–1987. Blood 1989;73(1):47–56.

88. Leibenhaut MH, Hoppe RT, Efron B, Halpern J, Nelsen T, Rosenberg SA: Prognostic indicators of laparotomy findings in clinical stage I-II supradiaphragmatic Hodgkin's disease. J Clin Oncol 1989;7(1):81–91.

89. Mauch P, Tarbell N, Weinstein H, et al: Stage IA and IIA supradiaphragmatic Hodgkin's disease: Prognostic factors in surgically staged patients treated with mantle and paraaortic irradiation. J Clin Oncol 1988;6(10):1576–1583.

90. Carde P, Burgers JM, Henry-Amar M, et al: Clinical stages I and II Hodgkin's disease: A specifically tailored therapy according to prognostic factors. J Clin Oncol 1988;6(2):239–252.

91. Hagenbeek A, Carde P, Noordjik EM, et al: Prognostic factor tailored treatment of early stage Hodgkin's disease. Results from a prospective randomized phase III clinical trial in 762 patients (H7 study) [abstract]. Blood 1997;90(Suppl 1):585.

92. Rostock RA, Giangreco A, Wharam MD, Lenhard R, Siegelman SS, Order SE: CT scan modification in the treatment of mediastinal Hodgkin's disease. Cancer 1982;49(11):2267–2275.

93. Carde P, Hagenbeek A, Hayat M, et al: Clinical staging versus laparotomy and combined modality with MOPP versus ABVD in early-stage Hodgkin's disease: The H6 twin randomized trials from the European Organization for Research and Treatment of Cancer Lymphoma Cooperative Group. J Clin Oncol 1993;11(11):2258–2272.

94. Shore T, Nelson N, Weinerman B: A meta-analysis of stages I and II Hodgkin's disease. Cancer 1990;65(5):1155–1160.

95. Santoro A, Bonfante V, Viviani S, et al: Subtotal nodal (STNI) vs. involved field (IFRT) irradiation after 4 cycles of ABVD in early stage Hodgkin's disease (HD) [abstract]. Proc Am Soc Clin Oncol 1996;15:415.

96. Klasa RJ, Connors JM, Fairey R, et al: Treatment of early stage Hodgkin's disease: Improved outcome with brief chemotherapy and radiotherapy without staging laparotomy [abstract]. Annal Oncol 1996;7(Suppl 3):21.

97. Tesch H, Sieber M, Ruffer JU, et al: 2 cycles of ABVD plus radiotherapy is more effective than radiotherapy alone in early stage Hodgkin's disease—Interim analysis of the HD7 trial of the GHSG [abstract 2001]. Blood 1998;92:485a.

98. Bodis S, Henry-Amar M, Bosq J, et al: Late relapse in early-stage Hodgkin's disease patients enrolled on European Organization for Research and Treatment of Cancer protocols. J Clin Oncol 1993;11(2):225–232.

99. Zittoun R, Audebert A, Hoerni B, et al: Extended versus involved fields irradiation combined with MOPP chemotherapy in early clinical stages of Hodgkin's disease. J Clin Oncol 1985;3(2):207–214.

100. Rosenberg SA, Kaplan HS: The evolution and summary results of the Stanford randomized clinical trials of the management of Hodgkin's disease: 1962–1984. Int J Radiat Oncol Biol Phys 1985;11(1):5–22.

101. Horning SJ, Hoppe RT, Hancock SL, Rosenberg SA: Vinblastine, bleomycin, and methotrexate: An effective adjuvant in favorable Hodgkin's disease. J Clin Oncol 1988;6(12):1822–1831.

102. Devita VT Jr, Serpick AA, Carbone PP: Combination chemotherapy in the treatment of advanced Hodgkin's disease. Ann Intern Med 1970;73(6):881–895.

103. Viviani S, Santoro A, Ragni G, Bonfante V, Bestetti O, Bonadonna G: Gonadal toxicity after combination chemotherapy for Hodgkin's disease. Comparative results of MOPP vs ABVD. Eur J Cancer Clin Oncol 1985;21(5):601–605.

104. Bonadonna G, Santoro A, Gianni AM, et al: Primary and salvage chemotherapy in advanced Hodgkin's disease: The Milan Cancer Institute experience. Ann Oncol 1991;2(Suppl 1):9–16.

105. Bonfante V, Santoro A, Viviani S, Valagussa P, Bonadonna G: ABVD in the treatment of Hodgkin's disease. Semin Oncol 1992;19(2 Suppl 5):38–44; discussion 44–45.

106. Santoro A, Bonadonna G, Valagussa P, et al: Long-term results of combined chemotherapy-radiotherapy approach in Hodgkin's disease: Superiority of ABVD plus radiotherapy versus MOPP plus radiotherapy. J Clin Oncol 1987;5(1):27–37.

107. Santoro A, Bonadonna G, Bonfante V, Valagussa P: Alternating drug combinations in the treatment of advanced Hodgkin's disease. N Engl J Med 1982;306:770–775.

108. Klimo P, Connors JM: MOPP/ABV hybrid program: Combination chemotherapy based on early introduction of seven effective drugs for advanced Hodgkin's disease. J Clin Oncol 1985;3(9):1174–1182.

109. Connors JM: Is cyclic chemotherapy better than standard four-drug chemotherapy for Hodgkin's disease? Yes. Important Adv Oncol 1993:189–195.

110. Bonadonna G, Valagussa P, Santoro A: Alternating non-cross-resistant combination chemotherapy or MOPP in stage IV

111. Glick JH, Tsiatis A: MOPP/ABVD chemotherapy for advanced Hodgkin's disease. Ann Intern Med 1986;104(6):876–878.

112. Longo DL, Duffey PL, DeVita VT Jr, et al: Treatment of advanced-stage Hodgkin's disease: Alternating noncrossresistant MOPP/CABS is not superior to MOPP. J Clin Oncol 1991;9(8):1409–1420.

113. Hancock BW, Vaughan Hudson G, Vaughan Hudson B, et al: LOPP alternating with EVAP is superior to LOPP alone in the initial treatment of advanced Hodgkin's disease: Results of a British National Lymphoma Investigation trial. J Clin Oncol 1992;10(8):1252–1258.

114. Somers R, Carde P, Henry-Amar M, et al: A randomized study in stage IIIB and IV Hodgkin's disease comparing eight courses of MOPP versus an alteration of MOPP with ABVD: A European Organization for Research and Treatment of Cancer Lymphoma Cooperative Group and Groupe Pierre-et-Marie-Curie controlled clinical trial. J Clin Oncol 1994;12(2):279–287.

115. Glick JH, Young ML, Harrington D, et al: MOPP/ABV hybrid chemotherapy for advanced Hodgkin's disease significantly improves failure-free and overall survival: The 8-year results of the intergroup trial. J Clin Oncol 1998;16:19–26.

116. Radford JA, Crowther D, Rohatiner AZ, et al: Results of a randomized trial comparing MVPP chemotherapy with a hybrid regimen, ChlVPP/EVA, in the initial treatment of Hodgkin's disease. J Clin Oncol 1995;13(9):2379–2385.

117. Santoro A, Bonfante V, Bonadonna G: Salvage chemotherapy with ABVD in MOPP-resistant Hodgkin's disease. Ann Intern Med 1982;96(2):139–143.

118. Santoro A, Viviani S, Villarreal CJ, et al: Salvage chemotherapy in Hodgkin's disease irradiation failures: Superiority of doxorubicin-containing regimens over MOPP. Cancer Treat Rep 1986;70(3):343–348.

119. Loeffler M, Brosteanu O, Hasenclever D, et al: Meta-analysis of chemotherapy versus combined modality treatment trials in Hodgkin's disease. International Database on Hodgkin's Disease Overview Study Group. J Clin Oncol 1998;16(3):818–829.

120. Raemaekers JMM, Aleman BMP, Henry-Amar M, Pinna A, Mandard AM: Involved field irradiation (IFRT) vs no further treatment in patients with stage III/IV Hodgkin's lymphoma in complete remission after MOPP/ABV: First results of the randomized EORTC trial # 20884 [abstract]. Leuk Lymphoma 2001;42(Suppl 2):14.

121. Diehl V, Loeffler M, Pfreundschuh M, et al: Further chemotherapy versus low-dose involved-field radiotherapy as consolidation of complete remission after six cycles of alternating chemotherapy in patients with advance Hodgkin's disease. German Hodgkins' Study Group (GHSG). Ann Oncol 1995;6(9):901–910.

122. Ferme C, Sebban C, Hennequin C, et al: Comparison of chemotherapy to radiotherapy as consolidation of complete or good partial response after six cycles of chemotherapy for patients with advanced Hodgkin's disease: Results of the groupe d'etudes des lymphomes de l'Adulte H89 trial. Blood 2000;95(7):2246–2252.

123. Weihrauch MR, Re D, Scheidhauer K, et al: Thoracic positron emission tomography using 18F-fluorodeoxyglucose for the evaluation of residual mediastinal Hodgkin disease. Blood 2001;98(10):2930–2934.

124. Bartlett NL, Rosenberg SA, Hoppe RT, Hancock SL, Horning SJ: Brief chemotherapy, Stanford V, and adjuvant radiotherapy for bulky or advanced-stage Hodgkin's disease: A preliminary report. J Clin Oncol 1995;13(5):1080–1088.

125. Horning SJ, Rosenberg SA, Hoppe RT: Brief chemotherapy (Stanford V) and adjuvant radiotherapy for bulky or advanced Hodgkin's disease: An update. Ann Oncol 1996;7(Suppl 4):105–108.

126. Horning SJ, Williams J, Bartlett NL, et al: Assessment of the Stanford V regimen and consolidative radiotherapy for bulky and advanced Hodgkin's disease: Eastern Cooperative Oncology Group pilot study E1492. J Clin Oncol 2000;18(5):972–980.

127. Horning SJ, Hoppe RT, Breslin S, Bartlett NL, Brown BW, Rosenberg SA: Stanford V and radiotherapy for locally extensive and advanced Hodgkin's disease: Mature results of a prospective clinical trial. J Clin Oncol 2002;20(3):630–637.

Hodgkin's disease. A report of 8-year results. Ann Intern Med 1986;104(6):739–746.

128. Chisesi T, Federico M, Levis A, et al: ABVD versus stanford V versus MEC in unfavourable Hodgkin's lymphoma: Results of a randomised trial. Ann Oncol 2002;13(Suppl 1):102–106.

129. Federico M: A randomized trial of high-dose therapy and autologous stem cell transplantation vs conventional therapy for patients with advanced Hodgkin's lymphoma responding to four courses of ABVD or ABVD-like regimens [abstract]. Leuk Lymphoma 2001;42(Suppl 2):16.

130. Proctor SJ, Mackie M, Dawson A, et al: A population-based study of intensive multi-agent chemotherapy with or without autotransplant for the highest risk Hodgkin's disease patients identified by the Scotland and Newcastle Lymphoma Group (SNLG) prognostic index. A Scotland and Newcastle Lymphoma Group study (SNLG HD III). Eur J Cancer 2002;38(6):795–806.

131. Valagussa P, Santoro A, Fossati-Bellani F, Banfi A, Bonadonna G: Second acute leukemia and other malignancies following treatment for Hodgkin's disease. J Clin Oncol 1986;4(6):830–837.

132. Valagussa P, Bonadonna G: Hodgkin's disease and the risk of acute leukemia in successfully treated patients. Haematologica 1998;83(9):769–770.

133. Aviles A, Neri N, Cuadra I, Alvarado I, Cleto S: Second lethal events associated with treatment for Hodgkin's disease: A review of 2980 patients treated in a single Mexican institute. Leuk Lymphoma 2000;39(3–4):311–319.

134. Biti G, Cellai E, Magrini SM, Papi MG, Ponticelli P, Boddi V: Second solid tumors and leukemia after treatment for Hodgkin's disease: An analysis of 1121 patients from a single institution. Int J Radiat Oncol Biol Phys 1994;29(1):25–31.

135. Cosset JM, Henry-Amar M, Meerwaldt JH: Long-term toxicity of early stages of Hodgkin's disease therapy: The EORTC experience. EORTC Lymphoma Cooperative Group. Ann Oncol 1991;2(Suppl 2):77–82.

136. Dores GM, Metayer C, Curtis RE, et al: Second malignant neoplasms among long-term survivors of Hodgkin's disease: A population-based evaluation over 25 years. J Clin Oncol 2002;20(16):3484–3494.

137. Henry-Amar M, Hayat M, Meerwaldt JH, et al: Causes of death after therapy for early stage Hodgkin's disease entered on EORTC protocols. EORTC Lymphoma Cooperative Group. Int J Radiat Oncol Biol Phys 1990;19(5):1155–1157.

138. Henry-Amar M: Second cancer after the treatment for Hodgkin's disease: A report from the International Database on Hodgkin's Disease. Ann Oncol 1992;3(Suppl 4):117–128.

139. Mauch PM, Kalish LA, Marcus KC, et al: Long term survival in Hodgkin's disease: Relative impact of mortality, second tumors, infection, and cardiovascular disease. Canc J Sci Amer 1995;1(1):33–42.

140. Mauch PM, Kalish LA, Marcus KC, et al: Second malignancies after treatment for laparotomy staged IA-IIIB Hodgkin's disease: Long-term analysis of risk factors and outcome. Blood 1996;87(9):3625–3632.

141. Ng AK, Bernardo MP, Weller E, et al: Long-term survival and competing causes of death in patients with early-stage Hodgkin's disease treated at age 50 or younger. J Clin Oncol 2002;20(8):2101–2108.

142. Ng AK, Bernardo MV, Weller E, et al: Second malignancy after Hodgkin disease treated with radiation therapy with or without chemotherapy: Long-term risks and risk factors. Blood 2002;100(6):1989–1996.

143. Salloum E, Doria R, Schubert W, et al: Second solid tumors in patients with Hodgkin's disease cured after radiation or chemotherapy plus adjuvant low-dose radiation. J Clin Oncol 1996;14(9):2435–2443.

144. Swerdlow AJ, Douglas AJ, Hudson GV, Hudson BV, Bennett MH, MacLennan KA: Risk of second primary cancers after Hodgkin's disease by type of treatment: Analysis of 2846 patients in the British National Lymphoma Investigation. BMJ 1992;304(6835):1137–1143.

145. Tucker MA, Coleman CN, Cox RS, Varghese A, Rosenberg SA: Risk of second cancers after treatment for Hodgkin's disease. N Engl J Med 1988;318(2):76–81.

146. van Leeuwen FE, Swerdlow AJ, Valagussa P, Tucker MA: Second cancers after treatment of Hodgkin's disease. In Mauch PM,

Armitage JO, Diehl V, Hoppe R, Weiss LM (eds): Hodgkin's Disease. Philadelphia, Lippincott Williams & Wilkins, 1999, pp 607–632.

147. Ferme C, Mounier N, Divine M, et al: Intensive salvage therapy with high-dose chemotherapy for patients with advanced Hodgkin's disease in relapse or failure after initial chemotherapy: Results of the Groupe d'Etudes des Lymphomes de l'Adulte H89 trial. J Clin Oncol 2002;20(2):467–475.

148. Sweetenham JW, Carella AM, Taghipour G, et al: High-dose therapy and autologous stem-cell transplantation for adult patients with Hodgkin's disease who do not enter remission after induction chemotherapy: Results in 175 patients reported to the European Group for Blood and Marrow Transplantation. Lymphoma Working Party. J Clin Oncol 1999;17(10):3101–3109.

149. Lazarus HM, Rowlings PA, Zhang MJ, et al: Autotransplants for Hodgkin's disease in patients never achieving remission: A report from the Autologous Blood and Marrow Transplant Registry. J Clin Oncol 1999;17(2):534–545.

150. Andre M, Henry-Amar M, Pico J-L, et al: Comparison of high-dose therapy and autologous stem-cell transplantation with conventional therapy for Hodgkin's disease induction failure: A case-control study. J Clin Oncol 1999;17:222–229.

151. Josting A, Katay I, Rueffer U, et al: Favorable outcome of patients with relapsed or refractory Hodgkin's disease treated with high-dose chemotherapy and stem cell rescue at the time of maximal response to conventional salvage therapy (Dex-BEAM). Ann Oncol 1998;9(3):289–295.

152. Yuen AR, Rosenberg SA, Hoppe RT, Halpern JD, Horning SJ: Comparison between conventional salvage therapy and high-dose therapy with autografting for recurrent or refractory Hodgkin's disease. Blood 1997;89(3):814–822.

153. Sweetenham JW, Taghipour G, Milligan D, et al: High-dose therapy and autologous stem cell rescue for patients with Hodgkin's disease in first relapse after chemotherapy: Results from the EBMT. Lymphoma Working Party of the European Group for Blood and Marrow Transplantation. Bone Marrow Transplant 1997;20(9):745–752.

154. Horning SJ, Chao NJ, Negrin RS, et al: High-dose therapy and autologous hematopoietic progenitor cell transplantation for recurrent or refractory Hodgkin's disease: Analysis of the Stanford University results and prognostic indices. Blood 1997;89(3):801–813.

155. Sweetenham JW, Taghipour G, Linch DC, Goldstone AH: Thirty percent of adult patients with primary refractory Hodgkin's disease are progression free at 5 years after high dose therapy and autologous stem cell transplantation: Data from 290 patients reported to the EBMT [abstract]. Blood 1996;88:486a.

156. Reece DE, Phillips GL: Intensive therapy and autologous stem cell transplantation for Hodgkin's disease in first relapse after combination chemotherapy. Leuk Lymphoma 1996;21(3–4):245–253.

157. Prince HM, Crump M, Imrie K, et al: Intensive therapy and autotransplant for patients with an incomplete response to front-line therapy for lymphoma. Ann Oncol 1996;7(10):1043–1049.

158. Carella AM, Prencipe E, Pungolino E, et al: Twelve years experience with high-dose therapy and autologous stem cell transplantation for high-risk Hodgkin's disease patients in first remission after MOPP/ABVD chemotherapy. Leuk Lymphoma 1996;21(1–2):63–70.

159. Bierman PJ, Anderson JR, Freeman MB, et al: High-dose chemotherapy followed by autologous hematopoietic rescue for Hodgkin's disease patients following first relapse after chemotherapy. Ann Oncol 1996;7(2):151–156.

160. Nademanee A, O'Donnell MR, Snyder DS, et al: High-dose chemotherapy with or without total body irradiation followed by autologous bone marrow and/or peripheral blood stem cell transplantation for patients with relapsed and refractory Hodgkin's disease: Results in 85 patients with analysis of prognostic factors. Blood 1995;85(5):1381–1390.

161. Reece DE, Connors JM, Spinelli JJ, et al: Intensive therapy with cyclophosphamide, carmustine, etoposide +/- cisplatin, and autologous bone marrow transplantation for Hodgkin's disease in first relapse after combination chemotherapy. Blood 1994;83(5):1193–1199.

162. Pfreundschuh MG, Rueffer U, Lathan B, et al: Dexa-BEAM in patients with Hodgkin's disease refractory to multidrug chemotherapy regimens: A trial of the German Hodgkin's Disease Study Group. J Clin Oncol 1994;12(3):580–586.

163. Crump M, Smith AM, Brandwein J, et al: High-dose etoposide and melphalan, and autologous bone marrow transplantation for patients with advanced Hodgkin's disease: Importance of disease status at transplant. J Clin Oncol 1993;11(4):704–711.

164. Chopra R, McMillan AK, Linch DC, et al: The place of high-dose BEAM therapy and autologous bone marrow transplantation in poor-risk Hodgkin's disease. A single-center eight-year study of 155 patients. Blood 1993;81(5):1137–1145.

165. Bierman PJ, Bagin RG, Jagannath S, et al: High dose chemotherapy followed by autologous hematopoietic rescue in Hodgkin's disease: Long-term follow-up in 128 patients. Ann Oncol 1993; 4(9):767–773.

166. Tourani JM, Levy R, Colonna P, et al: High-dose salvage chemotherapy without bone marrow transplantation for adult patients with refractory Hodgkin's disease. J Clin Oncol 1992;10(7):1086–1094.

167. Kessinger A, Bierman PJ, Vose JM, Armitage JO: High-dose cyclophosphamide, carmustine, and etoposide followed by autologous peripheral stem cell transplantation for patients with relapsed Hodgkin's disease. Blood 1991;77(11):2322–2325.

168. Longo DL, Duffey PL, Young RC, et al: Conventional-dose salvage combination chemotherapy in patients relapsing with Hodgkin's disease after combination chemotherapy: The low probability for cure. J Clin Oncol 1992;10(2):210–218.

169. Buzaid AC, Lippman SM, Miller TP: Salvage therapy of advanced Hodgkin's disease. Critical appraisal of curative potential. Am J Med 1987;83(3):523–532.

170. Bonfante V, Santoro A, Viviani S, et al: Outcome of patients with Hodgkin's disease failing after primary MOPP-ABVD. J Clin Oncol 1997;15(2):528–534.

171. Brada M, Eeles R, Ashley S, Nichols J, Horwich A: Salvage radiotherapy in recurrent Hodgkin's disease. Ann Oncol 1992;3(2):131–135.

172. Diehl LF, Perry DJ, Terebelo H, et al: Radiation as salvage therapy for patients with Hodgkin's disease relapsing after MOPP (mechlorethamine, vincristine, prednisone, and procarbazine) chemotherapy. Cancer Treat Rep 1983;67(9):827–829.

173. Fox KA, Lippman SM, Cassady JR, Heusinkveld RS, Miller TP: Radiation therapy salvage of Hodgkin's disease following chemotherapy failure. J Clin Oncol 1987;5(1):38–45.

174. Leigh BR, Fox KA, Mack CF, Baier M, Miller TP, Cassady JR: Radiation therapy salvage of Hodgkin's disease following chemotherapy failure. Int J Radiat Oncol Biol Phys 1993;27(4):855–862.

175. MacMillan CH, Bessell EM: The effectiveness of radiotherapy for localized relapse in patients with Hodgkin's disease (IIB-IVB) who obtained a complete response with chemotherapy alone as initial treatment. Clin Oncol (R Coll Radiol) 1994;6(3):147–150.

176. Mauch P, Tarbell N, Skarin A, Rosenthal D, Weinstein H: Wide-field radiation therapy alone or with chemotherapy for Hodgkin's disease in relapse from combination chemotherapy. J Clin Oncol 1987;5(4):544–549.

177. Pezner RD, Lipsett JA, Vora N, Forman SJ: Radical radiotherapy as salvage treatment for relapse of Hodgkin's disease initially treated by chemotherapy alone: Prognostic significance of the disease-free interval. Int J Radiat Oncol Biol Phys 1994;30(4):965–970.

178. Roach MD, Kapp DS, Rosenberg SA, Hoppe RT: Radiotherapy with curative intent: an option in selected patients relapsing after chemotherapy for advanced Hodgkin's disease. J Clin Oncol 1987;5(4):550–555.

179. Uematsu M, Tarbell NJ, Silver B, et al: Wide-field radiation therapy with or without chemotherapy for patients with Hodgkin disease in relapse after initial combination chemotherapy. Cancer 1993;72(1):207–212.

180. Wirth A, Corry J, Laidlaw C, Matthews J, Liew KH: Salvage radiotherapy for Hodgkin's disease following chemotherapy failure. Int J Radiat Oncol Biol Phys 1997;39(3):599–607.

181. Lohri A, Barnett M, Fairey RN, et al: Outcome of treatment of first relapse of Hodgkin's disease after primary chemotherapy: Identification of risk factors from the British Columbia experience 1970 to 1988. Blood 1991;77(10):2292–2298.

182. Korbling M, Holle R, Haas R, et al: Autologous blood stem-cell transplantation in patients with advanced Hodgkin's disease and prior radiation to the pelvic site. J Clin Oncol 1990;8(6):978–985.

183. Schmitz N, Linch DC, Dreger P, et al: Randomised trial of filgrastim-mobilised peripheral blood progenitor cell transplantation versus autologous bone-marrow transplantation in lymphoma patients. Lancet 1996;347(8998):353–357.

184. Smith TJ, Hillner BE, Schmitz N, et al: Economic analysis of a randomized clinical trial to compare filgrastim-mobilized peripheral-blood progenitor-cell transplantation and autologous bone marrow transplantation in patients with Hodgkin's and non-Hodgkin's lymphoma. J Clin Oncol 1997;15(1):5–10.

185. Wheeler C, Antin JH, Churchill WH, et al: Cyclophosphamide, carmustine, and etoposide with autologous bone marrow transplantation in refractory Hodgkin's disease and non-Hodgkin's lymphoma: A dose-finding study. J Clin Oncol 1990;8(4):648–656.

186. Crilley P, Lazarus H, Topolsky D, et al: Comparison of preparative transplantation regimens using carmustine/etoposide/cisplatin or busulfan/etoposide/cyclophosphamide in lymphoid malignancies. Semin Oncol 1993;20(4 Suppl 4):50–44.

187. Reece DE, Barnett MJ, Shepherd JD, et al: High-dose cyclophosphamide, carmustine (BCNU), and etoposide (VP16-213) with or without cisplatin (CBV +/- P) and autologous transplantation for patients with Hodgkin's disease who fail to enter a complete remission after combination chemotherapy. Blood 1995;86(2):451–456.

188. Reece DE, Nevill TJ, Sayegh A, et al: Regimen-related toxicity and non-relapse mortality with high-dose cyclophosphamide, carmustine (BCNU) and etoposide (VP16-213) (CBV) and CBV plus cisplatin (CBVP) followed by autologous stem cell transplantation in patients with Hodgkin's disease. Bone Marrow Transplant 1999;23(11):1131–1138.

189. Chopra R, Linch DC, McMillan AK, et al: Mini-BEAM followed by BEAM and ABMT for very poor risk Hodgkin's disease. Br J Haematol 1992;81(2):197–202.

190. Anderson JE, Litzow MR, Appelbaum FR, et al: Allogeneic, syngeneic, and autologous marrow transplantation for Hodgkin's disease: The 21-year Seattle experience. J Clin Oncol 1993;11(12):2342–2350.

191. Milpied N, Fielding AK, Pearce RM, Ernst P, Goldstone AH: Allogeneic bone marrow transplant is not better than autologous transplant for patients with relapsed Hodgkin's disease. European Group for Blood and Bone Marrow Transplantation. J Clin Oncol 1996;14(4):1291–1296.

192. Phillips GL, Reece DE, Barnett MJ, et al: Allogeneic marrow transplantation for refractory Hodgkin's disease. J Clin Oncol 1989;7(8):1039–1045.

193. Sureda A, Schmitz N: Role of allogeneic stem cell transplantation in relapsed or refractory Hodgkin's disease. Ann Oncol 2002;13(Suppl 1):128–132.

194. Gajewski JL, Phillips GL, Sobocinski KA, et al: Bone marrow transplants from HLA-identical siblings in advanced Hodgkin's disease. J Clin Oncol 1996;14(2):572–578.

195. Connors JM: Induction of secondary neoplasms by the treatment of malignant disease: Lessons from Hodgkin's disease. Prog Clin Biol Res 1990;354B:219–226.

196. Zucca E, Pinotti G, Roggero E, et al: High incidence of other neoplasms in patients with low-grade gastric MALT lymphoma. Ann Oncol 1995;6(7):726–728.

197. Bhatia S, Robison LL, Oberlin O, et al: Breast cancer and other second neoplasms after childhood Hodgkin's disease. N Engl J Med 1996;334(12):745–751.

198. Au WY, Gascoyne RD, Le N, et al: Incidence of second neoplasms in patients with MALT lymphoma: No increase in risk above the background population. Ann Oncol 1999;10(3):317–321.

199. Nichols CR, Breeden ES, Loehrer PJ, Williams SD, Einhorn LH: Secondary leukemia associated with a conventional dose of etoposide: Review of serial germ cell tumor protocols. J Natl Cancer Inst 1993;85(1):36–40.

200. Bokemeyer C, Schmoll HJ, Kuczyk MA, Beyer J, Siegert W: Risk of secondary leukemia following high cumulative doses of etoposide during chemotherapy for testicular cancer. J Natl Cancer Inst 1995;87(1):58–60.

201. Katato K, Flaherty L, Varterasian M: Secondary acute myelogenous leukemia following treatment with oral etoposide. Am J Hematol 1996;53(1):54-55.

202. Harris NL, Jaffe ES, Stein H, et al: A revised European-American classification of lymphoid neoplasms: A proposal from the International Lymphoma Study Group. Blood 1994;84(5):1361-1392.

203. Poppema S, Kaiserling E, Lennert K: Hodgkin's disease with lymphocytic predominance, nodular type (nodular paragranuloma) and progressively transformed germinal centres—A cytohistological study. Histopathology 1979;3(4):295-308.

204. Diehl V, Sextro M, Franklin J, et al: Clinical presentation, course, and prognostic factors in lymphocyte predominant Hodgkin's disease and lymphocyte-rich classical Hodgkin's disease: Report from the European Task Force on Lymphoma Project on Lymphocyte-Predominant Hodgkin's Disease. J Clin Oncol 1999;17(3):776-783.

205. Regula DP Jr, Hoppe RT, Weiss LM: Nodular and diffuse types of lymphocyte predominance Hodgkin's disease. N Engl J Med 1988;318(4):214-219.

206. Borg-Grech A, Radford JA, Crowther D, Swindell R, Harris M: A comparative study of the nodular and diffuse variants of lymphocyte predominant Hodgkin's disease. J Clin Oncol 1989;7(9):1303-1309.

207. Crennan E, D'Costa I, Liew KH, et al: Lymphocyte predominant Hodgkin's disease: A clinicopathologic comparative study of histologic and immunophenotypic subtypes. Int J Radiat Oncol Biol Phys 1995;31(2):333-337.

208. Pappa VI, Norton AJ, Gupta RK, Wilson AM, Rohatiner AZ, Lister TA: Nodular type of lymphocyte predominant Hodgkin's disease. A clinical study of 50 cases. Ann Oncol 1995;6(6):559-565.

209. Bodis S, Kraus MD, Pinkus G, et al: Clinical presentation and outcome in lymphocyte predominant Hodgkin's disease. J Clin Oncol 1997;15(9):3060-3066.

210. Anagnostopoulos I, Hansmann ML, Franssila K, et al: European Task Force on Lymphoma project on lymphocyte predominance Hodgkin disease: Histologic and immunohistologic analysis of submitted cases reveals 2 types of Hodgkin disease with a nodular growth pattern and abundant lymphocytes. Blood 2000;96(5):1889-1899.

211. Burns BF, Colby TV, Dorfman RF: Differential diagnostic features of nodular L & H Hodgkin's disease, including progressive transformation of germinal centers. Am J Surg Pathol 1984;8(4):253-261.

212. Osborne BM, Butler JJ: Clinical implications of progressive transformation of germinal centers. Am J Surg Pathol 1984;8(10):725-733.

213. Diehl V, Franklin J, Sextro M, Mauch PM: Clinical presentation and treatment of lymphocyte predominance Hodgkin's disease. In Armitage JO, Diehl V, Hoppe RT, Weiss LM (eds): Hodgkin's Disease. Philadelphia, Lippincott Williams & Wilkins, 1999, p 577.

214. Anselmo AP, Cavalieri E, Enrici RM, et al: Hodgkin's disease during pregnancy: Diagnostic and therapeutic management. Fetal Diagn Ther 1999;14(2):102-105.

215. Byram D, Foulstone P: Radiotherapy for Hodgkin's disease in pregnancy. Australas Radiol 1997;41(4):407-408.

216. Franceschi S, Bidoli E, La Vecchia C: Pregnancy and Hodgkin's disease. Int J Cancer 1994;58(3):465-466.

217. Gobbi PG, Attardo-Parrinello A, Danesino M, et al: Hodgkin's disease and pregnancy. Haematologica 1984;69(3):336-341.

218. Leung JT, Kuan R, Patel V: Radiotherapy for Hodgkin's disease in pregnancy. Australas Radiol 1996;40(2):146-148.

219. Lishner M, Zemlickis D, Degendorfer P, Panzarella T, Sutcliffe SB, Koren G: Maternal and foetal outcome following Hodgkin's disease in pregnancy. Br J Cancer 1992;65(1):114-117.

220. McCann SR, Daly H, Hanratty TD, Temperley IJ: Hodgkin's disease and pregnancy. Acta Haematol 1981;66(1):67-68.

221. Nisce LZ, Tome MA, He S, Lee BJ III, Kutcher GJ: Management of coexisting Hodgkin's disease and pregnancy. Am J Clin Oncol 1986;9(2):146-151.

222. Tawil E, Mercier JP, Dandavino A: Hodgkin's disease complicating pregnancy. J Can Assoc Radiol 1985;36(2):133-137.

223. Rapezzi D, Ugolini D, Ferraris AM, Racchi O, Gaetani GF: Histological subtypes of Hodgkin's disease in the setting of HIV infection. Ann Hematol 2001;80(6):340-344.

224. Tirelli U, Errante D, Dolcetti R, et al: Hodgkin's disease and human immunodeficiency virus infection: Clinicopathologic and virologic features of 114 patients from the Italian Cooperative Group on AIDS and Tumors. J Clin Oncol 1995;13(7):1758-1767.

225. Dolcetti R, Boiocchi M, Gloghini A, Carbone A: Pathogenetic and histogenetic features of HIV-associated Hodgkin's disease. Eur J Cancer 2001;37(10):1276-1287.

226. Powles T, Bower M: HIV-associated Hodgkin's disease. Int J STD AIDS 2000;11(8):492-494.

227. Levine AM, Li P, Cheung T, et al: Chemotherapy consisting of doxorubicin, bleomycin, vinblastine, and dacarbazine with granulocyte-colony-stimulating factor in HIV-infected patients with newly diagnosed Hodgkin's disease: A prospective, multi-institutional AIDS clinical trials group study (ACTG 149). J Acquir Immune Defic Syndr 2000;24(5):444-450.

228. Karcher DS: Clinically unsuspected Hodgkin disease presenting initially in the bone marrow of patients infected with the human immunodeficiency virus. Cancer 1993;71(4):1235-1238.

229. Errante D, Gabarre J, Ridolfo AL, et al: Hodgkin's disease in 35 patients with HIV infection: An experience with epirubicin, bleomycin, vinblastine and prednisone chemotherapy in combination with antiretroviral therapy and primary use of G-CSF. Ann Oncol 1999;10(2):189-195.

230. Vilchez RA, Finch CJ, Jorgensen JL, Butel JS: The clinical epidemiology of Hodgkin lymphoma in HIV-infected patients in the highly active antiretroviral therapy (HAART) era. Medicine (Baltimore) 2003;82(2):77-81.

231. Cimino G, Biti GP, Anselmo AP, et al: MOPP chemotherapy versus extended-field radiotherapy in the management of pathological stages I-IIA Hodgkin's disease. J Clin Oncol 1989;7(6):732-737.

232. Longo DL, Glatstein E, Duffey PL, et al: Radiation therapy versus combination chemotherapy in the treatment of early-stage Hodgkin's disease: Seven-year results of a prospective randomized trial. J Clin Oncol 1991;9(6):906-917.

233. Chau I, Harries M, Cunningham D, et al: Gemcitabine, cisplatin and methylprednisolone chemotherapy (GEM-P) is an effective regimen in patients with poor prognostic primary progressive or multiply relapsed Hodgkin's and non-Hodgkin's lymphoma. Br J Haematol 2003;120(6):970-977.

234. Zinzani PL, Bendandi M, Stefoni V, et al: Value of gemcitabine treatment in heavily pretreated Hodgkin's disease patients. Haematologica 2000;85(9):926-929.

235. Tesch H, Santoro A, Fiedler F, et al: Phase II study of gemcitabine in pretreated Hodgkin's disease results of a multicenter study [abstract 1514]. Blood 1997; 339a.

236. Sezer O, Eucker J, Jakob C, Kaufmann O, Schmid P, Possinger K: Achievement of complete remission in refractory Hodgkin's disease with prolonged infusion of gemcitabine. Invest New Drugs 2001;19(1):101-104.

237. Santoro A, Bredenfeld H, Devizzi L, et al: Gemcitabine in the treatment of refractory Hodgkin's disease: Results of a multicenter phase II study. J Clin Oncol 2000;18(13):2615-2619.

238. Crump M, Baetz T, Belch A, et al: Gemcitabine, dexamethasone, cisplatin (GDP) salvage chemotherapy for relapsed or refractory Hodgkin's disease (HD): A National Cancer Institute of Canada Clinical Trials Group study [abstract]. Blood 2002;100:570a.

239. Ekstrand BC, Lucas JB, Horwitz SM, et al: Rituximab in lymphocyte predominant Hodgkin's disease: Results of a phase II trial. Blood 2003;13:13.

240. Boulanger E, Meignin V, Leverger G, Solal-Celigny P: Rituximab monotherapy in nodular lymphocyte-predominant Hodgkin's disease. Ann Oncol 2003;14(1):171.

241. Lucas JB, Hoppe RT, Horwitz SM, Breslin S, Horning SJ: Rituximab is active in lymphocyte predominance Hodgkin's disease. Blood 2000;96:831a.

242. Keilholz U, Szelenyi H, Siehl J, Foss HD, Knauf W, Thiel E: Rapid regression of chemotherapy refractory lymphocyte predominant Hodgkin's disease after administration of rituximab (anti CD 20 mono-clonal antibody) and interleukin-2. Leuk Lymphoma 1999;35(5-6):641-642.

243. Rehwald U, Schulz H, Reiser M, et al: Treatment of relapsed CD20+

Hodgkin lymphoma with the monoclonal antibody rituximab is effective and well tolerated: Results of a phase 2 trial of the German Hodgkin Lymphoma Study Group. Blood 2003;101(2): 420–424.

244. Schnell R, Borchmann P, Schulz H, Engert A: Current strategies of antibody-based treatment in Hodgkin's disease. Ann Oncol 2002;13(Suppl 1):57–66.

245. Engert A, Diehl V, Schnell R, et al: A phase-I study of an anti-CD25 ricin A-chain immunotoxin (RFT5-SMPT- dgA) in patients with refractory Hodgkin's lymphoma. Blood 1997;89(2):403–410.

246. Schnell R, Staak O, Borchmann P, et al: A phase I study with an anti-CD30 ricin A-chain immunotoxin (Ki-4.dgA) in patients with refractory CD30+ Hodgkin's and non-Hodgkin's lymphoma. Clin Cancer Res 2002;8(6):1779–1786.

247. Schnell R, Vitetta E, Schindler J, et al: Treatment of refractory Hodgkin's lymphoma patients with an anti-CD25 ricin A-chain immunotoxin. Leukemia 2000;14(1):129–135.

248. Schnell R, Vitetta E, Schindler J, et al: Clinical trials with an anti-CD25 ricin A-chain experimental and immunotoxin (RFT5-SMPT-dgA) in Hodgkin's lymphoma. Leuk Lymphoma 1998;30(5–6):525–537.

249. Majolino I, Pearce R, Taghipour G, Goldstone AH: Peripheral-blood stem-cell transplantation versus autologous bone marrow transplantation in Hodgkin's and non-Hodgkin's lymphomas: A new matched-pair analysis of the European Group for Blood and Marrow Transplantation Registry Data. Lymphoma Working Party of the European Group for Blood and Marrow Transplantation. J Clin Oncol 1997;15(2):509–517.

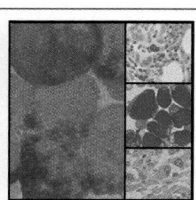

12 NON-HODGKIN'S LYMPHOMA

T. Andrew Lister

Bertrand Coiffier

James O. Armitage

SUMMARY OF KEY POINTS

INCIDENCE

- More than 56,000 cases occur each year in the United States (about 20 per 100,000 population). The WHO classification should be used for diagnosis. The most frequent subtypes are diffuse large B-cell (about one third of all lymphomas worldwide) and follicular lymphoma (about 30% of lymphomas in the United States, but there is considerable variability from country to country).
- The frequency of histologic subtypes with a poor prognosis is increasing.

ETIOLOGY AND BIOLOGY

- Association with specific infectious organisms is increasingly recognized. These include gastric mucosa-associated lymphoid tissue (MALT) lymphoma with *Helicobacter pylori*, post-transplant and CNS diffuse large B-cell lymphoma with EBV, Burkitt's lymphoma with EBV, adult T-cell lymphoma/leukemia with HTLV-1, aggressive B-cell lymphoma with HIV, and pleural effusion lymphoma with HHV-8.
- In the United States approximately 90% of lymphoma are of B-cell origin and 10% of T-cell origin.
- Certain genetic abnormalities are associated with specific lymphomas including: t(14;18) and bcl-2 with follicular lymphoma; t(8;14), t(2;8), t(8;22), and c-myc with Burkitt's lymphoma; t(11;14) and bcl-1 with mantle cell lymphoma; t(2;5) and ALK with an anaplastic T/null cell lymphoma; bcl-6 with diffuse large B-cell lymphoma; and t(11;18) and bcl-10 with MALT lymphoma.

DIFFERENTIAL DIAGNOSIS

- Any particular lymphoma can present as a solid tumor or as a leukemia. Those with the highest frequency of leukemic presentation are small lymphocytic/CLL, lymphoblastic, Burkitt's, splenic marginal zone, adult T-cell lymphoma/leukemia, cutaneous t-cell lymphoma and mantle cell.
- Distinguishing lymphoma from other lymph node pathology is usually straightforward.
- Follicular lymphoma is most likely to be confused with reactive follicular hyperplasia.
- Other lymphomas might be confused with infectious mononucleosis, cat scratch disease, lymphomatoid papulosis, granulocytic sarcoma, malignant melanoma, Hodgkin's disease, and plasmacytosis.
- To avoid confusion, the initial diagnosis should be based on a generous excisional biopsy reviewed by an experienced hematopathologist with fresh frozen tissue available for further study.

STAGING EVALUATION

- Evaluation should always include complete history and physical examination, hemogram, and chemistry studies including lactate dehydrogenase (LDH) levels, imaging studies of chest, retroperitoneum, and pelvis, and bone marrow biopsy.
- Additional studies should be performed as appropriate (e.g., lumbar puncture in patients at high risk for central nervous system (CNS) involvement such as those with lymphoblastic, Burkitt's, or testicular, sinus, or epidural involvement by diffuse large B-cell lymphoma).

PRIMARY THERAPY

- This is determined by the overall state of the patient, the histologic subtype, the stage and distribution of disease; the International Prognostic Index is utilized in many instances.
- Cure is possible with moderately intensive therapy for a proportion of patients with diffuse large B-cell lymphoma or anaplastic large T-cell lymphoma, and a smaller proportion with peripheral T-cell lymphoma; more intensive therapy is curative for some with precursor B and T lymphoblastic lymphoma and Burkitt's lymphoma.
- Prolonged survival may be achieved for the majority of those with follicular lymphoma, small lymphocytic lymphoma, and lymphoplasmacytoid lymphoma, but the curability of these subtypes is debated.
- Lymphomas of mucosa-associated lymphoid tissue (MALT) have a very long survival and probably are often cured. In the case of gastric MALT lymphoma, antibiotic therapy alone can induce remission. Radiotherapy or surgery is the treatment of choice in others.
- Mantle cell lymphoma is a therapeutic conundrum although new treatment approaches seem to have an improved outcome.

SECONDARY AND TERTIARY THERAPY

- This is very often appropriate, if only as palliation.
- A strategy of reinducing remission followed by consolidation with high-dose therapy may be curative for a significant proportion of patients.
- Many options are available and work repeatedly with survival advantage, particularly for follicular lymphoma.

INTRODUCTION

Non-Hodgkin's lymphoma is the generic term for a diverse group of disorders sharing in common a malignant process of the lymphoid system not microscopically characterized by Reed-Sternberg cells and the cellular admixture seen in Hodgkin's disease. The most common presentation, like that of Hodgkin's disease, is painless lymphadenopathy. Unlike Hodgkin's disease, multiple sites are much more frequently overtly involved and extranodal lesions are common, sometimes being the sole site of disease. Progression is much less orderly than in Hodgkin's disease, implying that the mode of dissemination is different. Without effective intervention death is almost always a consequence of the disease. Treatment available at the beginning of the 21st century has a powerful effect on the natural history of the disease, resulting in cure for a (smaller than large) proportion of patients and prolongation of pleasant life for many more.

INCIDENCE, EPIDEMIOLOGY, ETIOLOGY, AND INTERRELATIONSHIPS

Increasing Incidence

The non-Hodgkin's lymphomas are uncommon but not rare, and all evidence points to them becoming more common more rapidly than most other malignancies.[1] The increase in incidence appears to be occurring in all parts of the world, despite wide variations in the data from different continents, ranging from approximately 2 per 100,000 per year in Asia to nearly 10 per 100,000 in the United Kingdom[2,3] and approximately 20 per 100,000 per year in the United States.[4]

All the data suggest that the increase is most marked in the elderly[5] and occurs predominantly in diffuse large B-cell lymphoma (DLBCL). The incidence has been rising at a rate of approximately 4% a year, representing a 150% increase between the 1940s and the 1980s. In absolute numbers, there were more than 56,000 new cases of non-Hodgkin's lymphomas in the United States and about 20,000 deaths.[6] The increase is only in part due to age.[6] In the younger age groups, though the incidence is still rising, mortality is either stable or falling because of improvements in therapy. The reasons for the increase are not clear, although a number of etiologic factors can be implicated (Table 112-1). Artifactual increase due to different data reporting methods, or to diagnostic changes from non-Hodgkin's lymphoma from Hodgkin's disease, or from previously presumed nonmalignant conditions such as angioimmunoblastic lymphadenopathy with dysproteinemia (AILD) has been discounted.

Relevance of the Immune System

Non-Hodgkin's lymphomas develop against a background of both immune suppression and immune stimulation; considerably more attention is paid to immune-suppressive conditions. Both primary and secondary immunodeficiency states predispose to a high incidence of the disease, with substantial evidence supporting a role for the Epstein-Barr virus (EBV).[7] Most of the data come from patients with a genetic immune deficiency, HIV-induced immunodeficiency, or heart or renal transplant, or allogeneic bone marrow recipients receiving azathioprine or cyclosporine.[7,8,828-839] Despite predictions of an AIDS-related lymphoma epidemic, the increase in incidence over the past 40 years can clearly *not* be attributed to increased immunosuppression, by whatever mechanism.

Less well publicized, but also relevant to etiology, is the incidence of lymphoma in circumstances of chronic immune stimulation. A correlation exists between lymphoma and both sicca syndrome and rheumatoid arthritis.[9,10] In both, the risk is higher when immunosuppressive therapy is used. Additionally, the highest frequency of lymphoma in renal transplant recipients is found in those receiving more than one transplant.[10] Another more recently recognized example of the role of chronic immune stimulation in the genesis of lymphoma is that of MALT lymphoma in the stomach developing against a background of *Helicobacter pylori* infection.[11,12] Important though this may be, it is not likely that immune stimulation is responsible for the increasing incidence of lymphoma. Provocative data suggests that a similar example of such a mechanism may be found in the association of *Borrelia* with cutaneous MALT (mucosa-associated lymphoid tissue) lymphoma.[13]

Viruses

There is compelling evidence that viruses are implicated in the etiology of lymphoma in animals. They exert their effect either by direct insertion into the genome, leading

---

TABLE 112-1

 Factors Associated with an Increased Incidence of non-Hodgkin's Lymphoma

Altered Immunologic States

AIDS
Organ transplantation
Sicca syndrome
Rheumatoid arthritis
Inherited immune deficiencies

Viruses/Bacteria

HTLV
HIV
Epstein-Barr virus
HHV-8
Hepatitis C virus
H. Pylori

Chemical Exposure

Agriculture chemicals
Hair-darkening dyes

Miscellaneous

Treated Hodgkin's disease

AIDS, acquired immunodeficiency syndrome; HHV, human herpes virus; HIV, human immunodeficiency virus; HTLV, human T-cell leukemia/lymphoma virus.

to alteration of host gene expression, or by inducing increased proliferation of the lymphoid system. The situation is far from clear in humans, although close associations exist between at least three viruses—EBV, human T-cell leukemia/lymphoma virus 1 (HTLV-1), human herpes virus 8 (HHV8)—and lymphoma. The evidence for a "causative" role for EBV in immunocompromised patients and those with Burkitt's lymphoma was based first on serologic data but subsequently on the demonstration that viral genome was incorporated into the host DNA.[14] Burkitt's lymphoma in temperate zones (sporadic) is only associated with EBV in 30% of cases, however, compared with 95% in Africa (endemic). Different subtypes of Burkitt's lymphoma exist at the molecular level (see "Cytogenetics and Molecular Genetics"), allowing the hypothesis that EBV is relevant to some subtypes but not to others.

HTLV-1,[15] which is much less common, almost certainly plays a causative role in the genesis of the adult T-cell leukemia/lymphoma (ATL) syndrome.[16,17] ATL is most frequently seen in the southern islands of Japan and the Caribbean; carriers of HTLV-1 have an estimated lifetime chance of developing the illness of about 5%.[18] In all cases, the malignant cells contain integrated provirus.

HHV8 has recently been found to be associated with body cavity–based lymphoma (BCBL),[19] a rare B-cell lymphoma that occurs predominantly in patients with AIDS.[20] The virus was originally described in the tumoral lesions of AIDS-associated Kaposi's sarcoma.[21] Provocative data have recently been published about a putative role for simian virus 40 (SV40) also.[22,23] These important observations carry the promise of contributing to our understanding of the pathogenesis of this group of diseases. They do not suggest, however, that any of these viruses contribute to the increased incidence of non-Hodgkin's lymphoma, since EBV has been ubiquitous for years and HTLV is uncommon in the countries in which lymphoma is increasing the fastest.

Recently, the association of hepatitis C virus and lymphoplasmacytic lymphoma has been proposed.[24]

Environmental Factors

A multitude of epidemiologic studies have been carried out to determine the potential role of occupational and environmental factors.[25] It has been shown that agricultural workers have a high incidence of the disease.[26,27] Some authors have attributed this to pesticide exposure,[27,28,29] although alternative explanations have been postulated such as increased exposure to potentially oncogenic viruses, or at least to chronic antigenic stimulation. The accumulated data about pesticides, while not all compelling, led to a review of the overall potential adverse effects of herbicides by the National Academy of Sciences. This concluded that "evidence is sufficient that there is a positive association between exposure to herbicides (2,4-D; 2,4,5-T and its contaminants TCDD, cacodylic, and picloram) and non-Hodgkin's lymphoma."[30] The potential wider significance of the risk may be reflected in the fact that the domestic use of pesticides for lawns is increasing by more than 5% per year.[31]

The data about hair dyes, first identified as a possible risk in 1975, remain provocative.[32] There are more negative than positive studies. Two positive studies[33,34] allow the conclusion that a small proportion of those who use permanent hair-darkening dyes may be at increased risk of lymphoma. Like the issue of herbicides and lawns, this might be assumed to be important in light of the substantial number of people, at least in the United States, who dye their hair.

Summary

A considerable number of factors have been implicated in the etiology of lymphoma, the most prominent being abnormalities of the immune system, either suppression or stimulation. Exposure to certain viruses, agricultural work, pesticide exposure, and the use of hair dyes have been implicated. None of these factors alone satisfactorily explains the increase in incidence of non-Hodgkin's lymphoma over the past 30 to 40 years, since none of them has been shown to be increasing. The relevance of inherited genetic factors is as yet unclear.[35]

MAKING THE DIAGNOSIS

The diagnosis of non-Hodgkin's lymphoma rests entirely on biopsy of a lymph node or an affected extranodal site. This should be performed by an experienced surgeon, at a time of day when full attention may be paid to the specimen in the laboratory. The choice of site to biopsy when more than one node is involved should depend on the clinical circumstances. Usually the largest or most rapidly enlarging node is chosen because it is thought most likely to reveal the most aggressive histology (thereby influencing therapy) and because it will provide the most tissue. Multiple node biopsies may on occasion be indicated. Biopsy of nodes within the mediastinum and abdomen requires special caution. Thoracotomy may be required but should never be performed without particular attention to the patency of the airways and recognition of the risks of extubation. While excision biopsy is to be preferred, Trucut needle biopsy under computed tomographic (CT) or ultrasonographic guidance in the hands of an experienced radiologist may sometimes provide enough tissue to avoid open surgery, either in the chest or the abdomen.[36] The pathologic diagnosis of lymphomas is difficult, and it is a mistake to handicap one's pathologist with inadequate tissue. Fine-needle aspiration, for cytology only, should be used only when biopsy is impossible or when confirmation of previously established lymphoma is required. It does not allow the morphologic distinction between different types of lymphoma and may be misleading.

By following the contributions of the experienced physician who suspected the diagnosis, the experienced surgeon or invasive radiologist who provided the biopsy specimen, and the experienced technician who processed it, the experienced hematopathologist will be able to make the correct diagnosis with relative ease most of the time. This will involve distinguishing malignant from nonmalignant, lymphoma from carcinoma, non-Hodgkin's lymphoma from Hodgkin's disease, and finally giving a specific name in the locally accepted terminology. The criteria upon which the precise diagnosis is made are outside the scope of this chapter but are excellently reviewed elsewhere.[37-39]

The preceding diagnostic factors are most applicable to the initial presentation of the patient. Evaluation of the pathology at the time of treatment failure (either recurrence or progression) will depend on the influence that the findings may have on therapeutic decisions and the research interests of the physician. Repeat biopsy may reveal the same or altered lymphoma pathology. It may reveal another diagnosis. It should be performed as circumstances dictate, but it is always wise to perform a repeat biopsy if the patient was rendered disease-free by initial therapy.

CLASSIFICATION

The nomenclature surrounding the lymphomas has evolved since Hodgkin's disease was first described,[40] reflecting progress in the understanding of the processes involved and the development of increasingly sophisticated laboratory techniques for investigating the lymphoid system at the cellular and molecular levels. It is worth remembering that histopathology was fairly rudimentary in the middle of the 19th century, placing very much more emphasis on the clinical presentation of diseases and the macroscopic appearance of affected organs. It is refreshing to note that now, despite our ability to distinguish different lymphomas at the level of different associated gene rearrangements, terminology used by physicians is returning to that of the clinicopathologic syndrome; this is reflected in the new World Health Organization (WHO) classification.[41] The more attention that is paid to the illness, the better the patient is likely to be served. This simplistic statement conveniently ignores the effect of therapy. Because treatment is highly effective at least for a proportion of patients and because most patients with lymphoma are treated earlier rather than later, the natural history is inevitably obscured and the clinical course is revealed. The syndromes then become harder to describe and clinicopathologic correlates harder to make.

Morphology

The macroscropic and microscopic appearance of the involved tissue remains the most important component of the diagnosis.

It is still possible to trace the development of the pathologic classification of the lymphomas over the last one and a half centuries, to conclude that consistent progress has been made (even in terms of nomenclature), and to demonstrate the relevance of such progress today. The era of histopathology lasted more than 100 years and saw pathologists struggle to distinguish leukemia from lymphoma and to categorize the lymphomas on morphologic grounds. Virchow[42] (probably) coined the word *lymphosarcoma* as a generic term for all lymphomas,

and Kundrat[43] (probably) restricted it to what might be thought of as non-Hodgkin's lymphoma today, although his original cases were peculiar in that they were localized presentations. Not long after began the debates as to the origin of the lymphomas of large cells: were they tumors of mesenchymal tissue, or were they primitive lymphoid cells? Within the limitations of classic morphology, it was actually not possible to tell the difference. Ewing,[44] Oberling,[45] and Roulet[46] used the term *reticulum cell sarcoma*, clearly believing in the distinction, and the concept stuck. By 1940, however, it was being cogently argued that reticulum cell sarcoma included at least a proportion of malignancies (undoubtedly of highly immature lymphoid cells) called *stem cell lymphomas*, in contrast to clasmatocytic lymphoma, which was presumably of recticular origin. In their classification, Gall and Mallory[47] also recognized follicular lymphoma. This entity had first been described at the turn of the century[48,49] and again intermittently[50] until it finally achieved malignant status in 1938 when Symmers[51] reported his series of patients (in the context of a review of many others) and described a well-defined clinical entity. Using roughly the same terminology to document clearly overlapping clinical and pathologic entities for which the only therapy was palliation with surgery or modest irradiation, quite large series of cases were reported, demonstrating major survival differences among lymphocytic lymphosarcoma, reticulum cell sarcoma, and follicular lymphoma.[52] The classifications were of prognostic significance regardless of their scientific validity.

Rappaport[53] produced the last and possibly most widely acclaimed solely morphologic classification of the malignant lymphomas, based on two features: (1) that the malignant cell of any type of lymphoma might disrupt the nodal architecture in a nodular or diffuse manner; and (2) that lymphomas of histiocytic origin existed (and were in fact quite common). This classification, first mooted in an important paper concerning follicular lymphoma and how it should be distinguished from follicular hyperplasia,[53] and again 10 years later,[54] gained rapid and widespread acceptance in the United States and was, like its predecessors, shown to be "of prognostic significance." This fact, coupled with its descriptive precision, made it very readily acceptable to physicians. Application of the Rappaport classification was fairly simple in concept, as it divided lymphomas into those with large (i.e., incorrectly called histiocytes) or small cells, with or without a nodular (i.e., follicular) growth pattern.

Immunology

It is now clear that the immune phenotype may be critical for the accurate and prognostically relevant classification of lymphoma.

The era of immunology resulted in the demonstration that neither of the two major premises described previously were correct. The introduction of techniques using antibodies (initially raised in animals) to antigens on the surface of normally differentiating lymphoid cells and cytochemical assays[55,56] led to the incontrovertible demonstration that: (1) most non-Hodgkin's lymphomas were of B-cell origin; (2) all follicular or nodular lymphomas were of follicle center cell origin; and (3) the very great majority of lymphomas previously designated as reticulum cell sarcoma, clasmatocytic lymphoma, or histiocytic lymphoma had the immunologic characteristics of transformed lymphocytes.[55,57,59] Thus the 1970s saw the introduction of classifications based on the presumed source of the cell type in question and the grade of malignancy. The Kiel classification was based heavily on the work of Lennert and rapidly gained popularity in Europe.[58] That of Lukes and Collins,[59] conceptually very similar, was transiently used in North America but was superceded largely by the consensus Working Formulation.[60] This is not a classification per se but a means whereby descriptive groupings of lymphomas have been made according to their expectation of survival in the late 1970s. Like the Rappaport classification, the divisions are largely based on cell size (large versus small), cell shape (round versus not round), and growth pattern (follicular versus diffuse). It gained wide acceptance in North America but did not constitute an advance in our understanding of these disorders.

Cytogenetics and Molecular Genetics

Nonrandom chromosomal abnormalities associated with specific subtypes of lymphoma are being identified with increasing frequency (Table 112-2).

The current era of pathologic classification incorporates both cytogenetics and molecular findings, made possible by the explosion of new techniques presently available. It is now clear that, as in leukemia, many of the lymphomas are associated with nonrandom chromosomal abnormalities that reflect molecular rearrangements involving specific oncogenes and one of the immunoglobulin genes (in B-cell lymphoma). It was first demonstrated that Burkitt's lymphoma was associated with the translocation t(8;14)[61]; more recently it was shown that c-myc was the relevant oncogene.[62] Similarly the translocation t(14;18) occurs in approximately 85% of cases of follicular lymphoma,[63] the bcl-2 oncogene being transposed and becoming adjacent to the site of the immunoglobulin heavy chain gene.[64] The occurrence of a t(11;14)[65] translocation involving the bcl-1[66] gene in a subset of B-cell lymphomas has contributed to the recognition of mantle cell lymphoma (see "'New' Entities"). Further examples are shown in Table 112-3. While their practical relevance may at present lie predominantly in increasing understanding of the diseases and classification, it is to be hoped that they may in the future provide the rationale for better therapy.

Gene expression profiling has now made it possible to subcategorize the lymphomas according to whether certain genes, or groups of genes are upregulated or downregulated. This has already been shown to be prognostically significant: it may lead to detection of new therapeutic targets.[67,68]

"New" Entities

The advanced immunologic and genetic techniques, as well as increased experience in looking at these tumors,

has led to the recognition of a number of new syndromes that were not recognized in the Working Formulation[69] (Table 112-4). Lymphomas represent malignant transformation of lymphocytes, and any particular lymphoma can be related to the stage of lymphoid maturation and the corresponding location of the lymph node. Mantle cell lymphomas are not rare but are an important newly recognized entity in the United States, although they have been recognized in Europe as centrocytic lymphoma for some years.[58,70] These B-cell lymphomas of the lymphocytes that surround follicles are defined by a particular morphology, staining with CD5, and a translocation between chromosomes 11 and 14 involving the bcl-1 oncogene.[71-73] Although they are small cell lymphomas, these tumors pursue an aggressive and relentless clinical course.[74-76] When they are disseminated, complete remissions have been, until recently, unusual and rarely durable.

In contrast, marginal zone lymphomas tend to pursue an indolent course. They can be separated from the mantle zone lymphomas by their lack of staining with CD5. Marginal zone B-cell lymphomas may be extranodal or nodal, the former being represented by the spectrum of MALT lymphomas.[77-83] These present in extranodal sites, tend to remain localized, and can sometimes be cured with local excision.[80-83] Relapses and an indolent natural history are more characteristic, however. In at least one study, gastric MALT lymphomas were associated with infection by *Helicobacter pylori* and seemed to respond sometimes to bismuth and antibiotic therapy directed against the microorganism.[84] Nodal marginal zone B-cell lymphomas, sometimes called monocytoid B-cell lymphoma, presents with nodal disease. The rare splenic marginal zone lymphoma, presents with splenomegaly and minimal lymphadenopathy.[85]

The WHO classification recognizes several "new" relatively aggressive lymphomas. These include the mediastinal B-cell lymphomas, a variant of diffuse large B-cell lymphoma, which presents with mediastinal masses containing fibrosis.[86-95] Anaplastic large cell lymphomas are usually T-cell tumors and frequently present in extranodal sites. These tumors are recognized by staining with the CD30 or Ki-1 antigen (i.e., a characteristic of Reed-Sternberg cells) and the frequent appearance of a characteristic chromosomal translocation between chromosomes 2 and 5.[96-102]

Primary effusion lymphomas (PEL) are a rare subset of AIDS-related lymphomas that present as lymphomatous effusions without an identifiable tumor mass.[19] They are consistently associated with HHV8, the Kaposi's sarcoma–associated herpes virus.[21]

Many illnesses that would previously have been called angioimmunoblastic lymphadenopathy also seem to be T-cell lymphomas. Angiocentric processes such as lymphomatoid granulomatosis and facial/sinus processes that might have previously been called lethal midline granuloma also usually represent aggressive T-cell lymphomas.[103]

The Interface between Leukemia and Lymphoma and Semantic Problems

The distinction between lymphoma and leukemia is usually semantic. Without special stains, however, it is

TABLE 112-2

Typical Immunophenotypic and Genetic Abnormalities of the Major Subtypes of Non-Hodgkin's Lymphoma

	FOLLICULAR	SMALL LYMPHOCYTIC	MALT	MARGINAL ZONE, NODAL	MANTLE CELL	DIFFUSE LARGE B-CELL	MEDIASTINAL LARGE B-CELL	BURKITT'S	LYMPHOBLASTIC	PERIPHERAL T-CELL	ANAPLASTIC LARGE T/NULL CELL
Characteristic Immunophenotype	CD20+, CD3– CD10+, CD5–	CD20+, CD3– CD10–, CD5+ CD23+	CD20+, CD3– CD10–, CD5– CD23–	CD20+, CD3– CD10–, CD5– CD23–	CD20+, CD– CD10–, CD5+ CD24–, PRAD1+	CD20+, CD3–	CD20+, CD3–	CD20+, CD3– CD10–, CD5–	CD3–CD20–, CD3+ Tdt+ Tdt–	CD20–, CD3+	CD20–, CD3– CD30+, CD15– EMA+, ALK+
Most frequent cytogenetic abnormality	t(14;18) (q32q21)	del(13q), +12	t(11;18) (q21;q21) +3, +18	+3, +18	t(11;14) (q13;q32)	t(14;18) (q32;q21) t(8;14) (q24;q32) t(3;14) (q27;q32)	Variable	t(8;14) (q24;32) t(2;8) (p12;q24) t(8;22) (q24;q11)	Variable	Variable	t(2;5) (q23;q35)
Associated oncogenes	bcl-2	Unknown	bcl-10	Unknown	bcl-1 (PRAD1)	bcl-6 bcl-2 c-myc	Unknown	c-myc	tcl1-3	Unknown	alk

TABLE 112-3

Major Cytogenetic Translocations Associated with Non-Hodgkin's Lymphoma

TRANSLOCATION	USUAL HISTOLOGIC TYPE	KNOWN ONCOGENE INVOLVED	USUAL IMMUNOPHENOTYPE
t(11;14) (q24;q32)	Mantle cell	bcl-1	B
t(14;18) (q32;q21)	All follicular lymphomas and some diffuse large cell	bcl-2	B
t(9;14) (p13;q32)		pa ×5	B
t(3;–) (q27;q–)*	Diffuse large cell	bcl-6	B
t(2;5) (q23;q35)	Anaplastic large cell	alk	T
t(11;18)	MALT	bcl-10	B

*3q27 is involved in translocations to numerous other sites.

possible to confuse isolated granulocytic sarcoma with lymphoma.[104,105]

A number of non-Hodgkin's lymphomas can also present as a chronic lymphocytic leukemia[41,106,107] (Table 112-5). The most characteristic of these is small lymphocytic lymphoma, which more often presents as typical B-cell chronic lymphocytic leukemia. Lymphoplasmacytic lymphomas that produce excessive amounts of IgM and involve the blood and bone marrow may also be called Waldenström's macroglobulinemia.[108] Follicular lymphomas can present with blood involvement[109,110] and used to be called lymphosarcoma cell leukemia.[111] A similar process can occur with mantle cell lymphomas.[75,112,113] Chronic T-cell leukemias include blood involvement by mycosis fungoides, known as Sézary syndrome,[114,115,129,130] and a smoldering process associated with infection by HTLV-1.[116]

The Present

The last 10 years have seen the formulation, proposal, dissemination, testing, modification, and finally acceptance by both the pathology and clinical community of a new classification.[38] This has been a major achievement, incorporating histopathology, immunology, cytogenetics, and clinical data in a concerted attempt to subclassify the lymphomas as far as possible into clinically recognizable entities. It has to be recognized, of course, that limitations are placed on the identification of these entities, first because the overwhelmingly most common presentation of lymphoma is that of painless lymphadenopathy, and second because the natural history of the "condition" is obscured by the effects of therapy.

The new WHO classification (Table 112-6) represents the culmination of the efforts of the informal International Lymphoma Study Group to adjust the "REAL" classification,[38] after an international investigation to test its reproducibility, validity, and clinical relevance. Subsequent to a meeting at the National Cancer Institute in 1994, when it was first presented to clinicians, pathologic material and clinical data from 1403 patients treated at nine centers in eight countries were evaluated.[117] In essence, the study design involved "local" pathologists making material available and a team of visiting pathologists conducting reviews and rereviews, and arriving at a diagnosis with morphology alone, morphology with immunophenotyping, and further (mainly clinical) information. Outcome data were available on all patients.

Analysis of the results demonstrated conclusively that the new classification, which concentrated on "entities" and dispenses with "grade" (either as described in the Working Formulation, or the Kiel classification), was: (1) reproducible; (2) prognostically significant; and (3) therefore appropriate for the millennium because the

TABLE 112-4

Newly Recognized Clinical Subtypes of Non-Hodgkin's Lymphoma

NAME	IMMUNOPHENOTYPE	PECULIAR IMMUNOLOGIC/GENETIC CHARACTERISTICS	PACE OF DISEASE	CHEMOTHERAPHY-CURABLE WHEN DISSEMINATED
Mantle cell lymphoma	B	CD5 positive; t(11,14)	Aggressive	No or rarely

Marginal zone lymphomas
   MALToma
   Monocytoid B-cell
   Splenic marginal zone
	B	CD5 negative	Indolent	No or rarely

Mediastinal B-cell lymphoma	B	—	Aggressive	Yes
Anaplastic large cell lymphoma	Mostly T or null	CD30 positive; t(2;5)	Aggressive	Yes
AILD-like lymphomas	T	—	Aggressive	Yes
Angiocentric lymphomas	T	—	Aggressive	Yes

Specific Malignancies

III

TABLE 112-5

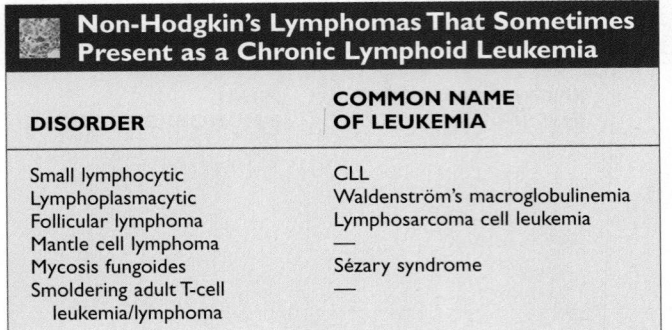

DISORDER	COMMON NAME OF LEUKEMIA
Small lymphocytic	CLL
Lymphoplasmacytic	Waldenström's macroglobulinemia
Follicular lymphoma	Lymphosarcoma cell leukemia
Mantle cell lymphoma	—
Mycosis fungoides	Sézary syndrome
Smoldering adult T-cell leukemia/lymphoma	—

prognostic significance took account of immunology, clinical features, and molecular considerations for the large proportion of cases. At a unique meeting of the WHO pathology panel, convened to include a clinical advisory committee, minor modifications were recom-

TABLE 112-6

WHO Classification of Non-Hodgkin's Lymphoma

B-CELL LYMPHOMAS

Precursor B-Cell Lymphoma

Precursor B lymphoblastic lymphoma/leukemia

Mature B-Cell Lymphoma

Chronic lymphocytic leukemia/small lymphocytic lymphoma
Lymphoplasmactic lymphoma
Splenic marginal zone lymphoma
Extranodal marginal zone B-cell lymphoma of mucosa-associated lymphoid tissue (MALT-lymphoma)
Nodal marginal zone B-cell lymphoma
Follicular lymphoma
Mantle cell lymphoma
Diffuse large B-cell lymphoma
   Mediastinal (thymic) large B-cell lymphoma
   Intravascular large B-cell lymphoma
   Primary effusion lymphoma
Burkitt lymphoma/leukemia

T/NK-CELL LYMPHOMA

Precursor T-Cell Lymphoma

Precursor T-cell lymphoblastic lymphoma

Mature T/NK Cell Lymphoma

Adult T-cell lymphoma/leukemia
Mycosis fungoides
   Sézary syndrome
Primary cutaneous anaplastic large cell lymphoma
Anaplastic large cell lymphoma
Peripheral T-cell lymphoma, unspecified
Angioimmunoblastic T-cell lymphoma
Extranodal NK/T cell lymphoma, nasal type
Enteropathy-type T-cell lymphoma
Hepatosplenic T-cell lymphoma
Subcutaneous panniculitis-like T-cell lymphoma
Blastic NK cell lymphoma

Adapted from Jaffe ES, Harris NL, Stein H, Vardiman JW (eds): World Health Organization Classification of Tumours. Pathology & Genetics. Tumours of Haematopoietic and Lymphoid Tissues. IARC Press, Lyon, 2001.

mended[118]: WHO classification has been published in a "Blue Book."[41] With luck and perseverance it will serve for at least a decade. Enthusiasm for it should be tempered by its somewhat lack of user friendliness. This arises predominantly from users' lack of familiarity with the structure and some of the nomenclature. It is hoped that this will be overcome.

The classification describes the lymphomas, dividing them first according to lineage, and second according to the stage of differentiation at which malignancy has occurred. Although there are many subtypes, in fact six account for 80% of cases. The WHO classification will be used throughout this chapter.

PRINCIPLES OF MANAGEMENT

History and Physical Examination

As with the management of most illnesses, the most important investigation is the full history complemented by examination. Questioning should particularly attempt to elicit whether symptoms suggest involvement or compromise of major organs or other extranodal sites and whether constitutional ("B") symptoms are present. From the point of view of therapeutic decision making, it is essential to know whether the patient is at particular risk of HIV infection and to ascertain the general state of health, with particular reference to cardiac, respiratory, and renal function. Many other factors may be of interest and may be usefully recorded, for example, previous history of immune disorder or treatment with immuno-suppressive drugs, use of hair dyes, and family history of lymphoma. Examination should be directed specifically at demonstrating clinical evidence of lymphoma, with particular attention given to the lymph node areas, the liver and spleen, the fauces (some recommend formal ear, nose, and throat evaluation), and the testes. The overall health of the patient should also be determined.

Further Investigations

By the end of the initial consultation, provided that the diagnosis has been confirmed, the physician should have a clear idea of which, if any, therapy is indicated. Little further information may be necessary for this immediate decision, although almost invariably many tests may be performed. The rationale behind the further investigation of those patients for whom therapy has already been selected is often fully justified and lies in the requirement for a baseline from which the response to therapy can be fully evaluated. It is rare for the patient with lymphoma to be grossly underinvestigated.

Concept of Staging

Classification of the lymphomas has traditionally involved both pathologic and distributional findings, which together have been used to predict patterns of survival. Staging of these illnesses has advanced in parallel with an

EVALUATION OF A NEW PATIENT WITH NON-HODGKIN'S LYMPHOMA

OBJECT OF EVALUATION	MANDATORY STUDIES	SOMETIMES APPROPRIATE STUDIES
Confirm diagnosis	*Adequate* biopsy reviewed by experienced hematopathologists	Immunophenotyping Cytogenetics Molecular studies
General overview	Careful history and physical examination Complete blood count (including platelet count) Chemistry screen (including liver and renal function studies) Chest radiograph	Blood coagulation studies Serum and viral protein studies Serum electrolytes, uric acid
Prognostic categorization	Serum LDH Serum albumin	Erythrocyte sedimentation rate Serum β_2-microglobulin Estimate of tumor growth fraction
Evaluate the abdomen and pelvis	CT scan	Ultrasonography Lymphangiogram MRI
Search for occult sites of involvement	Bone marrow biopsy	Chest CT scan Lumbar puncture Bone scan PET scan Biopsy of suspicious sites

understanding of pathology and now almost incorporates aspects of the latter by virtue of the use of immunologic and molecular tumor markers. Staging involves those studies that allow patients with a particular type of lymphoma to be divided into different groups with different prognoses or treatment requirements. It begins with a history and detailed physical examination and is complete after a spectrum of possible investigations directed at determining optimal management has been performed. The studies currently used are discussed later.

The clinical pattern of Hodgkin's disease (frequent contiguous spread) and potential curability when localized (with extended-field irradiation) made it the prototype for an anatomic staging classification. Techniques for detecting clinically impalpable lymphadenopathy have advanced over the past 25 years from plain radiography through whole-lung tomography, to lymphography and CT. Magnetic resonance imaging (MRI) may contribute under some circumstances, as may radiolabeled imaging.[119] Positron emission tomography is gaining in popularity and relevance. CT-guided biopsy, particularly of intra-abdominal masses, may obviate the need for open surgery. Bone marrow aspirate and biopsy, a critical investigation originally used to detect morphologic evidence of infiltration, may now reveal involvement immunologically at the level of 1 cell in 100 or 1000, or molecularly at the level of 1 cell in 100,000. Progress in detecting occult lymphoma has thus paralleled progress in understanding this group of diseases, allowing for the continuing refinement of both pathologic and staging classifications.

The Cotswold's modification of the Ann Arbor staging classification for Hodgkin's disease (Table 112-7) provides a framework for assigning an anatomic, clinically based stage and incorporates a designation for the presence of "bulk" disease (arbitrarily selected as denoting a mass of nodes with one diameter of greater than 10 cm or a mediastinal mass of greater than one third of the transthoracic width).[120] Even without this modification, it can be seen that the anatomic stage is a powerful predictor of prognosis (independent of histology) in a large series of patients treated according to the protocols in use during a 20-year period. An international survey of patients with intermediate/high-grade[60] (Working Formulation) or high-grade (Kiel)[58] histology (using defunct terminology) involving several large centers and cooperative groups, treated with similar protocols, yielded similar results and led to formulation of the International Prognostic Index.[121] For these reasons, it still seems entirely appropriate to retain the description of anatomic stage as an integral part of the information required for the selection of therapy in the 21st century.

While extranodal sites are accommodated in the anatomic classification by the suffix "E," the gastrointestinal tract (in the light of its natural history) may require special attention. The issue is compounded by the precision with which primary gastrointestinal tract lymphoma is defined. It is probably justifiable to define such lymphomas *relatively* loosely and to adjust the staging classification to accommodate their pattern of spread. A proposed modification of the Musshoff classification has been favored by some.[122]

The limitations of anatomic staging (or at least its relevance to non-Hodgkin's lymphoma) are based on the heterogeneous presentation of the different subtypes. While a modified Ann Arbor classification is applied by most investigators, it is clearly inappropriate for many other primary extranodal presentations. Furthermore anatomic staging classifications do not take the volume of tumor into account. The relevance of any staging classification is its contribution to therapeutic decisions, chemotherapy of differing intensity being now indicated for different circumstances; the latest step in "staging" has been the development of prognostic indices.

TABLE 112-7

Ann Arbor Staging Classification and the Cotswold Modifications

STAGE	FEATURES
I	Involvement of a single lymph node region or lymphoid structure (e.g., spleen, thymus, Waldeyer's ring)
II	Involvement of two or more lymph node regions on the same side of the diaphragm
III	Involvement of lymph regions or structures on both sides of the diaphragm
IV	Involvement of extranodal site(s) beyond that designated E
For all stages	
A	No symptoms
B	Fever (>38°C), drenching sweats, weight loss (10% body weight over 6 months)
For stages I to III	
E	Involvement of a single, extranodal site contiguous or proximal to known nodal site
Cotswold modifications	
(i)	Suffix X to designate bulky disease as > 1/3 widening of the mediastinum of > 10 cm maximum dimension of nodal mass
(ii)	The number of anatomic regions involved should be indicated by a subscript (e.g., II_3)
(iii)	Stage III: it may be subdivided into:
	III_1, with or without splenic, hilar, celiac, or portal nodes
	III_2, with para-aortic, iliac, mesenteric nodes
(iv)	Staging should be identified as clinical stage (CS) or pathologic stage (PS)
(v)	A new category of response to therapy, unconfirmed/uncertain complete remission (CR) should be introduced because of the persistent radiologic abnormalities of uncertain significance

As previously emphasized, the purpose of investigation and designation of "stage" is to ensure that the most appropriate treatment is prescribed. It has been clear for some time that other factors beyond histology and anatomic stage correlate with outcome. This has been most extensively studied in the aggressive non-Hodgkin's lymphomas (Working Formulation, high and intermediate grade; Kiel classification, high grade; WHO classification, mostly DLBC lymphoma). A number of studies have shown the importance of age, performance status, bulk, and other surrogate markers of tumor activity (particularly albumin, lactate dehydrogenase [LDH], and β2-microglobulin) and have allocated patients into good-, intermediate-, or bad-risk groups, according to the presence or absence of numbers of adverse factors.[123-128] These findings culminated in the study by Shipp and colleagues,[121] mentioned previously, that constructed an International Prognostic Index based on age, stage, number of extranodal sites, performance status, and serum lactate dehydrogenase (LDH) level[121] (Table 112-8). Such an approach provides a further refinement of the criteria for therapy decisions, allowing the identification of patients for whom different experimental approaches might be considered; it also facilitates comparison of results among different centers. Attempts have been made to do the same for the other lymphomas,[129-134] for which the International Prognostic Index also seems to work. A modification has been proposed for follicular lymphoma.[135]

Assessment of Response after Therapy

Response to therapy should be documented by physical findings and repeat testing of those parameters that were abnormal before therapy. Treatment strategies based on the rate of response may demand reevaluation during therapy. While theoretically attractive, this is often difficult to accomplish because of demands for CT scanning time and fiscal restraints. Delays in therapy may result. In addition, inconsistent evaluation may lead to artificial differences in response rates to the same treatment program.

The frequency and extent of investigations during follow-up after completion of therapy depend on the presumed risk of recurrence, on the belief (or not) in the concept that detection of early, or at least subclinical, recurrence may improve the outcome of subsequent therapy, and last but not least, on the research interests of the physician. No strong evidence shows that those who have achieved complete remission warrant any special investigation beyond physical examination and probably chest radiograph if they are asymptomatic. By contrast, patients who have achieved either an equivocal complete remission or partial remission (especially if shown by a persistent radiologic abnormality), for whom enthusiastic intervention is being considered in the face of progression, should be regularly monitored with CT scanning probably at 3-month intervals for at least 18 months. The "molecular monitoring" of remission, for example, by polymerase chain reaction (PCR) for the t(14;18) translocation in patients with follicular lymphoma, while of potential future importance,[136] is at present a research investigation.

In cases of overt recurrence, investigations are determined by what influence the results will have on therapy decisions. The automatic instinct to "reevaluate" should be resisted, while it must be remembered that important questions need to be answered about the prognosis from recurrence justifying extensive investigation at the time. For example, one thrust of research into curative therapy for recurrent disease revolves around the use of myeloablative therapy with either bone marrow or peripheral blood progenitor cell rescue in this setting. Early circumstantial evidence has suggested that some patients with follicular lymphoma may have benefited greatly from this treatment,[137-140] (see later discussion). The more data available on the total cohort of patients with recurrent

TABLE 112-8

Outcome According to Risk Group Defined by the International Index

RISK GROUP	NO. OF RISK FACTORS	DISTRIBUTION OF PATIENTS (%)	RATE (%)	COMPLETE RESPONSE	
				RELAPSE-FREE SURVIVAL (5-YEAR RATE, %)	SURVIVAL (5-YEAR RATE, %)
International index all patients (n = 2,031)					
Adverse factors (age >60 years, ↑ LDH, poor performance status, extranodal sites, Ann Arbor stage III or IV)					
Low	0 or 1	35	87	70	73
Low intermediate	2	27	67	50	51
High intermediate	3	22	55	49	43
High	4 or 5	16	44	40	26
Age-adjusted index patients ≤60 years old (n = 1,274)					
Adverse factors (↑ LDH, poor performance status, Ann Arbor stage III or IV)					
Low	0	22	92	86	83
Low intermediate	1	32	78	66	69
High intermediate	2	32	57	53	46
High	3	14	56	58	32
Age-adjusted index patients >60 years old (n = 761)					
Adverse factors (↑ LDH, poor performance status, Ann Arbor stage III or IV)					
Low	0	18	91	46	56
Low intermediate	1	31	71	45	44
High intermediate	2	35	56	41	37
High	3	16	36	37	21

disease and their outcomes, regardless of the treatment given, the easier it will be to demonstrate which, if any, should be treated experimentally. Thus the research arguments in favor of repeat biopsy and repetition of the investigations that were indicated at the original presentation are compelling. At the present time, no formal staging system or prognostic factor index for documenting symptoms at recurrence or progression exist. They are urgently required.

In 1998, a workshop was held under the auspices of the National Cancer Institute to define response criteria that could be standardized and universally applied, particularly in the context of clinical trials.[141] Of necessity some of the decisions were arbitrary, particularly in relation to what size of lymph node would be considered normal after therapy. Emphasis was placed upon the distinction between "measurability and assessability." It was concluded that complete remission required the patient to be in normal health without clinical evidence of lymphoma, and with no node larger than 1.5 cm in long axis on the CT scan (despite the recognition that this was larger than normal in a person without lymphoma). Unilateral bone marrow biopsy of at least 1-cm core in length had to be morphologically free of lymphoma. A new category, complete remission (uncertain) (CRU), which approximated that previously described as good partial remission (GPR), was introduced. This required greater than 75% reduction in the size of lymph nodes (bidimensional measurements). The spleen was to be treated as a lymph node and measured on CT scan rather than clinically, as were focal lesions. Focal lesions in the liver were considered measurable. Otherwise, partial remission (PR) required the same measurements as previously discussed, with a 50% reduction in size of lymph nodes.

The assessment of response to therapy was to be 1 to 2 months after completion of therapy unless progression occurred earlier. Thus in-treatment evaluation was to be ignored in terms of final outcome. It was recognized that there were other tests being used for research purposes, and that they would be documented but not taken into account.

Specific Imaging Studies

Supradiaphragmatic Studies

Plain x-ray of the chest, with lateral and posterolateral views (if routine CT scanning of the chest is not performed) yields valuable information on mediastinal and hilar nodes and the lung fields. Considerably more information, at more than three times the expense, may be obtained by CT, MRI, and gallium scanning.

Infradiaphragmatic Studies

CT is the investigation of choice for the abdomen and pelvis, first for determining the presence of clinically undetectable disease and second for allowing accurate measurement of its dimensions. As previously mentioned, it may be needed for guided needle biopsy. Liver and spleen enlargement can be shown on CT scanning, although this may not equate with infiltration. It has been suggested, at least for Hodgkin's disease, that focal defects presumed to be due to lymphoma should be confirmed with another imaging method. Although lymphography is excellent for delineating para-aortic lymphadenopathy, it is unsatisfactory for other sites, and in practice is not usually used in the investigation of non-Hodgkin's lymphoma. MRI may be used as an alternative to CT scanning; no convincing data yet show that it is superior for detecting nodal disease, although it may be better for examining the liver and bone marrow. Staging laparotomy is not indicated.

Other Sites

Both plain x-rays and CT scanning of the postnasal space and sinuses are indicated in patients with lymphoma arising in the head and neck, particularly to determine whether bony infiltration has occurred. MRI may be particularly helpful in this context. Some consider that barium studies of the gastrointestinal tract are indicated in patients with postnasal space or Waldeyer's ring lymphoma. Routine radiography of the skeletal system is not warranted, but is the investigation of first choice if a bony lesion is suspected. CT scanning with bone setting and MRI scanning are both more accurate than technetium scanning, although they require suspicion of specific sites. If clinically indicated, the central nervous system (CNS) is best investigated by MRI, CT scanning, and myelography, with examination of the cerebrospinal fluid (CSF).

PET Scanning

Over the past 10 years it has become clear that functional imaging is complementary to, if not a substitute for, anatomical imaging both for staging and post-treatment evaluation in patients with lymphoma. Positron Emission Tomography (PET) utilizes F-18 flurodeoxyglucose (FDG), which is taken up in hypermetabolic tissues, exploiting the increased FDS metabolism of malignant as opposed to nonmalignant cells.

It has been suggested in reviews of relatively small retrospective series that it has similar accuracy for nodal disease as CT,[142] and may be better in the central nervous system and abdomen. Similarly it is increasingly popular both for distinguishing persistent disease from scarring,[143-145] and predicting disease-free survival.[146-148]

Hematology

Peripheral blood count with examination of a peripheral blood smear is an essential investigation. Apart from nonspecific changes, it may reveal pancytopenia or circulating lymphoma cells. These may be demonstrated morphologically, more frequently immunologically, and even more frequently at the molecular level. The significance of findings beyond overt morphologic involvement has not yet been proved. In a patient with small lymphocytic lymphoma/chronic lymphocytic leukemia (CLL) who becomes anemic, a hemolysis screen may be advisable and should at least be considered.

Bone marrow aspiration and trephine biopsy are almost invariably performed and often advance the stage of patients, particularly those with follicular lymphoma, from stage III to stage IV. Bone marrow biopsy in patients with DLBC lymphoma can be positive by virtue of involvement by small lymphocytes in a paratrabecular fashion; this finding does not necessarily suggest a poor prognosis.[149] The frequency with which the investigation influences the decision of whether to treat with irradiation alone or not is, however, probably very low. Once again, this does not mean that bone marrow biopsy is unnecessary. It may be justified on the general grounds that it is important

to clarify marrow cellularity before instituting chemotherapy and that it is necessary for accurate restaging. It is also essential to know as much as possible about the state of the marrow if myeloablative therapy with either autologous bone marrow or peripheral blood progenitor cell rescue is being considered. The cerebrospinal fluid should be examined by cytospin in all those at serious risk of meningeal involvement.

Chemistry

Biochemical tests of liver and kidney function are essential investigations of the patient with non-Hodgkin's lymphoma. While none is definitive for staging, all are important for general management. For example, Adriamycin (doxorubicin, hydroxydaunorubicin) should never be prescribed without knowledge of bilirubin levels. At least as important is the fact that several biochemical tests have been shown to correlate closely with prognosis. Examples include serum albumin (very cheap), LDH (cheap), and β2-microglobulin (expensive). Although they are not necessary for all patients, serum electrophoresis and immunoglobulin quantitation should be performed in patients with any suggestion of lymphoplasmacytoid lymphoma. At the completion of those tests considered essential (properly completed within a week of the diagnosis and occasionally in a much shorter time), it should be possible to assign a modified Ann Arbor stage and also (at least for some types of lymphoma) a Prognostic Index and a complete basis upon which to decide on therapy.

Other Tests

The search for evidence of otherwise occult tumor cells can be carried out using various techniques; the presence of occult lymphoma cells in the blood or bone marrow might have prognostic significance and might make a patient a poor candidate for bone marrow or blood harvest in anticipation of high-dose therapy and autotransplantation. One method to search for a small population of tumor cells is flow cytometry on blood or marrow using antibodies to allow identification of the presence of monoclonal B cells. Another technique involves using PCR to search for cells with a specific genetic abnormality. The most popular approach has been to look for cells with bcl-2 gene rearrangements. In some studies, the presence of such cells in the blood or marrow has seemed to predict a poorer treatment outcome.[136,140,150] Circulating lymphocytes with bcl-2 gene[150] rearrangements are occasionally seen in normal individuals and are sometimes found in normal tonsils, however.[151-153] At the present time within the context of refinement of the techniques in use, the implications of finding circulating lymphocytes with bcl-2 gene rearrangements are sufficiently unclear that this is probably not an appropriate part of initial evaluation of a patient with B-cell lymphoma.

Summary

Investigations of the lymphoma patient at different time points in the disease have been presented previously. The basic recommendations are straightforward; the extras reflect an eye to the future. It cannot be overemphasized that the investigation to be undertaken is the one most appropriate for the patient in question; this decision lies rightly in the hands of the physician. When research and service go hand in hand, everyone's best interests are served. The objective is to make sure the best treatment is given.

TREATMENT

Background and Principles of Antilymphoma Therapy

Over the past 150 years, the malignant lymphomas have been discovered, "lumped," and "split" on the basis of the current techniques available for investigating them. Histopathology, immunology, cytogenetics, molecular biology, and radiology have all advanced mightily, providing the physician with an amazing array of information upon which to decide what advice to give the patient about therapy, which has also changed out of all recognition. More than 50 years ago radiation was proven to give symptomatic relief and possibly extend life. Chemotherapy, first as palliation and then with curative intent, has become established as the treatment of choice for most patients with non-Hodgkin's lymphoma. Myeloablative chemotherapy or chemotherapy in combination with radiation therapy (made increasingly feasible by the advent of hematopoietic growth factors, autologous bone marrow, and peripheral blood progenitor cell rescue) may now be used in those at high risk of failure using conventional dose therapy. Other biologic therapy, antibody therapy, whether alone or in combination with chemotherapy, has become "conventional" in certain circumstances in the form of delivering toxin via antibodies; allogeneic transplantation and vaccine are under investigation.

The objective of therapy is to return the patient to normal for as long as possible. When this is not possible, quality of life is obviously at a premium. A considerable array of options is available; with intelligent informed selection by the physician, and some good luck, much may be achieved for almost everyone with non-Hodgkin's lymphoma (needless to say, with great room for improvement). Choice of therapy will be mainly determined by the histologic subtype, the "extent of disease" (stage, and so forth), and the patient's general state of health. The decision, and the chances of success, will be greatly influenced by whether it is made at the initial presentation or later in the course of the illness when earlier strategies have failed.

In the year 2004, a minority of patients will be cured by the initial therapy; such therapy will quickly fail for another group, who will die early despite intervention. Most will face a remitting/recurring pattern and a rapidly diminishing probability of cure with the passage of time. This holds true for most subtypes of non-Hodgkin's lymphoma, although considerable differences exist between one and another. Not surprisingly, since repeated albeit incomplete regression of lymphadenopathy or infiltration of other organs is the rule rather than the

exception (even late in the disease), physicians are reluctant to "give up"; the conscious decision to treat with mild therapy, without anticipation of long-term benefit, may be hard to make. It must, however, be faced frequently and honestly; usually the cost-benefit ratio increases with the selection of less preferred and less well-tried options. The conscious decision to advise experimental therapy, with the obvious corollary that this may yield more benefit to future patients than to the individual in question, is difficult. The object of the exercise must be continually borne in mind.

The importance of appropriately (wholly, fully) informing the patient in general terms, at the onset of the illness, about what the future may hold cannot be overemphasized. The degree of frankness with which the situation is presented must of course be influenced by the perceived ability of the patient to comprehend and by the patient's cultural background. When the first treatment plan is made, the physician should present a balanced, and preferably not too detailed, indication of the probabilities of success and the relative risks. Mention should also be made of the experimental approaches currently in vogue, with reference to the circumstances under which they might be appropriate. Such full discussion, making it easy for the patient to approach the doctor later without embarrassment, cements the rapport between doctor and patient; such rapport is required to reach the degree of confidence necessary for facing the difficult decisions that may be ahead. A sympathetic presentation of the facts at the outset is enormously important, especially later, when treatment may not go as planned and chances of cure are gravely diminished. Such a presentation is particularly important for patients who may be sent to a secondary or tertiary referral center later and for the physicians who take on their care at that time.

Most attention is rightly given to the specific therapy of the non-Hodgkin's lymphomas, since elimination of the disease is sometimes possible and should always be the objective of the exercise. Supportive care, particularly moral support for both patient and family, is as important as the treatment. In general the attendance of as few doctors as possible is probably best; the skill required to determine who will benefit from referral to another "-ologist" or "-ist," particularly a psychiatrist, is considerable. At no time should the patient or relatives believe that "the doctors could do no more." That is *doctor,* not treatment, failure.

Specific Therapeutic Options

Surgery

Although surgery is often necessary to make the diagnosis of lymphoma and sometimes necessary to deal with complications of the disease or other therapies, it has not been considered an acceptable therapy, mostly because these malignancies are rarely localized. The one exception can be stage I MALT lymphomas. Although total gastrectomy for gastric MALT lymphomas is unnecessarily morbid, there are times when removal of skin, lung, and other MALT lymphoma is the simplest and most acceptable treatment.

Radiation Therapy

Irradiation was the first treatment to cause regression of lymph node masses in patients with lymphoma,[154,155] and early circumstantial evidence also showed that this effect might prolong life.[156] Megavoltage therapy may be used with expectation of cure, or certainly with long-term benefit in a small proportion of patients with stage I disease[157] and also at recurrence[158]; superficial beam therapy plays an integral part in the treatment of skin lymphoma; and in selected patients, total-body irradiation is used as part of myeloablative therapy, given with curative intent. In addition, radiation therapy may be an essential component of palliative therapy, often providing relief of pain, and also significant reduction of disease in awkward sites after chemotherapy has failed.[159] It may be vital if cord compression exists. Its place in elective combined-modality therapy is less clear. In patients with localized lymphomas, the use of involved-field radiation therapy allows a reduction in the amount of chemotherapy. With refinements in the equipment and delivery of radiation therapy, the potential side effects have been much reduced, although they are not to be neglected. Particularly important are mucositis and dryness in the mouth after irradiation to the head and neck, as well as sometimes very considerable gastrointestinal symptoms after abdominal irradiation. The risk of "radiation recall" with certain types of chemotherapy, particularly doxorubicin and methtrexate, must be remembered. In young patients, the delayed appearance of irradiation-induced solid tumors needs to be considered.

Chemotherapy

Single Agents. Cytotoxic chemotherapy was first introduced into the therapy of the non-Hodgkin's lymphomas half a century ago and is now the predominant mode of treatment for most patients. Chlorambucil[160] and cyclophosphamide,[161] both of which may be given orally, were evaluated soon after their synthesis; both drugs have approximately equivalent activity, with myelosuppression as the major toxicity.[162-170] These drugs remain popular as treatment for lymphomas for which cure is unlikely, a notable advantage being that both may be administered as tablets. If responses are to occur, they are generally apparent within 6 weeks.[163] Continuing administration (to patients in whom responses are seen) may result in further gradual regression of disease; complete remission has been documented as late as 18 months. The rate of response increases with increasing dose, but this may not confer a survival advantage. Responses occur much more frequently in follicular lymphoma than in other subtypes, although paradoxically, high doses of cyclophosphamide may be curative for some patients with Burkitt's lymphoma. The choice of dosage and schedule depend on the lymphoma being treated, whether or not the drug is given alone or in combination, and the whim of the physician. No evidence supports the indefinite prescription of alkylating agents, and they have considerable potential disadvantages. The major side effects are myelosuppression, infertility, and secondary acute myelogenous leukemia (AML). The risk of all these effects increases with the total dose, and evidence also suggests that the risk is worst with chronic administration.

The antimetabolites have been used in the treatment of hematologic malignancy since the demonstration in 1948 that they could induce complete remission of acute lymphoblastic leukemia in childhood.[171] They have been used in a variety of schedules, both orally and parenterally. The major attractions of methotrexate, the only one in frequent use, are that it may be used in very high doses, with the toxicity being reversed by citrovorum factor, and that it crosses the blood-brain barrier. Alone, therefore, it may be very useful in palliation, both of nodal and CNS disease. Its major drawbacks are myelosuppression and mucositis.

More recently the vinca alkaloids, particularly vincristine, were extracted from the periwinkle *Vinca rosea* and fortuitously demonstrated to have antitumor activity. Both objective and subjective responses were observed in about half the cases of lymphoma noted, with vincristine being given weekly by intravenous injection. The major dose-limiting side effect is neurotoxicity; myelosuppression is mild.[172-175] Much has been made of the possible dose-intensity effect of giving maximal doses of vincristine, in combination therapy; in practice, many patients, particularly the elderly, cannot tolerate even 1.4 mg/m^2 weekly for more than a few weeks. Many physicians cap the dose at a maximum of 2 mg; others deplore this practice. The level of responsiveness is probably not much higher than that achieved with vinblastine, but vincristine remains more popular, certainly in the therapy of non-Hodgkin's lymphoma, because the severe myelosuppression that may be seen with vinblastine makes its incorporation into combinations more difficult. Newer vinca alkaloids have not yet been shown to be better than vincristine.

It is rare for a patient with non-Hodgkin's lymphoma to die without having received corticosteroids for one reason or another. Responses are recorded for all types of lymphoma, with suggestions that very high doses may be particularly useful in follicular lymphoma.[176-182] Even in low doses they increase well-being and are specifically indicated during episodes of hemolysis and before or with irradiation for CNS disease. They are generally only given in the short term and, provided the prednisolone dose does not exceed 40 mg/day for a few weeks, the problems of chronic administration are limited. Attention must be paid to the potential risk of proximal muscle wasting, raised blood sugar, and psychological disturbance, particularly with high doses.

The anthracycline antibiotics have been extensively investigated in the treatment of non-Hodgkin's lymphoma. Single-agent data are remarkably sparse, relating almost exclusively to patients who had received a great deal of prior therapy, since the anthracyclines were discovered after the alkylating agents and (at least as important) after the concept of combination chemotherapy had been accepted.[183-185] Nonetheless they play a central role in almost every treatment program for aggressive advanced disease, despite the disadvantages of mucositis, myelosuppression, alopecia, and cumulative risk of cardiac failure. None of the newer DNA intercalating agents has yet been shown to be better than doxorubicin.

The single-agent data are possibly even weaker for the epipodophyllins.[186-188] Their popularity is not as great, but many programs for initial therapy of advanced large B-cell lymphoma employ them, and they are used by some physicians in high doses as part of myeloablative therapy. Both etoposide (VP-16) and teniposide (VM-26) may be used intravenously or orally; bioavailability is variable by mouth but is on the order of 50%. This is clearly a drawback if cure is the objective; but if palliation is sought, the capsules are very convenient. Substantial evidence in small cell lung cancer[189] and lymphoma[190] shows that administration over several days is best. The major toxicity is myelosuppression, and acute leukemias associated with translocations involving chromosome 11q23 and a specific gene have been reported.[191]

Cytosine arabinoside (cytarabine; a pyrimidine analog), one of the most effective drugs for the treatment of acute myeloid leukemia, causes rapid regression of diffuse large B-cell lymphoma or lymphoblastic lymphoma and "transformed" follicular lymphoma, even when the disease is refractory to previous therapy.[192-194] These responses may be very rapid, particularly if high doses are used. Unfortunately they are usually short-lived and regrowth of lymph node masses not infrequently occurs before the inevitable accompanying myelosuppression has resolved. Like methotrexate, this drug has a particular importance in the therapy of CNS disease, given both systemically at gram doses and intrathecally in milligram doses.

The most recent group of compounds to be evaluated comprises the purine analogs. Most data on lymphoma therapy relate to fludarabine, although both deoxyco-formycin (pentostatin) and 2-chlorodeoxy adenosine (cladribine) have proved highly effective for chronic lymphocytic leukemia and are now showing promise in lymphoma.[195,196] It appears that fludarabine is most effective for follicular lymphoma, with clinical responses reported in approximately 50% of patients.[197-203] Relatively few single agent data are presently available on efficacy in newly diagnosed cases; the information that does exist suggests that the response rate, both complete and partial, is higher.[204,205] The drug is very well tolerated in the doses now being used in phase II and III clinical trials. Almost no nausea or vomiting occurs, and alopecia is rarely recorded. The debilitating and potentially fatal neurotoxicity seen with high doses has been less evident with current doses and schedules. Considerable T-lymphocytic dysfunction has been reported, as well as undoubted incidences of opportunistic infection, not necessarily related to neutropenia (which is inevitable).[206] The drug is reasonably well absorbed if given orally, and the bioavailability of the tablet is about 50%.[207] Since fludarabine given alone appears to have considerable activity in diseases for which palliative therapy is required, the oral formulation has become popular in Europe.

Combination Therapy. Single-agent chemotherapy is, of course, rarely used for most patients as the treatment of first choice. The observation of high complete remission rates achieved with combination chemotherapy for Hodgkin's disease (and the subsequent demonstration that some of these remissions have become cures) led to attempts to improve therapy for non-Hodgkin's lymphoma in the same way.[208] Some, but less, success has been achieved.

Early studies suggested that combinations, particularly of cyclophosphamide, vincristine, and prednisolone, induced higher response rates than the drugs given alone, in all subtypes.[209] Some authors suggested very early that the higher the dose of drugs, the more obvious the advantage.[210] With the passage of time, and the increase in the number of drugs available, an almost infinite number of combinations of drugs in different schedules has been evaluated. Combining drugs with different modes of action and different toxicities (allowing maximization of the therapeutic ratio) has been difficult; use of most drugs is restricted by myelosuppression and mucositis. Hemopoietic growth factors undoubtedly aid marrow recovery; it remains to be seen whether enough benefit accrues to increase the number of cures or to make their use cost effective.

Combination chemotherapy has certainly resulted in more cures of aggressive lymphoma than single-agent therapy. It remains to be shown whether different therapies give different qualities of remission or whether there are just "many ways to skin a cat." No convincing evidence has yet shown that combination chemotherapy improves survival of patients with follicular lymphoma, small lymphocytic lymphoma, or lymphoplasmacytic lymphoma.

Myeloablative therapy, using either autologous bone marrow or peripheral blood progenitor cell support, is the most popular means of testing the more-is-better hypothesis. With both mortality and costs falling because of more rapid bone marrow reconstitution using the current techniques and better prevention of infection, many patients are receiving such therapy. No doubt most of the patients now being advised to receive this therapy will survive it and will return to normal. The major issues are whether or not it works, or is worth it (see main specific diseases); a lesser issue is how important in vitro manipulation of the marrow is before reinfusion. A case-matched comparison of the latter for patients reported to the European Blood and Marrow Transplant (EBMT) Registry showed no difference in hematologic engraftment or in the risk of treatment-related death. There was also no significant difference in progression-free survival.[211]

Biologic Therapy. There have been exciting recent developments in this area. Interferon-α (IFN-α) has been under investigation for more than 25 years. Regardless of source, it has been shown to induce partial remission rather slowly in 30% to 40% of patients with follicular lymphoma[212-220]; the results are the same regardless of the source of interferon. Many phase III clinical trials (discussion follows) have been conducted, and a meta-analysis suggests a survival advantage for patients receiving interferon in association with moderately intensive chemotherapy.[221] It may be the treatment of choice for certain cutaneous T-cell lymphomas.[222,223] In contrast to this there is as yet no demonstrated role for interleukin-2 (IL-2).[224-227]

Passive antibody therapy has been investigated over many years[227-230] but until relatively recently has been impeded by technical problems of production, inherent difficulties relating to antigenic modulation, and the risk of stimulating the development of human antimouse antibodies.[231] With the advent of recombinant DNA technology the field has changed dramatically,[232] with the first "humanized" antibody having been licenced for use in lymphoma.[233] Chemo-immunotherapy is already perceived by many as the therapy of choice for several lymphomas.[234,235] The prospect of targeting irradiation with antibodies[236-239] is also now a realistic possibility, with encouraging phase II trials (discussion to follow). Radio-immunoconjugates, with anti-CD20 delivering either I^{131} or Y^{90}, result in higher complete remission rates than antibody alone, and some long freedom from progression has been reported.[240-242] Conjugated immunotoxins showed promise in phase II trials,[243-246] but no benefit has been demonstrated in at least one phase III trial.[247]

Allogeneic bone marrow transplantation (which may be considered immunotherapy) has been used in a relatively small number of patients.[248] Current interest is focused on the use of nonmyeloablative regimens and subsequent administration of donor lymphocyte infusions, in the hope of harnessing the utility of conventional myeloablative therapy in the allogeneic setting (see later discussion).[249-256]

CHARACTERISTICS AND THERAPY OF SPECIFIC LYMPHOMAS

To provide optimal care, a patient with non-Hodgkin's lymphoma should not be approached as belonging to a broad category (e.g., low grade, intermediate grade, aggressive, indolent), but rather as having a specific type of lymphoma. As illustrated in Table 112-9, the clinical characteristics of patients with different lymphomas vary considerably. As presented in the following sections, the appropriate management can also vary widely. Excellent care for a patient with lymphoma requires an accurate and specific diagnosis.

In the following pages, the way to approach patients with the major subtypes of lymphoma is presented. The disorder is divided into those of mature B-cell origin, precursor B- or T-cell origin, and lymphoma of mature T-cell origin. Two lymphomas of mature T-cell origin (i.e., cutaneous T-cell lymphoma/mycosis fungoides and adult T-cell leukemia/lymphoma) are dealt with in separate chapters and will not be discussed here.

Lymphomas of Mature B-Cell Origin: Follicular Lymphoma

Follicular lymphoma accounts for approximately 20% to 30% of non-Hodgkin's lymphoma in North America

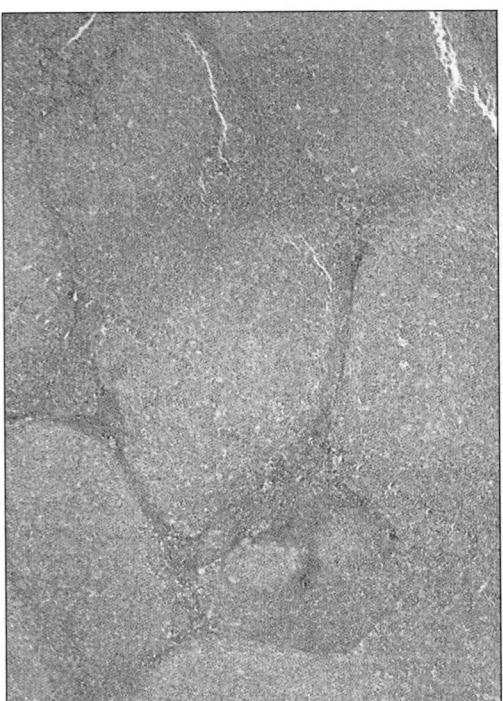

Figure 112-1. Nodular (follicular) lymphoma. The well-defined uniform follicles seen in this low-power photomicrograph are due to compression of reticulin around the neoplastic follicles. (From Dorfman DM, Skarin AT: Hodgkin's disease and non-Hodgkin's lymphoma. In Skarin AT [ed]: Atlas of Diagnostic Oncology, 3rd ed. St. Louis, Mosby, 2003, pp 475-553.)

and Western Europe.[41,117] It is graded according to the proportion of large cells present and the proportion of diffuse infiltration (Figs. 112-1, 112-2, and 112-3; see Table 112-9). Grade 3, particularly when characterized by large diffuse areas, is probably best treated like diffuse large B-cell lymphoma.[257] The most common presentation is that of a middle-aged to older well person, with painless lymphadenopathy usually in multiple sites. Investigation usually demonstrates further impalpable lymphadenopathy and, often, paratrabecular infiltration of bone marrow (Fig. 112-4). Extranodal location outside bone marrow often predicts an aggressive course.

Without intervention, progression, albeit often slow, is the rule. Spontaneous regression in the size of nodes, although rarely disappearance, is not infrequent.[258] To date there is abundant evidence that specific therapy is beneficial at some time for most patients. The median survival has increased over the last half century from 5 to 10 years. Specifically, there is little evidence that immediate intervention in the patient with asymptomatic, disseminated disease improves survival.[259,260] The appearance of monoclonal antibody therapy has changed our understanding on how to treat these patients but the precise role of the therapy is unclear.[233,261,262] In the light of these facts, outside the research setting, treatment is only undertaken if the disease is localized, the patient is "ill," or there is a large tumor mass, vital organ compromise, or unequivocal evidence of progression. There is

TABLE 112-9

Clinical Characteristics of the Major Subtypes of Non-Hodgkin's Lymphoma

	FOLLICULAR (%)	SMALL LYMPHOCYTIC (%)	MALT (%)	MARGINAL ZONE, NODAL (%)	MANTLE CELL (%)	DIFFUSE LARGE B-CELL (%)	MEDIASTINAL LARGE B-CELL (%)	BURKITT'S (%)	LYMPHOBLASTIC (%)	PERIPHERAL T-CELL (%)	ANAPLASTIC LARGE T/NULL CELL (%)
NHL Worldwide	22	7	8	2	6	31	2	4	2	7	2
NHL in North America	32	4	7	—	7	29	1	—	—	2	3
NHL in Europe	18	9	9	—	9	29	3	—	—	5	2
Median Age	59	65	60	58	63	64	37	31	28	61	34
Male	42	53	48	42	74	55	34	89	64	55	69
Stage I	16	4	0	13	10	12	10	25	0	1	16
IE	2	0	39	0	3	13	0	12	0	7	3
II	11	2	0	13	6	13	34	13	11	6	22
IIE	4	3	28	0	1	16	22	12	0	6	10
III	16	8	2	34	9	13	3	0	14	15	10
IV	51	83	31	40	71	33	31	38	75	65	39
B-symptoms	28	33	19	37	28	33	38	22	21	50	53
Elevated LDH	30	41	27	40	40	53	81	75	70	64	45
Karnofsky score ≤70	9	11	15	0	21	24	22	44	29	32	26
Tumor mass >10 cm	28	13	8	0	25	30	52	22	32	12	17
Any extranodal sites	64	80	98	47	81	71	56	78	82	82	59
>1 extranodal site	23	29	31	16	51	29	19	56	43	45	28
Bone marrow positive	42	72	14	32	64	16	3	33	50	36	13
GI tract positive	4	3	50	5	9	18	0	11	4	15	9
International Prognostic Index											
0/1	45	23	44	60	23	35	52	57	33	17	61
2/3	48	64	48	27	54	46	37	29	41	52	18
4/5	7	13	8	13	23	19	11	14	26	31	21

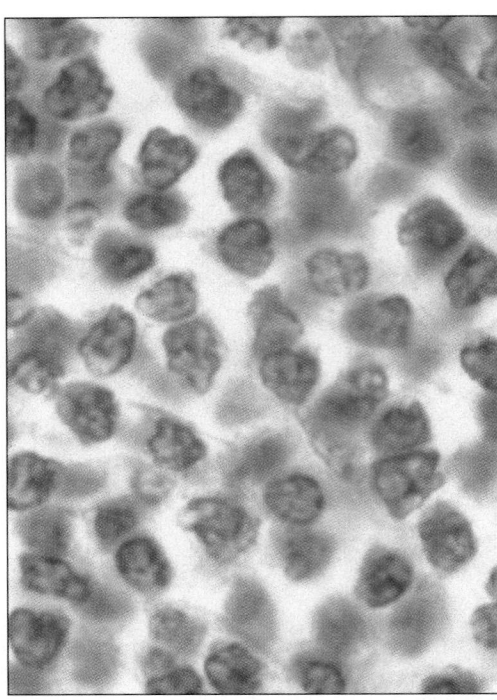

Figure 112-2. Follicular lymphoma, grade I. High-power microscopic section shows small cells with nuclear irregularity, including cleaves (notches) and indentations. (From Dorfman DM, Skarin AT: Hodgkin's disease and non-Hodgkin's lymphoma. In Skarin AT [ed]: Atlas of Diagnostic Oncology, 3rd ed. St. Louis, Mosby, 2003, pp 475–553.)

no uniformly acceptable indication for beginning therapy. The specific therapy is usually based predominantly on the stage of disease at the time. There is increasing evidence that the International Prognostic Index developed for more aggressive lymphoma might be more valuable, but a specific index for follicular lymphoma was recently developed.[131,132,263-265] FLIPI (Follicular Lymphoma International Prognostic Index) is based on five parameters: age, disease stage, number of nodal sites, hemoglobin level, and lactate dehydrogenase (LDH) level. Validation is awaited.

Despite responsiveness to chemotherapy, irradiation, and even to biologic therapy, death occurs, almost always as a consequence of the disease or its treatment.[266] In 40% of patients, at some point, evolution to a histological pattern very similar to that of DLBCL is diagnosed (histologic progression or transformation).[267,268] The pathologic changes are usually accompanied by rapid clinical progression and death, unless remission can be achieved and followed by high-dose therapy with autologous hematopoietic progenitor cell support, after which a proportion of patients will survive long term.[269] Transformation may occur early in the course of the illness, after several recurrences, 9 to 10 years after diagnosis, or never, and the frequency with which it occurs is the same, irrespective of whether treatment is started at the time of diagnosis or later.[267,270] Patients in whom a clinical complete response to first-line treatment was achieved, however, had less or later occurrence of

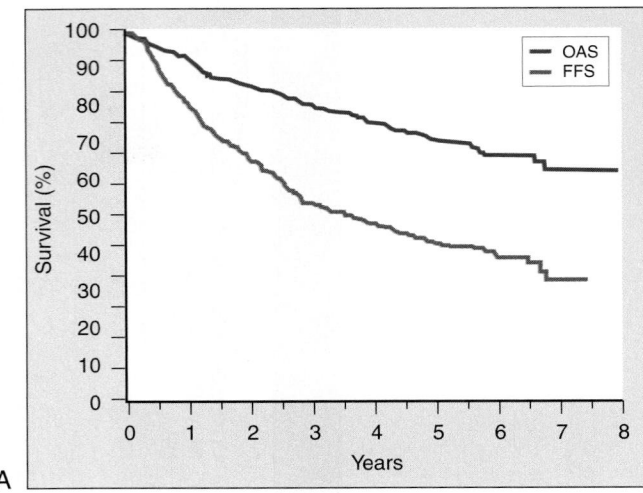

A

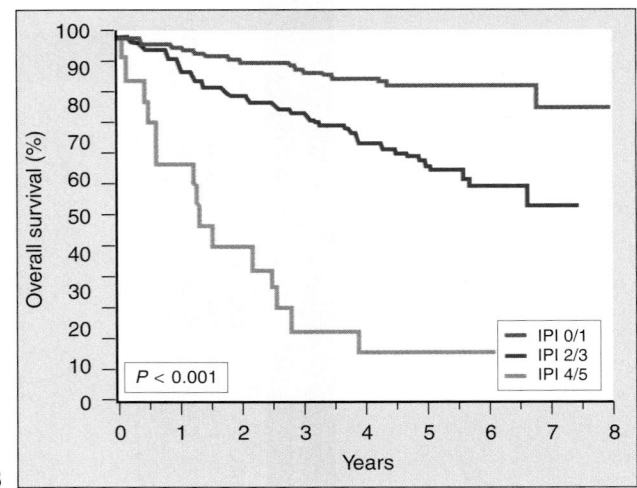

B

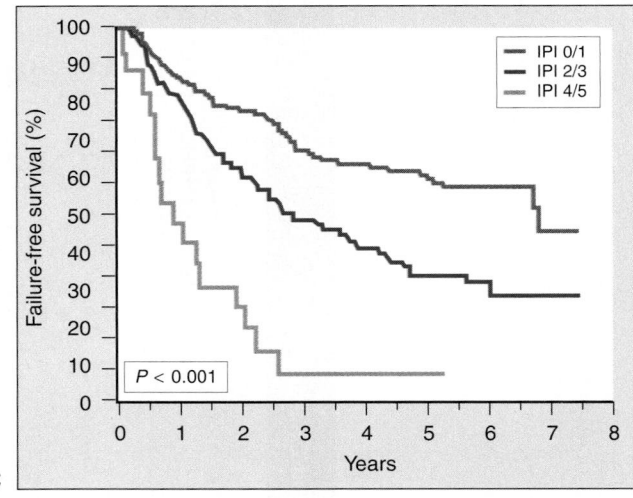

C

Figure 112-3. A, Overall survival (OAS) and failure-free survival (FFS) for an unselected group of patients with follicular lymphoma. **B,** OAS by International Prognostic Index score for patients with follicular lymphoma. **C,** FFS by International Prognostic Index score for patients with follicular lymphoma.

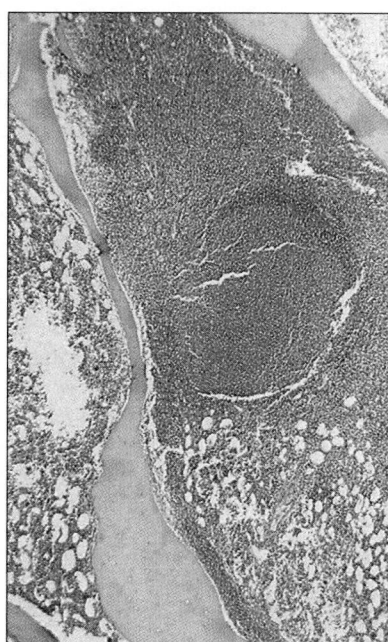

Figure 112-4. Bone marrow involvement in follicular lymphoma showing the typical paratrabecular location. (From Dorfman DM, Skarin AT: Hodgkin's disease and non-Hodgkin's lymphoma. In Skarin AT [ed]: Atlas of Diagnostic Oncology, 3rd ed. St. Louis, Mosby, 2003, pp 475-553.)

transformation.[132] Patients may also present with DLBCL but with evidence of a residual follicular pattern, suggesting that the tumor arose from follicular lymphoma (de novo transformation). Alternatively there may be discordance between a peripheral lymph node that shows follicular histology and, for example, an abdominal mass that on biopsy reveals DLBCL. It is also not unusual to find patients with DLBCL in large tumor masses and, concurrently, paratrabecular infiltration typical of follicular lymphoma in the bone marrow.[149] All these clinical presentations must be considered for a therapeutic point of view as primary DLBCL even if the biologic nature of the tumor is different.

There is now much information available about the cytogenetic and molecular changes that occur in association with transformation.[271-274] It is not unreasonable to envisage a time when these could become the target for therapeutic intervention. If transformation could be prevented, survival of a substantial proportion of patients with follicular lymphoma would certainly be prolonged.

Management

At Diagnosis. There is no definitive indication that patients with the different grades must be treated differently, except perhaps those with grade III or significant areas of diffuse large cell proliferation.[257] On the basis of accumulated data, particularly from Stanford, and two randomized trials, it is reasonable to manage asymptomatic patients expectantly until trouble arises.[259,260] The exception to this is the relatively uncommon circumstance in which the disease is of small volume and local-ized to one (stage I) or even less often to two sites (stage II). It is perceived that involved-field irradiation might be curative or result in such long periods of freedom from progression that it should be prescribed at diagnosis. A dose of 35 Gy, except at a site where local toxicity might be a problem, is the most popular choice. The overall survival curve is excellent, with 80% alive at 15 years, although disease-free survival is not so good.[266,275,276] It has been suggested that adjuvant chemotherapy might improve the results further, but with such long-term survival patterns, certainty about this is difficult. Disease-free survival may be a better end point.[277] Chemotherapy alone may well be as effective; the site of involvement and other general factors may dictate the choice. This strategy designed on data generated with nonprospective studies is certainly valuable, but the overall strategy for treating localized follicular lymphoma has to be reviewed with data generated by monoclonal antibodies. It must be stressed, however, that there are no randomized trials comparing excision surgery and expectant management with immediate intervention; open studies suggest that there may be no advantage to the latter. Failure to achieve complete remission with any intervention is rare; in many instances, the therapy is "adjuvant" to surgical remission. If the disease recurs, further investigation, including repeat biopsy (although this may be difficult to interpret after irradiation), should be undertaken if appropriate and the patient managed as if there were progressive systemic disease.

When Treatment Is First Indicated. In addition to the criteria of constitutional "B" symptoms, vital organ impairment, and unequivocal progression or large tumor, the philosophy of both the patient and the physician will determine when treatment is to begin, and what it will be.

The criteria having been fulfilled, it is disappointing to record that no better therapy than chlorambucil or cyclophosphamide has yet been convincingly demonstrated in randomized trials, but older studies have included all patients, with a need or not to be treated; thus these results may be questioned. Chlorambucil alone given for no more than 6 months as the initial therapy rarely causes symptoms, and even less rarely causes alopecia or admission to hospital.[266,278-280] This simple treatment results in rapid improvement for most patients. Clinical responses are seen in most, and complete remission in the minority. To a certain extent, survival correlates with response to therapy; that is, patients for whom the initial treatment fails live for the shortest time and patients who achieve a remission live longer.[132,266,281,282] Those who achieve a good partial remission or complete remission (CR) live longest. Twenty-five percent of patients who achieve a complete remission will remain in remission for 10 years or more.

Many attempts have been made to improve upon this regimen. In the 1970s, trials compared alkylating agents alone with cyclical combination chemotherapy, usually cyclophosphamide, vincristine, and prednisolone (CVP, COP), usually given six times at 3-weekly intervals.[283,284] Similar responses were achieved with low-dose total-body irradiation.[285] Increasing the number of drugs used or administering maintenance chemotherapy prolongs the freedom from progression time but not survival.

Analysis of a large retrospective series of patients, predominantly with follicular lymphoma treated by the Southwest Oncology Group (SWOG), showed that the addition of doxorubicin to CVP conferred no overall survival advantage, despite some suggestion that the small subset with grade III follicular lymphoma patients may benefit.[279] This approach may cause more rapid tumor regression.

These observations do not imply that alkylating agents are good treatment for follicular lymphoma. They reflect the facts that no chemotherapy regimen is regularly curative, and that the disease usually has a multiply progressing and regressing pattern, potentially eliminating any superficial advantage of an alternative therapy being introduced earlier. The intriguing concept of molecular remission in which cells with rearrangements of the bcl-2 gene consequent to the t(14;18) translocation are reduced to the level of 1 in 10^5 may perhaps introduce a surrogate marker for better therapy that will help discriminate between therapies that are otherwise superficially equivalent.[286]

Much attention has been given to determining whether IFN-α should be incorporated into the early management of follicular lymphoma, either in combination with chemotherapy or after it as maintenance. The results of randomized trials are conflicting, although a meta-analysis finds in its favor under specific circumstances.[287] The facts are as follows. Given alone, IFN-α induces remissions, usually incomplete, and an open phase II trial confirmed that it was feasible to combine IFN-α with chlorambucil in conventional doses.[288]

Following these observations, more than 10 randomized trials have been undertaken to determine whether or not IFN-α confers an advantage given either with chemotherapy as remission induction, with chemotherapy as maintenance, or as maintenance alone. Two of these trials reported both freedom from progression and survival advantages for patients receiving interferon.[289-292] In most of the other studies, the addition of interferon to chemotherapy showed freedom from progression advantages but not a survival advantage[293,294]; others were completely negative.[295] A meta-analysis has been performed on updated individual patient data from these studies. The analysis overall showed both a freedom from recurrence and survival advantage for the interferon arms of the trials, but there was substantial heterogeneity between trials. This was clarified by dividing the trials into those using more (or less) intensive initial chemotherapy. It was concluded that interferon was only beneficial if given in combination with a doxorubicin-containing regimen and in a sufficient dosage.[287]

Role of Purine Analogs. It is highly likely that these compounds will at the very least establish themselves as part of combination therapy within an algorithm of therapy for follicular lymphoma. Most data are available about fludarabine but more are appearing about cladribine. Phase II studies revealed fludarabine to have a response rate in recurrent and refractory follicular lymphoma of about 50%.[201,202] Limited experience in the first treatment setting suggests the overall response rate to be 65%, with approximately half of this being complete.[204] Toxicity is important, particularly with reference to life-threatening infection in heavily pretreated cases. Taken in isolation, these results do not suggest a curative potential for a drug with activity no greater than chlorambucil, but more dangerous toxicity. In the only randomized study comparing fludarabine with an anthracycline-containing combination chemotherapy regimen plus interferon in first-line elderly patients with follicular lymphoma, fludarabine was associated with worse outcome than the combination plus interferon.[296] In another randomized study in relapsing patients, fludarabine alone was associated with a longer progression-free survival and a higher toxicity than CVP, but an identical survival.[297] Thus fludarabine alone is not recommended for first-line treatment.

Combination of fludarabine with mitoxantrone or cyclophosphamide and dexamethasone (FND, FC) yielded better results.[298-300] Once again, the infectious complications must be emphasized, but the overall response rate in previously treated patients exceeded 90%, with 50% complete remissions. In a small number (so far) of patients receiving the therapy as first line, the complete remission rate exceeded 80%, better than anything reported before. If molecular response was observed in both peripheral blood and bone marrow, molecular remission was rare.[301] FND was compared with a complicatied alternating series of regimens, a regimen favored by the M.D. Anderson Cancer Center but not standard, and showed a nearly similar activity: ATT allowed a longer progression-free survival but was more toxic.[302] It must be stressed that there is concern about the long-term effect of fludarabine on the bone marrow, possibly compromising second- or third-line therapy should it not be curative.[303]

Rituximab and Other Monoclonal Antibodies (mAbs). It has been known for many years that anti-idiotype therapy (i.e., producing an antibody specific to the idiotype of the particular immunoglobin expressed by each lymphoma) may result in prolonged remission of lymphoma. It is logistically an unrealistic therapy for an illness that affects 4 per 100,000 people per year, however. Murine monoclonal antibodies were tested in the 1980s and were unsatisfactory, partly because of toxicity, partly because of antigenic modulation, and partly because of the development of human antimouse antibodies (HAMA), limiting repeated administration.[304]

The construction of a humanized anti-CD20 antibody (rituximab) led to its introduction into clinical trials.[305] Rituximab has now undergone a full development and is licensed for use in recurrent and refractory follicular lymphoma. Given in a schedule of four injections at weekly intervals, the antibody results in an overall response rate of 50–60%, only few being complete.[233] This result is achieved with minimal toxicity, apart from reactions to the first injection. Due to this efficacy, rituximab was tested as initial therapy; only 75% of patients responded and less than 50% with a complete response.[306,307] Moreover nearly all patients progressed between 1 and 3 years after treatment, even those with a molecular remission. This drug presumably having action through antibody-dependent cellular toxicity and complement-dependent cytolysis, response seems logically to depend on immunologic capability of the patients.[308,309] Some authors have tried to maintain this response with repeated infusions and showed significantly prolonged remissions.[310] Because of this relatively disappointing effect when used alone and because of a theoretical rationale for expecting synergy with chemotherapy,[311-313] it has been tested in open phase II studies in sequence with CHOP (cyclophosphamide, doxorubicin, vincristine, and prednisone); the response rate was 100% and median duration of response longer than 6 years.[314] Currently, various combinations of rituximab plus chemotherapy are tested in different randomized studies to define the best strategy of using this important drug. Other monoclonal antibodies are currently being developed.

When the First Treatment Fails.

Management at this time is influenced by: (1) how success and failure (i.e., PR, GPR, CR) are defined; (2) the manifestations of failure; (3) the available options; (4) the initial therapy; and (5) of course, the wishes of the patient. Failure, in follicular lymphoma, is usually considered to be the attainment of less than a good partial remission,[266,315] or progression after PR or CR as currently defined. Once again, the general circumstances of the patient will have a major bearing on the decision.

Failure to Achieve an Adequate Response in First Line or Later.

This is a serious situation, demanding further, this time effective, therapy if survival aim is to be longer than a year. Repeat lymph node biopsy of particularly suspicious sites should be undertaken (to show or eliminate a transformed lymphoma), as should formal restaging if further action is deemed wise. Combination chemotherapy, CHOP (cyclophosphamide, doxorubicin, vincristine, and prednisone), DHAP (dexamethasone, high-dose cytarabine, and cisplatin), or a fludarabine-containing combination are probably the first next choice of therapy in terms of proven efficacy today, provided there is no evidence of transformation. If not used before, combination with rituximab is suitable because of the potentiation of both effects.

If successful, many would argue that consolidation with high-dose therapy and peripheral blood progenitor cell rescue should be advised.[316] Further failure is an indication for more experimental therapy. Genuine chemorefractoriness so early in the course of the disease is uncommon; allogeneic bone marrow transplantation, either of the conventional or the nonmyeloablative type, may be considered in the younger, otherwise fit patient.[254,317] Palliation, either with irradiation or general support, must always be considered.

Progression after Remission (Recurrence) Not Necessarily First Time.

Provided that the response has been of reasonable duration, retreatment with the same therapy that had been used previously is likely to yield a similar response rate (if this regimen does not use drugs with known cumulative toxicity).[266,318] Thereafter remissions become shorter. While possibly adequate for the elderly and otherwise infirm, this is essentially an unsatisfactory outcome.

If biopsy at the time of progression or recurrence reveals transformation to an aggressive lymphoma, treatment as for the latter, with a doxorubicin-containing regimen (e.g., CHOP), is mandatory. In younger patients, this may appropriately be followed by high-dose therapy with peripheral blood progenitor support.[319]

Consolidation of Remission with Myeloablative Therapy and Hematopoietic Stem Cell Support.

This approach is being used increasingly, at least in Europe, peripheral blood progenitor cells having superceded bone marrow for supporting the treatment. The data may be summarized as follows. Employed in second or subsequent complete or good partial remission, this treatment yields very significantly longer remissions than had previously been achieved, if historical controls are to be accepted.[320-322] This treatment has been proven superior in a small randomized study, the CUP trial.[323] While the judicious use of antibiotics, platelet transfusion, and growth factors has reduced the early mortality to less than 5%, there is a worrying incidence of myelodsyplasia and acute myeloid leukemia, the precise etiology of which is not clear. Some encouragement may be taken from the fact that survival after failure of high-dose therapy does not result in a worse prognosis than failure after conventional therapy at the equivalent time.[324] Open phase II studies have tested the hypothesis that the best outcome might be obtained if the therapy were used in first remission.[325-327] Preliminary data of randomized phase III trials confirm the benefit associated with intensification in first-line young patients, but these studies were realized before the advent of monoclonal antibodies.[328]

Such data as there are concerning molecular remission lend strength to the hypothesis that it is worth attaining. Attempts to purge either autologous bone marrow or peripheral blood of contaminating lymphoma cells have been variously successful, interpretation of the results depending to a considerable extent on the PCR techniques used to detect cells bearing the bcl-2 rearrangement.[140,329,330] It seems probable that this is the best therapy under some circumstances for patients who have had more than one episode of follicular lymphoma.

Passive Immunotherapy.

Monoclonal antibodies such as rituximab have shown their activity in relapsing and refractory patients with follicular lymphoma. While 60% to 70% of the patients respond to this treatment, only 10% or less reach a complete response and the median duration of response is usually 18 months, this treatment is certainly recommended in relapsing patients before high-dose therapy.[262] While this response rate makes it unlikely that it will cure any patients with follicular lymphoma, it may well have a role in response induction for patient relapsing after chemotherapy. The extremely low toxicity profile of the therapy is certainly popular with patients.

Other monoclonal antibodies, such as epratuzumab (anti-CD22), are currently tested alone or in combination with rituximab.[331,332] A definitive advantage over rituximab remains to be defined.

Targeted Irradiation. Another exciting approach is the use of murine anti-CD20 to "deliver" iodine-131 (^{131}I; iodine I 131 tositumomab)[331] or Yttrium-90 (^{90}Y; yttrium-90 ibritumomab tiuxetan).[333] Smaller numbers of patients have been treated, but the results in heavily pretreated patients with low-dose irradiation seem superior to those obtained with rituximab, with the overall response rate being 90%, 50% of the responses being complete.[333-336] The duration of response, however, was not longer than with rituximab in a randomized trial available.[333] The therapy is complex to organize, but relatively simple to administer and with low immediate toxicity, provided the bone marrow is not heavily infiltrated. Cases of secondary myelodysplasia have been described and the exact risk is not yet well known.

Anti-CD20 ^{131}I has also been used in high doses, requiring hematopoietic stem cell support as an alternative to other myeloablative therapy.[337] Once again, the therapy is complex and requires admission to the hospital in lead-lined rooms while the patient is "hot." The results are most impressive, however. As with the "naked" antibody, it remains to be seen how this treatment could be incorporated into a curative or better palliative strategy of therapy for follicular lymphoma.

Active Immunotherapy. This is at a much more experimental stage. Suffice it to say, there are now many practicable ways in which the unique antigen of follicular lymphoma may be presented to the patient, whether as antigen itself, DNA, or via dendritic cells.[338,339] Preliminary clinical studies suggest that under the right conditions, humoral and cellular responses occur and that they correlate with outcome.[340] The inability of the host to recognize the antigen remains a stubborn problem that is being addressed in a number of ways.[341,342]

Antisense oligonucleotides to bcl-2 have been tested in a phase I trial,[343] the rationale being based on experiments in a murine model.[344]

It will be many years before it is clear whether this plethora of new therapies will alter the natural history of follicular lymphoma, but there is room for hope and the design of better nontoxic algorithms of therapy.

Small Lymphocytic Lymphoma B-Cell Chronic Lymphocytic Leukemia and Lymphoplasmacytoid Lymphoma

These B-cell lymphoid malignancies will be considered together, since they represent a spectrum of entities, the interrelationships of which have been redefined in the WHO classification. Both the Working Formulation and the Kiel classification recognized small lymphocytic lymphoma as the nodal counterpart of B-cell CLL.[58,60] The semantic problems surrounding this statement have often been repeated, being determined predominantly by the differences in referral patterns of patients with and without a leukemic blood picture and the relative infrequency of lymph node biopsy in patients with B-CLL.

At the other end of the spectrum, the lymphoplasmacytoid malignancies were much more precisely defined in the Kiel classification than in the Working Formulation. Originally designated as immunocytoma, they were subsequently subdivided into lymphoplasmacytoid, lymphoplasmacytic, and pleomorphic types, the former being by far the most common and the latter being by far the least frequent. In the WHO classification, the lymphoplasmacytoid subtype of immunocytoma of the Kiel classification becomes a variant of small lymphocytic lymphoma (SLL)/B-CLL because these tumors retain the immunophenotype of B-CLL. The lymphoplasmacytic subtype of the Kiel classification becomes a single, uncommon type of lymphoma (i.e., lymphoplasmacytoid lymphoma/immunocytoma in the WHO classification) and the pleomorphic type disappears. Some of these subtypes are in fact marginal zone lymphoma, the difference being detected only by the phenotype and the clinical presentation.

Half of Waldenström's macroglobulinemia[108,345,346] corresponds to the bone marrow counterpart of lymphoplasmacytic lymphomas that often present with splenomegaly, without lymphadenopathy, but with symptoms of increased viscosity or bone marrow failure, and may be characterized by the morphologic appearance in the bone marrow of either plasmacytoid or plasmacytic cells and a high circulating level of IgM, the other half being splenic marginal zone lymphoma.[347,348]

An accurate statement about the incidence of these subtypes depends upon the inclusion or exclusion of patients with leukemic presentations. The incidence of CLL displays considerable international variation, being between 2 and 5 per 100,000 in North America and Western Europe and much less frequent in Asia. In the international study, SLL and the lymphoplasmacytoid and lymphoplasmacytic lymphomas together represented only about 8% of cases reported.[117] It is to be hoped that the widespread adoption of the WHO classification will gradually allow better comparison of data sets about these closely related entities. Inevitably, as yet there is relatively little information, and experience from the past tends to emphasize the semantic issues.

The majority of patients with SLL/B-CLL lymphoplasmacytic subtype are older, and more likely to be men than women. They may present with generalized lymphadenopathy, sometimes of long standing, problems associated with bone marrow failure, hypergammaglobulinemia, or less commonly, with constitutional "B" symptoms. Early-stage disease is most uncommon. In patients with Waldenström's macroglobulinemia, the clinical picture is often dominated by symptoms of hyperviscosity (e.g., dizziness, tiredness, and a propensity for bleeding from the mucous membranes). There may also be symptoms due to cryoglobulinemia and cold agglutinin anemia. In addition, some patients develop peripheral neuropathy, renal disease, and amyloidosis.[349,350]

Twenty years ago, Pangelis described a series of cases of small lymphocytic lymphoma and B-CLL, comparing and contrasting their outcome.[351] While showing different clinical presentations and hematologic findings, it was concluded that the entities were histopathologically very similar, although it is noteworthy that there were some cases with monoclonal gammopathy. These cases might otherwise have been defined as lymphoplasmacytoid lymphoma in the Kiel classification, or the plasmacytoid variant of SLL in the WHO classification. No survival differences were demonstrated. Similar conclusions might be drawn from a series from the M.D. Anderson Cancer Center.[352] The earliest paper validating the prognostic significance of the Kiel classification from Kiel clearly demonstrated that if lymphoplasmacytoid lymphoma were equated with the earlier definition of immunocytoma, overall this group had a significantly worse prognosis than SLL.[74]

A large retrospective study from St. Bartholomew's Hospital analyzed the outcome for patients with immunocytoma and compared it with that of patients with B-CLL/SLL treated over the same period.[353] An attempt to reduce the risk of bias was made by conducting the analysis first to include all patients and then only those in whom lymph node biopsy had been performed as in the International Project. The results were the same for both groups. It was shown that the immunocytomas were a repeatedly remitting and recurring group of diseases, with fewer complete remissions and shorter progression-free survival than follicular lymphoma. There were significant differences in survival between the three subtypes, the smallest (now nonexistent!) group having by far the worst outcome. An interesting observation, revealed as a consequence of a rigorous repeat biopsy policy, was the frequency of transformation to more aggressive looking histology comparable with DLBC lymphoma. Comparison of overall survival between B-CLL/SLL and immunocytoma showed a significant difference. When the analysis extended to a comparison of SLL/B-CLL with the individual subtypes of immunocytoma, however, it became apparent that there was only a trend in difference between SLL and the lymphoplasmacytoid subtype. This would appear to justify the inclusion of lymphoplasmacytoid lymphoma (Kiel) within SLL, provided that it may be described as a variant. Similarly, the retention of the lymphoplasmacytic type as a distinct entity, albeit small, is warranted by its quite distinct pathologic features.

Management

The same principles of management are applied to these subtypes of lymphoma as to follicular lymphoma, with therapy being recommended only if it is clinically indicated. The patient population being generally older and more likely to have comorbid problems, there has to date been less enthusiasm for aggressive intervention.[354-358] Unfortunately, this philosophy has been reinforced by the failure of most recent attempts to improve the situation.

As with CLL, purine analogs (i.e., fludarabine, cladribine, and pentostatin) alone and in combination have held the greatest promise in terms of new chemotherapy for SLL/B-CLL and the lymphoplasmacytoid lymphomas. The efficacy of fludarabine alone (and cladribine) in previously treated B-CLL inevitably extended interest further, with response rates between 30% and 50%.[205,359-363]

Several studies investigating combinations of fludarabine with cyclophosphamide[364] or with mitoxantrone and high doses of dexamethasone[365] have been encouraging, although substantial toxicity has been seen. The combination of fludarabine with cyclophosphamide and rituximab has yielded a high proportion of complete remissions, previously a rare outcome in this disease.[366]

The relative seniority of many of the patients as well as the incompleteness of clearance of bone marrow infiltration makes high-dose therapy with hematopoietic stem cell support inappropriate for the majority. Hence the data about it are sparse and refer to highly selected patients. The declining mortality of the procedure, however, coupled with some encouraging early results certainly warrant further investigation. For those younger patients with an HLA-matched sibling, allogeneic transplantation with low-dose conditioning is finding increasing popularity within the research setting.[249-251] It will become clear when larger numbers of patients have been treated how relevant this will be. Monoclonal antibody therapy with rituximab has been evaluated in a single open phase II study in Europe with less impressive results than have been achieved in follicular lymphoma, the response being less than one third in patients with lymphoplasmacytoid lymphoma and less than one fifth in those with small lymphocytic lymphoma (specifically not CLL).[367] Studies in progress will elucidate whether the alternative antibody alemtuzumab directed at CD52 is any better.[368,369] Monoclonal antibodies targeted with radionuclide have not really been investigated in this disease because of the large bone marrow involvement.

In patients with Waldenström's macroglobulinemia, plasmapheresis rapidly reduces the level of IgM but needs to be used together with effective chemotherapy for the lymphoma. Until recently, therapy comprised chlorambucil and prednisolone.[370-372] The use of more intensive therapy has not improved survival.[363] Fludarabine and cladribine have resulted in high response rates[205,373,374] and fludarabine, mitoxantrone, and dexamethasone (FMD) is now being evaluated. Rituximab is also active.[375]

While cure remains a distant prospect for this relatively chronic group of diseases, evidence is accumulating about an increasing range of options that may be appropriate at different times during the clinical course. Without doubt also, supportive care in terms of antimicrobial therapy has led to an ability to improve quality of life.

Marginal Zone B-Cell Lymphoma

In 1983, Isaacson and Wright described a malignant lymphoma of mucosa-associated lymphoid tissue (i.e., MALT) that had a specific histologic pattern and equally specific clinical features.[376] The concept of the MALT lymphomas has since been characterized further and extended to include a spectrum of sites and different presentations.[377] It should be noted that the commonly used name *MALT lymphoma* can be confusing, since not all MALT lymphomas occur at mucosal sites. The nomenclature for other types of marginal zone B-cell lymphoma (MZL) is also somewhat confusing (Fig. 112-5; see Table 112-9). Most lymphomas derived from the marginal zone present in extranodal sites and have the features of MALT lymphomas. Regional lymph nodes may be involved (particularly in gastric and salivary gland MALT lymphomas), the involved lymph nodes have a characteristic appearance (monocytoid B-cell lymphoma), and it has been suggested that the latter represents the nodal variant of MALT lymphoma.

Splenic MZL has been considered as a variant of these MALT lymphoma but more and more data show that it is a different lymphoma.[347] Usually, it only involves spleen (which may be very large), blood, and bone marrow. An M-component or an autoimmune cytopenia is frequent. Some cases described as Waldenström macroglobulinemia were in fact splenic MZL. The disease is very indolent but may disseminate or transform as MALT lymphomas.

Extranodal B-Cell Lymphoma of MALT

MALT lymphomas are usually localized, and are seen most frequently in the stomach, lung, salivary gland, thyroid, and lacrimal gland.[378] They may less often involve the orbit, skin, conjunctiva, breast, bladder, kidney, thymus, or essentially and other epithelial site.[379] Apart from a swelling in the relevant area (in the case of salivary gland tumors), patients may be otherwise asymptomatic; these are slow-growing tumors. Recurrence may occur at the original site or at another MALT lymphoma–associated one. However, 30% of them are disseminated with two or more sites at diagnosis but with the same indolent course.[380]

The diagnosis of MALT lymphoma is usually applied to a small cell lymphoma. MALT lymphomas can undergo histologic progression to a large cell lymphoma, however. The term *high-grade MALT* is sometimes misused to describe this situation. These patients should not be confused with having a typical small cell MALT lymphoma and need to be treated like any other diffuse large B-cell lymphoma.

There is an association with autoimmune diseases: for example, MALT lymphomas of salivary glands are associated with Sjögren's syndrome[11]; MALT lymphoma of the thyroid is associated with Hashimoto's thyroiditis.[381,382] The development of gastric MALT lymphomas has been attributed to antigenic stimulation associated with chronic *Helicobacter pylori* gastritis.[383] Indeed, standard treatment for early-stage disease in the stomach is now antibiotic therapy to eradicate the infection. Regression of lymphoma then occurs in some patients.[84]

Management

Localized gastric MALT lymphomas are best treated initially with a combination of antibiotics and antiacid.[384] The chances for remission are inversely related to depth of invasion[385] and reduced by the presence of the t(11;18).[386] Even in complete responders there is often molecular evidence of persistence of monoclonal B-cells.[387] In patients not responding to antibiotics, radiotherapy usually will yield complete remission.[388,389] When disease

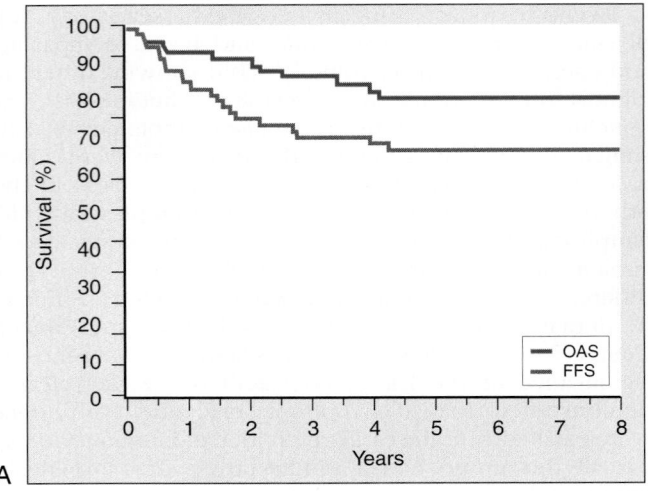

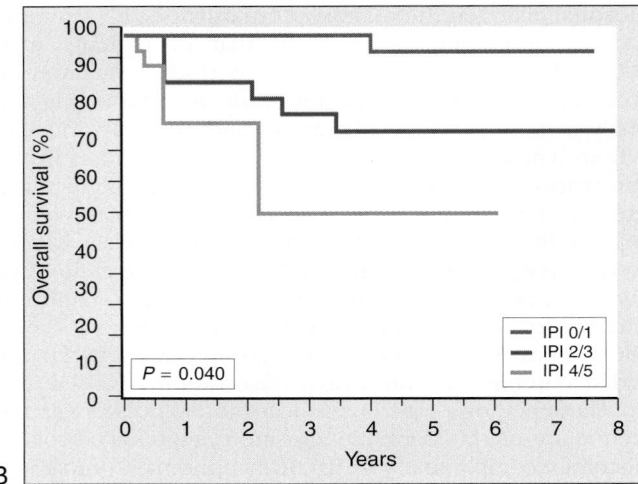

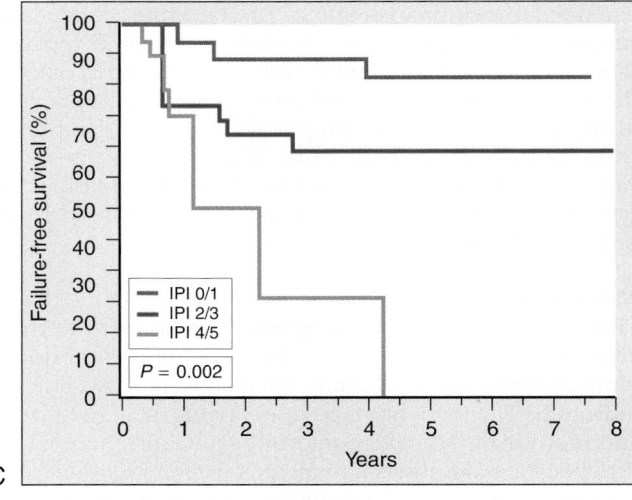

Figure 112-5. A, Overall survival (OAS) and failure-free survival (FFS) for an unselected group of patients with marginal zone (MALT) B-cell lymphoma. **B,** OAS by International Prognostic Index score for patients with marginal zone B-cell lymphoma. **C,** FFS by International Prognostic Index score for patients with marginal zone B-cell lymphoma, MALT type.

progresses, no standard treatment is recognized and several options are probably associated with the same outcome. Surgery is certainly too aggressive to be used early in the disease and radiation therapy or single agent chemotherapy should be favored. Multidrug regimens are only used after transformation.

For nongastric MALT lymphomas, there is no universally recommended therapy, several possibilities being associated with a good outcome. Surgical excision is often required to make the diagnosis. Further treatment may not be needed. Where the tumor has been incompletely excised, radiotherapy may be appropriate. Some would use adjuvant chlorambucil.[390-393]

In the few patients who present with more widespread disease, systemic chemotherapy and rituximab are effective; the precise regimen will depend on the pathology. The majority of MALT lymphomas respond to treatment as for follicular lymphoma (e.g., chlorambucil).[394] Evolution to DLBC lymphoma can occur, however, for which a doxorubicin-containing regimen is necessary.[377]

Nodal Marginal Zone B-Cell Lymphoma with Monocytoid B-Cells

This is a rare disease, mainly of older women. Most patients present with lymphadenopathy, often in the neck.[395] Histologically, these tumors are considered to be the lymphomatous counterpart of monocytoid B-cells but typical monocytoid B-cells may be absent. The latter are reactive cells described in association with infections (e.g., toxoplasmosis) and sometimes in the context of other subtypes of non-Hodgkin's lymphomas and Hodgkin's disease.

The relationship with MALT lymphomas is complex. As mentioned previously, they may occur in the context of a MALT lymphoma (e.g., lymph node involvement secondary to a gastric or parotid MALT lymphoma).[396] They may occur in the absence of extranodal disease and are often more aggressive than MALT lymphoma. The immunophenotype is characteristically indistinguishable from that of MALT lymphomas.[85]

There is little consensus about treatment, management being dictated by the site involved and the age of the patient. In general, however, the principles of therapy described for follicular lymphomas can be applied.

Splenic Marginal Zone Lymphoma

This entity includes that previously referred to as splenic lymphoma with villous lymphocytes. Typically, patients present with splenomegaly without lymphadenopathy. Histologically the appearance is somewhat similar to that of small lymphocytic lymphoma but the immunophenotype differs, the splenic lymphoma characteristically being CD5, CD23, and CD10 negative.[397,398] The cells are thought to derive from the cells of the normal splenic marginal zone. Bone marrow involvement is common; there may be a paraprotein.

A splenectomy is often required to establish the diagnosis, and remission afterwards may be prolonged.[399] After splenectomy, symptoms due to bone marrow infil-

tration usually supervene eventually. When this occurs, most patients have been treated as for chronic lymphocytic leukemia with chlorambucil and prednisolone. Rituximab has a great efficacy in this disease, however, and may be favored because of the little toxicity in these elderly patients. Multidrug regimens are kept for histologic transformation.[399]

Mantle Cell Lymphoma

Representing only 6% of the lymphomas,[400] mantle cell lymphoma has been the focus of much attention and undoubtedly reflects one of the major improvements of the WHO classification over the Working Formulation (see Table 112-9). The clinicopathologic entity has now been very precisely defined as predominantly an illness of older men, manifest by generalized lymphadenopathy, sometimes massive splenomegaly, with peripheral blood involvement and a predilection for diffuse polypoid lesions in the gastrointestinal tract.[76] It is an excellent example of the confusion generated by the different use of the term *grade* in the Kiel classification and the Working Formulation, being low grade (pathologic) in the former and intermediate grade (clinical) in the latter. The characteristic morphology has been precisely documented and is usually accompanied by the t(11;14) translocation and rearrangement of the cyclin D1 gene (bcl-1), now identifiable with monoclonal antibodies.[66,71,72,401,402]

There is, however, no doubt that this is the malignant lymphoma of which the natural history has been least influenced, at least until recently, by the advent of radiotherapy and chemotherapy. A multitude of reasonably sized retrospective analyses have shown the median survival to be about 3 years with very few long survivors,[403-410] the outcome being best in the small proportion of patients with localized disease. While there are also anecdotal patients with advanced disease who behave like those with chronic lymphocytic leukemia, for most it is an inevitably progressive illness, interrupted by partial remission of decreasing frequency and duration, and during which transformation may occur.[407]

Management

To date, the major problem remains the achievement of complete remission. Until 10 years ago, no chemotherapy regimen was associated with a longer event-free or overall survival, even if a doxorubicin-containing regimen gave a higher response rate. Until recently the best remission rates have been reached with a combination of CHOP plus rituximab.[411] More aggressive approaches have been piloted in selected younger patients. At the M.D. Anderson Cancer Center hyper-CVAD with rituximab has been reported to be tolerable and to have a much higher complete response rate than previously achieved.[412] In reasonably fit patients this regimen achieves complete remission in the majority.[413] High-dose chemoradiotherapy or chemotherapy with hematopoietic stem cell rescue has been evaluated at several transplant centers, mostly in patients responding to conventional therapy[414-419] The morbidity and mortality have been acceptable, and long-term disease-free survival seems achievable in some patients. In patients young and fit enough for the procedure, allogeneic transplant seems effective.

The expression of CD20 on the cell surface makes mantle cell lymphoma an obvious target for antibody therapy, particularly given its limited toxicity and the general state of health of many of the patients. Two phase II trials in Europe have tested anti-CD20 in both newly diagnosed and previously treated mantle cell lymphoma.[364,420] The overall response rate is between 35% and 40%, with 10% to 15% complete remissions. Given that the therapy comprises four injections at weekly intervals, this might be important, even if only as palliation.

Diffuse Large B-Cell Lymphoma

Diffuse large B-cell lymphoma (DLBCL) is the commonest of the non-Hodgkin's lymphomas accounting for approximately one third of cases in the WHO classification (Figs. 112-6, 112-7, and 112-8; see Table 112-9). DLBCL carries a significantly better prognosis than peripheral T-cell lymphoma, which was lumped with it in the Working Formulation.[117,421-423] It includes several subtypes not completely characterized and only recognizable by molecular analysis[424-426] Some entities such as primary mediastinal lymphoma or intravascular lymphoma have been described to be of different origin and to bear a different outcome, but currently they are treated with the same regimens as other DLBCLs. A significant number of patients are diagnosed at the time with DLBCL, but are in fact transformed indolent lymphomas, not previously diagnosed. This may be suspected because of bone marrow infiltration with the indolent lymphoma, a mixture of indolent lymphoma and DLBCL in lymph nodes, or the presence of specific genetic abnormalities. These patients must be treated as de novo DLBCL, however.

Management

Everything argues in favor of the urgent initiation of therapy with curative intent. The diagnosis having been established, investigations should be completed within 1 week and therapy begun. The best chance for cure is with the first-line treatment and thus precise treatment is essential. Only a minority of relapsing patients may be salvaged and even fewer refractory patients.

Localized Disease. Even though radiation therapy has been clearly shown to be curative for a selected, rather small proportion of those presenting with aggressive, clinically localized (i.e., stage I and minimal stage II) DLBCL, it is now rarely the therapy of first choice.[427-437] The question usually raised is whether adjuvant radiation therapy should be given after the apparently successful induction of remission with chemotherapy.

Early attempts to improve on the results with irradiation alone (for *all* patients with stage I and II disease) focused on the use of involved field or modestly extended-field irradiation followed by CVP, usually six cycles.[438-444] Several randomized trials showed that this regimen

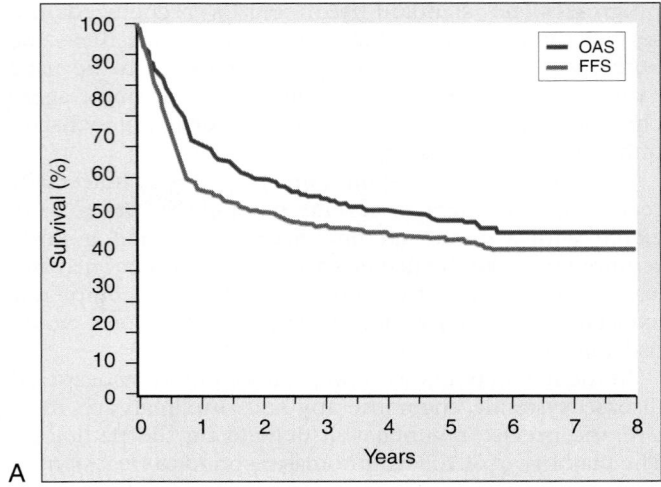

A

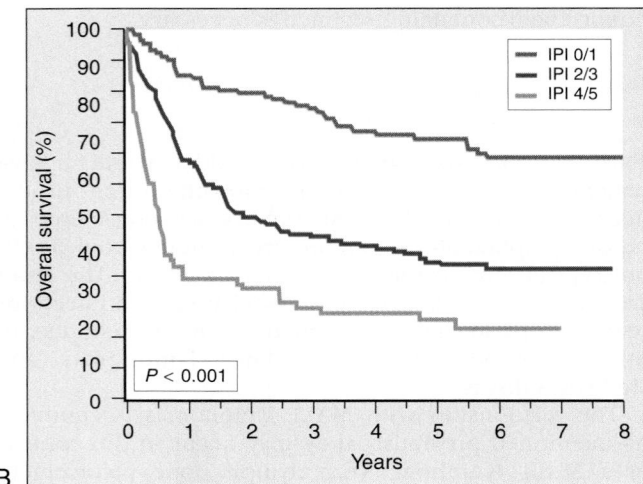

B

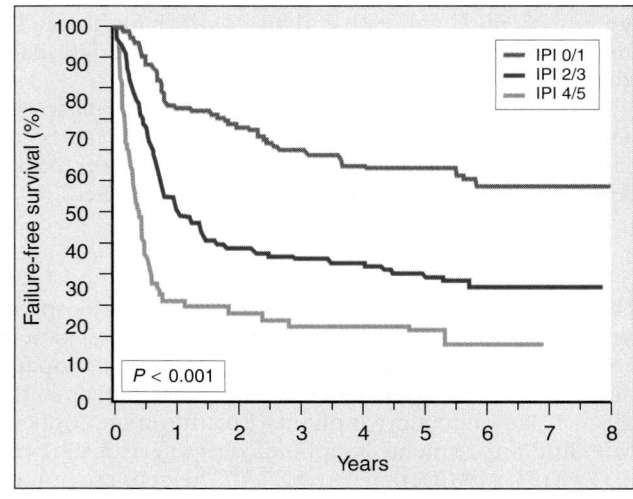

C

Figure 112-6. A, Overall survival (OAS) and failure-free survival (FFS) for an unselected group of patients with diffuse large B-cell lymphoma. **B,** OAS by International Prognostic Index score for patients with diffuse large B-cell lymphoma. **C,** FFS by International Prognostic Index score for patients with diffuse large B-cell lymphoma.

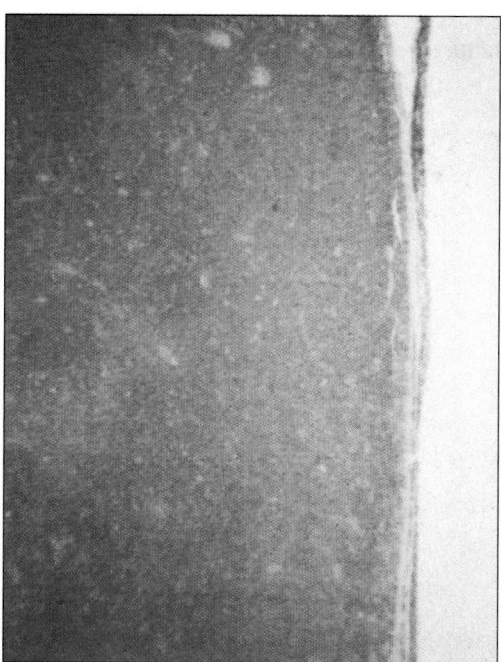

Figure 112-7. Low magnification of a diffuse lymphoma reveals complete effacement of the normal nodal architecture by a diffuse lymphomatous process. (From Dorfman DM, Skarin AT: Hodgkin's disease and non-Hodgkin's lymphoma. In Skarin AT [ed]: Atlas of Diagnostic Oncology, 3rd ed. St. Louis, Mosby, 2003, pp 475–553.)

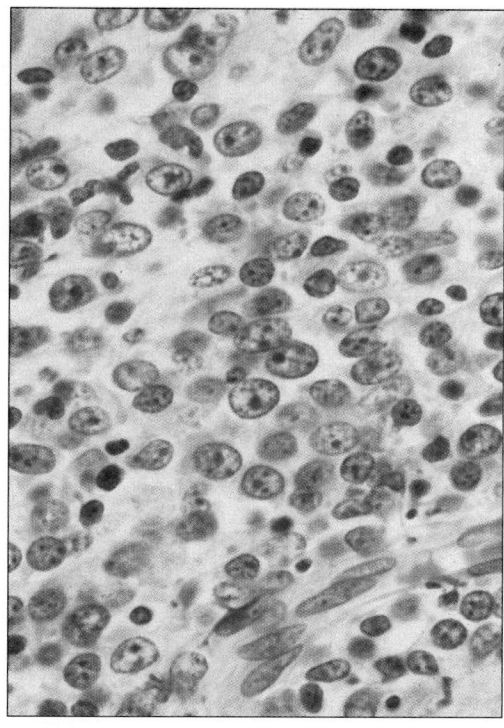

Figure 112-8. Large cell lymphoma: large noncleaved cell type, NCI subgroup G. High magnification reveals large cells with predominantly round nuclei, distinct nucleoli, and a moderate amount of cytoplasm. Small lymphocytes in the background allow size comparison. Note the lack of well-defined cell borders and an absence of an organized pattern, features more commonly associated with carcinomas. (From Dorfman DM, Skarin AT: Hodgkin's disease and non-Hodgkin's lymphoma. In Skarin AT [ed]: Atlas of Diagnostic Oncology, 3rd ed. St. Louis, Mosby, 2003, pp 475–553.)

improved the freedom from recurrence pattern. Advent of the doxorubicin-containing combination encouraged the evaluation of chemotherapy as the primary therapy for localized aggressive disease. This strategy was highly successful in preliminary reports.[445,446] These findings, coupled with the observation that recurrences after irradiation therapy were usually at distant sites, have led to the use of adjuvant irradiation after chemotherapy for localized aggressive disease. Circumstantial evidence from a number of trials supports this regimen; an 80% survival at 5 years for *all* patients with stage I and II disease, regardless of site or bulk of tumor, has been reported.[447–450] Certain issues remain, however, notably whether any irradiation is necessary. Most physicians have seen the benefit of such radiation in localized Hodgkin's lymphoma and are reluctant not to use it in DLBCL patients.

One trial found improved failure-free and overall survival with CHOP × 4 and involved field radiotherapy over CHOP × 8.[451] The advantage declined with long follow-up, however. Another study compared CHOP × 4 with CHOP × 4 followed by radiotherapy in patients older than 60 years of age.[452] There was no difference in outcome with CHOP alone except for a better overall survival in patients older than 70 years of age. Finally, a recently reported trial compared CHOP × 3 followed by radiotherapy with ACVBP alone and found significantly better disease-free and overall survival with ACVBP.[453]

It does appear that the amount of chemotherapy can be reduced by half if adjuvant irradiation is going to be given,

but is there clinical advantage in using radiation therapy given the higher long-term toxicity of combined treatment?[442,446,451]

The current recommendations for primary therapy of localized diffuse large B-cell disease may be disputed. Bulky stage I or stage II disease should be treated like advanced disease, with combination chemotherapy. Irradiation should only be given if complete remission is not achieved, when doubt exists, or if the physician prefers to deliver less chemotherapy. In the absence of specific indications, prophylactic intrathecal therapy is not indicated.

No evidence supports the use of maintenance therapy. Management of failure or recurrence is the same as that for recurrence in patients who initially presented advanced disease.

Advanced Disease: The Initial Decision. All reports indicate that combination chemotherapy should be instituted as a matter of urgency at the first presentation in all patients with advanced diffuse large B-cell lymphoma if normal long-term survival is the goal. For some elderly patients, an aggressive approach will be inappro-

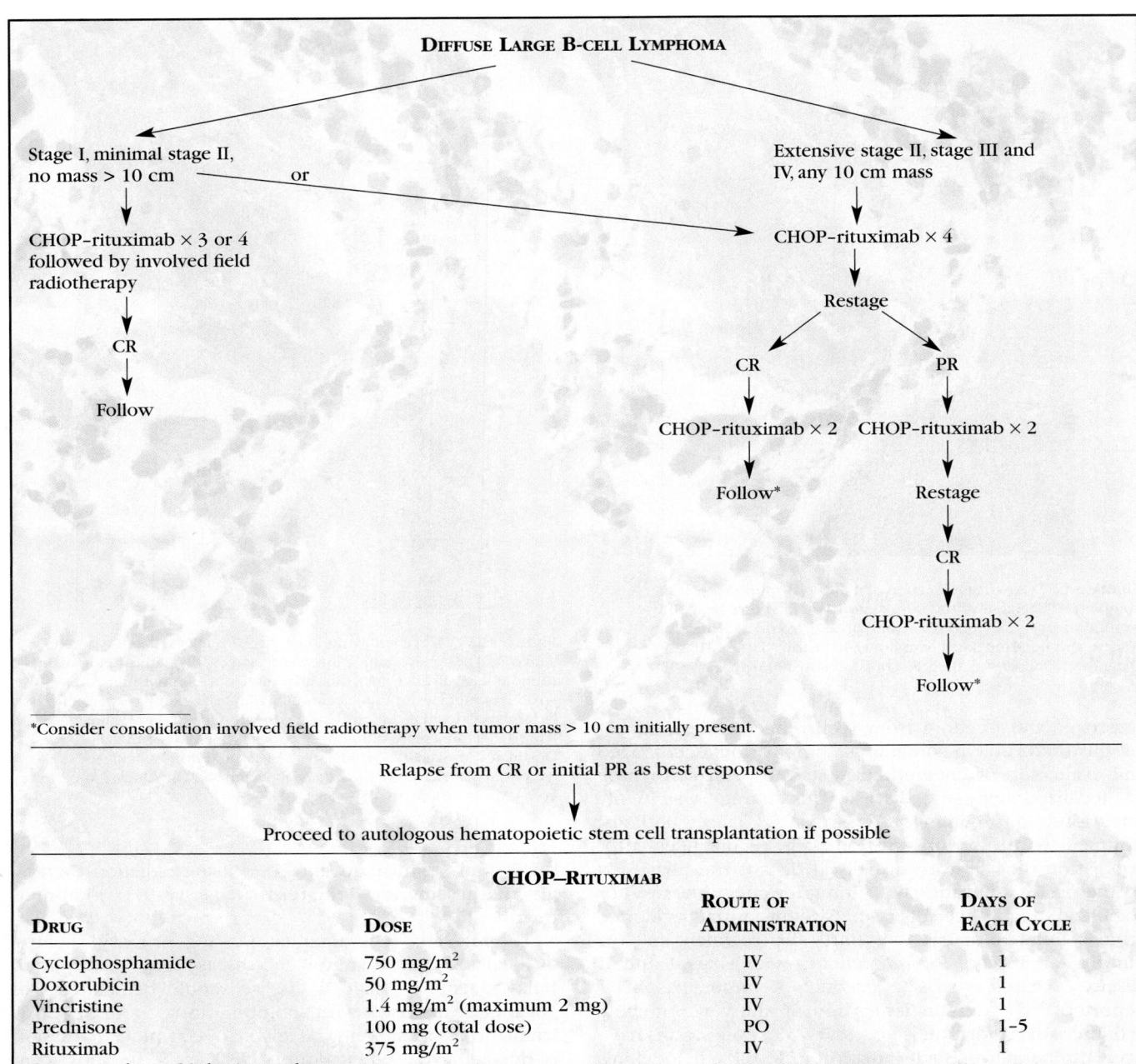

DIFFUSE LARGE B-CELL LYMPHOMA

Stage I, minimal stage II, no mass > 10 cm

or

Extensive stage II, stage III and IV, any 10 cm mass

CHOP–rituximab × 3 or 4 followed by involved field radiotherapy

CHOP–rituximab × 4

↓

Restage

CR

↓

Follow

CR   PR

CHOP–rituximab × 2   CHOP–rituximab × 2

Follow*   Restage

↓

CR

↓

CHOP–rituximab × 2

↓

Follow*

*Consider consolidation involved field radiotherapy when tumor mass > 10 cm initially present.

Relapse from CR or initial PR as best response

↓

Proceed to autologous hematopoietic stem cell transplantation if possible

CHOP–RITUXIMAB

DRUG	DOSE	ROUTE OF ADMINISTRATION	DAYS OF EACH CYCLE
Cyclophosphamide	750 mg/m^2	IV	1
Doxorubicin	50 mg/m^2	IV	1
Vincristine	1.4 mg/m^2 (maximum 2 mg)	IV	1
Prednisone	100 mg (total dose)	PO	1–5
Rituximab	375 mg/m^2	IV	1
Repeat cycles at 21-day intervals			

priate because of frailty or disinclination. Age alone should not be a reason to withhold potentially curative therapy, however.

The first evidence that the progress of this group of diseases might be cured came from two small studies of young patients treated at Yale[451] and the National Cancer Institute (NCI).[454] Approximately one half of those who achieved complete remission continued without recurrence for 2 years. During the time that these patients were being treated, the high responsiveness of aggressive non-Hodgkin's lymphoma to doxorubicin was being documented, leading to the development of CHOP in the mid 1970s.

Reports from the SWOG confirming the advantage of cyclophosphamide, vincristine, and prednisolone (COP) with doxorubicin (CHOP) over COP alone rapidly led to CHOP, given cyclically every 3 weeks for 6 to 8 cycles, becoming the treatment of choice.[455] Variations in dosage and timing were investigated; all appeared to result in a complete remission rate of approximately 50% to 60% and an overall survival at 5 years in about one third of patients with stage III and IV disease. All these studies included patients with a variety of aggressive lymphomas and not just diffuse large B-cell lymphoma. It is notable that almost all people can tolerate this treatment without admission to the hospital.

The most obvious drawback of the treatment (beyond alopecia, nausea, vomiting, and myelosuppression) is that it fails, either early or late, to cure lymphoma in a significant proportion of patients. This problem was addressed in three ways. The first was to add a nonmyelotoxic drug, most often bleomycin, to the 3-week schedule (CHOP-BLEO,[456] BACOP[457]). The second was to introduce a non-myelotoxic drug *between* cycles of CHOP or BACOP. Theoretically, the most interesting choice was that of high-dose methotrexate, reversed by folinic acid on day 10 (M-BACOD).[458] Another variation on this theme was the return to semicontinuous or weekly therapy, first used in the 1970s, using relatively small doses of myelosuppressive drugs, alternately, over a 12-week period with non-myelosuppressive drugs (MACOP-B).[459-461] The third was to give as many drugs as possible, as flexibly as possible (ProMACE-MOPP).[462] All these so-called third-generation treatments, the most widely used of which were M-BACOD (later modified, without influencing the results, to m-BACOD),[463] MACOP-B, and ProMACE-MOPP, later modified to ProMACE-CytaBOM,[464] were tested in open phase II trials; all yielded higher response rates and better freedom from recurrence than CHOP. At the same time outstanding results were being reported from the GELA group in France and Belgium using regimens based on the ACVB combination.[465,466] Many physicians accepted the results as a vindication of the more-is-better approach and adapted one or another combination as the treatment of choice. Almost without exception, preliminary results from other major centers, or from the "real world," were worse than those originally reported, with lower response rates and greater toxicity, sometimes in randomized trials. The interpretation of those conducting the studies and interested observers perhaps reflected their own bias, but a considerable body of opinion has suggested that the patients' prognostic characteristics may have been the most important variable.

Against this background, the SWOG initiated a randomized trial in 1986 in which patients with bulky stage II, stage III, and stage IV intermediate- or high-grade lymphoma (WF; high grade, Kiel) presumably 80% DLBC lymphoma in the WHO classification, were allocated to receive standard CHOP, M-BACOD, MACOP-B, or ProMACE-CytaBOM as described in the initial reports.[467] The trial comprised 1138 patients; 899 remained eligible after histology review. Stratification was undertaken to accommodate age, bulk, histology, and LDH level, and exhaustive multivariate analyses were performed. With a median follow-up time of almost 3 years (maximum, 6 years), no significant differences emerged between the four groups in terms of efficacy, but CHOP was the least toxic. Most important, no subgroup was identified that did better with the more intensive therapies. It was therefore concluded that none of the more complicated regimens was superior to CHOP.

This is only one of many randomized trials of different combination regimens in patients with aggressive disease.[468] A summation of all these studies suggested that no obvious superior therapy exists for patients with diffuse large B-cell lymphoma. However, this question was reopened with three directions[469]: the first one was to test high-dose therapy with autologous transplant in first line because of the remarkable efficacy in relapsing patients; the second looked at increasing dosage of the most important drugs, cyclophosphamide and doxorubicin, and shortening delay between cycles (to every 2 weeks); and the third added rituximab to chemotherapy.

Apart from age and stage, a number of other biologic observations can help in classifying or predicting the outcome of patients with lymphomas. In patients with diffuse large B-cell lymphoma, bcl-2 protein expression on immunohistochemical analysis is associated with an increased risk of recurrence.[470-474] Rearrangement of the bcl-6 gene,[475,476] important in germinal center formation,[477] is the genetic lesion most closely associated with DLBCL,[478,479] and in at least one series was correlated with a more favorable clinical outcome.[480] Tumor proliferative rate, as reflected by flow cytometric studies or studies with Ki-67, has predicted a poor treatment outcome in some but not all studies[481-484] Factors such as serum LDH and serum β2-microglobulin might be indirect reflections of tumor burden, tumor growth rate, or other metabolic characteristics.[485] The expression of HLA-DR on the tumor cell surface, the expression of various cell adhesion molecules, and the existence of infiltrating T lymphocytes in B-cell tumors might reflect the ability of the host immune system to recognize and respond to the lymphoma.[486] Finally, gene expression patterns offer a promising new approach to predicting outcome and, perhaps, choosing therapy.[424-426]

For some authors, whose preferred mode of investigating new therapy is the open phase II trial, relying heavily on historical controls and the construction of mathematical models of disease, prognostic factor analyses such as these have been essential. For those planning randomized trials to be conducted in particular subgroups, it is scarcely less important. In the forefront of these investigations have been the groups from Houston,[127] Lyon,[124,487] and Boston.[488] All have analyzed the relevance of many variables and then combined them to identify two or three groups within the total patient population with good, bad, or intermediate outcome using response to therapy, freedom from progression, and survival as end points. On the strength of these and other observations,[489-493] the International Non-Hodgkin's Lymphoma Prognostic Factor Project was founded, with the objective of developing a predictive model for aggressive disease. This included predominantly diffuse large B-cell lymphoma and peripheral T-cell lymphoma. Data from 3273 patients aged 16 to 92 years (median, 56) from 16 institutions and cooperative groups in North America and Europe were analyzed for presentation features and their impact upon survival and freedom from recurrence. Sadly, immunophenotype and maximum tumor diameter were not included in the analysis. The patients were all treated between 1982 and 1987 with doxorubicin-containing combination chemotherapy. With a minimum follow-up approaching 5 years, it was possible to identify four risk groups with predicted survivals at 5 years. When adjusted for the 1274 patients 60 years of age or younger, groups were also identifiable on the basis of stage, serum LDH, and performance status, with predicted survivals at

ACVB*				
Cycle	I	II	III	IV
Week	0	2	4	6
Drug Doses				

Drug Doses		
Doxorubicin	75 mg/m²	d1
Cyclophosphamide	1,200 mg/m²	d1
Vindesine	3 mg/m²	d1,d5
Bleomycin	15 mg	d1,d5
Prednisone	60 mg/m²	d1 to d5
Methotrexate intra-thecal	10 mg	d2
Filgrastim	5 µg/kg	d6 to d13

*This regimen is followed by an intensive consolidation regimen.

Figure 112-9. ACVB regimen as used by GELA for the last 20 years. (From Coiffier B: Fourteen years of high-dose CHOP [ACVB regimen]: Preliminary conclusions about the treatment of aggressive-lymphoma patients. Ann Oncol 1995;6:211–217.)

5 years of 83%, 69%, 46%, and 32%, respectively[121] (see Table 112-8). Both lower response rates and a higher recurrence rate contributed to the higher death rate in the worse-prognosis groups. These findings provided a reasonable background against which to select patients for whom more or very different therapy from CHOP should be prescribed.

Myeloablative chemotherapy or chemotherapy/ radiation therapy with autologous bone marrow transplantation (ABMT) has become accepted as indicated in younger patients with recurrent but demonstrably sensitive disease[494-502] (discussion to follow); it is thus being asked whether such treatment should be used as early as possible in newly diagnosed younger patients in the high- or higher-risk categories. The substitution of peripheral blood progenitor cells for ABMT has resulted in a marked shortening of time to bone marrow reconstitution. The approach has been tested in several randomized trials, of which some,[503,504] but not all,[505,506] lend strong supportive evidence in favor of high-dose therapy as a component of early therapy for patients with adverse risk factors.[507]

The GELA, GLSG, SWOG, and CALGB have run phase II studies and randomized studies (for the first two groups) comparing more intense chemotherapy to CHOP in young patients with diffuse large B-cell lymphoma. These dose-intense regimens were always associated with a higher hematological toxicity, however. The GELA has developed since 1984 a high-dose regimen called ACVBP plus sequential consolidation (Fig. 112-9) consisting of four cycles of ACVBP followed by four different drugs (high-dose methotrexate, ifosfamide, etoposide, and cytarabine) administered sequentially every 2 weeks for 4 months.[508] In several studies, this regimen was associated with a longer event-free survival and overall survival than usually observed with CHOP (Fig. 112-10). Two studies from the GELA showed a benefit in terms of overall survival and event-free survival for some patients. The first one compared ACVBP plus sequential therapy to M-BACOD in young patients and those with adverse prognostic

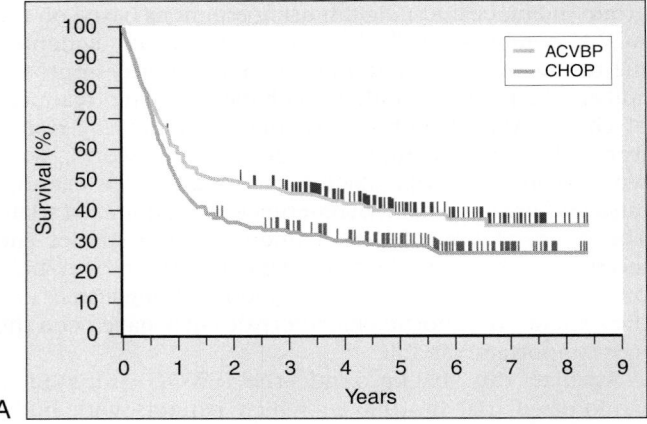

A

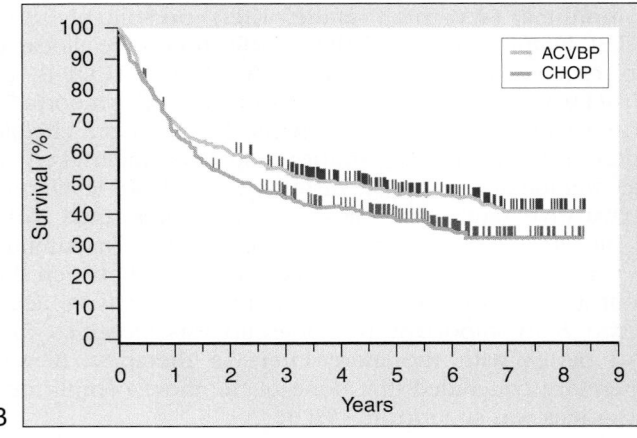

B

Figure 112-10. GELA study comparing ACVB + sequential therapy to CHOP regimen in elderly patients (60–90 years old) with aggressive lymphoma. **A,** Event-free survival (P = 0.005). **B,** Overall survival (P < 0.05). (From Coiffier B: Fourteen years of high-dose CHOP [ACVB regimen]: Preliminary conclusions about the treatment of aggressive-lymphoma patients. Ann Oncol 1995;6:211–217.)

parameters.[509] The second one compared ACVB plus sequential consolidation to CHOP in patients 60 to 70 years old. In the whole group, ACVB was associated with longer event-free and overall survivals, and particularly in patients younger than 65 years.[509]

The GLSG has used CHOEP (the drugs used in CHOP plus etoposide) and has observed in young patients a benefit in terms of survival.[510] Recently, CHOP done every 2 weeks was proven to be superior to a regimen of CHOP every 3 weeks in elderly patients.[511]

Finally, the most recent data showed that CHOP combined with rituximab was clearly superior to CHOP in elderly patients.[234] In this randomized study run by the GELA, 399 elderly patients with de novo DLBCL were entered; 50% were 70 years or older, 66% had high LDH levels, and 60% were a poor risk as defined by the International Prognostic Index (IPI). With a 3-year median survival, event-free survival and overall survival were at least 15% above CHOP and this benefit was observed for low-risk and high-risk patients (Fig. 112-11). It appears that benefit from the addition of rituximab may be

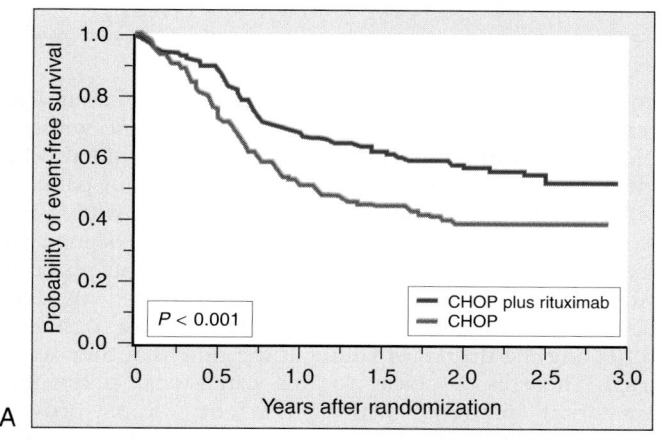

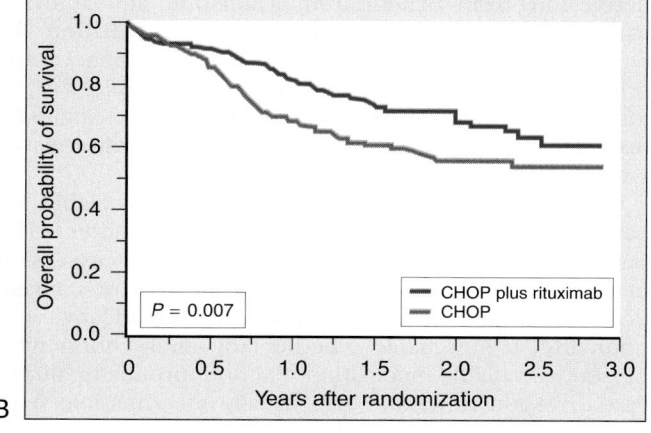

Figure 112-11. A, Event-free survival among 999 patients assigned to chemotherapy with cyolophosphamide, doxorubicin, vincristine, and prednisone (CHOP) or with CHOP + rituximab. **B,** Overall survival among 389 patients assigned to CHOP or with CHOP + rituximab. (From Coiffier B, Lepage E, Briére J et al: CHOP chemotherapy and Rituximab compared with CHOP alone in elderly patients with diffuse large B cell lymphoma. N Engl J Med 2002;346:235–242.)

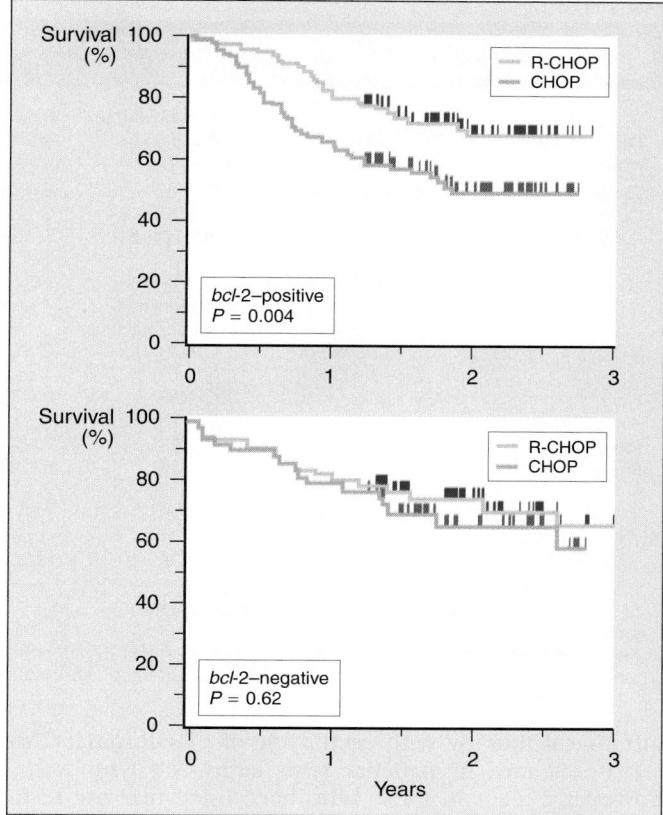

Figure 112-12. R-CHOP: Effect on *bcl*-2–related chemotherapy resistance (GELA). R-CHOP demonstrated a significant increase in overall survival and event-free survival in patients with *bcl*-2–positive diffuse large B-cell lymphoma. (From Mounier N, Briere J, Gisselbrecht C, Emile J-F, et al: Rituximab plus CHOP [R-CHOP] overcomes bcl-2-associated resistance to chemotherapy in elderly patients with diffuse large B-cell lymphoma [DLBCL] Blood 2003;101:4279–4284.)

confined to patients whose lymphomas overexpress bcl-2[512,513] (Fig. 112-12). Other randomized studies are ongoing and not reported to confirm the benefit in elderly or young patients of the combination of monoclonal antibodies and chemotherapy. The standard practice has implemented this regimen as the most used regimen in patients with DLBCL.

At the present time, then, CHOP is no longer the first choice for the newly diagnosed patient with advanced, aggressive non-Hodgkin's lymphoma. Table 112-10 lists 10 trials in which more intensive therapy led to better results.[234,507,509,511,514–518,531] The definitive standard regimen is not yet known but will certainly be a combination of rituximab (or another monoclonal antibody) with a dose-intense CHOP-like regimen. Due to this, an inclusion of patients in well-defined prospective trial remains the best clinical practice and certainly the best therapeutic option a physician may offer to patients.

CNS Prophylaxis. Opinions vary as to the requirement for central nervous system prophylaxis. It is reasonable to examine the CSF in patients with advanced aggressive lymphoma, and in some centers it is routine to administer

TABLE 112-10

Randomized Studies Showing a Statistically Significant Benefit over a Standard Arm Regimen in Aggressive Lymphomas*

REFERENCE	SETTING	STANDARD ARM	EXPERIMENTAL ARM	NO. OF PATIENTS	ENDPOINT	EFS (%)	OAS (%)
Carde[514]	Unfavorable subtypes	CHVmP	CHVmP-VB	141	5 years	—	29 vs. 53
Coiffier[234]	Elderly, DLCL	CHOP	CHOP-rituximab	399	2 years	38 vs. 57	57 vs. 70
Gianni[503]	Young, DLCL	MACOP-B	Sequential HDT	98	55 months	49 vs. 76 DFS	55 vs. 81 (P = 0.09)
Haioun[507]	Young, aaIPI = 2 or 3	ACVB—sequential consolidation	ACVB +CBV and autologous transplant	236	8 years	39 vs. 55	49 vs. 64
Intragumtornchai[515]	>56 years, aaIPI = 2 or 3	CHOP	CHOP, ESHAP, and HDT	58	4 years	15 vs. 38	30 vs. 51 (P = 0.25)
Linch[516]	Aggressive	CHOP	PACEBOM	459	8 years	—	CSS 49 vs 59
Pfreundschuh[517]	Aggressive, >60 years	CHOP	CHOP-14	738	49 months	39 vs. 47	45 vs. 59
Pfreundschuh[511]	Aggressive, young, low risk	CHOP	CHOEP	762	49 months	63 vs. 73	81 vs. 86 (P = 0.13)
Tilly[509]	60 to 69 years, aaIPI >0	CHOP	ACVB + sequential consolidation	635	5 years	29 vs. 39	38 vs. 46
Wolf[518]	Aggressive	CHOP	MACOP-B	236	6.5 years	30 vs. 42	41 vs. 54

CSS, cause-specific survival; DFS, disease-free survival; DLCl, diffuse large cell lymphoma; EFS, event-free survival; HDT, high-dose therapy with autotransplant; OAS, overall survival.
*Studies with longer event-free and overall survival rates are shaded. Event-free and overall survival are statistically significantly different, except when specified.

intrathecal therapy with each cycle of CHOP. Initial CNS relapse is rare in patients with large cell lymphoma, however, except in those who have bone marrow, testicular, epidural, sinus, or orbital involvement.[534] In a GELA study comparing CHOP without intrathecal methotrexate and ACVBP plus sequential consolidation, fewer CNS relapses were observed with ACVBP, but it may be secondary to the sequential consolidation and not the intrathecal methotrexate.[519] Overt disease should be treated with intrathecal chemotherapy concurrent with systemic chemotherapy, and if the systemic disease is controlled, encephalic irradiation should be considered.

Patients with Persisting Image Abnormalities but Otherwise Complete Response. Patients with diffuse large B-cell lymphoma with large masses in the mediastinum and retroperitoneum often have a residual mass at the completion of therapy. Whether this represents persistant disease or a slowly resolving fibrotic reaction is, obviously, an important distinction. Patients who have a dramatic reduction in size after two to four cycles of treatment, but little change thereafter are often really in complete remission. Biopsy of the mass is only definitive if tumor is found.

The ability to make this distinction has been helped by the use of gallium and PET scans. If the tumor is known to be abnormal on gallium or PET scan, no uptake in a residual mass seen on CT scan is good evidence that complete remission has been achieved.[520,521] The use of early normalization of gallium and PET scans has been suggested as an important predictor of treatment outcome.[520,521]

Failure. At the first sign of failure, urgent alternative action should be considered and undertaken if feasible and desired by the patient. If the patient was in complete remission, further treatment should not be done without biopsy proof of recurrence. Consideration should also be given to biopsy of new lesions, as a minority of patients will relapse with lymphoma of less aggressive histology.[522] A considerable number of salvage programs designed on the basis of preclinical evidence of activity and phase II single-agent studies have been tested.[523-529] Widely disparate results have been reported, almost certainly reflecting the degree of failure at the time that they were used. There is a caveat to this categorical statement: anecdotal patients with persistent, biopsy-proven lymphoma in a single site, often in the abdomen, may derive long-term benefit from irradiation; and adjuvant irradiation or perhaps complementary irradiation for patients with persistent mediastinal lymphoma of the sclerosing type has been suggested to be valuable.[90,91,95] It must be appreciated that, particularly in this diagnosis, persistent mediastinal widening is not necessarily equated with active lymphoma.[489,530]

A wide range of palliative options are available for patents no longer being treated with curative intent. The outcome for patients in whom there is overt progression of disease during or shortly after six cycles of conventional combination chemotherapy is statistically very poor, and it is arguable whether any intervention with presently available medication will do more than palliate. Partial responsiveness is also usually incompatible with long survival, but not entirely. There are two reasons for potential optimism in this setting. The first relates to the criteria for defining complete remission and the meaning of persistent radiologic abnormalities, within either the mediastinum or the abdomen. Such changes may only represent fibrosis, or at least an extent of disease amenable to irradiation or further chemotherapy. Second, it is becoming evident that partial remission may be converted to long-term complete remission with additional induction chemotherapy, followed by myeloablative therapy with hematopoietic stem cell rescue. There is a large number of salvage regimens that have been shown to be effective in patients with refractory or recurrent disease, which have been variously used to treat refractory disease or convert partial into complete remission. The disparity in their efficacy can almost certainly be accounted for by the clinical characterization of the patients in the different trials.

An aggressive approach to recurrence after complete remission is now conventional, based on the outcome of the Parma trial, which showed that both freedom from progression and overall survival were better for patients receiving reinduction therapy followed by high-dose consolidation with hematopoietic stem cell rescue than for those receiving only conventional dose therapy.[494,502,531] These results, combined with the very substantial body of single-center trials and registry data, indicate that perhaps a third of patients in whom a recurrence occurs and who are still responsive may have long-term survival. Outcome is better for those in complete remission than for those in partial remission,[532] and for those with follicular large cell lymphoma.[533]

There remains, however, little room for complacency. Large B-cell lymphoma remains a dangerous diagnosis, and is fatal for the majority of patients in whom it is diagnosed; relatively few cytotoxic drugs have recently shown exciting new promise. Immunologic approaches to date have been unimpressive, but there may be some ground for optimism with the advent of newer antibody approaches. The humanized antibody rituximab, investigated to date predominantly in follicular lymphoma,[233,534] has been shown to induce remission, mostly partial, in patients with large B-cell lymphoma.[420] However, most patients today receive rituximab as part of their primary therapy. As yet, few data are available about antibody-targeted irradiation; while alone it is unlikely to be curative for advanced disease, it might be a valuable adjunct to conventional or high-dose therapy. The relative lack of toxicity of both approaches makes them attractive to investigate. Other modifications of high-dose therapy may improve its efficacy. The subsequent use of IL-2 as immunotherapy has been promoted.[535] Despite its toxicity, allogeneic transplantation is now being reconsidered as an alternative in younger patients to high-dose therapy with autologous hematopoietic stem cell rescue.

Relatively little attention is given to the management of failure after high-dose therapy, which occurs in at least half of those treated. There may well be no indication for any specific intervention; the strategy will depend greatly on the enthusiasm of the physician and the patient, the overall state of health of the patient, the extent of the recurrence, and the interval between high-dose therapy and progression. Overall, the outcome is very poor. There is no doubt, nonetheless, that some interventional treatment, whether mild, moderate, or intensive, may be beneficial. Local irradiation may produce excellent relief of pain, and various chemotherapy programs may cause enough regression of disease to improve quality of life.[536,537] Recurrence in the meninges, or less commonly in the brain, is ominous and almost certainly means the patient is incurable. Every effort must be made, however, to deal with this situation effectively, to prevent the awful problems of base-of-skull infiltration. Usually, intrathecal therapy should be undertaken; this may reverse cranial nerve palsy. If any doubt exists, at least base-of-skull irradiation should be given. Corticosteroids may help. Once again, patients should never be told that the doctor can do nothing, and there are many exceptions proving this rule.[538,539]

There is still room for improvement.

Sclerosing B-Cell Lymphoma of the Mediastinum (Mediastinal Diffuse Large B-Cell Lymphoma)

It has for some time been recognized that a small proportion of patients with diffuse large B-cell lymphoma present with mediastinal widening and superior vena cava (SVC) obstruction,[540,541] and the pathologic appearance of the lymph node may be characterized by sclerosis (see Table 112-9).[117] The entity occurs more frequently in younger women and the distribution of extranodal sites is unusual, with not infrequent involvement of the kidneys.[90] Overall management is the same as for large B-cell lymphoma, and the outcome is superficially the same. The most common clinical problem is incomplete resolution of mediastinal widening after conventional chemotherapy. It has become conventional as the result of several reports to complement the intial therapy with mediastinal irradiation, particularly if the mediastinal mass is larger than 10 cm. The role of adjuvant high-dose therapy is debated.[542] The fact that the overall survival pattern is the same as that of large B-cell lymphoma masks the problem that failure of initial therapy is frequently fatal, and unpleasant because of the major site of disease.

Burkitt's Lymphoma

Burkitt's lymphoma is predominantly a disease of children and accounts for up to one third of all pediatric lymphomas in the United States (Figs. 112-13 and 112-14; see Table 112-9).[543] Abdominal presentations are the most frequent but it may also present in extranodal sites (e.g., the ovaries, breasts, kidney, or ileocecal region) in nonendemic areas, in contrast to the typical jaw presentation seen in West African children.[544] It is now also being seen more frequently in HIV-positive patients, and in some it may be the AIDS-defining illness.[545]

Most cases are associated with a t(8;14) translocation[546]; less often, a t(8;2) or t(8;22) is involved.[547] All the translocations involve the c-myc oncogene. EBV is associated with Burkitt's lymphoma in endemic regions but is less frequently involved in the United States and Europe.[548]

In previous lymphoma classifications, a subgroup of non-Hodgkin's lymphoma, variously termed *small noncleaved non-Burkitt's* or *Burkitt's-like*, has been recognized. At present it seems that this category was a mixture of patients with either diffuse large B-cell lymphoma or true

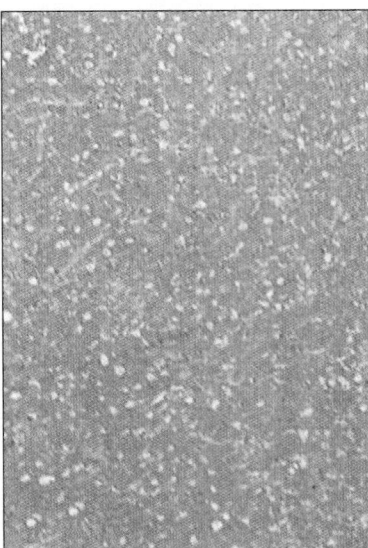

Figure 112-13. Burkitt's lymphoma, NCI subgroup J. Low-power photomicrograph reveals a "starry sky" appearance resulting from the presence of benign macrophages, which are active in the phagocytosis of necrotic cells and debris. This pattern is nonspecific and can be seen with any rapidly proliferating lymphoma. (From Dorfman DM, Skarin AT: Hodgkin's disease and non-Hodgkin's lymphoma. In Skarin AT [ed]: Atlas of Diagnostic Oncology, 3rd ed. St. Louis, Mosby, 2003, pp 475–553.)

Burkitt's lymphoma. Adults with this intermediate classification should probably be diagnosed as having diffuse large B-cell lymphoma, except perhaps those with extremely high growth fractions who should be diagnosed with Burkitt's lymphoma. Some have suggested that these

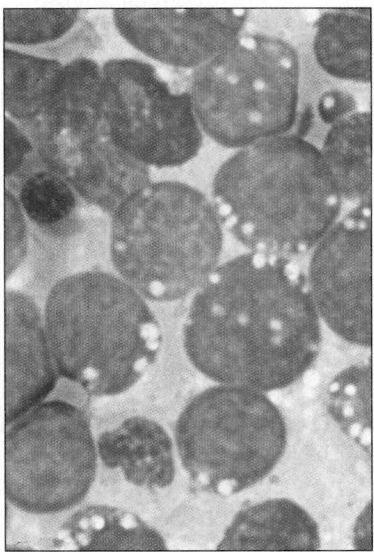

Figure 112-14. Burkitt's lymphoma, NCI subgroup J. Bone marrow aspirate shows small, immature cells with deep basophilic cytoplasm containing many vacuoles. Distinct nucleoli are seen in several of the cells. (From Dorfman DM, Skarin AT: Hodgkin's disease and non-Hodgkin's lymphoma. In Skarin AT [ed]: Atlas of Diagnostic Oncology, 3rd ed. St. Louis, Mosby, 2003, pp 475–553.)

patients should receive CNS prophylactic therapy in addition to systemic chemotherapy.

Management

In view of the high frequency of abdominal presentation, making the diagnosis itself often entails laparotomy. The LDH level is often very high, as is the urate level. The typical pathology may be confirmed by cytogenetics and helped by immunophenotyping. The cells express surface immunoglobulin and are terminal deoxynucleotidyl transferase (TdT) negative, in contrast to cells from other subtypes of acute lymphoblastic leukemia.

Burkitt's lymphoma is the fastest dividing lymphoma (100% of cells being in cell cycle at any time). Patients may therefore present with life-threatening gastrointestinal tract complications or renal failure. CNS involvement is not unusual. Attention must therefore first be paid to such potentially fatal problems before chemotherapy is instituted. However, starting chemotherapy in the presence of hyperuricemia and impaired urinary output in the context of acute tumor lysis syndrome, which results from the extremely high growth fraction and cell turnover rate of Burkitt's lymphoma, is likely to result in the death of the patient, due to hyperkalemia and renal failure. Biochemical abnormalities must therefore first be corrected and good urine flow established (or the patient dialyzed) before specific treatment is started. These are rare diseases; the number of patients in reported series is therefore relatively small.

It is now clear that the treatment protocols for acute lymphoblastic leukemia (whilst very successful as treatment for precursor B and T lymphoblastic lymphoma) are not sufficient as treatment for Burkitt's lymphoma. Specific protocols comprising high doses of cyclophosphamide, methotrexate, vincristine, anthracycline, epipodophyllotoxins, and cytarabine arabinoside have resulted in overall survival rates of 80% to 90% (Table 112-11).[549,550-552] CNS prophylaxis is essential.

There is no dispute that after recurrence, provided that second remission can be achieved, high-dose treatment with autologous hemopoietic progenitor cell support (or allogeneic BMT) is the only strategy with any chance of cure. The role of high-dose treatment with autologous hematopoietic stem cell transplantation in first remission is, however, less clear and probably not necessary when a complete remission is achieved. Rituximab appears to be very active and is being incorporated into primary treatment regimens.

Precursor B and T Neoplasms: Lymphomas of Precursor B-Cell or T-Cell Origin

Fundamental to the WHO classification is recognition of B- or T-cell lineage for each histologic subtype. The lymphoblastic lymphomas are therefore addressed separately in the classification according to cell of origin (see Table 112-6). However, they do have in common an exponential growth rate and the fact that without vigorous intervention they are invariably rapidly fatal.

Precursor B lymphoblastic lymphoma most often presents in children and younger adults (as does acute

TABLE 112-11

Results of Treatment for Lymphoblastic and Burkitt's Lymphoma in Adults

STUDY GROUP	NO. OF PATIENTS	CHEMOTHERAPY REGIMEN	CENTRAL NERVOUS SYSTEM PROPHYLAXIS	OTHER IRRADIATION	CR RATE (%)	DFS IN ALL PATIENTS [% SURVIVING (DURATION)]
Lymphoblastic Lymphoma						
Slater et al.[565]	51	Variable	Intrathecal methotrexate	—	78	45 (5 yr)
Coleman et al.[573]	44	Induction: cyclophosphamide, doxorubicin, vincristine, prednisone, asparaginase Maintenance: methotrexate, mercaptopurine	Intrathecal and high-dose methotrexate, cranial radiation therapy	—	95	56 (3 yr)
Solloum et al.[566]	34	Variable	Variable	Variable	74	30 (3 yr)
Voakes et al.[567]	32	Variable	Variable	Variable	53	—
Levine et al.[568]	15	Induction: cyclophosphamide, doxorubicin, vincristine, prednisone, cytarabine, thioguanine, asparaginase, lomustine Maintenance: thioguanine, methotrexate, cyclophosphamide, hydroxyurea, doxorubicin, lomustine, cytarabine, vincristine	Intrathecal methotrexate, cranial radiation therapy	To mediastinum	73	35 (5 yr)
Hoelzer et al.[559]		GMALL 04/89 and 05/93			93	51 (7 yr)
Thomas et al.[560]		Hyper-CVAD			94	78 (3 yr)
Sweetenham[563]		Multiple + auto BMT			—	56 (3 yr)
Burkitt's Lymphoma						
Lopez et al.[569]	44	Variable	Intrathecal methotrexate	—	80	60 (3 yr)
McMaster et al.[570]	20	Cyclophosphamide, etoposide, vincristine, bleomycin, doxorubicin, methotrexate, prednisone	Intrathecal methotrexate	—	85	60 (5 yr)
Lee et al.[551]		CALGB 9251			83	52 (5 yr)
Magrath et al.[550]		CODOX-M + IVAC			95	87 (2 yr)
Soussain et al.[552]		Pediatric LMB protocol			89	74 (3 yr)

CR, complete response; DFS, disease-free survival.

lymphoblastic leukemia) with lymphadenopathy, postnasal space, or bone involvement.[553,554] Primary cutaneous lymphoblastic lymphoma generally affects young children and has a less aggressive course (discussion follows).[555]

There may be abdominal lymph node enlargement and involvement of the liver or spleen. The great majority of patients present with stage III or IV disease. The bone marrow is frequently involved and bone marrow infiltration correlates with the presence of CNS involvement, which may be overt and symptomatic or covert (i.e., only picked up on examination of CSF). Immunophenotyping is helpful; the cells have an immature B-cell phenotype and express TdT.

Patients with precursor T-lymphoblastic lymphoma are generally boys or young men who present with a large mediastinal mass that is frequently associated with pleural effusions, SVC obstruction, tracheal obstruction, or a pericardial effusion.[556,557] There is often rapid progression to the bone marrow and the CNS.

Management

The principles of management are the same, irrespective of lineage. Until recently, B- or T-lymphoblastic lymphomas were associated with an appalling prognosis. With the advent of modern, very intensive regimens, this situation has changed dramatically. The initial treatment of choice, regardless of stage, is intensive systemic chemotherapy, accompanied by intrathecal.[549,558-562] Most treatment schedules contain large numbers of drugs given over as short a period of time as possible. Many patients with T-cell lymphoblastic lymphoma have received the same chemotherapy regimens as those used in acute lymphoblastic leukemia. Review of the literature suggests that approximately 50% may be cured with an intensive approach[559,562-572] (see Table 112-11). In the past, patients who presented with lymphoblastic lymphomas without bone marrow or CNS involvement or very bulky tumors had a much better outcome (i.e., durable complete remission rates of 75% or more) compared to patients who presented with any or all of these adverse risk factors, in whom the chance of cure was only 20% or less.[573] However, intensive multiagent regimens seem to overcome the adverse effect of these prognostic factors.[559,560] Autologous bone marrow transplantation in first remission led to a slightly better outcome in one study, but the initial chemotherapy regimens used were not always optimal.[563] Whether autologous transplants could add to the outcome in optimally treated patients is unclear. Patients who fail primary therapy can occasionally be salvaged with allogeneic or, less often, autologous transplantation. Allogeneic transplantation should be done rarely or not at all in adults in first remission.

Lysis of tumor is usually very rapid and care must be taken to prevent the tumor lysis syndrome, which can be fatal because of acute renal failure. Adequate hydration and high doses of allopurinol are essential; whenever possible, pretreatment hyperuricemia should be corrected before institution of cytoxic chemotherapy. While the overall treatment program must be intensive if cure is to be effected, the *very first injections* may need to be in low doses to avoid this potential toxicity.

Mature T-Cell Lymphoma

There are several major groups of lymphomas of mature T cells (i.e., peripheral T-cell lymphomas) recognized in the WHO system for lymphoma classification (see Table 112-6). These include mycosis fungoides/Sézary syndrome and adult T-cell lymphoma/leukemia, which have separate chapters in this text and will not be dealt with in this chapter.

Peripheral T-Cell Lymphoma

The diagnosis of peripheral T-cell lymphoma is typically applied to non-Hodgkin's lymphomas of mature T-cell immunophenotype that do not fit into the categories of mycosis fungoides/Sézary syndrome, adult T-cell lymphoma/leukemia, or anaplastic large T/null cell lymphoma (Fig. 112-15; see Table 112-9). Lymphomas included in this category represent a heterogenous group of malignancies, both histologically and clinically. These lymphomas are not rare and make up approximately 7% of all non-Hodgkin's lymphomas worldwide.[117] Their occurrence is not geographically uniform, however. In a recent international study, this category made up 10% of all non-Hodgkin's lymphomas seen in Hong Kong, but only 1% of non-Hodgkin's lymphomas seen in British Columbia.[574]

The fact that peripheral T-cell lymphomas occur much less frequently in Western countries than B-cell lymphomas probably contributes to increased difficulty in diagnosing peripheral T-cell lymphomas. Also, peripheral T-cell lymphomas often have a "mixed" histologic picture, with many of the cells in the tumor representing a reaction to the malignant cells.[575-578] Some previously described clinical entities frequently or usually represent T-cell lymphomas. These include angioimmunoblastic lymphadenopathy with dysproteinemia, and "malignant" histiocytosis.

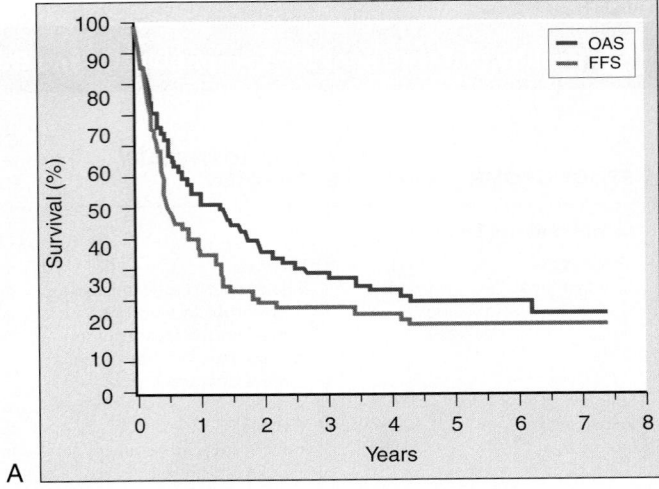

A

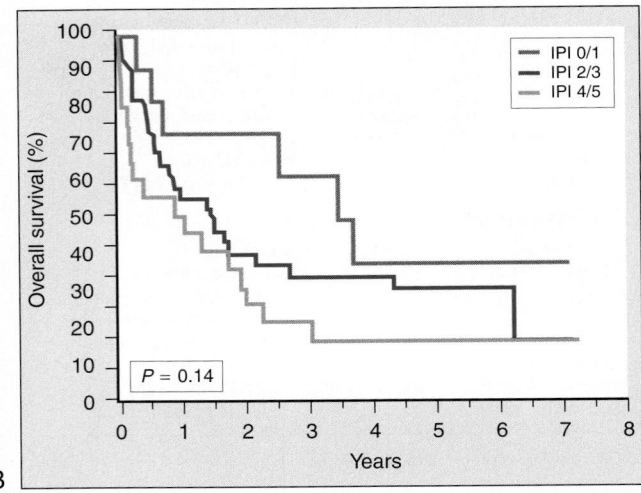

B

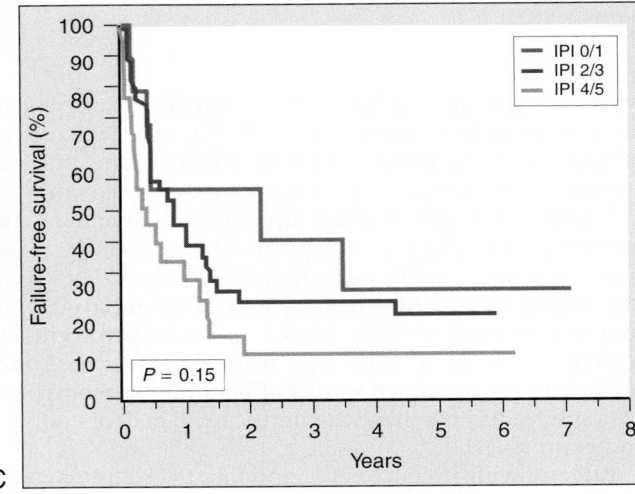

C

Figure 112-15. A, Overall survival (OAS) and failure-free survival (FFS) for an unselected group of patients with peripheral T-cell lymphoma. **B,** OAS by International Prognostic Index score for patients with peripheral T-cell lymphoma. **C,** FFS by International Prognostic Index score for patients with peripheral T-cell lymphoma.

Angioimmunoblastic lymphadenopathy with dysproteinemia describes a clinical entity characterized by lymphadenopathy, hepatosplenomegaly, skin rash, systemic symptoms, polyclonal hypergammaglobulinemia, hemolytic anemia, and a frequently fatal course despite the presumed "benign" histologic appearance of the disorder.[579,580] The histologic picture includes diffuse effacement of the lymph node architecture with a mixed cellular infiltrate involving lymphocytes, immunoblasts, plasma cells, and histiocytes accompanied by an unusual, "arborizing" vascular pattern. The condition was described first in the English literature in 1974.[581] Subsequent studies demonstrated the clonal nature of the process in most patients.[582,583] It is now clear that this entity often represents a peripheral T-cell lymphoma and the phrase *angioimmunoblastic T-cell lymphoma* has become widely used. As was demonstrated in one large study, these patients can be cured with combination chemotherapy.[584] All patients diagnosed as angioimmunoblastic lymphadenopathy with dysproteinemia do not have a rapidly fatal disorder, however, and therein lies the clinical problem. If there is no clonal T-cell population demonstrated and the diagnosis of lymphoma cannot be made with confidence, a therapeutic trial with steroids can be undertaken and is sometimes successful.[585]

Angiocentric lymphoid proliferations that represent forms of peripheral T-cell lymphoma have gone by such names as *lethal midline granuloma,*[586] *polymorphic reticulosis,*[586] *angiocentric lymphoproliferative lesion,*[587] and *angiocentric lymphoma.*[587] These clinically aggressive disorders should be recognized and treated in a manner appropriate for histologically aggressive non-Hodgkin's lymphoma.

The entity previously called *malignant histiocytosis* we now know usually represents a form of peripheral T-cell lymphoma typically referred to as *anaplastic large cell lymphoma.*[588] The characteristic chromosomal translocation involving chromosomes 2 and 5 once described for malignant histiocytosis is characteristic of this type of non-Hodgkin's lymphoma.[103] Anaplastic large cell lymphoma, previously sometimes known as *Ki-1 positive lymphoma,* responds to the same therapy as other histologically aggressive lymphoma[588] (see "Anaplastic Large T/Null Cell Lymphoma").

Lymphomas classified as peripheral T-cell lymphoma unspecified represent a wide variety of histologic and clinical entities. While many lymphomas cannot be put into any specific diagnostic grouping, there are several histologic and clinical syndromes that have been identified. The most common of these are angioimmunoblastic T-cell lymphoma and extranodal nasal T or natural killer (NK) cell lymphoma. As noted before, angioimmunoblastic T-cell lymphoma[589-595] represents most patients that used to be diagnosed as having angioimmunoblastic lymphadenopathy and dysproteinemia.[596,597]

Extranodal nasal T or NK cell lymphoma has an extraordinary geographic specificity and is predominantly seen in areas in Asia and South America.[598] The histologic appearance usually involves invasion of blood vessel walls by atypical cells.[599,600] This tumor probably represents most of the patients that were originally described as

having lethal midline granuloma and malignant midline reticulosis.[601-602] Aggressive therapy can sometimes produce long-term survival.[610,611] Unlike other aggressive lymphomas, patients with localized disease might have a better prognosis when radiotherapy precedes chemotherapy.[611]

Other clinicopathologic syndromes recognized in the peripheral T-cell lymphomas include the hepatosplenic gamma delta T-cell lymphoma.[612-615] The name describes the typical sites of presentation and the expression of the more primitive gamma delta T-cell receptor genes. Occasionally hepatosplenic lymphomas can express the alpha beta T-cell receptor and are thought to be phenotypic variants of the same entity. At presentation, B-symptoms, hepatosplenomegaly but not lymphadenopathy, and thrombocytopenia (and often pancytopenia) are typically present. Patients with this syndrome have infiltration of the liver, spleen, bone marrow, and sometimes other organs by atypical T cells. There are frequently no tumor masses, with diffuse infiltration of the involved organs. Such patients can be diagnostic dilemmas when presenting with systemic symptoms and organ dysfunction.

The enteropathy type intestinal T-cell lymphoma is most often seen in patients with celiac disease or gluten-sensitive enteropathy.[616-619] It is felt that the development of lymphoma in these patients might be prevented by treatment of the celiac disease. Patients present with abdominal pain, weight loss, diarrhea, and frequently bowel perforation. The histologic picture is usually one of multiple small bowel ulcers and infiltration by atypical T cells.

Another unusual peripheral T-cell lymphoma is a subcutaneous panniculitis-like T-cell lymphoma.[620-622] This rare disease presents with subcutaneous nodules that are often mistaken for lipomas. On histologic evaluation, the diagnosis can be atypical panniculitis. Histologic diagnosis is usually made with recognition of atypical T cells in the tumor and is more likely to be done in a timely manner when clinicians and pathologists are acquainted with this lymphoma.

Most patients with peripheral T-cell lymphoma present with adenopathy.[576] There are a number of unusual clinical syndromes that might lead to the diagnosis of peripheral T-cell lymphoma, however. These include the hemophagocytic syndrome,[623,624] the facial/nasal syndrome,[601-610] a systemic illness with organ infiltration,[612-616] and unexplained pulmonary infiltrates.[625] The occurrence of the hemophagocytic syndrome might be associated with other processes, but should also lead to the consideration of peripheral T-cell lymphoma.[623,624] Patients with peripheral T-cell lymphoma can also present with eosinophilia,[626] vasculitis,[626,627] bone marrow dysfunction,[628] granulomatous liver disease,[629] and unusual neurologic findings.[630] Patients with peripheral T-cell lymphoma frequently have a history of a preceding disorder of the immune system.[631] Immunophenotyping is necessary for an accurate diagnosis.[632]

The clinical characteristics in a large series of patients with peripheral T-cell lymphoma are presented in Table 112-9. In the absence of presentation as an unusual clinical syndrome as noted previously, patients with peripheral T-cell lymphoma will usually not be able to be distinguished clinically from those with an aggressive B-cell lymphoma. Whether the occurrence of a peripheral T-cell lymphoma has unique prognostic characteristics has been a point for debate. Some authors have felt that patients with peripheral T-cell lymphoma have a worse outlook than similar patients with B-cell lymphoma,[633-639] while others have found no difference in prognosis.[611,640-642] The predominance of the studies, however, report that patients with T-cell lymphomas have a worse outlook than those with similar B-cell lymphomas. In a recent international study, the overall survival of patients with peripheral T-cell lymphoma unspecified was approximately half that of patients with diffuse large B-cell lymphoma, despite similar treatment approaches.[117]

Factors found to predict treatment outcome in patients treated for peripheral T-cell lymphoma include performance status,[632,643] age,[643] bulky tumors,[643] bone marrow involvement,[643,644] liver involvement,[644] elevated serum LDH,[643] elevated serum b2 microglobulin,[643] and disseminated disease.[643,644] The most practical method to predict treatment outcome is the International Prognostic Index.[632,642,643]

The treatment for patients with peripheral T-cell lymphoma utilizes the same regimens and generally follows the same principles as outlined for diffuse large B-cell lymphoma. At the present time, there is no convincing evidence that one regimen is superior. A wide variety of regimens have been shown to be able to induce long-term disease-free survival.[633,645-648] Two studies have shown the superiority of an effective multiagent chemotherapy regimen utilizing full doses as the primary therapy. One study from Hong Kong demonstrated that patients who received a primary chemotherapy regimen such as BACOP had a higher complete response rate than patients who receive reduced-dose regimens (84% versus 19%) and a superior disease-free survival (80% versus 0% at 18 months).[645] In a German study of patients with angioimmunoblastic lymphadenopathy-like T-cell lymphoma, an initial combination chemotherapy regimen named COP-BLAM/IMBP-16 was compared with initial prednisone and aggressive chemotherapy only in patients who progressed on prednisone. Patients treated initially with a combination chemotherapy regimen had a superior complete response rate (64% versus 29%).[646]

Salvage therapy for patients failing primary treatment has been studied using a variety of approaches. Autologous bone marrow transplantation has been shown to be able to produce long-term disease-free survival in a significant proportion of patients with relapsed peripheral T-cell lymphoma.[649-651] In one study, patients with T-cell and B-cell aggressive lymphoma had similar outcomes with autotransplantation[649] and it has been suggested that transplantation in first remission might be a strategy to improve treatment outcome in high-risk patients.[651]

Standard salvage chemotherapy regimens can induce responses in some patients with peripheral T-cell lymphoma, but are rarely curative. Popular regimens include those utilizing cisplatin, such as DHAP (cisplatin, high-dose cytarabine, and dexamethasone).[652] Occasional good responses have been described using alternative approaches such as 13-cisretinoic acid,[653] cyclosporine,[654] and IFN-α.[655]

Anaplastic Large T/Null Cell Lymphoma

Anaplastic large T/null cell lymphoma is a recently recognized subtype of non-Hodgkin's lymphoma that has unique histologic, immunologic, genetic, and clinical characteristics (Fig. 112-16; see Table 112-9).[656-666] In the past, patients with this lymphoma were often felt to have disorders other than non-Hodgkin's lymphoma.[656] Many were considered to have undifferentiated malignant neoplasms or malignant histiocytosis.[657] The discovery of the Ki-1 or CD30 antigen led directly to the discovery of this lymphoma. The chromosomal abnormality commonly seen in these patients (i.e., t[2;5]) was previously thought to be characteristic of malignant histiocytosis. It is now clear, however, that this is a characteristic chromosomal abnormality of anaplastic large T/null cell lymphoma.[666-668] Overexpression of the alk oncogene is a product of this translocation and represents an important marker for this subtype of lymphoma.[669,670] alk protein overexpression is seen more often in younger than older patients and rarely in B-cell variants of anaplastic large cell lymphoma.[671] The presence of alk protein is an important factor in predicting treatment outcome, with patients expressing alk approximately twice as likely to be cured.[672]

The characteristic histologic appearance of anaplastic large T/null cell lymphoma is a proliferation of pleomorphic, large lymphoid cells with abundant cytoplasm and, sometimes, multiple nuclei. A cohesive growth pattern and a sinusoidal spread in lymph nodes has led to the diagnosis of an epithelial neoplasm rather than a lymphoma. There are small cell variants of this tumor, more commonly seen in children.[673,674]

B-cell variants of anaplastic large cell lymphoma also occur. It is now clear, however, that they have the same

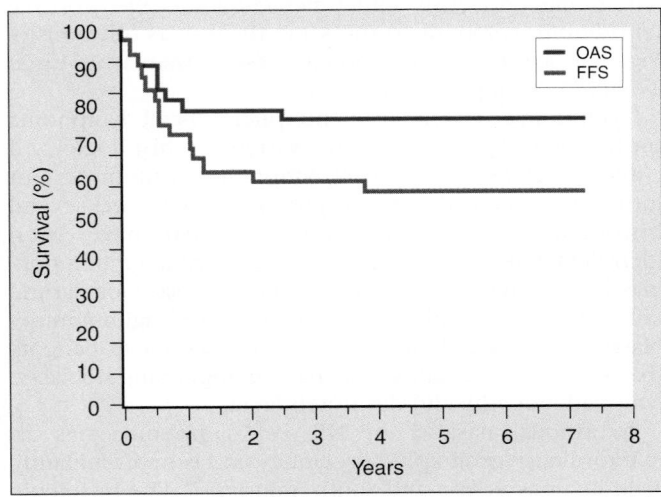

Figure 112-16. Overall survival (OAS) and failure-free survival (FFS) for an unselected group of patients with anaplastic large T/null cell lymphoma.

clinical characteristics and treatment outcome as other diffuse large B-cell lymphomas, and are not considered as a separate group.[117] There are also patients with lymphomas that are at the interface between Hodgkin's disease and anaplastic large T/null cell lymphoma. Some have proposed a separate category for these tumors.[675,676]

The diagnosis for anaplastic large T/null cell lymphoma can be difficult and confusing. Part of the confusion lies in the overlap of several different variables. These include the anaplastic appearance, expression of CD30, the t(2;5), overexpression of the alk protein, and a frequent occurrence in young patients. When all of these characteristics are found in an individual patient, the diagnosis is straightforward. There are subsets of patients with only one or two of these characteristics, however. Whether they represent the same disease has been a point for considerable debate. Recent studies suggest that the occurrence in younger patients and an excellent treatment outcome might correlate best with overexpression of the alk protein.[677,678]

Patients with anaplastic neoplasms involving only the skin, which express CD30, present a particular diagnostic problem. Some of these patients will have lymphomatoid papulosis (see "Atypical Lymphoid Proliferations Sometimes Confused with Lymphoma"). Other patients appear to have an indolent process that is different from patients with anaplastic large T/null cell lymphoma involving multiple sites or other organs.[38,679] Some have suggested that patients should be divided into subgroups representing either typical anaplastic large T/null cell lymphoma, lymphomatoid papulosis, or a cutaneous variant of anaplastic large T/null cell lymphoma that is not progressive.[679] These tumors are typically alk-negative.[680]

Characteristics of patients with anaplastic large T/null cell lymphoma are presented in Table 112-9. The most striking features are the young median age and the striking male predominance.[117,681] The therapy for these patients is not different from that for other types of diffuse aggressive lymphoma. The results are distinctly better in patients with anaplastic large T/ null cell lymphoma than for other aggressive T-cell lymphomas. The 5-year progression-free survival for all patients is more than 50% and the 5-year overall survival is more than 70%.[117,681,682] Factors predicting treatment outcome in addition to alk expression include the serum level of CD30 antigen[683] in addition to other factors reflecting disease extent.

LYMPHOMA AT EXTRANODAL SITES

Depending upon how it is defined, extranodal non-Hodgkin's lymphoma accounts for approximately 25% of cases. Twenty-five years ago, a retrospective regional cancer registry study identified 24% of 8000 cases as extranodal; 15% of the extranodal cases were tonsillar or in Waldeyer's ring.[684] A prospective population-based study in 1991 found almost the same incidence in a survey of 1257 newly diagnosed patients in West Jutland, Denmark.[685] In this study, the criteria for an extranodal diagnosis were initial presentation with lymphoma at one or more extranodal sites, either alone (i.e., primary solitary

extranodal disease) or with a minor accompanying nodal component, suggesting that the extranodal site was primary. Several important observations were made. First, the majority of patients had what would now be described as diffuse large B-cell (DLBC) lymphoma. Second, the most common sites for solitary extranodal lymphoma were stomach, skin, and brain. Survival correlated with histologic subtype; that is, the patterns of behavior overall mirrored that of nodal lymphoma. Another analysis showed that, stage for stage, the outcome was the same for extranodal as for nodal lymphoma.[686] It might be inferred from these data that primary extranodal presentations should therefore be investigated and treated like their nodal counterparts. This is quite likely to be an oversimplification; grouping all extranodal lymphomas together could disguise major differences between the extranodal and nodal forms. The staging evaluation may be the same. Should the results be presented in the same way, or should there be a different system of documentation for extranodal lymphoma? Furthermore, making the diagnosis may be difficult, first because specimens may be crushed, and second, particularly with T-cell lymphoma, because the distinction between malignant and nonmalignant may not be easy to make. In practice, the same guidelines are applied to the management of extranodal and primary nodal lymphoma. Caveats, however, must be applied. For example, patients with gastrointestinal lymphoma may present with weight loss due to malabsorption; this does not constitute a B symptom in the conventional sense. Special staging classifications may be appropriate for extranodal lymphoma at specific sites. Reevaluation may be difficult; the radiologic appearances after therapy for lymphoma in bone may continue to be abnormal even if cure has been effected. These and other problems should be borne in mind in interpreting the published data.

Major Sites

Gastrointestinal Tract Lymphoma
In most series of primary extranodal lymphomas, the gastrointestinal tract is the most common site, accounting for 30% to 40% of the total.[684] Lymphoma may arise anywhere in the gastrointestinal tract but is seen most frequently in the stomach, and then the small bowel.[687-689] Increasing evidence shows that some gastric lymphomas presenting like gastric carcinoma as well as some intestinal lymphomas are of MALT origin.[77,79] Some other intestinal lymphomas are either enteropathy associated and of the T-cell type, arising against a background of celiac disease, or (usually in patients from the Middle East) they are part of immunoproliferative small intestinal disease (IPSID) (previously termed Mediterranean B-cell lymphoma).[690,691] Clinically, the enteropathy-associated T-cell type and the IPSID type present predominantly with malabsorption, while the rest present with obstructive symptoms. Most patients with gastrointestinal lymphoma have diffuse large B-cell lymphoma, however.

Gastric Lymphoma
The clinical course of "low-grade" gastric lymphoma of MALT has changed dramatically, first because the use of

endoscopy as opposed to open surgery for diagnosing lesions within the gastrointestinal tract and second because of increased understanding of its pathophysiology. The published literature suggesting that 50% of those in whom the lymphoma is low grade and confined to the stomach may be cured with surgery alone[692-703] and that this cure fraction may be increased by chemotherapy[704-706] or irradiation[707-710] and that surgery may now happily be redundant.[711] The demonstration of the association *between Helicobacter pylori* infection and lymphoma[383] in the stomach has led to anti-Helicobacter therapy becoming the treatment of first choice *provided* the lymphoma is histologically of low grade. Several studies have shown that 10-day therapy with ampicillin with either metronidazole, tripotassium dicitrobismuthate, or omeprazole will result in complete or partial regression of lymphoma over many months, making it the treatment of first choice.[84,712-716] Critical to this dramatic change in management is strict adherence to 6-monthly follow-up with repeat endoscopy by an experienced endoscopist. It may well be appropriate to define the extent of disease with endoscopic ultrasonography.[717] Histological and endoscopic remission while in general inferring an excellent prognosis may not equate with cure: half of such remission may be associated with persistent "disease" at the molecular level.[716,718-720] It may be that those with t(11;18) (q21:q21) involving the AP12 gene may be antibiotic resistant.[721] Failure to eradicate *H. pylori* with first-line therapy should be followed by second-line antibiotics.

For the subset of patients with antibiotic resistance or evidence of *H. pylori* infection at presentation, relatively innocuous chemotherapy or irradiation yield excellent results.[722-724] Surgery holds little attraction.

Diffuse Large B-Cell (Either Primary or Transformed from Low-Grade MALT) Lymphoma. This should be managed with curative intent in the same way as nodal diffuse large B-cell (DLBC) lymphoma with similar prognostic factors, although there is data showing that in selected patients anti-Helicobacter therapy may yield remissions.[725-728] A large prospective study showed identical outcome for patients in which DLBC arose in the GI tract, and those in whom in was nodal.[729] Hence until recently combination chemotherapy with CHOP would have been the treatment of choice. It is likely that this will be superseded by CHOP-R, even though no randomized trial has been undertaken.

Intestinal Lymphomas

Bowel lymphomas are almost always aggressive, whether of T- or B-cell origin. The principles of management include countering the problems of malabsorption whenever possible, surgery, and adjuvant chemotherapy. Particular attention must be paid to the risk of perforation. Overall outcome correlates with the same factors as those for nodal lymphoma.[121] It has been reported that the first-year survival of those with aggressive T-cell intestinal lymphoma is only 25% compared with 75% for the relatively uncommon low-grade B-cell lymphomas.[730-732] Primary treatment of intestinal lymphoma is usually surgical. This may be followed by whole-abdominal radiation or, in the case of diffuse large B-cell lymphoma, a doxorubicin-containing regimen. There is little consensus as to the optimal treatment, however.

Those presenting with IPSID may well be unable to tolerate a conventional lymphoma approach because of general debility. It is therefore gratifying that antibiotics have been reported to induce remissions. The effect of antibiotics, however, seems to be confined to those patients in whom a monoclonal large cell lymphoma has not developed. Despite this success, as well as some success with chemotherapy, the overall outcome remains poor, survival being less than 50% at 5 years even for those with resectable localized tumors.[690,691,733,734] Surgical resection of the involved bowel is important in both large and small bowel tumors to reduce the chance of perforation with chemotherapy and its dire consequences.

The management of treatment failure is the same as for nodal lymphoma.

Pancreas

Pancreatic lymphomas, while extremely rare, deserve special comment. As pancreatic carcinoma has such a dismal outlook, many patients do not undergo biopsy, but a small proportion of pancreatic neoplasms will be diffuse large B-cell lymphomas. To fail to make this diagnosis eliminates the chance of cure.

Skin Lymphoma

Primary extranodal lymphomas arising in the skin present quite a different clinical problem from nodal lymphoma and must be distinguished from skin deposits of lymphoma that originated in the lymph nodes. Skin lymphomas may be of B- or T-cell type, are frequently indolent, and despite multiple recurrences after apparently successful therapy may remain confined to the skin for many years. The WHO classification does not distinguish between primary nodal and extranodal presentations of lymphoma. There is some debate about whether it is applicable to the skin.[735,736] Most discussion surrounds the primary cutaneous B-cell lymphomas (PCBCL)[737] which are much less common than their T-cell counterpart (see Chapter 113). It may well be that the EORTC classification is the more clinically relevant scheme for PCBCL.[735] It has been postulated that some, or many, are the cutaneous counterpart of the MALT lymphomas in the gastrointestinal tract.[726,727] Most critical is the fact that even if the histological appearance is aggressive the clinical course may not be, with the disease being confined to sites (they may be multiple) in the skin, repeated responsiveness to therapy and long survival being the rule rather than the exception.[738] Expectant management may be appropriate after excision biopsy. Radiotherapy is considered the treatment of choice,[728] although single agent and combination chemotherapy have their protagonists.[728,739] Anti-CD20 has been advocated[740,741] and there may be a theoretical indication for anti-Borrelia burgdorferi therapy in some cases associated with acrodermatitis chronica atrophicans.[742] The only probable indication for an intensive approach is when the presentation is on the leg.[743]

Primary Central Nervous System Lymphoma

Primary central nervous system lymphoma (PCNSL) is defined as lymphoma arising in, and confined to the neuraxis. It has in the past been recorded as accounting for 1% to 2% of all primary brain tumors, and 3% to 4% of extranodal lymphoma,[744,745] but is undoubtedly increasing in incidence. Data from the United States Surveillance, Epidemiology, and End Results (SEER) program indicate a 10-fold increase both in the immunocompetent and immunocompromised between 1973 and 1992.

The most common presentation is that of a patient who is in late middle age or elderly if immunocompetent, but younger if immunocompromised, with cognitive or personality changes for a few weeks. In many patients there are multiple lesions and there may be focal symptoms and signs. Seizures occur more commonly in the immunocompromised. The diagnosis is made by stereotactic biopsy; this is the only role for surgery. Optimal investigation includes gadolinium-enhanced cranial spinal MRI and cerebrospinal fluid cytology, complemented by routine staging for lymphoma and other sites.

The natural history as has been known for three quarters of a century is dismal. Even today, with current therapy, the prognosis for most people is very poor[746-775] although there may be glimmers of hope. Intervention often palliates successfully if only for months. Prolonged disease-free survival may be achieved for a proportion, but often at a severe price. Corticosteroids are always included, both reducing edema and having a direct lympholytic effect, strong enough that they should be withheld whenever possible until a suspected diagnosis has been confirmed.[747]

Radiotherapy has historically been the mainstay of treatment. Whole neuraxis irradiation is not usually undertaken, although including the posterior two thirds of the eye in the field is advisable. Whole brain irradiation at a dose of 40 to 50 Gy results in regression of symptoms and signs and radiological improvement in up to 80% of cases, but the responses are rarely durable.[748] Recurrences usually occur within the radiation field, and although they may be responsive to chemotherapy, the median survival does not exceed 18 months, and later neurotoxicity in survivors may be a problem.[749]

Many attempts have been made to improve upon these results by the introduction of chemotherapy into the initial treatment plan. Inconveniently most of the drugs effective in the management of systemic lymphoma do not cross the intact blood-brain barrier in tumorical doses, and are hence ineffective. Methotrexate, given intravenously in doses exceeding 1 g/m^2 (followed by folinic acid rescue) is a major exception, yielding results approximating to those of irradiation.[750-754] Sequential chemoradiotherapy has become accepted by many as being the treatment of choice at least for younger patients in the 21st century. Several relatively small single-center studies suggest that the overall response rate may approach 100% and that the median survival is much longer than with irradiation alone. In a multicenter study[755] of more than 100 patients, methotrexate at a dose of 2.5 g/m^2 was given every 3 weeks for a total of 5 doses with procarbazine and vincristine before whole brain radiotherapy. This was followed by two cycles of high-dose cytosine arabinoside. The median progression-free survival was 2 years, and 25% of patients were progression free at 5 years. The excellence of these results in contrast to historical controls must sadly be interpreted within the context of 15% long-term severe neurotoxicity. The issue of whether the irradiation could be omitted (initially) was addressed in a pilot study[756] of 25 patients who received methotrexate at a dose of 8 g/m^2 every 2 weeks as induction, followed by consolidation and then maintenance for a year. Irradiation was reserved for recurrence. While the progression-free survival was not as impressive as the combined modality treatment, the median survival had not yet been reached, and the neurotoxicity reported was much less. Hence the challenge lies in determining which group of patients is at high enough risk of the disease to justify the potential risk of very severe unpleasant debilitating morbidity.

Many questions remain to be answered: what is the optimal dose of methotrexate and how often should it be given; which if any other drugs will improve the response rate (possibly cytosine arabinoside); and in which circumstances can the irradiation be omitted.[757] The latter is probably the most important. The rarity of the condition makes the design of the relevant trials difficult. The opportunity and necessity of providing excellent palliative care for patients with cerebral lymphoma is enormous.

Orbital Lymphoma

These tumors are most often seen in older people. They present with ptosis, a conjunctival mass, or blurred vision.[758] Alternatively, they may present with swelling and proptosis of the eye with disturbance of eye movements.[759] A biopsy is essential to making the diagnosis. CT or MRI scans of the orbit are helpful in establishing the extent of disease. These tumors are usually localized. In terms of histologic subtype, most orbital lymphomas are of B-cell origin, usually being small lymphocytic, MALT, follicular, or mantle cell in histology, although diffuse large B-cell lymphomas also occur.[760]

Radiotherapy is very effective as treatment and results in local control for more than 95% of patients, although systemic chemotherapy should be used for diffuse large B-cell lymphoma.[761,762]

Extradural Lymphoma

Cord compression may be the presenting symptom of lymphoma or patients may develop an extradural lesion as a manifestation of recurrence. Most extradural lymphomas occur in the thoracic spine. Back pain is the most frequent symptom, and is usually followed by progressive neurologic dysfunction, starting with weakness, followed by sensory loss with a sensory level and, finally, impairment of sphincter function.

The diagnosis is usually suspected on the basis of a CT-myelogram and/or MRI scan but may often not be made until emergency decompression is accompanied by a biopsy. Pathology usually shows diffuse large B-cell lymphoma.[763] After decompression of the spinal cord, treatment usually comprises radiotherapy, but this is usually not sufficient. Thus surgery and radiotherapy should be followed by chemotherapy with a doxorubicin-containing regimen. The addition of the latter has been shown to improve survival.[764]

Head and Neck Lymphoma

Lymphomas arising within Waldeyer's ring, the sinuses, and the oropharynx are variously considered to be or not to be extranodal. The distinction is semantically important, since they account for perhaps 15% of all extranodal lymphomas. The most common single site is the tonsil. Histologically they are usually diffuse large B-cell lymphomas. Limited extended irradiation has been the most widely used treatment of first choice; cure rates between 25% and 60% have been reported, with the better rates for those with stage I presentations[765-767] Progression is usually outside the irradiation field. Some studies have shown that combined-modality therapy gives better results.[768-770] Few data exist for chemotherapy alone. Sinus presentations are usually of B-cell origin in the Western population,[771-773] although in the East, T-cell types occur.[117,769] While the results of irradiation for the former are similar to those for lymphoma arising in Waldeyer's ring,[768] control is more difficult to achieve and distant spread may occur.[769,770,774]

The salivary gland is the only head and neck extranodal site of lymphoma in which the histologic pattern is usually of the MALT type.[775] Treatment principles are the same as for other MALT lymphomas.

Thyroid

Thyroid lymphoma frequently arises against a background of Hashimoto's thyroiditis[776,777] and is usually a diffuse large B-cell lymphoma. Radiation therapy is curative for most patients,[775] but distant recurrences occur. This led to the use of combined-modality therapy for those considered at high risk[778,779]; chemotherapy alone has also been advocated.[780]

Testicle

Testicular lymphoma is also almost invariably a diffuse large B-cell lymphoma and requires special attention. The most common presentation is of a unilateral testicular swelling, but both testes may be involved. In addition, spread to the CNS has been suggested as a complication. Therapy comprises systemic chemotherapy (always), local irradiation to the opposite testicle, and CNS prophylaxis with intrathecal methotrexate.[781-786]

Other Sites

Lymphomas arising in other extranodal sites are rare. Reports tend to be anecdotal, since testicular lymphomas are likely to be referred to the urologist, bone lymphoma to the orthopedic surgeon, ovarian lymphoma to the gynecologist, and so on. An increasing body of evidence shows that some of them may be analogous to the MALT lymphomas arising in the gastrointestinal tract, particularly those occurring in the lung, breast, thyroid, salivary glands, and skin. Management has been based on the same principles as those applied to nodal lymphoma.

SPECIAL PROBLEMS

HIV-Associated Lymphoma

Lymphoma in Patients with HIV Infection

With the advent of antiretroviral therapy, there appeared to be an increase in the number of patients developing HIV-associated lymphoma.[787-789] Subsequently, the introduction of highly active antiretroviral therapy (HAART) has had a dramatic impact upon the length and quality of life of those with HIV infection living in countries where it is available. There has been a marked reduction in the incidence of HIV-associated lymphoma, particularly in the central nervous system.[790,791] It remains a significant risk for those on HAART, however, and an almost intractable problem if it develops in those not on HAART.

HIV-associated lymphoma may be the AIDS-defining illness, or develop during the course of AIDS. It is almost always B cell in origin, most commonly large B-cell lymphoma, and sometimes Burkitt's lymphoma. It has been postulated that the lymphoma develops as a consequence of HIV stimulation and reactivation of latent EBV infection.[792] Apart from the rare cases of primary effusion lymphoma[793] the majority of patients present with advanced disease, not infrequently involving extranodal sites. The bone marrow is often involved, and meningeal involvement may be asymptomatic. In general the workup is as for lymphoma in the immunocompetent, and must include examination of the cerebrospinal fluid, as meningeal involvement may be asymptomatic.

The overall management must be considered within the context of the overall situation, and will be markedly different for those being successfully treated with HAART from those who are not. The former may be treated with curative intent and some anticipation of success. Palliation is the only realistic goal for the large majority of the remainder. Close cooperation between oncologist and infectious disease specialist is vital.

Cyclical combination chemotherapy is the treatment of choice whenever possible; variations on a theme of CHOP, with intrathecal methotrexate, as CNS-directed therapy are favored by most. The prognosis correlates with the International Prognostic Index (IPI), with age younger than 35 years being the important cutoff.[794]

Excellent results have been achieved with combinations containing infusional etoposide,[795] most success being reported with EPOCH (etoposide, prednisolone, oncovorin, cyclophosphamide, hydroxydaunorubicin),[796] developed at the National Cancer Institute. It is recommended that HAART be withheld during the period of therapy, although with other regimens it may well be wise to continue it.[797]

It is fortunate that primary central nervous system lymphoma has become very rare in the context of HIV infection in the HAART era. When it occurs, it may be appropriate to treat aggressively as in the immunocompetent. If HAART is not available, whole brain irradiation may yield the best palliation.[798] Although not strictly the topic of this chapter, Hodgkin's disease occurs more frequently in the HIV setting than otherwise. If preliminary, data suggest moderately intensive chemotherapy may be successful.

Post-Transplant Lymphoproliferative Disorder

Uncommon in the practice of hemato-oncology as a whole, post-transplant lymphoproliferative disorder (PTLD) presents a significant problem for those undertaking allogeneic transplantation of solid organs.[799] The prognosis of renal and cardiac transplantation has improved: a recent study reported the relative risk of lymphoma in this patient population to be between 28 and 49.[800] The Epstein-Barr virus is thought to be critical in the large majority of cases. The risk is greatest in those who are EBV seronegative at the time of transplantation. Ninety percent of all episodes of PTLD occur within 5 years of transplantation, and half of them within the first 6 months. The presentation may be with lymphadenopathy and constitutional "B" symptoms or solitary nodal or extranodal masses.

Management begins with close liaison between oncologist and renal and cardiac transplant teams. Prophylaxis with acyclovir or ganciclovir may reduce the risk.[801,802] Once the diagnosis has been established, reduction of immunosuppression as far as is feasible is the first course of action and is likely, particularly in the first year post-transplant, to be successful initially, although the mortality remains quite high.[803] The longer the interval between transplant and PTLD the less favorable the outcome. Chemotherapy is reserved for patients when reducing the immunosuppression is not feasible or fails, as for some patients in whom it is not considered wise to wait.[804] Reasonable remission rates have been reported.

More interesting is immunotherapy. Data are accumulating about the potential role of anti-CD20 (rituximab) which has reported to result in a response rate similar to chemotherapy. Less practicable, but theoretically much more attractive is adoptive chemotherapy with EBV-specific cytotoxic T cells.[805-807]

Lymphoma in the Elderly

The incidence of lymphoma increases with advancing age and the life span is lengthening; at least in the "developed" world the management of older patients with lymphoma is becoming an increasing problem. Regardless of the age cutoff used to define *elderly*, the challenge is predominantly that of contending with patients who are at high risk of comorbidity and have social circumstances that may complicate the overall management plan. Clearly, for those patients with follicular lymphoma or the other lymphomas with a relatively long clinical course, an expectant policy or minimal intervention becomes the most appropriate course. Brief treatments such as targeted irradiation are attractive in these circumstances, also for those with large B-cell lymphoma.

For those with lymphomas for which prolonged survival is only possible if complete remission is achieved, philosophical as well as pragmatic issues come into play. It is gratifying that rituximab combined with CHOP has proved to be tolerable with a relatively low mortality in those "elderly" patients being treated with curative intent, and that the combination renders a significant proportion of patients disease free for prolonged periods. Data,

presented so far only in abstract form, indicate that with the judicious use of growth factors it is possible to administer CHOP at 14-day intervals as opposed to 21-day intervals and that this also results in improved outcome in the elderly. It remains to be determined whether the "best standard of care" at the beginning of 21st century will be CHOP-R or CHOP-14-R. Not surprisingly there is inevitable selection of older patients into clinical trials. A high proportion of cases will inevitably, and appropriately, receive individualized therapy, a multititude of factors beyond the IPI coming into play.

ATYPICAL LYMPHOID PROLIFERATIONS SOMETIMES CONFUSED WITH LYMPHOMA

All examples of disordered lymphoid proliferation do not represent lymphomas. These clinicopathologic entities can present confusing clinical problems, however. These conditions include benign lymphoid proliferations that can be confused with either T- or B-cell lymphomas. To confuse the picture further, these latter entities sometime evolve into lymphoma.

Of the atypical lymphoid proliferations confused with lymphoma, the most common are processes referred to as "reactive" or "atypical" lymphoid hyperplasia. These patients present with localized or disseminated lymphadenopathy associated with an underlying condition that may or may not be obvious. The patients sometimes have systemic symptoms, depending upon the associated illness. Problems underlying this condition include drugs (e.g., dilantin and carbamazepine),[808] autoimmune disorders (e.g., rheumatoid arthritis, systemic lupus erythematosus, and Sjögren's syndrome),[809-812] viral infections (e.g., cytomegalovirus, EBV, and varicella-zoster virus), and bacterial infections (e.g., cat scratch disease). The distinction between these entities and malignant lymphoma is tremendously important. Lymphadenopathy in these patients rarely evolves into malignant lymphoma, and successful treatment of the underlying condition usually resolves the problem. When no explanation can be found for atypical lymphadenopathy, observation of the patient is appropriate. On occasion, subsequent biopsies will demonstrate lymphoma.

An unusual clinical entity variously known as Castleman's disease, angiofollicular lymph node hyperplasia, and giant lymph node hyperplasia can be confused with malignant lymphoma. First described in 1956,[813] this entity can present with localized or disseminated lymphadenopathy involving essentially all lymph node bearing areas.[814] Lymphadenopathy is frequently accompanied by systemic symptoms such as fever, night sweats, or weight loss. The condition is found with an increased frequency in patients infected with HIV-1.[815] Castleman's disease can be found in patients with POEMS syndrome.[816] Biopsy of an involved lymph node reveals one of two histologic patterns. The more common pattern involves lymph node effacement by small hyaline, vascular follicles and interfollicular capillary proliferation, while in a few patients the histologic pattern is large hyperplastic lymphoid follicles with intervening sheets of plasma cells.[817] The patients often have anemia and polyclonal hypergammaglobulinemia. It is now known that many of the manifestations of this disorder seem to be mediated by excessive production of the cytokine IL-6, and the symptoms of the disease can sometimes be ameliorated by administration of a monoclonal antibody against interleukin IL-6.[818] Patients with Castleman's disease can die of the disorder or complications of therapy. Management is further complicated by the fact that some of these patients develop malignant lymphomas on follow-up. The successful management of patients who present with localized involvement can be accomplished with surgery or radiation therapy.[818] Patients with disseminated disease sometimes respond completely to therapy with glucocorticoids.[814] Symptomatic patients who do not respond completely are sometimes treated with chemotherapeutic agents in a manner similar to that used for malignant lymphoma. Successful treatment has been described with interferon,[819] monoclonal anit-IL-6 antibody,[820] rituximab,[821] autologous bone marrow transplantation,[822] and allogeneic bone marrow transplantation.[823] It should be remembered, however, that this disorder sometimes spontaneously remits, and a cause of death has been treatment-related complications.

Among the other, unusual disorders associated with atypical lymphadenopathy is sinus histiocytosis with massive lymphadenopathy (Rosai-Dorfman disease). First described in 1969,[824] this entity usually presents with bulky lymphadenopathy but can have extranodal sites of involvement.[825] This disorder is most commonly seen in children or young adults. Biopsy reveals lymph nodes with a distorted architecture due to a thickened fibrous capsule, distension of the lymphoid sinuses by histiocytes, and infiltration of the node by plasma cells. The histiocytes in this disorder are morphologically characteristic. The disease is usually nonprogressive and self-limiting. Occasional cases have associated autoimmune hemolytic anemias that can be severe or even fatal but should be treated like other autoimmune hemolytic anemias. Surgery or radiation therapy can be utilized to manage symptomatic, bulky disease sites.

Lymphomatoid papulosis represents a clinically benign cutaneous lymphoproliferative disorder that is often confused with anaplastic large cell lymphoma involving the skin.[826] This is because the cells of lymphomatoid papulosis are atypical and stain for the Ki-1 (CD30) antigen. This is an extremely important distinction that can only be effectively made when the clinician and pathologist communicate.[827] The key to the diagnosis is an accurate history. Patients with lymphomatoid papulosis have waxing and waning skin lesions that usually heal leaving small scars. Therapy appropriate for malignant lymphoma is contraindicated and dangerous. The clinical picture is complicated by the fact that patients with lymphomatoid papulosis sometimes develop malignant lymphomas.

CONCLUSIONS

The malignant non-Hodgkin's lymphomas offer a challenge to all branches of medicine. This chapter tried to give a broad perspective, with particular reference to the evolution of management, in an attempt to indicate how these lymphomas may best be treated today. We hope that the next edition of this book will reveal even greater progress than has been achieved so far.

REFERENCES

1. Weisenburger DD: Epidemiology of non-Hodgkin's lymphoma: Recent findings regarding an emerging epidemic. Ann Oncol 1994;5:S19.
2. Devesa SS, Silverman DT, et al: Cancer incidence and mortality trends among whites in the United States, 1947–1984. J Natl Cancer Inst 1987;79:701.
3. Leukaemia Research Fund: Leukaemia and Lymphoma: An Atlas of Distribution within Areas of England and Wales 1984–1988. London, Leukaemia Research Fund, 1990.
4. Hartge P, Devesa SS, Franmeni JF: Hodgkin's and non-Hodgkin's lymphomas. In Doll R, Franmeni J, Muir C (eds): Trends in Cancer Incidence and Mortality Cancer Surveys. Cold Spring Harbor, New York, Cold Spring Harbor Laboratory Press, 1994, p 423.
5. McNally RJQ, Rowland D, Roman E, et al: Age and sex distributions of hematological malignancies in the U.K. Haematol Oncol 1997;15:173.
6. Ries LAG, Miller BA, Hankey BF, et al (eds): SEER Cancer Statistics Review 1973–1991: Tables and Graphs. National Cancer Institute NIH Publication No. 942789. Bethesda, MD, U.S. Department of Health and Human Services, 1994.
7. Filipovich AH, Mathur A, et al: Primary immunodeficiencies: Genetic risk factors for lymphoma. Cancer Res 1992;52:5465s.
8. Perry GSI, Spector BD, et al: The Wiskott-Aldrich syndrome in the United States and Canada (1892–1979). J Paediatr 1980;97:72.
9. Kassan SS, Thomas TL, et al: Increased risk of lymphoma in Sicca syndrome. Ann Intern Med 1978;89:888.
10. Hoover RN: Lymphoma risks in populations with altered immunity: A search for mechanism. Cancer Res 1992;52:5477s.
11. Hussell T, Isaacson P, Crabtree J, et al: The response of cells from low-grade B-cell gastric lymphomas of mucosa-associated lymphoid tissue to Helicobacter pylori. Lancet 1993;342:571.
12. Zucca E, Bertoni F, Roggero E, et al: Molecular analysis of the progression from Helicobacter pylori–associated chronic gastritis to mucosa-associated lymphoid-tissue lymphoma of the stomach. N Engl J Med 1998;388:804.
13. Ferreri AJ, Guidoboni M, Ponzoni M, et al: Evidence for association between Chlamydia psittaci infection and ocular adnexal lymphoma. J Clin Oncol 2003;22: 565a.
14. Epstein MA, Achong BG, et al: Virus particles in cultured lymphoblasts from Burkitt's lymphoma. Lancet 1964;1:702.
15. Poiesz BJ, Ruscetti FW, Gazdar AF, et al: Detection and isolation of type C retrovirus particles from fresh and cultured lymphocyte of a patient with cutaneous T-cell lymphoma. Proc Natl Acad Sci USA 1980;77:7415.
16. Uchiyama T, Yodoi J, Sagawa X, et al: Adult T-cell leukemia: Clinical and hematologic features of 16 cases. Blood 1977;50:481.
17. Blattner WA, Blayney DW, Robert-Guroff M, et al: Epidemiology of human T-cell leukemia/lymphoma virus. J Infect Dis 1983;147:406.
18. Murphy EL, Hanchard B, Figueroa JP, et al: Modelling the risk of adult T cell leukaemia/lymphoma. Int J Cancer 1989;43:250.
19. Nador RG, Cesarman E, Chadburn A, et al: Primary effusion lymphoma: A distinct clinicopathologic entity associated with the Kaposi's sarcoma-associated herpes virus. Blood 1996;88:645.
20. Gessain A, Briere J, Angelin-Duclos C, et al: Human herpes virus 8 (Kaposi's sarcoma herpes virus) and malignant lymphoproliferations in France: A molecular study of 250 cases including two AIDS-associated body cavity based lymphomas. Leukemia 1997;11:266.
21. Chang Y, Cesarman E, Pessin MS, et al: Identification of herpesvirus-like DNA sequences in AIDS-associated Kaposi's sarcoma. Science 1994;266:1865.
22. Butel JS, Lednicky JA: Cell and molecular biology of simian virus 40: Implications for human infections and disease. J Natl Acad Sci USA 1999;91:119–134.

23. Vilchez RA, Madden CR, Kozinetz CA et al: Association between simian virus 40 and non-Hodgkin's lymphoma. Lancet 2002;359:817–823.

24. Turner NC, Dusheiko G, Jones A: Hepatitis C and B-cell lymphoma. Ann Oncol 2003;14:1341–1345.

25. Pearce N, Bethwaite P: Increasing incidence of non-Hodgkin's lymphoma: occupational and environmental factors. Cancer Res 1992;52:5496s.

26. Pearce NE, Smith AH, et al: Malignant lymphoma and multiple myeloma linked with agricultural occupations in New Zealand Cancer Registry–based study. Am J Epidemiol 1985;121:225.

27. Pearce NE, Reif JS: Epidemiologic studies of cancer in agricultural workers. Am J Ind Med 1990;18:133.

28. Hardell L: Malignant lymphoma of histiocytic type and exposure to phenoxyacetic acids or chlorophenols. Lancet 1979;1:55.

29. Dich J, Zahm SH, Hanberg A, et al: Pesticides and cancer. Cancer Causes Control 1997;8:420.

30. Veterans and Agent Orange: Health Effects of Herbicides Used in Vietnam. Washington, DC, National Acad of Sciences, 1994.

31. Zahm SH, Blair A: Pesticides and non-Hodgkin's lymphoma. Cancer Res 1992;52:5485s.

32. Ames BN, Kammen HO, Yamasaki E: Hair dyes are mutagenic: Identification of a variety of mitogenic ingredients. Proc Natl Acad Sci USA 1975;72:2423.

33. Cantor KP, Blair A, et al: Hair dye use and risk of leukemia and lymphoma. Am J Public Health 1988;78:570.

34. Zahm SH, Weisenberger DD, Babbitt PA, et al: Use of hair coloring products and the risk of lymphoma, multiple myeloma and chronic lymphocytic leukemia. Am J Public Health 1992;82:990.

35. Linet MS, Pottern LM: Familial aggregation of hematopoietic malignancies and risk of non-Hodgkin's lymphoma. Cancer Res 1992;52:5468s.

36. Pappa VI, Hussain HK, Reznek RH, et al: The role of image-guided core needle biopsy in the management of patients with lymphoma. J Clin Oncol 1996;14:2427.

37. Jaffe ES: Surgical Pathology of the Lymph Nodes and Related Organs. Philadelphia, WB Saunders, 1985.

38. Harris N, Jaffe ES, Stein H, et al: A revised European-American classification of lymphoid neoplasms: A proposal from the International Lymphoma Study Group. Blood 1994;84:1361.

39. Stansfeld AG, D'Ardenne AJ: Lymph Node Biopsy Interpretation. New York, Churchill Livingstone, 1992.

40. Hodgkin T: On some of the morbid appearances of the absorbent glands and spleen. Trans Med Chir Soc Lond 1832;17:68.

41. Jaffe ES, Harris NL, Stein H, Vardiman JW (eds): Pathology and Genetics: Tumours of Haematopoietic and Lymphoid Tissues. (WHO classification of tumours) Lyon, IARC Press, 2001.

42. Virchow R: Die Krankenhaften Geschwülste. Berlin, Herschwald, 1864.

43. Kundrat H: Uber Lymphosarcomatosis. Klin Wochenschr (Wien) 1893;6:211.

44. Ewing J: Reticulum cell sarcoma. J Med Res 1913;32:1.

45. Oberling C: Les reticulo-sarcoma et les reticulo-endothelio-sarcoma de la moelle ossense (sarcoma d'Ewing). Bull Assoc France Etude Cancer 1928;17:259.

46. Roulet F: Das priamare Retothelsarkom der Lymphknoten. Virchows Arch 1930;277:15.

47. Gall EA, Mallory TB: Malignant lymphoma: A clinicopathological survey of 618 cases. Am J Pathol 1942;18:381.

48. Becker E: Rein Betrag zur Lehr von den Lymphomen. Dtsch Med Wochenscr 1901;27:726.

49. Baehr G: The clinical and pathological picture of follicular lymphoblastoma. Trans Assoc Am Physicians 1932;47:330.

50. Symmers D: Follicular lymphadenopathy with splenomegaly: A newly recognised disease of the lymphatic system. Arch Pathol 1927;3:816.

51. Symmers D: Giant follicular lymphoma with or without splenomegaly. Arch Pathol 1938;26:603.

52. Rosenberg SA, Diamond HD, et al: Lymphosarcoma: A review of 1269 cases. Medicine (Baltimore) 1961;40:31.

53. Rappaport HW, Winter J, et al: Follicular lymphoma: A reevaluation of its place in the scheme of malignant lymphoma based on a survey of 253 cases. Cancer 1956;9:792.

54. Rappaport H: Malignant Lymphomas in Tumors of Hematopoietic System. (Publication 91) Washington, DC, Armed Forces Institute of Pathology, 1966.

55. Brouet JC, Preud'Homme JL, et al: Membrane markers in "histiocytic" lymphomas (reticulum cell sarcomas). J Natl Cancer Inst 1976;56:361.

56. Leech JH, Glick AD, et al: Malignant lymphomas of follicular center cell origin in man. I. Immunologic studies. J Natl Cancer Inst 1975;54:11.

57. Lennert K, Stein H, et al: Cytological and functional criteria for the classification of malignant lymphomata. Br J Cancer 1975;31 (Suppl II):29.

58. Gerard-Marchant R, Hamblin I, et al: Classification of non-Hodgkin's lymphoma. Lancet 1974;2:406.

59. Lukes RJ, Collins RD: Immunologic characterization of human malignant lymphomas. Cancer 1974;34:1488–1503.

60. National Cancer Institute: National Cancer Institute sponsored study of classifications of non-Hodgkin's lymphomas: Summary and description of a working formulation for clinical usage. Cancer 1982;49:2112.

61. Zech L, Harglund V, Nilsson K, et al: Characteristic chromosomal abnormalities in biopsies and lymphoid cell lines from patients with Burkitt's and non Burkitt's lymphoma: Int J Cancer 1976;17:47.

62. Dalla Favera R, Bregni M, Erikson J, et al: Human c-myc gene is located on the region of chromosome 8 and is translocated in Burkitt's lymphoma cells. Proc Natl Acad Sci USA 1982;79:7824.

63. Rowley JD: Chromosome studies in non-Hodgkin's lymphomas: The role of the t(14;18) translocation. J Clin Oncol 1988;6:919.

64. Cleary ML, Sklar J: Nucleotide sequence of a t(14;18) breakpoint cluster in follicular lymphoma and demonstration of a breakpoint cluster near a transcriptionally active locus on chromosome 18. Proc Natl Acad Sci USA 1985;82:7439.

65. Weisenburger DD, Sanger WG, Armitage JO, et al: Intermediate lymphocytic lymphoma: Immunophenotypic and cytogenetic findings. Blood 1987;69:1617.

66. Tsujimoto Y, Yunis J, Onorato-Showe L, et al: Molecular cloning of the chromosomal breakpoint of B-cell lymphomas and leukemias with the t(11;14) chromosome translocation. Science 1984;224:1403.

67. Alizadeth AA, Eisen MB, Davies RE, et al: Distinct types of large B cell lymphoma identified by gene expression profiling. Nature 2000;403:503.

68. Shipp MA, Ross K, Tamayo P, et al: Diffuse large B cell lymphoma outcome prediction by gene expression profiling and supervised learning. Nat Med 2002;8:1.

69. Pittaluga S, Bijnens L, Teodorovic I, et al: Clinical analysis of 670 cases in two trials of the European organization for the research and treatment of Cancer Lymphoma Cooperative Group subtyped according to the revised European-American classification of lymphoid neoplasms: A comparison with the Working Formulation. Blood 1996;87:4358.

70. Zucca E, Stein H, Coiffer B: European Lymphoma Task Force (ELTF): Report of the workshop on mantle cell lymphoma. Ann Oncol 1994;5:507.

71. Williams ME, Meeker TC, Swerdlow SH: Rearrangement of chromosome 11 bcl-1 locus in centrocytic lymphoma: Analysis with multiple breakpoint probes. A Southern blot study with four different bcl-1 probes showing two clusters of rearrangements 24 kb apart in 12 of 23 patients. Blood 1991;78:493.

72. Withers DA, Harvey RC, Faust JB, et al: Characterization of a candidate bcl-1 gene. Chromosome walking between the breakpoint and the first Hpa II tiny-fragment island, identifying the CDNA encoding a cyclin gene. Mol Cell Biol 1991;11:4846.

73. Rosenberg CI, Wong E, Petty EM, et al: PRADI, a candidate BCL1 oncogene: Mapping and expression in centrocytic lymphoma. Proc Natl Acad Sci USA 1991;88:9638.

74. Brittinger G, Bartels H, Common H, et al: Clinical and prognostic relevance of the Kiel classification of non-Hodgkin's lymphoma: Results of a prospective multicentre study by the Kiel Lymphoma Group. Hematol Oncol 1984;2:269.

75. Swerdlow SH, Habeshaw JA, Marray LJ, et al: Centrocytic lymphoma: A distinct clinicopathologic and immunologic entity. Am J Pathol 1983;113:181.

Specific Malignancies

III

76. Richards MA, Hall PA, Gregory WM, et al: Lymphoplasmacytoid and small cell centrocytic non-Hodgkin's lymphoma: A retrospective analysis from St. Bartholomew's Hospital 1972–1986. Hematol Oncol 1989;7:19.

77. Issacson P, Wright DH: Malignant lymphoma of mucosa associated lymphoid tissue. Cancer 1983;53:2515.

78. Isaacson PG: Lymphomas of mucosa-associated lymphoid tissue (MALT). Histopathology 1990;16:617.

79. Isaacson PG, Spencer J: Malignant lymphoma of mucosa-associated lymphoid tissue. Histopathology 1987;11:445.

80. Addis BJ, Hyjek E, Isaacson PG: Primary pulmonary lymphoma: A reappraisal of its histogenesis and its relationship to pseudolymphoma and lymphoid interstitial pneumonia. Histopathology 1988;13:1.

81. Hyjek E, Smith WJ, Isaacson PG: Primary B cell lymphoma of one salivary gland and its relationship to myoepithelial sialadenitis. Hum Pathol 1988;19:766.

82. Hyjek E, Isaacson PG: Primary B cell lymphoma of the thyroid and its relationship to Hashimoto's thyroiditis. Hum Pathol 1988;19:1315.

83. Medeiros LJ, Harris NL: Lymphoid infiltrates of the orbit and conjunctiva. Am J Surg Pathol 1989;13:459.

84. Wotherspoon AC, Doglinoni C, Diss TC, et al: Regression of primary low grade B cell lymphoma of mucosa-associated lymphoid tissue type after eradication of *Helicobacter pylori*. Lancet 1993;342:575.

85. Dierlamm J, Pittaluga S, Wlodarska I, et al: Marginal zone B-cell lymphomas of different sites share similar cytogenetic and morphologic features. Blood 1996;87:299.

86. Miller JB, Variakojis D, Bitran JD, et al: Diffuse histiocytic lymphoma with sclerosis: A clinicopathologic entity frequently causing superior venacaval obstruction. Cancer 1981;47:748.

87. Perron T, Frizzera G, Rosai J: Mediastinal diffuse large-cell lymphoma with sclerosis. A clinicopathologic study of 60 cases. Am J Surg Pathol 1986;10:176.

88. Lamarre L, Jacobson JO, Aisenberg AC, et al: Primary large cell lymphoma of the mediastinum: A histologic and immunophenotypic study of 29 cases. Am J Surg Pathol 1989;13:730.

89. Al-Sharabati M, Chittal S, Duga-Neeulat I, et al: Primary anterior mediastinal B-cell lymphoma: A clinicopathologic and immunohistochemical study of 16 cases. Cancer 1991;67:2579.

90. Jacobson JO, Aisenberg AC, Lamarre L, et al: Mediastinal large cell lymphoma: An uncommon subset of adult lymphoma curable with combined modality therapy. Cancer 1988;62:1893.

91. Todeschini G, Ambrosetti A, Meneghini G, et al: Mediastinal large-B-cell lymphoma with sclerosis: A clinical study of 21 patients. J Clin Oncol 1990;8:804.

92. Trump DL, Mann RB: Diffuse large cell and undifferentiated lymphomas with prominent mediastinal involvement: A poor prognostic subset of patients with non-Hodgkin's lymphoma. Cancer 1982;50:277.

93. Yousem SA, Weiss LM, Warnke RA: Primary mediastinal non-Hodgkin's lymphomas: A morphologic and immunologic study of 19 cases. Am J Clin Pathol 1985;83:676.

94. Menestrina F, Chilosi M, Bonetti F, et al: Mediastinal large-cell lymphoma of B-type, with sclerosis: Histopathological and immunohistochemical study of eight cases. Histopathology 1986;10:589.

95. Rohatiner AZS, Whelan JS, Ganjoo RK, et al: Mediastinal large cell lymphoma with sclerosis (MLCLS). Br J Cancer 1994;69:601.

96. Delsol G, Alsaati T, Gatter KL, et al: Coexpression of epithelial membrane antigen (EMA) Ki-1 and interlukin-2 receptor by anaplastic large cell lymphomas. Diagnostic value in so-called malignant histiocytosis. Am J Pathol 1988;130:59.

97. Agnarsson BA, Kadin ME: Ki-1 positive large cell lymphoma: A morphologic and immunologic study. Am J Surg Pathol 1988;12:264.

98. Carbone A, Gloghini A, De Re V, et al: Histopathologic, immunophenotyping and genotypic analysis of Ki-1 anaplastic large cell lymphomas express histiocyte-associated antigens. Cancer 1990;66:2547.

99. Stein H, Mason DY, Gerdes T, et al: The expression of the Hodgkin's disease-associated antigen Ki-1 in reactive and neoplastic lymphoid tissue: Evidence that Reed cells and histiocytic malignancies are derived from activated lymphoid cells. Blood 1985;66:848.

100. Ficher P, Nacheva E, Mason DY, et al: A KI-1 (CD30)–positive human cell line (Karpas 299) established from a high grade non-Hodgkin's lymphoma showing a 2:5 translocation and rearrangement of the T cell receptor chain gene. Blood 1988;72:234.

101. Rimokh R, Magaud JP, Berger R, et al: A translocation involving a specific breakpoint (q35) on chromosome 5 characteristic of anaplastic large cell lymphoma (Ki-1 lymphoma). Br J Haematol 1989;71:31.

102. Bitter MA, Franklin WA, Larson RA, et al: Morphology in Ki-1 (CD30)–positive non-Hodgkin's lymphoma is correlated with clinical features and the presence of a unique chromosomal abnormality. Am J Surg Pathol 1990;14:305.

103. Jaffe E: Pathologic and clinical spectrum of post-thymic T-cell malignancies. Cancer Invest 1984;2:413.

104. Eshghabadi M, Shojania AM, Carr I: Isolated granulocytic sarcoma: Report of a case and review of the literature. J Clin Oncol 1986;4:912.

105. Nieman RS, Barios M, Berard C, et al: Granulocyte sarcoma: A clinicopathological survey of 61 biopsed cases. Cancer 1981;46:1426.

106. Bennett JM, Catovsky D, Daniel MT, et al: The French American British (FAB) cogenerative group proposals for the classification of chronic (mature) B and T lymphoid leukemias. J Clin Pathol 1989;42:567.

107. Bennett JM, Cain KC, Glick JH, et al: The significance of bone marrow involvement in non-Hodgkin's lymphomas: The Eastern Cooperative Oncology experience. J Clin Oncol 1986;4:1462.

108. Waldenström J: Incipient myeloma or essential hyperglobulinaemia with fibrogenopenia: A new syndrome? Acta Med Scand 1944;117:216.

109. Spiro S, Galton DAG, Wiltshaw E, et al: Follicular lymphoma: A survey of 75 cases with specific relevance to the syndrome resembling chronic lymphocytic leukaemia. Br J Cancer 1975;31:60.

110. Melo JV, Robinson DSF, De Oliveira MP, et al: Morphology and immunology of circulating cells in leukaemic phase of follicular lymphoma. J Clin Pathol 1988;41:951.

111. Isaacs R: Lymphosarcoma cell leukemia. Ann Intern Med 1937;11:657.

112. Jaffe S, Bookman MA, Longo DL: Lymphocytic lymphoma of intermediate differentiation: Mantle zone lymphoma: a distinct of B cell lymphoma. Hum Pathol 1987;18:877.

113. Pombo DE, Oliveira MS, Jaffe H, et al: Leukemia phase of mantle-zone (intermediate) lymphoma: Its characterization in 11 cases. J Clin Pathol 1989;42:962.

114. Flandrin G, Brouet JC: The Sézary cell: Cytologic, cytochemical and immunologic studies. Mayo Clin Proc 1974;49:575.

115. Lutzner MA, Edelson RL, Schein P, et al: Cutaneous T-cell lymphomas: The Sézary syndrome, mycosis fungoides, and related disorders. Ann Intern Med 1975;83:534.

116. Abrams MB, Sidany M, Novich M: Smoldering HTLV-associated T cell leukemia. Arch Intern Med 1985;145:2257.

117. The Non-Hodgkin's Lymphoma Classification Project: A clinical evaluation of the International Lymphoma Study Group Classification of Non-Hodgkins Lymphoma. Blood 1997;89(11):3909–3918.

118. Harris NL, Jaffe ES, Diebold J, et al: World Health Organization Classification of neoplastic diseases of the haematopoietic and lymphoid tissues: Report of the Clinical Advisory Committee. JCO 17:1997;3835–3849.

119. Altehoefer C, Blum U, Bathmann J, et al: Comparative diagnostic accuracy of magnetic resonance imaging and immunoscintigraphy for detection of bone marrow involvement in patients with malignant lymphoma. J Clin Oncol 1997;15:1754.

120. Lister TA, Crowther D, Sutcliffe SB, et al: Report of a committee convened to discuss the evaluation and staging of patients with Hodgkin's disease. J Clin Oncol 1989;7:1650.

121. Shipp M, Harrington D, Anderson J, et al: Development of a predictive model for aggressive lymphoma: The International NHL Prognostic Factors Project. N Engl J Med 1993;329:997.

122. Rohatiner A, on behalf of d'Amore F, Coiffier B, Crowther D, et al: Report of a workshop convened to discuss the pathological and staging classifications of gastrointestinal tract lymphoma. Ann Oncol 1994;5:397.

123. Armitage JO, Dick FR, Corder MP, et al: Predicting therapeutic outcome in patients with diffuse histiocytic lymphoma treated with cyclophosphamide, Adriamycin, vincristine, and prednisolone (CHOP). Cancer 1982;50:1695.

124. Coiffier B, Gisselbrecht C, Vose J, et al: Prognostic factors in aggressive malignant lymphomas: Description and validation of a prognostic index that could identify patients requiring a more intensive therapy. J Clin Oncol 1991;9:211.

125. Cowan RA, Jones M, Harris M, et al: Prognostic factors in high and intermediate grade non-Hodgkin's lymphoma. Br J Cancer 1989;59:276.

126. Velasquez W, Jagannath S, Tucker S, et al: Risk classification as the basis for clinical staging of diffuse large-cell lymphoma derived from 10-year survival data. Blood 1989;74:551.

127. Jagannath S, Valasquez WS, Tucker SL, et al: Tumour burden assessment and its implication for a prognostic model in advanced diffuse large cell lymphoma. J Clin Oncol 1986; 4:859.

128. Non-Hodgkin's Lymphoma Classification Project: Effect of age on the characteristics and clinical behavior of non-Hodgkin's lymphoma patients. Ann Oncol 1997;8:973.

129. Coiffier B, Bastion Y, Berger F, et al: Prognostic factors in follicular lymphomas. Semin Oncol 1993;20:89.

130. Lopez-Guillermo A, Montserrat E, Bosch F, et al: Applicability of the International Index for aggressive lymphomas to patients with low-grade lymphomas. J Clin Oncol 1994;12:1343.

131. Bastion Y, Coiffier B: Is the International Prognostic Index for aggressive lymphoma patients useful for follicular lymphoma patients? (editorial) J Clin Oncol 1994;12:1340.

132. Bastion Y, Berger F, Bryon PA, Felman P, French M, Coiffier B: Follicular lymphomas: assessment of prognostic factors in 127 patients followed for 10 years. Ann Oncol 1991; 9(Suppl 2):123–129.

133. Decaudin D, Lepage E, Brousse N, et al: Low-grade stage III-IV follicular lymphoma: Multivariate analysis of prognostic factors in 484 patients. A study of the Groupe d'Etude des Lymphomes de l'Adulte. J Clin Oncol 1999;17(8):2499–2505.

134. Federico M, Vitolo U, Zinzani PL, et al: Prognosis of follicular lymphoma: A predictive model based on a retrospective analysis of 987 cases. Blood 2000;95(3):783–789.

135. Solal-Celigny P, Roy P: Follicular Lymphoma International Prognostic Index (FLIPI). Eighth International Conference on Malignant Lymphoma, Lugano, Switzerland, June 12–15, 2002. Ann Oncol 2002; 18.

136. Lopez-Guillermo A, Cabanillas F, McLaughlin P, et al: The clinical significance of molecular response in indolent follicular lymphomas. Blood 1998;91:2955.

137. Freedman AS, Ritz J, Neuberg D, et al: Autologous bone marrow transplantation in 69 patients with a history of low grade B-cell non-Hodgkin's lymphoma. Blood 1991;77:2524.

138. Colombat P, Binet C, Linassier C, et al: High dose chemotherapy with autologous bone marrow transplantation in follicular lymphoma. Leuk Lymphoma 1992;7:3.

139. Rohatiner A, Johnson P, Price C, et al: Myeloablative therapy with autologous bone marrow transplantation as consolidation therapy for recurrent follicular lymphoma. J Clin Oncol 1994;12(6): 1177–1184.

140. Gribben JG, Freedman AS, Neuberg D, et al: Immunologic purging of marrow assessed by PCR before ABMT for B-cell lymphoma. N Engl J Med 1991;325:1525.

141. Cheson BD, Horning SJ, Coiffier B, et al: Report of an international workshop to standardize response criteria for non-Hodgkin's lymphomas. J Clin Oncol 1999;17: 1244–1253.

142. Talbot JN, Haioun C, Rain JD, et al: 18-F-FDG positron imaging in clinical management of lymphoma patients. Crit Rev Oncol Hematol 2001;38:193–221.

143. Kostakoglu L, Goldsmith SJ: Fluorine-18-fluorodeoxyglucose positron emission tomography in the staging and follow-up of lymphoma: Is it time to shift gears? Eur J Nucl Med 2000;27:1564–1578.

144. Pro B, Romaguera J, Macapinlac A, et al: Positron emission tomography using Flurodeoxyglucose but not gallium-67 scintigraphy is a sensitive imaging modality in the staging of mantle cell lymphoma. American Society of Hematology 2002, 3041a, and poster presentation 461-III.

145. Bar-Shalom R, Mor M, Yefremov N, Goldsmith SJ: The value of Ga-67 scintigraphy and F-18 flurodeoxyglucose positron emission tomography in staging and monitoring the response of lymphoma to treatment. Semin Nucl Med 2001;31:177–190.

146. Jerusalem G, Beguin Y, Fassotte MF, et al: Persistent tumor 18F-FDG uptake after a few cycles of polychemotherapy is predictive of treatment failure in non-Hodgkin's lymphoma. Haematologica 2000;85:613–618.

147. Romer W, Hanauske AR, Ziegler S, et al: Positron emission tomography in non-Hodgkin's lymphoma: Assessment of chemotherapy with flurodeoxyglucose. Blood 1998;91: 4464–4471.

148. Trneny M, Jaeger U, Belohlavek O, Becherer A, Pytilik R, Skrabs C: Early whole body F-18 (FDG) positron emission tomography (PET) restaging has significant prognostic impact in diffuse large B-cell lymphomas (DLBCLs) and other aggressive lymphomas. American Society of Hematology 2002; 3038a and poster presentation 458-III.

149. Conlan MG, Bast M, Armitage JO, Weisenburger DD: Bone marrow involvement by non-Hodgkin's lymphoma: The clinical significance of morphologic discordance between the lymph node and bone marrow. J Clin Oncol 1990;8(7):1163–1172.

150. Hardingham JE, Kotasek D, Sage RE, et al: Significance of molecular marker-positive cells after autologous peripheral blood stem cell transplantation for non-Hodgkin's lymphoma. J Clin Oncol 1995;13:1073.

151. Limpens J, De Jong D, Van Krieken JH, et al: bcl-2/J_H rearrangements in benign lymphoid tissues with follicular hyperplasia. Oncogene 1991;6:2271.

152. Rauzy O, Galoin S, Chale J-J, et al: Detection of t(14;18) carrying cells in bone marrow and peripheral blood from patients affected by non-lymphoid diseases. J Clin Pathol Mol Pathol 1998;51:333.

153. Summers KE, Goff LK, Wilson AG, et al: Incidence and frequency of bcl-2/I_gH rearrangement in normal individuals: Implications for the monitoring of disease in patients with follicular lymphoma. J Clin Oncol 2001;19:420–424.

154. Pusey WA: Cases of sarcoma and of Hodgkin's disease treated by exposure to x-rays. JAMA 1902;38:166.

155. Senn A: Therapeutic value of roentgen ray in treatment of pseudoleukaemia. N Y Med 1902;106:467.

156. Sugarbaker ED, Craver LF: Lymphosarcoma: A study of 196 cases with biopsy. JAMA 1940;115:112.

157. MacManus MP, Hoppe RT: Is radiotherapy curative for stage I and II low-grade follicular lymphoma? Results of a long-term follow-up study of patients treated at Stanford University. J Clin Oncol 1996;14:1282.

158. Haas RLM, Poortmans PH, de Jong D, et al: High response rates and lasting remission after low-dose involved field radiotherapy in indolent lymphomas. J Clin Oncol 2003;21:2474-2480.

159. Sawyer EJ, Timothy AR: Low dose palliative radiotherapy in low grade non-Hodgkin's lymphoma. Radiother Oncol 1997;42:49.

160. Everett JL, Roberts JR, Ross WCJ: Aryl-2-halogenoalkylamines. Part VII. Some carboxyl derivation of NN-di-2-chlorethylandine. J Chem Soc 1953;3:3286.

161. Arnold H, Borseaux P: Synthese und abban cytostatish wirksamer cyclischt n-phosphadimester des bis (B-chlorethyl) amins. Angewandte Chemie 1958;17:539.

162. Altman SJ, Haut A, Cartwright GE, et al: Early experience with P-(NN di-2-chlorethyl) aminobutyric acid (CB 1438), a new chemotherapeutic agent in the treatment of chronic lymphatic leukemia. Cancer 1956;9:512.

163. Israels LG, Galton DAG, Till M, et al: Clinical evaluation of CB 1348 in malignant lymphoma and related diseases. Ann N Y Acad Sci 1958;68:915.

164. Miller DG, Diamond HM, Craver LF: The clinical use of chlorambucil. N Engl J Med 1959;261:11.

165. Scott JL: The effect of nitrogen mustard and maintenance chlorambucil in the treatment of Hodgkin's disease. Cancer Chemother Rep 1963;27:27.

166. Galton DAG, Wiltshaw E, Szur L, et al: The use of chlorambucil and steroids in the treatment of chronic lymphatic leukaemia. Br J Haematol 1961;7:73.

167. Lazlo J, Grizzle J, Jonsson U, et al: Comparative study of mannitol mustard cyclophosphamide and nitrogen mustard in malignant lymphomas. Cancer Chemother Rep 1962;16:247.

168. Jacobs EM, Peters FC, Luce JK, et al: Mechlorethamine HCl and cyclophosphamide in the treatment of Hodgkin's disease and the lymphomas. JAMA 1968;203:6.

169. Gold GL, Salvin LG, Schneider BI: A comparative study with the alkylating agents mechlorethamine cyclophosphamide and uracic mustard. Cancer Chemother Rep 1962;16:147.

170. Carbone PP, Spurr C, Schneiderman M, et al: Management of patients with malignant lymphoma: A comparative study with cyclophosphamide and vinca alkaloids. Cancer Res 1968;28:811.

171. Farber S, Diamond LK, Mercer RD, et al: Temporary remissions in leukemia in children produced by folic acid antagonist 4-aminopteroly-glutamic acid (aminopterin). N Engl J Med 1948;238:787.

172. Bohannon RA, Miller DG, Diamond HD: Vincristine in the treatment of leukaemias and lymphomas. Cancer Res 1962;23:613.

173. Whitelaw DM, Cowan DH, Cassidy FR, et al: Clinical experience with vincristine. Cancer Chemother 1963;30:13.

174. Gubisch NF, Norena D, Perlia CP, et al: Experience with vincristine in solid tumors. Cancer Chemother Rep 1963;32:19.

175. Whitelaw DM, Kim HS: Vincristine in the treatment of malignant disease. J Can Med Assoc 1964;90:1385.

176. Pearson OH, Eliel LP, Rawson RW, et al: ACTH and cortisone-induced regression of lymphoid tumors in man. Cancer 1949;2:943.

177. Pearson OH, Eliel LP: Use of pituitary adrenocorticotrophic hormone (ACTH) and cortisone in leukemia and lymphomas. JAMA 1950;144:1349.

178. Second report to the Medical Research Council by the panel on the haematological applications of ACTH and cortisone. Br Med J 1953;2:1401.

179. Kofman S, Perlia CP, Boesen E, et al: The role of corticosteroids in the treatment of malignant lymphomas. Cancer 1962;15:2.

180. Kyle RA, McParland CE, Damashek W: Large doses of prednisolone in the treatment of malignant lymphoproliferative disorders. Ann Intern Med 1962;57:5.

181. Hall TC, Choi OS, Abadi A, et al: High dose corticosteroid therapy in Hodgkin's disease and other lymphomas. Ann Intern Med 1967;66:6.

182. Ezdinli EZ, Stutzman L, Aungst CW, et al: Corticosteroid therapy for lymphoma and chronic lymphatic leukaemia. Cancer 1969;23:4.

183. Wang JJ, Cortes E, Sinks LF, et al: Therapeutic effect and toxicity of Adriamycin in patients with neoplastic disease. Cancer 1971;28:837.

184. Bonnadonna G, Monfardini S, De Lena M, et al: Phase I and preliminary phase II. evaluation of Adriamycin (NSC123129). Cancer Res 1970;30:2572.

185. Rozman C, Camps ES, Ribismundo M, et al: Clinical trials with Adriamycin. In Carter SK, Di Marco A, Ghiona M, et al (eds): International Symposium on Adriamycin. New York, Springer-Verlag, 1985, p 188.

186. Cavalli F: Etoposide: VP-16. Semin Oncol 1985;1:33.

187. O'Reilly SE, Klimo P, Connors JM: The evolving role of etoposide in the management of lymphoma and Hodgkin's disease. Cancer 1991;67(Suppl 1):271.

188. Young RC: Etoposide in the treatment of non-Hodgkin's lymphomas. Semin Oncol 1992;19:6.

189. Slevin ML, Clark PI, Joel SP, et al: A randomized trial to evaluate the effect of schedule on the activity of etoposide in small cell lung cancer. J Clin Oncol 1989;7:1333.

190. Hainsworth DJ, Johnson DH, Frazier SR, et al: Chronic daily administration of oral etoposide in refractory lymphoma. Engl J Cancer 1990;7:818.

191. Pedersen-Bjergaard J, Philips P, Larsen SO, et al: Chromosome aberrations and prognostic factors in therapy-related myelodysplasia and acute nonlymphocytic leukemia. Blood 1990;76:1083.

192. Kremer WB: Cytarabine. Ann Intern Med 1975;82:684.

193. Kantarjian H, Barlogie B, Plunkett W, et al: High dose cytosine arabinoside in non-Hodgkin's lymphoma. J Clin Oncol 1993;11:689.

194. Richards MA, Barnett MJ, Waxman JA, et al: The use of high dose cytosine arabinoside for non-Hodgkin's lymphoma. Semin Oncol 1985;3:223.

195. Kay AC, Saven A, Carrera CJ, et al: 2-Chlorodeoxy-adenosine treatment of low-grade lymphomas. J Clin Oncol 1992;10:371.

196. Hickish T, Serafinowski P, Cunningham D, et al: 2-Chlorodeoxyadenosine: Evaluation of a novel predominantly lymphocyte selective agent in lymphoid malignancies. Br J Cancer 1993;6:139.

197. Hochster HS, Kim KM, Green MD, et al: Activity of fludarabine in previously treated non-Hodgkin's low-grade lymphoma: Results of an Eastern Cooperative Oncology Group study. J Clin Oncol 1992;10:28.

198. Redman JR, Cabanillas F, Velasquez WS, et al: Phase II trial of fludarabine phosphate in lymphoma: An effective new agent in low-grade lymphoma. J Clin Oncol 1992;10:790.

199. Leiby JM, Snider KM, Kraut EH, et al: Phase II trial of 9-b-D-arabinosyl-2-fluoroadenine 5′-monophosphate in non-Hodgkin's lymphoma: Prospective comparison of response with deoxycytidine kinase activity. Cancer Res 1987;47:2719.

200. Whelan JS, Davis CL, Rule S, et al: Fludarabine phosphate for the treatment of low grade lymphoid malignancy. Br J Cancer 1991;64:120.

201. Pigaditou A, Rohatiner AZ, Whelan JS, et al: Fludarabine in low-grade lymphoma. Semin Oncol 1993;20(5 Suppl 7):24–27.

202. Zinzani PL, Lauria F, Rondelli D, et al: Fludarabine: An active agent in the treatment of previously treated and untreated low-grade non-Hodgkin's lymphoma. Ann Oncol 1993;4(7):575–578.

203. Hiddeman W, Unterhalt M, Pott C, et al: Fludarabine single-agent therapy for relapsed low-grade non-Hodgkin's lymphoma: a phase II study of the German low-grade Non-Hodgkin's Lymphoma Study Group. Semin Oncol 1993;20:28.

204. Solal-Celigny P, Brice P, Brousse N, et al: Phase II trial of fludarabine monophosphate as first-line treatment in patients with advanced follicular lymphoma: A multicenter study by the Group d'Etude des Lymphomes de l'Adulte. J Clin Oncol 1996;14:514.

205. Foran JM, Rohatiner AZS, Coiffier B, et al: A multicenter, phase II trial of intravenous fludarabine phosphate for patients with newly diagnosed lymphoplasmacytoid lymphoma, Waldenström's macroglobulinemia, and mantle cell lymphoma. J Clin Oncol 1999;17:546.

206. Schilling PJ, Vadhan-Raj S: Concurrent cytomegalovirus and pneumocystis pneumonia after fludarabine therapy for chronic lymphocytic leukemia. (letter) N Engl J Med 1990;323:833.

207. Foran JM, Oscier D, Orchard J, et al: A pharmacokinetic study of single doses of oral fludarabine phosphate. J Clin Oncol 1999;17:1574.

208. De Vita VT Jr, Serpick AA, Carbone PP: Combination chemotherapy in the treatment of Hodgkin's disease. Ann Intern Med 1970;73:881.

209. Bagley CH, De Vita VT, Berard CW, et al: Advanced lymphosarcoma: Intensive cyclic combination chemotherapy with cyclophosphamide vincristine and prednisolone. Ann Intern Med 1972;76:272.

210. Hoogstraten B, Owns A, Lenhard RE, et al: Combination chemotherapy in lymphosarcoma. Blood 1969;33:370.

211. Williams, CD, Goldstone AH, Pearce RM, et al: Purging of bone marrow in autologous bone marrow transplantation for non-Hodgkin's lymphoma: A case-matched comparison with unpurged cases by the European Blood and Marrow Transplant Lymphoma Registry. J Clin Oncol 1996;14:2454.

212. Louie AC, Gallagher JC, Sikora K, et al: Follow-up observations on the effect of human leukocyte interferon in non-Hodgkin's lymphoma. Blood 1981;58:712.

213. O'Connell MJ, Colgan JP, Oken MM, et al: Clinical trial of recombinant leukocyte A interferon as initial therapy for favorable histology non-Hodgkin's lymphomas and chronic lymphocytic leukemia. J Clin Oncol 1986;4:128.

214. Quesada GR, Hawkins M, Horning SJ, et al: Collaborative phase I-II study of recombinant DNA-produced leukocyte interferon

(clone A) in metastatic breast cancer, malignant lymphoma, and multiple myeloma. Am J Med 1984;77:427.

215. Wagstaff J, Loynds P, Crowther D: A phase II study of human recombinant DNAa2 interferon in patients with low-grade non-Hodgkin's lymphoma. Cancer Chemother Pharmacol 1986;18:54.

216. Gutterman JU, Blumenschein GR, Alexanian R: Leukocyte interferon-induced tumor regression in human metastatic breast cancer, multiple myeloma, and malignant lymphoma. Ann Intern Med 1980;93:399.

217. Foon KA, Roth MS, Bunn PA: Interferon therapy of non-Hodgkin's lymphoma. Cancer 1987;59:601.

218. Siegert W, Themal H, Fink W, et al: Treatment of non-Hodgkin's lymphoma of low grade malignancy with human fibroblast interferon. Anticancer Res 1982;2:193.

219. Horning S, Merigan TC, Itrown SE, et al: Human interferon alpha in malignant lymphoma and Hodgkin's disease: Results of the American Cancer Society trial. Cancer 1985;56:1305.

220. Leavitt RD, Ratanathara Thorn V, Ozer H, et al: Alfa-26 interferon in the treatment of Hodgkin's disease and non-Hodgkin's disease lymphoma. Semin Oncol 1987;14:18.

221. Rohatiner AZ, Gregory W, Beterson B, Smalley R, et al: A meta-analysis of randomized studies evaluating the role of interferon alpha as treatment for follicular lymphoma. Proc Am Soc Clin Oncol 2002;21:264a.

222. Bunn PA, Ihde DC, Foon KA: The role of recombinant interferon alpha-2a in the therapy of cutaneous T cell lymphoma. Cancer 1986;57:1689.

223. Olsen EA, Rosen ST, Vollmer RT, et al: Interferon alpha-2a in the treatment of cutaneous T cell lymphoma. J Am Acad Dermatol 1989;20:395.

224. Lotze MT, Chang AE, Seipp CA, et al: High dose recombinant interleukin 2 in the treatment of patients with disseminated cancer: Responses, treatment-recovered morbidity, and histologic findings. JAMA 1986;256:3117.

225. Allison MA, Jones SE, McGuffey P: Phase II trial of out-patient interleukin-2 in malignant lymphoma chronic lymphoma leukemia and selected solid tumors. J Clin Oncol 1989;7:75.

226. Paciucci PA, Haland JF, Glidewell O, et al: Recombinant interleukin-2 by continuous infusion and adoptive transfer of recombinant interleukin-2. Activated cells in patients with advanced cancer. J Clin Oncol 1989;7:869.

227. Rosenberg SA, Lotze MT, Muul LM, et al: A progress report on the treatment of 157 patients with advanced cancer using lymphokine activated killer cells and interleukin-2 or high dose interleukin-2 alone. N Engl J Med 1987;316:889.

228. Foon KA, Schroff RW, Bunn RA, et al: Effects of monoclonal antibody therapy in patients with chronic lymphatic leukemia. Blood 1984;64:1085.

229. Nadler LM, Stashenko P, Hardy R, et al: Serotherapy of a patient with a monoclonal antibody directed against a human leukemia associated antigen. Cancer Res 1980;40:3147.

230. Press OW, Applebaum F, Ledbetter JA, et al: Monoclonal antibody IF5 (anti-CD20) serotherapy of human B cell lymphomas. Blood 1987;69:584.

231. Grossbard ML, Press OW, Appelbaum FR, et al: Monoclonal antibody-based therapies of leukemia and lymphoma. Blood 1992;80:863.

232. Riechmann L, Clark M, Waldmann H, et al: Reshaping human antibodies for therapy. Nature 1988;332:323.

233. McLaughlin P, Grillo-Lopez AJ, Link BK, et al: Rituximab chimeric anti-CD20 monoclonal antibody therapy for relapsed indolent lymphoma: Half of patients respond to a four-dose treatment program. J Clin Oncol 1998;16(8):2825–2833.

234. Coiffier B, Lepage E, Briére J: CHOP chemotherapy and Rituximab compared with CHOP alone in elderly patients with diffuse large B cell lymphoma. N Engl J Med 2002;346:235–242.

235. Mounier N, Briere J, Gisselbrecht C, Emile J-F: Rituximab plus CHOP (R-CHOP) overcomes bcl-2-associated resistance to chemotherapy in elderly patients with diffuse large B-cell lymphoma (DLBCL). Blood 2003;101:4279–4284.

236. DeNardo GL, DeNardo SJ, O'Grady LF, et al: Fractionated radioimmunotherapy of B cell malignancies with ^{3}I Lym-1. Cancer Res 1990;50(Suppl 1):1014S.

237. Goldenberg DM, Horowitz JA, Sharkey RM, et al: Targeting, dosimetry, and radioimmunotherapy of B-cell lymphomas with iodine-131 labelled LL2 monoclonal antibody. J Clin Oncol 1991;9:548.

238. Kaminski MS, Zasadny KR, Francis IR, et al: Radioimmunotherapy of B cell lymphoma with ^{3}I anti-B1 (anti-CD20) antibody. N Engl J Med 1993;329:459.

239. Press OW, Eary JF, Frederick R, et al: Radio-labeled antibody therapy of B-cell lymphoma with autologous bone marrow support. N Engl J Med 1993;329:1219.

240. Kaminski MS, Zelenetz AD, Press OW: Pivotal study of iodine I^3 tositumomab for chemotherapy-refractory low-grade or transformed low-grade B-cell non-Hodgkin's lymphoma. J Clin Oncol 2001;19:3918–3928.

241. Press OW, Eary JF, Golley T: A phase I/II trial of iodine-131-tositumomab (anti-CD20), etoposide, cyclophosphamide, and autologous stem cell transplantation for relapsed B-cell lymphomas. Blood 2000;96:2934–2942.

242. Witzig TE, Gordon LI, Cabanillas F: Randomized controlled trial of yttrium-90-labeled ibritumomab tiuxetan radioimmunotherapy versus rituximab immunotherapy for patients with relapsed or refractory low-grade, follicular, or transformed B-cell non-Hodgkin's lymphoma. J Clin Oncol 2000;20:2453–2463.

243. Vitetta ES, Stone M, Amlot P, et al: Phase I immunotoxin trial in patients with B-cell lymphoma. Cancer Res 1991;512:4052.

244. Amlot PL, Stone MJ, Cunningham D, et al: A phase I study of an anti-CD22-deglycosylated ricin A chain immunotoxin in the treatment of B-cell lymphomas resistant to conventional therapy. Blood 1993;82:2624.

245. Grossbard ML, Freedman AS, Ritz J, et al: Serotherapy of B-cell neoplasms with anti-B4 blocked ricin: A phase I trial of a daily bolus infusion. Blood 1992;79:576.

246. Grossbard ML, Lambert JM, Goldmacher VS, et al: Anti-B4-blocked ricin: A phase I trial of 7-day continuous infusion in patients with B-cell neoplasms. J Clin Oncol 1993;11:726.

247. Grossbard ML, Niedzwiecki D, Nadler LM, et al: Anti-B4-blocked ricin (Anti-B4-bR) adjuvant therapy post–autologous bone marrow transplant (ABMT) (CALB 9254): A phase III intergroup study. Proc Am Soc Clin Oncol 1998;17:3a.

248. Toze CL, Barnett MJ: Allogeneic stem cell transplantation for non-Hodgkin's lymphoma: Best practice and research. Clin Haematol 2002;15(3):481–504.

249. Giralt S, Estey E, Albitar M, et al: Engraftment of allogeneic hematopoietic progenitor cells with purine analog-containing chemotherapy: Harnessing graft versus leukemia without myeloablative therapy. Blood 1997;89:4531.

250. Khouri IF, Keating M, Korbling M, et al: Transplant-lite: Induction of graft versus malignancy using fludarabine-based nonablative chemotherapy and allogeneic blood progenitor-cell transplantation as treatment for lymphoid malignancies. J Clin Oncol 1998;16:2817.

251. Slavin S, Nagler A, Naparstek E, et al: Non-myeloablative stem cell transplantation and cell therapy as an alternative to conventional bone marrow transplantation with lethal cytoreduction for the treatment of malignant and nonmalignant hematologic diseases. Blood 1998;91:756.

252. Branson K, Chopra R, Kottaridis PD, McQuaker G: Role of nonmyeloablative allogeneic stem cell transplantation after failure of autologous transplantation in patients with lymphoproliferative malignancies. J Clin Oncol 2002;20:4022–4031.

253. Robinson SP, Goldstone AH, Mackinnon S, Carella A, Russell N: Chemoresistant or aggressive lymphoma predicts for a poor outcome following reduced-intensity allogeneic progenitor cell transplantation: An analysis from the Lymphoma Working Party of the European Group for Blood and Bone Marrow Transplantation. Blood 100: 4310-4316. 2002;

254. Khouri IF, Saliba RM, Giralt SA, Lee M-S: Nonablative allogeneic hematopoietic transplantation as adoptive immunotherapy for indolent lymphoma: Low incidence of toxicity, acute graft versus host disease, and treatment-related mortality. Blood 2001;98:3595–3599.

255. Sykes M, Preffer F, McAfee S, Saidman SL: Mixed lymphohaemaopoietic chimerism and graft-versus-lymphoma effects after

nonmyeloablative therapy and HLA-mismatched bone marrow transplantation. Lancet 1999;353:1755–1759.

256. Carella AM, Cavaliere M, Lerma E, Ferrara R: Autografting followed by nonmyeloablative immunosuppressive chemotherapy and allogeneic peripheral-blood hematopoietic stem cell transplantation as treatment of resistant Hodgkin's disease and non-Hodgkin's lymphoma. J Clin Oncol 2000;18:3918–3924.

257. Hans CP, Weisenburger DD, Vose JM, et al: A significant diffuse component predicts for inferior survival in grade 3 follicular lymphoma, but cytologic subtypes do not predict survival. Blood 2003;101(6):2363–2367.

258. Horning SJ, Doggett RS, Warnke RA, Dorfman RF, Cox RS, Levy R: Clinical relevance of immunologic phenotype in diffuse large cell lymphoma. Blood 1984;63:1209–1215.

259. Portlock CS, Rosenberg SA: No initial therapy for stage III and IV non-Hodgkin's lymphomas of favorable histologic types. Ann Int Med 1979;90(1):10–13.

260. Brice P, Bastion Y, Lepage E, et al: Comparison in low-tumor-burden follicular lymphomas between an initial no-treatment policy, prednimustine, or interferon alfa: A randomized study from the Groupe d'Etude des Lymphomes Folliculaires. J Clin Oncol 1997;15(3):1110–1117.

261. Grillo-Lopez AJ, Hedrick E, Rashford M, Benyunes M: Rituximab: Ongoing and future clinical development. Semin Oncol 2002;29(1 Suppl 2):105–112.

262. Coiffier B: Monoclonal antibodies combined to chemotherapy for the treatment of patients with lymphoma. Blood Rev 2003;17(1):25–31.

263. Decaudin D, Lepage E, Brousse N, et al: Low-grade stage III-IV follicular lymphoma: Multivariate analysis of prognostic factors in 484 patients: A study of the Groupe d'Etude des Lymphomes de l'Adulte. J Clin Oncol 1999;17(8):2499–2505.

264. Federico M, Vitolo U, Zinzani PL, et al: Prognosis of follicular lymphoma: A predictive model based on a retrospective analysis of 987 cases. Blood 2000;95(3):783–789.

265. Solal-Celigny P, Roy P: Follicular Lymphoma International Prognostic Index (FLIPI). Eighth International Conference on Malignant Lymphoma, Lugano, Switzerland, June 12–15, 2002. Ann Oncol 2002;18.

266. Johnson P, Rohatiner A, Whelan JS, et al: Patterns of survival in patients with recurrent follicular lymphoma: A 20-year study from a single center. J Clin Oncol 1995;13(1):140–147.

267. Bastion Y, Sebban C, Berger F, et al: Incidence, predictive factors, and outcome of lymphoma transformation in follicular lymphoma patients. J Clin Oncol 1997;15(4):1587–1594.

268. Muller-Hermelink HK, Zettl A, Pfeifer W, Ott G: Pathology of lymphoma progression. Histopathology 2001;38(4):285–306.

269. Williams CD, Harrison CN, Lister TA, et al: High-dose therapy and autologous stem-cell support for chemosensitive transformed low-grade follicular non-Hodgkin's lymphoma: A case-matched study from the European bone marrow transplant registry. J Clin Oncol 2001;19(3):727–735.

270. Yuen AR, Kamel OW, Halpern J, Horning SJ: Long-term survival after histologic transformation of low-grade follicular lymphoma. J Clin Oncol 1995;13(7):1726–1733.

271. Lo Coco F, Gaidano G, Louie DC, Offit K, Chaganti RSK, Dalla-Favera R: p53 mutations are associated with histologic transformation of follicular lymphoma. Blood 1993;82(8):2289–2295.

272. Tilly H, Rossi A, Stamatoullas A, et al: Prognostic value of chromosomal abnormalities in follicular lymphoma. Blood 1994;84:1043.

273. Lossos IS, Alizadeh AA, Diehn M, et al: Transformation of follicular lymphoma to diffuse large-cell lymphoma: Alternative patterns with increased or decreased expression of c-myc and its regulated genes. Proc Natl Acad Sci USA 2002;99(13):8886–8891.

274. de Vos S, Hofmann WK, Grogan TM, et al: Gene expression profile of serial samples of transformed B-cell lymphomas. Lab Invest 2003;83(2):271–285.

275. Richards MA, Gregory WM, Hall PA, et al: Management of localized non-Hodgkin's lymphoma: The experience at St. Bartholomew's Hospital 1972–1985. Hematol Oncol 1989;7:1.

276. Paryani SB, Hoppe RT, Cox RS, et al: Analysis of non-Hodgkin's lymphomas with nodular and favorable histologies, stages I and II. Cancer 1983;52:2300.

277. Tsang RW, Gospodarowicz MK, O'Sullivan B: Staging and management of localized non-Hodgkin's lymphomas: Variations among experts in radiation oncology. Int J Radiat Oncol Biol Phys 2002;52(3):643–651.

278. Brandt L, Kimby E, Nygren P, Glimelius B: A systematic overview of chemotherapy effects in indolent non-Hodgkin's lymphoma. Acta Oncol 2001;40(2-3):213–223.

279. Dana BW, Dahlberg S, Nathwani BN, et al: Long-term follow-up of patients with low-grade malignant lymphomas treated with doxorubicin-based chemotherapy or chemoimmunotherapy. J Clin Oncol 1993;11(4):644–651.

280. Peterson BA, Petroni GR, Frizzera G, et al: Prolonged single-agent versus combination chemotherapy in indolent follicular lymphomas: A study of the Cancer and Leukemia Group. Br J Clin Oncol 2003;21(1):5–15.

281. Lepage E, Sebban D, Gisselbrecht C, et al: Treatment of low-grade non-Hodgkin's lymphomas: Assessment of doxorubicin in a controlled trial. Hematol Oncol 1990;8:31.

282. Cabanillas F, Smith T, Bodey CP, et al: Nodular malignant lymphomas: factors affecting complete response and survival. Cancer 1979;44:1983.

283. Lister TA, Cullen MH, Beard MEJ, et al: Comparison of combined and single agent chemotherapy in non-Hodgkin's lymphoma of favorable histological sub-type. Br Med J 1978;1:533.

284. Anderson T, DeVita VT, Simon RM, et al: Malignant lymphoma II: Prognostic factors and response to treatment of 473 patients at the National Cancer Institute. Cancer 1982;50:2708.

285. Murtha AD, Knox SJ, Hoppe RT, Rupnow BA, Hanson J: Long-term follow-up of patients with stage III follicular lymphoma treated with primary radiotherapy at Stanford University. Int J Radiat Oncol Biol Phys 2001;49(1):3–15.

286. Lopez-Guillermo A, Cabanillas F, McDonnell TI, et al: Correlation of bcl-2 rearrangement with clinical characteristics and outcome in indolent follicular lymphoma. Blood 1999;93(9):3081–3087.

287. Rohatiner AZ, Gregory W, Peterson B, et al: A meta-analysis of randomized studies evaluating the role of interferon alpha as treatment for follicular lymphoma (FL). (abstract 1053) Proc Am Soc Clin Oncol 2002;21:264a.

288. Rohatiner AZS, Richards MA, Barnett MJ, et al: Chlorambucil and interferon for low grade non-Hodgkin's lymphoma. Br J Cancer 1987;55:437.

289. Solal-Celigny P, Lepage E, Brousse N, et al: Recombinant interferon alfa-2b combined with a regimen containing doxorubicin in patients with advanced follicular lymphoma. Groupe d'Etude des Lymphomes de l'Adults. N Engl J Med 1993;329:1608.

290. Solal-Celigny P, Lepage E, Brousse N, et al: Doxorubicin-containing regimen with or without interferon alfa-2b for advanced follicular lymphomas: Final analysis of survival and toxicity in the Groupe d'Etude des Lymphomes Folliculaires–86 trial. J Clin Oncol 1998;16(7):2332–2338.

291. Smalley RV, Andersen JW, Hawkins MJ, et al: Interferon alfa combined with cytotoxic chemotherapy for patients with non-Hodgkin's lymphoma. N Engl J Med 1992;327:1336.

292. Smalley RV, Weller E, Hawkins MJ, et al: Final analysis of the ECOG I-COPA trial (E6484) in patients with non-Hodgkin's lymphoma treated with interferon alfa (IFN-alpha 2a) plus an anthracycline-based induction regimen. Leukemia 2001;15(7):1118–1122.

293. Hagenbeek A, Carde P, Meerwaldt JH, et al: Maintenance of remission with human recombinant interferon alfa-2a in patients with stages III and IV low-grade malignant non-Hodgkin's lymphoma. J Clin Oncol 1998;16(1):41–47.

294. Arranz R, Garcia-Alfonso P, Sobrino P, et al: Role of interferon alfa-2b in the induction and maintenance treatment of low-grade non-Hodgkin's lymphoma: Results from a prospective, multicenter trial with double randomization. J Clin Oncol 1998;16(4):1538–1546.

295. Fisher RI, Dana BW, LeBlanc M, et al: Interferon alfa consolidation after intensive chemotherapy does not prolong the progression-free survival of patients with low-grade non-Hodgkin's lymphoma: Results of the Southwest Oncology Group randomized phase III study 8809. J Clin Oncol 2000;18(10):2010–2016.

296. Coiffier B, Neidhardt-Berard EM, Tilly H, et al: Fludarabine alone compared to CHVP plus interferon in elderly patients with follicular lymphoma and adverse prognostic parameters: A GELA study. Ann Oncol 1999;10(10):1191–1197.

297. Klasa RJ, Meyer RM, Shustik C, et al: Randomized phase III study of fludarabine phosphate versus cyclophosphamide, vincristine, and prednisone in patients with recurrent low-grade non-Hodgkin's lymphoma previously treated with an alkylating agent or alkylator-containing regimen. J Clin Oncol 2002;20(24):4649–4654.

298. McLaughlin P, Hagemeister FB, Romaguera JE, et al: Fludarabine, mitoxantrone, and dexamethasone: An effective new regimen for indolent lymphoma. J Clin Oncol 1996;14(4):1262–1268.

299. Flinn IW, Byrd JC, Morrison C, et al: Fludarabine and cyclophosphamide with filgrastim support in patients with previously untreated indolent lymphoid malignancies. Blood 2000;96(1):71–75.

300. Lazzarino R, Orlandi E, Montillo M, et al: Fludarabine, cyclophosphamide, and dexamethasone (FluCyD) combination is effective in pretreated low-grade non-Hodgkin's lymphoma. Ann Oncol 1999;10(1):59–64.

301. Crawley CR, Foran JM, Gupta RK, et al: A phase II study to evaluate the combination of fludarabine, mitoxantrone, and dexamethasone (FMD) in patients with follicular lymphoma. Ann Oncol 2000;11(7):861–865.

302. Tsimberidou AM, McLaughlin P, Younes A, et al: Fludarabine, mitoxantrone, dexamethasone (FND) compared with an alternating triple therapy (ATT) regimen in patients with stage IV indolent lymphoma. Blood 2002;100(13):4351–4357.

303. Orchard JA, Bolam S, Oscier DG: Association of myelodysplastic changes with purine analogues. Br J Haematol 1998;100(4):677–679.

304. Miller RA, Maloney DG, Warnke R, Levy R: Treatment of B-cell lymphoma with monoclonal anti-idiotype antibody. N Engl J Med 1982;306(9):517–522.

305. Reff ME, Carner K, Chambers KS, et al: Depletion of B cells in vivo by a chimeric mouse human monoclonal antibody to CD20. Blood 1994;83(2):435–445.

306. Hainsworth JD, Burris HA, Morrissey LH, et al: Rituximab monoclonal antibody as initial systemic therapy for patients with low-grade non-Hodgkin's lymphoma. Blood 2000;95(10):3052–3056.

307. Colombat P, Salles G, Brousse N, et al: Rituximab (anti-CD20 monoclonal antibody) as single first-line therapy for patients with follicular lymphoma with a low tumor burden: Clinical and molecular evaluation. Blood 2001;97(1):101–106.

308. Cartron G, Dacheux L, Salles G, et al: Therapeutic activity of humanized anti-CD20 monoclonal antibody and polymorphism in IgG Fc receptor Fc gamma RIIIa gene. Blood 2002;99(3):754–758.

309. Bohen SP, Troyanskaya OG, Alter O, et al: Variation in gene expression patterns in follicular lymphoma and the response to rituximab. Proc Natl Acad Sci USA 2003;100(4):1926–1930.

310. Hainsworth JD, Litchy S, Burris HA, et al: Rituximab as first-line and maintenance therapy for patients with indolent non-Hodgkin's lymphoma. J Clin Oncol 2002;20(20):4261–4267.

311. Alas S, Bonavida B, Emmanouilides C: Potentiation of fludarabine cytotoxicity on non-Hodgkin's lymphoma by pentoxifylline and rituximab. Anticancer Res 2000;20(5A):2961–2966.

312. Alas S, Bonavida B: Rituximab inactivates signal transducer and activation of transcription 3 (STAT3) activity in B-non-Hodgkin's lymphoma through inhibition of the interleukin 10 autocrine/paracrine loop and results in downregulation of bcl-2 and sensitization to cytotoxic drugs. Cancer Res 2001;61(13):5137–5144.

313. Demidem A, Lam T, Alas S, Hariharan K, Hanna N, Bonavida B: Chimeric anti-CD20 (Idec-C2b8) monoclonal antibody sensitizes a B-cell lymphoma cell line to cell killing by cytotoxic drugs. Cancer Biother Radiopharm 1997;12(3):177–186.

314. Czuczman MS, Grillo-Lopez AJ, White CA, et al: Treatment of patients with low-grade B-cell lymphoma with the combination of chimeric anti-CD20 monoclonal antibody and CHOP chemotherapy. J Clin Oncol 1999;17(1):268–276.

315. Cheson BD, Horning SJ, Coiffier B, et al: Report of an international workshop to standardize response criteria for non-Hodgkin's lymphomas. J Clin Oncol 1999;17(4):1244–1253.

316. Apostolidis J, Gupta RK, Grenzelias D, et al: High-dose therapy with autologous bone marrow support as consolidation of remission in follicular lymphoma: Long-term clinical and molecular follow-up. J Clin Oncol 2000;18(3):527–536.

317. Schimmer AD, Jamal S, Messner H, et al: Allogeneic or autologous bone marrow transplantation (BMT) for non-Hodgkin's lymphoma (NHL): Results of a provincial strategy. Bone Marrow Transplant 2000;26(8):859–864.

318. Gallagher CJ, Gregory WM, Jones AE, et al: Follicular lymphoma: Prognostic factors for response and survival. J Clin Oncol 1986;4:1470–1480.

319. Williams CD, Harrison CN, Lister TA, et al: High-dose therapy and autologous stem-cell support for chemosensitive transformed low-grade follicular non-Hodgkin's lymphoma: A case-matched study from the European bone marrow transplant registry. J Clin Oncol 2001;19(3):727–735.

320. Freedman AS, Neuberg D, Mauch P, et al: Long-term follow-up of autologous bone marrow transplantation in patients with relapsed follicular lymphoma. Blood 1999;94(10):3325–3333.

321. Rohatiner A, Johnson P, Price C, et al: Myeloablative therapy with autologous bone marrow transplantation as consolidation therapy for recurrent follicular lymphoma. J Clin Oncol 1994;12(6):1177–1184.

322. Bierman PJ, Vose JM, Anderson JR, Bishop MR, Kessinger A, Armitage JO: High-dose therapy with autologous hematopoietic rescue for follicular low-grade non-Hodgkin's lymphoma. J Clin Oncol 1997;15(2):445–450.

323. Schouten HC, Qian W, Kvaloy S, et al: High-dose therapy improves progression-free survival and survival in relapsed follicular non-Hodgkin's lymphoma (NHL): Results from the randomized European CUP trial. J Clin Oncol 2003;21:3918–3927.

324. Apostolidis J, Foran JM, Johnson PWM, et al: Patterns of outcome following recurrence after myeloablative therapy with autologous bone marrow transplantation for follicular lymphoma. J Clin Oncol 1999;17(1):216–221.

325. Bastion Y, Brice P, Haioun C, et al: Intensive therapy with peripheral blood progenitor cell transplantation in 60 patients with poor-prognosis follicular lymphoma. Blood 1995;86(8):3257–3262.

326. Horning SJ, Negrin RS, Hoppe RT, et al: High-dose therapy and autologous bone marrow transplantation for follicular lymphoma in first complete or partial remission: Results of a phase II clinical trial. Blood 2001;97(2):404–409.

327. Brice P, Simon D, Bouabdallah R, et al: High-dose therapy with autologous stem-cell transplantation (ASCT) after first progression prolonged survival of follicular lymphoma patients included in the prospective GELF 86 protocol. Ann Oncol 2000;11(12):1585–1590.

328. Sebban C, Belanger C, Brice P, et al: A randomized controlled trial in follicular lymphoma comparing a standard chemotherapy regimen associated with interferon with four courses of CHOP regimen followed by an autologous stem cell transplantation with a TBI conditioning regimen: Results of the GELF 94 trial (GELA study group). Hematol J 2003;4(Suppl 2):150.

329. Di Nicola M, Siena S, Corradini P, et al: Elimination of bcl-2-IgH-positive follicular lymphoma cells from blood transplants with high recovery of hematopoietic progenitors by the Miltenyi CD34^P cell sorting system. Bone Marrow Transplant 1996;18:1117.

330. Nadler LM, Takvorian T, Botnick L, et al: Anti-B1 monoclonal antibody and complement treatment in autologous bone marrow transplantation for relapsed B-cell non-Hodgkin's lymphoma. Lancet 1984;2:427.

331. Leonard JP, Link BK: Immunotherapy of non-Hodgkin's lymphoma with hLL2 (epratuzumab, an anti-CD22 monoclonal antibody) and Hu1D10 (apolizumab). Semin Oncol 2002;29(1 Suppl 2):81–86.

332. Leonard JP, Coleman M, Ketas JC, et al: Phase I/II trial of epratuzumab (humanized anti-CD22 antibody) in indolent non-Hodgkin's lymphoma. J Clin Oncol 2003;21(16):5051–5059.

333. Witzig TE, Gordon LI, Cabanillas F, et al: Randomized controlled trial of yttrium-90-labeled ibritumomab tiuxetan radioimmunotherapy versus rituximab immunotherapy for patients with relapsed or refractory low-grade, follicular, or transformed B-cell non-Hodgkin's lymphoma. J Clin Oncol 2002;20(10):2453–2463.

334. Chanan-Khan A, Czuczman MS: Radioimmunotherapy in non-Hodgkin's lymphoma. Curr Opin Oncol 2002;14(5):484–489.

335. Cheson BD: Radioimmunotherapy of non-Hodgkin's lymphomas. (review) Blood 2003;101(2):391–398.

336. Dillman RO: Radio-labeled anti-CD20 monoclonal antibodies for the treatment of B-cell lymphoma. J Clin Oncol 2002;20(16):3545–3557.

337. Press OW, Eary JF, Gooley T, et al: A phase I/II trial of iodine-131-tositumomab (anti-CD20), etoposide, cyclophosphamide, and autologous stem cell transplantation for relapsed B-cell lymphomas. Blood 2000;96(9):2934–2942.

338. Kwak LW, Campbell MJ, Czerwinski BS, et al: Induction of immune responses in patients with B cell lymphoma against the surface-immunoglobulin idiotype expressed by their tumors. N Engl J Med 1992;327:1209.

339. Hsu FJ, Benika C, Fangoni F, et al: Vaccination of patients with B cell lymphoma using autologous pulsed dendritic cells. Nat Med 1996;2(1):52.

340. Hsu FJ, Caspar CB, Kwak LW, et al: Results of a trial of idiotype specific vaccine therapy for B-cell lymphoma. Blood 1986;10:273a.

341. Tao MH, Levy R: Idiotype/granulocyte colony stimulating factor fusion protein as a vaccine for B cell lymphoma. Nature 1993;263:755.

342. Shamash J, Davies DC, Salam A, et al: Induction of CD80 expression in low grade B cell lymphoma: A potential immunotherapeutic target. Leukemia 1995;9:1349.

343. Webb A, Cunningham D, Cotter F, et al: bcl-2 antisense therapy in patients with non-Hodgkin's lymphoma. Lancet 1997;349:1137.

344. Cotter FE, Johnson P, Hall P, et al: Antisense oligonucleotides suppress B-cell lymphoma growth in a SCID-hu mouse model. Oncogene 1994;9:3049.

345. Alexanian R: Blood volume in monoclonal gammopathy. Blood 1977;49:301.

346. Crawford J, Cox EB, Cohen HJ: Evaluation of hyperviscosity in monoclonal gammopathies. Am J Med 1985;79:13.

347. Thieblemont C, Felman P, Callet-Bauchu E, et al: Splenic marginal-zone lymphoma: A distinct clinical and pathological entity. Lancet Oncol 2003;4(2):95–103.

348. Johnson SA, Oscier DG, Leblond V: Waldenström's macroglobulinemia. Blood Rev 2002;16(3):175–184.

349. Dellagi K, Dupouey P, Brouet JC, et al: Waldenström's macroglobulinemia and peripheral neuropathy: A clinical and immunologic study of 25 patients. Blood 1983;62:280.

350. Kelly JJ, Adelman LS, Berkman E, et al: Polyneuropathies associated with IgM monoclonal gammopathies. Arch Neurol 1988;45:1355.

351. Pangalis GA, Nathwani BN, Rappaport H: Malignant lymphoma, well-differentiated lymphocytic: Its relationship with chronic lymphocytic leukemia and macroglobulinemia of Waldenström. Cancer 1977;39:999.

352. Evans HL, Butler JJ, Youness EL: Malignant lymphoma, small lymphocytic type. Cancer 1978;41:1440.

353. Papamichael D, Norton AJ, Foran JM, et al: Immunocytoma: A retrospective analysis from St. Bartholomew's Hospital—1972 to 1996. J Clin Oncol 1999;17(9):2847–2853.

354. Jones SE, Fuks Z, Bull M, et al: Non-Hodgkin's lymphoma IV: Clinicopathologic correlation in 405 cases. Cancer 1973;31:806.

355. Ezdinli EZ, Costello W, Lenhard R, et al: Survival of nodular versus diffuse pattern lymphocytic poorly differentiated lymphoma. Cancer 1978;41:1990.

356. Al-Katib A, Koziner B, Kurland E, et al: Treatment of diffuse poorly differentiated lymphocytic lymphoma. Cancer 1984;53:2402.

357. Offit K, Padilla M, Straus D, et al: Extended survival in patients with small cleaved diffuse lymphoma (SCCD) treated with anthracycline-containing chemotherapy: Follow-up at 8 years. Proc Am Soc Clin Oncol 1989;8:263.

358. Perry DA, Bast MA, Armitage JO, et al: Diffuse intermediate lymphocytic lymphoma: A clinicopathologic study and comparison with small lymphocytic lymphoma and diffuse small cleaved cell lymphoma. Cancer 1990;66:1995.

359. Pott-Hoeck C, Hiddemann W: Purine analogs in the treatment of low-grade lymphomas and chronic lymphocytic leukemia. Ann Oncol 1995;6:421.

360. Grever MR, Coltman CA, Files JL, et al: Fludarabine monophosphate in chronic lymphocytic leukemia. Blood 1986;68:223a.

361. Keating MJ, Kantarjian H, Talpaz M, et al: Fludarabine: A new agent with major activity against chronic lymphocytic leukemia. Blood 1989;74:19.

362. Keating MJ, Kantarjian HM, O'Brien S, et al: Fludarabine (FLU) prednisolone (PRED): A safe, effective combination in refractory chronic lymphocytic leukemia. Proc Am Soc Clin Oncol 1989;8:201.

363. Keating M, Kantarjian H, O'Brien S: Fludarabine: A new agent with marked cytoreductive activity in untreated chronic lymphocytic leukemia. J Clin Oncol 1991;9:44.

364. Klasa R, Connors J, Gascoyne R, et al: CPF (cyclophosphamide, prednisone, fludarabine) in advanced stage previously untreated low grade and mantle cell lymphoma. Blood 1997;90(S1):5429.

365. Zinzani PL, Bendandi M, Magagnoli M, et al: Fludarabine-mitoxantrone combination-containing regimen in recurrent low-grade non-Hodgkin's lymphoma. Ann Oncol 1997;8:379.

366. Keating MJ, Manshouri T, O'Brien S, et al: A high proportion of true complete remission can be obtained with a fludarabine, cyclophosphamide, rituximab combination (FCR) in contronic lymphocytic leukemia. Proc Am Soc Clin Oncol 2003;22:569(2289).

367. Foran JM, Rohatiner AZS, Cunningham D, et al: Immunotherapy of mantle cell lymphoma, lymphoplasmacytoid lymphoma, Waldenström's macroglobulinemia, and small lymphocytic lymphoma with rituximab (IDEC-C2B8): Preliminary results of an ongoing international multicenter trial. Proceedings of the ISH-EHA combined Congress. Br J Haematol 1998;102:586a.

368. Hale G, Dyer MJS, Clark MR, et al: Remission induction in non-Hodgkin's lymphoma with reshaped human monoclonal antibody CAMPATH-1H. Lancet 1988;2:1394.

369. Lundin J, Osterborg A, Brittinger G, et al: CAMPATH-1H monoclonal antibody in therapy for previously treated low-grade non-Hodgkin's lymphomas: A phase II multicenter study. J Clin Oncol 1998;16:3257.

370. Petrucci MT, Avvisati G, Tribalto M, et al: Waldenström's macroglobulinemia: results of a combined oral treatment in 34 newly diagnosed patients. J Intern Med 1989;226:443.

371. MacKenzie MR, Fudenberg HH: Macroglobulinemia: An analysis of 40 patients. Blood 1972;39:874.

372. McCallister BD, Bayrd ED, Harrison EG, et al: Primary macroglobulinemia. Am J Med 1967;43:394.

373. Dimopoulos MA, Weber D, Delasalle KB, et al: Treatment of Waldenström's macroglobulinemia resistant to standard therapy with 2-chlorodeoxyadenosine: identification of prognostic factors. Ann Oncol 1995;6:49.

374. Kantarjian HM, Alexanian R, Koller CA, et al: Fludarabine therapy in macroglobulinemic lymphoma. Blood 1990;75:1928.

375. Dimopoulos MA, Zervas C, Zomas A, et al: Treatment of Waldenström's macroglobulinemia with rituximab. J Clin Oncol 2002;20:2327–2333.

376. Isaacson P, Wright D: Malignant lymphoma of mucosa associated lymphoid tissue: A distinctive B-cell lymphoma. Cancer 1983;52:1410.

377. Zucca E: B-cell lymphoma of MALT type: A review with special emphasis on diagnostic and management problems of low-grade gastric tumours. Br J Haematol 1998;100:3.

378. Pelstring R, Essell J, Kurtin P, et al: Diversity of organ site involvement among malignant lymphomas of mucosa-associated tissues. Am J Clin Pathol 1991;96:738.

379. Parveen T, Navarro-Roman L, Medeiros L, et al: Low-grade B-cell lymphoma of mucosa-associated lymphois tissue arising in the kidney. Arch Pathol Lab Med 1993;117:780.

380. Thieblemont C, Berger F, Dumontet C, et al: Mucosa-associated lymphoid tissue lymphoma is a disseminated disease in one third of 158 patients analyzed. Blood 2000;95(3):802–806.

381. Holm LE, Blomgren H, Lowhagen T: Cancer risks in patients with chronic lymphocytic thyroiditis. N Engl J Med 1985;312:601.

382. Skarsgard ED, Connors JM, Robins RE: A current analysis of primary lymphoma of the thyroid. Arch Surg 1991;126:1199.

383. Wotherspoon AC, Ortiz HC, Falzon CR, et al: *Helicobacter pylori* associated gastritis and primary B-cell gastric lymphoma. (see comments) Lancet 1991;338:1175.

384. Isaacson PG, Diss TC, Wotherspoon AC, et al: Long-term follow-up of gastric MALT lymphoma treated by eradication of *H. pylori* with antibiotics. Gastroenterology 1999;117:750–751.

385. Sackmann M, Morgner A, Rudolph B, et al: Regression of gastric MALT lymphoma after eradication of *Helicobacter pylori* is predicted by endosonographic staging: MALT Lymphoma Study Group. Gastroenterology 1997;113:1087–1090.

386. Liu H, Ruskone-Fourmestrauz A, Lavergne-Slove A., et al: Resistance of t(11;18) positive gastric mucosa-associated lymphoid tissue lymphoma to *Helicobacter pylori* eradication therapy. Lancet 2001;357:39–40.

387. Thiede C, Wundisch T, Alpen B, et al: Long-term persistence of monoclonal B cells after cure of *Helicobacter pylori* infection and complete histologic remission in gastric mucosa-associated lymphoid tissue B-cell lymphoma. J Clin Oncol 2001;19:1600–1609.

388. Thieblemont C, Dumontet C, Bouafia F, et al: Outcome in relation to treatment modalities in 48 patients with localized gastric MALT lymphoma: A retrospective study of patients treated during 1976–2001. Leuk Lymphoma 2003;44:257–262.

389. Schechter NR, Portlock CS, Yahalom J: Treatment of mucosa-associated lymphoid tissue lymphoma of the stomach with radiation alone. J Clin Oncol 1998;16:1916–1921.

390. Hitchcock S, Ng AK, Fisher DC, et al: Treatment outcome of mucosa-associated lymphoid tissues/marginal zone non-Hodgkin's lymphoma. Int J Radiat Oncol Biol Phys 2002;52:1058–1066.

391. Tsang RW, Gospodarowicz MK, Pintilie M, et al: Stage I and II MALT lymphoma: Results of treatment with radiotherapy. Int J Radiat Oncol Biol Phys 2001;50:1258–1264.

392. Hammel P, Haioun C, Chaumette MT, et al: Efficacy of single-agent chemotherapy in low-grade B-cell mucosa-associated lymphoid tissue lymphoma with prominent gastric expression. J Clin Oncol 1995;13:2524–2529.

393. Conconi A, Martinelli G, Thieblemont C, et al: Clinical activity of rituximab in extramodal marginal zone B-cell lymphoma of MALT type. Blood 2003;102:2741–2745.

394. Hammel P, Haioun C, Chaumette MT, et al: Efficacy of single-agent chemotherapy in low-grade B-cell mucosa-associated lymphoid tissue lymphoma with prominent gastric expression. J Clin Oncol 1995;13:2524.

395. Sheibani K, Burke JS, Swartz WG, et al: Monocytoid B-cell lymphoma: Clinicopathologic study of 21 cases of a unique type of low-grade lymphoma. Cancer 1988;62:1531.

396. Cogliatti S, Lennert K, Hansmann M, et al: Monocytoid B-cell lymphoma: Clinical and prognostic features of 21 patients. J Clin Pathol 1990;43:619.

397. Schmid C, Kirkham N, Diss T, et al: Splenic marginal zone cell lymphoma. Am J Surg Pathol 1992;16:455.

398. Jadayel D, Matutes E, Dyer MJ, et al: Splenic lymphoma with villous lymphocytes: Analysis of bcl-1 rearrangements and expression of the cyclin D1 gene. Blood 1994;83:3664.

399. Thieblemont C, Felman P, Berger F, et al: Treatment of splenic marginal zone B-cell lymphoma: An analysis of 81 patients. Clin Lymphoma 2002;3(1):41–47.

400. Armitage JO, Weisenburger DD: New approach to classifying non-Hodgkin's lymphomas: Clinical features of the major histologic subtypes. J Clin Oncol 1998;16:2780.

401. Athan E, Foitl D, Knowles D: bcl-1 rearrangement: frequency and clinical significance among B-cell chronic lymphocytic leukemias and non-Hodgkin's lymphomas. Am J Pathol 1991;138:591.

402. Williams ME, Westermann CD, Swerdlow SH: Genotypic characterization of centrocytic lymphoma: Frequent rearrangement of the chromosome 11 bcl-1 locus. Blood 1990;76:1387.

403. Fisher RI, Dahlberg S, Nathwani BN, et al: A clinical analysis of two indolent lymphoma entities: Mantle cell lymphoma and marginal zone lymphoma: A Southwest Oncology Group study. Blood 1995;85:1075.

404. Berger F, Felman P, Sonet A, et al: Nonfollicular small B-cell lymphomas: A heterogeneous group of patients with distinct clinical features and outcome. Blood 1994;83:2829.

405. Weisenburger DD, Nathwani BN, Diamond LW, et al: Malignant lymphoma, intermediate lymphocytic type: A clinicopathologic study of 42 cases. Cancer 1981;48:1415.

406. Meusers P, Engelhard M, Bartels H, et al: Multicenter randomized therapeutic trial for advanced centrocytic lymphoma: Anthracycline does not improve the prognosis. Hematol Oncol 1989;7:365.

407. Norton AJ, Matthews J, Pappa V, et al: Mantle cell lymphoma: Natural history defined in a serially biopsied population over a 20-year period. Ann Oncol 1995;6:249.

408. Pittaluga S, Wlodarska I, Stul MS, et al: Mantle cell lymphoma: A clinicopathological study of 55 cases. Histopathology 1995;26:17.

409. Teodorovic I, Pittaluga S, Kluin-Nelemans JC, et al, for the European Organization for the Research and Treatment of Cancer Lymphoma Cooperative Group: Efficacy of four different regimens in 64 mantle cell lymphoma cases: Clinicopathologic comparison with 498 other non-Hodgkin's lymphoma subtypes. J Clin Oncol 1995;13:2816–2826.

410. Zucca E, Roggero E, Pinotti G, et al: Patterns of survival in mantle cell lymphoma. Ann Oncol 1995;6:257.

411. Howard OM, Gribben JG, Neuberg DS, et al: Rituximab and CHOP induction therapy for newly diagnosed mantle-cell lymphoma: Molecular complete responses are not predictive of progression-free survival. J Clin Oncol 2002;20:1288–1294.

412. Khouri IF, Romaguera J, Palmer JL, et al: Preliminary report of a new active regimen for aggressive mantle cell lymphoma. Proceedings ISH-EHA. Br J Haematol 1998;102:240a.

413. Romaguera J, Cabanillas F, Dang N, et al: Mantle cell lymphoma (MCL): Update on results after R-HCVAD without stem cell transplant (SCT). (abstract 24) Ann Oncol 2002;13(Suppl 2):8.

414. Stewart DA, Vose JM, Weisenburger DD, et al: The role of high-dose therapy and autologous hematopoietic stem cell transplantation for mantle cell lymphoma. Ann Oncol 1995;6:263.

415. Haas R, Brittinger G, Meusers P, et al: Myeloablative therapy with blood stem cell transplantation is effective in mantle cell lymphoma. Leukemia 1996;10:1975.

416. Dreger P, von Neuhoff N, Kuse R, et al: Sequential high-dose therapy and autologous stem cell transplantation for treatment of mantle cell lymphoma. Ann Oncol 1997;8:401.

417. Ketterer N, Salles G, Espinouse D, et al: Intensive therapy with peripheral stem cell transplantation in 16 patients with mantle cell lymphoma. Ann Oncol 1997;8:701.

418. Freedman AS, Neuberg D, Gribben JG, et al: High-dose chemoradiotherapy and anti-B-cell monoclonal antibody-purged autologous bone marrow transplantation in mantle cell lymphoma: No evidence for long-term remission. J Clin Oncol 1998;16:13.

419. Andersen NS, Donovan JW, Borus JS, et al: Failure of immunologic purging in mantle cell lymphoma assessed by polymerase chain reaction detection of minimal residual disease. Blood 1997;90:4212.

420. Coiffier B, Haioun C, Ketterer N, et al: Rituximab (anti-CD20 monoclonal antibody) for the treatment of patients with relapsing or refractory aggressive lymphoma: A multicenter phase II study. Blood 1998;92:1927.

421. Liang R, Todd D, Ho FCS: Aggressive non-Hodgkin's lymphoma: T-cell versus B-cell. Hematol Oncol 1996;14:1.

422. Melnyk A, Rodriguez A, Pugh WC, et al: Evaluation of the revised European-American lymphoma classification confirms the clinical relevance of immunophenotype in 560 cases of aggressive non-Hodgkin's lymphoma. Blood 1997;89:4514.

423. Lopez-Guillermo A, Cid J, Salar A, et al: Peripheral T-cell lymphomas: Initial features, natural history, and prognostic factors in a series of 174 patients diagnosed according to the REAL classification. Ann Oncol 1998;9:849.

424. Alizadeh AA, Eisen MD, David RE, et al: Distinct types of diffuse large B-cell lymphoma identified by gene expression profiling. Nature 2000;403:503–511.

425. Shipp MA, Ross KN, Tamayo P, et al: Diffuse large B-cell lymphoma outcome prediction by gene-expression profiling and supervised machine learning. Nat Med 2002;8:68–74.

426. Rosenwald A, Wright G, Chan WC, et al: The use of molecular profiling to predict survival after the chemotherapy for diffuse large B-cell lymphoma. N Engl J Med 2002;346(25):1937–1947.

427. Jones SE, Fuks Z, Kaplan KS, et al: Non-Hodgkin's lymphomas: Results of radiotherapy. Cancer 1973;32:682.

428. Peckman MJ, Guay JP, Kamlin IME, et al: Survival in localized nodal and extranodal non-Hodgkin's lymphoma. Br J Cancer 1975;31:413.

429. Hellman S, Chaffey JT, Rosenthal DS, et al: The place of radiation therapy in the treatment of non-Hodgkin's lymphomas. Cancer 1977;39:843.

Specific Malignancies

III

430. Chen MG, Prosnitz LR, Gonzales-Serva A, et al: Results of radiotherapy in control of stage I and II non-Hodgkin's lymphoma. Cancer 1979;443:1245.

431. Sweet DL, Kwziert J, Gacke MS, et al: Survival of patients with localized diffuse histocytic lymphoma. Blood 1981;58:1218.

432. Hoppe RT: The role of radiation therapy in the management of the non-Hodgkin's lymphomas. Cancer 1985;55:2176.

433. Sutcliffe SB, Gospodarowicz MK, Bush RS, et al: Role of radiation therapy in localized non-Hodgkin's lymphoma. Radiother Oncol 1985;4:211.

434. Levitt SH, Lee CKK, Bloomfield CD, et al: The role of radiation therapy in the treatment of early stage large cell lymphoma. Hematol Oncol 1985;3:33.

435. Vokes EE, Ultmann JE, Golomb KM, et al: Long-term survival of patients with localized diffuse histocytic lymphoma. J Clin Oncol 1985;3:1309.

436. Reddy S, Saxena VS, Pelletiere V, et al: Stage I and II non-Hodgkin's lymphomas: Long-term results of radiation therapy. Int J Radiat Oncol Biol Phys 1989;16:687.

437. Kallahan DE, Farah RE, Vokes EE, et al: The pattern of failure in patients with pathological stage I and II diffuse histocytic lymphoma treated with radiation therapy alone. Int J Radiat Oncol Biol Phys 1989;17:767.

438. Nissen NI, Ersboll J, Hansen HS, et al: A randomized study of radiotherapy plus chemotherapy in stage I and II non-Hodgkin's lymphoma. Cancer 1983;52:1.

439. Bonnadonna G, Lattuda A, Monfardini S, et al: Combined radiotherapy-chemotherapy in localized non-Hodgkin's lymphoma: 5-year results of a randomized study. II. In Jones SE, Salmon SE (eds): Adjuvant Therapy of Cancer II. New York, Grune & Stratton, 1979, p 145.

440. Cossett JM, Henry AMAR, Vuong T, et al: Alternating chemotherapy and radiotherapy combination for bulky stage I and II intermediate and high-grade non-Hodgkin's lymphoma: An update. Radiother Oncol 1991;20:30.

441. Mauch P, Leonard R, Skarin A, et al: Improved survival following combined radiation therapy and chemotherapy for unfavorable prognosis stage I and II non-Hodgkin's lymphoma. J Clin Oncol 1985;3:1301.

442. Connors JM, Klimo P, Fairey RN, et al: Brief chemotherapy and involved-field radiation therapy for limited stage histologically aggressive lymphoma. Ann Intern Med 1987;107:25.

443. Prestidge BR, Horning SJ, Hoppe RT: Combined modality therapy for stage I-II large cell lymphoma. Int J Radiat Oncol Biol Phys 1988;15:633.

444. Longo DL, Glatstein E, Duffey PL, et al: Treatment of localized aggressive lymphomas with combination chemotherapy followed by involved-field radiation therapy. J Clin Oncol 1989;7:1295.

445. Miller TP, Jones SE: Initial chemotherapy for clinically localized lymphomas of unfavorable histology. Blood 1983;62:413.

446. Jones SE, Miller TP, Connors JM: Long-term follow-up analysis for prognostic factors for patients with limited-stage diffuse large cell lymphoma treated with initial chemotherapy with or without adjuvant radiotherapy. J Clin Oncol 1989;7:1186.

447. Cabanillas F: Chemotherapy as definitive treatment of stage I-II large cell and diffuse mixed lymphomas. Hematol Oncol 1985;3:25.

448. Munck JN, Dhermain F, Koscielny S, et al: Alternating chemotherapy and radiotherapy for limited-stage intermediate and high-grade non-Hodgkin's lymphomas: Long-term results for 96 patients with tumors > 5 cm. Ann Oncol 1996;7:925.

449. Freilone R, Botto B, Vitolo U, et al: Combined modality treatment with a weekly brief chemotherapy (ACOP-B) followed by locoregional radiotherapy in localized-stage intermediate- to high-grade non-Hodgkin's lymphoma. Ann Oncol 1996;7:919.

450. Berd D, Cornog J, De Conti R, et al: Long-term remission in diffuse histocytic lymphoma treated with combination sequential chemotherapy. Cancer 1975;35:1050.

451. Levitt M, March JC, DeConti R, et al: Combination sequential chemotherapy in advanced reticulum cell sarcoma. Cancer 1972;29:630-636.

452. Fillet G, Bonnet C: Radiotherapy is unnecessary in elderly patients with localized aggressive non-Hodgkin's lymphoma: Results of the GELA LNH-93-4 Study. Blood 2002;100:92a.

453. Reyes F, Lepage E, et al: Superiority of chemotherapy alone with the ACVBP regimen over a combined treatment with three cycles of CHOP followed by involved field radiotherapy in patients with low-risk localized aggressive non-Hodgkin's lymphoma: Results of the LNH93-1 study. Blood 2002;100:93a.

454. DeVita VT, Chabner B, Hubbard SM, et al: Advanced diffuse histiocytic lymphoma, a potentially curable disease. Lancet 1975;1:248.

455. Jones SE, Grozea PN, Metz EN, et al: Superiority of Adriamycin-containing combination chemotherapy in the treatment of diffuse lymphoma: A Southwest Oncology Group study. Cancer 1979;43:417.

456. Rodriguez V, Cabanillas F, Burgess MA, et al: Combination chemotherapy (CHOP-Bleo) in advanced non-Hodgkin's lymphoma. Blood 1977;49:325.

457. Schein P, De Vita V, Hubbard S, et al: Bleomycin, Adriamycin, cyclophosphamide, vincristine, and prednisolone (BACOP) combination chemotherapy in the treatment of advanced diffuse histiocytic lymphoma. Ann Intern Med 1976;85:417.

458. Skarin AT, Canellos GP, Rosenthal DS, et al: Improved prognosis of diffuse histiocytic and undifferentiated lymphoma by use of high-dose methotrexate alternating with standard agents (M-BACOD). J Clin Oncol 1983;1:91.

459. Klimo P, Connors JM: MACOP-B chemotherapy for the treatment of diffuse large cell lymphoma. Ann Intern Med 1985;102:596.

460. Connors JM, Klimo P: Updated clinical experience with MACOP-B. Semin Hematol 1987;24(Suppl 1):26.

461. Schneider AM, Strauss DJ, Schluger AT, et al: Treatment results with an aggressive chemotherapeutic regimen (MACOP-B) for intermediate and some high grade non-Hodgkin's lymphomas. J Clin Oncol 1990;8:94.

462. Fisher RI, DeVita VT, Hubbard SM, et al: Diffuse aggressive lymphomas: Increased survival after alternating flexible sequences of Pro-MACE and MOPP chemotherapy. Ann Intern Med 1983;98:304.

463. Shipp M, Yeap B, Harrington D, et al: The m-BACOD combination chemotherapy regimen in large-cell lymphoma: Analysis of the completed trial and comparison with the M-BACOD regimen. J Clin Oncol 1990;8:84.

464. Miller T, Dahlberg S, Weick J, et al: Unfavorable histologies of non-Hodgkin's lymphoma treated with ProMace-CytaBOM: A Southwest Oncology Group study. J Clin Oncol 1990;8:1951.

465. Coiffier B, Bryon PA, Berger F, et al: Inventive and sequential combination chemotherapy for aggressive malignant lymphomas (protocol LNH-80). J Clin Oncol 1986;4:47.

466. Coiffier B, Gisselbrecht C, Herbrecht R, et al: LNH-84 study regimen and multicenter study of intensive therapy chemotherapy in 737 patients with aggressive malignant lymphoma. J Clin Oncol 1989;7:1018.

467. Fisher RI, Gaynor ER, Dahlberg S, et al: Comparison of a standard regimen (CHOP) with three intensive chemotherapy regimens for advanced non-Hodgkin's lymphoma. N Engl J Med 1993;328:1002.

468. Armitage JO, Mauch P, Harris N, Dalla-Favera R, Bierman P: Diffuse large B-cell lymphoma. In Mauch PM, Armitage JO, Harris NL, Coiffier B, Dalla-Favera R (eds): Non-Hodgkin's Lymphoma. Philadelphia, Lippincott Williams & Wilkins, 2003, pp 427-453.

469. Coiffier B: Increasing chemotherapy intensity in aggressive lymphomas: A renewal? J Clin Oncol 2003;21:2457-2459.

470. Hill ME, MacLennan KA, Cunningham DC, et al: Prognostic significance of bcl-2 expression and bcl-2 major breakpoint region rearrangement in diffuse large cell non-Hodgkin's lymphoma: A British National Lymphoma Investigation study. Blood 1996;88:1046.

471. Hermine O, Haioun C, Lepage E, et al: Prognostic significance of bcl-2 protein expression in aggressive non-Hodgkin's lymphoma. Blood 1996;87:265.

472. Kramer MHH, Hermans J, Parker J, et al: Clinical significance of bcl2 and p53 protein expression in diffuse large B-cell lymphoma: A population-based study. J Clin Oncol 1996;14:2131.

473. Gascoyne RD, Adomat SA, Krajewski S, et al: Prognostic significance of bcl-2 protein expression and bcl-2 gene rearrangement in diffuse aggressive non-Hodgkin's lymphoma. Blood 1997;90:244.

474. Zucca E, Bertoni F, Bosshard G, et al: Clinical significance of bcl-2 (MBR)J_H rearrangement in the peripheral blood of patients with diffuse large B-cell lymphomas. Ann Oncol 1996;7:1023.

475. Bastard C, Tilly H, Lenormand B, et al: Translocations involving band 3q27 and Ig gene regions in non-Hodgkin's lymphoma. Blood 1992;79:2527.

476. Ye BH, Lista F, Lo Coco F, et al: Alterations of a zinc finger-encoding gene, bcl-6, in diffuse large cell lymphoma. Science 1993;262:747.

477. Cattoretti G, Chang CC, Cechova K, et al: bcl-6 protein is expressed in germinal-center B cells. Blood 1995;86:45.

478. Lo Coco F, Ye BH, Lista F, et al: Rearrangements of the bcl-6 gene in diffuse large cell non-Hodgkin's lymphoma. Blood 1994;83:1757.

479. Gaidano G, Lo Coco F, Ye BH, et al: Rearrangements of the bcl-6 gene in acquired immunodeficiency syndrome–associated non-Hodgkin's lymphoma: Associated with diffuse large cell subtype. Blood 1994;84:397.

480. Offit K, Lo Coco F, Louie DC, et al: Rearrangement of the bcl-6 gene as a prognostic marker in diffuse large-cell lymphoma. N Engl J Med 1994;331:74.

481. Bauer KD, Merkel DE, Winter JN, et al: Prognostic implications of ploidy and proliferative activity in diffuse large cell lymphomas. Cancer Res 1986;46:3173–3178.

482. Wooldridge TN, Grierson HL, Weisenburger DD, et al: Association of DNA content and proliferative activity with clinical outcome in patients with diffuse mixed cell and large cell non-Hodgkin's lymphoma. Cancer Res 1988;48:6608–6613.

483. Grogan TM, Lippman SM, Spier CM, et al: Independent prognostic significance of a nuclear proliferation antigen in diffuse large cell lymphomas as determined by the monoclonal antibody Ki-67. Blood 1988;71:1157–1160.

484. Wilson WH, Teruya-Feldstein J, Fest T, et al: Relationship of p53, bcl-2, and tumor proliferation to clinical drug resistance in non-Hodgkin's lymphomas. Blood 1997;89:601–609.

485. Swan FJ, Velasquez WS, Tucker S, et al: A new serologic staging system for large cell lymphomas based on initial beta-2-microglobulin and lactate dehydrogenase levels. J Clin Onocol 1989;7:1518–1527.

486. Miller TP, Lippman SM, Spier CM, et al: HLA-DR (Ia) immune phenotype predicts outcome for patients with diffuse large cell lymphoma. J Clin Invest 1988;82:370–372.

487. Coiffier B, Lepage E: Prognosis of aggressive lymphomas: A study of five prognostic models with patients included in the LNH-84 regimen. Blood 1989;74:558.

488. Shipp M, Harrington DP, Klatt M, et al: Identification of major prognostic subgroups of patients with large cell lymphoma treated with m-BACOD or M-MACOD. Ann Intern Med 1986;104:757.

489. Dhaliwal HS, Rohatinter AZS, Gregory W, et al: Combination chemotherapy for intermediate and high grade non-Hodgkin's lymphoma. Br J Cancer 1993;684:767.

490. Koziner B, Little C, Passe S, et al: Treatment of advanced diffuse histiocytic lymphomas: An analysis of prognostic variables. Cancer 1982;49:1571.

491. Cowan RA, Jones M, Harris M, et al: Prognostic factors in high and intermediate grade non-Hodgkin's lymphoma. Br J Cancer 1989;59:276.

492. Daniel L, Wong G, Koziner B, et al: Predictive model for prognosis in advanced diffuse histiocytic lymphoma. Cancer Res 1986;46: 5372.

493. Swan F, Velasquez WS, Tucker S, et al: A new serologic staging system for large cell lymphomas based on initial beta-2-microglobulin and lactate dehydrogenase levels. J Clin Oncol 1989;7:1518.

494. Kessinger A, Armitage JO, Smith DM, et al: High-dose therapy and autologous peripheral blood stem cell transplantation for patients with lymphoma. Blood 1989;74:1260.

495. Philip T, Armitage JO, Spitzer G, et al: High dose therapy and autologous bone marrow transplantation after failure of conventional chemotherapy in adults with intermediate grade or high grade non-Hodgkin's lymphoma. N Engl J Med 1987;316:1493.

496. Takvorian T, Canellos G, Ritz J, et al: Prolonged disease-free survival after autologous bone marrow transplantation in patients with non-Hodgkin's lymphoma with a poor prognosis. N Engl J Med 1987;316:1499.

497. Phillips GL, Herzig RH, Lazarus HM, et al: Treatment of resistant malignant lymphoma with cyclophosphamide, total body irradiation, and transplantation of cryopreserved autologous marrow. N Engl J Med 1987;310:1557.

498. Vose JM, Anderson JR, Kessinger A, et al: High-dose chemotherapy and autologous hematopoietic stem cell transplantation for aggressive non-Hodgkin's lymphoma. J Clin Oncol 1993;11:1846.

499. Gulati SC, Shank B, Black P, et al: Autologous bone marrow transplantation for patients with poor prognosis lymphoma. J Clin Oncol 1988;6:1303.

500. Gribben JG, Goldstone AH, Linch DC, et al: Effectiveness of high dose combination chemotherapy and autologous bone marrow transplantation for patients with non-Hodgkin's lymphomas who are still responsive to conventional dose therapy. J Clin Oncol 1989;7:1621.

501. Petersen FB, Appelbaum FR, Hill R, et al: Autologous transplantation for malignant lymphoma: A report of 101 cases from Seattle. J Clin Oncol 1990;8:638.

502. Freedman AS, Takvorian T, Andersen KC, et al: Autologous bone marrow transplantation in B cell non-Hodgkin's lymphoma: Very low treatment related mortality in 100 patients in sensitive relapse. J Clin Oncol 1990;8:784.

503. Gianni AM, Bregni M, Siena S, et al: High dose chemotherapy and autologous bone marrow transplantation compared with MACOP-B in aggressive B-cell lymphoma. N Engl J Med 1997;337:711.

504. Pettengell R, Radford JA, Morgenstern GR, et al: Survival benefit from high-dose therapy with autologous blood progenitor cell transplantation in poor prognosis non-Hodgkin's lymphoma. J Clin Oncol 1996;14:586.

505. Verdonck LF, van Putten WL, Hagenbeek A, et al: Comparison of CHOP chemotherapy with autologous bone marrow transplantation for slowly responding patients with aggressive non-Hodgkin's lymphoma. N Engl J Med 1995;332:1045.

506. Martelli M, Vignetti M, Zinzani PL, et al: High-dose chemotherapy followed by autologus bone marrow transplantation versus dexamethasone, cisplatin, and cytarabine in aggressive non-Hodgkin's lymphoma with partial response to front-line chemotherapy: A prospective randomized Italian multicenter study. J Clin Oncol 1996;14:534.

507. Haioun C, Lepage E, Gisselbrecht C, et al: Survival benefit of high-dose therapy in poor-risk aggressive non-Hodgkin's lymphoma: Final analysis of the prospective LNH87-2 protocol. A Groupe d'Etude des Lymphomes de l'Adulte Study. J Clin Oncol 2000;18(16):3025–3030.

508. Coiffier B, Gisselbrecht C, Herbrecht R, et al: LNH-84 regimen: A multicenter study if intensive chemotherapy in 737 patients with aggressive malignant lymphoma. J Clin Oncol 1989;7:1018–1026.

509. Tilly H, Lepage E, Coiffier B, et al: A randomized comparison of ACVBP and CHOP in the treatment of advanced aggressive non-Hodgkin's lymphoma: The LNH 93-5 study. Blood 2000;96:832a.

510. Pfreundschuh M, Trumper L, Kloess M, et al: CHOEP (CHOP + etopside) is the new standard regimen for young patients with aggressive NHL. Ann Oncol 2002;13(Suppl 2):74.

511. Pfreundschuh M, Trumper L, Schmits R, et al: 2-weekly versus 3 weekly CHOP with and without etoposide in young patients with low-risk (low LDH) aggressive non-Hodgkin's lymphoma: Results of the completed non-Hodgkin's lymphoma-B-1 trial of the DSHNHL. Blood 2002;100(Suppl 1):110a.

512. Mounier N, Briere J, Gisselbrecht C, et al: Rituximab plus CHOP (R-CHOP) in the treatment of elderly patients with diffuse large B-cell lymphoma (DLBCL) overcomes Bcl1-associated chemotherapy resistance. (abstract 603) Blood 2002;100;161a.

513. Wilson WH, Pittaluga S, O'Connor P, et al: Rituximab may overcome Bcl-2-associated chemotherapy resistance in untreated diffuse large B-cell lymphomas. (abstract 1447) Blood 2001;98:343a.

514. Carde P, Meerwaldt JH, van Glabbeke M, et al: Superiority of second over first generation chemotherapy in a randomized trial for stage III-IV intermediate- and high-grade non-Hodgkin's lymphoma: The 1980–1985 EORTC trial. The EORTC Lymphoma Group. Ann Oncol 1991;2:431–435.

515. Intragumtornchai T, Wannakrairoj P, Chaimongkol B, et al:

Non-Hodgkin's lymphomas in Thailand: A retrospective pathologic and clinical analysis of 1391 cases. Cancer 1996;78(8):1813–1819.

516. Linch DC, Smith P, Hancock BW, et al: A randomized British National Lymphoma Investigation trial of CHOP versus a weekly multiagent regimen (PACEBOM) in patients with histologically aggressive non-Hodgkin's lymphoma. Ann Oncol 2000; 11(Suppl 1);87–90.

517. Pfreundschuh M, Trumper L, Kloess M, et al: 2 weekly versus 3 weekly CHOP with and without etoposide for patients > 60 years of age with aggressive non-Hodgkin's lymphoma: Results of the completed non-Hodgkin's lymphoma B-2 trial of the DSHNHL. Blood 2002;100(Suppl 1);774a.

518. Wolf M, Matthews JP, Stone J, Cooper IA, Robertson TOI, Fox RM: Long-term survival advantage of MACOP-B over CHOP in intermediate-grade non-Hodgkin's lymphoma. Ann Oncol 1997;8(Suppl 1):71–75.

519. Haioun C, Besson C, Lepage E, et al: Incidence and risk factors of central nervous system relapse in histologically aggressive non-Hodgkin's lymphoma uniformly treated and receiving intrathecal central nervous system prophylaxis: A GELA study on 974 pateints. Ann Oncol 200;11(6):685–690.

520. Mavromatis BH, Cheson BD: Pre- and post-treatment evaluation of non-Hodgkin's lymphoma. Best Pract Res Clin Haematol 200;15(3):429–447.

521. Naumann R, Vaic A, Beuthien-Baumann B, et al: Prognostic value of positron emission tomography in the evaluation of post-treatment residual mass in patients with Hodgkin's disease and non-Hodgkin's lymphoma. Br J Haematol 2001;115(4): 793–800.

522. Hoskins PJ, Le N, Gascoyne RD, et al: Advanced diffuse large cell lymphoma treated with 12 week combination chemotherapy: Natural history of relapse after initial complete response and prognostic variables defining outcome after relapse. Ann Oncol 1997;8:1125.

523. Cabanillas F, Hagemeister FB, McLaughlin P, et al: Results of MIME salvage regimen for recurrence of refractory lymphoma. J Clin Oncol 1987;5:407.

524. Herbrecht R, Garcirs JJ, Bergerat JP, et al: VP-16 ifosfamide and methotrexate combination chemotherapy for aggressive non-Hodgkin's lymphoma after failure of LNH 84 regimen. Cancer Chemother Pharmacol 1989;24:338.

525. Velasquez WS, Hagemeister G, McLaughlin P, et al: E-SHAP: An effective treatment for refractory and relapsing lymphoma. Proc Am Soc Clin Oncol 1992;11:326.

526. Johnson PWM, Whelan J, Longhurst S, et al: E-SHAP: Poor treatment for recurrent lymphoma. Ann Oncol 1993;4:63.

527. Velasquez WS, Cabanillas F, Salvador P: Effective salvage therapy for lymphoma with cis-platin in combination with high dose ara-C and dexamethasone (DHAP). Blood 1988;71:117.

528. Hickish T, Roldan A, Cunningham D, et al: EPIC: An effective low toxicity regimen for relapsing lymphoma. Br J Cancer 1993;68:599.

529. Wilson WH, Bryant G, Bates S, et al: EPOCH chemotherapy: Toxicity and efficacy in relapsed and refractory non-Hodgkin's lymphoma. J Clin Oncol 1993;11:1573.

530. Shipp MA, Klatt MM, Yeap B, et al: Patterns of relapse in large cell lymphoma patients with bulk disease: Implications for the use of adjuvant radiation therapy. J Clin Oncol 1989;7:613.

531. Philip T, Guglielmi C, Hagenbeek A, et al: Autologous bone marrow transplantation as compared with salvage chemotherapy in relapses of chemotherapy-sensitive non-Hodgkin's lymphoma. N Engl J Med 1995;333:1540.

532. Bosly A, Sonet A, Salles G, et al: Superiority of late over early intensification in relapsing/refractory aggressive non-Hodgkin's lymphoma: A randomized study from the GELA: LNH RP 93. Proceedings ISH-EHA, Amsterdam, July 1998. Br J Haematol 1998;102:148a.

533. Vose JM, Bierman PJ, Lynch JC, et al: Effect of follicularity on autologous transplantation for large cell non-Hodgkin's lymphoma. J Clin Oncol 1998;16:844.

534. Maloney DG, Grillo-Lopez AJ, White CA, et al: IDEC-C2B8 (Rituximab) anti-CD20 monoclonal antibody therapy in patients with relapsed low-grade non-Hodgkin's lymphoma. Blood 1997;90:2188.

535. Nagler A, Ackerstein A, Or R, et al: Immunotherapy with recombinant human interluekin-2 and recombinant interferon-alpha in lymphoma patients post–autologous marrow or stem cell transplantation. Blood 1997;89:3951.

536. Shamash J, Apostolidis J, Foran JM, et al: Low dose continuous chemotherapy in refractory lymphoma. Br J Haematol 1998;102:118a.

537. Salminen E, Nikkanen V, Lindholm L: Palliative chemotherapy in non-Hodgkin's lymphoma. Oncology 1997;54:108.

538. Fetscher S, Lubbert M, Kanz L, et al: Treatment of relapsed non-Hodgkin's lymphoma after BEAM chemotherapy and autologous transplantation by BU-CY chemotherapy and salvage transplantation. Bone Marrow Transplant 1997;19:527.

539. de Lima M, van Besien KW, Giralt SA, et al: Bone marrow transplantation after failure of autologous transplant for non-Hodgkin's lymphoma. Bone Marrow Transplant 1997;19:121.

540. Addis B, Isaacson P: Large cell lymphoma of the mediastinum: A B-cell tumor of probable thymic origin. Histopathology 1986;10:379.

541. Moller P, Moldenhauer G, Momburg F, et al: Mediastinal lymphoma of clear cell type is a tumor corresponding to terminal steps of B-cell differentiation. Blood 1987;69:1087.

542. Sehn LH, Antin JH, Shulman LN, et al: Primary diffuse large B-cell lymphoma of the mediastinum: Outcome following high-dose chemotherapy and autologous hematopoietic cell transplantation. Blood 1998;91:717.

543. Magrath I, Shiramizu B: Biology and treatment of small noncleaved cell lymphoma. Oncology 1989;3:41.

544. Burkitt DP: Geographical distribution. In Burkitt DP, Wright DH (eds): Burkitt's Lymphoma. Edinburgh, Churchill Livingstone, 1970, p 186.

545. Ballerini P, Gaidano G, Gong J, et al: Multiple genetic lesions in AIDS-related non-Hodgkin's lymphoma. Blood 1993;81:166.

546. Pelicci P, Knowles D, Magrath I, et al: Chromosomal breakpoints and structural alterations of the c-myc locus differ in endemic and sporadic forms of Burkitt's lymphoma. Proc Natl Acad Sci USA 1986;83:2984.

547. Yano T, van Krieken J, Magrath IT, et al: Histogenetic correlations between subcategories of small noncleaved cell lymphomas. Blood 1992;79:1282.

548. Dorfman RF: Childhood lymphosarcoma in St Louis, Missouri, clinically and histologically resembling Burkitt's lymphoma. Cancer 1965;18:418.

549. Patte C, Philip T, Radary C, et al: High cure rate in advanced B cell lymphoma and leukemia without CNS involvement with a short intensive polychemotherapy. J Clin Oncol 1991;9:123.

550. Magrath IT, Adde M, Shad A, et al: Adults and children with small noncleaved-cell lymphoma have a similar excellent outcome when treated with the same chemotherapy regimen. J Clin Oncol 1996;14:925.

551. Lee EJ, Petroni GR, Schiffer CA, et al: Brief-duration high-intensity chemotherapy for patients with small noncleaved-cell lymphoma or FAB L3 acute lymphocytic leukemia: Results of cancer and leukemia group B study 9251. J Clin Oncol 2001;19:4014–4022.

552. Soussain C, Patte C, Ostronoff M, et al: Small noncleaved cell lymphoma and leukemia in adults. A retrospective study of 65 adults treated with the LMB pediatric protocols. Blood 1995;85:664–674.

553. Borowitz M, Croker B, Metzgar R: Lymphoblastic lymphoma with the phenotype of common acute lymphoblastic leukemia. Am J Clin Pathol 1983;79:387.

554. Haddy TB, Kennan AM, Jaffe ES, et al: Bone involvement in young patients with non-Hodgkin's lymphoma: Efficacy of chemotherapy without local radiotherapy. Blood 1988;72:1141.

555. Sander C, Medeiros L, Abruzzo L, et al: Lymphoblastic lymphoma presenting in cutaneous sites: A clinicopathologic analysis of six cases. J Am Acad Dermatol 1991;25:1023.

556. Picozzi VJ, Coleman CN: Lymphoblastic lymphoma. Semin Oncol 1990;17:96.

557. Streuli RA, Kaneko Y, Variakojis D, et al: Lymphoblastic lymphoma in adults. Cancer 1981;47:2510.

558. Strauss DJ, Wong GH, Lik J, et al: Small noncleaved lymphoma (undifferentiated Burkitt's type) in American adults: Results with treatment designed for acute lymphoblastic leukaemia. Am J Med 1991;90:328.

559. Hoelzer D, Gokbuget N, Digel W, et al: Outcome of adult patients with T-lymphoblastic lymphoma treated according to protocols for acute lymphoblastic leukemia. Blood 2002;99:4379.

560. Thomas DA, Cortes J, O'Brien SM, et al: Improved outcome with the hyper-CVAD regimen in lymphoblastic lymphoma (LL). (abstract 3598) Blood 2000;96(Suppl 1):883a.

561. Kaiser U, Uebelacker I, Havemann K: Non-Hodgkin's lymphoma protocols in the treatment of patients with Burkitt's lymphoma and lymphoblastic lymphoma: A report on 58 patients. Leuk Lymphoma 1999;36:101.

562. Philip T: Lymphoblastic lymphoma and Burkitt's lymphoma in Caucasian adults: Please don't forget the pediatric experience. (editorial) Ann J Oncol 1995;6:414.

563. Sweetenham JW, Santini G, Quian W, et al: High-dose therapy and autologous stem-cell transplantation versus conventional-dose consolidation/maintenance therapy as postremission therapy for adult patients with lymphoblastic lymphoma: Results of a randomized trial of the European Group for Blood and Marrow Transplantation and the United Kingdom Lymphoma Group. J Clin Oncol 2001;19:2927.

564. Zinzani PL, Bendandi M, Visani G, et al: Adult lymphoblastic lymphoma: Clinical features and prognostic factors in 53 patients. Leuk Lymphoma 1996;23:577.

565. Slater DE, Mertelsmann R, Koziner B, et al: Lymphoblastic lymphoma in adults. J Clin Oncol 1986;4:57.

566. Salloum E, Henry-Amar M, Caillou B, et al: Lymphoblastic lymphoma in adults: A clinicopathological study of 34 cases treated at the Institute Gustave-Roussy. Eur J Cancer Clin Oncol 1988;24:1609.

567. Voakes JB, Jones SE, McKelvey EM: The chemotherapy of lymphoblastic lymphoma. Blood 1981;57:186.

568. Levine AM, Forman SJ, Meyer PR, et al: Successful therapy of convoluted T-lymphoblastic lymphoma in the adult. Blood 1983;61:92.

569. Lopez TM, Hagenmeister FB, McLaughlin P, et al: Small noncleaved cell lymphoma in adults: Superior results for stages III disease. J Clin Oncol 1990;8:615.

570. McMaster ML, Greer JP, Greco FA, et al: Effective treatment of small noncleaved cell lymphoma with high-density, brief-duration chemotherapy. J Clin Oncol 1991;9:941.

571. Bernstein JI, Coleman CN, Strickler JG, et al: Combined modality therapy for adults with small noncleaved cell lymphoma (Burkitt's and non-Burkitt's type). J Clin Oncol 1986;4:847.

572. Morel P, Legage E, Brice P, et al: Prognosis and treatment of lymphoblastic lymphoma in adults: A report on 80 patients. J Clin Oncol 1992;7:1078.

573. Coleman CN, Picozzi VJ Jr, Cox RS, et al: Treatment of lymphoblastic lymphoma in adults. J Clin Oncol 1986;4:1628.

574. Anderson JR, Armitage JO, Weisenberger DD, for the Non-Hodgkin's Lymphoma Classification Project: Epidemiology of the non-Hodgkin's lymphomas: Distributions of the major subtypes differ by geographic locations. Ann Oncol 1998;9:717.

575. Horning SJ, Weiss LM, Crabtree GS, et al: Clinical and phenotypic diversity of T-cell lymphomas. Blood 1986;67:1578.

576. Armitage JO, Greer JP, Levine AM, et al: Peripheral T-cell lymphoma. Cancer 1989;63:158.

577. Weisenburger DD, Astorino RN, Glassy FJ, et al: Peripheral T-cell lymphoma: A clinicopathologic study of a morphologically diverse entity. Cancer 1985;56:2061.

578. Coiffier B, Berger F, Bryon PA, et al: T-cell lymphomas: Immunologic, histologic, clinical, and therapeutic analysis of 63 cases. J. Clin Oncol 1988;6:1584.

579. Cullen MH, Stansfeld AG, Oliver RTD, et al: Angioimmunoblastic lymphadenopathy: Report of 10 cases and review of the literature. Q J Med 1979;189:151.

580. Ganesan TS, Dhaliwal HS, Dorreen MS, et al: Angioimmunoblastic lymphadenopathy: A clinical, immunological, and molecular study. Br J Cancer 1987;55:437.

581. Frizzera G, Moran EM, Rappaport H: Angioimmunoblastic lymphadenopathy with dysproteinemia. Lancet 1974;1:1070.

582. Lipford EH, Smith HR, Pittaluga S, et al: Clonality of angioimmunoblastic lymphadenopathy and implications for its evolution to malignant lymphoma. J Clin Invest 1987; 79:637.

583. Kaneko Y, Maseki N, Sakurai M, et al: Characteristic karyotypic pattern in T-cell lymphoproliferative disorders with reactive "angioimmunoblastic lymphadenopathy with dysproteinemia-type" features. Blood 1988;72:413.

584. Siegert W, Agthe A, Griesser H, et al: Treatment of angioimmunoblastic lymphadenopathy (AILD)–type T-cell lymphoma using prednisone with or without the COPBLAM/IMVP-16 regimen. Ann Intern Med 1992;117:364.

585. Freter CE, Cossman J: Angioimmunoblastic lymphadenopathy with dysproteinemia. Semin Oncol 1993;20:627.

586. Jaffe E: Pathologic and clinical spectrum of post-thymic T-cell malignancies. Cancer Invest 1984;2:413.

587. Lipford E, Margolick J, Longo D, et al: Angiocentric immunoproliferative lesions: A clinicopathologic spectrum of post-thymic T-cell proliferations. Blood 1988;72:1674.

588. Greer J, Kinney M, Collins R, et al: Clinical features of 31 patients with Ki-1 anaplastic large cell lymphoma. J Clin Oncol 1991;9:539.

589. Watanabe S, Sato Y, Shimoyama M, et al: Immunoblastic lymphadenopathy angioimmunoblastic lymphodemopathy, and IBL-like T-cell lymphoma. Cancer 1986;58:2224.

590. Weiss L, Strickler J, Dorfman R, et al: Clonal T-cell populations in angioimmunoblastic lymphadenopathy and angioimmunoblastic lymphadenopathy-like lymphoma. Am J Pathol 1986;122:392.

591. Tobinai K, Minato K, Ohtsu T, et al: Clinicopathologic, immunophenotypic, and immunogenetic analysis of immunoblastic lymphadenopathy-like T-cell lymphoma. Blood 1988;72:1000.

592. Siegert W, Nerl C, Agthe A, et al: Angioimmunoblastic lymphadenopathy (AILD)–type T-cell lymphoma: Prognostic impact of clinical observations and laboratory findings at presentation. Ann Oncol 1995;6:659.

593. Nathwani BN, Jaffe ES: Angioimmunoblastic lymphadenopathy (AILD) and AILD-like T-cell lymphomas. In Jaffe ES (ed): Surgical Pathology of the Lymph Nodes and Related Organs. Philadelphia, WB Saunders, 1995, p 390.

594. Anagnostopoulos I, Hummel M, Finn T, et al: Heterogeneous Epstein-Barr virus infection patterns in peripheral T-cell lymphoma of angioimmunoblastic lymphadenopathy type. Blood 1992;80:1804.

595. Schlegelberger B, Feller A, Godde W, Lennert K: Stepwise development of chromosomal abnormalities in angioimmunoblastic lymphadenopathy. Cancer Genet Cytogenet 1990; 50:15.

596. Frizzera G, Moran EM, Rappaport H: Angioimmunoblastic lymphadenopathy with dysproteinemia. Lancet 1974;1:1070.

597. Tobinai K, Minato K, Ohtsu T, et al: Clinicopathologic, immunophenotypic, and immunogenotypic analysis of immunoblastic lymphadenopathy-like T-cell lymphoma. Blood 1988;72:1000.

598. Weiss L: Primary nasal T-cell lymphoma. (abstract) Fifth International Conference on Malignant Lymphoma, Lugano, Switzerland, 1993;72:57.

599. Ferry J, Sklar J, Zukerberg L, Harris N: Nasal lymphoma: A clinicopathologic study with immunophenotypic and genotypic analysis. Am J Surg Pathol 1991;15:268.

600. Lipford E, Margolich J, Longo D, et al: Angiocentric immunoproliferative lesions: A clinicopathologic spectrum of post-thymic T cell proliferation. Blood 1988;5:1674.

601. Chan J, Ng C, Lau W, Ho S: Most nasal/nasopharyngeal lymphomas are peripheral T cell neoplasms. Am J Surg Pathol 1987;11:418.

602. Ho F, Choy D, Loke S, et al: Polymorphic reticulosis and conventional lymphomas of the nose and upper aerodigestive tract: A clinicopathologic study of 76 cases, and immunophenotypic studies in 16 cases. Hum Pathol 1990;21:1041.

603. Strickler JG, Meneses MF, Habermann TM, et al: Polymorphic reticulosis: A reappraisal. Hum Pathol 1994;25:659.

604. Lippman S, Grogan T, Spier C, et al: Lethal midline granuloma with a novel T-cell phenotype as found in peripheral T-cell lymphoma. Cancer 1987;59:936.

605. Aviles A, Rodriguez L, Guzman R, et al: Angiocentric T-cell lymphoma of the nose, paranasal sinuses, and hard palate. Hematol Oncol 1992;10:141.

606. Harabuchi Y, Yamanaka N, Kataura A, et al: Epstein-Barr virus in nasal T-cell lymphomas in patients with lethal midline granuloma. Lancet 1990;335:128.

607. Mishima K, Horiuchi K, Kojya S, et al: Epstein-Barr virus in patients with polymorphic reticulosis (lethal midline granuloma) from China and Japan. Cancer 1994;73:3041.

608. Chott A, Rappersberger K, Schlossarek W, Radaszkiewicz T: Peripheral T-cell lymphoma presenting primarily as lethal midline granuloma. Hum Pathol 1988;19:1093.

609. Soler J, Bordes R, Ortuni F, et al: Aggressive natural killer cell leukaemia/lymphoma in two patients with lethal midline granuloma. Br J Haematol 88;1994:659.

610. Liang R, Todd D, Chan TK, et al: Treatment outcome and prognostic factors for primary nasal lymphomas. J Clin Oncol 1995;13:666.

611. Liang R, Todd D, Ho F: Aggressive non-Hodgkin's lymphoma T-cell versus B-cell. Hematol Oncol 1996;14:1.

612. Farcet J, Gaulard P, Marolleau J, et al: Hepatosplenic T-cell lymphoma: Sinusal/sinusoidal localization of malignant cells expressing the T-cell receptors γδ. Blood 1990;75:2213.

613. Cooke BC, Krenacs L, Statler-Stevenson M, et al: Hepatosplenic T-Cell lymphoma: A distinct clinicopathologic entity of cytotoxic γδ T-cell origin. Blood 1996;88:4265.

614. Cooke C, Greiner T, Raffeld M, et al: T-cell lymphoma: A distinct clinicopathologic entity. Mod Pathol 1994;7:106A.

615. Wong KF, Chan JK, Matutes E: Hepatosplenic T cell lymphoma: A distinctive aggressive lymphoma type. Am J Surg Pathol 1995;19:718.

616. Isaacson P, O'Connor NT, Spencer J, et al: Malignant histiocytosis of the intestine: A T-call lymphoma. Lancet 1985;2:688.

617. O'Farrelly C, Feighery C, O'Briain DS, et al: Humoral response to wheat protein in patients with coeliac disease and enteropathy associated T-cell lymphoma. Br Med J 1986;293:908.

618. Spencer J, Cerf-Bensussan N, Jarry A, et al: Enteropathy-associated T-cell lymphoma is recognized by a monoclonal antibody (HML-1) that defines a membrane molecular on human mucosal lymphocytes. Am J Pathol 1988;132:1.

619. Isaacson P, Spencer J, Connolly C, et al: Malignant histiocytosis of the intestine: A T-cell lymphoma. Lancet 1985;ii:688.

620. Gonzalez C, Medeiros L, Braziel R, Jaffe E: T-cell lymphoma involving subcutaneous tissue: A clinicopathologic entity commonly associated with hemophagocytic syndrome. Am J Surg Pathol 1991;15:17.

621. Kumar S, Krenacs L, Medeiros J, et al: Subcutaneous panniculitic T-cell lymphoma is a tumor of cytotoxic T-lymphocytes. Hum Pathol 1998;29:397.

622. Salhany KE, Macon WR, Choi JK, et al: Subcutaneous panniculitis-like T-cell lymphoma: Clinicopathologic, immunophenotypic, and genotypic analysis of alpha/beta and gamma/delta subtypes. Am J Surg Pathol 1998;22:881.

623. Chan E, Chan G, Todd D, et al: Peripheral T-cell lymphoma presenting as hemophagocytic syndrome. Hematol Oncol 1989;7:275.

624. Falini B, Pileri S, DeSolas I, et al: Peripheral T-cell lymphoma associated with hemophagocytic syndrome. Blood 1990;75:434.

625. Harrison NK, Twelves C, Addis BJ, et al: Peripheral T-cell lymphoma presenting with angioedema and diffuse pulmonary infiltrate. Am Rev Respir Dis 1988;138:976.

626. O'Shea JJ, Jaffee ES, Lane HC, et al: Peripheral T-cell lymphoma presenting as hypereosinophilia with vasculitis. Am J Med 1987;82:539.

627. Foley JF, Linder J, Koh J, et al: Cutaneous necrotizing granulomatous vasculitis with evolution to T-cell lymphoma. Am J Med 1987;82:839.

628. Auger MJ, Nash JRG, Mackie MJ: Marrow involvement with T-cell lymphoma initially presenting as abnormal myelopoiesis. J Clin Pathol 1986;39:1134.

629. Saito K, Nakanuma Y, Ogawa S, et al: Extensive hepatic granulomas associated with peripheral T-cell lymphoma. Am J Gastroenterol 1991;86:1243.

630. Gherardi R, Gaulard P, Prost C, et al: T-cell lymphoma revealed by a peripheral neuropathy. Cancer 1986;58:2710.

631. Armitage JO, Greer JP, Levine AM, et al: Peripheral T-cell lymphoma. Cancer 1989;63:158.

632. Rudiger T, Weisenburger DD, Anderson JR, et al: Peripheral T-cell lymphoma (excluding anaplastic large cell lymphoma): Results from the Non-Hodgkin's Lymphoma Classification project. Ann Oncol 2002;13:140.

633. Armitage JO, Vose JM, Linder J, et al: Clinical significance of immunophenotyping in diffuse aggressive non-Hodgkin's lymphoma. J Clin Oncol 1989;7:1783.

634. Shimoyama M, Oyama A, Tajima K, et al: Differences in clinicopathological characteristics and major prognostic factors between B-lymphoma and peripheral T-lymphoma excluding adult T-cell leukemia/lymphoma. Leuk Lymphoma 1993;10:335.

635. Coiffier B, Brousse N, Peuchmaur M, et al: Peripheral T-cell lymphomas have a worse prognosis than B-cell lymphomas: A prospective study of 361 immunophenotyped patients treated with the LNH-84 regimen. The GELA (Groupe d'Etude des Lymphomes Agressives). Ann Oncol 1990;1:45.

636. Lippman SM, Miller TP, Spier CM, et al: The prognostic significance of the immunotype in diffuse large cell lymphoma: A comparative study of the T-cell and B-cell phenotype. Blood 1988;72:436.

637. Shimizu K, Hamajima N, Ohnishi K, et al: T-cell phenotype is associated with decreased survival in non-Hodgkin's lymphoma. Jpn J Cancer Res 1989;80:720.

638. Brown DC, Heryet A, Gatter KC, Mason DY: The prognostic significance of immunophenotype in high-grade non-Hodgkin's lymphoma. Histopathology 1989;14:621.

639. Karakas T, Bergmann L, Stutte HI, et al: Peripheral T-cell lymphomas respond well to vincristine, adriamycin, cyclophosphamide, prednisone, and etoposide (VACPE) and have a similar outcome as high-grade B-cell lymphomas. Leuk Lymphoma 1996;24:121.

640. Kwak L, Wilson M, Weiss L, et al: Similar outcome of treatment of B-cell and T-cell diffuse large cell lymphomas: The Stanford experience. J Clin Oncol 1991;9:1426.

641. Cheng AL, Chen YC, Wang CH, et al: Direct comparisons of peripheral T-cell lymphoma with diffuse B-cell lymphoma of comparable histological grades: Should peripheral T-cell lymphoma be considered separately? J Clin Oncol 1989;7:725.

642. Gisselbrecht C, Gaulard P, Lepage B, et al: Prognostic significance of T-cell phenotype in aggressive non-Hodgkin's lymphomas. Blood 1998;92:76.

643. Lopez-Guillermo A, Cid J, Salar A, et al: Peripheral T-cell lymphomas: Initial features, natural history, and prognostic factors in a series of 174 patients diagnosed according to the REAL classification. Ann Oncol 1998;9:849.

644. Ansell SM, Habermann TM, Kurtin PJ, et al: Predictive capacity of the International Prognostic Factor Index in patients with peripheral T-cell lymphoma. I. Clin Oncol 1997;15:2296.

645. Liang R, Todd D, Chan TK, et al: Intensive chemotherapy for peripheral T-cell lymphomas. Hematol Oncol 1992;10:155.

646. Siegert W, Agthe A, Griesser H: Treatment of angioimmunoblastic lymphadenopathy (AILD)–type T-cell lymphoma using prednisone with or without the COPBLAM/IMVP-16 regimen. Ann Intern Med 1992;117:364.

647. Greer JP, York JC, Cousar JB, et al: Peripheral T-cell lymphoma: A clinicopathologic study of 42 cases. J Clin Oncol 1984;2:788.

648. Haioun C, Gaulard P, Bourquelot P, et al: Clinical and biological analysis of peripheral T-cell lymphomas: A single-institution study. Leuk Lymphoma 1992;7:449.

649. Vose JM, Peterson C, Bierman PJ, et al: Comparison of high-dose therapy and autologous bone marrow transplantation for T-cell and B-cell non-Hodgkin's lymphomas. Blood 1990;76:424.

650. Gordon BC, Weisenburger DD, Warkentin PI, et al: Peripheral T-cell lymphoma in childhood and adolescence. Cancer 1993;71:257.

651. Rodriguez I, Munsell M, Yazji S, et al: Impact of high-dose chemotherapy on peripheral T-cell lymphomas. J Clin Oncol 2001;19:3766.

652. Philip T, Guglielmi C, Hagenbeek A, et al: Autologous bone marrow transplantation as compared with salvage chemotherapy in relapses of chemotherapy-sensitive non-Hodgkin's lymphoma. N Engl J Med 1995;333:1540–1545.

653. Cheng AL, Su IJ, Chen CC, et al: Use of retinoic acids in the treatment of peripheral T-cell lymphoma: A pilot study. J Clin Oncol 1994;12:1185.

654. Cooper DL, Braverman IM, Sarris AH, et al: Cyclosporine treatment of refractory T-cell lymphomas. Cancer 1993;71:2335.

655. Armitage JO, Coiffier B: Activity of interferon-alpha in relapsed patients with diffuse large B-cell and peripheral T-cell non-Hodgkin's lymphoma. Ann Oncol 2000;11:359.

656. Stein H, Mason DY, Gerdes J, et al: The expression of Hodgkin's disease associated antigen Ki-1 in reactive and neoplastic lymphoid tissue: Evidence that Reed-Stenberg cells and histiocytic malignancies are derived from activated lymphoid cells. Blood 1985;66:848.

657. Agnarsson B, Kaden M: Ki-1 positive large cell lymphoma: A morphologic and immunologic study of 19 cases. Am J Surg Pathol 1988;12:264.

658. Lokich J, Sherburne B: Ki-1 anaplastic large cell lymphoma in the differential diagnosis of unknown primary cancer. Cancer Invest 1998;16:309.

659. Kaudewitz P, Stein H, Dallenbach F, et al: Primary and secondary cutaneous Ki-1+ (CD30+) anaplastic large cell lymphomas. Am J Pathol 1989;135:359.

660. Mason D, Bastard C, Rimokh R, et al: CD30-positive large cell lymphomas (Ki-1 lymphome) are associated with a chromosomal translocation involving 5q35. Br J Haematol 1990;74:161.

661. Greer J, Kinney M, Collins R, et al: Clinical features of 31 patients with Ki-1 anaplastic large cell lymphoma. J Clin Oncol 1991;9:539.

662. DeBruin PC, Baljaards RC, van Heerde P, et al: Differences in clinical behavior and immunophenotype between primary cutaneous and primary nodal anaplastic large cell lymphoma of T-cell or null-cell phenotype. Histopathology 1993;23:127.

663. Shulman LN, Frisard B, Antin JH, et al: Primary Ki-1 anaplastic large cell lymphoma in adults: Clinical characteristics and therapeutic outcome. J Clin Oncol 1993;11:937.

664. Pileri S, Bocchia M, Baroni C, et al: Anaplastic large cell lymphoma (CD30+/Ki-1+): Results of a prospective clinicopathologic study of 69 cases. Br J Haematol 1994;86:513.

665. Romaguera J, Garcia-Foncillas J, Cabanillas F: Sixteen-year experience at M. D. Anderson Cancer Center with primary Ki-1 (CD30) antigen expression and anaplastic morphology in adult patients with diffuse large cell lymphoma. Leuk Lymphoma 1995;20:97.

666. Weisenburger DD, Gordon BG, Vose JM, et al: Occurrence of the t(2;5) (p23;q35) in non-Hodgkin's lymphoma. Blood 1996;87:3860.

667. Shiota M, Nakamura S, Ichinohasama R, et al: Anaplastic large cell lymphomas expressing the novel chimeric protein p80 NPM/ALK: A distinct clinicopathologic entity. Blood 1995;86:1954.

668. Sandlund J, Pui C-H, Roberts W, et al: Clinicopathologic features and treatment outcome of children with large cell lymphoma and the t(2;5) (p23;q35). Blood 1994;84:2467.

669. Pulford K, Lamant L, Morris S, et al: Detection of anaplastic lymphoma kinase (ALK) and nucleolar protein nucleophosmin (SPN)-ALD proteins in normal and neoplastic cells with the monoclonal antibody ALK1. Blood 1997;89:1394.

670. Pittaluga SP, Wolodarska I, Mason D, et al: ALK-1 antibody staining pattern in anaplastic large cell lymphoma (ALCL) and ALCL-Hodgkin's-like. Mod Pathol 1997;10:132A.

671. Delsol G, Lamant L, Mariame B, et al: A new subtype of large B-cell lymphoma expressing the ALK kinase and lacking the 2;5 translocation. Blood 1997;89:1483.

672. Fiorani C, Vinci G, Sacchi S, et al: Primary systemic anaplastic large-cell lymphoma (CD3O+): Advances in biology and current therapeutic approaches. Clin Lymphoma 2001;2:29.

673. Pileri S, Falinin B, Delsol G, et al: Lymphohistiocytic T-cell lymphoma (anaplastic large cell lymphoma CD30+/Kil+) with a high content of reactive histiocytes. Histopathology 1990;16:383.

674. Kinney M, Collins R, Greer J, et al: A small-cell-predominant variant of primary Ki-1 (CD30)+ T-cell lymphoma. Am J Surg Pathol 1993;17:859.

675. Pileri S, Bocchia M, Baroni C, et al: Anaplastic large cell lymphoma (CD30+/Ki-1+): Results of a prospective clinicopathologic study of 69 cases. Br J Haematol 1994;86:513.

676. Zinzani P, Bendandi M, Martelli M, et al: Anaplastic large cell lymphoma (Ki-1/CD30+): Clinical and prognostic evaluation of 90 adult patients. J Clin Oncol 1996;14:955.

677. Benharroch D, Meguerian-Bedoyan Z, Lamant L, et al: ALK-positive lymphoma: A single disease with a broad spectrum of morphology. Blood 1998;91:2076.

678. Skinnider BF, Connors JM, Sutcliffe SB, et al: Anaplastic large cell lymphoma: A clinicopathologic analysis. Hematol Oncol 1999;17:137.

679. Kadin ME: The spectrum of Ki-1+ cutaneous lymphoma. Curr Probl Dermatol 1990;19:132.

680. Beylot-Barry M, Groppi A, Vergier B, et al: Characterization of t(2:5) reciprocal transcripts and genomic breakpoints in CD30+ cutaneous lymphoproliferations. Blood 1998;91:4668.

681. Tilly H, Gaulard P, Lepage E, et al: Primary anaplastic large cell lymphoma in adults: Clinical presentation, immunophenotype, and outcome. Blood 1997;90:3727.

682. Zinzani PL, Martelli M, Magagnoli M, et al: Anaplastic large cell lymphoma Hodgkin's-like: A randomized trial of ABVD versus MACOP-B with and without radiation therapy. Blood 1998;92:790.

683. Zinzani PL, Pileri S, Bendandi M, et al: Clinical implications of serum levels of soluble CD30 in 70 adult anaplastic large-cell lymphoma patients. J Clin Oncol 1998;16:1532.

684. Freeman C, Berg JW, Culter SJ: Occurrence and prognosis of extranodal lymphomas. Cancer 1972;29:252.

685. d'Amore F, Christensen BE, Brincker H, et al: Clinicopathological features and prognostic factors in extranodal non-Hodgkin's lymphomas. Danish Lyfo Study Group. Eur J Cancer 1991;27:1201.

686. Sutcliffe CB, Gospodarowicz MK, Keating A, et al: Localized extranodal lymphomas. Hematol Oncol 1992;10:198.

687. Lewin KJ, Ranchod M, Dorfman RF: Lymphomas of the gastrointestinal tract: A study of 117 cases presenting with gastrointestinal disease. Cancer 1978;42:693.

688. Herrmann R, Panahon AM, Barcos MP, et al: Gastrointestinal involvement in non-Hodgkin's lymphoma. Cancer 1980;46:215.

689. Skudder PA, Schwartz SI: Primary lymphoma of the parainstestinal tract. Surg Gynecol Obstet 1985;160:5.

690. Khojasteh A, Haghshenass M, Haghighs P: Immunoproliferative small intestinal disease: A "third world" lesion. N Engl J Med 1983;308:1401.

691. Al-Mondhiry H: Primary lymphomas of the small intestine: East-West contrast. Am J Hematol 1986;22:89.

692. Nicoloff DM, Haynes LB, Wengensteen OM: Primary lymphosar-coma of the gastrointestinal tract. Surg Gynecol Obstet 1963;117:433.

693. Loehr WJ, Miyahead Z, Zahn FD, et al: Primary lymphoma of the gastrointestinal tract: A review of 100 cases. Ann Surg 1969;170:232.

694. Naque MS, Burrows L, Kark AE: Lymphoma of the gastrointestinal tract: Prognostic guides based on 162 cases. Ann Surg 1969;170:221.

695. Kahn LB, Selzer G, Kascular ROC: Primary gastrointestinal lymphoma: A clinicopathologic study of 57 cases. Am J Digest Dis 1972;17:219.

696. Brooks JJ, Enterline HT: Primary gastric lymphomas: A clinicopathology study of 58 cases with long-term follow-up and literature review. Cancer 1983;51:701.

697. Dragosics B, Bauer P, Radaszkiewicz T: Primary gastrointestinal non-Hodgkin's lymphomas: A retrospective clinicopathologic study of 150 cases. Cancer 1985;55:1060.

698. Taal BG, Burgers JMV, van Heerde P, et al: The clinical spectrum and treatment of primary non-Hodgkin's lymphoma of the stomach. Ann Oncol 1993;4:839.

699. Rosen CB, van Heerden JA, Martin JK, et al: Is an aggressive surgical approach to the patient with gastric lymphoma warranted? Ann Surg 1987;205:634.

700. Hockey MS, Powell J, Crocker J, et al: Primary gastric lymphoma. Br J Surg 1987;74:483.

701. Papadimitriou G, Papacharalampous N, Kittas C: Primary gastrointestinal malignant lymphomas. Cancer 1985;55:870.

702. Ravaioli A, Amadori M, Faedi M, et al: Primary gastric lymphoma: A review of 45 cases. Eur J Cancer Clin Oncol 1986;22:1461.

703. Weingrad DN, Decosse JJ, Sherlock P, et al: Primary gastrointestinal lymphoma: A 30 year review. Cancer 1982;48:1258.

704. Shepherd FA, Evans WK, Kutas G, et al: Chemotherapy following surgery for stages IE and IIE non-Hodgkin's lymphoma of the gastrointestinal tract. J Clin Oncol 1988;6:253.

705. Bellesi G, Alterini A, Messori A, et al: Combined surgery and chemotherapy for the treatment of primary gastrointestinal intermediate or high grade non-Hodgkin's lymphomas. Br J Cancer 1989;60:244.

706. Tondini C, Giardini R, Bozzetti F, et al: Combined modality therapy for primary gastrointestinal non-Hodgkin's lymphoma: The Milan Cancer Institute experience. Ann Oncol 1993;4:831.

707. Gospodarowicz MK, Sutcliffe SB, Clark RM, et al: Outcome analysis of localised gastrointestinal lymphoma treated with surgery and postoperative irradiation. Int J Radiat Oncol Biol Phys 1990;19:1351.

708. Gospodarowicz M, Bush R, Brown T, et al: Curability of gastrointestinal lymphoma with combined surgery and radiation. Int J Radiat Oncol Biol Phys 1983;9:3.

709. Maor MH, Maddux B, Osborne BM, et al: Stages IE and IIE non-Hodgkin's lymphomas of the stomach: Comparison of treatment modalities. Cancer 1984;54:2330.

710. Shiu MH, Nisce LZ, Pinna A, et al: Recent results of multimodal therapy of gastric lymphoma. Cancer 1986;58:1389.

711. Coiffier B, Salles G: Does surgery belong to medical history for gastric lymphoma? Ann Oncol 1997;8:419–421.

712. Roggero E, Zucca E, Pinotti G, et al: Eradication of Helicobacter pylori infection in primary low-grade gastric lymphoma of mucosa-associated lymphoid tissue. Ann Intern Med 1995;122:767.

713. Montabalan C, Manzanal A, Boixeda D et al: Helicobacter Pylori eradication for the treatment of low-grade gastric MALT lymphoma: Follow-up together with sequential molecular studies. Ann Oncol 1997;8(Suppl 2):37–40.

714. Ruskone-Fourmestraux A, Lavergne A, Aegerter PH, et al: Predictive factors for regression of gastric MALT lypmhoma after anti–Helicobater Pylori treatment. Gut 2001;48:297–303.

715. Zucca E, Roggero E, Delchier JC, et al: Interim evaluation of gastric MALT lymphoma response to antibiotics in the ongoing LY03 randomised cooperative trial of observation versus chlorambucil after anti-Helicobacter therapy. Proc Am Soc Clin Oncol 2000;19:5a.

716. Neubauer A, Thiede C, Morgner A, et al: Cure of Helicobacter pylori infection and duration of remission of low-grade gastric mucosa-associated lymphoid tissue lymphoma. J Natl Cancer Inst 1997;89:1350–1355.

717. Nakamura S, Matsumoto T, Suekane H, et al: Predictive value of endoscopic ultrasonography for regression of gastric low grade and high grade MALT lymphomas after cure by eradication of Helicobacter pylori. Gut 2001;48:454–460.

718. Savio A, Franzin G, Wotherspoon AC, et al: Diagnosis and post-treatment follow-up of Helicobacter pylori–positive gastric lymphoma of mucosa-associated lymphoma tissue: Histology, polymerase chain reaction, or both? Blood 1996;87:1255–1260.

719. Bertoni F, Conconi A, Capella C, et al: Molecular follow-up in gastric MALT lymphomas: Early analysis from the LY-03 cooperative trial. Blood 2002;99:2541–2544.

720. Isaacson PG, Diss TC, Wotherspoon AC, et al: Long-term follow-up of gastric MALT lymphoma treated by eradication of H. pylori with antibodies. Gastroenterology 1999;117:750–751.

721. Liu H, Ruskon-Fourmestraux A, Lavergne-Slove A, et al: Resistance of t(11;18) positive gastric mucosa-associated lymphoid tissue lymphoma to Helicobacter pylori eradication therapy. Lancet 2001;357:39–40.

722. Hammel P, Haioun C, Chaumette MT, et al: Efficacy of single-agent chemotherapy in low-grade B-cell mucosa-associated lymphoid tissue lymphoma with prominent gastric expression. J Clin Oncol 1995;13:2524–2529.

723. Pinotti G, Zucca E, Roggero E, et al: Clinical features, treatment, and outcome in a series of 93 patients with low-grade gastric MALT lymphoma. Leuk Lymphoma 1997;26:527–537.

724. Tsang RW, Gospodarowicz MK, Pintilie M, et al: Stage I and II MALT lymphoma: Results of treatment with radiotherapy. Int J Radiat Oncol Biol Phys 2001;50:1258–1264.

725. Seymour JF, Anderson RP, Bhathal PS: Regression of gastric lymphoma with therapy for Helicobacter Pylori infections. Ann Intern Med 1997;127:247.

726. Roggero E, Copie-Bergman C, Traullé C, et al: Regression of high-grade B-cell gastric lymphoma after eradication of Helicobacter Pylori infection. Ann Oncol 1999;10(Suppl 3):67.

727. Boot H, de Jong D, van Heerde P, Taal B: Role of Helicobater Pylori eradication in high-grade MALT lymphoma. Lancet 1995;346:448.

728. Morgner A, Miehlke S, Fischbach W, et al: Complete remission of primary high-grade B-cell gastric lymphoma after cure of Helicobacter pylori infection. J Clin Oncol. 2001;19:2041–2048.

729. Salles G, Herbrecht R, Tilly H, et al: Aggressive primary gastrointestinal lymphomas: Review of 91 patients treated with the LNH-83 regimen. A study of the GELA. Am J Med 1991;90:77–84.

730. Domizio P, Owen RA, Shepherd NA, et al: Primary lymphoma of the small intestine: A clinicopathologic study of 119 cases. Am J Surg Pathol 1993;17:429.

731. Morton JE, Leyland MJ, Vaughan Hudson G, et al: Primary gastrointestinal non-Hodgkin's lymphoma: A review of 175 British National Lymphoma Investigation cases. Br J Cancer 1993;67:776.

732. D'Amore F, Brincker M, Gronbaeck K, et al: Non-Hodgkin's lymphoma of the gastrointestinal tract: A population based analysis of incidence, geographic distribution, clinicopathological presentation features, and prognosis. J Clin Oncol 1994;12:1673.

733. Al-Bahrani Z, Al-Mohindry H, Bakir F: Clinical and pathological subtypes of primary intestinal lymphoma: Experience with 132 patients over a 14-year period. Cancer 1983;52:1666.

734. Salem P, Nassas VH, Shahid MJ, et al: Mediterranean abdominal lymphoma or immunoproliferative small intestinal disease. Part I. Clinical aspects. Cancer 1977;40:2941.

735. Willemze R, Kerl H, Sterry W, et al: EORTC classification for primary cutaneous lymphomas: A proposal from the cutaneous lymphoma study group of the European Organization for Research and Treatment of Cancer. Blood 1997;90:354–371.

736. Leonard JP, Link BK: Immunotherapy of non-Hodgkin's lymphoma with hLL2 (epratuzumab, an anti-CD22 monoclonal antibody) and Hu1D10 (apolizumab). Semin Oncol 2002;29(1 Suppl 2):81–86.

737. Pandolfino TL, Siegel RS, Kuzel TM, et al: Primary cutaneous B-cell lymphoma: Review and current concepts. J Clin Oncol 2000;18:2152–2168.

738. Wood GS, Burke JS, Horning S, et al: The immunologic and clinicopathologic heterogeneity of cutaneous lymphomas other than mycosis fungoides. Blood 1983;62:464.

739. Sarris AH, Braunschweig I, Medeiros LJ, et al: Primary cutaneous non-Hodgkin's lymphoma of Ann Arbor stage I: Preferential cutaneous relapses but high cure rate with doxorubicin-based therapy. J Clin Oncol 2001;19:398–405.

740. Paul T, Radny P, Krober SM, et al: Intralesional rituximab for cutaneous B-cell lymphoma. Br J Dermatol 2001;144:1239–1243.

741. Heinzerling LM, Urbanek M, Funk JO, et al: Reduction of tumor burden and stabilization of disease by systemic therapy with anti-CD20 antibody (rituximab) in patients with primary cutaneous B-cell lymphoma. Cancer 2000;89:1835–1844.

742. Roggero E, Zucca E, Mainetti C, et al: Eradication of Borrelia burgdorferi infection in primary marginal zone B-cell lymphoma of the skin. Human Pathol 2000;31:263–268.

743. Grange F, Bekkenk MW, Wechsler J, et al: Prognostic factors in primary cutaneous large B-cell lymphomas: A European multicenter study. J Clin Oncol 2001;19:3602–3610.

744. Statistical Report: Primary Brain Tumors in the United States, 1992–1997. Chicago, Central Brain Tumor Registry of the United States, 2002.

745. Eby NL, Grufferman S, Flannelly CM, et al: Increasing incidence of primary brain lymphoma in the U.S. Cancer 1988;62:2461–2465.

746. Bailey P: Intracranial sarcomatous tumours of leptomeningeal origin. Arch Surg 1929;18:1359.

747. Weller M: Glucocorticoid treatment of primary CNS lymphoma. J Neurol Oncol 1999;43:237–239.

748. Nelson DF, Martz KL, Bonner H, et al: Non-Hodgkin's lymphoma of the brain: Can high dose, large volume radiation therapy improve survival? Report on a prospective trial by the Radiation Therapy Oncology Group (RTOG): RTOG 8315. Int J Radiat Oncol Biol Phys 1992;23:9–17.

749. Abrey LE, Yahalom J, DeAngelis LM: Relapse and late neurotoxicity in primary central nervous system lymphoma (PCNSL). Neurology 1997;48:A18.

750. Cho B, Hochberg F, Loefflet J, et al: Methotrexate reinduction in patients with relapsed primary central nervous system lymphoma. Neurooncol 2001;3:356.

751. Ng S, Rosenthal MA, Ashley D, et al: High-dose methotrexate for primary CNS lymphomas in the elderly. Neuro-oncol 2000;2:40–44.

752. Gabbai AA, Hochberg FH, Linggood RM, et al: High-dose methotrexate for non-AIDS primary central nervous system lymphoma: Report of 13 cases. J Neurosurg 1989;70:190–194.

753. Glass J, Gruber ML, Cher L, et al: Preirradiation methotrexate chemotherapy of primary central nervous system lymphoma: Long-term outcome. J Neurosurg 1994;81:188–195.

754. O'Brien P, Roos D, Pratt G, et al: Phase II multicenter study of brief single-agent methotrexate followed by irradiation in primary CNS lymphoma. J Clin Oncol 2000;18:519–526.

755. DeAngelis LM, Seiferheld W, Schold SC, et al: Combination chemotherapy and radiotherapy for primary central nervous system lymphoma: Radiation Therapy Oncology Group Study 93-10. J Clin Oncol 2002;20:4643–4648.

756. Batchelor T, Carson K, O'Neill A, et al: Treatment of primary CNS lymphoma with methotrexate and deferred radiotherapy: A report of NABTT 96-07. J Clin Oncol 2003;21:1044–1049.

757. Fine HA: Primary central nervous system lymphoma: Time to ask the question. J Clin Oncol 2002;20:4615–4617.

758. Kim JH, Fayos JV: Primary orbital lymphoma: A radiotherapeutic experience. Int J Radiat Oncol Biol Phys 1976;1:1099.

759. Bessell EM, Henk JM, Wright JE, et al: Orbital and conjunctival lymphoma treatment and prognosis. Radiother Oncol 1988;13:237.

760. Letschert JG, Gonzalez GD, Oskam J, et al: Results of radiotherapy in patients with stage I orbital non-Hodgkin's lymphoma. Radiother Oncol 1991;22:36.

761. Jereb B, Lee H, Jakobiec FA, et al: Radiation therapy of conjunctival and orbital lymphoid tumors. Int J Radiat Oncol Biol Phys 1984;10:1013.

762. Reddy EK, Bhatia P, Evans RG: Primary orbital lymphomas. Int J Radiat Oncol Biol Phys 1988;15:1239.

763. Friedman M, Kim TH, Panahon AM: Spinal cord compression in malignant lymphoma: Treatment and results. Cancer 1976;37:1485.

764. Herman TS, Hammond N, Jones SE, et al: Involvement of the central nervous system by non-Hodgkin's lymphoma: The Southwest Oncology Group experience. Cancer 1979;43:390.

765. Wang CC: Primary malignant lymphoma of the oral cavity and paranasal sinuses. Radiology 1971;100:151.

766. Banfi A, Bonadonna G, Ricci SB, et al: Malignant lymphoma of Waldeyer's ring: Natural history and survival after radiotherapy. Br Med J 1972;3:140.

767. Hoppe RT, Burke JS, Glatstein E, et al: Non Hodgkin's lymphoma: Involvement of Waldeyer's ring. Cancer 1978;42:1096.

768. Liang R, Ng RP, Tod D, et al: Management of stage I-II diffuse aggressive non-Hodgkin's lymphoma of the Waldeyer's ring: Combined modality therapy versus radiotherapy alone. Hematol Oncol 1978;5:223.

769. Li YX, Coucke PA, Li JY, et al: Primary non-Hodgkin's lymphoma of the nasal cavity: Prognostic significance of paranasal extension and the role of radiotherapy and chemotherapy. Cancer 1998;83:449.

770. Hausdorff J, Davis E, Long G, et al: Non-Hodgkin's lymphoma of the paranasal sinuses: Clinical and pathological features, and response to combined-modality therapy. Cancer Sci Am 1997;3:303.

771. Abbondanzo SL, Wenig BM: Non-Hodgkin's lymphoma of the sinonasal tract: A clinicopathologic and immunophenotypic study of 120 cases. Cancer 1995;75:1281.

772. Frierson HF Jr, Innes DJ Jr, Mills SE, et al: Immunophenotypic analysis of sinonasal non-Hodgkin's lymphomas. Hum Pathol 1989;20:636.

773. Campo E, Cardesa A, Alos L, et al: Non-Hodgkin's lymphomas of nasal cavity and paranasal sinuses: An immunohistochemical study. Am J Clin Pathol 1991;96:184.

774. Itami J, Itam M, Mikata A, et al: Non-Hodgkin's lymphoma confined to the nasal cavity: Its relationship to the polymorphic reticulosis and results of radiation therapy. Int J Radiat Oncol Biol Phys 1991;20:797.

775. Blair TJ, Evans RG, Buskirk SJ, et al: Radiotherapeutic management of primary thyroid lymphoma. Int J Radiat Oncol Biol Phys 1985;11:365.

776. Hawkins RE, Zhu D, Ovecka M, et al: Idiotype vaccination against human B-cell lymphoma: Rescue of variable region gene sequences from biopsy material for assembly as single-chain F, personal vaccines. Blood 1994;83:3279.

777. Hyjek E, Isaacson PG: Primary B cell lymphoma of the thyroid and its relationship to Hashimoto's thyroiditis. Hum Pathol 1988;19:1315.

778. Doria R, Jekel JF, Cooper DL: Thyroid lymphoma: The case for combined modality therapy. Cancer 1994;73:200.

779. Tsang RW, Gospodarowicz MK, Sutcliffe SB: Non-Hodgkin's lymphoma of the thyroid gland: Prognostic factors and treatment outcome. The Princess Margaret Lymphoma Group. Int J Radiat Oncol Biol Phys 1993;27:599.

780. Leedman PJ, Sheridan WP, Downey WF, et al: Combination chemotherapy as single modality therapy for stage IE and IIE thyroid lymphoma. Med J Aust 1990;152:40.

781. Ferry JA, Harris NL, Young RH, et al: Malignant lymphoma of the testis, epididymis, and spermatic cord: A clinicopathologic study of 69 cases with immunophenotypic analysis. Am J Surg Pathol 1994;18:376.

782. Moller MB, d'Amore F, Christensen BE: Testicular lymphoma: A population-based study of incidence, clinicopathological correlations, and prognosis. The Danish Lymphoma Study Group. Eur J Cancer 1994;30A:1760.

783. Nonomura N, Aozasa K, Ueda T, et al: Malignant lymphoma of the testis: Histologic and immunohistological study of 28 cases. J Urol 1989;141:368.

784. Martenson JA Jr, Buskirk SJ, Ilstrup DM, et al: Patterns of failure in primary testicular non-Hodgkin's lymphoma. J Clin Oncol 1988;6:297.

785. Connors JM, Klimo P, Voss N, et al: Testicular lymphoma: improved outcome with early brief chemotherapy. J Clin Oncol 1988;6:776.

786. Touroutoglou N, Dimopoulos MA, Younes A, et al: Testicular lymphoma: Late relapses and poor outcome despite doxorubicin-based therapy. J Clin Oncol 1995;13:1361.

787. Moore RD, Kessler H, Richman DD, et al: Non-Hodgkin's lymphoma in patients with advanced HIV infection treated with zidovudine. JAMA 1991;265:2208.

788. Ziegler JL, Drew WL, Miner RL, et al: Outbreak of Burkitt's-like lymphoma in homosexual men. Lancet 1982;2:631.

789. Pluda JM, Yarchoan R, Jaffe ES, et al: Development of non-Hodgkin's lymphoma in a cohort of patients with severe human immunodeficient virus (HIV) infection on long-term antiviral therapy. Ann Intern Med 1990;113:276.

790. Beral V, Peterman T, Berkelman R, Jaffe H: AIDS-associated non-Hodgkin's lymphoma. Lancet 1991;337:805–809.

791. International Collaboration on HIV and Cancer: Highly active antiretroviral therapy and incidence of cancer in human immunodeficiency virus infected adults. J Natl Cancer Inst 2000;92:1823–1830.

792. Schnittman SM, Lane HC, Higgins SE, et al: Direct polyclonal activation of human B lymphocytes by the AIDS virus. Science 1896;233:1084–1086.

793. Nador RG, Cesarman E, Chadburn A, et al: Primary effusion lymphoma: A distinct clinicopathologic entity associated with the Kaposi's sarcoma–associated herpes virus. Blood 1996;88:645–656.

794. Levine AM, Seneviratne L, Espina BM, et al: Evolving characteristics of AIDS related lymphoma. Blood 2000;96:4084–4090.

795. Sparano JA, Wiernik PH, Hu X, et al: Pilot trial of effusional cyclophosphamide, doxorubicin, and octoposide plus didanosine and filgrastim in patients with HIV-associated non-Hodgkin's lymphoma. J Clin Oncol 1996;14:3026–3035.

796. Little R, Pearson D, Steinberg S, et al: Dose-adjusted EPOCH chemotherqapy in previously untreated HIV-associated non-Hodgkin's lymphoma. Proc Am Soc Clin Oncol 1999;18:10a.

797. Ratner L, Lee J, Tang S, et al: Chemotherapy for HIV-associated non-Hodgkin's lymphoma in combination with highly active antiretroviral therapy. J Clin Oncol 2001;19:2171–2178.

798. Levin AM, personal communication.

799. Opelz G, Henderson R: Incidence of non-Hodgkin's lymphoma in kidney and heart transplant recepients. Lancet 1993;342:1514–1516.

800. Boubenider S, Heisse C, Groupy C, et al: Incidence and consequences of post-transplantation lymphoproliferation disorders. J Nephrol 1997;10:136–145.

801. Davis CL, Harrison K, McVicar JP, et al: Antiviral prophylaxis and the Epstein-Barr virus–related post-transplant lymphoproliferative disorder. Clin Transplant 1995;9:53–59.

802. Darenkov IA, Marcarelli M, Basadonna GP, et al: Reduced incidence of Epstein-Barr virus associated post-transplant lymphoproliferative disorder using preemptive antiviral therapy. Transplantation 1997;64:848–852.

803. Nalesnik MA, Makowla L, Starlz TE: The diagnosis and treatment of post-transplant lymphoproliferative disorders. Curr Probl Surg 1988;25:367–472.

804. Gross TG, Hinrichs S, Winner J, et al: Treatment of post-transplant lymphoproliferative disease (PTLD) following solid organ transplantation with low-dose chemotherapy. Ann Oncol 1998;9:339–340.

805. Mipied N, Vasseur B, Parquet N, et al: Humanised anti-CD20 monoclonal antibody (rituximab) in post-transplant B-lymphoproliferative disorder: A retrospective analysis on 32 patients. Ann Oncol 2000;2 (Suppl 1):113–116.

806. Heslop HE, Brenner M, Rooney CM: Donor T cells to treat EBV-associated lymphoma. N Engl J Med 1994;331:679–680.

807. Rooney CM, Smith C, Ng CY, et al: Use of gene-modified virus-specific T lymphocytes to control Epstein-Barr virus–related lymphoproliferation. Lancet 1995;345:9–13.

808. Segal GH, Clough JD, Tubbs RR: Autoimmune and iatrogenic causes of lymphadenopathy. Semin Oncol 1993;20:611.

809. Frayha RA, Nasr FW, Mufarrij AA: Mixed connective tissue disease, Sjögren's syndrome, and abdominal pseudolymphoma. Br J Rheumatol 1985;24:70.

810. Fox RA, Rosahn PB: The lymph node in disseminated lupus erythematosus. Am J Pathol 1943;19:73.

811. Motulsky AG, Weinberg S, Saphir O, et al: Lymph nodes in rheumatoid arthritis. Arch Intern Med 1952;90:660.

812. Kondratowicz GM, Symmons DPM, Bacon PA, et al: Rheumatoid lymphadenopathy: A morphological and immunohistochemical study. J Clin Pathol 1990;143:106.

813. Castleman B, Iverson L, Menendex V: Localized mediastinal lymph node hyperplasia resembling thymoma. Cancer 1956;9:822.

814. Peterson BA, Frizzera G: Multicentric Castleman's disease. Semin Oncol 1993;20:636.

815. Oksenhendler B, Duarte M, Soulier J, et al: Multicentre Castleman's disease in HIV infection: A clinical and pathological study of 20 patients. AIDS 1996;10:61.

816. Case records of the Massachusetts General Hospital. Case 10-1987: A 59-year-old woman with progressive polyneuropathy and monoclonal gammopathy. N Engl J Med 1987;316:606.

817. Weisenburger DD, Nathwani BN, Winberg CD, et al: Multicentric angiofollicular lymph node hyperplasia. Hum Pathol 1985;16:162.

818. Weisenburger DD, DeGown RL, Gibson DP, et al: Remission of giant lymph node hyperplasia with anemia after radiotherapy. Cancer 1979;44:457.

819. Andres E, Maloisel F: Interferon-α as first-line therapy for treatment of multicentre Castleman's disease. Ann Oncol 2000;11:1613.

820. Beck JT, Hsu S-M, Wijdenes J, et al: Brief report: Alleviation of systemic manifestations of Castleman's disease by monoclonal anti-interleukin-6 antibody. N Engl J Med 1994;330:602–605.

821. Marcelin A-G, Aaron L, Mateus C, et al: Rituximab therapy for HIV-associated Castleman disease. Blood 2003;102:2786–2788.

822. Advani R, Warnke R, Rosenberg S: Treatment of multicentre Castleman's disease complicated by the development of non-Hodgkin's lymphoma with high-dose chemotherapy and autologous peripheral stem-cell support. Ann Oncol 1999;10:1207.

823. Jacobs P, Wood L, Jogessar V: Refractory Castleman's Disease. Hematology 1998;3:299.

824. Rosai J, Dorfman RF: Sinus histiocytosis with massive lymphadenopathy: A newly recognized benign clinicopathologic entity. Arch Pathol 1969;87:63.

825. Foucar E, Rosai J, Dorfman R: Sinus histiocytosis with massive lymphadenopathy (Rosai-Dorfman disease): Review of the entity. Semin Diagn Pathol 1990;7:19.

826. Willemze R, Meyer CJLM, van Vloten WA, et al: The clinical and histological spectrum of lymphomatoid papulosis. Br J Dermatol 1982;107:131.

827. Sarris AH, Luthra R, Papadimitracopoulou V, et al: Amplification of genomic DNA demonstrates the presence of the t(2;5) (p23;q35) in anaplastic large cell lymphoma, but not in other non-Hodgkin's lymphomas, Hodgkin's disease, or lymphomatoid papulosis. Blood 1996;88:1771.

828. Kinlen IJ: Immunosuppressive therapy and cancer. Cancer Surv 1982;1:565.

829. Kinlen IJ: Incidence of cancer in rheumatoid arthritis and other disorders after immunosuppressive treatment. Am J Med 1985;78:44.

830. Kinlen L: Immunosuppressive therapy and acquired immunological disorders. Cancer Res 1992;52:54s.

831. Ross RK, Dworsky RL, et al: Non-Hodgkin's lymphomas in never married men in Los Angeles. Br J Cancer 1985;52:785.

832. Centers for Disease Control: Revision of the case definition of acquired immunodeficiency syndrome for national reporting in the United States. Ann Intern Med 1985;103:402.

833. Morrell D, Cromartie E, et al: Mortality and cancer in 263 patients with ataxia telangiectasia. J Natl Cancer Inst 1968;77:89.

834. Cunningham-Rundles C, Siegal FP, et al: Incidence of cancer in 98 patients with common variable immunodeficiency. J Clin Immunol 1987;7:294.

835. Levine AM, Shibata D, et al: Epidemiological and biological study of acquired immunodeficiency syndrome–related lymphoma in the county of Los Angeles: Preliminary results. Cancer Res 1992;52:5482s.

836. Cohen JI: Epstein-Barr virus lymphoproliferative disease associated with acquired immunodeficiency. Medicine 1991;70:137.

837. Leblond V, Sutton L, Dorent R, et al: Lymphoproliferative disorders after organ transplantation: A report of 24 cases observed in a single center. J Clin Oncol 1995;13:961.

838. Bhatia S, Ramsay NKC, Steinbuch M, et al: Malignant neoplasms following bone marrow transplantation. Blood 1996;87:3633.

839. Deeg HJ, Socie G: Malignancies after hematopoietic stem cell transplantation: Many questions, some answers. Blood 1998;91:1833.

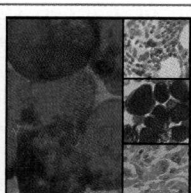

113

CUTANEOUS T-CELL LYMPHOMA AND CUTANEOUS B-CELL LYMPHOMA

Thomas M. Habermann

Mark R. Pittelkow

SUMMARY OF KEY POINTS

INCIDENCE
- There are 0.9 of 100,000 cases of cutaneous T-cell lymphoma (CTCL) in Rochester, Minnesota, and 0.4 in 100,000 cases per year in the Surveillance, Epidemiology, and End Results (SEER) program.
- Cutaneous B-cell non-Hodgkin's lymphoma represents about 10% of all primary cutaneous lymphomas. The average age at presentation is 50 to 60 years, but children and adolescents have been reported.

DIFFERENTIAL DIAGNOSIS
- Premalignant disorders that potentially evolve into CTCL are parapsoriasis, lymphomatoid papulosis, follicular mucinosis, pre–Sézary syndrome, atypical dermatitis, and dermal reticulosis.
- Histologic and clinical variants of CTCL include granulomatous, pustular, bullous, verrucous, hyperkeratotic, hypopigmented, papulomatous, purpuric, and angiocentric CTCL.

- CTCL should further be distinguished from adult T-cell leukemia/lymphoma, Ki-1+ anaplastic large cell lymphoma, peripheral T-cell non-Hodgkin's lymphoma, cutaneous B-cell lymphomas, T-cell chronic lymphocytic leukemia, leukemia cutis, cutaneous Hodgkin's disease, pseudolymphomas, cutaneous lymphoid hyperplasias, lymphomatoid contact reactions, and insect bites.

STAGING EVALUATION
- The initial evaluation should include complete history and physical examination, complete blood count (CBC), and differential to determine the presence of disease in the peripheral blood, chemistry studies, and chest radiography.
- The physical examination should describe the percentage of body surface area involved.
- Skin biopsy should be obtained for routine histology, immunohistochemistry analysis, and T-cell receptor

gene rearrangement studies at the time of the initial diagnosis.

PRIMARY THERAPY
- This is an indolent, extra-nodal lymphoma.
- Localized limited stage disease is potentially curable. All other presentations are incurable.
- Current initial therapies are tailored to extent, burden, and type of disease present and include topical corticosteroids, topical chemotherapy (nitrogen mustard or BCNU), phototherapy, psoralen ultraviolet A (PUVA), electron beam, photon irradiation, extracorporeal photochemotherapy, and chemotherapy.

SELECTIVE SECOND- AND THIRD-LINE THERAPIES
- Patients may respond to the same therapeutic modality on more than one occasion.
- Multiple other palliative therapeutic options are available as well.

INTRODUCTION

Primary cutaneous lymphomas represent the second most common extranodal site for non-Hodgkin's lymphoma.[1] Cutaneous T-cell lymphoma (CTCL) is a heterogeneous group of non-Hodgkin's lymphomas that represent about 80% of all primary cutaneous lymphomas. These disorders of malignant lymphocytes have a proclivity for the skin and epidermis. The diagnosis of CTCL is based on clinicopathologic criteria. This class of malignant lymphomas includes mycosis fungoides and Sézary syndrome. CTCL forms a group of clinically diverse disorders. In addition to CTCL, other malignant lymphoproliferative diseases that involve the skin include Ki-1+ anaplastic large cell lymphoma, peripheral T-cell lymphoma, cutaneous B-cell lymphoma, adult T-cell leukemia/lymphoma, T-cell chronic lymphoid leukemia (T-cell CLL), and cutaneous Hodgkin's disease (Table 113-1). However, CTCL can be separated from these other malignancies by

histologic, immunologic, and molecular features. This chapter reviews the clinicopathologic features of, and therapy for, CTCL, including mycosis fungoides and Sézary syndrome, as well as their variants and related disorders. Cutaneous B-cell lymphomas, localized or generalized, are much less common.

EPIDEMIOLOGY

The incidence of mycosis fungoides (MF) and Sézary syndrome in the well-defined population of Rochester, Minnesota, is 0.9 per 100,000 residents.[1] Epidemiologic data from the SEER program showed an increase in incidence of CTCL from 0.2 case per 100,000 in 1973 to 0.4 case per 100,000 in 1984.[2] From 1983 to 1994, there was no evidence of an increased incidence.[3] The incidence rate from 1973 to 1992 was 0.36 per 100,000 person years.[4] The incidence of CTCL increases with age. Most cases of CTCL are in adults. The average age

TABLE 113-1

Cutaneous T-Cell Lymphoma, Variants, Premalignant Dermatoses, Related Disorders, and Benign Lymphoid Reactions

Mycosis fungoides
Sézary syndrome
Variants
   Granulomatous slack skin disorder
   Pagetoid reticulosis (Woringer-Kolopp disease)
Premalignant disorders
   Large plaque (en plaque) parapsoriasis
   Poikiloderma atrophicans vasculare
   Lymphomatoid papulosis
   Follicular mucinosis
   Mucha-Habermann disease
Malignant lymphoma/leukemia with skin involvement
   Adult T-cell leukemia/lymphoma
   Ki-1+ anaplastic large cell lymphoma
   Peripheral T-cell lymphoma
   B-cell lymphoma
   Leukemia cutis
   T-cell chronic lymphoid leukemia
   Hodgkin's disease
Benign lymphocytic-lymphomatoid reactions with clinical or histologic reactions mimicking cutaneous T-cell lymphoma
   Lymphomatoid contact dermatitis
   Arthropod bites
   Drug eruptions
   Chronic actinic dermatitis, actinic reticuloid
   Lichenoid eruption
   Poikilodermatous disease
   Erythrodermas

at presentation is 50 to 60 years.[4-8] Cases of mycosis fungoides in children and adolescents have been reported, however.[9] CTCL is more likely to develop in males. Black populations are at higher risk of developing CTCL.[2] MF is the most common CTCL, representing 40% to 82% of new cases in two series.[10-11]

Although environmental factors have been implicated in the pathogenesis of CTCL, two case-controlled studies have not supported the concept that industrial or related exposures cause the disease.[12,13] Furthermore no significant differences were documented in cutaneous allergy to plants, metals, and cosmetics or in reactions to medications, foods, or insect bites between cases of mycosis fungoides and controls, indicating that in most cases prolonged exposure to contact allergens is not related to the development of CTCL.[13] In selected cases, however, patients with atopy, contact sensitivity, chronic dermatitis, or immunodeficiency may develop CTCL.[14-16] The majority of patients are human T-cell lymphotrophic virus type 1 (HTLV-1)-negative. CTCL has been documented after B-cell lymphoma, Hodgkin's lymphoma, and renal transplantation.[17-19] CTCL has been reported in the acquired immunodeficiency syndrome.[20-21]

CLASSIFICATION

Previous lymphoma classifications have not adequately characterized the cutaneous lymphomas. The most recent lymphoma classification is the World Health Organization classification (see Table 113-2).[22] The European Organiza-

tion for Research and Treatment of Cancer (EORTC) proposed a classification for these disorders that is divided into primary B-cell and T-cell lymphomas (see Table 113-2).[23] The T-cell entities described in both of the classifications are similar. CD30+ large cell lymphomas, primary cutaneous anaplastic large cell lymphomas in the WHO classification are characterized as cutaneous T-cell lymphomas CD30+ in the EORTC classification. The EORTC classification may also include CD30+ nonanaplastic large cell lymphoma that would be called peripheral T-cell lymphoma, unspecified in the WHO classification. Large cell CD30 negative cutaneous T-cell lymphoma and CTCL with pleomorphic small and medium cell types are characterized as aggressive in the EORTC classification and are classified as peripheral T-cell lymphomas, unspecified, in the WHO classification. Subcutaneous panniculitis-like T-cell lymphoma is a distinct entity in the WHO classification, but a provisional diagnosis in the EORTC classification. The WHO classification recognizes nasal-type T-NK(natural killer)-cell lymphomas, blastic NK-cell lymphomas, and gamma-delta T-cell lymphomas that the EORTC classification does not recognize. A series of 556 patients was assessed by the EORTC and the WHO classifications.[24] The estimated 5-year survival rates demonstrated nearly complete concordance in the indolent CTCL and the B-cell lymphomas. There were differences in the MF-associated follicular mucinosis and Sézary syndrome and in the entities not described by the EORTC classification including CD8+ epidermotropic cytotoxic T-cell lymphoma and primary cutaneous natural killer/T-cell lymphoma.

CLINICAL MANIFESTATIONS

The cutaneous clinical manifestations of cutaneous lymphoma are diverse, ranging from difficult to diagnose or indeterminate dermatitis-like lesions of skin to plaque-stage or tumor-stage CTCL. The most common CTCL is MF. The second most common cutaneous lymphoma is Sézary syndrome. Sézary syndrome usually arises without a previous history of MF. If MF evolves into SS, then the diagnosis should be "Sézary syndrome preceded by MF." Occasionally, atypical cutaneous lesions are eventually found to represent CTCL. Patients may have a premalignant phase with eczematous or dermatitic skin lesions for several years, or even decades, before the diagnosis of CTCL is established. The median duration of the preceding skin eruption is about 6 years.[8] Periodic skin examination and repeat skin biopsies as necessary are requisites in patients with suspicious cutaneous lesions. The spectrum of premalignant disorders includes various less common but distinctive lymphoid dermatoses, such as large-plaque parapsoriasis, poikiloderma atrophicans vasculare, follicular mucinosis (alopecia mucinosa), pityriasis lichenoides et varioliformis acuta (Mucha-Habermann disease), lymphomatoid papulosis, and other atypical lymphocytic infiltrates of the skin. Generally, no specific clinical or pathologic markers have been identified that clearly delineate those cases that will progress to CTCL.

The classic malignant phases of CTCL are manifested principally in the skin and include patch-stage CTCL, plaque-stage CTCL, tumor-stage CTCL, and erythrodermic CTCL (Fig. 113-1). Extracutaneous involvement, nodal or extranodal, of CTCL develops with disease progression.[5-7]

The patch stage of MF is characterized by cutaneous erythematous macules and slightly infiltrated patches of variable size, often located over the waist, trunk, or proximal extremities. Pruritus may be noted by the patient. Individual skin lesions occasionally exhibit superficial scale, whereas induration is minimal or absent. Pigmentation may be altered and, depending on the natural degree of pigment, hypopigmentation or hyperpigmentation may be observed. The lesions may be present for months to years before the plaque stage of CTCL develops (see Fig. 113-1).

Since the initial description of this disease by the French dermatologist Alibert during the early 1800s, the discrete plaque stage and tumor stages of CTCL have classically been defined as mycosis fungoides.[25] Clinically, plaque-stage lesions are characterized by sharply demarcated circular plaques that are infiltrated and elevated above the surrounding normal skin on the trunk and extremities. The plaques are erythematous or occasionally violaceous and may exhibit central involution. Individual patches may overlap, producing a geographic appearance. The lesions may be scaly or encrusted, occasionally exhibiting a papular quality (Fig. 113-1B). They rarely become vesicular, pustular, or have bullous features or a translucent granulomatous appearance. Patches evolve into a larger plaque stage with oval and well-demarcated lesions with elevated borders. The plaques may affect the face, and the dermal thickening on the face may evolve into the classical appearance of "leonine facies." Infiltration of the palms and soles leads to hyperkeratosis and fissuring. More extensive involvement of the scalp and other hair-bearing areas is often accompanied by alopecia (Fig. 113-1C). Pruritus may be significant; it can involve both lesional and nonlesional skin. Rarely, a solitary plaque or nodule of mycosis fungoides has been observed in the complete absence of other skin findings.[26]

Tumor-stage lesions of CTCL have variable growth rates and typically occur at sites of previous plaque-stage involvement. Progression likely reflects local proliferation and evolution of more aggressive clones of malignant cells. Multiple tumor-stage lesions of CTCL rarely arise de novo in the absence of patch-stage or plaque-stage CTCL but, when observed, have been reported as the *d'emblée* form of mycosis fungoides. The tumorous lesions may appear anywhere on the body but have a predilection for the body folds, including the groin, antecubital fossa, neck, axilla, and inframammary areas. The nodules and tumors are typically reddish brown or purplish and have a tendency to ulcerate (Fig. 113-1D). Multiple lobulated and coalescing lesions may develop on the face, resulting in a leonine facies (Fig. 113-1E). Tumor-stage CTCL is more clinically aggressive than patch-stage CTCL, probably owing to the evolution of a later stage of malignancy. Nodular lesions are infrequently pruritic and are more often painful and tender, especially after ulceration has occurred. Ulcerative lesions frequently become colonized

and purulent. Histologically, the lesions may be similar to plaque-stage disease, but they are denser and extend into the deep dermis and subcutaneous fat. Cellular composition may demonstrate lymphoid polymorphism and inflammation, or the lesions may be monomorphus, with almost exclusively less mature malignant T cells and minimal or absent epidermotropism. At presentation about 40% of patients have plaques on less than 10% of the body surface area, 30% have extensive plaques, 15% have a tumor phase, and 10% have an erythroderma phase.

The classic erythrodermic form of CTCL, Sézary syndrome, is a distinctive CTCL entity that derives its name from the descriptive studies and identification of unique blood cells by Sézary and Bouvrain during the 1930s.[27] Although this disease was initially reported in the late 19th century, Sézary and Bouvrain associated the malignant reticulemic (leukemic) erythroderma with circulating hyperchromatic mononuclear cells containing convoluted or cerebriform nuclei. These same cells infiltrate adenopathic lymph nodes. The cells were subsequently designated *Sézary cells*. The first description in the English literature of Sézary syndrome was by Taswell and Winkelmann in 1961.[28] The clinical presentation of this syndrome includes exfoliative erythroderma, lymphadenopathy, and keratoderma or thickening of the skin of the palms and soles that often cracks and fissures (palmoplantar hyperkeratosis) (Fig. 113-1F and G). Pruritus is a characteristic, often intense, symptom. Pruritus leads to excoriations, exudation, and crust formation. Nail dystrophy (onychodystrophy), ectropion of the (pulled down) lower eyelids, and alopecia are frequently observed.

Sézary syndrome is defined by the presence of Sézary cells in the peripheral blood and the characteristic clinical and histologic features of the skin mentioned above. Although mycosis fungoides uncommonly presents with erythroderma and similar clinical findings, Sézary cells are not detected in the peripheral blood by routine microscopic examination. These differences may distinguish rare cases of erythrodermic forms of mycosis fungoides from Sézary syndrome, both of which are classified as CTCL, but more sophisticated analysis of peripheral blood and skin by phenotypic and genotypic examination may indicate that separation of these classic forms of CTCL by clinical and morphologic examination alone may be arbitrary.

Extracutaneous disease involving sites beyond the blood and peripheral lymph nodes occurs in advanced CTCL. The reported range of extracutaneous involvement at autopsy is 54% to 100%, with almost every organ reported to be involved.[6,29-34] The histologic features of the malignant lymphoid population are similar to those of the skin.[31,32] Loss of epidermotropism may play a role as the disease disseminates.[35,36] With disease progression, extracutaneous involvement becomes more common.[37]

Clinical evidence of extracutaneous involvement of CTCL is classically manifested by peripheral lymphadenopathy.[37] Computed tomography (CT) demonstrates pelvic, abdominal, and axillary nodes that may not be palpable. Less commonly, thoracic nodal disease is recognized with this imaging technique. CT is not routinely used to stage

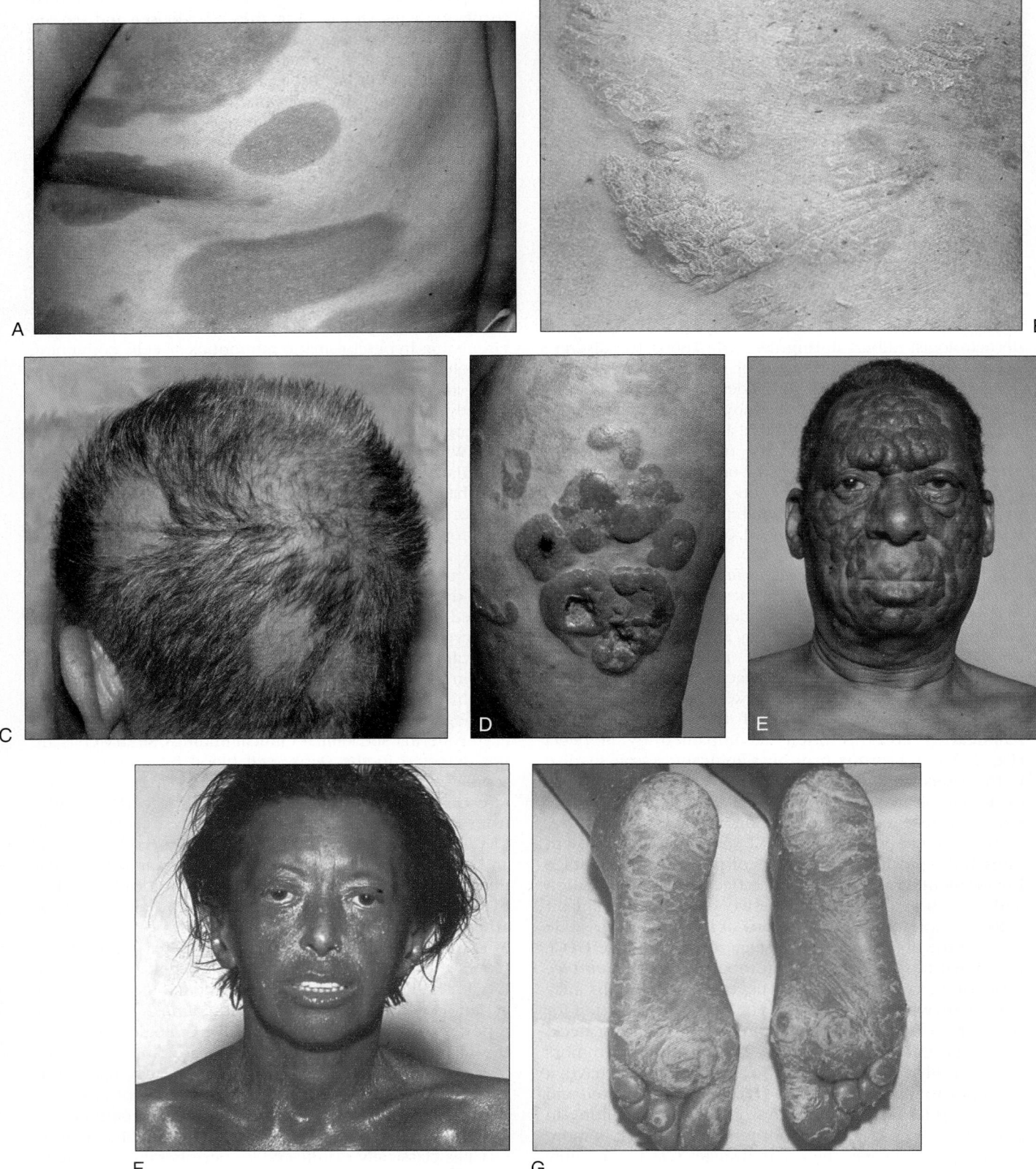

Figure 113-1. Cutaneous malignant phases and skin findings in cutaneous T-cell lymphoma. **A,** Patch stage. **B,** Plaque phase with scaling. **C,** Alopecia of scalp. **D,** Tumor stage. **E,** Leonine facies of tumor phase. **F,** Erythroderma of Sézary syndrome. **G,** Erythema, hyperkeratosis, and fissuring of soles in Sézary syndrome.

early CTCL, because the yield is low. In a retrospective review of 251 lymph nodes in 200 patients, Vonderheid and colleagues reported lymph node involvement to be associated with a poor prognosis and the survival of patients with small cell type (median survival, 40 months) to be better than that for other types (median survival, 20 months).[38] The Dutch Cutaneous Lymphoma Group reported that the presence of extracutaneous disease, the type and extent of cutaneous involvement, the response to initial therapy, and the presence of follicular mucinosis were associated with a higher rate of disease progression and mortality.[39]

Histologically, the paracortical T-cell regions are the areas of the lymph node involved initially. As the neoplastic lymphoid cells further infiltrate and replicate, the follicular centers are preserved, with effacement of the other areas of the node.[38,40-42] With disease progression, the abnormal cells become larger and more dysplastic.[38,40-42] Variable degrees of transformation are present in many nodes.[3,43,44] Complete histologic transformation may be present in up to 35% of nodes.[38,40,42,45] In the Sézary syndrome, the nodal effacement is produced by a more uniform small cell population, but transformation may occur.[41,42,44]

Bone marrow involvement may develop during progression of CTCL. In early studies, the antemortem incidence was less than 2.5%.[3,29,37,46] At autopsy, the incidence increased to 27% to 47%.[7,31,32,34] In more recent series, 7% to 13% of CTCL cases undergoing initial staging, including bone, had evidence of marrow involvement.[47,48] Bone marrow involvement by CTCL is subtle, requiring examination of aspirate and biopsy sections under oil immersion. Most patients with bone marrow involvement have concomitant nodal or organ involvement and shortened survival.[48]

Liver involvement by CTCL is documented by nodular lymphoid infiltration of the portal tracts on liver biopsy and has been reported in 8% to 16% of CTCL patients.[47,49,50] Occasionally, liver involvement is difficult to establish. In this case, the presence of abnormal cells in the hepatic sinusoids is not diagnostic of liver involvement.[50] In one series of patients who underwent formal staging laparotomy, splenic involvement was confirmed in 31% of cases.[49] Rarely, involvement of the central nervous system by CTCL has been documented by imaging studies on tissue biopsy or at autopsy.

TISSUE DIAGNOSIS

The diagnosis of CTCL is established by tissue biopsy. Punch biopsies, 4 to 6 mm, of involved skin are recommended for evaluation of patch-, plaque-, and tumor-stage lesions.[53,54] In selected tumor-stage cases, elliptic excision biopsies may be necessary. Several biopsies should be performed because multiple specimens are often required to demonstrate diagnostic pathologic findings. Tissue can be sectioned for separate analytic examinations before routine formalin or special fixation. Specimens for immunotyping and molecular genetic studies should be snap-frozen in liquid nitrogen and stored at –70°C.

Cell suspensions for flow cytometry and cytogenetic evaluation may be prepared from fresh tissue.[53]

Cutaneous Histopathology

The diagnosis of cutaneous lymphoproliferative disorders is complex.[54,55] The most recent classification of all lymphomas is the WHO classification.[22] The European Organization for Research and Treatment of Cancer (EORTC) proposed a classification for cutaneous lymphomas (Table 113-2).[23] The cell type involved in the pathogenesis of CTCL is the T lymphocyte. The histologic diagnosis of CTCL consists of abnormal lymphocyte morphology, a bandlike superficial dermal infiltrate, epidermotropism, and Pautrier's microabscesses.[32] These diagnostic criteria are uniformly accepted, but significant variability exists in the expression of these pathologic characteristics and the degree of the individual abnormalities[56-60] (Fig. 113-2A to C). There is significant intraobserver and interobserver variability.[61-63] In a study of 73 mycosis fungoides (MF) biopsies reviewed on two separate occasions by three expert hematopathologists, an accurate diagnosis was rendered on both readings about 50% of the time.[63] No single histopathologic criterion will establish the diagnosis. Lymphocytes within the epidermis that are larger than those within the dermis is an important feature of epidermatropism.[64] Pautrier's microabcesses are present in 4% to 37% of cases.[65,66]

By microscopic examination, the lymphocytes in CTCL (called mycosis cells or Sézary cells) have variable but usually ample cytoplasm. Nucleoli of the neoplastic cells are relatively large and hyperchromatic. Mycosis cells can be isolated from various tissue by touch preparation and microscopic examination. Sézary cells circulate in the blood and can be enriched by density centrifugation or immunophenotypic characteristics. The prominent characteristics of individual nuclei of Sézary cells are their irregularity, with prominent indentations or convolutions that have a cerebriform appearance (Fig. 113-3).[27,67] In 1968, Lutzner and Jordan further characterized the serpentine, or cerebriform, nuclei by electron microscopic examination[68] (Fig. 113-4). Reactive lymphoid cells infiltrating the skin in dermatitis, lichen planus, drug eruptions, psoriasis, and other dermatoses may have a similar nuclear morphology by light microscopy, but they have a normal nuclear diameter, nuclear-to-cytoplasm ratio, and nuclear contour index. A review of 222 biopsy specimens of MF/SS reported that CTCL produces the patterns for diagnosing inflammatory disease including superficial perivascular invasion with atypical lymphocytes in almost half of cases.[55] The cells that mimic mycosis cells or Sézary cells represent activated T lymphocytes and have been classified as Sézary-like cells.[69] Similar cells have been demonstrated in the peripheral blood of patients hospitalized for extensive dermatoses.[70] Therefore morphologic examination alone can result in misdiagnoses.[51,52,68] The limitation of light microscopy has led to the development of more sophisticated approaches to CTCL diagnosis.[60] Of interest, the EORTC reported that identification of epidermal lymphocytes with extremely convoluted nuclei was 100% specific and 92% sensitive in establishing the

TABLE 113-2

Comparison of EORTC and WHO Classification of CTCL

	EORTC	WHO
T-Cell Lymphomas	Indolent	
	Mycosis fungoides	Mycosis fungoides
	Mycosis fungoides-associated follicular mucinosis	Mycosis fungoides-associated follicular mucinosis
	Pagetoid reticulosis	Pagetoid reticulosis
	CTCL, large cell, CD30+	Primary cutaneous anaplastic large cell lymphoma
	Lymphomatoid papulosis	Lymphomatoid papulosis
	Aggressive	
	Sézary syndrome	Sézary syndrome
	CTCL, large-cell CD30–	Peripheral T-cell lymphoma, unspecified
	Provisional	
	Granulomatous slack skin	Granulomatous slack skin
	Pleomorphic small/medium-sized CTCL	Peripheral T-cell lymphoma, unspecified
	Subcutaneous panniculitis-like T-cell lymphoma	Subcutaneous panniculitis-like T-cell lymphoma
B-Cell Lymphomas	Indolent	
	Follicle center cell lymphoma	Follicular lymphoma and diffuse large B-cell lymphoma
	Immunocytoma (marginal zone B-cell lymphoma)	Extranodal marginal zone B-cell lymphoma
	Intermediate	
	Large B-cell lymphoma of the leg	Diffuse large B-cell lymphoma and follicular lymphoma
	Provisional	
	Intravascular large B-cell lymphoma	Intravascular large B-cell lymphoma
	Plasmacytoma	Plasmacytoma

CTCL, cutaneous T-cell lymphoma; EORTC, European Organization for Research and Treatment of Cancer; WHO, World Health Organization.

diagnosis.[63] Uniform criteria and training sessions can improve the concensus rate.[71]

The tumor stage of CTCL is characterized by a dense dermal infiltrate that often extends into the deep dermis and subcutis and becomes nonepidermotropic or less epidermotropic. The individual malignant cells are pleomorphic large cells with prominent nucleoli. Complete transformation to a large cell variant that resembles diffuse large cell lymphoma or anaplastic large cell lymphoma is typically seen in tumors and is occasionally present in plaques and erythroderma.[38,44,71-74]

Skin-biopsy specimens of Sézary syndrome, in contrast to those of MF, frequently lack prominent epidermotropism. Buechner and Winkelmann reported that 17% of skin biopsies of Sézary syndrome were nondiagnostic by light microscopic examination alone.[75] Patients whose skin-biopsy specimen demonstrated only a lichenoid or bandlike infiltrate without other criteria to establish MF or Sézary syndrome have been shown to have CTCL by other diagnostic and laboratory criteria.[59] Nonetheless the presence of abnormal lymphocytes and characteristic Pautrier's microabscesses are important for the diagnosis of MF and Sézary syndrome. The propensity to develop Pautrier's microabscesses in Sézary syndrome is less prominent, however, and may hinder confirmation of the diagnosis. The cellular composition and morphology of the dermal infiltrate in Sézary syndrome is similar to those of MF. In Sézary syndrome, the abnormal cells are characteristically present and reflect the presence of Sézary cells in the peripheral blood. Increased number of Sézary cells is a major criterion for establishing the diagnosis.[72-77] The propensity to develop Pautrier's microabscesses in

Sézary syndrome is less prominent and may hinder the confirmation of the diagnosis.[78-79]

Immunophenotype and Genotype Analysis

Antibodies against cell surface proteins as standardized in terms of a cluster designation (CD) system and identified by immunoperoxidase staining of frozen sections, fixed tissue, or flow cytometric analysis of cell suspensions have aided immensely in the diagnosis of CTCL. The cell line of origin in Sézary syndrome was confirmed as lymphocytic during the early 1970s.[80] The neoplastic cell was identified as a T cell in 1973.[81-82] In 1976, Broder and colleagues demonstrated that the T cell is usually of helper phenotype (CD4+) (Fig. 113-5A and B).[83] Most patients have a disease of mature post-thymic lymphocytes of T origin (CD2+, CD3+, CD5+, CD1–) and T-helper phenotype (CD4+, CD8–).[84-92] The T-helper lymphocyte population can be subdivided into helper-inducer and suppressor-inducer subtypes.[93] In mycosis fungoides, the neoplastic T cells represent memory T cells.[93-95] The suppressor T-cell phenotype has been described in selected cases of MF and Sézary syndrome but is rare.[44,89,96-99] Aberrant antigen expression of the malignant T-cell population is observed in MF and Sézary syndrome and is manifested as decreased or absent expression of pan-T-cell antigens (CD2, CD3, CD5), absent expression of subset antigens (CD4–, CD8–), or coexpression of T-cell antigens (CD4+, CD8+).[87-91,95,100,101] "Double negative" CTCL patients may have an aggressive course.[102] Characteristically, CD7 and Leu-8 are diminished or absent in all stages of CTCL, and activation-associated antigens (HLA-DR, CD25, CD30,

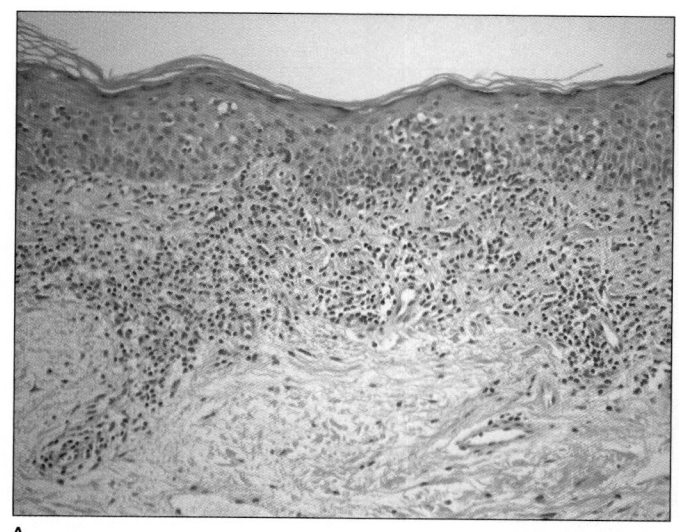

A

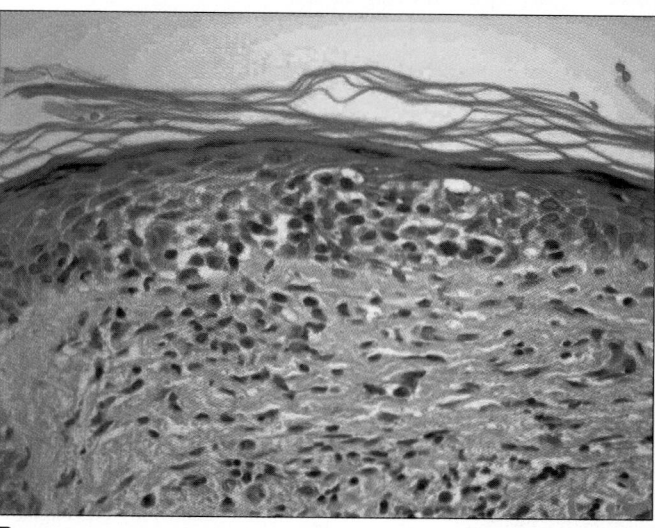

B

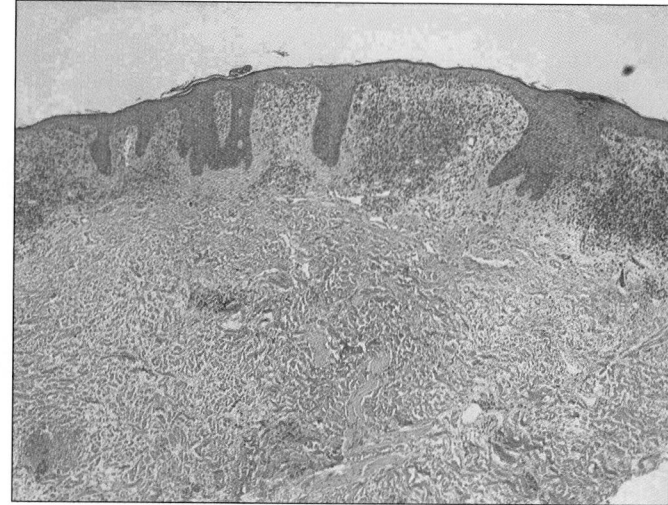

C

Figure 113-2. Skin biopsy specimens of cutaneous T-cell lymphoma. **A,** Mononuclear cell infiltrate in perivascular area and bandlike distribution of dermis with single cell exocytosis into epidermis of early mycosis fungoides (H&E; original magnification, ×40). **B,** Collections of lymphoid cells in the epidermis forming Pautrier's microabscess, and dermal infiltration of lymphocytes in plaque of mycosis fungoides (H&E; original magnification, ×40). **C,** Lichenoid dermatitis-like pattern with basal epidermal infiltration by atypical lymphocytes (H&E; original magnification, ×160).

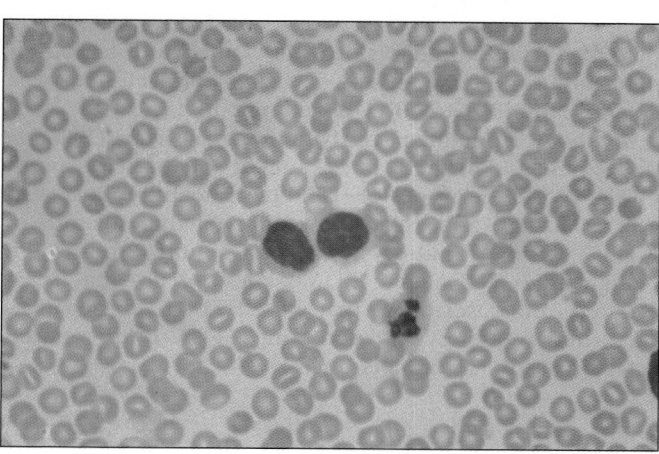

Figure 113-3. Peripheral blood smear demonstrating irregular Sézary cell nucleus with cerebriform appearance (Wright stain).

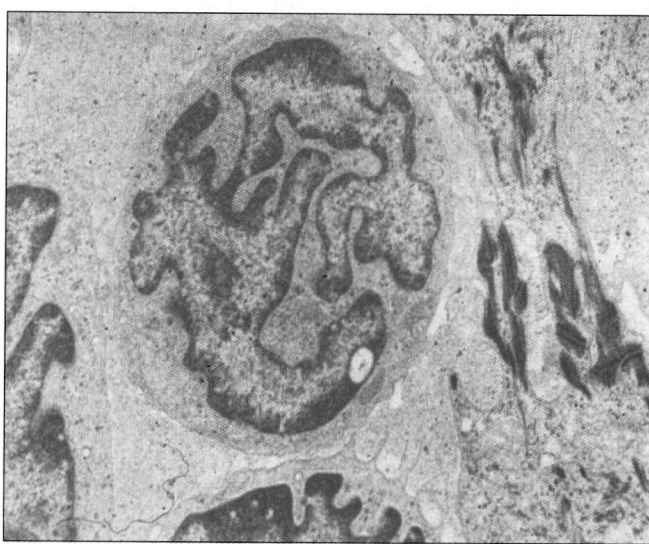

Figure 113-4. Electron photomicrograph of "serpentine," or cerebriform, nuclei of Sézary cells from peripheral blood.

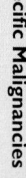

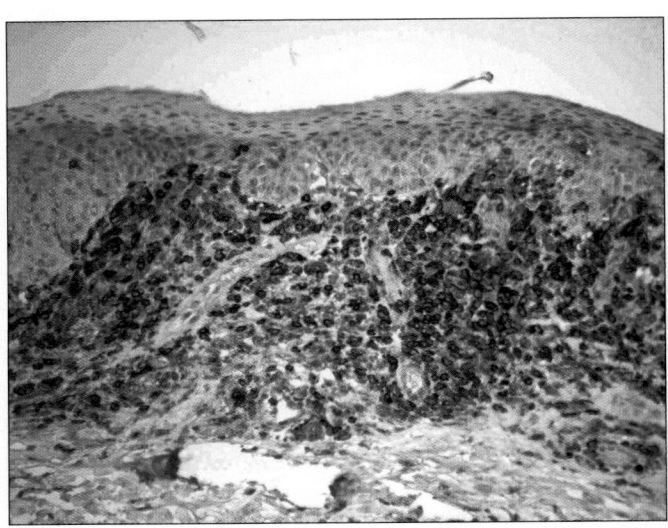 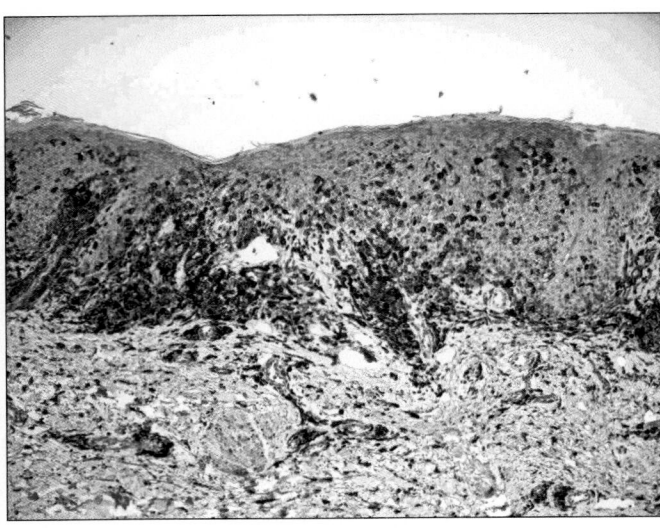

A   B

Figure 113-5. A, Uniform CD4+ cellular infiltrate in dense bandlike pattern in papillary dermis of Sézary syndrome. **B,** CD4+ cells forming a dense dermal infiltrate and Pautrier's microabscesses in mycosis fungoides (H&E; original magnification, ×160).

CD38) or proliferation-associated antigens (CD71, Ki-67) may be expressed by mycosis cells or Sézary cells in selected compartments (epidermis versus dermis) in patients with advanced disease.[44,103-105] IL-2 receptor (CD25) was present in 60% of cases. CTCL cells are skin homing, cutaneous lymphoid antigen (CLA)-expressing lymphocytes. Sézary syndrome is characterized by decreased cell-mediated cytotoxicity associated with defective production of IL-12. A synergistic enhancement of cell-mediated immunity by IL-12 plus IL-2 has been reported in vitro.[106] CTCL cells express alpha and beta integrin, CDC2, and BE-2.[107,108] Progressively transformed cells that express aberrant phenotypes acquire new proliferation and activation-associated antigens but retain their T-helper or suppressor phenotype and may produce diagnostic dilemmas. For example, transformed cells in mycosis fungoides or Sézary syndrome have been shown to acquire CD30 (Ki-1) antigens and may be confused with Ki-1+ large cell lymphoma or lymphomatoid papulosis. In other cases, neoplastic cells of CTCL may acquire Leu-M1 and be confused with Hodgkin's disease.[44,90,109-112]

Methods designed to identify the malignant cell population in mycosis fungoides and Sézary syndrome have been limited by the relative nonspecificity of phenotypic analysis of T-cell lymphocyte subsets.[113-116] No immunohistochemical techniques clearly demonstrate clonality of T-cell lymphoproliferative disorders. Despite the use of these special methods, a definitive diagnosis may not be possible in the patch stage of mycosis fungoides or in early Sézary syndrome. Monoclonal antibodies (mAbs) to the variable-region beta chain of the T-cell receptor (TCR) protein have been developed.[117] These reagents identify some cases, and the ultimate value of these antibodies has not been defined.[118] Further antibodies are being developed.

The early stages of CTCL are difficult to diagnose. The EORTC assessed the inter-rater and intra-rater agreement rates from 32 patients with early CTCL and 13 eczematous or psoriaform dermatitis. The percentage of false positive and false negative cases was nearly 50%.[65] Prospective histologic scores do not appear to correlate with stage of disease, clinical outcome, or response to diagnosis.[117] At this time, no clear benefit has been established in the early diagnosis of CTCL. Patients must be followed up.

Association of CTCL with expression of specific class I and II major histocompatibility antigens (AW31, AW32, B8, BW35, and DR5) has been described.[119-121] This association, however, has no clinical utility.

Cytogenetic abnormalities have been identified in CTCL. The most common numerical change is loss of chromosome 10.[122-131] Other reported abnormalities from skin, peripheral blood, lymph nodes, and bone marrow include complex translocations or deletions in chromosomes 1, 2, 6, 9, 11, 13, 14, and 17.[122-136] These abnormalities may cause activation of oncogenes, such as *erb* A, *K-ras,* *v-fps,* or *lck.*[92,132] *lck* is located on chromosome 1 and may enhance the clonal growth of T lymphocytes.[133] A mediator of apoptosis in T-cells is the *Fas* receptor. A splice variant of *Fas* was identified in 15 of 22 patients.[134] These findings provide further information for delineating the mechanisms of malignant T-cell neoplasia and susceptibility to CTCL development.

Antibodies to human T-cell lymphotropic virus-1 (HTLV-1) have been identified in a subset of patients with CTCL.[135,136] Other types of HTLV have been implicated in CTCL. Manzari and colleagues reported the isolation of HTLV-V from a patient with CTCL and other T-cell malignancies.[137] Deleted HTLV-1 provirus also has been isolated from cases of MF that were HTLV-1 seronegative, but the frequency of detecting HTLV-1 or related retroviruses in MF or SS is small.[138-142]

Molecular Studies

Molecular genetic studies represent a significant technologic advance that supplements the evaluation of CTCL by routine morphologic and immunohistochemical methods. Southern blot analysis to examine the T-cell antigen receptor (TCR) gene is among the most sensitive techniques for detecting an abnormal clone of lymphoid cells in the skin, blood, or lymph nodes.[143-144] Clonal TCR gene rearrangements are identified as nongermline bands on Southern blot analysis of DNA hybridized to TCR-beta, TCR-gamma, and TCR-delta chain molecular probes (Fig. 113-6A and B). In one series, 20 of 24 skin biopsy samples from patients with mycosis fungoides and 19 of 21 peripheral blood samples from patients with Sézary syndrome had a demonstrable clonal gene rearrangement.[145] Clonal rearrangements of the TCR-beta gene have been documented in most patients.[144-149] In early patch-stage MF, the number of infiltrating T cells is minimal and Southern blot analysis may not detect clonal T-cell populations.[128-129] Skin and blood samples were both required to identify the TCR gene rearrangement in a few cases of SS and MF. Biopsies from different sites usually have identical TCR gene rearrangement patterns, although deletions or additional rearrangements may develop as part of the neoplastic progression of CTCL. Serial studies have demonstrated the development of new clones over time, and it may be possible to monitor the extent of cell tumor burden and therapeutic response by serial examination of clonal TCR gene rearrangement.[150-151]

Potentially more sensitive methods have been examined for identifying clonal lymphoid cell populations among reactive inflammatory cell populations in the skin or for cells that represent an exceedingly small population in the circulating peripheral blood, bone marrow, lymph nodes, or other tissues. Using polymerase chain reaction (PCR) techniques to amplify specific genetic rearrange-

ments detected in the malignant T cells of Sézary syndrome, patient-specific molecular probes can be generated, and the sensitivity of identifying the neoplastic clone can be increased dramatically up to 1000-fold.[152] A PCR assay study revealed circulating clonal T cells in 26 of 45 MF patients with skin biopsy clones in 29 of 40 patients, 6 of 7 SS patients with skin biopsy clones in 3 of 4 patients, and 10 of 13 pleomorphic CTCL patients with skin biopsy clones in 12 of 12 patients.[153] On PCR analysis, up to 90% of MF skin biopsy samples have clonal cells.[154] The high frequency of identical clonal T cells in peripheral blood and skin is of clinical interest and supports the concept that CTCL is an early systemic disease.[155] The detection of circulating clonal cells is not likely an indicator of a worse prognosis. These technical advances provide the capability for improved monitoring of disease progression and treatment response and earlier detection of minimal residual disease, quiescent disease, or disease relapse.

Documented lymph node involvement by clonal TCR gene rearrangement has been associated with decreased survival.[156] Clonal TCR gene rearrangements are found in disorders that are not overtly malignant, however, including lymphomatoid papulosis, pityriasis lichenoides, and pagetoid reticulosis.[157-160] T-cell clonality has been reported in 6% to 24% of benign skin disorders that have a lymphoid infiltrate.[161-162] Therefore equating clonal gene rearrangement with malignancy may be presumptuous. Thirty-nine patients with 91 skin biopsies and 11 lymph node biopsies were studied via a PCR assay. Patients who had the same gene rearrangements at the time of diagnosis were more likely to have progressive disease than those who had different gene rearrangements via a PCR assay.[163] The most reasonable and prudent approach is to integrate the clinical history, physical examination, and histologic findings with the TCR gene rearrangement analysis and other laboratory results.[164]

Ancillary laboratory studies have provided additional perspectives on CTCL. Flow cytometry for DNA histography can detect cell populations containing the normal number of chromosomes (diploid) versus the abnormal number (aneuploid). The presence of aneuploidy has been associated with a more aggressive disease course.[165]

The density of epidermal Langerhans cells in biopsy samples has been reported to be a prognostic factor in CTCL. Langerhans cell concentration of greater than 90 cells/mm^2 correlated with a significantly lower risk of death from CTCL compared with patients bearing fewer epidermal dendritic cells.[166]

Bcl-2 was expressed in 22 of 26 cases.[167] This is consistent with a similar observation in the low-grade B-cell lymphoproliferative disorders. Expression profiling microarray studies are ongoing. Unsupervised hierarchic clustering has revealed two major classes of MF and deregulation of multiple genes involving the tumor necrosis factor (TNF) pathway.[168] Further studies will be required with different approaches including supervised machine-based learning.

The diagnosis of CTCL should include clinical history, light microscopy, immunohistochemistry, and molecular genetics.

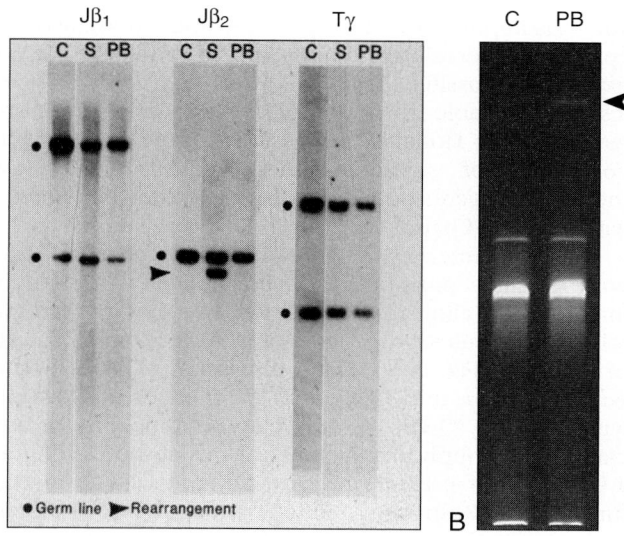

Figure 113-6. A, Immunogenotyping by Southern blot analysis of a patient with Sézary syndrome. Control (C), skin (S), and peripheral blood (PB) specimens. A distinct clonal rearranged band is identified (*arrow*) using probes that recognize the T-cell beta chain genes (Jβ2). Only germline bands are identified in the Jβ1 gene. **B,** Polymerase chain reaction (PCR) analysis of PB identified a distinct clonal rearranged band (*arrow*).

Specific Malignancies

III

CTCL VARIANTS, ASSOCIATED CONDITIONS, AND DIFFERENTIAL DIAGNOSIS

The clinical manifestations of Sézary syndrome and MF are diverse and range from indeterminate lesions to plaque-stage and tumor-stage disease. Patients may have a premalignant phase with eczematous skin lesions that persist for years before the diagnosis is made. The premalignant stages evolving to CTCL are encompassed within a range of lymphoid to lymphomatoid reactions that are observed in skin, including various forms of parapsoriasis, lymphomatoid papulosis, follicular mucinosis (alopecia mucinosa), pre–Sézary syndrome, atypical dermatitis, and dermal reticulosis.[169-172] Histologic or clinical variants of CTCL have been recognized and identified as granulomatous, pustular, bullous, verrucous, hyperkeratotic, hypopigmented, papillomatous (acanthosis nigricans–like), purpuric, and angiocentric CTCL.[169] Epidermotropic T-cell lymphomas that are variants of or closely related to CTCL include granulomatous slack skin disorder, pagetoid reticulosis (Woringer-Kolopp disease), and unilesional mycosis fungoides. These disorders must be differentiated from peripheral T-cell lymphoma, suppressor T-cell lymphoma, adult T-cell leukemia/lymphoma, CD30+ large cell lymphoma, lymphomatoid granulomatosis, Pseudolymphomas, cutaneous lymphoid hyperplasias, lymphomatoid contact reactions, and insect bite reactions also must be differentiated from CTCL. In addition, primary B-cell lymphoma of the skin is a distinct clinical entity.

The various forms of parapsoriasis are the most common of the premalignant lesions. These include acute and chronic guttate and plaque forms of parapsoriasis, retiform parapsoriasis, and poikiloderma atrophicans vasculare. The skin findings of erythema and atrophy are typically accompanied by pigmentation and telangiectasia. These lesions may persist for years before malignant features become evident.[170] They occur most commonly on the trunk, waist, and buttocks, often requiring multiple skin-biopsy specimens to establish the diagnosis. Large-plaque parapsoriasis has a clinical appearance similar to that of patch-stage mycosis fungoides; a predominance of CD4+ helper T cells and variably absent CD7 and Leu-8 expression.[173] Reports suggest that CTCL eventually develops in approximately 10% or more of patients with large-plaque parapsoriasis.[169] These eruptions may vary seasonally, over time, in intensity, and in the extent of disease present. The early eruption of poikiloderma atrophicans vasculare may resolve with exposure to sunlight.[174]

In the WHO and EORTC classification systems, lymphomatoid papulosis is an indolent disorder that is not considered malignant. It is characterized by recurrent, self-healing, erythematous, and papular to nodular lesions of less than 2.5 cm in size that may develop central necrosis and crust[175] (Fig. 113-7). Individual lesions typically develop and resolve over several weeks. The disease is most frequent in the third and fourth decades. The clinical course of the disease is unpredictable. The duration of

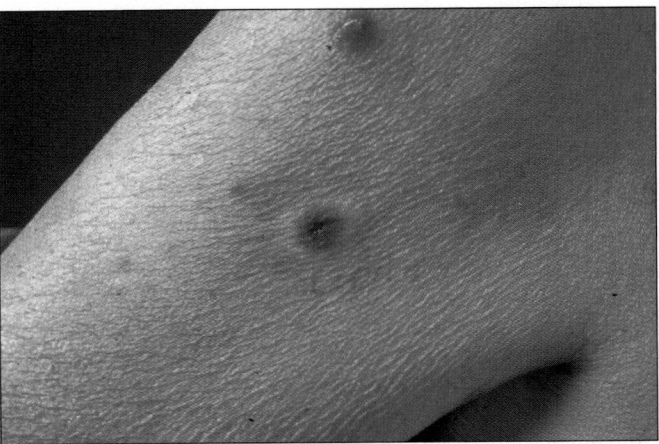

Figure 113-7. Erythematous papulonodules with crust and ulceration in lymphomatoid papulosis.

disease activity varies from a few months to more than 20 years. CTCL or other malignant lymphomas may develop in 10% to 20% of patients with lymphomatoid papulosis.[176-178] The median time to develop lymphoma was 12 years, with an absolute risk of 24% and a cumulative risk at 15 years of 80% plus or minus 18%.[45] The clonal nature of lymphomatoid papulosis has been demonstrated in some cases.[157] Clonality has not been shown to correlate uniformly with the development of malignant lymphoma, however. Histologic examination demonstrates a nonepidermatotropic wedge-shaped infiltrate with large atypical multilobulated cells in an inflammatory cell background. Dense dermal perivascular and interstitial wedge-shaped polymorphic cellular infiltrate composed of lymphocytes, histiocytes, and atypical pleomorphic lymphoid cells is characteristic. Neutrophils and eosinophils are also present, and spongiosis and epidermal necrosis are often seen. Morphologic patterns have been classified as type A and type B.[179,180] Type A lesions resemble those of Ki-1+ anaplastic large cell lymphoma or Hodgkin's disease, and type B lesions are composed of small lymphoid cells.[109,181-183] Most therapeutic agents do not substantially alter the course of lymphomatoid papulosis.

Follicular mucinosis is a disorder of localized alopecia with mucin deposition in the hair follicle, with variable inflammation clinically characterized by multiple grouped follicular papules with occasional formation of patches or nodules (Fig. 113-8). This disease may be associated with or evolve into CTCL in 15% of cases of Hodgkin's lymphoma.[184-187] This disease may be idiopathic or associated with lymphoma. Biopsy features do not distinguish a benign course from one that may progress to mycosis fungoides.[187] Response to initial treatment, risk of disease, progression, disease-specific survival, and overall survival of patients with follicular MF were worse than in classic MF patients.[188]

The erythematous papular to papulovesicular or necrotic lesions of acute guttate parapsoriasis (Mucha-Habermann disease) occur in crops, with some cases demonstrating a lymphomatoid histology. The T-cell

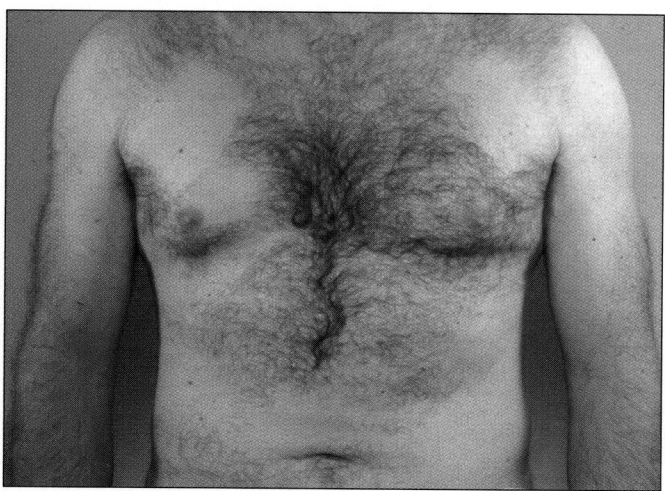

Figure 113-8. Follicular mucinosis manifested as patches of alopecia.

population is genotypically clonal in a significant percentage of the few cases in which TCR rearrangement analysis has been reported.[158]

Pagetoid reticulosis (Woringer-Kolopp disease) and granulomatous slack skin are two rare epidermotropic T-cell lymphomas that likely represent variants of mycosis fungoides. Pagetoid reticulosis, initially described in 1939, is a clonal T-cell process.[159,189] It is characterized by solitary slow-growing plaque or multiple skin lesions of the hands or feet that grow slowly and progress to disseminated skin lesions or, in some cases, to systemic disease. The solitary slow-growing lesion has a chronic course of years to decades.[190] Large atypical mononuclear cells infiltrate the epidermis, and individual cells exhibit variably shaped hyperchromatic nuclei and a pale cytoplasm, creating a halo appearance. The dermal lymphoid cell population appears to be benign and reactive without the distinctive cellular morphology of epidermal lymphoid cell populations. The epidermal lymphoid cells express CD4+ but may also express a T-suppressor (CD8+) phenotype.[190,191] TCR gene rearrangements have been documented in this entity.[159]

Granulomatous slack skin is a disorder characterized by excessive redundant folds of skin and plaques in the axilla and groin.[192] The infiltrate occupies both dermal and epidermal compartments.[193] Clonal proliferations of helper T cells have been documented. A striking granulomatous reaction and loss of dermal elastic tissue accompany the lymphocytic infiltrate, and the disease may progress to disseminated T-cell lymphoma.[193]

Gamma-delta T-cell phenotypic CTCL is associated with a trend in decreased survival.[194] This entity is not defined in the WHO or EORTC classifications.

CTCL must be distinguished from adult T-cell leukemia/lymphoma, Ki-1+ anaplastic large cell lymphomas, peripheral T-cell non-Hodgkin's lymphoma, cutaneous B-cell lymphomas, T-cell chronic lymphocytic leukemia, leukemia cutis, and cutaneous Hodgkin's disease. These types of malignant lymphomas and leukemias may cause similar cutaneous lesions; more infiltrative lesions destroy cutaneous structures and ulcerate.

PATHOBIOLOGY

Phenotypic and genotypic investigations have clearly established T lymphocytes as the malignant population in mycosis fungoides (MF) and Sézary syndrome. The biologic origins and progression of CTCL are less defined.

The cellular and tissue interactions among the malignant T lymphocytes, other hematopoietic cells, and the skin (including Langerhans cells and keratinocytes) are complex.[195] The development, clinical presentation, and progression of CTCL appear to be dependent on the interaction of the malignant T-lymphocyte population, immune system, and inflammatory cell populations with the skin. Observations about the molecules that regulate cell and tissue recognition, homing, and adhesion have significantly enhanced the understanding of the biology of CTCL. One class of cellular adhesion receptors, the integrins, are heterodimeric proteins composed of alpha- and beta-subunits that are involved in various cellular functions, including cell-cell recognition, cell-matrix interactions, cell migration, and tissue homing.[196,197] Other cell surface molecules, such as the intracellular adhesion molecules (ICAMs; e.g., ICAM-1), are counterreceptors or ligands expressed by keratinocytes that facilitate cellular association with lymphocytes that express integrins. LFA-1 is a member of the beta2-integrins expressed on lymphoid cells; it binds ICAM-1 and ICAM-2.[198-200] The epidermis and keratinocytes of patients with MF express ICAM-1. In MF, T cells in the epidermis strongly express LFA-1. Cases of Sézary syndrome that lack epidermotropism exhibit either low or no expression of ICAM-1 by keratinocytes.[201] Physical association between T lymphocytes and keratinocytes appears to be partially mediated by integrins and other cell adhesion molecules. Antibodies to ICAM-1 or LFA-1 partially block this interaction.[202-203]

It is likely that other integrins, their ligands, and additional cell adhesion molecules such as the cadherins are equally important in malignant T-cell homing to skin, endothelial adhesion, and dermal and/or epidermal tropism.[204-206] For example, LFA-3, VLA-1, and VLA-6 are also expressed by infiltrating cells in most cases of epidermotropic mycosis fungoides, but are absent in most other varieties of CTCL.[205] Furthermore infiltrating cells in Sézary syndrome express alpha3/beta1-integrin.[206] Future studies designed to identify and characterize the regulation of expression and activity of integrins and other adhesion molecules will undoubtedly lead to a clearer understanding of the pathogenesis of CTCL.

The molecular expression and regulation of cytokines by Sézary cells and mycosis cells demonstrate that these populations of malignant T lymphocytes are apparently distinct subsets within the CD4 lineage. Peripheral blood mononuclear cells from patients with CTCL respond better mitogenically to interleukin-4 (IL-4) than to IL-2 and produce greater amounts of IL-4 than interferon gamma.[207] As only a few cells (<5% Sézary syndrome cells) were identified in the peripheral blood of these patients with CTCL, the findings suggest that an imbalance in circulating Th1/Th2 cells is a consequence of CTCL, rather than a direct response by the malignant population. Sézary cells express IL-4 and IL-5. IL-4, IL-5, and IL-10 mRNA (messenger RNA) was detected by a polymerase chain reaction (PCR) assay in epidermal samples in patients with Sézary syndrome.[208] This suggests that the malignant helper T cell is a Th2 cell.[209-210] Possible autocrine (self-stimulated) growth of Sézary cells has also been investigated. IL-7 has been reported to function as a growth factor for Sézary lymphoma cells in culture and is produced by these same cells.[211]

Long-term prognosis may be related to the extent of host-infiltrating CD8 cytotoxic T-lymphocytes.[212] p53 gene mutation is not a critical in CTCL. In one series, only 2 of 37 biopsy specimens demonstrated p53 expression.[213]

STAGING AND PROGNOSIS

As in Hodgkin's and non-Hodgkin's lymphomas, the prognosis of CTCL is related to the stage of the disease (Fig. 113-9). The significant prognostic factors in CTCL are the extent and type of skin involvement. The Mycosis Fungoides Cooperative Group adopted a modified TNM (tumor, node, metastasis) classification in 1975, and this classification system was further modified by the Staging Committee at the International Workshop on Mycosis Fungoides[214] (Tables 113-3 and 113-4). The TNM classification system is not routinely utilized in clinical practice.

The greater the percentage of involvement of skin surface area by CTCL, the worse the prognosis.[7] Involvement of less than 10% of the body surface area by CTCL (stage IA) portends a better prognosis than that associated with stage IB, defined as a greater than 10% skin involvement. Patients with plaque-stage disease have a more favorable prognosis than do tumor-stage patients. In MF,

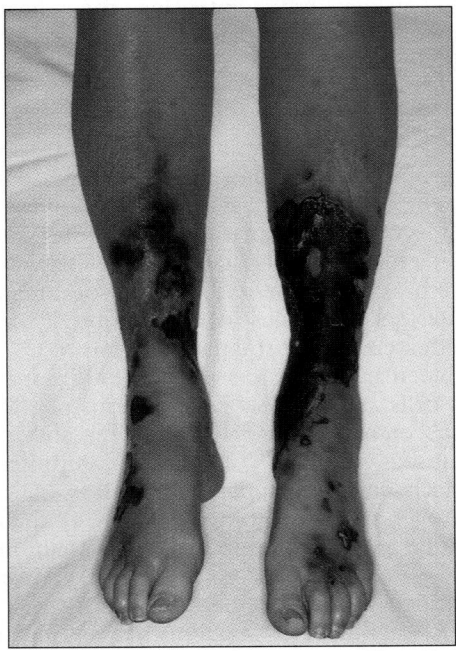

Figure 113-9. Subcutaneous T-cell lymphoma.

TABLE 113-3

Staging of Cutaneous T-Cell Lymphoma: TNM Classification

CLASSIFICATION	DESCRIPTION
T: Skin	
T0	Lesions clinically and/or histopathologically suggestive of CTCL
T1	Limited plaques, papules, or eczematous patches covering <10% of skin surface
T2	Generalized plaques, papules, or erythematous patches covering ≥10% of skin surface
T3	Tumors
T4	Generalized erythroderma
N: Lymph Nodes	
N0	No palpable adenopathy, lymph node pathology negative for CTCL
N1	Palpable adenopathy, lymph node pathology negative for CTCL
N2	No palpable adenopathy, lymph node pathology positive for CTCL
N3	Palpable adenopathy, lymph node pathology positive for CTCL
B: Peripheral Blood	
B0	Atypical circulating cells not present (<5%)
B1	Atypical circulating cells present (>5%)
M: Visceral Organs	
M0	No visceral organ involvement
M1	Visceral involvement (must have pathologic confirmation, and organ involved should be specified)

90% of patients with patch- or plaque-stage disease with less than 10% of skin surface involvement survived 15 years or longer.[215] Thirty-two percent of patients progressed and 2% of 122 patients with limited cutaneous disease died after 32 years.[216] Of 309 patients with MF, the 5-year disease-free survival was 100% with limited cutaneous disease, 80% with tumor phase disease, and 40% for lymph node phase disease.[217] Survival of tumor-stage patients is reported to be greater than that of patients with stage III or erythrodermic disease.[218,219] Stage IA

TABLE 113-4

Staging Classification of Cutaneous T-Cell Lymphoma

STAGING		CLASSIFICATION	
T	N	M	
IA	1	0	0
IB	2	0	0
IIA	1, 2	1	0
IIB	3	0, 1	0
III	4	0, 1	0
IVA	1–4	2, 3	0
IVB	1–4	0–3	1

B, peripheral blood; M, visceral organ; N, lymph node; T, skin.
Bunn PA Jr, Lamberg SI: Report of the Committee on Staging and Classification of Cutaneous T-Cell Lymphomas. Cancer Treat Rep 1979;63:725.

TABLE 113-5

Evaluation of a Patient with Cutaneous T-Cell Lymphoma

Complete history and physical examination
Whole body mapping of skin lesions with or without photography
Complete blood count, differential, and platelet count; Sézary cell count
Serum chemistries (liver and renal function tests, calcium, phosphorus, creatinine, and uric acid)
Chest radiography
Skin biopsy for routine histology and possible immunophenotyping/ T-cell receptor gene rearrangement analysis
Lymph node biopsy (palpable node from draining area—cervical before axillary before inguinal.
Evaluation of other organs if foregoing tests suggest involvement; computed tomographic scans, liver biopsies, and bone marrow biopsies only for patients with stages II, III, and IV disease

patients have plaques and no adenopathy, whereas stage IIB patients have tumors with or without adenopathy. Unequivocal histologic involvement in the lymph nodes is predictive of survival, with a median actuarial survival of 53 months if involved and 137 months if not involved.[220-221]

Peripheral blood involvement correlates with the stage of cutaneous involvement. Eight percent to 12% of patients with plaque-stage CTCL, 16% to 20% of those with tumor-stage CTCL, and more than 90% of patients with erythrodermic CTCL manifest peripheral blood involvement as noted by morphologic criteria alone.[47,222]

The past recommended staging procedures are outlined in Table 113-5[214] and serve as general guidelines for clinical trials. Skin involvement should be recorded by either mapping or photography. Lymphangiograms and liver biopsies are not indicated in the routine staging of these patients. The role of routine CT scans is controversial. Routine CT scanning does not improve detection of advanced disease, but may be clinically useful in early plaque-stage disease.[223,224]

A retrospective study of 152 patients evaluated at the National Cancer Institute (NCI) identified three risk groups.[225] Good-risk patients had a median survival of 12 years for plaque-exclusive skin disease. Intermediate-risk patients had a median survival of 5 years and no visceral involvement, but were found to have skin tumors, erythroderma, or plaque lesions with lymphadenopathy or peripheral blood involvement. Poor-risk patients had a median survival of 2.5 years and visceral involvement or complete effacement of lymph nodes. In the Stanford series, 112 of 434 patients had extracutaneous involvement at presentation with a median survival of 13 months.[226] In this series, at 20 years of follow-up from the time of initial diagnosis, the risk to progression to extracutaneous disease was 0% for limited patch/plaque disease, 10% for generalized patch/plaque disease, 35.5% for tumor disease, and 41% for erythrodermic disease. The International Society for Cutaneous Lymphomas defined three subsets of erythroderma: leukemic phase E-CTCL, erythrodermic MF (secondary E-CTCL developing in MF patients), and E-CTCL not otherwise defined.[227] Sézary syndrome has a worse survival than does MF,

with a 5-year survival of only 33.5%. Patients with zero to one of three criteria, which included periodic acid-Schiff (PAS)-positive cytoplasmic inclusions in circulating Sézary syndrome cells, CD7– phenotype, and histologic transformation to large circulating Sézary syndrome cells, had a 5-year survival of 58% versus 5% in patients with two or three of the criteria.[228]

At initial diagnosis, about 42% of patients have plaques covering less than 10% of the body surface (T1), 30% are characterized as T2, 16% have tumors (T3), and 12% have erythroderma (T4).[214,218,219]

Bone marrow involvement is less common. Morphologically, Salhany and colleagues demonstrated aggregates of lymphocytes with cerebriform nuclei in 21.7% of cases and abnormal lymphoid aggregates in 31.6%.[48] Infiltrative disease was associated with peripheral blood involvement. Clonal T-cell involvement in the bone marrow has been reported to be 75% and does not alter the prognosis.[229] Other prognosis experience has been reported.[234,237-240]

Transformation is defined as the presence of large cells exceeding 25% and represents an evolution of the original clone. The risk of transformation has been reported to be 12% to 23%, with reported median times from diagnosis to transformation of 12 months to 6.5 years and a median survival of 19 months to 22 months.[230-232] Age and extracutaneous involvement were associated with a worse prognosis.[232]

The long-term survival of early stage MF approaches that of the normal population.[233-234] The 5-year relative survival of MF has gone from 68% between 1973 and 1977 to 80% between 1978 and 1992.[235]

Prognostic factors have been reported. The absence or presence of greater than 1000 Sézary cells and a CD4+/CD7– phenotype double the risk of death.[236] Other prognostic factors include age of 60 or older, elevated LDH, and a low percentage of CD8+ cells in the lymph node.[212,237] Modified staging systems will lead to new modifications but will be more biologically orientated and simpler.[238,239]

SECOND CANCERS

The Finnish Cancer Registry and others have reported an increased overall risk of lung cancer, small cell lung cancer, Hodgkin's lymphoma, and non-Hodgkin's lymphoma.[240,241]

CAUSE OF DEATH

The most common cause of death in CTCL is infection, the most common organisms of which are *Staphylococcus aureus,* Enterobacteriaceae, and *Pseudomonas aeruginosa.*[242,243] Disseminated herpes and fungal infections may occur in patients with advanced disease. Up to 47% of deaths are caused by cardiopulmonary disease or secondary malignancy.[6,243] Patients with cutaneous tumors and erythroderma characteristically die of complications of progressive disease.

THERAPY

Therapeutically, CTCL is similar to low-grade non-Hodgkin's lymphoma in that only limited stage disease is potentially curable, and the diseases are remarkably responsive to many different therapeutic modalities despite eventual relapse. Patients with either type of lymphoma may respond to the same therapeutic modality on more than one occasion, and they survive for years after the initial diagnosis. Advanced disease is rarely curable, and both CTCL and low-grade non-Hodgkin's lymphoma may transform into higher-grade lymphoproliferative disorders. In the absence of a therapeutic approach that leads to long-term disease-free remissions and cure, current therapies are tailored to the extent, burden, and type of disease present. The primary goals of treatment are to control the cutaneous disease, obtain symptomatic relief, and attain complete clinical remission.

Therapies available for the treatment of CTCL are wide ranging and illustrate the distinctive presentation and disease course of this type of lymphoproliferative disorder, as well as the unique challenges that face clinicians and therapists in treating and managing patients with CTCL. Therapies broadly include skin-directed, biologic response modifiers, and cytotoxic therapy. Therapeutic options include topical treatments with corticosteroids, chemotherapy (nitrogen mustard or BCNU), ultraviolet B (UVB) phototherapy, photochemotherapy with psoralen ultraviolet A (PUVA), radiation therapy with electron beam or photon irradiation, systemic chemotherapy with either single or multiple agents, and combined modality therapy incorporating chemotherapy, electron beam radiation therapy, or other combinations. Newer therapies include extracorporeal photochemotherapy (ECP), interferons, monoclonal antibody therapy, retinoids, and the purine analogs used either alone or in combination. Other drugs or therapies that have received more limited evaluation but have been reported to provide a clinical response in selected CTCL patients include cyclosporine, acyclovir, IL-12, and autologous bone marrow transplantation (ABMT). These and newer therapies such as denileukin diftitox and alemtuzumab are outlined in Table 113-6.

Factors other than disease stage that require consideration in the therapeutic management of CTCL patients include the general health and age of the patient, the availability of various therapeutic options, and the extent and aggressiveness of the disease. In the discussion of therapeutic results and toxicities, it must be recognized that many of the published studies of CTCL are not prospective randomized trials with control groups. As CTCL is an uncommon disease, multicenter cooperative clinical trials have been limited and consensus on staging, treatment responses, and the most effective therapies is neither well defined nor uniformly accepted. Table 113-7 details specific options for different stages of MF and Sézary syndrome.

General Skin Care Measures

Nonspecific topical treatment of mycosis fungoides and Sézary syndrome includes supportive therapies that

TABLE 113-6

Stage-specific Options for Cutaneous T-Cell Lymphoma

Patch, Limited and Generalized Plaque

Primary therapy
  Topical corticosteroids
  PUVA photochemotherapy
  UVB phototherapy
  Bexarotene gel or capsule
  Nitrogen mustard
  Electron beam
Secondary therapy
  BCNU (carmustine)
  Imiquimod
  High-intensity UVA1 phototherapy

Tumorous Disease

Primary Therapy
  CHOP
  Denileukin diftitox
  Bexarotene capsule
Secondary Therapy
  Radiation therapy
  Purine nucleoside analogs
  Alemtuzumab (anti-CD52)

Erythroderma-Sézary Syndrome

Primary Therapy
  Extracorporeal photopheresis (ECP)
  Interferon alpha
  Bexarotene
Secondary Therapy
  Denileukin diftitox
  Interleukin-12
  Purine nucleoside analogs
  Bone marrow transplantation

Extracutaneous Disease

Primary Therapy
  CHOP
  Denileukin diftitox
Secondary Therapy
  Purine nucleoside analogs
  Alemtuzumab (anti-CD52)
  Bone marrow transplantation

minimize skin irritation, provide lubrication and adequate hydration, and ameliorate inflammatory reactions of the skin that accompany CTCL. After the diagnosis of CTCL has been established with skin biopsy, low-potency and mid-potency topical corticosteroid creams or ointments may be used to control the symptoms of pruritus and dermatitis.[244] Topical corticosteroids should be avoided or discontinued for several weeks before skin biopsy because these agents suppress cutaneous inflammatory responses and can potentially mask the histopathologic features of CTCL. Regular soaking baths and application of a lubricating cream to maintain skin hydration are also beneficial. Prompt treatment of infected areas of skin and colonized or purulent ulcers minimizes the potential for the development of more serious infections.[243]

Topical Therapies

Topical Chemotherapy

Topical corticosteroids are a mainstay in the management of CTCL. Topical class I steroids applied twice daily for

TABLE 113-7

Therapeutic Options for Cutaneous T-Cell Lymphoma

Topical
  Corticosteroid
  Nitrogen mustard
  BCNU (carmustine)
  Bexarotene gel
  Imiquimod
Ultraviolet B phototherapy
PUVA photochemotherapy
High-intensity UVA1 phototherapy
Photodynamic therapy (PDT)—5-ALA
Radiotherapy with electron beam
Photon irradiation
Single chemotherapy
  Single agents
    Low-dose
      Methotrexate
      Chlorambucil
    Standard
Combination chemotherapy
Combined-modality therapy
Extracorporeal phototherapy (ECP)
Cytokines
  Interferons
  Interleukin-12
  Thymopentin
Monoclonal antibody therapy
  Alemtuzumab (anti-CD52)
  Anti-CD4
Retinoids
  Isotretinoin
  Acitretin
  Bexarotene
Purine nucleoside analogs
  2′-deoxycoformycin (pentostatin)
  Fludarabine
  2-chlorodeoxyadenosine (cladrabine)
  Gemcitabine
Immunotoxins
  IL-2 fusion toxin (denileukin diftitox)
  Pseudomonas immunotoxin anti-Tac(Fv)-PE38 (LMB-2)
Depsipeptide (FR901228)-histone deactylase inhibitor
Vaccination-immunotherapy
Bone marrow transplantation
  Autologous
  Allogeneic

2 to 3 months are effective in MF plaque- and patch-stage disease and likely effect apoptosis. Skin atrophy and adrenal suppression are complications. In a series of 79 patients with a median follow-up of 9 months, 63% of patients achieved a complete remission and 31% a partial remission.[245]

Nitrogen mustard (mechlorethamine hydrochloride, HN2) was the first topical agent with demonstrated efficacy in CTCL.[216] Since its initial clinical use during the late 1940s at the Mayo Clinic, this alkylating drug has proved effective in controlling the progression and symptoms of cutaneous lesions of CTCL. The agent undergoes rapid degradation to an active ethylenimonium ion that has high antimitotic activity and a half-life of less than 10 minutes. Nitrogen mustard may be prepared and applied in several different ways. It is soluble in water and typically formulated at a concentration of 10 to 20 mg/dL. Alternatively, an alcoholic extract of nitrogen mustard can be suspended in an oil-water base such as aquaphor. This preparation is more stable than the solution in water and is estimated to remain active for longer than 1 month. Nitrogen mustard is routinely applied to the entire skin surface, except the eyelids, genitalia, rectum, and intertriginous areas where irritation limits its use. Application of the solution is performed daily by painting the skin with a soaked gauze or sponge or by applying the ointment. This may be increased to twice a day or the concentration can be doubled. The initial treatment program lasts 6 to 12 months, and maintenance therapy 3 times per week is continued for 1 to 2 years or longer. The agent does not cause cytopenias or secondary leukemias because it is not absorbed systemically. It is an efficient and conservative outpatient program in patients without large tumors or systemic involvement of disease.

Nitrogen mustard has been evaluated in several clinical series.[246-250] Vonderheid and colleagues reported on 324 patients with CTCL, with complete remission rates of 80% in stage IA disease, 68% in stage IB, 61% in stage IIA, 49% in stage IIB, and 60% in stage III.[249] Twenty percent of patients had complete remission of 4 years or more, and 11% had continuous complete remission. Other therapy was used in many patients, including local radiation, electron beam radiation therapy, psoralen ultraviolet A (PUVA), ultraviolet B (UVB) phototherapy, and chemotherapy. None of the 34 patients who were in long-term complete remission received electron beam radiation therapy or phototherapy, but nine patients received chemotherapy, including intravenous administration of methotrexate and nitrogen mustard. Therapy was discontinued within 6 months of complete remission in 10 of 34 patients who did not experience a relapse after 8 years.

Ramsay and colleagues reported on 117 CTCL patients who received treatment with nitrogen mustard.[248] These investigators found that the probability of achieving complete remission at 2 years for stage I disease was 75.8%; for stage II, 44.6%; and for stage III, 48.6%. The median time to complete remission was approximately 11 months. After therapy was discontinued and relapse occurred, a second complete remission was attained in 21 of 29 patients. Radiation therapy was the only other therapy given in this series.

Hoppe and colleagues reported on 123 patients who received an ointment-based nitrogen mustard in aquaphor or polyethylene gel with complete remission rates in T1 disease of 51%; T2, 26%; T3, 0%; and T4, 22%.[247] These patients received no other therapy. In 54% of the patients with relapse, complete remission was achieved with a second course. The freedom from relapse was 11%, and no relapse occurred after 8 years. This experience was updated.[250]

The treatment durations varied in these series. Hoppe and colleagues recommended treatment for 1 to 2 years after achieving a response. Ramsay and colleagues treated for 6 months after clearing and tapering over 1.5 years, and Vonderheid recommended only 6 months of therapy. Topical nitrogen mustard is effective in early plaque/patch disease. In all three of these reports, the earlier the stage at which patients began topical therapy, the greater the likelihood of remission.

The major toxic reaction of nitrogen mustard is allergic contact dermatitis that occurs in 35% to 67% of patients.[247-257,250] Patients can be desensitized.[256] Ointment-based preparations have a lower frequency of hypersensitivity.[247,255,257] Alternatively, the incidence may be decreased to less than 10% with nitrogen mustard dissolved in ointment. The response rates and relapse rates are similar for aqueous and ointment preparations. Avoidance of skin exposure to sunlight is recommended. Other toxic reactions include dry skin, irritant dermatitis, hyperpigmentation, bullous reactions, urticaria, Stevens-Johnson Syndrome, and telangiectasias.[247,251,258] There is an increased risk in the secondary tumors of squamous cell carcinoma and basal cell carcinoma.[247,249,251,258] However, most patients received multiple other therapies. In the Hoppe series, only 1 of 14 patients who were treated with nitrogen mustard alone developed a secondary cutaneous malignancy. Adverse outcomes of family members and health-care workers exposed to topical agents have not been documented. There are no available randomized comparative trials with adequate numbers of patients evaluating topical therapy versus other therapeutic modalities.

Carmustine (BCNU) applied at daily doses of 10 to 20 mg per day for 4 to 8 weeks is the other main drug used in the topical management of CTCL.[259-260] Zackheim and colleagues reported on 143 patients with complete remission rates for stage IA disease of 86%; stage IB, 47%; stage IIA, 55%; stage IIB, 17%; stage III, 21%; and stage IV, 0%.[260] Complete remission rates, relapse rates, and 5-year survival rates were similar to those for nitrogen mustard. In contrast to nitrogen mustard, bone marrow suppression occurred in 7.4% of patients treated with a 10- to 25-mg/day dose of BCNU for 3 to 17 weeks. Hypersensitivity reactions were observed in only 7% of patients. Chronic skin telangiectasias may occur.

Topical bexarotene 1% gel applied twice daily is the first synthetic retinoid approved by the FDA in the United States. For CTCL, the complete remission rates are 21% to 23% and overall response rates are 63%. The median time to progression was 149 days (range, 52 to 342 days).[261,262] The response rate was reported to be 45% at a 300 mg/m^2/day dose schedule in a series of 94 patients.[263] Rash was reported in 56% of patients and pruritus in 18%. The most frequent side effects are hypertriglyceridemia, pancreatitis, hypercholesterolemia, hypothyroidism, and headaches. Bexarotene induces apoptosis in CTCL.[264]

Other topical agents that have been evaluated include cytarabine, dianhydrogalactitol, dacarbazine, guanazole, teniposide, hydroxyurea, thiotepa, and methotrexate.[265,266]

Ultraviolet B Phototherapy and Ultraviolet A Photochemotherapy

Ultraviolet B (UVB) phototherapy has been used for years in the treatment of early patch-stage CTCL and the premalignant dermatosis, large-plaque parapsoriasis. This treatment is administered three times per week. A retrospective study has supported the clinical observations that UVB phototherapy provides favorable responses for clinical remission and lasting improvement in early

patch-stage CTCL.[267] UVB penetrates only the epidermis and the superficial dermis, however, and has no effect on more indurated plaque-stage or extensive forms of CTCL. UVB phototherapy in patients with darkly pigmented skin is less effective because melanin absorbs the ultraviolet radiation.[268] UVB phototherapy has a tendency to aggravate the erythroderma and pruritus of Sézary syndrome and should be avoided.

Treatment of CTCL with psoralen ultraviolet A (PUVA) with 8-methoxypsoralen preparations administered orally has been shown to be effective in the control of early disease. 8-Methoxypsoralen is a member of a family of photoactivated compounds that inhibit DNA synthesis through the formation of monofunctional or bifunctional adducts and crosslinks of nucleic acids resulting in apoptotic cell death.[269-270] PUVA has other biologic effects that may contribute to the responses in CTCL, including direct cytotoxic, anti-inflammatory, and immunomodulatory reactions.

Several formulations of 8-methoxypsoralen have been available. A dose of 0.6 mg/kg of 8-methoxypsoralen is given 2 hours before UVA treatment, or an encapsulated liquid form (Oxsoralen Ultra or Uvadex) is ingested 1 hour before treatment. The main toxicity is nausea and vomiting, which may be avoided by using 5-methoxypsoralen.[271] This drug is contraindicated in liver disease. The patient is then exposed to UVA lamps, which emit long UV (A-band) radiation in the wavelength range of 320 to 400 nm. An initial dose of 0.5 to 1.0 J/cm^3 that can be increased slowly with each treatment is administered three times per week. UV-protective eyeglasses are worn for 24 hours after treatment. This therapy is usually three times per week for 3 to 6 months followed by tapering.

The tissue containing the psoralen must be irradiated with UVA for a photodynamic reaction to develop. After the initial report by Gilchrest and colleagues,[272] multiple trials on the efficacy of PUVA in early-stage disease have been reported.[273-279]

In the series by Roenigk and colleagues with a mean follow-up of 45 months, 82% of patients had complete clearing of limited plaque disease, with 88% remaining in remission for a median duration of 13 months.[280] Of the patients with extensive plaque disease, 51.9% had complete clearing for a mean duration of 11 months, and no clearing was attained in patients with tumor-stage or nodal-stage disease. In erythrodermic CTCL, 46% of cases had clearing of the disease, but 75% had relapse. Hönigsmann and colleagues reported no recurrences in 55.6% of patients with stage IA disease and 38.5% of those with stage IIB.[281] Patients received no maintenance therapy and were followed for a mean of 44 months.

PUVA has been combined with topical nitrogen mustard, retinoids, aerosolized granulocyte-macrophage colony-stimulating factor, and interferon alfa-2a.[282-287] Retinoids have been reported to decrease the number of PUVA treatments and total UVA dose.[283] The total response rate in 39 patients with MF was 90% (62% complete remissions and 28% partial remissions) with a median response duration of 28 months. Eighty-three percent of patients (25 of 30) evaluated retrospectively achieved a complete remission after a median of 5 months treatment and median remission of 22 months with low-dose interferon alfa-2a.[287]

Contraindications to ultraviolet radiation therapy include systemic lupus erythematosus, skin cancer, porphyria, and genetic syndromes secondary to DNA repair defects.[271] Toxic reactions from PUVA therapy include nausea, vomiting, pruritus, erythema, xerosis, dry skin, blistering, and burns. Other less common or potential side effects include development of pigmented melanocytic macules of the skin, nail pigmentation, and cataract formation.[288-291] UV light blocking glasses should be worn for 24 hours after psoralen is administered. Long-term toxic reactions of more concern include squamous cell carcinoma of the skin or genitalia, photoaging, and amyloid deposition in the skin.[290,292-294]

Electron Beam Radiation Therapy

Electron beam radiation therapy was first used for malignant cutaneous lesions in 1953 and has been advocated for treatment of CTCL with both limited and extensive cutaneous involvement.[295] Electrons are delivered to a depth of several millimeters to 1 cm. Several series have been reported.[296-304]

Early experiences of the Stanford group suggested that complete clinical responses were high and long-lasting. Subsequent reports from this group—summarizing 192 patients receiving treatment with total skin electron beam between 1966 and 1987 to a total dose of more than 2000 cGy—showed complete remission rates in limited-plaque disease (T1) of 98% with a freedom from relapse of 50%; generalized plaque disease (T2), 71% with a freedom from relapse of 20%; tumor-stage disease, 36%; and erythroderma, 64%, with most relapses occurring in 5 years. The 10-year survival rate was 46%.[304] Others have reported an overall survival rate of 70%.[300-301] The total dose is usually 3000 to 3600 cGy delivered over 8 to 10 weeks of treatment.[296,301,304] The toxic reactions include desquamative skin reactions of the feet and toes, erythema, blister formation, exfoliation, dryness, extensive alopecia with eventual recovery, temporary nail loss, inability to sweat because of loss of sweat glands, hyperpigmentation, and telangiectasias.[300-304] The increased risk of squamous and basal cell carcinomas focuses in particular on those patients who have received multiple therapies, including irradiation, topical nitrogen mustard, and PUVA.[305] Most patients are treated with only a single course of this treatment. One study of 15 patients who were retreated, however, reported six complete remissions and eight partial remissions.[306] Adjuvant therapy may be utilized to decrease the risk of relapse with nitrogen mustard, PUVA, or extracorporeal photochemotherapy.[307]

Extracorporeal Photochemotherapy

Extracorporeal photochemotherapy (ECP), or photopheresis, is a systemic form of PUVA which combines leukapheresis with photochemotherapy. Early apheresis approaches to remove circulating Sézary cells in Sézary syndrome and therapeutic benefits derived from tradi-

tional PUVA photochemotherapy suggested that these two therapies could be used simultaneously to direct treatment to circulating lymphoid cell populations. The biologic mechanisms that mediate clinical responses to ECP in CTCL are not clearly defined. Direct effects on DNA synthesis and membrane alterations induced by psoralens and UVA may cause cytotoxicity, but the immunomodulatory effects and possible induction of immune responses to the malignant lymphoid cell population may also explain the clinical responses observed in treating CTCL with ECP.[308-310] The ECP process induces an anti-idiotypic cytotoxic T-cell response against circulating CTCL cells that subsequently undergo apoptosis. Patients ingest 8-methoxypsoralen and then undergo leukapheresis and cell separation. Cells of the mononuclear fraction are exposed to ultraviolet (UVA) radiation from lamps housed ex vivo in the apheresis device followed by reinfusion of the treated cells. This results in DNA crosslinking, apoptosis, and cell death. Activation of dendritic cells may stimulate antitumor CD8+ T-cells.[311] The process is usually performed on two consecutive days every 4 weeks.

The initial report by Edelson and colleagues demonstrated that 27 of 37 patients with resistant or refractory CTCL had a positive response, as manifested by a greater than 25% skin improvement.[312] Nine patients had complete or nearly complete responses. Eight of 10 patients had nodal involvement, and 24 of 29 had generalized erythroderma. Three of eight patients with extensive plaque disease had a positive response. Long-term follow-up evaluation of patients with CTCL treated with photopheresis revealed a median survival with erythroderma from diagnosis of 60.3 months, and a median survival from onset of treatment of 47.9 months. Complete remissions were observed in 6 of 29 patients (21%), and long-term complete remissions were observed in 4 patients, with the best responses in patients with lower CD4/CD8 ratios.[313] Clinical indications for favorable ECP are patients with erythrodermic CTCL or Sézary syndrome, patients with less than 2 years of widespread disease, and patients with near-normal CD8 cell counts.[310] Significant beneficial responses to photopheresis have not been demonstrated in patients with patch/plaque-stage or tumor-stage mycosis fungoides or with advanced CTCL, but this treatment may prolong remission in patients who had previously received radiation therapy.[314-316] After a minimum of six cycles of ECP, photopheresis is continued through clearing and for approximately 6 additional months of treatment.[312,314,315] A higher baseline lymphocyte count and a higher absolute Sézary cell count were associated with a decrease in skin score and response after 6 months.[317] Toxic reactions include nausea, fever, occasional erythematous flares after reinfusion, and hypotension during leukapheresis. Venous access has been a problem in some patients, requiring placement of indwelling central catheters. Septicemia has also developed in some patients; it is likely related to the immunocompromised state associated with CTCL and the propensity for infectious complications

Other series have confirmed the efficacy of ECP in CTCL.[318-320] Response rates have ranged from 54% to 75%, with 15% to 25% of patients achieving a complete response, but others have reported lower response rates.[321] In addition, concomitant or adjuvant therapies have been introduced. Low-dose methotrexate given orally was added to the photopheresis program of eight patients.[322] Five of eight patients who did not have a response to photopheresis alone had a response to this combined regimen. The maximum dose of methotrexate was 15 mg three times a month.[322] Studies have reported on combined interferon and extracorporeal photopheresis at doses of 3 million to 12 million units per day.[323-325] Combined immunomodulatory therapies are being evaluated.[326]

Interferons

Interferon (IFN) alfa (2a or 2b) has significant activity in mycosis fungoides and Sézary syndrome. Bunn and colleagues initially reported on 20 patients with advanced disease who were previously treated but no longer responsive to standard therapies.[321,327] Nine patients (45%) responded: three had complete remissions and six had partial remissions. The median duration of response was 5.5 months. The maximum tolerated dose of IFN-alfa-2a in this trial was 50×10^6 IU IM three times a week. The toxic reactions were significant because of the high doses administered. Kohn and colleagues treated 24 patients with refractory disease at a dose of 10×10^6 IU/m^2 on day 1, followed by 50×10^6 IU/m^2 on days 2 to 5 every 3 weeks, with a response rate of 29% and a median duration of remission of 8 months.[328]

The antitumor activity of IFN-alfa-2a at doses of 36×10^6 IU was been confirmed.[329-331] Olsen and colleagues attempted to compare treatment with low doses of 3×10^6 IU with escalating doses up to 36 million IU, but low accrual prevented completion.[332] However, the objective response rate was 11 of 14 (64%) in patients receiving high doses versus 3 of 8 in patients receiving low doses. The small sample populations prevented assessment of dose and clinical response. The optimal dose of recombinant IFN-alfa in the treatment of CTCL has not been determined. The overall response rates appear to be 60%.[333]

Intralesional interferon has been evaluated for the management of local skin involvement with CTCL. Injections with IFN-alfa-2a at a dose of 2×10^6 IU three times daily for 4 weeks cleared three of nine lesions and improved six of nine.[334] Injections with IFN-alfa-2b three times daily for 4 weeks at a dose of 1×10^6 IU resulted in complete clinical regression in 10 of 12 patients who received the drug compared with 1 of 12 lesions treated with placebo.[335]

Recombinant IFN-alfa is not currently approved for CTCL by the U.S. Food and Drug Administration (FDA). This limits the use of a drug that appears to offer significant activity in both early and advanced CTCL. The toxicity associated with IFN-alfa at a dose of 3 to 7.5×10^6 IU SC either daily or three times a week is not significant. The suggested initial dose is 3 million IU administered three times per week since no dose-response data has been demonstrated.[321] Initially, fever and chills develop with the first three doses, but then resolve. Leukopenia occurs early in the first 3 months of therapy but is usually of no clinical significance. Patients may experience chronic fatigue while receiving recombinant IFN-alfa therapy.

Systemic Chemotherapy

Chemotherapy administered orally or parenterally either as single or combined agents is utilized in patients with CTCL in whom refractory disease has developed, patients who have relapsed, and in patients who have transformed histologically. Patients with extracutaneous or extranodal disease and those enrolled in clinical trials have also received systemic chemotherapy.[336-351]

Results of chemotherapy trials have been reviewed.[4,5] Bunn reported on 528 patients treated with different single-agent chemotherapy regimens with a complete response rate of 32% and an objective response rate of 62%. The median duration of response ranged from 3 to 22 months. With combination chemotherapy, the complete remission rate in 331 total patients was 38%, with an overall response rate of 81%. The response duration was 5 to 41 months. The median duration of response was less than 1 year, however. The single agents evaluated included alkylating agents, methotrexate, cisplatin, etoposide, bleomycin, doxorubicin, vincristine, vinblastine, and oral corticosteroids. The regimen most commonly used for Sézary syndrome (erythrodermic CTCL) is oral chlorambucil and prednisone administered daily. Moderate doses of methotrexate (60 to 240 mg/m^2), followed by leucovorin calcium given orally, produced complete remission in 7 of 11 patients and partial remission in 2 of 11.[246] After this regimen, patients received maintenance doses of methotrexate orally for 6 to 30 months. A common intravenous regimen is the combination of cyclophosphamide, vincristine, and prednisone (CVP); doxorubicin (Adriamycin) added to CVP (CHOP); methotrexate; or occasionally other agents. A series of favorable clinical responses was reported by Zakem and colleagues.[255] Seven of 10 patients who received bleomycin, doxorubicin, methotrexate, and topical nitrogen mustard had complete remission with a median duration of 19 months. Three young splenectomized patients with stage IV disease had a continuous complete remission for more than 3 years. Gemcitabine at a dose of 1200 mg/m^2 on days 1, 8, and 15 of a 28-day cycle for 3 cycles is active in previously treated patients.[352] Pegylated doxorubicin resulted in a complete remission in 6 patients and partial remission in 2 patients in 10 treated patients with a response duration of 15 months.[353]

Valid interpretation of the efficacy of chemotherapy in treatment of CTCL is not possible, and the current role of this therapy in the management of CTCL compared with that of other therapies is difficult to determine. In published studies, patients had received multiple and variable previous treatments; the series have reported small numbers of patients; stage of disease was not reported; various stages of CTCL were included; pathologic documentation of extracutaneous disease was often lacking; and studies often combined patients with either MF or Sézary syndrome. No clinical trial has clearly demonstrated benefit to survival in patients receiving aggressive versus palliative treatment. Therefore more aggressive systemic chemotherapy should be reserved for clinical studies or should be used after topical regimens have failed or other therapies (e.g., photopheresis or interferon) no longer provide benefit.

Purine Nucleoside Analogs

The purine nucleoside analogs have been evaluated in several clinical trials of CTCL. This class of drugs includes deoxycoformycin or pentostatin, fludarabine, and cladribine. These agents are adenosine deaminase inhibitors. Their mechanism of action is different from that of other chemotherapeutic regimens. Grever and colleagues initially reported complete remissions in two of four patients treated with pentostatin.[354] In a follow-up trial of 19 patients conducted by Ho and colleagues, there was one complete remission and four partial remissions.[355] In an Eastern Cooperative Oncology Group trial, four of eight patients with CTCL had a partial remission. Of 94 patients treated with single agent pentostatin in five phase II studies, the complete remission rate was 7% with an overall response rate of 40% and a median time to progression of 1.3 to 8.3 months.[357] The Southwestern Oncology Group reported on 33 patients who received fludarabine, one of whom had complete remission; the overall response rate was 19%.[358] At 4-week intervals, cladribine is administered in a 7-day continuous intravenous infusion at a dose of 0.1 mg/kg daily. Saven and colleagues reported on six patients with mycosis fungoides and three with Sézary syndrome.[359] Of the patients with MF, one had complete remission of 1.5 months' duration and two had partial remission. No patient with Sézary syndrome had either partial or complete remission. Pancytopenia developed in two-thirds of cases. Myelosuppression with significant leukopenia and thrombocytopenia in CTCL was more common in the patients with MF and SS than in those with peripheral T-cell non-Hodgkin's lymphoma. Disseminated candidiasis developed in one patient with Sézary syndrome. Kuzel and colleagues reported on 12 patients with MF and SS who received cladribine.[360] Two of these patients achieved complete remission and two had partial remission. After a median of two cycles, four patients had significant neutropenia and one had significant thrombocytopenia that required transfusion. Future trials evaluating these agents in combination with other agents may result in higher response rates. Combination therapy with pentostatin and IFN-alfa-2a in a trial of 41 patients resulted in two complete remissions and 15 partial remissions with no responses in patients with visceral disease.[361]

Vitamin A Analogs

Retinoids are derivatives of vitamin A that have been reported to be effective in CTCL. Isotretinoin (Accutane) and acitretin (Soriatane) have moderate activity. Of 25 patients with stage T2 or greater disease, 11 (44%) had a response to isotretinoin (13-cisretinoic acid), with a median duration of 8 months.[362] The responses were only partial because three complete clinical responses showed histologic evidence of residual disease. The initial dose of 1 mg/kg/day orally was often altered because of mucocutaneous drying and irritation. An additional report confirmed the clinical activity of this drug.[362] A trial with the arotinoid Ro 13-6298 at a dose of 0.3 mg/day in five patients with refractory advanced CTCL showed one complete response and three objective responses.[364-365] As single agents, retinoids have limited clinical use. Side effects with larger doses of medication, including dry mucous membranes, skin fragility, arthralgias, myalgias, headache, fatigue, and increased levels of triglycerides, make this drug intolerable for most patients. A summary of the results of multiple studies suggests that the complete remission rate was 19% and the overall response rate was 58%.

Monoclonal Antibodies

Murine monoclonal antibodies (mAbs) have been used as unaltered immunoglobulin, conjugated to toxins or radioisotopes, or modified as chimeric antibodies. Each form has been used in the treatment of CTCL.[333,366-368] The responses were transient and minor. In 1981, Miller and Levy reported the clinical use of a murine hybridoma monoclonal anti-T-cell antibody directed against the Leu-1 determinate of mature human T cells in CTCL.[366] Of seven patients, five showed partial remission of short duration, and in four of the seven patients human antimouse immunoglobulin antibodies also developed accompanied by a relapse of the disease. Subsequent antibodies have been developed, including a chimeric murine/human anti-CD4 antibody. The use of antibodies to direct toxic or radioactive therapies has potential advantages and has been examined in CTCL.[369-371]

Anti-CD52 monoclonal antibody, alemtuzumab (Campath-1H) treatment has been reported.[372-374] In one series, this agent produced a complete remission rate of 23% with a higher response rate in erythroderma (59% overall response rate) than plaque or skin tumors (40% overall response rate) and a median time to treatment failure of 12 months.[374] 90Y-T101 treatment resulted in partial remissions in three of eight patients.[375,376] 90Y anti-CD25 and anti-Tac pseudomonas exotoxin immunoconjugates have been reported.[377]

Issues with monoclonal antibody therapy include: (1) the development of a host response and production of antibodies; (2) the evolution of malignant clones of cells that downregulate or no longer express the specific antigen to which the antibody binds; (3) myelosuppression and radiation injury of organs in which the conjugated antibodies localize or concentrate; and (4) hepatotoxicity or fluid retention caused by toxins released from the conjugated antibodies. Other reported side effects include fever, malaise, pruritus, urticaria, and dyspnea.

Bone Marrow Transplantation

Bone marrow transplantation has been evaluated in the therapy for advanced CTCL. Bigler and associates reported on six patients who underwent an autologous bone marrow transplant for refractory advanced CTCL.[378] Five of the six patients responded, but three of these responses lasted less than 100 days. Two patients received treatment with a preparatory regimen of carmustine, etoposide, and cisplatin and were alive without evidence of active disease at more than 1 year after transplantation. Nine patients were reported who were treated with a T-cell depleted peripheral blood stem cell transplant.[379] Seven patients relapsed at a median of 7 months (range 2 to 14 months), one patient did not engraft, and one patient died of sepsis. Allogeneic bone marrow transplantation has been reported with 3 patients alive and disease free 15 months to 4.5 years.[380,381] Another patient relapsed after allogeneic bone marrow transplantation but went into remission after withdrawal of cyclosporine.[382]

Interleukins and Recombinant Fusion Proteins

Bioactive recombinant interleukins and other cytokines have favorable prospects in the treatment of CTCL. Recombinant IL-2 was administered in four patients. All the patients had a response, and two of them had a complete response.[383] Approximately one half of patients with MF/SS have Il-2 receptors. An IL-2 genetically engineered fusion protein that is a hybrid of IL-2 and diphtheria toxin was developed, $DAB_{486}IL-2$.[384] Initial response rates were 21%. A smaller fusion protein was developed, $DAB_{389}IL-2$. A multi-institution trial reported responses in 13 of 35 IL-2 expressing MF patients.[385] The recombinant DNA-derived cytotoxic protein (ONTAK, Seragen) composed of the amino acid sequences for diphtheria toxin fragments A and B (Met_1-Thr_{387}) followed by the sequences for IL-2 ($IL-2; Ala_1-Thr_{133}$) administered intravenously at a dose of 9 or 18 mcg/kg/day for 5 days every 21 days is FDA approved. A randomized, double-blind study of 71 patients reported an objective response rate of 30% (10% complete remission, 20% partial remission). CD25 expression of greater than or equal to 20% of lymphocytes was required.[386] The median response was 6.9 months (range, 2.7 to 46.1 months). Side effects included flulike symptoms, acute infusion-related events (hypotension, chest pain, and back pain), vascular leak syndrome, elevated liver function tests (61%), and hypoalbuminemia (79%).

Other Therapies

Other biologic factors and pharmacologic agents have been tested and reported in CTCL in an attempt to identify better and safer therapies. One such therapy is antithymocyte globulin, administered in advanced mycosis fungoides and Sézary syndrome, for which it has produced transient responses.[387] Cyclosporine, the T-cell-selective immunosuppressant, has been reported to induce occasional brief responses in selected patients with CTCL, usually in earlier stages.[388,389] Cyclosporine may accelerate later stage disease. Acyclovir, the antiviral agent, has been reported to induce remission in tumor-stage mycosis fungoides when administered parentally.[390-392]

Combined Modality Therapy

Investigators have developed treatment regimens by combining two or more therapies to improve the results obtained with single agents. The various treatment programs developed include chemotherapy plus radiation therapy, chemotherapy plus radiation therapy followed by topical treatments, and recombinant IFN-alfa in combination with other topical or systemic treatments. Thus combined modality therapy has come to identify treatment programs beyond those of chemotherapy and radiation therapy alone. Some of these approaches have already been outlined in this chapter.

Griem and colleagues in 1979 reported on the combination of electron beam radiation therapy and local radiation therapy followed by combination chemotherapy in a nonrandomized pilot study and suggested that survival and remission duration might be improved.[393] The initial results have been updated.[394] An early difference in response rate and disease-free survival was noted in the group treated with combination therapy, but the number of patients was small. The 10-year follow-up results were reported for 21 patients treated with 3200 to 4000 cGy total skin electron beam irradiation followed by six monthly cycles of chemotherapy with COPP or MOPP. The complete response rate was 52% with a median disease-free survival of 12 months. All patients with plaque CTCL had relapse within 25 months and were subsequently managed with chemotherapy, PUVA, and topical nitrogen mustard. The 10-year survival rate was 40%. Braverman and colleagues at Yale reported on 50 nonrandomized patients who received total skin electron beam irradiation followed by combination chemotherapy with doxorubicin and cyclophosphamide.[395] The complete remission rate was 88%. Early-stage CTCL treated with combination chemotherapy had a significant increase in the duration of complete remission. There was no difference in advanced disease, however. Those patients in clinical remission frequently had karyotypic abnormalities in the peripheral blood. Skin biopsy also showed nonspecific inflammatory changes, but CTCL could not be confirmed.

Winkler and colleagues reported on 39 patients who received combined modality therapy.[396] Thirteen patients with stage I disease were given 3000 cGY total skin electron beam radiation therapy, followed by mechlorethamine administered intravenously. Twenty-six patients with stage II to IV disease received 2400 cGy total skin electron beam irradiation, followed by vinblastine, doxorubicin, and bleomycin given intravenously alternating with oral cyclophosphamide, methotrexate, and prednisone given orally every 3 weeks. With a median follow-up of 5 years, the disease-free survival in patients with stage I was greater, with 7 of 13 (54%) remaining disease free, than in patients with stage II to IV disease, only 20% of whom were disease free.

The first randomized clinical trial of 103 patients compared conservative sequential topical therapy with total electron beam radiation therapy.[397] Patients of all stages were eligible, and there were no restrictions on performance status. The sequential topical regimen was initiated with topical nitrogen mustard and was changed to PUVA if progression of CTCL or toxicity to topical nitrogen mustard occurred. For continued disease progression, the patient received total skin electron beam radiation therapy, followed by methotrexate given orally. If extracutaneous disease developed, systemic chemotherapy was administered. The combined therapy regimen consisted of 3000 cGy total skin electron beam radiation therapy, followed by cyclophosphamide, doxorubicin, etoposide, and vincristine administered intravenously. After a median follow-up of 75 months, the only significant difference was the complete remission rates of the two groups, 38% in the combined modality group and 10% in the topical group. No statistical difference was observed in the disease-free survival or overall survival as a group or by stage for the two arms. Toxicity was greater in the combined modality group and included myelosuppression, radiodermatitis, neuropathy, and congestive heart failure. Less than 10% of patients in both groups remained disease free.

Since these trials, newer agents have been incorporated into combined modality approaches. In a combined program using IFN-alfa with cisretinoic acid for 4 months, chemotherapy consisting of cyclophosphamide, methothrexate, etoposide, and decadron alternating with Adriamycin, bleomycin, and vinblastine followed electron beam therapy in stage III and IV patients with the same regimen in stage I and II patients without chemotherapy, the complete remission rate was 71% with a median failure-free survival of 8 months.[398] Combined modality therapy may offer the greatest promise for effective therapy in CTCL, because the other more traditional therapies that have been successfully implemented for other types of malignant lymphomas have proved less effective in the treatment or cure of CTCL.

PRIMARY CUTANEOUS B-CELL LYMPHOMA

Primary cutaneous B-cell lymphomas (PCBCLs) may compose up to 20% of cutaneous lymphomas (Figure 113-10).[399] This group of disorders must be distinguished from pseudolymphoma.[400] The major WHO histologic types include lymphoblastic lymphoma (<10%), follicular lymphoma, diffuse large B-cell lymphoma, and intravascular lymphoma.[22,401] Primary cutaneous follicular lymphoma may compose up to 39% of cases.[402] Primary cutaneous marginal zone lymphomas occur most commonly in sun-exposed areas and in females and account for 25% of the primary cutaneous B-cell lymphomas.[403] Primary cutaneous diffuse large B-cell lymphoma is the most common, comprising 34% to 46% of PCBCL cases.[402,404,405] The 5-year overall survival rate is over 90% with a relapse-free 4-year survival of 74%.[404] The location of diffuse large B-cell lymphoma (DLBCL) may be important. Primary cutaneous diffuse large cell lymphoma of the leg is more aggressive with a 5-year survival rate reported to be 58%. Multiagent chemotherapy is the treatment of choice.[405,406] Multicentric cutaneous large cell lymphoma with no other evidence of

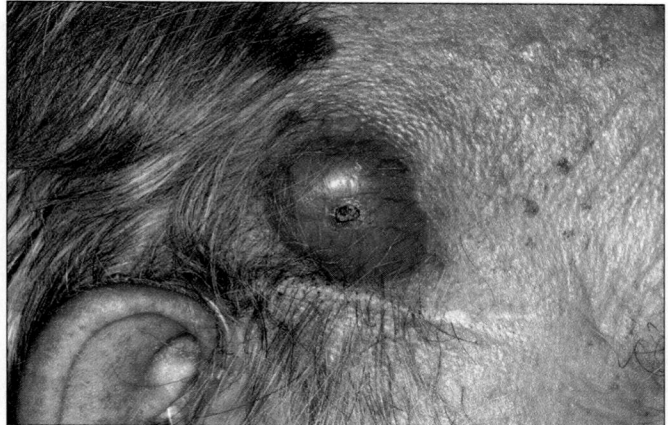

A

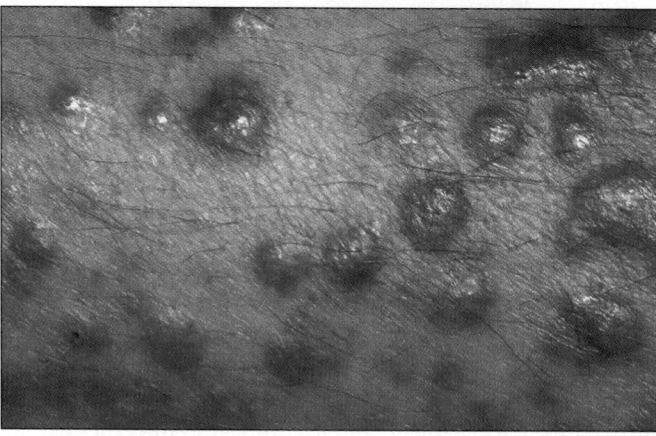

B

Figure 113-10. A, Unicentric cutaneous B-cell lymphoma (diffuse large B-cell lymphoma). **B,** Multicentric disseminated cutaneous B-cell lymphoma (diffuse large B-cell lymphoma).

disease has a poor prognosis if treated with local radiation therapy (Figure 113-11).[407]

This may be more important than the location on the leg. Intravascular large B-cell lymphomas are an aggressive subtype of extranodal DLBCL in the WHO classification and a provisional entity in the EORTC classification.

From a therapeutic intervention perspective, follicular and MALT-type PCBCLs that are stage IAE are usually treated with local radiation therapy. Diffuse large B-cell PCBCL that is stage IAE is treated either with CHOP chemotherapy for three cycles followed by radiation therapy versus radiation therapy alone (Table 113-8).[407-411] Future understanding of the biology of this disease will alter therapeutic approaches and will further refine the WHO and EORTC classifications.

CONCLUSION

Most patients with cutaneous lymphoma are not cured. Progress has been made in the classification of CTCL and PCBCL, and the characterization of the relationship of

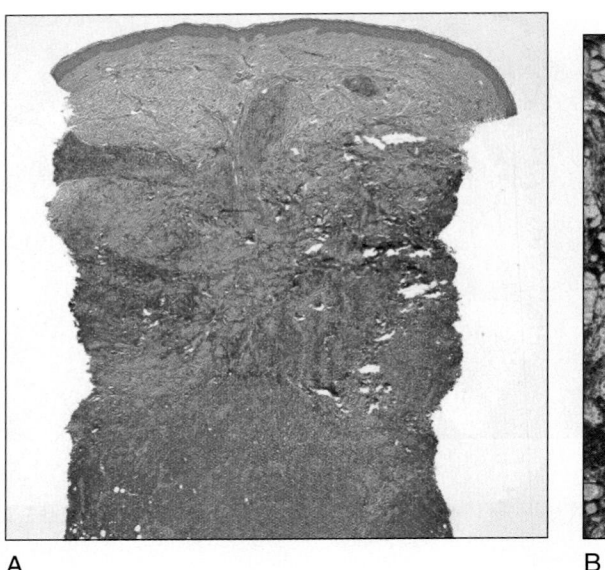

A

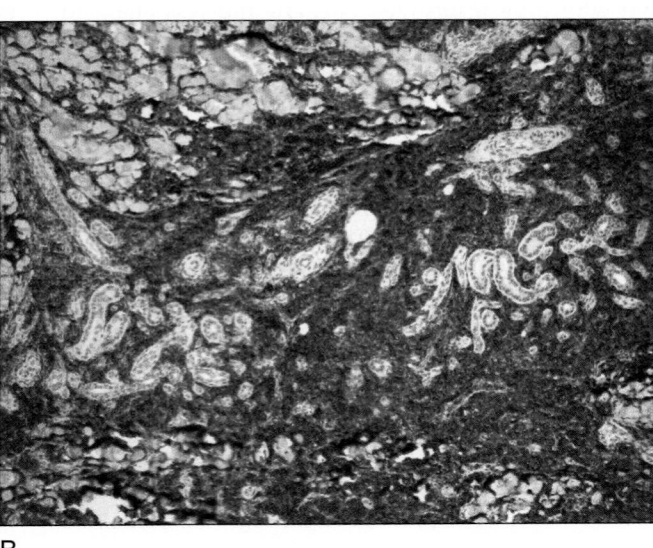

B

Figure 113-11. A, H&E stain of cutaneous B-cell lymphoma. **B,** CD20 stain of cutaneous B-cell lymphoma.

mycosis fungoides, Sézary syndrome, and other pre-malignant or associated conditions with CTCL and cutaneous B-cell lymphoma, and the understanding of the pathology of CTCL in skin, blood, or other organs and tissues. Survival and relapse data in CTCL have different implications for topical therapy and systemic therapy in this chronic disease. Recent advances in immunobiology, cell biology, and molecular biology have further identified and defined the malignant lymphoid population involved in CTCL and the mechanisms by which these cells may interact with skin and manifest the clinical features of CTCL. Although molecular genetic studies may provide an early diagnosis, early therapy has not been clearly shown to be beneficial. It is anticipated that with continued advances in our understanding of the pathobiology of CTCL and with the uncovering of potential targets in this disease, new therapeutic interventions will markedly improve the survival of patients with cutaneous B-cell lymphoma and CTCL.

TABLE 113-8

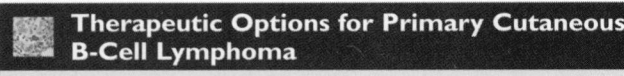

Therapeutic Options for Primary Cutaneous B-Cell Lymphoma

Radiotherapy
Surgical excision
Systemic chemotherapy
    CHOP
    CEVP
Systemic anti-CD20 monoclonal antibody (rituximab)

REFERENCES

1. Chuang T-Y, Su WP, Muller SA: Incidence of cutaneous T cell lymphoma and other rare skin cancers in a defined population. J Am Acad Dermatol 1990;23:254.
2. Weinstock MA, Horm JW: Mycosis fungoides in the United States: Increasing incidence and descriptive epidemiology. JAMA 1988;260:42.
3. Broder S, Bunn PA Jr: Cutaneous T-cell lymphomas. Semin Oncol 1980;7:310.
4. Weinstock MA, Horm JW: Mycosis fungoides in the United States: Increasing incidence and descriptive epidemiology. JAMA 2002;120:42.
5. Hamminga L, Hermans J, Noordijk EM, et al: Cutaneous T-cell lymphoma: Clinicopathological relationships, therapy and survival in 92 patients. Br J Dermatol 1982;107:145.
6. Hoppe RT, Wood GS, Abel EA: Mycosis fungoides and the Sézary syndrome: Pathology, staging, and treatment. Curr Probl Cancer 1990;14:293.
7. Epstein EH Jr, Levin DL, Croft JD Jr, Lutzner MA: Mycosis fungoides: Survival, prognostic features, response to therapy, and autopsy findings. Medicine (Baltimore) 1972;51:61.
8. Levi JA, Wiernik PH: Management of mycosis fungoides: Current status and future prospects. Medicine (Baltimore) 1974;54:73.
9. Peters MS, Thibodeau SN, White JW Jr, Winkelmann RK: Mycosis fungoides in children and adolescents. J Am Acad Dermatol 1990;22:1011.
10. Willemze R, Kerl H, Sterry W, et al: EORTC classification for primary cutaneous lymphomas: A proposal from the Cutaneous Lymphoma Study Group of the European Organization for Research and Treatment of Cancer. Blood 1997;90:354–371.
11. Zackheim HS, Vonderheid EC, Ramsay DL, et al: Relative frequency of various forms of primary cutaneous lymphomas. J Am Acad Dermatol 2000;43:793–796.
12. Tuyp E, Burgoyne A, Aitchison T, Mackie R: A case-control study of possible causative factors in mycosis fungoides. Arch Dermatol 1987;123:196.
13. Whittemore AS, Holley EA, Lee I-M, et al: Mycosis fungoides in relation to environmental exposures and immune response: A case-control study. J Natl Cancer Inst 1989;81:1560.

14. Rajka G, Winkelmann RK: Atopic dermatitis and Sézary syndrome. Arch Dermatol 1984;120:83.

15. Winkelmann RK, Buechner SA, Diaz-Perez JL: Pre-Sézary syndrome. J Am Acad Dermatol 1984;10:992.

16. Shupp DL, Winkelmann RK: Patch tests in Sézary syndrome and mycosis fungoides. Contact Dermatitis 1985;13:180.

17. Lambert WC: Premycotic eruptions. Dermatol Clin 1985;3:629.

18. Van der Akker TW, Van der Willigen AH, Van der Kwast TH, et al: Cutaneous T-cell lymphoma after successful treatment of follicular B-cell lymphoma Br J Dermatol 1990;123:266.

19. Kaufman D, Gordon LI, Variakojis D, et al: Successfully treated Hodgkin's disease followed by mycosis fungoides: Case report and review of the literature. Cutis 1987;39:291.

20. Nahass GT, Kraffert CA, Penneys NS: Cutaneous T-cell lymphoma associated with the acquired immunodeficiency syndrome. Arch Dermatol 1991;127:1020.

21. Crane GA, Variakojis D, Rosen ST, et al: Cutaneous T-cell lymphoma in patients with human immunodeficiency virus infection. Arch Dermatol 1991;127:989.

22. Harris NL, Jaffe ES, Diebold J, et al: World Health Organization classification of neoplastic diseases of the hematopoietic and lymphoid tissues: Report of the Clinical Advisory Committee meeting, Airlie, Virginia, November 1997. J Clin Oncol 1999;17: 3835–3849.

23. Willemze R, Kerl H, Sterry W, et al: EORTC classification for primary cutaneous lymphomas: A proposal from the Cutaneous Lymphoma Study Group of the European Organization for Research and Treatment of Cancer. Blood 1997;90:354–371.

24. Fink-Puches R, Zenahlik P, Back B, et al: Primary cutaneous lymphomas: applicability of current classification schemes (European Organization for Research and Treatment of Cancer, World Health Organization) based on clinicopathologic features observed in a large group of patients. Blood 2002;99:800–805.

25. Alibert JLM: Description des maladies de la peau. Observées à l'Hôpital Saint-Louis et exposition des meilleures méthodes suivies pour leur traitement. Paris, Barrois L'aine et Fils, 1806.

26. Oliver GF, Winkelmann RK: Unilesional mycosis fungoides: A distinct entity. J Am Acad Dermatol 1989;20:63.

27. Sézary A, Bouvrain Y: Erythrodermie avec présence de cellules monstreuses dans le derme et le sang circulant. Bull Soc Fr Dermatol Syphiligr 1938;45:254.

28. Taswell HF, Winkelmann RK: Sézary syndrome: A malignant reticulemic erythroderma. JAMA 1961;177:465.

29. Cyr DP, Geokas MC, Worsley GH: Mycosis fungoides: Hematologic findings and terminal course. Arch Dermatol 1966;94:558.

30. Fuks ZY, Bagshaw MA, Farber EM: Prognostic signs and the management of mycosis fungoides. Cancer 1973;32:1385.

31. Long JC, Mihm MC: Mycosis fungoides with extracutaneous dissemination: A distinct clinicopathologic entity. Cancer 1974;34:1745.

32. Rappaport H, Thomas LB: Mycosis fungoides: the pathology of extracutaneous involvement. Cancer 1974;34:1198.

33. Merlo CJ, Hoppe RT, Abel E, Cox RS: Extracutaneous mycosis fungoides. Cancer 1987;60:397.

34. Arai E, Katayama I, Ishihara K: Mycosis fungoides and Sézary syndrome in Japan: Clinicopathologic study of 107 autopsy cases. Pathol Res Pract 1991;187:451.

35. Edelson RL: Cutaneous T cell lymphoma: Mycosis fungoides, Sézary syndrome, and other variants. J Am Acad Dermatol 1980;2:89.

36. Murphy GF, Elder DE: Cutaneous lymphoproliferative tumors. In Atlas of Tumor Pathology, 3rd series, fascicle 1. Washington DC, Armed Forces Institute of Pathology, 1991, p 155.

37. Bunn PA Jr, Huberman MS, Whang-Peng J, et al: Prospective staging evaluation of patients with cutaneous T-cell lymphomas: Demonstration of a high frequency of extracutaneous dissemination. Ann Intern Med 1980;93:223.

38. Vonderheid EC, Diamond LW, Lai S-M, et al: Lymph node histopathologic findings in cutaneous T-cell lymphoma: A prognostic classification system based on morphologic assessment. Am J Clin Pathol 1992;97:121.

39. van Doorn R, van Haselen C, van Voorst V, et al: Mycosis fungoides: Disease evolution and prognosis of 309 Dutch patients. Arch Dermatol 2000;136(4):504–510.

40. Scheffer E, Meijer CJLM, van Vloten WA: Dermatopathic lymphadenopathy and lymph node involvement in mycosis fungoides. Cancer 1980;45:137.

41. Buzzanga J, Banks PM, Winkelmann RK: Lymph node histopathology in Sézary syndrome. J Am Acad Dermatol 1984;11:880.

42. Scheffer E, Meijer CJLM, van Vloten WA, Willemze R: A histologic study of lymph nodes from patients with the Sézary syndrome. Cancer 1986;57:2375.

43. Colby TV, Burke JS, Hoppe RT: Lymph node biopsy in mycosis fungoides. Cancer 1981;47:351.

44. Salhany KE, Cousar JB, Greer JP, et al: Transformation of cutaneous T cell lymphoma to large cell lymphoma: A clinicopathologic and immunologic study. Am J Pathol 1988;132:265.

45. Greer JP, Salhany KE, Coursar JB, et al: Clinical features associated with transformation of cerebriform T-cell lymphoma to a large cell process. Hematol Oncol 1990;8:215.

46. Edelson RL, Kirkpatrick CH, Shevach EM, et al: Preferential cutaneous infiltration by neoplastic thymus-derived lymphocytes: Morphologic and functional studies. Ann Intern Med 1974;80:685.

47. Sausville EA, Eddy JL, Makuch RW, et al: Histopathologic staging at initial diagnosis of mycosis fungoides and the Sézary syndrome: definition of three distinctive prognostic groups. Ann Intern Med 1988;109:372.

48. Salhany KE, Greer JP, Cousar JB, Collins RD: Marrow involvement in cutaneous T-cell lymphoma: a clinicopathologic study of 60 cases. Am J Clin Pathol 1989;92:747.

49. Variakojis D, Rosas-Uribe A, Rappaport H: Mycosis fungoides: pathologic findings in staging laparotomies. Cancer 1974;33:1589.

50. Huberman MS, Bunn PA Jr, Matthews MJ, et al: Hepatic involvement in the cutaneous T-cell lymphomas: results of percutaneous biopsy and peritoneoscopy. Cancer 1980;45:1683.

51. Sanchez JL, Ackerman AB: The patch stage of mycosis fungoides: criteria for histologic diagnosis. Am J Dermatopathol 1979;1:5.

52. Nickoloff BJ: Light-microscopic assessment of 100 patients with patch/plaque-stage mycosis fungoides. Am J Dermatopathol 1988;10:469.

53. Collins RD: Lymph node examination: what is an adequate workup? Arch Pathol Lab Med 1985;109:797.

54. Slater DN: Diagnostic difficulties in "non-mycotic" cutaneous lymphoproliferative diseases. Histopathology 1992;21:203.

55. Shapiro PE, Pinto FJ: The histologic spectrum of mycosis fungoides/ Sézary syndrome (cutaneous T-cell lymphoma). Am J Surg Pathol 1994;18:645.

56. Lever WF, Schaumberg-Lever G: Histopathology of the Skin, 5th ed. Philadelphia, JB Lippincott, 1975, p 696.

57. Winkelmann RK, Caro WA: Current problems in mycosis fungoides and Sézary syndrome. Annu Rev Med 1977;28:251.

58. Murphy GF, Elder DE: Cutaneous lymphoproliferative tumors. In Atlas of Tumor Pathology, 3rd series, fascicle 1. Washington DC, Armed Forces Institute of Pathology, 1991.

59. Oliver GF, Winkelmann RK, Muller SA: Lichenoid dermatitis: a clinicopathologic and immunopathologic review of sixty-two cases. J Am Acad Dermatol 1989;21:284.

60. Lefever WP, Robinson JK, Clendenning WE, et al: Attempt to enhance light microscopic diagnosis of cutaneous T-cell lymphoma (mycosis fungoides). Arch Dermatol 1981;117:498.

61. Burg G, Zwingers T, Staegemeir E, et al: Interrater and intrarater variabilities in the evaluation of cutaneous lymphoproliferative T-cell infiltrates. Dermatol Clin 1994;12:311.

62. Walsh NMG, Prokopetz R, Tron VA, et al: Histopathology in erythroderma: review of a series of cases by multiple observers. J Cutan Pathol 1994;12:419.

63. Santucci M, Burg G, Feller AC: Interrater and intrarater reliability of histologic criteria in early cutaneous T-cell lymphoma. Dermatol Clin 1994;12:323.

64. Glusac EJ: Of cells and architecture: new approaches to old criteria in mycosis fungoides. J Cutan Pathol 2001;28:169–173.

65. Smoller BR, Bishop K, Glusac EJ, et al: Reassessment of histologic parameters in the diagnosis of mycosis fungoides. Am J Surg Pathol 1995;19:1423.

66. Santucci M, Biggeri A, Feller AC, et al: Efficacy of histologic criteria for diagnosing early mycosis fungoides. An EORTC Cutaneous Lymphoma Study Group Investigation. Am J Surg Pathol 2000;24:40.

67. Lutzner MA, Hobbs JW, Horvath P: Ultrastructure of abnormal cells in Sézary syndrome, mycosis fungoides, and parapsoriasis en plaque. Arch Dermatol 1971;103:375.

68. Lutzner MA, Jordan HW: The ultrastructure of an abnormal cell in Sézary syndrome. Blood 1968;31:719.

69. Flaxman BA, Zelazny G, Van Scott EJ: Nonspecificity of characteristic cells in mycosis fungoides. Arch Dermatol 1971;104:141.

70. Duncan SC, Winkelmann RK: Circulating Sézary cells in hospitalized dermatology patients. Br J Dermatol 1978;99:171.

71. Guitart J, Kennedy J, Ronan S, et al: Histologic criteria for the diagnosis of mycosis fungoides: proposal for a grading system to standardize pathology reporting. J Cutaneous Pathology 2001;28:174-183.

72. Vonderheid EC, Tam DW, Johnson WC, et al: Prognostic significance of cytomorphology in the cutaneous T-cell lymphomas. Cancer 1981;47:119.

73. Kerl H, Cerroni L, Burg G: The morphologic spectrum of T-cell lymphomas of the skin: a proposal for a new classification. Semin Diagn Pathol 1991;8:55.

74. Dmitrovsky E, Matthews MJ, Bunn PA, et al: Cytologic transformation in cutaneous T cell lymphoma: a clinicopathologic entity associated with poor prognosis. J Clin Oncol 1987;5:208.

75. Buechner SA, Winkelmann RK: Sézary syndrome: a clinicopathologic study of 39 cases. Arch Dermatol 1983;119:979.

76. Willemze R, van Vloten WA, Hermans J, et al: Diagnostic criteria in Sézary syndrome: A multiparameter study of peripheral blood lymphocytes in 32 patients with erythroderma. J Invest Dermatol 1983;81:392.

77. Vonderheid EC, Sobel EL, Nowell PC, et al: Diagnostic and prognostic significance of Sézary cells in peripheral blood smears from patients with cutaneous T cell lymphoma. Blood 1985;66:358.

78. Smoller BR, Bishop D, Glusac E, et al: Reassessment of histologic parameters in the diagnosis of mycosis fungoides. Am J Surg Pathol 1995;19:1423-1430.

79. Cribier BJ: The myth of Pautrier's microabscesses. J Am Acad Dermatol 2003;48:796-797.

80. Crossen PE, Mellor JEL, Finley AG, et al: The Sézary syndrome: Cytogenetic studies and identification of the Sézary cell as an abnormal lymphocyte. Am J Med 1971;50:25.

81. Broome JD, Zucker-Franklin D, Weiner MS, et al: Leukemic cells with membrane properties of thymus-derived (T) lymphocytes in a case of Sézary's syndrome: Morphologic and immunologic studies. Clin Immunol Immunopathol 1973;1:319.

82. Brouet J-C, Flandrin G, Seligmann M: Indications of the thymus-derived nature of the proliferating cells in six patients with Sézary's syndrome. N Engl J Med 1973;289:341.

83. Broder S, Edelson RL, Lutzner MA, et al: The Sézary syndrome: A malignant proliferation of helper T cells. J Clin Invest 1976;58:1297.

84. Berger CL, Warburton D, Raafat J, et al: Cutaneous T-cell lymphoma: neoplasm of T cells with helper activity. Blood 1979;53:642.

85. Kung PC, Berger CL, Goldstein G, et al: Cutaneous T cell lymphoma: characterization by monoclonal antibodies. Blood 1981;57:261.

86. Haynes BF, Metzgar RS, Minna JD, Bunn PA: Phenotypic characterization of cutaneous T-cell lymphoma: Use of monoclonal antibodies to compare with other malignant T cells. N Engl J Med 1981;304:1319.

87. Willemze R, de Graaf-Reitsma CB, Cnossen J, et al: Characterization of T-cell subpopulations in skin and peripheral blood of patients with cutaneous T-cell lymphomas and benign inflammatory dermatoses. J Invest Dermatol 1983;80:60.

88. Chu A, Patterson J, Berger C, et al: In situ study of T-cell subpopulations in cutaneous T-cell lymphoma: Diagnostic criteria. Cancer 1984;54:2414.

89. Nasu K, Said J, Vonderheid E, et al: Immunopathology of cutaneous T-cell lymphomas. Am J Pathol 1985;119:436.

90. Ralfkiaer E, Wantzin GL, Mason DY, et al: Phenotypic characterization of lymphocyte subsets in mycosis fungoides: comparison with large plaque parapsoriasis and benign chronic dermatoses. Am J Clin Pathol 1985;84:610.

91. van der Putte SCJ, Toonstra J, van Wichen DF, et al: Aberrant immunophenotypes in mycosis fungoides. Arch Dermatol 1988;124:373.

92. Vonderheid EC, Tan E, Sobel EL, et al: Clinical implications of immunologic phenotyping in cutaneous T cell lymphoma. J Am Acad Dermatol 1987;17:40.

93. Sterry W, Mielke V: CD4+ cutaneous T-cell lymphomas show the phenotype of helper/inducer T cells (CD45RA-, CDw29+). J Invest Dermatol 1989;93:413.

94. Heald P, Yan SL, Edelson RL, et al: Skin selective homing mechanisms in the pathogenesis of leukemic cutaneous T-cell lymphoma. J Invest Dermatol 1993;101:222.

95. Haynes BF, Hensley LL, Jegasothy BV: Phenotypic characterization of skin-infiltrating T cells in cutaneous T-cell lymphoma: Comparison with benign cutaneous T-cell infiltrates. Blood 1982;60:463.

96. Bennett SR, Greer JP, Stein RS, et al: Death due to splenic rupture in suppressor cell mycosis fungoides: A case report. Am J Clin Pathol 1984;82:104.

97. Salmeron G, Hillman N, Paul CC, et al: Cutaneous T cell lymphoma with suppressor phenotype and function. South Med J 1989;82:520.

98. Agnarsson BA, Vonderheid EC, Kadin ME: Cutaneous T cell lymphoma with suppressor/cytotoxic (CD8) phenotype: identification of rapidly progressive and chronic subtypes. J Am Acad Dermatol 1990;22:569.

99. Ralfkiaer E: Immunohistological markers for the diagnosis of cutaneous lymphomas. Semin Diagn Pathol 1991;8:62.

100. Wood GS, Burke JS, Horning S, et al: The immunologic and clinicopathologic heterogeneity of cutaneous lymphomas other than mycosis fungoides. Blood 1983;62:464.

101. Wood GS, Deneau Degenerative, Miller RA, et al: Subtypes of cutaneous T-cell lymphoma defined by expression of Leu-1 and Ia. Blood 1982;59:876.

102. Jones D, Vega F, Sarris AH, et al: CD4- and CD8- "Double-negative" cutaneous T-cell lymphomas share common histologic features and an aggressive clinical course. Am J Surg Pathol 2002;26(2):225-231.

103. Wood GS, Abel EA, Hoppe R, et al: Leu-8 and Leu-9 antigen phenotypes: immunologic criteria for the distinction of mycosis fungoides from cutaneous inflammation. J Am Acad Dermatol 1986;14:1006.

104. Kung E, Meissner K, Loning T: Cutaneous T cell lymphoma: Immunocytochemical study on activation/proliferation and differentiation associated antigens in lymph nodes, skin, and peripheral blood. Virchows Arch A Pathol Anat Histopathol 1988;413:539.

105. Heald PW, Yan SL, Edelson RL, et al: Skin-selective lymphocyte homing mechanisms in the pathogenesis of leukemic cutaneous T-cell lymphoma. J Invest Dermatol 1993;101:222-226.

106. Zaki MH, Wysocka M, Everetts SE, et al: Synergistic enhancement of cell-mediated immunity by interleukin-12 plus interleukin-2: Basis for therapy of cutaneous T cell lymphoma. J Invest Dermatol 2002;118:366-371.

107. Simonitsch I, Volc-Platzer B, Mosberger I, et al: Expression of monoclonal antibody HML-1-defined alpha E beta 7 integrin in cutaneous T-cell lymphoma Am J Pathol 1994;145:1148-1158.

108. Heald PW, Berger CL, Yamamura T, et al: BE-2 antigen: Appearance in activation and long-term growth of T cells. J Invest Dermatol 1990;94:452-455.

109. Kaudewitz P, Stein H, Burg G, et al: Atypical cells in lymphomatoid papulosis express the Hodgkin cell-associated antigen Ki-1. J Invest Dermatol 1986;86:350.

110. Stein H, Mason DY, Gerdes J, et al: The expression of the Hodgkin's disease associated antigen Ki-1 in reactive and neoplastic lymphoid tissue: Evidence that Reed-Sternberg cells and histiocytic malignancies are derived from activated lymphoid cells. Blood 1985;66:848.

111. Wieczorek R, Suhrland M, Ramsay D, et al: Leu-M1 antigen expression in advanced (tumor) stage mycosis fungoides. Am J Clin Pathol 1986;S86:25.

112. Kaudewitz P, Stein H, Dallenbach F, et al: Primary and secondary cutaneous Ki-1+ (CD30+) anaplastic large cell lymphomas: Morphologic, immunohistologic and clinical characteristics. Am J Pathol 1989;135:359.

113. Piepkorn M, Marty J, Kjeldsberg CR: T cell subset heterogeneity in a series of patients with mycosis fungoides and Sézary syndrome. J Am Acad Dermatol 1984;11:427.

114. Samlowski WE, Conrath FC, Piepkorn MW, Kjeldsberg CR: Immunologic studies documenting the development of mycosis fungoides following successful therapy of a large-cell lymphoma. Arch Pathol Lab Med 1985;109:864.

115. Michie SA, Abel EA, Hoppe RT, et al: Expression of T-cell receptor antigens in mycosis fungoides and inflammatory skin lesions. J Invest Dermatol 1989;93:116.

116. Hastrup N, et al: Use of monoclonal antibodies for the diagnosis of T-cell malignancies: Applications and limitations. Leuk Lymphoma 1990;2:35.

117. Bagot M, Wechsler J, Lescs M-C, et al: Intraepidermal localization of the clone in cutaneous T-cell lymphoma. J Am Acad Dermatol 1992;27:589.

118. Olerud JE, Kulin PA, Chew DE, et al: Cutaneous T-cell lymphoma: Evaluation of pretreatment skin biopsy specimens by a panel of pathologists. Arch Dermatol 1992;128:501.

119. MacKie R, Dick HM, De Sousa MB: HLA and mycosis fungoides (letter). Lancet 1976;1:1179.

120. Safai B, Myskowski PL, Dupont B, Pollack MS: Association of HLA-DR5 with mycosis fungoides. J Invest Dermatol 1983;80:395.

121. Rosen ST, Radvany R, Roenigk H Jr, et al: Human leukocyte antigens in cutaneous T cell lymphoma. J Am Acad Dermatol 1985;12:531.

122. Edelson RL, Berger CL, Raafat J, Warburton D: Karyotype studies of cutaneous T cell lymphoma: Evidence for clonal origin. J Invest Dermatol 1979;73:548.

123. Shah-Reddy I, Mayeda K, Mirchandani I, Koppitch FC: Sézary syndrome with a 14:14 (q12:q31) translocation. Cancer 1982;49:75.

124. Nowell PC, Finan JB, Vonderheid EC: Clonal characteristics of cutaneous T cell lymphomas: Cytogenetic evidence from blood, lymph nodes, and skin. J Invest Dermatol 1982;78:69.

125. Whang-Peng J, Bunn PA Jr, Knutsen T, et al: Clinical implications of cytogenetic studies in cutaneous T-cell lymphoma (CTCL). Cancer 1982;50:1539.

126. Johnson GA, Dewald GW, Strand WA, Winkelmann RK: Chromosome studies in 17 patients with the Sézary syndrome. Cancer 1985;55:2426.

127. Mecucci C, Van Den Berghe H: OKT8-positive T-cell lymphoma associated with a chromosome rearrangement t(2;17) possibly involving the T8 locus (letter). N Engl J Med 1985;313:185.

128. Ralfkiaer E, O'Connor NTJ, Crick J, et al: Genotypic analysis of cutaneous T-cell lymphomas. J Invest Dermatol 1987;88:762.

129. Dosoka N, Tanaka T, Fugita M, et al: Southern blot analysis of clonal rearrangements of the T-cell receptor gene in plaque lesions of mycosis fungoides. J Invest Dermatol 1989;93:626.

130. Limon J, Nedoszytko B, Brozek I, et al: Chromosome aberrations, spontaneous SCE and growth kinetics in PHA-stimulated lymphocytes of five cases with the Sézary syndrome. Cancer Genet Cytogenet 1985;83:75.

131. Karenko L, Hyytinen E, Sarna S, et al: Chromosomal abnormalities in cutaneous T-cell lymphoma and in its premalignant conditions as detected by G-banding and interphase cytogenetic methods. J Invest Dermatol 1997;108:22.

132. Woloschak GE, Hooper WC, Doerge MJ, et al: Oncogene expression in T-cell lymphoproliferative disorders. Leuk Res 1988;12:327.

133. Koga Y, Kimura N, Minowada J, Mak TW: Expression of the human T-cell-specific tyrosine kinase YT16 (*lck*) message in leukemic T-cell lines. Cancer Res 1988;48:856.

134. van Doorn R, Dijkman R, Vermeer MH, et al: A novel splice variant of the *fas* gene in patients with cutaneous T-cell lymphoma. Cancer Research 2002;62:5389–5392.

135. Knobler RM, Rehle T, Grossman M, et al: Clinical evolution of cutaneous T cell lymphoma in a patient with antibodies to human T-lymphotropic virus type I. J Am Acad Dermatol 1987;17:903.

136. Wantzin GL, Thomsen K, Nissen NI, et al: Occurrence of human T cell lymphotropic virus (type I) antibodies in cutaneous T cell lymphoma. J Am Acad Dermatol 1986;15:598.

137. Manzari V, Gismondi A, Barillari G, et al: A new human retrovirus isolated in a tac-negative T-cell lymphoma/leukemia. Science 1987;238:1581.

138. Hall WW, Liu CR, Schneewind O, et al: Deleted HTLV-I provirus in blood and cutaneous lesions of patients with mycosis fungoides. Science 1991;253:317.

139. Whittaker SJ, Luzzatto L: HTLV-1 provirus and mycosis fungoides. Science 1993;259:1470.

140. Bazarbachi A, Saal F, Laroche L, et al: HTLV-1 provirus and mycosis fungoides. Science 1993;259:1470.

141. Zucker-Franklin D, Pancake BA: The role of human T-cell lymphotropic viruses (HTLV-I/II) in cutaneous T-cell lymphomas. Semin Dermatol 1994;13:160.

142. Pancake BA, Zucker-Franklin D, Coutavas EE: The cutaneous T-cell lymphoma, mycosis fungoides, in a human T-cell lymphotropic virus-associated disease: A study of 50 patients. J Clin Invest 1995;95:54.

143. Waldmann TA, Davis MM, Bongiovanni KF, Korsmeyer SJ: Rearrangements of genes for the antigen receptor on T cells as markers of lineage and clonality in human lymphoid neoplasms. N Engl J Med 1985;313:776.

144. Weiss LM, Hu E, Wood GS, et al: Clonal rearrangements of T-cell receptor genes in mycosis fungoides and dermatopathic lymphadenopathy. N Engl J Med 1985;313:539.

145. Zelickson BD, Peters MS, Muller SA, et al: T-cell receptor gene rearrangement analysis: Cutaneous T cell lymphoma, peripheral T cell lymphoma, and premalignant and benign cutaneous lymphoproliferative disorders. J Am Acad Dermatol 1991;25:787.

146. Ralfkiaer E, O'Connor NTJ, Crick J, et al: Genotypic analysis of cutaneous T-cell lymphomas. J Invest Dermatol 1987;88:762.

147. Weiss LM, Wood GS, Hu E, et al: Detection of clonal T-cell receptor gene rearrangements in the peripheral blood of patients with mycosis fungoides/Sézary syndrome. J Invest Dermatol 1989;92:601.

148. Whittaker SJ, Smith NP, Jones RR, Luzzatto L: Analysis of beta, gamma, and delta T-cell receptor genes in mycosis fungoides and Sézary syndrome. Cancer 1991;68:1572.

149. Wood GS: Recent advances in the molecular biology of cutaneous lymphomas and related disorders. Semin Dermatol 1991;10:172.

150. Berger C, Lee M, Tien J, et al: Loss of initial clone and emergence of a novel genotype in cutaneous T cell lymphoma treated with photochemotherapy (abstract). J Invest Dermatol 1990;94:506.

151. Zelickson B, Thibodeau SN, Peters M, et al: Serial T-cell receptor gene rearrangement analysis in Sézary syndrome (abstract). J Invest Dermatol 1990;94:594.

152. Lessin SR, Rook AH, Rovera G: Molecular diagnosis of cutaneous T-cell lymphoma: Polyermase chain reaction amplification of T-cell antigen receptor beta-chain gene rearrangements. J Invest Dermatol 1991;96:299.

153. Muche JM, Kukowsky A, Asadullah K, et al: Demonstration of frequent occurrence of clonal T cells in the peripheral blood of patients with primary cutaneous T-cell lymphoma. Blood 1997;90:1636.

154. Wood GS, Tung RM, Haeffner AC, et al: Detection of clonal T-cell receptor [gamma] gene arrangements in early mycosis fungoides/Sézary syndrome by polymerase chain reaction and denaturing gradient gel electrophoresis (PCR/DGGE) J Invest Dermatol 1994;103:34–41.

155. Laetsch B, Haeffner AC, Dobbeling U, et al: CD4+/CD7−T cell frequency and polymerase chain reaction-based clonality assay correlate with stage in cutaneous T cell lymphomas. J Invest Dermatol 2000;114:107–111.

156. Lynch JW Jr, Linoilla I, Sausville EA, et al: Prognostic implications of evaluation for lymph node involvement by T-cell antigen receptor gene rearrangement in mycosis fungoides. Blood 1992;79:3293.

157. Weiss LM, Wood GA, Trela M, et al: Clonal T-cell populations in lymphomatoid papulosis. Evidence of a lymphoproliferative origin for a clinically benign disease. N Engl J Med 1986;315:475.

158. Weiss LM, Wood GS, Ellisen LW, et al: Clonal T-cell populations in pityriasis lichenoides et varioliformis acuta (Mucha-Habermann disease). Am J Pathol 1987;126:417.

159. Wood GS, Weiss LM, Hu C-H, et al: T-cell antigen deficiencies and clonal rearrangement of T-cell receptor genes in pagetoid reticulosis (Woringer-Kolopp disease). N Engl J Med 1988;318:164.

Specific Malignancies

III

160. Kadin ME, Vonderheid EC, Sako D, et al: Clonal composition of T cells in lymphomatoid papulosis. Am J Pathol 1987;126:13.

161. Wood GS, Tung RM, Haeffner AC, et al: Detection of clonal T-cell receptor gamma gene rearrangements in early mycosis fungoides/Sézary syndrome by polymerase chain reactin and denaturing gradient gel electrophoresis (PCR/DGGE). J Invest Dermatol 1994;103:34–41.

162. Delfau-Larue MH, Laroche L, Wechsler J, et al: Diagnostic value of dominant T-cell clones in peripheral blood in 363 patients presenting consecutively with a clinical suspicion of cutaneous lymphoma. Blood 2000;96:2987–2992.

163. Vega F, Luthra R, Medeiros J, et al: Clonal heterogeneity in mycosis fungoides and its relationship to clinical course. Blood 2002;100:3369–3373.

164. Payne CM, Grogan TM, Spier CM, et al: A multidisciplinary approach to the diagnosis of cutaneous T-cell lymphomas. Ultrastruc Pathol 1992;16:99.

165. Bunn PA Jr, Whang-Peng J, Carney DN, et al: DNA content analysis by flow cytometry and cytogenetic analysis in mycosis fungoides and Sézary syndrome: Diagnostic and prognostic implications. J Clin Invest 1980;65:1440.

166. Meissner K, Michaelis K, Rehpenning W, Löning T: Epidermal Langerhans' cell densities influence survival in mycosis fungoides and Sézary syndrome. Cancer 1990;65:2069.

167. Dummer R, Michie S, Kell D, et al: Expressions of bcl-2 protein and ki-67 nuclear proliferation antigen in benign and malignant cutaneous T-cell infiltrates. J Cutan Pathol 1995;22:11.

168. Tracey L, Villuendas R, Dotor AM, et al: Mycosis fungoides shows concurrent deregulation of multiple genes involved in the TNF signaling pathway: An expression profile study. Blood 2003;102(3):1042–1050.

169. LeBoit PE: Variants of mycosis fungoides and related cutaneous T-cell lymphoma. Semin Diagn Pathol 1991;8:73.

170. Lambert WC, Everett MA: The nosology of parapsoriasis. J Am Acad Dermatol 1981;5:373.

171. Buechner SA, Winkelmann RK: Pre-Sézary erythroderma evolving to Sézary syndrome: A report of seven cases. Arch Dermatol 1983;119:285.

172. McNutt NS: Cutaneous lymphohistiocytic infiltrates simulating malignant lymphoma. In Murphy GF, Mihm MC (eds): Lymphoproliferative Disorders of the Skin. Stoneham, Mass, Butterworth, 1986, p 256.

173. Lindae ML, Abel EA, Hoppe RT, Wood GS: Poikilodermatous mycosis fungoides and atrophic large-plaque parapsoriasis exhibit similar abnormalities of T-cell antigen expression. Arch Dermatol 1988;124:366.

174. Watsky MS, Lynnfield YL: Poikiloderma vasculare atrophicans. Cutis 1976;17:938.

175. Macaulay WL: Lymphomatoid papulosis: A continuing self-healing eruption, clinically benign–histologically malignant. Arch Dermatol 1968;97:23.

176. Sanchez NP, Pittelkow MR, Muller SA, et al: The clinicopathologic spectrum of lymphomatoid papulosis: Study of 31 cases. J Am Acad Dermatol 1983;8:81.

177. Weinman VF, Ackerman AB: Lymphomatoid papulosis: A critical review and new findings. Am J Dermatopathol 1981;3:129.

178. Thomsen K, Wantzin GL: Lymphomatoid papulosis: A follow-up study of 30 patients. J Am Acad Dermatol 1987;17:632.

179. Willemze R, Scheffer E, Ruiter DJ, et al: Immunological, cytochemical and ultrastructural studies in lymphomatoid papulosis. Br J Dermatol 1983;108:381.

180. Willemze R, Meyer CJLM, van Vloten WA, Scheffer E: The clinical and histological spectrum of lymphomatoid papulosis. Br J Dermatol 1982;107:131.

181. Kadin M, Nasu K, Sako D, et al: Lymphomatoid papulosis: A cutaneous proliferation of activated helper T cells expressing Hodgkin's disease-associated antigens. Am J Pathol 1985;119:315.

182. Kinney MC, Greer JP, Glick AD, et al: Anaplastic large-cell Ki-1 malignant lymphomas: Recognition, biological and clinical implications. Pathol Annu 1991;26(part 1):1.

183. Kaudewitz P, Burg G: Lymphomatoid papulosis and Ki-1 (CD30)–positive cutaneous large cell lymphomas. Semin Diagn Pathol 1991;8:117.

184. Gibson LE, Muller SA, Leiferman KM, Peters MS: Follicular mucinosis: Clinical and histopathologic study. J Am Acad Dermatol 1989;20:441.

185. Plotnick H, Abbrecht M: Alopecia mucinosa and lymphoma: Report of two cases and review of the literature. Arch Dermatol 1965;92:137.

186. Mehregan DA, Gibson LE, Muller SA: Follicular mucinosis: Histopathologic review of 33 cases. Mayo Clin Proc 1991;66:387.

187. Cerroni L, Fink-Puches R, Back B, et al: Follicular mucinosis. Arch Dermatol 2002;138:182–189.

188. van Doorn R, Scheffer E, Willemze R, for the Dutch Cutaneous Lymphoma Group: Follicular mycosis fungoides, a distinct disease entity with or without associated follicular mucinosis: A clinicopathologic and follow-up study of 51 patients. Arch Dermatol 2002;138:191–198.

189. Braun-Falco O, Schmoeckel C, Burg G, Ryckmanns F: Pagetoid reticulosis: A further case report with a review of the literature. Acta Derm Venereol (Stockh) 1979;Suppl 85:11.

190. Deneau DG, Wood GS, Beckstead J, et al: Woringer-Kolopp disease (pagetoid reticulosis): Four cases with histopathologic, ultrastructural, and immunohistologic observations. Arch Dermatol 1984;120:1045.

191. Mielke V, Wolff HH, Winzer M, Sterry W: Localized and disseminated pagetoid reticulosis: Diagnostic immunophenotypical findings. Arch Dermatol 1989;125:402.

192. Helm KF, Cerio R, Winkelmann RK: Granulomatous slack skin: A clinicopathological and immunohistochemical study of three cases. Br J Dermatol 1992;126:142.

193. LeBoit PE, Zackheim HS, White CR Jr: Granulomatous variants of cutaneous T-cell lymphoma: The histopathology of granulomatous mycosis fungoides and granulomatous slack skin. Am J Surg Pathol 1988;12:83.

194. Toro JR, Liewehr DJ, Pabby N, et al: Gamma-delta T-cell phenotype is associated with significantly decreased survival in cutaneous T-cell lymphoma. Blood 2003;101(9):3407–3412.

195. Heald P, Edelson R: Immunology of cutaneous T-cell lymphoma. J Natl Cancer Inst 1991;83:400.

196. Hynes RO: Integrins: A family of cell surface receptors. Cell 1987;48:549.

197. Ruoslahti E: Integrins. J Clin Invest 1991;87:1.

198. Dustin ML, Rothlein R, Bahn AK, et al: Induction by IL-1 and interferon-gamma tissue distribution, biochemistry, and function of a natural adherence molecule (ICAM-1). J Immunol 1986;137:245.

199. Marlin SD, Springer TA: Purified intercellular adhesion molecule-1 (ICAM-1) is a ligand for lymphocyte function-associated antigen 1 (LFA-1). Cell 1987;51:813.

200. Staunton DE, Dustin ML, Springer TA: Functional cloning of ICAM-2, a cell adhesion ligand for LFA-1 homologous to ICAM-1. Nature 1989;339:61.

201. Nickoloff BJ, Griffiths CEM, Baadsgaard O, et al: Markedly diminished epidermal keratinocyte expression of intercellular adhesion molecule-1 (ICAM-1) in Sézary syndrome. JAMA 1989;261:2217.

202. Dustin ML, Singer KH, Tuck DT, Springer TA: Adhesion of T-lymphoblasts to epidermal keratinocytes is regulated by interferon gamma and is mediated by intercellular adhesion molecule 1 (ICAM-1). J Exp Med 1988;167:1323.

203. Nickoloff BJ, Mitra RS: Phorbol ester treatment enhances binding of mononuclear leukocytes to autologous and allogeneic gamma-interferon-treated keratinocytes, which is blocked by anti-LFA-1 monoclonal antibody. J Invest Dermatol 1988;90:684.

204. Takeichi M: Cadherin cell adhesion receptors as a morphogenetic regulator. Science 1991;251:1451.

205. Sterry W, Mielke V, Konter U, et al: Role of beta-1 integrins in epidermotropism of malignant T cells. Am J Pathol 1992;141:855.

206. Savoia P, Novelli M, Fierro MT, et al: Expression and role of integrin receptors in Sézary syndrome. J Invest Dermatol 1992;99:151.

207. Dummer R, Kohl O, Gillessen J, et al: Peripheral blood mononuclear cells in patients with nonleukemic cutaneous T-cell lymphoma: Reduced proliferation and preferential secretion of a T helper-2-like cytokine pattern on stimulation. Arch Dermatol 1993;129:433.

208. Vowels BR, Cassin M, Vonderheid EC, Rook AH: Aberrant cytokine production by Sézary syndrome patients: Cytokine secretion pattern resembles murine Th2 cells. J Invest Dermatol 1992;99:90.

209. Saed G, Fivenson DP, Naidu Y, et al: Mycosis fungoides exhibits a Th-1 type cell mediated cytokine profile whereas Sézary syndrome express Th-2 type profile. J Invest Dermatol 1994;103:29.

210. Vowels BF, Lessin SR, Cassin M, et al: Th 2 cytokine expression in skin cutaneous T-cell lymphoma. J invest Dermatol 1994;103:669.

211. Dalloul A, Laroche L, Bagot M, et al: Interleukin-7 is a growth factor for Sézary lymphoma cells. J Clin Invest 1992;90:1054.

212. Hoppe RT, Medeiros LJ, Warnke RA, et al: CD8-tumor-infiltrating lymphocytes influence survival of patients with mycosis fungoides. J Am Acad Dermatol 1995;32:448.

213. McGregor JM, Dublin EA, Levison DA, et al: p53 immunoreactivity is uncommon in primary cutaneous T-cell lymphoma. Br J Dermatol 1995;132:353.

214. Bunn PA Jr, Lamberg SI: Report of the Committee on Staging and Classification of Cutaneous T-Cell Lymphomas. Cancer Treat Rep 1979;63:725.

215. Kashi-Sabet M, McMillan A, Zackheim HS: A modified staging classification for cutaneous T-cell lymphoma. J Am Acad Dermatol 2001;45(5):700-706.

216. Kim YH, Chow S, Varghese A, et al: Clinical characteristics and long-term outcome of patients with generalized patch and/or plaque (T2) mycosis fungoides. Arch Dermatol 1999;135(1):26-32.

217. van Doorn R, van Haselen CW, van Voorst V, et al: Mycosis fungoides: Disease evolution and prognosis of 309 Dutch patients. Arch Dermatol 2000;136(4):504-510.

218. Lamberg SI, Green SB, Byar DP, et al: Status report of 376 mycosis fungoides patients at 4 years: Mycosis Fungoides Cooperative Group. Cancer Treat Rep 1979;63:701.

219. Lamberg SI, Green SB, Byar DP, et al: Clinical staging for cutaneous T-cell lymphoma. Ann Intern Med 1984;100:187.

220. Vonderheid EC, Diamond LW, Lai SM, et al: Lymph node histo-pathologic findings in cutaneous T-cell lymphoma. Am J Clin Pathol 1992;97:121.

221. Vonderheid EC, Diamond LW, van Vloten WA, et al: Lymph node classification systems in cutaneous T-cell lymphomas. Cancer 1994;73:207.

222. Schechter GP, Sausville EA, Fischmann AB, et al: Evaluation of circulating malignant cells provides prognostic information in cutaneous T cell lymphoma. Blood 1987;69:841.

223. Rosen S, Gore E. Brennan J, et al: Evaluation of computerized axial tomography and radionuclide scanning in the staging of cutaneous T-cell lymphoma. Arch Dermatol 1986;122:884.

224. Bass K, Korobkin M, Cooper K, et al: Cutaneous T-cell lymphoma: CT in evaluation and staging. Radiology 1993;186:273.

225. Levi JA, Rosen ST: Cutaneous T-cell lymphomas. In Moossa AR, Schimpff SC, Robson MC (eds): Comprehensive Textbook of Oncology, Vol. 2. Baltimore, Williams & Wilkins, 1991, p 1302.

226. de Coninck E, Kim YH, Varghese A, et al: Clinical characteristics and outcome of patients with extracutaneous mycosis fungoides. J Clin Oncol 2001;19(3):779-784.

227. Vonderheid EC, Bernengo MG, Burg G, et al: Update on erythrodermic cutaneous T-cell lymphoma: Report of the International Society for Cutaneous Lymphomas. J Am Acad Dermatol 2002;46(1):95-106.

228. Bernengo MG, Quaglino P, Novelli M, et al: Prognostic factors in Sézary syndrome: A multivariate analysis of clinical, haematological, and immunological features. Ann Oncol 1998;9(8):857-863.

229. Sibaud V, Beylot-Barry M, Thiebaut R, et al: Bone marrow histopathologic and molecular staging in epidermotropic T-cell lymphomas. Am J Clin Pathol 2003;119:414-423.

230. Dmitrovsky E, Matthews MJ, Bunn PA, et al: Cytologic transformation in cutaneous T-cell lymphoma: A clinicopathologic entity associated with poor prognosis. J clin Oncol 1987;5(2):208-215.

231. Diamandidou E, Colome-Grimmer M, Fayad L, et al: Transformation of mycosis fungoides/Sézary syndrome: Clinical characteristics and prognosis. Blood 1998;92(4):1150-1159.

232. Vergier B, de Muret A, Beylot-Barry M, et al: Transformation of mycosis fungoides: Clinicopathological and prognostic features of 45 cases. French Study Group of Cutaneous Lymphomas. Blood 2000;95(7):2212-2218.

233. Kim HK, Jensen RA, Watanabe GL, et al: Clinical stage IA (limited patch and plaque) mycosis fungoides: A long-term outcome and analysis. Arch Dermatol 1996;132:1309.

234. Zackheim HS, Amin S, Kashani-Sabet M, et al: Prognosis in cutaneous T-cell lymphoma by skin stage: Long-term survival in 489 patients. J Am Acad Dermatol 1999;40:418-425.

235. Weinstock MA, Horm JW: Population-based estimate of survival and determinants of prognosis in patients with mycosis fungoides. Cancer 1988;62:1658.

236. Kim YH, Bishop K, Varghese A, et al: Prognostic factors in erythrodermic mycosis fungoides and the Sézary syndrome. Arch Dermatol 1995;131:1003-1008.

237. Diamandidou E, Colome M, Fayad L, et al: Prognostic factor analysis in mycosis funcoides/Sézary syndrome. J Am Acad Dermatol 1999;40:914-924.

238. Kashani-Sabet M, McMillan A, Zackheim HS: A modified staging classification for cutaneous T-cell lymphoma. J Am Acad Dermatol 2001;45:700-706.

239. Vonderheid EC, Diamond LW, van Vloten WA, et al: Lymph node classification systems in cutaneous T-cell lymphoma: Evidence for the utility of the Working Formulation of Non-Hodgkin's Lymphomas for Clinical Usage. Cancer 1994;73:207-218.

240. Vakeva L, Pukkala E, Ranki A: Increased risk of secondary cancers in patients with primary cutaneous T-cell lymphoma. J Invest Dermatol 2000;115(1):62-65.

241. Kantor AF, Curtis RE, Vonderheid EC, et al: Risk of second malignancy after cutaneous T-cell lymphoma. Cancer 1989;63:1612.

242. Posner LE, Fossieck BE Jr, Eddy JL, Bunn PA Jr: Septicemic complications of the cutaneous T-cell lymphomas. Am J Med 1981;71:210.

243. Kuzel TM, Roenigk HH Jr, Rosen ST: Mycosis fungoides and the Sézary syndrome: A review of pathogenesis, diagnosis, and therapy. J Clin Oncol 1991;9:1298.

244. Farber EM, Zackheim HS, McClintock RP, et al: Treatment of mycosis fungoides. Arch Dermatol 1968;97:165.

245. Zackheim HS, Kashani-Sabet M, Amin S: Topical corticosteroids for mycosis fungoides: Experience in 79 patients. Arch Dermatol 1998;134:949-954.

246. Kierland RR, Watkins CH, Shullenberger CC: The use of nitrogen mustard in the treatment of mycosis fungoides. J Invest Dermatol 1947;9:195.

247. Hoppe RT, Abel EA, Deneau DG, Price NM: Mycosis fungoides: Management with topical nitrogen mustard. J Clin Oncol 1987;5:1796.

248. Ramsay DL, Halperin PS, Zeleniuch-Jacquotte A: Topical mechlorethamine therapy for early stage mycosis fungoides. J Am Acad Dermatol 1988;19:684.

249. Vonderheid EC, Tan ET, Kantor AF, et al: Long-term efficacy, curative potential, and carcinogenicity of topical mechlorethamine chemotherapy in cutaneous T cell lymphoma. J Am Acad Dermatol 1989;20:416.

250. Kim YH, Martinez G, Varghese A, et al: Topical nitrogen mustard in the management of mycosis fungoides: Update of the Stanford experience. Arch Dermatol 2003;139:165-173.

251. Vonderheid EC: Topical mechlorethamine chemotherapy: Considerations on its use in mycosis fungoides. Int J Dermatol 1984;23:180.

252. Van Scott EJ, Kalmanson JD: Complete remissions of mycosis fungoides lymphoma induced by total nitrogen mustard (HN2): Control of delayed hypersensitivity to HN2 by desensitization and by induction of specific immunologic tolerance. Cancer 1973;32:18.

253. Volden G, Larsen TE: Remissions of mycosis fungoides induced by nitrogen mustard (HN2). Dermatologica 1978;156:129.

254. Hamminga B, Noordijk EM, van Vloten WA: Treatment of mycosis fungoides: Total-skin electron-beam irradiation versus topical mechlorethamine therapy. Arch Dermatol 1982;118:150.

255. Price NM, Hoppe RT, Deneau DG: Ointment-based mechlorethamine treatment for mycosis fungoides. Cancer 1983;52:2214.

256. Constantine VS, Fuks ZY, Farber EM: Mechlorethamine desensitization in therapy for mycosis fungoides: Topical desensitization to mechlorethamine (nitrogen mustard) contact hypersensitivity. Arch Dermatol 1975;111:484.

257. Esteve E, Bagot M, Joly P, et al: A prospective study of cutaneous intolerance to topical mechlorethamine therapy in patients with cutaneous T-cell lymphomas. French Study Group of Cutaneous Lymphomas. Arch Dermatol 1999;135:1349-1353.

258. Lee LA, Fritz KA, Golitz L, et al: Second cutaneous malignancies in patients with mycosis fungoides treated with topical nitrogen mustard. J Am Acad Dermatol 1982;7:590.

259. Zackheim HS, Epstein EH Jr, McNutt NS, et al: Topical carmustine (BCNU) for mycosis fungoides and related disorders: A 10-year experience. J Am Acad Dermatol 1983;9:363.

260. Zackheim HS, Epstein EH Jr, Crain WR: Topical carmustine (BCNU) for cutaneous T cell lymphoma: A 15-year experience in 143 patients. J Am Acad Dermatol 1990;22:802.

261. Breneman D, Duvic M, Kuzel T, et al: Phase 1 and 2 trial of bexarotene gel for skin-directed treatment of patients with cutaneous T-cell lymphoma. Arch Dermatol 2002;138(3): 325-332.

262. Heald P: The treatment of cutaneous T-cell lymphoma with a novel retinoid. Clin Lymphoma 2000;1(Suppl 1):S45-49.

263. Duvic M, Hymes K, Heald P, et al: Bexarotene is effective and safe for treatment of refractory advanced-stage cutaneous T-cell lymphoma: Multinational phase II-III trial results. J Clin Oncol 2001;19(9):2456-2471.

264. Zhang C, Hazarika P, Xiao N, et al: Induction of apoptosis by bexarotene in cutaneous T-cell lymphoma cells. Clin Cancer Res 2002;8:1234-1240.

265. Argyropoulos CL, Lamberg SI, Clendenning WE, et al: Preliminary evaluation of 15 chemotherapeutic agents applied topically in the treatment of mycosis fungoides. Cancer Treat Rep 1979;63:619.

266. Zackheim HS: Treatment of mycosis fungoides with topical nitrosourea compounds. Arch Dermatol 1972;106:177.

267. Ramsay DL, Lish KM, Yalowitz CB, Soter NA: Ultraviolet-B phototherapy for early-stage cutaneous T-cell lymphoma. Arch Dermatol 1992;128:931.

268. Gathers, RC, Scherschun L, Malick F, et al: Narrowband UBV phototherapy for early-stage mycosis fungoides. J Am Acad Dermatol 2002;47:191-197.

269. Cech T, Pathak MA, Biswas RK: An electron microscopic study of the photochemical cross-linking of DNA in guinea pig epidermis by psoralen derivatives. Biochim Biophys Acta 1979;562:342.

270. Loveday KS, Donahue BA: Induction of sister chromatid exchanges and gene mutations in Chinese hamster ovary cells by psoralens. Natl Cancer Inst Monogr 1984;66:149.

271. British Photodermatology Group guidelines for PUVA. Br J Dermatol 1994;130:246-255.

272. Gilchrest BA, Parrish JA, Tanenbaum L, et al: Oral methoxsalen photochemotherapy of mycosis fungoides. Cancer 1976;38:683.

273. Gilchrest B: Methoxsalen photochemotherapy for mycosis fungoides. Cancer Treat Rep 1979;63:663.

274. Roenigk HH Jr: Photochemotherapy for mycosis fungoides: Long-term follow-up study. Cancer Treat Rep 1979;63:669.

275. Lowe NJ, Cripps DJ, Dufton PA, Vickers CFH: Photochemotherapy for mycosis fungoides: A clinical and histological study. Arch Dermatol 1979;115:50.

276. Powell FC, Spiegel GT, Muller SA: Treatment of parapsoriasis and mycosis fungoides: The role of psoralen and long-wave ultraviolet light A (PUVA). Mayo Clin Proc 1984;59:538.

277. Hönigsmann H, Tanew A, Wolff K: Treatment of mycosis fungoides with PUVA. Photodermatol 1987;4:55.

278. Rosenbaum MM, Roenigk HH Jr, Caro WA, Esker A: Photochemotherapy in cutaneous T cell lymphoma and parapsoriasis en plaques: Long-term follow-up in 43 patients. J Am Acad Dermatol 1985;13:613.

279. Abel EA, Sendagorta E, Hoppe RT, Hu C-H: PUVA treatment of erythrodermic and plaque-type mycosis fungoides: 10-year follow-up study. Arch Dermatol 1987;123:897.

280. Roenigk HH Jr, Kuzel TM, Skoutelis AP, et al: Photochemotherapy alone or combined with interferon alpha-2a in the treatment of cutaneous T-cell lymphoma. J Invest Dermatol 1990;95(Suppl): S198.

281. Hönigsmann H, Brenner W, Rauschmeier W, et al: Photochemotherapy for cutaneous T cell lymphoma: A follow-up study. J Am Acad Dermatol 1984;10:238.

282. DeVivier A, Vollum DI: Photochemotherapy and topical nitrogen mustard in the therapy of mycosis fungoides. Br J Dermatol 1980;102:319.

283. Thomsen K, Hammar H, Molin L, et al: Retinoids plus PUVA (RePUVA) and PUVA in mycosis fungoides, plaque state. Acta Derm Venereol 1989;69:536.

284. Bouwhuis S, Markovic SN, McEvoy MT, et al: Extracorporeal photopheresis and adjuvant aerosolized grand macrophage colony-stimulating factor for Sézary syndrome. Mayo Clinic Proc 2002;7(2):197-200.

285. Roenigk HH, Kuzel TM, Skoutelis AP, et al: Photochemotherapy alone or combined with interferon alpha-2a in the therapy of cutaneous T-cell lymphoma. J Invest Dermatol 1990;12:257.

286. Kuzel T, Roenigk H, Samuelson E, et al: Effectiveness of interferon-alpha-2a combined with phototherapy for mycosis fungoides and Sézary syndrome. J Clin Oncol 1995;13:257.

287. Kuzel TM, Gilyon K, Springer E, et al: Interferon alfa-2a combined with phototherapy in the treatment of cutaneous T-cell lymphoma. J Natl Cancer Inst 1990;82(3):203-207.

288. Gupta AK, Anderson TF: Psoralen photochemotherapy. J Am Acad Dermatol 1987;17:703.

289. Rhodes AR, Harrist TJ, Momtaz-T K: The PUVA-induced pigmented macule: A lentiginous proliferation of large, sometimes cytologically atypical, melanocytes. J Am Acad Dermatol 1983;9:47.

290. Greene I, Cox AJ: Amyloid deposition after psoriasis therapy with psoralen and long-wave ultraviolet light. Arch Dermatol 1979;115: 1200.

291. Trattner A, Ingber A, Sandbank M. Nail pigmentation resulting from PUVA treatment (letter). Int J Dermatol 1990;29:310.

292. Stern RS, Thibodeau LA, Kleinerman RA, et al: Risk of cutaneous carcinoma in patients treated with oral methoxsalen photochemotherapy for psoriasis. N Engl J Med 1979;300:809.

293. Stern RS, Laird N, Melski J, et al: Cutaneous squamous-cell carcinoma in patients treated with PUVA. N Engl J Med 1984;310:1156.

294. Stern RS, Members of the Photochemotherapy Follow-up Study: Genital tumors among men with psoriasis exposed to psoralens and ultraviolet A radiation (PUVA) and ultraviolet B radiation. N Engl J Med 1990;322:1093.

295. Trump JG, Wright KA, Evans WW, Anson JH: High energy electrons for the treatment of extensive superficial malignant lesions. Am J Roentgenol 1953;69:623.

296. Hoppe RT, Cox RS, Fuks Z, et al: Electron-beam therapy for mycosis fungoides: The Stanford University experience. Cancer Treat Rep 1979;63:691.

297. Lo TCM, Salzman FA, Moschella SL, et al: Whole body surface electron irradiation in the treatment of mycosis fungoides: An evaluation of 200 patients. Radiology 1979;130:453.

298. Nisce LZ, Safai B: Once weekly total-skin electron beam therapy for mycosis fungoides: Seven years' experience. Cancer Treat Rep 1979;63:633.

299. Nisce LZ, Safai B, Kim JH: Effectiveness of once weekly total skin electron beam therapy in mycosis fungoides and Sézary syndrome. Cancer 1981;47:870.

300. Tadros AAM, Tepperman BS, Hryniuk WM, et al: Total skin electron irradiation for mycosis fungoides: Failure analysis and prognostic factors. Int J Radiat Oncol Biol Phys 1983;9:1279.

301. van Vloten WA, de Vroome H, Noordijk EM: Total skin electron beam irradiation for cutaneous T-cell lymphoma (mycosis fungoides). Br J Dermatol 1985;112:697.

302. Le Bourgeois JP, Haddad E, Marinello G, et al: The indications for total cutaneous electron beam radiation therapy of mycosis fungoides. Int J Radiat Oncol Biol Phys 1987;13:189.

303. Micaily B, Moser C, Vonderheid EC, et al: The radiation therapy of early stage cutaneous T-cell lymphoma. Int J Radiat Oncol Biol Phys 1990;18:1333.

304. Hoppe RT: The management of mycosis fungoides at Stanford: Standard and innovative treatment programmes. Leukemia 1991;5(Suppl 1):46.

305. Abel EA, Sendagorta E, Hoppe RT: Cutaneous malignancies and

metastatic squamous cell carcinoma following topical therapies for mycosis fungoides. J Am Acad Dermatol 1986;14:1029.

306. Becker M, Hoppe RT, Knox SJ: Multiple courses of high-dose total skin electron beam therapy in the management of mycosis fungoides. Int J Radiat Oncol Biol Phys 1995;32:1445.

307. Wilson, DL, Licata AL, Braverman IM, et al: Systemic chemotherapy and extracorporeal photochemotherapy for T3 and T4 cutaneous T-cell lymphoma patients who have achieved a complete response to total skin electron beam therapy. Int J Radiat Oncol Biol Phys 1995;32:987.

308. Edelson RL: Light-activated drugs. Sci Am 1988;259:68.

309. Fossel ET, Fletcher JG, McDonagh J, Hui KKS: Selective cytotoxicity of low-density lipoprotein to helper T cells of cutaneous T-cell lymphoma after photoperoxidation with 8-methoxypsoralen. J Natl Cancer Inst 1991;83:1316.

310. Vowels BR, Cassin M, Boufal MH, et al: Extracorporeal photochemotherapy induces the production of tumor necrosis factor-alpha by monocytes: Implications for the treatment of cutaneous T-cell lymphoma and systemic sclerosis. J Invest Dermatol 1992;98:686.

311. Berger CL, Hanlon D, Kanada D, et al: Transimmunization, a novel approach for tumor immunotherapy. Transfus Apheresis Sci 2002;26:205–216.

312. Edelson RL, Berger C, Gasparro F, et al: Treatment of cutaneous T-cell lymphoma by extracorporeal photochemotherapy: Preliminary results. N Engl J Med 1987;316:297.

313. Heald P, Rook A, Perez M, et al: Treatment of erythrodermic cutaneous T-cell lymphoma with extracorporeal photochemotherapy. J Am Acad Dermatol 1992;27:427.

314. Edelson R, Heald P, Perez M, Rook A: Photopheresis update. Prog Dermatol 1991;25(3):1.

315. Heald PW, Perez MI, Christensen I, et al: Photopheresis therapy of cutaneous T-cell lymphoma: The Yale–New Haven Hospital experience. Yale J Biol Med 1989;62:629.

316. Edelson RL: Photopheresis: A new therapeutic concept. Yale J Biol Med 1989;62:565.

317. Evans AV, Wood BP, Scarisbrick JJ, et al: Extracorporeal photopheresis in Sézary syndrome: Hematologic parameters as predictors of response. Blood 2001;98(5):1298–1301.

318. Armus S, Keyes B, Cahill C, et al: Photopheresis for the treatment of cutaneous T-cell lymphoma. J Am Acad Dermatol 1990;23:898.

319. Marks DI, Rockman SP, Oziemski MA, et al: Mechanisms of lymphocytotoxicity induced by extracorporeal photochemo-therapy for cutaneous T-cell lymphoma. J Clin Invest 1990;86:2080.

320. Peterseim JM, Knster W, Gebauer H-J, et al: Cytogenetic effects during extracorporeal photopheresis treatment of two patients with cutaneous T-cell lymphoma. Arch Dermatol Res 1991;283:81.

321. Bunn PA Jr, Ihde DC, Foon KA: The role of recombinant interferon alpha-2a in the therapy of cutaneous T-cell lymphomas. Cancer 1986;57:1689.

322. Heald PW, Perez MI, Christensen I, et al: Photopheresis therapy of cutaneous T-cell lymphoma: The Yale–New Haven Hospital experience. Yale J Biol Med 1989;62:629.

323. Rook AH, Prystowsky MB, Cassin M, et al: Combined therapy for Sézary syndrome with extracorporeal photochemotherapy and low-dose interferon alfa therapy. Arch Dermatol 1991;127:1535.

324. Vonderheid EC, Bigler RD, Greenbery AS, et al: Extracorporeal photopheresis and recombinant interferon alfa 2b in Sézary syndrome. Am J Clin Oncol 1994;17:255.

325. Wollina U, Looks A, Meyer J, et al: Treatment of Stage II cutaneous T-cell lymphoma with interferon alfa-2a and extracorporeal photochemotherapy: A prospective controlled trial. J am Acad Dermatol 2001;44:253–260.

326. Suchin KR, Cucciara AJ, Gottleib SL, et al: Treatment of cutaneous T-cell lymphoma with combined immunomodulatory therapy: A 14-year experience at a single institution. Arch Dermatol 2002;138:1054–1060.

327. Bunn PA Jr, Foon KA, Idhe DC, et al: Recombinant leukocyte A interferon: An active agent in advanced cutaneous T-cell lymphomas. Ann Intern Med 1984;101:484.

328. Kohn EC, Steis RG, Sausville EA, et al: Phase II trial of intermittent high-dose recombinant interferon alfa-2a in mycosis fungoides and the Sézary syndrome. J Clin Oncol 1990;8:155.

329. Thestrup-Pedersen K, Hammer R, Kaltoft K, et al: Treatment of mycosis fungoides with recombinant interferon alfa 2a alone and in combination with etretinate. Br J Dermatol 1988;118:911.

330. Zachariae H, Thestrup-Pedersen K: Interferon alpha and etretinate combination treatment of cutaneous T-cell lymphoma. J Invest Dermatol 1990;95:S206.

331. Nicolas JF, Balblanc JC, Frappaz A, et al: Treatment of cutaneous T-cell lymphoma with intermediate doses of interferon alpha 2a. Dermatologica 1989;179:34.

332. Olsen EA, Rosen ST, Vollmer RT: Interferon alfa-2a in the treatment of cutaneous T-cell lymphoma. J Am Acad Dermatol 1989;20:395.

333. Bunn PA Jr, Norris DA: The therapeutic role of interferons and monoclonal antibodies in cutaneous T-cell lymphomas. J Invest Dermatol 1990;95:S209.

334. Wolff JM, Zitelli JA, Rabin BS, et al: Intralesional interferon in the treatment of early mycosis fungoides. J Am Acad Dermatol 1985;13:604.

335. Vonderheid EC, Thompson R, Smiles KA, Lattanand A: Recombinant inteferon alfa-2b in plaque-phase mycosis fungoides: Intralesional and low-dose intramuscular therapy. Arch Dermatol 1987;123:757.

336. Van Scott EJ, Grekin DA, Kalmanson JD, et al: Frequent low doses of intravenous mechlorethamine for late-stage mycosis fungoides lymphoma. Cancer 1975;36:1613.

337. Grozea PN, Jones SE, McKelvey EM, et al: Combination chemotherapy for mycosis fungoides: A Southwest Oncology Group study. Cancer Treat Rep 1979;63:647.

338. Levi JA, Diggs CH, Wiernik PH: Adriamycin therapy in advanced mycosis fungoides. Cancer 1977;39:1967.

339. McDonald CJ, Bertino JR: Treatment of mycosis fungoides lymphoma: Effectiveness of infusions of methotrexate followed by oral citrovorum factor. Cancer Treat Rep 1978;62:1009.

340. Molin L, Thomsen K, Volden G, et al: Epipodophyllotoxin (VP-16-23) in mycosis fungoides: A report for the Scandinavian Mycosis Fungoides Group. Acta Derm Venereol Suppl (Stockh) 1979;59:84.

341. Thomsen K: Scandinavian Mycosis Fungoides Trial. Cancer Treat Rep 1979;63:709.

342. Witman G, Cadman E, Braverman I: Cisplatin treatment of cutaneous T-cell lymphoma (letter). Cancer Treat Rep 1981;65:920.

343. Molin L, Thomsen K, Volden G, et al: Combination chemotherapy in the tumour stage of mycosis fungoides with cyclophosphamide, vincristine, VP-16, Adriamycin and prednisolone (COP, CHOP, CAVOP): A report from the Scandinavian Mycosis Fungoides Study Group. Acta Derm Venereol Suppl (Stockh) 1980;60:542.

344. Tirelli U, Carbone A, Veronesi A, et al: Combination chemotherapy with cyclophosphamide, vincristine, and prednisone (CVP) in TNM-classified stage IV mycosis fungoides. Cancer Treat Rep 1982;66:167.

345. Holmes RC, McGibbon DH, Black MM: Mycosis fungoides: progression towards Sézary syndrome reversed with chlorambucil. Clin Exp Dermatol 1983;8:429.

346. Case DC Jr: Combination chemotherapy for mycosis fungoides with cyclophosphamide, vincristine, methotrexate, and prednisone. Am J Clin Oncol 1984;7:453.

347. Tirelli U, Carbone U, Zagonel V, et al: Staging and treatment with cyclophosphamide, vincristine, and prednisone (CVP) in advanced cutaneous T-cell lymphomas. Hematol Oncol 1986;4:83.

348. Zakem MH, Davis BR, Adelstein DJ, Hines JD: Treatment of advanced stage mycosis fungoides with bleomycin, doxorubicin, and methotrexate with topical nitrogen mustard (BAM-M). Cancer 1986;58:2611.

349. Doberauer C, Öhl S: Advanced mycosis fungoides: Chemotherapy with etoposide, methotrexate, bleomycin, and prednimustine. Acta Dermatol Venereol Suppl (Stockh) 1989;69:538.

350. Zackheim HS, Epstein EH, Jr.: Low-dose methotrexate for the Sézary syndrome. J Am Acad Dermatol 1989;21:757.

351. Sorio R, Tirelli U, Zagonel V, et al: Phase II study of teniposide (VM26) in cutaneous T-cell lymphomas. Am J Clin Oncol 1990;13:14.

352. Zinzani PL, Baliva G, Magagnoli M, et al: Gemcitabine treatment in pretreated cutaneous T-cell lymphoma: Experience in 44 patients. J Clin Oncol 2000;18(13), 2603–2606.

353. Wollina U, Graefe T, Kaatz M: Pegylated doxorubicin for primary cutaneous T-cell lymphoma: A report on 10 patients with follow-up. Jour Cancer Res and Clin Onc 2001;127(2),128–134.

354. Grever MR, Bisaccia E, Scarborough DA, et al: An investigation of 2'deoxycoformycin in the treatment of cutaneous T-cell lymphoma. Blood 1983;61:279.

355. Ho AD, Thaler J, Willemze R, et al: Pentostatin (2'deoxycoformycin) for the treatment of lymphoid neoplasms. Cancer Treat Rev 1990;17:213.

356. Cummings FJ, Kim K, Neiman RS, et al: Phase II trial of pentostatin in refractory lymphomas and cutaneous T-cell disease. J Clin Oncol 1991;9:565.

357. Foss FM: Activity of pentostatin (Nipent) in cutaneous T-cell lymphoma: Single-agent and combination studies. Semin Oncol 2000;27(2):58–63.

358. von Hoff DD, Dahlberg S, Hartstock RJ, et al: Activity of fludarabine monophosphate in patients with advanced mycosis fungoides: A Southwest Oncology Group study. J Natl Cancer Inst 1990;82:1353.

359. Saven A, Carrera CJ, Carson DA, et al: 2-chlorodeoxyadenosine: An active agent in the treatment of cutaneous T-cell lymphoma. Blood 1992;80:587.

360. Kuzel T, Samuelson E, Roenigk H, et al: Phase II trial of 2-chlorodeoxyadenosine (2-CDA) for the treatment of mycosis fungoides or the Sézary syndrome (MF/SS). Proc Am Soc Clin Oncol 1992;11:321.

361. Foss FM, Ihde DC, Breneman DL, et al: Phase II study of pentostatin and intermittent high-dose recombinant interferon alfa-2a in advanced mycosis fungoides/Sézary syndrome. J Clin Oncol 1992;10:1907.

362. Kessler JF, Jones SE, Levine N, et al: Isotretinoin and cutaneous helper T-cell lymphoma (mycosis fungoides). Arch Dermatol 1987;123:201.

363. Thomsen K, Molin L, Volden G, et al: 13-cis-Retinoic acid effective in mycosis fungoides: A report from the Scandinavian Mycosis Fungoides Group. Acta Derm Venerol Suppl (Stockh) 1984;64:563.

364. Tousignant J, Raymond GP, Light MJ: Treatment of cutaneous T-cell lymphoma with the arotinoid Ro 13-6298. J Am Acad Dermatol 1987;16:167.

365. Hoting E, Meissner K: Arotinoid-ethylester: Effectiveness in refractory cutaneous T-cell lymphoma. Cancer 1988;62;1044.

366. Miller RA, Levy R: Response of cutaneous T cell lymphoma to therapy with hybridoma monoclonal antibody. Lancet 1981;2:226.

367. Dillman RO, Shawler DL, Dillman JB, et al: Therapy of chronic lymphocytic leukemia and cutaneous T-cell lymphoma with T101 monoclonal antibody. J Clin Oncol 1984;2:881.

368. Bertram JH, Gill PS, Levine AM, et al: Monoclonal antibody T101 in T-cell malignancies: A clinical, pharmacokinetic, and immunologic correlation. Blood 1986;68:752.

369. Boven E, Lindmo, T, Mitchell JB, et al: Selective cytotoxicity of ^{125}I-labeled monoclonal antibody T101 in human malignant T cell lines. Blood 1986;67:429.

370. Rosen ST, Zimmer AM, Goldman-Leikin R, et al: Radioimmuno-detection and radioimmunotherapy of cutaneous T-cell lymphomas using an ^{131}I-labeled monoclonal antibody: An Illinois Cancer Council study. J Clin Oncol 1987;5:562.

371. LeMaistre CF, Rosen S, Frankel A, et al: Phase I trial of H65-RTA imunoconjugate in patients with cutaneous T-cell lymphoma. Blood 1991;78:1173.

372. Vonderheid EC, Bernengo MG, Burg G, et al: Update on erythrodermic cutaneous T-cell lymphoma: Report of the International Society for Cutaneous Lymphomas. J Am Acad Dermatol 2002;46(1):95–106.

373. Lundin J, Osterborg A, Brittinger G, et al: CAMPATH-1H monoclonal antibody in therapy for previously treated low-grade non-Hodgkin's lymphomas, a Phase II multicenter study. European Study Group of CAMPATH-1H Treatment in Low-Grade Non-Hodgkin's Lymphoma. J Clin Oncol 1998;16(10):3257–3263.

374. Lundin J, Hagberg H, Repp R, et al: Phase I study of alemtuzumab (anti-CD52 monoclonal antibody) in patients with advanced mycosis fungoides/Sézary syndrome. Blood 2003;101(11): 4267–4272.

375. Foss FM, Raubitscheck A, Mulshine JL, et al: Phase I study of the pharmacokinetics of a radioimmunoconjugate, 90Y-T101, in patients with CD5-expressing leukemia and lymphoma. Clin Cancer Res 1998;4(11):2691–2700.

376. Rosen ST, Zimmer AM, Goldman-Leiken R, et al: Radioimmuno-detection and radioimmunotherapy of cutaneous T-cell lymphomas using an 131I-labeled monoclonal antibody: An Illinois Cancer Council study. J Clin Oncol 1987;5(4): 562–573.

377. Kreitman RJ, Wilson WH, White JD, et al: Phase I trial of recombinant immunotoxin anti-Tac(Fv)-PE38 (LMB-2) in patients with hematologic malignancies. J Clin Oncol 2000;18(8):1622–1636.

378. Bigler RD, Crilley P, Micaily B, et al: Autologous bone marrow transplantation for advanced stage mycosis fungoides. Bone Marrow Transplant 1991;7:133.

379. Olavarria E, Child F, Woolford A, et al: T-cell depletion and autologous stem cell transplantation in the management of tumour stage mycosis fungoides with peripheral blood involvement. Br J Haematol 2001;114:624–631.

380. Guitart J, Wickless SC, Oyama Y, et al: Long-term remission after allogeneic hematopoietic stem cell transplantation for refractory cutaneous T-cell lymphoma. Arch Dermatol 2002;138:1359–1365.

381. Masood N, Russell KJ, Olerud JE, et al: Induction of complete remission of advanced stage mycosis fungoides by allogeneic hematopoietic stem cell transplantation. J Am Acad Dermatol 2002;47:140–145.

382. Burt RK, Guitart J, Traynor A, et al: Allogeneic hematopoietic stem cell transplantation for advanced mycosis fungoides: Evidence of a graft-versus-tumor effect. Bone Marrow Transplant 2000;25: 111–113.

383. Gisselbrecht C, Maraninchi D, Pico JL, et al: Interleukine 2 (IL2) in lymphoma: A phase II multicentric study. Proc Annu Meet Am Assoc Cancer Res 1992;33:227.

384. Hesketh P, Caguioa P, Bulger K, et al: Complete response of a cutaneous T-cell lymphoma to an IL-2-dophtheria hybrid toxin (DAB486IL-2). Proc Am Soc Clin Oncol 1991;10:998A.

385. Kuzel T, Foss F, LeMaistre C, et al: Phase I trial of a diphtheria toxin (DT) fusion rpotein (DAB389IL-2) for the treatment of interleukin-2 receptor (IL02R) expressing hematologic neoplasms. Blood 1995;86:274a.

386. Olsen E, Divic M, Frankel A, et al: Pivotal Phase III trial of two dose levels of denileukin diftitox for the treatment of cutaneous T-cell lymphoma. J Clin Oncol 2001;19(2):376–388.

387. Edelson RL, Raafat J, Berger CL, et al: Antithymocyte globulin in the management of cutaneous T-cell lymphoma. Cancer Treat Rep 1979;63:675.

388. Street ML, Muller SA, Pittelkow MR: Cyclosporine in the treatment of cutaneous T-cell lymphoma. J Am Acad Dermatol 1990;23:1084.

389. Kreis W, Budman DR, Shapiro PE: Cyclosporin A (cyclosporine) in the treatment of cutaneous T-cell lymphoma (mycosis fungoides) (letter). J Am Acad Dermatol 1988;18:1139.

390. Resnick L, Schleider-Kushner N, Horowitz SN, et al: Remission of tumor-stage mycosis fungoides following intravenously administered acyclovir. JAMA 1984;251:1571.

391. Burg G, Klepzig K, Kaudewitz P, et al: Acyclovir in lymphomatoid papilosis and mycosis fungoides. JAMA 1986;256:214.

392. Scheman AJ, Steinberg I, Taddeini L: Abatement of Sézary syndrome lesions following treatment with acyclovir. Am J Med 1986;80:1199.

393. Griem ML, Tokars RP, Petras V, et al: Combined therapy for patients with mycosis fungoides. Cancer Treat Rep 1979;63:655.

394. Hallahan DE, Griem ML, Griem SF, et al: Combined modality therapy for tumor stage mycosis fungoides: Results of a 10-year follow-up. J Clin Oncol 1988;6:1177.

395. Braverman IM, Yager NB, Chen M, et al: Combined total body electron beam irradiation and chemotherapy for mycosis fungoides. J Am Acad Dermatol 1987;16:45.

396. Winkler CF, Sausville EA, Ihde DC, et al: Combined modality treatment of cutaneous T cell lymphoma: Results of a six-year follow-up. J Clin Oncol 1986;4:1094.

397. Kaye FJ, Bunn PA Jr, Steinberg SM, et al: A randomized trial comparing combination electron-beam radiation and chemotherapy with topical therapy in the initial treatment of mycosis fungoides. N Engl J Med 1989;321:1784.

398. Duvic M, Lemak NA, Redman JR, et al: Combined modality therapy for cutaneous T-cell lymphoma. J Am Acad Dermatol 1996;34:1022.

399. Zackheim HS, Vonderheid EC, Ransay DL, et al: Relative frequency of various forms of primary cutaneous lymphomas. J Am Acad Dermatol 2000;43:793–796.

400. Burg G, Kerl H, Schmoeckel C: Differentiation between malignant B-cell lymphomas and pseudolymphomas of the skin. J Dermatol Surg Oncol 1984;10:271–275.

401. Fink-Puches R, Zenahlik P, Back B, et al: Primary cutaneous lymphomas: Applicability of current classification schemes (European Organization for Research and Treatment of Cancer and World Health Organization) based on clinicopathologic features observed in a large group of patients. Blood 2002;99:800–805.

402. Yang B, Tubbs RR, Finn W, et al: Clinicopathologic reassessment of primary cutaneous B-cell lymphomas with immunophenotypic and molecular genetic characterization. Am J Surg Pathol 2000;24:694–702.

403. Baldassano MF, Bailey EM, Ferry JA, et al: Cutaneous lymphoid hyperplasia and cutaneous marginal zone lymphoma: Comparison of morphologic and immunophenotypic features. Am J Surg Pathol 1999;23:88–96.

404. Tembury TA, Lee B, Gascoyne RD, et al: Primary cutaneous diffuse large B-cell lymphoma: A clinicopathologic study of 15 cases. Am J Clin Pathol 2002;117:574–580.

405. Wechsler J, Bagot M: Primary cutaneous large B-cell lymphomas. Semin Cutan Med Surg 2000;19:130–132.

406. Vermeer MH, Geelen FA, van Haselen CW, et al: Primary cutaneous large B-cell lymphoma with an intermediate prognosis. Dutch Cutaneous Lymphoma Working Group. Arch Dermatol 1996;132:1304–1308.

407. Kurtin PH, DiCaudo DJ, Habermann TM, et al: Primary cutaneous large cell lymphomas: Morphologic, immunophenotypic, and clinical features of 20 cases. Am J Surg Pathol 1994;18:1183–1191.

408. Joly P, Charlotte F, Leibowitch M, et al: Cutaneous lymphomas other than mycosis fungoides: Follow-up study of 52 patients. J Clin Oncol 1991;9(11):1994–2001.

409. Rijlaarsdam JU, Toonstra J, Meijer OW, et al: Treatment of primary cutaneous B-cell lymphomas of follicle center cell origin: A clinical follow-up study of 55 patients treated with radiotherapy or polychemotherapy. J Clin Oncol 1996;14(2):549–555.

410. Pandolfino TL, Siegel RS, Kuzel TM, et al: Primary cutaneous B-cell lymphoma: Review and current concepts. J Clin Oncol 2000;18(10):2152–2168.

411. Sarris AH, Braunschweig I, Medeiros LJ, et al: Primary cutaneous non-Hodgkin's lymphoma of Ann Arbor Stage I: Preferential cutaneous relapses but high cure rate with doxorubicin-based therapy. J Clin Oncol 2001;19(2):398–405.

Specific Malignancies

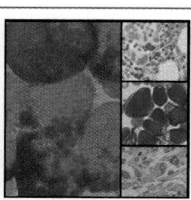

ADULT T-CELL
LEUKEMIA-LYMPHOMA

Kensei Tobinai

Toshiki Watanabe

SUMMARY OF KEY POINTS

BACKGROUND
Adult T-cell leukemia-lymphoma (ATL) is a distinct peripheral T-cell malignancy associated with human T-cell leukemia virus type I (HTLV-I).

VIROLOGY
- HTLV-I is reverse-transcribed into DNA and integrated into the host cell.
- The HTLV-I genome does not contain an oncogene, but it encodes two unique regulatory proteins—Tax and Rex—that are responsible for viral expression and cellular transformation. Tax transactivates viral and cellular genes that could be involved in the pathogenesis of ATL.

EPIDEMIOLOGY
- The major cluster of HTLV-I-infected individuals and patients with ATL exists in Japan, where approximately 1.2 million people are infected with the virus.
- Other clusters have been noted in the Caribbean islands (African), tropical Africa (African), South America (Mongoloid), and northern Oceania (Melanesian).

- HTLV-I is transmitted by mother to child through breast-feeding, by sexual contact, and by blood-borne transmission.
- The estimated cumulative risk of the development of ATL in HTLV-I-positive individuals is 2.5%.

CLINICAL MANIFESTATIONS
- Patients with ATL show diverse clinical features, and four clinical subtypes have been recognized: acute, lymphoma, chronic, and smoldering types.
- The typical manifestations of acute-type ATL include circulating neoplastic cells in the peripheral blood, generalized lymph node swelling, hepatosplenomegaly, skin involvement, and hypercalcemia.

HISTOPATHOLOGY
- Leukemic cells in the peripheral blood characteristically show markedly polylobated nuclei, the so-called "flower cells." Their immunophenotypes are CD4+ and CD8- T cell in most cases.
- All histopathologic specimens show the findings of diffuse non-Hodgkin's lymphoma (NHL) of various subtypes.

DIAGNOSIS
- ATL is suspected when the aforementioned characteristic clinical manifestations and/or the cytologic findings of leukemic cells in the peripheral blood are recognized.
- An immunophenotypic analysis of neoplastic cells and a serological assay against HTLV-I are required for the clinical diagnosis of ATL.
- The demonstration of the monoclonal integration of HTLV-I proviral DNA in the tumor cells can lead to a definite diagnosis of ATL.

TREATMENT
- An accurate diagnosis of the clinical subtype is vital for appropriate decisions regarding treatment.
- Combination chemotherapies used in the treatment of NHL are usually given to patients with the acute or lymphoma subtype of ATL; however, most patients with ATL are not curable with current chemotherapy regimens.
- Further efforts to incorporate new, innovative treatment modalities, such as new anticancer agents, monoclonal antibody therapy, molecular-targeting therapy, and allogeneic hematopoietic stem cell transplantation, are needed.

INTRODUCTION

Adult T-cell leukemia-lymphoma (ATL) was first recognized in Japan by Takatsuki and colleagues in 1977.[1-3] The disease was characterized as leukemia of peripheral T cells, generalized lymphadenopathy, hepatosplenomegaly, and skin involvement. Due to its unusual geographic clustering in southwestern Japan, it was postulated that some infectious agent(s) had causative roles. Using interleukin-2 (IL-2), human T-lymphotropic virus (HTLV) was first isolated by Gallo and associates[4] in the United States from cultured cells from one patient with an aggressive variant of mycosis fungoides and from one with Sézary syndrome. Although both patients were diagnosed clinically as having cutaneous T-cell lymphoma (CTCL) at the time of reporting, their clinical features were later found to closely resemble those of Japanese patients with ATL.

In 1980, Miyoshi and coworkers[5] established the first cell line (MT-1) derived from neoplastic cells in an ATL patient. They cocultured neoplastic cells from an ATL patient with normal human cord blood lymphocytes and established the cell line MT-2 (derived from cord blood lymphocytes), which produced high amounts of type C retrovirus.[6] Using the MT-1 cell line, Hinuma and colleagues[7] found that patients with ATL had antibodies against the virus-associated antigen (ATL virus-associated antigen, ATLA) in their sera. The "ATL virus" was then isolated and characterized as an RNA retrovirus.[8-10] As HTLV and ATL virus were found to be identical by a DNA sequence analysis, this virus was designated human T-cell leukemia virus type I or human T-lymphotropic virus type I (HTLV-I).[11]

The etiological association of HTLV-I and ATL is based on the following findings:

- The areas of high incidence of patients with ATL closely correspond with those of a high prevalence of HTLV-I carriers.[12,13]
- HTLV-I immortalizes T cells in vitro.[14]
- HTLV-I proviral DNA is detected in the neoplastic cells of ATL.[15,16]
- Almost all patients with ATL have antibodies against HTLV-I in their sera.

HTLV-I is the first retrovirus that was found to be associated with a malignant neoplasm in humans.

VIROLOGY[17-19] AND PATHOGENESIS

HTLV-I is reverse-transcribed into DNA and integrated as a proviral DNA in the host cell. The HTLV-I provirus is 9.0 kilobases (kb) long and has structural genes in the order 5'-gag-pol-env-3'. Both ends of the HTLV-I proviral DNA contain repeats called long terminal repeats (LTRs). No specific integration sites of the HTLV-I provirus in the host cellular chromosomes have been identified.[20] A unique feature of the viral structure of HTLV-I provirus is the presence of a long sequence between env and 3'LTR. One product of this pX gene, p40tax, acts on the LTRs for the transactivation of the viral gene.[9,10,21,22]

The HTLV-I gene encodes three structural proteins—group antigen (gag), reverse transcriptase (pol), and envelope (env) proteins. The full-length mRNA is used for synthesis of gag and pol gene products. The gag protein is synthesized as a precursor polypeptide of 55 kDa that is proteolytically cleaved into the individual gag proteins p19, p24, and p15. The protease is encoded in a different reading frame that spans the 3' part of the gag region and the 5' part of the pol region. The pol region encodes the reverse transcriptase (RT), integrase, and RNaseH. The env gene encodes two proteins made from a singly spliced mRNA. It is then cleaved intracellularly into an extracellular glycosylated protein (gp46) and a transmembrane (gp21). It is postulated that two regulatory proteins, Tax and Rex, are essential for HTLV-I expression.

The life cycle of a retrovirus begins with the binding of the virus to specific receptors on the cell surface via viral envelope proteins. The putative gene encoding the cellular receptor for HTLV-I was found to localize at chromosome 17.[23] The HTLV-I enters the cell through a membrane-to-membrane fusion mechanism. Sagara and associates[24] proposed that 71 kDa heat shock cognate protein (HSC70) on the target cell surface acts as a cellular acceptor to gp46 on the HTLV-I-infected cell for syncytium formation, thereby leading to cell-to-cell transmission of HTLV-I.

Mechanisms of Pathogenesis

Role of Tax

The onset of ATL is preceded by a long period of clinical latency, frequently lasting more than 4 decades. In addition, less than 5% of all infected individuals with HTLV-I develop ATL. The promoter insertion model was rejected as the leukemogenic mechanism because integration sites of the provirus were random depending on the patient.[20] Consequently, a trans-acting viral factor, Tax, was proposed to be responsible for leukemogenesis.[21,22,25,26] Tax is a 40-kDa phosphoprotein mainly located in the nucleus. Tax mediates potent activation of viral transcription through interaction with three 21-bp repeats in the LTR, each containing a cyclic AMP response element (CRE) core flanked by 5' G-rich and 3' C-rich sequences. The CREs are bound by the cellular basic domain-leucine zipper (bZip) transcription factors CREB and ATF-1, which, in turn, recruit Tax into stable ternary complexes in which Tax binds the basic domains of CREB/ATF-1 and makes contacts with the flanking GC-rich sequences.[27] Tax further recruits the coactivators CREB binding protein (CBP), p300, and a CBP-associated factor (P/CAF) for potent transcriptional activation. Tax also transcriptionally regulates cellular genes by interaction with enhancer-binding proteins such as CREB, NF-κB, and serum response factor (SRF), and by tethering coactivators to the DNA bound transcription factors.[28-32] If Tax shows a low affinity with a specific transcription factor, however, it represses the gene expression driven by that factor through interaction competition with coactivators.[33]

Among the cellular genes that are the targets of Tax are those with growth-promoting capacities, such as interleukin-6 (IL-6) and lymphokine receptors such as IL-2-receptor α-chain (IL-2Rα), and oncogenes such as c-fos.[34-36] Genes with growth-retarding functions (e.g., p18^{INK4C} and Lck) are included among those transrepressed, however.[37,38] Thus, transcriptional deregulation by Tax will lead to efficient proliferation of infected cells.[39]

Tax interacts and activates specific components of growth factor signal transduction pathways, such as IKK-IkB-NF-kB, RAS/mitogen-activated protein kinase, and protein kinase A (PKA) and PKC.[40,41] Interaction with IKKγ, a component of IKK complex, results in constitutive activation of this kinase complex.[42] Constitutive activation of the JAK-STAT pathway in HTLV-I transformed cells has also been reported, although the mechanisms are not well understood.[43] Thus, HTLV-I infection results in aberrant activation of growth-promoting signaling pathways. Tax also induces cell cycle progression by inhibiting negative cell cycle regulators such as p53 and p16^{INK4A} and stimulates positive cell cycle regulators such as cdk4/6, D-type cyclins, and E2F.[44] The effects of Tax on apoptosis depend on the experimental systems in which Tax was shown to induce or to inhibit apoptosis. Tax-induced resistance to apoptosis supports its role as a transforming factor. The oncogenic capacity of Tax has been reported in various systems; however, cellular transformation by HTLV-I in vivo is a multistage process, and viral gene expression is absent in ATL cells in vivo.[45,46] Moreover, proviruses integrated in ATL cells are frequently defective, have mutations in the coding region of Tax, and/or are methylated in the 5′ and 5′ LTR regions.[47-49] Thus, in addition to promoting growth directly, Tax should endow the infected T cells with capacities that aid the progression to transformed phenotypes in the absence of Tax. In this context, induction of a mutator phenotype by Tax in the infected cells appears to play an important role.[50]

Tax impairs the cell's ability to repair DNA damage. Tax appears to suppress base excision repair (BER) through repression of human DNA polymerase-β and to inhibit cellular nucleotide excision repair (NER) by suppression of DNA polymerase δ activity.[51-53] Induction of BclxL by Tax might also contribute to the suppression of homologous recombination through inhibition of the RAD51 recombination pathway.[54,55] Functional inactivation of p53 by Tax allows HTLV-I-infected cells to survive and proliferate in the presence of unrepaired genomic damage.[56,57] Thus, Tax not only stimulates proliferation of cells but also induces DNA damage in HTLV-I-infected cells, which could constitute a basis for multistep leukemogenesis rendering a mutator phenotype. The roles of HTLV-I Tax in the multistep leukemogenesis of ATL are illustrated in Figure 114-1.

It is assumed that in addition to the critical role of Tax in the leukemogenesis of ATL, additional cellular events have some roles in the development of ATL. Fas antigen (Apo-1/CD95) is an apoptosis-signaling cell surface receptor that belongs to the tumor necrosis factor (TNF) receptor superfamily. Sugahara and associates[58] found that the membrane isoform (mFas) was strongly expressed in ATL cells and that the soluble isoform (sFas) levels were higher in sera from patients with ATL. Several Fas gene mutations were reported in primary samples from patients with ATL.[59] Maeda and coworkers[60] found that the ATL cell line KOB carries heterozygous Fas gene mutation and acquires Fas resistance. Moreover, by transferring the mutant Fas gene to Fas-negative Jurkat cells, these researchers observed that the aberrant Fas antigen functions as a dominant negative interfering Fas signal. These results suggest that abnormality of Fas function could be one of the important steps in the progression of ATL.

Role of Chromosomal Abnormalities

Various karyotypic abnormalities have been reported in neoplastic cells of ATL; however, no specific karyotypic abnormality has been found. In general, the chromosomal abnormalities are more complex in the acute type compared with those in the chronic type. Recently, Itoyama and colleagues[61] reported the results of cytogenetic analysis of 50 cases of ATL and found aneuploidy and multiple breaks more frequently in acute and lymphoma types. Multiple breaks and partial loss of chromosomes correlated with shorter survival. The authors claim that one model of an oncogenic mechanism—activation of a proto-oncogene by translocation of a T-cell receptor (TCR) gene—might not be applicable to the main pathway of development of ATL and that a multistep process of leukemogenesis is required.

In a study by Tsukasaki and associates,[62] 64 patients with ATL were analyzed usng comparative genomic hybridization (CGH). The most frequent observations were gains at chromosomes 14q, 7q, and 3p and losses at chromosomes 6q and 13q. Chromosome imbalances, losses, and gains were observed more frequently in acute or lymphoma types. An increased number of chromosomal imbalances were associated with a shorter survival. Paired samples (i.e., samples obtained at different sites from four patients) and sequential samples from 13 patients (from six during both chronic phase and acute crisis and from seven during both acute onset and relapse) were examined by CGH and Southern blotting for HTLV-I. All but two paired samples showed differences on CGH assessment. Two chronic/crisis samples showed distinct results regarding both CGH and HTLV-I integration sites, suggesting clonal changes in ATL at crisis. In 11 patients, the finding of identical HTLV-I sites and clonally related CGH results suggested a common origin of sequential samples. In contrast to chronic/crisis samples, CGH results with all acute/relapse sample pairs showed the presence of clonally related but not evolutional subclones at relapse (i.e., alterations consisted of imbalances common for both phases and those unique for each phase, thereby suggesting marked chromosomal instability). It was concluded that clonal diversity is common during progression of ATL, and that CGH alterations are associated with clinical course.

Role of p53 and Other Tumor Suppressor Genes

p53 is a nuclear phosphoprotein that functions as a tumor suppressor gene. A loss of normally functioning *p53* through mutation or allelic loss has been found in

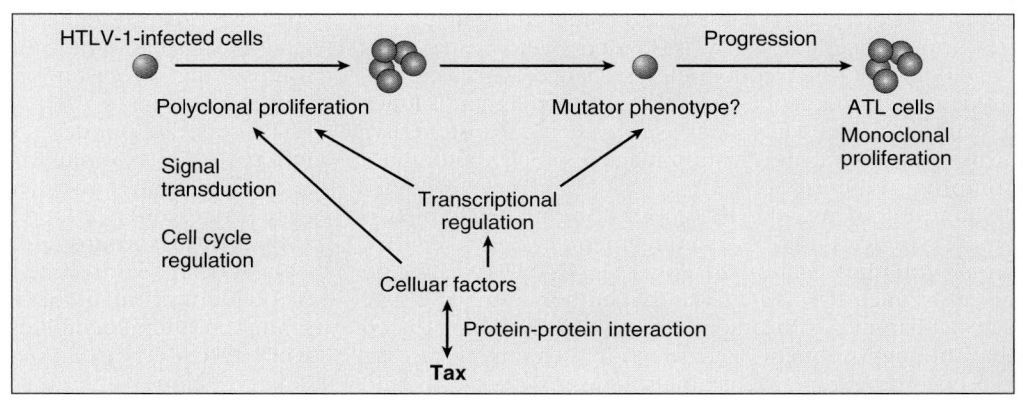

Figure 114-1. Roles of HTLV-I Tax in the multistep leukemogenesis of ATL. Tax exerts its biological effects mainly through protein-protein interaction, resulting in deregulation of transcription, cell cycle control, and signal transduction. It also impairs the cell's ability to repair DNA damage, which can lead to the mutator phenotype of the infected cells.

Specific Malignancies

III

several kinds of malignant neoplasms. Mutations of the *p53* gene have also been found in some patients with ATL.[63,64] According to the study by Cesarman and coworkers,[64] no *p53* mutations were detected in samples from 11 patients with the chronic type-ATL, whereas 9 (28%) of 28 samples from patients with the acute type-ATL exhibited *p53* mutations. In one patient, a tumor sample obtained during the chronic phase did not have a mutation of the *p53* gene, but subsequently the mutation was detected in a sample obtained at crisis. These results suggest that alterations of the p53 gene might contribute to disease progression in a fraction of patients with ATL.

Other putative tumor suppressor genes, *p15[INK4B]* and *p16[INK4A]*, were reported to be associated with ATL.[65-67] Yamada and associates[66] reported that 28 (25%) of 114 patients with ATL showed homozygous deletions of the *p15* and/or *p16* genes. These results correlated well with the clinical subtypes of ATL. In addition, the patients with deleted *p15* and/or *p16* genes showed significantly shorter survival than those in whom both genes were preserved ($P < 0.0001$). Moreover, three of the five chronic-type patients who progressed to acute-type lost the *p16* gene alone or both genes at their exacerbation phase. These results suggest that the deletions of *p15* and/or *p16* genes play a key role in the disease progression of some patients with ATL. Uchida and colleagues[67] found the point mutation of the *p16* gene in 3 (7%) of 44 patients with ATL. It is suggested that the *p16* gene is inactivated not only by homozygous deletion but also by point mutation.

Role of HTLV-I Provirus

The implications of the integration pattern of HTLV-I provirus in the disease progression of ATL have been analyzed by several investigators.[47,68] It is known that the neoplastic cells of ATL have one copy of complete HTLV-I provirus per cell in some patients (complete-type), while others have multiple complete copies of the virus per cell (multiple-type). The HTLV-I proviruses in the remaining patients do not have the complete genome but rather a defective genome (defective-type). Tsukasaki and associates[68] found that the median survival times (MST) for patients were 6.8 months, 24.4 months, and 33.3 months for defective-type, complete-type, and multiple-type ATL, respectively ($P = 0.006$). Among 52 sequentially examined patients, the HTLV-I integration patterns changed in four patients (7.5%). In three of these four, the rearrangements of the TCR-β gene changed concomitantly, suggesting the appearance of a new ATL clone. The researchers concluded that the frequent clonal change of ATL at crisis reflects the emergence of multiple premalignant clones in viral leukemogenesis, as suggested in Epstein-Barr virus (EBV)–associated lymphomagenesis in the immuno-compromised host.

Tamiya and coworkers[47] reported the presence of two types of defective virus. Among them, type 2 defective virus with the deletion that includes 5′-LTR was found more frequently in acute and lymphoma types (39%, 21/54) than in the chronic type (6%, 1/18). It is postulated that the high frequency of the type 2 defective viruses is caused by the genetic instability of HTLV-I provirus, and

that this defective virus is selected because it escapes from the immune surveillance system in the host.

HTLV-I is an etiologic agent not only in ATL but also in the neurologic disorder known as tropical spastic paraparesis (TSP) among Caribbean patients or as HTLV-I-associated myelopathy (HAM) among Japanese patients.[69,70] In TSP/HAM, the HTLV-I provirus remains randomly integrated, whereas in ATL the provirus is monoclonally integrated.

EPIDEMIOLOGY OF HTLV-I AND ATL

Southwestern Japan has the highest recorded prevalence of HTLV-I infection and the highest incidence of patients with ATL in the world.[12,13,71-74] A high prevalence of HTLV-I is also found in the Caribbean islands (African), tropical Africa (African), South America (Mongoloid), and northern Oceania (Melanesian).[71-76] Many patients who have been diagnosed as having ATL in Western countries are immigrants from the West Indies and tropical Africa. The world map of the distribution of HTLV-I and HTLV-II and the presumed routes of spread are shown in Figure 114-2.[73] The geographic clustering of HTLV-I carriers is suggested to be strongly associated with a high frequency of mother-to-child transmission of the virus under closed conditions in particular groups.[3,77]

A population-based nationwide survey of HTLV-I seroprevalence in adult populations in Japan showed characteristic geographical variations from 0.2% in low-endemic areas to 13% in highly endemic areas.[12] It has been estimated that approximately 1.2 million HTLV-I-infected individuals reside in Japan, and the annual incidence of ATL has been estimated to be approximately 700 in Japan.[13] The annual rate of ATL development among HTLV-I carriers older than 40 years is estimated at 1.5/1,000 in males and 0.5/1,000 in females, and the cumulative risk of ATL development among the HTLV-I carriers is estimated to be 2.5% over the course of a 70-year lifespan.[78]

In a national survey in Japan, the mean age of patients with ATL has been estimated at 57.6 years, and this age appears to have increased over time.[13] It has been reported that the age of patients with ATL in areas outside Japan is somewhat lower, with an overall mean age in the mid-forties.[79] In endemic areas, there is a marked increase in HTLV-I prevalence with age until age 70, and an increased prevalence among females compared with males. Transmission occurs via sexual and blood-borne routes. A major reason for the increase in seroprevalence with age appears to be the decreasing prevalence of HTLV-I in the population over time, at least in Japan, where it has been most extensively studied.[80-83] Yamaguchi and coworkers[83] reported that the HTLV-I carrier rates among blood donors in Japan had fallen since 1986 in all age groups under 50 years and in both genders. This decrease in HTLV-I carriers among younger blood donors might be explained by improvements in sanitation, and general lifestyle changes in recent years, as well as the decrease in hepatitis B virus infection rates in Japan. A shorter duration of breast-feeding, the increasing

Figure 114-2. World map of HTLV distribution and its presumed routes of spread. (From Blattner WA, Gallo RC: Epidemiology of HTLV-I and HTLV-II infection. In Takatsuki K [ed]: Adult T-cell Leukaemia. Oxford, Oxford University Press, 1994, p 45. Prepared by Dr. Robert J Biggar, National Cancer Institute, USA).

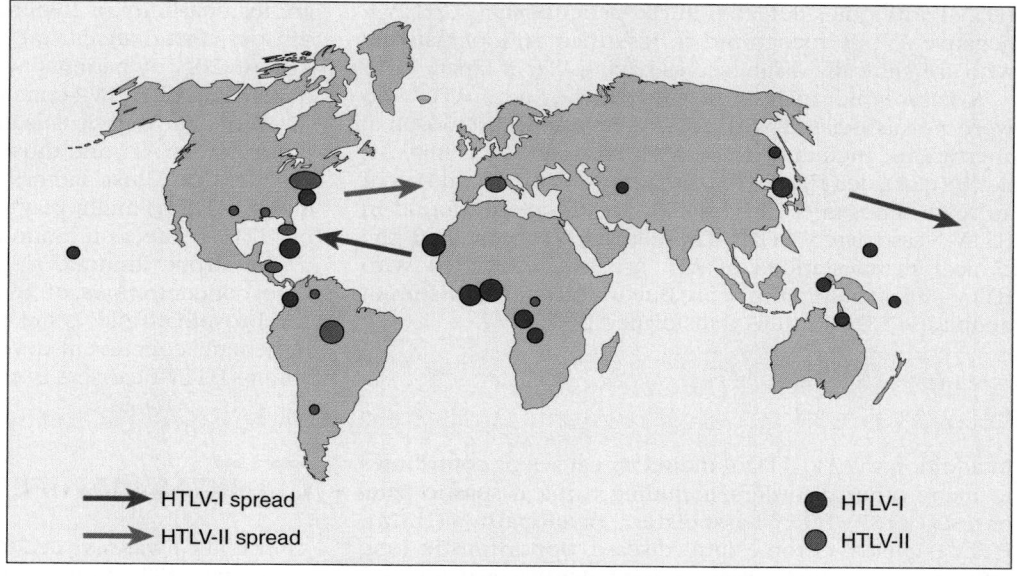

HTLV-I spread

HTLV-II spread

HTLV-I

HTLV-II

use of artificial feeding for babies, and decreasing family size are also likely to be factors for the recent decline in the vertical transmission rates of HTLV-I.[3,83] Overall, there is a slight male predominance of ATL cases, with the male-to-female ratio ranging from 1.1 to 1.5. This is in contrast to TSP and HAM, which affect females more frequently than males.

It has been shown that HTLV-I is transmitted by at least three routes:

1. Mother-to child-transmission, mainly by HTLV-I-positive lymphocytes in breast milk.[84-86]
2. Sexual transmission, more commonly from males to females.
3. Blood-borne transmission, including blood transfusions and sharing of needles by intravenous drug abusers.[87-91]

The first route is vertical transmission from mother to child via HTLV-I-positive lymphocytes in breast milk. The overall infection rate of HTLV-I in children by seropositive mothers has been estimated to be 10% to 30%. HTLV-I infection has also been reported in children who had not been breast-fed, however, which suggests the possibility of intrauterine or transvaginal infection. Several kinds of intervention trials are being conducted in HTLV-I-endemic areas in Japan, where seropositive pregnant women are advised not to breast-feed.[77,92]

The second route is transmission through sexual contact. Transmission of HTLV-I frequently occurs from male to female, but rarely from female to male. HTLV-I has been isolated in semen. It appears likely that the risk of development of ATL after HTLV-I infection by this route of transmission is not high.

To prevent HTLV-I transmission through blood transfusions, serological screening of all blood donors for HTLV-I has been conducted in Japan since November 1986.[87-89] Inaba and coworkers[90] reviewed the effectiveness of the donor screening in preventing transmission of HTLV-I through blood transfusion in Japan. Patients who

received transfusions in Japan from 1990 to 1997 were analyzed. Seroconversion was found in only 1 of 4672 transfused patients, but the donor was confirmed to be negative for anti-HTLV-I antibody and virus genome by nested polymerase chain reaction. A total of 23,323 red cell concentrates and 17,237 platelet concentrates were transfused to these 4,672 patients. Therefore, the anti-HTLV-I prevalence in blood for transfusion after screening was estimated at 1 in 45,560 [0.0022%; the upper 95% confidence interval (CI) was 0.0080%]. This study confirmed that the present donor screening program for HTLV-I can almost completely prevent virus transmission by transfusion in Japan. In contrast to red cell and platelet concentrates, fresh-frozen plasma and plasma fractions have never been shown to transmit HTLV-I.

From the viewpoint of the epidemiological aspects of HTLV-I and ATL, several points can be made in ATL leukemogenesis:

1. Viral infection alone is not adequate for the expression of the malignant phenotype.
2. The timing and/or length of viral exposure is critical.
3. The long latency period suggests that the disease progression is a multistep process.[93] This is in contrast to TSP/HAM, which can occur with a shorter latency period, especially among recipients of blood transfusions.

HTLV-I Negative ATL

Shimoyama and colleagues[94-98] reported the occurrence of ATL among patients not associated with HTLV-I. These patients showed the typical clinical manifestations, including generalized lymphadenopathy, hepatosplenomegaly, skin involvement, hypercalcemia, and elevated lactate dehydrogenase (LDH), typical cell morphology, and immunophenotypes of ATL, but HTLV-I proviral DNA was not detected by Southern blot analysis, nor were anti-

HTLV-I antibodies detected in the patients' sera.[95] HTLV-I-negative ATL is recognized in less than 10% of patients who are clinically diagnosed as having ATL in Japan.

A karyotypic analysis of the patients with ATL who were not associated with HTLV-I revealed chromosomal aberrations, including trisomy 3, trisomy 7, trisomy 21, del(6)(q21), del(10)(p13), 14q11 translocation, and loss of an X chromosome, all of which are frequently found in HTLV-I–associated ATL.[96] These results suggest that the clinical manifestations of ATL are not associated with HTLV-I itself, but that they are due to the characteristics of neoplastic CD4+ T cells transformed by HTLV-I.

HTLV-I–associated Diseases Other Than ATL

In addition to ATL, HTLV-I indirectly causes or contributes to many other disorders, including tropical spastic paraparesis (TSP)/HTLV-I-associated myelopathy (HAM), HTLV-I uveitis, chronic lung disease, opportunistic lung infections, strongyloidiasis, lymphadenitis, arthropathy, and infectious dermatitis (in Jamaican children).[69,70,99-104]

TSP was first found to be associated with HTLV-I by Gessain and associates.[69] Independently, Osame and colleagues[70] revealed an association between HTLV-I and spastic paraparesis (HAM). TSP and HAM were suggested to be identical, and more than 1000 cases have been reported worldwide. A nationwide survey in Japan identified more than 700 cases of TSP/HAM. The endemic area of TSP/HAM corresponds well with those of ATL and HTLV-I carriers. The main neurologic features of TSP/HAM are leg spasticity or hyper-reflexia, leg muscle weakness, sensory disturbances, and urinary bladder disturbances. Almost 20% of patients with TSP/HAM have received a transfusion of HTLV-I-contaminated blood.

Given that the virus isolated from the lymphocytes in patients with ATL and those with TSP/HAM were found to be identical, host factors (including human leukocyte antigen [HLA]) might play some role in the manifestations of HTLV-I infection. Sonoda and colleagues[105] reported that a strong immune response to the virus, shown by high concentrations of HTLV-I antibodies in serum and cerebrospinal fluid, is linked to specific HLA haplotypes. In general, concurrent development of ATL and TSP/HAM among HTLV-I carriers is rare.

CLINICAL MANIFESTATIONS

After HTLV-I was revealed to be associated with ATL, it was found that ATL shows a marked diversity in its clinical manifestations.[106-111] ATL cases have been subdivided into four distinct clinicopathologic entities: acute, lymphoma, chronic, and smoldering types. The recognition of the four clinical subtypes is important in understanding the natural history, clinical features, treatment strategy, and leukemogenesis of ATL. Based on the nationwide survey of 854 patients with ATL who were diagnosed between 1983 and 1987 in Japan, the Lymphoma Study Group proposed the diagnostic criteria of the four clinical subtypes (Table 114-1).[112]

TABLE 114-1

Diagnostic Criteria for Clinical Subtypes of ATL

	SMOLDERING	CHRONIC	LYMPHOMA	ACUTE
Anti-HTLV-I antibody	+	+	+	+
Lymphocyte (× 10^3/μL)	<4	≥4[‡]	<4	*
Abnormal T lymphocytes	≥5%[‖]	+[§]	≤1%	+[§]
"Flower cells" with T-cell marker	[†]	[†]	No	+
LDH	≤1.5N	≤2N	*	*
Corrected Ca^{2+} (mEq/L)	<5.5	<5.5	*	*
Histology-proven				
Lymphadenopathy	No	*	+	*
Tumor lesion				
Skin and/or lung	*	*	*	*
Lymph node	No	*	Yes	*
Liver	No	*	*	*
Spleen	No	*	*	*
Central nervous system	No	*	*	*
Bone	No	No	*	*
Ascites	No	No	*	*
Pleural effusion	No	No	*	*
Gastrointestinal tract	No	No	*	*

ATL, adult T-cell leukemia-lymphoma; HTLV-I, human T-lymphotropic virus type I; LDH, lactate dehydrogenase; N normal upper limit.
*No essential qualification except terms required for other subtype(s).
[†]Typical "flower cells" may be seen occasionally.
[‡]Accompanied by T lymphocytosis (3.5×10^3/μL or more).
[§]If abnormal T lymphocytes are less than 5% in peripheral blood, histologically proven tumor lesion is required.
[‖]Histologically proven skin and/or pulmonary lesion(s) is required if there are fewer than 5% abnormal T lymphocytes in peripheral blood.
From Shimoyama M, and members of the Lymphoma Study Group (1984–1987): Diagnostic criteria and classification of clinical subtypes of adult T-cell leukemia-lymphoma. Br J Haematol 1991;79:428.

- The acute type shows a rapidly progressive clinical course and most of the characteristic features of ATL: generalized lymphadenopathy, hepatomegaly, splenomegaly, skin involvement, hypercalcemia, and organ infiltration (lung, gastrointestinal tract, etc.). The symptoms and signs include abdominal pain, diarrhea, ascites, pleural effusion, cough, sputum, and chest x-ray abnormalities.

- The smoldering type shows an indolent clinical course and only a small percentage of leukemic cells, but it also can include skin involvement.[108,112]

- The chronic type, with a high percentage of leukemic cells, is occasionally associated with skin involvement, lymphadenopathy, and hepatosplenomegaly and also shows an indolent clinical course.

- The lymphoma type includes patients who present with the manifestations of non-Hodgkin's lymphoma (NHL) without circulating malignant cells in the peripheral blood.[112,113] When patients with ATL are staged according to the Ann Arbor classification, most patients are categorized as stage IV, because leukemic cells are recognized even in clinically indolent forms such as the smoldering type and chronic type. Therefore, in ATL, the clinical subtype is more important than the Ann Arbor stage for predicting prognosis and determining appropriate treatment strategies for individual patients.

ATL, particularly the aggressive forms (acute and lymphoma types), has been found to infiltrate the stomach and the intestines in 29% and 25% of patients, respectively, at autopsy.[114] The involvement may be focal as an isolated gastric lesion or so diffuse as to involve the entire gastrointestinal tract.[114,115] Extensive infiltration of the intestines can lead to moderate to severe diarrhea and malabsorption. Patients with ATL suffer from a variety of abdominal symptoms (e.g., nausea, vomiting, abdominal fullness, and diarrhea), which might be attributable to infiltration by neoplastic cells, but because of the associated immunodeficiency, various opportunistic infections such as *Strongyloidiasis* can complicate cases.

Hepatic involvement of ATL cells can be found in up to one fourth of patients with acute and lymphoma subtypes and not infrequently manifests with jaundice and hepatic transaminase elevations. Yamada and coworkers[116] examined 111 patients with acute-type or lymphoma-type ATL and compared them with 106 patients with NHL other than ATL. Among patients with ATL there was more frequent palpable hepatomegaly, higher total bilirubin, hepatic transaminase, LDH, and alkaline phosphatase values than among other NHL patients. Autopsy liver samples disclosed that the portal area was most frequently infiltrated with ATL cells. The researchers also noted a tendency for patients with ATL who also had impaired hepatic function to have shorter survival times.

Pulmonary complications, which are common in ATL, are due to leukemic infiltration in one half of patients and to infections with a variety of bacterial and opportunistic organisms in the other half.[117] Of 854 Japanese patients with ATL, 26% had active infections at the time of diagnosis.[112] The incidence was highest among patients with the chronic and smoldering types (36%) and lower

for patients with the acute (27%) and lymphoma (11%) subtypes. The infections encountered were bacterial (pneumonias, sepsis, and tuberculosis) in 43%, fungal in 31%, protozoal in 18%, and viral in 8% of patients with ATL (see Table 114-2). The immunodeficiency at presentation in ATL can be exacerbated by the neutropenia produced by cytotoxic chemotherapy, leading to an extremely high risk of infection throughout the course of therapy. Infections are responsible for the patient's death in about half of the cases.

Central nervous system (CNS) involvement occurs in approximately 10% of patients with ATL. Teshima and associates[118] identified 15 instances of CNS involvement in 10 of 99 patients with ATL. Leptomeningeal involvement was present in 9 of 10 patients, intracerebral infiltration was noted in 3, and the spinal cord was involved in 2. The initial symptoms included muscle weakness (47%), altered mental status (47%), paresthesias (40%), headache (33%), and urinary incontinence (27%). Signs included nuchal rigidity (33%) and cranial nerve palsies (13%). Hyponatremia secondary to the syndrome of inappropriate secretion of antidiuretic hormone was observed in four patients. CNS involvement frequently occurs in association with a systemic progression of disease.

LABORATORY FINDINGS

Laboratory findings also depend on the clinical subtype of ATL (see Table 114-1).[112] Leukocytosis is found among patients with the acute or chronic subtype at presentation, exhibiting characteristic atypical lymphoid cells with markedly lobated nuclei, termed *flower cells*. Although not all patients present with a leukemic feature, peripheral blood involvement develops in most patients at some time during the course of their disease. Most patients with the acute or lymphoma subtype of ATL have elevated serum LDH levels.

The most striking laboratory finding in patients with ATL is hypercalcemia, which was evident in 32% of Japanese patients with ATL.[112] Multiple factors have been suggested to contribute to the development of hypercalcemia. Lytic bone lesions have been described in some patients; however, examinations of bone obtained at autopsy or from bone marrow biopsies usually reveal activated osteoclasts with increased bone resorption; infiltrating neoplastic T cells are rarely found. Patients with ATL have low phosphates, hypercalciuria, high levels of nephrogenous cyclic adenosine monophosphate (cAMP), and low levels of 1,25-dihydroxyvitamin D. This pattern suggests the presence of humoral hypercalcemia of malignancy, which was found to be secondary to the production of a parathyroid hormone (PTH)-like molecule by malignant cells. HTLV-I-infected cells were found to produce a protein with PTH-like activity, such as PTH-related peptide (PTHrP).[119-123] The constitutive expression of the PTHrP gene was detected in peripheral blood mononuclear cells from HTLV-I carriers and in patients with TSP/HAM, in addition to patients with ATL.[123] Another suggested contributor to hypercalcemia in patients with ATL is cytokine production by the tumor cells. Osteoclast-

Specific Malignancies

III

activating factor was first discovered in supernatants of cultured neoplastic T cells.[124,125] HTLV-I–infected cell lines and fresh ATL cells from hypercalcemic patients produce TNF-α, TNF-β, IL-1α, and IL-1β.[126-129] Each of these cytokines can enhance osteoclast activity and bone-resorbing activity in animal models. Ishibashi and colleagues[130] demonstrated elevated serum levels of TNF-β in seven of eight patients with ATL who had complications of hypercalcemia and in none of 28 patients with ATL who had normal serum calcium levels.

Recently, Nosaka and coworkers[131] analyzed the expression of various genes that were suggested to regulate serum calcium levels in ATL and reported that the overexpression of the receptor activator of NF-κB (RANK) ligand gene correlated with hypercalcemia. ATL cells from patients with hypercalcemia, which highly expressed the transcripts of the RANK ligand (RANKL) gene, induced the differentiation of human hematopoietic precursor cells (HPCs) into osteoclasts in vitro in the presence of macrophage colony-stimulating factor (M-CSF). In contrast, ATL cells from patients without hypercalcemia did not induce such differentiation, suggesting that the induction of the differentiation correlated with the expression of the RANKL gene in ATL cells. Cell differentiation was suppressed by osteoprotegerin/Fc, an inhibitor of RANKL, suggesting that such differentiation occurred through the RANK-RANKL pathway. In addition, direct contact between ATL cells and HPCs was essential for the differentiation, suggesting that membrane-bound RANKL rather than the soluble form plays a role in this process. The authors claimed that ATL cells induce the differentiation of HPCs to osteoclasts through RANKL expressed on their surface, in cooperation with M-CSF, and that they ultimately cause hypercalcemia. The etiology of hypercalcemia in ATL is likely to be multifactorial and in individual patients is probably due to some combination of the factors just described.

Elevated serum levels of soluble interleukin-2 receptor (sIL-2R) in patients with ATL, especially in those with the acute or lymphoma subtype, have been noted in several studies.[132,133] The serum level of sIL-2R is suggested to be one of the useful markers for evaluating the clinical aggressiveness of the disease and for monitoring the response to therapy in patients with ATL.

Histopathology

The circulating cells in the peripheral blood have markedly polylobated nuclei with homogeneous and condensed chromatin, small or absent nucleoli, and agranular and basophilic cytoplasm—the so-called "flower cells" that are characteristic of ATL (Fig. 114-3).[112] A considerable diversity of morphology among ATL cells has been recognized, however. Tsukasaki and associates[134] investigated the morphology of ATL cells in 36 acute cases and 14 chronic cases. Chronic lymphocytic leukemia (CLL)–like morphology with round nuclei was more frequent in the chronic type than in the acute type. In contrast, unusual morphology (lymphoblastic, vacuolated, granular pleomorphic, or large cells) was more frequent in the acute type than in the chronic type.

The swollen lymph nodes in patients with ATL show diffuse NHL of various histologic subtypes, including pleomorphic, large-cell, mixed-cell, or medium-sized cell types.[135-140] Figure 114-4 shows the histology of a biopsied swollen lymph node from a patient with lymphoma-type ATL. The pleomorphic pattern (i.e., a mixture of various-sized lymphoma cells from small cells to giant cells) and nuclear polymorphism are recognized. Lymph nodes from some patients in the incipient or early neoplastic phase of ATL histologically resemble those found in Hodgkin's lymphoma.[141,142] This pattern is recognized in the WHO classification as a morphological variant.[143] Similar Reed-Sternberg–like cells have been described in other forms of peripheral T-cell lymphoma, most commonly in angio-immunoblastic T-cell lymphoma.[144] No correlation between histologic subtype and clinical behavior has been recognized.

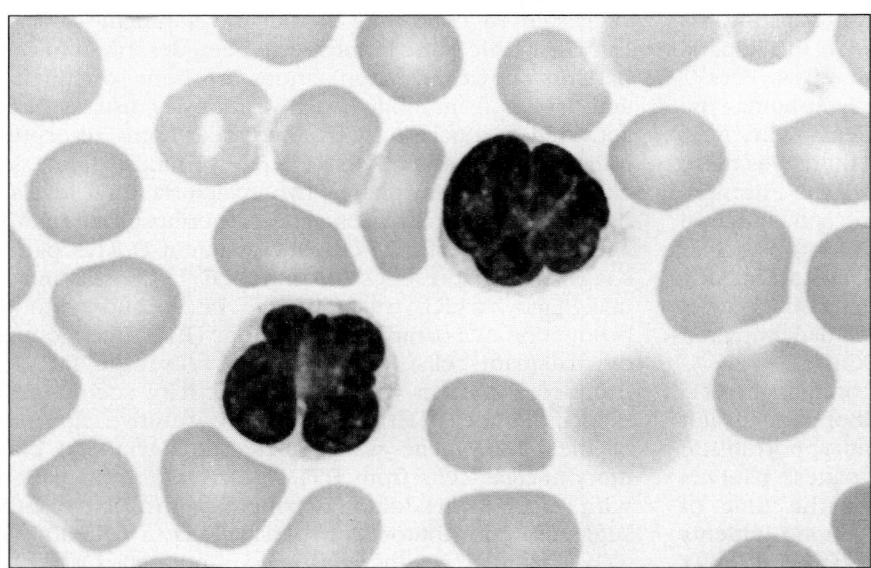

A

Figure 114-3. A–C, Leukemic cells (the so-called *flower cells*) showing characteristic polymorphic nuclei in a peripheral blood smear from a patient with acute-type ATL.

Figure 114-3, *cont'd.*

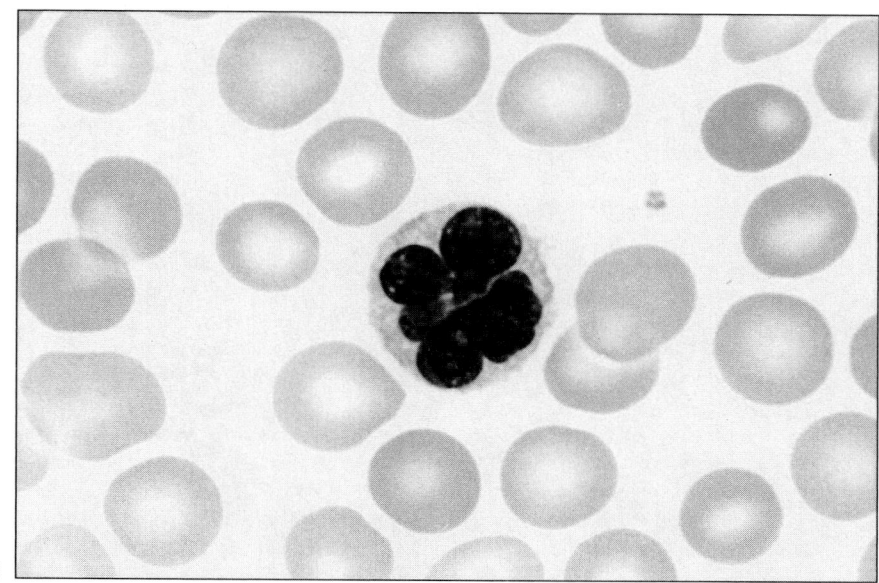

B

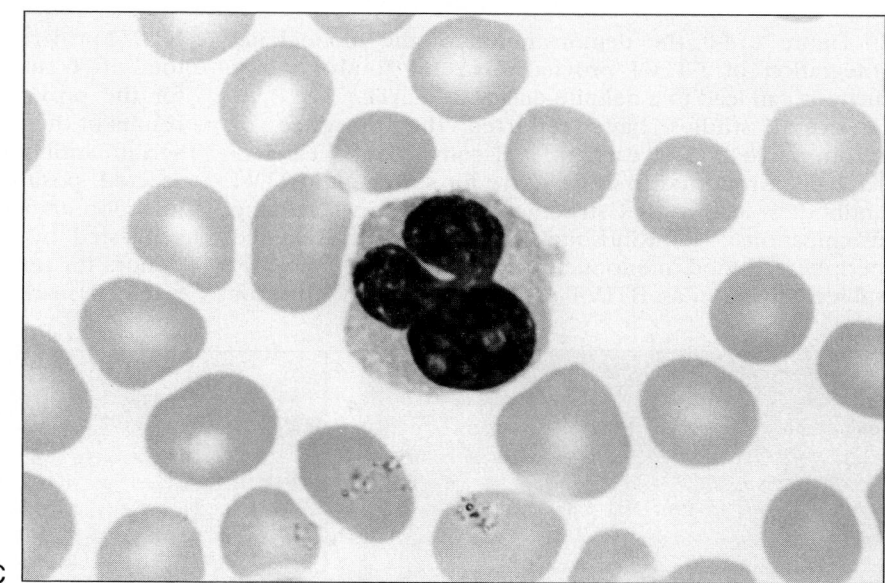

C

ATL cells frequently involve the skin. Generalized nodular or papulonodular eruptions, as shown in Figure 114-5A, are common; however, tumorous lesions are also recognized in some patients. Erythematous plaque formation and sometimes nodular tumors are other cutaneous manifestations.[139,145] Histologically, diffuse or patchy infiltration of atypical lymphoid cells—usually small or medium in size with polymorphic nuclear contours in the upper dermis, sometimes with an intraepidermal infiltration—is noted (Fig. 114-5B). Large-nuclear cells with highly irregular or cerebriform features are intermingled in some cases.

One of the difficult issues in the diagnosis of ATL is its relationship with other peripheral T-cell malignancies not associated with HTLV-I. The clinical diagnosis of ATL is suspected by the unique combination of its clinical and pathologic features. One of the T-cell malignancies that is likely to be confused with ATL is mycosis fungoides-Sézary syndrome (MF/SS). Because cutaneous involvement is frequent in ATL, the differentiation of smoldering-type ATL from MF/SS is often difficult based on the clinical manifestations alone. In the differential diagnosis of ATL and other peripheral T-cell malignancies, HTLV-I serology and the molecular detection of the monoclonal integration of HTLV-I proviral DNA are important.[15,16,146,147] Various kinds of serological assays have been used, including the immunofluorescence assay, the particle agglutination (PA) assay, the enzyme-linked immunosorbent assay (ELISA), and the Western blot assay.[7,89,146-148] In general, a particle agglutination assay or ELISA is useful as a screening test, and Western blotting is used for the confirmation of the presence of serum antibody to HTLV-I.[148] As shown

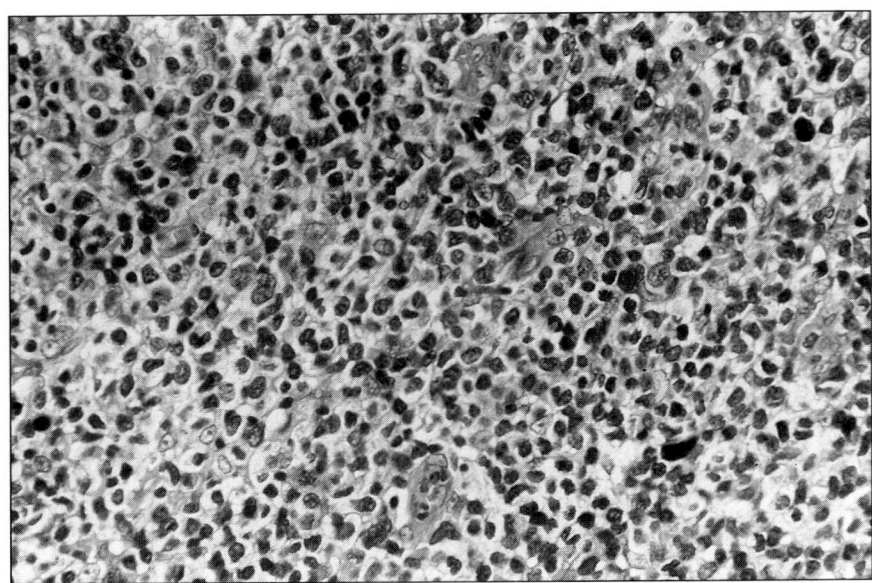

Figure 114-4. Histology of a swollen lymph node from a patient with lymphoma-type ATL, showing diffuse non-Hodgkin's lymphoma of the pleomorphic type. Lymphoma cells of various sizes—small cells, medium-size cells, large cells, and giant cells—are present. Nuclear polymorphism is present in most lymphoma cells.

in Figure 114-6, the demonstration of the monoclonal integration of HTLV-I proviral DNA by Southern blot analysis can lead to a definite diagnosis of ATL.

Several studies have reported the presence of seronegative HTLV-I carriers, and some HTLV-I carriers have been reported to be negative for serum anti-HTLV-I antibodies against viral structural proteins on screening examinations.[149-151] Kinoshita and associates[152] examined peripheral blood mononuclear cells from 209 healthy subjects living in an HTLV-I–endemic district in Japan for

HTLV-I provirus, using polymerase chain reaction (PCR). A total of 76 subjects were positive and 133 were negative for the provirus, showing a close correlation with the results of the previously mentioned assays for anti-HTLV-I serum antibodies. None of the seronegative subjects reacted positively in PCR analysis. Infrequent HTLV-I infection among seronegative subjects in Japan was also suggested by the finding that the screening of blood donors for serum HTLV-I antibodies by the PA assay has reduced markedly the risk of HTLV-I transmission by

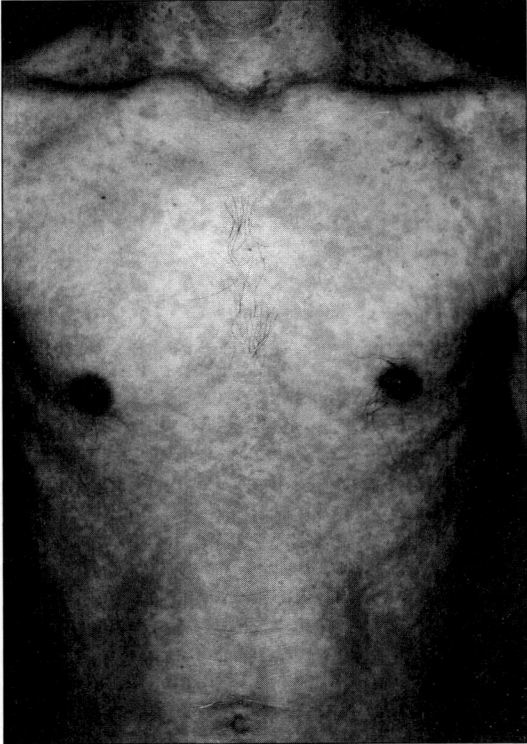

A

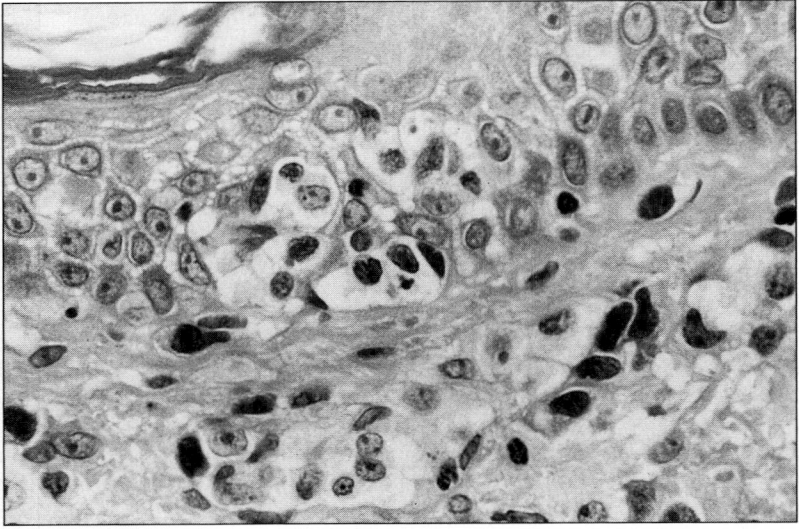

B

Figure 114-5. Skin involvement of ATL. **A**, Photograph of skin lesions in a patient with acute-type ATL. **B**, Histology of skin infiltration of ATL cells in the same patient; infiltrating leukemic cells are present in the epidermis.

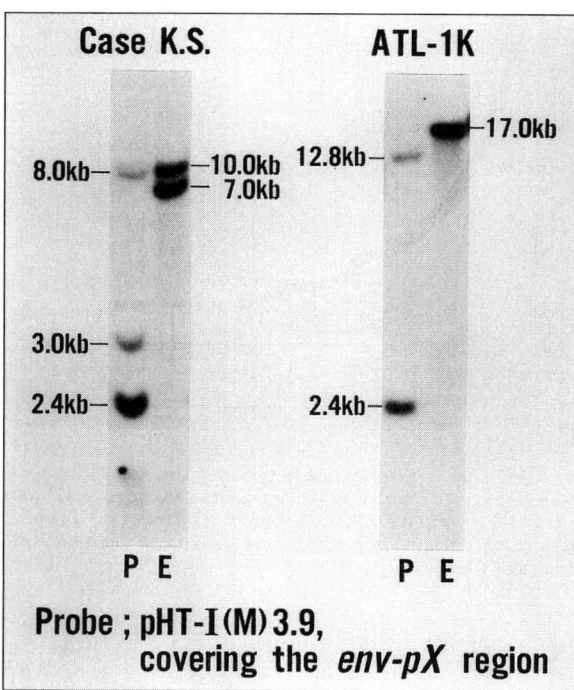

Figure 114-6. Southern blot analysis of HTLV-I proviral DNA in peripheral blood mononuclear cells from an ATL patient. The genomic probe, pHT-I (M) 3.9, covering the *env-pX* region, was used. ATL-1K, a cultured cell line from ATL, was used as a positive control. The restriction enzymes Pst I (P) and EcoRI (E) were used. In the cellular DNA from this patient, two bands are present in the EcoRI digest, indicating the monoclonal integration of HTLV-I proviral DNA.

blood transfusions.[153,154] Furthermore, using PCR analysis, the absence of seronegative HTLV-I carriers among blood donors and healthy junior high-school students in Japan was confirmed.[155,156] These observations suggest that seronegative HTLV-I carriers are extremely rare, although the possibility of their existence remains.

In Western countries, it has been reported that the HTLV-I viral genome was detected in the genomic DNA from patients with MF/SS, and a causal relation between HTLV-I and MF/SS was proposed.[157,158] An opposite conclusion was reached in a Japanese study; using PCR with four sets of primers (including *gag, pol, env,* and *pX* regions of HTLV-I), Kikuchi and colleagues[159] investigated both fresh and cultured T cells (128 specimens) derived from 50 Japanese patients with CTCL. In their study, none of the 128 DNA samples revealed positive results for HTLV-I. They concluded that CTCL, which does not include HTLV-I, is present in Japan. The absence of a correlation between HTLV-I and CTCL was also confirmed by an international cooperative study reported by Bazarbachi and coworkers.[160] These researchers analyzed 128 patients (85 with MF, 28 with SS, 5 with Sézary cell leukemia, 4 with lymphomatoid papulosis, and 5 with unspecified CTCL) originating from Europe (France, Spain, United Kingdom, Portugal) or from the United States (California) for the presence of HTLV-I infection markers, using a serological analysis for antibody to HTLV-I, a reverse transcriptase assay, and a molecular

analysis with PCR-amplified specimens. The results of this international study from five different countries suggest that MF and SS are not associated with HTLV-I infection.

HTLV-I can infect lymphoid cells of different cell lineages in vitro, but the neoplastic cells in the great majority of ATL cases exhibit the phenotype of mature CD4+ T cells.[161,162] Malignant cells from the peripheral blood or from involved lymph nodes express CD2, CD3, CD4, CD5, the αβ-chains of the TCR, CD25 (IL-2Rα), CD45, CD29, and HLA-DR.[147,163-171] It is known that the expression of the CD3/TCR complex is decreased in ATL cells.[172] Most ATL cells lack CD7. Considerable phenotypic heterogeneity has been found in the neoplastic cells of ATL. Although the most common phenotype is CD4+/CD8-, some patients with ATL exhibit a CD4+/CD8+, CD4-/CD8+, or CD4-/CD8- phenotype.[166,169] In addition, some patients with ATL show phenotypic changes throughout the course of their disease, although the integration patterns of HTLV-I proviral DNA and/or the rearrangement patterns of TCR genes do not change.[173,174] Despite the expression of CD4, the great majority of ATL cells exhibit a suppressor function when tested in an assay of pokeweed mitogen-induced immunoglobulin production by normal B cells.[165,168,170,171,175]

One of the remarkable features of ATL cells (and of most HTLV-I-infected cells) is the expression of IL-2R. Both the α- and β-chains of IL-2R are expressed on the surface of ATL cells.[170] It is postulated that IL-2 and IL-2R are implicated in the pathogenesis of ATL. IL-2R is expected to be an excellent target for monoclonal antibody therapy.[176-180]

CLINICAL COURSE AND TREATMENT

ATL most often pursues the prototypic acute course originally described by Takatsuki and colleagues[1,2,181]; however, approximately one fourth of patients show a more indolent course (chronic and smoldering types), with disease limited predominantly to the peripheral blood and/or skin. These patients might experience multiple infections but can remain remarkably free of disease progression for many years.[112] These indolent diseases frequently progress to full-blown acute or lymphomatous ATL, an event that is sometimes called the "crisis." Some studies have reported that various kinds of infectious episodes might predispose to the transformation from an indolent to an aggressive disease course. At present, however, it is impossible to identify patients at the highest risk of transformation.

Most patients with ATL are not curable with current treatment modalities, even at the early stage of disease. In addition, no treatment has been shown to prevent disease progression to a more aggressive disease. Patients with chronic- or smoldering-type ATL should be watched carefully for the development of infectious complications and for signs of disease progression to acute or lymphomatous ATL.

Without treatment, most previously untreated patients with aggressive forms (acute or lymphoma type) of ATL die within weeks or months of diagnosis. The treatment of patients with acute or lymphomatous ATL has not been very successful. Figure 114-7 shows the overall survival of 818 patients with ATL regardless of disease subtype, and Figure 114-8 presents their survival curves according to the four clinical subtypes.[112] Some 85% of the patients received chemotherapy with one of a variety of different regimens. Most of the patients with the smoldering type of ATL lived well without chemotherapy for a long period. Approximately two thirds of the chronic-type patients died within about 2.5 years from diagnosis. Patients with the lymphoma type of ATL had poor prognoses, with an MST of 10.2 months. The most aggressive type of ATL was the acute type, with an MST of 6.2 months. The projected 4-year survival rates of patients with the lymphoma and acute types were only 5%. The clinical subtype clearly determines the prognosis of each patient, suggesting that it can be used as a prognostic indicator for patients with ATL.[112]

The prognostic factors for each subtype of ATL have been analyzed by the Lymphoma Study Group in Japan.[182-184] In all cases of ATL, advanced age (40 years or greater), poor performance status, high serum LDH, hypercalcemia and four or more involved lesions were unfavorable prognostic factors. For patients with chronic-type ATL, the major prognostic factors were the serum values of LDH, albumin, and blood urea nitrogen (BUN). Patients with chronic-type ATL and normal values for the three factors (30% of patients with chronic type disease) showed a prognosis as good as those with smoldering-type ATL. Thus, patients with the favorable chronic type with normal LDH, albumin, and BUN values need not be treated immediately and can be placed on follow-up without treatment, whereas patients with the unfavorable

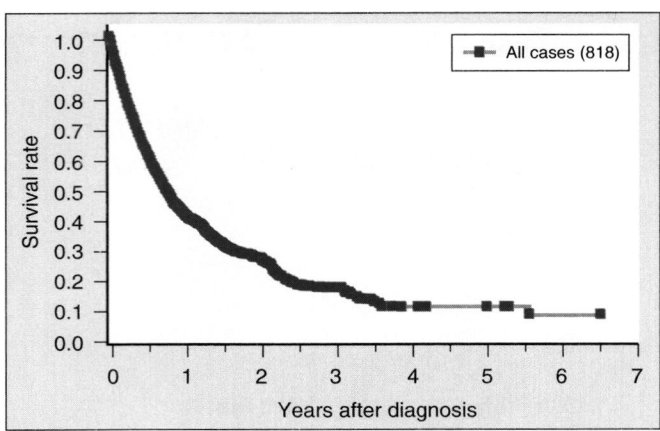

Figure 114-7. Survival curves of 818 patients with ATL. Numbers in parentheses indicate number of patients. (From Shimoyama M and members of the Lymphoma Study Group, 1984–1987: Diagnostic criteria and classification of clinical subtypes of adult T-cell leukemia-lymphoma. Br J Haematol 1991;79:428.)

chronic type having an abnormal value in at least one of the three factors are candidates for cytotoxic chemotherapy.[184]

ATL Clinical Trials by the Lymphoma Study Group of the Japan Clinical Oncology Group

Six consecutive chemotherapy trials focusing on ATL have been conducted by the Japan Clinical Oncology Group (JCOG)-LSG since 1978.[185-191] The first trial, called LSG1 protocol (1978–1980), utilized "VEPA" therapy, which consisted of vincristine (VCR), cyclophosphamide (CPA), prednisolone (PSL), and doxorubicin (DOX). In this study, patients with NHL (including ATL) at an advanced stage were enrolled. The complete remission (CR) rate

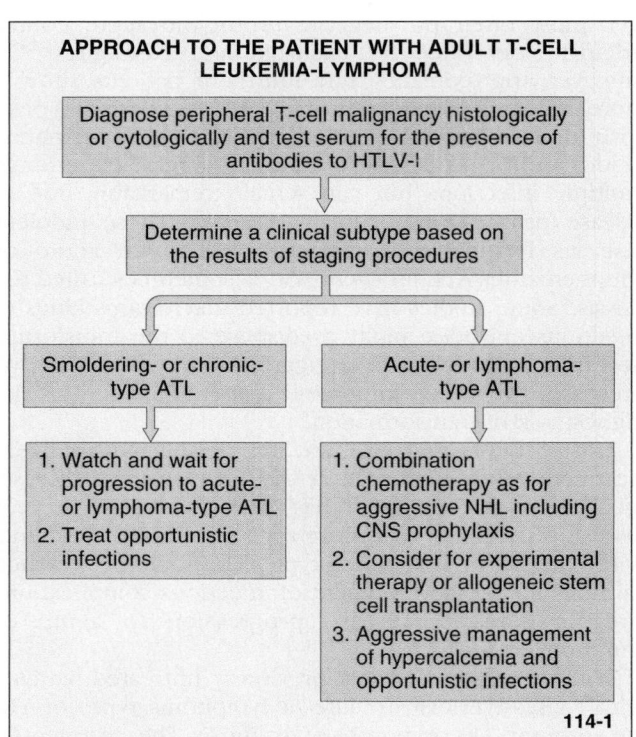

APPROACH TO THE PATIENT WITH ADULT T-CELL LEUKEMIA-LYMPHOMA

Diagnose peripheral T-cell malignancy histologically or cytologically and test serum for the presence of antibodies to HTLV-I

Determine a clinical subtype based on the results of staging procedures

Smoldering- or chronic-type ATL

Acute- or lymphoma-type ATL

1. Watch and wait for progression to acute- or lymphoma-type ATL
2. Treat opportunistic infections

1. Combination chemotherapy as for aggressive NHL including CNS prophylaxis
2. Consider for experimental therapy or allogeneic stem cell transplantation
3. Aggressive management of hypercalcemia and opportunistic infections

114-1

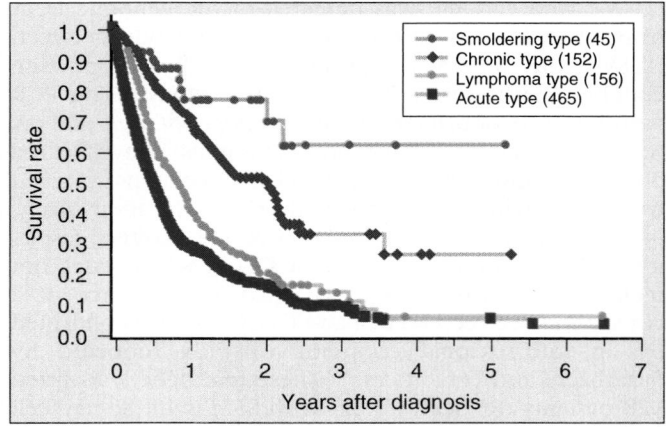

Figure 114-8. Survival curves of 818 patients with ATL according to four clinical subtypes defined by the diagnostic criteria. Numbers in parentheses indicate number of patients. (From Shimoyama M and members of the Lymphoma Study Group, 1984–1987: Diagnostic criteria and classification of clinical subtypes of adult T-cell leukemia-lymphoma. Br J Haematol 1991;79:428.)

MANAGEMENT STRATEGY FOR PATIENTS WITH ATL

When oncologists diagnose patients suspected of lymphoid malignancy, it is important to consider the possibility of ATL. A routine check for serum HTLV-I antibody is recommended at initial diagnosis. The following three points are essential for the diagnosis of ATL:

1. Cytologically or histologically proven lymphoid malignancy
2. Mature T-cell phenotype, mostly CD4+, determined by flow cytometry or immunohistochemistry
3. Positive for anti-HTLV-I antibody

When a patient is diagnosed with ATL, it is important to determine the clinical subtype for the sake of optimizing treatment strategy. For patients with smoldering- or chronic-type ATL, close observation is recommended. Careful monitoring for opportunistic infections—including bacterial, fungal, or *Pneumocystis carinii* infection—is also needed.

For patients with acute- or lymphoma-type ATL, serum calcium level should be checked immediately. For those with complications of hypercalcemia, prompt management includes fluid therapy, bisphosphonate, and chemotherapy. Patients with acute- or lymphoma-type ATL requiring therapy should be enrolled in clinical trials if these are available. When there is no active clinical trial, or if a patient is ineligible for the trial, chemotherapy for aggressive NHL should be considered. For such patients, we usually give biweekly CHOP therapy (CHOP every 2 weeks with the prophylactic use of G-CSF) and prophylactic intrathecal administration of MTX. Because most patients with ATL are not curable with current chemotherapy regimens, it is reasonable to consider the applicability of allogeneic stem cell transplantation for patients who have responded to chemotherapy. For relapsed or refractory patients, consider allogeneic stem cell transplantation or enrollment in a clinical trial of a new chemotherapeutic agent.

---

was lowest (18%) for ATL, intermediate (36%) for peripheral non-ATL T-lymphoma (PNTL), and highest (64%) for B-cell lymphoma.[185,186] Between 1981 and 1983, the JCOG-LSG conducted a randomized phase III trial using LSG1-VEPA vs. LSG2-VEPA-M (VEPA + methotrexate) against advanced NHL, including ATL.[187,188] Patients' sera were examined for anti-HTLV-I antibody to distinguish ATL from PNTL.[192] The CR rate for patients given LSG2-VEPA-M for ATL (37%) was higher than that for patients given LSG1-VEPA (17%) (P = 0.09). In the LSG1/LSG2 trial, however, the CR rate was significantly lower for ATL than for B-cell lymphoma and PNTL (P < 0.001). The MST of the 54 patients with ATL treated with LSG1/LSG2 was 6 months, and the estimated 4-year survival rate was only 8%.[187,188] These results suggest that first-generation combination chemotherapy was not very effective against ATL.

Between 1987 and 1991, the JCOG-LSG conducted a combination phase II study (JCOG8701) of a new second-generation combination chemotherapy against advanced aggressive NHL (including ATL). This combination chemotherapy, called LSG4 protocol, consisted of three different regimens:

1. VEPA-B—VCR, CPA, PSL, DOX and bleomycin (BLM)
2. M-FEPA—methotrexate (MTX), vindesine (VDS), CPA, PSL and DOX
3. VEPP-B—VCR, etoposide (ETP), procarbazine (PCZ), PSL, and BLM[189]

The CR rate (72%) for the LSG4 protocol among aggressive NHL patients was significantly higher than that for the LSG1/LSG2 trial (57%) (P < 0.05). The CR rate for ATL was improved from 28% (LSG1/LSG2) to 43% (LSG4). On the other hand, the CR rate for LSG4 was significantly lower for ATL than for B lymphoma and PNTL (P < 0.01). The patients with ATL still showed a poor prognosis, with an MST of 8 months and a 4-year survival rate of 12%; however, the continued CR rate was increased to 12% (5/43) compared with 4% (2/54) in the LSG1/LSG2 trial (P = 0.13). A multivariate analysis of the 267 patients

with advanced aggressive NHL who were treated with the LSG4 protocol demonstrated that the clinical diagnosis of ATL was the most significant unfavorable prognostic factor (relative risk, 3185; P = 0.0001) for aggressive NHL patients in Japan.[189]

The disappointing results with conventional chemotherapies have led to the search for new active agents. 2′-Deoxycoformycin (DCF, pentostatin), which is an irreversible inhibitor of adenosine deaminase, has been shown to be effective in a number of lymphoid malignancies. In 1984, Daenen and colleagues[193] reported a CR in a female with acute-type ATL following multiple intravenous administrations of DCF at 5 mg/m²/week. Based on the promising results of some single-institute studies of DCF against ATL, multicenter phase I and phase II studies of DCF as a single agent were conducted against ATL in Japan.[184,193-196] The phase II study of DCF revealed a response rate of 32% (10/31) in relapsed or refractory ATL, using the weekly intravenous administration of 5 mg/m². Two patients achieved CR, and eight achieved PR.[184] These encouraging results prompted the Japanese investigators to conduct a DCF-containing combination phase II trial (JCOG9109; LSG11 protocol) as initial chemotherapy for ATL.[190] Patients with the acute, lymphoma, and unfavorable chronic types of ATL were eligible for this trial. Between 1991 and 1993, 62 previously untreated patients with ATL (34 patients with acute, 21 with lymphoma, and 7 with chronic subtypes) were enrolled, but 2 of them were ineligible because they were judged to be of the favorable chronic type. VCR (1 mg/m² intravenously on days 1 and 8), DOX (40 mg/m² intravenously on day 1), ETP (100 mg/m² intravenously on days 1 through 3), PSL (40 mg/m² orally on days 1 and 2), and DCF (5 mg/m² intravenously on days 8, 15, and 22) were administered every 28 days for 10 cycles unless disease progression or toxic complications occurred. Among the 61 patients evaluable for toxicity, 4 patients (7%) died of fatal infections (2 of sepsis and 2 of cytomegalovirus [CMV] pneumonia). No other fatal nonhematologic toxicities occurred. In the 60 eligible patients, 17 (28%; 95% CI 19%–41%) achieved CR, while 14 achieved PR (response rate 52%; 95% CI 39%–64%). After a median observation time of 27 months, the MST was 7.4 months, and the estimated 2-year survival was 17%—findings that were identical to those for the 43 patients with ATL who were treated with the previous LSG4 protocol (JCOG8701).[189,190] Two conclusions were reached based on the JCOG9109 study. First, patients with ATL who were treated with a DCF-containing five-drug regimen (the LSG11 protocol) showed survival comparable with those treated with a nine-drug regimen (the LSG4 protocol). Second, the prognosis of the patients with ATL remained poor even though they were treated with a DCF-containing combination chemotherapy.

In 1994, JCOG-LSG initiated a new multiagent combination phase II study (JCOG9303; LSG15 protocol): a nine-drug regimen consisting of VCR, CPA, DOX, PSL, nimustine (MCNU), VDS, ETP, and carboplatin (CBDCA) with the intrathecal administration of MTX and PSL, for untreated patients with ATL.[191] In this study, the elevation of relative dose intensity was attempted with the prophylactic use of granulocyte colony-stimulating factor (G-CSF). In addition, non–cross-resistant agents such as MCNU and CBDCA were incorporated into the regimens. Ninety-six previously untreated patients with aggressive ATL were enrolled: 58 with acute type, 28 with lymphoma type, and 10 with unfavorable chronic type. Of the 93 eligible patients, 81% responded (75/93), with 33 patients (35%) achieving CR and 42 (45%) achieving PR. Patients with lymphoma-type ATL showed a better CR rate (67%, 18/27) than patients with acute-type ATL (20%, 11/56) and patients with unfavorable chronic-type ATL (40%, 4/10). The overall survival of 93 eligible patients at 2 years was estimated to be 31% (Fig. 114-9). The MST was 13 months,

and the median follow-up duration of the 20 surviving patients was 4.2 years. A trend toward better survival for patients with lymphoma-type ATL (MST, 20 months) compared with patients with acute-type ATL (MST, 11 months) was recognized (hazard ratio, 1.65). Grade 4 hematologic toxicities of neutropenia and thrombocytopenia were observed in 65% and 53% of the patients, respectively, but grade 4 nonhematologic toxicity was observed in only one patient. It was concluded that the LSG15 protocol was feasible with mild nonhematologic toxicity and that it improved the clinical outcome of patients with ATL. To confirm whether the LSG15 is a new standard for the treatment of aggressive patients with ATL, JCOG-LSG is presently conducting a randomized phase III study comparing the LSG15 and biweekly CHOP (CPA, DOX, VCR, PSL) with the prophylactic use of G-CSF and intrathecal administration of MTX and PSL.

Development of New Agents for Therapy of ATL

In addition to DCF, several types of new agents against ATL have been investigated.

Sobuzoxane (MST-16)

Sobuzoxane (MST-16) is a bis(2,6-dioxopiperazine) analog that inhibits topoisomerase II. Sobuzoxane is bioavailable following oral administration and has myelosuppression as its dose-limiting toxicity (DLT). In a phase I–II study of sobuzoxane, which was administered orally at 1200 to 2800 mg/day for 7 days, the response rate among 23 patients with ATL was reported to be 44%, including two patients achieving CR and eight achieving PR.[197] Unfortunately, the duration of remission was generally short.

Irinotecan Hydrochloride (CPT-11)

Irinotecan hydrochloride (CPT-11) is a semisynthetic analog of camptothecin with inhibitory activity against topoisomerase I. Preclinical studies of CPT-11 have suggested a lack of cross-resistance between topoisomerase I inhibitors and other anticancer agents. Phase II studies of CPT-11 conducted in Japan have demonstrated definitive activity against various kinds of solid tumors. Multicenter early- and late-phase II studies of CPT-11 have been conducted against relapsed or refractory NHL in Japan.[198,199] In this study, 9 patients achieved CR, and 17 patients achieved PR (response rate 38% [26/69]), using a weekly intravenous administration of 40 mg/m^2/day for 3 consecutive days. Within this group, 5 of 13 patients with ATL (38%) showed a response to CPT-11 (1 patient achieving CR and 4 achieving PR).[199,200] The major toxicities of CPT-11 were leukopenia, diarrhea, and nausea and/or vomiting. Subsequently, to develop a new effective chemotherapy regimen against NHL and ATL, we conducted two kinds of phase I/II studies of CPT-11 in combination with CBDCA or ETP for patients with relapsed or refractory NHL.[201,202] In both studies, however, dose escalation was halted because of hematologic toxicity (in combination with CBDCA) and hepatotoxicity (in combination with ETP).

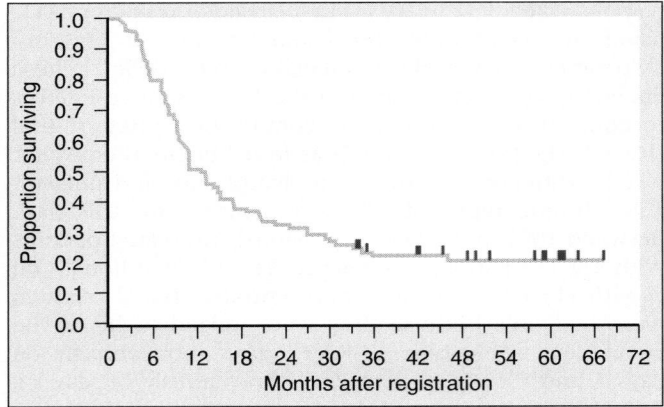

Figure 114-9. Kaplan-Meier estimate of the overall survival (OS) for the 93 eligible patients with aggressive ATL. OS was defined as the time from registration until death from any cause or until the last follow-up evaluation for patients who were still alive (20 patients). (From Yamada Y, Tomonaga M, Fukuda H, et al: A new G-CSF-supported combination chemotherapy, LSG15, for adult T-cell leukemia-lymphoma [ATL]: Japan Clinical Oncology Group (JCOG) Study 9303. Br J Haematol 2001;113:375.)

High-Dose Interferon-α

Based on preliminary documentation of the efficacy of interferon-α against ATL, two kinds of phase II trials of high-dose interferon-α (intravenous administration and subcutaneous administration) have been conducted; however, the results have not been impressive. In 1995, Gill and associates[203] in the United States reported that 11 of 19 patients with acute- or lymphoma-type ATL achieved major responses (5 CR and 6 PR) by the combination therapy of interferon-α and zidovudine. The efficacy of this combination was also observed in a French study; major objective responses were obtained in all five patients with ATL (four with acute type and one with smoldering type).[204] Although the results of this combination are encouraging, the overall survival of previously untreated patients with ATL was relatively short (4.8 months) compared with the survival of those in the chemotherapy trials conducted by the JCOG-LSG (7 to 8 months).[187-190,203,205] Furthermore, the CR-rate associated with the use of interferon-α and zidovudine among previously untreated patients (25%, 3/12) was not superior to the CR rates among those treated with the JCOG-LSG chemotherapy protocols (28%–42%). In 2001, White and colleagues[206] reported the results of this combination used for 18 patients with ATL; only three patients showed objective responses (one CR and two PRs). Seventeen patients died with an MST after initiation of therapy of 6 months. To evaluate the role of this combination in ATL, further studies are needed.

Cladribine (2-chlorodeoxyadenosine, 2-CdA)

Cladribine (2-chlorodeoxyadenosine, 2-CdA) is a chlorinated purine analog that resists degradation by adenosine deaminase. Cladribine has been found to be effective against various B-cell malignancies such as hairy cell leukemia, B-CLL, and indolent B-cell NHL. It is known that deoxycytidine kinase is rich in T cells, and an in vitro study showed the sensitivity of T-lymphoblastoid cell lines to cladribine.[207] In addition, cladribine was reported to be effective against CTCL. Therefore, cladribine could have some benefit in the treatment of ATL. With the aim of establishing an effective treatment against ATL, clinical trials of cladribine were conducted in Japan. In the Japanese phase I study of cladribine, one patient with ATL who relapsed after receiving sobuzoxane achieved PR by cladribine administration.[208,209] Based on this encouraging result, a multicenter phase II study of cladribine against ATL was conducted in Japan.[210] Cladribine was administered as 0.09 mg/kg/day by 7-day continuous intravenous infusion every 28 days up to 6 courses. When the planned interim analysis revealed that only 1 of the 15 eligible patients showed PR (response rate 7%; 90% CI 0-28%), however, patient entry into the phase II study was discontinued.

Monoclonal Antibodies

Because most ATL cells express the α-chain of IL-2R (CD25), Waldmann and colleagues have treated patients with ATL with monoclonal antibodies to CD25.[176-180] Anti-Tac (anti-CD25) is a murine monoclonal IgG2a antibody that does not fix human complement, nor does it mediate antibody-dependent cell-mediated cytotoxicity (ADCC). Anti-Tac has been shown to prevent the growth of certain cell lines in vitro, however, even in the absence of complement, by blocking IL-2 from gaining access to its receptor.[211,212] Six of 19 patients (32%) who were treated with anti-Tac showed PR (4 patients) or CR (2 patients) lasting from 9 weeks to more than 3 years.[178] One of the significant impediments to this approach is that a quantity of soluble IL-2R is shed by the tumor cells into the circulation. The soluble IL-2R can bind to anti-Tac and inhibit binding to the tumor cell.

Other strategies using IL-2R as a target for the treatment of ATL are conjugation with an immunotoxin (*Pseudomonas* exotoxin) or radioisotope (yttrium-90 [⁹⁰Y]). Anti-Tac coupled with *Pseudomonas* exotoxin, which inhibits protein synthesis, has been administered to patients with ATL.[177,213] Although relatively low doses were used, tumor regression was observed in some patients. The action of immunotoxins depends on the expression of the target antigen on all malignant cells and on the cell's ability to internalize the antigen-antibody-complex containing the toxin. To circumvent findings that not all malignant cells express the target antigen and that not all cells internalize bound substances, radiolabeled monoclonal antibodies (radioimmunoconjugates) were developed. Radioimmunoconjugates have the advantage of killing adjacent antigen-negative neoplastic cells or cells that fail to internalize the antigen-antibody complex. Waldmann and associates[179] have developed a stable conjugate of anti-Tac with ⁹⁰Y. They have treated 18 patients with ATL using this radioimmunoconjugate. Among the 16 patients who received 5- to 15-mCi doses, 9 (56%) showed objective responses (2 CR and 7 PR). The duration of response was longer than the previous results with unconjugated anti-Tac. Grade 3 or greater toxicities were limited largely to hematologic toxicities. The researchers claim that ⁹⁰Y-labeled anti-Tac might provide a useful approach for the treatment of ATL.

Prolonged circulation of radioimmunoconjugate irradiates normal tissues and radiosensitive bone marrow, producing DLTs (including myelosuppression), which limit the radiation dose that can be administered safely. In addition, the large size of the antibodies yields only slow access to tumor cells in bulky masses, precluding the use of short-lived radionuclides. In the "pretargeting" system, antibody and radionuclides are administered separately, and radioactivity rapidly and selectively accumulates in tumors, with a parallel reduction of radioactivity in normal tissues. Several molecular pairs with a high binding affinity, such as avidin and biotin, can be utilized for this purpose. "Pretargeting" is a novel technique in radioimmunotherapy that might offer means to deliver higher doses of radioimmunoconjugates in a way that significantly reduces exposure to normal tissues.[214,215]

One of the potentially promising strategies for developing a new treatment against ATL is to overcome drug resistance.[216-218] Kuwazuru and colleagues[216] analyzed the expression of p-glycoprotein (P-gp) in samples from 25 patients with ATL, by immunoblotting with a monoclonal antibody against P-gp. All six patients at the relapsed stage were P-gp positive. More important, neoplastic cells from

8 of 20 patients with ATL expressed P-gp at initial presentation. These results suggest that the expression of multidrug-resistant (mdr1)/P-gp might correlate with the refractory nature of ATL cells to cytotoxic chemotherapy. Subsequently, Lau and coworkers[218] reported the results of their investigation of the presence of an active multidrug-resistance phenotype in freshly isolated peripheral blood mononuclear cells from asymptomatic HTLV-I carriers, patients with TSP/HAM, and patients with ATL. Significant P-gp-mediated efflux activity and enhanced *mdr1* mRNA expression were observed in CD3+ T-cell populations from 9 of 10 subjects. Furthermore, it was found that *mdr1* gene promoter is transcriptionally activated by the HTLV-I Tax protein. These observations suggest the possibility of new chemotherapeutic strategies against ATL through the use of P-gp inhibitors.

Arsenic Trioxide (As2O3)

Arsenic trioxide (As2O3) is an effective agent for acute promyelocytic leukemia. Ishitsuka and associates[219] examined the suppressing effect of As2O3 on in vitro growth of HTLV-I-infected T-cell lines and fresh ATL cells. Proliferation of four HTLV-I-infected T-cell lines was reduced significantly by As2O3. The authors claimed that As2O3 has therapeutic potential for the treatment of ATL. Bazarbachi and colleagues[220] tested the effects of the combination of As2O3 and interferon-α on cell proliferation, cell cycle phase distribution, and apoptosis in ATL-derived T-cell lines; they found a synergistic effect between both.

Allogeneic Hematopoietic Stem Cell Transplantation

There have been at least five studies on allogenic hematopoietic stem cell transplantation (allo-HSCT) for patients with ATL.[221-225] Recently, the results of allo-HSCT for 10 patients with ATL was reported by Utsunomiya and associates.[224] The patients tolerated well the conditioning regimens, which included total body irradiation, and engraftment occurred in all cases. The median disease-free survival (DFS) after allo-HSCT was 17.5+ months (range, 3.7–34.4+). Six of 10 patients developed acute graft-versus-host disease (GVHD) (one case each with grade I, III or IV, and three cases with grade II), and three patients developed extensive chronic GVHD. Four patients died during the study period from acute GVHD (grade IV), pneumonitis, gastrointestinal bleeding, or renal insufficiency. Two of 10 cases with no symptoms of GVHD relapsed. These results suggest that allo-HSCT might improve survival in a fraction of patients with ATL if a controlled degree of GVHD develops. In addition to the conventional

TABLE 114-2

Infectious Complications at Diagnosis in 818 Japanese Patients with ATL

INFECTION	NO. OF PATIENTS*				
	ACUTE	LYMPHOMA	CHRONIC	SMOLDERING	TOTAL
Bacterial infection	(55)	(9 + 1)[†]	(25)	(4)	(93)
Pneumonia	35[‡]	1	14	4	54
Pyoderma	1	1	3	0	5
Septicemia	6	0	1	0	7
Tuberculosis	7	1	3	0	11
Other	6	6	4	0	16
Fungal infection[§]	(36 + 2)[‡]	(6)	(16)	(8)	(66)
Cutaneous	26	5[†]	12	5	48
Oral	2	0	0	0	2
Esophageal	2	0	2	1	5
Pulmonary	5	1	1	0	7
Meningitis	1	0	1	2	4
Protozoal infection[§]	(22)	(2)	(10)	(4)	(38)
Strongyloidiasis	13[‡]	2	5	1	21
Giardiasis	1	0	0	0	1
Pneumocystis carinii	8	0	5	3	16
Viral infection[§]	(13)	(0)	(3)	(0)	(16)
Herpes zoster	7	0	2	0	9
CMV pneumonia	3	0	0	0	3
Pneumonitis	2	0	1	0	3
Condyloma acuminatum	1	0	0	0	1
No infection[‖]	339	139	98	29	605
Total	465	156	152	45	818

ATL, adult T-cell leukemia; CMV, cytomegalovirus.
*Numbers in parentheses indicate total number of patients in each category.
[†]One patient had leprosy.
[‡]One patient each suffered from oral candidiasis.
[§]P <0.05.
[‖]P <0.01.
From Shimoyama M, and members of the Lymphoma Study Group (1984–1987): Diagnostic criteria and classification of clinical subtypes of adult T-cell leukemia-lymphoma. Br J Haematol 1991;79:428.

allo-HSCT, a multicenter study of nonmyeloablative allo-HSCT against ATL is presently being conducted in Japan.[225]

Treatment of Complications

Hypercalcemia, which eventually occurs in most patients with ATL, usually responds poorly to treatment by natriuresis and corticosteroids but can be controlled with antitumor therapy and the appropriate use of other calcium-lowering agents.

Another major obstacle for the successful treatment of ATL is T-cell immunodeficiency. Patients with ATL often have infectious complications at diagnosis. As shown in Table 114-2, 26% had infections at initial presentation, more than half of which were fungal, protozoal, and viral infections.[112] This finding could be due to a profound T-cell immunodeficiency that occurs with this disease. Other frequently encountered opportunistic infections in patients with ATL include *Pneumocystis carinii* infection, tuberculosis, and adenovirus type 11-induced hemorrhagic cystitis.[173]

Subclinical immunodeficiency was also evident among healthy carriers of HTLV-I.[226] Strongyloidiasis is frequently associated with both smoldering type-ATL and an intermediate state between the healthy carrier state and smoldering-type ATL.[101,227] HTLV-I is known to induce the suppression or alteration of T-cell function.[228,229] Recently, Yasunaga and coworkers,[230] in a study of peripheral blood mononuclear cells from HTLV-I-infected individuals, found a decrease in naive T cells and decreased levels of TCR gene rearrangement excision circles (TRECs, generated by DNA recombination during early T lymphopoiesis) and an increase in EBV DNA. It was suggested that the low number of naive T cells was due to suppressed production of T cells in the thymus, which might account for immuno-deficiency in HTLV-I-infected individuals. Patients with ATL require some supportive or preventive therapies for fungal, protozoal, and viral infections. A low dose of cotri-mexazole and an oral antifungal agent are recommended for use, together with cytotoxic chemotherapy.

There are case reports of B-cell NHL and Hodgkin's lymphoma associated with EBV and of Kaposi's sarcoma in patients with ATL.[173,231,232] The profound immuno-deficient state in patients with ATL might allow the emergence of such opportunistic tumors.

REFERENCES

1. Takatsuki K, Uchiyama T, Sagawa K, Yodoi J: Adult T cell leukemia in Japan. In Seno S, Takaku F, Irino S (eds): Topics in Hematology. Amsterdam, Excerpta Medica, 1977, p 73.
2. Uchiyama T, Yodoi J, Sagawa K, et al: Adult T-cell leukemia: Clinical and hematologic features of 16 cases. Blood 1977;50:481.
3. Yamaguchi K: Human T-lymphotropic virus type I in Japan. Lancet 1994;343:213.
4. Poiesz BJ, Ruscetti FW, Gazdar AF, et al: Detection and isolation of type C retrovirus particles from fresh and cultured lymphocytes of a patient with cutaneous T-cell lymphoma. Proc Natl Acad Sci USA 1980;77:7415.
5. Miyoshi I, Kubonishi I, Sumida M, et al: A novel T-cell line derived from adult T-cell leukemia. Jpn J Cancer Res 1980;71:155.
6. Miyoshi I, Kubonishi I, Yoshimoto S, et al: Type C virus particles in a cord T-cell line derived by co-cultivating normal human cord leukocytes and human leukaemic T cells. Nature 1981;294:770.
7. Hinuma Y, Nagata K, Hanaoka M, et al: Adult T-cell leukemia: Antigen in adult T-cell leukemia cell line and detection of antibodies to the antigen in human sera. Proc Natl Acad Sci USA 1981;78:6476.
8. Yoshida M, Miyoshi I, Hinuma Y: Isolation and characterization of retrovirus from cell lines of human adult T cell leukemia and its implication in the disease. Proc Natl Acad Sci USA 1982;79:2031.
9. Seiki M, Hattori S, Yoshida M: Human adult T-cell leukemia virus: Molecular cloning of the provirus DNA and the unique terminal structure. Proc Natl Acad Sci USA 1982;79:6899.
10. Seiki M, Hattori S, Hirayama M, et al: Human adult T-cell leukemia virus: Complete nucleotide sequence of the provirus genome integrated in leukemic cell DNA. Proc Natl Acad Sci USA 1983;80:3618.
11. Watanabe T, Seiki M, Yoshida M: ATLV (Japanese isolated) and HTLV (US isolated) are the same strain of retrovirus. Virology 1984;133:238.
12. Maeda Y, Fukuhara M, Takehara Y, et al: Prevalence of possible adult T-cell leukemia virus carriers among volunteer blood donors in Japan: A nationwide study. Int J Cancer 1984;33:717.
13. Tajima K and T- and B-cell Malignancy Study Group: The 4th nationwide study of adult T-cell leukemia/lymphoma (ATL) in Japan: Estimates of risk of ATL and its geographical and clinical features. Int J Cancer 1990;45:237.
14. Akagi T, Ono H, Shimotohno K: Characterization of T cells immortalized by Tax1 of human T-cell leukemia virus type 1. Blood 1995;86:4243.
15. Yoshida M, Seiki M, Yamaguchi K, Takatsuki K: Monoclonal integration of human T-cell leukemia provirus in all primary tumors of adult T-cell leukemia suggests causative role of human T-cell leukemia virus in the disease. Proc Natl Acad Sci USA 1984;81:2534.
16. Yamaguchi K, Seiki M, Yoshida M, et al: The detection of human T-cell leukemia virus proviral DNA and its application for classification and diagnosis of T-cell malignancy. Blood 1984;63:1235.
17. Hollsberg P, Hafler DA: Pathogenesis of diseases induced by human lymphotropic virus type I infection. N Engl J Med 1993;328:1173.
18. Yoshida M, Suzuki T, Hirai H, et al: Regulation of HTLV-I gene expression and its roles in ATL development. In Takatsuki K (ed): Adult T-cell Leukaemia. Oxford, Oxford University Press, 1994, p 28.
19. Franchini G: Molecular mechanisms of human T-cell leukemia/lymphotropic virus type I infection. Blood 1995;86:3619.
20. Seiki M, Eddy R, Shows TB, Yoshida M: Nonspecific integration of the HTLV-I provirus genome into adult T-cell leukemia. Nature 1984;309:640.
21. Seiki M, Hikikoshi A, Taniguchi T, Yoshida, M: Expression of the pX gene of HTLV-I: General splicing mechanism in the HTLV-I family. Science 1985;228:1532.
22. Fujisawa J, Seiki M, Kiyokawa T, Yoshida, M: Functional activation of the long terminal repeat of human T-cell leukemia virus type I by a trans-activating factor. Proc Natl Acad Sci USA 1985;82:2277.
23. Sommerfelt MA, Williams BP, Clapham PR, et al: Human T cell leukemia viruses use a receptor determined by human chromosome 17. Science 1988;242:1557.
24. Sagara Y, Ishida C, Inoue Y, et al: 71-kilodalton heat shock cognate protein acts as a cellular receptor for syncytium formation induced by human T-cell lymphotropic virus type 1. J Virol 1998;72:535.
25. Cann AJ, Rosenblatt JD, Wachsman W, et al: Identification of the gene responsible for human T-cell leukaemia virus transcriptional regulation. Nature 1985;318:571.
26. Sodroski JG, Rosen CA, Haseltine WA: Trans-acting transcriptional activation of the long terminal repeat of human T lymphotropic viruses in infected cells. Science 1984;225:381.
27. Wagner S, Green MR: HTLV-I Tax protein stimulation of DNA binding of bZIP proteins by enhancing dimerization. Science 1993;262:395.

28. Zhao LJ, Giam CZ: Human T-cell lymphotropic virus type I (HTLV-I) transcriptional activator, Tax, enhances CREB binding to HTLV-I 21-base-pair repeats by protein-protein interaction. Proc Natl Acad Sci USA 1992;89:7070.

29. Suzuki T, Hirai H, Yoshida M: Tax protein of HTLV-1 interacts with the Rel homology domain of NF-kappa B p65 and c-Rel proteins bound to the NF-kappa B binding site and activates transcription. Oncogene 1994;9:3099.

30. Fujii M, Tsuchiya H, Chuhjo T, et al: Interaction of HTLV-1 Tax1 with p67SRF causes the aberrant induction of cellular immediate early genes through CArG boxes. Genes Dev 1992;6:2066.

31. Giebler HA, Loring JE, van Orden K, et al: Anchoring of CREB binding protein to the human T-cell leukemia virus type 1 promoter: A molecular mechanism of Tax transactivation. Mol Cell Biol 1997;17:5156.

32. Kwok RP, Laurance ME, Lundblad JR, et al: Control of cAMP-regulated enhancers by the viral transactivator Tax through CREB and the co-activator CBP. Nature 1996;380:642.

33. Van Orden K, Yan JP, Ulloa A, et al: Binding of the human T-cell leukemia virus Tax protein to the coactivator CBP interferes with CBP-mediated transcriptional control. Oncogene 1999;18:3766.

34. Mori N, Shirakawa F, Shimizu H, et al: Transcriptional regulation of the human interleukin-6 gene promoter in human T-cell leukemia virus type I-infected T-cell lines: Evidence for the involvement of NF-kappa B. Blood 1994;84:2904.

35. Inoue J, Seiki M, Taniguchi T, et al: Induction of interleukin 2 receptor gene expression by p40x encoded by human T-cell leukemia virus type 1. EMBO J 1986;5:2883.

36. Fujii M, Sassone-Corsi P, Verma IM: c-fos promoter trans-activation by the tax1 protein of human T-cell leukemia virus type I. Proc Natl Acad Sci USA 1988;85:8526.

37. Suzuki T, Narita T, Uchida-Toita M, et al: Down-regulation of the INK4 family of cyclin-dependent kinase inhibitors by tax protein of HTLV-1 through two distinct mechanisms. Virology 1999;259:384.

38. Lemasson I, Robert-Hebmann V, Hamaia S, et al: Transrepression of lck gene expression by human T-cell leukemia virus type 1-encoded p40tax. J Virol 1997;71:1975.

39. Yoshida M: Multiple viral strategies of HTLV-1 for dysregulation of cell growth control. Annu Rev Immunol 2001;19:475.

40. Pozzatti R, Vogel J, Jay G: The human T-lymphotropic virus type I tax gene can cooperate with the ras oncogene to induce neoplastic transformation of cells. Mol Cell Biol 1990;10:413.

41. Kadison P, Poteat HT, Klein KM, et al: Role of protein kinase A in tax transactivation of the human T-cell leukemia virus type I long terminal repeat. J Virol 1990;64:2141.

42. Harhaj EW, Sun SC: IKKgamma serves as a docking subunit of the IkappaB kinase (IKK) and mediates interaction of IKK with the human T-cell leukemia virus Tax protein. J Biol Chem 1999;274:22911.

43. Migone TS, Lin JX, Cereseto A, et al: Constitutively activated Jak-STAT pathway in T cells transformed with HTLV-I. Science 1995;269:79.

44. Mesnard JM, Devaux C: Multiple control levels of cell proliferation by human T-cell leukemia virus type 1 Tax protein. Virology 1999;257:277.

45. Franchini G, Wong-Staal F, Gallo RC: Human T-cell leukemia virus (HTLV-I) transcripts in fresh and cultured cells of patients with adult T-cell leukemia. Proc Natl Acad Sci USA 1984;81:6207.

46. Kozuru M, Uike N, Takeichi N, et al: The possible mode of escape of adult T-cell leukaemia cells from antibody-dependent cellular cytotoxicity. Br J Haematol 1989;72:502.

47. Tamiya S, Matsuoka M, Etoh K, et al: Two types of defective human T-lymphotropic virus type I provirus in adult T-cell leukemia. Blood 1996;88:3065.

48. Kitamura T, Takano M, Hoshino H, et al: Methylation pattern of human T-cell leukemia virus in vivo and in vitro: pX and LTR regions are hypomethylated in vivo. Int J Cancer 1985;35:629.

49. Koiwa T, Usami-Hamano A, Ishida T, et al: 5'-LTR-selective CpG methylation of latent HTLV-1 provirus in vitro and in vivo. J Virol 2002;76:9389.

50. Loeb LA: A mutator phenotype in cancer. Cancer Res 2001;61:3230.

51. Jeang KT, Widen SG, Semmes OJT, et al: HTLV-I trans-activator protein, tax, is a trans-repressor of the human beta-polymerase gene. Science 1990;247:1082.

52. Philpott SM, Buehring GC: Defective DNA repair in cells with human T-cell leukemia/bovine leukemia viruses: Role of tax gene. J Natl Cancer Inst 1999;91:933.

53. Kao SY, Marriott SJ: Disruption of nucleotide excision repair by the human T-cell leukemia virus type 1 Tax protein. J Virol 1999;73:4299.

54. Nicot C, Mahieux R, Takemoto S, et al: Bcl-X(L) is up-regulated by HTLV-I and HTLV-II in vitro and in ex vivo ATLL samples. Blood 2000;96:275.

55. Saintigny Y, Dumay A, Lambert S, et al: A novel role for the Bcl-2 protein family: Specific suppression of the RAD51 recombination pathway. Embo J 2001;20:2596.

56. Cereseto A, Diella F, Mulloy JC, et al: p53 functional impairment and high p21waf1/cip1 expression in human T-cell lymphotropic/leukemia virus type I-transformed T cells. Blood 1996;88:1551.

57. Reid RL, Lindholm PF, Mireskandari A, et al: Stabilization of wild-type p53 in human T-lymphocytes transformed by HTLV-I. Oncogene 1993;8:3029.

58. Sugahara K, Yamada Y, Hiragata Y, et al: Soluble and membrane isoforms of Fas/CD95 in fresh adult T-cell leukemia (ATL) cells and ATL-cell lines. Int J Cancer 1997;72:128.

59. Tamiya S, Etoh K, Suzushima H, et al: Mutation of CD95 (Fas/Apo-1) gene in adult T-cell leukemia cells. Blood 1998;91:3935.

60. Maeda T, Yamada Y, Moriuchi R, et al: Fas gene mutation in the progression of adult T cell leukemia. J Exp Med 1999;189:1063.

61. Itoyama T, Chaganti RS, Yamada Y, et al: Cytogenetic analysis and clinical significance in adult T-cell leukemia/lymphoma: A study of 50 cases from the human T-cell leukemia virus type-1 endemic area, Nagasaki. Blood 2001;97:3612.

62. Tsukasaki K, Krebs J, Nagai K, et al: Comparative genomic hybridization analysis in adult T-cell leukemia/lymphoma: Correlation with clinical course. Blood 2001;97:3875.

63. Nagai H, Kinoshita T, Imamura J, et al: Genetic alteration of p53 in some patients with adult T-cell leukemia. Jpn J Cancer Res 1991;82:1421.

64. Cesarman E, Chadburn A, Inghirami G, et al: Structural and functional analysis of oncogenes and tumor suppressor genes in adult T-cell leukemia/lymphoma shows frequent p53 mutations. Blood 1992;80:3205.

65. Hatta Y, Hirama T, Miller CW, et al: Homozygous deletions of the p15 (MTS-2) and p16 (CDKN2/MTS1) genes in adult T-cell leukemia. Blood 1995;85:2699.

66. Yamada Y, Hatta Y, Murata K, et al: Deletions of p15 and/or p16 genes as a poor-prognosis factor in adult T-cell leukemia. J Clin Oncol 1997;15:1778.

67. Uchida T, Kinoshita T, Watanabe T, et al: The CDKN2 gene alterations in various types of adult T-cell leukaemia. Br J Haematol 1996;94:665.

68. Tsukasaki K, Tsushima H, Yamamura M, et al: Integration patterns of HTLV-I provirus in relation to the clinical course of ATL: Frequent clonal change at crisis from indolent disease. Blood 1997;89:948.

69. Gessain A, Barin F, Vernant JC, et al: Antibodies to human T-lymphotropic virus type-I in patients with tropical spastic paraparesis. Lancet 1985;ii:407.

70. Osame M, Usuku K, Izumo S, et al: HTLV-I associated myelopathy, A new clinical entity. Lancet 1986;1:1031.

71. Tajima K, Hinuma Y: Epidemiology of HTLV-I/II in Japan and the world. In Takatsuki K, Hinuma Y, Yoshida M (eds): Advances in Adult T-cell Leukemia and HTLV-I Research. Gann Monogr on Cancer Research No. 39. Tokyo, Japanese Scientific Society Press, 1992, p 129.

72. Tajima K, Inoue M, Takezaki T et al: Ethnoepidemiology of ATL in Japan with special reference to the Mongoloid dispersal. In Takatsuki K (ed): Adult T-cell Leukaemia. Oxford, Oxford University Press, 1994, p 91.

73. Blattner WA, Gallo RC: Epidemiology of HTLV-I and HTLV-II infection. In Takatsuki K (ed): Adult T-cell Leukaemia. Oxford, Oxford University Press, 1994, p 45.

74. Takezaki T, Hirose K, Hamajima N, et al: Estimation of adult T-cell leukemia incidence in Kyushu district from vital statistics Japan between 1983 and 1992: Comparison with a nationwide survey. Jpn J Clin Oncol 1997;27:140.

75. Tsugane S, Watanabe S, Sugimura H, et al: Infectious states of human T lymphotropic virus type I and hepatitis B virus among Japanese immigrants in the Republic of Bolivia. Am J Epidemiol 1988;128:1153.

76. Levine PH, Cleghorn F, Manns A, et al: Adult T-cell leukemia/ lymphoma: A working point-score classification for epidemiological studies. Int J Cancer 1994;59:491.

77. Tajima K: HTLV-I/II related disease with special reference to its distribution among Mongoloids. In Tajima K, Sonoda S (eds): Gann Monograph on Cancer Research, No. 44, Ethnoepidemiology of Cancer. Tokyo, Japanese Scientific Society Press, 1996, p 123.

78. Kondo T, Kondo H, Miyamoto N, et al: Age- and sex-specific cumulative rate and risk of ATLL for HTLV-I carriers. Int J Cancer 1989;43:1061.

79. Clark JW, Blattner WA, Gallo RC: Human T-cell leukemia virus. In Mendelsohn J, Petersdorf RG, Adams RD, et al (eds): Principles of Internal Medicine. New York, McGraw-Hill, 1986, p 29.

80. Oguma S, Imamura Y, Kusomoto Y, et al: Accelerated declining tendency of human T-cell leukemia virus type I carrier rates among younger blood donors in Kumamoto, Japan. Cancer Res 192;52:2620.

81. Ho GY, Nomura AM, Nelson K, et al: Declining seroprevalence and transmission of HTLV-I in Japanese families who immigrated to Hawaii. Am J Epidemiol 1991;134:981.

82. Ueda K, Kusuhara K, Tokugawa K, et al: Cohort effect on HTLV-I seroprevalence in southern Japan. Lancet 1989;ii:979.

83. Yamaguchi K, Nishimura Y, Kusumoto Y, et al: Declining trends of HTLV-I prevalence among blood donors in Kumamoto, Japan. J AIDS 1992;5:533.

84. Kinoshita K, Hino S, Amagasaki T, et al: Demonstration of adult T-cell leukemia virus antigen in milk from three seropositive mothers. Jpn J Cancer Res 1984;75:103.

85. Hino S, Yamaguchi K, Katamine S, et al: Mother-to-child transmission of human T-cell leukemia virus type-I. Jpn J Cancer Res 1985;76:474.

86. Tsuji Y, Doi H, Yamabe T, et al: Prevention of mother-to-child transmission of human T-lymphotropic virus type-I. Pediatrics 1990;86:11.

87. Okochi K, Sato H, Hinuma Y: A retrospective study on transmission of adult T-cell leukemia virus by blood transfusion: Seroconversion in recipients. Vox Sang 1984;46:245.

88. Sato H, Okochi K: Transmission of human T-cell leukemia virus (HTLV-I) by blood transfusion: Demonstration of proviral DNA in recipients' blood lymphocytes. Int J Cancer 1986;37:395.

89. Tobinai K, Minato K, Shimoyama M, et al: Antibodies to human immunodeficiency virus and human T-cell leukemia virus type I in Japanese patients with hematologic malignancies. Jpn J Cancer Res 1986;77:1207.

90. Inaba S, Okochi K, Sato H, et al: Efficacy of donor screening for HTLV-I and the natural history of transfusion-transmitted infection. Transfusion 1999;39:1104.

91. Brown LS Jr, Chu A, Allain JP, et al: Seroepidemiology and clinical aspects of human T-cell lymphotropic virus type I/II infection in a cohort of intravenous drug users in New York City. NY State J Med 1991;91:93.

92. Takezaki T, Tajima K, Ito M, et al: Short-term breast-feeding may reduce the risk of vertical transmission of HTLV-I. Leukemia 1997;11(Suppl 3):60.

93. Okamoto T, Ohno Y, Tsugane S, et al: Multi-step carcinogenesis model for adult T-cell leukemia. Jpn J Cancer Res 1989;80:191.

94. Shimoyama M, Minato K, Tobinai K, et al: Anti-ATLA (antibody to adult T-cell leukemia-lymphoma virus-associated antigen)-negative adult T-cell leukemia-lymphoma. Jpn J Clin Oncol 1983;13:245.

95. Shimoyama M, Kagami Y, Shimotohno K, et al: Adult T-cell leukemia/lymphoma not associated with human T-cell leukemia virus type I. Proc Natl Acad Sci USA 1986;83:4524.

96. Shimoyama M, Abe T, Miyamoto K, et al: Chromosome aberrations and clinical features of adult T cell leukemia-lymphoma not associated with human T cell leukemia virus type I. Blood 1987;69:984.

97. Miyamoto K, Kagami Y, Shimoyama M et al: A unique T-cell line derived from an HTLV-I-negative adult T-cell leukemia. Jpn J Cancer Res 1987;78:1031–1035.

98. Kagami Y, Tobinai K, Kinoshita T, et al: Novel interleukin-2 dependent T-cell line derived from adult T-cell leukemia not associated with human T-cell leukemia virus type I. Jpn J Cancer Res 1993;84:371.

99. Mochizuki M, Watanabe T, Yamaguchi K, et al: HTLV-I uveitis: A distinct clinical entity by HTLV-I. Jpn J Cancer Res 1992;83:236.

100. Mochizuki M, Watanabe T, Yamaguchi K, et al: Uveitis associated with human T-lymphotropic virus type I. Am J Ophthalmol 1992;114:123.

101. Nakada K, Yamaguchi K, Furugen S, et al: Monoclonal integration of HTLV-I proviral DNA in patients with strongyloidiasis. Int J Cancer 1987;40:145.

102. Oshima K, Kikuchi M, Masuda Y, et al: HTLV-I-associated lymphadenopathy. Cancer 1992;69:239.

103. Nishioka K, Maruyama I, Sato K, et al: Chronic inflammatory arthropathy associated with HTLV-I [letter]. Lancet 1989;i:441.

104. LaGrenade L, Hanchard B, Fletcher V, et al: Infective dermatitis of Jamaican children: A marker for HTLV-I infection. Lancet 1990;i:1345.

105. Sonoda S, Yashiki S, Fujiyoshi T, et al: Immunogenetic factors involved in the pathogenesis of adult T-cell leukemia and HTLV-I-associated myelopathy. In Takatsuki K, Hinuma Y, Yoshida M (eds.): Advances in Adult T-cell Leukemia and HTLV-I Research. Gann Monograph on Cancer Research, No. 39. Tokyo, Japanese Scientific Society Press, 1992, p 81.

106. Shimoyama M, Minato K, Saito H, et al: Comparisons of clinical, morphologic and immunologic characteristics of adult T-cell leukemia-lymphoma and cutaneous T-cell lymphoma. Jpn J Clin Oncol 1979;9(Suppl 1):357.

107. Shimoyama M, Minato K, Tobinai K, et al: Atypical adult T-cell leukemia-lymphoma: Diverse clinical manifestations of adult T-cell leukemia-lymphoma. Jpn J Clin Oncol 1983;13(Suppl 2):165.

108. Yamaguchi K, Nishimura H, Kohrogi H, et al: A proposal for smoldering adult T-cell leukemia: A clinicopathologic study of five cases. Blood 1983;62:758.

109. Kinoshita K, Amagasaki T, Ikeda S, et al: Preleukemic state of adult T cell leukemia: Abnormal T lymphocytosis induced by human adult T cell leukemia-lymphoma virus. Blood 1985;66:120.

110. Kawano F, Yamaguchi K, Nishimura H, et al: Variation in the clinical courses of adult T-cell leukemia. Cancer 1985;55:851.

111. Takatsuki K, Yamaguchi K, Kawano F, et al: Clinical diversity in adult T-cell leukemia-lymphoma. Cancer Res 1985;45(Suppl):4644.

112. Shimoyama M and members of the Lymphoma Study Group (1984-1987): Diagnostic criteria and classification of clinical subtypes of adult T-cell leukemia-lymphoma. Br J Haematol 1991;79:428.

113. Yamaguchi K, Yoshioka R, Kiyokawa T, et al: Lymphoma type adult T-cell leukemia: a clinicopathologic study of HTLV related T-cell type malignant lymphoma. Hematol Oncol 1986;4:59.

114. Utsunomiya A, Hanada S, Terada, A et al: Adult T-cell leukemia with leukemia cell infiltration into the gastrointestinal tract. Cancer 1988;61:824.

115. Cappell MS, Chow J: HTLV-I-associated lymphoma involving the entire alimentary tract and presenting with an acquired immune deficiency. Am J Med 1987;82:649.

116. Yamada Y, Kamihira S, Murata K, et al: Frequent hepatic involvement in adult T-cell leukemia: Comparison with non-Hodgkin's lymphoma. Leuk Lymphoma 1997;26:327.

117. Yoshioka R, Yamaguchi K, Yoshinaga T, et al: Pulmonary complications in patients with adult T-cell leukemia. Cancer 1985;55:2491.

118. Teshima T, Akashi K, Shibuya T, et al: Central nervous system involvement in adult T-cell leukemia/lymphoma. Cancer 1990;65:327.

119. Fukumoto S, Matsumoto T, Ikeda K, et al: Clinical evaluation of calcium metabolism in adult T-cell leukemia/lymphoma. Arch Intern Med 1988;148:921.

120. Fukumoto S, Matsumoto T, Watanabe T, et al: Secretion of parathyroid hormone-like activity from human T-cell lymphotropic virus type I-infected lymphocytes. Cancer Res 1989;49:3849.

121. Honda S, Yamaguchi K, Miyake Y, et al: Production of parathyroid hormone-related protein in adult T-cell leukemia cells. Jpn J Cancer Res 1988;79:1264.

122. Motokura T, Fukumoto S, Matsumoto T, et al: Parathyroid hormone-related protein in adult T-cell leukemia/lymphoma. Ann Intern Med 1989;111:484.

123. Watanabe T, Yamaguchi K, Takatsuki K, et al: Constitutive expression of parathyroid hormone-related protein gene in human T cell leukemia virus type 1 (HTLV-1) carriers and adult T cell leukemia patients that can be trans-activated by HTLV-1 *tax* gene. J Exp Med 1990;172:759.

124. Breslau NA, McGuire JL, Zerwelk JE, et al: Hypercalcemia associated with increased serum calcitrol levels in three patients with lymphoma. Ann Intern Med 1984;100:1.

125. Grossman B, Schechter GP, Horton JE, et al: Hypercalcemia associated with T-cell lymphoma-leukemia. Am J Clin Pathol 1981;75:149.

126. Yamashita U, Shirakawa F, Nakamura H: Production of interleukin 1 by adult T cell leukemia (ATL) cell lines. J Immunol 1987;138:3284.

127. Wano Y, Hattori T, Matsuoka M, et al: Interleukin 1 gene expression in adult T cell leukemia. J Clin Invest 1987;80:911.

128. Shirakawa F, Yamashita U, Tanaka Y, et al: Production of bone-resorbing activity corresponding to interleukin-1a by adult T-cell leukemia cells in humans. Cancer 1988;48:4284.

129. Tschachler E, Robert-Guroff M, Gallo R, et al: Human T-lymphotropic virus I-infected T cells constitutively express lymphotoxin in vitro. Blood 1989;73:194.

130. Ishibashi K, Ishitsuka K, Chuman Y, et al: Tumor necrosis factor-β in the serum of adult T-cell leukemia with hypercalcemia. Blood 1991;77:2451.

131. Nosaka K, Miyamoto T, Sakai T, et al: Mechanism of hypercalcemia in adult T-cell leukemia: Overexpression of receptor activator of nuclear factor kappaB ligand on adult T-cell leukemia cells. Blood 2002;99:634.

132. Marcon L, Rubin LA, Kurman CC, et al: Elevated serum levels of soluble Tac peptide in adult T-cell leukemia: correlation with clinical status during chemotherapy. Ann Intern Med 1988;109:274.

133. Kamihira S, Atogami S, Sohda H, et al: Significance of soluble interleukin-2 receptor levels for evaluation of the progression of adult T-cell leukemia. Cancer 1994;73:2753.

134. Tsukasaki K, Imaizumi Y, Tawara M, et al: Diversity of leukaemic cell morphology in ATL correlates with prognostic factors, aberrant immunophenotype and defective HTLV-1 genotype. Br J Haematol 1999;105:369.

135. Suchi T, Tajima K, Nanba K, et al: Some problems on histopathological diagnosis of non–Hodgkin's malignant lymphoma: Proposal of a new type. Acta Pathol Jpn 1979;29:755.

136. Jaffe ES, Blattner WA, Blayney DW, et al: The pathologic spectrum of adult T-cell leukemia/lymphoma in the United States. Am J Surg Pathol 1984;8:263.

137. Kikuchi M, Mitsui T, Takeshita M, et al: Virus-associated adult T-cell leukemia (ATL) in Japan: Clinical, histological and immunological studies. Hematol Oncol 1986;4:67.

138. Sato E, Tokunaga M, Hasui K, et al: Pathoepidemiological features of adult T-cell lymphoma/leukemia in an endemic area: Kagoshima, Japan. Cancer Detect Prev 1990;14:423.

139. Kikuchi M, Takeshita M, Ohshima K, et al: Pathology of adult T-cell leukemia/lymphoma and HTLV-I associated organopathies. In Takatsuki K, Hinuma Y, Yoshida M (eds): Gann Monograph on Cancer Research, No. 39, Advances in Adult T-cell Leukemia and HTLV-I Research. Tokyo, Japanese Scientific Society Press, 1992, p 81.

140. Watanabe S: Adult T cell leukemia/lymphoma. In Knowles DM (ed): Neoplastic Hematopathology, 2nd ed. Philadelphia, Lippincott Williams & Wilkins, 2001, p 1603.

141. Ohshima K, Suzumiya J, Kato A, et al: Clonal HTLV-I-infected CD4+ T-lymphocytes and non-clonal non-HTLV-I- infected giant cells in incipient ATLL with Hodgkin-like histologic features. Int J Cancer 1997;72:592.

142. Duggan D, Ehrlich G, Davey F, et al: HTLV-I induced lymphoma mimicking Hodgkin's disease: Diagnosis by polymerase chain reaction amplification of specific HTLV-I sequences in tumor DNA. Blood 1988;71:1027.

143. Kikuchi M, Jaffe ES, Ralfkiaer E: In Jaffe ES, Harris NL, Stein H, Vardiman J (eds): Pathology and Genetics of Tumours of Haematopoietic and Lymphoid Tissues. World Health Organization Classification of Tumours. Lyon, France, IARC Press, 2001, p 200.

144. Quintanilla-Martinez L, Fend F, Moguel LR, et al: Peripheral T-cell lymphoma with Reed-Sternberg-like cells of B-cell phenotype and genotype associated with Epstein-Barr virus infection. Am J Surg Pathol 1999;23:1233.

145. Nagatani T, Matsuzaki T, Iemoto G, et al: Comparative study of cutaneous T-cell lymphoma and adult T-cell leukemia/lymphoma. Cancer 1990;66:2380.

146. Ikeda M, Fujino R, Matsui T, et al: A new agglutination test for serum antibodies to adult T-cell leukemia virus. Jpn J Cancer Res 1984;75:845.

147. Tobinai K, Nagai M, Setoya T, et al: Anti-ATLA (antibody to adult T-cell leukemia virus-associated antigen), highly positive in OKT4-positive mature T-cell malignancies. Jpn J Clin Oncol 1983;13(Suppl 2):237.

148. Ohtsu T, Tsugane S, Tobinai K, et al: Prevalence of antibodies to human T-cell leukemia/lymphoma virus type I and human immunodeficiency virus in Japanese immigrant colonies in Bolivia and Bolivian natives. Jpn J Cancer Res 1987;78:1347.

149. Saito S, Ando Y, Furuki K, et al: Detection of HTLV-I genome in seronegative infants born to HTLV-I seropositive mothers by polymerase chain reaction. Jpn J Cancer Res 1989;80:808.

150. Kajiyama W, Kashiwagi S, Hayashi J, et al: Study of seroconversion of antibody to human T-cell lymphotropic virus type-I in children of Okinawa, Japan. Microbiol Immunol 1990;34:259.

151. Ehrlich GD, Glayser JB, Abbott MA, et al: Detection of anti-HTLV-I Tax antibodies in HTLV-I enzyme-linked immunosorbent assay-negative individuals. Blood 1989;74:1066.

152. Kinoshita T, Imamura J, Nagai H, et al: Absence of HTLV-I infection among seronegative subjects in an endemic area of Japan. Int J Cancer 1993;54:16.

153. Inaba S, Sato H, Okochi K, et al: Prevention of transmission of human T-lymphotropic virus type I (HTLV-I) through transfusion, by donor screening with antibody to the virus. One year experience. Transfusion 1989;29:7.

154. Yamaguchi K, Nishimura Y, Fukuyoshi Y, et al: Decrease of HTLV-I infection in haemodialyis patients after donor screening. Lancet 1990;ii:1070.

155. Matsumoto C, Mitsunaga S, Oguchi T, et al: Detection of human T-cell leukemia virus type I (HTLV-I) provirus in an infected cell line and in peripheral mononuclear cells of blood donors by the nested double polymerase chain reaction method: Comparison with HTLV-I antibody test. J Virol 1990;64:5290.

156. Nagashima M, Itagaki A, Yamada O, et al: Evidence against a seronegative HTLV-I carrier rate among children. AIDS Res Hum Retroviruses 1990;6:1057.

157. Hall WW, Liu CR, Schneewind O, et al: Deleted HTLV-I provirus in blood and cutaneous lesions of patients with mycosis fungoides. Science 1991;253:317.

158. Pancake BA, Zucker-Franklin D, Coutavas EE: The cutaneous T-cell lymphoma, mycosis fungoides is a human T cell lymphotropic virus-associated disease. J Clin Invest 1995;95:547.

159. Kikuchi A, Nishikawa T, Ikeda Y, et al: Absence of human T-lymphotropic virus type I in Japanese patients with cutaneous T-cell lymphoma. Blood 1997;89:1529.

160. Bazarbachi A, Soriano V, Pawson R, et al: Mycosis fungoides and Sezary syndrome are not associated with HTLV-I infection: An international study. Br J Haematol 1997;98:927.

161. Longo DL, Gelmann EP, Cossman J, et al: Isolation of HTLV-I transformed B-lymphocyte clone from a patient with HTLV-I associated adult T-cell leukaemia. Nature 1984;310:505.

162. Dhawan S, Streicher HZ, Wahl LM, et al: Model for studying virus attachment. II. binding of biotinylated human T cell leukemia virus type I to human blood mononuclear cells: potential targets for human T cell leukemia virus type I infection. J Immunol 1991;147:102.

163. Hattori T, Uchiyama T, Toibana T, et al: Surface phenotype of Japanese adult T-cell leukemia cells characterized by monoclonal antibodies. Blood 1981;58:645.

164. Tobinai K, Hirose M, Yamada H, et al: Cellular origin of human lymphoid malignancies as based on immunologic analysis of membrane differentiation antigens. Jpn J Clin Oncol 1982;12:73.

165. Yamada Y: Phenotypic and functional analysis of leukemic cells from 16 patients with adult T-cell leukemia/lymphoma. Blood 1983;61:192.

166. Yamada Y, Kamihira S, Amagasaki T, et al: Changes of adult T cell leukemia cell surface antigens at relapse or at exacerbation phase after chemotherapy defined by use of monoclonal antibodies. Blood 1984;64:440.

167. Yamada Y, Kamihira S, Amagasaki T, et al: Adult T cell leukemia with atypical surface phenotypes: Clinical correlation. J Clin Oncol 1985;3:782.

168. Yamada Y, Ichimaru M, Shiku H: Adult T cell leukaemia cells are of CD4+ CDw29+ T cell origin and secrete a B-cell differentiation factor. Br J Haematol 1989;72:370.

169. Kodaka T, Uchiyama T, Ishikawa T, et al: Interleukin-2 receptor β-chain (p70) expressed on leukemic cells from adult T cell leukemia patients. Jpn J Cancer Res 1990;81:902.

170. Waldmann TA, Greene WC, Sarin PS, et al: Functional and phenotypic comparison of human T cell leukemia/lymphoma virus positive adult T cell leukemia with human T cell leukemia/lymphoma virus negative Sezary leukemia, and their distinction using anti-TAC monoclonal antibody identifying the human receptor for T cell growth factor. J Clin Invest 1984;73:1711.

171. Morimoto C, Matsuyama T, Oshige C, et al: Functional and phenotypic studies of Japanese adult T cell leukemia cells. J Clin Invest 1985;75:836.

172. Tsuda H, Takatsuki K: Specific decrease in T3 antigen density in adult T-cell leukemia cells: I. Flow microfluorometric analysis. Br J Cancer 1984;50:843.

173. Tobinai K, Ohtsu T, Hayashi M, et al: Epstein-Barr virus (EBV) genome carrying monoclonal B-cell lymphoma in a patient with adult T-cell leukemia-lymphoma. Leuk Res 1991;15:837.

174. Joh T, Yamada Y, Seto M, et al: Expression of CD8b and alteration of cell surface phenotype in adult T-cell leukemia. Br J Haematol 1997;98:151.

175. Uchiyama T, Sagawa K, Takatsuki K, et al: Effect of adult T-cell leukemia cells on pokeweed mitogen-induced normal B-cell differentiation. Clin Immunol Immunopathol 1978;10:24.

176. Waldmann TA: Multichain interleukin-2 receptor: A target for immunotherapy in lymphoma. J Natl Cancer Inst 1989;81:914.

177. Waldmann TA, Pastan IH, Gansow OA, et al: The multichain interleukin-2 receptor: A target for immunotherapy. Ann Intern Med 1992;116:148.

178. Waldmann TA, White JD, Goldman CK, et al: The interleukin-2 receptor: A target for monoclonal antibody treatment of human T-cell lymphotropic virus I-induced adult T-cell leukemia. Blood 1993;82:1701.

179. Waldmann TA, White JD, Carrasquillo JA, et al: Radioimmunotherapy of interleukin-2Ra-expressing adult T-cell leukemia with yttrium-90-labeled anti-Tac. Blood 1995;86:4063.

180. Waldmann TA: The IL-2/IL-15 receptor systems: Targets for immunotherapy. J Clin Immunol 2002;22:51.

181. Takatsuki K, Matsuoka M, Yamaguchi K: ATL and HTLV-I-related disease. In Takatsuki K (ed): Adult T-cell Leukaemia. Oxford, Oxford University Press, 1994, p 1.

182. Lymphoma Study Group: Major prognostic factors of patients with adult T-cell leukemia-lymphoma: A cooperative study. Leuk Res 1991;15:81.

183. Shimoyama M: Treatment of patients with adult T-cell leukemia-lymphoma: An overview. In Takatsuki K, Hinuma S, Yoshida M (eds): Advances in Adult T-cell Leukemia and HTLV-I Research. Gann Monograph on Cancer Research, No. 39. Tokyo, Japanese Scientific Society Press, 1992, p 43.

184. Shimoyama M: Chemotherapy of ATL. In Takatsuki K (ed): Adult T-cell Leukaemia. Oxford, Oxford University Press, 1994, p 221.

185. Lymphoma Study Group: Combination chemotherapy with vincristine, cyclophosphamide (Endoxan), prednisolone and adriamycin (VEPA) in advanced adult non–Hodgkin's lymphoid malignancies: Relation between T-cell or non-T-cell phenotype and response. Jpn J Clin Oncol 1979;9(Suppl):397.

186. Lymphoma Study Group: Final results of cooperative study of VEPA [vincristine, cyclophosphamide (Endoxan), prednisolone and adriamycin] therapy in advanced adult non–Hodgkin's lymphoma: Relation between T- or B-cell phenotype and response. Jpn J Clin Oncol 1982;12:227.

187. Shimoyama M, Ota K, Kikuchi M, et al: Chemotherapeutic results and prognostic factors of patients with advanced non–Hodgkin's lymphoma treated with VEPA or VEPA-M. J Clin Oncol 1988;6:128.

188. Shimoyama M, Ota K, Kikuchi M, et al: Major prognostic factors of adult patients with advanced T-cell lymphoma/leukemia. J Clin Oncol 1988;6:1088.

189. Tobinai K, Shimoyama M, Minato K, et al: Japan Clinical Oncology Group phase II trial of second-generation "LSG4 protocol" in aggressive T- and B-lymphoma: A new predictive model for T-and B-lymphoma [abstract]. Proc Am Soc Clin Oncol 1994;13:378.

190. Tsukasaki K, Tobinai K, Shimoyama M, et al: Deoxycoformycin-containing combination chemotherapy for adult T-cell leukemia-lymphoma: Japan Clinical Oncology Group Study (JCOG9109). Int J Hematol 2003;77:164.

191. Yamada Y, Tomonaga M, Fukuda H, et al: A new G-CSF-supported combination chemotherapy, LSG15, for adult T-cell leukemia-lymphoma (ATL): Japan Clinical Oncology Group (JCOG) Study 9303. Br J Haematol 2001;113:375.

192. Shimoyama M, Oyama A, Tajima K, et al: Differences in clinicopathological characteristics and major prognostic factors between B-lymphoma and peripheral T-lymphoma excluding adult T-cell leukemia/lymphoma. Leuk Lymphoma 1993;10:335.

193. Daenen S, Rojer RA, Smit JW, et al: Successful chemotherapy with deoxycoformycin in adult T-cell lymphoma-leukaemia. Br J Haematol 1984;58:723.

194. Yamaguchi K, Yul LS, Oda T, et al: Clinical consequences of 2′-deoxycoformycin treatment in patients with refractory adult T-cell leukaemia. Leukemia Res 1986;10:989.

195. Lofters W, Campbell M, Gibbs WN, et al: 2′-Deoxycoformycin therapy in adult T-cell leukemia/lymphoma. Cancer 1987;60:2605.

196. Tobinai K, Shimoyama M, Inoue S, et al: Phase I study of YK-176 (2′-deoxycoformycin) in patients with adult T-cell leukemia-lymphoma. Jpn J Clin Oncol 1992;22:164.

197. Ohno R, Masaoka T, Shirakawa S, et al: Treatment of adult T-cell leukemia/lymphoma with MST-16, a new oral antitumor drug and a derivative of bis(2,6-dioxopiperazine). Cancer 1993;71:2217.

198. Ohno R, Okada K, Masaoka T, et al: An early phase II study of CPT-11: A new derivative of camptothecin, for the treatment of leukemia and lymphoma. J Clin Oncol 1990;8:1907.

199. Tsuda H, Takatsuki K, Ohno R, et al: A late phase II trial of a potent topoisomerase inhibitor, CPT-11, in malignant lymphoma [abstract]. Proc Am Soc Clin Oncol 1992;11:316.

200. Tsuda H, Takatsuki K, Ohno R, et al: Treatment of adult T-cell leukemia-lymphoma with irinotecan hydrochloride. Br J Cancer 1994;70:771.

201. Tobinai K, Hotta T, Saito H, et al: Combination phase I/II study of irinotecan hydrochloride and carboplatin in relapsed or refractory non-Hodgkin's lymphoma. Jpn J Clin Oncol 1996;26:455.

202. Ohtsu T, Sasaki Y, Igarashi T, et al: Unexpected hepatotoxicities in patients with non–Hodgkin's lymphoma treated with irinotecan (CPT-11) and etoposide. Jpn J Clin Oncol 1998;28:502.

203. Gill PS, Harrington W, Kaplan MH, et al: Treatment of adult T-cell leukemia-lymphoma with a combination of interferon alfa and zidovudine. N Engl J Med 1995;332:1744.

204. Hermine O, Bouscary D, Gessain A, et al: Treatment of adult T-cell leukemia-lymphoma with zidovudine and interferon alfa. N Engl J Med 1995;332:1749.

205. Tobinai K, Kobayashi Y, Shimoyama M [letter] and Gill PS, Harrington W, Levine AM [the authors' reply]: Interferon alfa and zidovudine in adult T-cell leukemia-lymphoma [correspndence]. N Engl J Med 1995;333:1285.

206. White JD, Wharfe G, Stewart DM, et al: The combination of zidovudine and interferon alpha-2B in the treatment of adult T-cell leukemia/lymphoma. Leuk Lymphoma 2001;40:287.

207. Seto S, Carrera CJ, Kubota M, et al: Mechanism of deoxyadenosine and 2-chlorodeoxyadnosine toxicity to nondividing human lymphocytes. J Clin Invest 1985;75:377.

208. Tobinai K, Ogura M, Hotta T, et al: Phase I study of cladribine (2-chlorodeoxyadenosine) in lymphoid malignancies. Jpn J Clin Oncol 1997;27:146.

209. Uike N, Choi I, Tokoro A, et al: Adult T-cell leukemia-lymphoma successfully treated with 2-chlorodeoxyadenosine. Intern Med 1998;37:411.

210. Tobinai K, Uike N, Saburi Y, et al: Phase II study of cladribine (2-chlorodeoxyadenosine) in relapsed or refractory adult T-cell leukemia-lymphoma. Int J Hematol 2003;77:512.

211. Uchiyama T, Broder S, Waldmann TA: A monoclonal antibody (anti-Tac) reactive with activated and functionally mature human T-cells. I. Production of anti-Tac monoclonal antibody and distribution of Tac+ cells. J Immunol 1981;126:1393.

212. Uchiyama T, Hori T, Tsudo M, et al: Interleukin-2 receptor (Tac antigen) expressed on adult T-cell leukemia cells. J Clin Invest 1985;76:446.

213. Kreitman RJ, Wilson WH, White JD, et al: Phase I trial of recombinant immunotoxin anti-Tac(Fv)-PE38 (LMB-2) in patients with hematologic malignancies. J Clin Oncol 2000;18:1622.

214. Meredith R, Lobuglio AI, Knox S, et al: A phase I study evaluating the pharmacokinetics of anti-CD20 fusion protein, synthetic clearing agent and ^{90}yttrium DOTA-biotin [abstract]. Proc Am Soc Clin Oncol 2002;21:3a.

215. Zhang M, Yao Z, Garmestani K, et al: Pretargeting radioimmuno-therapy of a murine model of adult T-cell leukemia with the a-emitting radionuclide, bismuth 213. Blood 2002;100:208.

216. Kuwazuru Y, Hanada S, Furukawa T, et al: Expression of p-glycoprotein in adult T-cell leukemia cells. Blood 1990; 76:2065.

217. Kato S, Nishimura J, Muta K, et al: Overexpression of P-glycoprotein in adult T-cell leukemia. Lancet 1990;336:573.

218. Lau A, Nightingale S, Taylor GP, et al: Enhanced MDR1 gene expression in human T-cell leukemia virus-I-infected patients offers new prospects for therapy. Blood 1998;91:2467.

219. Ishitsuka K, Hanada S, Suzuki S, et al: Arsenic trioxide inhibits growth of human T-cell leukaemia virus type I infected T-cell lines more effectively than retinoic acids. Br J Haematol 1998; 103:721.

220. Bazarbachi A, El-Sabban ME, Nasr R, et al: Arsenic trioxide and interferon-alpha synergize to induce cell cycle arrest and apoptosis in human T-cell lymphotropic virus type I-transformed cells. Blood 1999;93:278.

221. Sobue R, Yamauchi T, Miyamura K, et al: Treatment of adult T cell leukemia with mega-dose cyclophosphamide and total body irradiation followed by allogeneic bone marrow transplantation. Bone Marrow Transplant 1987;2:441.

222. Ljungman P, Lawler M, Asjo B, et al: Infection of donor lymphocytes with human T lymphotropic virus type I following allogeneic bone marrow transplantation for HTLV-I positive adult T-cell leukaemia. Br J Haematol 1994;88:403.

223. Borg A, Liu Yin JA, Johnson PRE, et al: Successful treatment of HTLV-I-associated acute adult T-cell leukaemia lymphoma by allogeneic bone marrow transplantation. Br J Haematol 1996;94:713.

224. Utsunomiya A, Miyazaki Y, Takatsuka Y, et al: Improved outcome of adult T cell leukemia/lymphoma with allogeneic hematopoietic stem cell transplantation. Bone Marrow Transplant 2001;27:15.

225. Abe Y, Yashiki S, Choi I, et al: Eradication of virus-infected T-cells in a case of adult T-cell leukemia/lymphoma by nonmyeloablative peripheral blood stem cell transplantation with conditioning consisting of low-dose total body irradiation and pentostatin. Int J Hematol 2002;76:91.

226. Katsuki T, Katsuki K, Imai J, Hinuma Y: Immune suppression in healthy carriers of adult T-cell leukemia retrovirus (HTLV-I): Impairment of T-cell control of Epstein-Barr virus-infected B-cells. Jpn J Cancer Res 1987;78:639.

227. Yamaguchi K, Kiyokawa T, Nakada K, et al: Polyclonal integration of HTLV-I proviral DNA in lymphocytes from HTLV-I seropositive individuals: An intermediate state between the healthy carrier state and smouldering ATL. Br J Haematol 1988;68:169.

228. Popovic M, Flomenberg N, Volkman DJ, et al: Alterations of T-cell functions by infection with HTLV-I or HTLV-II. Science 1984;226:459.

229. DeVecchis L, Graziani G, Macchi B, et al: Decline of natural cytotoxicity of human lymphocytes following infection with human T-cell leukemia/lymphoma virus (HTLV). Leuk Res 1985;9:349.

230. Yasunaga J, Sakai T, Nosaka K, et al: Impaired production of naive T lymphocytes in human T-cell leukemia virus type I-infected individuals: Its implications in the immunodeficient state. Blood 2001;97:3177.

231. Sadahira Y, Nishihara H, Shimizu M, et al: Epstein-Barr virus-associated Hodgkin's disease in HTLV-I seropositive patients: A report of two cases. Pathol Int 1998;48:67.

232. Greenberg SJ, Jaffe ES, Ehrlich GD, et al: Kaposi's sarcoma in human T-cell leukemia virus type I-associated adult T-cell leukemia. Blood 1990;76:971.

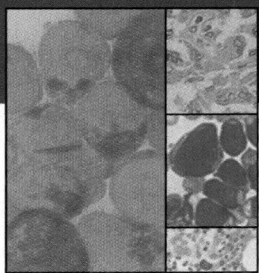

INDEX

Note: Page numbers followed by f and t indicate figures and tables, respectively. Page numbers followed by b indicate boxed material.

A33 (monoclonal antibody), radiolabeled, 668
A 79175 (lipoxygenase inhibitor), in chemoprevention, of lung cancer, 1673–1674
AA-861 (lipoxygenase inhibitor), 1674
AACR. *See* American Association for Cancer Research (AACR)
AAV. *See* Adenoassociated virus (AAV)
Abarelix, and reproductive function, 1274
ABCD mnemonic, for melanoma, 1566
ABCM therapy, for multiple myeloma, 2966
Abdominal complications, 1025–1043
  of bone marrow transplantation, 1036–1038
  in childhood lymphomas, 2775
Abdominal fat aspiration, for primary amyloidosis, 2975
Abdominal hysterectomy, surgical alternatives to, 2233–2234
Abdominal pain, in acute abdomen, 1026
Abdominal radiotherapy, and reproductive function, 1274
Abdominoperineal resection, and reproductive function, 1272
Ablative therapy
  for liver metastases, 1141
  superficial, for cervical cancer, 2232
ABL gene, as therapeutic target, 624, 624t
ABMTR. *See* Autologous Blood and Bone Marrow Transplant Registry
Abortion, and gestational trophoblastic disease, 2348
Absolute ethanol injection, for liver metastases, 1141
Absolute risk, 409
AC133, in angiogenesis, 155t
Access to Cancer Clinical Trials Act of 2001, 397
Accutane. *See* Isotretinoin (Accutane)
Acetabulum, Ewing's sarcoma of, 2525
Acetowhitening, for cervical cancer diagnosis, 2226
Acetylation phenotype, 492
Achalasia, and esophageal cancer, 1789
Achlorhydria, and gastric cancer, 1820
Acitretin (Soriatane), for cutaneous T-cell lymphoma, 3095
Aclarubicin, intrapericardial, for pericardial effusion, 1198
aCML. *See* Atypical chronic myelogenous leukemia; Atypical chronic myeloid leukemia
ACOS-OG. *See* American College of Surgeons Oncology Group
Acoustic neuroma, 1399–1401
  clinical considerations with, 1399
  pathology of, 1399
  radiation therapy for, 1400–1401, 1400f
  surgery for, 1399–1400

Acquired immunodeficiency syndrome (AIDS). *See* HIV-infected (AIDS) patients
Acral erythema, 796t, 801–803. *See also* Palmar-plantar dysesthesia and erythrodysesthesia syndrome
  with graft-versus-host disease, 803
  in liver disease, 803
Acridinylaniside. *See* Amsacrine (AMSA)
Acrosclerosis, 796t
ACT-D. *See* Dactinomycin (Cosmegen)
ACTH. *See* Adrenocorticotropic hormone (corticotropin, ACTH)
Actinic keratoses
  inflamed, 796t
  management of, 451
  photodynamic therapy for, 641, 650
  and skin cancer risk, 449
  and squamous cell carcinoma
    of conjunctiva, 1473
    of eyelid, 1472
Actinium-225, in radioimmunotherapy, 666t
Actinomycin D. *See also* Dactinomycin (Cosmegen)
  for gestational trophoblastic disease, 2359–2363
  for ovarian cancer, 2337
  pigmentation reaction caused by, 804
  and testicular function, in children, 1276
Activation loop, 21, 22
Activin(s), 31, 1270
Activities of daily living, in geriatric assessment, 1321–1322
Activity level, cancer-related fatigue and, 837
Acupressure, 699
Acupuncture, 699–700
  adverse effects and side effects of, 707
  certification in, 700
  needles for, 700
  regulation of, 700
  for xerostomia, 784
Acute abdomen, 1025–1027, 1026t
Acute erythroblastic leukemia, immunologic classification of, 2737–2738, 2737t
Acute erythroid leukemia, morphology of, 2831, 2831f
Acute erythroleukemia, immunologic classification of, 2737–2738, 2737t
Acute granulocytic leukemia, chemotherapy for, 492
Acute lymphoblastic (lymphocytic, lymphoid) leukemia (ALL)
  in adults, 2793–2817
    biology of, 2800–2804
    chemotherapy for, 2806–2809, 2807t
    clinical manifestations of, 2804
    CNS prophylaxis in, 2809–2810
    cytogenetics of, 2801, 2801t
    differential diagnosis of, 2804–2805, 2805t
    epidemiology of, 2794
    FAB classification of, 2796–2797, 2796f, 2797t

lymphoblasts in, 2796–2797, 2796f, 2797t
    minimal residual disease in, 307–308, 308f, 2811–2812
    morphologic and cytochemical classification of, 2796–2797, 2796f, 2797t
    newly diagnosed, management of, 2815b
    pathology of, 2795–2800
    prognosis for, 2805–2806
    remission induction in, 2806–2808
    risk factors for, 2795
    salvage therapy for, 2812–2814
    stem cell transplantation in, 2810–2811, 2813–2814
    survival rates for, 2800
    treatment of, 2806–2812, 2807t, 2816
    work-up for, 2804, 2805t
  ALL-precursor, chromosomal abnormalities in, 316t
  B-cell
    antigen expression in, 2738
    in children, 2733
    immunologic markers in, 2797–2799, 2798t
    subtypes of, defined by global gene expression, 2740
  biphenotypic, scoring system for, 2800, 2800t
  bone marrow transplantation in, 596
  chemotherapy for, 492
    and second malignant neoplasms, 1301, 1302f
  chromosomal abnormalities in
    numerical, 2801
    structural, 2801–2803
  classification of, 2724
  common, 2798
  comparison with lymphoblastic lymphoma, 2770, 2804
  congenital disorders associated with, 2732, 2732t, 2795
  cytogenetics of, 307, 2738–2741, 2739f, 2797–2798, 2799f, 2801, 2801t
  diagnostic criteria for, 2796
  etiology of, 2794–2795
  flow cytometry in, 2797–2798, 2799f
  gene expression profiling in, 2803–2804
  genetic factors in, 2795
  hyperdiploid, 2801
  hypodiploid, 2801
  immunoglobulin gene rearrangements in, 2798t, 2800
  immunophenotyping of, 2797–2798, 2798t, 2799f
  incidence of, 2825
  infections in, 926
  intrauterine metastasis of, 2732
  laboratory tests in, 323b
  mature B-cell, 2814
    epidemiology of, 2814
    treatment of, 2814–2815
  mature pre-B-ALL, 2798–2799, 2798t
  mixed-lineage, immunologic markers in, 2799–2800
  molecularly targeted therapy for, 624, 624t

molecular pathogenesis of, 2733, 2800–2801
  non-B, non-T-ALL, 2798
  null, 2798
  pediatric
    age distribution of, 2732
    B-cell, 2736, 2736t
    with BCR-ABL rearrangements, 2740
    biology of, 2800
    clinical features of, 2734
    with c-MYC rearrangements, 2740
    CNS prophylaxis and treatment in, 2747
    cytogenetic and molecular classification of, 2738–2741, 2739f
    differential diagnosis of, 2734, 2804–2805, 2805t
    with E2A-PBX1 and E2A-HLF rearrangements, 2739
    early pre-B ALL, 2735–2736, 2736t
    epidemiology of, 2732, 2794
    hyperdiploid, 2738–2739
    immunologic classification of, 2735–2737, 2736t
    laboratory findings in, 2734
    minimal residual disease in, 307–308, 2752–2754, 2753f
    with MLL rearrangements, 2739–2740
    pre-B ALL, 2736, 2736t
    prognosis for, 314, 2743–2744, 2743f
    racial distribution of, 2732, 2794
    relapse of, 2742–2743
    remission induction in, 2745–2746
    risk factors for, 2733
    survivors of, endocrine complications in, 1289
    with TEL-AML1 rearrangements, 2739
    T-lineage, 2736–2737, 2736t
    transitional (late) pre-B ALL, 2736, 2736t
    treatment of, 2744–2748, 2745t, 2754
  Philadelphia chromosome (Ph)-positive, 2816
  pre-B-ALL, 2798, 2798t, 2802
  pre-pre-B-ALL, 2798, 2802
  pro-B-ALL, 2798, 2798t
  radiation-related, 2795
  radiation therapy for, and second malignant neoplasms, 1299, 1299f, 1350
  radioimmunotherapy for, 667
  seasonality of, 2795
  T-cell, 2770–2771
    antigen expression in, 2738
    in children, 2732
    genetic abnormalities in, 2740–2741
    immunologic markers in, 2797–2798, 2798t, 2799
  T-cell receptor gene rearrangements in, 2800, 2803
  transitional pre-B-ALL, 2798, 2798t
  treatment of
    bispecific MAbs with cellular immunoconjugates in, 669
    second malignancy after, 2574